Peterson's®
Graduate Programs in the Biological/Biomedical Sciences & Health-Related Medical Professions

2017

About Peterson's®

Peterson's®, a Nelnet company, has been your trusted educational publisher for over 50 years. It's a milestone we're quite proud of, as we continue to offer the most accurate, dependable, high-quality education content in the field, providing you with everything you need to succeed. No matter where you are on your academic or professional path, you can rely on Peterson's publications and its online information at **www.petersons.com** for the most up-to-date education exploration data, expert test-prep tools, and the highest quality career success resources—everything you need to achieve your educational goals.

For more information, contact Peterson's Publishing, 3 Columbia Circle, Suite 205, Albany, NY 12203-5158; 800-338-3282 Ext. 54229; or find us on the World Wide Web at www.petersons.com.

ISSN 1093-8443
ISBN: 978-0-7689-4094-7

Printed in the United States of America

10 9 8 7 6 5 4 3 2 1   19 18 17

Fifty-First Edition

CONTENTS

CONTENTS

**ACADEMIC AND PROFESSIONAL PROGRAMS
IN THE MEDICAL PROFESSIONS AND
SCIENCES**

A Note from the Peterson's Editors

The six volumes of Peterson's *Graduate and Professional Programs*, the only annually updated reference work of its kind, provide wide-ranging information on the graduate and professional programs offered by accredited colleges and universities in the United States, U.S. territories, and Canada and by those institutions outside the United States that are accredited by U.S. accrediting bodies. More than 44,000 individual academic and professional programs at more than 2,200 institutions are listed. Peterson's *Graduate and Professional Programs* have been used for more than fifty years by prospective graduate and professional students, placement counselors, faculty advisers, and all others interested in postbaccalaureate education.

Graduate & Professional Programs: An Overview contains information on institutions as a whole, while the other books in the series are devoted to specific academic and professional fields:

* *Graduate Programs In the Biological/Biomedical Sciences & Health-Related Medical Professions*

* *Graduate Programs in Business, Education, Information Studies, Law & Social Work*

* *Graduate Programs in Engineering & Applied Sciences*

* *Graduate Programs in the Humanities, Arts & Social Sciences*

* *Graduate Programs in the Physical Sciences, Mathematics, Agricultural Sciences, the Environment & Natural Resources*

The books may be used individually or as a set. For example, if you have chosen a field of study but do not know what institution you want to attend or if you have a college or university in mind but have not chosen an academic field of study, it is best to begin with the Overview guide.

Graduate & Professional Programs: An Overview presents several directories to help you identify programs of study that might interest you; you can then research those programs further in the other books in the series by using the Directory of Graduate and Professional Programs by Field, which lists 500 fields and gives the names of those institutions that offer graduate degree programs in each.

For geographical or financial reasons, you may be interested in attending a particular institution and will want to know what it has to offer. You should turn to the Directory of Institutions and Their Offerings, which lists the degree programs available at each institution. As in the Directory of Graduate and Professional Programs by Field, the level of degrees offered is also indicated.

All books in the series include advice on graduate education, including topics such as admissions tests, financial aid, and accreditation. **The Graduate Adviser** includes two essays and information about accreditation. The first essay, "The Admissions Process," discusses general admission requirements, admission tests, factors to consider when selecting a graduate school or program, when and how to apply, and how admission decisions are made. Special information for international students and tips for minority students are also included. The second essay, "Financial Support," is an overview of the broad range of support available at the graduate level. Fellowships, scholarships, and grants; assistantships and internships; federal and private loan programs, as well as Federal Work-Study; and the GI bill are detailed. This essay concludes with advice on applying for need-based financial aid. "Accreditation and Accrediting Agencies" gives information on accreditation and its purpose and lists institutional accrediting agencies first and then specialized accrediting agencies relevant to each volume's specific fields of study.

With information on more than 40,000 graduate programs in more than 500 disciplines, Peterson's *Graduate and Professional Programs* give you all the information you need about the programs that are of interest to you in three formats: **Profiles** (capsule summaries of basic information), **Displays** (information that an institution or program wants to emphasize), and **Close-Ups** (written by administrators, with more expansive information than the **Profiles**, emphasizing different aspects of the programs). By using these various formats of program information, coupled with **Appendixes** and **Indexes** covering directories and subject areas for all six books, you will find that these guides provide the most comprehensive, accurate, and up-to-date graduate study information available.

Peterson's publishes a full line of resources with information you need to guide you through the graduate admissions process. Peterson's publications can be found at college libraries and career centers and your local bookstore or library—or visit us on the Web at www.petersons.com.

Colleges and universities will be pleased to know that Peterson's helped you in your selection. Admissions staff members are more than happy to answer questions, address specific problems, and help in any way they can. The editors at Peterson's wish you great success in your graduate program search!

THE GRADUATE ADVISER

The Admissions Process

Generalizations about graduate admissions practices are not always helpful because each institution has its own set of guidelines and procedures. Nevertheless, some broad statements can be made about the admissions process that may help you plan your strategy.

Factors Involved in Selecting a Graduate School or Program

Selecting a graduate school and a specific program of study is a complex matter. Quality of the faculty; program and course offerings; the nature, size, and location of the institution; admission requirements; cost; and the availability of financial assistance are among the many factors that affect one's choice of institution. Other considerations are job placement and achievements of the program's graduates and the institution's resources, such as libraries, laboratories, and computer facilities. If you are to make the best possible choice, you need to learn as much as you can about the schools and programs you are considering before you apply.

The following steps may help you narrow your choices.

- Talk to alumni of the programs or institutions you are considering to get their impressions of how well they were prepared for work in their fields of study.
- Remember that graduate school requirements change, so be sure to get the most up-to-date information possible.
- Talk to department faculty members and the graduate adviser at your undergraduate institution. They often have information about programs of study at other institutions.
- Visit the websites of the graduate schools in which you are interested to request a graduate catalog. Contact the department chair in your chosen field of study for additional information about the department and the field.
- Visit as many campuses as possible. Call ahead for an appointment with the graduate adviser in your field of interest and be sure to check out the facilities and talk to students.

General Requirements

Graduate schools and departments have requirements that applicants for admission must meet. Typically, these requirements include undergraduate transcripts (which provide information about undergraduate grade point average and course work applied toward a major), admission test scores, and letters of recommendation. Most graduate programs also ask for an essay or personal statement that describes your personal reasons for seeking graduate study. In some fields, such as art and music, portfolios or auditions may be required in addition to other evidence of talent. Some institutions require that the applicant have an undergraduate degree in the same subject as the intended graduate major.

Most institutions evaluate each applicant on the basis of the applicant's total record, and the weight accorded any given factor varies widely from institution to institution and from program to program.

The Application Process

You should begin the application process at least one year before you expect to begin your graduate study. Find out the application deadline for each institution (many are provided in the **Profile** section of this guide). Go to the institution's website and find out if you can apply online. If not, request a paper application form. Fill out this form thoroughly and neatly. Assume that the school needs all the information it is requesting and that the admissions officer will be sensitive to the neatness and overall quality of what you submit. Do not supply more information than the school requires.

The institution may ask at least one question that will require a three- or four-paragraph answer. Compose your response on the assumption that the admissions officer is interested in both what you think and how you express yourself. Keep your statement brief and to the point, but, at the same time, include all pertinent information about your past experiences and your educational goals. Individual statements vary greatly in style and content, which helps admissions officers differentiate among applicants. Many graduate departments give considerable weight to the statement in making their admissions decisions, so be sure to take the time to prepare a thoughtful and concise statement.

If recommendations are a part of the admissions requirements, carefully choose the individuals you ask to write them. It is generally best to ask current or former professors to write the recommendations, provided they are able to attest to your intellectual ability and motivation for doing the work required of a graduate student. It is advisable to provide stamped, preaddressed envelopes to people being asked to submit recommendations on your behalf.

Completed applications, including references, transcripts, and admission test scores, should be received at the institution by the specified date.

Be advised that institutions do not usually make admissions decisions until all materials have been received. Enclose a self-addressed postcard with your application, requesting confirmation of receipt. Allow at least ten days for the return of the postcard before making further inquiries.

If you plan to apply for financial support, it is imperative that you file your application early.

ADMISSION TESTS

The major testing program used in graduate admissions is the Graduate Record Examinations (GRE®) testing program, sponsored by the GRE Board and administered by Educational Testing Service, Princeton, New Jersey.

The Graduate Record Examinations testing program consists of a General Test and eight Subject Tests. The General Test measures critical thinking, verbal reasoning, quantitative reasoning, and analytical writing skills. It is offered as an Internet-based test (iBT) in the United States, Canada, and many other countries.

The GRE® revised General Test's questions were designed to reflect the kind of thinking that students need to do in graduate or business school and demonstrate that students are indeed ready for graduate-level work.

- **Verbal Reasoning**—Measures ability to analyze and evaluate written material and synthesize information obtained from it, analyze relationships among component parts of sentences, and recognize relationships among words and concepts.
- **Quantitative Reasoning**—Measures problem-solving ability, focusing on basic concepts of arithmetic, algebra, geometry, and data analysis.
- **Analytical Writing**—Measures critical thinking and analytical writing skills, specifically the ability to articulate and support complex ideas clearly and effectively.

The computer-delivered GRE® revised General Test is offered year-round at Prometric™ test centers and on specific dates at testing locations outside of the Prometric test center network. Appointments are scheduled on a first-come, first-served basis. The GRE® revised General Test is also offered as a paper-based test three times a year in areas where computer-based testing is not available.

You can take the computer-delivered GRE® revised General Test once every twenty-one days, up to five times within any continuous rolling twelve-month period (365 days)—even if you canceled your scores on a previously taken test. You may take the paper-delivered GRE® revised General Test as often as it is offered.

Three scores are reported on the revised General Test:

1. A **Verbal Reasoning score** is reported on a 130–170 score scale, in 1-point increments.

2. A **Quantitative Reasoning score** is reported on a 130–170 score scale, in 1-point increments.

3. An **Analytical Writing score** is reported on a 0–6 score level, in half-point increments.

The GRE® Subject Tests measure achievement and assume undergraduate majors or extensive background in the following eight disciplines:

- Biochemistry, Cell and Molecular Biology
- Biology
- Chemistry
- Computer Science
- Literature in English
- Mathematics
- Physics
- Psychology

The Subject Tests are available three times per year as paper-based administrations around the world. Testing time is approximately 2 hours and 50 minutes. You can obtain more information about the GRE® by visiting the ETS website at www.ets.org or consulting the GRE® *Information and Registration Bulletin*. The *Bulletin* can be obtained at many undergraduate colleges. You can also download it from the ETS website or obtain it by contacting Graduate Record Examinations, Educational Testing Service, P.O. Box 6000, Princeton, NJ 08541-6000; phone: 609-771-7670.

If you expect to apply for admission to a program that requires any of the GRE® tests, you should select a test date well in advance of the application deadline. Scores on the computer-based General Test are reported within ten to fifteen days; scores on the paper-based Subject Tests are reported within six weeks.

Another testing program, the Miller Analogies Test® (MAT®), is administered at more than 500 Controlled Testing Centers, licensed by Harcourt Assessment, Inc., in the United States, Canada, and other countries. The MAT® computer-based test is now available. Testing time is 60 minutes. The test consists of 120 partial analogies. You can obtain the *Candidate Information Booklet,* which contains a list of test centers and instructions for taking the test, from http://www.milleranalogies.com or by calling 800-328-5999 (toll-free).

Check the specific requirements of the programs to which you are applying.

How Admission Decisions Are Made

The program you apply to is directly involved in the admissions process. Although the final decision is usually made by the graduate dean (or an associate) or the faculty admissions committee, recommendations from faculty members in your intended field are important. At some institutions, an interview is incorporated into the decision process.

A Special Note for International Students

In addition to the steps already described, there are some special considerations for international students who intend to apply for graduate study in the United States. All graduate schools require an indication of competence in English. The purpose of the Test of English as a Foreign Language (TOEFL®) is to evaluate the English proficiency of people who are nonnative speakers of English and want to study at colleges and universities where English is the language of instruction. The TOEFL® is administered by Educational Testing Service (ETS) under the general direction of a policy board established by the College Board and the Graduate Record Examinations Board.

The TOEFL® iBT assesses the four basic language skills: listening, reading, writing, and speaking. It was administered for the first time in September 2005, and ETS continues to introduce the TOEFL® iBT in selected cities. The Internet-based test is administered at secure, official test centers. The testing time is approximately 4 hours. Because the TOEFL® iBT includes a speaking section, the Test of Spoken English (TSE) is no longer needed.

The TOEFL® is also offered in the paper-based format in areas of the world where Internet-based testing is not available. The paper-based TOEFL® consists of three sections—listening comprehension, structure and written expression, and reading comprehension. The testing time is approximately 3 hours. The Test of Written English (TWE®) is also given. The TWE® is a 30-minute essay that measures the examinee's ability to compose in English. Examinees receive a TWE® score separate from their TOEFL® score. The *Information Bulletin* contains information on local fees and registration procedures.

The TOEFL® paper-based test (TOEFL® PBT) began being phased out in mid-2012. For those who may have taken the TOEFL® PBT, scores remain valid for two years after the test date. The Test of Written English (TWE®) is also given. The TWE® is a 30-minute essay that measures the examinee's ability to compose in English. Examinees receive a TWE® score separate from their TOEFL® score. The Information Bulletin contains information on local fees and registration procedures.

Additional information and registration materials are available from TOEFL® Services, Educational Testing Service, P.O. Box 6151, Princeton, New Jersey 08541-6151. Phone: 609-771-7100. Website: www.toefl.org.

International students should apply especially early because of the number of steps required to complete the admissions process. Furthermore, many United States graduate schools have a limited number of spaces for international students, and many more students apply than the schools can accommodate.

International students may find financial assistance from institutions very limited. The U.S. government requires international applicants to submit a certification of support, which is a statement attesting to the applicant's financial resources. In addition, international students *must* have health insurance coverage.

Tips for Minority Students

Indicators of a university's values in terms of diversity are found both in its recruitment programs and its resources directed to student success. Important questions: Does the institution vigorously recruit minorities for its graduate programs? Is there funding available to help with the costs associated with visiting the school? Are minorities represented in the institution's brochures or website or on their faculty rolls? What campus-based resources or services (including assistance in locating housing or career counseling and placement) are available? Is funding available to members of underrepresented groups?

At the program level, it is particularly important for minority students to investigate the "climate" of a program under consideration. How many minority students are enrolled and how many have graduated? What opportunities are there to work with diverse faculty and mentors whose research interests match yours? How are conflicts resolved or concerns addressed? How interested are faculty in building strong and supportive relations with students? "Climate" concerns should be addressed by posing questions to various individuals, including faculty members, current students, and alumni.

Information is also available through various organizations, such as the Hispanic Association of Colleges & Universities (HACU), and publications such as *Diverse Issues in Higher Education* and *Hispanic Outlook* magazine. There are also books devoted to this topic, such as *The Multicultural Student's Guide to Colleges* by Robert Mitchell.

Financial Support

The range of financial support at the graduate level is very broad. The following descriptions will give you a general idea of what you might expect and what will be expected of you as a financial support recipient.

Fellowships, Scholarships, and Grants

These are usually outright awards of a few hundred to many thousands of dollars with no service to the institution required in return. Fellowships and scholarships are usually awarded on the basis of merit and are highly competitive. Grants are made on the basis of financial need or special talent in a field of study. Many fellowships, scholarships, and grants not only cover tuition, fees, and supplies but also include stipends for living expenses with allowances for dependents. However, the terms of each should be examined because some do not permit recipients to supplement their income with outside work. Fellowships, scholarships, and grants may vary in the number of years for which they are awarded.

In addition to the availability of these funds at the university or program level, many excellent fellowship programs are available at the national level and may be applied for before and during enrollment in a graduate program. A listing of many of these programs can be found at the Council of Graduate Schools' website: http://www.cgsnet.org. There is a wealth of information in the "Programs" and "Awards" sections.

Assistantships and Internships

Many graduate students receive financial support through assistantships, particularly involving teaching or research duties. It is important to recognize that such appointments should not be viewed simply as employment relationships but rather should constitute an integral and important part of a student's graduate education. As such, the appointments should be accompanied by strong faculty mentoring and increasingly responsible apprenticeship experiences. The specific nature of these appointments in a given program should be considered in selecting that graduate program.

TEACHING ASSISTANTSHIPS

These usually provide a salary and full or partial tuition remission and may also provide health benefits. Unlike fellowships, scholarships, and grants, which require no service to the institution, teaching assistantships require recipients to provide the institution with a specific amount of undergraduate teaching, ideally related to the student's field of study. Some teaching assistants are limited to grading papers, compiling bibliographies, taking notes, or monitoring laboratories. At some graduate schools, teaching assistants must carry lighter course loads than regular full-time students.

RESEARCH ASSISTANTSHIPS

These are very similar to teaching assistantships in the manner in which financial assistance is provided. The difference is that recipients are given basic research assignments in their disciplines rather than teaching responsibilities. The work required is normally related to the student's field of study; in most instances, the assistantship supports the student's thesis or dissertation research.

ADMINISTRATIVE INTERNSHIPS

These are similar to assistantships in application of financial assistance funds, but the student is given an assignment on a part-time basis, usually as a special assistant with one of the university's administrative offices. The assignment may not necessarily be directly related to the recipient's discipline.

RESIDENCE HALL AND COUNSELING ASSISTANTSHIPS

These assistantships are frequently assigned to graduate students in psychology, counseling, and social work, but they may be offered to students in other disciplines, especially if the student has worked in this capacity during his or her undergraduate years. Duties can vary from being available in a dean's office for a specific number of hours for consultation with undergraduates to living in campus residences and being responsible for both counseling and administrative tasks or advising student activity groups. Residence hall assistantships often include a room and board allowance and, in some cases, tuition assistance and stipends. Contact the Housing and Student Life Office for more information.

Health Insurance

The availability and affordability of health insurance is an important issue and one that should be considered in an applicant's choice of institution and program. While often included with assistantships and fellowships, this is not always the case and, even if provided, the benefits may be limited. It is important to note that the U.S. government requires international students to have health insurance.

The GI Bill

This provides financial assistance for students who are veterans of the United States armed forces. If you are a veteran, contact your local Veterans Administration office to determine your eligibility and to get full details about benefits. There are a number of programs that offer educational benefits to current military enlistees. Some states have tuition assistance programs for members of the National Guard. Contact the VA office at the college for more information.

Federal Work-Study Program (FWS)

Employment is another way some students finance their graduate studies. The federally funded Federal Work-Study Program provides eligible students with employment opportunities, usually in public and private nonprofit organizations. Federal funds pay up to 75 percent of the wages, with the remainder paid by the employing agency. FWS is available to graduate students who demonstrate financial need. Not all schools have these funds, and some only award them to undergraduates. Each school sets its application deadline and workstudy earnings limits. Wages vary and are related to the type of work done. You must file the Free Application for Federal Student Aid (FAFSA) to be eligible for this program.

Loans

Many graduate students borrow to finance their graduate programs when other sources of assistance (which do not have to be repaid) prove insufficient. You should always read and understand the terms of any loan program before submitting your application.

FEDERAL DIRECT LOANS

Federal Direct Loans. The Federal Direct Loan Program offers a variable-fixed interest rate loan to graduate students with the Department of Education acting as the lender. Students receive a new rate with each new loan, but that rate is fixed for the life of the loan. Beginning with loans made on or after July 1, 2013, the interest rate for loans made each July 1st to June 30th period are determined based on the last 10-year Treasury note auction prior to June 1st of that year, plus an added percentage. The interest rate can be no higher than 9.5%.

Beginning July 1, 2012, the Federal Direct Loan for graduate students is an unsubsidized loan. Under the *unsubsidized* program, the grad borrower pays the interest on the loan from the day proceeds are issued and is responsible for paying interest during all periods. If the borrower chooses not to pay the interest while in school, or during the grace periods, deferment, or forbearance, the interest accrues and will be capitalized.

Graduate students may borrow up to $20,500 per year through the Direct Loan Program, up to a cumulative maximum of $138,500, including undergraduate borrowing. No more than $65,000 of the $138,500 can be from subsidized loans, including loans the grad borrower may have received for periods of enrollment that began before July 1, 2012, or for prior undergraduate borrowing. You may borrow up to the cost of attendance at the school in which you are enrolled or will attend, minus estimated financial assistance from other federal, state, and private sources, up to a maximum of $20,500. Grad borrowers who reach the aggregate loan limit over the course of their education cannot receive additional loans; however, if they repay some of their loans to bring the outstanding balance below the aggregate limit, they could be eligible to borrow again, up to that limit.

For Unsubsidized loans first disbursed on or after July 1, 2015, and before July 1, 2016, the interest rate was 5.84%. For those first disbursed on or after July 1, 2016, and before July 1, 2017, the interest rate is 5.31%.

A fee is deducted from the loan proceeds upon disbursement. Loans with a first disbursement on or after July 1, 2010 but before July 1, 2012, have a borrower origination fee of 1 percent. For loans disbursed after July 1, 2012, these fee deductions no longer apply. The Budget Control Act of 2011, signed into law on August 2, 2011, eliminated Direct Subsidized Loan eligibility for graduate and professional students for periods of enrollment beginning on or after July 1, 2012, and terminated the authority of the Department of Education to offer most repayment incentives to Direct Loan borrowers for loans disbursed on or after July 1, 2012.

Under the *subsidized* Federal Direct Loan Program, repayment begins six months after your last date of enrollment on at least a half-time basis. Under the *unsubsidized* program, repayment of interest begins within thirty days from disbursement of the loan proceeds, and repayment of the principal begins six months after your last enrollment on at least a half-time basis. Some borrowers may choose to defer interest payments while they are in school. The accrued interest is added to the loan balance when the borrower begins repayment. There are several repayment options.

Federal Perkins Loans. The Federal Perkins Loan is available to students demonstrating financial need and is administered directly by the school. Not all schools have these funds, and some may award them to undergraduates only. Eligibility is determined from the information you provide on the FAFSA. The school will notify you of your eligibility.

Eligible graduate students may borrow up to $8,000 per year, up to a maximum of $60,000, including undergraduate borrowing (even if your previous Perkins Loans have been repaid). The interest rate for Federal Perkins Loans is 5 percent, and no interest accrues while you remain in school at least half-time. Students who are attending less than half-time need to check with their school to determine the length of their grace period. There are no guarantee, loan, or disbursement fees. Repayment begins nine months after your last date of enrollment on at least a half-time basis and may extend over a maximum of ten years with no prepayment penalty.

Federal Direct Graduate PLUS Loans. Effective July 1, 2006, graduate and professional students are eligible for Graduate PLUS loans. This program allows students to borrow up to the cost of attendance, less any other aid received. These loans have a fixed interest rate, and interest begins to accrue at the time of disbursement. Beginning with loans made on or after July 1, 2013, the interest rate for loans made each July 1st to June 30th period are determined based on the last 10-year Treasury note auction prior to June 1st of that year. The interest rate can be no higher than 10.5%. The PLUS loans do involve a credit check; a PLUS borrower may obtain a loan with a cosigner if his or her credit is not good enough. Grad PLUS loans may be deferred while a student is in school and for the six months following a drop below half-time

enrollment. For more information, you should contact a representative in your college's financial aid office.

Deferring Your Federal Loan Repayments. If you borrowed under the Federal Direct Loan Program, Federal Direct PLUS Loan Program, or the Federal Perkins Loan Program for previous undergraduate or graduate study, your payments may be deferred when you return to graduate school, depending on when you borrowed and under which program.

There are other deferment options available if you are temporarily unable to repay your loan. Information about these deferments is provided at your entrance and exit interviews. If you believe you are eligible for a deferment of your loan payments, you must contact your lender or loan servicer to request a deferment. The deferment must be filed prior to the time your payment is due, and it must be re-filed when it expires if you remain eligible for deferment at that time.

SUPPLEMENTAL (PRIVATE) LOANS

Many lending institutions offer supplemental loan programs and other financing plans, such as the ones described here, to students seeking additional assistance in meeting their education expenses. Some loan programs target all types of graduate students; others are designed specifically for business, law, or medical students. In addition, you can use private loans not specifically designed for education to help finance your graduate degree.

If you are considering borrowing through a supplemental or private loan program, you should carefully consider the terms and be sure to read the fine print. Check with the program sponsor for the most current terms that will be applicable to the amounts you intend to borrow for graduate study. Most supplemental loan programs for graduate study offer unsubsidized, credit-based loans. In general, a credit-ready borrower is one who has a satisfactory credit history or no credit history at all. A creditworthy borrower generally must pass a credit test to be eligible to borrow or act as a cosigner for the loan funds.

Many supplemental loan programs have minimum and maximum annual loan limits. Some offer amounts equal to the cost of attendance minus any other aid you will receive for graduate study. If you are planning to borrow for several years of graduate study, consider whether there is a cumulative or aggregate limit on the amount you may borrow. Often this cumulative or aggregate limit will include any amounts you borrowed and have not repaid for undergraduate or previous graduate study.

The combination of the annual interest rate, loan fees, and the repayment terms you choose will determine how much you will repay over time. Compare these features in combination before you decide which loan program to use. Some loans offer interest rates that are adjusted monthly, quarterly, or annually. Some offer interest rates that are lower during the in-school, grace, and deferment periods and then increase when you begin repayment. Some programs include a loan origination fee, which is usually deducted from the principal amount you receive when the loan is disbursed and must be repaid along with the interest and other principal when you graduate, withdraw from school, or drop below half-time study. Sometimes the loan fees are reduced if you borrow with a qualified cosigner. Some programs allow you to defer interest and/or principal payments while you are enrolled in graduate school. Many programs allow you to capitalize your interest payments; the interest due on your loan is added to the outstanding balance of your loan, so you don't have to repay immediately, but this increases the amount you owe. Other programs allow you to pay the interest as you go, which reduces the amount you later have to repay. The private loan market is very competitive, and your financial aid office can help you evaluate these programs.

Applying for Need-Based Financial Aid

Schools that award federal and institutional financial assistance based on need will require you to complete the FAFSA and, in some cases, an institutional financial aid application.

If you are applying for federal student assistance, you **must** complete the FAFSA. A service of the U.S. Department of Education, the FAFSA is free to all applicants. Most applicants apply online at www.fafsa.ed.gov. Paper applications are available at the financial aid office of your local college.

After your FAFSA information has been processed, you will receive a Student Aid Report (SAR). If you provided an e-mail address on the FAFSA, this will be sent to you electronically; otherwise, it will be mailed to your home address.

Follow the instructions on the SAR if you need to correct information reported on your original application. If your situation changes after you file your FAFSA, contact your financial aid officer to discuss amending your information. You can also appeal your financial aid award if you have extenuating circumstances.

If you would like more information on federal student financial aid, visit the FAFSA website or download the most recent version of *Funding Education Beyond High School: The Guide to Federal Student Aid* at http://studentaid.ed.gov/students/publications/student_guide/index.html. This guide is also available in Spanish.

The U.S. Department of Education also has a toll-free number for questions concerning federal student aid programs. The number is 1-800-4-FED AID (1-800-433-3243). If you are hearing impaired, call toll-free, 1-800-730-8913.

Summary

Remember that these are generalized statements about financial assistance at the graduate level. Because each institution allots its aid differently, you should communicate directly with the school and the specific department of interest to you. It is not unusual, for example, to find that an endowment vested within a specific department supports one or more fellowships. You may fit its requirements and specifications precisely.

Accreditation and Accrediting Agencies

Colleges and universities in the United States, and their individual academic and professional programs, are accredited by nongovernmental agencies concerned with monitoring the quality of education in this country. Agencies with both regional and national jurisdictions grant accreditation to institutions as a whole, while specialized bodies acting on a nationwide basis—often national professional associations—grant accreditation to departments and programs in specific fields.

Institutional and specialized accrediting agencies share the same basic concerns: the purpose an academic unit—whether university or program—has set for itself and how well it fulfills that purpose, the adequacy of its financial and other resources, the quality of its academic offerings, and the level of services it provides. Agencies that grant institutional accreditation take a broader view, of course, and examine university-wide or college-wide services with which a specialized agency may not concern itself.

Both types of agencies follow the same general procedures when considering an application for accreditation. The academic unit prepares a self-evaluation, focusing on the concerns mentioned above and usually including an assessment of both its strengths and weaknesses; a team of representatives of the accrediting body reviews this evaluation, visits the campus, and makes its own report; and finally, the accrediting body makes a decision on the application. Often, even when accreditation is granted, the agency makes a recommendation regarding how the institution or program can improve. All institutions and programs are also reviewed every few years to determine whether they continue to meet established standards; if they do not, they may lose their accreditation.

Accrediting agencies themselves are reviewed and evaluated periodically by the U.S. Department of Education and the Council for Higher Education Accreditation (CHEA). Recognized agencies adhere to certain standards and practices, and their authority in matters of accreditation is widely accepted in the educational community.

This does not mean, however, that accreditation is a simple matter, either for schools wishing to become accredited or for students deciding where to apply. Indeed, in certain fields the very meaning and methods of accreditation are the subject of a good deal of debate. For their part, those applying to graduate school should be aware of the safeguards provided by regional accreditation, especially in terms of degree acceptance and institutional longevity. Beyond this, applicants should understand the role that specialized accreditation plays in their field, as this varies considerably from one discipline to another. In certain professional fields, it is necessary to have graduated from a program that is accredited in order to be eligible for a license to practice, and in some fields the federal government also makes this a hiring requirement. In other disciplines, however, accreditation is not as essential, and there can be excellent programs that are not accredited. In fact, some programs choose not to seek accreditation, although most do.

Institutions and programs that present themselves for accreditation are sometimes granted the status of candidate for accreditation, or what is known as "preaccreditation." This may happen, for example, when an academic unit is too new to have met all the requirements for accreditation. Such status signifies initial recognition and indicates that the school or program in question is working to fulfill all requirements; it does not, however, guarantee that accreditation will be granted.

Institutional Accrediting Agencies—Regional

MIDDLE STATES ASSOCIATION OF COLLEGES AND SCHOOLS

Accredits institutions in Delaware, District of Columbia, Maryland, New Jersey, New York, Pennsylvania, Puerto Rico, and the Virgin Islands.

Dr. Elizabeth Sibolski, President
Middle States Commission on Higher Education
3624 Market Street, Second Floor West
Philadelphia, Pennsylvania 19104
Phone: 267-284-5000
Fax: 215-662-5501
E-mail: info@msche.org
Website: www.msche.org

NEW ENGLAND ASSOCIATION OF SCHOOLS AND COLLEGES

Accredits institutions in Connecticut, Maine, Massachusetts, New Hampshire, Rhode Island, and Vermont.

Dr. Barbara E. Brittingham, President/Director
Commission on Institutions of Higher Education
3 Burlington Woods Drive, Suite 100
Burlington, Massachusetts 01803-4531
Phone: 855-886-3272 or 781-425-7714
Fax: 781-425-1001
E-mail: cihe@neasc.org
Website: http://cihe.neasc.org

THE HIGHER LEARNING COMMISSION

Accredits institutions in Arizona, Arkansas, Colorado, Illinois, Indiana, Iowa, Kansas, Michigan, Minnesota, Missouri, Nebraska, New Mexico, North Dakota, Ohio, Oklahoma, South Dakota, West Virginia, Wisconsin, and Wyoming.

Dr. Barbara Gellman-Danley, President
The Higher Learning Commission
230 South LaSalle Street, Suite 7-500
Chicago, Illinois 60604-1413
Phone: 800-621-7440 or 312-263-0456
Fax: 312-263-7462
E-mail: info@hlcommission.org
Website: www.hlcommission.org

NORTHWEST COMMISSION ON COLLEGES AND UNIVERSITIES

Accredits institutions in Alaska, Idaho, Montana, Nevada, Oregon, Utah, and Washington.

Dr. Sandra E. Elman, President
8060 165th Avenue, NE, Suite 100
Redmond, Washington 98052
Phone: 425-558-4224
Fax: 425-376-0596
E-mail: selman@nwccu.org
Website: www.nwccu.org

SOUTHERN ASSOCIATION OF COLLEGES AND SCHOOLS

Accredits institutions in Alabama, Florida, Georgia, Kentucky, Louisiana, Mississippi, North Carolina, South Carolina, Tennessee, Texas, and Virginia.

Dr. Belle S. Wheelan, President
Commission on Colleges
1866 Southern Lane
Decatur, Georgia 30033-4097
Phone: 404-679-4500 Ext. 4504
Fax: 404-679-4558
E-mail: questions@sacscoc.org
Website: www.sacscoc.org

WESTERN ASSOCIATION OF SCHOOLS AND COLLEGES

Accredits institutions in California, Guam, and Hawaii.

Dr. Mary Ellen Petrisko, President
Accrediting Commission for Senior Colleges and Universities
985 Atlantic Avenue, Suite 100
Alameda, California 94501
Phone: 510-748-9001
Fax: 510-748-9797
E-mail: wasc@wascsenior.org
Website: http://www.wascsenior.org/

Institutional Accrediting Agencies—Other

ACCREDITING COUNCIL FOR INDEPENDENT COLLEGES AND SCHOOLS
Anthony S. Bieda, Executive in Charge
750 First Street, NE, Suite 980
Washington, DC 20002-4241
Phone: 202-336-6780
Fax: 202-842-2593
E-mail: info@acics.org
Website: www.acics.org

DISTANCE EDUCATION AND ACCREDITING COMMISSION (DEAC)
Accrediting Commission
Leah Matthews, Executive Director
1101 17th Street, NW, Suite 808
Washington, DC 20036-4704
Phone: 202-234-5100
Fax: 202-332-1386
E-mail: info@deac.org
Website: www.deac.org

Specialized Accrediting Agencies

ACUPUNCTURE AND ORIENTAL MEDICINE
Mark S. McKenzie, LAc MsOM DiplOM, Executive Director
Accreditation Commission for Acupuncture and Oriental Medicine
8941 Aztec Drive
Eden Prairie, Minnesota 55347
Phone: 952-212-2434
Fax: 301-313-0912
E-mail: coordinator@acaom.org
Website: www.acaom.org

ALLIED HEALTH
Kathleen Megivern, Executive Director
Commission on Accreditation of Allied Health Education Programs (CAAHEP)
25400 US Hwy 19 North, Suite 158
Clearwater, Florida 33763
Phone: 727-210-2350
Fax: 727-210-2354
E-mail: mail@caahep.org
Website: www.caahep.org

ART AND DESIGN
Karen P. Moynahan, Executive Director
National Association of Schools of Art and Design (NASAD)
Commission on Accreditation
11250 Roger Bacon Drive, Suite 21
Reston, Virginia 20190-5248
Phone: 703-437-0700
Fax: 703-437-6312
E-mail: info@arts-accredit.org
Website: http://nasad.arts-accredit.org

ATHLETIC TRAINING EDUCATION
Micki Cuppett, Executive Director
Commission on Accreditation of Athletic Training Education (CAATE)
6850 Austin Center Blvd., Suite 100
Austin, Texas 78731-3184
Phone: 512-733-9700
E-mail: micki@caate.net
Website: www.caate.net

AUDIOLOGY EDUCATION
Doris Gordon, Executive Director
Accreditation Commission for Audiology Education (ACAE)
11480 Commerce Park Drive, Suite 220
Reston, Virginia 20191
Phone: 202-986-9550
Fax: 202-986-9500
E-mail: info@acaeaccred.org
Website: www.acaeaccred.org

AVIATION
Dr. Gary J. Northam, Executive Director
Aviation Accreditation Board International (AABI)
3410 Skyway Drive
Auburn, Alabama 36830
Phone: 334-844-2431
Fax: 334-844-2432
E-mail: bayenva@auburn.edu
Website: www.aabi.aero

BUSINESS
Robert D. Reid, Executive Vice President and Chief Accreditation Officer
AACSB International—The Association to Advance Collegiate Schools of Business
777 South Harbour Island Boulevard, Suite 750
Tampa, Florida 33602
Phone: 813-769-6500
Fax: 813-769-6559
E-mail: bob@aacsb.edu
Website: www.aacsb.edu

BUSINESS EDUCATION
Dennis N. Gash, President and Chief Executive Officer
International Assembly for Collegiate Business Education (IACBE)
11257 Strang Line Road
Lenexa, Kansas 66215
Phone: 913-631-3009
Fax: 913-631-9154
E-mail:iacbe@iacbe.org
Website: www.iacbe.org

CHIROPRACTIC
Craig S. Little, President
Council on Chiropractic Education (CCE)
Commission on Accreditation
8049 North 85th Way
Scottsdale, Arizona 85258-4321
Phone: 480-443-8877 or 888-443-3506
Fax: 480-483-7333
E-mail: cce@cce-usa.org
Website: www.cce-usa.org

CLINICAL LABORATORY SCIENCES
Dianne M. Cearlock, Ph.D., Chief Executive Officer
National Accrediting Agency for Clinical Laboratory Sciences
5600 North River Road, Suite 720
Rosemont, Illinois 60018-5119
Phone: 773-714-8880 or 847-939-3597
Fax: 773-714-8886
E-mail: info@naacls.org
Website: www.naacls.org

CLINICAL PASTORAL EDUCATION
Trace Haythorn, Executive Director
Association for Clinical Pastoral Education, Inc.
1549 Clairmont Road, Suite 103
Decatur, Georgia 30033-4611
Phone: 404-320-1472
Fax: 404-320-0849
E-mail: acpe@acpe.edu
Website: www.acpe.edu

DANCE
Karen P. Moynahan, Executive Director
National Association of Schools of Dance (NASD)
Commission on Accreditation
11250 Roger Bacon Drive, Suite 21
Reston, Virginia 20190-5248
Phone: 703-437-0700
Fax: 703-437-6312
E-mail: info@arts-accredit.org
Website: http://nasd.arts-accredit.org

DENTISTRY
Dr. Sherin Tooks, Director
Commission on Dental Accreditation
American Dental Association
211 East Chicago Avenue, Suite 1900
Chicago, Illinois 60611
Phone: 312-440-4643 or 800-621-8099
E-mail: accreditation@ada.org
Website: www.ada.org

DIETETICS AND NUTRITION
Mary B. Gregoire, Ph.D., Executive Director; RD, FADA, FAND
Academy of Nutrition and Dietetics
Accreditation Council for Education in Nutrition and Dietetics (ACEND)
120 South Riverside Plaza, Suite 2000
Chicago, Illinois 60606-6995
Phone: 800-877-1600 Ext. 5400 or 312-899-0040
Fax: 312-899-4817
E-mail: acend@eatright.org
Website: www.eatright.org/ACEND

EDUCATION PREPARATION
Christopher Koch, President
Council for the Accreditation of Education Preparation (CAEP)
1140 19th Street NW, Suite 400
Washington, DC 20036
Phone: 202-223-0077
Fax: 202-296-6620
E-mail: caep@caepnet.org
Website: www.caepnet.org

ENGINEERING
Michael Milligan, Ph.D., PE, Executive Director
Accreditation Board for Engineering and Technology, Inc. (ABET)
415 North Charles Street
Baltimore, Maryland 21201
Phone: 410-347-7700
E-mail: accreditation@abet.org
Website: www.abet.org

FORENSIC SCIENCES
Nancy J. Jackson, Director of Development and Accreditation
American Academy of Forensic Sciences (AAFS)
Forensic Science Education Program Accreditation Commission (FEPAC)
410 North 21st Street
Colorado Springs, Colorado 80904
Phone: 719-636-1100
Fax: 719-636-1993
E-mail: njackson@aafs.org
Website: www.fepac-edu.org

FORESTRY
Carol L. Redelsheimer
Director of Science and Education
Society of American Foresters
5400 Grosvenor Lane
Bethesda, Maryland 20814-2198
Phone: 301-897-8720 or 866-897-8720
Fax: 301-897-3690
E-mail: redelsheimerc@safnet.org
Website: www.safnet.org

HEALTHCARE MANAGEMENT
Commission on Accreditation of Healthcare Management Education (CAHME)
Anthony Stanowski, President and CEO
1700 Rockville Pike
Suite 400
Rockville, Maryland 20852
Phone: 301-998-6101
E-mail: info@cahme.org
Website: www.cahme.org

HEALTH INFORMATICS AND HEALTH MANAGEMENT
Claire Dixon-Lee, Executive Director
Commission on Accreditation for Health Informatics and Information Management Education (CAHIIM)
233 North Michigan Avenue, 21st Floor
Chicago, Illinois 60601-5800
Phone: 312-233-1100
Fax: 312-233-1948
E-mail:E-mall: claire.dixon-lee@cahiim.org
Website: www.cahiim.org

HUMAN SERVICE EDUCATION
Dr. Elaine Green, President
Council for Standards in Human Service Education (CSHSE)
3337 Duke Street
Alexandria, Virginia 22314
Phone: 571-257-3959
E-mail: info@cshse.org
Web: http://www.cshse.org

INTERIOR DESIGN
Holly Mattson, Executive Director
Council for Interior Design Accreditation
206 Grandview Avenue, Suite 350
Grand Rapids, Michigan 49503-4014
Phone: 616-458-0400
Fax: 616-458-0460
E-mail: info@accredit-id.org
Website: www.accredit-id.org

JOURNALISM AND MASS COMMUNICATIONS
Susanne Shaw, Executive Director
Accrediting Council on Education in Journalism and Mass Communications (ACEJMC)
School of Journalism
Stauffer-Flint Hall
University of Kansas
1435 Jayhawk Boulevard
Lawrence, Kansas 66045-7575
Phone: 785-864-3973
Fax: 785-864-5225
E-mail: sshaw@ku.edu
Website: http://www2.ku.edu/~acejmc/

LANDSCAPE ARCHITECTURE
Kristopher D. Pritchard, Executive Director
Landscape Architectural Accreditation Board (LAAB)
American Society of Landscape Architects (ASLA)
636 Eye Street, NW
Washington, DC 20001-3736
Phone: 202-216-2359
Fax: 202-898-1185
E-mail: info@asla.org
Website: www.asla.org

LAW
Barry Currier, Managing Director of Accreditation & Legal Education
American Bar Association
321 North Clark Street, 21st Floor
Chicago, Illinois 60654
Phone: 312-988-6738
Fax: 312-988-5681
E-mail: legaled@americanbar.org
Website: http://www.americanbar.org/groups/legal_education/
    resources/accreditation.html

LIBRARY
Karen O'Brien, Director
Office for Accreditation
American Library Association
50 East Huron Street
Chicago, Illinois 60611-2795
Phone: 312-280-2432
Fax: 312-280-2433
E-mail: accred@ala.org
Website: www.ala.org/accreditation/

MARRIAGE AND FAMILY THERAPY
Tanya A. Tamarkin, Director of Educational Affairs
Commission on Accreditation for Marriage and Family Therapy
    Education (COAMFTE)
American Association for Marriage and Family Therapy
112 South Alfred Street
Alexandria, Virginia 22314-3061
Phone: 703-838-9808
Fax: 703-838-9805
E-mail: coa@aamft.org
Website: www.aamft.org

MEDICAL ILLUSTRATION
Kathleen Megivern, Executive Director
Commission on Accreditation of Allied Health Education Programs
    (CAAHEP)
1361 Park Street
Clearwater, Florida 33756
Phone: 727-210-2350
Fax: 727-210-2354
E-mail: mail@caahep.org
Website: www.caahep.org

MEDICINE
Liaison Committee on Medical Education (LCME)
Robert B. Hash, M.D., LCME Secretary
American Medical Association
Council on Medical Education
330 North Wabash Avenue, Suite 39300
Chicago, Illinois 60611-5885
Phone: 312-464-4933
E-mail: lcme@aamc.org
Website: www.ama-assn.org

Liaison Committee on Medical Education (LCME)
Heather Lent, M.A., Director
Accreditation Services
Association of American Medical Colleges
655 K Street, NW
Washington, DC 20001-2399
Phone: 202-828-0596
E-mail: lcme@aamc.org
Website: www.lcme.org

MUSIC
Karen P. Moynahan, Executive Director
National Association of Schools of Music (NASM)
Commission on Accreditation
11250 Roger Bacon Drive, Suite 21
Reston, Virginia 20190-5248
Phone: 703-437-0700
Fax: 703-437-6312
E-mail: info@arts-accredit.org
Website: http://nasm.arts-accredit.org/

NATUROPATHIC MEDICINE
Daniel Seitz, J.D., Ed.D., Executive Director
Council on Naturopathic Medical Education
P.O. Box 178
Great Barrington, Massachusetts 01230
Phone: 413-528-8877
E-mail: www.cnme.org/contact.html
Website: www.cnme.org

NURSE ANESTHESIA
Francis R.Gerbasi, Ph.D., CRNA, COA Executive Director
Council on Accreditation of Nurse Anesthesia Educational Programs
    (CoA-NAEP)
American Association of Nurse Anesthetists
222 South Prospect Avenue, Suite 304
Park Ridge, Illinois 60068-4010
Phone: 847-655-1160
Fax: 847-692-7137
E-mail: accreditation@coa.us.com
Website: http://home.coa.us.com

NURSE EDUCATION
Jennifer L. Butlin, Executive Director
Commission on Collegiate Nursing Education (CCNE)
One Dupont Circle, NW, Suite 530
Washington, DC 20036-1120
Phone: 202-887-6791
Fax: 202-887-8476
E-mail: jbutlin@aacn.nche.edu
Website: www.aacn.nche.edu/accreditation

Marsal P. Stoll, Chief Executive Officer
Accreditation Commission for Education in Nursing (ACEN)
3343 Peachtree Road, NE, Suite 850
Atlanta, Georgia 30326
Phone: 404-975-5000
Fax: 404-975-5020
E-mail: mstoll@acenursing.org
Website: www.acenursing.org

NURSE MIDWIFERY
Heather L. Maurer, M.A., Executive Director
Accreditation Commission for Midwifery Education (ACME)
American College of Nurse-Midwives
8403 Colesville Road, Suite 1550
Silver Spring, Maryland 20910
Phone: 240-485-1800
Fax: 240-485-1818
E-mail: info@acnm.org
Website: www.midwife.org/Program-Accreditation

NURSE PRACTITIONER
Gay Johnson, CEO
National Association of Nurse Practitioners in Women's Health
Council on Accreditation
505 C Street, NE
Washington, DC 20002
Phone: 202-543-9693 Ext. 1
Fax: 202-543-9858
E-mail: info@npwh.org
Website: www.npwh.org

NURSING
Marsal P. Stoll, Chief Executive Director
Accreditation Commission for Education in Nursing (ACEN)
3343 Peachtree Road, NE, Suite 850
Atlanta, Georgia 30326
Phone: 404-975-5000
Fax: 404-975-5020
E-mail: info@acenursing.org
Website: www.acenursing.org

OCCUPATIONAL THERAPY
Heather Stagliano, DHSc, OTR/L, Executive Director
The American Occupational Therapy Association, Inc.
4720 Montgomery Lane, Suite 200
Bethesda, Maryland 20814-3449
Phone: 301-652-6611 Ext. 2682
TDD: 800-377-8555
Fax: 240-762-5150
E-mail: accred@aota.org
Website: www.aoteonline.org

OPTOMETRY
Joyce L. Urbeck, Administrative Director
Accreditation Council on Optometric Education (ACOE)
American Optometric Association
243 North Lindbergh Boulevard
St. Louis, Missouri 63141-7881
Phone: 314-991-4100, Ext. 4246
Fax: 314-991-4101
E-mail: accredit@aoa.org
Website: www.theacoe.org

OSTEOPATHIC MEDICINE
Director, Department of Accreditation
Commission on Osteopathic College Accreditation (COCA)
American Osteopathic Association
142 East Ontario Street
Chicago, Illinois 60611
Phone: 312-202-8048
Fax: 312-202-8202
E-mail: predoc@osteopathic.org
Website: www.aoacoca.org

PHARMACY
Peter H. Vlasses, PharmD, Executive Director
Accreditation Council for Pharmacy Education
135 South LaSalle Street, Suite 4100
Chicago, Illinois 60603-4810
Phone: 312-664-3575
Fax: 312-664-4652
E-mail: csinfo@acpe-accredit.org
Website: www.acpe-accredit.org

PHYSICAL THERAPY
Sandra Wise, Senior Director
Commission on Accreditation in Physical Therapy Education (CAPTE)
American Physical Therapy Association (APTA)
1111 North Fairfax Street
Alexandria, Virginia 22314-1488
Phone: 703-706-3245
Fax: 703-706-3387
E-mail: accreditation@apta.org
Website: www.capteonline.org

PHYSICIAN ASSISTANT STUDIES
Sharon L. Luke, Executive Director
Accredittion Review Commission on Education for the Physician Assistant, Inc. (ARC-PA)
12000 Findley Road, Suite 150
Johns Creek, Georgia 30097
Phone: 770-476-1224
Fax: 770-476-1738
E-mail: arc-pa@arc-pa.org
Website: www.arc-pa.org

PLANNING
Ms. Shonagh Merits, Executive Director
American Institute of Certified Planners/Association of Collegiate Schools of Planning/American Planning Association
Planning Accreditation Board (PAB)
2334 West Lawrence Avenue, Suite 209
Chicago, Illinois 60625
Phone: 773-334-7200
E-mail: smerits@planningaccreditationboard.org
Website: www.planningaccreditationboard.org

PODIATRIC MEDICINE
Alan R. Tinkleman, M.P.A., Executive Director
Council on Podiatric Medical Education (CPME)
American Podiatric Medical Association (APMA)
9312 Old Georgetown Road
Bethesda, Maryland 20814-1621
Phone: 301-581-9200
Fax: 301-571-4903
Website: www.cpme.org

PSYCHOLOGY AND COUNSELING
Jacqueline Remondet Wall, CEO of the Accrediting Unit,
Office of Program Consultation and Accreditation
American Psychological Association
750 First Street, NE
Washington, DC 20002-4202
Phone: 202-336-5979 or 800-374-2721
TDD/TTY: 202-336-6123
Fax: 202-336-5978
E-mail: apaaccred@apa.org
Website: www.apa.org/ed/accreditation

Carol L. Bobby, Ph.D., Executive Director
Council for Accreditation of Counseling and Related Educational Programs (CACREP)
1001 North Fairfax Street, Suite 510
Alexandria, Virginia 22314
Phone: 703-535-5990
Fax: 703-739-6209
E-mail: cacrep@cacrep.org
Website: www.cacrep.org

Richard M. McFall, Executive Director
Psychological Clinical Science Accreditation System (PCSAS)
1101 East Tenth Street
IU Psychology Building
Bloomington, Indiana 47405-7007
Phone: 812-856-2570
Fax: 812-322-5545
E-mail: rmmcfall@pcsas.org
Website: www.pcsas.org

PUBLIC HEALTH
Laura Rasar King, M.P.H., MCHES, Executive Director
Council on Education for Public Health
1010 Wayne Avenue, Suite 220
Silver Spring, Maryland 20910
Phone: 202-789-1050
Fax: 202-789-1895
E-mail: Lking@ceph.org
Website: www.ceph.org

PUBLIC POLICY, AFFAIRS AND ADMINISTRATION
Crystal Calarusse, Chief Accreditation Officer
Commission on Peer Review and Accreditation
Network of Schools of Public Policy, Affairs, and Administration (NASPAA-COPRA)
1029 Vermont Avenue, NW, Suite 1100
Washington, DC 20005
Phone: 202-628-8965
Fax: 202-626-4978
E-mail: copra@naspaa.org
Website: www.naspaa.org

RADIOLOGIC TECHNOLOGY
Leslie Winter, Chief Executive Officer Joint Review Committee on Education in Radiologic Technology (JRCERT)
20 North Wacker Drive, Suite 2850
Chicago, Illinois 60606-3182
Phone: 312-704-5300
Fax: 312-704-5304
E-mail: mail@jrcert.org
Web: www.jrcert.org

REHABILITATION EDUCATION
Frank Lane, Ph.D., Executive Director
Council on Rehabilitation Education (CORE)
Commission on Standards and Accreditation
1699 Woodfield Road, Suite 300
Schaumburg, Illinois 60173
Phone: 847-944-1345
Fax: 847-944-1346
E-mail: flane@core-rehab.org
Website: www.core-rehab.org

RESPIRATORY CARE
Thomas Smalling, Executive Director
Commission on Accreditation for Respiratory Care (CoARC)
1248 Harwood Road
Bedford, Texas 76021-4244
Phone: 817-283-2835
Fax: 817-354-8519
E-mail: tom@coarc.com
Website: www.coarc.com

SOCIAL WORK
Dr. Stacey Borasky, Director of Accreditation
Office of Social Work Accreditation
Council on Social Work Education
1701 Duke Street, Suite 200
Alexandria, Virginia 22314
Phone: 703-683-8080
Fax: 703-519-2078
E-mail: info@cswe.org
Website: www.cswe.org

SPEECH-LANGUAGE PATHOLOGY AND AUDIOLOGY
Patrima L. Tice, Accreditation Executive Director
American Speech-Language-Hearing Association
Council on Academic Accreditation in Audiology and Speech-Language Pathology
2200 Research Boulevard #310
Rockville, Maryland 20850-3289
Phone: 301-296-5700
Fax: 301-296-8750
E-mail: accreditation@asha.org
Website: http://caa.asha.org

TEACHER EDUCATION
Christopher A. Koch, President
National Council for Accreditation of Teacher Education (NCATE)
Teacher Education Accreditation Council (TEAC)
1140 19th Street, Suite 400
Washington, DC 20036
Phone: 202-223-0077
Fax: 202-296-6620
E-mail: caep@caepnet.org
Website: www.ncate.org

TECHNOLOGY
Michale S. McComis, Ed.D., Executive Director
Accrediting Commission of Career Schools and Colleges
2101 Wilson Boulevard, Suite 302
Arlington, Virginia 22201
Phone: 703-247-4212
Fax: 703-247-4533
E-mail: mccomis@accsc.org
Website: www.accsc.org

TECHNOLOGY, MANAGEMENT, AND APPLIED ENGINEERING
Kelly Schild, Director of Accreditation
The Association of Technology, Management, and Applied Engineering (ATMAE)
275 N. York Street, Suite 401
Elmhurst, Illinois 60126
Phone: 630-433-4514
Fax: 630-563-9181
E-mail: Kelly@atmae.org
Website: www.atmae.org

THEATER
Karen P. Moynahan, Executive Director
National Association of Schools of Theatre Commission on Accreditation
11250 Roger Bacon Drive, Suite 21
Reston, Virginia 20190
Phone: 703-437-0700
Fax: 703-437-6312
E-mail: info@arts-accredit.org
Website: http://nast.arts-accredit.org/

THEOLOGY
Dr. Bernard Fryshman, Executive VP
Emeritus and Interim Executive Director
Association of Advanced Rabbinical and Talmudic Schools (AARTS)
Accreditation Commission
11 Broadway, Suite 405
New York, New York 10004
Phone: 212-363-1991
Fax: 212-533-5335
E-mail: office.aarts@gmail.com

Daniel O. Aleshire, Executive Director
Association of Theological Schools in the United States and Canada (ATS)
Commission on Accrediting
10 Summit Park Drive
Pittsburgh, Pennsylvania 15275
Phone: 412-788-6505
Fax: 412-788-6510
E-mail: ats@ats.edu
Website: www.ats.edu

Dr. Timothy Eaton, Interim President
Transnational Association of Christian Colleges and Schools (TRACS)
Accreditation Commission
15935 Forest Road
Forest, Virginia 24551
Phone: 434-525-9539
Fax: 434-525-9538
E-mail: info@tracs.org
Website: www.tracs.org

VETERINARY MEDICINE
Dr. Karen Brandt, Director of Education and Research
American Veterinary Medical Association (AVMA)
Council on Education
1931 North Meacham Road, Suite 100
Schaumburg, Illinois 60173-4360
Phone: 847-925-8070 Ext. 6674
Fax: 847-285-5732
E-mail: info@avma.org
Website: www.avma.org

How to Use These Guides

As you identify the particular programs and institutions that interest you, you can use both the *Graduate & Professional Programs: An Overview* volume and the specialized volumes in the series to obtain detailed information.

- *Graduate Programs in the Biological/Biomedical Sciences & Health-Related Professions*
- *Graduate Programs in Business, Education, Information Studies, Law & Social Work*
- *Graduate Programs in Engineering & Applied Sciences*
- *Graduate Programs the Humanities, Arts & Social Sciences*
- *Graduate Programs in the Physical Sciences, Mathematics, Agricultural Sciences, the Environment & Natural Resources*

Each of the specialized volumes in the series is divided into sections that contain one or more directories devoted to programs in a particular field. If you do not find a directory devoted to your field of interest in a specific volume, consult "Directories and Subject Areas" (located at the end of each volume). After you have identified the correct volume, consult the "Directories and Subject Areas in This Book" index, which shows (as does the more general directory) what directories cover subjects not specifically named in a directory or section title.

Each of the specialized volumes in the series has a number of general directories. These directories have entries for the largest unit at an institution granting graduate degrees in that field. For example, the general Engineering and Applied Sciences directory in the *Graduate Programs in Engineering & Applied Sciences* volume consists of **Profiles** for colleges, schools, and departments of engineering and applied sciences.

General directories are followed by other directories, or sections, that give more detailed information about programs in particular areas of the general field that has been covered. The general Engineering and Applied Sciences directory, in the previous example, is followed by nineteen sections with directories in specific areas of engineering, such as Chemical Engineering, Industrial/Management Engineering, and Mechanical Engineering.

Because of the broad nature of many fields, any system of organization is bound to involve a certain amount of overlap. Environmental studies, for example, is a field whose various aspects are studied in several types of departments and schools. Readers interested in such studies will find information on relevant programs in the *Graduate Programs in the Biological/Biomedical Sciences & Health-Related Professions* volume under Ecology and Environmental Biology and Environmental and Occupational Health; in the *Graduate Programs in the Physical Sciences, Mathematics, Agricultural Sciences, the Environment & Natural Resources* volume under Environmental Management and Policy and Natural Resources; and in the *Graduate Programs in Engineering & Applied Sciences* volume under Energy Management and Policy and Environmental Engineering. To help you find all of the programs of interest to you, the introduction to each section within the specialized volumes includes, if applicable, a paragraph suggesting other sections and directories with information on related areas of study.

Directory of Institutions with Programs in the Biological/Biomedical Sciences & Health-Related Medical Professions

This directory lists institutions in alphabetical order and includes beneath each name the academic fields in which each institution offers graduate programs. The degree level in each field is also indicated, provided that the institution has supplied that information in response to Peterson's Annual Survey of Graduate and Professional Institutions.

An M indicates that a master's degree program is offered; a D indicates that a doctoral degree program is offered; a P indicates that the first professional degree is offered; an O signifies that other advanced degrees (e.g., certificates or specialist degrees) are offered; and an * (asterisk) indicates that a **Close-Up** and/or **Display** is located in this volume. See the index, "Close-Ups and Displays," for the specific page number.

Profiles of Academic and Professional Programs in the Specialized Volumes

Each section of **Profiles** has a table of contents that lists the Program Directories, **Displays**, and **Close-Ups.** Program Directories consist of the **Profiles** of programs in the relevant fields, with **Displays** following if programs have chosen to include them. **Close-Ups,** which are more individualized statements, are also listed for those graduate schools or programs that have chosen to submit them.

The **Profiles** found in the 500 directories in the specialized volumes provide basic data about the graduate units in capsule form for quick reference. To make these directories as useful as possible, **Profiles** are generally listed for an institution's smallest academic unit within a subject area. In other words, if an institution has a College of Liberal Arts that administers many related programs, the **Profile** for the individual program (e.g., Program in History), not the entire College, appears in the directory.

There are some programs that do not fit into any current directory and are not given individual **Profiles.** The directory structure is reviewed annually in order to keep this number to a minimum and to accommodate major trends in graduate education.

The following outline describes the **Profile** information found in the guides and explains how best to use that information. Any item that does not apply to or was not provided by a graduate unit is omitted from its listing. The format of the **Profiles** is constant, making it easy to compare one institution with another and one program with another.

A ★ graphic next to the school's name indicates the institution has additional detailed information in a "Premium Profile" on Petersons.com. After reading their information here, you can learn more about the school by visiting www.petersons.com and searching for that particular college or university's graduate program.

Identifying Information. The institution's name, in boldface type, is followed by a complete listing of the administrative structure for that field of study. (For example, University of Akron, Buchtel College of Arts and Sciences, Department of Theoretical and Applied Mathematics, Program in Mathematics.) The last unit listed is the one to which all information in the **Profile** pertains. The institution's city, state, and zip code follow.

Offerings. Each field of study offered by the unit is listed with all postbaccalaureate degrees awarded. Degrees that are not preceded by a specific concentration are awarded in the general field listed in the unit name. Frequently, fields of study are broken down into subspecializations, and those appear following the degrees awarded; for example, "Offerings in secondary education (M.Ed.), including English education, mathematics education, science education." Students enrolled in the M.Ed. program would be able to specialize in any of the three fields mentioned.

Professional Accreditation. Some **Profiles** indicate whether a program is professionally accredited. Because it is possible for a program to receive or lose professional accreditation at any time, students entering fields in which accreditation is important to a career should verify the status of programs by contacting either the chairperson or the appropriate accrediting association.

Jointly Offered Degrees. Explanatory statements concerning programs that are offered in cooperation with other institutions are included in the list of degrees offered. This occurs most commonly on a regional basis (for example, two state universities offering a cooperative Ph.D. in special education) or where the specialized nature of the institutions encourages joint efforts (a J.D./M.B.A. offered by a law school at an institution with no formal business programs and an institution with a business school but lacking a law school). Only programs that are truly cooperative are listed; those involving only limited course work at another institution are not. Interested students should contact the heads of such units for further information.

Program Availability. This may include the following: part-time, evening/weekend, online only, 100% online, blended/hybrid learning, and/or minimal on-campus study, When information regarding the availability of part-time or evening/weekend study appears in the **Profile**, it means that students are able to earn a degree exclusively through such study. Blended/hybrid learning describe those courses in which some traditional in-class time has been replaced by online learning activities. Hybrid courses take advantage of the best features of both face-to-face and online learning.

Faculty. Figures on the number of faculty members actively involved with graduate students through teaching or research are separated into full- and part-time as well as men and women whenever the information has been supplied.

Students. Figures for the number of students enrolled in graduate and professional programs pertain to the semester of highest enrollment from the 2015–16 academic year. These figures are broken down into full- and part-time and men and women whenever the data have been supplied. Information on the number of matriculated students enrolled in the unit who are members of a minority group or are international students appears here. The average age of the matriculated students is followed by the number of applicants, the percentage accepted, and the number enrolled for fall 2015.

Degrees Awarded. The number of degrees awarded in the calendar year is listed. Many doctoral programs offer a terminal master's degree if students leave the program after completing only part of the requirements for a doctoral degree; that is indicated here. All degrees are classified into one of four types: master's, doctoral, first professional, and other advanced degrees. A unit may award one or several degrees at a given level; however, the data are only collected by type and may therefore represent several different degree programs.

Degree Requirements. The information in this section is also broken down by type of degree, and all information for a degree level pertains to all degrees of that type unless otherwise specified. Degree requirements are collected in a simplified form to provide some very basic information on the nature of the program and on foreign language, thesis or dissertation, comprehensive exam, and registration requirements. Many units also provide a short list of additional requirements, such as fieldwork or an internship. For complete information on graduation requirements, contact the graduate school or program directly.

Entrance Requirements. Entrance requirements are broken down into the four degree levels of master's, doctoral, first professional, and other advanced degrees. Within each level, information may be provided in two basic categories: entrance exams and other requirements. The entrance exams are identified by the standard acronyms used by the testing agencies, unless they are not well known. Other entrance requirements are quite varied, but they often contain an undergraduate or graduate grade point average (GPA). Unless otherwise stated, the GPA is calculated on a 4.0 scale and is listed as a minimum required for admission. Additional exam requirements/recommendations for international students may be listed here. Application deadlines for domestic and international students, the application fee, and whether electronic applications are accepted may be listed here. Note that the deadline should be used for reference only; these dates are subject to change, and students interested in applying should always contact the graduate unit directly about application procedures and deadlines.

Expenses. The typical cost of study for the 2016–2017 academic year (2015–16 if 2016–17 figures were not available) is given in two basic categories: tuition and fees. Cost of study may be quite complex at a graduate institution. There are often sliding scales for part-time study, a different cost for first-year students, and other variables that make it impossible to completely cover the cost of study for each graduate program. To provide the most usable information, figures are given for full-time study for a full year where available and for part-time study in terms of a per-unit rate (per credit, per semester hour, etc.). Occasionally, variances may be noted in tuition and fees for reasons such as the type of program, whether courses are taken during the day or evening, whether courses are at the master's or doctoral level, or other institution-specific reasons. Respondents were also given the opportunity to provide more specific and detailed tuition and fees information at the unit level. When provided, this information will appear in place of any typical costs entered elsewhere on the university-level survey. Expenses are usually subject to change; for exact costs at any given time, contact your chosen schools and programs directly. Keep in mind that the tuition of Canadian institutions is usually given in Canadian dollars.

Financial Support. This section contains data on the number of awards administered by the institution and given to graduate students during the 2015–16 academic year. The first figure given represents the total number of students receiving financial support enrolled in that unit. If the unit has provided information on graduate appointments, these are broken down into three major categories: fellowships give money to graduate students to cover the cost of study and living expenses and are not based on a work obligation or research commitment, research assistantships provide stipends to graduate students for assistance in a formal research project with a faculty member, and teaching assistantships provide stipends to graduate students for teaching or for assisting faculty members in teaching undergraduate classes. Within each category, figures are given for the total number of awards, the average yearly amount per award, and whether full or partial tuition reimbursements are awarded. In addition to graduate appointments, the availability of several other financial aid sources is covered in this section. Tuition waivers are routinely part of a graduate appointment, but units sometimes waive part or all of a student's tuition even if a graduate appointment is not available. Federal WorkStudy is made available to students who demonstrate need and meet the federal guidelines; this form of aid normally includes 10 or more hours of work per week in an office of the institution. Institutionally sponsored loans are low-interest loans available to graduate students to cover both educational and living expenses. Career-related internships or fieldwork offer money to students who are participating in a formal off-campus research project or practicum. Grants, scholarships, traineeships, unspecified assistantships, and other awards may also be noted. The availability of financial support to part-time students is also indicated here.

Some programs list the financial aid application deadline and the forms that need to be completed for students to be eligible for financial awards. There are two forms: FAFSA, the Free Application for Federal Student Aid, which is required for federal aid, and the CSS PROFILE®.

Faculty Research. Each unit has the opportunity to list several keyword phrases describing the current research involving faculty members and graduate students. Space limitations prevent the unit from listing complete information on all research programs. The total expenditure for funded research from the previous academic year may also be included.

Unit Head and Application Contact. The head of the graduate program for each unit may be listed with academic title, phone and fax numbers, and e-mail address. In addition to the unit head's contact information, many graduate programs also list a separate contact for application and admission information, followed by the graduate school, program, or department's website. If no unit head or application contact is given, you should contact the overall institution for information on graduate admissions.

Displays and Close-Ups

The **Displays** and **Close-Ups** are supplementary insertions submitted by deans, chairs, and other administrators who wish to offer an additional, more individualized statement to readers. A number of graduate school and program administrators have attached a **Display** ad near the **Profile** listing. Here you will find information that an institution or program wants to emphasize. The **Close-Ups** are by their very nature more expansive and flexible than the **Profiles**, and the administrators who have written them may emphasize different aspects of their programs. All of the **Close-Ups** are organized in the same way (with the exception of a few that describe research and training opportunities instead of degree programs), and in each one you will find information on the same basic topics, such as programs of study, research facilities, tuition and fees, financial aid, and application procedures. If an institution or program has submitted a **Close-Up**, a boldface cross-reference appears below its **Profile**. As with the **Displays**, all of the **Close-Ups** in the guides have been submitted by choice; the absence of a **Display** or **Close-Up** does not reflect any type of editorial judgment on the part of Peterson's, and their presence in the guides should not be taken as an indication of status, quality, or approval. Statements regarding a university's objectives and accomplishments are a reflection of its own beliefs and are not the opinions of the Peterson's editors.

Appendixes

This section contains two appendixes. The first, "Institutional Changes Since the 2016 Edition," lists institutions that have closed, merged, or changed their name or status since the last edition of the guides. The second, "Abbreviations Used in the Guides," gives abbreviations of degree names, along with what those abbreviations stand for. These appendixes are identical in all six volumes of *Peterson's Graduate and Professional Programs*.

Indexes

There are three indexes presented here. The first index, "Close-Ups and Displays," gives page references for all programs that have chosen to place **Close-Ups** and **Displays** in this volume. It is arranged alphabetically by institution; within institutions, the arrangement is alphabetical by subject area. It is not an index to all programs in the book's directories of **Profiles**; readers must refer to the directories themselves for **Profile** information on programs that have not submitted the additional, more individualized statements. The second index, "Directories and Subject Areas in Other Books in This Series", gives book references for the directories in the specialized volumes and also includes cross-references for subject area names not used in the directory structure, for example, "Computing Technology (see Computer Science)." The third index, "Directories and Subject Areas in This Book," gives page references for the directories in this volume and cross-references for subject area names not used in this volume's directory structure.

Data Collection Procedures

The information published in the directories and Profiles of all the books is collected through Peterson's Annual Survey of Graduate and Professional Institutions. The survey is sent each spring to more than 2,200 institutions offering postbaccalaureate degree programs, including accredited institutions in the United States, U.S. territories, and Canada and those institutions outside the United States that are accredited by U.S. accrediting bodies. Deans and other administrators complete these surveys, providing information on programs in the 500 academic and professional fields covered in the guides as well as overall institutional information. While every effort has been made to ensure the

accuracy and completeness of the data, information is sometimes unavailable or changes occur after publication deadlines. All usable information received in time for publication has been included. The omission of any particular item from a directory or Profile signifies either that the item is not applicable to the institution or program or that information was not available. Profiles of programs scheduled to begin during the 2016–17 academic year cannot, obviously, include statistics on enrollment or, in many cases, the number of faculty members. If no usable data were submitted by an institution, its name, address, and program name appear in order to indicate the availability of graduate work.

Criteria for Inclusion in This Guide

To be included in this guide, an institution must have full accreditation or be a candidate for accreditation (preaccreditation) status by an institutional or specialized accrediting body recognized by the U.S. Department of Education or the Council for Higher Education Accreditation (CHEA). Institutional accrediting bodies, which review each institution as a whole, include the six regional associations of schools and colleges (Middle States, New England, North Central, Northwest, Southern, and Western), each of which is responsible for a specified portion of the United States and its territories. Other institutional accrediting bodies are national in scope and accredit specific kinds of institutions (e.g., Bible colleges, independent colleges, and rabbinical and Talmudic schools). Program registration by the New York State Board of Regents is considered to be the equivalent of institutional accreditation, since the board requires that all programs offered by an institution meet its standards before recognition is granted. A Canadian institution must be chartered and authorized to grant degrees by the provincial government, affiliated with a chartered institution, or accredited by a recognized U.S. accrediting body. This guide also includes institutions outside the United States that are accredited by these U.S. accrediting bodies. There are recognized specialized or professional accrediting bodies in more than fifty different fields, each of which is authorized to accredit institutions or specific programs in its particular field. For specialized institutions that offer programs in one field only, we designate this to be the equivalent of institutional accreditation. A full explanation of the accrediting process and complete information on recognized institutional (regional and national) and specialized accrediting bodies can be found online at www.chea.org or at www.ed.gov/admins/finaid/accred/index.html.

DIRECTORY OF INSTITUTIONS WITH PROGRAMS IN THE BIOLOGICAL/BIOMEDICAL SCIENCES & HEALTH-RELATED MEDICAL PROFESSIONS

ABILENE CHRISTIAN UNIVERSITY
Communication Disorders — M
Nutrition — O
Occupational Therapy — M

ACADEMY FOR FIVE ELEMENT ACUPUNCTURE
Acupuncture and Oriental Medicine — M

ACADEMY OF CHINESE CULTURE AND HEALTH SCIENCES
Acupuncture and Oriental Medicine — M

ACADIA UNIVERSITY
Biological and Biomedical Sciences—General — M

ACUPUNCTURE & INTEGRATIVE MEDICINE COLLEGE, BERKELEY
Acupuncture and Oriental Medicine — M

ACUPUNCTURE AND MASSAGE COLLEGE
Acupuncture and Oriental Medicine — M

ADELPHI UNIVERSITY
Adult Nursing — M
Biological and Biomedical Sciences—General — M
Communication Disorders — M,D
Community Health — M,O
Health Services Management and Hospital Administration — M
Nursing and Healthcare Administration — M,O
Nursing—General — D
Nutrition — M,D,O
Public Health—General — M,O

ADLER UNIVERSITY
Biopsychology — M,D,O

ADVENTIST UNIVERSITY OF HEALTH SCIENCES
Nurse Anesthesia — M

ALABAMA AGRICULTURAL AND MECHANICAL UNIVERSITY
Biological and Biomedical Sciences—General — M,D
Communication Disorders — M
Nutrition — M

ALABAMA STATE UNIVERSITY
Allied Health—General — M,D
Biological and Biomedical Sciences—General — M,D
Occupational Therapy — M
Physical Therapy — D
Rehabilitation Sciences — M

ALASKA PACIFIC UNIVERSITY
Health Services Management and Hospital Administration — M

ALBANY COLLEGE OF PHARMACY AND HEALTH SCIENCES
Cell Biology — M
Clinical Laboratory Sciences/Medical Technology — M
Health Services Research — M,D
Molecular Biology — M
Pharmaceutical Sciences — M,D
Pharmacology — M,D
Pharmacy — M,D

ALBANY MEDICAL COLLEGE
Allopathic Medicine — D
Bioethics — M,D,O
Cardiovascular Sciences — M,D
Cell Biology — M,D
Immunology — M,D
Microbiology — M,D
Molecular Biology — M,D
Neuroscience — M,D
Nurse Anesthesia — M
Pharmacology — M,D
Physician Assistant Studies — M

ALBANY STATE UNIVERSITY
Family Nurse Practitioner Studies — M
Health Services Management and Hospital Administration — M
Nursing Education — M
Nursing—General — M

ALBERT EINSTEIN COLLEGE OF MEDICINE
Allopathic Medicine — D
Anatomy — D
Biochemistry — D
Biological and Biomedical Sciences—General — D
Biophysics — D
Cell Biology — D
Clinical Research — D
Computational Biology — D
Developmental Biology — D
Genetics — D
Genomic Sciences — D
Immunology — D
Microbiology — D
Molecular Biology — D
Molecular Genetics — D
Molecular Pharmacology — D
Neurobiology — D
Pathology — D
Physiology — D
Systems Biology — D

ALCORN STATE UNIVERSITY
Biological and Biomedical Sciences—General — M
Nursing—General — M

ALDERSON BROADDUS UNIVERSITY
Physician Assistant Studies — M

ALLEN COLLEGE
Acute Care/Critical Care Nursing — M,D,O

Adult Nursing — M,D,O
Community Health Nursing — M,D,O
Family Nurse Practitioner Studies — M,D,O
Gerontological Nursing — M,D,O
Nursing and Healthcare Administration — M,D,O
Nursing—General — M,D,O
Occupational Therapy — M,D,O
Psychiatric Nursing — M,D,O
Public Health—General — M,D,O

ALLIANT INTERNATIONAL UNIVERSITY–SAN DIEGO
Neuroscience — M,D,O

ALLIANT INTERNATIONAL UNIVERSITY–SAN FRANCISCO
Pharmacology — M

ALVERNIA UNIVERSITY
Occupational Therapy — M

ALVERNO COLLEGE
Family Nurse Practitioner Studies — M
Nursing—General — M
Psychiatric Nursing — M

AMERICAN COLLEGE OF ACUPUNCTURE AND ORIENTAL MEDICINE
Acupuncture and Oriental Medicine — M

AMERICAN COLLEGE OF HEALTHCARE SCIENCES
Allied Health—General — M,O
Nutrition — M,O

AMERICAN INTERCONTINENTAL UNIVERSITY ONLINE
Health Services Management and Hospital Administration — M

AMERICAN INTERNATIONAL COLLEGE
Family Nurse Practitioner Studies — M
Nursing and Healthcare Administration — M
Nursing Education — M
Nursing—General — M
Occupational Therapy — M
Physical Therapy — M

AMERICAN MUSEUM OF NATURAL HISTORY–RICHARD GILDER GRADUATE SCHOOL
Biological and Biomedical Sciences—General — D

AMERICAN PUBLIC UNIVERSITY SYSTEM
Health Services Management and Hospital Administration — M
Public Health—General — M

AMERICAN SENTINEL UNIVERSITY
Health Services Management and Hospital Administration — M
Nursing—General — M

AMERICAN UNIVERSITY
Biopsychology — M,D,O
Health Promotion — M
Neuroscience — M,D,O
Nutrition — M,O

AMERICAN UNIVERSITY OF ARMENIA
Public Health—General — M

AMERICAN UNIVERSITY OF BEIRUT
Allopathic Medicine — M,D
Anatomy — M,D
Biochemistry — M,D
Biological and Biomedical Sciences—General — M,D
Cell Biology — M,D
Community Health — M
Environmental and Occupational Health — M
Epidemiology — M
Genetics — M,D
Health Promotion — M
Health Services Management and Hospital Administration — M
Immunology — M,D
Microbiology — M,D
Molecular Biology — M,D
Neuroscience — M,D
Nursing—General — M
Nutrition — M
Pharmacology — M,D
Psychiatric Nursing — M
Toxicology — M,D

AMERICAN UNIVERSITY OF HEALTH SCIENCES
Clinical Research — M

ANDREWS UNIVERSITY
Allied Health—General — M
Biological and Biomedical Sciences—General — M
Communication Disorders — M
Nursing—General — M,D
Nutrition — M,O
Physical Therapy — D
Public Health—General — M,O

ANGELO STATE UNIVERSITY
Biological and Biomedical Sciences—General — M
Family Nurse Practitioner Studies — M
Nursing Education — M
Nursing—General — M
Physical Therapy — D

ANNA MARIA COLLEGE
Environmental and Occupational Health — M

ANTIOCH UNIVERSITY NEW ENGLAND
Conservation Biology — M

AOMA GRADUATE SCHOOL OF INTEGRATIVE MEDICINE
Acupuncture and Oriental Medicine — M,D

APPALACHIAN COLLEGE OF PHARMACY
Pharmacy — D

APPALACHIAN STATE UNIVERSITY
Biological and Biomedical Sciences—General — M
Cell Biology — M
Communication Disorders — M
Molecular Biology — M
Nutrition — M
Rehabilitation Sciences — M

AQUINAS COLLEGE (MI)
Health Services Management and Hospital Administration — M

AQUINAS COLLEGE (TN)
Nursing Education — M
Nursing—General — M

AQUINAS INSTITUTE OF THEOLOGY
Health Services Management and Hospital Administration — M,D,O

ARCADIA UNIVERSITY
Community Health — M
Physical Therapy — D
Physician Assistant Studies — M
Public Health—General — M

ARGOSY UNIVERSITY, ATLANTA
Biopsychology — M,D,O
Health Services Management and Hospital Administration — M,D
Public Health—General — M

ARGOSY UNIVERSITY, CHICAGO
Health Services Management and Hospital Administration — M,D
Neuroscience — D
Public Health—General — M

ARGOSY UNIVERSITY, DALLAS
Health Services Management and Hospital Administration — M,D
Public Health—General — M

ARGOSY UNIVERSITY, DENVER
Health Services Management and Hospital Administration — M,D
Public Health—General — M

ARGOSY UNIVERSITY, HAWAI'I
Health Services Management and Hospital Administration — M,D,O
Pharmacology — M,O
Public Health—General — M

ARGOSY UNIVERSITY, INLAND EMPIRE
Health Services Management and Hospital Administration — M,D
Public Health—General — M

ARGOSY UNIVERSITY, LOS ANGELES
Health Services Management and Hospital Administration — M,D
Public Health—General — M

ARGOSY UNIVERSITY, NASHVILLE
Health Services Management and Hospital Administration — M,D
Public Health—General — M

ARGOSY UNIVERSITY, ORANGE COUNTY
Health Services Management and Hospital Administration — M,D,O
Public Health—General — M

ARGOSY UNIVERSITY, PHOENIX
Health Services Management and Hospital Administration — M,D
Neuroscience — M,D
Public Health—General — M

ARGOSY UNIVERSITY, SALT LAKE CITY
Health Services Management and Hospital Administration — M,D
Public Health—General — M

ARGOSY UNIVERSITY, SAN DIEGO
Public Health—General — M

ARGOSY UNIVERSITY, SAN FRANCISCO BAY AREA
Health Services Management and Hospital Administration — M,D
Public Health—General — M

ARGOSY UNIVERSITY, SARASOTA
Health Services Management and Hospital Administration — M,D,O
Public Health—General — M

ARGOSY UNIVERSITY, SCHAUMBURG
Health Services Management and Hospital Administration — M,D,O
Public Health—General — M

ARGOSY UNIVERSITY, SEATTLE
Health Services Management and Hospital Administration — M,D
Public Health—General — M

ARGOSY UNIVERSITY, TAMPA
Health Services Management and Hospital Administration — M,D
Neuroscience — M,D
Public Health—General — M

ARGOSY UNIVERSITY, TWIN CITIES
Biopsychology — M,D,O
Health Services Management and Hospital Administration — M,D
Public Health—General — M

ARGOSY UNIVERSITY, WASHINGTON DC
Health Services Management and Hospital Administration — M,D,O
Public Health—General — M

ARIZONA SCHOOL OF ACUPUNCTURE AND ORIENTAL MEDICINE
Acupuncture and Oriental Medicine — M

ARIZONA STATE UNIVERSITY AT THE TEMPE CAMPUS
Animal Behavior — M,D
Biochemistry — M,D
Biological and Biomedical Sciences—General — M,D
Cell Biology — M,D
Communication Disorders — M,D
Community Health — M,D,O
Conservation Biology — M,D
Evolutionary Biology — M,D
Family Nurse Practitioner Studies — M,D,O
Gerontological Nursing — M,D,O
Health Promotion — M,D
Health Services Management and Hospital Administration — M,D
International Health — M,D,O
Microbiology — M,D
Molecular Biology — M,D
Neuroscience — M,D
Nursing and Healthcare Administration — M,D,O
Nursing Education — M,D,O
Nursing—General — M,D,O
Nutrition — M,D
Plant Biology — M,D
Psychiatric Nursing — M,D,O
Public Health—General — M,D,O

ARKANSAS STATE UNIVERSITY
Biological and Biomedical Sciences—General — M,O
Communication Disorders — M,O
Health Services Management and Hospital Administration — M,D,O
Molecular Biology — M,D
Nurse Anesthesia — M,D,O
Nursing—General — M,D,O
Occupational Therapy — D
Physical Therapy — D

ARKANSAS TECH UNIVERSITY
Nursing—General — M

ARMSTRONG STATE UNIVERSITY
Adult Nursing — M,O
Communication Disorders — M
Family Nurse Practitioner Studies — M,O
Gerontological Nursing — M,O
Health Services Management and Hospital Administration — M
Nursing—General — M,O
Physical Therapy — D
Public Health—General — M

ASHWORTH COLLEGE
Health Services Management and Hospital Administration — M

ASSUMPTION COLLEGE
Health Services Management and Hospital Administration — M,O

ATHABASCA UNIVERSITY
Allied Health—General — M,O
Nursing and Healthcare Administration — M,O
Nursing—General — M,O

ATLANTIC INSTITUTE OF ORIENTAL MEDICINE
Acupuncture and Oriental Medicine — M,D

A.T. STILL UNIVERSITY
Allied Health—General — M,D
Biological and Biomedical Sciences—General — M,D
Communication Disorders — M,D
Dentistry — D
Health Services Management and Hospital Administration — M,D
Occupational Therapy — M,D
Oral and Dental Sciences — M,D,O
Osteopathic Medicine — M,D
Physical Therapy — M,D
Physician Assistant Studies — M,D
Public Health—General — M,D

AUBURN UNIVERSITY
Anatomy — M,D
Biochemistry — M,D
Biological and Biomedical Sciences—General — M,D
Botany — M,D
Cell Biology — M,D
Communication Disorders — M,D
Entomology — M,D
Health Promotion — M,D,O
Molecular Biology — M,D
Nursing Education — M
Nursing—General — M
Nutrition — M,D,O
Pathobiology — M,D
Pharmaceutical Sciences — M,D
Pharmacology — M,D
Pharmacy — D
Plant Pathology — M,D
Radiation Biology — M,D
Veterinary Medicine — D
Veterinary Sciences — M,D
Zoology — M,D

AUBURN UNIVERSITY AT MONTGOMERY
Health Services Management and Hospital Administration — M,D,O
Nursing Education — M
Nursing—General — M

Public Health—General	M,D,O

AUGSBURG COLLEGE

Family Nurse Practitioner Studies	M,D
Nursing—General	M,D
Physician Assistant Studies	M
Transcultural Nursing	M,D

AUGUSTA UNIVERSITY

Acute Care/Critical Care Nursing	D
Allopathic Medicine	D
Anatomy	D
Biochemistry	D
Cancer Biology/Oncology	D
Cardiovascular Sciences	D
Cell Biology	D
Clinical Research	M
Dentistry	D
Environmental and Occupational Health	M
Family Nurse Practitioner Studies	M,D,O
Genomic Sciences	M,D
Gerontological Nursing	D
Molecular Medicine	D
Neuroscience	D
Nurse Anesthesia	D
Nursing and Healthcare Administration	M
Nursing—General	D
Occupational Therapy	M
Oral and Dental Sciences	M,D
Pediatric Nursing	M,D,O
Pharmacology	D
Physical Therapy	D
Physician Assistant Studies	M
Physiology	D
Psychiatric Nursing	D
Public Health—General	M

AURORA UNIVERSITY

Nursing—General	M

AUSTIN PEAY STATE UNIVERSITY

Biological and Biomedical Sciences—General	M
Clinical Laboratory Sciences/Medical Technology	M
Family Nurse Practitioner Studies	M
Nursing and Healthcare Administration	M
Nursing Education	M
Nursing Informatics	M
Nursing—General	M
Public Health—General	M

AVILA UNIVERSITY

Health Services Management and Hospital Administration	M

AZUSA PACIFIC UNIVERSITY

Nursing Education	M,D
Nursing—General	M,D
Physical Therapy	D

BAKER COLLEGE CENTER FOR GRADUATE STUDIES–ONLINE

Health Services Management and Hospital Administration	M,D

BALDWIN WALLACE UNIVERSITY

Communication Disorders	M
Health Services Management and Hospital Administration	M
Physician Assistant Studies	M

BALL STATE UNIVERSITY

Biological and Biomedical Sciences—General	M,D
Communication Disorders	M,D
Family Nurse Practitioner Studies	M,D,O
Gerontological Nursing	M,D,O
Health Promotion	M
Neuroscience	M,D,O
Nursing Education	M,D,O
Nursing—General	M,D,O
Nutrition	M
Physiology	M

BANK STREET COLLEGE OF EDUCATION

Maternal and Child Health	M

BARRY UNIVERSITY

Acute Care/Critical Care Nursing	M,O
Anatomy	M
Biological and Biomedical Sciences—General	M
Communication Disorders	M
Family Nurse Practitioner Studies	M,O
Health Services Management and Hospital Administration	M,O
Nurse Anesthesia	M
Nursing and Healthcare Administration	M,D,O
Nursing Education	M,O
Nursing—General	M,D,O
Occupational Therapy	M
Physician Assistant Studies	M
Podiatric Medicine	D
Public Health—General	M

BARUCH COLLEGE OF THE CITY UNIVERSITY OF NEW YORK

Health Services Management and Hospital Administration	M

BASTYR UNIVERSITY

Acupuncture and Oriental Medicine	M,D,O
Naturopathic Medicine	D
Nurse Midwifery	M,O
Nutrition	M,O

BAYLOR COLLEGE OF MEDICINE

Allopathic Medicine	D
Biochemistry	D
Biological and Biomedical Sciences—General	M,D
Biophysics	D
Cancer Biology/Oncology	D
Cardiovascular Sciences	D
Cell Biology	D
Clinical Laboratory Sciences/Medical Technology	M,D
Computational Biology	D
Developmental Biology	D
Genetics	D
Human Genetics	D
Immunology	D
Microbiology	D
Molecular Biology	D
Molecular Biophysics	D
Molecular Medicine	D
Molecular Physiology	D
Neuroscience	D
Nurse Anesthesia	D
Pathology	D
Pharmacology	D
Physician Assistant Studies	M
Structural Biology	D
Translational Biology	D
Virology	D

BAYLOR UNIVERSITY

Allied Health—General	M,D
Biological and Biomedical Sciences—General	M,D
Communication Disorders	M
Community Health	M,D
Ecology	D
Emergency Medical Services	D
Environmental Biology	M,D
Family Nurse Practitioner Studies	M,D
Health Promotion	M
Health Services Management and Hospital Administration	M
Maternal and Child/Neonatal Nursing	M,D
Nurse Midwifery	M,D
Nursing—General	M,D
Nutrition	M
Physical Therapy	D

BAY PATH UNIVERSITY

Occupational Therapy	M
Physician Assistant Studies	M

BELHAVEN UNIVERSITY (MS)

Health Services Management and Hospital Administration	M

BELLARMINE UNIVERSITY

Family Nurse Practitioner Studies	M,D
Nursing and Healthcare Administration	M,D
Nursing Education	M,D
Nursing—General	M,D
Physical Therapy	M,D

BELLEVUE UNIVERSITY

Health Services Management and Hospital Administration	M

BELLIN COLLEGE

Family Nurse Practitioner Studies	M
Nursing Education	M
Nursing—General	M

BELMONT UNIVERSITY

Allied Health—General	M,D
Health Services Management and Hospital Administration	M
Nursing—General	M,D
Occupational Therapy	M,D
Pharmacy	D
Physical Therapy	M,D

BEMIDJI STATE UNIVERSITY

Biological and Biomedical Sciences—General	M

BENEDICTINE UNIVERSITY

Health Promotion	M
Health Services Management and Hospital Administration	M
Nursing—General	M
Nutrition	M
Public Health—General	M

BENNINGTON COLLEGE

Allied Health—General	O

BETHEL COLLEGE

Nursing—General	M

BETHEL UNIVERSITY (MN)

Nurse Midwifery	M,D,O
Nursing Education	M,D,O
Nursing—General	M,D,O
Physician Assistant Studies	M,D,O

BETHEL UNIVERSITY (TN)

Physician Assistant Studies	M

BINGHAMTON UNIVERSITY, STATE UNIVERSITY OF NEW YORK

Biological and Biomedical Sciences—General	M,D
Biopsychology	D
Health Services Management and Hospital Administration	M,D
Nursing—General	M,D,O

BIOLA UNIVERSITY

Communication Disorders	M,O

BLACK HILLS STATE UNIVERSITY

Genomic Sciences	M

BLESSING-RIEMAN COLLEGE OF NURSING

Nursing—General	M

BLESSING–RIEMAN COLLEGE OF NURSING AND HEALTH SCIENCES

Nursing and Healthcare Administration	M
Nursing Education	M
Nursing—General	M

BLOOMSBURG UNIVERSITY OF PENNSYLVANIA

Adult Nursing	M
Biological and Biomedical Sciences—General	M,D
Communication Disorders	M,D
Community Health	M
Family Nurse Practitioner Studies	M
Nurse Anesthesia	M
Nursing and Healthcare Administration	M
Nursing—General	M

BLUFFTON UNIVERSITY

Health Services Management and Hospital Administration	M

BOISE STATE UNIVERSITY

Biological and Biomedical Sciences—General	M,D
Environmental and Occupational Health	M,O
Gerontological Nursing	M,D,O
Health Promotion	M,O
Molecular Biology	M,D
Nursing—General	M,D,O
Public Health—General	M,D,O

BOSTON COLLEGE

Adult Nursing	M,D
Biochemistry	M,D
Biological and Biomedical Sciences—General	D
Forensic Nursing	M,D
Gerontological Nursing	M,D
Maternal and Child/Neonatal Nursing	M,D
Nurse Anesthesia	M,D
Nursing—General	M,D
Pediatric Nursing	M,D
Psychiatric Nursing	M,D
Women's Health Nursing	M,D

BOSTON UNIVERSITY

Allied Health—General	M,D
Allopathic Medicine	D
Anatomy	M,D
Biochemistry	M,D
Biological and Biomedical Sciences—General	M,D
Biophysics	M,D
Biopsychology	M
Cell Biology	M,D
Clinical Research	M
Communication Disorders	M,D
Community Health	M,D
Dental Hygiene	M,D,O
Environmental and Occupational Health	M,D
Epidemiology	M,D
Genetics	D
Genomic Sciences	D
Health Services Management and Hospital Administration	M,D
Immunology	D
International Health	M,D
Medical Imaging	M
Molecular Biology	M,D
Molecular Medicine	D
Neurobiology	M,D
Neuroscience	D
Nutrition	M,D
Occupational Therapy	D
Oral and Dental Sciences	M,D,O
Pathology	D
Pharmaceutical Sciences	M,D
Pharmacology	M,D
Physical Therapy	D
Physician Assistant Studies	M
Physiology	M,D
Public Health—General	M,D,O
Rehabilitation Sciences	D

BOWIE STATE UNIVERSITY

Family Nurse Practitioner Studies	M
Nursing and Healthcare Administration	M
Nursing Education	M
Nursing—General	M

BOWLING GREEN STATE UNIVERSITY

Biological and Biomedical Sciences—General	M,D
Communication Disorders	M,D
Nutrition	M
Public Health—General	M

BRADLEY UNIVERSITY

Biochemistry	M
Biological and Biomedical Sciences—General	M
Nursing and Healthcare Administration	M,D,O
Nursing Education	M,D,O
Nursing—General	M,D,O
Physical Therapy	D

BRANDEIS UNIVERSITY

Biochemistry	D
Biological and Biomedical Sciences—General	M,D,O
Biophysics	D
Cell Biology	M,D
Genetics	M,D
Health Services Management and Hospital Administration	M
International Health	M,D
Microbiology	M,D
Molecular Biology	M,D
Neurobiology	M,D
Neuroscience	M,D

BRANDMAN UNIVERSITY

Health Services Management and Hospital Administration	M

BRENAU UNIVERSITY

Family Nurse Practitioner Studies	M
Health Services Management and Hospital Administration	M
Nursing and Healthcare Administration	M
Nursing Education	M
Occupational Therapy	M

BRIAR CLIFF UNIVERSITY

Nursing—General	M

BRIDGEWATER STATE UNIVERSITY

Health Promotion	M

BRIGHAM YOUNG UNIVERSITY

Biochemistry	M,D
Biological and Biomedical Sciences—General	M,D
Communication Disorders	M
Developmental Biology	M,D
Family Nurse Practitioner Studies	M
Health Promotion	M,D
Microbiology	M,D
Molecular Biology	M,D
Neuroscience	M,D
Nursing—General	M
Nutrition	M
Physiology	M,D

BROADVIEW UNIVERSITY–WEST JORDAN

Health Services Management and Hospital Administration	M

BROCK UNIVERSITY

Allied Health—General	M,D
Biological and Biomedical Sciences—General	M,D
Neuroscience	M,D

BROOKLYN COLLEGE OF THE CITY UNIVERSITY OF NEW YORK

Biological and Biomedical Sciences—General	M
Communication Disorders	M,D
Community Health	M
Health Services Management and Hospital Administration	M
Nutrition	M
Public Health—General	M

BROWN UNIVERSITY

Allopathic Medicine	D
Biochemistry	M,D
Biological and Biomedical Sciences—General	M,D
Cell Biology	M,D
Community Health	M,D
Ecology	D
Epidemiology	M,D
Evolutionary Biology	D
Health Services Research	D
Molecular Biology	M,D
Molecular Pharmacology	M,D
Neuroscience	D
Pathobiology	M,D
Physiology	M,D
Public Health—General	M

BRYAN COLLEGE OF HEALTH SCIENCES

Nurse Anesthesia	M

BUCKNELL UNIVERSITY

Animal Behavior	M
Biological and Biomedical Sciences—General	M

BUFFALO STATE COLLEGE, STATE UNIVERSITY OF NEW YORK

Biological and Biomedical Sciences—General	M
Communication Disorders	M

BUTLER UNIVERSITY

Pharmaceutical Sciences	M,D
Pharmacy	M,D
Physician Assistant Studies	M,D

CABARRUS COLLEGE OF HEALTH SCIENCES

Occupational Therapy	M

CALIFORNIA BAPTIST UNIVERSITY

Adult Nursing	M
Communication Disorders	M
Family Nurse Practitioner Studies	M
Health Promotion	M
Health Services Management and Hospital Administration	M
Nursing Education	M
Nursing—General	M,D
Physician Assistant Studies	M
Public Health—General	M

CALIFORNIA COAST UNIVERSITY

Health Services Management and Hospital Administration	M

CALIFORNIA INSTITUTE OF INTEGRAL STUDIES

Acupuncture and Oriental Medicine	M,D
Ecology	M,D

CALIFORNIA INSTITUTE OF TECHNOLOGY

Biochemistry	M,D

---

*M—masters degree; D—doctorate; O—other advanced degree; *—Close-Up and/or Display*

Biological and Biomedical Sciences—General D
Biophysics D
Cell Biology D
Developmental Biology D
Genetics D
Immunology D
Molecular Biology D
Molecular Biophysics M,D
Neurobiology D
Neuroscience M,D

CALIFORNIA INTERCONTINENTAL UNIVERSITY
Health Services Management and Hospital Administration M,D

CALIFORNIA POLYTECHNIC STATE UNIVERSITY, SAN LUIS OBISPO
Biochemistry M
Biological and Biomedical Sciences—General M

CALIFORNIA SCHOOL OF PODIATRIC MEDICINE AT SAMUEL MERRITT UNIVERSITY
Podiatric Medicine D

CALIFORNIA STATE POLYTECHNIC UNIVERSITY, POMONA
Biological and Biomedical Sciences—General M
Nutrition M

CALIFORNIA STATE UNIVERSITY, BAKERSFIELD
Biological and Biomedical Sciences—General M
Health Services Management and Hospital Administration M

CALIFORNIA STATE UNIVERSITY, CHICO
Biological and Biomedical Sciences—General M
Communication Disorders M
Health Services Management and Hospital Administration M
Nursing—General M
Nutrition M

CALIFORNIA STATE UNIVERSITY, DOMINGUEZ HILLS
Biological and Biomedical Sciences—General M
Nursing—General M
Occupational Therapy M

CALIFORNIA STATE UNIVERSITY, EAST BAY
Biochemistry M
Biological and Biomedical Sciences—General M
Communication Disorders M
Health Services Management and Hospital Administration M

CALIFORNIA STATE UNIVERSITY, FRESNO
Biological and Biomedical Sciences—General M
Communication Disorders M
Family Nurse Practitioner Studies M
Health Promotion M
Health Services Management and Hospital Administration M
Nursing Education M
Nursing—General M
Physical Therapy M,D
Public Health—General M

CALIFORNIA STATE UNIVERSITY, FULLERTON
Biological and Biomedical Sciences—General M
Communication Disorders M
Nurse Anesthesia M,D
Nursing and Healthcare Administration M,D
Nursing Education M,D
Nursing—General M,D
Public Health—General M
Women's Health Nursing M,D

CALIFORNIA STATE UNIVERSITY, LONG BEACH
Biochemistry M
Biological and Biomedical Sciences—General M
Communication Disorders M
Health Services Management and Hospital Administration M
Microbiology M
Nursing—General M,D
Nutrition M
Physical Therapy D

CALIFORNIA STATE UNIVERSITY, LOS ANGELES
Biochemistry M
Biological and Biomedical Sciences—General M
Communication Disorders M
Health Services Management and Hospital Administration M,O
Nursing—General M,O
Nutrition M,O

CALIFORNIA STATE UNIVERSITY, NORTHRIDGE
Biochemistry M
Biological and Biomedical Sciences—General M
Communication Disorders M
Environmental and Occupational Health

Health Services Management and Hospital Administration M
Industrial Hygiene M
Physical Therapy M
Public Health—General M

CALIFORNIA STATE UNIVERSITY, SACRAMENTO
Biological and Biomedical Sciences—General M
Cell Biology M
Communication Disorders M
Conservation Biology M
Developmental Biology M
Molecular Biology M
Nursing—General M

CALIFORNIA STATE UNIVERSITY, SAN BERNARDINO
Biological and Biomedical Sciences—General M
Health Services Management and Hospital Administration M
Nursing—General M
Public Health—General M

CALIFORNIA STATE UNIVERSITY, SAN MARCOS
Biological and Biomedical Sciences—General M
Communication Disorders M

CALIFORNIA STATE UNIVERSITY, STANISLAUS
Conservation Biology M
Ecology M
Gerontological Nursing M
Nursing Education M
Nursing—General M

CALIFORNIA UNIVERSITY OF PENNSYLVANIA
Communication Disorders M
Nursing and Healthcare Administration M
Rehabilitation Sciences M

CAMBRIDGE COLLEGE
Health Services Management and Hospital Administration M
School Nursing M,D,O

CAMPBELL UNIVERSITY
Pharmaceutical Sciences M,D
Pharmacy M,D
Physical Therapy M,D
Physician Assistant Studies M,D

CANADIAN COLLEGE OF NATUROPATHIC MEDICINE
Naturopathic Medicine O

CANADIAN MEMORIAL CHIROPRACTIC COLLEGE
Acupuncture and Oriental Medicine O
Chiropractic D,O

CANISIUS COLLEGE
Allied Health—General M,O
Communication Disorders M,O
Community Health M,O
Nutrition M,O
Zoology M

CAPELLA UNIVERSITY
Environmental and Occupational Health M,D
Epidemiology D
Gerontological Nursing M
Health Services Management and Hospital Administration M,D
Nursing and Healthcare Administration M
Nursing Education M,D
Nursing—General M,D

CAPITAL UNIVERSITY
Nursing and Healthcare Administration M
Nursing—General M

CARDINAL STRITCH UNIVERSITY
Nursing—General M

CARIBBEAN UNIVERSITY
Gerontological Nursing M,D
Pediatric Nursing M,D

CARLETON UNIVERSITY
Biological and Biomedical Sciences—General M,D
Neuroscience M,D

CARLOS ALBIZU UNIVERSITY
Communication Disorders M,D

CARLOS ALBIZU UNIVERSITY, MIAMI CAMPUS
Communication Disorders M,D

CARLOW UNIVERSITY
Family Nurse Practitioner Studies M,O
Health Services Management and Hospital Administration M
Nursing and Healthcare Administration M
Nursing Education M
Nursing—General D

CARNEGIE MELLON UNIVERSITY
Biochemistry M,D
Biological and Biomedical Sciences—General M,D
Biophysics M,D
Biopsychology D
Cell Biology M,D
Computational Biology M,D
Developmental Biology M,D
Genetics M,D

Health Services Management and Hospital Administration M
Molecular Biology M,D
Molecular Biophysics M
Neurobiology M,D
Neuroscience D
Structural Biology M,D

CARROLL UNIVERSITY
Physical Therapy M,D
Physician Assistant Studies M

CARSON-NEWMAN UNIVERSITY
Family Nurse Practitioner Studies M
Nursing Education M
Nursing—General M

CASE WESTERN RESERVE UNIVERSITY
Acute Care/Critical Care Nursing M
Allopathic Medicine D
Anatomy M
Anesthesiologist Assistant Studies M
Biochemistry M,D
Bioethics M
Biological and Biomedical Sciences—General M,D
Biophysics M,D
Cancer Biology/Oncology D
Cell Biology M,D
Clinical Research M
Communication Disorders M,D
Dentistry D
Epidemiology M,D
Family Nurse Practitioner Studies M
Genetics D
Genomic Sciences D
Gerontological Nursing M
Health Services Management and Hospital Administration M
Health Services Research M,D
Human Genetics D
Immunology M,D
Maternal and Child/Neonatal Nursing M
Microbiology D
Molecular Biology D
Molecular Medicine D
Molecular Physiology M,D
Neuroscience D
Nurse Anesthesia M
Nurse Midwifery M
Nursing Education M
Nursing—General M,D
Nutrition M,D
Oncology Nursing M
Oral and Dental Sciences M,O
Pathology M,D
Pediatric Nursing M
Pharmacology D
Physician Assistant Studies M
Physiology M,D
Psychiatric Nursing M
Public Health—General M
Virology D
Women's Health Nursing M

THE CATHOLIC UNIVERSITY OF AMERICA
Biological and Biomedical Sciences—General M,D
Cell Biology M,D
Clinical Laboratory Sciences/Medical Technology M,D
Microbiology M,D
Nursing—General M,D,O

CEDAR CREST COLLEGE
Nursing and Healthcare Administration M
Nursing Education M
Nursing—General M
Nutrition O

CEDARS-SINAI MEDICAL CENTER
Biological and Biomedical Sciences—General D
Translational Biology D

CEDARVILLE UNIVERSITY
Family Nurse Practitioner Studies M,D
International Health M,D
Pharmacy M,D

CENTRAL CONNECTICUT STATE UNIVERSITY
Biological and Biomedical Sciences—General M,O
Molecular Biology M,O
Nurse Anesthesia M,O

CENTRAL METHODIST UNIVERSITY
Nursing and Healthcare Administration M
Nursing Education M
Nursing—General M

CENTRAL MICHIGAN UNIVERSITY
Biological and Biomedical Sciences—General M
Communication Disorders M,D
Conservation Biology M
Health Services Management and Hospital Administration M,D,O
International Health M,D,O
Neuroscience M,D
Nutrition M,D,O
Physical Therapy M,D
Physician Assistant Studies M,D
Rehabilitation Sciences M,D

CENTRAL WASHINGTON UNIVERSITY
Biological and Biomedical Sciences—General M
Nutrition M

CHAMPLAIN COLLEGE
Health Services Management and Hospital Administration M

CHAPMAN UNIVERSITY
Communication Disorders M
Nutrition M
Pharmaceutical Sciences M,D
Pharmacy M,D
Physical Therapy D

CHARLES R. DREW UNIVERSITY OF MEDICINE AND SCIENCE
Allopathic Medicine D
Public Health—General M

CHATHAM UNIVERSITY
Biological and Biomedical Sciences—General M
Environmental Biology M
Nursing and Healthcare Administration M,D
Nursing Education M,D
Nursing—General M,D
Occupational Therapy M,D
Physical Therapy D
Physician Assistant Studies M

CHICAGO STATE UNIVERSITY
Biological and Biomedical Sciences—General M
Nursing—General M
Occupational Therapy M
Pharmacy D
Public Health—General M

CHRISTIAN BROTHERS UNIVERSITY
Physician Assistant Studies M

THE CITADEL, THE MILITARY COLLEGE OF SOUTH CAROLINA
Biological and Biomedical Sciences—General M

CITY COLLEGE OF THE CITY UNIVERSITY OF NEW YORK
Biochemistry M,D
Biological and Biomedical Sciences—General M,D

CLAREMONT GRADUATE UNIVERSITY
Botany M,D
Computational Biology M,D
Health Promotion M,D
Public Health—General M,D

CLARION UNIVERSITY OF PENNSYLVANIA
Communication Disorders M
Family Nurse Practitioner Studies M,D,O
Nursing Education M,D,O
Nursing—General M,D
Rehabilitation Sciences M

CLARK ATLANTA UNIVERSITY
Biological and Biomedical Sciences—General M,D

CLARKE UNIVERSITY
Family Nurse Practitioner Studies D
Nursing—General D
Physical Therapy D

CLARKSON COLLEGE
Adult Nursing M,O
Family Nurse Practitioner Studies M,O
Nursing and Healthcare Administration M,O
Nursing Education M,O
Nursing—General M,O

CLARKSON UNIVERSITY
Bioethics M,O
Health Services Management and Hospital Administration M,O
Health Services Research M
Occupational Therapy M
Physical Therapy D
Physician Assistant Studies M

CLARK UNIVERSITY
Biochemistry M,D
Biological and Biomedical Sciences—General M,D

CLAYTON STATE UNIVERSITY
Biological and Biomedical Sciences—General M
Family Nurse Practitioner Studies M
Nursing—General M

CLEARY UNIVERSITY
Health Services Management and Hospital Administration M,O

CLEMSON UNIVERSITY
Biochemistry D
Biological and Biomedical Sciences—General M,D
Clinical Research M,D,O
Ecology M,D
Entomology M,D
Environmental and Occupational Health M
Evolutionary Biology M,D
Genetics M,D
Microbiology M,D
Molecular Biology D
Nursing—General M,D
Nutrition M
Plant Biology M,D
Public Health—General M,D,O
Veterinary Sciences M,D

CLEVELAND STATE UNIVERSITY
Allied Health—General M
Bioethics M,O
Biological and Biomedical Sciences—General M,D
Communication Disorders M
Community Health Nursing M,D
Forensic Nursing M,D
Health Services Management and Hospital Administration M,O

Medical Imaging	M
Medical Physics	M
Molecular Medicine	M,D
Nursing Education	M,D
Nursing—General	M,D
Occupational Therapy	M
Physical Therapy	D
Physician Assistant Studies	M
Public Health—General	M

CLEVELAND UNIVERSITY–KANSAS CITY

Chiropractic	D
Health Promotion	M

COLD SPRING HARBOR LABORATORY

Biological and Biomedical Sciences—General	D

THE COLLEGE AT BROCKPORT, STATE UNIVERSITY OF NEW YORK

Biological and Biomedical Sciences—General	M,O
Health Services Management and Hospital Administration	M,O

COLLEGE OF CHARLESTON

Marine Biology	M

COLLEGE OF MOUNT SAINT VINCENT

Adult Nursing	M,O
Family Nurse Practitioner Studies	M,O
Gerontological Nursing	M,O
Nursing and Healthcare Administration	M,O
Nursing Education	M,O
Nursing—General	M,O

THE COLLEGE OF NEW JERSEY

Nursing—General	M,O

THE COLLEGE OF NEW ROCHELLE

Acute Care/Critical Care Nursing	M,O
Family Nurse Practitioner Studies	M,O
Nursing and Healthcare Administration	M,O
Nursing Education	M,O
Nursing—General	M,O

COLLEGE OF SAINT ELIZABETH

Health Services Management and Hospital Administration	M
Nursing—General	M
Nutrition	M,O

COLLEGE OF SAINT MARY

Nursing—General	M
Occupational Therapy	M

THE COLLEGE OF SAINT ROSE

Communication Disorders	M

THE COLLEGE OF ST. SCHOLASTICA

Nursing—General	M,O
Occupational Therapy	M
Physical Therapy	D

COLLEGE OF STATEN ISLAND OF THE CITY UNIVERSITY OF NEW YORK

Adult Nursing	M,O
Biological and Biomedical Sciences—General	M
Family Nurse Practitioner Studies	D
Gerontological Nursing	M,O
Neuroscience	M
Nursing—General	M,D,O
Physical Therapy	D

THE COLLEGE OF WILLIAM AND MARY

Biological and Biomedical Sciences—General	M
Clinical Laboratory Sciences/Medical Technology	M,D
Computational Biology	M,D
Medical Physics	M,D
Neuroscience	M,D

COLORADO HEIGHTS UNIVERSITY

Health Services Management and Hospital Administration	M

COLORADO MESA UNIVERSITY

Family Nurse Practitioner Studies	M,D,O
Nursing Education	M,D,O
Nursing—General	M,D,O

COLORADO SCHOOL OF TRADITIONAL CHINESE MEDICINE

Acupuncture and Oriental Medicine	M

COLORADO STATE UNIVERSITY

Biochemistry	M,D
Biological and Biomedical Sciences—General	M,D
Botany	M,D
Cell Biology	M,D
Conservation Biology	M,D
Ecology	M,D
Entomology	M,D
Environmental and Occupational Health	M,D
Immunology	M,D
Microbiology	M,D
Molecular Biology	M,D
Neuroscience	D
Nutrition	M,D
Occupational Therapy	M,D
Pathology	M,D
Plant Pathology	M,D
Radiation Biology	M,D
Toxicology	M,D
Veterinary Medicine	D
Veterinary Sciences	M,D
Zoology	M,D

COLORADO STATE UNIVERSITY–GLOBAL CAMPUS

Health Services Management and Hospital Administration	M

COLORADO STATE UNIVERSITY–PUEBLO

Biochemistry	M
Biological and Biomedical Sciences—General	M
Nursing—General	M

COLUMBIA SOUTHERN UNIVERSITY

Environmental and Occupational Health	M
Health Services Management and Hospital Administration	M

COLUMBIA UNIVERSITY

Acute Care/Critical Care Nursing	M,O
Adult Nursing	M,O
Allopathic Medicine	M,D
Anatomy	M,D
Biochemistry	M,D
Bioethics	M
Biological and Biomedical Sciences—General	M,D,O*
Biophysics	M,D
Cell Biology	M,D
Community Health	M,D
Conservation Biology	M,D
Dentistry	D
Developmental Biology	M,D
Ecology	M,D
Environmental and Occupational Health	M,D
Epidemiology	M,D
Evolutionary Biology	M,D
Family Nurse Practitioner Studies	M,O
Genetics	M,D
Gerontological Nursing	M,O
Health Services Management and Hospital Administration	M
Maternal and Child Health	M,D
Medical Physics	M,D
Microbiology	M,D
Molecular Biology	D
Neurobiology	D
Nurse Anesthesia	M,O
Nurse Midwifery	M
Nursing—General	M,D,O
Nutrition	M,D
Occupational Therapy	M,D
Oral and Dental Sciences	M,D,O
Pathobiology	M,D
Pathology	M,O
Pediatric Nursing	M,O
Pharmaceutical Administration	M
Pharmacology	M,D
Physical Therapy	D
Physiology	M,D
Psychiatric Nursing	M,O
Public Health—General	M,D
Structural Biology	D
Toxicology	M,D

COLUMBUS STATE UNIVERSITY

Family Nurse Practitioner Studies	M
Health Services Management and Hospital Administration	M
Nursing and Healthcare Administration	M
Nursing Education	M
Nursing Informatics	M
Nursing—General	M

THE COMMONWEALTH MEDICAL COLLEGE

Allied Health—General	D
Biological and Biomedical Sciences—General	M

CONCORDIA UNIVERSITY (CANADA)

Biological and Biomedical Sciences—General	M,D,O
Genomic Sciences	M,D,O

CONCORDIA UNIVERSITY, ST. PAUL

Health Services Management and Hospital Administration	M
Physical Therapy	M,D,O

CONCORDIA UNIVERSITY WISCONSIN

Family Nurse Practitioner Studies	M
Gerontological Nursing	M
Health Services Management and Hospital Administration	M
Nursing Education	M
Nursing—General	M
Occupational Therapy	M
Physical Therapy	M,D
Rehabilitation Sciences	M

CONCORD UNIVERSITY

Health Promotion	M

CONNECTICUT COLLEGE

Biopsychology	M
Neuroscience	M

COPENHAGEN BUSINESS SCHOOL

Health Services Management and Hospital Administration	M,D

COPPIN STATE UNIVERSITY

Family Nurse Practitioner Studies	M,O
Nursing—General	M,O

CORNELL UNIVERSITY

Anatomy	D
Animal Behavior	D
Biochemistry	M,D
Biological and Biomedical Sciences—General	M,D
Biophysics	D

Biopsychology	D
Cell Biology	D
Computational Biology	D
Conservation Biology	M,D
Developmental Biology	M,D
Ecology	M,D
Entomology	M,D
Epidemiology	M,D
Evolutionary Biology	D
Genetics	D
Genomic Sciences	D
Health Services Management and Hospital Administration	M,D
Immunology	M,D
Infectious Diseases	M,D
Microbiology	D
Molecular Biology	M,D
Molecular Medicine	M,D
Neurobiology	D
Nutrition	M,D
Pharmacology	M,D
Physiology	M,D
Plant Biology	M,D
Plant Molecular Biology	M,D
Plant Pathology	M,D
Plant Physiology	M,D
Reproductive Biology	M,D
Structural Biology	M,D
Toxicology	M,D
Veterinary Medicine	D
Zoology	D

COX COLLEGE

Family Nurse Practitioner Studies	M
Nursing and Healthcare Administration	M
Nursing Education	M
Nursing—General	M

CREIGHTON UNIVERSITY

Adult Nursing	M,D,O
Allied Health—General	M,D
Allopathic Medicine	D
Anatomy	M
Biological and Biomedical Sciences—General	M,D
Dentistry	D
Emergency Medical Services	M
Family Nurse Practitioner Studies	M,D,O
Gerontological Nursing	M,D,O
Immunology	M,D
Maternal and Child/Neonatal Nursing	M,D,O
Medical Microbiology	M,D
Nursing and Healthcare Administration	M,D,O
Nursing—General	M,D,O
Occupational Therapy	D
Pediatric Nursing	M,D,O
Pharmaceutical Sciences	M,D
Pharmacology	M,D
Pharmacy	D
Physical Therapy	D
Psychiatric Nursing	M,D,O

CURRY COLLEGE

Nursing—General	M

DAEMEN COLLEGE

Adult Nursing	M,D,O
Community Health	M
Epidemiology	M
Health Services Management and Hospital Administration	M
Medical/Surgical Nursing	M,D,O
Nursing and Healthcare Administration	M,D,O
Nursing Education	M,D,O
Nursing—General	M,D,O
Physical Therapy	D,O
Physician Assistant Studies	M
Public Health—General	M

DALHOUSIE UNIVERSITY

Allopathic Medicine	M,D
Anatomy	M,D
Biochemistry	M,D
Biological and Biomedical Sciences—General	M,D
Biophysics	M,D
Botany	M
Communication Disorders	M,D
Community Health	M
Ecology	M
Environmental Biology	M
Epidemiology	M
Health Services Management and Hospital Administration	M,D
Immunology	M,D
Microbiology	M,D
Neurobiology	M,D
Neuroscience	M,D
Nursing—General	M,D
Occupational Therapy	M
Oral and Dental Sciences	M
Pathology	M,D
Pharmacology	M,D
Physical Therapy	M
Physiology	M,D
Plant Pathology	M
Plant Physiology	M

DALLAS BAPTIST UNIVERSITY

Health Services Management and Hospital Administration	M

DARTMOUTH COLLEGE

Allopathic Medicine	D
Biochemistry	M,D
Biological and Biomedical Sciences—General	D
Cell Biology	D
Ecology	D

Evolutionary Biology	D
Genetics	D
Health Services Management and Hospital Administration	M,D
Health Services Research	M,D
Immunology	D
Microbiology	D
Molecular Biology	D
Molecular Medicine	
Molecular Pathogenesis	D
Neuroscience	D
Public Health—General	M

DAVENPORT UNIVERSITY

Health Services Management and Hospital Administration	M
Public Health—General	M

DEFIANCE COLLEGE

Health Services Management and Hospital Administration	M

DELAWARE STATE UNIVERSITY

Biological and Biomedical Sciences—General	M
Neuroscience	M,D
Nursing—General	M

DELTA STATE UNIVERSITY

Biological and Biomedical Sciences—General	M
Family Nurse Practitioner Studies	M,D
Health Services Management and Hospital Administration	M,D
Nursing Education	M,D
Nursing—General	M,D

DEPAUL UNIVERSITY

Biological and Biomedical Sciences—General	M,D
Family Nurse Practitioner Studies	M,D
Health Services Management and Hospital Administration	M
Nursing—General	M
Public Health—General	M

DESALES UNIVERSITY

Family Nurse Practitioner Studies	M,D,O
Health Services Management and Hospital Administration	M
Nurse Anesthesia	M,D,O
Nurse Midwifery	M,D,O
Nursing and Healthcare Administration	M,D,O
Nursing Education	M,D,O
Nursing—General	M,D,O

DES MOINES UNIVERSITY

Anatomy	M
Biological and Biomedical Sciences—General	M
Health Services Management and Hospital Administration	M
Osteopathic Medicine	D
Physical Therapy	D
Physician Assistant Studies	M
Podiatric Medicine	D
Public Health—General	M

DOMINICAN COLLEGE

Allied Health—General	M,D
Family Nurse Practitioner Studies	M,D
Health Services Management and Hospital Administration	M
Occupational Therapy	M
Physical Therapy	M,D

DOMINICAN UNIVERSITY OF CALIFORNIA

Biological and Biomedical Sciences—General	M
Clinical Laboratory Sciences/Medical Technology	M
Occupational Therapy	M

DONGGUK UNIVERSITY LOS ANGELES

Acupuncture and Oriental Medicine	M

DRAKE UNIVERSITY

Pharmacy	D

DREW UNIVERSITY

Biological and Biomedical Sciences—General	M,D,O
Health Services Management and Hospital Administration	M,D,O

DREXEL UNIVERSITY

Acute Care/Critical Care Nursing	M
Allied Health—General	M,D,O
Allopathic Medicine	D
Biochemistry	M,D
Biological and Biomedical Sciences—General	M,D,O
Biopsychology	M,D
Cell Biology	M,D
Emergency Medical Services	M
Epidemiology	M,D,O
Family Nurse Practitioner Studies	M,D
Genetics	M,D
Immunology	M,D
Microbiology	M,D
Molecular Biology	M,D
Molecular Medicine	M,D
Neuroscience	M,D
Nurse Anesthesia	M
Nursing and Healthcare Administration	M
Nursing Education	M
Nursing—General	M,D
Nutrition	M
Pathobiology	M,D
Pediatric Nursing	M
Pharmaceutical Sciences	M
Pharmacology	M,D

*M—masters degree; D—doctorate; O—other advanced degree; *—Close-Up and/or Display*

Physical Therapy — M,D,O
Physician Assistant Studies — M
Psychiatric Nursing — M
Public Health—General — M,D,O
Veterinary Sciences — M
Women's Health Nursing — M

DUKE UNIVERSITY
Acute Care/Critical Care Nursing — M,D,O
Adult Nursing — M,D,O
Allopathic Medicine — D
Anatomy — D
Biochemistry — D
Bioethics — M
Biological and Biomedical
  Sciences—General — M,D
Biopsychology — D
Cancer Biology/Oncology — D
Cell Biology — D,O
Clinical Laboratory
  Sciences/Medical Technology — M
Clinical Research — M
Computational Biology — D,O
Developmental Biology — O
Ecology — D,O
Environmental and Occupational
  Health — O
Family Nurse Practitioner Studies — M,D,O
Genetics — D
Genomic Sciences — D
Gerontological Nursing — M,D,O
Health Services Management and
  Hospital Administration — M,O
Immunology — D
International Health — M
Maternal and Child/Neonatal
  Nursing — M,D,O
Medical Physics — M,D
Microbiology — D
Molecular Biology — D,O
Molecular Biophysics — O
Molecular Genetics — D
Neurobiology — D
Neuroscience — D,O
Nurse Anesthesia — M,D,O
Nursing and Healthcare
  Administration — M,D,O
Nursing Education — M,D,O
Nursing Informatics — M,D,O
Nursing—General — D
Pathology — M,D
Pediatric Nursing — M,D,O
Pharmacology — D
Physical Therapy — D
Physician Assistant Studies — M
Structural Biology — O
Toxicology — O
Women's Health Nursing — M,D,O

DUQUESNE UNIVERSITY
Allied Health—General — M,D,O
Bioethics — M,D,O
Biological and Biomedical
  Sciences—General — D
Communication Disorders — M,D
Family Nurse Practitioner Studies — M,O
Forensic Nursing — M,O
Health Services Management and
  Hospital Administration — M,D
Medicinal and Pharmaceutical
  Chemistry — M,D
Nursing Education — M,O
Nursing—General — M,D,O
Occupational Therapy — M,D
Pharmaceutical Administration — M
Pharmaceutical Sciences — M,D
Pharmacology — M,D
Pharmacy — D
Physical Therapy — M,D
Physician Assistant Studies — M,D
Rehabilitation Sciences — M,D

D'YOUVILLE COLLEGE
Chiropractic — D
Family Nurse Practitioner Studies — M,D,O
Health Services Management and
  Hospital Administration — M,D,O
Nursing—General — M,D,O
Nutrition — M
Occupational Therapy — M
Pharmacy — D
Physical Therapy — D,O
Physician Assistant Studies — M

EAST CAROLINA UNIVERSITY
Allied Health—General — M,D,O
Allopathic Medicine — D
Anatomy — D
Biochemistry — M,D
Biological and Biomedical
  Sciences—General — M,D
Biophysics — M,D
Cell Biology — D
Communication Disorders — M,D
Community Health — M,O
Dentistry — D
Environmental and Occupational
  Health — M,D
Health Physics/Radiological Health — M
Health Promotion — M
Immunology — M,D
Maternal and Child Health — M,D
Medical Physics — M,D
Microbiology — M,D
Molecular Biology — M,D
Nursing—General — M,D,O
Nutrition — M
Occupational Therapy — M,D,O
Pharmacology — D
Physical Therapy — D
Physician Assistant Studies — M
Physiology — D
Public Health—General — M
Rehabilitation Sciences — M,D,O

EASTERN ILLINOIS UNIVERSITY
Biological and Biomedical
  Sciences—General — M
Communication Disorders — M
Nutrition — M

EASTERN KENTUCKY UNIVERSITY
Allied Health—General — M
Biological and Biomedical
  Sciences—General — M
Communication Disorders — M
Community Health — M
Ecology — M
Environmental and Occupational
  Health — M
Family Nurse Practitioner Studies — M
Health Promotion — M
Health Services Management and
  Hospital Administration — M
Nursing—General — M
Nutrition — M
Occupational Therapy — M

EASTERN MENNONITE UNIVERSITY
Biological and Biomedical
  Sciences—General — M
Health Services Management and
  Hospital Administration — M
Nursing and Healthcare
  Administration — M
Nursing—General — M
School Nursing — M

EASTERN MICHIGAN UNIVERSITY
Adult Nursing — M,O
Biological and Biomedical
  Sciences—General — M
Cell Biology — M
Clinical Research — M,O
Communication Disorders — M
Ecology — M
Health Promotion — M,O
Health Services Management and
  Hospital Administration — M,O
Molecular Biology — M
Nursing and Healthcare
  Administration — M,O
Nursing Education — M,O
Nutrition — M
Occupational Therapy — M
Physician Assistant Studies — M
Physiology — M

EASTERN NEW MEXICO UNIVERSITY
Biochemistry — M
Biological and Biomedical
  Sciences—General — M
Botany — M
Cell Biology — M
Communication Disorders — M
Ecology — M
Microbiology — M
Molecular Biology — M
Nursing—General — M
Zoology — M

EASTERN UNIVERSITY
Health Services Management and
  Hospital Administration — M
School Nursing — M,O

EASTERN VIRGINIA MEDICAL SCHOOL
Allopathic Medicine — D
Biological and Biomedical
  Sciences—General — M,D
Medical/Surgical Nursing — M
Physician Assistant Studies — M
Public Health—General — M
Reproductive Biology — M
Vision Sciences — O

EASTERN WASHINGTON UNIVERSITY
Biological and Biomedical
  Sciences—General — M
Communication Disorders — M
Dental Hygiene — M
Occupational Therapy — M
Physical Therapy — D

EAST STROUDSBURG UNIVERSITY OF PENNSYLVANIA
Biological and Biomedical
  Sciences—General — M
Communication Disorders — M
Physiology — M
Public Health—General — M
Rehabilitation Sciences — M

EAST TENNESSEE STATE UNIVERSITY
Allied Health—General — M,D,O
Allopathic Medicine — D
Anatomy — D
Biochemistry — D
Biological and Biomedical
  Sciences—General — M,D
Communication Disorders — M,D
Environmental and Occupational
  Health — M,D
Family Nurse Practitioner Studies — M,D,O
Health Services Management and
  Hospital Administration — M,O
Microbiology — D
Nursing—General — M,D,O
Nutrition — M
Pharmaceutical Sciences — D
Pharmacology — D
Pharmacy — D
Physical Therapy — D
Physiology — D
Public Health—General — M,D,O

EAST WEST COLLEGE OF NATURAL MEDICINE
Acupuncture and Oriental Medicine — M

EDGEWOOD COLLEGE
Nursing and Healthcare
  Administration — M,D
Nursing Education — M,D
Nursing—General — M,D

EDINBORO UNIVERSITY OF PENNSYLVANIA
Communication Disorders — M
Family Nurse Practitioner Studies — M
Nursing Education — M,D
Nursing—General — M,D

EDP UNIVERSITY OF PUERTO RICO–SAN SEBASTIAN
Nursing—General — M

EDWARD VIA COLLEGE OF OSTEOPATHIC MEDICINE–VIRGINIA CAMPUS
Osteopathic Medicine — D

EDWARD VIA COLLEGE OF OSTEOPATHIC MEDICINE–CAROLINAS CAMPUS
Osteopathic Medicine — D

ELIZABETH CITY STATE UNIVERSITY
Biological and Biomedical
  Sciences—General — M

ELIZABETHTOWN COLLEGE
Occupational Therapy — M

ELLIS UNIVERSITY
Health Services Management and
  Hospital Administration — M

ELMEZZI GRADUATE SCHOOL OF MOLECULAR MEDICINE
Molecular Medicine — D

ELMHURST COLLEGE
Communication Disorders — M
Nursing—General — M
Public Health—General — M

ELMS COLLEGE
Communication Disorders — M,O
Health Services Management and
  Hospital Administration — M
Nursing and Healthcare
  Administration — M,D
Nursing Education — M,D
Nursing—General — M,D

ELON UNIVERSITY
Physical Therapy — D
Physician Assistant Studies — M

EMBRY-RIDDLE AERONAUTICAL UNIVERSITY–PRESCOTT
Environmental and Occupational
  Health — M

EMBRY-RIDDLE AERONAUTICAL UNIVERSITY–WORLDWIDE
Environmental and Occupational
  Health — M

EMERSON COLLEGE
Communication Disorders — M

EMMANUEL COLLEGE (UNITED STATES)
Nursing and Healthcare
  Administration — M,O
Nursing Education — M,O
Nursing—General — M,O

EMORY UNIVERSITY
Adult Nursing — M
Allied Health—General — M,D
Allopathic Medicine — D
Anesthesiologist Assistant Studies — M
Animal Behavior — D
Biochemistry — D
Bioethics — M
Biological and Biomedical
  Sciences—General — D
Biophysics — D
Cancer Biology/Oncology — D
Cell Biology — D
Clinical Research — M
Developmental Biology — D
Ecology — D
Environmental and Occupational
  Health — M,D
Epidemiology — M,D
Evolutionary Biology — D
Family Nurse Practitioner Studies — M
Genetics — D
Health Promotion — M
Health Services Management and
  Hospital Administration — M,D
Health Services Research — M,D
Human Genetics — M
Immunology — D
International Health — M
Microbiology — D
Molecular Biology — D
Molecular Genetics — D
Molecular Pathogenesis — D
Neuroscience — D
Nurse Midwifery — M
Nursing and Healthcare
  Administration — M
Nursing—General — M,D
Nutrition — M,D
Pediatric Nursing — M
Pharmacology — D
Physical Therapy — D
Physician Assistant Studies — M
Public Health—General — M,D
Women's Health Nursing — M

EMPEROR'S COLLEGE OF TRADITIONAL ORIENTAL MEDICINE
Acupuncture and Oriental Medicine — M,D

EMPORIA STATE UNIVERSITY
Biological and Biomedical
  Sciences—General — M
Botany — M
Cell Biology — M
Environmental Biology — M
Microbiology — M
Nursing Informatics — M
Zoology — M

ENDICOTT COLLEGE
Nursing—General — M,D

EVERGLADES UNIVERSITY
Public Health—General — M

EXCELSIOR COLLEGE
Health Services Management and
  Hospital Administration — M,O
Nursing and Healthcare
  Administration — M
Nursing Education — M
Nursing Informatics — M
Nursing—General — M
Public Health—General — M,O

FAIRFIELD UNIVERSITY
Family Nurse Practitioner Studies — M,D
Nurse Anesthesia — M,D
Nursing and Healthcare
  Administration — M,D
Nursing—General — M,D
Psychiatric Nursing — M,D

FAIRLEIGH DICKINSON UNIVERSITY, COLLEGE AT FLORHAM
Biological and Biomedical
  Sciences—General — M
Health Services Management and
  Hospital Administration — M
Pharmacology — M,O

FAIRLEIGH DICKINSON UNIVERSITY, METROPOLITAN CAMPUS
Biological and Biomedical
  Sciences—General — M
Clinical Laboratory
  Sciences/Medical Technology — M
Health Services Management and
  Hospital Administration — M
Nursing—General — M,D,O
Pharmaceutical Administration — M,O

FAIRMONT STATE UNIVERSITY
Health Promotion — M

FAYETTEVILLE STATE UNIVERSITY
Biological and Biomedical
  Sciences—General — M

FELICIAN UNIVERSITY
Adult Nursing — M,O
Family Nurse Practitioner Studies — M,O
Gerontological Nursing — M,O
Health Services Management and
  Hospital Administration — M
Nursing and Healthcare
  Administration — M,D,O
Nursing Education — M,O
Nursing—General — M,D,O
School Nursing — M,O

FERRIS STATE UNIVERSITY
Allied Health—General — M
Nursing and Healthcare
  Administration — M
Nursing Education — M
Nursing Informatics — M
Nursing—General — M
Optometry — D
Pharmacy — D

FIELDING GRADUATE UNIVERSITY
Neuroscience — M,D,O

FISK UNIVERSITY
Biological and Biomedical
  Sciences—General — M

FITCHBURG STATE UNIVERSITY
Biological and Biomedical
  Sciences—General — M,O
Forensic Nursing — M,O

FIVE BRANCHES UNIVERSITY
Acupuncture and Oriental Medicine — M,D

FLORIDA AGRICULTURAL AND MECHANICAL UNIVERSITY
Allied Health—General — M,D
Health Services Research — M,D
Medicinal and Pharmaceutical
  Chemistry — M,D
Nursing and Healthcare
  Administration — M,D
Nursing—General — M,D
Occupational Therapy — M
Pharmaceutical Administration — M,D
Pharmaceutical Sciences — M,D
Pharmacology — M,D
Pharmacy — D
Physical Therapy — D
Public Health—General — M,D
Toxicology — M,D

FLORIDA ATLANTIC UNIVERSITY
Biological and Biomedical
  Sciences—General — M
Communication Disorders — M
Health Promotion — M
Neuroscience — D
Nursing and Healthcare
  Administration — M,D,O
Nursing—General — M,D,O

FLORIDA COLLEGE OF INTEGRATIVE MEDICINE
Acupuncture and Oriental Medicine — M

FLORIDA GULF COAST UNIVERSITY
Allied Health—General — M,D
Nurse Anesthesia — M
Occupational Therapy — M
Physical Therapy — D

FLORIDA INSTITUTE OF TECHNOLOGY
Biochemistry — M
Biological and Biomedical
  Sciences—General — M,D
Cell Biology — M,D
Conservation Biology — M
Ecology — M,D
Health Services Management and
  Hospital Administration — M
Marine Biology — M,D
Molecular Biology — M,D

FLORIDA INTERNATIONAL UNIVERSITY
Allopathic Medicine — M,D
Biological and Biomedical
  Sciences—General — M,D
Communication Disorders — M
Environmental and Occupational
  Health — M,D
Epidemiology — M,D
Health Promotion — M,D
Health Services Management and
  Hospital Administration — M,D
Neuroscience — M,D
Nursing—General — M,D
Nutrition — M,D
Occupational Therapy — D
Physical Therapy — D
Physician Assistant Studies — M
Public Health—General — M,D

FLORIDA NATIONAL UNIVERSITY
Family Nurse Practitioner Studies — M
Health Services Management and
  Hospital Administration — M
Nursing and Healthcare
  Administration — M
Nursing Education — M
Nursing—General — M

FLORIDA SOUTHERN COLLEGE
Adult Nursing — M
Gerontological Nursing — M
Nursing and Healthcare
  Administration — M
Nursing Education — M
Nursing—General — M

FLORIDA STATE UNIVERSITY
Biochemistry — M,D
Biological and Biomedical
  Sciences—General — M,D
Cell Biology — M,D
Communication Disorders — M,D
Computational Biology — D
Ecology — M,D
Evolutionary Biology — M,D
Family Nurse Practitioner Studies — M,D,O
Molecular Biology — M,D
Molecular Biophysics — D
Neuroscience — M,D
Nursing and Healthcare
  Administration — M,D,O
Nursing Education — M,D,O
Nursing—General — M,D,O
Nutrition — M,D
Plant Biology — M,D
Public Health—General — M
Structural Biology — M,D

FONTBONNE UNIVERSITY
Communication Disorders — M

FORDHAM UNIVERSITY
Biological and Biomedical
  Sciences—General — M,D,O
Clinical Research — M,D
Conservation Biology — M,D,O

FORT HAYS STATE UNIVERSITY
Biological and Biomedical
  Sciences—General — M
Communication Disorders — M
Nursing—General — M

FORT VALLEY STATE UNIVERSITY
Environmental and Occupational
  Health — M
Public Health—General — M

FRAMINGHAM STATE UNIVERSITY
Health Services Management and
  Hospital Administration — M
Nursing and Healthcare
  Administration — M
Nursing Education — M
Nursing—General — M
Nutrition — M

FRANCISCAN UNIVERSITY OF STEUBENVILLE
Nursing—General — M

FRANCIS MARION UNIVERSITY
Family Nurse Practitioner Studies — M
Health Services Management and
  Hospital Administration — M
Nursing Education — M
Nursing—General — M
Physician Assistant Studies — M

FRANKLIN PIERCE UNIVERSITY
Health Services Management and
  Hospital Administration — M,D,O
Nursing and Healthcare
  Administration — M,D,O
Nursing Education — M,D,O
Physical Therapy — M,D,O
Physician Assistant Studies — M,D,O

FRESNO PACIFIC UNIVERSITY
Family Nurse Practitioner Studies — M
Nursing—General — M

FRIENDS UNIVERSITY
Health Services Management and
  Hospital Administration — M

FRONTIER NURSING UNIVERSITY
Family Nurse Practitioner Studies — M,D,O
Nurse Midwifery — M,D,O
Nursing—General — M,D,O
Women's Health Nursing — M,D,O

FROSTBURG STATE UNIVERSITY
Biological and Biomedical
  Sciences—General — M
Conservation Biology — M
Ecology — M
Nursing and Healthcare
  Administration — M
Nursing Education — M
Nursing—General — M

GALLAUDET UNIVERSITY
Communication Disorders — M,D,O
Neuroscience — M,D,O

GANNON UNIVERSITY
Environmental and Occupational
  Health — M
Family Nurse Practitioner Studies — M,O
Nurse Anesthesia — M,O
Nursing and Healthcare
  Administration — M,D
Nursing—General — M,D
Occupational Therapy — M,D
Physical Therapy — D
Physician Assistant Studies — M

GARDNER-WEBB UNIVERSITY
Nursing—General — M,D
Physician Assistant Studies — M

GENEVA COLLEGE
Cardiovascular Sciences — M

GEORGE FOX UNIVERSITY
Physical Therapy — D

GEORGE MASON UNIVERSITY
Biochemistry — M,D
Biological and Biomedical
  Sciences—General — M,D,O
Community Health — M,O
Ecology — M,D
Epidemiology — M,O
Health Promotion — M,D,O
Health Services Management and
  Hospital Administration — M,D
International Health — M,O
Neuroscience — M,D,O
Nursing—General — M,D,O
Nutrition — M
Public Health—General — M,O
Rehabilitation Sciences — D,O

GEORGETOWN UNIVERSITY
Acute Care/Critical Care Nursing — M,D
Allopathic Medicine — D
Biochemistry — M,D
Biological and Biomedical
  Sciences—General — M,D
Epidemiology — M,O
Family Nurse Practitioner Studies — M,D
Health Physics/Radiological Health — M
Health Promotion — M,D
Immunology — M,D
Infectious Diseases — M,D
International Health — M,D
Microbiology — M,D
Molecular Biology — M,D
Neuroscience — D
Nurse Anesthesia — M,D
Nurse Midwifery — M,D
Nursing Education — M,D
Nursing—General — M,D
Pharmacology — M,D
Physiology — M,D
Public Health—General — M,D
Radiation Biology — M

THE GEORGE WASHINGTON UNIVERSITY
Adult Nursing — M,D,O
Allopathic Medicine — D
Biochemistry — D
Biological and Biomedical
  Sciences—General — M,D
Communication Disorders — M
Community Health — M,D
Environmental and Occupational
  Health — D
Epidemiology — M
Family Nurse Practitioner Studies — M,D,O
Health Services Management and
  Hospital Administration — M,D,O
Health Services Research — M,D,O
Immunology — D
Infectious Diseases — M,D,O
International Health — M,D
Microbiology — M,D,O
Molecular Medicine — D
Nursing and Healthcare
  Administration — M,D,O
Nursing Education — M,D,O
Nursing—General — M,D,O
Physical Therapy — D
Physician Assistant Studies — M
Public Health—General — M,D
Systems Biology — D
Toxicology — M,O

GEORGIA CAMPUS–PHILADELPHIA COLLEGE OF OSTEOPATHIC MEDICINE
Osteopathic Medicine — D
Pharmacy — D*

GEORGIA COLLEGE & STATE UNIVERSITY
Biological and Biomedical
  Sciences—General — M
Health Promotion — M
Nursing—General — M,D

GEORGIA INSTITUTE OF TECHNOLOGY
Biological and Biomedical
  Sciences—General — M,D
Health Physics/Radiological Health — M,D
Health Services Management and
  Hospital Administration — M
Physiology — M,D

GEORGIA SOUTHERN UNIVERSITY
Allied Health—General — M,D,O
Biological and Biomedical
  Sciences—General — M
Community Health — M,D
Environmental and Occupational
  Health — M,D,O
Epidemiology — M,D
Family Nurse Practitioner Studies — M
Health Services Management and
  Hospital Administration — M,D,O
Nursing Education — O
Nursing—General — D
Nutrition — O
Psychiatric Nursing — M
Public Health—General — M,D

GEORGIA STATE UNIVERSITY
Adult Nursing — M,D,O
Allied Health—General — M
Biochemistry — M,D
Biological and Biomedical
  Sciences—General — M,D*
Cell Biology — M,D
Communication Disorders — M,D
Environmental Biology — M,D
Family Nurse Practitioner Studies — M,D,O
Health Services Management and
  Hospital Administration — M,D,O
Microbiology — M,D
Molecular Biology — M,D
Molecular Genetics — M,D
Neurobiology — M,D
Neuroscience — D
Nursing and Healthcare
  Administration — M,D,O
Nursing Informatics — M,D,O
Nursing—General — M,D,O
Nutrition — M
Pediatric Nursing — M,D,O
Physical Therapy — D
Physiology — M,D
Psychiatric Nursing — M,D,O
Public Health—General — M,D,O
Women's Health Nursing — M,D,O

GERSTNER SLOAN KETTERING GRADUATE SCHOOL OF BIOMEDICAL SCIENCES
Biological and Biomedical
  Sciences—General — D
Cancer Biology/Oncology — D*

GLOBE UNIVERSITY–WOODBURY
Health Services Management and
  Hospital Administration — M

GODDARD COLLEGE
Health Promotion — M

GOLDEY-BEACOM COLLEGE
Health Services Management and
  Hospital Administration — M

GOLDFARB SCHOOL OF NURSING AT BARNES-JEWISH COLLEGE
Acute Care/Critical Care Nursing — M
Adult Nursing — M
Gerontological Nursing — M
Health Services Management and
  Hospital Administration — M
Nurse Anesthesia — M
Nursing Education — M
Nursing—General — M

GONZAGA UNIVERSITY
Nursing—General — M,D
Physiology — M,D

GOSHEN COLLEGE
Family Nurse Practitioner Studies — M
Nursing—General — M

GOUCHER COLLEGE
Biological and Biomedical
  Sciences—General — O

GOVERNORS STATE UNIVERSITY
Communication Disorders — M
Environmental Biology — M
Health Services Management and
  Hospital Administration — M
Nursing—General — M
Occupational Therapy — M
Physical Therapy — M,D

GRACELAND UNIVERSITY (IA)
Family Nurse Practitioner Studies — M,D,O
Nursing Education — M,D,O
Nursing—General — M,D,O

THE GRADUATE CENTER, CITY UNIVERSITY OF NEW YORK
Biochemistry — D

Biological and Biomedical
  Sciences—General — D
Biopsychology — D
Communication Disorders — D
Neuroscience — D
Nursing—General — D
Physical Therapy — D
Public Health—General — D

GRAMBLING STATE UNIVERSITY
Family Nurse Practitioner Studies — M,O
Health Services Management and
  Hospital Administration — M
Nursing—General — M,O

GRAND CANYON UNIVERSITY
Acute Care/Critical Care Nursing — M,O
Family Nurse Practitioner Studies — M,O
Health Services Management and
  Hospital Administration — M,O
Nursing Education — M,O
Nursing—General — M,O
Public Health—General — M

GRAND VALLEY STATE UNIVERSITY
Allied Health—General — M,D
Biological and Biomedical
  Sciences—General — M
Cell Biology — M
Communication Disorders — M
Health Services Management and
  Hospital Administration — M,D
Molecular Biology — M
Nursing and Healthcare
  Administration — M,D
Nursing Education — M,D
Nursing—General — M,D
Occupational Therapy — M
Physical Therapy — D
Physician Assistant Studies — M
Public Health—General — M

GRAND VIEW UNIVERSITY
Nursing—General — M

GRANTHAM UNIVERSITY
Health Services Management and
  Hospital Administration — M
Nursing and Healthcare
  Administration — M
Nursing Education — M
Nursing Informatics — M

GWYNEDD MERCY UNIVERSITY
Adult Nursing — M,D
Family Nurse Practitioner Studies — M,D
Gerontological Nursing — M,D
Health Services Management and
  Hospital Administration — M
Nursing Education — M,D
Nursing—General — M,D
Oncology Nursing — M,D
Pediatric Nursing — M,D

HAMPTON UNIVERSITY
Adult Nursing — M,D
Allied Health—General — M
Biological and Biomedical
  Sciences—General — M
Communication Disorders — M
Community Health Nursing — M,D
Environmental Biology — M
Gerontological Nursing — M,D
Medical Physics — M,D
Nursing—General — M,D
Pediatric Nursing — M,D
Pharmacy — D
Physical Therapy — D
Psychiatric Nursing — M,D
Women's Health Nursing — M,D

HARDING UNIVERSITY
Allied Health—General — M,D
Communication Disorders — M
Health Services Management and
  Hospital Administration — M
Pharmacy — D
Physical Therapy — D
Physician Assistant Studies — M

HARDIN-SIMMONS UNIVERSITY
Family Nurse Practitioner Studies — M
Maternal and Child/Neonatal
  Nursing — M
Nursing—General — M
Physical Therapy — D

HARRISBURG UNIVERSITY OF SCIENCE AND TECHNOLOGY
Health Services Management and
  Hospital Administration — M

HARVARD UNIVERSITY
Allopathic Medicine — D
Biochemistry — D
Biological and Biomedical
  Sciences—General — M,D,O
Biophysics — D*
Biopsychology — D
Cell Biology — D
Computational Biology — M,D,O
Dentistry — M,D,O
Environmental and Occupational
  Health — M,D
Epidemiology — M,D
Evolutionary Biology — D
Genetics — D
Genomic Sciences — D
Health Promotion — M,D
Health Services Management and
  Hospital Administration — M,D
International Health — M,D
Medical Physics — D
Microbiology — D
Molecular Biology — D

M—masters degree; D—doctorate; O—other advanced degree; *—Close-Up and/or Display

Molecular Genetics — D
Molecular Pharmacology — D
Neurobiology — D
Neuroscience — D
Nutrition — D
Oral and Dental Sciences — M,D,O
Pathology — D
Physiology — M,D
Public Health—General — M,D*
Structural Biology — D
Systems Biology — D

HAWAI'I PACIFIC UNIVERSITY
Nursing—General — M

HERZING UNIVERSITY ONLINE
Health Services Management and
   Hospital Administration — M
Nursing and Healthcare
   Administration — M
Nursing Education — M
Nursing—General — M

HILBERT COLLEGE
Health Services Management and
   Hospital Administration — M

HODGES UNIVERSITY
Health Services Management and
   Hospital Administration — M

HOFSTRA UNIVERSITY
Allopathic Medicine — D
Biological and Biomedical
   Sciences—General — M,D,O
Communication Disorders — M,D
Community Health — M
Health Services Management and
   Hospital Administration — M,O
Medical Physics — M
Molecular Medicine — D
Physician Assistant Studies — M
Public Health—General — M

HOLY FAMILY UNIVERSITY
Health Services Management and
   Hospital Administration — M
Nursing and Healthcare
   Administration — M
Nursing Education — M
Nursing—General — M

HOLY NAMES UNIVERSITY
Community Health Nursing — M,O
Family Nurse Practitioner Studies — M,O
Nursing and Healthcare
   Administration — M,O
Nursing Education — M,O
Nursing—General — M,O

HOOD COLLEGE
Biological and Biomedical
   Sciences—General — M,O*
Environmental Biology — M
Immunology — M,O
Microbiology — M,O
Molecular Biology — M,O

HOWARD UNIVERSITY
Allopathic Medicine — D
Anatomy — M,D
Biochemistry — M,D
Biological and Biomedical
   Sciences—General — M,D
Biophysics — D
Biopsychology — M,D
Communication Disorders — M,D
Dentistry — D,O
Family Nurse Practitioner Studies — M,O
Microbiology — D
Molecular Biology — M,D
Nursing—General — M,O
Nutrition — M,D
Oral and Dental Sciences — D,O
Pharmacology — M,D
Pharmacy — D
Physiology — D
Public Health—General — M

HUMBOLDT STATE UNIVERSITY
Biological and Biomedical
   Sciences—General — M
Physical Therapy — D

HUNTER COLLEGE OF THE CITY UNIVERSITY OF NEW YORK
Adult Nursing — M
Biochemistry — M,D
Biological and Biomedical
   Sciences—General — M,D
Communication Disorders — M
Community Health Nursing — M
Community Health — M
Environmental and Occupational
   Health — M
Epidemiology — M
Gerontological Nursing — M
Health Services Management and
   Hospital Administration — M
Nursing—General — M,O
Nutrition — M
Psychiatric Nursing — M,O
Public Health—General — M

HUNTINGTON COLLEGE OF HEALTH SCIENCES
Nutrition — M,D

HUSSON UNIVERSITY
Community Health Nursing — M,O
Family Nurse Practitioner Studies — M,O
Health Services Management and
   Hospital Administration — M
Nursing Education — M,O
Nursing—General — M,O
Occupational Therapy — M
Pharmacy — D
Physical Therapy — D

Psychiatric Nursing — M,O

ICAHN SCHOOL OF MEDICINE AT MOUNT SINAI
Allopathic Medicine — D
Bioethics — M
Biological and Biomedical
   Sciences—General — M,D
Clinical Research — M,D
Community Health — M,D
Neuroscience — M,D

IDAHO STATE UNIVERSITY
Allied Health—General — M,D,O
Biological and Biomedical
   Sciences—General — M,D
Communication Disorders — M,D,O
Community Health — O
Dental Hygiene — M
Dentistry — O
Health Physics/Radiological Health — M,D
Medical Microbiology — M,D
Medicinal and Pharmaceutical
   Chemistry — M,D
Microbiology — M,D
Nursing—General — M,O
Nutrition — M,O
Occupational Therapy — M
Oral and Dental Sciences — O
Pharmaceutical Administration — M,D
Pharmaceutical Sciences — M,D
Pharmacology — M,D
Pharmacy — M,D
Physical Therapy — D
Physician Assistant Studies — M
Public Health—General — M,O

ILLINOIS COLLEGE OF OPTOMETRY
Optometry — M

ILLINOIS INSTITUTE OF TECHNOLOGY
Biochemistry — M,D
Biological and Biomedical
   Sciences—General — M,D
Cell Biology — M,D
Health Physics/Radiological Health — M,D
Medical Imaging — M,D
Microbiology — M,D
Molecular Biology — M,D
Molecular Biophysics — M,D

ILLINOIS STATE UNIVERSITY
Animal Behavior — M,D
Bacteriology — M,D
Biochemistry — M,D
Biological and Biomedical
   Sciences—General — M,D
Biophysics — M,D
Botany — M,D
Cell Biology — M,D
Communication Disorders — M
Conservation Biology — M,D
Developmental Biology — M,D
Ecology — M,D
Entomology — M,D
Evolutionary Biology — M,D
Family Nurse Practitioner Studies — M,D,O
Genetics — M,D
Immunology — M,D
Microbiology — M,D
Molecular Biology — M,D
Molecular Genetics — M,D
Neurobiology — M,D
Neuroscience — M,D
Nursing—General — M,D,O
Parasitology — M,D
Physiology — M,D
Plant Biology — M,D
Plant Molecular Biology — M,D
Structural Biology — M,D
Zoology — M,D

IMMACULATA UNIVERSITY
Health Promotion — M
Neuroscience — M,D,O
Nursing and Healthcare
   Administration — M
Nursing Education — M
Nursing—General — M
Nutrition — M

INDEPENDENCE UNIVERSITY
Community Health Nursing — M
Community Health — M
Gerontological Nursing — M
Health Promotion — M
Health Services Management and
   Hospital Administration — M
Nursing and Healthcare
   Administration — M
Nursing—General — M
Public Health—General — M

INDIANA STATE UNIVERSITY
Biological and Biomedical
   Sciences—General — M,D
Cell Biology — M,D
Communication Disorders — M,D,O
Ecology — M,D
Environmental and Occupational
   Health — M
Evolutionary Biology — M,D
Family Nurse Practitioner Studies — M,D
Molecular Biology — M,D
Nursing and Healthcare
   Administration — M,D
Nursing Education — M,D
Nursing—General — M,D
Occupational Therapy — M,D
Physical Therapy — M,D
Physician Assistant Studies — M,D
Physiology — M,D

INDIANA TECH
Health Services Management and
   Hospital Administration — M

INDIANA UNIVERSITY BLOOMINGTON
Biochemistry — M,D
Biological and Biomedical
   Sciences—General — M,D
Cell Biology — M,D
Communication Disorders — M,D
Community Health — M,D
Ecology — M,D,O
Environmental and Occupational
   Health — M,D
Epidemiology — M,D
Evolutionary Biology — M,D
Genetics — M,D
Health Promotion — M,D
Health Services Management and
   Hospital Administration — M,D
Medical Physics — M,D
Microbiology — M,D
Molecular Biology — M,D
Neuroscience — D
Nutrition — M,D
Optometry — M,D
Plant Biology — M,D
Public Health—General — M,D
Toxicology — M,D,O
Zoology — M,D

INDIANA UNIVERSITY EAST
Nursing—General — M

INDIANA UNIVERSITY KOKOMO
Health Services Management and
   Hospital Administration — M,O
Nursing and Healthcare
   Administration — M
Nursing Education — M
Nursing—General — M

INDIANA UNIVERSITY NORTHWEST
Health Services Management and
   Hospital Administration — M,O

INDIANA UNIVERSITY OF PENNSYLVANIA
Biological and Biomedical
   Sciences—General — M
Communication Disorders — M
Environmental and Occupational
   Health — M,D
Health Services Management and
   Hospital Administration — M,D
Nursing and Healthcare
   Administration — M
Nursing Education — M
Nursing—General — D
Nutrition — M

INDIANA UNIVERSITY–PURDUE UNIVERSITY FORT WAYNE
Adult Nursing — M,O
Biological and Biomedical
   Sciences—General — M,O
Family Nurse Practitioner Studies — M,O
Gerontological Nursing — M,O
Nursing and Healthcare
   Administration — M,O
Nursing Education — M,O
Nursing—General — M,O

INDIANA UNIVERSITY–PURDUE UNIVERSITY INDIANAPOLIS
Allopathic Medicine — M,D
Anatomy — M,D
Biochemistry — M,D
Bioethics — M,O
Biological and Biomedical
   Sciences—General — M,D
Biopsychology — M,D
Cell Biology — M,D
Community Health — M,D
Dentistry — M,D,O
Environmental and Occupational
   Health — M,D,O
Epidemiology — M,D
Health Services Management and
   Hospital Administration — M,D
Immunology — M,D
Microbiology — M,D
Molecular Biology — M,D
Molecular Genetics — M,D
Neurobiology — D
Nursing and Healthcare
   Administration — M,O
Nursing Education — M,O
Nursing—General — M,D,O
Nutrition — M,D
Occupational Therapy — M,D
Pathology — M,D
Pharmacology — M,D
Physical Therapy — M,D
Public Health—General — M,D
Rehabilitation Sciences — M,D
Toxicology — M,D

INDIANA UNIVERSITY SOUTH BEND
Family Nurse Practitioner Studies — M
Nursing—General — M

INDIANA WESLEYAN UNIVERSITY
Health Services Management and
   Hospital Administration — M,O
Nursing and Healthcare
   Administration — M,O
Nursing Education — M
Nursing—General — M

INSTITUTE OF CLINICAL ACUPUNCTURE AND ORIENTAL MEDICINE
Acupuncture and Oriental Medicine — M

INSTITUTE OF PUBLIC ADMINISTRATION
Health Services Management and
   Hospital Administration — M,O

INSTITUT FRANCO-EUROP• DE CHIROPRAXIE
Chiropractic — D

INSTITUTO TECNOLOGICO DE SANTO DOMINGO
Allopathic Medicine — M,D
Bioethics — M,O
Health Promotion — M,O
Maternal and Child Health — M,O
Nutrition — M,O

INTER AMERICAN UNIVERSITY OF PUERTO RICO, ARECIBO CAMPUS
Acute Care/Critical Care Nursing — M
Medical/Surgical Nursing — M
Nurse Anesthesia — M
Nursing—General — M

INTER AMERICAN UNIVERSITY OF PUERTO RICO, BAYAMÓN CAMPUS
Ecology — M

INTER AMERICAN UNIVERSITY OF PUERTO RICO, METROPOLITAN CAMPUS
Clinical Laboratory
   Sciences/Medical Technology — M
Microbiology — M
Molecular Biology — M

INTER AMERICAN UNIVERSITY OF PUERTO RICO SCHOOL OF OPTOMETRY
Optometry — D

IONA COLLEGE
Communication Disorders — M
Health Services Management and
   Hospital Administration — M,O

IOWA STATE UNIVERSITY OF SCIENCE AND TECHNOLOGY
Biological and Biomedical
   Sciences—General — M,D
Biophysics — M,D
Cell Biology — M,D
Computational Biology — M,D
Developmental Biology — M,D
Ecology — M,D
Entomology — M,D
Evolutionary Biology — M,D
Genetics — M,D
Immunology — M,D
Microbiology — M,D
Molecular Biology — M,D
Molecular Genetics — M,D
Neuroscience — M,D
Nutrition — M,D
Pathology — M,D
Plant Biology — M,D
Plant Pathology — M,D
Structural Biology — M,D
Toxicology — M,D
Veterinary Medicine — M,D
Veterinary Sciences — M,D

IRELL & MANELLA GRADUATE SCHOOL OF BIOLOGICAL SCIENCES
Biochemistry — D
Biological and Biomedical
   Sciences—General — D*
Cancer Biology/Oncology — D
Cell Biology — D
Developmental Biology — D
Genetics — D
Immunology — D
Molecular Biology — D
Neuroscience — D
Pharmaceutical Sciences — D

ITHACA COLLEGE
Allied Health—General — M,D
Communication Disorders — M
Occupational Therapy — M
Physical Therapy — D

JACKSON STATE UNIVERSITY
Biological and Biomedical
   Sciences—General — M,D
Communication Disorders — M

JACKSONVILLE STATE UNIVERSITY
Biological and Biomedical
   Sciences—General — M
Nursing—General — M

JACKSONVILLE UNIVERSITY
Allied Health—General — M
Communication Disorders — M
Nursing—General — M,D
Oral and Dental Sciences — O

JAMES MADISON UNIVERSITY
Biological and Biomedical
   Sciences—General — M
Communication Disorders — M,D
Family Nurse Practitioner Studies — M,D
Gerontological Nursing — M,D
Nurse Midwifery — M,D
Nursing and Healthcare
   Administration — M,D
Nursing—General — M,D
Nutrition — M
Occupational Therapy — M
Physician Assistant Studies — M
Physiology — M

JEFFERSON COLLEGE OF HEALTH SCIENCES
Nursing and Healthcare
   Administration — M
Nursing Education — M
Nursing—General — M
Occupational Therapy — M
Physician Assistant Studies — M

JOHN CARROLL UNIVERSITY
Biological and Biomedical
Sciences—General | M

JOHNS HOPKINS UNIVERSITY
Allopathic Medicine | D
Anatomy | D
Biochemistry | M,D
Bioethics | M,D
Biological and Biomedical
Sciences—General | M,D
Biophysics | D
Cardiovascular Sciences | M,D
Cell Biology | D
Clinical Research | M,D
Community Health | M,D
Developmental Biology | D
Environmental and Occupational
Health | M,D
Epidemiology | M,D
Evolutionary Biology | D
Genetics | M,D
Health Services Management and
Hospital Administration | M,D,O
Health Services Research | D
Human Genetics | D
Immunology | M,D
Infectious Diseases | M,D
International Health | M,D
Microbiology | M,D
Molecular Biology | M,D
Molecular Medicine | D
Neuroscience | D
Nursing—General | M,D,O
Nutrition | M,D
Pathobiology | D
Pathology | D
Pharmaceutical Sciences | M
Pharmacology | D
Physiology | M,D
Public Health—General | M,D
Toxicology | M,D

JOHNSON & WALES UNIVERSITY
Physician Assistant Studies | M

KANSAS CITY UNIVERSITY OF MEDICINE AND BIOSCIENCES
Bioethics | M
Biological and Biomedical
Sciences—General | M
Osteopathic Medicine | D

KANSAS STATE UNIVERSITY
Biochemistry | M,D
Biological and Biomedical
Sciences—General | M,D
Communication Disorders | M,O
Entomology | M,D
Genetics | M,D
Nutrition | M,D
Pathobiology | M,D
Physiology | D
Plant Pathology | M,D
Public Health—General | M,D,O
Veterinary Medicine | D
Veterinary Sciences | M,O

KAPLAN UNIVERSITY, DAVENPORT CAMPUS
Health Services Management and
Hospital Administration | M,O
Nursing and Healthcare
Administration | M
Nursing Education | M
Nursing—General | M

KEAN UNIVERSITY
Communication Disorders | M
Community Health Nursing | M
Health Services Management and
Hospital Administration | M
Nursing and Healthcare
Administration | M,D
Nursing—General | M
Occupational Therapy | M
School Nursing | M

KECK GRADUATE INSTITUTE
Biological and Biomedical
Sciences—General | M,D,O
Pharmacy | D

KEENE STATE COLLEGE
Environmental and Occupational
Health | M,O

KEISER UNIVERSITY
Health Services Management and
Hospital Administration | M
Nursing—General | M
Physician Assistant Studies | M

KENNESAW STATE UNIVERSITY
Biochemistry | M
Biological and Biomedical
Sciences—General | M
Health Services Management and
Hospital Administration | M
Nursing—General | M,D

KENT STATE UNIVERSITY
Adult Nursing | M,D,O
Biological and Biomedical
Sciences—General | M,D
Cell Biology | M,D
Communication Disorders | M,D,O
Ecology | M,D
Family Nurse Practitioner Studies | M,D,O
Genetics | M,D
Gerontological Nursing | M,D,O
Health Promotion | M,D
Molecular Biology | M,D
Neuroscience | M,D

Nursing and Healthcare
Administration | M,D,O
Nursing Education | M,D,O
Nursing—General | M,D,O
Nutrition | M
Pediatric Nursing | M,D,O
Pharmacology | M,D
Physiology | M,D
Podiatric Medicine | D
Psychiatric Nursing | M,D,O
Public Health—General | M,D
Women's Health Nursing | M,D,O

KENTUCKY STATE UNIVERSITY
Nursing—General | M,D

KETTERING COLLEGE
Physician Assistant Studies | M

KEUKA COLLEGE
Gerontological Nursing | M
Nursing—General | M
Occupational Therapy | M

KING'S COLLEGE
Health Services Management and
Hospital Administration | M
Physician Assistant Studies | M

KING UNIVERSITY
Health Services Management and
Hospital Administration | M

LAKE ERIE COLLEGE
Health Services Management and
Hospital Administration | M

LAKE ERIE COLLEGE OF OSTEOPATHIC MEDICINE
Biological and Biomedical
Sciences—General | M,D,O
Osteopathic Medicine | M,D,O
Pharmacy | M,D,O

LAKE FOREST GRADUATE SCHOOL OF MANAGEMENT
Health Services Management and
Hospital Administration | M

LAKEHEAD UNIVERSITY
Biological and Biomedical
Sciences—General | M
Health Services Research | M

LAKELAND UNIVERSITY
Health Services Management and
Hospital Administration | M

LAMAR UNIVERSITY
Biological and Biomedical
Sciences—General | M
Communication Disorders | M,D
Health Services Management and
Hospital Administration | M
Nursing and Healthcare
Administration | M
Nursing Education | M
Nursing—General | M
Public Health—General | M

LANDER UNIVERSITY
Nursing—General | M

LANGSTON UNIVERSITY
Physical Therapy | D

LA ROCHE COLLEGE
Nurse Anesthesia | M
Nursing and Healthcare
Administration | M
Nursing Education | M
Nursing—General | M

LA SALLE UNIVERSITY
Adult Nursing | M,D,O
Communication Disorders | M
Community Health Nursing | M,D,O
Family Nurse Practitioner Studies | M,D,O
Gerontological Nursing | M,D,O
Nurse Anesthesia | M,D,O
Nursing and Healthcare
Administration | M,D,O
Nursing Education | M,D,O
Nursing—General | M,D,O
Public Health—General | M
School Nursing | M,D,O

LASELL COLLEGE
Health Services Management and
Hospital Administration | M,O
Rehabilitation Sciences | M

LAURENTIAN UNIVERSITY
Biochemistry | M
Biological and Biomedical
Sciences—General | M,D
Ecology | M,D
Nursing—General | M
Public Health—General | D

LEBANESE AMERICAN UNIVERSITY
Pharmacy | D

LEBANON VALLEY COLLEGE
Health Services Management and
Hospital Administration | M
Physical Therapy | D

LEE UNIVERSITY
Biological and Biomedical
Sciences—General | M,O

LEHIGH UNIVERSITY
Biochemistry | M,D
Biological and Biomedical
Sciences—General | M,D
Cell Biology | M,D

Health Services Management and
Hospital Administration | M
Molecular Biology | M,D

LEHMAN COLLEGE OF THE CITY UNIVERSITY OF NEW YORK
Adult Nursing | M
Biological and Biomedical
Sciences—General | M
Communication Disorders | M
Gerontological Nursing | M
Health Promotion | M
Maternal and Child/Neonatal
Nursing | M
Nursing—General | M
Nutrition | M
Pediatric Nursing | M

LE MOYNE COLLEGE
Gerontological Nursing | M,O
Nursing and Healthcare
Administration | M,O
Nursing Education | M,O
Nursing Informatics | M,O
Nursing—General | M,O
Occupational Therapy | M
Physician Assistant Studies | M

LENOIR-RHYNE UNIVERSITY
Health Services Management and
Hospital Administration | M
Nursing and Healthcare
Administration | M
Nursing Education | M
Nursing—General | M
Occupational Therapy | M
Physician Assistant Studies | M
Public Health—General | M

LESLEY UNIVERSITY
Ecology | M,D,O

LETOURNEAU UNIVERSITY
Health Services Management and
Hospital Administration | M

LEWIS & CLARK COLLEGE
Communication Disorders | M

LEWIS UNIVERSITY
Adult Nursing | M,D
Environmental and Occupational
Health | M
Health Services Management and
Hospital Administration | M
Nursing and Healthcare
Administration | M,D
Nursing Education | M,D
Nursing—General | M,D

LIBERTY UNIVERSITY
Biological and Biomedical
Sciences—General | M,O
Family Nurse Practitioner Studies | M,D
Health Promotion | M,D,O
Health Services Management and
Hospital Administration | M,D,O
International Health | M,O
Nursing and Healthcare
Administration | M,D
Nursing Education | M,D
Nursing—General | M,D
Nutrition | M,O
Osteopathic Medicine | D

LIFE CHIROPRACTIC COLLEGE WEST
Chiropractic | D

LIFE UNIVERSITY
Chiropractic | D
Nutrition | M

LINCOLN MEMORIAL UNIVERSITY
Family Nurse Practitioner Studies | M
Nurse Anesthesia | M
Nursing—General | M
Osteopathic Medicine | D
Psychiatric Nursing | M

LINDENWOOD UNIVERSITY
Communication Disorders | M,D,O
Health Promotion | M
Health Services Management and
Hospital Administration | M,O
Nursing—General | M

LINDENWOOD UNIVERSITY–BELLEVILLE
Health Services Management and
Hospital Administration | M

LIPSCOMB UNIVERSITY
Health Services Management and
Hospital Administration | M,O
Molecular Biology | M
Nutrition | M
Pharmacy | M,D

LOCK HAVEN UNIVERSITY OF PENNSYLVANIA
Health Promotion | M
Health Services Management and
Hospital Administration | M
Physician Assistant Studies | M

LOGAN UNIVERSITY
Chiropractic | M,D
Nutrition | M,D
Rehabilitation Sciences | M,D

LOMA LINDA UNIVERSITY
Adult Nursing | M
Allied Health—General | M,D
Allopathic Medicine | M,D
Anatomy | D
Biochemistry | M,D
Bioethics | M,O

Communication Disorders | M,D
Dentistry | M,D,O
Environmental and Occupational
Health | M
Epidemiology | M,D
Gerontological Nursing | M
Health Services Management and
Hospital Administration | M
International Health | M
Microbiology | M,D
Nursing and Healthcare
Administration | M
Nursing Education | M
Nursing—General | D
Nutrition | M,D
Occupational Therapy | M,D
Oral and Dental Sciences | M,O
Pathology | D
Pediatric Nursing | M
Pharmacology | D
Pharmacy | D
Physical Therapy | M,D
Physician Assistant Studies | M
Physiology | D
Public Health—General | M,D
Rehabilitation Sciences | M,D

LONDON METROPOLITAN UNIVERSITY
Biological and Biomedical
Sciences—General | M,D
Health Services Management and
Hospital Administration | M,D
Immunology | M,D
Nutrition | M,D
Pharmacology | M,D
Public Health—General | M,D

LONG ISLAND UNIVERSITY–HUDSON AT ROCKLAND
Pharmaceutical Sciences | M,O

LONG ISLAND UNIVERSITY–HUDSON AT WESTCHESTER
Health Services Management and
Hospital Administration | M,O

LONG ISLAND UNIVERSITY–LIU BROOKLYN
Adult Nursing | M,O
Biological and Biomedical
Sciences—General | M,D,O
Communication Disorders | M,D,O
Family Nurse Practitioner Studies | M,O
Health Services Management and
Hospital Administration | M,O
Nursing Education | M,O
Nursing—General | M,O
Occupational Therapy | M,D
Pharmaceutical Sciences | M,D
Pharmacology | M,D
Pharmacy | M,D
Physical Therapy | M,D
Physician Assistant Studies | M,D
Public Health—General | M,D
Toxicology | M,D

LONG ISLAND UNIVERSITY–LIU POST
Allied Health—General | M
Biological and Biomedical
Sciences—General | M,O
Cancer Biology/Oncology | M,O
Communication Disorders | M,D,O
Family Nurse Practitioner Studies | M,O
Infectious Diseases | M,O
Microbiology | M,O
Nursing and Healthcare
Administration | M,O
Nursing Education | M,O
Nutrition | M,O

LONGWOOD UNIVERSITY
Communication Disorders | M

LOUISIANA STATE UNIVERSITY AND AGRICULTURAL & MECHANICAL COLLEGE
Biochemistry | M,D
Biological and Biomedical
Sciences—General | M,D
Biopsychology | M,D
Communication Disorders | M,D
Entomology | M,D
Medical Physics | M,D
Plant Pathology | M,D
Toxicology | M,D
Veterinary Medicine | D
Veterinary Sciences | M,D

LOUISIANA STATE UNIVERSITY HEALTH SCIENCES CENTER
Allopathic Medicine | M,D
Anatomy | D
Biological and Biomedical
Sciences—General | D
Cell Biology | D
Communication Disorders | M,D
Community Health Nursing | M,D,O
Community Health | M,D
Dentistry | D
Developmental Biology | D
Environmental and Occupational
Health | M,D
Epidemiology | M,D,O
Family Nurse Practitioner Studies | M,D,O
Gerontological Nursing | M,D,O
Health Services Management and
Hospital Administration | M,D
Human Genetics | D
Immunology | D
Maternal and Child/Neonatal
Nursing | M,D,O
Microbiology | D
Neurobiology | D

M—masters degree; D—doctorate; O—other advanced degree; *—Close-Up and/or Display

Neuroscience — D
Nurse Anesthesia — M,D,O
Nursing and Healthcare Administration — M,D,O
Nursing Education — M,D,O
Nursing—General — M,D,O
Occupational Therapy — M
Parasitology — D
Pharmacology — D
Physical Therapy — D
Physician Assistant Studies — M
Physiology — D
Public Health—General — M,D

LOUISIANA STATE UNIVERSITY HEALTH SCIENCES CENTER AT SHREVEPORT
Allopathic Medicine — D
Anatomy — M,D
Biochemistry — M,D
Biological and Biomedical Sciences—General — M
Cell Biology — M,D
Immunology — M,D
Microbiology — M,D
Molecular Biology — M,D
Pharmacology — M,D
Physiology — M,D

LOUISIANA STATE UNIVERSITY IN SHREVEPORT
Biological and Biomedical Sciences—General — M
Health Services Management and Hospital Administration — M
Public Health—General — M

LOUISIANA TECH UNIVERSITY
Biological and Biomedical Sciences—General — M
Communication Disorders — M,D
Molecular Biology — M
Nutrition — M

LOURDES UNIVERSITY
Nurse Anesthesia — M
Nursing and Healthcare Administration — M
Nursing Education — M

LOYOLA MARYMOUNT UNIVERSITY
Bioethics — M

LOYOLA UNIVERSITY CHICAGO
Adult Nursing — M,D,O
Biochemistry — M,D
Bioethics — D,O
Biological and Biomedical Sciences—General — M,D
Cancer Biology/Oncology — M,D,O
Cell Biology — M,D
Clinical Research — M
Family Nurse Practitioner Studies — M,D,O
Gerontological Nursing — M,D,O
Health Services Management and Hospital Administration — M,O
Immunology — M,D
Infectious Diseases — M,D
Microbiology — M,D
Molecular Biology — M,D
Molecular Pharmacology — M,D
Molecular Physiology — M,D
Neuroscience — M,D
Nursing and Healthcare Administration — M,D,O
Nursing—General — M,D,O
Nutrition — M,D,O
Physiology — M,D
Public Health—General — M
Women's Health Nursing — M,D,O

LOYOLA UNIVERSITY MARYLAND
Communication Disorders — M

LOYOLA UNIVERSITY NEW ORLEANS
Health Services Management and Hospital Administration — M,D
Nursing—General — M,D

LYNCHBURG COLLEGE
Nursing and Healthcare Administration — M
Nursing—General — M
Physical Therapy — D

MADONNA UNIVERSITY
Adult Nursing — M
Health Services Management and Hospital Administration — M
Hospice Nursing — M
Nursing and Healthcare Administration — M
Nursing—General — M

MALONE UNIVERSITY
Family Nurse Practitioner Studies — M
Nursing—General — M

MANCHESTER UNIVERSITY
Pharmacy — D

MANHATTANVILLE COLLEGE
Health Promotion — M,O

MANSFIELD UNIVERSITY OF PENNSYLVANIA
Nursing—General — M

MARIAN UNIVERSITY (IN)
Osteopathic Medicine — D

MARIAN UNIVERSITY (WI)
Adult Nursing — M
Nursing Education — M
Nursing—General — M

MARIETTA COLLEGE
Physician Assistant Studies — M

MARQUETTE UNIVERSITY
Acute Care/Critical Care Nursing — M,D,O
Adult Nursing — M,D,O
Biological and Biomedical Sciences—General — M,D
Cardiovascular Sciences — M
Cell Biology — M,D
Communication Disorders — M,O
Dentistry — D
Developmental Biology — M,D
Ecology — M,D
Family Nurse Practitioner Studies — M,D,O
Genetics — M,D
Gerontological Nursing — M,D,O
Microbiology — M,D
Molecular Biology — M,D
Neuroscience — M,D
Nurse Midwifery — M,D,O
Nursing and Healthcare Administration — M,D,O
Nursing—General — M,D,O
Oral and Dental Sciences — M,O
Pediatric Nursing — M,D,O
Physical Therapy — D
Physician Assistant Studies — M
Physiology — M,D
Rehabilitation Sciences — M,D

MARSHALL B. KETCHUM UNIVERSITY
Optometry — M,D
Vision Sciences — M,D

MARSHALL UNIVERSITY
Allopathic Medicine — D
Biological and Biomedical Sciences—General — M,D
Communication Disorders — M
Health Services Management and Hospital Administration — M
Nurse Anesthesia — D
Nursing—General — M
Nutrition — M
Pharmacy — D
Physical Therapy — D
Public Health—General — M

MARYLAND UNIVERSITY OF INTEGRATIVE HEALTH
Acupuncture and Oriental Medicine — M,O

MARYLHURST UNIVERSITY
Health Services Management and Hospital Administration — M

MARYMOUNT UNIVERSITY
Allied Health—General — M,D,O
Family Nurse Practitioner Studies — M,D,O
Health Promotion — M
Health Services Management and Hospital Administration — M
Nursing—General — M,D,O
Physical Therapy — D

MARYVILLE UNIVERSITY OF SAINT LOUIS
Acute Care/Critical Care Nursing — M,D
Adult Nursing — M,D
Allied Health—General — M,D
Family Nurse Practitioner Studies — M,D
Gerontological Nursing — M,D
Health Services Management and Hospital Administration — M,O
Nursing—General — M,D
Occupational Therapy — M
Pediatric Nursing — M,D
Physical Therapy — D

MARYWOOD UNIVERSITY
Communication Disorders — M
Health Services Management and Hospital Administration — M
Nutrition — M,O
Physician Assistant Studies — M

MASSACHUSETTS INSTITUTE OF TECHNOLOGY
Biochemistry — D
Biological and Biomedical Sciences—General — M,D
Cell Biology — D
Communication Disorders — M,D
Computational Biology — D
Developmental Biology — D
Environmental Biology — M,D,O
Genetics — D
Genomic Sciences — M,D
Immunology — D
Medical Physics — M,D
Microbiology — D
Molecular Biology — D
Molecular Toxicology — D
Neurobiology — D
Neuroscience — D
Structural Biology — D
Systems Biology — D
Toxicology — M,D

MAYO GRADUATE SCHOOL
Biochemistry — D
Biological and Biomedical Sciences—General — D
Cancer Biology/Oncology — D
Cell Biology — D
Genetics — D
Immunology — D
Molecular Biology — D
Molecular Pharmacology — D
Neuroscience — D
Structural Biology — D
Virology — D

MAYO MEDICAL SCHOOL
Allopathic Medicine — D

MAYO SCHOOL OF HEALTH SCIENCES
Nurse Anesthesia — D
Physical Therapy — D

MCGILL UNIVERSITY
Allopathic Medicine — M,D
Anatomy — M,D
Biochemistry — M,D
Bioethics — M,D,O
Biological and Biomedical Sciences—General — M,D
Cell Biology — M,D
Communication Disorders — M,D
Community Health — M,D,O
Dentistry — M,D,O
Entomology — M,D
Environmental and Occupational Health — M,D
Epidemiology — M,D,O
Family Nurse Practitioner Studies — M,D,O
Health Services Management and Hospital Administration — M,D,O
Human Genetics — M,D
Immunology — M,D
Medical Physics — M,D
Microbiology — M,D
Neuroscience — M,D
Nursing—General — M,D,O
Nutrition — M,D,O
Oral and Dental Sciences — M,D,O
Parasitology — M,D,O
Pathology — M,D
Pharmacology — M,D
Physiology — M,D
Rehabilitation Sciences — M,D,O

MCKENDREE UNIVERSITY
Nursing and Healthcare Administration — M
Nursing Education — M
Nursing—General — M

MCMASTER UNIVERSITY
Biochemistry — M,D
Biological and Biomedical Sciences—General — M,D
Cancer Biology/Oncology — M,D
Cardiovascular Sciences — M,D
Cell Biology — M,D
Genetics — M,D
Health Physics/Radiological Health — M,D
Health Services Research — M,D
Immunology — M,D
Medical Physics — M,D
Molecular Biology — M,D
Neuroscience — M,D
Nursing—General — M,D
Nutrition — M,D
Occupational Therapy — M
Pharmacology — M,D
Physical Therapy — M
Physiology — M,D
Rehabilitation Sciences — M,D
Virology — M,D

MCMURRY UNIVERSITY
Family Nurse Practitioner Studies — M
Nursing Education — M
Nursing—General — M

MCNEESE STATE UNIVERSITY
Family Nurse Practitioner Studies — M,O
Health Promotion — M
Nursing and Healthcare Administration — M,O
Nursing Education — M
Nursing—General — M,O
Nutrition — M
Psychiatric Nursing — M,O

MCPHS UNIVERSITY
Acupuncture and Oriental Medicine — M
Health Services Management and Hospital Administration — M
Nursing—General — M
Pharmaceutical Sciences — M,D
Pharmacology — M,D
Pharmacy — D
Physician Assistant Studies — M

MEDICAL COLLEGE OF WISCONSIN
Allopathic Medicine — D
Biochemistry — D
Bioethics — M,O
Biological and Biomedical Sciences—General — M,D,O
Biophysics — D
Clinical Laboratory Sciences/Medical Technology — M,D
Clinical Research — M
Community Health — M,D,O
Epidemiology — M,D,O
Medical Imaging — D
Microbiology — M,D
Molecular Genetics — M,D
Neuroscience — D
Pharmacology — D
Physiology — D
Public Health—General — M,D,O
Toxicology — D

MEDICAL UNIVERSITY OF SOUTH CAROLINA
Adult Nursing — M,D
Allied Health—General — M,D
Allopathic Medicine — D
Biochemistry — M,D
Biological and Biomedical Sciences—General — M,D
Cancer Biology/Oncology — D
Cardiovascular Sciences — D
Cell Biology — D
Clinical Research — M
Dentistry — D
Developmental Biology — D
Epidemiology — M,D
Family Nurse Practitioner Studies — M,D
Genetics — D
Gerontological Nursing — M,D

Health Services Management and Hospital Administration — M,D
Immunology — M,D
International Health — M
Maternal and Child/Neonatal Nursing — M,D
Medical Imaging — D
Medicinal and Pharmaceutical Chemistry — D
Microbiology — M,D
Molecular Biology — M,D
Molecular Pharmacology — M,D
Neuroscience — M,D
Nurse Anesthesia — M
Nursing and Healthcare Administration — M
Nursing Education — M
Nursing—General — D
Occupational Therapy — M
Pathobiology — D
Pathology — M,D
Pharmacy — D
Physical Therapy — D
Physician Assistant Studies — M
Rehabilitation Sciences — D
Toxicology — D

MEHARRY MEDICAL COLLEGE
Allopathic Medicine — D
Biological and Biomedical Sciences—General — D
Cancer Biology/Oncology — D
Community Health — M
Dentistry — D
Environmental and Occupational Health — M
Health Services Management and Hospital Administration — M
Immunology — D
Microbiology — D
Neuroscience — D
Pharmacology — D

MEMORIAL UNIVERSITY OF NEWFOUNDLAND
Biochemistry — M,D
Biological and Biomedical Sciences—General — M,D,O
Biopsychology — M,D
Cancer Biology/Oncology — M,D
Cardiovascular Sciences — M,D
Clinical Research — M
Community Health — M,D,O
Epidemiology — M,D,O
Human Genetics — M,D
Immunology — M,D
Neuroscience — M,D
Nursing—General — M,D
Pharmaceutical Sciences — M,D

MERCER UNIVERSITY
Allopathic Medicine — M,D
Environmental and Occupational Health — M,D
Gerontological Nursing — M,D,O
Nursing—General — M,D,O
Pharmaceutical Sciences — D
Pharmacy — D
Physical Therapy — M,D
Physician Assistant Studies — M,D
Public Health—General — M,D

MERCY COLLEGE
Allied Health—General — M,D
Communication Disorders — M
Health Services Management and Hospital Administration — M
Nursing and Healthcare Administration — M
Nursing Education — M
Nursing—General — M
Occupational Therapy — M
Physical Therapy — D
Physician Assistant Studies — M

MERCYHURST UNIVERSITY
Physician Assistant Studies — M

MEREDITH COLLEGE
Nutrition — M,O

MERRIMACK COLLEGE
Community Health — M
Health Promotion — M

MESSIAH COLLEGE
Nursing Education — M

METHODIST UNIVERSITY
Physician Assistant Studies — M

METROPOLITAN COLLEGE OF NEW YORK
Health Services Management and Hospital Administration — M

METROPOLITAN STATE UNIVERSITY
Nursing and Healthcare Administration — M,D
Nursing Education — M,D
Nursing—General — M,D
Oral and Dental Sciences — M,D

MGH INSTITUTE OF HEALTH PROFESSIONS
Communication Disorders — M,O
Gerontological Nursing — M,D,O
Nursing Education — M,D,O
Nursing—General — M,D,O
Occupational Therapy — D
Pediatric Nursing — M,D,O
Physical Therapy — M,D,O
Physician Assistant Studies — M
Psychiatric Nursing — M,D,O
Women's Health Nursing — M,D,O

MIAMI UNIVERSITY
Biochemistry — M,D

Biological and Biomedical Sciences—General	M,D
Communication Disorders	M
Microbiology	M,D

MICHIGAN STATE UNIVERSITY

Allopathic Medicine	D
Biochemistry	M,D
Biological and Biomedical Sciences—General	M,D
Cell Biology	M,D
Clinical Laboratory Sciences/Medical Technology	M
Communication Disorders	M,D
Ecology	D
Entomology	M,D
Epidemiology	M,D
Evolutionary Biology	D
Genetics	M,D
Microbiology	M,D
Molecular Biology	M,D
Molecular Genetics	M,D
Neuroscience	M,D
Nursing—General	M,D
Nutrition	M,D
Osteopathic Medicine	D
Pathobiology	M,D
Pathology	M,D
Pharmacology	M,D
Physiology	M,D
Plant Biology	M,D
Plant Pathology	M,D
Public Health—General	D
Structural Biology	D
Systems Biology	D
Toxicology	M,D
Veterinary Medicine	D
Veterinary Sciences	M,D
Zoology	M,D

MICHIGAN TECHNOLOGICAL UNIVERSITY

Biochemistry	M,D,O
Biological and Biomedical Sciences—General	M,D
Ecology	M,D
Molecular Biology	M,D,O
Plant Molecular Biology	M,D

MIDAMERICA NAZARENE UNIVERSITY

Nursing and Healthcare Administration	M
Nursing Education	M
Public Health—General	M

MIDDLE GEORGIA STATE UNIVERSITY

Gerontological Nursing	M

MIDDLE TENNESSEE SCHOOL OF ANESTHESIA

Nurse Anesthesia	M,D

MIDDLE TENNESSEE STATE UNIVERSITY

Biological and Biomedical Sciences—General	M
Family Nurse Practitioner Studies	M,O
Molecular Biology	D
Nursing and Healthcare Administration	M
Nursing Education	M
Nursing—General	M,O

MIDWEST COLLEGE OF ORIENTAL MEDICINE

Acupuncture and Oriental Medicine	M,O

MIDWESTERN STATE UNIVERSITY

Biological and Biomedical Sciences—General	M
Community Health	M,O
Family Nurse Practitioner Studies	M
Health Physics/Radiological Health	M
Health Services Management and Hospital Administration	M,O
Nursing Education	M
Nursing—General	M
Psychiatric Nursing	M

MIDWESTERN UNIVERSITY, DOWNERS GROVE CAMPUS

Allied Health—General	D
Biological and Biomedical Sciences—General	M
Dentistry	D
Occupational Therapy	M
Osteopathic Medicine	D
Pharmacy	D
Physical Therapy	D
Physician Assistant Studies	M

MIDWESTERN UNIVERSITY, GLENDALE CAMPUS

Allied Health—General	M,D
Biological and Biomedical Sciences—General	M
Cardiovascular Sciences	M
Dentistry	D
Nurse Anesthesia	M
Occupational Therapy	M
Optometry	D
Osteopathic Medicine	D
Pharmacy	D
Physical Therapy	D
Physician Assistant Studies	M
Podiatric Medicine	D

MIDWIVES COLLEGE OF UTAH

Nurse Midwifery	M

MILLERSVILLE UNIVERSITY OF PENNSYLVANIA

Family Nurse Practitioner Studies	M
Nursing Education	M

Nursing—General	M

MILLIGAN COLLEGE

Occupational Therapy	M

MILLIKIN UNIVERSITY

Nurse Anesthesia	M,D
Nursing Education	M,D
Nursing—General	M,D

MILLS COLLEGE

Biological and Biomedical Sciences—General	O

MILWAUKEE SCHOOL OF ENGINEERING

Cardiovascular Sciences	M
Clinical Laboratory Sciences/Medical Technology	M
Health Services Management and Hospital Administration	M
Nursing and Healthcare Administration	M
Perfusion	M*

MINNESOTA STATE UNIVERSITY MANKATO

Allied Health—General	M,D,O
Biological and Biomedical Sciences—General	M
Communication Disorders	M
Community Health	M,O
Family Nurse Practitioner Studies	M,D
Nursing—General	M

MINNESOTA STATE UNIVERSITY MOORHEAD

Communication Disorders	M,O
Health Services Management and Hospital Administration	M,O
Nursing—General	M,O

MINOT STATE UNIVERSITY

Communication Disorders	M

MISERICORDIA UNIVERSITY

Allied Health—General	M,D
Communication Disorders	M
Health Services Management and Hospital Administration	M
Nursing—General	M,D
Occupational Therapy	M,D
Physical Therapy	D

MISSISSIPPI COLLEGE

Biochemistry	M
Biological and Biomedical Sciences—General	M
Health Services Management and Hospital Administration	M

MISSISSIPPI STATE UNIVERSITY

Biochemistry	M,D
Biological and Biomedical Sciences—General	M,D
Entomology	M,D
Genetics	M,D
Health Promotion	M,D
Molecular Biology	M,D
Nutrition	M,D
Plant Pathology	M,D
Veterinary Medicine	D
Veterinary Sciences	M,D

MISSISSIPPI UNIVERSITY FOR WOMEN

Communication Disorders	M,O
Nursing—General	M,O

MISSOURI SOUTHERN STATE UNIVERSITY

Dental Hygiene	M
Nursing—General	M

MISSOURI STATE UNIVERSITY

Biological and Biomedical Sciences—General	M
Cell Biology	M
Family Nurse Practitioner Studies	M,D
Health Services Management and Hospital Administration	M
Molecular Biology	M
Nurse Anesthesia	D
Nursing Education	M,D
Nursing—General	M,D
Nutrition	M,D,O
Occupational Therapy	M
Physical Therapy	D
Physician Assistant Studies	M
Public Health—General	M

MISSOURI UNIVERSITY OF SCIENCE AND TECHNOLOGY

Biological and Biomedical Sciences—General	M
Environmental Biology	M

MISSOURI WESTERN STATE UNIVERSITY

Biological and Biomedical Sciences—General	M
Nursing and Healthcare Administration	M,O
Nursing Education	M,O
Nursing—General	M,O

MOLLOY COLLEGE

Adult Nursing	M,D,O
Biological and Biomedical Sciences—General	M,O
Communication Disorders	M
Family Nurse Practitioner Studies	M,D,O
Gerontological Nursing	M,D,O
Health Services Management and Hospital Administration	M
Nursing and Healthcare Administration	M,D,O

Nursing Education	M,D,O
Nursing—General	M,D,O
Pediatric Nursing	M,D,O
Psychiatric Nursing	M,D,O

MONMOUTH UNIVERSITY

Adult Nursing	M,D,O
Communication Disorders	M,O
Family Nurse Practitioner Studies	M,D,O
Forensic Nursing	M,D,O
Gerontological Nursing	M,D,O
Nursing and Healthcare Administration	M,D,O
Nursing Education	M,D,O
Nursing—General	M,D,O
Physician Assistant Studies	M,D,O
Psychiatric Nursing	M,D,O
School Nursing	M,D,O

MONROE COLLEGE

Public Health—General	M

MONTANA STATE UNIVERSITY

Biochemistry	M,D
Biological and Biomedical Sciences—General	M,D
Ecology	M,D
Family Nurse Practitioner Studies	M,D,O
Immunology	M,D
Infectious Diseases	M,D
Microbiology	M,D
Neuroscience	M,D
Nursing and Healthcare Administration	M,D,O
Nursing Education	M,D,O
Plant Pathology	M,D
Psychiatric Nursing	M,D,O

MONTANA STATE UNIVERSITY BILLINGS

Health Services Management and Hospital Administration	M

MONTANA TECH OF THE UNIVERSITY OF MONTANA

Industrial Hygiene	M

MONTCLAIR STATE UNIVERSITY

Biochemistry	M
Biological and Biomedical Sciences—General	M
Communication Disorders	M,D
Ecology	M
Evolutionary Biology	M
Marine Biology	M
Molecular Biology	M,O
Nutrition	M,O
Pharmacology	M
Physiology	M
Public Health—General	M

MORAVIAN COLLEGE

Allied Health—General	M
Health Services Management and Hospital Administration	M
Nursing and Healthcare Administration	M
Nursing Education	M
Nursing—General	M

MOREHEAD STATE UNIVERSITY

Biological and Biomedical Sciences—General	M

MOREHOUSE SCHOOL OF MEDICINE

Allopathic Medicine	D
Biological and Biomedical Sciences—General	M,D
Clinical Research	M
Public Health—General	M

MORGAN STATE UNIVERSITY

Biological and Biomedical Sciences—General	M,D
Environmental Biology	D
Nursing—General	M
Public Health—General	M,D

MOUNT ALLISON UNIVERSITY

Biological and Biomedical Sciences—General	M

MOUNT ALOYSIUS COLLEGE

Health Services Management and Hospital Administration	M

MOUNT CARMEL COLLEGE OF NURSING

Acute Care/Critical Care Nursing	M,D
Adult Nursing	M,D
Family Nurse Practitioner Studies	M,D
Gerontological Nursing	M,D
Nursing and Healthcare Administration	M,D
Nursing Education	M,D
Nursing—General	M,D

MOUNT IDA COLLEGE

Health Services Management and Hospital Administration	M

MOUNT MARTY COLLEGE

Nurse Anesthesia	M
Nursing—General	M

MOUNT MARY UNIVERSITY

Nursing and Healthcare Administration	M
Nutrition	M
Occupational Therapy	M,D

MOUNT MERCY UNIVERSITY

Nursing and Healthcare Administration	M
Nursing Education	M
Nursing—General	M

MOUNT ST. JOSEPH UNIVERSITY

Health Promotion	M,O
Health Services Management and Hospital Administration	D
Nursing and Healthcare Administration	M
Nursing Education	M
Nursing—General	M,D
Physical Therapy	D

MOUNT SAINT MARY COLLEGE

Adult Nursing	M,O
Family Nurse Practitioner Studies	M,O
Nursing and Healthcare Administration	M,O
Nursing Education	M,O
Nursing—General	M,O

MOUNT SAINT MARY'S UNIVERSITY (CA)

Health Services Management and Hospital Administration	M,D,O
Nursing—General	M,D,O
Physical Therapy	M,D,O

MOUNT ST. MARY'S UNIVERSITY (MD)

Health Services Management and Hospital Administration	M

MOUNT SAINT VINCENT UNIVERSITY

Nutrition	M

MURRAY STATE UNIVERSITY

Biological and Biomedical Sciences—General	M,D
Communication Disorders	M
Environmental and Occupational Health	M
Family Nurse Practitioner Studies	M
Industrial Hygiene	M
Nurse Anesthesia	M
Nursing—General	M

NATIONAL COLLEGE OF MIDWIFERY

Nurse Midwifery	M,D

NATIONAL COLLEGE OF NATURAL MEDICINE

Acupuncture and Oriental Medicine	M
Naturopathic Medicine	M,D

NATIONAL UNIVERSITY

Biological and Biomedical Sciences—General	M,O
Communication Disorders	M,O
Forensic Nursing	M,D,O
Health Promotion	M,D,O
Health Services Management and Hospital Administration	M,D,O
Nurse Anesthesia	M,D,O
Nursing and Healthcare Administration	M,D,O
Nursing Informatics	M,D,O
Nursing—General	M,D,O
Public Health—General	M,D,O

NATIONAL UNIVERSITY OF HEALTH SCIENCES

Chiropractic	M,D

NAZARETH COLLEGE OF ROCHESTER

Communication Disorders	M
Physical Therapy	D

NEBRASKA METHODIST COLLEGE

Health Promotion	M
Health Services Management and Hospital Administration	M
Nursing and Healthcare Administration	M
Nursing Education	M
Nursing—General	M

NEBRASKA WESLEYAN UNIVERSITY

Nursing—General	M

NEUMANN UNIVERSITY

Gerontological Nursing	M
Nursing Education	M
Nursing—General	M
Physical Therapy	D

NEW CHARTER UNIVERSITY

Health Services Management and Hospital Administration	M

NEW ENGLAND COLLEGE

Health Services Management and Hospital Administration	M

NEW ENGLAND COLLEGE OF OPTOMETRY

Optometry	M,D
Vision Sciences	M,D

NEW ENGLAND INSTITUTE OF TECHNOLOGY

Occupational Therapy	M

NEW JERSEY CITY UNIVERSITY

Allied Health—General	M
Community Health	M
Health Services Management and Hospital Administration	M

NEW JERSEY INSTITUTE OF TECHNOLOGY

Biological and Biomedical Sciences—General	M,D,O
Computational Biology	M,D,O
Health Services Management and Hospital Administration	M,D
Medicinal and Pharmaceutical Chemistry	M
Pharmaceutical Administration	M,D
Pharmacology	M,D

*M—masters degree; D—doctorate; O—other advanced degree; *—Close-Up and/or Display*

NEWMAN UNIVERSITY
Nurse Anesthesia — M

NEW MEXICO INSTITUTE OF MINING AND TECHNOLOGY
Biological and Biomedical Sciences—General — M,D

NEW MEXICO STATE UNIVERSITY
Biological and Biomedical Sciences—General — M,D
Communication Disorders — M,D,O
Community Health Nursing — M,D
Entomology — M,D
Family Nurse Practitioner Studies — M,D
Gerontological Nursing — M,D
Molecular Biology — M,D
Nursing and Healthcare Administration — M,D
Nursing—General — M
Nutrition — M
Plant Pathology — M
Psychiatric Nursing — M,D
Public Health—General — M,O

NEW YORK ACADEMY OF ART
Anatomy — M

NEW YORK CHIROPRACTIC COLLEGE
Acupuncture and Oriental Medicine — M
Anatomy — M
Chiropractic — D*
Nutrition — M

NEW YORK COLLEGE OF HEALTH PROFESSIONS
Acupuncture and Oriental Medicine — M

NEW YORK COLLEGE OF PODIATRIC MEDICINE
Podiatric Medicine — D

NEW YORK COLLEGE OF TRADITIONAL CHINESE MEDICINE
Acupuncture and Oriental Medicine — M

NEW YORK INSTITUTE OF TECHNOLOGY
Nutrition — M
Occupational Therapy — M
Osteopathic Medicine — M,D
Physical Therapy — M
Physician Assistant Studies — M

NEW YORK MEDICAL COLLEGE
Allopathic Medicine — D
Anatomy — M,D
Biochemistry — M,D
Biological and Biomedical Sciences—General — M,D
Cell Biology — M,D
Communication Disorders — M
Environmental and Occupational Health — M,O
Epidemiology — M
Health Promotion — M,O
Health Services Management and Hospital Administration — M,D,O
Immunology — M,D
Industrial Hygiene — O
International Health — O
Microbiology — M,D
Molecular Biology — M,D
Pathology — M,D
Pharmacology — M,D
Physical Therapy — D
Physiology — M,D
Public Health—General — M,D,O

NEW YORK UNIVERSITY
Acute Care/Critical Care Nursing — M,D,O
Adult Nursing — M,D,O
Allopathic Medicine — M,D
Bioethics — M
Biological and Biomedical Sciences—General — M,D,O
Cancer Biology/Oncology — M,D
Cell Biology — D
Clinical Research — M
Communication Disorders — M,D
Community Health — M,D
Computational Biology — D
Dentistry — D
Developmental Biology — M,D
Environmental and Occupational Health — M,D*
Epidemiology — M,D
Family Nurse Practitioner Studies — M,D,O
Genetics — M,D
Genomic Sciences — D
Gerontological Nursing — M,O
Health Promotion — M,D,O
Health Services Management and Hospital Administration — M,D,O
Immunology — M,D
International Health — M,D
Medical Imaging — D
Microbiology — M,D
Molecular Biology — M,D
Molecular Biophysics — D
Molecular Genetics — M,D
Molecular Pharmacology — D
Molecular Toxicology — M,D
Neurobiology — M,D
Neuroscience — D
Nurse Midwifery — M,D,O
Nursing Education — M,O
Nursing Informatics — M,O
Nursing—General — M,D,O
Nutrition — M,D
Occupational Therapy — M,D
Oral and Dental Sciences — M,D,O
Pathobiology — M,D
Pediatric Nursing — M,D,O
Physical Therapy — M,D,O
Physiology — D
Plant Biology — M,D

Psychiatric Nursing — M,D,O
Public Health—General — M,D
Rehabilitation Sciences — M,D
Structural Biology — D
Toxicology — M,D

NIAGARA UNIVERSITY
Health Services Management and Hospital Administration — M

NICHOLLS STATE UNIVERSITY
Environmental Biology — M
Family Nurse Practitioner Studies — M
Marine Biology — M
Nursing and Healthcare Administration — M
Nursing Education — M
Nursing—General — M
Psychiatric Nursing — M

NORTH CAROLINA AGRICULTURAL AND TECHNICAL STATE UNIVERSITY
Biological and Biomedical Sciences—General — M
Environmental and Occupational Health — M
Nutrition — M

NORTH CAROLINA CENTRAL UNIVERSITY
Biological and Biomedical Sciences—General — M
Communication Disorders — M

NORTH CAROLINA STATE UNIVERSITY
Biochemistry — D
Biological and Biomedical Sciences—General — M,D,O
Botany — M,D
Cell Biology — M,D
Entomology — M,D
Epidemiology — M,D
Genetics — M,D
Genomic Sciences — M,D
Immunology — M,D
Infectious Diseases — M,D
Microbiology — M,D
Molecular Toxicology — M,D
Nutrition — M,D
Pathology — M,D
Pharmacology — M,D
Physiology — M,D
Plant Biology — M,D
Plant Pathology — M,D
Toxicology — M,D
Veterinary Medicine — M,D
Veterinary Sciences — M,D
Zoology — M,D

NORTH DAKOTA STATE UNIVERSITY
Biochemistry — M,D
Biological and Biomedical Sciences—General — M,D
Botany — M,D
Cell Biology — M,D
Ecology — M,D
Entomology — M,D
Genomic Sciences — M,D
Health Promotion — M,D
Microbiology — M,D
Molecular Biology — M,D
Molecular Pathogenesis — M,D
Nursing—General — M,D
Nutrition — M,D
Pathology — M,D
Pharmacy — M,D
Plant Pathology — M,D
Public Health—General — M,D
Zoology — M,D

NORTHEASTERN ILLINOIS UNIVERSITY
Biological and Biomedical Sciences—General — M

NORTHEASTERN STATE UNIVERSITY
Communication Disorders — M
Environmental and Occupational Health — M
Nursing Education — M
Occupational Therapy — M
Optometry — D

NORTHEASTERN UNIVERSITY
Acute Care/Critical Care Nursing — M,D,O
Allied Health—General — M,D,O
Biological and Biomedical Sciences—General — M,D
Communication Disorders — M,D,O
Community Health — M,D,O
Ecology — M,D
Evolutionary Biology — M,D
Family Nurse Practitioner Studies — M,D,O
Gerontological Nursing — M,D,O
Marine Biology — M,D
Maternal and Child/Neonatal Nursing — M,D,O
Medicinal and Pharmaceutical Chemistry — M,D,O
Nurse Anesthesia — M,D,O
Nursing and Healthcare Administration — M,D,O
Nursing—General — M,D,O
Nutrition — M
Pediatric Nursing — M,D,O
Pharmaceutical Sciences — M,D,O
Pharmacology — M,D,O
Pharmacy — M,D,O
Physical Therapy — M,D,O
Physician Assistant Studies — M,D,O
Psychiatric Nursing — M,D,O

NORTHEAST OHIO MEDICAL UNIVERSITY
Allopathic Medicine — D
Bioethics — M,D,O
Health Services Management and Hospital Administration — M,D,O

Pharmaceutical Administration — M,D,O
Pharmaceutical Sciences — M,D,O
Pharmacy — D
Public Health—General — M,D,O

NORTHERN ARIZONA UNIVERSITY
Allied Health—General — M,D,O
Biological and Biomedical Sciences—General — M,D
Communication Disorders — M
Family Nurse Practitioner Studies — M,D,O
Nursing—General — M,D,O
Physical Therapy — D
Physician Assistant Studies — M

NORTHERN ILLINOIS UNIVERSITY
Biological and Biomedical Sciences—General — M,D
Communication Disorders — M,D
Nursing—General — M
Nutrition — M
Physical Therapy — M,D
Public Health—General — M

NORTHERN KENTUCKY UNIVERSITY
Allied Health—General — M
Nursing—General — M,D,O

NORTHERN MICHIGAN UNIVERSITY
Biochemistry — M
Biological and Biomedical Sciences—General — M
Clinical Laboratory Sciences/Medical Technology — M
Family Nurse Practitioner Studies — M,D
Molecular Genetics — M
Nursing—General — M,D

NORTH PARK UNIVERSITY
Adult Nursing — M
Nursing and Healthcare Administration — M
Nursing—General — M

NORTHWESTERN HEALTH SCIENCES UNIVERSITY
Acupuncture and Oriental Medicine — M
Chiropractic — D

NORTHWESTERN STATE UNIVERSITY OF LOUISIANA
Health Physics/Radiological Health — M
Nursing—General — M

NORTHWESTERN UNIVERSITY
Allopathic Medicine — D
Biochemistry — D
Biological and Biomedical Sciences—General — D
Biophysics — D
Biopsychology — D
Cell Biology — D
Clinical Laboratory Sciences/Medical Technology — M
Clinical Research — M,O
Communication Disorders — M,D
Developmental Biology — D
Epidemiology — D
Health Services Management and Hospital Administration — M,D
Health Services Research — D
International Health — M
Molecular Biology — D
Neurobiology — M,D
Neuroscience — D
Physical Therapy — D
Physiology — M
Plant Biology — M,D
Public Health—General — M
Rehabilitation Sciences — D
Structural Biology — D
Systems Biology — D

NORTHWEST MISSOURI STATE UNIVERSITY
Biological and Biomedical Sciences—General — M

NORTHWEST NAZARENE UNIVERSITY
Health Services Management and Hospital Administration — M
Nursing and Healthcare Administration — M

NORWICH UNIVERSITY
Nursing and Healthcare Administration — M
Nursing Education — M
Nursing—General — M

NOVA SOUTHEASTERN UNIVERSITY
Allied Health—General — M,D
Anesthesiologist Assistant Studies — M,D
Biological and Biomedical Sciences—General — M,D,O
Communication Disorders — M,D
Dentistry — M,D
Marine Biology — M,D,O
Nursing—General — M,D
Occupational Therapy — M,D
Optometry — M,D
Osteopathic Medicine — M,D,O
Pharmaceutical Administration — D
Pharmacy — D*
Physical Therapy — M,D
Physician Assistant Studies — M,D
Public Health—General — M,D,O

OAKLAND UNIVERSITY
Allied Health—General — M,D,O
Biological and Biomedical Sciences—General — M,D,O
Environmental and Occupational Health — M
Family Nurse Practitioner Studies — M,O
Gerontological Nursing — M,O
Maternal and Child Health — D,O
Medical Physics — M,D

Nurse Anesthesia — M,O
Nursing—General — M,D,O
Physical Therapy — D,O

OCCIDENTAL COLLEGE
Biological and Biomedical Sciences—General — M

OHIO DOMINICAN UNIVERSITY
Health Services Management and Hospital Administration — M
Physician Assistant Studies — M

OHIO NORTHERN UNIVERSITY
Pharmacy — D

THE OHIO STATE UNIVERSITY
Allied Health—General — M
Allopathic Medicine — D
Anatomy — M,D
Biochemistry — M,D
Biological and Biomedical Sciences—General — M,D
Biophysics — M,D
Cell Biology — M,D
Communication Disorders — M,D
Dental Hygiene — M,D
Dentistry — M,D
Developmental Biology — M,D
Ecology — M,D
Entomology — M,D
Evolutionary Biology — M,D
Genetics — M,D
Health Services Management and Hospital Administration — M,D
Microbiology — M,D
Molecular Biology — M,D
Molecular Genetics — M,D
Neuroscience — D
Nursing—General — M,D
Nutrition — M,D
Occupational Therapy — M,D
Optometry — M,D
Oral and Dental Sciences — M,D
Pharmaceutical Administration — M,D
Pharmacology — M,D
Pharmacy — D
Physical Therapy — D
Plant Pathology — M,D
Public Health—General — M,D
Rehabilitation Sciences — D
Veterinary Sciences — M,D

OHIO UNIVERSITY
Acute Care/Critical Care Nursing — M
Biochemistry — M,D
Biological and Biomedical Sciences—General — M,D
Cell Biology — M,D
Communication Disorders — M,D
Ecology — M,D
Environmental Biology — M,D
Evolutionary Biology — M,D
Family Nurse Practitioner Studies — M
Health Services Management and Hospital Administration — M,D
Microbiology — M,D
Molecular Biology — M,D
Neuroscience — M,D
Nursing and Healthcare Administration — M
Nursing Education — M
Nursing—General — M
Nutrition — M
Osteopathic Medicine — D
Physical Therapy — D
Physiology — M,D
Plant Biology — M,D
Public Health—General — M

OKLAHOMA BAPTIST UNIVERSITY
Nursing Education — M
Nursing—General — M

OKLAHOMA CHRISTIAN UNIVERSITY
Health Services Management and Hospital Administration — M

OKLAHOMA CITY UNIVERSITY
Nursing Education — M,D
Nursing—General — M,D

OKLAHOMA STATE UNIVERSITY
Biochemistry — M,D
Biological and Biomedical Sciences—General — M,D
Botany — M,D
Communication Disorders — M
Ecology — M,D
Entomology — M,D
Evolutionary Biology — M,D
Microbiology — M,D
Molecular Biology — M,D
Molecular Genetics — M,D
Nutrition — M,D
Plant Biology — M,D
Plant Pathology — M,D
Veterinary Medicine — D
Veterinary Sciences — M,D

OKLAHOMA STATE UNIVERSITY CENTER FOR HEALTH SCIENCES
Biological and Biomedical Sciences—General — M,D
Health Services Management and Hospital Administration — M
Osteopathic Medicine — D
Toxicology — M

OKLAHOMA WESLEYAN UNIVERSITY
Nursing and Healthcare Administration — M
Nursing Education — M

OLD DOMINION UNIVERSITY
Adult Nursing — M
Allied Health—General — M,D
Biochemistry — M,D

Biological and Biomedical Sciences—General M,D
Communication Disorders M
Community Health M
Dental Hygiene M
Ecology D
Family Nurse Practitioner Studies M,D
Gerontological Nursing M
Health Promotion M
Health Services Research D
Maternal and Child/Neonatal Nursing M
Nurse Anesthesia M
Nurse Midwifery M,D
Nursing and Healthcare Administration M,D
Nursing Education M
Nursing—General M,D
Pediatric Nursing M
Physical Therapy M,D

OREGON COLLEGE OF ORIENTAL MEDICINE
Acupuncture and Oriental Medicine M,D

OREGON HEALTH & SCIENCE UNIVERSITY
Allopathic Medicine D
Biochemistry M,D
Biological and Biomedical Sciences—General M,D,O
Biopsychology D
Cancer Biology/Oncology D
Cell Biology D
Clinical Research M,O
Community Health Nursing M,O
Dentistry D,O
Developmental Biology D
Family Nurse Practitioner Studies M,D,O
Genetics D
Gerontological Nursing M,D,O
Health Services Management and Hospital Administration M,O
Immunology D
Microbiology D
Molecular Biology M,D
Neuroscience D
Nurse Anesthesia M
Nurse Midwifery M,D,O
Nursing Education M,O
Nursing—General M,D,O
Nutrition M,O
Oral and Dental Sciences M,D,O
Pediatric Nursing M,D,O
Pharmacology D
Physician Assistant Studies M
Physiology D
Psychiatric Nursing M,O

OREGON STATE UNIVERSITY
Allied Health—General M,D
Biochemistry M,D
Bioethics M
Biological and Biomedical Sciences—General M,D
Biophysics M,D
Botany M,D
Cell Biology M,D
Conservation Biology M,D
Developmental Biology M,D
Ecology M,D
Environmental and Occupational Health M,D
Epidemiology M,D
Genomic Sciences M,D
Health Physics/Radiological Health M,D
Health Promotion M,D
Health Services Management and Hospital Administration M,D
Immunology M,D
International Health M,D
Medical Physics M,D
Medicinal and Pharmaceutical Chemistry M,D
Microbiology M,D
Molecular Biology D
Molecular Pathogenesis D
Nutrition M,D
Parasitology M,D
Pharmaceutical Sciences M,D
Pharmacology M,D
Pharmacy D
Plant Molecular Biology D
Plant Pathology M,D
Public Health—General M,D
Structural Biology D
Toxicology M,D
Veterinary Medicine D
Virology M,D
Zoology M,D

OTTERBEIN UNIVERSITY
Family Nurse Practitioner Studies M,D,O
Nurse Anesthesia M,D,O
Nursing and Healthcare Administration M,D,O
Nursing Education M,D,O
Nursing—General M,D,O

OUR LADY OF THE LAKE COLLEGE
Health Services Management and Hospital Administration M
Nurse Anesthesia M
Nursing and Healthcare Administration M
Nursing Education M
Nursing—General M
Physician Assistant Studies M

OUR LADY OF THE LAKE UNIVERSITY OF SAN ANTONIO
Communication Disorders M

Health Services Management and Hospital Administration M

PACE UNIVERSITY
Biochemistry M
Biological and Biomedical Sciences—General M,O
Family Nurse Practitioner Studies M,D,O
Health Services Management and Hospital Administration M
Molecular Biology M
Nursing and Healthcare Administration M,D,O
Nursing Education M,D,O
Nursing—General M,D,O
Physician Assistant Studies M

PACIFIC COLLEGE OF ORIENTAL MEDICINE
Acupuncture and Oriental Medicine M,D

PACIFIC COLLEGE OF ORIENTAL MEDICINE–CHICAGO
Acupuncture and Oriental Medicine M

PACIFIC COLLEGE OF ORIENTAL MEDICINE-NEW YORK
Acupuncture and Oriental Medicine M

PACIFIC LUTHERAN UNIVERSITY
Family Nurse Practitioner Studies D
Nursing—General M,D

PACIFIC UNIVERSITY
Communication Disorders M,D
Health Services Management and Hospital Administration M
Occupational Therapy D
Optometry M,D
Pharmacy D
Physical Therapy M,D
Physician Assistant Studies M
Vision Sciences M,D

PALM BEACH ATLANTIC UNIVERSITY
Family Nurse Practitioner Studies M,D
Nursing and Healthcare Administration M,D
Nursing—General M,D
Pharmacy D

PALMER COLLEGE OF CHIROPRACTIC
Anatomy M
Chiropractic D
Clinical Research M

PALO ALTO UNIVERSITY
Biopsychology D

PARKER UNIVERSITY
Chiropractic D

PARK UNIVERSITY
Health Services Management and Hospital Administration M,O
International Health M,O

PENN STATE GREAT VALLEY
Health Services Management and Hospital Administration M,O

PENN STATE HARRISBURG
Health Services Management and Hospital Administration M,D,O

PENN STATE HERSHEY MEDICAL CENTER
Allopathic Medicine M,D
Anatomy M,D
Biochemistry M,D
Biological and Biomedical Sciences—General M,D
Cell Biology D
Developmental Biology D
Health Services Research M
Immunology M,D
Infectious Diseases D
Molecular Genetics M,D
Molecular Medicine D
Molecular Toxicology D
Neurobiology D
Neuroscience M,D
Public Health—General M,D
Veterinary Sciences M
Virology M,D

PENN STATE UNIVERSITY PARK
Biochemistry M,D
Biological and Biomedical Sciences—General M,D
Biopsychology M,D
Cell Biology M,D
Communication Disorders M,D,O
Ecology M,D
Entomology M,D
Health Services Management and Hospital Administration M,D
Microbiology M,D
Molecular Biology M,D
Nursing—General M,D
Nutrition M,D
Pathobiology M,D
Physiology M,D
Plant Biology M,D
Plant Pathology M,D

PENNSYLVANIA COLLEGE OF HEALTH SCIENCES
Health Services Management and Hospital Administration M
Nursing and Healthcare Administration M
Nursing Education M

PFEIFFER UNIVERSITY
Health Services Management and Hospital Administration M

PHILADELPHIA COLLEGE OF OSTEOPATHIC MEDICINE
Biological and Biomedical Sciences—General M
Biopsychology M,D,O
Osteopathic Medicine D
Physician Assistant Studies M*

PHILADELPHIA UNIVERSITY
Nurse Midwifery M,O
Occupational Therapy M,D
Physician Assistant Studies M

PITTSBURG STATE UNIVERSITY
Biological and Biomedical Sciences—General M
Nursing—General M

PLYMOUTH STATE UNIVERSITY
Biological and Biomedical Sciences—General M
Health Promotion M

POINT LOMA NAZARENE UNIVERSITY
Biological and Biomedical Sciences—General M
Family Nurse Practitioner Studies M,O
Gerontological Nursing M,O
Health Services Management and Hospital Administration M
Maternal and Child/Neonatal Nursing M,O
Nursing—General M,O
Psychiatric Nursing M,O

PONCE HEALTH SCIENCES UNIVERSITY
Allopathic Medicine D
Biological and Biomedical Sciences—General D
Epidemiology M,D
Public Health—General M,D

PONTIFICAL CATHOLIC UNIVERSITY OF PUERTO RICO
Biological and Biomedical Sciences—General M
Clinical Laboratory Sciences/Medical Technology O
Medical/Surgical Nursing M
Nursing—General M
Psychiatric Nursing M

PONTIFICIA UNIVERSIDAD CATOLICA MADRE Y MAESTRA
Allopathic Medicine D

PORTLAND STATE UNIVERSITY
Biological and Biomedical Sciences—General M,D
Communication Disorders M
Health Promotion M,D,O
Health Services Management and Hospital Administration M,D
Public Health—General M,D,O

POST UNIVERSITY
Health Services Management and Hospital Administration M

PRAIRIE VIEW A&M UNIVERSITY
Family Nurse Practitioner Studies M
Nursing and Healthcare Administration M
Nursing Education M
Nursing—General M

PRINCETON UNIVERSITY
Computational Biology D
Ecology D
Evolutionary Biology D
Marine Biology D
Molecular Biology D
Neuroscience D

PURDUE UNIVERSITY
Allied Health—General M,D
Anatomy M,D
Biochemistry M,D
Biological and Biomedical Sciences—General M,D
Biophysics M,D
Botany D
Cancer Biology/Oncology M,D
Cell Biology M,D
Communication Disorders M,D
Developmental Biology M,D
Ecology M,D
Entomology M,D
Environmental and Occupational Health M,D
Epidemiology M,D
Evolutionary Biology M,D
Genetics D
Genomic Sciences D
Health Physics/Radiological Health M,D
Immunology M,D
Medical Physics M,D
Medicinal and Pharmaceutical Chemistry D
Microbiology M,D
Molecular Biology M,D
Molecular Pharmacology D
Neurobiology M,D
Neuroscience D
Nutrition M,D
Pathobiology M,D
Pathology M,D
Pharmaceutical Administration M,D,O
Pharmaceutical Sciences M,D
Pharmacology M,D
Pharmacy D

Physiology M,D
Plant Pathology M,D
Plant Physiology M,D
Public Health—General M
Systems Biology D
Toxicology M,D
Veterinary Medicine D
Veterinary Sciences M,D
Virology M,D

PURDUE UNIVERSITY NORTHWEST
Acute Care/Critical Care Nursing M
Adult Nursing M
Biological and Biomedical Sciences—General M
Family Nurse Practitioner Studies M
Nursing and Healthcare Administration M
Nursing—General M

QUEENS COLLEGE OF THE CITY UNIVERSITY OF NEW YORK
Biological and Biomedical Sciences—General M,O
Communication Disorders M
Neuroscience M,O
Nutrition M,O

QUEEN'S UNIVERSITY AT KINGSTON
Allopathic Medicine D
Anatomy M,D
Biochemistry M,D
Biological and Biomedical Sciences—General M,D
Cancer Biology/Oncology M,D
Cardiovascular Sciences M,D
Cell Biology M,D
Epidemiology M,D
Family Nurse Practitioner Studies M,D,O
Health Services Management and Hospital Administration M,D
Immunology M,D
Microbiology M,D
Molecular Biology M,D
Molecular Medicine M,D
Neurobiology M,D
Neuroscience M,D
Nursing—General M,D,O
Occupational Therapy M,D
Pathology M,D
Pediatric Nursing M,D,O
Pharmaceutical Sciences M,D
Pharmacology M,D
Physical Therapy M,D
Physiology M,D
Public Health—General M,D
Rehabilitation Sciences M,D
Reproductive Biology M,D
Toxicology M,D
Women's Health Nursing M,D,O

QUEENS UNIVERSITY OF CHARLOTTE
Nursing and Healthcare Administration M
Nursing Education M
Nursing—General M

QUINNIPIAC UNIVERSITY
Adult Nursing M,D
Allied Health—General M
Allopathic Medicine D
Anesthesiologist Assistant Studies M
Cardiovascular Sciences M
Cell Biology M
Clinical Laboratory Sciences/Medical Technology M
Community Health D
Family Nurse Practitioner Studies M,D
Health Physics/Radiological Health M
Health Services Management and Hospital Administration M
Molecular Biology M
Nurse Anesthesia D
Nursing and Healthcare Administration D
Nursing—General M,D
Pathology M
Perfusion M
Physician Assistant Studies M

RADFORD UNIVERSITY
Communication Disorders M
Nursing—General D
Occupational Therapy M
Physical Therapy D

RAMAPO COLLEGE OF NEW JERSEY
Nursing Education M
Nursing—General M

REGENT UNIVERSITY
Health Services Management and Hospital Administration M,D,O

REGIS COLLEGE (MA)
Biological and Biomedical Sciences—General M,D,O
Family Nurse Practitioner Studies M,D,O
Health Services Management and Hospital Administration M,D,O
Nursing Education M,D,O
Nursing—General M,D,O
Occupational Therapy M,D,O

REGIS UNIVERSITY
Allied Health—General M,D,O
Biological and Biomedical Sciences—General M
Environmental Biology M
Family Nurse Practitioner Studies M,D,O
Health Services Management and Hospital Administration M,D,O
Maternal and Child/Neonatal Nursing M,D,O

M—masters degree; D—doctorate; O—other advanced degree; *—Close-Up and/or Display

Nursing Education	M,D,O
Pharmacy	M,D,O
Physical Therapy	M,D,O

RENSSELAER POLYTECHNIC INSTITUTE

Biochemistry	M,D
Biological and Biomedical Sciences—General	M,D
Biophysics	M,D

RESEARCH COLLEGE OF NURSING

Adult Nursing	M
Family Nurse Practitioner Studies	M
Gerontological Nursing	M
Nursing and Healthcare Administration	M
Nursing—General	M

RESURRECTION UNIVERSITY

Nursing—General	M

RHODE ISLAND COLLEGE

Biological and Biomedical Sciences—General	M,O
Nursing—General	M

RICE UNIVERSITY

Biochemistry	M,D
Cell Biology	M,D
Ecology	M,D
Evolutionary Biology	M,D
Health Services Management and Hospital Administration	M

RIVIER UNIVERSITY

Family Nurse Practitioner Studies	M
Nursing Education	M
Nursing—General	M
Psychiatric Nursing	M

ROBERT MORRIS UNIVERSITY

Nursing—General	M,D

ROBERT MORRIS UNIVERSITY ILLINOIS

Health Services Management and Hospital Administration	M

ROBERTS WESLEYAN COLLEGE

Health Services Management and Hospital Administration	M
Nursing and Healthcare Administration	M
Nursing Education	M
Nursing—General	M

ROCHESTER INSTITUTE OF TECHNOLOGY

Biological and Biomedical Sciences—General	M
Environmental and Occupational Health	M
Health Services Management and Hospital Administration	M,O
Occupational Therapy	M

THE ROCKEFELLER UNIVERSITY

Biological and Biomedical Sciences—General	M,D*

ROCKHURST UNIVERSITY

Communication Disorders	M
Health Services Management and Hospital Administration	M,O
Occupational Therapy	M
Physical Therapy	D

ROCKY MOUNTAIN COLLEGE

Physician Assistant Studies	M

ROCKY MOUNTAIN UNIVERSITY OF HEALTH PROFESSIONS

Communication Disorders	D
Family Nurse Practitioner Studies	D
Occupational Therapy	D
Physical Therapy	D
Physician Assistant Studies	M
Physiology	D

ROCKY VISTA UNIVERSITY

Osteopathic Medicine	D

ROGER WILLIAMS UNIVERSITY

Health Services Management and Hospital Administration	M

ROLLINS COLLEGE

Health Services Management and Hospital Administration	M

ROOSEVELT UNIVERSITY

Pharmacy	D

ROSALIND FRANKLIN UNIVERSITY OF MEDICINE AND SCIENCE

Allied Health—General	M,D,O
Allopathic Medicine	D
Anatomy	D
Biochemistry	D
Biological and Biomedical Sciences—General	M,D
Biophysics	M,D
Cell Biology	D
Health Promotion	M
Health Services Management and Hospital Administration	M,O
Immunology	D
Microbiology	D
Molecular Biology	D
Molecular Pharmacology	M,D
Neuroscience	D
Nurse Anesthesia	D
Nutrition	M
Pathology	M
Pharmacy	D
Physical Therapy	M,D
Physician Assistant Studies	M
Physiology	M,D
Podiatric Medicine	D

ROSEMAN UNIVERSITY OF HEALTH SCIENCES

Dentistry	M,D,O
Pharmacy	D

ROWAN UNIVERSITY

Biological and Biomedical Sciences—General	M
Health Promotion	M
Nursing—General	M
Osteopathic Medicine	D
Pharmaceutical Sciences	M
School Nursing	M,D,O

ROYAL ROADS UNIVERSITY

Health Services Management and Hospital Administration	O

RUSH UNIVERSITY

Adult Nursing	D
Allopathic Medicine	D
Anatomy	M,D
Biochemistry	M,D
Cell Biology	M,D
Clinical Laboratory Sciences/Medical Technology	M
Communication Disorders	M,D
Community Health Nursing	D
Family Nurse Practitioner Studies	D
Gerontological Nursing	D
Health Services Management and Hospital Administration	M,D
Immunology	M,D
Maternal and Child/Neonatal Nursing	D,O
Medical Physics	M,D
Microbiology	M,D
Neuroscience	M,D
Nurse Anesthesia	D
Nursing and Healthcare Administration	M
Nursing—General	M,D,O
Nutrition	M
Occupational Therapy	M
Pediatric Nursing	D,O
Perfusion	M
Pharmaceutical Sciences	M,D
Pharmacology	M,D
Physical Therapy	M
Physician Assistant Studies	M
Physiology	D
Psychiatric Nursing	D
Virology	M,D

RUTGERS UNIVERSITY–CAMDEN

Biological and Biomedical Sciences—General	M
Computational Biology	M,D
Health Services Management and Hospital Administration	M,O
Physical Therapy	D
Public Health—General	M,O

RUTGERS UNIVERSITY–NEWARK

Adult Nursing	M,D,O
Allied Health—General	M,D,O
Allopathic Medicine	D
Biochemistry	M,D
Biological and Biomedical Sciences—General	M,D,O
Biopsychology	D
Cancer Biology/Oncology	D,O
Cell Biology	D
Clinical Laboratory Sciences/Medical Technology	M
Computational Biology	M
Dentistry	M,D,O
Developmental Biology	D,O
Epidemiology	M,O
Family Nurse Practitioner Studies	M,D,O
Health Physics/Radiological Health	M
Health Services Management and Hospital Administration	M,D,O
Immunology	D
Infectious Diseases	D,O
Medical Imaging	M
Microbiology	D
Molecular Biology	M,D
Molecular Genetics	D
Molecular Medicine	D
Molecular Pathology	D
Neuroscience	D
Nurse Anesthesia	M,D,O
Nursing Informatics	M
Nursing—General	M,D,O
Nutrition	M,D,O
Occupational Health Nursing	M,D,O
Oral and Dental Sciences	M,D,O
Pathology	D
Pharmaceutical Administration	M
Pharmacology	D
Physical Therapy	D
Physician Assistant Studies	M
Physiology	D
Public Health—General	M,O
Transcultural Nursing	M,D,O
Women's Health Nursing	M,D,O

RUTGERS UNIVERSITY–NEW BRUNSWICK

Allopathic Medicine	D
Biochemistry	M,D
Biological and Biomedical Sciences—General	M,D
Biopsychology	D
Cancer Biology/Oncology	M,D
Cell Biology	M,D
Clinical Laboratory Sciences/Medical Technology	M
Computational Biology	M,D
Developmental Biology	M,D
Ecology	M,D
Entomology	M,D
Environmental and Occupational Health	M,D,O
Environmental Biology	M,D

Epidemiology	M,D,O
Evolutionary Biology	M,D
Genetics	M,D
Health Services Management and Hospital Administration	M,D,O
Immunology	M,D
Marine Biology	M,D
Medical Microbiology	M,D
Medicinal and Pharmaceutical Chemistry	M,D
Microbiology	M,D
Molecular Biology	M,D
Molecular Biophysics	D
Molecular Genetics	M,D
Molecular Pharmacology	M,D
Molecular Physiology	M,D
Neuroscience	M,D
Nutrition	M,D
Pharmaceutical Sciences	M,D
Pharmacy	M,D
Physiology	M,D
Plant Biology	M,D
Plant Molecular Biology	M,D
Plant Pathology	M,D
Public Health—General	M,D
Reproductive Biology	M,D
Systems Biology	D
Toxicology	M,D
Translational Biology	M
Virology	M,D

SACRED HEART UNIVERSITY

Communication Disorders	M
Family Nurse Practitioner Studies	M,D,O
Nursing and Healthcare Administration	M,D,O
Nursing Education	M,D,O
Nursing—General	M,D,O
Nutrition	M
Occupational Therapy	M
Physical Therapy	D,O

SAGE GRADUATE SCHOOL

Adult Nursing	M,D,O
Family Nurse Practitioner Studies	M,O
Gerontological Nursing	M,O
Health Services Management and Hospital Administration	M,D,O
Nursing Education	D
Nursing—General	M,D,O
Nutrition	M,O
Occupational Therapy	M
Physical Therapy	D
Psychiatric Nursing	M,O

SAGINAW VALLEY STATE UNIVERSITY

Family Nurse Practitioner Studies	M,D
Health Services Management and Hospital Administration	M
Nursing and Healthcare Administration	M
Nursing—General	M
Occupational Therapy	M

ST. AMBROSE UNIVERSITY

Communication Disorders	M
Health Services Management and Hospital Administration	M,D
Nursing—General	M
Occupational Therapy	M
Physical Therapy	D

SAINT ANTHONY COLLEGE OF NURSING

Nursing—General	M

ST. CATHERINE UNIVERSITY

Adult Nursing	M,D
Gerontological Nursing	M,D
Health Services Management and Hospital Administration	M
Maternal and Child/Neonatal Nursing	M,D
Nursing Education	M,D
Nursing—General	M,D
Occupational Therapy	M,D
Pediatric Nursing	M,D
Physical Therapy	D
Physician Assistant Studies	M
Public Health—General	M

ST. CLOUD STATE UNIVERSITY

Biological and Biomedical Sciences—General	M
Communication Disorders	M

SAINT FRANCIS MEDICAL CENTER COLLEGE OF NURSING

Family Nurse Practitioner Studies	M,D,O
Gerontological Nursing	M,D,O
Maternal and Child/Neonatal Nursing	M,D,O
Medical/Surgical Nursing	M,D,O
Nursing and Healthcare Administration	M,D,O
Nursing Education	M,D,O
Nursing—General	M,D,O
Psychiatric Nursing	M,D,O

SAINT FRANCIS UNIVERSITY

Biological and Biomedical Sciences—General	M
Occupational Therapy	M
Physical Therapy	D
Physician Assistant Studies	M

ST. FRANCIS XAVIER UNIVERSITY

Biological and Biomedical Sciences—General	M

ST. JOHN FISHER COLLEGE

Family Nurse Practitioner Studies	M,O
Nursing—General	M,D,O
Pharmacy	D

ST. JOHN'S UNIVERSITY (NY)

Biological and Biomedical Sciences—General	M,D

Communication Disorders	M,D
Pharmaceutical Administration	M
Pharmaceutical Sciences	M,D
Public Health—General	M
Toxicology	M

ST. JOSEPH'S COLLEGE, LONG ISLAND CAMPUS

Health Services Management and Hospital Administration	M
Nursing—General	M

ST. JOSEPH'S COLLEGE, NEW YORK

Health Services Management and Hospital Administration	M
Nursing—General	M

SAINT JOSEPH'S COLLEGE OF MAINE

Family Nurse Practitioner Studies	M,O
Health Services Management and Hospital Administration	M
Nursing and Healthcare Administration	M,O
Nursing Education	M,O
Nursing—General	M,O

SAINT JOSEPH'S UNIVERSITY

Biological and Biomedical Sciences—General	M
Environmental and Occupational Health	M
Health Services Management and Hospital Administration	M,O
Nurse Anesthesia	M
Nursing and Healthcare Administration	M
School Nursing	M

SAINT LEO UNIVERSITY

Health Services Management and Hospital Administration	M

ST. LOUIS COLLEGE OF PHARMACY

Pharmacy	D*

SAINT LOUIS UNIVERSITY

Allied Health—General	M,D,O
Allopathic Medicine	D
Anatomy	M,D
Biochemistry	D
Bioethics	D,O
Biological and Biomedical Sciences—General	M,D
Communication Disorders	M
Community Health	M
Dentistry	M
Health Services Management and Hospital Administration	M,D
Immunology	D
Microbiology	D
Molecular Biology	D
Nursing—General	M,D,O
Nutrition	M*
Occupational Therapy	M
Oral and Dental Sciences	M
Pathology	D
Pharmacology	D
Physical Therapy	M,D
Physician Assistant Studies	M
Physiology	D
Public Health—General	M,D

SAINT MARY'S COLLEGE

Communication Disorders	M
Nursing—General	M

SAINT MARY'S UNIVERSITY OF MINNESOTA

Environmental and Occupational Health	M
Health Services Management and Hospital Administration	M
Nurse Anesthesia	M

ST. NORBERT COLLEGE

Health Services Management and Hospital Administration	M

SAINT PETER'S UNIVERSITY

Adult Nursing	M,D,O
Health Services Management and Hospital Administration	M
Nursing and Healthcare Administration	M,D,O
Nursing—General	M,D,O

ST. THOMAS UNIVERSITY

Health Services Management and Hospital Administration	M,O

SAINT VINCENT COLLEGE

Nurse Anesthesia	M,D

SAINT XAVIER UNIVERSITY

Communication Disorders	M
Health Services Management and Hospital Administration	M,O
Nursing—General	M,O

SALEM STATE UNIVERSITY

Gerontological Nursing	M
Nursing and Healthcare Administration	M
Nursing Education	M
Nursing—General	M
Occupational Therapy	M

SALISBURY UNIVERSITY

Biological and Biomedical Sciences—General	M
Family Nurse Practitioner Studies	D
Nursing and Healthcare Administration	M,D
Nursing Education	M
Nursing—General	M,D
Physiology	M

SALUS UNIVERSITY

Communication Disorders	D
Optometry	D

Physician Assistant Studies	M
Public Health—General	M
Rehabilitation Sciences	M,O
Vision Sciences	M,O

SALVE REGINA UNIVERSITY

Health Services Management and Hospital Administration	M,O
Nursing—General	D

SAMFORD UNIVERSITY

Biological and Biomedical Sciences—General	M,D,O
Communication Disorders	M,D
Family Nurse Practitioner Studies	M,D
Health Services Management and Hospital Administration	M,D
Nurse Anesthesia	M,D
Nursing and Healthcare Administration	M,D
Nursing Education	M,D
Nursing—General	M,D
Pharmacy	D
Physical Therapy	M,D
Public Health—General	M

SAM HOUSTON STATE UNIVERSITY

Allied Health—General	M
Biological and Biomedical Sciences—General	M
Nutrition	M

SAMUEL MERRITT UNIVERSITY

Family Nurse Practitioner Studies	M,D,O
Nurse Anesthesia	M,D,O
Nursing and Healthcare Administration	M,D,O
Nursing—General	M,D,O
Occupational Therapy	M
Physical Therapy	D
Physician Assistant Studies	M

SAN DIEGO STATE UNIVERSITY

Biochemistry	M,D
Biological and Biomedical Sciences—General	M,D
Cell Biology	M,D
Communication Disorders	M,D
Ecology	M,D
Emergency Medical Services	M,D
Environmental and Occupational Health	M,D
Epidemiology	M,D
Health Physics/Radiological Health	M
Health Promotion	M,D
Health Services Management and Hospital Administration	M,D
International Health	M,D
Microbiology	M
Molecular Biology	M,D
Nursing—General	M
Nutrition	M
Pharmaceutical Administration	D
Physical Therapy	D
Public Health—General	M,D
Toxicology	M,D

SANFORD BURNHAM PREBYS MEDICAL DISCOVERY INSTITUTE

Biological and Biomedical Sciences—General	D

SAN FRANCISCO STATE UNIVERSITY

Acute Care/Critical Care Nursing	M,O
Biochemistry	M
Biological and Biomedical Sciences—General	M
Cell Biology	M
Communication Disorders	M
Community Health Nursing	M,O
Developmental Biology	M
Ecology	M
Family Nurse Practitioner Studies	M,O
Health Services Management and Hospital Administration	M
Marine Biology	M
Microbiology	M
Molecular Biology	M
Nursing and Healthcare Administration	M,O
Nursing—General	M,O
Pediatric Nursing	M,O
Physical Therapy	D
Physiology	M
Public Health—General	M
Women's Health Nursing	M,O

SAN JOSE STATE UNIVERSITY

Biological and Biomedical Sciences—General	M,O
Communication Disorders	M,D,O
Ecology	M,O
Molecular Biology	M,O
Nutrition	M,O
Occupational Therapy	M,O
Physiology	M,O
Public Health—General	M,O

SARAH LAWRENCE COLLEGE

Human Genetics	M
Public Health—General	M

SAYBROOK UNIVERSITY

Nutrition	M,D,O

THE SCRIPPS RESEARCH INSTITUTE

Biological and Biomedical Sciences—General	D

SEATTLE INSTITUTE OF ORIENTAL MEDICINE

Acupuncture and Oriental Medicine	M

SEATTLE PACIFIC UNIVERSITY

Adult Nursing	M,O
Family Nurse Practitioner Studies	M,O
Gerontological Nursing	M,O
Nursing and Healthcare Administration	M,O
Nursing Education	M,O
Nursing Informatics	M,O
Nursing—General	M,O

SEATTLE UNIVERSITY

Adult Nursing	M
Community Health Nursing	M
Family Nurse Practitioner Studies	M
Gerontological Nursing	M
Nurse Midwifery	M
Nursing—General	M,D
Psychiatric Nursing	M

SETON HALL UNIVERSITY

Adult Nursing	M,D
Allied Health—General	D
Biochemistry	M,D
Biological and Biomedical Sciences—General	M,D
Communication Disorders	M
Gerontological Nursing	M,D
Health Services Management and Hospital Administration	M,D,O
International Health	M,O
Microbiology	M,D
Molecular Biology	M,D
Neuroscience	M,D
Nursing and Healthcare Administration	M,D
Nursing Education	M,D
Nursing—General	M
Occupational Therapy	M
Pediatric Nursing	M,D
Physical Therapy	D
Physician Assistant Studies	M
School Nursing	M,D

SETON HILL UNIVERSITY

Oral and Dental Sciences	M,O
Physician Assistant Studies	M

SHAWNEE STATE UNIVERSITY

Occupational Therapy	M

SHENANDOAH UNIVERSITY

Allied Health—General	M,D,O
Family Nurse Practitioner Studies	M,D,O
Health Services Management and Hospital Administration	M,O
Nurse Midwifery	M,D,O
Nursing and Healthcare Administration	M,D,O
Nursing Education	M,D,O
Nursing—General	M,D,O
Occupational Therapy	M
Pharmacy	D
Physical Therapy	D
Physician Assistant Studies	M
Psychiatric Nursing	M,D,O

SHERMAN COLLEGE OF CHIROPRACTIC

Chiropractic	D*

SHIPPENSBURG UNIVERSITY OF PENNSYLVANIA

Biological and Biomedical Sciences—General	M

SIENA HEIGHTS UNIVERSITY

Health Services Management and Hospital Administration	M,O

SIMMONS COLLEGE

Family Nurse Practitioner Studies	M,D,O
Health Promotion	M,D,O
Health Services Management and Hospital Administration	M
Nursing—General	M,D,O
Nutrition	M,D,O
Physical Therapy	M,D,O

SIMON FRASER UNIVERSITY

Biochemistry	M,D,O
Biological and Biomedical Sciences—General	M,D,O
Entomology	M,D,O
International Health	M,D,O
Molecular Biology	M,D,O
Public Health—General	M,D,O
Toxicology	M,D,O

SLIPPERY ROCK UNIVERSITY OF PENNSYLVANIA

Physical Therapy	D

SMITH COLLEGE

Biological and Biomedical Sciences—General	M

SONOMA STATE UNIVERSITY

Biochemistry	M
Biological and Biomedical Sciences—General	M
Cell Biology	M
Ecology	M
Environmental Biology	M
Evolutionary Biology	M
Family Nurse Practitioner Studies	M
Health Promotion	M
Molecular Biology	M
Nursing—General	M
Occupational Therapy	M
Physical Therapy	M

SOUTH BAYLO UNIVERSITY

Acupuncture and Oriental Medicine	M

SOUTH CAROLINA STATE UNIVERSITY

Allied Health—General	M

Biological and Biomedical Sciences—General	M
Communication Disorders	M
Nutrition	M

SOUTH COLLEGE

Physician Assistant Studies	M

SOUTH DAKOTA STATE UNIVERSITY

Biological and Biomedical Sciences—General	M,D
Microbiology	M,D
Nursing—General	M,D
Nutrition	M,D
Pharmaceutical Sciences	M,D
Pharmacy	D
Veterinary Sciences	M,D

SOUTHEASTERN LOUISIANA UNIVERSITY

Biological and Biomedical Sciences—General	M
Communication Disorders	M

SOUTHEASTERN OKLAHOMA STATE UNIVERSITY

Environmental and Occupational Health	M

SOUTHEAST MISSOURI STATE UNIVERSITY

Biological and Biomedical Sciences—General	M
Communication Disorders	M
Health Services Management and Hospital Administration	M
Nursing—General	M
Nutrition	M

SOUTHERN ADVENTIST UNIVERSITY

Acute Care/Critical Care Nursing	M
Adult Nursing	M
Family Nurse Practitioner Studies	M
Health Services Management and Hospital Administration	M
Nursing and Healthcare Administration	M
Nursing—General	M

SOUTHERN ARKANSAS UNIVERSITY–MAGNOLIA

Psychiatric Nursing	M

SOUTHERN CALIFORNIA UNIVERSITY OF HEALTH SCIENCES

Acupuncture and Oriental Medicine	M,D
Chiropractic	D

SOUTHERN COLLEGE OF OPTOMETRY

Optometry	D

SOUTHERN CONNECTICUT STATE UNIVERSITY

Biological and Biomedical Sciences—General	M
Communication Disorders	M
Family Nurse Practitioner Studies	M
Nursing Education	M
Nursing—General	M
Public Health—General	M

SOUTHERN ILLINOIS UNIVERSITY CARBONDALE

Biochemistry	M,D
Biological and Biomedical Sciences—General	M,D
Communication Disorders	M
Community Health	M
Health Services Management and Hospital Administration	M
Medical Physics	M
Microbiology	M,D
Molecular Biology	M,D
Nutrition	M
Pharmacology	M,D
Physician Assistant Studies	M
Physiology	M,D
Plant Biology	M,D
Zoology	M,D

SOUTHERN ILLINOIS UNIVERSITY EDWARDSVILLE

Biological and Biomedical Sciences—General	M
Communication Disorders	M
Dentistry	D
Family Nurse Practitioner Studies	M,D,O
Nurse Anesthesia	D
Nursing and Healthcare Administration	M,O
Nursing Education	M,O
Nursing—General	M,D,O
Pharmacy	D

SOUTHERN METHODIST UNIVERSITY

Biological and Biomedical Sciences—General	M,D
Cell Biology	M,D
Molecular Biology	M,D
Physiology	M

SOUTHERN NAZARENE UNIVERSITY

Health Services Management and Hospital Administration	M
Nursing and Healthcare Administration	M
Nursing Education	M
Nursing—General	M

SOUTHERN NEW HAMPSHIRE UNIVERSITY

Community Health	M,O
Health Services Management and Hospital Administration	M,O

SOUTHERN UNIVERSITY AND AGRICULTURAL AND MECHANICAL COLLEGE

Biochemistry	M
Biological and Biomedical Sciences—General	M
Family Nurse Practitioner Studies	M,D,O
Gerontological Nursing	M,D,O
Nursing and Healthcare Administration	M,D,O
Nursing Education	M,D,O
Nursing—General	M,D,O

SOUTH UNIVERSITY (AL)

Health Services Management and Hospital Administration	M
Nursing—General	M

SOUTH UNIVERSITY

Family Nurse Practitioner Studies	M
Health Services Management and Hospital Administration	M
Nursing—General	M
Occupational Therapy	D

SOUTH UNIVERSITY

Adult Nursing	M
Family Nurse Practitioner Studies	M
Health Services Management and Hospital Administration	M
Nursing Education	M
Nursing—General	M
Physician Assistant Studies	M

SOUTH UNIVERSITY (GA)

Anesthesiologist Assistant Studies	M
Health Services Management and Hospital Administration	M
Nursing Education	M
Nursing—General	M
Pharmacy	
Physician Assistant Studies	M

SOUTH UNIVERSITY (MI)

Nursing—General	M

SOUTH UNIVERSITY (SC)

Health Services Management and Hospital Administration	M
Nursing—General	M
Pharmacy	D

SOUTH UNIVERSITY

Nursing—General	M

SOUTH UNIVERSITY

Family Nurse Practitioner Studies	M
Nursing—General	M

SOUTHWEST ACUPUNCTURE COLLEGE

Acupuncture and Oriental Medicine	M

SOUTHWEST BAPTIST UNIVERSITY

Health Services Management and Hospital Administration	M
Physical Therapy	D

SOUTHWEST COLLEGE OF NATUROPATHIC MEDICINE AND HEALTH SCIENCES

Naturopathic Medicine	D

SOUTHWESTERN OKLAHOMA STATE UNIVERSITY

Allied Health—General	M
Microbiology	M
Pharmacy	D

SPALDING UNIVERSITY

Adult Nursing	M,D,O
Family Nurse Practitioner Studies	M,D,O
Nursing and Healthcare Administration	M,D,O
Nursing—General	M,D,O
Occupational Therapy	M
Pediatric Nursing	M,D,O

SPRING ARBOR UNIVERSITY

Nursing—General	M

SPRINGFIELD COLLEGE

Health Promotion	M,D
Occupational Therapy	M
Physical Therapy	D
Physician Assistant Studies	M

SPRING HILL COLLEGE

Nursing and Healthcare Administration	M,O
Nursing—General	M,O

STANFORD UNIVERSITY

Allopathic Medicine	D
Biochemistry	D
Biological and Biomedical Sciences—General	M,D
Biophysics	D
Clinical Research	M,D
Developmental Biology	M,D
Ecology	M,D
Epidemiology	M,D
Genetics	D
Health Services Research	M,D
Immunology	D*
Microbiology	D
Physiology	D
Structural Biology	D
Systems Biology	D

STATE UNIVERSITY OF NEW YORK AT FREDONIA

Biological and Biomedical Sciences—General	M
Communication Disorders	M

*M—masters degree; D—doctorate; O—other advanced degree; *—Close-Up and/or Display*

STATE UNIVERSITY OF NEW YORK AT NEW PALTZ
Communication Disorders	M

STATE UNIVERSITY OF NEW YORK AT PLATTSBURGH
Communication Disorders	M

STATE UNIVERSITY OF NEW YORK COLLEGE AT CORTLAND
Community Health	M

STATE UNIVERSITY OF NEW YORK COLLEGE AT ONEONTA
Biological and Biomedical Sciences—General	M
Nutrition	M

STATE UNIVERSITY OF NEW YORK COLLEGE AT POTSDAM
Community Health	M

STATE UNIVERSITY OF NEW YORK COLLEGE OF ENVIRONMENTAL SCIENCE AND FORESTRY
Biochemistry	M,D
Conservation Biology	M,D
Ecology	M,D
Entomology	M,D
Environmental Biology	M,D
Plant Pathology	M,D

STATE UNIVERSITY OF NEW YORK COLLEGE OF OPTOMETRY
Optometry	D
Vision Sciences	M,D

STATE UNIVERSITY OF NEW YORK COLLEGE OF TECHNOLOGY AT DELHI
Nursing Education	M

STATE UNIVERSITY OF NEW YORK DOWNSTATE MEDICAL CENTER
Allopathic Medicine	M,D
Biological and Biomedical Sciences—General	M,D
Cell Biology	D
Community Health	M
Family Nurse Practitioner Studies	M,O
Medical/Surgical Nursing	M,O
Molecular Biology	D
Neuroscience	D
Nurse Anesthesia	M
Nurse Midwifery	M,O
Nursing—General	M,O
Public Health—General	M

STATE UNIVERSITY OF NEW YORK EMPIRE STATE COLLEGE
Nursing Education	M

STATE UNIVERSITY OF NEW YORK POLYTECHNIC INSTITUTE
Family Nurse Practitioner Studies	M,O
Nursing and Healthcare Administration	M
Nursing Education	M,O

STATE UNIVERSITY OF NEW YORK UPSTATE MEDICAL UNIVERSITY
Allopathic Medicine	D
Anatomy	M,D
Biochemistry	M,D
Biological and Biomedical Sciences—General	M,D
Cell Biology	M,D
Clinical Laboratory Sciences/Medical Technology	M
Family Nurse Practitioner Studies	M,O
Immunology	M,D
Microbiology	M,D
Molecular Biology	M,D
Neuroscience	D
Nursing—General	M,O
Pharmacology	D
Physical Therapy	D
Physiology	M,D

STEPHEN F. AUSTIN STATE UNIVERSITY
Biological and Biomedical Sciences—General	M
Communication Disorders	M

STEVENS INSTITUTE OF TECHNOLOGY
Biochemistry	M,D,O
Pharmaceutical Sciences	M,O

STEVENSON UNIVERSITY
Biological and Biomedical Sciences—General	M
Health Services Management and Hospital Administration	M
Nursing Education	M
Nursing—General	M

STOCKTON UNIVERSITY
Communication Disorders	M
Nursing—General	M
Occupational Therapy	M
Physical Therapy	D

STONY BROOK UNIVERSITY, STATE UNIVERSITY OF NEW YORK
Adult Nursing	M,D,O
Allopathic Medicine	D
Anatomy	D
Biochemistry	M,D
Bioethics	
Biological and Biomedical Sciences—General	M,D,O
Biophysics	D
Cell Biology	M,D
Community Health	M,D,O
Dentistry	D,O
Developmental Biology	M,D
Ecology	M,D
Evolutionary Biology	M,D
Family Nurse Practitioner Studies	M,D,O

Genetics	D
Gerontological Nursing	M,D,O
Health Services Management and Hospital Administration	M,D,O
Immunology	M,D
Maternal and Child/Neonatal Nursing	M,D,O
Medical Physics	M,D
Microbiology	D
Molecular Biology	M,D
Molecular Genetics	D
Molecular Physiology	D
Neuroscience	M,D
Nurse Midwifery	M,D,O
Nursing and Healthcare Administration	M,O
Nursing Education	M,O
Nursing—General	M,D,O
Nutrition	M,O
Occupational Therapy	M,D,O
Oral and Dental Sciences	M,D,O
Pathology	M,D
Pediatric Nursing	M,D,O
Pharmacology	D
Physical Therapy	M,D,O
Physician Assistant Studies	M,D,O
Physiology	D
Psychiatric Nursing	M,D,O
Public Health—General	M,O
Structural Biology	D
Women's Health Nursing	M,D,O

STRATFORD UNIVERSITY (VA)
Health Services Management and Hospital Administration	M,D

STRAYER UNIVERSITY
Health Services Management and Hospital Administration	M

SUFFOLK UNIVERSITY
Health Services Management and Hospital Administration	M,O

SUL ROSS STATE UNIVERSITY
Biological and Biomedical Sciences—General	M

SWEDISH INSTITUTE, COLLEGE OF HEALTH SCIENCES
Acupuncture and Oriental Medicine	M

SYRACUSE UNIVERSITY
Biochemistry	D
Biological and Biomedical Sciences—General	M,D,O
Biophysics	D
Communication Disorders	M,D
Environmental and Occupational Health	O
Health Services Management and Hospital Administration	O
International Health	M
Neuroscience	M,D
Nutrition	M
Physiology	M
Public Health—General	M
Structural Biology	D
Toxicology	M,O

TARLETON STATE UNIVERSITY
Biological and Biomedical Sciences—General	M
Clinical Laboratory Sciences/Medical Technology	M
Nursing and Healthcare Administration	M
Nursing Education	M
Nursing—General	M
Public Health—General	M

TEACHERS COLLEGE, COLUMBIA UNIVERSITY
Biological and Biomedical Sciences—General	M,D
Communication Disorders	M,D,O
Community Health	M,D,O
Neuroscience	M,D
Nursing and Healthcare Administration	M,D
Nursing Education	M,D,O
Nutrition	M,D,O
Physiology	M,D

TEMPLE UNIVERSITY
Adult Nursing	D
Allied Health—General	M,D
Allopathic Medicine	D
Biological and Biomedical Sciences—General	M,D
Communication Disorders	M,D
Dentistry	D
Family Nurse Practitioner Studies	D
Health Services Management and Hospital Administration	M
Medicinal and Pharmaceutical Chemistry	M,D
Nursing—General	D
Occupational Therapy	M,D
Oral and Dental Sciences	M,O
Pharmaceutical Administration	M
Pharmaceutical Sciences	M,D
Physical Therapy	D
Podiatric Medicine	D
Public Health—General	M,D
Rehabilitation Sciences	M,D

TENNESSEE STATE UNIVERSITY
Allied Health—General	M,D,O
Biological and Biomedical Sciences—General	D
Communication Disorders	M
Family Nurse Practitioner Studies	M,O
Nursing—General	M,O
Occupational Therapy	M
Physical Therapy	D
Public Health—General	M

TENNESSEE TECHNOLOGICAL UNIVERSITY
Biological and Biomedical Sciences—General	M,D
Family Nurse Practitioner Studies	M
Health Promotion	M
Nursing and Healthcare Administration	M
Nursing Education	M
Nursing Informatics	M
Nursing—General	M

TEXAS A&M INTERNATIONAL UNIVERSITY
Biological and Biomedical Sciences—General	M
Family Nurse Practitioner Studies	M
Nursing—General	M

TEXAS A&M UNIVERSITY
Allied Health—General	M,D
Biochemistry	M,D
Biological and Biomedical Sciences—General	M,D
Community Health	M,D
Dentistry	M,D,O
Entomology	M,D
Family Nurse Practitioner Studies	M
Health Physics/Radiological Health	M,D
Health Promotion	M,D
Health Services Management and Hospital Administration	M,D
Health Services Research	M,D
Microbiology	M,D
Nursing Education	M
Nursing—General	M
Nutrition	M,D
Pharmacy	D
Plant Pathology	M,D
Public Health—General	M,D
Veterinary Medicine	M,D
Veterinary Sciences	M,D

TEXAS A&M UNIVERSITY AT GALVESTON
Marine Biology	M,D

TEXAS A&M UNIVERSITY–CORPUS CHRISTI
Biological and Biomedical Sciences—General	M
Family Nurse Practitioner Studies	M
Health Services Management and Hospital Administration	M
Nursing and Healthcare Administration	M
Nursing Education	M
Nursing—General	M

TEXAS A&M UNIVERSITY–KINGSVILLE
Biological and Biomedical Sciences—General	M
Communication Disorders	M

TEXAS A&M UNIVERSITY–SAN ANTONIO
Health Services Management and Hospital Administration	M

TEXAS CHIROPRACTIC COLLEGE
Chiropractic	D

TEXAS CHRISTIAN UNIVERSITY
Adult Nursing	M,O
Allied Health—General	M,D,O
Biochemistry	M,D
Biological and Biomedical Sciences—General	M
Biophysics	M,D
Communication Disorders	M
Gerontological Nursing	M,O
Neuroscience	M,D
Nurse Anesthesia	D
Nursing and Healthcare Administration	M,D,O
Nursing Education	M,O
Nursing—General	M,D,O
Pediatric Nursing	M,O

TEXAS HEALTH AND SCIENCE UNIVERSITY
Health Services Management and Hospital Administration	M,D

TEXAS SOUTHERN UNIVERSITY
Biological and Biomedical Sciences—General	M
Health Services Management and Hospital Administration	M
Pharmaceutical Sciences	M,D
Pharmacy	D
Toxicology	M,D

TEXAS STATE UNIVERSITY
Allied Health—General	M,D
Biochemistry	M
Biological and Biomedical Sciences—General	M
Communication Disorders	M
Conservation Biology	M
Family Nurse Practitioner Studies	M
Health Services Management and Hospital Administration	M
Marine Biology	M,D
Nutrition	M
Physical Therapy	D

TEXAS TECH UNIVERSITY
Biological and Biomedical Sciences—General	M,D
Health Services Management and Hospital Administration	M,D
Microbiology	M,D
Nutrition	M,D
Toxicology	M,D
Zoology	M,D

TEXAS TECH UNIVERSITY HEALTH SCIENCES CENTER
Acute Care/Critical Care Nursing	M,D,O
Allopathic Medicine	D
Biological and Biomedical Sciences—General	M,D
Cell Biology	M,D
Communication Disorders	M,D
Family Nurse Practitioner Studies	M,D,O
Gerontological Nursing	M,D,O
Health Services Management and Hospital Administration	M
Molecular Pathology	M
Nursing and Healthcare Administration	M,D,O
Nursing Education	M,D,O
Nursing—General	M,D,O
Occupational Therapy	M
Pediatric Nursing	M,D,O
Pharmaceutical Sciences	M,D
Physical Therapy	D
Physician Assistant Studies	M
Rehabilitation Sciences	D

TEXAS WESLEYAN UNIVERSITY
Nurse Anesthesia	M,D

TEXAS WOMAN'S UNIVERSITY
Acute Care/Critical Care Nursing	M,D
Adult Nursing	M,D
Allied Health—General	M,D
Biological and Biomedical Sciences—General	M,D
Communication Disorders	M
Family Nurse Practitioner Studies	M,D
Health Services Management and Hospital Administration	M,D
Molecular Biology	M,D
Nursing and Healthcare Administration	M,D
Nursing Education	M,D
Nursing—General	M,D
Nutrition	M
Occupational Therapy	M,D
Pediatric Nursing	M,D
Physical Therapy	D
Women's Health Nursing	M,D

THOMAS EDISON STATE UNIVERSITY
Epidemiology	O
Nursing Education	O
Nursing—General	M,D

THOMAS JEFFERSON UNIVERSITY
Allopathic Medicine	D
Biochemistry	D
Biological and Biomedical Sciences—General	M,D,O
Cancer Biology/Oncology	D
Cell Biology	M,D
Clinical Laboratory Sciences/Medical Technology	M
Clinical Research	M,O
Developmental Biology	M,D
Genetics	D
Genomic Sciences	D
Health Physics/Radiological Health	M
Health Services Management and Hospital Administration	M,D,O
Health Services Research	M,D,O
Immunology	D
Infectious Diseases	O
Microbiology	M,D
Molecular Pharmacology	D
Neuroscience	D
Nursing—General	M,D
Occupational Therapy	M,D
Pharmacology	M
Pharmacy	D
Physical Therapy	D
Physician Assistant Studies	M
Public Health—General	M,O
Toxicology	M

THOMAS UNIVERSITY
Nursing—General	M

TIFFIN UNIVERSITY
Health Services Management and Hospital Administration	M

TOURO COLLEGE
Communication Disorders	M,D
Occupational Therapy	M,D
Physical Therapy	M,D
Physician Assistant Studies	M,D

TOURO UNIVERSITY CALIFORNIA
Osteopathic Medicine	M,D
Pharmacy	D
Public Health—General	M,D

TOWSON UNIVERSITY
Allied Health—General	M
Biological and Biomedical Sciences—General	M
Communication Disorders	M,D
Environmental and Occupational Health	D
Health Services Management and Hospital Administration	M,O
Nursing Education	M,O
Nursing—General	M,O
Occupational Therapy	M
Physician Assistant Studies	M

TRENT UNIVERSITY
Biological and Biomedical Sciences—General	M,D

TREVECCA NAZARENE UNIVERSITY
Physician Assistant Studies	M

TRIDENT UNIVERSITY INTERNATIONAL
Clinical Research	M,D,O
Environmental and Occupational Health	M,D,O

Health Services Management and
  Hospital Administration   M,D,O
International Health   M,D,O
Nursing and Healthcare
  Administration   M,D,O
Public Health—General   M,D,O

TRINITY INTERNATIONAL UNIVERSITY
Bioethics   M

TRINITY UNIVERSITY
Health Services Management and
  Hospital Administration   M

TRINITY WASHINGTON UNIVERSITY
Public Health—General   M

TRINITY WESTERN UNIVERSITY
Health Services Management and
  Hospital Administration   M,O
Nursing—General   M

TRI-STATE COLLEGE OF ACUPUNCTURE
Acupuncture and Oriental Medicine   M,O

TROPICAL AGRICULTURE RESEARCH AND HIGHER EDUCATION CENTER
Conservation Biology   M,D

TROY UNIVERSITY
Adult Nursing   M,D,O
Biological and Biomedical
  Sciences—General   M,O
Family Nurse Practitioner Studies   M,D,O
Health Services Management and
  Hospital Administration   M
Maternal and Child Health   M,D,O
Nursing Informatics   M,D,O
Nursing—General   M,D,O

TRUMAN STATE UNIVERSITY
Biological and Biomedical
  Sciences—General   M
Communication Disorders   M

TUFTS UNIVERSITY
Allopathic Medicine   D
Biochemistry   D
Biological and Biomedical
  Sciences—General   M,D,O
Cancer Biology/Oncology   D
Cell Biology   D
Clinical Research   M,D,O
Dentistry   D
Developmental Biology   D
Environmental and Occupational
  Health   M,D
Epidemiology   M,D,O
Genetics   D
Health Services Management and
  Hospital Administration   M,D,O
Immunology   D
Infectious Diseases   M,D
International Health   M,D
Microbiology   D
Molecular Biology   D
Molecular Medicine   D
Neuroscience   M,D
Nutrition   M,D,O
Occupational Therapy   M,D,O
Oral and Dental Sciences   M,O
Pathology   M,D
Pharmacology   M,D
Physician Assistant Studies   M,D,O
Public Health—General   M,D,O
Reproductive Biology   M,D
Structural Biology   D
Veterinary Medicine   M,D

TULANE UNIVERSITY
Allopathic Medicine   D
Biochemistry   M
Biological and Biomedical
  Sciences—General   M,D
Cell Biology   M,D
Community Health   M,D
Ecology   M,D
Environmental and Occupational
  Health   M,D
Epidemiology   M,D
Evolutionary Biology   M,D
Health Services Management and
  Hospital Administration   M,D
Human Genetics   M
Immunology   M
International Health   M,D
Microbiology   M
Molecular Biology   M,D
Neuroscience   M,D
Parasitology   M,D,O
Pharmacology   M
Physiology   M
Public Health—General   M,D
Structural Biology   M,D

TUSKEGEE UNIVERSITY
Biological and Biomedical
  Sciences—General   M,D
Nutrition   M
Occupational Therapy   M
Veterinary Medicine   M,D
Veterinary Sciences   M,D

UNIFORMED SERVICES UNIVERSITY OF THE HEALTH SCIENCES
Biological and Biomedical
  Sciences—General   M,D
Cell Biology   M,D
Environmental and Occupational
  Health   M,D
Family Nurse Practitioner Studies   M,D
Gerontological Nursing   M,D
Health Services Management and
  Hospital Administration   M,D

Immunology   D
Infectious Diseases   D*
International Health   M,D
Molecular Biology   M,D*
Neuroscience   D*
Nurse Anesthesia   M,D
Nursing—General   M,D
Psychiatric Nursing   M,D
Public Health—General   M,D
Women's Health Nursing   M,D
Zoology   M,D

UNION COLLEGE (NE)
Physician Assistant Studies   M

UNION INSTITUTE & UNIVERSITY
Health Promotion   M

UNION UNIVERSITY
Family Nurse Practitioner Studies   M,D,O
Nurse Anesthesia   M,D,O
Nursing and Healthcare
  Administration   M,D,O
Nursing Education   M,D,O
Nursing—General   M,D,O

UNITED STATES UNIVERSITY
Family Nurse Practitioner Studies   M

UNIVERSIDAD ADVENTISTA DE LAS ANTILLAS
Medical/Surgical Nursing   M

UNIVERSIDAD AUTONOMA DE GUADALAJARA
Allopathic Medicine   D
Environmental and Occupational
  Health   M,D

UNIVERSIDAD CENTRAL DEL CARIBE
Allopathic Medicine   M,D
Anatomy   M,D
Biochemistry   M,D
Biological and Biomedical
  Sciences—General   M,D
Cell Biology   M,D
Immunology   M,D
Microbiology   M,D
Molecular Biology   M,D
Pharmacology   M,D
Physiology   M,D

UNIVERSIDAD CENTRAL DEL ESTE
Allopathic Medicine   D
Dentistry   D

UNIVERSIDAD DE CIENCIAS MEDICAS
Allopathic Medicine   M,D,O
Anatomy   M,D,O
Biological and Biomedical
  Sciences—General   M,D,O
Community Health   M,D,O
Environmental and Occupational
  Health   M,D,O
Health Services Management and
  Hospital Administration   M,D,O
Pharmacy   M,D,O

UNIVERSIDAD DE IBEROAMERICA
Acute Care/Critical Care Nursing   M,D
Allopathic Medicine   M,D
Health Services Management and
  Hospital Administration   M,D
Neuroscience   M,D

UNIVERSIDAD DE LAS AMÉRICAS PUEBLA
Clinical Laboratory
  Sciences/Medical Technology   M

UNIVERSIDAD DEL TURABO
Adult Nursing   M,O
Communication Disorders   M
Environmental Biology   M,D
Family Nurse Practitioner Studies   M
Health Promotion   M
Naturopathic Medicine   D

UNIVERSIDAD IBEROAMERICANA
Allopathic Medicine   M
Dentistry   M,D

UNIVERSIDAD METROPOLITANA
Nursing and Healthcare
  Administration   M,O
Nursing—General   M,O
Oncology Nursing   M,O

UNIVERSIDAD NACIONAL PEDRO HENRIQUEZ URENA
Allopathic Medicine   D
Dentistry   D
Ecology   M

UNIVERSITÉ DE MONCTON
Biochemistry   M
Biological and Biomedical
  Sciences—General   M
Nutrition   M

UNIVERSITÉ DE MONTRÉAL
Allopathic Medicine   D
Biochemistry   M,D,O
Bioethics   M,D,O
Biological and Biomedical
  Sciences—General   M,D
Cell Biology   M,D
Communication Disorders   M,D
Community Health   M,D,O
Dental Hygiene   O
Environmental and Occupational
  Health   O
Genetics   M
Health Services Management and
  Hospital Administration   M,O
Immunology   M,D

Microbiology   M,D
Molecular Biology   M,D
Neuroscience   M,D
Nursing—General   M,D,O
Nutrition   M,D,O
Occupational Therapy   O
Optometry   D
Oral and Dental Sciences   M,O
Pathology   M,D,O
Pharmaceutical Sciences   M,D,O
Pharmacology   M,D
Physiology   M,D
Public Health—General   M,D,O
Rehabilitation Sciences   O
Toxicology   M,D
Veterinary Medicine   D
Veterinary Sciences   M,D
Virology   D
Vision Sciences   M,O

UNIVERSITÉ DE SHERBROOKE
Allopathic Medicine   D
Biochemistry   M,D
Biological and Biomedical
  Sciences—General   M,D,O
Biophysics   M,D
Cell Biology   M,D
Clinical Laboratory
  Sciences/Medical Technology   M,D
Immunology   M,D
Microbiology   M,D
Pharmacology   M,D
Physiology   M,D
Radiation Biology   M,D

UNIVERSITÉ DU QUÉBEC À CHICOUTIMI
Genetics   M,D

UNIVERSITÉ DU QUÉBEC À MONTRÉAL
Biological and Biomedical
  Sciences—General   M,D
Environmental and Occupational
  Health   O

UNIVERSITÉ DU QUÉBEC À RIMOUSKI
Nursing—General   M,O

UNIVERSITÉ DU QUÉBEC À TROIS-RIVIÈRES
Biophysics   M,D
Chiropractic   D
Nursing—General   M,O

UNIVERSITÉ DU QUÉBEC EN ABITIBI-TÉMISCAMINGUE
Biological and Biomedical
  Sciences—General   M,D

UNIVERSITÉ DU QUÉBEC EN OUTAOUAIS
Nursing—General   M,O

UNIVERSITÉ DU QUÉBEC, INSTITUT NATIONAL DE LA RECHERCHE SCIENTIFIQUE
Biological and Biomedical
  Sciences—General   M,D
Immunology   M,D
Medical Microbiology   M,D
Microbiology   M,D
Virology   M,D

UNIVERSITÉ LAVAL
Allopathic Medicine   D,O
Anatomy   O
Anesthesiologist Assistant Studies   O
Biochemistry   M,D,O
Biological and Biomedical
  Sciences—General   M,D,O
Cancer Biology/Oncology   O
Cardiovascular Sciences   O
Cell Biology   M,D
Communication Disorders   M
Community Health   M,D,O
Dentistry   D,O
Emergency Medical Services   O
Environmental and Occupational
  Health   O
Epidemiology   M,D
Health Physics/Radiological Health   O
Immunology   M,D
Infectious Diseases   O
Microbiology   M,D
Molecular Biology   M,D
Neurobiology   M,D
Nursing—General   M,D,O
Nutrition   M,D
Oral and Dental Sciences   M,O
Pathology   O
Pharmaceutical Sciences   M,D,O
Physiology   M,D
Plant Biology   M,D

UNIVERSITY AT ALBANY, STATE UNIVERSITY OF NEW YORK
Biological and Biomedical
  Sciences—General   M,D
Cell Biology   M,D
Conservation Biology   M
Developmental Biology   D
Ecology   D
Environmental and Occupational
  Health   M,D
Epidemiology   M,D
Evolutionary Biology   D
Health Services Management and
  Hospital Administration   M,D,O
Immunology   M,D
Molecular Biology   D
Neurobiology   D
Neuroscience   M,D
Public Health—General   M,D
Structural Biology   M,D
Toxicology   M,D

Microbiology   M,D
Molecular Biology   M,D
Neuroscience   M,D
Nursing—General   M,D,O
Nutrition   M,D,O
Occupational Therapy   O
Optometry   D
Oral and Dental Sciences   M,O
Pathology   M,D,O
Pharmaceutical Sciences   M,D,O
Pharmacology   M,D
Physiology   M,D
Public Health—General   M,D,O
Rehabilitation Sciences   O
Toxicology   M,D
Veterinary Medicine   D
Veterinary Sciences   M,D
Virology   D
Vision Sciences   M,O

UNIVERSITY AT BUFFALO, THE STATE UNIVERSITY OF NEW YORK
Adult Nursing   M,D,O
Allied Health—General   M,D,O
Allopathic Medicine   D
Anatomy   M,D
Biochemistry   M,D
Biological and Biomedical
  Sciences—General   M,D
Biophysics   M,D
Cancer Biology/Oncology   M
Cell Biology   D
Clinical Laboratory
  Sciences/Medical Technology   M
Communication Disorders   M,D
Community Health   M,D
Dentistry   D
Ecology   M,D,O
Epidemiology   M,D
Evolutionary Biology   M,D,O
Family Nurse Practitioner Studies   M,D,O
Genetics   M,D
Genomic Sciences   M,D
Gerontological Nursing   M,D,O
Health Services Management and
  Hospital Administration   M,D,O
Immunology   M,D
Medical Physics   M,D
Medicinal and Pharmaceutical
  Chemistry   M,D
Microbiology   M,D
Molecular Biology   D
Molecular Biophysics   M,D
Molecular Pharmacology   D
Neuroscience   M,D
Nurse Anesthesia   M,D,O
Nursing and Healthcare
  Administration   M,D,O
Nursing—General   M,D,O
Nutrition   M,D,O
Occupational Therapy   M
Oral and Dental Sciences   M,D,O
Pathology   M,D
Pharmaceutical Sciences   M,D
Pharmacology   M,D
Pharmacy   D
Physical Therapy   D
Physiology   M,D
Psychiatric Nursing   M,D,O
Public Health—General   M,D
Rehabilitation Sciences   M,D,O
Structural Biology   M,D
Toxicology   M,D

THE UNIVERSITY OF AKRON
Biological and Biomedical
  Sciences—General   M,D
Communication Disorders   M,D
Health Services Management and
  Hospital Administration   M
Nursing—General   M,D
Public Health—General   M,D

THE UNIVERSITY OF ALABAMA
Biological and Biomedical
  Sciences—General   M,D
Communication Disorders   M
Community Health   M
Health Promotion   M,D
Nursing—General   M,D
Nutrition   M

THE UNIVERSITY OF ALABAMA AT BIRMINGHAM
Allied Health—General   M,D,O
Allopathic Medicine   D
Biochemistry   D
Biological and Biomedical
  Sciences—General   M,D
Cancer Biology/Oncology   D
Cell Biology   D
Clinical Laboratory
  Sciences/Medical Technology   M,D
Community Health   M
Dentistry   D
Developmental Biology   D
Environmental and Occupational
  Health   M,D
Epidemiology   M,D
Genetics   D
Genomic Sciences   D
Health Promotion   D
Health Services Management and
  Hospital Administration   M,D
Health Services Research   M,D
Industrial Hygiene   M,D
Maternal and Child Health   M,D
Microbiology   D
Molecular Biology   D
Molecular Medicine   D
Neurobiology   D
Neuroscience   M,D
Nurse Anesthesia   M,D
Nursing—General   M,D
Nutrition   M,D
Occupational Therapy   M,O
Optometry   D
Oral and Dental Sciences   M
Pathobiology   D
Pharmacology   D
Physical Therapy   D
Physician Assistant Studies   M
Public Health—General   M,D
Rehabilitation Sciences   D
Structural Biology   D
Toxicology   M,D
Vision Sciences   M,D

THE UNIVERSITY OF ALABAMA IN HUNTSVILLE
Acute Care/Critical Care Nursing   M,D,O

---

*M—masters degree; D—doctorate; O—other advanced degree; *—Close-Up and/or Display*

Biological and Biomedical
  Sciences—General — M,D
Family Nurse Practitioner Studies — M,D,O
Gerontological Nursing — M,D,O
Health Services Management and
  Hospital Administration — M,D,O
Nursing Education — M,D,O
Nursing—General — M,D,O

UNIVERSITY OF ALASKA ANCHORAGE
Biological and Biomedical
  Sciences—General — M
Nursing—General — M
Public Health—General — M

UNIVERSITY OF ALASKA FAIRBANKS
Biochemistry — M,D
Marine Biology — M,D
Neuroscience — M,D

UNIVERSITY OF ALBERTA
Biochemistry — M,D
Biological and Biomedical
  Sciences—General — M,D
Cancer Biology/Oncology — M,D
Cell Biology — M,D
Clinical Laboratory
  Sciences/Medical Technology — M,D
Communication Disorders — M,D
Community Health — M,D
Conservation Biology — M,D
Dental Hygiene — O
Dentistry — D
Ecology — M,D
Environmental and Occupational
  Health — M,D
Environmental Biology — M,D
Epidemiology — M,D
Evolutionary Biology — M,D
Genetics — M,D
Health Physics/Radiological Health — M,D
Health Promotion — M,O
Health Services Management and
  Hospital Administration — M,D
Health Services Research — M,D
Immunology — M,D
International Health — M,D
Maternal and Child/Neonatal
  Nursing — D
Medical Microbiology — M,D
Medical Physics — M,D
Microbiology — M,D
Molecular Biology — M,D
Neuroscience — M,D
Nursing—General — M,D
Occupational Therapy — M,D
Oral and Dental Sciences — M,D
Pathology — M,D
Pharmaceutical Sciences — M,D
Pharmacology — M,D
Pharmacy — M,D
Physical Therapy — M,D
Physiology — M,D
Plant Biology — M,D
Public Health—General — M,D
Rehabilitation Sciences — D
Vision Sciences — M,D

THE UNIVERSITY OF ARIZONA
Allopathic Medicine — M,D
Biochemistry — M,D
Biological and Biomedical
  Sciences—General — M,D
Cancer Biology/Oncology — D
Cell Biology — M,D,O
Communication Disorders — M,D,O
Ecology — M,D
Entomology — M,D
Epidemiology — M,D
Evolutionary Biology — M,D
Family Nurse Practitioner Studies — M,D,O
Genetics — M,D
Immunology — D
Medical Physics — M
Microbiology — D
Molecular Biology — M,D,O
Molecular Medicine — M,D
Neuroscience — D
Nursing—General — M,D,O
Nutrition — M,D
Perfusion — M,D
Pharmaceutical Sciences — M,D
Pharmacology — M,D
Pharmacy — D
Physiology — M,D
Plant Pathology — M,D
Public Health—General — M,D

UNIVERSITY OF ARKANSAS
Biological and Biomedical
  Sciences—General — M,D
Cell Biology — M,D
Communication Disorders — M
Community Health — M,D
Entomology — M,D
Health Promotion — M,D
Molecular Biology — M,D
Nursing—General — M
Plant Pathology — M

UNIVERSITY OF ARKANSAS AT LITTLE ROCK
Biological and Biomedical
  Sciences—General — M

UNIVERSITY OF ARKANSAS FOR MEDICAL SCIENCES
Allopathic Medicine — D
Biochemistry — M,D,O
Biological and Biomedical
  Sciences—General — M,D,O
Communication Disorders — M,D
Environmental and Occupational
  Health — M,D,O
Epidemiology — M,D,O
Health Physics/Radiological Health — M,D

Health Promotion — M,D,O
Health Services Management and
  Hospital Administration — M,D,O
Health Services Research — M,D,O
Immunology — M,D,O
Microbiology — M,D,O
Molecular Biology — M,D,O
Molecular Biophysics — M,D,O
Neurobiology — M,D,O
Nursing—General — D
Nutrition — M,D,O
Pharmacology — M,D,O
Pharmacy — M,D
Physician Assistant Studies — M,D
Physiology — M,D,O
Public Health—General — M,D,O
Toxicology — M,D,O

UNIVERSITY OF BALTIMORE
Health Services Management and
  Hospital Administration — M

UNIVERSITY OF BRIDGEPORT
Acupuncture and Oriental Medicine — M
Chiropractic — D
Dental Hygiene — M
Naturopathic Medicine — D
Nutrition — M
Physician Assistant Studies — M

THE UNIVERSITY OF BRITISH COLUMBIA
Allopathic Medicine — M,D
Biochemistry — M,D
Biopsychology — M,D
Botany — M,D
Cell Biology — M,D
Communication Disorders — M,D
Dentistry — D
Developmental Biology — M,D
Environmental and Occupational
  Health — M,D
Epidemiology — M,D
Genetics — M,D
Health Services Management and
  Hospital Administration — M,D
Immunology — M,D
Microbiology — M,D
Molecular Biology — M,D
Neuroscience — M,D
Nurse Anesthesia — M,D
Nursing—General — M,D
Nutrition — M,D
Occupational Therapy — M
Oral and Dental Sciences — M,D,O
Pathology — M,D
Pharmaceutical Sciences — M,D
Pharmacology — M,D
Pharmacy — M,D
Public Health—General — M,D
Rehabilitation Sciences — M,D
Reproductive Biology — M,D
Zoology — M,D

UNIVERSITY OF CALGARY
Allopathic Medicine — D
Biochemistry — M,D
Biological and Biomedical
  Sciences—General — M,D
Cancer Biology/Oncology — M,D
Cardiovascular Sciences — M,D
Community Health — M,D
Genetics — M,D
Immunology — M,D
Infectious Diseases — M,D
Microbiology — M,D
Molecular Biology — M,D
Molecular Genetics — M,D
Neuroscience — M,D
Nursing—General — M,D,O
Pathology — M,D
Physiology — M,D

UNIVERSITY OF CALIFORNIA, BERKELEY
Allopathic Medicine
Biochemistry — D
Biological and Biomedical
  Sciences—General — D
Biophysics — D
Cell Biology — D
Clinical Research — O
Environmental and Occupational
  Health — M,D
Epidemiology — M,D
Health Services Management and
  Hospital Administration — D
Immunology — D
Infectious Diseases — M,D
Microbiology — D
Molecular Biology — D
Molecular Toxicology — D
Neuroscience — D
Nutrition — D
Optometry — D,O
Physiology — M,D
Plant Biology — D
Public Health—General — M,D
Vision Sciences — M,D

UNIVERSITY OF CALIFORNIA, DAVIS
Allopathic Medicine
Animal Behavior — D
Biochemistry — M,D
Biophysics — M,D
Cell Biology — M,D
Clinical Research — M
Developmental Biology — M,D
Ecology — M,D
Entomology — M,D
Epidemiology — M,D
Evolutionary Biology — D
Genetics — M,D
Immunology — M,D
Maternal and Child Health — M
Microbiology — M,D

Molecular Biology — M,D
Neuroscience — D
Nutrition — M,D
Pathology — M,D
Pharmacology — M,D
Physiology — M,D
Plant Biology — M,D
Plant Pathology — M,D
Toxicology — M,D
Veterinary Medicine — D
Veterinary Sciences — M,O
Zoology — M

UNIVERSITY OF CALIFORNIA, IRVINE
Allopathic Medicine
Anatomy — M,D
Biochemistry — M,D
Biological and Biomedical
  Sciences—General — M,D
Biophysics — D
Cell Biology — M,D
Computational Biology — D
Developmental Biology — M,D
Ecology — M,D
Environmental and Occupational
  Health — M,D
Epidemiology — M,D
Evolutionary Biology — M,D
Genetics — D
Health Services Management and
  Hospital Administration — M
Medicinal and Pharmaceutical
  Chemistry — D
Microbiology — M,D
Molecular Biology — M,D
Molecular Genetics — M,D
Neurobiology — M,D
Neuroscience — D
Nursing—General — M
Pathology — D
Pharmaceutical Sciences — D
Physiology — D
Public Health—General — M,D
Systems Biology — D
Toxicology — M,D
Translational Biology — M

UNIVERSITY OF CALIFORNIA, LOS ANGELES
Allopathic Medicine — D
Anatomy — M,D
Biochemistry — M,D
Biological and Biomedical
  Sciences—General — M,D
Cell Biology — M,D
Clinical Research — M
Community Health — M,D
Dentistry — D,O
Developmental Biology — M,D
Ecology — M,D
Environmental and Occupational
  Health — M,D
Epidemiology — M,D
Evolutionary Biology — M,D
Health Services Management and
  Hospital Administration — M,D
Human Genetics — M,D
Immunology — M,D
Medical Physics — M,D
Microbiology — M,D
Molecular Biology — M,D
Molecular Genetics — M,D
Molecular Physiology — M,D
Molecular Toxicology — D
Neurobiology — M,D
Neuroscience — D
Nursing—General — M,D
Oral and Dental Sciences — M,D
Pathology — M,D
Pharmacology — M,D
Physiology — M,D
Public Health—General — M,D
Toxicology — D

UNIVERSITY OF CALIFORNIA, MERCED
Biochemistry — M,D
Biological and Biomedical
  Sciences—General — M,D
Systems Biology — M,D

UNIVERSITY OF CALIFORNIA, RIVERSIDE
Biochemistry — M,D
Biological and Biomedical
  Sciences—General — M,D
Botany — M,D
Cell Biology — M,D
Developmental Biology — M,D
Entomology — M,D
Evolutionary Biology — M,D
Genetics — D
Genomic Sciences — D
Microbiology — M,D
Molecular Biology — M,D
Neuroscience — D
Plant Biology — M,D
Plant Molecular Biology — M,D
Plant Pathology — M,D
Toxicology — M,D

UNIVERSITY OF CALIFORNIA, SAN DIEGO
Allopathic Medicine — D
Biochemistry — M,D
Biological and Biomedical
  Sciences—General — M,D*
Biophysics — D
Clinical Laboratory
  Sciences/Medical Technology — M,D
Clinical Research — M
Communication Disorders — D
Epidemiology — D
Health Services Management and
  Hospital Administration — M
International Health — D

Molecular Biology — M,D
Neuroscience — D
Nutrition — M,D
Pathology — M,D
Pharmacology — M,D
Physiology — M,D
Plant Biology — M,D
Plant Pathology — M,D
Toxicology — M,D
Veterinary Medicine — D
Veterinary Sciences — M,O
Zoology — M

UNIVERSITY OF CALIFORNIA, SAN FRANCISCO
Allopathic Medicine — D
Biochemistry — D
Biological and Biomedical
  Sciences—General — D
Biophysics — D
Cell Biology — D
Dentistry — D
Developmental Biology — D
Genetics — D
Genomic Sciences — D
Medical Imaging — M
Medicinal and Pharmaceutical
  Chemistry — D
Molecular Biology — D
Neuroscience — D
Nursing—General — M,D
Oral and Dental Sciences — M,D
Pharmaceutical Sciences — D
Pharmacology — D
Pharmacy — D*
Physical Therapy — D

UNIVERSITY OF CALIFORNIA, SANTA BARBARA
Biochemistry — D
Biophysics — D
Cell Biology — M,D
Developmental Biology — M,D
Ecology — M,D
Evolutionary Biology — M,D
Marine Biology — M,D
Molecular Biology — M,D
Neuroscience — D

UNIVERSITY OF CALIFORNIA, SANTA CRUZ
Biochemistry — M,D
Cell Biology — M,D
Developmental Biology — M,D
Ecology — M,D
Environmental Biology — M,D
Evolutionary Biology — M,D
Molecular Biology — M,D
Toxicology — M,D

UNIVERSITY OF CENTRAL ARKANSAS
Adult Nursing — M,O
Biological and Biomedical
  Sciences—General — M
Communication Disorders — M,D
Family Nurse Practitioner Studies — M,O
Nursing and Healthcare
  Administration — M,O
Nursing Education — M,O
Nursing—General — M,O
Occupational Therapy — M
Physical Therapy — D

UNIVERSITY OF CENTRAL FLORIDA
Allopathic Medicine — M,D
Biological and Biomedical
  Sciences—General — M,D
Communication Disorders — M,D,O
Conservation Biology — M,D,O
Health Services Management and
  Hospital Administration — M,O
Nursing—General — M,D,O
Physical Therapy — D
Physiology — M

UNIVERSITY OF CENTRAL MISSOURI
Biological and Biomedical
  Sciences—General — M,D,O
Communication Disorders — M,D,O
Environmental and Occupational
  Health — M,D,O
Industrial Hygiene — M,D,O
Nursing—General — M,D,O

UNIVERSITY OF CENTRAL OKLAHOMA
Biological and Biomedical
  Sciences—General — M
Communication Disorders — M
Health Promotion — M
Nursing—General — M
Nutrition — M

UNIVERSITY OF CHARLESTON
Pharmacy — D
Physician Assistant Studies — M

UNIVERSITY OF CHICAGO
Allopathic Medicine — D
Anatomy — D
Biochemistry — D
Biological and Biomedical
  Sciences—General — D
Biophysics — D
Cancer Biology/Oncology — D
Cell Biology — D
Developmental Biology — D
Ecology — D
Evolutionary Biology — D
Genetics — D
Genomic Sciences — D
Health Promotion — M,D
Health Services Management and
  Hospital Administration — M,O
Human Genetics — D
Immunology — D
Medical Physics — D
Microbiology — D
Molecular Biology — D
Molecular Biophysics — D
Neurobiology — D
Neuroscience — D
Nutrition — D
Systems Biology — D
Zoology — D

UNIVERSITY OF CINCINNATI

Acute Care/Critical Care Nursing	M,D
Adult Nursing	M,D
Allopathic Medicine	D
Biochemistry	M,D
Biological and Biomedical Sciences—General	M,D,O
Biophysics	D
Cancer Biology/Oncology	D
Cell Biology	D
Communication Disorders	M,D,O
Community Health Nursing	M,D
Developmental Biology	D
Environmental and Occupational Health	M,D
Epidemiology	M,D
Genomic Sciences	M,D
Health Physics/Radiological Health	M
Health Services Research	M
Immunology	M,D
Industrial Hygiene	M,D
Maternal and Child/Neonatal Nursing	M,D
Medical Imaging	M,D
Medical Physics	M
Microbiology	M,D
Molecular Biology	M,D
Molecular Genetics	M,D
Molecular Medicine	D
Molecular Toxicology	M,D
Neuroscience	D
Nurse Anesthesia	M,D
Nurse Midwifery	M,D
Nursing and Healthcare Administration	M,D
Nursing—General	M
Nutrition	M
Occupational Health Nursing	M,D
Pathobiology	D
Pathology	D
Pediatric Nursing	M,D
Pharmaceutical Sciences	D
Pharmacology	D
Pharmacy	D
Physiology	D
Psychiatric Nursing	M,D
Rehabilitation Sciences	D
Women's Health Nursing	M,D

UNIVERSITY OF COLORADO BOULDER

Animal Behavior	M,D
Biochemistry	M,D
Cell Biology	M,D
Communication Disorders	M,D
Developmental Biology	M,D
Ecology	M,D
Evolutionary Biology	M,D
Genetics	M,D
Marine Biology	M,D
Medical Physics	M,D
Microbiology	M,D
Molecular Biology	M,D
Neurobiology	M,D
Physiology	M,D

UNIVERSITY OF COLORADO COLORADO SPRINGS

Adult Nursing	M,D
Gerontological Nursing	M,D
Nursing—General	M,D

UNIVERSITY OF COLORADO DENVER

Adult Nursing	M,D
Allopathic Medicine	D
Anatomy	M,D
Anesthesiologist Assistant Studies	M
Animal Behavior	M,D
Biochemistry	D
Biological and Biomedical Sciences—General	M,D
Biophysics	M,D
Cancer Biology/Oncology	D
Cell Biology	M,D
Clinical Laboratory Sciences/Medical Technology	M,D
Clinical Research	M,D
Community Health	M,D
Computational Biology	M,D
Dentistry	M,D
Developmental Biology	M,D
Ecology	M,D
Environmental and Occupational Health	M,D
Epidemiology	M,D
Evolutionary Biology	M,D
Family Nurse Practitioner Studies	M,D
Genetics	M,D
Health Services Management and Hospital Administration	M,D
Health Services Research	M,D
Immunology	D
International Health	M
Microbiology	M,D
Molecular Biology	M,D
Molecular Genetics	D
Neurobiology	M,D
Neuroscience	D
Nurse Midwifery	M,D
Nursing and Healthcare Administration	M,D
Nursing—General	M,D
Oral and Dental Sciences	M,D
Pediatric Nursing	M,D
Pharmaceutical Sciences	D
Pharmacology	D
Physical Therapy	D
Physician Assistant Studies	M
Physiology	D
Psychiatric Nursing	M,D
Public Health—General	M,D
Rehabilitation Sciences	D

Toxicology	D
Women's Health Nursing	M,D

UNIVERSITY OF CONNECTICUT

Biopsychology	M,D
Botany	M,D
Communication Disorders	M,D
Ecology	M,D
Environmental and Occupational Health	O
Genomic Sciences	M
Health Services Management and Hospital Administration	M,D
Medicinal and Pharmaceutical Chemistry	M,D
Neurobiology	M,D
Neuroscience	M,D
Nursing—General	M,D,O
Nutrition	M,D
Pathobiology	M,D
Pharmaceutical Sciences	M,D
Pharmacology	M,D
Pharmacy	D
Physical Therapy	D
Physiology	M,D*
Toxicology	M,D

UNIVERSITY OF CONNECTICUT HEALTH CENTER

Allopathic Medicine	D
Biochemistry	D
Biological and Biomedical Sciences—General	D*
Cell Biology	D*
Clinical Research	M
Dentistry	D,O
Developmental Biology	D
Genetics	D*
Immunology	D*
Molecular Biology	D*
Neuroscience	D*
Oral and Dental Sciences	M,D*
Public Health—General	M

UNIVERSITY OF DALLAS

Health Services Management and Hospital Administration	M,D

UNIVERSITY OF DAYTON

Biological and Biomedical Sciences—General	M,D
Physical Therapy	D
Physician Assistant Studies	M

UNIVERSITY OF DELAWARE

Adult Nursing	M,O
Biochemistry	M,D
Biological and Biomedical Sciences—General	M,D
Cancer Biology/Oncology	M,D
Cell Biology	M,D
Developmental Biology	M,D
Ecology	M,D
Entomology	M,D
Evolutionary Biology	M,D
Family Nurse Practitioner Studies	M,O
Genetics	M,D
Gerontological Nursing	M,O
Health Promotion	M
HIV/AIDS Nursing	M,O
Maternal and Child/Neonatal Nursing	M,O
Microbiology	M,D
Molecular Biology	M,D
Neuroscience	D
Nursing and Healthcare Administration	M,O
Nursing—General	M,O
Nutrition	M
Oncology Nursing	M,O
Pediatric Nursing	M,O
Physical Therapy	D
Physiology	M,D
Psychiatric Nursing	M,O
Women's Health Nursing	M,O

UNIVERSITY OF DENVER

Biological and Biomedical Sciences—General	M,D
Cell Biology	M,D
Ecology	M,D
Evolutionary Biology	M,D
International Health	M,D,O
Molecular Biology	M,D

UNIVERSITY OF DETROIT MERCY

Allied Health—General	M,D,O
Dentistry	M,D,O
Family Nurse Practitioner Studies	M,D,O
Health Services Management and Hospital Administration	M,D,O
Nurse Anesthesia	M,D,O
Nursing Education	M,D,O
Nursing—General	M,D,O
Oral and Dental Sciences	M,D,O
Physician Assistant Studies	M,D,O

UNIVERSITY OF EVANSVILLE

Health Services Management and Hospital Administration	M
Physical Therapy	D

THE UNIVERSITY OF FINDLAY

Health Services Management and Hospital Administration	M,D
Occupational Therapy	M,D
Pharmacy	M,D
Physical Therapy	M,D
Physician Assistant Studies	M,D

UNIVERSITY OF FLORIDA

Allied Health—General	M,D,O
Allopathic Medicine	D
Biochemistry	D

Biological and Biomedical Sciences—General	M,D
Botany	M,D
Cell Biology	M,D
Clinical Laboratory Sciences/Medical Technology	M,D
Clinical Research	M,D,O
Communication Disorders	M,D
Dentistry	D,O
Ecology	M,D,O
Environmental and Occupational Health	M,D,O
Epidemiology	M,D,O
Genetics	D
Health Services Management and Hospital Administration	M,D
Health Services Research	D
Immunology	D
International Health	M,D
Medical Physics	M,D,O
Medicinal and Pharmaceutical Chemistry	M,D
Microbiology	M,D
Molecular Biology	M,D
Molecular Genetics	M
Neuroscience	D
Nursing—General	M,D
Nutrition	M,D
Occupational Therapy	M
Oral and Dental Sciences	M,D,O
Pharmaceutical Administration	M,D
Pharmaceutical Sciences	M,D
Pharmacology	M,D
Pharmacy	M,D
Physical Therapy	D
Physician Assistant Studies	M
Physiology	M,D
Plant Biology	M,D
Plant Molecular Biology	M,D
Plant Pathology	M,D
Public Health—General	M,D,O
Rehabilitation Sciences	D
Toxicology	M,D,O
Veterinary Medicine	D
Veterinary Sciences	M,D,O
Zoology	M,D

UNIVERSITY OF GEORGIA

Anatomy	M
Biochemistry	M,D
Biological and Biomedical Sciences—General	D
Cell Biology	M,D
Communication Disorders	M,D,O
Ecology	M,D
Entomology	M,D
Environmental and Occupational Health	M
Genetics	M,D
Genomic Sciences	M,D
Health Promotion	M,D
Health Services Management and Hospital Administration	M
Infectious Diseases	M,D
Microbiology	M,D
Molecular Biology	M,D
Neuroscience	D
Nutrition	M,D
Pathology	M,D
Pharmaceutical Administration	D
Pharmaceutical Sciences	D
Pharmacology	M,D
Pharmacy	M,D,O
Physiology	M,D
Plant Biology	M,D
Plant Pathology	M,D
Public Health—General	D
Veterinary Medicine	M,D
Veterinary Sciences	M

UNIVERSITY OF GUAM

Biological and Biomedical Sciences—General	M
Marine Biology	M

UNIVERSITY OF GUELPH

Acute Care/Critical Care Nursing	M,D,O
Anatomy	M,D
Anesthesiologist Assistant Studies	M,D,O
Biochemistry	M,D
Biological and Biomedical Sciences—General	M,D
Biophysics	M,D
Botany	M,D
Cardiovascular Sciences	M,D,O
Cell Biology	M,D
Ecology	M,D
Emergency Medical Services	M,D,O
Entomology	M,D
Environmental Biology	M,D
Epidemiology	M,D
Evolutionary Biology	M,D
Immunology	M,D,O
Infectious Diseases	M,D,O
Medical Imaging	M,D,O
Microbiology	M,D
Molecular Biology	M,D
Molecular Genetics	M,D
Neuroscience	M,D,O
Nutrition	M,D
Pathology	M,D,O
Pharmacology	M,D
Physiology	M,D
Plant Pathology	M,D
Toxicology	M,D
Veterinary Medicine	M,D,O
Veterinary Sciences	M,D,O
Vision Sciences	M,D,O
Zoology	M,D

Biological and Biomedical Sciences—General	M,D
Botany	M,D
Cell Biology	M,D
Clinical Laboratory Sciences/Medical Technology	M,D
Clinical Research	M,D,O
Communication Disorders	M,D
Dentistry	D,O
Ecology	M,D,O
Environmental and Occupational Health	M,D,O
Epidemiology	M,D,O
Genetics	D
Health Services Management and Hospital Administration	M,D
Health Services Research	D
Immunology	D
International Health	M,D
Medical Physics	M,D,O
Medicinal and Pharmaceutical Chemistry	M,D
Microbiology	M,D
Molecular Biology	M,D
Molecular Genetics	M
Neuroscience	D
Nursing—General	M,D
Nutrition	M,D
Occupational Therapy	M
Oral and Dental Sciences	M,D,O
Pharmaceutical Administration	M,D
Pharmaceutical Sciences	M,D
Pharmacology	M,D
Pharmacy	M,D
Physical Therapy	D
Physician Assistant Studies	M
Physiology	M,D
Plant Biology	M,D
Plant Molecular Biology	M,D
Plant Pathology	M,D
Public Health—General	M,D,O
Rehabilitation Sciences	D
Toxicology	M,D,O
Veterinary Medicine	D
Veterinary Sciences	M,D,O
Zoology	M,D

UNIVERSITY OF HARTFORD

Biological and Biomedical Sciences—General	M
Community Health Nursing	M
Neuroscience	M
Nursing Education	M
Nursing—General	M
Physical Therapy	M,D

UNIVERSITY OF HAWAII AT HILO

Conservation Biology	M
Marine Biology	M
Nursing—General	D
Pharmaceutical Sciences	D*
Pharmacology	D
Pharmacy	D

UNIVERSITY OF HAWAII AT MANOA

Adult Nursing	M,D,O
Allopathic Medicine	D
Biological and Biomedical Sciences—General	M,D
Botany	M,D
Communication Disorders	M
Community Health Nursing	M,D,O
Developmental Biology	M,D
Entomology	M,D
Epidemiology	D
Family Nurse Practitioner Studies	M,D,O
Genetics	M,D
Marine Biology	M,D
Medical Microbiology	M,D
Microbiology	M,D
Molecular Biology	M,D
Nursing and Healthcare Administration	M,D,O
Nursing—General	M,D,O
Nutrition	M,D
Physiology	M,D
Plant Pathology	M,D
Public Health—General	M,D,O
Reproductive Biology	M,D
Zoology	M,D

UNIVERSITY OF HOUSTON

Biochemistry	M,D
Biological and Biomedical Sciences—General	M,D
Communication Disorders	M
Family Nurse Practitioner Studies	M
Nursing and Healthcare Administration	M
Nursing Education	M
Nursing—General	M
Nutrition	M,D
Optometry	D
Pharmaceutical Administration	M,D
Pharmaceutical Sciences	M,D
Pharmacology	M,D
Pharmacy	M,D
Vision Sciences	M,D

UNIVERSITY OF HOUSTON—CLEAR LAKE

Biological and Biomedical Sciences—General	M
Health Services Management and Hospital Administration	M

UNIVERSITY OF HOUSTON—VICTORIA

Biological and Biomedical Sciences—General	M

UNIVERSITY OF IDAHO

Biochemistry	M,D
Biological and Biomedical Sciences—General	M,D
Computational Biology	M,D
Entomology	M,D
Microbiology	M,D
Neuroscience	M,D
Veterinary Sciences	M,D

UNIVERSITY OF ILLINOIS AT CHICAGO

Acute Care/Critical Care Nursing	M,O
Adult Nursing	M,O
Allied Health—General	M,D,O
Allopathic Medicine	D
Anatomy	M
Biochemistry	D
Biological and Biomedical Sciences—General	M,D
Biophysics	M,D
Cell Biology	M,D
Community Health Nursing	M,O
Community Health	M,D
Dentistry	D
Environmental and Occupational Health	M,D
Epidemiology	M,D
Family Nurse Practitioner Studies	M,O
Genetics	D
Gerontological Nursing	M,O
Health Services Management and Hospital Administration	M,D
Health Services Research	M,D
Immunology	D
Maternal and Child/Neonatal Nursing	M,O
Microbiology	D
Molecular Biology	D
Molecular Genetics	D
Neuroscience	M,D
Nurse Midwifery	M,O
Nursing and Healthcare Administration	M,O
Nursing—General	M,D,O
Nutrition	M,D
Occupational Health Nursing	M,O
Occupational Therapy	M,D
Oral and Dental Sciences	M,D
Pediatric Nursing	M,O
Pharmaceutical Administration	M,D

Pharmaceutical Sciences	M,D
Pharmacology	D
Pharmacy	M,D
Physical Therapy	M,D
Physiology	M,D
Public Health—General	M,D
School Nursing	M,O
Toxicology	M
Women's Health Nursing	M,O

UNIVERSITY OF ILLINOIS AT SPRINGFIELD

Biological and Biomedical Sciences—General	M
Community Health	M,O
Epidemiology	M,O
Public Health—General	M,O

UNIVERSITY OF ILLINOIS AT URBANA–CHAMPAIGN

Allopathic Medicine	
Biochemistry	M,D
Biological and Biomedical Sciences—General	M,D
Biophysics	M,D
Cell Biology	D
Communication Disorders	M,D
Community Health	M,D
Computational Biology	M,D
Conservation Biology	M,D
Developmental Biology	D
Ecology	M,D
Entomology	M,D
Evolutionary Biology	M,D
Health Services Management and Hospital Administration	M,D
Microbiology	M,D
Molecular Physiology	M,D
Neuroscience	D
Nutrition	M,D
Pathobiology	M,D
Physiology	M,D
Plant Biology	M,D
Public Health—General	M,D
Rehabilitation Sciences	M,D
Veterinary Medicine	D
Veterinary Sciences	M,D
Zoology	M,D

UNIVERSITY OF INDIANAPOLIS

Biological and Biomedical Sciences—General	M
Family Nurse Practitioner Studies	M,D
Maternal and Child/Neonatal Nursing	M,D
Nurse Midwifery	M,D
Nursing and Healthcare Administration	M,D
Nursing Education	M,D
Nursing—General	M,D
Occupational Therapy	M,D
Physical Therapy	M,D
Public Health—General	M
Women's Health Nursing	M,D

THE UNIVERSITY OF IOWA

Allopathic Medicine	D
Anatomy	D
Bacteriology	M,D
Biochemistry	M,D
Biological and Biomedical Sciences—General	M,D
Biophysics	M,D
Cell Biology	M,D
Clinical Research	M,D
Communication Disorders	M,D
Community Health	M,D
Computational Biology	M,D,O
Dentistry	M,D,O
Environmental and Occupational Health	M,D,O
Epidemiology	M,D
Evolutionary Biology	M,D
Genetics	M,D
Health Services Management and Hospital Administration	M,D
Immunology	M,D
Industrial Hygiene	M,D,O
Medicinal and Pharmaceutical Chemistry	M,D
Microbiology	M,D
Molecular Biology	D
Neurobiology	M,D
Neuroscience	D
Nursing—General	M,D
Oral and Dental Sciences	M,D,O
Pathology	M
Pharmaceutical Sciences	M,D
Pharmacology	M,D
Pharmacy	M,D
Physical Therapy	M,D
Physician Assistant Studies	M
Physiology	M,D
Public Health—General	M,D,O
Radiation Biology	M
Rehabilitation Sciences	M,D
Toxicology	M,D
Translational Biology	M,D
Virology	M,D

UNIVERSITY OF JAMESTOWN

Physical Therapy	D

THE UNIVERSITY OF KANSAS

Adult Nursing	M,D,O
Allied Health—General	M,D,O
Allopathic Medicine	D
Anatomy	M,D
Biochemistry	M,D
Biological and Biomedical Sciences—General	D*
Biophysics	M,D
Botany	M,D
Cell Biology	M,D
Clinical Research	M
Communication Disorders	

Community Health Nursing	M,D,O
Computational Biology	D
Developmental Biology	M,D
Ecology	M,D
Entomology	M,D
Environmental and Occupational Health	M
Epidemiology	M
Evolutionary Biology	M,D
Gerontological Nursing	M,D,O
Health Services Management and Hospital Administration	M,D
Medicinal and Pharmaceutical Chemistry	M,D
Microbiology	M,D
Molecular Biology	M,D
Neuroscience	M,D
Nurse Anesthesia	D
Nurse Midwifery	M,D,O
Nursing and Healthcare Administration	M,D,O
Nursing—General	M,D,O
Nutrition	M,D,O
Occupational Therapy	M,D
Pathology	D
Pharmaceutical Sciences	M
Pharmacology	M,D
Physical Therapy	D
Physiology	D
Psychiatric Nursing	M,D,O
Public Health—General	M
Rehabilitation Sciences	M,D
Toxicology	M,D

UNIVERSITY OF KENTUCKY

Allied Health—General	M,D
Allopathic Medicine	D
Anatomy	D
Biochemistry	D
Biological and Biomedical Sciences—General	M,D
Clinical Research	M
Communication Disorders	M
Dentistry	D
Entomology	M,D
Epidemiology	D
Health Physics/Radiological Health	M
Health Promotion	M,D
Health Services Management and Hospital Administration	M
Immunology	D
Medical Physics	M
Microbiology	D
Neurobiology	D
Nursing—General	D
Nutrition	M,D
Oral and Dental Sciences	M
Pharmaceutical Sciences	M,D
Pharmacology	D
Pharmacy	D
Physical Therapy	D
Physician Assistant Studies	M
Physiology	D
Plant Pathology	M,D
Public Health—General	M,D
Rehabilitation Sciences	D
Toxicology	M,D
Veterinary Sciences	M,D

UNIVERSITY OF LA VERNE

Health Services Management and Hospital Administration	M,D,O
Health Services Research	M

UNIVERSITY OF LETHBRIDGE

Biochemistry	M,D
Biological and Biomedical Sciences—General	M,D
Molecular Biology	M,D
Neuroscience	M,D
Nursing—General	M,D

UNIVERSITY OF LOUISIANA AT LAFAYETTE

Biological and Biomedical Sciences—General	M,D
Communication Disorders	M,D
Environmental Biology	M,D
Evolutionary Biology	M,D
Nursing—General	M

UNIVERSITY OF LOUISIANA AT MONROE

Biological and Biomedical Sciences—General	M
Communication Disorders	M
Occupational Therapy	M
Pharmacy	D
Toxicology	D

UNIVERSITY OF LOUISVILLE

Allopathic Medicine	D
Anatomy	M,D
Biochemistry	M,D
Biological and Biomedical Sciences—General	M,D
Biophysics	M,D
Clinical Research	M,D
Communication Disorders	M,D
Community Health	M
Dentistry	M,D
Environmental and Occupational Health	M,D
Environmental Biology	M,D
Epidemiology	M,D
Family Nurse Practitioner Studies	M,D
Gerontological Nursing	M,D
Health Promotion	M,D
Health Services Management and Hospital Administration	M
Immunology	M,D
Maternal and Child/Neonatal Nursing	M,D
Microbiology	M,D
Molecular Biology	M,D
Neurobiology	M,D

Nursing and Healthcare Administration	M,D
Nursing Education	M,D
Nursing—General	M,D
Oral and Dental Sciences	M,D
Pharmacology	M,D
Physiology	M,D
Psychiatric Nursing	M,D
Public Health—General	M,D
Toxicology	M,D
Women's Health Nursing	M,D

UNIVERSITY OF MAINE

Biological and Biomedical Sciences—General	M,D
Botany	M,D
Communication Disorders	M
Ecology	M,D
Entomology	M,D
Family Nurse Practitioner Studies	M,O
Marine Biology	M,D
Microbiology	M,D
Molecular Biology	M,D
Nursing Education	M,O
Nursing—General	M,O
Nutrition	M,D,O
Plant Pathology	M,D
Zoology	M,D

UNIVERSITY OF MANAGEMENT AND TECHNOLOGY

Health Services Management and Hospital Administration	M

THE UNIVERSITY OF MANCHESTER

Biochemistry	M,D
Biological and Biomedical Sciences—General	M,D
Biophysics	M,D
Cancer Biology/Oncology	M,D
Cell Biology	M,D
Communication Disorders	M,D
Dentistry	M,D
Developmental Biology	M,D
Ecology	M,D
Environmental Biology	M,D
Evolutionary Biology	M,D
Genetics	M,D
Immunology	M,D
Microbiology	M,D
Molecular Biology	M,D
Molecular Genetics	M,D
Neurobiology	M,D
Neuroscience	M,D
Nurse Midwifery	M,D
Nursing—General	M,D
Optometry	M,D
Oral and Dental Sciences	M,D
Pharmaceutical Sciences	M,D
Pharmacology	M,D
Pharmacy	M,D
Physiology	M,D
Public Health—General	M,D
Structural Biology	M,D
Toxicology	M,D
Vision Sciences	M,D

UNIVERSITY OF MANITOBA

Anatomy	M,D
Biochemistry	M,D
Biological and Biomedical Sciences—General	M,D,O
Botany	M,D
Cancer Biology/Oncology	M
Community Health	M,D,O
Dentistry	D
Ecology	M,D
Entomology	M,D
Human Genetics	M,D
Immunology	M,D
Medical Microbiology	M,D
Microbiology	M,D
Nursing—General	M
Nutrition	M,D
Occupational Therapy	M,D
Oral and Dental Sciences	M,D
Pathology	M,D
Pharmaceutical Sciences	M,D
Pharmacology	M,D
Physical Therapy	M,D
Physiology	M,D
Plant Physiology	M,D
Rehabilitation Sciences	M,D
Zoology	M,D

UNIVERSITY OF MARY

Bioethics	M
Cardiovascular Sciences	M
Family Nurse Practitioner Studies	M,D
Health Services Management and Hospital Administration	M
Nursing and Healthcare Administration	M,D
Nursing Education	M,D
Nursing—General	M,D
Occupational Therapy	M,D
Physical Therapy	D

UNIVERSITY OF MARY HARDIN-BAYLOR

Family Nurse Practitioner Studies	M,O
Nursing and Healthcare Administration	M,O
Nursing Education	M,O
Nursing—General	M,O
Physical Therapy	D

UNIVERSITY OF MARYLAND, BALTIMORE

Allopathic Medicine	D
Biochemistry	M,D
Biological and Biomedical Sciences—General	M,D
Cancer Biology/Oncology	M,D
Cell Biology	M,D
Clinical Laboratory Sciences/Medical Technology	M

Clinical Research	M,D,O
Community Health Nursing	M
Dentistry	D,O
Epidemiology	M,D
Genomic Sciences	M,D
Gerontological Nursing	M
Health Services Research	M,D
Human Genetics	M,D
Immunology	D
Maternal and Child/Neonatal Nursing	M
Medical/Surgical Nursing	M
Microbiology	D
Molecular Biology	M,D
Molecular Medicine	M,D
Neurobiology	D
Neuroscience	D
Nurse Midwifery	M
Nursing and Healthcare Administration	M
Nursing Education	M
Nursing—General	M,D,O
Oral and Dental Sciences	M,D,O
Pathology	M
Pediatric Nursing	M
Pharmaceutical Administration	M,D
Pharmaceutical Sciences	D
Pharmacology	M,D
Pharmacy	M,D
Physical Therapy	D
Psychiatric Nursing	M
Rehabilitation Sciences	D
Toxicology	M,D

UNIVERSITY OF MARYLAND, BALTIMORE COUNTY

Biochemistry	M,D,O
Biological and Biomedical Sciences—General	M,D,O
Cell Biology	D
Epidemiology	M,O
Health Services Management and Hospital Administration	M,D,O
Molecular Biology	M,D
Neuroscience	D

UNIVERSITY OF MARYLAND, COLLEGE PARK

Biochemistry	M,D
Biological and Biomedical Sciences—General	M,D
Biophysics	D
Cell Biology	M,D
Communication Disorders	M,D
Computational Biology	D
Conservation Biology	M
Ecology	M,D
Entomology	M,D
Environmental and Occupational Health	M
Epidemiology	M,D
Evolutionary Biology	M,D
Genomic Sciences	D
Health Services Management and Hospital Administration	M,D
Maternal and Child Health	M,D
Molecular Biology	D
Molecular Genetics	M,D
Neuroscience	M,D
Nutrition	M,D
Plant Biology	M,D
Public Health—General	M,D
Veterinary Medicine	D
Veterinary Sciences	M,D

UNIVERSITY OF MARYLAND EASTERN SHORE

Physical Therapy	D
Rehabilitation Sciences	M
Toxicology	M,D

UNIVERSITY OF MARYLAND UNIVERSITY COLLEGE

Health Services Management and Hospital Administration	M,O

UNIVERSITY OF MASSACHUSETTS AMHERST

Adult Nursing	M,D
Animal Behavior	M,D
Biochemistry	M,D
Biological and Biomedical Sciences—General	M,D
Cell Biology	M,D
Communication Disorders	M,D
Community Health Nursing	M,D
Community Health	M,D
Developmental Biology	D
Environmental and Occupational Health	M,D
Environmental Biology	M,D
Epidemiology	M,D
Evolutionary Biology	M,D
Family Nurse Practitioner Studies	M,D
Genetics	M,D
Gerontological Nursing	M,D
Health Services Management and Hospital Administration	M,D
Microbiology	M,D*
Molecular Biophysics	D
Neuroscience	M,D
Nursing and Healthcare Administration	M,D
Nursing—General	M,D
Nutrition	M,D
Physiology	M,D
Plant Biology	M,D
Plant Molecular Biology	M,D
Plant Physiology	M,D
Public Health—General	M,D

UNIVERSITY OF MASSACHUSETTS BOSTON

Biological and Biomedical Sciences—General	M,D
Nursing—General	M,D

Vision Sciences — M

UNIVERSITY OF MASSACHUSETTS DARTMOUTH
Adult Nursing — M,D
Biochemistry — M,D
Biological and Biomedical Sciences—General — M
Clinical Laboratory Sciences/Medical Technology — M,D
Community Health Nursing — M,D
Health Services Management and Hospital Administration — M
Marine Biology — M
Nursing—General — M,D

UNIVERSITY OF MASSACHUSETTS LOWELL
Allied Health—General — M,D
Biochemistry — M,D
Biological and Biomedical Sciences—General — M
Clinical Laboratory Sciences/Medical Technology — M
Family Nurse Practitioner Studies — M
Gerontological Nursing — M
Health Physics/Radiological Health — M
Health Promotion — D
Nursing—General — M,D
Physical Therapy — D

UNIVERSITY OF MASSACHUSETTS MEDICAL SCHOOL
Adult Nursing — M,D,O
Allopathic Medicine — D
Biochemistry — M,D
Biological and Biomedical Sciences—General — M,D
Cancer Biology/Oncology — M,D
Cell Biology — M,D
Clinical Research — M,D
Community Health — M,D,O
Computational Biology — M,D
Family Nurse Practitioner Studies — M,D,O
Gerontological Nursing — M,D,O
Health Services Research — M,D
Immunology — M,D
Microbiology — M,D
Molecular Pharmacology — M,D
Neuroscience — M,D
Nursing and Healthcare Administration — M,D,O
Nursing Education — M,D,O
Nursing—General — M,D,O
Translational Biology — M,D

UNIVERSITY OF MEMPHIS
Biological and Biomedical Sciences—General — M,D
Communication Disorders — M,D
Environmental and Occupational Health — M
Epidemiology — M
Family Nurse Practitioner Studies — M,O
Health Services Management and Hospital Administration — M
Nursing and Healthcare Administration — M,O
Nursing Education — M,O
Nursing—General — M,O
Public Health—General — M

UNIVERSITY OF MIAMI
Acute Care/Critical Care Nursing — M,D
Adult Nursing — M,D
Allopathic Medicine — D
Biochemistry — D
Biological and Biomedical Sciences—General — M,D
Biophysics — D
Cancer Biology/Oncology — D
Cell Biology — D
Community Health — D
Developmental Biology — D
Environmental and Occupational Health — M
Epidemiology — M,D
Evolutionary Biology — M,D
Family Nurse Practitioner Studies — M,D
Genetics — D
Immunology — D
Marine Biology — M,D
Microbiology — D
Molecular Biology — D
Neuroscience — M,D
Nurse Anesthesia — M,D
Nurse Midwifery — M,D
Nursing—General — M,D
Nutrition — M
Pharmacology — D
Physical Therapy — D
Physiology — D
Public Health—General — M,D

UNIVERSITY OF MICHIGAN
Allopathic Medicine — D
Biochemistry — M,D
Biological and Biomedical Sciences—General — M,D
Biophysics — D
Biopsychology — D
Cancer Biology/Oncology — M,D
Cell Biology — M,D
Clinical Research — M
Dental Hygiene — M
Dentistry — D
Developmental Biology — M,D
Ecology — M,D
Environmental and Occupational Health — M,D
Epidemiology — M,D
Evolutionary Biology — M,D
Health Physics/Radiological Health — M,D,O

Health Promotion — M,D
Health Services Management and Hospital Administration — M,D
Human Genetics — M,D
Immunology — M,D
Industrial Hygiene — M,D
International Health — M,D
Medicinal and Pharmaceutical Chemistry — D
Microbiology — M,D
Molecular Biology — M,D
Molecular Pathology — D
Neuroscience — D
Nursing—General — M,D,O
Nutrition — M,D
Oral and Dental Sciences — M,D
Pathology — D
Pediatric Nursing — M,D,O
Pharmaceutical Administration — D
Pharmaceutical Sciences — D
Pharmacology — M,D
Pharmacy — D
Physiology — M,D
Public Health—General — M,D
Toxicology — M,D

UNIVERSITY OF MICHIGAN–FLINT
Biological and Biomedical Sciences—General — M
Family Nurse Practitioner Studies — M,D,O
Health Services Management and Hospital Administration — M
Neuroscience — D,O
Nurse Anesthesia — M,D
Nursing—General — M,D,O
Physical Therapy — D,O
Psychiatric Nursing — M,D,O
Public Health—General — M

UNIVERSITY OF MINNESOTA, DULUTH
Allopathic Medicine — D
Biochemistry — M,D
Biological and Biomedical Sciences—General — M,D
Biophysics — M,D
Communication Disorders — M
Immunology — M,D
Medical Microbiology — M,D
Molecular Biology — M,D
Pharmacology — M,D
Pharmacy — M,D
Physiology — M,D
Toxicology — M,D

UNIVERSITY OF MINNESOTA, TWIN CITIES CAMPUS
Adult Nursing — M
Allopathic Medicine — M,D
Animal Behavior — M,D
Biochemistry — D
Biological and Biomedical Sciences—General — M
Biophysics — M,D
Biopsychology — D
Cancer Biology/Oncology — D
Cell Biology — M,D
Clinical Laboratory Sciences/Medical Technology — M
Clinical Research — M
Communication Disorders — M,D
Community Health Nursing — M
Community Health — M
Conservation Biology — M,D
Dentistry — D
Developmental Biology — M,D
Ecology — M,D
Entomology — M,D
Environmental and Occupational Health — M,D,O
Epidemiology — M,D
Evolutionary Biology — M,D
Family Nurse Practitioner Studies — M
Genetics — M,D
Gerontological Nursing — M
Health Services Management and Hospital Administration — M,D
Health Services Research — M,D
Immunology — D
Industrial Hygiene — M,D
Infectious Diseases — M,D
International Health — M,D
Maternal and Child Health — M
Medical Physics — M,D
Medicinal and Pharmaceutical Chemistry — M,D
Microbiology — D
Molecular Biology — M,D
Neurobiology — M,D
Neuroscience — M,D
Nurse Anesthesia — M
Nurse Midwifery — M
Nursing and Healthcare Administration — M
Nursing—General — M,D
Nutrition — M,D
Occupational Health Nursing — M,D
Oral and Dental Sciences — M,D,O
Pediatric Nursing — M
Pharmaceutical Administration — M,D
Pharmaceutical Sciences — M,D
Pharmacology — M,D
Pharmacy — M,D
Physical Therapy — M,D
Physiology — D
Plant Biology — M,D
Plant Pathology — M,D
Psychiatric Nursing — M
Public Health—General — M,D,O
Structural Biology — D
Toxicology — M,D
Veterinary Medicine — D
Veterinary Sciences — M,D

Virology — D
Women's Health Nursing — M

UNIVERSITY OF MISSISSIPPI
Biological and Biomedical Sciences—General — M,D
Communication Disorders — M,D
Health Promotion — M,D
Nutrition — M,D
Pharmacy — M,D

UNIVERSITY OF MISSISSIPPI MEDICAL CENTER
Allied Health—General — M
Allopathic Medicine — D
Anatomy — M,D
Biochemistry — D
Biological and Biomedical Sciences—General — M,D
Biophysics — D
Dentistry — M,D
Microbiology — D
Neuroscience — D
Nursing—General — M,D
Occupational Therapy — M
Oral and Dental Sciences — M,D
Pathology — D
Pharmacology — D
Physical Therapy — M
Physiology — D
Toxicology — D

UNIVERSITY OF MISSOURI
Adult Nursing — M,D,O
Allopathic Medicine — D
Anatomy — M
Biochemistry — M,D
Biological and Biomedical Sciences—General — M,D
Communication Disorders — M,D
Community Health — M,D
Conservation Biology — M,D
Ecology — M,D
Entomology — M,D
Evolutionary Biology — M,D
Family Nurse Practitioner Studies — M,D,O
Genetics — D
Gerontological Nursing — M,D,O
Health Physics/Radiological Health — M
Health Promotion — M,O
Health Services Management and Hospital Administration — M,D,O
Immunology — D
International Health — M,O
Microbiology — D
Neuroscience — M,D,O
Nursing and Healthcare Administration — M,D,O
Nursing—General — M,D,O
Nutrition — M,D
Occupational Therapy — M
Pathobiology — M
Pathology — M
Pediatric Nursing — M,D,O
Pharmacology — M,D
Physical Therapy — D
Physiology — M,D
Plant Biology — M,D
Psychiatric Nursing — M,D,O
Public Health—General — M,O
Veterinary Medicine — M,D
Veterinary Sciences — M,D

UNIVERSITY OF MISSOURI–KANSAS CITY
Adult Nursing — M,D
Allopathic Medicine — M,D
Anesthesiologist Assistant Studies — M,D
Biochemistry — D
Biological and Biomedical Sciences—General — M,D
Biophysics — D
Cell Biology — D
Dental Hygiene — M,D,O
Dentistry — M,D,O
Family Nurse Practitioner Studies — M,D
Gerontological Nursing — M,D
Maternal and Child/Neonatal Nursing — M,D
Molecular Biology — D
Nursing and Healthcare Administration — M,D
Nursing Education — M,D
Nursing—General — M,D
Oral and Dental Sciences — M,D,O
Pediatric Nursing — M,D
Pharmaceutical Sciences — D
Pharmacology — D
Pharmacy — D
Physician Assistant Studies — M,D
Toxicology — D
Women's Health Nursing — M,D

UNIVERSITY OF MISSOURI–ST. LOUIS
Adult Nursing — M,D,O
Biochemistry — M,D
Biological and Biomedical Sciences—General — M,D,O
Family Nurse Practitioner Studies — M,D,O
Gerontological Nursing — M,D,O
Neuroscience — M,D,O
Nursing Education — M,D,O
Nursing—General — M,D,O
Optometry — D
Pediatric Nursing — M,D,O
Psychiatric Nursing — M,D,O
Women's Health Nursing — M,D,O

UNIVERSITY OF MOBILE
Nursing—General — M

UNIVERSITY OF MONTANA
Animal Behavior — M,D,O

Biochemistry — D
Biological and Biomedical Sciences—General — M,D
Cell Biology — D
Community Health — M
Developmental Biology — M
Ecology — M,D
Immunology — D
Medicinal and Pharmaceutical Chemistry — M,D
Microbiology — D
Molecular Biology — D
Neuroscience — M,D
Pharmaceutical Sciences — M,D
Pharmacy — M,D
Physical Therapy — D
Public Health—General — M,O
Toxicology — M,D
Zoology — M,D

UNIVERSITY OF MONTEVALLO
Communication Disorders — M

UNIVERSITY OF MOUNT UNION
Physician Assistant Studies — M

UNIVERSITY OF NEBRASKA AT KEARNEY
Biological and Biomedical Sciences—General — M
Communication Disorders — M

UNIVERSITY OF NEBRASKA AT OMAHA
Biological and Biomedical Sciences—General — M,O
Communication Disorders — M

UNIVERSITY OF NEBRASKA–LINCOLN
Biochemistry — M,D
Biological and Biomedical Sciences—General — M,D
Biopsychology — M,D
Communication Disorders — M,D
Entomology — M,D
Health Promotion — M,D
Nutrition — M,D
Toxicology — M,D
Veterinary Sciences — M,D

UNIVERSITY OF NEBRASKA MEDICAL CENTER
Allied Health—General — M,D,O
Allopathic Medicine — D,O
Anatomy — M,D
Biochemistry — M,D
Biological and Biomedical Sciences—General — M,D
Cancer Biology/Oncology — D
Cell Biology — M,D
Clinical Laboratory Sciences/Medical Technology — M,O
Environmental and Occupational Health — D
Epidemiology — D
Genetics — M,D
Health Promotion — D
Health Services Research — D
Microbiology — M,D
Molecular Biology — M,D
Neuroscience — D
Nursing—General — O
Nutrition — O
Pathology — M,D
Perfusion — M
Pharmaceutical Sciences — M,D
Pharmacology — D
Pharmacy — D
Physical Therapy — D
Physician Assistant Studies — M
Physiology — M,D
Public Health—General — M
Toxicology — D

UNIVERSITY OF NEVADA, LAS VEGAS
Allied Health—General — M,D,O
Biochemistry — M,D
Biological and Biomedical Sciences—General — M,D
Community Health — M,D
Dentistry — M,D
Family Nurse Practitioner Studies — M,D
Health Physics/Radiological Health — M,D,O
Health Services Management and Hospital Administration — M
Nursing—General — M,D,O
Nutrition — M,D
Oral and Dental Sciences — M,D
Physical Therapy — D
Public Health—General — M,D

UNIVERSITY OF NEVADA, RENO
Biochemistry — M,D
Biological and Biomedical Sciences—General — M
Cell Biology — M,D
Communication Disorders — M,D
Conservation Biology — D
Ecology — D
Environmental and Occupational Health — M,D
Evolutionary Biology — D
Molecular Biology — M,D
Molecular Pharmacology — D
Nursing—General — M,D
Nutrition — M
Physiology — D
Public Health—General — M,D

UNIVERSITY OF NEW BRUNSWICK FREDERICTON
Biological and Biomedical Sciences—General — M,D
Health Services Research — M
Nursing Education — M

M—masters degree; D—doctorate; O—other advanced degree; *—Close-Up and/or Display

Nursing—General — M

UNIVERSITY OF NEW BRUNSWICK SAINT JOHN
Biological and Biomedical
   Sciences—General — M,D

UNIVERSITY OF NEW ENGLAND
Biological and Biomedical
   Sciences—General — M
Dentistry — D
Nurse Anesthesia — M
Occupational Therapy — M
Pharmacy — D
Physical Therapy — D
Physician Assistant Studies — M

UNIVERSITY OF NEW HAMPSHIRE
Biochemistry — M,D
Biological and Biomedical
   Sciences—General — M,D
Communication Disorders — M
Conservation Biology — M
Evolutionary Biology — D
Family Nurse Practitioner Studies — M,D,O
Genetics — M,D
Marine Biology — M,D,O
Microbiology — M,D
Nursing—General — M,D,O
Nutrition — M,D
Occupational Therapy — M,O
Public Health—General — M,O

UNIVERSITY OF NEW HAVEN
Cell Biology — M,O
Ecology — M,O
Environmental and Occupational
   Health — M,O
Health Services Management and
   Hospital Administration — M,O
Molecular Biology — M,O
Nutrition — M,O

UNIVERSITY OF NEW MEXICO
Allied Health—General — M,D,O
Allopathic Medicine — D
Biochemistry — M,D
Biological and Biomedical
   Sciences—General — M,D
Cell Biology — M,D
Clinical Laboratory
   Sciences/Medical Technology — M,O
Communication Disorders — M
Community Health — M
Dental Hygiene — M
Epidemiology — M
Genetics — M,D
Health Services Management and
   Hospital Administration — M
Microbiology — M,D
Molecular Biology — M,D
Neuroscience — M,D
Nursing—General — M,D
Nutrition — M
Occupational Therapy — M
Pathology — M,D
Pharmaceutical Sciences — M,D
Pharmacy — D
Physical Therapy — D
Physician Assistant Studies — M
Physiology — M,D
Public Health—General — M
Toxicology — M,D

UNIVERSITY OF NEW ORLEANS
Biological and Biomedical
   Sciences—General — M,D
Health Services Management and
   Hospital Administration — M

UNIVERSITY OF NORTH ALABAMA
Environmental and Occupational
   Health — M
Health Promotion — M
Health Services Management and
   Hospital Administration — M
Nursing—General — M

THE UNIVERSITY OF NORTH CAROLINA AT CHAPEL HILL
Adult Nursing — M,D,O
Allied Health—General — M,D
Allopathic Medicine — D
Biochemistry — M,D
Biological and Biomedical
   Sciences—General — M,D
Biophysics — M,D
Biopsychology — D
Botany — M,D
Cell Biology — M,D
Communication Disorders — M,D
Computational Biology — D
Dental Hygiene — M,D
Dentistry — D
Developmental Biology — M,D
Ecology — M,D
Environmental and Occupational
   Health — M,D
Epidemiology — M,D
Evolutionary Biology — M,D
Family Nurse Practitioner Studies — M,D,O
Genetics — M,D
Gerontological Nursing — M,D,O
Health Promotion — M
Health Services Management and
   Hospital Administration — M,D
Immunology — M,D
Industrial Hygiene — M,D
Maternal and Child Health — M,D
Microbiology — M,D
Molecular Biology — M,D
Molecular Physiology — D
Neurobiology — D
Neuroscience — D
Nursing and Healthcare
   Administration — M,D,O
Nursing Education — M,D,O

Nursing Informatics — M,D,O
Nursing—General — M,D,O
Nutrition — M,D
Occupational Health Nursing — M
Occupational Therapy — M,D
Oral and Dental Sciences — M,D
Pathology — D
Pediatric Nursing — M,D,O
Pharmaceutical Administration — M,D
Pharmaceutical Sciences — M,D
Pharmacology — D
Physical Therapy — M,D
Psychiatric Nursing — M,D,O
Public Health—General — M,D
Toxicology — M,D

THE UNIVERSITY OF NORTH CAROLINA AT CHARLOTTE
Acute Care/Critical Care Nursing — M,D,O
Biological and Biomedical
   Sciences—General — M,D
Community Health Nursing — M,D,O
Community Health — M,D,O
Family Nurse Practitioner Studies — M,D,O
Gerontological Nursing — M,D,O
Health Services Management and
   Hospital Administration — M,D,O
Health Services Research — D
Nurse Anesthesia — M,D,O
Nursing and Healthcare
   Administration — M,D,O
Nursing Education — M,D,O
Nursing—General — M,D,O
Public Health—General — M,D,O

THE UNIVERSITY OF NORTH CAROLINA AT GREENSBORO
Adult Nursing — M,D,O
Biochemistry — M
Biological and Biomedical
   Sciences—General — M
Communication Disorders — M,D
Community Health — M,D
Gerontological Nursing — M,D,O
Nurse Anesthesia — M,D,O
Nursing and Healthcare
   Administration — M,D,O
Nursing Education — M,D,O
Nursing—General — M,D,O
Nutrition — M,D

THE UNIVERSITY OF NORTH CAROLINA AT PEMBROKE
Nursing and Healthcare
   Administration — M
Nursing Education — M
Nursing—General — M

THE UNIVERSITY OF NORTH CAROLINA WILMINGTON
Biological and Biomedical
   Sciences—General — M,D
Clinical Research — M,O
Family Nurse Practitioner Studies — M,O
Marine Biology — M,D
Nursing—General — M,O

UNIVERSITY OF NORTH DAKOTA
Allopathic Medicine — D
Anatomy — M,D
Biochemistry — M,D
Biological and Biomedical
   Sciences—General — M,D
Botany — M,D
Cell Biology — M,D
Clinical Laboratory
   Sciences/Medical Technology — M
Communication Disorders — M,D
Community Health Nursing — M,D
Ecology — M,D
Entomology — M,D
Environmental Biology — M,D
Family Nurse Practitioner Studies — M,D
Genetics — M,D
Gerontological Nursing — M,D
Immunology — M,D
Microbiology — M,D
Molecular Biology — M,D
Nurse Anesthesia — M,D
Nursing Education — M,D
Nursing—General — M,D
Occupational Therapy — M
Pharmacology — M,D
Physical Therapy — M,D
Physician Assistant Studies — M
Physiology — M,D
Psychiatric Nursing — M,D
Public Health—General — M,D
Zoology — M,D

UNIVERSITY OF NORTHERN BRITISH COLUMBIA
Community Health — M,D,O

UNIVERSITY OF NORTHERN COLORADO
Biological and Biomedical
   Sciences—General — M
Communication Disorders — M,D
Family Nurse Practitioner Studies — M,D
Nursing Education — M,D
Nursing—General — M,D
Public Health—General — M,D

UNIVERSITY OF NORTHERN IOWA
Allied Health—General — M,D
Biological and Biomedical
   Sciences—General — M
Communication Disorders — M
Community Health — M
Health Promotion — M

UNIVERSITY OF NORTH FLORIDA
Adult Nursing — M,D,O
Allied Health—General — M,D,O
Biological and Biomedical
   Sciences—General — M

Communication Disorders — M
Community Health — M,O
Family Nurse Practitioner Studies — M,D,O
Health Services Management and
   Hospital Administration — M,O
Nurse Anesthesia — M,D,O
Nursing and Healthcare
   Administration — M,D,O
Nursing—General — M,D,O
Nutrition — M
Physical Therapy — M,D
Public Health—General — M,O

UNIVERSITY OF NORTH GEORGIA
Family Nurse Practitioner Studies — M,O
Physical Therapy — D

UNIVERSITY OF NORTH TEXAS
Biochemistry — M,D,O
Biological and Biomedical
   Sciences—General — M,D,O
Communication Disorders — M,D,O
Health Services Management and
   Hospital Administration — M,D,O
Molecular Biology — M,D,O

UNIVERSITY OF NORTH TEXAS HEALTH SCIENCE CENTER AT FORT WORTH
Anatomy — M,D
Biochemistry — M,D
Biological and Biomedical
   Sciences—General — M,D
Community Health — M,D
Environmental and Occupational
   Health — M,D
Epidemiology — M,D
Genetics — M,D
Health Services Management and
   Hospital Administration — M,D
Immunology — M,D
Microbiology — M,D
Molecular Biology — M,D
Osteopathic Medicine — M,D
Pharmacology — M,D
Physician Assistant Studies — M
Physiology — M,D
Public Health—General — M,D

UNIVERSITY OF NOTRE DAME
Biochemistry — M,D
Biological and Biomedical
   Sciences—General — M,D
Cell Biology — M,D
Ecology — M,D
Evolutionary Biology — M,D
Genetics — M,D
Molecular Biology — M,D
Parasitology — M,D
Physiology — M,D

UNIVERSITY OF OKLAHOMA
Biochemistry — M,D
Biological and Biomedical
   Sciences—General — M,D
Ecology — D
Evolutionary Biology — M,D
Health Promotion — M,D
Health Services Management and
   Hospital Administration — M,O
Microbiology — M,D
Neurobiology — D
Plant Biology — M,D

UNIVERSITY OF OKLAHOMA HEALTH SCIENCES CENTER
Allied Health—General — M,D,O
Allopathic Medicine — D
Biochemistry — M,D
Biological and Biomedical
   Sciences—General — M,D
Biopsychology — M,D
Cell Biology — M,D
Communication Disorders — M,D,O
Dentistry — D,O
Environmental and Occupational
   Health — M,D
Epidemiology — M,D
Health Physics/Radiological Health — M,D
Health Promotion — M,D
Health Services Management and
   Hospital Administration — M,D
Immunology — M,D
Medical Physics — M,D
Microbiology — M,D
Molecular Biology — M,D
Neuroscience — M,D
Nursing—General — M
Nutrition — M
Occupational Therapy — M
Oral and Dental Sciences — M
Pathology — D
Pharmaceutical Sciences — M,D
Pharmacy — D
Physical Therapy — M
Physician Assistant Studies — M
Physiology — M,D
Public Health—General — M,D
Radiation Biology — M,D
Rehabilitation Sciences — M

UNIVERSITY OF OREGON
Biochemistry — M,D
Biological and Biomedical
   Sciences—General — M,D
Biopsychology — M,D
Ecology — M,D
Evolutionary Biology — M,D
Genetics — M,D
Marine Biology — M,D
Molecular Biology — M,D
Neuroscience — M,D
Physiology — M,D

UNIVERSITY OF OTTAWA
Allopathic Medicine — M,D
Biochemistry — M,D

Biological and Biomedical
   Sciences—General — M,D
Cell Biology — M,D
Communication Disorders — M
Community Health — M,D,O
Epidemiology — M
Health Services Management and
   Hospital Administration — M,O
Health Services Research — D,O
Immunology — M,D
Microbiology — M,D
Molecular Biology — M,D
Nursing—General — M,D,O
Public Health—General — D
Rehabilitation Sciences — M

UNIVERSITY OF PENNSYLVANIA
Acute Care/Critical Care Nursing — M
Adult Nursing — M
Allopathic Medicine — D
Biochemistry — D
Bioethics — M
Biological and Biomedical
   Sciences—General — M,D
Cancer Biology/Oncology — D
Cell Biology — D
Clinical Laboratory
   Sciences/Medical Technology — M
Computational Biology — D
Dentistry — D
Developmental Biology — D
Environmental and Occupational
   Health — M
Epidemiology — M
Family Nurse Practitioner Studies — M,O
Genetics — D
Genomic Sciences — D
Gerontological Nursing — M
Health Services Management and
   Hospital Administration — M,D
Health Services Research — M
Human Genetics — M
Immunology — D
International Health — M
Maternal and Child/Neonatal
   Nursing — M
Medical Physics — M,D
Microbiology — D
Molecular Biology — D
Molecular Biophysics — D
Neuroscience — D
Nurse Anesthesia — M
Nurse Midwifery — M
Nursing and Healthcare
   Administration — M,D
Nursing—General — M,D,O
Pediatric Nursing — M
Pharmacology — D
Physiology — D
Psychiatric Nursing — M
Public Health—General — M
Veterinary Medicine — D
Virology — D
Women's Health Nursing — M

UNIVERSITY OF PHOENIX–ATLANTA CAMPUS
Health Services Management and
   Hospital Administration — M
Nursing Education — M
Nursing—General — M

UNIVERSITY OF PHOENIX–AUGUSTA CAMPUS
Health Services Management and
   Hospital Administration — M
Nursing Education — M
Nursing—General — M

UNIVERSITY OF PHOENIX–BAY AREA CAMPUS
Gerontological Nursing — M,D
Health Services Management and
   Hospital Administration — M,D
Nursing and Healthcare
   Administration — M,D
Nursing Education — M,D
Nursing Informatics — M,D
Nursing—General — M,D

UNIVERSITY OF PHOENIX–CENTRAL VALLEY CAMPUS
Community Health — M
Health Services Management and
   Hospital Administration — M
Nursing—General — M

UNIVERSITY OF PHOENIX–CHARLOTTE CAMPUS
Health Services Management and
   Hospital Administration — M
Nursing Education — M
Nursing Informatics — M
Nursing—General — M

UNIVERSITY OF PHOENIX–COLORADO CAMPUS
Health Services Management and
   Hospital Administration — M
Nursing—General — M

UNIVERSITY OF PHOENIX–COLORADO SPRINGS DOWNTOWN CAMPUS
Health Services Management and
   Hospital Administration — M
Nursing—General — M

UNIVERSITY OF PHOENIX–COLUMBUS GEORGIA CAMPUS
Nursing—General — M

UNIVERSITY OF PHOENIX–HAWAII CAMPUS
Community Health — M
Family Nurse Practitioner Studies — M
Health Services Management and
   Hospital Administration — M

Nursing Education — M
Nursing—General — M

UNIVERSITY OF PHOENIX–HOUSTON CAMPUS
Health Services Management and
   Hospital Administration — M
Nursing—General — M

UNIVERSITY OF PHOENIX–LAS VEGAS CAMPUS
Allied Health—General — M

UNIVERSITY OF PHOENIX–NEW MEXICO CAMPUS
Health Services Management and
   Hospital Administration — M
Nursing Education — M
Nursing—General — M

UNIVERSITY OF PHOENIX–NORTH FLORIDA CAMPUS
Health Services Management and
   Hospital Administration — M
Nursing Education — M
Nursing—General — M

UNIVERSITY OF PHOENIX–ONLINE CAMPUS
Family Nurse Practitioner Studies — M,O
Health Services Management and
   Hospital Administration — M,D,O
Nursing Education — M,O
Nursing—General — M,D,O

UNIVERSITY OF PHOENIX–PHOENIX CAMPUS
Family Nurse Practitioner Studies — M,O
Gerontological Nursing — M,O
Health Services Management and
   Hospital Administration — M,O
Nursing Education — M,O
Nursing Informatics — M,O
Nursing—General — M,O

UNIVERSITY OF PHOENIX–SACRAMENTO VALLEY CAMPUS
Family Nurse Practitioner Studies — M
Health Services Management and
   Hospital Administration — M
Nursing Education — M
Nursing—General — M

UNIVERSITY OF PHOENIX–SAN ANTONIO CAMPUS
Health Services Management and
   Hospital Administration — M
Nursing—General — M

UNIVERSITY OF PHOENIX–SAN DIEGO CAMPUS
Nursing Education — M
Nursing—General — M

UNIVERSITY OF PHOENIX–SOUTHERN CALIFORNIA CAMPUS
Family Nurse Practitioner Studies — M,O
Health Services Management and
   Hospital Administration — M
Nursing Education — M,O
Nursing Informatics — M,O
Nursing—General — M,O

UNIVERSITY OF PHOENIX–SOUTH FLORIDA CAMPUS
Health Services Management and
   Hospital Administration — M
Nursing Education — M
Nursing—General — M

UNIVERSITY OF PHOENIX–UTAH CAMPUS
Nursing Education — M
Nursing—General — M

UNIVERSITY OF PHOENIX–WASHINGTON D.C. CAMPUS
Health Services Management and
   Hospital Administration — M,D
Nursing and Healthcare
   Administration — M,D
Nursing Education — M,D
Nursing Informatics — M,D
Nursing—General — M,D

UNIVERSITY OF PIKEVILLE
Osteopathic Medicine — D

UNIVERSITY OF PITTSBURGH
Acute Care/Critical Care Nursing — M,D
Allopathic Medicine — D
Bioethics — M
Biological and Biomedical
   Sciences—General — D
Cell Biology — D
Clinical Laboratory
   Sciences/Medical Technology — D
Clinical Research — M,O
Communication Disorders — M,D
Community Health — M,D,O
Computational Biology — D
Dentistry — M,D,O
Developmental Biology — D
Ecology — D
Environmental and Occupational
   Health — M,D
Epidemiology — M,D
Evolutionary Biology — D
Family Nurse Practitioner Studies — M,D
Gerontological Nursing — M,D
Health Services Management and
   Hospital Administration — M,D,O
Human Genetics — M,D,O
Immunology — D

Infectious Diseases — M,D
Maternal and Child/Neonatal
   Nursing — M,D
Microbiology — M,D
Molecular Biology — D
Molecular Biophysics — D
Molecular Genetics — D
Molecular Pathology — D
Molecular Pharmacology — D
Molecular Physiology — D
Neurobiology — D
Neuroscience — D
Nurse Anesthesia — M,D
Nursing and Healthcare
   Administration — M,D
Nursing Informatics — M,D
Nursing—General — D
Nutrition — M
Occupational Therapy — M
Oral and Dental Sciences — M,D,O
Pathology — D
Pediatric Nursing — M,D
Pharmaceutical Sciences — M,D
Pharmacy — D
Physical Therapy — M,D
Physician Assistant Studies — M
Psychiatric Nursing — M,D
Public Health—General — M,D,O
Rehabilitation Sciences — M,D
Structural Biology — D
Systems Biology — D
Virology — D
Vision Sciences — M,D

UNIVERSITY OF PORTLAND
Family Nurse Practitioner Studies — M,D
Health Services Management and
   Hospital Administration — M
Nursing Education — M,D
Nursing—General — M,D

UNIVERSITY OF PRINCE EDWARD ISLAND
Anatomy — M,D
Bacteriology — M,D
Biological and Biomedical
   Sciences—General — M
Epidemiology — M,D
Immunology — M,D
Parasitology — M,D
Pathology — M,D
Pharmacology — M,D
Physiology — M,D
Toxicology — M,D
Veterinary Medicine — D
Veterinary Sciences — M,D
Virology — M,D

UNIVERSITY OF PUERTO RICO, MAYAGÜEZ CAMPUS
Biological and Biomedical
   Sciences—General — M

UNIVERSITY OF PUERTO RICO, MEDICAL SCIENCES CAMPUS
Acute Care/Critical Care Nursing — M
Adult Nursing — M
Allied Health—General — M,D,O
Allopathic Medicine — D
Anatomy — M,D
Biochemistry — M,D
Biological and Biomedical
   Sciences—General — M,D
Clinical Laboratory
   Sciences/Medical Technology — M,O
Clinical Research — M,O
Communication Disorders — M,D
Community Health Nursing — M
Dentistry — D
Environmental and Occupational
   Health — M,D
Epidemiology — M
Family Nurse Practitioner Studies — M
Gerontological Nursing — M
Health Promotion — O
Health Services Management and
   Hospital Administration — M
Health Services Research — M
Industrial Hygiene — M
Maternal and Child Health — M
Maternal and Child/Neonatal
   Nursing — M
Microbiology — M,D
Nurse Midwifery — M,O
Nursing—General — M
Nutrition — M,D,O
Occupational Therapy — M
Oral and Dental Sciences — O
Pediatric Nursing — M
Pharmaceutical Sciences — M,D
Pharmacology — M,D
Pharmacy — M,D
Physical Therapy — M
Physiology — M,D
Psychiatric Nursing — M
Toxicology — M,D

UNIVERSITY OF PUERTO RICO, RÍO PIEDRAS CAMPUS
Biological and Biomedical
   Sciences—General — M,D
Cell Biology — M,D
Ecology — M,D
Evolutionary Biology — M,D
Genetics — M,D
Molecular Biology — M,D
Neuroscience — M,D
Nutrition — M

UNIVERSITY OF PUGET SOUND
Occupational Therapy — M,D
Physical Therapy — D

UNIVERSITY OF REDLANDS
Communication Disorders — M

UNIVERSITY OF REGINA
Biochemistry — M,D
Biological and Biomedical
   Sciences—General — M,D
Biophysics — M,D
Cancer Biology/Oncology — M,D
Health Services Management and
   Hospital Administration — M,D,O
Nursing—General — M

UNIVERSITY OF RHODE ISLAND
Acute Care/Critical Care Nursing — M,D
Biochemistry — M,D
Biological and Biomedical
   Sciences—General — M,D
Cell Biology — M,D
Clinical Laboratory
   Sciences/Medical Technology — M,D
Communication Disorders — M
Family Nurse Practitioner Studies — M,D
Gerontological Nursing — M,D
Health Services Management and
   Hospital Administration — M,D
Medicinal and Pharmaceutical
   Chemistry — M,D
Microbiology — M,D
Molecular Biology — M,D
Molecular Genetics — M,D
Nursing Education — M,D
Nursing—General — M,D
Nutrition — M,D
Pharmaceutical Sciences — M,D
Pharmacology — M,D
Pharmacy — M,D
Physical Therapy — D
Toxicology — M,D

UNIVERSITY OF ROCHESTER
Acute Care/Critical Care Nursing — M,D
Allopathic Medicine — D
Anatomy — D
Biochemistry — D
Biological and Biomedical
   Sciences—General — M,D
Biophysics — D
Clinical Research — M
Computational Biology — D
Epidemiology — D
Family Nurse Practitioner Studies — M,D
Genetics — D
Genomic Sciences — D
Gerontological Nursing — M,D
Health Services Management and
   Hospital Administration — M,D
Health Services Research — M,D
Immunology — M,D
Maternal and Child/Neonatal
   Nursing — M,D
Microbiology — M,D
Molecular Biology — D
Neurobiology — D
Neuroscience — D
Nursing and Healthcare
   Administration — M,D
Nursing Education — M,D
Nursing—General — M,D
Oral and Dental Sciences — M
Pathology — D
Pediatric Nursing — M,D
Pharmacology — M,D
Physiology — M,D
Psychiatric Nursing — M,D
Public Health—General — M
Structural Biology — D
Toxicology — D

UNIVERSITY OF ST. AUGUSTINE FOR HEALTH SCIENCES
Occupational Therapy — M,D
Physical Therapy — D

UNIVERSITY OF ST. FRANCIS (IL)
Family Nurse Practitioner Studies — M,D,O
Health Services Management and
   Hospital Administration — M
Nursing and Healthcare
   Administration — M,D,O
Nursing Education — M,D,O
Nursing—General — M,D,O
Physician Assistant Studies — M,O
Psychiatric Nursing — M,D,O

UNIVERSITY OF SAINT FRANCIS (IN)
Environmental and Occupational
   Health — M
Family Nurse Practitioner Studies — M,O
Health Services Management and
   Hospital Administration — M
Nursing—General — M,O
Physician Assistant Studies — M

UNIVERSITY OF SAINT JOSEPH
Biochemistry — M
Biological and Biomedical
   Sciences—General — M
Family Nurse Practitioner Studies — M,D
Nursing Education — M,D
Nursing—General — M,D
Nutrition — M
Pharmacy — D
Psychiatric Nursing — M,D

UNIVERSITY OF SAINT MARY
Health Services Management and
   Hospital Administration — M
Nursing and Healthcare
   Administration — M
Nursing Education — M
Nursing—General — M
Physical Therapy — D

UNIVERSITY OF ST. THOMAS (MN)
Health Services Management and
   Hospital Administration — M

UNIVERSITY OF SAN DIEGO
Adult Nursing — M,D
Communication Disorders — M
Family Nurse Practitioner Studies — M,D
Gerontological Nursing — M,D
Nursing and Healthcare
   Administration — M,D
Nursing—General — M,D
Psychiatric Nursing — M,D

UNIVERSITY OF SAN FRANCISCO
Biological and Biomedical
   Sciences—General — M
Family Nurse Practitioner Studies — D
Health Services Management and
   Hospital Administration — M
Nursing and Healthcare
   Administration — M,D
Nursing—General — M,D
Psychiatric Nursing — D
Public Health—General — M

UNIVERSITY OF SASKATCHEWAN
Allopathic Medicine — D
Anatomy — M,D
Biochemistry — M,D
Biological and Biomedical
   Sciences—General — M,D
Cell Biology — M,D
Community Health — M,D
Dentistry — D
Epidemiology — M,D
Health Services Management and
   Hospital Administration — M
Immunology — M,D
Microbiology — M,D
Nursing—General — M
Pathology — M,D
Pharmaceutical Sciences — M,D
Pharmacology — M,D
Physiology — M,D
Reproductive Biology — M,D
Toxicology — M,D,O
Veterinary Medicine — M,D
Veterinary Sciences — M,D

THE UNIVERSITY OF SCRANTON
Biochemistry — M
Family Nurse Practitioner Studies — M,D,O
Health Services Management and
   Hospital Administration — M
Nurse Anesthesia — M,D,O
Nursing and Healthcare
   Administration — M,D,O
Nursing—General — M,D,O
Occupational Therapy — M
Physical Therapy — D

UNIVERSITY OF SIOUX FALLS
Health Services Management and
   Hospital Administration — M

UNIVERSITY OF SOUTH AFRICA
Acute Care/Critical Care Nursing — M,D
Health Services Management and
   Hospital Administration — M,D
Maternal and Child/Neonatal
   Nursing — M,D
Medical/Surgical Nursing — M,D
Nurse Midwifery — M,D
Public Health—General — M,D

UNIVERSITY OF SOUTH ALABAMA
Allied Health—General — M,D
Allopathic Medicine — D
Biological and Biomedical
   Sciences—General — M,D
Communication Disorders — M,D
Environmental and Occupational
   Health — M
Nursing and Healthcare
   Administration — M,D,O
Nursing Education — M,D,O
Nursing—General — M,D,O
Occupational Therapy — M
Physical Therapy — D
Physician Assistant Studies — M
Toxicology — M

UNIVERSITY OF SOUTH CAROLINA
Acute Care/Critical Care Nursing — M,O
Adult Nursing — M
Allopathic Medicine — D
Biochemistry — M,D
Biological and Biomedical
   Sciences—General — M,D,O
Cell Biology — M,D
Communication Disorders — M,D
Community Health Nursing — M
Developmental Biology — M,D
Ecology — M,D
Environmental and Occupational
   Health — M,D
Epidemiology — M,D
Evolutionary Biology — M,D
Family Nurse Practitioner Studies — M
Health Promotion — M,D,O
Health Services Management and
   Hospital Administration — M,D
Industrial Hygiene — M,D
Medical/Surgical Nursing — M
Molecular Biology — M,D
Nurse Anesthesia — M
Nursing and Healthcare
   Administration — M
Nursing—General — M,O
Pediatric Nursing — M
Pharmaceutical Sciences — M,D
Pharmacy — D

M—masters degree; D—doctorate; O—other advanced degree; *—Close-Up and/or Display

Psychiatric Nursing — M,O
Public Health—General — M
Rehabilitation Sciences — M,O
Women's Health Nursing — M

THE UNIVERSITY OF SOUTH DAKOTA
Allied Health—General — M,D,O
Allopathic Medicine — D
Biological and Biomedical Sciences—General — M,D
Cardiovascular Sciences — M,D
Cell Biology — M,D
Communication Disorders — M,D
Health Services Management and Hospital Administration — M
Immunology — M,D
Microbiology — M,D
Molecular Biology — M,D
Neuroscience — M,D
Occupational Therapy — M,D
Pharmacology — M,D
Physical Therapy — D
Physician Assistant Studies — M
Physiology — M,D

UNIVERSITY OF SOUTHERN CALIFORNIA
Allopathic Medicine — D
Biochemistry — M
Biological and Biomedical Sciences—General — M,D,O
Biophysics — M
Cancer Biology/Oncology — D
Cell Biology — M,D
Clinical Research — M,D,O
Computational Biology — D
Dentistry — D
Developmental Biology — D
Environmental and Occupational Health — M
Environmental Biology — M,D
Epidemiology — M,D
Evolutionary Biology — D
Genomic Sciences — D
Health Promotion — M
Health Services Management and Hospital Administration — M,O
Health Services Research — D
Immunology — M
International Health — M,O
Marine Biology — M,D
Medical Imaging — M,D
Medical Microbiology — D
Microbiology — M
Molecular Biology — M,D
Molecular Pharmacology — M,D
Neurobiology — D
Neuroscience — M,D
Occupational Therapy — M,D
Oral and Dental Sciences — M,D,O
Pathology — M,D
Pharmaceutical Administration — M
Pharmaceutical Sciences — M,D,O
Pharmacy — D
Physical Therapy — M,D
Physician Assistant Studies — M
Physiology — M
Public Health—General — M,D
Toxicology — M,D

UNIVERSITY OF SOUTHERN INDIANA
Health Services Management and Hospital Administration — M
Nursing—General — M,D
Occupational Therapy — M

UNIVERSITY OF SOUTHERN MAINE
Adult Nursing — M,D,O
Biological and Biomedical Sciences—General — M
Family Nurse Practitioner Studies — M,D
Gerontological Nursing — M,D,O
Health Services Management and Hospital Administration — M
Immunology — M
Molecular Biology — M
Nursing and Healthcare Administration — M,D,O
Nursing Education — M,D,O
Nursing—General — M,D,O
Occupational Therapy — M
Psychiatric Nursing — M,D,O
Public Health—General — M,O

UNIVERSITY OF SOUTHERN MISSISSIPPI
Biochemistry — M
Biological and Biomedical Sciences—General — M,D
Clinical Laboratory Sciences/Medical Technology — M
Communication Disorders — M,D
Environmental Biology — M,D
Epidemiology — M,D
Family Nurse Practitioner Studies — M,D,O
Health Services Management and Hospital Administration — M
Marine Biology — M,D
Maternal and Child/Neonatal Nursing — M,D,O
Microbiology — M,D
Molecular Biology — M,D
Nursing—General — M,D,O
Nutrition — M,D
Psychiatric Nursing — M,D,O
Public Health—General — M,D

UNIVERSITY OF SOUTH FLORIDA
Acute Care/Critical Care Nursing — M,D,O
Adult Nursing — M,D,O
Allopathic Medicine — M,D
Anatomy — M,D
Bioethics — O
Biological and Biomedical Sciences—General — M,D
Biophysics — M,D
Cancer Biology/Oncology — M,D
Cardiovascular Sciences — O
Cell Biology — M,D
Clinical Research — M,D,O
Communication Disorders — M,D,O
Community Health — M,D,O
Computational Biology — M,D
Ecology — M,D
Environmental and Occupational Health — M,D,O
Environmental Biology — M,D
Epidemiology — M,D,O
Evolutionary Biology — M,D
Family Nurse Practitioner Studies — M,D,O
Gerontological Nursing — M,D,O
Health Services Management and Hospital Administration — M,D,O
Immunology — M,D
International Health — M,D,O
Maternal and Child Health — O
Medical Microbiology — M,D
Medical Physics — M,D
Microbiology — M,D
Molecular Biology — M,D
Molecular Medicine — M,D
Molecular Pharmacology — M,D
Neuroscience — M,D,O
Nurse Anesthesia — M,D,O
Nursing and Healthcare Administration — M,D,O
Nursing Education — M,D,O
Nursing—General — M,D,O
Nutrition — M,D,O
Occupational Health Nursing — M,D,O
Oncology Nursing — M,D,O
Pathology — M,D
Pediatric Nursing — M,D,O
Pharmaceutical Sciences — M,D
Pharmacology — M,D
Pharmacy — M,D,O
Physical Therapy — D
Physiology — M,D
Public Health—General — M,D,O*
Rehabilitation Sciences — D

THE UNIVERSITY OF TAMPA
Adult Nursing — M
Family Nurse Practitioner Studies — M
Nursing—General — M
Nutrition — M

THE UNIVERSITY OF TENNESSEE
Anatomy — M,D
Animal Behavior — M,D
Biochemistry — M,D
Bioethics — M,D
Biological and Biomedical Sciences—General — M,D
Communication Disorders — M,D,O
Community Health — M,D
Ecology — M,D
Entomology — M,D
Evolutionary Biology — M,D
Genetics — M,D
Genomic Sciences — M,D
Health Promotion — M
Health Services Management and Hospital Administration — M
Microbiology — M,D
Nursing—General — M,D
Nutrition — M
Physiology — M,D
Plant Pathology — M,D
Plant Physiology — M,D
Public Health—General — M
Veterinary Medicine — D

THE UNIVERSITY OF TENNESSEE AT CHATTANOOGA
Family Nurse Practitioner Studies — M,D,O
Nurse Anesthesia — M,D,O
Nursing and Healthcare Administration — M,D,O
Nursing Education — M,D,O
Nursing—General — M,D,O
Physical Therapy — D

THE UNIVERSITY OF TENNESSEE AT MARTIN
Nutrition — M

THE UNIVERSITY OF TENNESSEE HEALTH SCIENCE CENTER
Allied Health—General — M,D
Allopathic Medicine — D
Biological and Biomedical Sciences—General — M,D
Clinical Laboratory Sciences/Medical Technology — M,D
Communication Disorders — M,D
Dentistry — D
Epidemiology — M,D
Gerontological Nursing — M,D,O
Health Services Research — M,D
Nursing and Healthcare Administration — M,D,O
Nursing—General — M,D,O
Occupational Therapy — M,D
Oral and Dental Sciences — M,D
Pathology — M,D
Pharmaceutical Sciences — M,D
Pharmacology — M,D
Pharmacy — M,D
Physical Therapy — M,D
Physician Assistant Studies — M,D

THE UNIVERSITY OF TENNESSEE–OAK RIDGE NATIONAL LABORATORY
Biological and Biomedical Sciences—General — M,D
Genomic Sciences — M,D

THE UNIVERSITY OF TEXAS AT ARLINGTON
Biological and Biomedical Sciences—General — M,D
Family Nurse Practitioner Studies — M,D
Health Services Management and Hospital Administration — M
Nursing and Healthcare Administration — M,D
Nursing Education — M,D
Nursing—General — M,D

THE UNIVERSITY OF TEXAS AT AUSTIN
Adult Nursing — M,D
Animal Behavior — D
Biochemistry — D
Biological and Biomedical Sciences—General — M,D
Biopsychology — D
Cell Biology — D
Clinical Laboratory Sciences/Medical Technology — M,D
Communication Disorders — M,D
Community Health Nursing — M,D
Ecology — D
Evolutionary Biology — D
Family Nurse Practitioner Studies — M,D
Gerontological Nursing — M,D
Maternal and Child/Neonatal Nursing — M,D
Medicinal and Pharmaceutical Chemistry — M,D
Microbiology — D
Molecular Biology — D
Neurobiology — D
Neuroscience — D
Nursing and Healthcare Administration — M,D
Nursing Education — M,D
Nursing—General — M,D
Nutrition — M,D
Pediatric Nursing — M,D
Pharmaceutical Sciences — M,D
Pharmacology — M,D
Pharmacy — D
Plant Biology — M,D
Psychiatric Nursing — M,D
Toxicology — M,D

THE UNIVERSITY OF TEXAS AT DALLAS
Biological and Biomedical Sciences—General — M,D
Cell Biology — M,D
Communication Disorders — M,D
Health Services Management and Hospital Administration — M,D
Molecular Biology — M,D
Neuroscience — M,D

THE UNIVERSITY OF TEXAS AT EL PASO
Allied Health—General — D
Biological and Biomedical Sciences—General — M,D
Communication Disorders — M
Family Nurse Practitioner Studies — M,D,O
Health Services Management and Hospital Administration — M,D,O
Nursing and Healthcare Administration — M,D,O
Nursing Education — M,D,O
Nursing—General — M,D,O
Occupational Therapy — M
Physical Therapy — D

THE UNIVERSITY OF TEXAS AT SAN ANTONIO
Biological and Biomedical Sciences—General — M,D
Cell Biology — M,D
Molecular Biology — M,D
Neurobiology — M,D
Translational Biology — M,D

THE UNIVERSITY OF TEXAS AT TYLER
Biological and Biomedical Sciences—General — M
Environmental and Occupational Health — M
Family Nurse Practitioner Studies — M,D
Health Services Management and Hospital Administration — M
Nursing and Healthcare Administration — M,D
Nursing Education — M,D
Nursing—General — M,D

THE UNIVERSITY OF TEXAS HEALTH SCIENCE CENTER AT HOUSTON
Allopathic Medicine — D
Biochemistry — M,D
Biological and Biomedical Sciences—General — M,D
Cancer Biology/Oncology — M,D
Cell Biology — M,D
Dentistry — M,D
Developmental Biology — M,D
Genetics — M,D
Human Genetics — M,D
Immunology — M,D
Medical Physics — M,D
Microbiology — M,D
Molecular Biology — M,D
Molecular Genetics — M,D
Molecular Pathology — M,D
Neuroscience — M,D
Nursing—General — M,D
Public Health—General — M,D,O
Virology — M,D

THE UNIVERSITY OF TEXAS HEALTH SCIENCE CENTER AT SAN ANTONIO
Acute Care/Critical Care Nursing — M,D,O
Allopathic Medicine — M,D
Biochemistry — M,D
Biological and Biomedical Sciences—General — D
Cell Biology — M,D
Clinical Laboratory Sciences/Medical Technology — D
Clinical Research — M
Communication Disorders — M,D
Community Health Nursing — M,D,O
Dentistry — M,D,O
Family Nurse Practitioner Studies — M,D,O
Gerontological Nursing — M,D,O
Immunology — M,D
Medical Physics — D
Microbiology — M,D
Molecular Medicine — M,D
Neuroscience — D
Nursing and Healthcare Administration — M,D
Nursing Education — M,D
Nursing—General — M,D
Occupational Therapy — M,D
Pediatric Nursing — M,D,O
Pharmacology — D
Physical Therapy — M,D
Physician Assistant Studies — M,D
Psychiatric Nursing — M,D,O
Structural Biology — M
Toxicology — M

THE UNIVERSITY OF TEXAS MD ANDERSON CANCER CENTER
Genetics — M

THE UNIVERSITY OF TEXAS MEDICAL BRANCH
Allied Health—General — M,D
Allopathic Medicine — D
Bacteriology — D
Biochemistry — D
Biological and Biomedical Sciences—General — M,D
Biophysics — D
Cell Biology — D
Clinical Laboratory Sciences/Medical Technology — M,D
Community Health — M,D
Computational Biology — D
Genetics — D
Immunology — M,D
Infectious Diseases — D
Microbiology — M,D
Molecular Biophysics — M,D
Neuroscience — D
Nursing—General — M,D
Occupational Therapy — M
Pathology — D
Pharmacology — M,D
Physical Therapy — M,D
Physician Assistant Studies — M
Physiology — D
Public Health—General — M
Rehabilitation Sciences — M,D
Structural Biology — D
Toxicology — M,D
Virology — D

THE UNIVERSITY OF TEXAS OF THE PERMIAN BASIN
Biological and Biomedical Sciences—General — M

THE UNIVERSITY OF TEXAS RIO GRANDE VALLEY
Adult Nursing — M
Allopathic Medicine — D
Biological and Biomedical Sciences—General — M
Communication Disorders — M
Family Nurse Practitioner Studies — M
Nursing—General — M
Occupational Therapy — M

THE UNIVERSITY OF TEXAS SOUTHWESTERN MEDICAL CENTER
Allopathic Medicine — D
Biochemistry — D
Biological and Biomedical Sciences—General — M,D
Cancer Biology/Oncology — D
Cell Biology — D
Developmental Biology — D
Genetics — D
Immunology — D
Microbiology — D
Molecular Biophysics — D
Neuroscience — D
Nutrition — M
Physical Therapy — D
Physician Assistant Studies — M

UNIVERSITY OF THE CUMBERLANDS
Physician Assistant Studies — M

UNIVERSITY OF THE DISTRICT OF COLUMBIA
Cancer Biology/Oncology — M
Communication Disorders — M
Nutrition — M

UNIVERSITY OF THE INCARNATE WORD
Biological and Biomedical Sciences—General — M
Health Promotion — M
Health Services Management and Hospital Administration — M
Nursing and Healthcare Administration — M,D
Nursing—General — M,D
Nutrition — M
Optometry — D
Pharmacy — D

UNIVERSITY OF THE PACIFIC
Biological and Biomedical Sciences—General — M
Communication Disorders — M
Dentistry — M,D,O
Pharmaceutical Sciences — M,D
Pharmacy — D
Physical Therapy — M,D

UNIVERSITY OF THE SACRED HEART
Environmental and Occupational Health	M
Occupational Health Nursing	M

UNIVERSITY OF THE SCIENCES
Biochemistry	M,D
Cell Biology	M
Health Services Management and Hospital Administration	M,D
Medicinal and Pharmaceutical Chemistry	M,D
Occupational Therapy	M,D
Pharmaceutical Administration	M
Pharmaceutical Sciences	M,D
Pharmacology	M,D
Pharmacy	D
Physical Therapy	D
Physician Assistant Studies	M
Public Health—General	M
Toxicology	M,D

THE UNIVERSITY OF TOLEDO
Biochemistry	M,D
Biological and Biomedical Sciences—General	M,D,O
Cancer Biology/Oncology	M,D
Cardiovascular Sciences	M,D
Communication Disorders	M,D
Community Health Nursing	M,O
Ecology	M,D
Environmental and Occupational Health	M,O
Epidemiology	M,O
Family Nurse Practitioner Studies	M,O
Genomic Sciences	M,O
Health Promotion	M,D,O
Health Services Management and Hospital Administration	M,O
Immunology	M,D
Industrial Hygiene	M,O
International Health	M,O
Medical Physics	M,D
Medicinal and Pharmaceutical Chemistry	M,D
Neuroscience	M,D
Nursing and Healthcare Administration	M,O
Nursing Education	M,O
Nursing—General	M,D,O
Nutrition	M,O
Occupational Therapy	M,D
Oral and Dental Sciences	M
Pathology	M,O
Pediatric Nursing	M,O
Pharmaceutical Administration	M
Pharmaceutical Sciences	M
Pharmacology	M,D
Physical Therapy	M,D
Physician Assistant Studies	M
Public Health—General	M,O

UNIVERSITY OF TORONTO
Allopathic Medicine	M,D
Biochemistry	M,D
Bioethics	M,D
Biophysics	M,D
Cell Biology	M,D
Communication Disorders	M,D
Community Health	M,D
Dentistry	D
Ecology	M,D
Environmental and Occupational Health	M,D
Epidemiology	M,D
Evolutionary Biology	M,D
Health Physics/Radiological Health	M,D
Health Promotion	M,D
Health Services Management and Hospital Administration	M
Immunology	M,D
Molecular Genetics	M,D
Nursing—General	M,D
Nutrition	M,D
Occupational Therapy	M
Oral and Dental Sciences	M,D
Pathobiology	M,D
Pharmaceutical Sciences	M,D
Pharmacology	M,D
Physical Therapy	M
Physiology	M,D
Public Health—General	M,D
Rehabilitation Sciences	M,D
Systems Biology	M,D

THE UNIVERSITY OF TULSA
Biochemistry	M
Biological and Biomedical Sciences—General	M,D
Communication Disorders	M

UNIVERSITY OF UTAH
Allopathic Medicine	D
Anatomy	D
Biochemistry	M,D
Biological and Biomedical Sciences—General	M,D,O
Cancer Biology/Oncology	M,D
Clinical Laboratory Sciences/Medical Technology	M
Communication Disorders	D
Dentistry	D
Gerontological Nursing	M,O
Health Promotion	M,D
Health Services Management and Hospital Administration	M,D
Health Services Research	M,D
Human Genetics	M,D
Medical Physics	M,D
Medicinal and Pharmaceutical Chemistry	M,D
Molecular Biology	D

UNIVERSITY OF VERMONT
Neurobiology	D
Neuroscience	D
Nursing—General	M,D
Nutrition	M,D
Occupational Therapy	M,D
Pathology	M,D
Pharmaceutical Administration	M,D
Pharmaceutical Sciences	M,D
Pharmacology	D
Pharmacy	D
Physical Therapy	D
Physician Assistant Studies	M
Physiology	M,D
Public Health—General	M,D
Rehabilitation Sciences	D
Toxicology	D

UNIVERSITY OF VERMONT
Allied Health—General	M,D
Biological and Biomedical Sciences—General	M,D,O
Cell Biology	D
Clinical Laboratory Sciences/Medical Technology	M,D,O
Communication Disorders	M
Molecular Biology	D
Neuroscience	D
Nursing—General	M,D
Nutrition	M,D
Pathology	M
Pharmacology	M,D
Physical Therapy	D
Plant Biology	M,D

UNIVERSITY OF VICTORIA
Biochemistry	M,D
Biological and Biomedical Sciences—General	M,D
Family Nurse Practitioner Studies	M,D
Medical Physics	M,D
Microbiology	M,D
Nursing and Healthcare Administration	M,D
Nursing Education	M,D
Nursing—General	M,D

UNIVERSITY OF VIRGINIA
Acute Care/Critical Care Nursing	M,D
Allopathic Medicine	M,D
Biochemistry	D
Biological and Biomedical Sciences—General	M,D
Biophysics	M,D
Cell Biology	D
Clinical Research	M
Communication Disorders	M
Community Health	M,D
Health Services Management and Hospital Administration	M
Health Services Research	M
Microbiology	D
Molecular Genetics	D
Molecular Physiology	M,D
Neuroscience	D
Nursing and Healthcare Administration	M,D
Nursing—General	M,D
Pathology	D
Pharmacology	D
Physiology	D
Psychiatric Nursing	M,D
Public Health—General	M,D

UNIVERSITY OF WASHINGTON
Allopathic Medicine	D
Animal Behavior	D
Bacteriology	D
Biochemistry	D
Bioethics	M
Biological and Biomedical Sciences—General	M,D
Biophysics	D
Cell Biology	D*
Clinical Laboratory Sciences/Medical Technology	M
Clinical Research	M,D
Communication Disorders	M,D
Community Health	D
Dentistry	D
Ecology	M,D
Environmental and Occupational Health	M,D
Epidemiology	M,D
Genetics	M,D
Genomic Sciences	D
Health Services Management and Hospital Administration	M
Health Services Research	M,D
Immunology	D
International Health	M,D
Maternal and Child Health	M,D
Medicinal and Pharmaceutical Chemistry	D
Microbiology	D
Molecular Biology	D
Molecular Medicine	D
Neurobiology	D
Nursing—General	M,D,O
Nutrition	M,D
Occupational Therapy	M,D
Oral and Dental Sciences	M,D,O
Parasitology	D
Pathobiology	D
Pathology	D
Pharmaceutical Sciences	D
Pharmacology	D
Pharmacy	M,D
Physical Therapy	M,D
Physiology	D
Public Health—General	M
Rehabilitation Sciences	M,D
Structural Biology	D

UNIVERSITY OF WASHINGTON, BOTHELL
Nursing—General	M

UNIVERSITY OF WASHINGTON, TACOMA
Community Health Nursing	M
Nursing and Healthcare Administration	M
Nursing Education	M
Nursing—General	M

UNIVERSITY OF WATERLOO
Biochemistry	M,D
Biological and Biomedical Sciences—General	M,D
Optometry	M,D
Public Health—General	M,D
Vision Sciences	M,D

THE UNIVERSITY OF WESTERN ONTARIO
Allopathic Medicine	M,D
Anatomy	M,D
Biochemistry	M,D
Biological and Biomedical Sciences—General	M,D
Biophysics	M,D
Cell Biology	M,D
Communication Disorders	M
Dentistry	D
Epidemiology	M,D
Health Services Management and Hospital Administration	M,D
Immunology	M,D
Microbiology	M,D
Neuroscience	M,D
Nursing—General	M
Occupational Therapy	M
Oral and Dental Sciences	M
Pathology	M,D
Physical Therapy	M,O
Physiology	M,D

UNIVERSITY OF WESTERN STATES
Chiropractic	D*

UNIVERSITY OF WEST FLORIDA
Biochemistry	M
Biological and Biomedical Sciences—General	M
Community Health	M
Environmental and Occupational Health	M
Environmental Biology	M
Nursing and Healthcare Administration	M
Nursing—General	M
Public Health—General	M

UNIVERSITY OF WEST GEORGIA
Biological and Biomedical Sciences—General	M,O
Communication Disorders	M,D,O
Health Services Management and Hospital Administration	M,D,O
Nursing Education	M,D,O
Nursing—General	M,D,O

UNIVERSITY OF WINDSOR
Biochemistry	M,D
Biological and Biomedical Sciences—General	M,D
Biopsychology	M,D
Nursing—General	M

UNIVERSITY OF WISCONSIN–EAU CLAIRE
Adult Nursing	M,D
Communication Disorders	M
Family Nurse Practitioner Studies	M,D
Gerontological Nursing	M,D
Nursing and Healthcare Administration	M,D
Nursing Education	M,D
Nursing—General	M,D

UNIVERSITY OF WISCONSIN–GREEN BAY
Nursing and Healthcare Administration	M

UNIVERSITY OF WISCONSIN–LA CROSSE
Biological and Biomedical Sciences—General	M
Cancer Biology/Oncology	M
Cell Biology	M
Community Health	M
Medical Microbiology	M
Microbiology	M
Molecular Biology	M
Nurse Anesthesia	M
Occupational Therapy	M
Physical Therapy	D
Physician Assistant Studies	M
Physiology	M
Rehabilitation Sciences	M

UNIVERSITY OF WISCONSIN–MADISON
Adult Nursing	M
Allopathic Medicine	D
Bacteriology	M
Biochemistry	M,D
Biological and Biomedical Sciences—General	
Biophysics	D
Biopsychology	D
Botany	M,D
Cancer Biology/Oncology	D
Cell Biology	D

Ursuline College (continued)
Toxicology	M,D
Veterinary Sciences	M

Clinical Research	M,D
Communication Disorders	M,D
Community Health	M,D*
Conservation Biology	M
Ecology	M
Entomology	M,D
Environmental Biology	M,D
Epidemiology	M,D
Genetics	M,D
Gerontological Nursing	D
Medical Microbiology	D
Medical Physics	M,D
Microbiology	D
Molecular Biology	D
Molecular Pathology	D
Neuroscience	D
Nursing—General	D
Nutrition	M,D
Occupational Therapy	M,D
Pathology	D
Pediatric Nursing	D
Pharmaceutical Administration	M,D
Pharmaceutical Sciences	M,D
Pharmacology	D
Pharmacy	D
Physical Therapy	D
Physician Assistant Studies	M
Physiology	M,D
Plant Pathology	M,D
Psychiatric Nursing	D
Public Health—General	M
Toxicology	M,D
Veterinary Medicine	M,D
Veterinary Sciences	M,D
Zoology	M,D

UNIVERSITY OF WISCONSIN–MILWAUKEE
Allied Health—General	M,D,O
Biological and Biomedical Sciences—General	M,D
Cancer Biology/Oncology	M
Communication Disorders	M,O
Environmental and Occupational Health	D
Family Nurse Practitioner Studies	M,D,O
Health Promotion	M,D,O
Immunology	M
Microbiology	M
Nursing—General	M,D,O
Occupational Therapy	M,D,O
Pharmacology	M
Physical Therapy	D
Public Health—General	M,D,O
Toxicology	M

UNIVERSITY OF WISCONSIN–OSHKOSH
Adult Nursing	M
Biological and Biomedical Sciences—General	M
Botany	M
Family Nurse Practitioner Studies	M
Health Services Management and Hospital Administration	M
Microbiology	M
Nursing—General	M
Zoology	M

UNIVERSITY OF WISCONSIN–PARKSIDE
Molecular Biology	M

UNIVERSITY OF WISCONSIN–RIVER FALLS
Communication Disorders	M

UNIVERSITY OF WISCONSIN–STEVENS POINT
Communication Disorders	M,D
Health Promotion	M
Nutrition	M

UNIVERSITY OF WISCONSIN–STOUT
Conservation Biology	M
Industrial Hygiene	M
Nutrition	M

UNIVERSITY OF WISCONSIN–WHITEWATER
Communication Disorders	M
Environmental and Occupational Health	M

UNIVERSITY OF WYOMING
Botany	M,D
Cell Biology	D
Communication Disorders	M
Community Health	M,D
Computational Biology	D
Ecology	M,D
Entomology	M,D
Genetics	D
Health Promotion	M
Health Services Management and Hospital Administration	M,D
Microbiology	D
Molecular Biology	M,D
Nursing—General	M
Nutrition	M
Pathobiology	M
Pharmacy	M,D
Physiology	M,D
Reproductive Biology	M,D
Zoology	M,D

URBANA UNIVERSITY
Nursing—General	M

URSULINE COLLEGE
Adult Nursing	M,D
Family Nurse Practitioner Studies	M,D
Gerontological Nursing	M,D
Medical/Surgical Nursing	M,D
Nursing Education	M,D
Nursing—General	M,D

---

*M—masters degree; D—doctorate; O—other advanced degree; *—Close-Up and/or Display*

UTAH STATE UNIVERSITY

Biochemistry	M,D
Biological and Biomedical Sciences—General	M,D
Communication Disorders	M,D,O
Ecology	M,D
Nutrition	M,D
Toxicology	M,D
Veterinary Sciences	M,D

UTAH VALLEY UNIVERSITY

Nursing—General	M

UTICA COLLEGE

Health Services Management and Hospital Administration	M
Occupational Therapy	M
Physical Therapy	D

VALDOSTA STATE UNIVERSITY

Health Services Management and Hospital Administration	M

VALPARAISO UNIVERSITY

Health Services Management and Hospital Administration	M
Nursing Education	M,D,O
Nursing—General	M,D,O
Public Health—General	M,D,O

VAN ANDEL INSTITUTE GRADUATE SCHOOL

Genetics	D
Molecular Genetics	D

VANDERBILT UNIVERSITY

Acute Care/Critical Care Nursing	M,D,O
Adult Nursing	M,D,O
Allopathic Medicine	M,D
Biochemistry	M,D
Biological and Biomedical Sciences—General	M,D
Biophysics	M,D
Cancer Biology/Oncology	M,D
Cell Biology	M,D
Clinical Research	M
Communication Disorders	M,D
Developmental Biology	M,D
Family Nurse Practitioner Studies	M,D,O
Gerontological Nursing	M,D,O
Health Physics/Radiological Health	M,D
Health Services Management and Hospital Administration	M
Human Genetics	D
Immunology	M,D
Maternal and Child/Neonatal Nursing	M,D,O
Microbiology	M,D
Molecular Biology	M,D
Molecular Physiology	M,D
Nurse Midwifery	M,D,O
Nursing and Healthcare Administration	M,D,O
Nursing Informatics	M,D,O
Nursing—General	M,D,O
Pathology	D
Pediatric Nursing	M,D,O
Pharmacology	D
Psychiatric Nursing	M,D,O
Public Health—General	M
Women's Health Nursing	M,D,O

VANGUARD UNIVERSITY OF SOUTHERN CALIFORNIA

Nursing—General	M

VILLANOVA UNIVERSITY

Adult Nursing	M,D,O
Biological and Biomedical Sciences—General	M
Family Nurse Practitioner Studies	M,D,O
Health Services Management and Hospital Administration	M
Nurse Anesthesia	M,D,O
Nursing Education	M,D,O
Nursing—General	M,D,O
Pediatric Nursing	M,D,O

VIRGINIA COLLEGE IN BIRMINGHAM

Health Services Management and Hospital Administration	M

VIRGINIA COMMONWEALTH UNIVERSITY

Adult Nursing	M,D,O
Allied Health—General	D
Allopathic Medicine	D
Anatomy	D,O
Biochemistry	M,D,O
Biological and Biomedical Sciences—General	M,D,O
Biopsychology	D
Clinical Laboratory Sciences/Medical Technology	M,D
Community Health	M,D
Dentistry	M,D
Epidemiology	M,D
Family Nurse Practitioner Studies	M,O
Genetics	M,D
Health Physics/Radiological Health	D
Health Services Management and Hospital Administration	M,D
Health Services Research	D
Human Genetics	M,D,O
Immunology	M,D
Medical Physics	M,D
Medicinal and Pharmaceutical Chemistry	M,D
Microbiology	M,D,O
Molecular Biology	M,D
Neurobiology	D
Neuroscience	M,D,O
Nurse Anesthesia	M,D
Nursing and Healthcare Administration	M,D,O
Nursing Education	M,D,O
Nursing—General	M,D,O

Occupational Therapy	M,D
Pathology	D
Pediatric Nursing	M,D,O
Pharmaceutical Administration	M,D,O
Pharmaceutical Sciences	M,D
Pharmacology	M,D,O
Pharmacy	D
Physical Therapy	M,D
Physiology	M,D,O
Psychiatric Nursing	M,D,O
Public Health—General	M,D
Rehabilitation Sciences	D
Systems Biology	D
Toxicology	M,D,O
Women's Health Nursing	M,D

VIRGINIA INTERNATIONAL UNIVERSITY

Health Services Management and Hospital Administration	M,O

VIRGINIA POLYTECHNIC INSTITUTE AND STATE UNIVERSITY

Biological and Biomedical Sciences—General	M,D
Entomology	M,D
Genetics	M,D
Nutrition	M,D
Plant Pathology	M,D
Plant Physiology	M,D
Public Health—General	M,D,O
Veterinary Medicine	M,D,O
Veterinary Sciences	M,D,O

VIRGINIA STATE UNIVERSITY

Biological and Biomedical Sciences—General	M
Community Health	M,D

VITERBO UNIVERSITY

Health Services Management and Hospital Administration	M
Nursing—General	D

WAGNER COLLEGE

Health Services Management and Hospital Administration	M
Microbiology	M

WAKE FOREST UNIVERSITY

Allopathic Medicine	D
Anatomy	D
Biochemistry	D
Biological and Biomedical Sciences—General	M,D
Cancer Biology/Oncology	D
Genomic Sciences	D
Health Services Research	M
Human Genetics	D
Immunology	D
Microbiology	D
Molecular Biology	D
Molecular Genetics	D
Molecular Medicine	M,D
Neurobiology	D
Neuroscience	D
Pathobiology	M,D
Pharmacology	D
Physiology	D

WALDEN UNIVERSITY

Adult Nursing	M,D,O
Clinical Research	M,D,O
Community Health	M,D,O
Epidemiology	M,D,O
Family Nurse Practitioner Studies	M,D,O
Gerontological Nursing	M,D,O
Health Promotion	M,D,O
Health Services Management and Hospital Administration	M,D,O
International Health	M,D,O
Nursing and Healthcare Administration	M,D,O
Nursing Education	M,D,O
Nursing Informatics	M,D,O
Nursing—General	M,D,O
Public Health—General	M,D,O

WALLA WALLA UNIVERSITY

Biological and Biomedical Sciences—General	M

WALSH UNIVERSITY

Health Services Management and Hospital Administration	M,O
Nursing and Healthcare Administration	M,D
Nursing Education	M,D
Nursing—General	M,D
Physical Therapy	D

WASHBURN UNIVERSITY

Nursing and Healthcare Administration	M,D,O
Nursing—General	M,D,O

WASHINGTON ADVENTIST UNIVERSITY

Health Services Management and Hospital Administration	M
Nursing and Healthcare Administration	M
Nursing Education	M
Nursing—General	M

WASHINGTON STATE UNIVERSITY

Biochemistry	M,D
Bioethics	M,D,O
Biological and Biomedical Sciences—General	M,D
Biophysics	M,D
Cell Biology	M,D
Communication Disorders	M
Community Health	M,D,O
Entomology	M,D
Epidemiology	M,D
Family Nurse Practitioner Studies	M,D,O
Genetics	M,D
Health Services Management and Hospital Administration	M

Immunology	M,D
Microbiology	M,D
Neuroscience	M,D
Nursing—General	M,D,O
Nutrition	M
Pharmacy	M,D
Plant Pathology	M,D
Psychiatric Nursing	M,D,O
Veterinary Medicine	D
Veterinary Sciences	M,D

WASHINGTON UNIVERSITY IN ST. LOUIS

Allopathic Medicine	D
Biochemistry	D
Bioethics	M
Biological and Biomedical Sciences—General	D
Cell Biology	D
Clinical Research	M
Communication Disorders	M,D
Computational Biology	D
Developmental Biology	D
Ecology	D
Environmental Biology	D
Epidemiology	M,D,O
Evolutionary Biology	D
Genetics	M,D
Genomic Sciences	M
Health Services Research	M,O
Human Genetics	D
Immunology	D
International Health	M,D,O
Microbiology	D
Molecular Biology	D
Molecular Biophysics	D
Molecular Genetics	D
Molecular Pathogenesis	D
Neuroscience	D
Occupational Therapy	M,D
Physical Therapy	D
Plant Biology	D
Public Health—General	M,D,O
Rehabilitation Sciences	D
Systems Biology	D

WAYLAND BAPTIST UNIVERSITY

Health Services Management and Hospital Administration	M,D

WAYNESBURG UNIVERSITY

Health Services Management and Hospital Administration	M,D
Nursing and Healthcare Administration	M,D
Nursing Education	M,D
Nursing Informatics	M,D
Nursing—General	M,D

WAYNE STATE UNIVERSITY

Acute Care/Critical Care Nursing	D,O
Adult Nursing	D
Allopathic Medicine	D
Anatomy	D
Biochemistry	M,D
Biological and Biomedical Sciences—General	M,D
Biopsychology	D
Cancer Biology/Oncology	D
Communication Disorders	M,D
Computational Biology	M,D,O
Evolutionary Biology	M,D
Family Nurse Practitioner Studies	D
Genomic Sciences	M,D
Gerontological Nursing	D
Health Services Management and Hospital Administration	M,D
Immunology	M,D
Maternal and Child/Neonatal Nursing	M,D
Medical Imaging	M,D,O
Medical Physics	M,D
Medicinal and Pharmaceutical Chemistry	M,D
Microbiology	M,D
Molecular Biology	M,D
Molecular Genetics	M,D,O
Molecular Medicine	M,D,O
Neurobiology	M,D
Neuroscience	M,D
Nurse Anesthesia	M,O
Nurse Midwifery	M,D,O
Nursing Education	O
Nursing—General	D
Nutrition	M,D,O
Occupational Therapy	M
Pathology	D
Pediatric Nursing	M,D,O
Pharmaceutical Sciences	M,D
Pharmacology	M,D
Pharmacy	M,D
Physical Therapy	D
Physician Assistant Studies	M
Physiology	M,D
Psychiatric Nursing	M,O
Public Health—General	M,O
Toxicology	M,D

WEBER STATE UNIVERSITY

Health Physics/Radiological Health	M
Health Services Management and Hospital Administration	M
Nursing—General	M

WEBSTER UNIVERSITY

Communication Disorders	M
Health Services Management and Hospital Administration	M
Nurse Anesthesia	M
Nursing and Healthcare Administration	M
Nursing Education	M
Nursing—General	M

WEILL CORNELL MEDICINE

Biochemistry	M,D

Biological and Biomedical Sciences—General	M,D
Biophysics	M,D
Cell Biology	M,D
Computational Biology	D
Epidemiology	M
Health Services Research	M
Immunology	M,D
Molecular Biology	M,D
Neuroscience	M,D
Pharmacology	M,D
Physician Assistant Studies	M
Physiology	M,D
Structural Biology	M,D
Systems Biology	M,D

WESLEYAN UNIVERSITY

Biochemistry	D
Biological and Biomedical Sciences—General	D
Cell Biology	D
Developmental Biology	D
Ecology	D
Evolutionary Biology	D
Genetics	D
Genomic Sciences	D
Molecular Biology	D
Molecular Biophysics	D
Molecular Genetics	D
Neurobiology	D

WESLEY COLLEGE

Nursing—General	M

WEST CHESTER UNIVERSITY OF PENNSYLVANIA

Biological and Biomedical Sciences—General	M,O
Communication Disorders	M
Community Health	M,O
Environmental and Occupational Health	M,O
Gerontological Nursing	M,D,O
Health Services Management and Hospital Administration	M,O
Nursing Education	M,D,O
Nursing—General	M,D,O
Public Health—General	M,O
School Nursing	M,D,O

WEST COAST UNIVERSITY

Family Nurse Practitioner Studies	M,D
Health Services Management and Hospital Administration	M,D
Nursing—General	M,D
Occupational Therapy	M,D
Pharmacy	M,D
Physical Therapy	M,D

WESTERN CAROLINA UNIVERSITY

Biological and Biomedical Sciences—General	M
Communication Disorders	M
Health Services Management and Hospital Administration	M
Nursing—General	M,D,O
Physical Therapy	M

WESTERN CONNECTICUT STATE UNIVERSITY

Adult Nursing	M,D
Biological and Biomedical Sciences—General	M
Gerontological Nursing	M,D
Health Services Management and Hospital Administration	M
Nursing Education	D
Nursing—General	M,D

WESTERN GOVERNORS UNIVERSITY

Health Services Management and Hospital Administration	M
Nursing and Healthcare Administration	M
Nursing Education	M

WESTERN ILLINOIS UNIVERSITY

Biological and Biomedical Sciences—General	M,O
Communication Disorders	M
Ecology	D
Health Services Management and Hospital Administration	M,O
Marine Biology	M,O
Zoology	M,O

WESTERN KENTUCKY UNIVERSITY

Biological and Biomedical Sciences—General	M
Communication Disorders	M
Health Services Management and Hospital Administration	M
Nursing—General	M
Physical Therapy	M
Public Health—General	M

WESTERN MICHIGAN UNIVERSITY

Biological and Biomedical Sciences—General	M,D,O
Communication Disorders	M,D
Health Services Management and Hospital Administration	M,D,O
Nursing—General	M
Occupational Therapy	M
Physician Assistant Studies	M
Physiology	M
Rehabilitation Sciences	M

WESTERN NEW ENGLAND UNIVERSITY

Pharmacy	D

WESTERN NEW MEXICO UNIVERSITY

Occupational Therapy	M

WESTERN UNIVERSITY OF HEALTH SCIENCES

Allied Health—General	M,D

Biological and Biomedical Sciences—General	M
Dentistry	D
Family Nurse Practitioner Studies	M
Nursing and Healthcare Administration	M
Nursing—General	M,D
Optometry	D
Osteopathic Medicine	D
Pharmaceutical Sciences	M
Pharmacy	D
Physical Therapy	D
Physician Assistant Studies	M
Veterinary Medicine	D

WESTERN WASHINGTON UNIVERSITY

Biological and Biomedical Sciences—General	M
Communication Disorders	M

WESTMINSTER COLLEGE (UT)

Family Nurse Practitioner Studies	M
Nurse Anesthesia	M
Nursing Education	M
Nursing—General	M
Public Health—General	M

WEST TEXAS A&M UNIVERSITY

Biological and Biomedical Sciences—General	M
Communication Disorders	M
Family Nurse Practitioner Studies	M
Nursing—General	M

WEST VIRGINIA SCHOOL OF OSTEOPATHIC MEDICINE

Osteopathic Medicine	D

WEST VIRGINIA UNIVERSITY

Allopathic Medicine	D
Biochemistry	M,D
Biological and Biomedical Sciences—General	M,D
Cancer Biology/Oncology	M,D
Cell Biology	M,D
Communication Disorders	M,D
Community Health	M,D
Dentistry	D
Developmental Biology	M,D
Entomology	M,D
Environmental and Occupational Health	D
Environmental Biology	M,D
Evolutionary Biology	M,D
Genetics	M,D
Genomic Sciences	M,D
Health Promotion	M,D
Human Genetics	M,D
Immunology	M,D
Industrial Hygiene	M
Medicinal and Pharmaceutical Chemistry	M,D
Microbiology	M,D
Molecular Biology	M,D
Neurobiology	M,D
Neuroscience	D
Nursing—General	M,D,O
Nutrition	M
Occupational Therapy	M
Oral and Dental Sciences	M
Pharmaceutical Administration	M,D
Pharmaceutical Sciences	M,D
Pharmacology	M,D
Pharmacy	M,D
Physical Therapy	D
Physiology	M,D
Plant Pathology	M,D
Public Health—General	M,D
Reproductive Biology	M,D

Teratology	M,D
Toxicology	M,D

WEST VIRGINIA WESLEYAN COLLEGE

Family Nurse Practitioner Studies	M,O
Nurse Midwifery	M,O
Nursing and Healthcare Administration	M,O
Nursing Education	M,O
Nursing—General	M,O
Psychiatric Nursing	M,O

WHEELING JESUIT UNIVERSITY

Nursing—General	M
Physical Therapy	D

WICHITA STATE UNIVERSITY

Allied Health—General	M,D
Biological and Biomedical Sciences—General	M
Communication Disorders	M,D
Nursing—General	M,D
Physical Therapy	D
Physician Assistant Studies	M

WIDENER UNIVERSITY

Health Services Management and Hospital Administration	M
Nursing—General	M,D,O
Physical Therapy	M,D

WILFRID LAURIER UNIVERSITY

Biological and Biomedical Sciences—General	M
Health Promotion	M
Neuroscience	M,D

WILKES UNIVERSITY

Health Services Management and Hospital Administration	M
Nursing—General	M,D
Pharmacy	D

WILLIAM CAREY UNIVERSITY

Nursing—General	M

WILLIAM JAMES COLLEGE

Community Health	M,D,O
International Health	M,D,O

WILLIAM PATERSON UNIVERSITY OF NEW JERSEY

Biological and Biomedical Sciences—General	M,D
Communication Disorders	M,D
Nursing—General	M,D

WILLIAM WOODS UNIVERSITY

Health Services Management and Hospital Administration	M,D,O

WILMINGTON UNIVERSITY

Adult Nursing	M,D
Family Nurse Practitioner Studies	M,D
Gerontological Nursing	M,D
Health Services Management and Hospital Administration	M,D
Nursing and Healthcare Administration	M,D
Nursing—General	M,D

WILSON COLLEGE

Health Services Management and Hospital Administration	M
Nursing and Healthcare Administration	M
Nursing Education	M
Nursing—General	M

WINGATE UNIVERSITY

Pharmacy	D

WINONA STATE UNIVERSITY

Adult Nursing	M,D,O
Family Nurse Practitioner Studies	M,D,O
Nursing and Healthcare Administration	M,D,O
Nursing Education	M,D,O
Nursing—General	M,D,O

WINSTON-SALEM STATE UNIVERSITY

Family Nurse Practitioner Studies	M,D
Health Services Management and Hospital Administration	M
Nursing Education	M,D
Nursing—General	M,D
Occupational Therapy	M
Physical Therapy	D

WINTHROP UNIVERSITY

Biological and Biomedical Sciences—General	M
Nutrition	M,O

WON INSTITUTE OF GRADUATE STUDIES

Acupuncture and Oriental Medicine	M,O

WOODS HOLE OCEANOGRAPHIC INSTITUTION

Marine Biology	D

WORCESTER POLYTECHNIC INSTITUTE

Biochemistry	M,D
Biological and Biomedical Sciences—General	M,D
Computational Biology	M,D

WORCESTER STATE UNIVERSITY

Communication Disorders	M
Community Health Nursing	M
Health Services Management and Hospital Administration	M
Nursing Education	M
Occupational Therapy	M

WORLD MEDICINE INSTITUTE

Acupuncture and Oriental Medicine	M

WRIGHT STATE UNIVERSITY

Acute Care/Critical Care Nursing	M
Adult Nursing	M
Allopathic Medicine	D
Anatomy	M
Biochemistry	M
Biological and Biomedical Sciences—General	M,D
Biophysics	M
Community Health Nursing	M
Family Nurse Practitioner Studies	M
Health Promotion	M
Health Services Management and Hospital Administration	M
Immunology	M
Medical Physics	M
Microbiology	M
Molecular Biology	M
Nursing and Healthcare Administration	M
Nursing—General	M
Pediatric Nursing	M
Pharmacology	M
Physiology	M
Public Health—General	M
School Nursing	M
Toxicology	M

XAVIER UNIVERSITY

Health Services Management and Hospital Administration	M*
Nursing—General	M,D,O
Occupational Therapy	M

XAVIER UNIVERSITY OF LOUISIANA

Pharmacy	D

YALE UNIVERSITY

Allopathic Medicine	D
Biochemistry	D
Biological and Biomedical Sciences—General	D
Biophysics	D
Cancer Biology/Oncology	D
Cell Biology	D
Computational Biology	D
Developmental Biology	D
Ecology	D
Environmental and Occupational Health	M,D
Epidemiology	M,D
Evolutionary Biology	D
Genetics	D
Genomic Sciences	D
Health Services Management and Hospital Administration	M,D
Immunology	D
Infectious Diseases	D
International Health	M,D
Microbiology	D
Molecular Biology	D
Molecular Biophysics	D
Molecular Medicine	D
Molecular Pathology	D
Molecular Physiology	D
Neurobiology	D
Neuroscience	D
Nursing—General	M,D,O
Pathobiology	D
Pathology	M,D
Pharmacology	D
Physician Assistant Studies	M
Physiology	D
Plant Biology	D
Public Health—General	M,D
Virology	D

YESHIVA UNIVERSITY

Communication Disorders	M,D

YORK COLLEGE OF PENNSYLVANIA

Adult Nursing	M,D
Gerontological Nursing	M,D
Health Services Management and Hospital Administration	M
Nurse Anesthesia	M,D
Nursing and Healthcare Administration	M,D
Nursing Education	M,D
Nursing—General	M,D

YORK UNIVERSITY

Biological and Biomedical Sciences—General	M,D
Nursing—General	M

YO SAN UNIVERSITY OF TRADITIONAL CHINESE MEDICINE

Acupuncture and Oriental Medicine	M

YOUNGSTOWN STATE UNIVERSITY

Anatomy	M
Biochemistry	M
Biological and Biomedical Sciences—General	M
Environmental Biology	M
Health Services Management and Hospital Administration	M
Microbiology	M
Molecular Biology	M
Nursing—General	M
Physical Therapy	D
Physiology	M

M—masters degree; D—doctorate; O—other advanced degree; *—Close-Up and/or Display

ACADEMIC AND PROFESSIONAL PROGRAMS IN THE BIOLOGICAL AND BIOMEDICAL SCIENCES

Section 1
Biological and Biomedical Sciences

This section contains a directory of institutions offering graduate work in biological and biomedical sciences, followed by in-depth entries submitted by institutions that chose to prepare detailed program descriptions. Additional information about programs listed in the directory but not augmented by an in-depth entry may be obtained by writing directly to the dean of a graduate school or chair of a department at the address given in the directory.

Programs in fields related to the biological and biomedical sciences may be found throughout this book. In the other guides in this series:

Graduate Programs in the Humanities, Arts & Social Sciences

See *Psychology and Counseling* and *Sociology, Anthropology, and Archaeology*

Graduate Programs in the Physical Sciences, Mathematics, Agricultural Sciences, the Environment & Natural Resources

See *Chemistry, Marine Sciences and Oceanography,* and *Mathematical Sciences*

Graduate Programs in Engineering & Applied Sciences

See *Agricultural Engineering and Bioengineering, Biomedical Engineering and Biotechnology, Civil and Environmental Engineering, Management of Engineering and Technology,* and *Ocean Engineering*

CONTENTS

Biological and Biomedical Sciences—General

Acadia University, Faculty of Pure and Applied Science, Department of Biology, Wolfville, NS B4P 2R6, Canada. Offers M Sc. *Degree requirements:* For master's, comprehensive exam, thesis. *Entrance requirements:* For master's, minimum B-average in last 2 years of major. Additional exam requirements/recommendations for international students: Required—TOEFL (minimum score 580 paper-based; 93 iBT), IELTS (minimum score 6.5). *Faculty research:* Respiration physiology, estuaries and fisheries, limnology, plant biology, conservation biology.

Adelphi University, College of Arts and Sciences, Department of Biology, Garden City, NY 11530-0701. Offers MS. *Program availability:* Part-time, evening/weekend. *Degree requirements:* For master's, thesis or alternative. *Entrance requirements:* For master's, bachelor's degree in biology or allied sciences, essay, 3 letters of recommendation, official transcripts. Additional exam requirements/recommendations for international students: Required—TOEFL (minimum score 550 paper-based; 80 iBT). Electronic applications accepted. *Faculty research:* Plant-animal interactions, physiology (plant, cornea), reproductive behavior, topics in evolution, fish biology.

Alabama Agricultural and Mechanical University, School of Graduate Studies, College of Agricultural, Life and Natural Sciences, Department of Biological and Environmental Sciences, Huntsville, AL 35811. Offers biology (MS, PhD); plant and soil science (MS, PhD). *Program availability:* Evening/weekend. Terminal master's awarded for partial completion of doctoral program. *Degree requirements:* For master's, thesis optional; for doctorate, one foreign language, thesis/dissertation optional. *Entrance requirements:* For master's, GRE General Test, BS in agriculture; for doctorate, GRE General Test, master's degree. Additional exam requirements/recommendations for international students: Required—TOEFL (minimum score 500 paper-based; 61 iBT). Electronic applications accepted. *Faculty research:* Plant breeding, cytogenetics, crop production, soil chemistry and fertility, remote sensing.

Alabama State University, College of Science, Mathematics and Technology, Department of Biological Sciences, Montgomery, AL 36101-0271. Offers MS, PhD. *Faculty:* 13 full-time (4 women), 7 part-time/adjunct (4 women). *Students:* 2 full-time (0 women), 22 part-time (9 women); includes 19 minority (18 Black or African American, non-Hispanic/Latino; 1 Asian, non-Hispanic/Latino), 4 international. Average age 33. 20 applicants, 30% accepted, 1 enrolled. In 2015, 2 master's, 3 doctorates awarded. *Degree requirements:* For master's, one foreign language, comprehensive exam, thesis; for doctorate, 3 foreign languages, thesis/dissertation. *Entrance requirements:* For master's, GRE General Test, GRE Subject Test, writing competency test. Additional exam requirements/recommendations for international students: Required—TOEFL (minimum score 500 paper-based). *Application deadline:* For fall admission, 7/15 for domestic students; for spring admission, 12/15 for domestic students. Applications are processed on a rolling basis. Application fee: $25. *Expenses: Tuition, area resident:* Full-time $3087; part-time $2744 per credit. Tuition, nonresident: full-time $6174; part-time $5488 per credit. *Required fees:* $2284; $1142 per credit. $571 per semester. Tuition and fees vary according to class time, course level, course load, degree level, program and student level. *Financial support:* Research assistantships and scholarships/grants available. Financial award application deadline: 6/30. *Faculty research:* Salmonella pseudomonas, cancer cells. *Unit head:* Dr. Boakai K. Robertson, Chair, 334-229-4467, Fax: 334-229-1007, E-mail: bkrobertson@alasu.edu. *Application contact:* Dr. William Person, Dean of Graduate Studies, 334-229-4274, Fax: 334-229-4928, E-mail: wperson@alasu.edu.
Website: http://www.alasu.edu/academics/colleges—departments/science-mathematics-technology/biological-sciences-department/index.aspx

Albert Einstein College of Medicine, Graduate Division of Biomedical Sciences, Bronx, NY 10461. Offers PhD, MD/PhD. *Faculty:* 12 full-time, 17 part-time/adjunct. *Students:* 393 full-time; includes 45 minority (13 Black or African American, non-Hispanic/Latino; 24 Asian, non-Hispanic/Latino; 8 Hispanic/Latino), 101 international. Average age 25. In 2015, 37 doctorates awarded. *Degree requirements:* For doctorate, thesis/dissertation. *Entrance requirements:* For doctorate, GRE General Test. Additional exam requirements/recommendations for international students: Required—TOEFL. *Application deadline:* For fall admission, 12/15 for domestic students. Applications are processed on a rolling basis. Application fee: $75. Electronic applications accepted. *Financial support:* In 2015–16, 229 fellowships were awarded. *Unit head:* Dr. Victoria H. Freedman, Assistant Dean for Graduate Studies, 718-430-2345, Fax: 718-430-8655. *Application contact:* Salvatore Calabro, Assistant Director of Admissions, 718-430-2345, Fax: 718-430-8655, E-mail: phd@einstein.yu.edu.
Website: https://www.einstein.yu.edu/phd

Albert Einstein College of Medicine, Medical Scientist Training Program, Bronx, NY 10461. Offers MD/PhD.

Alcorn State University, School of Graduate Studies, School of Arts and Sciences, Department of Biology, Lorman, MS 39096-7500. Offers MS.

American Museum of Natural History–Richard Gilder Graduate School, Program in Comparative Biology, New York, NY 10024. Offers PhD. *Degree requirements:* For doctorate, thesis/dissertation, qualifying examination. *Entrance requirements:* For doctorate, GRE General Test (taken within the past five years); GRE Subject Test (recommended), BA, BS, or equivalent degree from accredited institution; official transcripts; essay;. Additional exam requirements/recommendations for international students: Required—TOEFL (minimum score 600 paper-based; 100 iBT), IELTS (minimum score 7).

American University of Beirut, Graduate Programs, Faculty of Arts and Sciences, Beirut, Lebanon. Offers anthropology (MA); Arab and Middle Eastern history (PhD); Arabic language and literature (MA, PhD); archaeology (MA); biology (MS); cell and molecular biology (PhD); chemistry (MS); clinical psychology (MA); computational sciences (MS); computer science (MS); economics (MA); English language (MA); English literature (MA); environmental policy planning (MS); financial economics (MAFE); geology (MS); history (MA); mathematics (MA, MS); media studies (MA); Middle Eastern studies (MA); physics (MS); political studies (MA); psychology (MA); public administration (MA); sociology (MA); statistics (MA, MS); theoretical physics (PhD); transnational American studies (MA). *Program availability:* Part-time. *Faculty:* 114 full-time (36 women), 4 part-time/adjunct (2 women). *Students:* 258 full-time (190 women), 207 part-time (142 women). Average age 27. 241 applicants, 71% accepted, 98 enrolled. In 2015, 47 master's, 3 doctorates awarded. *Degree requirements:* For master's, one foreign language, comprehensive exam, thesis (for some programs); for doctorate, one foreign language, comprehensive exam, thesis/dissertation. *Entrance requirements:* For master's, GRE (for some MA, MS programs), letter of recommendation; for doctorate, GRE, letters of recommendation. Additional exam requirements/recommendations for international students: Required—TOEFL (minimum score 600 paper-based; 97 iBT), IELTS (minimum score 7). *Application deadline:* For fall admission, 4/1 for domestic and international students; for spring admission, 11/1 for

domestic and international students. Application fee: $50. Electronic applications accepted. *Expenses: Tuition, area resident:* Full-time $16,254; part-time $903 per credit. *Required fees:* $699. Tuition and fees vary according to course load and program. *Financial support:* Research assistantships, career-related internships or fieldwork, institutionally sponsored loans, scholarships/grants, health care benefits, and unspecified assistantships available. Financial award application deadline: 2/4; financial award applicants required to submit FAFSA. *Faculty research:* Analysis and algebra; software engineering; machine learning and big data analysis; philosophy of mind and political philosophy; anthropology of art, anthropology of migration and medical anthropology; sociology of knowledge, sociology of migration, critical theory; sociology of education; hybrid solid materials; photocatalysis; human creativity. *Total annual research expenditures:* $680,360. *Unit head:* Dr. Patrick McGreevy, Dean, 961-1374374 Ext. 3800, Fax: 961-1744461, E-mail: pm07@aub.edu.lb. *Application contact:* Dr. Salim Kanaan, Director, Admissions Office, 961-1350000 Ext. 2590, Fax: 961-1750775, E-mail: sk00@aub.edu.lb.
Website: http://www.aub.edu.lb/fas/

American University of Beirut, Graduate Programs, Faculty of Medicine, Beirut, Lebanon. Offers anatomy, cell biology and human morphology (MS); biochemistry and medical genetics (MS); biomedical sciences (PhD); experimental pathology, immunology and microbiology (MS); medicine (MD); neuroscience (MS); pharmacology and toxicology (MS). *Program availability:* Part-time. *Faculty:* 302 full-time (95 women), 64 part-time/adjunct (11 women). *Students:* 381 full-time (173 women), 61 part-time (51 women). Average age 23. In 2015, 14 master's awarded. *Degree requirements:* For master's, one foreign language, comprehensive exam, thesis (for some programs); for doctorate, one foreign language, comprehensive exam, thesis/dissertation. *Entrance requirements:* For master's, letter of recommendation; for doctorate, MCAT, bachelor's degree. Additional exam requirements/recommendations for international students: Required—TOEFL (minimum score 600 paper-based; 100 iBT), IELTS (minimum score 7.5). *Application deadline:* For fall admission, 4/30 for domestic and international students; for spring admission, 11/1 for domestic and international students. Application fee: $50. Electronic applications accepted. *Expenses: Tuition, area resident:* Full-time $16,254; part-time $903 per credit. *Required fees:* $699. Tuition and fees vary according to course load and program. *Financial support:* In 2015–16, 273 students received support, including 45 teaching assistantships (averaging $9,000 per year); career-related internships or fieldwork, institutionally sponsored loans, scholarships/grants, health care benefits, and unspecified assistantships also available. Financial award application deadline: 2/2. *Faculty research:* Cancer research (targeted therapy, mechanisms of leukemogenesis, tumor cell extravasation and metastasis, cancer stem cells), stem cell research (regenerative medicine, drug discovery), genetic research (neurogenetics, hereditary cardiomyopathy, hemoglobinopathies, pharmacogenomics, proteomics), neuroscience research (pain, neurodegenerative disorder), metabolism (inflammation and metabolism, metabolic disorder, diabetes mellitus), vascular and renal biology, signal transduction. *Total annual research expenditures:* $2.6 million. *Unit head:* Dr. Mohamed Sayegh, Dean, 961-1350000 Ext. 4700, Fax: 961-1744464, E-mail: msayegh@aub.edu.lb. *Application contact:* Dr. Salim Kanaan, Director, Admissions Office, 961-1350000 Ext. 2594, Fax: 961-1750775, E-mail: sk00@aub.edu.lb.
Website: http://www.aub.edu.lb/fm/fm_home/Pages/index.aspx

Andrews University, School of Graduate Studies, College of Arts and Sciences, Department of Biology, Berrien Springs, MI 49104. Offers MAT, MS. *Faculty:* 7 full-time (3 women). *Students:* 6 full-time (all women), 2 international. Average age 30. 7 applicants, 43% accepted, 3 enrolled. In 2015, 2 master's awarded. *Degree requirements:* For master's, comprehensive exam, thesis. *Entrance requirements:* For master's, GRE Subject Test. Additional exam requirements/recommendations for international students: Required—TOEFL (minimum score 550 paper-based). *Application deadline:* Applications are processed on a rolling basis. Application fee: $40. *Financial support:* Fellowships, research assistantships, teaching assistantships, career-related internships or fieldwork, Federal Work-Study, and institutionally sponsored loans available. Financial award application deadline: 3/15. *Faculty research:* Manatee habitat characterization, seabird habitat dynamics. *Unit head:* Dr. Thomas Goodwin, Chairman, 269-471-3243. *Application contact:* Monica Wringer, Supervisor of Graduate Admission, 800-253-2874, Fax: 269-471-6321, E-mail: graduate@andrews.edu.

Angelo State University, College of Graduate Studies, College of Arts and Sciences, Department of Biology, San Angelo, TX 76909. Offers MS. *Program availability:* Part-time, evening/weekend. *Degree requirements:* For master's, comprehensive exam, thesis optional. *Entrance requirements:* For master's, GRE General Test, essay. Additional exam requirements/recommendations for international students: Required—TOEFL or IELTS. *Application deadline:* For fall admission, 7/15 priority date for domestic students, 6/10 for international students; for spring admission, 12/1 priority date for domestic students, 11/1 for international students. Applications are processed on a rolling basis. Application fee: $40 ($50 for international students). Electronic applications accepted. *Expenses: Tuition, area resident:* Full-time $3726; part-time $2484 per year. Tuition, state resident: full-time $3726; part-time $2484 per year. Tuition, nonresident: full-time $10,746; part-time $7164 per year. International tuition: $10,746 full-time. *Required fees:* $2538; $1702 per unit. *Financial support:* Research assistantships, teaching assistantships, career-related internships or fieldwork, Federal Work-Study, scholarships/grants, and unspecified assistantships available. Support available to part-time students. Financial award application deadline: 3/1. *Faculty research:* Texas poppy-mallow project, Chisos hedgehog cactus, skunks, reptiles, amphibians, rodents, seed germination, mammals. *Unit head:* Dr. Russell Wilke, Chair, 325-486-6638, Fax: 325-942-2184, E-mail: russell.wilke@angelo.edu. *Application contact:* Dr. Bonnie B. Amos, Graduate Advisor, 325-486-6656, Fax: 325-942-2184, E-mail: bonnie.amos@angelo.edu.
Website: http://www.angelo.edu/dept/biology/

Appalachian State University, Cratis D. Williams Graduate School, Department of Biology, Boone, NC 28608. Offers cell and molecular biology (MS); general biology (MS). *Program availability:* Part-time. *Degree requirements:* For master's, comprehensive exam, thesis. *Entrance requirements:* For master's, GRE General Test, 3 letters of recommendation. Additional exam requirements/recommendations for international students: Required—TOEFL (minimum score 570 paper-based; 79 iBT), IELTS (minimum score 6.5). Electronic applications accepted. *Faculty research:* Aquatic and terrestrial ecology, animal and plant physiology, behavior and systematics, immunology and cell biology, molecular biology and microbiology.

Arizona State University at the Tempe campus, College of Liberal Arts and Sciences, School of Life Sciences, Tempe, AZ 85287-4601. Offers animal behavior (PhD); applied ethics (biomedical and health ethics) (MA); biology (MS, PhD), including biology, biology and society, complex adaptive systems science (PhD), plant biology and conservation

(MS); environmental life sciences (PhD); evolutionary biology (PhD); history and philosophy of science (PhD); human and social dimensions of science and technology (PhD); microbiology (PhD); molecular and cellular biology (PhD); neuroscience (PhD). Terminal master's awarded for partial completion of doctoral program. *Degree requirements:* For master's, thesis (for some programs), interactive Program of Study (iPOS) submitted before completing 50 percent of required credit hours; for doctorate, variable foreign language requirement, comprehensive exam, thesis/dissertation, interactive Program of Study (iPOS) submitted before completing 50 percent of required credit hours. *Entrance requirements:* For master's and doctorate, GRE, minimum GPA of 3.0 or equivalent in last 2 years of work leading to bachelor's degree. Additional exam requirements/recommendations for international students: Required—TOEFL (minimum score 600 paper-based; 100 iBT). Electronic applications accepted.

Arkansas State University, Graduate School, College of Sciences and Mathematics, Department of Biological Sciences, State University, AR 72467. Offers biological sciences (MA); biology (MS); biology education (MSE, SCCT); biotechnology (PSM). *Program availability:* Part-time. *Faculty:* 22 full-time (7 women). *Students:* 13 full-time (5 women), 24 part-time (9 women); includes 2 minority (1 Black or African American, non-Hispanic/Latino; 1 Hispanic/Latino), 3 international. Average age 27. 42 applicants, 33% accepted, 13 enrolled. In 2015, 9 master's awarded. *Degree requirements:* For master's, comprehensive exam, thesis (for some programs); for SCCT, comprehensive exam. *Entrance requirements:* For master's, GRE General Test, appropriate bachelor's degree, letters of reference, interview, official transcripts, immunization records, statement of educational objectives and career goals, teaching certificate (for MSE); for SCCT, GRE General Test or MAT, interview, master's degree, letters of reference, official transcript, personal statement, immunization records. Additional exam requirements/recommendations for international students: Required—TOEFL (minimum score 550 paper-based; 79 iBT), IELTS (minimum score 6), PTE (minimum score 56). *Application deadline:* For fall admission, 7/1 for domestic and international students; for spring admission, 11/15 for domestic students, 11/14 for international students. Applications are processed on a rolling basis. Application fee: $30 ($40 for international students). Electronic applications accepted. *Expenses:* Tuition, state resident: full-time $4572; part-time $254 per credit hour. Tuition, nonresident: full-time $9144; part-time $508 per credit hour. *International tuition:* $9844 full-time. *Required fees:* $1188; $66 per credit hour. $25 per term. Tuition and fees vary according to course load and program. *Financial support:* In 2015–16, 19 students received support. Research assistantships, career-related internships or fieldwork, scholarships/grants, and unspecified assistantships available. Financial award application deadline: 7/1; financial award applicants required to submit FAFSA. *Unit head:* Dr. Thomas Risch, Chair, 870-972-3082, Fax: 870-972-2638, E-mail: trisch@astate.edu. *Application contact:* Vickey Ring, Graduate Admissions Coordinator, 870-972-2737, Fax: 870-972-3917, E-mail: vickeyring@astate.edu.
Website: http://www.astate.edu/college/sciences-and-mathematics/departments/biology/

A.T. Still University, Kirksville College of Osteopathic Medicine, Kirksville, MO 63501. Offers biomedical sciences (MS); osteopathic medicine (DO). *Accreditation:* AOsA. *Faculty:* 40 full-time (7 women), 32 part-time/adjunct (4 women). *Students:* 724 full-time (302 women), 7 part-time (1 woman); includes 129 minority (18 Black or African American, non-Hispanic/Latino; 2 American Indian or Alaska Native, non-Hispanic/Latino; 49 Asian, non-Hispanic/Latino; 31 Hispanic/Latino; 29 Two or more races, non-Hispanic/Latino), 3 international. Average age 26. 5,061 applicants, 8% accepted, 188 enrolled. In 2015, 12 master's, 156 doctorates awarded. *Degree requirements:* For master's, thesis; for doctorate, Level 1 and 2 COMLEX-PE and CE exams. *Entrance requirements:* For master's, GRE, MCAT, or DAT, minimum undergraduate GPA of 2.65 (cumulative and science); for doctorate, MCAT, bachelor's degree with minimum GPA of 2.8 (cumulative and science) or 90 semester hours with minimum GPA of 3.5 (cumulative and science). Additional exam requirements/recommendations for international students: Recommended—TOEFL. *Application deadline:* For fall admission, 2/1 for domestic students; for summer admission, 2/1 for domestic students. Applications are processed on a rolling basis. Application fee: $70. Electronic applications accepted. Application fee is waived when completed online. *Expenses:* Contact institution. *Financial support:* In 2015–16, 243 students received support, including 25 fellowships with full tuition reimbursements available (averaging $52,320 per year); Federal Work-Study and scholarships/grants also available. Financial award application deadline: 5/1; financial award applicants required to submit FAFSA. *Faculty research:* Practice-based research network, antibiotic resistance, staphylococcus aureus, bacterial virulence and environmental survival, excitability of the exercise pressor reflex, clinical trials. *Total annual research expenditures:* $164,130. *Unit head:* Dr. Margaret Wilson, Dean, 660-626-2354, Fax: 660-626-2080, E-mail: mwilson@atsu.edu. *Application contact:* Donna Sparks, Associate Director, Admissions Processing, 660-626-2117, Fax: 660-626-2969, E-mail: admissions@atsu.edu.
Website: http://www.atsu.edu/kcom/

Auburn University, College of Veterinary Medicine and Graduate School, Graduate Programs in Veterinary Medicine, Auburn University, AL 36849. Offers biomedical sciences (MS, PhD), including anatomy, physiology and pharmacology (MS); biomedical sciences (PhD); clinical sciences (MS); large animal surgery and medicine (MS); pathobiology (MS); radiology (MS); small animal surgery and medicine (MS); DVM/MS. *Program availability:* Part-time. *Faculty:* 97 full-time (40 women), 4 part-time/adjunct (2 women). *Students:* 19 full-time (11 women), 54 part-time (34 women); includes 10 minority (2 Black or African American, non-Hispanic/Latino; 2 American Indian or Alaska Native, non-Hispanic/Latino; 2 Asian, non-Hispanic/Latino; 4 Hispanic/Latino), 23 international. Average age 31. 39 applicants, 59% accepted, 14 enrolled. In 2015, 12 master's, 6 doctorates awarded. *Degree requirements:* For doctorate, thesis/dissertation. *Entrance requirements:* For master's, GRE General Test; for doctorate, GRE General Test, GRE Subject Test. *Application deadline:* Applications are processed on a rolling basis. Application fee: $50 ($60 for international students). Electronic applications accepted. *Expenses:* Tuition, state resident: full-time $8802; part-time $489 per credit hour. Tuition, nonresident: full-time $26,406; part-time $1467 per credit hour. *Required fees:* $808 per semester. Tuition and fees vary according to degree level and program. *Financial support:* Research assistantships, teaching assistantships, and Federal Work-Study available. Support available to part-time students. Financial award application deadline: 3/15; financial award applicants required to submit FAFSA. *Unit head:* Dr. Calvin Johnson, Acting Dean, 334-844-2650. *Application contact:* Dr. George Flowers, Dean of the Graduate School, 334-844-2125.

Auburn University, Graduate School, College of Sciences and Mathematics, Department of Biological Sciences, Auburn University, AL 36849. Offers botany (MS); zoology (MS). *Faculty:* 39 full-time (14 women). *Students:* 57 full-time (36 women), 54 part-time (29 women); includes 14 minority (5 Black or African American, non-Hispanic/Latino; 4 Asian, non-Hispanic/Latino; 2 Hispanic/Latino; 3 Two or more races, non-Hispanic/Latino), 12 international. Average age 27. 83 applicants, 43% accepted, 28 enrolled. In 2015, 10 master's, 4 doctorates awarded. *Entrance requirements:* For master's and doctorate, GRE General Test. Additional exam requirements/recommendations for international students: Required—TOEFL. Application fee: $50 ($60 for international students). Electronic applications accepted. *Expenses:* Tuition, state resident: full-time $8802; part-time $489 per credit hour. Tuition, nonresident: full-time $26,406; part-time $1467 per credit hour. *Required fees:* $808 per semester. Tuition and fees vary according to degree level and program. *Financial support:* Research assistantships and teaching assistantships available. Financial award applicants required to submit FAFSA. *Unit head:* Dr. Jack W. Feminella, Chair, 334-844-3906, Fax: 334-844-1645. *Application contact:* Dr. George Flowers, Dean of the Graduate School, 334-844-2125.

Austin Peay State University, College of Graduate Studies, College of Science and Mathematics, Department of Biology, Clarksville, TN 37044. Offers clinical laboratory science (MS). *Program availability:* Part-time. *Faculty:* 11 full-time (5 women). *Students:* 3 full-time (1 woman), 26 part-time (16 women); includes 4 minority (1 Black or African American, non-Hispanic/Latino; 3 Two or more races, non-Hispanic/Latino). Average age 26. 56 applicants, 27% accepted, 13 enrolled. In 2015, 9 master's awarded. *Degree requirements:* For master's, comprehensive exam, thesis optional. *Entrance requirements:* For master's, GRE General Test, 3 letters of recommendation, minimum undergraduate GPA of 2.75. Additional exam requirements/recommendations for international students: Required—TOEFL (minimum score 500 paper-based). *Application deadline:* For fall admission, 8/3 priority date for domestic students. Applications are processed on a rolling basis. Application fee: $25. Electronic applications accepted. *Expenses:* Tuition, state resident: full-time $8080; part-time $404 per credit hour. Tuition, nonresident: full-time $21,680; part-time $1084 per credit hour. *Required fees:* $1453; $72.65 per credit hour. *Financial support:* In 2015–16, research assistantships with full tuition reimbursements (averaging $5,184 per year) were awarded; career-related internships or fieldwork, Federal Work-Study, institutionally sponsored loans, scholarships/grants, and unspecified assistantships also available. Support available to part-time students. Financial award application deadline: 3/1; financial award applicants required to submit FAFSA. *Faculty research:* Molecular basis of microbial pathogenesis, avian ecology, aquatic toxicology, endocrinology, aquatic biology. *Unit head:* Dr. Don Dailey, Chair, 931-221-7781, Fax: 931-221-6323, E-mail: daileyd@apsu.edu. *Application contact:* June D. Lee, Graduate Coordinator, 800-859-4723, Fax: 931-221-7641, E-mail: gradadmissions@apsu.edu.
Website: http://www.apsu.edu/biology

Ball State University, Graduate School, College of Sciences and Humanities, Department of Biology, Program in Biology, Muncie, IN 47306. Offers MA, MS. *Program availability:* Part-time. *Students:* 17 full-time (9 women), 30 part-time (14 women); includes 5 minority (1 Black or African American, non-Hispanic/Latino; 1 Asian, non-Hispanic/Latino; 3 Hispanic/Latino), 4 international. Average age 24. 37 applicants, 73% accepted, 18 enrolled. In 2015, 16 master's awarded. *Entrance requirements:* For master's, minimum baccalaureate GPA of 2.75 or 3.0 in latter half of baccalauareate, transcripts of all prior coursework, three letters of recommendation. Additional exam requirements/recommendations for international students: Required—TOEFL (minimum score 550 paper-based; 79 iBT), IELTS (minimum score 6.5). *Application deadline:* Applications are processed on a rolling basis. Application fee: $60. Electronic applications accepted. *Expenses: Tuition, area resident:* Full-time $6948; part-time $2316 per semester. Tuition, state resident: full-time $10,422; part-time $3474 per semester. Tuition, nonresident: full-time $19,062; part-time $6354 per semester. *Required fees:* $651 per semester. Tuition and fees vary according to campus/location, program and reciprocity agreements. *Financial support:* In 2015–16, 31 students received support, including 4 research assistantships with partial tuition reimbursements available (averaging $15,528 per year), 25 teaching assistantships with partial tuition reimbursements available (averaging $11,697 per year); unspecified assistantships also available. Financial award application deadline: 3/1; financial award applicants required to submit FAFSA. *Unit head:* Dr. Kemuel Badger, Chairman, 765-285-8820, Fax: 765-285-8804, E-mail: kbadger@bsu.edu. *Application contact:* Dr. David LeBlanc, Graduate Advisor, 765-285-8832, Fax: 765-285-8820, E-mail: dleblanc@bsu.edu.
Website: http://www.bsu.edu/biology

Ball State University, Graduate School, College of Sciences and Humanities, Interdepartmental Program in Environmental Sciences, Muncie, IN 47306. Offers environmental science (PhD), including biology, chemistry, geological sciences. *Program availability:* Part-time. *Students:* 3 full-time (0 women), 9 part-time (3 women), 4 international. Average age 31. 4 applicants, 25% accepted, 1 enrolled. In 2015, 2 doctorates awarded. *Degree requirements:* For doctorate, thesis/dissertation. *Entrance requirements:* For doctorate, GRE General Test, minimum cumulative GPA of 3.0 (chemistry), 3.2 (biology and geological sciences); acknowledged arrangement for doctoral environmental sciences research with faculty mentor; three letters of recommendation. Additional exam requirements/recommendations for international students: Required—TOEFL (minimum score 550 paper-based; 79 iBT), IELTS (minimum score 6.5). *Application deadline:* Applications are processed on a rolling basis. Application fee: $60. Electronic applications accepted. *Expenses: Tuition, area resident:* Full-time $6948; part-time $2316 per semester. Tuition, state resident: full-time $10,422; part-time $3474 per semester. Tuition, nonresident: full-time $19,062; part-time $6354 per semester. *Required fees:* $651 per semester. Tuition and fees vary according to campus/location, program and reciprocity agreements. *Financial support:* In 2015–16, 9 students received support, including 5 research assistantships with partial tuition reimbursements available (averaging $13,866 per year), 4 teaching assistantships with partial tuition reimbursements available (averaging $15,142 per year). Financial award application deadline: 3/1; financial award applicants required to submit FAFSA. *Unit head:* Dr. E. Michael Perdue, Director, 765-285-8096, Fax: 765-285-6505, E-mail: emperdue@bsu.edu.
Website: http://cms.bsu.edu/Academics/CollegesandDepartments/EnvironmentalScience.aspx

Barry University, College of Health Sciences, Programs in Biology and Biomedical Sciences, Miami Shores, FL 33161-6695. Offers biology (MS); biomedical sciences (MS). *Program availability:* Part-time, evening/weekend. *Degree requirements:* For master's, comprehensive exam, thesis (for some programs). *Entrance requirements:* For master's, GRE General Test or Florida Teacher's Certification Exam (biology); GRE General Test, MCAT, or DAT (biomedical sciences). Electronic applications accepted. *Faculty research:* Genetics, immunology, anthropology.

Baylor College of Medicine, Graduate School of Biomedical Sciences, Houston, TX 77030-3498. Offers MS, PhD, MD/PhD. Terminal master's awarded for partial completion of doctoral program. *Degree requirements:* For master's, thesis; for doctorate, thesis/dissertation, public defense. *Entrance requirements:* For doctorate, GRE General Test, GRE Subject Test (strongly recommended), minimum GPA of 3.0. Additional exam requirements/recommendations for international students: Required—TOEFL. Electronic applications accepted. *Faculty research:* Cell and molecular biology of cardiac muscle, structural biophysics, gene expression and regulation, human genomes, viruses.

Baylor University, Graduate School, College of Arts and Sciences, Department of Biology, Waco, TX 76798. Offers biology (MA, MS, PhD); environmental biology (MS); limnology (MS). *Program availability:* Part-time. *Degree requirements:* For master's, thesis (for some programs); for doctorate, thesis/dissertation. *Entrance requirements:* For master's and doctorate, GRE General Test. Additional exam requirements/recommendations for international students: Required—TOEFL. *Faculty research:* Terrestrial ecology, aquatic ecology, genetics.

Biological and Biomedical Sciences—General

Baylor University, Graduate School, Institute of Biomedical Studies, Waco, TX 76798. Offers MS, PhD. *Faculty:* 17 part-time/adjunct (3 women). *Students:* 28 full-time (9 women), 1 part-time (0 women); includes 5 minority (1 Black or African American, non-Hispanic/Latino; 2 Asian, non-Hispanic/Latino; 2 Hispanic/Latino), 14 international. Average age 24. 69 applicants, 10% accepted, 5 enrolled. In 2015, 5 doctorates awarded. *Degree requirements:* For master's, thesis (for some programs); for doctorate, thesis/dissertation. *Entrance requirements:* For master's and doctorate, GRE General Test. Additional exam requirements/recommendations for international students: Required—TOEFL (minimum score 550 paper-based). *Application deadline:* Applications are processed on a rolling basis. Application fee: $25. *Financial support:* In 2015–16, 22 students received support, including 11 research assistantships (averaging $20,000 per year), 11 teaching assistantships (averaging $20,000 per year); tuition waivers also available. *Unit head:* Dr. Chris Kearney, Graduate Program Director, 254-710-2131, Fax: 254-710-3878, E-mail: chris_kearney@baylor.edu. *Application contact:* Rhonda Bellert, Administrative Assistant, 254-710-2514, Fax: 254-710-2199, E-mail: rhonda_bellert@baylor.edu.
Website: http://www.baylor.edu/biomedical/

Bemidji State University, School of Graduate Studies, Bemidji, MN 56601. Offers biology (MS); education (MS); English (MA, MS); environmental studies (MS); mathematics (MS); mathematics (elementary and middle level education) (MS); special education (M Sp Ed). *Program availability:* Part-time, online learning. *Degree requirements:* For master's, comprehensive exam, thesis (for some programs). *Entrance requirements:* For master's, GRE; GMAT, letters of recommendation, letters of interest. Additional exam requirements/recommendations for international students: Required—TOEFL (minimum score 550 paper-based; 80 iBT). Electronic applications accepted. *Expenses:* Contact institution. *Faculty research:* Human performance, sport, and health: physical education teacher education, continuum models, spiritual health, intellectual health, resiliency, health priorities; psychology: health psychology, college student drinking behavior, micro-aggressions, infant cognition, false memories, leadership assessment; biology: structure and dynamics of forest communities, aquatic and riverine ecology, interaction between animal populations and aquatic environments, cellular motility.

Binghamton University, State University of New York, Graduate School, School of Arts and Sciences, Department of Biological Sciences, Binghamton, NY 13902-6000. Offers MA, MS, PhD. *Program availability:* Part-time. *Faculty:* 27 full-time (11 women), 8 part-time/adjunct (2 women). *Students:* 74 full-time (35 women), 1 (woman) part-time; includes 20 minority (3 Black or African American, non-Hispanic/Latino; 1 American Indian or Alaska Native, non-Hispanic/Latino; 9 Asian, non-Hispanic/Latino; 5 Hispanic/Latino; 2 Native Hawaiian or other Pacific Islander, non-Hispanic/Latino), 10 international. Average age 27. 97 applicants, 39% accepted, 27 enrolled. In 2015, 11 master's, 5 doctorates awarded. Terminal master's awarded for partial completion of doctoral program. *Degree requirements:* For master's, thesis; for doctorate, comprehensive exam, thesis/dissertation. *Entrance requirements:* For master's and doctorate, GRE General Test. Additional exam requirements/recommendations for international students: Required—TOEFL (minimum score 550 paper-based; 100 iBT). *Application deadline:* For fall admission, 1/15 priority date for domestic and international students; for spring admission, 10/15 priority date for domestic and international students. Application fee: $75. Electronic applications accepted. *Financial support:* In 2015–16, 46 students received support, including 3 research assistantships with full tuition reimbursements available (averaging $19,000 per year), 37 teaching assistantships with full tuition reimbursements available (averaging $17,500 per year); career-related internships or fieldwork, Federal Work-Study, institutionally sponsored loans, scholarships/grants, health care benefits, tuition waivers (full and partial), and unspecified assistantships also available. Financial award applicants required to submit FAFSA. *Unit head:* Dr. Curt M. Pueschel, Chairperson, 607-777-2602, E-mail: curtp@binghamton.edu. *Application contact:* Kishan Zuber, Recruiting and Admissions Coordinator, 607-777-2151, Fax: 607-777-2501, E-mail: kzuber@binghamton.edu.

Bloomsburg University of Pennsylvania, School of Graduate Studies, College of Science and Technology, Department of Biological and Allied Health Sciences, Program in Biology, Bloomsburg, PA 17815-1301. Offers MS. *Degree requirements:* For master's, thesis optional. *Entrance requirements:* For master's, minimum QPA of 3.0, 2 letters of recommendation, personal statement, undergraduate degree in biology. Additional exam requirements/recommendations for international students: Required—TOEFL (minimum score 550 paper-based). Electronic applications accepted.

Boise State University, College of Arts and Sciences, Department of Biological Sciences, Boise, ID 83725-1515. Offers biology (MA, MS); biomolecular sciences (PhD); raptor biology (MS). *Program availability:* Part-time. *Faculty:* 26. *Students:* 51 full-time (23 women), 10 part-time (5 women); includes 7 minority (1 Black or African American, non-Hispanic/Latino; 1 American Indian or Alaska Native, non-Hispanic/Latino; 1 Asian, non-Hispanic/Latino; 3 Hispanic/Latino; 1 Native Hawaiian or other Pacific Islander, non-Hispanic/Latino), 6 international. Average age 30. 45 applicants, 27% accepted, 10 enrolled. In 2015, 13 master's awarded. *Degree requirements:* For master's, thesis. *Entrance requirements:* For master's, GRE General Test, minimum GPA of 3.0. Additional exam requirements/recommendations for international students: Required—TOEFL (minimum score 550 paper-based; 80 iBT), IELTS (minimum score 6). *Application deadline:* For fall admission, 1/15 for domestic and international students; for spring admission, 10/1 for domestic and international students. Application fee: $65 ($95 for international students). Electronic applications accepted. *Expenses:* Tuition, state resident: full-time $6058; part-time $358 per credit hour. Tuition, nonresident: full-time $20,108; part-time $608 per credit hour. *Required fees:* $2108. Tuition and fees vary according to program. *Financial support:* In 2015–16, 6 students received support, including 18 research assistantships (averaging $7,534 per year), 29 teaching assistantships (averaging $8,918 per year); institutionally sponsored loans and unspecified assistantships also available. Financial award application deadline: 1/15; financial award applicants required to submit FAFSA. *Faculty research:* Soil and stream microbial ecology, avian ecology. *Unit head:* Dr. Kevin Feris, Chair, 208-426-5498, E-mail: kevinferis@boisestate.edu. *Application contact:* Dr. Julie Heath, Graduate Coordinator, 208-426-3208, E-mail: julieheath@boisestate.edu.
Website: http://biology.boisestate.edu/graduate-programs/

Boston College, Graduate School of Arts and Sciences, Department of Biology, Chestnut Hill, MA 02467. Offers PhD, MBA/MS. *Faculty:* 26 full-time. *Students:* 43 full-time (24 women); includes 3 minority (1 Black or African American, non-Hispanic/Latino; 1 Asian, non-Hispanic/Latino; 1 Two or more races, non-Hispanic/Latino), 9 international. 85 applicants, 16% accepted, 2 enrolled. In 2015, 11 doctorates awarded. *Degree requirements:* For doctorate, thesis/dissertation. *Entrance requirements:* For doctorate, GRE General Test, GRE Subject Test. Additional exam requirements/recommendations for international students: Required—TOEFL (minimum score 600 paper-based; 100 iBT), IELTS (minimum score 8). *Application deadline:* For fall admission, 1/2 priority date for domestic students, 1/2 for international students. Application fee: $75. Electronic applications accepted. Tuition and fees vary according to program. *Financial support:* In 2015–16, 43 students received support, including fellowships with full tuition reimbursements available (averaging $30,000 per year), research assistantships with full tuition reimbursements available (averaging $30,000

per year), teaching assistantships with full tuition reimbursements available (averaging $30,000 per year); Federal Work-Study, scholarships/grants, health care benefits, and unspecified assistantships also available. Support available to part-time students. Financial award application deadline: 1/2. *Faculty research:* Molecular cell biology and genetics, cell cycle, neurobiology, developmental biology, structural and cellular biochemistry, vector biology, infectious disease, bioinformatics. *Unit head:* Dr. Welkin Johnson, Chairperson, 617-552-4223, E-mail: welkin.johnson@bc.edu. *Application contact:* Dr. Charlie Hoffman, Graduate Program Director, 617-552-2779, E-mail: charles.hoffman@bc.edu.
Website: http://www.bc.edu/biology

Boston University, Graduate School of Arts and Sciences, Department of Biology, Boston, MA 02215. Offers MA, PhD. *Students:* 71 full-time (42 women), 1 part-time (0 women); includes 7 minority (1 Black or African American, non-Hispanic/Latino; 4 Asian, non-Hispanic/Latino; 1 Hispanic/Latino; 1 Two or more races, non-Hispanic/Latino), 8 international. Average age 29. 218 applicants, 15% accepted, 15 enrolled. In 2015, 10 master's, 11 doctorates awarded. Terminal master's awarded for partial completion of doctoral program. *Degree requirements:* For master's, one foreign language, thesis (for some programs); for doctorate, one foreign language, comprehensive exam, thesis/dissertation. *Entrance requirements:* For master's and doctorate, GRE General Test, GRE Subject Test (recommended), 3 letters of recommendation, transcripts, personal statement, curriculum vitae. Additional exam requirements/recommendations for international students: Required—TOEFL (minimum score 550 paper-based; 84 iBT). *Application deadline:* For fall admission, 12/7 for domestic and international students. Application fee: $95. Electronic applications accepted. *Financial support:* In 2015–16, 54 students received support, including 6 fellowships with full tuition reimbursements available (averaging $21,000 per year), 20 research assistantships with full tuition reimbursements available (averaging $21,000 per year), 28 teaching assistantships with full tuition reimbursements available (averaging $21,000 per year); Federal Work-Study, scholarships/grants, traineeships, and health care benefits also available. Financial award application deadline: 12/7. *Unit head:* Thomas Gilmore, Chair, 617-353-5444, Fax: 617-353-6340, E-mail: gilmore@bu.edu. *Application contact:* Christina Honeycutt, Academic Administrator, 617-353-2432, Fax: 617-353-6340, E-mail: cjhoney@bu.edu.
Website: http://www.bu.edu/biology/

Boston University, School of Medicine, Division of Graduate Medical Sciences, Program in Biomedical Sciences (Pub's), Boston, MA 02118. Offers PhD. *Entrance requirements:* For doctorate, GRE. *Financial support:* In 2015–16, fellowships (averaging $30,500 per year), research assistantships (averaging $30,500 per year), teaching assistantships (averaging $30,500 per year) were awarded. *Unit head:* Dr. Linda Hyman, Associate Provost, 617-638-5255, Fax: 617-638-5740. *Application contact:* GMS Office of Admissions, 617-638-5255, E-mail: askgms@bu.edu.
Website: http://www.bumc.bu.edu/gms/gateway/prospective/program-in-biomedical-sciences-track/

Bowling Green State University, Graduate College, College of Arts and Sciences, Department of Biological Sciences, Bowling Green, OH 43403. Offers MAT, MS, PhD. *Program availability:* Part-time. *Degree requirements:* For master's, thesis or alternative; for doctorate, comprehensive exam, thesis/dissertation. *Entrance requirements:* For master's and doctorate, GRE General Test. Additional exam requirements/recommendations for international students: Required—TOEFL. Electronic applications accepted. *Faculty research:* Aquatic ecology, endocrinology and neurophysiology, nitrogen fixation, photosynthesis.

Bradley University, Graduate School, College of Liberal Arts and Sciences, Department of Biology, Peoria, IL 61625-0002. Offers MS. *Program availability:* Part-time. *Degree requirements:* For master's, comprehensive exam, thesis. *Entrance requirements:* For master's, GRE. Additional exam requirements/recommendations for international students: Required—TOEFL (minimum score 550 paper-based; 79 iBT), IELTS (minimum score 6.5). Electronic applications accepted.

Brandeis University, Graduate School of Arts and Sciences, Department of Physics, Waltham, MA 02454-9110. Offers physics (MS, PhD); quantitative biology (PhD). *Program availability:* Part-time. *Faculty:* 15 full-time (3 women), 1 part-time/adjunct (0 women). *Students:* 47 full-time (12 women); includes 2 minority (1 Asian, non-Hispanic/Latino; 1 Hispanic/Latino), 19 international. 147 applicants, 14% accepted, 7 enrolled. In 2015, 3 master's, 10 doctorates awarded. Terminal master's awarded for partial completion of doctoral program. *Degree requirements:* For master's, thesis optional, qualifying exam, 1-year residency; for doctorate, comprehensive exam, thesis/dissertation, qualifying and advanced exams. *Entrance requirements:* For master's and doctorate, GRE General Test; GRE Subject Test (recommended), resume, 2 letters of recommendation, statement of purpose, transcript(s). Additional exam requirements/recommendations for international students: Required—TOEFL (minimum score 600 paper-based; 100 iBT); Recommended—IELTS (minimum score 7), TSE (minimum score 68). *Application deadline:* For fall admission, 1/15 priority date for domestic students. Application fee: $75. Electronic applications accepted. *Financial support:* In 2015–16, 56 students received support, including 22 fellowships with full tuition reimbursements available (averaging $26,000 per year), 22 research assistantships with full tuition reimbursements available (averaging $26,000 per year), 12 teaching assistantships with partial tuition reimbursements available (averaging $2,500 per year); Federal Work-Study, scholarships/grants, health care benefits, and tuition waivers (full and partial) also available. Support available to part-time students. Financial award application deadline: 1/15; financial award applicants required to submit FAFSA. *Faculty research:* Astrophysics, condensed-matter and biophysics, high energy and gravitational theory, particle physics, microfluidics, radio astronomy, string theory. *Unit head:* Dr. Jane Kondev, Department Chair, 781-736-2800, E-mail: kondev@brandeis.edu. *Application contact:* Catherine Broderick, Department Administrator, 781-736-2800, E-mail: cbroderi@brandeis.edu.
Website: http://www.brandeis.edu/gsas

Brandeis University, Graduate School of Arts and Sciences, Post-Baccalaureate Premedical Program, Waltham, MA 02454-9110. Offers Postbaccalaureate Certificate. *Students:* 8 full-time (5 women), 2 part-time (both women); includes 3 minority (1 Black or African American, non-Hispanic/Latino; 2 Asian, non-Hispanic/Latino). 37 applicants, 59% accepted, 8 enrolled. In 2015, 3 Postbaccalaureate Certificates awarded. *Entrance requirements:* For degree, GRE, ACT, or SAT, resume with paid and/or volunteer work relevant to field of medicine, letters of recommendation, transcript(s), statement of purpose. *Application deadline:* For fall admission, 5/15 for domestic students. Application fee: $75. Electronic applications accepted. *Expenses:* $8,400 per semester. *Financial support:* Applicants required to submit FAFSA. *Faculty research:* Health profession preparation, pre-medical, pre-veterinary, pre-dental, pre-optometry, pre-osteopathic. *Unit head:* Abby Voss, Assistant Director of Pre-Health Advising, 781-736-3493, Fax: 781-736-3469, E-mail: avoss@brandeis.edu.
Website: http://www.brandeis.edu/gsas

Brandeis University, Graduate School of Arts and Sciences, Program in Biochemistry and Biophysics, Waltham, MA 02454. Offers biochemistry and biophysics (PhD); quantitative biology (PhD). *Faculty:* 10 full-time (3 women). *Students:* 38 full-time (16 women); includes 3 minority (1 Asian, non-Hispanic/Latino; 1 Hispanic/Latino; 1 Two or more races, non-Hispanic/Latino), 12 international. 70 applicants, 29% accepted, 5

enrolled. In 2015, 4 doctorates awarded. Terminal master's awarded for partial completion of doctoral program. *Degree requirements:* For doctorate, thesis/dissertation, qualifying exams. *Entrance requirements:* For doctorate, GRE General Test, resume, 3 letters of recommendation, statement of purpose, transcript(s). Additional exam requirements/recommendations for international students: Required—TOEFL (minimum score 600 paper-based; 100 iBT); Recommended—IELTS (minimum score 7), TSE (minimum score 68). *Application deadline:* For fall admission, 12/15 priority date for domestic students. Application fee: $75. Electronic applications accepted. *Financial support:* In 2015–16, 31 students received support, including 14 fellowships with full tuition reimbursements available (averaging $30,500 per year), 17 research assistantships with full tuition reimbursements available (averaging $30,500 per year); Federal Work-Study, scholarships/grants, health care benefits, and tuition waivers (full and partial) also available. Financial award application deadline: 4/15; financial award applicants required to submit FAFSA. *Faculty research:* Macromolecular chemistry, structure and function, biochemistry, biophysics, biological macromolecules. *Unit head:* Prof. Dagmar Ringe, Director of Graduate Studies, 781-736-2300, Fax: 781-736-2349, E-mail: scigradoffice@brandeis.edu. *Application contact:* 781-736-2300, E-mail: scigradoffice@brandeis.edu.
Website: http://www.brandeis.edu/gsas

Brandeis University, Graduate School of Arts and Sciences, Program in Molecular and Cell Biology, Waltham, MA 02454-9110. Offers genetics (PhD); microbiology (PhD); molecular and cell biology (MS, PhD); molecular biology (PhD); neurobiology (PhD); quantitative biology (PhD). *Faculty:* 26 full-time (12 women), 4 part-time/adjunct (2 women). *Students:* 60 full-time (30 women); includes 5 minority (1 Black or African American, non-Hispanic/Latino; 1 American Indian or Alaska Native, non-Hispanic/Latino; 1 Asian, non-Hispanic/Latino; 2 Hispanic/Latino), 25 international. 183 applicants, 27% accepted, 12 enrolled. In 2015, 13 master's, 7 doctorates awarded. Terminal master's awarded for partial completion of doctoral program. *Degree requirements:* For master's, thesis optional, research project, research lab, or project lab; for doctorate, comprehensive exam, thesis/dissertation, journal clubs; research seminar; colloquia; qualifying exam. *Entrance requirements:* For master's, GRE General Test, official transcript(s), resume, 2 letters of recommendation, statement of purpose; for doctorate, GRE General Test, official transcript(s), resume, 3 letters of recommendation, statement of purpose, list of previous research experience. Additional exam requirements/recommendations for international students: Required—TOEFL (minimum score 600 paper-based; 100 iBT); Recommended—IELTS (minimum score 7), TSE (minimum score 68). *Application deadline:* For fall admission, 12/15 priority date for domestic students. Application fee: $75. Electronic applications accepted. *Financial support:* In 2015–16, 35 students received support, including 16 fellowships with full tuition reimbursements available (averaging $30,500 per year), 19 research assistantships with full tuition reimbursements available (averaging $30,500 per year); scholarships/grants and tuition waivers (partial) also available. Financial award application deadline: 4/15; financial award applicants required to submit FAFSA. *Faculty research:* Molecular biology, genetics and development; structural and cell biology; neurobiology. *Unit head:* Dr. Maria Miara, Director of Graduate Studies, 781-736-2300, Fax: 781-736-3107, E-mail: scigradoffice@brandeis.edu. *Application contact:* Dr. Maryanna Aldrich, Department Administrator, 781-736-2300, Fax: 781-736-3107, E-mail: scigradoffice@brandeis.edu.
Website: http://www.brandeis.edu/gsas

Brandeis University, Graduate School of Arts and Sciences, Program in Neuroscience, Waltham, MA 02454-9110. Offers neuroscience (MS, PhD); quantitative biology (PhD). *Faculty:* 21 full-time (9 women). *Students:* 58 full-time (24 women), 1 (woman) part-time; includes 14 minority (1 Black or African American, non-Hispanic/Latino; 1 American Indian or Alaska Native, non-Hispanic/Latino; 6 Asian, non-Hispanic/Latino; 6 Hispanic/Latino), 9 international. 192 applicants, 23% accepted, 15 enrolled. In 2015, 10 master's, 6 doctorates awarded. Terminal master's awarded for partial completion of doctoral program. *Degree requirements:* For master's, thesis optional, research project; for doctorate, comprehensive exam, thesis/dissertation, qualifying exams, teaching experience, journal club, research seminars. *Entrance requirements:* For master's, GRE General Test, official transcript(s), statement of purpose, resume, 2 letters of recommendation; for doctorate, GRE General Test, official transcript(s), statement of purpose, resume, 3 letters of recommendation, listing of previous research experience. Additional exam requirements/recommendations for international students: Required—TOEFL (minimum score 600 paper-based; 100 iBT); Recommended—IELTS (minimum score 7), TSE (minimum score 68). *Application deadline:* For fall admission, 12/15 priority date for domestic students. Application fee: $75. Electronic applications accepted. *Financial support:* In 2015–16, 49 students received support, including 32 fellowships with full tuition reimbursements available (averaging $30,500 per year), 17 research assistantships with full tuition reimbursements available (averaging $30,500 per year); Federal Work-Study, scholarships/grants, health care benefits, and tuition waivers (full and partial) also available. Financial award application deadline: 4/15; financial award applicants required to submit FAFSA. *Faculty research:* Behavioral/cognitive neuroscience, cellular and molecular neuroscience, computational neuroscience and systems neuroscience, and developmental neuroscience. *Unit head:* Dr. Don Katz, Director of Graduate Studies, 781-736-3100, Fax: 781-736-3107, E-mail: dbkatz@brandeis.edu. *Application contact:* Dr. Maryanna Aldrich, Department Administrator, 781-736-2300, Fax: 781-736-3107, E-mail: scigradoffice@brandeis.edu.
Website: http://www.brandeis.edu/gsas

Brigham Young University, Graduate Studies, College of Life Sciences, Department of Biology, Provo, UT 84602. Offers biological science education (MS); biology (MS, PhD). *Faculty:* 22 full-time (2 women). *Students:* 42 full-time (18 women); includes 3 minority (2 Hispanic/Latino; 1 Native Hawaiian or other Pacific Islander, non-Hispanic/Latino), 5 international. Average age 29. 27 applicants, 56% accepted, 15 enrolled. In 2015, 10 master's, 6 doctorates awarded. *Degree requirements:* For master's, comprehensive exam, thesis, prospectus, defense of research, defense of thesis; for doctorate, comprehensive exam, thesis/dissertation, prospectus, defense of research, defense of dissertation. *Entrance requirements:* For master's and doctorate, GRE General Test, minimum cumulative GPA of 3.0 for undergraduate degree. Additional exam requirements/recommendations for international students: Required—TOEFL (minimum score 580 paper-based; 85 iBT). *Application deadline:* For fall admission, 1/15 for domestic and international students. Application fee: $50. Electronic applications accepted. *Financial support:* In 2015–16, 31 students received support, including 6 fellowships with tuition reimbursements available (averaging $22,500 per year), 25 research assistantships with tuition reimbursements available (averaging $6,250 per year), 28 teaching assistantships with tuition reimbursements available (averaging $6,989 per year); career-related internships or fieldwork, institutionally sponsored loans, scholarships/grants, health care benefits, tuition waivers (full and partial), and unspecified assistantships also available. Financial award application deadline: 3/1; financial award applicants required to submit FAFSA. *Faculty research:* Systematics, bioinformatics, ecology, evolution. *Total annual research expenditures:* $1.6 million. *Unit head:* Dr. Dennis K. Shiozawa, Chair, 801-422-4972, Fax: 801-422-0004, E-mail: dennis_shiozawa@byu.edu. *Application contact:* Gentri Glaittli, Graduate Secretary, 801-422-7137, Fax: 801-422-0004, E-mail: biogradsec@byu.edu.
Website: http://biology.byu.edu/

Brock University, Faculty of Graduate Studies, Faculty of Mathematics and Science, Program in Biological Sciences, St. Catharines, ON L2S 3A1, Canada. Offers M Sc, PhD. *Program availability:* Part-time. *Degree requirements:* For master's, thesis; for doctorate, thesis/dissertation. *Entrance requirements:* For master's, honors B Sc in biology, minimum undergraduate GPA of 3.0; for doctorate, M Sc. Additional exam requirements/recommendations for international students: Required—TOEFL (minimum score 550 paper-based; 80 iBT), IELTS (minimum score 6.5), TWE (minimum score 4). Electronic applications accepted. *Faculty research:* Viticulture, neurobiology, ecology, molecular biology, molecular genetics.

Brooklyn College of the City University of New York, School of Education, Program in Middle Childhood Science Education, Brooklyn, NY 11210-2889. Offers biology (MA); chemistry (MA); earth science (MA); general science (MA); physics (MA). *Program availability:* Part-time, evening/weekend. *Entrance requirements:* For master's, LAST, interview, previous course work in education and mathematics, resume, 2 letters of recommendation, essay. Additional exam requirements/recommendations for international students: Required—TOEFL (minimum score 500 paper-based; 61 iBT). Electronic applications accepted. *Faculty research:* Geometric thinking, mastery of basic facts, problem-solving strategies, history of mathematics.

Brooklyn College of the City University of New York, School of Natural and Behavioral Sciences, Department of Biology, Brooklyn, NY 11210-2889. Offers MA. *Degree requirements:* For master's, one foreign language, comprehensive exam, thesis. *Entrance requirements:* For master's, minimum GPA of 3.0, 2 letters of recommendation. Additional exam requirements/recommendations for international students: Required—TOEFL (minimum score 500 paper-based; 61 iBT). Electronic applications accepted. *Faculty research:* Evolutionary biology, molecular biology of development, cell biology, comparative endocrinology, ecology.

Brown University, Graduate School, Division of Biology and Medicine, Providence, RI 02912. Offers AM, M Sc, MA, MPH, Sc M, MD, PhD, MD/PhD. *Program availability:* Part-time. Terminal master's awarded for partial completion of doctoral program. *Degree requirements:* For doctorate, thesis/dissertation. *Entrance requirements:* For master's and doctorate, GRE General Test. Additional exam requirements/recommendations for international students: Required—TOEFL. Electronic applications accepted.

Bucknell University, Graduate Studies, College of Arts and Sciences, Department of Biology, Lewisburg, PA 17837. Offers MS. *Degree requirements:* For master's, thesis. *Entrance requirements:* For master's, GRE General Test, GRE Subject Test, minimum GPA of 3.0. Additional exam requirements/recommendations for international students: Required—TOEFL (minimum score 600 paper-based).

Buffalo State College, State University of New York, The Graduate School, Faculty of Natural and Social Sciences, Department of Biology, Buffalo, NY 14222-1095. Offers biology (MA); secondary education (MS Ed), including biology. *Program availability:* Evening/weekend. *Degree requirements:* For master's, thesis (for some programs), project. *Entrance requirements:* For master's, minimum GPA of 2.75. Additional exam requirements/recommendations for international students: Required—TOEFL (minimum score 550 paper-based).

California Institute of Technology, Division of Biology, Pasadena, CA 91125-0001. Offers biochemistry and molecular biophysics (PhD); cell biology and biophysics (PhD); developmental biology (PhD); genetics (PhD); immunology (PhD); molecular biology (PhD); neurobiology (PhD). *Degree requirements:* For doctorate, thesis/dissertation, qualifying exam. *Entrance requirements:* For doctorate, GRE General Test. Additional exam requirements/recommendations for international students: Required—TOEFL. Electronic applications accepted. *Faculty research:* Molecular genetics of differentiation and development, structure of biological macromolecules, molecular and integrative neurobiology.

California Polytechnic State University, San Luis Obispo, College of Science and Mathematics, Department of Biological Sciences, San Luis Obispo, CA 93407. Offers MA, MS. *Program availability:* Part-time. *Faculty:* 9 full-time (3 women). *Students:* 20 full-time (15 women), 16 part-time (10 women); includes 6 minority (3 Asian, non-Hispanic/Latino; 3 Hispanic/Latino), 1 international. Average age 25. 66 applicants, 32% accepted, 13 enrolled. In 2015, 13 master's awarded. *Degree requirements:* For master's, comprehensive exam (for some programs), thesis (for some programs). *Application deadline:* For fall admission, 2/1 for domestic and international students. Applications are processed on a rolling basis. Application fee: $55. Electronic applications accepted. *Expenses:* Tuition, state resident: full-time $6738; part-time $3906 per year. Tuition, nonresident: full-time $15,666; part-time $8370 per year. *Required fees:* $3528; $3075 per unit. $1025 per term. *Financial support:* Fellowships, research assistantships, teaching assistantships, career-related internships or fieldwork, and Federal Work-Study available. Support available to part-time students. Financial award application deadline: 3/2; financial award applicants required to submit FAFSA. *Faculty research:* Ancient fossil DNA, restoration ecology microbe biodiversity indices, biological inventories. *Unit head:* Dr. Emily Taylor, Graduate Coordinator, 805-756-2616, Fax: 805-756-1419, E-mail: etaylor@calpoly.edu.
Website: http://bio.calpoly.edu/

California State Polytechnic University, Pomona, Program in Biological Sciences, Pomona, CA 91768-2557. Offers MS. *Program availability:* Part-time. *Students:* 24 full-time (16 women), 50 part-time (28 women); includes 41 minority (2 Black or African American, non-Hispanic/Latino; 13 Asian, non-Hispanic/Latino; 24 Hispanic/Latino; 2 Two or more races, non-Hispanic/Latino), 5 international. Average age 25. 39 applicants, 44% accepted, 13 enrolled. In 2015, 15 master's awarded. *Degree requirements:* For master's, thesis. *Entrance requirements:* For master's, GRE General Test. *Application deadline:* For fall admission, 5/1 priority date for domestic students; for winter admission, 10/15 priority date for domestic students; for spring admission, 1/20 priority date for domestic students. Applications are processed on a rolling basis. Application fee: $55. Electronic applications accepted. *Expenses:* Tuition, state resident: full-time $6738. Tuition, nonresident: full-time $13,434. *Required fees:* $1504. Tuition and fees vary according to course load, degree level and program. *Financial support:* Career-related internships or fieldwork, Federal Work-Study, and institutionally sponsored loans available. Support available to part-time students. Financial award application deadline: 3/2; financial award applicants required to submit FAFSA. *Unit head:* Dr. Robert J. Talmadge, Graduate Coordinator, 909-869-3025, Fax: 909-869-4078, E-mail: rjtalmadge@cpp.edu.
Website: http://www.cpp.edu/~sci/biological-sciences/graduate-studies/index.shtml

California State University, Bakersfield, Division of Graduate Studies, School of Natural Sciences, Mathematics, and Engineering, Program in Biology, Bakersfield, CA 93311. Offers MS. *Entrance requirements:* For master's, GRE, minimum undergraduate GPA of 3.0 in last 90 quarter units, 3 letters of recommendation. Additional exam requirements/recommendations for international students: Required—TOEFL. *Application deadline:* Applications are processed on a rolling basis. *Expenses:* Tuition, area resident: Full-time $2246; part-time $1302 per semester. Tuition, state resident: full-time $2246; part-time $1302 per semester. *Financial support:* Teaching assistantships available. *Unit head:* Dr. Anna L. Jacobsen, Director, 661-654-2572, E-mail: ajacobsen@csub.edu. *Application contact:* Debbie Blowers, Assistant Director of Admissions, 661-664-3381, E-mail: dblowers@csub.edu.
Website: http://www.csub.edu/biology/index.html

Biological and Biomedical Sciences—General

California State University, Chico, Office of Graduate Studies, College of Natural Sciences, Department of Biological Sciences, Chico, CA 95929-0722. Offers biological sciences (MS). *Degree requirements:* For master's, thesis, independent research project resulting in a thesis. *Entrance requirements:* For master's, GRE, two letters of recommendation, statement of purpose, resume. Additional exam requirements/recommendations for international students: Required—TOEFL (minimum score 550 paper-based; 80 iBT), IELTS (minimum score 6.5), PTE (minimum score 59). *Application deadline:* For fall admission, 3/1 priority date for domestic students, 3/1 for international students; for spring admission, 9/15 priority date for domestic students, 9/15 for international students. Application fee: $55. Electronic applications accepted. *Expenses: Tuition,* area resident: Full-time $4146; part-time $2730. *Financial support:* Fellowships, research assistantships, teaching assistantships, career-related internships or fieldwork, and scholarships/grants available. Financial award application deadline: 3/1; financial award applicants required to submit FAFSA. *Unit head:* Dr. Jeffrey Bell, Chair, 530-898-5356, Fax: 530-898-5060, E-mail: biol@csuchico.edu. *Application contact:* Judy L. Rice, Graduate Admissions Coordinator, 530-898-5356, Fax: 530-898-3342, E-mail: jlrice@csuchico.edu. Website: http://www.csuchico.edu/biol/

California State University, Dominguez Hills, College of Natural and Behavioral Sciences, Department of Biology, Carson, CA 90747-0001. Offers MS. *Program availability:* Part-time, evening/weekend. *Degree requirements:* For master's, thesis. *Entrance requirements:* For master's, minimum GPA of 2.75. Additional exam requirements/recommendations for international students: Required—TOEFL (minimum score 550 paper-based). *Application deadline:* For fall admission, 6/1 for domestic students, 5/1 for international students; for spring admission, 12/15 for domestic students, 10/1 for international students. Application fee: $55. Electronic applications accepted. *Faculty research:* Cancer biology, infectious diseases, ecology of native plants, remediation, community ecology. *Unit head:* Dr. Helen Chun, Chair, 310-243-3397, Fax: 310-243-2350, E-mail: hchun@csudh.edu. *Application contact:* Dr. Getachew Kidane, Graduate Program Coordinator, 310-243-3564, Fax: 310-243-2350, E-mail: gkidane@csudh.edu. Website: http://www4.csudh.edu/biology/

California State University, East Bay, Office of Graduate Studies, College of Science, Department of Biological Sciences, Hayward, CA 94542-3000. Offers biological sciences (MS); marine science (MS). *Program availability:* Part-time. *Students:* 17 full-time (9 women), 11 part-time (10 women); includes 12 minority (3 Black or African American, non-Hispanic/Latino; 3 Asian, non-Hispanic/Latino; 3 Hispanic/Latino; 3 Two or more races, non-Hispanic/Latino), 4 international. Average age 29. 36 applicants, 25% accepted, 4 enrolled. In 2015, 10 master's awarded. *Degree requirements:* For master's, thesis. *Entrance requirements:* For master's, GRE General and Subject Tests, minimum GPA of 3.0 in field, 2.75 overall; 3 letters of reference; statement of purpose. Additional exam requirements/recommendations for international students: Required—TOEFL (minimum score 550 paper-based). *Application deadline:* For fall admission, 4/15 for domestic and international students. Applications are processed on a rolling basis. Application fee: $55. Electronic applications accepted. *Financial support:* Fellowships, teaching assistantships, career-related internships or fieldwork, Federal Work-Study, institutionally sponsored loans, and scholarships/grants available. Support available to part-time students. Financial award application deadline: 3/2; financial award applicants required to submit FAFSA. *Unit head:* Dr. Donald Gailey, Chair, 510-885-3471, Fax: 510-885-4747, E-mail: donald.gailey@csueastbay.edu. *Application contact:* Prof. Maria Nieto, Interim Graduate Coordinator, 510-885-4757, Fax: 510-885-4747, E-mail: maria.nieto@csueastbay.edu. Website: http://www20.csueastbay.edu/csci/departments/biology/

California State University, Fresno, Division of Graduate Studies, College of Science and Mathematics, Department of Biology, Fresno, CA 93740-8027. Offers biology (MA); biotechnology (MBT). *Program availability:* Part-time, evening/weekend. *Degree requirements:* For master's, thesis. *Entrance requirements:* For master's, GRE General Test, GRE Subject Test, minimum GPA of 2.5 in last 60 units. Additional exam requirements/recommendations for international students: Required—TOEFL. Electronic applications accepted. *Faculty research:* Genome neuroscience, ecology conflict resolution, biomechanics, cell death, vibrio cholerae.

California State University, Fullerton, Graduate Studies, College of Natural Science and Mathematics, Department of Biological Science, Fullerton, CA 92834-9480. Offers biology (MS); biotechnology (MBT). *Program availability:* Part-time. *Degree requirements:* For master's, thesis. *Entrance requirements:* For master's, GRE General and Subject Tests, MCAT, or DAT, minimum GPA of 3.0 in biology. *Faculty research:* Glycosidase release and the block to polyspermy in ascidian eggs.

California State University, Long Beach, Graduate Studies, College of Natural Sciences and Mathematics, Department of Biological Sciences, Long Beach, CA 90840. Offers biology (MS); microbiology (MS). *Program availability:* Part-time. *Entrance requirements:* For master's, GRE Subject Test, minimum GPA of 3.0. Electronic applications accepted.

California State University, Los Angeles, Graduate Studies, College of Natural and Social Sciences, Department of Biological Sciences, Los Angeles, CA 90032-8530. Offers biology (MS). *Program availability:* Part-time, evening/weekend. *Degree requirements:* For master's, comprehensive exam or thesis. *Entrance requirements:* Additional exam requirements/recommendations for international students: Required—TOEFL (minimum score 500 paper-based). *Application deadline:* For fall admission, 5/1 for domestic and international students. Applications are processed on a rolling basis. Application fee: $55. *Financial support:* Federal Work-Study available. Support available to part-time students. Financial award application deadline: 3/1. *Faculty research:* Ecology, environmental biology, cell and molecular biology, physiology, medical microbiology. Website: http://www.calstatela.edu/academic/biol/

California State University, Northridge, Graduate Studies, College of Science and Mathematics, Department of Biology, Northridge, CA 91330. Offers MS. *Faculty:* 28 full-time (12 women), 69 part-time/adjunct (42 women). *Students:* 32 full-time (19 women), 46 part-time (24 women); includes 17 minority (1 Black or African American, non-Hispanic/Latino; 4 Asian, non-Hispanic/Latino; 9 Hispanic/Latino; 3 Two or more races, non-Hispanic/Latino), 3 international. Average age 28. 79 applicants, 35% accepted, 22 enrolled. *Degree requirements:* For master's, thesis, seminar. *Entrance requirements:* For master's, GRE Subject Test, GRE General Test. Additional exam requirements/recommendations for international students: Required—TOEFL. *Application deadline:* For fall admission, 3/15 priority date for domestic students; for spring admission, 10/15 priority date for domestic students. Application fee: $55. *Financial support:* Research assistantships, teaching assistantships, Federal Work-Study, institutionally sponsored loans, tuition waivers (partial), and unspecified assistantships available. Support available to part-time students. Financial award applicants required to submit FAFSA. *Faculty research:* Cell adhesion, cancer research, fishery research. *Unit head:* Dr. Larry Allen, Chair, 818-677-3356. Website: http://www.csun.edu/~hfbio002/

California State University, Sacramento, Office of Graduate Studies, College of Natural Sciences and Mathematics, Department of Biological Sciences, Sacramento, CA 95819. Offers biological conservation (MS); molecular and cellular biology (MS); stem cell (MA). *Program availability:* Part-time. *Degree requirements:* For master's, thesis, writing proficiency exam. *Entrance requirements:* For master's, GRE, bachelor's degree in biology or equivalent; minimum GPA of 3.0 in biology, 2.75 overall during last 2 years of course work. Additional exam requirements/recommendations for international students: Required—TOEFL. Electronic applications accepted.

California State University, San Bernardino, Graduate Studies, College of Natural Sciences, Program in Biology, San Bernardino, CA 92407. Offers MS. *Program availability:* Part-time. *Students:* 9 full-time (4 women), 17 part-time (7 women); includes 13 minority (2 Asian, non-Hispanic/Latino; 11 Hispanic/Latino). 17 applicants, 41% accepted, 7 enrolled. In 2015, 2 master's awarded. *Application deadline:* For fall admission, 5/1 for domestic students; for winter admission, 10/16 for domestic students; for spring admission, 1/22 for domestic students. Application fee: $55. *Expenses:* Tuition, state resident: full-time $7843; part-time $5011.20 per year. Tuition and fees vary according to course load, degree level, program and reciprocity agreements. *Faculty research:* Ecology, molecular biology, physiology, cell biology, neurobiology. *Unit head:* Dr. Michael Chao, Chair, 909-537-5388, E-mail: mchao@csusb.edu. *Application contact:* Dr. Jeffrey Thompson, Dean of Graduate Studies, 909-537-5058, E-mail: jthompso@csusb.edu.

California State University, San Marcos, College of Science and Mathematics, Program in Biological Sciences, San Marcos, CA 92096-0001. Offers MS. *Program availability:* Part-time. *Degree requirements:* For master's, thesis. *Entrance requirements:* For master's, GRE General Test, minimum GPA of 2.75 in mathematics and science or 3.0 in last 35 units of mathematics and science, bachelor's degree in the biological or related sciences. Additional exam requirements/recommendations for international students: Required—TOEFL, TWE. *Faculty research:* Gene regulation of life states, carbon cycling, genetic markers of viral infection, neurobiology.

Carleton University, Faculty of Graduate Studies, Faculty of Science, Department of Biology, Ottawa, ON K1S 5B6, Canada. Offers M Sc, PhD. Programs offered jointly with University of Ottawa. *Degree requirements:* For master's, thesis, seminar; for doctorate, comprehensive exam, thesis/dissertation, seminar. *Entrance requirements:* For master's, honors degree in science; for doctorate, M Sc. Additional exam requirements/recommendations for international students: Required—TOEFL. *Faculty research:* Biochemical, structural, and genetic regulation in cells; behavioral ecology; insect taxonomy; physiology of cells.

Carnegie Mellon University, Mellon College of Science, Department of Biological Sciences, Pittsburgh, PA 15213-3891. Offers biochemistry (PhD); biophysics (PhD); cell and developmental biology (PhD); computational biology (MS, PhD); genetics (PhD); molecular biology (PhD); neuroscience (PhD); structural biology (PhD). *Degree requirements:* For doctorate, comprehensive exam, thesis/dissertation. *Entrance requirements:* For doctorate, GRE General Test, GRE Subject Test, interview. Electronic applications accepted. *Faculty research:* Genetic structure, function, and regulation; protein structure and function; biological membranes; biological spectroscopy.

Case Western Reserve University, School of Graduate Studies, Department of Biology, Cleveland, OH 44106. Offers MS, PhD. *Program availability:* Part-time. *Faculty:* 24 full-time (12 women), 9 part-time/adjunct (4 women). *Students:* 70 full-time (29 women), 6 part-time (3 women); includes 10 minority (3 Black or African American, non-Hispanic/Latino; 4 Asian, non-Hispanic/Latino; 3 Hispanic/Latino), 27 international. Average age 26. 95 applicants, 44% accepted, 23 enrolled. In 2015, 10 master's, 8 doctorates awarded. Terminal master's awarded for partial completion of doctoral program. *Degree requirements:* For master's, thesis or alternative; for doctorate, thesis/dissertation. *Entrance requirements:* For master's and doctorate, GRE General Test, GRE Subject Test, statement of objectives; three letters of recommendation. Additional exam requirements/recommendations for international students: Required—TOEFL (minimum score 577 paper-based; 90 iBT); Recommended—IELTS (minimum score 7). *Application deadline:* For fall admission, 1/9 priority date for domestic students. Applications are processed on a rolling basis. Application fee: $50. Electronic applications accepted. *Expenses: Tuition,* area resident: Full-time $41,137; part-time $1714 per credit hour. Required fees: $32. Tuition and fees vary according to course load and program. *Financial support:* Fellowships, research assistantships, teaching assistantships, career-related internships or fieldwork, Federal Work-Study, scholarships/grants, tuition waivers, unspecified assistantships, and stipends available. Financial award application deadline: 1/9; financial award applicants required to submit CSS PROFILE or FAFSA. *Faculty research:* Cellular, developmental, and molecular biology; genetics; genetic engineering; biotechnology; ecology. *Unit head:* Mark Willis, Professor and Chair, Department of Biology, 216-368-4358, Fax: 216-368-4762, E-mail: mark.willis@case.edu. *Application contact:* Julia Brown-Allen, Graduate Coordinator/Graduate Recruiter, 216-368-3556, Fax: 216-368-4672, E-mail: julia.brown@case.edu. Website: http://biology.case.edu/

Case Western Reserve University, School of Medicine and School of Graduate Studies, Graduate Programs in Medicine, Biomedical Sciences Training Program, Cleveland, OH 44106. Offers PhD. *Degree requirements:* For doctorate, thesis/dissertation. *Entrance requirements:* For doctorate, GRE General Test. Additional exam requirements/recommendations for international students: Required—TOEFL. Electronic applications accepted. *Expenses: Tuition,* area resident: Full-time $41,137; part-time $1714 per credit hour. Required fees: $32. Tuition and fees vary according to course load and program. *Faculty research:* Biochemistry, molecular biology, immunology, genetics, neurosciences.

Case Western Reserve University, School of Medicine and School of Graduate Studies, Graduate Programs in Medicine, Department of Biochemistry, Program in RNA Biology, Cleveland, OH 44106. Offers PhD. *Degree requirements:* For doctorate, comprehensive exam, thesis/dissertation. *Entrance requirements:* For doctorate, GRE. Additional exam requirements/recommendations for international students: Required—TOEFL (minimum score 550 paper-based). *Expenses: Tuition,* area resident: Full-time $41,137; part-time $1714 per credit hour. Required fees: $32. Tuition and fees vary according to course load and program.

Case Western Reserve University, School of Medicine, Medical Scientist Training Program, Cleveland, OH 44106. Offers MD/PhD. Electronic applications accepted. *Expenses: Tuition,* area resident: Full-time $41,137; part-time $1714 per credit hour. Required fees: $32. Tuition and fees vary according to course load and program. *Faculty research:* Biomedical research.

The Catholic University of America, School of Arts and Sciences, Department of Biology, Washington, DC 20064. Offers biotechnology (MS); cell and microbial biology (MS, PhD), including cell biology; clinical laboratory science (MS, PhD); MSLS/MS. *Program availability:* Part-time. *Faculty:* 9 full-time (4 women), 7 part-time/adjunct (1 woman). *Students:* 29 full-time (18 women), 36 part-time (22 women); includes 8 minority (3 Black or African American, non-Hispanic/Latino; 2 Asian, non-Hispanic/Latino; 1 Hispanic/Latino; 2 Two or more races, non-Hispanic/Latino), 44 international.

Average age 30. 68 applicants, 38% accepted, 13 enrolled. In 2015, 21 master's, 1 doctorate awarded. *Degree requirements:* For master's and doctorate, comprehensive exam. *Entrance requirements:* For master's and doctorate, GRE General Test, GRE Subject Test, statement of purpose, official copies of academic transcripts, three letters of recommendation. Additional exam requirements/recommendations for international students: Required—TOEFL (minimum score 550 paper-based; 80 iBT). *Application deadline:* For fall admission, 7/15 priority date for domestic students, 7/1 for international students; for spring admission, 11/15 priority date for domestic students, 11/1 for international students. Applications are processed on a rolling basis. Application fee: $55. Electronic applications accepted. *Expenses:* $20,700 per semester full-time tuition, $200 per semester full-time fees; $1,650 per credit hour part-time tuition, $145 per semester part-time fees. *Financial support:* Fellowships, research assistantships, teaching assistantships, Federal Work-Study, scholarships/grants, tuition waivers (full and partial), and unspecified assistantships available. Financial award application deadline: 2/1; financial award applicants required to submit FAFSA. *Faculty research:* Virus structure and assembly, hepatic and epithelial cell biology, drug resistance and genome stabilization in yeast, biophysics of ion-conductive nanostructures, eukaryotic gene regulation, cancer and vaccine research. *Total annual research expenditures:* $2.2 million. *Unit head:* Dr. Venigalla Rao, Chair, 202-319-5271, Fax: 202-319-5721, E-mail: rao@cua.edu. *Application contact:* Director of Graduate Admissions, 202-319-5057, Fax: 202-319-6533, E-mail: cua-admissions@cua.edu.
Website: http://biology.cua.edu/

Cedars-Sinai Medical Center, Graduate Program in Biomedical Sciences and Translational Medicine, Los Angeles, CA 90048. Offers PhD. *Degree requirements:* For doctorate, comprehensive exam, thesis/dissertation. *Entrance requirements:* For doctorate, GRE, 3 letters of recommendation. Additional exam requirements/recommendations for international students: Required—TOEFL (minimum score 550 paper-based; 80 iBT), IELTS (minimum score 6.5). Electronic applications accepted. *Faculty research:* Immunology and infection, neuroscience, cardiovascular science, cancer, human genetics.

Central Connecticut State University, School of Graduate Studies, School of Engineering, Science and Technology, Department of Biology, New Britain, CT 06050-4010. Offers biological sciences (MA, MS), including anesthesia (MS), ecology and environmental sciences (MA), general biology (MA), health sciences (MS), professional education (MS); biology (Certificate). *Program availability:* Part-time, evening/weekend. *Faculty:* 7 full-time (2 women), 2 part-time/adjunct (both women). *Students:* 113 full-time (69 women), 12 part-time (9 women); includes 24 minority (10 Black or African American, non-Hispanic/Latino; 9 Asian, non-Hispanic/Latino; 2 Hispanic/Latino; 3 Two or more races, non-Hispanic/Latino), 1 international. Average age 31. 20 applicants, 60% accepted, 2 enrolled. In 2015, 43 master's, 1 other advanced degree awarded. *Degree requirements:* For master's, comprehensive exam, thesis or alternative; for Certificate, qualifying exam. *Entrance requirements:* For master's and Certificate, minimum undergraduate GPA of 2.7, essay, letters of recommendation. Additional exam requirements/recommendations for international students: Required—TOEFL (minimum score 550 paper-based; 79 iBT). *Application deadline:* For fall admission, 6/1 for domestic students, 5/1 for international students; for spring admission, 11/1 for domestic and international students. Applications are processed on a rolling basis. Application fee: $50. Electronic applications accepted. *Expenses:* Tuition, area resident: Full-time $6188. Tuition, state resident: full-time $9284; part-time $577 per credit. Tuition, nonresident: full-time $17,240; part-time $592 per credit. *Required fees:* $4266; $234 per credit. *Financial support:* In 2015–16, 6 students received support, including 1 research assistantship; career-related internships or fieldwork, Federal Work-Study, scholarships/grants, and unspecified assistantships also available. Support available to part-time students. Financial award application deadline: 3/1; financial award applicants required to submit FAFSA. *Faculty research:* Environmental science, anesthesia, health sciences, zoology, animal behavior. *Unit head:* Dr. Douglas Carter, Chair, 860-832-2645, E-mail: carterd@ccsu.edu. *Application contact:* Patricia Gardner, Associate Director of Graduate Studies, 860-832-2350, Fax: 860-832-2362, E-mail: graduateadmissions@ccsu.edu.
Website: http://web.ccsu.edu/biodept/

Central Michigan University, College of Graduate Studies, College of Science and Technology, Department of Biology, Mount Pleasant, MI 48859. Offers biology (MS); conservation biology (MS). *Program availability:* Part-time. *Degree requirements:* For master's, thesis or alternative. *Entrance requirements:* For master's, GRE, bachelor's degree with a major in biological science, minimum GPA of 3.0. Electronic applications accepted. *Faculty research:* Conservation biology, morphology and taxonomy of aquatic plants, molecular biology and genetics, microbials and invertebrate ecology, vertebrates.

Central Washington University, Graduate Studies and Research, College of the Sciences, Department of Biological Sciences, Ellensburg, WA 98926. Offers MS. *Program availability:* Part-time. *Degree requirements:* For master's, thesis. *Entrance requirements:* For master's, GRE General Test, minimum GPA of 3.0. Additional exam requirements/recommendations for international students: Required—TOEFL (minimum score 550 paper-based; 79 iBT). Electronic applications accepted.

Chatham University, Program in Biology, Pittsburgh, PA 15232-2826. Offers environmental biology (MS); human biology (MS). *Program availability:* Part-time. *Faculty:* 1 (woman) full-time, 1 (woman) part-time/adjunct. *Students:* 52 full-time (33 women), 11 part-time (7 women); includes 20 minority (11 Black or African American, non-Hispanic/Latino; 4 Asian, non-Hispanic/Latino; 5 Hispanic/Latino), 7 international. Average age 25. 149 applicants, 66% accepted, 42 enrolled. In 2015, 35 master's awarded. *Degree requirements:* For master's, thesis optional. *Entrance requirements:* For master's, 3 letters of recommendation. Additional exam requirements/recommendations for international students: Required—TOEFL (minimum score 600 paper-based; 100 iBT), IELTS (minimum score 7), TWE. *Application deadline:* For fall admission, 4/1 priority date for domestic and international students; for spring admission, 11/1 priority date for domestic students, 10/1 priority date for international students. Applications are processed on a rolling basis. Application fee: $45. Electronic applications accepted. Application fee is waived when completed online. *Expenses: Tuition, area resident:* Full-time $15,786; part-time $877 per credit hour. *Required fees:* $468; $26 per credit hour. *Financial support:* Applicants required to submit FAFSA. *Faculty research:* Molecular evolution of iron homeostasis, characteristics of soil bacterial communities, gene flow through seed movement, role of gonadotropins in spermatogonial proliferation, phosphatid/linositol metabolism in epithelial cells. *Unit head:* Dr. Lisa Lambert, Director, 412-365-1217, E-mail: lambert@chatham.edu. *Application contact:* Ashlee Bartko, Senior Assistant Director of Graduate Admission, 412-365-1115, Fax: 412-365-1609, E-mail: gradadmissions@chatham.edu.
Website: http://www.chatham.edu/departments/sciences/graduate/biology

Chicago State University, School of Graduate and Professional Studies, College of Arts and Sciences, Department of Biological Sciences, Chicago, IL 60628. Offers MS. *Program availability:* Part-time, evening/weekend. *Degree requirements:* For master's, thesis. *Entrance requirements:* For master's, minimum GPA of 3.0, 15 credit hours in biological sciences. *Faculty research:* Molecular genetics of gene complexes,

mammalian immune cell function, genetics of agriculturally important microbes, environmental toxicology, neuromuscular physiology.

The Citadel, The Military College of South Carolina, Citadel Graduate College, Department of Biology, Charleston, SC 29409. Offers MA. *Accreditation:* NCATE. *Program availability:* Part-time, evening/weekend. *Faculty:* 4 full-time (1 woman). *Students:* 10 part-time (6 women); includes 2 minority (both Black or African American, non-Hispanic/Latino). Average age 26. In 2015, 7 master's awarded. *Entrance requirements:* For master's, GRE (minimum combined score of 290 verbal and quantitative) or MAT (minimum raw score of 396), minimum undergraduate GPA of 2.5. Additional exam requirements/recommendations for international students: Required—TOEFL (minimum score 550 paper-based). *Application deadline:* Applications are processed on a rolling basis. Application fee: $40. Electronic applications accepted. *Expenses:* Tuition, state resident: part-time $551 per credit hour. Tuition, nonresident: part-time $927 per credit hour. *Required fees:* $90 per term. *Financial support:* Health care benefits and unspecified assistantships available. Support available to part-time students. Financial award application deadline: 3/15; financial award applicants required to submit FAFSA. *Faculty research:* Genetic control of parasite-host interactions, mechanisms of development of antibiotic resistance in pseudomonas aeruginosa, interaction of visual and vocal signals in avian mate choice and competition, effects of pollutants on salt marsh animals, structure and function of mitochondrial histone H3 protein, development of cardiac conduction tissue in tadpoles with left-right axis perturbation, evolution and ecology of barnacles and marine hosts. *Unit head:* Dr. John E. Weinstein, Department Head, 843-953-5203, Fax: 843-953-7264, E-mail: john.weinstein@citadel.edu. *Application contact:* Dr. Robert H. McNamara, Associate Provost, The Citadel Graduate College, 843-953-5089, Fax: 843-953-7630, E-mail: cgc@citadel.edu.
Website: http://www.citadel.edu/root/biology

City College of the City University of New York, Graduate School, Division of Science, Department of Biology, New York, NY 10031-9198. Offers MS, PhD. PhD program offered jointly with Graduate School and University Center of the City University of New York. *Program availability:* Part-time. Terminal master's awarded for partial completion of doctoral program. *Degree requirements:* For master's, thesis or alternative; for doctorate, one foreign language, thesis/dissertation, teaching experience. *Entrance requirements:* For doctorate, GRE General Test. Additional exam requirements/recommendations for international students: Required—TOEFL (minimum score 500 paper-based; 61 iBT). *Application deadline:* For fall admission, 5/1 for domestic and international students; for spring admission, 11/15 for domestic and international students. Applications are processed on a rolling basis. Application fee: $125. Electronic applications accepted. Tuition and fees vary according to course load, degree level and program. *Financial support:* Fellowships, research assistantships, teaching assistantships, career-related internships or fieldwork, and scholarships/grants available. Financial award applicants required to submit FAFSA. *Faculty research:* Animal behavior, ecology, genetics, neurobiology, molecular biology. *Unit head:* Prof. Mark Pezzano, Chair, 212-650-8559, E-mail: biology@sci.ccny.cuny.edu. *Application contact:* 216-650-6977, E-mail: gradadm@ccny.cuny.edu.
Website: http://www.ccny.cuny.edu/biology/

Clark Atlanta University, School of Arts and Sciences, Department of Biology, Atlanta, GA 30314. Offers MS, PhD. *Program availability:* Part-time. *Faculty:* 8 full-time (3 women), 1 part-time/adjunct (0 women). *Students:* 21 full-time (13 women), 10 part-time (7 women); includes 19 minority (all Black or African American, non-Hispanic/Latino), 11 international. Average age 30. 60 applicants, 50% accepted, 1 enrolled. In 2015, 1 doctorate awarded. Terminal master's awarded for partial completion of doctoral program. *Degree requirements:* For master's, one foreign language, thesis; for doctorate, 2 foreign languages, thesis/dissertation. *Entrance requirements:* For master's, GRE General Test, minimum GPA of 2.5; for doctorate, GRE General Test, minimum graduate GPA of 3.0. Additional exam requirements/recommendations for international students: Required—TOEFL (minimum score 500 paper-based; 61 iBT). *Application deadline:* For fall admission, 4/1 for domestic and international students; for spring admission, 11/1 for domestic and international students. Applications are processed on a rolling basis. Application fee: $40 ($55 for international students). Electronic applications accepted. *Expenses:* Tuition, area resident: Full-time $15,498; part-time $861 per credit hour. *Required fees:* $1006; $1006 per unit. Tuition and fees vary according to course load. *Financial support:* Research assistantships, career-related internships or fieldwork, Federal Work-Study, scholarships/grants, traineeships, and unspecified assistantships available. Support available to part-time students. Financial award application deadline: 4/30; financial award applicants required to submit FAFSA. *Faculty research:* Regulation of amino-DNA, cellular regulations. *Unit head:* Dr. Jaideep Chaudhary, Interim Chairperson, 404-880-6821, E-mail: jchaudhary@cau.edu. *Application contact:* Graduate Program Admissions, 404-880-8483, E-mail: graduateadmissions@cau.edu.

Clark University, Graduate School, Department of Biology, Worcester, MA 01610-1477. Offers MS, PhD. *Faculty:* 10 full-time (3 women), 2 part-time/adjunct (0 women). *Students:* 31 full-time (16 women), 2 part-time (1 woman); includes 3 minority (2 Asian, non-Hispanic/Latino; 1 Hispanic/Latino), 8 international. Average age 26. 26 applicants, 69% accepted, 15 enrolled. In 2015, 3 master's, 1 doctorate awarded. *Degree requirements:* For master's, thesis; for doctorate, thesis/dissertation. *Entrance requirements:* For master's and doctorate, GRE General Test. Additional exam requirements/recommendations for international students: Required—TOEFL. *Application deadline:* For fall admission, 1/15 priority date for domestic students. Applications are processed on a rolling basis. Application fee: $75. Electronic applications accepted. *Expenses:* Tuition, area resident: Full-time $41,590; part-time $1300 per credit hour. *Required fees:* $80. Tuition and fees vary according to course load and program. *Financial support:* In 2015–16, 4 research assistantships with full tuition reimbursements (averaging $20,225 per year), 12 teaching assistantships with full tuition reimbursements (averaging $20,225 per year) were awarded; fellowships, scholarships/grants, and tuition waivers (full and partial) also available. *Faculty research:* Nitrogen assimilation in marine algae, polyporale taxonomies, fungal evolutionary history, drug discovery, taste sensitivities, biodiversity inventories. *Total annual research expenditures:* $1 million. *Unit head:* Dr. Susan Foster, Chair, 508-793-7204. *Application contact:* Paula Kupstas, Department Secretary, 508-793-7173, Fax: 528-793-7174, E-mail: pkupstas@clarku.edu.
Website: http://www.clarku.edu/departments/biology/phd/index.cfm

Clayton State University, School of Graduate Studies, College of Arts and Sciences, Program in Education, Morrow, GA 30260-0285. Offers biology (MAT); English (MAT); history (MAT); mathematics (MAT). *Accreditation:* NCATE. *Entrance requirements:* For master's, GRE, GACE, 2 official copies of transcripts, 3 recommendation letters, statement of purpose. Additional exam requirements/recommendations for international students: Required—TOEFL (minimum score 550 paper-based). *Application deadline:* For fall admission, 6/15 priority date for domestic students, 5/1 for international students; for spring admission, 10/15 priority date for domestic students. Applications are processed on a rolling basis. Application fee: $75. Electronic applications accepted. *Expenses:* Tuition, state resident: full-time $3528; part-time $196 per credit hour. Tuition, nonresident: full-time $13,176; part-time $732 per credit hour. *Required fees:*

SECTION 1: BIOLOGICAL AND BIOMEDICAL SCIENCES

Biological and Biomedical Sciences—General

$1454; $1454 per semester. $727 per semester. Tuition and fees vary according to campus/location and program. *Unit head:* Dr. Mari Ann Roberts, Program Director, Master of Arts in Teaching, 678-466-4720, E-mail: mariroberts@clayton.edu.

Clemson University, Graduate School, College of Science, Department of Biological Sciences, Program in Biological Sciences, Clemson, SC 29634. Offers MS, PhD. *Program availability:* Part-time. *Faculty:* 9 full-time (2 women). *Students:* 31 full-time (20 women); includes 1 minority (Two or more races, non-Hispanic/Latino), 8 international. Average age 28. 45 applicants, 31% accepted, 6 enrolled. In 2015, 1 master's, 5 doctorates awarded. *Degree requirements:* For master's, thesis; for doctorate, comprehensive exam, thesis/dissertation. *Entrance requirements:* For master's and doctorate, GRE General Test, unofficial transcripts, letters of recommendation. Additional exam requirements/recommendations for international students: Required—TOEFL (minimum score 100 iBT), IELTS (minimum score 7.5), PTE (minimum score 7). *Application deadline:* For fall admission, 1/5 for domestic and international students. Application fee: $80 ($90 for international students). Electronic applications accepted. *Expenses:* $4,060 per semester full-time resident, $8,103 per semester full-time non-resident, $448 per credit hour part-time resident, $898 per credit hour part-time non-resident. *Financial support:* In 2015–16, 31 students received support, including 1 fellowship with partial tuition reimbursement available (averaging $5,000 per year), 2 research assistantships with partial tuition reimbursements available (averaging $21,600 per year), 29 teaching assistantships with partial tuition reimbursements available (averaging $26,656 per year); career-related internships or fieldwork and health care benefits also available. Financial award application deadline: 1/5. *Faculty research:* Cell and developmental biology, evolutionary biology, ecology, molecular biology. *Unit head:* Dr. Robert Cohen, Department Chair, 864-656-1112, Fax: 864-656-0435, E-mail: rscohen@clemson.edu. *Application contact:* Jay Lyn Martin, Student Services Program Coordinator, 864-656-3587, Fax: 864-656-0435, E-mail: jaylyn@clemson.edu. Website: http://www.clemson.edu/cafls/departments/biosci/

Clemson University, Graduate School, College of Science, Department of Biological Sciences, Program in Biological Sciences for Science Educators, Clemson, SC 29364. Offers MBS. *Program availability:* Part-time/evening/weekend, online only, 100% online. *Faculty:* 12 full-time (6 women). *Students:* 7 full-time (5 women), 195 part-time (132 women); includes 28 minority (10 Black or African American, non-Hispanic/Latino; 5 Asian, non-Hispanic/Latino; 5 Hispanic/Latino; 1 Native Hawaiian or other Pacific Islander, non-Hispanic/Latino; 7 Two or more races, non-Hispanic/Latino). Average age 36. 131 applicants, 85% accepted, 112 enrolled. In 2015, 32 master's awarded. *Entrance requirements:* For master's, GRE General Test (waived for teachers with 1 or more years' teaching experience), unofficial transcripts, letters of recommendation, resume. Additional exam requirements/recommendations for international students: Required—TOEFL (minimum score 550 paper-based; 80 iBT), IELTS (minimum score 6.5). *Application deadline:* For fall admission, 8/1 for domestic students; for spring admission, 12/15 for domestic students; for summer admission, 5/1 for domestic students. Applications are processed on a rolling basis. Application fee: $80 ($90 for international students). Electronic applications accepted. *Expenses:* $394 per credit hour, $10 per credit hour technology fee, $39 per session fees. *Financial support:* Tuition waiver for state of SC employees available. *Unit head:* Dr. Robert Cohen, Department Chair, 864-656-1112, E-mail: rscohen@clemson.edu. *Application contact:* Dr. Robert Ballard, Program Coordinator, 864-656-3579, E-mail: ballard@clemson.edu. Website: http://www.clemson.edu/cafls/departments/biosci/biol_online_masters/index.html

Cleveland State University, College of Graduate Studies, College of Sciences and Health Professions, Department of Biological, Geological, and Environmental Sciences, Cleveland, OH 44115. Offers biology (MS); environmental science (MS); regulatory biology (PhD). *Program availability:* Part-time. *Faculty:* 18 full-time (5 women), 54 part-time/adjunct (22 women). *Students:* 53 full-time (28 women), 15 part-time (10 women); includes 6 minority (2 Black or African American, non-Hispanic/Latino; 4 Asian, non-Hispanic/Latino), 35 international. Average age 30. 40 applicants, 63% accepted, 9 enrolled. In 2015, 6 master's, 12 doctorates awarded. Terminal master's awarded for partial completion of doctoral program. *Degree requirements:* For master's, comprehensive exam (for some programs), thesis (for some programs), thesis defense; for doctorate, comprehensive exam, thesis/dissertation, dissertation defense. *Entrance requirements:* For master's, GRE General Test, 3 letters of recommendation; for doctorate, GRE General Test, 3 letters of recommendation; 1-2 page essay; statement of career goals and research interests. Additional exam requirements/recommendations for international students: Required—TOEFL (minimum score 550 paper-based; 78 iBT), IELTS. *Application deadline:* For fall admission, 7/1 priority date for domestic students, 5/15 priority date for international students; for spring admission, 11/15 priority date for domestic students, 11/1 for international students; for summer admission, 4/1 for domestic students, 3/15 for international students. Applications are processed on a rolling basis. Application fee: $30. Electronic applications accepted. *Expenses:* Tuition, state resident: full-time $9565. Tuition, nonresident: full-time $17,980. Tuition and fees vary according to program. *Financial support:* In 2015–16, 33 students received support, including 1 fellowship with full tuition reimbursement available (averaging $21,000 per year), 16 research assistantships with full tuition reimbursements available (averaging $21,000 per year), 31 teaching assistantships with full tuition reimbursements available (averaging $21,000 per year); tuition waivers and unspecified assistantships also available. Financial award applicants required to submit FAFSA. *Faculty research:* Cardiopulmonary pathology, signaling pathways and RNA interference, toxoplasmosis, plant ecology, biology and biochemistry of nitric oxide. *Unit head:* Dr. Crystal M. Weyman, Chairperson/Professor, 216-687-6971, Fax: 216-687-6972, E-mail: c.weyman@csuohio.edu. *Application contact:* Dr. Girish C. Shukla, Associate Professor and Graduate Program Director, 216-687-2395, Fax: 216-687-6972, E-mail: g.shukla@csuohio.edu. Website: http://www.csuohio.edu/sciences/bges

Cold Spring Harbor Laboratory, Watson School of Biological Sciences, Cold Spring Harbor, NY 11724. Offers biological sciences (PhD). *Faculty:* 48 full-time (11 women). *Students:* 42 full-time (22 women); includes 4 minority (1 Black or African American, non-Hispanic/Latino; 1 Asian, non-Hispanic/Latino; 2 Hispanic/Latino), 25 international. Average age 27. 310 applicants, 9% accepted, 7 enrolled. In 2015, 7 doctorates awarded. *Degree requirements:* For doctorate, comprehensive exam, thesis/dissertation, lab rotations, teaching experience, qualifying exam, postdoctoral proposals. *Entrance requirements:* For doctorate, GRE (recommended). Additional exam requirements/recommendations for international students: Required—TOEFL or IELTS. *Application deadline:* For fall admission, 12/1 for domestic and international students. Application fee: $60. Electronic applications accepted. *Financial support:* In 2015–16, 42 students received support, including 42 fellowships with full tuition reimbursements available (averaging $33,000 per year); health care benefits and tuition waivers (full) also available. Financial award application deadline: 12/1. *Faculty research:* Genetics and genomics, neurobiology, cancer, plant biology, molecular biology, quantitative biology, bioinformatics. *Application contact:* E-mail: gradschool@cshl.edu. Website: http://www.cshl.edu/gradschool

The College at Brockport, State University of New York, School of Education and Human Services, Department of Education and Human Development, Program in Inclusive Generalist Education, Brockport, NY 14420-2997. Offers biology (MS Ed, AGC); chemistry (MS Ed, AGC); English (MS Ed, Advanced Certificate); mathematics (MS Ed, Advanced Certificate); science (MS Ed, Advanced Certificate); social studies (MS Ed, Advanced Certificate). *Students:* 27 full-time (16 women), 24 part-time (16 women); includes 13 minority (4 Black or African American, non-Hispanic/Latino; 3 Asian, non-Hispanic/Latino; 2 Hispanic/Latino; 4 Two or more races, non-Hispanic/Latino). 23 applicants, 57% accepted, 10 enrolled. In 2015, 13 master's, 1 AGC awarded. *Degree requirements:* For master's, thesis or alternative. *Entrance requirements:* For master's, minimum GPA of 3.0, letters of recommendation, statement of objectives, academic major (or equivalent) in program discipline, current resume. Additional exam requirements/recommendations for international students: Required—TOEFL (minimum score 550 paper-based; 79 iBT), IELTS (minimum score 6.5). *Application deadline:* For fall admission, 3/15 priority date for domestic and international students; for spring admission, 10/15 priority date for domestic and international students; for summer admission, 3/15 for domestic and international students. Application fee: $80. Electronic applications accepted. *Expenses:* $11,840 per academic year. *Financial support:* Federal Work-Study, scholarships/grants, and unspecified assistantships available. Support available to part-time students. Financial award application deadline: 3/15; financial award applicants required to submit FAFSA. *Unit head:* Dr. Sue Robb, Chairperson, 585-395-5935, Fax: 585-395-2171, E-mail: awalton@brockport.edu. *Application contact:* Anne Walton, Coordinator of Certification and Graduate Advisement, 585-395-2326, Fax: 585-395-2172, E-mail: awalton@brockport.edu. Website: http://www.brockport.edu/ehd/

The College at Brockport, State University of New York, School of Science and Mathematics, Department of Biology, Brockport, NY 14420-2997. Offers MS, PSM. *Program availability:* Part-time. *Faculty:* 5 full-time (1 woman). *Students:* 9 full-time (4 women), 6 part-time (5 women); includes 3 minority (1 Black or African American, non-Hispanic/Latino; 1 Asian, non-Hispanic/Latino; 1 Hispanic/Latino). 15 applicants, 40% accepted, 4 enrolled. In 2015, 7 master's awarded. *Degree requirements:* For master's, comprehensive exam, thesis or alternative. *Entrance requirements:* For master's, letters of recommendation, minimum GPA of 3.0, scientific writing sample, statement of objectives. Additional exam requirements/recommendations for international students: Required—TOEFL (minimum score 550 paper-based; 79 iBT), IELTS (minimum score 6.5). *Application deadline:* For fall admission, 7/15 priority date for domestic and international students; for spring admission, 11/15 priority date for domestic and international students; for summer admission, 6/15 priority date for domestic and international students. Application fee: $50. Electronic applications accepted. *Expenses:* $11,840 per academic year. *Financial support:* In 2015–16, 8 teaching assistantships with full tuition reimbursements (averaging $6,000 per year) were awarded; Federal Work-Study, scholarships/grants, and unspecified assistantships also available. Support available to part-time students. Financial award applicants required to submit FAFSA. *Faculty research:* Microbiology, molecular genetics, cellular biology, developmental biology, animal physiology. *Unit head:* Dr. Rey Sia, Chairperson, 585-395-2783, Fax: 585-395-2741, E-mail: rsia@brockport.edu. *Application contact:* Dr. Adam Rich, Graduate Program Director, 585-395-5740, Fax: 585-395-2741, E-mail: arich@brockport.edu. Website: http://www.brockport.edu/biology/graduate/

College of Staten Island of the City University of New York, Graduate Programs, Division of Science and Technology, Program in Biology, Staten Island, NY 10314-6600. Offers MS. *Program availability:* Part-time, evening/weekend. *Faculty:* 10 full-time, 5 part-time/adjunct. *Students:* 11 full-time, 17 part-time. Average age 27. 33 applicants, 61% accepted, 16 enrolled. In 2015, 3 master's awarded. *Entrance requirements:* For master's, GRE General Test, GRE Subject Test (biology), BS in biology from accredited college; minimum overall GPA of 2.75, 3.0 in undergraduate science and mathematics courses; two letters of recommendation. Additional exam requirements/recommendations for international students: Required—TOEFL (minimum score 550 paper-based; 79 iBT), IELTS (minimum score 6.5). *Application deadline:* For fall admission, 4/15 for domestic and international students; for spring admission, 11/25 for domestic and international students. Applications are processed on a rolling basis. Application fee: $125. Electronic applications accepted. *Expenses:* Tuition, state resident: full-time $10,130; part-time $425 per credit. Tuition, nonresident: full-time $18,720; part-time $780 per credit. *Required fees:* $181.10 per semester. Tuition and fees vary according to program. *Financial support:* Applicants required to submit FAFSA. *Unit head:* Dr. Shaibal Mira, Graduate Program Coordinator, General Biology Track, 718-982-3858, Fax: 718-982-3852, E-mail: shaibal.mitra@csi.cuny.edu. *Application contact:* Sasha Spence, Associate Director for Graduate Admissions, 718-982-2019, Fax: 718-982-2500, E-mail: sasha.spence@csi.cuny.edu. Website: http://www.csi.cuny.edu/departments/biology/graduate.html

College of Staten Island of the City University of New York, Graduate Programs, School of Education, Program in Adolescence Education, Staten Island, NY. 10314-6600. Offers biology (MS Ed). *Program availability:* Part-time, evening/weekend. *Faculty:* 20 full-time, 7 part-time/adjunct. *Students:* 8 full-time, 97 part-time. Average age 28. 59 applicants, 47% accepted, 27 enrolled. In 2015, 38 master's awarded. *Degree requirements:* For master's, 2 foreign languages, thesis, educational research project; minimum of 33-38 credits distributed among 11 courses or minimum of 46-53 credits. *Entrance requirements:* For master's, relevant bachelor's degree, minimum overall GPA of 3.0, two letters of recommendation, one- or two-page personal statement. Additional exam requirements/recommendations for international students: Required—TOEFL (minimum score 550 paper-based; 79 iBT), IELTS (minimum score 6.5). *Application deadline:* For fall admission, 4/25 for domestic and international students; for spring admission, 11/25 for domestic and international students. Applications are processed on a rolling basis. Application fee: $125. Electronic applications accepted. *Expenses:* Tuition, state resident: full-time $10,130; part-time $425 per credit. Tuition, nonresident: full-time $18,720; part-time $780 per credit. *Required fees:* $181.10 per semester. Tuition and fees vary according to program. *Financial support:* Applicants required to submit FAFSA. *Faculty research:* Development and assessment of TPACK (technological pedagogical content knowledge), technology and differentiation in stem classrooms, teacher effectiveness and student achievement, teacher knowledge, knowledge transfer from college to classroom. *Unit head:* Dr. Bethany Rogers, Graduate Program Director, 718-982-4147, E-mail: bethany.rogers@csi.cuny.edu. *Application contact:* Sasha Spence, Associate Director for Graduate Admissions, 718-982-2019, Fax: 718-982-2500, E-mail: sasha.spence@csi.cuny.edu. Website: http://www.csi.cuny.edu/catalog/graduate/graduate-programs-in-education.htm#o2608

The College of William and Mary, Faculty of Arts and Sciences, Department of Biology, Williamsburg, VA 23187-8795. Offers MS. *Faculty:* 28 full-time (11 women). *Students:* 20 full-time (13 women); includes 2 minority (both Hispanic/Latino), 2 international. Average age 25. 73 applicants, 15% accepted, 9 enrolled. In 2015, 7 master's awarded. *Degree requirements:* For master's (for some programs). *Entrance requirements:* For master's, GRE Subject Test (recommended for students who have not earned bachelor's degree in biology), GRE General Test, minimum GPA of 3.0. Additional exam requirements/recommendations for international students: Required—TOEFL. *Application deadline:* For fall admission, 2/1

priority date for domestic and international students. *Application fee:* $45. Electronic applications accepted. *Expenses:* Tuition, state resident: full-time $8009; part-time $450 per credit hour. Tuition, nonresident: full-time $23,752; part-time $1160 per credit hour. *Required fees:* $4162. One-time fee: $400 full-time. *Financial support:* In 2015–16, 15 teaching assistantships with full tuition reimbursements (averaging $13,500 per year) were awarded; Federal Work-Study, institutionally sponsored loans, and unspecified assistantships also available. Financial award application deadline: 2/1; financial award applicants required to submit FAFSA. *Faculty research:* Cellular and molecular biology, genetics, ecology, organismal biology, physiology. *Total annual research expenditures:* $225,000. *Unit head:* Dr. Eric L. Bradley, Chair, 757-221-2220, E-mail: elbrad@wm.edu. *Application contact:* Dr. Matthew Wawersik, Graduate Director, 757-221-2237, E-mail: mjwawe@wm.edu.
Website: http://www.wm.edu/biology/

Colorado State University, College of Natural Sciences, Department of Biology, Fort Collins, CO 80523-1878. Offers botany (MS, PhD); zoology (MS, PhD). *Faculty:* 29 full-time (9 women), 4 part-time/adjunct (3 women). *Students:* full-time (8 women), 22 part-time (13 women); includes 5 minority (4 Asian, non-Hispanic/Latino; 1 Hispanic/Latino), 6 international. Average age 30. 18 applicants, 94% accepted, 11 enrolled. In 2015, 7 master's, 2 doctorates awarded. Terminal master's awarded for partial completion of doctoral program. *Degree requirements:* For master's, comprehensive exam, thesis; for doctorate, comprehensive exam, thesis/dissertation. *Entrance requirements:* For master's and doctorate, GRE General Test (minimum scores above 70th percentile), transcripts, 3 letters of recommendation, statement of purpose, minimum GPA of 3.0. Additional exam requirements/recommendations for international students: Required—TOEFL (minimum score 550 paper-based; 80 iBT), IELTS (minimum score 6.5). *Application deadline:* For fall admission, 1/15 priority date for domestic and international students; for spring admission, 11/1 priority date for domestic and international students. Applications are processed on a rolling basis. Application fee: $60 ($70 for international students). Electronic applications accepted. *Expenses:* Tuition, state resident: full-time $9348. Tuition, nonresident: full-time $22,916. *Required fees:* $2174; $473.72 per credit hour. $236.86 per semester. Tuition and fees vary according to course load and program. *Financial support:* In 2015–16, 21 fellowships (averaging $42,613 per year), 12 research assistantships with full tuition reimbursements (averaging $18,531 per year), 66 teaching assistantships with full tuition reimbursements (averaging $17,703 per year) were awarded; career-related internships or fieldwork, Federal Work-Study, scholarships/grants, traineeships, and unspecified assistantships also available. Financial award application deadline: 1/1; financial award applicants required to submit FAFSA. *Faculty research:* Global ecological change; organismal interactions in infectious disease; stream ecology; muscle protein structure; plant biotechnology. *Total annual research expenditures:* $7.8 million. *Unit head:* Dr. Michael F. Antolin, Department Chair, 970-491-7011, Fax: 970-491-0649, E-mail: michael.antolin@colostate.edu. *Application contact:* Dorothy Ramirez, Graduate Coordinator, 970-491-1923, Fax: 970-491-0649, E-mail: dramirez@colostate.edu.
Website: http://www.biology.colostate.edu/

Colorado State University, College of Veterinary Medicine and Biomedical Sciences, Department of Biomedical Sciences, Fort Collins, CO 80523-1680. Offers MS, PhD. *Faculty:* 38 full-time (18 women), 2 part-time/adjunct (1 woman). *Students:* 82 full-time (52 women), 34 part-time (17 women); includes 21 minority (3 Black or African American, non-Hispanic/Latino; 2 American Indian or Alaska Native, non-Hispanic/Latino; 3 Asian, non-Hispanic/Latino; 6 Hispanic/Latino; 7 Two or more races, non-Hispanic/Latino), 6 international. Average age 26. 260 applicants, 32% accepted, 76 enrolled. In 2015, 47 master's, 2 doctorates awarded. *Degree requirements:* For master's, comprehensive exam (for some programs), thesis (for some programs); for doctorate, comprehensive exam (for some programs), thesis/dissertation (for some programs). *Entrance requirements:* For master's, GRE General Test, MCAT, or DAT, bachelor's degree, minimum GPA of 3.0; for doctorate, GRE General Test, MCAT, or DAT, bachelor's or professional degree, minimum GPA of 3.0. Additional exam requirements/recommendations for international students: Required—TOEFL (minimum score 550 paper-based; 80 iBT), IELTS (minimum score 6.5). *Application deadline:* For fall admission, 4/1 priority date for domestic and international students; for spring admission, 9/1 priority date for domestic and international students; for summer admission, 1/1 priority date for domestic and international students. Application fee: $60 ($70 for international students). Electronic applications accepted. *Expenses:* Contact institution. *Financial support:* In 2015–16, 40 students received support, including 13 fellowships with full tuition reimbursements available (averaging $44,022 per year), 19 research assistantships with full tuition reimbursements available (averaging $21,857 per year), 7 teaching assistantships with full tuition reimbursements available (averaging $18,240 per year); scholarships/grants and unspecified assistantships also available. Financial award application deadline: 4/1; financial award applicants required to submit FAFSA. *Faculty research:* Cardiovascular physiology, reproductive physiology, neurobiology, equine reproduction, assisted reproductive technologies. *Total annual research expenditures:* $9 million. *Unit head:* Dr. Colin M. Clay, Professor and Department Head, 970-491-7571, Fax: 970-491-3557, E-mail: colin.clay@colostate.edu. *Application contact:* Erin Bisenius, Graduate Education Coordinator, 970-491-6188, Fax: 970-491-7569, E-mail: erin.bisenius@colostate.edu.
Website: http://csu-cvmbs.colostate.edu/academics/bms/Pages/default.aspx

Colorado State University–Pueblo, College of Science and Mathematics, Pueblo, CO 81001-4901. Offers applied natural science (MS), including biochemistry, biology, chemistry. *Program availability:* Part-time, evening/weekend. *Degree requirements:* For master's, comprehensive exam (for some programs), thesis (for some programs), internship report (if non-thesis). *Entrance requirements:* For master's, GRE General Test (minimum score 1000), 2 letters of reference, minimum GPA of 3.0. Additional exam requirements/recommendations for international students: Required—TOEFL (minimum score 500 paper-based), IELTS (minimum score 5). *Faculty research:* Fungal cell walls, molecular biology, bioactive materials synthesis, atomic force microscopy-surface chemistry, nanoscience.

Columbia University, College of Physicians and Surgeons, New York, NY 10032. Offers M Phil, MA, MS, DN Sc, DPT, Ed D, MD, PhD, Adv C, MBA/MS, MD/DDS, MD/MPH, MD/MS, MD/PhD, MPH/MS. *Program availability:* Part-time. *Entrance requirements:* For master's, GRE General Test. Additional exam requirements/recommendations for international students: Required—TOEFL. *Expenses:* Contact institution.

★ **Columbia University,** Graduate School of Arts and Sciences, Department of Biological Sciences, New York, NY 10027. Offers PhD. *Degree requirements:* For doctorate, comprehensive exam, thesis/dissertation, teaching experience. *Entrance requirements:* For doctorate, GRE General Test, GRE Subject Test (recommended), letters of recommendation. Additional exam requirements/recommendations for international students: Required—TOEFL (minimum score 600 paper-based; 100 iBT). *Application deadline:* For fall admission, 1/4 for domestic students. Application fee: $100. *Financial support:* Fellowships, teaching assistantships, Federal Work-Study, institutionally sponsored loans, and health care benefits available. Support available to part-time students. Financial award application deadline: 12/1;

financial award applicants required to submit FAFSA. *Unit head:* Sarah Kim Fein, Program Coordinator, 212-854-2313, Fax: 212-865-8246, E-mail: sarah@biology.columbia.edu. *Application contact:* Robert Furno, Assistant Dean for Admissions, 212-854-4738, Fax: 212-854-2863, E-mail: ref8@columbia.edu.
Website: http://biology.columbia.edu/

See Display on next page and Close-Up on page 105.

The Commonwealth Medical College, Graduate Programs in Medicine, Scranton, PA 18509. Offers biomedical sciences (MBS). *Program availability:* Part-time, evening/weekend. *Students:* 55 full-time (26 women), 3 part-time (0 women). *Entrance requirements:* For master's, MCAT, DAT, GRE, bachelor's degree; coursework in biology with lab, organic chemistry with lab, inorganic chemistry with lab, physics with lab, and English; official transcripts; three letters of recommendation. *Application deadline:* Applications are processed on a rolling basis. Application fee: $55. Electronic applications accepted. *Financial support:* Application deadline: 3/1; applicants required to submit FAFSA. *Application contact:* Jillian Golaszewski, Enrollment Management Recruiter, 570-504-7000, Fax: 570-504-2794, E-mail: jgolaszewski@tcmc.edu.
Website: http://www.tcmc.edu/mbs

Concordia University, School of Graduate Studies, Faculty of Arts and Science, Department of Biology, Montréal, QC H3G 1M8, Canada. Offers biology (M Sc, PhD); biotechnology and genomics (Diploma). *Degree requirements:* For master's, thesis; for doctorate, thesis/dissertation, pedagogical training. *Entrance requirements:* For master's, honors degree in biology; for doctorate, M Sc in life science. *Application deadline:* For fall admission, 1/15 priority date for domestic students; for winter admission, 8/31 for domestic students. Application fee: $50. Tuition and fees vary according to course load, degree level and program. *Faculty research:* Cell biology, animal physiology, ecology, microbiology/molecular biology, plant physiology/biochemistry and biotechnology. *Unit head:* Patrick Gulick, Chair, 514-848-2424 Ext. 3407, Fax: 514-848-2881. *Application contact:* Selvadurai Dayanandan, Graduate Program Director, 514-848-2424 Ext. 3414, Fax: 514-848-2881.
Website: http://www.concordia.ca/artsci/biology.html

Cornell University, Graduate School, Graduate Fields of Comparative Biomedical Sciences, Field of Comparative Biomedical Sciences, Ithaca, NY 14853-0001. Offers cellular and molecular medicine (MS, PhD); developmental and reproductive biology (MS, PhD); infectious diseases (MS, PhD); population medicine and epidemiology (MS, PhD); structural and functional biology (MS, PhD). *Degree requirements:* For master's, thesis; for doctorate, comprehensive exam, thesis/dissertation. *Entrance requirements:* For master's and doctorate, GRE General Test, 2 letters of recommendation. Additional exam requirements/recommendations for international students: Required—TOEFL (minimum score 550 paper-based; 77 iBT). Electronic applications accepted. *Faculty research:* Receptors and signal transduction, viral and bacterial infectious diseases, tumor metastasis, clinical sciences/nutritional disease, developmental/neurological disorders.

Creighton University, School of Medicine and Graduate School, Graduate Programs in Medicine, Department of Biomedical Sciences, Omaha, NE 68178-0001. Offers MS, PhD, MD/PhD. Terminal master's awarded for partial completion of doctoral program. *Degree requirements:* For master's, thesis; for doctorate, thesis/dissertation. *Entrance requirements:* For master's, GRE General Test (minimum 50th percentile), three recommendations; for doctorate, GRE General Test (minimum score: 50th percentile), three recommendations. Additional exam requirements/recommendations for international students: Required—TOEFL. Electronic applications accepted. *Expenses:* Tuition, area resident: Full-time $14,400; part-time $800 per credit hour. *Required fees:* $158 per semester. Tuition and fees vary according to course load, campus/location, program, reciprocity agreements and student's religious affiliation. *Faculty research:* Molecular biology and gene transfection.

Dalhousie University, Faculty of Graduate Studies and Faculty of Medicine, Graduate Programs in Medicine, Halifax, NS B3H 4R2, Canada. Offers M Sc, PhD. *Degree requirements:* For master's, thesis; for doctorate, thesis/dissertation. *Entrance requirements:* Additional exam requirements/recommendations for international students: Required—1 of 5 approved tests: TOEFL, IELTS, CANTEST, CAEL, Michigan English Language Assessment Battery. Electronic applications accepted. *Expenses:* Contact institution.

Dalhousie University, Faculty of Science, Department of Biology, Halifax, NS B3H 4R2, Canada. Offers M Sc, PhD. Terminal master's awarded for partial completion of doctoral program. *Degree requirements:* For master's, thesis; for doctorate, thesis/dissertation. *Entrance requirements:* Additional exam requirements/recommendations for international students: Required—TOEFL, IELTS, CANTEST, CAEL, or Michigan English Language Assessment Battery. Electronic applications accepted. *Faculty research:* Marine biology, ecology, animal physiology, plant physiology, microbiology (cell, molecular, genetics, development).

Dartmouth College, Graduate Program in Molecular and Cellular Biology, Department of Biological Sciences, Hanover, NH 03755. Offers PhD, MBA/PhD, MD/PhD. *Faculty:* 19 full-time (7 women). *Students:* 45 full-time (23 women); includes 7 minority (1 Asian, non-Hispanic/Latino; 5 Hispanic/Latino; 1 Two or more races, non-Hispanic/Latino), 11 international. Average age 27. *Entrance requirements:* For doctorate, GRE General Test, letters of recommendation. Additional exam requirements/recommendations for international students: Required—TOEFL (minimum score paper-based 550, iBT 100) or IELTS (7.0). *Application deadline:* For fall admission, 12/1 for domestic students. Application fee: $75. Electronic applications accepted. *Expenses:* Tuition, area resident: Full-time $48,120. *Required fees:* $296. One-time fee: $50 full-time. *Financial support:* In 2015–16, fellowships with full tuition reimbursements (averaging $28,200 per year) were awarded; health care benefits also available. *Unit head:* Dr. Thomas Jack, Chair and Professor, 603-646-2378, E-mail: biology@dartmouth.edu. *Application contact:* Janet Cheney, Program Coordinator, 603-650-1612, Fax: 603-650-1006, E-mail: mcb@dartmouth.edu.
Website: http://www.dartmouth.edu/~mcb/

Delaware State University, Graduate Programs, Department of Biological Sciences, Program in Biological Sciences, Dover, DE 19901-2277. Offers MS. *Entrance requirements:* For master's, GRE, prerequisite undergraduate courses. Additional exam requirements/recommendations for international students: Required—TOEFL.

Delta State University, Graduate Programs, College of Arts and Sciences, Division of Biological and Physical Sciences, Cleveland, MS 38733-0001. Offers natural sciences (MSNS). *Program availability:* Part-time. *Degree requirements:* For master's, research project or thesis. *Entrance requirements:* For master's, GRE General Test.

DePaul University, College of Science and Health, Chicago, IL 60614. Offers applied mathematics (MS); applied statistics (MS); biological sciences (MA, MS); chemistry (MS); mathematics education (MA); mathematics for teaching (MS); nursing (MS); nursing practice (DNP); physics (MS); psychology (MS); pure mathematics (MS); science education (MS); MA/PhD. Electronic applications accepted.

Des Moines University, College of Osteopathic Medicine, Program in Biomedical Sciences, Des Moines, IA 50312-4104. Offers MS.

Biological and Biomedical Sciences—General

Dominican University of California, School of Health and Natural Sciences, Program in Biological Sciences, San Rafael, CA 94901-2298. Offers MS. *Faculty:* 5 full-time (2 women), 6 part-time/adjunct (4 women). *Students:* 20 full-time (13 women), 1 part-time (0 women); includes 12 minority (1 Black or African American, non-Hispanic/Latino; 5 Asian, non-Hispanic/Latino; 5 Hispanic/Latino; 1 Two or more races, non-Hispanic/Latino), 4 international. Average age 25. 14 applicants, 93% accepted, 12 enrolled. *Degree requirements:* For master's, thesis. *Entrance requirements:* For master's, GRE, BS in biology, biological sciences or biomedical sciences; minimum GPA of 3.0 in last 60 units. Additional exam requirements/recommendations for international students: Required—TOEFL (minimum score 550 paper-based; 80 iBT), IELTS (minimum score 6.5). *Application deadline:* For fall admission, 3/15 priority date for domestic and international students. Applications are processed on a rolling basis. Electronic applications accepted. Application fee is waived when completed online. *Expenses:* Contact institution. *Financial support:* Research assistantships, career-related internships or fieldwork, and scholarships/grants available. Financial award application deadline: 3/2; financial award applicants required to submit FAFSA. *Unit head:* Dr. Maggie Louie, Program Director, 415-485-3248, E-mail: maggie.louie@dominican.edu. *Application contact:* Shannon Lovelace-White, Assistant Vice President, Graduate and Adult Admissions, 415-485-3204, Fax: 415-485-3214, E-mail: shannon.lovelace-white@dominican.edu.
Website: http://www.dominican.edu/academics/hns/sciencemath/graduate/copy_of_msbio

Drew University, Caspersen School of Graduate Studies, Madison, NJ 07940-1493. Offers conflict resolution and leadership (Certificate), including community leadership, moderation, peace building; history and culture (MA, PhD), including American history, book history, British history, European history, Holocaust and genocide (M Litt, MA, D Litt, PhD), intellectual history, Irish history, print culture, public history; K-12 education (MAT), including art, biology, chemistry, elementary education, English, French, Italian, math, secondary education, special education, teacher of students with disabilities; liberal studies (M Litt, D Litt), including history, Holocaust and genocide (M Litt, MA, D Litt, PhD), Irish/Irish-American studies, literature (M Litt, MMH, D Litt, DMH, CMH), religion, spirituality, teaching in the two-year college, writing; medical humanities (MMH, DMH, CMH), including arts, health, healthcare, literature (M Litt, MMH, D Litt, DMH, CMH), scientific research; poetry and poetry in translation (MFA). *Program availability:* Part-time, evening/weekend. *Faculty:* 1 full-time, 26 part-time/adjunct. *Students:* 125 full-time (82 women), 261 part-time (164 women); includes 34 minority (17 Black or African American, non-Hispanic/Latino; 6 Asian, non-Hispanic/Latino; 11 Hispanic/Latino), 6 international. Average age 42. 120 applicants, 90% accepted, 76 enrolled. In 2015, 54 master's, 36 doctorates, 9 other advanced degrees awarded. Terminal master's awarded for partial completion of doctoral program. *Degree requirements:* For master's and other advanced degree, thesis (for some programs); for doctorate, one foreign language, comprehensive exam (for some programs), thesis/dissertation. *Entrance requirements:* For master's, GRE (MA in history and culture), PRAXIS Core and Subject Area tests (MAT), resume, transcripts, writing sample, personal statement, letters of recommendation; for doctorate, GRE (PhD in history and culture), resume, transcripts, writing sample, personal statement, letters of recommendation. Additional exam requirements/recommendations for international students: Required—TOEFL (minimum score 587 paper-based; 94 iBT), IELTS (minimum score 7), TWE (minimum score 4). *Application deadline:* Applications are processed on a rolling basis. Application fee: $35. Tuition and fees vary according to program. *Financial support:* In 2015–16, 214 students received support. Fellowships, research assistantships, teaching assistantships, career-related internships or fieldwork, Federal Work-Study, scholarships/grants, and unspecified assistantships available. Support available to part-time students. Financial award applicants required to submit FAFSA. *Unit head:* Dr.

Robert Ready, Dean, 973-408-3285, Fax: 973-408-3040, E-mail: gsdean@drew.edu. *Application contact:* Leanne Horinko, Interim Director of Admissions, 973-408-3110, Fax: 973-408-3110, E-mail: gradm@drew.edu.
Website: http://www.drew.edu/graduate

Drexel University, College of Arts and Sciences, Department of Biology, Philadelphia, PA 19104-2875. Offers biological sciences (MS, PhD); human nutrition (MS). *Program availability:* Part-time. *Degree requirements:* For doctorate, thesis/dissertation. *Entrance requirements:* For master's and doctorate, GRE General Test. Additional exam requirements/recommendations for international students: Required—TOEFL. Electronic applications accepted. *Faculty research:* Genetic engineering, physiological ecology.

Drexel University, College of Medicine, Biomedical Graduate Programs, Philadelphia, PA 19129. Offers MLAS, MMS, MS, PhD, Certificate, MD/PhD. *Program availability:* Part-time. Terminal master's awarded for partial completion of doctoral program. *Degree requirements:* For master's, comprehensive exam; for doctorate, thesis/dissertation, qualifying exam. *Entrance requirements:* For master's and doctorate, GRE General Test. Additional exam requirements/recommendations for international students: Required—TOEFL. Electronic applications accepted. *Expenses:* Contact institution.

Drexel University, College of Medicine, MD/PhD Program, Philadelphia, PA 19104-2875. Offers MD/PhD. Electronic applications accepted.

Drexel University, School of Biomedical Engineering, Science and Health Systems, Program in Biomedical Science, Philadelphia, PA 19104-2875. Offers MS, PhD. *Degree requirements:* For master's, thesis (for some programs); for doctorate, thesis/dissertation. Electronic applications accepted.

Duke University, Graduate School, Department of Biology, Durham, NC 27708. Offers PhD. *Degree requirements:* For doctorate, one foreign language, thesis/dissertation. *Entrance requirements:* For doctorate, GRE General Test, GRE Subject Test (recommended). Additional exam requirements/recommendations for international students: Required—TOEFL (minimum score 577 paper-based; 90 iBT) or IELTS (minimum score 7). Electronic applications accepted.

Duke University, School of Medicine, Program in Biomedical Sciences, Durham, NC 27710. Offers MS. *Faculty:* 16 full-time (9 women), 1 part-time/adjunct (0 women). *Students:* 34 full-time (13 women); includes 18 minority (7 Black or African American, non-Hispanic/Latino; 5 Asian, non-Hispanic/Latino; 2 Hispanic/Latino; 4 Two or more races, non-Hispanic/Latino), 1 international. 190 applicants, 23% accepted, 33 enrolled. *Entrance requirements:* For master's, GRE, BS from accredited institution; minimum GPA of 3.2. *Application deadline:* For fall admission, 1/31 priority date for domestic students. Applications are processed on a rolling basis. Application fee: $75. Electronic applications accepted. *Financial support:* In 2015–16, 13 students received support. Scholarships/grants available. Financial award application deadline: 5/1; financial award applicants required to submit FAFSA. *Unit head:* Dr. Linda S. Lee, Associate Professor, 919-684-6351, Fax: 919-681-0720, E-mail: linda.s.lee@duke.edu. *Application contact:* Christie T. McCray, Administrative Coordinator, 919-684-6351, Fax: 919-681-0720, E-mail: christie.mccray@duke.edu.
Website: https://medschool.duke.edu/education/degree-programs-and-admissions/master-biomedical-sciences

Duquesne University, Bayer School of Natural and Environmental Sciences, Department of Biological Sciences, Pittsburgh, PA 15282-0001. Offers PhD. *Faculty:* 14 full-time (4 women), 2 part-time/adjunct (0 women). *Students:* 28 full-time (16 women), 2 part-time (both women); includes 2 minority (1 Asian, non-Hispanic/Latino; 1 Two or more races, non-Hispanic/Latino), 9 international. Average age 29. 42 applicants, 24% accepted, 9 enrolled. In 2015, 7 doctorates awarded. *Median time to degree:* Of those

COLUMBIA UNIVERSITY
DEPARTMENT OF BIOLOGICAL SCIENCES

The Department of Biological Sciences at Columbia University offers training leading to Ph.D. degrees with concentrations in cellular, molecular, developmental, computational, and structural biology as well as genetics, biophysics, and neurobiology. The mentors in the Ph.D. program include twelve members of the National Academy of Sciences, seven members of the Institute of Medicine, three Nobel Laureates, and a Lasker Award winner. The program provides each student with a solid background in contemporary molecularly oriented biology and an in-depth knowledge of one or more of the above areas. Acceptance to the program is determined by a student's academic background as well as consideration of prior research experience, GRE scores, and letters of recommendation.

Tuition, fees, health insurance, and a generous stipend are paid for all graduate students accepted to the program. These benefits ensure that students have the time and resources necessary to focus on study and research. Most students live in University-owned, subsidized apartments or dorms within easy walking distance of the laboratories. In addition, both the Morningside and Health Sciences campuses are easily reached by public transportation from all areas of the city.

Applications for admission to the program for the fall term will be reviewed in the order in which they are received, starting in early December of the previous year. All applications submitted by the first Monday after January 1 will be considered, but applicants applying earlier are more likely to receive an invitation to one of two Open House recruiting events that typically are held in late January and early March.

For more information, please contact:
Graduate Student Adviser
Department of Biological Sciences
Graduate School of Arts and Sciences
Columbia University
Sherman Fairchild Center, 1212 Amsterdam Avenue, Mailcode 2402
New York, NY 10027
biology@columbia.edu
http://biology.columbia.edu/

who began their doctoral program in fall 2007, 100% received their degree in 8 years or less. *Degree requirements:* For doctorate, thesis/dissertation. *Entrance requirements:* For doctorate, GRE General Test; GRE Subject Test in biology, biochemistry, or cell and molecular biology (recommended), BS or MS in biological sciences or related field, 3 letters of recommendation, statement of purpose, official transcripts. Additional exam requirements/recommendations for international students: Required—TOEFL (minimum score 95 iBT) or IELTS. *Application deadline:* For fall admission, 1/15 for domestic and international students. Applications are processed on a rolling basis. Application fee: $0. Electronic applications accepted. *Expenses:* $1,218 per credit. *Financial support:* In 2015–16, 25 students received support, including 1 fellowship with full tuition reimbursement available (averaging $25,200 per year), 3 research assistantships with full tuition reimbursements available (averaging $24,200 per year), 21 teaching assistantships with full tuition reimbursements available (averaging $24,200 per year); scholarships/grants, tuition waivers (partial), and unspecified assistantships also available. Financial award application deadline: 5/31. *Faculty research:* Cell and developmental biology, molecular biology and genetics, evolution, ecology, physiology and microbiology. *Total annual research expenditures:* $813,716. *Unit head:* Dr. Joseph McCormick, Chair, 412-396-4775, Fax: 412-396-5907, E-mail: mccormick@duq.edu. *Application contact:* Heather Costello, Graduate Academic Advisor, 412-396-6339, E-mail: costelloh@duq.edu. Website: http://www.duq.edu/academics/schools/natural-and-environmental-sciences/academic-programs/biological-sciences

East Carolina University, Brody School of Medicine, Department of Biochemistry and Molecular Biology, Greenville, NC 27858-4353. Offers biochemistry and molecular biology (PhD); biomedical science (MS). *Students:* 7 full-time (4 women), 1 international. Average age 24. 15 applicants, 33% accepted, 4 enrolled. In 2015, 6 master's awarded. *Degree requirements:* For doctorate, comprehensive exam, thesis/dissertation. *Entrance requirements:* For doctorate, GRE General Test. Additional exam requirements/recommendations for international students: Required—TOEFL. *Application deadline:* For fall admission, 6/1 priority date for domestic students. Applications are processed on a rolling basis. *Financial support:* Fellowships with tuition reimbursements available. Financial award application deadline: 6/1. *Faculty research:* Gene regulation, development and differentiation, contractility and motility, macromolecular interactions, cancer. *Unit head:* Dr. Phillip H. Pekala, Chairman, 252-744-2684, Fax: 252-744-3383, E-mail: pekalap@ecu.edu. Website: http://www.ecu.edu/cs-dhs/biochemistry/gradProgram.cfm

East Carolina University, Graduate School, Thomas Harriot College of Arts and Sciences, Department of Biology, Greenville, NC 27858-4353. Offers biology (MS); molecular biology and biotechnology (MS). *Program availability:* Part-time. *Students:* 41 full-time (22 women), 13 part-time (7 women); includes 6 minority (2 Black or African American, non-Hispanic/Latino; 2 Asian, non-Hispanic/Latino; 1 Hispanic/Latino; 1 Two or more races, non-Hispanic/Latino). Average age 26. 67 applicants, 51% accepted, 26 enrolled. In 2015, 12 master's awarded. *Degree requirements:* For master's, one foreign language, comprehensive exam, thesis. *Entrance requirements:* For master's, GRE General Test, GRE Subject Test. Additional exam requirements/recommendations for international students: Required—TOEFL. *Application deadline:* For fall admission, 6/1 priority date for domestic students; for spring admission, 10/15 for domestic students. Applications are processed on a rolling basis. Application fee: $50. *Financial support:* Fellowships with partial tuition reimbursements, research assistantships with partial tuition reimbursements, teaching assistantships with partial tuition reimbursements, career-related internships or fieldwork, Federal Work-Study, scholarships/grants, and unspecified assistantships available. Support available to part-time students. Financial award application deadline: 6/1. *Faculty research:* Biochemistry, microbiology, cell biology. *Unit head:* Dr. Jeff McKinnon, Chair, 252-328-6718, E-mail: mckinnonj@ecu.edu. *Application contact:* Dean of Graduate School, 252-328-6012, Fax: 252-328-6071, E-mail: gradschool@ecu.edu. Website: http://www.ecu.edu/cs-cas/biology/graduate.cfm

Eastern Illinois University, Graduate School, College of Sciences, Department of Biological Sciences, Charleston, IL 61920. Offers MS. *Program availability:* Part-time, evening/weekend. *Degree requirements:* For master's, comprehensive exam (for some programs), thesis (for some programs). *Entrance requirements:* For master's, GMAT or GRE. Additional exam requirements/recommendations for international students: Required—TOEFL (minimum score 500 paper-based; 61 iBT), IELTS (minimum score 6). Electronic applications accepted.

Eastern Kentucky University, The Graduate School, College of Arts and Sciences, Department of Biological Sciences, Richmond, KY 40475-3102. Offers biological sciences (MS); ecology (MS). *Program availability:* Part-time. *Degree requirements:* For master's, thesis. *Entrance requirements:* For master's, GRE General Test, minimum GPA of 2.5. *Faculty research:* Systematics, ecology, and biodiversity; animal behavior; protein structure and molecular genetics; biomonitoring and aquatic toxicology; pathogenesis of microbes and parasites.

Eastern Mennonite University, Program in Biomedicine, Harrisonburg, VA 22802-2462. Offers MA. *Application deadline:* For fall admission, 7/31 for domestic students; for spring admission, 11/30 for domestic students. Applications are processed on a rolling basis. Application fee: $50. Electronic applications accepted. *Expenses: Tuition,* area resident: Part-time $600 per credit hour. *Required fees:* $25 per unit. Part-time tuition and fees vary according to course load and program. *Unit head:* Dr. Roman J. Miller, Director, 540-432-4412, E-mail: millerrj@emu.edu. *Application contact:* Don A. Yoder, Director of Seminary and Graduate Admissions, 540-432-4257, Fax: 540-432-4598, E-mail: yoderda@emu.edu. Website: http://www.emu.edu/ma-biomed/

Eastern Michigan University, Graduate School, College of Arts and Sciences, Department of Biology, Ypsilanti, MI 48197. Offers cell and molecular biology (MS); community college biology teaching (MS); ecology and organismal biology (MS); general biology (MS); water resources (MS). *Program availability:* Part-time, evening/weekend, online learning. *Faculty:* 26 full-time (8 women). *Students:* 15 full-time (9 women), 33 part-time (19 women); includes 8 minority (3 Black or African American, non-Hispanic/Latino; 2 Asian, non-Hispanic/Latino; 2 Hispanic/Latino; 1 Two or more races, non-Hispanic/Latino), 3 international. Average age 27. 47 applicants, 51% accepted, 19 enrolled. In 2015, 14 master's awarded. *Entrance requirements:* For master's, GRE General Test, GRE Subject Test. Additional exam requirements/recommendations for international students: Required—TOEFL. *Application deadline:* Applications are processed on a rolling basis. Application fee: $45. *Financial support:* Fellowships, research assistantships with full tuition reimbursements, teaching assistantships with full tuition reimbursements, career-related internships or fieldwork, Federal Work-Study, institutionally sponsored loans, scholarships/grants, tuition waivers (partial), and unspecified assistantships available. Support available to part-time students. Financial award applicants required to submit FAFSA. *Unit head:* Dr. Daniel Clemans, Department Head, 734-487-4242, Fax: 734-487-9235, E-mail: dclemans@emich.edu. *Application contact:* Dr. David Kass, Graduate Coordinator, 734-487-4242, Fax: 734-487-9235, E-mail: dkass@emich.edu. Website: http://www.emich.edu/biology

Eastern New Mexico University, Graduate School, College of Liberal Arts and Sciences, Department of Biology, Portales, NM 88130. Offers applied ecology (MS); botany (MS); cell, molecular biology and biotechnology (MS); microbiology (MS); zoology (MS). *Program availability:* Part-time. *Degree requirements:* For master's, comprehensive exam, thesis optional. *Entrance requirements:* For master's, GRE, minimum GPA of 3.0, 2 letters of recommendation, statement of research interest, bachelor's degree related to field of study or proof of common knowledge. Additional exam requirements/recommendations for international students: Required—TOEFL (minimum score 550 paper-based; 79 iBT), IELTS (minimum score 6). Electronic applications accepted.

Eastern Virginia Medical School, Doctoral Program in Biomedical Sciences, Norfolk, VA 23501-1980. Offers PhD. *Degree requirements:* For doctorate, thesis/dissertation. *Entrance requirements:* For doctorate, GRE General Test. Additional exam requirements/recommendations for international students: Required—TOEFL. Electronic applications accepted. *Expenses:* Contact institution.

Eastern Virginia Medical School, Master's Program in Biomedical Sciences Research, Norfolk, VA 23501-1980. Offers MS. *Degree requirements:* For master's, comprehensive exam (for some programs), thesis optional. *Entrance requirements:* For master's, GRE. Additional exam requirements/recommendations for international students: Required—TOEFL. Electronic applications accepted. *Expenses:* Contact institution.

Eastern Virginia Medical School, Master's Program in Clinical Embryology and Andrology, Norfolk, VA 23501-1980. Offers MS. *Program availability:* Online learning. *Entrance requirements:* Additional exam requirements/recommendations for international students: Required—TOEFL (minimum score 550 paper-based; 80 iBT). Electronic applications accepted. *Expenses:* Contact institution.

Eastern Virginia Medical School, Medical Master's Program in Biomedical Sciences, Norfolk, VA 23501-1980. Offers MS. *Entrance requirements:* For master's, MCAT. Electronic applications accepted. *Expenses:* Contact institution.

Eastern Washington University, Graduate Studies, College of Science, Health and Engineering, Department of Biology, Cheney, WA 99004-2431. Offers MS. *Degree requirements:* For master's, comprehensive exam, thesis. *Entrance requirements:* For master's, GRE General Test, minimum GPA of 3.0. *Faculty research:* Ecology of Eastern Washington Channeled Scablands, Columbia River fisheries, biotechnology applied to vaccines, role of mycorrhiza in plant nutrition, exercise and estrous cycles.

East Stroudsburg University of Pennsylvania, Graduate College, College of Arts and Sciences, Department of Biological Sciences, East Stroudsburg, PA 18301-2999. Offers biology (M Ed). *Program availability:* Part-time, evening/weekend. *Degree requirements:* For master's, comprehensive exam, thesis or alternative. *Entrance requirements:* For master's, GRE, resume, undergraduate major in life science (or equivalent), completion of organic chemistry (minimum two semesters), 3 letters of recommendation, letter of intent. Additional exam requirements/recommendations for international students: Required—TOEFL (minimum score 560 paper-based; 83 iBT) or IELTS. *Application deadline:* For fall admission, 7/31 for domestic students, 6/30 priority date for international students; for spring admission, 11/30 for domestic students, 10/31 for international students. Applications are processed on a rolling basis. Application fee: $50. Electronic applications accepted. *Expenses: Tuition,* area resident: Full-time $8460; part-time $5640 per year. Tuition, state resident: full-time $8460; part-time $5640 per year. Tuition, nonresident: full-time $12,690; part-time $8460 per year. *International tuition:* $15,368 full-time. *Required fees:* $2462; $1630 per unit. $815 per semester. Tuition and fees vary according to course load, campus/location and program. *Financial support:* Research assistantships with tuition reimbursements, Federal Work-Study, and institutionally sponsored loans available. Financial award application deadline: 3/1; financial award applicants required to submit FAFSA. *Unit head:* Maria Kitchens-Kintz, Chair, 570-422-3723, Fax: 570-422-3724, E-mail: mkitchens@esu.edu. *Application contact:* Kevin Quintero, Graduate Admission Coordinator, 570-422-3536, Fax: 570-422-3711, E-mail: kquintero@esu.edu. Website: http://www4.esu.edu/academics/departments/biology/graduate_programs/index.cfm

East Tennessee State University, James H. Quillen College of Medicine, Department of Biomedical Sciences, Johnson City, TN 37614. Offers anatomy (PhD); biochemistry (PhD); microbiology (PhD); pharmaceutical sciences (PhD); pharmacology (PhD); physiology (PhD); quantitative biosciences (PhD). *Faculty:* 30 full-time (6 women). *Students:* 35 full-time (17 women), 2 part-time (1 woman); includes 13 minority (9 Black or African American, non-Hispanic/Latino; 4 Asian, non-Hispanic/Latino), 13 international. Average age 29. 53 applicants, 17% accepted, 8 enrolled. In 2015, 8 doctorates awarded. *Degree requirements:* For doctorate, thesis/dissertation, comprehensive qualifying exam. *Entrance requirements:* For doctorate, GRE General Test, GRE Subject Test, 3 letters of recommendation. Additional exam requirements/recommendations for international students: Required—TOEFL (minimum score 550 paper-based; 79 iBT). *Application deadline:* For fall admission, 3/15 priority date for domestic students, 3/1 priority date for international students. Application fee: $35 ($45 for international students). Electronic applications accepted. *Expenses:* Contact institution. *Financial support:* In 2015–16, 30 students received support, including 27 research assistantships with full tuition reimbursements available (averaging $20,000 per year); career-related internships or fieldwork, institutionally sponsored loans, scholarships/grants, and unspecified assistantships also available. Financial award application deadline: 7/1; financial award applicants required to submit FAFSA. *Faculty research:* Cardiovascular, infectious disease, neurosciences, cancer, immunology. *Unit head:* Dr. Mitchell E. Robinson, Associate Dean/Program Director, 423-439-2031, Fax: 423-439-2140, E-mail: robinson@etsu.edu. *Application contact:* Shella Bennett, Graduate Specialist, 423-439-4708, Fax: 423-439-5624, E-mail: bennetsg@etsu.edu. Website: http://www.etsu.edu/com/dbms/

East Tennessee State University, School of Graduate Studies, College of Arts and Sciences, Department of Biological Sciences, Johnson City, TN 37614. Offers paleontology (MS). *Faculty:* 21 full-time (4 women). *Students:* 33 full-time (15 women), 4 part-time (1 woman); includes 1 minority (Black or African American, non-Hispanic/Latino), 18 international. Average age 26. 67 applicants, 42% accepted, 18 enrolled. In 2015, 14 master's awarded. *Degree requirements:* For master's, comprehensive exam, thesis. *Entrance requirements:* For master's, GRE General Test or GRE Subject Test, minimum GPA of 3.0, undergraduate degree in life or physical sciences, two letters of recommendation. Additional exam requirements/recommendations for international students: Required—TOEFL (minimum score 550 paper-based; 79 iBT). *Application deadline:* For fall admission, 4/1 for domestic students, 2/1 for international students; for spring admission, 9/1 for domestic students, 7/1 for international students. Application fee: $35 ($45 for international students). Electronic applications accepted. *Financial support:* In 2015–16, 36 students received support, including 28 teaching assistantships with full tuition reimbursements available (averaging $8,000 per year); institutionally sponsored loans, scholarships/grants, and unspecified assistantships also available. Financial award application deadline: 7/1; financial award applicants required to submit FAFSA. *Faculty research:* Neuroethology, chronobiology, molecular biology, behavioral ecology, systematics, paleobotany. *Unit head:* Dr. Joseph Bidwell, Chair, 423-439-4329,

Biological and Biomedical Sciences—General

Fax: 423-439-5958, E-mail: bidwell@etsu.edu. *Application contact:* Angela Edwards, Graduate Specialist, 423-439-4703, Fax: 423-439-5624, E-mail: edwardag@etsu.edu. Website: http://www.etsu.edu/cas/biology/

Elizabeth City State University, School of Mathematics, Science and Technology, Master of Science in Biology/Biological Science Program, Elizabeth City, NC 27909-7806. Offers biological sciences (MS); biology education (MS). *Program availability:* Part-time, evening/weekend. *Degree requirements:* For master's, thesis. *Entrance requirements:* For master's, GRE, minimum GPA of 3.0, 3 letters of recommendation, 2 official transcripts from all undergraduate/graduate schools attended, typewritten one-page expository description of student educational preparation, research interests and career aspirations. Additional exam requirements/recommendations for international students: Required—TOEFL (minimum score 550 paper-based, 80 iBT) or IELTS (minimum score 6.5). Electronic applications accepted. *Faculty research:* Apoptosis and cancer, plant bioengineering, development of biofuels, microbial degradation, developmental toxicology.

Emory University, Laney Graduate School, Division of Biological and Biomedical Sciences, Atlanta, GA 30322-1100. Offers PhD. *Degree requirements:* For doctorate, comprehensive exam, thesis/dissertation. *Entrance requirements:* For doctorate, GRE General Test, minimum GPA of 3.0 in science course work (recommended). Additional exam requirements/recommendations for international students: Required—TOEFL. Electronic applications accepted. *Expenses:* Contact institution. *Faculty research:* Biochemistry; cancer; genetics; immunology and microbiology; neuroscience and pharmacology; nutrition; population biology and ecology.

Emporia State University, Department of Biological Sciences, Emporia, KS 66801-5415. Offers botany (MS); environmental biology (MS); general biology (MS); microbial and cellular biology (MS); zoology (MS). *Program availability:* Part-time. *Faculty:* 14 full-time (3 women), 1 part-time/adjunct (0 women). *Students:* 26 full-time (13 women), 15 part-time (7 women); includes 1 minority (Two or more races, non-Hispanic/Latino), 24 international. 16 applicants, 100% accepted, 11 enrolled. In 2015, 17 master's awarded. *Degree requirements:* For master's, comprehensive exam or thesis. *Entrance requirements:* For master's, GRE, appropriate undergraduate degree, interview, letters of reference. Additional exam requirements/recommendations for international students: Required—TOEFL (minimum score 520 paper-based; 68 iBT). *Application deadline:* For fall admission, 8/15 priority date for domestic students. Applications are processed on a rolling basis. Application fee: $30 ($75 for international students). Electronic applications accepted. *Expenses:* Tuition, state resident: full-time $5640; part-time $235 per credit hour. Tuition, nonresident: full-time $17,544; part-time $731 per credit hour. *Required fees:* $1848; $77 per credit hour. *Financial support:* In 2015–16, 7 research assistantships with full tuition reimbursements (averaging $7,344 per year), 12 teaching assistantships with full tuition reimbursements (averaging $7,844 per year) were awarded; career-related internships or fieldwork, Federal Work-Study, institutionally sponsored loans, health care benefits, and unspecified assistantships also available. Financial award application deadline: 3/15; financial award applicants required to submit FAFSA. *Faculty research:* Fisheries, range, and wildlife management; aquatic, plant, grassland, vertebrate, and invertebrate ecology; mammalian and plant systematics, taxonomy, and evolution; immunology, virology, and molecular biology. *Unit head:* Dr. Yixin Eric Yang, Chair, 620-341-5311, Fax: 620-341-5608, E-mail: yyang@emporia.edu. Website: http://www.emporia.edu/info/degrees-courses/grad/biology

Fairleigh Dickinson University, College at Florham, Maxwell Becton College of Arts and Sciences, Department of Biological and Allied Health Sciences, Program in Biology, Madison, NJ 07940-1099. Offers MS.

Fairleigh Dickinson University, Metropolitan Campus, University College: Arts, Sciences, and Professional Studies, School of Natural Sciences, Program in Biology, Teaneck, NJ 07666-1914. Offers MS.

Fayetteville State University, Graduate School, Department of Biological Sciences, Fayetteville, NC 28301-4298. Offers MS. *Program availability:* Part-time, evening/weekend. *Faculty:* 11 full-time (4 women), 2 part-time/adjunct (1 woman). *Students:* 1 (woman) full-time; minority (Hispanic/Latino). Average age 27. 1 applicant, 100% accepted, 1 enrolled. In 2015, 4 master's awarded. *Degree requirements:* For master's, comprehensive exam, thesis, internship. *Entrance requirements:* For master's, GRE General Test. Additional exam requirements/recommendations for international students: Required—TOEFL. *Application deadline:* For fall admission, 4/15 for domestic students; for spring admission, 10/15 for domestic students. Applications are processed on a rolling basis. Application fee: $40. Electronic applications accepted. *Financial support:* Application deadline: 3/1; applicants required to submit FAFSA. *Faculty research:* Genetic and Quantitative Trait Loci (QTL) mapping of important agronomic traits in soybean and other plant species as disease resistance, yield, and phyto-pharmaceuticals; dinosaur paleo biology, dinosaur systematic, and the evolution/creation controversy; coral reef toxins in education; animal behavior and physiology; forensic science, DNA fingerprinting, and latent evidence. *Total annual research expenditures:* $170,000. *Unit head:* Dr. Kassem Abdelmajid, Chairperson, 910-672-1695, Fax: 910-672-1159, E-mail: mkassem@uncfsu.edu. *Application contact:* Deborah Keller, Administrative Support Associate, 910-672-1695, Fax: 910-672-1159, E-mail: dkeller@uncfsu.edu.

Fisk University, Division of Graduate Studies, Department of Biology, Nashville, TN 37208-3051. Offers MA. *Program availability:* Part-time. *Degree requirements:* For master's, comprehensive exam, thesis. *Entrance requirements:* For master's, GRE. Electronic applications accepted. *Faculty research:* Cell biology, topographical imaging, serotonin receptors in rats, enzyme assays, developmental biology.

Fitchburg State University, Division of Graduate and Continuing Education, Programs in Biology and Teaching Biology (Secondary Level), Fitchburg, MA 01420-2697. Offers MA, MAT, Certificate. *Accreditation:* NCATE. *Program availability:* Part-time, evening/weekend. *Students:* 1 full-time (0 women), 6 part-time (4 women). Average age 37. 5 applicants, 100% accepted, 5 enrolled. In 2015, 1 master's awarded. *Entrance requirements:* Additional exam requirements/recommendations for international students: Required—TOEFL (minimum score 500 paper-based; 79 iBT). *Application deadline:* For fall admission, 7/15 for international students; for spring admission, 12/1 for international students. Applications are processed on a rolling basis. Application fee: $25 ($50 for international students). Electronic applications accepted. *Expenses:* Tuition, state resident: full-time $3006; part-time $1002 per year. Tuition, nonresident: full-time $3006; part-time $1002 per year. *Required fees:* $2468. *Financial support:* In 2015–16, research assistantships with partial tuition reimbursements (averaging $5,500 per year) were awarded; Federal Work-Study, scholarships/grants, and unspecified assistantships also available. Support available to part-time students. Financial award application deadline: 3/1; financial award applicants required to submit FAFSA. *Unit head:* Dr. Lisa Grimm, Chair, 978-665-3174, Fax: 978-665-3658, E-mail: gce@fitchburgstate.edu. *Application contact:* Sean Ganas, Director of Admissions, 978-665-3144, Fax: 978-665-4540, E-mail: admissions@fitchburgstate.edu. Website: http://www.fitchburgstate.edu

Florida Atlantic University, Charles E. Schmidt College of Medicine, Boca Raton, FL 33431-0991. Offers biomedical science (MS). *Program availability:* Part-time. *Degree requirements:* For master's, thesis (for some programs). *Entrance requirements:* For

master's, GRE, minimum GPA of 3.0. *Application deadline:* For fall admission, 5/1 for domestic students, 3/15 for international students; for spring admission, 10/1 for domestic and international students. Application fee: $30. Electronic applications accepted. *Expenses:* Tuition, area resident: Full-time $7392; part-time $369.82 per credit hour. Tuition, state resident: full-time $7392; part-time $369.82 per credit hour. Tuition, nonresident: full-time $19,432; part-time $1024.81 per credit hour. *Financial support:* Fellowships and research assistantships available. Financial award applicants required to submit FAFSA. *Faculty research:* Osteoarthritis, aging, breast cancer, HIV/AIDS, cardiometabolic risk in psychiatry. Website: http://med.fau.edu/

Florida Atlantic University, Charles E. Schmidt College of Science, Department of Biological Sciences, Boca Raton, FL 33431-0991. Offers biology (MS, MST). *Program availability:* Part-time. *Degree requirements:* For master's, thesis (for some programs). *Entrance requirements:* For master's, GRE General Test, minimum GPA of 3.0. Additional exam requirements/recommendations for international students: Required—TOEFL (minimum score 500 paper-based; 61 iBT), IELTS (minimum score 6). *Application deadline:* For fall admission, 3/15 for domestic and international students; for spring admission, 10/1 for domestic and international students. Application fee: $30. *Expenses:* Tuition, area resident: Full-time $7392; part-time $369.82 per credit hour. Tuition, state resident: full-time $7392; part-time $369.82 per credit hour. Tuition, nonresident: full-time $19,432; part-time $1024.81 per credit hour. *Financial support:* Fellowships, research assistantships, teaching assistantships, career-related internships or fieldwork, and Federal Work-Study available. *Faculty research:* Ecology of the Everglades, molecular biology and biotechnology, marine biology. Website: http://www.science.fau.edu/biology/

Florida Institute of Technology, College of Science, Program in Biological Sciences, Melbourne, FL 32901-6975. Offers biological science (PhD); biotechnology (MS); cell and molecular biology (MS); ecology (MS); marine biology (MS). *Program availability:* Part-time. *Students:* 65 full-time (39 women), 10 part-time (3 women); includes 4 minority (2 Asian, non-Hispanic/Latino; 1 Two or more races, non-Hispanic/Latino), 38 international. Average age 26. 230 applicants, 24% accepted, 21 enrolled. In 2015, 23 master's, 3 doctorates awarded. *Degree requirements:* For master's, thesis (for some programs), research, seminar, internship, or summer lab; for doctorate, comprehensive exam, thesis/dissertation, dissertations seminar, publications. *Entrance requirements:* For master's, GRE General Test, 3 letters of recommendation; statement of objectives; bachelor's degree in biology, chemistry, biochemistry or equivalent; for doctorate, GRE General Test, resume, 3 letters of recommendation, minimum GPA of 3.2, statement of objectives. Additional exam requirements/recommendations for international students: Required—TOEFL (minimum score 550 paper-based; 79 iBT). *Application deadline:* For fall admission, 3/1 for domestic students, 4/1 for international students; for spring admission, 9/1 for domestic and international students. Applications are processed on a rolling basis. Electronic applications accepted. *Expenses:* Tuition, area resident: Full-time $21,690; part-time $1205 per credit hour. *Required fees:* $500. Tuition and fees vary according to degree level, campus/location and program. *Financial support:* Career-related internships or fieldwork, institutionally sponsored loans, tuition waivers (partial), unspecified assistantships, and tuition remissions available. Support available to part-time students. Financial award application deadline: 3/1; financial award applicants required to submit FAFSA. *Faculty research:* Initiation of protein synthesis in eukaryotic cells, fixation of radioactive carbon, changes in DNA molecule, endangered or threatened avian and mammalian species, hydroacoustics and feeding preference of the West Indian manatee. *Unit head:* Dr. Richard B. Aronson, Department Head, 321-674-8034, Fax: 321-674-7238, E-mail: raronson@fit.edu. *Application contact:* Cheryl A. Brown, Associate Director of Graduate Admissions, 321-674-7581, Fax: 321-723-9468, E-mail: cbrown@fit.edu. Website: http://cos.fit.edu/biology/

Florida International University, College of Arts, Sciences, and Education, Department of Biological Sciences, Miami, FL 33199. Offers MS, PhD. *Program availability:* Part-time. *Faculty:* 46 full-time (16 women), 36 part-time/adjunct (19 women). *Students:* 109 full-time (56 women), 18 part-time (7 women); includes 32 minority (1 Black or African American, non-Hispanic/Latino; 2 Asian, non-Hispanic/Latino; 23 Hispanic/Latino; 6 Two or more races, non-Hispanic/Latino), 44 international. Average age 29. 99 applicants, 19% accepted, 18 enrolled. In 2015, 3 master's, 16 doctorates awarded. *Degree requirements:* For master's, thesis; for doctorate, comprehensive exam, thesis/dissertation. *Entrance requirements:* For master's, GRE General Test, 2 letters of recommendation, minimum GPA of 3.0, faculty sponsor; for doctorate, GRE General Test, 3 letters of recommendation, faculty sponsor with dissertation advisor status, minimum GPA of 3.0. Additional exam requirements/recommendations for international students: Required—TOEFL (minimum score 550 paper-based; 80 iBT). *Application deadline:* For fall admission, 2/1 priority date for domestic and international students; for spring admission, 8/1 priority date for domestic and international students. Applications are processed on a rolling basis. Application fee: $30. Electronic applications accepted. *Expenses:* Tuition, state resident: full-time $10,708; part-time $455.64 per credit hour. Tuition, nonresident: full-time $23,816; part-time $1001.69 per credit hour. *Required fees:* $390; $195 per semester. Tuition and fees vary according to program. *Financial support:* Institutionally sponsored loans and scholarships/grants available. Financial award application deadline: 3/1; financial award applicants required to submit FAFSA. *Unit head:* Dr. Steven Oberbauer, Chair, 305-348-2580, E-mail: steven.oberbauer@fiu.edu. *Application contact:* Nanett Rojas, Manager, Graduate Operations, 305-348-7442, Fax: 305-348-7441, E-mail: gradadm@fiu.edu. Website: http://casbiology.fiu.edu/biology/

Florida State University, The Graduate School, College of Arts and Sciences, Department of Biological Science, Tallahassee, FL 32306-4295. Offers cell and molecular biology (MS, PhD); ecology and evolutionary biology (MS, PhD); neuroscience (MS, PhD); plant biology (MS, PhD); science teaching (MST), including community college science teaching; structural biology (MS, PhD). *Faculty:* 45 full-time (14 women). *Students:* 106 full-time (53 women); includes 13 minority (3 Black or African American, non-Hispanic/Latino; 1 Asian, non-Hispanic/Latino; 9 Hispanic/Latino), 27 international. Average age 28. 191 applicants, 18% accepted, 16 enrolled. In 2015, 4 master's, 12 doctorates awarded. Terminal master's awarded for partial completion of doctoral program. *Degree requirements:* For master's, comprehensive exam, thesis, teaching experience, seminar presentations; for doctorate, comprehensive exam, thesis/dissertation, teaching experience; seminar presentations. *Entrance requirements:* For master's and doctorate, GRE General Test, minimum upper-division GPA of 3.0. Additional exam requirements/recommendations for international students: Required—TOEFL (minimum score 600 paper-based; 92 iBT). *Application deadline:* For fall admission, 12/1 for domestic and international students. Application fee: $30. Electronic applications accepted. *Expenses:* Tuition, area resident: Full-time $7263; part-time $403.50 per credit hour. Tuition, nonresident: full-time $18,087; part-time $1004.85 per credit hour. *Required fees:* $1365; $75.81 per credit hour. $20 per semester. Tuition and fees vary according to campus/location. *Financial support:* In 2015–16, 113 students received support, including 8 fellowships with full tuition reimbursements available (averaging $30,000 per year), 29 research assistantships with full tuition reimbursements available (averaging $21,500 per year), 76 teaching assistantships with

full tuition reimbursements available (averaging $21,500 per year); scholarships/grants, traineeships, and unspecified assistantships also available. Financial award application deadline: 12/1; financial award applicants required to submit FAFSA. *Faculty research:* Cell and molecular biology and genetics, ecology and evolutionary biology, plant science, structural biology. *Unit head:* Dr. Thomas A. Houpt, Professor and Associate Chair, 850-644-4906, Fax: 850-644-4907, E-mail: houpt@neuro.fsu.edu. *Application contact:* Dr. Michael B. Miller, Academic Program Specialist, 850-644-3023, Fax: 850-644-9829, E-mail: gradinfo@bio.fsu.edu.
Website: http://www.bio.fsu.edu/

Florida State University, The Graduate School, College of Arts and Sciences, Department of Mathematics, Tallahassee, FL 32306-4510. Offers applied computational mathematics (MS, PhD); biomathematics (MS, PhD); financial mathematics (MS, PhD); pure mathematics (MS, PhD). *Program availability:* Part-time. *Faculty:* 34 full-time (4 women). *Students:* 145 full-time (43 women), 4 part-time (1 woman); includes 18 minority (2 Black or African American, non-Hispanic/Latino; 5 Asian, non-Hispanic/Latino; 2 Hispanic/Latino; 9 Two or more races, non-Hispanic/Latino), 87 international. 300 applicants, 41% accepted, 39 enrolled. In 2015, 44 master's, 14 doctorates awarded. Terminal master's awarded for partial completion of doctoral program. *Degree requirements:* For master's, comprehensive exam (for some programs), thesis optional; for doctorate, comprehensive exam (for some programs), thesis/dissertation, candidacy exam (including written qualifying examinations which differ by degree concentration). *Entrance requirements:* For master's and doctorate, GRE General Test, minimum upper-division GPA of 3.0, 4-year bachelor's degree. Additional exam requirements/recommendations for international students: Required—TOEFL (minimum score 550 paper-based; 80 iBT), IELTS (minimum score 6.5). *Application deadline:* For fall admission, 1/15 priority date for domestic and international students. Applications are processed on a rolling basis. Application fee: $30. Electronic applications accepted. *Expenses: Tuition, area resident:* Full-time $7263; part-time $403.50 per credit hour. Tuition, nonresident: full-time $18,087; part-time $1004.85 per credit hour. *Required fees:* $1365; $75.81 per credit hour. $20 per semester. Tuition and fees vary according to campus/location. *Financial support:* In 2015–16, 106 students received support, including 1 fellowship with full tuition reimbursement available (averaging $22,600 per year), 11 research assistantships with full tuition reimbursements available (averaging $22,000 per year), 83 teaching assistantships with full tuition reimbursements available (averaging $20,650 per year); career-related internships or fieldwork, institutionally sponsored loans, scholarships/grants, health care benefits, tuition waivers (full and partial), and unspecified assistantships also available. Financial award application deadline: 1/30. *Faculty research:* Low-dimensional and geometric topology, mathematical modeling in neuroscience, computational stochastics and Monte Carlo methods, mathematical physics, applied analysis. *Total annual research expenditures:* $1.4 million. *Unit head:* Dr. Xiaoming Wang, Chairperson, 850-645-3338, Fax: 850-644-4053, E-mail: wxm@math.fsu.edu. *Application contact:* Kari Aime, Graduate Advisor and Admissions Coordinator, 850-644-2278, Fax: 850-644-4053, E-mail: aime@math.fsu.edu.
Website: http://www.math.fsu.edu/

Florida State University, The Graduate School, College of Arts and Sciences, Department of Scientific Computing, Tallahassee, FL 32306-4120. Offers computational science (MS, PhD), including atmospheric science (PhD), biochemistry (PhD), biological science (PhD), computational science (PhD), geological science (PhD), materials science (PhD), physics (PhD). *Program availability:* Part-time. *Faculty:* 14 full-time (2 women). *Students:* 32 full-time (4 women), 7 part-time (1 woman); includes 14 minority (9 Asian, non-Hispanic/Latino; 3 Hispanic/Latino; 2 Two or more races, non-Hispanic/Latino). Average age 27. 28 applicants, 43% accepted, 7 enrolled. In 2015, 9 master's, 7 doctorates awarded. *Degree requirements:* For master's, thesis (for some programs); for doctorate, comprehensive exam, thesis/dissertation. *Entrance requirements:* For master's and doctorate, GRE General Test, knowledge of at least one object-oriented computing language, 3 letters of recommendation, resume, statement of purpose. Additional exam requirements/recommendations for international students: Required—TOEFL (minimum score 550 paper-based; 80 iBT). *Application deadline:* For fall admission, 1/15 for domestic and international students. Application fee: $30. Electronic applications accepted. *Expenses: Tuition, area resident:* Full-time $7263; part-time $403.50 per credit hour. Tuition, nonresident: full-time $18,087; part-time $1004.85 per credit hour. *Required fees:* $1365; $75.81 per credit hour. $20 per semester. Tuition and fees vary according to campus/location. *Financial support:* In 2015–16, 33 students received support, including 10 research assistantships with full tuition reimbursements available (averaging $20,000 per year), 23 teaching assistantships with full tuition reimbursements available (averaging $20,000 per year); scholarships/grants and unspecified assistantships also available. Financial award application deadline: 1/15. *Faculty research:* Morphometrics, mathematical and systems biology, mining proteomic and metabolic data, computational materials research, advanced 4-D Var data-assimilation methods in dynamic meteorology and oceanography, computational fluid dynamics, astrophysics. *Unit head:* Dr. Gordon Erlebacher, Chair, 850-644-7024, E-mail: gerlebacher@fsu.edu. *Application contact:* Mark Howard, Academic Program Specialist, 850-644-0143, Fax: 850-644-0098, E-mail: mlhoward@fsu.edu.
Website: http://www.sc.fsu.edu

Fordham University, Graduate School of Arts and Sciences, Department of Biological Sciences, New York, NY 10458. Offers biological sciences (MS, PhD); conservation biology (Graduate Certificate). *Program availability:* Part-time, evening/weekend. *Faculty:* 18 full-time (2 women). *Students:* 43 full-time (20 women), 10 part-time (8 women); includes 3 minority (1 Black or African American, non-Hispanic/Latino; 2 Asian, non-Hispanic/Latino), 13 international. Average age 29. 123 applicants, 24% accepted, 13 enrolled. In 2015, 8 master's, 3 doctorates, 4 other advanced degrees awarded. Terminal master's awarded for partial completion of doctoral program. *Degree requirements:* For master's, one foreign language, comprehensive exam, thesis optional; for doctorate, one foreign language, comprehensive exam, thesis/dissertation. *Entrance requirements:* For master's and doctorate, GRE General Test, GRE Subject Test (recommended). Additional exam requirements/recommendations for international students: Required—TOEFL (minimum score 550 paper-based). *Application deadline:* For fall admission, 1/4 priority date for domestic students; for spring admission, 11/1 for domestic students. Application fee: $70. Electronic applications accepted. *Financial support:* In 2015–16, 28 students received support, including 4 fellowships with tuition reimbursements available (averaging $31,000 per year), 42 teaching assistantships with tuition reimbursements available (averaging $29,270 per year); Federal Work-Study, institutionally sponsored loans, scholarships/grants, tuition waivers (full and partial), and unspecified assistantships also available. Support available to part-time students. Financial award application deadline: 1/4; financial award applicants required to submit FAFSA. *Faculty research:* Avian ecology, behavioral ecology, and conservation biology; plant, community and ecosystem responses to invasive organisms; neurobiology and ion channel disorders; biochemical, physiological and morphological basis of pattern formation; behavioral, physiological and biochemical adaptations of mammals to extreme environments; evolutionary ecology, functional morphology and ichthyology; genotypic response to biogeographic and anthropogenic factors; community-based sustainable resource use. *Total annual research expenditures:* $1.5 million. *Unit head:* Dr. James Lewis, Chair, 718-817-3642, Fax: 718-817-3645, E-mail: jdlewis@

fordham.edu. *Application contact:* Bernadette Valentino-Morrison, Director of Graduate Admissions, 718-817-4419, Fax: 718-817-3566, E-mail: valentinomor@fordham.edu.

Fort Hays State University, Graduate School, College of Health and Life Sciences, Department of Biological Sciences, Program in Biology, Hays, KS 67601-4099. Offers MS. *Program availability:* Part-time. *Degree requirements:* For master's, comprehensive exam, thesis optional. *Entrance requirements:* Additional exam requirements/recommendations for international students: Required—TOEFL (minimum score 550 paper-based). Electronic applications accepted.

Frostburg State University, Graduate School, College of Liberal Arts and Sciences, Department of Biology, Frostburg, MD 21532-1099. Offers applied ecology and conservation biology (MS); fisheries and wildlife management (MS). *Program availability:* Part-time, evening/weekend. *Degree requirements:* For master's, thesis. *Entrance requirements:* For master's, GRE General Test, resume. Additional exam requirements/recommendations for international students: Required—TOEFL. Electronic applications accepted. *Faculty research:* Molecular and morphological evolution, ecology and behavior of birds, conservation genetics of amphibians and fishes, biology of endangered species.

George Mason University, College of Science, School of Systems Biology, Manassas, VA 22030. Offers systems biology (PhD). *Faculty:* 8 full-time (1 woman), 1 part-time/adjunct (0 women). *Students:* 94 full-time (49 women), 76 part-time (43 women); includes 49 minority (4 Black or African American, non-Hispanic/Latino; 32 Asian, non-Hispanic/Latino; 10 Hispanic/Latino; 3 Two or more races, non-Hispanic/Latino), 39 international. Average age 31. 155 applicants, 61% accepted, 52 enrolled. In 2015, 5 doctorates, 2 other advanced degrees awarded. *Degree requirements:* For doctorate, comprehensive exam, thesis/dissertation. *Entrance requirements:* For doctorate, GRE, self-assessment form; resume; 3 letters of recommendation; expanded goals statement; 2 copies of official transcripts; bachelor's degree in related field with minimum GPA of 3.0 in last 60 hours; for Certificate, resume; 2 copies of official transcripts. Additional exam requirements/recommendations for international students: Required—TOEFL (minimum score 575 paper-based; 88 iBT), IELTS (minimum score 6.5), PTE (minimum score 59). Application fee: $75 ($80 for international students). Electronic applications accepted. *Financial support:* In 2015–16, 56 students received support, including 6 fellowships (averaging $12,519 per year), 11 research assistantships with tuition reimbursements available (averaging $16,971 per year), 36 teaching assistantships with tuition reimbursements available (averaging $14,299 per year); career-related internships or fieldwork, Federal Work-Study, scholarships/grants, unspecified assistantships, and health care benefits (for full-time research or teaching assistantship recipients) also available. Support available to part-time students. Financial award application deadline: 3/1; financial award applicants required to submit FAFSA. *Faculty research:* Functional genomics of chronic human diseases, ecology of vector-borne infectious diseases, neurogenetics, molecular biology, computational modeling, proteomics, chronic metabolic diseases, nanotechnology. *Total annual research expenditures:* $1.4 million. *Unit head:* Dr. James D. Willett, Director, 703-993-8311, Fax: 703-993-8976, E-mail: jwillett@gmu.edu. *Application contact:* Diane St. Germain, Graduate Student Services Coordinator, 703-993-4263, Fax: 703-993-8976, E-mail: dstgerma@gmu.edu.
Website: http://ssb.gmu.edu/

George Mason University, School of Policy, Government, and International Affairs, Program in Biodefense, Arlington, VA 22201. Offers MS, PhD. *Faculty:* 3 full-time (1 woman), 6 part-time/adjunct. *Students:* 18 full-time (10 women), 42 part-time (26 women); includes 14 minority (2 Black or African American, non-Hispanic/Latino; 5 Asian, non-Hispanic/Latino; 5 Hispanic/Latino; 2 Two or more races, non-Hispanic/Latino), 1 international. Average age 31. 56 applicants, 52% accepted, 19 enrolled. In 2015, 14 master's, 3 doctorates awarded. *Entrance requirements:* For master's, GRE (taken in the past five years), transcripts from all previous institutions attended in the U.S.; goals statement; two letters of recommendation; current resume; writing sample; for doctorate, GRE (taken in the past five years), official transcript from all colleges and universities attended; current resume; two letters of recommendation; statement of goals (not to exceed 500 words); writing sample (approximately 10-25 pages in length). Additional exam requirements/recommendations for international students: Required—TOEFL (minimum score 575 paper-based; 88 iBT), IELTS (minimum score 6.5), PTE (minimum score 59). *Application deadline:* For fall admission, 2/1 priority date for domestic students. Application fee: $75 ($80 for international students). Electronic applications accepted. *Financial support:* In 2015–16, 2 research assistantships with tuition reimbursements (averaging $20,500 per year) were awarded; career-related internships or fieldwork, Federal Work-Study, scholarships/grants, unspecified assistantships, and health care benefits (for full-time research or teaching assistantship recipients) also available. Support available to part-time students. *Unit head:* Gregory Koblentz, 703-993-1266, Fax: 703-993-1399, E-mail: gkoblent@gmu.edu. *Application contact:* Morgan Fisher, Associate Director of Graduate Admissions, 703-993-4478, E-mail: mfisherb@gmu.edu.
Website: http://spgia.gmu.edu/programs/graduate-degrees/ms-in-biodefense/

George Mason University, School of Policy, Government, and International Affairs, Program in Public Administration, Arlington, VA 22201. Offers administration of justice (Certificate); biodefense (MS, PhD); political science (MA); public administration (MPA). *Accreditation:* NASPAA (one or more programs are accredited). *Faculty:* 18 full-time (6 women), 13 part-time/adjunct (5 women). *Students:* 54 full-time (22 women), 204 part-time (119 women); includes 79 minority (31 Black or African American, non-Hispanic/Latino; 13 Asian, non-Hispanic/Latino; 29 Hispanic/Latino; 6 Two or more races, non-Hispanic/Latino), 5 international. Average age 32. 151 applicants, 73% accepted, 62 enrolled. In 2015, 98 master's awarded. *Entrance requirements:* For degree, expanded goals statement; 3 letters of recommendation; official transcripts; resume. Additional exam requirements/recommendations for international students: Required—TOEFL, IELTS, PTE. *Application deadline:* For fall admission, 2/1 priority date for domestic students. Application fee: $75 ($80 for international students). Electronic applications accepted. *Expenses:* Contact institution. *Financial support:* In 2015–16, 5 research assistantships with tuition reimbursements (averaging $12,600 per year), 1 teaching assistantship with tuition reimbursement (averaging $2,900 per year) were awarded; career-related internships or fieldwork, Federal Work-Study, scholarships/grants, unspecified assistantships, and health care benefits (for full-time research or teaching assistantship recipients) also available. Support available to part-time students. Financial award application deadline: 3/1; financial award applicants required to submit FAFSA. *Unit head:* Paul Posner, Director, 703-993-8138, Fax: 703-993-1399, E-mail: pposner@gmu.edu. *Application contact:* Travis Major, Director of Graduate Admissions, 703-993-3183, Fax: 703-993-4876, E-mail: tmajor@gmu.edu.
Website: http://spgia.gmu.edu/programs/graduate-degrees/mpa-in-public-administration/

Georgetown University, GeorgeSquared Special Master's Program, Washington, DC 20057. Offers MS. Program offered jointly with George Mason University.

Georgetown University, Graduate School of Arts and Sciences, Department of Biology, Washington, DC 20057. Offers PhD. Terminal master's awarded for partial completion of doctoral program. *Degree requirements:* For doctorate, comprehensive exam, thesis/dissertation. *Entrance requirements:* For doctorate, GRE General Test,

Biological and Biomedical Sciences—General

GRE Subject Test (biology). Additional exam requirements/recommendations for international students: Required—TOEFL (minimum score 550 paper-based). Electronic applications accepted. *Faculty research:* Parasitology, ecology, evaluation and behavior, neuroscience and development, cell and molecular biology, immunology.

Georgetown University, National Institutes of Health Sponsored Programs, GU-NIH Graduate Partnership Programs in Biomedical Sciences, Washington, DC 20057. Offers MS, PhD, MD/PhD, MS/PhD. *Entrance requirements:* For doctorate, GRE General Test. Additional exam requirements/recommendations for international students: Required—TOEFL.

The George Washington University, Columbian College of Arts and Sciences, Department of Biological Sciences, Washington, DC 20052. Offers MS, PhD. *Program availability:* Part-time, evening/weekend. *Faculty:* 26 full-time (8 women), 5 part-time/adjunct (1 woman). *Students:* 16 full-time (6 women), 24 part-time (14 women); includes 9 minority (1 Black or African American, non-Hispanic/Latino; 4 Asian, non-Hispanic/Latino; 3 Hispanic/Latino; 1 Two or more races, non-Hispanic/Latino), 14 international. Average age 28. 94 applicants, 27% accepted, 11 enrolled. In 2015, 4 master's, 4 doctorates awarded. Terminal master's awarded for partial completion of doctoral program. *Degree requirements:* For master's, comprehensive exam; for doctorate, thesis/dissertation, general exam. *Entrance requirements:* For master's and doctorate, GRE General Test, minimum GPA of 3.0. Additional exam requirements/ recommendations for international students: Required—TOEFL (minimum score 550 paper-based; 80 iBT). *Application deadline:* For fall admission, 1/2 priority date for domestic and international students; for spring admission, 10/1 priority date for domestic and international students. Applications are processed on a rolling basis. Application fee: $75. Electronic applications accepted. *Financial support:* In 2015–16, 25 students received support. Fellowships with full tuition reimbursements available, teaching assistantships with full tuition reimbursements available, Federal Work-Study, and tuition waivers available. Financial award application deadline: 1/2. *Faculty research:* Systematics, evolution, ecology, developmental biology, cell/molecular biology. *Total annual research expenditures:* $900,000. *Unit head:* Dr. Diana Lipscomb, Chair, 202-994-5828, Fax: 202-994-6100, E-mail: biodl@gwu.edu.

The George Washington University, Columbian College of Arts and Sciences, Institute for Biomedical Sciences, Washington, DC 20037. Offers biochemistry and systems biology (PhD); microbiology and immunology (PhD); molecular medicine (PhD), including molecular and cellular oncology, neurosciences, pharmacology and physiology. *Program availability:* Part-time, evening/weekend. *Faculty:* 26 full-time (8 women), 5 part-time/adjunct (1 woman). *Students:* 103 full-time (67 women), 86 part-time (52 women); includes 62 minority (6 Black or African American, non-Hispanic/Latino; 1 American Indian or Alaska Native, non-Hispanic/Latino; 31 Asian, non-Hispanic/Latino; 13 Hispanic/Latino; 11 Two or more races, non-Hispanic/Latino), 47 international. Average age 28. 673 applicants, 31% accepted, 83 enrolled. In 2015, 11 doctorates awarded. *Degree requirements:* For doctorate, thesis/dissertation. *Entrance requirements:* For doctorate, GRE General Test, minimum GPA of 3.0. Additional exam requirements/recommendations for international students: Required—TOEFL (minimum score 600 paper-based; 80 iBT). *Application deadline:* For fall admission, 12/15 priority date for domestic and international students. Applications are processed on a rolling basis. Application fee: $60. Electronic applications accepted. *Financial support:* In 2015–16, 24 students received support. Fellowships with full tuition reimbursements available, Federal Work-Study, institutionally sponsored loans, and tuition waivers available. *Unit head:* Dr. Linda L. Werling, Director, 202-994-2918, Fax: 202-994-0967, E-mail: lwerling@gwu.edu. *Application contact:* 202-994-2179, Fax: 202-994-0967, E-mail: gwibs@gwu.edu.
Website: http://smhs.gwu.edu/ibs/

Georgia College & State University, Graduate School, College of Arts and Sciences, Department of Biology, Milledgeville, GA 31061. Offers MS. *Program availability:* Part-time. *Students:* 21 full-time (13 women), 6 part-time (3 women); includes 5 minority (3 Black or African American, non-Hispanic/Latino; 2 Two or more races, non-Hispanic/Latino), 4 international. Average age 26. 16 applicants, 100% accepted, 10 enrolled. In 2015, 13 master's awarded. *Degree requirements:* For master's, thesis optional, minimum GPA of 3.0. *Entrance requirements:* For master's, GRE (minimum score of 800 under the old system and 286 under the new scoring system), 30 hours of undergraduate course work in biological science, 2 transcripts, certificate of immunization. Additional exam requirements/recommendations for international students: Recommended—TOEFL (minimum score 550 paper-based; 79 iBT). *Application deadline:* For fall admission, 7/1 priority date for domestic students, 4/1 for international students; for spring admission, 11/1 priority date for domestic students, 9/1 for international students; for summer admission, 4/1 priority date for domestic students. Applications are processed on a rolling basis. Application fee: $40. Electronic applications accepted. *Expenses:* $7,174 per year full-time in-state tuition and fees, $20,476 per year full-time out-of-state tuition and fees. *Financial support:* Unspecified assistantships available. Support available to part-time students. Financial award application deadline: 3/1; financial award applicants required to submit FAFSA. *Faculty research:* Molecular genetics, cell biology, environmental microbiology, microbial ecology. *Unit head:* Dr. Indiren Pillay, Chair, 478-445-0809, E-mail: indiren.pillayll@gcsu.edu. *Application contact:* Dr. Chris Skelton, Graduate Coordinator, 478-445-2440, E-mail: chris.skelton@gcsu.edu.

Georgia Institute of Technology, Graduate Studies, College of Sciences, School of Biological Sciences, Atlanta, GA 30332-0001. Offers applied physiology (PhD); biology (MS, PhD); prosthetics and orthotics (MS). *Program availability:* Part-time. Terminal master's awarded for partial completion of doctoral program. *Degree requirements:* For master's, thesis; for doctorate, thesis/dissertation, qualifying exam. *Entrance requirements:* For master's and doctorate, GRE General Test. Additional exam requirements/recommendations for international students: Required—TOEFL (minimum score 600 paper-based; 100 iBT). *Application deadline:* For fall admission, 1/1 priority date for domestic and international students. Applications are processed on a rolling basis. Application fee: $75. Electronic applications accepted. *Financial support:* Fellowships, research assistantships, teaching assistantships, career-related internships or fieldwork, Federal Work-Study, institutionally sponsored loans, tuition waivers (partial), and unspecified assistantships available. Support available to part-time students. Financial award application deadline: 5/1. *Faculty research:* Microbiology, molecular and cell biology, ecology.
Website: http://biosci.gatech.edu/

Georgia Southern University, Jack N. Averitt College of Graduate Studies, College of Science and Mathematics, Program in Biology, Statesboro, GA 30460. Offers biology (MS). *Program availability:* Part-time. *Students:* 38 full-time (17 women), 16 part-time (7 women); includes 4 minority (1 Black or African American, non-Hispanic/Latino; 3 Hispanic/Latino; 1 Two or more races, non-Hispanic/Latino). Average age 25. 35 applicants, 37% accepted, 12 enrolled. In 2015, 13 master's awarded. *Degree requirements:* For master's, comprehensive exam, thesis optional, terminal exam. *Entrance requirements:* For master's, GRE General Test, GRE Subject Test (preferred), minimum GPA of 2.8, BS in biology, 2 letters of reference. Additional exam requirements/recommendations for international students: Required—TOEFL (minimum score 550 paper-based; 80 iBT), IELTS (minimum score 6). *Application deadline:* For fall

admission, 3/1 priority date for domestic and international students; for spring admission, 10/1 priority date for domestic students, 10/1 for international students. Applications are processed on a rolling basis. Application fee: $50. Electronic applications accepted. *Expenses:* Tuition, state resident: full-time $7236; part-time $277 per semester hour. Tuition, nonresident: full-time $27,118; part-time $1105 per semester hour. *Required fees:* $2092. *Financial support:* In 2015–16, 44 students received support, including 13 research assistantships with full tuition reimbursements available (averaging $10,000 per year), 31 teaching assistantships with full tuition reimbursements available (averaging $10,000 per year); career-related internships or fieldwork, Federal Work-Study, scholarships/grants, tuition waivers (full), and unspecified assistantships also available. Support available to part-time students. Financial award application deadline: 4/15; financial award applicants required to submit FAFSA. *Faculty research:* Behavior, evolution and ecology, molecular biology, physiology, parasitology, vector-borne diseases, natural resources, coastal plain science. *Total annual research expenditures:* $420,563. *Unit head:* Dr. Checo Colon-Gaud, Program Coordinator, 912-478-0053, Fax: 912-478-0845, E-mail: jccolongaud@georgiasouthern.edu.
Website: http://www.bio.georgiasouthern.edu

Georgia State University, College of Arts and Sciences, Department of Biology, Atlanta, GA 30302-3083. Offers applied and environmental microbiology (MS, PhD), including applied and environmental microbiology, bioinformatics (MS); cellular and molecular biology and physiology (MS, PhD), including bioinformatics (MS), cellular and molecular biology and physiology; molecular genetics and biochemistry (MS, PhD), including bioinformatics (MS), molecular genetics and biochemistry; neurobiology and behavior (MS, PhD), including bioinformatics (MS), neurobiology and behavior. *Program availability:* Part-time. *Faculty:* 28 full-time (14 women). *Students:* 247 full-time (153 women), 36 part-time (24 women); includes 119 minority (54 Black or African American, non-Hispanic/Latino; 32 Asian, non-Hispanic/Latino; 21 Hispanic/Latino; 1 Native Hawaiian or other Pacific Islander, non-Hispanic/Latino; 11 Two or more races, non-Hispanic/Latino), 77 international. Average age 28. 193 applicants, 47% accepted, 57 enrolled. In 2015, 89 master's, 12 doctorates awarded. Terminal master's awarded for partial completion of doctoral program. *Degree requirements:* For master's, comprehensive exam (for some programs), thesis optional; for doctorate, comprehensive exam, thesis/dissertation. *Entrance requirements:* For master's, GRE. Additional exam requirements/recommendations for international students: Required—TOEFL (minimum score 550 paper-based; 82 iBT) or IELTS (minimum score 7). *Application deadline:* For fall admission, 6/1 priority date for domestic and international students; for spring admission, 10/1 priority date for domestic and international students. Applications are processed on a rolling basis. Application fee: $50. Electronic applications accepted. *Expenses:* Tuition, state resident: full-time $6876; part-time $382 per credit hour. Tuition, nonresident: full-time $22,374; part-time $1243 per credit hour. *Required fees:* $2128; $2128 per term. $1064 per term. Part-time tuition and fees vary according to course load and program. *Financial support:* In 2015–16, fellowships with full tuition reimbursements (averaging $2,200 per year), research assistantships with full tuition reimbursements (averaging $20,000 per year), teaching assistantships with full tuition reimbursements (averaging $5,400 per year) were awarded; unspecified assistantships also available. Financial award application deadline: 3/1; financial award applicants required to submit FAFSA. *Faculty research:* Applied and environmental microbiology, cell biology and immunology, molecular pathogenesis, protein modeling, neurobiology and behavior. *Unit head:* Dr. Charles Derby, Director of Graduate Studies, 404-413-5393, E-mail: cderby@gsu.edu.
Website: http://biology.gsu.edu/

See Display on next page and Close-Up on page 107.

Georgia State University, College of Arts and Sciences, MD/PhD Program, Atlanta, GA 30302-3083. Offers MD/PhD. *Expenses:* Tuition, state resident: full-time $6876; part-time $382 per credit hour. Tuition, nonresident: full-time $22,374; part-time $1243 per credit hour. *Required fees:* $2128; $2128 per term. $1064 per term. Part-time tuition and fees vary according to course load and program. *Unit head:* Dr. William J. Long, Dean, 404-413-5114, Fax: 404-413-5117, E-mail: long@gsu.edu. *Application contact:* Amber Amari, Director, Graduate and Scheduling Services, 404-413-5037, E-mail: aamari@gsu.edu.

Georgia State University, College of Education, Department of Middle and Secondary Education, Atlanta, GA 30302-3083. Offers curriculum and instruction (Ed D); English education (MAT); mathematics education (M Ed, MAT); middle level education (MAT); reading, language and literacy education (M Ed, MAT), including reading instruction (M Ed); science education (M Ed, MAT), including biology (MAT), broad field science (MAT), chemistry (MAT), earth science (MAT), physics (MAT); social studies education (M Ed, MAT), including economics (MAT), geography (MAT), history (MAT), political science (MAT); teaching and learning (PhD), including language and literacy, mathematics education, music education, science education, social studies education, teaching and teacher education. *Accreditation:* NCATE. *Program availability:* Part-time, evening/weekend, online learning. *Faculty:* 19 full-time (15 women). *Students:* 153 full-time (109 women), 174 part-time (122 women); includes 145 minority (112 Black or African American, non-Hispanic/Latino; 1 American Indian or Alaska Native, non-Hispanic/Latino; 10 Asian, non-Hispanic/Latino; 17 Hispanic/Latino; 5 Two or more races, non-Hispanic/Latino), 9 international. Average age 35. 68 applicants, 75% accepted, 38 enrolled. In 2015, 63 master's awarded. *Degree requirements:* For master's, comprehensive exam (for some programs), thesis or alternative, exit portfolio; for doctorate, comprehensive exam, thesis/dissertation. *Entrance requirements:* For master's, GRE; GACE I (for initial teacher preparation programs), baccalaureate degree or equivalent, resume, goals statement, two letters of recommendation, minimum undergraduate GPA of 2.5; proof of initial teacher certification in the content area (for M Ed); for doctorate, GRE, resume, goals statement, writing sample, two letters of recommendation, minimum graduate GPA of 3.3, interview. Additional exam requirements/recommendations for international students: Required—TOEFL (minimum score 550 paper-based; 79 iBT) or IELTS (minimum score 6.5). *Application deadline:* For fall admission, 1/15 priority date for domestic and international students; for spring admission, 10/1 for domestic and international students. Application fee: $50. Electronic applications accepted. *Expenses:* Tuition, state resident: full-time $6876; part-time $382 per credit hour. Tuition, nonresident: full-time $22,374; part-time $1243 per credit hour. *Required fees:* $2128; $2128 per term. $1064 per term. Part-time tuition and fees vary according to course load and program. *Financial support:* In 2015–16, fellowships with full tuition reimbursements (averaging $19,667 per year), research assistantships with full tuition reimbursements (averaging $5,436 per year), teaching assistantships with full tuition reimbursements (averaging $2,779 per year) were awarded; career-related internships or fieldwork, Federal Work-Study, scholarships/grants, health care benefits, tuition waivers (full and partial), and unspecified assistantships also available. Financial award application deadline: 3/15. *Faculty research:* Teacher education in language and literacy, mathematics, science, and social studies in urban middle and secondary school settings; learning technologies in school, community, and corporate settings; multicultural education and education for social justice; urban education; international education. *Unit head:* Dr. Dana L. Fox, Chair, 404-413-8060, Fax: 404-413-8063, E-mail: dfox@gsu.edu. *Application contact:* Bobbie Turner, Administrative Coordinator I,

404-413-8405, Fax: 404-413-8063, E-mail: bnturner@gsu.edu. Website: http://mse.education.gsu.edu/

Gerstner Sloan Kettering Graduate School of Biomedical Sciences, Program in Cancer Biology, New York, NY 10021. Offers PhD. *Degree requirements:* For doctorate, thesis/dissertation. *Entrance requirements:* For doctorate, GRE, transcripts, three letters of recommendation. Additional exam requirements/recommendations for international students: Required—TOEFL. Electronic applications accepted. *Faculty research:* Structural biology, computational biology, genomics, immunology, chemical biology.

See Display on page 174 and Close-Up on page 221.

Goucher College, Post-Baccalaureate Premedical Program, Baltimore, MD 21204-2794. Offers Certificate. *Faculty:* 11 full-time (5 women). *Students:* 31 full-time (18 women); includes 5 minority (1 Black or African American, non-Hispanic/Latino; 3 Asian, non-Hispanic/Latino; 1 Hispanic/Latino). Average age 25. 339 applicants, 12% accepted, 30 enrolled. *Entrance requirements:* For degree, GRE, SAT or ACT. *Application deadline:* Applications are processed on a rolling basis. Application fee: $60. Electronic applications accepted. *Expenses:* Contact institution. *Financial support:* In 2015–16, 6 students received support, including 8 fellowships (averaging $4,000 per year); institutionally sponsored loans and scholarships/grants also available. Financial award application deadline: 3/1; financial award applicants required to submit FAFSA. *Unit head:* Betsy Merideth, Director, 800-414-3437, Fax: 410-337-6461, E-mail: bmerideth@goucher.edu. *Application contact:* Theresa Reifsnider, Program Assistant, 800-414-3437, Fax: 410-337-6461, E-mail: pbpm@goucher.edu. Website: http://www.goucher.edu/postbac/

The Graduate Center, City University of New York, Graduate Studies, Program in Biology, New York, NY 10016-4039. Offers PhD. *Degree requirements:* For doctorate, thesis/dissertation, teaching experience. *Entrance requirements:* For doctorate, GRE General Test. Additional exam requirements/recommendations for international students: Required—TOEFL. Electronic applications accepted.

Grand Valley State University, College of Liberal Arts and Sciences, Biology Department, Allendale, MI 49401-9403. Offers MS. *Program availability:* Part-time. *Faculty:* 10 full-time (4 women). *Students:* 37 full-time (18 women), 18 part-time (12 women); includes 4 minority (2 Black or African American, non-Hispanic/Latino; 1 American Indian or Alaska Native, non-Hispanic/Latino; 1 Asian, non-Hispanic/Latino), 2 international. Average age 26. 33 applicants, 52% accepted, 17 enrolled. In 2015, 13 master's awarded. *Degree requirements:* For master's, comprehensive exam, thesis or alternative. *Entrance requirements:* For master's, GRE General Test, 3 letters of reference. Additional exam requirements/recommendations for international students: Required—TOEFL. *Application deadline:* For winter admission, 1/15 priority date for domestic students. Applications are processed on a rolling basis. Application fee: $30. Electronic applications accepted. *Financial support:* In 2015–16, 27 students received support, including 1 fellowship (averaging $530 per year), 26 research assistantships with tuition reimbursements available (averaging $11,394 per year). Financial award application deadline: 1/15. *Faculty research:* Natural resources conservation biology, aquatic sciences, terrestrial ecology, behavioral biology. *Unit head:* Dr. Neil MacDonald, Director, 616-331-2697, E-mail: macdonan@gvsu.edu. *Application contact:* Dr. Mark Luttenton, Graduate Program Director, 616-331-2503, E-mail: luttentm@gvsu.edu.

Grand Valley State University, College of Liberal Arts and Sciences, Department of Biomedical Sciences, Allendale, MI 49401-9403. Offers MHS. *Program availability:* Part-time. *Faculty:* 23 full-time (6 women). *Students:* 21 full-time (12 women), 14 part-time (8 women); includes 5 minority (2 Black or African American, non-Hispanic/Latino; 2 Asian, non-Hispanic/Latino; 1 Two or more races, non-Hispanic/Latino). Average age 26. 26 applicants, 38% accepted, 10 enrolled. In 2015, 3 master's awarded. *Degree requirements:* For master's, thesis, qualifying exam. *Entrance requirements:* For

master's, GRE General Test, minimum GPA of 3.0. Additional exam requirements/recommendations for international students: Required—TOEFL. *Application deadline:* For fall admission, 2/1 priority date for domestic and international students. Applications are processed on a rolling basis. Application fee: $30. Electronic applications accepted. *Financial support:* In 2015–16, 4 students received support, including 1 fellowship (averaging $750 per year), 3 research assistantships (averaging $10,602 per year); scholarships/grants and unspecified assistantships also available. Financial award application deadline: 2/1. *Faculty research:* Cell regulation, neurobiology, parasitology, virology, microbial pathogenicity. *Unit head:* Dr. Daniel Bergman, Chair, 616-331-8837, Fax: 616-331-2090, E-mail: bergmand@gvsu.edu. *Application contact:* Dr. Debra Burg, Director, 616-331-3721, Fax: 616-331-2090, E-mail: burgd@gvsu.edu.

Hampton University, School of Science, Department of Biological Sciences, Hampton, VA 23668. Offers biology (MS); environmental science (MS); medical science (MS). *Program availability:* Part-time. *Degree requirements:* For master's, comprehensive exam (for some programs), thesis optional. *Entrance requirements:* For master's, GRE General Test. Additional exam requirements/recommendations for international students: Required—TOEFL (minimum score 525 paper-based) or IELTS (6.5). Electronic applications accepted. *Expenses: Tuition, area resident:* Full-time $10,263; part-time $522 per credit hour. *Required fees:* $35. Tuition and fees vary according to course load and program. *Faculty research:* Molecular mechanisms responsible for initiation, promotion, and progression of breast, colon, prostate, thyroid, and skin cancers; isolation and characterization of bacteria in natural and contaminated environments and study of probable uses in biocontrol, diabetes, and hypertension.

Harvard University, Extension School, Cambridge, MA 02138-3722. Offers applied sciences (CAS); biotechnology (ALM); educational technologies (ALM); educational technology (CET); English for graduate and professional studies (DGP); environmental management (ALM, CEM); information technology (ALM); journalism (ALM); liberal arts (ALM); management (ALM, CM); mathematics for teaching (ALM); museum studies (ALM); premedical studies (Diploma); publication and communication (CPC). *Program availability:* Part-time, evening/weekend. *Degree requirements:* For master's, thesis. *Entrance requirements:* For master's, 3 completed graduate courses with grade of B or higher. Additional exam requirements/recommendations for international students: Required—TOEFL (minimum score 600 paper-based), TWE (minimum score 5). *Expenses:* Contact institution.

Harvard University, Graduate School of Arts and Sciences, Department of Organismic and Evolutionary Biology, Cambridge, MA 02138. Offers biology (PhD). *Degree requirements:* For doctorate, 2 foreign languages, public presentation of thesis research, exam. *Entrance requirements:* For doctorate, GRE General Test, GRE Subject Test (recommended), 7 courses in biology, chemistry, physics, mathematics, computer science, or geology. Additional exam requirements/recommendations for international students: Required—TOEFL.

Harvard University, Graduate School of Arts and Sciences, Division of Medical Sciences, Boston, MA 02115. Offers biological chemistry and molecular pharmacology (PhD); cell biology (PhD); genetics (PhD); microbiology and molecular genetics (PhD); pathology (PhD), including experimental pathology. *Degree requirements:* For doctorate, thesis/dissertation. *Entrance requirements:* For doctorate, GRE General Test, GRE Subject Test. Additional exam requirements/recommendations for international students: Required—TOEFL.

Harvard University, Harvard T.H. Chan School of Public Health, PhD Program in Biological Sciences in Public Health, Boston, MA 02115. Offers PhD. *Faculty:* 28 full-time (11 women), 13 part-time/adjunct (2 women). *Students:* 48 full-time (33 women); includes 16 minority (5 Black or African American, non-Hispanic/Latino; 5 Asian, non-Hispanic/Latino; 4 Hispanic/Latino; 2 Two or more races, non-Hispanic/Latino), 9

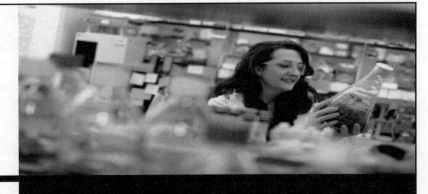

international. Average age 25. 249 applicants, 14% accepted, 27 enrolled. In 2015, 7 doctorates awarded. *Degree requirements:* For doctorate, qualifying examination, dissertation/defense. *Entrance requirements:* For doctorate, GRE General Test. Additional exam requirements/recommendations for international students: Recommended—TOEFL (minimum score 600 paper-based; 100 iBT), IELTS (minimum score 7). *Application deadline:* For fall admission, 12/8 for domestic students. Electronic applications accepted. *Financial support:* In 2015–16, 48 students received support. Fellowships, research assistantships, teaching assistantships, institutionally sponsored loans, health care benefits, and tuition waivers (full) available. Financial award application deadline: 1/1. *Faculty research:* Nutrition biochemistry, molecular and cellular toxicology, cardiovascular disease, cancer biology, immunology and infectious diseases, environmental health physiology. *Unit head:* Carole Knapp, Administrator, 617-432-2932.
Website: http://www.hsph.harvard.edu/admissions/degree-programs/doctor-of-philosophy/phd-in-biological-sciences-and-public-health/

See Display on page 789 and Close-Up on page 849.

Hofstra University, College of Liberal Arts and Sciences, Programs in Biology, Hempstead, NY 11549. Offers biology (MA, MS); urban ecology (MA, MS). *Program availability:* Part-time, evening/weekend. *Students:* 15 full-time (9 women), 8 part-time (5 women); includes 4 minority (1 Black or African American, non-Hispanic/Latino; 2 Hispanic/Latino; 1 Two or more races, non-Hispanic/Latino). Average age 26. 24 applicants, 75% accepted, 7 enrolled. In 2015, 6 master's awarded. *Degree requirements:* For master's, thesis, minimum GPA of 3.0. *Entrance requirements:* For master's, GRE, bachelor's degree in biology or equivalent, 2 letters of recommendation, essay. Additional exam requirements/recommendations for international students: Required—TOEFL (minimum score 550 paper-based; 80 iBT). *Application deadline:* Applications are processed on a rolling basis. Application fee: $70 ($75 for international students). Electronic applications accepted. *Financial support:* In 2015–16, 16 students received support, including 11 fellowships with tuition reimbursements available (averaging $5,859 per year); research assistantships with tuition reimbursements available, Federal Work-Study, institutionally sponsored loans, scholarships/grants, and tuition waivers (full and partial) also available. Support available to part-time students. Financial award applicants required to submit FAFSA. *Faculty research:* Genomic, hormonal and neurobiological bases for behavior; applied and environmental microbiology; developmental genetics, tissue-specific gene regulation; plant and soil ecology, urbanization, global environmental change; systematics and biology of marine polychaete worms and crustaceans. *Unit head:* Dr. Maureen K. Krause, Program Director, 516-463-6178, Fax: 516-463-5112, E-mail: biomkk@hofstra.edu. *Application contact:* Sunil Samuel, Assistant Vice President of Admissions, 516-463-4723, Fax: 516-463-4664, E-mail: graduateadmission@hofstra.edu.
Website: http://www.hofstra.edu/hclas

Hofstra University, School of Education, Programs in Teacher Education, Hempstead, NY 11549. Offers bilingual education (MA), including biology (MA, MS Ed); geology; business education (MS Ed); early childhood and childhood education (MS Ed), including French; early childhood education (MA); education technology (Advanced Certificate); elementary education (MA), including science, technology, engineering, and mathematics (STEM); English education (MS Ed); fine arts education (MS Ed), including biology (MA, MS Ed); foreign language and TESOL (MS Ed); learning and teaching (Ed D), including applied linguistics, art education, arts and humanities, early childhood education, English education, human development, math education, math, science, and technology, multicultural education, physical education, science education, social studies education, special education; mathematics education (MA, MS Ed); secondary education (Advanced Certificate); social studies education (MA, MS Ed). *Program*

availability: Part-time, evening/weekend, online learning. *Students:* 141 full-time (111 women), 119 part-time (84 women); includes 58 minority (13 Black or African American, non-Hispanic/Latino; 14 Asian, non-Hispanic/Latino; 28 Hispanic/Latino; 1 Native Hawaiian or other Pacific Islander, non-Hispanic/Latino; 2 Two or more races, non-Hispanic/Latino), 18 international. Average age 30. 301 applicants, 87% accepted, 112 enrolled. In 2015, 133 master's, 5 doctorates, 28 other advanced degrees awarded. *Degree requirements:* For master's, comprehensive exam, thesis (for some programs), exit project, student teaching, fieldwork, electronic portfolio, curriculum project, minimum GPA of 3.0; for doctorate, thesis/dissertation; for Advanced Certificate, 3 foreign languages, comprehensive exam (for some programs), thesis project. *Entrance requirements:* For master's, 2 letters of recommendation, portfolio, teacher certification (MA), interview, essay; for doctorate, GMAT, GRE, LSAT, or MAT; for Advanced Certificate, 2 letters of recommendation, essay, interview and/or portfolio, teaching certificate. Additional exam requirements/recommendations for international students: Required—TOEFL (minimum score 550 paper-based; 80 iBT). *Application deadline:* Applications are processed on a rolling basis. Application fee: $70 ($75 for international students). Electronic applications accepted. *Financial support:* In 2015–16, 153 students received support, including 60 fellowships with tuition reimbursements available (averaging $5,084 per year), 4 research assistantships with tuition reimbursements available (averaging $7,095 per year); Federal Work-Study, institutionally sponsored loans, scholarships/grants, health care benefits, and tuition waivers (full and partial) also available. Support available to part-time students. Financial award applicants required to submit FAFSA. *Faculty research:* Appropriate content in secondary school disciplines, lesson development across content, interdisciplinary curriculum, multicultural education. *Unit head:* Dr. Eustace Thompson, Chairperson, 516-463-5749, Fax: 516-463-6275, E-mail: edaegt@hofstra.edu. *Application contact:* Sunil Samuel, Assistant Vice President of Admissions, 516-463-4723, Fax: 516-463-4664, E-mail: graduateadmission@hofstra.edu.
Website: http://www.hofstra.edu/education/

 Hood College, Graduate School, Program in Biomedical Science, Frederick, MD 21701-8575. Offers bioinformatics (Certificate); biomedical science (MS), including biotechnology/molecular biology, microbiology/immunology/virology, regulatory compliance. *Program availability:* Part-time, evening/weekend. *Degree requirements:* For master's, comprehensive exam, thesis or alternative. *Entrance requirements:* For master's, bachelor's degree in biology; minimum GPA of 2.75; undergraduate course work in cell biology, chemistry, organic chemistry, and genetics. Additional exam requirements/recommendations for international students: Required—TOEFL (minimum score 575 paper-based; 89 iBT), IELTS (minimum score 6.5). *Application deadline:* For fall admission, 7/15 priority date for domestic students, 7/15 for international students; for spring admission, 12/1 priority date for domestic students, 12/1 for international students. Applications are processed on a rolling basis. Application fee: $35. Electronic applications accepted. Application fee is waived when completed online. *Expenses: Tuition, area resident:* Part-time $450 per credit hour. *Required fees:* $105 per term. Part-time tuition and fees vary according to degree level, campus/location and program. *Financial support:* Research assistantships with full tuition reimbursements, tuition waivers (partial), and unspecified assistantships available. Financial award applicants required to submit FAFSA.
Website: http://www.hood.edu/graduate

See Display below and Close-Up on page 109.

Howard University, Graduate School, Department of Biology, Washington, DC 20059-0002. Offers MS, PhD. *Program availability:* Part-time. *Degree requirements:* For master's, thesis, qualifying exams; for doctorate, thesis/dissertation, qualifying exams. *Entrance requirements:* For master's and doctorate, GRE General Test, minimum GPA of 3.0. Additional exam requirements/recommendations for international students: Required—TOEFL. Electronic applications accepted. *Faculty research:* Physiology, molecular biology, cell biology, microbiology, environmental biology.

Humboldt State University, Academic Programs, College of Natural Resources and Sciences, Department of Biological Sciences, Arcata, CA 95521-8299. Offers MS. *Degree requirements:* For master's, project or thesis. *Entrance requirements:* For master's, GRE General Test, appropriate bachelor's degree, minimum GPA of 2.5, 3 letters of recommendation. Additional exam requirements/recommendations for international students: Required—TOEFL (minimum score 500 paper-based). *Application deadline:* For fall admission, 2/15 for domestic and international students. Applications are processed on a rolling basis. Application fee: $55. *Financial support:* Application deadline: 3/1; applicants required to submit FAFSA. *Faculty research:* Plant ecology, DNA sequencing, invertebrates. Website: http://www.humboldt.edu/biosci/programs/grad.html

Hunter College of the City University of New York, Graduate School, School of Arts and Sciences, Department of Biological Sciences, New York, NY 10065-5085. Offers MA, PhD. PhD offered jointly with The Graduate Center, City University of New York. *Program availability:* Part-time. *Faculty:* 6 full-time (2 women). *Students:* 2 full-time (1 woman), 8 part-time (5 women); includes 4 minority (2 Asian, non-Hispanic/Latino; 2 Hispanic/Latino), 2 international. Average age 27. 27 applicants, 33% accepted, 3 enrolled. In 2015, 18 master's awarded. Terminal master's awarded for partial completion of doctoral program. *Degree requirements:* For master's, one foreign language, comprehensive exam or thesis. *Entrance requirements:* For master's, GRE, 1 year of course work in organic chemistry (including laboratory), college physics, and calculus; undergraduate major in biology, botany, physiology, zoology, chemistry or physics. Additional exam requirements/recommendations for international students: Required—TOEFL. *Application deadline:* For fall admission, 4/1 for domestic students, 2/1 for international students; for spring admission, 11/1 for domestic students, 9/1 for international students. *Financial support:* Fellowships, research assistantships, teaching assistantships, scholarships/grants, and tuition waivers (partial) available. Support available to part-time students. *Faculty research:* Analysis of prokaryotic and eukaryotic DNA, protein structure, mammalian DNA replication, oncogene expression, neuroscience. *Unit head:* Dr. Shirley Raps, Chairperson, 212-772-5293, E-mail: raps@genectr.hunter.cuny.edu. *Application contact:* William Zlata, Director for Graduate Admissions, 212-772-4482, Fax: 212-650-3336, E-mail: admissions@hunter.cuny.edu.

Icahn School of Medicine at Mount Sinai, Graduate School of Biomedical Sciences, New York, NY 10029-6504. Offers biomedical sciences (MS, PhD); clinical research education (MS, PhD); community medicine (MPH); genetic counseling (MS); neurosciences (PhD); MD/PhD. Terminal master's awarded for partial completion of doctoral program. *Degree requirements:* For master's, thesis; for doctorate, comprehensive exam, thesis/dissertation. *Entrance requirements:* For master's, GRE General Test; for doctorate, GRE General Test, GRE Subject Test, 3 years of college pre-med course work. Additional exam requirements/recommendations for international students: Required—TOEFL. Electronic applications accepted. *Faculty research:* Cancer, genetics and genomics, immunology, neuroscience, developmental and stem cell biology, translational research.

Idaho State University, Office of Graduate Studies, College of Science and Engineering, Department of Biological Sciences, Pocatello, ID 83209-8007. Offers biology (MNS, MS, DA, PhD); clinical laboratory science (MS); microbiology (MS). *Accreditation:* NAACLS. *Program availability:* Part-time. *Degree requirements:* For master's, comprehensive exam, thesis; for doctorate, comprehensive exam, thesis/dissertation, 9 credits of internship (for DA). *Entrance requirements:* For master's, GRE General Test, minimum GPA of 3.0 in all upper division classes; for doctorate, GRE General Test, GRE Subject Test (biology), diagnostic exam (DA), minimum GPA of 3.0 in all upper division classes. Additional exam requirements/recommendations for international students: Required—TOEFL (minimum score 550 paper-based; 80 iBT). Electronic applications accepted. *Faculty research:* Ecology, plant and animal physiology, plant and animal developmental biology, immunology, molecular biology, bioinfomatics.

Illinois Institute of Technology, Graduate College, College of Science, Department of Biological Sciences, Chicago, IL 60616. Offers biochemistry (MS); biology (MS, PhD); cell and molecular biology (MS); microbiology (MS); molecular biochemistry and biophysics (MS, PhD). *Program availability:* Part-time, evening/weekend, online learning. Terminal master's awarded for partial completion of doctoral program. *Degree requirements:* For master's, comprehensive exam, thesis (for some programs); for doctorate, comprehensive exam, thesis/dissertation. *Entrance requirements:* For master's, GRE General Test (minimum score 300 Quantitative and Verbal, 2.5 Analytical Writing), minimum undergraduate GPA of 3.0; for doctorate, GRE General Test (minimum score 310 Quantitative and Verbal, 3.0 Analytical Writing); GRE Subject Test (strongly recommended), minimum undergraduate GPA of 3.0. Additional exam requirements/recommendations for international students: Required—TOEFL (minimum score 550 paper-based; 80 iBT). Electronic applications accepted. *Faculty research:* Macromolecular crystallography, insect immunity and basic cell biology, improvement of bacterial strains for enhanced biodesulfurization of petroleum, programmed cell death in cancer cells.

Illinois State University, Graduate School, College of Arts and Sciences, Department of Biological Sciences, Normal, IL 61790-2200. Offers animal behavior (MS); bacteriology (MS); biochemistry (MS); biological sciences (MS); biology (PhD); biophysics (MS); biotechnology (MS); botany (MS, PhD); cell biology (MS); conservation biology (MS); developmental biology (MS); ecology (MS, PhD); entomology (MS); evolutionary biology (MS); genetics (MS, PhD); immunology (MS); microbiology (MS, PhD); molecular biology (MS); molecular genetics (MS); neurobiology (MS); neuroscience (MS); parasitology (MS); physiology (MS, PhD); plant biology (MS); plant molecular biology (MS); plant sciences (MS); structural biology (MS); zoology (MS, PhD). *Program availability:* Part-time. *Degree requirements:* For master's, thesis or alternative; for doctorate, variable foreign language requirement, thesis/dissertation, 2 terms of residency. *Entrance requirements:* For master's, GRE General Test, minimum GPA of 2.6 in last 60 hours of course work; for doctorate, GRE General Test. *Application deadline:* Applications are processed on a rolling basis. Application fee: $40. *Financial support:* Research assistantships, teaching assistantships, Federal Work-Study, tuition waivers (full), and unspecified assistantships available. Financial award application deadline: 4/1. *Faculty research:* Redoc balance and drug development in schistosoma mansoni, control of the growth of listeria monocytogenes at low temperature, regulation of cell expansion and microtubule function by SPRI, CRUI: physiology and fitness consequences of different life history phenotypes. *Application contact:* Steven Juliano, Graduate Coordinator, E-mail: sajulian@ilstu.edu. Website: http://www.bio.ilstu.edu/

Indiana State University, College of Graduate and Professional Studies, College of Arts and Sciences, Department of Biology, Terre Haute, IN 47809. Offers cellular and molecular biology (PhD); ecology, systematics and evolution (PhD); life sciences (MS); physiology (PhD); science education (MS). *Degree requirements:* For master's, thesis optional; for doctorate, comprehensive exam, thesis/dissertation. *Entrance*

requirements: For master's and doctorate, GRE General Test. Electronic applications accepted.

Indiana University Bloomington, University Graduate School, College of Arts and Sciences, Department of Biology, Bloomington, IN 47405. Offers biology teaching (MAT); biotechnology (MA); evolution, ecology, and behavior (MA, PhD); genetics (PhD); microbiology (MA, PhD); molecular, cellular, and developmental biology (PhD); plant sciences (MA, PhD); zoology (MA, PhD). Terminal master's awarded for partial completion of doctoral program. *Degree requirements:* For master's, thesis, oral defense; for doctorate, thesis/dissertation, oral defense. *Entrance requirements:* For master's and doctorate, GRE General Test. Additional exam requirements/recommendations for international students: Required—TOEFL (minimum score 100 iBT). Electronic applications accepted. *Faculty research:* Evolution, ecology and behavior; microbiology; molecular biology and genetics; plant biology.

Indiana University of Pennsylvania, School of Graduate Studies and Research, College of Natural Sciences and Mathematics, Department of Biology, Program in Biology, Indiana, PA 15705-1087. Offers MS. *Program availability:* Part-time. *Faculty:* 12 full-time (3 women). *Students:* 20 full-time (11 women), 9 part-time (3 women); includes 2 minority (1 Black or African American, non-Hispanic/Latino; 1 Asian, non-Hispanic/Latino), 6 international. Average age 28. 47 applicants, 45% accepted, 10 enrolled. In 2015, 14 master's awarded. *Degree requirements:* For master's, comprehensive exam, thesis optional. *Entrance requirements:* For master's, 2 letters of recommendation. Additional exam requirements/recommendations for international students: Required—TOEFL (minimum score 550 paper-based). *Application deadline:* Applications are processed on a rolling basis. Application fee: $50. Electronic applications accepted. *Financial support:* In 2015–16, 11 research assistantships with tuition reimbursements (averaging $3,735 per year) were awarded; fellowships with full tuition reimbursements, career-related internships or fieldwork, Federal Work-Study, scholarships/grants, and unspecified assistantships also available. Financial award application deadline: 4/15; financial award applicants required to submit FAFSA. *Unit head:* Dr. Josiah Townsend, Graduate Coordinator, 724-357-2587, E-mail: josiah.townsend@iup.edu. Website: http://www.iup.edu/grad/biology/default.aspx

Indiana University–Purdue University Fort Wayne, College of Arts and Sciences, Department of Biology, Fort Wayne, IN 46805-1499. Offers MS. *Program availability:* Part-time, evening/weekend. *Faculty:* 13 full-time (2 women), 1 (woman) part-time/adjunct. *Students:* 18 full-time (10 women), 25 part-time (19 women); includes 4 minority (2 Asian, non-Hispanic/Latino; 1 Hispanic/Latino; 1 Two or more races, non-Hispanic/Latino), 8 international. Average age 25. 19 applicants, 100% accepted, 13 enrolled. In 2015, 11 master's awarded. *Degree requirements:* For master's, thesis optional. *Entrance requirements:* For master's, GRE General Test, minimum GPA of 3.0, major or minor in biology, three letters of recommendation. Additional exam requirements/recommendations for international students: Required—TOEFL (minimum score 550 paper-based; 79 iBT), TWE. *Application deadline:* For fall admission, 4/15 priority date for domestic students, 2/15 priority date for international students; for spring admission, 8/15 priority date for domestic and international students. Applications are processed on a rolling basis. Application fee: $55 ($60 for international students). Electronic applications accepted. *Financial support:* In 2015–16, 10 research assistantships with partial tuition reimbursements (averaging $13,522 per year), 18 teaching assistantships with partial tuition reimbursements (averaging $13,522 per year) were awarded; scholarships/grants and unspecified assistantships also available. Support available to part-time students. Financial award application deadline: 3/1; financial award applicants required to submit FAFSA. *Faculty research:* Photosynthates, unicellular green algae, Chinook salmon. *Total annual research expenditures:* $278,441. *Unit head:* Dr. Frank Paladino, Chair/Professor, 260-481-6304, Fax: 260-481-6087, E-mail: paladino@ipfw.edu. Website: http://www.ipfw.edu/biology

Indiana University–Purdue University Indianapolis, School of Science, Department of Biology, Indianapolis, IN 46202. Offers MS, PhD. PhD offered jointly with Purdue University. *Program availability:* Part-time, evening/weekend. Terminal master's awarded for partial completion of doctoral program. *Degree requirements:* For master's, thesis (for some programs); for doctorate, thesis/dissertation. *Entrance requirements:* For master's and doctorate, GRE General Test. *Faculty research:* Cell and model membranes, cell and molecular biology, immunology, oncology, developmental biology.

Iowa State University of Science and Technology, Department of Biomedical Sciences, Ames, IA 50011. Offers MS, PhD. *Entrance requirements:* For master's and doctorate, GRE General Test. Additional exam requirements/recommendations for international students: Required—TOEFL (minimum score 590 paper-based; 79 iBT), IELTS (minimum score 6.5). Electronic applications accepted. *Faculty research:* Cerebella research; endocrine physiology; memory, learning and associated diseases; ion-channels and dry resistance; glia-neuron signaling; neurobiology of pain.

Irell & Manella Graduate School of Biological Sciences, Graduate Program, Duarte, CA 91010. Offers brain metastatic cancer (PhD); cancer and stem cell metabolism (PhD); cancer biology (PhD); cancer biology and developmental therapeutics (PhD); cell biology (PhD); chemical biology (PhD); chromosomal break repair (PhD); diabetes and pancreatic progenitor cell biology (PhD); DNA repair and cancer biology (PhD); germline epigenetic remodeling and endocrine disruptors (PhD); hematology and hematopoietic cell transplantation (PhD); hematology and immunology (PhD); inflammation and cancer (PhD); micrornas and gene regulation in cardiovascular disease (PhD); mixed chimrism for reversal of autoimmunity (PhD); molecular and cellular biology (PhD); molecular biology and genetics (PhD); nanoparticle mediated twist1 silencing in metastatic cancer (PhD); neuro-oncology and stem cell biology (PhD); neuroscience (PhD); rna directed therapies for hiv-1 (PhD); small rna-induced transcriptional gene activation (PhD); stem cell regulation by the microenvironment (PhD); translational oncology and pharmaceutical sciences (PhD); tumor biology (PhD). *Faculty:* 70 full-time (18 women). *Students:* 75 full-time (40 women); includes 28 minority (2 Black or African American, non-Hispanic/Latino; 8 Asian, non-Hispanic/Latino; 10 Hispanic/Latino; 2 Native Hawaiian or other Pacific Islander, non-Hispanic/Latino; 4 Two or more races, non-Hispanic/Latino), 15 international. Average age 26. 197 applicants, 12% accepted, 19 enrolled. In 2015, 12 doctorates awarded. *Degree requirements:* For doctorate, comprehensive exam, thesis/dissertation, qualifying exams, two advanced courses. *Entrance requirements:* For doctorate, GRE General Test; GRE Subject Test (recommended), 2 years of course work in chemistry (general and organic); 1 year of course work each in biochemistry, general biology, and general physics; 2 semesters of course work in mathematics; significant research laboratory experience. Additional exam requirements/recommendations for international students: Required—TOEFL. *Application deadline:* For fall admission, 1/1 priority date for domestic and international students. Application fee: $0. Electronic applications accepted. Full-time tuition and fees vary according to class time, course level, course load, degree level, campus/location, program and student level. *Financial support:* In 2015–16, 12 students received support, including 35 fellowships with full tuition reimbursements available (averaging $32,000 per year); teaching assistantships, health care benefits, and tuition waivers (full) also available. Financial award applicants required to submit FAFSA. *Faculty research:* Cancer biology, diabetes, stem cell biology, neuroscience, immunology. *Unit head:* Dr. John J. Rossi, Dean, 877-715-GRAD, Fax: 626-471-3901, E-mail: gradschool@coh.org.

Biological and Biomedical Sciences—General

Application contact: Dr. Kate Sleeth, Interim Associate Dean of Administration and Student Development, 626-218-1742, Fax: 626-471-3901, E-mail: gradschool@coh.org. Website: http://cityofhope.org/gradschool

See Display on this page and Close-Up on page 111.

Jackson State University, Graduate School, College of Science, Engineering and Technology, Department of Biology, Jackson, MS 39217. Offers environmental science (MS, PhD). *Program availability:* Part-time, evening/weekend. *Degree requirements:* For master's, comprehensive exam, thesis (alternative accepted for MST); for doctorate, comprehensive exam, thesis/dissertation. *Entrance requirements:* For master's, GRE General Test; for doctorate, MAT. Additional exam requirements/recommendations for international students: Required—TOEFL (minimum score 520 paper-based; 67 iBT). *Faculty research:* Comparative studies on the carbohydrate composition of marine macroalgae, host-parasite relationship between the spruce budworm and entomepathogen fungus.

Jacksonville State University, College of Graduate Studies and Continuing Education, College of Arts and Sciences, Department of Biology, Jacksonville, AL 36265-1602. Offers MS. *Program availability:* Part-time, evening/weekend. *Faculty:* 10 full-time (1 woman). *Students:* 5 full-time (all women), 24 part-time (14 women); includes 5 minority (3 Black or African American, non-Hispanic/Latino; 1 Asian, non-Hispanic/Latino; 1 Hispanic/Latino), 4 international. Average age 27. 21 applicants, 86% accepted, 10 enrolled. In 2015, 8 master's awarded. *Degree requirements:* For master's, comprehensive exam, thesis (for some programs). *Entrance requirements:* For master's, GRE General Test or MAT. Additional exam requirements/recommendations for international students: Required—TOEFL (minimum score 500 paper-based; 61 iBT). *Application deadline:* Applications are processed on a rolling basis. Application fee: $35. Electronic applications accepted. *Financial support:* In 2015–16, 23 students received support. Available to part-time students. Application deadline: 4/1; applicants required to submit FAFSA. *Unit head:* Dr. Ted Klimasewski, Acting Head, 256-782-5813, E-mail: tedk@jsu.edu. *Application contact:* Dr. Jean Pugliese, Associate Dean, 256-782-8278, Fax: 256-782-5321, E-mail: pugliese@jsu.edu.

James Madison University, The Graduate School, College of Science and Mathematics, Program in Biology, Harrisonburg, VA 22807. Offers MS. *Program availability:* Part-time. *Faculty:* 51 full-time (20 women), 1 part-time/adjunct (0 women). *Students:* 16 full-time (8 women), 3 part-time (1 woman); includes 4 minority (1 Black or African American, non-Hispanic/Latino; 2 Asian, non-Hispanic/Latino; 1 Hispanic/Latino). Average age 30. 28 applicants, 43% accepted, 7 enrolled. In 2015, 9 master's awarded. Application fee: $55. Electronic applications accepted. *Financial support:* In 2015–16, 14 students received support, including 1 fellowship; Federal Work-Study, unspecified assistantships, and 14 assistantships (averaging $7530) also available. Financial award application deadline: 3/1; financial award applicants required to submit FAFSA. *Faculty research:* Evolutionary ecology, gene regulation, microbial ecology, plant development, biomechanics. *Unit head:* Dr. Joanna B. Mott, Department Head, E-mail: mottjb@jmu.edu. *Application contact:* Lynette D. Michael, Director of Graduate Admissions and Student Records, 540-568-6131 Ext. 6395, E-mail: michaeld@jmu.edu. Website: http://www.jmu.edu/biology/index.shtml

John Carroll University, Graduate School, Department of Biology, University Heights, OH 44118-4581. Offers MA, MS. *Program availability:* Part-time. *Degree requirements:* For master's, essay or thesis, seminar. *Entrance requirements:* For master's, undergraduate major in biology, 1 semester of biochemistry, minimum 2.5 GPA. Electronic applications accepted. *Faculty research:* Algal ecology, systematics, molecular genetics, neurophysiology, behavioral ecology.

Johns Hopkins University, National Institutes of Health Sponsored Programs, Baltimore, MD 21218. Offers biology (PhD), including biochemistry, biophysics, cell biology, developmental biology, genetic biology, molecular biology; cell, molecular, and developmental biology and biophysics (PhD). *Degree requirements:* For doctorate, comprehensive exam, thesis/dissertation. *Entrance requirements:* For doctorate, GRE General Test. Additional exam requirements/recommendations for international students: Required—TOEFL (minimum score 600 paper-based), TWE. Electronic applications accepted. *Faculty research:* Protein and nucleic acid biochemistry and biophysical chemistry, molecular biology and development.

Johns Hopkins University, School of Education, Master's Programs in Education, Baltimore, MD 21218. Offers counseling (MS), including clinical mental health counseling, school counseling; education (MS), including educational studies, gifted education, reading, school administration and supervision, technology for educators; elementary education (MAT); health professions (M Ed); intelligence analysis (MS); organizational leadership (MS); secondary education (MAT), including biology, chemistry, earth/space science, English, mathematics, physics, science, social studies; special education (MS), including early childhood special education, general special education studies, mild to moderate disabilities, severe disabilities. *Program availability:* Part-time, evening/weekend, 100% online, blended/hybrid learning. *Students:* 302 full-time (241 women), 1,472 part-time (1,106 women); includes 710 minority (313 Black or African American, non-Hispanic/Latino; 6 American Indian or Alaska Native, non-Hispanic/Latino; 133 Asian, non-Hispanic/Latino; 167 Hispanic/Latino; 11 Native Hawaiian or other Pacific Islander, non-Hispanic/Latino; 80 Two or more races, non-Hispanic/Latino), 46 international. Average age 28. 1,717 applicants, 69% accepted, 904 enrolled. In 2015, 623 master's awarded. *Degree requirements:* For master's, comprehensive exam (for some programs), portfolio, capstone project and/or internship; PRAXIS II Core (for teacher preparation programs that lead to licensure). *Entrance requirements:* For master's, GRE (for full-time programs only); PRAXIS I or state approved alternative (for teacher preparation programs that lead to licensure), minimum of a bachelor's degree from regionally- or nationally-accredited institution; minimum GPA of 3.0 in all previous programs of study; official transcripts from all post-secondary institutions attended; essay; curriculum vitae/resume; letters of recommendation (3 for full-time, 2 for part-time). Additional exam requirements/recommendations for international students: Required—TOEFL (minimum score 600 paper-based; 100 iBT), IELTS (minimum score 7). *Application deadline:* For fall admission, 4/1 for domestic and international students; for spring admission, 10/1 for domestic and international students; for summer admission, 2/1 for domestic and international students. Application fee: $80. Electronic applications accepted. *Expenses:* Contact institution. *Financial support:* Applicants required to submit FAFSA. *Unit head:* Dr. Mariale M. Hardiman, Interim Dean, 410-516-7820, Fax: 410-516-6697, E-mail: mmhardiman@jhu.edu. *Application contact:* Rhodri Evans, Director of Enrollment Services, 410-516-0741, Fax: 410-516-6697, E-mail: revans@jhu.edu.

Johns Hopkins University, School of Medicine, Graduate Programs in Medicine, Baltimore, MD 21218. Offers MA, PhD, MD/PhD. *Degree requirements:* For doctorate, thesis/dissertation. *Entrance requirements:* Additional exam requirements/recommendations for international students: Required—TOEFL. Electronic applications accepted. *Expenses:* Contact institution.

Johns Hopkins University, Zanvyl Krieger School of Arts and Sciences, Chemistry-Biology Interface Program, Baltimore, MD 21218. Offers PhD. Terminal master's awarded for partial completion of doctoral program. *Degree requirements:* For doctorate, comprehensive exam, thesis/dissertation, 8 one-semester courses, research proposal, graduate board oral exam. *Entrance requirements:* For doctorate, GRE General Test, GRE Subject Test in biochemistry, cell and molecular biology, biology or chemistry (strongly recommended), 3 letters of recommendation, transcripts, statement of purpose, interview. Additional exam requirements/recommendations for international students: Required—TOEFL. Electronic applications accepted. *Faculty research:* Enzyme mechanisms, inhibitors, and metabolic pathways; DNA replication, damaged, and repair; using small molecules to probe signal transduction, gene regulation, angiogenesis, and other biological processes; synthetic methods and medicinal chemistry; synthetic modeling of metalloenzymes.

Johns Hopkins University, Zanvyl Krieger School of Arts and Sciences, Department of Biology, Baltimore, MD 21218. Offers PhD. Terminal master's awarded for partial completion of doctoral program. *Degree requirements:* For doctorate, comprehensive exam, thesis/dissertation. *Entrance requirements:* For doctorate, GRE General Test. Additional exam requirements/recommendations for international students: Required—TOEFL (minimum score 600 paper-based), IELTS, TWE. Electronic applications accepted. *Faculty research:* Cell biology, molecular biology and development, biochemistry, developmental biology, biophysics, genetics.

Kansas City University of Medicine and Biosciences, College of Biosciences, Kansas City, MO 64106-1453. Offers bioethics (MA); biomedical sciences (MS). *Program availability:* Part-time. *Degree requirements:* For master's, comprehensive exam, thesis (for some programs). *Entrance requirements:* For master's, MCAT, GRE.

Kansas State University, Graduate School, College of Arts and Sciences, Division of Biology, Manhattan, KS 66506. Offers biology (MS). Terminal master's awarded for partial completion of doctoral program. *Degree requirements:* For master's, thesis; for doctorate, thesis/dissertation. *Entrance requirements:* For master's, GRE General Test, minimum undergraduate GPA of 3.0; for doctorate, GRE General Test, minimum GPA of 3.0. Additional exam requirements/recommendations for international students: Required—TOEFL (minimum score 550 paper-based). Electronic applications accepted. *Faculty research:* Ecology, genetics, developmental biology, microbiology, cell biology.

Kansas State University, Graduate School, College of Veterinary Medicine, Department of Diagnostic Medicine/Pathobiology, Manhattan, KS 66506. Offers biomedical science (MS); diagnostic medicine/pathobiology (PhD). Terminal master's awarded for partial completion of doctoral program. *Degree requirements:* For doctorate, thesis/dissertation. *Entrance requirements:* For master's and doctorate, interviews. Additional exam requirements/recommendations for international students: Required—TOEFL (minimum score 550 paper-based). Electronic applications accepted. *Faculty research:* Infectious disease of animals, food safety and security, epidemiology and public health, toxicology, pathology.

Keck Graduate Institute, School of Applied Life Sciences, Claremont, CA 91711. Offers applied life sciences (PhD); bioscience (MBS); bioscience management (Certificate). *Degree requirements:* For master's, comprehensive exam, project. *Entrance requirements:* For master's, GRE General Test or MCAT. Additional exam requirements/recommendations for international students: Required—TOEFL. Electronic applications accepted. *Faculty research:* Computational biology, drug discovery and development, molecular and cellular biology, biomedical engineering, biomaterials and tissue engineering.

Kennesaw State University, College of Science and Mathematics, Program in Integrative Biology, Kennesaw, GA 30144. Offers MS. *Degree requirements:* For master's, thesis. *Entrance requirements:* For master's, GRE, two letters of recommendation, official transcript, statement of interest. Additional exam requirements/recommendations for international students: Required—TOEFL (minimum score 550 paper-based; 80 iBT), IELTS (minimum score 6.5). Electronic applications accepted.

Kennesaw State University, Leland and Clarice C. Bagwell College of Education, Program in Teaching, Kennesaw, GA 30144. Offers art education (MAT); biology (MAT); chemistry (MAT); foreign language education (Chinese and Spanish) (MAT); physics (MAT); secondary English (MAT); secondary mathematics (MAT); special education (MAT); teaching English to speakers of other languages (MAT). *Program availability:* Part-time, evening/weekend. *Entrance requirements:* For master's, GRE, GACE I (state certificate exam), minimum GPA of 2.75, 2 recommendations, resume. Additional exam requirements/recommendations for international students: Required—TOEFL (minimum score 550 paper-based; 80 iBT), IELTS (minimum score 6.5). Electronic applications accepted.

Kent State University, College of Arts and Sciences, Department of Biological Sciences, Kent, OH 44242-0001. Offers biological sciences (MS, PhD), including ecology, physiology. *Program availability:* Part-time. *Faculty:* 37 full-time (12 women). *Students:* 52 full-time (33 women), 15 part-time (9 women); includes 7 minority (3 Black or African American, non-Hispanic/Latino; 2 Asian, non-Hispanic/Latino; 2 Two or more races, non-Hispanic/Latino), 20 international. Average age 30. 142 applicants, 27% accepted, 24 enrolled. In 2015, 15 master's, 9 doctorates awarded. *Degree requirements:* For master's, thesis (for some programs); for doctorate, thesis/dissertation. *Entrance requirements:* For master's and doctorate, GRE General Test, minimum GPA of 3.0, transcript, resume, statement of purpose, 3 letters of recommendation. Additional exam requirements/recommendations for international students: Required—TOEFL (minimum score: paper-based 525, iBT 71), Michigan English Language Assessment Battery (minimum score of 75), IELTS (minimum score of 6.0), PTE Academic (minimum score of 48), or completion of ELS level 112 Intensive Program. *Application deadline:* For fall admission, 12/15 for domestic students, 12/5 for international students; for spring admission, 11/29 for domestic and international students. Application fee: $45 ($70 for international students). Electronic applications accepted. *Expenses:* Tuition, state resident: full-time $10,864; part-time $495 per credit hour. Tuition, nonresident: full-time $18,380; part-time $837 per credit hour. *Financial support:* Research assistantships with full tuition reimbursements, teaching assistantships with full tuition reimbursements, career-related internships or fieldwork, Federal Work-Study, scholarships/grants, and unspecified assistantships available. Financial award application deadline: 2/1. *Unit head:* Dr. James L. Blank, Dean, 330-672-2650, E-mail: jblank@kent.edu. *Application contact:* Dr. Heather K. Caldwell, Associate Professor and Graduate Coordinator, 330-672-3636, E-mail: hcaldwel@kent.edu.
Website: http://www.kent.edu/biology/

Kent State University, College of Arts and Sciences, School of Biomedical Sciences, Kent, OH 44242-0001. Offers biological anthropology (PhD); cellular and molecular biology (PhD), including cellular biology and structures, molecular biology and genetics; neurosciences (PhD); pharmacology (MS); physiology (PhD). *Students:* 76 full-time (46 women), 1 (woman) part-time; includes 6 minority (1 Black or African American, non-Hispanic/Latino; 2 Asian, non-Hispanic/Latino; 1 Hispanic/Latino; 2 Two or more races, non-Hispanic/Latino), 28 international. Average age 29. 223 applicants, 13% accepted, 22 enrolled. In 2015, 5 master's, 7 doctorates awarded. Terminal master's awarded for partial completion of doctoral program. *Degree requirements:* For master's, thesis; for doctorate, thesis/dissertation, candidacy exam. *Entrance requirements:* For master's and doctorate, GRE General Test, minimum GPA of 3.0, transcript, goal statement, resume, 3 letters of recommendation. Additional exam requirements/recommendations for international students: Required—TOEFL (minimum score: paper-based 525, iBT

71), Michigan English Language Assessment Battery (minimum score of 75), IELTS (minimum score of 6.0), PTE Academic (minimum score of 48), or completion of ELS level 112 Intensive Program. *Application deadline:* For fall admission, 1/1 for domestic students. Application fee: $45 ($70 for international students). Electronic applications accepted. *Expenses:* Tuition, state resident: full-time $10,864; part-time $495 per credit hour. Tuition, nonresident: full-time $18,380; part-time $837 per credit hour. *Financial support:* In 2015–16, 76 students received support. Research assistantships with full tuition reimbursements available, teaching assistantships, career-related internships or fieldwork, Federal Work-Study, and unspecified assistantships available. Financial award application deadline: 1/1. *Unit head:* Dr. Eric Mintz, Director, 330-672-2263, E-mail: emintz@kent.edu. *Application contact:* 330-672-2263, Fax: 330-672-9391, E-mail: jwearden@kent.edu.
Website: http://www.kent.edu/biomedical/

Lake Erie College of Osteopathic Medicine, Professional Programs, Erie, PA 16509-1025. Offers biomedical sciences (Postbaccalaureate Certificate); medical education (MS); osteopathic medicine (DO); pharmacy (Pharm D). *Accreditation:* ACPE; AOsA. *Degree requirements:* For doctorate, comprehensive exam, National Osteopathic Medical Licensing Exam, Levels 1 and 2; for Postbaccalaureate Certificate, comprehensive exam, North American Pharmacist Licensure Examination (NAPLEX). *Entrance requirements:* For doctorate, MCAT, minimum GPA of 3.2, letters of recommendation; for Postbaccalaureate Certificate, PCAT, letters of recommendation, minimum GPA of 3.5. Electronic applications accepted. *Faculty research:* Cardiac smooth and skeletal muscle mechanics, chemotherapeutics and vitamins, osteopathic manipulation.

Lakehead University, Graduate Studies, Faculty of Social Sciences and Humanities, Department of Biology, Thunder Bay, ON P7B 5E1, Canada. Offers M Sc. *Program availability:* Part-time, evening/weekend. *Degree requirements:* For master's, thesis, department seminary, oral examination. *Entrance requirements:* For master's, minimum B average. Additional exam requirements/recommendations for international students: Required—TOEFL. *Faculty research:* Systematics and biogeography, wildlife parasitology, plant physiology and biochemistry, plant ecology, fishery biology.

Lamar University, College of Graduate Studies, College of Arts and Sciences, Department of Biology, Beaumont, TX 77710. Offers MS. *Program availability:* Part-time, evening/weekend. *Faculty:* 6 full-time (1 woman). *Students:* 4 full-time (3 women), 7 part-time (4 women); includes 3 minority (1 Black or African American, non-Hispanic/Latino; 1 Asian, non-Hispanic/Latino; 1 Hispanic/Latino), 4 international. Average age 28. 11 applicants, 82% accepted, 5 enrolled. In 2015, 8 master's awarded. *Degree requirements:* For master's, thesis. *Entrance requirements:* For master's, GRE General Test, minimum GPA of 2.5 in last 60 hours of undergraduate course work. Additional exam requirements/recommendations for international students: Required—TOEFL (minimum score 550 paper-based; 79 iBT), IELTS (minimum score 6.5). *Application deadline:* For fall admission, 8/10 for domestic students, 7/1 for international students; for spring admission, 1/5 for domestic students, 12/1 for international students. Applications are processed on a rolling basis. Application fee: $25 ($50 for international students). Electronic applications accepted. *Expenses:* Tuition, area resident: Full-time $6720; part-time $4032. Tuition, nonresident: full-time $14,880; part-time $8928. *Required fees:* $1900; $950 $784. *Financial support:* Teaching assistantships available. Financial award application deadline: 4/1. *Faculty research:* Microbiology, limnology, vertebrate ecology, invertebrate hemoglobin, ornithology. *Unit head:* Dr. Paul Nicoletto, Chair, 409-880-8262, Fax: 409-880-7147. *Application contact:* Melissa Gallien, Director, Admissions and Academic Services, 409-880-8888, Fax: 409-880-7419, E-mail: gradmissions@lamar.edu.
Website: http://artssciences.lamar.edu/biology

Laurentian University, School of Graduate Studies and Research, Programme in Biology, Sudbury, ON P3E 2C6, Canada. Offers biology (M Sc); boreal ecology (PhD). *Program availability:* Part-time. *Degree requirements:* For master's, thesis. *Entrance requirements:* For master's, honors degree with second class or better. *Faculty research:* Recovery of acid-stressed lakes, effects of climate change, origin and maintenance of biocomplexity, radionuclide dynamics, cytogenetic studies of plants.

Lee University, Program in Education, Cleveland, TN 37320-3450. Offers art (MAT); curriculum and instruction (M Ed, Ed S); early childhood (MAT); educational leadership (M Ed, Ed S); elementary education (MAT); English and math (MAT); English and science (MAT); English and social studies (MAT); higher education administration (MS); history (MAT); history and economics (MAT); math and science (MAT); math and social studies (MAT); middle grades (MAT); science and social studies (MASW); secondary education (MAT); Spanish (MAT); special education (M Ed, MAT); TESOL (MAT). *Accreditation:* NCATE. *Program availability:* Part-time. *Faculty:* 12 full-time (6 women), 7 part-time/adjunct (2 women). *Students:* 39 full-time (28 women), 57 part-time (37 women); includes 13 minority (7 Black or African American, non-Hispanic/Latino; 4 Hispanic/Latino; 1 Native Hawaiian or other Pacific Islander, non-Hispanic/Latino; 1 Two or more races, non-Hispanic/Latino), 5 international. Average age 30. 46 applicants, 76% accepted, 29 enrolled. In 2015, 45 master's, 10 other advanced degrees awarded. *Degree requirements:* For master's, variable foreign language requirement, thesis optional, internship. *Entrance requirements:* For master's, MAT or GRE General Test, minimum undergraduate GPA of 2.75, 3 letters of recommendation, interview, writing sample, official transcripts, background check; for Ed S, minimum undergraduate and master's GPA of 2.75, official transcripts for undergraduate and master's degrees. Additional exam requirements/recommendations for international students: Required—TOEFL (minimum score 450 paper-based). *Application deadline:* For fall admission, 6/1 priority date for domestic and international students; for spring admission, 11/1 priority date for domestic and international students; for summer admission, 4/1 priority date for domestic and international students. Applications are processed on a rolling basis. Application fee: $25. Electronic applications accepted. *Expenses:* Tuition, area resident: Full-time $10,800; part-time $600 per credit hour. *Required fees:* $35 per term. One-time fee: $25. Tuition and fees vary according to program. *Financial support:* In 2015–16, 52 students received support. Career-related internships or fieldwork, Federal Work-Study, institutionally sponsored loans, scholarships/grants, and unspecified assistantships available. Financial award application deadline: 3/1; financial award applicants required to submit FAFSA. *Unit head:* Dr. William Kamm, Director, 423-614-8544, E-mail: wkamm@leeuniversity.edu. *Application contact:* Crystal Keeter, Graduate Education Secretary, 423-614-8544, E-mail: ckeeter@leeuniversity.edu.
Website: http://www.leeuniversity.edu/academics/graduate/education

Lehigh University, College of Arts and Sciences, Department of Biological Sciences, Bethlehem, PA 18015. Offers biochemistry (PhD); cell and molecular biology (PhD); integrative biology (PhD); molecular biology (MS). *Program availability:* Part-time, 100% online. *Faculty:* 19 full-time (9 women). *Students:* 38 full-time (22 women), 21 part-time (15 women); includes 13 minority (5 Black or African American, non-Hispanic/Latino; 1 American Indian or Alaska Native, non-Hispanic/Latino; 6 Hispanic/Latino; 1 Two or more races, non-Hispanic/Latino), 5 international. Average age 27. 38 applicants, 50% accepted, 10 enrolled. In 2015, 6 master's, 1 doctorate awarded. Terminal master's awarded for partial completion of doctoral program. *Degree requirements:* For master's, thesis optional; for doctorate, comprehensive exam, thesis/dissertation. *Entrance requirements:* For doctorate, GRE General Test. Additional exam requirements/

Biological and Biomedical Sciences—General

recommendations for international students: Required—TOEFL (minimum score 85 iBT). *Application deadline:* For fall admission, 12/15 for domestic and international students. Application fee: $75. *Expenses:* $1,185 per credit hour tuition (PhD); $925 per credit hour tuition (MS). *Financial support:* In 2015–16, 34 students received support, including 8 fellowships with full tuition reimbursements available (averaging $29,667 per year), 6 research assistantships with full tuition reimbursements available (averaging $27,000 per year), 19 teaching assistantships with full tuition reimbursements available (averaging $27,000 per year); scholarships/grants also available. Financial award application deadline: 12/15. *Faculty research:* Gene expression, cytoskeleton and cell structure, cell cycle and growth regulation, neuroscience, animal behavior, microbiology. *Total annual research expenditures:* $1.9 million. *Unit head:* Dr. Murray Itzkowitz, Chairperson, 610-758-3680, Fax: 610-758-4004, E-mail: mi00@lehigh.edu. *Application contact:* Dr. Mary Kathryn Iovine, Graduate Coordinator, 610-758-6981, Fax: 610-758-4004, E-mail: mki3@lehigh.edu.
Website: http://www.lehigh.edu/~inbios/

Lehman College of the City University of New York, School of Natural and Social Sciences, Department of Biological Sciences, Program in Biology, Bronx, NY 10468-1589. Offers MA.

Liberty University, School of Health Sciences, Lynchburg, VA 24515. Offers biomedical sciences (MS); global health (MPH); health promotion (MPH); healthcare management (Certificate); nutrition (MPH). *Program availability:* Part-time, online learning. *Students:* 435 full-time (342 women), 609 part-time (489 women); includes 301 minority (238 Black or African American, non-Hispanic/Latino; 6 American Indian or Alaska Native, non-Hispanic/Latino; 25 Asian, non-Hispanic/Latino; 12 Hispanic/Latino; 1 Native Hawaiian or other Pacific Islander, non-Hispanic/Latino; 19 Two or more races, non-Hispanic/Latino; 71 international. Average age 33. 1,433 applicants, 43% accepted, 295 enrolled. In 2015, 50 master's, 8 other advanced degrees awarded. *Degree requirements:* For master's, thesis (for some programs). *Entrance requirements:* Additional exam requirements/recommendations for international students: Required—TOEFL (minimum score 600 paper-based; 100 iBT). Application fee: $50. *Unit head:* Dr. Ralph Linstra, Dean. *Application contact:* Jay Bridge, Director of Admissions, 800-424-9595, Fax: 800-628-7977, E-mail: gradadmissions@liberty.edu.

London Metropolitan University, Graduate Programs, London, United Kingdom. Offers applied psychology (M Sc); architecture (MA); biomedical science (M Sc); blood science (M Sc); cancer pharmacology (M Sc); computer networking and cyber security (M Sc); computing and information systems (M Sc); conference interpreting (MA); counter-terrorism studies (M Sc); creative, digital and professional writing (MA); crime, violence and prevention (M Sc); criminology (M Sc); curating contemporary art (MA); data analytics (M Sc); digital media (MA); early childhood studies (MA); education (MA, Ed D); financial services law, regulation and compliance (LL M); food science (M Sc); forensic psychology (M Sc); health and social care management and policy (M Sc); human nutrition (M Sc); human resource management (MA); human rights and international conflict (MA); information technology (M Sc); intelligence and security studies (M Sc); international oil, gas and energy law (LL M); international relations (MA); interpreting (MA); learning and teaching in higher education (MA); legal practice (LL M); media and entertainment law (LL M); organizational and consumer psychology (M Sc); psychological therapy (M Sc); psychology of mental health (M Sc); public health (M Sc); public policy and management (MPA); security studies (M Sc); social work (M Sc); spatial planning and urban design (MA); sports therapy (M Sc); supporting older children and young people with dyslexia (MA); teaching languages (MA), including Arabic, English; translation (MA); woman and child abuse (MA).

Long Island University–LIU Brooklyn, Richard L. Conolly College of Liberal Arts and Sciences, Brooklyn, NY 11201-8423. Offers biology (MA); chemistry (MS); clinical psychology (PhD); communication sciences and disorders (MS); creative writing (MFA); English (MA); media arts (MA, MFA); political science (MA); psychology (MA); social science (MS); speech-language pathology (MS); United Nations (Advanced Certificate); urban studies (MA); writing and production for television (MFA). *Program availability:* Part-time, evening/weekend, blended/hybrid learning. *Faculty:* 90 full-time (35 women), 125 part-time/adjunct (67 women). *Students:* 382 full-time (288 women), 223 part-time (154 women); includes 257 minority (129 Black or African American, non-Hispanic/Latino; 33 Asian, non-Hispanic/Latino; 80 Hispanic/Latino; 1 Native Hawaiian or other Pacific Islander, non-Hispanic/Latino; 14 Two or more races, non-Hispanic/Latino; 93 international. Average age 33. 801 applicants, 44% accepted, 169 enrolled. In 2015, 163 master's, 16 doctorates, 9 other advanced degrees awarded. *Degree requirements:* For doctorate, thesis/dissertation. *Entrance requirements:* Additional exam requirements/recommendations for international students: Required—TOEFL (minimum score 550 paper-based; 79 iBT). *Application deadline:* Applications are processed on a rolling basis. Application fee: $50. Electronic applications accepted. *Expenses:* $1,155 per credit tuition, $934 per term full-time fees, $442 per term part-time fees. *Financial support:* In 2015–16, 221 students received support, including 135 fellowships with full tuition reimbursements available (averaging $23,986 per year), 29 research assistantships with partial tuition reimbursements available (averaging $13,860 per year), 185 teaching assistantships with full tuition reimbursements available (averaging $20,790 per year). Financial award application deadline: 2/15; financial award applicants required to submit FAFSA. *Faculty research:* Nanocrystal polymerization of cellulose using electron microscopy. *Unit head:* Dr. David Cohen, Dean, 718-488-1003, E-mail: david.cohen@liu.edu. *Application contact:* Richard Sunday, Dean of Admissions, 718-488-1011, Fax: 718-780-6110, E-mail: bkln-admissions@liu.edu.

Long Island University–LIU Post, College of Liberal Arts and Sciences, Brookville, NY 11548-1300. Offers applied mathematics (MS); behavior analysis (MA); biology (MS); criminal justice (MS); earth science (MS); English (MA); environmental studies (MS); environmental sustainability (MS); genetic counseling (MS); gerontology (Advanced Certificate); health care administration (MPA); history (MA); interdisciplinary studies (MA, MS); mathematics for secondary school teachers (MS); mobile GIS application development (Advanced Certificate); non-profit management (Advanced Certificate); political science (MA); psychology (MA); public administration (MPA). *Program availability:* Part-time, evening/weekend, online learning. *Faculty:* 77 full-time (35 women), 36 part-time/adjunct (17 women). *Students:* 254 full-time (178 women), 177 part-time (134 women); includes 104 minority (40 Black or African American, non-Hispanic/Latino; 27 Asian, non-Hispanic/Latino; 28 Hispanic/Latino; 1 Native Hawaiian or other Pacific Islander, non-Hispanic/Latino; 8 Two or more races, non-Hispanic/Latino; 44 international. Average age 31. 686 applicants, 47% accepted, 138 enrolled. In 2015, 135 master's awarded. *Degree requirements:* For master's, comprehensive exam (for some programs), thesis (for some programs). *Entrance requirements:* Additional exam requirements/recommendations for international students: Required—TOEFL (minimum score 550 paper-based; 79 iBT), IELTS (minimum score 6.5). *Application deadline:* Applications are processed on a rolling basis. Application fee: $50. Electronic applications accepted. *Expenses:* $1,155 per credit; $934 full-time fees; $442 part-time fees. *Financial support:* In 2015–16, 48 fellowships (averaging $12,637 per year), 5 research assistantships with full tuition reimbursements were awarded; Federal Work-Study and institutionally sponsored loans also available. Support available to part-time students. Financial award application deadline: 2/15; financial award applicants required to submit FAFSA. *Faculty research:* Biology, criminal justice, earth and

environmental science, English, health care and public administration, history, mathematics, political science, psychology, Spanish. *Unit head:* Dr. Nicholas J. Ramer, Acting Dean, 516-299-2233, Fax: 516-299-4140, E-mail: nicholas.ramer@liu.edu. *Application contact:* Carol Zerah, Director of Graduate Admissions, 516-299-2900 Ext. 3952, Fax: 516-299-2137, E-mail: enroll@cwpost.liu.edu.
Website: http://liu.edu/CWPost/Academics/Schools/CLAS

Long Island University–LIU Post, School of Health Professions and Nursing, Brookville, NY 11548-1300. Offers biomedical sciences (MS), including applied laboratory medicine, cancer biology, medical and molecular immunology, microbiology/infectious diseases; cardiovascular perfusion (MS); dietetic internship (Advanced Certificate); family nurse practitioner (MS); forensic social work (Advanced Certificate); nursing education (MS); social work (MSW). *Program availability:* Part-time, evening/weekend, blended/hybrid learning. *Faculty:* 16 full-time (14 women), 46 part-time/adjunct (33 women). *Students:* 190 full-time (139 women), 181 part-time (157 women); includes 141 minority (51 Black or African American, non-Hispanic/Latino; 46 Asian, non-Hispanic/Latino; 41 Hispanic/Latino; 3 Two or more races, non-Hispanic/Latino; 47 international. Average age 36. 422 applicants, 64% accepted, 141 enrolled. In 2015, 96 master's, 28 other advanced degrees awarded. *Degree requirements:* For master's, comprehensive exam (for some programs), thesis (for some programs). *Entrance requirements:* Additional exam requirements/recommendations for international students: Required—TOEFL, IELTS. *Application deadline:* Applications are processed on a rolling basis. Application fee: $50. Electronic applications accepted. *Expenses:* $1,155 per credit, $934 per term full-time university fee, $442 per term part-time university fee. *Financial support:* In 2015–16, 6 research assistantships with partial tuition reimbursements were awarded; career-related internships or fieldwork, Federal Work-Study, institutionally sponsored loans, tuition waivers (partial), and unspecified assistantships also available. Support available to part-time students. Financial award application deadline: 2/15; financial award applicants required to submit FAFSA. *Faculty research:* Breast cancer, childhood obesity, dietary beverage consumption, emotional distress, histone modification, interprofessional practice, interstitial cystitis, lung cancer, pancreatic cancer, pediatric pain management, post-traumatic growth, poverty, renal nutrition, social ethics, yeast and bacterial drug resistance. *Total annual research expenditures:* $15,000. *Unit head:* Dr. Stacy Gropack, Acting Dean, 516-299-2486, Fax: 516-299-2527, E-mail: post-shpn@liu.edu. *Application contact:* Carol Zerah, Director of Graduate and International Admissions, 516-299-2900 Ext. 3952, Fax: 516-299-2137, E-mail: post-enroll@liu.edu.
Website: http://liu.edu/post/health

Louisiana State University and Agricultural & Mechanical College, Graduate School, College of Science, Department of Biological Sciences, Baton Rouge, LA 70803. Offers biochemistry (MS, PhD); biological science (MS, PhD); science (MNS).

Louisiana State University Health Sciences Center, School of Graduate Studies in New Orleans, New Orleans, LA 70112-2223. Offers PhD, MD/PhD. *Faculty:* 159 full-time (45 women). *Students:* 70 full-time (36 women), 2 part-time (1 woman); includes 17 minority (5 Black or African American, non-Hispanic/Latino; 8 Asian, non-Hispanic/Latino; 4 Hispanic/Latino), 14 international. Average age 26. 75 applicants, 28% accepted, 15 enrolled. In 2015, 21 doctorates awarded. Terminal master's awarded for partial completion of doctoral program. *Degree requirements:* For doctorate, comprehensive exam, thesis/dissertation. *Entrance requirements:* For doctorate, GRE General Test. Additional exam requirements/recommendations for international students: Recommended—TOEFL (minimum score 90 iBT), IELTS (minimum score 7). *Application deadline:* For fall admission, 4/1 for domestic and international students. Applications are processed on a rolling basis. Application fee: $30. *Financial support:* Unspecified assistantships available. *Unit head:* Dr. Joseph M. Moerschbaecher, III, Head, 504-568-2211, Fax: 504-568-2361. *Application contact:* Leigh A. Smith-Vaniz, Coordinator of Student Affairs, 504-568-2211, Fax: 504-568-5588, E-mail: lsmi30@lsuhsc.edu.

Louisiana State University Health Sciences Center at Shreveport, Master of Science in Biomedical Sciences Program, Shreveport, LA 71130-3932. Offers MS. Terminal master's awarded for partial completion of doctoral program. *Degree requirements:* For master's, thesis, seminar and journal club presentations, research component. *Entrance requirements:* For master's, GRE. Additional exam requirements/recommendations for international students: Required—TOEFL, IELTS. *Faculty research:* Cardiovascular, cancer, neuroscience, genetics, virology, immunology.

Louisiana State University in Shreveport, College of Arts and Sciences, Program in Biological Sciences, Shreveport, LA 71115-2399. Offers MS. *Program availability:* Part-time, evening/weekend. *Students:* 28 full-time (21 women), 13 part-time (6 women); includes 19 minority (14 Black or African American, non-Hispanic/Latino; 3 Asian, non-Hispanic/Latino; 2 Hispanic/Latino), 4 international. Average age 26. 127 applicants, 94% accepted, 20 enrolled. In 2015, 3 master's awarded. *Degree requirements:* For master's, comprehensive exam (for some programs), thesis optional. *Entrance requirements:* For master's, GRE. Additional exam requirements/recommendations for international students: Required—TOEFL (minimum score 550 paper-based; 61 iBT). *Application deadline:* For fall admission, 6/30 for domestic and international students; for spring admission, 11/30 for domestic and international students; for summer admission, 4/30 for domestic and international students. Applications are processed on a rolling basis. Application fee: $20 ($30 for international students). Electronic applications accepted. *Expenses:* Tuition, state resident: part-time $325 per credit hour. Tuition, nonresident: part-time $1019 per credit hour. *Required fees:* $52 per credit hour. Tuition and fees vary according to program. *Financial support:* Applicants required to submit FAFSA. *Unit head:* Dr. Stephen Banks, Director, 318-797-5220, E-mail: stephen.banks@lsus.edu. *Application contact:* David Stanford, Director of Admissions, 318-795-2403, Fax: 318-797-5286, E-mail: david.stanford@lsus.edu.
Website: http://www.lsus.edu/academics/graduate-studies/graduate-programs/master-of-science-in-biological-sciences

Louisiana Tech University, Graduate School, College of Applied and Natural Sciences, School of Biological Sciences, Ruston, LA 71272. Offers biology (MS); molecular sciences and nanotechnology (MS). *Program availability:* Part-time. *Degree requirements:* For master's, thesis or alternative. *Entrance requirements:* For master's, GRE General Test, GRE Subject Test. *Application deadline:* For fall admission, 7/29 priority date for domestic students; for spring admission, 2/3 for domestic students. Applications are processed on a rolling basis. Application fee: $20 ($30 for international students). *Financial support:* Fellowships, research assistantships, and teaching assistantships available. Financial award application deadline: 2/1. *Faculty research:* Genetics, animal biology, plant biology. *Unit head:* Dr. William J. Campbell, Director, 318-257-4573, Fax: 318-257-4574, E-mail: campbell@latech.edu.
Website: http://ans.latech.edu/bls.html

Loyola University Chicago, Graduate School, Department of Biology, Chicago, IL 60660. Offers biology (MS); medical sciences (MA). *Faculty:* 21 full-time (8 women). *Students:* 83 full-time (43 women); includes 34 minority (6 Black or African American, non-Hispanic/Latino; 22 Asian, non-Hispanic/Latino; 4 Hispanic/Latino; 2 Two or more races, non-Hispanic/Latino), 2 international. Average age 25. 228 applicants, 67% accepted, 61 enrolled. In 2015, 59 master's awarded. *Degree requirements:* For master's, thesis. *Entrance requirements:* For master's, GRE General Test, 3 letters of

recommendation. Additional exam requirements/recommendations for international students: Required—TOEFL. *Application deadline:* For fall admission, 6/1 for domestic and international students. Applications are processed on a rolling basis. Application fee: $50. Electronic applications accepted. *Expenses: Tuition, area resident:* Full-time $18,054; part-time $9027 per credit hour. *Required fees:* $832; $284 per credit hour. Part-time tuition and fees vary according to course load, degree level and program. *Financial support:* In 2015–16, 7 students received support, including 7 fellowships with full tuition reimbursements available (averaging $16,000 per year); Federal Work-Study and institutionally sponsored loans also available. Financial award application deadline: 2/1; financial award applicants required to submit FAFSA. *Faculty research:* Evolution and systematics, development, aquatic biology, molecular biology and genetics, cell biology, neurobiology. *Total annual research expenditures:* $2.5 million. *Unit head:* Dr. Terry Grande, Graduate Program Director, 773-583-5649, Fax: 773-508-3646, E-mail: tgrande@luc.edu. *Application contact:* Ron Martin, Assistant Director of Enrollment Management, 312-915-8950, Fax: 312-915-8905, E-mail: gradapp@luc.edu.
Website: http://www.luc.edu/biology/

Loyola University Chicago, Graduate School, Integrated Program in Biomedical Sciences, Maywood, IL 60153. Offers biochemistry and molecular biology (MS, PhD); cell and molecular physiology (PhD); infectious disease and immunology (MS); integrative cell biology (PhD); medical physiology (MS); microbiology and immunology (MS, PhD); molecular pharmacology and therapeutics (MS, PhD); neuroscience (MS, PhD). *Students:* 135 full-time (65 women), 1 part-time (0 women); includes 28 minority (5 Black or African American, non-Hispanic/Latino; 15 Asian, non-Hispanic/Latino; 6 Hispanic/Latino; 2 Two or more races, non-Hispanic/Latino), 16 international. Average age 28. 442 applicants, 23% accepted, 55 enrolled. In 2015, 40 master's, 17 doctorates awarded. *Expenses: Tuition, area resident:* Full-time $18,054; part-time $9027 per credit hour. *Required fees:* $832; $284 per credit hour. Part-time tuition and fees vary according to course load, degree level and program. *Unit head:* Dr. Samuel Attoh, Dean, 773-508-3459, Fax: 773-508-2460, E-mail: sattoh@luc.edu. *Application contact:* Ron Martin, Associate Director of Enrollment Management, 312-915-8950, Fax: 312-915-8905, E-mail: gradapp@luc.edu.
Website: http://ssom.luc.edu/graduate_school/degree-programs/ipbsphd/

Marquette University, Graduate School, College of Arts and Sciences, Department of Biology, Milwaukee, WI 53201-1881. Offers cell biology (MS, PhD); developmental biology (MS, PhD); ecology (MS, PhD); epithelial physiology (MS, PhD); genetics (MS, PhD); microbiology (MS, PhD); molecular biology (MS, PhD); muscle and exercise physiology (MS, PhD); neuroscience (PhD). *Faculty:* 22 full-time (7 women), 3 part-time/adjunct (2 women). *Students:* 28 full-time (11 women), 12 part-time (4 women); includes 4 minority (1 Asian, non-Hispanic/Latino; 1 Hispanic/Latino; 2 Two or more races, non-Hispanic/Latino), 11 international. Average age 27. 72 applicants, 28% accepted, 5 enrolled. In 2015, 2 master's, 4 doctorates awarded. Terminal master's awarded for partial completion of doctoral program. *Degree requirements:* For master's, comprehensive exam, thesis, 1 year of teaching experience or equivalent; for doctorate, thesis/dissertation, 1 year of teaching experience or equivalent, qualifying exam. *Entrance requirements:* For master's and doctorate, GRE General Test, GRE Subject Test, official transcripts from all current and previous colleges/universities except Marquette, statement of professional goals and aspirations, three letters of recommendation. Additional exam requirements/recommendations for international students: Required—TOEFL (minimum score 530 paper-based). *Application deadline:* For fall admission, 12/15 for domestic and international students. Application fee: $50. Electronic applications accepted. *Financial support:* In 2015–16, 39 students received support, including 6 fellowships (averaging $1,208 per year), 4 research assistantships with full tuition reimbursements available (averaging $21,750 per year), 29 teaching assistantships with full tuition reimbursements available (averaging $21,750 per year); scholarships/grants, health care benefits, tuition waivers (full and partial), and unspecified assistantships also available. Support available to part-time students. Financial award application deadline: 2/15. *Faculty research:* Neurobiology, neuroendocrinology, epithelial physiology, neuropeptide interactions, synaptic transmission. *Total annual research expenditures:* $1.2 million. *Unit head:* Dr. Ed Blumenthal, Chair, 414-288-1748. *Application contact:* Dr. Michael Schlappi, Recruiting Contact, 414-288-1467.
Website: http://www.marquette.edu/biology/

Marshall University, Academic Affairs Division, College of Science, Department of Biological Science, Huntington, WV 25755. Offers MA, MS. *Students:* 24 full-time (14 women), 5 part-time (3 women); includes 3 minority (1 Black or African American, non-Hispanic/Latino; 1 Asian, non-Hispanic/Latino; 1 Native Hawaiian or other Pacific Islander, non-Hispanic/Latino), 1 international. Average age 24. In 2015, 13 master's awarded. *Degree requirements:* For master's, thesis (for some programs). *Entrance requirements:* For master's, GRE General Test. Application fee: $40. *Financial support:* Career-related internships or fieldwork available. *Unit head:* Dr. David Mallory, Chairperson, 304-696-2353, E-mail: mallory@marshall.edu. *Application contact:* Information Contact, 304-746-1900, Fax: 304-746-1902, E-mail: services@marshall.edu.

Marshall University, Joan C. Edwards School of Medicine and Academic Affairs Division, Program in Biomedical Sciences, Huntington, WV 25755. Offers MS, PhD. Terminal master's awarded for partial completion of doctoral program. *Degree requirements:* For master's, comprehensive exam, thesis optional; for doctorate, thesis/dissertation, written and oral qualifying exams. *Entrance requirements:* For master's, GRE General Test or MCAT (medical science), 1 year of course work in biology, physics, chemistry, and organic chemistry and associated labs; for doctorate, GRE General Test, 1 year of course work in biology, physics, chemistry, and organic chemistry and associated labs. Additional exam requirements/recommendations for international students: Required—TOEFL (minimum score 525 paper-based). *Expenses:* Contact institution. *Faculty research:* Neurosciences, cardiopulmonary science, molecular biology, toxicology, endocrinology.

Massachusetts Institute of Technology, School of Engineering, Harvard-MIT Health Sciences and Technology Program, Cambridge, MA 02139. Offers health sciences and technology (SM, PhD, Sc D), including bioastronautics (PhD, Sc D), bioinformatics and integrative genomics (PhD, Sc D), medical engineering and medical physics (PhD, Sc D), speech and hearing bioscience and technology (PhD, Sc D). *Faculty:* 125 full-time (20 women). *Students:* 271 full-time (111 women), 15 part-time (4 women); includes 79 minority (2 Black or African American, non-Hispanic/Latino; 1 American Indian or Alaska Native, non-Hispanic/Latino; 61 Asian, non-Hispanic/Latino; 12 Hispanic/Latino; 3 Two or more races, non-Hispanic/Latino), 51 international. Average age 26. 265 applicants, 11% accepted, 21 enrolled. In 2015, 3 master's, 25 doctorates awarded. Terminal master's awarded for partial completion of doctoral program. *Degree requirements:* For master's, thesis; for doctorate, comprehensive exam, thesis/dissertation. *Entrance requirements:* For doctorate, GRE General Test (for medical engineering and medical physics). Additional exam requirements/recommendations for international students: Required—TOEFL (minimum score 600 paper-based; 100 iBT), IELTS (minimum score 7). *Application deadline:* For fall admission, 12/15 for domestic and international students. Application fee: $75. Electronic applications accepted. *Expenses: Tuition:* Full-time $46,400; part-time $725 per credit. One-time fee: $304 full-

time. Full-time tuition and fees vary according to course load and program. *Financial support:* In 2015–16, 128 students received support, including 57 fellowships (averaging $38,200 per year), 52 research assistantships (averaging $34,200 per year), 1 teaching assistantship (averaging $19,500 per year); Federal Work-Study, institutionally sponsored loans, scholarships/grants, traineeships, health care benefits, and unspecified assistantships also available. Support available to part-time students. Financial award application deadline: 4/15; financial award applicants required to submit FAFSA. *Faculty research:* Signal processing, biomedical imaging, drug delivery, medical devices, medical diagnostics, regenerative biomedical technologies. *Unit head:* Emery N. Brown, Director, 617-452-4091. *Application contact:* 617-253-3609, Fax: 617-253-6692, E-mail: hst-phd-admissions@mit.edu.
Website: http://hst.mit.edu/

Massachusetts Institute of Technology, School of Science, Department of Biology, Cambridge, MA 02139. Offers biochemistry (PhD); biological oceanography (PhD); biology (PhD); biophysical chemistry and molecular structure (PhD); cell biology (PhD); computational and systems biology (PhD); developmental biology (PhD); genetics (PhD); immunology (PhD); microbiology (PhD); molecular biology (PhD); neurobiology (PhD). *Faculty:* 57 full-time (14 women). *Students:* 283 full-time (137 women); includes 83 minority (3 Black or African American, non-Hispanic/Latino; 1 American Indian or Alaska Native, non-Hispanic/Latino; 38 Asian, non-Hispanic/Latino; 31 Hispanic/Latino; 10 Two or more races, non-Hispanic/Latino), 48 international. Average age 26. 673 applicants, 14% accepted, 46 enrolled. In 2015, 32 doctorates awarded. *Degree requirements:* For doctorate, comprehensive exam, thesis/dissertation, teaching assistantship during two semesters. *Entrance requirements:* For doctorate, GRE General Test. Additional exam requirements/recommendations for international students: Required—TOEFL (minimum score 577 paper-based), IELTS. *Application deadline:* For fall admission, 12/1 for domestic and international students. Application fee: $75. Electronic applications accepted. *Expenses: Tuition:* Full-time $46,400; part-time $725 per credit. One-time fee: $304 full-time. Full-time tuition and fees vary according to course load and program. *Financial support:* In 2015–16, 235 students received support, including 118 fellowships (averaging $37,500 per year), 163 research assistantships (averaging $38,900 per year), 1 teaching assistantship; Federal Work-Study, institutionally sponsored loans, scholarships/grants, traineeships, health care benefits, and unspecified assistantships also available. Support available to part-time students. Financial award application deadline: 4/15; financial award applicants required to submit FAFSA. *Faculty research:* Cellular, developmental and molecular (plant and animal) biology; biochemistry, bioengineering, biophysics and structural biology; classical and molecular genetics, stem cell and epigenetics; immunology and microbiology; cancer biology, molecular medicine, neurobiology and human disease; computational and systems biology. *Total annual research expenditures:* $42.8 million. *Unit head:* Prof. Alan Grossman, Department Head, 617-253-4701. *Application contact:* Biology Education Office, 617-253-3717, Fax: 617-258-9329, E-mail: gradbio@mit.edu.
Website: https://biology.mit.edu/

Mayo Graduate School, Graduate Programs in Biomedical Sciences, Rochester, MN 55905. Offers PhD, MD/PhD. *Degree requirements:* For doctorate, oral defense of dissertation, qualifying oral and written exam. *Entrance requirements:* For doctorate, GRE, 1 year of chemistry, biology, calculus, and physics. Additional exam requirements/recommendations for international students: Required—TOEFL. Electronic applications accepted.

McGill University, Faculty of Graduate and Postdoctoral Studies, Faculty of Medicine, Department of Medicine, Montréal, QC H3A 2T5, Canada. Offers experimental medicine (M Sc, PhD), including bioethics (M Sc), experimental medicine.

McGill University, Faculty of Graduate and Postdoctoral Studies, Faculty of Science, Department of Biology, Montréal, QC H3A 2T5, Canada. Offers bioinformatics (M Sc, PhD); environment (M Sc, PhD); neo-tropical environment (M Sc, PhD).

McMaster University, Faculty of Health Sciences, Department of Biochemistry and Biomedical Sciences, Hamilton, ON L8S 4M2, Canada. Offers M Sc, PhD. Terminal master's awarded for partial completion of doctoral program. *Degree requirements:* For master's, thesis; for doctorate, comprehensive exam, thesis/dissertation. *Entrance requirements:* For master's and doctorate, minimum B+ average. Additional exam requirements/recommendations for international students: Required—TOEFL (minimum score 550 paper-based). *Faculty research:* Molecular and cell biology, biomolecular structure and function, molecular pharmacology and toxicology.

McMaster University, Faculty of Health Sciences and School of Graduate Studies, Program in Medical Sciences, Hamilton, ON L8S 4M2, Canada. Offers blood and vascular (M Sc, PhD); genetics and cancer (M Sc, PhD); immunity and infection (M Sc, PhD); metabolism and nutrition (M Sc, PhD); neurosciences and behavioral sciences (M Sc, PhD); physiology/pharmacology (M Sc, PhD); MD/PhD. *Degree requirements:* For master's, thesis; for doctorate, comprehensive exam, thesis/dissertation. *Entrance requirements:* For master's, honors B Sc, B+ average in related field; for doctorate, M Sc, minimum B+ average. Additional exam requirements/recommendations for international students: Required—TOEFL (minimum score 580 paper-based; 92 iBT).

McMaster University, School of Graduate Studies, Faculty of Science, Department of Biology, Hamilton, ON L8S 4M2, Canada. Offers M Sc, PhD. *Program availability:* Part-time. *Degree requirements:* For master's, thesis; for doctorate, comprehensive exam, thesis/dissertation. *Entrance requirements:* Additional exam requirements/recommendations for international students: Required—TOEFL (minimum score 550 paper-based).

Medical College of Wisconsin, Graduate School of Biomedical Sciences, Milwaukee, WI 53226-0509. Offers MA, MPH, MS, PhD, Graduate Certificate, MD/PhD. *Program availability:* Part-time, evening/weekend, online learning. *Degree requirements:* For master's, comprehensive exam (for some programs), thesis (for some programs); for doctorate, comprehensive exam, thesis/dissertation. *Entrance requirements:* For master's and doctorate, GRE General Test. Additional exam requirements/recommendations for international students: Required—TOEFL. Electronic applications accepted. *Faculty research:* Clinical and translational science, genomics and proteomics, cancer.

Medical College of Wisconsin, Interdisciplinary Program in Biomedical Sciences, Milwaukee, WI 53226-0509. Offers PhD.

Medical University of South Carolina, College of Graduate Studies, Charleston, SC 29425. Offers MS, PhD, DMD/PhD, MD/PhD, Pharm D/PhD. Terminal master's awarded for partial completion of doctoral program. *Degree requirements:* For master's, thesis; for doctorate, thesis/dissertation, oral and written exams. *Entrance requirements:* For doctorate, GRE General Test, interview. Additional exam requirements/recommendations for international students: Required—TOEFL (minimum score 600 paper-based; 100 iBT). Electronic applications accepted. *Expenses:* Contact institution. *Faculty research:* Cell signaling and cancer biology, drug discovery and toxicology, biochemistry and genetics, macromolecular structure, neurosciences, microbiology and immunology.

Meharry Medical College, School of Graduate Studies, Program in Biomedical Sciences, Nashville, TN 37208-9989. Offers cancer biology (PhD); microbiology and

Biological and Biomedical Sciences—General

immunology (PhD); neuroscience (PhD); pharmacology (PhD); MD/PhD. *Degree requirements:* For doctorate, comprehensive exam, thesis/dissertation. *Entrance requirements:* For doctorate, GRE General Test, GRE Subject Test. *Application deadline:* For fall admission, 6/1 for domestic students. Applications are processed on a rolling basis. Application fee: $65. *Financial support:* Fellowships and research assistantships available. Financial award application deadline: 4/15; financial award applicants required to submit FAFSA.

Memorial University of Newfoundland, Faculty of Medicine and School of Graduate Studies, Graduate Programs in Medicine, St. John's, NL A1C 5S7, Canada. Offers M Sc, PhD, Diploma, MD/PhD. *Program availability:* Part-time. *Degree requirements:* For master's, thesis; for doctorate, comprehensive exam, thesis/dissertation, oral defense of thesis. *Entrance requirements:* For master's, MD or B Sc; for doctorate, MD or M Sc; for Diploma, bachelor's degree in health-related field. Additional exam requirements/recommendations for international students: Required—TOEFL (minimum score 550 paper-based). Electronic applications accepted. *Expenses: Tuition, area resident:* Full-time $2199 Canadian dollars. *International tuition:* $2859 Canadian dollars full-time. *Faculty research:* Human genetics, community health, clinical epidemial, cancer, immunology, cardiovascular and immol sciences, applied health services research, neuroscience.

Memorial University of Newfoundland, School of Graduate Studies, Department of Biology, St. John's, NL A1C 5S7, Canada. Offers biology (M Sc, PhD). *Program availability:* Part-time. *Degree requirements:* For master's, thesis; for doctorate, comprehensive exam, thesis/dissertation, oral defense of thesis. *Entrance requirements:* For master's, honors degree (minimum 2nd class standing) in related field; for doctorate, M Sc. *Application deadline:* For fall and spring admission, 1/31 for domestic and international students. Applications are processed on a rolling basis. Application fee: $50 Canadian dollars ($100 Canadian dollars for international students). Electronic applications accepted. *Expenses: Tuition, area resident:* Full-time $2199 Canadian dollars. *International tuition:* $2859 Canadian dollars full-time. *Financial support:* Fellowships, research assistantships, and teaching assistantships available. *Faculty research:* Northern flora and fauna, especially cold ocean and boreal environments. *Unit head:* Dr. Paul Marino, Head, 709-864-7498, Fax: 709-864-3018, E-mail: pmarino@mun.ca. *Application contact:* Dr. Brian Staveley, Graduate Officer, 709-864-4317, E-mail: bestave@mun.ca.
Website: http://www.mun.ca/biology/

Miami University, College of Arts and Science, Department of Biology, Oxford, OH 45056. Offers MA, MAT, MS, PhD. *Program availability:* Part-time, blended/hybrid learning. *Students:* 89 full-time (44 women), 747 part-time (635 women); includes 86 minority (10 Black or African American, non-Hispanic/Latino; 1 American Indian or Alaska Native, non-Hispanic/Latino; 14 Asian, non-Hispanic/Latino; 34 Hispanic/Latino; 1 Native Hawaiian or other Pacific Islander, non-Hispanic/Latino; 26 Two or more races, non-Hispanic/Latino), 35 international. Average age 33. In 2015, 156 master's, 11 doctorates awarded. *Entrance requirements:* For master's and doctorate, GRE General Test, names and contact information of three people who will write letters of recommendation; official copies of transcripts; resume/curriculum vitae; statement about area of specialization and career objectives. Additional exam requirements/recommendations for international students: Recommended—TOEFL (minimum score 80 iBT), IELTS (minimum 6.5), TSE (minimum score 54). *Application deadline:* For fall admission, 1/1 for domestic and international students. Application fee: $50. Electronic applications accepted. *Expenses:* Tuition, state resident: full-time $12,888; part-time $537 per credit hour. Tuition, nonresident: full-time $29,022; part-time $1209 per credit hour. *Required fees:* $530; $24 per credit hour. $30 per semester. Part-time tuition and fees vary according to course load and program. *Financial support:* Application deadline: 2/15; applicants required to submit FAFSA. *Unit head:* Dr. Thomas Crist, Chair, 513-529-3100, E-mail: biology@miamioh.edu.
Website: http://miamioh.edu/cas/academics/departments/biology/

Michigan State University, College of Human Medicine and The Graduate School, Graduate Programs in Human Medicine, East Lansing, MI 48824. Offers biochemistry and molecular biology (MS, PhD); epidemiology (MS, PhD); microbiology (MS); microbiology and molecular genetics (PhD); pharmacology and toxicology (MS, PhD); physiology (MS, PhD); public health (MPH). *Entrance requirements:* Additional exam requirements/recommendations for international students: Required—TOEFL.

Michigan State University, College of Osteopathic Medicine and The Graduate School, Graduate Studies in Osteopathic Medicine, East Lansing, MI 48824. Offers biochemistry and molecular biology (MS, PhD); microbiology (MS); microbiology and molecular genetics (PhD); pharmacology and toxicology (MS, PhD), including integrative pharmacology (MS), pharmacology and toxicology, pharmacology and toxicology-environmental toxicology (PhD); physiology (MS, PhD).

Michigan State University, College of Veterinary Medicine and The Graduate School, Graduate Programs in Veterinary Medicine, Program in Comparative Medicine and Integrative Biology, East Lansing, MI 48824. Offers comparative medicine and integrative biology (MS, PhD); comparative medicine and integrative biology-environmental toxicology (PhD). *Entrance requirements:* Additional exam requirements/recommendations for international students: Required—TOEFL. Electronic applications accepted.

Michigan Technological University, Graduate School, College of Sciences and Arts, Department of Biological Sciences, Houghton, MI 49931. Offers MS, PhD. *Program availability:* Part-time. *Faculty:* 31 full-time (12 women), 15 part-time/adjunct. *Students:* 29 full-time (11 women), 11 part-time (6 women); includes 5 minority (1 Black or African American, non-Hispanic/Latino; 1 Asian, non-Hispanic/Latino; 1 Hispanic/Latino; 2 Two or more races, non-Hispanic/Latino), 10 international. Average age 29. 103 applicants, 15% accepted, 12 enrolled. In 2015, 4 master's, 3 doctorates awarded. Terminal master's awarded for partial completion of doctoral program. *Degree requirements:* For master's, comprehensive exam (for some programs), thesis (for some programs); for doctorate, comprehensive exam, thesis/dissertation. *Entrance requirements:* For master's and doctorate, GRE, statement of purpose, personal statement, official transcripts, 2 letters of recommendation, resume/curriculum vitae. Additional exam requirements/recommendations for international students: Required—TOEFL (minimum score 85 iBT) or IELTS. *Application deadline:* For fall admission, 1/15 priority date for domestic and international students. Applications are processed on a rolling basis. Electronic applications accepted. *Expenses:* Tuition, state resident: full-time $15,507; part-time $861.50 per credit. Tuition, nonresident: full-time $15,507; part-time $861.50 per credit. *Required fees:* $240; $240. Tuition and fees vary according to course load and program. *Financial support:* In 2015–16, 29 students received support, including 3 fellowships with tuition reimbursements available (averaging $14,516 per year), 10 research assistantships with tuition reimbursements available (averaging $14,516 per year), 6 teaching assistantships with tuition reimbursements available (averaging $14,516 per year); career-related internships or fieldwork, Federal Work-Study, scholarships/grants, health care benefits, unspecified assistantships, and cooperative program also available. Financial award applicants required to submit FAFSA. *Faculty research:* Aquatic ecology, biological control, predator-prey interactions, environmental microbiology, microbial and plant biochemistry. *Total annual research expenditures:* $1 million. *Unit head:* Dr. Chandrashekhar P. Joshi, Chair, 906-487-2738, Fax: 906-487-

3167, E-mail: cpjoshi@mtu.edu. *Application contact:* Dr. Nancy Auer, Director of Graduate Studies, 906-487-2353, Fax: 906-487-3167, E-mail: naauer@mtu.edu.
Website: http://www.mtu.edu/biological/

Middle Tennessee State University, College of Graduate Studies, College of Basic and Applied Sciences, Department of Biology, Murfreesboro, TN 37132. Offers MS. *Program availability:* Part-time, evening/weekend, online learning. *Degree requirements:* For master's, comprehensive exam, thesis. *Entrance requirements:* For master's, GRE. Additional exam requirements/recommendations for international students: Required—TOEFL (minimum score 525 paper-based; 71 iBT) or IELTS (minimum score 6). Electronic applications accepted. *Faculty research:* Molecular biosciences.

Midwestern State University, Billie Doris McAda Graduate School, College of Science and Mathematics, Department of Biology, Wichita Falls, TX 76308. Offers MS. *Program availability:* Part-time, evening/weekend. *Degree requirements:* For master's, comprehensive exam, thesis. *Entrance requirements:* For master's, GRE General Test, MAT or GMAT. Additional exam requirements/recommendations for international students: Required—TOEFL (minimum score 550 paper-based). Electronic applications accepted. *Faculty research:* Molecular analysis of flora and fauna, mineral toxicity in plants, embryonic patterning and cell signaling, animal physiology, mammology.

Midwestern University, Downers Grove Campus, College of Health Sciences, Illinois Campus, Master of Arts Program in Biomedical Sciences, Downers Grove, IL 60515-1235. Offers MA. *Entrance requirements:* For master's, GRE General Test, MCAT, PCAT, DAT, OAT or other professional exam, bachelor's degree, minimum cumulative GPA of 2.75.

Midwestern University, Downers Grove Campus, College of Health Sciences, Illinois Campus, Program in Biomedical Sciences, Downers Grove, IL 60515-1235. Offers MBS. *Program availability:* Part-time. *Entrance requirements:* For master's, GRE General Test, MCAT or PCAT, 2 letters of recommendation.

Midwestern University, Glendale Campus, College of Health Sciences, Arizona Campus, MA Program in Biomedical Sciences, Glendale, AZ 85308. Offers MA. *Entrance requirements:* For master's, GRE General Test, MCAT, or other professional exam, bachelor's degree, minimum cumulative GPA of 2.75.

Midwestern University, Glendale Campus, College of Health Sciences, Arizona Campus, MBS Program in Biomedical Sciences, Glendale, AZ 85308. Offers MBS. *Expenses:* Contact institution.

Mills College, Graduate Studies, Pre-Medical Studies Program, Oakland, CA 94613-1000. Offers Certificate. *Program availability:* Part-time. *Faculty:* 5 full-time (2 women). *Students:* 49 full-time (35 women), 8 part-time (6 women); includes 21 minority (3 Black or African American, non-Hispanic/Latino; 1 American Indian or Alaska Native, non-Hispanic/Latino; 11 Asian, non-Hispanic/Latino; 3 Hispanic/Latino; 3 Two or more races, non-Hispanic/Latino), 3 international. Average age 26. 140 applicants, 61% accepted, 24 enrolled. In 2015, 26 Certificates awarded. *Entrance requirements:* For degree, SAT/ACT or GRE General Test, bachelor's degree in a non-science area. Additional exam requirements/recommendations for international students: Required—TOEFL (minimum score 550 paper-based; 80 iBT) or IELTS (minimum score 6). *Application deadline:* For fall admission, 2/1 priority date for domestic students, 12/15 for international students. Applications are processed on a rolling basis. Application fee: $50. Electronic applications accepted. *Expenses:* Contact institution. *Financial support:* In 2015–16, 42 students received support, including 10 teaching assistantships with tuition reimbursements available (averaging $69,489 per year); fellowships with tuition reimbursements available, institutionally sponsored loans, and scholarships/grants also available. Support available to part-time students. Financial award application deadline: 2/1; financial award applicants required to submit FAFSA. *Faculty research:* Antifungal compounds and their modes of action, organic chemistry-spectroscopy and organic chemistry reaction mechanisms, oceanography, physics and chemistry education, cell-cell and cell-extracellular matrix interactions. *Total annual research expenditures:* $277,899. *Unit head:* Dr. John Brabson, Chair of Pre-Medical Program, 510-430-2203, Fax: 510-430-2159, E-mail: johnb@mills.edu. *Application contact:* Shrim Bathey, Director of Graduate Admission, 510-430-3309, Fax: 510-430-2159, E-mail: grad-admission@mills.edu.
Website: http://www.mills.edu/premed

Minnesota State University Mankato, College of Graduate Studies and Research, College of Science, Engineering and Technology, Department of Biological Sciences, Mankato, MN 56001. Offers biology (MS); biology education (MS); environmental sciences (MS). *Program availability:* Part-time. *Degree requirements:* For master's, one foreign language, comprehensive exam, thesis or alternative. *Entrance requirements:* For master's, minimum GPA of 3.0 during previous 2 years of course work. Additional exam requirements/recommendations for international students: Required—TOEFL. Electronic applications accepted. *Faculty research:* Limnology, enzyme analysis, membrane engineering, converters.

Mississippi College, Graduate School, College of Arts and Sciences, School of Science and Mathematics, Department of Biological Sciences, Clinton, MS 39058. Offers biological science (M Ed); biology (MCS); biology-biological sciences (MS); biology-medical sciences (MS). *Program availability:* Part-time. *Degree requirements:* For master's, comprehensive exam, thesis optional. *Entrance requirements:* For master's, GRE General Test, minimum GPA of 2.5. Additional exam requirements/recommendations for international students: Recommended—TOEFL, IELTS. Electronic applications accepted.

Mississippi State University, College of Arts and Sciences, Department of Biological Sciences, Mississippi State, MS 39762. Offers MS, PhD. MS offered online only. *Program availability:* Online learning. *Faculty:* 15 full-time (6 women), 2 part-time/adjunct (0 women). *Students:* 41 full-time (23 women), 48 part-time (31 women); includes 7 minority (4 Black or African American, non-Hispanic/Latino; 1 Hispanic/Latino; 2 Two or more races, non-Hispanic/Latino), 14 international. Average age 32. 78 applicants, 47% accepted, 33 enrolled. In 2015, 34 master's, 1 doctorate awarded. Terminal master's awarded for partial completion of doctoral program. *Median time to degree:* Of those who began their doctoral program in fall 2007, 60% received their degree in 8 years or less. *Degree requirements:* For master's, one foreign language, thesis, comprehensive oral or written exam; for doctorate, one foreign language, thesis/dissertation, comprehensive oral or written exam. *Entrance requirements:* For master's, GRE General Test, minimum GPA of 2.75 on last 60 hours of undergraduate courses; for doctorate, GRE General Test. Additional exam requirements/recommendations for international students: Required—TOEFL (minimum score 550 paper-based; 79 iBT); Recommended—IELTS (minimum score 6.5). *Application deadline:* For fall admission, 7/1 for domestic students, 5/1 for international students; for spring admission, 11/1 for domestic students, 9/1 for international students. Applications are processed on a rolling basis. Application fee: $60. Electronic applications accepted. *Expenses: Tuition, area resident:* Full-time $7502; part-time $833.74 per credit hour. Tuition, nonresident: full-time $20,142; part-time $2238.24 per credit hour. *Financial support:* In 2015–16, 4 research assistantships with tuition reimbursements (averaging $16,039 per year), 36 teaching assistantships with tuition reimbursements (averaging $15,616 per year) were awarded; Federal Work-Study, institutionally sponsored loans, scholarships/grants, and unspecified assistantships also available. Financial award applicants required to submit

FAFSA. *Faculty research:* Botany, zoology, microbiology, ecology. *Total annual research expenditures:* $5.9 million. *Unit head:* Dr. Walter Diehl, Interim Department Head, 662-325-7577, Fax: 662-325-7939, E-mail: wdiehl@biology.msstate.edu. *Application contact:* Meredith Nagel, Admissions Assistant, 662-325-9077, E-mail: mnagel@grad.msstate.edu.
Website: http://www.biology.msstate.edu

Missouri State University, Graduate College, College of Natural and Applied Sciences, Department of Biology, Springfield, MO 65897. Offers biology (MS); natural and applied science (MNAS), including biology (MNAS, MS Ed); secondary education (MS Ed), including biology (MNAS, MS Ed). *Faculty:* 18 full-time (3 women), 7 part-time/adjunct (2 women). *Students:* 15 full-time (11 women), 27 part-time (15 women); includes 2 minority (1 Asian, non-Hispanic/Latino; 1 Two or more races, non-Hispanic/Latino), 6 international. Average age 26. 34 applicants, 41% accepted, 10 enrolled. In 2015, 19 master's awarded. *Degree requirements:* For master's, comprehensive exam, thesis or alternative. *Entrance requirements:* For master's, GRE (MS, MNAS), 24 hours of course work in biology (MS); minimum GPA of 3.0 (MS, MNAS), 9-12 teacher certification (MS Ed). Additional exam requirements/recommendations for international students: Required—TOEFL (minimum score 550 paper-based; 79 iBT), IELTS (minimum score 6). *Application deadline:* For fall admission, 7/20 priority date for domestic students, 5/1 for international students; for spring admission, 12/20 priority date for domestic students, 9/1 for international students; for summer admission, 5/20 priority date for domestic students. Applications are processed on a rolling basis. Application fee: $35 ($50 for international students). Electronic applications accepted. *Expenses:* Tuition, state resident: full-time $5500. Tuition, nonresident: full-time $10,108. *Required fees:* $1000. *Financial support:* In 2015–16, 2 research assistantships with full tuition reimbursements (averaging $10,573 per year), 26 teaching assistantships with full tuition reimbursements (averaging $9,746 per year) were awarded; Federal Work-Study, institutionally sponsored loans, scholarships/grants, and unspecified assistantships also available. Financial award application deadline: 3/31; financial award applicants required to submit FAFSA. *Faculty research:* Hibernation physiology of bats, behavioral ecology of salamanders, mussel conservation, plant evolution and systematics, cellular/molecular mechanisms involved in migraine pathology. *Unit head:* Dr. S. Alicia Mathis, Head, 417-836-5126, Fax: 417-836-6934, E-mail: biology@missouristate.edu. *Application contact:* Michael Edwards, Coordinator of Graduate Admissions, 417-836-5330, Fax: 417-836-6200, E-mail: michaeledwards@missouristate.edu.
Website: http://biology.missouristate.edu/

Missouri University of Science and Technology, Graduate School, Department of Biological Sciences, Rolla, MO 65409. Offers applied and environmental biology (MS). *Faculty:* 10 full-time (3 women). *Students:* 10 full-time (6 women), 6 part-time (5 women); includes 1 minority (Hispanic/Latino), 6 international. Average age 28. 19 applicants, 68% accepted, 7 enrolled. In 2015, 8 master's awarded. *Entrance requirements:* For master's, GRE (minimum score 600 quantitative, 4 writing). Additional exam requirements/recommendations for international students: Required—TOEFL (minimum score 570 paper-based). Application fee: $50. *Expenses:* Tuition, state resident: full-time $10,536. Tuition, nonresident: full-time $27,015. Full-time tuition and fees vary according to course load. *Financial support:* In 2015–16, 6 research assistantships (averaging $1,810 per year), 1 teaching assistantship (averaging $1,814 per year) were awarded; institutionally sponsored loans and unspecified assistantships also available. *Total annual research expenditures:* $306,173. *Unit head:* Dr. Robert Aronstam, Chair, 573-341-4819, Fax: 573-341-4821, E-mail: aronstam@mst.edu. *Application contact:* Debbie Schwertz, Admissions Coordinator, 573-341-6013, Fax: 573-341-6271, E-mail: schwertz@mst.edu.
Website: http://biosci.mst.edu/

Missouri Western State University, Program in Applied Science, St. Joseph, MO 64507-2294. Offers chemistry (MAS); engineering technology management (MAS); human factors and usability testing (MAS); industrial life science (MAS); information technology management (MAS); sport and fitness management (MAS). *Program availability:* Part-time. *Students:* 40 full-time (14 women), 38 part-time (12 women); includes 9 minority (8 Black or African American, non-Hispanic/Latino; 1 Asian, non-Hispanic/Latino), 19 international. Average age 29. 36 applicants, 92% accepted, 25 enrolled. In 2015, 28 master's awarded. *Entrance requirements:* Additional exam requirements/recommendations for international students: Recommended—TOEFL (minimum score 79 iBT), IELTS (minimum score 6). *Application deadline:* For fall admission, 7/15 for domestic and international students; for spring admission, 11/1 for domestic students, 10/15 for international students; for summer admission, 4/29 for domestic students. Applications are processed on a rolling basis. Application fee: $45 ($50 for international students). Electronic applications accepted. *Expenses:* Tuition, state resident: full-time $6290; part-time $314 per credit hour. Tuition, nonresident: full-time $11,490; part-time $574 per credit hour. *Required fees:* $542; $99 per credit hour. $176 per semester. One-time fee: $45. Tuition and fees vary according to course load and program. *Financial support:* Scholarships/grants and unspecified assistantships available. Support available to part-time students. *Unit head:* Dr. Benjamin D. Caldwell, Dean of the Graduate School, 816-271-4394, Fax: 816-271-4525, E-mail: graduate@missouriwestern.edu.

Molloy College, Graduate Education Program, Rockville Centre, NY 11571-5002. Offers adolescent education in biology (MS Ed); adolescent special education (Advanced Certificate); bilingual extension (Advanced Certificate); childhood education (MS Ed); childhood special education (Advanced Certificate); early childhood education (MS Ed); English (MS Ed); mathematics (MS Ed); social studies (MS Ed); Spanish (MS Ed); special education on both childhood and adolescent levels (MS Ed); teaching English to speakers of other languages (TESOL) in grades Pre-K to 12 (MS Ed); TESOL (Advanced Certificate). *Accreditation:* NCATE. *Program availability:* Part-time, evening/weekend. *Faculty:* 18 full-time (16 women), 29 part-time/adjunct (26 women). *Students:* 84 full-time (66 women), 176 part-time (133 women); includes 35 minority (8 Black or African American, non-Hispanic/Latino; 4 Asian, non-Hispanic/Latino; 23 Hispanic/Latino). Average age 27. 116 applicants, 79% accepted, 83 enrolled. In 2015, 85 master's, 5 Advanced Certificates awarded. *Entrance requirements:* Additional exam requirements/recommendations for international students: Required—TOEFL (minimum score 550 paper-based; 79 iBT). *Application deadline:* Applications are processed on a rolling basis. Application fee: $60. Electronic applications accepted. *Expenses:* Tuition, area resident: Full-time $18,450; part-time $1025 per credit. *Required fees:* $900; $740 per unit. Tuition and fees vary according to course load. *Financial support:* Applicants required to submit FAFSA. *Faculty research:* TESOL education, bilingual education, meeting the needs of students with disabilities, teacher collaboration, public policy issues. *Unit head:* Joanne O'Brien, Associate Dean/Director, 516-323-3116, E-mail: jobrien@molloy.edu. *Application contact:* Jaclyn Machowicz, Assistant Director for Admissions, 516-323-4010, E-mail: jmachowicz@molloy.edu.

Montana State University, The Graduate School, College of Letters and Science, Department of Cell Biology and Neuroscience, Bozeman, MT 59717. Offers biological sciences (PhD); neuroscience (MS, PhD). *Program availability:* Part-time. *Degree requirements:* For master's, comprehensive exam; for doctorate, comprehensive exam, thesis/dissertation. *Entrance requirements:* For master's and doctorate, GRE General Test. Additional exam requirements/recommendations for international students:

Required—TOEFL (minimum score 550 paper-based). Electronic applications accepted. *Faculty research:* Development of the nervous system, neuronal mechanisms of visual perception, ion channel biophysics, mechanisms of sensory coding, neuroinformatics.

Montclair State University, The Graduate School, College of Science and Mathematics, Program in Biology, Montclair, NJ 07043-1624. Offers biological science/education (MS); biology (MS); ecology and evolution (MS); physiology (MS). *Students:* 10 full-time (7 women), 35 part-time (27 women); includes 9 minority (6 Asian, non-Hispanic/Latino; 2 Hispanic/Latino; 1 Two or more races, non-Hispanic/Latino). Average age 28. 23 applicants, 57% accepted, 12 enrolled. In 2015, 18 master's awarded. *Expenses:* Tuition, state resident: part-time $553 per credit. Tuition, nonresident: part-time $854 per credit. *Required fees:* $91 per credit. Tuition and fees vary according to program. *Unit head:* Dr. Liza C. Hazard, Chairperson, 973-655-4397, E-mail: hazardl@mail.montclair.edu. *Application contact:* Amy Aiello, Director of Graduate Admissions and Operations, 973-655-5147, Fax: 973-655-7869, E-mail: graduate.school@montclair.edu.

Morehead State University, Graduate Programs, College of Science and Technology, Department of Biology and Chemistry, Morehead, KY 40351. Offers biology (MS); biology regional analysis (MS). *Program availability:* Part-time. *Degree requirements:* For master's, comprehensive exam, thesis optional, oral and written final exams. *Entrance requirements:* For master's, GRE General Test, minimum GPA of 3.0 in biology, 2.5 overall; undergraduate major/minor in biology, environmental science, or equivalent. Additional exam requirements/recommendations for international students: Required—TOEFL (minimum score 525 paper-based). Electronic applications accepted. *Faculty research:* Atherosclerosis, RNA evolution, cancer biology, water quality/ecology, immunoparasitology.

Morehouse School of Medicine, Graduate Programs in Biomedical Sciences, Atlanta, GA 30310-1495. Offers biomedical research (MS); biomedical sciences (PhD); biomedical technology (MS); medical sciences (MS). *Degree requirements:* For master's, thesis (for some programs); for doctorate, thesis/dissertation. *Entrance requirements:* For doctorate, GRE General Test. Additional exam requirements/recommendations for international students: Required—TOEFL (minimum score 550 paper-based). *Application deadline:* For fall admission, 10/1 for domestic and international students; for spring admission, 2/1 for domestic and international students. Application fee: $50. Electronic applications accepted. *Expenses:* Contact institution. *Financial support:* Fellowships with tuition reimbursements, career-related internships or fieldwork, institutionally sponsored loans, scholarships/grants, traineeships, health care benefits, and tuition waivers (full) available. Financial award application deadline: 5/1; financial award applicants required to submit FAFSA. *Unit head:* Dr. Douglas Paulsen, Associate Dean for Graduate Studies, 404-752-1559. *Application contact:* Brandon Hunter, Director of Admissions, 404-752-1650, Fax: 404-752-1512, E-mail: phdadmissions@msm.edu.
Website: http://www.msm.edu/Education/GEBS/index.php

Morgan State University, School of Graduate Studies, School of Computer, Mathematical, and Natural Sciences, Department of Biology, Baltimore, MD 21251. Offers bioenvironmental science (PhD); biology (MS); science education (MS). *Degree requirements:* For master's, comprehensive exam, thesis. *Entrance requirements:* For master's, minimum GPA of 3.0.

Mount Allison University, Department of Biology, Sackville, NB E4L 1E4, Canada. Offers M Sc. *Degree requirements:* For master's, thesis. *Entrance requirements:* For master's, honors degree. *Faculty research:* Ecology, evolution, physiology, behavior, biochemistry.

Murray State University, College of Science, Engineering and Technology, Program in Biological Sciences, Murray, KY 42071. Offers MAT, MS, PhD. PhD offered jointly with University of Louisville. *Program availability:* Part-time. *Degree requirements:* For master's, comprehensive exam, thesis optional. *Entrance requirements:* For master's, GRE General Test. Additional exam requirements/recommendations for international students: Required—TOEFL. *Faculty research:* Aquatic and terrestrial ecology, molecular systematics, micro ecology, cell biology and metabolism, palentology.

National University, Academic Affairs, College of Letters and Sciences, La Jolla, CA 92037-1011. Offers applied linguistics (MA); biology (MS); counseling psychology (MA), including licensed professional clinical counseling, marriage and family therapy; creative writing (MFA); English (MA), including Gothic studies, rhetoric; film studies (MA); forensic and crime science (Certificate); forensic studies (MFS), including criminalistics, investigation; history (MA); human behavior (MA); mathematics for educators (MS); performance psychology (MA); strategic communications (MA). *Program availability:* Part-time, evening/weekend, 100% online, blended/hybrid learning. *Faculty:* 75 full-time (39 women), 87 part-time/adjunct (39 women). *Students:* 689 full-time (493 women), 318 part-time (230 women); includes 508 minority (137 Black or African American, non-Hispanic/Latino; 5 American Indian or Alaska Native, non-Hispanic/Latino; 50 Asian, non-Hispanic/Latino; 248 Hispanic/Latino; 10 Native Hawaiian or other Pacific Islander, non-Hispanic/Latino; 58 Two or more races, non-Hispanic/Latino), 5 international. Average age 34. In 2015, 470 master's awarded. *Degree requirements:* For master's, thesis (for some programs). *Entrance requirements:* For master's, interview, minimum GPA of 2.5. Additional exam requirements/recommendations for international students: Required—TOEFL (minimum score 550 paper-based; 79 iBT), IELTS (minimum score 6). *Application deadline:* Applications are processed on a rolling basis. Application fee: $60 ($65 for international students). Electronic applications accepted. *Financial support:* Career-related internships or fieldwork, institutionally sponsored loans, scholarships/grants, and tuition waivers (partial) available. Support available to part-time students. Financial award application deadline: 6/30; financial award applicants required to submit FAFSA. *Unit head:* College of Letters and Sciences, 800-628-8648, E-mail: cols@nu.edu. *Application contact:* Brandon Jouganatos, Interim Vice President for Enrollment Services, 800-628-8648, E-mail: advisor@nu.edu.
Website: http://www.nu.edu/OurPrograms/CollegeOfLettersAndSciences.html

New Jersey Institute of Technology, College of Science and Liberal Arts, Newark, NJ 07102. Offers applied mathematics (MS); applied physics (M Sc, PhD); applied statistics (MS, Certificate); biology (MS, PhD); biostatistics (MS); chemistry (MS, PhD); computational biology (MS); environmental science (MS, PhD); history (MA, MAT); materials science and engineering (MS, PhD); mathematical and computational finance (MS); mathematics science (PhD); pharmaceutical chemistry (MS); practice of technical communications (Certificate); professional and technical communications (MS). *Program availability:* Part-time, evening/weekend. *Faculty:* 153 full-time (35 women), 100 part-time/adjunct (40 women). *Students:* 212 full-time (82 women), 94 part-time (37 women); includes 72 minority (22 Black or African American, non-Hispanic/Latino; 25 Asian, non-Hispanic/Latino; 19 Hispanic/Latino; 6 Two or more races, non-Hispanic/Latino), 164 international. Average age 29. 519 applicants, 62% accepted, 104 enrolled. In 2015, 98 master's, 21 doctorates, 3 other advanced degrees awarded. Terminal master's awarded for partial completion of doctoral program. *Degree requirements:* For master's, thesis optional; for doctorate, thesis/dissertation. *Entrance requirements:* For master's, GRE General Test; for doctorate, GRE General Test, minimum graduate GPA of 3.5. Additional exam requirements/recommendations for international students: Required—TOEFL (minimum score 550 paper-based; 79 iBT). *Application deadline:* For

Biological and Biomedical Sciences—General

fall admission, 6/1 priority date for domestic students, 5/1 priority date for international students; for spring admission, 11/15 priority date for domestic and international students. Applications are processed on a rolling basis. Application fee: $75. Electronic applications accepted. *Expenses:* $28,800 per year non-resident full-time. *Financial support:* In 2015–16, 56 research assistantships with full tuition reimbursements (averaging $17,711 per year), 52 teaching assistantships with full tuition reimbursements (averaging $17,914 per year) were awarded; fellowships with full tuition reimbursements also available. Financial award application deadline: 1/15. *Total annual research expenditures:* $23.1 million. *Unit head:* Dr. Kevin Belfield, Dean, 973-596-3676, Fax: 973-565-0586, E-mail: kevin.d.belfield@njit.edu. *Application contact:* Stephen Eck, Director of Admissions, 973-596-3300, Fax: 973-596-3461, E-mail: admissions@njit.edu.
Website: http://csla.njit.edu/

New Mexico Institute of Mining and Technology, Center for Graduate Studies, Department of Biology, Socorro, NM 87801. Offers biology (MS); geobiology (PhD). *Program availability:* Part-time. *Degree requirements:* For master's, thesis. *Entrance requirements:* For master's, GRE General Test. Additional exam requirements/recommendations for international students: Required—TOEFL (minimum score 540 paper-based). Electronic applications accepted. *Expenses:* Tuition, state resident: full-time $5811; part-time $322.81 per credit. Tuition, nonresident: full-time $19,220; part-time $1067.79 per credit. *Required fees:* $1030. Tuition and fees vary according to course load. *Faculty research:* Molecular biology, evolution and evolutionary ecology, immunology, endocrinology.

New Mexico State University, College of Arts and Sciences, Department of Biology, Las Cruces, NM 88003-8001. Offers biology (MS, PhD); biotechnology (MS). *Program availability:* Part-time. *Faculty:* 22 full-time (10 women). *Students:* 54 full-time (28 women), 10 part-time (7 women); includes 17 minority (1 Black or African American, non-Hispanic/Latino; 1 American Indian or Alaska Native, non-Hispanic/Latino; 3 Asian, non-Hispanic/Latino; 12 Hispanic/Latino), 19 international. Average age 32. 39 applicants, 46% accepted, 11 enrolled. In 2015, 9 master's, 5 doctorates awarded. *Degree requirements:* For master's, thesis (for some programs), defense or oral exam; for doctorate, comprehensive exam, thesis/dissertation, qualifying exam. *Entrance requirements:* For master's and doctorate, GRE. Additional exam requirements/recommendations for international students: Required—TOEFL (minimum score 550 paper-based; 79 iBT), IELTS (minimum score 6.5). *Application deadline:* For fall admission, 1/15 priority date for domestic students, 1/15 for international students; for spring admission, 10/4 priority date for domestic students, 10/4 for international students. Applications are processed on a rolling basis. Application fee: $40 ($50 for international students). Electronic applications accepted. *Expenses:* $274.50 per credit hour for in-state students, and all students enrolled in six or fewer credits; $839.30 per credit hour for out-of-state and international students enrolled in at least seven hours. *Financial support:* In 2015–16, 50 students received support, including 3 fellowships (averaging $4,088 per year), 15 research assistantships (averaging $19,052 per year), 30 teaching assistantships (averaging $18,374 per year); career-related internships or fieldwork, Federal Work-Study, scholarships/grants, traineeships, health care benefits, and unspecified assistantships also available. Support available to part-time students. Financial award application deadline: 3/1. *Faculty research:* Microbiology, cell and organismal physiology, ecology and ethology, evolution, genetics, developmental biology. *Total annual research expenditures:* $2.7 million. *Unit head:* Dr. Ralph Preszler, Department Head, 575-646-3611, Fax: 575-646-5665, E-mail: rpreszle@nmsu.edu. *Application contact:* Dr. Angus Dawe, Associate Professor, 575-646-3611, Fax: 575-646-5665, E-mail: biologygrads@nmsu.edu.
Website: http://bio.nmsu.edu

New York Medical College, Graduate School of Basic Medical Sciences, Valhalla, NY 10595-1691. Offers MS, PhD, MD/PhD. *Program availability:* Part-time, evening/weekend. Terminal master's awarded for partial completion of doctoral program. *Degree requirements:* For master's, thesis; for doctorate, comprehensive exam, thesis/dissertation. *Entrance requirements:* For master's, GRE General Test, MCAT, or DAT; for doctorate, GRE General Test. Additional exam requirements/recommendations for international students: Required—TOEFL. Electronic applications accepted. *Expenses: Tuition, area resident:* Full-time $44,355; part-time $1025 per credit. *Required fees:* $500; $95 per year. One-time fee: $140 part-time. Tuition and fees vary according to course load and program. *Faculty research:* Cardiovascular science, infectious diseases, neuroscience, cancer, cell signaling.

New York University, Graduate School of Arts and Science, Department of Biology, New York, NY 10012-1019. Offers biology (PhD); biomedical journalism (MS); cancer and molecular biology (PhD); computational biology (PhD); computers in biological research (MS); developmental genetics (PhD); general biology (MS); immunology and microbiology (PhD); molecular genetics (PhD); neurobiology (PhD); oral biology (MS); plant biology (PhD); recombinant DNA technology (MS); MS/MBA. *Program availability:* Part-time. Terminal master's awarded for partial completion of doctoral program. *Degree requirements:* For master's, thesis or alternative, qualifying paper; for doctorate, comprehensive exam, thesis/dissertation. *Entrance requirements:* For master's and doctorate, GRE General Test. Additional exam requirements/recommendations for international students: Required—TOEFL. *Faculty research:* Genomics, molecular and cell biology, development and molecular genetics, molecular evolution of plants and animals.

New York University, Graduate School of Arts and Science, Department of Environmental Medicine, New York, NY 10012-1019. Offers environmental health sciences (MS, PhD), including biostatistics (PhD), environmental hygiene (MS), epidemiology (PhD), ergonomics and biomechanics (PhD), exposure assessment and health effects (PhD), molecular toxicology/carcinogenesis (PhD), toxicology. *Program availability:* Part-time. Terminal master's awarded for partial completion of doctoral program. *Degree requirements:* For master's, thesis or alternative; for doctorate, one foreign language, thesis/dissertation, oral and written exams. *Entrance requirements:* For master's and doctorate, GRE General Test, minimum GPA of 3.0; bachelor's degree in biological, physical, or engineering science. Additional exam requirements/recommendations for international students: Required—TOEFL.

See Close-Up on page 851.

New York University, School of Medicine and Graduate School of Arts and Science, Medical Scientist Training Program, New York, NY 10012-1019. Offers MD/MS, MD/PhD. Students must be accepted by both the School of Medicine and the Graduate School of Arts and Science. Electronic applications accepted. *Expenses:* Contact institution. *Faculty research:* Neurosciences, cell biology and molecular genetics, structural biology, microbial pathogenesis and host defense.

New York University, Steinhardt School of Culture, Education, and Human Development, Department of Teaching and Learning, New York, NY 10003. Offers clinically rich integrated science (MA), including clinically rich integrated science, teaching biology grades 7-12, teaching chemistry 7-12, teaching physics 7-12; early childhood and childhood education (MA), including childhood education, early childhood education, early childhood education/early childhood special education; English education (MA, PhD, Advanced Certificate), including clinically-based English education, grades 7-12 (MA), English education (PhD, Advanced Certificate), English education, grades 7-12 (MA); environmental conservation education (MA); literacy education (MA), including literacy 5-12, literacy B-6; mathematics education (MA), including teachers of mathematics 7-12; multilingual/multicultural studies (MA, PhD, Advanced Certificate), including bilingual education, foreign language education (MA), teaching English to speakers of other languages (MA, PhD), teaching foreign languages, 7-12 (MA), teaching French as a foreign language (MA), teaching Spanish as a foreign language (MA); social studies education (MA), including teaching art/social studies 7-12, teaching social studies 7-12; special education (MA), including childhood, early childhood; teaching and learning (Ed D, PhD). *Program availability:* Part-time. *Degree requirements:* For doctorate, thesis/dissertation. *Entrance requirements:* For doctorate, GRE General Test, interview; for Advanced Certificate, master's degree. Additional exam requirements/recommendations for international students: Required—TOEFL (minimum score 100 iBT). Electronic applications accepted. *Faculty research:* Cultural contexts for literacy learning, school restructuring, parenting and education, teacher learning, language assessment.

North Carolina Agricultural and Technical State University, School of Graduate Studies, College of Arts and Sciences, Department of Biology, Greensboro, NC 27411. Offers biology (MS); biology education (MAT). *Program availability:* Part-time, evening/weekend. *Degree requirements:* For master's, comprehensive exam, thesis (for some programs), qualifying exam. *Entrance requirements:* For master's, GRE General Test, personal statement. *Faculty research:* Physical ecology, cytochemistry, botany, parasitology, microbiology.

North Carolina Central University, College of Science and Technology, Department of Biology, Durham, NC 27707-3129. Offers MS. *Degree requirements:* For master's, one foreign language, comprehensive exam, thesis. *Entrance requirements:* For master's, GRE, minimum GPA of 3.0 in major, 2.5 overall. Additional exam requirements/recommendations for international students: Required—TOEFL.

North Carolina State University, College of Veterinary Medicine, Program in Comparative Biomedical Sciences, Raleigh, NC 27695. Offers cell biology (MS, PhD); infectious disease (MS, PhD); pathology (MS, PhD); pharmacology (MS, PhD); population medicine (MS, PhD). *Program availability:* Part-time. *Degree requirements:* For master's, thesis; for doctorate, thesis/dissertation. *Entrance requirements:* For master's and doctorate, GRE General Test. Additional exam requirements/recommendations for international students: Required—TOEFL (minimum score 550 paper-based). Electronic applications accepted. *Expenses:* Contact institution. *Faculty research:* Infectious diseases, cell biology, pharmacology and toxicology, genomics, pathology and population medicine.

North Carolina State University, Graduate School, College of Agriculture and Life Sciences, Raleigh, NC 27695. Offers M Tox, MAE, MB, MBAE, MFG, MFM, MFS, MG, MMB, MN, MP, MS, MZS, Ed D, PhD, Certificate. *Program availability:* Part-time. Electronic applications accepted.

North Dakota State University, College of Graduate and Interdisciplinary Studies, College of Science and Mathematics, Department of Biological Sciences, Fargo, ND 58102. Offers biology (MS); botany (MS, PhD); cellular and molecular biology (PhD); genomics (PhD); zoology (MS, PhD). *Degree requirements:* For master's, thesis; for doctorate, thesis/dissertation. *Entrance requirements:* For master's and doctorate, GRE General Test. Additional exam requirements/recommendations for international students: Required—TOEFL. *Application deadline:* For fall admission, 1/15 for domestic students. Applications are processed on a rolling basis. Application fee: $35. Electronic applications accepted. *Financial support:* Fellowships with full tuition reimbursements, research assistantships with full tuition reimbursements, teaching assistantships with full tuition reimbursements, career-related internships or fieldwork, Federal Work-Study, institutionally sponsored loans, scholarships/grants, tuition waivers (full), and unspecified assistantships available. Support available to part-time students. Financial award application deadline: 4/15; financial award applicants required to submit FAFSA. *Faculty research:* Comparative endocrinology, physiology, behavioral ecology, plant cell biology, aquatic biology. *Unit head:* Dr. Wendy Reed, Head, 701-231-5921, E-mail: wendy.reed@ndsu.edu. *Application contact:* Elizabeth Worth, Marketing, Recruitment, and Public Relations Coordinator, 701-231-8476, Fax: 701-231-6524, E-mail: elizabeth.worth@ndsu.edu.
Website: http://www.ndsu.edu/biology/

Northeastern Illinois University, College of Graduate Studies and Research, College of Arts and Sciences, Program in Biology, Chicago, IL 60625-4699. Offers MS. *Program availability:* Part-time, evening/weekend. *Degree requirements:* For master's, comprehensive exam, thesis optional. *Entrance requirements:* For master's, minimum GPA of 2.75. Additional exam requirements/recommendations for international students: Required—TOEFL (minimum score 550 paper-based; 79 iBT). Electronic applications accepted. *Faculty research:* Paleoecology and freshwater biology, protein biosynthesis and targeting, microbial growth and physiology, molecular biology of antibody production, reptilian neurobiology.

Northeastern University, College of Science, Boston, MA 02115-5096. Offers applied mathematics (MS); bioinformatics (MS); biology (PhD); biotechnology (MS); chemistry (MS, PhD); ecology, evolution, and marine biology (PhD); marine biology (MS); mathematics (MS, PhD); network science (PhD); operations research (MSOR); physics (MS, PhD); psychology (PhD). *Program availability:* Part-time. *Faculty:* 216 full-time (70 women), 62 part-time/adjunct (20 women). *Students:* 517 full-time (252 women), 80 part-time (39 women). In 2015, 94 master's, 46 doctorates awarded. Terminal master's awarded for partial completion of doctoral program. *Degree requirements:* For master's, comprehensive exam (for some programs), thesis; for doctorate, comprehensive exam (for some programs), thesis/dissertation. *Entrance requirements:* For master's, GRE General Test. *Application deadline:* Applications are processed on a rolling basis. Application fee: $75. Electronic applications accepted. *Expenses:* $1,325 per credit; $1,170 per credit (for marine biology). *Financial support:* Fellowships with tuition reimbursements, research assistantships with tuition reimbursements, teaching assistantships with tuition reimbursements, career-related internships or fieldwork, scholarships/grants, health care benefits, tuition waivers (full and partial), and unspecified assistantships available. Support available to part-time students. Financial award applicants required to submit FAFSA. *Unit head:* Dr. Jonathan Tilly, Interim Dean. *Application contact:* Graduate Student Services, 617-373-4275, E-mail: gradcos@neu.edu.
Website: http://www.northeastern.edu/cos/

Northern Arizona University, Graduate College, College of Engineering, Forestry, and Natural Sciences, Department of Biological Sciences, Flagstaff, AZ 86011. Offers MS, PhD. *Degree requirements:* For master's, thesis, oral exam; for doctorate, thesis/dissertation. *Entrance requirements:* For master's and doctorate, GRE General Test. Additional exam requirements/recommendations for international students: Required—TOEFL (minimum score 550 paper-based; 80 iBT), IELTS (minimum score 7). *Application deadline:* For fall admission, 2/15 priority date for domestic and international students. Application fee: $65. Electronic applications accepted. *Expenses: Tuition, area resident:* Full-time $8710. Tuition, nonresident: full-time $20,350. *Required fees:* $896. *Financial support:* Fellowships, research assistantships with full tuition reimbursements,

teaching assistantships with full tuition reimbursements, Federal Work-Study, scholarships/grants, traineeships, health care benefits, tuition waivers (full and partial), and unspecified assistantships available. Financial award applicants required to submit FAFSA. *Faculty research:* Genetic levels of trophic levels, plant hybrid zones, insect biodiversity, natural history and cognition of wild jays. *Unit head:* Jason Wilder, Chair, 928-523-5286, Fax: 928-523-7500, E-mail: jason.wilder@nau.edu. *Application contact:* Judi Irons, Administrative Assistant, 928-523-0896, Fax: 928-523-7500, E-mail: judith.irons@nau.edu.
Website: http://nau.edu/cefns/natsci/biology/

Northern Illinois University, Graduate School, College of Liberal Arts and Sciences, Department of Biological Sciences, De Kalb, IL 60115-2854. Offers MS, PhD. *Program availability:* Part-time. *Faculty:* 30 full-time (6 women), 7 part-time/adjunct (1 woman). *Students:* 55 full-time (26 women), 15 part-time (11 women); includes 6 minority (1 Asian, non-Hispanic/Latino; 5 Hispanic/Latino), 17 international. Average age 31. 84 applicants, 36% accepted, 9 enrolled. In 2015, 15 master's, 5 doctorates awarded. Terminal master's awarded for partial completion of doctoral program. *Degree requirements:* For master's, comprehensive exam, thesis optional; for doctorate, thesis/dissertation, candidacy exam, dissertation defense. *Entrance requirements:* For master's, GRE General Test, bachelor's degree in related field, minimum GPA of 2.75; for doctorate, GRE General Test, bachelor's or master's degree in related field; minimum undergraduate GPA of 2.75, graduate 3.2. Additional exam requirements/recommendations for international students: Required—TOEFL (minimum score 550 paper-based). *Application deadline:* For fall admission, 6/1 for domestic students, 5/1 for international students; for spring admission, 11/1 for domestic students, 10/1 for international students. Applications are processed on a rolling basis. Application fee: $40. Electronic applications accepted. *Financial support:* In 2015–16, 9 research assistantships with full tuition reimbursements, 39 teaching assistantships with full tuition reimbursements were awarded; fellowships with full tuition reimbursements, career-related internships or fieldwork, Federal Work-Study, scholarships/grants, tuition waivers (full), and unspecified assistantships also available. Support available to part-time students. Financial award applicants required to submit FAFSA. *Faculty research:* Plant molecular biology, neurosecretory control, ethnobotany, organellar genomes, carbon metabolism. *Unit head:* Dr. Barrie P. Bode, Chair, 815-753-1753, Fax: 815-753-0461, E-mail: bodebp@niu.edu. *Application contact:* Dr. Thomas Sims, Director of Graduate Studies, 815-753-7873.
Website: http://www.bios.niu.edu/

Northern Michigan University, Office of Graduate Education and Research, College of Arts and Sciences, Department of Biology, Marquette, MI 49855-5301. Offers biochemistry (MS); biology (MS). *Program availability:* Part-time. *Degree requirements:* For master's, thesis. *Entrance requirements:* For master's, GRE, minimum GPA of 3.0; references; coursework in biology and other sciences; faculty member as mentor. Additional exam requirements/recommendations for international students: Required—TOEFL (minimum score 550 paper-based; 79 iBT), IELTS (minimum score 6.5). Electronic applications accepted. *Faculty research:* Evolutionary genetics, neurobiology, conservation biology, fisheries and wildlife, microbiology.

Northwestern University, Feinberg School of Medicine, Combined MD/PhD Medical Scientist Training Program, Evanston, IL 60208. Offers MD/PhD. Application must be made to both The Graduate School and the Medical School. *Accreditation:* LCME/AMA. Electronic applications accepted. *Faculty research:* Cardiovascular epidemiology, cancer epidemiology, nutritional interventions for the prevention of cardiovascular disease and cancer, women's health, outcomes research.

Northwestern University, Feinberg School of Medicine and Interdepartmental Programs, Integrated Graduate Programs in the Life Sciences, Chicago, IL 60611. Offers biostatistics (PhD); epidemiology (PhD); health and biomedical informatics (PhD); health services and outcomes research (PhD); healthcare quality and patient safety (PhD); translational outcomes in science (PhD). *Degree requirements:* For doctorate, comprehensive exam, thesis/dissertation, written and oral qualifying exams. *Entrance requirements:* For doctorate, GRE General Test. Additional exam requirements/recommendations for international students: Required—TOEFL (minimum score 600 paper-based). Electronic applications accepted.

Northwestern University, The Graduate School, Interdisciplinary Biological Sciences Program (IBiS), Evanston, IL 60208. Offers biochemistry (PhD); bioengineering and biotechnology (PhD); biotechnology (PhD); cell and molecular biology (PhD); developmental and systems biology (PhD); nanotechnology (PhD); neurobiology (PhD); structural biology and biophysics (PhD). *Degree requirements:* For doctorate, thesis/dissertation, qualifying exam. *Entrance requirements:* For doctorate, GRE General Test. Additional exam requirements/recommendations for international students: Required—TOEFL (minimum score 600 paper-based). Electronic applications accepted. *Faculty research:* Biophysics/structural biology, cell/molecular biology, synthetic biology, developmental systems biology, chemical biology/nanotechnology.

Northwest Missouri State University, Graduate School, College of Arts and Sciences, Department of Natural Sciences, Maryville, MO 64468-6001. Offers biology (MS); teaching: science (MS Ed). *Program availability:* Part-time. *Students:* 5 full-time (4 women). *Degree requirements:* For master's, comprehensive exam, thesis. *Entrance requirements:* For master's, GRE General Test, minimum GPA of 3.0 in last 60 hours or 2.75 overall, writing sample. Additional exam requirements/recommendations for international students: Required—TOEFL (minimum score 550 paper-based). *Application deadline:* For fall admission, 7/1 for domestic and international students; for spring admission, 11/15 for domestic and international students. Applications are processed on a rolling basis. Application fee: $0 ($50 for international students). *Expenses:* Tuition, state resident: part-time $359 per credit hour. Tuition, nonresident: part-time $612 per credit hour. *Required fees:* $106 per credit hour. *Financial support:* Teaching assistantships with full tuition reimbursements and tutorial assistantships available. Financial award application deadline: 4/1; financial award applicants required to submit FAFSA. *Unit head:* Dr. Mark Corson, Chair, 660-562-1672.
Website: http://www.nwmissouri.edu/naturalsciences/

Nova Southeastern University, College of Medical Sciences, Fort Lauderdale, FL 33314-7796. Offers biomedical sciences (MBS). *Students:* 44 full-time (19 women); includes 20 minority (4 Black or African American, non-Hispanic/Latino; 4 Asian, non-Hispanic/Latino; 10 Hispanic/Latino; 2 Two or more races, non-Hispanic/Latino). Average age 25. In 2015, 4 master's awarded. *Degree requirements:* For master's, thesis. *Entrance requirements:* For master's, MCAT, DAT, minimum GPA of 2.5. *Application deadline:* For fall admission, 4/15 for domestic students. Applications are processed on a rolling basis. Application fee: $50. *Expenses:* Contact institution. *Financial support:* Application deadline: 4/15; applicants required to submit FAFSA. *Faculty research:* Neurophysiology, mucosal immunology, allergies involving the lungs, cardiovascular physiology parasitology. *Unit head:* Dr. Harold E. Laubach, Dean, 954-262-1303, Fax: 954-262-1802, E-mail: harold@nova.edu. *Application contact:* Lori B. Dribin, PhD, Assistant Dean for Student Affairs, 954-262-1341, Fax: 954-262-1802, E-mail: lorib@nova.edu.

Nova Southeastern University, Halmos College of Natural Sciences and Oceanography, Fort Lauderdale, FL 33314-7796. Offers biological sciences (MS);

coastal studies (Certificate); coastal zone management (MS); marine and coastal climate change (Certificate); marine and coastal studies (MA); marine biology (MS); marine biology and oceanography (PhD), including marine biology, oceanography; marine environmental sciences (MS). *Program availability:* Part-time, evening/weekend, 100% online, blended/hybrid learning. *Faculty:* 17 full-time (3 women), 22 part-time/adjunct (11 women). *Students:* 100 full-time (57 women), 114 part-time (76 women); includes 32 minority (6 Black or African American, non-Hispanic/Latino; 1 American Indian or Alaska Native, non-Hispanic/Latino; 6 Asian, non-Hispanic/Latino; 10 Hispanic/Latino; 9 Two or more races, non-Hispanic/Latino), 5 international. Average age 30. 85 applicants, 60% accepted, 39 enrolled. In 2015, 47 master's, 2 doctorates, 9 other advanced degrees awarded. *Degree requirements:* For master's, thesis; for doctorate, comprehensive exam, thesis/dissertation, departmental qualifying exam. *Entrance requirements:* For master's, GRE General Test, 3 letters of recommendation, BS/BA in natural science (for marine biology program), BS/BA in biology (for biological sciences program), minor in the natural sciences or equivalent (for coastal zone management and marine environmental sciences); for doctorate, GRE General Test, master's degree. Additional exam requirements/recommendations for international students: Required—TOEFL (minimum score 550 paper-based). *Application deadline:* Applications are processed on a rolling basis. Application fee: $50. Electronic applications accepted. *Expenses:* $34,749 per year (for PhD); $3,738 per course (for MS and Graduate Certificate). *Financial support:* In 2015–16, 157 students received support, including 14 fellowships with tuition reimbursements available (averaging $25,000 per year), 42 research assistantships with tuition reimbursements available (averaging $19,000 per year); teaching assistantships, career-related internships or fieldwork, Federal Work-Study, scholarships/grants, health care benefits, tuition waivers (full and partial), and unspecified assistantships also available. Support available to part-time students. Financial award application deadline: 4/15; financial award applicants required to submit FAFSA. *Faculty research:* Physical oceanography, biological oceanography, molecular and microbiology, ecology and evolution, coral reefs. *Total annual research expenditures:* $5 million. *Unit head:* Dr. Richard Dodge, Dean, 954-262-3600, Fax: 954-262-4020, E-mail: dodge@nsu.nova.edu. *Application contact:* Dr. Bernhard Riegl, Chair, Department of Marine and Environmental Sciences, 954-262-3600, Fax: 954-262-4020, E-mail: rieglb@nova.edu.
Website: http://cnso.nova.edu

Oakland University, Graduate Study and Lifelong Learning, College of Arts and Sciences, Department of Biological Sciences, Rochester, MI 48309-4401. Offers biology (MA, MS); biomedical sciences (Graduate Certificate); biomedical sciences: biomedical communication (PhD). *Faculty:* 16 full-time (8 women), 1 (woman) part-time/adjunct. *Students:* 41 full-time (21 women), 6 part-time (1 woman); includes 1 minority (Asian, non-Hispanic/Latino), 6 international. Average age 26. 97 applicants, 32% accepted, 21 enrolled. In 2015, 4 master's awarded. *Degree requirements:* For master's, thesis. *Entrance requirements:* For master's, GRE Subject Test, GRE General Test, minimum GPA of 3.0. Additional exam requirements/recommendations for international students: Required—TOEFL (minimum score 550 paper-based). *Application deadline:* Applications are processed on a rolling basis. Application fee: $0. Electronic applications accepted. *Expenses:* Contact institution. *Financial support:* Federal Work-Study, institutionally sponsored loans, and tuition waivers (full) available. Financial award application deadline: 3/1; financial award applicants required to submit FAFSA. *Unit head:* Dr. Doug Wendall, Chair, 248-370-4457, Fax: 248-370-4225, E-mail: wendall@oakland.edu. *Application contact:* Dr. Doug Wendell, Associate Professor, 248-370-4457, E-mail: wendell@oakland.edu.
Website: http://www2.oakland.edu/biology

Occidental College, Graduate Studies, Department of Biology, Los Angeles, CA 90041-3314. Offers MA. *Program availability:* Part-time. *Degree requirements:* For master's, thesis, final exam. *Entrance requirements:* For master's, GRE General Test, GRE Subject Test, minimum GPA of 3.0. Additional exam requirements/recommendations for international students: Required—TOEFL (minimum score 625 paper-based). *Expenses:* Contact institution.

The Ohio State University, College of Medicine, School of Biomedical Science, Biomedical Sciences Graduate Program, Columbus, OH 43210. Offers PhD. *Students:* 114 full-time (55 women); includes 34 minority (6 Black or African American, non-Hispanic/Latino; 1 American Indian or Alaska Native, non-Hispanic/Latino; 11 Asian, non-Hispanic/Latino; 12 Hispanic/Latino; 1 Native Hawaiian or other Pacific Islander, non-Hispanic/Latino; 3 Two or more races, non-Hispanic/Latino), 3 international. Average age 27. In 2015, 21 doctorates awarded. *Degree requirements:* For doctorate, thesis/dissertation. *Entrance requirements:* For doctorate, GRE General Test. Additional exam requirements/recommendations for international students: Required—TOEFL (minimum score 600 paper-based; 100 iBT), Michigan English Language Assessment Battery (minimum score 86); Recommended—IELTS (minimum score 8). *Application deadline:* For fall admission, 12/1 for domestic students, 11/1 for international students; for summer admission, 12/1 priority date for domestic students, 11/1 priority date for international students. Applications are processed on a rolling basis. Application fee: $60 ($70 for international students). Electronic applications accepted. *Financial support:* Fellowships with full tuition reimbursements, research assistantships with full tuition reimbursements, scholarships/grants, and unspecified assistantships available. Financial award application deadline: 1/15. *Unit head:* Dr. Joanna Groden, Co-Director, 614-688-4301, Fax: 614-292-6226, E-mail: ibgp@osumc.edu. *Application contact:* Graduate and Professional Admissions, 614-292-9444, Fax: 614-292-3895, E-mail: gpadmissions@osu.edu.
Website: http://medicine.osu.edu/bsgp

The Ohio State University, Graduate School, College of Arts and Sciences, Division of Natural and Mathematical Sciences, Department of Mathematics, Columbus, OH 43210. Offers computational sciences (MMS); mathematical biosciences (MMS); mathematics (PhD); mathematics for educators (MMS). *Degree requirements:* For master's, thesis optional; for doctorate, one foreign language, thesis/dissertation. *Entrance requirements:* For master's, GRE General Test; for doctorate, GRE General Test (recommended), GRE Subject Test (mathematics). Additional exam requirements/recommendations for international students: Required—TOEFL (minimum score 550 paper-based; 79 iBT), Michigan English Language Assessment Battery (minimum score 82); Recommended—IELTS (minimum score 7). Electronic applications accepted.

Ohio University, Graduate College, College of Arts and Sciences, Department of Biological Sciences, Athens, OH 45701-2979. Offers biological sciences (MS, PhD); cell biology and physiology (MS, PhD); ecology and evolutionary biology (MS, PhD); exercise physiology and muscle biology (MS, PhD); microbiology (MS, PhD); neuroscience (MS, PhD). Terminal master's awarded for partial completion of doctoral program. *Degree requirements:* For master's, comprehensive exam, thesis, 1 quarter of teaching experience; for doctorate, comprehensive exam, thesis/dissertation, 2 quarters of teaching experience. *Entrance requirements:* For master's, GRE General Test, names of three faculty members whose research interests most closely match the applicant's interest; for doctorate, GRE General Test, essay concerning prior training, research interest and career goals, plus names of three faculty members whose research interests most closely match the applicant's interest. Additional exam requirements/recommendations for international students: Required—TOEFL (minimum

Biological and Biomedical Sciences—General

score 620 paper-based; 105 iBT) or IELTS (minimum score 7.5). Electronic applications accepted. *Faculty research:* Ecology and evolutionary biology, exercise physiology and muscle biology, neurobiology, cell biology, physiology.

Oklahoma State University, College of Arts and Sciences, Department of Integrative Biology, Stillwater, OK 74078. Offers MS, PhD. *Faculty:* 28 full-time (13 women), 3 part-time/adjunct (2 women). *Students:* 7 full-time (5 women), 65 part-time (32 women); includes 14 minority (2 Black or African American, non-Hispanic/Latino; 3 Asian, non-Hispanic/Latino; 5 Hispanic/Latino; 4 Two or more races, non-Hispanic/Latino), 7 international. Average age 29. 27 applicants, 78% accepted, 15 enrolled. In 2015, 5 master's, 5 doctorates awarded. *Degree requirements:* For master's, thesis; for doctorate, comprehensive exam, thesis/dissertation. *Entrance requirements:* For master's and doctorate, GRE General Test. Additional exam requirements/recommendations for international students: Required—TOEFL (minimum score 550 paper-based; 79 iBT). *Application deadline:* For fall admission, 3/1 priority date for international students; for spring admission, 8/1 priority date for international students. Applications are processed on a rolling basis. Application fee: $40 ($75 for international students). Electronic applications accepted. *Expenses:* Tuition, state resident: full-time $3528; part-time $196 per credit hour. Tuition, nonresident: full-time $14,144; part-time $785.75 per credit hour. *Required fees:* $1895; $105.25 per credit hour. Tuition and fees vary according to campus/location. *Financial support:* In 2015–16, 18 research assistantships (averaging $23,507 per year), 49 teaching assistantships (averaging $21,604 per year) were awarded; career-related internships or fieldwork, Federal Work-Study, scholarships/grants, health care benefits, tuition waivers (partial), and unspecified assistantships also available. Support available to part-time students. Financial award application deadline: 3/1; financial award applicants required to submit FAFSA. *Unit head:* Dr. Loren Smith, Department Head, 405-744-5555, Fax: 405-744-7824, E-mail: loren.smith@okstate.edu.
Website: http://integrativebiology.okstate.edu/

Oklahoma State University Center for Health Sciences, Program in Biomedical Sciences, Tulsa, OK 74107-1898. Offers MS, PhD, DO/PhD. *Faculty:* 38 full-time (8 women), 1 part-time/adjunct (0 women). *Students:* 44 full-time (18 women); includes 11 minority (2 Black or African American, non-Hispanic/Latino; 3 American Indian or Alaska Native, non-Hispanic/Latino; 4 Asian, non-Hispanic/Latino; 1 Hispanic/Latino; 1 Two or more races, non-Hispanic/Latino), 5 international. Average age 26. 33 applicants, 61% accepted, 15 enrolled. In 2015, 6 master's, 2 doctorates awarded. *Degree requirements:* For master's, thesis; for doctorate, thesis/dissertation, comprehensive, oral and written exam. *Entrance requirements:* For master's, GRE General Test, minimum GPA of 3.0; for doctorate, GRE General Test, MCAT, minimum GPA of 3.0. Additional exam requirements/recommendations for international students: Required—TOEFL (minimum score 79 iBT). *Application deadline:* For fall admission, 1/15 for domestic and international students. Application fee: $50 ($75 for international students). Electronic applications accepted. *Expenses:* Contact institution. *Financial support:* In 2015–16, 14 students received support, including 12 research assistantships with full tuition reimbursements available (averaging $21,180 per year), 2 teaching assistantships with full tuition reimbursements available (averaging $21,180 per year); Federal Work-Study, health care benefits, and tuition waivers (full) also available. Financial award application deadline: 4/1; financial award applicants required to submit FAFSA. *Faculty research:* Neuroscience, cell biology, cell signaling, infectious disease, virology, neurotoxicology. *Unit head:* Dr. Randall L. Davis, Director, 918-561-8408, Fax: 918-561-8276. *Application contact:* Patrick Anderson, Coordinator of Graduate Admissions, 800-677-1972, Fax: 918-561-8243, E-mail: patrick.anderson@okstate.edu.
Website: http://www.healthsciences.okstate.edu/biomedical/

Old Dominion University, College of Sciences, Master of Science in Biology Program, Norfolk, VA 23529. Offers MS. *Program availability:* Part-time. *Faculty:* 22 full-time (4 women), 23 part-time/adjunct (2 women). *Students:* 16 full-time (10 women), 10 part-time (5 women); includes 2 minority (1 Black or African American, non-Hispanic/Latino; 1 Asian, non-Hispanic/Latino). Average age 27. 25 applicants, 48% accepted, 10 enrolled. In 2015, 16 master's awarded. *Degree requirements:* For master's, comprehensive exam, thesis optional. *Entrance requirements:* For master's, GRE General Test, MCAT, minimum GPA of 3.0. Additional exam requirements/recommendations for international students: Required—TOEFL (minimum score 550 paper-based; 79 iBT). *Application deadline:* For fall admission, 2/1 priority date for domestic and international students; for winter admission, 6/1 priority date for domestic and international students; for spring admission, 10/1 priority date for domestic and international students. Application fee: $50. Electronic applications accepted. *Expenses:* Tuition, state resident: full-time $11,136; part-time $464 per credit hour. Tuition, nonresident: full-time $27,840; part-time $1160 per credit hour. *Required fees:* $64 per semester. Tuition and fees vary according to campus/location, program and reciprocity agreements. *Financial support:* In 2015–16, 2 fellowships (averaging $6,575 per year), 10 research assistantships with partial tuition reimbursements (averaging $15,000 per year), 8 teaching assistantships with partial tuition reimbursements (averaging $15,000 per year) were awarded; career-related internships or fieldwork and scholarships/grants also available. Support available to part-time students. Financial award application deadline: 2/1; financial award applicants required to submit FAFSA. *Faculty research:* Wetland ecology, systematics and ecology of vertebrates, marine biology, molecular and cellular microbiology, cell biology, immunology, physiological and reproductive biology. *Total annual research expenditures:* $2 million. *Unit head:* Dr. Robert Ratzlaff, Graduate Program Director, 757-683-4361, Fax: 757-683-5283, E-mail: biolgpd@odu.edu. *Application contact:* William Heffelfinger, Director of Graduate Admissions, 757-683-5554, Fax: 757-683-3255, E-mail: gradadmit@odu.edu.
Website: http://sci.odu.edu/biology/academics/bio-ms.shtml

Old Dominion University, College of Sciences, Program in Biomedical Sciences, Norfolk, VA 23529. Offers PhD. Program offered jointly with Eastern Virginia Medical School. *Faculty:* 29 full-time (8 women). *Students:* 12 full-time (5 women), 7 part-time (4 women); includes 5 minority (2 Black or African American, non-Hispanic/Latino; 1 Hispanic/Latino; 2 Two or more races, non-Hispanic/Latino), 9 international. Average age 33. 18 applicants, 22% accepted, 4 enrolled. In 2015, 5 doctorates awarded. *Degree requirements:* For doctorate, comprehensive exam, thesis/dissertation. *Entrance requirements:* For doctorate, GRE General Test, minimum GPA of 3.0. Additional exam requirements/recommendations for international students: Required—TOEFL (minimum score 79 iBT). *Application deadline:* For fall admission, 2/1 priority date for domestic and international students. Application fee: $50. Electronic applications accepted. *Expenses:* Tuition, state resident: full-time $11,136; part-time $464 per credit hour. Tuition, nonresident: full-time $27,840; part-time $1160 per credit hour. *Required fees:* $64 per semester. Tuition and fees vary according to campus/location, program and reciprocity agreements. *Financial support:* In 2015–16, 2 fellowships with full tuition reimbursements (averaging $18,000 per year), 2 research assistantships with full tuition reimbursements (averaging $18,000 per year), 4 teaching assistantships with full tuition reimbursements (averaging $15,000 per year) were awarded; career-related internships or fieldwork, scholarships/grants, tuition waivers (partial), and unspecified assistantships also available. Support available to part-time students. Financial award application deadline: 2/15; financial award applicants required to submit FAFSA. *Faculty research:* Systems biology and biophysics, pure and applied biomedical sciences, biological chemistry, clinical chemistry, cell biology and molecular

pathogenesis. *Total annual research expenditures:* $3.7 million. *Unit head:* Dr. Robert Ratzlaff, Graduate Program Director, 757-683-4361, Fax: 757-683-5283, E-mail: bimdgpd@odu.edu. *Application contact:* William Heffelfinger, Director of Graduate Admissions, 757-683-5554, Fax: 757-683-3255, E-mail: gradadmit@odu.edu.
Website: http://sci.odu.edu/biology/academics/phdmed.shtml

Oregon Health & Science University, School of Medicine, Graduate Programs in Medicine, Portland, OR 97239-3098. Offers MBA, MCR, MPAS, MS, MSCNU, PhD, Certificate. *Program availability:* Part-time. *Faculty:* 333 full-time (124 women), 605 part-time/adjunct (187 women). *Students:* 317 full-time (186 women), 459 part-time (257 women); includes 182 minority (19 Black or African American, non-Hispanic/Latino; 4 American Indian or Alaska Native, non-Hispanic/Latino; 95 Asian, non-Hispanic/Latino; 43 Hispanic/Latino; 2 Native Hawaiian or other Pacific Islander, non-Hispanic/Latino; 19 Two or more races, non-Hispanic/Latino), 51 international. Average age 33. 2,451 applicants, 17% accepted, 26 enrolled. Terminal master's awarded for partial completion of doctoral program. *Degree requirements:* For master's, thesis (for some programs), thesis or capstone experience; for doctorate, comprehensive exam, thesis/dissertation, qualifying exam. *Entrance requirements:* For master's, GRE General Test (minimum scores: 153 Verbal/148 Quantitative/4.5 Analytical), MCAT or GMAT (for some programs); for doctorate, GRE General Test (minimum scores: 153 Verbal/148 Quantitative/4.5 Analytical). Additional exam requirements/recommendations for international students: Required—IELTS or TOEFL. *Application deadline:* Applications are processed on a rolling basis. Application fee: $70. Electronic applications accepted. *Expenses:* Contact institution. *Financial support:* Fellowships, research assistantships, teaching assistantships, scholarships/grants, health care benefits, and full tuition and stipends (for PhD students) available. *Unit head:* Dr. Allison Fryer, Associate Dean for Graduate Studies, 503-494-6222, E-mail: somgrad@ohsu.edu. *Application contact:* Lorie Gookin, Admissions Coordinator, 503-494-6222, E-mail: somgrad@ohsu.edu.

Oregon State University, Interdisciplinary/Institutional Programs, Program in Comparative Health Sciences, Corvallis, OR 97331. Offers biomedical sciences (MS, PhD); clinical sciences (MS, PhD). *Faculty:* 19 full-time (9 women), 3 part-time/adjunct (2 women). *Students:* 16 full-time (11 women), 2 part-time (1 woman); includes 2 minority (1 Black or African American, non-Hispanic/Latino; 1 Asian, non-Hispanic/Latino), 4 international. Average age 29. 24 applicants, 38% accepted, 8 enrolled. *Entrance requirements:* For master's and doctorate, GRE. Additional exam requirements/recommendations for international students: Required—TOEFL (minimum score 80 iBT), IELTS (minimum score 6.5). *Application deadline:* For fall admission, 12/10 for domestic students. Application fee: $75 ($85 for international students). *Expenses:* Tuition, state resident: full-time $12,150; part-time $450 per credit. Tuition, nonresident: full-time $20,952; part-time $776 per credit. *Required fees:* $1572; $1443 per unit. One-time fee: $350. Tuition and fees vary according to course load, campus/location and program. *Unit head:* Dr. Luiz E. Bermudez, Department Head/Professor. *Application contact:* Beth Chamblin, E-mail: beth.chamblin@oregonstate.edu.

Pace University, School of Education, New York, NY 10038. Offers adolescent education (MST), including biology, business education, chemistry, earth science, English, foreign languages, mathematics, physics, social studies, visual arts; childhood education (MST); early childhood development, learning and intervention (MST); educational technology studies (MS); inclusive adolescent education (MST), including biology, business education, chemistry, earth science, English, foreign languages, mathematics, physics, social studies, visual arts; integrated instruction for educational technology (Certificate); integrated instruction for literacy and technology (Certificate); literacy (MS Ed); special education (MS Ed). *Accreditation:* NCATE. *Program availability:* Part-time, evening/weekend. *Faculty:* 19 full-time (13 women), 86 part-time/adjunct (49 women). *Students:* 112 full-time (95 women), 432 part-time (306 women); includes 179 minority (89 Black or African American, non-Hispanic/Latino; 1 American Indian or Alaska Native, non-Hispanic/Latino; 24 Asian, non-Hispanic/Latino; 55 Hispanic/Latino; 10 Two or more races, non-Hispanic/Latino), 9 international. Average age 30. 181 applicants, 78% accepted, 72 enrolled. In 2015, 261 master's, 11 other advanced degrees awarded. *Degree requirements:* For master's, internship. *Entrance requirements:* For master's, interview, teaching certificate. Additional exam requirements/recommendations for international students: Required—TOEFL (minimum score 88 iBT), IELTS or PTE. *Application deadline:* For fall admission, 8/1 priority date for domestic students, 6/1 for international students; for spring admission, 12/1 priority date for domestic students, 10/1 for international students. Applications are processed on a rolling basis. Application fee: $70. Electronic applications accepted. *Expenses:* Contact institution. *Financial support:* In 2015–16, 17 students received support, including 17 research assistantships with partial tuition reimbursements available (averaging $6,020 per year); career-related internships or fieldwork and Federal Work-Study also available. Financial award application deadline: 2/15; financial award applicants required to submit FAFSA. *Faculty research:* STEM education, TESOL, teacher education, special education, language and literary development. *Total annual research expenditures:* $290,153. *Unit head:* Dr. Xiao-Lei Wang, Dean, School of Education, 914-773-3876, E-mail: xwang@pace.edu. *Application contact:* Susan Ford-Goldschein, Director of Graduate Admissions, 212-346-1531, Fax: 212-346-1585, E-mail: graduateadmission@pace.edu.
Website: http://www.pace.edu/school-of-education

Penn State Hershey Medical Center, College of Medicine, Graduate School Programs in the Biomedical Sciences, Hershey, PA 17033. Offers MPH, MS, Dr PH, PhD, MD/PhD, PhD/MBA. Terminal master's awarded for partial completion of doctoral program. *Degree requirements:* For master's, thesis or alternative; for doctorate, comprehensive exam, thesis/dissertation, oral exam. *Entrance requirements:* For master's, GRE; for doctorate, GRE, minimum GPA of 3.0. Additional exam requirements/recommendations for international students: Required—TOEFL (minimum score 550 paper-based; 81 iBT). *Application deadline:* Applications are processed on a rolling basis. Application fee: $65. Electronic applications accepted. *Expenses:* Contact institution. *Financial support:* In 2015–16, 3 fellowships with full tuition reimbursements (averaging $27,250 per year), 30 research assistantships with full tuition reimbursements (averaging $26,196 per year) were awarded; career-related internships or fieldwork, scholarships/grants, health care benefits, tuition waivers (full), and unspecified assistantships also available. *Unit head:* Dr. Charles Lang, Associate Dean of Graduate Studies, 717-531-8892, Fax: 717-531-0786, E-mail: grad-hmc@psu.edu. *Application contact:* Kristin E. Smith, Director of Graduate Admissions, 717-531-1045, Fax: 717-531-0786, E-mail: kec17@psu.edu.
Website: http://www.pennstatehershey.org/web/gsa/home

Penn State University Park, Graduate School, Eberly College of Science, Department of Biology, University Park, PA 16802. Offers biology (MS, PhD). *Unit head:* Dr. Douglas R. Cavener, Dean, 814-865-9591, Fax: 814-865-3634. *Application contact:* Lori Stania, Director, Graduate Student Services, 814-865-1795, Fax: 814-863-4627, E-mail: l-gswww@lists.psu.edu.
Website: http://bio.psu.edu/

Penn State University Park, Graduate School, Intercollege Graduate Programs, Program in Molecular, Cellular, and Integrative Biosciences, University Park, PA 16802. Offers molecular, cellular, and integrative biosciences (MS, PhD). *Unit head:* Dr. Regina Vasilatos-Younken, Dean, 814-865-2516, Fax: 814-863-4627. *Application contact:* Lori

Stania, Director, Graduate Student Services, 814-865-1795, Fax: 814-863-4627, E-mail: l-gswww@lists.psu.edu.

Philadelphia College of Osteopathic Medicine, Graduate and Professional Programs, Graduate Programs in Biomedical Sciences, Philadelphia, PA 19131-1694. Offers MS. *Program availability:* Evening/weekend. *Degree requirements:* For master's, thesis optional. *Entrance requirements:* For master's, GRE, MCAT, DAT, OAT, PCAT, pre-medical prerequisite coursework; biochemistry (recommended). Additional exam requirements/recommendations for international students: Required—TOEFL (minimum score 79 iBT). Electronic applications accepted. *Faculty research:* Neuroscience and neurodegenerative disorders, inflammation and allergic response to food allergens, cardiovascular function and disease, bone and joint disorders, cancer biology.

Pittsburg State University, Graduate School, College of Arts and Sciences, Department of Biology, Pittsburg, KS 66762. Offers MS. *Students:* 12 (9 women), 4 international. In 2015, 5 master's awarded. *Degree requirements:* For master's, thesis or alternative. *Entrance requirements:* For master's, letter of intent. Additional exam requirements/recommendations for international students: Required—TOEFL (minimum score 520 paper-based; 68 iBT), IELTS (minimum score 6), PTE (minimum score 47). *Application deadline:* For fall admission, 6/1 for international students; for spring admission, 10/15 for international students; for summer admission, 4/1 for international students. Applications are processed on a rolling basis. *Application fee:* $35 ($60 for international students). Electronic applications accepted. *Expenses:* $305 per credit for residents; $711 per credit for non-residents. *Financial support:* In 2015–16, 5 teaching assistantships with full tuition reimbursements (averaging $5,500 per year) were awarded; research assistantships, career-related internships or fieldwork, Federal Work-Study, and unspecified assistantships also available. Financial award application deadline: 2/1; financial award applicants required to submit FAFSA. *Unit head:* Dr. Dixie Smith, Chairperson, 620-235-4741, E-mail: dsmith@pittstate.edu. *Application contact:* Lisa Allen, Assistant Director, 620-235-4223, Fax: 620-235-4219, E-mail: lallen@pittstate.edu.

Plymouth State University, College of Graduate Studies, Graduate Studies in Education, Program in Science, Plymouth, NH 03264-1595. Offers applied meteorology (MS); biology (MS); clinical mental health counseling (MS); environmental science and policy (MS); science education (MS).

Point Loma Nazarene University, Department of Biology, San Diego, CA 92106-2899. Offers MA, MS. *Program availability:* Part-time. *Faculty:* 4 full-time (2 women). *Students:* 19 part-time (16 women); includes 6 minority (1 Black or African American, non-Hispanic/Latino; 2 Asian, non-Hispanic/Latino; 2 Hispanic/Latino; 1 Two or more races, non-Hispanic/Latino). Average age 33. 5 applicants, 100% accepted, 3 enrolled. In 2015, 7 master's awarded. *Degree requirements:* For master's, comprehensive exam (for some programs), thesis (for some programs). *Entrance requirements:* For master's, major field test in biology or GRE Subject Test (biology), BA/BS in science field, letters of recommendation, essay, interview. Additional exam requirements/recommendations for international students: Required—TOEFL. *Application deadline:* For fall admission, 7/26 priority date for domestic students; for spring admission, 11/29 priority date for domestic students; for summer admission, 5/23 priority date for domestic students. Application fee: $50. *Expenses:* Contact institution. *Financial support:* Available to part-time students. Applicants required to submit FAFSA. *Faculty research:* Biology education, immunology, angiogenesis, population genetics. *Unit head:* Dr. Dianne Anderson, Director of Master's Program in Biology, 619-849-2705, E-mail: dianneanderson@pointloma.edu. *Application contact:* Laura Leinweber, Graduate Enrollment Counselor, 866-692-4723, E-mail: lauraleinweber@pointloma.edu. Website: http://gps.pointloma.edu/m-biology

Ponce Health Sciences University, Program in Biomedical Sciences, Ponce, PR 00732-7004. Offers PhD. *Degree requirements:* For doctorate, one foreign language, comprehensive exam, thesis/dissertation. *Entrance requirements:* For doctorate, GRE General Test, proficiency in Spanish and English, minimum overall GPA of 3.0, 3 letters of recommendation, minimum of 35 credits in science.

Pontifical Catholic University of Puerto Rico, College of Sciences, Department of Biology, Ponce, PR 00717-0777. Offers environmental sciences (MS). *Degree requirements:* For master's, thesis. *Entrance requirements:* For master's, GRE, 2 letters of recommendation, interview, minimum GPA of 2.75.

Portland State University, Graduate Studies, College of Liberal Arts and Sciences, Department of Biology, Portland, OR 97201-0751. Offers MA, MS, PhD. *Faculty:* 31 full-time (13 women), 5 part-time/adjunct (3 women). *Students:* 34 full-time (19 women), 44 part-time (22 women); includes 6 minority (1 American Indian or Alaska Native, non-Hispanic/Latino; 1 Asian, non-Hispanic/Latino; 4 Hispanic/Latino), 2 international. Average age 31. 97 applicants, 68% accepted, 47 enrolled. In 2015, 7 master's, 4 doctorates awarded. *Degree requirements:* For master's, one foreign language, thesis; for doctorate, thesis/dissertation. *Entrance requirements:* For master's, GRE General Test, GRE Subject Test, minimum GPA of 3.0 in upper-division course work or 2.75 overall, 2 letters of reference; for doctorate, GRE General Test, GRE Subject Test, minimum GPA of 3.5 in science. Additional exam requirements/recommendations for international students: Required—TOEFL (minimum score 550 paper-based; 80 iBT). *Application deadline:* For fall admission, 2/15 for domestic and international students; for winter admission, 9/1 for domestic students, 7/1 for international students; for spring admission, 11/1 for domestic and international students. Application fee: $50. *Expenses:* $11,490 per year. *Financial support:* In 2015–16, 4 research assistantships with tuition reimbursements (averaging $6,000 per year), 44 teaching assistantships with tuition reimbursements (averaging $6,000 per year) were awarded; Federal Work-Study, scholarships/grants, tuition waivers (partial), and unspecified assistantships also available. Support available to part-time students. Financial award application deadline: 3/1; financial award applicants required to submit FAFSA. *Faculty research:* Genetic diversity and natural population, vertebrate temperature regulation, water balance and sensory physiology, trace elements and aquatic ecology, molecular genetics. *Total annual research expenditures:* $2.1 million. *Unit head:* Dr. Jason Podrabsky, Chair, 503-725-5772, E-mail: jpod@pdx.edu. *Application contact:* Leah Tuor, Program Manager, 503-725-8758, Fax: 503-725-3888, E-mail: leaht@pdx.edu. Website: http://www.bio.pdx.edu/

Purdue University, Graduate School, Biomedical Sciences Interdisciplinary Graduate Program, West Lafayette, IN 47907. Offers PhD. Program offered jointly by School of Veterinary Medicine and Weldon School of Biomedical Engineering. *Degree requirements:* For doctorate, thesis/dissertation, seminars, teaching experience. *Entrance requirements:* For doctorate, GRE General Test (minimum scores: verbal 550, quantitative 700), minimum undergraduate GPA of 3.0. Additional exam requirements/recommendations for international students: Required—TOEFL (minimum score 550 paper-based; 77 iBT); Recommended—TWE. Electronic applications accepted.

Purdue University, Graduate School, College of Science, Department of Biological Sciences, West Lafayette, IN 47907. Offers biochemistry (PhD); biophysics (PhD); cell and developmental biology (PhD); ecology, evolutionary and population biology (MS, PhD), including ecology, evolutionary biology, population biology; genetics (MS, PhD); microbiology (MS, PhD); molecular biology (PhD); neurobiology (MS, PhD); plant physiology (PhD). Terminal master's awarded for partial completion of doctoral program.

Degree requirements: For master's, thesis (for some programs); for doctorate, thesis/dissertation, seminars, teaching experience. *Entrance requirements:* For master's, GRE General Test (minimum analytical writing score of 3.5), minimum undergraduate GPA of 3.0; for doctorate, GRE General Test (minimum analytical writing score of 3.5), minimum undergraduate GPA of 3.5. Additional exam requirements/recommendations for international students: Required—TOEFL (minimum score 600 paper-based; 107 iBT for MS, 80 iBT for PhD). Electronic applications accepted.

Purdue University, Graduate School, PULSe - Purdue University Life Sciences Program, West Lafayette, IN 47907. Offers biomolecular structure and biophysics (PhD); biotechnology (PhD); chemical biology (PhD); chromatin and regulation of gene expression (PhD); integrative neuroscience (PhD); integrative plant sciences (PhD); membrane biology (PhD); microbiology (PhD); molecular evolutionary and cancer biology (PhD); molecular evolutionary genetics (PhD); molecular virology (PhD). *Entrance requirements:* For doctorate, GRE, minimum undergraduate GPA of 3.0. Additional exam requirements/recommendations for international students: Required—TOEFL (minimum score 550 paper-based; 77 iBT). Electronic applications accepted.

Purdue University Northwest, Graduate Studies Office, School of Engineering, Mathematics, and Science, Department of Biological Sciences, Hammond, IN 46323-2094. Offers biology (MS); biology teaching (MS); biotechnology (MS). *Entrance requirements:* For master's, GRE. Additional exam requirements/recommendations for international students: Required—TOEFL. Electronic applications accepted. *Faculty research:* Cell biology, molecular biology, genetics, microbiology, neurophysiology.

Queens College of the City University of New York, Division of Education, Department of Secondary Education and Youth Services, Flushing, NY 11367-1597. Offers adolescent biology (MAT); art (MS Ed); biology (MS Ed, AC); chemistry (MS Ed, AC); earth sciences (MS Ed, AC); English (MS Ed, AC); French (MS Ed, AC); Italian (MS Ed, AC); literacy education (MS Ed); mathematics (MS Ed, AC); music (MS Ed, AC); physics (MS Ed, AC); social studies (MS Ed, AC); Spanish (MS Ed, AC). *Program availability:* Part-time, evening/weekend. *Faculty:* 22 full-time (14 women), 35 part-time/adjunct (22 women). *Students:* 20 full-time (11 women), 462 part-time (334 women); includes 160 minority (42 Black or African American, non-Hispanic/Latino; 1 American Indian or Alaska Native, non-Hispanic/Latino; 46 Asian, non-Hispanic/Latino; 71 Hispanic/Latino), 9 international. Average age 30. 309 applicants, 73% accepted, 154 enrolled. In 2015, 134 master's, 63 other advanced degrees awarded. *Degree requirements:* For master's, research project; for AC, thesis optional. *Entrance requirements:* For master's, minimum GPA of 3.0. Additional exam requirements/recommendations for international students: Required—TOEFL, IELTS. *Application deadline:* For fall admission, 4/1 for domestic students; for spring admission, 11/1 for domestic students. Applications are processed on a rolling basis. Application fee: $125. Electronic applications accepted. *Expenses:* Tuition, state resident: full-time $5065; part-time $425 per credit. Tuition, nonresident: part-time $780 per credit. *Required fees:* $522. Part-time tuition and fees vary according to course load and program. *Financial support:* Career-related internships or fieldwork available. Financial award application deadline: 4/1; financial award applicants required to submit FAFSA. *Unit head:* Dr. Eleanor Armour-Thomas, Chairperson, 718-997-5150, E-mail: armourthomas@yahoo.com.

Queens College of the City University of New York, Mathematics and Natural Sciences Division, Department of Biology, Flushing, NY 11367-1597. Offers biology (MA). *Program availability:* Part-time. *Faculty:* 18 full-time (6 women), 25 part-time/adjunct (12 women). *Students:* 31 part-time (20 women); includes 11 minority (4 Black or African American, non-Hispanic/Latino; 2 Asian, non-Hispanic/Latino; 5 Hispanic/Latino), 1 international. Average age 29. 26 applicants, 42% accepted, 6 enrolled. In 2015, 19 master's awarded. *Degree requirements:* For master's, comprehensive exam, thesis or alternative, qualifying exam. *Entrance requirements:* For master's, minimum GPA of 3.0. Additional exam requirements/recommendations for international students: Required—TOEFL (minimum score 100 iBT), IELTS (minimum score 7). *Application deadline:* For fall admission, 4/1 for domestic students; for spring admission, 11/1 for domestic students. Applications are processed on a rolling basis. Application fee: $125. Electronic applications accepted. *Expenses:* Tuition, state resident: full-time $5065; part-time $425 per credit. Tuition, nonresident: part-time $780 per credit. *Required fees:* $522. Part-time tuition and fees vary according to course load and program. *Financial support:* Career-related internships or fieldwork, Federal Work-Study, institutionally sponsored loans, tuition waivers (partial), and unspecified assistantships available. Support available to part-time students. Financial award application deadline: 4/1; financial award applicants required to submit FAFSA. *Unit head:* Dr. Pokay Ma, Chairperson, 718-997-3412, E-mail: pokay.ma@qc.cuny.edu.

Queen's University at Kingston, School of Graduate Studies, Faculty of Arts and Sciences, Department of Biology, Kingston, ON K7L 3N6, Canada. Offers M Sc, PhD. *Program availability:* Part-time. *Degree requirements:* For master's, thesis; for doctorate, comprehensive exam, thesis/dissertation. *Entrance requirements:* Additional exam requirements/recommendations for international students: Required—TOEFL. *Faculty research:* Limnology, plant morphogenesis, nitrogen fixation, cell cycle, genetics.

Regis College, School of Nursing and Health Sciences, Weston, MA 02493. Offers applied behavior analysis (MS); biomedical sciences (MS); counseling psychology (MA); health administration (MS); molecular imaging and therapeutics (MS); nurse practitioner (Certificate); nursing (MS, DNP); nursing education (Certificate); occupational therapy (MS). *Accreditation:* ACEN. *Program availability:* Part-time, evening/weekend. *Degree requirements:* For master's, thesis. *Entrance requirements:* For master's, GRE General Test or MAT, minimum GPA of 3.0; for doctorate, MAT or GRE if GPA from master's lower than 3.5. Additional exam requirements/recommendations for international students: Required—TOEFL (minimum score 550 paper-based). *Application deadline:* Applications are processed on a rolling basis. Application fee: $50. Electronic applications accepted. *Financial support:* Research assistantships, Federal Work-Study, scholarships/grants, traineeships, and unspecified assistantships available. Support available to part-time students. Financial award applicants required to submit FAFSA. *Faculty research:* Health policy, education, aging, job satisfaction, psychiatric nursing, critical thinking. *Application contact:* Shelagh Tomaino, Associate Director, Graduate Admission, 781-768-7188, Fax: 781-768-7071, E-mail: shelagh.tomaino@regiscollege.edu.

Regis College, Regis College, Denver, CO 80221-1099. Offers biomedical sciences (MS); development practice (MA); environmental biology (MS). *Accreditation:* Teacher Education Accreditation Council. *Program availability:* Part-time. *Faculty:* 2 full-time (1 woman), 22 part-time/adjunct (12 women). *Students:* 60 full-time (38 women), 11 part-time (8 women); includes 13 minority (4 Asian, non-Hispanic/Latino; 7 Hispanic/Latino; 2 Two or more races, non-Hispanic/Latino), 2 international. Average age 27. 390 applicants, 71% accepted, 45 enrolled. In 2015, 29 master's awarded. *Degree requirements:* For master's, thesis (for some programs), capstone presentation. *Entrance requirements:* For master's, official transcript reflecting baccalaureate degree awarded from U.S.-based regionally-accredited college or university. Additional exam requirements/recommendations for international students: Required—TOEFL (minimum score 550 paper-based; 82 iBT). *Application deadline:* For fall admission, 5/15 priority date for domestic students, 4/1 priority date for international students; for spring admission, 12/15 priority date for domestic students. Applications are processed on a

Biological and Biomedical Sciences—General

rolling basis. Application fee: $75. Electronic applications accepted. *Expenses:* Contact institution. *Financial support:* Federal Work-Study and scholarships/grants available. Financial award application deadline: 4/15; financial award applicants required to submit FAFSA. *Unit head:* Dr. Thomas Bowie, Academic Dean. *Application contact:* Sarah Engel, Director of Admissions, 303-458-4900, Fax: 303-964-5534, E-mail: ruadmissions@regis.edu.
Website: http://www.regis.edu/RC.aspx

Rensselaer Polytechnic Institute, Graduate School, School of Science, Program in Biology, Troy, NY 12180-3590. Offers MS, PhD. *Faculty:* 19 full-time (7 women), 3 part-time/adjunct (2 women). *Students:* 30 full-time (13 women), 1 part-time (0 women); includes 2 minority (both Black or African American, non-Hispanic/Latino), 7 international. Average age 26. 89 applicants, 30% accepted, 10 enrolled. In 2015, 1 master's, 5 doctorates awarded. Terminal master's awarded for partial completion of doctoral program. *Degree requirements:* For master's, comprehensive exam, thesis optional; for doctorate, comprehensive exam, thesis/dissertation. *Entrance requirements:* For master's and doctorate, GRE. Additional exam requirements/recommendations for international students: Required—TOEFL (minimum score 570 paper-based; 88 iBT), IELTS (minimum score 6.5), PTE (minimum score 60). *Application deadline:* For fall admission, 1/1 priority date for domestic and international students. Applications are processed on a rolling basis. Application fee: $75. Electronic applications accepted. *Financial support:* In 2015–16, research assistantships (averaging $21,500 per year), teaching assistantships (averaging $21,500 per year) were awarded; fellowships also available. Financial award application deadline: 1/1. *Faculty research:* Biochemistry; bioinformatics; biophysics; cancer biology; computational biology; ecology and environmental sciences; microbiology; molecular, cell, and developmental biology; neuroscience; stem cells; structural biology. *Unit head:* Dr. Doug Swank, Graduate Program Director, 518-276-4174, E-mail: swankd@rpi.edu. *Application contact:* Office of Graduate Admissions, 518-276-6216, E-mail: gradadmissions@rpi.edu.
Website: http://www.rpi.edu/dept/bio/

Rhode Island College, School of Graduate Studies, Faculty of Arts and Sciences, Department of Biology, Providence, RI 02908-1991. Offers biology (MA); modern biological sciences (CGS). *Program availability:* Part-time. *Faculty:* 7 full-time (6 women). *Students:* 1 full-time (0 women), 4 part-time (1 woman). Average age 32. In 2015, 2 master's awarded. *Degree requirements:* For master's, thesis. *Entrance requirements:* For master's, GRE General and Subject Tests. Additional exam requirements/recommendations for international students: Recommended—TOEFL (minimum score 550 paper-based; 79 iBT). *Application deadline:* For fall admission, 3/1 for domestic students. Applications are processed on a rolling basis. Application fee: $50. Electronic applications accepted. *Expenses:* Tuition, state resident: full-time $8928; part-time $372 per credit. Tuition, nonresident: full-time $17,376; part-time $724 per credit. *Required fees:* $604; $22 per credit. One-time fee: $74. *Financial support:* In 2015–16, 3 teaching assistantships with full tuition reimbursements (averaging $2,042 per year) were awarded; career-related internships or fieldwork, Federal Work-Study, scholarships/grants, health care benefits, and unspecified assistantships also available. Support available to part-time students. Financial award application deadline: 5/15; financial award applicants required to submit FAFSA. *Unit head:* Dr. Lloyd Matsumoto, Chair, 401-456-8010, E-mail: biology@ric.edu. *Application contact:* Graduate Studies, 401-456-8700.
Website: http://www.ric.edu/biology/index.php

Rochester Institute of Technology, Graduate Enrollment Services, College of Science, School of Life Sciences, Rochester, NY 14623. Offers MS. *Program availability:* Part-time. *Students:* 23 full-time (12 women), 20 part-time (12 women); includes 5 minority (2 Black or African American, non-Hispanic/Latino; 2 Hispanic/Latino; 1 Two or more races, non-Hispanic/Latino), 8 international. Average age 27. 45 applicants, 38% accepted, 12 enrolled. In 2015, 7 master's awarded. *Degree requirements:* For master's, thesis or alternative. *Entrance requirements:* For master's, GRE (for some programs), minimum GPA of 3.0 (recommended). Additional exam requirements/recommendations for international students: Required—PTE (minimum score 58), TOEFL (minimum score 550 paper-based, 79 iBT) or IELTS (minimum score 6.5). *Application deadline:* For fall admission, 2/15 priority date for domestic and international students; for spring admission, 12/15 priority date for domestic and international students. Applications are processed on a rolling basis. Application fee: $60. Electronic applications accepted. *Expenses: Tuition, area resident:* Full-time $41,084; part-time $1742 per credit hour. *Required fees:* $274. Tuition and fees vary according to course load and program. *Financial support:* In 2015–16, 31 students received support. Research assistantships with partial tuition reimbursements available, teaching assistantships with partial tuition reimbursements available, career-related internships or fieldwork, scholarships/grants, and unspecified assistantships available. Support available to part-time students. Financial award applicants required to submit FAFSA. *Faculty research:* Bioinformatics software development, bioscience, biomedical research, environmental research examining the human relationship to nature and developing solutions that prevent or reverse environmental deterioration. *Unit head:* Dr. Larry Buckley, School Head, 585-475-7507, E-mail: ljbsbi@rit.edu. *Application contact:* Diane Ellison, Associate Vice President, Graduate Enrollment Services, 585-475-2229, Fax: 585-475-7164, E-mail: gradinfo@rit.edu.
Website: http://www.rit.edu/science/gsols

★ **The Rockefeller University,** Graduate Program in Biomedical Sciences, New York, NY 10021-6399. Offers MS, PhD. *Faculty:* 72 full-time (11 women). *Students:* 209 full-time (84 women); includes 38 minority (3 Black or African American, non-Hispanic/Latino; 18 Asian, non-Hispanic/Latino; 17 Hispanic/Latino), 78 international. Average age 25. 755 applicants, 10% accepted, 22 enrolled. In 2015, 9 master's, 28 doctorates awarded. Terminal master's awarded for partial completion of doctoral program. *Degree requirements:* For master's, thesis; for doctorate, thesis/dissertation. *Entrance requirements:* For doctorate, GRE General Test; GRE Subject Test (strongly recommended), three letters of recommendation, official college or university transcripts, personal essay. Additional exam requirements/recommendations for international students: Required—TOEFL. *Application deadline:* For fall and winter admission, 12/1 for domestic and international students. Application fee: $50. Electronic applications accepted. Application fee is waived when completed online. *Financial support:* In 2015–16, 209 students received support. Fellowships with full tuition reimbursements available, institutionally sponsored loans, scholarships/grants, traineeships, and health care benefits available. *Unit head:* Dr. Sidney Strickland, Dean of Graduate and Postgraduate Studies/Vice President, 212-327-8086, Fax: 212-327-8505, E-mail: phd@rockefeller.edu. *Application contact:* Kristen Cullen, Graduate Admissions Administrator/Registrar, 212-327-8086, Fax: 212-327-8505, E-mail: phd@rockefeller.edu.
Website: http://www.rockefeller.edu/graduate/
See Display on this page and Close-Up on page 113.

Rosalind Franklin University of Medicine and Science, College of Health Professions, Department of Interprofessional Healthcare Studies, Biomedical Sciences Program, North Chicago, IL 60064-3095. Offers MS. *Entrance requirements:* For master's, MCAT, DAT, OAT, PCAT or GRE, BS in chemistry, physics, biology.

SCIENCE FOR THE BENEFIT OF HUMANITY

The David Rockefeller Graduate Program
Ph.D. Program in the Biological Sciences

The Rockefeller University is a world-renowned center for research and graduate education in the biomedical sciences. The university's Ph.D. program, whose hallmark is learning science by doing science, offers:

• a flexible academic experience with freedom to explore different areas of science

• interdisciplinary research and collaboration

• close mentoring by faculty

• unique environment without academic departments

• modern facilities and state-of-the-art research support in its more than 70 labs.

Graduate students receive a yearly stipend, free health and dental insurance, subsidized housing on or adjacent to the university's lush 14-acre campus and an annual research allowance for travel and lab support.

Founded by John D. Rockefeller in 1901 as the nation's first institute for medical research, the university's world-class faculty, with innovative approaches to scientific discovery, have produced pioneering achievements in biology and medicine. Numerous prestigious awards have been given to Rockefeller faculty, including 24 Nobel Prizes—most recently, to the late Ralph Steinman, the 2011 recipient in Physiology and Medicine.

Additional exam requirements/recommendations for international students: Required—TOEFL.

Rosalind Franklin University of Medicine and Science, School of Graduate and Postdoctoral Studies - Interdisciplinary Graduate Program in Biomedical Sciences, North Chicago, IL 60064-3095. Offers MS, PhD, DPM/PhD, MD/PhD. Terminal master's awarded for partial completion of doctoral program. *Degree requirements:* For master's, comprehensive exam, thesis, publication; for doctorate, comprehensive exam, thesis/dissertation. *Entrance requirements:* For master's and doctorate, GRE General Test. Additional exam requirements/recommendations for international students: Required—TOEFL, TWE. Electronic applications accepted. *Expenses:* Contact institution. *Faculty research:* Extracellular matrix, nutrition and mood, neuropsychopharmacology, membrane transport, brain metabolism.

Rowan University, Graduate School, College of Science and Mathematics, Department of Biological Science, Glassboro, NJ 08028-1701. Offers MS. Electronic applications accepted. *Expenses: Tuition,* area resident: full-time $8710; part-time $871 per credit. Tuition, state resident: full-time $8710; part-time $871 per credit. Tuition, nonresident: full-time $8710; part-time $871 per credit. *International tuition:* $8710 full-time. *Required fees:* $1510; $151 per credit.

Rutgers University–Camden, Graduate School of Arts and Sciences, Program in Biology, Camden, NJ 08102. Offers MS. *Program availability:* Part-time, evening/weekend. *Degree requirements:* For master's, comprehensive exam, thesis (for some programs), 30 credits. *Entrance requirements:* For master's, GRE General Test, GRE Subject Test (recommended), 3 letters of recommendation; statement of personal, professional and academic goals; biology or related undergraduate degree (preferred). Additional exam requirements/recommendations for international students: Required—TOEFL, IELTS. Electronic applications accepted. *Faculty research:* Neurobiology, biochemistry, ecology, developmental biology, biological signaling mechanisms.

Rutgers University–Newark, Graduate School of Biomedical Sciences, Newark, NJ 07107. Offers biodefense (Certificate); biomedical engineering (PhD); biomedical sciences (multidisciplinary) (PhD); cellular biology, neuroscience and physiology (PhD), including neuroscience, physiology, biophysics, cardiovascular biology, molecular pharmacology, stem cell biology; infection, immunity and inflammation (PhD), including immunology, infectious disease, microbiology, oral biology; molecular biology, genetics and cancer (PhD), including biochemistry, molecular genetics, cancer biology, radiation biology, bioinformatics; neuroscience (Certificate); pharmacological sciences (Certificate); stem cell (Certificate); DMD/PhD; MD/PhD. PhD in biomedical engineering offered jointly with New Jersey Institute of Technology. *Program availability:* Part-time, evening/weekend. Terminal master's awarded for partial completion of doctoral program. *Degree requirements:* For doctorate, thesis/dissertation, qualifying exam. *Entrance requirements:* For doctorate, GRE General Test. Additional exam requirements/recommendations for international students: Required—TOEFL. Electronic applications accepted.

Rutgers University–Newark, Graduate School, Program in Biology, Newark, NJ 07102. Offers MS, PhD. *Program availability:* Part-time, evening/weekend. Terminal master's awarded for partial completion of doctoral program. *Degree requirements:* For master's, comprehensive exam, thesis optional; for doctorate, thesis/dissertation, qualifying exam. *Entrance requirements:* For master's, GRE General Test, minimum undergraduate B average; for doctorate, GRE General Test, GRE Subject Test, minimum B average. Electronic applications accepted. *Faculty research:* Cell-cytoskeletal elements, development and regeneration in the nervous system, cellular trafficking, environmental stressors and their impact on development, opportunistic parasitic infections in AIDS.

Rutgers University–Newark, Graduate School, Program in Computational Biology, Newark, NJ 07102. Offers MS. Program offered jointly with New Jersey Institute of Technology. *Entrance requirements:* For master's, GRE, minimum undergraduate B average. Additional exam requirements/recommendations for international students: Required—TOEFL.

Rutgers University–New Brunswick, Graduate School-New Brunswick, BioMaPS Institute for Quantitative Biology, Piscataway, NJ 08854-8097. Offers computational biology and molecular biophysics (PhD). *Degree requirements:* For doctorate, comprehensive exam, thesis/dissertation. *Entrance requirements:* For doctorate, GRE. Additional exam requirements/recommendations for international students: Required—TOEFL. Electronic applications accepted. *Faculty research:* Structural biology, systems biology, bioinformatics, translational medicine, genomics.

Rutgers University–New Brunswick, Graduate School of Biomedical Sciences, Piscataway, NJ 08854-5635. Offers biochemistry and molecular biology (MS, PhD); biomedical engineering (MS, PhD); biomedical science (MS); cellular and molecular pharmacology (MS, PhD); clinical and translational science (MS); environmental sciences/exposure assessment (PhD); molecular genetics, microbiology and immunology (MS, PhD); neuroscience (MS, PhD); physiology and integrative biology (MS, PhD); toxicology (MS, PhD); MD/PhD. Terminal master's awarded for partial completion of doctoral program. *Degree requirements:* For master's, thesis (for some programs), ethics training; for doctorate, comprehensive exam, thesis/dissertation, ethics training. *Entrance requirements:* For master's, GRE General Test, MCAT, DAT; for doctorate, GRE General Test. Additional exam requirements/recommendations for international students: Required—TOEFL. Electronic applications accepted.

St. Cloud State University, School of Graduate Studies, College of Science and Engineering, Department of Biology, St. Cloud, MN 56301-4498. Offers MA, MS. *Degree requirements:* For master's, comprehensive exam (for some programs), thesis or alternative. *Entrance requirements:* For master's, GRE General Test, minimum GPA of 2.75. Additional exam requirements/recommendations for international students: Recommended—TOEFL (minimum score 550 paper-based), IELTS (minimum score 6.5). Electronic applications accepted.

Saint Francis University, Medical Science Program, Loretto, PA 15940-0600. Offers MMS. *Program availability:* Part-time, evening/weekend, online learning. *Degree requirements:* For master's, thesis or alternative, successful completion of affiliate PA program, minimum GPA of 2.8 in program. *Entrance requirements:* For master's, enrollment in affiliate PA program, bachelor's degree with minimum GPA of 2.5, resume, transcript. Additional exam requirements/recommendations for international students: Recommended—TOEFL (minimum score 80 iBT). *Application deadline:* For fall admission, 6/15 for domestic students; for spring admission, 11/15 for domestic students; for summer admission, 3/15 for domestic students. Applications are processed on a rolling basis. Application fee: $0. Electronic applications accepted. *Expenses:* Contact institution. *Financial support:* Available to part-time students. Applicants required to submit FAFSA. *Faculty research:* Health care policy, physician assistant practice roles, health promotion/disease prevention, public health epidemiology. *Application contact:* Jean A. Kline, Administrative Assistant, 814-472-3357, Fax: 814-472-3066, E-mail: jkline@francis.edu.
Website: http://francis.edu/master-of-medical-science/

St. Francis Xavier University, Graduate Studies, Department of Biology, Antigonish, NS B2G 2W5, Canada. Offers M Sc. *Degree requirements:* For master's, thesis.

Entrance requirements: For master's, 2 letters of recommendation. Additional exam requirements/recommendations for international students: Required—TOEFL (minimum score 580 paper-based). *Faculty research:* Cellular, whole organism, and population levels; marine photosynthesis; biophysical mechanisms; aquatic biology.

St. John's University, St. John's College of Liberal Arts and Sciences, Department of Biological Sciences, Queens, NY 11439. Offers MS, PhD. *Program availability:* Part-time, evening/weekend. *Degree requirements:* For master's, comprehensive exam, thesis optional, residency; for doctorate, comprehensive exam, thesis/dissertation, residency. *Entrance requirements:* For master's, GRE, minimum GPA of 3.0, 2 letters of recommendation, transcript, bachelor's degree; for doctorate, GRE General Test, GRE Subject Test, minimum GPA of 3.0 (undergraduate), 3.5 (graduate); 3 letters of recommendation; writing sample; MS in biology; transcript. Additional exam requirements/recommendations for international students: Required—TOEFL (minimum score 600 paper-based; 100 iBT), IELTS (minimum score 7). Electronic applications accepted. *Faculty research:* Regulation of gene transcription, immunology and inflammation, cancer research, infectious diseases, molecular control of developmental processes, signal transduction, neurobiology and neurodegenerative diseases.

Saint Joseph's University, College of Arts and Sciences, Department of Biology, Philadelphia, PA 19131-1395. Offers MA, MS. *Program availability:* Part-time. *Degree requirements:* For master's, comprehensive exam (for some programs), thesis (for some programs), minimum GPA of 3.0, completion of degree within 5 years. *Entrance requirements:* For master's, GRE, 2 letters of recommendation, transcript, personal statement, resume. Additional exam requirements/recommendations for international students: Required—TOEFL (minimum score 550 paper-based; 80 iBT), IELTS (minimum score 6.5). Electronic applications accepted. *Faculty research:* Life science; undergraduate science education, telomere biology; bridging the gap in racial disparities in colorectal cancer; understanding the origins of genetic disorders through experiential learning; science education; outreach into K-12 schools; genetic, ecological, and evolutionary aspects of animal behavior.

Saint Louis University, Graduate Education, College of Arts and Sciences and Graduate Education, Department of Biology, St. Louis, MO 63103. Offers MS, MS-R, PhD. *Degree requirements:* For master's, comprehensive exam, thesis (for some programs); for doctorate, thesis/dissertation, preliminary exams. *Entrance requirements:* For master's, GRE General Test, letters of recommendation, resume; for doctorate, GRE General Test, letters of recommendation, resumé, statement, transcripts. Additional exam requirements/recommendations for international students: Required—TOEFL (minimum score 550 paper-based). Electronic applications accepted. *Faculty research:* Systematics, speciation, evolution, community ecology, conservation biology, molecular signaling.

Saint Louis University, Graduate Education and School of Medicine, Graduate Program in Biomedical Sciences, St. Louis, MO 63103. Offers MS-R, PhD. *Degree requirements:* For doctorate, comprehensive exam, thesis/dissertation. *Entrance requirements:* For doctorate, GRE. Additional exam requirements/recommendations for international students: Required—TOEFL. Electronic applications accepted. *Faculty research:* Biochemistry and molecular biology, physiology and pharmacology, virology, pathology, immunology.

Salisbury University, Department of Biological Sciences, Salisbury, MD 21801-6837. Offers applied biology (MS). *Program availability:* Part-time. *Faculty:* 7 full-time (4 women). *Students:* 8 full-time (2 women), 1 (woman) part-time. Average age 25. 10 applicants, 60% accepted, 5 enrolled. In 2015, 4 master's awarded. *Degree requirements:* For master's, comprehensive exam, thesis optional. *Entrance requirements:* For master's, GRE (with scores at or above 50th percentile), undergraduate degree in biology or related field with minimum cumulative GPA of 3.0; completion of prerequisite courses in chemistry; 3 letters of recommendation; personal statement; meeting with and endorsement of graduate advisor. Additional exam requirements/recommendations for international students: Required—TOEFL (minimum score 550 paper-based, 79 iBT) or IELTS (6.5). *Application deadline:* For fall admission, 3/1 priority date for domestic and international students; for spring admission, 10/1 priority date for domestic and international students. Application fee: $65. Electronic applications accepted. *Expenses:* $370 per credit hour resident; $659 per credit hour non-resident; $78 per credit hour fees. *Financial support:* In 2015–16, 1 research assistantship with full tuition reimbursement (averaging $14,000 per year) was awarded; career-related internships or fieldwork, institutionally sponsored loans, scholarships/grants, and unspecified assistantships also available. Support available to part-time students. Financial award application deadline: 3/1; financial award applicants required to submit FAFSA. *Faculty research:* Animal behavior; soil biology; microbiology and genetics; ecology; evolution. *Unit head:* Dr. Dana Price, Graduate Program Director, Applied Biology, 410-543-6498, Fax: 410-543-6433, E-mail: dlprice@salisbury.edu. *Application contact:* Valerie Butler, Administrative Assistant, 410-543-6490, Fax: 410-543-6433, E-mail: vwbutler@salisbury.edu.
Website: http://www.salisbury.edu/gsr/gradstudies/MSBIOpage.html

Samford University, Orlean Bullard Beeson School of Education, Birmingham, AL 35229. Offers early childhood/elementary education (MS Ed); educational leadership (MS Ed, Ed D); elementary education (MS Ed); gifted education (MS Ed, Certificate); instructional design and technology (MS Ed); instructional leadership (MS Ed, Certificate, Ed S); K-12 collaborative special education (MS Ed); secondary education (MS Ed), including biology, general science, general social science, history, mathematics, physical education, Spanish; teacher leader (Ed S). *Accreditation:* NCATE. *Program availability:* Part-time, evening/weekend, blended/hybrid learning. *Faculty:* 20 full-time (14 women), 41 part-time/adjunct (32 women). *Students:* 194 full-time (146 women), 98 part-time (69 women); includes 61 minority (54 Black or African American, non-Hispanic/Latino; 4 American Indian or Alaska Native, non-Hispanic/Latino; 1 Asian, non-Hispanic/Latino; 2 Hispanic/Latino), 1 international. Average age 36. 113 applicants, 96% accepted, 80 enrolled. In 2015, 60 master's, 19 doctorates, 3 Certificates awarded. *Degree requirements:* For master's, comprehensive exam (for some programs); for doctorate, comprehensive exam, thesis/dissertation; for other advanced degree, comprehensive exam. *Entrance requirements:* For master's, GRE (minimum score of 295) or MAT (minimum score of 396); Alabama Educator Certification Testing Program (AECTP); PRAXIS, transcripts, essays, recommendations; for doctorate, professional resume, writing sample, letter of recommendation, original copy of all transcripts, interview; for other advanced degree, letter of recommendation, original copy of all transcripts. Additional exam requirements/recommendations for international students: Required—TOEFL (minimum score 90 iBT), IELTS (minimum score 6.5). *Application deadline:* For fall admission, 7/15 for domestic students, 7/1 for international students; for spring admission, 11/15 for domestic and international students; for summer admission, 4/15 for domestic and international students. Application fee: $35. Electronic applications accepted. *Expenses: Tuition,* area resident: Full-time $18,673; part-time $766 per credit hour. *Required fees:* $550. Tuition and fees vary according to course load, degree level and student level. *Financial support:* In 2015–16, 229 students received support. Scholarships/grants available. Financial award application deadline: 3/1; financial award applicants required to submit FAFSA. *Faculty research:* Computer-mediated learning, educational administration assessment and accreditation, gifted children, contributions to the

Biological and Biomedical Sciences—General

Alabama Veterans to state history. *Total annual research expenditures:* $11,000. *Unit head:* Dr. Jean Box, Dean, 205-726-2565, Fax: 205-726-4233, E-mail: jabox@samford.edu. *Application contact:* Brooke Karr, Graduate Admissions Coordinator, 205-729-2783, Fax: 205-726-4233, E-mail: kbgilrea@samford.edu. Website: http://www.samford.edu/education/

Sam Houston State University, College of Sciences, Department of Biological Sciences, Huntsville, TX 77341. Offers MA, MS. *Program availability:* Part-time. *Degree requirements:* For master's, comprehensive exam, thesis (for some programs). *Entrance requirements:* For master's, GRE General Test, letters of recommendation, statement of purpose. Additional exam requirements/recommendations for international students: Required—TOEFL (minimum score 550 paper-based; 78 iBT), IELTS (minimum score 6.5). Electronic applications accepted.

San Diego State University, Graduate and Research Affairs, College of Sciences, Department of Biology, San Diego, CA 92182. Offers biology (MA, MS), including ecology (MS), molecular biology (MS), physiology (MS), systematics/evolution (MS); cell and molecular biology (PhD); ecology (MS, PhD); microbiology (MS). Terminal master's awarded for partial completion of doctoral program. *Degree requirements:* For master's, thesis; for doctorate, thesis/dissertation. *Entrance requirements:* For master's, GRE General Test, GRE Subject Test, resume or curriculum vitae, 2 letters of recommendation. Additional exam requirements/recommendations for international students: Required—TOEFL. Electronic applications accepted.

Sanford Burnham Prebys Medical Discovery Institute, Graduate School of Biomedical Sciences, La Jolla, CA 92037. Offers PhD.

San Francisco State University, Division of Graduate Studies, College of Science and Engineering, Department of Biology, San Francisco, CA 94132-1722. Offers cell and molecular biology (MS); ecology, evolution, and conservation biology (MS); marine biology (MS); marine science (MS); microbiology (MS); physiology and behavioral biology (MS); science (PSM), including biotechnology, stem cell science. *Application deadline:* Applications are processed on a rolling basis. *Expenses:* Tuition, state resident: full-time $6738. Tuition, nonresident: full-time $15,666. *Required fees:* $1004. *Unit head:* Dr. Michael A. Goldman, Chair, 415-338-1549, Fax: 415-338-2295, E-mail: goldman@sfsu.edu. *Application contact:* Dr. Diana Chu, Graduate Coordinator, 415-405-3487, Fax: 415-338-2295, E-mail: chud@sfsu.edu. Website: http://biology.sfsu.edu/

San Jose State University, Graduate Studies and Research, College of Science, San Jose, CA 95192-0001. Offers biological sciences (MA, MS), including molecular biology and microbiology (MS), organismal biology, conservation and ecology (MS), physiology (MS); chemistry (MA, MS); computer science (MS); cybersecurity (Certificate); cybersecurity: core technologies (Certificate); geology (MS); marine science (MS); master biotechnology (MBT); mathematics (MA, MS), including mathematics education (MA), science; meteorology (MS); physics (MS), including computational physics, modern optics, science (MA, MS); science education (MA); statistics (MS); Unix system administration (Certificate). *Program availability:* Part-time, evening/weekend. *Students:* 118 full-time (68 women), 52 part-time (25 women); includes 125 minority (5 Black or African American, non-Hispanic/Latino; 97 Asian, non-Hispanic/Latino; 23 Hispanic/Latino), 121 international. Average age 27. 1,236 applicants, 21% accepted, 171 enrolled. In 2015, 168 master's awarded. *Entrance requirements:* For master's, GRE. *Application deadline:* For fall admission, 6/29 for domestic students; for spring admission, 11/30 for domestic students. Applications are processed on a rolling basis. Application fee: $55. Electronic applications accepted. *Financial support:* Teaching assistantships, career-related internships or fieldwork, Federal Work-Study, and institutionally sponsored loans available. Support available to part-time students. Financial award applicants required to submit FAFSA. *Faculty research:* Radiochemistry/environmental analysis, health physics, radiation effects. *Unit head:* J. Michael Parrish, Dean, 408-924-4800, Fax: 408-924-4815. *Application contact:* 408-924-2480, Fax: 408-924-2477. Website: http://www.science.sjsu.edu/

The Scripps Research Institute, Kellogg School of Science and Technology, La Jolla, CA 92037. Offers chemical and biological sciences (PhD). *Degree requirements:* For doctorate, thesis/dissertation. *Entrance requirements:* For doctorate, GRE General Test, GRE Subject Test, 3 letters of recommendation, official transcripts. Additional exam requirements/recommendations for international students: Required—TOEFL. Electronic applications accepted. *Faculty research:* Molecular structure and function, plant biology, immunology, bioorganic chemistry and molecular design, synthetic organic chemistry and natural product synthesis.

Seton Hall University, College of Arts and Sciences, Department of Biological Sciences, South Orange, NJ 07079-2697. Offers biology (MS); biology/business administration (MS); microbiology (MS); molecular bioscience (PhD); molecular bioscience/neuroscience (PhD). *Program availability:* Part-time, evening/weekend. *Degree requirements:* For master's, thesis optional; for doctorate, comprehensive exam, thesis/dissertation. *Entrance requirements:* For master's, GRE or undergraduate degree (BS in biological sciences) with minimum GPA of 3.0 from accredited U.S. institution; for doctorate, GRE. Additional exam requirements/recommendations for international students: Required—TOEFL. Electronic applications accepted. *Faculty research:* Neurobiology, genetics, immunology, molecular biology, cellular physiology, toxicology, microbiology, bioinformatics.

Shippensburg University of Pennsylvania, School of Graduate Studies, College of Arts and Sciences, Department of Biology, Shippensburg, PA 17257-2299. Offers MS. *Program availability:* Part-time, evening/weekend. *Faculty:* 11 full-time (4 women). *Students:* 19 full-time (12 women), 17 part-time (11 women); includes 2 minority (1 Black or African American, non-Hispanic/Latino; 1 Hispanic/Latino), 4 international. Average age 28. 36 applicants, 67% accepted, 13 enrolled. In 2015, 12 master's awarded. *Degree requirements:* For master's, thesis, oral thesis defense, seminar, minimum QPA of 3.0. *Entrance requirements:* For master's, minimum GPA of 2.75; essay; 500-word statement of purpose; 33 credits of course work in biology; minimum of 3 courses with labs including both inorganic and organic chemistry or biochemistry; completion of math through calculus (including a statistics course) and two lab courses in physics. Additional exam requirements/recommendations for international students: Required—TOEFL (minimum score 80 iBT); Recommended—IELTS (minimum score 6.5). *Application deadline:* For fall admission, 4/30 for international students; for spring admission, 9/30 for international students. Applications are processed on a rolling basis. Application fee: $45. Electronic applications accepted. *Expenses:* Tuition, state resident: part-time $470 per credit. Tuition, nonresident: part-time $705 per credit. *Required fees:* $137 per credit. *Financial support:* In 2015–16, 12 students received support, including 13 research assistantships (averaging $5,000 per year); career-related internships or fieldwork, scholarships/grants, unspecified assistantships, resident hall director and student payroll positions also available. Support available to part-time students. Financial award application deadline: 3/1; financial award applicants required to submit FAFSA. *Unit head:* Dr. Theo S. Light, Professor and Program Coordinator, 717-477-1401, Fax: 717-477-4064, E-mail: tsligh@ship.edu. *Application contact:* Jeremy R. Goshorn, Assistant Dean of Graduate Admissions, 717-477-1231, Fax: 717-477-4016, E-mail: jrgoshorn@ship.edu. Website: http://www.ship.edu/biology/

Simon Fraser University, Office of Graduate Studies, Faculty of Science, Department of Biological Sciences, Burnaby, BC V5A 1S6, Canada. Offers bioinformatics (Graduate Diploma); biological sciences (M Sc, PhD); environmental toxicology (MET); pest management (MPM). *Degree requirements:* For master's, thesis; for doctorate, thesis/dissertation, candidacy exam. *Entrance requirements:* For Graduate Diploma, practicum. *Entrance requirements:* For master's, minimum GPA of 3.0 (on scale of 4.33), or 3.33 based on last 60 credits of undergraduate courses; for doctorate, minimum GPA of 3.5 (on scale of 4.33); for Graduate Diploma, minimum GPA of 2.5 (on scale of 4.33), or 2.67 based on the last 60 credits of undergraduate courses. Additional exam requirements/recommendations for international students: Recommended—TOEFL (minimum score 580 paper-based; 93 iBT), IELTS (minimum score 7), TWE (minimum score 5). Electronic applications accepted. *Faculty research:* Cell biology, wildlife ecology, environmental and evolutionary physiology, environmental toxicology, pest management.

Smith College, Graduate and Special Programs, Department of Biological Sciences, Northampton, MA 01063. Offers MAT, MS. *Program availability:* Part-time-only. *Students:* 1 (woman) full-time, 8 part-time (all women); includes 2 minority (1 Black or African American, non-Hispanic/Latino; 1 Asian, non-Hispanic/Latino), 1 international. Average age 23. 7 applicants, 86% accepted, 5 enrolled. In 2015, 5 master's awarded. *Degree requirements:* For master's, one foreign language, thesis (for some programs). *Entrance requirements:* For master's, GRE General Test (for MS). Additional exam requirements/recommendations for international students: Required—TOEFL (minimum score 595 paper-based; 97 iBT), IELTS. *Application deadline:* For fall admission, 1/15 for domestic and international students; for spring admission, 12/1 for domestic students. Application fee: $60. *Expenses:* Tuition, area resident: Full-time $34,560; part-time $1440 per credit. Tuition and fees vary according to course load and program. *Financial support:* In 2015–16, 9 students received support, including 7 research assistantships with full tuition reimbursements available (averaging $13,710 per year); fellowships with full tuition reimbursements available and scholarships/grants also available. Support available to part-time students. Financial award application deadline: 1/15; financial award applicants required to submit CSS PROFILE or FAFSA. *Unit head:* Jesse Bellemare, Graduate Student Advisor, 413-585-3812, E-mail: jbellema@smith.edu. *Application contact:* Ruth Morgan, Program Assistant, 413-585-3050, Fax: 413-585-3054, E-mail: rmorgan@smith.edu. Website: http://www.smith.edu/biology/

Sonoma State University, School of Science and Technology, Department of Biology, Rohnert Park, CA 94928. Offers biochemistry (MA); ecology (MS); environmental biology (MS); evolutionary biology (MS); functional morphology (MS); molecular and cell biology (MS); organismal biology (MS). *Program availability:* Part-time. *Degree requirements:* For master's, thesis or alternative, oral exam. *Entrance requirements:* For master's, GRE General Test, GRE Subject Test, minimum GPA of 3.0. Additional exam requirements/recommendations for international students: Required—TOEFL (minimum score 500 paper-based). *Faculty research:* Plant physiology, comparative physiology, community ecology, restoration ecology, marine ecology, conservation genetics, primate behavior, behavioral ecology, developmental biology, plant and animal systematics.

South Carolina State University, College of Graduate and Professional Studies, Department of Education, Orangeburg, SC 29117-0001. Offers early childhood education (MAT); education (M Ed); elementary education (M Ed, MAT); English (MAT); general science/biology (MAT); mathematics (MAT); secondary education (M Ed), including biology education, business education, counselor education, English education, home economics education, industrial education, mathematics education, science education, social studies education; special education (M Ed), including emotionally handicapped, learning disabilities, mentally handicapped. *Accreditation:* NCATE. *Program availability:* Part-time, evening/weekend. *Faculty:* 17 full-time (12 women), 3 part-time/adjunct (1 woman). *Students:* 30 full-time (20 women), 32 part-time (23 women); all minorities (all Black or African American, non-Hispanic/Latino). Average age 31. 22 applicants, 95% accepted, 19 enrolled. In 2015, 13 master's awarded. *Degree requirements:* For master's, thesis optional, departmental qualifying exam. *Entrance requirements:* For master's, GRE General Test, NTE, interview, teaching certificate. *Application deadline:* For fall admission, 6/15 priority date for domestic students, 6/15 for international students; for spring admission, 11/1 for domestic and international students. Applications are processed on a rolling basis. Application fee: $25. Electronic applications accepted. *Expenses:* Tuition, state resident: full-time $8906; part-time $495 per credit hour. Tuition, nonresident: full-time $18,674; part-time $1037 per credit hour. *Required fees:* $2497; $66 per credit hour. *Financial support:* Fellowships, career-related internships or fieldwork, Federal Work-Study, and scholarships/grants available. Financial award application deadline: 6/1. *Unit head:* Dr. Charlie Spell, Interim Chair, Department of Education, 803-536-8963, Fax: 803-516-4568, E-mail: cspell@scsu.edu. *Application contact:* Curtis Foskey, Coordinator of Graduate Studies, 803-536-8419, Fax: 803-536-8812, E-mail: cfoskey@scsu.edu.

South Dakota State University, Graduate School, College of Agriculture and Biological Sciences, Department of Animal and Range Sciences, Brookings, SD 57007. Offers animal science (MS, PhD); biological sciences (PhD). *Program availability:* Part-time. *Degree requirements:* For master's, thesis, oral exam; for doctorate, comprehensive exam, thesis/dissertation, preliminary oral and written exams. *Entrance requirements:* Additional exam requirements/recommendations for international students: Required—TOEFL (minimum score 550 paper-based; 79 iBT). *Faculty research:* Ruminant and nonruminant nutrition, meat science, reproductive physiology, range utilization, ecology genetics, muscle biology, animal production.

South Dakota State University, Graduate School, College of Agriculture and Biological Sciences, Department of Biology and Microbiology, Brookings, SD 57007. Offers biological sciences (MS, PhD). *Program availability:* Part-time. *Degree requirements:* For master's, thesis (for some programs), oral exam; for doctorate, comprehensive exam, thesis/dissertation, oral exam. *Entrance requirements:* For master's and doctorate, GRE General Test. Additional exam requirements/recommendations for international students: Required—TOEFL (minimum score 600 paper-based; 100 iBT). *Faculty research:* Ecosystem ecology; plant, animal and microbial genomics; animal infectious disease, microbial bioproducts.

South Dakota State University, Graduate School, College of Agriculture and Biological Sciences, Department of Dairy Science, Brookings, SD 57007. Offers animal sciences (MS, PhD); biological sciences (MS, PhD). *Program availability:* Part-time. *Degree requirements:* For master's, thesis, oral exam; for doctorate, comprehensive exam, thesis/dissertation, preliminary oral and written exams. *Entrance requirements:* Additional exam requirements/recommendations for international students: Required—TOEFL (minimum score 550 paper-based). *Faculty research:* Dairy cattle nutrition, energy metabolism, food safety, dairy processing technology.

South Dakota State University, Graduate School, College of Agriculture and Biological Sciences, Department of Veterinary and Biomedical Sciences, Brookings, SD 57007. Offers biological sciences (MS, PhD). *Program availability:* Part-time, evening/weekend. *Degree requirements:* For master's, thesis (for some programs), oral exam; for doctorate, comprehensive exam, thesis/dissertation, preliminary oral and written exams. *Entrance requirements:* Additional exam requirements/recommendations for international students: Required—TOEFL (minimum score 525 paper-based; 71 iBT). *Faculty research:* Infectious disease, food animal, virology, immunology.

South Dakota State University, Graduate School, College of Engineering, Department of Agricultural and Biosystems Engineering, Brookings, SD 57007. Offers biological sciences (MS, PhD); engineering (MS). PhD offered jointly with Iowa State University of Science and Technology. *Program availability:* Part-time. *Degree requirements:* For master's, thesis (for some programs), oral exam; for doctorate, thesis/dissertation, preliminary oral and written exams. *Entrance requirements:* For master's and doctorate, engineering degree. Additional exam requirements/recommendations for international students: Required—TOEFL (minimum score 550 paper-based; 79 iBT). *Faculty research:* Water resources, food engineering, natural resources engineering, machine design, bioprocess engineering.

South Dakota State University, Graduate School, College of Pharmacy, Department of Pharmaceutical Sciences, Brookings, SD 57007. Offers biological science (MS); pharmaceutical sciences (PhD). *Degree requirements:* For master's, thesis, oral exam; for doctorate, comprehensive exam, thesis/dissertation, oral exam. *Entrance requirements:* For master's and doctorate, GRE General Test. Additional exam requirements/recommendations for international students: Required—TOEFL (minimum score 550 paper-based). *Faculty research:* Drugs of abuse, anti-cancer drugs, sustained drug delivery, drug metabolism.

Southeastern Louisiana University, College of Science and Technology, Department of Biological Sciences, Hammond, LA 70402. Offers biology (MS). *Program availability:* Part-time. *Faculty:* 15 full-time (4 women), 1 part-time/adjunct (0 women). *Students:* 18 full-time (8 women), 7 part-time (5 women); includes 3 minority (all Hispanic/Latino), 1 international. Average age 32. 19 applicants, 63% accepted, 11 enrolled. In 2015, 1 master's awarded. *Degree requirements:* For master's, comprehensive exam, thesis (for some programs). *Entrance requirements:* For master's, GRE General Test (minimum score 1000), minimum GPA of 3.0; 30 hours of undergraduate biology courses; two letters of recommendation; curriculum vitae; letter of intent. Additional exam requirements/recommendations for international students: Required—TOEFL (minimum score 500 paper-based; 61 iBT). *Application deadline:* For fall admission, 7/15 priority date for domestic students, 6/1 priority date for international students; for spring admission, 12/1 priority date for domestic students, 10/1 priority date for international students. Applications are processed on a rolling basis. Application fee: $20 ($30 for international students). Electronic applications accepted. *Expenses: Tuition, area resident:* Full-time $5551; part-time $436 per credit hour. Tuition, nonresident: full-time $18,115; part-time $1129 per credit hour. *Required fees:* $1559. *Financial support:* In 2015–16, 4 research assistantships (averaging $9,383 per year), 10 teaching assistantships (averaging $10,100 per year) were awarded; career-related internships or fieldwork, Federal Work-Study, institutionally sponsored loans, scholarships/grants, traineeships, and unspecified assistantships also available. Support available to part-time students. Financial award application deadline: 5/1; financial award applicants required to submit FAFSA. *Faculty research:* Evolutionary biology, ecology, molecular biology, morphology and physiology, microbiology and immunology. *Total annual research expenditures:* $103,448. *Unit head:* Dr. Christopher Beachy, Department Head, 985-549-3740, Fax: 985-549-3851, E-mail: christopher.beachy@selu.edu. *Application contact:* Amanda Harper, Graduate Admissions Analyst, 985-549-5620, Fax: 985-549-5632, E-mail: admissions@selu.edu.
Website: http://www.selu.edu/acad_research/depts/biol

Southeast Missouri State University, School of Graduate Studies, Department of Biology, Cape Girardeau, MO 63701-4799. Offers MNS. *Program availability:* Part-time. *Faculty:* 15 full-time (4 women). *Students:* 16 full-time (6 women), 24 part-time (10 women); includes 1 minority (Asian, non-Hispanic/Latino), 8 international. Average age 27. 31 applicants, 35% accepted, 11 enrolled. In 2015, 15 master's awarded. *Degree requirements:* For master's, comprehensive exam (for some programs), thesis (for some programs), thesis and oral defense, or research paper and comprehensive exam. *Entrance requirements:* For master's, GRE General Test, minimum undergraduate GPA of 2.5, 2.75 in last 30 hours of undergraduate course work in science and mathematics; 2 letters of recommendation; faculty sponsor agreement. Additional exam requirements/recommendations for international students: Required—TOEFL (minimum score 550 paper-based; 79 iBT), IELTS (minimum score 6), PTE (minimum score 53). *Application deadline:* For fall admission, 4/1 for domestic and international students; for spring admission, 10/1 for domestic and international students; for summer admission, 4/1 for domestic students. Applications are processed on a rolling basis. Application fee: $30 ($40 for international students). Electronic applications accepted. *Expenses: Tuition, state resident:* part-time $260.80 per credit hour. Tuition, nonresident: part-time $486.80 per credit hour. *Required fees:* $33.70 per credit hour. *Financial support:* In 2015–16, 26 students received support, including 6 research assistantships with full tuition reimbursements available (averaging $8,467 per year), 25 teaching assistantships with full tuition reimbursements available (averaging $8,467 per year); career-related internships or fieldwork, Federal Work-Study, scholarships/grants, traineeships, tuition waivers (full), and unspecified assistantships also available. Financial award application deadline: 6/30; financial award applicants required to submit FAFSA. *Faculty research:* Evolutionary ecology, animal behavior and ecology, case-based learning, plant systematics and physiology, genetics. *Total annual research expenditures:* $964,517. *Unit head:* Dr. James E. Champine, Department of Biology Chair/Professor, 573-651-2171, Fax: 573-651-2382, E-mail: jchampine@semo.edu. *Application contact:* Dr. Dustin Siegel, Department of Biology Graduate Coordinator, 573-651-2171, Fax: 573-651-2382, E-mail: dsiegel@semo.edu.
Website: http://www.semo.edu/biology/

Southern Connecticut State University, School of Graduate Studies, School of Arts and Sciences, Department of Biology, New Haven, CT 06515-1355. Offers MS. *Program availability:* Part-time, evening/weekend. *Faculty:* 6 full-time (3 women). *Students:* 5 full-time (2 women), 18 part-time (9 women); includes 2 minority (1 Asian, non-Hispanic/Latino; 1 Hispanic/Latino), 1 international. Average age 29. 27 applicants, 33% accepted, 8 enrolled. In 2015, 6 master's awarded. *Degree requirements:* For master's, thesis optional. *Entrance requirements:* For master's, previous course work in biology, chemistry, and mathematics; interview. *Application deadline:* Applications are processed on a rolling basis. Application fee: $50. Electronic applications accepted. *Expenses:* Tuition, state resident: full-time $4968; part-time $494 per credit hour. Tuition, nonresident: full-time $16,078; part-time $509 per credit hour. *Required fees:* $4632; $55 per semester. Tuition and fees vary according to program. *Financial support:* Career-related internships or fieldwork, scholarships/grants, and unspecified assistantships available. Financial award application deadline: 4/15; financial award applicants required to submit FAFSA. *Unit head:* Dr. Sean Grace, Chairperson, 203-392-6216, Fax: 203-392-5364, E-mail: graces2@southernct.edu. *Application contact:* Lisa Galvin, Director of Graduate Admissions, 203-392-5240, Fax: 203-392-5235, E-mail: galvinl1@southernct.edu.

Southern Illinois University Carbondale, Graduate School, College of Science, Biological Sciences Program, Carbondale, IL 62901-4701. Offers MS. *Students:* 8 full-time (6 women); includes 7 minority (6 Black or African American, non-Hispanic/Latino; 1 Hispanic/Latino), 1 international. Average age 25. 3 applicants. *Degree requirements:* For master's, thesis or alternative. *Entrance requirements:* For master's, GRE General Test, minimum GPA of 2.7. Additional exam requirements/recommendations for international students: Required—TOEFL. *Application deadline:* For summer admission,

5/1 for domestic students. Applications are processed on a rolling basis. Application fee: $65. *Financial support:* In 2015–16, 2 students received support, including 2 teaching assistantships with full tuition reimbursements available; fellowships with full tuition reimbursements available, research assistantships with full tuition reimbursements available, Federal Work-Study, institutionally sponsored loans, and tuition waivers (full) also available. Support available to part-time students. *Faculty research:* Molecular mechanisms of mutagenesis, reproductive endocrinology, avian energetics and nutrition, developmental plant physiology. *Unit head:* Linda Herrold, Assistant Dean, 618-453-1460, E-mail: lherrold@siumed.edu. *Application contact:* Dr. Anneke Metz, Interim Director, 618-453-1650, E-mail: ametz@siumed.edu.

Southern Illinois University Carbondale, Graduate School, Graduate Programs in Medicine, Carbondale, IL 62901-4701. Offers molecular, cellular and systemic physiology (MS); molecular, cellular, and systemic physiology (PhD); pharmacology (MS, PhD); physician assistant studies (MSPA). *Faculty:* 31 full-time (5 women). *Students:* 83 full-time (59 women); includes 3 minority (1 Black or African American, non-Hispanic/Latino; 1 American Indian or Alaska Native, non-Hispanic/Latino; 1 Asian, non-Hispanic/Latino), 50 international. 48 applicants, 23% accepted, 6 enrolled. In 2015, 33 master's, 6 doctorates awarded. Terminal master's awarded for partial completion of doctoral program. *Degree requirements:* For master's, thesis; for doctorate, thesis/dissertation. *Entrance requirements:* For master's, GRE, minimum GPA of 3.0; for doctorate, GRE, minimum GPA of 3.25. Additional exam requirements/recommendations for international students: Required—TOEFL. *Application deadline:* For fall admission, 1/15 for domestic students. Application fee: $65. *Financial support:* In 2015–16, 29 students received support, including 3 fellowships with full tuition reimbursements available, 22 research assistantships with full tuition reimbursements available, 4 teaching assistantships with full tuition reimbursements available; institutionally sponsored loans and tuition waivers (full) also available. *Faculty research:* Cardiovascular physiology, neurophysiology of hearing. *Unit head:* Dr. J. Kevin Dorsey, Dean, 217-545-3625, E-mail: kdorsey@siumed.edu.

Southern Illinois University Edwardsville, Graduate School, College of Arts and Sciences, Department of Biological Sciences, Program in Biology, Edwardsville, IL 62026-0001. Offers MA, MS. *Program availability:* Part-time, evening/weekend. *Faculty:* 19. *Students:* 21 full-time (11 women), 35 part-time (21 women); includes 10 minority (3 Black or African American, non-Hispanic/Latino; 1 Asian, non-Hispanic/Latino; 4 Hispanic/Latino; 2 Two or more races, non-Hispanic/Latino), 3 international. 31 applicants, 84% accepted, 21 enrolled. *Degree requirements:* For master's, thesis (for some programs). *Entrance requirements:* For master's, GRE. Additional exam requirements/recommendations for international students: Required—TOEFL (minimum score 550 paper-based; 79 iBT), IELTS (minimum score 6.5). *Application deadline:* For fall admission, 7/22 for domestic students, 7/15 for international students; for spring admission, 12/9 for domestic students, 11/15 for international students; for summer admission, 4/29 for domestic students, 4/15 for international students. Applications are processed on a rolling basis. Application fee: $30. Electronic applications accepted. *Expenses:* Tuition, state resident: full-time $5026; part-time $837 per course. Tuition, nonresident: full-time $12,566; part-time $2094 per course. *Required fees:* $1682; $474 per course. Tuition and fees vary according to course load, campus/location and program. *Financial support:* In 2015–16, 32 students received support, including 3 research assistantships with full tuition reimbursements available, 27 teaching assistantships with full tuition reimbursements available; fellowships with full tuition reimbursements available, career-related internships or fieldwork, institutionally sponsored loans, scholarships/grants, and unspecified assistantships also available. Financial award application deadline: 3/1; financial award applicants required to submit FAFSA. *Unit head:* Dr. Rick Essner, Director, 618-650-3468, E-mail: ressner@siue.edu. *Application contact:* Melissa K. Mace, Coordinator of International and Graduate Recruitment, 618-650-3705, Fax: 618-650-3618, E-mail: graduateadmissions@siue.edu.
Website: http://www.siue.edu/artsandsciences/biologicalsciences/

Southern Methodist University, Dedman College of Humanities and Sciences, Department of Biological Sciences, Dallas, TX 75275. Offers molecular and cellular biology (MA, MS, PhD). Terminal master's awarded for partial completion of doctoral program. *Degree requirements:* For master's, thesis (for MS), oral exam; for doctorate, thesis/dissertation, qualifying exam. *Entrance requirements:* For master's, GRE General Test (minimum score 1200), minimum GPA of 3.0; for doctorate, GRE General Test (minimum score: 1200), minimum GPA of 3.0. Additional exam requirements/recommendations for international students: Required—TOEFL (minimum score 550 paper-based). Electronic applications accepted. *Faculty research:* Free radicals and aging, protein structure, chromatin structure, signal processes, retroviral pathogenesis.

Southern University and Agricultural and Mechanical College, Graduate School, College of Sciences, Department of Biology, Baton Rouge, LA 70813. Offers MS. *Degree requirements:* For master's, comprehensive exam, thesis. *Entrance requirements:* For master's, GRE General Test. Additional exam requirements/recommendations for international students: Required—TOEFL (minimum score 525 paper-based). *Faculty research:* Toxicology, neuroendocrinology, mycotoxin, virology.

Stanford University, School of Humanities and Sciences, Department of Biology, Stanford, CA 94305-9991. Offers MS, PhD. Terminal master's awarded for partial completion of doctoral program. *Degree requirements:* For doctorate, thesis/dissertation, oral exam. *Entrance requirements:* For master's, GRE General Test; for doctorate, GRE General Test, GRE Subject Test. Additional exam requirements/recommendations for international students: Required—TOEFL. Electronic applications accepted. *Expenses: Tuition, area resident:* Full-time $45,729. *Required fees:* $591.

Stanford University, School of Medicine, Graduate Programs in Medicine, Stanford, CA 94305-9991. Offers MS, PhD. Terminal master's awarded for partial completion of doctoral program. *Degree requirements:* For master's, thesis; for doctorate, thesis/dissertation. *Entrance requirements:* For master's, GRE General Test or MCAT. Additional exam requirements/recommendations for international students: Required—TOEFL. Electronic applications accepted. *Expenses: Tuition, area resident:* Full-time $45,729. *Required fees:* $591.

State University of New York at Fredonia, College of Liberal Arts and Sciences, Fredonia, NY 14063. Offers biology (MS); interdisciplinary studies (MS); speech pathology (MS); MA/MS. *Program availability:* Part-time, evening/weekend. *Degree requirements:* For master's, comprehensive exam (for some programs), thesis (for some programs). *Entrance requirements:* For master's, GRE. Additional exam requirements/recommendations for international students: Required—TOEFL (minimum score 79 iBT), IELTS (minimum score 6.5), Cambridge English Advanced (minimum score: 52) recommended. Electronic applications accepted. *Expenses:* Tuition, state resident: full-time $10,870; part-time $453 per credit. Tuition, nonresident: full-time $22,210; part-time $925 per credit. *Required fees:* $1604; $66.70 per credit. *Faculty research:* Immunology/microbiology, applied human physiology, ecology and evolution, invertebrate biology, molecular biology, biochemistry, physiology, animal behavior, science education, vertebrate physiology, cell biology, plant biology, developmental biology, aquatic ecology, bilingual language acquisition, bilingual language acquisition and disorders, augmentative and alternate communication with ALS, World War I, Zweig, environmental literature, editing, adolescent literature, pedagogy.

Biological and Biomedical Sciences—General

State University of New York College at Oneonta, Graduate Education, Department of Biology, Oneonta, NY 13820-4015. Offers MA. *Program availability:* Part-time, evening/weekend. *Degree requirements:* For master's, comprehensive exam. *Entrance requirements:* For master's, GRE General Test, GRE Subject Test.

State University of New York Downstate Medical Center, School of Graduate Studies, Brooklyn, NY 11203-2098. Offers MS, PhD, MD/PhD. *Degree requirements:* For doctorate, thesis/dissertation. *Entrance requirements:* For doctorate, GRE. Additional exam requirements/recommendations for international students: Required—TOEFL. *Faculty research:* Cellular and molecular neurobiology, role of oncogenes in early cardiogenesis, mechanism of gene regulation, cardiovascular physiology, yeast molecular genetics.

State University of New York Upstate Medical University, College of Graduate Studies, Syracuse, NY 13210-2334. Offers MS, PhD, MD/PhD. Terminal master's awarded for partial completion of doctoral program. *Degree requirements:* For master's, thesis; for doctorate, comprehensive exam, thesis/dissertation. *Entrance requirements:* For master's, GRE General Test, interview; for doctorate, GRE General Test, telephone interview. Additional exam requirements/recommendations for international students: Required—TOEFL. Electronic applications accepted. *Faculty research:* Cancer, disorders of the nervous system, infectious diseases, diabetes/metabolic disorders/cardiovascular diseases.

Stephen F. Austin State University, Graduate School, College of Sciences and Mathematics, Department of Biology, Nacogdoches, TX 75962. Offers MS. *Degree requirements:* For master's, comprehensive exam, thesis optional. *Entrance requirements:* For master's, GRE General Test, minimum GPA of 2.8 in last 60 hours, 2.5 overall. Additional exam requirements/recommendations for international students: Required—TOEFL.

Stevenson University, Program in Forensic Science, Owings Mills, MD 21117. Offers biology (MS); chemistry (MS); crime scene investigation (MS). Program offered in partnership with Maryland State Police Forensic Sciences Division. *Program availability:* Part-time. *Faculty:* 4 full-time (3 women), 5 part-time/adjunct (2 women). *Students:* 20 full-time (14 women), 23 part-time (18 women); includes 19 minority (18 Black or African American, non-Hispanic/Latino; 1 Hispanic/Latino). Average age 27. 28 applicants, 71% accepted, 16 enrolled. In 2015, 23 master's awarded. *Degree requirements:* For master's, capstone course. *Entrance requirements:* For master's, bachelor's degree in a natural science from regionally-accredited institution; official college transcripts from all previous academic work; minimum cumulative GPA of 3.0 in past academic work. Additional exam requirements/recommendations for international students: Required—TOEFL (minimum score 550 paper-based), IELTS (minimum score 6.5). *Application deadline:* Applications are processed on a rolling basis. Application fee: $0. Electronic applications accepted. *Expenses:* $670 per credit, $125 fee per semester. *Financial support:* Applicants required to submit FAFSA. *Unit head:* John Tobin, PhD, Coordinator, 443-352-4142, Fax: 443-394-0538, E-mail: jtobin@stevenson.edu. *Application contact:* William Wellein, Enrollment Counselor, 443-352-5843, Fax: 443-394-0538, E-mail: wwellein@stevenson.edu.
Website: http://www.stevenson.edu

Stony Brook University, State University of New York, Stony Brook Medicine, School of Medicine and Graduate School, Graduate Programs in Medicine, Stony Brook, NY 11794. Offers MS, PhD, Advanced Certificate. *Students:* 124 full-time (55 women), 9 part-time (4 women); includes 42 minority (12 Black or African American, non-Hispanic/Latino; 18 Asian, non-Hispanic/Latino; 11 Hispanic/Latino; 1 Two or more races, non-Hispanic/Latino), 20 international. 225 applicants, 38% accepted, 53 enrolled. In 2015, 32 master's, 9 doctorates awarded. *Degree requirements:* For doctorate, thesis/dissertation, exam. *Entrance requirements:* For doctorate, GRE General Test. Additional exam requirements/recommendations for international students: Required—TOEFL. *Application deadline:* For fall admission, 1/15 for domestic students; for spring admission, 10/1 for domestic students. Application fee: $100. Electronic applications accepted. *Expenses:* $12,421 full-time resident tuition and fees, $453 per credit hour; $23,761 full-time nonresident tuition and fees, $925 per credit hour. *Financial support:* Fellowships, research assistantships, teaching assistantships, career-related internships or fieldwork, and Federal Work-Study available. Financial award application deadline: 3/15. *Unit head:* Dr. Kenneth Kaushansky, Dean and Senior Vice President of Health Sciences, 631-444-2113, Fax: 631-444-6032. *Application contact:* Melissa Jordan, Assistant Dean, 631-632-9712, Fax: 631-632-7243, E-mail: melissa.jordan@stonybrook.edu.

Stony Brook University, State University of New York, Stony Brook Medicine, School of Medicine, Medical Scientist Training Program, Stony Brook, NY 11794. Offers MD/PhD. *Entrance requirements:* Additional exam requirements/recommendations for international students: Required—TOEFL. *Application deadline:* For fall admission, 1/15 for domestic students. *Expenses:* Tuition, state resident: full-time $10,870; part-time $453 per credit hour. Tuition, nonresident: full-time $22,210; part-time $925 per credit hour. *Financial support:* Tuition waivers (full) available. *Unit head:* Dr. Michael A. Frohman, Director, Medical Scientist Training Program, 631-444-3219, Fax: 631-444-6229, E-mail: michael.frohman@stonybrook.edu. *Application contact:* Carron Allen, Program Administrator, 631-444-3219, Fax: 631-444-3492, E-mail: carron.kaufman@stonybrook.edu.
Website: http://www.pharm.stonybrook.edu/mstp/

Sul Ross State University, College of Arts and Sciences, Department of Biology, Alpine, TX 79832. Offers MS. *Program availability:* Part-time. *Students:* 10 full-time (6 women), 8 part-time (4 women); includes 8 minority (1 Black or African American, non-Hispanic/Latino; 6 Hispanic/Latino; 1 Two or more races, non-Hispanic/Latino), 1 international. Average age 26. *Degree requirements:* For master's, thesis optional. *Entrance requirements:* For master's, GRE General Test, minimum GPA of 2.5 in last 60 hours of undergraduate work. *Application deadline:* Applications are processed on a rolling basis. Application fee: $0 ($50 for international students). *Financial support:* Research assistantships, teaching assistantships, career-related internships or fieldwork, Federal Work-Study, and institutionally sponsored loans available. Support available to part-time students. Financial award application deadline: 5/1; financial award applicants required to submit FAFSA. *Faculty research:* Plant-animal interaction, Chihuahuan desert biology, insect biological control, plant and animal systematics, wildlife biology. *Unit head:* Dr. Chris Ritzi, Chair, 432-837-8420, Fax: 432-837-8682, E-mail: critzi@sulross.edu. *Application contact:* Lonora Hunt, Department Secretary, 432-837-8112, Fax: 432-837-8682, E-mail: lhunt@sulross.edu.
Website: http://www.sulross.edu/section/33/biology

Syracuse University, College of Arts and Sciences, Programs in Biology, Syracuse, NY 13244. Offers biology (MS, PhD), including biology (MS), neuroscience (PhD). *Program availability:* Part-time. *Students:* Average age 26. In 2015, 2 master's, 3 doctorates awarded. Terminal master's awarded for partial completion of doctoral program. *Degree requirements:* For master's, thesis; for doctorate, thesis/dissertation. *Entrance requirements:* For master's and doctorate, GRE General Test, GRE Subject Test (recommended), BS or BA, at least a minimal background in both physical and biological sciences, three letters of recommendation, personal statement, transcripts. Additional exam requirements/recommendations for international students: Required—TOEFL

(minimum score 100 iBT). *Application deadline:* For fall admission, 12/15 priority date for domestic and international students. Application fee: $75. Electronic applications accepted. *Expenses: Tuition, area resident:* Full-time $25,974; part-time $1443 per credit hour. *Required fees:* $802; $50 per course. Tuition and fees vary according to course load and program. *Financial support:* Fellowships with full tuition reimbursements, research assistantships with tuition reimbursements, teaching assistantships with tuition reimbursements, and scholarships/grants available. Financial award application deadline: 1/1; financial award applicants required to submit FAFSA. *Faculty research:* Cell signaling, plant ecosystem ecology, aquatic ecology, genetics and molecular biology of color vision, ion transport by cell membranes. *Unit head:* Dr. Steve Dorus, Graduate Program Director, 315-443-7091, E-mail: biology@syr.edu. *Application contact:* Lynn Fall, Graduate Program Administrator, 315-443-9154, E-mail: biology@syr.edu.
Website: http://biology.syr.edu/

Syracuse University, College of Arts and Sciences, Programs in Forensic Science, Syracuse, NY 13244. Offers firearm and tool mark examination (CAS); forensic science (MS), including advanced, biology, biomedical forensic sciences, crime scene investigation, forensic anthropology, general, impressions evidence, jurisprudence, linguistics, medicolegal death investigation, national security science, nuclear forensics, psychiatry and behavioral science, regulatory science, toxicology; medicolegal death investigation (CAS); MS/JD. *Program availability:* Part-time. *Students:* Average age 25. In 2015, 15 master's awarded. *Degree requirements:* For master's, internship. *Entrance requirements:* For master's, GRE General Test, personal statement, three letters of recommendation, transcripts, telephone interview. Additional exam requirements/recommendations for international students: Required—TOEFL (minimum score 100 iBT). *Application deadline:* For fall admission, 2/15 priority date for domestic and international students; for summer admission, 2/15 for domestic students, 2/16 priority date for international students. Applications are processed on a rolling basis. Application fee: $75. Electronic applications accepted. *Expenses: Tuition, area resident:* Full-time $25,974; part-time $1443 per credit hour. *Required fees:* $802; $50 per course. Tuition and fees vary according to course load and program. *Financial support:* Fellowships with full tuition reimbursements, research assistantships, teaching assistantships, and scholarships/grants available. Financial award application deadline: 1/1; financial award applicants required to submit FAFSA. *Faculty research:* Chemical analysis, molecular genetics, forensic biochemical analysis, forensic entomology, human osteology. *Unit head:* Dr. Michael M. Sponsler, Director of Curricular Programs for the Forensic and National Security Sciences Institute, 315-443-4347, E-mail: sponsler@syr.edu. *Application contact:* Cassidy Perreault, Administrative Specialist, 315-443-2875, E-mail: forensics@syr.edu.
Website: http://forensics.syr.edu/index.html

Syracuse University, School of Education, Programs in Science Education, Syracuse, NY 13244. Offers biology (MS, PhD); chemistry (MS, PhD); earth science (MS, PhD); physics (MS, PhD). *Program availability:* Part-time. *Students:* Average age 38. In 2015, 4 doctorates awarded. *Degree requirements:* For doctorate, comprehensive exam, thesis/dissertation. *Entrance requirements:* For master's, official transcripts from previous academic institutions, 3 letters of recommendation (preferably from faculty), personal statement that makes a clear and compelling argument for why applicant wants to teach secondary science; for doctorate, GRE General Test or MAT, master's degree, interview. Additional exam requirements/recommendations for international students: Required—TOEFL (minimum score 100 iBT). *Application deadline:* For fall admission, 1/15 priority date for domestic and international students; for spring admission, 10/15 priority date for domestic and international students. Applications are processed on a rolling basis. Application fee: $75. Electronic applications accepted. *Expenses: Tuition, area resident:* Full-time $25,974; part-time $1443 per credit hour. *Required fees:* $802; $50 per course. Tuition and fees vary according to course load and program. *Financial support:* Fellowships with full tuition reimbursements, research assistantships with tuition reimbursements, teaching assistantships with tuition reimbursements, and scholarships/grants available. Financial award application deadline: 1/15. *Faculty research:* Diverse field experiences and theoretical and practical knowledge in research-based science teaching, biology, chemistry, earth science, and physics. *Unit head:* Dr. John Tillotson, Program Coordinator, 315-443-9137, E-mail: jwtillot@syr.edu. *Application contact:* Speranza Migliore, Graduate Admissions Recruiter, 315-443-2505, E-mail: gradrcrt@syr.edu.
Website: http://soeweb.syr.edu/

Tarleton State University, College of Graduate Studies, College of Science and Technology, Department of Biological Sciences, Stephenville, TX 76402. Offers biology (MS). *Program availability:* Part-time, evening/weekend. *Faculty:* 11 full-time (2 women), 1 (woman) part-time/adjunct. *Students:* 9 full-time (6 women), 9 part-time (2 women); includes 2 minority (1 Black or African American, non-Hispanic/Latino; 1 Hispanic/Latino). 6 applicants, 67% accepted, 2 enrolled. In 2015, 8 master's awarded. *Degree requirements:* For master's, comprehensive exam, thesis (for some programs). *Entrance requirements:* For master's, GRE General Test, minimum GPA of 3.0. Additional exam requirements/recommendations for international students: Required—TOEFL (minimum score 550 paper-based; 80 iBT). *Application deadline:* For fall admission, 8/15 priority date for domestic students; for spring admission, 1/7 for domestic students. Applications are processed on a rolling basis. Application fee: $45 ($145 for international students). Electronic applications accepted. *Expenses:* Tuition, state resident: part-time $204 per credit hour. Tuition, nonresident: part-time $594 per credit hour. *Required fees:* $1994 per unit. *Financial support:* Research assistantships, teaching assistantships, career-related internships or fieldwork, and Federal Work-Study available. Support available to part-time students. Financial award application deadline: 5/1; financial award applicants required to submit FAFSA. *Unit head:* Dr. Allan Nelson, Department Head, 254-968-9158, E-mail: nelson@tarleton.edu. *Application contact:* Information Contact, 254-968-9104, Fax: 254-968-9670, E-mail: gradoffice@tarleton.edu.
Website: http://www.tarleton.edu/degrees/masters/ms-biology/

Teachers College, Columbia University, Department of Mathematics, Science and Technology, New York, NY 10027-6696. Offers biology 7-12 (MA); chemistry 7-12 (MA); communication and education (MA); communications (Ed M); communications and education (Ed D); computing in education (MA); computing in education-distant learning (MA); earth science 7-12 (MA); instructional technology and media (Ed M, MA, Ed D); mathematics education (Ed M, MA, Ed D, Ed DCT, PhD); physics 7-12 (MA); science and dental education (MA); science education (Ed M, MS, Ed DCT, PhD); supervisor/teacher of science education (MA); technology specialist (MA). *Program availability:* Part-time, evening/weekend. *Students:* 134 full-time (89 women), 285 part-time (168 women); includes 219 minority (49 Black or African American, non-Hispanic/Latino; 124 Asian, non-Hispanic/Latino; 31 Hispanic/Latino; 15 Two or more races, non-Hispanic/Latino), 29 international. Terminal master's awarded for partial completion of doctoral program. *Degree requirements:* For doctorate, thesis/dissertation. *Expenses:* Tuition, area resident: Full-time $1454 per credit. *Required fees:* $428 per semester. One-time fee: $475 full-time. Full-time tuition and fees vary according to course load. *Unit head:* Dr. O. Roger Anderson, Chair, 212-678-3405, Fax: 212-678-8129, E-mail: ora@ldeo.columbia.edu. *Application contact:* David Estrella, Director of Admission, E-mail: estrella@tc.columbia.edu.
Website: http://www.tc.columbia.edu/mathematics-science-and-technology/

Temple University, College of Science and Technology, Department of Biology, Philadelphia, PA 19122. Offers biology (MS, PMS, PhD); biotechnology (MS). *Faculty:* 34 full-time (14 women), 3 part-time/adjunct (1 woman). *Students:* 60 full-time (36 women), 17 part-time (11 women); includes 26 minority (5 Black or African American, non-Hispanic/Latino; 14 Asian, non-Hispanic/Latino; 5 Hispanic/Latino; 2 Two or more races, non-Hispanic/Latino), 15 international. 104 applicants, 48% accepted, 36 enrolled. In 2015, 5 master's, 5 doctorates awarded. Terminal master's awarded for partial completion of doctoral program. *Degree requirements:* For master's, comprehensive exam (for some programs), thesis (for some programs); for doctorate, comprehensive exam (for some programs), thesis/dissertation. *Entrance requirements:* For master's and doctorate, GRE General Test, minimum GPA of 3.0. Additional exam requirements/recommendations for international students: Required—TOEFL (minimum score 550 paper-based; 79 iBT). *Application deadline:* For fall admission, 1/15 for domestic students, 12/15 for international students; for spring admission, 10/15 for domestic students, 8/1 for international students. Applications are processed on a rolling basis. Application fee: $60. *Financial support:* Fellowships, research assistantships, teaching assistantships, Federal Work-Study, and tuition waivers (full) available. Financial award application deadline: 1/15; financial award applicants required to submit FAFSA. *Faculty research:* Membrane proteins, genetics, molecular biology, neuroscience, aquatic biology. *Unit head:* Dr. Allen Nicholson, Chair, 215-204-9048, Fax: 215-204-6646, E-mail: biology@temple.edu. *Website:* https://bio.cst.temple.edu/

Temple University, School of Medicine, Philadelphia, PA 19122-6096. Offers biomedical sciences (MS); MD/MA; MD/MBA; MD/MPH; MD/PhD. *Faculty:* 29 full-time (13 women), 1 (woman) part-time/adjunct. *Students:* 1,025 full-time (488 women), 19 part-time (14 women); includes 354 minority (47 Black or African American, non-Hispanic/Latino; 188 Asian, non-Hispanic/Latino; 87 Hispanic/Latino; 2 Native Hawaiian or other Pacific Islander, non-Hispanic/Latino; 30 Two or more races, non-Hispanic/Latino), 36 international. 170 applicants, 27% accepted, 32 enrolled. In 2015, 18 master's, 227 doctorates awarded. Terminal master's awarded for partial completion of doctoral program. *Degree requirements:* For master's, thesis optional; for doctorate, thesis/dissertation (for some programs), research seminars (for PhD). *Entrance requirements:* For master's, GRE General Test, minimum undergraduate GPA of 3.0; for doctorate, GRE General Test (for PhD); MCAT (for MD), minimum undergraduate GPA of 3.0. Additional exam requirements/recommendations for international students: Required—TOEFL. *Application deadline:* For fall admission, 2/15 for domestic and international students. Application fee: $60. Electronic applications accepted. *Expenses:* Contact institution. *Financial support:* In 2015–16, 70 fellowships with full tuition reimbursements (averaging $26,500 per year), 41 research assistantships with full tuition reimbursements (averaging $26,500 per year) were awarded; scholarships/grants and health care benefits also available. Financial award application deadline: 2/15; financial award applicants required to submit FAFSA. *Faculty research:* Translational medicine, molecular biology and immunology of autoimmune disease and cancer, cardiovascular and pulmonary disease pathophysiology, biology of substance abuse, causes and consequences of obesity, molecular mechanisms of neurological dysfunction. *Unit head:* Dr. Scott K. Shore, Associate Dean, 215-707-2423, Fax: 215-707-5072, E-mail: sks@temple.edu. *Application contact:* Tracy Burton, Office of Admissions, 215-707-2423, E-mail: tusmgrad@temple.edu. *Website:* http://www.temple.edu/medicine/

Tennessee State University, The School of Graduate Studies and Research, College of Agriculture, Human and Natural Sciences, Department of Biological Sciences, Nashville, TN 37209-1561. Offers PhD. *Degree requirements:* For doctorate, thesis/dissertation. *Entrance requirements:* For doctorate, GRE General Test, GRE Subject Test. *Application deadline:* For fall admission, 4/1 priority date for domestic and international students. Applications are processed on a rolling basis. Application fee: $25. *Financial support:* Fellowships, research assistantships, and unspecified assistantships available. Support available to part-time students. *Faculty research:* Cellular and molecular biology and agrobiology. *Unit head:* Dr. Terrance Johnson, Head, 615-963-5681, E-mail: tjohnson@tnstate.edu. *Application contact:* Dr. Terrance Johnson, Head, 615-963-5681, E-mail: tjohnson@tnstate.edu. *Website:* http://www.tnstate.edu/biology/

Tennessee Technological University, College of Graduate Studies, College of Arts and Sciences, Department of Biology, Cookeville, TN 38505. Offers fish, game, and wildlife management (MS). *Program availability:* Part-time. *Faculty:* 22 full-time (2 women). *Students:* 4 full-time (3 women), 17 part-time (9 women); includes 2 minority (1 Black or African American, non-Hispanic/Latino; 1 Hispanic/Latino). Average age 25. 19 applicants, 16% accepted, 3 enrolled. In 2015, 6 master's awarded. *Degree requirements:* For master's, thesis. *Entrance requirements:* For master's, GRE. Additional exam requirements/recommendations for international students: Required—TOEFL (minimum score 527 paper-based; 71 iBT), IELTS (minimum score 5.5), PTE (minimum score 48), or TOEIC (Test of English as an International Communication). *Application deadline:* For fall admission, 8/1 for domestic students, 5/1 for international students; for spring admission, 12/1 for domestic students, 10/1 for international students; for summer admission, 5/1 for domestic students, 2/1 for international students. Applications are processed on a rolling basis. Application fee: $35 ($40 for international students). Electronic applications accepted. *Expenses:* Tuition, state resident: full-time $8961; part-time $6132 per credit hour. Tuition, nonresident: full-time $23,121; part-time $14,608 per credit hour. *Financial support:* In 2015–16, 17 research assistantships (averaging $9,000 per year), 8 teaching assistantships (averaging $7,500 per year) were awarded. Financial award application deadline: 4/1. *Faculty research:* Aquatics, environmental studies. *Unit head:* Dr. Robert Kissell, Chairperson, 931-372-3134, Fax: 931-372-6257, E-mail: rkissell@tntech.edu. *Application contact:* Shelia K. Kendrick, Coordinator of Graduate Studies, 931-372-3808, Fax: 931-372-3497, E-mail: skendrick@tntech.edu.

Tennessee Technological University, College of Graduate Studies, School of Environmental Studies, Department of Environmental Sciences, Cookeville, TN 38505. Offers biology (PhD); chemistry (PhD). *Program availability:* Part-time. *Students:* 4 full-time (0 women), 12 part-time (5 women), 7 international. 13 applicants, 38% accepted, 2 enrolled. In 2015, 5 doctorates awarded. *Degree requirements:* For doctorate, comprehensive exam, thesis/dissertation. *Entrance requirements:* For doctorate, GRE. Additional exam requirements/recommendations for international students: Required—TOEFL (minimum score 527 paper-based; 71 iBT), IELTS (minimum score 5.5), PTE (minimum score 48), or TOEIC (Test of English as an International Communication). *Application deadline:* For fall admission, 8/1 for domestic students, 5/1 for international students; for spring admission, 12/1 for domestic students, 10/2 for international students; for summer admission, 5/1 for domestic students, 2/1 for international students. Applications are processed on a rolling basis. Application fee: $35 ($40 for international students). Electronic applications accepted. *Expenses:* Tuition, state resident: full-time $8961; part-time $6132 per credit hour. Tuition, nonresident: full-time $23,121; part-time $14,608 per credit hour. *Financial support:* In 2015–16, 5 research assistantships (averaging $10,000 per year), 3 teaching assistantships (averaging $10,000 per year) were awarded; fellowships also available. Financial award application deadline: 4/1. *Unit head:* Dr. Hayden Mattingly, Interim Director, 931-372-6246, E-mail:

hmattingly@tntech.edu. *Application contact:* Shelia K. Kendrick, Coordinator of Graduate Studies, 931-372-3808, Fax: 931-372-3497, E-mail: skendrick@tntech.edu.

Texas A&M International University, Office of Graduate Studies and Research, College of Arts and Sciences, Department of Biology and Chemistry, Laredo, TX 78041-1900. Offers biology (MS). *Degree requirements:* For master's, comprehensive exam, thesis (for some programs). *Entrance requirements:* Additional exam requirements/recommendations for international students: Required—TOEFL (minimum score 79 iBT).

Texas A&M University, College of Science, Department of Biology, College Station, TX 77843. Offers biology (MS, PhD); microbiology (MS, PhD). *Faculty:* 37. *Students:* 97 full-time (58 women), 4 part-time (2 women); includes 13 minority (2 Black or African American, non-Hispanic/Latino; 1 American Indian or Alaska Native, non-Hispanic/Latino; 2 Asian, non-Hispanic/Latino; 7 Hispanic/Latino; 1 Two or more races, non-Hispanic/Latino), 52 international. Average age 28. 97 applicants, 24% accepted, 12 enrolled. In 2015, 3 master's, 7 doctorates awarded. *Degree requirements:* For master's, thesis or alternative; for doctorate, comprehensive exam, thesis/dissertation. *Entrance requirements:* For master's and doctorate, GRE General Test. Additional exam requirements/recommendations for international students: Required—TOEFL. *Application deadline:* For fall admission, 1/15 for domestic students. Applications are processed on a rolling basis. Application fee: $50 ($90 for international students). Electronic applications accepted. *Expenses:* Contact institution. *Financial support:* In 2015–16, 102 students received support, including 7 fellowships with tuition reimbursements available (averaging $23,990 per year), 29 research assistantships with tuition reimbursements available (averaging $8,464 per year), 63 teaching assistantships with tuition reimbursements available (averaging $8,222 per year); career-related internships or fieldwork, institutionally sponsored loans, scholarships/grants, traineeships, health care benefits, tuition waivers (full and partial), and unspecified assistantships also available. Support available to part-time students. Financial award application deadline: 4/1; financial award applicants required to submit FAFSA. *Faculty research:* Biological clocks, cell, molecular and developmental biology, ecology and evolutionary biology, genetics and genomics, microbiology. *Unit head:* Dr. Tom McKnight, Department Head, 979-845-3896, Fax: 979-845-2891, E-mail: mcknight@bio.tamu.edu. *Application contact:* Dr. Arne Lekven, Graduate Advisor, 979-458-3461, Fax: 979-845-2891, E-mail: alekven@bio.tamu.edu. *Website:* http://www.bio.tamu.edu/index.html

Texas A&M University–Corpus Christi, College of Graduate Studies, College of Science and Engineering, Program in Biology, Corpus Christi, TX 78412-5503. Offers MS. *Program availability:* Part-time, evening/weekend. *Students:* 11 full-time (9 women), 8 part-time (3 women); includes 2 minority (1 Asian, non-Hispanic/Latino; 1 Hispanic/Latino). Average age 29. 11 applicants, 36% accepted, 3 enrolled. In 2015, 5 master's awarded. *Degree requirements:* For master's, comprehensive exam, thesis (for some programs), thesis or project. *Entrance requirements:* For master's, GRE General Test (taken within 5 years), essay (up to 1000 words), 3 letters of recommendation. Additional exam requirements/recommendations for international students: Required—TOEFL (minimum score 550 paper-based; 79 iBT), IELTS (minimum score 6.5). *Application deadline:* For fall admission, 2/1 priority date for domestic and international students; for spring admission, 8/1 priority date for domestic students, 6/1 priority date for international students; for summer admission, 2/1 priority date for domestic and international students. Applications are processed on a rolling basis. Application fee: $50 ($70 for international students). Electronic applications accepted. *Financial support:* Research assistantships, teaching assistantships, institutionally sponsored loans, scholarships/grants, health care benefits, and unspecified assistantships available. Support available to part-time students. Financial award application deadline: 3/15. *Unit head:* Dr. Kim Withers, Coordinator, 361-825-3259, Fax: 361-825-2742, E-mail: david.moury@tamucc.edu. *Application contact:* Graduate Admissions Coordinator, 361-825-2177, Fax: 361-825-2755, E-mail: gradweb@tamucc.edu. *Website:* http://www.biol.tamucc.edu/ms/

Texas A&M University–Kingsville, College of Graduate Studies, College of Arts and Sciences, Department of Biological and Health Sciences, Kingsville, TX 78363. Offers biology (MS). *Faculty:* 12 full-time (2 women). *Students:* 21 full-time (10 women), 8 part-time (6 women); includes 10 minority (all Hispanic/Latino), 16 international. Average age 25. 16 applicants, 100% accepted, 8 enrolled. In 2015, 6 master's awarded. *Entrance requirements:* Additional exam requirements/recommendations for international students: Required—TOEFL (minimum score 550 paper-based; 79 iBT); Recommended—IELTS (minimum score 6). *Application deadline:* Applications are processed on a rolling basis. Application fee: $35 ($50 for international students). Electronic applications accepted. *Unit head:* Glenn Perrigo, Interim Chair, Department of Biological and Health Sciences, 361-593-4170, Fax: 361-593-3800, E-mail: glenn-perrigo@tamuk.edu.

Texas Christian University, College of Science and Engineering, Department of Biology, Fort Worth, TX 76129. Offers MA, MS. *Program availability:* Part-time. *Faculty:* 11 full-time (3 women). *Students:* 12 full-time (10 women); includes 2 minority (1 Hispanic/Latino; 1 Two or more races, non-Hispanic/Latino). Average age 24. 20 applicants, 65% accepted, 7 enrolled. In 2015, 4 master's awarded. *Degree requirements:* For master's, thesis (for some programs). *Entrance requirements:* For master's, GRE General Test. Additional exam requirements/recommendations for international students: Required—TOEFL (minimum score 560 paper-based). *Application deadline:* For fall admission, 2/1 priority date for domestic students, 1/15 for international students; for spring admission, 9/1 priority date for domestic students, 8/15 for international students. Applications are processed on a rolling basis. Application fee: $60. Electronic applications accepted. *Expenses: Tuition, area resident:* Full-time $26,640; part-time $1480 per credit hour. *Required fees:* $48; $48 per unit. Tuition and fees vary according to program. *Financial support:* In 2015–16, 13 students received support, including 13 teaching assistantships with full tuition reimbursements available (averaging $16,000 per year). Financial award application deadline: 2/1. *Faculty research:* Invasive species, anthrax, mercury contamination in food webs, ecological impacts of wind turbines, toxicology. *Total annual research expenditures:* $729,849. *Unit head:* Dr. Ray Drenner, Chairperson, 817-257-7165, E-mail: r.drenner@tcu.edu. *Application contact:* Dr. Amanda Hale, Associate Professor, 817-257-6182, E-mail: a.hale@tcu.edu. *Website:* http://www.bio.tcu.edu/

Texas Southern University, School of Science and Technology, Department of Biology, Houston, TX 77004-4584. Offers MS. *Program availability:* Part-time, evening/weekend. *Degree requirements:* For master's, one foreign language, comprehensive exam, thesis. *Entrance requirements:* For master's, GRE General Test, minimum GPA of 2.5. Additional exam requirements/recommendations for international students: Required—TOEFL. Electronic applications accepted. *Faculty research:* Microbiology, cell and molecular biology, biochemistry, biochemical virology, biophysics.

Texas State University, The Graduate College, College of Science and Engineering, Program in Biology, San Marcos, TX 78666. Offers MA, MS. *Program availability:* Part-time. *Faculty:* 12 full-time (4 women), 1 part-time/adjunct (0 women). *Students:* 33 full-time (20 women), 14 part-time (9 women); includes 11 minority (1 Black or African American, non-Hispanic/Latino; 10 Hispanic/Latino), 9 international. Average age 29. 31

Biological and Biomedical Sciences—General

applicants, 55% accepted, 13 enrolled. In 2015, 20 master's awarded. *Degree requirements:* For master's, comprehensive exam, thesis (for some programs). *Entrance requirements:* For master's, GRE General Test (recommended minimum score in at least the 50th percentile on both the verbal and quantitative portions), baccalaureate degree in biology or related discipline from regionally-accredited university with minimum GPA of 3.0 on last 60 undergraduate semester hours, current curriculum vitae, statement of purpose, 3 letters of recommendation, letter of intent to mentor from faculty member of Biology Department. Additional exam requirements/recommendations for international students: Required—TOEFL (minimum score 550 paper-based; 78 iBT). *Application deadline:* For fall admission, 2/1 priority date for domestic and international students; for spring admission, 10/15 for domestic students, 10/1 for international students; for summer admission, 4/15 for domestic students, 3/15 for international students. Applications are processed on a rolling basis. Application fee: $40 ($90 for international students). Electronic applications accepted. *Expenses:* $3,615 in-state tuition (for 12 semester credit hours/1 full-time semester), $974 in-state fees. *Financial support:* In 2015–16, 31 students received support, including 4 research assistantships (averaging $12,826 per year), 31 teaching assistantships (averaging $13,584 per year); Federal Work-Study, institutionally sponsored loans, scholarships/grants, health care benefits, and unspecified assistantships also available. Support available to part-time students. Financial award application deadline: 3/1; financial award applicants required to submit FAFSA. *Faculty research:* Pax6 as a mediator of ocular development in Texas Blind and San Marcos Salamander, improving teacher quality, using an extensively documented and validated habitat suitability model, characterization of new arabidopsis mutants with altered response. *Total annual research expenditures:* $420,662. *Unit head:* Dr. David Lemke, Graduate Advisor, 512-245-2178, E-mail: dl10@txstate.edu. *Application contact:* Dr. Andrea Golato, Dean of the Graduate School, 512-245-2581, Fax: 512-245-8365, E-mail: jw02@swt.edu.
Website: http://www.bio.txstate.edu/

Texas Tech University, Graduate School, College of Arts and Sciences, Department of Biological Sciences, Lubbock, TX 79409-3131. Offers biology (MS, PhD); environmental sustainability and natural resources management (PSM); microbiology (MS); zoology (MS, PhD). *Program availability:* Part-time, blended/hybrid learning. *Faculty:* 41 full-time (12 women), 2 part-time/adjunct (1 woman). *Students:* 94 full-time (51 women), 5 part-time (3 women); includes 6 minority (1 American Indian or Alaska Native, non-Hispanic/Latino; 1 Asian, non-Hispanic/Latino; 3 Hispanic/Latino; 1 Two or more races, non-Hispanic/Latino), 53 international. Average age 29. 92 applicants, 39% accepted, 21 enrolled. In 2015, 7 master's, 9 doctorates awarded. *Degree requirements:* For master's, thesis or alternative; for doctorate, thesis/dissertation. *Entrance requirements:* For master's and doctorate, GRE General Test. Additional exam requirements/recommendations for international students: Required—TOEFL (minimum score 550 paper-based; 79 iBT). *Application deadline:* For fall admission, 6/1 priority date for domestic students, 1/15 priority date for international students; for spring admission, 9/1 priority date for domestic students, 6/15 priority date for international students. Applications are processed on a rolling basis. Application fee: $60. Electronic applications accepted. *Expenses:* Tuition, state resident: full-time $6477; part-time $269.89 per credit hour. Tuition, nonresident: full-time $15,837; part-time $659.89 per credit hour. *Required fees:* $2751; $36.50 per credit hour. $937.50 per semester. Tuition and fees vary according to course level. *Financial support:* In 2015–16, 98 students received support, including 79 fellowships (averaging $1,515 per year), 36 research assistantships (averaging $6,272 per year), 98 teaching assistantships (averaging $13,936 per year). Financial award application deadline: 4/15; financial award applicants required to submit FAFSA. *Faculty research:* Biodiversity, genomics and evolution, climate change in arid ecosystems, plant biology and biotechnology, animal communication and behavior, zoonotic and emerging diseases. *Total annual research expenditures:* $1.4 million. *Unit head:* Dr. Ron Chesser, Chair, 806-834-0121, Fax: 806-742-2963, E-mail: ron.chesser@ttu.edu. *Application contact:* Dr. Lou Densmore, Graduate Adviser, 806-834-6479, Fax: 806-742-2963, E-mail: lou.densmore@ttu.edu. Website: http://www.depts.ttu.edu/biology/

Texas Tech University Health Sciences Center, Graduate School of Biomedical Sciences, Lubbock, TX 79430-0002. Offers MS, PhD, MD/PhD, MS/PhD. Terminal master's awarded for partial completion of doctoral program. *Degree requirements:* For master's, thesis; for doctorate, thesis/dissertation. *Entrance requirements:* For master's and doctorate, GRE General Test, minimum GPA of 3.0. Additional exam requirements/recommendations for international students: Required—TOEFL (minimum score 550 paper-based). Electronic applications accepted. *Faculty research:* Genetics of neurological disorders, hemodynamics to prevent DVT, toxin A synthesis, DA neurons, peroxidases.

Texas Woman's University, Graduate School, College of Arts and Sciences, Department of Biology, Denton, TX 76201. Offers biology (MS); molecular biology (PhD). *Program availability:* Part-time. Terminal master's awarded for partial completion of doctoral program. *Degree requirements:* For master's, comprehensive exam, thesis; for doctorate, comprehensive exam, thesis/dissertation, residency. *Entrance requirements:* For master's, GRE General Test (preferred minimum score 149 [425 old version] verbal, 141 [425 old version] quantitative), 3 letters of reference; letter of interest; for doctorate, GRE General Test (preferred minimum score 153 [500 old version] verbal, 144 [500 old version] quantitative), 3 letters of reference, letter of interest. Additional exam requirements/recommendations for international students: Required—TOEFL (minimum score 550 paper-based; 79 iBT). *Application deadline:* For fall admission, 2/1 priority date for domestic students, 2/1 for international students. Applications are processed on a rolling basis. Application fee: $50 ($75 for international students). Electronic applications accepted. *Expenses:* Tuition, state resident: full-time $4380; part-time $243 per credit hour. Tuition, nonresident: full-time $11,400; part-time $633 per credit hour. *International tuition:* $11,465 full-time. *Required fees:* $1778; $99 per credit hour. $283 per semester. One-time fee: $50. Tuition and fees vary according to course load and program. *Financial support:* Research assistantships, career-related internships or fieldwork, Federal Work-Study, institutionally sponsored loans, scholarships/grants, traineeships, health care benefits, and unspecified assistantships available. Support available to part-time students. Financial award application deadline: 3/1; financial award applicants required to submit FAFSA. *Faculty research:* Computational biology, protein-protein interactions, chromatin structure and regulation, regulation of RNA synthesis, virus-host interactions, regulation of axon growth and guidance in neurons, estrogen compounds in plants, regulation of gene expression in male reproductive tissues, female gonadal hormones in the development of anxiety and depression, electron microscopy. *Unit head:* Dr. DiAnna Hynds, Interim Co-Chair, 940-898-2359, Fax: 940-898-2382, E-mail: dhynds@twu.edu. *Application contact:* Dr. Samuel Wheeler, Assistant Director of Admissions, 940-898-3188, Fax: 940-898-3081, E-mail: wheelersr@twu.edu.
Website: http://www.twu.edu/biology

Thomas Jefferson University, Jefferson College of Biomedical Sciences, Philadelphia, PA 19107. Offers MS, PhD, Certificate, MD/PhD. *Program availability:* Part-time, evening/weekend. *Faculty:* 190 full-time (53 women), 37 part-time/adjunct (15 women). *Students:* 124 full-time (69 women), 78 part-time (42 women); includes 42 minority (10 Black or African American, non-Hispanic/Latino; 22 Asian, non-Hispanic/Latino; 10 Hispanic/Latino), 27 international. 277 applicants, 38% accepted, 77 enrolled. In 2015,

36 master's, 18 doctorates, 3 other advanced degrees awarded. Terminal master's awarded for partial completion of doctoral program. *Degree requirements:* For master's, thesis; for doctorate, comprehensive exam, thesis/dissertation. *Entrance requirements:* For master's, GRE or MCAT; for doctorate, GRE or MCAT, minimum GPA of 3.2. Additional exam requirements/recommendations for international students: Required—TOEFL (minimum score 100 iBT), IELTS (minimum score 7). *Application deadline:* Applications are processed on a rolling basis. Application fee: $50. Electronic applications accepted. *Financial support:* Fellowships, Federal Work-Study, institutionally sponsored loans, scholarships/grants, and traineeships available. Support available to part-time students. Financial award application deadline: 5/1; financial award applicants required to submit FAFSA. *Unit head:* Dr. Gerald B. Grunwald, Dean, 215-503-4191, Fax: 215-503-6690, E-mail: gerald.grunwald@jefferson.edu. *Application contact:* Marc E. Stearns, Director of Admissions, 215-503-0155, Fax: 215-503-3433, E-mail: jgsbs-info@jefferson.edu.
Website: http://www.jefferson.edu/university/biomedical-sciences.html

Towson University, Program in Biology, Towson, MD 21252-0001. Offers MS. *Program availability:* Part-time, evening/weekend. *Students:* 20 full-time (11 women), 24 part-time (12 women); includes 11 minority (7 Black or African American, non-Hispanic/Latino; 3 Asian, non-Hispanic/Latino; 1 Two or more races, non-Hispanic/Latino), 2 international. *Degree requirements:* For master's, thesis optional. *Entrance requirements:* For master's, GRE General Test (for thesis students), minimum GPA of 3.0; 24 credits in related course work; 3 letters of recommendation; minimum 24 units in biology; coursework in chemistry, organic chemistry, and physics; personal statement; official transcripts. Application fee: $45. Electronic applications accepted. *Expenses:* Tuition, state resident: full-time $7440; part-time $372 per unit. Tuition, nonresident: full-time $15,400; part-time $770 per unit. *Required fees:* $2360; $118 per year. $354 per term. *Financial support:* Application deadline: 4/1. *Unit head:* Dr. John Lapolla, Graduate Program Co-Director, 410-704-3121, E-mail: jlapolla@towson.edu. *Application contact:* Alicia Arkell-Kleis, University Admissions, 410-704-2113, Fax: 410-704-3030, E-mail: grads@towson.edu.
Website: http://grad.towson.edu/program/master/biol-ms/

Trent University, Graduate Studies, Program in Applications of Modeling in the Natural and Social Sciences, Peterborough, ON K9J 7B8, Canada. Offers applications of modeling in the natural and social sciences (MA); biology (M Sc, PhD); chemistry (M Sc); computer studies (M Sc); geography (M Sc, PhD); physics (M Sc). *Program availability:* Part-time. *Degree requirements:* For master's, thesis. *Entrance requirements:* For master's, honours degree. *Faculty research:* Computation of heat transfer, atmospheric physics, statistical mechanics, stress and coping, evolutionary ecology.

Trent University, Graduate Studies, Program in Environmental and Life Sciences and Program in Applications of Modeling in the Natural and Social Sciences, Department of Biology, Peterborough, ON K9J 7B8, Canada. Offers M Sc, PhD. *Program availability:* Part-time. *Degree requirements:* For master's, thesis; for doctorate, thesis/dissertation. *Entrance requirements:* For master's, honours degree; for doctorate, master's degree. *Faculty research:* Aquatic and behavioral ecology, hydrology and limnology, human impact on ecosystems, behavioral ecology of birds, ecology of fish.

Troy University, Graduate School, College of Arts and Sciences, Program in Biomedical Sciences, Troy, AL 36082. Offers MS, Certificate. *Program availability:* Part-time, evening/weekend. *Faculty:* 8 full-time (2 women). *Students:* 13 full-time (6 women), 10 part-time (4 women); includes 18 minority (7 Black or African American, non-Hispanic/Latino; 11 Two or more races, non-Hispanic/Latino). Average age 26. 30 applicants, 93% accepted. In 2015, 3 master's awarded. *Degree requirements:* For master's, comprehensive exam. *Entrance requirements:* For master's, GRE (minimum score of 850 on old exam or 290 on new exam), MAT (minimum score of 385), or GMAT (minimum score of 380), baccalaureate degree, official transcripts, two letters of recommendation, 500-word personal statement. Additional exam requirements/recommendations for international students: Required—TOEFL (minimum score 523 paper-based; 70 iBT), IELTS (minimum score 6). *Application deadline:* For fall admission, 6/1 for international students; for spring admission, 10/15 for international students. Applications are processed on a rolling basis. Application fee: $50. Electronic applications accepted. *Expenses:* Tuition, state resident: full-time $7146; part-time $397 per credit hour. Tuition, nonresident: full-time $14,292; part-time $794 per credit hour. *Required fees:* $802. Tuition and fees vary according to campus/location and program. *Financial support:* Fellowships, career-related internships or fieldwork, and scholarships/grants available. Support available to part-time students. Financial award applicants required to submit FAFSA. *Unit head:* Prof. Janet Gaston, Health Professional Advisor. *Application contact:* Jessica A. Kimbro, Director of Graduate Admissions, 334-670-3178, E-mail: jacord@troy.edu.

Troy University, Graduate School, College of Arts and Sciences, Program in Environmental and Biological Sciences, Troy, AL 36082. Offers biological science (MS); environmental policy (MS); environmental science (MS). *Program availability:* Part-time, evening/weekend, 100% online, blended/hybrid learning. *Faculty:* 9 full-time (6 women), 1 (woman) part-time/adjunct. *Students:* 14 full-time (7 women), 28 part-time (16 women); includes 10 minority (6 Black or African American, non-Hispanic/Latino; 2 Asian, non-Hispanic/Latino; 1 Hispanic/Latino; 1 Two or more races, non-Hispanic/Latino). Average age 28. 35 applicants, 91% accepted, 9 enrolled. In 2015, 10 master's awarded. *Degree requirements:* For master's, comprehensive exam (for some programs), thesis (for some programs), comprehensive exam or thesis, minimum GPA of 3.0, admission to candidacy. *Entrance requirements:* For master's, GRE (minimum score of 850 on old exam or 290 on new exam), MAT (minimum score of 385) or GMAT (minimum score of 380), bachelor's degree; minimum undergraduate GPA of 2.5 or 3.0 on last 30 semester hours. Additional exam requirements/recommendations for international students: Required—TOEFL (minimum score 523 paper-based; 70 iBT), IELTS (minimum score 6). *Application deadline:* Applications are processed on a rolling basis. Application fee: $50. Electronic applications accepted. *Expenses:* Tuition, state resident: full-time $7146; part-time $397 per credit hour. Tuition, nonresident: full-time $14,292; part-time $794 per credit hour. *Required fees:* $802. Tuition and fees vary according to campus/location and program. *Financial support:* Fellowships, career-related internships or fieldwork, and scholarships/grants available. Support available to part-time students. *Unit head:* Dr. Glenn Cohen, Divisional Chairman, 334-670-3660, Fax: 334-670-3401, E-mail: gcohen@troy.edu. *Application contact:* Jessica A. Kimbro, Director of Graduate Admissions, 334-670-3178, E-mail: jacord@troy.edu.

Truman State University, Graduate School, School of Arts and Letters, Program in Biology, Kirksville, MO 63501-4221. Offers MS. *Degree requirements:* For master's, comprehensive exam, thesis. *Entrance requirements:* For master's, GRE General Test, minimum GPA of 3.0. Additional exam requirements/recommendations for international students: Required—TOEFL (minimum score 550 paper-based). *Application deadline:* For fall admission, 6/1 for domestic and international students; for spring admission, 11/1 for domestic and international students; for summer admission, 4/1 for domestic and international students. Applications are processed on a rolling basis. Application fee: $40. Electronic applications accepted. *Expenses:* Tuition, state resident: full-time $6870; part-time $343.50 per credit hour. Tuition, nonresident: full-time $11,790; part-time $589.50 per credit hour. Tuition and fees vary according to course load and program. *Financial support:* Research assistantships with tuition reimbursements, teaching assistantships with tuition reimbursements, career-related internships or fieldwork, and Federal Work-Study available. Financial award application deadline: 5/1; financial award applicants required to submit FAFSA. *Unit head:* Dr. Laura Fielden-Rechav, Director, 660-785-4624. *Application contact:* Stephanie Rudolph, Graduate Office Secretary, 660-785-4109, Fax: 660-785-7460, E-mail: sdunn@truman.edu.

Tufts University, Cummings School of Veterinary Medicine, North Grafton, MA 01536. Offers animals and public policy (MS); biomedical sciences (PhD), including digestive diseases, infectious diseases, neuroscience and reproductive biology, pathology; conservation medicine (MS); veterinary medicine (DVM); DVM/MPH; DVM/MS. *Accreditation:* AVMA (one or more programs are accredited). *Degree requirements:* For master's, thesis (for some programs); for doctorate, comprehensive exam, thesis/dissertation (for some programs). *Entrance requirements:* For master's and doctorate, GRE General Test. Additional exam requirements/recommendations for international students: Required—TOEFL or IELTS. Electronic applications accepted. *Expenses:* Contact institution. *Faculty research:* Oncology, veterinary ethics, international veterinary medicine, veterinary genomics, pathogenesis of Clostridium difficile, wildlife fertility control.

Tufts University, Graduate School of Arts and Sciences, Department of Biology, Medford, MA 02155. Offers biology (MS, PhD); soft materials robotics (PhD). *Program availability:* Part-time. Terminal master's awarded for partial completion of doctoral program. *Degree requirements:* For master's, thesis (for some programs); for doctorate, thesis/dissertation. *Entrance requirements:* For master's and doctorate, GRE General Test. Additional exam requirements/recommendations for international students: Required—TOEFL (minimum score 550 paper-based; 80 iBT), IELTS (minimum score 6.5). Electronic applications accepted. *Expenses: Tuition, area resident:* Full-time $48,412; part-time $1210 per credit hour. *Required fees:* $806. Full-time tuition and fees vary according to degree level, program and student level. Part-time tuition and fees vary according to course load.

Tufts University, Sackler School of Graduate Biomedical Sciences, Boston, MA 02111. Offers MS, PhD, Certificate, DVM/PhD, MD/PhD. *Faculty:* 200 full-time (60 women). *Students:* 228 full-time (140 women), 3 part-time (1 woman); includes 55 minority (10 Black or African American, non-Hispanic/Latino; 29 Asian, non-Hispanic/Latino; 8 Hispanic/Latino; 8 Two or more races, non-Hispanic/Latino), 41 international. Average age 33. 623 applicants, 14% accepted, 46 enrolled. In 2015, 7 master's, 28 doctorates, 4 other advanced degrees awarded. Terminal master's awarded for partial completion of doctoral program. *Degree requirements:* For master's, comprehensive exam (for some programs), thesis; for doctorate, thesis/dissertation. *Entrance requirements:* For doctorate, GRE General Test, 3 letters of reference. Additional exam requirements/recommendations for international students: Required—TOEFL (minimum score 600 paper-based; 100 iBT). *Application deadline:* For fall admission, 12/15 priority date for domestic and international students. Application fee: $70. Electronic applications accepted. *Expenses:* $19,626 per year tuition. *Financial support:* In 2015–16, 175 research assistantships with full tuition reimbursements (averaging $32,000 per year) were awarded; traineeships and health care benefits also available. Financial award application deadline: 12/15. *Unit head:* Dr. Naomi Rosenberg, Dean, 617-636-6767, Fax: 617-636-0375, E-mail: naomi.rosenberg@tufts.edu. *Application contact:* Dr. Elizabeth Storrs, Registrar/Director of Enrollment Services, 617-636-6767, Fax: 617-636-0375, E-mail: sackler-school@tufts.edu.
Website: http://sackler.tufts.edu/

Tulane University, School of Medicine and School of Liberal Arts, Graduate Programs in Biomedical Sciences, New Orleans, LA 70118-5669. Offers MS, PhD, MD/PhD. *Degree requirements:* For doctorate, thesis/dissertation. *Entrance requirements:* For master's, GRE General Test, minimum B average in undergraduate course work; for doctorate, GRE General Test. Additional exam requirements/recommendations for international students: Required—TOEFL. *Application deadline:* For fall admission, 2/1 for domestic and international students. Application fee: $61. *Expenses:* Contact institution. *Financial support:* Fellowships, research assistantships, teaching assistantships, career-related internships or fieldwork, Federal Work-Study, institutionally sponsored loans, scholarships/grants, traineeships, tuition waivers (full), and unspecified assistantships available. Financial award application deadline: 2/1; financial award applicants required to submit FAFSA.

Tuskegee University, Graduate Programs, College of Arts and Sciences, Department of Biology, Tuskegee, AL 36088. Offers MS. *Degree requirements:* For master's, thesis. *Entrance requirements:* For master's, GRE General Test, GRE Subject Test. Additional exam requirements/recommendations for international students: Required—TOEFL (minimum score 500 paper-based).

Tuskegee University, Graduate Programs, Program in Integrative Biosciences, Tuskegee, AL 36088. Offers PhD. *Degree requirements:* For doctorate, thesis/dissertation. *Entrance requirements:* For doctorate, GRE General Test, GRE Subject Test, minimum cumulative GPA of 3.0, 3.4 in upper-division courses; 3 letters of recommendation; resume or curriculum vitae. Additional exam requirements/recommendations for international students: Required—TOEFL (minimum score 500 paper-based). Electronic applications accepted.

Uniformed Services University of the Health Sciences, F. Edward Hebert School of Medicine, Graduate Programs in the Biomedical Sciences and Public Health, Bethesda, MD 20814. Offers emerging infectious diseases (PhD); medical and clinical psychology (PhD), including clinical psychology, medical psychology; medicine (MS, PhD), including health professions education; molecular and cell biology (MS, PhD); neuroscience (PhD); preventive medicine and biometrics (MPH, MS, MSPH, MTMH, Dr PH, PhD), including environmental health sciences (PhD), healthcare administration and policy (MS), medical zoology (PhD), public health (MPH, MSPH, Dr PH), tropical medicine and hygiene (MTMH). *Faculty:* 372 full-time (119 women), 4,044 part-time/adjunct (908 women). *Students:* 240 full-time (133 women); includes 40 minority (15 Black or African American, non-Hispanic/Latino; 13 Asian, non-Hispanic/Latino; 12 Hispanic/Latino), 30 international. Average age 25. 598 applicants, 17% accepted, 77 enrolled. In 2015, 19 master's, 50 doctorates awarded. Terminal master's awarded for partial completion of doctoral program. *Degree requirements:* For master's, comprehensive exam, thesis or alternative; for doctorate, comprehensive exam, thesis/dissertation, qualifying exam. *Entrance requirements:* For master's, GRE General Test; for doctorate, GRE General Test, minimum GPA of 3.0. *Application deadline:* For fall admission, 12/15 priority date for domestic students. Applications are processed on a rolling basis. Application fee: $0. Electronic applications accepted. *Financial support:* In 2015–16, 50 fellowships (averaging $43,000 per year) were awarded; research assistantships, career-related internships or fieldwork, scholarships/grants, health care benefits, and tuition waivers (full) also available. *Unit head:* Dr. Gregory Mueller, Associate Dean, 301-295-3507, E-mail: gregory.mueller@usuhs.edu. *Application contact:* Tina Finley, Administrative Officer, 301-295-3642, Fax: 301-295-6772, E-mail: netina.finley@usuhs.edu.
Website: http://www.usuhs.mil/graded

Universidad Central del Caribe, School of Medicine, Program in Biomedical Sciences, Bayamón, PR 00960-6032. Offers anatomy and cell biology (MA, MS); biochemistry (MS); biomedical sciences (MA); cellular and molecular biology (PhD); microbiology and immunology (MA, MS); pharmacology (MS); physiology (MS).

Universidad de Ciencias Medicas, Graduate Programs, San Jose, Costa Rica. Offers dermatology (SP); family health (MS); health service center administration (MHA); human anatomy (MS); medical and surgery (MD); occupational medicine (MS); pharmacy (Pharm D). *Program availability:* Part-time. *Degree requirements:* For master's, thesis; for doctorate and SP, comprehensive exam. *Entrance requirements:* For master's, MD or bachelor's degree; for doctorate, admissions test; for SP, admissions test, MD.

Université de Moncton, Faculty of Sciences, Department of Biology, Moncton, NB E1A 3E9, Canada. Offers M Sc. *Degree requirements:* For master's, one foreign language, thesis. *Entrance requirements:* For master's, minimum GPA of 3.0. Electronic applications accepted. *Faculty research:* Terrestrial ecology, aquatic ecology, marine biology, aquaculture, ethology, biotechnology.

Université de Montréal, Faculty of Arts and Sciences, Department of Biological Sciences, Montréal, QC H3C 3J7, Canada. Offers M Sc, PhD. *Program availability:* Part-time. *Degree requirements:* For master's, thesis; for doctorate, thesis/dissertation, general exam. *Entrance requirements:* For doctorate, MS in biology or related field. Electronic applications accepted. *Faculty research:* Fresh water ecology, plant biotechnology, neurobiology, genetics, cell physiology.

Université de Montréal, Faculty of Medicine, Programs in Biomedical Sciences, Montréal, QC H3C 3J7, Canada. Offers M Sc, PhD. *Degree requirements:* For master's, thesis; for doctorate, thesis/dissertation, general exam. *Entrance requirements:* For master's and doctorate, proficiency in French, knowledge of English. Electronic applications accepted.

Université de Sherbrooke, Faculty of Medicine and Health Sciences, Graduate Programs in Medicine, Sherbrooke, QC J1H 5N4, Canada. Offers M Sc, PhD. *Program availability:* Part-time. Terminal master's awarded for partial completion of doctoral program. *Degree requirements:* For master's, thesis; for doctorate, thesis/dissertation. Electronic applications accepted. *Expenses:* Contact institution.

Université de Sherbrooke, Faculty of Sciences, Department of Biology, Sherbrooke, QC J1K 2R1, Canada. Offers M Sc, PhD, Diploma. *Degree requirements:* For master's, thesis; for doctorate, comprehensive exam, thesis/dissertation. *Entrance requirements:* For doctorate, master's degree. Electronic applications accepted. *Faculty research:* Microbiology, ecology, molecular biology, cell biology, biotechnology.

Université du Québec à Montréal, Graduate Programs, Program in Biology, Montréal, QC H3C 3P8, Canada. Offers M Sc, PhD. *Program availability:* Part-time. *Degree requirements:* For master's, thesis; for doctorate, thesis/dissertation. *Entrance requirements:* For master's, appropriate bachelor's degree or equivalent, proficiency in French; for doctorate, appropriate master's degree or equivalent, proficiency in French.

Université du Québec en Abitibi-Témiscamingue, Graduate Programs, Program in Environmental Sciences, Rouyn-Noranda, QC J9X 5E4, Canada. Offers biology (MS); environmental sciences (PhD); sustainable forest ecosystem management (MS).

Université du Québec, Institut National de la Recherche Scientifique, Graduate Programs, Research Center–INRS–Institut Armand-Frappier, Laval, QC H7V 1B7, Canada. Offers applied microbiology (M Sc); biology (PhD); experimental health sciences (M Sc); virology and immunology (M Sc, PhD). *Program availability:* Part-time. *Degree requirements:* For master's, thesis; for doctorate, thesis/dissertation. *Entrance requirements:* For master's, appropriate bachelor's degree, proficiency in French; for doctorate, appropriate master's degree, proficiency in French. Electronic applications accepted. *Faculty research:* Immunity, infection and cancer; toxicology and environmental biotechnology; molecular pharmacochemistry.

Université Laval, Faculty of Medicine, Graduate Programs in Medicine, Québec, QC G1K 7P4, Canada. Offers M Sc, PhD, Diploma. *Degree requirements:* For doctorate, comprehensive exam, thesis/dissertation. *Entrance requirements:* For doctorate, knowledge of French, comprehension of written English; for Diploma, knowledge of French. Electronic applications accepted.

Université Laval, Faculty of Sciences and Engineering, Department of Biology, Programs in Biology, Québec, QC G1K 7P4, Canada. Offers M Sc, PhD. Terminal master's awarded for partial completion of doctoral program. *Degree requirements:* For master's, thesis; for doctorate, comprehensive exam, thesis/dissertation. *Entrance requirements:* For master's and doctorate, knowledge of French and English. Electronic applications accepted.

University at Albany, State University of New York, College of Arts and Sciences, Department of Biological Sciences, Albany, NY 12222-0001. Offers biodiversity, conservation, and policy (MS); ecology and evolutionary biology (PhD); forensic biology (MS); molecular, cellular, developmental, and neural biology (PhD). *Degree requirements:* For master's, one foreign language; for doctorate, one foreign language, thesis/dissertation. *Entrance requirements:* For master's and doctorate, GRE General Test. Additional exam requirements/recommendations for international students: Required—TOEFL (minimum score 550 paper-based). Electronic applications accepted. *Faculty research:* Interferon, neural development, RNA self-splicing, behavioral ecology, DNA repair enzymes.

University at Albany, State University of New York, School of Public Health, Department of Biomedical Sciences, Albany, NY 12222-0001. Offers immunobiology and infectious diseases (MS, PhD); neuroscience (MS, PhD); structural and cell biology (MS, PhD). *Degree requirements:* For master's, thesis; for doctorate, comprehensive exam, thesis/dissertation. *Entrance requirements:* For master's and doctorate, GRE General Test, 3 letters of reference. Additional exam requirements/recommendations for international students: Required—TOEFL (minimum score 600 paper-based). Electronic applications accepted. *Faculty research:* Geno expression; RNA processing; membrane transport; immune response regulation; etiology of AIDS, Lyme disease, epilepsy.

University at Buffalo, the State University of New York, Graduate School, College of Arts and Sciences, Department of Biological Sciences, Buffalo, NY 14260. Offers MA, MS, PhD. Terminal master's awarded for partial completion of doctoral program. *Degree requirements:* For master's, thesis, research rotation, seminar; for doctorate, comprehensive exam, thesis/dissertation, oral candidacy exam, research, seminar. *Entrance requirements:* For master's and doctorate, GRE General Test, 2 semesters of course work in calculus, course work in chemistry through organic chemistry, strong biology background. Additional exam requirements/recommendations for international students: Required—TOEFL (minimum score 600 paper-based; 100 iBT). Electronic applications accepted. *Faculty research:* Biochemistry, bioinformatics, biophysics, biotechnology, botany, cell biology, developmental biology, evolutionary biology, genetics, genomics, molecular biology, microbiology, neuroscience, physiology, plant physiology, plant sciences, structural biology, virology, zoology.

University at Buffalo, the State University of New York, Graduate School, School of Medicine and Biomedical Sciences, Graduate Programs in Medicine and Biomedical Sciences, Buffalo, NY 14260. Offers MA, MS, PhD, MD/PhD. *Faculty:* 245 full-time (63 women), 6 part-time/adjunct (1 woman). *Students:* 215 full-time (114 women); includes 63 minority (12 Black or African American, non-Hispanic/Latino; 2 American Indian or

Biological and Biomedical Sciences—General

Alaska Native, non-Hispanic/Latino; 39 Asian, non-Hispanic/Latino; 7 Hispanic/Latino; 3 Two or more races, non-Hispanic/Latino; 64 international. 575 applicants, 20% accepted, 52 enrolled. In 2015, 33 master's, 22 doctorates awarded. Terminal master's awarded for partial completion of doctoral program. *Degree requirements:* For master's, comprehensive exam (for some programs), thesis (for some programs); for doctorate, comprehensive exam, thesis/dissertation. *Entrance requirements:* For master's, GRE General Test; for doctorate, GRE General Test, 3 letters of recommendation. Additional exam requirements/recommendations for international students: Required—TOEFL (minimum score 600 paper-based; 100 iBT). *Application deadline:* For fall admission, 2/1 for domestic and international students. Applications are processed on a rolling basis. Application fee: $85. Electronic applications accepted. *Expenses:* Contact institution. *Financial support:* In 2015–16, 41 students received support, including 11 fellowships with full tuition reimbursements available (averaging $13,083 per year), 85 research assistantships with full tuition reimbursements available (averaging $24,843 per year), 8 teaching assistantships with full tuition reimbursements available (averaging $19,967 per year); career-related internships or fieldwork, Federal Work-Study, institutionally sponsored loans, scholarships/grants, traineeships, health care benefits, and unspecified assistantships also available. Financial award application deadline: 2/1; financial award applicants required to submit FAFSA. *Faculty research:* Neuroscience; molecular, cell, and structural biology; microbial pathogenesis; cardiopulmonary physiology; biochemistry, biotechnology and clinical laboratory science. *Total annual research expenditures:* $31.6 million. *Unit head:* Dr. Anthony Campagnari, Senior Associate Dean for Research and Graduate Education, 716-829-3398, Fax: 716-829-2437, E-mail: aac@buffalo.edu. *Application contact:* Elizabeth A. White, Administrative Director, 716-829-3399, Fax: 716-829-2437, E-mail: bethw@buffalo.edu.

University at Buffalo, the State University of New York, Graduate School, School of Medicine and Biomedical Sciences, PhD Program in Biomedical Sciences, Buffalo, NY 14260. Offers PhD. *Students:* 15 full-time (14 women); includes 3 minority (1 Black or African American, non-Hispanic/Latino; 2 Asian, non-Hispanic/Latino), 1 international. 305 applicants, 12% accepted, 15 enrolled. *Degree requirements:* For doctorate, comprehensive exam, thesis/dissertation. *Entrance requirements:* For doctorate, GRE General Test, 3 letters of recommendation. Additional exam requirements/recommendations for international students: Required—TOEFL (minimum score 600 paper-based; 100 iBT), IELTS (minimum score 7.5). *Application deadline:* For fall admission, 1/10 priority date for domestic and international students. Applications are processed on a rolling basis. Application fee: $85. Electronic applications accepted. *Financial support:* In 2015–16, 15 students received support, including 3 fellowships (averaging $5,000 per year), 15 research assistantships with full tuition reimbursements available (averaging $27,000 per year); scholarships/grants and health care benefits also available. Financial award application deadline: 1/10. *Faculty research:* Molecular, cell and structural biology; pharmacology and toxicology; neurosciences; microbiology; pathogenesis and disease. *Unit head:* Dr. Mark Sutton, Director, 716-829-3398, Fax: 716-829-2437, E-mail: smbs-gradprog@buffalo.edu. *Application contact:* Elizabeth A. White, Administrative Director, 716-829-3399, Fax: 716-829-2437, E-mail: bethw@buffalo.edu.
Website: http://medicine.buffalo.edu/phdprogram

The University of Akron, Graduate School, Buchtel College of Arts and Sciences, Department of Biology, Akron, OH 44325. Offers biology (MS); integrated bioscience (PhD). *Program availability:* Part-time. *Faculty:* 17 full-time (4 women), 9 part-time/adjunct (4 women). *Students:* 67 full-time (27 women), 3 part-time (1 woman); includes 12 minority (3 Black or African American, non-Hispanic/Latino; 3 Asian, non-Hispanic/Latino; 3 Hispanic/Latino; 3 Two or more races, non-Hispanic/Latino), 14 international. Average age 28. 40 applicants, 40% accepted, 15 enrolled. In 2015, 9 master's, 6 doctorates awarded. *Degree requirements:* For master's, thesis optional, oral defense of thesis, oral exam, seminars; for doctorate, thesis/dissertation, oral defense of dissertation, seminars. *Entrance requirements:* For master's, GRE, baccalaureate degree in biology or the equivalent; minimum GPA of 3.0 overall and in biology; letter of interest; letter from potential biology adviser; for doctorate, GRE, minimum overall GPA of 3.0, letters of recommendation, personal statement of career goals and research interest. Additional exam requirements/recommendations for international students: Required—TOEFL (minimum score 550 paper-based; 79 iBT), IELTS (minimum score 6.5). *Application deadline:* Applications are processed on a rolling basis. Application fee: $45 ($70 for international students). Electronic applications accepted. *Expenses:* Tuition, state resident: full-time $7958; part-time $442 per credit hour. Tuition, nonresident: full-time $13,464; part-time $748 per credit hour. *Required fees:* $1404. *Financial support:* In 2015–16, 3 research assistantships with full tuition reimbursements, 15 teaching assistantships with full tuition reimbursements were awarded. Financial award application deadline: 1/10. *Faculty research:* Behavior/neuroscience, ecology-evolution, genetics, molecular biology, physiology. *Total annual research expenditures:* $1.3 million. *Unit head:* Dr. Stephen Weeks, Interim Chair, 330-972-7156, E-mail: scweeks@uakron.edu. *Application contact:* Dr. Todd Blackledge, Graduate Director, 330-972-4264, E-mail: blackledge@uakron.edu.
Website: http://www.uakron.edu/biology/

The University of Alabama, Graduate School, College of Arts and Sciences, Department of Biological Sciences, Tuscaloosa, AL 35487. Offers MS, PhD. *Faculty:* 32 full-time (16 women). *Students:* 68 full-time (28 women), 3 part-time (all women); includes 10 minority (4 Black or African American, non-Hispanic/Latino; 1 Asian, non-Hispanic/Latino; 2 Hispanic/Latino; 3 Two or more races, non-Hispanic/Latino), 23 international. Average age 28. 89 applicants, 21% accepted, 10 enrolled. In 2015, 13 master's, 10 doctorates awarded. Terminal master's awarded for partial completion of doctoral program. *Degree requirements:* For master's, comprehensive exam, thesis optional; for doctorate, comprehensive exam, thesis/dissertation, written and oral candidacy exams. *Entrance requirements:* For master's and doctorate, GRE General Test, minimum GPA of 3.0. Additional exam requirements/recommendations for international students: Required—TOEFL (minimum score 550 paper-based; 80 iBT). *Application deadline:* For fall admission, 12/5 priority date for domestic and international students; for spring admission, 12/5 priority date for domestic students, 9/5 priority date for international students. Applications are processed on a rolling basis. Application fee: $50 ($60 for international students). Electronic applications accepted. *Expenses:* Tuition, state resident: full-time $10,170. Tuition, nonresident: full-time $25,950. *Financial support:* In 2015–16, 23 fellowships with full tuition reimbursements (averaging $18,000 per year), 21 research assistantships with full tuition reimbursements (averaging $21,000 per year), 44 teaching assistantships with full tuition reimbursements (averaging $17,000 per year) were awarded; scholarships/grants, health care benefits, and unspecified assistantships also available. Financial award application deadline: 7/1; financial award applicants required to submit FAFSA. *Faculty research:* Molecular and cellular biology, developmental genetics, ecology, evolutionary biology, systematics. *Total annual research expenditures:* $2.8 million. *Unit head:* Dr. Patrica A. Sobecky, Chair, 205-348-1807, Fax: 205-348-1786, E-mail: psobecky@as.ua.edu. *Application contact:* Dr. Stevan Marcus, Graduate Program Director, 205-348-8094, Fax: 205-348-1786, E-mail: smarcus@as.ua.edu.
Website: http://bsc.ua.edu

The University of Alabama at Birmingham, College of Arts and Sciences, Program in Biology, Birmingham, AL 35294. Offers MS, PhD. Terminal master's awarded for partial completion of doctoral program. *Degree requirements:* For master's, comprehensive exam (for some programs), thesis (for some programs); for doctorate, thesis/dissertation. *Entrance requirements:* For master's and doctorate, GRE General Test, previous course work in biology, calculus, organic chemistry, and physics; letters of recommendation. Additional exam requirements/recommendations for international students: Required—TOEFL, TWE. Electronic applications accepted. *Expenses:* Tuition, state resident: full-time $7340. Tuition, nonresident: full-time $16,628. Full-time tuition and fees vary according to course load and program.

The University of Alabama at Birmingham, Graduate Programs in Joint Health Sciences, Program in Basic Medical Sciences, Birmingham, AL 35294. Offers MSBMS. *Entrance requirements:* For master's, GRE. Electronic applications accepted. *Expenses:* Tuition, state resident: full-time $7340. Tuition, nonresident: full-time $16,628. Full-time tuition and fees vary according to course load and program. *Unit head:* Dr. David A. Schneider, Associate Dean for Graduate Biomedical Sciences, 205-934-2845, E-mail: dschneid@uab.edu. *Application contact:* Holly Hebard, 205-996-2583, E-mail: hghebard@uab.edu.
Website: http://www.uab.edu/gbs/home/

The University of Alabama in Huntsville, School of Graduate Studies, College of Science, Department of Biological Sciences, Huntsville, AL 35899. Offers biology (MS); biotechnology science and engineering (PhD); education (MS). *Program availability:* Part-time, evening/weekend. *Degree requirements:* For master's, comprehensive exam, thesis or alternative, oral and written exams. *Entrance requirements:* For master's, GRE General Test, previous course work in biochemistry and organic chemistry, minimum GPA of 3.0. Additional exam requirements/recommendations for international students: Required—TOEFL (minimum score 550 paper-based; 80 iBT), IELTS (minimum score 6.5). *Application deadline:* For fall admission, 7/15 priority date for domestic students, 4/1 priority date for international students; for spring admission, 11/30 for domestic students, 9/1 priority date for international students. Applications are processed on a rolling basis. Application fee: $50. Electronic applications accepted. *Expenses: Tuition, area resident:* Full-time $9548; part-time $547 per credit hour. Tuition, state resident: full-time $9548; part-time $547 per credit hour. Tuition, nonresident: full-time $21,402; part-time $1224 per credit hour. *International tuition:* $21,402 full-time. *Financial support:* Fellowships with full tuition reimbursements, research assistantships, teaching assistantships with tuition reimbursements, career-related internships or fieldwork, Federal Work-Study, institutionally sponsored loans, scholarships/grants, health care benefits, tuition waivers (full and partial), and unspecified assistantships available. Support available to part-time students. Financial award application deadline: 4/1; financial award applicants required to submit FAFSA. *Faculty research:* Physiology, microbiology, genomics and protemics, ecology and evolution, drug discovery. *Unit head:* Dr. Debra M. Moriarity, Chair, 256-824-6045, Fax: 256-824-6305, E-mail: moriard@uah.edu. *Application contact:* Kim Gray, Graduate Studies Admissions Manager, 256-824-6002, Fax: 256-824-6405, E-mail: deangrad@uah.edu.
Website: http://www.uah.edu/science/departments/biology

University of Alaska Anchorage, College of Arts and Sciences, Department of Biological Sciences, Anchorage, AK 99508. Offers MS. *Program availability:* Part-time. *Degree requirements:* For master's, comprehensive exam, thesis. *Entrance requirements:* For master's, GRE General Test, GRE Subject Test, bachelor's degree in biology, chemistry or equivalent science. Additional exam requirements/recommendations for international students: Required—TOEFL (minimum score 550 paper-based). *Faculty research:* Taxonomy and vegetative analysis in Alaskan ecosystems, fish environment and seafood, biochemistry, arctic ecology, vertebrate ecology.

University of Alberta, Faculty of Graduate Studies and Research, Department of Biological Sciences, Edmonton, AB T6G 2E1, Canada. Offers environmental biology and ecology (M Sc, PhD); microbiology and biotechnology (M Sc, PhD); molecular biology and genetics (M Sc, PhD); physiology and cell biology (M Sc, PhD); plant biology (M Sc, PhD); systematics and evolution (M Sc, PhD). Terminal master's awarded for partial completion of doctoral program. *Degree requirements:* For master's, thesis; for doctorate, thesis/dissertation. *Entrance requirements:* Additional exam requirements/recommendations for international students: Required—TOEFL.

University of Alberta, Faculty of Medicine and Dentistry and Faculty of Graduate Studies and Research, Graduate Programs in Medicine, Edmonton, AB T6G 2E1, Canada. Offers M Sc, MD, PhD. *Program availability:* Part-time. *Degree requirements:* For doctorate, thesis/dissertation (for some programs). *Faculty research:* Basic, clinical, and applied biomedicine.

The University of Arizona, College of Agriculture and Life Sciences, School of Animal and Comparative Biomedical Sciences, Tucson, AZ 85721. Offers MS, PhD. *Degree requirements:* For master's, thesis; for doctorate, comprehensive exam, thesis/dissertation. *Entrance requirements:* For master's and doctorate, GRE, minimum GPA of 3.0, 3 letters of recommendation, letter of intent. Additional exam requirements/recommendations for international students: Required—TOEFL (minimum score 550 paper-based; 79 iBT). *Application deadline:* For fall admission, 2/28 for domestic students, 12/1 for international students. Application fee: $75. Electronic applications accepted. *Financial support:* Research assistantships, teaching assistantships, health care benefits, and unspecified assistantships available. Financial award application deadline: 3/22. *Unit head:* Dr. Andre-Denis Wright, Head, 520-621-0868, E-mail: adwright@email.arizona.edu. *Application contact:* Kathryn Johansen, Administrative Assistant, 520-621-4507, E-mail: millerk@email.arizona.edu.
Website: http://acbs.cals.arizona.edu/

University of Arkansas, Graduate School, J. William Fulbright College of Arts and Sciences, Department of Biological Sciences, Fayetteville, AR 72701-1201. Offers MA, MS, PhD. *Students:* 5 full-time (3 women), 51 part-time (28 women); includes 2 minority (both Two or more races, non-Hispanic/Latino), 9 international. In 2015, 2 master's, 3 doctorates awarded. *Degree requirements:* For doctorate, one foreign language, thesis/dissertation. *Entrance requirements:* For master's and doctorate, GRE Subject Test. *Application deadline:* For fall admission, 4/1 for international students; for spring admission, 10/1 for international students. Applications are processed on a rolling basis. Application fee: $40 ($50 for international students). Electronic applications accepted. *Financial support:* In 2015–16, 27 research assistantships, 8 teaching assistantships were awarded; fellowships with full tuition reimbursements, career-related internships or fieldwork, and Federal Work-Study also available. Support available to part-time students. Financial award application deadline: 4/1; financial award applicants required to submit FAFSA. *Unit head:* Dr. Steve Beaupre, Department Chairperson, 479-575-3251, Fax: 479-575-4010, E-mail: sbeaupre@uark.edu. *Application contact:* Dr. David McNabb, Graduate Coordinator, 479-575-3797, Fax: 479-575-4010, E-mail: dmcnabb@uark.edu.
Website: http://biology.uark.edu/

University of Arkansas at Little Rock, Graduate School, College of Arts, Letters, and Sciences, Department of Biology, Little Rock, AR 72204-1099. Offers MS. *Expenses:* Tuition, state resident: part-time $300 per credit hour. Tuition, nonresident: part-time $690 per credit hour. *Required fees:* $100 per credit hour. One-time fee: $40 full-time.

University of Arkansas for Medical Sciences, Graduate School, Little Rock, AR 72205. Offers biochemistry and molecular biology (MS, PhD); bioinformatics (MS, PhD); cellular physiology and molecular biophysics (MS, PhD); clinical nutrition (MS); interdisciplinary biomedical sciences (MS, PhD, Certificate); interdisciplinary toxicology (MS); microbiology and immunology (PhD); neurobiology and developmental sciences (PhD); pharmacology (PhD); MD/PhD. Bioinformatics programs hosted jointly with the University of Arkansas at Little Rock. *Program availability:* Part-time. Terminal master's awarded for partial completion of doctoral program. *Degree requirements:* For master's, comprehensive exam (for some programs), thesis (for some programs); for doctorate, thesis/dissertation. *Entrance requirements:* For master's and doctorate, GRE. Additional exam requirements/recommendations for international students: Required—TOEFL. Electronic applications accepted. *Expenses:* Contact institution.

University of Calgary, Cumming School of Medicine and Faculty of Graduate Studies, Medical Science Graduate Program, Calgary, AB T2N 1N4, Canada. Offers cancer biology (M Sc, PhD); critical care medicine (M Sc, PhD); joint injury and arthritis (M Sc, PhD); molecular and medical genetics (M Sc, PhD); mountain medicine and high altitude physiology (M Sc, PhD); pathologists' assistant (M Sc, PhD). *Degree requirements:* For master's, thesis; for doctorate, thesis/dissertation, candidacy exam. *Entrance requirements:* For master's, minimum undergraduate GPA of 3.2; for doctorate, minimum graduate GPA of 3.2. Additional exam requirements/recommendations for international students: Required—TOEFL (minimum score 600 paper-based). Electronic applications accepted. *Faculty research:* Cancer biology, immunology, joint injury and arthritis, medical education, population genomics.

University of Calgary, Faculty of Graduate Studies, Faculty of Science, Department of Biological Sciences, Calgary, AB T2N 1N4, Canada. Offers M Sc, PhD. *Program availability:* Part-time. *Degree requirements:* For master's, thesis; for doctorate, thesis/dissertation, candidacy exam. *Entrance requirements:* Additional exam requirements/recommendations for international students: Required—TOEFL. Electronic applications accepted. *Faculty research:* Biochemistry; cellular, molecular, and microbial biology; botany; ecology; zoology.

University of California, Berkeley, Graduate Division, College of Letters and Science, Department of Integrative Biology, Berkeley, CA 94720-1500. Offers PhD. *Degree requirements:* For doctorate, thesis/dissertation, oral qualifying exam. *Entrance requirements:* For doctorate, GRE General Test, GRE Subject Test, 3 letters of recommendation. Additional exam requirements/recommendations for international students: Required—TOEFL. *Faculty research:* Morphology, physiology, development of plants and animals, behavior, ecology.

University of California, Irvine, Francisco J. Ayala School of Biological Sciences, Irvine, CA 92697. Offers MS, PhD, MD/PhD. *Students:* 290 full-time (151 women), 2 part-time (1 woman); includes 114 minority (5 Black or African American, non-Hispanic/Latino; 1 American Indian or Alaska Native, non-Hispanic/Latino; 57 Asian, non-Hispanic/Latino; 38 Hispanic/Latino; 1 Native Hawaiian or other Pacific Islander, non-Hispanic/Latino; 12 Two or more races, non-Hispanic/Latino), 36 international. Average age 27. 837 applicants, 19% accepted, 82 enrolled. In 2015, 34 master's, 36 doctorates awarded. *Degree requirements:* For doctorate, thesis/dissertation. *Entrance requirements:* For master's and doctorate, GRE General Test, GRE Subject Test, minimum GPA of 3.0. Additional exam requirements/recommendations for international students: Required—TOEFL (minimum score 550 paper-based). *Application deadline:* For fall admission, 12/15 for domestic and international students. Applications are processed on a rolling basis. Application fee: $90 ($110 for international students). Electronic applications accepted. *Financial support:* Fellowships with full tuition reimbursements, research assistantships with full tuition reimbursements, teaching assistantships with full tuition reimbursements, career-related internships or fieldwork, institutionally sponsored loans, scholarships/grants, traineeships, health care benefits, and unspecified assistantships available. Financial award application deadline: 3/1; financial award applicants required to submit FAFSA. *Faculty research:* Molecular biology and biochemistry, developmental and cell biology, physiology and biophysics, neurosciences, ecology and evolutionary biology. *Unit head:* Prof. Frank Laferla, Dean, 949-824-5315, Fax: 949-824-3035, E-mail: laferla@uci.edu. *Application contact:* Prof. R. Michael Mulligan, Associate Dean, 949-824-8433, Fax: 949-824-4709, E-mail: rmmullig@uci.edu.
Website: http://www.bio.uci.edu/

University of California, Los Angeles, David Geffen School of Medicine and Graduate Division, Graduate Programs in Medicine, Los Angeles, CA 90095. Offers MS, PhD, MD/PhD. Terminal master's awarded for partial completion of doctoral program. *Degree requirements:* For doctorate, thesis/dissertation, written and oral qualifying exams. Electronic applications accepted. *Expenses:* Contact institution.

University of California, Los Angeles, Graduate Division, College of Letters and Science, Department of Ecology and Evolutionary Biology, Los Angeles, CA 90095. Offers MA, PhD. Terminal master's awarded for partial completion of doctoral program. *Degree requirements:* For master's, comprehensive exam or thesis; for doctorate, thesis/dissertation, oral and written qualifying exams; 3 quarters of teaching experience. *Entrance requirements:* For master's and doctorate, GRE General Test, GRE Subject Test (biology), bachelor's degree; minimum undergraduate GPA of 3.0 (or its equivalent if letter grade system not used). Additional exam requirements/recommendations for international students: Required—TOEFL. Electronic applications accepted.

University of California, Merced, Graduate Division, School of Natural Sciences, Merced, CA 95343. Offers applied mathematics (MS, PhD); chemistry and chemical biology (MS, PhD); physics (MS, PhD); quantitative and systems biology (MS, PhD). *Faculty:* 63 full-time (25 women). *Students:* 156 full-time (64 women); includes 58 minority (3 Black or African American, non-Hispanic/Latino; 23 Asian, non-Hispanic/Latino; 22 Hispanic/Latino; 1 Native Hawaiian or other Pacific Islander, non-Hispanic/Latino; 9 Two or more races, non-Hispanic/Latino), 37 international. Average age 27. 199 applicants, 57% accepted, 45 enrolled. In 2015, 12 master's, 11 doctorates awarded. Terminal master's awarded for partial completion of doctoral program. *Degree requirements:* For master's, variable foreign language requirement, comprehensive exam, thesis or alternative; for doctorate, variable foreign language requirement, comprehensive exam, thesis/dissertation. *Entrance requirements:* For master's and doctorate, GRE. Additional exam requirements/recommendations for international students: Required—TOEFL (minimum score 550 paper-based; 80 iBT); Recommended—IELTS (minimum score 7). *Application deadline:* For fall admission, 1/15 for domestic and international students. Application fee: $90 ($110 for international students). Electronic applications accepted. *Expenses:* $11,220 per year resident tuition, $15,102 per year non-resident tuition. *Financial support:* In 2015–16, 151 students received support, including 12 fellowships with full tuition reimbursements available (averaging $23,614 per year), 37 research assistantships with full tuition reimbursements available (averaging $18,842 per year), 127 teaching assistantships with full tuition reimbursements available (averaging $18,538 per year); scholarships/grants, traineeships, and health care benefits also available. Financial award application deadline: 1/15. *Faculty research:* Computational science, soft matter physics, neurobiology, genomics, biochemistry. *Total annual research expenditures:* $5.3 million. *Unit head:* Dr. Juan C. Meza, Dean, 209-228-4487, Fax: 209-228-4060, E-mail: jcmeza@ucmerced.edu. *Application contact:* Tsu Ya, Director of Graduate Admissions and Academic Services, 209-228-4521, Fax: 209-228-6906, E-mail: tya@ucmerced.edu.

University of California, Riverside, Graduate Division, Department of Biology, Riverside, CA 92521-0102. Offers evolution, ecology and organismal biology (MS, PhD). Terminal master's awarded for partial completion of doctoral program. *Degree requirements:* For master's, thesis, oral defense of thesis; for doctorate, thesis/dissertation, 3 quarters of teaching experience, qualifying exams. *Entrance requirements:* For master's and doctorate, GRE General Test, minimum GPA of 3.2. Additional exam requirements/recommendations for international students: Required—TOEFL (minimum score 550 paper-based, 80 iBT) or IELTS. Electronic applications accepted. *Expenses: Tuition, area resident:* Full-time $16,665.50; part-time $11,055.54. Tuition, state resident: full-time $16,665.50; part-time $11,055.54. Tuition, nonresident: full-time $31,768. *International tuition:* $31,767.50 full-time. *Required fees:* $16,665.50; $11,055.54 per quarter. Tuition and fees vary according to program. *Faculty research:* Ecology, evolutionary biology, physiology, quantitative genetics, conservation biology.

University of California, Riverside, Graduate Division, Program in Biomedical Sciences, Riverside, CA 92521-0102. Offers PhD. *Degree requirements:* For doctorate, thesis/dissertation, qualifying exams. *Entrance requirements:* For doctorate, GRE General Test, minimum GPA of 3.2. Additional exam requirements/recommendations for international students: Required—TOEFL (minimum score 550 paper-based; 80 iBT). *Application deadline:* For fall admission, 12/15 priority date for domestic students, 5/1 for international students. Application fee: $80 ($100 for international students). Electronic applications accepted. *Expenses: Tuition, area resident:* Full-time $16,665.50; part-time $11,055.54. Tuition, state resident: full-time $16,665.50; part-time $11,055.54. Tuition, nonresident: full-time $31,768. *International tuition:* $31,767.50 full-time. *Required fees:* $16,665.50; $11,055.54 per quarter. Tuition and fees vary according to program. *Financial support:* Fellowships with tuition reimbursements, research assistantships with tuition reimbursements, teaching assistantships with tuition reimbursements, and scholarships/grants available. Financial award application deadline: 2/1; financial award applicants required to submit FAFSA. *Faculty research:* Cancer cell biology; chronic inflammatory and autoimmune disease; cytokine, chemokine and endocrine biology in health and disease; microbiology, parasitology and vector borne diseases; neurodegeneration.
Website: http://medschool.ucr.edu/graduate/

University of California, San Diego, Graduate Division, Department of Physics, La Jolla, CA 92093. Offers biophysics (PhD); multi-scale biology (PhD); physics (MS, PhD). *Students:* 154 full-time (18 women); includes 26 minority (3 Black or African American, non-Hispanic/Latino; 15 Asian, non-Hispanic/Latino; 8 Hispanic/Latino), 52 international. 481 applicants, 13% accepted, 17 enrolled. In 2015, 13 master's, 27 doctorates awarded. *Degree requirements:* For doctorate, comprehensive exam, thesis/dissertation, 1-quarter teaching assistantship. *Entrance requirements:* For doctorate, GRE General Test, GRE Subject Test. Additional exam requirements/recommendations for international students: Required—TOEFL (minimum score 550 paper-based; 80 iBT), IELTS (minimum score 7). *Application deadline:* For fall admission, 12/23 for domestic students. Application fee: $90 ($110 for international students). Electronic applications accepted. *Expenses:* Tuition, state resident: full-time $11,220. Tuition, nonresident: full-time $26,322. *Required fees:* $1800. *Financial support:* Fellowships, research assistantships, teaching assistantships, scholarships/grants, and unspecified assistantships available. Financial award applicants required to submit FAFSA. *Faculty research:* Astrophysics/astronomy, biological physics, condensed matter/material science, elementary particles, plasma physics. *Unit head:* Benjamin Grinstein, Chair, 858-534-6857, E-mail: chair@physics.ucsd.edu. *Application contact:* Sharmila Poddar, Graduate Coordinator, 858-822-1074, E-mail: shpoddar@ucsd.edu.
Website: http://physics.ucsd.edu/

University of California, San Diego, Graduate Division, Division of Biological Sciences, La Jolla, CA 92093. Offers anthropogeny (PhD); bioinformatics (PhD); biology (PhD); interdisciplinary environmental research (PhD); multi-scale biology (PhD); quantitative biology (PhD). PhD in biology offered jointly with San Diego State University. *Students:* 287 full-time (160 women), 5 part-time (2 women); includes 117 minority (5 Black or African American, non-Hispanic/Latino; 82 Asian, non-Hispanic/Latino; 29 Hispanic/Latino; 1 Native Hawaiian or other Pacific Islander, non-Hispanic/Latino), 81 international. 679 applicants, 25% accepted, 99 enrolled. In 2015, 24 doctorates awarded. *Degree requirements:* For doctorate, comprehensive exam, thesis/dissertation, 3 quarters of teaching assistantship. *Entrance requirements:* For doctorate, GRE General Test; GRE Subject Test (recommended: biology, biochemistry, cell and molecular biology, chemistry). Additional exam requirements/recommendations for international students: Required—TOEFL (minimum score 550 paper-based; 80 iBT), IELTS (minimum score 7). *Application deadline:* For fall admission, 12/1 for domestic students. Electronic applications accepted. *Expenses:* Tuition, state resident: full-time $11,220. Tuition, nonresident: full-time $26,322. *Required fees:* $1800. *Financial support:* Fellowships, research assistantships, teaching assistantships, scholarships/grants, traineeships, and unspecified assistantships available. Financial award applicants required to submit FAFSA. *Faculty research:* Molecular, cellular and developmental biology, genetics, behavior and evolution; microbiology; bioinformatics; signal transduction; quantitative biology, neurobiology. *Unit head:* Dr. Jens Lykke-Andersen, Graduate Director, 858-534-2580, E-mail: jlykkeandersen@ucsd.edu. *Application contact:* Brandon Keith, Graduate Admissions Coordinator, 858-534-8983, E-mail: biogradprog@ucsd.edu.
Website: http://biology.ucsd.edu/

See Close-Up on page 115.

University of California, San Diego, School of Medicine and Graduate Division, Graduate Studies in Biomedical Sciences, La Jolla, CA 92093-0685. Offers anthropogony (PhD); bioinformatics (PhD); biomedical sciences (PhD); multi-scale biology (PhD). *Students:* 172 full-time (94 women), 5 part-time (1 woman); includes 75 minority (7 Black or African American, non-Hispanic/Latino; 2 American Indian or Alaska Native, non-Hispanic/Latino; 48 Asian, non-Hispanic/Latino; 18 Hispanic/Latino), 2 international. 427 applicants, 18% accepted, 25 enrolled. In 2015, 28 doctorates awarded. *Degree requirements:* For doctorate, comprehensive exam, thesis/dissertation, 1-quarter teaching assistantship. *Entrance requirements:* For doctorate, GRE General Test; GRE Subject Test in either biology, biochemistry, cell and molecular biology or chemistry (recommended). Additional exam requirements/recommendations for international students: Required—TOEFL (minimum score 550 paper-based; 80 iBT), IELTS (minimum score 7). *Application deadline:* For fall admission, 12/1 for domestic students. Application fee: $90 ($110 for international students). Electronic applications accepted. *Expenses:* Tuition, state resident: full-time $11,220. Tuition, nonresident: full-time $26,322. *Required fees:* $1800. *Financial support:* Fellowships, research assistantships, teaching assistantships, scholarships/grants, traineeships, unspecified assistantships, and stipends available. Financial award applicants required to submit FAFSA. *Faculty research:* Genetics, microbiology and immunology, molecular cell biology, molecular pharmacology, molecular pathology. *Unit head:* Deborah Spector, Chair, 858-822-4003, E-mail: dspector@ucsd.edu. *Application contact:* Leanne

Biological and Biomedical Sciences—General

Nordeman, Graduate Coordinator, 858-534-3982, E-mail: biomedsci@ucsd.edu. Website: http://biomedsci.ucsd.edu

University of California, San Diego, School of Medicine, Medical Scientist Training Program, La Jolla, CA 92093. Offers MD/PhD. *Application deadline:* For fall admission, 9/30 for domestic students. *Expenses:* Tuition, state resident: full-time $11,220. Tuition, nonresident: full-time $26,322. *Required fees:* $1800. *Financial support:* Fellowships, research assistantships, scholarships/grants, and traineeships available. Financial award applicants required to submit FAFSA. *Unit head:* Paul A. Insel, Director, 858-534-2295. *Application contact:* Mary Alice Kiisel, Assistant, 858-534-0689, E-mail: mstp@ucsd.edu.

University of California, San Francisco, Graduate Division, Biomedical Sciences Graduate Program, San Francisco, CA 94143. Offers PhD. *Degree requirements:* For doctorate, thesis/dissertation. *Entrance requirements:* For doctorate, GRE General Test, three letters of recommendation, official transcripts. Additional exam requirements/recommendations for international students: Required—TOEFL, IELTS. *Faculty research:* Cancer biology and cell signaling, developmental and stem cell biology, human genetics, immunology, neurobiology, tissue/organ biology and endocrinology, vascular and cardiac biology, virology and microbial pathogenesis.

University of California, San Francisco, School of Medicine, San Francisco, CA 94143-0410. Offers MD, PhD, MD/MPH, MD/MS, MD/PhD. *Accreditation:* LCME/AMA (one or more programs are accredited). *Faculty:* 2,035 full-time (871 women), 368 part-time/adjunct (195 women). *Students:* 647 full-time (330 women); includes 354 minority (47 Black or African American, non-Hispanic/Latino; 2 American Indian or Alaska Native, non-Hispanic/Latino; 156 Asian, non-Hispanic/Latino; 94 Hispanic/Latino; 9 Native Hawaiian or other Pacific Islander, non-Hispanic/Latino; 46 Two or more races, non-Hispanic/Latino). Average age 24. 7,453 applicants, 4% accepted, 149 enrolled. In 2015, 163 doctorates awarded. *Entrance requirements:* For doctorate, MCAT (for MD), interview (for MD). *Application deadline:* For fall admission, 10/15 for domestic students. Applications are processed on a rolling basis. Application fee: $80 ($100 for international students). Electronic applications accepted. *Expenses:* $32,751 in-state tuition, $44,996 out-of-state tuition, $4,593 student fees. *Financial support:* In 2015–16, 517 students received support. Federal Work-Study, institutionally sponsored loans, scholarships/grants, and tuition waivers (partial) available. Financial award application deadline: 2/1; financial award applicants required to submit FAFSA. *Faculty research:* Neurosciences, human genetics, developmental biology, social/behavioral/policy sciences, immunology. *Total annual research expenditures:* $495.6 million. *Unit head:* Dr. Talmadge E. King, Jr., Dean, 415-476-2342, Fax: 415-476-0689. *Application contact:* Hallen Chung, Director of Admissions, 415-476-8090, Fax: 415-476-5490, E-mail: hallen.chung@ucsf.edu.
Website: http://medschool.ucsf.edu/

University of Central Arkansas, Graduate School, College of Natural Sciences and Math, Department of Biological Science, Conway, AR 72035-0001. Offers MS. *Program availability:* Part-time. *Degree requirements:* For master's, comprehensive exam, thesis optional. *Entrance requirements:* For master's, GRE General Test, minimum GPA of 2.7. Additional exam requirements/recommendations for international students: Required—TOEFL (minimum score 550 paper-based; 80 iBT). Electronic applications accepted.

University of Central Florida, College of Education and Human Performance, School of Teaching, Learning, and Leadership, Program in Teacher Education, Orlando, FL 32816. Offers art education (MAT); English language (MAT); mathematics education (MAT); middle school mathematics (MAT); science education (MAT), including biology, chemistry, physics; social science education (MAT). *Accreditation:* NCATE. *Program availability:* Part-time, evening/weekend. *Students:* 25 full-time (16 women), 43 part-time (32 women); includes 19 minority (5 Black or African American, non-Hispanic/Latino; 2 Asian, non-Hispanic/Latino; 10 Hispanic/Latino; 2 Two or more races, non-Hispanic/Latino). Average age 30. In 2015, 88 master's awarded. *Entrance requirements:* For master's, GRE General Test. Additional exam requirements/recommendations for international students: Required—TOEFL. *Application deadline:* For fall admission, 7/15 for domestic students; for spring admission, 12/1 for domestic students. Application fee: $30. Electronic applications accepted. *Expenses:* Tuition, state resident: part-time $288.16 per credit hour. Tuition, nonresident: part-time $1071.31 per credit hour. *Financial support:* Fellowships, research assistantships, teaching assistantships, career-related internships or fieldwork, Federal Work-Study, institutionally sponsored loans, tuition waivers (partial), and unspecified assistantships available. Financial award application deadline: 3/1; financial award applicants required to submit FAFSA. *Unit head:* Dr. Michael Hynes, Director, 407-823-2005, E-mail: mychael.hynes@ucf.edu. *Application contact:* Director, Admissions and Student Support, 407-823-2766, Fax: 407-823-6442, E-mail: gradadmissions@ucf.edu.

University of Central Florida, College of Medicine, Burnett School of Biomedical Sciences, Orlando, FL 32816. Offers biomedical sciences (MS, PhD); biotechnology (MS). *Faculty:* 13 full-time (4 women), 1 (woman) part-time/adjunct. *Students:* 80 full-time (44 women), 6 part-time (4 women); includes 23 minority (8 Black or African American, non-Hispanic/Latino; 10 Asian, non-Hispanic/Latino; 4 Hispanic/Latino; 1 Two or more races, non-Hispanic/Latino), 19 international. Average age 27. 118 applicants, 47% accepted, 30 enrolled. In 2015, 19 master's, 8 doctorates awarded. Electronic applications accepted. *Expenses:* Tuition, state resident: part-time $288.16 per credit hour. Tuition, nonresident: part-time $1071.31 per credit hour. *Financial support:* In 2015–16, 55 students received support, including 16 fellowships with partial tuition reimbursements available (averaging $3,500 per year), 48 research assistantships with partial tuition reimbursements available (averaging $8,000 per year), 44 teaching assistantships with partial tuition reimbursements available (averaging $6,500 per year). *Unit head:* Dr. Griffith Parks, Director, 407-226-1000, E-mail: griffith.parks@ucf.edu. *Application contact:* Director, Admissions and Student Services, 407-823-2766, Fax: 407-823-6442, E-mail: gradadmissions@ucf.edu.
Website: http://www.biomed.ucf.edu

University of Central Missouri, The Graduate School, Warrensburg, MO 64093. Offers accountancy (MA); accounting (MBA); applied mathematics (MS); aviation safety (MA); biology (MS); business administration (MBA); career and technical education leadership (MS); college student personnel administration (MS); communication (MA); computer science (MS); counseling (MS); criminal justice (MS); educational leadership (Ed D); educational technology (MS); elementary and early childhood education (MSE); English (MA); environmental studies (MS); finance (MBA); history (MA); human services/educational technology (Ed S); human services/learning resources (Ed S); human services/professional counseling (Ed S); industrial hygiene (MS); industrial management (MS); information systems (MBA); information technology (MS); kinesiology (MS); library science and information services (MS); literacy education (MSE); marketing (MBA); mathematics (MA); music (MA); occupational safety management (MS); psychology (MS); rural family nursing (MS); school administration (MSE); social gerontology (MS); sociology (MA); special education (MSE); speech language pathology (MS); superintendency (Ed S); teaching (MAT); teaching English as a second language (MA); technology (MS); technology management (PhD); theatre (MA). *Program availability:* Part-time, 100% online, blended/hybrid learning. *Faculty:* 336 full-time (145 women), 39 part-time/adjunct (25 women). *Students:* 2,161 full-time (723 women), 2,077 part-time (1,061 women); includes 188 minority (93 Black or African American, non-Hispanic/

Latino; 4 American Indian or Alaska Native, non-Hispanic/Latino; 15 Asian, non-Hispanic/Latino; 32 Hispanic/Latino; 1 Native Hawaiian or other Pacific Islander, non-Hispanic/Latino; 43 Two or more races, non-Hispanic/Latino), 2,514 international. Average age 28. 3,454 applicants, 68% accepted, 1632 enrolled. In 2015, 1,530 master's, 53 other advanced degrees awarded. *Degree requirements:* For master's and Ed S, comprehensive exam (for some programs), thesis (for some programs). *Entrance requirements:* Additional exam requirements/recommendations for international students: Required—TOEFL (minimum score 550 paper-based; 79 iBT). *Application deadline:* For fall admission, 6/1 priority date for domestic and international students; for spring admission, 10/1 priority date for domestic and international students; for summer admission, 4/1 priority date for domestic and international students. Applications are processed on a rolling basis. Application fee: $30 ($75 for international students). Electronic applications accepted. *Expenses:* Tuition, state resident: full-time $6683; part-time $278.45 per credit hour. Tuition, nonresident: full-time $13,366; part-time $556.90 per credit hour. *Required fees:* $701; $29.20 per credit hour. Tuition and fees vary according to degree level and campus/location. *Financial support:* In 2015–16, 97 students received support, including 146 research assistantships with partial tuition reimbursements available (averaging $7,500 per year), 73 teaching assistantships with partial tuition reimbursements available (averaging $7,500 per year); career-related internships or fieldwork, Federal Work-Study, scholarships/grants, and administrative and laboratory assistantships also available. Support available to part-time students. Financial award application deadline: 3/1; financial award applicants required to submit FAFSA. *Unit head:* Tina Church-Hockett, Director of Graduate School and International Admissions, 660-543-4621, Fax: 660-543-4778, E-mail: church@ucmo.edu. *Application contact:* Brittany Lawrence, Graduate Student Services Coordinator, 660-543-4621, Fax: 660-543-4778, E-mail: gradinfo@ucmo.edu.
Website: http://www.ucmo.edu/graduate/

University of Central Oklahoma, The Jackson College of Graduate Studies, College of Mathematics and Science, Department of Biology, Edmond, OK 73034-5209. Offers MS. *Program availability:* Part-time. *Degree requirements:* For master's, thesis. *Entrance requirements:* For master's, GRE General Test, GRE Subject Test (biology), faculty commitment to mentor. Additional exam requirements/recommendations for international students: Required—TOEFL (minimum score 550 paper-based; 79 iBT), IELTS (minimum score 6.5). Electronic applications accepted.

University of Chicago, Division of the Biological Sciences, The Interdisciplinary Scientist Training Program, Chicago, IL 60637-1513. Offers PhD. *Students:* 48 full-time (22 women); includes 16 minority (4 Black or African American, non-Hispanic/Latino; 8 Asian, non-Hispanic/Latino; 2 Hispanic/Latino; 2 Two or more races, non-Hispanic/Latino). Average age 27. In 2015, 2 doctorates awarded. *Degree requirements:* For doctorate, thesis/dissertation, ethics class, 2 teaching assistantships. *Entrance requirements:* For doctorate, GRE General Test. Additional exam requirements/recommendations for international students: Required—TOEFL (minimum score 600 paper-based; 104 iBT), IELTS (minimum score 7). *Application deadline:* For fall admission, 12/1 for domestic and international students. Application fee: $90. Electronic applications accepted. *Financial support:* In 2015–16, 2 students received support, including fellowships (averaging $29,781 per year), research assistantships (averaging $29,781 per year); institutionally sponsored loans, scholarships/grants, traineeships, and health care benefits also available. Financial award applicants required to submit FAFSA. *Unit head:* Dr. Daniel Margoliash, Program Director, 773-702-3224, Fax: 773-702-0037. *Application contact:* Diane Hall, Student Contact, E-mail: djh8@uchicago.edu.
Website: https://pritzker.uchicago.edu/jointdegrees/mstp/ISTP.shtml

University of Cincinnati, Graduate School, College of Medicine, Biomedical Sciences Flex Option Program, Cincinnati, OH 45221. Offers PhD. *Degree requirements:* For doctorate, thesis/dissertation, qualifying exam. *Entrance requirements:* For doctorate, GRE, 2 letters of recommendation. Additional exam requirements/recommendations for international students: Required—TOEFL. Electronic applications accepted. *Faculty research:* Environmental health, developmental biology, cell and molecular biology, immunobiology, molecular genetics.

University of Cincinnati, Graduate School, College of Medicine, Graduate Programs in Biomedical Sciences, Cincinnati, OH 45221. Offers MS, PhD, Graduate Certificate. Terminal master's awarded for partial completion of doctoral program. *Degree requirements:* For master's, thesis; for doctorate, thesis/dissertation, qualifying exam. *Entrance requirements:* For master's and doctorate, GRE General Test. Additional exam requirements/recommendations for international students: Required—TOEFL (minimum score 600 paper-based; 100 iBT). Electronic applications accepted. *Expenses:* Contact institution. *Faculty research:* Cancer, cardiovascular, metabolic disorders, neuroscience, computational medicine.

University of Cincinnati, Graduate School, College of Medicine, Physician Scientist Training Program, Cincinnati, OH 45221. Offers MD/PhD. *Entrance requirements:* Additional exam requirements/recommendations for international students: Required—TOEFL. Electronic applications accepted.

University of Cincinnati, Graduate School, McMicken College of Arts and Sciences, Department of Biological Sciences, Cincinnati, OH 45221-0006. Offers MS, PhD. *Program availability:* Part-time. Terminal master's awarded for partial completion of doctoral program. *Degree requirements:* For master's, thesis; for doctorate, comprehensive exam, thesis/dissertation. *Entrance requirements:* For master's and doctorate, GRE General Test, BS in biology, chemistry, or equivalent. Additional exam requirements/recommendations for international students: Required—TOEFL (minimum score 600 paper-based; 100 iBT). Electronic applications accepted. *Faculty research:* Physiology and development, cell and molecular, ecology and evolutionary.

University of Colorado Denver, College of Liberal Arts and Sciences, Department of Integrative and Systems Biology, Denver, CO 80217. Offers animal behavior (MS); biology (MS); cell and developmental biology (MS); ecology (MS); evolutionary biology (MS); genetics (MS); integrative and systems biology (PhD); microbiology (MS); molecular biology (MS); neurobiology (MS); plant systematics (MS). *Program availability:* Part-time. *Faculty:* 21 full-time (8 women), 3 part-time/adjunct (1 woman). *Students:* 31 full-time (19 women), 7 part-time (3 women); includes 8 minority (1 Black or African American, non-Hispanic/Latino; 1 Asian, non-Hispanic/Latino; 3 Hispanic/Latino; 3 Two or more races, non-Hispanic/Latino), 1 international. Average age 28. 34 applicants, 29% accepted, 8 enrolled. In 2015, 6 master's awarded. *Degree requirements:* For master's, comprehensive exam, thesis, 30-32 credit hours; for doctorate, comprehensive exam, thesis/dissertation. *Entrance requirements:* For master's, GRE General Test (minimum score in 50th percentile in each section), BA/BS from accredited institution awarded within the last 10 years; minimum undergraduate GPA 3.0; prerequisite courses: 1 year each of general biology and general chemistry; 1 semester each of general genetics, general ecology, and cell biology; and a structure/function course; for doctorate, GRE, minimum undergraduate GPA of 3.2, three letters of recommendation, official transcripts from all universities and colleges attended. Additional exam requirements/recommendations for international students: Required—TOEFL (minimum score 537 paper-based; 75 iBT); Recommended—IELTS (minimum score 6.5). *Application deadline:* For fall admission, 1/15 for domestic and international students. Application fee: $50 ($75 for international students). Electronic applications accepted. *Financial support:* In 2015–16, 32 students received support. Fellowships, research assistantships, teaching assistantships, Federal Work-Study, institutionally sponsored loans, scholarships/grants, and traineeships available. Financial award application deadline: 4/1; financial award applicants required to submit FAFSA. *Faculty research:* Molecular developmental biology; quantitative ecology, biogeography, and population dynamics; environmental signaling and endocrine disruption; speciation, the evolution of reproductive isolation, and hybrid zones; evolutionary, behavioral, and conservation ecology. *Unit head:* Dr. John Swallow, Chair, 303-556-6154, E-mail: john.swallow@ucdenver.edu. *Application contact:* Dr. Michael Wunder, Graduate Advisor, 303-556-8870, E-mail: michael.wunder@ucdenver.edu. Website: http://www.ucdenver.edu/academics/colleges/CLAS/Departments/biology/Programs/MasterofScience/Pages/BiologyMasterOfScience.aspx

University of Colorado Denver, School of Medicine, Biomedical Sciences Program, Aurora, CO 80045. Offers MS, PhD. *Students:* 24 full-time (14 women), 1 (woman) part-time; includes 6 minority (2 Asian, non-Hispanic/Latino; 2 Hispanic/Latino; 2 Two or more races, non-Hispanic/Latino), 4 international. Average age 26. 169 applicants, 14% accepted, 22 enrolled. In 2015, 8 master's awarded. Terminal master's awarded for partial completion of doctoral program. *Degree requirements:* For master's and doctorate, comprehensive exam. *Entrance requirements:* For master's, GRE, three letters of recommendation; for doctorate, GRE, minimum undergraduate GPA of 3.0; prerequisite coursework in organic chemistry, biology, biochemistry, physics, and calculus; letters of recommendation; interview. Additional exam requirements/recommendations for international students: Required—TOEFL (minimum score 550 paper-based; 80 iBT). *Application deadline:* For fall admission, 12/1 for domestic students, 11/1 for international students. Application fee: $50 ($75 for international students). Electronic applications accepted. *Expenses:* Contact institution. *Financial support:* In 2015–16, 11 students received support. Fellowships, research assistantships, teaching assistantships, Federal Work-Study, institutionally sponsored loans, scholarships/grants, traineeships, health care benefits, tuition waivers (full), and unspecified assistantships available. Financial award applicants required to submit FAFSA. *Unit head:* Heide Ford, Director, 303-724-3509, E-mail: heide.ford@ucdenver.edu. *Application contact:* Elizabeth Bowen, Program Administrator, 303-724-3565, E-mail: elizabeth.bowen@ucdenver.edu. Website: http://www.ucdenver.edu/academics/colleges/Graduate-School/academic-programs/Biomedical/Pages/home.aspx

University of Connecticut Health Center, Graduate School and School of Medicine, Combined Degree Program in Biomedical Sciences, Farmington, CT 06030. Offers MD/PhD. *Entrance requirements:* Additional exam requirements/recommendations for international students: Required—TOEFL (minimum score 600 paper-based). *Expenses:* Contact institution.

★ **University of Connecticut Health Center,** Graduate School, Programs in Biomedical Sciences, Farmington, CT 06030. Offers PhD, DMD/PhD, MD/PhD. *Degree requirements:* For doctorate, comprehensive exam, thesis/dissertation. *Entrance requirements:* For doctorate, GRE General Test. Additional exam requirements/recommendations for international students: Required—TOEFL (minimum score 600 paper-based).
See Display below and Close-Up on page 117.

University of Connecticut Health Center, Graduate School, Programs in Biomedical Sciences - Integrated, Farmington, CT 06030. Offers PhD, DMD/PhD, MD/PhD. *Degree requirements:* For doctorate, comprehensive exam, thesis/dissertation. *Entrance requirements:* For doctorate, GRE General Test. Additional exam requirements/recommendations for international students: Required—TOEFL (minimum score 600 paper-based). Electronic applications accepted.

University of Dayton, Department of Biology, Dayton, OH 45469. Offers MS, PhD. *Faculty:* 16 full-time (6 women). *Students:* 18 full-time (11 women), 1 part-time (0 women); includes 2 minority (both Asian, non-Hispanic/Latino), 8 international. Average age 26. 63 applicants, 8% accepted, 5 enrolled. In 2015, 3 master's, 5 doctorates awarded. Terminal master's awarded for partial completion of doctoral program. *Degree requirements:* For master's, thesis; for doctorate, thesis/dissertation. *Entrance requirements:* For master's and doctorate, GRE General Test, minimum undergraduate GPA of 3.0. Additional exam requirements/recommendations for international students: Required—TOEFL (minimum score 550 paper-based; 80 iBT). *Application deadline:* For fall admission, 1/31 priority date for domestic and international students. Applications are processed on a rolling basis. Application fee: $0 ($50 for international students). Electronic applications accepted. *Financial support:* In 2015–16, 3 research assistantships with full tuition reimbursements (averaging $18,760 per year), 15 teaching assistantships with full tuition reimbursements (averaging $18,760 per year) were awarded; institutionally sponsored loans, health care benefits, and unspecified assistantships also available. Financial award applicants required to submit FAFSA. *Faculty research:* Invasive species, regeneration, developmental genetics, microbial metabolism, neuropharmacology. *Total annual research expenditures:* $75,000. *Unit head:* Dr. Mark G. Nielsen, Chair, 937-229-2521, Fax: 937-229-2021, E-mail: mnielsen1@udayton.edu. *Application contact:* Dr. Amit Singh, Director, Biology Graduate Programs, 937-229-2894, Fax: 937-229-2021, E-mail: asingh1@udayton.edu. Website: https://www.udayton.edu/artssciences/academics/biology/grad/index.php

University of Delaware, College of Arts and Sciences, Department of Biological Sciences, Newark, DE 19716. Offers biotechnology (MS); cancer biology (MS, PhD); cell and extracellular matrix biology (MS, PhD); cell and systems physiology (MS, PhD); developmental biology (MS, PhD); ecology and evolution (MS, PhD); microbiology (MS, PhD); molecular biology and genetics (MS, PhD). Terminal master's awarded for partial completion of doctoral program. *Degree requirements:* For master's, thesis, preliminary exam; for doctorate, comprehensive exam, thesis/dissertation, preliminary exam. *Entrance requirements:* For master's and doctorate, GRE General Test. Additional exam requirements/recommendations for international students: Required—TOEFL (minimum score 600 paper-based); Recommended—TWE. Electronic applications accepted. *Faculty research:* Microorganisms, bone, cancer metastasis, developmental biology, cell biology, DNA.

University of Denver, Division of Natural Sciences and Mathematics, Department of Biological Sciences, Denver, CO 80208. Offers biology, ecology and evolution (MS, PhD); biomedical sciences (PSM); cell and molecular biology (MS, PhD). *Program availability:* Part-time. *Faculty:* 23 full-time (7 women), 2 part-time/adjunct (both women). *Students:* 8 full-time (all women), 27 part-time (21 women); includes 4 minority (2 Black or African American, non-Hispanic/Latino; 2 Hispanic/Latino), 6 international. Average age 26. 77 applicants, 38% accepted, 21 enrolled. In 2015, 6 master's, 3 doctorates awarded. Terminal master's awarded for partial completion of doctoral program. *Degree requirements:* For master's, comprehensive exam (for some programs), thesis; for doctorate, one foreign language, comprehensive exam (for some programs), thesis/dissertation. *Entrance requirements:* For master's and doctorate, GRE General Test, bachelor's degree in biology or related field, transcripts, personal statement, three letters of recommendation. Additional exam requirements/recommendations for international students: Required—TOEFL (minimum score 550 paper-based; 80 iBT). *Application deadline:* For fall admission, 1/1 priority date for domestic and international students. Applications are processed on a rolling basis. Application fee: $65. Electronic applications accepted. *Expenses:* $30,477. *Financial support:* In 2015–16, 35 students received support, including 8 research assistantships with tuition reimbursements available (averaging $15,834 per year), 23 teaching assistantships with tuition reimbursements available (averaging $17,210 per year); Federal Work-Study,

institutionally sponsored loans, scholarships/grants, and unspecified assistantships also available. Support available to part-time students. Financial award application deadline: 2/15; financial award applicants required to submit FAFSA. *Faculty research:* Molecular biology, cell biology, neurobiology, ecology, molecular evolution. *Unit head:* Dr. Joseph Angleson, Associate Professor and Chair, 303-871-3463, Fax: 303-871-3471, E-mail: jangleso@du.edu. *Application contact:* Randi Flageolle, Assistant to the Chair, 303-871-3457, Fax: 303-871-3471, E-mail: rflageol@du.edu.
Website: http://www.du.edu/nsm/departments/biologicalsciences

University of Florida, College of Medicine and Graduate School, Interdisciplinary Program in Biomedical Sciences, Gainesville, FL 32610-0229. Offers MS, PhD, MD/PhD. *Degree requirements:* For doctorate, comprehensive exam, thesis/dissertation. *Entrance requirements:* For doctorate, GRE General Test, minimum GPA of 3.0, biochemistry before enrollment. Additional exam requirements/recommendations for international students: Required—TOEFL, IELTS. Electronic applications accepted. *Expenses:* Contact institution.

University of Georgia, Biomedical and Health Sciences Institute, Athens, GA 30602. Offers neuroscience (PhD). *Entrance requirements:* For doctorate, GRE, official transcripts, 3 letters of recommendation, statement of interest. Additional exam requirements/recommendations for international students: Required—TOEFL.

University of Guam, Office of Graduate Studies, College of Natural and Applied Sciences, Program in Biology, Mangilao, GU 96923. Offers tropical marine biology (MS). *Degree requirements:* For master's, comprehensive exam, thesis. *Entrance requirements:* For master's, GRE General Test, GRE Subject Test. Additional exam requirements/recommendations for international students: Required—TOEFL. *Faculty research:* Maintenance and ecology of coral reefs.

University of Guelph, Graduate Studies, College of Biological Science, Guelph, ON N1G 2W1, Canada. Offers M Sc, PhD. *Program availability:* Part-time. *Degree requirements:* For master's, thesis (for some programs); for doctorate, comprehensive exam (for some programs), thesis/dissertation. *Entrance requirements:* Additional exam requirements/recommendations for international students: Required—TOEFL (minimum score 550 paper-based). Electronic applications accepted.

University of Hartford, College of Arts and Sciences, Department of Biology, West Hartford, CT 06117-1599. Offers biology (MS); neuroscience (MS). *Program availability:* Part-time, evening/weekend. *Degree requirements:* For master's, comprehensive exam, thesis optional, oral exams. *Entrance requirements:* For master's, GRE or MCAT. Additional exam requirements/recommendations for international students: Required—TOEFL (minimum score 550 paper-based). Electronic applications accepted. *Faculty research:* Neurobiology of aging, central actions of neural steroids, neuroendocrine control of reproduction, retinopathies in sharks, plasticity in the central nervous system.

University of Hawaii at Manoa, John A. Burns School of Medicine and Graduate Division, Graduate Programs in Biomedical Sciences, Honolulu, HI 96822. Offers MS, PhD. *Program availability:* Part-time. *Faculty:* 17 full-time (10 women), 1 part-time/adjunct (0 women). *Students:* 9 full-time (7 women), 6 part-time (5 women); includes 7 minority (2 Black or African American, non-Hispanic/Latino; 2 Asian, non-Hispanic/Latino; 1 Native Hawaiian or other Pacific Islander, non-Hispanic/Latino; 2 Two or more races, non-Hispanic/Latino), 3 international. Average age 42. 1 applicant, 100% accepted, 1 enrolled. In 2015, 1 master's, 3 doctorates awarded. Terminal master's awarded for partial completion of doctoral program. *Degree requirements:* For master's, thesis optional; for doctorate, comprehensive exam, thesis/dissertation. *Entrance requirements:* For master's and doctorate, GRE General Test. Additional exam requirements/recommendations for international students: Required—TOEFL (minimum score 500 paper-based; 61 iBT), IELTS (minimum score 5). *Application deadline:* For fall admission, 6/1 for domestic and international students. Application fee: $100. *Expenses:* Contact institution. *Financial support:* In 2015–16, 1 fellowship (averaging $18,126 per year), 1 research assistantship (averaging $23,022 per year) were awarded; career-related internships or fieldwork, Federal Work-Study, institutionally sponsored loans, and tuition waivers (full and partial) also available. Support available to part-time students. *Total annual research expenditures:* $989,000. *Unit head:* Dr. Jerris R. Hedges, Dean, 808-692-0881. *Application contact:* Rosanne Harrigan, Graduate Chairperson, 808-692-0904, Fax: 808-692-1247, E-mail: harrigan@hawaii.edu. Website: http://www2.hawaii.edu/~mscr/

University of Houston, College of Natural Sciences and Mathematics, Department of Biology and Biochemistry, Houston, TX 77204. Offers biochemistry (MA, PhD); biology (MA). Terminal master's awarded for partial completion of doctoral program. *Degree requirements:* For master's, comprehensive exam (for some programs), thesis optional; for doctorate, comprehensive exam (for some programs), thesis/dissertation. *Entrance requirements:* For master's and doctorate, GRE. Additional exam requirements/recommendations for international students: Required—TOEFL (minimum score 550 paper-based; 79 iBT), IELTS (minimum score 6.5). Electronic applications accepted. *Faculty research:* Cell and molecular biology, ecology and evolution, biochemical and biophysical sciences, chemical biology.

University of Houston–Clear Lake, School of Science and Computer Engineering, Program in Biological Sciences, Houston, TX 77058-1002. Offers MS. *Program availability:* Part-time, evening/weekend. *Entrance requirements:* For master's, GRE General Test. Additional exam requirements/recommendations for international students: Required—TOEFL (minimum score 550 paper-based).

University of Houston–Victoria, School of Arts and Sciences, Program in Biomedical Sciences, Victoria, TX 77901-4450. Offers biological sciences (MS); biomedical sciences (MS); forensic science (MS).

University of Idaho, College of Graduate Studies, College of Science, Department of Biological Sciences, Moscow, ID 83844-3051. Offers biology (MS, PhD); microbiology, molecular biology and biochemistry (PhD); neuroscience (MS). *Faculty:* 18 full-time. *Students:* 25 full-time, 2 part-time. Average age 29. In 2015, 5 doctorates awarded. *Degree requirements:* For doctorate, one foreign language, thesis/dissertation. *Entrance requirements:* For master's, GRE, minimum GPA of 2.8; for doctorate, GRE, minimum undergraduate GPA of 2.8, 3.0 graduate. Additional exam requirements/recommendations for international students: Required—TOEFL. *Application deadline:* For fall admission, 8/1 for domestic students; for spring admission, 12/15 for domestic students. Applications are processed on a rolling basis. Application fee: $60. Electronic applications accepted. *Expenses:* Tuition, state resident: full-time $6205; part-time $399 per credit hour. Tuition, nonresident: full-time $20,209; part-time $1177 per credit hour. *Required fees:* $2017; $58 per credit hour. Full-time tuition and fees vary according to course load and reciprocity agreements. *Financial support:* Research assistantships and teaching assistantships available. Financial award applicants required to submit FAFSA. *Faculty research:* Animal behavior development, germ cell development, evolutionary biology, fish reproductive biology, molecular mechanisms. *Unit head:* Dr. James J. Nagler, Interim Department Chair, 208-885-6280, E-mail: biosci@uidaho.edu. *Application contact:* Sean Scoggin, Graduate Recruitment Coordinator, 208-885-4723, Fax: 208-885-4406, E-mail: graduateadmissions@uidaho.edu. Website: http://www.uidaho.edu/sci/biology

University of Illinois at Chicago, College of Liberal Arts and Sciences, Department of Biological Sciences, Chicago, IL 60607-7128. Offers MS, PhD. *Faculty:* 39 full-time (15 women), 5 part-time/adjunct (4 women). *Students:* 97 full-time (63 women), 9 part-time (4 women); includes 21 minority (6 Black or African American, non-Hispanic/Latino; 5 Asian, non-Hispanic/Latino; 8 Hispanic/Latino; 2 Two or more races, non-Hispanic/Latino), 30 international. Average age 29. *Degree requirements:* For master's, thesis; for doctorate, thesis/dissertation, preliminary exam. *Entrance requirements:* For master's and doctorate, GRE General Test, GRE Subject Test, previous course work in physics, calculus, and organic chemistry; minimum GPA of 2.75. Additional exam requirements/recommendations for international students: Required—TOEFL. *Application deadline:* For fall admission, 1/1 for domestic and international students. Applications are processed on a rolling basis. Application fee: $60. Electronic applications accepted. *Expenses:* Contact institution. *Financial support:* In 2015–16, 1 fellowship with full tuition reimbursement was awarded; research assistantships with full tuition reimbursements, teaching assistantships with full tuition reimbursements, career-related internships or fieldwork, Federal Work-Study, scholarships/grants, traineeships, tuition waivers (full), and unspecified assistantships also available. Financial award application deadline: 3/1; financial award applicants required to submit FAFSA. *Faculty research:* Classical and molecular genetic analysis, modulation of synaptic transmission, molecular ecology, landscape genetics, conservation biology, ecophysiology, plant nutrition and global climate change, predator-prey interactions and urban wildlife, genetic studies of Drosophila, glutamate signaling in Drosophila, molecular mechanisms of exocytosis and endocytosis, global change biology, plant and ecosystem physiology, isotope ecology, respiration, community. *Unit head:* Prof. Brian K. Kay, Head, 312-996-4249, E-mail: bkay@uic.edu. *Application contact:* Prof. Aixa Alfonso, Director of Graduate Studies, 312-355-0318, E-mail: aalfonso@uic.edu. Website: http://www.uic.edu/depts/bios/

University of Illinois at Chicago, College of Medicine and Graduate College, Graduate Programs in Medicine, Chicago, IL 60607-7128. Offers MHPE, MS, PhD, MD/MS, MD/PhD. *Program availability:* Part-time. *Faculty:* 20 full-time (12 women), 42 part-time/adjunct (32 women). *Students:* 130 full-time (85 women), 103 part-time (72 women); includes 40 minority (9 Black or African American, non-Hispanic/Latino; 14 Asian, non-Hispanic/Latino; 10 Hispanic/Latino; 7 Two or more races, non-Hispanic/Latino), 75 international. Average age 33. Terminal master's awarded for partial completion of doctoral program. *Degree requirements:* For master's, thesis; for doctorate, thesis/dissertation. *Entrance requirements:* For master's and doctorate, GRE General Test. *Application deadline:* For fall admission, 3/1 priority date for domestic students, 2/15 for international students. Application fee: $60. *Expenses:* Contact institution. *Financial support:* In 2015–16, 14 fellowships with full tuition reimbursements were awarded; research assistantships with full tuition reimbursements, teaching assistantships with full tuition reimbursements, career-related internships or fieldwork, Federal Work-Study, institutionally sponsored loans, scholarships/grants, traineeships, tuition waivers (full), and unspecified assistantships also available. Financial award application deadline: 3/1; financial award applicants required to submit FAFSA. *Unit head:* Dr. Dimitri T. Azar, Head, 312-996-3500, Fax: 312-996-9006, E-mail: dtazar@uic.edu. *Application contact:* Jackie Ryan, Graduate College Receptionist, 312-413-2550, Fax: 312-413-0185, E-mail: gradcoll@uic.edu. Website: http://www.medicine.uic.edu/

University of Illinois at Springfield, Graduate Programs, College of Liberal Arts and Sciences, Program in Biology, Springfield, IL 62703-5407. Offers MS. *Program availability:* Part-time, evening/weekend. *Faculty:* 3 full-time (1 woman). *Students:* 5 full-time (3 women), 3 part-time (all women); includes 1 minority (Hispanic/Latino). Average age 28. 28 applicants, 29% accepted, 5 enrolled. In 2015, 7 master's awarded. *Degree requirements:* For master's, oral presentation of the written thesis or non-thesis comprehensive examination. *Entrance requirements:* For master's, GRE General Test, GRE Subject Test (biology), minimum undergraduate GPA of 3.0; letter that discusses academic and career goals including how goals fit with departmental specialties; 2 letters of reference. Additional exam requirements/recommendations for international students: Required—TOEFL (minimum score 500 paper-based; 61 iBT). *Application deadline:* Applications are processed on a rolling basis. Application fee: $60 ($75 for international students). Electronic applications accepted. *Expenses:* Tuition, state resident: part-time $329 per credit hour. Tuition, nonresident: part-time $675 per credit hour. *Financial support:* In 2015–16, fellowships with full tuition reimbursements (averaging $9,900 per year), research assistantships with full tuition reimbursements (averaging $9,956 per year), teaching assistantships with full tuition reimbursements (averaging $9,956 per year) were awarded; career-related internships or fieldwork, Federal Work-Study, scholarships/grants, health care benefits, and unspecified assistantships also available. Support available to part-time students. Financial award application deadline: 11/15; financial award applicants required to submit FAFSA. *Unit head:* Dr. Hua Chen, Program Administrator, 217-206-6630, Fax: 217-206-7205, E-mail: hchen40@uis.edu. *Application contact:* Dr. Lynn Pardie, Office of Graduate Studies, 800-252-8533, Fax: 217-206-7623, E-mail: lpard1@uis.edu. Website: http://www.uis.edu/biology

University of Illinois at Urbana–Champaign, Graduate College, College of Liberal Arts and Sciences, School of Chemical Sciences, Champaign, IL 61820. Offers MA, MS, PhD, MS/JD, MS/MBA. *Expenses:* Contact institution.

University of Illinois at Urbana–Champaign, Graduate College, College of Liberal Arts and Sciences, School of Integrative Biology, Champaign, IL 61820. Offers MS, MST, PSM, PhD. *Program availability:* Part-time, online learning.

University of Indianapolis, Graduate Programs, College of Arts and Sciences, Department of Biology, Indianapolis, IN 46227-3697. Offers human biology (MS). *Program availability:* Part-time, evening/weekend. *Degree requirements:* For master's, thesis. *Entrance requirements:* For master's, GRE General Test, 3 letters of recommendation; minimum GPA of 3.0; BA/BS in anthropology, biology, human biology or closely-related field; resume. Additional exam requirements/recommendations for international students: Required—TOEFL (minimum score 550 paper-based).

The University of Iowa, Graduate College, College of Liberal Arts and Sciences, Department of Biology, Iowa City, IA 52242-1324. Offers biology (MS, PhD); cell and developmental biology (MS, PhD); evolution (MS, PhD); genetics (MS, PhD); neurobiology (MS, PhD). Terminal master's awarded for partial completion of doctoral program. *Degree requirements:* For master's, thesis optional, exam; for doctorate, comprehensive exam, thesis/dissertation. *Entrance requirements:* For master's and doctorate, GRE General Test, minimum GPA of 3.0. Additional exam requirements/recommendations for international students: Required—TOEFL (minimum score 600 paper-based; 100 iBT). Electronic applications accepted. *Faculty research:* Neurobiology, evolutionary biology, genetics, cell and developmental biology.

The University of Iowa, Roy J. and Lucille A. Carver College of Medicine and Graduate College, Graduate Programs in Medicine, Iowa City, IA 52242-1316. Offers MA, MPAS, MS, DPT, PhD, JD/MHA, MBA/MHA, MD/JD, MD/PhD, MHA/MA, MHA/MS, MPH/MHA, MS/MA, MS/MS. *Program availability:* Part-time. *Degree requirements:* For doctorate, thesis/dissertation. Electronic applications accepted. *Expenses:* Contact institution.

The University of Iowa, Roy J. and Lucille A. Carver College of Medicine and Graduate College, Medical Scientist Training Program, Iowa City, IA 52242-1316. Offers MD/PhD. Electronic applications accepted. Application fee is waived when completed online. *Faculty research:* Structure and function of ion channels, molecular genetics of human disease, neurobiology of pain, viral immunology and immunopathology, epidemiology of aging and cancer, human learning and memory, structural enzymology.

The University of Kansas, University of Kansas Medical Center, School of Medicine, Interdisciplinary Graduate Program in Biomedical Sciences (IGPBS), Kansas City, KS 66160. Offers PhD, MD/PhD. *Students:* 14 full-time (7 women); includes 1 minority (Black or African American, non-Hispanic/Latino), 6 international. Average age 26. 115 applicants, 13% accepted, 14 enrolled. Terminal master's awarded for partial completion of doctoral program. *Degree requirements:* For doctorate, comprehensive exam, thesis/dissertation. *Entrance requirements:* For doctorate, GRE. Additional exam requirements/recommendations for international students: Required—TOEFL. *Application deadline:* For fall admission, 12/1 priority date for domestic and international students. Applications are processed on a rolling basis. Application fee: $60. Electronic applications accepted. *Financial support:* In 2015–16, 3 research assistantships with full tuition reimbursements (averaging $24,000 per year), 18 teaching assistantships with full tuition reimbursements (averaging $24,000 per year) were awarded; scholarships/grants and unspecified assistantships also available. Financial award application deadline: 3/1; financial award applicants required to submit FAFSA. *Faculty research:* Cardiovascular biology, neurosciences, signal transduction and cancer biology, molecular biology and genetics, developmental biology. *Unit head:* Dr. Michael J. Werle, Director, 913-588-7491, Fax: 913-588-2710, E-mail: mwerle@kumc.edu. *Application contact:* Martin J. Graham, Coordinator, 913-588-2719, Fax: 913-588-5242, E-mail: mgraham4@kumc.edu. Website: http://www.kumc.edu/igpbs.html

See Display below and Close-Up on page 119.

University of Kentucky, Graduate School, College of Arts and Sciences, Program in Biology, Lexington, KY 40506-0032. Offers MS, PhD. *Degree requirements:* For master's, comprehensive exam, thesis optional; for doctorate, comprehensive exam, thesis/dissertation. *Entrance requirements:* For master's, GRE General Test, minimum undergraduate GPA of 2.75; for doctorate, GRE General Test, minimum graduate GPA of 3.0. Additional exam requirements/recommendations for international students: Required—TOEFL (minimum score 550 paper-based). Electronic applications accepted. *Faculty research:* General biology, microbiology, &ITDrosophila&RO molecular genetics, molecular virology, multiple loci inheritance.

University of Kentucky, Graduate School, Graduate School Programs from the College of Medicine, Lexington, KY 40506-0032. Offers MS, PhD, MD/PhD. *Degree requirements:* For master's, comprehensive exam, thesis (for some programs); for doctorate, comprehensive exam, thesis/dissertation. *Entrance requirements:* For master's, GRE General Test, minimum undergraduate GPA of 2.75; for doctorate, GRE General Test, minimum undergraduate GPA of 3.0. Additional exam requirements/recommendations for international students: Required—TOEFL (minimum score 550 paper-based). Electronic applications accepted.

University of Lethbridge, School of Graduate Studies, Lethbridge, AB T1K 3M4, Canada. Offers addictions counseling (M Sc); agricultural biotechnology (M Sc); agricultural studies (M Sc, MA); anthropology (MA); archaeology (M Sc, MA); art (MA, MFA); biochemistry (M Sc); biological sciences (M Sc); biomolecular science (PhD); biosystems and biodiversity (PhD); Canadian studies (MA); chemistry (M Sc); computer science (M Sc); computer science and geographical information science (M Sc); counseling (MC); counseling psychology (M Ed); dramatic arts (MA); earth, space, and physical science (PhD); economics (MA); education (MA, PhD); educational leadership

(M Ed); English (MA); environmental science (M Sc); evolution and behavior (PhD); exercise science (M Sc); French (MA); French/German (MA); French/Spanish (MA); general education (M Ed); geography (M Sc, MA); German (MA); health sciences (M Sc); individualized multidisciplinary (M Sc, MA); kinesiology (M Sc, MA); management (M Sc), including accounting, finance, human resource management and labor relations, information systems, international management, marketing, policy and strategy; mathematics (M Sc); music (M Mus, MA); Native American studies (MA); neuroscience (M Sc, PhD); new media (MA, MFA); nursing (M Sc, MN); philosophy (MA); physics (M Sc); political science (MA); psychology (M Sc, MA); religious studies (MA); sociology (MA); theatre and dramatic arts (MFA); theoretical and computational science (PhD); urban and regional studies (MA); women and gender studies (MA). *Program availability:* Part-time, evening/weekend. *Students:* 448 full-time (249 women), 110 part-time (64 women). Average age 32. 285 applicants, 36% accepted, 96 enrolled. In 2015, 154 master's, 11 doctorates awarded. *Degree requirements:* For master's, thesis (for some programs); for doctorate, comprehensive exam, thesis/dissertation. *Entrance requirements:* For master's, GMAT (for M Sc in management), bachelor's degree in related field, minimum GPA of 3.0 during previous 20 graded semester courses, 2 years' teaching or related experience (M Ed); for doctorate, master's degree, minimum graduate GPA of 3.5. Additional exam requirements/recommendations for international students: Required—TOEFL (minimum score 580 paper-based; 93 iBT). Application fee: $100 Canadian dollars ($140 Canadian dollars for international students). Electronic applications accepted. *Financial support:* Fellowships, research assistantships, teaching assistantships, scholarships/grants, health care benefits, and unspecified assistantships available. *Faculty research:* Movement and brain plasticity, gibberellin physiology, photosynthesis, carbon cycling, molecular properties of main-group ring components. *Unit head:* Kathleen Schrage, Manager, School of Graduate Studies, 403-329-2121, E-mail: schrage@uleth.ca. *Application contact:* School of Graduate Studies, 403-329-5194, E-mail: sgsinquiries@uleth.ca. Website: http://www.uleth.ca/graduate-studies/

University of Louisiana at Lafayette, College of Sciences, Department of Biology, Lafayette, LA 70504. Offers biology (MS); environmental and evolutionary biology (PhD). Terminal master's awarded for partial completion of doctoral program. *Degree requirements:* For master's, thesis; for doctorate, 2 foreign languages, comprehensive exam, thesis/dissertation. *Entrance requirements:* For master's, GRE General Test, minimum GPA of 2.75; for doctorate, GRE General Test, GRE Subject Test, minimum GPA of 3.0. Additional exam requirements/recommendations for international students: Required—TOEFL (minimum score 550 paper-based). Electronic applications accepted. *Faculty research:* Structure and ultrastructure, system biology, ecology, processes, environmental physiology.

University of Louisiana at Monroe, Graduate School, College of Arts, Education, and Sciences, Department of Biology, Monroe, LA 71209-0001. Offers MS. *Degree requirements:* For master's, thesis optional. *Entrance requirements:* For master's, GRE General Test, minimum GPA of 2.5. Additional exam requirements/recommendations for international students: Required—TOEFL (minimum score 500 paper-based; 61 iBT); Recommended—IELTS (minimum score 5.5). Electronic applications accepted. *Faculty research:* Fish systematics and zoogeography, taxonomy and distribution of Louisiana plants, aquatic biology, secondary succession, microbial ecology.

University of Louisville, Graduate School, College of Arts and Sciences, Department of Biology, Louisville, KY 40292-0001. Offers biology (MS); environmental biology (PhD). *Program availability:* Part-time. *Students:* 52 full-time (29 women), 2 part-time (0 women); includes 4 minority (1 Black or African American, non-Hispanic/Latino; 1 Asian, non-Hispanic/Latino; 1 Hispanic/Latino; 1 Two or more races, non-Hispanic/Latino), 11 international. Average age 29. 35 applicants, 54% accepted, 15 enrolled. In 2015, 3 master's, 1 doctorate awarded. Terminal master's awarded for partial completion of

Biological and Biomedical Sciences—General

doctoral program. *Degree requirements:* For master's, comprehensive exam, thesis (for some programs); for doctorate, comprehensive exam, thesis/dissertation. *Entrance requirements:* For master's, GRE, MCAT, or DAT; for doctorate, GRE. Additional exam requirements/recommendations for international students: Required—TOEFL (minimum score 550 paper-based, 83 iBT) or IELTS (6.5). *Application deadline:* For fall admission, 1/31 priority date for domestic and international students; for spring admission, 12/1 for domestic and international students; for summer admission, 4/15 for domestic and international students. Applications are processed on a rolling basis. Application fee: $60. Electronic applications accepted. *Expenses:* Tuition, state resident: full-time $11,664; part-time $649 per credit hour. Tuition, nonresident: full-time $24,274; part-time $1350 per credit hour. *Required fees:* $196. Tuition and fees vary according to program and reciprocity agreements. *Financial support:* In 2015–16, 415,878 students received support, including 2 fellowships with full tuition reimbursements available (averaging $22,000 per year), 2 research assistantships with full tuition reimbursements available (averaging $22,000 per year), 24 teaching assistantships with full tuition reimbursements available (averaging $22,000 per year); Federal Work-Study and unspecified assistantships also available. Financial award application deadline: 1/31. *Faculty research:* Molecular, microbiology, ecology, animal behavior, evolution. *Total annual research expenditures:* $717,917. *Unit head:* Dr. Ronald Fell, Chair, 502-852-6771, Fax: 502-852-0725, E-mail: rdfell@louisville.edu. *Application contact:* Libby Leggett, Director, Graduate Admissions, 502-852-3101, Fax: 502-852-6536, E-mail: gradadm@louisville.edu.
Website: http://louisville.edu/biology

University of Maine, Graduate School, College of Natural Sciences, Forestry, and Agriculture, Department of Molecular and Biomedical Sciences, Orono, ME 04469. Offers microbiology (PhD). *Faculty:* 30 full-time (6 women), 20 part-time/adjunct (4 women). *Students:* 22 full-time (12 women); includes 2 minority (1 Asian, non-Hispanic/Latino; 1 Two or more races, non-Hispanic/Latino), 3 international. Average age 30. 40 applicants, 28% accepted, 6 enrolled. In 2015, 7 master's, 3 doctorates awarded. *Degree requirements:* For master's, thesis (for some programs); for doctorate, comprehensive exam, thesis/dissertation. *Entrance requirements:* For master's and doctorate, GRE General Test. Additional exam requirements/recommendations for international students: Required—TOEFL. *Application deadline:* For fall admission, 2/1 priority date for domestic students. Applications are processed on a rolling basis. Application fee: $65. Electronic applications accepted. *Financial support:* In 2015–16, 20 students received support, including 8 research assistantships with full tuition reimbursements available (averaging $16,800 per year), 12 teaching assistantships with full tuition reimbursements available (averaging $19,000 per year); tuition waivers (full and partial) also available. Financial award application deadline: 3/1. *Total annual research expenditures:* $242,844. *Unit head:* Dr. Robert Gundersen, Chair, 207-581-2802, Fax: 207-581-2801. *Application contact:* Scott G. Delcourt, Assistant Vice President for Graduate Studies and Senior Associate Dean, 207-581-3291, Fax: 207-581-3232, E-mail: graduate@maine.edu.
Website: http://umaine.edu/biomed/

University of Maine, Graduate School, College of Natural Sciences, Forestry, and Agriculture, School of Biology and Ecology, Orono, ME 04469. Offers biological sciences (PhD); botany and plant pathology (MS); ecology and environmental science (MS, PhD); entomology (MS); plant science (PhD); zoology (MS, PhD). *Program availability:* Part-time. *Faculty:* 24 full-time (12 women), 34 part-time/adjunct (13 women). *Students:* 64 full-time (36 women), 1 part-time (0 women); includes 4 minority (1 American Indian or Alaska Native, non-Hispanic/Latino; 1 Asian, non-Hispanic/Latino; 1 Hispanic/Latino; 1 Two or more races, non-Hispanic/Latino), 8 international. Average age 29. 52 applicants, 25% accepted, 11 enrolled. In 2015, 7 master's, 8 doctorates awarded. Terminal master's awarded for partial completion of doctoral program. *Degree requirements:* For master's, thesis (for some programs); for doctorate, comprehensive exam, thesis/dissertation. *Entrance requirements:* For master's and doctorate, GRE General Test. Additional exam requirements/recommendations for international students: Required—TOEFL. *Application deadline:* For fall admission, 2/1 priority date for domestic students. Applications are processed on a rolling basis. Application fee: $65. Electronic applications accepted. *Financial support:* In 2015–16, 14 students received support, including 6 research assistantships with full tuition reimbursements available (averaging $14,600 per year), 8 teaching assistantships with full tuition reimbursements available (averaging $14,600 per year); career-related internships or fieldwork, Federal Work-Study, institutionally sponsored loans, and tuition waivers (full and partial) also available. Financial award application deadline: 3/1. *Faculty research:* Ecology and evolution (aquatic, terrestrial, paleo); development and genetics; biomedical research; ecophysiology and stress; invasion ecology and pest management. *Total annual research expenditures:* $3.2 million. *Unit head:* Dr. Andrei Aloykhin, Director, 207-581-2977, Fax: 207-581-2537. *Application contact:* Scott G. Delcourt, Assistant Vice President for Graduate Studies and Senior Associate Dean, 207-581-3291, Fax: 207-581-3232, E-mail: graduate@maine.edu.
Website: http://sbe.umaine.edu/

University of Maine, Graduate School, Graduate School of Biomedical Science and Engineering, Orono, ME 04469. Offers bioinformatics (PSM); biomedical engineering (PhD); biomedical science (PhD). *Faculty:* 151 full-time (45 women). *Students:* 41 full-time (24 women), 2 part-time (both women); includes 2 minority (both Two or more races, non-Hispanic/Latino), 12 international. Average age 31. 69 applicants, 19% accepted, 12 enrolled. In 2015, 2 master's, 2 doctorates awarded. *Degree requirements:* For doctorate, comprehensive exam, thesis/dissertation. *Entrance requirements:* For doctorate, GRE General Test, master's degree. Additional exam requirements/recommendations for international students: Required—TOEFL. *Application deadline:* For fall admission, 12/31 for domestic students. Application fee: $65. *Financial support:* In 2015–16, 28 students received support, including 1 fellowship with full tuition reimbursement available (averaging $20,000 per year), 22 research assistantships with full tuition reimbursements available (averaging $23,000 per year), 5 teaching assistantships (averaging $7,500 per year). Financial award application deadline: 3/1. *Faculty research:* Molecular and cellular biology, neuroscience, biomedical engineering, toxicology, bioinformatics and computational biology. *Total annual research expenditures:* $62 million. *Unit head:* Dr. David Neivandt, Director, 207-581-2803. *Application contact:* Scott G. Delcourt, Assistant Vice President for Graduate Studies and Senior Associate Dean, 207-581-3291, Fax: 207-581-3232, E-mail: graduate@maine.edu.
Website: http://gsbse.umaine.edu/

The University of Manchester, Faculty of Life Sciences, Manchester, United Kingdom. Offers adaptive organismal biology (M Phil, PhD); animal biology (M Phil, PhD); biochemistry (M Phil, PhD); bioinformatics (M Phil, PhD); biomolecular sciences (M Phil, PhD); biotechnology (M Phil, PhD); cell biology (M Phil, PhD); cell matrix research (M Phil, PhD); channels and transporters (M Phil, PhD); developmental biology (M Phil, PhD); Egyptology (M Phil, PhD); environmental biology (M Phil, PhD); evolutionary biology (M Phil, PhD); gene expression (M Phil, PhD); genetics (M Phil, PhD); history of science, technology and medicine (M Phil, PhD); immunology (M Phil, PhD); integrative neurobiology and behavior (M Phil, PhD); membrane trafficking (M Phil, PhD); microbiology (M Phil, PhD); molecular and cellular neuroscience (M Phil, PhD); molecular biology (M Phil, PhD); molecular cancer studies (M Phil, PhD); neuroscience

(M Phil, PhD); ophthalmology (M Phil, PhD); optometry (M Phil, PhD); organelle function (M Phil, PhD); pharmacology (M Phil, PhD); physiology (M Phil, PhD); plant sciences (M Phil, PhD); stem cell research (M Phil, PhD); structural biology (M Phil, PhD); systems neuroscience (M Phil, PhD); toxicology (M Phil, PhD).

The University of Manchester, School of Chemical Engineering and Analytical Science, Manchester, United Kingdom. Offers biocatalysis (M Phil, PhD); chemical engineering (M Phil, PhD); chemical engineering and analytical science (M Phil, D Eng, PhD); colloids, crystals, interfaces and materials (M Phil, PhD); environment and sustainable technology (M Phil, PhD); instrumentation (M Phil, PhD); multi-scale modeling (M Phil, PhD); process integration (M Phil, PhD); systems biology (M Phil, PhD).

The University of Manchester, School of Materials, Manchester, United Kingdom. Offers advanced aerospace materials engineering (M Sc); advanced metallic systems (PhD); biomedical materials (M Phil, M Sc, PhD); ceramics and glass (M Phil, M Sc, PhD); composite materials (M Sc, PhD); corrosion and protection (M Phil, M Sc, PhD); materials (M Phil, PhD); metallic materials (M Phil, M Sc, PhD); nanostructural materials (M Phil, M Sc, PhD); paper science (M Phil, M Sc, PhD); polymer science and engineering (M Phil, M Sc, PhD); technical textiles (M Sc); textile design, fashion and management (M Phil, M Sc, PhD); textile science and technology (M Phil, M Sc, PhD); textiles (M Phil, PhD); textiles and fashion (M Ent).

The University of Manchester, School of Medicine, Manchester, United Kingdom. Offers M Phil, PhD.

University of Manitoba, Faculty of Graduate Studies, Faculty of Science, Department of Biological Sciences, Winnipeg, MB R3T 2N2, Canada. Offers botany (M Sc, PhD); ecology (M Sc, PhD); zoology (M Sc, PhD).

University of Manitoba, Faculty of Medicine and Faculty of Graduate Studies, Graduate Programs in Medicine, Winnipeg, MB R3T 2N2, Canada. Offers M Sc, MPH, PhD, G Dip, MD/PhD. *Accreditation:* LCME/AMA. *Program availability:* Part-time. *Expenses:* Contact institution.

University of Maryland, Baltimore, Graduate School, Graduate Program in Life Sciences, Baltimore, MD 21201. Offers biochemistry and molecular biology (MS, PhD), including biochemistry; epidemiology (PhD); gerontology (PhD); molecular medicine (MS, PhD), including cancer biology (PhD), cell and molecular physiology (PhD), human genetics and genomic medicine (PhD), molecular medicine (MS), molecular toxicology and pharmacology (PhD); molecular microbiology and immunology (PhD); neuroscience (PhD); physical rehabilitation science (PhD); toxicology (MS, PhD); MD/MS; MD/PhD. *Degree requirements:* For master's, comprehensive exam (for some programs), thesis (for some programs); for doctorate, comprehensive exam, thesis/dissertation. *Entrance requirements:* For master's and doctorate, GRE. Additional exam requirements/recommendations for international students: Required—TOEFL (minimum score 550 paper-based; 80 iBT); Recommended—IELTS (minimum score 7). Electronic applications accepted. Tuition and fees vary according to program. *Faculty research:* Cancer, reproduction, cardiovascular, immunology.

University of Maryland, Baltimore County, The Graduate School, College of Arts, Humanities and Social Sciences, Department of Education, Program in Teaching, Baltimore, MD 21250. Offers early childhood education (MAT); elementary education (MAT); teaching (MAT), including art, biology, chemistry, choral music, classical foreign language, dance, earth/space science, English, instrumental music, mathematics, modern foreign language, physical science, physics, social studies, theatre. *Program availability:* Part-time, evening/weekend. *Faculty:* 24 full-time (18 women), 25 part-time/adjunct (19 women). *Students:* 43 full-time (34 women), 40 part-time (27 women); includes 29 minority (9 Black or African American, non-Hispanic/Latino; 10 Asian, non-Hispanic/Latino; 9 Hispanic/Latino; 1 Two or more races, non-Hispanic/Latino), 1 international. Average age 30. 54 applicants, 69% accepted, 35 enrolled. In 2015, 106 master's awarded. *Degree requirements:* For master's, comprehensive exam (for some programs), thesis (for some programs). *Entrance requirements:* For master's, PRAXIS Core Examination or GRE (minimum score of 1000), minimum GPA of 3.0. Additional exam requirements/recommendations for international students: Required—TOEFL. *Application deadline:* For fall admission, 6/1 for domestic and international students; for spring admission, 11/1 for domestic and international students. Applications are processed on a rolling basis. Application fee: $50. Electronic applications accepted. *Expenses:* Tuition, state resident: full-time $12,816. Tuition, nonresident: full-time $19,710. *Financial support:* In 2015–16, 6 students received support, including teaching assistantships with tuition reimbursements available (averaging $12,000 per year); career-related internships or fieldwork, Federal Work-Study, scholarships/grants, tuition waivers, and unspecified assistantships also available. Financial award application deadline: 3/1. *Faculty research:* STEM teacher education, culturally sensitive pedagogy, ESOL/bilingual education, early childhood education, language, literacy and culture. *Unit head:* Dr. Susan M. Blunck, Graduate Program Director, 410-455-2869, Fax: 410-455-3986, E-mail: blunck@umbc.edu. *Application contact:* Cheryl Johnson, MAT Program Specialist, 410-455-3388, E-mail: blackwel@umbc.edu.
Website: http://www.umbc.edu/education/

University of Maryland, Baltimore County, The Graduate School, College of Natural and Mathematical Sciences, Department of Biological Sciences, Baltimore, MD 21250. Offers applied molecular biology (MS); biological sciences (MS, PhD); biotechnology (MPS), including biotechnology, biotechnology (Graduate Certificate), including biotechnology management; molecular and cell biology (PhD); neuroscience and cognitive sciences (PhD). *Faculty:* 26 full-time (11 women). *Students:* 70 full-time (39 women), 25 part-time (17 women); includes 31 minority (8 Black or African American, non-Hispanic/Latino; 19 Asian, non-Hispanic/Latino; 4 Hispanic/Latino), 22 international. Average age 27. 137 applicants, 24% accepted, 20 enrolled. In 2015, 23 master's, 10 doctorates awarded. Terminal master's awarded for partial completion of doctoral program. *Degree requirements:* For master's, thesis; for doctorate, thesis/dissertation. *Entrance requirements:* For master's and doctorate, GRE General Test, minimum GPA of 3.0. Additional exam requirements/recommendations for international students: Required—TOEFL (minimum score 80 iBT). *Application deadline:* For fall admission, 1/1 priority date for domestic and international students. Application fee: $50. Electronic applications accepted. *Expenses:* Tuition, state resident: full-time $12,816. Tuition, nonresident: full-time $19,710. *Financial support:* In 2015–16, 49 students received support, including 9 fellowships with full tuition reimbursements available (averaging $24,000 per year), 11 research assistantships with full tuition reimbursements available (averaging $24,000 per year), 31 teaching assistantships with full tuition reimbursements available (averaging $23,500 per year); career-related internships or fieldwork and health care benefits also available. *Unit head:* Dr. Philip Farabaugh, Chairman, 410-455-3081, Fax: 410-455-3875, E-mail: farabaug@umbc.edu. *Application contact:* Dr. Hua Lu, Director, 410-455-5972, Fax: 410-455-3875, E-mail: biograd@umbc.edu.
Website: http://biology.umbc.edu/

University of Maryland, College Park, Academic Affairs, College of Computer, Mathematical and Natural Sciences, Department of Biology, PhD Program in Biological Sciences, College Park, MD 20742. Offers behavior, ecology, evolution, and systematics (PhD); computational biology, bioinformatics, and genomics (PhD);

molecular and cellular biology (PhD); physiological systems (PhD). *Degree requirements:* For doctorate, comprehensive exam, thesis/dissertation, thesis work presentation in seminar. *Entrance requirements:* For doctorate, GRE General Test; GRE Subject Test in biology (recommended), academic transcripts, statement of purpose/ research interests, 3 letters of recommendation. Additional exam requirements/ recommendations for international students: Required—TOEFL. Electronic applications accepted.

University of Maryland, College Park, Academic Affairs, College of Computer, Mathematical and Natural Sciences, Department of Biology, Program in Biology, College Park, MD 20742. Offers MS, PhD. *Program availability:* Part-time, evening/ weekend. Terminal master's awarded for partial completion of doctoral program. *Degree requirements:* For master's, comprehensive exam, thesis optional; for doctorate, thesis/ dissertation, oral exam.

University of Maryland, College Park, Academic Affairs, College of Computer, Mathematical and Natural Sciences, Program in Life Sciences, College Park, MD 20742. Offers MLS. *Degree requirements:* For master's, scholarly paper. *Entrance requirements:* For master's, 1 year of teaching experience, letters of recommendation. Electronic applications accepted. *Faculty research:* Genetic engineering, gene therapy, ecology, biocomplexity.

University of Massachusetts Amherst, Graduate School, College of Natural Sciences, Department of Animal Biotechnology and Biomedical Sciences, Amherst, MA 01003. Offers MS, PhD. *Program availability:* Part-time. Terminal master's awarded for partial completion of doctoral program. *Degree requirements:* For master's, thesis or alternative; for doctorate, comprehensive exam, thesis/dissertation. *Entrance requirements:* For doctorate, GRE General Test. Additional exam requirements/ recommendations for international students: Required—TOEFL (minimum score 550 paper-based; 80 iBT), IELTS (minimum score 6.5). Electronic applications accepted.

University of Massachusetts Boston, College of Science and Mathematics, Program in Biology, Boston, MA 02125-3393. Offers MS, PhD. *Program availability:* Part-time, evening/weekend. *Faculty:* 35 full-time (12 women), 16 part-time/adjunct (10 women). *Students:* 35 full-time (17 women), 29 part-time (17 women); includes 8 minority (2 Black or African American, non-Hispanic/Latino; 3 Asian, non-Hispanic/Latino; 2 Hispanic/ Latino; 1 Two or more races, non-Hispanic/Latino), 12 international. 82 applicants, 17% accepted, 9 enrolled. In 2015, 6 master's, 2 doctorates awarded. *Degree requirements:* For master's, thesis, oral exams. *Entrance requirements:* For master's, GRE General Test, GRE Subject Test, minimum GPA of 2.75. *Application deadline:* For fall admission, 3/1 for domestic students; for spring admission, 11/1 for domestic students. *Expenses:* Tuition, state resident: full-time $2590. Tuition, nonresident: full-time $9758. *Required fees:* $13,525. *Financial support:* Research assistantships with full tuition reimbursements, teaching assistantships with full tuition reimbursements, career-related internships or fieldwork, Federal Work-Study, and unspecified assistantships available. Support available to part-time students. Financial award application deadline: 3/1; financial award applicants required to submit FAFSA. *Faculty research:* Microbial ecology, population and conservation genetics energetics of insect locomotion, science education, evolution and ecology of marine invertebrates. *Unit head:* Dr. Greg Beck, Director, 617-287-6600. *Application contact:* Peggy Roldan Patel, Graduate Admissions Coordinator, 617-287-6400, Fax: 617-287-6236, E-mail: bos.gadm@dpc.umassp.edu.

University of Massachusetts Boston, College of Science and Mathematics, Program in Biotechnology and Biomedical Sciences, Boston, MA 02125-3393. Offers MS. *Program availability:* Part-time, evening/weekend. *Students:* 1 (woman) full-time, 2 part-time (1 woman). 39 applicants, 3% accepted. In 2015, 2 master's awarded. *Degree requirements:* For master's, comprehensive exam, thesis optional, oral exams. *Entrance requirements:* For master's, GRE General Test, GRE Subject Test, minimum GPA of 2.75, 3.0 in science and math. *Application deadline:* For fall admission, 3/1 for domestic students; for spring admission, 11/1 for domestic students. *Expenses:* Tuition, state resident: full-time $2590. Tuition, nonresident: full-time $9758. *Required fees:* $13,525. *Financial support:* Research assistantships with full tuition reimbursements, teaching assistantships with full tuition reimbursements, career-related internships or fieldwork, Federal Work-Study, and unspecified assistantships available. Support available to part-time students. Financial award application deadline: 3/1; financial award applicants required to submit FAFSA. *Faculty research:* Evolutionary and molecular immunology, molecular genetics, tissue culture, computerized laboratory technology. *Unit head:* Dr. Greg Beck, Director, 617-287-6600. *Application contact:* Peggy Roldan Patel, Graduate Admissions Coordinator, 617-287-6400, Fax: 617-287-6236, E-mail: bos.gadm@ dpc.umassp.edu.

University of Massachusetts Dartmouth, Graduate School, College of Arts and Sciences, Department of Biology, North Dartmouth, MA 02747-2300. Offers biology (MS); marine biology (MS). *Program availability:* Part-time. *Faculty:* 19 full-time (8 women), 2 part-time/adjunct (both women). *Students:* 11 full-time (8 women), 9 part-time (6 women); includes 2 minority (1 Hispanic/Latino; 1 Two or more races, non-Hispanic/ Latino). Average age 26. 20 applicants, 65% accepted, 6 enrolled. In 2015, 5 master's awarded. *Degree requirements:* For master's, thesis. *Entrance requirements:* For master's, GRE, statement of purpose (minimum of 300 words), resume, official transcripts, 3 letters of recommendation. Additional exam requirements/ recommendations for international students: Required—TOEFL (minimum score 533 paper-based; 72 iBT). *Application deadline:* For fall admission, 2/15 priority date for domestic students, 1/15 priority date for international students. Applications are processed on a rolling basis. Application fee: $60. Electronic applications accepted. *Expenses:* Tuition, state resident: full-time $2071; part-time $86.29 per credit. Tuition, nonresident: full-time $8099; part-time $337.46 per credit. *Required fees:* $18,074; $762.08 per credit. Tuition and fees vary according to course load and reciprocity agreements. *Financial support:* In 2015–16, 1 research assistantship (averaging $16,000 per year), 8 teaching assistantships (averaging $16,000 per year) were awarded; career-related internships or fieldwork and unspecified assistantships also available. Support available to part-time students. Financial award application deadline: 3/1; financial award applicants required to submit FAFSA. *Faculty research:* Shark biology, marine mammal biology, domestication of fish, cell body, fish biology. *Total annual research expenditures:* $1.9 million. *Unit head:* Whitney Hable, Graduate Program Director, 508-999-8206, E-mail: whable@umassd.edu. *Application contact:* Steven Briggs, Director of Recruitment and Marketing for Graduate Studies, 508-999-8604, Fax: 508-999-8183, E-mail: graduate@umassd.edu.
Website: http://www.umassd.edu/cas/biology/

University of Massachusetts Lowell, College of Sciences, Department of Biological Sciences, Lowell, MA 01854. Offers biological sciences (MS). *Program availability:* Part-time. *Degree requirements:* For master's, thesis. *Entrance requirements:* For master's, GRE General Test. *Application deadline:* For fall admission, 4/1 priority date for domestic students; for spring admission, 10/1 for domestic students. Applications are processed on a rolling basis. Application fee: $20 ($35 for international students). Electronic applications accepted. *Expenses:* Tuition, state resident: full-time $14,304. Tuition, nonresident: full-time $25,853. *Required fees:* $375. Full-time tuition and fees vary according to campus/location and reciprocity agreements. *Financial support:* Research assistantships with full tuition reimbursements, teaching assistantships with full tuition reimbursements, career-related internships or fieldwork, Federal Work-Study,

institutionally sponsored loans, scholarships/grants, and traineeships available. Support available to part-time students. Financial award application deadline: 4/1.

University of Massachusetts Medical School, Graduate School of Biomedical Sciences, Worcester, MA 01655-0115. Offers biomedical sciences (PhD), including biochemistry and molecular pharmacology, bioinformatics and computational biology, cancer biology, cell biology, immunology and microbiology, interdisciplinary, neuroscience, translational science; biomedical sciences (millennium program) (PhD); clinical and population health research (PhD); clinical investigation (MS). *Faculty:* 1,339 full-time (521 women), 301 part-time/adjunct (189 women). *Students:* 363 full-time (184 women); includes 58 minority (13 Black or African American, non-Hispanic/Latino; 30 Asian, non-Hispanic/Latino; 15 Hispanic/Latino), 141 international. Average age 29. 661 applicants, 26% accepted, 51 enrolled. In 2015, 10 master's, 58 doctorates awarded. Terminal master's awarded for partial completion of doctoral program. *Degree requirements:* For master's, comprehensive exam, thesis; for doctorate, comprehensive exam, thesis/dissertation. *Entrance requirements:* For master's, MD, PhD, DVM, or PharmD; for doctorate, GRE General Test, bachelor's degree. Additional exam requirements/recommendations for international students: Required—TOEFL (minimum score 100 iBT) or IELTS (minimum score 7.5). *Application deadline:* For fall admission, 12/15 for domestic and international students; for spring admission, 5/15 for domestic students. Application fee: $80. Electronic applications accepted. *Expenses:* $6,966 resident per year; $14,182 non-resident per year. *Financial support:* In 2015–16, 383 students received support, including research assistantships with full tuition reimbursements available (averaging $30,600 per year); scholarships/grants, health care benefits, tuition waivers (full), and unspecified assistantships also available. Financial award application deadline: 5/16. *Faculty research:* RNA interference, cell/ molecular/developmental biology, bioinformatics, clinical/translational research, infectious disease. *Total annual research expenditures:* $250.3 million. *Unit head:* Dr. Anthony Carruthers, Dean, 508-856-4135, E-mail: anthony.carruthers@umassmed.edu. *Application contact:* Dr. Kendall Knight, Assistant Vice Provost for Admissions, 508-856-5628, Fax: 508-856-3659, E-mail: kendall.knight@umassmed.edu.
Website: http://www.umassmed.edu/gsbs/

University of Memphis, Graduate School, College of Arts and Sciences, Department of Biology, Memphis, TN 38152. Offers MS, PhD. *Faculty:* 15 full-time (3 women), 2 part-time/adjunct (1 woman). *Students:* 22 full-time (14 women), 21 part-time (15 women); includes 5 minority (1 Black or African American, non-Hispanic/Latino; 1 Asian, non-Hispanic/Latino; 2 Hispanic/Latino; 1 Two or more races, non-Hispanic/Latino), 11 international. Average age 29. 24 applicants, 54% accepted, 5 enrolled. In 2015, 4 master's, 4 doctorates awarded. Terminal master's awarded for partial completion of doctoral program. *Degree requirements:* For master's, comprehensive exam, thesis (for some programs); for doctorate, one foreign language, comprehensive exam, thesis/ dissertation. *Entrance requirements:* For master's, GRE General Test; for doctorate, GRE General Test, master's degree. Additional exam requirements/recommendations for international students: Required—TOEFL (minimum score 550 paper-based; 79 iBT). *Application deadline:* For fall admission, 2/1 for domestic and international students; for spring admission, 10/15 for domestic and international students. Applications are processed on a rolling basis. Application fee: $35 ($60 for international students). Electronic applications accepted. *Financial support:* In 2015–16, 16 students received support. Research assistantships with full tuition reimbursements available, teaching assistantships with full tuition reimbursements available, Federal Work-Study, scholarships/grants, and unspecified assistantships available. Financial award application deadline: 2/15; financial award applicants required to submit FAFSA. *Faculty research:* Protein trafficking and signal transduction; animal behavior and communication, neurobiology, and circadian clock function; phylogenetics, evolution, and ecology; causation and prevention of cancer; reproductive biology. *Unit head:* Dr. Randall Bayer, Chairman, 901-678-2596, Fax: 901-678-4746, E-mail: rbayer@ memphis.edu. *Application contact:* Dr. Melvin Beck, Professor and Graduate Studies Coordinator, 901-678-2970, Fax: 901-678-4457, E-mail: mbeck@memphis.edu.
Website: http://www.memphis.edu/biology/

University of Miami, Graduate School, College of Arts and Sciences, Department of Biology, Coral Gables, FL 33124. Offers biology (MS, PhD); genetics and evolution (MS, PhD). Terminal master's awarded for partial completion of doctoral program. *Degree requirements:* For master's, comprehensive exam (for some programs), thesis (for some programs); for doctorate, thesis/dissertation, oral and written qualifying exam. *Entrance requirements:* For master's, GRE General Test, 3 letters of recommendation, research papers; for doctorate, GRE General Test, 3 letters of recommendation, research papers, sponsor letter. Additional exam requirements/recommendations for international students: Required—TOEFL (minimum score 550 paper-based; 59 iBT). Electronic applications accepted. *Faculty research:* Neuroscience to ethology; plants, vertebrates and mycorrhizae; phylogenies, life histories and species interactions; molecular biology, gene expression and populations; cells, auditory neurons and vertebrate locomotion.

University of Michigan, Medical School and Rackham Graduate School, Medical Scientist Training Program, Ann Arbor, MI 48109. Offers MD/PhD. *Accreditation:* LCME/ AMA. *Students:* 92 full-time (39 women); includes 44 minority (2 Black or African American, non-Hispanic/Latino; 1 American Indian or Alaska Native, non-Hispanic/ Latino; 38 Asian, non-Hispanic/Latino; 3 Hispanic/Latino). 337 applicants, 11% accepted, 10 enrolled. *Application deadline:* For fall admission, 10/15 for domestic students. Applications are processed on a rolling basis. Application fee: $160. Electronic applications accepted. *Financial support:* In 2015–16, 92 students received support, including 81 fellowships with full tuition reimbursements available (averaging $29,025 per year), 7 research assistantships with full tuition reimbursements available (averaging $29,025 per year), 4 teaching assistantships with full tuition reimbursements available (averaging $29,025 per year); scholarships/grants, traineeships, and health care benefits also available. *Unit head:* Dr. Ronald J. Koenig, Director, 734-764-6176, Fax: 734-764-8180, E-mail: rkoenig@umich.edu. *Application contact:* Laurie Koivupalo, Administrative Associate, 734-764-6176, Fax: 734-764-8180, E-mail: lkoivupl@ umich.edu.
Website: http://www.med.umich.edu/medschool/mstp/

University of Michigan, Rackham Graduate School, Program in Biomedical Sciences (PIBS), Ann Arbor, MI 48109-5619. Offers MS, PhD. *Faculty:* 513 full-time. *Students:* 66 full-time (37 women); includes 18 minority (3 Black or African American, non-Hispanic/ Latino; 4 Asian, non-Hispanic/Latino; 9 Hispanic/Latino; 2 Two or more races, non-Hispanic/Latino), 11 international. Average age 25. 754 applicants, 24% accepted, 67 enrolled. *Degree requirements:* For doctorate, thesis/dissertation, oral defense of dissertation, preliminary exam. *Entrance requirements:* For doctorate, GRE General Test, 3 letters of recommendation, research experience. Additional exam requirements/ recommendations for international students: Required—TOEFL (minimum score 84 iBT). *Application deadline:* For fall admission, 12/1 for domestic and international students. Application fee: $75 ($90 for international students). Electronic applications accepted. *Financial support:* In 2015–16, 66 students received support, including 66 fellowships with full tuition reimbursements available (averaging $29,025 per year); scholarships/grants, health care benefits, tuition waivers (full), and unspecified assistantships also available. Financial award application deadline: 12/1. *Faculty research:* Genetics, cellular and molecular biology, microbial pathogenesis, cancer

Biological and Biomedical Sciences—General

biology, neuroscience. *Unit head:* Dr. Scott Barolo, Associate Professor, Cell and Developmental Biology/Director of the Program in Biomedical Sciences, 734-615-7005, Fax: 734-647-7022, E-mail: sbarolo@umich.edu. *Application contact:* Michelle DiMondo, Academic Affairs and Student Success Coordinator, 734-647-5773, Fax: 734-647-7022, E-mail: mdimondo@umich.edu.
Website: http://medicine.umich.edu/phd

University of Michigan–Flint, College of Arts and Sciences, Program in Biology, Flint, MI 48502-1950. Offers MS. *Program availability:* Part-time. *Faculty:* 20 full-time (10 women), 5 part-time/adjunct (3 women). *Students:* 11 full-time (7 women), 10 part-time (5 women); includes 3 minority (1 Black or African American, non-Hispanic/Latino; 1 Asian, non-Hispanic/Latino; 1 Two or more races, non-Hispanic/Latino), 2 international. Average age 30. 17 applicants, 59% accepted, 6 enrolled. In 2015, 7 master's awarded. *Degree requirements:* For master's, thesis optional. *Entrance requirements:* For master's, bachelor's degree in biology or related life science from accredited institution; minimum overall undergraduate GPA of 3.0 and in prerequisite courses; completion of following prerequisites at an accredited university: cell biology, ecology, general physics, and genetics. Additional exam requirements/recommendations for international students: Required—TOEFL (minimum score 560 paper-based; 84 iBT), IELTS (minimum score 6.5). *Application deadline:* For fall admission, 8/1 for domestic students, 5/1 for international students; for winter admission, 11/15 for domestic students, 9/1 for international students; for spring admission, 3/15 for domestic students, 1/1 for international students; for summer admission, 5/15 for domestic students. Applications are processed on a rolling basis. Application fee: $55. Electronic applications accepted. *Financial support:* Federal Work-Study, scholarships/grants, and unspecified assistantships available. Support available to part-time students. Financial award application deadline: 3/1; financial award applicants required to submit FAFSA. *Faculty research:* Research and assisting with the capture of invasive feral swine in Michigan. *Unit head:* Dr. Joseph Sucic, Director, 810-762-3360, Fax: 810-762-3310, E-mail: jsucic@umflint.edu. *Application contact:* Bradley T. Maki, Director of Graduate Admissions, 810-762-3171, Fax: 810-766-6789, E-mail: bmaki@umflint.edu.
Website: https://www.umflint.edu/graduateprograms/biology

University of Minnesota, Duluth, Graduate School, Swenson College of Science and Engineering, Department of Biology, Integrated Biosciences Program, Duluth, MN 55812-2496. Offers MS, PhD. Terminal master's awarded for partial completion of doctoral program. *Degree requirements:* For master's, thesis, seminar; for doctorate, comprehensive exam, thesis/dissertation, written and oral exam, seminar, written thesis. *Entrance requirements:* For master's, GRE, 1 year of biology, physics, and chemistry; 1 semester of calculus; for doctorate, GRE, 1 year each of chemistry, biology, physics, calculus, and advanced chemistry. Additional exam requirements/recommendations for international students: Required—TOEFL (minimum score 550 paper-based; 79 iBT). Electronic applications accepted. *Faculty research:* Ecology, organizational and population biology; cell, molecular and physiological biology.

University of Minnesota, Twin Cities Campus, Graduate School, College of Biological Sciences, Biological Science Program, Minneapolis, MN 55455-0213. Offers MBS. *Program availability:* Part-time, evening/weekend. *Entrance requirements:* For master's, 2 years of work experience. Electronic applications accepted. *Expenses:* Contact institution.

University of Minnesota, Twin Cities Campus, Graduate School, Stem Cell Biology Graduate Program, Minneapolis, MN 55455-3007. Offers MS. *Degree requirements:* For master's, thesis. *Entrance requirements:* For master's, GRE, BS, BA, or foreign equivalent in biological sciences or related field; minimum undergraduate GPA of 3.2. Additional exam requirements/recommendations for international students: Required—TOEFL (minimum score 580 paper-based, with a minimum score of 4 in the TWE, or 94 Internet-based, with a minimum score of 22 on each of the reading and listening, 26 on the speaking, and 26 on the writing section. *Faculty research:* Stem cell and developmental biology; embryonic stem cells; iPS cells; muscle satellite cells; hematopoietic stem cells; neuronal stem cells; cardiovascular, kidney and limb development; regenerating systems.

University of Mississippi, Graduate School, College of Liberal Arts, University, MS 38677. Offers anthropology (MA); biology (MS, PhD); chemistry (MS, PhD); clinical psychology (PhD); economics (MA, PhD); English (MA, MFA, PhD); experimental psychology (PhD); history (MA, PhD); mathematics (MS, PhD); modern languages (MA); music (MM, PhD); philosophy (MA); physics (MA, MS, PhD); political science (MA, PhD); sociology (MA); studio art (MFA). *Program availability:* Part-time. *Faculty:* 446 full-time (186 women), 84 part-time/adjunct (36 women). *Students:* 475 full-time (233 women), 79 part-time (37 women); includes 83 minority (42 Black or African American, non-Hispanic/Latino; 9 Asian, non-Hispanic/Latino; 19 Hispanic/Latino; 13 Two or more races, non-Hispanic/Latino), 107 international. *Degree requirements:* For doctorate, thesis/dissertation. *Entrance requirements:* For master's, GRE General Test, minimum GPA of 3.0; for doctorate, GRE General Test. Additional exam requirements/recommendations for international students: Required—TOEFL. *Application deadline:* For fall admission, 4/1 for domestic students; for spring admission, 10/1 for domestic students. Applications are processed on a rolling basis. Application fee: $40. Electronic applications accepted. *Financial support:* Fellowships, research assistantships, teaching assistantships, career-related internships or fieldwork, Federal Work-Study, institutionally sponsored loans, scholarships/grants, and unspecified assistantships available. Financial award application deadline: 3/1; financial award applicants required to submit FAFSA. *Unit head:* Dean, 662-915-7177, Fax: 662-915-5792, E-mail: libarts@olemiss.edu. *Application contact:* Dr. Christy M. Wyandt, Associate Dean of Graduate School, 662-915-7474, Fax: 662-915-7577, E-mail: cwyandt@olemiss.edu.

University of Mississippi Medical Center, School of Graduate Studies in the Health Sciences, Jackson, MS 39216-4505. Offers MS, PhD, MD/PhD. *Program availability:* Part-time. Terminal master's awarded for partial completion of doctoral program. *Degree requirements:* For master's, thesis (for some programs); for doctorate, comprehensive exam, thesis/dissertation, first authored publication. *Entrance requirements:* For master's and doctorate, GRE. Additional exam requirements/recommendations for international students: Required—TOEFL (minimum score 550 paper-based; 79 iBT), IELTS (minimum score 6.5), PTE (minimum score 53). *Faculty research:* Immunology; protein chemistry and biosynthesis; cardiovascular, renal, and endocrine physiology; rehabilitation therapy on immune system/hypothalamic/adrenal axis interaction.

University of Missouri, College of Veterinary Medicine and Office of Research and Graduate Studies, Graduate Programs in Veterinary Medicine, Department of Biomedical Sciences, Columbia, MO 65211. Offers biomedical sciences (MS, PhD); comparative medicine (MS); veterinary medicine and surgery (MS); DVM/PhD. *Degree requirements:* For master's, thesis; for doctorate, comprehensive exam, thesis/dissertation. *Entrance requirements:* For master's, GRE General Test, minimum GPA of 3.0; 10 hrs biology, 3 hrs physics, 3 hrs biochemistry, 10 hrs chemistry, 3 hrs calculus; for doctorate, GRE General Test (V+B = 300 if taken after 8/1/11); 3.5 analytical, minimum GPA of 3.0; 10 hrs biology, 3 hrs physics, 3 hrs biochemistry, 10 hrs chemistry, 3 hrs calculus. Additional exam requirements/recommendations for international students: Required—TOEFL (minimum score 600 paper-based; 100 iBT). *Application deadline:* For fall admission, 2/1 for domestic and international students; for winter admission, 9/1 for domestic and international students. Application fee: $65 ($90 for

international students). Electronic applications accepted. *Financial support:* Fellowships with full tuition reimbursements, research assistantships with full tuition reimbursements, teaching assistantships with full tuition reimbursements, institutionally sponsored loans, scholarships/grants, traineeships, health care benefits, and unspecified assistantships available. Support available to part-time students. Financial award applicants required to submit FAFSA. *Faculty research:* Anatomy (gross or microscopic); physiology/pharmacology (molecular, cellular and integrative); biochemistry/molecular biology; endocrinology; toxicology; exercise biology including cardiac, vascular and muscle biology; cardiovascular biology including neuroendocrine regulation; membrane transport biology including cystic fibrosis and cardiac disease; reproductive biology.
Website: http://biomed.missouri.edu/

University of Missouri, Office of Research and Graduate Studies, College of Arts and Science, Division of Biological Sciences, Columbia, MO 65211. Offers evolutionary biology and ecology (MA, PhD). Terminal master's awarded for partial completion of doctoral program. *Degree requirements:* For master's, thesis; for doctorate, comprehensive exam, thesis/dissertation. *Entrance requirements:* For master's and doctorate, GRE General Test (minimum score 1200 verbal and quantitative), minimum GPA of 3.0. Additional exam requirements/recommendations for international students: Required—TOEFL (minimum score 600 paper-based; 100 iBT). *Application deadline:* For fall admission, 12/15 priority date for domestic and international students. Applications are processed on a rolling basis. Application fee: $55 ($75 for international students). Electronic applications accepted. *Financial support:* Fellowships with full tuition reimbursements, research assistantships with full tuition reimbursements, teaching assistantships with full tuition reimbursements, institutionally sponsored loans, traineeships, health care benefits, and unspecified assistantships available.
Website: http://biology.missouri.edu/graduate-studies/

University of Missouri, School of Medicine and Office of Research and Graduate Studies, Graduate Programs in Medicine, Columbia, MO 65211. Offers family and community medicine (MS); health administration (MS); medical pharmacology and physiology (MS, PhD); molecular microbiology and immunology (MS, PhD); pathology and anatomical sciences (MS). *Program availability:* Part-time. *Degree requirements:* For doctorate, thesis/dissertation. *Entrance requirements:* For master's and doctorate, GRE General Test, minimum GPA of 3.0. Additional exam requirements/recommendations for international students: Required—TOEFL. *Application deadline:* Applications are processed on a rolling basis. Application fee: $55 ($75 for international students). *Expenses:* Contact institution. *Financial support:* Fellowships, research assistantships, teaching assistantships, career-related internships or fieldwork, and institutionally sponsored loans available.
Website: http://som.missouri.edu/departments.shtml

University of Missouri–Kansas City, School of Biological Sciences, Kansas City, MO 64110-2499. Offers biology (MA); cell biology and biophysics (PhD); cellular and molecular biology (MS); molecular biology and biochemistry (PhD). PhD (interdisciplinary) offered through the School of Graduate Studies. *Program availability:* Part-time, evening/weekend. *Faculty:* 31 full-time (9 women), 3 part-time/adjunct (2 women). *Students:* 5 full-time (3 women), 12 part-time (3 women); includes 6 minority (1 Black or African American, non-Hispanic/Latino; 2 Asian, non-Hispanic/Latino; 2 Hispanic/Latino; 1 Two or more races, non-Hispanic/Latino), 1 international. Average age 26. 66 applicants, 26% accepted, 10 enrolled. In 2015, 22 master's awarded. *Degree requirements:* For doctorate, comprehensive exam, thesis/dissertation. *Entrance requirements:* For master's, GRE, minimum GPA of 3.0; for doctorate, GRE General Test. Additional exam requirements/recommendations for international students: Required—TOEFL (minimum score 550 paper-based; 80 iBT). *Application deadline:* For fall admission, 2/15 priority date for domestic and international students. Applications are processed on a rolling basis. Application fee: $45 ($50 for international students). *Financial support:* In 2015–16, 11 research assistantships with full tuition reimbursements (averaging $24,189 per year), 17 teaching assistantships with full tuition reimbursements (averaging $15,312 per year) were awarded; Federal Work-Study, institutionally sponsored loans, scholarships/grants, tuition waivers (full and partial), and unspecified assistantships also available. Support available to part-time students. Financial award application deadline: 3/1; financial award applicants required to submit FAFSA. *Faculty research:* Structural biology, molecular genetics. *Unit head:* Dr. Theodore White, Dean, 816-235-2538, Fax: 816-235-5158, E-mail: whitetc@umkc.edu. *Application contact:* Information Contact, 816-235-1330, Fax: 816-235-5158, E-mail: sbsgradrecruit@umkc.edu.
Website: http://sbs.umkc.edu/

University of Missouri–St. Louis, College of Arts and Sciences, Department of Biology, St. Louis, MO 63121. Offers MS, PhD, Certificate. *Program availability:* Part-time. *Faculty:* 22 full-time (9 women), 9 part-time/adjunct (3 women). *Students:* 37 full-time (24 women), 21 part-time (15 women); includes 6 minority (2 Black or African American, non-Hispanic/Latino; 1 Asian, non-Hispanic/Latino; 2 Hispanic/Latino; 1 Two or more races, non-Hispanic/Latino), 24 international. 44 applicants, 52% accepted, 14 enrolled. *Degree requirements:* For master's, thesis or alternative; for doctorate, thesis/dissertation, 1 semester of teaching experience. *Entrance requirements:* For master's, 3 letters of recommendation; for doctorate, GRE General Test, 3 letters of recommendation. Additional exam requirements/recommendations for international students: Required—TOEFL (minimum score 79 iBT), IELTS (minimum score 6.5). *Application deadline:* For fall admission, 12/15 priority date for domestic and international students; for spring admission, 12/1 for domestic and international students. Application fee: $50 ($40 for international students). Electronic applications accepted. *Financial support:* Fellowships with full tuition reimbursements, research assistantships with tuition reimbursements, teaching assistantships with tuition reimbursements, career-related internships or fieldwork, and Federal Work-Study available. Support available to part-time students. Financial award application deadline: 2/1. *Faculty research:* Molecular biology, microbial genetics, animal behavior, tropical ecology, plant systematics. *Unit head:* Dr. Teresa Thiel, Director of Graduate Studies, 314-516-6208, Fax: 314-516-6233, E-mail: thiel@umsl.edu. *Application contact:* 314-516-5458, Fax: 314-516-7015, E-mail: gradadm@umsl.edu.
Website: http://www.umsl.edu/~biology/

University of Montana, Graduate School, College of Health Professions and Biomedical Sciences, Skaggs School of Pharmacy, Department of Biomedical and Pharmaceutical Sciences, Missoula, MT 59812-0002. Offers biomedical sciences (PhD); medicinal chemistry (MS, PhD); molecular and cellular toxicology (MS, PhD); neuroscience (PhD); pharmaceutical sciences (MS). *Accreditation:* ACPE. *Degree requirements:* For master's, oral defense of thesis; for doctorate, research dissertation defense. *Entrance requirements:* For master's and doctorate, GRE General Test. Additional exam requirements/recommendations for international students: Required—TOEFL (minimum score 540 paper-based). Electronic applications accepted. *Faculty research:* Cardiovascular pharmacology, medicinal chemistry, neuroscience, environmental toxicology, pharmacogenetics, cancer.

University of Montana, Graduate School, College of Humanities and Sciences, Division of Biological Sciences, Missoula, MT 59812-0002. Offers cellular, molecular and microbial biology (PhD), including cellular and developmental biology, microbial evolution and ecology, microbiology and immunology, molecular biology and biochemistry; organismal biology and ecology (MS, PhD); systems ecology (MS, PhD). Terminal master's awarded for partial completion of doctoral program. *Degree requirements:* For master's, thesis; for doctorate, thesis/dissertation. *Entrance requirements:* For master's and doctorate, GRE General Test. Additional exam requirements/recommendations for international students: Required—TOEFL. *Faculty research:* Biochemistry/microbiology, organismal biology, ecology.

University of Nebraska at Kearney, Graduate Studies and Research, College of Natural and Social Sciences, Department of Biology, Kearney, NE 68849. Offers biology (MS); science/math education (MA Ed). *Program availability:* Part-time, evening/weekend, 100% online. *Faculty:* 17 full-time (6 women). *Students:* 32 full-time (24 women), 203 part-time (133 women); includes 35 minority (10 Black or African American, non-Hispanic/Latino; 1 American Indian or Alaska Native, non-Hispanic/Latino; 3 Asian, non-Hispanic/Latino; 17 Hispanic/Latino; 4 Two or more races, non-Hispanic/Latino), 2 international. Average age 31. 76 applicants, 89% accepted, 45 enrolled. In 2015, 74 master's awarded. *Degree requirements:* For master's, comprehensive exam, thesis optional. *Entrance requirements:* For master's, GRE (for thesis option and for online program applicants if undergraduate GPA is below 2.75), letter of interest. Additional exam requirements/recommendations for international students: Recommended—TOEFL (minimum score 550 paper-based; 79 iBT), IELTS (minimum score 6.5). *Application deadline:* For fall admission, 6/15 for domestic students, 5/15 for international students; for spring admission, 10/15 for domestic and international students; for summer admission, 3/15 for domestic and international students. Application fee: $45. Electronic applications accepted. *Expenses: Tuition, area resident:* Full-time $3965; part-time $220.25 per credit hour. Tuition, nonresident: full-time $8699; part-time $483.25 per credit hour. *Required fees:* $677; $21 per credit hour. $174. Part-time tuition and fees vary according to course load and program. *Financial support:* In 2015–16, 9 students received support, including 1 research assistantship with full tuition reimbursement available (averaging $11,500 per year), 8 teaching assistantships with full tuition reimbursements available (averaging $11,500 per year); career-related internships or fieldwork, scholarships/grants, health care benefits, and unspecified assistantships also available. Support available to part-time students. Financial award application deadline: 2/28; financial award applicants required to submit FAFSA. *Faculty research:* Pollution injury, molecular biology-viral gene expression, prairie range condition modeling, evolution of symbiotic nitrogen fixation. *Unit head:* Dr. Julie Shaffer, Graduate Program Chair, 308-865-8661, E-mail: shafferjj@unk.edu. *Application contact:* Brian Peterson, Graduate Studies and Research Director, 308-865-1589, E-mail: msbiology@unk.edu.
Website: http://unkcms.unk.edu/academics/biology/index.php

University of Nebraska at Omaha, Graduate Studies, College of Arts and Sciences, Department of Biology, Omaha, NE 68182. Offers biology (MS); business for bioscientists (Certificate). *Program availability:* Part-time. *Faculty:* 11 full-time (5 women). *Students:* 7 full-time (5 women), 16 part-time (9 women); includes 1 minority (Hispanic/Latino), 2 international. Average age 27. 19 applicants, 47% accepted, 7 enrolled. In 2015, 11 master's awarded. *Degree requirements:* For master's, comprehensive exam (for some programs), thesis (for some programs). *Entrance requirements:* For master's, GRE General Test, minimum GPA of 3.0, transcripts, 24 undergraduate biology hours, 3 letters of recommendation, statement of purpose. Additional exam requirements/recommendations for international students: Required—TOEFL, IELTS, PTE. *Application deadline:* For fall admission, 2/15 priority date for domestic and international students; for spring admission, 10/15 priority date for domestic and international students; for summer admission, 2/15 priority date for domestic and international students. Applications are processed on a rolling basis. Application fee: $45. Electronic applications accepted. *Financial support:* In 2015–16, 18 students received support, including 1 research assistantship with tuition reimbursement available, 17 teaching assistantships with tuition reimbursements available; fellowships, Federal Work-Study, institutionally sponsored loans, scholarships/grants, health care benefits, tuition waivers (partial), and unspecified assistantships also available. Support available to part-time students. Financial award application deadline: 3/1; financial award applicants required to submit FAFSA. *Unit head:* Dr. William Tapprich, Chairperson, 402-554-2341, E-mail: graduate@unomaha.edu. *Application contact:* Dr. John McCarty, Graduate Program Chair, 402-554-2341, E-mail: graduate@unomaha.edu.

University of Nebraska–Lincoln, Graduate College, College of Agricultural Sciences and Natural Resources, School of Veterinary Medicine and Biomedical Sciences, Lincoln, NE 68588. Offers veterinary science (MS). MS, PhD offered jointly with University of Nebraska Medical Center. *Program availability:* Online learning. *Degree requirements:* For master's, thesis optional; for doctorate, comprehensive exam, thesis/dissertation. *Entrance requirements:* For master's, GRE General Test; for doctorate, GRE General Test, MCAT, or VCAT. Additional exam requirements/recommendations for international students: Required—TOEFL (minimum score 550 paper-based). Electronic applications accepted. *Faculty research:* Virology, immunobiology, molecular biology, mycotoxins, ocular degeneration.

University of Nebraska–Lincoln, Graduate College, College of Arts and Sciences, School of Biological Sciences, Lincoln, NE 68588. Offers MA, MS, PhD. *Degree requirements:* For master's, thesis optional; for doctorate, comprehensive exam, thesis/dissertation. *Entrance requirements:* For master's and doctorate, GRE General Test. Additional exam requirements/recommendations for international students: Required—TOEFL (minimum score 550 paper-based). Electronic applications accepted. *Faculty research:* Behavior, botany, and zoology; ecology and evolutionary biology; genetics; cellular and molecular biology; microbiology.

University of Nebraska Medical Center, Medical Sciences Interdepartmental Area, Omaha, NE 68198. Offers genetics, cell biology and anatomy (MS); internal medicine (MS). *Program availability:* Part-time. *Faculty:* 195 full-time, 20 part-time/adjunct. *Students:* 49 full-time (28 women), 40 part-time (27 women); includes 10 minority (1 Black or African American, non-Hispanic/Latino; 6 Asian, non-Hispanic/Latino; 3 Hispanic/Latino), 16 international. Average age 32. 46 applicants, 41% accepted, 19 enrolled. In 2015, 12 master's, 17 doctorates awarded. Terminal master's awarded for partial completion of doctoral program. *Degree requirements:* For master's, comprehensive exam, thesis; for doctorate, comprehensive exam, thesis/dissertation. *Entrance requirements:* For master's, GRE General Test; for doctorate, GRE General Test, MCAT or DCAT. Additional exam requirements/recommendations for international students: Required—TOEFL (minimum score 550 paper-based; 80 iBT). *Application deadline:* For fall admission, 4/1 for domestic and international students; for spring admission, 8/1 for domestic and international students; for summer admission, 1/1 for domestic and international students. Applications are processed on a rolling basis. Application fee: $45. Electronic applications accepted. *Expenses:* Tuition, state resident: full-time $7830; part-time $3915 per credit hour. Tuition, nonresident: full-time $22,410; part-time $11,205 per credit hour. *Required fees:* $521. *Financial support:* In 2015–16, 3 fellowships with full tuition reimbursements (averaging $23,100 per year), 4 research assistantships with full tuition reimbursements (averaging $23,100 per year) were awarded; teaching assistantships and scholarships/grants also available. Support available to part-time students. Financial award application deadline: 2/15; financial award applicants required to submit FAFSA. *Faculty research:* Molecular genetics, oral

biology, veterinary pathology, newborn medicine, immunology, clinical research. *Unit head:* Dr. Laura Bilek, Graduate Committee Chair, 402-559-6923, E-mail: lbilek@unmc.edu.
Website: http://www.unmc.edu/gradstudies/programs/msia/

University of Nevada, Las Vegas, Graduate College, College of Sciences, School of Life Sciences, Las Vegas, NV 89154-4004. Offers biological sciences (MS, PhD). *Program availability:* Part-time. *Faculty:* 13 full-time (3 women). *Students:* 40 full-time (20 women), 9 part-time (5 women); includes 16 minority (1 Black or African American, non-Hispanic/Latino; 2 Asian, non-Hispanic/Latino; 7 Hispanic/Latino; 6 Two or more races, non-Hispanic/Latino), 5 international. Average age 30. 34 applicants, 47% accepted, 14 enrolled. In 2015, 1 doctorate awarded. *Degree requirements:* For master's, thesis; for doctorate, one foreign language, comprehensive exam, thesis/dissertation. *Entrance requirements:* For master's and doctorate, GRE General Test. Additional exam requirements/recommendations for international students: Required—TOEFL (minimum score 550 paper-based; 80 iBT), IELTS (minimum score 7). *Application deadline:* For fall admission, 1/15 for domestic students, 5/1 for international students. Application fee: $60 ($95 for international students). Electronic applications accepted. *Expenses:* $264 per credit state resident full-time and part-time; $6,955 per semester, $264 per credit nonresident full-time; $555 per credit nonresident part-time. *Financial support:* In 2015–16, 44 students received support, including 2 fellowships with full tuition reimbursements available (averaging $15,000 per year), 14 research assistantships with partial tuition reimbursements available (averaging $16,440 per year), 28 teaching assistantships with partial tuition reimbursements available (averaging $18,142 per year); institutionally sponsored loans, scholarships/grants, health care benefits, and unspecified assistantships also available. Financial award application deadline: 3/1. *Faculty research:* Environmental and medical microbiology; biodiversity, evolution, and ecological sustainability; cell and molecular biology; integrative physiology. Total annual research expenditures: $2.2 million. *Unit head:* Dr. Dennis Bazylinski, Director/Professor, 702-895-2053, Fax: 702-895-3956, E-mail: dennis.bazylinski@unlv.edu. *Application contact:* Graduate College Admissions Evaluator, 702-895-3367, Fax: 702-895-4180, E-mail: gradadmissions@unlv.edu.
Website: http://sols.unlv.edu/

University of Nevada, Reno, Graduate School, College of Science, Department of Biology, Reno, NV 89557. Offers MS. *Degree requirements:* For master's, thesis optional. *Entrance requirements:* For master's, GRE General Test, minimum GPA of 2.75. Additional exam requirements/recommendations for international students: Required—TOEFL (minimum score 500 paper-based; 61 iBT), IELTS (minimum score 6). Electronic applications accepted. *Faculty research:* Gene expression, stress protein genes, secretory proteins, conservation biology, behavioral ecology.

University of New Brunswick Fredericton, School of Graduate Studies, Faculty of Science, Department of Biology, Fredericton, NB E3B 5A3, Canada. Offers M Sc, PhD. *Program availability:* Part-time. *Faculty:* 25 full-time (8 women), 27 part-time/adjunct (9 women). *Students:* 51 full-time (32 women), 7 part-time (5 women). In 2015, 2 master's, 8 doctorates awarded. *Degree requirements:* For master's, thesis; for doctorate, thesis/dissertation. *Entrance requirements:* For master's, minimum GPA of 3.0; undergraduate degree (B Sc or equivalent preferred); for doctorate, minimum GPA of 3.0; undergraduate and/or master's degree in related discipline. Additional exam requirements/recommendations for international students: Required—TWE (minimum score 4), TOEFL (minimum score 600 paper-based) or IELTS (minimum score 7). *Application deadline:* For fall admission, 3/1 for domestic students. Applications are processed on a rolling basis. Application fee: $50 Canadian dollars. Electronic applications accepted. *Financial support:* Fellowships, research assistantships with tuition reimbursements, and teaching assistantships available. *Faculty research:* Evolutionary biology, aquatic ecology, wildlife and conservation biology, marine biology, algae and plant biology. *Unit head:* Dr. Les C. Cwynar, Director of Graduate Studies, 506-452-6197, Fax: 506-453-3583, E-mail: biodogs@unb.ca. *Application contact:* Heidi Stewart, Graduate Secretary, 506-458-7488, E-mail: scigrad@unb.ca.
Website: http://go.unb.ca/gradprograms

University of New Brunswick Saint John, Department of Biology, Saint John, NB E2L 4L5, Canada. Offers M Sc, PhD. *Program availability:* Part-time. *Faculty:* 12 full-time (4 women), 19 part-time/adjunct (4 women). *Students:* 41 full-time (24 women), 6 part-time (3 women). In 2015, 8 master's, 1 doctorate awarded. *Degree requirements:* For master's, thesis; for doctorate, comprehensive exam, thesis/dissertation. *Entrance requirements:* For master's, B Sc, minimum GPA of 3.0; for doctorate, M Sc, minimum GPA of 3.0. Additional exam requirements/recommendations for international students: Required—TOEFL (minimum score 600 paper-based), TWE (minimum score 4). *Application deadline:* For fall admission, 2/15 for domestic and international students. Applications are processed on a rolling basis. Application fee: $50 Canadian dollars. Electronic applications accepted. *Financial support:* Fellowships, research assistantships, teaching assistantships, scholarships/grants, and unspecified assistantships available. *Faculty research:* Marine and environmental biology (including assessing impacts of anthropogenic stressors on aquatic and terrestrial systems using molecular through ecological endpoints), evolution, natural products chemistry. *Unit head:* Dr. Kate Frego, Acting Director of Graduate Studies, 506-648-5967, Fax: 506-648-5811, E-mail: jeffhoul@unb.ca. *Application contact:* Kim Banks, Secretary, 506-648-5605, Fax: 506-648-5811, E-mail: kbanks@unb.ca.
Website: http://go.unb.ca/gradprograms

University of New England, College of Arts and Sciences, Program in Biological Science, Biddeford, ME 04005-9526. Offers MS. *Faculty:* 20 full-time (10 women), 4 part-time/adjunct (3 women). *Students:* 7 full-time (4 women), 1 international. Average age 23. 9 applicants, 44% accepted, 4 enrolled. *Degree requirements:* For master's, thesis. *Entrance requirements:* For master's, GRE. *Application deadline:* For fall admission, 2/1 for domestic students. Application fee: $40. Tuition and fees vary according to degree level and program. *Financial support:* Application deadline: 5/1; applicants required to submit FAFSA. *Unit head:* Dr. A. Christine Brown, Chair/Professor, 207-602-2617, E-mail: sbrown@une.edu. *Application contact:* Scott Steinberg, Dean of University Admission, 207-221-4224, Fax: 207-523-1925, E-mail: ssteinberg@une.edu.
Website: http://www.une.edu/cas/biology/graduate/index.cfm

University of New Hampshire, Graduate School, College of Life Sciences and Agriculture, Department of Biological Sciences, Durham, NH 03824. Offers agricultural sciences (MS, PhD); integrative and organismal biology (MS, PhD). *Program availability:* Part-time. *Degree requirements:* For doctorate, thesis/dissertation. *Entrance requirements:* For master's and doctorate, GRE General Test. Additional exam requirements/recommendations for international students: Required—TOEFL (minimum score 550 paper-based; 80 iBT). *Application deadline:* For fall admission, 6/1 for domestic students, 4/1 for international students; for spring admission, 12/1 for domestic students. Applications are processed on a rolling basis. Application fee: $65. Electronic applications accepted. *Expenses:* Tuition, state resident: full-time $13,840; part-time $770 per credit hour. Tuition, nonresident: full-time $27,130; part-time $1175 per credit hour. *Required fees:* $2080; $1040. Tuition and fees vary according to degree level and program. *Financial support:* Fellowships, research assistantships, and teaching assistantships available. *Unit head:* Larry Harris, Chair, 603-862-3897. *Application*

Biological and Biomedical Sciences—General

contact: Diane Lavalliere, Senior Academic/Student Support Assistant, 603-862-2100, Fax: 603-862-0275, E-mail: grad.school@unh.edu. Website: http://www.colsa.unh.edu/dbs

University of New Mexico, Graduate Studies, College of Arts and Sciences, Program in Biology, Albuquerque, NM 87131. Offers MS, PhD. *Faculty:* 34 full-time (7 women), 1 part-time/adjunct (0 women). *Students:* 59 full-time (32 women), 44 part-time (28 women); includes 24 minority (2 American Indian or Alaska Native, non-Hispanic/Latino; 3 Asian, non-Hispanic/Latino; 17 Hispanic/Latino; 2 Two or more races, non-Hispanic/Latino), 10 international. Average age 32. 88 applicants, 23% accepted, 19 enrolled. In 2015, 9 master's, 6 doctorates awarded. *Degree requirements:* For master's, comprehensive exam, thesis optional; for doctorate, comprehensive exam, thesis/dissertation. *Entrance requirements:* For master's and doctorate, GRE General Test, minimum GPA of 3.2, letters of recommendation. Additional exam requirements/recommendations for international students: Required—TOEFL (minimum score 550 paper-based; 79 iBT). *Application deadline:* For fall admission, 1/3 priority date for domestic and international students. Applications are processed on a rolling basis. Application fee: $50. Electronic applications accepted. *Financial support:* Fellowships with full tuition reimbursements, research assistantships with full tuition reimbursements, teaching assistantships with full tuition reimbursements, Federal Work-Study, scholarships/grants, health care benefits, and unspecified assistantships available. Financial award application deadline: 1/3; financial award applicants required to submit FAFSA. *Faculty research:* Aquatic ecology, behavioral ecology, botany, cell biology, comparative biology, conservation biology, developmental biology, ecology, evolutionary biology, genetics, genomics, global change biology, immunology, invertebrate biology, mathematical biology, microbiology, molecular evolution, paleobiology, parasitology, physiological ecology, plant biology, systematics, vertebrate biology. *Total annual research expenditures:* $10.8 million. *Unit head:* Dr. Robert D. Miller, Chair, 505-277-2496, Fax: 505-277-0304, E-mail: rdmiller@unm.edu. *Application contact:* Cheryl Martin, Graduate Program Coordinator, 505-277-1712, Fax: 505-277-0304, E-mail: cherylm@unm.edu.
Website: http://biology.unm.edu/

University of New Mexico, Graduate Studies, Health Sciences Center, Program in Biomedical Sciences, Albuquerque, NM 87131-5196. Offers biochemistry and molecular biology (MS, PhD); cell biology and physiology (MS, PhD); molecular genetics and microbiology (MS, PhD); neuroscience (MS, PhD); pathology (MS, PhD); toxicology (MS, PhD). *Program availability:* Part-time. *Faculty:* 18 full-time (10 women), 1 part-time/adjunct (0 women). *Students:* 31 full-time (17 women), 45 part-time (26 women); includes 29 minority (1 American Indian or Alaska Native, non-Hispanic/Latino; 3 Asian, non-Hispanic/Latino; 22 Hispanic/Latino; 2 Native Hawaiian or other Pacific Islander, non-Hispanic/Latino; 1 Two or more races, non-Hispanic/Latino), 18 international. Average age 30. 98 applicants, 11% accepted, 11 enrolled. In 2015, 11 master's, 14 doctorates awarded. Terminal master's awarded for partial completion of doctoral program. *Degree requirements:* For master's, thesis; for doctorate, comprehensive exam, thesis/dissertation, qualifying exam at the end of year 1/core curriculum. *Entrance requirements:* For master's and doctorate, GRE General Test, minimum undergraduate GPA of 3.0. Additional exam requirements/recommendations for international students: Required—TOEFL. *Application deadline:* For fall admission, 3/1 priority date for domestic and international students. Applications are processed on a rolling basis. Application fee: $50. Electronic applications accepted. *Financial support:* Fellowships with tuition reimbursements, research assistantships with full tuition reimbursements, teaching assistantships, career-related internships or fieldwork, Federal Work-Study, institutionally sponsored loans, scholarships/grants, traineeships, health care benefits, and unspecified assistantships available. Financial award application deadline: 1/1; financial award applicants required to submit FAFSA. *Faculty research:* Infectious disease/immunity, cancer biology, cardiovascular and metabolic diseases, brain and behavioral illness, environmental health. *Unit head:* Dr. Helen J. Hathaway, Program Director, 505-272-1887, Fax: 505-272-2412, E-mail: hhathaway@salud.unm.edu. *Application contact:* Mary Fenton, Admissions Coordinator, 505-272-1887, Fax: 505-272-2412, E-mail: mfenton@salud.unm.edu.

University of New Orleans, Graduate School, College of Sciences, Department of Biological Sciences, New Orleans, LA 70148. Offers MS, PhD. *Degree requirements:* For master's, one foreign language, thesis. *Entrance requirements:* For master's, GRE General Test. Additional exam requirements/recommendations for international students: Required—TOEFL (minimum score 550 paper-based; 79 iBT), IELTS (minimum score 6.5). Electronic applications accepted. *Faculty research:* Biochemistry, genetics, vertebrate and invertebrate systematics and ecology, cell and mammalian physiology, morphology.

The University of North Carolina at Chapel Hill, Graduate School, College of Arts and Sciences, Department of Biology, Chapel Hill, NC 27599. Offers botany (MA, MS, PhD); cell biology, development, and physiology (MA, MS, PhD); cell motility and cytoskeleton (PhD); ecology and behavior (MA, MS, PhD); genetics and molecular biology (MA, MS, PhD); morphology, systematics, and evolution (MA, MS, PhD). Terminal master's awarded for partial completion of doctoral program. *Degree requirements:* For master's, comprehensive exam, thesis (for some programs); for doctorate, comprehensive exam, thesis/dissertation. *Entrance requirements:* For master's, GRE General Test, GRE Subject Test, 2 semesters of calculus or statistics; 3 semesters of physics, organic chemistry; 3 semesters of biology; for doctorate, GRE General Test, GRE Subject Test, 2 semesters calculus or statistics, 2 semesters physics, organic chemistry, 3 semesters of biology. Additional exam requirements/recommendations for international students: Required—TOEFL (minimum score 550 paper-based). Electronic applications accepted. *Faculty research:* Gene expression, biomechanics, yeast genetics, plant ecology, plant molecular biology.

The University of North Carolina at Chapel Hill, School of Medicine and Graduate School, Graduate Programs in Medicine, Chapel Hill, NC 27599. Offers allied health sciences (MPT, MS, Au D, DPT, PhD), including human movement science (MS, PhD), occupational science (MS, PhD), physical therapy (MPT, MS, DPT), rehabilitation counseling and psychology (MS), speech and hearing sciences (MS, Au D, PhD); biochemistry and biophysics (MS, PhD); bioinformatics and computational biology (PhD); biomedical engineering (MS, PhD); cell and developmental biology (PhD); cell and molecular physiology (PhD); genetics and molecular biology (PhD); microbiology and immunology (MS, PhD), including immunology, microbiology, neurobiology (PhD); pathology and laboratory medicine (PhD), including experimental pathology; pharmacology (PhD); MD/PhD. *Program availability:* Online learning. Terminal master's awarded for partial completion of doctoral program. *Degree requirements:* For master's, comprehensive exam; for doctorate, thesis/dissertation. Electronic applications accepted. *Expenses:* Contact institution.

The University of North Carolina at Charlotte, College of Liberal Arts and Sciences, Department of Biological Sciences, Charlotte, NC 28223-0001. Offers MA, MS, PhD. *Program availability:* Part-time. *Faculty:* 22 full-time (7 women). *Students:* 26 full-time (13 women), 14 part-time (11 women); includes 6 minority (1 Black or African American, non-Hispanic/Latino; 2 Asian, non-Hispanic/Latino; 1 Hispanic/Latino; 2 Two or more races, non-Hispanic/Latino), 6 international. Average age 29. 28 applicants, 43% accepted, 8 enrolled. In 2015, 7 master's, 5 doctorates awarded. Terminal master's

awarded for partial completion of doctoral program. *Degree requirements:* For master's, comprehensive exam, thesis or project; for doctorate, thesis/dissertation. *Entrance requirements:* For master's and doctorate, GRE General Test, BS or BA from accredited university; minimum overall GPA of 3.0. Additional exam requirements/recommendations for international students: Required—TOEFL (minimum score 557 paper-based, 83 iBT) or IELTS (minimum score 6.5). *Application deadline:* For fall admission, 1/15 for domestic and international students; for spring admission, 10/1 for domestic and international students. Application fee: $75. Electronic applications accepted. *Expenses:* Tuition, state resident: full-time $4128. Tuition, nonresident: full-time $16,799. *Required fees:* $2904. Tuition and fees vary according to course load and program. *Financial support:* In 2015–16, 33 students received support, including 5 fellowships (averaging $41,566 per year), 6 research assistantships (averaging $8,917 per year), 22 teaching assistantships (averaging $8,604 per year); career-related internships or fieldwork, institutionally sponsored loans, scholarships/grants, and unspecified assistantships also available. Support available to part-time students. Financial award application deadline: 3/1; financial award applicants required to submit FAFSA. *Faculty research:* The role of the neuropeptide substance P in microbially-induced central nervous system (CNS) inflammation, the mechanism of enhanced metastasis induced by arthritis, the use of plant-derived vaccines. *Total annual research expenditures:* $1.5 million. *Unit head:* Dr. Pinku Mukherjee, Chair, 704-687-5465, E-mail: pmukherj@uncc.edu. *Application contact:* Kathy B. Giddings, Director of Graduate Admissions, 704-687-5503, Fax: 704-687-1668, E-mail: gradadm@uncc.edu. Website: http://biology.uncc.edu/

The University of North Carolina at Greensboro, Graduate School, College of Arts and Sciences, Department of Biology, Greensboro, NC 27412-5001. Offers MS. *Degree requirements:* For master's, thesis. *Entrance requirements:* For master's, GRE General Test, GRE Subject Test. Additional exam requirements/recommendations for international students: Required—TOEFL. Electronic applications accepted. *Faculty research:* Environmental biology, biochemistry, animal ecology, vertebrate reproduction.

The University of North Carolina Wilmington, College of Arts and Sciences, Department of Biology and Marine Biology, Wilmington, NC 28403-3297. Offers biology (MS); marine biology (MS, PhD). *Program availability:* Part-time. *Faculty:* 38 full-time (11 women). *Students:* 2 full-time (1 woman), 65 part-time (36 women); includes 10 minority (1 Black or African American, non-Hispanic/Latino; 2 Asian, non-Hispanic/Latino; 6 Hispanic/Latino; 1 Two or more races, non-Hispanic/Latino), 4 international. Average age 31. 89 applicants, 17 enrolled. In 2015, 14 master's, 1 doctorate awarded. *Degree requirements:* For master's, comprehensive exam, thesis; for doctorate, comprehensive exam, thesis/dissertation. *Entrance requirements:* For master's, GRE General Test, minimum B average in undergraduate work, 3 recommendations, resume, statement of interest, bachelor's degree in field of biology; for doctorate, GRE General Test, minimum B average in undergraduate and graduate work, resume, summary of MS thesis research, master's degree, statement of interest. Additional exam requirements/recommendations for international students: Required—TOEFL (minimum score 79 iBT), IELTS (minimum score 6.5). *Application deadline:* For fall admission, 6/15 for domestic students; for spring admission, 11/30 for domestic students. Applications are processed on a rolling basis. Application fee: $60. Electronic applications accepted. *Expenses:* $8,854 in-state full-time per year; $20,945 out-of-state full-time per year. *Financial support:* Research assistantships with tuition reimbursements, teaching assistantships with tuition reimbursements, and scholarships/grants available. Support available to part-time students. Financial award application deadline: 3/15; financial award applicants required to submit FAFSA. *Faculty research:* Ecology, physiology, cell and molecular biology, systematics, biomechanics. *Unit head:* Dr. Chris Finelli, Chair, 910-962-3487, E-mail: finellic@uncw.edu. *Application contact:* Dr. Stephen Kinsey, Graduate Coordinator, 910-962-7398, Fax: 910-962-4066, E-mail: kinseys@uncw.edu. Website: http://www.uncw.edu/bio/graduate.html

University of North Dakota, Graduate School, College of Arts and Sciences, Department of Biology, Grand Forks, ND 58202. Offers botany (MS, PhD); ecology (MS, PhD); entomology (MS, PhD); environmental biology (MS, PhD); fisheries/wildlife (MS, PhD); genetics (MS, PhD); zoology (MS, PhD). Terminal master's awarded for partial completion of doctoral program. *Degree requirements:* For master's, thesis, final exam; for doctorate, comprehensive exam, thesis/dissertation, final exam. *Entrance requirements:* For master's, GRE General Test, GRE Subject Test, minimum GPA of 3.0; for doctorate, GRE General Test, GRE Subject Test, minimum GPA of 3.5. Additional exam requirements/recommendations for international students: Required—TOEFL (minimum score 550 paper-based; 79 iBT), IELTS (minimum score 6.5). Electronic applications accepted. *Faculty research:* Population biology, wildlife ecology, RNA processing, hormonal control of behavior.

University of Northern Colorado, Graduate School, College of Natural and Health Sciences, School of Biological Sciences, Program in Biology, Greeley, CO 80639. Offers MS. *Program availability:* Part-time. *Degree requirements:* For master's, comprehensive exam. *Entrance requirements:* For master's, GRE General Test, 3 letters of recommendation. Electronic applications accepted.

University of Northern Iowa, Graduate College, College of Humanities, Arts and Sciences, Department of Biology, Cedar Falls, IA 50614. Offers MS. *Program availability:* Part-time. *Students:* 17 full-time (7 women), 19 part-time (7 women); includes 1 minority (Two or more races, non-Hispanic/Latino), 1 international. 14 applicants, 43% accepted, 6 enrolled. In 2015, 5 master's awarded. *Degree requirements:* For master's, comprehensive exam (for some programs), thesis or alternative. *Entrance requirements:* For master's, minimum GPA of 3.0; 3 letters of recommendation. Additional exam requirements/recommendations for international students: Required—TOEFL (minimum score 500 paper-based; 61 iBT). *Application deadline:* For fall admission, 8/1 priority date for domestic students. Applications are processed on a rolling basis. Application fee: $50 ($70 for international students). Electronic applications accepted. *Financial support:* Scholarships/grants available. Financial award application deadline: 2/1. *Unit head:* Dr. David Saunders, Department Head, 319-273-2456, Fax: 319-273-7125, E-mail: david.saunders@uni.edu. *Application contact:* Laurie S. Russell, Record Analyst, 319-273-2623, Fax: 319-273-2885, E-mail: laurie.russell@uni.edu.
Website: http://www.uni.edu/biology/graduate-programs

University of North Florida, College of Arts and Sciences, Department of Biology, Jacksonville, FL 32224. Offers MA, MS. *Program availability:* Part-time. *Faculty:* 16 full-time (7 women). *Students:* 16 full-time (11 women), 14 part-time (11 women); includes 3 minority (1 Asian, non-Hispanic/Latino; 1 Hispanic/Latino; 1 Two or more races, non-Hispanic/Latino). Average age 27. 37 applicants, 35% accepted, 8 enrolled. In 2015, 12 master's awarded. *Degree requirements:* For master's, thesis (for some programs). *Entrance requirements:* For master's, GRE General Test, minimum GPA of 3.0 in last 60 hours, letters of recommendation. Additional exam requirements/recommendations for international students: Required—TOEFL (minimum score 570 paper-based). Application fee: $30. Electronic applications accepted. *Expenses:* Tuition, state resident: part-time $408.10 per credit hour. Tuition, nonresident: part-time $932.61 per credit hour. *Required fees:* $111.81 per credit hour. Tuition and fees vary according to course load, campus/location and program. *Financial support:* In 2015–16, 10 students received support, including 1 research assistantship (averaging $4,928 per year);

teaching assistantships, Federal Work-Study, scholarships/grants, and unspecified assistantships also available. Support available to part-time students. Financial award application deadline: 4/1; financial award applicants required to submit FAFSA. *Total annual research expenditures:* $474,019. *Unit head:* Dr. Daniel Moon, Chair, 904-620-2239, Fax: 904-620-3885, E-mail: dmoon@unf.edu. *Application contact:* Dr. Amanda Pascale, Director, The Graduate School, 904-620-1360, Fax: 904-620-1362, E-mail: graduateschool@unf.edu.
Website: http://www.unf.edu/coas/biology/

University of North Texas, Robert B. Toulouse School of Graduate Studies, Denton, TX 76203-5459. Offers accounting (MS); applied anthropology (MA, MS); applied behavior analysis (Certificate); applied geography (MA); applied technology and performance improvement (M Ed, MS); art education (MA); art history (MA); art museum education (Certificate); arts leadership (Certificate); audiology (Au D); behavior analysis (MS); behavioral science (PhD); biochemistry and molecular biology (MS); biology (MA, MS); biomedical engineering (MS); business analysis (MS); chemistry (MS); clinical health psychology (PhD); communication studies (MA, MS); computer engineering (MS); computer science (MS); counseling (M Ed, MS), including clinical mental health counseling (MS), college and university counseling, elementary school counseling, secondary school counseling; creative writing (MA); criminal justice (MS); curriculum and instruction (M Ed); decision sciences (MBA); design (MA, MFA), including fashion design (MFA), innovation studies, interior design (MFA); early childhood studies (MS); economics (MS); educational leadership (M Ed, Ed D); educational psychology (MS, PhD), including family studies (MS), gifted and talented (MS), human development (MS), learning and cognition (MS), research, measurement and evaluation (MS); electrical engineering (MS); emergency management (MPA); engineering technology (MS); English (MA); English as a second language (MA); environmental science (MS); finance (MBA, MS); financial management (MPA); French (MA); health services management (MBA); higher education (M Ed, Ed D); history (MA); hospitality management (MS); human resources management (MPA); information science (MS); information systems (PhD); information technologies (MBA); interdisciplinary studies (MA, MS); international studies (MA); international sustainable tourism (MS); jazz studies (MM); journalism (MA, MJ, Graduate Certificate), including interactive and virtual digital communication (Graduate Certificate), narrative journalism (Graduate Certificate), public relations (Graduate Certificate); kinesiology (MS); linguistics (MA); local government management (MPA); logistics (PhD); logistics and supply chain management (MBA); long-term care, senior housing, and aging services (MA); management (PhD); marketing (MBA); mathematics (MA, MS); mechanical and energy engineering (MS, PhD); music (MA), including ethnomusicology, music theory, musicology, performance; music composition (PhD); music education (MM Ed, PhD); nonprofit management (MPA); operations and supply chain management (MBA); performance (MM, DMA); philosophy (MA); political science (MA); professional and technical communication (MA); radio, television and film (MA, MFA); rehabilitation counseling (Certificate); sociology (MA); Spanish (MA); special education (M Ed); speech-language pathology (MA); strategic management (MBA); studio art (MFA); teaching (M Ed); MBA/MS. *Program availability:* Part-time, evening/weekend, online learning. Terminal master's awarded for partial completion of doctoral program. *Degree requirements:* For master's, variable foreign language requirement, comprehensive exam (for some programs), thesis (for some programs); for doctorate, variable foreign language requirement, comprehensive exam (for some programs), thesis/dissertation; for other advanced degree, variable foreign language requirement, comprehensive exam (for some programs). *Entrance requirements:* For master's and doctorate, GRE, GMAT. Additional exam requirements/recommendations for international students: Required—TOEFL (minimum score 550 paper-based; 79 iBT). Electronic applications accepted.

University of North Texas Health Science Center at Fort Worth, Graduate School of Biomedical Sciences, Fort Worth, TX 76107-2699. Offers anatomy and cell biology (MS, PhD); biochemistry and molecular biology (MS, PhD); biomedical sciences (MS, PhD); biotechnology (MS); forensic genetics (MS); integrative physiology (MS, PhD); medical science (MS); microbiology and immunology (MS, PhD); pharmacology (MS, PhD); science education (MS); DO/MS; DO/PhD. Terminal master's awarded for partial completion of doctoral program. *Degree requirements:* For master's, thesis; for doctorate, thesis/dissertation. *Entrance requirements:* For master's and doctorate, GRE General Test. Additional exam requirements/recommendations for international students: Required—TOEFL. *Expenses:* Contact institution. *Faculty research:* Alzheimer's disease, aging, eye diseases, cancer, cardiovascular disease.

University of Notre Dame, Graduate School, College of Science, Department of Biological Sciences, Notre Dame, IN 46556. Offers aquatic ecology, evolution and environmental biology (MS, PhD); cellular and molecular biology (MS, PhD); genetics (MS, PhD); physiology (MS, PhD); vector biology and parasitology (MS, PhD). Terminal master's awarded for partial completion of doctoral program. *Degree requirements:* For master's, comprehensive exam, thesis; for doctorate, comprehensive exam, thesis/dissertation, candidacy exam. *Entrance requirements:* For master's and doctorate, GRE General Test. Additional exam requirements/recommendations for international students: Required—TOEFL (minimum score 600 paper-based; 80 iBT). Electronic applications accepted. *Faculty research:* Tropical disease, molecular genetics, neurobiology, evolutionary biology, aquatic biology.

University of Oklahoma, College of Arts and Sciences, Department of Biology, Program in Biology, Norman, OK 73019. Offers bioinformatics (MS, PhD); biology (MS, PhD). *Students:* 8 full-time (3 women), 19 part-time (9 women); includes 2 minority (both Asian, non-Hispanic/Latino), 4 international. Average age 27. 26 applicants, 15% accepted, 4 enrolled. In 2015, 2 master's, 1 doctorate awarded. *Degree requirements:* For master's, thesis, course in biostatistics; for doctorate, comprehensive exam, thesis/dissertation, course in biostatistics; 2 semesters as a teaching assistant. *Entrance requirements:* For master's and doctorate, GRE General Test, transcripts, 3 letters of recommendation, personal statement, curriculum vitae. Additional exam requirements/recommendations for international students: Required—TOEFL (minimum score 79 iBT) or IELTS (minimum score 6.5). *Application deadline:* For fall admission, 12/15 for domestic and international students. Application fee: $50 ($100 for international students). Electronic applications accepted. *Expenses:* Tuition, state resident: full-time $4577; part-time $190.70 per credit hour. Tuition, nonresident: full-time $17,758; part-time $739.90 per credit hour. *Required fees:* $3060; $115.70 per credit hour. $141.50 per semester. *Financial support:* In 2015–16, 23 students received support. Fellowships, research assistantships, teaching assistantships, scholarships/grants, health care benefits, unspecified assistantships, and assistantships (with tuition waivers and health insurance), supplementary scholarship funding available. Financial award application deadline: 6/1; financial award applicants required to submit FAFSA. *Faculty research:* Geographical ecology; biology of behavior; cellular and behavioral neurobiology; evolutionary and molecular genetics; evolution of development. *Unit head:* Dr. Richard Broughton, Professor and Chair, 405-325-6200, Fax: 405-325-6202, E-mail: biology@ou.edu. *Application contact:* Dianna Wilson, Academic Counselor, 405-325-9139, Fax: 405-325-6202, E-mail: biologygrad@ou.edu.
Website: http://www.ou.edu/cas/biology

University of Oklahoma Health Sciences Center, College of Medicine and Graduate College, Graduate Programs in Medicine, Oklahoma City, OK 73190. Offers

biochemistry and molecular biology (MS, PhD), including biochemistry, molecular biology; cell biology (MS, PhD); medical sciences (MS); microbiology and immunology (MS, PhD), including immunology, microbiology; neuroscience (MS, PhD); pathology (PhD); physiology (MS, PhD); psychiatry and behavioral sciences (MS, PhD), including biological psychology; radiological sciences (MS, PhD), including medical radiation physics; MD/PhD. *Program availability:* Part-time. Terminal master's awarded for partial completion of doctoral program. *Degree requirements:* For doctorate, thesis/dissertation. *Entrance requirements:* For doctorate, GRE General Test, 3 letters of recommendation. Additional exam requirements/recommendations for international students: Required—TOEFL. *Expenses:* Contact institution. *Faculty research:* Behavior and drugs, structure and function of endothelium, genetics and behavior, gene structure and function, action of antibiotics.

University of Oregon, Graduate School, College of Arts and Sciences, Department of Biology, Eugene, OR 97403. Offers ecology and evolution (MA, MS, PhD); marine biology (MA, MS, PhD); molecular, cellular and genetic biology (PhD); neuroscience and development (PhD). Terminal master's awarded for partial completion of doctoral program. *Degree requirements:* For master's, thesis (for some programs); for doctorate, thesis/dissertation. *Entrance requirements:* For master's and doctorate, GRE General Test, minimum GPA of 3.2. Additional exam requirements/recommendations for international students: Required—TOEFL. *Faculty research:* Developmental neurobiology; evolution, population biology, and quantitative genetics; regulation of gene expression; biochemistry of marine organisms.

University of Ottawa, Faculty of Graduate and Postdoctoral Studies, Faculty of Science, Ottawa-Carleton Institute of Biology, Ottawa, ON K1N 6N5, Canada. Offers M Sc, PhD. M Sc, PhD offered jointly with Carleton University. *Program availability:* Part-time. *Degree requirements:* For master's, thesis, seminar; for doctorate, comprehensive exam, thesis/dissertation, seminar. *Entrance requirements:* For master's, honors B Sc degree or equivalent, minimum B average; for doctorate, honors B Sc with minimum B+ average or M Sc with minimum B+ average. Electronic applications accepted. *Faculty research:* Physiology/biochemistry, cellular and molecular biology, ecology, behavior and systematics.

University of Pennsylvania, Perelman School of Medicine, Biomedical Graduate Studies, Philadelphia, PA 19104. Offers MS, PhD, MD/PhD, VMD/PhD. *Faculty:* 949. *Students:* 800 full-time (417 women), 106 part-time (70 women); includes 275 minority (29 Black or African American, non-Hispanic/Latino; 4 American Indian or Alaska Native, non-Hispanic/Latino; 140 Asian, non-Hispanic/Latino; 66 Hispanic/Latino; 2 Native Hawaiian or other Pacific Islander, non-Hispanic/Latino; 34 Two or more races, non-Hispanic/Latino), 106 international. 1,290 applicants, 20% accepted, 104 enrolled. In 2015, 81 master's, 115 doctorates awarded. Terminal master's awarded for partial completion of doctoral program. *Entrance requirements:* Additional exam requirements/recommendations for international students: Required—TOEFL. *Application deadline:* For fall admission, 12/1 priority date for domestic students, 12/1 for international students. Applications are processed on a rolling basis. Application fee: $80. Electronic applications accepted. *Expenses: Tuition,* area resident: Full-time $31,068; part-time $5762 per course. *Required fees:* $3200; $336 per course. Full-time tuition and fees vary according to degree level, program and student level. Part-time tuition and fees vary according to course load, degree level and program. *Financial support:* In 2015–16, 740 students received support. *Unit head:* Dr. Michael Nusbaum, Director, 215-898-1585, E-mail: nusbaum@mail.med.upenn.edu. *Application contact:* Aislinn Wallace, Admissions Coordinator, 215-746-6349, E-mail: aislinnw@mail.med.upenn.edu.
Website: http://www.med.upenn.edu/bgs/

University of Pennsylvania, School of Arts and Sciences, Graduate Group in Biology, Philadelphia, PA 19104. Offers PhD. *Faculty:* 42 full-time (10 women), 6 part-time/adjunct (1 woman). *Students:* 50 full-time (19 women); includes 10 minority (6 Asian, non-Hispanic/Latino; 2 Hispanic/Latino; 2 Two or more races, non-Hispanic/Latino), 19 international. Average age 28. 159 applicants, 10% accepted, 5 enrolled. In 2015, 6 doctorates awarded. *Expenses: Tuition,* area resident: Full-time $31,068; part-time $5762 per course. *Required fees:* $3200; $336 per course. Full-time tuition and fees vary according to degree level, program and student level. Part-time tuition and fees vary according to course load, degree level and program.
Website: http://www.bio.upenn.edu

University of Pittsburgh, Dietrich School of Arts and Sciences, Department of Biological Sciences, Pittsburgh, PA 15260. Offers ecology and evolution (PhD); molecular, cellular, and developmental biology (PhD). *Faculty:* 26 full-time (7 women). *Students:* 51 full-time (29 women); includes 3 minority (1 Black or African American, non-Hispanic/Latino; 1 Asian, non-Hispanic/Latino; 1 Hispanic/Latino), 10 international. Average age 23. 136 applicants, 24% accepted, 10 enrolled. In 2015, 7 doctorates awarded. *Degree requirements:* For doctorate, comprehensive exam, thesis/dissertation, completion of research integrity module. *Entrance requirements:* For doctorate, GRE General Test, GRE Subject Test. Additional exam requirements/recommendations for international students: Required—TOEFL (minimum score 90 iBT). *Application deadline:* For fall admission, 1/3 priority date for domestic students, 12/9 priority date for international students. Applications are processed on a rolling basis. Application fee: $0 ($50 for international students). Electronic applications accepted. *Expenses:* $33,000 per year in-state, $53,526 per year out-of-state. *Financial support:* In 2015–16, 41 fellowships with full tuition reimbursements (averaging $33,193 per year), 76 research assistantships with full tuition reimbursements (averaging $27,585 per year), 32 teaching assistantships with full tuition reimbursements (averaging $26,779 per year) were awarded; Federal Work-Study, traineeships, health care benefits, and tuition waivers (full) also available. *Faculty research:* Molecular biology; ecology and evolution; microbiology; biochemistry; structural biology. *Total annual research expenditures:* $7.4 million. *Unit head:* Dr. Paula J. Grabowski, Professor and Chair, 412-624-4350, Fax: 412-624-4349, E-mail: pag4@pitt.edu. *Application contact:* Cathleen M. Barr, Graduate Administrator, 412-624-4268, Fax: 412-624-4349, E-mail: cbarr@pitt.edu.
Website: http://www.biology.pitt.edu

University of Pittsburgh, Dietrich School of Arts and Sciences, Program in Computational Modeling and Simulation, Pittsburgh, PA 15260. Offers biological science (PhD); chemistry (PhD); computer science (PhD); economics (PhD); mathematics (PhD); physics and astronomy (PhD); psychology (PhD); statistics (PhD). *Program availability:* Part-time. *Faculty:* 3 full-time (0 women). *Students:* 3 full-time (1 woman); includes 2 minority (both Asian, non-Hispanic/Latino). Average age 23. 13 applicants, 31% accepted, 2 enrolled. *Degree requirements:* For doctorate, comprehensive exam, thesis/dissertation, preliminary exam. *Entrance requirements:* For doctorate, GRE, statement of purpose, transcripts for all college-level institutions attended, three letters of reference. Additional exam requirements/recommendations for international students: Required—TOEFL (minimum score 90 iBT), IELTS (minimum score 7). *Application deadline:* For fall admission, 1/15 for domestic and international students. Applications are processed on a rolling basis. Application fee: $0 ($50 for international students). Electronic applications accepted. Tuition and fees vary according to program. *Financial support:* In 2015–16, 3 students received support, including 2 fellowships with full tuition reimbursements available (averaging $27,000 per year), 1 research assistantship with full tuition reimbursement available (averaging $21,500 per year); tuition waivers (full)

Biological and Biomedical Sciences—General

also available. Financial award application deadline: 4/15. *Faculty research:* Econometric modeling, developing reduced-scaling first principles approaches for expedited predictions of molecular and materials properties, developing computational models to quantitatively describe origins of reactivity and selectivity in organocatalytic reactions. *Unit head:* Dr. Kathleen Blee, Associate Dean, Graduate Studies and Research, 412-624-3939, Fax: 412-624-6855. *Application contact:* Wendy G. Janocha, Graduate Administrator, 412-648-7251, E-mail: wgj1@pitt.edu.
Website: http://cmsp.pitt.edu/

University of Pittsburgh, School of Medicine, Graduate Programs in Medicine, Interdisciplinary Biomedical Graduate Program, Pittsburgh, PA 15260. Offers PhD. *Faculty:* 302 full-time (81 women). *Students:* 25 full-time (9 women); includes 8 minority (1 Black or African American, non-Hispanic/Latino; 4 Asian, non-Hispanic/Latino; 3 Hispanic/Latino). Average age 24. 386 applicants, 17% accepted, 25 enrolled. *Degree requirements:* For doctorate, comprehensive exam, thesis/dissertation. *Entrance requirements:* For doctorate, GRE General Test, GRE Subject Test, minimum QPA of 3.0. Additional exam requirements/recommendations for international students: Required—TOEFL (minimum score 600 paper-based; 100 iBT), IELTS (minimum score 7). *Application deadline:* For fall admission, 12/1 priority date for domestic and international students. Application fee: $50. Electronic applications accepted. Tuition and fees vary according to program. *Financial support:* In 2015–16, 25 students received support, including 25 research assistantships with full tuition reimbursements available (averaging $27,000 per year); fellowships, teaching assistantships, scholarships/grants, traineeships, and health care benefits also available. *Faculty research:* Cell biology and molecular physiology, cellular and molecular pathology, immunology, molecular genetics and developmental biology, molecular pharmacology and molecular virology and microbiology. *Unit head:* Dr. John P. Horn, Director, 412-648-8957, Fax: 412-648-1077, E-mail: gradstudies@medschool.pitt.edu. *Application contact:* Carol Williams, Admissions and Recruiting Manager, 412-648-8957, Fax: 412-648-1077, E-mail: gradstudies@medschool.pitt.edu.
Website: http://www.gradbiomed.pitt.edu/

University of Prince Edward Island, Faculty of Science, Charlottetown, PE C1A 4P3, Canada. Offers biology (M Sc); chemistry (M Sc). *Degree requirements:* For master's, thesis. *Entrance requirements:* Additional exam requirements/recommendations for international students: Required—TOEFL (minimum score 550 paper-based; 80 iBT), Canadian Academic English Language Assessment, Michigan English Language Assessment Battery, Canadian Test of English for Scholars and Trainees. *Faculty research:* Ecology and wildlife biology, molecular, genetics and biotechnology, organametallic, bio-organic, supramolecular and synthetic organic chemistry, neurobiology and stoke materials science.

University of Puerto Rico, Mayagüez Campus, Graduate Studies, College of Arts and Sciences, Department of Biology, Mayagüez, PR 00681-9000. Offers MS. *Program availability:* Part-time. *Degree requirements:* For master's, one foreign language, comprehensive exam, thesis. *Entrance requirements:* For master's, GRE General Test, BS in biology or its equivalent; minimum GPA of 3.0 in biology courses. Additional exam requirements/recommendations for international students: Required—TOEFL. *Faculty research:* Herpetology, entomology, microbiology, immunology, botany.

University of Puerto Rico, Medical Sciences Campus, School of Medicine, Biomedical Sciences Graduate Program, San Juan, PR 00936-5067. Offers MS, PhD. Terminal master's awarded for partial completion of doctoral program. *Degree requirements:* For master's, one foreign language, thesis; for doctorate, one foreign language, comprehensive exam, thesis/dissertation. *Entrance requirements:* For master's and doctorate, GRE General Test, GRE Subject Test, interview, 3 letters of recommendation, minimum GPA of 3.0. Electronic applications accepted. *Expenses:* Contact institution.

University of Puerto Rico, Río Piedras Campus, College of Natural Sciences, Department of Biology, San Juan, PR 00931-3300. Offers ecology/systematics (MS, PhD); evolution/genetics (MS, PhD); molecular/cellular biology (MS, PhD); neuroscience (MS, PhD). *Program availability:* Part-time. *Degree requirements:* For master's, one foreign language, comprehensive exam, thesis; for doctorate, one foreign language, comprehensive exam, thesis/dissertation. *Entrance requirements:* For master's, GRE Subject Test, interview, minimum GPA of 3.0, letter of recommendation; for doctorate, GRE Subject Test, interview, master's degree, minimum GPA of 3.0, letter of recommendation. *Faculty research:* Environmental, poblational and systematic biology.

University of Regina, Faculty of Graduate Studies and Research, Faculty of Science, Department of Biology, Regina, SK S4S 0A2, Canada. Offers M Sc, PhD. *Program availability:* Part-time. *Degree requirements:* For master's, thesis; for doctorate, comprehensive exam, thesis/dissertation. *Entrance requirements:* Additional exam requirements/recommendations for international students: Required—TOEFL (minimum score 580 paper-based; 80 iBT), IELTS (minimum score 6.5), PTE (minimum score 59). Electronic applications accepted. *Faculty research:* Aquatic and terrestrial ecology, molecular and population genetics, developmental biology, microbiology, plant physiology and morphology.

University of Rhode Island, Graduate School, College of the Environment and Life Sciences, Department of Biological Sciences, Kingston, RI 02881. Offers MS, PhD. *Program availability:* Part-time. *Faculty:* 17 full-time (8 women), 4 part-time/adjunct (3 women). *Students:* 93 full-time (61 women), 14 part-time (10 women); includes 5 minority (1 Black or African American, non-Hispanic/Latino; 1 Asian, non-Hispanic/Latino; 2 Hispanic/Latino; 1 Two or more races, non-Hispanic/Latino), 9 international. In 2015, 14 master's, 3 doctorates awarded. *Degree requirements:* For master's, comprehensive exam (for some programs), thesis optional; for doctorate, comprehensive exam, thesis/dissertation. *Entrance requirements:* For master's and doctorate, GRE, 2 letters of recommendation. Additional exam requirements/recommendations for international students: Required—TOEFL (minimum score 550 paper-based). *Application deadline:* For fall admission, 4/15 for domestic students, 1/15 for international students. Application fee: $65. Electronic applications accepted. *Expenses:* Tuition, state resident: full-time $11,796; part-time $655 per credit. Tuition, nonresident: full-time $24,206; part-time $1345 per credit. *Required fees:* $1546; $44 per credit. One-time fee: $155 full-time; $35 part-time. *Financial support:* In 2015–16, 3 research assistantships with tuition reimbursements (averaging $13,507 per year), 8 teaching assistantships with tuition reimbursements (averaging $13,305 per year) were awarded. Financial award application deadline: 1/15; financial award applicants required to submit FAFSA. *Faculty research:* Physiological constraints on predators in the Antarctic, effects of CO2 absorption in salt water particularly as it impacts pteropods. *Total annual research expenditures:* $1.2 million. *Unit head:* Dr. Marian Goldsmith, Chairperson, 401-874-2637, Fax: 401-874-2065, E-mail: mrgoldsmith@uri.edu.
Website: http://web.uri.edu/bio/

University of Rochester, School of Arts and Sciences, Department of Biology, Rochester, NY 14627. Offers MS, PhD. *Faculty:* 21 full-time (6 women). *Students:* 45 full-time (18 women), 1 part-time (0 women); includes 4 minority (1 Asian, non-Hispanic/Latino; 1 Hispanic/Latino; 2 Two or more races, non-Hispanic/Latino), 25 international. 95 applicants, 23% accepted, 8 enrolled. In 2015, 8 master's, 7 doctorates awarded. Terminal master's awarded for partial completion of doctoral program. *Degree*

requirements: For doctorate, thesis/dissertation, qualifying exam. *Entrance requirements:* For master's and doctorate, GRE General Test, GRE Subject Test (highly recommended). Additional exam requirements/recommendations for international students: Required—TOEFL. *Application deadline:* For fall admission, 1/1 priority date for domestic and international students. Application fee: $50. Electronic applications accepted. *Expenses: Tuition, area resident:* Full-time $47,450; part-time $1482 per credit hour. *Required fees:* $528. Tuition and fees vary according to program. *Financial support:* Fellowships, research assistantships, teaching assistantships, and tuition scholarships (for PhD students) available. Financial award application deadline: 1/1. *Faculty research:* Molecular, cellular, and developmental biology; genetics, ecology and evolutionary biology. *Unit head:* Gloria Culver, Chair, 585-276-3602. *Application contact:* Cindy Landry, Graduate Program Administrative Assistant, 585-275-7991.
Website: http://www.rochester.edu/College/BIO/graduate.html

University of Rochester, School of Medicine and Dentistry, Graduate Programs in Medicine and Dentistry, Interdepartmental Program in Translational Biomedical Science, Rochester, NY 14627. Offers PhD. *Expenses: Tuition, area resident:* Full-time $47,450; part-time $1482 per credit hour. *Required fees:* $528. Tuition and fees vary according to program.

University of Saint Joseph, Department of Biology, West Hartford, CT 06117-2700. Offers MS. *Program availability:* Part-time, online learning. *Degree requirements:* For master's, comprehensive exam, thesis or alternative. *Entrance requirements:* For master's, 2 letters of recommendation. *Application deadline:* Applications are processed on a rolling basis. Application fee: $50. Electronic applications accepted. Application fee is waived when completed online. *Financial support:* Unspecified assistantships available. Support available to part-time students. Financial award applicants required to submit FAFSA.
Website: http://www.usj.edu/index.php/academics/schools/school-of-health-natural-sciences/biology

University of San Francisco, College of Arts and Sciences, Program in Biology, San Francisco, CA 94117-1080. Offers MS. *Faculty:* 5 full-time (2 women). *Students:* 5 full-time (4 women), 1 (woman) part-time; includes 3 minority (2 Asian, non-Hispanic/Latino; 1 Two or more races, non-Hispanic/Latino), 2 international. Average age 26. 37 applicants, 8% accepted, 1 enrolled. In 2015, 3 master's awarded. *Degree requirements:* For master's, thesis. *Entrance requirements:* For master's, GRE General Test, GRE Subject Test, BS in biology or the equivalent. Additional exam requirements/recommendations for international students: Required—TOEFL, IELTS, PTE. *Application deadline:* For fall admission, 3/15 for domestic and international students; for spring admission, 10/15 for domestic and international students. Application fee: $55 ($65 for international students). *Expenses: Tuition, area resident:* Full-time $22,410; part-time $1245 per credit. Tuition and fees vary according to course load, degree level and campus/location. *Financial support:* In 2015–16, 6 students received support. Teaching assistantships, career-related internships or fieldwork, Federal Work-Study, institutionally sponsored loans, and tuition waivers available. Financial award application deadline: 3/2; financial award applicants required to submit FAFSA. *Unit head:* Dr. James Sikes, Chair, 415-422-6755, Fax: 415-422-6363. *Application contact:* Mark Landerghini, Information Contact, 415-422-5101, Fax: 415-422-2217, E-mail: asgraduate@usfca.edu.
Website: http://www.usfca.edu/artsci/biog/

University of Saskatchewan, College of Graduate Studies and Research, College of Arts and Science, Department of Biology, Saskatoon, SK S7N 5A2, Canada. Offers M Sc, PhD. *Degree requirements:* For master's, thesis (for some programs); for doctorate, comprehensive exam (for some programs), thesis/dissertation. *Entrance requirements:* Additional exam requirements/recommendations for international students: Required—TOEFL (minimum score 80 iBT); Recommended—IELTS (minimum score 6.5). Electronic applications accepted.

University of Saskatchewan, Western College of Veterinary Medicine and College of Graduate Studies and Research, Graduate Programs in Veterinary Medicine, Department of Veterinary Biomedical Sciences, Saskatoon, SK S7N 5A2, Canada. Offers veterinary anatomy (M Sc); veterinary biomedical sciences (M Vet Sc); veterinary physiological sciences (M Sc, PhD). *Degree requirements:* For master's, thesis; for doctorate, comprehensive exam (for some programs), thesis/dissertation. *Entrance requirements:* Additional exam requirements/recommendations for international students: Required—TOEFL (minimum score 80 iBT); Recommended—IELTS (minimum score 6.5). Electronic applications accepted. *Faculty research:* Toxicology, animal reproduction, pharmacology, chloride channels, pulmonary pathobiology.

University of South Alabama, College of Arts and Sciences, Department of Biological Sciences, Mobile, AL 36688. Offers MS. *Program availability:* Part-time. *Faculty:* 6 full-time (2 women). *Students:* 7 full-time (2 women), 2 part-time (1 woman). Average age 25. 19 applicants, 11% accepted, 2 enrolled. *Degree requirements:* For master's, one foreign language, comprehensive exam, thesis optional. *Entrance requirements:* For master's, GRE Subject Test (or MCAT with minimum score of 24 for applicants to a cellular/molecular area), minimum GPA of 3.0. Additional exam requirements/recommendations for international students: Required—TOEFL (minimum score 600 paper-based). *Application deadline:* For fall admission, 7/1 priority date for domestic students, 6/1 priority date for international students; for spring admission, 12/1 priority date for domestic students, 11/1 priority date for international students; for summer admission, 5/1 priority date for domestic students. Applications are processed on a rolling basis. Application fee: $35. Electronic applications accepted. *Expenses:* Tuition, state resident: full-time $9480; part-time $395 per credit hour. Tuition, nonresident: full-time $18,960; part-time $790 per credit hour. *Financial support:* Fellowships, research assistantships, teaching assistantships, career-related internships or fieldwork, Federal Work-Study, institutionally sponsored loans, scholarships/grants, and unspecified assistantships available. Support available to part-time students. Financial award application deadline: 5/31; financial award applicants required to submit FAFSA. *Faculty research:* Aquatic and marine biology, molecular biochemistry, plant and animal taxonomy. *Unit head:* Dr. Tim Sherman, Chair, Biology, 251-460-7529, E-mail: tsherman@southalabama.edu. *Application contact:* Dr. Brian Axsmith, Graduate Coordinator, Biology, 251-460-7528, E-mail: baxsmith@southalabama.edu.
Website: http://www.southalabama.edu/biology/index.html

University of South Alabama, College of Medicine and Graduate School, Interdisciplinary Graduate Program in Basic Medical Sciences, Mobile, AL 36688-0002. Offers PhD. *Faculty:* 26 full-time (5 women). *Students:* 43 full-time (23 women), 6 part-time (3 women); includes 5 minority (3 Black or African American, non-Hispanic/Latino; 1 Asian, non-Hispanic/Latino; 1 Hispanic/Latino), 6 international. Average age 30. 32 applicants, 25% accepted, 8 enrolled. In 2015, 5 doctorates awarded. *Degree requirements:* For doctorate, comprehensive exam, thesis/dissertation. *Entrance requirements:* For doctorate, GRE, three semesters or quarters of undergraduate work in physics, general chemistry, organic chemistry, biology, English composition, and mathematics (including statistics and calculus) with minimum GPA of 3.0. Additional exam requirements/recommendations for international students: Required—TOEFL (minimum score 600 paper-based; 100 iBT). *Application deadline:* For fall admission, 3/31 for domestic and international students. Application fee: $25. Electronic applications accepted. *Expenses:* Contact institution. *Financial support:* Fellowships, research

---

96 www.petersons.com

assistantships, teaching assistantships, career-related internships or fieldwork, Federal Work-Study, institutionally sponsored loans, scholarships/grants, and unspecified assistantships available. Support available to part-time students. Financial award application deadline: 5/31; financial award applicants required to submit FAFSA. *Faculty research:* Microcirculation, molecular biology, cell biology, growth control. *Unit head:* Dr. Thomas Rich, Director of College of Medicine Graduate Studies, 251-460-6153, Fax: 251-460-6071, E-mail: trich@southalabama.edu. *Application contact:* Lanett Flagge, Academic Advisor, 251-460-6153, Fax: 251-461-6071, E-mail: lflagge@southalabama.edu.

University of South Carolina, The Graduate School, College of Arts and Sciences, Department of Biological Sciences, Columbia, SC 29208. Offers biology (MS, PhD); biology education (IMA, MAT); ecology, evolution and organismal biology (MS, PhD); molecular, cellular, and developmental biology (MS, PhD). IMA and MAT offered in cooperation with the College of Education. Terminal master's awarded for partial completion of doctoral program. *Degree requirements:* For master's, one foreign language, thesis (for some programs); for doctorate, one foreign language, thesis/dissertation. *Entrance requirements:* For master's and doctorate, GRE General Test, minimum GPA of 3.0 in science. Electronic applications accepted. *Faculty research:* Marine ecology, population and evolutionary biology, molecular biology and genetics, development.

University of South Carolina, School of Medicine and The Graduate School, Graduate Programs in Medicine, Columbia, SC 29208. Offers biomedical science (MBS, PhD); genetic counseling (MS); nurse anesthesia (MNA); rehabilitation counseling (MRC, Certificate), including psychiatric rehabilitation (Certificate), rehabilitation counseling (MRC). Terminal master's awarded for partial completion of doctoral program. *Degree requirements:* For master's, comprehensive exam, thesis (for some programs), practicum; for doctorate, comprehensive exam, thesis/dissertation. *Entrance requirements:* For master's, doctorate, and Certificate, GRE General Test. Electronic applications accepted. *Expenses:* Contact institution. *Faculty research:* Cardiovascular diseases, oncology, neuroscience, psychiatric rehabilitation, genetics.

University of South Carolina, School of Medicine and The Graduate School, Graduate Programs in Medicine, Graduate Program in Biomedical Science, Doctoral Program in Biomedical Science, Columbia, SC 29208. Offers PhD. *Degree requirements:* For doctorate, comprehensive exam, thesis/dissertation. *Entrance requirements:* For doctorate, GRE General Test. Electronic applications accepted. *Faculty research:* Cancer, neuroscience, cardiovascular, reproductive, immunology.

University of South Carolina, School of Medicine and The Graduate School, Graduate Programs in Medicine, Graduate Program in Biomedical Science, Master's Program in Biomedical Science, Columbia, SC 29208. Offers MBS. *Degree requirements:* For master's, comprehensive exam, thesis. *Entrance requirements:* For master's, GRE General Test. Electronic applications accepted. *Faculty research:* Cardiovascular diseases, oncology, reproductive biology, neuroscience, microbiology.

The University of South Dakota, Graduate School, College of Arts and Sciences, Department of Biology, Vermillion, SD 57069-2390. Offers MA, MS, PhD. *Degree requirements:* For master's, comprehensive exam (for some programs), thesis (for some programs); for doctorate, comprehensive exam, thesis/dissertation. *Entrance requirements:* For master's, GRE Subject Test, GRE General Test, minimum GPA of 2.7; for doctorate, GRE General Test, GRE Subject Test, minimum GPA of 2.7. Additional exam requirements/recommendations for international students: Required—TOEFL (minimum score 550 paper-based; 70 iBT). *Application deadline:* Applications are processed on a rolling basis. Application fee: $35. Electronic applications accepted. *Financial support:* Fellowships with partial tuition reimbursements, research assistantships with partial tuition reimbursements, teaching assistantships with partial tuition reimbursements, Federal Work-Study, and unspecified assistantships available. Support available to part-time students. Financial award applicants required to submit FAFSA. *Faculty research:* Evolutionary and ecological informatics, neuroscience, stress physiology. *Unit head:* Dr. Kaius Helenurm, Chair, 605-677-6174, E-mail: kaius.helenurm@usd.edu. *Application contact:* 605-677-5211, Fax: 605-677-6557, E-mail: biology@usd.edu.
Website: http://www.usd.edu/biology

The University of South Dakota, Graduate School, Sanford School of Medicine and Graduate School, Biomedical Sciences Graduate Program, Vermillion, SD 57069-2390. Offers cardiovascular research (MS, PhD); cellular and molecular biology (MS, PhD); molecular microbiology and immunology (MS, PhD); neuroscience (MS, PhD); physiology and pharmacology (MS, PhD). *Students:* Average age 26. Terminal master's awarded for partial completion of doctoral program. *Degree requirements:* For master's, thesis; for doctorate, comprehensive exam, thesis/dissertation. *Entrance requirements:* For master's and doctorate, GRE General Test, minimum GPA of 3.0. Additional exam requirements/recommendations for international students: Required—TOEFL (minimum score 550 paper-based; 80 iBT), IELTS (minimum score 6). *Application deadline:* For fall admission, 4/15 priority date for domestic students, 3/15 for international students. Applications are processed on a rolling basis. Application fee: $35. Electronic applications accepted. *Expenses:* Contact institution. *Financial support:* In 2015–16, 44 students received support. Fellowships with partial tuition reimbursements available, research assistantships with tuition reimbursements available, teaching assistantships, and unspecified assistantships available. Financial award application deadline: 4/15; financial award applicants required to submit FAFSA. *Faculty research:* Molecular biology, microbiology, neuroscience, cellular biology, physiology. *Total annual research expenditures:* $7.4 million. *Unit head:* 605-658-6322, Fax: 605-677-6381, E-mail: biomed@usd.edu.
Website: http://www.usd.edu/medicine/basic-biomedical-sciences/graduate

The University of South Dakota, Graduate School, School of Education, Division of Curriculum and Instruction, Program in Elementary Education, Vermillion, SD 57069-2390. Offers elementary education (MA), including early childhood education, English language learning, reading specialist/literacy coach, science, technology or math (STM). *Accreditation:* NCATE. *Program availability:* Part-time, 100% online, blended/hybrid learning. *Degree requirements:* For master's, comprehensive exam, thesis or alternative. *Entrance requirements:* For master's, GRE General Test, MAT, minimum GPA of 2.7. Additional exam requirements/recommendations for international students: Required—TOEFL (minimum score 550 paper-based; 79 iBT). *Application deadline:* Applications are processed on a rolling basis. Application fee: $35. Electronic applications accepted. *Financial support:* Research assistantships with partial tuition reimbursements, teaching assistantships with partial tuition reimbursements, career-related internships or fieldwork, Federal Work-Study, and unspecified assistantships available. Financial award applicants required to submit FAFSA. *Unit head:* Dr. Nicholas Shudak, Division Chair, 605-677-5207, Fax: 605-677-3102, E-mail: nicholas.shudak@usd.edu. *Application contact:* Graduate School, 605-658-6140, Fax: 605-677-6118, E-mail: cde@usd.edu.
Website: http://www.usd.edu/education/curriculum-and-instruction/graduate

The University of South Dakota, Graduate School, School of Education, Division of Curriculum and Instruction, Program in Secondary Education, Vermillion, SD 57069-

2390. Offers secondary education (MA), including English language learning, science, technology or math (STM), secondary education plus certification. *Accreditation:* NCATE. *Program availability:* Part-time, online learning. *Degree requirements:* For master's, comprehensive exam, thesis or alternative. *Entrance requirements:* For master's, GRE General Test, MAT, minimum GPA of 2.7. Additional exam requirements/recommendations for international students: Required—TOEFL (minimum score 550 paper-based; 79 iBT). *Application deadline:* Applications are processed on a rolling basis. Application fee: $35. Electronic applications accepted. *Financial support:* Research assistantships with partial tuition reimbursements, teaching assistantships with partial tuition reimbursements, career-related internships or fieldwork, Federal Work-Study, and unspecified assistantships available. Financial award applicants required to submit FAFSA. *Unit head:* Dr. Nicholas Shudak, Division Chair, 605-677-5207, Fax: 605-677-3102, E-mail: nicholas.shudak@usd.edu.
Website: http://www.usd.edu/education/curriculum-and-instruction/graduate

University of Southern California, Graduate School, Dana and David Dornsife College of Letters, Arts and Sciences, Department of Biological Sciences, Los Angeles, CA 90089. Offers biology (MS); computational molecular biology (MS); integrative and evolutionary biology (PhD); marine biology and biological oceanography (MS, PhD), including marine and environmental biology (MS), marine biology and biological oceanography (PhD); molecular and computational biology (PhD), including biology, computational biology and bioinformatics, molecular biology; neurobiology (PhD). Terminal master's awarded for partial completion of doctoral program. *Degree requirements:* For master's, comprehensive exam (for some programs), research paper; for doctorate, thesis/dissertation, qualifying examination, dissertation defense. *Entrance requirements:* For master's, GRE, 3 letters of recommendation, personal statement, resume, minimum GPA of 3.0; for doctorate, GRE, 3 letters of recommendation, resume, minimum GPA of 3.0. Additional exam requirements/recommendations for international students: Required—TOEFL (minimum score 600 paper-based; 100 iBT). Electronic applications accepted. *Faculty research:* Microarray data analysis, microbial ecology and genetics, integrative organismal and behavioral biology and ecology, stem cell pluipotency, cancer cell biology.

University of Southern California, Keck School of Medicine and Graduate School, Graduate Programs in Medicine, Los Angeles, CA 90089. Offers MPAP, MPH, MS, PhD, Certificate. *Faculty:* 420 full-time (128 women), 20 part-time/adjunct (9 women). *Students:* 841 full-time (560 women), 44 part-time (27 women); includes 393 minority (46 Black or African American, non-Hispanic/Latino; 2 American Indian or Alaska Native, non-Hispanic/Latino; 226 Asian, non-Hispanic/Latino; 108 Hispanic/Latino; 5 Native Hawaiian or other Pacific Islander, non-Hispanic/Latino; 6 Two or more races, non-Hispanic/Latino), 204 international. Average age 25. 1,966 applicants, 29% accepted, 366 enrolled. In 2015, 311 master's, 15 doctorates awarded. Terminal master's awarded for partial completion of doctoral program. *Entrance requirements:* For master's, GRE General Test, minimum GPA of 3.0; for doctorate, GRE General Test (minimum combined Verbal and Quantitative score of 1000), minimum GPA of 3.0. Additional exam requirements/recommendations for international students: Required—TOEFL (minimum score 600 paper-based; 100 iBT). *Application deadline:* Applications are processed on a rolling basis. Application fee: $85. Electronic applications accepted. *Expenses:* Contact institution. *Financial support:* In 2015–16, 28 fellowships with tuition reimbursements (averaging $32,000 per year), 82 research assistantships with tuition reimbursements (averaging $32,000 per year), 43 teaching assistantships with tuition reimbursements (averaging $32,000 per year) were awarded; career-related internships or fieldwork, Federal Work-Study, institutionally sponsored loans, scholarships/grants, traineeships, health care benefits, and unspecified assistantships also available. Support available to part-time students. Financial award application deadline: 5/4; financial award applicants required to submit CSS PROFILE or FAFSA. *Unit head:* Dr. Peggy Farnham, Associate Dean for Graduate Affairs, 323-442-8015, Fax: 323-442-7739, E-mail: pfarnham@usc.edu. *Application contact:* Marisela Zuniga, Administrative Coordinator, 323-442-1607, Fax: 323-442-1199, E-mail: mzuniga@usc.edu.
Website: http://keck.usc.edu/

University of Southern Maine, College of Science, Technology, and Health, Program in Biology, Portland, ME 04103. Offers MS. *Expenses: Tuition, area resident:* Full-time $6840; part-time $380 per credit hour. *Tuition, state resident:* full-time $10,260; part-time $570 per credit hour. *Tuition, nonresident:* full-time $18,468; part-time $1026 per credit hour. *Required fees:* $830; $83 per credit hour. Tuition and fees vary according to course load and program. *Faculty research:* Salt marsh plant ecology, marine microbial ecology, brain development, ecophysiology of marine cyanobacteria, evolution of mammalian social behavior.

University of Southern Mississippi, Graduate School, College of Science and Technology, Department of Biological Sciences, Hattiesburg, MS 39406-0001. Offers environmental biology (MS); marine biology (MS); microbiology (MS, PhD); molecular biology (MS, PhD). Terminal master's awarded for partial completion of doctoral program. *Degree requirements:* For master's, comprehensive exam, thesis; for doctorate, comprehensive exam, thesis/dissertation. *Entrance requirements:* For master's, GRE General Test, minimum GPA of 3.0 on last 60 hours; for doctorate, GRE General Test, minimum GPA of 3.5. Additional exam requirements/recommendations for international students: Required—TOEFL, IELTS.

University of South Florida, College of Arts and Sciences, Department of Cell Biology, Microbiology, and Molecular Biology, Tampa, FL 33620-9951. Offers biology (MS), including cell and molecular biology; cancer biology (PhD); cell and molecular biology (PhD); microbiology (MS). *Faculty:* 21 full-time (7 women). *Students:* 41 full-time (6 women), 45 part-time (2 women); includes 11 minority (1 Black or African American, non-Hispanic/Latino; 2 Asian, non-Hispanic/Latino; 5 Hispanic/Latino; 3 Two or more races, non-Hispanic/Latino), 22 international. Average age 27. 171 applicants, 14% accepted, 18 enrolled. In 2015, 22 master's, 14 doctorates awarded. *Degree requirements:* For master's, thesis or alternative; for doctorate, comprehensive exam, thesis/dissertation. *Entrance requirements:* For master's and doctorate, GRE General Test, minimum GPA of 3.0, extensive background in biology or chemistry. Additional exam requirements/recommendations for international students: Required—TOEFL (minimum score 570 paper-based; 79 iBT) or IELTS (minimum score 6.5). *Application deadline:* For fall admission, 2/1 for domestic students, 1/1 for international students. Application fee: $30. *Financial support:* Career-related internships or fieldwork, health care benefits, and unspecified assistantships available. Financial award application deadline: 4/1. *Faculty research:* Cell biology, microbiology and molecular biology: basic and applied science in bacterial pathogenesis, genome integrity and mechanisms of aging, structural and computational biology; cancer biology: immunology, cancer control, signal transduction, drug discovery, genomics. *Total annual research expenditures:* $1.9 million. *Unit head:* Dr. James Garey, Professor/Chair, 813-974-7103, Fax: 813-974-1614, E-mail: garey@usf.edu. *Application contact:* Dr. Kenneth Wright, Associate Professor of Cancer Biology, H. Lee Moffitt Cancer Center and Research Institute, 813-745-3918, Fax: 813-974-1614, E-mail: ken.wright@moffitt.org.
Website: http://biology.usf.edu/cmmb/

University of South Florida, College of Arts and Sciences, Department of Integrative Biology, Tampa, FL 33620-9951. Offers biology (MS), including ecology and evolution (MS, PhD), environmental and ecological microbiology (MS, PhD), physiology and

Biological and Biomedical Sciences—General

morphology (MS, PhD); integrative biology (PhD), including ecology and evolution (MS, PhD), environmental and ecological microbiology (MS, PhD), physiology and morphology (MS, PhD). *Program availability:* Part-time. *Faculty:* 14 full-time (6 women). *Students:* 48 full-time (30 women), 6 part-time (3 women); includes 10 minority (1 American Indian or Alaska Native, non-Hispanic/Latino; 1 Asian, non-Hispanic/Latino; 7 Hispanic/Latino; 1 Two or more races, non-Hispanic/Latino), 3 international. Average age 30. 43 applicants, 37% accepted, 12 enrolled. In 2015, 8 master's, 3 doctorates awarded. *Degree requirements:* For master's, comprehensive exam, thesis (for some programs); for doctorate, comprehensive exam, thesis/dissertation. *Entrance requirements:* For master's and doctorate, GRE General Test, minimum GPA of 3.0 in last 60 hours of BS. Additional exam requirements/recommendations for international students: Required—TOEFL (minimum score 570 paper-based; 88 iBT). *Application deadline:* For fall admission, 2/15 priority date for domestic students, 1/2 for international students; for spring admission, 8/1 for domestic students, 6/1 for international students. Application fee: $30. Electronic applications accepted. *Financial support:* Research assistantships, teaching assistantships, and unspecified assistantships available. Financial award application deadline: 6/30; financial award applicants required to submit FAFSA. *Faculty research:* Marine ecology, ecosystem responses to urbanization, biomechanical and physiological mechanisms of animal movement, population biology and conservation, microbial ecology and public health microbiology, natural diversity of parasites and herbivores; ecosystems, vertebrates, disturbance ecology, functional and ecological morphology of feeding in fishes, rare amphibians and reptiles, genomics in ecological experiments, ecotoxicology, global carbon cycle, plant-animal interactions. *Total annual research expenditures:* $1.3 million. *Unit head:* Dr. Valerie Harwood, Professor and Chair, 813-974-1524, Fax: 813-974-3263, E-mail: vharwood@usf.edu. *Application contact:* Dr. Lynn Martin, Associate Professor and Graduate Program Director, 813-974-0157, Fax: 813-974-3263, E-mail: lbmartin@usf.edu. Website: http://biology.usf.edu/ib/grad/

University of South Florida, Morsani College of Medicine and College of Graduate Studies, Graduate Programs in Medical Sciences, Tampa, FL 33620-9951. Offers advanced athletic training (MS); athletic training (MS); bioinformatics and computational biology (MSBCB); biotechnology (MSB); health informatics (MSHI); medical sciences (MSMS, PhD), including aging and neuroscience (MSMS), allergy, immunology and infectious disease (PhD), anatomy, athletic training (MSMS), clinical and translational research, health informatics (MSMS), health sciences (MSMS), interdisciplinary medical sciences (MSMS), medical microbiology and immunology (MSMS), metabolic and nutritional medicine (MSMS), molecular medicine, molecular pharmacology and physiology (PhD), neurology (PhD), pathology and laboratory medicine (PhD), pharmacology and therapeutics (PhD), physiology and biophysics (PhD), women's health (MSMS). *Students:* 510 full-time (261 women), 318 part-time (208 women); includes 360 minority (108 Black or African American, non-Hispanic/Latino; 3 American Indian or Alaska Native, non-Hispanic/Latino; 101 Asian, non-Hispanic/Latino; 124 Hispanic/Latino; 1 Native Hawaiian or other Pacific Islander, non-Hispanic/Latino; 23 Two or more races, non-Hispanic/Latino), 52 international. Average age 26. 6,567 applicants, 13% accepted, 469 enrolled. In 2015, 216 master's awarded. Terminal master's awarded for partial completion of doctoral program. *Degree requirements:* For master's, comprehensive exam, thesis; for doctorate, comprehensive exam, thesis/dissertation. *Entrance requirements:* For master's, GRE General Test or GMAT, bachelor's degree or equivalent from regionally-accredited university with minimum GPA of 3.0 in upper-division sciences coursework; prerequisites in general biology, general chemistry, general physics, organic chemistry, quantitative analysis, and integral and differential calculus; for doctorate, GRE General Test, bachelor's degree from regionally-accredited university with minimum GPA of 3.0 in upper-division sciences coursework; 3 letters of recommendation; personal interview; 1-2 page personal statement; prerequisites in biology, chemistry, physics, organic chemistry, quantitative analysis, and integral/differential calculus. Additional exam requirements/recommendations for international students: Required—TOEFL (minimum score 550 paper-based; 79 iBT) or IELTS (minimum score 6.5). *Application deadline:* For fall admission, 2/15 for domestic students, 1/2 for international students. Application fee: $30. *Expenses:* Contact institution. *Faculty research:* Anatomy, biochemistry, cancer biology, cardiovascular disease, cell biology, immunology, microbiology, molecular biology, neuroscience, pharmacology, physiology. *Unit head:* Dr. Michael Barber, Professor/Associate Dean for Graduate and Postdoctoral Affairs, 813-974-9908, Fax: 813-974-4317, E-mail: mbarber@health.usf.edu. *Application contact:* Dr. Eric Bennett, Graduate Director, PhD Program in Medical Sciences, 813-974-1545, Fax: 813-974-4317, E-mail: esbennet@health.usf.edu.
Website: http://health.usf.edu/nocms/medicine/graduatestudies/

The University of Tennessee, Graduate School, College of Arts and Sciences, Program in Life Sciences, Knoxville, TN 37996. Offers genome science and technology (MS, PhD); plant physiology and genetics (MS, PhD). *Degree requirements:* For doctorate, one foreign language, thesis/dissertation. *Entrance requirements:* For master's and doctorate, GRE General Test, minimum GPA of 2.7. Additional exam requirements/recommendations for international students: Required—TOEFL. Electronic applications accepted.

The University of Tennessee, Graduate School, Intercollegiate Programs, Program in Comparative and Experimental Medicine, Knoxville, TN 37996. Offers MS, PhD. *Degree requirements:* For master's, thesis; for doctorate, thesis/dissertation. *Entrance requirements:* For master's and doctorate, GRE General Test, minimum GPA of 2.7. Additional exam requirements/recommendations for international students: Required— TOEFL. Electronic applications accepted.

The University of Tennessee Health Science Center, College of Graduate Health Sciences, Memphis, TN 38163-0002. Offers biomedical engineering (MS, PhD); biomedical sciences (PhD); dental sciences (MDS); epidemiology (MS); health outcomes and policy research (PhD); laboratory research and management (MS); nursing science (PhD); pharmaceutical sciences (PhD); pharmacology (MS); speech and hearing science (PhD); DDS/PhD; DNP/PhD; MD/PhD; Pharm D/PhD. Terminal master's awarded for partial completion of doctoral program. *Degree requirements:* For master's, comprehensive exam, thesis; for doctorate, comprehensive exam, thesis/ dissertation, oral and written preliminary and comprehensive exams. *Entrance requirements:* For master's and doctorate, GRE General Test, minimum GPA of 3.0. Additional exam requirements/recommendations for international students: Required— TOEFL (minimum score 79 iBT); Recommended—IELTS (minimum score 6.5). Electronic applications accepted.

The University of Tennessee–Oak Ridge National Laboratory, Graduate Program in Genome Science and Technology, Knoxville, TN 37966. Offers life sciences (MS, PhD). *Degree requirements:* For master's, thesis; for doctorate, comprehensive exam, thesis/ dissertation. *Entrance requirements:* For master's and doctorate, GRE General Test. Additional exam requirements/recommendations for international students: Required— TOEFL. Electronic applications accepted. *Faculty research:* Genetics/genomics, structural biology/proteomics, computational biology/bioinformatics, bioanalytical technologies.

The University of Texas at Arlington, Graduate School, College of Science, Department of Biology, Arlington, TX 76019. Offers biology (MS); quantitative biology (PhD). *Program availability:* Part-time, evening/weekend. *Degree requirements:* For master's, thesis, oral defense of thesis; for doctorate, comprehensive exam, thesis/ dissertation, oral defense of dissertation. *Entrance requirements:* For master's and doctorate, GRE General Test. Additional exam requirements/recommendations for international students: Required—TOEFL (minimum score 550 paper-based; 79 iBT). Electronic applications accepted. *Faculty research:* Cellular and microbiology, comparative genomics, evolution and ecology.

The University of Texas at Austin, Graduate School, College of Natural Sciences, School of Biological Sciences, Austin, TX 78712-1111. Offers ecology, evolution and behavior (PhD); microbiology (PhD); plant biology (MA, PhD). *Entrance requirements:* For master's and doctorate, GRE General Test. Electronic applications accepted.

The University of Texas at Dallas, School of Natural Sciences and Mathematics, Department of Biological Sciences, Richardson, TX 75080. Offers bioinformatics and computational biology (MS); biotechnology (MS); molecular and cell biology (MS, PhD). *Program availability:* Part-time, evening/weekend. *Faculty:* 22 full-time (4 women), 1 part-time/adjunct (0 women). *Students:* 114 full-time (71 women), 13 part-time (6 women); includes 15 minority (1 Black or African American, non-Hispanic/Latino; 9 Asian, non-Hispanic/Latino; 4 Hispanic/Latino; 1 Two or more races, non-Hispanic/ Latino), 90 international. Average age 27. 359 applicants, 25% accepted, 40 enrolled. In 2015, 32 master's, 4 doctorates awarded. *Degree requirements:* For master's, thesis optional; for doctorate, thesis/dissertation, publishable paper. *Entrance requirements:* For master's and doctorate, GRE (minimum combined score of 1000 on verbal and quantitative). Additional exam requirements/recommendations for international students: Required—TOEFL (minimum score 550 paper-based; 80 iBT). *Application deadline:* For fall admission, 7/15 for domestic students, 5/1 priority date for international students; for spring admission, 11/15 for domestic students, 9/1 priority date for international students. Applications are processed on a rolling basis. Application fee: $50 ($100 for international students). *Expenses:* Tuition, state resident: full-time $11,940; part-time $663 per semester hour. Tuition, nonresident: full-time $22,786; part-time $1266 per semester hour. Tuition and fees vary according to course load. *Financial support:* In 2015–16, 71 students received support, including 2 fellowships with partial tuition reimbursements available (averaging $350 per year), 18 research assistantships with partial tuition reimbursements available (averaging $23,800 per year), 53 teaching assistantships with partial tuition reimbursements available (averaging $17,134 per year); career-related internships or fieldwork, Federal Work-Study, institutionally sponsored loans, scholarships/grants, and unspecified assistantships also available. Support available to part-time students. Financial award application deadline: 4/30; financial award applicants required to submit FAFSA. *Faculty research:* Role of mitochondria in neurodegenerative diseases, protein-DNA interactions in site-specific recombination, eukaryotic gene expression, bio-nanotechnology, sickle cell research. *Unit head:* Dr. Stephen Spiro, Department Head, 972-883-6032, Fax: 972-883-2409, E-mail: stephen.spiro@utdallas.edu. *Application contact:* Dr. Lawrence Reitzer, Graduate Advisor, 972-883-2502, Fax: 972-883-2409, E-mail: reitzer@ utdallas.edu.
Website: http://www.utdallas.edu/biology/

The University of Texas at El Paso, Graduate School, College of Science, Department of Biological Sciences, El Paso, TX 79968-0001. Offers bioinformatics (MS); biological sciences (MS, PhD). *Program availability:* Part-time, evening/weekend. *Degree requirements:* For master's, thesis; for doctorate, thesis/dissertation. *Entrance requirements:* For master's, GRE, minimum GPA of 3.0, letters of recommendation; for doctorate, GRE, statement of purpose, letters of recommendation. Additional exam requirements/recommendations for international students: Required—TOEFL; Recommended—IELTS. Electronic applications accepted.

The University of Texas at San Antonio, College of Sciences, Department of Biology, San Antonio, TX 78249-0617. Offers biology (MS); biotechnology (MS); cell and molecular biology (PhD); neurobiology (PhD). *Faculty:* 36 full-time (10 women), 1 part-time/adjunct (0 women). *Students:* 96 full-time (53 women), 60 part-time (28 women); includes 73 minority (5 Black or African American, non-Hispanic/Latino; 1 American Indian or Alaska Native, non-Hispanic/Latino; 7 Asian, non-Hispanic/Latino; 54 Hispanic/ Latino; 1 Native Hawaiian or other Pacific Islander, non-Hispanic/Latino; 5 Two or more races, non-Hispanic/Latino), 28 international. Average age 28. 147 applicants, 46% accepted, 40 enrolled. In 2015, 43 master's, 8 doctorates awarded. Terminal master's awarded for partial completion of doctoral program. *Degree requirements:* For master's, comprehensive exam, thesis or alternative; for doctorate, comprehensive exam, thesis/ dissertation. *Entrance requirements:* For master's, GRE General Test, bachelor's degree with 18 credit hours in field of study or in another appropriate field of study; for doctorate, GRE General Test, 3 letters of recommendation, statement of purpose, resume. Additional exam requirements/recommendations for international students: Required—TOEFL (minimum score 500 paper-based; 100 iBT), IELTS (minimum score 5). *Application deadline:* For fall admission, 7/1 for domestic students, 4/1 for international students; for spring admission, 11/1 for domestic students, 9/1 for international students. Application fee: $45 ($80 for international students). Electronic applications accepted. *Faculty research:* Development of human and veterinary vaccines against a fungal disease, mammalian germ cells and stem cells, dopamine neuron physiology and addiction, plant biochemistry, dendritic computation and synaptic plasticity. *Unit head:* Dr. Garry Sunter, Chair, 210-458-5479, E-mail: garry.sunter@ utsa.edu. *Application contact:* Rene Munguia, Jr., Senior Program Coordinator, 210-458-4642, Fax: 210-458-5658, E-mail: rene.munguia@utsa.edu.
Website: http://bio.utsa.edu/

The University of Texas at Tyler, College of Arts and Sciences, Department of Biology, Tyler, TX 75799-0001. Offers biology (MS); interdisciplinary studies (MSIS). *Degree requirements:* For master's, comprehensive exam, thesis, oral qualifying exam, thesis defense. *Entrance requirements:* For master's, GRE General Test, GRE Subject Test, bachelor's degree in biology or equivalent. Additional exam requirements/ recommendations for international students: Required—TOEFL. Electronic applications accepted. *Faculty research:* Phenotypic plasticity and heritability of life history traits, invertebrate ecology and genetics, systematics and phylogenetics of reptiles, hibernation physiology in turtles, landscape ecology, host-microbe interaction, outer membrane proteins in bacteria.

The University of Texas Health Science Center at Houston, Graduate School of Biomedical Sciences, Houston, TX 77225-0036. Offers MS, MD, MD/PhD. Terminal master's awarded for partial completion of doctoral program. *Degree requirements:* For master's, thesis; for doctorate, thesis/dissertation. *Entrance requirements:* For master's and doctorate, GRE General Test. Additional exam requirements/recommendations for international students: Required—TOEFL. Electronic applications accepted. *Faculty research:* Biomedical sciences.

The University of Texas Health Science Center at San Antonio, Graduate School of Biomedical Sciences, Integrated Biomedical Sciences Program, San Antonio, TX 78229-3900. Offers PhD. *Degree requirements:* For doctorate, comprehensive exam, thesis/dissertation.

The University of Texas Medical Branch, Graduate School of Biomedical Sciences, Galveston, TX 77555. Offers MA, MMS, MPH, MS, PhD, MD/PhD. Terminal master's awarded for partial completion of doctoral program. *Degree requirements:* For master's, comprehensive exam (for some programs), thesis or alternative; for doctorate, comprehensive exam, thesis/dissertation. *Entrance requirements:* For master's and doctorate, GRE General Test, 3 letters of recommendation. Additional exam requirements/recommendations for international students: Required—TOEFL (minimum score 550 paper-based; 80 iBT), IELTS (minimum score 6.5). Electronic applications accepted. *Expenses:* Contact institution.

The University of Texas of the Permian Basin, Office of Graduate Studies, College of Arts and Sciences, Department of Biology, Odessa, TX 79762-0001. Offers MS. *Program availability:* Part-time, evening/weekend. *Degree requirements:* For master's, comprehensive exam, thesis or alternative. *Entrance requirements:* For master's, GRE General Test. Additional exam requirements/recommendations for international students: Required—TOEFL (minimum score 550 paper-based).

The University of Texas Rio Grande Valley, College of Sciences, Department of Biology, Edinburg, TX 78539. Offers MS. *Program availability:* Part-time, evening/weekend. *Degree requirements:* For master's, comprehensive exam, thesis optional, minimum GPA of 3.0 overall and in all higher biology courses. *Entrance requirements:* For master's, GRE General Test, 24 hours of undergraduate courses in biological sciences or closely-related disciplines with minimum GPA of 3.0. Additional exam requirements/recommendations for international students: Required—TOEFL (minimum score 500 paper-based; 61 iBT); Recommended—IELTS (minimum score 5.5). Electronic applications accepted. Tuition and fees vary according to course load and program. *Faculty research:* Flora and fauna of South Padre Island, plant taxonomy of Rio Grande Valley.

The University of Texas Southwestern Medical Center, Southwestern Graduate School of Biomedical Sciences, Clinical Science Program, Dallas, TX 75390. Offers MCS, MSCS. *Program availability:* Part-time. *Degree requirements:* For master's, 1-year clinical research project. *Entrance requirements:* For master's, graduate degree in biomedical science. Electronic applications accepted.

The University of Texas Southwestern Medical Center, Southwestern Graduate School of Biomedical Sciences, Division of Basic Science, Dallas, TX 75390. Offers biological chemistry (PhD); biomedical engineering (MS, PhD); cancer biology (PhD); cell regulation (PhD); genetics and development (PhD); immunology (PhD); integrative biology (PhD); molecular biophysics (PhD); molecular microbiology (PhD); neuroscience (PhD); MD/PhD. *Degree requirements:* For doctorate, thesis/dissertation, qualifying exam. *Entrance requirements:* For doctorate, GRE General Test, research experience. Additional exam requirements/recommendations for international students: Required—TOEFL. Electronic applications accepted.

The University of Texas Southwestern Medical Center, Southwestern Graduate School of Biomedical Sciences, Medical Scientist Training Program, Dallas, TX 75390. Offers PhD, MD/PhD. Electronic applications accepted.

University of the Incarnate Word, School of Graduate Studies and Research, School of Mathematics, Science, and Engineering, Program in Biology, San Antonio, TX 78209-6397. Offers MA, MS. *Program availability:* Part-time, evening/weekend. *Faculty:* 8 full-time (4 women), 1 (woman) part-time/adjunct. *Students:* 10 full-time (8 women), 5 part-time (4 women); includes 7 minority (all Hispanic/Latino), 7 international. Average age 25. 57 applicants, 84% accepted, 4 enrolled. In 2015, 1 master's awarded. *Degree requirements:* For master's, comprehensive exam (for MA); thesis defense (for MS). *Entrance requirements:* For master's, GRE Subject Test (biology), minimum GPA of 3.0 in biology or GRE (minimum combined score 1000 Verbal and Quantitative), 8 hours of principles of chemistry, 6 hours of organic chemistry, 12 upper-division hours in biology. Additional exam requirements/recommendations for international students: Required—TOEFL (minimum score 560 paper-based; 83 iBT). *Application deadline:* Applications are processed on a rolling basis. Application fee: $20. Electronic applications accepted. *Expenses: Tuition, area resident:* Part-time $885 per credit hour. *Required fees:* $40 per credit hour. Tuition and fees vary according to course load, degree level, campus/location, program and student level. *Financial support:* Federal Work-Study, scholarships/grants, tuition waivers (partial), and unspecified assistantships available. Financial award applicants required to submit FAFSA. *Faculty research:* Regeneration of nervous system elements, social behaviors of electric fish, gene expression in human cells, transmission of pathogenic protozoa, human DNA response to cancer fighting molecules. *Total annual research expenditures:* $1.2 million. *Unit head:* Dr. David Foglesong, Graduate Program Director, 210-283-5033, Fax: 210-829-3153, E-mail: davidf@uiwtx.edu. *Application contact:* Johnny Garcia, Graduate Admissions Counselor, 210-805-3554, Fax: 210-829-3921, E-mail: admis@uiwtx.edu. Website: http://www.uiw.edu/biology/graduate_program.htm

University of the Pacific, College of the Pacific, Department of Biological Sciences, Stockton, CA 95211-0197. Offers MS. *Degree requirements:* For master's, thesis. *Entrance requirements:* For master's, GRE General Test, GRE Subject Test. Additional exam requirements/recommendations for international students: Required—TOEFL.

The University of Toledo, College of Graduate Studies, College of Medicine and Life Sciences, Interdepartmental Programs, Toledo, OH 43606-3390. Offers bioinformatics and proteomics/genomics (MSBS); biomarkers and bioinformatics (Certificate); biomarkers and diagnostics (PSM); human donation sciences (MSBS); medical sciences (MSBS); MD/MSBS. *Degree requirements:* For master's, thesis or alternative. *Entrance requirements:* For master's, GRE, minimum undergraduate GPA of 3.0, three letters of recommendation, statement of purpose, transcripts from all prior institutions attended, resume; for Certificate, minimum undergraduate GPA of 3.0, three letters of recommendation, statement of purpose, transcripts from all prior institutions attended, resume. Additional exam requirements/recommendations for international students: Required—TOEFL (minimum score 550 paper-based; 80 iBT). Electronic applications accepted.

The University of Toledo, College of Graduate Studies, College of Natural Sciences and Mathematics, Department of Biological Sciences, Toledo, OH 43606-3390. Offers biology (MS, PhD). *Program availability:* Part-time. *Degree requirements:* For master's, thesis or alternative; for doctorate, thesis/dissertation. *Entrance requirements:* For master's and doctorate, GRE General Test, GRE Subject Test, minimum cumulative point-hour ratio of 2.7 for all previous academic work, three letters of recommendation, statement of purpose, transcripts from all prior institutions attended. Additional exam requirements/recommendations for international students: Required—TOEFL (minimum score 550 paper-based; 80 iBT). Electronic applications accepted. *Faculty research:* Biochemical parasitology, physiological ecology, animal physiology.

The University of Toledo, College of Graduate Studies, College of Natural Sciences and Mathematics, Department of Environmental Sciences, Toledo, OH 43606-3390. Offers biology (MS, PhD), including ecology; geology (MS), including earth surface processes. *Program availability:* Part-time. *Degree requirements:* For master's, thesis or alternative. *Entrance requirements:* For master's, GRE General Test, minimum cumulative point-hour ratio of 2.7 for all previous academic work, three letters of recommendation, statement of purpose, transcripts from all prior institutions attended. Additional exam requirements/recommendations for international students: Required—TOEFL (minimum score 550 paper-based; 80 iBT). Electronic applications accepted.

Faculty research: Environmental geochemistry, geophysics, petrology and mineralogy, paleontology, geohydrology.

The University of Tulsa, Graduate School, College of Engineering and Natural Sciences, Department of Biological Science, Tulsa, OK 74104-3189. Offers MS, MTA, PhD, JD/MS. *Program availability:* Part-time. *Faculty:* 12 full-time (2 women). *Students:* 15 full-time (6 women), 6 part-time (4 women); includes 5 minority (4 American Indian or Alaska Native, non-Hispanic/Latino; 1 Hispanic/Latino), 6 international. Average age 31. 28 applicants, 18% accepted, 3 enrolled. In 2015, 2 master's, 1 doctorate awarded. Terminal master's awarded for partial completion of doctoral program. *Degree requirements:* For master's, thesis, oral exams; for doctorate, comprehensive exam, thesis/dissertation. *Entrance requirements:* For master's and doctorate, GRE General Test. Additional exam requirements/recommendations for international students: Required—TOEFL (minimum score 550 paper-based; 80 iBT), IELTS (minimum score 6). *Application deadline:* Applications are processed on a rolling basis. Application fee: $55. Electronic applications accepted. *Expenses: Tuition, area resident:* Full-time $22,230; part-time $1176 per credit hour. *Required fees:* $590 per semester. Tuition and fees vary according to course load. *Financial support:* In 2015–16, 22 students received support, including 14 fellowships with full tuition reimbursements available (averaging $8,677 per year), 3 research assistantships with full tuition reimbursements available (averaging $13,541 per year), 10 teaching assistantships with full tuition reimbursements available (averaging $12,502 per year); career-related internships or fieldwork, Federal Work-Study, scholarships/grants, health care benefits, tuition waivers (full and partial), and unspecified assistantships also available. Support available to part-time students. Financial award application deadline: 2/1; financial award applicants required to submit FAFSA. *Faculty research:* Aerobiology, animal behavior and behavioral ecology, cell and molecular biology, ecology, developmental biology, genetics, herpetology, glycobiology, immunology, microbiology, morphology, mycology, ornithology, molecular systematic and virology. *Total annual research expenditures:* $232,593. *Unit head:* Dr. Estelle Levetin, Chairperson, 918-631-2764, Fax: 918-631-2762, E-mail: estelle-levetin@utulsa.edu. *Application contact:* Dr. Harrington Wells, Advisor, 918-631-3071, Fax: 918-631-2762, E-mail: harrington-wells@utulsa.edu. Website: http://engineering.utulsa.edu/academics/biological-science/

The University of Tulsa, Graduate School, Kendall College of Arts and Sciences, School of Urban Education, Program in Teaching Arts, Tulsa, OK 74104-3189. Offers art (MTA); biology (MTA); English (MTA); history (MTA); mathematics (MTA). *Program availability:* Part-time. *Students:* 1 (woman) full-time. Average age 25. In 2015, 1 master's awarded. *Entrance requirements:* For master's, GRE General Test. Additional exam requirements/recommendations for international students: Required—TOEFL (minimum score 577 paper-based), IELTS (minimum score 6.5). *Application deadline:* Applications are processed on a rolling basis. Application fee: $55. Electronic applications accepted. *Expenses: Tuition, area resident:* Full-time $22,230; part-time $1176 per credit hour. *Required fees:* $590 per semester. Tuition and fees vary according to course load. *Financial support:* In 2015–16, 2 students received support, including 1 teaching assistantship with full tuition reimbursement available (averaging $13,410 per year); fellowships with tuition reimbursements available, research assistantships with tuition reimbursements available, career-related internships or fieldwork, Federal Work-Study, scholarships/grants, health care benefits, tuition waivers (full and partial), and unspecified assistantships also available. Support available to part-time students. Financial award application deadline: 2/1; financial award applicants required to submit FAFSA. *Unit head:* Dr. Sharon Baker, Chair, 918-631-2238, Fax: 918-631-3721, E-mail: sharon-baker@utulsa.edu. *Application contact:* Dr. David Brown, Advisor, 918-631-2719, Fax: 918-631-2133, E-mail: david-brown@utulsa.edu.

University of Utah, Graduate School, College of Science, Department of Biology, Salt Lake City, UT 84112. Offers MS, PhD. *Program availability:* Part-time. *Faculty:* 44 full-time (10 women), 27 part-time/adjunct (14 women). *Students:* 62 full-time (26 women), 14 part-time (3 women); includes 8 minority (1 Black or African American, non-Hispanic/Latino; 3 Asian, non-Hispanic/Latino; 2 Hispanic/Latino; 2 Two or more races, non-Hispanic/Latino), 19 international. Average age 28. 135 applicants, 13% accepted, 12 enrolled. In 2015, 4 master's, 10 doctorates awarded. Terminal master's awarded for partial completion of doctoral program. *Degree requirements:* For master's, comprehensive exam, thesis; for doctorate, comprehensive exam, thesis/dissertation. *Entrance requirements:* For master's and doctorate, GRE General Test, minimum GPA of 3.0. Additional exam requirements/recommendations for international students: Required—TOEFL (minimum score 500 paper-based; 80 iBT). *Application deadline:* For fall admission, 1/4 for domestic and international students. Electronic applications accepted. Application fee is waived when completed online. *Expenses:* $3,861.48 per semester; $12,334.93 per semester (international); $2,000 per year health insurance. *Financial support:* In 2015–16, 76 students received support, including 19 fellowships with full tuition reimbursements available (averaging $26,000 per year), 19 research assistantships with full tuition reimbursements available (averaging $26,000 per year), 38 teaching assistantships with full tuition reimbursements available (averaging $22,000 per year); career-related internships or fieldwork, scholarships/grants, traineeships, and health care benefits also available. Financial award application deadline: 3/15; financial award applicants required to submit FAFSA. *Faculty research:* Ecology, evolutionary biology, cell and developmental biology, physiology and organismal biology, molecular biology, biochemistry, microbiology, plant biology, neurobiology, genetics. *Total annual research expenditures:* $9.2 million. *Unit head:* Dr. M. Denise Dearing, Department Chair, 801-585-1298, E-mail: denise.dearing@utah.edu. *Application contact:* Shannon Nielsen, Administrative Program Coordinator, 801-581-5636, Fax: 801-581-4668, E-mail: shannon.nielsen@bioscience.utah.edu. Website: http://www.biology.utah.edu

University of Utah, School of Medicine and Graduate School, Graduate Programs in Medicine, Salt Lake City, UT 84112-1107. Offers M Phil, M Stat, MPAS, MPH, MS, MSPH, PhD, Certificate. *Program availability:* Part-time. *Degree requirements:* For doctorate, thesis/dissertation. *Entrance requirements:* For doctorate, MCAT. Electronic applications accepted. *Faculty research:* Molecular biology, biochemistry, cell biology, immunology, bioengineering.

University of Vermont, College of Medicine and Graduate College, Graduate Programs in Medicine, Burlington, VT 05405. Offers MS, PhD, Certificate. *Degree requirements:* For master's, thesis; for doctorate, thesis/dissertation. *Entrance requirements:* For master's and doctorate, GRE General Test. Additional exam requirements/recommendations for international students: Required—TOEFL (minimum score 550 paper-based; 80 iBT). *Application deadline:* For fall admission, 4/1 priority date for domestic students, 4/1 for international students. Applications are processed on a rolling basis. Application fee: $65. Electronic applications accepted. *Financial support:* Fellowships, research assistantships, teaching assistantships, traineeships, and analytical assistantships available. Financial award application deadline: 3/1.

University of Vermont, Graduate College, Cellular, Molecular and Biomedical Sciences Program, Burlington, VT 05405. Offers PhD. *Degree requirements:* For doctorate, thesis/dissertation. *Entrance requirements:* For doctorate, GRE General Test. Additional exam requirements/recommendations for international students: Required—TOEFL (minimum score 550 paper-based; 80 iBT). *Application deadline:* For fall admission, 12/

Biological and Biomedical Sciences—General

1 priority date for domestic students, 12/1 for international students. Application fee: $65. Electronic applications accepted. *Financial support:* Fellowships, research assistantships, teaching assistantships, and career-related internships or fieldwork available. Financial award application deadline: 3/1. *Unit head:* Dr. Matthew Poynter, 802-656-9673, E-mail: cmb@uvm.edu. *Application contact:* Dr. Matthew Poynter, 802-656-9673, E-mail: cmb@uvm.edu.

University of Vermont, Graduate College, College of Arts and Sciences, Department of Biology, Burlington, VT 05405. Offers biology (MS, PhD); biology education (MST). *Degree requirements:* For master's, thesis; for doctorate, thesis/dissertation. *Entrance requirements:* For master's and doctorate, GRE General Test. Additional exam requirements/recommendations for international students: Required—TOEFL (minimum score 550 paper-based; 80 iBT). *Application deadline:* For fall admission, 12/15 priority date for domestic students, 12/15 for international students. Applications are processed on a rolling basis. Application fee: $65. Electronic applications accepted. *Financial support:* Fellowships, research assistantships, and teaching assistantships available. Financial award application deadline: 3/1. *Application contact:* Dr. Judith Van Houten, Coordinator, 802-656-2922, E-mail: judith.vanhouten@uvm.edu.

University of Victoria, Faculty of Graduate Studies, Faculty of Science, Department of Biology, Victoria, BC V8W 2Y2, Canada. Offers M Sc, PhD. *Degree requirements:* For master's, thesis, seminar; for doctorate, thesis/dissertation, seminar, candidacy exam. *Entrance requirements:* For master's and doctorate, GRE General Test, minimum B+ average in previous 2 years of biology course work. Additional exam requirements/recommendations for international students: Required—TOEFL (minimum score 575 paper-based), IELTS (minimum score 7). Electronic applications accepted. *Faculty research:* Neurobiology of vertebrates and invertebrates, physiology, reproduction and tissue culture of forest trees, evolution and ecology, cell and molecular biology, molecular biology of environmental health.

University of Virginia, College and Graduate School of Arts and Sciences, Department of Biology, Charlottesville, VA 22903. Offers MA, MS, PhD. *Degree requirements:* For master's, thesis; for doctorate, thesis/dissertation. *Entrance requirements:* For master's and doctorate, GRE General Test, GRE Subject Test (recommended), 2 letters of recommendation. Additional exam requirements/recommendations for international students: Required—TOEFL (minimum score 600 paper-based; 90 iBT), IELTS (minimum score 7). Electronic applications accepted. *Faculty research:* Ecology and evolution, neurobiology and behavior, molecular genetics, cell development.

University of Virginia, School of Medicine, Department of Molecular Physiology and Biological Physics, Program in Biological and Physical Sciences, Charlottesville, VA 22903. Offers MS. *Entrance requirements:* For master's, GRE General Test. Additional exam requirements/recommendations for international students: Required—TOEFL. Electronic applications accepted.

University of Washington, Graduate School, College of Arts and Sciences, Department of Biology, Seattle, WA 98195. Offers PhD.

University of Washington, Graduate School, School of Medicine, Graduate Programs in Medicine, Seattle, WA 98195. Offers MA, MOT, MPO, MS, DPT, PhD. *Program availability:* Part-time. *Degree requirements:* For doctorate, thesis/dissertation. *Entrance requirements:* For doctorate, GRE. Electronic applications accepted. *Expenses:* Contact institution.

University of Waterloo, Graduate Studies, Faculty of Science, Department of Biology, Waterloo, ON N2L 3G1, Canada. Offers M Sc, PhD. *Program availability:* Part-time. *Degree requirements:* For master's, thesis, seminar; for doctorate, comprehensive exam, thesis/dissertation, seminar. *Entrance requirements:* For master's, honor's degree; for doctorate, master's degree. Additional exam requirements/recommendations for international students: Required—TOEFL, IELTS, PTE. Application fee: $100 Canadian dollars. Electronic applications accepted. *Financial support:* In 2015–16, 15 students received support. Research assistantships, teaching assistantships, and career-related internships or fieldwork available. *Faculty research:* Biosystematics, ecology and limnology, molecular and cellular biology, biochemistry, physiology. Website: https://uwaterloo.ca/biology/

The University of Western Ontario, Faculty of Graduate Studies, Biosciences Division, Department of Biology, London, ON N6A 5B8, Canada. Offers M Sc, PhD. *Degree requirements:* For master's, thesis; for doctorate, thesis/dissertation. *Entrance requirements:* For doctorate, M Sc or equivalent. Additional exam requirements/recommendations for international students: Required—TOEFL. *Faculty research:* Ecology systematics, plant biochemistry and physiology, yeast genetics, molecular biology.

University of West Florida, College of Science and Engineering, School of Allied Health and Life Sciences, Department of Biology, Pensacola, FL 32514-5750. Offers biological chemistry (MS); biology (MS); biology education (MST); biotechnology (MS); coastal zone studies (MS); environmental biology (MS). *Degree requirements:* For master's, thesis. *Entrance requirements:* For master's, GRE (minimum score: verbal 450, quantitative 550), official transcripts; BS in biology or related field; letter of interest; relevant past experience; three letters of recommendation from individuals who can evaluate applicant's academic ability. Additional exam requirements/recommendations for international students: Required—TOEFL (minimum score 550 paper-based).

University of West Georgia, College of Science and Mathematics, Carrollton, GA 30118. Offers biology (MS); computer science (MS); geographic information systems (Postbaccalaureate Certificate); mathematics (MS). *Program availability:* Part-time, evening/weekend, 100% online. *Faculty:* 54 full-time (19 women). *Students:* 20 full-time (8 women), 69 part-time (18 women); includes 15 minority (10 Black or African American, non-Hispanic/Latino; 2 Asian, non-Hispanic/Latino; 1 Hispanic/Latino; 1 Native Hawaiian or other Pacific Islander, non-Hispanic/Latino; 1 Two or more races, non-Hispanic/Latino), 9 international. Average age 35. 75 applicants, 88% accepted, 53 enrolled. In 2015, 21 master's, 4 other advanced degrees awarded. *Entrance requirements:* Additional exam requirements/recommendations for international students: Required—TOEFL (minimum score 523 paper-based; 69 iBT); Recommended—IELTS (minimum score 6.5). *Application deadline:* For fall admission, 6/1 for domestic and international students; for spring admission, 11/15 for domestic students, 10/15 for international students; for summer admission, 4/1 for domestic students, 3/30 for international students. Applications are processed on a rolling basis. Application fee: $40. Electronic applications accepted. *Expenses:* Contact institution. *Financial support:* Fellowships, research assistantships, teaching assistantships, career-related internships or fieldwork, Federal Work-Study, institutionally sponsored loans, scholarships/grants, and unspecified assistantships available. Support available to part-time students. Financial award application deadline: 4/1; financial award applicants required to submit FAFSA. *Unit head:* Dr. Scott Gordon, Interim Dean, 678-839-5190, Fax: 678-839-5191, E-mail: sgordon@westga.edu. *Application contact:* Dr. Toby Ziglar, Director of Graduate Studies and International Admissions, 678-839-1394, Fax: 678-839-1395, E-mail: graduate@westga.edu. Website: http://www.westga.edu/cosm

University of Windsor, Faculty of Graduate Studies, Faculty of Science, Department of Biological Sciences, Windsor, ON N9B 3P4, Canada. Offers M Sc, PhD. *Program availability:* Part-time. *Degree requirements:* For master's, thesis; for doctorate, comprehensive exam, thesis/dissertation. *Entrance requirements:* For master's and doctorate, minimum B average. Additional exam requirements/recommendations for international students: Required—TOEFL (minimum score 560 paper-based). Electronic applications accepted. *Faculty research:* Great Lakes Institute: aquatic ecotoxicology, regulation and development of the olfactory system, mating system evolution, signal transduction, aquatic ecology.

University of Wisconsin–La Crosse, College of Science and Health, Department of Biology, La Crosse, WI 54601-3742. Offers aquatic sciences (MS); biology (MS); cellular and molecular biology (MS); clinical microbiology (MS); microbiology (MS); nurse anesthesia (MS); physiology (MS). *Program availability:* Part-time. *Students:* 19 full-time (12 women), 50 part-time (26 women); includes 4 minority (3 Asian, non-Hispanic/Latino; 1 Hispanic/Latino), 1 international. Average age 29. 44 applicants, 75% accepted, 27 enrolled. In 2015, 27 master's awarded. *Degree requirements:* For master's, comprehensive exam, thesis. *Entrance requirements:* For master's, GRE General Test, minimum GPA of 2.85. Additional exam requirements/recommendations for international students: Required—TOEFL (minimum score 550 paper-based; 79 iBT). *Application deadline:* For fall admission, 2/1 priority date for domestic and international students; for spring admission, 1/4 priority date for domestic and international students. Applications are processed on a rolling basis. Electronic applications accepted. *Financial support:* Research assistantships with partial tuition reimbursements, Federal Work-Study, scholarships/grants, health care benefits, and tuition waivers (partial) available. Support available to part-time students. Financial award application deadline: 3/15; financial award applicants required to submit FAFSA. *Unit head:* Dr. Mark Sandheinrich, Department Chair, 608-785-8261, E-mail: msandheinrich@uwlax.edu. *Application contact:* Brandon Schaller, Senior Graduate Student Status Examiner, 608-785-8941, E-mail: admissions@uwlax.edu. Website: http://uwlax.edu/biology/

University of Wisconsin–Madison, School of Medicine and Public Health, Medical Scientist Training Program, Madison, WI 53705-2221. Offers MD/PhD. *Accreditation:* LCME/AMA. *Faculty:* 380 full-time (80 women). *Students:* 73 full-time (28 women); includes 19 minority (5 Black or African American, non-Hispanic/Latino; 1 American Indian or Alaska Native, non-Hispanic/Latino; 10 Asian, non-Hispanic/Latino; 3 Hispanic/Latino). 308 applicants, 11% accepted, 10 enrolled. *Application deadline:* For fall admission, 12/1 for domestic students. Applications are processed on a rolling basis. Application fee: $54. Electronic applications accepted. *Expenses:* Contact institution. *Financial support:* In 2015–16, 73 students received support, including fellowships with full tuition reimbursements available (averaging $28,000 per year), research assistantships with full tuition reimbursements available (averaging $28,000 per year); traineeships and health care benefits also available. *Unit head:* Dr. Anna Huttenlocher, Director, 608-265-4642, Fax: 608-262-8418, E-mail: huttenlocher@wisc.edu. *Application contact:* Paul Cook, Program Coordinator, 608-262-0736, Fax: 608-262-4226, E-mail: chanewall@wisc.edu. Website: http://mstp.med.wisc.edu/

University of Wisconsin–Milwaukee, Graduate School, College of Health Sciences, PhD Program in Health Sciences, Milwaukee, WI 53201-0413. Offers PhD. *Faculty:* 8 full-time (4 women), 1 part-time/adjunct (0 women). *Students:* 20 full-time (13 women), 8 part-time (6 women); includes 5 minority (1 Black or African American, non-Hispanic/Latino; 3 Asian, non-Hispanic/Latino; 1 Two or more races, non-Hispanic/Latino), 11 international. Average age 34. 15 applicants, 73% accepted, 7 enrolled. In 2015, 3 doctorates awarded. *Degree requirements:* For doctorate, comprehensive exam, thesis/dissertation. *Entrance requirements:* For doctorate, GRE. Additional exam requirements/recommendations for international students: Required—TOEFL (minimum score 600 paper-based), IELTS (minimum score 6.5). Application fee: $56 ($96 for international students). *Financial support:* In 2015–16, 4 fellowships, 5 research assistantships, 3 teaching assistantships were awarded; project assistantships also available. *Unit head:* Paula M. Rhyner, PhD, Program Representative, 414-229-4878, E-mail: prhyner@uwm.edu. *Application contact:* Roger O. Smith, General Information Contact, 414-229-6697, Fax: 414-229-6697, E-mail: smithro@uwm.edu. Website: http://www4.uwm.edu/chs/academics/phd_health_sciences/

University of Wisconsin–Milwaukee, Graduate School, College of Health Sciences, Program in Biomedical Sciences, Milwaukee, WI 53211. Offers cancer (MS); immunology (MS); microbiology (MS); neurodegenerative disease (MS); pharmacology and toxicology (MS); photobiomodulation (MS). *Accreditation:* NAACLS. *Program availability:* Part-time. *Faculty:* 8 full-time (4 women). *Students:* 8 full-time (7 women), 3 part-time (1 woman); includes 1 minority (Two or more races, non-Hispanic/Latino), 2 international. Average age 29. 42 applicants, 14% accepted, 4 enrolled. In 2015, 7 master's awarded. *Degree requirements:* For master's, thesis. *Entrance requirements:* For master's, GRE General Test. Additional exam requirements/recommendations for international students: Required—TOEFL (minimum score 550 paper-based; 79 iBT), IELTS (minimum score 6.5). *Application deadline:* For fall admission, 1/1 priority date for domestic students; for spring admission, 9/1 for domestic students. Applications are processed on a rolling basis. Application fee: $56 ($96 for international students). *Financial support:* In 2015–16, 6 teaching assistantships were awarded; fellowships, research assistantships, career-related internships or fieldwork, and unspecified assistantships also available. Support available to part-time students. Financial award application deadline: 4/15. *Unit head:* Raymond Fleming, Representative, 414-229-3980, E-mail: mundo@uwm.edu. *Application contact:* Roger O. Smith, General Information Contact, 414-229-6697, Fax: 414-229-6697, E-mail: smithro@uwm.edu. Website: http://www4.uwm.edu/chs/academics/biomedical_sciences/bms_masters/

University of Wisconsin–Milwaukee, Graduate School, College of Letters and Science, Department of Biological Sciences, Milwaukee, WI 53201-0413. Offers MS, PhD. *Faculty:* 31 full-time (10 women). *Students:* 36 full-time (21 women), 21 part-time (11 women); includes 3 minority (1 Asian, non-Hispanic/Latino; 2 Two or more races, non-Hispanic/Latino), 14 international. Average age 30. 97 applicants, 21% accepted, 11 enrolled. In 2015, 3 master's, 8 doctorates awarded. *Degree requirements:* For master's, thesis; for doctorate, thesis/dissertation, 1 foreign language or data analysis proficiency. *Entrance requirements:* For master's and doctorate, GRE General Test. Additional exam requirements/recommendations for international students: Required—TOEFL (minimum score 550 paper-based; 79 iBT), IELTS (minimum score 6.5). *Application deadline:* For fall admission, 3/1 priority date for domestic students. Applications are processed on a rolling basis. Application fee: $56 ($96 for international students). *Financial support:* In 2015–16, 3 fellowships, 9 research assistantships, 67 teaching assistantships were awarded; career-related internships or fieldwork, unspecified assistantships, and project assistantships also available. Support available to part-time students. Financial award application deadline: 4/15; financial award applicants required to submit FAFSA. *Unit head:* R. David Heathcote, Department Chair, 414-229-6471, E-mail: rdh@uwm.edu. *Application contact:* General Information Contact, 414-229-4982, Fax: 414-229-6967, E-mail: gradschool@uwm.edu. Website: https://uwm.edu/biology/

University of Wisconsin–Oshkosh, Graduate Studies, College of Letters and Science, Department of Biology and Microbiology, Oshkosh, WI 54901. Offers biology (MS), including botany, microbiology, zoology. *Degree requirements:* For master's, comprehensive exam, thesis. *Entrance requirements:* For master's, GRE General Test, minimum GPA of 3.0, BS in biology. Additional exam requirements/recommendations for international students: Required—TOEFL (minimum score 550 paper-based; 79 iBT). Electronic applications accepted.

Utah State University, School of Graduate Studies, College of Science, Department of Biology, Logan, UT 84322. Offers biology (MS, PhD); ecology (MS, PhD). *Program availability:* Part-time. *Degree requirements:* For master's, thesis; for doctorate, thesis/dissertation. *Entrance requirements:* For master's and doctorate, GRE General Test, minimum GPA of 3.0. Additional exam requirements/recommendations for international students: Required—TOEFL (minimum score 575 paper-based). *Faculty research:* Plant, insect, microbial, and animal biology.

Vanderbilt University, Department of Biological Sciences, Nashville, TN 37240-1001. Offers MS, PhD, MD/PhD. *Faculty:* 20 full-time (3 women), 1 part-time/adjunct. *Students:* 49 full-time (27 women); includes 9 minority (2 Black or African American, non-Hispanic/Latino; 4 Asian, non-Hispanic/Latino; 2 Hispanic/Latino; 1 Two or more races, non-Hispanic/Latino), 13 international. Average age 26. 133 applicants, 6% accepted, 5 enrolled. In 2015, 1 master's, 11 doctorates awarded. Terminal master's awarded for partial completion of doctoral program. *Degree requirements:* For master's, thesis; for doctorate, thesis/dissertation, final and qualifying exams. *Entrance requirements:* For master's and doctorate, GRE General Test. Additional exam requirements/recommendations for international students: Required—TOEFL (minimum score 570 paper-based; 88 iBT). *Application deadline:* For fall admission, 1/15 for domestic and international students. Electronic applications accepted. *Financial support:* Fellowships with tuition reimbursements, research assistantships with full tuition reimbursements, teaching assistantships with full tuition reimbursements, Federal Work-Study, institutionally sponsored loans, scholarships/grants, traineeships, and health care benefits available. Financial award application deadline: 1/15; financial award applicants required to submit CSS PROFILE or FAFSA. *Faculty research:* Protein structure and function, protein transport, membrane ion channels and receptors, signal transduction, posttranscriptional control of gene expression, DNA replication and recombination, biological clocks, development, neurobiology, vector biology, insect physiology, ecology and evolution, bioinformatics. *Unit head:* Dr. Katherine Friedman, Director of Graduate Studies, 615-322-2008, Fax: 615-343-6707, E-mail: donna.webb@vanderbilt.edu. *Application contact:* Leslie L. Maxwell, Program Coordinator, 615-343-3076, Fax: 615-343-6707, E-mail: leslie.l.maxwell@vanderbilt.edu.
Website: http://sitemason.vanderbilt.edu/biosci/grad/

Villanova University, Graduate School of Liberal Arts and Sciences, Department of Biology, Villanova, PA 19085-1699. Offers MA, MS. *Program availability:* Part-time, evening/weekend. *Faculty:* 11. *Students:* 46 full-time (23 women), 4 part-time (3 women); includes 10 minority (4 Asian, non-Hispanic/Latino; 4 Hispanic/Latino; 2 Two or more races, non-Hispanic/Latino), 6 international. Average age 27. 33 applicants, 70% accepted, 14 enrolled. In 2015, 20 master's awarded. *Degree requirements:* For master's, comprehensive exam (for some programs), thesis (for some programs). *Entrance requirements:* For master's, GRE General Test, minimum GPA of 3.0, 3 recommendation letters. *Application deadline:* For fall admission, 3/1 priority date for domestic students, 5/1 for international students; for spring admission, 11/15 priority date for domestic students, 10/15 for international students; for summer admission, 5/1 for domestic students, 4/1 for international students. Applications are processed on a rolling basis. Application fee: $50. Electronic applications accepted. *Financial support:* Research assistantships with tuition reimbursements, teaching assistantships with tuition reimbursements, scholarships/grants, health care benefits, and unspecified assistantships available. Financial award applicants required to submit FAFSA. *Unit head:* Dr. John Olson, Chair, 610-519-4830, E-mail: john.olson@villanova.edu.
Website: http://www1.villanova.edu/villanova/artsci/biology/academics/graduate.html

Virginia Commonwealth University, Graduate School, College of Humanities and Sciences, Department of Biology, Richmond, VA 23284-9005. Offers MS. *Program availability:* Part-time. *Degree requirements:* For master's, thesis. *Entrance requirements:* For master's, GRE General Test, BS in biology or related field. Additional exam requirements/recommendations for international students: Required—TOEFL (minimum score 600 paper-based; 100 iBT) or IELTS (minimum score 6.5). *Faculty research:* Molecular and cellular biology, terrestrial and aquatic ecology, systematics, physiology and developmental biology.

Virginia Commonwealth University, Graduate School, School of Life Sciences, Richmond, VA 23284-9005. Offers M Env Sc, MB, MS, PhD. *Entrance requirements:* For master's and doctorate, GRE. Additional exam requirements/recommendations for international students: Required—TOEFL (minimum score 600 paper-based; 100 iBT). Electronic applications accepted.

Virginia Commonwealth University, Medical College of Virginia-Professional Programs, School of Medicine, School of Medicine Graduate Programs, Richmond, VA 23284-9005. Offers MPH, MS, PhD, Certificate, MD/MPH, MD/PhD. *Program availability:* Part-time. Terminal master's awarded for partial completion of doctoral program. *Degree requirements:* For doctorate, thesis/dissertation, comprehensive oral and written exams. *Entrance requirements:* For doctorate, GRE General Test, MCAT.

Virginia Commonwealth University, Program in Pre-Medical Basic Health Sciences, Richmond, VA 23284-9005. Offers anatomy (CBHS); biochemistry (CBHS); human genetics (CBHS); microbiology (CBHS); pharmacology (CBHS); physiology (CBHS). *Entrance requirements:* For degree, GRE, MCAT or DAT, course work in organic chemistry, minimum undergraduate GPA of 2.8. Additional exam requirements/recommendations for international students: Required—TOEFL (minimum score 600 paper-based). Electronic applications accepted.

Virginia Polytechnic Institute and State University, Graduate School, College of Science, Blacksburg, VA 24061. Offers biological sciences (MS, PhD); biomedical technology development and management (MS); chemistry (MS, PhD); economics (MA, PhD); geosciences (MS, PhD); mathematics (MS, PhD); physics (MS, PhD); psychology (MS, PhD); statistics (MS, PhD). *Degree requirements:* For master's, comprehensive exam (for some programs), thesis (for some programs); for doctorate, comprehensive exam (for some programs), thesis/dissertation (for some programs). *Entrance requirements:* For master's and doctorate, GRE/GMAT (may vary by department). Additional exam requirements/recommendations for international students: Required—TOEFL (minimum score 550 paper-based). Electronic applications accepted.

Virginia State University, College of Graduate Studies, College of Natural and Health Sciences, Department of Biology, Petersburg, VA 23806-0001. Offers MS. *Degree requirements:* For master's, one foreign language, thesis. *Entrance requirements:* For master's, GRE General Test. *Application deadline:* For fall admission, 5/1 priority date for domestic students. Applications are processed on a rolling basis. Application fee: $25. *Financial support:* Application deadline: 5/1.
Website: http://www.cnhs.vsu.edu/departments/biology/

Wake Forest University, Graduate School of Arts and Sciences, Department of Biology, Winston-Salem, NC 27109. Offers MS, PhD. *Program availability:* Part-time. *Degree requirements:* For master's, one foreign language, thesis; for doctorate, 2 foreign languages, comprehensive exam, thesis/dissertation. *Entrance requirements:* For master's and doctorate, GRE General Test. Additional exam requirements/

recommendations for international students: Required—TOEFL (minimum score 79 iBT). Electronic applications accepted. *Faculty research:* Cell biology, ecology, parasitology, immunology.

Wake Forest University, School of Medicine and Graduate School of Arts and Sciences, Graduate Programs in Medicine, Winston-Salem, NC 27109. Offers MS, PhD, MD/PhD. *Degree requirements:* For master's, thesis; for doctorate, thesis/dissertation. *Entrance requirements:* For master's and doctorate, GRE General Test. Additional exam requirements/recommendations for international students: Required—TOEFL. Electronic applications accepted. *Expenses:* Contact institution. *Faculty research:* Atherosclerosis, cardiovascular physiology, pharmacology, neuroanatomy, endocrinology.

Walla Walla University, Graduate School, Department of Biological Sciences, College Place, WA 99324-1198. Offers biology (MS). *Degree requirements:* For master's, thesis. *Entrance requirements:* For master's, GRE General Test, GRE Subject Test, minimum GPA of 2.75. Additional exam requirements/recommendations for international students: Required—TOEFL (minimum score 550 paper-based; 79 iBT). Electronic applications accepted. *Faculty research:* Marine biology, plant development, neurobiology, animal physiology, behavior.

Washington State University, College of Arts and Sciences, School of Biological Sciences, Pullman, WA 99164-4236. Offers MS, PhD. Programs are offered at the Pullman campus. *Degree requirements:* For master's, comprehensive exam (for some programs), thesis, oral exam; for doctorate, comprehensive exam, thesis/dissertation, oral exam. *Entrance requirements:* For master's and doctorate, GRE General Test, GRE Subject Test (recommended), three letters of recommendation, official transcripts from each university-level school attended, minimum GPA of 3.0. Additional exam requirements/recommendations for international students: Required—TOEFL, IELTS.

Washington University in St. Louis, Graduate School of Arts and Sciences, Division of Biology and Biomedical Sciences, St. Louis, MO 63130-4899. Offers biochemistry (PhD); computational and molecular biophysics (PhD); computational and systems biology (PhD); developmental, regenerative, and stem cell biology (PhD); evolution, ecology and population biology (PhD), including ecology, environmental biology, evolutionary biology, genetics; human and statistical genetics (PhD); immunology (PhD); molecular cell biology (PhD); molecular genetics and genomics (PhD); molecular microbiology and microbial pathogenesis (PhD); neurosciences (PhD); plant and microbial biosciences (PhD); MD/PhD. *Students:* 542 full-time (246 women); includes 106 minority (27 Black or African American, non-Hispanic/Latino; 5 American Indian or Alaska Native, non-Hispanic/Latino; 60 Asian, non-Hispanic/Latino; 11 Hispanic/Latino; 3 Two or more races, non-Hispanic/Latino), 115 international. 1,085 applicants, 21% accepted, 77 enrolled. In 2015, 87 doctorates awarded. *Degree requirements:* For doctorate, thesis/dissertation. *Entrance requirements:* For doctorate, GRE General Test, GRE Subject Test. Additional exam requirements/recommendations for international students: Required—TOEFL. *Application deadline:* For fall admission, 12/1 for domestic students. Application fee: $0. Electronic applications accepted. *Financial support:* Fellowships, research assistantships, and tuition waivers (full) available. Financial award application deadline: 1/15. *Unit head:* Dr. John Russell, Associate Dean, 314-747-0840. *Application contact:* Rebecca Riney, 314-474-4648, E-mail: dbbsphdadmissions@wusm.wustl.edu.
Website: http://dbbs.wustl.edu/

Wayne State University, College of Liberal Arts and Sciences, Department of Biological Sciences, Detroit, MI 48202. Offers biological sciences (MA, MS); cell development and neurobiology (PhD); evolution and organismal biology (PhD); molecular biology and biotechnology (PhD); molecular biotechnology (MS). PhD and MS programs admit for fall only. *Faculty:* 27. *Students:* 56 full-time (31 women), 8 part-time (2 women); includes 5 minority (2 Black or African American, non-Hispanic/Latino; 2 Asian, non-Hispanic/Latino; 1 Two or more races, non-Hispanic/Latino), 37 international. Average age 29. 210 applicants, 9% accepted, 7 enrolled. In 2015, 5 master's, 10 doctorates awarded. *Degree requirements:* For master's, thesis (for some programs); for doctorate, thesis/dissertation. *Entrance requirements:* For master's, GRE (for MS applicants), minimum GPA of 3.0; adequate preparation in biological sciences and supporting courses in chemistry, physics and mathematics; curriculum vitae; personal statement; three letters of recommendation (two for MA); for doctorate, GRE, curriculum vitae, statement of goals and career objectives, three letters of reference, bachelor's or master's degree in biological or other science. Additional exam requirements/recommendations for international students: Required—TOEFL (minimum score 550 paper-based; 79 iBT), TWE (minimum score 5.5), Michigan English Language Assessment Battery (minimum score 85); Recommended—IELTS (minimum score 6.5). Application fee: $0. Electronic applications accepted. *Expenses:* Tuition, state resident: full-time $14,165; part-time $590.20 per credit hour. Tuition, nonresident: full-time $30,682; part-time $1278.40 per credit hour. *Required fees:* $1688; $47.45 per credit hour. $274.60 per semester. Tuition and fees vary according to course load and program. *Financial support:* In 2015–16, 55 students received support, including 3 fellowships with tuition reimbursements available (averaging $16,000 per year), 8 research assistantships with tuition reimbursements available (averaging $19,506 per year), 45 teaching assistantships with tuition reimbursements available (averaging $19,536 per year); scholarships/grants and unspecified assistantships also available. Financial award application deadline: 3/31; financial award applicants required to submit FAFSA. *Faculty research:* Transcription and chromatin remodeling, genomic and developmental evolution, community and landscape ecology and environmental degradation, microbiology and virology, cell and neurobiology. *Total annual research expenditures:* $2.1 million. *Unit head:* Dr. David Njus, Professor and Chair, 313-577-3105, E-mail: dnjus@wayne.edu. *Application contact:* Rose Mary Priest, Graduate Secretary, 313-577-6818, E-mail: rpriest@wayne.edu.
Website: http://clas.wayne.edu/Biology/

Weill Cornell Medicine, Weill Cornell Graduate School of Medical Sciences, New York, NY 10065. Offers MS, PhD. Terminal master's awarded for partial completion of doctoral program. *Degree requirements:* For master's, comprehensive exam, thesis (for some programs); for doctorate, thesis/dissertation, final exam. *Entrance requirements:* For doctorate, GRE General Test. Additional exam requirements/recommendations for international students: Required—TOEFL. Electronic applications accepted. *Expenses:* Contact institution.

Weill Cornell Medicine, Weill Cornell/Rockefeller/Sloan-Kettering Tri-Institutional MD-PhD Program, New York, NY 10065. Offers MD/PhD. Offered jointly with The Rockefeller University and Sloan-Kettering Institute. Electronic applications accepted. *Expenses:* Contact institution. *Faculty research:* Neuroscience, pharmacology, immunology, structural biology, genetics.

Wesleyan University, Graduate Studies, Department of Biology, Middletown, CT 06459. Offers cell and developmental biology (PhD); evolution and ecology (PhD); genetics and genomics (PhD), including bioinformatics; neurobiology and behavior (PhD). *Faculty:* 14 full-time (5 women). *Students:* 26 full-time (12 women); includes 5 minority (2 Black or African American, non-Hispanic/Latino; 3 Asian, non-Hispanic/Latino), 5 international. In 2015, 3 doctorates awarded. Terminal master's awarded for partial completion of doctoral program. *Degree requirements:* For doctorate,

Biological and Biomedical Sciences—General

comprehensive exam, thesis/dissertation, public seminar. *Entrance requirements:* For doctorate, GRE. Additional exam requirements/recommendations for international students: Required—TOEFL or IELTS. *Application deadline:* For fall admission, 1/15 for domestic and international students. Application fee: $0. Electronic applications accepted. *Financial support:* Stipends available. *Faculty research:* Evolution and ecology, neurobiology and behavior, cell and developmental biology, genetics, genomics and bioinformatics. *Unit head:* Dr. John Kirn, Chair/Professor, 860-685-3494, E-mail: jrkirn@wesleyan.edu. *Application contact:* Marjorie Fitzgibbons, Administrative Assistant, 860-685-2157, E-mail: mfitzgibbons@wesleyan.edu.
Website: http://www.wesleyan.edu/bio/

West Chester University of Pennsylvania, College of Arts and Sciences, Department of Biology, West Chester, PA 19383. Offers biology (MS, Teaching Certificate). *Program availability:* Part-time, evening/weekend. *Faculty:* 9 full-time (1 woman). *Students:* 9 full-time (6 women), 19 part-time (15 women); includes 1 minority (Hispanic/Latino), 2 international. Average age 29. 25 applicants, 76% accepted, 11 enrolled. In 2015, 8 master's, 1 other advanced degree awarded. *Degree requirements:* For master's, comprehensive exam, thesis (for some programs). *Entrance requirements:* For master's, two letters of reference. Additional exam requirements/recommendations for international students: Required—TOEFL or IELTS. *Application deadline:* For fall admission, 5/15 for international students; for spring admission, 10/15 for international students. Applications are processed on a rolling basis. Application fee: $50. Electronic applications accepted. *Expenses:* Tuition, state resident: full-time $8460; part-time $470 per credit. Tuition, nonresident: full-time $12,690; part-time $705 per credit. *Required fees:* $2312; $126.75 per credit. Tuition and fees vary according to campus/location and program. *Financial support:* Scholarships/grants and unspecified assistantships available. Financial award application deadline: 2/15; financial award applicants required to submit FAFSA. *Faculty research:* Medical microbiology, molecular genetics and physiology of living systems, mammalian biomechanics, invertebrate and vertebrate animal systems, aquatic and terrestrial ecology. *Unit head:* Dr. Jack Waber, Chair, 610-436-2319, E-mail: jwaber@wcupa.edu. *Application contact:* Dr. Xin Fan, Graduate Coordinator, 610-436-2281, E-mail: xfan@wcupa.edu.
Website: http://bio.wcupa.edu/biology/index.php

Western Carolina University, Graduate School, College of Arts and Sciences, Department of Biology, Cullowhee, NC 28723. Offers MS. *Program availability:* Part-time, evening/weekend. *Degree requirements:* For master's, thesis. *Entrance requirements:* For master's, GRE General Test, appropriate undergraduate degree, 3 letters of recommendation. Additional exam requirements/recommendations for international students: Required—TOEFL (minimum score 550 paper-based; 79 iBT). *Application deadline:* For fall admission, 5/1 priority date for domestic students; for spring admission, 9/1 priority date for domestic students. Applications are processed on a rolling basis. Application fee: $50. *Financial support:* Fellowships, research assistantships with tuition reimbursements, teaching assistantships with tuition reimbursements, career-related internships or fieldwork, institutionally sponsored loans, scholarships/grants, and unspecified assistantships available. Financial award application deadline: 3/31; financial award applicants required to submit FAFSA. *Faculty research:* Pathogen interactions, gene expression, plant community ecology, restoration ecology, ornithology, herpetology.
Website: http://www.wcu.edu/as/biology/index.html

Western Connecticut State University, Division of Graduate Studies, Maricostas School of Arts and Sciences, Department of Biological and Environmental Sciences, Danbury, CT 06810-6885. Offers MAT. *Program availability:* Part-time. *Degree requirements:* For master's, comprehensive exam or thesis, completion of program in 6 years. *Entrance requirements:* For master's, minimum GPA of 2.5. Additional exam requirements/recommendations for international students: Recommended—TOEFL (minimum score 550 paper-based; 79 iBT), IELTS (minimum score 6). *Expenses:* Contact institution. *Faculty research:* Biology, taxonomy and evolution of aquatic flowering plants; aquatic plant reproductive systems, the spread of invasive aquatic plants, aquatic plant structure, and the taxonomy of water starworts (Callitrichaceae) and riverweeds (Podostemaceae).

Western Illinois University, School of Graduate Studies, College of Arts and Sciences, Department of Biological Sciences, Macomb, IL 61455-1390. Offers biological sciences (MS); environmental geographic information systems (Certificate); zoo and aquarium studies (Certificate). *Program availability:* Part-time. *Students:* 57 full-time (40 women), 32 part-time (23 women); includes 5 minority (2 Black or African American, non-Hispanic/Latino; 1 Hispanic/Latino; 2 Two or more races, non-Hispanic/Latino), 25 international. Average age 28. 56 applicants, 84% accepted, 30 enrolled. In 2015, 15 master's, 11 other advanced degrees awarded. *Degree requirements:* For master's, thesis or alternative. *Entrance requirements:* Additional exam requirements/recommendations for international students: Required—TOEFL (minimum score 550 paper-based; 80 iBT); Recommended—IELTS. *Application deadline:* Applications are processed on a rolling basis. Application fee: $30. Electronic applications accepted. *Financial support:* In 2015–16, 15 research assistantships with full tuition reimbursements (averaging $7,544 per year), 15 teaching assistantships with full tuition reimbursements (averaging $8,688 per year) were awarded; unspecified assistantships also available. Financial award applicants required to submit FAFSA. *Unit head:* Dr. Charles Lydeard, Chairperson, 309-298-1546. *Application contact:* Dr. Nancy Parsons, Associate Provost and Director of Graduate Studies, 309-298-1806, Fax: 309-298-2345, E-mail: grad-office@wiu.edu.
Website: http://wiu.edu/biology

Western Kentucky University, Graduate Studies, Ogden College of Science and Engineering, Department of Biology, Bowling Green, KY 42101. Offers MS. *Program availability:* Online learning. *Degree requirements:* For master's, comprehensive exam, thesis optional, research tool. *Entrance requirements:* For master's, GRE General Test, minimum GPA of 2.75. Additional exam requirements/recommendations for international students: Required—TOEFL (minimum score 555 paper-based; 79 iBT). *Faculty research:* Phytoremediation, culturing of salt water organisms, PCR-based standards, biological monitoring (water) bioremediation, genetic diversity.

Western Michigan University, Graduate College, College of Arts and Sciences, Department of Biological Sciences, Kalamazoo, MI 49008. Offers MS, PhD. *Degree requirements:* For master's, thesis; for doctorate, thesis/dissertation.

Western Michigan University, Graduate College, College of Arts and Sciences, Department of Interdisciplinary Arts and Sciences, Kalamazoo, MI 49008. Offers science education (MA, PhD), including biological sciences (PhD), chemistry (PhD), geosciences (PhD), physical geography (PhD), physics (PhD), science education (PhD). *Degree requirements:* For doctorate, thesis/dissertation.

Western University of Health Sciences, Graduate College of Biomedical Sciences, Master of Science in Biomedical Sciences Program, Pomona, CA 91766-1854. Offers MS. *Faculty:* 5 full-time (0 women), 4 part-time/adjunct (1 woman). *Students:* 11 full-time (5 women); includes 8 minority (3 Asian, non-Hispanic/Latino; 4 Hispanic/Latino; 1 Two or more races, non-Hispanic/Latino). Average age 26. 34 applicants, 53% accepted, 8 enrolled. In 2015, 6 master's awarded. *Degree requirements:* For master's, comprehensive exam (for some programs), thesis. *Entrance requirements:* For master's,

GRE, MCAT, or DAT, minimum overall GPA of 3.0; letters of recommendation; personal statement; resume; BS in pharmacy, chemistry, biology or related scientific area. Additional exam requirements/recommendations for international students: Required—TOEFL (minimum score 92 iBT). *Application deadline:* For fall admission, 11/1 for domestic and international students; for spring admission, 6/1 for domestic and international students. Application fee: $50. Electronic applications accepted. *Expenses:* $748 per unit tuition. *Financial support:* Scholarships/grants available. Financial award application deadline: 3/2; financial award applicants required to submit FAFSA. *Unit head:* Dr. Guru Betageri, Associate Dean, Graduate College of Biomedical Sciences, 909-469-5682, E-mail: gbetageri@westernu.edu. *Application contact:* Kathryn Ford, Director of Admission, 909-469-5335, Fax: 909-469-5570, E-mail: admissions@westernu.edu.
Website: https://www.westernu.edu/biomedical-sciences/biomedical-sciences-academics/biomedical-sciences-msbs/

Western University of Health Sciences, Graduate College of Biomedical Sciences, Master of Science in Medical Sciences Program, Pomona, CA 91766-1854. Offers MS. *Faculty:* 2 full-time (1 woman). *Students:* 29 full-time (21 women); includes 26 minority (2 Black or African American, non-Hispanic/Latino; 15 Asian, non-Hispanic/Latino; 8 Hispanic/Latino; 1 Two or more races, non-Hispanic/Latino). Average age 26. 268 applicants, 11% accepted, 27 enrolled. In 2015, 32 master's awarded. *Degree requirements:* For master's, comprehensive exam (for some programs). *Entrance requirements:* For master's, GRE, MCAT, OAT, or DAT, minimum overall GPA of 2.5; letters of recommendation; personal statement; resume; transcripts; bachelor's degree. Additional exam requirements/recommendations for international students: Required—TOEFL (minimum score 89 iBT). *Application deadline:* For fall admission, 2/1 for domestic and international students. Application fee: $50. Electronic applications accepted. *Expenses:* $24,388 tuition; $40 student body fees; $350 graduation fee. *Financial support:* Scholarships/grants available. Financial award application deadline: 3/2; financial award applicants required to submit FAFSA. *Unit head:* Marcos Villa, Director, Master of Medical Sciences Program, Fax: 909-469-5577, E-mail: mvilla@westernu.edu. *Application contact:* Kathryn Ford, Director of Admission, 909-469-5335, Fax: 909-469-5570, E-mail: admissions@westernu.edu.
Website: http://prospective.westernu.edu/medical-sciences/welcome-4/

Western Washington University, Graduate School, College of Sciences and Technology, Department of Biology, Bellingham, WA 98225-5996. Offers MS. *Program availability:* Part-time. *Degree requirements:* For master's, thesis. *Entrance requirements:* For master's, GRE General Test, GRE Subject Test (biology), minimum GPA of 3.0 in last 60 semester hours or last 90 quarter hours. Additional exam requirements/recommendations for international students: Required—TOEFL (minimum score 567 paper-based). Electronic applications accepted. *Faculty research:* Organismal biology, ecology and evolutionary biology, marine biology, cell and molecular biology, developmental biology, larval ecology, microzoo planton, symbiosis.

West Texas A&M University, College of Agriculture, Science and Engineering, Department of Life, Earth, and Environmental Sciences, Program in Biology, Canyon, TX 79016-0001. Offers MS. *Program availability:* Part-time. *Degree requirements:* For master's, comprehensive exam, thesis optional. *Entrance requirements:* For master's, GRE General Test. Additional exam requirements/recommendations for international students: Required—TOEFL (minimum score 550 paper-based). Electronic applications accepted. *Faculty research:* Aeroallergen concentration, scorpions, kangaroo mice, seed anatomy with light and scanning electron microscope.

West Virginia University, Eberly College of Arts and Sciences, Department of Biology, Morgantown, WV 26506. Offers cell and molecular biology (MS, PhD); environmental and evolutionary biology (MS, PhD); forensic biology (MS, PhD); genomic biology (MS, PhD); neurobiology (MS, PhD). Terminal master's awarded for partial completion of doctoral program. *Degree requirements:* For master's, thesis, final exam; for doctorate, thesis/dissertation, preliminary and final exams. *Entrance requirements:* For master's, GRE General Test, GRE Subject Test, minimum GPA of 3.0; for doctorate, GRE General Test, minimum GPA of 3.0. Additional exam requirements/recommendations for international students: Required—TOEFL. *Expenses:* Tuition, state resident: full-time $8568. Tuition, nonresident: full-time $22,140. Tuition and fees vary according to program. *Faculty research:* Environmental biology, genetic engineering, developmental biology, global change, biodiversity.

West Virginia University, School of Medicine, Graduate Programs at the Health Sciences Center, Morgantown, WV 26506. Offers MS, PhD, MD/PhD. *Program availability:* Part-time, evening/weekend, online learning. *Expenses:* Contact institution.

Wichita State University, Graduate School, Fairmount College of Liberal Arts and Sciences, Department of Biological Sciences, Wichita, KS 67260. Offers MS. *Program availability:* Part-time. *Students:* 25 (15 women). In 2015, 10 master's awarded. *Application deadline:* For fall admission, 3/1 for domestic and international students; for spring admission, 10/1 for domestic students, 8/1 for international students. Application fee: $50 ($65 for international students). *Unit head:* Dr. William J. Hendry, III, Chair, 316-978-3111, Fax: 316-978-3772, E-mail: william.hendry@wichita.edu. *Application contact:* Jordan Oleson, Admissions Coordinator, 316-978-3095, E-mail: jordan.oleson@wichita.edu.
Website: http://www.wichita.edu/biology

Wilfrid Laurier University, Faculty of Graduate and Postdoctoral Studies, Faculty of Science, Department of Biology, Waterloo, ON N2L 3C5, Canada. Offers integrative biology (M Sc). *Degree requirements:* For master's, thesis. *Entrance requirements:* For master's, honours BA in last two years of undergraduate studies with a minimum B average. Additional exam requirements/recommendations for international students: Required—TOEFL (minimum score 89 iBT). Electronic applications accepted. *Faculty research:* Genetic/development, anatomy/physiology, ecology/environment, evolution.

William Paterson University of New Jersey, College of Science and Health, Wayne, NJ 07470-8420. Offers biology (MS); biotechnology (MS); communication disorders (MS); exercise and sports studies (MS); nursing (MSN); nursing practice (DNP). *Program availability:* Part-time, evening/weekend. *Faculty:* 25 full-time (11 women), 13 part-time/adjunct (4 women). *Students:* 73 full-time (58 women), 208 part-time (183 women); includes 111 minority (18 Black or African American, non-Hispanic/Latino; 40 Asian, non-Hispanic/Latino; 50 Hispanic/Latino; 3 Two or more races, non-Hispanic/Latino), 5 international. Average age 34. 495 applicants, 27% accepted, 74 enrolled. In 2015, 63 master's, 10 doctorates awarded. *Degree requirements:* For master's, comprehensive exam (for some programs), thesis (for some programs), non-thesis internship/practicum (for some programs). *Entrance requirements:* For master's, GRE/MAT, minimum GPA of 3.0; 2 or 3 letters of recommendation; personal statement; work experience (for some programs); for doctorate, GRE/MAT, minimum GPA of 3.3; work experience; 3 letters of recommendation; interview; master's degree in nursing. Additional exam requirements/recommendations for international students: Required—TOEFL (minimum score 550 paper-based; 79 iBT), IELTS (minimum score 6). *Application deadline:* For fall admission, 6/1 for domestic students, 3/1 for international students; for spring admission, 11/1 for domestic students, 10/1 for international students. Applications are processed on a rolling basis. Application fee: $50. Electronic applications accepted. *Expenses:* Tuition, state resident: full-time $11,544; part-time

$577.21 per credit. Tuition, nonresident: full-time $19,024; part-time $951.21 per credit. *Required fees:* $1916; $95.79 per credit. $62.50 per semester. Tuition and fees vary according to course load and degree level. *Financial support:* Research assistantships with full tuition reimbursements, career-related internships or fieldwork, Federal Work-Study, scholarships/grants, and unspecified assistantships available. Support available to part-time students. Financial award application deadline: 4/1; financial award applicants required to submit FAFSA. *Faculty research:* Human biomechanics, autism, nanomaterials, health and environment, neurophysiology and neurobiology. *Unit head:* Dr. Kenneth Wolf, Dean, 973-720-2194, Fax: 973-720-3414, E-mail: wolfk@wpunj.edu. *Application contact:* Christina Aiello, Assistant Director, Graduate Admissions, 973-720-2506, Fax: 973-720-2035, E-mail: aielloc@wpunj.edu. Website: http://www.wpunj.edu/cosh

Winthrop University, College of Arts and Sciences, Department of Biology, Rock Hill, SC 29733. Offers MS. *Program availability:* Part-time. *Faculty:* 6 full-time, 1 part-time/adjunct. *Students:* 12 full-time (9 women), 6 part-time (1 woman); includes 2 minority (both Hispanic/Latino). Average age 28. In 2015, 7 master's awarded. *Degree requirements:* For master's, thesis optional. *Entrance requirements:* For master's, GRE General Test. Additional exam requirements/recommendations for international students: Required—TOEFL (minimum score 550 paper-based; 79 iBT). *Application deadline:* For fall admission, 7/15 priority date for domestic students; for spring admission, 12/1 for domestic students. Applications are processed on a rolling basis. Application fee: $50. Electronic applications accepted. *Expenses: Tuition, area resident:* Part-time $579 per credit hour. Tuition, state resident: full-time $13,828. Tuition, nonresident: full-time $26,638; part-time $1114 per credit hour. *Financial support:* Research assistantships with full tuition reimbursements, Federal Work-Study, scholarships/grants, and unspecified assistantships available. Support available to part-time students. Financial award application deadline: 2/1; financial award applicants required to submit FAFSA. *Faculty research:* Bone biology, bone biomechanics; development of the visual system; cancer research, prostate cancer metastasis; new monkey species in rainforest in Peru. *Unit head:* Dr. Dwight Dimaculangan, Department Chair, 803-323-2111, Fax: 803-323-2246, E-mail: dimaculangad@winthrop.edu. *Application contact:* 800-411-7041, Fax: 803-323-2292, E-mail: gradschool@winthrop.edu. Website: http://www.winthrop.edu/graduate-studies/biology.htm

Worcester Polytechnic Institute, Graduate Studies and Research, Department of Biology and Biotechnology, Worcester, MA 01609-2280. Offers biology and biotechnology (MS); biotechnology (PhD). *Faculty:* 11 full-time (6 women). *Students:* 18 full-time (8 women), 4 international. 58 applicants, 24% accepted, 5 enrolled. In 2015, 3 master's, 4 doctorates awarded. Terminal master's awarded for partial completion of doctoral program. *Degree requirements:* For master's, thesis; for doctorate, comprehensive exam, thesis/dissertation, qualifying exam. *Entrance requirements:* For master's and doctorate, GRE General Test, 3 letters of recommendation, statement of purpose. Additional exam requirements/recommendations for international students: Required—TOEFL (minimum score 563 paper-based; 84 iBT), IELTS (minimum score 7). *Application deadline:* For fall admission, 1/1 priority date for domestic and international students. Application fee: $70. Electronic applications accepted. *Financial support:* Research assistantships, teaching assistantships, career-related internships or fieldwork, institutionally sponsored loans, scholarships/grants, and unspecified assistantships available. Financial award application deadline: 1/1; financial award applicants required to submit FAFSA. *Unit head:* Dr. Joseph Duffy, Head, 508-831-4111, Fax: 508-831-5936, E-mail: jduffy@wpi.edu. *Application contact:* Dr. Reeta Rao, Graduate Coordinator, 508-831-5538, Fax: 508-831-5936, E-mail: rpr@wpi.edu. Website: http://www.wpi.edu/Academics/Depts/BBT/

Wright State University, School of Graduate Studies, College of Science and Mathematics, Department of Biological Sciences, Dayton, OH 45435. Offers biological sciences (MS); environmental sciences (MS). *Degree requirements:* For master's, thesis optional. *Entrance requirements:* Additional exam requirements/recommendations for international students: Required—TOEFL.

Wright State University, School of Graduate Studies, College of Science and Mathematics and School of Medicine, Program in Biomedical Sciences, Dayton, OH 45435. Offers PhD. *Degree requirements:* For doctorate, thesis/dissertation. *Entrance requirements:* For doctorate, GRE General Test. Additional exam requirements/recommendations for international students: Required—TOEFL.

Yale University, School of Medicine and Graduate School of Arts and Sciences, Combined Program in Biological and Biomedical Sciences (BBS), New Haven, CT 06520. Offers PhD, MD/PhD. *Degree requirements:* For doctorate, thesis/dissertation. *Entrance requirements:* For doctorate, GRE General Test. Additional exam requirements/recommendations for international students: Required—TOEFL. Electronic applications accepted. *Expenses:* Contact institution.

York University, Faculty of Graduate Studies, Faculty of Science, Program in Biology, Toronto, ON M3J 1P3, Canada. Offers M Sc, PhD. *Program availability:* Part-time, evening/weekend. *Degree requirements:* For master's, thesis or alternative; for doctorate, comprehensive exam, thesis/dissertation, preliminary exam. Electronic applications accepted.

Youngstown State University, Graduate School, College of Science, Technology, Engineering and Mathematics, Department of Biological Sciences, Youngstown, OH 44555-0001. Offers environmental biology (MS); molecular biology, microbiology, and genetic (MS); physiology and anatomy (MS). *Program availability:* Part-time. *Degree requirements:* For master's, comprehensive exam, thesis, oral review. *Entrance requirements:* For master's, GRE General Test, minimum GPA of 2.7. Additional exam requirements/recommendations for international students: Required—TOEFL. *Faculty research:* Cell biology, neurophysiology, molecular biology, neurobiology, gene regulation.

COLUMBIA UNIVERSITY
Graduate School of Arts and Sciences
Department of Biological Sciences

 For more information, visit http://petersons.to/columbiabiologicalsciences

Program of Study

The Department offers training leading to a Ph.D. in cellular, molecular, developmental, computational, and structural biology as well as genetics, biophysics, and neurobiology. The graduate program provides each student with a solid background in contemporary biology and an in-depth knowledge of one or more of the above areas. The specific nature and scheduling of courses taken during the first two graduate years are determined by the student's consultation with the graduate student adviser, taking into account the background and specific research interests of the student. During the first year, all students take an intensive core course that provides a solid background in structural biology, cell biology, genetics, molecular biology, and bioinformatics.

Beginning in the first year, graduate students attend advanced seminar courses, including the preresearch seminar, which is a forum for faculty-student research discussion. Important components of graduate education include the ability to analyze critically the contemporary research literature and to present such analyses effectively through oral and written presentations. Students acquire training in these skills through participation in advanced-level seminars and journal clubs, as well as through presentation and defense of original research proposals during the spring semester of the second year of graduate study or the fall semester of the third year.

Beginning in the first year of graduate work, students also engage in research training. Students may choose laboratories in the Department of Biological Sciences on Columbia's main Morningside Heights Campus or in about twenty-five other laboratories, including many at Columbia's Health Sciences Campus. To inform incoming students of research opportunities, faculty members discuss ongoing research projects with them in the preresearch seminar held in the autumn term of the first year. All students are required to participate in ongoing research in up to three different laboratories during the first year. The choice of a dissertation sponsor is made after consultation between the student and potential faculty advisers, and intensive research begins following the spring term of the student's first year. Each student is assigned a Ph.D. Advisory Committee made up of the student's sponsor and 2 other faculty members.

Research Facilities

The Department of Biological Sciences is located in the Sherman Fairchild Center for the Life Sciences. The building provides nearly 78,000 square feet of laboratory space for the Department's laboratories, as well as extensive shared instrument facilities, including extensive sophisticated microscopy, X-ray diffraction, fluorescence-activated cell sorting (FACS), real-time PCR analysis, mass spectrometry, infrared scanning, phosphorimaging, and microinjection, as well as housing and care of research animals, including transgenic mice. In addition, several laboratories are located in the nearby new state-of-the-art Northwest Corner interdisciplinary science building.

Financial Aid

All accepted students receive generous stipends, complete tuition exemption, and medical insurance. Special fellowships with larger stipends are also available (e.g., to members of minority groups).

Cost of Study

Tuition and fees are paid for all graduate students accepted into the Department.

Living and Housing Costs

Most students live in University-owned, subsidized apartments within easy walking distance of the laboratories. In addition, both the Morningside and Health Sciences Campuses are easily reached by public transportation from all areas of the city.

Student Group

There are about 100 graduate students and 60 postdoctoral fellows in the Department.

Location

New York is the cultural center of the country and offers unrivaled opportunities for attending concerts, operas, plays, and sporting events, for visiting outstanding museums, and for varied, affordable dining. Many excellent beaches, ski slopes, and state and national parks are within reasonable driving distance.

The University and The Department

Columbia was established as King's College in 1754 and has grown into one of the major universities of the world. The Department is located on the beautiful main campus in Morningside Heights, which combines the advantages of an urban setting and a peaceful college-town atmosphere.

Applying

Undergraduate training in one of the natural or physical sciences is recommended, although successful students have come from computer science or engineering backgrounds, as well. It is desirable for students to have had at least one year of calculus, as well as courses in organic and physical chemistry, physics, genetics, biochemistry, and cell biology. Any deficiencies may be made up while in graduate school. The Graduate Record Examinations (GRE) is required, as is the Test of English as a Foreign Language (TOEFL) for international applicants whose native language is not English and who do not hold an undergraduate degree from a U.S. college. The GRE Subject Test in biology, biochemistry, chemistry, computer science, or physics is highly recommended. Completed applications should be returned by January 4 for admission to the fall semester. Applications will be reviewed in the order received, so those submitting complete applications earlier have a better chance of being invited for an interview. Application forms and additional information can be obtained from the Department's website.

Columbia University is an Equal Opportunity/Affirmative Action institution.

Correspondence and Information

Graduate Student Adviser
Department of Biological Sciences
Columbia University
1212 Amsterdam Avenue, Mail Code 2402
Sherman Fairchild Center, Room 600
New York, New York 10027
United States
Phone: 212-854-2313
Fax: 212-865-8246
E-mail: biology@columbia.edu
Website: http://biology.columbia.edu

Columbia University

THE FACULTY AND THEIR RESEARCH

J. Chloë Bulinski, Professor; Ph.D., Wisconsin, 1980. Dynamics and functions of microtubules during myogenic differentiation and cell-cycle progression.

Harmen Bussemaker, Professor; Ph.D., Utrecht (Netherlands), 1995. Data-driven modeling of transcriptional and posttranscriptional networks based on biophysical principles.

Martin Chalfie, Professor; Ph.D., Harvard, 1977; Member, National Academy of Sciences and Nobel Laureate in Chemistry 2008. Developmental genetics of identified nerve cells in *Caenorhabditis elegans;* genetic analysis of cell differentiation, mechanosensory transduction, synapse specification, and aging.

Lawrence A. Chasin, Professor; Ph.D., MIT, 1967. Pre-mRNA splicing in cultured mammalian cells.

Lars Dietrich, Assistant Professor, Ph.D., Heidelberg (Germany), 2004. Bacterial models for biological shape and pattern formation.

Julio Fernandez, Professor; Ph.D., Berkeley, 1982. Study of the cellular events that lead to the release of histamine or catecholamine-containing secretory granules from single, isolated mast cells or chromaffin cells; analysis of single-protein elasticity by atomic force microscopy (AFM).

Stuart Firestein, Professor; Ph.D., Berkeley, 1988. Cellular and molecular physiology of transduction; coding and neuronal regeneration in the vertebrate olfactory system.

Joachim Frank, Professor and Howard Hughes Medical Institute Investigator; Ph.D., Munich Technical, 1970; Member, National Academy of Sciences. Cryoelectron microscopy and three-dimensional reconstruction for the study of the mechanism of protein biosynthesis.

Iva Greenwald, Professor and Howard Hughes Medical Institute Investigator; Ph.D., MIT, 1982; Member, National Academy of Sciences. Development and cell-cell interactions.

Tulle Hazelrigg, Professor; Ph.D., Indiana, 1982. mRNA localization in *Drosophila* oocytes.

Oliver Hobert, Professor and Howard Hughes Medical Institute Investigator; Ph.D., Max Planck Institute for Biochemistry, Martinsried, Germany, 1995. Nervous system development and function.

John F. Hunt, Professor; Ph.D., Yale, 1993. Structural genomics and biophysical studies of the molecular mechanism of transmembrane transport.

Songtao Jia, Associate Professor; Ph.D., UCLA, 2003. Epigenetic regulation of the genome.

Daniel D. Kalderon, Professor; Ph.D., London, 1984. Molecular mechanisms of cellular interactions mediated by cAMP-dependent protein kinase (PKA) in *Drosophila;* roles of PKA in hedgehog signaling and in generating anterior/posterior polarity in oocytes.

Darcy B. Kelley, Professor and Howard Hughes Medical Institute Professor; Ph.D., Rockefeller, 1975. Sexual differentiation of the nervous system; molecular analyses of androgen-regulated development in neurons and muscle; neuroethology of vocal communication; evolution of the nuclear receptor family.

Laura Landweber, Professor; Ph.D., Harvard, 1993. Molecular evolution and RNA-mediated epigenetic inheritance.

James L. Manley, Professor; Ph.D., SUNY at Stony Brook, 1976. Regulation of mRNA synthesis in animal cells; biochemical and genetic analysis of mechanisms and control of mRNA transcription, splicing, and polyadenylation; developmental control of gene expression.

Joseph Pickrell, Adjunct Assistant Professor; Ph.D., Chicago, 2011. Computational genomics to develop novel statistical approaches to transform large-scale genomic data into improved understanding of human biology and history.

Carol L. Prives, Professor; Ph.D., McGill, 1968; Member, National Academy of Sciences and National Institute of Medicine. Structure and function of the p53 tumor suppressor protein and p53 family members; studies on cell cycle and apoptosis; stress-activated signaling and control of proteolysis.

Ron Prywes, Professor; Ph.D., MIT, 1984. Normal and cancerous mechanisms of regulation of cellular proliferation and gene expression; signal transduction and activation of transcription factors; activation of transcription by the ER stress/unfolded protein response.

Molly Przeworski, Professor; Ph.D., Chicago, 2000. Population genetics, evolutionary genetics, meiotic recombination.

Ozgur Sahin, Associate Professor of Biological Sciences and Physics; Ph.D., Stanford, 2005. Mechanical investigations of biological systems for energy, environment, and biological research.

Guy Sella, Associate Professor; Ph.D., Tel Aviv (Israel), 2001. Evolutionary genetics of adaptation, disease risk and other quantitative traits.

Brent Stockwell, Professor and Howard Hughes Medical Institute Investigator; Ph.D., Harvard, 1997. Diagramming disease networks with chemical and biological tools.

Raju Tomer, Assistant Professor; Ph.D. European Molecular Biology Laboratory, 2010. Developing and applying molecular, optical, and data analytic methods for multi-scale understanding of complex biological systems.

Liang Tong, Professor; Ph.D., Berkeley, 1989. Structural biology of proteins involved in human diseases (obesity, diabetes, cancer); structural biology of proteins involved in pre-mRNA 3'-end processing.

Alexander A. Tzagoloff, Professor of Biological Sciences; Ph.D., Columbia, 1962. Energy-coupling mechanisms; structure of membrane enzymes; biogenesis of mitochondria; genetics of mitochondria in yeast.

Jian Yang, Professor; Ph.D., Washington (Seattle), 1991. Structure and function of ion channels; molecular mechanisms of ion channel regulation and localization.

Rafael Yuste, Professor and Howard Hughes Medical Institute Investigator; M.D., Madrid, 1987; Ph.D., Rockefeller, 1992. Development and function of the cortical microcircuitry.

Additional Faculty Sponsors for Ph.D. Research

Cory Abate-Shen, Urology, Medicine, Systems Biology, and Pathology and Cell Biology. Computational and preclinical analyses of mouse models of prostate and bladder cancer.

Dimitris Anastassiou, Electrical Engineering. Data mining of large biological datasets—cancer research.

Richard Axel, Biochemistry and Molecular Biophysics/Pathology and Cell Biology; Howard Hughes Medical Institute Investigator and Nobel Laureate in Physiology or Medicine 2004; Member, National Academy of Sciences. Central and peripheral organization of the olfactory system.

Richard J. Baer, Pathology and Cell Biology. The pathogenesis of hereditary breast cancer.

Andrea Califano, Biomedical Informatics. Study of gene regulatory and signaling networks in mammalian cellular contexts using computational methods.

Virginia Cornish, Chemistry. Development of in vivo selection strategies for evolving proteins with novel catalytic properties.

Franklin D. Costantini, Genetics and Development. Genetics of kidney development in the mouse; cellular and genetic basis of epithelial branching morphogenesis.

Riccardo Dalla-Favera, Genetics and Development, and Microbiology and Immunology. Molecular genetics of cancer; molecular pathogenesis of lymphoma and leukemia.

Jonathan E. Dworkin, Microbiology and Immunology. Bacterial signaling and interactions with the host.

Jean Gautier, Genetics and Development/Institute for Cancer Genetics. Cell cycle and cell death during early development.

Ruben L. Gonzalez Jr., Chemistry. Single molecule biophysics.

Eric C. Greene, Biochemistry and Molecular Biophysics; Howard Hughes Medical Institute Investigator. Molecular mechanisms of DNA recombination and repair; single-molecule fluorescence microscopy and other biochemical approaches.

Lloyd Greene, Pathology and Cell Biology. Mechanisms of neuronal differentiation and degeneration and their regulation by external growth factors.

Wesley Grueber, Physiology and Cellular Biophysics/Neuroscience. Molecular basis of nervous system development and function in *Drosophila.*

Wei Gu, Pathology and Cell Biology. P53 in tumor suppression and aging.

René Hen, Pharmacology. Serotonin receptors and behavior.

Wayne Hendrickson, Biochemistry and Molecular Biophysics; Howard Hughes Medical Institute Investigator; Member, National Academy of Sciences. Macromolecular structure; X-ray crystallography.

Thomas Jessell, Biochemistry and Molecular Biophysics; Howard Hughes Medical Institute Investigator; Member, National Academy of Sciences. Molecular mechanisms of neural differentiation.

Laura Johnston, Genetics and Development. Control of growth and cell division during development.

Eric Kandel, Physiology and Cellular Biophysics/Psychiatry/Biochemistry and Molecular Biophysics; Howard Hughes Medical Institute Investigator and Nobel Laureate in Physiology or Medicine 2000; Member, National Academy of Sciences. Cell and molecular mechanisms of associative and nonassociative learning.

Richard Mann, Biochemistry and Molecular Biophysics. Transcriptional control.

Ann McDermott, Chemistry/Biological Sciences/Chemical Engineering; Member, National Academy of Sciences. Solid-state NMR of enzyme active sites and model systems.

Arthur G. Palmer, Biochemistry and Molecular Biophysics. Biomolecular dynamics, structure, and function; NMR spectroscopy.

Liam Paninski, Statistics. Statistical analysis of neural and imaging data.

Virginia Papaioannou, Genetics and Development. Genetic control of mammalian development in the peri-implantation period.

Itsik Pe'er, Computer Science. Novel computational methods in human genetics.

Rodney Rothstein, Genetics and Development. Yeast genetics; mechanisms of genetic recombination; control of genome stability; functional genomics.

Christian Schindler, Microbiology/Medicine. JAK-STAT signaling and immune response.

Steve Siegelbaum, Pharmacology; Howard Hughes Medical Institute Investigator. Molecular studies of ion channel structure and function; synaptic transmission and plasticity in the mammalian brain.

Gary Struhl, Genetics and Development; Howard Hughes Medical Institute Investigator; Member, National Academy of Sciences. Developmental genetics in *Drosophila.*

Lorraine Symington, Microbiology. Homologous recombination in the yeast *Saccharomyces cerevisiae.*

Richard Vallee, Pathology and Cell Biology. Motor proteins in axonal transport, brain developmental disease, and synaptic function.

Charles Zuker, Biochemistry and Molecular Biophysics/Neuroscience. Signal processing, information transfer, and coding mechanisms in sensory systems.

GEORGIA STATE UNIVERSITY
Department of Biology

 For more information, visit http://petersons.to/gsu-biology

Georgia State University.

Programs of Study

The mission of Georgia State University's Department of Biology is three-fold: to provide undergraduate and graduate students with training and education in the biological sciences; to conduct cutting-edge research that advances the understanding and/or application of biological principles; and to use faculty and student expertise and outreach programs to support community needs.

A large faculty and dedicated staff strive to carry out the Department's mission. The talented Biology faculty comprises both tenure track and non-tenure track members. Tenure-track faculty (professors) are involved in both research and education at the graduate and undergraduate levels. The non-tenure track faculty includes lecturers and academic professionals who focus on undergraduate education, and research professors who focus on scientific investigations. An enthusiastic staff provides administrative support and assistance to faculty and students.

The Department of Biology offers several graduate degree programs including a Master of Science (thesis and non-thesis) and a Doctor of Philosophy. Each degree offers the possibility to concentrate in a specific area of biology. Non-degree programs are also available. Students can choose from a wide range of courses and internships. Multiple research opportunities exist and two interdisciplinary areas of focus—the Molecular Basis of Disease program and the Brains and Behavior program—provide competitive fellowships, seminars, and symposia to support biology undergraduate and graduate researchers. The Department also offers students the unique opportunity to participate in community outreach through the Bio-Bus program, which sends a mobile teaching laboratory to primary and secondary schools throughout Metro Atlanta. The surgical anatomy course is taught through partnership with Atlanta Medical Center, utilizing a medical school–level anatomy laboratory that is equipped with human cadavers for surgical dissection.

The Doctor of Philosophy (Ph.D.) program has four areas of emphasis: Applied and Environmental Biology; Cellular Molecular Biology and Physiology; Molecular Genetics and Biochemistry; and Neurobiology and Behavior. Students are asked to prioritize their choices among the four areas of emphasis. Generally third-year students take a written and oral examination. Upon passing the qualifying examinations, students begin work on dissertations. More information about the Ph.D. program is available at http://biology.gsu.edu/phdprogram/.

The Master of Science (M.S.) program has six areas of emphasis: Applied and Environmental Microbiology; Bioinformatics; Biotechnology; Cellular Molecular Biology and Physiology; Molecular Genetics and Biochemistry; and Neurobiology and Behavior.

Students may choose to apply under a specific area/concentration; however, a concentration is not required. A non-thesis (curriculum-based) or thesis (research-based) course of study may be pursued. It is possible to complete the master's program within one year; however, most students choose to complete the program in about two years.

Students must complete at least 40 semester credit hours of approved course work. More information can be found at http://biology.gsu.edu/masters-program/.

The Department of Biology also offers a non-degree program in graduate studies for students who want to take graduate-level courses (up to 9 hours of course work), but who are not pursuing a graduate degree. More details can be found online at http://biology.gsu.edu/non-degree-program/.

Several study-abroad opportunities are offered that allow Department of Biology graduate students to enroll in science courses taught in Argentina, Taiwan, and Italy.

Research

Research in the Department of Biology reflects the diversity of the field, with faculty interests ranging from the structure and function of a molecule to the organization and evolution of behavior. For the practical purpose of graduate training and administration, members of the Graduate Faculty are grouped into four overlapping primary concentrations: Cell and Molecular Biology and Physiology (CMBP), Neurobiology and Behavior (NB&B), Molecular Genetics and Biochemistry (MGB), and Applied Environmental Microbiology (AEM). Most members of the Graduate Faculty also belong to centers and/or institutes that focus on a specific problem or area in the Biological Sciences.

The Faculty

Faculty in the Department of Biology conduct basic, translational, and collaborative clinical research. Georgia State University is among 10 national universities that have shown notable substantial changes in funding over the past decade (NPR analysis of NIH data). Researchers received $81.7 million from external agencies in fiscal year 2014, marking the third straight year of record-breaking research funding. Department of Biology researchers received $6.5 million from external agencies in fiscal year 2014 making it the highest funded department in the University. Teaching faculty use novel, evidence-based teaching methods that include active learning, problem-based learning, and case studies that ensure that classrooms are student-centered and dynamic.

The Georgia State University Department of Biology consists of 55 full-time faculty, 20 part-time faculty, 9 adjunct faculty, and 3 emeritus faculty. Of the 32 full-time tenure-track faculty, 4 are assistant professors, 13 are associate professors, and 15 are professors with primary appointments in one of the four research disciplines (5 faculty in Applied and Environmental Microbiology, 8 faculty in Cellular Molecular Biology and Physiology, 11 faculty in Molecular Genetics and Biochemistry, and 8 faculty in Neurobiology and Behavior). Of the 23 full-time non-tenure track faculty, 17 are lecturers and 6 are academic professionals dedicated solely to undergraduate education.

Financial Aid

Graduate have access to a wide variety of funding sources, including a limited number of graduate teaching, research, and laboratory assistantships. Assistantships provide stipends and tuition waivers for up to 20 hours or service each week. Students with graduate assistantships also participate in the student health insurance program, for which the university and the college provide premium cost offsets each term. Prospective and current students interested in pursuing graduate assistant positions should contact their program director.

Graduate fellowships are offered through several of the university's interdisciplinary area of focus programs. For more information, please visit the program website or contact the program director(s). The college and many of its departments and institutes have endowed fellowships and awards for their students. In the biology department, these include the Ahmed T. Abdelal Fellowships in Molecular Genetics and Biotechnology, the Donald Ahearn Endowed Fellowship in Applied and Environmental Microbiology, the Neurobiology and Behavior Graduate Fellowship, and the William G. Nolan Memorial Scholarship Award.

Georgia State University

Other forms of financial aid, such as unsubsidized loans and Grad Plus loans, are also available.

Costs

The most current information on tuition and fees is available online at http://sfs.gsu.edu/tuition-fees/what-it-costs/tuition-and-fees/.

Student Group

The Master of Science degree program consists of 205 graduate students who are seeking M.S. degrees (thesis or non-thesis) with concentrations in one of the four research disciplines as well as Bioinformatics and Biotechnology.

The Ph.D. degree program currently consists of 103 graduate students who are seeking a doctorate degree in a number of interdisciplinary research initiatives that are organized within one of four areas of research, each corresponding to one of four different Ph.D. disciplines within the department.

Information on Georgia State's Biology Graduate Student Association (BGSA) can be found at http://sites.gsu.edu/bgsa/#.V5E5HqITWzB.

The University

Located in the heart of downtown Atlanta, Georgia State University has approximately 32,000 undergraduate and graduate students. Georgia State offers full-time and part-time educational opportunities as well as over 250 degree programs. It is a nationally known research institution and ranks within the top 100 public universities for awarding doctoral degrees.

Location

Georgia State University is located in Atlanta, the capital of Georgia. A number of other academic and research institutes are located in Atlanta, including Georgia Institute for Technology, Emory University, Morehouse College, Clark Atlantic University, and the Centers for Disease Control and Prevention. While located in the South, Atlanta has become the cultural and economic hub of an increasingly diverse and multicultural metropolitan area.

The Department of Biology has many internship opportunities available every semester with Zoo Atlanta, Serenbe Farms, and the Georgia Aquarium.

Admission Requirements

An undergraduate grade point average of at least 3.0 is encouraged but not required. GRE scores should fall in at least the 40th percentile in 2 out of 3 areas. Be aware, however, that these are guidelines for scores and are not strict cutoffs points.

All interested students are encouraged to apply. Doctor of Philosophy applicants should contact the Doctor of Philosophy Coordinator at 404-413-5300.

Applying

For fall semester, Master's applications and supporting materials are due July 1. Doctor of Philosophy applications are due by March 15, with a priority deadline of December 6.

For spring semester, Master's applications and supporting materials are due November 15. Doctor of Philosophy applications are accepted for fall semester only.

The application can be filled out online at http://cas.gsu.edu/graduate-studies/admissions/. Required materials include the online application, an application fee, a statement of goals, 3 letters of recommendation, official GRE scores, official TOEFL/IELTS/G-STEP scores (for international students), and officials transcripts of all undergraduate courses.

Correspondence and Information

Department of Biology
Georgia State University
100 Piedmont Avenue, Suite 495
Atlanta, Georgia 30303
United States
Phone: 404-413-5300
Fax: 404-413-5301
E-mail: biology@gsu.edu
Website: www.biology.gsu.edu

HOOD COLLEGE

College of the Arts and Sciences
Program in Biology

 For more information, visit http://petersons.to/hoodcollege-biomedsci

HOOD
C O L L E G E
GRADUATE SCHOOL

Programs of Study

The Biomedical Science program at Hood College Graduate School is designed for the working professional with an undergraduate degree in cell biology, molecular biology, or biochemistry who is ready to move up the career ladder. Tailored specifically to the demands of the region's growing hub of life science research employers, it answers the call for relevant curriculum and evening classes.

The Master of Science (M.S.) in Biomedical Science is a 33-credit program and is designed primarily for individuals who work in government or private-sector laboratories and are seeking a part-time program. It has concentrations in immunology and virology, microbiology, molecular biology, and regulatory compliance. Course work begins with molecular biology, biochemistry, and bioinformatics, after which students select a track in molecular biology or microbiology.

The program's curriculum has a thesis option, which is best suited for students who plan to continue their education beyond the master's degree or pursue research careers. These students typically complete the laboratory research thesis at their places of employment under the supervision of advisers approved by the Graduate School. The thesis option includes 12 credits of core courses, 12 credits of elective courses, 3 credits for a research seminar, and 6 credits for the thesis (including an oral defense of the thesis).

Students who don't have working relationships with laboratories are encouraged to pursue the alternative option, which includes the following: 12 credits of core courses, 18 credits of elective courses, and 3 credits for a research seminar that involves creating a mock grant proposal and providing an oral defense of it.

The Master of Science (M.S.) in Bioinformatics program addresses the cross-cutting core subject areas and skill sets identified by the International Society for Computational Biology as essential for bioinformaticians. With the advent of "big data," bioinformatics has become one of the major growth opportunities in the life sciences. The program meets the growing demand for desk- and bench-based science professionals to demonstrate expertise in the experimental design, data handling and data analysis of biology studies that examine genes— genomics, proteins—proteomics, and metabolites—metabolomics. The 33-credit M.S. program can be completed in as little as two years or longer on a less accelerated schedule. Evening classes accommodate working professionals and are held on the Hood College campus.

A dual-gateway approach allows individuals from both biology and computer backgrounds to enter the program successfully by beginning with different foundation courses. It also ensures that students receive the cross-disciplinary training necessary in today's bioinformatics job market. Students are strongly encouraged to pursue experiential learning with local research labs and biotechnology companies. Course work emphasizes the leadership and project management training needed in the team-based environment of bioinformatics research today. In addition, students have access to a laboratory information management system with features that support modern laboratory operations.

Students benefit from small classes taught by faculty who are highly qualified in computer science, biology and bioinformatics and have experience with top R&D and biotechnology firms and federal and private laboratories. Their professional connections are instrumental in establishing and maintaining relevant partnerships that provide practical learning opportunities.

The 15-credit Bioinformatics Certificate program is designed for individuals with backgrounds in biomedical science, biotechnology, and the life sciences. Students can earn the certificate in one year of full-time study. They acquire the skills to effectively apply appropriate tools concerning genomics, proteomics, and structural biology; communicate effectively in the field; construct and manage bioinformatics data sets; manipulate and configure bioinformatics for downstream analysis; and perform statistical analyses of bioinformatics problems.

Hood's proximity to Fort Detrick and the burgeoning biotech corridor make it the convenient choice for the area's large population of lab and science employees. Strategic location also affords the programs strong relationships with top R&D firms, biotech and pharmaceutical companies, and nearby federal and private laboratories. In addition to highly qualified full-time faculty, students benefit from the knowledge of adjunct instructors who are leaders at NCI, USAMRIID and other major research organizations.

Research Facilities

The Biology Department is housed on the first floor of the Hodson Science and Technology Center, a $20-million complex that opened in 2002. Classrooms and labs are designed to engage students in a rich variety of learning activities. All classrooms are equipped with the latest in multimedia teaching tools. Specially designed and equipped labs for ecology, microbiology, molecular biology, cell culture, physiology, and animal behavior are available for course work and student-faculty research collaborations.

Financial Aid

Hood College offers students an affordable education and the following financial aid options: Federal Direct Unsubsidized and Grad PLUS loans, graduate assistantships, institutional scholarships, state scholarships, veterans' benefits, and workshops.

Students may also receive financial assistance through employer tuition reimbursement programs. In addition, Hood College offers a tuition payment plan that allows students to pay tuition and fees over a four- or five-month period.

Costs

The cost of attendance for graduate students may vary. Tuition and fees are determined by the degree program and the number of enrolled credits per semester. The most current information on tuition and fees can be found online at http://www.hood.edu/Campus-Services/Accounting-Services/Tuition-and-Fees-2016-17.html.

Faculty and Students

Hood College's faculty members are accomplished scholars and experienced practitioners who bring real-world experience to their classrooms. As a result, students from more than 25 countries receive instruction grounded in theoretical understanding and practical application. They learn in small classes that emphasize collaboration, promote a vigorous exchange of ideas, and provide information about different cultures and perspectives on world events.

Location

One of the largest cities in Maryland, Frederick is steeped in history yet firmly rooted in the 21st century. Restaurants, shops, art galleries and museums abound in the cosmopolitan downtown. Suburban neighborhoods, the countryside and smaller towns outside the city offer comfortable living and recreational opportunities.

Hood College

Graduate School classes are held on Hood College's picturesque 50-acre campus, located in a quiet residential area just a 10-minute walk to historic downtown Frederick. The campus is situated in a historic yet growing center of business and industry at the top of the I-270 technology corridor, just an hour from both Washington, D.C., and Baltimore.

The College's location provides access to the greatest concentration of biological scientists, doctoral scientists, engineers, health care providers, mathematical scientists, and technical professionals in the United States. It also maintains an extensive and established network of businesses, government institutions, and military installations. The College boasts close ties with top industries including the aerospace, biomedical, engineering, information technology, life science, and research and development (R&D) industries. These resources provide many academic, internship, networking, and workshop opportunities.

The College and the Graduate School

Hood, a private liberal arts college, consistently ranks among the nation's best colleges, and the same enduring commitment to high quality education prevails at the graduate level.

The Graduate School at Hood College is among the best graduate schools in the nation for high quality education, advanced resources, and convenient scheduling. It has 17 master's programs including the Master of Science in Biomedical Science and 11 post-baccalaureate certificate and education certification programs as well as doctorates in organizational leadership and business administration.

The College's well-regarded faculty and caring support staff provide a quality education at the undergraduate and graduate levels in a small-college environment that integrates the liberal arts with professional studies and experiential learning. Hood's core values and traditions, its commitment to continuous improvement, comparative excellence, and exceeding student expectations have made it a treasured institution to current students and to more than 23,000 graduates living in the United States and around the world.

Hood College prepares students to excel in meeting the personal, professional and global challenges of the future. Hood is committed to the integration of the liberal arts, the professions and technology, to the exploration of values, a sense of community, and to the preparation of students for lives of responsibility, leadership and service.

Applying

The Graduate School at Hood College welcomes applications from qualified candidates holding a minimum of a bachelor's degree from an accredited institution with at least a 2.75 grade point average (GPA) on a 4.0 scale. GRE or GMAT exams are not required. Students with a GPA between 2.5 and 2.7 may be considered for possible provisional admission. Applicants can visit www.hood.edu/gradapply to complete the online application and review required admission materials. Students should review admission requirements for the program in which they are interested in for any additional application requirements.

To ensure timely review of applications and enrollment, Graduate School candidates are encouraged to apply and submit all required supplemental documents by July 15 for the fall semester, December 1 for the spring semester, and May 1 for summer terms. After these dates, completed applications will continue to be accepted, reviewed and considered on a space-available basis. Students applying for an F-1 visa should have their documentation postmarked for fall admission; otherwise, such requests will be deferred for the spring semester.

Correspondence and Information

Hood College
401 Rosemont Avenue
Frederick, Maryland 21701
United States
Phone: 301-696-3600
E-mail: gofurther@hood.edu
Website: www.hood.edu/graduate

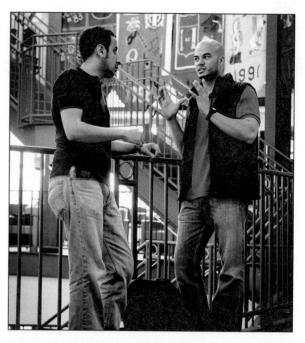

Hood College graduate students in the Whitaker Campus Center, a 24/7 gathering place for the entire campus community.

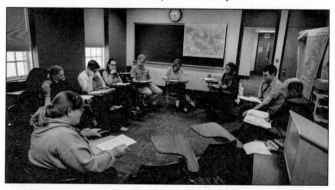

A Hood College graduate school class engages in a group discussion in Rosenstock Hall. Hood's small classes and an emphasis on collaboration stimulate lively exchanges of ideas and information.

Erin George, Ph.D., Assistant Professor of Economics, lectures and leads a class discussion. Hood faculty members bring both scholarly and real-world experience to the classroom, affording students instruction that is grounded in academic knowledge and practical application.

IRELL & MANELLA GRADUATE SCHOOL OF BIOLOGICAL SCIENCES

City of Hope National Medical Center
Beckman Research Institute

Programs of Study

The mission of the City of Hope Graduate School of Biological Sciences is to train students to be outstanding research scientists in chemical, molecular, and cellular biology. Graduates of this program are awarded the degree of Doctor of Philosophy in biological sciences and are equipped to address fundamental questions in the life sciences and biomedicine for careers in academia, industry, and government. The time spent in the program is devoted to full-time study and research. During the first year, the student completes the core curriculum and three laboratory rotations (eight to ten weeks each). The core curriculum contains biochemistry, molecular biology, cell biology, and biostatistics/bioinformatics. After the first year, the student prepares and orally defends a research proposal based on an original topic not related to previous work conducted by the student, and in the second year students prepare and defend a research proposal based on their actual thesis topic. Two additional Advanced Topics courses are required after the first year and students are required to take a literature-based journal club every year after the first year. Students also participate in courses on scientific communication and on the responsible conduct of research. After successfully completing the core curriculum and research proposal, students concentrate the majority of their time on their individual dissertation laboratory research project. The written thesis/dissertation must be presented by the student for examination by 3 members of the City of Hope staff and 1 qualified member from an outside institution.

Research Facilities

City of Hope is a premier medical center, one of sixty-nine National Cancer Institute–designated Comprehensive Cancer Centers. Its Beckman Research Institute launched the biotech industry by creating the first human recombinant gene products, insulin and growth hormone, which are now used by millions of people worldwide. State-of-the-art facilities include mass spectrometry, NMR, molecular modeling, cell sorting, DNA sequencing, molecular pathology, scanning and transmission electron microscopy, confocal microscopy, and molecular imaging. The Lee Graff Medical and Scientific Library allows access to the latest biomedical information via its journal and book collection, document delivery, interlibrary loans, and searches of online databases.

Financial Aid

All students in the Graduate School receive a fellowship of $33,000 per year as well as paid health and dental insurance.

Cost of Study

There are no tuition charges. A student services fee of $50 per semester ($150 per year) is the student's only financial obligation to City of Hope.

Living and Housing Costs

The School has limited, low-cost housing available. Living in student housing provides easy access to campus resources and a connection to the vibrant campus community. Additional housing is available within the immediate area at an average cost of $700 to $1,000 per month.

Student Group

The Graduate School faculty consists of 84 of City of Hope's investigators. Eighty-eight graduate students were working toward the Ph.D. degree in biological sciences in 2015–16.

Student Outcomes

Graduates have gone on to work as postdoctoral fellows at California Institute of Technology; Harvard University; Scripps Research Institute; Stanford University; University of California, Los Angeles; University of California, San Diego; University of California, Irvine; Genentech; University of Southern California; and Washington University in St. Louis. Graduates have also found positions with Wyeth-Ayerst Research; Allergan, Inc.; and the U.S. Biodefense and its subsidary, Stem Cell Research Institute of California, Inc.

Location

City of Hope is located 25 miles northeast of downtown Los Angeles, minutes away from Pasadena and close to beaches, mountains, and many recreational and cultural activities.

The Medical Center and The Institute

City of Hope was founded in 1913, initially as a tuberculosis sanatorium. Research programs were initiated in 1951, and, in 1983, the Beckman Research Institute of City of Hope was established with support from the Arnold and Mabel Beckman Foundation. The Institute comprises basic science research groups within the Divisions of Biology, Immunology, Molecular Medicine, and Neurosciences, among others.

Applying

The deadline for application is January 1 for classes starting in August. Applying early is advisable. Candidates must submit transcripts, three letters of recommendation, and take the Graduate Record Examination (General Test required, Subject Test recommended). For further information and an application, students should contact the School at the address listed in this description.

Correspondence and Information

City of Hope
Irell & Manella Graduate School of Biological Sciences
1500 East Duarte Road
Duarte, California 91010
United States
Phone: 877-715-GRAD or 626-256-4723
Fax: 626-471-3901
E-mail: gradschool@coh.org
Website: http://www.cityofhope.org/gradschool

Irell & Manella Graduate School of Biological Sciences

THE FACULTY AND THEIR RESEARCH

Professors

Karen S. Aboody, M.D. Neural stem cells—therapeutic applications

David K. Ann, Ph.D. Signal transduction, metabolism, genomic integrity, tumorigenesis and progression.

Behnam Badie, M.D., FACS. Development of minimally invasive techniques for treatment of benign and malignant brain tumors.

Michael E. Barish, Ph.D. Physiological and imaging studies of brain tumors.

Edouard M. Cantin, Ph.D. Herpes simplex virus infections in the nervous system.

Wing-Chun (John) Chan, M.D. The functional genomics of lymphoma.

Saswati Chatterjee, Ph.D. Adeno-associated virus vectors for stem-cell gene therapy.

Shiuan Chen, Ph.D. Hormones and cancer.

Yuan Chen, Ph.D. Ubiquitin-like modifications.

Warren Chow, M.D. Cell signaling and cancer.

David Colcher, Ph.D. Immunodiagnostics and immuno-therapeutics.

Don J. Diamond, Ph.D. Translational research in cancer vaccines.

Richard W. Ermel, D.V.M., M.P.V.M., Ph.D. Comparative medicine.

Stephen J. Forman, M.D., FACP. T-Cell immunotherapy for treatment of cancer.

David Horne, Ph.D. Developing natural products as novel anti-cancer agents.

Keiichi Itakura, Ph.D. Functions of Mrf-1 and Mrf-2.

Markus Kalkum, Dr. Rer. Nat. (Ph.D.). Emerging infectious diseases, vaccines, and advanced diagnostics.

Larry W. Kwak, M.D., Ph.D. Hematologic malignancies and stem cell transplantation institute.

Peter P. Lee, Ph.D. The impact of cancer on immune system.

Ren-Jang Lin, Ph.D. RNA splicing, microRNA, and gene screening.

Linda Malkas, Ph.D. The selective targeting of cancer cells.

Marcia M. Miller, Ph.D. Molecular immunogenetics.

Kevin V. Morris, Ph.D. Center for gene therapy.

Rama Natarajan, Ph.D. Diabetic vascular complications.

Susan Neuhausen, Ph.D. Genetic epidemiology of complex diseases.

Timothy R. O'Connor, Ph.D. DNA repair.

Gerd P. Pfeifer, Ph.D. Molecular mechanisms of cancer.

Arthur D. Riggs, Ph.D. Epigenetics, chromatin structure, and gene regulation.

Bart O. Roep, Ph.D. Translating cause to cure of type 1 diabetes.

Steven T. Rosen, M.D. Developing novel therapies for treatment of hematologic malignancies.

John J. Rossi, Ph.D. The biology and applications of small RNAs.

Paul M. Salvaterra, Ph.D. Modeling Alzheimer-type neurodegeneration.

Victoria Seewaldt, M.D. Wellness and breast cancer prevention.

Binghui Shen, Ph.D. DNA replication, repair, and apoptosis nucleases in genome stability and cancer.

Yanhong Shi, Ph.D. Stem cell–based disease modeling and therapeutic development.

John E. Shively, Ph.D. Structure, function, and regulation of carcinoembryonic antigen genes.

Steven S. Smith, Ph.D. Cancer epigenetics.

Cy A. Stein, M.D., Ph.D. Cellular delivery of therapeutic oligonucleotides.

Zijie (ZJ) Sun, M.D., Ph.D. Transcriptional regulation, cell signaling, and hormone action in oncogenesis and development.

Zuoming Sun, Ph.D. Mechanisms regulating T cell-mediated immunity.

John Termini, Ph.D. Mutagenesis and carcinogenesis.

Debbie C. Thurmond, Ph.D. Insulin action and insulin secretion dysfunction in diabetes.

Nagarajan Vaidehi, Ph.D. Predicting protein structure and dynamics for drug discovery.

Jeffrey N. Weitzel, M.D. Genetic predisposition to cancer.

Xiaochun Yu, M.D., Ph.D. DNA damage response, epigenetic modifications and their roles in tumorigenesis.

Jiing-Kuan Yee, Ph.D. Vectors for gene therapy.

Hua Yu, Ph.D. Stat 3: from basic discoveries to the clinic.

John A. Zaia, M.D. Anti-HIV/AIDS gene therapy.

Associate and Assistant Professors

Adam M. Bailis, Ph.D. Homologous recombination governs genome dynamics and tumor suppression.

Jacob Berlin, Ph.D. Nanoparticles for the diagnosis and treatment of cancer.

Mark Boldin, M.D., Ph.D. Control of mammalian hematopoiesis, immunity, and cancer by regulatory RNAs.

John Burnett, Ph.D. Development of gene and RNA therapies for acquired diseases and genetic disorders.

Angelo Cardoso, M.D., Ph.D. Leukemia cells and the bone marrow microenvironment.

Ching-Cheng Chen, Ph.D. Cellular and molecular characterization of the hematopoietic niche.

Mike Y. Chen, M.D., Ph.D. CBX mediated epigenetic control of glioblastoma epithelial to mesenchymal cell transition.

WenYong Chen, Ph.D. Epigenetics, cancer, and aging.

Zhen (Jen) Chen, B.Med., Ph.D. Non-coding RNA in epigenetic control and endothelial stress responses.

Jessica Clague DeHart, Ph.D., M.P.H. Identifying molecular mechanisms of exercise for cancer prevention.

Thanh Dellinger, M.D. Innovative gene therapy for ovarian cancer.

Patrick Fueger, Ph.D. Identifying molecular mechanisms regulating homeostasis during health and disease.

Carlotta A. Glackin, Ph.D. Understanding gene regulation from stem cells.

Robert Hickey, Ph.D. Identification and clinical translation of molecular signatures of disease.

Wendong Huang, Ph.D. Metabolic regulation, cancer, and aging.

Janice M. Huss, Ph.D. The role of orphan nuclear receptors in cardiac and skeletal muscle biology.

Rahul Jandial, M.D, Ph.D. Breast metastatic cancer.

Jeremy Jones, Ph.D. The androgen receptor in human disease.

Tijana Jovanovic-Talisman, Ph.D. Super-resolution imaging in drug discovery.

Mei Kong, Ph.D. Signal transduction and cancer metabolism.

Marcin Kortylewski, Ph.D. Immune cells as targets for cancer therapy.

Hsun Teresa Ku, Ph.D. Pancreatic stem cells.

Ya-Huei Kuo, Ph.D. Molecular genetics of hematopoietic stem cells and leukemia stem cells.

Yilun Liu, Ph.D. Human RECQ helicases in aging and cancer prevention.

Qiang Lu, Ph.D. Understanding the mechanisms that control self-renewal and differentiation of neural progenitor/stem cells.

Edwin R. Manuel, Ph.D. Methods to enhance anti-tumor responses.

Edward M. Newman, Ph.D. Biochemical pharmacology of anti-metabolites.

Vu Ngo, Ph.D. Molecular targets in lymphoid malignancies.

Russell Rockne, Ph.D. Mathematical oncology.

Andrei S. Rodin, Ph.D. Computational biology, large data, and molecular evolution.

Dustin E. Schones, Ph.D. Chromatin, gene regulation, gene by environment interactions.

Ben Hung Ping Shih, Ph.D. Stem cell biology and organogenesis.

Jeremy M. Stark, Ph.D. Factors and pathways that influence mammalian chromosomal stability.

Timothy W. Synold, Pharm.D. Pharmacokinetics and pharmacodynamics of anti-cancer drugs.

John C. Williams, Ph.D. Structural biology and biophysics.

Yanzhong (Frankie) Yang, M.D., Ph.D. Epigenetic regulation of gene expression and genome stability.

Defu Zeng, M.D. Transplantation immune tolerance.

THE ROCKEFELLER UNIVERSITY

Graduate Programs

 For more information, visit http://petersons.to/rockefellerbiomedicalsciences

Programs of Study

Graduate education leading to the Ph.D. is offered to outstanding students regarded as potential leaders in their scientific fields. The University's research covers a wide range of biomedical and related sciences, including chemical and structural biology; genetics and genomics; immunology, virology, and microbiology; medical sciences, systems physiology and human genetics; molecular and cell biology; neurosciences and behavior; organismal biology, evolution, ethology, and ecology; physical, mathematical, and computational biology; and stem cells, development, regeneration, and aging, as summarized by the faculty list in this description. Students work closely with a faculty of active scientists and are encouraged to learn through a combination of course work, tutorial guidance, and apprenticeship in research laboratories. Graduate Fellows spend the first two years engaged in a flexible combination of courses geared toward academic qualification while conducting research in laboratories pertaining to their area of scientific interest. They choose a laboratory for thesis research by the end of the first year and devote their remaining time to pursuit of significant experimental or theoretical research, culminating in a dissertation and thesis defense. Students can spend full time in research; there are no teaching or other service obligations.

The faculties of the Rockefeller University, Weill Medical College of Cornell University, the Weill Graduate School of Medical Sciences of Cornell University, and Sloan Kettering Institute collaborate in offering a combined M.D./Ph.D. program in the biomedical sciences to about 120 students. This program, conducted on the adjacent campuses of these three institutions in New York City, normally requires six or seven years of study and leads to an M.D. degree conferred by Cornell University and a Ph.D. degree conferred by either the Rockefeller University or the Weill Graduate School of Cornell University, depending upon the organizational affiliation of the student's adviser.

Research Facilities

The University and its affiliate Howard Hughes Medical Institute maintain a full range of laboratories and services for the research activities of the professional staff and students. Facilities include clinical and animal research centers on campus, a library, computing services, a field research center in Dutchess County, the Aaron Diamond AIDS Research Center (ADARC), as well as new centers for human genetics, studies in physics and biology, biochemistry and structural biology, immunology and immune diseases, sensory neuroscience, and Alzheimer's disease research.

Financial Aid

Each student accepted into the Ph.D. program receives a stipend ($38,200 in 2016–17) that is adequate to meet all living expenses. Students also receive an annual budget of $1,500 that can be used for travel, books and journals, computer purchases, and lab supplies.

Cost of Study

The University provides full remission of all tuition and fees for all accepted students.

Living and Housing Costs

On-campus housing is available for all students at subsidized rates. The stipend is designed to cover the cost of food, housing, and other basic living expenses. Students may elect to live off campus, but rents in the vicinity are very high.

Student Group

There are 194 graduate students, of whom 164 are enrolled in the Ph.D. program and 30 in the Ph.D. phase of the combined M.D./Ph.D. program. It is the policy of the Rockefeller University to support equality of educational opportunity. No individual is denied admission to the University or otherwise discriminated against with respect to any program of the University because of creed, color, national or ethnic origin, race, sex, or disability.

Student Outcomes

Graduates of the Rockefeller University have excelled in their professions. Two graduates have been awarded the Nobel Prize, and 31 graduates are members of the National Academy of Sciences. Most Ph.D. graduates move to postdoctoral positions at academic and research centers and subsequently have careers in academics, biotechnology, and the pharmaceutical industry. A few have pursued careers in medicine, law, and business. Almost all M.D./Ph.D. graduates first complete residencies in medical specialties, and most become medical scientists at major academic and medical research centers.

Location

The University is situated between 62nd and 68th streets in Manhattan, overlooking the East River. Despite its central metropolitan location, the 15-acre campus has a distinctive nonurban character, featuring gardens, picnic areas, fountains, and a tennis court. In addition to administrative and residential buildings, there are seven large laboratory buildings and a forty-bed hospital that serves as a clinical research center. Immediate neighbors are the New York Hospital, the Weill Medical College of Cornell University, Memorial Hospital, and the Sloan-Kettering Institute for Cancer Research. The wide range of institutions in New York City affords unlimited opportunities in research specialties, library facilities, and cultural resources.

The University

The Rockefeller University is dedicated to benefiting humankind through scientific research and its application. Founded in 1901 by John D. Rockefeller as the Rockefeller Institute for Medical Research, it rapidly became a source of major scientific innovation in treating and preventing human disease. Since 1954, the institute has extended its function by offering graduate work at the doctoral level to a select group of qualified students.

Laboratories, rather than departments, are the fundamental units of the University. The absence of departmental barriers between laboratories encourages interdisciplinary, problem-oriented approaches to research and facilitates intellectual interaction and collaboration. The collegial atmosphere fosters independence and initiative in students. In addition to the 194 doctoral students, there are 315 postdoctoral associates and fellows and a faculty of 78 full, associate, and assistant professors on campus who head laboratories.

Applying

Applications for the M.D./Ph.D. program must be completed by September 30; those for the Ph.D. program must be completed by December 1. Applicants are required to submit a personal statement describing research experience and goals as well as reasons for pursuing graduate study at The Rockefeller University. Also required are official transcripts and at least three letters of recommendation. Official GRE General Test scores are required and Subject Test scores are highly recommended for admission to the Ph.D. program. MCAT scores are required for the M.D./Ph.D. program. Further information about each program and details on application procedures may be obtained from the programs' respective websites. This information is also available on the University website, from which application forms and instructions can be downloaded (https://graduateapplication.rockefeller.edu).

Correspondence and Information

Kristen E. Cullen, M.A.
Graduate Admissions Administrator and Registrar
The David Rockefeller Graduate Program
The Rockefeller University
1230 York Avenue, Box 177
New York, New York 10065
Phone: 212-327-8086
E-mail: phd@rockefeller.edu
Website: http://www.rockefeller.edu/graduate
        https://www.facebook.com/rockefelleruniversity
        https://twitter.com/rockefelleruniv

LABORATORY HEADS AND THEIR RESEARCH

C. David Allis, Ph.D. (Chromatin Biology and Epigenetics). Studies the role of DNA packaging proteins in gene expression and DNA replication and repair.

Gregory Alushin, Ph.D. (Biophysics). Using cryo-electron microscopy to determine how molecules change their structure in response to pushing or pulling forces.

Cori Bargmann, Ph.D. (Neural Circuits and Behavior). Studies the relationship between genes, neural circuits and behavior in *C. elegans*.

Paul Bieniasz, Ph.D. (Retrovirology) Studies the biology and evolution of retroviruses, including HIV, and genetics of host-virus interactions.

Kivanc Birsoy, Ph.D. (Cancer Cell Metabolism). Investigating cellular metabolism with an emphasis on cancer and metabolic disorders.

Günter Blobel, M.D., Ph.D. (Cell Biology). Uses genetic, biochemical, and ultrastructural methods to elucidate mechanisms of protein production and regulation.

Sean Brady, Ph.D. (Genetically Encoded Small Molecules). Discovers and characterizes new small molecules from microbial sources.

Jan L. Breslow, M.D. (Biochemical Genetics and Metabolism). Investigates the genetic basis of atherosclerotic disease.

Ali Brivanlou, Ph.D. (Stem Cell Biology and Molecular Embryology).Researches the molecular events and cellular interactions that establish cell fate in vertebrate embryogenesis.

The Rockefeller University

Jean-Laurent Casanova, M.D., Ph.D. (Human Genetics of Infectious Diseases). Researches the genetic basis of pediatric infectious diseases.

Brian T. Chait, D.Phil. (Mass Spectrometry and Gaseous Ion Chemistry). Uses mass spectrometry as a tool for studying biomolecules and protein interactions.

Jue Chen, Ph.D. (Membrane Biology and Biophysics). Combines structural and function techniques to study ABC membrane transporter proteins in health and disease.

Nam-Hai Chua, Ph.D. (Plant Molecular Biology). Studies molecular signaling pathways involved in plants' response to stress, light and infection.

Joel Cohen, Ph.D., Dr.P.H. (Populations). Studies interactions among groups of living beings in order to develop concepts helpful for understanding populations.

Paul Cohen, M.D., Ph.D. (Molecular Metabolism). Investigates the molecular basis for metabolic disease related to obesity.

Barry Coller, M.D. (Blood and Vascular Biology). Investigates the role of blood platelets and the mechanisms of blood cell adhesion in vascular disease.

Frederick P. Cross, Ph.D. (Cell Cycle Genetics). Investigates the molecular basis of cell cycle control.

Robert B. Darnell, M.D., Ph.D. (Molecular Neuro-Oncology). Works to understand human autoimmune responses to cancer and neurologic disease.

Seth Darst, Ph.D. (Molecular Biophysics). Investigates the structure, function and regulation of the bacterial transcription machinery.

Titia de Lange, Ph.D. (Cell Biology and Genetics). Studies how telomeres protect chromosome ends from the DNA damage response.

Mitchell J. Feigenbaum, Ph.D. (Mathematical Physics). Develops mathematical descriptions and predictions of natural events that exhibit erratic behavior.

Vincent A. Fischetti, Ph.D. (Bacterial Pathogenesis and Immunology). Investigates bacterial infectious disease and the use of phage enzymes to block infection.

Winrich Freiwald, Ph.D. (Neural Systems). Researches the neural processes of object recognition and attention.

Jeffrey M. Friedman, M.D., Ph.D. (Molecular Genetics). Studies the molecular mechanisms that regulate food intake and body weight.

Elaine Fuchs, Ph.D. (Mammalian Cell Biology and Development). Investigates molecular mechanisms of skin stem cells, how they make and repair tissues, and how cancers develop.

Hinonori Funabiki, Ph.D. (Chromosome and Cell Biology). Studies signaling events in chromosome segregation in mitosis.

David C. Gadsby, Ph.D. (Cardiac and Membrane Physiology). Works to understand how ion transport proteins function in cells.

Charles D. Gilbert, M.D., Ph.D. (Neurobiology). Studies neural mechanisms of visual perception, learning and memory.

Konstantin A. Goulianos, Ph.D. (Experimental High-Energy Physics). Studies interactions among basic constituents of matter in order to explore the evolution and fate of the universe.

Paul Greengard, Ph.D. (Molecular and Cellular Neuroscience). Researches the molecular basis of communication between neurons in the mammalian brain.

Howard C. Hang, Ph.D. (Chemical Biology and Microbial Pathogenesis). Develops chemical tools for the study of microbe-host interaction.

Mary E. Hatten, Ph.D. (Developmental Neurobiology). Investigates mechanisms of neuronal differentiation and migration during embryonic development.

Nathaniel Heintz, Ph.D. (Molecular Biology). Investigates histological and functional aspects of the mammalian brain in health and disease.

David D. Ho, M.D. (Dynamics of HIV/SIV Replication). Pursues the development of drugs and vaccines to prevent HIV transmission.

A. James Hudspeth, M.D., Ph.D. (Sensory Neuroscience). Studies neural mechanisms of hearing and pursues treatments for hearing loss.

Erich Jarvis, Ph.D. (Neurobiology). Studies the mechanisms behind vocal learning, with an emphasis on the molecules that guide neuronal connections from motor learning pathways to vocal neurons.

Tarun Kapoor, Ph.D. (Chemistry and Cell Biology). Investigates molecular and physical mechanisms of cell division.

Sebastian Klinge, Ph.D. (Protein and Nucleic Acid Chemistry). Studies the structure and function of macromolecular complexes involved in eukaryotic ribosome assembly.

Bruce W. Knight Jr. (Biophysics). Develops mathematical descriptions of the nerve networks involved in visual perception.

Mary Jeanne Kreek, M.D. (Biology of Addictive Diseases). Investigates the genetic basis of, and novel treatments for, addictive diseases.

Daniel Kronauer, Ph.D. (Insect Social Evolution). Studies evolution in insect societies at the level of the gene, individual, and colony.

James G. Krueger, M.D., Ph.D. (Investigative Dermatology). Uses psoriasis as a model to investigate the pathogenesis of inflammatory disease and autoimmunity.

Stanislas Leibler, Ph.D. (Living Matter). Conducts quantitative analyses of microbial systems on cellular and population levels.

Albert J. Libchaber, Ph.D. (Experimental Condensed-Matter Physics). Applies mathematical models to biological systems at organismal, cellular, and molecular levels.

Shixin Liu, Ph.D. (Nanoscale Biophysics and Biochemistry). Investigates the interactions between biological machines, such as the transcription and translation apparatuses in bacteria.

Roderick MacKinnon, M.D. (Molecular Neurobiology and Biophysics). Studies principles underlying electricity in biology, particularly the passage of ions across cell membranes.

Marcelo Magnasco, Ph.D. (Mathematical Physics). Creates computational and mathematical models to describe neurophysiological systems and living organisms.

Gaby Maimon, Ph.D. (Integrative Brain Function). Studies electrical activity and computation underlying behavior in *Drosophila*.

Luciano Marraffini, Ph.D. (Bacteriology). Investigates the exchange of genetic material among bacteria.

Bruce S. McEwen, Ph.D. (Neuroendocrinology). Studies molecular mechanisms underlying effects of stress and sex hormones on the brain.

Daniel Mucida, Ph.D. (Mucosal Immunology). Investigates mechanisms of immune activity and tolerance in intestinal mucosa.

Fernando Nottebohm, Ph.D. (Animal Behavior). Investigates the biology of vocal learning and neuronal replacement in songbirds.

Michel C. Nussenzweig, M.D., Ph.D. (Molecular Immunology). Studies molecular aspects of adaptive and innate immune responses.

Michael O'Donnell, Ph.D. (DNA Replication). Studies molecular mechanisms of DNA replication, recombination, and repair.

F. Nina Papavasiliou, Ph.D. (Lymphocyte Biology). Studies RNA editing and DNA mutation as creators of information diversity in biological systems.

Donald W. Pfaff, Ph.D. (Neurobiology and Behavior). Studies steroid hormone effects on nerve cells regulating specific natural behaviors and overall CNS arousal.

Priya Rajasethupathy, Ph.D. (Neurobiology). Investigates genetic and circuit level mechanisms that underlie disturbances in memory processing.

Jeffrey V. Ravetch, M.D., Ph.D. (Molecular Genetics and Immunology). Investigates mechanisms of the functional diversity of antibodies in host defense and immunotherapy.

George N. Reeke Jr., Ph.D. (Biological Modeling). Uses computational modeling to understand complex biological or neurological functions.

Charles Rice, Ph.D. (Virology). Investigates mechanisms of hepatitis C virus infection and replication.

Robert G. Roeder, Ph.D. (Biochemistry and Molecular Biology). Studies the proteins and enzymes that execute and regulate gene transcription.

Michael P. Rout, Ph.D. (Cellular and Structural Cell Biology). Researches the structure of nuclear pore complexes and their role in oncogenic and developmental defects.

Vanessa Ruta, Ph.D. (Neurophysiology and Behavior). Investigates neural circuits that underlie innate and learned behaviors.

Thomas P. Sakmar, M.D. (Chemical Biology and Signal Transduction). Conducts biological and chemical investigations of G protein coupled receptors.

Shai Shaham, Ph.D. (Developmental Genetics). Investigates the role of glial cells in nervous system development and function.

Eric Siggia, Ph.D. (Theoretical Condensed-Matter Physics). Uses bioinformatics to study regulatory patterns in gene expression.

Sanford M. Simon, Ph.D. (Cellular Biophysics). Uses imaging techniques and other biophysical tools to study single events in biological systems.

Agata Smogorzewska, M.D., Ph.D. (Genome Maintenance). Uses Fanconia anemia as a backdrop to investigate DNA repair mechanisms in aging and cancer.

C. Erec Stebbins, Ph.D. (Structural Microbiology). Examines the targeting of host machineries by bacterial virulence factors.

Hermann Steller, Ph.D. (Apoptosis and Cancer Biology). Investigates signaling pathways underlying apoptosis.

Sidney Strickland, Ph.D. (Neurobiology and Genetics). Investigates neurovascular dysfunction in Alzheimer's disease and hemorrhagic stroke.

Alexander Tarakhovsky, M.D., Ph.D. (Immune Cell Epigenetics and Signaling). Investigates the epigenetic control of immune gene expression.

Sohail Tavazoie, M.D., Ph.D. (Systems Cancer Biology). Uses a variety of laboratory and clinical approaches to study the processes of cancer metastasis.

Marc Tessier-Lavigne, Ph.D. (Brain Development and Repair). Investigates nerve circuit formation and regeneration and the mechanisms underlying nerve cell death.

Alexander Tomasz, Ph.D. (Microbiology and Infectious Diseases). Tracks and studies mechanisms of bacterial antibiotic resistance.

Thomas Tuschl, Ph.D. (RNA Molecular Biology). Investigates gene regulatory mechanisms triggered by double-stranded RNA and RNA-binding proteins.

Alipasha Vaziri, Ph.D. (Neurotechnology and Biophysics). Develops and applies new optical imaging techniques with the goal of creating functional images of neural circuits.

Gabriel Victora, Ph.D. (Lymphocyte Dynamics). Investigates the molecular mechanisms behind the immune response.

Leslie Vosshall, Ph.D. (Neurogenetics and Behavior). Investigates how odor stimuli are processed and perceived.

Thomas Walz, Ph.D. (Structural Biology). Using cryo-electron microscopy to understand how the protein structure of membranes enables them to perform their functions.

Michael W. Young, Ph.D. (Genetics). Investigates the genetic regulation of biological clocks that underlie many activities of living organisms.

Li Zhao, Ph.D. (Evolutionary Biology). Using CRISPR-Cas 9 genome editing to investigate the biological func-tion of de novo genes; Investigates the role of natural selection in the origin of genes.

UNIVERSITY OF CALIFORNIA, SAN DIEGO
College of the Arts and Sciences
Program in Biology

UC San Diego

 For more information, visit http:/petersons.to/uc-sandiego_biosci

Programs of Study

The University of California, San Diego (UC San Diego), Division of Biological Sciences, in association with the Salk Institute for Biological Studies, offers a program of graduate studies leading to the Ph.D. degree in biology. The program provides an extraordinary setting for highly motivated students interested in training with distinguished faculty members. The major areas of faculty research are biochemistry and biophysics; bioinformatics; cell and developmental biology; ecology, behavior, and evolution; genetics; immunology, virology, and cancer biology; molecular biology; neurobiology; plant molecular biology; plant systems biology; and signal transduction.

The goal of the program is to enable highly talented individuals to develop the skills and experience necessary to become successful world-class scientists, in a supportive and stimulating environment. The program includes training in writing research papers and grant applications, presentation of lectures, the ethical conduct of research, and professional skill development to enhance career options. These skills allow graduates to pursue a broad range of careers that involve the use of science to increase the quality of life everywhere.

The educational philosophy of the Biological Sciences doctoral program is to provide a supportive and stimulating environment for highly talented individuals to develop skills and experience necessary to become research leaders in academic and biotechnology, biomedical, or pharmaceutical industries. The program recognizes that graduate students have various career goals and that training and advising requires a broad range of information. Ph.D.'s graduating from the program will have sought after skills and experiences suited to a broad range of career paths, ranging from faculty positions at research universities and teaching colleges through positions in private industry to leadership roles in science communication and policy.

Students must complete the course requirements for one of the program's curricular tracks. Most course work is completed during the first year. All incoming doctoral students take Graduate Boot Camp and Graduate School Fundamentals courses during their first quarter.

Lectures in molecular biology, cell biology, and genetics that provide an advanced foundation in these fundamental disciplines are complemented by small group discussions with faculty moderators focused on the critical evaluation of the primary scientific literature. Flexibility for each student to pursue individual interests during the first year is provided not only through rotations, but also through elective courses. Once the core course load is completed, students are encouraged to take other courses that enhance their education and research experience.

Building synergies with special and often interdisciplinary training programs is a hallmark of the Ph.D. program. These programs help students develop a broad set of research and professional skills and create vibrant intellectual communities.

Research Facilities

Students have access to more than 100 modern and fully equipped research laboratories in the Division of Biological Sciences and the Salk Institute. The division is also associated with three organized research groups: the Center for Molecular Genetics, the Kavli Institute for Brain and Mind, and the San Diego Center for Molecular Agriculture. Campus research facilities and tools include the San Diego Supercomputer Center; the Biomedical Genomics Microarray Center; the Protein Sequencing Facility; the Biomolecular Mass Spectrometry Facility; a DNA sequencer; and confocal, electron, and photon microscopes. The campus also houses the $115-million San Diego Consortium for Regenerative Medicine facility dedicated to stem cell research.

Biology faculty head several campuswide interdisciplinary initiatives that include other on-campus and off-campus units. These centers create critical research mass well-suited to tackle big research challenges and to jointly propose innovative solutions. Other facilities where students may be involved with research efforts include the Biomedical Genomics Laboratory, the Center for Circadian Biology, the Center for Neural Circuits and Behavior, the California Center for Algae Biotechnology, the San Diego Center for systems Biology, the UC San Diego Natural Reserve system, the UC San Diego Stem Cell Initiative, and Food & Fuel for the 21st Century.

Financial Aids

The Division of Biological Sciences supports all Ph.D. students with an annual stipend. The stipend is funded by federal and state grants and private sources. The stipend is provided in the form of research and teaching assistantships, fellowships, and NIH training grant appointments. International students receive the same level of support as domestic students.

The Program will pay only 1 year of nonresident tuition for U.S. citizens who are non-California residents. It is the responsibility of the nonresident student to become an official resident of the State of California by the end of their first year in order to be exempt from out-of-state tuition in subsequent years.

Students are expected to apply for extramural predoctoral fellowships such as those offered by the National Science Foundation, Ford Foundation, etc., in addition to those administered by the University. If the student is successful and receives funding outside of UC San Diego in the form of a fellowship (e.g., AHA, NIH, Merck, Ford Foundation, home country) that provides stipend and/or fee support, the student may be eligible for a bonus of up to $3,000 above the standard biology graduate stipend.

Housing

All full-time graduate students are eligible for Associated Residential Community Housing. More information is available at http://hdh.ucsd.edu/arch/pages/FAQ.html. Students may also choose to seek their own off-campus housing.

The Faculty

The Division of Biological Science's outstanding faculty and research programs attract the best and brightest students, who want to learn from researchers working at the cutting edge of their respective fields. This concentration of many of the best scientific minds in the world creates truly invaluable learning opportunities for students, providing a scientific breadth and diversity that is tremendously beneficial to their education. A complete listing of faculty members and their areas of research is available online at http://biology.ucsd.edu/publicinfo/dwc?action=faculty_research_list.

Location

UC San Diego and the Salk Institute are located on the Torrey Pines Mesa, along the San Diego coast, overlooking the Pacific Ocean. The campus is also an easy drive from several mountain and desert locales. Along with San Diego's dry, temperate climate, UC San Diego is ideally situated to offer its students year-round outdoor recreational opportunities. The area also shares a rich heritage with its neighbor, Mexico, and supports many cultural events.

University of California, San Diego

The Torrey Pines Mesa is the setting of a world-class scientific and research community as well. This community includes the UC San Diego School of Medicine, the Scripps Institution of Oceanography, the Scripps Research Institute, the Neurosciences Institute, the La Jolla Institute for Allergy and Immunology, the Burnham Institute for Medical Research, the Sidney Kimmel Cancer Center, and hundreds of biotechnology research firms.

The University

UC San Diego is one of the nation's most accomplished research universities, widely acknowledged for its local impact, national influence, and global reach. A leader in climate science research, UC San Diego is one of the greenest universities in the U.S. and works with communities, governments, businesses, and organizations to promote sustainability solutions throughout the region and the world.

With a majestic view of the Pacific Ocean, this distinctively beautiful campus is both a magnet and a catalyst for acclaimed institutes and Nobel laureates. The University's award-winning scholars are experts at the forefront of their fields, with an impressive track record for achieving scientific, medical, and technological breakthroughs. Renowned for its collaborative, diverse, and cross-disciplinary ethos that transcends traditional boundaries in science, arts, and the humanities, UC San Diego attracts like-minded faculty and staff members and stellar students.

Applying

Admission to UC San Diego's Ph.D. program in Biology is highly competitive with only 35–40 students joining the doctoral program each year. New students are admitted for fall quarter only. Competitive applicants must demonstrate excellent undergraduate training in the biological sciences and a strong commitment to research.

Students with exceptional achievement and diverse backgrounds are encouraged to apply. UCSD does not discriminate on the basis of nationality, race, socioeconomic status, sexual orientation, sex, citizenship or disability.

Approximately 30 percent of each incoming class consists of international students. As such, qualified international applicants are also encouraged to apply.

Prospective students should use the UCSC Application for Graduation Admission online. In addition to the application forms, applicants must submit a copy of their GRE test scores, 3 letters of recommendation, a copy of their most recent academic transcripts, and a statement of purpose. It is recommended that applications be submitted well before the deadline to be considered for on-campus interviews.

Applications are processed in order in which they are submitted. Screening of applications will begin in late November. Applications are evaluated by the Admissions Committee (which is comprised of representatives from both the faculty and graduate students) November through January. Important factors in the evaluation of an application include: the nature and quality of the applicant's undergraduate degree program; past academic performance; preparation in the physical sciences and mathematics; previous laboratory and/or field research experience; statement of purpose; letters of recommendation; scores on the Graduate Record Exam; and scores on the English Proficiency Exams (international applicants only).

Selected applicants will be invited to visit the campus and participate in faculty interviews in February. The interviews consist of meetings with both faculty and graduate students, as well as the opportunity to visit the UCSD campus and the surrounding research community. Based on the results of the interviews, offers of admission in most cases will be made before the end of February. All applicants will be notified of the Division's decision no later than March 15.

Correspondence and Information

Dr. Jens Lykke-Andersen, Graduate Director
Division of Biological Sciences
University of California, San Diego
9500 Gilman Drive
La Jolla, California 92093
United States
Phone: 858-534-2580
E-mail: biogradprog@ucsd.edu
Website: https://biology.ucsd.edu/education/grad/current/index.html

UCONN HEALTH
Graduate Programs in Biomedical Sciences

UCONN
HEALTH

 For more information, visit http://petersons.to/uconnhealth_biomed

Programs of Study

Work leading to the Ph.D. degree in biomedical sciences and master's degrees in dental sciences, public health, and clinical and translational research is offered through Graduate School faculty members associated with the Schools of Medicine and Dental Medicine at the UConn Health in Farmington. A combined-degree program with the School of Medicine offers an M.D./Ph.D. degree to qualified students interested in academic medicine and research. The School of Dental Medicine offers a D.M.D./Ph.D. and a Combined Certificate Training Ph.D. program for students with advanced dental degrees. In addition, the Schools of Medicine and Dental Medicine, in conjunction with the Public Health Program, offer a combined program leading to the M.D./M.P.H. or D.M.D./M.P.H. Ph.D. students apply to the Integrated Admissions Mode, which offers a first year of study in the basic science curriculum prior to the selection of an area of concentration in which to pursue the Ph.D. thesis work.

Research Facilities

Programs are located at UConn Health in Farmington. A wide range of general and specialized equipment and expertise in the biological, biochemical, and biophysical sciences is available. Students have access to all facilities and equipment necessary for the pursuit of their research programs. In addition, major institutional resources include central small-animal facilities and the Lyman Maynard Stowe Library that contains approximately 200,000 volumes and 450 CAI programs and subscribes to more than 1,700 current periodicals.

Financial Aid

Support for biomedical science doctoral students engaged in full-time degree programs at UConn Health is provided on a competitive basis. Graduate research assistantships for 2016–17 provide a stipend of $29,000 per year, which includes a waiver of tuition/most University fees for the fall and spring semesters and the option of participating in a student health insurance plan. While financial aid is offered competitively, UConn Health makes every possible effort to address the financial needs of all doctoral students during their period of training.

Cost of Study

For 2016–17, tuition is $14,310 per year for full-time students who are Connecticut residents and $35,346 per year for full-time students who are out-of-state residents. General University fees are added to the cost of tuition for students who do not receive a tuition waiver. These costs are usually met by traineeships or research assistantships for doctoral students.

Living and Housing Costs

There is a wide range of affordable housing options in the greater Hartford area within easy commuting distance of the campus, including an extensive complex that is adjacent to UConn Health. Costs range from $700 to $1,000 per month for a one-bedroom unit; 2 or more students sharing an apartment usually pay less. University housing is not available on campus.

Student Group

Approximately 550 students in the Schools of Medicine and Dental Medicine, 400 graduate students in the Ph.D. and master's programs, and numerous postdoctoral fellows use the facilities in Farmington.

Location

UConn Health is located in the historic town of Farmington, Connecticut. Set in the beautiful New England countryside on a hill overlooking the Farmington Valley, it is close to ski areas, hiking trails, and facilities for boating, fishing, and swimming. Connecticut's capital city of Hartford, 7 miles east of Farmington, is the center of an urban region of approximately 800,000 people. The beaches of the Long Island Sound are about 50 minutes away to the south, and the beautiful Berkshires are a short drive to the northwest. New York City and Boston can be reached within 2½ hours by car. Hartford is the home of the acclaimed Hartford Stage Company, TheatreWorks, the Hartford Symphony and Chamber orchestras, two ballet companies, an opera company, the Wadsworth Athenaeum (the oldest public art museum in the nation), the Mark Twain house, the Hartford Civic Center, and many other interesting cultural and recreational facilities. The area is also home to several branches of the University of Connecticut, Trinity College, and the

University of Hartford, which includes the Hartt School of Music. Bradley International Airport (about 30 minutes from campus) serves the Hartford/Springfield area with frequent airline connections to major cities in this country and abroad. Frequent bus and rail service is also available from Hartford.

The UConn Health Campus

The 200-acre UConn Health campus at Farmington houses a division of the University of Connecticut Graduate School, as well as the Schools of Medicine and Dental Medicine. The campus also includes the John Dempsey Hospital, associated clinics, and extensive medical research facilities, all in a centralized facility with more than 1 million square feet of floor space. The Academic Research Building, built in 1999, is an impressive eleven-story structure providing 170,000 square feet of laboratory space and renovations are underway in the main Laboratory building, converting existing lab space into state-of-the-art open lab areas. In addition, the Jackson Laboratory for Genomic Medicine opened its 189,000-square-foot facility on the UConn Health campus in fall 2014. There are more than 260 full-time members at UConn Health. The institution has a strong commitment to graduate study within an environment that promotes social and intellectual interaction among the various educational programs. Graduate students are represented on various administrative committees concerned with curricular affairs, and the Graduate Student Organization (GSO) represents graduate students' needs and concerns to the faculty and administration, in addition to fostering social contact among graduate students at UConn Health.

Applying

Prospective students should check with their degree program of interest for specific admission requirements. For the biomedical science Ph.D. program, applications for admission should be submitted via the online application system and should be filed together with transcripts, three letters of recommendation, a personal statement, and recent results from the General Test of the Graduate Record Examinations. International students must take the Test of English as a Foreign Language (TOEFL) to satisfy Graduate School requirements. The deadline for completed applications and receipt of all supplemental materials is **December 1** for the Ph.D. in Biomedical Science program. Note that GRE and TOEFL exams taken after the due date will not be accepted for consideration for admission. In accordance with the laws of the state of Connecticut and of the United States, UConn Health does not discriminate against any person in its educational and employment activities on the grounds of race, color, creed, national origin, sex, age, or physical disability. Details and contact information for additional degree programs is available online at grad.uchc.edu.

Correspondence and Information

Graduate Admissions Office
Ph.D. in Biomedical Science Program
UConn Health
263 Farmington Ave., MC 3906
Farmington, Connecticut 06030-3906
United States
Phone: 860-679-4509
E-mail: BiomedSciAdmissions@uchc.edu
Website: http://health.uconn.edu/graduate-school/academics/programs/
      ph-d-biomedical-science/

FACULTY AND RESEARCH AREAS

Biomedical Science Ph.D. Research Areas:

UConn Health's graduate faculty of more than 150 members is drawn from both the basic and clinical departments of the Schools of Medicine and Dental Medicine.

Cell Analysis and Modeling (CAM). This program is designed to train students from diverse disciplinary backgrounds in the cutting-edge research techniques that comprise the interdisciplinary research of modern cell biology. Faculty members associated with this area explore complex biological systems using computational cell biology, optical imaging, and other quantitative approaches to analyze processes in living cells. The CAM program is particularly strong in the following areas of research: cellular modeling (analysis and simulation, data integration, modeling movies boundaries, modularity and multistate complexes, molecular flux in crowded spaces, stochastic modeling and discrete particles); biophysics (biological signaling platforms, in vivo nanofabrication); optical imaging (fluorescent correlation spectroscopy, optical probe development, second harmonic generation, single-molecule imaging); cell biology (cellular tissues and development, cytoskeletal dynamics, RNA trafficking, signal transduction, molecular medicine). John H. Carson, Professor of Molecular, Microbial, and Structural Biology and Program Director.

Cell Biology. This interdisciplinary program offers the student the opportunity to bring modern molecular and physical techniques to bear on problems in cell biology. Faculty members' research spans a broad range of interests in the areas of eukaryotic cell biology and related clinical aspects. The program is particularly strong in the following areas of research: angiogenesis, cancer biology, gene expression, molecular medicine, reproductive biology, signal transduction, vascular biology, optical methods, proteomics, and computer modeling of complex biological systems. Guo-Hua Fong, Associate Professor of Cell Biology and Center for Vascular Biology and Program Director.

Genetics and Developmental Biology. This program emphasizes cellular and molecular bases of differentiation and development and includes opportunities in molecular human genetics. Research opportunities are available in the biology of human embryonic stem cells, mapping and cloning of genes responsible for human disease, RNA processing (including RNA editing, alternative splicing, antisense regulation, and RNA interference), the molecular mechanisms of aging, signal transduction pathways, microbial pathogenesis, developmental neurobiology, cell differentiation, musculoskeletal development, morphogenesis and pattern formation, reproductive biology, and endocrinology. Blanka Rogina, Associate Professor of Genetics and Developmental Biology and Program Director.

Immunology. The central focus of this program is to train the student to become an independent investigator and educator who will provide research and educational contributions to basic, applied, or clinical immunology through lectures, seminars, laboratory rotations, research presentations, and a concentration on laboratory research. Research in the program is focused on the cellular and molecular aspects of immune system structure and function in animal models and in humans. Areas of emphasis include molecular immunology (mechanisms of antigen presentation, major histocompatibility complex genetics and function, cytokines and cytokine receptors, and tumor antigens), cellular immunology (biochemical mechanisms and biological aspects of signal transduction of lymphocytes and granulocytes; cellular and molecular requirements for thymic T-lymphocyte development, selection, and activation; cytokines in B- and T-cell development; regulation of antitumor immunity; immunoparasitology, including parasite genetics and immune recognition of parasite antigens; and mechanisms of inflammation), organ-based immunology (immune effector mechanisms of the intestine, lymphocyte interactions in the lung, and immune regulation of the eye), immunity to infectious agents (viruses, bacteria, and parasites, including vector-borne organisms), and autoimmunity (animal models of autoimmune disease and effector mechanisms in human autoimmunity). H. Leonardo Aguila, Associate Professor of Immunology and Program Director.

Molecular Biology and Biochemistry. This program uniquely bridges modern molecular biology, microbiology, biochemistry, cell biology, and structural biology. Research in this program is directed toward explaining biological phenomena at the molecular level. The program includes four major areas of concentration and research: relation of the structure of macromolecules to their function, biosynthesis of macromolecules, biochemical genetics, and assembly of macromolecules into complex cellular structures. Kimberly Dodge-Kafka, Associate Professor in the Department of Cell Biology and Program Director.

Neuroscience. This interdepartmental program offers comprehensive conceptual and experimental training in molecular, systems, and behavioral neuroscience. The faculty members of the neuroscience program engage in research that involves cellular, molecular, and developmental neurobiology; neuroanatomy; neuroimaging; neurophysiology; neurochemistry; neuroendocrinology; neuropharmacology; and neuropathology. Royce Mohan, Associate Professor of Neuroscience and Program Director.

Skeletal Biology and Regeneration. This program offers interdisciplinary research training in the areas of skeletal, craniofacial, and oral biology, emphasizing contemporary research technologies in cell, molecular, and developmental biology; genetics; and biochemistry. Areas of research include regulation of the formation, outgrowth, and patterning of the developing limb; control of cartilage differentiation, endochondral ossification, osteogenesis, and joint formation; molecular regulation of gene expression in bone; homeobox gene regulation of osteoblast differentiation; gene therapy of bone diseases; hormonal and cytokine regulation of bone growth, formation, and remodeling; control of craniofacial skeletogenesis and tooth development; signal transduction and intracellular signaling pathways; cellular and molecular aspects of the pathogenesis of inflammatory disease;

microbiology, pathogenesis, and immunology of caries and periodontal disease; neural structure and function in the gustatory system; biomaterial development for tissue engineering; bone cell–implant interactions; differentiation of human embryonic stem cells into skeletal tissues; and analysis of oral and mucosal function and disease. Anne Delany, Associate Professor of Medicine and Program Director.

Combined Degree Programs:
Combined M.D./Ph.D. Program. This program is designed for students interested in careers in medical research and academic medicine. It enables students to acquire competence in both the basic science and clinical aspects of their chosen fields. The program allows a student to combine the curricula of two schools in a way that meets the specific degree requirements of each, and yet it allows the completion of both in a period less than that needed if the two curricula were taken in sequence. Entry into the program is limited to a small number of unusually well qualified students who are either currently enrolled in the medical school or who have been accepted into the first-year class. Carol Pilbeam, Professor of Medicine and Program Director.

Combined D.M.D./Ph.D. Program. This program is designed for students interested in careers in dental research and academic dental medicine. It enables students to acquire competence in both the basic science and clinical aspects of their chosen fields. The program allows a student to combine the curricula of two schools in a way that meets the specific degree requirements of each, and yet it allows the completion of both in a period less than that needed if the two curricula were taken in sequence. Entry into the program is limited to a small number of unusually well qualified students who are either currently enrolled in the dental school or who have been accepted into the first-year class. Mina Mina, Professor of Orthodontics, Oral and Maxillofacial Surgery, Pediatric Dentistry, and Advanced Education and Program Director.

Combined M.D./M.P.H. or D.M.D./M.P.H. Program. A joint-degree program leading to the Master of Public Health in addition to the Doctor of Medicine or the Doctor of Dental Medicine is sponsored by the Graduate Program in Public Health and the Schools of Medicine and Dental Medicine. The joint-degree program has been developed to prepare future physicians and dentists to deal creatively with the rapidly changing environment of medicine and health care. It is possible to complete the degree requirements for both programs during the four years of medical or dental school. David Gregorio, Professor of Community Medicine and Health Care and Program Director.

Other Degree Programs:
Clinical and Translational Research. The Master of Science degree program in clinical and translational research is administered in the Department of Medicine and stresses clinical research methods and research practicum in order to provide practical research training in preparation for independent research. The program is offered to individuals who have a health-related terminal degree (M.D., D.M.D., or Ph.D.) or who are involved in an M.D., D.M.D., or Ph.D. program in a health-related field and are in good standing. The master's program is based on both course work and research experience, but no research thesis is required. Students are required to sit for a final examination, which may entail the oral defense of a grant application and a manuscript. Administrator: Lisa Godin (godin@nso.uchc.edu).

Dental Science. The Master of Dental Science degree program is an interdepartmental program whose primary objective is to provide instruction in dental science that will enhance the student's ability to instruct and undertake research in dental schools. This program provides an opportunity for cooperative study and research between dentistry, the basic sciences, and allied health fields. Both M.Dent.Sc. and oral biology Ph.D. students may combine their work in these programs with advanced clinical training in endodontics, orthodontics, oral pathology, pedodontics, periodontics, oral medicine, oral radiology, and oral and maxillofacial surgery. Administrator: Suan Garthwait (garthwait@uchc.edu).

Public Health. This multidisciplinary master's program, accredited by the Council for Education in Public Health, is based in the Department of Community Medicine and Health Care. It offers a core curriculum in epidemiology, biostatistics, health administration, environmental health, the sociomedical sciences, health law, and electives in these and related areas. A Ph.D. program in public health is also offered. David Gregorio, Professor of Community Medicine and Health Care and Program Director.

THE UNIVERSITY OF KANSAS MEDICAL CENTER

Interdisciplinary Graduate Program in Biomedical Sciences

 For more information, visit http://petersons.to/kansasubiomedicalsciences

Programs of Study

At the University of Kansas Medical Center (KUMC), students pursue graduate studies on the cutting edge of biomedical research. Students have the opportunity to develop research skills and earn a Ph.D. degree in a broad range of biomedical research areas, including neuroscience; protein structure and function; pharmacology and toxicology; cancer; and viral, microbial, molecular, cellular, developmental, reproductive, immunological, renal, and physiological biology. Research also includes many clinically related studies that focus on a wide range of human diseases. The graduate program is a partnership between KUMC (http://www.kumc.edu/igpbs) and the nearby Stowers Institute for Medical Research (http://www.stowers-institute.org); students may conduct their research at either institution.

Graduate students pursuing a Ph.D. degree in biomedical sciences are admitted through the Interdisciplinary Graduate Program in Biomedical Sciences (IGPBS). This program is responsible for the first-year, highly integrated curriculum that allows each student to experience current areas of biomedical science before selecting a laboratory in which to carry out his or her doctoral research. In addition to the fundamental principles essential to the biomedical sciences, students receive an introduction to practical aspects of research, including biographics, bioethics, appropriate use of animals in research, laboratory safety, and procedures for human studies research. Faculty members also present their research programs to students through a research seminar series, giving students the opportunity to evaluate each research program. Following this introduction, each student selects three laboratory rotations that are completed during the first year. Laboratory rotations expose students to potential research advisers and to the principles and procedures of cutting-edge laboratory techniques, and they allow students to decide which laboratory best fits their needs. At the beginning of the second year, each student selects a research adviser for their doctoral research. At this time, the student also enters one of eight graduate programs.

Research Facilities

State-of-the-art technology and equipment is available through a variety of core research facilities, including DNA microarray technology, laser capture microdissection, rodent behavioral testing facilities, bioinformatics, transgenic mouse laboratories, fluorescence-activated cell sorting, molecular neurobiology, mass spectrometry, a highly automated histological and immunohistochemistry core, FT-IR microspectroscopy, electron microscopy, confocal microscopes for live cell imaging and spectral separation, noninvasive magnetic resonance spectroscopy, functional magnetic resonance imaging, and magnetoencephalography.

Areas of Research

Faculty members at KUMC have the following areas of research emphasis:

- Bacterial and viral pathogenesis
- Biophysics
- Cancer biology
- Cardiovascular biology
- Cell and developmental biology
- Imaging
- Immunology
- Liver biology
- Metabolism in health and disease
- Molecular biology and genetics
- Musculoskeletal biology
- Neurosciences
- Personalized medicine
- Pharmacological sciences
- Renal biology
- Reproductive biology
- Signal transduction
- Stem cell biology
- Structural biology
- Toxicology and environmental health
- Transcription, chromatin, and epigenetics
- Translational medicine

Financial Aid

Teaching and research assistantships are available. Students admitted into the IGPBS are awarded $24,000 in financial support and given a tuition waiver. Student travel awards are also available.

Cost of Study

Students accepted into the IGPBS receive a tuition waiver upon meeting enrollment requirements. Students are responsible for campus and library fees, estimated at $473 per academic year. International students will pay an international student fee.

Living and Housing Costs

Multiple options are available near the KUMC campus. Current housing costs are between $450 and $800 per month.

Student Group

Twenty-five percent of the students enrolled in the IGPBS are from international locales. The age range of students generally falls between 22 and 32 years.

Student Outcomes

Upon graduation from KUMC, students can expect to obtain a position in the biotechnology, academic, or governmental career fields.

The University of Kansas Medical Center

Location

The University of Kansas Medical Center is located at 39th Avenue and Rainbow Boulevard in Kansas City, Kansas. It is on the border of Kansas and Missouri, with quick access to Westport, the Country Club Plaza, the Nelson-Atkins Museum of Art, and the Kansas City Art Institute.

The Graduate Program

The Interdisciplinary Graduate Program in Biomedical Sciences is an educational program within the School of Medicine at the University of Kansas Medical Center. It consists of eight degree-granting departments or programs. The IGPBS is made up of the Departments of Anatomy and Cell Biology; Biochemistry and Molecular Biology; Microbiology, Molecular Genetics, and Immunology; Pathology and Laboratory Medicine; Molecular and Integrative Physiology; Pharmacology, Toxicology, and Therapeutics; the Neuroscience Graduate Program; the Training Program in Environmental Toxicology; and Cancer Biology.

Applying

Students who are interested in the IGPBS may apply online at http://www.kumc.edu/igpbs. Applications must be received by December 1, although applications received after that date will be considered until the class is filled.

Correspondence and Information

Michael J. Werle, Ph.D., Director
Interdisciplinary Graduate Program in Biomedical Sciences
5015 Wescoe, MS3025
The University of Kansas Medical Center
3901 Rainbow Boulevard
Kansas City, Kansas 66160-7836
Phone: 913-588-2719
      800-408-2039 (toll-free)
Fax: 913-588-5242
E-mail: igpbs@kumc.edu
Website: http://www.kumc.edu/igpbs

Section 2
Anatomy

This section contains a directory of institutions offering graduate work in anatomy. Additional information about programs listed in the directory may be obtained by writing directly to the dean of a graduate school or chair of a department at the address given in the directory.

For programs offering related work, see also in this book *Allied Health; Biomedical Sciences; Cell, Molecular, and Structural Biology; Dentistry and Dental Sciences; Genetics, Developmental Biology, and Reproductive Biology; Neuroscience and Neurobiology; Pathology and Pathobiology; Physiology; Veterinary Medicine and Sciences;* and *Zoology.* In another guide in this series:

Graduate Programs in the Humanities, Arts & Social Sciences
See *Sociology, Anthropology, and Archaeology*

CONTENTS

Anatomy

Albert Einstein College of Medicine, Graduate Division of Biomedical Sciences, Department of Anatomy and Structural Biology, Bronx, NY 10461. Offers anatomy (PhD); cell and developmental biology (PhD); MD/PhD. *Degree requirements:* For doctorate, thesis/dissertation. *Entrance requirements:* For doctorate, GRE General Test. Additional exam requirements/recommendations for international students: Required—TOEFL. Electronic applications accepted. *Faculty research:* Cell motility, cell membranes and membrane-cytoskeletal interactions as applied to processing of pancreatic hormones, mechanisms of secretion.

American University of Beirut, Graduate Programs, Faculty of Medicine, Beirut, Lebanon. Offers anatomy, cell biology and human morphology (MS); biochemistry and medical genetics (MS); biomedical sciences (PhD); experimental pathology, immunology and microbiology (MS); medicine (MD); neuroscience (MS); pharmacology and toxicology (MS). *Program availability:* Part-time. *Faculty:* 302 full-time (95 women), 64 part-time/adjunct (11 women). *Students:* 381 full-time (173 women), 61 part-time (51 women). Average age 23. In 2015, 14 master's awarded. *Degree requirements:* For master's, one foreign language, comprehensive exam, thesis (for some programs); for doctorate, one foreign language, comprehensive exam, thesis/dissertation. *Entrance requirements:* For master's, letter of recommendation; for doctorate, MCAT, bachelor's degree. Additional exam requirements/recommendations for international students: Required—TOEFL (minimum score 600 paper-based; 100 iBT), IELTS (minimum score 7.5). *Application deadline:* For fall admission, 4/30 for domestic and international students; for spring admission, 11/1 for domestic and international students. Application fee: $50. Electronic applications accepted. *Expenses: Tuition, area resident:* Full-time $16,254; part-time $903 per credit. *Required fees:* $699. Tuition and fees vary according to course load and program. *Financial support:* In 2015–16, 273 students received support, including 45 teaching assistantships (averaging $9,000 per year); career-related internships or fieldwork, institutionally sponsored loans, scholarships/grants, health care benefits, and unspecified assistantships also available. Financial award application deadline: 2/2. *Faculty research:* Cancer research (targeted therapy, mechanisms of leukemogenesis, tumor cell extravasation and metastasis, cancer stem cells), stem cell research (regenerative medicine, drug discovery), genetic research (neurogenetics, hereditary cardiomyopathy, hemoglobinopathies, pharmacogenomics, proteomics), neuroscience research (pain, neurodegenerative disorder), metabolism (inflammation and metabolism, metabolic disorder, diabetes mellitus), vascular and renal biology, signal transduction. *Total annual research expenditures:* $2.6 million. *Unit head:* Dr. Mohamed Sayegh, Dean, 961-1350000 Ext. 4700, Fax: 961-1744464, E-mail: msayegh@aub.edu.lb. *Application contact:* Dr. Salim Kanaan, Director, Admissions Office, 961-1350000 Ext. 2594, Fax: 961-1750775, E-mail: sk00@aub.edu.lb. Website: http://www.aub.edu.lb/fm/fm_home/Pages/index.aspx

Auburn University, College of Veterinary Medicine and Graduate School, Graduate Programs in Veterinary Medicine, Auburn University, AL 36849. Offers biomedical sciences (MS, PhD), including anatomy, physiology and pharmacology (MS); biomedical sciences (PhD); clinical sciences (MS); large animal surgery and medicine (MS); pathobiology (MS); radiology (MS); small animal surgery and medicine (MS); DVM/MS. *Program availability:* Part-time. *Faculty:* 97 full-time (40 women), 4 part-time/adjunct (2 women). *Students:* 19 full-time (11 women), 54 part-time (34 women); includes 10 minority (2 Black or African American, non-Hispanic/Latino; 2 American Indian or Alaska Native, non-Hispanic/Latino; 2 Asian, non-Hispanic/Latino; 4 Hispanic/Latino), 23 international. Average age 31. 39 applicants, 59% accepted, 14 enrolled. In 2015, 12 master's, 6 doctorates awarded. *Degree requirements:* For doctorate, thesis/dissertation. *Entrance requirements:* For master's, GRE General Test; for doctorate, GRE General Test, GRE Subject Test. *Application deadline:* Applications are processed on a rolling basis. Application fee: $50 ($60 for international students). Electronic applications accepted. *Expenses: Tuition, state resident:* full-time $8802; part-time $489 per credit hour. Tuition, nonresident: full-time $26,406; part-time $1467 per credit hour. *Required fees:* $808 per semester. Tuition and fees vary according to degree level and program. *Financial support:* Research assistantships, teaching assistantships, and Federal Work-Study available. Support available to part-time students. Financial award application deadline: 3/15; financial award applicants required to submit FAFSA. *Unit head:* Dr. Calvin Johnson, Acting Dean, 334-844-2650. *Application contact:* Dr. George Flowers, Dean of the Graduate School, 334-844-2125.

Augusta University, The Graduate School, Program in Cellular Biology and Anatomy, Augusta, GA 30912. Offers PhD. *Degree requirements:* For doctorate, comprehensive exam, thesis/dissertation. *Entrance requirements:* For doctorate, GRE General Test. Additional exam requirements/recommendations for international students: Required—TOEFL (minimum score 550 paper-based; 79 iBT). *Application deadline:* For fall admission, 1/15 for domestic and international students. Applications are processed on a rolling basis. Application fee: $50. *Financial support:* Fellowships with partial tuition reimbursements, research assistantships with partial tuition reimbursements, teaching assistantships with partial tuition reimbursements, Federal Work-Study, institutionally sponsored loans, and scholarships/grants available. Support available to part-time students. Financial award application deadline: 5/31; financial award applicants required to submit FAFSA. *Faculty research:* Eye disease, developmental biology, cell injury and death, stroke and neurotoxicity, diabetic complications. *Unit head:* Dr. Sylvia B. Smith, Chair and Professor, 706-721-3731, Fax: 706-721-6120, E-mail: sbsmith@augusta.edu. *Application contact:* Dr. Mark Hamrick, Director, 706-721-1958. Website: http://www.augusta.edu/mcg/cba/

Barry University, School of Podiatric Medicine, Program in Anatomy, Miami Shores, FL 33161-6695. Offers MS. *Entrance requirements:* For master's, GRE.

Boston University, College of Health and Rehabilitation Sciences: Sargent College, Department of Health Sciences, Programs in Human Physiology, Boston, MA 02215. Offers MS, PhD. *Faculty:* 10 full-time (9 women), 5 part-time/adjunct (2 women). *Students:* 10 full-time (4 women), 7 part-time (5 women); includes 5 minority (1 Black or African American, non-Hispanic/Latino; 1 Asian, non-Hispanic/Latino; 2 Hispanic/Latino; 1 Two or more races, non-Hispanic/Latino), 3 international. Average age 24. 40 applicants, 30% accepted, 9 enrolled. In 2015, 9 master's awarded. Terminal master's awarded for partial completion of doctoral program. *Degree requirements:* For master's, thesis or alternative; for doctorate, comprehensive exam, thesis/dissertation. *Entrance requirements:* For master's, GRE General Test, minimum GPA of 3.0; for doctorate, GRE General Test. Additional exam requirements/recommendations for international students: Required—TOEFL (minimum score 550 paper-based; 84 iBT). *Application deadline:* For fall admission, 1/15 priority date for domestic and international students; for spring admission, 10/1 for domestic and international students. Applications are processed on a rolling basis. Application fee: $80. Electronic applications accepted. *Expenses:* $1,537 per credit. *Financial support:* In 2015–16, 9 students received support, including 2 research assistantships with full tuition reimbursements available (averaging $21,000 per year); career-related internships or fieldwork, Federal Work-

Study, institutionally sponsored loans, and scholarships/grants also available. Support available to part-time students. Financial award application deadline: 2/15; financial award applicants required to submit FAFSA. *Faculty research:* Skeletal muscle, neural systems, smooth muscle, muscular dystrophy. *Total annual research expenditures:* $1.9 million. *Unit head:* Dr. Paula Quatromoni, Chair, 617-353-5797, Fax: 617-353-7567, E-mail: paulaq@bu.edu. *Application contact:* Sharon Sankey, Director, Student Services, 617-353-2713, Fax: 617-353-7500, E-mail: ssankey@bu.edu.

Boston University, School of Medicine, Division of Graduate Medical Sciences, Department of Anatomy and Neurobiology, Boston, MA 02118. Offers MA, PhD, MD/PhD. *Program availability:* Part-time. Terminal master's awarded for partial completion of doctoral program. *Degree requirements:* For master's, thesis; for doctorate, thesis/dissertation. *Application deadline:* For fall admission, 1/15 for domestic students; for spring admission, 10/15 for domestic students. *Unit head:* Dr. Mark Moss, Chairman, 617-638-4200, Fax: 617-638-4216. *Application contact:* GMS Admissions Office, 617-638-5255, E-mail: askgms@bu.edu. Website: http://www.bumc.bu.edu/anatneuro/

Case Western Reserve University, School of Medicine and School of Graduate Studies, Graduate Programs in Medicine, Department of Anatomy, Cleveland, OH 44106. Offers applied anatomy (MS); biological anthropology (MS); cellular biology (MS); MD/MS. *Program availability:* Part-time. *Degree requirements:* For master's, comprehensive exam, thesis (for some programs). *Entrance requirements:* For master's, GRE General Test. Additional exam requirements/recommendations for international students: Required—TOEFL. *Expenses: Tuition, area resident:* Full-time $41,137; part-time $1714 per credit hour. *Required fees:* $32. Tuition and fees vary according to course load and program. *Faculty research:* Hypoxia, cell injury, biochemical aberration occurrences in ischemic tissue, human functional morphology, evolutionary morphology.

Columbia University, College of Physicians and Surgeons, Department of Anatomy and Cell Biology, New York, NY 10032. Offers anatomy (M Phil, MA, PhD); anatomy and cell biology (PhD); MD/PhD. Only candidates for the PhD are admitted. Terminal master's awarded for partial completion of doctoral program. *Degree requirements:* For doctorate, thesis/dissertation, oral exam. *Entrance requirements:* For master's and doctorate, GRE General Test. Additional exam requirements/recommendations for international students: Required—TOEFL. *Faculty research:* Protein sorting, membrane biophysics, muscle energetics, neuroendocrinology, developmental biology, cytoskeleton, transcription factors.

Cornell University, Graduate School, Graduate Fields of Agriculture and Life Sciences, Field of Zoology and Wildlife Conservation, Ithaca, NY 14853-0001. Offers animal cytology (PhD); comparative and functional anatomy (PhD); developmental biology (PhD); ecology (PhD); histology (PhD); wildlife conservation (PhD). *Degree requirements:* For doctorate, comprehensive exam, thesis/dissertation, 2 semesters of teaching experience. *Entrance requirements:* For doctorate, GRE General Test, GRE Subject Test (biology), 2 letters of recommendation. Additional exam requirements/recommendations for international students: Required—TOEFL (minimum score 550 paper-based; 77 iBT). Electronic applications accepted. *Faculty research:* Organismal biology, functional morphology, biomechanics, comparative vertebrate anatomy, comparative invertebrate anatomy, paleontology.

Creighton University, School of Medicine and Graduate School, Graduate Programs in Medicine, Program in Clinical Anatomy, Omaha, NE 68178-0001. Offers MS. *Degree requirements:* For master's, comprehensive exam, thesis or alternative. *Entrance requirements:* For master's, GRE, MCAT or DAT. Additional exam requirements/recommendations for international students: Required—TOEFL. Electronic applications accepted. *Expenses: Tuition, area resident:* Full-time $14,400; part-time $800 per credit hour. *Required fees:* $158 per semester. Tuition and fees vary according to course load, campus/location, program, reciprocity agreements and student's religious affiliation. *Faculty research:* Neural crest cell migration; ontogenetic and phylogenetic nervous system development; skeletal biology.

Dalhousie University, Faculty of Graduate Studies and Faculty of Medicine, Graduate Programs in Medicine, Department of Anatomy and Neurobiology, Halifax, NS B3H 4R2, Canada. Offers M Sc, PhD. *Degree requirements:* For master's, thesis; for doctorate, thesis/dissertation. *Entrance requirements:* For master's and doctorate, GRE (recommended), minimum A- average. Additional exam requirements/recommendations for international students: Required—1 of 5 approved tests: TOEFL, IELTS, CANTEST, CAEL, Michigan English Language Assessment Battery. Electronic applications accepted. *Faculty research:* Neuroscience histology, cell biology, neuroendocrinology, evolutionary biology.

Des Moines University, College of Osteopathic Medicine, Program in Anatomy, Des Moines, IA 50312-4104. Offers MS.

Duke University, Graduate School, Department of Evolutionary Anthropology, Durham, NC 27708. Offers cellular and molecular biology (PhD); gross anatomy and physical anthropology (PhD), including comparative morphology of human and non-human primates, primate social behavior, vertebrate paleontology; neuroanatomy (PhD). *Degree requirements:* For doctorate, one foreign language, thesis/dissertation. *Entrance requirements:* For doctorate, GRE General Test. Additional exam requirements/recommendations for international students: Required—TOEFL (minimum score 577 paper-based; 90 iBT) or IELTS (minimum score 7). Electronic applications accepted.

East Carolina University, Brody School of Medicine, Department of Anatomy and Cell Biology, Greenville, NC 27858-4353. Offers PhD. *Students:* 11 full-time (7 women); includes 2 minority (1 Black or African American, non-Hispanic/Latino; 1 Asian, non-Hispanic/Latino), 2 international. Average age 27. 6 applicants, 50% accepted, 3 enrolled. In 2015, 2 doctorates awarded. *Degree requirements:* For doctorate, comprehensive exam, thesis/dissertation. *Entrance requirements:* For doctorate, GRE General Test. Additional exam requirements/recommendations for international students: Required—TOEFL. *Application deadline:* For fall admission, 6/1 priority date for domestic students. Applications are processed on a rolling basis. *Financial support:* Fellowships with full tuition reimbursements and health care benefits available. Financial award application deadline: 6/1. *Faculty research:* Kinesin motors during slow mitogenesis, mitochondria and peroxisomes in obesity, ovarian innervation, tight junction function and regulation. *Unit head:* Dr. Cheryl Knudson, Chairman, 252-744-2852, Fax: 252-744-2850, E-mail: knudsonc@ecu.edu. *Application contact:* Dr. Ron Dudek, Senior Director of Graduate Studies, 252-744-2863, Fax: 252-744-2850, E-mail: dudekr@ecu.edu. Website: http://www.ecu.edu/cs-dhs/anatomy/gradProg.cfm

East Tennessee State University, James H. Quillen College of Medicine, Department of Biomedical Sciences, Johnson City, TN 37614. Offers anatomy (PhD); biochemistry (PhD); microbiology (PhD); pharmaceutical sciences (PhD); pharmacology (PhD);

physiology (PhD); quantitative biosciences (PhD). *Faculty:* 30 full-time (6 women). *Students:* 35 full-time (17 women), 2 part-time (1 woman); includes 13 minority (9 Black or African American, non-Hispanic/Latino; 4 Asian, non-Hispanic/Latino; 13 international. Average age 29. 53 applicants, 17% accepted, 8 enrolled. In 2015, 8 doctorates awarded. *Degree requirements:* For doctorate, thesis/dissertation, comprehensive qualifying exam. *Entrance requirements:* For doctorate, GRE General Test, GRE Subject Test, 3 letters of recommendation. Additional exam requirements/recommendations for international students: Required—TOEFL (minimum score 550 paper-based; 79 iBT). *Application deadline:* For fall admission, 3/15 priority date for domestic students, 3/1 priority date for international students. Application fee: $35 ($45 for international students). Electronic applications accepted. *Expenses:* Contact institution. *Financial support:* In 2015–16, 30 students received support, including 27 research assistantships with full tuition reimbursements available (averaging $20,000 per year); career-related internships or fieldwork, institutionally sponsored loans, scholarships/grants, and unspecified assistantships also available. Financial award application deadline: 7/1; financial award applicants required to submit FAFSA. *Faculty research:* Cardiovascular, infectious disease, neurosciences, cancer, immunology. *Unit head:* Dr. Mitchell E. Robinson, Associate Dean/Program Director, 423-439-2031, Fax: 423-439-2140, E-mail: robinson@etsu.edu. *Application contact:* Shella Bennett, Graduate Specialist, 423-439-4708, Fax: 423-439-5624, E-mail: bennetsg@etsu.edu. Website: http://www.etsu.edu/com/dbms/

Howard University, Graduate School, Department of Anatomy, Washington, DC 20059-0002. Offers MS, PhD. *Degree requirements:* For master's, comprehensive exam, thesis, teaching experience; for doctorate, comprehensive exam, thesis/dissertation, teaching experience. *Entrance requirements:* For master's and doctorate, GRE General Test, minimum GPA of 3.0. Additional exam requirements/recommendations for international students: Required—TOEFL (minimum score 550 paper-based). Electronic applications accepted. *Faculty research:* Neural control of function, mammalian evolution and paleontology, cellular differentiation, cellular and neuronal communication, development, cell biology, molecular biology, anatomy.

Indiana University–Purdue University Indianapolis, Indiana University School of Medicine, Department of Anatomy and Cell Biology, Indianapolis, IN 46202. Offers MS, PhD, MD/PhD. *Degree requirements:* For master's, thesis or alternative; for doctorate, thesis/dissertation. *Entrance requirements:* For master's and doctorate, GRE General Test. *Faculty research:* Acoustic reflex control, osteoarthritis and bone disease, diabetes, kidney diseases, cellular and molecular neurobiology.

Johns Hopkins University, School of Medicine, Graduate Programs in Medicine, Center for Functional Anatomy and Evolution, Baltimore, MD 21218. Offers PhD. *Degree requirements:* For doctorate, comprehensive exam, thesis/dissertation, oral exams. *Entrance requirements:* For doctorate, GRE. Additional exam requirements/recommendations for international students: Required—TOEFL. *Faculty research:* Vertebrate evolution, functional anatomy, primate evolution, vertebrate paleobiology, vertebrate morphology.

Loma Linda University, School of Medicine, Programs in Pathology and Human Anatomy, Loma Linda, CA 92350. Offers human anatomy (PhD); pathology (PhD). *Program availability:* Part-time. Terminal master's awarded for partial completion of doctoral program. *Degree requirements:* For doctorate, 2 foreign languages, thesis/dissertation. *Entrance requirements:* For doctorate, GRE General Test. Additional exam requirements/recommendations for international students: Required—TOEFL (minimum score 550 paper-based). *Application deadline:* For fall admission, 7/1 for domestic students. Applications are processed on a rolling basis. Application fee: $60. *Financial support:* Tuition waivers (full and partial) available. Support available to part-time students. *Faculty research:* Neuroendocrine system, histochemistry and image analysis, effect of age and diabetes on PNS, electron microscopy, histology. *Application contact:* Admissions Office, 909-651-5029, Fax: 909-558-4879, E-mail: admissions.app@llu.edu.

Louisiana State University Health Sciences Center, School of Graduate Studies in New Orleans, Department of Cell Biology and Anatomy, New Orleans, LA 70112-2223. Offers cell biology and anatomy (PhD), including clinical anatomy, development, cell, and neurobiology; MD/PhD. *Faculty:* 17 full-time (2 women). *Students:* 5 full-time (4 women), 1 international. 2 applicants, 100% accepted, 2 enrolled. *Degree requirements:* For doctorate, comprehensive exam, thesis/dissertation. *Entrance requirements:* For doctorate, GRE General Test, minimum undergraduate GPA of 3.0. Additional exam requirements/recommendations for international students: Recommended—TOEFL, IELTS. *Application deadline:* For fall admission, 3/1 priority date for domestic students, 3/1 for international students. Applications are processed on a rolling basis. Application fee: $30. *Financial support:* In 2015–16, 6 students received support. Unspecified assistantships available. Financial award application deadline: 4/1. *Faculty research:* Visual system organization, neural development, plasticity of sensory systems, information processing through the nervous system, visuomotor integration. *Total annual research expenditures:* $900,000. *Unit head:* Dr. Samuel McClugage, Head, 504-568-4011, Fax: 504-568-2165, E-mail: smcclu@lsuhsc.edu. *Application contact:* Dr. R. John Cork, Graduate Coordinator and Professor, 504-568-7177, E-mail: jcork@lsuhsc.edu.
Website: http://www.medschool.lsuhsc.edu/cell_biology/

Louisiana State University Health Sciences Center at Shreveport, Department of Cellular Biology and Anatomy, Shreveport, LA 71130-3932. Offers MS, PhD, MD/PhD. Terminal master's awarded for partial completion of doctoral program. *Degree requirements:* For master's, thesis; for doctorate, thesis/dissertation. *Entrance requirements:* For master's and doctorate, GRE General Test. Additional exam requirements/recommendations for international students: Required—TOEFL. *Faculty research:* Cancer biology, redox biology, neurosciences, immunobiology, cardiovascular sciences.

McGill University, Faculty of Graduate and Postdoctoral Studies, Faculty of Medicine, Department of Anatomy and Cell Biology, Montréal, QC H3A 2T5, Canada. Offers M Sc, PhD.

New York Academy of Art, Master of Fine Arts Program, New York, NY 10013-2911. Offers drawing (MFA), including anatomy, printmaking; painting (MFA), including anatomy, printmaking; sculpture (MFA), including anatomy, printmaking. *Accreditation:* NASAD. *Degree requirements:* For master's, thesis. *Entrance requirements:* For master's, slide portfolio, two letters of recommendation, essay, official undergraduate transcripts. Additional exam requirements/recommendations for international students: Required—TOEFL, IELTS. Application fee is waived when completed online.

New York Chiropractic College, Program in Clinical Anatomy, Seneca Falls, NY 13148-0800. Offers MS. *Degree requirements:* For master's, thesis. *Entrance requirements:* For master's, minimum GPA of 3.0, DC, bachelor's degree or equivalent. Electronic applications accepted. *Faculty research:* Bone histology, biomechanics, craniofacial growth and anatomy, skeletal morphology.

New York Chiropractic College, Program in Human Anatomy and Physiology Instruction, Seneca Falls, NY 13148-0800. Offers MS. *Program availability:* Online learning.

New York Medical College, Graduate School of Basic Medical Sciences, Cell Biology and Anatomy - Master's Program, Valhalla, NY 10595-1691. Offers MS, MD/PhD. *Program availability:* Part-time, evening/weekend. *Degree requirements:* For master's, thesis. *Entrance requirements:* For master's, GRE General Test, MCAT, or DAT. Additional exam requirements/recommendations for international students: Required—TOEFL. Electronic applications accepted. *Expenses: Tuition, area resident:* Full-time $44,355; part-time $1025 per credit. *Required fees:* $500; $95 per year. One-time fee: $140 part-time. Tuition and fees vary according to course load and program. *Faculty research:* Mechanisms of growth control in skeletal muscle, cartilage differentiation, cytoskeletal functions, signal transduction pathways, neuronal development and plasticity.

New York Medical College, Graduate School of Basic Medical Sciences, Integrated PhD Program, Valhalla, NY 10595-1691. Offers biochemistry and molecular biology (PhD); cell biology and anatomy (PhD); microbiology and immunology (PhD); pathology (PhD); pharmacology (PhD); physiology (PhD). *Degree requirements:* For doctorate, comprehensive exam, thesis/dissertation. *Entrance requirements:* For doctorate, GRE General Test. Additional exam requirements/recommendations for international students: Required—TOEFL. Electronic applications accepted. *Expenses: Tuition, area resident:* Full-time $44,355; part-time $1025 per credit. *Required fees:* $500; $95 per year. One-time fee: $140 part-time. Tuition and fees vary according to course load and program. *Faculty research:* Cardiovascular sciences, infectious diseases, neuroscience, cancer and cell signaling.

The Ohio State University, College of Medicine, School of Health and Rehabilitation Sciences, Program in Anatomy, Columbus, OH 43210. Offers MS, PhD. *Faculty:* 13. *Students:* 28 full-time (18 women), 1 (woman) part-time. Average age 27. In 2015, 8 master's, 1 doctorate awarded. Terminal master's awarded for partial completion of doctoral program. *Degree requirements:* For master's, thesis (for some programs); for doctorate, thesis/dissertation. *Entrance requirements:* For master's and doctorate, GRE General Test (suggested minimum score in 50th percentile). Additional exam requirements/recommendations for international students: Required—TOEFL (minimum score 600 paper-based; 100 iBT), Michigan English Language Assessment Battery (minimum score 86); Recommended—IELTS (minimum score 8). *Application deadline:* For fall admission, 12/1 priority date for domestic students, 11/1 priority date for international students. Applications are processed on a rolling basis. Application fee: $60 ($70 for international students). Electronic applications accepted. *Financial support:* Fellowships with tuition reimbursements, research assistantships with tuition reimbursements, teaching assistantships with tuition reimbursements, and Federal Work-Study available. Financial award application deadline: 1/10. *Faculty research:* Cell biology, biomechanical trauma, computer-assisted instruction. *Unit head:* Dr. Kirk McHugh, Graduate Studies Committee Chair, E-mail: mchugh.57@osu.edu. *Application contact:* Graduate and Professional Admissions, 614-292-9444, Fax: 614-292-3895, E-mail: gpadmissions@osu.edu.
Website: http://medicine.osu.edu/hrs/anatomy

Palmer College of Chiropractic, Division of Graduate Studies, Davenport, IA 52803-5287. Offers clinical research (MS). *Faculty:* 8 full-time (3 women), 3 part-time/adjunct (2 women). *Students:* 7 full-time (2 women), 1 (woman) part-time; includes 1 minority (Black or African American, non-Hispanic/Latino). 3 applicants, 100% accepted, 3 enrolled. In 2015, 5 master's awarded. *Degree requirements:* For master's, 2 mentored practicum projects. *Entrance requirements:* For master's, GRE General Test, minimum GPA of 2.5, bachelor's and doctoral-level health professions degrees. Additional exam requirements/recommendations for international students: Required—TOEFL. *Application deadline:* For fall admission, 8/1 for domestic and international students; for spring admission, 5/28 for domestic students. Applications are processed on a rolling basis. Application fee: $50. Electronic applications accepted. *Expenses:* Contact institution. *Financial support:* In 2015–16, 7 students received support, including 7 research assistantships with full tuition reimbursements available (averaging $30,000 per year), teaching assistantships with tuition reimbursements available (averaging $6,269 per year); tuition waivers (full) and unspecified assistantships also available. Financial award application deadline: 8/1; financial award applicants required to submit FAFSA. *Faculty research:* Chiropractic clinical research. *Unit head:* Dr. Dan Weinert, Interim Vice President for Academic Affairs, 563-884-5761, Fax: 563-884-5624, E-mail: weinert_d@palmer.edu. *Application contact:* Lori Byrd, Program Coordinator, 563-884-5198, Fax: 563-884-5227, E-mail: lori.byrd@plamer.edu.

Penn State Hershey Medical Center, College of Medicine, Graduate School Programs in the Biomedical Sciences, Program in Anatomy, Hershey, PA 17033. Offers MS, PhD. *Students:* 15 full-time (10 women); includes 3 minority (all Asian, non-Hispanic/Latino). 21 applicants, 24% accepted, 5 enrolled. In 2015, 2 master's, 1 doctorate awarded. Terminal master's awarded for partial completion of doctoral program. *Degree requirements:* For master's, thesis or alternative; for doctorate, comprehensive exam, thesis/dissertation. *Entrance requirements:* For master's and doctorate, GRE General Test or MCAT, minimum GPA of 3.0. Additional exam requirements/recommendations for international students: Required—TOEFL (minimum score 500 paper-based). *Application deadline:* For fall admission, 1/31 priority date for domestic students, 2/1 priority date for international students. Applications are processed on a rolling basis. Application fee: $65. Electronic applications accepted. *Financial support:* In 2015–16, research assistantships with full tuition reimbursements (averaging $26,196 per year) were awarded; fellowships with full tuition reimbursements, scholarships/grants, health care benefits, and unspecified assistantships also available. Financial award applicants required to submit FAFSA. *Faculty research:* Developmental biology, stem cell, cancer-basic science and clinical application, wound healing, angiogenesis. *Unit head:* Dr. Patricia J. McLaughlin, Program Director, 717-531-0003, Fax: 717-531-0306, E-mail: anat-grad-hmc@psu.edu. *Application contact:* Dee Clarke, Program Assistant, 717-531-0003, Fax: 717-531-0306, E-mail: anat-grad-hmc@psu.edu.
Website: http://www.pennstatehershey.org/web/anatomy/home

Purdue University, School of Veterinary Medicine and Graduate School, Graduate Programs in Veterinary Medicine, Department of Basic Medical Sciences, West Lafayette, IN 47907. Offers anatomy (MS, PhD); pharmacology (MS, PhD); physiology (MS, PhD). *Program availability:* Part-time. Terminal master's awarded for partial completion of doctoral program. *Degree requirements:* For master's, thesis; for doctorate, thesis/dissertation. *Entrance requirements:* For master's and doctorate, GRE General Test. Additional exam requirements/recommendations for international students: Required—TOEFL. Electronic applications accepted. *Faculty research:* Development and regeneration, tissue injury and shock, biomedical engineering, ovarian function, bone and cartilage biology, cell and molecular biology.

Queen's University at Kingston, School of Graduate Studies, Faculty of Health Sciences, Department of Anatomy and Cell Biology, Kingston, ON K7L 3N6, Canada. Offers biology of reproduction (M Sc, PhD); cancer (M Sc, PhD); cardiovascular pathophysiology (M Sc, PhD); cell and molecular biology (M Sc, PhD); drug metabolism (M Sc, PhD); endocrinology (M Sc, PhD); motor control (M Sc, PhD); neural regeneration (M Sc, PhD); neurophysiology (M Sc, PhD). *Program availability:* Part-time. *Degree requirements:* For master's, thesis; for doctorate, one foreign language, comprehensive exam, thesis/dissertation. *Entrance requirements:* Additional exam requirements/recommendations for international students: Required—TOEFL.

Anatomy

Electronic applications accepted. *Faculty research:* Human kinetics, neuroscience, reproductive biology, cardiovascular.

Rosalind Franklin University of Medicine and Science, School of Graduate and Postdoctoral Studies - Interdisciplinary Graduate Program in Biomedical Sciences, Department of Cell Biology and Anatomy, North Chicago, IL 60064-3095. Offers PhD, MD/PhD. Terminal master's awarded for partial completion of doctoral program. *Degree requirements:* For doctorate, comprehensive exam, thesis/dissertation, original research project. *Entrance requirements:* For doctorate, GRE General Test, minimum GPA of 3.0. Additional exam requirements/recommendations for international students: Required—TOEFL, TWE. *Faculty research:* Neuroscience, molecular biology.

Rush University, Graduate College, Division of Anatomy and Cell Biology, Chicago, IL 60612-3832. Offers MS, PhD, MD/MS, MD/PhD. Terminal master's awarded for partial completion of doctoral program. *Degree requirements:* For master's, thesis; for doctorate, comprehensive exam, thesis/dissertation, preliminary exam, dissertation proposal. *Entrance requirements:* For master's, GRE General Test, minimum GPA of 3.0, bachelor's degree in biology or chemistry (preferred), interview; for doctorate, GRE General Test, minimum GPA of 3.0, interview. Additional exam requirements/recommendations for international students: Required—TOEFL. Electronic applications accepted. *Faculty research:* Incontinence following vaginal distension, knee replacement, biomimetic materials, injured spinal motoneurons, implant fixation.

Saint Louis University, Graduate Education and School of Medicine, Graduate Program in Biomedical Sciences and Graduate Education, Center for Anatomical Science and Education, St. Louis, MO 63103. Offers anatomy (MS-R, PhD). *Degree requirements:* For master's, comprehensive exam, thesis; for doctorate, comprehensive exam, thesis/dissertation, departmental qualifying exams. *Entrance requirements:* For master's, GRE General Test, letters of recommendation, resume; for doctorate, GRE General Test, letters of recommendation, resumé, goal statement, transcripts. Additional exam requirements/recommendations for international students: Required—TOEFL (minimum score 525 paper-based). *Faculty research:* Neurodegenerative diseases, cerebellar cortical circuitry, neurogenesis, evolutionary anatomy.

State University of New York Upstate Medical University, College of Graduate Studies, Program in Cell and Developmental Biology, Syracuse, NY 13210-2334. Offers anatomy (MS, PhD); MD/PhD. Terminal master's awarded for partial completion of doctoral program. *Degree requirements:* For master's, thesis; for doctorate, comprehensive exam, thesis/dissertation. *Entrance requirements:* For master's, GRE General Test, interview; for doctorate, GRE General Test, telephone interview. Additional exam requirements/recommendations for international students: Required—TOEFL. Electronic applications accepted. *Faculty research:* Cancer, disorders of the nervous system, infectious diseases, diabetes/metabolic disorders/cardiovascular diseases.

Stony Brook University, State University of New York, Stony Brook Medicine, School of Medicine and Graduate School, Graduate Programs in Medicine, Department of Anatomical Sciences, Stony Brook, NY 11794. Offers PhD. *Faculty:* 15 full-time (6 women), 1 part-time/adjunct. *Students:* 6 full-time (3 women), 1 part-time (0 women), 1 international. Average age 27. 11 applicants, 18% accepted, 1 enrolled. *Degree requirements:* For doctorate, comprehensive exam, thesis/dissertation. *Entrance requirements:* For doctorate, GRE General Test, GRE Subject Test, BA in life sciences, minimum GPA of 3.0. Additional exam requirements/recommendations for international students: Required—TOEFL. *Application deadline:* For fall admission, 1/15 for domestic students; for spring admission, 10/1 for domestic students. Application fee: $100. *Expenses:* $12,421 full-time resident tuition and fees, $453 per credit hour; $23,761 full-time nonresident tuition and fees, $925 per credit hour. *Financial support:* In 2015–16, 6 research assistantships were awarded; fellowships, teaching assistantships, and Federal Work-Study also available. Financial award application deadline: 3/15. *Faculty research:* Anatomy, bioimaging, paleontology, paleobiology, anatomical systems or sites. *Total annual research expenditures:* $762,929. *Unit head:* Dr. Randall Susman, Professor and Chairman, 631-444-3125, Fax: 631-444-3947, E-mail: randall.susman@stonybrook.edu. *Application contact:* Christine Johnson, Coordinator, 631-444-3114, Fax: 631-444-3947, E-mail: christine.johnson@stonybrook.edu.
Website: http://www.anat.stonybrook.edu/

Universidad Central del Caribe, School of Medicine, Program in Biomedical Sciences, Bayamón, PR 00960-6032. Offers anatomy and cell biology (MA, MS); biochemistry (MS); biomedical sciences (MA); cellular and molecular biology (PhD); microbiology and immunology (MA, MS); pharmacology (MS); physiology (MS).

Universidad de Ciencias Medicas, Graduate Programs, San Jose, Costa Rica. Offers dermatology (SP); family health (MS); health service center administration (MHA); human anatomy (MS); medical and surgery (MD); occupational medicine (MS); pharmacy (Pharm D). *Program availability:* Part-time. *Degree requirements:* For master's, thesis; for doctorate and SP, comprehensive exam. *Entrance requirements:* For master's, MD or bachelor's degree; for doctorate, admissions test; for SP, admissions test, MD.

Université Laval, Faculty of Medicine, Post-Professional Programs in Medical Studies, Québec, QC G1K 7P4, Canada. Offers anatomy–pathology (DESS); anesthesiology (DESS); cardiology (DESS); care of older people (Diploma); clinical research (DESS); community health (DESS); dermatology (DESS); diagnostic radiology (DESS); emergency medicine (Diploma); family medicine (DESS); general surgery (DESS); geriatrics (DESS); hematology (DESS); internal medicine (DESS); maternal and fetal medicine (Diploma); medical biochemistry (DESS); medical microbiology and infectious diseases (DESS); medical oncology (DESS); nephrology (DESS); neurology (DESS); neurosurgery (DESS); obstetrics and gynecology (DESS); ophthalmology (DESS); orthopedic surgery (DESS); oto-rhino-laryngology (DESS); palliative medicine (Diploma); pediatrics (DESS); plastic surgery (DESS); psychiatry (DESS); pulmonary medicine (DESS); radiology–oncology (DESS); thoracic surgery (DESS); urology (DESS). *Degree requirements:* For other advanced degree, comprehensive exam. *Entrance requirements:* For degree, knowledge of French. Electronic applications accepted.

University at Buffalo, the State University of New York, Graduate School, School of Medicine and Biomedical Sciences, Graduate Programs in Medicine and Biomedical Sciences, Department of Pathology and Anatomical Sciences, Buffalo, NY 14214. Offers anatomical sciences (MA, PhD); pathology (MA, PhD). *Program availability:* Part-time. *Faculty:* 17 full-time (6 women). *Students:* 9 full-time (3 women); includes 1 minority (Asian, non-Hispanic/Latino) 1 international. Average age 29. 14 applicants, 14% accepted, 2 enrolled. In 2015, 2 master's, 1 doctorate awarded. *Degree requirements:* For master's, thesis; for doctorate, comprehensive exam, thesis/dissertation. *Entrance requirements:* For master's and doctorate, GRE, MCAT, or DAT, 3 letters of recommendation. Additional exam requirements/recommendations for international students: Required—TOEFL (minimum score 600 paper-based; 100 iBT). *Application deadline:* For fall admission, 5/1 priority date for domestic students, 3/1 priority date for international students. Application fee: $85. *Financial support:* In 2015–16, 2 students received support, including 1 research assistantship with full tuition reimbursement available (averaging $24,900 per year), 1 teaching assistantship with full tuition reimbursement available (averaging $24,900 per year); health care benefits also available. Financial award application deadline: 2/1; financial award applicants required to submit FAFSA. *Faculty research:* Immunopathology-immunobiology, experimental hypertension, neuromuscular disease, molecular pathology, cell motility and cytoskeleton. *Unit head:* Dr. John E. Tomaszewski, Department Chair, 716-829-2846, Fax: 716-829-2911, E-mail: johntoma@buffalo.edu. *Application contact:* Graduate Program Coordinator, 716-829-2846, Fax: 716-829-2911, E-mail: upbathad@buffalo.edu.
Website: http://wings.buffalo.edu/smbs/path/

University of California, Irvine, School of Medicine and Francisco J. Ayala School of Biological Sciences, Department of Anatomy and Neurobiology, Irvine, CA 92697. Offers biological sciences (MS, PhD); MD/PhD. *Faculty:* 26 full-time (13 women), 2 part-time/adjunct (1 woman). *Students:* 19 full-time (12 women), 2 part-time (both women); includes 8 minority (all Asian, non-Hispanic/Latino), 3 international. Average age 28. In 2015, 1 master's, 5 doctorates awarded. *Degree requirements:* For master's, thesis; for doctorate, thesis/dissertation. *Entrance requirements:* For master's and doctorate, GRE General Test, GRE Subject Test. Additional exam requirements/recommendations for international students: Required—TOEFL (minimum score 550 paper-based). *Application deadline:* For fall admission, 1/15 priority date for domestic students, 1/15 for international students. Applications are processed on a rolling basis. Application fee: $90 ($110 for international students). Electronic applications accepted. *Financial support:* Fellowships, research assistantships with full tuition reimbursements, teaching assistantships, institutionally sponsored loans, traineeships, health care benefits, and unspecified assistantships available. Financial award application deadline: 3/1; financial award applicants required to submit FAFSA. *Faculty research:* Neurotransmitter immunocytochemistry, intracellular physiology, molecular neurobiology, forebrain organization and development, structure and function of sensory and motor systems. *Unit head:* Prof. Christine Gall, Interim Chair, 949-824-8652, Fax: 949-824-1255, E-mail: cmgall@uci.edu. *Application contact:* David Lyon, Director of Graduate Studies, 949-824-0447, E-mail: dclyon@uci.edu.

University of California, Los Angeles, David Geffen School of Medicine and Graduate Division, Graduate Programs in Medicine, Department of Neurobiology, Los Angeles, CA 90095. Offers MS, PhD. Terminal master's awarded for partial completion of doctoral program. *Degree requirements:* For master's, comprehensive exam; for doctorate, thesis/dissertation, oral and written qualifying exams; 2 quarters of teaching experience. *Entrance requirements:* For doctorate, GRE General Test; GRE Subject Test, bachelor's degree; minimum undergraduate GPA of 3.0 (or its equivalent if letter grade system not used). Additional exam requirements/recommendations for international students: Required—TOEFL. Electronic applications accepted.

University of Chicago, Division of the Biological Sciences, Department of Organismal Biology and Anatomy, Chicago, IL 60637. Offers integrative biology (PhD). *Students:* 22 full-time (13 women); includes 3 minority (1 Asian, non-Hispanic/Latino; 2 Hispanic/Latino), 2 international. Average age 27. 17 applicants, 35% accepted, 4 enrolled. *Degree requirements:* For doctorate, thesis/dissertation, ethics class, 2 teaching assistantships. *Entrance requirements:* For doctorate, GRE General Test. Additional exam requirements/recommendations for international students: Required—TOEFL (minimum score 600 paper-based; 104 iBT), IELTS (minimum score 7). *Application deadline:* For fall admission, 12/1 for domestic and international students. Application fee: $90. Electronic applications accepted. *Financial support:* In 2015–16, 12 students received support, including fellowships with tuition reimbursements available (averaging $29,781 per year), research assistantships with tuition reimbursements available (averaging $29,781 per year); institutionally sponsored loans, scholarships/grants, traineeships, and health care benefits also available. Financial award applicants required to submit FAFSA. *Faculty research:* Ecological physiology, evolution of fossil reptiles, vertebrate paleontology. *Unit head:* Dr. Robert Ho, Chairman, 773-834-8423, Fax: 773-702-0037, E-mail: rkh@uchicago.edu.
Website: http://pondside.uchicago.edu/oba/

University of Colorado Denver, School of Medicine, Program in Cell Biology, Stem Cells, and Developmental Biology, Aurora, CO 80045. Offers cell biology, stem cells, and developmental biology (PhD); modern human anatomy (MS). *Students:* 29 full-time (13 women); includes 7 minority (1 Asian, non-Hispanic/Latino; 4 Hispanic/Latino; 2 Two or more races, non-Hispanic/Latino), 3 international. Average age 29. 42 applicants, 7% accepted, 3 enrolled. In 2015, 1 doctorate awarded. *Degree requirements:* For doctorate, comprehensive exam, thesis/dissertation, at least 30 credit hours of coursework and 30 credit hours of thesis research; laboratory rotations. *Entrance requirements:* For doctorate, GRE, minimum GPA of 3.0; 3 letters of reference; prerequisite coursework in organic chemistry, biology, biochemistry, physics and calculus; research experience (highly recommended). Additional exam requirements/recommendations for international students: Required—TOEFL (minimum score 550 paper-based; 80 iBT). *Application deadline:* For fall admission, 12/1 for domestic students, 11/1 priority date for international students. Application fee: $50 ($75 for international students). Electronic applications accepted. *Expenses:* Contact institution. *Financial support:* In 2015–16, 29 students received support. Fellowships, research assistantships, teaching assistantships, Federal Work-Study, institutionally sponsored loans, scholarships/grants, traineeships, health care benefits, and tuition waivers (full) available. Financial award application deadline: 3/15; financial award applicants required to submit FAFSA. *Faculty research:* Development and repair of the vertebrate nervous system; molecular, genetic and developmental mechanisms involved in the patterning of the early spinal cord (neural plate) during vertebrate embryogenesis; structural analysis of protein glycosylation using NMR and mass spectrometry; small RNAs and post-transcriptional gene regulation during nematode gametogenesis and early development; diabetes-mediated changes in cardiovascular gene expression and functional exercise capacity. *Total annual research expenditures:* $5.7 million. *Unit head:* Dr. Bruce Appel, Director, 303-724-3465, E-mail: bruce.appel@ucdenver.edu. *Application contact:* Kenton Owsley, Program Administrator, 303-724-3468, Fax: 303-724-3420, E-mail: kenton.owsley@ucdenver.edu.
Website: http://www.ucdenver.edu/academics/colleges/medicalschool/programs/CSD/Pages/CSD.aspx

University of Georgia, College of Veterinary Medicine, Department of Veterinary Anatomy and Radiology, Athens, GA 30602. Offers veterinary anatomy (MS). *Degree requirements:* For master's, thesis. *Entrance requirements:* For master's, GRE General Test. Electronic applications accepted.

University of Guelph, Ontario Veterinary College and Graduate Studies, Graduate Programs in Veterinary Sciences, Department of Biomedical Sciences, Guelph, ON N1G 2W1, Canada. Offers morphology (M Sc, DV Sc, PhD); neuroscience (M Sc, DV Sc, PhD); pharmacology (M Sc, DV Sc, PhD); physiology (M Sc, DV Sc, PhD); toxicology (M Sc, DV Sc, PhD). *Program availability:* Part-time. *Degree requirements:* For master's, thesis; for doctorate, comprehensive exam, thesis/dissertation. *Entrance requirements:* For master's, honors B Sc, minimum 75% average in last 20 courses; for doctorate, M Sc with thesis from accredited institution. Additional exam requirements/recommendations for international students: Required—TOEFL (minimum score 550 paper-based; 89 iBT). Electronic applications accepted. *Faculty research:* Cellular morphology; endocrine, vascular and reproductive physiology; clinical pharmacology; veterinary toxicology; developmental biology, neuroscience.

University of Illinois at Chicago, College of Medicine and Graduate College, Graduate Programs in Medicine, Department of Anatomy and Cell Biology, Chicago, IL 60607. Offers MS, MD/PhD. *Faculty:* 15 full-time (6 women), 21 part-time/adjunct (12 women). *Students:* 6 full-time (4 women); includes 1 minority (Black or African American, non-Hispanic/Latino), 2 international. Average age 27. *Degree requirements:* For master's, preliminary oral examination, dissertation and oral defense. *Entrance requirements:* For master's, GRE General Test, minimum GPA of 2.75, 3 letters of recommendation. Additional exam requirements/recommendations for international students: Required—TOEFL (minimum score 550 paper-based). *Application deadline:* For fall admission, 5/15 for domestic students, 2/15 for international students. Applications are processed on a rolling basis. Application fee: $60. Electronic applications accepted. *Expenses:* Tuition, state resident: full-time $11,480; part-time $3826 per credit. Tuition, nonresident: full-time $23,720; part-time $7906 per credit. *Required fees:* $1333 per semester. Part-time tuition and fees vary according to course load and program. *Financial support:* Research or teaching assistantships with stipend of $24,000 per year, plus a tuition waiver available. *Faculty research:* Synapses, axonal transport, neurodegenerative diseases. *Unit head:* Prof. Scott T. Brady, Head, 312-996-3313, Fax: 312-413-0354, E-mail: stbrady@uic.edu. *Application contact:* Dr. Ernesto R. Bongarzone, Associate Professor/Director of Graduate Studies, 312-996-6791, Fax: 312-413-0354, E-mail: ebongarz@uic.edu.
Website: http://www.anatomy.uic.edu/

The University of Iowa, Roy J. and Lucille A. Carver College of Medicine and Graduate College, Graduate Programs in Medicine, Department of Anatomy and Cell Biology, Iowa City, IA 52242-1316. Offers PhD. *Degree requirements:* For doctorate, comprehensive exam, thesis/dissertation. *Entrance requirements:* For doctorate, GRE General Test, minimum GPA of 3.0. Additional exam requirements/recommendations for international students: Required—TOEFL (minimum score 600 paper-based; 100 iBT). Electronic applications accepted. *Faculty research:* Biology of differentiation and transformation, developmental and vascular cell biology, neurobiology.

The University of Kansas, University of Kansas Medical Center, School of Medicine, Department of Anatomy and Cell Biology, Kansas City, KS 66160. Offers MS, PhD, MD/PhD. *Faculty:* 28 full-time (11 women), 9 part-time/adjunct (6 women). *Students:* 12 full-time (6 women), 6 international. Average age 28. In 2015, 6 doctorates awarded. Terminal master's awarded for partial completion of doctoral program. *Degree requirements:* For master's, thesis; for doctorate, comprehensive exam, thesis/dissertation. *Entrance requirements:* For master's and doctorate, GRE. Additional exam requirements/recommendations for international students: Required—TOEFL. *Application deadline:* For fall admission, 1/15 priority date for domestic students. Applications are processed on a rolling basis. Application fee: $0. Electronic applications accepted. *Financial support:* In 2015–16, 16 research assistantships with full tuition reimbursements (averaging $24,500 per year), 3 teaching assistantships with full tuition reimbursements (averaging $24,500 per year) were awarded; fellowships, institutionally sponsored loans, scholarships/grants, health care benefits, and unspecified assistantships also available. Financial award application deadline: 3/1; financial award applicants required to submit FAFSA. *Faculty research:* Development of the synapse and neuromuscular junction, pain perception and diabetic neuropathies, cardiovascular and kidney development, reproductive immunology, post-fertilization signaling events. *Total annual research expenditures:* $11 million. *Unit head:* Dr. Dale R. Abrahamson, Chairman, 913-588-0702, Fax: 913-588-2710, E-mail: dabrahamson@kumc.edu. *Application contact:* Dr. Julie A. Christianson, Assistant Professor, 913-945-6430, Fax: 913-588-5677, E-mail: jchristianson@kumc.edu.
Website: http://www.kumc.edu/school-of-medicine/anatomy-and-cell-biology.html

University of Kentucky, Graduate School, Graduate School Programs from the College of Medicine, Program in Anatomy and Neurobiology, Lexington, KY 40506-0032. Offers PhD. *Degree requirements:* For doctorate, comprehensive exam, thesis/dissertation. *Entrance requirements:* For doctorate, GRE General Test, minimum undergraduate GPA of 2.75. Additional exam requirements/recommendations for international students: Required—TOEFL (minimum score 550 paper-based). Electronic applications accepted. *Faculty research:* Neuroendocrinology, developmental neurobiology, neurotrophic substances, neural plasticity and trauma, neurobiology of aging.

University of Louisville, School of Medicine, Department of Anatomical Sciences and Neurobiology, Louisville, KY 40292-0001. Offers MS, PhD, MD/PhD. *Students:* 21 full-time (10 women), 7 part-time (4 women); includes 5 minority (2 Hispanic/Latino; 3 Two or more races, non-Hispanic/Latino), 2 international. Average age 28. 43 applicants, 23% accepted, 7 enrolled. In 2015, 1 master's, 2 doctorates awarded. Terminal master's awarded for partial completion of doctoral program. *Degree requirements:* For master's, thesis; for doctorate, comprehensive exam, thesis/dissertation. *Entrance requirements:* For master's and doctorate, GRE General Test (minimum score of 1000 verbal and quantitative), minimum GPA of 3.0. Additional exam requirements/recommendations for international students: Required—TOEFL. *Application deadline:* For fall admission, 1/15 priority date for domestic students; for spring admission, 4/15 priority date for domestic and international students. Applications are processed on a rolling basis. Application fee: $60. Electronic applications accepted. *Expenses:* Tuition, state resident: full-time $11,664; part-time $649 per credit hour. Tuition, nonresident: full-time $24,274; part-time $1350 per credit hour. *Required fees:* $196. Tuition and fees vary according to program and reciprocity agreements. *Financial support:* In 2015–16, 235,179 students received support. Fellowships with full tuition reimbursements available, research assistantships with full tuition reimbursements available, health care benefits, and unspecified assistantships available. Financial award application deadline: 4/15. *Faculty research:* Human adult neural stem cells, development and plasticity of the nervous system, organization of the dorsal thalamus, electrophysiology/neuroanatomy of central neurons mediating control of reproductive and pelvic organs, normal neural mechanisms and plasticity following injury and/or chronic pain, differentiation and regeneration of motor neurons and oligodendrocytes. *Total annual research expenditures:* $3.5 million. *Unit head:* Dr. William Guido, Chair, 502-852-6227, Fax: 502-852-6228, E-mail: w0guid01@gwise.louisville.edu. *Application contact:* Dr. Charles Hubscher, Director of Graduate Studies, 502-852-3058, Fax: 502-852-6228, E-mail: chhub01@louisville.edu.
Website: http://louisville.edu/medicine/departments/anatomy

University of Manitoba, Faculty of Medicine and Faculty of Graduate Studies, Graduate Programs in Medicine, Department of Human Anatomy and Cell Science, Winnipeg, MB R3T 2N2, Canada. Offers M Sc, PhD. *Degree requirements:* For master's, thesis; for doctorate, one foreign language, thesis/dissertation.

University of Mississippi Medical Center, School of Graduate Studies in the Health Sciences, Department of Anatomy, Jackson, MS 39216-4505. Offers clinical anatomy (MS, PhD); MD/PhD. *Degree requirements:* For doctorate, comprehensive exam, thesis/dissertation, first authored publication. *Entrance requirements:* For doctorate, GRE General Test, minimum GPA of 3.0, personal statement. Additional exam requirements/recommendations for international students: Required—TOEFL. *Faculty research:* Systems neuroscience with emphasis on motor and sensory, cell biology with emphasis on cell-matrix interactions, development of cardiovascular system, biology of glial cells.

University of Missouri, School of Medicine and Office of Research and Graduate Studies, Graduate Programs in Medicine, Department of Pathology and Anatomical Sciences, Columbia, MO 65211. Offers MS. *Entrance requirements:* For master's, GRE (minimum Verbal and Analytical score of 1250), letters of recommendation, minimum GPA of 3.5. Additional exam requirements/recommendations for international students: Required—TOEFL. Application fee: $55 ($75 for international students). Electronic applications accepted.
Website: http://pathology-anatomy.missouri.edu/

University of Nebraska Medical Center, Department of Genetics, Cell Biology and Anatomy, Omaha, NE 68198. Offers MS, PhD. *Faculty:* 22 full-time (5 women), 1 (woman) part-time/adjunct. *Students:* 41 full-time (17 women); includes 6 minority (2 Black or African American, non-Hispanic/Latino; 1 American Indian or Alaska Native, non-Hispanic/Latino; 2 Asian, non-Hispanic/Latino; 1 Hispanic/Latino), 9 international. Average age 25. 19 applicants, 32% accepted, 6 enrolled. In 2015, 14 master's, 7 doctorates awarded. Terminal master's awarded for partial completion of doctoral program. *Degree requirements:* For master's, comprehensive exam, thesis; for doctorate, comprehensive exam, thesis/dissertation. *Entrance requirements:* For master's and doctorate, GRE General Test. Additional exam requirements/recommendations for international students: Required—TOEFL (minimum score 550 paper-based; 80 iBT). *Application deadline:* For fall admission, 4/1 priority date for domestic and international students; for spring admission, 8/1 for domestic and international students; for summer admission, 1/1 for domestic and international students. Applications are processed on a rolling basis. Application fee: $45. Electronic applications accepted. *Expenses:* Tuition, state resident: full-time $7830; part-time $3915 per credit hour. Tuition, nonresident: full-time $22,410; part-time $11,205 per credit hour. *Required fees:* $521. *Financial support:* In 2015–16, 1 fellowship with full tuition reimbursement (averaging $23,100 per year), 1 research assistantship with full tuition reimbursement (averaging $24,000 per year) were awarded; scholarships/grants also available. Support available to part-time students. Financial award application deadline: 3/1; financial award applicants required to submit FAFSA. *Faculty research:* Hematology, immunology, developmental biology, genetics cancer biology, neuroscience. *Unit head:* Dr. Karen Gould, Graduate Committee Chair, 402-559-2456, E-mail: kagould@unmc.edu. *Application contact:* Bryan Katafiasa, Administrative Associate, 402-559-4031, Fax: 402-559-7328, E-mail: bkatafiasz@unmc.edu.
Website: http://www.unmc.edu/genetics/

University of Nebraska Medical Center, Medical Sciences Interdepartmental Area, Omaha, NE 68198. Offers genetics, cell biology and anatomy (MS); internal medicine (MS). *Program availability:* Part-time. *Faculty:* 195 full-time, 20 part-time/adjunct. *Students:* 49 full-time (28 women), 40 part-time (27 women); includes 10 minority (1 Black or African American, non-Hispanic/Latino; 6 Asian, non-Hispanic/Latino; 3 Hispanic/Latino), 16 international. Average age 32. 46 applicants, 41% accepted, 19 enrolled. In 2015, 12 master's, 17 doctorates awarded. Terminal master's awarded for partial completion of doctoral program. *Degree requirements:* For master's, comprehensive exam, thesis; for doctorate, comprehensive exam, thesis/dissertation. *Entrance requirements:* For master's, GRE General Test; for doctorate, GRE General Test, MCAT or DCAT. Additional exam requirements/recommendations for international students: Required—TOEFL (minimum score 550 paper-based; 80 iBT). *Application deadline:* For fall admission, 4/1 for domestic and international students; for spring admission, 8/1 for domestic and international students; for summer admission, 1/1 for domestic and international students. Applications are processed on a rolling basis. Application fee: $45. Electronic applications accepted. *Expenses:* Tuition, state resident: full-time $7830; part-time $3915 per credit hour. Tuition, nonresident: full-time $22,410; part-time $11,205 per credit hour. *Required fees:* $521. *Financial support:* In 2015–16, 3 fellowships with full tuition reimbursements (averaging $23,100 per year), 4 research assistantships with full tuition reimbursements (averaging $23,100 per year) were awarded; teaching assistantships and scholarships/grants also available. Support available to part-time students. Financial award application deadline: 2/15; financial award applicants required to submit FAFSA. *Faculty research:* Molecular genetics, oral biology, veterinary pathology, newborn medicine, immunology, clinical research. *Unit head:* Dr. Laura Bilek, Graduate Committee Chair, 402-559-6923, E-mail: lbilek@unmc.edu.
Website: http://www.unmc.edu/gradstudies/programs/msia/

University of North Dakota, Graduate School and Graduate School, Graduate Programs in Medicine, Department of Anatomy and Cell Biology, Grand Forks, ND 58202. Offers MS, PhD. *Degree requirements:* For master's, thesis, final exam; for doctorate, comprehensive exam, thesis/dissertation, final exam. *Entrance requirements:* For master's and doctorate, GRE General Test, minimum GPA of 3.0. Additional exam requirements/recommendations for international students: Required—TOEFL (minimum score 550 paper-based; 79 iBT), IELTS (minimum score 6.5). Electronic applications accepted. *Faculty research:* Coronary vessel, vasculogenesis, acellular glomerular and retinal microvessel membranes, ependymal cells, cardiac muscle.

University of North Texas Health Science Center at Fort Worth, Graduate School of Biomedical Sciences, Fort Worth, TX 76107-2699. Offers anatomy and cell biology (MS, PhD); biochemistry and molecular biology (MS, PhD); biomedical sciences (MS, PhD); biotechnology (MS); forensic genetics (MS); integrative physiology (MS, PhD); medical science (MS); microbiology and immunology (MS, PhD); pharmacology (MS, PhD); science education (MS); DO/MS; DO/PhD. Terminal master's awarded for partial completion of doctoral program. *Degree requirements:* For master's, thesis; for doctorate, thesis/dissertation. *Entrance requirements:* For master's and doctorate, GRE General Test. Additional exam requirements/recommendations for international students: Required—TOEFL. *Expenses:* Contact institution. *Faculty research:* Alzheimer's disease, aging, eye diseases, cancer, cardiovascular disease.

University of Prince Edward Island, Atlantic Veterinary College, Graduate Program in Veterinary Medicine, Charlottetown, PE C1A 4P3, Canada. Offers anatomy (M Sc, PhD); bacteriology (M Sc, PhD); clinical pharmacology (M Sc, PhD); clinical sciences (M Sc, PhD); epidemiology (M Sc, PhD), including reproduction; fish health (M Sc, PhD); food animal nutrition (M Sc, PhD); immunology (M Sc, PhD); microanatomy (M Sc, PhD); parasitology (M Sc, PhD); pathology (M Sc, PhD); pharmacology (M Sc, PhD); physiology (M Sc, PhD); toxicology (M Sc, PhD); veterinary science (M Vet Sc); virology (M Sc, PhD). *Program availability:* Part-time. *Degree requirements:* For master's, thesis; for doctorate, thesis/dissertation. *Entrance requirements:* For master's, DVM, B Sc honors degree, or equivalent; for doctorate, M Sc. Additional exam requirements/recommendations for international students: Required—TOEFL (minimum score 550 paper-based; 80 iBT). *Expenses:* Contact institution. *Faculty research:* Animal health management, infectious diseases, fin fish and shellfish health, basic biomedical sciences, ecosystem health.

University of Puerto Rico, Medical Sciences Campus, School of Medicine, Biomedical Sciences Graduate Program, Department of Anatomy and Neurobiology, San Juan, PR 00936-5067. Offers anatomy (MS, PhD). *Degree requirements:* For master's, one foreign language, comprehensive exam, thesis; for doctorate, one foreign language, comprehensive exam, thesis/dissertation. *Entrance requirements:* For master's and doctorate, GRE General Test, GRE Subject Test, interview, minimum GPA of 3.0, 3 letters of recommendation. Electronic applications accepted. *Faculty research:* Neurobiology, primatology, visual system, muscle structure.

Anatomy

University of Rochester, School of Medicine and Dentistry, Graduate Programs in Medicine and Dentistry, Department of Neurobiology and Anatomy, Programs in Neurobiology and Anatomy, Rochester, NY 14627. Offers PhD, MD/MS. *Degree requirements:* For doctorate, thesis/dissertation, qualifying exam. *Entrance requirements:* For doctorate, GRE General Test. *Expenses: Tuition,* area resident: Full-time $47,450; part-time $1482 per credit hour. *Required fees:* $528. Tuition and fees vary according to program.

University of Saskatchewan, College of Medicine, Department of Anatomy and Cell Biology, Saskatoon, SK S7N 5A2, Canada. Offers M Sc, PhD. *Degree requirements:* For master's, thesis; for doctorate, thesis/dissertation. *Entrance requirements:* Additional exam requirements/recommendations for international students: Required—TOEFL.

University of Saskatchewan, Western College of Veterinary Medicine and College of Graduate Studies and Research, Graduate Programs in Veterinary Medicine, Department of Veterinary Biomedical Sciences, Saskatoon, SK S7N 5A2, Canada. Offers veterinary anatomy (M Sc); veterinary biomedical sciences (M Vet Sc); veterinary physiological sciences (M Sc, PhD). *Degree requirements:* For master's, thesis; for doctorate, comprehensive exam (for some programs), thesis/dissertation. *Entrance requirements:* Additional exam requirements/recommendations for international students: Required—TOEFL (minimum score 80 iBT); Recommended—IELTS (minimum score 6.5). Electronic applications accepted. *Faculty research:* Toxicology, animal reproduction, pharmacology, chloride channels, pulmonary pathobiology.

University of South Florida, Morsani College of Medicine and College of Graduate Studies, Graduate Programs in Medical Sciences, Tampa, FL 33620-9951. Offers advanced athletic training (MS); athletic training (MS); bioinformatics and computational biology (MSBCB); biotechnology (MSB); health informatics (MSHI); medical sciences (MSMS, PhD), including aging and neuroscience (MSMS); allergy, immunology and infectious disease (PhD), anatomy, athletic training (MSMS), clinical and translational research, health informatics (MSMS), health science (MSMS); interdisciplinary medical sciences (MSMS), medical microbiology and immunology (MSMS), metabolic and nutritional medicine (MSMS), molecular medicine, molecular pharmacology and physiology (PhD), neurology (PhD), pathology and laboratory medicine (PhD), pharmacology and therapeutics (PhD), physiology and biophysics (PhD), women's health (MSMS). *Students:* 510 full-time (261 women), 318 part-time (208 women); includes 360 minority (108 Black or African American, non-Hispanic/Latino; 3 American Indian or Alaska Native, non-Hispanic/Latino; 101 Asian, non-Hispanic/Latino; 124 Hispanic/Latino; 1 Native Hawaiian or other Pacific Islander, non-Hispanic/Latino; 23 Two or more races, non-Hispanic/Latino), 52 international. Average age 26. 6,567 applicants, 13% accepted, 469 enrolled. In 2015, 216 master's awarded. Terminal master's awarded for partial completion of doctoral program. *Degree requirements:* For master's, comprehensive exam, thesis; for doctorate, comprehensive exam, thesis/dissertation. *Entrance requirements:* For master's, GRE General Test or GMAT, bachelor's degree or equivalent from regionally-accredited university with minimum GPA of 3.0 in upper-division sciences coursework; prerequisites in general biology, general chemistry, general physics, organic chemistry, quantitative analysis, and integral and differential calculus; for doctorate, GRE General Test, bachelor's degree from regionally-accredited university with minimum GPA of 3.0 in upper-division sciences coursework; 3 letters of recommendation; personal interview; 1-2 page personal statement; prerequisites in biology, chemistry, physics, organic chemistry, quantitative analysis, and integral/differential calculus. Additional exam requirements/recommendations for international students: Required—TOEFL (minimum score 550 paper-based; 79 iBT) or IELTS (minimum score 6.5). *Application deadline:* For fall admission, 2/15 for domestic students, 1/2 for international students. Application fee: $30. *Expenses:* Contact institution. *Faculty research:* Anatomy, biochemistry, cancer biology, cardiovascular disease, cell biology, immunology, microbiology, molecular biology, neuroscience, pharmacology, physiology. *Unit head:* Dr. Michael Barber, Professor/Associate Dean for Graduate and Postdoctoral Affairs, 813-974-9908, Fax: 813-974-4317, E-mail: mbarber@health.usf.edu. *Application contact:* Dr. Eric Bennett, Graduate Director, PhD Program in Medical Sciences, 813-974-1545, Fax: 813-974-4317, E-mail: esbennet@health.usf.edu.
Website: http://health.usf.edu/nocms/medicine/graduatestudies/

The University of Tennessee, Graduate School, College of Agricultural Sciences and Natural Resources, Department of Animal Science, Knoxville, TN 37996. Offers animal anatomy (PhD); breeding (MS, PhD); management (MS, PhD); nutrition (MS, PhD); physiology (MS, PhD). *Program availability:* Part-time. *Degree requirements:* For master's, thesis; for doctorate, thesis/dissertation. *Entrance requirements:* For master's and doctorate, GRE General Test, minimum GPA of 2.7. Additional exam requirements/recommendations for international students: Required—TOEFL. Electronic applications accepted.

University of Utah, School of Medicine and Graduate School, Graduate Programs in Medicine, Department of Neurobiology and Anatomy, Salt Lake City, UT 84112-1107. Offers PhD. *Program availability:* Part-time. Terminal master's awarded for partial completion of doctoral program. *Degree requirements:* For doctorate, comprehensive exam, thesis/dissertation. *Entrance requirements:* For doctorate, GRE General Test.

Additional exam requirements/recommendations for international students: Required—TOEFL. *Faculty research:* Neuroscience, neuroanatomy, developmental neurobiology, neurogenetics.

The University of Western Ontario, Faculty of Graduate Studies, Biosciences Division, Department of Anatomy and Cell Biology, London, ON N6A 5B8, Canada. Offers anatomy and cell biology (M Sc, PhD); clinical anatomy (M Sc). *Degree requirements:* For master's, thesis; for doctorate, comprehensive exam, thesis/dissertation. *Entrance requirements:* For master's, honors degree or equivalent in biological sciences; for doctorate, master's degree. Additional exam requirements/recommendations for international students: Required—TOEFL. *Faculty research:* Cell and molecular biology, developmental biology, neuroscience, immunobiology and cancer.

Virginia Commonwealth University, Medical College of Virginia-Professional Programs, School of Medicine, School of Medicine Graduate Programs, Department of Anatomy and Neurobiology, Program in Anatomy and Neurobiology, Richmond, VA 23284-9005. Offers PhD. *Accreditation:* APTA. *Degree requirements:* For doctorate, thesis/dissertation. *Entrance requirements:* For doctorate, GRE, MCAT or DAT. Electronic applications accepted.

Virginia Commonwealth University, Program in Pre-Medical Basic Health Sciences, Richmond, VA 23284-9005. Offers anatomy (CBHS); biochemistry (CBHS); human genetics (CBHS); microbiology (CBHS); pharmacology (CBHS); physiology (CBHS). *Entrance requirements:* For degree, GRE, MCAT or DAT, course work in organic chemistry, minimum undergraduate GPA of 2.8. Additional exam requirements/recommendations for international students: Required—TOEFL (minimum score 600 paper-based). Electronic applications accepted.

Wake Forest University, School of Medicine and Graduate School of Arts and Sciences, Graduate Programs in Medicine, Department of Neurobiology and Anatomy, Winston-Salem, NC 27109. Offers PhD, MD/PhD. *Degree requirements:* For doctorate, thesis/dissertation. *Entrance requirements:* For doctorate, GRE General Test. Additional exam requirements/recommendations for international students: Required—TOEFL. Electronic applications accepted. *Faculty research:* Sensory neurobiology, reproductive endocrinology, regulatory processes in cell biology.

Wayne State University, School of Medicine, Office of Biomedical Graduate Programs, Department of Anatomy and Cell Biology, Detroit, MI 48202. Offers anatomy (PhD); MD/PhD. Admission to the master's degree program is limited and based on special circumstances. *Faculty:* 24. *Students:* 14 full-time (5 women), 1 (woman) part-time; includes 5 minority (1 Black or African American, non-Hispanic/Latino; 1 Asian, non-Hispanic/Latino; 3 Hispanic/Latino), 6 international. Average age 28. 18 applicants, 28% accepted, 4 enrolled. In 2015, 2 doctorates awarded. *Degree requirements:* For doctorate, thesis/dissertation. *Entrance requirements:* For doctorate, GRE General Test, minimum GPA of 3.0 undergraduate, in life science coursework, and overall; research experience beyond coursework laboratory assignments; three letters of faculty recommendation; personal statement; resume; interview. Additional exam requirements/recommendations for international students: Required—TOEFL (minimum score 100 iBT). *Application deadline:* For fall admission, 3/1 priority date for domestic and international students. Applications are processed on a rolling basis. Application fee: $0. Electronic applications accepted. *Expenses:* $17,645 annual resident tuition, $33,311 non-resident tuition; $735.20 per credit hour resident tuition, $1,387.95 per credit hour non-resident tuition; fees include $47.45 per credit hour student services fee and $274.60 per semester registration fee. *Financial support:* In 2015–16, 12 students received support, including 2 fellowships with tuition reimbursements available (averaging $29,149 per year), 12 research assistantships with tuition reimbursements available (averaging $26,781 per year); Federal Work-Study, scholarships/grants, health care benefits, and unspecified assistantships also available. Financial award application deadline: 3/31; financial award applicants required to submit FAFSA. *Faculty research:* Vision science, neuroscience, molecular cell and developmental biology. *Unit head:* Dr. Paul Walker, Director, 313-577-5678, E-mail: pdwalker@med.wayne.edu.
Website: http://www.anatomy.med.wayne.edu/phdprogram.php

Wright State University, School of Graduate Studies, College of Science and Mathematics, Department of Neuroscience, Cell Biology, and Physiology, Dayton, OH 45435. Offers anatomy (MS); physiology and biophysics (MS). *Degree requirements:* For master's, thesis optional. *Entrance requirements:* Additional exam requirements/recommendations for international students: Required—TOEFL. *Faculty research:* Reproductive cell biology, neurobiology of pain, neurohistochemistry.

Youngstown State University, Graduate School, College of Science, Technology, Engineering and Mathematics, Department of Biological Sciences, Youngstown, OH 44555-0001. Offers environmental biology (MS); molecular biology, microbiology, and genetic (MS); physiology and anatomy (MS). *Program availability:* Part-time. *Degree requirements:* For master's, comprehensive exam, thesis, oral review. *Entrance requirements:* For master's, GRE General Test, minimum GPA of 2.7. Additional exam requirements/recommendations for international students: Required—TOEFL. *Faculty research:* Cell biology, neurophysiology, molecular biology, neurobiology, gene regulation.

Section 3
Biochemistry

This section contains a directory of institutions offering graduate work in biochemistry. Additional information about programs listed in the directory may be obtained by writing directly to the dean of a graduate school or chair of a department at the address given in the directory.

For programs offering related work, see also in this book *Allied Health; Biological and Biomedical Sciences; Biophysics; Botany and Plant Biology; Cell, Molecular, and Structural Biology; Genetics, Developmental Biology, and Reproductive Biology; Microbiological Sciences; Neuroscience and Neurobiology; Nutrition; Pathology and Pathobiology; Pharmacology and Toxicology; Pharmacy and Pharmaceutical Sciences;* and *Physiology.* In the other guides in this series:

Graduate Programs in the Physical Sciences, Mathematics, Agricultural Sciences, the Environment & Natural Resources

See *Agricultural and Food Sciences, Chemistry,* and *Physics*

Graduate Programs in Engineering & Applied Sciences

See *Agricultural Engineering and Bioengineering, Biomedical Engineering and Biotechnology, Chemical Engineering,* and *Materials Sciences and Engineering*

CONTENTS

Biochemistry

Albert Einstein College of Medicine, Graduate Division of Biomedical Sciences, Department of Biochemistry, Bronx, NY 10461-1602. Offers PhD, MD/PhD. *Degree requirements:* For doctorate, thesis/dissertation. *Entrance requirements:* For doctorate, GRE General Test. Additional exam requirements/recommendations for international students: Required—TOEFL. *Faculty research:* Biochemical mechanisms, enzymology, protein chemistry, bio-organic chemistry, molecular genetics.

American University of Beirut, Graduate Programs, Faculty of Medicine, Beirut, Lebanon. Offers anatomy, cell biology and human morphology (MS); biochemistry and medical genetics (MS); biomedical sciences (PhD); experimental pathology, immunology and microbiology (MS); medicine (MD); neuroscience (MS); pharmacology and toxicology (MS). *Program availability:* Part-time. *Faculty:* 302 full-time (95 women), 64 part-time/adjunct (11 women). *Students:* 381 full-time (173 women), 61 part-time (51 women). Average age 23. In 2015, 14 master's awarded. *Degree requirements:* For master's, one foreign language, comprehensive exam, thesis (for some programs); for doctorate, one foreign language, comprehensive exam, thesis/dissertation. *Entrance requirements:* For master's, letter of recommendation; for doctorate, MCAT, bachelor's degree. Additional exam requirements/recommendations for international students: Required—TOEFL (minimum score 600 paper-based; 100 iBT), IELTS (minimum score 7.5). *Application deadline:* For fall admission, 4/30 for domestic and international students; for spring admission, 11/1 for domestic and international students. Application fee: $50. Electronic applications accepted. *Expenses: Tuition, area resident:* Full-time $16,254; part-time $903 per credit. *Required fees:* $699. Tuition and fees vary according to course load and program. *Financial support:* In 2015–16, 273 students received support, including 45 teaching assistantships (averaging $9,000 per year); career-related internships or fieldwork, institutionally sponsored loans, scholarships/grants, health care benefits, and unspecified assistantships also available. Financial award application deadline: 2/2. *Faculty research:* Cancer research (targeted therapy, mechanisms of leukemogenesis, tumor cell extravasation and metastasis, cancer stem cells), stem cell research (regenerative medicine, drug discovery), genetic research (neurogenetics, hereditary cardiomyopathy, hemoglobinopathies, pharmacogenomics, proteomics), neuroscience research (pain, neurodegenerative disorder), metabolism (inflammation and metabolism, metabolic disorder, diabetes mellitus), vascular and renal biology, signal transduction. *Total annual research expenditures:* $2.6 million. *Unit head:* Dr. Mohamed Sayegh, Dean, 961-1350000 Ext. 4700, Fax: 961-1744464, E-mail: msayegh@aub.edu.lb. *Application contact:* Dr. Salim Kanaan, Director, Admissions Office, 961-1350000 Ext. 2594, Fax: 961-1750775, E-mail: sk00@aub.edu.lb. Website: http://www.aub.edu.lb/fm/fm_home/Pages/index.aspx

Arizona State University at the Tempe campus, College of Liberal Arts and Sciences, Department of Chemistry and Biochemistry, Tempe, AZ 85287-1604. Offers biochemistry (MS, PhD); chemistry (MS, PhD); nanoscience (PSM). Terminal master's awarded for partial completion of doctoral program. *Degree requirements:* For master's, thesis, interactive Program of Study (iPOS) submitted before completing 50 percent of required credit hours; for doctorate, comprehensive exam, thesis/dissertation, interactive Program of Study (iPOS) submitted before completing 50 percent of required credit hours. *Entrance requirements:* For master's and doctorate, GRE, minimum GPA of 3.0 or equivalent in last 2 years of work leading to bachelor's degree. Additional exam requirements/recommendations for international students: Required—TOEFL, IELTS, or PTE. Electronic applications accepted.

Auburn University, Graduate School, College of Sciences and Mathematics, Department of Chemistry and Biochemistry, Auburn University, AL 36849. Offers analytical chemistry (MS, PhD); biochemistry (MS, PhD); inorganic chemistry (MS, PhD); organic chemistry (MS, PhD); physical chemistry (MS, PhD). *Program availability:* Part-time. *Faculty:* 27 full-time (4 women), 2 part-time/adjunct (0 women). *Students:* 45 full-time (17 women), 26 part-time (15 women); includes 9 minority (7 Black or African American, non-Hispanic/Latino; 1 American Indian or Alaska Native, non-Hispanic/Latino; 1 Asian, non-Hispanic/Latino), 38 international. Average age 27. 33 applicants, 52% accepted, 16 enrolled. In 2015, 1 master's, 6 doctorates awarded. *Degree requirements:* For master's, thesis (for some programs); for doctorate, thesis/dissertation, oral and written exams. *Entrance requirements:* For master's and doctorate, GRE General Test. *Application deadline:* Applications are processed on a rolling basis. Application fee: $50 ($60 for international students). Electronic applications accepted. *Expenses:* Tuition, state resident: full-time $8802; part-time $489 per credit hour. Tuition, nonresident: full-time $26,406; part-time $1467 per credit hour. *Required fees:* $808 per semester. Tuition and fees vary according to degree level and program. *Financial support:* Fellowships, research assistantships, and teaching assistantships available. Financial award application deadline: 3/15; financial award applicants required to submit FAFSA. *Unit head:* Dr. Curtis Shannon, Chair, 334-844-4043, Fax: 334-844-4043. *Application contact:* Dr. George Flowers, Dean of the Graduate School, 334-844-2125.
Website: http://www.auburn.edu/cosam/departments/chemistry/

Augusta University, The Graduate School, Program in Biochemistry and Cancer Biology, Augusta, GA 30912. Offers PhD. *Faculty:* 2 full-time. *Degree requirements:* For doctorate, comprehensive exam, thesis/dissertation. *Entrance requirements:* For doctorate, GRE General Test. Additional exam requirements/recommendations for international students: Required—TOEFL (minimum score 550 paper-based; 79 iBT). *Application deadline:* For fall admission, 1/15 for domestic and international students. Application fee: $50. Electronic applications accepted. *Financial support:* Research assistantships with partial tuition reimbursements, Federal Work-Study, institutionally sponsored loans, and scholarships/grants available. Support available to part-time students. Financial award application deadline: 5/31; financial award applicants required to submit FAFSA. *Faculty research:* Bacterial pathogenesis, eye diseases, vitamins and amino acid transporters, transcriptional control and molecular oncology, tumor biology. *Unit head:* Dr. Vinata Lokeshwar, Chair, 706-721-7652, Fax: 706-721-9947, E-mail: vlokeshwar@augusta.edu. *Application contact:* Dr. Darren Browning, Director, 706-721-7658, E-mail: dbrowning@augusta.edu.
Website: http://www.augusta.edu/cancer/students/

Baylor College of Medicine, Graduate School of Biomedical Sciences, Department of Biochemistry and Molecular Biology, Houston, TX 77030-3498. Offers PhD, MD/PhD. *Degree requirements:* For doctorate, thesis/dissertation, public defense. *Entrance requirements:* For doctorate, GRE General Test, GRE Subject Test (strongly recommended), minimum GPA of 3.0. Additional exam requirements/recommendations for international students: Required—TOEFL. Electronic applications accepted. *Faculty research:* DNA repair, homologous recombination, gene therapy, trinucleotide repeat diseases, retinitis pigmentosa.

Baylor College of Medicine, Graduate School of Biomedical Sciences, Interdepartmental Program in Cell and Molecular Biology, Houston, TX 77030-3498.

Offers biochemistry (PhD); cell and molecular biology (PhD); genetics (PhD); human genetics (PhD); immunology (PhD); microbiology (PhD); virology (PhD); MD/PhD. *Degree requirements:* For doctorate, thesis/dissertation, public defense. *Entrance requirements:* For doctorate, GRE General Test, GRE Subject Test (strongly recommended), minimum GPA of 3.0. Additional exam requirements/recommendations for international students: Required—TOEFL. Electronic applications accepted. *Faculty research:* Molecular and cellular biology; cancer, aging and stem cells; genomics and proteomics; microbiome, molecular microbiology; infectious disease, immunology and translational research.

Boston College, Graduate School of Arts and Sciences, Department of Chemistry, Chestnut Hill, MA 02467. Offers biochemistry (PhD); inorganic chemistry (PhD); organic chemistry (PhD); physical chemistry (PhD); science education (MST). *Faculty:* 21 full-time. *Students:* 121 full-time (57 women); includes 9 minority (6 Asian, non-Hispanic/Latino; 3 Hispanic/Latino), 53 international. 222 applicants, 50% accepted, 43 enrolled. In 2015, 2 master's, 11 doctorates awarded. *Degree requirements:* For doctorate, thesis/dissertation, qualifying exam. *Entrance requirements:* For doctorate, GRE General Test, GRE Subject Test. Additional exam requirements/recommendations for international students: Required—TOEFL (minimum score 600 paper-based; 100 iBT), IELTS (minimum score 8). *Application deadline:* For fall admission, 1/2 for domestic and international students. Application fee: $75. Electronic applications accepted. Tuition and fees vary according to program. *Financial support:* In 2015–16, 121 students received support, including fellowships with full tuition reimbursements available (averaging $30,000 per year), research assistantships with full tuition reimbursements available (averaging $30,000 per year), teaching assistantships with full tuition reimbursements available (averaging $30,000 per year); Federal Work-Study, scholarships/grants, health care benefits, and unspecified assistantships also available. Support available to part-time students. Financial award application deadline: 1/2. *Faculty research:* Organic and organometallic chemistry, chemical biology and biochemistry, physical and theoretical chemistry, inorganic chemistry. *Unit head:* Dr. Amir Hoveyda, Chairperson, 617-552-1735, E-mail: amir.hoveyda@bc.edu. *Application contact:* Dr. Jianmin Gao, Graduate Program Director, 617-552-0326, Fax: 617-552-0833, E-mail: gaojc@bc.edu.
Website: http://www.bc.edu/chemistry

Boston University, Graduate School of Arts and Sciences, Molecular Biology, Cell Biology, and Biochemistry Program (MCBB), Boston, MA 02215. Offers MA, PhD. *Students:* 32 full-time (14 women), 3 part-time (2 women); includes 10 minority (3 Black or African American, non-Hispanic/Latino; 2 Asian, non-Hispanic/Latino; 4 Hispanic/Latino; 1 Two or more races, non-Hispanic/Latino), 8 international. Average age 29. 139 applicants, 11% accepted, 3 enrolled. In 2015, 16 master's, 3 doctorates awarded. Terminal master's awarded for partial completion of doctoral program. *Degree requirements:* For master's, one foreign language, thesis (for some programs); for doctorate, one foreign language, comprehensive exam, thesis/dissertation. *Entrance requirements:* For master's and doctorate, GRE General Test, GRE Subject Test (recommended), 3 letters of recommendation, transcripts, personal statement. Additional exam requirements/recommendations for international students: Required—TOEFL (minimum score 550 paper-based; 84 iBT). *Application deadline:* For fall admission, 12/7 for domestic and international students. Application fee: $95. Electronic applications accepted. *Financial support:* In 2015–16, 30 students received support, including 2 fellowships with full tuition reimbursements available (averaging $21,000 per year), 15 research assistantships with full tuition reimbursements available (averaging $21,000 per year), 12 teaching assistantships with full tuition reimbursements available (averaging $21,000 per year); Federal Work-Study, scholarships/grants, traineeships, and health care benefits also available. Financial award application deadline: 12/7; financial award applicants required to submit FAFSA. *Unit head:* Dr. Ulla Hansen, Director, 617-353-2432, Fax: 617-353-6340, E-mail: uhansen@bu.edu. *Application contact:* Christina Honeycutt, Academic Administrator, 617-353-2432, Fax: 617-353-6340, E-mail: cjhoney@bu.edu.
Website: http://www.bu.edu/mcbb/

Bradley University, Graduate School, College of Liberal Arts and Sciences, Department of Chemistry and Biochemistry, Peoria, IL 61625-0002. Offers chemistry (MS). *Program availability:* Part-time, evening/weekend. *Degree requirements:* For master's, comprehensive exam, thesis. *Entrance requirements:* Additional exam requirements/recommendations for international students: Required—TOEFL (minimum score 550 paper-based; 79 iBT), IELTS (minimum score 6.5). Electronic applications accepted.

Brandeis University, Graduate School of Arts and Sciences, Program in Biochemistry and Biophysics, Waltham, MA 02454. Offers biochemistry and biophysics (PhD); quantitative biology (PhD). *Faculty:* 10 full-time (3 women). *Students:* 38 full-time (16 women); includes 3 minority (1 Asian, non-Hispanic/Latino; 1 Hispanic/Latino; 1 Two or more races, non-Hispanic/Latino), 12 international. 70 applicants, 29% accepted, 5 enrolled. In 2015, 4 doctorates awarded. Terminal master's awarded for partial completion of doctoral program. *Degree requirements:* For doctorate, thesis/dissertation, qualifying exams. *Entrance requirements:* For doctorate, GRE General Test, resume, 3 letters of recommendation, statement of purpose, transcript(s). Additional exam requirements/recommendations for international students: Required—TOEFL (minimum score 600 paper-based; 100 iBT); Recommended—IELTS (minimum score 7), TSE (minimum score 68). *Application deadline:* For fall admission, 12/15 priority date for domestic students. Application fee: $75. Electronic applications accepted. *Financial support:* In 2015–16, 31 students received support, including 14 fellowships with full tuition reimbursements available (averaging $30,500 per year), 17 research assistantships with full tuition reimbursements available (averaging $30,500 per year); Federal Work-Study, scholarships/grants, health care benefits, and tuition waivers (full and partial) also available. Financial award application deadline: 4/15; financial award applicants required to submit FAFSA. *Faculty research:* Macromolecular chemistry, structure and function, biochemistry, biophysics, biological macromolecules. *Unit head:* Prof. Dagmar Ringe, Director of Graduate Studies, 781-736-2300, Fax: 781-736-2349, E-mail: scigradoffice@brandeis.edu. *Application contact:* 781-736-2300, E-mail: scigradoffice@brandeis.edu.
Website: http://www.brandeis.edu/gsas

Brigham Young University, Graduate Studies, College of Physical and Mathematical Sciences, Department of Chemistry and Biochemistry, Provo, UT 84602. Offers biochemistry (MS, PhD); chemistry (MS, PhD). *Faculty:* 30 full-time (1 woman). *Students:* 92 full-time (32 women); includes 5 minority (2 Asian, non-Hispanic/Latino; 2 Hispanic/Latino; 1 Native Hawaiian or other Pacific Islander, non-Hispanic/Latino), 47 international. Average age 28. 52 applicants, 50% accepted, 17 enrolled. In 2015, 1 master's, 14 doctorates awarded. *Degree requirements:* For master's, thesis; for doctorate, comprehensive exam, thesis/dissertation, qualifying exam. *Entrance*

requirements: For master's and doctorate, GRE General Test, minimum GPA of 3.0. Additional exam requirements/recommendations for international students: Required—TOEFL (minimum score 580 paper-based; 85 iBT), IELTS (minimum score 7); Recommended—TWE. *Application deadline:* For fall admission, 2/1 priority date for domestic and international students. Applications are processed on a rolling basis. Application fee: $50. Electronic applications accepted. *Financial support:* In 2015–16, 90 students received support, including 13 fellowships with full tuition reimbursements available (averaging $21,250 per year), 39 research assistantships with full tuition reimbursements available (averaging $21,250 per year), 38 teaching assistantships with full tuition reimbursements available (averaging $21,250 per year); institutionally sponsored loans, scholarships/grants, health care benefits, unspecified assistantships, and supplementary awards also available. Financial award application deadline: 2/1. *Faculty research:* Separation science, molecular recognition, organic synthesis and biomedical application, biochemistry and molecular biology, molecular spectroscopy. *Total annual research expenditures:* $2.2 million. *Unit head:* Dr. Gregory F. Burton, Chair, 801-422-4917, Fax: 801-422-0153, E-mail: gburton@byu.edu. *Application contact:* Dr. Paul B. Farnsworth, Graduate Coordinator, 801-422-6502, Fax: 801-422-0153, E-mail: pbfarnsw@byu.edu.
Website: http://www.chem.byu.edu/

Brown University, Graduate School, Division of Biology and Medicine, Department of Molecular Biology, Cell Biology, and Biochemistry, Providence, RI 02912. Offers MA, PhD. *Program availability:* Part-time. Terminal master's awarded for partial completion of doctoral program. *Degree requirements:* For master's, thesis (for some programs); for doctorate, one foreign language, thesis/dissertation, preliminary exam. *Entrance requirements:* For master's and doctorate, GRE General Test, GRE Subject Test. Additional exam requirements/recommendations for international students: Required—TOEFL. Electronic applications accepted. *Faculty research:* Molecular genetics, gene regulation.

California Institute of Technology, Division of Biology and Division of Chemistry and Chemical Engineering, Biochemistry and Molecular Biophysics Graduate Option, Pasadena, CA 91125-0001. Offers PhD. *Degree requirements:* For doctorate, thesis/dissertation, qualifying exam. *Entrance requirements:* For doctorate, GRE General Test. Additional exam requirements/recommendations for international students: Required—TOEFL. Electronic applications accepted.

California Institute of Technology, Division of Chemistry and Chemical Engineering, Pasadena, CA 91125-0001. Offers biochemistry and molecular biophysics (MS, PhD); chemical engineering (MS, PhD); chemistry (MS, PhD). *Faculty:* 41 full-time (7 women). *Students:* 309 full-time (98 women); includes 1 minority (Black or African American, non-Hispanic/Latino). Average age 26. 710 applicants, 21% accepted, 59 enrolled. In 2015, 14 master's, 59 doctorates awarded. Terminal master's awarded for partial completion of doctoral program. *Degree requirements:* For master's, thesis; for doctorate, thesis/dissertation. *Entrance requirements:* For doctorate, GRE, BS. Additional exam requirements/recommendations for international students: Required—TOEFL; Recommended—IELTS, TWE. *Application deadline:* For fall admission, 12/15 for domestic and international students. Application fee: $100. Electronic applications accepted. *Financial support:* In 2015–16, 309 students received support, including fellowships (averaging $31,000 per year), research assistantships (averaging $25,900 per year), teaching assistantships (averaging $5,100 per year); Federal Work-Study, institutionally sponsored loans, scholarships/grants, traineeships, health care benefits, and unspecified assistantships also available. Financial award application deadline: 12/15. *Unit head:* Prof. Jacqueline K. Barton, Chair, Division of Chemistry and Chemical Engineering, 626-395-3646, Fax: 626-395-6948, E-mail: jkbarton@caltech.edu. *Application contact:* Natalie Gilmore, Graduate Office, 626-395-3812, Fax: 626-577-9246, E-mail: ngilmore@its.caltech.edu.
Website: http://www.cce.caltech.edu/

California Polytechnic State University, San Luis Obispo, College of Science and Mathematics, Department of Chemistry and Biochemistry, San Luis Obispo, CA 93407. Offers polymers and coating science (MS). *Program availability:* Part-time. *Faculty:* 3 full-time (0 women). *Students:* 8 full-time (4 women), 8 part-time (4 women); includes 4 minority (3 Asian, non-Hispanic/Latino; 1 Hispanic/Latino), 2 international. Average age 24. 14 applicants, 50% accepted, 5 enrolled. In 2015, 3 master's awarded. *Degree requirements:* For master's, comprehensive exam (for some programs), thesis (for some programs). *Application deadline:* For fall admission, 4/1 for domestic and international students; for winter admission, 11/1 for domestic students, 6/30 for international students; for spring admission, 2/1 for domestic students. Applications are processed on a rolling basis. Application fee: $55. Electronic applications accepted. *Expenses:* Tuition, state resident: full-time $6738; part-time $3906 per year. Tuition, nonresident: full-time $15,666; part-time $8370 per year. *Required fees:* $3528; $3075 per unit. $1025 per term. *Financial support:* Fellowships, research assistantships, career-related internships or fieldwork, Federal Work-Study, and scholarships/grants available. Support available to part-time students. Financial award application deadline: 3/2; financial award applicants required to submit FAFSA. *Faculty research:* Polymer physical chemistry and analysis, polymer synthesis, coatings formulation.
Website: http://www.chemistry.calpoly.edu/

California State University, East Bay, Office of Graduate Studies, College of Science, Department of Chemistry and Biochemistry, Hayward, CA 94542-3000. Offers chemistry (MS), including biochemistry. *Students:* 11 full-time (7 women), 21 part-time (11 women); includes 19 minority (1 Black or African American, non-Hispanic/Latino; 15 Asian, non-Hispanic/Latino; 3 Hispanic/Latino), 5 international. Average age 30. 44 applicants, 52% accepted, 8 enrolled. In 2015, 12 master's awarded. *Degree requirements:* For master's, comprehensive exam or thesis. *Entrance requirements:* For master's, minimum GPA of 2.6 in field during previous 2 years of course work. Additional exam requirements/recommendations for international students: Required—TOEFL (minimum score 550 paper-based). *Application deadline:* For fall admission, 6/30 for domestic and international students. Application fee: $55. Electronic applications accepted. *Financial support:* Fellowships, career-related internships or fieldwork, Federal Work-Study, institutionally sponsored loans, and scholarships/grants available. Support available to part-time students. Financial award application deadline: 3/2; financial award applicants required to submit FAFSA. *Unit head:* Dr. Ann McPartland, Chair, 510-885-3452, Fax: 510-885-4675, E-mail: ann.mcpartland@csueastbay.edu. *Application contact:* Prof. Chul Kim, Chemistry Graduate Advisor, 510-885-3490, Fax: 510-885-4675, E-mail: chul.kim@csueastbay.edu.
Website: http://www20.csueastbay.edu/csci/departments/chemistry

California State University, Long Beach, Graduate Studies, College of Natural Sciences and Mathematics, Department of Chemistry and Biochemistry, Long Beach, CA 90840. Offers biochemistry (MS); chemistry (MS). *Program availability:* Part-time. *Degree requirements:* For master's, thesis, departmental qualifying exam. Electronic applications accepted. *Faculty research:* Enzymology, organic synthesis, molecular modeling, environmental chemistry, reaction kinetics.

California State University, Los Angeles, Graduate Studies, College of Natural and Social Sciences, Department of Chemistry and Biochemistry, Los Angeles, CA 90032-8530. Offers analytical chemistry (MS). *Program availability:* Part-time, evening/weekend. *Degree requirements:* For master's, one foreign language, comprehensive

exam or thesis. *Entrance requirements:* Additional exam requirements/recommendations for international students: Required—TOEFL. *Application deadline:* For fall admission, 5/1 for domestic and international students. Applications are processed on a rolling basis. Application fee: $55. *Financial support:* Federal Work-Study available. Support available to part-time students. Financial award application deadline: 3/1. *Faculty research:* Intercalation of heavy metal, carborane chemistry, conductive polymers and fabrics, titanium reagents, computer modeling and synthesis.
Website: http://www.calstatela.edu/dept/chem/index.htm

California State University, Northridge, Graduate Studies, College of Science and Mathematics, Department of Chemistry and Biochemistry, Northridge, CA 91330. Offers biochemistry (MS); chemistry (MS), including chemistry, environmental chemistry. *Faculty:* 14 full-time (4 women), 30 part-time/adjunct (10 women). *Students:* 2 full-time (1 woman), 30 part-time (12 women); includes 15 minority (1 Black or African American, non-Hispanic/Latino; 7 Asian, non-Hispanic/Latino; 7 Hispanic/Latino), 3 international. Average age 26. 69 applicants, 23% accepted, 8 enrolled. *Degree requirements:* For master's, thesis. *Entrance requirements:* For master's, GRE General Test or minimum GPA of 3.0. Additional exam requirements/recommendations for international students: Required—TOEFL. *Application deadline:* For fall admission, 11/30 for domestic students. Application fee: $55. Electronic applications accepted. *Financial support:* Teaching assistantships available. Support available to part-time students. Financial award application deadline: 3/1. *Unit head:* Eric Kelson, Chair, 818-677-3381.
Website: http://www.csun.edu/chemistry/

Carnegie Mellon University, Mellon College of Science, Department of Biological Sciences, Pittsburgh, PA 15213-3891. Offers biochemistry (PhD); biophysics (PhD); cell and developmental biology (PhD); computational biology (MS, PhD); genetics (PhD); molecular biology (PhD); neuroscience (PhD); structural biology (PhD). *Degree requirements:* For doctorate, comprehensive exam, thesis/dissertation. *Entrance requirements:* For doctorate, GRE General Test, GRE Subject Test, interview. Electronic applications accepted. *Faculty research:* Genetic structure, function, and regulation; protein structure and function; biological membranes; biological spectroscopy.

Carnegie Mellon University, Mellon College of Science, Department of Chemistry, Pittsburgh, PA 15213-3891. Offers atmospheric chemistry (PhD); bioinorganic chemistry (PhD); bioorganic chemistry and chemical biology (PhD); biophysical chemistry (PhD); catalysis (PhD); green and environmental chemistry (PhD); materials and nanoscience (PhD); renewable energy (PhD); sensors, probes, and imaging (PhD); spectroscopy and single molecule analysis (PhD); theoretical and computational chemistry (PhD). *Program availability:* Part-time. Terminal master's awarded for partial completion of doctoral program. *Degree requirements:* For doctorate, thesis/dissertation, departmental qualifying and oral exams, teaching experience. *Entrance requirements:* For doctorate, GRE General Test, GRE Subject Test. Additional exam requirements/recommendations for international students: Required—TOEFL. Electronic applications accepted. *Faculty research:* Physical and theoretical chemistry, chemical synthesis, biophysical/bioinorganic chemistry.

Case Western Reserve University, School of Medicine and School of Graduate Studies, Graduate Programs in Medicine, Department of Biochemistry, Cleveland, OH 44106. Offers biochemical research (MS); biochemistry (MS, PhD); RNA biology (PhD); MD/PhD. *Program availability:* Part-time. Terminal master's awarded for partial completion of doctoral program. *Degree requirements:* For master's, thesis (for some programs); for doctorate, thesis/dissertation. *Entrance requirements:* For master's and doctorate, GRE General Test. Additional exam requirements/recommendations for international students: Required—TOEFL. Electronic applications accepted. *Expenses:* Tuition, area resident: Full-time $41,137; part-time $1714 per credit hour. *Required fees:* $32. Tuition and fees vary according to course load and program. *Faculty research:* Regulation of metabolism, regulation of gene expression and protein synthesis, cell biology, molecular biology, structural biology.

Case Western Reserve University, School of Medicine and School of Graduate Studies, Graduate Programs in Medicine, Department of Nutrition, Cleveland, OH 44106-4954. Offers dietetics (MS); nutrition (MS, PhD), including molecular nutrition (PhD), nutrition and biochemistry (PhD); public health nutrition (MS). *Program availability:* Part-time. Terminal master's awarded for partial completion of doctoral program. *Degree requirements:* For master's, thesis (for some programs); for doctorate, thesis/dissertation. *Entrance requirements:* For master's, GRE General Test; for doctorate, GRE General Test, GRE Subject Test. Additional exam requirements/recommendations for international students: Required—TOEFL. *Expenses:* Tuition, area resident: Full-time $41,137; part-time $1714 per credit hour. *Required fees:* $32. Tuition and fees vary according to course load and program. *Faculty research:* Fatty acid metabolism, application of gene therapy to nutritional problems, dietary intake methodology, nutrition and physical fitness, metabolism during infancy and pregnancy.

City College of the City University of New York, Graduate School, Division of Science, Department of Chemistry, Program in Biochemistry, New York, NY 10031-9198. Offers MS, PhD. PhD program offered jointly with Graduate School and University Center of the City University of New York. Terminal master's awarded for partial completion of doctoral program. *Degree requirements:* For doctorate, one foreign language, thesis/dissertation. *Entrance requirements:* For doctorate, GRE. Additional exam requirements/recommendations for international students: Required—TOEFL (minimum score 550 paper-based; 79 iBT). *Application deadline:* For fall admission, 5/1 for domestic and international students; for spring admission, 11/15 for domestic and international students. Applications are processed on a rolling basis. Application fee: $125. Electronic applications accepted. Tuition and fees vary according to course load, degree level and program. *Financial support:* Scholarships/grants available. Financial award application deadline: 6/1; financial award applicants required to submit FAFSA. *Faculty research:* Fatty acid metabolism, lectins, gene structure. *Unit head:* Dr. Daniel L. Akins, Chair, 212-650-8402.

Clark University, Graduate School, Gustav H. Carlson School of Chemistry, Worcester, MA 01610-1477. Offers biochemistry (MS, PhD); chemistry (MS, PhD). *Faculty:* 10 full-time (1 woman), 1 (woman) part-time/adjunct. *Students:* 17 full-time (6 women), 2 part-time (1 woman); includes 4 minority (2 Asian, non-Hispanic/Latino; 2 Hispanic/Latino), 9 international. Average age 27. 52 applicants, 23% accepted, 5 enrolled. In 2015, 5 master's awarded. Terminal master's awarded for partial completion of doctoral program. *Degree requirements:* For master's, thesis or alternative; for doctorate, one foreign language, thesis/dissertation. *Entrance requirements:* For master's and doctorate, GRE General Test. Additional exam requirements/recommendations for international students: Required—TOEFL. *Application deadline:* For fall admission, 1/15 priority date for domestic students. Applications are processed on a rolling basis. Application fee: $75. *Expenses:* Tuition, area resident: Full-time $41,590; part-time $1300 per credit hour. *Required fees:* $80. Tuition and fees vary according to course load and program. *Financial support:* In 2015–16, fellowships with full tuition reimbursements (averaging $21,875 per year), 11 teaching assistantships with full tuition reimbursements (averaging $21,875 per year) were awarded; research assistantships with full tuition reimbursements and tuition waivers (full) also available. *Faculty research:* Nuclear chemistry, molecular biology simulation, NMR studies, biochemistry, protein folding mechanisms. *Total annual research expenditures:* $25,000.

Biochemistry

Unit head: Dr. Luis Smith, Chair, 508-793-7753. *Application contact:* Rene Baril, Managerial Secretary, 508-793-7130, Fax: 528-793-7117, E-mail: mbaril@clarku.edu. Website: http://www.clarku.edu/departments/chemistry/graduate/index.cfm

Clemson University, Graduate School, College of Science, Department of Genetics and Biochemistry, Program in Biochemistry and Molecular Biology, Clemson, SC 29634. Offers PhD. *Faculty:* 28 full-time (14 women), 1 (woman) part-time/adjunct. *Students:* 15 full-time (8 women); includes 1 minority (Asian, non-Hispanic/Latino), 7 international. Average age 29. 24 applicants, 25% accepted, 1 enrolled. In 2015, 5 doctorates awarded. *Degree requirements:* For doctorate, comprehensive exam, thesis/dissertation. *Entrance requirements:* For doctorate, GRE General Test, unofficial transcripts, letters of recommendation. Additional exam requirements/recommendations for international students: Required—TOEFL (minimum score 80 iBT), IELTS (minimum score 6.5). *Application deadline:* For fall admission, 1/1 for domestic and international students; for spring admission, 9/1 for domestic and international students. Application fee: $80 ($90 for international students). Electronic applications accepted. *Expenses:* $4,060 per semester full-time resident, $8,103 per semester full-time non-resident, $448 per credit hour part-time resident, $898 per credit hour part-time non-resident. *Financial support:* In 2015–16, 15 students received support, including 3 fellowships with partial tuition reimbursements available (averaging $3,333 per year), 5 research assistantships with partial tuition reimbursements available (averaging $21,881 per year), 9 teaching assistantships with partial tuition reimbursements available (averaging $21,044 per year); health care benefits also available. Financial award application deadline: 1/1. *Faculty research:* Cell and developmental biology, microbial pathogenesis, protein structure and function, plant biochemistry. *Unit head:* Dr. William Marcotte, Jr., Department Chair, 864-656-3586, Fax: 864-656-6879, E-mail: marcotw@clemson.edu. *Application contact:* Nicole Clark-Mount, Administrative Assistant, 864-656-6237, Fax: 864-656-6879, E-mail: hluo@clemson.edu. Website: http://www.clemson.edu/genbiochem/graduate_programs/

Colorado State University, College of Natural Sciences, Department of Biochemistry and Molecular Biology, Fort Collins, CO 80523-1870. Offers biochemistry (MS, PhD). *Program availability:* Part-time. *Faculty:* 25 full-time (11 women), 3 part-time/adjunct (all women). *Students:* 20 full-time (7 women), 26 part-time (13 women); includes 3 minority (1 Hispanic/Latino; 2 Two or more races, non-Hispanic/Latino), 8 international. Average age 26. 31 applicants, 35% accepted, 11 enrolled. In 2015, 4 master's, 4 doctorates awarded. Terminal master's awarded for partial completion of doctoral program. *Degree requirements:* For master's, comprehensive exam, thesis optional; for doctorate, comprehensive exam, thesis/dissertation, preliminary exam, teaching experience, faculty evaluation. *Entrance requirements:* For master's, GRE, 3 letters of recommendation, resume/curriculum vitae, statement of purpose, transcripts; for doctorate, GRE, BS/BA with minimum GPA of 3.0, statement of purpose, research interests, 3 letters of recommendation, resume. Additional exam requirements/recommendations for international students: Required—TOEFL (minimum score 550 paper-based; 80 iBT), IELTS (minimum score 6.5). *Application deadline:* For fall admission, 1/1 priority date for domestic and international students. Applications are processed on a rolling basis. Application fee: $60 ($70 for international students). Electronic applications accepted. *Expenses:* Tuition: state resident: full-time $9348. Tuition, nonresident: full-time $22,916. *Required fees:* $2174; $473.72 per credit hour. $236.86 per semester. Tuition and fees vary according to course load and program. *Financial support:* In 2015–16, 5 students received support, including 3 fellowships with full tuition reimbursements available (averaging $37,709 per year), 26 research assistantships with full tuition reimbursements available (averaging $28,328 per year), 11 teaching assistantships with full tuition reimbursements available (averaging $25,335 per year); career-related internships or fieldwork, scholarships/grants, and unspecified assistantships also available. Financial award application deadline: 1/1. *Faculty research:* Structural biology, gene expression, cellular biochemistry. *Total annual research expenditures:* $4.9 million. *Unit head:* Dr. P. Shing Ho, Professor and Chair, 970-491-0569, Fax: 970-491-0494, E-mail: shing.ho@colostate.edu. *Application contact:* Neda Amidon, Graduate Program Assistant, 970-491-6841, Fax: 970-491-0494, E-mail: neda.amidon@colostate.edu. Website: http://www.bmb.colostate.edu/

Colorado State University–Pueblo, College of Science and Mathematics, Pueblo, CO 81001-4901. Offers applied natural science (MS), including biochemistry, biology, chemistry. *Program availability:* Part-time, evening/weekend. *Degree requirements:* For master's, comprehensive exam (for some programs), thesis (for some programs), internship report (if non-thesis). *Entrance requirements:* For master's, GRE General Test (minimum score 1000), 2 letters of reference, minimum GPA of 3.0. Additional exam requirements/recommendations for international students: Required—TOEFL (minimum score 500 paper-based), IELTS (minimum score 5). *Faculty research:* Fungal cell walls, molecular biology, bioactive materials synthesis, atomic force microscopy-surface chemistry, nanoscience.

Columbia University, College of Physicians and Surgeons, Department of Biochemistry and Molecular Biophysics, New York, NY 10032. Offers biochemistry and molecular biophysics (M Phil, PhD); biophysics (PhD); MD/PhD. Only candidates for the PhD are admitted. *Degree requirements:* For doctorate, one foreign language, thesis/dissertation. *Entrance requirements:* For master's and doctorate, GRE General Test. Additional exam requirements/recommendations for international students: Required—TOEFL.

Cornell University, Graduate School, Graduate Fields of Agriculture and Life Sciences, Field of Biochemistry, Molecular and Cell Biology, Ithaca, NY 14853-0001. Offers biochemistry (PhD); biophysics (PhD); cell biology (PhD); molecular biology (PhD). *Degree requirements:* For doctorate, comprehensive exam, thesis/dissertation, 2 semesters of teaching experience. *Entrance requirements:* For doctorate, GRE General Test, GRE Subject Test (biology, chemistry, physics, biochemistry, cell and molecular biology), 3 letters of recommendation. Additional exam requirements/recommendations for international students: Required—TOEFL (minimum score 600 paper-based; 77 iBT). Electronic applications accepted. *Faculty research:* Biophysics, structural biology.

Cornell University, Graduate School, Graduate Fields of Agriculture and Life Sciences, Field of Plant Biology, Ithaca, NY 14853-0001. Offers cytology (MS, PhD); paleobotany (MS, PhD); plant biochemistry (MS, PhD); plant cell biology (MS, PhD); plant ecology (MS, PhD); plant molecular biology (MS, PhD); plant morphology, anatomy and biomechanics (MS, PhD); plant physiology (MS, PhD); systematic botany (MS, PhD). *Degree requirements:* For doctorate, comprehensive exam, thesis/dissertation. *Entrance requirements:* For doctorate, GRE General Test, GRE Subject Test in biology (recommended), 3 letters of recommendation. Additional exam requirements/recommendations for international students: Required—TOEFL (minimum score 610 paper-based; 77 iBT). Electronic applications accepted. *Faculty research:* Plant cell biology/cytology; plant molecular biology; plant morphology/anatomy/biomechanics; plant physiology, systematic botany, paleobotany; plant ecology, ethnobotany, plant biochemistry, photosynthesis.

Cornell University, Graduate School, Graduate Fields of Arts and Sciences, Field of Chemistry and Chemical Biology, Ithaca, NY 14853-0001. Offers analytical chemistry (PhD); bio-organic chemistry (PhD); biophysical chemistry (PhD); chemical biology (PhD); chemical physics (PhD); inorganic chemistry (PhD); materials chemistry (PhD); organic chemistry (PhD); organometallic chemistry (PhD); physical chemistry (PhD); polymer chemistry (PhD); theoretical chemistry (PhD). *Degree requirements:* For doctorate, comprehensive exam, thesis/dissertation. *Entrance requirements:* For doctorate, GRE General Test, GRE Subject Test (chemistry), 3 letters of recommendation. Additional exam requirements/recommendations for international students: Required—TOEFL (minimum score 600 paper-based; 77 iBT). Electronic applications accepted. *Faculty research:* Analytical, organic, inorganic, physical, materials, chemical biology.

Dalhousie University, Faculty of Medicine, Department of Biochemistry and Molecular Biology, Halifax, NS B3H 4R2, Canada. Offers M Sc, PhD. *Degree requirements:* For master's, thesis, demonstrating/teaching experience, oral defense, seminar; for doctorate, comprehensive exam, thesis/dissertation, demonstrating/teaching experience, oral defense, seminar, 2 short grant proposals in year 3. *Entrance requirements:* For master's and doctorate, GRE. Additional exam requirements/recommendations for international students: Required—1 of 5 approved tests: TOEFL, IELTS, CANTEST, CAEL, Michigan English Language Assessment Battery. Electronic applications accepted. *Expenses:* Contact institution. *Faculty research:* Gene expression and cell regulation; lipids, lipoproteins, and membranes; molecular evolution; proteins, molecular cell biology and molecular genetics; structure, function, and metabolism of biomolecules.

Dartmouth College, Arts and Sciences Graduate Programs, Department of Chemistry, Hanover, NH 03755. Offers biophysical chemistry (MS); chemistry (PhD). *Faculty:* 19 full-time (4 women), 1 (woman) part-time/adjunct. *Students:* 47 full-time (22 women); includes 8 minority (1 American Indian or Alaska Native, non-Hispanic/Latino; 4 Asian, non-Hispanic/Latino; 3 Two or more races, non-Hispanic/Latino), 15 international. Average age 26. 97 applicants, 12% accepted, 9 enrolled. In 2015, 3 master's, 6 doctorates awarded. *Degree requirements:* For doctorate, thesis/dissertation, departmental qualifying exams, research proposal, research seminar, teaching. *Entrance requirements:* For doctorate, GRE General Test, GRE Subject Test. Additional exam requirements/recommendations for international students: Required—TOEFL. *Application deadline:* For fall admission, 1/4 for domestic students. Application fee: $45. Electronic applications accepted. *Expenses: Tuition, area resident:* Full-time $48,120. *Required fees:* $296. One-time fee: $50 full-time. *Financial support:* Fellowships with full tuition reimbursements, research assistantships with full tuition reimbursements, teaching assistantships with full tuition reimbursements, institutionally sponsored loans, scholarships/grants, traineeships, tuition waivers (full), and unspecified assistantships available. Financial award application deadline: 4/1; financial award applicants required to submit CSS PROFILE or FAFSA. *Faculty research:* Organic and polymer synthesis, bioinorganic chemistry, magnetic resonance parameters. *Unit head:* Dr. Dale F. Mierke, Chair, 603-646-1154. *Application contact:* Deborah Carr, Administrative Assistant, 603-646-2189, E-mail: deborah.a.carr@dartmouth.edu. Website: http://www.dartmouth.edu/~chem/

Dartmouth College, Graduate Program in Molecular and Cellular Biology, Department of Biochemistry, Hanover, NH 03755. Offers PhD, MBA/PhD, MD/PhD. *Program availability:* 15 full-time (2 women), 1 part-time/adjunct (0 women). *Students:* 36 full-time (20 women); includes 3 minority (1 Hispanic/Latino; 2 Two or more races, non-Hispanic/Latino), 9 international. Average age 27. In 2015, 8 doctorates awarded. *Entrance requirements:* For doctorate, GRE General Test, letters of recommendation, minimum GPA of 3.0. Additional exam requirements/recommendations for international students: Required—TOEFL (minimum score paper-based 550, iBT 100) or IELTS (7.0). *Application deadline:* For fall admission, 12/1 for domestic students. Application fee: $75. Electronic applications accepted. *Expenses: Tuition, area resident:* Full-time $48,120. *Required fees:* $296. One-time fee: $50 full-time. *Financial support:* In 2015–16, fellowships with full tuition reimbursements (averaging $28,200 per year) were awarded; health care benefits also available. *Unit head:* Dr. Charles Barlowe, Chair and Professor, 603-650-1616, Fax: 603-650-1128, E-mail: biochemistry@dartmouth.edu. *Application contact:* Janet Cheney, Program Coordinator, 603-650-1612, Fax: 603-650-1006, E-mail: mcb@dartmouth.edu. Website: http://dms.dartmouth.edu/biochem/

Drexel University, College of Medicine, Biomedical Graduate Programs, Program in Biochemistry, Philadelphia, PA 19104-2875. Offers MS, PhD, MD/PhD. *Program availability:* Part-time. Terminal master's awarded for partial completion of doctoral program. *Degree requirements:* For master's, comprehensive exam, thesis; for doctorate, thesis/dissertation, qualifying exam. *Entrance requirements:* For master's, GRE General Test, minimum GPA of 2.75; for doctorate, GRE General Test, minimum GPA of 3.0. Additional exam requirements/recommendations for international students: Required—TOEFL. Electronic applications accepted.

Duke University, Graduate School, Department of Biochemistry, Durham, NC 27710. Offers crystallography of macromolecules (PhD); enzyme mechanisms (PhD); lipid biochemistry (PhD); membrane structure and function (PhD); molecular genetics (PhD); neurochemistry (PhD); nucleic acid structure and function (PhD); protein structure and function (PhD). *Degree requirements:* For doctorate, thesis/dissertation. *Entrance requirements:* For doctorate, GRE General Test, GRE Subject Test (recommended). Additional exam requirements/recommendations for international students: Required—TOEFL (minimum score 577 paper-based; 90 iBT) or IELTS (minimum score 7). Electronic applications accepted.

East Carolina University, Brody School of Medicine, Department of Biochemistry and Molecular Biology, Greenville, NC 27858-4353. Offers biochemistry and molecular biology (PhD); biomedical science (MS). *Students:* 7 full-time (4 women), 1 international. Average age 24. 15 applicants, 33% accepted, 4 enrolled. In 2015, 6 master's awarded. *Degree requirements:* For doctorate, comprehensive exam, thesis/dissertation. *Entrance requirements:* For doctorate, GRE General Test. Additional exam requirements/recommendations for international students: Required—TOEFL. *Application deadline:* For fall admission, 6/1 priority date for domestic students. Applications are processed on a rolling basis. *Financial support:* Fellowships with tuition reimbursements available. Financial award application deadline: 6/1. *Faculty research:* Gene regulation, development and differentiation, contractility and motility, macromolecular interactions, cancer. *Unit head:* Dr. Phillip H. Pekala, Chairman, 252-744-2684, Fax: 252-744-3383, E-mail: pekalap@ecu.edu. Website: http://www.ecu.edu/cs-dhs/biochemistry/gradProgram.cfm

Eastern New Mexico University, Graduate School, College of Liberal Arts and Sciences, Department of Physical Sciences, Portales, NM 88130. Offers chemistry (MS), including analytical, biochemistry, inorganic, organic, physical. *Program availability:* Part-time. *Degree requirements:* For master's, thesis optional, seminar, oral and written comprehensive exams. *Entrance requirements:* For master's, ACS placement examination, minimum GPA of 3.0; 2 letters of recommendation; personal statement of career goals; bachelor's degree with one year minimum each of general, organic, and analytical chemistry. Additional exam requirements/recommendations for international students: Required—TOEFL (minimum score 550 paper-based; 79 iBT), IELTS (minimum score 6). Electronic applications accepted. *Faculty research:* Synfuel, electrochemistry, protein chemistry.

East Tennessee State University, James H. Quillen College of Medicine, Department of Biomedical Sciences, Johnson City, TN 37614. Offers anatomy (PhD); biochemistry (PhD); microbiology (PhD); pharmaceutical sciences (PhD); pharmacology (PhD); physiology (PhD); quantitative biosciences (PhD). *Faculty:* 30 full-time (6 women). *Students:* 35 full-time (17 women), 2 part-time (1 woman); includes 13 minority (9 Black or African American, non-Hispanic/Latino; 4 Asian, non-Hispanic/Latino), 13 international. Average age 29. 53 applicants, 17% accepted, 8 enrolled. In 2015, 8 doctorates awarded. *Degree requirements:* For doctorate, thesis/dissertation, comprehensive qualifying exam. *Entrance requirements:* For doctorate, GRE General Test, GRE Subject Test, 3 letters of recommendation. Additional exam requirements/recommendations for international students: Required—TOEFL (minimum score 550 paper-based; 79 iBT). *Application deadline:* For fall admission, 3/15 priority date for domestic students, 3/1 priority date for international students. Application fee: $35 ($45 for international students). Electronic applications accepted. *Expenses:* Contact institution. *Financial support:* In 2015–16, 30 students received support, including 27 research assistantships with full tuition reimbursements available (averaging $20,000 per year); career-related internships or fieldwork, institutionally sponsored loans, scholarships/grants, and unspecified assistantships also available. Financial award application deadline: 7/1; financial award applicants required to submit FAFSA. *Faculty research:* Cardiovascular, infectious disease, neurosciences, cancer, immunology. *Unit head:* Dr. Mitchell E. Robinson, Associate Dean/Program Director, 423-439-2031, Fax: 423-439-2140, E-mail: robinson@etsu.edu. *Application contact:* Shella Bennett, Graduate Specialist, 423-439-4708, Fax: 423-439-5624, E-mail: bennetsg@etsu.edu.
Website: http://www.etsu.edu/com/dbms/

Emory University, Laney Graduate School, Division of Biological and Biomedical Sciences, Program in Biochemistry, Cell and Developmental Biology, Atlanta, GA 30322. Offers PhD. *Degree requirements:* For doctorate, comprehensive exam, thesis/dissertation. *Entrance requirements:* For doctorate, GRE General Test, minimum GPA of 3.0 in science course work (recommended). Additional exam requirements/recommendations for international students: Required—TOEFL. Electronic applications accepted. *Faculty research:* Signal transduction, molecular biology, enzymes and cofactors, receptor and ion channel function, membrane biology.

Florida Institute of Technology, College of Science, Program in Biochemistry, Melbourne, FL 32901-6975. Offers MS. *Program availability:* Part-time. *Students:* 4 full-time (3 women), 2 part-time (0 women), all international. Average age 28. 32 applicants, 63% accepted, 2 enrolled. In 2015, 1 master's awarded. *Degree requirements:* For master's, thesis optional, research proposal, oral examination in defense of the thesis, or final program examination and research project, 30 credit hours. *Entrance requirements:* For master's, undergraduate degree in biochemistry, chemistry, or related area. Additional exam requirements/recommendations for international students: Required—TOEFL (minimum score 550 paper-based; 79 iBT). *Application deadline:* For fall admission, 4/4 for international students; for spring admission, 9/30 for international students. Applications are processed on a rolling basis. Electronic applications accepted. *Expenses: Tuition, area resident:* Full-time $21,690; part-time $1205 per credit hour. *Required fees:* $500. Tuition and fees vary according to degree level, campus/location and program. *Financial support:* Applicants required to submit FAFSA. *Faculty research:* Energy storage applications, marine and organic chemistry, stereochemistry, medicinal chemistry, environmental chemistry. *Unit head:* Dr. Michael Freund, Department Head, 321-674-7153, E-mail: msfreund@fit.edu. *Application contact:* Cheryl A. Brown, Associate Director of Graduate Admissions, 321-674-7581, Fax: 321-723-9468, E-mail: cbrown@fit.edu.
Website: http://www.fit.edu/programs/

Florida State University, The Graduate School, College of Arts and Sciences, Department of Chemistry and Biochemistry, Tallahassee, FL 32306-4390. Offers analytical chemistry (MS, PhD); biochemistry (MS, PhD); inorganic chemistry (MS, PhD); materials chemistry (PhD); organic chemistry (MS, PhD); physical chemistry (MS, PhD). *Faculty:* 40 full-time (6 women), 4 part-time/adjunct (2 women). *Students:* 162 full-time (56 women); includes 37 minority (8 Black or African American, non-Hispanic/Latino; 6 Asian, non-Hispanic/Latino; 18 Hispanic/Latino; 1 Native Hawaiian or other Pacific Islander, non-Hispanic/Latino; 4 Two or more races, non-Hispanic/Latino), 54 international. Average age 28. 182 applicants, 47% accepted, 31 enrolled. In 2015, 6 master's, 18 doctorates awarded. Terminal master's awarded for partial completion of doctoral program. *Median time to degree:* Of those who began their doctoral program in fall 2007, 100% received their degree in 8 years or less. *Degree requirements:* For master's, thesis (for some programs); for doctorate, thesis/dissertation. *Entrance requirements:* For master's and doctorate, GRE General Test (minimum scores: 150 verbal, 151 quantitative; 1100 total on the old scale), minimum GPA of 3.1 in undergraduate course work. Additional exam requirements/recommendations for international students: Required—TOEFL (minimum score 90 iBT). *Application deadline:* For fall admission, 12/15 priority date for domestic and international students. Application fee: $30. Electronic applications accepted. *Expenses: Tuition, area resident:* Full-time $7263; part-time $403.50 per credit hour. Tuition, nonresident: full-time $18,087; part-time $1004.85 per credit hour. *Required fees:* $1365; $75.81 per credit hour. $20 per semester. Tuition and fees vary according to campus/location. *Financial support:* In 2015–16, 162 students received support, including 4 fellowships with tuition reimbursements available (averaging $22,000 per year), 51 research assistantships with full tuition reimbursements available (averaging $22,809 per year), 67 teaching assistantships with full tuition reimbursements available (averaging $22,809 per year). Financial award application deadline: 12/15; financial award applicants required to submit FAFSA. *Faculty research:* Bioanalytical chemistry, including separations, microfluidics, petroleomics; materials chemistry, including magnets, polymers, catalysts, nanomaterials; spectroscopy, including NMR and EPR, ultrafast, Raman, and mass spectrometry; organic synthesis, natural products, photochemistry, and supramolecular chemistry; biochemistry, with focus on structural biology, metabolomics, and anticancer drugs. *Total annual research expenditures:* $3.5 million. *Unit head:* Dr. Timothy Logan, Chairman, 850-644-3810, Fax: 850-644-8281, E-mail: gradinfo@chem.fsu.edu. *Application contact:* Dr. Geoffrey Strouse, Associate Chair for Graduate Studies, 850-445-9042, Fax: 850-644-8281, E-mail: gradinfo@chem.fsu.edu.
Website: http://www.chem.fsu.edu/

Florida State University, The Graduate School, College of Arts and Sciences, Department of Scientific Computing, Tallahassee, FL 32306-4120. Offers computational science (MS, PhD), including atmospheric science (PhD), biological science (PhD), computational science (PhD), geological science (PhD), materials science (PhD), physics (PhD). *Program availability:* Part-time. *Faculty:* 14 full-time (2 women). *Students:* 32 full-time (4 women), 7 part-time (1 woman); includes 14 minority (9 Asian, non-Hispanic/Latino; 3 Hispanic/Latino; 2 Two or more races, non-Hispanic/Latino). Average age 27. 28 applicants, 43% accepted, 7 enrolled. In 2015, 9 master's, 3 doctorates awarded. *Degree requirements:* For master's, thesis (for some programs); for doctorate, comprehensive exam, thesis/dissertation. *Entrance requirements:* For master's and doctorate, GRE General Test, knowledge of at least one object-oriented computing language, 3 letters of recommendation, resume, statement of purpose. Additional exam requirements/recommendations for international students: Required—TOEFL (minimum score 550 paper-based; 80 iBT). *Application deadline:* For fall admission, 1/15 for domestic and international students. Application fee: $30. Electronic

applications accepted. *Expenses: Tuition, area resident:* Full-time $7263; part-time $403.50 per credit hour. Tuition, nonresident: full-time $18,087; part-time $1004.85 per credit hour. *Required fees:* $1365; $75.81 per credit hour. $20 per semester. Tuition and fees vary according to campus/location. *Financial support:* In 2015–16, 33 students received support, including 10 research assistantships with full tuition reimbursements available (averaging $20,000 per year), 23 teaching assistantships with full tuition reimbursements available (averaging $20,000 per year); scholarships/grants and unspecified assistantships also available. Financial award application deadline: 1/15. *Faculty research:* Morphometrics, mathematical and systems biology, mining proteomic and metabolic data, computational materials research, advanced 4-D Var data-assimilation methods in dynamic meteorology and oceanography, computational fluid dynamics, astrophysics. *Unit head:* Dr. Gordon Erlebacher, Chair, 850-644-7024, E-mail: gerlebacher@fsu.edu. *Application contact:* Mark Howard, Academic Program Specialist, 850-644-0143, Fax: 850-644-0098, E-mail: mlhoward@fsu.edu.
Website: http://www.sc.fsu.edu

George Mason University, College of Science, Department of Chemistry and Biochemistry, Fairfax, VA 22030. Offers chemistry (MS); chemistry and biochemistry (PhD). *Faculty:* 16 full-time (5 women), 6 part-time/adjunct (4 women). *Students:* 30 full-time (20 women), 25 part-time (12 women); includes 23 minority (8 Black or African American, non-Hispanic/Latino; 7 Asian, non-Hispanic/Latino; 6 Hispanic/Latino; 2 Two or more races, non-Hispanic/Latino), 6 international. Average age 30. 41 applicants, 49% accepted, 10 enrolled. In 2015, 14 master's, 2 doctorates awarded. *Degree requirements:* For master's, thesis or alternative; for doctorate, comprehensive exam, thesis/dissertation, exit seminar. *Entrance requirements:* For master's, GRE, bachelor's degree in related field; 2 official copies of transcripts; expanded goals statement; 3 letters of recommendation; resume for those whose bachelor's degree is 5 years or older; for doctorate, GRE, undergraduate degree in related field; BS with minimum GPA of 3.0; 3 letters of recommendation; 2 copies of official transcripts; expanded goals statement; resume. Additional exam requirements/recommendations for international students: Required—TOEFL (minimum score 575 paper-based; 88 iBT), IELTS (minimum 6.5), PTE (minimum score 59). Application fee: $75 ($80 for international students). Electronic applications accepted. *Financial support:* In 2015–16, 27 students received support, including 2 fellowships with tuition reimbursements available (averaging $12,897 per year), 5 research assistantships with tuition reimbursements available (averaging $16,420 per year), 20 teaching assistantships with tuition reimbursements available (averaging $12,752 per year); career-related internships or fieldwork, Federal Work-Study, scholarships/grants, unspecified assistantships, and health care benefits (for full-time research or teaching assistantship recipients) also available. Support available to part-time students. Financial award application deadline: 3/1; financial award applicants required to submit FAFSA. *Faculty research:* Electroanalytical techniques for the study of toxic species in the environment, problems associated with the solid-gas interface, applying peptide/protein engineering principles to investigate biomolecules, enzymes, isoprene biosynthesis, contaminants in the aquatic environment, radioactivity, middle distillate fuels. *Total annual research expenditures:* $155,380. *Unit head:* John A. Schreifels, Chair, 703-993-1082, Fax: 703-993-1055, E-mail: jschreif@gmu.edu. *Application contact:* Robert Honeychuck, Graduate Coordinator, 703-993-1076, Fax: 703-993-1055, E-mail: rhoneych@gmu.edu.
Website: http://chemistry.gmu.edu/

Georgetown University, Graduate School of Arts and Sciences, Department of Biochemistry and Molecular and Cellular Biology, Washington, DC 20057. Offers MS, PhD. *Degree requirements:* For doctorate, comprehensive exam, thesis/dissertation. *Entrance requirements:* For doctorate, GRE General Test. Additional exam requirements/recommendations for international students: Required—TOEFL.

Georgetown University, Graduate School of Arts and Sciences, Department of Chemistry, Washington, DC 20057. Offers analytical chemistry (PhD); biochemistry (PhD); computational chemistry (PhD); inorganic chemistry (PhD); materials chemistry (PhD); organic chemistry (PhD); theoretical chemistry (PhD). Terminal master's awarded for partial completion of doctoral program. *Degree requirements:* For doctorate, comprehensive exam, thesis/dissertation. *Entrance requirements:* For doctorate, GRE General Test. Additional exam requirements/recommendations for international students: Required—TOEFL.

The George Washington University, Columbian College of Arts and Sciences, Institute for Biomedical Sciences, Program in Biochemistry and Systems Biology, Washington, DC 20037. Offers PhD. *Students:* 5 full-time (2 women), 8 part-time (3 women); includes 5 minority (3 Asian, non-Hispanic/Latino; 1 Hispanic/Latino; 1 Two or more races, non-Hispanic/Latino), 3 international. Average age 32. Terminal master's awarded for partial completion of doctoral program. *Degree requirements:* For doctorate, thesis/dissertation, general exam. *Entrance requirements:* For doctorate, GRE General Test, interview, minimum GPA of 3.0. Additional exam requirements/recommendations for international students: Required—TOEFL (minimum score 600 paper-based). *Application deadline:* For fall admission, 12/15 priority date for domestic and international students; for spring admission, 10/1 priority date for domestic and international students. Applications are processed on a rolling basis. Application fee: $75. Electronic applications accepted. *Financial support:* In 2015–16, 3 students received support. Fellowships, Federal Work-Study, institutionally sponsored loans, and tuition waivers available. Financial award application deadline: 2/1; financial award applicants required to submit FAFSA. *Unit head:* Dr. Eric Hoffman, Director, 202-476-6029, E-mail: ehoffman@cnmcresearch.org. *Application contact:* Information Contact, 202-994-7120, Fax: 202-994-6100, E-mail: genetics@gwu.edu.
Website: http://smhs.gwu.edu/

Georgia State University, College of Arts and Sciences, Department of Biology, Program in Molecular Genetics and Biochemistry, Atlanta, GA 30302-3083. Offers bioinformatics (MS); molecular genetics and biochemistry (MS, PhD). *Program availability:* Part-time. Terminal master's awarded for partial completion of doctoral program. *Degree requirements:* For master's, comprehensive exam (for some programs), thesis optional; for doctorate, comprehensive exam, thesis/dissertation. *Entrance requirements:* For master's and doctorate, GRE. Additional exam requirements/recommendations for international students: Required—TOEFL (minimum score 550 paper-based; 82 iBT) or IELTS (minimum score 7). *Application deadline:* For fall admission, 7/1 priority date for domestic students, 6/1 priority date for international students; for spring admission, 11/15 priority date for domestic students, 10/15 priority date for international students. Applications are processed on a rolling basis. Application fee: $50. Electronic applications accepted. *Expenses:* Tuition, state resident: full-time $6876; part-time $382 per credit hour. Tuition, nonresident: full-time $22,374; part-time $1243 per credit hour. *Required fees:* $2128; $2128 per term. $1064 per term. Part-time tuition and fees vary according to course load and program. *Financial support:* In 2015–16, fellowships with full tuition reimbursements (averaging $22,000 per year), research assistantships with full tuition reimbursements (averaging $20,000 per year) were awarded. Financial award application deadline: 12/3. *Faculty research:* Gene regulation, microbial pathogenesis, molecular transport, protein modeling, viral pathogenesis. *Unit head:* Dr. Charles Derby, Director of Graduate Studies, 404-413-5393, Fax: 404-413-5446, E-mail: cderby@gsu.edu.
Website: http://biology.gsu.edu/

Biochemistry

Georgia State University, College of Arts and Sciences, Department of Chemistry, Atlanta, GA 30302-3083. Offers analytical chemistry (MS, PhD); biochemistry (MS, PhD); bioinformatics (MS, PhD); biophysical chemistry (PhD); computational chemistry (MS, PhD); geochemistry (PhD); organic/medicinal chemistry (MS, PhD); physical chemistry (MS). PhD in geochemistry offered jointly with Department of Geosciences. *Program availability:* Part-time. *Faculty:* 26 full-time (4 women). *Students:* 158 full-time (53 women), 4 part-time (all women); includes 43 minority (22 Black or African American, non-Hispanic/Latino; 1 American Indian or Alaska Native, non-Hispanic/Latino; 9 Asian, non-Hispanic/Latino; 7 Hispanic/Latino; 4 Two or more races, non-Hispanic/Latino), 81 international. Average age 28. 117 applicants, 50% accepted, 42 enrolled. In 2015, 28 master's, 15 doctorates awarded. Terminal master's awarded for partial completion of doctoral program. *Degree requirements:* For master's, one foreign language, comprehensive exam (for some programs), thesis (for some programs); for doctorate, one foreign language, comprehensive exam, thesis/dissertation. *Entrance requirements:* For master's and doctorate, GRE. Additional exam requirements/recommendations for international students: Required—TOEFL (minimum score 550 paper-based; 80 iBT) or IELTS (minimum score 6.5). *Application deadline:* For fall admission, 7/1 priority date for domestic and international students; for winter admission, 11/15 priority date for domestic and international students; for spring admission, 4/15 priority date for domestic and international students. Applications are processed on a rolling basis. Application fee: $50. Electronic applications accepted. *Expenses:* Tuition, state resident: full-time $6876; part-time $382 per credit hour. Tuition, nonresident: full-time $22,374; part-time $1243 per credit hour. *Required fees:* $2128; $2128 per term. $1064 per term. Part-time tuition and fees vary according to course load and program. *Financial support:* Fellowships with full tuition reimbursements, research assistantships with full tuition reimbursements, and teaching assistantships with full tuition reimbursements available. Financial award applicants required to submit FAFSA. *Faculty research:* Analytical chemistry, biological/biochemistry, biophysical/computational chemistry, chemical education, organic/medicinal chemistry. *Unit head:* Dr. Peng George Wang, Department Chair, 404-413-3591, Fax: 404-413-5505, E-mail: pwang11@gsu.edu. *Website:* http://chemistry.gsu.edu/

The Graduate Center, City University of New York, Graduate Studies, Program in Biochemistry, New York, NY 10016-4039. Offers PhD. *Degree requirements:* For doctorate, thesis/dissertation, field experience. *Entrance requirements:* For doctorate, GRE General Test. Additional exam requirements/recommendations for international students: Required—TOEFL. Electronic applications accepted.

Harvard University, Graduate School of Arts and Sciences, Department of Chemistry and Chemical Biology, Cambridge, MA 02138. Offers biochemical chemistry (PhD); inorganic chemistry (PhD); organic chemistry (PhD); physical chemistry (PhD). *Degree requirements:* For doctorate, thesis/dissertation, cumulative exams. *Entrance requirements:* For doctorate, GRE General Test, GRE Subject Test. Additional exam requirements/recommendations for international students: Required—TOEFL.

Harvard University, Graduate School of Arts and Sciences, Division of Medical Sciences, Boston, MA 02115. Offers biological chemistry and molecular pharmacology (PhD); cell biology (PhD); genetics (PhD); microbiology and molecular genetics (PhD); pathology (PhD), including experimental pathology. *Degree requirements:* For doctorate, thesis/dissertation. *Entrance requirements:* For doctorate, GRE General Test, GRE Subject Test. Additional exam requirements/recommendations for international students: Required—TOEFL.

Howard University, College of Medicine, Department of Biochemistry and Molecular Biology, Washington, DC 20059-0002. Offers biochemistry and molecular biology (PhD); biotechnology (MS); MD/PhD. *Program availability:* Part-time. *Degree requirements:* For master's, externship; for doctorate, comprehensive exam, thesis/dissertation. *Entrance requirements:* For master's and doctorate, GRE General Test, minimum GPA of 3.0. *Faculty research:* Cellular and molecular biology of olfaction, gene regulation and expression, enzymology, NMR spectroscopy of molecular structure, hormone regulation/metabolism.

Howard University, Graduate School, Department of Chemistry, Washington, DC 20059-0002. Offers analytical chemistry (MS, PhD); atmospheric (MS, PhD); biochemistry (MS, PhD); environmental (MS, PhD); inorganic chemistry (MS, PhD); organic chemistry (MS, PhD); physical chemistry (MS, PhD). Terminal master's awarded for partial completion of doctoral program. *Degree requirements:* For master's, comprehensive exam, thesis, teaching experience; for doctorate, comprehensive exam, thesis/dissertation, teaching experience. *Entrance requirements:* For master's, GRE General Test, minimum GPA of 2.7; for doctorate, GRE General Test, minimum GPA of 3.0. Additional exam requirements/recommendations for international students: Required—TOEFL. Electronic applications accepted. *Faculty research:* Synthetic organics, materials, natural products, mass spectrometry.

Hunter College of the City University of New York, Graduate School, School of Arts and Sciences, Department of Chemistry, Program in Biochemistry, New York, NY 10065-5085. Offers MA, PhD. *Program availability:* Part-time. *Faculty:* 6 full-time (2 women). *Students:* 8 part-time (5 women); includes 3 minority (1 Asian, non-Hispanic/Latino; 2 Hispanic/Latino), 2 international. Average age 27. 8 applicants, 38% accepted, 2 enrolled. In 2015, 1 master's awarded. *Degree requirements:* For master's, comprehensive exam or thesis. *Entrance requirements:* For master's, GRE General Test, 1 year of course work in chemistry, quantitative analysis, organic chemistry, physical chemistry, biology, biochemistry lecture and laboratory. Additional exam requirements/recommendations for international students: Required—TOEFL. *Application deadline:* For fall admission, 4/1 for domestic students; for spring admission, 11/1 for domestic students. *Financial support:* Teaching assistantships, Federal Work-Study, scholarships/grants, and tuition waivers (partial) available. Support available to part-time students. *Faculty research:* Protein/nucleic acid interactions, physical properties of iron-sulfur proteins, neurotransmitter receptors and ion channels, Drosophila melanogaster, requirements of DNA synthesis, oncogenes. *Unit head:* Yuiia Xu, Adviser, 212-772-4310. *Application contact:* William Zlata, Director for Graduate Admissions, 212-772-4482, Fax: 212-650-3336, E-mail: admissions@hunter.cuny.edu.

Illinois Institute of Technology, Graduate College, College of Science, Department of Biological Sciences, Chicago, IL 60616. Offers biochemistry (MS); biology (MS, PhD); cell and molecular biology (MS); microbiology (MS); molecular biochemistry and biophysics (MS, PhD). *Program availability:* Part-time, evening/weekend, online learning. Terminal master's awarded for partial completion of doctoral program. *Degree requirements:* For master's, comprehensive exam, thesis (for some programs); for doctorate, comprehensive exam, thesis/dissertation. *Entrance requirements:* For master's, GRE General Test (minimum score 300 Quantitative and Verbal, 2.5 Analytical Writing), minimum undergraduate GPA of 3.0; for doctorate, GRE General Test (minimum score 310 Quantitative and Verbal, 3.0 Analytical Writing); GRE Subject Test (strongly recommended), minimum undergraduate GPA of 3.0. Additional exam requirements/recommendations for international students: Required—TOEFL (minimum score 550 paper-based; 80 iBT). Electronic applications accepted. *Faculty research:* Macromolecular crystallography, insect immunity and basic cell biology, improvement of

bacterial strains for enhanced biodesulfurization of petroleum, programmed cell death in cancer cells.

Illinois State University, Graduate School, College of Arts and Sciences, Department of Biological Sciences, Normal, IL 61790-2200. Offers animal behavior (MS); bacteriology (MS); biochemistry (MS); biological sciences (MS); biology (PhD); biophysics (MS); biotechnology (MS); botany (MS, PhD); cell biology (MS); conservation biology (MS); developmental biology (MS); ecology (MS, PhD); entomology (MS); evolutionary biology (MS); genetics (MS, PhD); immunology (MS); microbiology (MS, PhD); molecular biology (MS); molecular genetics (MS); neurobiology (MS); neuroscience (MS); parasitology (MS); physiology (MS, PhD); plant biology (MS); plant molecular biology (MS); plant sciences (MS); structural biology (MS); zoology (MS, PhD). *Program availability:* Part-time. *Degree requirements:* For master's, thesis or alternative; for doctorate, variable foreign language requirement, thesis/dissertation, 2 terms of residency. *Entrance requirements:* For master's, GRE General Test, minimum GPA of 2.6 in last 60 hours of course work; for doctorate, GRE General Test. *Application deadline:* Applications are processed on a rolling basis. Application fee: $40. *Financial support:* Research assistantships, teaching assistantships, Federal Work-Study, tuition waivers (full), and unspecified assistantships available. Financial award application deadline: 4/1. *Faculty research:* Redoc balance and drug development in schistosoma mansoni, control of the growth of listeria monocytogenes at low temperature, regulation of cell expansion and microtubule function by SPRI, CRUI: physiology and fitness consequences of different life history phenotypes. *Application contact:* Steven Juliano, Graduate Coordinator, E-mail: sajulian@ilstu.edu. *Website:* http://www.bio.ilstu.edu/

Indiana University Bloomington, University Graduate School, College of Arts and Sciences, Department of Chemistry, Bloomington, IN 47405. Offers analytical chemistry (PhD); chemical biology (PhD); chemistry (MAT); inorganic chemistry (PhD); materials chemistry (PhD); organic chemistry (PhD); physical chemistry (PhD); MSES/MS. Terminal master's awarded for partial completion of doctoral program. *Degree requirements:* For master's, thesis; for doctorate, thesis/dissertation. *Entrance requirements:* For master's and doctorate, GRE General Test, GRE Subject Test. Additional exam requirements/recommendations for international students: Required—TOEFL. Electronic applications accepted. *Faculty research:* Synthesis of complex natural products, organic reaction mechanisms, organic electrochemistry, transitive-metal chemistry, solid-state and surface chemistry.

Indiana University Bloomington, University Graduate School, College of Arts and Sciences, Interdisciplinary Biochemistry Graduate Program, Bloomington, IN 47405. Offers PhD. Terminal master's awarded for partial completion of doctoral program. *Degree requirements:* For doctorate, comprehensive exam, thesis/dissertation, Test of English Proficiency for International Associate Instructor Candidates (TEPAIC)(for international students). *Entrance requirements:* For doctorate, GRE. Additional exam requirements/recommendations for international students: Required—TOEFL (minimum score 550 paper-based; 79 iBT). Electronic applications accepted. *Expenses:* Contact institution. *Faculty research:* Biochemistry of genes and genomes, microbial biochemistry and virology, structural biology, chemical biology, cellular and medicinal biochemistry, plant biochemistry.

Indiana University–Purdue University Indianapolis, Indiana University School of Medicine, Department of Biochemistry and Molecular Biology, Indianapolis, IN 46202. Offers MS, PhD, MD/MS, MD/PhD. Terminal master's awarded for partial completion of doctoral program. *Degree requirements:* For master's, thesis; for doctorate, thesis/dissertation. *Entrance requirements:* For master's and doctorate, GRE General Test, GRE Subject Test (recommended), previous course work in organic chemistry. Additional exam requirements/recommendations for international students: Required—TOEFL. Electronic applications accepted. *Faculty research:* Metabolic regulation, enzymology, peptide and protein chemistry, cell biology, signal transduction.

Indiana University–Purdue University Indianapolis, School of Science, Department of Chemistry and Chemical Biology, Indianapolis, IN 46202. Offers MS, PhD, MD/PhD. MD/PhD offered jointly with Indiana University School of Medicine and Purdue University. *Program availability:* Part-time, evening/weekend. Terminal master's awarded for partial completion of doctoral program. *Degree requirements:* For master's, thesis (for some programs); for doctorate, comprehensive exam, thesis/dissertation. *Entrance requirements:* For master's and doctorate, minimum GPA of 3.0. Additional exam requirements/recommendations for international students: Required—TOEFL (minimum score 106 iBT). Electronic applications accepted. *Faculty research:* Analytical, biological, inorganic, organic, and physical chemistry.

Irell & Manella Graduate School of Biological Sciences, Graduate Program, Duarte, CA 91010. Offers brain metastatic cancer (PhD); cancer and stem cell metabolism (PhD); cancer biology (PhD); cancer biology and developmental therapeutics (PhD); cell biology (PhD); chemical biology (PhD); chromosomal break repair (PhD); diabetes and pancreatic progenitor cell biology (PhD); DNA repair and cancer biology (PhD); germline epigenetic remodeling and endocrine disruptors (PhD); hematology and hematopoietic cell transplantation (PhD); hematology and immunology (PhD); inflammation and cancer (PhD); micrornas and gene regulation in cardiovascular disease (PhD); mixed chimrism for reversal of autoimmunity (PhD); molecular and cellular biology (PhD); molecular biology and genetics (PhD); nanoparticle mediated twist1 silencing in metastatic cancer (PhD); neuro-oncology and stem cell biology (PhD); neuroscience (PhD); rna directed therapies for hiv-1 (PhD); small rna-induced transcriptional gene activation (PhD); stem cell regulation by the microenvironment (PhD); translational oncology and pharmaceutical sciences (PhD); tumor biology (PhD). *Faculty:* 70 full-time (18 women). *Students:* 75 full-time (40 women); includes 28 minority (2 Black or African American, non-Hispanic/Latino; 10 Asian, non-Hispanic/Latino; 10 Hispanic/Latino; 2 Native Hawaiian or other Pacific Islander, non-Hispanic/Latino; 4 Two or more races, non-Hispanic/Latino), 15 international. Average age 26. 197 applicants, 12% accepted, 19 enrolled. In 2015, 12 doctorates awarded. *Degree requirements:* For doctorate, comprehensive exam, thesis/dissertation, qualifying exams, two advanced courses. *Entrance requirements:* For doctorate, GRE General Test; GRE Subject Test (recommended), 2 years of course work in chemistry (general and organic); 1 year of course work each in biochemistry, general biology, and general physics; 2 semesters of course work in mathematics; significant research laboratory experience. Additional exam requirements/recommendations for international students: Required—TOEFL. *Application deadline:* For fall admission, 1/1 priority date for domestic and international students. Application fee: $0. Electronic applications accepted. Full-time tuition and fees vary according to class time, course level, course load, degree level, campus/location, program and student level. *Financial support:* In 2015–16, 12 students received support, including 35 fellowships with full tuition reimbursements available (averaging $32,000 per year); teaching assistantships, health care benefits, and tuition waivers (full) also available. Financial award applicants required to submit FAFSA. *Faculty research:* Cancer biology, diabetes, stem cell biology, neuroscience, immunology. *Unit head:* Dr. John J. Rossi, Dean, 877-715-GRAD, Fax: 626-471-3901, E-mail: gradschool@coh.org. *Application contact:* Dr. Kate Sleeth, Interim Associate Dean of Administration and Student Development, 626-218-1742, Fax: 626-471-3901, E-mail: gradschool@coh.org. *Website:* http://cityofhope.org/gradschool

See Display on page 66 and Close-Up on page 111.

Johns Hopkins University, Bloomberg School of Public Health, Department of Biochemistry and Molecular Biology, Baltimore, MD 21205. Offers MHS, Sc M, PhD. *Program availability:* Part-time. *Degree requirements:* For master's, thesis; for doctorate, comprehensive exam, thesis/dissertation, oral and written exams. *Entrance requirements:* For master's, MCAT or GRE, 3 letters of recommendation, curriculum vitae; for doctorate, GRE General Test, 3 letters of recommendation, curriculum vitae. Additional exam requirements/recommendations for international students: Required—TOEFL (minimum score 600 paper-based). Electronic applications accepted. *Faculty research:* DNA replication, repair, structure, carcinogenesis, protein structure, enzyme catalysts, reproductive biology.

Johns Hopkins University, National Institutes of Health Sponsored Programs, Baltimore, MD 21218. Offers biology (PhD), including biochemistry, biophysics, cell biology, developmental biology, genetic biology, molecular biology; cell, molecular, and developmental biology and biophysics (PhD). *Degree requirements:* For doctorate, comprehensive exam, thesis/dissertation. *Entrance requirements:* For doctorate, GRE General Test. Additional exam requirements/recommendations for international students: Required—TOEFL (minimum score 600 paper-based), TWE. Electronic applications accepted. *Faculty research:* Protein and nucleic acid biochemistry and biophysical chemistry, molecular biology and development.

Johns Hopkins University, School of Medicine, Graduate Programs in Medicine, Department of Biological Chemistry, Baltimore, MD 21205. Offers PhD. *Degree requirements:* For doctorate, thesis/dissertation. *Entrance requirements:* For doctorate, GRE General Test. Additional exam requirements/recommendations for international students: Required—TOEFL. Electronic applications accepted. *Faculty research:* Cell adhesion, genetics, signal transduction and RNA metabolism, enzyme structure and function, gene expression.

Johns Hopkins University, School of Medicine, Graduate Programs in Medicine, Program in Biochemistry, Cellular and Molecular Biology, Baltimore, MD 21205. Offers PhD. *Degree requirements:* For doctorate, comprehensive exam, thesis/dissertation. *Entrance requirements:* For doctorate, GRE General Test. Additional exam requirements/recommendations for international students: Required—TOEFL. Electronic applications accepted. *Faculty research:* Developmental biology, genomics/proteomics, protein targeting, signal transduction, structural biology.

Kansas State University, Graduate School, College of Arts and Sciences, Department of Biochemistry and Molecular Biophysics, Manhattan, KS 66506. Offers MS, PhD. *Degree requirements:* For master's, thesis; for doctorate, thesis/dissertation, preliminary exam. *Entrance requirements:* For master's, GRE General Test, minimum GPA of 3.0 for junior and senior year; for doctorate, GRE General Test, minimum undergraduate GPA of 3.0 or an excellent postgraduate record. Additional exam requirements/recommendations for international students: Required—TOEFL (minimum score 550 paper-based; 79 iBT). Electronic applications accepted. *Faculty research:* Protein structure/function, insect biochemistry, computational biochemistry, molecular mechanisms in cancer, membrane and lipids biochemistry.

Kansas State University, Graduate School, College of Arts and Sciences, Department of Chemistry, Manhattan, KS 66506. Offers analytical chemistry (MS); biological chemistry (MS); inorganic chemistry (MS); materials chemistry (MS); organic chemistry (MS); physical chemistry (MS). Terminal master's awarded for partial completion of doctoral program. *Degree requirements:* For master's, thesis; for doctorate, thesis/dissertation. *Entrance requirements:* For master's and doctorate, GRE, minimum GPA of 3.0. Additional exam requirements/recommendations for international students: Required—TOEFL (minimum score 550 paper-based). Electronic applications accepted. *Faculty research:* Inorganic chemistry, organic and biological chemistry, analytical chemistry, physical chemistry, materials chemistry and nanotechnology.

Kennesaw State University, College of Science and Mathematics, Program in Chemical Sciences, Kennesaw, GA 30144. Offers biochemistry (MS); chemistry (MS). *Degree requirements:* For master's, thesis. *Entrance requirements:* For master's, GRE. Additional exam requirements/recommendations for international students: Required—TOEFL (minimum score 550 paper-based; 80 iBT), IELTS (minimum score 6.5). Electronic applications accepted.

Laurentian University, School of Graduate Studies and Research, Programme in Chemistry and Biochemistry, Sudbury, ON P3E 2C6, Canada. Offers analytical chemistry (M Sc); biochemistry (M Sc); environmental chemistry (M Sc); organic chemistry (M Sc); physical/theoretical chemistry (M Sc). *Program availability:* Part-time. *Degree requirements:* For master's, thesis or alternative. *Entrance requirements:* For master's, honors degree with minimum second class. *Faculty research:* Cell cycle checkpoints, kinetic modeling, toxicology to metal stress, quantum chemistry, biogeochemistry metal speciation.

Lehigh University, College of Arts and Sciences, Department of Biological Sciences, Bethlehem, PA 18015. Offers biochemistry (PhD); cell and molecular biology (PhD); integrative biology (PhD); molecular biology (PhD). *Program availability:* Part-time, 100% online. *Faculty:* 19 full-time (9 women). *Students:* 38 full-time (22 women), 21 part-time (15 women); includes 13 minority (5 Black or African American, non-Hispanic/Latino; 1 American Indian or Alaska Native, non-Hispanic/Latino; 6 Hispanic/Latino; 1 Two or more races, non-Hispanic/Latino), 5 international. Average age 27. 38 applicants, 50% accepted, 10 enrolled. In 2015, 6 master's, 1 doctorate awarded. Terminal master's awarded for partial completion of doctoral program. *Degree requirements:* For master's, thesis optional; for doctorate, comprehensive exam, thesis/dissertation. *Entrance requirements:* For doctorate, GRE General Test. Additional exam requirements/recommendations for international students: Required—TOEFL (minimum score 85 iBT). *Application deadline:* For fall admission, 12/15 for domestic and international students. Application fee: $75. *Expenses:* $1,185 per credit hour tuition (PhD); $925 per credit hour tuition (MS). *Financial support:* In 2015–16, 34 students received support, including 8 fellowships with full tuition reimbursements available (averaging $29,667 per year), 6 research assistantships with full tuition reimbursements available (averaging $27,000 per year), 19 teaching assistantships with full tuition reimbursements available (averaging $27,000 per year); scholarships/grants also available. Financial award application deadline: 12/15. *Faculty research:* Gene expression, cytoskeleton and cell structure, cell cycle and growth regulation, neuroscience, animal behavior, microbiology. *Total annual research expenditures:* $1.9 million. *Unit head:* Dr. Murray Itzkowitz, Chairperson, 610-758-3680, Fax: 610-758-4004, E-mail: mi00@lehigh.edu. *Application contact:* Dr. Mary Kathryn Iovine, Graduate Coordinator, 610-758-6981, Fax: 610-758-4004, E-mail: mki3@lehigh.edu.
Website: http://www.lehigh.edu/~inbios/

Loma Linda University, School of Medicine, Programs in Biochemistry and Microbiology, Loma Linda, CA 92350. Offers biochemistry (MS, PhD); microbiology (PhD). *Program availability:* Part-time. *Degree requirements:* For master's, thesis or alternative; for doctorate, thesis/dissertation. *Entrance requirements:* For master's and doctorate, GRE General Test. Additional exam requirements/recommendations for international students: Required—TOEFL (minimum score 550 paper-based). *Application deadline:* For fall admission, 7/1 for domestic students. Applications are processed on a rolling basis. Application fee: $60. *Financial support:* Tuition waivers (full and partial) available. Support available to part-time students. *Faculty research:*

Physical chemistry of macromolecules, biochemistry of endocrine system, biochemical mechanism of bone volume regulation. *Unit head:* Dr. Hansel Fletcher, Vice Chair, 909-558-8497. *Application contact:* Admissions Office, 909-651-5029, Fax: 909-558-4879, E-mail: admissions.app@llu.edu.

Louisiana State University and Agricultural & Mechanical College, Graduate School, College of Science, Department of Biological Sciences, Baton Rouge, LA 70803. Offers biochemistry (MS, PhD); biological science (MS, PhD); science (MNS).

Louisiana State University Health Sciences Center at Shreveport, Department of Biochemistry and Molecular Biology, Shreveport, LA 71130-3932. Offers MS, PhD, MD/PhD. *Faculty:* 13 full-time (3 women). *Students:* 12 full-time (6 women), 10 international. Average age 28. 16 applicants, 31% accepted, 3 enrolled. In 2015, 1 master's, 3 doctorates awarded. *Degree requirements:* For master's, thesis; for doctorate, thesis/dissertation. *Entrance requirements:* For master's and doctorate, GRE General Test. Additional exam requirements/recommendations for international students: Required—TOEFL (minimum score 100 iBT), IELTS (minimum score 7). *Application deadline:* For fall admission, 3/15 for domestic and international students. Applications are processed on a rolling basis. Electronic applications accepted. *Expenses:* Contact institution. *Financial support:* In 2015–16, 3 fellowships (averaging $28,000 per year), 9 research assistantships (averaging $26,000 per year) were awarded. *Faculty research:* Yeast genetics, prostate cancer, cell biology, mTOR signaling, Parkinson's Disease, transcriptional mechanisms, chromatin, DNA repair and damage response, protein synthesis, neuroscience, diabetes, cell cycle regulation, tRNA synthetases, stress response, glucose transporters, transmigration and wound repair. *Unit head:* Dr. Stephan N. Witt, Interim Head, 318-675-5161, Fax: 318-675-5180. *Application contact:* April Coutee, Coordinator, 318-675-5160, Fax: 318-675-5180, E-mail: admissions-bmb@lsuhsc.edu.

Loyola University Chicago, Graduate School, Integrated Program in Biomedical Sciences, Maywood, IL 60153. Offers biochemistry and molecular biology (MS, PhD); cell and molecular physiology (PhD); infectious disease and immunology (MS); integrative cell biology (PhD); medical physiology (MS); microbiology and immunology (MS, PhD); molecular pharmacology and therapeutics (PhD); neuroscience (MS, PhD). *Students:* 135 full-time (65 women), 1 part-time (0 women); includes 28 minority (5 Black or African American, non-Hispanic/Latino; 15 Asian, non-Hispanic/Latino; 6 Hispanic/Latino; 2 Two or more races, non-Hispanic/Latino), 16 international. Average age 28. 442 applicants, 23% accepted, 55 enrolled. In 2015, 40 master's, 17 doctorates awarded. *Expenses:* Tuition, area resident: Full-time $18,054; part-time $9027 per credit hour. *Required fees:* $832; $284 per credit hour. Part-time tuition and fees vary according to course load, degree level and program. *Unit head:* Dr. Samuel Attoh, Dean, 773-508-3459, Fax: 773-508-2460, E-mail: sattoh@luc.edu. *Application contact:* Ron Martin, Associate Director of Enrollment Management, 312-915-8950, Fax: 312-915-8905, E-mail: gradapp@luc.edu.
Website: http://ssom.luc.edu/graduate_school/degree-programs/ipbsphd/

Massachusetts Institute of Technology, School of Science, Department of Biology, Cambridge, MA 02139. Offers biochemistry (PhD); biological oceanography (PhD); biology (PhD); biophysical chemistry and molecular structure (PhD); cell biology (PhD); computational and systems biology (PhD); developmental biology (PhD); genetics (PhD); immunology (PhD); microbiology (PhD); molecular biology (PhD); neurobiology (PhD). *Faculty:* 57 full-time (14 women). *Students:* 283 full-time (137 women); includes 83 minority (3 Black or African American, non-Hispanic/Latino; 1 American Indian or Alaska Native, non-Hispanic/Latino; 38 Asian, non-Hispanic/Latino; 31 Hispanic/Latino; 10 Two or more races, non-Hispanic/Latino), 48 international. Average age 26. 673 applicants, 14% accepted, 46 enrolled. In 2015, 32 doctorates awarded. *Degree requirements:* For doctorate, comprehensive exam, thesis/dissertation, teaching assistantship during two semesters. *Entrance requirements:* For doctorate, GRE General Test. Additional exam requirements/recommendations for international students: Required—TOEFL (minimum score 577 paper-based), IELTS. *Application deadline:* For fall admission, 12/1 for domestic and international students. Application fee: $75. Electronic applications accepted. *Expenses: Tuition:* Full-time $46,400; part-time $725 per credit. One-time fee: $304 full-time. Full-time tuition and fees vary according to course load and program. *Financial support:* In 2015–16, 235 students received support, including 118 fellowships (averaging $37,500 per year), 163 research assistantships (averaging $38,900 per year), 1 teaching assistantship; Federal Work-Study, institutionally sponsored loans, scholarships/grants, traineeships, health care benefits, and unspecified assistantships also available. Support available to part-time students. Financial award application deadline: 4/15; financial award applicants required to submit FAFSA. *Faculty research:* Cellular, developmental and molecular (plant and animal) biology; biochemistry, bioengineering, biophysics and structural biology; classical and molecular genetics, stem cell and epigenetics; immunology and microbiology; cancer biology, molecular medicine, neurobiology and human disease; computational and systems biology. *Total annual research expenditures:* $42.8 million. *Unit head:* Prof. Alan Grossman, Department Head, 617-253-4701. *Application contact:* Biology Education Office, 617-253-3717, Fax: 617-258-9329, E-mail: gradbio@mit.edu.
Website: https://biology.mit.edu/

Massachusetts Institute of Technology, School of Science, Department of Chemistry, Cambridge, MA 02139. Offers biological chemistry (PhD); inorganic chemistry (PhD); organic chemistry (PhD); physical chemistry (PhD). *Faculty:* 29 full-time (6 women). *Students:* 236 full-time (81 women); includes 51 minority (2 Black or African American, non-Hispanic/Latino; 1 American Indian or Alaska Native, non-Hispanic/Latino; 30 Asian, non-Hispanic/Latino; 12 Hispanic/Latino; 6 Two or more races, non-Hispanic/Latino), 83 international. Average age 26. 591 applicants, 18% accepted, 38 enrolled. In 2015, 40 doctorates awarded. *Degree requirements:* For doctorate, comprehensive exam, thesis/dissertation, teaching assistantship during two semesters. *Entrance requirements:* For doctorate, GRE General Test. Additional exam requirements/recommendations for international students: Required—TOEFL (minimum score 600 paper-based), IELTS (minimum score 7). *Application deadline:* For fall admission, 12/15 for domestic and international students. Application fee: $75. Electronic applications accepted. *Expenses: Tuition:* Full-time $46,400; part-time $725 per credit. One-time fee: $304 full-time. Full-time tuition and fees vary according to course load and program. *Financial support:* In 2015–16, 218 students received support, including 62 fellowships (averaging $45,800 per year), 129 research assistantships (averaging $37,000 per year), 43 teaching assistantships (averaging $38,300 per year); Federal Work-Study, institutionally sponsored loans, scholarships/grants, traineeships, health care benefits, and unspecified assistantships also available. Support available to part-time students. Financial award application deadline: 4/15; financial award applicants required to submit FAFSA. *Faculty research:* Synthetic organic and organometallic chemistry including catalysis; biological chemistry including bioorganic chemistry; physical chemistry including chemical dynamics, theoretical chemistry and biophysical chemistry; inorganic chemistry including synthesis, catalysis, bioinorganic and physical inorganic chemistry; materials chemistry including surface science, nanoscience and polymers. *Total annual research expenditures:* $30.3 million. *Unit head:* Prof. Timothy F. Jamison, Department Head, 617-253-1803, Fax: 617-258-7500. *Application contact:* Graduate Administrator, 617-253-1845, Fax: 617-258-0241, E-mail: chemgradeducation@mit.edu.
Website: http://web.mit.edu/chemistry/

Biochemistry

Mayo Graduate School, Graduate Programs in Biomedical Sciences, Programs in Biochemistry, Structural Biology, Cell Biology, and Genetics, Rochester, MN 55905. Offers biochemistry and structural biology (PhD); cell biology and genetics (PhD); molecular biology (PhD). *Degree requirements:* For doctorate, oral defense of dissertation, qualifying oral and written exam. *Entrance requirements:* For doctorate, GRE, 1 year of chemistry, biology, calculus, and physics. Additional exam requirements/recommendations for international students: Required—TOEFL. Electronic applications accepted. *Faculty research:* Gene structure and function, membranes and receptors/cytoskeleton, oncogenes and growth factors, protein structure and function, steroid hormonal action.

McGill University, Faculty of Graduate and Postdoctoral Studies, Faculty of Medicine, Department of Biochemistry, Montréal, QC H3A 2T5, Canada. Offers M Sc, PhD.

McGill University, Faculty of Graduate and Postdoctoral Studies, Faculty of Science, Department of Chemistry, Montréal, QC H3A 2T5, Canada. Offers chemical biology (M Sc, PhD); chemistry (M Sc, PhD).

McMaster University, Faculty of Health Sciences, Department of Biochemistry and Biomedical Sciences, Hamilton, ON L8S 4M2, Canada. Offers M Sc, PhD. Terminal master's awarded for partial completion of doctoral program. *Degree requirements:* For master's, thesis; for doctorate, comprehensive exam, thesis/dissertation. *Entrance requirements:* For master's and doctorate, minimum B+ average. Additional exam requirements/recommendations for international students: Required—TOEFL (minimum score 550 paper-based). *Faculty research:* Molecular and cell biology, biomolecular structure and function, molecular pharmacology and toxicology.

Medical College of Wisconsin, Graduate School of Biomedical Sciences, Department of Biochemistry, Milwaukee, WI 53226-0509. Offers PhD, MD/PhD. *Degree requirements:* For doctorate, comprehensive exam, thesis/dissertation. *Entrance requirements:* For doctorate, GRE, official transcripts, three letters of recommendation. Additional exam requirements/recommendations for international students: Required—TOEFL. *Faculty research:* Enzymology, macromolecular structure and synthesis, nucleic acids, molecular and cell biology.

Medical University of South Carolina, College of Graduate Studies, Department of Biochemistry and Molecular Biology, Charleston, SC 29425. Offers MS, PhD, MD/PhD. Terminal master's awarded for partial completion of doctoral program. *Degree requirements:* For master's, thesis, oral exam/thesis defense; for doctorate, thesis/dissertation, oral and written exams/dissertation defense. *Entrance requirements:* For master's, GRE General Test; for doctorate, GRE General Test, interview, minimum GPA of 3.0. Additional exam requirements/recommendations for international students: Required—TOEFL (minimum score 600 paper-based; 100 iBT). Electronic applications accepted. *Faculty research:* Lipid biochemistry, DNA replication, nucleic acids, protein structure.

Memorial University of Newfoundland, School of Graduate Studies, Department of Biochemistry, St. John's, NL A1C 5S7, Canada. Offers biochemistry (M Sc, PhD); food science (M Sc, PhD). *Program availability:* Part-time. *Degree requirements:* For master's, thesis; for doctorate, comprehensive exam, thesis/dissertation, oral defense of thesis. *Entrance requirements:* For master's, 2nd class degree in related field; for doctorate, M Sc. *Application deadline:* For fall admission, 3/1 for domestic and international students; for winter admission, 7/1 for domestic and international students; for spring admission, 11/1 for domestic and international students. Applications are processed on a rolling basis. Application fee: $50 Canadian dollars ($100 Canadian dollars for international students). Electronic applications accepted. *Expenses:* Tuition, area resident: Full-time $2199 Canadian dollars. *International tuition:* $2859 Canadian dollars full-time. *Financial support:* Fellowships, research assistantships, and teaching assistantships available. *Faculty research:* Toxicology, cell and molecular biology, food engineering, marine biotechnology, lipid biology. *Total annual research expenditures:* $1.1 million. *Unit head:* Dr. Mark D. Berry, Head, 709-864-8529, E-mail: biochead@mun.ca. *Application contact:* Dr. Robert Bertolo, Graduate Officer, 709-864-7954, Fax: 709-864-2422, E-mail: biochem@mun.ca.
Website: http://www.mun.ca/biochem

Miami University, College of Arts and Science, Department of Chemistry and Biochemistry, Oxford, OH 45056. Offers MS, PhD. *Students:* 54 full-time (26 women), 1 part-time (0 women); includes 6 minority (3 Black or African American, non-Hispanic/Latino; 3 Hispanic/Latino), 21 international. Average age 27. In 2015, 5 master's, 10 doctorates awarded. *Entrance requirements:* For master's and doctorate, GRE General Test; GRE Subject Test (recommended), bachelor's degree in chemistry from accredited college or university; personal statement; three letters of recommendation. Additional exam requirements/recommendations for international students: Recommended—TOEFL (minimum score 80 iBT), IELTS (minimum score 6.5), TSE (minimum score 54). *Application deadline:* Applications are processed on a rolling basis. Application fee: $50. Electronic applications accepted. *Expenses:* Tuition, state resident: full-time $12,888; part-time $537 per credit hour. Tuition, nonresident: full-time $29,022; part-time $1209 per credit hour. *Required fees:* $530; $24 per credit hour. $30 per semester. Part-time tuition and fees vary according to course load and program. *Financial support:* Application deadline: 2/15; applicants required to submit FAFSA. *Unit head:* Dr. Michael Crowder, Professor and Chair, 513-529-2813, E-mail: crowdemw@miamioh.edu. *Application contact:* Dr. David Tierney, Professor, 513-529-3731, E-mail: tiernedl@miamioh.edu.
Website: http://www.miamioh.edu/cas/academics/departments/chemistry-biochemistry/

Michigan State University, College of Human Medicine and The Graduate School, Graduate Programs in Human Medicine, East Lansing, MI 48824. Offers biochemistry and molecular biology (MS, PhD); epidemiology (MS, PhD); microbiology (MS); microbiology and molecular genetics (PhD); pharmacology and toxicology (MS, PhD); physiology (MS, PhD); public health (MPH). *Entrance requirements:* Additional exam requirements/recommendations for international students: Required—TOEFL.

Michigan State University, College of Osteopathic Medicine and The Graduate School, Graduate Studies in Osteopathic Medicine, East Lansing, MI 48824. Offers biochemistry and molecular biology (MS, PhD); microbiology (MS); microbiology and molecular genetics (PhD); pharmacology and toxicology (MS, PhD), including integrative pharmacology (MS), pharmacology and toxicology, pharmacology and toxicology-environmental toxicology (PhD); physiology (MS, PhD).

Michigan State University, The Graduate School, College of Agriculture and Natural Resources, MSU-DOE Plant Research Laboratory, East Lansing, MI 48824. Offers biochemistry and molecular biology (PhD); cellular and molecular biology (PhD); crop and soil sciences (PhD); genetics (PhD); microbiology and molecular genetics (PhD); plant biology (PhD); plant physiology (PhD). Offered jointly with the Department of Energy. *Degree requirements:* For doctorate, comprehensive exam, thesis/dissertation, laboratory rotation, defense of dissertation. *Entrance requirements:* For doctorate, GRE General Test, acceptance into one of the affiliated department programs; 3 letters of recommendation; bachelor's degree or equivalent in life sciences, chemistry, biochemistry, or biophysics; research experience. Electronic applications accepted. *Faculty research:* Role of hormones in the regulation of plant development and physiology, molecular mechanisms associated with signal recognition, development and application of genetic methods and materials, protein routing and function.

Michigan State University, The Graduate School, College of Natural Science and Graduate Programs in Human Medicine and Graduate Studies in Osteopathic Medicine, Department of Biochemistry and Molecular Biology, East Lansing, MI 48824. Offers biochemistry and molecular biology (MS, PhD); biochemistry and molecular biology/environmental toxicology (PhD). *Entrance requirements:* Additional exam requirements/recommendations for international students: Required—TOEFL. Electronic applications accepted.

Michigan Technological University, Graduate School, Interdisciplinary Programs, Houghton, MI 49931. Offers atmospheric sciences (PhD); biochemistry and molecular biology (PhD); computational science and engineering (PhD); data science (MS, Graduate Certificate); engineering (M Eng); environmental engineering (PhD); international profile (Graduate Certificate); nanotechnology (Graduate Certificate); sustainability (Graduate Certificate); sustainable water resources systems (Graduate Certificate). *Program availability:* Part-time. *Faculty:* 53 full-time (22 women), 10 part-time/adjunct. *Students:* 53 full-time (22 women), 10 part-time; includes 2 minority (1 Asian, non-Hispanic/Latino; 1 Two or more races, non-Hispanic/Latino), 44 international. Average age 30. 300 applicants, 19% accepted, 17 enrolled. In 2015, 3 master's, 7 doctorates, 4 other advanced degrees awarded. Terminal master's awarded for partial completion of doctoral program. *Degree requirements:* For master's, comprehensive exam (for some programs), thesis (for some programs); for doctorate, comprehensive exam, thesis/dissertation. *Entrance requirements:* For master's, doctorate, and Graduate Certificate, GRE, statement of purpose, personal statement, official transcripts, 2-3 letters of recommendation. Additional exam requirements/recommendations for international students: Required—TOEFL or IELTS. *Application deadline:* Applications are processed on a rolling basis. Electronic applications accepted. *Expenses:* Tuition, state resident: full-time $15,507; part-time $861.50 per credit. Tuition, nonresident: full-time $15,507; part-time $861.50 per credit. *Required fees:* $248; $248. Tuition and fees vary according to course load and program. *Financial support:* In 2015–16, 41 students received support, including 7 fellowships with tuition reimbursements available (averaging $14,516 per year), 16 research assistantships with tuition reimbursements available (averaging $14,516 per year), 9 teaching assistantships with tuition reimbursements available (averaging $14,516 per year); career-related internships or fieldwork, Federal Work-Study, scholarships/grants, health care benefits, unspecified assistantships, and cooperative program also available. Financial award applicants required to submit FAFSA. *Faculty research:* Big data, atmospheric sciences, bioinformatics and systems biology, molecular dynamics, environmental studies. *Unit head:* Dr. Jacqueline E. Huntoon, Provost and Vice President for Academic Affairs, 906-487-2440, Fax: 906-487-2284, E-mail: jeh@mtu.edu. *Application contact:* Carol T. Wingerson, Administrative Aide, 906-487-2328, Fax: 906-487-2284, E-mail: gradadms@mtu.edu.

Mississippi College, Graduate School, College of Arts and Sciences, School of Science and Mathematics, Department of Chemistry and Biochemistry, Clinton, MS 39058. Offers MCS, MS. *Program availability:* Part-time. *Degree requirements:* For master's, comprehensive exam, thesis (for some programs). *Entrance requirements:* For master's, GRE. Additional exam requirements/recommendations for international students: Recommended—TOEFL, IELTS. Electronic applications accepted.

Mississippi State University, College of Agriculture and Life Sciences, Department of Biochemistry, Molecular Biology, Entomology and Plant Pathology, Mississippi State, MS 39762. Offers agriculture life sciences (MS), including biochemistry (MS, PhD), entomology (MS, PhD), plant pathology (MS, PhD); life science (PhD), including biochemistry (MS, PhD), entomology (MS, PhD), plant pathology (MS, PhD); molecular biology (PhD). *Faculty:* 32 full-time (6 women), 2 part-time/adjunct (1 woman). *Students:* 44 full-time (20 women), 11 part-time (6 women); includes 6 minority (3 Black or African American, non-Hispanic/Latino; 1 Asian, non-Hispanic/Latino; 1 Hispanic/Latino; 1 Two or more races, non-Hispanic/Latino), 12 international. Average age 29. 35 applicants, 40% accepted, 12 enrolled. In 2015, 12 master's, 7 doctorates awarded. Terminal master's awarded for partial completion of doctoral program. *Degree requirements:* For master's, thesis (for some programs), final oral exam; for doctorate, thesis/dissertation, preliminary oral and written exam. *Entrance requirements:* For master's, GRE General Test, minimum GPA of 2.75; for doctorate, GRE. Additional exam requirements/recommendations for international students: Required—TOEFL (minimum score 500 paper-based; 61 iBT); Recommended—IELTS (minimum score 5.5). *Application deadline:* For fall admission, 7/1 for domestic students, 5/1 for international students; for spring admission, 11/1 for domestic students, 9/1 for international students. Applications are processed on a rolling basis. Application fee: $60. Electronic applications accepted. *Expenses: Tuition, area resident:* Full-time $7502; part-time $833.74 per credit hour. Tuition, nonresident: full-time $20,142; part-time $2238.24 per credit hour. *Financial support:* In 2015–16, 40 research assistantships with full tuition reimbursements (averaging $16,730 per year) were awarded; Federal Work-Study, institutionally sponsored loans, and unspecified assistantships also available. Financial award application deadline: 4/1; financial award applicants required to submit FAFSA. *Faculty research:* Fish nutrition, plant and animal molecular biology, plant biochemistry, enzymology, lipid metabolism, chromatin, cell wall synthesis in rice, a model grass bioenergy species and the source of rice Stover residues using reverse genetic and functional genomic and proteomic approaches. *Unit head:* Dr. Jeffrey Dean, Professor and Department Head, 662-325-0643, Fax: 662-325-8664, E-mail: jd1891@msstate.edu. *Application contact:* Marina Hunt, Admissions Assistant, 662-325-5188, E-mail: mhunt@grad.msstate.edu.
Website: http://www.biochemistry.msstate.edu

Montana State University, The Graduate School, College of Letters and Science, Department of Chemistry and Biochemistry, Bozeman, MT 59717. Offers biochemistry (MS, PhD); chemistry (MS, PhD). *Program availability:* Part-time. *Degree requirements:* For master's, comprehensive exam, thesis (for some programs); for doctorate, comprehensive exam, thesis/dissertation. *Entrance requirements:* For master's and doctorate, GRE General Test, transcripts, letter of recommendation. Additional exam requirements/recommendations for international students: Required—TOEFL (minimum score 550 paper-based). Electronic applications accepted. *Faculty research:* Proteomics, nano-materials chemistry, computational chemistry, optical spectroscopy, photochemistry.

Montclair State University, The Graduate School, College of Science and Mathematics, Program in Pharmaceutical Biochemistry, Montclair, NJ 07043-1624. Offers MS. *Program availability:* Part-time, evening/weekend. *Students:* 6 full-time (5 women), 2 part-time (0 women); includes 2 minority (1 Black or African American, non-Hispanic/Latino; 1 Hispanic/Latino), 4 international. Average age 24. 8 applicants, 63% accepted, 4 enrolled. *Entrance requirements:* For master's, GRE General Test, 24 undergraduate credits in chemistry, 2 letters of recommendation, essay. *Application deadline:* Applications are processed on a rolling basis. Application fee: $60. Electronic applications accepted. *Expenses:* Tuition, state resident: part-time $553 per credit. Tuition, nonresident: part-time $854 per credit. *Required fees:* $91 per credit. Tuition and fees vary according to program. *Financial support:* Federal Work-Study, scholarships/grants, and unspecified assistantships available. Support available to part-time students. Financial award application deadline: 3/1. *Faculty research:* Enzyme kinetics, enzyme expression, pharmaceutical biochemistry, medicinal chemistry,

biophysical chemistry. *Unit head:* Dr. Marc Kasner, Chair, 973-655-6864. *Application contact:* Amy Aiello, Executive Director of The Graduate School, 973-655-5147, E-mail: graduate.school@montclair.edu.
Website: http://www.montclair.edu/graduate/programs-of-study/pharmaceutical-biochemistry/

New York Medical College, Graduate School of Basic Medical Sciences, Biochemistry and Molecular Biology - Master's Program, Valhalla, NY 10595-1691. Offers MS, MD/PhD. *Program availability:* Part-time, evening/weekend. *Degree requirements:* For master's, thesis. *Entrance requirements:* For master's, GRE General Test, MCAT, or DAT. Additional exam requirements/recommendations for international students: Required—TOEFL. Electronic applications accepted. *Expenses: Tuition, area resident:* Full-time $44,355; part-time $1025 per credit. *Required fees:* $500; $95 per year. One-time fee: $140 part-time. Tuition and fees vary according to course load and program. *Faculty research:* Expression, mechanisms of hormone action and cell signaling, enzymology, mechanisms of DNA replication and repair, cell cycle regulation, control of cell growth, molecular biology of cancer cells and the cancer process, mechanisms of nutrition and cancer prevention, molecular neurobiology and studies of neurodegenerative disorders, the aging process.

New York Medical College, Graduate School of Basic Medical Sciences, Integrated PhD Program, Valhalla, NY 10595-1691. Offers biochemistry and molecular biology (PhD); cell biology and anatomy (PhD); microbiology and immunology (PhD); pathology (PhD); pharmacology (PhD); physiology (PhD). *Degree requirements:* For doctorate, comprehensive exam, thesis/dissertation. *Entrance requirements:* For doctorate, GRE General Test. Additional exam requirements/recommendations for international students: Required—TOEFL. Electronic applications accepted. *Expenses: Tuition, area resident:* Full-time $44,355; part-time $1025 per credit. *Required fees:* $500; $95 per year. One-time fee: $140 part-time. Tuition and fees vary according to course load and program. *Faculty research:* Cardiovascular sciences, infectious diseases, neuroscience, cancer and cell signaling.

North Carolina State University, Graduate School, College of Agriculture and Life Sciences, Department of Biochemistry, Raleigh, NC 27695. Offers PhD. *Degree requirements:* For doctorate, thesis/dissertation. *Entrance requirements:* For doctorate, GRE General Test. Additional exam requirements/recommendations for international students: Required—TOEFL. Electronic applications accepted. *Faculty research:* Regulation of gene expression, structure and function of proteins and nucleic acids, molecular biology, high-field NMR, bioinorganic chemistry.

North Dakota State University, College of Graduate and Interdisciplinary Studies, College of Science and Mathematics, Department of Chemistry and Biochemistry, Program in Biochemistry, Fargo, ND 58102. Offers MS, PhD. *Program availability:* Part-time. *Degree requirements:* For master's, thesis; for doctorate, thesis/dissertation. *Entrance requirements:* Additional exam requirements/recommendations for international students: Required—TOEFL (minimum score 550 paper-based). *Application deadline:* For fall admission, 3/1 priority date for domestic and international students; for spring admission, 9/1 priority date for domestic and international students. Applications are processed on a rolling basis. Application fee: $35. Electronic applications accepted. *Financial support:* Research assistantships with full tuition reimbursements, teaching assistantships with full tuition reimbursements, career-related internships or fieldwork, Federal Work-Study, and institutionally sponsored loans available. Financial award application deadline: 4/15. *Unit head:* Dr. Gregory Cook, Chair, 701-231-7413, Fax: 701-231-8831, E-mail: gregory.cook@ndsu.edu. *Application contact:* Elizabeth Worth, Marketing, Recruitment, and Public Relations Coordinator, 701-231-8476, Fax: 701-231-6524, E-mail: elizabeth.worth@ndsu.edu.

Northern Michigan University, Office of Graduate Education and Research, College of Arts and Sciences, Department of Biology, Marquette, MI 49855-5301. Offers biochemistry (MS); biology (MS). *Program availability:* Part-time. *Degree requirements:* For master's, thesis. *Entrance requirements:* For master's, GRE, minimum GPA of 3.0; references; coursework in biology and other sciences; faculty member as mentor. Additional exam requirements/recommendations for international students: Required—TOEFL (minimum score 550 paper-based; 79 iBT), IELTS (minimum score 6.5). Electronic applications accepted. *Faculty research:* Evolutionary genetics, neurobiology, conservation biology, fisheries and wildlife, microbiology.

Northwestern University, The Graduate School, Interdisciplinary Biological Sciences Program (IBiS), Evanston, IL 60208. Offers biochemistry (PhD); bioengineering and biotechnology (PhD); biotechnology (PhD); cell and molecular biology (PhD); developmental and systems biology (PhD); nanotechnology (PhD); neurobiology (PhD); structural biology and biophysics (PhD). *Degree requirements:* For doctorate, thesis/dissertation, qualifying exam. *Entrance requirements:* For doctorate, GRE General Test. Additional exam requirements/recommendations for international students: Required—TOEFL (minimum score 600 paper-based). Electronic applications accepted. *Faculty research:* Biophysics/structural biology, cell/molecular biology, synthetic biology, developmental systems biology, chemical biology/nanotechnology.

The Ohio State University, Graduate School, College of Arts and Sciences, Division of Natural and Mathematical Sciences, Biochemistry Program, Columbus, OH 43210. Offers PhD. *Students:* 77 full-time (34 women), 1 part-time (0 women); includes 5 minority (1 Black or African American, non-Hispanic/Latino; 3 Asian, non-Hispanic/Latino; 1 Hispanic/Latino), 19 international. Average age 26. In 2015, 15 doctorates awarded. Terminal master's awarded for partial completion of doctoral program. *Degree requirements:* For doctorate, thesis/dissertation. *Entrance requirements:* For doctorate, GRE General Test. Additional exam requirements/recommendations for international students: Required—TOEFL (minimum score 620 paper-based; 105 iBT); Recommended—IELTS (minimum score 8). *Application deadline:* For fall admission, 12/15 priority date for domestic students, 12/1 priority date for international students. Applications are processed on a rolling basis. Application fee: $60 ($70 for international students). Electronic applications accepted. *Financial support:* Fellowships with tuition reimbursements, research assistantships with tuition reimbursements, and teaching assistantships with tuition reimbursements available. *Unit head:* Dr. Thomas Magliery, Program Director, 614-292-2120, Fax: 614-292-6511, E-mail: ibba.1@osu.edu. *Application contact:* Graduate and Professional Admissions, 614-292-9444, Fax: 614-292-3895, E-mail: gpadmissions@osu.edu.
Website: http://osbp.osu.edu/

The Ohio State University, Graduate School, College of Arts and Sciences, Division of Natural and Mathematical Sciences, Department of Chemistry and Biochemistry, Columbus, OH 43210. Offers biochemistry (MS); chemistry (MS, PhD). *Faculty:* 48. *Students:* 227 full-time (88 women); includes 27 minority (8 Black or African American, non-Hispanic/Latino; 1 American Indian or Alaska Native, non-Hispanic/Latino; 7 Asian, non-Hispanic/Latino; 7 Hispanic/Latino; 4 Two or more races, non-Hispanic/Latino), 115 international. Average age 26. In 2015, 25 master's, 27 doctorates awarded. *Degree requirements:* For master's, thesis optional; for doctorate, thesis/dissertation. *Entrance requirements:* For master's and doctorate, GRE General Test. Additional exam requirements/recommendations for international students: Required—TOEFL (minimum score 550 paper-based; 79 iBT), Michigan English Language Assessment Battery (minimum score 82); Recommended—IELTS (minimum score 7). *Application deadline:*

For fall admission, 12/15 for domestic and international students. Applications are processed on a rolling basis. Application fee: $60 ($70 for international students). Electronic applications accepted. *Financial support:* Fellowships, research assistantships, teaching assistantships, Federal Work-Study, and institutionally sponsored loans available. Support available to part-time students. *Unit head:* Dr. Susan V. Olesik, Chair, 614-292-0733, E-mail: chair@chemistry.ohio-state.edu. *Application contact:* Graduate and Professional Admissions, 614-292-9444, Fax: 614-292-3895, E-mail: gpadmissions@osu.edu.
Website: https://chemistry.osu.edu/

Ohio University, Graduate College, College of Arts and Sciences, Department of Chemistry and Biochemistry, Athens, OH 45701-2979. Offers MS, PhD. *Degree requirements:* For master's, comprehensive exam, thesis, exam; for doctorate, comprehensive exam, thesis/dissertation, exam. *Entrance requirements:* For master's and doctorate, GRE. Additional exam requirements/recommendations for international students: Required—TOEFL (minimum score 550 paper-based; 80 iBT) or IELTS (minimum score 6.5). Electronic applications accepted. *Faculty research:* Materials, RNA, synthesis, carbohydrate, mass spectrometry.

Oklahoma State University, College of Agricultural Science and Natural Resources, Department of Biochemistry and Molecular Biology, Stillwater, OK 74078. Offers MS, PhD. *Faculty:* 18 full-time (6 women). *Students:* 5 full-time (2 women), 19 part-time (7 women); includes 4 minority (1 American Indian or Alaska Native, non-Hispanic/Latino; 1 Asian, non-Hispanic/Latino; 2 Hispanic/Latino), 12 international. Average age 29. 25 applicants, 36% accepted, 4 enrolled. In 2015, 3 master's, 5 doctorates awarded. *Degree requirements:* For master's, thesis, oral exam; for doctorate, comprehensive exam, thesis/dissertation. *Entrance requirements:* For master's and doctorate, GRE or GMAT. Additional exam requirements/recommendations for international students: Required—TOEFL (minimum score 550 paper-based, 79 iBT). *Application deadline:* For fall admission, 3/1 priority date for international students; for spring admission, 8/1 priority date for international students. Applications are processed on a rolling basis. Application fee: $40 ($75 for international students). Electronic applications accepted. *Expenses:* Tuition, state resident: full-time $3528; part-time $196 per credit hour. Tuition, nonresident: full-time $14,144; part-time $785.75 per credit hour. *Required fees:* $1895; $105.25 per credit hour. Tuition and fees vary according to campus/location. *Financial support:* In 2015–16, 23 research assistantships (averaging $19,619 per year), 2 teaching assistantships (averaging $19,722 per year) were awarded; career-related internships or fieldwork, Federal Work-Study, scholarships/grants, health care benefits, tuition waivers (partial), and unspecified assistantships also available. Support available to part-time students. Financial award application deadline: 3/1; financial award applicants required to submit FAFSA. *Unit head:* Dr. John Gustafson, Department Head, 405-744-6189, Fax: 405-744-7799, E-mail: john.gustafson@okstate.edu.
Website: http://biochemistry.okstate.edu/

Old Dominion University, College of Sciences, Program in Chemistry, Norfolk, VA 23529. Offers analytical (MS, PhD); biochemistry (MS, PhD); environmental (MS, PhD); inorganic (MS, PhD); organic (MS, PhD); physical (MS, PhD). *Program availability:* Part-time, evening/weekend. *Faculty:* 19 full-time (5 women). *Students:* 35 full-time (17 women), 6 part-time (2 women); includes 5 minority (4 Black or African American, non-Hispanic/Latino; 1 Two or more races, non-Hispanic/Latino), 16 international. Average age 27. 20 applicants, 55% accepted, 4 enrolled. In 2015, 9 master's, 9 doctorates awarded. *Degree requirements:* For master's, comprehensive exam, thesis (for some programs); for doctorate, comprehensive exam, thesis/dissertation. *Entrance requirements:* For master's and doctorate, GRE General Test, minimum GPA of 3.0 in major, 2.5 overall, transcripts, essay, three letters of recommendation, resume. Additional exam requirements/recommendations for international students: Required—TOEFL. *Application deadline:* For fall admission, 7/1 for domestic students, 1/15 for international students; for spring admission, 11/1 for domestic students, 8/15 for international students. Applications are processed on a rolling basis. Application fee: $50. Electronic applications accepted. *Expenses:* $464 per credit in-state tuition; $1,160 per credit out-of-state tuition. *Financial support:* In 2015–16, 42 students received support, including 2 fellowships with full tuition reimbursements available (averaging $18,000 per year), 10 research assistantships with full tuition reimbursements available (averaging $18,000 per year), 33 teaching assistantships with full tuition reimbursements available (averaging $18,000 per year); career-related internships or fieldwork, institutionally sponsored loans, scholarships/grants, health care benefits, and unspecified assistantships also available. Financial award application deadline: 2/15; financial award applicants required to submit FAFSA. *Faculty research:* Biogeochemistry, materials chemistry, computational chemistry, organic chemistry, biofuels. *Total annual research expenditures:* $2.6 million. *Unit head:* Dr. John R. Donat, Graduate Program Director, 757-683-4098, Fax: 757-683-4628, E-mail: chemgpd@odu.edu. *Application contact:* Kristi Rehrauer, Graduate Program Assistant, 757-683-6979, Fax: 757-683-4628, E-mail: krehraue@odu.edu.

Oregon Health & Science University, School of Medicine, Graduate Programs in Medicine, Department of Environmental and Biomolecular Systems, Portland, OR 97239-3098. Offers biochemistry and molecular biology (MS, PhD); environmental science and engineering (MS, PhD). *Program availability:* Part-time. *Faculty:* 13 full-time (4 women). *Students:* 19 full-time (16 women), 2 part-time (1 woman); includes 8 minority (2 Black or African American, non-Hispanic/Latino; 3 Asian, non-Hispanic/Latino; 2 Hispanic/Latino; 1 Two or more races, non-Hispanic/Latino), 4 international. Average age 26. 42 applicants, 33% accepted, 7 enrolled. In 2015, 10 master's, 5 doctorates awarded. Terminal master's awarded for partial completion of doctoral program. *Degree requirements:* For master's, thesis (for some programs); for doctorate, comprehensive exam, thesis/dissertation, qualifying exam. *Entrance requirements:* For master's and doctorate, GRE General Test (minimum scores: 153 Verbal/148 Quantitative/4.5 Analytical) or MCAT (for some programs). Additional exam requirements/recommendations for international students: Required—TOEFL. *Application deadline:* For fall admission, 7/15 for domestic students, 5/15 for international students; for winter admission, 10/15 for domestic students, 9/15 for international students; for spring admission, 1/15 for domestic students, 12/15 for international students. Applications are processed on a rolling basis. Application fee: $70. Electronic applications accepted. *Financial support:* Health care benefits and full tuition and stipends (for PhD students) available. *Faculty research:* Metalloprotein biochemistry, molecular microbiology, environmental microbiology, environmental chemistry, biogeochemistry. *Unit head:* Dr. Bradley Tebo, Program Director, 503-346-3438, E-mail: tebob@ohsu.edu. *Application contact:* Vanessa Green, Program Coordinator, 503-346-3411, E-mail: greenva@ohsu.edu.

Oregon Health & Science University, School of Medicine, Graduate Programs in Medicine, Program in Molecular and Cellular Biosciences, Department of Biochemistry and Molecular Biology, Portland, OR 97239-3098. Offers PhD. *Faculty:* 12 full-time (3 women), 21 part-time/adjunct (3 women). *Students:* 7 full-time (3 women), 1 international. Average age 27. *Degree requirements:* For doctorate, comprehensive exam, thesis/dissertation, qualifying exam. *Entrance requirements:* For doctorate, GRE General Test (minimum scores: 153 Verbal/148 Quantitative/4.5 Analytical). Additional exam requirements/recommendations for international students: Required—TOEFL. *Application deadline:* For fall admission, 12/1 for domestic and international students.

Biochemistry

Application fee: $70. Electronic applications accepted. *Financial support:* Health care benefits, tuition waivers (full), and full tuition and stipends (for PhD students) available. *Faculty research:* Leishmania, parasites, structure and function of G proteins, cystic fibrosis, genomic instability, biology of ion channels. *Unit head:* Dr. David Farrens, Program Director, 503-494-7781, E-mail: farrensd@ohsu.edu. *Application contact:* Lola Bichler, Administrative Coordinator, 503-494-5824, E-mail: bichler@ohsu.edu. Website: http://www.ohsu.edu/som-biochem/

Oregon State University, College of Science, Program in Biochemistry and Biophysics, Corvallis, OR 97331. Offers biochemistry (MA, MS, PhD); biophysics (MA, MS, PhD). *Faculty:* 15 full-time (4 women), 2 part-time/adjunct (0 women). *Students:* 27 full-time (13 women), 1 part-time (0 women); includes 3 minority (1 Black or African American, non-Hispanic/Latino; 2 Asian, non-Hispanic/Latino), 5 international. Average age 28. 43 applicants, 26% accepted, 6 enrolled. In 2015, 2 master's, 3 doctorates awarded. *Degree requirements:* For master's, thesis optional; for doctorate, thesis/dissertation, exams. *Entrance requirements:* For master's and doctorate, GRE, minimum GPA of 3.0. Additional exam requirements/recommendations for international students: Required—TOEFL (minimum score 600 paper-based; 100 iBT), IELTS (minimum score 7). *Application deadline:* For fall admission, 12/15 priority date for domestic students. Application fee: $75 ($85 for international students). *Expenses:* Tuition, state resident: full-time $12,150; part-time $450 per credit. Tuition, nonresident: full-time $20,952; part-time $776 per credit. *Required fees:* $1572; $1443 per unit. One-time fee: $350. Tuition and fees vary according to course load, campus/location and program. *Financial support:* Research assistantships, teaching assistantships, and institutionally sponsored loans available. Support available to part-time students. Financial award application deadline: 12/15. *Faculty research:* DNA and deoxy ribonucleotide metabolism, cell growth control, receptors and membranes, protein structure and function. *Unit head:* Dr. Andy Karplus, Professor and Chair. *Application contact:* Graduate Program Coordinator, 541-737-4511, E-mail: bboffice@oregonstate.edu. Website: http://biochem.science.oregonstate.edu/

Oregon State University, Interdisciplinary/Institutional Programs, Program in Environmental Sciences, Corvallis, OR 97331. Offers biogeochemistry (MS, PhD); ecology (MS, PhD); environmental education (MS, PhD); environmental sciences (PSM); natural resources (MS, PhD); quantitative analysis (MS, PhD); social science (MS, PhD); water resources (MS, PhD). *Program availability:* Part-time. *Students:* 17 full-time (12 women), 12 part-time (6 women); includes 7 minority (1 Black or African American, non-Hispanic/Latino; 2 Asian, non-Hispanic/Latino; 2 Hispanic/Latino; 2 Two or more races, non-Hispanic/Latino), 3 international. Average age 34. 42 applicants, 19% accepted, 3 enrolled. In 2015, 6 master's, 4 doctorates awarded. *Entrance requirements:* For master's and doctorate, GRE. Additional exam requirements/recommendations for international students: Required—TOEFL (minimum score 80 iBT), IELTS (minimum score 6.5). *Application deadline:* For fall admission, 1/15 for domestic students. Application fee: $75 ($85 for international students). *Expenses:* Contact institution. *Unit head:* Dr. Carolyn Fonyo Boggess, Interim Director, E-mail: carolyn.fonyo@oregonstate.edu. Website: http://envsci.science.oregonstate.edu/

Pace University, Dyson College of Arts and Sciences, Program in Biochemistry and Molecular Biology, New York, NY 10038. Offers MS. *Program availability:* Part-time, evening/weekend. *Students:* 11 full-time (6 women); includes 4 minority (2 Black or African American, non-Hispanic/Latino; 2 Hispanic/Latino). Average age 24. 22 applicants, 86% accepted, 11 enrolled. *Degree requirements:* For master's, thesis. *Entrance requirements:* For master's, official transcripts, two letters of recommendation, personal statement. Additional exam requirements/recommendations for international students: Required—TOEFL (minimum score 88 iBT), IELTS (minimum score 7) or PTE (minimum score 60). *Application deadline:* For fall admission, 4/15 priority date for domestic students. Applications are processed on a rolling basis. Application fee: $70. Electronic applications accepted. *Expenses: Tuition, area resident:* Part-time $1195 per credit. *Required fees:* $260 per semester. Tuition and fees vary according to degree level, campus/location and program. *Financial support:* 3 credit scholarships for full-time students with minimum GPA of 3.5 available. Financial award application deadline: 2/15; financial award applicants required to submit FAFSA. *Unit head:* Dr. Nigel Yarlett, Director, MS in Biochemistry and Molecular Biology, 212-346-1853, E-mail: nyarlett@pace.edu. *Application contact:* Susan Ford-Goldschein, Director of Admissions, 212-346-1531, Fax: 212-346-1585, E-mail: graduateadmission@pace.edu. Website: http://www.pace.edu/dyson/programs/ms-biochemistry-molecular-biology-nyc

Penn State Hershey Medical Center, College of Medicine, Graduate School Programs in the Biomedical Sciences, Graduate Program in Biomedical Sciences, Hershey, PA 17033. Offers biochemistry and molecular genetics (MS, PhD); biomedical sciences (MS, PhD); translational therapeutics (MS, PhD); virology and immunology (MS, PhD); MD/PhD; PhD/MBA. *Students:* 79 full-time (43 women); includes 27 minority (7 Black or African American, non-Hispanic/Latino; 15 Asian, non-Hispanic/Latino; 4 Hispanic/Latino; 1 Native Hawaiian or other Pacific Islander, non-Hispanic/Latino), 17 international. 275 applicants, 16% accepted, 17 enrolled. Terminal master's awarded for partial completion of doctoral program. *Degree requirements:* For master's, thesis (for some programs); for doctorate, comprehensive exam, thesis/dissertation, candidacy exam. *Entrance requirements:* For doctorate, GRE General Test. Additional exam requirements/recommendations for international students: Required—TOEFL (minimum score 550 paper-based; 81 iBT). *Application deadline:* For fall admission, 1/1 for domestic and international students. Applications are processed on a rolling basis. Application fee: $65. Electronic applications accepted. *Expenses:* Contact institution. *Financial support:* In 2015–16, 79 students received support, including 79 research assistantships with full tuition reimbursements available (averaging $26,196 per year); fellowships, scholarships/grants, health care benefits, and unspecified assistantships also available. *Unit head:* Dr. Ralph L. Keil, Chair, 717-531-8595, Fax: 717-531-0786, E-mail: rlk9@psu.edu. *Application contact:* Kristin E. Smith, Director of Graduate Admissions, 717-531-1045, Fax: 717-531-0786, E-mail: kec17@psu.edu. Website: http://med.psu.edu/bms

Penn State University Park, Graduate School, Eberly College of Science, Department of Biochemistry and Molecular Biology, University Park, PA 16802. Offers biochemistry, microbiology, and molecular biology (MS, PhD); biotechnology (MBIOT). *Unit head:* Dr. Douglas R. Cavener, Dean, 814-865-9591, Fax: 814-865-3634. *Application contact:* Lori Stania, Director, Graduate Student Services, 814-865-1795, Fax: 814-863-4627, E-mail: l-gswww@lists.psu.edu. Website: http://bmb.psu.edu/

Purdue University, College of Pharmacy and Pharmacal Sciences and Graduate School, Graduate Programs in Pharmacy and Pharmacal Sciences, Department of Medicinal Chemistry and Molecular Pharmacology, West Lafayette, IN 47907. Offers biophysical and computational chemistry (PhD); cancer research (PhD); immunology and infectious disease (PhD); medicinal biochemistry and molecular biology (PhD); medicinal chemistry and chemical biology (PhD); molecular pharmacology (PhD); neuropharmacology, neurodegeneration, and neurotoxicity (PhD); systems biology and functional genomics (PhD). *Degree requirements:* For doctorate, thesis/dissertation. *Entrance requirements:* For doctorate, GRE General Test; GRE Subject Test in biology, biochemistry, and chemistry (recommended), minimum undergraduate GPA of 3.0.

Additional exam requirements/recommendations for international students: Required—TOEFL (minimum score 550 paper-based; 77 iBT); Recommended—TWE. Electronic applications accepted. *Faculty research:* Drug design and development, cancer research, drug synthesis and analysis, chemical pharmacology, environmental toxicology.

Purdue University, Graduate School, College of Agriculture, Department of Biochemistry, West Lafayette, IN 47907. Offers MS, PhD. Terminal master's awarded for partial completion of doctoral program. *Degree requirements:* For doctorate, thesis/dissertation, preliminary and qualifying exams. *Entrance requirements:* For doctorate, GRE General Test, minimum undergraduate GPA of 3.0 or equivalent. Additional exam requirements/recommendations for international students: Required—TOEFL (minimum score 600 paper-based; 77 iBT). Electronic applications accepted. *Faculty research:* Molecular biology and post-translational modifications of neuropeptides, membrane transport proteins.

Purdue University, Graduate School, PULSe - Purdue University Life Sciences Program, West Lafayette, IN 47907. Offers biomolecular structure and biophysics (PhD); biotechnology (PhD); chemical biology (PhD); chromatin and regulation of gene expression (PhD); integrative neuroscience (PhD); integrative plant sciences (PhD); membrane biology (PhD); microbiology (PhD); molecular evolutionary and cancer biology (PhD); molecular evolutionary genetics (PhD); molecular virology (PhD). *Entrance requirements:* For doctorate, GRE, minimum undergraduate GPA of 3.0. Additional exam requirements/recommendations for international students: Required—TOEFL (minimum score 550 paper-based; 77 iBT). Electronic applications accepted.

Queen's University at Kingston, School of Graduate Studies, Faculty of Health Sciences, Department of Biochemistry, Kingston, ON K7L 3N6, Canada. Offers M Sc, PhD. *Program availability:* Part-time. *Degree requirements:* For master's, thesis, research proposal; for doctorate, comprehensive exam, thesis/dissertation, research proposal. *Entrance requirements:* For master's, GRE (if undergraduate degree is not from a Canadian University); for doctorate, GRE required if undergraduate degree is not from a Canadian University. Additional exam requirements/recommendations for international students: Required—TOEFL (minimum score 580 paper-based). Electronic applications accepted. *Faculty research:* Gene expression, protein structure, enzyme activity, signal transduction.

Rensselaer Polytechnic Institute, Graduate School, School of Science, Program in Biochemistry and Biophysics, Troy, NY 12180-3590. Offers MS, PhD. *Faculty:* 6 full-time (3 women), 2 part-time/adjunct (0 women). *Students:* 15 full-time (8 women); includes 2 minority (1 Asian, non-Hispanic/Latino; 1 Two or more races, non-Hispanic/Latino), 1 international. Average age 24. 36 applicants, 22% accepted, 1 enrolled. In 2015, 2 doctorates awarded. Terminal master's awarded for partial completion of doctoral program. *Degree requirements:* For master's, thesis optional; for doctorate, comprehensive exam, thesis/dissertation. *Entrance requirements:* For master's and doctorate, GRE. Additional exam requirements/recommendations for international students: Required—TOEFL (minimum score 600 paper-based; 100 iBT), IELTS (minimum score 7), PTE (minimum score 68). *Application deadline:* For fall admission, 1/1 priority date for domestic and international students; for spring admission, 8/15 priority date for domestic and international students. Applications are processed on a rolling basis. Application fee: $75. Electronic applications accepted. *Financial support:* In 2015–16, research assistantships (averaging $21,500 per year), teaching assistantships (averaging $21,500 per year) were awarded; fellowships also available. Financial award application deadline: 1/1. *Faculty research:* Biochemistry; bioinformatics; biophysics; cancer biology; computational biology; molecular, cell, and developmental biology; neuroscience; protein folding; stem cells; structural biology. *Unit head:* Dr. Chunyu Wang, Graduate Program Director, 518-276-3497, E-mail: wangc5@rpi.edu. *Application contact:* Office of Graduate Admissions, 518-276-6216, E-mail: gradadmissions@rpi.edu. Website: http://www.rpi.edu/dept/bcbp/

Rice University, Graduate Programs, Wiess School of Natural Sciences, Department of Biochemistry and Cell Biology, Houston, TX 77251-1892. Offers MA, PhD. Terminal master's awarded for partial completion of doctoral program. *Degree requirements:* For master's, thesis; for doctorate, thesis/dissertation. *Entrance requirements:* For master's and doctorate, GRE. Additional exam requirements/recommendations for international students: Required—TOEFL (minimum score 600 paper-based; 90 iBT). Electronic applications accepted. *Expenses:* Contact institution. *Faculty research:* Steroid metabolism, protein structure NMR, biophysics, cell growth and movement.

Rosalind Franklin University of Medicine and Science, School of Graduate and Postdoctoral Studies - Interdisciplinary Graduate Program in Biomedical Sciences, Department of Biochemistry and Molecular Biology, North Chicago, IL 60064-3095. Offers PhD, MD/PhD. Terminal master's awarded for partial completion of doctoral program. *Degree requirements:* For doctorate, comprehensive exam, thesis/dissertation. *Entrance requirements:* For doctorate, GRE General Test, minimum GPA of 3.0. Additional exam requirements/recommendations for international students: Required—TOEFL, TWE. Electronic applications accepted. *Faculty research:* Structure of control enzymes, extracellular matrix, glucose metabolism, gene expression, ATP synthesis.

Rush University, Graduate College, Division of Biochemistry, Chicago, IL 60612-3832. Offers MS, PhD, MD/PhD. *Degree requirements:* For doctorate, thesis/dissertation, preliminary exam. *Entrance requirements:* For doctorate, GRE General Test. Additional exam requirements/recommendations for international students: Required—TOEFL. Electronic applications accepted. *Faculty research:* Biochemistry of extracellular matrix, connective tissue biosynthesis and degradation, molecular biology of connective tissue components, cartilage, arthritis.

Rutgers University–Newark, Graduate School of Biomedical Sciences, Department of Biochemistry and Molecular Biology, Newark, NJ 07107. Offers MS, PhD. *Degree requirements:* For master's, thesis; for doctorate, thesis/dissertation, qualifying exam. *Entrance requirements:* For master's and doctorate, GRE General Test. Additional exam requirements/recommendations for international students: Required—TOEFL. Electronic applications accepted.

Rutgers University–Newark, Graduate School, Program in Chemistry, Newark, NJ 07102. Offers analytical chemistry (MS, PhD); biochemistry (MS, PhD); inorganic chemistry (MS, PhD); organic chemistry (MS, PhD); physical chemistry (MS, PhD). *Program availability:* Part-time, evening/weekend. Terminal master's awarded for partial completion of doctoral program. *Degree requirements:* For master's, thesis optional, cumulative exams; for doctorate, thesis/dissertation, exams, research proposal. *Entrance requirements:* For master's and doctorate, GRE General Test, minimum undergraduate B average. Additional exam requirements/recommendations for international students: Required—TOEFL. Electronic applications accepted. *Faculty research:* Medicinal chemistry, natural products, isotope effects, biophysics and bioorganic approaches to enzyme mechanisms, organic and organometallic synthesis.

Rutgers University–New Brunswick, Graduate School-New Brunswick, Department of Chemistry and Chemical Biology, Piscataway, NJ 08854-8097. Offers biological chemistry (MS, PhD); inorganic chemistry (MS, PhD); organic chemistry (MS, PhD); physical chemistry (MS, PhD). *Program availability:* Part-time, evening/weekend.

Terminal master's awarded for partial completion of doctoral program. *Degree requirements:* For master's, thesis or alternative, exam; for doctorate, thesis/dissertation, 1 year residency. *Entrance requirements:* For master's and doctorate, GRE General Test, GRE Subject Test. Additional exam requirements/recommendations for international students: Required—TOEFL. Electronic applications accepted. *Faculty research:* Biophysical organic/bioorganic, inorganic/bioinorganic, theoretical, and solid-state/surface chemistry.

Rutgers University–New Brunswick, Graduate School-New Brunswick, Programs in the Molecular Biosciences, Piscataway, NJ 08854-8097. Offers biochemistry (PhD); cell and developmental biology (MS, PhD); microbiology and molecular genetics (MS, PhD), including applied microbiology, clinical microbiology (MS), clinical mircobiology (PhD), computational molecular biology (PhD), immunology, microbial biochemistry, molecular genetics, virology. MS, PhD offered jointly with University of Medicine and Dentistry of New Jersey.

Rutgers University–New Brunswick, Graduate School of Biomedical Sciences, Program in Biochemistry, Piscataway, NJ 08854-5635. Offers MS, PhD, MD/PhD. PhD, MS offered jointly with Rutgers, The State University of New Jersey, New Brunswick. Terminal master's awarded for partial completion of doctoral program. *Degree requirements:* For master's, thesis, qualifying exam; for doctorate, thesis/dissertation, qualifying exam. *Entrance requirements:* For master's and doctorate, GRE General Test. Additional exam requirements/recommendations for international students: Required—TOEFL. Electronic applications accepted. *Faculty research:* Signal transduction, regulation of RNA, polymerase II transcribed genes, developmental gene expression.

Saint Louis University, Graduate Education and School of Medicine, Graduate Program in Biomedical Sciences and Graduate Education, Department of Biochemistry and Molecular Biology, St. Louis, MO 63103. Offers PhD. *Degree requirements:* For doctorate, comprehensive exam, thesis/dissertation, departmental qualifying exams. *Entrance requirements:* For doctorate, GRE General Test, GRE Subject Test (optional), letters of recommendation, resume, interview. Additional exam requirements/recommendations for international students: Required—TOEFL (minimum score 525 paper-based). Electronic applications accepted. *Faculty research:* Transcription, chromatin modification and regulation of gene expression; structure/function of proteins and enzymes, including x-ray crystallography; inflammatory mediators in pathenogenesis of diabetes and arteriosclerosis; cellular signaling in response to growth factors, opiates and angiogenic mediators; genomics and proteomics of Cryptococcus neoformans.

San Diego State University, Graduate and Research Affairs, College of Sciences, Department of Chemistry and Biochemistry, San Diego, CA 92182. Offers MA, MS, PhD. PhD offered jointly with University of California, San Diego. Terminal master's awarded for partial completion of doctoral program. *Degree requirements:* For doctorate, thesis/dissertation. *Entrance requirements:* For master's, GRE General Test, bachelor's degree in related field, 3 letters of reference; for doctorate, GRE General Test, GRE Subject Test. Additional exam requirements/recommendations for international students: Required—TOEFL. Electronic applications accepted. *Faculty research:* Nonlinear, laser, and electrochemistry; surface reaction dynamics; catalysis, synthesis, and organometallics; proteins, enzymology, and gene expression regulation.

San Francisco State University, Division of Graduate Studies, College of Science and Engineering, Department of Chemistry and Biochemistry, San Francisco, CA 94132-1722. Offers biochemistry (MS); chemistry and biochemistry (MS). *Program availability:* Part-time. *Application deadline:* Applications are processed on a rolling basis. Electronic applications accepted. *Expenses:* Tuition, state resident: full-time $6738. Tuition, nonresident: full-time $15,666. *Required fees:* $1004. *Unit head:* Dr. Jane DeWitt, Chair, 415-338-1895, Fax: 415-338-2384, E-mail: dewitt@sfsu.edu. *Application contact:* Dr. Andrew Ichimura, Graduate Coordinator, 415-405-0721, Fax: 415-338-2384, E-mail: ichimura@sfsu.edu.
Website: http://www.chembiochem.sfsu.edu/0home/0layout.php

Seton Hall University, College of Arts and Sciences, Department of Chemistry and Biochemistry, South Orange, NJ 07079-2697. Offers analytical chemistry (MS, PhD); biochemistry (MS, PhD); chemistry (MS); inorganic chemistry (MS, PhD); organic chemistry (MS, PhD); physical chemistry (MS, PhD). *Program availability:* Part-time, evening/weekend. Terminal master's awarded for partial completion of doctoral program. *Degree requirements:* For master's, thesis optional; for doctorate, comprehensive exam, thesis/dissertation. *Entrance requirements:* Additional exam requirements/recommendations for international students: Required—TOEFL. Electronic applications accepted. *Faculty research:* DNA metal reactions; chromatography; bioinorganic, biophysical, organometallic, polymer chemistry; heterogeneous catalyst; synthetic organic and carbohydrate chemistry.

Simon Fraser University, Office of Graduate Studies, Faculty of Science, Department of Molecular Biology and Biochemistry, Burnaby, BC V5A 1S6, Canada. Offers bioinformatics (Graduate Diploma); molecular biology and biochemistry (M Sc, PhD). *Degree requirements:* For master's, thesis; for doctorate, thesis/dissertation; for Graduate Diploma, practicum. *Entrance requirements:* For master's, minimum GPA of 3.0 (on scale of 4.33), or 3.33 based on last 60 credits of undergraduate courses; for doctorate, minimum GPA of 3.5; for Graduate Diploma, minimum GPA of 2.5 (on scale of 4.33), or 2.67 based on the last 60 credits of undergraduate courses. Additional exam requirements/recommendations for international students: Recommended—TOEFL (minimum score 580 paper-based; 100 iBT), IELTS (minimum score 7.5), TWE (minimum score 5). Electronic applications accepted. *Faculty research:* Genomics and bioinformatics, cell and developmental biology, structural biology/biochemistry, immunology, nucleic acid function.

Sonoma State University, School of Science and Technology, Department of Biology, Rohnert Park, CA 94928. Offers biochemistry (MA); ecology (MS); environmental biology (MS); evolutionary biology (MS); functional morphology (MS); molecular and cell biology (MS); organismal biology (MS). *Program availability:* Part-time. *Degree requirements:* For master's, thesis or alternative, oral exam. *Entrance requirements:* For master's, GRE General Test, GRE Subject Test, minimum GPA of 3.0. Additional exam requirements/recommendations for international students: Required—TOEFL (minimum score 500 paper-based). *Faculty research:* Plant physiology, comparative physiology, community ecology, restoration ecology, marine ecology, conservation genetics, primate behavior, behavioral ecology, developmental biology, plant and animal systematics.

Southern Illinois University Carbondale, Graduate School, College of Science, Department of Chemistry and Biochemistry, Carbondale, IL 62901-4701. Offers MS, PhD. *Program availability:* Part-time. *Faculty:* 18 full-time (1 woman), 2 part-time/adjunct (0 women). *Students:* 39 full-time (19 women), 13 part-time (6 women); includes 2 minority (both Asian, non-Hispanic/Latino), 34 international. Average age 25. 31 applicants, 29% accepted, 5 enrolled. In 2015, 4 master's, 9 doctorates awarded. Terminal master's awarded for partial completion of doctoral program. *Degree requirements:* For master's, one foreign language, thesis; for doctorate, variable foreign language requirement, thesis/dissertation. *Entrance requirements:* For master's, GRE, minimum GPA of 2.7; for doctorate, GRE General Test, minimum GPA of 3.25. Additional exam requirements/recommendations for international students: Required—

TOEFL. *Application deadline:* For fall admission, 1/2 for domestic students; for spring admission, 6/30 for domestic students. Applications are processed on a rolling basis. Application fee: $65. *Financial support:* In 2015–16, 38 students received support, including 8 research assistantships with full tuition reimbursements available, 30 teaching assistantships with full tuition reimbursements available; fellowships with full tuition reimbursements available, Federal Work-Study, institutionally sponsored loans, and tuition waivers (full) also available. Support available to part-time students. *Faculty research:* Materials, separations, computational chemistry, synthetics. *Total annual research expenditures:* $1 million. *Unit head:* Gary Kinsel, Chair, 618-453-6482, Fax: 618-453-6408. *Application contact:* Andrea Steen, Office Manager, 618-453-6413, E-mail: asteen@siu.edu.

Southern Illinois University Carbondale, Graduate School, College of Science, Program in Molecular Biology, Microbiology, and Biochemistry, Carbondale, IL 62901-4701. Offers MS, PhD. *Faculty:* 16 full-time (2 women). *Students:* 38 full-time (28 women), 29 part-time (13 women); includes 5 minority (2 Black or African American, non-Hispanic/Latino; 3 Asian, non-Hispanic/Latino), 43 international. Average age 25. 83 applicants, 17% accepted, 612 enrolled. In 2015, 9 master's, 13 doctorates awarded. *Degree requirements:* For master's, thesis; for doctorate, thesis/dissertation. *Entrance requirements:* For master's, GRE, minimum GPA of 2.7; for doctorate, GRE, minimum GPA of 3.25. Additional exam requirements/recommendations for international students: Required—TOEFL. *Application deadline:* Applications are processed on a rolling basis. Application fee: $65. *Financial support:* In 2015–16, 49 students received support, including 42 research assistantships with full tuition reimbursements available, 7 teaching assistantships with full tuition reimbursements available; fellowships with full tuition reimbursements available, Federal Work-Study, and institutionally sponsored loans also available. Support available to part-time students. Financial award application deadline: 3/1. *Faculty research:* Prokaryotic gene regulation and expression; eukaryotic gene regulation; microbial, phylogenetic, and metabolic diversity; immune responses to tumors, pathogens, and autoantigens; protein folding and structure. *Unit head:* Dr. Judy Davie, Director, 618-453-5002, E-mail: jdavie@siumed.edu. *Application contact:* Donna K. Mueller, Office Manager, 618-453-8911, E-mail: mueller1@siu.edu.
Website: http://mbmb.siu.edu/

Southern University and Agricultural and Mechanical College, Graduate School, College of Sciences, Department of Chemistry, Baton Rouge, LA 70813. Offers analytical chemistry (MS); biochemistry (MS); environmental sciences (MS); inorganic chemistry (MS); organic chemistry (MS); physical chemistry (MS). *Degree requirements:* For master's, thesis. *Entrance requirements:* For master's, GMAT or GRE General Test. Additional exam requirements/recommendations for international students: Required—TOEFL (minimum score 525 paper-based). *Faculty research:* Synthesis of macrocyclic ligands, latex accelerators, anticancer drugs, biosensors, absorption isotheums, isolation of specific enzymes from plants.

Stanford University, School of Medicine, Graduate Programs in Medicine, Department of Biochemistry, Stanford, CA 94305-9991. Offers PhD. *Degree requirements:* For doctorate, thesis/dissertation. *Entrance requirements:* For doctorate, GRE General Test, GRE Subject Test (biology or chemistry). Additional exam requirements/recommendations for international students: Required—TOEFL. Electronic applications accepted. *Expenses:* Tuition, area resident: Full-time $45,729. *Required fees:* $591. *Faculty research:* DNA replication, recombination, and gene regulation; methods of isolating, analyzing, and altering genes and genomes; protein structure, protein folding, and protein processing; protein targeting and transport in the cell; intercellular signaling.

Stanford University, School of Medicine, Graduate Programs in Medicine, Department of Chemical and Systems Biology, Stanford, CA 94305-9991. Offers PhD. *Degree requirements:* For doctorate, thesis/dissertation, qualifying examination. *Entrance requirements:* For doctorate, GRE General Test, GRE Subject Test. Additional exam requirements/recommendations for international students: Required—TOEFL. Electronic applications accepted. *Expenses:* Tuition, area resident: Full-time $45,729. *Required fees:* $591. *Faculty research:* Action of drugs such as epinephrine, cell differentiation and development, microsomal enzymes, neuropeptide gene expression.

State University of New York College of Environmental Science and Forestry, Department of Chemistry, Syracuse, NY 13210-2779. Offers biochemistry (MPS, MS, PhD); environmental chemistry (MPS, MS, PhD); organic chemistry of natural products (MPS, MS, PhD); polymer chemistry (MPS, MS, PhD). *Faculty:* 17 full-time (2 women), 1 part-time/adjunct (0 women). *Students:* 33 full-time (13 women), 5 part-time (2 women); includes 2 minority (1 Black or African American, non-Hispanic/Latino; 1 Asian, non-Hispanic/Latino), 10 international. 55 applicants, 67% accepted, 12 enrolled. In 2015, 4 master's, 7 doctorates awarded. *Degree requirements:* For master's, thesis; for doctorate, comprehensive exam, thesis/dissertation. *Entrance requirements:* For master's and doctorate, GRE General Test, GRE Subject Test, minimum GPA of 3.0. Additional exam requirements/recommendations for international students: Required—TOEFL (minimum score 550 paper-based; 80 iBT), IELTS (minimum score 6). *Application deadline:* For fall admission, 2/1 priority date for domestic and international students; for spring admission, 11/1 priority date for domestic and international students. Applications are processed on a rolling basis. Application fee: $60. Electronic applications accepted. *Expenses:* Tuition, state resident: full-time $10,870; part-time $453 per credit. Tuition, nonresident: full-time $22,210; part-time $925 per credit. *Required fees:* $1075; $89.22 per credit. *Financial support:* In 2015–16, 40 students received support, including 5 fellowships with full tuition reimbursements available (averaging $4,000 per year), 19 research assistantships with full tuition reimbursements available (averaging $20,000 per year), 44 teaching assistantships with full tuition reimbursements available (averaging $21,300 per year); Federal Work-Study, institutionally sponsored loans, scholarships/grants, health care benefits, unspecified assistantships, and departmental tuition assistance also available. Financial award application deadline: 6/30; financial award applicants required to submit FAFSA. *Faculty research:* Polymer chemistry, biochemistry, environmental chemistry, natural products chemistry. *Total annual research expenditures:* $1.8 million. *Unit head:* Prof. Ivan Gitsov, Chair, 315-470-6851, Fax: 315-470-6856, E-mail: igivanov@syr.edu. *Application contact:* Scott Shannon, Associate Provost for Instruction/Dean of the Graduate School, 315-470-6599, Fax: 315-470-6978, E-mail: sshannon@esf.edu.
Website: http://www.esf.edu/chemistry

State University of New York Upstate Medical University, College of Graduate Studies, Program in Biochemistry and Molecular Biology, Syracuse, NY 13210-2334. Offers biochemistry (MS); biochemistry and molecular biology (PhD); MD/PhD. Terminal master's awarded for partial completion of doctoral program. *Degree requirements:* For master's, thesis; for doctorate, comprehensive exam, thesis/dissertation. *Entrance requirements:* For master's, GRE General Test, interview; for doctorate, GRE General Test, telephone interview. Additional exam requirements/recommendations for international students: Required—TOEFL. Electronic applications accepted. *Faculty research:* Enzymology, membrane structure and functions, developmental biology.

Stevens Institute of Technology, Graduate School, Charles V. Schaefer Jr. School of Engineering, Department of Chemistry, Chemical Biology and Biomedical Engineering, Program in Chemical Biology, Hoboken, NJ 07030. Offers MS, PhD, Certificate. *Program availability:* Part-time, evening/weekend. *Students:* 22 full-time (14 women); includes 3 minority (2 Black or African American, non-Hispanic/Latino; 1 Asian, non-

Biochemistry

Hispanic/Latino), 17 international. Average age 26. 51 applicants, 53% accepted, 4 enrolled. In 2015, 6 master's, 1 doctorate awarded. *Entrance requirements:* Additional exam requirements/recommendations for international students: Required—TOEFL (minimum score 74 iBT). *Application deadline:* For fall admission, 6/1 for domestic students, 4/15 for international students; for spring admission, 11/30 for domestic students, 11/1 for international students. Applications are processed on a rolling basis. Application fee: $60. Electronic applications accepted. *Expenses: Tuition, area resident:* Full-time $32,200; part-time $1450 per credit. *Required fees:* $1150; $550 per unit. $275 per semester. *Financial support:* Fellowships, research assistantships, teaching assistantships, career-related internships or fieldwork, Federal Work-Study, scholarships/grants, and unspecified assistantships available. Financial award application deadline: 2/15; financial award applicants required to submit FAFSA. *Unit head:* Patricia Muisener, Program Director, 201-216-3715, Fax: 201-216-8240, E-mail: patricia.muisener@stevens.edu. *Application contact:* Graduate Admissions, 888-783-8367, Fax: 888-511-1306, E-mail: graduate@stevens.edu.

Stony Brook University, State University of New York, Graduate School, College of Arts and Sciences, Department of Biochemistry and Cell Biology, Biochemistry and Cell Biology Program, Stony Brook, NY 11794. Offers MS. *Program availability:* Part-time. *Students:* 17 full-time (6 women), 4 part-time (1 woman); includes 5 minority (1 Black or African American, non-Hispanic/Latino; 2 Asian, non-Hispanic/Latino; 2 Hispanic/Latino), 4 international. 76 applicants, 34% accepted, 14 enrolled. In 2015, 11 master's awarded. *Degree requirements:* For master's, thesis. *Entrance requirements:* For master's, three letters of recommendation, BS or BA in a life science related field with minimum B average, personal statement. Additional exam requirements/recommendations for international students: Required—TOEFL (minimum score 550 paper-based; 90 iBT). *Application deadline:* For fall admission, 4/1 for domestic and international students. Applications are processed on a rolling basis. Electronic applications accepted. *Expenses:* $12,421 full-time resident tuition and fees, $453 per credit hour; $23,761 full-time non-resident tuition and fees, $925 per credit hour. *Unit head:* Prof. Aaron Neiman, Chair, 631-632-1543, Fax: 631-632-9730, E-mail: aaron.neiman@stonybrook.edu. *Application contact:* Pam Wolfskill, Coordinator, 631-632-8585, Fax: 631-632-8575, E-mail: carol.juliano@stonybrook.edu. Website: http://www.stonybrook.edu/commcms/biochem/education/graduate/overview.html

Stony Brook University, State University of New York, Graduate School, College of Arts and Sciences, Department of Biochemistry and Cell Biology, Molecular and Cellular Biology Program, Stony Brook, NY 11794. Offers biochemistry and molecular biology (PhD); biological sciences (MA); immunology and pathology (PhD); molecular and cellular biology (PhD). *Faculty:* 22 full-time (7 women). *Students:* 66 full-time (41 women); includes 11 minority (2 Black or African American, non-Hispanic/Latino; 6 Asian, non-Hispanic/Latino; 3 Hispanic/Latino), 38 international. Average age 28. 175 applicants, 16% accepted, 8 enrolled. In 2015, 11 doctorates awarded. *Degree requirements:* For doctorate, comprehensive exam, thesis/dissertation, teaching experience. *Entrance requirements:* For doctorate, GRE General Test, GRE Subject Test. Additional exam requirements/recommendations for international students: Required—TOEFL. *Application deadline:* For fall admission, 1/15 for domestic students; for spring admission, 10/1 for domestic students. Application fee: $100. *Expenses:* $12,421 per year full-time resident tuition and fees, $453 per credit hour; $23,761 per year full-time non-resident tuition and fees, $925 per credit hour. *Financial support:* In 2015–16, 4 fellowships, 33 research assistantships, 8 teaching assistantships were awarded; Federal Work-Study also available. *Unit head:* Prof. Aaron Neiman, Chair, 631-632-1543, E-mail: aaron.neiman@stonybrook.edu. *Application contact:* Pam Wolfskill, Administrative Specialist/Program Administrator, 631-632-8585, Fax: 631-632-9730, E-mail: pamela.wolfskill@stonybrook.edu.

Stony Brook University, State University of New York, Graduate School, College of Arts and Sciences, Department of Biochemistry and Cell Biology, Program in Biochemistry and Structural Biology, Stony Brook, NY 11794. Offers PhD. *Students:* 32 full-time (14 women); includes 5 minority (1 Black or African American, non-Hispanic/Latino; 1 Asian, non-Hispanic/Latino; 2 Hispanic/Latino; 1 Native Hawaiian or other Pacific Islander, non-Hispanic/Latino), 15 international. Average age 27. 49 applicants, 33% accepted, 4 enrolled. In 2015, 5 doctorates awarded. *Entrance requirements:* For doctorate, GRE. Additional exam requirements/recommendations for international students: Required—TOEFL (minimum score 90 iBT). *Application deadline:* For fall admission, 1/15 for domestic students; for spring admission, 10/1 for domestic students. Application fee: $100. *Expenses:* $12,421 per year full-time resident tuition and fees, $453 per credit hour; $23,761 per year full-time non-resident tuition and fees, $925 per credit hour. *Financial support:* In 2015–16, 2 fellowships, 18 research assistantships, 8 teaching assistantships were awarded. *Unit head:* Prof. Robert Haltiwanger, Chair, 631-632-7336, Fax: 631-632-9730, E-mail: robert.haltiwanger@stonybrook.edu. *Application contact:* Joann DeLucia-Conlon, Graduate Program Assistant, 631-632-8613, Fax: 631-632-8575, E-mail: joann.delucia-conlon@stonybrook.edu. Website: http://www.stonybrook.edu/commcms/biochem/education/graduate/overview.html

Syracuse University, College of Arts and Sciences, Ph.D. Program in Structural Biology, Biochemistry and Biophysics, Syracuse, NY 13244. Offers structural biology, biochemistry, and biophysics (PhD). *Students:* Average age 28. *Degree requirements:* For doctorate, comprehensive exam, thesis/dissertation. *Entrance requirements:* For doctorate, GRE General Test, GRE Subject Test, three letters of recommendation, resume, personal statement, transcripts. Additional exam requirements/recommendations for international students: Required—TOEFL (minimum score 100 iBT). *Application deadline:* For fall admission, 12/15 priority date for domestic and international students. Application fee: $75. Electronic applications accepted. *Expenses: Tuition, area resident:* Full-time $25,974; part-time $1443 per credit hour. *Required fees:* $802; $50 per course. Tuition and fees vary according to course load and program. *Financial support:* Fellowships with full tuition reimbursements, research assistantships with tuition reimbursements, teaching assistantships with tuition reimbursements, scholarships/grants, and tuition waivers available. Financial award application deadline: 1/1. *Faculty research:* Biochemistry, genetic engineering, biomolecular modeling, methods for computerized simulation of molecules, ethical conduct of science. *Unit head:* Prof. Liviu Movileanu, Associate Professor, Physics, 315-443-9154, Fax: 315-443-2012, E-mail: lmovilea@syr.edu. *Application contact:* Patty Whitmore, Academic Program Coordinator, 315-443-5958, E-mail: pawhitmo@syr.edu. Website: http://sb3.syr.edu/

Texas A&M University, College of Agriculture and Life Sciences, Department of Biochemistry and Biophysics, College Station, TX 77843. Offers biochemistry (MS, PhD). *Faculty:* 28. *Students:* 142 full-time (64 women), 8 part-time (3 women); includes 18 minority (3 Black or African American, non-Hispanic/Latino; 1 American Indian or Alaska Native, non-Hispanic/Latino; 3 Asian, non-Hispanic/Latino; 10 Hispanic/Latino; 1 Two or more races, non-Hispanic/Latino), 65 international. Average age 28. 166 applicants, 27% accepted, 37 enrolled. In 2015, 7 master's, 17 doctorates awarded. *Entrance requirements:* For master's and doctorate, GRE General Test. Additional exam requirements/recommendations for international students: Required—TOEFL (minimum score 550 paper-based; 80 iBT), IELTS (minimum score 6), PTE (minimum score 53).

Application deadline: For fall admission, 2/1 priority date for domestic students, 12/1 priority date for international students. Applications are processed on a rolling basis. Application fee: $50 ($90 for international students). Electronic applications accepted. *Expenses:* Contact institution. *Financial support:* In 2015–16, 147 students received support, including 14 fellowships with tuition reimbursements available (averaging $12,243 per year), 104 research assistantships with tuition reimbursements available (averaging $9,598 per year), 36 teaching assistantships with tuition reimbursements available (averaging $7,819 per year); career-related internships or fieldwork, institutionally sponsored loans, scholarships/grants, traineeships, health care benefits, tuition waivers (full and partial), and unspecified assistantships also available. Support available to part-time students. Financial award application deadline: 3/15; financial award applicants required to submit FAFSA. *Faculty research:* Enzymology, gene expression, protein structure, plant biochemistry. *Unit head:* Dr. Gregory D. Reinhart, Department Head, 979-862-5032, Fax: 979-845-9274, E-mail: gdr@tamu.edu. *Application contact:* Rafael Almanzar, Graduate Advisor, 979-845-1779, Fax: 979-845-9274, E-mail: r.almanzar1@tamu.edu. Website: http://biochemistry.tamu.edu/

Texas Christian University, College of Science and Engineering, Department of Chemistry and Biochemistry, Fort Worth, TX 76129. Offers MA, MS, PhD. *Program availability:* Part-time. *Faculty:* 12 full-time (3 women). *Students:* 22 full-time (12 women), 2 part-time (0 women); includes 4 minority (2 Asian, non-Hispanic/Latino; 1 Hispanic/Latino; 1 Two or more races, non-Hispanic/Latino), 11 international. Average age 27. 18 applicants, 33% accepted, 4 enrolled. In 2015, 1 master's, 4 doctorates awarded. Terminal master's awarded for partial completion of doctoral program. *Degree requirements:* For master's, thesis; for doctorate, thesis/dissertation, literature seminar, cumulative exams, research progress report, independent research proposal, teaching of undergraduate labs. *Entrance requirements:* For master's and doctorate, GRE General Test. Additional exam requirements/recommendations for international students: Required—TOEFL (minimum score 80 iBT). *Application deadline:* For fall admission, 2/1 for domestic and international students; for spring admission, 9/1 for domestic and international students. Application fee: $60. Electronic applications accepted. *Expenses: Tuition, area resident:* Full-time $26,640; part-time $1480 per credit hour. *Required fees:* $48; $48 per unit. Tuition and fees vary according to program. *Financial support:* In 2015–16, 18 students received support, including 18 fellowships with full tuition reimbursements available (averaging $21,000 per year); scholarships/grants, tuition waivers, and unspecified assistantships also available. Support available to part-time students. Financial award application deadline: 2/1. *Faculty research:* Bioinorganic and materials chemistry, protein folding, aggregation and transport phenomena, synthetic methodology and total synthesis, synthetic switches for sensing applications, electronic structure approximations. *Unit head:* Dr. Eric Simanek, Chair/Professor, 817-257-5355, Fax: 817-257-5851, E-mail: e.simanek@tcu.edu. *Application contact:* Dr. Benjamin G Janesko, Director of Graduate Studies/Associate Professor, 817-257-6202, Fax: 817-257-5851, E-mail: b.janesko@tcu.edu. Website: http://www.chm.tcu.edu/

Texas State University, The Graduate College, College of Science and Engineering, Program in Biochemistry, San Marcos, TX 78666. Offers MS. *Program availability:* Part-time. *Faculty:* 6 full-time (3 women). *Students:* 16 full-time (10 women), 4 part-time (all women); includes 10 minority (3 Black or African American, non-Hispanic/Latino; 1 Asian, non-Hispanic/Latino; 5 Hispanic/Latino; 1 Two or more races, non-Hispanic/Latino), 2 international. Average age 27. 22 applicants, 45% accepted, 5 enrolled. In 2015, 7 master's awarded. *Degree requirements:* For master's, comprehensive exam, thesis. *Entrance requirements:* For master's, GRE (minimum preferred score of 300), baccalaureate degree in chemistry, biochemistry or closely-related field from regionally-accredited university with minimum GPA of 3.0 on last 60 undergraduate semester hours, 2 letters of recommendation, statement of purpose. Additional exam requirements/recommendations for international students: Required—TOEFL (minimum score 550 paper-based; 78 iBT). *Application deadline:* For fall admission, 2/1 priority date for domestic and international students; for spring admission, 10/15 for domestic students, 10/1 for international students. Applications are processed on a rolling basis. Application fee: $40 ($90 for international students). Electronic applications accepted. *Expenses:* $3,615 in-state tuition (for 12 semester credit hour/1 full-time semester), $974 in-state fees. *Financial support:* In 2015–16, 10 students received support, including 12 research assistantships (averaging $13,197 per year), 7 teaching assistantships (averaging $13,557 per year); Federal Work-Study, institutionally sponsored loans, scholarships/grants, health care benefits, and unspecified assistantships also available. Support available to part-time students. Financial award application deadline: 3/1; financial award applicants required to submit FAFSA. *Faculty research:* Synthesis and characterization of Tetrapods to support quantum materials, responsive hydrogels based on binary nucleic acid probes for molecular detection, quantitative description of phosphorylation effects on disordered protein structure, non-dispersive reaction and separation processes for pharmaceutical synthesis, interfaces in materials research triangle. *Total annual research expenditures:* $1.5 million. *Unit head:* Dr. Chad Booth, Graduate Advisor, 512-245-8789, Fax: 512-245-2374, E-mail: cb31@txstate.edu. *Application contact:* Dr. Andrea Golato, Dean of Graduate School, 512-245-2581, Fax: 512-245-8365, E-mail: gradcollege@txstate.edu. Website: http://www.txstate.edu/chemistry/

Thomas Jefferson University, Jefferson College of Biomedical Sciences, PhD Program in Biochemistry and Molecular Pharmacology, Philadelphia, PA 19107. Offers PhD. *Faculty:* 68 full-time (19 women), 1 (woman) part-time/adjunct. *Students:* 36 full-time (23 women); includes 9 minority (1 Black or African American, non-Hispanic/Latino; 8 Asian, non-Hispanic/Latino), 10 international. 25 applicants, 36% accepted, 6 enrolled. In 2015, 4 doctorates awarded. *Degree requirements:* For doctorate, comprehensive exam, thesis/dissertation. *Entrance requirements:* For doctorate, GRE General Test or MCAT, minimum GPA of 3.2. Additional exam requirements/recommendations for international students: Required—TOEFL, IELTS (minimum score 7). *Application deadline:* For fall admission, 12/15 priority date for domestic and international students. Applications are processed on a rolling basis. Application fee: $50. Electronic applications accepted. *Financial support:* In 2015–16, 36 students received support, including 36 fellowships with full tuition reimbursements available (averaging $56,298 per year); Federal Work-Study, institutionally sponsored loans, scholarships/grants, traineeships, and stipends also available. Financial award application deadline: 5/1; financial award applicants required to submit FAFSA. *Faculty research:* Signal transduction and molecular genetics, translational biochemistry, human mitochondrial genetics, molecular biology of protein-RNA interaction, mammalian mitochondrial biogenesis and function. *Unit head:* Dr. Michael J. Root, MD, Program Director, 215-503-4564, Fax: 215-923-2117, E-mail: michael.root@jefferson.edu. *Application contact:* Marc E. Stearns, Director of Admissions, 215-503-0155, Fax: 215-503-3433, E-mail: jgsbs-info@jefferson.edu. Website: http://www.jefferson.edu/university/biomedical-sciences/degrees-programs/phd-programs/biochemistry-pharmacology.html

Tufts University, Sackler School of Graduate Biomedical Sciences, Cell, Molecular, and Developmental Biology Program, Medford, MA 02155. Offers cancer biology (PhD); developmental and regenerative biology (PhD); molecular and cellular medicine (PhD); structural and chemical biology (PhD). *Faculty:* 45 full-time (15 women). *Students:* 36

full-time (18 women); includes 13 minority (2 Black or African American, non-Hispanic/Latino; 9 Asian, non-Hispanic/Latino; 1 Hispanic/Latino; 1 Two or more races, non-Hispanic/Latino), 4 international. Average age 28. 189 applicants, 7% accepted, 6 enrolled. In 2015, 2 doctorates awarded. Terminal master's awarded for partial completion of doctoral program. *Degree requirements:* For doctorate, comprehensive exam, thesis/dissertation. *Entrance requirements:* For doctorate, GRE General Test, 3 letters of reference. Additional exam requirements/recommendations for international students: Required—TOEFL (minimum score 600 paper-based; 100 iBT). *Application deadline:* For fall admission, 12/15 priority date for domestic and international students. Application fee: $70. Electronic applications accepted. *Expenses: Tuition, area resident:* Full-time $48,412; part-time $1210 per credit hour. *Required fees:* $806. Full-time tuition and fees vary according to degree level, program and student level. Part-time tuition and fees vary according to course load. *Financial support:* In 2015–16, 36 students received support, including 36 research assistantships with full tuition reimbursements available (averaging $32,000 per year); health care benefits also available. *Faculty research:* Reproduction and hormone action, control of gene expression, cell-matrix and cell-cell interactions, growth control and tumorigenesis, cytoskeleton and contractile proteins. *Unit head:* Dr. Ira Herman, Program Director, 617-636-2991, Fax: 617-636-0375. *Application contact:* Dr. Elizabeth Storrs, Registrar/Director of Academic Services, 617-636-6767, Fax: 617-636-0375, E-mail: sackler-school@tufts.edu. Website: http://sackler.tufts.edu/Academics/CMDB-Welcome

Tulane University, School of Medicine and School of Liberal Arts, Graduate Programs in Biomedical Sciences, Department of Biochemistry and Molecular Biology, New Orleans, LA 70118-5669. Offers MS. MS and PhD offered through the Graduate School. *Degree requirements:* For master's, thesis. *Entrance requirements:* For master's, GRE General Test, GRE Subject Test, minimum B average in undergraduate course work. Additional exam requirements/recommendations for international students: Required—TOEFL. *Application deadline:* For fall admission, 2/1 for domestic students. Application fee: $45. Electronic applications accepted. *Expenses: Tuition, area resident:* Full-time $47,658; part-time $2648 per credit hour. *Required fees:* $1980; $44.50 per credit hour. $550 per term. Tuition and fees vary according to course load, degree level and program. *Financial support:* Fellowships with full tuition reimbursements, research assistantships with full tuition reimbursements, and tuition waivers (full) available. Financial award application deadline: 2/1. *Faculty research:* Nucleic acid chemistry, complex carbohydrates biochemistry.

Universidad Central del Caribe, School of Medicine, Program in Biomedical Sciences, Bayamón, PR 00960-6032. Offers anatomy and cell biology (MA, MS); biochemistry (MS); biomedical sciences (MA); cellular and molecular biology (PhD); microbiology and immunology (MA, MS); pharmacology (MS); physiology (MS).

Université de Moncton, Faculty of Sciences, Department of Chemistry and Biochemistry, Moncton, NB E1A 3E9, Canada. Offers biochemistry (M Sc); chemistry (M Sc). *Program availability:* Part-time. *Degree requirements:* For master's, one foreign language, thesis. *Entrance requirements:* For master's, minimum GPA of 3.0. Electronic applications accepted. *Faculty research:* Environmental contaminants, natural products synthesis, nutraceutical, organic catalysis, molecular biology of cancer.

Université de Montréal, Faculty of Medicine, Department of Biochemistry, Montréal, QC H3C 3J7, Canada. Offers biochemistry (M Sc, PhD); clinical biochemistry (DEPD). Terminal master's awarded for partial completion of doctoral program. *Degree requirements:* For master's, thesis; for doctorate, thesis/dissertation, general exam. *Entrance requirements:* For master's and doctorate, proficiency in French, knowledge of English; for DEPD, proficiency in French. Electronic applications accepted.

Université de Sherbrooke, Faculty of Medicine and Health Sciences, Graduate Programs in Medicine, Department of Biochemistry, Sherbrooke, QC J1H 5N4, Canada. Offers M Sc, PhD. Terminal master's awarded for partial completion of doctoral program. *Degree requirements:* For master's, thesis; for doctorate, thesis/dissertation. Electronic applications accepted. *Faculty research:* RNA structure-function, chromatin and gene expression, genetic diseases.

Université Laval, Faculty of Medicine, Post-Professional Programs in Medical Studies, Québec, QC G1K 7P4, Canada. Offers anatomy–pathology (DESS); anesthesiology (DESS); cardiology (DESS); care of older people (Diploma); clinical research (DESS); community health (DESS); dermatology (DESS); diagnostic radiology (DESS); emergency medicine (Diploma); family medicine (DESS); general surgery (DESS); geriatrics (DESS); hematology (DESS); internal medicine (DESS); maternal and fetal medicine (Diploma); medical biochemistry (DESS); medical microbiology and infectious diseases (DESS); medical oncology (DESS); nephrology (DESS); neurology (DESS); neurosurgery (DESS); obstetrics and gynecology (DESS); ophthalmology (DESS); orthopedic surgery (DESS); oto-rhino-laryngology (DESS); palliative medicine (Diploma); pediatrics (DESS); plastic surgery (DESS); psychiatry (DESS); pulmonary medicine (DESS); radiology–oncology (DESS); thoracic surgery (DESS); urology (DESS). *Degree requirements:* For other advanced degree, comprehensive exam. *Entrance requirements:* For degree, knowledge of French. Electronic applications accepted.

Université Laval, Faculty of Sciences and Engineering, Department of Biochemistry and Microbiology, Programs in Biochemistry, Québec, QC G1K 7P4, Canada. Offers M Sc, PhD. Terminal master's awarded for partial completion of doctoral program. *Degree requirements:* For master's, thesis; for doctorate, comprehensive exam, thesis/dissertation. *Entrance requirements:* For master's and doctorate, knowledge of French, comprehension of written English. Electronic applications accepted.

University at Buffalo, the State University of New York, Graduate School, School of Medicine and Biomedical Sciences, Graduate Programs in Medicine and Biomedical Sciences, Department of Biochemistry, Buffalo, NY 14260. Offers MA, PhD. *Faculty:* 22 full-time (7 women), 1 (woman) part-time/adjunct. *Students:* 36 full-time (19 women); includes 3 minority (1 American Indian or Alaska Native, non-Hispanic/Latino; 2 Hispanic/Latino), 18 international. Average age 27. 17 applicants, 71% accepted, 7 enrolled. In 2015, 5 master's, 4 doctorates awarded. Terminal master's awarded for partial completion of doctoral program. *Degree requirements:* For master's, thesis optional; for doctorate, comprehensive exam, thesis/dissertation. *Entrance requirements:* For master's, GRE General Test; for doctorate, GRE General Test, 3 letters of recommendation. Additional exam requirements/recommendations for international students: Required—TOEFL (minimum score 79 iBT). *Application deadline:* For fall admission, 2/1 priority date for domestic and international students. Applications are processed on a rolling basis. Application fee: $85. Electronic applications accepted. *Expenses:* Contact institution. *Financial support:* In 2015–16, 2 fellowships with full tuition reimbursements (averaging $22,900 per year), 25 research assistantships with full tuition reimbursements (averaging $27,000 per year) were awarded; Federal Work-Study, institutionally sponsored loans, scholarships/grants, health care benefits, and unspecified assistantships also available. Financial award application deadline: 2/1; financial award applicants required to submit FAFSA. *Faculty research:* Gene expression, proteins and metalloenzymes, biochemical endocrinology. *Total annual research expenditures:* $2.8 million. *Unit head:* Dr. Mark R. O'Brian, Chair, 716-829-3200, Fax: 716-829-2725, E-mail: mrobrian@buffalo.edu. *Application contact:* Dr. Lee Ann Sinha, Director of Graduate Studies, 716-881-7995, Fax: 716-829-2725, E-mail: leesinha@buffalo.edu. Website: http://www.smbs.buffalo.edu/bch/

The University of Alabama at Birmingham, Graduate Programs in Joint Health Sciences, Biochemistry, Structural and Stem Cell Biology Program, Birmingham, AL 35294-0024. Offers PhD. *Students:* 34 full-time (11 women); includes 7 minority (4 Black or African American, non-Hispanic/Latino; 2 Hispanic/Latino; 1 Two or more races, non-Hispanic/Latino), 5 international. Average age 26. *Degree requirements:* For doctorate, comprehensive exam, thesis/dissertation. *Entrance requirements:* For doctorate, GRE (minimum combined verbal/quantitative score of 300, 1100 on old exam), interview, letters of recommendation, minimum GPA of 3.0, research experience. Additional exam requirements/recommendations for international students: Required—TOEFL (minimum score 600 paper-based; 100 iBT). *Application deadline:* For fall admission, 12/1 priority date for domestic students, 1/15 for international students. Application fee: $60 ($60 for international students). Electronic applications accepted. *Expenses:* Tuition, state resident: full-time $7340. Tuition, nonresident: full-time $16,628. Full-time tuition and fees vary according to course load and program. *Financial support:* In 2015–16, fellowships with full tuition reimbursements (averaging $29,000 per year) were awarded. *Faculty research:* Enzymology, chromatin structure, gene expression, cell signaling, protein structure. *Unit head:* Dr. Thomas Ryan, Program Director, 205-996-2175, E-mail: tryan@uab.edu. *Application contact:* Holly Hebard, Director of Student and Academic Services, 205-996-5696, E-mail: hghebard@uab.edu. Website: http://www.uab.edu/gbs/bssb/

University of Alaska Fairbanks, College of Natural Sciences and Mathematics, Department of Chemistry and Biochemistry, Fairbanks, AK 99775-6160. Offers biochemistry and neuroscience (PhD); chemistry (MA, MS), including chemistry (MS); environmental chemistry (PhD). *Program availability:* Faculty: 10 full-time (3 women). *Students:* 31 full-time (17 women), 4 part-time (3 women); includes 3 minority (1 Asian, non-Hispanic/Latino; 2 Two or more races, non-Hispanic/Latino), 9 international. Average age 29. 27 applicants, 30% accepted, 7 enrolled. In 2015, 4 master's, 1 doctorate awarded. *Degree requirements:* For master's, comprehensive exam, thesis (for some programs), oral defense of project or thesis; for doctorate, comprehensive exam, thesis/dissertation, oral defense of dissertation. *Entrance requirements:* For master's, GRE General Test (for MS), bachelor's degree from accredited institution with minimum cumulative undergraduate and major GPA of 3.0; for doctorate, GRE General Test, minimum cumulative GPA of 3.0. Additional exam requirements/recommendations for international students: Required—TOEFL (minimum score 550 paper-based; 79 iBT), TWE. *Application deadline:* For fall admission, 6/1 for domestic students, 3/1 for international students; for spring admission, 10/15 for domestic students, 9/1 for international students. Applications are processed on a rolling basis. Application fee: $60. Electronic applications accepted. *Expenses:* Tuition, state resident: full-time $7614; part-time $423 per credit. Tuition, nonresident: full-time $15,552; part-time $864 per credit. *Required fees:* $38 per credit. $187 per semester. Tuition and fees vary according to course level, course load, program and reciprocity agreements. *Financial support:* In 2015–16, 14 research assistantships with full tuition reimbursements (averaging $16,421 per year), 14 teaching assistantships with full tuition reimbursements (averaging $17,322 per year) were awarded; fellowships with full tuition reimbursements, Federal Work-Study, scholarships/grants, health care benefits, and unspecified assistantships also available. Support available to part-time students. Financial award application deadline: 7/1; financial award applicants required to submit FAFSA. *Faculty research:* Atmospheric aerosols, cold adaptation, hibernation and neuroprotection, liganogated ion channels, arctic contaminants. *Unit head:* Bill Simpson, Department Chair, 907-474-5510, Fax: 907-474-5640, E-mail: uaf-chem-biochem@alaska.edu. *Application contact:* Mary Kreta, Director of Admissions, 907-474-7500, Fax: 907-474-7097, E-mail: admissions@uaf.edu. Website: http://www.uaf.edu/chem

University of Alberta, Faculty of Medicine and Dentistry and Faculty of Graduate Studies and Research, Graduate Programs in Medicine, Department of Biochemistry, Edmonton, AB T6G 2E1, Canada. Offers M Sc, PhD. Terminal master's awarded for partial completion of doctoral program. *Degree requirements:* For master's, thesis; for doctorate, thesis/dissertation. *Entrance requirements:* For master's and doctorate, minimum GPA of 3.3. Additional exam requirements/recommendations for international students: Required—TOEFL (minimum score 550 paper-based). *Faculty research:* Proteins, nucleic acids, membranes, regulation of gene expression, receptors.

The University of Arizona, College of Science, Department of Chemistry and Biochemistry, Tucson, AZ 85721. Offers biochemistry (PhD). *Program availability:* Part-time. *Degree requirements:* For doctorate, comprehensive exam, thesis/dissertation. *Entrance requirements:* For doctorate, GRE General Test, 3 letters of recommendation, statement of purpose. Additional exam requirements/recommendations for international students: Required—TOEFL (minimum score 550 paper-based; 79 iBT). *Application deadline:* For fall admission, 2/1 for domestic students, 1/1 for international students; for spring admission, 10/15 for domestic and international students. Applications are processed on a rolling basis. Application fee: $75. Electronic applications accepted. *Financial support:* Research assistantships, teaching assistantships, institutionally sponsored loans, scholarships/grants, health care benefits, tuition waivers (partial), and unspecified assistantships available. Financial award applicants required to submit FAFSA. *Faculty research:* Analytical, inorganic, organic, physical chemistry, biological chemistry. *Unit head:* Dr. Roger L. Miesfeld, Department Head, 520-626-2343, Fax: 520-621-8407, E-mail: rlm@email.arizona.edu. *Application contact:* Dr. Kriss Pope, Director, Finance and Administration, 520-621-6345, E-mail: kpope@email.arizona.edu. Website: http://www.chem.arizona.edu/

University of Arkansas for Medical Sciences, Graduate School, Little Rock, AR 72205. Offers biochemistry and molecular biology (MS, PhD); bioinformatics (MS, PhD); cellular physiology and molecular biophysics (MS, PhD); clinical nutrition (MS); interdisciplinary biomedical sciences (MS, PhD, Certificate); interdisciplinary toxicology (MS); microbiology and immunology (PhD); neurobiology and developmental sciences (PhD); pharmacology (PhD); MD/PhD. Bioinformatics programs hosted jointly with the University of Arkansas at Little Rock. *Program availability:* Part-time. Terminal master's awarded for partial completion of doctoral program. *Degree requirements:* For master's, comprehensive exam (for some programs), thesis (for some programs); for doctorate, thesis/dissertation. *Entrance requirements:* For master's and doctorate, GRE. Additional exam requirements/recommendations for international students: Required—TOEFL. Electronic applications accepted. *Expenses:* Contact institution.

The University of British Columbia, Faculty of Medicine, Department of Biochemistry and Molecular Biology, Vancouver, BC V6T 1Z1, Canada. Offers M Sc, PhD. *Degree requirements:* For master's, thesis; for doctorate, comprehensive exam, thesis/dissertation. *Entrance requirements:* For master's, first class B Sc; for doctorate, master's or first class honors bachelor's degree in biochemistry. Additional exam requirements/recommendations for international students: Required—TOEFL (minimum score 625 paper-based). Electronic applications accepted. *Faculty research:* Membrane biochemistry, protein structure/function, signal transduction, biochemistry.

University of Calgary, Cumming School of Medicine and Faculty of Graduate Studies, Department of Biochemistry and Molecular Biology, Calgary, AB T2N 1N4, Canada. Offers M Sc, PhD. *Degree requirements:* For master's, thesis; for doctorate, thesis/dissertation, candidacy exam. *Entrance requirements:* For master's and doctorate, GRE General Test, minimum GPA of 3.2. Additional exam requirements/recommendations for

Biochemistry

international students: Required—TOEFL. Electronic applications accepted. *Faculty research:* Molecular and developmental genetics; molecular biology of disease; genomics, proteomics and bioinformatics; cell signaling and structure.

University of California, Berkeley, Graduate Division, Group in Comparative Biochemistry, Berkeley, CA 94720-1500. Offers PhD. *Degree requirements:* For doctorate, thesis/dissertation, qualifying exam. *Entrance requirements:* For doctorate, GRE General Test, GRE Subject Test, minimum GPA of 3.0, 3 letters of recommendation. Additional exam requirements/recommendations for international students: Required—TOEFL.

University of California, Davis, Graduate Studies, Graduate Group in Biochemistry and Molecular Biology, Davis, CA 95616. Offers MS, PhD. Terminal master's awarded for partial completion of doctoral program. *Degree requirements:* For master's, comprehensive exam (for some programs), thesis (for some programs); for doctorate, thesis/dissertation. *Entrance requirements:* For master's and doctorate, GRE General Test, GRE Subject Test. Additional exam requirements/recommendations for international students: Required—TOEFL (minimum score 550 paper-based). Electronic applications accepted. *Faculty research:* Gene expression, protein structure, molecular virology, protein synthesis, enzymology, membrane transport and structural biology.

University of California, Irvine, Francisco J. Ayala School of Biological Sciences, Department of Molecular Biology and Biochemistry, Irvine, CA 92697. Offers biological science (MS); biological sciences (PhD); biotechnology (MS); biotechnology management (MS); MD/PhD. *Students:* 43 full-time (19 women), 1 part-time (0 women); includes 16 minority (2 Black or African American, non-Hispanic/Latino; 9 Asian, non-Hispanic/Latino; 5 Hispanic/Latino), 3 international. Average age 28. In 2015, 1 master's, 16 doctorates awarded. *Degree requirements:* For doctorate, thesis/dissertation. *Entrance requirements:* For master's, GRE, minimum GPA of 3.0; for doctorate, GRE General Test, GRE Subject Test, minimum GPA of 3.0. Additional exam requirements/recommendations for international students: Required—TOEFL (minimum score 550 paper-based). *Application deadline:* For fall admission, 12/15 priority date for domestic students, 12/15 for international students. Applications are processed on a rolling basis. Application fee: $90 ($110 for international students). Electronic applications accepted. *Financial support:* Fellowships, research assistantships with full tuition reimbursements, teaching assistantships, institutionally sponsored loans, traineeships, health care benefits, and unspecified assistantships available. Financial award application deadline: 3/1; financial award applicants required to submit FAFSA. *Faculty research:* Structure and synthesis of nucleic acids and proteins, regulation, virology, biochemical genetics, gene organization. *Unit head:* Prof. Christopher Hughes, Chair, 949-824-8771, Fax: 949-824-8551, E-mail: cchughes@uci.edu. *Application contact:* Morgan Oldham, Student Affairs Assistant, 949-826-6034, Fax: 949-824-8551, E-mail: morgano@uci.edu. Website: http://www.bio.uci.edu/

University of California, Irvine, Francisco J. Ayala School of Biological Sciences and School of Medicine, Interdisciplinary Graduate Program in Cellular and Molecular Biosciences, Irvine, CA 92697. Offers PhD. *Students:* 26 full-time (14 women); includes 11 minority (5 Asian, non-Hispanic/Latino; 3 Hispanic/Latino; 3 Two or more races, non-Hispanic/Latino), 2 international. Average age 25. 322 applicants, 18% accepted, 25 enrolled. *Degree requirements:* For doctorate, thesis/dissertation, teaching assignment, preliminary exam. *Entrance requirements:* For doctorate, GRE General Test, three letters of recommendation, interview. Additional exam requirements/recommendations for international students: Required—TOEFL or IELTS. *Application deadline:* For fall admission, 12/8 for domestic and international students. Application fee: $90 ($110 for international students). Electronic applications accepted. *Expenses:* Contact institution. *Financial support:* Fellowships with full tuition reimbursements, institutionally sponsored loans, scholarships/grants, tuition waivers (full), unspecified assistantships, and stipends available. Financial award application deadline: 1/1; financial award applicants required to submit FAFSA. *Faculty research:* Cellular biochemistry; gene structure and expression; protein structure, function, and design; molecular genetics; pathogenesis and inherited disease. *Unit head:* Melanie Cocco, Director, 949-824-4487, Fax: 949-824-1965, E-mail: mcocco@uci.edu. *Application contact:* Renee Frigo, Administrator, 949-824-8145, Fax: 949-824-1965, E-mail: rfrigo@uci.edu. Website: http://cmb.uci.edu/

University of California, Irvine, School of Medicine and Francisco J. Ayala School of Biological Sciences, Department of Biological Chemistry, Irvine, CA 92697. Offers biological sciences (MS, PhD). *Students:* 18 full-time (6 women); includes 10 minority (4 Black or African American, non-Hispanic/Latino; 2 Asian, non-Hispanic/Latino; 4 Hispanic/Latino), 3 international. Average age 28. In 2015, 4 doctorates awarded. *Degree requirements:* For doctorate, thesis/dissertation. *Entrance requirements:* For master's, minimum GPA of 3.0; for doctorate, GRE General Test, GRE Subject Test, minimum GPA of 3.0. Additional exam requirements/recommendations for international students: Required—TOEFL (minimum score 550 paper-based). *Application deadline:* For fall admission, 1/15 priority date for domestic students, 1/15 for international students. Application fee: $90 ($110 for international students). Electronic applications accepted. *Financial support:* Fellowships, research assistantships with full tuition reimbursements, teaching assistantships, institutionally sponsored loans, traineeships, health care benefits, and unspecified assistantships available. Financial award application deadline: 3/1; financial award applicants required to submit FAFSA. *Faculty research:* RNA splicing, mammalian chromosomal organization, membrane-hormone interactions, regulation of protein synthesis, molecular genetics of metabolic processes. *Unit head:* Peter Kaiser, Chair/Professor, 949-824-9442, Fax: 949-824-2688, E-mail: pkaiser@uci.edu. *Application contact:* Andrew Komoto, Graduate Coordinator, 949-824-6051, Fax: 949-824-2688, E-mail: akomoto@uci.edu. Website: http://www.bio.uci.edu/

University of California, Los Angeles, David Geffen School of Medicine and Graduate Division, Graduate Programs in Medicine, Department of Biological Chemistry, Los Angeles, CA 90095. Offers MS, PhD. Terminal master's awarded for partial completion of doctoral program. *Degree requirements:* For master's, comprehensive exam or thesis; for doctorate, thesis/dissertation, oral and written qualifying exams; 2 quarters of teaching experience. *Entrance requirements:* For master's and doctorate, GRE General Test, bachelor's degree; minimum undergraduate GPA of 3.0 (or its equivalent if letter grade system not used). Additional exam requirements/recommendations for international students: Required—TOEFL. Electronic applications accepted.

University of California, Los Angeles, Graduate Division, College of Letters and Science, Department of Chemistry and Biochemistry, Program in Biochemistry and Molecular Biology, Los Angeles, CA 90095. Offers MS, PhD. Terminal master's awarded for partial completion of doctoral program. *Degree requirements:* For master's, comprehensive exam or thesis; for doctorate, thesis/dissertation, oral and written qualifying exams; 3 quarters of teaching experience. *Entrance requirements:* For doctorate, GRE General Test, GRE Subject Test (recommended), bachelor's degree; minimum undergraduate GPA of 3.0 (or its equivalent if letter grade system not used). Additional exam requirements/recommendations for international students: Required—TOEFL. Electronic applications accepted.

University of California, Los Angeles, Graduate Division, College of Letters and Science and David Geffen School of Medicine, UCLA ACCESS to Programs in the Molecular, Cellular and Integrative Life Sciences, Los Angeles, CA 90095. Offers biochemistry and molecular biology (PhD); biological chemistry (PhD); cellular and molecular pathology (PhD); human genetics (PhD); microbiology, immunology, and molecular genetics (PhD); molecular biology (PhD); molecular toxicology (PhD); molecular, cellular and integrative physiology (PhD); neurobiology (PhD); oral biology (PhD); physiology (PhD). *Degree requirements:* For doctorate, thesis/dissertation, oral and written qualifying exams. *Entrance requirements:* For doctorate, GRE General Test, bachelor's degree; minimum undergraduate GPA of 3.0 (or its equivalent if letter grade system not used). Additional exam requirements/recommendations for international students: Required—TOEFL. Electronic applications accepted.

University of California, Merced, Graduate Division, School of Natural Sciences, Merced, CA 95343. Offers applied mathematics (MS, PhD); chemistry and chemical biology (MS, PhD); physics (MS, PhD); quantitative and systems biology (MS, PhD). *Faculty:* 63 full-time (25 women). *Students:* 156 full-time (64 women); includes 58 minority (3 Black or African American, non-Hispanic/Latino; 23 Asian, non-Hispanic/Latino; 22 Hispanic/Latino; 1 Native Hawaiian or other Pacific Islander, non-Hispanic/Latino; 9 Two or more races, non-Hispanic/Latino), 37 international. Average age 27. 199 applicants, 57% accepted, 45 enrolled. In 2015, 12 master's, 11 doctorates awarded. Terminal master's awarded for partial completion of doctoral program. *Degree requirements:* For master's, variable foreign language requirement, comprehensive exam, thesis or alternative; for doctorate, variable foreign language requirement, comprehensive exam, thesis/dissertation. *Entrance requirements:* For master's and doctorate, GRE. Additional exam requirements/recommendations for international students: Required—TOEFL (minimum score 550 paper-based; 80 iBT); Recommended—IELTS (minimum score 7). *Application deadline:* For fall admission, 1/15 for domestic and international students. Application fee: $90 ($110 for international students). Electronic applications accepted. *Expenses:* $11,220 per year resident tuition, $15,102 per year non-resident tuition. *Financial support:* In 2015–16, 151 students received support, including 12 fellowships with full tuition reimbursements available (averaging $23,614 per year), 37 research assistantships with full tuition reimbursements available (averaging $18,842 per year), 127 teaching assistantships with full tuition reimbursements available (averaging $18,538 per year); scholarships/grants, traineeships, and health care benefits also available. Financial award application deadline: 1/15. *Faculty research:* Computational science, soft matter physics, neurobiology, genomics, biochemistry. Total annual research expenditures: $5.3 million. *Unit head:* Dr. Juan C. Meza, Dean, 209-228-4487, Fax: 209-228-4060, E-mail: jcmeza@ucmerced.edu. *Application contact:* Tsu Ya, Director of Graduate Admissions and Academic Services, 209-228-4521, Fax: 209-228-6906, E-mail: tya@ucmerced.edu.

University of California, Riverside, Graduate Division, Department of Biochemistry and Molecular Biology, Riverside, CA 92521-0102. Offers biochemistry and molecular biology (MS, PhD). *Program availability:* Part-time. Terminal master's awarded for partial completion of doctoral program. *Degree requirements:* For master's, thesis (for some programs), comprehensive exam or thesis; for doctorate, comprehensive exam, thesis/dissertation, 2 quarters of teaching experience, written exam, oral qualifying exam. *Entrance requirements:* For master's, GRE General Test, minimum GPA of 3.0; for doctorate, GRE General Test, minimum GPA of 3.25. Additional exam requirements/recommendations for international students: Required—TOEFL (minimum score 550 paper-based; 80 iBT). *Application deadline:* For fall admission, 1/5 priority date for domestic and international students; for winter admission, 12/1 for domestic students, 7/1 for international students; for spring admission, 3/1 for domestic students, 10/1 for international students. Application fee: $80 ($100 for international students). Electronic applications accepted. *Expenses:* Tuition, area resident: Full-time $16,665.50; part-time $11,055.54. Tuition, state resident: full-time $16,665.50; part-time $11,055.54. Tuition, nonresident: full-time $31,768. International tuition: $31,767.50 full-time. *Required fees:* $16,665.50; $11,055.54 per quarter. $3685.18 per quarter. Tuition and fees vary according to program. *Financial support:* Fellowships with full tuition reimbursements, research assistantships with full tuition reimbursements, teaching assistantships with full tuition reimbursements, career-related internships or fieldwork, institutionally sponsored loans, and scholarships/grants available. Financial award application deadline: 1/5; financial award applicants required to submit FAFSA. *Faculty research:* Structural biology and molecular biophysics, signal transduction, plant biochemistry and molecular biology, gene expression and metabolic regulation, molecular toxicology and pathogenesis. Website: http://www.biochemistry.ucr.edu/

University of California, San Diego, Graduate Division, Department of Chemistry and Biochemistry, La Jolla, CA 92093. Offers chemistry (MS, PhD). PhD offered jointly with San Diego State University. *Students:* 285 full-time (102 women), 5 part-time (1 woman); includes 99 minority (9 Black or African American, non-Hispanic/Latino; 3 American Indian or Alaska Native, non-Hispanic/Latino; 60 Asian, non-Hispanic/Latino; 26 Hispanic/Latino; 1 Native Hawaiian or other Pacific Islander, non-Hispanic/Latino), 52 international. 640 applicants, 34% accepted, 85 enrolled. In 2015, 54 master's, 44 doctorates awarded. *Degree requirements:* For master's, comprehensive exam (for some programs), thesis (for some programs); for doctorate, comprehensive exam, thesis/dissertation. *Entrance requirements:* For master's, GRE General Test; for doctorate, GRE General Test, GRE Subject Test. Additional exam requirements/recommendations for international students: Required—TOEFL (minimum score 550 paper-based; 80 iBT), IELTS. *Application deadline:* For fall admission, 12/15 priority date for domestic students. Application fee: $90 ($110 for international students). Electronic applications accepted. *Expenses:* Tuition, state resident: full-time $11,220. Tuition, nonresident: full-time $26,322. *Required fees:* $1800. *Financial support:* Fellowships, research assistantships, teaching assistantships, scholarships/grants, and traineeships available. Financial award applicants required to submit FAFSA. *Faculty research:* Analytical and atmospheric chemistry, biochemistry & biophysics, cellular and systems biochemistry, chemical biology, inorganic chemistry, organic chemistry, physical chemistry, quantitative biology, structural biology, theoretical and computational chemistry. *Unit head:* Partho Ghosh, Chair, 858-822-1339, E-mail: pghosh@ucsd.edu. *Application contact:* Jeff Rances, Admissions Coordinator, 858-534-9728, Fax: 858-534-7687, E-mail: chemgradinfo@ucsd.edu. Website: http://chemistry.ucsd.edu

University of California, San Francisco, Graduate Division and School of Medicine, Tetrad Graduate Program, Biochemistry and Molecular Biology Track, San Francisco, CA 94143. Offers PhD, MD/PhD. *Degree requirements:* For doctorate, thesis/dissertation. *Entrance requirements:* For doctorate, GRE General Test, GRE Subject Test. Additional exam requirements/recommendations for international students: Required—TOEFL. *Expenses:* Contact institution. *Faculty research:* Structural biology, genetics, cell biology, cell physiology, metabolism.

University of California, San Francisco, School of Pharmacy and Graduate Division, Chemistry and Chemical Biology Graduate Program, San Francisco, CA 94143. Offers PhD. *Degree requirements:* For doctorate, thesis/dissertation. *Entrance requirements:* For doctorate, GRE General Test, minimum GPA of 3.0, bachelor's degree. Additional exam requirements/recommendations for international students: Required—TOEFL (minimum score 550 paper-based; 80 iBT). Electronic applications accepted. *Faculty research:* Macromolecular structure function and dynamics, computational chemistry and biology, biological chemistry and synthetic biology, chemical biology and molecular design, nanomolecular design.

University of California, Santa Barbara, Graduate Division, College of Letters and Sciences, Division of Mathematics, Life, and Physical Sciences, Interdepartmental Graduate Program in Biomolecular Science and Engineering, Santa Barbara, CA 93106-2014. Offers biochemistry and molecular biology (PhD), including biochemistry and molecular biology, biophysics and bioengineering. *Faculty:* 35 full-time (3 women), 3 part-time/adjunct (all women). *Students:* 27 full-time (9 women); includes 7 minority (5 Asian, non-Hispanic/Latino; 2 Hispanic/Latino), 1 international. Average age 26. 105 applicants, 21% accepted, 11 enrolled. In 2015, 8 doctorates awarded. Terminal master's awarded for partial completion of doctoral program. *Degree requirements:* For doctorate, thesis/dissertation. *Entrance requirements:* For doctorate, GRE General Test. Additional exam requirements/recommendations for international students: Required—TOEFL (minimum score 630 paper-based; 109 iBT), IELTS (minimum score 7). *Application deadline:* For fall admission, 12/15 for domestic and international students. Application fee: $90 ($110 for international students). Electronic applications accepted. *Financial support:* In 2015–16, 28 students received support, including 16 fellowships with tuition reimbursements available, 31 research assistantships with tuition reimbursements available, 16 teaching assistantships with tuition reimbursements available; Federal Work-Study, traineeships, health care benefits, tuition waivers (full and partial), and unspecified assistantships also available. Financial award application deadline: 12/15; financial award applicants required to submit FAFSA. *Faculty research:* Biochemistry and molecular biology, biophysics, biomaterials, bioengineering, systems biology. *Unit head:* Prof. Omar A. Saleh, Director/Professor, 805-893-8814, E-mail: saleh@engineering.ucsb.edu. *Application contact:* Lauren Baker, Graduate Program Assistant, 805-893-3011, E-mail: bmse-gradasst@lifesci.ucsb.edu.
Website: http://www.bmse.ucsb.edu/

University of California, Santa Cruz, Division of Graduate Studies, Division of Physical and Biological Sciences, Department of Chemistry and Biochemistry, Santa Cruz, CA 95064. Offers MS, PhD. *Degree requirements:* For master's, thesis optional; for doctorate, one foreign language, thesis/dissertation, qualifying exam. *Entrance requirements:* For master's and doctorate, GRE General Test, GRE Subject Test. Additional exam requirements/recommendations for international students: Required—TOEFL (minimum score 570 paper-based; 89 iBT); Recommended—IELTS (minimum score 8). Electronic applications accepted. *Faculty research:* Marine chemistry; biochemistry; inorganic, organic, and physical chemistry.

University of Chicago, Division of the Biological Sciences, Department of Biochemistry and Molecular Biophysics, Chicago, IL 60637. Offers PhD, MD/PhD. *Students:* 28 full-time (14 women); includes 4 minority (2 Asian, non-Hispanic/Latino; 2 Hispanic/Latino), 6 international. Average age 28. 64 applicants, 28% accepted, 6 enrolled. In 2015, 4 doctorates awarded. *Degree requirements:* For doctorate, thesis/dissertation, ethics class, 2 teaching assistantships. *Entrance requirements:* For doctorate, GRE General Test. Additional exam requirements/recommendations for international students: Required—TOEFL (minimum score 600 paper-based; 104 iBT), IELTS (minimum score 7). *Application deadline:* For fall admission, 12/1 for domestic and international students. Application fee: $90. Electronic applications accepted. *Financial support:* In 2015–16, 26 students received support, including fellowships with tuition reimbursements available (averaging $29,781 per year), research assistantships with tuition reimbursements available (averaging $29,781 per year); institutionally sponsored loans, scholarships/grants, traineeships, and health care benefits also available. Financial award applicants required to submit FAFSA. *Faculty research:* Molecular biology, gene expression, and DNA-protein interactions; membrane biochemistry, molecular endocrinology, and transmembrane signaling; enzyme mechanisms, physical biochemistry, and structural biology. *Total annual research expenditures:* $5 million. *Unit head:* Dr. Tobin Sosnick, Chair. *Application contact:* Lisa Anderson, Graduate Student Administrator, 773-834-3586, Fax: 773-702-0439, E-mail: landerso@bsd.uchicago.edu.
Website: http://bmb.uchospitals.edu/

University of Cincinnati, Graduate School, College of Medicine, Graduate Programs in Biomedical Sciences, Department of Molecular Genetics, Biochemistry and Microbiology, Cincinnati, OH 45221. Offers MS, PhD. Terminal master's awarded for partial completion of doctoral program. *Degree requirements:* For master's, thesis or alternative; for doctorate, thesis/dissertation, qualifying exam. *Entrance requirements:* For master's and doctorate, GRE General Test. Additional exam requirements/recommendations for international students: Required—TOEFL (minimum score 600 paper-based; 100 iBT), TWE. Electronic applications accepted. *Faculty research:* Cancer biology and developmental genetics, gene regulation and chromosome structure, microbiology and pathogenic mechanisms, structural biology, membrane biochemistry and signal transduction.

University of Cincinnati, Graduate School, McMicken College of Arts and Sciences, Department of Chemistry, Cincinnati, OH 45221. Offers analytical chemistry (MS, PhD); biochemistry (MS, PhD); inorganic chemistry (MS, PhD); organic chemistry (MS, PhD); physical chemistry (MS, PhD); polymer chemistry (MS, PhD); sensors (PhD). *Program availability:* Part-time, evening/weekend. Terminal master's awarded for partial completion of doctoral program. *Degree requirements:* For master's, thesis optional; for doctorate, comprehensive exam, thesis/dissertation. *Entrance requirements:* For master's and doctorate, GRE General Test. Additional exam requirements/recommendations for international students: Required—TOEFL (minimum score 580 paper-based). Electronic applications accepted. *Faculty research:* Biomedical chemistry, laser chemistry, surface science, chemical sensors, synthesis.

University of Colorado Boulder, Graduate School, College of Arts and Sciences, Department of Chemistry and Biochemistry, Boulder, CO 80309. Offers biochemistry (PhD); chemistry (MS). *Faculty:* 46 full-time (9 women). *Students:* 222 full-time (78 women), 3 part-time (2 women); includes 33 minority (8 Asian, non-Hispanic/Latino; 18 Hispanic/Latino; 7 Two or more races, non-Hispanic/Latino), 37 international. Average age 26. 574 applicants, 27% accepted, 51 enrolled. In 2015, 9 master's, 44 doctorates awarded. Terminal master's awarded for partial completion of doctoral program. *Degree requirements:* For master's, comprehensive exam or thesis; for doctorate, comprehensive exam, thesis/dissertation, cumulative exam. *Entrance requirements:* For master's, GRE General Test, GRE Subject Test, minimum undergraduate GPA of 2.75; for doctorate, GRE General Test, GRE Subject Test, minimum GPA of 3.0. *Application deadline:* For fall admission, 12/15 for domestic and international students. Applications are processed on a rolling basis. Application fee: $50 ($70 for international students). Electronic applications accepted. Application fee is waived when completed online. *Financial support:* In 2015–16, 529 students received support, including 25 fellowships (averaging $4,975 per year), 126 research assistantships with tuition reimbursements available (averaging $33,604 per year), 98 teaching assistantships with tuition reimbursements available (averaging $33,154 per year); institutionally sponsored loans, scholarships/grants, health care benefits, and unspecified assistantships also available. Financial award applicants required to submit FAFSA. *Faculty research:* Biochemistry; physical chemistry, biochemistry: proteins, catalysis/kinetics, biochemistry: nucleic acid.

Total annual research expenditures: $24.7 million. *Application contact:* E-mail: chemgrad@colorado.edu.
Website: http://chem.colorado.edu

University of Colorado Denver, School of Medicine, Biochemistry Program, Aurora, CO 80045. Offers biochemistry (PhD); biochemistry and molecular genetics (PhD). *Students:* 14 full-time (4 women); includes 3 minority (2 Asian, non-Hispanic/Latino; 1 Hispanic/Latino). Average age 28. 24 applicants, 17% accepted, 4 enrolled. In 2015, 2 doctorates awarded. *Degree requirements:* For doctorate, comprehensive exam, thesis/dissertation, 30 credit hours each of coursework and thesis research. *Entrance requirements:* For doctorate, GRE, minimum of three letters of recommendation from qualified referees. Additional exam requirements/recommendations for international students: Required—TOEFL (minimum score 550 paper-based; 80 iBT). *Application deadline:* For fall admission, 12/1 for domestic students. Applications are processed on a rolling basis. Application fee: $50 ($75 for international students). Electronic applications accepted. *Expenses:* Contact institution. *Financial support:* In 2015–16, 14 students received support. Fellowships, research assistantships, teaching assistantships, Federal Work-Study, institutionally sponsored loans, scholarships/grants, traineeships, health care benefits, tuition waivers (full), and unspecified assistantships available. Financial award application deadline: 3/15; financial award applicants required to submit FAFSA. *Faculty research:* DNA damage, cancer and neurodegeneration, molecular mechanisms of pro-MRNA splicing, yeast RNA polymerases, DNA replication. *Total annual research expenditures:* $8.6 million. *Unit head:* Dr. Mark Johnston, Professor and Chair, 303-724-3203, Fax: 303-724-3215, E-mail: mark.johnston@ucdenver.edu. *Application contact:* Sue Brozowski, Department Contact, 303-724-3202, Fax: 303-724-3215, E-mail: sue.brozowski@ucdenver.edu.
Website: http://www.ucdenver.edu/academics/colleges/medicalschool/departments/biochemistry/Pages/Home.aspx

University of Connecticut Health Center, Graduate School, Programs in Biomedical Sciences, Graduate Program in Molecular Biology and Biochemistry, Farmington, CT 06030. Offers PhD, DMD/PhD, MD/PhD. *Degree requirements:* For doctorate, comprehensive exam, thesis/dissertation. *Entrance requirements:* For doctorate, GRE General Test. Additional exam requirements/recommendations for international students: Required—TOEFL (minimum score 600 paper-based). Electronic applications accepted. *Faculty research:* Molecular biology, structural biology, protein biochemistry, microbial physiology and pathogenesis.

See Display on page 208 and Close-Up on page 229.

University of Delaware, College of Arts and Sciences, Department of Chemistry and Biochemistry, Newark, DE 19716. Offers biochemistry (MA, MS, PhD); chemistry (MA, MS, PhD). *Program availability:* Part-time. Terminal master's awarded for partial completion of doctoral program. *Degree requirements:* For master's, one foreign language, thesis (for some programs); for doctorate, one foreign language, thesis/dissertation, cumulative exam. *Entrance requirements:* For master's and doctorate, GRE General Test. Additional exam requirements/recommendations for international students: Required—TOEFL (minimum score 600 paper-based). Electronic applications accepted. *Faculty research:* Micro-organisms, bone, cancer metastosis, developmental biology, cell biology, molecular biology.

University of Florida, College of Medicine and Graduate School, Interdisciplinary Program in Biomedical Sciences, Concentration in Biochemistry and Molecular Biology, Gainesville, FL 32611. Offers PhD. *Degree requirements:* For doctorate, thesis/dissertation. *Entrance requirements:* For doctorate, GRE General Test, minimum GPA of 3.0, biochemistry before enrollment. Additional exam requirements/recommendations for international students: Required—TOEFL. Electronic applications accepted. *Faculty research:* Gene expression, metabolic regulation, structural biology, enzyme mechanism, membrane transporters.

University of Georgia, Franklin College of Arts and Sciences, Department of Biochemistry and Molecular Biology, Athens, GA 30602. Offers MS, PhD. *Degree requirements:* For master's, one foreign language, thesis; for doctorate, one foreign language, thesis/dissertation. *Entrance requirements:* For master's and doctorate, GRE General Test. Additional exam requirements/recommendations for international students: Required—TOEFL. Electronic applications accepted.

University of Guelph, Graduate Studies, College of Biological Science, Department of Molecular and Cellular Biology, Guelph, ON N1G 2W1, Canada. Offers biochemistry (M Sc, PhD); biophysics (M Sc, PhD); botany (M Sc, PhD); microbiology (M Sc, PhD); molecular biology and genetics (M Sc, PhD). *Degree requirements:* For master's, thesis, research proposal; for doctorate, comprehensive exam, thesis/dissertation, research proposal. *Entrance requirements:* For master's, minimum B-average during previous 2 years of coursework; for doctorate, minimum A-average. Additional exam requirements/recommendations for international students: Required—TOEFL (minimum score 550 paper-based), IELTS (minimum score 6.5). Electronic applications accepted. *Faculty research:* Physiology, structure, genetics, and ecology of microbes; virology and microbial technology.

University of Guelph, Graduate Studies, College of Physical and Engineering Science, Guelph-Waterloo Centre for Graduate Work in Chemistry and Biochemistry, Guelph, ON N1G 2W1, Canada. Offers M Sc, PhD. M Sc, PhD offered jointly with University of Waterloo. *Program availability:* Part-time. *Degree requirements:* For master's, thesis; for doctorate, thesis/dissertation. *Faculty research:* Inorganic, analytical, biological, physical/theoretical, polymer, and organic chemistry.

University of Houston, College of Natural Sciences and Mathematics, Department of Biology and Biochemistry, Houston, TX 77204. Offers biochemistry (MA, PhD); biology (MA). Terminal master's awarded for partial completion of doctoral program. *Degree requirements:* For master's, comprehensive exam (for some programs), thesis optional; for doctorate, comprehensive exam (for some programs), thesis/dissertation. *Entrance requirements:* For master's and doctorate, GRE. Additional exam requirements/recommendations for international students: Required—TOEFL (minimum score 550 paper-based; 79 iBT), IELTS (minimum score 6.5). Electronic applications accepted. *Faculty research:* Cell and molecular biology, ecology and evolution, biochemical and biophysical sciences, chemical biology.

University of Idaho, College of Graduate Studies, College of Science, Department of Biological Sciences, Moscow, ID 83844-3051. Offers biology (MS, PhD); microbiology, molecular biology and biochemistry (PhD); neuroscience (MS, PhD). *Faculty:* 18 full-time. *Students:* 25 full-time, 2 part-time. Average age 29. In 2015, 5 doctorates awarded. *Degree requirements:* For doctorate, one foreign language, thesis/dissertation. *Entrance requirements:* For master's, GRE, minimum GPA of 2.8; for doctorate, GRE, minimum undergraduate GPA of 2.8, 3.0 graduate. Additional exam requirements/recommendations for international students: Required—TOEFL. *Application deadline:* For fall admission, 8/1 for domestic students; for spring admission, 12/15 for domestic students. Applications are processed on a rolling basis. Application fee: $60. Electronic applications accepted. *Expenses:* Tuition, state resident: full-time $6205; part-time $399 per credit hour. Tuition, nonresident: full-time $20,209; part-time $1177 per credit hour. *Required fees:* $2017; $58 per credit hour. Full-time tuition and fees vary according to course load and reciprocity agreements. *Financial support:* Research assistantships

Biochemistry

and teaching assistantships available. Financial award applicants required to submit FAFSA. *Faculty research:* Animal behavior development, germ cell development, evolutionary biology, fish reproductive biology, molecular mechanisms. *Unit head:* Dr. James J. Nagler, Interim Department Chair, 208-885-6280, E-mail: biosci@uidaho.edu. *Application contact:* Sean Scoggin, Graduate Recruitment Coordinator, 208-885-4723, Fax: 208-885-4406, E-mail: graduateadmissions@uidaho.edu.
Website: http://www.uidaho.edu/sci/biology

University of Illinois at Chicago, College of Medicine and Graduate College, Graduate Programs in Medicine, Department of Biochemistry and Molecular Genetics, Chicago, IL 60607-7128. Offers PhD, MD/PhD. *Faculty:* 31 full-time (12 women), 19 part-time/adjunct (9 women). *Students:* 22 full-time (12 women); includes 5 minority (1 Black or African American, non-Hispanic/Latino; 3 Asian, non-Hispanic/Latino; 1 Hispanic/Latino), 9 international. Average age 29. Terminal master's awarded for partial completion of doctoral program. *Degree requirements:* For doctorate, thesis/dissertation. *Entrance requirements:* For doctorate, GRE General Test. Additional exam requirements/recommendations for international students: Required—TOEFL. *Application deadline:* For fall admission, 3/1 priority date for domestic students, 2/15 for international students. Applications are processed on a rolling basis. Application fee: $60. Electronic applications accepted. *Expenses:* Tuition, state resident: full-time $11,480; part-time $3826 per credit. Tuition, nonresident: full-time $23,720; part-time $7906 per credit. *Required fees:* $1333 per semester. Part-time tuition and fees vary according to course load and program. *Financial support:* Fellowships with full tuition reimbursements, research assistantships with full tuition reimbursements, teaching assistantships with full tuition reimbursements, career-related internships or fieldwork, Federal Work-Study, institutionally sponsored loans, traineeships, tuition waivers (full), and unspecified assistantships available. Financial award application deadline: 3/1; financial award applicants required to submit FAFSA. *Faculty research:* Signal transduction, cell cycle regulation, membrane biology, regulation of gene function and development, protein and nucleic acid structure and function, cancer biology. *Unit head:* Dr. Jack Kaplan, Head, 312-355-2732, Fax: 312-413-0353, E-mail: kaplanj@uic.edu. *Application contact:* Dr. Karen Colley, Co-Director of Graduate Studies, 312-996-7756. Website: http://www.uic.edu/com/bcmg/

University of Illinois at Urbana–Champaign, Graduate College, College of Liberal Arts and Sciences, School of Chemical Sciences, Champaign, IL 61820. Offers MA, MS, PhD, MS/JD, MS/MBA. *Expenses:* Contact institution.

University of Illinois at Urbana–Champaign, Graduate College, College of Liberal Arts and Sciences, School of Molecular and Cellular Biology, Department of Biochemistry, Champaign, IL 61820. Offers MS, PhD.

The University of Iowa, Roy J. and Lucille A. Carver College of Medicine and Graduate College, Graduate Programs in Medicine, Department of Biochemistry, Iowa City, IA 52242. Offers MS, PhD, MD/PhD. Terminal master's awarded for partial completion of doctoral program. *Degree requirements:* For master's, thesis; for doctorate, comprehensive exam, thesis/dissertation. *Entrance requirements:* For master's, GRE General Test. Additional exam requirements/recommendations for international students: Required—TOEFL (minimum score 600 paper-based; 100 iBT). Electronic applications accepted. *Faculty research:* Regulation of gene expression, protein structure, membrane structure/function, DNA structure and replication.

The University of Kansas, Graduate Studies, College of Liberal Arts and Sciences, Department of Molecular Biosciences, Lawrence, KS 66044. Offers biochemistry and biophysics (MA, PhD); microbiology (MA, PhD); molecular, cellular, and developmental biology (MA, PhD). *Students:* 57 full-time (34 women), 4 part-time (1 woman); includes 9 minority (5 Asian, non-Hispanic/Latino; 2 Hispanic/Latino; 2 Two or more races, non-Hispanic/Latino), 23 international. Average age 27. 78 applicants, 46% accepted, 18 enrolled. In 2015, 3 master's, 7 doctorates awarded. Terminal master's awarded for partial completion of doctoral program. *Entrance requirements:* For master's and doctorate, GRE General Test. Additional exam requirements/recommendations for international students: Required—TOEFL or IELTS. *Application deadline:* For fall admission, 12/15 for domestic and international students. Application fee: $65 ($85 for international students). Electronic applications accepted. *Financial support:* Fellowships, research assistantships, teaching assistantships, health care benefits, and unspecified assistantships available. Financial award application deadline: 3/1. *Faculty research:* Structure and function of proteins, genetics of organism development, molecular genetics, neurophysiology, molecular virology and pathogenics, developmental biology, cell biology. *Unit head:* Susan M. Egan, Chair, 785-864-4294, E-mail: sme@ku.edu. *Application contact:* John Connolly, Graduate Admissions Contact, 785-864-4311, E-mail: jconnolly@ku.edu. Website: http://www.molecularbiosciences.ku.edu/

The University of Kansas, University of Kansas Medical Center, School of Medicine, Department of Biochemistry and Molecular Biology, Kansas City, KS 66160. Offers PhD, MD/PhD. *Faculty:* 22. *Students:* 7 full-time (4 women), 3 international. Average age 27. In 2015, 3 doctorates awarded. Terminal master's awarded for partial completion of doctoral program. *Degree requirements:* For doctorate, thesis/dissertation, comprehensive oral and written exam. *Entrance requirements:* For doctorate, GRE. Additional exam requirements/recommendations for international students: Required—TOEFL. *Application deadline:* For fall admission, 12/1 for domestic and international students. Applications are processed on a rolling basis. Application fee: $60. Electronic applications accepted. Application fee is waived when completed online. *Financial support:* In 2015–16, 3 research assistantships with partial tuition reimbursements, 4 teaching assistantships with partial tuition reimbursements were awarded; fellowships, traineeships, health care benefits, and unspecified assistantships also available. Financial award application deadline: 3/1; financial award applicants required to submit FAFSA. *Faculty research:* Determination of portion structure, underlying bases for interaction of proteins with their target, mapping allosteric circuiting within proteins, mechanism of action of transcription factors, renal signal transduction. *Total annual research expenditures:* $1.5 million. *Unit head:* Dr. Gerald M. Carlson, Chairman, 913-588-7005, Fax: 913-588-9896, E-mail: gcarlson@kumc.edu. *Application contact:* Dr. Liskin Swint-Kruse, Associate Professor, 913-588-0399, Fax: 913-588-9896, E-mail: lswint-kruse@kumc.edu.
Website: http://www.kumc.edu/school-of-medicine/biochemistry-and-molecular-biology.html

University of Kentucky, Graduate School, Graduate School Programs from the College of Medicine, Program in Molecular and Cellular Biochemistry, Lexington, KY 40506-0032. Offers PhD, MD/PhD. *Degree requirements:* For doctorate, comprehensive exam, thesis/dissertation. *Entrance requirements:* For doctorate, GRE General Test, minimum undergraduate GPA of 2.75. Additional exam requirements/recommendations for international students: Required—TOEFL (minimum score 550 paper-based). Electronic applications accepted.

University of Lethbridge, School of Graduate Studies, Lethbridge, AB T1K 3M4, Canada. Offers addictions counseling (M Sc); agricultural biotechnology (M Sc); agricultural studies (M Sc, MA); anthropology (MA); archaeology (M Sc, MA); art (MA, MFA); biochemistry (M Sc); biological sciences (M Sc); biomolecular science (PhD); biosystems and biodiversity (PhD); Canadian studies (MA); chemistry (M Sc); computer science (M Sc); computer science and geographical information science (M Sc); counseling (MC); counseling psychology (M Ed); dramatic arts (MA); earth, space, and physical science (PhD); economics (MA); education (MA, PhD); educational leadership (M Ed); English (MA); environmental science (M Sc); evolution and behavior (PhD); exercise science (M Sc); French (MA); French/German (MA); French/Spanish (MA); general education (M Ed); geography (M Sc, MA); German (MA); health sciences (M Sc); individualized multidisciplinary (M Sc, MA); kinesiology (M Sc, MA); management (M Sc), including accounting, finance, human resource management and labor relations, information systems, international management, marketing, policy and strategy; mathematics (M Sc); music (M Mus, MA); Native American studies (MA); neuroscience (M Sc, PhD); new media (MA, MFA); nursing (M Sc, MN); philosophy (MA); physics (M Sc); political science (MA); psychology (M Sc, MA); religious studies (MA); sociology (MA); theatre and dramatic arts (MFA); theoretical and computational science (PhD); urban and regional studies (MA); women and gender studies (MA). *Program availability:* Part-time, evening/weekend. *Students:* 448 full-time (249 women), 110 part-time (64 women). Average age 32. 285 applicants, 36% accepted, 96 enrolled. In 2015, 154 master's, 11 doctorates awarded. *Degree requirements:* For master's, thesis (for some programs); for doctorate, comprehensive exam, thesis/dissertation. *Entrance requirements:* For master's, GMAT (for M Sc in management), bachelor's degree in related field, minimum GPA of 3.0 during previous 20 graded semester courses, 2 years' teaching or related experience (M Ed); for doctorate, master's degree, minimum graduate GPA of 3.5. Additional exam requirements/recommendations for international students: Required—TOEFL (minimum score 580 paper-based; 93 iBT). Application fee: $100 Canadian dollars ($140 Canadian dollars for international students). Electronic applications accepted. *Financial support:* Fellowships, research assistantships, teaching assistantships, scholarships/grants, health care benefits, and unspecified assistantships available. *Faculty research:* Movement and brain plasticity, gibberellin physiology, photosynthesis, carbon cycling, molecular properties of main-group ring components. *Unit head:* Kathleen Schrage, Manager, School of Graduate Studies, 403-329-2121, E-mail: schrage@uleth.ca. *Application contact:* School of Graduate Studies, 403-329-5194, E-mail: sgsinquiries@uleth.ca.
Website: http://www.uleth.ca/graduate-studies/

University of Louisville, Graduate School, College of Arts and Sciences, Department of Chemistry, Louisville, KY 40292-0001. Offers analytical chemistry (MS, PhD); biochemistry (MS, PhD); chemical physics (PhD); inorganic chemistry (MS, PhD); organic chemistry (MS, PhD); physical chemistry (MS, PhD). *Students:* 46 full-time (16 women), 8 part-time (1 woman); includes 3 minority (1 Black or African American, non-Hispanic/Latino; 1 Asian, non-Hispanic/Latino; 1 Two or more races, non-Hispanic/Latino), 36 international. Average age 29. 51 applicants, 22% accepted, 6 enrolled. In 2015, 2 master's, 1 doctorate awarded. Terminal master's awarded for partial completion of doctoral program. *Degree requirements:* For master's, variable foreign language requirement, comprehensive exam, thesis optional; for doctorate, variable foreign language requirement, comprehensive exam, thesis/dissertation. *Entrance requirements:* For master's and doctorate, GRE General Test, BA or BS coursework. Additional exam requirements/recommendations for international students: Required—TOEFL (minimum score 550 paper-based; 79 iBT). *Application deadline:* For fall admission, 3/15 for domestic students, 5/1 priority date for international students; for winter admission, 9/15 for domestic and international students; for spring admission, 11/1 priority date for international students; for summer admission, 4/1 priority date for international students. Applications are processed on a rolling basis. Application fee: $60. Electronic applications accepted. *Expenses:* Tuition, state resident: full-time $11,664; part-time $649 per credit hour. Tuition, nonresident: full-time $24,274; part-time $1350 per credit hour. *Required fees:* $196. Tuition and fees vary according to program and reciprocity agreements. *Financial support:* In 2015–16, 757,720 students received support. Fellowships with full tuition reimbursements available, research assistantships with full tuition reimbursements available, teaching assistantships with full tuition reimbursements available, career-related internships or fieldwork, scholarships/grants, traineeships, health care benefits, and unspecified assistantships available. Support available to part-time students. Financial award application deadline: 3/15. *Faculty research:* Computational chemistry, biophysics nuclear magnetic resonance, synthetic organic chemistry, synthetic inorganic chemistry, medicinal chemistry, protein chemistry, enzymology, nano chemistry, electrochemistry, analytical chemistry, synthetic biology, bioinformatics. *Total annual research expenditures:* $2.4 million. *Unit head:* Dr. Richard J. Wittebort, Professor/Chair, 502-852-6613. *Application contact:* Libby Leggett, Director, Graduate Admissions, 502-852-3101, Fax: 502-852-6536, E-mail: gradadm@louisville.edu.
Website: http://louisville.edu/chemistry

University of Louisville, School of Medicine, Department of Biochemistry and Molecular Biology, Louisville, KY 40292-0001. Offers MS, PhD, MD/PhD. *Students:* 24 full-time (13 women), 7 part-time (2 women); includes 3 minority (2 Black or African American, non-Hispanic/Latino; 1 Asian, non-Hispanic/Latino), 8 international. Average age 29. 39 applicants, 18% accepted, 5 enrolled. In 2015, 9 master's, 1 doctorate awarded. Terminal master's awarded for partial completion of doctoral program. *Degree requirements:* For master's, thesis; for doctorate, comprehensive exam, thesis/dissertation, one first-author publication. *Entrance requirements:* For master's and doctorate, GRE General Test (minimum score of 1000 verbal and quantitative), minimum GPA of 3.0. Additional exam requirements/recommendations for international students: Required—TOEFL. *Application deadline:* For fall admission, 4/15 for domestic and international students. Applications are processed on a rolling basis. Application fee: $60. Electronic applications accepted. *Expenses:* Tuition, state resident: full-time $11,664; part-time $649 per credit hour. Tuition, nonresident: full-time $24,274; part-time $1350 per credit hour. *Required fees:* $196. Tuition and fees vary according to program and reciprocity agreements. *Financial support:* In 2015–16, 246,603 students received support, including 12 fellowships with full tuition reimbursements available (averaging $22,000 per year), 23 research assistantships with full tuition reimbursements available (averaging $22,000 per year); teaching assistantships with tuition reimbursements available, scholarships/grants, traineeships, tuition waivers (full and partial), and unspecified assistantships also available. Financial award application deadline: 4/15. *Faculty research:* Genetic regulatory mechanisms, microRNAs, vesicular trafficking in cancer metastasis and angiogenesis, ribosome biogenesis and disease, regulation of foreign compound metabolism/lipid and steroid metabolism. *Total annual research expenditures:* $2.4 million. *Unit head:* Dr. Ronald G. Gregg, Chair, 502-852-5217, Fax: 502-852-6222, E-mail: rggreg02@gwise.louisville.edu. *Application contact:* Dr. William L. Dean, Information Contact, 502-852-5227, Fax: 502-852-6222, E-mail: wldean01@gwise.louisville.edu.

The University of Manchester, Faculty of Life Sciences, Manchester, United Kingdom. Offers adaptive organismal biology (M Phil, PhD); animal biology (M Phil, PhD); biochemistry (M Phil, PhD); bioinformatics (M Phil, PhD); biomolecular sciences (M Phil, PhD); biotechnology (M Phil, PhD); cell biology (M Phil, PhD); cell matrix research (M Phil, PhD); channels and transporters (M Phil, PhD); developmental biology (M Phil, PhD); Egyptology (M Phil, PhD); environmental biology (M Phil, PhD); evolutionary biology (M Phil, PhD); gene expression (M Phil, PhD); genetics (M Phil, PhD); history of science, technology and medicine (M Phil, PhD); immunology (M Phil, PhD); integrative neurobiology and behavior (M Phil, PhD); membrane trafficking (M Phil, PhD);

microbiology (M Phil, PhD); molecular and cellular neuroscience (M Phil, PhD); molecular biology (M Phil, PhD); molecular cancer studies (M Phil, PhD); neuroscience (M Phil, PhD); ophthalmology (M Phil, PhD); optometry (M Phil, PhD); organelle function (M Phil, PhD); pharmacology (M Phil, PhD); physiology (M Phil, PhD); plant sciences (M Phil, PhD); stem cell research (M Phil, PhD); structural biology (M Phil, PhD); systems neuroscience (M Phil, PhD); toxicology (M Phil, PhD).

The University of Manchester, School of Chemistry, Manchester, United Kingdom. Offers biological chemistry (PhD); chemistry (M Ent, M Phil, M Sc, D Ent, PhD); inorganic chemistry (PhD); materials chemistry (PhD); nanoscience (PhD); nuclear fission (PhD); organic chemistry (PhD); physical chemistry (PhD); theoretical chemistry (PhD).

University of Manitoba, Faculty of Medicine and Faculty of Graduate Studies, Graduate Programs in Medicine, Department of Biochemistry and Medical Genetics, Winnipeg, MB R3T 2N2, Canada. Offers M Sc, PhD. Terminal master's awarded for partial completion of doctoral program. *Degree requirements:* For master's, thesis; for doctorate, thesis/dissertation. *Faculty research:* Cancer, gene expression, membrane lipids, metabolic control, genetic diseases.

University of Maryland, Baltimore, Graduate School, Graduate Program in Life Sciences, Program in Biochemistry and Molecular Biology, Baltimore, MD 21201. Offers biochemistry (MS, PhD); MD/PhD. *Degree requirements:* For doctorate, comprehensive exam, thesis/dissertation. *Entrance requirements:* For doctorate, GRE General Test. Additional exam requirements/recommendations for international students: Required—TOEFL (minimum score 550 paper-based; 80 iBT); Recommended—IELTS (minimum score 7). Electronic applications accepted. Tuition and fees vary according to program. *Faculty research:* Membrane transport, hormonal regulation, protein structure, molecular virology.

University of Maryland, Baltimore County, The Graduate School, College of Natural and Mathematical Sciences, Department of Chemistry and Biochemistry, Baltimore, MD 21250. Offers biochemistry (PhD); chemistry (MS, PhD); chemistry and biochemistry (Postbaccalaureate Certificate). *Program availability:* Part-time. *Faculty:* 21 full-time (5 women), 4 part-time/adjunct (1 woman). *Students:* 44 full-time (23 women), 1 part-time (0 women); includes 11 minority (6 Black or African American, non-Hispanic/Latino; 1 American Indian or Alaska Native, non-Hispanic/Latino; 2 Asian, non-Hispanic/Latino; 2 Hispanic/Latino), 6 international. Average age 26. 59 applicants, 25% accepted, 9 enrolled. In 2015, 4 master's, 4 doctorates awarded. Terminal master's awarded for partial completion of doctoral program. *Degree requirements:* For master's, comprehensive exam (for some programs), thesis (for some programs); for doctorate, comprehensive exam, thesis/dissertation. *Entrance requirements:* For master's, GRE General Test, minimum GPA of 3.0; for doctorate, GRE General Test, GRE Subject Test (recommended), minimum GPA of 3.0. Additional exam requirements/recommendations for international students: Required—TOEFL (minimum score 550 paper-based, 80 iBT) or IELTS. *Application deadline:* For fall admission, 6/1 priority date for domestic students, 1/1 priority date for international students; for spring admission, 11/1 priority date for domestic students, 5/1 for international students. Applications are processed on a rolling basis. Application fee: $50. Electronic applications accepted. Application fee is waived when completed online. *Expenses:* Tuition, state resident: full-time $12,816. Tuition, nonresident: full-time $19,710. *Financial support:* In 2015–16, 44 students received support, including 7 fellowships with full tuition reimbursements available (averaging $24,000 per year), 12 research assistantships with full tuition reimbursements available (averaging $23,166 per year), 25 teaching assistantships with full tuition reimbursements available (averaging $23,166 per year); health care benefits also available. *Faculty research:* Protein structures, bio-organic chemistry, enzyme catalysis, molecular biology, metabolism, nanotechnology. *Total annual research expenditures:* $4.4 million. *Unit head:* Dr. Zeev Rosenzweig, Chairman, 410-455-2521, Fax: 410-455-2608, E-mail: chemgrad@umbc.edu. *Application contact:* Patricia Gagne, Graduate Coordinator, 866-PHD-UMBC, Fax: 410-455-2608, E-mail: pgagne1@umbc.edu.
Website: http://chemistry.umbc.edu

University of Maryland, College Park, Academic Affairs, College of Computer, Mathematical and Natural Sciences, Department of Chemistry and Biochemistry, Biochemistry Program, College Park, MD 20742. Offers MS, PhD. *Program availability:* Part-time, evening/weekend. Terminal master's awarded for partial completion of doctoral program. *Degree requirements:* For master's, thesis or alternative; for doctorate, thesis/dissertation, 2 seminar presentations, oral exam. *Entrance requirements:* For master's and doctorate, GRE General Test, GRE Subject Test (recommended), minimum GPA of 3, 3 letters of recommendation. Additional exam requirements/recommendations for international students: Required—TOEFL. Electronic applications accepted. *Faculty research:* Analytical biochemistry, immunochemistry, drug metabolism, biosynthesis of proteins, mass spectrometry.

University of Massachusetts Amherst, Graduate School, College of Natural Sciences, Department of Biochemistry and Molecular Biology, Amherst, MA 01003. Offers MS, PhD. *Program availability:* Part-time. Terminal master's awarded for partial completion of doctoral program. *Degree requirements:* For master's, thesis or alternative; for doctorate, comprehensive exam, thesis/dissertation. *Entrance requirements:* Additional exam requirements/recommendations for international students: Required—TOEFL (minimum score 550 paper-based; 80 iBT), IELTS (minimum score 6.5). Electronic applications accepted.

University of Massachusetts Amherst, Graduate School, Interdisciplinary Programs, Program in Molecular and Cellular Biology, Amherst, MA 01003. Offers biological chemistry and molecular biophysics (PhD); biomedicine (PhD); cellular and developmental biology (PhD). *Program availability:* Part-time. Terminal master's awarded for partial completion of doctoral program. *Degree requirements:* For doctorate, comprehensive exam, thesis/dissertation. *Entrance requirements:* For doctorate, GRE General Test. Additional exam requirements/recommendations for international students: Required—TOEFL (minimum score 550 paper-based; 80 iBT), IELTS (minimum score 6.5). Electronic applications accepted.

University of Massachusetts Amherst, Graduate School, Interdisciplinary Programs, Program in Plant Biology, Amherst, MA 01003. Offers biochemistry and metabolism (MS, PhD); cell biology and physiology (MS, PhD); environmental, ecological and integrative biology (MS, PhD); genetics and evolution (MS, PhD). *Degree requirements:* For master's, thesis; for doctorate, 2 foreign languages, comprehensive exam, thesis/dissertation. *Entrance requirements:* For master's and doctorate, GRE General Test. Additional exam requirements/recommendations for international students: Required—TOEFL (minimum score 550 paper-based; 80 iBT), IELTS (minimum score 6.5). Electronic applications accepted.

University of Massachusetts Dartmouth, Graduate School, College of Arts and Sciences, Department of Chemistry and Biochemistry, North Dartmouth, MA 02747-2300. Offers chemistry (MS, PhD). *Program availability:* Part-time. *Faculty:* 18 full-time (6 women), 4 part-time/adjunct (2 women). *Students:* 21 full-time (9 women), 17 part-time (9 women); includes 4 minority (1 Black or African American, non-Hispanic/Latino; 3 Asian, non-Hispanic/Latino), 20 international. Average age 27. 31 applicants, 84% accepted, 11 enrolled. In 2015, 8 master's awarded. *Degree requirements:* For master's,

thesis or project; for doctorate, comprehensive exam, thesis/dissertation. *Entrance requirements:* For master's, GRE (recommended), statement of purpose (minimum of 300 words), resume, official transcripts, 2 letters of recommendation; for doctorate, GRE, statement of purpose (minimum of 300 words), resume, official transcripts, 2 letters of recommendation. Additional exam requirements/recommendations for international students: Required—TOEFL (minimum score 533 paper-based; 72 iBT). *Application deadline:* For fall admission, 3/15 priority date for domestic students, 2/15 priority date for international students; for spring admission, 11/1 priority date for domestic students, 10/1 priority date for international students. Applications are processed on a rolling basis. Application fee: $60. Electronic applications accepted. *Expenses:* Tuition, state resident: full-time $2071; part-time $86.29 per credit. Tuition, nonresident: full-time $8099; part-time $337.46 per credit. *Required fees:* $18,074; $762.08 per credit. Tuition and fees vary according to course load and reciprocity agreements. *Financial support:* In 2015–16, 2 fellowships (averaging $21,000 per year), 4 research assistantships (averaging $11,250 per year), 17 teaching assistantships (averaging $11,294 per year) were awarded; Federal Work-Study and unspecified assistantships also available. Support available to part-time students. Financial award application deadline: 3/1; financial award applicants required to submit FAFSA. *Total annual research expenditures:* $1.3 million. *Unit head:* Yuegang Zuo, Graduate Program Director, 508-999-8959, E-mail: yzuo@umassd.edu. *Application contact:* Steven Briggs, Director of Recruitment and Marketing for Graduate Studies, 508-999-8604, Fax: 508-999-8183, E-mail: graduate@umassd.edu.
Website: http://www.umassd.edu/cas/chemistry/

University of Massachusetts Lowell, College of Sciences, Department of Chemistry, Lowell, MA 01854. Offers analytical chemistry (PhD); biochemistry (PhD); chemistry (MS, PhD); environmental studies (PhD); green chemistry (PhD); inorganic chemistry (PhD); organic chemistry (PhD); polymer science (MS). Terminal master's awarded for partial completion of doctoral program. *Degree requirements:* For master's, thesis; for doctorate, 2 foreign languages, thesis/dissertation. *Entrance requirements:* For master's and doctorate, GRE General Test. *Application deadline:* For fall admission, 4/1 priority date for domestic students; for spring admission, 10/1 for domestic students. Applications are processed on a rolling basis. Application fee: $20 ($35 for international students). Electronic applications accepted. *Expenses:* Tuition, state resident: full-time $14,304. Tuition, nonresident: full-time $25,853. *Required fees:* $375. Full-time tuition and fees vary according to campus/location and reciprocity agreements. *Financial support:* Fellowships, research assistantships with full tuition reimbursements, teaching assistantships with full tuition reimbursements, career-related internships or fieldwork, scholarships/grants, and traineeships available. Financial award application deadline: 4/1.

University of Massachusetts Medical School, Graduate School of Biomedical Sciences, Worcester, MA 01655-0115. Offers biomedical sciences (PhD), including biochemistry and molecular pharmacology, bioinformatics and computational biology, cancer biology, cell biology, immunology and microbiology, interdisciplinary, neuroscience, translational science; biomedical sciences (millennium program) (PhD); clinical and population health research (PhD); clinical investigation (MS). *Faculty:* 1,339 full-time (521 women), 301 part-time (189 women). *Students:* 363 full-time (184 women); includes 58 minority (13 Black or African American, non-Hispanic/Latino; 30 Asian, non-Hispanic/Latino; 15 Hispanic/Latino), 141 international. Average age 29. 661 applicants, 26% accepted, 51 enrolled. In 2015, 10 master's, 58 doctorates awarded. Terminal master's awarded for partial completion of doctoral program. *Degree requirements:* For master's, comprehensive exam, thesis; for doctorate, comprehensive exam, thesis/dissertation. *Entrance requirements:* For master's, MD, PhD, DVM, or PharmD; for doctorate, GRE General Test, bachelor's degree. Additional exam requirements/recommendations for international students: Required—TOEFL (minimum score 100 iBT) or IELTS (minimum score 7.5). *Application deadline:* For fall admission, 12/15 for domestic and international students; for spring admission, 5/15 for domestic students. Application fee: $80. Electronic applications accepted. *Expenses:* $6,966 resident per year; $14,182 non-resident per year. *Financial support:* In 2015–16, 383 students received support, including research assistantships with full tuition reimbursements available (averaging $30,600 per year); scholarships/grants, health care benefits, tuition waivers (full), and unspecified assistantships also available. Financial award application deadline: 5/16. *Faculty research:* RNA interference, cell/molecular/developmental biology, bioinformatics, clinical/translational research, infectious disease. *Total annual research expenditures:* $250.3 million. *Unit head:* Dr. Anthony Carruthers, Dean, 508-856-4135, E-mail: anthony.carruthers@umassmed.edu. *Application contact:* Dr. Kendall Knight, Assistant Vice Provost for Admissions, 508-856-5628, Fax: 508-856-3659, E-mail: kendall.knight@umassmed.edu.
Website: http://www.umassmed.edu/gsbs/

University of Miami, Graduate School, Miller School of Medicine, Graduate Programs in Medicine, Department of Biochemistry and Molecular Biology, Coral Gables, FL 33124. Offers PhD, MD/PhD. *Degree requirements:* For doctorate, comprehensive exam, thesis/dissertation, proposition exams. *Faculty research:* Macromolecule metabolism, molecular genetics, protein folding and 3-D structure, regulation of gene expression and enzyme function, signal transduction and developmental biology.

University of Michigan, Rackham Graduate School, College of Literature, Science, and the Arts, Department of Chemistry, Ann Arbor, MI 48109-1055. Offers analytical (PhD); chemical biology (PhD); inorganic (PhD); materials (PhD); organic (PhD); physical (PhD). *Faculty:* 38 full-time (9 women), 9 part-time/adjunct (3 women). *Students:* 264 full-time (113 women). 535 applicants, 31% accepted, 54 enrolled. In 2015, 45 doctorates awarded. *Degree requirements:* For doctorate, comprehensive exam, thesis/dissertation, oral defense of dissertation, organic cumulative proficiency exams. *Entrance requirements:* For doctorate, GRE General Test, GRE Subject Test (recommended), 3 letters of recommendation. Additional exam requirements/recommendations for international students: Required—TOEFL (minimum score 560 paper-based; 84 iBT). *Application deadline:* For fall admission, 12/15 for domestic and international students. Applications are processed on a rolling basis. Application fee: $0 ($90 for international students). Electronic applications accepted. *Financial support:* In 2015–16, 264 students received support, including 40 fellowships with full tuition reimbursements available (averaging $29,000 per year), 78 research assistantships with full tuition reimbursements available (averaging $29,025 per year), 146 teaching assistantships with full tuition reimbursements available (averaging $29,025 per year); career-related internships or fieldwork, scholarships/grants, traineeships, health care benefits, and unspecified assistantships also available. *Faculty research:* Biological catalysis, protein engineering, chemical sensors, de novo metalloprotein design, supramolecular architecture. *Unit head:* Dr. Robert Kennedy, Professor of Chemistry/Chair, 734-763-9681, Fax: 734-647-4847. *Application contact:* Elizabeth Oxford, Graduate Program Coordinator, 734-764-7278, Fax: 734-647-4865, E-mail: chemadmissions@umich.edu.
Website: http://www.lsa.umich.edu/chem/

University of Michigan, Rackham Graduate School, Program in Biomedical Sciences (PIBS), Department of Biological Chemistry, Ann Arbor, MI 48109. Offers MS, PhD. *Faculty:* 39 full-time (9 women), 3 part-time/adjunct (0 women). *Students:* 24 full-time (9 women); includes 5 minority (2 Black or African American, non-Hispanic/Latino; 3 Asian,

Biochemistry

non-Hispanic/Latino), 1 international. Average age 27. 63 applicants, 22% accepted, 2 enrolled. In 2015, 10 master's, 12 doctorates awarded. Terminal master's awarded for partial completion of doctoral program. *Degree requirements:* For master's, thesis; for doctorate, comprehensive exam, thesis/dissertation. *Entrance requirements:* For master's, bachelor's degree; for doctorate, GRE, bachelor's degree. Additional exam requirements/recommendations for international students: Required—TOEFL (minimum score 84 iBT). *Application deadline:* For fall admission, 12/1 for domestic and international students. Application fee: $75 ($90 for international students). Electronic applications accepted. *Expenses:* Contact institution. *Financial support:* In 2015–16, 2 students received support, including 2 fellowships with full tuition reimbursements available (averaging $29,280 per year), 21 research assistantships with full tuition reimbursements available (averaging $29,025 per year), 8 teaching assistantships with tuition reimbursements available; traineeships, health care benefits, tuition waivers (full), and unspecified assistantships also available. *Faculty research:* Biochemical signaling, structural enzymology, protein processing and folding, regulation of gene expression. *Total annual research expenditures:* $5.7 million. *Unit head:* Sherry Cogswell, Chief Department Administrator, 734-763-0185, Fax: 734-763-4581, E-mail: shercogs@umich.edu. *Application contact:* Elizabeth L. Goodwin, Graduate Program Manager, 734-764-8594, Fax: 734-763-4581, E-mail: egoodwin@umich.edu.
Website: http://www.biochem.med.umich.edu/

University of Michigan, Rackham Graduate School, Program in Chemical Biology, Ann Arbor, MI 48109. Offers cancer chemical biology (MS); chemical biology (PhD). *Faculty:* 46 full-time (13 women). *Students:* 58 full-time (21 women), 2 part-time (1 woman); includes 17 minority (5 Black or African American, non-Hispanic/Latino; 1 American Indian or Alaska Native, non-Hispanic/Latino; 4 Asian, non-Hispanic/Latino; 4 Hispanic/Latino; 3 Two or more races, non-Hispanic/Latino), 10 international. 117 applicants, 62% accepted, 29 enrolled. In 2015, 7 master's, 10 doctorates awarded. *Degree requirements:* For doctorate, thesis/dissertation. *Entrance requirements:* Additional exam requirements/recommendations for international students: Required—TOEFL (minimum score 600 paper-based; 102 iBT). *Application deadline:* For fall admission, 12/15 priority date for domestic and international students. Applications are processed on a rolling basis. Application fee: $75 ($90 for international students). Electronic applications accepted. *Financial support:* In 2015–16, 47 students received support, including fellowships with full tuition reimbursements available (averaging $29,025 per year), research assistantships with full tuition reimbursements available (averaging $29,025 per year); career-related internships or fieldwork, scholarships/grants, traineeships, and unspecified assistantships also available. *Faculty research:* Chemical genetics, structural enzymology, signal transduction, biological catalysis, biomolecular structure, function and recognition. *Unit head:* Prof. Anna Mapp, Program Director, 734-763-7175, Fax: 734-615-1252, E-mail: chemicalbiology@umich.edu. *Application contact:* Admissions Office, 734-764-8129, E-mail: rackadmis@umich.edu.
Website: http://www.chembio.umich.edu/

University of Minnesota, Duluth, Graduate School, Swenson College of Science and Engineering, Department of Chemistry and Biochemistry, Duluth, MN 55812-2496. Offers MS. *Program availability:* Part-time. *Degree requirements:* For master's, thesis. *Entrance requirements:* For master's, bachelor's degree in chemistry, minimum GPA of 3.0. Additional exam requirements/recommendations for international students: Required—TOEFL (minimum score 550 paper-based; 79 iBT), IELTS (minimum score 6.5). *Faculty research:* Physical, inorganic, organic, and analytical chemistry; biochemistry and molecular biology.

University of Minnesota, Duluth, Medical School, Department of Biochemistry, Molecular Biology and Biophysics, Duluth, MN 55812-2496. Offers biochemistry, molecular biology and biophysics (MS); biology and biophysics (PhD); social, administrative, and clinical pharmacy (MS, PhD); toxicology (MS, PhD). Terminal master's awarded for partial completion of doctoral program. *Degree requirements:* For master's, comprehensive exam, thesis; for doctorate, comprehensive exam, thesis/dissertation. *Entrance requirements:* For master's and doctorate, GRE General Test. Additional exam requirements/recommendations for international students: Required—TOEFL. Electronic applications accepted. *Faculty research:* Intestinal cancer biology; hepatotoxins and mitochondriopathies; toxicology; cell cycle regulation in stem cells; neurobiology of brain development, trace metal function and blood-brain barrier; hibernation biology.

University of Minnesota, Twin Cities Campus, Graduate School, College of Biological Sciences, Biochemistry, Molecular Biology and Biophysics Graduate Program, Minneapolis, MN 55455-0213. Offers MS, PhD. *Degree requirements:* For doctorate, thesis/dissertation. *Entrance requirements:* For doctorate, GRE, 3 letters of recommendation, more than 1 semester of laboratory experience. Additional exam requirements/recommendations for international students: Required—TOEFL (minimum score 625 paper-based; 108 iBT with writing subsection 25 and reading subsection 25) or IELTS (minimum score 7). Electronic applications accepted. *Faculty research:* Microbial biochemistry, biotechnology, molecular biology, regulatory biochemistry, structural biology and biophysics, physical biochemistry, enzymology, physiological chemistry.

University of Mississippi Medical Center, School of Graduate Studies in the Health Sciences, Department of Biochemistry, Jackson, MS 39216-4505. Offers PhD, MD/PhD. *Degree requirements:* For doctorate, thesis/dissertation, first authored publication. *Entrance requirements:* For doctorate, GRE General Test, minimum GPA of 3.0. Additional exam requirements/recommendations for international students: Required—TOEFL. *Faculty research:* Structural biology, regulation of gene expression, enzymology of redox reactions, mechanism of anti cancer drugs, function of nuclear substructure.

University of Missouri, Office of Research and Graduate Studies, College of Agriculture, Food and Natural Resources, Department of Biochemistry, Columbia, MO 65211. Offers MS, PhD. Terminal master's awarded for partial completion of doctoral program. *Degree requirements:* For master's, thesis; for doctorate, comprehensive exam, thesis/dissertation. *Entrance requirements:* For master's and doctorate, GRE, minimum GPA of 3.0; undergraduate research; 3 letters of reference; 500-word personal statement. Additional exam requirements/recommendations for international students: Required—TOEFL (minimum score 620 paper-based; 95 iBT). *Application deadline:* For fall admission, 1/15 priority date for domestic students, 1/15 for international students. Application fee: $55 ($75 for international students). Electronic applications accepted. *Financial support:* Fellowships with tuition reimbursements, research assistantships with tuition reimbursements, teaching assistantships with tuition reimbursements, institutionally sponsored loans, scholarships/grants, health care benefits, and unspecified assistantships available. Support available to part-time students. *Faculty research:* Gene expression; molecular medicine; plant sciences; receptors and signaling; macromolecular synthesis, assembly and localization; structural and chemical biology; proteomics, genomics and combinatorial chemistry; enzymology, nutrition and metabolism.
Website: http://biochem.missouri.edu/grad-program/index.php

University of Missouri–Kansas City, School of Biological Sciences, Program in Molecular Biology and Biochemistry, Kansas City, MO 64110-2499. Offers PhD. Offered through the School of Graduate Studies. *Faculty:* 31 full-time (9 women), 3 part-time/adjunct (2 women). *Students:* 5 full-time (3 women), 12 part-time (3 women); includes 6 minority (1 Black or African American, non-Hispanic/Latino; 2 Asian, non-Hispanic/

Latino; 2 Hispanic/Latino; 1 Two or more races, non-Hispanic/Latino), 1 international. Average age 26. 33 applicants, 33% accepted, 10 enrolled. *Degree requirements:* For master's, comprehensive exam, thesis/dissertation. *Entrance requirements:* For doctorate, GRE General Test, bachelor's degree in chemistry, biology, or a related discipline; minimum GPA of 3.0. Additional exam requirements/recommendations for international students: Required—TOEFL (minimum score 550 paper-based; 80 iBT). *Application deadline:* For fall admission, 2/15 priority date for domestic and international students. Application fee: $45 ($50 for international students). *Financial support:* In 2015–16, 11 research assistantships with full tuition reimbursements (averaging $24,189 per year), 17 teaching assistantships with tuition reimbursements (averaging $15,312 per year) were awarded; scholarships/grants, tuition waivers (full and partial), and unspecified assistantships also available. Financial award application deadline: 3/1; financial award applicants required to submit FAFSA. *Unit head:* Dr. Xiao-Qiang Yu, Interim Head, 816-235-6379, E-mail: yux@umkc.edu. *Application contact:* Karen Bame, Graduate Programs Officer, 816-235-2243, Fax: 816-235-5595, E-mail: bamek@umkc.edu.
Website: http://sbs.umkc.edu/

University of Missouri–St. Louis, College of Arts and Sciences, Department of Chemistry and Biochemistry, St. Louis, MO 63121. Offers biochemistry and biotechnology (MS); chemistry (MS, PhD). *Program availability:* Part-time, evening/weekend. *Faculty:* 21 full-time (3 women), 3 part-time/adjunct (1 woman). *Students:* 37 full-time (24 women), 21 part-time (15 women); includes 8 minority (1 Black or African American, non-Hispanic/Latino; 3 Asian, non-Hispanic/Latino; 3 Hispanic/Latino; 1 Native Hawaiian or other Pacific Islander, non-Hispanic/Latino), 20 international. 39 applicants, 64% accepted, 16 enrolled. Terminal master's awarded for partial completion of doctoral program. *Degree requirements:* For master's, thesis optional; for doctorate, thesis/dissertation. *Entrance requirements:* For master's, 2 letters of recommendation; for doctorate, GRE General Test, 3 letters of recommendation. Additional exam requirements/recommendations for international students: Required—TOEFL (minimum score 550 paper-based; 79 iBT), IELTS (minimum score 6.5). *Application deadline:* For fall admission, 7/1 priority date for domestic and international students; for spring admission, 12/1 priority date for domestic and international students. Applications are processed on a rolling basis. Application fee: $50 ($40 for international students). Electronic applications accepted. *Financial support:* Fellowships with tuition reimbursements, research assistantships with tuition reimbursements, and teaching assistantships with tuition reimbursements available. *Faculty research:* Metalloborane chemistry, serum transferrin chemistry, natural products chemistry, organic synthesis. *Unit head:* Cynthia Dupureur, Interim Chair, 314-516-4392, Fax: 314-516-5342, E-mail: cdup@umsl.edu. *Application contact:* Graduate Admissions, 314-516-5458, Fax: 314-516-6996, E-mail: gradadm@umsl.edu.
Website: http://www.umsl.edu/chemistry/

University of Montana, Graduate School, College of Humanities and Sciences, Division of Biological Sciences, Program in Cellular, Molecular and Microbial Biology, Missoula, MT 59812-0002. Offers cellular and developmental biology (PhD); microbial evolution and ecology (PhD); microbiology and immunology (PhD); molecular biology and biochemistry (PhD). Terminal master's awarded for partial completion of doctoral program. *Degree requirements:* For doctorate, variable foreign language requirement, thesis/dissertation. *Entrance requirements:* For doctorate, GRE General Test. *Faculty research:* Ribosome structure, medical microbiology/pathogenesis, microbial ecology/environmental microbiology.

University of Nebraska–Lincoln, Graduate College, College of Agricultural Sciences and Natural Resources and College of Arts and Sciences, Department of Biochemistry, Lincoln, NE 68588. Offers MS, PhD. Terminal master's awarded for partial completion of doctoral program. *Degree requirements:* For master's, thesis optional; for doctorate, comprehensive exam, thesis/dissertation. *Entrance requirements:* For master's and doctorate, GRE General Test, GRE Subject Test. Additional exam requirements/recommendations for international students: Required—TOEFL (minimum score 550 paper-based). Electronic applications accepted. *Faculty research:* Molecular genetics, enzymology, photosynthesis, molecular virology, structural biology.

University of Nebraska–Lincoln, Graduate College, College of Arts and Sciences, Department of Chemistry, Lincoln, NE 68588. Offers analytical chemistry (PhD); biochemistry (PhD); chemistry (MS); inorganic chemistry (PhD); materials chemistry (PhD); organic chemistry (PhD); physical chemistry (PhD). *Degree requirements:* For master's, one foreign language, thesis optional, departmental qualifying exam; for doctorate, one foreign language, comprehensive exam, thesis/dissertation, departmental qualifying exams. *Entrance requirements:* For master's and doctorate, GRE. Additional exam requirements/recommendations for international students: Required—TOEFL (minimum score 550 paper-based). Electronic applications accepted. *Faculty research:* Bioorganic and bioinorganic chemistry, biophysical and bioanalytical chemistry, structure-function of DNA and proteins, organometallics, mass spectrometry.

University of Nebraska Medical Center, Department of Biochemistry and Molecular Biology, Omaha, NE 68198. Offers MS, PhD. *Faculty:* 32 full-time (8 women). *Students:* 42 full-time (23 women); includes 3 minority (1 Asian, non-Hispanic/Latino; 1 Hispanic/Latino; 1 Two or more races, non-Hispanic/Latino), 26 international. Average age 28. 18 applicants, 33% accepted, 6 enrolled. In 2015, 4 doctorates awarded. Terminal master's awarded for partial completion of doctoral program. *Degree requirements:* For master's, comprehensive exam, thesis; for doctorate, comprehensive exam, thesis/dissertation. *Entrance requirements:* For master's, GRE General Test; for doctorate, GRE General Test, MCAT, PCAT, DCAT. Additional exam requirements/recommendations for international students: Required—TOEFL (minimum score 550 paper-based). *Application deadline:* For fall admission, 3/1 for domestic students, 4/1 for international students; for spring admission, 8/1 for domestic and international students; for summer admission, 1/1 for domestic and international students. Application fee: $45. Electronic applications accepted. *Expenses:* Tuition, state resident: full-time $7830; part-time $3915 per credit hour. Tuition, nonresident: full-time $22,410; part-time $11,205 per credit hour. *Required fees:* $521. *Financial support:* In 2015–16, 13 students received support, including 4 fellowships with full tuition reimbursements available (averaging $23,100 per year), 7 research assistantships with full tuition reimbursements available (averaging $23,100 per year); scholarships/grants, health care benefits, and unspecified assistantships also available. Support available to part-time students. Financial award application deadline: 2/15; financial award applicants required to submit FAFSA. *Faculty research:* Recombinant DNA, cancer biology, diabetes and drug metabolism, biochemical endocrinology. *Unit head:* Dr. Paul Sorgen, Chairman, Graduate Committee, 402-559-7557, Fax: 402-559-6650, E-mail: psorgen@unmc.edu. *Application contact:* Karen Hankins, Office Associate, 402-559-4417, E-mail: karen.hankins@unmc.edu.
Website: http://www.unmc.edu/biochemistry/

University of Nevada, Las Vegas, Graduate College, College of Sciences, Department of Chemistry and Biochemistry, Las Vegas, NV 89154-4003. Offers biochemistry (MS); chemistry (MS, PhD); radiochemistry (PhD). *Program availability:* Part-time. *Faculty:* 16 full-time (3 women). *Students:* 45 full-time (23 women), 6 part-time (1 woman); includes 12 minority (4 Black or African American, non-Hispanic/Latino; 5 Asian, non-Hispanic/Latino; 3 Hispanic/Latino), 4 international. Average age 29. 39 applicants, 31%

accepted, 8 enrolled. In 2015, 1 master's, 7 doctorates awarded. *Degree requirements:* For master's, thesis, departmental seminar; for doctorate, comprehensive exam (for some programs), thesis/dissertation. *Entrance requirements:* For master's and doctorate, GRE General Test. Additional exam requirements/recommendations for international students: Required—TOEFL (minimum score 550 paper-based; 80 iBT), IELTS (minimum score 7). *Application deadline:* For fall admission, 2/1 for domestic students, 5/1 for international students; for spring admission, 10/1 for domestic and international students. Application fee: $60 ($95 for international students). Electronic applications accepted. *Expenses:* $264 per credit state resident full-time and part-time; $6,955 per semester, $264 per credit nonresident full-time; $555 per credit nonresident part-time. *Financial support:* In 2015–16, 44 students received support, including 24 research assistantships with partial tuition reimbursements available (averaging $19,528 per year), 20 teaching assistantships with partial tuition reimbursements available (averaging $19,031 per year); institutionally sponsored loans, scholarships/grants, health care benefits, and unspecified assistantships also available. Financial award application deadline: 3/1. *Faculty research:* Material science, biochemistry, chemical education, physical chemistry and theoretical computation, analytical and organic chemistry. *Total annual research expenditures:* $3 million. *Unit head:* Dr. David Hatchett, Chair/Associate Professor, 702-895-4226, Fax: 702-895-4072, E-mail: david.hatchett@unlv.edu. *Application contact:* Graduate College Admissions Evaluator, 702-895-3367, Fax: 702-895-4180, E-mail: gradadmissions@unlv.edu.
Website: http://www.unlv.edu/chemistry

University of Nevada, Reno, Graduate School, College of Agriculture, Biotechnology and Natural Resources, Program in Biochemistry, Reno, NV 89557. Offers MS, PhD. Terminal master's awarded for partial completion of doctoral program. *Degree requirements:* For master's, thesis; for doctorate, thesis/dissertation. *Entrance requirements:* For master's, GRE General Test, minimum GPA of 2.75; for doctorate, GRE General Test, minimum GPA of 3.0. Additional exam requirements/recommendations for international students: Required—TOEFL (minimum score 500 paper-based; 61 iBT), IELTS (minimum score 6). Electronic applications accepted. *Faculty research:* Cancer research, insect biochemistry, plant biochemistry, enzymology.

University of New Hampshire, Graduate School, College of Life Sciences and Agriculture, Department of Molecular, Cellular and Biomedical Sciences, Program in Biochemistry, Durham, NH 03824. Offers MS, PhD. *Program availability:* Part-time. Terminal master's awarded for partial completion of doctoral program. *Degree requirements:* For master's, thesis; for doctorate, one foreign language, thesis/dissertation. *Entrance requirements:* For master's and doctorate, GRE General Test. Additional exam requirements/recommendations for international students: Required—TOEFL (minimum score 550 paper-based; 80 iBT). *Application deadline:* For fall admission, 1/15 priority date for domestic students. Applications are processed on a rolling basis. Application fee: $65. Electronic applications accepted. *Expenses:* Tuition, state resident: full-time $13,840; part-time $770 per credit hour. Tuition, nonresident: full-time $27,130; part-time $1175 per credit hour. *Required fees:* $2080; $1040. Tuition and fees vary according to degree level and program. *Financial support:* Fellowships, research assistantships, teaching assistantships, career-related internships or fieldwork, Federal Work-Study, scholarships/grants, and tuition waivers (full and partial) available. Support available to part-time students. Financial award application deadline: 2/15. *Faculty research:* General areas of molecular biology, cellular biology, and biochemistry, with specific research programs in eukaryotic gene regulation; reproductive physiology; molecular population genetics; macromolecular interactions; cell signaling pathways in cancer and leukemia; evolution of eukaryotic genomes; glycobiology; protein kinases and phosphatases in plant signaling; mass spectrometry-based proteomics; chromatin biology; DNA repair mechanisms; etiology of vascular disease; sensory transduction. *Unit head:* Dr. Feixia Chu, Director, 603-862-2436. *Application contact:* Flora Joyal, Administrative Assistant, 603-862-2103, E-mail: flora.joyal@unh.edu.
Website: http://colsa.unh.edu/mcbs/grad/biochemistry/

University of New Mexico, Graduate Studies, Health Sciences Center, Program in Biomedical Sciences, Albuquerque, NM 87131-5196. Offers biochemistry and molecular biology (MS, PhD); cell biology and physiology (MS, PhD); molecular genetics and microbiology (MS, PhD); neuroscience (MS, PhD); pathology (MS, PhD); toxicology (MS, PhD). *Program availability:* Part-time. *Faculty:* 18 full-time (10 women), 1 part-time/adjunct (0 women). *Students:* 31 full-time (17 women), 45 part-time (26 women); includes 29 minority (1 American Indian or Alaska Native, non-Hispanic/Latino; 3 Asian, non-Hispanic/Latino; 22 Hispanic/Latino; 2 Native Hawaiian or other Pacific Islander, non-Hispanic/Latino; 1 Two or more races, non-Hispanic/Latino), 18 international. Average age 30. 98 applicants, 11% accepted, 11 enrolled. In 2015, 11 master's, 14 doctorates awarded. Terminal master's awarded for partial completion of doctoral program. *Degree requirements:* For master's, thesis; for doctorate, comprehensive exam, thesis/dissertation, qualifying exam at the end of year 1/core curriculum. *Entrance requirements:* For master's and doctorate, GRE General Test, minimum undergraduate GPA of 3.0. Additional exam requirements/recommendations for international students: Required—TOEFL. *Application deadline:* For fall admission, 3/1 priority date for domestic and international students. Applications are processed on a rolling basis. Application fee: $50. Electronic applications accepted. *Financial support:* Fellowships with tuition reimbursements, research assistantships with full tuition reimbursements, teaching assistantships, career-related internships or fieldwork, Federal Work-Study, institutionally sponsored loans, scholarships/grants, traineeships, health care benefits, and unspecified assistantships available. Financial award application deadline: 1/1; financial award applicants required to submit FAFSA. *Faculty research:* Infectious disease/immunity, cancer biology, cardiovascular and metabolic diseases, brain and behavioral illness, environmental health. *Unit head:* Dr. Helen J. Hathaway, Program Director, 505-272-1887, Fax: 505-272-2412, E-mail: hhathaway@salud.unm.edu. *Application contact:* Mary Fenton, Admissions Coordinator, 505-272-1887, Fax: 505-272-2412, E-mail: mfenton@salud.unm.edu.

The University of North Carolina at Chapel Hill, School of Medicine and Graduate School, Graduate Programs in Medicine, Department of Biochemistry and Biophysics, Chapel Hill, NC 27599. Offers MS, PhD. Terminal master's awarded for partial completion of doctoral program. *Degree requirements:* For master's, comprehensive exam, thesis; for doctorate, comprehensive exam, thesis/dissertation. *Entrance requirements:* For master's and doctorate, GRE General Test, GRE Subject Test (recommended), minimum GPA of 3.0. Additional exam requirements/recommendations for international students: Required—TOEFL. Electronic applications accepted.

The University of North Carolina at Greensboro, Graduate School, College of Arts and Sciences, Department of Chemistry and Biochemistry, Greensboro, NC 27412-5001. Offers biochemistry (MS); chemistry (MS). *Degree requirements:* For master's, one foreign language, thesis. *Entrance requirements:* For master's, GRE General Test. Additional exam requirements/recommendations for international students: Required—TOEFL. Electronic applications accepted. *Faculty research:* Synthesis of novel cyclopentadienes, molybdenum hydroxylase-cata ladder polymers, vinyl silicones.

University of North Dakota, Graduate School and Graduate School, Graduate Programs in Medicine, Department of Biochemistry and Molecular Biology, Grand Forks, ND 58202. Offers MS, PhD. *Degree requirements:* For master's, thesis, final exam; for doctorate, comprehensive exam, thesis/dissertation, final exam. *Entrance requirements:* For master's and doctorate, GRE General Test, minimum GPA of 3.0. Additional exam requirements/recommendations for international students: Required—TOEFL (minimum score 550 paper-based; 79 iBT), IELTS (minimum score 6.5). Electronic applications accepted. *Faculty research:* Glucose-6-phosphatase, guanine nucleotides, carbohydrate and lipid metabolism, cytoskeletal proteins, chromatin structure.

University of North Texas, Robert B. Toulouse School of Graduate Studies, Denton, TX 76203-5459. Offers accounting (MS); applied anthropology (MA, MS); applied behavior analysis (Certificate); applied geography (MA); applied technology and performance improvement (M Ed, MS); art education (MA); art history (MA); art museum education (Certificate); arts leadership (Certificate); audiology (Au D); behavior analysis (MS); behavioral science (PhD); biochemistry and molecular biology (MS); biology (MA, MS); biomedical engineering (MS); business analysis (MS); chemistry (MS); clinical health psychology (PhD); communication studies (MA, MS); computer engineering (MS); computer science (MS); counseling (M Ed, MS), including clinical mental health counseling (MS), college and university counseling, elementary school counseling, secondary school counseling; creative writing (MA); criminal justice (MS); curriculum and instruction (M Ed); decision sciences (MBA); design (MA, MFA), including fashion design (MFA), innovation studies, interior design (MFA); early childhood studies (MS); economics (MS); educational leadership (M Ed, Ed D); educational psychology (MS, PhD), including family studies (MS), gifted and talented (MS), human development (MS), learning and cognition (MS), research, measurement and evaluation (MS); electrical engineering (MS); emergency management (MPA); engineering technology (MS); English (MA); English as a second language (MA); environmental science (MS); finance (MBA, MS); financial management (MPA); French (MA); health services management (MBA); higher education (M Ed, Ed D); history (MA, MS); hospitality management (MS); human resources management (MPA); information science (MS); information systems (PhD); information technologies (MBA); interdisciplinary studies (MA, MS); international studies (MA); international sustainable tourism (MS); jazz studies (MM); journalism (MA, MJ, Graduate Certificate), including interactive and virtual digital communication (Graduate Certificate), narrative journalism (Graduate Certificate), public relations (Graduate Certificate); kinesiology (MS); linguistics (MA); local government management (MPA); logistics (PhD); logistics and supply chain management (MBA); long-term care, senior housing, and aging services (MA); management (PhD); marketing (MBA); mathematics (MA, MS); mechanical and energy engineering (MS, PhD); music (MA), including ethnomusicology, music theory, musicology, performance; music composition (PhD); music education (MM Ed, PhD); nonprofit management (MPA); operations and supply chain management (MBA); performance (MM, DMA); philosophy (MA); political science (MA); professional and technical communication (MA); radio, television and film (MA, MFA); rehabilitation counseling (Certificate); sociology (MA); Spanish (MA); special education (M Ed); speech-language pathology (MA); strategic management (MBA); studio art (MFA); teaching (M Ed); MBA/MS. *Program availability:* Part-time, evening/weekend, online learning. Terminal master's awarded for partial completion of doctoral program. *Degree requirements:* For master's, variable foreign language requirement, comprehensive exam (for some programs), thesis (for some programs); for doctorate, variable foreign language requirement, comprehensive exam (for some programs), thesis/dissertation; for other advanced degree, variable foreign language requirement, comprehensive exam (for some programs). *Entrance requirements:* For master's and doctorate, GRE, GMAT. Additional exam requirements/recommendations for international students: Required—TOEFL (minimum score 550 paper-based; 79 iBT). Electronic applications accepted.

University of North Texas Health Science Center at Fort Worth, Graduate School of Biomedical Sciences, Fort Worth, TX 76107-2699. Offers anatomy and cell biology (MS, PhD); biochemistry and molecular biology (MS, PhD); biomedical sciences (MS, PhD); biotechnology (MS); forensic genetics (MS); integrative physiology (MS, PhD); medical science (MS); microbiology and immunology (MS, PhD); pharmacology (MS, PhD); science education (MS); DO/MS. DO/PhD. Terminal master's awarded for partial completion of doctoral program. *Degree requirements:* For master's, thesis; for doctorate, thesis/dissertation. *Entrance requirements:* For master's and doctorate, GRE General Test. Additional exam requirements/recommendations for international students: Required—TOEFL. *Expenses:* Contact institution. *Faculty research:* Alzheimer's disease, aging, eye diseases, cancer, cardiovascular disease.

University of Notre Dame, Graduate School, College of Science, Department of Chemistry and Biochemistry, Notre Dame, IN 46556. Offers biochemistry (MS, PhD); inorganic chemistry (MS, PhD); organic chemistry (MS, PhD); physical chemistry (MS, PhD). Terminal master's awarded for partial completion of doctoral program. *Degree requirements:* For master's, comprehensive exam, thesis; for doctorate, thesis/dissertation, qualifying exam. *Entrance requirements:* For master's and doctorate, GRE General Test, GRE Subject Test (strongly recommended). Additional exam requirements/recommendations for international students: Required—TOEFL (minimum score 600 paper-based; 80 iBT). Electronic applications accepted. *Faculty research:* Reaction design and mechanistic studies; reactive intermediates; synthesis, structure and reactivity of organometallic cluster complexes and biologically active natural products; bioorganic chemistry; enzymology.

University of Oklahoma, College of Arts and Sciences, Department of Chemistry and Biochemistry, Norman, OK 73019. Offers bioinformatics (MS, PhD); chemistry (MS, PhD). *Program availability:* Part-time. *Faculty:* 30 full-time (10 women). *Students:* 65 full-time (24 women), 35 part-time (17 women); includes 14 minority (2 Black or African American, non-Hispanic/Latino; 1 American Indian or Alaska Native, non-Hispanic/Latino; 3 Asian, non-Hispanic/Latino; 7 Hispanic/Latino; 1 Two or more races, non-Hispanic/Latino), 35 international. Average age 26. 75 applicants, 36% accepted, 27 enrolled. In 2015, 16 master's, 7 doctorates awarded. Terminal master's awarded for partial completion of doctoral program. *Degree requirements:* For master's, comprehensive exam (for some programs), thesis (for some programs); for doctorate, comprehensive exam, thesis/dissertation, general exam. *Entrance requirements:* For master's and doctorate, GRE. Additional exam requirements/recommendations for international students: Required—TOEFL (minimum score 79 iBT). *Application deadline:* For fall admission, 3/1 priority date for domestic students, 3/1 for international students; for spring admission, 9/1 for domestic and international students. Application fee: $50 ($100 for international students). Electronic applications accepted. *Expenses:* Tuition, state resident: full-time $4577; part-time $190.70 per credit hour. Tuition, nonresident: full-time $17,758; part-time $739.90 per credit hour. *Required fees:* $3060; $115.70 per credit hour. $141.50 per semester. *Financial support:* In 2015–16, 92 students received support, including 4 fellowships with full tuition reimbursements available (averaging $4,375 per year), 26 research assistantships with full tuition reimbursements available (averaging $16,499 per year), 72 teaching assistantships with full tuition reimbursements available (averaging $16,613 per year); institutionally sponsored loans, scholarships/grants, health care benefits, unspecified assistantships, and full tuition with qualifying graduate assistantship also available. Support available to part-time students. Financial award application deadline: 6/1; financial award applicants required to submit FAFSA. *Faculty research:* Structural biology, synthesis and catalysis, natural products, membrane biochemistry, genomics. *Total annual research expenditures:* $7 million. *Unit head:* Dr. Ronald L. Halterman, Professor and Chair, 405-325-4812, Fax: 405-325-6111, E-mail: rhalterman@ou.edu. *Application contact:* Angelika Tietz, Graduate Program

Biochemistry

Assistant, 405-325-4811 Ext. 62946, Fax: 405-325-6111, E-mail: atietz@ou.edu.
Website: http://www.ou.edu/cas/chemistry

University of Oklahoma Health Sciences Center, College of Medicine and Graduate College, Graduate Programs in Medicine, Department of Biochemistry and Molecular Biology, Oklahoma City, OK 73190. Offers biochemistry (MS, PhD); molecular biology (MS, PhD). *Program availability:* Part-time. Terminal master's awarded for partial completion of doctoral program. *Degree requirements:* For master's, thesis; for doctorate, thesis/dissertation. *Entrance requirements:* For master's, GRE General Test, 2 letters of recommendation; for doctorate, GRE General Test, 3 letters of recommendation. Additional exam requirements/recommendations for international students: Required—TOEFL. *Faculty research:* Gene expression, regulation of transcription, enzyme evolution, melanogenesis, signal transduction.

University of Oregon, Graduate School, College of Arts and Sciences, Department of Chemistry, Eugene, OR 97403. Offers biochemistry (MA, MS, PhD); chemistry (MA, MS, PhD). Terminal master's awarded for partial completion of doctoral program. *Degree requirements:* For doctorate, thesis/dissertation. *Entrance requirements:* For master's and doctorate, GRE General Test, minimum GPA of 3.0. Additional exam requirements/recommendations for international students: Required—TOEFL. *Faculty research:* Organic chemistry, organometallic chemistry, inorganic chemistry, physical chemistry, materials science, biochemistry, chemical physics, molecular or cell biology.

University of Ottawa, Faculty of Graduate and Postdoctoral Studies, Faculty of Medicine, Department of Biochemistry, Microbiology and Immunology, Ottawa, ON K1N 6N5, Canada. Offers biochemistry (M Sc, PhD); microbiology and immunology (M Sc, PhD). *Degree requirements:* For master's, thesis; for doctorate, comprehensive exam, thesis/dissertation, seminar. *Entrance requirements:* For master's, honors degree or equivalent, minimum B average; for doctorate, master's degree, minimum B+ average. Electronic applications accepted. *Faculty research:* General biochemistry, molecular biology, microbiology, host biology, nutrition and metabolism.

University of Pennsylvania, Perelman School of Medicine, Biomedical Graduate Studies, Graduate Group in Biochemistry and Molecular Biophysics, Philadelphia, PA 19104. Offers PhD, MD/PhD, VMD/PhD. *Faculty:* 91. *Students:* 94 full-time (42 women); includes 26 minority (1 Black or African American, non-Hispanic/Latino; 1 American Indian or Alaska Native, non-Hispanic/Latino; 13 Asian, non-Hispanic/Latino; 11 Hispanic/Latino), 11 international. 82 applicants, 34% accepted, 14 enrolled. In 2015, 8 doctorates awarded. *Degree requirements:* For doctorate, thesis/dissertation. *Entrance requirements:* Additional exam requirements/recommendations for international students: Required—TOEFL. *Application deadline:* For fall admission, 12/1 priority date for domestic students, 12/1 for international students. Applications are processed on a rolling basis. Application fee: $80. *Expenses: Tuition, area resident:* Full-time $31,068; part-time $5762 per course. *Required fees:* $3200; $336 per course. Full-time tuition and fees vary according to degree level, program and student level. Part-time tuition and fees vary according to course load, degree level and program. *Financial support:* In 2015–16, 94 students received support. Fellowships, research assistantships, scholarships/grants, traineeships, and unspecified assistantships available. *Faculty research:* Biochemistry of cell differentiation, tissue culture, intermediary metabolism, structure of proteins and nucleic acids, biochemical genetics. *Unit head:* Dr. Kim Sharp, Chairperson, 215-573-3506. *Application contact:* Kelli McKenna, Coordinator, 215-898-4639.
Website: http://www.med.upenn.edu/bmbgrad/

University of Puerto Rico, Medical Sciences Campus, School of Medicine, Biomedical Sciences Graduate Program, Department of Biochemistry, San Juan, PR 00936-5067. Offers MS, PhD. *Degree requirements:* For master's, thesis; for doctorate, comprehensive exam, thesis/dissertation. *Entrance requirements:* For master's and doctorate, GRE General Test, GRE Subject Test, interview, minimum GPA of 3.0. Electronic applications accepted. *Faculty research:* Genetics, cell and molecular biology, cancer biology, protein structure/function, glycosilation of proteins.

University of Regina, Faculty of Graduate Studies and Research, Faculty of Science, Department of Chemistry and Biochemistry, Regina, SK S4S 0A2, Canada. Offers analytical/environmental chemistry (M Sc, PhD); biophysics of biological interfaces (M Sc, PhD); enzymology/chemical biology (M Sc, PhD); inorganic/organometallic chemistry (M Sc, PhD); signal transduction and mechanisms of cancer cell regulation (M Sc, PhD); supramolecular organic photochemistry and photophysics (M Sc, PhD); synthetic organic chemistry (M Sc, PhD); theoretical/computational chemistry (M Sc, PhD). *Degree requirements:* For master's, thesis; for doctorate, thesis/dissertation. *Entrance requirements:* Additional exam requirements/recommendations for international students: Required—TOEFL (minimum score 580 paper-based; 80 iBT), IELTS (minimum score 6.5), PTE (minimum score 59). Electronic applications accepted. *Faculty research:* Asymmetric synthesis and methodology, theoretical and computational chemistry, biophysical biochemistry, analytical and environmental chemistry, chemical biology.

University of Rhode Island, Graduate School, College of the Environment and Life Sciences, Department of Cell and Molecular Biology, Kingston, RI 02881. Offers biochemistry (MS, PhD); clinical laboratory sciences (MS), including biotechnology, clinical laboratory science, cytopathology; microbiology (MS, PhD); molecular genetics (MS, PhD). *Program availability:* Part-time. *Faculty:* 11 full-time (4 women), 1 (woman) part-time/adjunct. *Students:* 12 full-time (6 women), 36 part-time (27 women); includes 10 minority (4 Black or African American, non-Hispanic/Latino; 3 Asian, non-Hispanic/Latino; 2 Hispanic/Latino; 1 Two or more races, non-Hispanic/Latino), 8 international. In 2015, 19 master's, 1 doctorate awarded. *Degree requirements:* For master's, comprehensive exam (for some programs), thesis optional; for doctorate, comprehensive exam, thesis/dissertation. *Entrance requirements:* For master's and doctorate, GRE, 2 letters of recommendation. Additional exam requirements/recommendations for international students: Required—TOEFL (minimum score 530 paper-based). *Application deadline:* For fall admission, 7/15 for domestic students, 2/1 for international students; for spring admission, 11/15 for domestic students, 7/15 for international students. Application fee: $65. Electronic applications accepted. *Expenses:* Tuition, state resident: full-time $11,796; part-time $655 per credit. Tuition, nonresident: full-time $24,206; part-time $1345 per credit. *Required fees:* $1546; $44 per credit. One-time fee: $155 full-time; $35 part-time. *Financial support:* In 2015–16, 3 research assistantships with tuition reimbursements (averaging $13,507 per year), 8 teaching assistantships with tuition reimbursements (averaging $13,305 per year) were awarded; traineeships also available. Financial award application deadline: 2/1; financial award applicants required to submit FAFSA. *Faculty research:* Genomics. *Total annual research expenditures:* $6.7 million. *Unit head:* Dr. Gongqing Sun, Chairperson, 401-874-5937, Fax: 401-874-2202, E-mail: gsun@mail.uri.edu. *Application contact:* Graduate Admissions, 401-874-2872, E-mail: gradadm@etal.uri.edu.
Website: http://cels.uri.edu/cmb/

University of Rochester, School of Medicine and Dentistry, Graduate Programs in Medicine and Dentistry, Department of Biochemistry and Biophysics, Programs in Biochemistry, Rochester, NY 14627. Offers biochemistry and molecular biology (PhD). Terminal master's awarded for partial completion of doctoral program. *Degree requirements:* For doctorate, thesis/dissertation, qualifying exam. *Entrance*

requirements: For doctorate, GRE General Test. *Expenses: Tuition, area resident:* Full-time $47,450; part-time $1482 per credit hour. *Required fees:* $528. Tuition and fees vary according to program.

University of Saint Joseph, Department of Chemistry, West Hartford, CT 06117-2700. Offers biochemistry (MS); chemistry (MS). *Program availability:* Part-time, evening/weekend, online learning. *Degree requirements:* For master's, comprehensive exam, thesis optional. *Entrance requirements:* For master's, 2 letters of recommendation, official undergraduate transcript. *Application deadline:* Applications are processed on a rolling basis. Application fee: $50. Electronic applications accepted. Application fee is waived when completed online. *Financial support:* Career-related internships or fieldwork and unspecified assistantships available. Support available to part-time students. Financial award applicants required to submit FAFSA.
Website: http://www.usj.edu/academics/schools/school-of-health-natural-sciences/chemistry/

University of Saskatchewan, College of Medicine, Department of Biochemistry, Saskatoon, SK S7N 5A2, Canada. Offers M Sc, PhD. *Degree requirements:* For master's, thesis; for doctorate, thesis/dissertation. *Entrance requirements:* Additional exam requirements/recommendations for international students: Required—TOEFL.

The University of Scranton, College of Arts and Sciences, Department of Chemistry, Program in Biochemistry, Scranton, PA 18510. Offers MS. *Program availability:* Part-time, evening/weekend. *Students:* 7 full-time (2 women), 7 part-time (3 women); includes 1 minority (Hispanic/Latino), 1 international. Average age 23. 27 applicants, 52% accepted, 11 enrolled. *Degree requirements:* For master's, comprehensive exam (for some programs), thesis (for some programs), capstone experience. *Entrance requirements:* For master's, minimum GPA of 3.0, three letters of reference. Additional exam requirements/recommendations for international students: Required—TOEFL (minimum score 500 paper-based; 80 iBT), IELTS (minimum score 6.5). *Application deadline:* For fall admission, 6/1 for international students; for spring admission, 11/1 for international students; for summer admission, 3/1 for international students. Applications are processed on a rolling basis. Application fee: $0. Electronic applications accepted. *Financial support:* Applicants required to submit FAFSA. *Unit head:* Dr. Joan Wasilewski, Director, 570-941-7705, Fax: 570-941-7510, E-mail: joan.wasilewski@scranton.edu. *Application contact:* Dr. Christopher A. Baumann, Director, 570-941-6389, Fax: 570-941-7510, E-mail: cab@scranton.edu.

University of South Carolina, The Graduate School, College of Arts and Sciences, Department of Chemistry and Biochemistry, Columbia, SC 29208. Offers IMA, MAT, MS, PhD. IMA and MAT offered in cooperation with the College of Education. *Program availability:* Part-time. Terminal master's awarded for partial completion of doctoral program. *Degree requirements:* For master's, comprehensive exam, thesis; for doctorate, comprehensive exam, thesis/dissertation. *Entrance requirements:* For master's and doctorate, GRE General Test. Additional exam requirements/recommendations for international students: Required—TOEFL. Electronic applications accepted. *Faculty research:* Spectroscopy, crystallography, organic and organometallic synthesis, analytical chemistry, materials.

University of Southern California, Keck School of Medicine and Graduate School, Graduate Programs in Medicine, Department of Biochemistry and Molecular Biology, Los Angeles, CA 90089. Offers MS. *Faculty:* 22 full-time (4 women). *Students:* 45 full-time (31 women); includes 6 minority (4 Asian, non-Hispanic/Latino; 2 Hispanic/Latino), 37 international. Average age 24. 76 applicants, 58% accepted, 28 enrolled. In 2015, 17 master's awarded. Terminal master's awarded for partial completion of doctoral program. *Degree requirements:* For master's, thesis. *Entrance requirements:* For master's, GRE General Test, minimum GPA of 3.0. Additional exam requirements/recommendations for international students: Required—TOEFL (minimum score 600 paper-based; 100 iBT). *Application deadline:* For fall admission, 4/15 priority date for domestic and international students. Applications are processed on a rolling basis. Application fee: $85. Electronic applications accepted. *Expenses:* Contact institution. *Financial support:* Application deadline: 5/4; applicants required to submit CSS PROFILE or FAFSA. *Faculty research:* Molecular genetics, gene expression, membrane biochemistry, metabolic regulation, cancer biology. *Total annual research expenditures:* $7.4 million. *Unit head:* Dr. Michael R. Stallcup, Chair, 323-442-1145, Fax: 323-442-1224, E-mail: stallcup@usc.edu. *Application contact:* Janet Stoeckert, Administrative Director, Basic Science Departments, 323-442-3568, Fax: 323-442-1610, E-mail: janet.stoeckert@usc.edu.
Website: http://keck.usc.edu/en/Education/Academic_Department_and_Divisions/Department_of_Biochemistry_and_Molecular_Biology.aspx

University of Southern Mississippi, Graduate School, College of Science and Technology, Department of Chemistry and Biochemistry, Hattiesburg, MS 39406-0001. Offers inorganic chemistry (MS); organic chemistry (MS); physical chemistry (MS). *Degree requirements:* For master's, comprehensive exam, thesis; for doctorate, comprehensive exam, thesis/dissertation. *Entrance requirements:* For master's, GRE General Test, minimum GPA of 2.75 in last 60 hours; for doctorate, GRE General Test, minimum GPA of 3.5. Additional exam requirements/recommendations for international students: Required—TOEFL, IELTS. *Faculty research:* Plant biochemistry, photo chemistry, polymer chemistry, x-ray analysis, enzyme chemistry.

The University of Tennessee, Graduate School, College of Arts and Sciences, Department of Biochemistry, Cellular and Molecular Biology, Knoxville, TN 37996. Offers MS, PhD. Terminal master's awarded for partial completion of doctoral program. *Degree requirements:* For master's, thesis; for doctorate, thesis/dissertation. *Entrance requirements:* For master's and doctorate, GRE General Test, minimum GPA of 2.7. Additional exam requirements/recommendations for international students: Required—TOEFL. Electronic applications accepted.

The University of Texas at Austin, Graduate School, College of Natural Sciences, Department of Chemistry and Biochemistry, Program in Biochemistry, Austin, TX 78712-1111. Offers PhD. *Entrance requirements:* For doctorate, GRE General Test.

The University of Texas Health Science Center at Houston, Graduate School of Biomedical Sciences, Program in Biochemistry and Molecular Biology, Houston, TX 77225-0036. Offers MS, PhD, MD/PhD. Terminal master's awarded for partial completion of doctoral program. *Degree requirements:* For master's, thesis; for doctorate, thesis/dissertation. *Entrance requirements:* For master's and doctorate, GRE General Test. Additional exam requirements/recommendations for international students: Required—TOEFL. Electronic applications accepted. *Faculty research:* Biochemistry, membrane biology, macromolecular structure, structural biophysics, molecular models of human disease, molecular biology of the cell.

The University of Texas Health Science Center at San Antonio, Graduate School of Biomedical Sciences, Department of Biochemistry, San Antonio, TX 78229. Offers MS, PhD. *Degree requirements:* For master's, thesis; for doctorate, comprehensive exam, thesis/dissertation.

The University of Texas Medical Branch, Graduate School of Biomedical Sciences, Program in Biochemistry and Molecular Biology, Galveston, TX 77555. Offers biochemistry (PhD); bioinformatics (PhD); biophysics (PhD); cell biology (PhD); computational biology (PhD); structural biology (PhD). *Degree requirements:* For doctorate, thesis/dissertation. *Entrance requirements:* Additional exam requirements/ recommendations for international students: Required—TOEFL (minimum score 550 paper-based). Electronic applications accepted.

The University of Texas Southwestern Medical Center, Southwestern Graduate School of Biomedical Sciences, Division of Basic Science, Program in Biological Chemistry, Dallas, TX 75390. Offers PhD. *Degree requirements:* For doctorate, thesis/ dissertation, qualifying exam. *Entrance requirements:* For doctorate, GRE General Test, minimum GPA of 3.0. Additional exam requirements/recommendations for international students: Required—TOEFL. Electronic applications accepted. *Faculty research:* Regulation of gene expression, protein trafficking, molecular neurobiology, protein structure and function, metabolic regulation.

University of the Sciences, Program in Chemistry, Biochemistry and Pharmacognosy, Philadelphia, PA 19104-4495. Offers biochemistry (MS, PhD); chemistry (MS, PhD); pharmacognosy (MS, PhD). *Program availability:* Part-time. *Degree requirements:* For master's, thesis, qualifying exams; for doctorate, comprehensive exam, thesis/ dissertation, qualifying exams. *Entrance requirements:* For master's and doctorate, GRE General Test, GRE Subject Test. Additional exam requirements/recommendations for international students: Required—TOEFL, TWE. *Application deadline:* For fall admission, 5/1 for international students; for winter admission, 10/1 for international students; for spring admission, 3/1 for international students. Applications are processed on a rolling basis. Application fee: $50. *Expenses:* Contact institution. *Financial support:* Fellowships with full tuition reimbursements, research assistantships with full tuition reimbursements, teaching assistantships with full tuition reimbursements, institutionally sponsored loans, scholarships/grants, and tuition waivers (full) available. Financial award application deadline: 5/1. *Unit head:* Dr. James R. McKee, Director, 215-596-8847, E-mail: j.mckee@usciences.edu. *Application contact:* Dr. James R. McKee, Director, 215-596-8847, E-mail: j.mckee@usciences.edu.

The University of Toledo, College of Graduate Studies, College of Natural Sciences and Mathematics, Department of Chemistry, Toledo, OH 43606-3390. Offers analytical chemistry (MS, PhD); biological chemistry (MS, PhD); inorganic chemistry (MS, PhD); organic chemistry (MS, PhD); physical chemistry (MS, PhD). *Program availability:* Part-time. *Degree requirements:* For master's, thesis or alternative; for doctorate, thesis/ dissertation. *Entrance requirements:* For master's and doctorate, GRE General Test, GRE Subject Test, minimum cumulative point-hour ratio of 2.7 for all previous academic work, three letters of recommendation, statement of purpose, transcripts from all prior institutions attended. Additional exam requirements/recommendations for international students: Required—TOEFL (minimum score 550 paper-based; 80 iBT). Electronic applications accepted. *Faculty research:* Enzymology, materials chemistry, crystallography, theoretical chemistry.

The University of Toledo, College of Graduate Studies, College of Pharmacy and Pharmaceutical Sciences, Program in Medicinal and Biological Chemistry, Toledo, OH 43606-3390. Offers MS, PhD. Terminal master's awarded for partial completion of doctoral program. *Degree requirements:* For master's, thesis; for doctorate, thesis/ dissertation. *Entrance requirements:* For master's and doctorate, GRE General Test. Additional exam requirements/recommendations for international students: Required— TOEFL (minimum score 550 paper-based; 80 iBT). Electronic applications accepted. *Faculty research:* Neuroscience, molecular modeling, immunotoxicology, organic synthesis, peptide biochemistry.

University of Toronto, Faculty of Medicine, Department of Biochemistry, Toronto, ON M5S 1A1, Canada. Offers M Sc, PhD. *Degree requirements:* For master's, thesis, oral examination of thesis; for doctorate, thesis/dissertation, oral defense of thesis. *Entrance requirements:* For master's, B Sc in biochemistry or molecular biology, minimum B+ average, letters of reference. Additional exam requirements/recommendations for international students: Required—TOEFL (minimum score 580 paper-based; 93 iBT), TWE (minimum score 5). Electronic applications accepted.

The University of Tulsa, Graduate School, College of Engineering and Natural Sciences, Department of Chemistry and Biochemistry, Program in Biochemistry, Tulsa, OK 74104-3189. Offers MS. *Program availability:* Part-time. *Faculty:* 2 full-time (0 women). *Students:* 3 full-time (all women), all international. Average age 25. 5 applicants. In 2015, 1 master's awarded. *Degree requirements:* For master's, thesis (for some programs). *Entrance requirements:* For master's, GRE General Test. Additional exam requirements/recommendations for international students: Required—TOEFL (minimum score 550 paper-based; 80 iBT), IELTS (minimum score 6). *Application deadline:* Applications are processed on a rolling basis. Application fee: $55. Electronic applications accepted. *Expenses:* Tuition, area resident: Full-time $22,230; part-time $1176 per credit hour. *Required fees:* $590 per semester. Tuition and fees vary according to course load. *Financial support:* In 2015–16, 3 students received support, including 3 teaching assistantships with full tuition reimbursements available (averaging $11,175 per year); fellowships, career-related internships or fieldwork, Federal Work-Study, scholarships/grants, health care benefits, and unspecified assistantships also available. Support available to part-time students. Financial award application deadline: 2/1; financial award applicants required to submit FAFSA. *Unit head:* Dr. Dale C. Teeters, Chairperson, 918-631-2515, Fax: 918-631-3404, E-mail: dale-teeters@utulsa.edu. *Application contact:* Dr. Robert Sheaff, Advisor, 918-631-2319, Fax: 918-631-3404, E-mail: robert-sheaff@utulsa.edu.

University of Utah, School of Medicine and Graduate School, Graduate Programs in Medicine, Department of Biochemistry, Salt Lake City, UT 84112-1107. Offers MS, PhD. Terminal master's awarded for partial completion of doctoral program. *Degree requirements:* For master's, thesis; for doctorate, thesis/dissertation. *Entrance requirements:* For doctorate, GRE Subject Test, minimum GPA of 3.0. Additional exam requirements/recommendations for international students: Required—TOEFL. Electronic applications accepted. *Faculty research:* Protein structure and function, nucleic acid structure and function, nucleic acid enzymology, RNA modification, protein turnover.

University of Victoria, Faculty of Graduate Studies, Faculty of Science, Department of Biochemistry and Microbiology, Victoria, BC V8W 2Y2, Canada. Offers biochemistry (M Sc, PhD); microbiology (M Sc, PhD). *Degree requirements:* For master's, thesis, seminar; for doctorate, thesis/dissertation, seminar, candidacy exam. *Entrance requirements:* For master's, GRE General Test, minimum B+ average; for doctorate, GRE General Test, minimum B+ average, M Sc. Additional exam requirements/ recommendations for international students: Required—TOEFL (minimum score 600 paper-based). Electronic applications accepted. *Faculty research:* Molecular pathogenesis, prokaryotic, eukaryotic, macromolecular interactions, microbial surfaces, virology, molecular genetics.

University of Virginia, School of Medicine, Department of Biochemistry and Molecular Genetics, Charlottesville, VA 22903. Offers biochemistry (PhD); MD/PhD. *Degree requirements:* For doctorate, thesis/dissertation, written research proposal and defense. *Entrance requirements:* For doctorate, GRE General Test, 3 letters of recommendation. Additional exam requirements/recommendations for international students: Recommended—TOEFL (minimum score 630 paper-based; 90 iBT). Electronic applications accepted.

University of Washington, Graduate School, School of Medicine, Graduate Programs in Medicine, Department of Biochemistry, Seattle, WA 98195. Offers PhD. *Degree requirements:* For doctorate, thesis/dissertation. *Entrance requirements:* For doctorate, GRE General Test, GRE Subject Test (biology, chemistry, biochemistry, or cell and molecular biology), minimum GPA of 3.0. Additional exam requirements/ recommendations for international students: Required—TOEFL. Electronic applications accepted. *Faculty research:* Blood coagulation, structure and function of enzymes, fertilization events, interaction of plants with bacteria, protein structure.

University of Waterloo, Graduate Studies, Faculty of Science, Guelph-Waterloo Centre for Graduate Work in Chemistry and Biochemistry, Waterloo, ON N2L 3G1, Canada. Offers M Sc, PhD offered jointly with University of Guelph. *Program availability:* Part-time. *Degree requirements:* For master's and doctorate, project or thesis. *Entrance requirements:* For master's, GRE, honors degree, minimum B average; for doctorate, GRE, master's degree, minimum B average. Additional exam requirements/recommendations for international students: Required—TOEFL, IELTS, PTE. *Application deadline:* Applications are processed on a rolling basis. Application fee: $100 Canadian dollars. Electronic applications accepted. *Financial support:* Research assistantships, teaching assistantships, and scholarships/grants available. *Faculty research:* Polymer, physical, inorganic, organic, and theoretical chemistry. *Unit head:* E-mail: gwc@uwaterloo.ca. *Application contact:* E-mail: gwc@uoguelph.ca. Website: http://www.gwc2.on.ca/

The University of Western Ontario, Faculty of Graduate Studies, Biosciences Division, Department of Biochemistry, London, ON N6A 5B8, Canada. Offers M Sc, PhD. *Degree requirements:* For master's, thesis; for doctorate, thesis/dissertation. *Entrance requirements:* For master's, minimum B+ average in last 2 years of undergraduate study; for doctorate, M Sc or an external scholarship winner.

University of West Florida, College of Science and Engineering, School of Allied Health and Life Sciences, Department of Biology, Pensacola, FL 32514-5750. Offers biological chemistry (MS); biology (MS); biology education (MST); biotechnology (MS); coastal zone studies (MS); environmental biology (MS). *Degree requirements:* For master's, thesis. *Entrance requirements:* For master's, GRE (minimum score: verbal 450, quantitative 550), official transcripts; BS in biology or related field; letter of interest; relevant past experience; three letters of recommendation from individuals who can evaluate applicant's academic ability. Additional exam requirements/recommendations for international students: Required—TOEFL (minimum score 550 paper-based).

University of Windsor, Faculty of Graduate Studies, Faculty of Science, Department of Chemistry and Biochemistry, Windsor, ON N9B 3P4, Canada. Offers M Sc, PhD. *Program availability:* Part-time. *Degree requirements:* For master's, thesis; for doctorate, comprehensive exam, thesis/dissertation. *Entrance requirements:* For master's and doctorate, minimum B average. Additional exam requirements/recommendations for international students: Required—TOEFL (minimum score 560 paper-based). Electronic applications accepted. *Faculty research:* Molecular biology/recombinant DNA techniques (PCR, cloning mutagenesis), No/02 detectors, western immunoblotting and detection, CD/NMR protein/peptide structure determination, confocal/electron microscopes.

University of Wisconsin–Madison, Graduate School, College of Agricultural and Life Sciences, Department of Biochemistry, Madison, WI 53706. Offers PhD. Terminal master's awarded for partial completion of doctoral program. *Degree requirements:* For doctorate, thesis/dissertation. *Entrance requirements:* For doctorate, GRE General Test, GRE Subject Test (recommended). Additional exam requirements/recommendations for international students: Required—TOEFL. Electronic applications accepted. *Expenses:* Tuition, state resident: full-time $5364. Tuition, nonresident: full-time $12,027. *Required fees:* $571. Tuition and fees vary according to campus/location, program and reciprocity agreements. *Faculty research:* Molecular structure of vitamins and hormones, enzymology, NMR spectroscopy, protein structure, molecular genetics.

University of Wisconsin–Madison, School of Medicine and Public Health, Integrated Program in Biochemistry, Madison, WI 53706. Offers MS, PhD. Terminal master's awarded for partial completion of doctoral program. *Expenses:* Tuition, state resident: full-time $5364. Tuition, nonresident: full-time $12,027. *Required fees:* $571. Tuition and fees vary according to campus/location, program and reciprocity agreements. Website: https://ipib.wisc.edu/

Utah State University, School of Graduate Studies, College of Science, Department of Chemistry and Biochemistry, Logan, UT 84322. Offers biochemistry (MS, PhD); chemistry (MS, PhD). *Program availability:* Part-time. Terminal master's awarded for partial completion of doctoral program. *Degree requirements:* For master's, thesis, oral and written exams; for doctorate, thesis/dissertation, oral and written exams. *Entrance requirements:* For master's and doctorate, GRE General Test, minimum GPA of 3.0. Additional exam requirements/recommendations for international students: Required— TOEFL. *Faculty research:* Analytical, inorganic, organic, and physical chemistry; iron in asbestos chemistry and carcinogenicity; dicopper complexes; photothermal spectrometry; metal molecule clusters.

Vanderbilt University, School of Medicine, Department of Biochemistry, Nashville, TN 37240-1001. Offers MS, MD/PhD. *Faculty:* 19 full-time (1 woman). *Students:* 35 full-time (19 women); includes 9 minority (3 Black or African American, non-Hispanic/ Latino; 4 Hispanic/Latino; 2 Two or more races, non-Hispanic/Latino), 3 international. Average age 27. In 2015, 1 master's, 5 doctorates awarded. Terminal master's awarded for partial completion of doctoral program. *Degree requirements:* For master's, thesis; for doctorate, thesis/dissertation, preliminary, qualifying, and final exams. *Entrance requirements:* For master's, GRE General Test; for doctorate, GRE General Test, GRE Subject Test (recommended). Additional exam requirements/recommendations for international students: Required—TOEFL (minimum score 570 paper-based; 88 iBT). *Application deadline:* For fall admission, 1/15 for domestic and international students. Application fee: $0. Electronic applications accepted. *Financial support:* Fellowships with full tuition reimbursements, research assistantships with full tuition reimbursements, Federal Work-Study, institutionally sponsored loans, scholarships/grants, traineeships, and tuition waivers (partial) available. Financial award application deadline: 1/15; financial award applicants required to submit CSS PROFILE or FAFSA. *Faculty research:* Protein chemistry, carcinogenesis, metabolism, toxicology, receptors and signaling, DNA recognition and transcription. *Unit head:* Dr. Charles Sanders, Director of Graduate Studies, 615-322-3315, Fax: 615-322-4349, E-mail: chuck.sanders@vanderbilt.edu. *Application contact:* Walter B. Bieschke, Program Coordinator for Graduate Admissions, 615-342-0236, E-mail: vandygrad@vanderbilt.edu. Website: https://medschool.vanderbilt.edu/biochemistry/

Vanderbilt University, School of Medicine, Program in Chemical and Physical Biology, Nashville, TN 37240-1001. Offers PhD. *Students:* 34 full-time (15 women); includes 8 minority (1 Black or African American, non-Hispanic/Latino; 2 Asian, non-Hispanic/ Latino; 5 Hispanic/Latino), 5 international. Average age 29. In 2015, 13 doctorates awarded. *Degree requirements:* For doctorate, comprehensive exam, thesis/ dissertation, dissertation defense. *Entrance requirements:* For doctorate, GRE, 3 letters of recommendation, official transcripts. Additional exam requirements/recommendations for international students: Required—TOEFL. *Application deadline:* For fall admission, 1/15 priority date for domestic students, 1/15 for international students. Applications are

Biochemistry

processed on a rolling basis. Application fee: $0. Electronic applications accepted. *Financial support:* Fellowships with full tuition reimbursements, traineeships, health care benefits, and tuition waivers (full) available. *Faculty research:* Mathematical modeling, enzyme kinetics, structural biology, genomics, proteomics and mass spectrometry. *Unit head:* Dr. Bruce Damon, Director of Graduate Studies, 615-322-4235, Fax: 615-343-0490, E-mail: bruce.damon@vanderbilt.edu. *Application contact:* Patricia Muller, Coordinator, 615-322-8727, E-mail: patricia.l.mueller@vanderbilt.edu.

Virginia Commonwealth University, Medical College of Virginia-Professional Programs, School of Medicine, School of Medicine Graduate Programs, Department of Biochemistry, Richmond, VA 23284-9005. Offers biochemistry (MS, PhD); molecular biology (MS, PhD); MD/PhD. *Degree requirements:* For master's, thesis; for doctorate, thesis/dissertation, comprehensive oral and written exams. *Entrance requirements:* For master's and doctorate, GRE, MCAT or DAT. Electronic applications accepted. *Faculty research:* Molecular biology, peptide/protein chemistry, neurochemistry, enzyme mechanisms, macromolecular structure determination.

Virginia Commonwealth University, Program in Pre-Medical Basic Health Sciences, Richmond, VA 23284-9005. Offers anatomy (CBHS); biochemistry (CBHS); human genetics (CBHS); microbiology (CBHS); pharmacology (CBHS); physiology (CBHS). *Entrance requirements:* For degree, GRE, MCAT or DAT, course work in organic chemistry, minimum undergraduate GPA of 2.8. Additional exam requirements/recommendations for international students: Required—TOEFL (minimum score 600 paper-based). Electronic applications accepted.

Wake Forest University, School of Medicine and Graduate School of Arts and Sciences, Graduate Programs in Medicine, Department of Biochemistry, Winston-Salem, NC 27109. Offers PhD, MD/PhD. *Degree requirements:* For doctorate, thesis/dissertation. *Entrance requirements:* For doctorate, GRE General Test. Additional exam requirements/recommendations for international students: Required—TOEFL. Electronic applications accepted. *Faculty research:* Biomembranes, cancer, biophysics.

Washington State University, College of Veterinary Medicine, Program in Molecular Biosciences, Pullman, WA 99164. Offers molecular biology (PhD), including genetics, microbiology; molecular biosciences (PSM, PhD), including biochemistry (PhD), cell biology (PhD). *Program availability:* Online learning. *Faculty:* 30 full-time (12 women), 17 part-time/adjunct (5 women). *Students:* 47 full-time (26 women), 14 part-time (11 women); includes 13 minority (1 Black or African American, non-Hispanic/Latino; 1 American Indian or Alaska Native, non-Hispanic/Latino; 4 Asian, non-Hispanic/Latino; 5 Hispanic/Latino; 2 Two or more races, non-Hispanic/Latino), 1 international. Average age 28. 61 applicants, 23% accepted, 14 enrolled. In 2015, 5 master's, 8 doctorates awarded. Terminal master's awarded for partial completion of doctoral program. *Degree requirements:* For master's, thesis or alternative, oral exam; for doctorate, comprehensive exam, thesis/dissertation, oral exam, written exam. *Entrance requirements:* For master's and doctorate, GRE General Test, minimum GPA of 3.0. Additional exam requirements/recommendations for international students: Required—TOEFL (minimum score 100 iBT). *Application deadline:* For fall admission, 12/15 for domestic and international students. Application fee: $75. Electronic applications accepted. *Financial support:* In 2015–16, 5 fellowships with full tuition reimbursements (averaging $23,316 per year), 24 research assistantships with full tuition reimbursements (averaging $23,316 per year), 17 teaching assistantships with full tuition reimbursements (averaging $23,316 per year) were awarded; career-related internships or fieldwork, Federal Work-Study, traineeships, health care benefits, and unspecified assistantships also available. Financial award application deadline: 4/1; financial award applicants required to submit FAFSA. *Faculty research:* Gene regulation, signal transduction, protein export, reproductive biology, DNA repair. *Total annual research expenditures:* $5.8 million. *Unit head:* Dr. Jonathan Jones, Director, 509-335-8724, Fax: 509-335-9688, E-mail: jcr.jones@vetmed.wsu.edu. *Application contact:* Tami Breske, Coordinator, 509-335-4318, E-mail: tbreske@vetmed.wsu.edu. Website: http://www.smb.wsu.edu

Washington University in St. Louis, Graduate School of Arts and Sciences, Division of Biology and Biomedical Sciences, Program in Biochemistry, St. Louis, MO 63130-4899. Offers PhD. *Students:* 31 full-time (14 women); includes 5 minority (all Black or African American, non-Hispanic/Latino), 9 international. 75 applicants, 21% accepted, 6 enrolled. In 2015, 2 doctorates awarded. *Degree requirements:* For doctorate, thesis/dissertation. *Entrance requirements:* For doctorate, GRE General Test, GRE Subject Test. Additional exam requirements/recommendations for international students: Required—TOEFL. *Application deadline:* For fall admission, 12/1 for domestic students. Application fee: $0. Electronic applications accepted. *Financial support:* Fellowships and research assistantships available. Financial award application deadline: 1/15. *Faculty research:* Metabolic regulation, signal transduction, receptors, membrane channels and transporters, membrane structure and dynamics, membrane trafficking, cholesterol and lipid metabolism, nucleic acid-protein structure interactions and function, DNA replication and repair, recombination, transcription, translation, enzyme kinetics, cancer biology, cell cycle regulation, apoptosis, cell motility, cytoskeleton, cell division, extracellular matrix, vascular biology, aging, senescence, telomere biology. *Unit head:* Stacia Burd, Coordinator, 314-362-3364. *Application contact:* Rebecca Riney, 314-747-4648, E-mail: dbbsphdadmissions@wusm.wustl.edu.

Wayne State University, College of Liberal Arts and Sciences, Department of Chemistry, Detroit, MI 48202. Offers analytical chemistry (PhD); biochemistry (PhD); chemistry (MA, MS); inorganic chemistry (PhD); organic chemistry (PhD); physical chemistry (PhD). *Faculty:* 29. *Students:* 146 full-time (61 women); includes 9 minority (2 Asian, non-Hispanic/Latino; 3 Hispanic/Latino; 4 Two or more races, non-Hispanic/Latino), 95 international. Average age 28. 280 applicants, 19% accepted, 28 enrolled. In 2015, 4 master's, 22 doctorates awarded. *Degree requirements:* For master's, thesis (for some programs), oral exam; for doctorate, thesis/dissertation, oral exam. *Entrance requirements:* For master's, GRE (strongly recommended), 1 year of physics, math through calculus, general chemistry (8 credits), organic chemistry (8 credits), physical chemistry (6 credits), quantitative analysis (4 credits), advanced chemistry (3 credits), minimum undergraduate GPA of 2.75 in chemistry and cognate sciences, statement of interest, three letters of recommendation; for doctorate, GRE (strongly recommended), minimum undergraduate GPA of 3.0 in chemistry and cognate sciences. Additional exam requirements/recommendations for international students: Required—TOEFL (minimum score 90 iBT), IELTS (minimum score 6.5), TWE (minimum score 5.5). *Application deadline:* For fall admission, 12/1 priority date for domestic and international students. Applications are processed on a rolling basis. Application fee: $0. Electronic applications accepted. *Expenses:* Tuition, state resident: full-time $14,165; part-time $590.20 per credit hour. Tuition, nonresident: full-time $30,682; part-time $1278.40 per credit hour. *Required fees:* $1688; $47.45 per credit hour. $274.60 per semester. Tuition and fees vary according to course load and program. *Financial support:* In 2015–16, 141 students received support, including 10 fellowships with tuition reimbursements available (averaging $23,000 per year), 54 research assistantships with tuition reimbursements available (averaging $21,609 per year), 73 teaching assistantships with tuition reimbursements available (averaging $21,363 per year); scholarships/grants and unspecified assistantships also available. Financial award application deadline: 3/31; financial award applicants required to submit FAFSA. *Faculty research:* Natural products synthesis, molecular biology, molecular mechanics calculations, organometallic chemistry, experimental physical chemistry. *Total annual research expenditures:* $7.4 million. *Unit head:* Dr. James Rigby, Chair, 313-577-3472, E-mail: jhr@chem.wayne.edu. *Application contact:* Melissa Barton, Graduate Academic Services Officer, E-mail: melissa@chem.wayne.edu. Website: http://chem.wayne.edu/

Wayne State University, School of Medicine, Office of Biomedical Graduate Programs, Department of Biochemistry and Molecular Biology, Detroit, MI 48202. Offers MS, PhD, MD/PhD. *Faculty:* 11. *Students:* 27 full-time (15 women), 2 part-time (1 woman); includes 3 minority (1 Black or African American, non-Hispanic/Latino; 2 Asian, non-Hispanic/Latino), 12 international. Average age 28. 143 applicants, 9% accepted, 9 enrolled. In 2015, 1 master's, 2 doctorates awarded. *Degree requirements:* For master's, research project; for doctorate, thesis/dissertation. *Entrance requirements:* For master's, GRE, BA or BS in biology, chemistry, or (if approved) physics or mathematics with minimum GPA of 2.6 from accredited university; three letters of recommendation; personal statement; for doctorate, GRE, BA or BS in biology, chemistry, or (if approved) physics or mathematics with minimum GPA of 3.0 from accredited university; three letters of recommendation; personal statement; copies of any abstracts or papers on which the applicant is a co-author. Additional exam requirements/recommendations for international students: Required—TOEFL (minimum score 100 iBT). *Application deadline:* For fall admission, 2/1 priority date for domestic and international students. Applications are processed on a rolling basis. Application fee: $0. Electronic applications accepted. *Expenses:* $17,645 per year resident tuition, $33,311 non-resident tuition; $735.20 per credit hour resident tuition, $1,387.95 per credit hour non-resident tuition; fees include $47.45 per credit hour student services fee and $274.60 per semester registration fee. *Financial support:* In 2015–16, 27 students received support, including 3 fellowships with tuition reimbursements available (averaging $26,909 per year), 12 research assistantships with tuition reimbursements available (averaging $26,716 per year); scholarships/grants, health care benefits, and unspecified assistantships also available. Financial award application deadline: 3/31. *Faculty research:* Structural biology, cellular homeostasis and drug resistance, molecular biology and cancer, molecular and cellular bioenergetics, enzymology. *Unit head:* Dr. David Evans, 313-577-1016, E-mail: drevans@med.wayne.edu. *Application contact:* Dr. Zhe Yang, PhD, Program in Biochemistry and Molecular Biology Director, 313-577-1514, E-mail: zyang@med.wayne.edu. Website: http://www.biochem.med.wayne.edu/phd/

Weill Cornell Medicine, Weill Cornell Graduate School of Medical Sciences, Biochemistry, Cell and Molecular Biology Allied Program, New York, NY 10065. Offers MS, PhD. Terminal master's awarded for partial completion of doctoral program. *Degree requirements:* For master's, comprehensive exam; for doctorate, thesis/dissertation, final exam. *Entrance requirements:* For doctorate, GRE General Test, background in genetics, molecular biology, chemistry, or biochemistry. Additional exam requirements/recommendations for international students: Required—TOEFL. Electronic applications accepted. *Faculty research:* Molecular structure determination, protein structure, gene structure, stem cell biology, control of gene expression, DNA replication, chromosome maintenance, RNA biosynthesis.

Weill Cornell Medicine, Weill Cornell Graduate School of Medical Sciences, Cornell/Rockefeller/Sloan Kettering Tri-Institutional PhD Program in Chemical Biology, New York, NY 10065. Offers PhD. Program offered jointly with The Rockefeller University and Sloan Kettering Institute. *Degree requirements:* For doctorate, comprehensive exam, thesis/dissertation. *Entrance requirements:* For doctorate, GRE General Test; GRE Subject Test in chemistry (recommended), 3 letters of recommendation. Additional exam requirements/recommendations for international students: Required—TOEFL (minimum score 600 paper-based; 90 iBT). Electronic applications accepted. *Faculty research:* Bioreactive small molecules, macromolecular structure and function, chemical cell biology, biotechnology, computational chemistry.

Wesleyan University, Graduate Studies, Department of Chemistry, Middletown, CT 06459. Offers biochemistry (PhD); chemical physics (PhD); inorganic chemistry (PhD); organic chemistry (PhD); physical chemistry (PhD); theoretical chemistry (PhD). *Faculty:* 13 full-time (3 women), 3 part-time/adjunct (2 women). *Students:* 20 full-time (10 women), 2 part-time (0 women); includes 4 minority (1 Black or African American, non-Hispanic/Latino; 3 Asian, non-Hispanic/Latino), 8 international. Average age 25. In 2015, 6 doctorates awarded. Terminal master's awarded for partial completion of doctoral program. *Degree requirements:* For doctorate, thesis/dissertation, proposal. *Entrance requirements:* For doctorate, GRE General Test, 3 recommendations. Additional exam requirements/recommendations for international students: Required—TOEFL, IELTS. *Application deadline:* 2/15 for domestic and international students; for summer admission, 2/15 for domestic and international students. Applications are processed on a rolling basis. Application fee: $0. Electronic applications accepted. *Financial support:* In 2015–16, 4 research assistantships with full tuition reimbursements, 21 teaching assistantships with full tuition reimbursements were awarded; institutionally sponsored loans and health care benefits also available. Financial award application deadline: 4/15; financial award applicants required to submit FAFSA. *Faculty research:* The synthesis of noble metal and noble metal alloy nanoparticles with well-defined shapes and catalytically-active high-energy surfaces; inorganic chemistry; materials science; scanning electron microscopy (SEM). *Unit head:* Michael Calter, Chair, 860-685-2633, E-mail: mcalter@wesleyan.edu. *Application contact:* Roslyn Brault, Administrative Assistant/Graduate Program Coordinator, 860-685-2573, Fax: 860-685-2211, E-mail: rbrault@wesleyan.edu. Website: http://www.wesleyan.edu/chem

Wesleyan University, Graduate Studies, Department of Molecular Biology and Biochemistry, Middletown, CT 06459. Offers biochemistry (PhD); molecular biology (PhD); molecular biophysics (PhD); molecular genetics (PhD). *Faculty:* 8 full-time (3 women), 1 (woman) part-time/adjunct. *Students:* 18 full-time (9 women); includes 4 minority (2 Asian, non-Hispanic/Latino; 1 Hispanic/Latino; 1 Two or more races, non-Hispanic/Latino), 11 international. Average age 24. 28 applicants, 14% accepted, 1 enrolled. Terminal master's awarded for partial completion of doctoral program. *Degree requirements:* For doctorate, comprehensive exam, thesis/dissertation. *Entrance requirements:* For doctorate, GRE General Test, GRE Subject Test. Additional exam requirements/recommendations for international students: Required—TOEFL. *Application deadline:* For fall admission, 1/15 for domestic and international students. Application fee: $0. Electronic applications accepted. *Financial support:* Research assistantships with full tuition reimbursements, teaching assistantships with full tuition reimbursements, and institutionally sponsored loans available. Financial award application deadline: 4/15; financial award applicants required to submit FAFSA. *Faculty research:* The olfactory system and new frontiers in genome research, chromosome structure and gene expression, gene co-regulation, crystallographic and spectroscopic analysis, DNA replication and repair. *Unit head:* Scott Holmes, Chair, 860-685-2443, E-mail: sholmes@wesleyan.edu. *Application contact:* Anika Dane, Administrative Assistant, 860-685-2404, E-mail: adane@wesleyan.edu. Website: http://www.wesleyan.edu/mbb/

West Virginia University, School of Medicine, Graduate Programs at the Health Sciences Center, Interdisciplinary Graduate Programs in Biomedical Sciences, Program in Biochemistry and Molecular Biology, Morgantown, WV 26506. Offers MS, PhD, MD/

PhD. *Degree requirements:* For doctorate, comprehensive exam, thesis/dissertation. *Entrance requirements:* For doctorate, GRE General Test, minimum GPA of 3.0. Additional exam requirements/recommendations for international students: Required—TOEFL. Electronic applications accepted. *Expenses:* Tuition, state resident: full-time $8568. Tuition, nonresident: full-time $22,140. Tuition and fees vary according to program. *Faculty research:* Regulation of gene expression, cell survival mechanisms, signal transduction, regulation of metabolism, sensory neuroscience.

Worcester Polytechnic Institute, Graduate Studies and Research, Department of Chemistry and Biochemistry, Worcester, MA 01609-2280. Offers biochemistry (MS, PhD); chemistry (MS, PhD). *Program availability:* Evening/weekend. *Faculty:* 7 full-time (1 woman). *Students:* 16 full-time (8 women), 8 international. 44 applicants, 16% accepted, 3 enrolled. In 2015, 2 master's awarded. *Degree requirements:* For master's, thesis; for doctorate, comprehensive exam, thesis/dissertation. *Entrance requirements:* For master's and doctorate, GRE General Test, 3 letters of recommendation, statement of purpose. Additional exam requirements/recommendations for international students: Required—TOEFL (minimum score 563 paper-based; 84 iBT), IELTS (minimum score 7). *Application deadline:* For fall admission, 1/1 priority date for domestic and international students; for spring admission, 10/1 priority date for domestic and international students. Applications are processed on a rolling basis. Application fee: $70. Electronic applications accepted. *Financial support:* Research assistantships, teaching assistantships, career-related internships or fieldwork, institutionally sponsored loans, scholarships/grants, and unspecified assistantships available. Financial award application deadline: 1/1; financial award applicants required to submit FAFSA. *Unit head:* Dr. Arne Gericke, Department Head, 508-831-5371, Fax: 508-831-5933, E-mail: agericke@wpi.edu. *Application contact:* Dr. Shawn Burdette, Graduate Coordinator, 508-831-5371, Fax: 508-831-5933, E-mail: scburdette@wpi.edu. Website: http://www.wpi.edu/academics/cbc/gradprograms.html

Wright State University, School of Graduate Studies, College of Science and Mathematics, Department of Biochemistry and Molecular Biology, Dayton, OH 45435. Offers MS. *Degree requirements:* For master's, thesis. *Entrance requirements:* Additional exam requirements/recommendations for international students: Required—TOEFL. *Faculty research:* Regulation of gene expression, macromolecular structural function, NMR imaging, visual biochemistry.

Yale University, Graduate School of Arts and Sciences, Department of Geology and Geophysics, New Haven, CT 06520. Offers biogeochemistry (PhD); climate dynamics (PhD); geochemistry (PhD); geophysics (PhD); meteorology (PhD); oceanography (PhD); paleontology (PhD); paleooceanography (PhD); petrology (PhD); tectonics (PhD). *Degree requirements:* For doctorate, thesis/dissertation. *Entrance requirements:* For doctorate, GRE General Test. Additional exam requirements/recommendations for international students: Required—TOEFL.

Yale University, Graduate School of Arts and Sciences, Department of Molecular Biophysics and Biochemistry, New Haven, CT 06520. Offers PhD. *Degree requirements:* For doctorate, thesis/dissertation. *Entrance requirements:* For doctorate, GRE General Test, GRE Subject Test.

Yale University, Graduate School of Arts and Sciences, Department of Molecular, Cellular, and Developmental Biology, Program in Biochemistry, Molecular Biology and Chemical Biology, New Haven, CT 06520. Offers PhD. *Degree requirements:* For doctorate, thesis/dissertation. *Entrance requirements:* For doctorate, GRE General Test, GRE Subject Test.

Yale University, School of Medicine and Graduate School of Arts and Sciences, Combined Program in Biological and Biomedical Sciences (BBS), Molecular Biophysics and Biochemistry Track, New Haven, CT 06520. Offers PhD, MD/PhD. *Degree requirements:* For doctorate, thesis/dissertation. *Entrance requirements:* For doctorate, GRE General Test. Additional exam requirements/recommendations for international students: Required—TOEFL. Electronic applications accepted.

Youngstown State University, Graduate School, College of Science, Technology, Engineering and Mathematics, Department of Chemistry, Youngstown, OH 44555-0001. Offers analytical chemistry (MS); biochemistry (MS); chemistry education (MS); inorganic chemistry (MS); organic chemistry (MS); physical chemistry (MS). *Program availability:* Part-time. *Degree requirements:* For master's, thesis. *Entrance requirements:* For master's, bachelor's degree in chemistry, minimum GPA of 2.7. Additional exam requirements/recommendations for international students: Required—TOEFL. *Faculty research:* Analysis of antioxidants, chromatography, defects and disorder in crystalline oxides, hydrogen bonding, novel organic and organometallic materials.

Section 4
Biophysics

This section contains a directory of institutions offering graduate work in biophysics, followed by an in-depth entry submitted by an institution that chose to prepare a detailed program description. Additional information about programs listed in the directory but not augmented by an in-depth entry may be obtained by writing directly to the dean of a graduate school or chair of a department at the address given in the directory.

For programs offering related work, see also in this book *Allied Health; Biochemistry; Biological and Biomedical Sciences; Cell, Molecular, and Structural Biology; Optometry and Vision Sciences; Neuroscience and Neurobiology; Physiology;* and *Public Health.* In the other guides in this series:

Graduate Programs in the Physical Sciences, Mathematics, Agricultural Sciences, the Environment & Natural Resources

See *Chemistry* and *Physics*

Graduate Programs in Engineering & Applied Sciences

See *Agricultural Engineering* and *Bioengineering* and *Biomedical Engineering* and *Biotechnology*

CONTENTS

Biophysics

Albert Einstein College of Medicine, Graduate Division of Biomedical Sciences, Department of Physiology and Biophysics, Bronx, NY 10461. Offers PhD, MD/PhD. *Degree requirements:* For doctorate, thesis/dissertation. *Entrance requirements:* For doctorate, GRE General Test. Additional exam requirements/recommendations for international students: Required—TOEFL. *Faculty research:* Biophysical and biochemical basis of body function at the subcellular, cellular, organ, and whole-body level.

Baylor College of Medicine, Graduate School of Biomedical Sciences, Department of Molecular Physiology and Biophysics, Houston, TX 77030-3498. Offers cardiovascular sciences (PhD); molecular physiology and biophysics (PhD); MD/PhD. *Degree requirements:* For doctorate, thesis/dissertation, public defense. *Entrance requirements:* For doctorate, GRE General Test, GRE Subject Test (strongly recommended), minimum GPA of 3.0. Additional exam requirements/recommendations for international students: Required—TOEFL. Electronic applications accepted. *Faculty research:* Cardiovascular disease; skeletal muscle disease (myasthenia gravis, muscular dystrophy, malignant hyperthermia, central core disease); cancer; Alzheimer's disease; developmental diseases of the nervous system, eye and heart; diabetes; motor neuron disease (amyotrophic lateral sclerosis and spinal muscular atrophy); asthma; autoimmune diseases.

Boston University, School of Medicine, Division of Graduate Medical Sciences, Department of Physiology and Biophysics, Boston, MA 02118. Offers MA, PhD, MD/PhD. *Program availability:* Part-time. Terminal master's awarded for partial completion of doctoral program. *Degree requirements:* For master's, thesis; for doctorate, thesis/dissertation. *Application deadline:* For fall admission, 1/15 for domestic students; for spring admission, 10/15 for domestic students. *Faculty research:* X-ray scattering, NMR spectroscopy, protein crystallography, structural electron. *Unit head:* Dr. David Atkinson, Chairman, 617-638-4015, Fax: 617-638-4041, E-mail: atkinson@bu.edu. *Application contact:* GMS Admissions Office, 617-638-5255, E-mail: askgms@bu.edu. Website: http://www.bumc.bu.edu/phys-biophys/

Brandeis University, Graduate School of Arts and Sciences, Program in Biochemistry and Biophysics, Waltham, MA 02454. Offers biochemistry and biophysics (PhD); quantitative biology (PhD). *Faculty:* 10 full-time (3 women). *Students:* 38 full-time (16 women); includes 3 minority (1 Asian, non-Hispanic/Latino; 1 Hispanic/Latino; 1 Two or more races, non-Hispanic/Latino), 12 international. 70 applicants, 29% accepted, 5 enrolled. In 2015, 4 doctorates awarded. Terminal master's awarded for partial completion of doctoral program. *Degree requirements:* For doctorate, thesis/dissertation, qualifying exams. *Entrance requirements:* For doctorate, GRE General Test, resume, 3 letters of recommendation, statement of purpose, transcript(s). Additional exam requirements/recommendations for international students: Required—TOEFL (minimum score 600 paper-based; 100 iBT); Recommended—IELTS (minimum score 7), TSE (minimum score 68). *Application deadline:* For fall admission, 12/15 priority date for domestic students. Application fee: $75. Electronic applications accepted. *Financial support:* In 2015–16, 31 students received support, including 14 fellowships with full tuition reimbursements available (averaging $30,500 per year), 17 research assistantships with full tuition reimbursements available (averaging $30,500 per year); Federal Work-Study, scholarships/grants, health care benefits, and tuition waivers (full and partial) also available. Financial award application deadline: 4/15; financial award applicants required to submit FAFSA. *Faculty research:* Macromolecular chemistry, structure and function, biochemistry, biophysics, biological macromolecules. *Unit head:* Prof. Dagmar Ringe, Director of Graduate Studies, 781-736-2300, Fax: 781-736-2349, E-mail: scigradoffice@brandeis.edu. *Application contact:* 781-736-2300, E-mail: scigradoffice@brandeis.edu. Website: http://www.brandeis.edu/gsas

California Institute of Technology, Division of Biology, Program in Cell Biology and Biophysics, Pasadena, CA 91125-0001. Offers PhD. *Degree requirements:* For doctorate, thesis/dissertation, qualifying exam. *Entrance requirements:* For doctorate, GRE General Test.

Carnegie Mellon University, Mellon College of Science, Department of Biological Sciences, Pittsburgh, PA 15213-3891. Offers biochemistry (PhD); biophysics (PhD); cell and developmental biology (PhD); computational biology (MS, PhD); genetics (PhD); molecular biology (PhD); neuroscience (PhD); structural biology (PhD). *Degree requirements:* For doctorate, comprehensive exam, thesis/dissertation. *Entrance requirements:* For doctorate, GRE General Test, GRE Subject Test, interview. Electronic applications accepted. *Faculty research:* Genetic structure, function, and regulation; protein structure and function; biological membranes; biological spectroscopy.

Case Western Reserve University, School of Medicine and School of Graduate Studies, Graduate Programs in Medicine, Department of Physiology and Biophysics, Cleveland, OH 44106. Offers cell and molecular physiology (MS); cell physiology (PhD); molecular/cellular biophysics (PhD); physiology and biophysics (PhD); systems physiology (PhD); MD/PhD. Terminal master's awarded for partial completion of doctoral program. *Degree requirements:* For master's, thesis; for doctorate, thesis/dissertation. *Entrance requirements:* For master's, GRE General Test, minimum GPA of 3.28; for doctorate, GRE General Test, minimum GPA of 3.6. Additional exam requirements/recommendations for international students: Required—TOEFL. Electronic applications accepted. *Expenses: Tuition,* area resident: Full-time $41,137; part-time $1714 per credit hour. *Required fees:* $32. Tuition and fees vary according to course load and program. *Faculty research:* Cardiovascular physiology, calcium metabolism, epithelial cell biology.

Columbia University, College of Physicians and Surgeons, Department of Biochemistry and Molecular Biophysics, New York, NY 10032. Offers biochemistry and molecular biophysics (M Phil, PhD); biophysics (PhD); MD/PhD. Only candidates for the PhD are admitted. *Degree requirements:* For doctorate, one foreign language, thesis/dissertation. *Entrance requirements:* For master's and doctorate, GRE General Test. Additional exam requirements/recommendations for international students: Required—TOEFL.

Columbia University, College of Physicians and Surgeons, Department of Physiology and Cellular Biophysics, New York, NY 10032. Offers M Phil, MA, PhD, MD/PhD. Only candidates for the PhD are admitted. Terminal master's awarded for partial completion of doctoral program. *Degree requirements:* For doctorate, thesis/dissertation. *Entrance requirements:* For master's and doctorate, GRE General Test. Additional exam requirements/recommendations for international students: Required—TOEFL. *Faculty research:* Membrane physiology, cellular biology, cardiovascular physiology, neurophysiology.

Columbia University, College of Physicians and Surgeons, Integrated Program in Cellular, Molecular, Structural and Genetic Studies, New York, NY 10032. Offers PhD. Terminal master's awarded for partial completion of doctoral program. *Degree requirements:* For doctorate, thesis/dissertation. *Entrance requirements:* For doctorate, GRE General Test, GRE Subject Test. Additional exam requirements/recommendations for international students: Required—TOEFL. *Expenses:* Contact institution. *Faculty research:* Transcription, macromolecular sorting, gene expression during development, cellular interaction.

Cornell University, Graduate School, Graduate Fields of Agriculture and Life Sciences, Field of Biochemistry, Molecular and Cell Biology, Ithaca, NY 14853-0001. Offers biochemistry (PhD); biophysics (PhD); cell biology (PhD); molecular biology (PhD). *Degree requirements:* For doctorate, comprehensive exam, thesis/dissertation, 2 semesters of teaching experience. *Entrance requirements:* For doctorate, GRE General Test, GRE Subject Test (biology, chemistry, physics, biochemistry, cell and molecular biology), 3 letters of recommendation. Additional exam requirements/recommendations for international students: Required—TOEFL (minimum score 600 paper-based; 77 iBT). Electronic applications accepted. *Faculty research:* Biophysics, structural biology.

Cornell University, Graduate School, Graduate Fields of Agriculture and Life Sciences, Field of Biophysics, Ithaca, NY 14853-0001. Offers PhD. *Degree requirements:* For doctorate, comprehensive exam, thesis/dissertation. *Entrance requirements:* For doctorate, GRE General Test, GRE Subject Test (physics or chemistry preferred), 3 letters of recommendation. Additional exam requirements/recommendations for international students: Required—TOEFL (minimum score 550 paper-based; 77 iBT). Electronic applications accepted. *Faculty research:* Protein structure and function, biomolecular and cellular function, membrane biophysics, signal transduction, computational biology.

Dalhousie University, Faculty of Medicine, Department of Physiology and Biophysics, Halifax, NS B3H 1X5, Canada. Offers M Sc, PhD, M Sc/PhD. *Degree requirements:* For master's, thesis; for doctorate, thesis/dissertation. *Entrance requirements:* For master's and doctorate, GRE Subject Test (for international students). Additional exam requirements/recommendations for international students: Required—1 of 5 approved tests: TOEFL, IELTS, CANTEST, CAEL, Michigan English Language Assessment Battery. Electronic applications accepted. *Faculty research:* Computer modeling, reproductive and endocrine physiology, cardiovascular physiology, neurophysiology, membrane biophysics.

East Carolina University, Graduate School, Thomas Harriot College of Arts and Sciences, Department of Physics, Greenville, NC 27858-4353. Offers applied physics (MS); biomedical physics (PhD); health physics (MS); medical physics (MS). *Program availability:* Part-time. *Students:* 28 full-time (5 women), 8 part-time (3 women); includes 10 minority (4 Black or African American, non-Hispanic/Latino; 3 Asian, non-Hispanic/Latino; 1 Hispanic/Latino; 2 Two or more races, non-Hispanic/Latino), 5 international. Average age 29. 48 applicants, 60% accepted, 8 enrolled. In 2015, 6 master's, 1 doctorate awarded. *Degree requirements:* For master's, one foreign language, comprehensive exam. *Entrance requirements:* For master's, GRE General Test. Additional exam requirements/recommendations for international students: Required—TOEFL. *Application deadline:* Applications are processed on a rolling basis. Application fee: $50. *Financial support:* Research assistantships with partial tuition reimbursements, teaching assistantships with partial tuition reimbursements, and Federal Work-Study available. Support available to part-time students. Financial award application deadline: 6/1. *Unit head:* Dr. John Sutherland, Chair, 252-328-6739, E-mail: sutherlandj@ecu.edu. *Application contact:* Dean of Graduate School, 252-328-6012, Fax: 252-328-6071, E-mail: gradschool@ecu.edu. Website: http://www.ecu.edu/cs-cas/physics/Graduate-Program.cfm#

Emory University, Laney Graduate School, Department of Physics, Atlanta, GA 30322-1100. Offers biophysics (PhD); experimental condensed matter physics (PhD); theoretical and computational statistical physics (PhD); MS/PhD. *Degree requirements:* For doctorate, thesis/dissertation, qualifier proposal. *Entrance requirements:* For doctorate, GRE General Test, minimum GPA of 3.0. Additional exam requirements/recommendations for international students: Required—TOEFL (minimum score 600 paper-based). Electronic applications accepted. *Faculty research:* Experimental studies of the structure and function of metalloproteins, soft condensed matter, granular materials, biophotonics and fluorescence correlation spectroscopy, single molecule studies of DNA-protein systems.

Harvard University, Graduate School of Arts and Sciences, Committee on Biophysics, Cambridge, MA 02138. Offers PhD. *Degree requirements:* For doctorate, thesis/dissertation, exam, qualifying paper. *Entrance requirements:* For doctorate, GRE General Test, GRE Subject Test (recommended). Additional exam requirements/recommendations for international students: Required—TOEFL. *Faculty research:* Structural molecular biology, cell and membrane biophysics, molecular genetics, physical biochemistry, mathematical biophysics.

See Display on next page and Close-Up on page 161.

Howard University, Graduate School, Department of Physiology and Biophysics, Washington, DC 20059-0002. Offers biophysics (PhD); physiology (PhD). *Degree requirements:* For doctorate, comprehensive exam, thesis/dissertation. *Entrance requirements:* For doctorate, GRE General Test, minimum B average in field. *Faculty research:* Cardiovascular physiology, pulmonary physiology, renal physiology, neurophysiology, endocrinology.

Illinois State University, Graduate School, College of Arts and Sciences, Department of Biological Sciences, Normal, IL 61790-2200. Offers animal behavior (MS); bacteriology (MS); biochemistry (MS); biological sciences (MS); biology (PhD); biophysics (MS); biotechnology (MS); botany (MS, PhD); cell biology (MS); conservation biology (MS); developmental biology (MS); ecology (MS, PhD); entomology (MS); evolutionary biology (MS); genetics (MS, PhD); immunology (MS); microbiology (MS, PhD); molecular biology (MS); molecular genetics (MS); neurobiology (MS); neuroscience (MS); parasitology (MS); physiology (MS, PhD); plant biology (MS); plant molecular biology (MS); plant sciences (MS); structural biology (MS, PhD); zoology (MS, PhD). *Program availability:* Part-time. *Degree requirements:* For master's, thesis or alternative; for doctorate, variable foreign language requirement, thesis/dissertation, 2 terms of residency. *Entrance requirements:* For master's, GRE General Test, minimum GPA of 2.6 in last 60 hours of course work; for doctorate, GRE General Test. *Application deadline:* Applications are processed on a rolling basis. Application fee: $40. *Financial support:* Research assistantships, teaching assistantships, Federal Work-Study, tuition waivers (full), and unspecified assistantships available. Financial award application deadline: 4/1. *Faculty research:* Redox balance and drug development in schistosoma

Harvard University
Graduate Program in Biophysics

Initiated in 1959, the Committee on Higher Degrees in Biophysics at Harvard University has a long history of important research achievements.

Designed to nurture independent, creative scientists, the program is for students with sound preliminary training in a physical or quantitative science; such as chemistry, physics, mathematics, or computer science. The primary objective of the program is to educate and train individuals with this background to apply the concepts and methods of the physical sciences to the solution of biological problems.

Structural Biology
- X-ray crystallography
- NMR
- Electron microscopy
- Computational chemistry

Imaging
- Medical Imaging
  fMRI
  Magnetoencephalography
- Cellular Imaging
  Confocal microscopy
  Multiphoton microscopy
  Advance sub-Rayleigh approaches
- Molecular imaging
  Single molecule methods

Computational Biology
- Bioinformatics
- Genomics
- Proteomics

Computational Modeling
- Molecules
- Networks

Neurobiology
- Molecular
- Cellular
- Systems

Biophysics Program
HMS Campus, 240 Longwood Ave, Boston, MA 02115
Phone: 617-495-3360 Fax: 617-432-4360
http://www.fas.harvard.edu/~biophys/

Application Information:
http://www.gsas.harvard.edu/

---

mansoni, control of the growth of listeria monocytogenes at low temperature, regulation of cell expansion and microtubule function by SPRI, CRUI: physiology and fitness consequences of different life history phenotypes. *Application contact:* Steven Juliano, Graduate Coordinator, E-mail: sajulian@ilstu.edu. Website: http://www.bio.ilstu.edu/

Iowa State University of Science and Technology, Program in Biophysics, Ames, IA 50011. Offers MS, PhD. *Entrance requirements:* For master's, GRE. Additional exam requirements/recommendations for international students: Required—TOEFL (minimum score 550 paper-based; 79 iBT), IELTS (minimum score 6.5). Electronic applications accepted.

Johns Hopkins University, National Institutes of Health Sponsored Programs, Baltimore, MD 21218. Offers biology (PhD), including biochemistry, biophysics, cell biology, developmental biology, genetic biology, molecular biology; cell, molecular, and developmental biology and biophysics (PhD). *Degree requirements:* For doctorate, comprehensive exam, thesis/dissertation. *Entrance requirements:* For doctorate, GRE General Test. Additional exam requirements/recommendations for international students: Required—TOEFL (minimum score 600 paper-based), TWE. Electronic applications accepted. *Faculty research:* Protein and nucleic acid biochemistry and biophysical chemistry, molecular biology and development.

Johns Hopkins University, Zanvyl Krieger School of Arts and Sciences, Thomas C. Jenkins Department of Biophysics, Baltimore, MD 21218. Offers PhD. *Degree requirements:* For doctorate, comprehensive exam, thesis/dissertation. *Entrance requirements:* For doctorate, GRE General Test. Additional exam requirements/recommendations for international students: Required—TOEFL (minimum score 600 paper-based); IELTS; Recommended—TWE. Electronic applications accepted. *Faculty research:* Application of thermodynamics and kinetics, NMR spectroscopy, X-ray crystallography and computational methods to examine the function and structural and physical properties of proteins and nucleic acids.

Medical College of Wisconsin, Graduate School of Biomedical Sciences, Department of Biophysics, Milwaukee, WI 53226-0509. Offers PhD.

Medical College of Wisconsin, Graduate School of Biomedical Sciences, Program in Biophysics, Milwaukee, WI 53226-0509. Offers PhD, MD/PhD. *Program availability:* Part-time. *Degree requirements:* For doctorate, thesis/dissertation, oral exam. *Entrance requirements:* For doctorate, GRE General Test. Additional exam requirements/recommendations for international students: Required—TOEFL. Electronic applications accepted. *Faculty research:* X-ray crystallography, electron spin resonance and membrane structure, protein and membrane dynamics, magnetic resonance imaging, free radical biology.

Northwestern University, The Graduate School, Interdisciplinary Biological Sciences Program (IBiS), Evanston, IL 60208. Offers biochemistry (PhD); bioengineering and biotechnology (PhD); biotechnology (PhD); cell and molecular biology (PhD); developmental and systems biology (PhD); nanotechnology (PhD); neurobiology (PhD); structural biology and biophysics (PhD). *Degree requirements:* For doctorate, thesis/dissertation, qualifying exam. *Entrance requirements:* For doctorate, GRE General Test. Additional exam requirements/recommendations for international students: Required—TOEFL (minimum score 600 paper-based). Electronic applications accepted. *Faculty research:* Biophysics/structural biology, cell/molecular biology, synthetic biology, developmental systems biology, chemical biology/nanotechnology.

The Ohio State University, Graduate School, College of Arts and Sciences, Division of Natural and Mathematical Sciences, Program in Biophysics, Columbus, OH 43210. Offers MS, PhD. *Degree requirements:* For master's, thesis optional; for doctorate, thesis/dissertation. *Entrance requirements:* For master's and doctorate, GRE General Test (minimum 50th percentile on each section). Additional exam requirements/recommendations for international students: Required—TOEFL (minimum score 600 paper-based; 100 iBT), Michigan English Language Assessment Battery (minimum score 86); Recommended—IELTS (minimum score 8). Electronic applications accepted.

Oregon State University, College of Science, Program in Biochemistry and Biophysics, Corvallis, OR 97331. Offers biochemistry (MA, MS, PhD); biophysics (MA, MS, PhD). *Faculty:* 15 full-time (4 women), 2 part-time/adjunct (0 women). *Students:* 27 full-time (13 women), 1 part-time (0 women); includes 3 minority (1 Black or African American, non-Hispanic/Latino; 2 Asian, non-Hispanic/Latino), 5 international. Average age 28. 43 applicants, 26% accepted, 6 enrolled. In 2015, 2 master's, 3 doctorates awarded. *Degree requirements:* For master's, thesis optional; for doctorate, thesis/dissertation, exams. *Entrance requirements:* For master's and doctorate, GRE, minimum GPA of 3.0. Additional exam requirements/recommendations for international students: Required—TOEFL (minimum score 600 paper-based; 100 iBT), IELTS (minimum score 7). *Application deadline:* For fall admission, 12/15 priority date for domestic students. Application fee: $75 ($85 for international students). *Expenses:* Tuition, state resident: full-time $12,150; part-time $450 per credit. Tuition, nonresident: full-time $20,952; part-time $776 per credit. *Required fees:* $1572; $1443 per unit. One-time fee: $350. Tuition and fees vary according to course load, campus/location and program. *Financial support:* Research assistantships, teaching assistantships, and institutionally sponsored loans available. Support available to part-time students. Financial award application deadline: 12/15. *Faculty research:* DNA and deoxy ribonucleotide metabolism, cell growth control, receptors and membranes, protein structure and function. *Unit head:* Dr. Andy Karplus, Professor and Chair. *Application contact:* Graduate Program Coordinator, 541-737-4511, E-mail: bboffice@oregonstate.edu. Website: http://biochem.science.oregonstate.edu/

Purdue University, Graduate School, College of Science, Department of Biological Sciences, West Lafayette, IN 47907. Offers biochemistry (PhD); biophysics (PhD); cell and developmental biology (PhD); ecology, evolutionary and population biology (MS, PhD), including ecology, evolutionary biology, population biology; genetics (MS, PhD); microbiology (MS, PhD); molecular biology (PhD); neurobiology (MS, PhD); plant physiology (PhD). Terminal master's awarded for partial completion of doctoral program. *Degree requirements:* For master's, thesis (for some programs); for doctorate, thesis/dissertation, seminars, teaching experience. *Entrance requirements:* For master's, GRE General Test (minimum analytical writing score of 3.5), minimum undergraduate GPA of 3.0; for doctorate, GRE General Test (minimum analytical writing score of 3.5), minimum undergraduate GPA of 3.5. Additional exam requirements/recommendations for international students: Required—TOEFL (minimum score 600 paper-based; 107 iBT for MS, 80 iBT for PhD). Electronic applications accepted.

Purdue University, Graduate School, PULSe - Purdue University Life Sciences Program, West Lafayette, IN 47907. Offers biomolecular structure and biophysics (PhD); biotechnology (PhD); chemical biology (PhD); chromatin and regulation of gene expression (PhD); integrative neuroscience (PhD); integrative plant sciences (PhD); membrane biology (PhD); microbiology (PhD); molecular evolutionary and cancer biology (PhD); molecular evolutionary genetics (PhD); molecular virology (PhD). *Entrance requirements:* For doctorate, GRE, minimum undergraduate GPA of 3.0. Additional exam requirements/recommendations for international students: Required—TOEFL (minimum score 550 paper-based; 77 iBT). Electronic applications accepted.

Biophysics

Rensselaer Polytechnic Institute, Graduate School, School of Science, Program in Biochemistry and Biophysics, Troy, NY 12180-3590. Offers MS, PhD. *Faculty:* 6 full-time (3 women), 2 part-time/adjunct (0 women). *Students:* 15 full-time (8 women); includes 2 minority (1 Asian, non-Hispanic/Latino; 1 Two or more races, non-Hispanic/Latino), 1 international. Average age 24. 36 applicants, 22% accepted, 1 enrolled. In 2015, 2 doctorates awarded. Terminal master's awarded for partial completion of doctoral program. *Degree requirements:* For master's, thesis optional; for doctorate, comprehensive exam, thesis/dissertation. *Entrance requirements:* For master's and doctorate, GRE. Additional exam requirements/recommendations for international students: Required—TOEFL (minimum score 600 paper-based; 100 iBT), IELTS (minimum score 7), PTE (minimum score 68). *Application deadline:* For fall admission, 1/1 priority date for domestic and international students; for spring admission, 8/15 priority date for domestic and international students. Applications are processed on a rolling basis. Application fee: $75. Electronic applications accepted. *Financial support:* In 2015–16, research assistantships (averaging $21,500 per year), teaching assistantships (averaging $21,500 per year) were awarded; fellowships also available. Financial award application deadline: 1/1. *Faculty research:* Biochemistry; bioinformatics; biophysics; cancer biology; computational biology; molecular, cell, and developmental biology; neuroscience; protein folding; stem cells; structural biology. *Unit head:* Dr. Chunyu Wang, Graduate Program Director, 518-276-3497, E-mail: wangc5@rpi.edu. *Application contact:* Office of Graduate Admissions, 518-276-6216, E-mail: gradadmissions@rpi.edu.
Website: http://www.rpi.edu/dept/bcbp/

Rosalind Franklin University of Medicine and Science, School of Graduate and Postdoctoral Studies - Interdisciplinary Graduate Program in Biomedical Sciences, Department of Physiology and Biophysics, North Chicago, IL 60064-3095. Offers MS, PhD, MD/PhD. Terminal master's awarded for partial completion of doctoral program. *Degree requirements:* For master's, comprehensive exam, thesis; for doctorate, comprehensive exam, thesis/dissertation. *Entrance requirements:* For master's and doctorate, GRE General Test. Additional exam requirements/recommendations for international students: Required—TOEFL, TWE. *Faculty research:* Membrane transport, mechanisms of cellular regulation, brain metabolism, peptide metabolism.

Stanford University, School of Humanities and Sciences, Program in Biophysics, Stanford, CA 94305-9991. Offers PhD. *Degree requirements:* For doctorate, thesis/dissertation, oral exam. *Entrance requirements:* For doctorate, GRE General Test, GRE Subject Test. Additional exam requirements/recommendations for international students: Required—TOEFL. Electronic applications accepted. *Expenses:* Tuition, area resident: Full-time $45,729. *Required fees:* $591.

Stony Brook University, State University of New York, Stony Brook Medicine, School of Medicine and Graduate School, Graduate Programs in Medicine, Department of Physiology and Biophysics, Stony Brook, NY 11794. Offers PhD. *Faculty:* 17 full-time (6 women). *Students:* 33 full-time (15 women), 1 part-time (0 women); includes 18 minority (6 Black or African American, non-Hispanic/Latino; 6 Asian, non-Hispanic/Latino; 5 Hispanic/Latino; 1 Two or more races, non-Hispanic/Latino), 6 international. Average age 25. 5 applicants. In 2015, 3 doctorates awarded. *Degree requirements:* For doctorate, comprehensive exam, thesis/dissertation. *Entrance requirements:* For doctorate, GRE General Test, GRE Subject Test, BS in related field, minimum GPA of 3.0, recommendation. Additional exam requirements/recommendations for international students: Required—TOEFL (minimum score 550 paper-based). *Application deadline:* For fall admission, 1/15 for domestic students; for spring admission, 10/1 for domestic students. Application fee: $100. *Expenses:* $12,421 full-time resident tuition and fees, $453 per credit hour; $23,761 full-time nonresident tuition and fees, $925 per credit hour. *Financial support:* In 2015–16, 2 research assistantships were awarded; fellowships, teaching assistantships, and Federal Work-Study also available. Financial award application deadline: 3/15. *Faculty research:* Biophysics, physiology, neuropharmacology, neurophysiology, neuroscience. *Total annual research expenditures:* $5.2 million. *Unit head:* Dr. Todd Miller, Chair, 631-444-3533, Fax: 631-444-3432, E-mail: todd.miller@stonybrook.edu. *Application contact:* Odalis Hernandez, Coordinator, 631-444-3057, Fax: 631-444-3432, E-mail: odalis.hernandez@stonybrook.edu.
Website: http://pnb.informatics.stonybrook.edu/

Syracuse University, College of Arts and Sciences, Ph.D. Program in Structural Biology, Biochemistry and Biophysics, Syracuse, NY 13244. Offers structural biology, biochemistry, and biophysics (PhD). *Students:* Average age 28. *Degree requirements:* For doctorate, comprehensive exam, thesis/dissertation. *Entrance requirements:* For doctorate, GRE General Test, GRE Subject Test, three letters of recommendation, resume, personal statement, transcripts. Additional exam requirements/recommendations for international students: Required—TOEFL (minimum score 100 iBT). *Application deadline:* For fall admission, 12/15 priority date for domestic and international students. Application fee: $75. Electronic applications accepted. *Expenses:* Tuition, area resident: Full-time $25,974; part-time $1443 per credit hour. *Required fees:* $802; $50 per course. Tuition and fees vary according to course load and program. *Financial support:* Fellowships with full tuition reimbursements, research assistantships with tuition reimbursements, teaching assistantships with tuition reimbursements, scholarships/grants, and tuition waivers available. Financial award application deadline: 1/1. *Faculty research:* Biochemistry, genetic engineering, biomolecular modeling, methods for computerized simulation of molecules, ethical conduct of science. *Unit head:* Prof. Liviu Movileanu, Associate Professor, Physics, 315-443-9154, Fax: 315-443-2012, E-mail: lmovilea@syr.edu. *Application contact:* Patty Whitmore, Academic Program Coordinator, 315-443-5958, E-mail: pawhitmo@syr.edu.
Website: http://sb3.syr.edu/

Texas Christian University, College of Science and Engineering, Department of Physics and Astronomy, Fort Worth, TX 76129. Offers physics (MA, MS, PhD), including astrophysics (PhD), biophysics (PhD); PhD/MBA. *Program availability:* Part-time. *Faculty:* 8 full-time (2 women). *Students:* 15 full-time (5 women); includes 2 minority (both Hispanic/Latino), 9 international. Average age 32. 20 applicants, 30% accepted, 4 enrolled. In 2015, 3 master's, 2 doctorates awarded. Terminal master's awarded for partial completion of doctoral program. *Degree requirements:* For master's, one foreign language, comprehensive exam, thesis or alternative; for doctorate, comprehensive exam, thesis/dissertation. *Entrance requirements:* For master's and doctorate, GRE. Additional exam requirements/recommendations for international students: Required—TOEFL (minimum score 80 iBT). *Application deadline:* For fall admission, 2/1 for domestic and international students; for spring admission, 9/1 for domestic and international students. Applications are processed on a rolling basis. Application fee: $60. Electronic applications accepted. *Expenses:* Contact institution. *Financial support:* In 2015–16, 14 students received support, including 1 research assistantship with full tuition reimbursement available (averaging $23,000 per year), 13 teaching assistantships with full tuition reimbursements available (averaging $20,500 per year); scholarships/grants and unspecified assistantships also available. Financial award application deadline: 2/1. *Faculty research:* Nanomaterials, computer simulations of biophysical processes, nonlinear dynamics, spectra of local stellar populations, spectroscopy and fluorescence of biomolecules. *Unit head:* Dr. Yuri M. Strzhemechny, Associate Professor/Chair, 817-257-5793, Fax: 817-257-7742, E-mail: y.strzhemechny@tcu.edu. *Application contact:* Dr. Peter M. Frinchaboy, III, Associate Professor, 817-257-6387, Fax: 817-257-7742, E-mail: p.frinchaboy@tcu.edu.
Website: http://physics.tcu.edu/

Université de Sherbrooke, Faculty of Medicine and Health Sciences, Graduate Programs in Medicine, Department of Physiology and Biophysics, Sherbrooke, QC J1H 5N4, Canada. Offers M Sc, PhD. Terminal master's awarded for partial completion of doctoral program. *Degree requirements:* For master's, thesis; for doctorate, thesis/dissertation. Electronic applications accepted. *Faculty research:* Ion channels, neurological basis of pain, insulin resistance, obesity.

Université du Québec à Trois-Rivières, Graduate Programs, Program in Biophysics and Cellular Biology, Trois-Rivières, QC G9A 5H7, Canada. Offers M Sc, PhD. *Program availability:* Part-time. *Degree requirements:* For master's, thesis; for doctorate, thesis/dissertation. *Entrance requirements:* For master's, appropriate bachelor's degree, proficiency in French; for doctorate, appropriate master's degree, proficiency in French.

University at Buffalo, the State University of New York, Graduate School, Graduate Programs in Cancer Research and Biomedical Sciences at Roswell Park Cancer Institute, Department of Molecular and Cellular Biophysics and Biochemistry at Roswell Park Cancer Institute, Buffalo, NY 14260. Offers PhD. *Faculty:* 24 full-time (3 women). *Students:* 20 full-time (11 women); includes 3 minority (1 Black or African American, non-Hispanic/Latino; 2 Asian, non-Hispanic/Latino), 4 international. 15 applicants, 33% accepted, 3 enrolled. In 2015, 2 doctorates awarded. *Degree requirements:* For doctorate, comprehensive exam, thesis/dissertation, oral defense of dissertation. *Entrance requirements:* For doctorate, GRE General Test. Additional exam requirements/recommendations for international students: Required—TOEFL (minimum score 79 iBT). *Application deadline:* For fall admission, 1/5 priority date for domestic and international students. Application fee: $75. Electronic applications accepted. *Financial support:* In 2015–16, 20 students received support, including 20 research assistantships with full tuition reimbursements available (averaging $25,000 per year); scholarships/grants, health care benefits, and unspecified assistantships also available. Financial award application deadline: 1/5. *Faculty research:* MRI research, structural and function of biomolecules, photodynamic therapy, DNA damage and repair, heat-shock proteins and vaccine research. *Unit head:* Dr. Eugene Kandel, Director of Graduate Studies, 716-845-3530, E-mail: eugene.kandel@roswellpark.org. *Application contact:* Dr. Norman J. Karin, Associate Dean, 716-845-2339, Fax: 716-845-8178, E-mail: norman.karin@roswellpark.edu.
Website: http://www.roswellpark.edu/education/phd-programs/molecular-cellular-biophysics-and-biochemistry

University at Buffalo, the State University of New York, Graduate School, School of Medicine and Biomedical Sciences, Graduate Programs in Medicine and Biomedical Sciences, Department of Physiology and Biophysics, Buffalo, NY 14214. Offers biophysics (MS, PhD), including medical physics; physiology (MA, PhD). *Faculty:* 28 full-time (4 women). *Students:* 64 full-time (28 women); includes 34 minority (4 Black or African American, non-Hispanic/Latino; 26 Asian, non-Hispanic/Latino; 1 Hispanic/Latino; 3 Two or more races, non-Hispanic/Latino), 20 international. Average age 28. 62 applicants, 18% accepted, 8 enrolled. In 2015, 7 master's, 4 doctorates awarded. Terminal master's awarded for partial completion of doctoral program. *Degree requirements:* For master's, comprehensive exam, thesis optional, oral exam, project; for doctorate, comprehensive exam, thesis/dissertation, oral and written qualifying exam or 2 research proposals. *Entrance requirements:* For master's, GRE General Test, unofficial transcripts, 3 letters of recommendation, personal statement, curriculum vitae; for doctorate, GRE General Test or MCAT, unofficial transcripts, 3 letters of recommendation, personal statement, curriculum vitae. Additional exam requirements/recommendations for international students: Required—TOEFL (minimum score 550 paper-based; 79 iBT). *Application deadline:* Applications are processed on a rolling basis. Application fee: $85. Electronic applications accepted. *Financial support:* In 2015–16, 5 students received support, including 1 research assistantship with full tuition reimbursement available (averaging $25,000 per year); Federal Work-Study, institutionally sponsored loans, health care benefits, and unspecified assistantships also available. Financial award applicants required to submit FAFSA. *Faculty research:* Neurosciences, ion channels, cardiac physiology, renal/epithelial transport, cardiopulmonary exercise. *Total annual research expenditures:* $2.7 million. *Unit head:* Dr. Perry M. Hogan, Chair, 716-829-2738, Fax: 716-829-2344, E-mail: phogan@buffalo.edu. *Application contact:* Kara M. Rickicki, Graduate Programs Coordinator, 716-829-2417, Fax: 716-829-2344, E-mail: rickicki@buffalo.edu.
Website: http://www.smbs.buffalo.edu/phb/

University of California, Berkeley, Graduate Division, College of Letters and Science, Group in Biophysics, Berkeley, CA 94720-1500. Offers PhD. *Degree requirements:* For doctorate, thesis/dissertation, qualifying exam. *Entrance requirements:* For doctorate, GRE General Test, minimum GPA of 3.0, 3 letters of recommendation.

University of California, Davis, Graduate Studies, Graduate Group in Biophysics, Davis, CA 95616. Offers MS, PhD. *Degree requirements:* For doctorate, thesis/dissertation. *Entrance requirements:* For master's and doctorate, GRE General Test, GRE Subject Test. Additional exam requirements/recommendations for international students: Required—TOEFL (minimum score 550 paper-based). Electronic applications accepted. *Faculty research:* Molecular structure, protein structure/function relationships, spectroscopy.

University of California, Irvine, School of Medicine and Francisco J. Ayala School of Biological Sciences, Department of Physiology and Biophysics, Irvine, CA 92697. Offers biological sciences (PhD); MD/PhD. *Students:* 10 full-time (3 women); includes 5 minority (4 Asian, non-Hispanic/Latino; 1 Hispanic/Latino), 2 international. Average age 29. In 2015, 1 doctorate awarded. *Degree requirements:* For doctorate, thesis/dissertation. *Entrance requirements:* For doctorate, GRE General Test, GRE Subject Test, minimum GPA of 3.0. Additional exam requirements/recommendations for international students: Required—TOEFL (minimum score 550 paper-based). *Application deadline:* For fall admission, 1/15 priority date for domestic students, 1/15 for international students. Application fee: $80 ($100 for international students). Electronic applications accepted. *Financial support:* Fellowships, research assistantships with full tuition reimbursements, teaching assistantships, institutionally sponsored loans, traineeships, health care benefits, and unspecified assistantships available. Financial award application deadline: 3/1; financial award applicants required to submit FAFSA. *Faculty research:* Membrane physiology, exercise physiology, regulation of hormone biosynthesis and action, endocrinology, ion channels and signal transduction. *Unit head:* Prof. Michael Cahalan, Chair, 949-824-7776, Fax: 949-824-3143, E-mail: mcahalan@uci.edu. *Application contact:* Janita Parpana, Chief Administrative Officer, 949-824-6833, Fax: 949-824-8540, E-mail: jparpana@uci.edu.
Website: http://www.physiology.uci.edu/

University of California, San Diego, Graduate Division, Department of Physics, La Jolla, CA 92093. Offers biophysics (PhD); multi-scale biology (PhD); physics (MS, PhD). *Students:* 154 full-time (18 women); includes 26 minority (3 Black or African American, non-Hispanic/Latino; 15 Asian, non-Hispanic/Latino; 8 Hispanic/Latino), 52 international. 481 applicants, 13% accepted, 17 enrolled. In 2015, 13 master's, 27 doctorates awarded. *Degree requirements:* For doctorate, comprehensive exam, thesis/

dissertation, 1-quarter teaching assistantship. *Entrance requirements:* For doctorate, GRE General Test, GRE Subject Test. Additional exam requirements/recommendations for international students: Required—TOEFL (minimum score 550 paper-based; 80 iBT), IELTS (minimum score 7). *Application deadline:* For fall admission, 12/23 for domestic students. Application fee: $90 ($110 for international students). Electronic applications accepted. *Expenses:* Tuition, state resident: full-time $11,220. Tuition, nonresident: full-time $26,322. *Required fees:* $1800. *Financial support:* Fellowships, research assistantships, teaching assistantships, scholarships/grants, and unspecified assistantships available. Financial award applicants required to submit FAFSA. *Faculty research:* Astrophysics/astronomy, biological physics, condensed matter/material science, elementary particles, plasma physics. *Unit head:* Benjamin Grinstein, Chair, 858-534-6857, E-mail: chair@physics.ucsd.edu. *Application contact:* Sharmila Poddar, Graduate Coordinator, 858-822-1074, E-mail: shpoddar@ucsd.edu.
Website: http://physics.ucsd.edu/

University of California, San Francisco, School of Pharmacy and School of Medicine, Program in Biophysics, San Francisco, CA 94143. Offers PhD. *Degree requirements:* For doctorate, thesis/dissertation. *Entrance requirements:* For doctorate, GRE General Test; GRE Subject Test (recommended), bachelor's degree with minimum GPA of 3.0. Additional exam requirements/recommendations for international students: Required—TOEFL. Electronic applications accepted. *Faculty research:* Structural biology, proteomics and genomics, biophysical approaches to cell biology, complex biological systems, computational and theoretical biophysics, membrane biophysics, protein engineering and synthetic biology.

University of California, Santa Barbara, Graduate Division, College of Letters and Sciences, Division of Mathematics, Life, and Physical Sciences, Interdepartmental Graduate Program in Biomolecular Science and Engineering, Santa Barbara, CA 93106-2014. Offers biochemistry and molecular biology (PhD), including biochemistry and molecular biology, biophysics and bioengineering. *Faculty:* 35 full-time (3 women), 4 part-time/adjunct (all women). *Students:* 27 full-time (9 women); includes 7 minority (5 Asian, non-Hispanic/Latino; 2 Hispanic/Latino), 1 international. Average age 26. 105 applicants, 21% accepted, 11 enrolled. In 2015, 8 doctorates awarded. Terminal master's awarded for partial completion of doctoral program. *Degree requirements:* For doctorate, thesis/dissertation. *Entrance requirements:* For doctorate, GRE General Test. Additional exam requirements/recommendations for international students: Required—TOEFL (minimum score 630 paper-based; 109 iBT), IELTS (minimum score 7). *Application deadline:* For fall admission, 12/15 for domestic and international students. Application fee: $90 ($110 for international students). Electronic applications accepted. *Financial support:* In 2015–16, 28 students received support, including 16 fellowships with tuition reimbursements available, 31 research assistantships with tuition reimbursements available, 16 teaching assistantships with tuition reimbursements available; Federal Work-Study, traineeships, health care benefits, tuition waivers (full and partial), and unspecified assistantships also available. Financial award application deadline: 12/15; financial award applicants required to submit FAFSA. *Faculty research:* Biochemistry and molecular biology, biophysics, biomaterials, bioengineering, systems biology. *Unit head:* Prof. Omar A. Saleh, Director/Professor, 805-893-8814, E-mail: saleh@engineering.ucsb.edu. *Application contact:* Lauren Baker, Graduate Program Assistant, 805-893-3011, E-mail: bmse-gradasst@lifesci.ucsb.edu.
Website: http://www.bmse.ucsb.edu/

University of Chicago, Division of the Physical Sciences, Graduate Program in Biophysical Science, Chicago, IL 60637. Offers PhD. *Degree requirements:* For doctorate, comprehensive exam, thesis/dissertation, ethics class, 2 teaching assistantships. *Entrance requirements:* Additional exam requirements/recommendations for international students: Required—IELTS (minimum score 7); Recommended—TOEFL (minimum score 600 paper-based; 104 iBT). Electronic applications accepted. *Faculty research:* Physical probes of biological systems, ultrafast dynamics and nonequilibrium theory of biological systems, computational simulation of large-scale biodynamics, protein design and protein-lipid interactions, epigenetics and genomics.

University of Cincinnati, Graduate School, College of Medicine, Graduate Programs in Biomedical Sciences, Department of Pharmacology and Cell Biophysics, Cincinnati, OH 45221. Offers cell biophysics (PhD); pharmacology (PhD). *Degree requirements:* For doctorate, thesis/dissertation, qualifying exam. *Entrance requirements:* For doctorate, GRE General Test. Additional exam requirements/recommendations for international students: Required—TOEFL. Electronic applications accepted. *Faculty research:* Lipoprotein research, enzyme regulation, electrophysiology, gene actuation.

University of Colorado Denver, School of Medicine, Graduate Program in Genetic Counseling, Aurora, CO 80045. Offers biophysics and genetics (MS, PhD). *Students:* 12 full-time (all women); includes 2 minority (1 Asian, non-Hispanic/Latino; 1 Hispanic/Latino). Average age 26. 118 applicants, 5% accepted, 6 enrolled. In 2015, 3 master's awarded. *Degree requirements:* For master's, 44 core semester hours, project or thesis; for doctorate, comprehensive exam, thesis/dissertation, 30 hours each of didactic course work and research credits. *Entrance requirements:* For master's, GRE, minimum undergraduate GPA of 3.0; 4 letters of recommendation; prerequisite coursework in biology, general chemistry, general biochemistry, general genetics, general psychology; experience in counseling and laboratory settings and strong understanding of genetic counseling field (highly recommended); for doctorate, GRE, three letters of recommendation, laboratory research experience and solid undergraduate foundation in mathematics and biological sciences. Additional exam requirements/recommendations for international students: Required—TOEFL (minimum score 570 paper-based; 89 iBT). *Application deadline:* For fall admission, 1/1 for domestic, 12/1 for international students. Application fee: $50 ($75 for international students). Electronic applications accepted. *Expenses:* Contact institution. *Financial support:* In 2015–16, 12 students received support. Fellowships, research assistantships, teaching assistantships, career-related internships or fieldwork, Federal Work-Study, institutionally sponsored loans, scholarships/grants, traineeships, and unspecified assistantships available. Financial award application deadline: 4/1; financial award applicants required to submit FAFSA. *Faculty research:* Psychosocial aspects of genetic counseling, clinical cytogenetics and molecular genetics, human inborn errors of metabolism, congenital malformations and disorders of the newborn, cancer genetics and genetic counseling. *Application contact:* Kenton Owsley, Program Administrator, 303-724-3468, E-mail: somadmin@ucdenver.edu.
Website: http://www.ucdenver.edu/academics/colleges/Graduate-School/academic-programs/genetic-counseling/Pages/default.aspx

University of Guelph, Graduate Studies, Biophysics Interdepartmental Group, Guelph, ON N1G 2W1, Canada. Offers M Sc, PhD. *Degree requirements:* For master's, thesis; for doctorate, comprehensive exam, thesis/dissertation. *Entrance requirements:* For master's, minimum B average during previous 2 years of course work; for doctorate, minimum B+ average. Additional exam requirements/recommendations for international students: Required—TOEFL (minimum score 550 paper-based). Electronic applications accepted. *Faculty research:* Molecular, cellular, structural, and computational biophysics.

University of Guelph, Graduate Studies, College of Biological Science, Department of Molecular and Cellular Biology, Guelph, ON N1G 2W1, Canada. Offers biochemistry

(M Sc, PhD); biophysics (M Sc, PhD); botany (M Sc, PhD); microbiology (M Sc, PhD); molecular biology and genetics (M Sc, PhD). *Degree requirements:* For master's, thesis, research proposal; for doctorate, thesis/dissertation, research proposal. *Entrance requirements:* For master's, minimum B-average during previous 2 years of coursework; for doctorate, minimum A-average. Additional exam requirements/recommendations for international students: Required—TOEFL (minimum score 550 paper-based), IELTS (minimum score 6.5). Electronic applications accepted. *Faculty research:* Physiology, structure, genetics, and ecology of microbes; virology and microbial technology.

University of Illinois at Chicago, College of Medicine and Graduate College, Graduate Programs in Medicine, Department of Physiology and Biophysics, Chicago, IL 60607-7128. Offers MS, PhD. *Faculty:* 19 full-time (5 women), 3 part-time/adjunct (1 woman). *Students:* 8 full-time (3 women); includes 1 minority (Hispanic/Latino). Average age 28. Terminal master's awarded for partial completion of doctoral program. *Degree requirements:* For master's, thesis; for doctorate, thesis/dissertation. *Entrance requirements:* For master's and doctorate, GRE General Test. Additional exam requirements/recommendations for international students: Required—TOEFL. *Application deadline:* For fall admission, 1/15 priority date for domestic students, 2/15 for international students. Applications are processed on a rolling basis. Application fee: $60. Electronic applications accepted. *Expenses:* Tuition, state resident: full-time $11,480; part-time $3826 per credit. Tuition, nonresident: full-time $23,720; part-time $7906 per credit. *Required fees:* $1333 per semester. Part-time tuition and fees vary according to course load and program. *Financial support:* In 2015–16, 5 fellowships with full tuition reimbursements were awarded; research assistantships with full tuition reimbursements, teaching assistantships with full tuition reimbursements, Federal Work-Study, traineeships, and tuition waivers (full) also available. Financial award application deadline: 3/1; financial award applicants required to submit FAFSA. *Faculty research:* Neuroscience, endocrinology and reproduction, cell physiology, exercise physiology, NMR, cardiovascular physiology and metabolism, cytoskeleton and vascular biology, gastrointestinal and epithelial cell biology, reproductive and endocrine sciences. *Unit head:* Prof. R. John Solaro, Department Head, 312-996-7620, Fax: 312-996-1414, E-mail: solarorj@uic.edu. *Application contact:* Jackie Perry, Graduate College Receptionist, 312-413-2550, Fax: 312-413-0185, E-mail: gradcoll@uic.edu.
Website: http://www.physiology.uic.edu/

University of Illinois at Urbana–Champaign, Graduate College, College of Liberal Arts and Sciences, School of Molecular and Cellular Biology, Center for Biophysics and Computational Biology, Champaign, IL 61820. Offers MS, PhD.

The University of Iowa, Roy J. and Lucille A. Carver College of Medicine and Graduate College, Graduate Programs in Medicine, Department of Molecular Physiology and Biophysics, Iowa City, IA 52242. Offers MS, PhD. *Degree requirements:* For master's, comprehensive exam; for doctorate, comprehensive exam, thesis/dissertation. *Entrance requirements:* For master's, GRE General Test; for doctorate, GRE. Additional exam requirements/recommendations for international students: Required—TOEFL. Electronic applications accepted. *Faculty research:* Cellular and molecular endocrinology, membrane structure and function, cardiac cell electrophysiology, regulation of gene expression, neurophysiology.

The University of Kansas, Graduate Studies, College of Liberal Arts and Sciences, Department of Molecular Biosciences, Lawrence, KS 66044. Offers biochemistry and biophysics (MA, PhD); microbiology (MA, PhD); molecular, cellular, and developmental biology (MA, PhD). *Students:* 57 full-time (34 women), 4 part-time (1 woman); includes 9 minority (5 Asian, non-Hispanic/Latino; 2 Hispanic/Latino; 2 Two or more races, non-Hispanic/Latino), 23 international. Average age 27. 78 applicants, 46% accepted, 18 enrolled. In 2015, 3 master's, 7 doctorates awarded. Terminal master's awarded for partial completion of doctoral program. *Entrance requirements:* For master's and doctorate, GRE General Test. Additional exam requirements/recommendations for international students: Required—TOEFL or IELTS. *Application deadline:* For fall admission, 12/15 for domestic and international students. Application fee: $65 ($85 for international students). Electronic applications accepted. *Financial support:* Fellowships, research assistantships, teaching assistantships, health care benefits, and unspecified assistantships available. Financial award application deadline: 3/1. *Faculty research:* Structure and function of proteins, genetics of organism development, molecular genetics, neurophysiology, molecular virology and pathogenics, developmental biology, cell biology. *Unit head:* Susan M. Egan, Chair, 785-864-4294, E-mail: sme@ku.edu. *Application contact:* John Connolly, Graduate Admissions Contact, 785-864-4311, E-mail: jconnolly@ku.edu.
Website: http://www.molecularbiosciences.ku.edu/

University of Louisville, School of Medicine, Department of Physiology and Biophysics, Louisville, KY 40292-0001. Offers MS, PhD, MD/PhD. *Students:* 36 full-time (15 women), 11 part-time (1 woman); includes 12 minority (3 Black or African American, non-Hispanic/Latino; 4 Asian, non-Hispanic/Latino; 3 Hispanic/Latino; 2 Two or more races, non-Hispanic/Latino), 9 international. Average age 28. 47 applicants, 51% accepted, 20 enrolled. In 2015, 5 master's awarded. *Median time to degree:* Of those who began their doctoral program in fall 2007, 85% received their degree in 8 years or less. *Degree requirements:* For doctorate, comprehensive exam, thesis/dissertation. *Entrance requirements:* For master's and doctorate, GRE General Test (minimum score of 1000 verbal and quantitative), minimum GPA of 3.0. Additional exam requirements/recommendations for international students: Required—TOEFL (minimum score 550 paper-based). *Application deadline:* For fall admission, 1/15 for domestic students; for winter admission, 2/15 for international students; for spring admission, 2/15 for domestic students. Applications are processed on a rolling basis. Application fee: $60. Electronic applications accepted. *Expenses:* Tuition, state resident: full-time $11,664; part-time $649 per credit hour. Tuition, nonresident: full-time $24,274; part-time $1350 per credit hour. *Required fees:* $196. Tuition and fees vary according to program and reciprocity agreements. *Financial support:* In 2015–16, 4 fellowships with full tuition reimbursements (averaging $23,500 per year) were awarded; health care benefits also available. Financial award application deadline: 4/15. *Faculty research:* Vascular remodeling; cerebral microcirculation; renal vasculature; cardiac regeneration. *Total annual research expenditures:* $300,388. *Unit head:* Dr. Irving G. Joshua, Chair, 502-852-5371, Fax: 502-852-6239, E-mail: igjosh01@louisville.edu. *Application contact:* Dr. William Wead, Director of Admissions, 502-852-7571, Fax: 502-852-6849, E-mail: wbwead01@gwise.louisville.edu.
Website: http://louisville.edu/medicine/departments/physiology

The University of Manchester, School of Physics and Astronomy, Manchester, United Kingdom. Offers astronomy and astrophysics (M Sc, PhD); biological physics (M Sc, PhD); condensed matter physics (M Sc, PhD); nonlinear and liquid crystals physics (M Sc, PhD); nuclear physics (M Sc, PhD); particle physics (M Sc, PhD); photon physics (M Sc, PhD); physics (M Sc, PhD); theoretical physics (M Sc, PhD).

University of Maryland, College Park, Academic Affairs, College of Computer, Mathematical and Natural Sciences, Department of Biology, PhD Program in Biological Sciences, College Park, MD 20742. Offers behavior, ecology, evolution, and systematics (PhD); computational biology, bioinformatics, and genomics (PhD); molecular and cellular biology (PhD); physiological systems (PhD). *Degree requirements:* For doctorate, comprehensive exam, thesis/dissertation, thesis work

Biophysics

presentation in seminar. *Entrance requirements:* For doctorate, GRE General Test; GRE Subject Test in biology (recommended), academic transcripts, statement of purpose/research interests, 3 letters of recommendation. Additional exam requirements/recommendations for international students: Required—TOEFL. Electronic applications accepted.

University of Maryland, College Park, Academic Affairs, College of Computer, Mathematical and Natural Sciences, Institute for Physical Science and Technology, Program in Biophysics, College Park, MD 20742. Offers PhD.

University of Miami, Graduate School, Miller School of Medicine, Graduate Programs in Medicine, Department of Physiology and Biophysics, Coral Gables, FL 33124. Offers PhD, MD/PhD. *Degree requirements:* For doctorate, thesis/dissertation, qualifying exam. *Entrance requirements:* For doctorate, GRE General Test, minimum GPA of 3.0 in sciences. Additional exam requirements/recommendations for international students: Required—TOEFL. *Faculty research:* Cell and membrane physiology, cell-to-cell communication, molecular neurobiology, neuroimmunology, neural development.

University of Michigan, Rackham Graduate School, College of Literature, Science, and the Arts, Department of Biophysics, Ann Arbor, MI 48109. Offers biophysics (PhD). *Faculty:* 42 full-time (12 women). *Students:* 33 full-time (11 women); includes 5 minority (2 Black or African American, non-Hispanic/Latino; 2 Asian, non-Hispanic/Latino; 1 Hispanic/Latino), 5 international. Average age 22. 31 applicants, 39% accepted, 3 enrolled. In 2015, 5 doctorates awarded. *Degree requirements:* For doctorate, thesis/dissertation, oral defense of dissertation, preliminary exam. *Entrance requirements:* For doctorate, GRE General Test. Additional exam requirements/recommendations for international students: Required—TOEFL (minimum score 84 iBT). *Application deadline:* For fall admission, 12/1 for domestic and international students. Application fee: $75 ($90 for international students). Electronic applications accepted. Application fee is waived when completed online. *Financial support:* In 2015–16, 10 fellowships with full tuition reimbursements (averaging $29,025 per year), 10 research assistantships with full tuition reimbursements (averaging $29,025 per year), 7 teaching assistantships with full tuition reimbursements (averaging $29,025 per year) were awarded; scholarships/grants, traineeships, health care benefits, and unspecified assistantships also available. Financial award application deadline: 3/15. *Faculty research:* Structural biology, computational biophysics, physical chemistry, cellular biophysics, membrane biophysics. *Unit head:* Dr. Charles Brooks, III, Program Director, 734-764-1146, E-mail: brookscl@umich.edu. *Application contact:* Sara Grosky, Student Services Administrator, 734-763-6722, E-mail: saramin@umich.edu.
Website: https://www.lsa.umich.edu/biophysics

University of Minnesota, Duluth, Medical School, Department of Biochemistry, Molecular Biology and Biophysics, Duluth, MN 55812-2496. Offers biochemistry, molecular biology and biophysics (MS); biology and biophysics (PhD); social, administrative, and clinical pharmacy (MS, PhD); toxicology (MS, PhD). Terminal master's awarded for partial completion of doctoral program. *Degree requirements:* For master's, comprehensive exam, thesis; for doctorate, comprehensive exam, thesis/dissertation. *Entrance requirements:* For master's and doctorate, GRE General Test. Additional exam requirements/recommendations for international students: Required—TOEFL. Electronic applications accepted. *Faculty research:* Intestinal cancer biology; hepatotoxins and mitochondriopathies; toxicology; cell cycle regulation in stem cells; neurobiology of brain development, trace metal function and blood-brain barrier; hibernation biology.

University of Minnesota, Twin Cities Campus, Graduate School, College of Biological Sciences, Biochemistry, Molecular Biology and Biophysics Graduate Program, Minneapolis, MN 55455-0213. Offers PhD. *Degree requirements:* For doctorate, thesis/dissertation. *Entrance requirements:* For doctorate, GRE, 3 letters of recommendation, more than 1 semester of laboratory experience. Additional exam requirements/recommendations for international students: Required—TOEFL (minimum score 625 paper-based; 108 iBT with writing subsection 25 and reading subsection 25) or IELTS (minimum score 7). Electronic applications accepted. *Faculty research:* Microbial biochemistry, biotechnology, molecular biology, regulatory biochemistry, structural biology and biophysics, physical biochemistry, enzymology, physiological chemistry.

University of Minnesota, Twin Cities Campus, Graduate School, Program in Biophysical Sciences and Medical Physics, Minneapolis, MN 55455-0213. Offers MS, PhD. *Program availability:* Part-time. *Degree requirements:* For master's, thesis optional, research paper, oral exam; for doctorate, thesis/dissertation, oral/written preliminary exam, oral final exam. *Faculty research:* Theoretical biophysics, radiological physics, cellular and molecular biophysics.

University of Mississippi Medical Center, School of Graduate Studies in the Health Sciences, Department of Physiology and Biophysics, Jackson, MS 39216-4505. Offers PhD, MD/PhD. *Degree requirements:* For doctorate, thesis/dissertation, first authored publication. *Entrance requirements:* For doctorate, GRE General Test, minimum GPA of 3.0. *Faculty research:* Cardiovascular, renal, endocrine, and cellular neurophysiology; molecular physiology.

University of Missouri–Kansas City, School of Biological Sciences, Program in Cell Biology and Biophysics, Kansas City, MO 64110-2499. Offers PhD. Offered through the School of Graduate Studies. *Faculty:* 31 full-time (9 women), 3 part-time/adjunct (2 women). *Students:* 2 full-time (both women), 7 part-time (1 woman); includes 1 minority (Hispanic/Latino), 4 international. Average age 31. 8 applicants, 25% accepted. *Degree requirements:* For doctorate, comprehensive exam, thesis/dissertation. *Entrance requirements:* For doctorate, GRE General Test, bachelor's degree in chemistry, biology or related field; minimum GPA of 3.0. Additional exam requirements/recommendations for international students: Required—TOEFL (minimum score 550 paper-based; 80 iBT). *Application deadline:* For fall admission, 2/15 priority date for domestic and international students. Applications are processed on a rolling basis. Application fee: $45 ($50 for international students). Electronic applications accepted. *Financial support:* In 2015–16, 11 research assistantships with full tuition reimbursements (averaging $24,189 per year), 17 teaching assistantships with tuition reimbursements (averaging $15,312 per year) were awarded; fellowships with full tuition reimbursements, scholarships/grants, tuition waivers (full and partial), and unspecified assistantships also available. Financial award application deadline: 3/1; financial award applicants required to submit FAFSA. *Unit head:* Dr. Marilyn Yoder, Interim Head, 816-235-1986, E-mail: sbsgradrecruit@umkc.edu. *Application contact:* Mary Flores, Information Contact, 816-235-5247, Fax: 816-235-5158, E-mail: sbsgradrecruit@umkc.edu.
Website: http://sbs.umkc.edu/

The University of North Carolina at Chapel Hill, School of Medicine and Graduate School, Graduate Programs in Medicine, Department of Biochemistry and Biophysics, Chapel Hill, NC 27599. Offers MS, PhD. Terminal master's awarded for partial completion of doctoral program. *Degree requirements:* For master's, comprehensive exam, thesis; for doctorate, comprehensive exam, thesis/dissertation. *Entrance requirements:* For master's and doctorate, GRE General Test, GRE Subject Test (recommended), minimum GPA of 3.0. Additional exam requirements/recommendations for international students: Required—TOEFL. Electronic applications accepted.

University of Regina, Faculty of Graduate Studies and Research, Faculty of Science, Department of Chemistry and Biochemistry, Regina, SK S4S 0A2, Canada. Offers

analytical/environmental chemistry (M Sc, PhD); biophysics of biological interfaces (M Sc, PhD); enzymology/chemical biology (M Sc, PhD); inorganic/organometallic chemistry (M Sc, PhD); signal transduction and mechanisms of cancer cell regulation (M Sc, PhD); supramolecular organic photochemistry and photophysics (M Sc, PhD); synthetic organic chemistry (M Sc, PhD); theoretical/computational chemistry (M Sc, PhD). *Degree requirements:* For master's, thesis; for doctorate, thesis/dissertation. *Entrance requirements:* Additional exam requirements/recommendations for international students: Required—TOEFL (minimum score 580 paper-based; 80 iBT), IELTS (minimum score 6.5), PTE (minimum score 59). Electronic applications accepted. *Faculty research:* Asymmetric synthesis and methodology, theoretical and computational chemistry, biophysical biochemistry, analytical and environmental chemistry, chemical biology.

University of Rochester, School of Medicine and Dentistry, Graduate Programs in Medicine and Dentistry, Department of Biochemistry and Biophysics, Programs in Biophysics, Rochester, NY 14627. Offers biophysics, structural and computational biology (PhD). Terminal master's awarded for partial completion of doctoral program. *Degree requirements:* For doctorate, thesis/dissertation, qualifying exam. *Entrance requirements:* For doctorate, GRE General Test. *Expenses: Tuition, area resident:* Full-time $47,450; part-time $1482 per credit hour. *Required fees:* $528. Tuition and fees vary according to program.

University of Southern California, Keck School of Medicine and Graduate School, Graduate Programs in Medicine, Department of Physiology and Biophysics, Los Angeles, CA 90089. Offers MS. *Faculty:* 13 full-time (2 women). *Students:* 3 full-time (all women); includes 2 minority (1 Asian, non-Hispanic/Latino; 1 Hispanic/Latino). Average age 22. 7 applicants, 43% accepted, 3 enrolled. *Degree requirements:* For master's, thesis optional. *Entrance requirements:* For master's, GRE General Test, minimum GPA of 3.0. Additional exam requirements/recommendations for international students: Required—TOEFL (minimum score 600 paper-based; 100 iBT). *Application deadline:* For fall admission, 12/1 priority date for domestic and international students. Applications are processed on a rolling basis. Application fee: $85. Electronic applications accepted. *Expenses:* Contact institution. *Financial support:* Application deadline: 4/15. *Faculty research:* Endocrinology and metabolism, neurophysiology, mathematical modeling, cell transport, autoimmunity and cancer immunotherapy. *Unit head:* Dr. Berislav Zlokovic, Chair, 323-442-2566, Fax: 323-442-2230, E-mail: zlokovic@usc.edu. *Application contact:* Jim Lee, Student Services Advisor, 323-442-0230, Fax: 323-442-1610, E-mail: jim.lee@med.usc.edu.

University of South Florida, Morsani College of Medicine and College of Graduate Studies, Graduate Programs in Medical Sciences, Tampa, FL 33620-9951. Offers advanced athletic training (MS); athletic training (MS); bioinformatics and computational biology (MSBCB); biotechnology (MSB); health informatics (MSHI); medical sciences (MSMS, PhD), including aging and neuroscience (MSMS), allergy, immunology and infectious disease (PhD), anatomy, athletic training (MSMS), clinical and translational research, health informatics (MSMS), health science (MSMS), interdisciplinary medical sciences (MSMS), medical microbiology and immunology (MSMS), metabolic and nutritional medicine (MSMS), molecular medicine, molecular pharmacology and physiology (PhD), neurology (PhD), pathology and laboratory medicine (PhD), pharmacology and therapeutics (PhD), physiology and biophysics (PhD), women's health (MSMS). *Students:* 510 full-time (261 women), 318 part-time (208 women); includes 360 minority (108 Black or African American, non-Hispanic/Latino; 3 American Indian or Alaska Native, non-Hispanic/Latino; 101 Asian, non-Hispanic/Latino; 124 Hispanic/Latino; 1 Native Hawaiian or other Pacific Islander, non-Hispanic/Latino; 23 Two or more races, non-Hispanic/Latino), 52 international. Average age 26. 6,567 applicants, 13% accepted, 469 enrolled. In 2015, 216 master's awarded. Terminal master's awarded for partial completion of doctoral program. *Degree requirements:* For master's, comprehensive exam, thesis; for doctorate, comprehensive exam, thesis/dissertation. *Entrance requirements:* For master's, GRE General Test or GMAT, bachelor's degree or equivalent from regionally-accredited university with minimum GPA of 3.0 in upper-division sciences coursework; prerequisites in general biology, general chemistry, general physics, organic chemistry, quantitative analysis, and integral and differential calculus; for doctorate, GRE General Test, bachelor's degree from regionally-accredited university with minimum GPA of 3.0 in upper-division sciences coursework; 3 letters of recommendation; personal interview; 1-2 page personal statement; prerequisites in biology, chemistry, physics, organic chemistry, quantitative analysis, and integral/differential calculus. Additional exam requirements/recommendations for international students: Required—TOEFL (minimum score 550 paper-based; 79 iBT) or IELTS (minimum score 6.5). *Application deadline:* For fall admission, 2/15 for domestic students, 1/2 for international students. Application fee: $30. *Expenses:* Contact institution. *Faculty research:* Anatomy, biochemistry, cancer biology, cardiovascular disease, cell biology, immunology, microbiology, molecular biology, neuroscience, pharmacology, physiology. *Unit head:* Dr. Michael Barber, Professor/Associate Dean for Graduate and Postdoctoral Affairs, 813-974-9908, Fax: 813-974-4317, E-mail: mbarber@health.usf.edu. *Application contact:* Dr. Eric Bennett, Graduate Director, PhD Program in Medical Sciences, 813-974-1545, Fax: 813-974-4317, E-mail: esbennet@health.usf.edu.
Website: http://health.usf.edu/nocms/medicine/graduatestudies/

The University of Texas Medical Branch, Graduate School of Biomedical Sciences, Program in Biochemistry and Molecular Biology, Galveston, TX 77555. Offers biochemistry (PhD); bioinformatics (PhD); biophysics (PhD); cell biology (PhD); computational biology (PhD); structural biology (PhD). *Degree requirements:* For doctorate, thesis/dissertation. *Entrance requirements:* Additional exam requirements/recommendations for international students: Required—TOEFL (minimum score 550 paper-based). Electronic applications accepted.

University of Toronto, Faculty of Medicine, Department of Medical Biophysics, Toronto, ON M5S 1A1, Canada. Offers M Sc, PhD. *Degree requirements:* For master's, thesis; for doctorate, thesis/dissertation. *Entrance requirements:* For master's and doctorate, resume, 2 letters of reference. Additional exam requirements/recommendations for international students: Required—TOEFL (minimum score 620 paper-based), TWE (minimum score 5). Electronic applications accepted.

University of Virginia, School of Medicine, Department of Molecular Physiology and Biological Physics, Charlottesville, VA 22903. Offers biological and physical sciences (MS); physiology (PhD); MD/PhD. *Entrance requirements:* For doctorate, GRE General Test, GRE Subject Test. Additional exam requirements/recommendations for international students: Required—TOEFL. Electronic applications accepted.

University of Virginia, School of Medicine, Interdisciplinary Program in Biophysics, Charlottesville, VA 22908. Offers PhD. *Degree requirements:* For doctorate, thesis/dissertation, research proposal, oral defense. *Entrance requirements:* For doctorate, GRE General Test, GRE Subject Test (recommended), 2 or more letters of recommendation. Additional exam requirements/recommendations for international students: Required—TOEFL. Electronic applications accepted. *Faculty research:* Structural biology and structural genomics, structural biology of membrane proteins and membrane biophysics, spectroscopy and thermodynamics of macromolecular interactions, high resolution imaging and cell biophysics.

University of Washington, Graduate School, School of Medicine, Graduate Programs in Medicine, Department of Physiology and Biophysics, Seattle, WA 98195. Offers PhD. *Degree requirements:* For doctorate, thesis/dissertation. *Entrance requirements:* Required—TOEFL (minimum score 580 paper-based; 70 iBT). *Faculty research:* Membrane and cell biophysics, neuroendocrinology, cardiovascular and respiratory physiology, systems neurophysiology and behavior, molecular physiology.

The University of Western Ontario, Faculty of Graduate Studies, Biosciences Division, Department of Medical Biophysics, London, ON N6A 5B8, Canada. Offers M Sc, PhD. *Degree requirements:* For master's, thesis; for doctorate, thesis/dissertation. *Entrance requirements:* Additional exam requirements/recommendations for international students: Required—TOEFL. *Faculty research:* Haemodynamics and cardiovascular biomechanics, microcirculation, orthopedic biomechanics, radiobiology, medical imaging.

University of Wisconsin–Madison, Graduate School, Program in Biophysics, Madison, WI 53706. Offers PhD. *Faculty:* 44 full-time (12 women). *Students:* 35 full-time (15 women); includes 6 minority (1 Black or African American, non-Hispanic/Latino; 1 American Indian or Alaska Native, non-Hispanic/Latino; 1 Asian, non-Hispanic/Latino; 3 Hispanic/Latino), 15 international. Average age 26. 66 applicants, 42% accepted, 8 enrolled. In 2015, 3 doctorates awarded. *Degree requirements:* For doctorate, comprehensive exam, thesis/dissertation. *Entrance requirements:* For doctorate, GRE General Test, minimum GPA of 3.0. Additional exam requirements/recommendations for international students: Required—TOEFL (minimum score 580 paper-based; 92 iBT). *Application deadline:* For fall admission, 12/15 priority date for domestic and international students. Applications are processed on a rolling basis. Application fee: $56. Electronic applications accepted. *Expenses:* Tuition, state resident: full-time $5364. Tuition, nonresident: full-time $12,027. *Required fees:* $571. Tuition and fees vary according to campus/location, program and reciprocity agreements. *Financial support:* In 2015–16, 35 students received support, including 35 research assistantships with full tuition reimbursements available (averaging $26,000 per year); traineeships and health care benefits also available. Financial award application deadline: 12/15. *Faculty research:* NMR spectroscopy, high-speed automated DNA sequencing, x-ray crystallography, neuronal signaling and exocytosis, protein structure. Total annual research expenditures: $10 million. *Unit head:* Dr. Meyer Jackson, Chair, 608-262-9111, Fax: 608-262-7414, E-mail: mjackson@physiology.wics.edu. *Application contact:* Dr. Kim R. Voss, Administrator, 608-262-9880, Fax: 608-262-7414, E-mail: krvoss@wisc.edu.
Website: http://biophysics.wisc.edu/

Vanderbilt University, School of Medicine, Department of Molecular Physiology and Biophysics, Nashville, TN 37240-1001. Offers MS, PhD, MD/PhD. *Faculty:* 31 full-time (4 women). *Students:* 44 full-time (25 women); includes 7 minority (2 Black or African American, non-Hispanic/Latino; 1 Asian, non-Hispanic/Latino; 3 Hispanic/Latino; 1 Two or more races, non-Hispanic/Latino), 2 international. Average age 26. In 2015, 8 doctorates awarded. *Degree requirements:* For doctorate, comprehensive exam, thesis/ dissertation, preliminary, qualifying, and final exams. *Entrance requirements:* For doctorate, GRE General Test, GRE Subject Test (recommended). Additional exam requirements/recommendations for international students: Required—TOEFL (minimum score 570 paper-based; 88 iBT). *Application deadline:* For fall admission, 1/15 for domestic and international students. Application fee: $0. Electronic applications accepted. *Financial support:* Fellowships with full tuition reimbursements, research assistantships with full tuition reimbursements, Federal Work-Study, institutionally sponsored loans, scholarships/grants, traineeships, health care benefits, and tuition waivers (partial) available. Financial award application deadline: 1/15; financial award applicants required to submit CSS PROFILE or FAFSA. *Faculty research:* Biophysics, cell signaling and gene regulation, human genetics, diabetes and obesity, neuroscience. *Unit head:* Dr. Alyssa Hasty, Director of Graduate Studies, 615-322-7000, Fax: 615-343-0490, E-mail: alyssa.hasty@vanderbilt.edu. *Application contact:* Walter B. Bieschke, Program Coordinator for Graduate Admissions, 615-342-0236, E-mail: walter.bieschke@vanderbilt.edu.
Website: http://www.mc.vanderbilt.edu/root/vumc.php?site-MPB

Vanderbilt University, School of Medicine, Program in Chemical and Physical Biology, Nashville, TN 37240-1001. Offers PhD. *Students:* 34 full-time (15 women); includes 8 minority (1 Black or African American, non-Hispanic/Latino; 2 Asian, non-Hispanic/Latino; 5 Hispanic/Latino), 5 international. Average age 29. In 2015, 13 doctorates awarded. *Degree requirements:* For doctorate, comprehensive exam, thesis/ dissertation, dissertation defense. *Entrance requirements:* For doctorate, GRE, 3 letters of recommendation, official transcripts. Additional exam requirements/recommendations for international students: Required—TOEFL. *Application deadline:* For fall admission, 1/ 15 priority date for domestic students, 1/15 for international students. Applications are processed on a rolling basis. Application fee: $0. Electronic applications accepted. *Financial support:* Fellowships with full tuition reimbursements, traineeships, health care benefits, and tuition waivers (full) available. *Faculty research:* Mathematical modeling, enzyme kinetics, structural biology, genomics, proteomics and mass spectrometry. *Unit head:* Dr. Bruce Damon, Director of Graduate Studies, 615-322-4235, Fax: 615-343-0490, E-mail: bruce.damon@vanderbilt.edu. *Application contact:* Patricia Muller, Coordinator, 615-322-8727, E-mail: patricia.l.mueller@vanderbilt.edu.

Washington State University, College of Veterinary Medicine, Program in Molecular Biosciences, Pullman, WA 99164. Offers molecular biology (PhD), including genetics, microbiology; molecular biosciences (PSM, PhD), including biochemistry (PhD), cell biology (PhD). *Program availability:* Online learning. *Faculty:* 30 full-time (12 women), 17 part-time/adjunct (5 women). *Students:* 47 full-time (26 women), 14 part-time (11 women); includes 13 minority (1 Black or African American, non-Hispanic/Latino; 1 American Indian or Alaska Native, non-Hispanic/Latino; 4 Asian, non-Hispanic/Latino; 5 Hispanic/Latino; 2 Two or more races, non-Hispanic/Latino), 1 international. Average age 28. 61 applicants, 23% accepted, 14 enrolled. In 2015, 5 master's, 8 doctorates awarded. Terminal master's awarded for partial completion of doctoral program. *Degree requirements:* For master's, thesis or alternative, oral exam; for doctorate, comprehensive exam, thesis/dissertation, oral exam, written exam. *Entrance requirements:* For master's and doctorate, GRE General Test, minimum GPA of 3.0. Additional exam requirements/recommendations for international students: Required— TOEFL (minimum score 100 iBT). *Application deadline:* For fall admission, 12/15 for domestic and international students. Application fee: $75. Electronic applications accepted. *Financial support:* In 2015–16, 5 fellowships with full tuition reimbursements (averaging $23,316 per year), 24 research assistantships with full tuition reimbursements (averaging $23,316 per year), 17 teaching assistantships with full tuition reimbursements (averaging $23,316 per year) were awarded; career-related internships or fieldwork, Federal Work-Study, traineeships, health care benefits, and unspecified assistantships also available. Financial award application deadline: 4/1; financial award applicants required to submit FAFSA. *Faculty research:* Gene regulation, signal transduction, protein export, reproductive biology, DNA repair. *Total annual research expenditures:* $5.8 million. *Unit head:* Dr. Jonathan Jones, Director, 509-335-8724, Fax: 509-335-9688, E-mail: jcr.jones@vetmed.wsu.edu. *Application contact:* Tami Breske, Coordinator, 509-335-4318, E-mail: tbreske@vetmed.wsu.edu.
Website: http://www.smb.wsu.edu

Weill Cornell Medicine, Weill Cornell Graduate School of Medical Sciences, Physiology, Biophysics and Systems Biology Program, New York, NY 10065. Offers MS, PhD. Terminal master's awarded for partial completion of doctoral program. *Degree requirements:* For master's, comprehensive exam; for doctorate, thesis/dissertation, final exam. *Entrance requirements:* For doctorate, GRE General Test, introductory courses in biology, inorganic and organic chemistry, physics, and mathematics. Additional exam requirements/recommendations for international students: Required— TOEFL. *Faculty research:* Receptor-mediated regulation of cell function, molecular properties of channels or receptors, bioinformatics, mathematical modeling.

Wright State University, School of Graduate Studies, College of Science and Mathematics, Department of Neuroscience, Cell Biology, and Physiology, Dayton, OH 45435. Offers anatomy (MS); physiology and biophysics (MS). *Degree requirements:* For master's, thesis optional. *Entrance requirements:* Additional exam requirements/ recommendations for international students: Required—TOEFL. *Faculty research:* Reproductive cell biology, neurobiology of pain, neurohistochemistry.

Yale University, Graduate School of Arts and Sciences, Department of Molecular Biophysics and Biochemistry, New Haven, CT 06520. Offers PhD. *Degree requirements:* For doctorate, thesis/dissertation. *Entrance requirements:* For doctorate, GRE General Test, GRE Subject Test.

Molecular Biophysics

Baylor College of Medicine, Graduate School of Biomedical Sciences, Program in Structural and Computational Biology and Molecular Biophysics, Houston, TX 77030-3498. Offers PhD, MD/PhD. MD/PhD offered jointly with Rice University and University of Houston. *Degree requirements:* For doctorate, thesis/dissertation, public defense. *Entrance requirements:* For doctorate, GRE General Test, GRE Subject Test (strongly recommended), minimum GPA of 3.0. Additional exam requirements/recommendations for international students: Required—TOEFL. Electronic applications accepted. *Faculty research:* Computational biology, structural biology, biophysics.

California Institute of Technology, Division of Biology and Division of Chemistry and Chemical Engineering, Biochemistry and Molecular Biophysics Graduate Option, Pasadena, CA 91125-0001. Offers PhD. *Degree requirements:* For doctorate, thesis/ dissertation, qualifying exam. *Entrance requirements:* For doctorate, GRE General Test. Additional exam requirements/recommendations for international students: Required— TOEFL. Electronic applications accepted.

California Institute of Technology, Division of Chemistry and Chemical Engineering, Pasadena, CA 91125-0001. Offers biochemistry and molecular biophysics (MS, PhD); chemical engineering (MS, PhD); chemistry (MS, PhD). *Faculty:* 41 full-time (7 women). *Students:* 309 full-time (98 women); includes 1 minority (Black or African American, non-Hispanic/Latino). Average age 26. 710 applicants, 21% accepted, 59 enrolled. In 2015, 14 master's, 59 doctorates awarded. Terminal master's awarded for partial completion of doctoral program. *Degree requirements:* For master's, thesis; for doctorate, thesis/ dissertation. *Entrance requirements:* For doctorate, GRE, BS. Additional exam requirements/recommendations for international students: Required—TOEFL; Recommended—IELTS, TWE. *Application deadline:* For fall admission, 12/15 for domestic and international students. Application fee: $100. Electronic applications accepted. *Financial support:* In 2015–16, 309 students received support, including fellowships (averaging $31,000 per year), research assistantships (averaging $25,900 per year), teaching assistantships (averaging $5,100 per year); Federal Work-Study, institutionally sponsored loans, scholarships/grants, traineeships, health care benefits, and unspecified assistantships also available. Financial award application deadline: 12/

15. *Unit head:* Prof. Jacqueline K. Barton, Chair, Division of Chemistry and Chemical Engineering, 626-395-3646, Fax: 626-395-6948, E-mail: jkbarton@caltech.edu. *Application contact:* Natalie Gilmore, Graduate Office, 626-395-3812, Fax: 626-577-9246, E-mail: ngilmore@its.caltech.edu.
Website: http://www.cce.caltech.edu/

Carnegie Mellon University, Mellon College of Science, Joint Pitt + CMU Molecular Biophysics and Structural Biology Graduate Program, Pittsburgh, PA 15213-3891. Offers PhD. Program offered jointly with University of Pittsburgh. *Degree requirements:* For doctorate, comprehensive exam, thesis/dissertation. *Entrance requirements:* For doctorate, GRE General Test. Additional exam requirements/recommendations for international students: Required—TOEFL (minimum score 600 paper-based; 100 iBT), IELTS (minimum score 7). Electronic applications accepted. *Faculty research:* Structural biology, protein dynamics and folding, computational biophysics, molecular informatics, membrane biophysics and ion channels, NMR, x-ray crystallography cryaelectron microscopy.

Duke University, Graduate School, University Program in Structural Biology and Biophysics, Durham, NC 27710. Offers Certificate. Students must be enrolled in a participating PhD program (biochemistry, cell biology, chemistry, molecular genetics, neurobiology, pharmacology). *Entrance requirements:* For degree, GRE General Test. Additional exam requirements/recommendations for international students: Required— TOEFL (minimum score 577 paper-based; 90 iBT) or IELTS (minimum score 7).

Florida State University, The Graduate School, College of Arts and Sciences, Program in Molecular Biophysics, Tallahassee, FL 32306. Offers molecular biophysics (PhD); structural biology and computational biophysics (PhD). *Faculty:* 34 full-time (7 women). *Students:* 19 full-time (5 women); includes 2 minority (both Hispanic/Latino), 8 international. Average age 29. 14 applicants, 36% accepted, 2 enrolled. In 2015, 5 doctorates awarded. *Degree requirements:* For doctorate, comprehensive exam, thesis/ dissertation, teaching 1 term in professor's major department. *Entrance requirements:* For doctorate, GRE General Test. Additional exam requirements/recommendations for

Molecular Biophysics

international students: Required—TOEFL (minimum score 600 paper-based; 90 iBT). *Application deadline:* For fall admission, 12/15 for domestic and international students. Application fee: $30. Electronic applications accepted. *Expenses:* Tuition, area resident: Full-time $7263; part-time $403.50 per credit hour. Tuition, nonresident: full-time $18,087; part-time $1004.85 per credit hour. *Required fees:* $1365; $75.81 per credit hour. $20 per semester. Tuition and fees vary according to campus/location. *Financial support:* In 2015–16, 23 students received support, including 1 fellowship with tuition reimbursement available (averaging $34,200 per year), 20 research assistantships with tuition reimbursements available (averaging $24,200 per year), 2 teaching assistantships with tuition reimbursements available (averaging $24,200 per year); scholarships/grants, health care benefits, and unspecified assistantships also available. *Faculty research:* Protein and nucleic acid structure and function, membrane protein structure, computational biophysics, 3-D image reconstruction. *Total annual research expenditures:* $2.3 million. *Unit head:* Dr. Hong Li, Director, 850-644-6785, Fax: 850-644-7244, E-mail: hli4@fsu.edu. *Application contact:* Katie Mikusak, Academic Coordinator, Graduate Programs, 850-644-1012, Fax: 850-644-7244, E-mail: kmikusak@chem.fsu.edu.
Website: http://www.biophysics.fsu.edu/graduate-program

Illinois Institute of Technology, Graduate College, College of Science, Department of Biological Sciences, Chicago, IL 60616. Offers biochemistry (MS); biology (MS, PhD); cell and molecular biology (MS); microbiology (MS); molecular biochemistry and biophysics (MS, PhD). *Program availability:* Part-time, evening/weekend, online learning. Terminal master's awarded for partial completion of doctoral program. *Degree requirements:* For master's, comprehensive exam, thesis (for some programs); for doctorate, comprehensive exam, thesis/dissertation. *Entrance requirements:* For master's, GRE General Test (minimum score 300 Quantitative and Verbal, 2.5 Analytical Writing), minimum undergraduate GPA of 3.0; for doctorate, GRE General Test (minimum score 310 Quantitative and Verbal, 3.0 Analytical Writing); GRE Subject Test (strongly recommended), minimum undergraduate GPA of 3.0. Additional exam requirements/recommendations for international students: Required—TOEFL (minimum score 550 paper-based; 80 iBT). Electronic applications accepted. *Faculty research:* Macromolecular crystallography, insect immunity and basic cell biology, improvement of bacterial strains for enhanced biodesulfurization of petroleum, programmed cell death in cancer cells.

New York University, School of Medicine and Graduate School of Arts and Science, Sackler Institute of Graduate Biomedical Sciences, Program in Molecular Biophysics, New York, NY 10012-1019. Offers PhD. *Degree requirements:* For doctorate, comprehensive exam, thesis/dissertation, qualifying examination. *Faculty research:* Receptor tyrosine kinases, biophysics of t-cell activation, ion transport and cell-cell interactions.

Rutgers University–New Brunswick, Graduate School-New Brunswick, BioMaPS Institute for Quantitative Biology, Piscataway, NJ 08854-8097. Offers computational biology and molecular biophysics (PhD). *Degree requirements:* For doctorate, comprehensive exam, thesis/dissertation. *Entrance requirements:* For doctorate, GRE. Additional exam requirements/recommendations for international students: Required—TOEFL. Electronic applications accepted. *Faculty research:* Structural biology, systems biology, bioinformatics, translational medicine, genomics.

University at Buffalo, the State University of New York, Graduate School, Graduate Programs in Cancer Research and Biomedical Sciences at Roswell Park Cancer Institute, Buffalo, NY 14263. Offers cancer pathology and prevention (PhD); cellular and molecular biology (PhD); immunology (PhD); interdisciplinary natural sciences (MS); molecular and cellular biophysics and biochemistry (PhD); molecular pharmacology and cancer therapeutics (PhD). *Faculty:* 126 full-time (36 women). *Students:* 115 full-time (63 women); includes 12 minority (5 Black or African American, non-Hispanic/Latino; 2 Asian, non-Hispanic/Latino; 4 Hispanic/Latino; 1 Native Hawaiian or other Pacific Islander, non-Hispanic/Latino), 31 international. 166 applicants, 33% accepted, 28 enrolled. In 2015, 25 master's, 12 doctorates awarded. Terminal master's awarded for partial completion of doctoral program. *Degree requirements:* For master's, thesis, oral defense of thesis; for doctorate, comprehensive exam, thesis/dissertation, oral defense of dissertation. *Entrance requirements:* For master's and doctorate, GRE General Test. Additional exam requirements/recommendations for international students: Required—TOEFL (minimum score 79 iBT). *Application deadline:* For fall admission, 1/5 priority date for domestic and international students. Application fee: $75. Electronic applications accepted. *Financial support:* In 2015–16, 94 students received support, including 94 research assistantships with full tuition reimbursements available (averaging $25,000 per year); scholarships/grants, health care benefits, and unspecified assistantships also available. Financial award application deadline: 1/5. *Faculty research:* Basic and biomedical cancer research, cell and molecular biology, biophysics, drug design, immunology, genetics, experimental pathology, biochemistry, molecular pharmacology, cancer therapeutics. *Unit head:* Dr. Norman J. Karin, Associate Dean, 716-845-2339, Fax: 716-845-8178, E-mail: norman.karin@roswellpark.edu. *Application contact:* Dr. Norman J. Karin, Associate Dean, 716-845-2339, Fax: 716-845-8178, E-mail: norman.karin@roswellpark.edu.
Website: http://www.roswellpark.edu/education

University of Arkansas for Medical Sciences, Graduate School, Little Rock, AR 72205. Offers biochemistry and molecular biology (MS, PhD); bioinformatics (MS, PhD); cellular physiology and molecular biophysics (MS, PhD); clinical nutrition (MS); interdisciplinary biomedical sciences (MS, PhD, Certificate); interdisciplinary toxicology (MS); microbiology and immunology (PhD); neurobiology and developmental sciences (PhD); pharmacology (PhD); MD/PhD. Bioinformatics programs hosted jointly with the University of Arkansas at Little Rock. *Program availability:* Part-time. Terminal master's awarded for partial completion of doctoral program. *Degree requirements:* For master's, comprehensive exam (for some programs), thesis (for some programs); for doctorate, thesis/dissertation. *Entrance requirements:* For master's and doctorate, GRE. Additional exam requirements/recommendations for international students: Required—TOEFL. Electronic applications accepted. *Expenses:* Contact institution.

University of Chicago, Division of the Biological Sciences, Department of Biochemistry and Molecular Biophysics, Chicago, IL 60637. Offers PhD, MD/PhD. *Students:* 28 full-time (14 women); includes 4 minority (2 Asian, non-Hispanic/Latino; 2 Hispanic/Latino), 6 international. Average age 28. 64 applicants, 28% accepted, 6 enrolled. In 2015, 4 doctorates awarded. *Degree requirements:* For doctorate, thesis/dissertation, ethics class, 2 teaching assistantships. *Entrance requirements:* For doctorate, GRE General Test. Additional exam requirements/recommendations for international students: Required—TOEFL (minimum score 600 paper-based; 104 iBT), IELTS (minimum score 7). *Application deadline:* For fall admission, 12/1 for domestic and international students. Application fee: $90. Electronic applications accepted. *Financial support:* In 2015–16, 26 students received support, including fellowships with tuition reimbursements available (averaging $29,781 per year), research assistantships with tuition reimbursements available (averaging $29,781 per year); institutionally sponsored loans, scholarships/grants, traineeships, and health care benefits also available. Financial award applicants required to submit FAFSA. *Faculty research:* Molecular biology, gene expression, and DNA-protein interactions; membrane biochemistry, molecular endocrinology, and transmembrane signaling; enzyme mechanisms, physical

biochemistry, and structural biology. *Total annual research expenditures:* $5 million. *Unit head:* Dr. Tobin Sosnick, Chair. *Application contact:* Lisa Anderson, Graduate Student Administrator, 773-834-3586, Fax: 773-702-0439, E-mail: landerso@bsd.uchicago.edu. Website: http://bmb.uchospitals.edu/

University of Massachusetts Amherst, Graduate School, Interdisciplinary Programs, Program in Molecular and Cellular Biology, Amherst, MA 01003. Offers biological chemistry and molecular biophysics (PhD); biomedicine (PhD); cellular and developmental biology (PhD). *Program availability:* Part-time. Terminal master's awarded for partial completion of doctoral program. *Degree requirements:* For doctorate, comprehensive exam, thesis/dissertation. *Entrance requirements:* For doctorate, GRE General Test. Additional exam requirements/recommendations for international students: Required—TOEFL (minimum score 550 paper-based; 80 iBT), IELTS (minimum score 6.5). Electronic applications accepted.

University of Pennsylvania, Perelman School of Medicine, Biomedical Graduate Studies, Graduate Group in Biochemistry and Molecular Biophysics, Philadelphia, PA 19104. Offers PhD, MD/PhD, VMD/PhD. *Faculty:* 91. *Students:* 94 full-time (42 women); includes 26 minority (1 Black or African American, non-Hispanic/Latino; 1 American Indian or Alaska Native, non-Hispanic/Latino; 13 Asian, non-Hispanic/Latino; 11 Hispanic/Latino), 11 international. 82 applicants, 34% accepted, 14 enrolled. In 2015, 8 doctorates awarded. *Degree requirements:* For doctorate, thesis/dissertation. *Entrance requirements:* Additional exam requirements/recommendations for international students: Required—TOEFL. *Application deadline:* For fall admission, 12/1 priority date for domestic students, 12/1 for international students. Applications are processed on a rolling basis. Application fee: $80. *Expenses: Tuition, area resident:* Full-time $31,068; part-time $5762 per course. *Required fees:* $3200; $336 per course. Full-time tuition and fees vary according to degree level, program and student level. Part-time tuition and fees vary according to course load, degree level and program. *Financial support:* In 2015–16, 94 students received support. Fellowships, research assistantships, scholarships/grants, traineeships, and unspecified assistantships available. *Faculty research:* Biochemistry of cell differentiation, tissue culture, intermediary metabolism, structure of proteins and nucleic acids, biochemical genetics. *Unit head:* Dr. Kim Sharp, Chairperson, 215-573-3506. *Application contact:* Kelli McKenna, Coordinator, 215-898-4639.
Website: http://www.med.upenn.edu/bmbgrad/

University of Pittsburgh, School of Medicine and Dietrich School of Arts and Sciences, Molecular Biophysics and Structural Biology Graduate Program, Pittsburgh, PA 15260. Offers PhD. PhD jointly offered with Carnegie Mellon University. *Faculty:* 51 full-time (13 women). *Students:* 10 full-time (6 women); includes 1 minority (Hispanic/Latino), 2 international. Average age 26. 46 applicants, 22% accepted. In 2015, 4 doctorates awarded. *Degree requirements:* For doctorate, comprehensive exam, thesis/dissertation. *Entrance requirements:* For doctorate, GRE General Test. Additional exam requirements/recommendations for international students: Required—TOEFL (minimum score 600 paper-based; 100 iBT), IELTS (minimum score 7). *Application deadline:* For fall admission, 12/1 priority date for domestic and international students. Application fee: $50. Electronic applications accepted. Tuition and fees vary according to program. *Financial support:* In 2015–16, 10 students received support, including 2 fellowships with full tuition reimbursements available (averaging $27,000 per year), 8 research assistantships with full tuition reimbursements available (averaging $27,000 per year); teaching assistantships, scholarships/grants, traineeships, and health care benefits also available. *Faculty research:* Structural biology, protein dynamics and folding, computational biophysics, molecular informatics, membrane biophysics and ion channels, x-ray crystallography cryaelectron microscopy. *Unit head:* Dr. James Conway, Director, 412-648-8957, Fax: 412-648-1077, E-mail: mbsbinfo@medschool.pitt.edu. *Application contact:* Lauren Zielinski, Student Affairs Specialist, 412-383-7866, E-mail: mbsbinfo@medschool.pitt.edu.
Website: http://www.mbsb.pitt.edu

The University of Texas Medical Branch, Graduate School of Biomedical Sciences, Program in Cellular Physiology and Molecular Biophysics, Galveston, TX 77555. Offers MS, PhD. *Degree requirements:* For master's, thesis or alternative; for doctorate, thesis/dissertation. *Entrance requirements:* For master's and doctorate, GRE General Test. Additional exam requirements/recommendations for international students: Required—TOEFL (minimum score 550 paper-based). Electronic applications accepted.

The University of Texas Southwestern Medical Center, Southwestern Graduate School of Biomedical Sciences, Division of Basic Science, Program in Molecular Biophysics, Dallas, TX 75390. Offers PhD. *Degree requirements:* For doctorate, thesis/dissertation, qualifying exam. *Entrance requirements:* For doctorate, GRE General Test, minimum GPA of 3.0. Additional exam requirements/recommendations for international students: Required—TOEFL. Electronic applications accepted. *Faculty research:* Optical spectroscopy, x-ray crystallography, protein chemistry, ion channels, contractile and cytoskeletal proteins.

Washington University in St. Louis, Graduate School of Arts and Sciences, Division of Biology and Biomedical Sciences, Program in Computational and Molecular Biophysics, St. Louis, MO 63130-4899. Offers PhD. *Students:* 18 full-time (2 women); includes 1 minority (Asian, non-Hispanic/Latino), 5 international. 30 applicants, 33% accepted, 2 enrolled. In 2015, 1 doctorate awarded. *Degree requirements:* For doctorate, thesis/dissertation. *Entrance requirements:* For doctorate, GRE General Test, GRE Subject Test. Additional exam requirements/recommendations for international students: Required—TOEFL. *Application deadline:* For fall admission, 12/1 priority date for domestic students. Application fee: $0. Electronic applications accepted. *Financial support:* Research assistantships and teaching assistantships available. Financial award application deadline: 1/15. *Faculty research:* Structural biology, protein and nucleic acid kinetics and thermodynamics, single-molecule enzymology, motor proteins, biophysical pathogenesis, protein design, nanoscience, ion channels and lipid membranes, computational biophysics. *Unit head:* Stacia Burd, Coordinator, 314-362-3364. *Application contact:* Rebecca Riney, 314-474-4648, E-mail: dbbsphdadmissions@wusm.wustl.edu.
Website: http://dbbs.wustl.edu/divprograms/biophysics/Pages/ComputationalAndMolecularBiophysics.aspx

Wesleyan University, Graduate Studies, Department of Molecular Biology and Biochemistry, Middletown, CT 06459. Offers biochemistry (PhD); molecular biology (PhD); molecular biophysics (PhD); molecular genetics (PhD). *Faculty:* 8 full-time (3 women), 1 (woman) part-time/adjunct. *Students:* 18 full-time (9 women); includes 4 minority (2 Asian, non-Hispanic/Latino; 1 Hispanic/Latino; 1 Two or more races, non-Hispanic/Latino), 11 international. Average age 24. 28 applicants, 14% accepted, 1 enrolled. Terminal master's awarded for partial completion of doctoral program. *Degree requirements:* For doctorate, comprehensive exam, thesis/dissertation. *Entrance requirements:* For doctorate, GRE General Test, GRE Subject Test. Additional exam requirements/recommendations for international students: Required—TOEFL. *Application deadline:* For fall admission, 1/15 for domestic and international students. Application fee: $0. Electronic applications accepted. *Financial support:* Research assistantships with full tuition reimbursements, teaching assistantships with full tuition reimbursements, and institutionally sponsored loans available. Financial award application deadline: 4/15; financial award applicants required to submit FAFSA. *Faculty* *research:* The olfactory system and new frontiers in genome research, chromosome structure and gene expression, gene co-regulation, crystallographic and spectroscopic analysis, DNA replication and repair. *Unit head:* Scott Holmes, Chair, 860-685-2443, E-mail: sholmes@wesleyan.edu. *Application contact:* Anika Dane, Administrative Assistant, 860-685-2404, E-mail: adane@wesleyan.edu. Website: http://www.wesleyan.edu/mbb/

Yale University, School of Medicine and Graduate School of Arts and Sciences, Combined Program in Biological and Biomedical Sciences (BBS), Molecular Biophysics and Biochemistry Track, New Haven, CT 06520. Offers PhD, MD/PhD. *Degree requirements:* For doctorate, thesis/dissertation. *Entrance requirements:* For doctorate, GRE General Test. Additional exam requirements/recommendations for international students: Required—TOEFL. Electronic applications accepted.

Radiation Biology

Auburn University, College of Veterinary Medicine and Graduate School, Graduate Programs in Veterinary Medicine, Auburn University, AL 36849. Offers biomedical sciences (MS, PhD), including anatomy, physiology and pharmacology (MS), biomedical sciences (PhD), clinical sciences (MS), large animal surgery and medicine (MS), pathobiology (MS), radiology (MS), small animal surgery and medicine (MS); DVM/MS. *Program availability:* Part-time. *Faculty:* 97 full-time (40 women), 4 part-time/adjunct (2 women). *Students:* 19 full-time (11 women), 54 part-time (34 women); includes 10 minority (2 Black or African American, non-Hispanic/Latino; 2 American Indian or Alaska Native, non-Hispanic/Latino; 2 Asian, non-Hispanic/Latino; 4 Hispanic/Latino), 23 international. Average age 31. 39 applicants, 59% accepted, 14 enrolled. In 2015, 12 master's, 0 doctorates awarded. *Degree requirements:* For doctorate, thesis/dissertation. *Entrance requirements:* For master's, GRE General Test; for doctorate, GRE General Test, GRE Subject Test. *Application deadline:* Applications are processed on a rolling basis. Application fee: $50 ($60 for international students). Electronic applications accepted. *Expenses:* Tuition, state resident: full-time $8802; part-time $489 per credit hour. Tuition, nonresident: full-time $26,406; part-time $1467 per credit hour. *Required fees:* $808 per semester. Tuition and fees vary according to degree level and program. *Financial support:* Research assistantships, teaching assistantships, and Federal Work-Study available. Support available to part-time students. Financial award application deadline: 3/15; financial award applicants required to submit FAFSA. *Unit head:* Dr. Calvin Johnson, Acting Dean, 334-844-2650. *Application contact:* Dr. George Flowers, Dean of the Graduate School, 334-844-2125.

Colorado State University, College of Veterinary Medicine and Biomedical Sciences, Department of Environmental and Radiological Health Sciences, Fort Collins, CO 80523-1681. Offers environmental health (MS, PhD); radiological health sciences (MS, PhD); toxicology (MS, PhD). *Program availability:* Part-time. *Faculty:* 31 full-time (13 women), 6 part-time/adjunct (3 women). *Students:* 100 full-time (48 women), 40 part-time (21 women); includes 20 minority (2 Black or African American, non-Hispanic/Latino; 1 American Indian or Alaska Native, non-Hispanic/Latino; 4 Asian, non-Hispanic/Latino; 12 Hispanic/Latino; 1 Two or more races, non-Hispanic/Latino), 9 international. Average age 29. 117 applicants, 83% accepted, 69 enrolled. In 2015, 35 master's, 5 doctorates awarded. Terminal master's awarded for partial completion of doctoral program. *Degree requirements:* For master's, comprehensive exam (for some programs), thesis (for some programs); for doctorate, comprehensive exam, thesis/dissertation. *Entrance requirements:* For master's, GRE, minimum GPA of 3.0; for doctorate, GRE, minimum GPA of 3.0, MS or proof of research. Additional exam requirements/recommendations for international students: Recommended—TOEFL (minimum score 550 paper-based; 80 iBT), IELTS (minimum score 6.5). *Application deadline:* For fall admission, 7/1 for domestic students, 5/1 for international students; for spring admission, 7/1 for domestic students, 5/1 for international students. Applications are processed on a rolling basis. Application fee: $60 ($70 for international students). Electronic applications accepted. *Expenses:* Contact institution. *Financial support:* In 2015–16, 4 students received support, including 16 fellowships with full tuition reimbursements available (averaging $48,116 per year), 21 research assistantships with full tuition reimbursements available (averaging $21,807 per year), 3 teaching assistantships with full tuition reimbursements available (averaging $13,680 per year); scholarships/grants, traineeships, unspecified assistantships, and hourly employment positions also available. Financial award application deadline: 2/1. *Faculty research:* Chromosomes and telomeres in cancer and other human disease states, ambient environmental exposures, radiation physics and dosimetry, cellular toxicity, noise exposure assessment. *Total annual research expenditures:* $8.4 million. *Unit head:* Dr. Jac A. Nickoloff, Professor/Department Head, 970-491-6674, Fax: 970-491-0623, E-mail: j.nickoloff@colostate.edu. *Application contact:* Jeanne A. Brockway, Graduate Program Coordinator, 970-491-5003, Fax: 970-491-2940, E-mail: jeanne.brockway@colostate.edu.
Website: http://csu-cvmbs.colostate.edu/academics/erhs/Pages/graduate-studies.aspx

Georgetown University, Graduate School of Arts and Sciences, Department of Health Physics and Radiation Protection, Washington, DC 20057. Offers health physics (MS); nuclear nonproliferation (MS). *Degree requirements:* For master's, thesis. *Entrance requirements:* Additional exam requirements/recommendations for international students: Required—TOEFL.

Université de Sherbrooke, Faculty of Medicine and Health Sciences, Graduate Programs in Medicine, Program in Radiobiology, Sherbrooke, QC J1H 5N4, Canada. Offers M Sc, PhD. Terminal master's awarded for partial completion of doctoral program. *Degree requirements:* For master's, thesis; for doctorate, thesis/dissertation. Electronic applications accepted. *Faculty research:* DNA repair, physiochemical actions of radiation, radiopharmacy, phototherapy, imaging.

The University of Iowa, Roy J. and Lucille A. Carver College of Medicine and Graduate College, Graduate Programs in Medicine, Program in Free Radical and Radiation Biology, Iowa City, IA 52242-1316. Offers MS. *Program availability:* Part-time. *Degree requirements:* For master's, thesis. *Entrance requirements:* For master's, GRE. Additional exam requirements/recommendations for international students: Required—TOEFL. *Faculty research:* Radiation injury and cellular repair, cell proliferation kinetics, free radical biology, tumor control, positron emission tomography (PET) imaging, electron paramagnetic resonance (EPR).

University of Oklahoma Health Sciences Center, College of Medicine and Graduate College, Graduate Programs in Medicine, Department of Radiological Sciences, Oklahoma City, OK 73190. Offers medical radiation physics (MS, PhD), including diagnostic radiology, nuclear medicine, radiation therapy, ultrasound. *Program availability:* Part-time. Terminal master's awarded for partial completion of doctoral program. *Degree requirements:* For master's, thesis; for doctorate, thesis/dissertation. *Entrance requirements:* For master's, GRE General Test; for doctorate, GRE General Test, 3 letters of recommendation. Additional exam requirements/recommendations for international students: Required—TOEFL. *Faculty research:* Monte Carlo applications in radiation therapy, observer-performed studies in diagnostic radiology, error analysis in gated cardiac nuclear medicine studies, nuclear medicine absorbed fraction determinations.

HARVARD UNIVERSITY
Biophysics Program

 For more information visit http://petersons.to/harvardbiophysics

Program of Study

The Committee on Higher Degrees in Biophysics offers a program of study leading to the Ph.D. degree. The committee comprises senior representatives of the Departments of Chemistry and Chemical Biology, Physics, and Molecular and Cellular Biology; the School of Engineering and Applied Sciences; and the Division of Medical Sciences. Students receive sufficient training in physics, biology, and chemistry to enable them to apply the concepts and methods of the physical sciences to the solution of biological problems.

An initial goal of the Biophysics Program is to provide an introduction through courses and seminars to several of the diverse areas of biophysics, such as structural molecular biology, cell and membrane biophysics, neurobiology, molecular genetics, physical biochemistry, and theoretical biophysics. The program is flexible, and special effort has been devoted to minimizing course work and other formal requirements. Students engage in several research rotations during their first two years. The qualifying examination is taken at the end of the second year to determine admission to candidacy. Students undertake dissertation research as early as possible in the field and subject of their choice. Opportunities for dissertation research are available in a number of special fields. The Ph.D. requires not less than three years devoted to advanced studies, including dissertation research and the dissertation. The Committee on Higher Degrees in Biophysics anticipates that it takes an average of five years, with the maximum being six years, to complete this program.

Research Facilities

Many more of the University's modern research facilities are available to the biophysics student because of the interdepartmental nature of the program. Research programs may be pursued in the Departments of Chemistry and Chemical Biology, Molecular and Cellular Biology, Applied Physics, and Engineering Sciences in Cambridge as well as in the Departments of Biological Chemistry and Molecular Pharmacology, Genetics, Microbiology, Neurobiology, and Cell Biology in the Harvard Medical School Division of Medical Sciences. Research may also be pursued in the Harvard School of Public Health, the Dana Farber Cancer Institute, Children's Hospital, Massachusetts General Hospital, Beth Israel Hospital, and more than ten other Harvard-affiliated institutions located throughout the cities.

Financial Aid

In 2016–17, all graduate students receive a stipend ($36,720 for twelve months) and full tuition and health fees ($47,014). A semester of teaching is required in the second year. Students are strongly encouraged to apply for fellowships from such sources as the National Science Foundation, the NDSEG, the Hertz Foundation, and the Ford Foundation. Full-time Ph.D. candidates in good academic standing are guaranteed full financial support through their sixth year of study or throughout their academic program if less than six years.

Cost of Study

Tuition and health fees for the 2016–17 academic year are $47,014. After two years in residence, students are eligible for a reduced rate (currently $14,976).

Living and Housing Costs

Accommodations in graduate residence halls are available at rents ranging from $6,872 to $10,794 per academic year. In addition, there are approximately 1,500 apartments available for graduate students in Harvard-owned buildings. Applications may be obtained from the Harvard University Housing Office, which also maintains a list of available private rooms, houses, and apartments in the vicinity.

Student Group

On average, the program enrolls roughly 56 students annually. Currently, 12 women and 9 international students are enrolled in the program. Biophysics students intermingle in both their research and their social life with graduate students from the many other departments where research in the biophysical sciences is carried out.

Location

The Biophysics Program maintains a dual-campus orientation in the neighboring cities of Cambridge and Boston. Their proximity provides for a wide range of academic, cultural, extracurricular, and recreational opportunities, and the large numbers of theaters, museums, libraries, and universities contribute to enrich the scientific and cultural life of students. Because New England is compact in area, it is easy to reach countryside, mountains, and seacoast for winter and summer sports or just for a change of scenery.

The University

Established in 1636 in the Massachusetts Bay Colony, Harvard has grown to become a complex of many facilities whose educational vitality, social commitment, and level of cultural achievement contribute to make the University a leader in the academic world. Comprising more than 15,000 students and 3,000 faculty members, Harvard appeals to self-directed, resourceful students of diverse beliefs and backgrounds.

Applying

Students must apply by December 1, 2016, to be considered for admission in September 2017. Scores on the General Test of the Graduate Record Examinations are required except in rare circumstances. GRE Subject Tests are recommended. Due to the early application deadline, applicants should plan to take the GRE test no later than October to ensure that original scores are received by December 1. Information about Graduate School fellowships and scholarships, admission procedures, and graduate study at Harvard may be obtained by writing to the Admissions Office.

Correspondence and Information

For information on the program:
Harvard Biophysics Program
Building C2, Room 122
Harvard Medical School Campus
240 Longwood Avenue
Boston, Massachusetts 02115
United States
E-mail: biophys@fas.harvard.edu
Website: http://fas.harvard.edu/~biophys

For application forms for admission and financial aid (applications accepted online only):
Admissions Office
Graduate School of Arts and Sciences
Holyoke Center
Harvard University
1350 Massachusetts Avenue
Cambridge, Massachusetts 02138
United States
E-mail: admiss@fas.harvard.edu
Website: http://www.gsas.harvard.edu

THE FACULTY AND THEIR RESEARCH

The following faculty members accept students for degree work in biophysics. Thesis research with other faculty members is possible by arrangement.

Mark L. Andermann, Ph.D., Assistant Professor of Medicine. Cognitive networks mediating hunger-dependent attention to food cues.

John Assad, Ph.D., Professor of Neurobiology. Mechanisms of visual processing in the visual cortex of awake behaving monkeys.

Frederick M. Ausubel, Ph.D., Professor of Genetics. Molecular biology of microbial pathogenesis in plants and animals.

Brian J. Bacskai, M.D., Ph.D., Professor of Neurology. Using multi-photon microscopy to address fundamental questions in Alzheimer's disease research.

Stephen C. Blacklow, M.D., Ph.D., Gustavus Adolphus Pfeiffer Professor of Biological Chemistry and Molecular Pharmacology. Molecular basis for specificity in protein folding and protein-protein interactions.

Martha L. Bulyk, Ph.D., Associate Professor of Medicine and Health Sciences and Technology and of Pathology. Computational methods; genomic and proteomic technologies in the study of DNA-protein interactions.

James J. Chou, Ph.D., Associate Professor of Biological Chemistry and Molecular Pharmacology. NMR spectroscopy on membrane-associated proteins and peptides.

George McDonald Church, Ph.D., Professor of Genetics. Human and microbial functional genomics; genotyping; gene expression regulatory network models.

Lee Stirling Churchman, Ph.D., Assistant Professor of Genetics. Regulation of the RNA polymerase motor mechanism in vivo.

SECTION 4: BIOPHYSICS

Harvard University

David E. Clapham, M.D., Ph.D., Professor of Pediatrics and of Neurobiology. Intracellular signal transduction.

Adam E. Cohen, Ph.D., Assistant Professor of Chemistry and Chemical Biology and of Physics. Analysis of structure and function of nicotinic acetylcholine receptors.

Jonathan B. Cohen, Ph.D., Professor of Neurobiology. Structure and function of ligand-gated ion channels.

David P. Corey, Ph.D., Professor of Neurobiology. Ion channels in neural cell membranes.

Vladimir Denic, Ph.D., Assistant Professor of Molecular and Cellular Biology. Structural diversification of very long-chain fatty acids.

Michael M. Desai, Ph.D., Assistant Professor of Organismic and Evolutionary Biology and of Physics. Theoretical and experimental approaches to study genetic variation within populations.

Michael J. Eck, M.D., Ph.D., Professor of Biological Chemistry and Molecular Pharmacology. Structural studies of proteins involved in signal transduction pathways.

Florian Engert, Ph.D., Associate Professor of Molecular and Cellular Biology. Synaptic plasticity and neuronal networks.

Conor L. Evans, Ph.D., Assistant Professor of Dermatology. Development and application of optical detection, treatment, and monitoring approaches targeting major human diseases.

Ethan C. Garner, Ph.D., Assistant Professor of Molecular and Cellular Biology. Organization, structure, and dynamics of the prokaryotic cytoplasm.

Rachelle Gaudet, Ph.D., Associate Professor of Molecular and Cellular Biology. Structural studies of the stereochemistry of signaling and transport through biological membranes.

David E. Golan, M.D., Ph.D., Professor of Biological Chemistry and Molecular Pharmacology and of Medicine. Membrane dynamics; membrane structure; cellular adhesion.

Stephen C. Harrison, Ph.D., Professor of Biological Chemistry and Molecular Pharmacology. Structure of viruses and viral membranes; protein-DNA interactions; structural aspects of signal transduction and membrane traffic; X-ray diffraction.

Lene V. Hau, Ph.D., Mallinckrodt Professor of Physics and Applied Physics. Light-matter interactions, nanoscience, and molecular and synthetic biology.

James M. Hogle, Ph.D., Professor of Biological Chemistry and Molecular Pharmacology. Structure and function of viruses and virus-related proteins; X-ray crystallography.

Sun Hur, Ph.D., Assistant Professor of Biological Chemistry and Molecular Pharmacology. Principles of self versus nonself RNA discrimination by the immune system.

Donald E. Ingber, M.D., Ph.D., Professor of Bioengineering and Judah Folkman Professor of Vascular Biology. Research in integrin signaling, cytoskeleton, and control of angiogenesis.

Tomas Kirchhausen, Ph.D., Professor of Cell Biology. Molecular mechanisms of membrane traffic; X-ray crystallography; chemical genetics.

Andrew J. M. Kiruluta, Ph.D., Associate Professor of Radiology. Novel theory and experiments in NMR spectroscopy.

Nancy Kleckner, Ph.D., Herchel Smith Professor of Molecular Biology. Chromosome metabolism in bacteria and yeast.

Roberto G. Kolter, Ph.D., Professor of Microbiology and Molecular Genetics. DNA protection from oxidative damage; cell-cell communication in biofilms; microbial evolution.

Gabriel Kreiman, Ph.D., Assistant Professor of Neurology. Transcriptional regulatory circuits and neuronal circuits in visual recognition.

Andrew C. Kruse, Ph.D., Assistant Professor of Biological Chemistry and Molecular Pharmacology. Studying the molecular basis of cell signaling through biochemical and biophysical techniques.

Galit Lahav, Ph.D., Associate Professor of Systems Biology. Dynamics of network motifs in single living human cells.

Erel Levine, Ph.D., Assistant Professor of Physics. Communication in and between cells and organisms.

David R. Liu, Ph.D., Professor of Chemistry and Chemical Biology. Organic chemistry and chemical biology.

Jun S. Liu, Ph.D., Professor of Statistics. Stochastic processes, probability theory, and statistical inference.

Joseph J. Loparo, Ph.D., Assistant Professor of Biological Chemistry and Molecular Pharmacology. Developing novel single-molecule methods to study multiprotein complexes.

Jarrod Marto, Ph.D., Assistant Professor of Biological Chemistry and Molecular Pharmacology. Quantitative proteomics of cancer progression.

Keith W. Miller, Ph.D., Mallinckrodt Professor of Pharmacology, Department of Anesthesia. Molecular mechanisms of regulatory conformation changes and drug action on membrane receptors and channels, using rapid kinetics, time-resolved photolabeling, and spectroscopy (EPR, fluorescence, NMR); characterization of lipid-protein interactions in membrane proteins.

Timothy Mitchison, Ph.D., Hasib Sabbagh Professor of Systems Biology. Cytoskeleton dynamics; mechanism of mitosis and cell locomotion; small-molecule inhibitors.

Danesh Moazed, Ph.D., Professor of Cell Biology. Studies on the assembly and stable propagation of epigenetic chromatin domains.

Andrew W. Murray, Ph.D., Herchel Smith Professor of Molecular Genetics. Regulation of mitosis.

Venkatesh N. Murthy, Ph.D., Professor of Molecular and Cellular Biology. Mechanisms of synaptic transmission and plasticity.

Daniel J. Needleman, Ph.D., Assistant Professor of Applied Physics. Physics of macromolecular assemblies and subcellular organization.

Bence P. Olveczky, Ph.D., Assistant Professor of Organismic and Evolutionary Biology. Neurobiology of vocal learning.

Erin K. O'Shea, Ph.D., Professor of Molecular and Cellular Biology and of Chemistry and Chemical Biology. Quantitative analysis of regulatory networks.

David Pellman, M.D., Professor of Cell Biology. The mechanics and regulation of mitosis.

Mara Prentiss, Ph.D., Professor of Physics. Exploitation of optical manipulation to measure adhesion properties, including virus cell binding.

Sharad Ramanathan, Ph.D., Associate Professor of Molecular and Cellular Biology. Decision-making in cells and organisms.

Tom A. Rapoport, Ph.D., Professor of Cell Biology. Mechanism of how proteins are transported across the endoplasmic reticulum membrane.

Gary Ruvkun, Ph.D., Professor of Genetics. Genetic control of developmental timing, neurogenesis, and neural function.

Bernardo L. Sabatini, Ph.D., Associate Professor of Neurobiology. Regulation of synaptic transmission and dendritic function in the mammalian brain.

Aravinthan D. T. Samuel, Ph.D., Associate Professor of Physics. Topics in biophysics, neurobiology, and animal behavior.

Stuart L. Schreiber, Ph.D., Morris Loeb Professor of Chemistry and Chemical Biology. Forward and reverse chemical genetics: using small molecules to explore biology.

Brian Seed, Ph.D., Professor of Genetics. Genetic analysis of signal transduction in the immune system.

Jagesh V. Shah, Ph.D., Assistant Professor of Systems Biology, Assistant Professor of Health Sciences and Technology, and Assistant Professor of Medicine. Quantitative models of cellular behavior to investigate protein function.

Eugene Shakhnovich, Ph.D., Professor of Chemistry and Chemical Biology. Theory and experiments in protein folding and design; theory of molecular evolution; rational drug design and physical chemistry of protein-ligand interactions; theory of complex systems.

William Shih, Ph.D., Associate Professor of Biological Chemistry and Molecular Pharmacology. Biomolecular nanotechnology.

Steven E. Shoelson, M.D., Ph.D., Professor of Medicine. Structural and cellular biology of insulin signal transduction, insulin, resistance, diabetes, and obesity.

Pamela Silver, Ph.D., Professor of Systems Biology. Nucleocytoplasmic transport; RNA-protein interactions; protein methylation; cell-based small-molecule screens.

Poitrek Sliz, Ph.D., Associate Professor of Biological Chemistry and Molecular Pharmacology. Using structural biology and computing as robust tools to dissect mechanisms of disease.

Timothy A. Springer, Ph.D., Latham Family Professor of Pathology. Molecular biology of immune cell interactions.

Hanno Steen, Ph.D., Assistant Professor of Pathology. Cell cycle studies using mass spectrometric and proteomic technology.

Shamil R. Sunyaev, Ph.D., Associate Professor of Genetics. Population genetic variation and genomic divergence, with a focus on protein coding regions.

Jack W. Szostak, Ph.D., Professor of Genetics. Directed evolution; information content and molecular function; self-replicating systems.

Naoshige Uchida, Ph.D., Associate Professor of Molecular and Cellular Biology. Sensory information in neuronal processes.

Gregory L. Verdine, Ph.D., Erving Professor of Chemistry. Protein–nucleic acid interactions; transcriptional regulation; X-ray crystallography.

Gerhard Wagner, Ph.D., Elkan Blout Professor of Biological Chemistry and Molecular Pharmacology. Protein and nucleic acid structure, interaction, and mobility; NMR spectroscopy.

John R. Wakeley, Ph.D., Professor of Organismic and Evolutionary Biology. Theoretical population genetics.

Johannes C. Walter, Ph.D., Professor of Biological Chemistry and Molecular Pharmacology. Maintenance of genome stability in S phase.

George M. Whitesides, Ph.D., Mallinckrodt Professor of Chemistry. Molecular pharmacology; biosurface chemistry; virology.

Wesley P. Wong, Ph.D., Assistant Professor of Biological Chemistry and Molecular Pharmacology. Understanding physical basis of how biological systems work at the nanoscale, focused on the role of mechanical force.

Hao Wu, Ph.D., Asa and Patricia Springer Professor of Structural Biology. Elucidating the molecular mechanism of signal transduction by immune receptors.

Kai Wucherpfennig, M.D., Ph.D., Professor of Neurology. Basic mechanisms of T cell mediated autoimmune diseases.

Xiaoliang Sunney Xie, Ph.D., Mallinckrodt Professor of Chemistry and Chemical Biology. Single-molecule spectroscopy and dynamics; molecular interaction and chemical dynamics in biological systems.

Gary Yellen, Ph.D., Professor of Neurobiology. Molecular physiology of ion channels: functional motions, drug interactions, and electrophysiological mechanisms.

Xaiowei Zhuang, Ph.D., Professor of Chemistry and Chemical Biology and of Physics. Single-molecule biophysics.

Section 5
Botany and Plant Biology

This section contains a directory of institutions offering graduate work in botany and plant biology. Additional information about programs listed in the directory may be obtained by writing directly to the dean of a graduate school or chair of a department at the address given in the directory.

For programs offering related work, see also in this book *Biochemistry; Biological and Biomedical Sciences; Cell, Molecular, and Structural Biology; Ecology, Environmental Biology, and Evolutionary Biology; Entomology; Genetics, Developmental Biology, and Reproductive Biology;* and *Microbiological Sciences.* In the other guides in this series:

Graduate Programs in the Humanities, Arts & Social Sciences
See *Architecture (Landscape Architecture)* and *Economics (Agricultural Economics and Agribusiness)*

Graduate Programs in the Physical Sciences, Mathematics, Agricultural Sciences, the Environment & Natural Resources
See *Agricultural and Food Sciences*

Graduate Programs in Engineering & Applied Sciences
See *Agricultural Engineering* and *Bioengineering*

CONTENTS

Program Directories

Botany

Auburn University, Graduate School, College of Sciences and Mathematics, Department of Biological Sciences, Auburn University, AL 36849. Offers botany (MS); zoology (MS). *Faculty:* 39 full-time (14 women). *Students:* 57 full-time (36 women), 54 part-time (29 women); includes 14 minority (5 Black or African American, non-Hispanic/Latino; 4 Asian, non-Hispanic/Latino; 2 Hispanic/Latino; 3 Two or more races, non-Hispanic/Latino), 12 international. Average age 27. 83 applicants, 43% accepted, 28 enrolled. In 2015, 10 master's, 4 doctorates awarded. *Entrance requirements:* For master's and doctorate, GRE General Test. Additional exam requirements/recommendations for international students: Required—TOEFL. Application fee: $50 ($60 for international students). Electronic applications accepted. *Expenses:* Tuition, state resident: full-time $8802; part-time $489 per credit hour. Tuition, nonresident: full-time $26,406; part-time $1467 per credit hour. *Required fees:* $808 per semester. Tuition and fees vary according to degree level and program. *Financial support:* Research assistantships and teaching assistantships available. Financial award applicants required to submit FAFSA. *Unit head:* Dr. Jack W. Feminella, Chair, 334-844-3906, Fax: 334-844-1645. *Application contact:* Dr. George Flowers, Dean of the Graduate School, 334-844-2125.

Claremont Graduate University, Graduate Programs, Program in Botany, Claremont, CA 91711-6160. Offers MS, PhD. *Program availability:* Part-time. *Faculty:* 4 full-time (2 women). *Students:* 9 full-time (6 women), 4 part-time (1 woman); includes 3 minority (1 American Indian or Alaska Native, non-Hispanic/Latino; 2 Hispanic/Latino), 2 international. Average age 32. In 2015, 4 master's, 4 doctorates awarded. Terminal master's awarded for partial completion of doctoral program. *Entrance requirements:* For master's and doctorate, GRE General Test. Additional exam requirements/recommendations for international students: Required—TOEFL (minimum score 75 iBT). *Application deadline:* For fall admission, 2/1 priority date for domestic and international students. Applications are processed on a rolling basis. Application fee: $80. Electronic applications accepted. *Expenses: Tuition,* area resident: Full-time $43,032; part-time $1793 per unit. *Required fees:* $600; $300 per semester. $300 per semester. Tuition and fees vary according to course load and program. *Financial support:* Fellowships, research assistantships, Federal Work-Study, institutionally sponsored loans, scholarships/grants, and tuition waivers (full) available. Support available to part-time students. Financial award application deadline: 2/15; financial award applicants required to submit FAFSA. *Unit head:* Lucinda McDade, Director of Research/Chair, 909-625-8767 Ext. 234, Fax: 909-626-3489, E-mail: lucinda.mcdade@cgu.edu. *Application contact:* Frances Lehman, Program Coordinator, 909-625-8767 Ext. 241, Fax: 909-626-3489, E-mail: botany@cgu.edu.
Website: http://www.cgu.edu/pages/1311.asp

Colorado State University, College of Natural Sciences, Department of Biology, Fort Collins, CO 80523-1878. Offers botany (MS, PhD); zoology (MS, PhD). *Faculty:* 29 full-time (9 women), 4 part-time/adjunct (3 women). *Students:* 18 full-time (8 women), 22 part-time (13 women); includes 5 minority (4 Asian, non-Hispanic/Latino; 1 Hispanic/Latino), 6 international. Average age 30. 18 applicants, 94% accepted, 11 enrolled. In 2015, 7 master's, 2 doctorates awarded. Terminal master's awarded for partial completion of doctoral program. *Degree requirements:* For master's, comprehensive exam, thesis; for doctorate, comprehensive exam, thesis/dissertation. *Entrance requirements:* For master's and doctorate, GRE General Test (minimum scores above 70th percentile), transcripts, 3 letters of recommendation, statement of purpose, minimum GPA of 3.0. Additional exam requirements/recommendations for international students: Required—TOEFL (minimum score 550 paper-based; 80 iBT), IELTS (minimum score 6.5). *Application deadline:* For fall admission, 1/15 priority date for domestic and international students; for spring admission, 11/1 priority date for domestic and international students. Applications are processed on a rolling basis. Application fee: $60 ($70 for international students). Electronic applications accepted. *Expenses:* Tuition, state resident: full-time $9348. Tuition, nonresident: full-time $22,916. *Required fees:* $2174; $473.72 per credit hour. $236.86 per semester. Tuition and fees vary according to course load and program. *Financial support:* In 2015–16, 21 fellowships (averaging $42,613 per year), 12 research assistantships with full tuition reimbursements (averaging $18,531 per year), 66 teaching assistantships with full tuition reimbursements (averaging $17,703 per year) were awarded; career-related internships or fieldwork, Federal Work-Study, scholarships/grants, traineeships, and unspecified assistantships also available. Financial award application deadline: 1/1; financial award applicants required to submit FAFSA. *Faculty research:* Global ecological change; organismal interactions in infectious disease; stream ecology; muscle protein structure; plant biotechnology. *Total annual research expenditures:* $7.8 million. *Unit head:* Dr. Michael F. Antolin, Department Chair, 970-491-7011, Fax: 970-491-0649, E-mail: michael.antolin@colostate.edu. *Application contact:* Dorothy Ramirez, Graduate Coordinator, 970-491-1923, Fax: 970-491-0649, E-mail: dramirez@colostate.edu.
Website: http://www.biology.colostate.edu/

Dalhousie University, Faculty of Agriculture, Halifax, NS B3H 4R2, Canada. Offers agriculture (M Sc), including air quality, animal behavior, animal molecular genetics, animal nutrition, animal technology, aquaculture, botany, crop management, crop physiology, ecology, environmental microbiology, food science, horticulture, nutrient management, pest management, physiology, plant biotechnology, plant pathology, soil chemistry, soil fertility, waste management and composting, water quality. *Program availability:* Part-time. *Degree requirements:* For master's, thesis, ATC Exam Teaching Assistantship. *Entrance requirements:* For master's, honors B Sc, minimum GPA of 3.0. Additional exam requirements/recommendations for international students: Required—TOEFL (minimum score 580 paper-based; 92 iBT), IELTS, Michigan English Language Assessment Battery, CanTEST, CAEL. *Faculty research:* Bio-product development, organic agriculture, nutrient management, air and water quality, agricultural biotechnology.

Eastern New Mexico University, Graduate School, College of Liberal Arts and Sciences, Department of Biology, Portales, NM 88130. Offers applied ecology (MS); botany (MS); cell, molecular biology and biotechnology (MS); microbiology (MS); zoology (MS). *Program availability:* Part-time. *Degree requirements:* For master's, comprehensive exam, thesis optional. *Entrance requirements:* For master's, GRE, minimum GPA of 3.0, 2 letters of recommendation, statement of research interest, bachelor's degree related to field of study or proof of common knowledge. Additional exam requirements/recommendations for international students: Required—TOEFL (minimum score 550 paper-based; 79 iBT), IELTS (minimum score 6). Electronic applications accepted.

Emporia State University, Department of Biological Sciences, Emporia, KS 66801-5415. Offers botany (MS); environmental biology (MS); general biology (MS); microbial and cellular biology (MS); zoology (MS). *Program availability:* Part-time. *Faculty:* 14 full-time (3 women), 1 part-time/adjunct (0 women). *Students:* 26 full-time (13 women), 15 part-time (7 women); includes 1 minority (Two or more races, non-Hispanic/Latino), 24 international. 16 applicants, 100% accepted, 11 enrolled. In 2015, 17 master's awarded. *Degree requirements:* For master's, comprehensive exam or thesis. *Entrance requirements:* For master's, GRE, appropriate undergraduate degree, interview, letters of reference. Additional exam requirements/recommendations for international students: Required—TOEFL (minimum score 520 paper-based; 68 iBT). *Application deadline:* For fall admission, 8/15 priority date for domestic students. Applications are processed on a rolling basis. Application fee: $30 ($75 for international students). Electronic applications accepted. *Expenses:* Tuition, state resident: full-time $5640; part-time $235 per credit hour. Tuition, nonresident: full-time $17,544; part-time $731 per credit hour. *Required fees:* $1848; $77 per credit hour. *Financial support:* In 2015–16, 7 research assistantships with full tuition reimbursements (averaging $7,344 per year), 12 teaching assistantships with full tuition reimbursements (averaging $7,844 per year) were awarded; career-related internships or fieldwork, Federal Work-Study, institutionally sponsored loans, health care benefits, and unspecified assistantships also available. Financial award application deadline: 3/15; financial award applicants required to submit FAFSA. *Faculty research:* Fisheries, range, and wildlife management; aquatic, plant, grassland, vertebrate, and invertebrate ecology; mammalian and plant systematics, taxonomy, and evolution; immunology, virology, and molecular biology. *Unit head:* Dr. Yixin Eric Yang, Chair, 620-341-5311, Fax: 620-341-5608, E-mail: yyang@emporia.edu. Website: http://www.emporia.edu/info/degrees-courses/grad/biology

Illinois State University, Graduate School, College of Arts and Sciences, Department of Biological Sciences, Normal, IL 61790-2200. Offers animal behavior (MS); bacteriology (MS); biochemistry (MS); biological sciences (MS); biology (PhD); biophysics (MS); biotechnology (MS); botany (MS, PhD); cell biology (MS); conservation biology (MS); developmental biology (MS); ecology (MS, PhD); entomology (MS); evolutionary biology (MS); genetics (MS, PhD); immunology (MS); microbiology (MS, PhD); molecular biology (MS); molecular genetics (MS); neurobiology (MS); neuroscience (MS); parasitology (MS); physiology (MS, PhD); plant biology (MS); plant molecular biology (MS); plant sciences (MS); structural biology (MS); zoology (MS, PhD). *Program availability:* Part-time. *Degree requirements:* For master's, thesis or alternative; for doctorate, variable foreign language requirement, thesis/dissertation, 2 terms of residency. *Entrance requirements:* For master's, GRE General Test, minimum GPA of 2.6 in last 60 hours of course work; for doctorate, GRE General Test. *Application deadline:* Applications are processed on a rolling basis. Application fee: $40. *Financial support:* Research assistantships, teaching assistantships, Federal Work-Study, tuition waivers (full), and unspecified assistantships available. Financial award application deadline: 4/1. *Faculty research:* Redoc balance and drug development in schistosoma mansoni, control of the growth of listeria monocytogenes at low temperature, regulation of cell expansion and microtubule function by SPRI, CRUI: physiology and fitness consequences of different life history phenotypes. *Application contact:* Steven Juliano, Graduate Coordinator, E-mail: sajulian@ilstu.edu.
Website: http://www.bio.ilstu.edu/

North Carolina State University, Graduate School, College of Agriculture and Life Sciences, Department of Plant Biology, Raleigh, NC 27695. Offers MS, PhD. *Program availability:* Part-time. Terminal master's awarded for partial completion of doctoral program. *Degree requirements:* For master's, thesis (for some programs); for doctorate, thesis/dissertation. *Entrance requirements:* For master's and doctorate, GRE. Additional exam requirements/recommendations for international students: Required—TOEFL. Electronic applications accepted. *Faculty research:* Plant molecular and cell biology, aquatic ecology, community ecology, restoration, systematics plant pathogen and environmental interactions.

North Dakota State University, College of Graduate and Interdisciplinary Studies, College of Science and Mathematics, Department of Biological Sciences, Fargo, ND 58102. Offers biology (MS); botany (MS, PhD); cellular and molecular biology (PhD); genomics (PhD); zoology (MS, PhD). *Degree requirements:* For master's, thesis; for doctorate, thesis/dissertation. *Entrance requirements:* For master's and doctorate, GRE General Test. Additional exam requirements/recommendations for international students: Required—TOEFL. *Application deadline:* For fall admission, 1/15 for domestic students. Applications are processed on a rolling basis. Application fee: $35. Electronic applications accepted. *Financial support:* Fellowships with full tuition reimbursements, research assistantships with full tuition reimbursements, teaching assistantships with full tuition reimbursements, career-related internships or fieldwork, Federal Work-Study, institutionally sponsored loans, scholarships/grants, tuition waivers (full), and unspecified assistantships available. Support available to part-time students. Financial award application deadline: 4/15; financial award applicants required to submit FAFSA. *Faculty research:* Comparative endocrinology, physiology, behavioral ecology, plant cell biology, aquatic biology. *Unit head:* Dr. Wendy Reed, Head, 701-231-5921, E-mail: wendy.reed@ndsu.edu. *Application contact:* Elizabeth Worth, Marketing, Recruitment, and Public Relations Coordinator, 701-231-8476, Fax: 701-231-6524, E-mail: elizabeth.worth@ndsu.edu.
Website: http://www.ndsu.edu/biology/

Oklahoma State University, College of Arts and Sciences, Department of Plant Biology, Ecology, and Evolution, Stillwater, OK 74078. Offers botany (MS); environmental science (MS, PhD); plant science (PhD). *Faculty:* 14 full-time (5 women). *Students:* 8 part-time (3 women); includes 4 minority (1 Asian, non-Hispanic/Latino; 1 Hispanic/Latino; 2 Two or more races, non-Hispanic/Latino). Average age 32. 3 applicants, 67% accepted. In 2015, 3 master's awarded. *Degree requirements:* For master's, thesis; for doctorate, comprehensive exam, thesis/dissertation. *Entrance requirements:* For master's and doctorate, GRE or GMAT. Additional exam requirements/recommendations for international students: Required—TOEFL (minimum score 550 paper-based; 79 iBT). *Application deadline:* For fall admission, 3/1 priority date for international students; for spring admission, 8/1 priority date for international students. Applications are processed on a rolling basis. Application fee: $40 ($75 for international students). Electronic applications accepted. *Expenses:* Tuition, state resident: full-time $3528; part-time $196 per credit hour. Tuition, nonresident: full-time $14,144; part-time $785.75 per credit hour. *Required fees:* $1895; $105.25 per credit hour. Tuition and fees vary according to campus/location. *Financial support:* In 2015–16, 1 research assistantship (averaging $18,504 per year), 12 teaching assistantships (averaging $20,754 per year) were awarded; career-related internships or fieldwork, Federal Work-Study, scholarships/grants, health care benefits, tuition waivers (partial), and unspecified assistantships also available. Support available to part-time students. Financial award application deadline: 3/1; financial award applicants required to submit FAFSA. *Faculty research:* Ethnobotany, developmental genetics of arabidopsis, biological roles of plasmodesmata, community ecology and biodiversity, nutrient cycling in grassland ecosystems. *Unit head:* Dr. Linda Watson, Department Head, 405-744-5559, Fax: 405-744-7074, E-mail: linda.watson10@okstate.edu.
Website: http://plantbio.okstate.edu

Oregon State University, College of Agricultural Sciences, Program in Botany and Plant Pathology, Corvallis, OR 97331. Offers M Ag, MA, MS, PhD. *Faculty:* 23 full-time (4 women), 3 part-time/adjunct (0 women). *Students:* 39 full-time (18 women), 1 part-time (0 women); includes 4 minority (1 Black or African American, non-Hispanic/Latino; 1 Hispanic/Latino; 2 Two or more races, non-Hispanic/Latino), 5 international. Average age 29. 58 applicants, 28% accepted, 8 enrolled. In 2015, 8 master's, 3 doctorates awarded. *Entrance requirements:* For master's and doctorate, GRE. *Application deadline:* For fall admission, 12/1 for domestic and international students. Application fee: $75 ($85 for international students). *Expenses:* Tuition, state resident: full-time $12,150; part-time $450 per credit. Tuition, nonresident: full-time $20,952; part-time $776 per credit. *Required fees:* $1572; $1443 per unit. One-time fee: $350. Tuition and fees vary according to course load, campus/location and program. *Financial support:* Application deadline: 12/15. *Unit head:* Dr. Lynda M. Ciuffetti, Professor and Department Head.
Website: http://bpp.oregonstate.edu/

Purdue University, Graduate School, College of Agriculture, Department of Botany and Plant Pathology, West Lafayette, IN 47907. Offers MS, PhD. *Program availability:* Part-time. Terminal master's awarded for partial completion of doctoral program. *Degree requirements:* For master's, thesis; for doctorate, thesis/dissertation. *Entrance requirements:* For master's, GRE General Test, minimum undergraduate GPA of 3.0 or equivalent; for doctorate, GRE, minimum undergraduate GPA of 3.0 or equivalent. Additional exam requirements/recommendations for international students: Required—TOEFL (minimum score 550 paper-based; 77 iBT); Recommended—TWE. Electronic applications accepted. *Faculty research:* Biotechnology, plant growth, weed control, crop improvement, plant physiology.

The University of British Columbia, Faculty of Science, Department of Botany, Vancouver, BC V6T 1Z1, Canada. Offers M Sc, PhD. *Degree requirements:* For master's, thesis; for doctorate, comprehensive exam, thesis/dissertation. *Entrance requirements:* Additional exam requirements/recommendations for international students: Required—TOEFL. Electronic applications accepted. *Faculty research:* Plant ecology, evolution and systematics, cell and developmental biology, plant physiology/biochemistry, genetics.

University of California, Riverside, Graduate Division, Department of Botany and Plant Sciences, Riverside, CA 92521-0102. Offers plant biology (MS, PhD), including plant cell, molecular, and developmental biology (PhD), plant ecology (PhD), plant genetics (PhD). *Program availability:* Part-time. Terminal master's awarded for partial completion of doctoral program. *Degree requirements:* For master's, comprehensive exams or thesis; for doctorate, thesis/dissertation, qualifying exams. *Entrance requirements:* For master's and doctorate, GRE General Test, minimum GPA of 3.2. Additional exam requirements/recommendations for international students: Required—TOEFL (minimum score 550 paper-based; 80 iBT). Electronic applications accepted. *Expenses: Tuition,* area resident: Full-time $16,665.50; part-time $11,055.54. Tuition, state resident: full-time $16,665.50; part-time $11,055.54. Tuition, nonresident: full-time $31,768. *International tuition:* $31,767.50 full-time. *Required fees:* $16,665.50; $11,055.54 per quarter. $3685.18 per quarter. Tuition and fees vary according to program. *Faculty research:* Agricultural plant biology; biochemistry and physiology; cellular, molecular and developmental biology; ecology, evolution, systematics and ethnobotany; genetics, genomics and bioinformatics.

University of Connecticut, Graduate School, College of Liberal Arts and Sciences, Department of Ecology and Evolutionary Biology, Storrs, CT 06269. Offers botany (MS, PhD). Terminal master's awarded for partial completion of doctoral program. *Degree requirements:* For master's, comprehensive exam; for doctorate, thesis/dissertation. *Entrance requirements:* For master's and doctorate, GRE General Test, GRE Subject Test. Additional exam requirements/recommendations for international students: Required—TOEFL (minimum score 550 paper-based). *Application deadline:* For fall admission, 2/1 priority date for domestic and international students; for spring admission, 11/1 for domestic students, 10/1 for international students. Applications are processed on a rolling basis. Application fee: $55. Electronic applications accepted. *Financial support:* Fellowships, research assistantships with full tuition reimbursements, teaching assistantships with full tuition reimbursements, Federal Work-Study, scholarships/grants, health care benefits, and unspecified assistantships available. Financial award application deadline: 2/1; financial award applicants required to submit FAFSA.
Website: http://www.eeb.uconn.edu/

University of Florida, Graduate School, College of Liberal Arts and Sciences, Department of Biology, Gainesville, FL 32611. Offers botany (MS, MST, PhD), including botany, tropical conservation and development, wetland sciences; zoology (MS, MST, PhD), including animal molecular and cellular biology (PhD), tropical conservation and development, wetland sciences, zoology. *Faculty:* 9 full-time, 9 part-time/adjunct. *Students:* 96 full-time (41 women), 6 part-time (3 women); includes 9 minority (4 Asian, non-Hispanic/Latino; 5 Hispanic/Latino), 35 international. 77 applicants, 30% accepted, 16 enrolled. In 2015, 8 master's, 15 doctorates awarded. *Degree requirements:* For master's, comprehensive exam (for some programs), thesis; for doctorate, comprehensive exam, thesis/dissertation. *Entrance requirements:* For master's and doctorate, GRE General Test, minimum GPA of 3.0. Additional exam requirements/recommendations for international students: Required—TOEFL (minimum score 550 paper-based; 80 iBT), IELTS (minimum score 6). *Application deadline:* For fall admission, 12/1 for domestic and international students. Applications are processed on a rolling basis. Application fee: $30. Electronic applications accepted. *Financial support:* In 2015–16, 9 fellowships, 36 research assistantships, 62 teaching assistantships were awarded; unspecified assistantships also available. Financial award application deadline: 12/15; financial award applicants required to submit FAFSA. *Faculty research:* Ecology of natural populations, plant and animal genome evolution, biodiversity, plant biology, behavior. *Total annual research expenditures:* $3.6 million. *Unit head:* Dr. Marta Wayne, PhD, Professor and Chair, 352-392-9925, E-mail: mlwayne@ufl.edu. *Application contact:* William T. Barbazuk, PhD, Associate Professor/Graduate Coordinator, 352-273-8624, Fax: 352-392-3704, E-mail: bbarbazuk@ufl.edu.
Website: http://www.biology.ufl.edu/

University of Guelph, Graduate Studies, College of Biological Science, Department of Integrative Biology, Botany and Zoology, Guelph, ON N1G 2W1, Canada. Offers botany (M Sc, PhD); zoology (M Sc, PhD). *Program availability:* Part-time. *Degree requirements:* For master's, thesis, research proposal; for doctorate, thesis/dissertation, research proposal, qualifying exams. *Entrance requirements:* For master's, minimum B average during previous 2 years of course work. Additional exam requirements/recommendations for international students: Required—TOEFL (minimum score 550 paper-based), IELTS (minimum score 6.5). Electronic applications accepted. *Faculty research:* Aquatic science, environmental physiology, parasitology, wildlife biology, management.

University of Guelph, Graduate Studies, College of Biological Science, Department of Molecular and Cellular Biology, Guelph, ON N1G 2W1, Canada. Offers biochemistry (M Sc, PhD); biophysics (M Sc, PhD); botany (M Sc, PhD); microbiology (M Sc, PhD); molecular biology and genetics (M Sc, PhD). *Degree requirements:* For master's, thesis, research proposal; for doctorate, comprehensive exam, thesis/dissertation, research proposal. *Entrance requirements:* For master's, minimum B-average during previous 2 years of coursework; for doctorate, minimum A-average. Additional exam requirements/recommendations for international students: Required—TOEFL (minimum score 550 paper-based), IELTS (minimum score 6.5). Electronic applications accepted. *Faculty research:* Physiology, structure, genetics, and ecology of microbes; virology and microbial technology.

University of Hawaii at Manoa, Graduate Division, College of Natural Sciences, Department of Botany, Honolulu, HI 96822. Offers MS, PhD. *Program availability:* Part-time. *Faculty:* 23 full-time (8 women), 6 part-time/adjunct (0 women). *Students:* 31 full-time (21 women), 4 part-time (2 women); includes 14 minority (1 Asian, non-Hispanic/Latino; 3 Hispanic/Latino; 1 Native Hawaiian or other Pacific Islander, non-Hispanic/Latino; 9 Two or more races, non-Hispanic/Latino), 3 international. Average age 33. 35 applicants, 20% accepted, 6 enrolled. In 2015, 10 master's, 4 doctorates awarded. Terminal master's awarded for partial completion of doctoral program. *Degree requirements:* For master's, one foreign language, thesis optional, presentation; for doctorate, one foreign language, comprehensive exam, thesis/dissertation, presentation. *Entrance requirements:* For master's and doctorate, GRE General Test, GRE Subject Test (biology). Additional exam requirements/recommendations for international students: Required—TOEFL (minimum score 540 paper-based; 76 iBT), IELTS (minimum score 5). *Application deadline:* For fall admission, 2/1 for domestic students, 1/15 for international students. Application fee: $100. *Financial support:* In 2015–16, 2 students received support, including 15 fellowships (averaging $1,563 per year), 18 research assistantships (averaging $20,869 per year), 14 teaching assistantships (averaging $16,409 per year); tuition waivers (full and partial) also available. *Faculty research:* Plant ecology, evolution, systematics, conservation biology, ethnobotany. *Total annual research expenditures:* $14.3 million. *Unit head:* William Ditto, Dean, 808-956-6451, E-mail: wditto@hawaii.edu. *Application contact:* Tom Ranker, Graduate Field Chair, 808-956-3930, Fax: 808-956-3923, E-mail: ranker@hawaii.edu.
Website: http://www.botany.hawaii.edu/

The University of Kansas, Graduate Studies, College of Liberal Arts and Sciences, Department of Ecology and Evolutionary Biology, Lawrence, KS 66045. Offers botany (MA, PhD); ecology and evolutionary biology (MA, PhD); entomology (MA, PhD). *Students:* 69 full-time (35 women), 1 part-time (0 women); includes 8 minority (1 Black or African American, non-Hispanic/Latino; 1 Asian, non-Hispanic/Latino; 4 Native Hawaiian or other Pacific Islander, non-Hispanic/Latino; 2 Two or more races, non-Hispanic/Latino), 22 international. Average age 28. 66 applicants, 39% accepted, 20 enrolled. In 2015, 3 master's, 5 doctorates awarded. Terminal master's awarded for partial completion of doctoral program. *Degree requirements:* For master's, comprehensive exam, thesis (for some programs), 30-36 credits, thesis presentation; for doctorate, comprehensive exam, thesis/dissertation, residency, responsible scholarship and research skills, final exam, dissertation defense. *Entrance requirements:* For master's, GRE General Test, bachelor's degree with minimum undergraduate GPA of 3.0; for doctorate, GRE General Test, bachelor's degree; minimum undergraduate/graduate GPA of 3.0. Additional exam requirements/recommendations for international students: Required—TOEFL or IELTS. *Application deadline:* For fall admission, 12/1 for domestic and international students; for spring admission, 9/15 for domestic and international students. Application fee: $65 ($85 for international students). Electronic applications accepted. *Financial support:* Fellowships, research assistantships, teaching assistantships, scholarships/grants, traineeships, health care benefits, and unspecified assistantships available. Financial award application deadline: 12/1. *Faculty research:* Ecology and global change, diversity and macroevolution, evolutionary mechanisms, systematics/phylogenetics, biogeography. *Unit head:* Dr. Christopher H. Haufler, Chair, 785-864-3255, E-mail: vulgare@ku.edu. *Application contact:* Aagje Ashe, Graduate Coordinator, 785-864-2362, Fax: 785-864-5860, E-mail: a4ashe@ku.edu.
Website: http://eeb.ku.edu/

University of Maine, Graduate School, College of Natural Sciences, Forestry, and Agriculture, School of Biology and Ecology, Orono, ME 04469. Offers biological sciences (PhD); botany and plant pathology (MS); ecology and environmental sciences (MS, PhD); entomology (MS); plant science (PhD); zoology (MS, PhD). *Program availability:* Part-time. *Faculty:* 24 full-time (12 women), 34 part-time/adjunct (13 women). *Students:* 64 full-time (36 women), 1 part-time (0 women); includes 4 minority (1 American Indian or Alaska Native, non-Hispanic/Latino; 1 Asian, non-Hispanic/Latino; 1 Hispanic/Latino; 1 Two or more races, non-Hispanic/Latino), 8 international. Average age 29. 52 applicants, 25% accepted, 11 enrolled. In 2015, 7 master's, 8 doctorates awarded. Terminal master's awarded for partial completion of doctoral program. *Degree requirements:* For master's, thesis (for some programs); for doctorate, comprehensive exam, thesis/dissertation. *Entrance requirements:* For master's and doctorate, GRE General Test. Additional exam requirements/recommendations for international students: Required—TOEFL. *Application deadline:* For fall admission, 2/1 priority date for domestic students. Applications are processed on a rolling basis. Application fee: $65. Electronic applications accepted. *Financial support:* In 2015–16, 14 students received support, including 6 research assistantships with full tuition reimbursements available (averaging $14,600 per year), 8 teaching assistantships with full tuition reimbursements available (averaging $14,600 per year); career-related internships or fieldwork, Federal Work-Study, institutionally sponsored loans, and tuition waivers (full and partial) also available. Financial award application deadline: 3/1. *Faculty research:* Ecology and evolution (aquatic, terrestrial, paleo); development and genetics; biomedical research; ecophysiology and stress; invasion ecology and pest management. *Total annual research expenditures:* $3.2 million. *Unit head:* Dr. Andrei Aloykhin, Director, 207-581-2977, Fax: 207-581-2537. *Application contact:* Scott G. Delcourt, Assistant Vice President for Graduate Studies and Senior Associate Dean, 207-581-3291, Fax: 207-581-3232, E-mail: graduate@maine.edu.
Website: http://sbe.umaine.edu/

University of Manitoba, Faculty of Graduate Studies, Faculty of Science, Department of Biological Sciences, Winnipeg, MB R3T 2N2, Canada. Offers botany (M Sc, PhD); ecology (M Sc, PhD); zoology (M Sc, PhD).

The University of North Carolina at Chapel Hill, Graduate School, College of Arts and Sciences, Department of Biology, Chapel Hill, NC 27599. Offers botany (MA, MS, PhD); cell biology, development, and physiology (MA, MS, PhD); cell motility and cytoskeleton (PhD); ecology and behavior (MA, MS, PhD); genetics and molecular biology (MA, MS, PhD); morphology, systematics, and evolution (MA, MS, PhD). Terminal master's awarded for partial completion of doctoral program. *Degree requirements:* For master's, comprehensive exam, thesis (for some programs); for doctorate, comprehensive exam, thesis/dissertation. *Entrance requirements:* For master's, GRE General Test, GRE Subject Test, 2 semesters of calculus or statistics; 2 semesters of physics, organic chemistry; 3 semesters of biology; for doctorate, GRE General Test, GRE Subject Test, 2 semesters calculus or statistics, 2 semesters physics, organic chemistry, 3 semesters of biology. Additional exam requirements/recommendations for international students: Required—TOEFL (minimum score 550 paper-based). Electronic applications accepted. *Faculty research:* Gene expression, biomechanics, yeast genetics, plant ecology, plant molecular biology.

Botany

University of North Dakota, Graduate School, College of Arts and Sciences, Department of Biology, Grand Forks, ND 58202. Offers botany (MS, PhD); ecology (MS, PhD); entomology (MS, PhD); environmental biology (MS, PhD); fisheries/wildlife (MS, PhD); genetics (MS, PhD); zoology (MS, PhD). Terminal master's awarded for partial completion of doctoral program. *Degree requirements:* For master's, thesis, final exam; for doctorate, comprehensive exam, thesis/dissertation, final exam. *Entrance requirements:* For master's, GRE General Test, GRE Subject Test, minimum GPA of 3.0; for doctorate, GRE General Test, GRE Subject Test, minimum GPA of 3.5. Additional exam requirements/recommendations for international students: Required—TOEFL (minimum score 550 paper-based; 79 iBT), IELTS (minimum score 6.5). Electronic applications accepted. *Faculty research:* Population biology, wildlife ecology, RNA processing, hormonal control of behavior.

University of Wisconsin–Madison, Graduate School, College of Letters and Science, Department of Botany, Madison, WI 53706-1380. Offers MS, PhD. *Program availability:* Part-time. Terminal master's awarded for partial completion of doctoral program. *Degree requirements:* For master's, thesis; for doctorate, one foreign language, thesis/dissertation. *Entrance requirements:* For master's and doctorate, GRE General Test. Electronic applications accepted. *Expenses:* Tuition, state resident: full-time $5364. Tuition, nonresident: full-time $12,027. *Required fees:* $571. Tuition and fees vary

according to campus/location, program and reciprocity agreements. *Faculty research:* Taxonomy and systematics; ecology; structural botany; physiological, cellular, and molecular biology.

University of Wisconsin–Oshkosh, Graduate Studies, College of Letters and Science, Department of Biology and Microbiology, Oshkosh, WI 54901. Offers biology (MS), including botany, microbiology, zoology. *Degree requirements:* For master's, comprehensive exam, thesis. *Entrance requirements:* For master's, GRE General Test, minimum GPA of 3.0, BS in biology. Additional exam requirements/recommendations for international students: Required—TOEFL (minimum score 550 paper-based; 79 iBT). Electronic applications accepted.

University of Wyoming, College of Arts and Sciences, Department of Botany, Laramie, WY 82071. Offers botany (MS, PhD); botany/water resources (MS). *Program availability:* Part-time. Terminal master's awarded for partial completion of doctoral program. *Degree requirements:* For master's, thesis; for doctorate, thesis/dissertation. *Entrance requirements:* For master's and doctorate, GRE General Test, minimum GPA of 3.0. Additional exam requirements/recommendations for international students: Required—TOEFL. Electronic applications accepted. *Faculty research:* Ecology, systematics, physiology, mycology, genetics.

Plant Biology

Arizona State University at the Tempe campus, College of Liberal Arts and Sciences, School of Life Sciences, Tempe, AZ 85287-4601. Offers animal behavior (PhD); applied ethics (biomedical and health ethics) (MA); biology (MS, PhD), including biology, biology and society, complex adaptive systems science (PhD), plant biology and conservation (MS); environmental life sciences (PhD); evolutionary biology (PhD); history and philosophy of science (PhD); human and social dimensions of science and technology (PhD); microbiology (PhD); molecular and cellular biology (PhD); neuroscience (PhD). Terminal master's awarded for partial completion of doctoral program. *Degree requirements:* For master's, thesis (for some programs), interactive Program of Study (iPOS) submitted before completing 50 percent of required credit hours; for doctorate, variable foreign language requirement, comprehensive exam, thesis/dissertation, interactive Program of Study (iPOS) submitted before completing 50 percent of required credit hours. *Entrance requirements:* For master's and doctorate, GRE, minimum GPA of 3.0 or equivalent in last 2 years of work leading to bachelor's degree. Additional exam requirements/recommendations for international students: Required—TOEFL (minimum score 600 paper-based; 100 iBT). Electronic applications accepted.

Clemson University, Graduate School, College of Agriculture, Forestry and Life Sciences, Department of Plant and Environmental Sciences, Program in Plant and Environmental Sciences, Clemson, SC 29634. Offers MS, PhD. *Faculty:* 5 full-time (2 women). *Students:* 30 full-time (9 women), 16 part-time (5 women); includes 1 minority (Two or more races, non-Hispanic/Latino), 21 international. Average age 30. 27 applicants, 33% accepted, 7 enrolled. In 2015, 12 master's, 8 doctorates awarded. *Degree requirements:* For master's, thesis; for doctorate, comprehensive exam, thesis/dissertation. *Entrance requirements:* For master's and doctorate, GRE General Test, unofficial transcripts, letters of recommendation. Additional exam requirements/recommendations for international students: Required—TOEFL (minimum score 550 paper-based; 80 iBT), IELTS (minimum score 6.5), PTE (minimum score 54). *Application deadline:* For fall admission, 4/15 for domestic and international students; for spring admission, 11/15 for domestic and international students. Applications are processed on a rolling basis. Application fee: $80 ($90 for international students). Electronic applications accepted. *Expenses:* $4,060 per semester full-time resident, $8,103 per semester full-time non-resident, $448 per credit hour part-time resident, $898 per credit hour part-time non-resident. *Financial support:* In 2015–16, 33 students received support, including 3 fellowships with partial tuition reimbursements available (averaging $5,000 per year), 20 research assistantships with partial tuition reimbursements available (averaging $17,289 per year), 10 teaching assistantships with partial tuition reimbursements available (averaging $16,581 per year); career-related internships or fieldwork and health care benefits also available. Financial award application deadline: 4/15. *Faculty research:* Agronomy, horticulture, plant pathology, plant physiology, entomology. *Unit head:* Dr. Patricia Zungoli, Department Head, 864-656-5041, Fax: 864-656-4960, E-mail: pzngl@clemson.edu. *Application contact:* Dr. Paula Agudelo, Graduate Program Coordinator, 864-656-5741, E-mail: pagudel@clemson.edu.
Website: http://www.clemson.edu/graduate/academics/program-details.html?m_id=Plant-Environmental-Sciences

Cornell University, Graduate School, Graduate Fields of Agriculture and Life Sciences, Field of Plant Biology, Ithaca, NY 14853-0001. Offers cytology (MS, PhD); paleobotany (MS, PhD); plant biochemistry (MS, PhD); plant cell biology (MS, PhD); plant ecology (MS, PhD); plant molecular biology (MS, PhD); plant morphology, anatomy and biomechanics (MS, PhD); plant physiology (MS, PhD); systematic botany (MS, PhD). *Degree requirements:* For doctorate, comprehensive exam, thesis/dissertation. *Entrance requirements:* For doctorate, GRE General Test, GRE Subject Test in biology (recommended), 3 letters of recommendation. Additional exam requirements/recommendations for international students: Required—TOEFL (minimum score 610 paper-based; 77 iBT). Electronic applications accepted. *Faculty research:* Plant cell biology/cytology; plant molecular biology; plant morphology/anatomy/biomechanics; plant physiology, systematic botany, paleobotany; plant ecology, ethnobotany, plant biochemistry, photosynthesis.

Florida State University, The Graduate School, College of Arts and Sciences, Department of Biological Science, Specialization in Plant Biology, Tallahassee, FL 32304-4295. Offers MS, PhD. *Faculty:* 10 full-time (5 women). *Students:* 13 full-time (6 women); includes 2 minority (both Hispanic/Latino), 5 international. In 2015, 1 master's, 2 doctorates awarded. Terminal master's awarded for partial completion of doctoral program. *Degree requirements:* For master's, comprehensive exam, thesis, teaching experience, seminar presentation; for doctorate, comprehensive exam, thesis/dissertation, teaching experience, seminar presentation. *Entrance requirements:* For master's and doctorate, GRE General Test, minimum upper-division GPA of 3.0. Additional exam requirements/recommendations for international students: Required—TOEFL (minimum score 600 paper-based; 92 iBT). *Application deadline:* For fall admission, 12/1 for domestic and international students. Application fee: $30. Electronic applications accepted. *Expenses: Tuition, area resident:* Full-time $7263; part-time $403.50 per credit hour. *Tuition, nonresident:* full-time $18,087; part-time $1004.85 per credit hour. *Required fees:* $1365; $75.81 per credit hour. $20 per semester. Tuition and fees vary according to campus/location. *Financial support:* In 2015–16, 13 students

received support, including 5 research assistantships with full tuition reimbursements available (averaging $21,500 per year), 8 teaching assistantships with full tuition reimbursements available (averaging $21,500 per year). Financial award application deadline: 12/1; financial award applicants required to submit FAFSA. *Faculty research:* Plant cell and molecular biology; plant population ecology and evolution; meiosis in higher plants; plant systematics, evolution, ecology, and biogeography; plant-environment interaction; community ecology; plant-insect interactions; rhizobial/plant symbiotic interactions; cell fate specification and reprogramming in plants; evolutionary and developmental biology; plant-environment interaction. *Unit head:* Dr. Thomas A. Houpt, Professor and Associate Chair, 850-644-4907, Fax: 850-644-8447, E-mail: houpt@neuro.fsu.edu. *Application contact:* Dr. Michael B. Miller, Coordinator, Graduate Affairs, 850-644-3023, Fax: 850-644-9829, E-mail: gradinfo@bio.fsu.edu.
Website: http://bio.fsu.edu

Illinois State University, Graduate School, College of Arts and Sciences, Department of Biological Sciences, Normal, IL 61790-2200. Offers animal behavior (MS); bacteriology (MS); biochemistry (MS); biological sciences (MS); biology (PhD); biophysics (MS); biotechnology (MS); botany (MS, PhD); cell biology (MS); conservation biology (MS); developmental biology (MS); ecology (MS, PhD); entomology (MS); evolutionary biology (MS); genetics (MS, PhD); immunology (MS); microbiology (MS, PhD); molecular biology (MS); molecular genetics (MS); neurobiology (MS); neuroscience (MS); parasitology (MS); physiology (MS, PhD); plant biology (MS); plant molecular biology (MS); plant sciences (MS); structural biology (MS); zoology (MS, PhD). *Program availability:* Part-time. *Degree requirements:* For master's, thesis or alternative; for doctorate, variable foreign language requirement, thesis/dissertation, 2 terms of residency. *Entrance requirements:* For master's, GRE General Test, minimum GPA of 2.6 in last 60 hours of course work; for doctorate, GRE General Test. *Application deadline:* Applications are processed on a rolling basis. Application fee: $40. *Financial support:* Research assistantships, teaching assistantships, Federal Work-Study, tuition waivers (full), and unspecified assistantships available. Financial award application deadline: 4/1. *Faculty research:* Redoc balance and drug development in schistosoma mansoni, control of the growth of listeria monocytogenes at low temperature, regulation of cell expansion and microtubule function by SPRI, CRUI: physiology and fitness consequences of different life history phenotypes. *Application contact:* Steven Juliano, Graduate Coordinator, E-mail: sajulian@ilstu.edu.
Website: http://www.bio.ilstu.edu/

Indiana University Bloomington, University Graduate School, College of Arts and Sciences, Department of Biology, Bloomington, IN 47405. Offers biology teaching (MAT); biotechnology (MA); evolution, ecology, and behavior (MA, PhD); genetics (PhD); microbiology (MA, PhD); molecular, cellular, and developmental biology (PhD); plant sciences (MA, PhD); zoology (MA, PhD). Terminal master's awarded for partial completion of doctoral program. *Degree requirements:* For master's, thesis, oral defense; for doctorate, thesis/dissertation, oral defense. *Entrance requirements:* For master's and doctorate, GRE General Test. Additional exam requirements/recommendations for international students: Required—TOEFL (minimum score 100 iBT). Electronic applications accepted. *Faculty research:* Evolution, ecology and behavior; microbiology; molecular biology and genetics; plant biology.

Iowa State University of Science and Technology, Program in Plant Biology, Ames, IA 50011. Offers MS, PhD. *Degree requirements:* For master's, thesis; for doctorate, thesis/dissertation. *Entrance requirements:* For master's and doctorate, GRE General Test. Additional exam requirements/recommendations for international students: Required—TOEFL (minimum score 550 paper-based; 79 iBT), IELTS (minimum score 6.5). Electronic applications accepted.

Michigan State University, The Graduate School, College of Agriculture and Natural Resources, MSU-DOE Plant Research Laboratory, East Lansing, MI 48824. Offers biochemistry and molecular biology (PhD); cellular and molecular biology (PhD); crop and soil sciences (PhD); genetics (PhD); microbiology and molecular genetics (PhD); plant biology (PhD); plant physiology (PhD). Offered jointly with the Department of Energy. *Degree requirements:* For doctorate, comprehensive exam, thesis/dissertation, laboratory rotation, defense of dissertation. *Entrance requirements:* For doctorate, GRE General Test, acceptance into one of the affiliated department programs; 3 letters of recommendation; bachelor's degree or equivalent in life sciences, chemistry, biochemistry, or biophysics; research experience. Electronic applications accepted. *Faculty research:* Role of hormones in the regulation of plant development and physiology, molecular mechanisms associated with signal recognition, development and application of genetic methods and materials, protein routing and function.

Michigan State University, The Graduate School, College of Natural Science and College of Agriculture and Natural Resources, Department of Plant Biology, East Lansing, MI 48824. Offers plant biology (MS, PhD); plant breeding, genetics and biotechnology - plant biology (MS, PhD). *Entrance requirements:* Additional exam requirements/recommendations for international students: Required—TOEFL. Electronic applications accepted. *Faculty research:* Physiological, molecular, and biochemical mechanisms; systematics; inheritance; ecology and geohistory.

New York University, Graduate School of Arts and Science, Department of Biology, New York, NY 10012-1019. Offers biology (PhD); biomedical journalism (MS); cancer and molecular biology (PhD); computational biology (PhD); computers in biological research (MS); developmental genetics (PhD); general biology (MS); immunology and microbiology (PhD); molecular genetics (PhD); neurobiology (PhD); oral biology (MS); plant biology (PhD); recombinant DNA technology (MS); MS/MBA. *Program availability:* Part-time. Terminal master's awarded for partial completion of doctoral program. *Degree requirements:* For master's, thesis or alternative, qualifying paper; for doctorate, comprehensive exam, thesis/dissertation. *Entrance requirements:* For master's and doctorate, GRE General Test. Additional exam requirements/recommendations for international students: Required—TOEFL. *Faculty research:* Genomics, molecular and cell biology, development and molecular genetics, molecular evolution of plants and animals.

North Carolina State University, Graduate School, College of Agriculture and Life Sciences, Department of Plant Biology, Raleigh, NC 27695. Offers MS, PhD. *Program availability:* Part-time. Terminal master's awarded for partial completion of doctoral program. *Degree requirements:* For master's, thesis (for some programs); for doctorate, thesis/dissertation. *Entrance requirements:* For master's and doctorate, GRE. Additional exam requirements/recommendations for international students: Required—TOEFL. Electronic applications accepted. *Faculty research:* Plant molecular and cell biology, aquatic ecology, community ecology, restoration, systematics plant pathogen and environmental interactions.

Northwestern University, The Graduate School, Judd A. and Marjorie Weinberg College of Arts and Sciences, Program in Plant Biology and Conservation, Evanston, IL 60208. Offers MA, PhD. Program held jointly with Chicago Botanic Garden.

Ohio University, Graduate College, College of Arts and Sciences, Department of Environmental and Plant Biology, Athens, OH 45701-2979. Offers MS, PhD. *Program availability:* Part-time. *Degree requirements:* For master's, thesis, 2 terms of teaching experience; for doctorate, comprehensive exam, thesis/dissertation, 2 terms of teaching experience. *Entrance requirements:* For master's, GRE General Test, minimum GPA of 3.0; for doctorate, GRE General Test, minimum GPA of 3.2. Additional exam requirements/recommendations for international students: Required—TOEFL (minimum score 620 paper-based; 105 iBT) or IELTS (minimum score 7.5). Electronic applications accepted. *Faculty research:* Eastern deciduous forest ecology, evolutionary developmental plant biology, phylogenetic systematics, plant cell wall biotechnology.

Oklahoma State University, College of Arts and Sciences, Department of Plant Biology, Ecology, and Evolution, Stillwater, OK 74078. Offers botany (MS); environmental science (MS, PhD); plant science (PhD). *Faculty:* 14 full-time (5 women). *Students:* 8 part-time (2 women); includes 4 minority (1 Asian, non-Hispanic/Latino; 1 Hispanic/Latino; 2 Two or more races, non-Hispanic/Latino). Average age 32. 3 applicants, 67% accepted. In 2015, 3 master's awarded. *Degree requirements:* For master's, thesis; for doctorate, comprehensive exam, thesis/dissertation. *Entrance requirements:* For master's and doctorate, GRE or GMAT. Additional exam requirements/recommendations for international students: Required—TOEFL (minimum score 550 paper-based; 79 iBT). *Application deadline:* For fall admission, 3/1 priority date for international students; for spring admission, 8/1 priority date for international students. Applications are processed on a rolling basis. Application fee: $40 ($75 for international students). Electronic applications accepted. *Expenses:* Tuition, state resident: full-time $3528; part-time $196 per credit hour. Tuition, nonresident: full-time $14,144; part-time $785.75 per credit hour. *Required fees:* $1895; $105.25 per credit hour. Tuition and fees vary according to campus/location. *Financial support:* In 2015–16, 1 research assistantship (averaging $18,504 per year), 12 teaching assistantships (averaging $20,754 per year) were awarded; career-related internships or fieldwork, Federal Work-Study, scholarships/grants, health care benefits, tuition waivers (partial), and unspecified assistantships also available. Support available to part-time students. Financial award application deadline: 3/1; financial award applicants required to submit FAFSA. *Faculty research:* Ethnobotany, developmental genetics of arabidopsis, biological roles of plasmodesmata, community ecology and biodiversity, nutrient cycling in grassland ecosystems. *Unit head:* Dr. Linda Watson, Department Head, 405-744-5559, Fax: 405-744-7074, E-mail: linda.watson10@okstate.edu. Website: http://plantbio.okstate.edu

Penn State University Park, Graduate School, Intercollege Graduate Programs, Intercollege Graduate Program in Plant Biology, University Park, PA 16802. Offers plant biology (MS, PhD). *Unit head:* Dr. Regina Vasilatos-Younken, Dean, 814-865-2516, Fax: 814-863-4627. *Application contact:* Lori Stania, Director, Graduate Student Services, 814-865-1795, Fax: 814-863-4627, E-mail: l-gswww@lists.psu.edu.

Rutgers University–New Brunswick, Graduate School-New Brunswick, Program in Plant Biology, Piscataway, NJ 08854-8097. Offers horticulture and plant technology (MS, PhD); molecular and cellular biology (MS, PhD); organismal and population biology (MS, PhD); plant pathology (MS, PhD). *Program availability:* Part-time. Terminal master's awarded for partial completion of doctoral program. *Degree requirements:* For master's, comprehensive exam, thesis or alternative; for doctorate, comprehensive exam, thesis/dissertation. *Entrance requirements:* For master's and doctorate, GRE General Test, GRE Subject Test (recommended). Additional exam requirements/recommendations for international students: Required—TOEFL (minimum score 600 paper-based). Electronic applications accepted. *Faculty research:* Molecular biology and biochemistry of plants, plant development and genomics, plant protection, plant improvement, plant management of horticultural and field crops.

Southern Illinois University Carbondale, Graduate School, College of Science, Department of Plant Biology, Carbondale, IL 62901-4701. Offers MS, PhD. *Faculty:* 13 full-time (2 women). *Students:* 5 full-time (3 women), 15 part-time (7 women); includes 5 minority (2 Black or African American, non-Hispanic/Latino; 1 Asian, non-Hispanic/Latino; 2 Hispanic/Latino), 13 international. Average age 25. 20 applicants, 35% accepted, 3 enrolled. In 2015, 8 master's, 4 doctorates awarded. *Degree requirements:* For master's, thesis; for doctorate, one foreign language, thesis/dissertation. *Entrance requirements:* For master's, GRE General Test, minimum GPA of 2.7; for doctorate, GRE General Test, minimum GPA of 3.25. Additional exam requirements/recommendations for international students: Required—TOEFL (minimum score 80 iBT). *Application deadline:* Applications are processed on a rolling basis. Application fee: $65. *Financial support:* In 2015–16, 23 students received support, including 1 fellowship with full tuition reimbursement available, 6 research assistantships with full tuition reimbursements available, 16 teaching assistantships with full tuition reimbursements available; Federal Work-Study, institutionally sponsored loans, and tuition waivers (full) also available. Support available to part-time students. *Faculty research:* Algal toxins, ethnobotany, community and wetland ecology, morphogenesis, systematics and evolution. *Total annual research expenditures:* $524,140. *Unit head:* Dr. Stephen Ebbs, Chair, 618-453-3226, E-mail: sebbs@plant.siu.edu. *Application contact:* David Gibson, Director of Graduate Studies, 618-453-3231, E-mail: dgibson@plant.siu.edu.

Université Laval, Faculty of Agricultural and Food Sciences, Program in Plant Biology, Québec, QC G1K 7P4, Canada. Offers M Sc, PhD. Terminal master's awarded for partial completion of doctoral program. *Degree requirements:* For master's, thesis (for some programs); for doctorate, comprehensive exam, thesis/dissertation. *Entrance requirements:* For master's and doctorate, knowledge of French and English. Electronic applications accepted.

University of Alberta, Faculty of Graduate Studies and Research, Department of Biological Sciences, Edmonton, AB T6G 2E1, Canada. Offers environmental biology and ecology (M Sc, PhD); microbiology and biotechnology (M Sc, PhD); molecular biology and genetics (M Sc, PhD); physiology and cell biology (M Sc, PhD); plant biology (M Sc, PhD); systematics and evolution (M Sc, PhD). Terminal master's awarded for partial completion of doctoral program. *Degree requirements:* For master's, thesis; for doctorate, thesis/dissertation. *Entrance requirements:* Additional exam requirements/recommendations for international students: Required—TOEFL.

University of California, Berkeley, Graduate Division, College of Natural Resources, Department of Plant and Microbial Biology, Berkeley, CA 94720-1500. Offers plant biology (PhD). *Degree requirements:* For doctorate, thesis/dissertation, qualifying exam, seminar presentation. *Entrance requirements:* For doctorate, GRE General Test, minimum GPA of 3.0, 3 letters of recommendation. *Faculty research:* Development, molecular biology, genetics, microbial biology, mycology.

University of California, Davis, Graduate Studies, Graduate Group in Plant Biology, Davis, CA 95616. Offers MS, PhD. *Degree requirements:* For master's, comprehensive exam (for some programs), thesis (for some programs); for doctorate, thesis/dissertation. *Entrance requirements:* For master's, GRE General Test, GRE Subject Test (biology), minimum GPA of 3.0; for doctorate, GRE General Test, GRE Subject Test (biology). Additional exam requirements/recommendations for international students: Required—TOEFL (minimum score 550 paper-based). Electronic applications accepted. *Faculty research:* Cell and molecular biology, ecology, systematics and evolution, integrative plant and crop physiology, plant development and structure.

University of California, Riverside, Graduate Division, Department of Botany and Plant Sciences, Riverside, CA 92521-0102. Offers plant biology (MS, PhD), including plant cell, molecular, and developmental biology (PhD), plant ecology (PhD), plant genetics (PhD). *Program availability:* Part-time. Terminal master's awarded for partial completion of doctoral program. *Degree requirements:* For master's, comprehensive exams or thesis; for doctorate, thesis/dissertation, qualifying exams. *Entrance requirements:* For master's and doctorate, GRE General Test, minimum GPA of 3.2. Additional exam requirements/recommendations for international students: Required—TOEFL (minimum score 550 paper-based; 80 iBT). Electronic applications accepted. *Expenses:* Tuition, area resident: Full-time $16,665.50; part-time $11,055.54. Tuition, state resident: full-time $16,665.50; part-time $11,055.54. Tuition, nonresident: full-time $31,768. International tuition: $31,767.50 full-time. *Required fees:* $16,665.50; $11,055.54 per quarter. $3685.18 per quarter. Tuition and fees vary according to program. *Faculty research:* Agricultural plant biology; biochemistry and physiology; cellular, molecular and developmental biology; ecology, evolution, systematics and ethnobotany; genetics, genomics and bioinformatics.

University of Florida, Graduate School, College of Agricultural and Life Sciences and College of Liberal Arts and Sciences, Program in Plant Molecular and Cellular Biology, Gainesville, FL 32611. Offers plant molecular and cellular biology (MS, PhD), including toxicology (PhD). *Faculty:* 41. *Students:* 27 full-time (9 women), 1 part-time; includes 3 minority (1 Black or African American, non-Hispanic/Latino; 1 Asian, non-Hispanic/Latino; 1 Hispanic/Latino), 15 international. Average age 28. 33 applicants, 24% accepted, 6 enrolled. In 2015, 5 doctorates awarded. *Degree requirements:* For master's, thesis; for doctorate, comprehensive exam, thesis/dissertation, first author peer-reviewed publication. *Entrance requirements:* For master's and doctorate, GRE General Test, minimum GPA of 3.0. Additional exam requirements/recommendations for international students: Required—TOEFL (minimum score 550 paper-based; 80 iBT), IELTS (minimum score 6). *Application deadline:* For fall admission, 1/3 priority date for domestic students, 1/3 for international students; for spring admission, 8/1 for domestic and international students. Applications are processed on a rolling basis. Application fee: $30. Electronic applications accepted. *Financial support:* In 2015–16, 3 fellowships, 21 research assistantships, 2 teaching assistantships were awarded; unspecified assistantships also available. Financial award applicants required to submit FAFSA. *Faculty research:* The understanding of molecular and cellular mechanisms that mediate plant development, adaptation, and evolution including bioinformatics, genomics, proteomics, genetics, biochemistry, breeding, physiology and molecular and cellular biology. *Unit head:* A. Mark Settles, PhD, Director, 352-392-7571, Fax: 352-392-4726, E-mail: settles@ufl.edu. *Application contact:* Anna-Lisa Paul, PhD, Graduate Coordinator, 352-273-4855, E-mail: alp@ufl.edu. Website: http://pmcb.ifas.ufl.edu/

University of Georgia, Franklin College of Arts and Sciences, Department of Plant Biology, Athens, GA 30602. Offers MS, PhD. *Degree requirements:* For master's, thesis; for doctorate, one foreign language, thesis/dissertation. *Entrance requirements:* For master's and doctorate, GRE General Test. Electronic applications accepted.

University of Illinois at Urbana–Champaign, Graduate College, College of Liberal Arts and Sciences, School of Integrative Biology, Department of Plant Biology, Champaign, IL 61820. Offers plant biology (MS, PhD); plant biotechnology (PSM).

University of Maryland, College Park, Academic Affairs, College of Computer, Mathematical and Natural Sciences, Department of Cell Biology and Molecular Genetics, College Park, MD 20742. Offers cell biology and molecular genetics (MS, PhD); molecular and cellular biology (MS, PhD); plant biology (MS, PhD). *Program availability:* Part-time, evening/weekend. Terminal master's awarded for partial completion of doctoral program. *Degree requirements:* For master's, thesis; for doctorate, thesis/dissertation. *Entrance requirements:* For master's, GRE General Test, minimum GPA of 3.0, 3 letters of recommendation; for doctorate, GRE General Test. Additional exam requirements/recommendations for international students: Required—TOEFL. Electronic applications accepted. *Faculty research:* Cytoskeletal activity, membrane biology, cell division, genetics and genomics, virology.

University of Massachusetts Amherst, Graduate School, Interdisciplinary Programs, Program in Plant Biology, Amherst, MA 01003. Offers biochemistry and metabolism (MS, PhD); cell biology and physiology (MS, PhD); environmental, ecological and integrative biology (MS, PhD); genetics and evolution (MS, PhD). *Degree requirements:* For master's, thesis; for doctorate, 2 foreign languages, comprehensive exam, thesis/dissertation. *Entrance requirements:* For master's and doctorate, GRE General Test. Additional exam requirements/recommendations for international students: Required—TOEFL (minimum score 550 paper-based; 80 iBT), IELTS (minimum score 6.5). Electronic applications accepted.

University of Minnesota, Twin Cities Campus, Graduate School, College of Biological Sciences, Program in Plant Biological Sciences, Minneapolis, MN 55455-0213. Offers MS, PhD. *Program availability:* Part-time. Terminal master's awarded for partial completion of doctoral program. *Degree requirements:* For master's, thesis or alternative; for doctorate, thesis/dissertation, written and oral preliminary exams. *Entrance requirements:* For master's and doctorate, GRE General Test. Additional exam requirements/recommendations for international students: Required—TOEFL. Electronic applications accepted. *Faculty research:* Cell and molecular biology; plant physiology; plant structure, diversity, and development; ecology, systematics, plant evolution and genomics.

Plant Biology

University of Missouri, Office of Research and Graduate Studies, College of Agriculture, Food and Natural Resources, Division of Plant Insect Microbial Sciences, Columbia, MO 65211. Offers crop, soil and pest management (MS, PhD); entomology (MS, PhD); horticulture (MS, PhD); plant biology and genetics (MS, PhD); plant stress biology (MS, PhD). Terminal master's awarded for partial completion of doctoral program. *Degree requirements:* For master's, thesis; for doctorate, comprehensive exam, thesis/dissertation. *Entrance requirements:* For master's and doctorate, GRE General Test, minimum GPA of 3.0; bachelor's degree from accredited college. Additional exam requirements/recommendations for international students: Required—TOEFL (minimum score 500 paper-based; 61 iBT), IELTS (minimum score 5.5). *Application deadline:* For fall admission, 1/15 priority date for domestic students, 1/15 for international students. Applications are processed on a rolling basis. Application fee: $65 ($90 for international students). Electronic applications accepted. *Financial support:* Fellowships with tuition reimbursements, research assistantships with tuition reimbursements, teaching assistantships with tuition reimbursements, institutionally sponsored loans, scholarships/grants, health care benefits, and unspecified assistantships available. Support available to part-time students. *Faculty research:* Crop, soil and pest management; entomology; horticulture; plant biology and genetics; plant microbiology and pathology.
Website: http://plantsci.missouri.edu/graduate/

University of Oklahoma, College of Arts and Sciences, Department of Microbiology and Plant Biology, Program in Plant Biology, Norman, OK 73019. Offers MS, PhD. *Students:* 12 full-time (4 women), 13 part-time (8 women); includes 6 minority (2 American Indian or Alaska Native, non-Hispanic/Latino; 1 Asian, non-Hispanic/Latino; 2 Hispanic/Latino; 1 Two or more races, non-Hispanic/Latino), 9 international. Average age 29. 4 applicants, 50% accepted, 1 enrolled. In 2015, 3 master's awarded. Terminal master's awarded for partial completion of doctoral program. *Degree requirements:* For master's, thesis; for doctorate, comprehensive exam, thesis/dissertation. *Entrance requirements:* For master's and doctorate, GRE, 3 recommendation letters, letter of intent, bachelor's degree. Additional exam requirements/recommendations for international students: Required—TOEFL (minimum score 80 iBT). *Application deadline:* For fall admission, 3/1 for domestic and international students; for spring admission, 9/1 for domestic and international students; for summer admission, 9/1 for domestic and international students. Application fee: $50 ($100 for international students). Electronic applications accepted. *Expenses:* Tuition, state resident: full-time $4577; part-time $190.70 per credit hour. Tuition, nonresident: full-time $17,758; part-time $739.90 per credit hour. *Required fees:* $3060; $115.70 per credit hour. $141.50 per semester. *Financial support:* In 2015–16, 18 students received support. Research assistantships with full tuition reimbursements available, teaching assistantships with full tuition reimbursements available, Federal Work-Study, institutionally sponsored loans, scholarships/grants, health care benefits, and unspecified assistantships available. Support available to part-time students. Financial award application deadline: 6/1; financial award applicants required to submit FAFSA. *Faculty research:* Ecology, evolution, and systematics of plants; molecular biology of plant stress and reproduction;

global change biology and ecosystem modeling; plant structure and development; science education. *Unit head:* Dr. Anne K. Dunn, Interim Department Chair/Associate Professor of Microbiology, 405-325-4321, Fax: 405-325-7619, E-mail: akdunn@ou.edu. *Application contact:* Adell Hopper, Staff Assistant, 405-325-4322, Fax: 405-325-7619, E-mail: ahopper@ou.edu.
Website: http://mpbio.ou.edu/

The University of Texas at Austin, Graduate School, College of Natural Sciences, School of Biological Sciences, Program in Plant Biology, Austin, TX 78712-1111. Offers MA, PhD. *Entrance requirements:* For master's and doctorate, GRE General Test, minimum GPA of 3.0. Additional exam requirements/recommendations for international students: Required—TOEFL. Electronic applications accepted. *Faculty research:* Systematics, plant molecular biology, psychology, ecology, evolution.

University of Vermont, Graduate College, College of Agriculture and Life Sciences, Department of Plant Biology, Burlington, VT 05405. Offers field naturalist (MS); plant biology (MS, PhD). *Entrance requirements:* For master's and doctorate, GRE. Additional exam requirements/recommendations for international students: Required—TOEFL (minimum score 550 paper-based; 80 iBT). *Application deadline:* For fall admission, 12/1 priority date for domestic students, 12/1 for international students. Application fee: $65. Electronic applications accepted. *Unit head:* Dr. Jill Preston, 802-656-0434, E-mail: jill.preston@uvm.edu. *Application contact:* Dr. Jill Preston, 802-656-0434, E-mail: jill.preston@uvm.edu.

Washington University in St. Louis, Graduate School of Arts and Sciences, Division of Biology and Biomedical Sciences, Program in Plant and Microbial Biosciences, St. Louis, MO 63130-4899. Offers PhD. *Students:* 15 full-time (9 women); includes 4 minority (1 Black or African American, non-Hispanic/Latino; 3 Asian, non-Hispanic/Latino), 1 international. 55 applicants, 24% accepted, 4 enrolled. In 2015, 1 doctorate awarded. *Degree requirements:* For doctorate, thesis/dissertation. *Entrance requirements:* For doctorate, GRE General Test, GRE Subject Test. Additional exam requirements/recommendations for international students: Required—TOEFL. *Application deadline:* For fall admission, 12/1 for domestic students. Application fee: $0. Electronic applications accepted. *Financial support:* Fellowships, research assistantships, and teaching assistantships available. Financial award application deadline: 1/15. *Faculty research:* Cell biology; development; physiology, signaling, development, metabolic regulation, photosynthesis, bioenergy, protein structure-function, synthetic biology, biogeochemistry, environmental microbiology, ecology, population genetics and molecular evolution. *Unit head:* Stacia Burd, Coordinator, 314-362-3364. *Application contact:* Rebecca Riney, 314-747-4648, E-mail: dbbsphdadmissions@wusm.wustl.edu.

Yale University, Graduate School of Arts and Sciences, Department of Molecular, Cellular, and Developmental Biology, Program in Plant Sciences, New Haven, CT 06520. Offers PhD. *Degree requirements:* For doctorate, thesis/dissertation. *Entrance requirements:* For doctorate, GRE General Test, GRE Subject Test.

Plant Molecular Biology

Cornell University, Graduate School, Graduate Fields of Agriculture and Life Sciences, Field of Plant Biology, Ithaca, NY 14853-0001. Offers cytology (MS, PhD); paleobotany (MS, PhD); plant biochemistry (MS, PhD); plant cell biology (MS, PhD); plant ecology (MS, PhD); plant molecular biology (MS, PhD); plant morphology, anatomy and biomechanics (MS, PhD); plant physiology (MS, PhD); systematic botany (MS, PhD). *Degree requirements:* For doctorate, comprehensive exam, thesis/dissertation. *Entrance requirements:* For doctorate, GRE General Test, GRE Subject Test in biology (recommended), 3 letters of recommendation. Additional exam requirements/recommendations for international students: Required—TOEFL (minimum score 610 paper-based; 77 iBT). Electronic applications accepted. *Faculty research:* Plant cell biology/cytology; plant molecular biology; plant morphology/anatomy/biomechanics; plant physiology, systematic botany, paleobotany; plant ecology, ethnobotany, plant biochemistry, photosynthesis.

Illinois State University, Graduate School, College of Arts and Sciences, Department of Biological Sciences, Normal, IL 61790-2200. Offers animal behavior (MS); bacteriology (MS); biochemistry (MS); biological sciences (MS); biology (PhD); biophysics (MS); biotechnology (MS); botany (MS); cell biology (MS); conservation biology (MS); developmental biology (MS); ecology (MS, PhD); entomology (MS); evolutionary biology (MS); genetics (MS, PhD); immunology (MS); microbiology (MS, PhD); molecular biology (MS); molecular genetics (MS); neurobiology (MS); neuroscience (MS); parasitology (MS); physiology (MS, PhD); plant biology (MS); plant molecular biology (MS); plant sciences (MS); structural biology (MS); zoology (MS, PhD). *Program availability:* Part-time. *Degree requirements:* For master's, thesis or alternative; for doctorate, variable foreign language requirement, thesis/dissertation, 2 terms of residency. *Entrance requirements:* For master's, GRE General Test, minimum GPA of 2.6 in last 60 hours of course work; for doctorate, GRE General Test. *Application deadline:* Applications are processed on a rolling basis. Application fee: $40. *Financial support:* Research assistantships, teaching assistantships, Federal Work-Study, tuition waivers (full), and unspecified assistantships available. Financial award application deadline: 4/1. *Faculty research:* Redoc balance and drug development in schistosoma mansoni, control of the growth of listeria monocytogenes at low temperature, regulation of cell expansion and microtubule function by SPRI, CRUI: physiology and fitness consequences of different life history phenotypes. *Application contact:* Steven Juliano, Graduate Coordinator, E-mail: sajulian@ilstu.edu.
Website: http://www.bio.ilstu.edu/

Michigan Technological University, Graduate School, School of Forest Resources and Environmental Science, Houghton, MI 49931. Offers applied ecology (MS); forest ecology and management (MS); forest molecular genetics and biotechnology (MS, PhD); forest science (PhD); forestry (MF, MS); geographic information science (MGIS). *Accreditation:* SAF. *Program availability:* Part-time. *Faculty:* 41 full-time (11 women), 52 part-time/adjunct (18 women). *Students:* 58 full-time (24 women), 23 part-time (6 women); includes 2 minority (both Two or more races, non-Hispanic/Latino), 19 international. Average age 31. 92 applicants, 51% accepted, 32 enrolled. In 2015, 16 master's, 5 doctorates awarded. Terminal master's awarded for partial completion of doctoral program. *Degree requirements:* For master's, thesis (for some programs), comprehensive exam (for non-research degrees); for doctorate, comprehensive exam, thesis/dissertation. *Entrance requirements:* For master's and doctorate, GRE, statement of purpose, personal statement, official transcripts, 3 letters of recommendation, resume/curriculum vitae. Additional exam requirements/recommendations for international students: Required—TOEFL (recommended score 79 iBT) or IELTS.

Application deadline: Applications are processed on a rolling basis. Electronic applications accepted. *Expenses:* Tuition, state resident: full-time $15,507; part-time $861.50 per credit. Tuition, nonresident: full-time $15,507; part-time $861.50 per credit. *Required fees:* $248; $248. Tuition and fees vary according to course load and program. *Financial support:* In 2015–16, 51 students received support, including 6 fellowships with tuition reimbursements available (averaging $14,516 per year), 17 research assistantships with tuition reimbursements available (averaging $14,516 per year), 6 teaching assistantships with tuition reimbursements available (averaging $14,516 per year); career-related internships or fieldwork, Federal Work-Study, scholarships/grants, health care benefits, unspecified assistantships, and cooperative program also available. Financial award applicants required to submit FAFSA. *Faculty research:* Forest ecology and management, forest molecular genetics and biotechnology, forest biomaterials, restoration ecology, wildlife ecology and management. *Total annual research expenditures:* $3.7 million. *Unit head:* Dr. Terry Sharik, Dean, 906-487-2352, Fax: 906-487-2915, E-mail: tlsharik@mtu.edu. *Application contact:* Dr. Andrew J. Storer, Associate Dean, 906-487-3470, Fax: 906-487-2915, E-mail: storer@mtu.edu.
Website: http://www.mtu.edu/forest/

Oregon State University, Interdisciplinary/Institutional Programs, Program in Molecular and Cellular Biology, Corvallis, OR 97331. Offers bioinformatics (PhD); biotechnology (PhD); cell biology (PhD); developmental biology (PhD); genome biology (PhD); molecular biology (PhD); molecular pathogenesis (PhD); molecular virology (PhD); plant molecular biology (PhD); structural biology (PhD). *Students:* 28 full-time (14 women), 2 part-time (1 woman); includes 4 minority (2 Asian, non-Hispanic/Latino; 2 Hispanic/Latino), 10 international. Average age 29. 104 applicants, 5% accepted, 5 enrolled. In 2015, 5 doctorates awarded. *Degree requirements:* For doctorate, thesis/dissertation, oral and written qualifying exams. *Entrance requirements:* For doctorate, GRE. Additional exam requirements/recommendations for international students: Required—TOEFL (minimum score 80 iBT), IELTS (minimum score 6.5). *Application deadline:* For fall admission, 8/1 for domestic students, 4/1 for international students; for winter admission, 12/1 for domestic students, 7/1 for international students; for spring admission, 2/1 for domestic students, 10/1 for international students; for summer admission, 5/1 for domestic students, 1/1 for international students. Application fee: $75 ($85 for international students). *Expenses:* Tuition, state resident: full-time $12,150; part-time $450 per credit. Tuition, nonresident: full-time $20,952; part-time $776 per credit. *Required fees:* $1572; $1443 per unit. One-time fee: $350. Tuition and fees vary according to course load, campus/location and program. *Financial support:* Fellowships, career-related internships or fieldwork, Federal Work-Study, and institutionally sponsored loans available. Support available to part-time students. Financial award application deadline: 1/1. *Unit head:* Dr. Dee Denver, Director, Molecular and Cellular Biology Graduate Program, 541-737-3698. *Application contact:* Kristin Carroll, Assistant Director, 541-737-5259, E-mail: kristin.carroll@oregonstate.edu.
Website: http://www.mcb.oregonstate.edu/

Rutgers University–New Brunswick, Graduate School-New Brunswick, Program in Plant Biology, Piscataway, NJ 08854-8097. Offers horticulture and plant technology (MS, PhD); molecular and cellular biology (MS, PhD); organismal and population biology (MS, PhD); plant pathology (MS, PhD). *Program availability:* Part-time. Terminal master's awarded for partial completion of doctoral program. *Degree requirements:* For master's, comprehensive exam, thesis or alternative; for doctorate, comprehensive exam, thesis/dissertation. *Entrance requirements:* For master's and doctorate, GRE

General Test, GRE Subject Test (recommended). Additional exam requirements/recommendations for international students: Required—TOEFL (minimum score 600 paper-based). Electronic applications accepted. *Faculty research:* Molecular biology and biochemistry of plants, plant development and genomics, plant protection, plant improvement, plant management of horticultural and field crops.

University of California, Riverside, Graduate Division, Department of Botany and Plant Sciences, Riverside, CA 92521-0102. Offers plant biology (MS, PhD), including plant cell, molecular, and developmental biology (PhD), plant ecology (PhD), plant genetics (PhD). *Program availability:* Part-time. Terminal master's awarded for partial completion of doctoral program. *Degree requirements:* For master's, comprehensive exams or thesis; for doctorate, thesis/dissertation, qualifying exams. *Entrance requirements:* For master's and doctorate, GRE General Test, minimum GPA of 3.2. Additional exam requirements/recommendations for international students: Required—TOEFL (minimum score 550 paper-based; 80 iBT). Electronic applications accepted. *Expenses: Tuition, area resident:* Full-time $16,665.50; part-time $11,055.54. *Tuition, state resident:* full-time $16,665.50; part-time $11,055.54. *Tuition, nonresident:* full-time $31,768. *International tuition:* $31,767.50 full-time. *Required fees:* $16,665.50; $11,055.54 per quarter. $3685.18 per quarter. Tuition and fees vary according to program. *Faculty research:* Agricultural plant biology; biochemistry and physiology; cellular, molecular and developmental biology; ecology, evolution, systematics and ethnobotany; genetics, genomics and bioinformatics.

University of Florida, Graduate School, College of Agricultural and Life Sciences and College of Liberal Arts and Sciences, Program in Plant Molecular and Cellular Biology, Gainesville, FL 32611. Offers plant molecular and cellular biology (MS, PhD), including toxicology (PhD). *Faculty:* 41. *Students:* 27 full-time (9 women), 1 part-time; includes 3 minority (1 Black or African American, non-Hispanic/Latino; 1 Asian, non-Hispanic/Latino; 1 Hispanic/Latino), 15 international. Average age 28. 33 applicants, 24%

accepted, 6 enrolled. In 2015, 5 doctorates awarded. *Degree requirements:* For master's, thesis; for doctorate, comprehensive exam, thesis/dissertation, first author peer-reviewed publication. *Entrance requirements:* For master's and doctorate, GRE General Test, minimum GPA of 3.0. Additional exam requirements/recommendations for international students: Required—TOEFL (minimum score 550 paper-based; 80 iBT), IELTS (minimum score 6). *Application deadline:* For fall admission, 1/3 priority date for domestic students, 1/3 for international students; for spring admission, 8/1 for domestic and international students. Applications are processed on a rolling basis. Application fee: $30. Electronic applications accepted. *Financial support:* In 2015–16, 3 fellowships, 21 research assistantships, 2 teaching assistantships were awarded; unspecified assistantships also available. Financial award applicants required to submit FAFSA. *Faculty research:* The understanding of molecular and cellular mechanisms that mediate plant development, adaptation, and evolution including bioinformatics, genomics, proteomics, genetics, biochemistry, breeding, physiology and molecular and cellular biology. *Unit head:* A. Mark Settles, PhD, Director, 352-392-7571, Fax: 352-392-4726, E-mail: settles@ufl.edu. *Application contact:* Anna-Lisa Paul, PhD, Graduate Coordinator, 352-273-4855, E-mail: alp@ufl.edu.
Website: http://pmcb.ifas.ufl.edu/

University of Massachusetts Amherst, Graduate School, Interdisciplinary Programs, Program in Plant Biology, Amherst, MA 01003. Offers biochemistry and metabolism (MS, PhD); cell biology and physiology (MS, PhD); environmental, ecological and integrative biology (MS, PhD); genetics and evolution (MS, PhD). *Degree requirements:* For master's, thesis; for doctorate, 2 foreign languages, comprehensive exam, thesis/dissertation. *Entrance requirements:* For master's and doctorate, GRE General Test. Additional exam requirements/recommendations for international students: Required—TOEFL (minimum score 550 paper-based; 80 iBT), IELTS (minimum score 6.5). Electronic applications accepted.

Plant Pathology

Auburn University, Graduate School, College of Agriculture, Department of Entomology and Plant Pathology, Auburn University, AL 36849. Offers entomology (M Ag, MS, PhD); plant pathology (M Ag, MS, PhD). *Program availability:* Part-time. *Faculty:* 16 full-time (6 women). *Students:* 27 full-time (15 women), 10 part-time (1 woman); includes 2 minority (1 Black or African American, non-Hispanic/Latino; 1 Hispanic/Latino), 23 international. Average age 26. 28 applicants, 50% accepted, 13 enrolled. In 2015, 3 master's, 3 doctorates awarded. *Degree requirements:* For master's, thesis (for some programs); for doctorate, one foreign language, thesis/dissertation. *Entrance requirements:* For master's, GRE General Test; for doctorate, GRE General Test, GRE Subject Test, master's degree with thesis. *Application deadline:* Applications are processed on a rolling basis. Application fee: $50 ($60 for international students). Electronic applications accepted. *Expenses:* Tuition, state resident: full-time $8802; part-time $489 per credit hour. Tuition, nonresident: full-time $26,406; part-time $1467 per credit hour. *Required fees:* $808 per semester. Tuition and fees vary according to degree level and program. *Financial support:* Research assistantships, teaching assistantships, and Federal Work-Study available. Support available to part-time students. Financial award application deadline: 3/15; financial award applicants required to submit FAFSA. *Faculty research:* Pest management, biological control, systematics, medical entomology. *Unit head:* Dr. Nannan Liu, Chair, 334-844-4266. *Application contact:* Dr. George Flowers, Dean of the Graduate School, 334-844-2125.

Colorado State University, College of Agricultural Sciences, Department of Bioagricultural Sciences and Pest Management, Fort Collins, CO 80523-1177. Offers entomology (MS, PhD); pest management (MS); plant pathology and weed science (MS, PhD). *Program availability:* Part-time, evening/weekend. *Faculty:* 18 full-time (6 women), 5 part-time/adjunct (2 women). *Students:* 22 full-time (12 women), 13 part-time (7 women); includes 2 minority (both Two or more races, non-Hispanic/Latino), 8 international. Average age 28. 15 applicants, 100% accepted, 13 enrolled. In 2015, 3 master's, 4 doctorates awarded. *Degree requirements:* For master's, comprehensive exam, thesis; for doctorate, comprehensive exam, thesis/dissertation. *Entrance requirements:* For master's and doctorate, GRE General Test, minimum GPA of 3.0, letters of recommendation, essay, transcripts. Additional exam requirements/recommendations for international students: Required—TOEFL (minimum score 550 paper-based; 80 iBT), IELTS (minimum score 6.5). *Application deadline:* For fall admission, 1/15 priority date for domestic and international students; for spring admission, 9/1 priority date for domestic and international students. Applications are processed on a rolling basis. Application fee: $60 ($70 for international students). Electronic applications accepted. *Expenses:* Tuition, state resident: full-time $9348. Tuition, nonresident: full-time $22,916. *Required fees:* $2174; $473.72 per credit hour. $236.86 per semester. Tuition and fees vary according to course load and program. *Financial support:* In 2015–16, 4 fellowships with full tuition reimbursements (averaging $39,950 per year), 20 research assistantships with full tuition reimbursements (averaging $20,192 per year), 8 teaching assistantships with full tuition reimbursements (averaging $16,403 per year) were awarded. Financial award application deadline: 1/15. *Faculty research:* Genomics and molecular biology, ecology and biodiversity, biology and management of invasive species, integrated pest management. *Total annual research expenditures:* $3.3 million. *Unit head:* Dr. Louis Bjostad, Department Head, 970-491-3612, Fax: 970-491-3862, E-mail: louis.bjostad@colostate.edu. *Application contact:* Janet Dill, Graduate Coordinator, 970-491-0402, Fax: 970-491-3862, E-mail: janet.dill@colostate.edu.
Website: http://bspm.agsci.colostate.edu/

Cornell University, Graduate School, Graduate Fields of Agriculture and Life Sciences, Field of Plant Pathology and Plant-Microbe Biology, Ithaca, NY 14853-0001. Offers fungal and oomycete biology (MPS, MS, PhD); plant microbe biology (MPS, MS, PhD); plant pathology (MPS, MS, PhD). *Degree requirements:* For master's, thesis (MS), project paper (MPS); for doctorate, comprehensive exam, thesis/dissertation. *Entrance requirements:* For master's and doctorate, GRE General Test, GRE Subject Test (biology recommended), 3 letters of recommendation. Additional exam requirements/recommendations for international students: Required—TOEFL (minimum score 550 paper-based; 77 iBT). Electronic applications accepted. *Faculty research:* Plant pathology; mycology; molecular plant pathology; plant disease epidemiology, ecological and environmental plant pathology; plant disease epidemiology and simulation modeling.

Dalhousie University, Faculty of Agriculture, Halifax, NS B3H 4R2, Canada. Offers agriculture (M Sc), including air quality, animal behavior, animal molecular genetics, animal nutrition, animal technology, aquaculture, botany, crop management, crop physiology, ecology, environmental microbiology, food science, horticulture, nutrient

management, pest management, physiology, plant biotechnology, plant pathology, soil chemistry, soil fertility, waste management and composting, water quality. *Program availability:* Part-time. *Degree requirements:* For master's, thesis, ATC Exam Teaching Assistantship. *Entrance requirements:* For master's, honors B Sc, minimum GPA of 3.0. Additional exam requirements/recommendations for international students: Required—TOEFL (minimum score 580 paper-based; 92 iBT), IELTS, Michigan English Language Assessment Battery, CanTEST, CAEL. *Faculty research:* Bio-product development, organic agriculture, nutrient management, air and water quality, agricultural biotechnology.

Iowa State University of Science and Technology, Department of Plant Pathology, Ames, IA 50011. Offers MS, PhD. *Entrance requirements:* For master's and doctorate, GRE General Test, resume. Additional exam requirements/recommendations for international students: Required—TOEFL (minimum score 550 paper-based; 79 iBT), IELTS (minimum score 6.5). Electronic applications accepted.

Kansas State University, Graduate School, College of Agriculture, Department of Plant Pathology, Manhattan, KS 66506. Offers genetics (MS, PhD); plant pathology (MS, PhD). Terminal master's awarded for partial completion of doctoral program. *Degree requirements:* For master's, thesis, oral exam; for doctorate, thesis/dissertation, preliminary exams. *Entrance requirements:* For master's and doctorate, minimum undergraduate GPA of 3.0. Additional exam requirements/recommendations for international students: Required—TOEFL (minimum score 550 paper-based; 79 iBT). Electronic applications accepted. *Faculty research:* Applied microbiology, microbial genetics, microbial ecology/epidemiology, integrated pest management, plant genetics/genomics/molecular biology.

Louisiana State University and Agricultural & Mechanical College, Graduate School, College of Agriculture, Department of Plant Pathology and Crop Physiology, Baton Rouge, LA 70803. Offers plant health (MS, PhD).

Michigan State University, The Graduate School, College of Agriculture and Natural Resources and College of Natural Science, Department of Plant Pathology, East Lansing, MI 48824. Offers MS, PhD. *Entrance requirements:* Additional exam requirements/recommendations for international students: Required—TOEFL.

Mississippi State University, College of Agriculture and Life Sciences, Department of Biochemistry, Molecular Biology, Entomology and Plant Pathology, Mississippi State, MS 39762. Offers agriculture life sciences (MS), including biochemistry (MS, PhD), entomology (MS, PhD), plant pathology (MS, PhD); life science (PhD), including biochemistry (MS, PhD), entomology (MS, PhD), plant pathology (MS, PhD); molecular biology (PhD). *Faculty:* 32 full-time (6 women), 2 part-time/adjunct (1 woman). *Students:* 44 full-time (20 women), 11 part-time (6 women); includes 6 minority (3 Black or African American, non-Hispanic/Latino; 1 Asian, non-Hispanic/Latino; 1 Hispanic/Latino; 1 Two or more races, non-Hispanic/Latino), 12 international. Average age 29. 35 applicants, 40% accepted, 12 enrolled. In 2015, 12 master's, 7 doctorates awarded. Terminal master's awarded for partial completion of doctoral program. *Degree requirements:* For master's, thesis (for some programs), final oral exam; for doctorate, thesis/dissertation, preliminary oral and written exam. *Entrance requirements:* For master's, GRE General Test, minimum GPA of 2.75; for doctorate, GRE. Additional exam requirements/recommendations for international students: Required—TOEFL (minimum score 500 paper-based; 61 iBT); Recommended—IELTS (minimum score 5.5). *Application deadline:* For fall admission, 7/1 for domestic students, 5/1 for international students; for spring admission, 11/1 for domestic students, 9/1 for international students. Applications are processed on a rolling basis. Application fee: $60. Electronic applications accepted. *Expenses:* Tuition, area resident: Full-time $7502; part-time $833.74 per credit hour. Tuition, nonresident: full-time $20,142; part-time $2238.24 per credit hour. *Financial support:* In 2015–16, 40 research assistantships with full tuition reimbursements (averaging $16,730 per year) were awarded; Federal Work-Study, institutionally sponsored loans, and unspecified assistantships also available. Financial award application deadline: 4/1; financial award applicants required to submit FAFSA. *Faculty research:* Fish nutrition, plant and animal molecular biology, plant biochemistry, enzymology, lipid metabolism, chromatin, cell wall synthesis in rice, a model grass bioenergy species and the source of rice Stover residues using reverse genetic and functional genomic and proteomic approaches. *Unit head:* Dr. Jeffrey Dean, Professor and Department Head, 662-325-0643, Fax: 662-325-8664, E-mail: jd1891@msstate.edu. *Application contact:* Marina Hunt, Admissions Assistant, 662-325-5188, E-mail: mhunt@grad.msstate.edu.
Website: http://www.biochemistry.msstate.edu

Plant Pathology

Montana State University, The Graduate School, College of Agriculture, Department of Plant Sciences and Plant Pathology, Bozeman, MT 59717. Offers plant pathology (MS); plant sciences (MS, PhD), including plant genetics (PhD), plant pathology (PhD). *Program availability:* Part-time. *Degree requirements:* For master's, comprehensive exam; for doctorate, comprehensive exam, thesis/dissertation. *Entrance requirements:* For master's, GRE General Test, minimum GPA of 3.0; for doctorate, GRE General Test. Additional exam requirements/recommendations for international students: Required—TOEFL (minimum score 550 paper-based). Electronic applications accepted. *Faculty research:* Plant genetics, plant metabolism, plant microbe interactions, plant pathology, entomology research.

New Mexico State University, College of Agricultural, Consumer and Environmental Sciences, Department of Entomology, Plant Pathology and Weed Science, Las Cruces, NM 88003-8001. Offers MS. *Program availability:* Part-time. *Faculty:* 10 full-time (1 woman). *Students:* 8 full-time (3 women), 3 part-time (all women); includes 3 minority (1 American Indian or Alaska Native, non-Hispanic/Latino; 2 Hispanic/Latino), 4 international. Average age 29. 4 applicants, 75% accepted, 3 enrolled. In 2015, 6 master's awarded. *Degree requirements:* For master's, comprehensive exam, thesis. *Entrance requirements:* For master's, GRE General Test. Additional exam requirements/recommendations for international students: Required—TOEFL (minimum score 550 paper-based; 79 iBT), IELTS (minimum score 6.5). *Application deadline:* For fall admission, 7/1 priority date for domestic students; for spring admission, 11/1 priority date for domestic students. Applications are processed on a rolling basis. Application fee: $40 ($50 for international students). Electronic applications accepted. *Expenses:* $274.50 per credit hour for in-state students, and all students enrolled in six or fewer credits; $839.30 per credit hour for out-of-state and international students enrolled in at least seven hours. *Financial support:* In 2015–16, 10 students received support, including 6 research assistantships (averaging $21,962 per year), 3 teaching assistantships (averaging $16,022 per year); career-related internships or fieldwork, Federal Work-Study, scholarships/grants, traineeships, health care benefits, and unspecified assistantships also available. Support available to part-time students. Financial award application deadline: 3/1. *Faculty research:* Entomology, nematology, plant pathology, weed science. *Total annual research expenditures:* $2.3 million. *Unit head:* Dr. Gerald K. Sims, Department Head, 575-646-3225, Fax: 575-646-8087, E-mail: gksims@nmsu.edu. *Application contact:* Belinda Williams, 575-646-3225, Fax: 575-646-8087.
Website: http://eppws.nmsu.edu/

North Carolina State University, Graduate School, College of Agriculture and Life Sciences, Department of Plant Pathology, Raleigh, NC 27695. Offers MS, PhD. Terminal master's awarded for partial completion of doctoral program. *Degree requirements:* For master's, thesis (for some programs); for doctorate, thesis/dissertation. *Entrance requirements:* For master's and doctorate, GRE. Additional exam requirements/recommendations for international students: Required—TOEFL. Electronic applications accepted. *Faculty research:* Microbe-plant interactions, biology of plant pathogens, pathogen evaluation, host-plant resistance, genomics.

North Dakota State University, College of Graduate and Interdisciplinary Studies, College of Agriculture, Food Systems, and Natural Resources, Department of Plant Pathology, Fargo, ND 58102. Offers MS, PhD. *Program availability:* Part-time. *Degree requirements:* For master's, thesis; for doctorate, thesis/dissertation. *Entrance requirements:* Additional exam requirements/recommendations for international students: Required—TOEFL (minimum score 550 paper-based; 79 iBT). *Application deadline:* For fall admission, 5/1 for international students; for winter admission, 8/1 for international students. Applications are processed on a rolling basis. Application fee: $35. Electronic applications accepted. *Financial support:* Research assistantships with full tuition reimbursements, Federal Work-Study, and institutionally sponsored loans available. Financial award application deadline: 4/15. *Faculty research:* Electron microscopy, disease physiology, molecular biology, genetic resistance, tissue culture. *Unit head:* Dr. Jack Rasmussen, Chair, 701-231-7058, Fax: 701-231-7851, E-mail: jack.rasmussen@ndsu.edu. *Application contact:* Elizabeth Worth, Marketing, Recruitment, and Public Relations Coordinator, 701-231-8476, Fax: 701-231-6524, E-mail: elizabeth.worth@ndsu.edu.
Website: http://www.ag.ndsu.edu/plantpath/

The Ohio State University, Graduate School, College of Food, Agricultural, and Environmental Sciences, Department of Plant Pathology, Columbus, OH 43210. Offers MPHM, MS, PhD. MPHM offered jointly with Department of Entomology. *Students:* 43 full-time (22 women), 6 part-time (1 woman); includes 4 minority (1 Black or African American, non-Hispanic/Latino; 2 Hispanic/Latino; 1 Two or more races, non-Hispanic/Latino), 22 international. Average age 28. In 2015, 9 master's, 3 doctorates awarded. *Degree requirements:* For master's, thesis optional; for doctorate, thesis/dissertation. *Entrance requirements:* For master's and doctorate, GRE General Test. Additional exam requirements/recommendations for international students: Required—TOEFL (minimum score 550 paper-based; 79 iBT), Michigan English Language Assessment Battery (minimum score 82); Recommended—IELTS (minimum score 7). *Application deadline:* For fall admission, 12/13 priority date for domestic students, 11/30 priority date for international students; for spring admission, 10/17 for domestic students, 9/1 for international students; for summer admission, 2/13 for domestic students, 1/31 for international students. Applications are processed on a rolling basis. Application fee: $60 ($70 for international students). Electronic applications accepted. *Financial support:* Fellowships with tuition reimbursements, research assistantships with tuition reimbursements, teaching assistantships with tuition reimbursements, Federal Work-Study, and institutionally sponsored loans available. Support available to part-time students. *Unit head:* Dr. Laurence Madden, Acting Chair, 330-263-3839, E-mail: madden.1@osu.edu. *Application contact:* Graduate and Professional Admissions, 614-292-9444, Fax: 614-292-3895, E-mail: gpadmissions@osu.edu.
Website: http://plantpath.osu.edu/

Oklahoma State University, College of Agricultural Science and Natural Resources, Department of Entomology and Plant Pathology, Stillwater, OK 74078. Offers entomology (PhD); entomology and plant pathology (MS); plant pathology (PhD). *Faculty:* 29 full-time (10 women), 1 part-time/adjunct (0 women). *Students:* 6 full-time (4 women), 33 part-time (20 women); includes 3 minority (1 American Indian or Alaska Native, non-Hispanic/Latino; 2 Two or more races, non-Hispanic/Latino), 14 international. Average age 30. 13 applicants, 62% accepted, 4 enrolled. In 2015, 10 master's, 1 doctorate awarded. *Degree requirements:* For master's, thesis or alternative; for doctorate, comprehensive exam, thesis/dissertation. *Entrance requirements:* For master's and doctorate, GRE or GMAT. Additional exam requirements/recommendations for international students: Required—TOEFL (minimum score 550 paper-based; 79 iBT). *Application deadline:* For fall admission, 3/1 priority date for international students; for spring admission, 8/1 priority date for international students. Applications are processed on a rolling basis. Application fee: $40 ($75 for international students). Electronic applications accepted. *Expenses:* Tuition, state resident: full-time $3528; part-time $196 per credit hour. Tuition, nonresident: full-time $14,144; part-time $785.75 per credit hour. *Required fees:* $1895; $105.25 per credit hour. Tuition and fees vary according to campus/location. *Financial support:* In 2015–16, 30 research assistantships (averaging $18,582 per year), 2 teaching assistantships (averaging

$17,046 per year) were awarded; career-related internships or fieldwork, Federal Work-Study, scholarships/grants, health care benefits, tuition waivers (partial), and unspecified assistantships also available. Support available to part-time students. Financial award application deadline: 3/1; financial award applicants required to submit FAFSA. *Unit head:* Dr. Phillip Mulder, Jr., Department Head, 405-744-5527, Fax: 405-744-6039, E-mail: phil.mulder@okstate.edu. *Application contact:* Dr. Bob Hunger, Graduate Coordinator, 405-744-9958, Fax: 405-744-6039, E-mail: bob.hunger@okstate.edu.
Website: http://entoplp.okstate.edu/

Oregon State University, College of Agricultural Sciences, Program in Botany and Plant Pathology, Corvallis, OR 97331. Offers M Ag, MA, MS, PhD. *Faculty:* 23 full-time (4 women), 3 part-time/adjunct (0 women). *Students:* 39 full-time (18 women), 1 part-time (0 women); includes 4 minority (1 Black or African American, non-Hispanic/Latino; 1 Hispanic/Latino; 2 Two or more races, non-Hispanic/Latino), 5 international. Average age 29. 58 applicants, 28% accepted, 8 enrolled. In 2015, 8 master's, 3 doctorates awarded. *Entrance requirements:* For master's and doctorate, GRE. *Application deadline:* For fall admission, 12/1 for domestic and international students. Application fee: $75 ($85 for international students). *Expenses:* Tuition, state resident: full-time $12,150; part-time $450 per credit. Tuition, nonresident: full-time $20,952; part-time $776 per credit. *Required fees:* $1572; $1443 per unit. One-time fee: $350. Tuition and fees vary according to course load, campus/location and program. *Financial support:* Application deadline: 12/15. *Unit head:* Dr. Lynda M. Ciuffetti, Professor and Department Head.
Website: http://bpp.oregonstate.edu/

Penn State University Park, Graduate School, College of Agricultural Sciences, Department of Plant Pathology and Environmental Microbiology, University Park, PA 16802. Offers plant pathology (MS, PhD). *Unit head:* Dr. Richard T. Roush, Dean, 814-865-2541, Fax: 814-865-3103. *Application contact:* Lori Stania, Director, Graduate Student Services, 814-865-1795, Fax: 814-863-4627, E-mail: l-gswww@lists.psu.edu.
Website: http://plantpath.psu.edu/

Purdue University, Graduate School, College of Agriculture, Department of Botany and Plant Pathology, West Lafayette, IN 47907. Offers MS, PhD. *Program availability:* Part-time. Terminal master's awarded for partial completion of doctoral program. *Degree requirements:* For master's, thesis; for doctorate, thesis/dissertation. *Entrance requirements:* For master's, GRE General Test, minimum undergraduate GPA of 3.0 or equivalent; for doctorate, GRE, minimum undergraduate GPA of 3.0 or equivalent. Additional exam requirements/recommendations for international students: Required—TOEFL (minimum score 550 paper-based; 77 iBT); Recommended—TWE. Electronic applications accepted. *Faculty research:* Biotechnology, plant growth, weed control, crop improvement, plant physiology.

Rutgers University–New Brunswick, Graduate School-New Brunswick, Program in Plant Biology, Piscataway, NJ 08854-8097. Offers horticulture and plant technology (MS, PhD); molecular and cellular biology (MS, PhD); organismal and population biology (MS, PhD); plant pathology (MS, PhD). *Program availability:* Part-time. Terminal master's awarded for partial completion of doctoral program. *Degree requirements:* For master's, comprehensive exam, thesis or alternative; for doctorate, comprehensive exam, thesis/dissertation. *Entrance requirements:* For master's and doctorate, GRE General Test, GRE Subject Test (recommended). Additional exam requirements/recommendations for international students: Required—TOEFL (minimum score 600 paper-based). Electronic applications accepted. *Faculty research:* Molecular biology and biochemistry of plants, plant development and genomics, plant protection, plant improvement, plant management of horticultural and field crops.

State University of New York College of Environmental Science and Forestry, Department of Environmental and Forest Biology, Syracuse, NY 13210-2779. Offers applied ecology (MPS); chemical ecology (MPS, MS, PhD); conservation biology (MPS, MS, PhD); ecology (MPS, MS, PhD); entomology (MPS, MS, PhD); environmental interpretation (MPS, MS, PhD); environmental physiology (MPS, MS, PhD); fish and wildlife biology and management (MPS, MS, PhD); forest pathology and mycology (MPS, MS, PhD); plant biotechnology (MPS); plant science and biotechnology (MPS, MS, PhD). *Faculty:* 29 full-time (9 women), 4 part-time/adjunct (3 women). *Students:* 81 full-time (47 women), 57 part-time (24 women); includes 9 minority (1 Black or African American, non-Hispanic/Latino; 2 American Indian or Alaska Native, non-Hispanic/Latino; 1 Asian, non-Hispanic/Latino; 3 Hispanic/Latino; 2 Two or more races, non-Hispanic/Latino), 15 international. Average age 28. 47 applicants, 49% accepted, 15 enrolled. In 2015, 15 master's, 7 doctorates awarded. *Degree requirements:* For master's, thesis (for some programs), capstone seminar; for doctorate, comprehensive exam, thesis/dissertation, capstone seminar. *Entrance requirements:* For master's and doctorate, GRE General Test, minimum GPA of 3.0. Additional exam requirements/recommendations for international students: Required—TOEFL (minimum score 550 paper-based; 80 iBT), IELTS (minimum score 6). *Application deadline:* For fall admission, 2/1 priority date for domestic and international students; for spring admission, 11/1 priority date for domestic and international students. Applications are processed on a rolling basis. Application fee: $60. *Expenses:* Tuition, state resident: full-time $10,870; part-time $453 per credit. Tuition, nonresident: full-time $22,210; part-time $925 per credit. *Required fees:* $1075; $89.22 per credit. *Financial support:* In 2015–16, 4 fellowships with tuition reimbursements, 36 research assistantships with tuition reimbursements, 39 teaching assistantships with tuition reimbursements (averaging $11,490 per year) were awarded; Federal Work-Study, institutionally sponsored loans, scholarships/grants, health care benefits, and unspecified assistantships also available. Financial award application deadline: 6/30. *Faculty research:* Ecology, conservation biology, fish and wildlife biology and management, plant science, entomology. *Total annual research expenditures:* $4.1 million. *Unit head:* Dr. Donald J. Leopold, Chair, 315-470-6760, Fax: 315-470-6934, E-mail: djleopold@esf.edu. *Application contact:* Dr. Danilo D. Fernando, Director, Graduate Program/Associate Professor, 315-470-6746, Fax: 315-470-6934, E-mail: dfernando@esf.edu.
Website: http://www.esf.edu/efb/grad/default.asp

Texas A&M University, College of Agriculture and Life Sciences, Department of Plant Pathology and Microbiology, College Station, TX 77843. Offers plant pathology (MS, PhD). *Program availability:* Part-time, blended/hybrid learning. *Faculty:* 14. *Students:* 32 full-time (12 women), 2 part-time (1 woman); includes 8 minority (1 Black or African American, non-Hispanic/Latino; 3 Asian, non-Hispanic/Latino; 3 Hispanic/Latino; 1 Two or more races, non-Hispanic/Latino), 10 international. Average age 28. 26 applicants, 27% accepted, 5 enrolled. In 2015, 4 master's, 3 doctorates awarded. *Degree requirements:* For master's, comprehensive exam (for some programs), thesis; for doctorate, comprehensive exam, thesis/dissertation. *Entrance requirements:* For master's and doctorate, GRE General Test, letters of recommendation, BS/BA in biological sciences. Additional exam requirements/recommendations for international students: Required—TOEFL (minimum score 550 paper-based; 80 iBT), IELTS (minimum score 6), PTE (minimum score 53). *Application deadline:* Applications are processed on a rolling basis. Application fee: $50 ($90 for international students). Electronic applications accepted. *Expenses:* Contact institution. *Financial support:* In 2015–16, 34 students received support, including 8 fellowships with tuition reimbursements available (averaging $16,028 per year), 17 research assistantships with

tuition reimbursements available (averaging $5,227 per year), 14 teaching assistantships with tuition reimbursements available (averaging $4,912 per year); career-related internships or fieldwork, institutionally sponsored loans, scholarships/grants, traineeships, health care benefits, tuition waivers (full and partial), and unspecified assistantships also available. Support available to part-time students. Financial award application deadline: 3/15; financial award applicants required to submit FAFSA. *Faculty research:* Plant disease control, population biology of plant pathogens, disease epidemiology, molecular genetics of host/parasite interactions. *Unit head:* Dr. Leland S. Pierson, III, Professor and Department Head, 979-845-8288, Fax: 979-845-6483, E-mail: lspierson@tamu.edu. *Application contact:* Dr. Heather H. Wilkinson, Associate Department Head for Academics, 979-845-1491, E-mail: h-wilkinson@tamu.edu.
Website: http://plantpathology.tamu.edu/

The University of Arizona, College of Agriculture and Life Sciences, School of Plant Sciences, Tucson, AZ 85721. Offers plant pathology (MS, PhD). *Program availability:* Part-time. *Degree requirements:* For master's, thesis or alternative; for doctorate, thesis/dissertation. *Entrance requirements:* For master's, GRE General Test, GRE Subject Test (biology or chemistry recommended), minimum GPA of 3.0, academic resume, 3 letters of recommendation; for doctorate, GRE General Test, GRE Subject Test (biology or chemistry recommended), minimum GPA of 3.0, academic resume, statement of interest, 3 letters of recommendation. Additional exam requirements/recommendations for international students: Required—TOEFL (minimum score 550 paper-based; 79 iBT). *Application deadline:* For fall admission, 12/1 for domestic and international students; for spring admission, 6/1 for domestic and international students. Applications are processed on a rolling basis. Application fee: $75. Electronic applications accepted. *Financial support:* Research assistantships, teaching assistantships, career-related internships or fieldwork, Federal Work-Study, scholarships/grants, health care benefits, tuition waivers (partial), and unspecified assistantships available. *Faculty research:* Molecular/cell biology, plant genetics and physiology, agronomic and horticultural production (including turf and ornamentals). *Unit head:* Dr. Karen Schumaker, Director, E-mail: schumake@ag.arizona.edu. *Application contact:* 520-621-1945.
Website: http://cals.arizona.edu/spls/

University of Arkansas, Graduate School, Dale Bumpers College of Agricultural, Food and Life Sciences, Department of Plant Pathology, Fayetteville, AR 72701-1201. Offers MS. *Students:* 7 part-time (3 women); includes 1 minority (Black or African American, non-Hispanic/Latino), 1 international. In 2015, 3 master's awarded. *Degree requirements:* For master's, thesis. *Application deadline:* For fall admission, 4/1 for international students; for spring admission, 10/1 for international students. Applications are processed on a rolling basis. Application fee: $40 ($50 for international students). Electronic applications accepted. *Financial support:* In 2015–16, 10 research assistantships were awarded; fellowships, teaching assistantships, career-related internships or fieldwork, and Federal Work-Study also available. Support available to part-time students. Financial award application deadline: 4/1; financial award applicants required to submit FAFSA. *Unit head:* Dr. Ken Korth, Department Head, 479-575-2445, E-mail: kkorth@uark.edu. *Application contact:* Dr. Ken Korth, Graduate Coordinator, 479-575-2445, E-mail: kkorth@uark.edu.
Website: http://plantpathology.uark.edu/

University of California, Davis, Graduate Studies, Program in Plant Pathology, Davis, CA 95616. Offers MS, PhD. Terminal master's awarded for partial completion of doctoral program. *Degree requirements:* For master's, comprehensive exam (for some programs), thesis (for some programs); for doctorate, thesis/dissertation. *Entrance requirements:* For master's and doctorate, GRE General Test. Additional exam requirements/recommendations for international students: Required—TOEFL (minimum score 550 paper-based). Electronic applications accepted. *Faculty research:* Soil microbiology; diagnosis etiology and control of plant diseases; genomics and molecular biology of plant microbe interactions; biotechnology, ecology of plant pathogens and epidemiology of diseases in agricultural and native ecosystems.

University of California, Riverside, Graduate Division, Department of Plant Pathology, Riverside, CA 92521-0102. Offers MS, PhD. Terminal master's awarded for partial completion of doctoral program. *Degree requirements:* For master's, comprehensive exams or thesis; for doctorate, thesis/dissertation, qualifying exams. *Entrance requirements:* For master's and doctorate, GRE General Test (minimum score 1100 or approximately 300 on new scoring scale), minimum GPA of 3.2. Additional exam requirements/recommendations for international students: Required—TOEFL (minimum score 550 paper-based; 80 iBT). *Application deadline:* For fall admission, 5/1 for domestic students, 2/1 for international students; for winter admission, 9/1 for domestic students, 7/1 for international students; for spring admission, 12/1 for domestic students, 10/1 for international students. Applications are processed on a rolling basis. Application fee: $85 ($100 for international students). Electronic applications accepted. *Expenses: Tuition, area resident:* Full-time $16,665.50; part-time $11,055.54. *Tuition, state resident:* full-time $16,665.50; part-time $11,055.54. *Tuition, nonresident:* full-time $31,768. *International tuition:* $31,767.50 full-time. *Required fees:* $16,665.50; $11,055.54 per quarter. $3685.18 per quarter. Tuition and fees vary according to program. *Financial support:* Fellowships with tuition reimbursements, research assistantships with tuition reimbursements, teaching assistantships with tuition reimbursements, career-related internships or fieldwork, institutionally sponsored loans, scholarships/grants, health care benefits, tuition waivers (full and partial), and unspecified assistantships available. *Faculty research:* Host-pathogen interactions, biological control and integrated approaches to disease management, fungicide behavior, molecular genetics.
Website: http://www.plantpathology.ucr.edu/

University of Florida, Graduate School, College of Agricultural and Life Sciences, Department of Plant Pathology, Gainesville, FL 32611. Offers plant pathology (MS, PhD), including toxicology (PhD). *Program availability:* Part-time. *Faculty:* 26 full-time, 4 part-time/adjunct. *Students:* 48 full-time (26 women), 4 part-time (1 woman); includes 8 minority (1 Black or African American, non-Hispanic/Latino; 3 Asian, non-Hispanic/Latino; 4 Hispanic/Latino), 27 international. Average age 30. 36 applicants, 42% accepted, 10 enrolled. In 2015, 6 master's, 5 doctorates awarded. Terminal master's awarded for partial completion of doctoral program. *Degree requirements:* For master's, comprehensive exam (for some programs), thesis optional; for doctorate, comprehensive exam, thesis/dissertation. *Entrance requirements:* For master's and doctorate, GRE General Test, minimum GPA of 3.0. Additional exam requirements/recommendations for international students: Required—TOEFL (minimum score 550 paper-based; 80 iBT), IELTS (minimum score 6). *Application deadline:* For fall admission, 2/1 priority date for domestic students, 2/1 for international students; for winter admission, 2/1 for domestic and international students; for spring admission, 10/1 for domestic students, 9/1 for international students. Applications are processed on a rolling basis. Application fee: $30. Electronic applications accepted. *Financial support:* In 2015–16, 1 fellowship, 33 research assistantships were awarded; teaching assistantships and career-related internships or fieldwork also available. Financial award application deadline: 2/1; financial award applicants required to submit FAFSA. *Faculty research:* Epidemiology, molecular biology of host-parasite interactions, bacteriology, virology, post-harvest diseases. *Total annual research expenditures:* $3.9

million. *Unit head:* Rosemary Loria, PhD, Chair, 352-273-4634, Fax: 352-392-6532, E-mail: loria@ufl.edu. *Application contact:* Jeffrey B. Jones, PhD, Graduate Coordinator, 352-273-4673 Ext. 213, Fax: 352-392-6532, E-mail: jbjones@ufl.edu.
Website: http://plantpath.ifas.ufl.edu/

University of Georgia, College of Agricultural and Environmental Sciences, Department of Plant Pathology, Athens, GA 30602. Offers MS, PhD. *Degree requirements:* For master's, thesis (MS); for doctorate, one foreign language, thesis/dissertation. *Entrance requirements:* For master's and doctorate, GRE General Test. Electronic applications accepted.

University of Guelph, Graduate Studies, Ontario Agricultural College, Department of Environmental Biology, Guelph, ON N1G 2W1, Canada. Offers entomology (M Sc, PhD); environmental microbiology and biotechnology (M Sc, PhD); environmental toxicology (M Sc, PhD); plant and forest systems (M Sc, PhD); plant pathology (M Sc, PhD). *Program availability:* Part-time. *Degree requirements:* For master's, thesis; for doctorate, comprehensive exam, thesis/dissertation. *Entrance requirements:* For master's, minimum 75% during previous 2 years of course work; for doctorate, minimum 75% average. Additional exam requirements/recommendations for international students: Required—TOEFL or IELTS. Electronic applications accepted. *Faculty research:* Entomology, environmental microbiology and biotechnology, environmental toxicology, forest ecology, plant pathology.

University of Hawaii at Manoa, Graduate Division, College of Tropical Agriculture and Human Resources, Department of Plant and Environmental Protection Sciences, Program in Tropical Plant Pathology, Honolulu, HI 96822. Offers MS, PhD. *Program availability:* Part-time. *Faculty:* 34 full-time (6 women), 10 part-time/adjunct (5 women). *Students:* 16 full-time (7 women), 4 part-time (2 women); includes 9 minority (3 Asian, non-Hispanic/Latino; 3 Hispanic/Latino; 3 Two or more races, non-Hispanic/Latino), 8 international. Average age 34. 9 applicants, 78% accepted, 6 enrolled. In 2015, 2 master's awarded. *Degree requirements:* For master's, thesis optional; for doctorate, comprehensive exam, thesis/dissertation. *Entrance requirements:* For master's and doctorate, GRE General Test. Additional exam requirements/recommendations for international students: Required—TOEFL (minimum score 540 paper-based; 76 iBT), IELTS (minimum score 5). *Application deadline:* For fall admission, 3/1 for domestic and international students; for spring admission, 9/1 for domestic and international students. Application fee: $100. *Financial support:* In 2015–16, 2 fellowships (averaging $2,237 per year), 8 research assistantships (averaging $17,609 per year) were awarded. *Total annual research expenditures:* $1.8 million. *Unit head:* Dr. J. Kenneth Grace, Chair, 808-956-7076, Fax: 808-956-2428. *Application contact:* Dr. Brent Sipes, Graduate Chairperson, 808-956-7076, Fax: 808-956-2832, E-mail: sipes@hawaii.edu.
Website: http://www.hawaii.edu/graduatestudies/fields/html/departments/pr/plantpath/plantpath.htm

University of Kentucky, Graduate School, College of Agriculture, Food and Environment, Program in Plant Pathology, Lexington, KY 40506-0032. Offers MS, PhD. *Degree requirements:* For master's, comprehensive exam, thesis; for doctorate, comprehensive exam, thesis/dissertation. *Entrance requirements:* For master's, GRE General Test, minimum undergraduate GPA of 2.75; for doctorate, GRE General Test, minimum graduate GPA of 3.0. Additional exam requirements/recommendations for international students: Required—TOEFL (minimum score 550 paper-based). Electronic applications accepted. *Faculty research:* Molecular biology of viruses and fungi, biochemistry and physiology of disease resistance, plant transformation, disease ecology, forest pathology.

University of Maine, Graduate School, College of Natural Sciences, Forestry, and Agriculture, School of Biology and Ecology, Orono, ME 04469. Offers biological sciences (PhD); botany and plant biology (MS); ecology and environmental science (MS, PhD); entomology (MS); plant science (PhD); zoology (MS, PhD). *Program availability:* Part-time. *Faculty:* 24 full-time (12 women), 34 part-time/adjunct (13 women). *Students:* 64 full-time (36 women), 1 part-time (0 women); includes 4 minority (1 American Indian or Alaska Native, non-Hispanic/Latino; 1 Asian, non-Hispanic/Latino; 1 Hispanic/Latino; 1 Two or more races, non-Hispanic/Latino), 8 international. Average age 29. 52 applicants, 25% accepted, 11 enrolled. In 2015, 7 master's, 8 doctorates awarded. Terminal master's awarded for partial completion of doctoral program. *Degree requirements:* For master's, thesis (for some programs); for doctorate, comprehensive exam, thesis/dissertation. *Entrance requirements:* For master's and doctorate, GRE General Test. Additional exam requirements/recommendations for international students: Required—TOEFL. *Application deadline:* For fall admission, 2/1 priority date for domestic students. Applications are processed on a rolling basis. Application fee: $65. Electronic applications accepted. *Financial support:* In 2015–16, 14 students received support, including 6 research assistantships with full tuition reimbursements available (averaging $14,600 per year), 8 teaching assistantships with full tuition reimbursements available (averaging $14,600 per year); career-related internships or fieldwork, Federal Work-Study, institutionally sponsored loans, and tuition waivers (full and partial) also available. Financial award application deadline: 3/1. *Faculty research:* Ecology and evolution (aquatic, terrestrial, paleo); development and genetics; biomedical research; ecophysiology and stress; invasion ecology and pest management. *Total annual research expenditures:* $3.2 million. *Unit head:* Dr. Andrei Aloykhin, Director, 207-581-2977, Fax: 207-581-2537. *Application contact:* Scott G. Delcourt, Assistant Vice President for Graduate Studies and Senior Associate Dean, 207-581-3291, Fax: 207-581-3232, E-mail: graduate@maine.edu.
Website: http://sbe.umaine.edu/

University of Minnesota, Twin Cities Campus, Graduate School, College of Food, Agricultural and Natural Resource Sciences, Department of Plant Pathology, St. Paul, MN 55108. Offers MS, PhD. *Program availability:* Part-time. Terminal master's awarded for partial completion of doctoral program. *Degree requirements:* For master's, comprehensive exam, thesis; for doctorate, comprehensive exam, thesis/dissertation. *Entrance requirements:* For master's and doctorate, GRE General Test. Additional exam requirements/recommendations for international students: Required—TOEFL (minimum score 550 paper-based; 79 iBT), IELTS (minimum score 6.5). Electronic applications accepted. *Faculty research:* Plant disease management, disease resistance, product deterioration, international agriculture, molecular biology.

The University of Tennessee, Graduate School, College of Agricultural Sciences and Natural Resources, Department of Entomology and Plant Pathology, Knoxville, TN 37996. Offers entomology (MS, PhD); integrated pest management and bioactive natural products (PhD); plant pathology (MS, PhD). *Program availability:* Part-time. *Degree requirements:* For master's, thesis, seminar. *Entrance requirements:* For master's, GRE General Test, minimum GPA of 2.7, 3 reference letters, letter of intent; for doctorate, GRE General Test, minimum GPA of 2.7, 3 reference letters, letter of intent, proposed dissertation research. Additional exam requirements/recommendations for international students: Required—TOEFL. Electronic applications accepted.

University of Wisconsin–Madison, Graduate School, College of Agricultural and Life Sciences, Department of Plant Pathology, Madison, WI 53706-1380. Offers MS, PhD. *Program availability:* Part-time. Terminal master's awarded for partial completion of doctoral program. *Degree requirements:* For master's, thesis; for doctorate, thesis/dissertation. *Entrance requirements:* For master's and doctorate, GRE. Additional exam

Plant Pathology

requirements/recommendations for international students: Required—TOEFL. Electronic applications accepted. *Expenses:* Tuition, state resident: full-time $5364. Tuition, nonresident: full-time $12,027. *Required fees:* $571. Tuition and fees vary according to campus/location, program and reciprocity agreements. *Faculty research:* Plant disease, plant health, plant-microbe interactions, plant disease management, biological control.

Virginia Polytechnic Institute and State University, Graduate School, College of Agriculture and Life Sciences, Blacksburg, VA 24061. Offers agricultural and applied economics (MS); agricultural and life sciences (MS); animal and poultry science (MS, PhD); crop and soil environmental sciences (MS, PhD); dairy science (MS); entomology (PhD); horticulture (MS, PhD); human nutrition, foods and exercise (MS, PhD); life sciences (MS, PhD); plant pathology, physiology and weed science (PhD). *Degree requirements:* For master's, comprehensive exam (for some programs), thesis (for some programs); for doctorate, comprehensive exam (for some programs), thesis/dissertation (for some programs). *Entrance requirements:* For master's and doctorate, GRE/GMAT (may vary by department). Additional exam requirements/recommendations for international students: Required—TOEFL (minimum score 550 paper-based). Electronic applications accepted.

Washington State University, College of Agricultural, Human, and Natural Resource Sciences, Department of Plant Pathology, Pullman, WA 99164. Offers MS, PhD. Programs offered at the Pullman campus. Terminal master's awarded for partial completion of doctoral program. *Degree requirements:* For master's, comprehensive exam (for some programs), thesis (for some programs); for doctorate, comprehensive exam, thesis/dissertation, oral exam. *Entrance requirements:* For master's and doctorate, GRE, statement of purpose. Additional exam requirements/recommendations for international students: Required—TOEFL (minimum score 550 paper-based), IELTS. Electronic applications accepted. *Faculty research:* Biology of fungi, bacteria, and viruses; diseases of plants; genetics of fungi, bacteria, and viruses.

West Virginia University, Davis College of Agriculture, Forestry and Consumer Sciences, Division of Plant and Soil Sciences, Morgantown, WV 26506. Offers agricultural sciences (PhD), including animal and food sciences, plant and soil sciences; agronomy (MS); entomology (MS); environmental microbiology (MS); horticulture (MS); plant pathology (MS). *Degree requirements:* For master's, thesis. *Entrance requirements:* For master's, GRE, minimum GPA of 2.5. Additional exam requirements/recommendations for international students: Required—TOEFL. *Expenses:* Tuition, state resident: full-time $8568. Tuition, nonresident: full-time $22,140. Tuition and fees vary according to program. *Faculty research:* Water quality, reclamation of disturbed land, crop production, pest control, environmental protection.

Plant Physiology

Cornell University, Graduate School, Graduate Fields of Agriculture and Life Sciences, Field of Plant Biology, Ithaca, NY 14853-0001. Offers cytology (MS, PhD); paleobotany (MS, PhD); plant biochemistry (MS, PhD); plant cell biology (MS, PhD); plant ecology (MS, PhD); plant molecular biology (MS, PhD); plant morphology, anatomy and biomechanics (MS, PhD); plant physiology (MS, PhD); systematic botany (MS, PhD). *Degree requirements:* For doctorate, comprehensive exam, thesis/dissertation. *Entrance requirements:* For doctorate, GRE General Test, GRE Subject Test in biology (recommended), 3 letters of recommendation. Additional exam requirements/recommendations for international students: Required—TOEFL (minimum score 610 paper-based; 77 iBT). Electronic applications accepted. *Faculty research:* Plant cell biology/cytology; plant molecular biology; plant morphology/anatomy/biomechanics; plant physiology, systematic botany, paleobotany; plant ecology, ethnobotany, plant biochemistry, photosynthesis.

Dalhousie University, Faculty of Agriculture, Halifax, NS B3H 4R2, Canada. Offers agriculture (M Sc), including air quality, animal behavior, animal molecular genetics, animal nutrition, animal technology, aquaculture, botany, crop management, crop physiology, ecology, environmental microbiology, food science, horticulture, nutrient management, pest management, physiology, plant biotechnology, plant pathology, soil chemistry, soil fertility, waste management and composting, water quality. *Program availability:* Part-time. *Degree requirements:* For master's, thesis, ATC Exam Teaching Assistantship. *Entrance requirements:* For master's, honors B Sc, minimum GPA of 3.0. Additional exam requirements/recommendations for international students: Required—TOEFL (minimum score 580 paper-based; 92 iBT), IELTS, Michigan English Language Assessment Battery, CanTEST, CAEL. *Faculty research:* Bio-product development, organic agriculture, nutrient management, air and water quality, agricultural biotechnology.

Purdue University, Graduate School, College of Science, Department of Biological Sciences, West Lafayette, IN 47907. Offers biochemistry (PhD); biophysics (PhD); cell and developmental biology (PhD); ecology, evolutionary and population biology (MS, PhD), including ecology, evolutionary biology, population biology; genetics (MS, PhD); microbiology (MS, PhD); molecular biology (PhD); neurobiology (MS, PhD); plant physiology (PhD). Terminal master's awarded for partial completion of doctoral program. *Degree requirements:* For master's, thesis (for some programs); for doctorate, thesis/dissertation, seminars, teaching experience. *Entrance requirements:* For master's, GRE General Test (minimum analytical writing score of 3.5), minimum undergraduate GPA of 3.0; for doctorate, GRE General Test (minimum analytical writing score of 3.5), minimum undergraduate GPA of 3.5. Additional exam requirements/recommendations for

international students: Required—TOEFL (minimum score 600 paper-based; 107 iBT for MS, 80 iBT for PhD). Electronic applications accepted.

University of Manitoba, Faculty of Graduate Studies, Faculty of Agricultural and Food Sciences, Department of Plant Science, Winnipeg, MB R3T 2N2, Canada. Offers agronomy and plant protection (M Sc, PhD); horticulture (M Sc, PhD); plant breeding and genetics (M Sc, PhD); plant physiology-biochemistry (M Sc, PhD). *Degree requirements:* For master's, thesis; for doctorate, one foreign language, thesis/dissertation.

University of Massachusetts Amherst, Graduate School, Interdisciplinary Programs, Program in Plant Biology, Amherst, MA 01003. Offers biochemistry and metabolism (MS, PhD); cell biology and physiology (MS, PhD); environmental, ecological and integrative biology (MS, PhD); genetics and evolution (MS, PhD). *Degree requirements:* For master's, thesis; for doctorate, 2 foreign languages, comprehensive exam, thesis/dissertation. *Entrance requirements:* For master's and doctorate, GRE General Test. Additional exam requirements/recommendations for international students: Required—TOEFL (minimum score 550 paper-based; 80 iBT), IELTS (minimum score 6.5). Electronic applications accepted.

The University of Tennessee, Graduate School, College of Arts and Sciences, Program in Life Sciences, Knoxville, TN 37996. Offers genome science and technology (MS, PhD); plant physiology and genetics (MS, PhD). *Degree requirements:* For doctorate, one foreign language, thesis/dissertation. *Entrance requirements:* For master's and doctorate, GRE General Test, minimum GPA of 2.7. Additional exam requirements/recommendations for international students: Required—TOEFL. Electronic applications accepted.

Virginia Polytechnic Institute and State University, Graduate School, College of Agriculture and Life Sciences, Blacksburg, VA 24061. Offers agricultural and applied economics (MS); agricultural and life sciences (MS); animal and poultry science (MS, PhD); crop and soil environmental sciences (MS, PhD); dairy science (MS); entomology (PhD); horticulture (MS, PhD); human nutrition, foods and exercise (MS, PhD); life sciences (MS, PhD); plant pathology, physiology and weed science (PhD). *Degree requirements:* For master's, comprehensive exam (for some programs), thesis (for some programs); for doctorate, comprehensive exam (for some programs), thesis/dissertation (for some programs). *Entrance requirements:* For master's and doctorate, GRE/GMAT (may vary by department). Additional exam requirements/recommendations for international students: Required—TOEFL (minimum score 550 paper-based). Electronic applications accepted.

Section 6
Cell, Molecular, and Structural Biology

This section contains a directory of institutions offering graduate work in cell, molecular, and structural biology, followed by in-depth entries submitted by institutions that chose to prepare detailed program descriptions. Additional information about programs listed in the directory but not augmented by an in-depth entry may be obtained by writing directly to the dean of a graduate school or chair of a department at the address given in the directory.

For programs offering related work, see also in this book *Anatomy; Biochemistry; Biological and Biomedical Sciences; Biophysics; Botany and Plant Biology; Genetics, Developmental Biology, and Reproductive Biology; Microbiological Sciences; Pathology and Pathobiology; Pharmacology and Toxicology; Pharmacy and Pharmaceutical Sciences; Physiology;* and *Veterinary Medicine and Sciences.* In the other guides in this series:

Graduate Programs in the Physical Sciences, Mathematics, Agricultural Sciences, the Environment & Natural Resources
See *Chemistry*
Graduate Programs in Engineering & Applied Sciences
See *Agricultural Engineering and Bioengineering* and *Biomedical Engineering and Biotechnology*

CONTENTS

Program Directories

Displays and Close-Ups

See also:

Cancer Biology/Oncology

Augusta University, The Graduate School, Program in Biochemistry and Cancer Biology, Augusta, GA 30912. Offers PhD. *Faculty:* 2 full-time. *Degree requirements:* For doctorate, comprehensive exam, thesis/dissertation. *Entrance requirements:* For doctorate, GRE General Test. Additional exam requirements/recommendations for international students: Required—TOEFL (minimum score 550 paper-based; 79 iBT). *Application deadline:* For fall admission, 1/15 for domestic and international students. Application fee: $50. Electronic applications accepted. *Financial support:* Research assistantships with partial tuition reimbursements, Federal Work-Study, institutionally sponsored loans, and scholarships/grants available. Support available to part-time students. Financial award application deadline: 5/31; financial award applicants required to submit FAFSA. *Faculty research:* Bacterial pathogenesis, eye diseases, vitamins and amino acid transporters, transcriptional control and molecular oncology, tumor biology. *Unit head:* Dr. Vinata Lokeshwar, Chair, 706-721-7652, Fax: 706-721-9947, E-mail: vlokeshwar@augusta.edu. *Application contact:* Dr. Darren Browning, Director, 706-721-7658, E-mail: dbrowning@augusta.edu.
Website: http://www.augusta.edu/cancer/students/

Baylor College of Medicine, Graduate School of Biomedical Sciences, Program in Translational Biology and Molecular Medicine, Houston, TX 77030-3498. Offers PhD. *Degree requirements:* For doctorate, thesis/dissertation, public defense. *Entrance requirements:* For doctorate, GRE, minimum GPA of 3.0. Additional exam requirements/recommendations for international students: Required—TOEFL. Electronic applications accepted. *Faculty research:* Molecular medicine, translational biology, human disease biology and therapy.

Case Western Reserve University, School of Medicine and School of Graduate Studies, Graduate Programs in Medicine, Programs in Molecular and Cellular Basis of Disease/Pathology, Cancer Biology Training Program, Cleveland, OH 44106. Offers PhD, MD/PhD. *Degree requirements:* For doctorate, comprehensive exam, thesis/dissertation. *Entrance requirements:* For doctorate, GRE. Additional exam requirements/recommendations for international students: Required—TOEFL (minimum score 550 paper-based). *Expenses:* Tuition, area resident: Full-time $41,137; part-time $1714 per credit hour. *Required fees:* $32. Tuition and fees vary according to course load and program.

Duke University, Graduate School, University Program in Molecular Cancer Biology, Durham, NC 27710. Offers PhD. *Degree requirements:* For doctorate, thesis/dissertation. *Entrance requirements:* For doctorate, GRE General Test, GRE Subject Test in biology or biochemistry, cell and molecular biology (recommended). Additional exam requirements/recommendations for international students: Required—TOEFL (minimum score 577 paper-based; 90 iBT) or IELTS (minimum score 7). Electronic applications accepted.

Emory University, Laney Graduate School, Division of Biological and Biomedical Sciences, Program in Cancer Biology, Atlanta, GA 30322. Offers PhD. *Degree requirements:* For doctorate, comprehensive exam, thesis/dissertation. *Entrance requirements:* For doctorate, GRE General Test, minimum GPA of 3.0 in science course work (recommended). Additional exam requirements/recommendations for international students: Required—TOEFL. Electronic applications accepted. *Expenses:* Contact institution. *Faculty research:* Basic and translational cancer research, molecular and cellular biology, genetics and epigenetics, signal transduction, genetic engineering and nanotechnologies.

Gerstner Sloan Kettering Graduate School of Biomedical Sciences, Program in Cancer Biology, New York, NY 10021. Offers PhD. *Degree requirements:* For doctorate, thesis/dissertation. *Entrance requirements:* For doctorate, GRE, transcripts, three letters of recommendation. Additional exam requirements/recommendations for international students: Required—TOEFL. Electronic applications accepted. *Faculty research:* Structural biology, computational biology, genomics, immunology, chemical biology.
See Display below and Close-Up on page 221.

Irell & Manella Graduate School of Biological Sciences, Graduate Program, Duarte, CA 91010. Offers brain metastatic cancer (PhD); cancer and stem cell metabolism (PhD); cancer biology (PhD); cancer biology and developmental therapeutics (PhD); cell biology (PhD); chemical biology (PhD); chromosomal break repair (PhD); diabetes and pancreatic progenitor cell biology (PhD); DNA repair and cancer biology (PhD); germline epigenetic remodeling and endocrine disruptors (PhD); hematology and hematopoietic cell transplantation (PhD); hematology and immunology (PhD); inflammation and cancer (PhD); micrornas and gene regulation in cardiovascular disease (PhD); mixed chimrism for reversal of autoimmunity (PhD); molecular and cellular biology (PhD); molecular biology and genetics (PhD); nanoparticle mediated twist1 silencing in metastatic cancer (PhD); neuro-oncology and stem cell biology (PhD); neuroscience (PhD); rna directed therapies for hiv-1 (PhD); small rna-induced transcriptional gene activation (PhD); stem cell regulation by the microenvironment (PhD); translational oncology and pharmaceutical sciences (PhD); tumor biology (PhD). *Faculty:* 70 full-time (18 women). *Students:* 75 full-time (40 women); includes 28 minority (2 Black or African American, non-Hispanic/Latino; 10 Asian, non-Hispanic/Latino; 10 Hispanic/Latino; 2 Native Hawaiian or other Pacific Islander, non-Hispanic/Latino; 4 Two or more races, non-Hispanic/Latino), 15 international. Average age 26. 197 applicants, 12% accepted, 19 enrolled. In 2015, 12 doctorates awarded. *Degree requirements:* For doctorate, comprehensive exam, thesis/dissertation, qualifying exams, two advanced courses. *Entrance requirements:* For doctorate, GRE General Test; GRE Subject Test (recommended), 2 years of course work in chemistry (general and organic); 1 year of course work each in biochemistry, general biology, and general physics; 2 semesters of course work in mathematics; significant research laboratory experience. Additional exam requirements/recommendations for international students: Required—TOEFL. *Application deadline:* For fall admission, 1/1 priority date for domestic and international students. Application fee: $0. Electronic applications accepted. Full-time tuition and fees vary according to class time, course level, course load, degree level, campus/location, program and student level. *Financial support:* In 2015–16, 12 students received support, including 35 fellowships with full tuition reimbursements available (averaging $32,000 per year); teaching assistantships, health care benefits, and tuition waivers (full) also available. Financial award applicants required to submit FAFSA. *Faculty research:* Cancer biology, diabetes, stem cell biology, neuroscience, immunology. *Unit head:* Dr. John J. Rossi, Dean, 877-715-GRAD, Fax: 626-471-3901, E-mail: gradschool@coh.org. *Application contact:* Dr. Kate Sleeth, Interim Associate Dean of Administration and Student Development, 626-218-1742, Fax: 626-471-3901, E-mail: gradschool@coh.org.
Website: http://cityofhope.org/gradschool
See Display on page 66 and Close-Up on page 111.

We offer the next generation of basic scientists a program to study the biological sciences through the lens of cancer — while giving students the tools they will need to put them in the vanguard of research that can be applied in any area of human disease.

Visit us at **www.sloankettering.edu** to learn how to apply, for application deadlines, and for more information about our PhD program.

Gerstner Sloan Kettering Graduate School of Biomedical Sciences
Memorial Sloan Kettering Cancer Center
New York City

gradstudies@sloankettering.edu
646.888.6639

PhD Program in Cancer Biology

An internationally recognized research faculty in:

- Cancer genetics
- Genomic integrity
- Cell signaling and regulation
- Structural biology
- Immunology
- Chemical biology
- Developmental biology
- Computational biology
- Experimental therapeutics
- Experimental pathology
- Imaging and radiation sciences
- Oncology
- Genomics
- Animal models of disease

An innovative, integrated curriculum provides a fundamental understanding of:

- The nature of genes and gene expression
- Cellular organization
- Tissue and organ formation
- Cell-cell interactions
- Cellular response to the environment
- Enzyme activity

All matriculated students receive a full fellowship package for the duration of study.

Long Island University–LIU Post, School of Health Professions and Nursing, Brookville, NY 11548-1300. Offers biomedical sciences (MS), including applied laboratory medicine, cancer biology, medical and molecular immunology, microbiology/infectious diseases; cardiovascular perfusion (MS); dietetic internship (Advanced Certificate); family nurse practitioner (MS); forensic social work (Advanced Certificate); nursing education (MS); social work (MSW). *Program availability:* Part-time, evening/weekend, blended/hybrid learning. *Faculty:* 16 full-time (14 women), 46 part-time/adjunct (33 women). *Students:* 190 full-time (139 women), 181 part-time (157 women); includes 141 minority (51 Black or African American, non-Hispanic/Latino; 46 Asian, non-Hispanic/Latino; 41 Hispanic/Latino; 3 Two or more races, non-Hispanic/Latino), 47 international. Average age 36. 422 applicants, 64% accepted, 141 enrolled. In 2015, 96 master's, 28 other advanced degrees awarded. *Degree requirements:* For master's, comprehensive exam (for some programs), thesis (for some programs). *Entrance requirements:* Additional exam requirements/recommendations for international students: Required—TOEFL, IELTS. *Application deadline:* Applications are processed on a rolling basis. Application fee: $50. Electronic applications accepted. *Expenses:* $1,155 per credit, $934 per term full-time university fee, $442 per term part-time university fee. *Financial support:* In 2015–16, 6 research assistantships with partial tuition reimbursements were awarded; career-related internships or fieldwork, Federal Work-Study, institutionally sponsored loans, tuition waivers (partial), and unspecified assistantships also available. Support available to part-time students. Financial award application deadline: 2/15; financial award applicants required to submit FAFSA. *Faculty research:* Breast cancer, childhood obesity, dietary beverage consumption, emotional distress, histone modification, interprofessional practice, interstitial cystitis, lung cancer, pancreatic cancer, pediatric pain management, post-traumatic growth, poverty, renal nutrition, social ethics, yeast and bacterial drug resistance. *Total annual research expenditures:* $15,000. *Unit head:* Dr. Stacy Gropack, Acting Dean, 516-299-2486, Fax: 516-299-2527, E-mail: post-shpn@liu.edu. *Application contact:* Carol Zerah, Director of Graduate and International Admissions, 516-299-2900 Ext. 3952, Fax: 516-299-2137, E-mail: post-enroll@liu.edu.
Website: http://liu.edu/post/health

Loyola University Chicago, Graduate School, Marcella Niehoff School of Nursing, Maywood, IL 60153. Offers adult gerontology acute care clinical nurse specialist (MSN), including emergency care (MSN, Certificate); adult gerontology acute care nurse practitioner (MSN), including oncology (MSN, Certificate); adult gerontology clinical nurse specialist (MSN), including oncology (MSN, Certificate); adult gerontology nursing (Certificate), including oncology (MSN, Certificate); adult nurse practitioner (Certificate); dietetics (MS); family nurse practitioner (MSN, Certificate), including emergency care; informatics (MSN); leadership (DNP), including healthcare quality using education in safety and technology, infection prevention; nursing science (PhD); women's health nurse practitioner (MSN); women's health nursing (Certificate). *Accreditation:* AACN. *Program availability:* Part-time, blended/hybrid learning. *Faculty:* 27 full-time (25 women), 12 part-time/adjunct (10 women). *Students:* 174 full-time (161 women), 232 part-time (221 women); includes 95 minority (19 Black or African American, non-Hispanic/Latino; 2 American Indian or Alaska Native, non-Hispanic/Latino; 38 Asian, non-Hispanic/Latino; 28 Hispanic/Latino; 2 Native Hawaiian or other Pacific Islander, non-Hispanic/Latino; 6 Two or more races, non-Hispanic/Latino), 3 international. Average age 35. 209 applicants, 52% accepted, 83 enrolled. In 2015, 78 master's, 10 doctorates, 17 other advanced degrees awarded. *Degree requirements:* For master's, comprehensive exam; for doctorate, thesis/dissertation, qualifying examination (for PhD); capstone project (for DNP). *Entrance requirements:* For master's, BSN, minimum nursing GPA of 3.0, Illinois RN license, 3 letters of recommendation, 1000 hours of experience in area of specialty prior to starting clinical rotations, personal statement; for doctorate, GRE General Test (for PhD), BSN or MSN, minimum GPA of 3.0, professional nursing license, 3 letters of recommendation, personal statement. Additional exam requirements/recommendations for international students: Required—TOEFL (minimum score 550 paper-based; 79 iBT), IELTS (minimum score 6.5). *Application deadline:* For fall admission, 6/1 priority date for domestic and international students; for spring admission, 11/15 priority date for domestic and international students; for summer admission, 3/15 priority date for domestic and international students. Applications are processed on a rolling basis. Application fee: $50. Electronic applications accepted. Application fee is waived when completed online. *Expenses:* $1,081 per credit hour. *Financial support:* In 2015–16, 10 students received support, including 3 research assistantships with full tuition reimbursements available (averaging $18,000 per year), 1 teaching assistantship with full tuition reimbursement available (averaging $18,000 per year); scholarships/grants, unspecified assistantships, and nurse faculty loan program also available. Financial award application deadline: 5/1; financial award applicants required to submit FAFSA. *Faculty research:* Epigenetics and social determinants of health, women's health, vitamin D, interprofessional education, prevention and self-management of chronic disease. *Total annual research expenditures:* $649,606. *Unit head:* Dr. Vicky Keough, Dean, 708-216-5448, Fax: 708-216-9555, E-mail: vkeough@luc.edu. *Application contact:* Toni Topalova, Enrollment Advisor, 708-216-3751, Fax: 708-216-9555, E-mail: atopalova@luc.edu.
Website: http://www.luc.edu/nursing/

Mayo Graduate School, Graduate Programs in Biomedical Sciences, Program in Tumor Biology, Rochester, MN 55905. Offers PhD. *Degree requirements:* For doctorate, oral defense of dissertation, qualifying oral and written exam. *Entrance requirements:* For doctorate, GRE, 1 year of chemistry, biology, calculus, and physics. Additional exam requirements/recommendations for international students: Required—TOEFL. Electronic applications accepted.

McMaster University, Faculty of Health Sciences and School of Graduate Studies, Program in Medical Sciences, Genetics and Cancer Area, Hamilton, ON L8S 4M2, Canada. Offers M Sc, PhD, MD/PhD. *Degree requirements:* For master's, thesis; for doctorate, comprehensive exam, thesis/dissertation. *Entrance requirements:* For master's, honors B Sc, B+ average in related field; for doctorate, M Sc, minimum B+ average, students with proven research experience and an A average may be admitted with a B Sc degree. Additional exam requirements/recommendations for international students: Required—TOEFL (minimum score 580 paper-based; 92 iBT).

Medical University of South Carolina, College of Graduate Studies, Program in Molecular and Cellular Biology and Pathobiology, Charleston, SC 29425. Offers cancer biology (PhD); cardiovascular biology (PhD); cardiovascular imaging (PhD); cell regulation (PhD); craniofacial biology (PhD); genetics and development (PhD); marine biomedicine (PhD); DMD/PhD; MD/PhD. *Degree requirements:* For doctorate, thesis/dissertation, oral and written exams. *Entrance requirements:* For doctorate, GRE General Test, interview, minimum GPA of 3.0. Additional exam requirements/recommendations for international students: Required—TOEFL (minimum score 600 paper-based; 100 iBT). Electronic applications accepted.

Meharry Medical College, School of Graduate Studies, Program in Biomedical Sciences, Cancer Biology Emphasis, Nashville, TN 37208-9989. Offers PhD, MD/PhD. *Degree requirements:* For doctorate, comprehensive exam, thesis/dissertation. *Entrance requirements:* For doctorate, GRE. *Application deadline:* For fall admission, 6/1 for domestic students. Applications are processed on a rolling basis. Application fee: $65. *Financial support:* Fellowships available. Financial award application deadline: 4/

15. *Faculty research:* Regulation of metabolism, enzymology, signal transduction, physical biochemistry.

Memorial University of Newfoundland, Faculty of Medicine and School of Graduate Studies, Graduate Programs in Medicine, Division of Biomedical Sciences, St. John's, NL A1C 5S7, Canada. Offers cancer (M Sc, PhD); cardiovascular (M Sc, PhD); immunology (M Sc, PhD); neuroscience (M Sc, PhD). *Program availability:* Part-time. *Degree requirements:* For master's, thesis; for doctorate, comprehensive exam, thesis/dissertation, oral defense of thesis. *Entrance requirements:* For master's, MD or B Sc; for doctorate, MD or M Sc. Additional exam requirements/recommendations for international students: Required—TOEFL. *Expenses: Tuition, area resident:* Full-time $2199 Canadian dollars. *International tuition:* $2859 Canadian dollars full-time. *Faculty research:* Neuroscience, immunology, cardiovascular, and cancer.

New York University, Graduate School of Arts and Science, Department of Biology, New York, NY 10012-1019. Offers biology (PhD); biomedical journalism (MS); cancer and molecular biology (PhD); computational biology (PhD); computers in biological research (MS); developmental genetics (PhD); general biology (MS); immunology and microbiology (PhD); molecular genetics (PhD); neurobiology (PhD); oral biology (MS); plant biology (PhD); recombinant DNA technology (MS); MS/MBA. *Program availability:* Part-time. Terminal master's awarded for partial completion of doctoral program. *Degree requirements:* For master's, thesis or alternative, qualifying paper; for doctorate, comprehensive exam, thesis/dissertation. *Entrance requirements:* For master's and doctorate, GRE General Test. Additional exam requirements/recommendations for international students: Required—TOEFL. *Faculty research:* Genomics, molecular and cell biology, development and molecular genetics, molecular evolution of plants and animals.

New York University, School of Medicine and Graduate School of Arts and Science, Sackler Institute of Graduate Biomedical Sciences, Program in Molecular Oncology and Tumor Immunology, New York, NY 10012-1019. Offers immunology (PhD); molecular oncology (PhD). *Degree requirements:* For doctorate, one foreign language, comprehensive exam, thesis/dissertation, qualifying exam. *Faculty research:* Stem cells, immunology, genome instability, DNA damage checkpoints.

Oregon Health & Science University, School of Medicine, Graduate Programs in Medicine, Program in Molecular and Cellular Biosciences, Cancer Biology Program, Portland, OR 97239-3098. Offers PhD. *Faculty:* 55 part-time/adjunct (17 women). *Students:* 19 full-time (8 women); includes 2 minority (both Asian, non-Hispanic/Latino), 4 international. Average age 29. *Degree requirements:* For doctorate, comprehensive exam, thesis/dissertation, qualifying exam. *Entrance requirements:* For doctorate, GRE General Test (minimum scores: 158 Verbal/148 Quantitative/4.5 Analytical). Additional exam requirements/recommendations for international students: Required—IELTS or TOEFL. *Application deadline:* For fall admission, 12/1 for domestic and international students. Application fee: $70. Electronic applications accepted. *Financial support:* Health care benefits and full tuition and stipends (for PhD students) available. *Faculty research:* Signal transduction, apoptosis, carcinogenesis, genome integrity, tumor micro-environment. *Unit head:* Dr. Matthew Thayer, Program Leader, 503-494-2447, E-mail: thayerm@ohsu.edu. *Application contact:* Lola Bichler, Program Coordinator, 503-494-5824, E-mail: bichler@ohsu.edu.
Website: http://www.ohsu.edu/cancerbio

Purdue University, Graduate School, PULSe - Purdue University Life Sciences Program, West Lafayette, IN 47907. Offers biomolecular structure and biophysics (PhD); biotechnology (PhD); chemical biology (PhD); chromatin and regulation of gene expression (PhD); integrative neuroscience (PhD); integrative plant sciences (PhD); membrane biology (PhD); microbiology (PhD); molecular evolutionary and cancer biology (PhD); molecular evolutionary genetics (PhD); molecular virology (PhD). *Entrance requirements:* For doctorate, GRE, minimum undergraduate GPA of 3.0. Additional exam requirements/recommendations for international students: Required—TOEFL (minimum score 550 paper-based; 77 iBT). Electronic applications accepted.

Queen's University at Kingston, School of Graduate Studies, Faculty of Health Sciences, Department of Anatomy and Cell Biology, Kingston, ON K7L 3N6, Canada. Offers biology of reproduction (M Sc, PhD); cancer (M Sc, PhD); cardiovascular pathophysiology (M Sc, PhD); cell and molecular biology (M Sc, PhD); drug metabolism (M Sc, PhD); endocrinology (M Sc, PhD); motor control (M Sc, PhD); neural regeneration (M Sc, PhD); neurophysiology (M Sc, PhD). *Program availability:* Part-time. *Degree requirements:* For master's, thesis; for doctorate, one foreign language, comprehensive exam, thesis/dissertation. *Entrance requirements:* Additional exam requirements/recommendations for international students: Required—TOEFL. Electronic applications accepted. *Faculty research:* Human kinetics, neuroscience, reproductive biology, cardiovascular.

Rutgers University–Newark, Graduate School of Biomedical Sciences, Newark, NJ 07107. Offers biodefense (Certificate); biomedical engineering (PhD); biomedical sciences (multidisciplinary) (PhD); cellular biology, neuroscience and physiology (PhD), including neuroscience, physiology, biophysics, cardiovascular biology, molecular pharmacology, stem cell biology; infection, immunity and inflammation (PhD), including immunology, infectious disease, microbiology, oral biology; molecular biology, genetics and cancer (PhD), including biochemistry, molecular genetics, cancer biology, radiation biology, bioinformatics; neuroscience (Certificate); pharmacological sciences (Certificate); stem cell (Certificate); DMD/PhD; MD/PhD. PhD in biomedical engineering offered jointly with New Jersey Institute of Technology. *Program availability:* Part-time, evening/weekend. Terminal master's awarded for partial completion of doctoral program. *Degree requirements:* For doctorate, thesis/dissertation, qualifying exam. *Entrance requirements:* For doctorate, GRE General Test. Additional exam requirements/recommendations for international students: Required—TOEFL. Electronic applications accepted.

Rutgers University–New Brunswick, Graduate School-New Brunswick, Program in Endocrinology and Animal Biosciences, Piscataway, NJ 08854-8097. Offers MS, PhD. Terminal master's awarded for partial completion of doctoral program. *Degree requirements:* For master's, thesis; for doctorate, comprehensive exam, thesis/dissertation. *Entrance requirements:* For master's and doctorate, GRE General Test. Additional exam requirements/recommendations for international students: Required—TOEFL. Electronic applications accepted. *Faculty research:* Comparative and behavioral endocrinology, epigenetic regulation of the endocrine system, exercise physiology and immunology, fetal and neonatal developmental programming, mammary gland biology and breast cancer, neuroendocrinology and alcohol studies, reproductive and developmental toxicology.

Thomas Jefferson University, Jefferson College of Biomedical Sciences, PhD Program in Genetics, Genomics and Cancer Biology, Philadelphia, PA 19107. Offers PhD. *Faculty:* 48 full-time (16 women), 4 part-time/adjunct (3 women). *Students:* 21 full-time (12 women); includes 3 minority (1 Asian, non-Hispanic/Latino; 2 Hispanic/Latino), 3 international. 46 applicants, 11% accepted, 4 enrolled. In 2015, 1 doctorate awarded. *Degree requirements:* For doctorate, comprehensive exam, thesis/dissertation. *Entrance requirements:* For doctorate, GRE General Test, minimum GPA of 3.2. Additional exam requirements/recommendations for international students: Required—TOEFL, IELTS (minimum score 7). *Application deadline:* For fall admission, 12/15

Cancer Biology/Oncology

priority date for domestic and international students. Applications are processed on a rolling basis. Application fee: $50. Electronic applications accepted. *Financial support:* In 2015–16, 21 students received support, including 21 fellowships with full tuition reimbursements available (averaging $56,298 per year); Federal Work-Study, institutionally sponsored loans, scholarships/grants, traineeships, and stipends also available. Support available to part-time students. Financial award application deadline: 5/1; financial award applicants required to submit FAFSA. *Faculty research:* Functional genomics, cancer susceptibility, cell cycle, regulation oncogenes and tumor suppressor genes, genetics of neoplastic disease. *Unit head:* Dr. Lucia Languino, Program Director, 215-503-3442, E-mail: lucia.languino@jefferson.edu. *Application contact:* Marc E. Stearns, Director of Admissions, 215-503-0155, Fax: 215-503-3433, E-mail: jgsbs-info@jefferson.edu.
Website: http://www.jefferson.edu/university/biomedical-sciences/degrees-programs/phd-programs/genetics.html

Tufts University, Sackler School of Graduate Biomedical Sciences, Cell, Molecular, and Developmental Biology Program, Medford, MA 02155. Offers cancer biology (PhD); developmental and regenerative biology (PhD); molecular and cellular medicine (PhD); structural and chemical biology (PhD). *Faculty:* 45 full-time (15 women). *Students:* 36 full-time (18 women); includes 13 minority (2 Black or African American, non-Hispanic/Latino; 9 Asian, non-Hispanic/Latino; 1 Hispanic/Latino; 1 Two or more races, non-Hispanic/Latino), 4 international. Average age 28. 189 applicants, 7% accepted, 6 enrolled. In 2015, 2 doctorates awarded. Terminal master's awarded for partial completion of doctoral program. *Degree requirements:* For doctorate, comprehensive exam, thesis/dissertation. *Entrance requirements:* For doctorate, GRE General Test, 3 letters of reference. Additional exam requirements/recommendations for international students: Required—TOEFL (minimum score 600 paper-based; 100 iBT). *Application deadline:* For fall admission, 12/15 priority date for domestic and international students. Application fee: $70. Electronic applications accepted. *Expenses:* Tuition, area resident: Full-time $48,412; part-time $1210 per credit hour. *Required fees:* $806. Full-time tuition and fees vary according to degree level, program and student level. Part-time tuition and fees vary according to course load. *Financial support:* In 2015–16, 36 students received support, including 36 research assistantships with full tuition reimbursements available (averaging $32,000 per year); health care benefits also available. *Faculty research:* Reproduction and hormone action, control of gene expression, cell-matrix and cell-cell interactions, growth control and tumorigenesis, cytoskeleton and contractile proteins. *Unit head:* Dr. Ira Herman, Program Director, 617-636-2991, Fax: 617-636-0375. *Application contact:* Dr. Elizabeth Storrs, Registrar/Director of Academic Services, 617-636-6767, Fax: 617-636-0375, E-mail: sackler-school@tufts.edu.
Website: http://sackler.tufts.edu/Academics/CMDB-Welcome

Université Laval, Faculty of Medicine, Post-Professional Programs in Medical Studies, Québec, QC G1K 7P4, Canada. Offers anatomy–pathology (DESS); anesthesiology (DESS); cardiology (DESS); care of older people (Diploma); clinical research (DESS); community health (DESS); dermatology (DESS); diagnostic radiology (DESS); emergency medicine (Diploma); family medicine (DESS); general surgery (DESS); geriatrics (DESS); hematology (DESS); internal medicine (DESS); maternal and fetal medicine (Diploma); medical biochemistry (DESS); medical microbiology and infectious diseases (DESS); medical oncology (DESS); nephrology (DESS); neurology (DESS); neurosurgery (DESS); obstetrics and gynecology (DESS); ophthalmology (DESS); orthopedic surgery (DESS); oto-rhino-laryngology (DESS); palliative medicine (Diploma); pediatrics (DESS); plastic surgery (DESS); psychiatry (DESS); pulmonary medicine (DESS); radiology–oncology (DESS); thoracic surgery (DESS); urology (DESS). *Degree requirements:* For other advanced degree, comprehensive exam. *Entrance requirements:* For degree, knowledge of French. Electronic applications accepted.

University at Buffalo, the State University of New York, Graduate School, Graduate Programs in Cancer Research and Biomedical Sciences at Roswell Park Cancer Institute, Interdisciplinary Master of Science Program at Roswell Park Cancer Institute, Buffalo, NY 14260. Offers MS. *Program availability:* Part-time. *Faculty:* 126 full-time (36 women). *Students:* 21 full-time (8 women); includes 3 minority (1 Black or African American, non-Hispanic/Latino; 1 Asian, non-Hispanic/Latino; 1 Hispanic/Latino), 8 international. 28 applicants, 64% accepted, 9 enrolled. In 2015, 25 master's awarded. *Degree requirements:* For master's, thesis, oral defense of thesis based on research project. *Entrance requirements:* For master's, GRE General Test. Additional exam requirements/recommendations for international students: Required—TOEFL (minimum score 79 iBT). *Application deadline:* For fall admission, 3/1 priority date for domestic and international students. Application fee: $75. Electronic applications accepted. *Faculty research:* Biochemistry, oncology, pathology, biophysics, pharmacology, molecular biology, cellular biology, genetics, bioinformatics, immunology, therapeutic development, epidemiology. *Unit head:* Dr. Norman J. Karin, Associate Dean, 716-845-2339, Fax: 716-845-8178, E-mail: norman.karin@roswellpark.edu. *Application contact:* Dr. Norman J. Karin, Associate Dean, 716-845-2339, Fax: 716-845-8178, E-mail: norman.karin@roswellpark.edu.
Website: http://www.roswellpark.edu/education/interdisciplinary-masters

The University of Alabama at Birmingham, Graduate Programs in Joint Health Sciences, Cancer Biology Program, Birmingham, AL 35294. Offers PhD. *Degree requirements:* For doctorate, comprehensive exam, thesis/dissertation. *Entrance requirements:* For doctorate, GRE (minimum score of 1100 old test; 300 new test), minimum GPA of 3.0, minimum 6 months of research in a bench/lab setting, baccalaureate degree in biological or physical sciences, references. Additional exam requirements/recommendations for international students: Required—TOEFL (minimum score 600 paper-based; 100 iBT), IELTS (minimum score 6.5). Electronic applications accepted. *Expenses:* Tuition, state resident: full-time $7340. Tuition, nonresident: full-time $16,628. Full-time tuition and fees vary according to course load and program.

University of Alberta, Faculty of Medicine and Dentistry and Faculty of Graduate Studies and Research, Graduate Programs in Medicine, Department of Oncology, Edmonton, AB T6G 2E1, Canada. Offers M Sc, PhD. Terminal master's awarded for partial completion of doctoral program. *Degree requirements:* For master's, thesis; for doctorate, thesis/dissertation. *Entrance requirements:* For master's and doctorate, minimum GPA of 7.0 on a 9.0 scale, B SC. Additional exam requirements/recommendations for international students: Required—TOEFL (minimum score 600 paper-based). Electronic applications accepted. *Faculty research:* Experimental oncology, radiation oncology, medical physics, medical oncology.

The University of Arizona, Graduate Interdisciplinary Programs, Graduate Interdisciplinary Program in Cancer Biology, Tucson, AZ 85721. Offers PhD. *Degree requirements:* For doctorate, comprehensive exam, thesis/dissertation. *Entrance requirements:* For doctorate, GRE General Test, 3 letters of recommendation. Additional exam requirements/recommendations for international students: Required—TOEFL (minimum score 550 paper-based; 79 iBT). *Application deadline:* For fall admission, 12/1 for domestic and international students. Applications are processed on a rolling basis. Application fee: $75. Electronic applications accepted. *Financial support:* Research assistantships, institutionally sponsored loans, scholarships/grants, traineeships, health care benefits, tuition waivers (full), and unspecified assistantships available. *Faculty research:* Differential gene expression, DNA-protein cross linking, cell growth regulation

steroid, receptor proteins. *Unit head:* Dr. Margaret Briehl, Co-Chair, 520-626-7479, E-mail: mmbriehl@pathology.arizona.edu. *Application contact:* Anne Cione, Senior Program Coordinator, 520-626-7479, Fax: 520-626-4979, E-mail: acione@azcc.arizona.edu.
Website: http://www.azcc.arizona.edu/academics/cbio

University of Calgary, Cumming School of Medicine and Faculty of Graduate Studies, Medical Science Graduate Program, Calgary, AB T2N 1N4, Canada. Offers cancer biology (M Sc, PhD); critical care medicine (M Sc, PhD); joint injury and arthritis (M Sc, PhD); molecular and medical genetics (M Sc, PhD); mountain medicine and high altitude physiology (M Sc, PhD); pathologists' assistant (M Sc, PhD). *Degree requirements:* For master's, thesis; for doctorate, thesis/dissertation, candidacy exam. *Entrance requirements:* For master's, minimum undergraduate GPA of 3.2; for doctorate, minimum graduate GPA of 3.2. Additional exam requirements/recommendations for international students: Required—TOEFL (minimum score 600 paper-based). Electronic applications accepted. *Faculty research:* Cancer biology, immunology, joint injury and arthritis, medical education, population genomics.

University of Chicago, Division of the Biological Sciences, Committee on Cancer Biology, Chicago, IL 60637. Offers PhD. *Students:* 32 full-time (15 women); includes 5 minority (3 Asian, non-Hispanic/Latino; 2 Hispanic/Latino), 9 international. Average age 28. 117 applicants, 14% accepted, 9 enrolled. In 2015, 4 doctorates awarded. *Degree requirements:* For doctorate, thesis/dissertation, ethics class, 2 teaching assistantships. *Entrance requirements:* For doctorate, GRE General Test. Additional exam requirements/recommendations for international students: Required—TOEFL (minimum score 600 paper-based; 104 iBT), IELTS (minimum score 7). *Application deadline:* For fall admission, 12/1 for domestic and international students. Application fee: $90. Electronic applications accepted. *Financial support:* In 2015–16, 25 students received support, including fellowships with full tuition reimbursements available (averaging $29,781 per year), research assistantships with full tuition reimbursements available (averaging $29,781 per year); institutionally sponsored loans and traineeships also available. Financial award applicants required to submit FAFSA. *Faculty research:* Cancer genetics, apoptosis, signal transduction, tumor biology, cell cycle regulation. *Total annual research expenditures:* $58 million. *Application contact:* Emily Traw, Administrative Director, E-mail: biomed@bsd.uchicago.edu.
Website: http://biomedsciences.uchicago.edu/page/cancer-biology

University of Cincinnati, Graduate School, College of Medicine, Graduate Programs in Biomedical Sciences, Cancer and Cell Biology Graduate Program, Cincinnati, OH 45267. Offers PhD. *Degree requirements:* For doctorate, thesis/dissertation, qualifying exam. *Entrance requirements:* For doctorate, GRE General Test. Additional exam requirements/recommendations for international students: Required—TOEFL. Electronic applications accepted. *Faculty research:* Cancer biology, cell and molecular biology, breast cancer, pancreatic cancer, drug discovery.

University of Colorado Denver, School of Medicine, Program in Cancer Biology, Aurora, CO 80045. Offers PhD. *Students:* 34 full-time (25 women); includes 12 minority (4 Asian, non-Hispanic/Latino; 5 Hispanic/Latino; 1 Native Hawaiian or other Pacific Islander, non-Hispanic/Latino; 2 Two or more races, non-Hispanic/Latino), 4 international. Average age 27. 58 applicants, 9% accepted, 5 enrolled. In 2015, 3 doctorates awarded. *Degree requirements:* For doctorate, comprehensive exam, thesis/dissertation, 3 laboratory rotations. *Entrance requirements:* For doctorate, GRE General Test, interview, minimum undergraduate GPA of 3.0. Additional exam requirements/recommendations for international students: Required—TOEFL (minimum score 550 paper-based; 80 iBT). *Application deadline:* For fall admission, 12/1 for domestic students, 11/1 priority date for international students. Application fee: $50 ($75 for international students). Electronic applications accepted. *Expenses:* Contact institution. *Financial support:* In 2015–16, 30 students received support. Fellowships with full tuition reimbursements available, research assistantships, teaching assistantships, Federal Work-Study, institutionally sponsored loans, scholarships/grants, traineeships, health care benefits, tuition waivers (full), and unspecified assistantships available. Financial award application deadline: 3/15; financial award applicants required to submit FAFSA. *Faculty research:* Signal transduction by tyrosine kinases, estrogen and progesterone receptors in breast cancer, mechanism of mitochondrial DNA replication in the mammalian cell. *Total annual research expenditures:* $9 million. *Unit head:* Dr. Mary Reyland, Director, Cancer Biology Program, 303-724-4572, E-mail: mary.reyland@ucdenver.edu. *Application contact:* Sabrena Heilman, Program Administrator, 303-724-3245, E-mail: sabrena.heilman@ucdenver.edu.
Website: http://www.ucdenver.edu/academics/colleges/Graduate-School/academic-programs/cancerbiology/Pages/cancerbiologyprogram.aspx

University of Delaware, College of Arts and Sciences, Department of Biological Sciences, Newark, DE 19716. Offers biotechnology (MS); cancer biology (MS, PhD); cell and extracellular matrix biology (MS, PhD); cell and systems physiology (MS, PhD); developmental biology (MS, PhD); ecology and evolution (MS, PhD); microbiology (MS, PhD); molecular biology and genetics (MS, PhD). Terminal master's awarded for partial completion of doctoral program. *Degree requirements:* For master's, thesis, preliminary exam; for doctorate, comprehensive exam, thesis/dissertation, preliminary exam. *Entrance requirements:* For master's and doctorate, GRE General Test. Additional exam requirements/recommendations for international students: Required—TOEFL (minimum score 600 paper-based); Recommended—TWE. Electronic applications accepted. *Faculty research:* Microorganisms, bone, cancer metastasis, developmental biology, cell biology, DNA.

The University of Manchester, Faculty of Life Sciences, Manchester, United Kingdom. Offers adaptive organismal biology (M Phil, PhD); animal biology (M Phil, PhD); biochemistry (M Phil, PhD); bioinformatics (M Phil, PhD); biomolecular sciences (M Phil, PhD); biotechnology (M Phil, PhD); cell biology (M Phil, PhD); cell matrix research (M Phil, PhD); channels and transporters (M Phil, PhD); developmental biology (M Phil, PhD); Egyptology (M Phil, PhD); environmental biology (M Phil, PhD); evolutionary biology (M Phil, PhD); gene expression (M Phil, PhD); genetics (M Phil, PhD); history of science, technology and medicine (M Phil, PhD); immunology (M Phil, PhD); integrative neurobiology and behavior (M Phil, PhD); membrane trafficking (M Phil, PhD); microbiology (M Phil, PhD); molecular and cellular neuroscience (M Phil, PhD); molecular biology (M Phil, PhD); molecular cancer studies (M Phil, PhD); neuroscience (M Phil, PhD); ophthalmology (M Phil, PhD); optometry (M Phil, PhD); organelle function (M Phil, PhD); pharmacology (M Phil, PhD); physiology (M Phil, PhD); plant sciences (M Phil, PhD); stem cell research (M Phil, PhD); structural biology (M Phil, PhD); systems neuroscience (M Phil, PhD); toxicology (M Phil, PhD).

The University of Manchester, School of Dentistry, Manchester, United Kingdom. Offers basic dental sciences (cancer studies) (M Phil, PhD); basic dental sciences (molecular genetics) (M Phil, PhD); basic dental sciences (stem cell biology) (M Phil, PhD); biomaterials sciences and dental technology (M Phil, PhD); dental public health/community dentistry (M Phil, PhD); dental science (clinical) (PhD); endodontology (M Phil, PhD); fixed and removable prosthodontics (M Phil, PhD); operative dentistry (M Phil, PhD); oral and maxillofacial surgery (M Phil, PhD); oral radiology (M Phil, PhD); orthodontics (M Phil, PhD); restorative dentistry (M Phil, PhD).

University of Manitoba, Faculty of Graduate Studies, Faculty of Nursing, Winnipeg, MB R3T 2N2, Canada. Offers cancer nursing (MN); nursing (MN). *Degree requirements:* For master's, thesis.

University of Maryland, Baltimore, Graduate School, Graduate Program in Life Sciences, Program in Molecular Medicine, Baltimore, MD 21201. Offers cancer biology (PhD); cell and molecular physiology (PhD); human genetics and genomic medicine (PhD); molecular medicine (MS); molecular toxicology and pharmacology (PhD); MD/PhD. *Degree requirements:* For doctorate, comprehensive exam, thesis/dissertation. *Entrance requirements:* For master's and doctorate, GRE. Additional exam requirements/recommendations for international students: Required—TOEFL (minimum score 600 paper-based; 100 iBT); Recommended—IELTS (minimum score 7). Electronic applications accepted. Tuition and fees vary according to program.

University of Massachusetts Medical School, Graduate School of Biomedical Sciences, Worcester, MA 01655-0115. Offers biomedical sciences (PhD), including biochemistry and molecular pharmacology, bioinformatics and computational biology, cancer biology, cell biology, immunology and microbiology, interdisciplinary, neuroscience, translational science; biomedical sciences (millennium program) (PhD); clinical and population health research (PhD); clinical investigation (MS). *Faculty:* 1,339 full-time (521 women), 301 part-time/adjunct (189 women). *Students:* 363 full-time (184 women); includes 58 minority (13 Black or African American, non-Hispanic/Latino; 30 Asian, non-Hispanic/Latino; 15 Hispanic/Latino), 141 international. Average age 29. 661 applicants, 26% accepted, 51 enrolled. In 2015, 10 master's, 58 doctorates awarded. Terminal master's awarded for partial completion of doctoral program. *Degree requirements:* For master's, comprehensive exam, thesis; for doctorate, comprehensive exam, thesis/dissertation. *Entrance requirements:* For master's, MD, PhD, DVM, or PharmD; for doctorate, GRE General Test, bachelor's degree. Additional exam requirements/recommendations for international students: Required—TOEFL (minimum score 100 iBT) or IELTS (minimum score 7.5). *Application deadline:* For fall admission, 12/15 for domestic and international students; for spring admission, 5/15 for domestic students. Application fee: $80. Electronic applications accepted. *Expenses:* $6,966 resident per year; $14,182 non-resident per year. *Financial support:* In 2015–16, 383 students received support, including research assistantships with full tuition reimbursements available (averaging $30,600 per year); scholarships/grants, health care benefits, tuition waivers (full), and unspecified assistantships also available. Financial award application deadline: 5/16. *Faculty research:* RNA interference, cell/molecular/developmental biology, bioinformatics, clinical/translational research, infectious disease. *Total annual research expenditures:* $250.3 million. *Unit head:* Dr. Anthony Carruthers, Dean, 508-856-4135, E-mail: anthony.carruthers@umassmed.edu. *Application contact:* Dr. Kendall Knight, Assistant Vice Provost for Admissions, 508-856-5628, Fax: 508-856-3659, E-mail: kendall.knight@umassmed.edu.
Website: http://www.umassmed.edu/gsbs/

University of Miami, Graduate School, Miller School of Medicine, Program in Cancer Biology, Coral Gables, FL 33124. Offers PhD, MD/PhD.

University of Michigan, Rackham Graduate School, Program in Biomedical Sciences (PIBS), Doctoral Program in Cancer Biology, Ann Arbor, MI 48109. Offers PhD. *Faculty:* 40 full-time (11 women). *Students:* 16 full-time (12 women); includes 7 minority (1 Black or African American, non-Hispanic/Latino; 2 Asian, non-Hispanic/Latino; 3 Hispanic/Latino; 1 Native Hawaiian or other Pacific Islander, non-Hispanic/Latino), 3 international. Average age 27. 40 applicants, 35% accepted, 3 enrolled. In 2015, 1 doctorate awarded. *Degree requirements:* For doctorate, thesis/dissertation, preliminary examination, oral defense of dissertation. *Entrance requirements:* For doctorate, GRE General Test, three letters of recommendation, research experience, personal and research statements. Additional exam requirements/recommendations for international students: Required—TOEFL (minimum score 84 iBT). *Application deadline:* For fall admission, 12/1 for domestic students. Application fee: $75. Electronic applications accepted. *Expenses:* $10,340 in-state tuition and fees, $20,885 out-of-state. *Financial support:* In 2015–16, 15 students received support, including 6 fellowships with full tuition reimbursements available (averaging $29,025 per year), 9 research assistantships with full tuition reimbursements available (averaging $29,025 per year); scholarships/grants, health care benefits, tuition waivers (full), and unspecified assistantships also available. Financial award application deadline: 12/1. *Faculty research:* Tumor immunology, viral oncogenesis, cell biology, genetics, epidemiology, pathology, bioinformatics. *Unit head:* Dr. Elizabeth Lawlor, Professor of Pediatric Oncology/Associate Director for Education and Training, UM Comprehensive Cancer Center/Director, Cancer Biology Program, 734-615-4814, Fax: 734-764-9017, E-mail: elawlor@umich.edu. *Application contact:* Michelle S. Melis, Director of Student Life, Programs in Biomedical Sciences (PIBS), 734-615-6538, Fax: 734-647-7022, E-mail: msmtegan@umich.edu.
Website: http://cancerbio.medicine.umich.edu/

University of Michigan, Rackham Graduate School, Program in Chemical Biology, Ann Arbor, MI 48109. Offers cancer chemical biology (MS); chemical biology (PhD). *Faculty:* 46 full-time (13 women). *Students:* 58 full-time (21 women), 2 part-time (1 woman); includes 17 minority (5 Black or African American, non-Hispanic/Latino; 1 American Indian or Alaska Native, non-Hispanic/Latino; 4 Asian, non-Hispanic/Latino; 4 Hispanic/Latino; 3 Two or more races, non-Hispanic/Latino), 10 international. 117 applicants, 62% accepted, 29 enrolled. In 2015, 7 master's, 10 doctorates awarded. *Degree requirements:* For doctorate, thesis/dissertation. *Entrance requirements:* Additional exam requirements/recommendations for international students: Required—TOEFL (minimum score 600 paper-based; 102 iBT). *Application deadline:* For fall admission, 12/15 priority date for domestic and international students. Applications are processed on a rolling basis. Application fee: $75 ($90 for international students). Electronic applications accepted. *Financial support:* In 2015–16, 47 students received support, including fellowships with full tuition reimbursements available (averaging $29,025 per year), research assistantships with full tuition reimbursements available (averaging $29,025 per year); career-related internships or fieldwork, scholarships/grants, traineeships, and unspecified assistantships also available. *Faculty research:* Chemical genetics, structural enzymology, signal transduction, biological catalysis, biomolecular structure, function and recognition. *Unit head:* Prof. Anna Mapp, Program Director, 734-763-7175, Fax: 734-615-1252, E-mail: chemicalbiology@umich.edu. *Application contact:* Admissions Office, 734-764-8129, E-mail: rackadmis@umich.edu.
Website: http://www.chembio.umich.edu/

University of Minnesota, Twin Cities Campus, Graduate School, PhD Program in Microbiology, Immunology and Cancer Biology, Minneapolis, MN 55455-0213. Offers PhD. *Degree requirements:* For doctorate, thesis/dissertation. *Entrance requirements:* For doctorate, GRE General Test. Additional exam requirements/recommendations for international students: Required—TOEFL (minimum score 600 paper-based). Electronic applications accepted. *Faculty research:* Virology, microbiology, cancer biology, immunology.

University of Nebraska Medical Center, Program in Cancer Research, Omaha, NE 68198. Offers PhD. *Faculty:* 35 full-time (8 women), 3 part-time/adjunct (0 women). *Students:* 31 full-time (19 women), 1 (woman) part-time; includes 4 minority (2 Black or African American, non-Hispanic/Latino; 2 Hispanic/Latino), 7 international. Average age 27. 32 applicants, 19% accepted, 6 enrolled. In 2015, 8 doctorates awarded. Terminal master's awarded for partial completion of doctoral program. *Degree requirements:* For

doctorate, comprehensive exam, thesis/dissertation. *Entrance requirements:* For doctorate, GRE, 3 letters of reference; course work in chemistry, biology, physics and mathematics. Additional exam requirements/recommendations for international students: Required—TOEFL (minimum score 550 paper-based; 90 iBT). *Application deadline:* For fall admission, 7/1 for domestic and international students; for spring admission, 11/1 for domestic and international students; for summer admission, 4/1 for domestic and international students. Applications are processed on a rolling basis. Application fee: $45. Electronic applications accepted. *Expenses:* Tuition, state resident: full-time $7830; part-time $3915 per credit hour. Tuition, nonresident: full-time $22,410; part-time $11,205 per credit hour. *Required fees:* $521. *Financial support:* In 2015–16, 41 students received support, including 1 fellowship with full tuition reimbursement available (averaging $23,100 per year), 7 research assistantships with full tuition reimbursements available (averaging $23,100 per year); unspecified assistantships also available. Financial award application deadline: 2/15; financial award applicants required to submit FAFSA. *Faculty research:* Cancer genetics, cancer development and metastasis, cell signaling, tumor immunology, molecular therapies for cancer. *Unit head:* Dr. Joyce Solheim, Graduate Committee Chair, 402-559-4539, Fax: 402-559-8270, E-mail: jsolheim@unmc.edu. *Application contact:* Misty Pocwierz, Education and Project Associate, 402-559-4092, E-mail: misty.pocwierz@unmc.edu.
Website: http://www.unmc.edu/eppley/education/crgp.html

University of Pennsylvania, Perelman School of Medicine, Biomedical Graduate Studies, Graduate Group in Cell and Molecular Biology, Philadelphia, PA 19104. Offers cancer biology (PhD); cell biology, physiology, and metabolism (PhD); developmental stem cell regenerative biology (PhD); gene therapy and vaccines (PhD); genetics and gene regulation (PhD); microbiology, virology, and parasitology (PhD); MD/PhD; VMD/PhD. *Faculty:* 317. *Students:* 339 full-time (189 women); includes 100 minority (7 Black or African American, non-Hispanic/Latino; 2 American Indian or Alaska Native, non-Hispanic/Latino; 45 Asian, non-Hispanic/Latino; 34 Hispanic/Latino; 1 Native Hawaiian or other Pacific Islander, non-Hispanic/Latino; 11 Two or more races, non-Hispanic/Latino), 52 international. 493 applicants, 22% accepted, 37 enrolled. In 2015, 51 doctorates awarded. *Degree requirements:* For doctorate, thesis/dissertation. *Entrance requirements:* For doctorate, GRE General Test. Additional exam requirements/recommendations for international students: Required—TOEFL. *Application deadline:* For fall admission, 12/1 priority date for domestic and international students. Applications are processed on a rolling basis. Application fee: $80. Electronic applications accepted. *Expenses: Tuition, area resident:* Full-time $31,068; part-time $5762 per course. *Required fees:* $3200; $336 per course. Full-time tuition and fees vary according to degree level, program and student level. Part-time tuition and fees vary according to course load, degree level and program. *Financial support:* In 2015–16, 339 students received support. Fellowships, research assistantships, scholarships/grants, traineeships, and unspecified assistantships available. *Unit head:* Dr. Daniel Kessler, Graduate Group Chair, 215-898-1478. *Application contact:* Meagan Schofer, Coordinator, 215-898-4360.
Website: http://www.med.upenn.edu/camb/

University of Regina, Faculty of Graduate Studies and Research, Faculty of Science, Department of Chemistry and Biochemistry, Regina, SK S4S 0A2, Canada. Offers analytical/environmental chemistry (M Sc, PhD); biophysics of biological interfaces (M Sc, PhD); enzymology/chemical biology (M Sc, PhD); inorganic/organometallic chemistry (M Sc, PhD); signal transduction and mechanisms of cancer cell regulation (M Sc, PhD); supramolecular organic photochemistry and photophysics (M Sc, PhD); synthetic organic chemistry (M Sc, PhD); theoretical/computational chemistry (M Sc, PhD). *Degree requirements:* For master's, thesis; for doctorate, thesis/dissertation. *Entrance requirements:* Additional exam requirements/recommendations for international students: Required—TOEFL (minimum score 580 paper-based; 80 iBT), IELTS (minimum score 6.5), PTE (minimum score 59). Electronic applications accepted. *Faculty research:* Asymmetric synthesis and methodology, theoretical and computational chemistry, biophysical biochemistry, analytical and environmental chemistry, chemical biology.

University of Southern California, Keck School of Medicine, Program in Cancer Biology and Genomics, Los Angeles, CA 90089. Offers cancer biology and genomics (PhD). *Faculty:* 43 full-time (10 women). *Students:* 15 full-time (11 women); includes 5 minority (4 Asian, non-Hispanic/Latino; 1 Hispanic/Latino), 8 international. Average age 28. 3 applicants, 100% accepted, 3 enrolled. *Degree requirements:* For doctorate, comprehensive exam, thesis/dissertation. *Entrance requirements:* For doctorate, GRE, minimum GPA of 3.0. Additional exam requirements/recommendations for international students: Required—TOEFL (minimum score 600 paper-based; 100 iBT), IELTS (minimum score 7), PTE. *Application deadline:* For fall admission, 12/1 priority date for domestic and international students. Application fee: $85. Electronic applications accepted. *Financial support:* In 2015–16, 15 students received support, including 2 fellowships with full tuition reimbursements available (averaging $32,000 per year), 13 research assistantships with full tuition reimbursements available (averaging $32,000 per year); institutionally sponsored loans, scholarships/grants, traineeships, health care benefits, and unspecified assistantships also available. Financial award application deadline: 5/4; financial award applicants required to submit CSS PROFILE or FAFSA. *Unit head:* Dr. Baruch Frenkel, Director, 323-442-1475, Fax: 323-442-1199, E-mail: frenkel@med.usc.edu. *Application contact:* Dr. Joyce Perez, Manager of Student Programs, 323-442-1645, Fax: 323-442-1199, E-mail: jpperez@med.usc.edu.
Website: http://pibbs.usc.edu/research-and-programs/phd-programs/

University of South Florida, College of Arts and Sciences, Department of Cell Biology, Microbiology, and Molecular Biology, Tampa, FL 33620-9951. Offers biology (MS), including cell and molecular biology; cancer biology (PhD); cell and molecular biology (PhD); microbiology (MS). *Faculty:* 21 full-time (7 women). *Students:* 41 full-time (6 women), 45 part-time (2 women); includes 11 minority (1 Black or African American, non-Hispanic/Latino; 2 Asian, non-Hispanic/Latino; 5 Hispanic/Latino; 3 Two or more races, non-Hispanic/Latino), 22 international. Average age 27. 171 applicants, 14% accepted, 18 enrolled. In 2015, 22 master's, 14 doctorates awarded. *Degree requirements:* For master's, thesis or alternative; for doctorate, comprehensive exam, thesis/dissertation. *Entrance requirements:* For master's and doctorate, GRE General Test, minimum GPA of 3.0, extensive background in biology or chemistry. Additional exam requirements/recommendations for international students: Required—TOEFL (minimum score 570 paper-based; 79 iBT) or IELTS (minimum score 6.5). *Application deadline:* For fall admission, 2/1 for domestic students, 1/1 for international students. Application fee: $30. *Financial support:* Career-related internships or fieldwork, health care benefits, and unspecified assistantships available. Financial award application deadline: 4/1. *Faculty research:* Cell biology, microbiology and molecular biology: basic and applied science in bacterial pathogenesis, genome integrity and mechanisms of aging, structural and computational biology; cancer biology: immunology, cancer control, signal transduction, drug discovery, genomics. *Total annual research expenditures:* $1.9 million. *Unit head:* Dr. James Garey, Professor/Chair, 813-974-7103, Fax: 813-974-1614, E-mail: garey@usf.edu. *Application contact:* Dr. Kenneth Wright, Associate Professor of Cancer Biology, H. Lee Moffitt Cancer Center and Research Institute, 813-745-3918, Fax: 813-974-1614, E-mail: ken.wright@moffitt.org.
Website: http://biology.usf.edu/cmmb/

Cancer Biology/Oncology

The University of Texas Health Science Center at Houston, Graduate School of Biomedical Sciences, Program in Cancer Biology, Houston, TX 77225-0036. Offers MS, PhD, MD/PhD. Terminal master's awarded for partial completion of doctoral program. *Degree requirements:* For master's, thesis; for doctorate, thesis/dissertation. *Entrance requirements:* For master's and doctorate, GRE General Test. Additional exam requirements/recommendations for international students: Required—TOEFL. Electronic applications accepted. *Faculty research:* Cancer metastasis, signal transduction, therapeutic resistance, cell cycle deregulation, cancer markers and target.

The University of Texas Health Science Center at Houston, Graduate School of Biomedical Sciences, Program in Molecular Carcinogenesis, Houston, TX 77225-0036. Offers MS, PhD, MD/PhD. Terminal master's awarded for partial completion of doctoral program. *Degree requirements:* For master's, thesis; for doctorate, thesis/dissertation. *Entrance requirements:* For master's and doctorate, GRE General Test. Additional exam requirements/recommendations for international students: Required—TOEFL. Electronic applications accepted. *Faculty research:* Carcinogenesis, mutagenesis, epigenetics, mouse models, cancer prevention.

The University of Texas Southwestern Medical Center, Southwestern Graduate School of Biomedical Sciences, Division of Basic Science, Program in Cancer Biology, Dallas, TX 75390. Offers PhD. *Degree requirements:* For doctorate, thesis/dissertation, qualifying examination.

University of the District of Columbia, College of Arts and Sciences, Program in Cancer Biology, Prevention and Control, Washington, DC 20008-1175. Offers MS. Program offered in partnership with Lombardi Comprehensive Cancer Center at Georgetown University. Application fee: $50.
Website: http://www.udc-lccc.org/

The University of Toledo, College of Graduate Studies, College of Medicine and Life Sciences, Department of Biochemistry and Cancer Biology, Toledo, OH 43606-3390. Offers cancer biology (MSBS, PhD); MD/MSBS; MD/PhD. Terminal master's awarded for partial completion of doctoral program. *Degree requirements:* For master's, thesis, qualifying exam; for doctorate, thesis/dissertation, qualifying exam. *Entrance requirements:* For master's and doctorate, GRE, minimum undergraduate GPA of 3.0, three letters of recommendation, statement of purpose, transcripts from all prior institutions attended; resume. Additional exam requirements/recommendations for international students: Required—TOEFL (minimum score 550 paper-based; 80 iBT). Electronic applications accepted.

University of Utah, School of Medicine and Graduate School, Graduate Programs in Medicine, Department of Oncological Sciences, Salt Lake City, UT 84112-1107. Offers M Phil, MS, PhD. Terminal master's awarded for partial completion of doctoral program. *Degree requirements:* For master's, thesis (for some programs); for doctorate, thesis/dissertation. *Entrance requirements:* For master's and doctorate, GRE General Test, GRE Subject Test, minimum GPA of 3.0. Additional exam requirements/recommendations for international students: Required—TOEFL. *Faculty research:* Molecular basis of cell growth and differences, regulation of gene expression, biochemical mechanics of DNA replication, molecular biology and biochemistry of signal transduction, somatic cell genetics.

University of Wisconsin–La Crosse, College of Science and Health, Department of Health Professions, Program in Medical Dosimetry, La Crosse, WI 54601-3742. Offers MS. *Program availability:* Online learning. *Students:* 48 full-time (28 women), 1 (woman) part-time; includes 13 minority (2 Black or African American, non-Hispanic/Latino; 7 Asian, non-Hispanic/Latino; 2 Hispanic/Latino; 2 Two or more races, non-Hispanic/Latino). Average age 31. 44 applicants, 48% accepted, 21 enrolled. In 2015, 14 master's awarded. *Entrance requirements:* For master's, American Registry of Radiologic Technologists test, Medical Dosimetrist Certification Board Exam. Additional exam requirements/recommendations for international students: Required—TOEFL (minimum score 600 paper-based; 100 iBT). *Application deadline:* For fall admission, 12/1 priority date for domestic students, 11/1 priority date for international students. Application fee: $50. Electronic applications accepted. *Expenses:* Contact institution. *Financial support:* Federal Work-Study and scholarships/grants available. Support available to part-time students. Financial award applicants required to submit FAFSA. *Unit head:* Nishele Lenards, Program Director, 608-785-8470, E-mail: nlenards@uwlax.edu. *Application contact:* Brandon Schaller, Senior Graduate Student Status Examiner, 608-785-8941, E-mail: admissions@uwlax.edu.
Website: http://www.uwlax.edu/md/

University of Wisconsin–Madison, School of Medicine and Public Health, Cancer Biology Graduate Program, Madison, WI 53706. Offers PhD. *Faculty:* 51 full-time (15 women). *Students:* 24 full-time (10 women); includes 5 minority (2 Asian, non-Hispanic/Latino; 3 Hispanic/Latino), 4 international. 176 applicants, 9% accepted, 4 enrolled. In 2015, 8 doctorates awarded. *Degree requirements:* For doctorate, comprehensive exam, thesis/dissertation. *Entrance requirements:* For doctorate, GRE General Test. Additional exam requirements/recommendations for international students: Required—TOEFL (minimum score 580 paper-based; 92 iBT). *Application deadline:* For fall admission, 12/1 priority date for domestic and international students. Application fee: $56. Electronic applications accepted. *Expenses:* Tuition, state resident: full-time $5364. Tuition, nonresident: full-time $12,027. *Required fees:* $571. Tuition and fees vary according to campus/location, program and reciprocity agreements. *Financial support:* In 2015–16, 24 students received support, including fellowships with full tuition reimbursements available (averaging $26,000 per year), research assistantships with full tuition reimbursements available (averaging $26,000 per year), traineeships, health care benefits, and unspecified assistantships also available. Support available to part-time students. Financial award application deadline: 12/1. *Faculty research:* Cancer genetics, tumor virology, chemical carcinogenesis, signal transduction, cell cycle. *Total annual research expenditures:* $18 million. *Unit head:* Dr. Paul F. Lambert, Director, 608-262-8533, Fax: 608-262-2824, E-mail: lambert@oncology.wisc.edu. *Application contact:* Jenny M. Schroeder, Administrative Program Manager, 608-262-4682, Fax: 608-262-2824, E-mail: jmschroeder2@oncology.wisc.edu.
Website: http://www.cancerbiology.wisc.edu/

University of Wisconsin–Milwaukee, Graduate School, College of Health Sciences, Program in Biomedical Sciences, Milwaukee, WI 53211. Offers cancer (MS); immunology (MS); microbiology (MS); neurodegenerative disease (MS); pharmacology and toxicology (MS); photobiomodulation (MS). *Accreditation:* NAACLS. *Program availability:* Part-time. *Faculty:* 8 full-time (4 women). *Students:* 8 full-time (7 women), 3 part-time (1 woman); includes 1 minority (Two or more races, non-Hispanic/Latino), 2 international. Average age 29. 42 applicants, 14% accepted, 4 enrolled. In 2015, 7 master's awarded. *Degree requirements:* For master's, thesis. *Entrance requirements:* For master's, GRE General Test. Additional exam requirements/recommendations for international students: Required—TOEFL (minimum score 550 paper-based; 79 iBT), IELTS (minimum score 6.5). *Application deadline:* For fall admission, 1/1 priority date for domestic students; for spring admission, 9/1 for domestic students. Applications are processed on a rolling basis. Application fee: $56 ($96 for international students). *Financial support:* In 2015–16, 6 teaching assistantships were awarded; fellowships, research assistantships, career-related internships or fieldwork, and unspecified assistantships also available. Support available to part-time students. Financial award application deadline: 4/15. *Unit head:* Raymond Fleming, Representative, 414-229-3980, E-mail: mundo@uwm.edu. *Application contact:* Roger O. Smith, General Information Contact, 414-229-6697, Fax: 414-229-6697, E-mail: smithro@uwm.edu.
Website: http://www4.uwm.edu/chs/academics/biomedical_sciences/bms_masters/

Vanderbilt University, Department of Cancer Biology, Nashville, TN 37240-1001. Offers MS, PhD, MD/PhD. *Faculty:* 11 full-time (6 women). *Students:* 31 full-time (22 women); includes 10 minority (4 Black or African American, non-Hispanic/Latino; 3 Asian, non-Hispanic/Latino; 2 Hispanic/Latino; 1 Two or more races, non-Hispanic/Latino), 2 international. Average age 27. In 2015, 1 master's, 10 doctorates awarded. *Degree requirements:* For doctorate, thesis/dissertation, final and qualifying exams. *Entrance requirements:* For master's and doctorate, GRE General Test. Additional exam requirements/recommendations for international students: Required—TOEFL (minimum score 570 paper-based; 88 iBT). *Application deadline:* For fall admission, 1/15 for domestic and international students. Application fee: $0. Electronic applications accepted. *Financial support:* Fellowships with tuition reimbursements, research assistantships with tuition reimbursements, Federal Work-Study, institutionally sponsored loans, scholarships/grants, traineeships, and health care benefits available. Financial award application deadline: 1/15; financial award applicants required to submit CSS PROFILE or FAFSA. *Faculty research:* Micro environmental influences on cellular phenotype, in particular as it relates to host/tumor interactions, tumor-stroma interactions, angiogenesis, growth factor and cytokine signaling, oncogenes, tumor suppressors, matrix and matrix degradation, cell adhesion, metastasis. *Unit head:* Dr. Jin Chen, Director of Graduate Studies, 615-322-0375, Fax: 615-936-2911, E-mail: jin.chen@vanderbilt.edu. *Application contact:* Tracy Tveit, Graduate Program Coordinator, 615-936-2910, Fax: 615-936-2911, E-mail: tracy.s.tveit@vanderbilt.edu.
Website: https://medschool.vanderbilt.edu/cancer-biology/

Wake Forest University, School of Medicine and Graduate School of Arts and Sciences, Graduate Programs in Medicine, Department of Cancer Biology, Winston-Salem, NC 27109. Offers PhD, MD/PhD. *Degree requirements:* For doctorate, thesis/dissertation. *Entrance requirements:* For doctorate, GRE General Test. Additional exam requirements/recommendations for international students: Required—TOEFL. Electronic applications accepted. *Faculty research:* Cancer research, mechanisms of carcinogenesis, signal transduction and regulation of cell growth.

Wayne State University, School of Medicine, Office of Biomedical Graduate Programs, Cancer Biology Graduate Program, Detroit, MI 48202. Offers PhD. *Students:* 26 full-time (12 women); includes 4 minority (1 Black or African American, non-Hispanic/Latino; 1 Asian, non-Hispanic/Latino; 1 Hispanic/Latino; 1 Two or more races, non-Hispanic/Latino). Average age 26. 55 applicants, 7% accepted, 4 enrolled. In 2015, 7 doctorates awarded. *Degree requirements:* For doctorate, thesis/dissertation. *Entrance requirements:* For doctorate, GRE General Test, statement of purpose, detailed description of research experience, curriculum vitae or resume, three letters of recommendation, background in one of the chemical or biological sciences, bachelor's or master's degree with minimum GPA of 3.0. Additional exam requirements/recommendations for international students: Required—TOEFL (minimum score 100 iBT), TWE, Michigan English Language Assessment Battery (minimum score 85); Recommended—IELTS. *Application deadline:* For fall admission, 1/15 for domestic and international students. Application fee: $0. Electronic applications accepted. *Expenses:* $16,444 annual resident tuition, $32,915 non-resident tuition; $685.00 per credit hour resident tuition, $1,371.45 per credit hour non-resident tuition; fees include $47.45 per credit hour student services fee and $274.60 per semester registration fee. *Financial support:* In 2015–16, 25 students received support, including 12 fellowships with tuition reimbursements available (averaging $26,705 per year), 12 research assistantships with tuition reimbursements available (averaging $26,705 per year); scholarships/grants, health care benefits, and unspecified assistantships also available. Financial award application deadline: 3/31. *Faculty research:* Molecular therapeutics, molecular imaging and diagnostics, tumor microenvironment, population studies. *Unit head:* Dr. George Brush, Director, 313-578-4300, E-mail: brushg@karmanos.org. *Application contact:* E-mail: cancerbio@karmanos.org.
Website: http://cancerbiologyprogram.med.wayne.edu/program-description.php

West Virginia University, Davis College of Agriculture, Forestry and Consumer Sciences, Interdisciplinary Program in Genetics and Developmental Biology, Morgantown, WV 26506. Offers animal breeding (MS, PhD); biochemical and molecular genetics (MS, PhD); cytogenetics (MS, PhD); descriptive embryology (MS, PhD); developmental genetics (MS); experimental morphogenesis/teratology (MS); human genetics (MS, PhD); immunogenetics (MS, PhD); life cycles of animals and plants (MS, PhD); molecular aspects of development (MS, PhD); mutagenesis (MS, PhD); oncology (MS, PhD); plant genetics (MS, PhD); population and quantitative genetics (MS, PhD); regeneration (MS, PhD); teratology (PhD); toxicology (MS, PhD). *Degree requirements:* For master's, thesis; for doctorate, comprehensive exam, thesis/dissertation. *Entrance requirements:* For master's, GRE or MCAT, minimum GPA of 2.75. Additional exam requirements/recommendations for international students: Required—TOEFL. *Expenses:* Tuition, state resident: full-time $8568. Tuition, nonresident: full-time $22,140. Tuition and fees vary according to program.

West Virginia University, School of Medicine, Graduate Programs at the Health Sciences Center, Interdisciplinary Graduate Programs in Biomedical Sciences, Program in Cancer Cell Biology, Morgantown, WV 26506. Offers PhD, MD/PhD. *Degree requirements:* For doctorate, comprehensive exam, thesis/dissertation. *Entrance requirements:* For doctorate, GRE General Test, minimum GPA of 3.0. Additional exam requirements/recommendations for international students: Required—TOEFL. Electronic applications accepted. *Expenses:* Tuition, state resident: full-time $8568. Tuition, nonresident: full-time $22,140. Tuition and fees vary according to program. *Faculty research:* Cellular signaling, tumor microenvironment, cancer therapeutics.

Yale University, School of Medicine and Graduate School of Arts and Sciences, Combined Program in Biological and Biomedical Sciences (BBS), Pharmacological Sciences and Molecular Medicine Track, New Haven, CT 06520. Offers PhD, MD/PhD. *Degree requirements:* For doctorate, thesis/dissertation. *Entrance requirements:* For doctorate, GRE General Test. Additional exam requirements/recommendations for international students: Required—TOEFL. Electronic applications accepted.

Cell Biology

Albany College of Pharmacy and Health Sciences, School of Arts and Sciences, Albany, NY 12208. Offers clinical laboratory sciences (MS); cytotechnology and molecular cytology (MS); molecular biosciences (MS). *Degree requirements:* For master's, thesis. *Entrance requirements:* For master's, GRE, minimum GPA of 3.0. Additional exam requirements/recommendations for international students: Required—TOEFL (minimum score 84 iBT). Electronic applications accepted.

Albany Medical College, Center for Cell Biology and Cancer Research, Albany, NY 12208-3479. Offers MS, PhD. *Program availability:* Part-time. Terminal master's awarded for partial completion of doctoral program. *Degree requirements:* For master's, thesis; for doctorate, comprehensive exam, thesis/dissertation. *Entrance requirements:* For master's and doctorate, GRE General Test, all transcripts, letters of recommendation. Additional exam requirements/recommendations for international students: Required—TOEFL. *Faculty research:* Cancer cell biology, tissue remodeling, signal transduction, gene regulation, cell adhesion, angiogenesis.

Albert Einstein College of Medicine, Graduate Division of Biomedical Sciences, Department of Anatomy and Structural Biology, Bronx, NY 10461. Offers anatomy (PhD); cell and developmental biology (PhD); MD/PhD. *Degree requirements:* For doctorate, thesis/dissertation. *Entrance requirements:* For doctorate, GRE General Test. Additional exam requirements/recommendations for international students: Required—TOEFL. Electronic applications accepted. *Faculty research:* Cell motility, cell membranes and membrane-cytoskeletal interactions as applied to processing of pancreatic hormones, mechanisms of secretion.

Albert Einstein College of Medicine, Graduate Division of Biomedical Sciences, Department of Cell Biology, Bronx, NY 10461. Offers PhD, MD/PhD. *Degree requirements:* For doctorate, thesis/dissertation. *Entrance requirements:* For doctorate, GRE General Test. Additional exam requirements/recommendations for international students: Required—TOEFL. *Faculty research:* Molecular and genetic basis of gene expression in animal cells; expression of differentiated traits of albumin, hemoglobin, myosin, and immunoglobin.

American University of Beirut, Graduate Programs, Faculty of Arts and Sciences, Beirut, Lebanon. Offers anthropology (MA); Arab and Middle Eastern history (PhD); Arabic language and literature (MA, PhD); archaeology (MA); biology (MS); cell and molecular biology (PhD); chemistry (MS); clinical psychology (MA); computational sciences (MS); computer science (MS); economics (MA); English language (MA); English literature (MA); environmental policy planning (MS); financial economics (MAFE); geology (MS); history (MA); mathematics (MA, MS); media studies (MA); Middle Eastern studies (MA); physics (MS); political studies (MA); psychology (MA); public administration (MA); sociology (MA); statistics (MA, MS); theoretical physics (PhD); transnational American studies (MA). *Program availability:* Part-time. *Faculty:* 114 full-time (36 women), 4 part-time/adjunct (2 women). *Students:* 258 full-time (190 women), 207 part-time (142 women). Average age 27. 241 applicants, 71% accepted, 98 enrolled. In 2015, 47 master's, 3 doctorates awarded. *Degree requirements:* For master's, one foreign language, comprehensive exam, thesis (for some programs); for doctorate, one foreign language, comprehensive exam, thesis/dissertation. *Entrance requirements:* For master's, GRE (for some MA, MS programs), letter of recommendation; for doctorate, GRE, letters of recommendation. Additional exam requirements/recommendations for international students: Required—TOEFL (minimum score 600 paper-based; 97 iBT), IELTS (minimum score 7). *Application deadline:* For fall admission, 4/1 for domestic and international students; for spring admission, 11/1 for domestic and international students. Application fee: $50. Electronic applications accepted. *Expenses: Tuition, area resident:* Full-time $16,254; part-time $903 per credit. *Required fees:* $699. Tuition and fees vary according to course load and program. *Financial support:* Research assistantships, career-related internships or fieldwork, institutionally sponsored loans, scholarships/grants, health care benefits, and unspecified assistantships available. Financial award application deadline: 2/4; financial award applicants required to submit FAFSA. *Faculty research:* Analysis and algebra; software engineering; machine learning and big data analysis; philosophy of mind and political philosophy; anthropology of art, anthropology of migration and medical anthropology; sociology of knowledge, sociology of migration, critical theory; sociology of education; hybrid solid materials; photocatalysis; human creativity. *Total annual research expenditures:* $680,360. *Unit head:* Dr. Patrick McGreevy, Dean, 961-1374374 Ext. 3800, Fax: 961-1744461, E-mail: pm07@aub.edu.lb. *Application contact:* Dr. Salim Kanaan, Director, Admissions Office, 961-1350000 Ext. 2590, Fax: 961-1750775, E-mail: sk00@aub.edu.lb.
Website: http://www.aub.edu.lb/fas/

American University of Beirut, Graduate Programs, Faculty of Medicine, Beirut, Lebanon. Offers anatomy, cell biology and human morphology (MS); biochemistry and medical genetics (MS); biomedical sciences (PhD); experimental pathology, immunology and microbiology (MS); medicine (MD); neuroscience (MS); pharmacology and toxicology (MS). *Program availability:* Part-time. *Faculty:* 302 full-time (95 women), 64 part-time/adjunct (11 women). *Students:* 381 full-time (173 women), 61 part-time (51 women). Average age 23. In 2015, 14 master's awarded. *Degree requirements:* For master's, one foreign language, comprehensive exam, thesis (for some programs); for doctorate, one foreign language, comprehensive exam, thesis/dissertation. *Entrance requirements:* For master's, letter of recommendation; for doctorate, MCAT, bachelor's degree. Additional exam requirements/recommendations for international students: Required—TOEFL (minimum score 600 paper-based; 100 iBT), IELTS (minimum score 7.5). *Application deadline:* For fall admission, 4/30 for domestic and international students; for spring admission, 11/1 for domestic and international students. Application fee: $50. Electronic applications accepted. *Expenses: Tuition, area resident:* Full-time $16,254; part-time $903 per credit. *Required fees:* $699. Tuition and fees vary according to course load and program. *Financial support:* In 2015–16, 273 students received support, including 45 teaching assistantships (averaging $9,000 per year); career-related internships or fieldwork, institutionally sponsored loans, scholarships/grants, health care benefits, and unspecified assistantships also available. Financial award application deadline: 2/2. *Faculty research:* Cancer research (targeted therapy, mechanisms of leukemogenesis, tumor cell extravasation and metastasis, cancer stem cells), stem cell research (regenerative medicine, drug discovery), genetic research (neurogenetics, hereditary cardiomyopathy, hemoglobinopathies, pharmacogenomics, proteomics), neuroscience research (pain, neurodegenerative disorder), metabolism (inflammation and metabolism, metabolic disorder, diabetes mellitus), vascular and renal biology, signal transduction. *Total annual research expenditures:* $2.6 million. *Unit head:* Dr. Mohamed Sayegh, Dean, 961-1350000 Ext. 4700, Fax: 961-1744464, E-mail: msayegh@aub.edu.lb. *Application contact:* Dr. Salim Kanaan, Director, Admissions Office, 961-1350000 Ext. 2594, Fax: 961-1750775, E-mail: sk00@aub.edu.lb.
Website: http://www.aub.edu.lb/fm/fm_home/Pages/index.aspx

Appalachian State University, Cratis D. Williams Graduate School, Department of Biology, Boone, NC 28608. Offers cell and molecular biology (MS); general biology (MS). *Program availability:* Part-time. *Degree requirements:* For master's, comprehensive exam, thesis. *Entrance requirements:* For master's, GRE General Test, 3 letters of recommendation. Additional exam requirements/recommendations for international students: Required—TOEFL (minimum score 570 paper-based; 79 iBT), IELTS (minimum score 6.5). Electronic applications accepted. *Faculty research:* Aquatic and terrestrial ecology, animal and plant physiology, behavior and systematics, immunology and cell biology, molecular biology and microbiology.

Arizona State University at the Tempe campus, College of Liberal Arts and Sciences, School of Life Sciences, Tempe, AZ 85287-4601. Offers animal behavior (PhD); applied ethics (biomedical and health ethics) (MA); biology (MS, PhD), including biology, biology and society, complex adaptive systems science (PhD), plant biology and conservation (MS); environmental life sciences (PhD); evolutionary biology (PhD); history and philosophy of science (PhD); human and social dimensions of science and technology (PhD); microbiology (PhD); molecular and cellular biology (PhD); neuroscience (PhD). Terminal master's awarded for partial completion of doctoral program. *Degree requirements:* For master's, thesis (for some programs), interactive Program of Study (iPOS) submitted before completing 50 percent of required credit hours; for doctorate, variable foreign language requirement, comprehensive exam, thesis/dissertation, interactive Program of Study (iPOS) submitted before completing 50 percent of required credit hours. *Entrance requirements:* For master's and doctorate, GRE, minimum GPA of 3.0 or equivalent in last 2 years of work leading to bachelor's degree. Additional exam requirements/recommendations for international students: Required—TOEFL (minimum score 600 paper-based; 100 iBT). Electronic applications accepted.

Auburn University, Graduate School, Interdepartmental Programs, Auburn University, AL 36849. Offers applied economics (PhD); cell and molecular biology (PhD); real estate development (MRED); sociology and rural sociology (MA, MS), including rural sociology (MS), sociology. *Program availability:* Part-time. *Students:* 35 full-time (18 women), 44 part-time (11 women); includes 15 minority (13 Black or African American, non-Hispanic/Latino; 1 Asian, non-Hispanic/Latino; 1 Hispanic/Latino), 30 international. Average age 34. 62 applicants, 50% accepted, 24 enrolled. In 2015, 18 master's, 4 doctorates awarded. *Entrance requirements:* For master's, GRE General Test. *Application deadline:* Applications are processed on a rolling basis. Application fee: $50 ($60 for international students). Electronic applications accepted. *Expenses:* Tuition, state resident: full-time $8802; part-time $489 per credit hour. Tuition, nonresident: full-time $26,406; part-time $1467 per credit hour. *Required fees:* $808 per semester. Tuition and fees vary according to degree level and program. *Financial support:* Fellowships, research assistantships, teaching assistantships, and Federal Work-Study available. Support available to part-time students. Financial award application deadline: 3/15; financial award applicants required to submit FAFSA. *Application contact:* Dr. George Flowers, Dean of the Graduate School, 334-844-2125.

Augusta University, The Graduate School, Program in Cellular Biology and Anatomy, Augusta, GA 30912. Offers PhD. *Degree requirements:* For doctorate, comprehensive exam, thesis/dissertation. *Entrance requirements:* For doctorate, GRE General Test. Additional exam requirements/recommendations for international students: Required—TOEFL (minimum score 550 paper-based; 79 iBT). *Application deadline:* For fall admission, 1/15 for domestic and international students. Applications are processed on a rolling basis. Application fee: $50. *Financial support:* Fellowships with partial tuition reimbursements, research assistantships with partial tuition reimbursements, teaching assistantships with partial tuition reimbursements, Federal Work-Study, institutionally sponsored loans, and scholarships/grants available. Support available to part-time students. Financial award application deadline: 5/31; financial award applicants required to submit FAFSA. *Faculty research:* Eye disease, developmental biology, cell injury and death, stroke and neurotoxicity, diabetic complications. *Unit head:* Dr. Sylvia B. Smith, Chair and Professor, 706-721-3731, Fax: 706-721-6120, E-mail: sbsmith@augusta.edu. *Application contact:* Dr. Mark Hamrick, Director, 706-721-1958.
Website: http://www.augusta.edu/mcg/cba/

Baylor College of Medicine, Graduate School of Biomedical Sciences, Department of Molecular and Cellular Biology, Houston, TX 77030-3498. Offers PhD, MD/PhD. *Degree requirements:* For doctorate, thesis/dissertation, public defense, qualifying exam. *Entrance requirements:* For doctorate, GRE General Test, GRE Subject Test (strongly recommended), minimum GPA of 3.0. Additional exam requirements/recommendations for international students: Required—TOEFL. Electronic applications accepted. *Faculty research:* Hormone action, development, cancer, gene therapy, neurobiology.

Baylor College of Medicine, Graduate School of Biomedical Sciences, Interdepartmental Program in Cell and Molecular Biology, Houston, TX 77030-3498. Offers biochemistry (PhD); cell and molecular biology (PhD); genetics (PhD); human genetics (PhD); immunology (PhD); microbiology (PhD); virology (PhD); MD/PhD. *Degree requirements:* For doctorate, thesis/dissertation, public defense. *Entrance requirements:* For doctorate, GRE General Test, GRE Subject Test (strongly recommended), minimum GPA of 3.0. Additional exam requirements/recommendations for international students: Required—TOEFL. Electronic applications accepted. *Faculty research:* Molecular and cellular biology; cancer, aging and stem cells; genomics and proteomics; microbiome, molecular microbiology; infectious disease, immunology and translational research.

Baylor College of Medicine, Graduate School of Biomedical Sciences, Program in Developmental Biology, Houston, TX 77030-3498. Offers PhD, MD/PhD. *Degree requirements:* For doctorate, thesis/dissertation, public defense. *Entrance requirements:* For doctorate, GRE General Test, GRE Subject Test (strongly recommended), minimum GPA of 3.0. Additional exam requirements/recommendations for international students: Required—TOEFL. Electronic applications accepted. *Faculty research:* Stem cells, cancer, neurobiology, organogenesis, genetics of model organisms.

Boston University, Graduate School of Arts and Sciences, Molecular Biology, Cell Biology, and Biochemistry Program (MCBB), Boston, MA 02215. Offers MA, PhD. *Students:* 32 full-time (14 women), 3 part-time (2 women); includes 10 minority (3 Black or African American, non-Hispanic/Latino; 2 Asian, non-Hispanic/Latino; 4 Hispanic/Latino; 1 Two or more races, non-Hispanic/Latino), 8 international. Average age 29. 139 applicants, 11% accepted, 3 enrolled. In 2015, 16 master's, 3 doctorates awarded. Terminal master's awarded for partial completion of doctoral program. *Degree requirements:* For master's, one foreign language, thesis (for some programs); for doctorate, one foreign language, comprehensive exam, thesis/dissertation. *Entrance requirements:* For master's and doctorate, GRE General Test, GRE Subject Test (recommended), 3 letters of recommendation, transcripts, personal statement. Additional exam requirements/recommendations for international students: Required—TOEFL (minimum score 550 paper-based; 84 iBT). *Application deadline:* For fall

admission, 12/7 for domestic and international students. Application fee: $95. Electronic applications accepted. *Financial support:* In 2015–16, 30 students received support, including 2 fellowships with full tuition reimbursements available (averaging $21,000 per year), 15 research assistantships with full tuition reimbursements available (averaging $21,000 per year), 12 teaching assistantships with full tuition reimbursements available (averaging $21,000 per year); Federal Work-Study, scholarships/grants, traineeships, and health care benefits also available. Financial award application deadline: 12/7; financial award applicants required to submit FAFSA. *Unit head:* Dr. Ulla Hansen, Director, 617-353-2432, Fax: 617-353-6340, E-mail: uhansen@bu.edu. *Application contact:* Christina Honeycutt, Academic Administrator, 617-353-2432, Fax: 617-353-6340, E-mail: cjhoney@bu.edu.
Website: http://www.bu.edu/mcbb/

Boston University, School of Medicine, Division of Graduate Medical Sciences, Department of Biochemistry, Boston, MA 02118. Offers MA, PhD, MD/PhD. *Program availability:* Part-time. Terminal master's awarded for partial completion of doctoral program. *Degree requirements:* For master's, thesis or alternative; for doctorate, thesis/dissertation. *Application deadline:* For fall admission, 1/15 for domestic students; for spring admission, 10/15 for domestic students. *Unit head:* Dr. David A. Harris, Chair, 617-638-5090. *Application contact:* GMS Admissions Office, 617-638-5255, E-mail: askgms@bu.edu.
Website: http://www.bumc.bu.edu/biochemistry/

Boston University, School of Medicine, Division of Graduate Medical Sciences, Program in Cell and Molecular Biology, Boston, MA 02118. Offers PhD. *Degree requirements:* For doctorate, thesis/dissertation. *Application deadline:* For fall admission, 1/15 for domestic students; for spring admission, 10/15 for domestic students. *Financial support:* Scholarships/grants and traineeships available. Financial award applicants required to submit FAFSA. *Unit head:* Dr. Vickery Trinkaus-Randall, Director, 617-638-6099, Fax: 617-638-5337, E-mail: vickery@bu.edu. *Application contact:* GMS Admissions Office, 617-638-5255, E-mail: askgms@bu.edu.
Website: http://www.bumc.bu.edu/cmbio/

Brandeis University, Graduate School of Arts and Sciences, Program in Molecular and Cell Biology, Waltham, MA 02454-9110. Offers genetics (PhD); microbiology (PhD); molecular and cell biology (MS, PhD); molecular biology (PhD); neurobiology (PhD); quantitative biology (PhD). *Faculty:* 26 full-time (12 women), 4 part-time/adjunct (2 women). *Students:* 60 full-time (30 women); includes 5 minority (1 Black or African American, non-Hispanic/Latino; 1 American Indian or Alaska Native, non-Hispanic/Latino; 1 Asian, non-Hispanic/Latino; 2 Hispanic/Latino), 25 international. 183 applicants, 27% accepted, 12 enrolled. In 2015, 13 master's, 7 doctorates awarded. Terminal master's awarded for partial completion of doctoral program. *Degree requirements:* For master's, thesis optional, research project, research lab, or project lab; for doctorate, comprehensive exam, thesis/dissertation, journal clubs; research seminar; colloquia; qualifying exam. *Entrance requirements:* For master's, GRE General Test, official transcript(s), resume, 2 letters of recommendation, statement of purpose; for doctorate, GRE General Test, official transcript(s), resume, 3 letters of recommendation, statement of purpose, list of previous research experience. Additional exam requirements/recommendations for international students: Required—TOEFL (minimum score 600 paper-based; 100 iBT); Recommended—IELTS (minimum score 7), TSE (minimum score 68). *Application deadline:* For fall admission, 12/15 priority date for domestic students. Application fee: $75. Electronic applications accepted. *Financial support:* In 2015–16, 35 students received support, including 16 fellowships with full tuition reimbursements available (averaging $30,500 per year), 19 research assistantships with full tuition reimbursements available (averaging $30,500 per year); scholarships/grants and tuition waivers (partial) also available. Financial award application deadline: 4/15; financial award applicants required to submit FAFSA. *Faculty research:* Molecular biology, genetics and development; structural and cell biology; neurobiology. *Unit head:* Dr. Maria Miara, Director of Graduate Studies, 781-736-2300, Fax: 781-736-3107, E-mail: scigradoffice@brandeis.edu. *Application contact:* Dr. Maryanna Aldrich, Department Administrator, 781-736-2300, Fax: 781-736-3107, E-mail: scigradoffice@brandeis.edu.
Website: http://www.brandeis.edu/gsas

Brown University, Graduate School, Division of Biology and Medicine, Department of Molecular Biology, Cell Biology, and Biochemistry, Providence, RI 02912. Offers MA, PhD. *Program availability:* Part-time. Terminal master's awarded for partial completion of doctoral program. *Degree requirements:* For master's, thesis (for some programs); for doctorate, one foreign language, thesis/dissertation, preliminary exam. *Entrance requirements:* For master's and doctorate, GRE General Test, GRE Subject Test. Additional exam requirements/recommendations for international students: Required—TOEFL. Electronic applications accepted. *Faculty research:* Molecular genetics, gene regulation.

California Institute of Technology, Division of Biology, Program in Cell Biology and Biophysics, Pasadena, CA 91125-0001. Offers PhD. *Degree requirements:* For doctorate, thesis/dissertation, qualifying exam. *Entrance requirements:* For doctorate, GRE General Test.

California State University, Sacramento, Office of Graduate Studies, College of Natural Sciences and Mathematics, Department of Biological Sciences, Sacramento, CA 95819. Offers biological conservation (MS); molecular and cellular biology (MS); stem cell (MA). *Program availability:* Part-time. *Degree requirements:* For master's, thesis, writing proficiency exam. *Entrance requirements:* For master's, GRE, bachelor's degree in biology or equivalent; minimum GPA of 3.0 in biology, 2.75 overall during last 2 years of course work. Additional exam requirements/recommendations for international students: Required—TOEFL. Electronic applications accepted.

Carnegie Mellon University, Mellon College of Science, Department of Biological Sciences, Pittsburgh, PA 15213-3891. Offers biochemistry (PhD); biophysics (PhD); cell and developmental biology (PhD); computational biology (MS, PhD); genetics (PhD); molecular biology (PhD); neuroscience (PhD); structural biology (PhD). *Degree requirements:* For doctorate, comprehensive exam, thesis/dissertation. *Entrance requirements:* For doctorate, GRE General Test, GRE Subject Test, interview. Electronic applications accepted. *Faculty research:* Genetic structure, function, and regulation; protein structure and function; biological membranes; biological spectroscopy.

Case Western Reserve University, School of Medicine and School of Graduate Studies, Graduate Programs in Medicine, Department of Anatomy, Cleveland, OH 44106. Offers applied anatomy (MS); biological anthropology (MS); cellular biology (MS); MD/MS. *Program availability:* Part-time. *Degree requirements:* For master's, comprehensive exam, thesis (for some programs). *Entrance requirements:* For master's, GRE General Test. Additional exam requirements/recommendations for international students: Required—TOEFL. *Expenses: Tuition, area resident:* Full-time $41,137; part-time $1714 per credit hour. *Required fees:* $32. Tuition and fees vary according to course load and program. *Faculty research:* Hypoxia, cell injury, biochemical aberration occurrences in ischemic tissue, human functional morphology, evolutionary morphology.

Case Western Reserve University, School of Medicine and School of Graduate Studies, Graduate Programs in Medicine, Department of Molecular Biology and Microbiology, Cleveland, OH 44106-4960. Offers cellular biology (PhD); microbiology (PhD); molecular biology (PhD); molecular virology (PhD); MD/PhD. Students are admitted to an integrated Biomedical Sciences Training Program involving 11 basic science programs at Case Western Reserve University. *Degree requirements:* For doctorate, thesis/dissertation. *Entrance requirements:* For doctorate, GRE General Test, GRE Subject Test. Additional exam requirements/recommendations for international students: Required—TOEFL. Electronic applications accepted. *Expenses: Tuition, area resident:* Full-time $41,137; part-time $1714 per credit hour. *Required fees:* $32. Tuition and fees vary according to course load and program. *Faculty research:* Gene expression in eukaryotic and prokaryotic systems; microbial physiology; intracellular transport and signaling; mechanisms of oncogenesis; molecular mechanisms of RNA processing, editing, and catalysis.

Case Western Reserve University, School of Medicine and School of Graduate Studies, Graduate Programs in Medicine, Program in Cell Biology, Cleveland, OH 44106. Offers PhD. *Degree requirements:* For doctorate, thesis/dissertation. *Entrance requirements:* For doctorate, GRE General Test, GRE Subject Test, previous course work in biochemistry. Additional exam requirements/recommendations for international students: Required—TOEFL. Electronic applications accepted. *Expenses: Tuition, area resident:* Full-time $41,137; part-time $1714 per credit hour. *Required fees:* $32. Tuition and fees vary according to course load and program. *Faculty research:* Macromolecular transport, membrane traffic, signal transduction, nuclear organization, lipid metabolism.

Case Western Reserve University, School of Medicine and School of Graduate Studies, Graduate Programs in Medicine, Programs in Molecular and Cellular Basis of Disease/Pathology, Cleveland, OH 44106. Offers cancer biology (PhD); cell biology (MS, PhD); immunology (MS, PhD); pathology (MS, PhD); MD/PhD. Terminal master's awarded for partial completion of doctoral program. *Degree requirements:* For master's, thesis; for doctorate, thesis/dissertation. *Entrance requirements:* For master's and doctorate, GRE General Test, GRE Subject Test. Additional exam requirements/recommendations for international students: Required—TOEFL (minimum score 550 paper-based). Electronic applications accepted. *Expenses: Tuition, area resident:* Full-time $41,137; part-time $1714 per credit hour. *Required fees:* $32. Tuition and fees vary according to course load and program. *Faculty research:* Neurobiology, molecular biology, cancer biology, biomaterials, biocompatibility.

The Catholic University of America, School of Arts and Sciences, Department of Biology, Washington, DC 20064. Offers biotechnology (MS); cell and microbial biology (MS, PhD), including cell biology; clinical laboratory science (MS, PhD); MSLS/MS. *Program availability:* Part-time. *Faculty:* 9 full-time (4 women), 7 part-time/adjunct (1 woman). *Students:* 29 full-time (18 women), 36 part-time (22 women); includes 8 minority (3 Black or African American, non-Hispanic/Latino; 2 Asian, non-Hispanic/Latino; 1 Hispanic/Latino; 2 Two or more races, non-Hispanic/Latino), 44 international. Average age 30. 68 applicants, 38% accepted, 13 enrolled. In 2015, 21 master's, 1 doctorate awarded. *Degree requirements:* For master's and doctorate, comprehensive exam. *Entrance requirements:* For master's and doctorate, GRE General Test, GRE Subject Test, statement of purpose, official copies of academic transcripts, three letters of recommendation. Additional exam requirements/recommendations for international students: Required—TOEFL (minimum score 550 paper-based; 80 iBT). *Application deadline:* For fall admission, 7/15 priority date for domestic students, 7/1 for international students; for spring admission, 11/15 priority date for domestic students, 11/1 for international students. Applications are processed on a rolling basis. Application fee: $55. Electronic applications accepted. *Expenses:* $20,700 per semester full-time tuition, $200 per semester full-time fees; $1,650 per credit hour part-time tuition, $145 per semester part-time fees. *Financial support:* Fellowships, research assistantships, teaching assistantships, Federal Work-Study, scholarships/grants, tuition waivers (full and partial), and unspecified assistantships available. Financial award application deadline: 2/1; financial award applicants required to submit FAFSA. *Faculty research:* Virus structure and assembly, hepatic and epithelial cell biology, drug resistance and genome stabilization in yeast, biophysics of ion-conductive nanostructures, eukaryotic gene regulation, cancer and vaccine research. *Total annual research expenditures:* $2.2 million. *Unit head:* Dr. Venigalla Rao, Chair, 202-319-5271, Fax: 202-319-5721, E-mail: rao@cua.edu. *Application contact:* Director of Graduate Admissions, 202-319-5057, Fax: 202-319-6533, E-mail: cua-admissions@cua.edu.
Website: http://biology.cua.edu/

Colorado State University, Interdisciplinary College, Program in Cell and Molecular Biology, Fort Collins, CO 80523-1618. Offers MS, PhD. *Students:* 31 full-time (22 women), 44 part-time (25 women); includes 8 minority (2 Black or African American, non-Hispanic/Latino; 1 Asian, non-Hispanic/Latino; 4 Hispanic/Latino; 1 Two or more races, non-Hispanic/Latino), 25 international. Average age 30. 10 applicants, 70% accepted, 7 enrolled. In 2015, 4 master's, 10 doctorates awarded. Terminal master's awarded for partial completion of doctoral program. *Degree requirements:* For master's, comprehensive exam (for some programs), thesis; for doctorate, comprehensive exam, thesis/dissertation, preliminary exam. *Entrance requirements:* For master's and doctorate, GRE General Test, GRE Subject Test in biology (strongly recommended), minimum GPA of 3.0; BA/BS in biology, biochemistry, or physics; calculus sequence; letters of recommendation; transcript; personal statement; curriculum vitae. Additional exam requirements/recommendations for international students: Required—TOEFL (minimum score 625 paper-based; 107 iBT). *Application deadline:* For fall admission, 1/1 priority date for domestic and international students. Applications are processed on a rolling basis. Application fee: $60 ($70 for international students). Electronic applications accepted. *Expenses:* Tuition, state resident: full-time $9348. Tuition, nonresident: full-time $22,916. *Required fees:* $2174; $473.72 per credit hour. $236.86 per semester. Tuition and fees vary according to course load and program. *Financial support:* In 2015–16, 10 research assistantships with full tuition reimbursements (averaging $24,000 per year), 3 teaching assistantships with full tuition reimbursements (averaging $23,328 per year) were awarded. Financial award application deadline: 1/1. *Faculty research:* Cancer biology and infectious diseases; genomics and computational biology; metabolic regulation and regulation of gene expression; neuroscience and molecular physiology; reproductive and developmental biology. *Unit head:* Dr. Howard Liber, Program Director, 970-491-0580, Fax: 970-491-2194, E-mail: howard.liber@colostate.edu. *Application contact:* Lori Williams, Program Coordinator, 970-491-0241, Fax: 970-491-2194, E-mail: lori.williams@colostate.edu.
Website: http://cmb.colostate.edu/

Columbia University, College of Physicians and Surgeons, Department of Anatomy and Cell Biology, New York, NY 10032. Offers anatomy (M Phil, MA, PhD); anatomy and cell biology (PhD); MD/PhD. Only candidates for the PhD are admitted. Terminal master's awarded for partial completion of doctoral program. *Degree requirements:* For doctorate, thesis/dissertation, oral exam. *Entrance requirements:* For master's and doctorate, GRE General Test. Additional exam requirements/recommendations for international students: Required—TOEFL. *Faculty research:* Protein sorting, membrane biophysics, muscle energetics, neuroendocrinology, developmental biology, cytoskeleton, transcription factors.

Columbia University, College of Physicians and Surgeons, Integrated Program in Cellular, Molecular, Structural and Genetic Studies, New York, NY 10032. Offers PhD. Terminal master's awarded for partial completion of doctoral program. *Degree* *requirements:* For doctorate, thesis/dissertation. *Entrance requirements:* For doctorate, GRE General Test, GRE Subject Test. Additional exam requirements/recommendations for international students: Required—TOEFL. *Expenses:* Contact institution. *Faculty research:* Transcription, macromolecular sorting, gene expression during development, cellular interaction.

Cornell University, Graduate School, Graduate Fields of Agriculture and Life Sciences, Field of Biochemistry, Molecular and Cell Biology, Ithaca, NY 14853-0001. Offers biochemistry (PhD); biophysics (PhD); cell biology (PhD); molecular biology (PhD). *Degree requirements:* For doctorate, comprehensive exam, thesis/dissertation, 2 semesters of teaching experience. *Entrance requirements:* For doctorate, GRE General Test, GRE Subject Test (biology, chemistry, physics, biochemistry, cell and molecular biology), 3 letters of recommendation. Additional exam requirements/recommendations for international students: Required—TOEFL (minimum score 600 paper-based; 77 iBT). Electronic applications accepted. *Faculty research:* Biophysics, structural biology.

Cornell University, Graduate School, Graduate Fields of Agriculture and Life Sciences, Field of Computational Biology, Ithaca, NY 14853-0001. Offers computational behavioral biology (PhD); computational biology (PhD); computational cell biology (PhD); computational ecology (PhD); computational genetics (PhD); computational macromolecular biology (PhD); computational organismal biology (PhD). *Degree requirements:* For doctorate, comprehensive exam, thesis/dissertation, 2 semesters of teaching experience. *Entrance requirements:* For doctorate, GRE General Test, GRE Subject Test (biology), 2 letters of recommendation. Additional exam requirements/recommendations for international students: Required—TOEFL (minimum score 550 paper-based; 77 iBT). Electronic applications accepted. *Faculty research:* Computational behavioral biology, computational biology, computational cell biology, computational ecology, computational genetics, computational macromolecular biology, computational organismal biology.

Cornell University, Graduate School, Graduate Fields of Agriculture and Life Sciences, Field of Zoology and Wildlife Conservation, Ithaca, NY 14853-0001. Offers animal cytology (PhD); comparative and functional anatomy (PhD); developmental biology (PhD); ecology (PhD); histology (PhD); wildlife conservation (PhD). *Degree requirements:* For doctorate, comprehensive exam, thesis/dissertation, 2 semesters of teaching experience. *Entrance requirements:* For doctorate, GRE General Test, GRE Subject Test (biology), 2 letters of recommendation. Additional exam requirements/recommendations for international students: Required—TOEFL (minimum score 550 paper-based; 77 iBT). Electronic applications accepted. *Faculty research:* Organismal biology, functional morphology, biomechanics, comparative vertebrate anatomy, comparative invertebrate anatomy, paleontology.

Dartmouth College, Graduate Program in Molecular and Cellular Biology, Hanover, NH 03755. Offers PhD, MBA/PhD, MD/PhD. *Faculty:* 72 full-time (19 women), 4 part-time/adjunct (1 woman). *Students:* 98 full-time (52 women); includes 17 minority (7 Asian, non-Hispanic/Latino; 9 Hispanic/Latino; 1 Two or more races, non-Hispanic/Latino), 28 international. Average age 27. 193 applicants, 38% accepted, 30 enrolled. In 2015, 16 doctorates awarded. *Entrance requirements:* For doctorate, GRE General Test, letters of recommendation, minimum GPA of 3.0. Additional exam requirements/recommendations for international students: Required—TOEFL (minimum score paper-based 550, iBT 100) or IELTS (7.0). *Application deadline:* For fall admission, 12/1 for domestic students. Applications are processed on a rolling basis. Application fee: $75. Electronic applications accepted. *Expenses: Tuition, area resident:* Full-time $48,120. *Required fees:* $296. One-time fee: $50 full-time. *Financial support:* In 2015–16, fellowships with full tuition reimbursements (averaging $28,200 per year) were awarded; health care benefits also available. *Unit head:* Dr. Patrick J. Dolph, Chair, 603-650-1092, E-mail: mcb@dartmouth.edu. *Application contact:* Janet Cheney, Program Coordinator, 603-650-1612, Fax: 603-650-1006, E-mail: mcb@dartmouth.edu. Website: http://dms.dartmouth.edu/mcb/

Drexel University, College of Medicine, Biomedical Graduate Programs, Interdisciplinary Program in Molecular and Cell Biology and Genetics, Philadelphia, PA 19104-2875. Offers MS, PhD, MD/PhD. Terminal master's awarded for partial completion of doctoral program. *Degree requirements:* For master's, comprehensive exam, thesis; for doctorate, thesis/dissertation, qualifying exam. *Entrance requirements:* For master's, GRE General Test, minimum GPA of 2.75; for doctorate, GRE General Test, minimum GPA of 3.0. Additional exam requirements/recommendations for international students: Required—TOEFL. Electronic applications accepted. *Faculty research:* Molecular anatomy, biochemistry, medical biotechnology, molecular pathology, microbiology and immunology.

Duke University, Graduate School, Department of Cell Biology, Durham, NC 27710. Offers PhD. *Degree requirements:* For doctorate, thesis/dissertation. *Entrance requirements:* For doctorate, GRE General Test, GRE Subject Test in biology, chemistry, cell and molecular biology (recommended). Additional exam requirements/recommendations for international students: Required—TOEFL (minimum score 577 paper-based; 90 iBT) or IELTS (minimum score 7). Electronic applications accepted.

Duke University, Graduate School, Department of Evolutionary Anthropology, Durham, NC 27708. Offers cellular and molecular biology (PhD); gross anatomy and physical anthropology (PhD), including comparative morphology of human and non-human primates, primate social behavior, vertebrate paleontology; neuroanatomy (PhD). *Degree requirements:* For doctorate, one foreign language, thesis/dissertation. *Entrance requirements:* For doctorate, GRE General Test. Additional exam requirements/recommendations for international students: Required—TOEFL (minimum score 577 paper-based; 90 iBT) or IELTS (minimum score 7). Electronic applications accepted.

Duke University, Graduate School, Program in Cell and Molecular Biology, Durham, NC 27710. Offers Certificate. Students must be enrolled in a participating PhD program (biology, cell biology, immunology, molecular genetics, neurobiology, pathology, pharmacology). *Entrance requirements:* Additional exam requirements/recommendations for international students: Required—TOEFL (minimum score 577 paper-based; 90 iBT) or IELTS (minimum score 7). Electronic applications accepted.

East Carolina University, Brody School of Medicine, Department of Anatomy and Cell Biology, Greenville, NC 27858-4353. Offers PhD. *Students:* 11 full-time (7 women); includes 2 minority (1 Black or African American, non-Hispanic/Latino; 1 Asian, non-Hispanic/Latino), 2 international. Average age 27. 6 applicants, 50% accepted, 3 enrolled. In 2015, 2 doctorates awarded. *Degree requirements:* For doctorate, comprehensive exam, thesis/dissertation. *Entrance requirements:* For doctorate, GRE General Test. Additional exam requirements/recommendations for international students: Required—TOEFL. *Application deadline:* For fall admission, 6/1 priority date for domestic students. Applications are processed on a rolling basis. *Financial support:* Fellowships with full tuition reimbursements and health care benefits available. Financial award application deadline: 6/1. *Faculty research:* Kinesin motors during slow mitogenesis, mitochondria and peroxisomes in obesity, ovarian innervation, tight junction function and regulation. *Unit head:* Dr. Cheryl Knudson, Chairman, 252-744-2852, Fax: 252-744-2850, E-mail: knudsonc@ecu.edu. *Application contact:* Dr. Ron Dudek, Senior Director of Graduate Studies, 252-744-2863, Fax: 252-744-2850, E-mail: dudekr@ecu.edu. Website: http://www.ecu.edu/cs-dhs/anatomy/gradProg.cfm

Eastern Michigan University, Graduate School, College of Arts and Sciences, Department of Biology, Ypsilanti, MI 48197. Offers cell and molecular biology (MS); community college biology teaching (MS); ecology and organismal biology (MS); general biology (MS); water resources (MS). *Program availability:* Part-time, evening/weekend, online learning. *Faculty:* 26 full-time (8 women). *Students:* 15 full-time (9 women), 33 part-time (19 women); includes 8 minority (3 Black or African American, non-Hispanic/Latino; 2 Asian, non-Hispanic/Latino; 2 Hispanic/Latino; 1 Two or more races, non-Hispanic/Latino), 3 international. Average age 27. 47 applicants, 51% accepted, 19 enrolled. In 2015, 14 master's awarded. *Entrance requirements:* For master's, GRE General Test, GRE Subject Test. Additional exam requirements/recommendations for international students: Required—TOEFL. *Application deadline:* Applications are processed on a rolling basis. Application fee: $45. *Financial support:* Fellowships, research assistantships with full tuition reimbursements, teaching assistantships with full tuition reimbursements, career-related internships or fieldwork, Federal Work-Study, institutionally sponsored loans, scholarships/grants, tuition waivers (partial), and unspecified assistantships available. Support available to part-time students. Financial award applicants required to submit FAFSA. *Unit head:* Dr. Daniel Clemans, Department Head, 734-487-4242, Fax: 734-487-9235, E-mail: dclemans@emich.edu. *Application contact:* Dr. David Kass, Graduate Coordinator, 734-487-4242, Fax: 734-487-9235, E-mail: dkass@emich.edu. Website: http://www.emich.edu/biology

Eastern New Mexico University, Graduate School, College of Liberal Arts and Sciences, Department of Biology, Portales, NM 88130. Offers applied ecology (MS); botany (MS); cell, molecular biology and biotechnology (MS); microbiology (MS); zoology (MS). *Program availability:* Part-time. *Degree requirements:* For master's, comprehensive exam, thesis optional. *Entrance requirements:* For master's, GRE, minimum GPA of 3.0, 2 letters of recommendation, statement of research interest, bachelor's degree related to field of study or proof of common knowledge. Additional exam requirements/recommendations for international students: Required—TOEFL (minimum score 550 paper-based; 79 iBT), IELTS (minimum score 6). Electronic applications accepted.

Emory University, Laney Graduate School, Division of Biological and Biomedical Sciences, Program in Biochemistry, Cell and Developmental Biology, Atlanta, GA 30322. Offers PhD. *Degree requirements:* For doctorate, comprehensive exam, thesis/dissertation. *Entrance requirements:* For doctorate, GRE General Test, minimum GPA of 3.0 in science course work (recommended). Additional exam requirements/recommendations for international students: Required—TOEFL. Electronic applications accepted. *Faculty research:* Signal transduction, molecular biology, enzymes and cofactors, receptor and ion channel function, membrane biology.

Emporia State University, Department of Biological Sciences, Emporia, KS 66801-5415. Offers botany (MS); environmental biology (MS); general biology (MS); microbial and cellular biology (MS); zoology (MS). *Program availability:* Part-time. *Faculty:* 14 full-time (3 women), 1 part-time/adjunct (0 women). *Students:* 26 full-time (13 women), 15 part-time (7 women); includes 1 minority (Two or more races, non-Hispanic/Latino), 24 international. 16 applicants, 100% accepted, 11 enrolled. In 2015, 17 master's awarded. *Degree requirements:* For master's, comprehensive exam or thesis. *Entrance requirements:* For master's, GRE, appropriate undergraduate degree, interview, letters of reference. Additional exam requirements/recommendations for international students: Required—TOEFL (minimum score 520 paper-based; 68 iBT). *Application deadline:* For fall admission, 8/15 priority date for domestic students. Applications are processed on a rolling basis. Application fee: $30 ($75 for international students). Electronic applications accepted. *Expenses:* Tuition, state resident: full-time $5640; part-time $235 per credit hour. Tuition, nonresident: full-time $17,544; part-time $731 per credit hour. *Required fees:* $1848; $77 per credit hour. *Financial support:* In 2015–16, 7 research assistantships with full tuition reimbursements (averaging $7,344 per year), 12 teaching assistantships with full tuition reimbursements (averaging $7,844 per year) were awarded; career-related internships or fieldwork, Federal Work-Study, institutionally sponsored loans, health care benefits, and unspecified assistantships also available. Financial award application deadline: 3/15; financial award applicants required to submit FAFSA. *Faculty research:* Fisheries, range, and wildlife management; aquatic, plant, grassland, vertebrate, and invertebrate ecology; mammalian and plant systematics, taxonomy, and evolution; immunology, virology, and molecular biology. *Unit head:* Dr. Yixin Eric Yang, Chair, 620-341-5311, Fax: 620-341-5608, E-mail: yyang@emporia.edu. Website: http://www.emporia.edu/info/degrees-courses/grad/biology

Florida Institute of Technology, College of Science, Program in Biological Sciences, Melbourne, FL 32901-6975. Offers biological science (PhD); biotechnology (MS); cell and molecular biology (MS); ecology (MS); marine biology (MS). *Program availability:* Part-time. *Students:* 65 full-time (39 women), 10 part-time (3 women); includes 4 minority (2 Asian, non-Hispanic/Latino; 1 Hispanic/Latino; 1 Two or more races, non-Hispanic/Latino), 38 international. Average age 26. 230 applicants, 24% accepted, 21 enrolled. In 2015, 23 master's, 3 doctorates awarded. *Degree requirements:* For master's, thesis (for some programs), research, seminar, internship, or summer lab; for doctorate, comprehensive exam, thesis/dissertation, dissertations seminar, publications. *Entrance requirements:* For master's, GRE General Test, 3 letters of recommendation; statement of objectives; bachelor's degree in biology, chemistry, biochemistry or equivalent; for doctorate, GRE General Test, resume, 3 letters of recommendation, minimum GPA of 3.2, statement of objectives. Additional exam requirements/recommendations for international students: Required—TOEFL (minimum score 550 paper-based; 79 iBT). *Application deadline:* For fall admission, 3/1 for domestic students, 4/1 for international students; for spring admission, 9/1 for domestic and international students. Applications are processed on a rolling basis. Electronic applications accepted. *Expenses: Tuition, area resident:* Full-time $21,690; part-time $1205 per credit hour. *Required fees:* $500. Tuition and fees vary according to degree level, campus/location and program. *Financial support:* Career-related internships or fieldwork, institutionally sponsored loans, tuition waivers (partial), unspecified assistantships, and tuition remissions available. Support available to part-time students. Financial award application deadline: 3/1; financial award applicants required to submit FAFSA. *Faculty research:* Initiation of protein synthesis in eukaryotic cells, fixation of radioactive carbon, changes in DNA molecule, endangered or threatened avian and mammalian species, hydroacoustics and feeding preference of the West Indian manatee. *Unit head:* Dr. Richard B. Aronson, Department Head, 321-674-8034, Fax: 321-674-7238, E-mail: raronson@fit.edu. *Application contact:* Cheryl A. Brown, Associate Director of Graduate Admissions, 321-674-7581, Fax: 321-723-9468, E-mail: cbrown@fit.edu. Website: http://cos.fit.edu/biology/

Florida State University, The Graduate School, College of Arts and Sciences, Department of Biological Science, Specialization in Cell and Molecular Biology, Tallahassee, FL 32306-4295. Offers MS, PhD. *Faculty:* 25 full-time (7 women). *Students:* 62 full-time (28 women); includes 7 minority (1 Black or African American, non-Hispanic/Latino; 1 Asian, non-Hispanic/Latino; 5 Hispanic/Latino), 23 international. 113 applicants, 20% accepted, 9 enrolled. In 2015, 1 master's, 3 doctorates awarded. Terminal master's awarded for partial completion of doctoral program. *Degree requirements:* For master's, comprehensive exam, thesis, teaching experience, seminar

Cell Biology

presentation; for doctorate, comprehensive exam, thesis/dissertation, teaching experience; seminar presentation. *Entrance requirements:* For master's and doctorate, GRE General Test, minimum upper-division GPA of 3.0. Additional exam requirements/recommendations for international students: Required—TOEFL (minimum score 600 paper-based; 92 iBT). *Application deadline:* For fall admission, 12/1 for domestic and international students. Application fee: $30. Electronic applications accepted. *Expenses: Tuition, area resident:* Full-time $7263; part-time $403.50 per credit hour. Tuition, nonresident: full-time $18,087; part-time $1004.85 per credit hour. *Required fees:* $1365; $75.81 per credit hour. $20 per semester. Tuition and fees vary according to campus/location. *Financial support:* In 2015–16, 62 students received support, including 2 fellowships with full tuition reimbursements available (averaging $30,000 per year), 17 research assistantships with full tuition reimbursements available (averaging $21,500 per year), 43 teaching assistantships with full tuition reimbursements available (averaging $21,500 per year); scholarships/grants and unspecified assistantships also available. Financial award application deadline: 12/1; financial award applicants required to submit FAFSA. *Faculty research:* Molecular biology; genetics and genomics; developmental biology and gene expression; cell structure, function, and motility; cellular and organismal physiology; biophysical and structural biology. *Unit head:* Dr. Thomas A. Houpt, Professor and Associate Chair, 850-644-4907, Fax: 850-644-8447, E-mail: houpt@neuro.fsu.edu. *Application contact:* Dr. Michael B. Miller, Coordinator, Graduate Affairs, 850-644-3023, Fax: 850-644-8447, E-mail: gradinfo@bio.fsu.edu. Website: http://www.bio.fsu.edu/cmb/

Georgia State University, College of Arts and Sciences, Department of Biology, Program in Cellular and Molecular Biology and Physiology, Atlanta, GA 30302-3083. Offers bioinformatics (MS); cellular and molecular biology and physiology (MS, PhD). *Program availability:* Part-time. Terminal master's awarded for partial completion of doctoral program. *Degree requirements:* For master's, comprehensive exam (for some programs), thesis optional; for doctorate, comprehensive exam, thesis/dissertation. *Entrance requirements:* For master's and doctorate, GRE. Additional exam requirements/recommendations for international students: Required—TOEFL (minimum score 550 paper-based; 82 iBT) or IELTS (minimum score 7). *Application deadline:* For fall admission, 7/1 priority date for domestic students, 6/1 priority date for international students; for spring admission, 11/15 priority date for domestic students, 10/15 priority date for international students. Applications are processed on a rolling basis. Application fee: $50. Electronic applications accepted. *Expenses:* Tuition, state resident: full-time $6876; part-time $382 per credit hour. Tuition, nonresident: full-time $22,374; part-time $1243 per credit hour. *Required fees:* $2128; $2128 per term. $1064 per term. Part-time tuition and fees vary according to course load and program. *Financial support:* In 2015–16, fellowships with full tuition reimbursements (averaging $22,000 per year), research assistantships with full tuition reimbursements (averaging $20,000 per year) were awarded. Financial award application deadline: 12/3. *Faculty research:* Membrane transport, viral infection, molecular immunology, protein modeling, gene regulation. *Unit head:* Dr. Charles Derby, Director of Graduate Studies, 404-413-5393, Fax: 404-413-5446, E-mail: cderby@gsu.edu. Website: http://biology.gsu.edu/

Grand Valley State University, College of Liberal Arts and Sciences, Program in Cell and Molecular Biology, Allendale, MI 49401-9403. Offers MS. *Faculty:* 9 full-time (6 women). *Students:* 25 full-time (17 women), 32 part-time (19 women); includes 4 minority (1 Black or African American, non-Hispanic/Latino; 2 Asian, non-Hispanic/Latino; 1 Hispanic/Latino), 14 international. Average age 27. 26 applicants, 85% accepted, 22 enrolled. In 2015, 11 master's awarded. *Entrance requirements:* For master's, minimum GPA of 3.0. Application fee: $30. *Financial support:* In 2015–16, 22 students received support, including 2 fellowships (averaging $2,833 per year), 21 research assistantships with tuition reimbursements (averaging $4,969 per year); unspecified assistantships also available. *Faculty research:* Plant cell biology, plant development, cell/signal integration. *Unit head:* Dr. Mark Staves, Associate Professor/Coordinator, 616-331-2473, E-mail: stavesm@gvsu.edu. *Application contact:* Dr. Tim Born, Coordinator, 616-331-8643, E-mail: bornt@gvsu.edu.

Harvard University, Graduate School of Arts and Sciences, Department of Molecular and Cellular Biology, Cambridge, MA 02138. Offers PhD. *Degree requirements:* For doctorate, thesis/dissertation, oral exam. *Entrance requirements:* For doctorate, GRE General Test, GRE Subject Test (recommended). Additional exam requirements/recommendations for international students: Required—TOEFL.

Harvard University, Graduate School of Arts and Sciences, Division of Medical Sciences, Boston, MA 02115. Offers biological chemistry and molecular pharmacology (PhD); cell biology (PhD); genetics (PhD); microbiology and molecular genetics (PhD); pathology (PhD), including experimental pathology. *Degree requirements:* For doctorate, thesis/dissertation. *Entrance requirements:* For doctorate, GRE General Test, GRE Subject Test. Additional exam requirements/recommendations for international students: Required—TOEFL.

Illinois Institute of Technology, Graduate College, College of Science, Department of Biological Sciences, Chicago, IL 60616. Offers biochemistry (MS); biology (MS, PhD); cell and molecular biology (MS); microbiology (MS); molecular biochemistry and biophysics (MS, PhD). *Program availability:* Part-time, evening/weekend, online learning. Terminal master's awarded for partial completion of doctoral program. *Degree requirements:* For master's, comprehensive exam, thesis (for some programs); for doctorate, comprehensive exam, thesis/dissertation. *Entrance requirements:* For master's, GRE General Test (minimum score 300 Quantitative and Verbal, 2.5 Analytical Writing), minimum undergraduate GPA of 3.0; for doctorate, GRE General Test (minimum score 310 Quantitative and Verbal, 3.0 Analytical Writing); GRE Subject Test (strongly recommended), minimum undergraduate GPA of 3.0. Additional exam requirements/recommendations for international students: Required—TOEFL (minimum score 550 paper-based; 80 iBT). Electronic applications accepted. *Faculty research:* Macromolecular crystallography, insect immunity and basic cell biology, improvement of bacterial strains for enhanced biodesulfurization of petroleum, programmed cell death in cancer cells.

Illinois State University, Graduate School, College of Arts and Sciences, Department of Biological Sciences, Normal, IL 61790-2200. Offers animal behavior (MS); bacteriology (MS); biochemistry (MS); biological sciences (MS); biology (PhD); biophysics (MS); biotechnology (MS); botany (MS, PhD); cell biology (MS); conservation biology (MS); developmental biology (MS); ecology (MS, PhD); entomology (MS); evolutionary biology (MS); genetics (MS, PhD); immunology (MS); microbiology (MS, PhD); molecular biology (MS); molecular genetics (MS); neurobiology (MS); neuroscience (MS); parasitology (MS); physiology (MS, PhD); plant biology (MS); plant molecular biology (MS); plant sciences (MS); structural biology (MS); zoology (MS, PhD). *Program availability:* Part-time. *Degree requirements:* For master's, thesis or alternative; for doctorate, variable foreign language requirement, thesis/dissertation, 2 terms of residency. *Entrance requirements:* For master's, GRE General Test, minimum GPA of 2.6 in last 60 hours of course work; for doctorate, GRE General Test. *Application deadline:* Applications are processed on a rolling basis. Application fee: $40. *Financial support:* Research assistantships, teaching assistantships, Federal Work-Study, tuition waivers (full), and unspecified assistantships available. Financial award application deadline: 4/1. *Faculty research:* Redoc balance and drug development in schistosoma

mansoni, control of the growth of listeria monocytogenes at low temperature, regulation of cell expansion and microtubule function by SPRI, CRUI: physiology and fitness consequences of different life history phenotypes. *Application contact:* Steven Juliano, Graduate Coordinator, E-mail: sajulian@ilstu.edu. Website: http://www.bio.ilstu.edu/

Indiana State University, College of Graduate and Professional Studies, College of Arts and Sciences, Department of Biology, Terre Haute, IN 47809. Offers cellular and molecular biology (PhD); ecology, systematics and evolution (PhD); life sciences (MS); physiology (PhD); science education (MS). *Degree requirements:* For master's, thesis optional; for doctorate, comprehensive exam, thesis/dissertation. *Entrance requirements:* For master's and doctorate, GRE General Test. Electronic applications accepted.

Indiana University Bloomington, University Graduate School, College of Arts and Sciences, Department of Biology, Bloomington, IN 47405. Offers biology teaching (MAT); biotechnology (MA); evolution, ecology, and behavior (MA, PhD); genetics (PhD); microbiology (MA, PhD); molecular, cellular, and developmental biology (PhD); plant sciences (MA, PhD); zoology (MA, PhD). Terminal master's awarded for partial completion of doctoral program. *Degree requirements:* For master's, thesis, oral defense; for doctorate, thesis/dissertation, oral defense. *Entrance requirements:* For master's and doctorate, GRE General Test. Additional exam requirements/recommendations for international students: Required—TOEFL (minimum score 100 iBT). Electronic applications accepted. *Faculty research:* Evolution, ecology and behavior; microbiology; molecular biology and genetics; plant biology.

Indiana University–Purdue University Indianapolis, Indiana University School of Medicine, Department of Anatomy and Cell Biology, Indianapolis, IN 46202. Offers MS, PhD, MD/PhD. *Degree requirements:* For master's, thesis or alternative; for doctorate, thesis/dissertation. *Entrance requirements:* For master's and doctorate, GRE General Test. *Faculty research:* Acoustic reflex control, osteoarthritis and bone disease, diabetes, kidney diseases, cellular and molecular neurobiology.

Iowa State University of Science and Technology, Program in Molecular, Cellular, and Developmental Biology, Ames, IA 50011. Offers MS, PhD. *Entrance requirements:* For master's and doctorate, GRE General Test. Additional exam requirements/recommendations for international students: Required—TOEFL (minimum score 580 paper-based; 85 iBT), IELTS (minimum score 7). Electronic applications accepted.

Irell & Manella Graduate School of Biological Sciences, Graduate Program, Duarte, CA 91010. Offers brain metastatic cancer (PhD); cancer and stem cell metabolism (PhD); cancer biology (PhD); cancer biology and developmental therapeutics (PhD); cell biology (PhD); chemical biology (PhD); chromosomal break repair (PhD); diabetes and pancreatic progenitor cell biology (PhD); DNA repair and cancer biology (PhD); germline epigenetic remodeling and endocrine disruptors (PhD); hematology and hematopoietic cell transplantation (PhD); hematology and immunology (PhD); inflammation and cancer (PhD); micrornas and gene regulation in cardiovascular disease (PhD); mixed chimrism for reversal of autoimmunity (PhD); molecular and cellular biology (PhD); molecular biology and genetics (PhD); nanoparticle mediated twist1 silencing in metastatic cancer (PhD); neuro-oncology and stem cell biology (PhD); neuroscience (PhD); rna directed therapies for hiv-1 (PhD); small rna-induced transcriptional gene activation (PhD); stem cell regulation by the microenvironment (PhD); translational oncology and pharmaceutical sciences (PhD); tumor biology (PhD). *Faculty:* 70 full-time (18 women). *Students:* 75 full-time (40 women); includes 28 minority (2 Black or African American, non-Hispanic/Latino; 10 Asian, non-Hispanic/Latino; 10 Hispanic/Latino; 2 Native Hawaiian or other Pacific Islander, non-Hispanic/Latino; 4 Two or more races, non-Hispanic/Latino), 15 international. Average age 26. 197 applicants, 12% accepted, 19 enrolled. In 2015, 12 doctorates awarded. *Degree requirements:* For doctorate, comprehensive exam, thesis/dissertation, qualifying exams, two advanced courses. *Entrance requirements:* For doctorate, GRE General Test; GRE Subject Test (recommended), 2 years of course work in chemistry (general and organic); 1 year of course work each in biochemistry, general biology, and general physics; 2 semesters of course work in mathematics; significant research laboratory experience. Additional exam requirements/recommendations for international students: Required—TOEFL. *Application deadline:* For fall admission, 1/1 priority date for domestic and international students. Application fee: $0. Electronic applications accepted. Full-time tuition and fees vary according to class time, course level, course load, degree level, campus/location, program and student level. *Financial support:* In 2015–16, 12 students received support, including 35 fellowships with full tuition reimbursements available (averaging $32,000 per year); teaching assistantships, health care benefits, and tuition waivers (full) also available. Financial award applicants required to submit FAFSA. *Faculty research:* Cancer biology, diabetes, stem cell biology, neuroscience, immunology. *Unit head:* Dr. John J. Rossi, Dean, 877-715-GRAD, Fax: 626-471-3901, E-mail: gradschool@coh.org. *Application contact:* Dr. Kate Sleeth, Interim Associate Dean of Administration and Student Development, 626-218-1742, Fax: 626-471-3901, E-mail: gradschool@coh.org. Website: http://cityofhope.org/gradschool

See Display on page 66 and Close-Up on page 111.

Johns Hopkins University, National Institutes of Health Sponsored Programs, Baltimore, MD 21218. Offers biology (PhD), including biochemistry, biophysics, cell biology, developmental biology, genetic biology, molecular biology; cell, molecular, and developmental biology and biophysics (PhD). *Degree requirements:* For doctorate, comprehensive exam, thesis/dissertation. *Entrance requirements:* For doctorate, GRE General Test. Additional exam requirements/recommendations for international students: Required—TOEFL (minimum score 600 paper-based), TWE. Electronic applications accepted. *Faculty research:* Protein and nucleic acid biochemistry and biophysical chemistry, molecular biology and development.

Johns Hopkins University, School of Medicine, Graduate Programs in Medicine, Graduate Program in Cellular and Molecular Medicine, Baltimore, MD 21218. Offers PhD. *Degree requirements:* For doctorate, comprehensive exam, thesis/dissertation, oral exam. *Entrance requirements:* For doctorate, GRE. Additional exam requirements/recommendations for international students: Required—TOEFL. Electronic applications accepted. *Faculty research:* Cellular and molecular basis of disease.

Johns Hopkins University, School of Medicine, Graduate Programs in Medicine, Program in Biochemistry, Cellular and Molecular Biology, Baltimore, MD 21205. Offers PhD. *Degree requirements:* For doctorate, comprehensive exam, thesis/dissertation. *Entrance requirements:* For doctorate, GRE General Test. Additional exam requirements/recommendations for international students: Required—TOEFL. Electronic applications accepted. *Faculty research:* Developmental biology, genomics/proteomics, protein targeting, signal transduction, structural biology.

Kent State University, College of Arts and Sciences, School of Biomedical Sciences, Kent, OH 44242-0001. Offers biological anthropology (PhD); cellular and molecular biology (PhD), including cellular biology and structures, molecular biology and genetics; neurosciences (PhD); pharmacology (MS); physiology (PhD). *Students:* 76 full-time (46 women), 1 (woman) part-time; includes 6 minority (1 Black or African American, non-Hispanic/Latino; 2 Asian, non-Hispanic/Latino; 1 Hispanic/Latino; 2 Two or more races, non-Hispanic/Latino), 28 international. Average age 29. 223 applicants, 13% accepted,

22 enrolled. In 2015, 5 master's, 7 doctorates awarded. Terminal master's awarded for partial completion of doctoral program. *Degree requirements:* For master's, thesis; for doctorate, thesis/dissertation, candidacy exam. *Entrance requirements:* For master's and doctorate, GRE General Test, minimum GPA of 3.0, transcript, goal statement, resume, 3 letters of recommendation. Additional exam requirements/recommendations for international students: Required—TOEFL (minimum score: paper-based 525, iBT 71), Michigan English Language Assessment Battery (minimum score of 75), IELTS (minimum score of 6.0), PTE Academic (minimum score of 48), or completion of ELS level 112 Intensive Program. *Application deadline:* For fall admission, 1/1 for domestic students. Application fee: $45 ($70 for international students). Electronic applications accepted. *Expenses:* Tuition, state resident: full-time $10,864; part-time $495 per credit hour. Tuition, nonresident: full-time $18,380; part-time $837 per credit hour. *Financial support:* In 2015–16, 76 students received support. Research assistantships with full tuition reimbursements available, teaching assistantships, career-related internships or fieldwork, Federal Work-Study, and unspecified assistantships available. Financial award application deadline: 1/1. *Unit head:* Dr. Eric Mintz, Director, 330-672-2263, E-mail: emintz@kent.edu. *Application contact:* 330-672-2263, Fax: 330-672-9391, E-mail: jwearden@kent.edu.
Website: http://www.kent.edu/biomedical/

Lehigh University, College of Arts and Sciences, Department of Biological Sciences, Bethlehem, PA 18015. Offers biochemistry (PhD); cell and molecular biology (PhD); integrative biology (PhD); molecular biology (MS). *Program availability:* Part-time, 100% online. *Faculty:* 19 full-time (9 women). *Students:* 38 full-time (22 women), 21 part-time (15 women); includes 13 minority (5 Black or African American, non-Hispanic/Latino; 1 American Indian or Alaska Native, non-Hispanic/Latino; 6 Hispanic/Latino; 1 Two or more races, non-Hispanic/Latino), 5 international. Average age 27. 38 applicants, 50% accepted, 10 enrolled. In 2015, 6 master's, 1 doctorate awarded. Terminal master's awarded for partial completion of doctoral program. *Degree requirements:* For master's, thesis optional; for doctorate, comprehensive exam, thesis/dissertation. *Entrance requirements:* For doctorate, GRE General Test. Additional exam requirements/recommendations for international students: Required—TOEFL (minimum score 85 iBT). *Application deadline:* For fall admission, 12/15 for domestic and international students. Application fee: $75. *Expenses:* $1,185 per credit hour tuition (PhD); $925 per credit hour tuition (MS). *Financial support:* In 2015–16, 34 students received support, including 8 fellowships with full tuition reimbursements available (averaging $29,667 per year), 6 research assistantships with full tuition reimbursements available (averaging $27,000 per year), 19 teaching assistantships with full tuition reimbursements available (averaging $27,000 per year); scholarships/grants also available. Financial award application deadline: 12/15. *Faculty research:* Gene expression, cytoskeleton and cell structure, cell cycle and growth regulation, neuroscience, animal behavior, microbiology. *Total annual research expenditures:* $1.9 million. *Unit head:* Dr. Murray Itzkowitz, Chairperson, 610-758-3680, Fax: 610-758-4004, E-mail: mi00@lehigh.edu. *Application contact:* Dr. Mary Kathryn Iovine, Graduate Coordinator, 610-758-6981, Fax: 610-758-4004, E-mail: mki3@lehigh.edu.
Website: http://www.lehigh.edu/~inbios/

Louisiana State University Health Sciences Center, School of Graduate Studies in New Orleans, Department of Cell Biology and Anatomy, New Orleans, LA 70112-2223. Offers cell biology and anatomy (PhD), including clinical anatomy, development, cell, and neurobiology; MD/PhD. *Faculty:* 17 full-time (2 women). *Students:* 5 full-time (2 women), 1 international. 2 applicants, 100% accepted, 2 enrolled. *Degree requirements:* For doctorate, comprehensive exam, thesis/dissertation. *Entrance requirements:* For doctorate, GRE General Test, minimum undergraduate GPA of 3.0. Additional exam requirements/recommendations for international students: Recommended—TOEFL, IELTS. *Application deadline:* For fall admission, 3/1 priority date for domestic students, 3/1 for international students. Applications are processed on a rolling basis. Application fee: $30. *Financial support:* In 2015–16, 6 students received support. Unspecified assistantships available. Financial award application deadline: 4/1. *Faculty research:* Visual system organization, neural development, plasticity of sensory systems, information processing through the nervous system, visuomotor integration. *Total annual research expenditures:* $900,000. *Unit head:* Dr. Samuel McClugage, Head, 504-568-4011, Fax: 504-568-2165, E-mail: smcclu@lsuhsc.edu. *Application contact:* Dr. R. John Cork, Graduate Coordinator and Professor, 504-568-7177, E-mail: jcork@lsuhsc.edu.
Website: http://www.medschool.lsuhsc.edu/cell_biology/

Louisiana State University Health Sciences Center at Shreveport, Department of Cellular Biology and Anatomy, Shreveport, LA 71130-3932. Offers MS, PhD, MD/PhD. Terminal master's awarded for partial completion of doctoral program. *Degree requirements:* For master's, thesis; for doctorate, thesis/dissertation. *Entrance requirements:* For master's and doctorate, GRE General Test. Additional exam requirements/recommendations for international students: Required—TOEFL. *Faculty research:* Cancer biology, redox biology, neurosciences, immunobiology, cardiovascular sciences.

Loyola University Chicago, Graduate School, Integrated Program in Biomedical Sciences, Maywood, IL 60153. Offers biochemistry and molecular biology (MS, PhD); cell and molecular physiology (PhD); infectious disease and immunology (MS); integrative cell biology (PhD); medical physiology (MS); microbiology and immunology (MS, PhD); molecular pharmacology and therapeutics (MS, PhD); neuroscience (MS, PhD). *Students:* 135 full-time (65 women), 1 part-time (0 women); includes 28 minority (5 Black or African American, non-Hispanic/Latino; 15 Asian, non-Hispanic/Latino; 6 Hispanic/Latino; 2 Two or more races, non-Hispanic/Latino), 16 international. Average age 28. 442 applicants, 23% accepted, 55 enrolled. In 2015, 40 master's, 17 doctorates awarded. *Expenses:* Tuition, area resident: Full-time $18,054; part-time $9027 per credit hour. *Required fees:* $832; $284 per credit hour. Part-time tuition and fees vary according to course load, degree level and program. *Unit head:* Dr. Samuel Attoh, Dean, 773-508-3459, Fax: 773-508-2460, E-mail: sattoh@luc.edu. *Application contact:* Ron Martin, Associate Director of Enrollment Management, 312-915-8950, Fax: 312-915-8905, E-mail: gradapp@luc.edu.
Website: http://ssom.luc.edu/graduate_school/degree-programs/ipbsphd/

Marquette University, Graduate School, College of Arts and Sciences, Department of Biology, Milwaukee, WI 53201-1881. Offers cell biology (MS, PhD); developmental biology (MS, PhD); ecology (MS, PhD); epithelial physiology (MS, PhD); genetics (MS, PhD); microbiology (MS, PhD); molecular biology (MS, PhD); muscle and exercise physiology (MS, PhD); neuroscience (PhD). *Faculty:* 22 full-time (7 women), 3 part-time/adjunct (2 women). *Students:* 28 full-time (11 women), 12 part-time (4 women); includes 4 minority (1 Asian, non-Hispanic/Latino; 1 Hispanic/Latino; 2 Two or more races, non-Hispanic/Latino), 11 international. Average age 27. 72 applicants, 28% accepted, 5 enrolled. In 2015, 2 master's, 4 doctorates awarded. Terminal master's awarded for partial completion of doctoral program. *Degree requirements:* For master's, comprehensive exam, thesis, 1 year of teaching experience or equivalent; for doctorate, thesis/dissertation, 1 year of teaching experience or equivalent, qualifying exam. *Entrance requirements:* For master's and doctorate, GRE General Test, GRE Subject Test, official transcripts from all current and previous colleges/universities except Marquette, statement of professional goals and aspirations, three letters of recommendation. Additional exam requirements/recommendations for international students: Required—TOEFL (minimum score 530 paper-based). *Application deadline:* For fall admission, 12/15 for domestic and international students. Application fee: $50. Electronic applications accepted. *Financial support:* In 2015–16, 39 students received support, including 6 fellowships (averaging $1,208 per year), 4 research assistantships with full tuition reimbursements available (averaging $21,750 per year), 29 teaching assistantships with full tuition reimbursements available (averaging $21,750 per year); scholarships/grants, health care benefits, tuition waivers (full and partial), and unspecified assistantships also available. Support available to part-time students. Financial award application deadline: 2/15. *Faculty research:* Neurobiology, neuroendocrinology, epithelial physiology, neuropeptide interactions, synaptic transmission. *Total annual research expenditures:* $1.2 million. *Unit head:* Dr. Ed Blumenthal, Chair, 414-288-1748. *Application contact:* Dr. Michael Schlappi, Recruiting Contact, 414-288-1467.
Website: http://www.marquette.edu/biology/

Massachusetts Institute of Technology, School of Science, Department of Biology, Cambridge, MA 02139. Offers biochemistry (PhD); biological oceanography (PhD); biology (PhD); biophysical chemistry and molecular structure (PhD); cell biology (PhD); computational and systems biology (PhD); developmental biology (PhD); genetics (PhD); immunology (PhD); microbiology (PhD); molecular biology (PhD); neurobiology (PhD). *Faculty:* 57 full-time (14 women). *Students:* 283 full-time (137 women); includes 83 minority (3 Black or African American, non-Hispanic/Latino; 1 American Indian or Alaska Native, non-Hispanic/Latino; 38 Asian, non-Hispanic/Latino; 31 Hispanic/Latino; 10 Two or more races, non-Hispanic/Latino), 48 international. Average age 26. 673 applicants, 14% accepted, 46 enrolled. In 2015, 32 doctorates awarded. *Degree requirements:* For doctorate, comprehensive exam, thesis/dissertation, teaching assistantship during two semesters. *Entrance requirements:* For doctorate, GRE General Test. Additional exam requirements/recommendations for international students: Required—TOEFL (minimum score 577 paper-based), IELTS. *Application deadline:* For fall admission, 12/1 for domestic and international students. Application fee: $75. Electronic applications accepted. *Expenses:* Tuition: Full-time $46,400; part-time $725 per credit. One-time fee: $304 full-time. Full-time tuition and fees vary according to course load and program. *Financial support:* In 2015–16, 235 students received support, including 118 fellowships (averaging $37,500 per year), 163 research assistantships (averaging $38,900 per year), 1 teaching assistantship; Federal Work-Study, institutionally sponsored loans, scholarships/grants, traineeships, health care benefits, and unspecified assistantships also available. Support available to part-time students. Financial award application deadline: 4/15; financial award applicants required to submit FAFSA. *Faculty research:* Cellular, developmental and molecular (plant and animal) biology; biochemistry, bioengineering, biophysics and structural biology; classical and molecular genetics, stem cell and epigenetics; immunology and microbiology; cancer biology, molecular medicine, neurobiology and human disease; computational and systems biology. *Total annual research expenditures:* $42.8 million. *Unit head:* Prof. Alan Grossman, Department Head, 617-253-4701. *Application contact:* Biology Education Office, 617-253-3717, Fax: 617-258-9329, E-mail: gradbio@mit.edu.
Website: https://biology.mit.edu/

Mayo Graduate School, Graduate Programs in Biomedical Sciences, Programs in Biochemistry, Structural Biology, Cell Biology, and Genetics, Rochester, MN 55905. Offers biochemistry and structural biology (PhD); cell biology and genetics (PhD); molecular biology (PhD). *Degree requirements:* For doctorate, oral defense of dissertation, qualifying oral and written exam. *Entrance requirements:* For doctorate, GRE, 1 year of chemistry, biology, calculus, and physics. Additional exam requirements/recommendations for international students: Required—TOEFL. Electronic applications accepted. *Faculty research:* Gene structure and function, membranes and receptors/cytoskeleton, oncogenes and growth factors, protein structure and function, steroid hormonal action.

McGill University, Faculty of Graduate and Postdoctoral Studies, Faculty of Medicine, Department of Anatomy and Cell Biology, Montréal, QC H3A 2T5, Canada. Offers M Sc, PhD.

McMaster University, Faculty of Health Sciences and School of Graduate Studies, Program in Medical Sciences, Metabolism and Nutrition Area, Hamilton, ON L8S 4M2, Canada. Offers M Sc, PhD, MD/PhD. *Degree requirements:* For master's, thesis; for doctorate, comprehensive exam, thesis/dissertation. *Entrance requirements:* For master's, honors B Sc, B+ average in related field; for doctorate, M Sc, minimum B+ average, students with proven research experience and an A average may be admitted with a B Sc degree. Additional exam requirements/recommendations for international students: Required—TOEFL (minimum score 580 paper-based; 92 iBT).

Medical University of South Carolina, College of Graduate Studies, Program in Molecular and Cellular Biology and Pathobiology, Charleston, SC 29425. Offers cancer biology (PhD); cardiovascular biology (PhD); cardiovascular imaging (PhD); cell regulation (PhD); craniofacial biology (PhD); genetics and development (PhD); marine biomedicine (PhD); DMD/PhD; MD/PhD. *Degree requirements:* For doctorate, thesis/dissertation, oral and written exams. *Entrance requirements:* For doctorate, GRE General Test, interview, minimum GPA of 3.0. Additional exam requirements/recommendations for international students: Required—TOEFL (minimum score 600 paper-based; 100 iBT). Electronic applications accepted.

Michigan State University, The Graduate School, College of Agriculture and Natural Resources, MSU-DOE Plant Research Laboratory, East Lansing, MI 48824. Offers biochemistry and molecular biology (PhD); cellular and molecular biology (PhD); crop and soil sciences (PhD); genetics (PhD); microbiology and molecular genetics (PhD); plant biology (PhD); plant physiology (PhD). Offered jointly with the Department of Energy. *Degree requirements:* For doctorate, comprehensive exam, thesis/dissertation, laboratory rotation, defense of dissertation. *Entrance requirements:* For doctorate, GRE General Test, acceptance into one of the affiliated department programs; 3 letters of recommendation; bachelor's degree or equivalent in life sciences, chemistry, biochemistry, or biophysics; research experience. Electronic applications accepted. *Faculty research:* Role of hormones in the regulation of plant development and physiology, molecular mechanisms associated with signal recognition, development and application of genetic methods and materials, protein routing and function.

Michigan State University, The Graduate School, College of Natural Science, Program in Cell and Molecular Biology, East Lansing, MI 48824. Offers cell and molecular biology (MS, PhD); cell and molecular biology/environmental toxicology (PhD). *Entrance requirements:* Additional exam requirements/recommendations for international students: Required—TOEFL. Electronic applications accepted.

Missouri State University, Graduate College, College of Health and Human Services, Department of Biomedical Sciences, Program in Cell and Molecular Biology, Springfield, MO 65897. Offers MS. *Program availability:* Part-time. *Students:* 9 full-time (5 women), 3 part-time (2 women); includes 2 minority (1 Asian, non-Hispanic/Latino; 1 Hispanic/Latino), 2 international. Average age 25. 21 applicants, 43% accepted, 7 enrolled. In 2015, 4 master's awarded. *Degree requirements:* For master's, thesis or alternative, oral and written exams. *Entrance requirements:* For master's, GRE General Test, 2 semesters of course work in organic chemistry and physics, 1 semester of course work

Cell Biology

in calculus, minimum GPA of 3.0 in last 60 hours of course work. Additional exam requirements/recommendations for international students: Required—TOEFL (minimum score 550 paper-based; 79 iBT), IELTS (minimum score 6). *Application deadline:* For fall admission, 7/20 priority date for domestic students, 5/1 for international students; for spring admission, 12/20 priority date for domestic students, 9/1 for international students. Applications are processed on a rolling basis. Application fee: $35 ($50 for international students). Electronic applications accepted. *Expenses:* Tuition, state resident: full-time $5500. Tuition, nonresident: full-time $10,108. *Required fees:* $1000. *Financial support:* In 2015–16, 11 research assistantships (averaging $8,600 per year) were awarded; career-related internships or fieldwork, Federal Work-Study, institutionally sponsored loans, scholarships/grants, and unspecified assistantships also available. Support available to part-time students. Financial award application deadline: 3/31; financial award applicants required to submit FAFSA. *Faculty research:* Extracellular matrix membrane protein, P2 nucleotide receptors, double stranded RNA viruses. *Unit head:* Dr. Scott Zimmerman, Program Director, 417-836-5478, Fax: 417-836-5588, E-mail: scottzimmerman@missouristate.edu. *Application contact:* Michael Edwards, Coordinator of Graduate Admissions, 417-836-5033, Fax: 417-836-6200, E-mail: michaeledwards@missouristate.edu.
Website: http://www.missouristate.edu/bms/CMB/

New York Medical College, Graduate School of Basic Medical Sciences, Cell Biology and Anatomy - Master's Program, Valhalla, NY 10595-1691. Offers MS, MD/PhD. *Program availability:* Part-time, evening/weekend. *Degree requirements:* For master's, thesis. *Entrance requirements:* For master's, GRE General Test, MCAT, or DAT. Additional exam requirements/recommendations for international students: Required—TOEFL. Electronic applications accepted. *Expenses: Tuition, area resident:* Full-time $44,355; part-time $1025 per credit. *Required fees:* $500; $95 per year. One-time fee: $140 part-time. Tuition and fees vary according to course load and program. *Faculty research:* Mechanisms of growth control in skeletal muscle, cartilage differentiation, cytoskeletal functions, signal transduction pathways, neuronal development and plasticity.

New York Medical College, Graduate School of Basic Medical Sciences, Integrated PhD Program, Valhalla, NY 10595-1691. Offers biochemistry and molecular biology (PhD); cell biology and anatomy (PhD); microbiology and immunology (PhD); pathology (PhD); pharmacology (PhD); physiology (PhD). *Degree requirements:* For doctorate, comprehensive exam, thesis/dissertation. *Entrance requirements:* For doctorate, GRE General Test. Additional exam requirements/recommendations for international students: Required—TOEFL. Electronic applications accepted. *Expenses: Tuition, area resident:* Full-time $44,355; part-time $1025 per credit. *Required fees:* $500; $95 per year. One-time fee: $140 part-time. Tuition and fees vary according to course load and program. *Faculty research:* Cardiovascular sciences, infectious diseases, neuroscience, cancer and cell signaling.

New York University, School of Medicine and Graduate School of Arts and Science, Sackler Institute of Graduate Biomedical Sciences, Program in Cellular and Molecular Biology, New York, NY 10012-1019. Offers PhD. *Degree requirements:* For doctorate, comprehensive exam, thesis/dissertation, qualifying exam. *Faculty research:* Membrane and organelle structure and biogenesis, intracellular transport and processing of proteins, cellular recognition and cell adhesion, oncogene structure and function, action of growth factors.

North Carolina State University, College of Veterinary Medicine, Program in Comparative Biomedical Sciences, Raleigh, NC 27695. Offers cell biology (MS, PhD); infectious disease (MS, PhD); pathology (MS, PhD); pharmacology (MS, PhD); population medicine (MS, PhD). *Program availability:* Part-time. *Degree requirements:* For master's, thesis; for doctorate, thesis/dissertation. *Entrance requirements:* For master's and doctorate, GRE General Test. Additional exam requirements/recommendations for international students: Required—TOEFL (minimum score 550 paper-based). Electronic applications accepted. *Expenses:* Contact institution. *Faculty research:* Infectious diseases, cell biology, pharmacology and toxicology, genomics, pathology and population medicine.

North Dakota State University, College of Graduate and Interdisciplinary Studies, College of Science and Mathematics, Department of Biological Sciences, Fargo, ND 58102. Offers biology (MS); botany (MS, PhD); cellular and molecular biology (PhD); genomics (PhD); zoology (MS, PhD). *Degree requirements:* For master's, thesis; for doctorate, thesis/dissertation. *Entrance requirements:* For master's and doctorate, GRE General Test. Additional exam requirements/recommendations for international students: Required—TOEFL. *Application deadline:* For fall admission, 1/15 for domestic students. Applications are processed on a rolling basis. Application fee: $35. Electronic applications accepted. *Financial support:* Fellowships with full tuition reimbursements, research assistantships with full tuition reimbursements, teaching assistantships with full tuition reimbursements, career-related internships or fieldwork, Federal Work-Study, institutionally sponsored loans, scholarships/grants, tuition waivers (full), and unspecified assistantships available. Support available to part-time students. Financial award application deadline: 4/15; financial award applicants required to submit FAFSA. *Faculty research:* Comparative endocrinology, physiology, behavioral ecology, plant cell biology, aquatic biology. *Unit head:* Dr. Wendy Reed, Head, 701-231-5921, E-mail: wendy.reed@ndsu.edu. *Application contact:* Elizabeth Worth, Marketing, Recruitment, and Public Relations Coordinator, 701-231-8476, Fax: 701-231-6524, E-mail: elizabeth.worth@ndsu.edu.
Website: http://www.ndsu.edu/biology/

North Dakota State University, College of Graduate and Interdisciplinary Studies, Interdisciplinary Program in Cellular and Molecular Biology, Fargo, ND 58102. Offers PhD. Program offered in cooperation with 11 departments in the university. *Degree requirements:* For doctorate, thesis/dissertation. *Entrance requirements:* For doctorate, GRE. Additional exam requirements/recommendations for international students: Required—TOEFL (minimum score 525 paper-based; 71 iBT). *Application deadline:* Applications are processed on a rolling basis. Application fee: $35. Electronic applications accepted. *Financial support:* Fellowships with full tuition reimbursements, research assistantships with full tuition reimbursements, teaching assistantships with full tuition reimbursements, and unspecified assistantships available. Financial award application deadline: 3/15. *Faculty research:* Plant and animal cell biology, gene regulation, molecular genetics, plant and animal virology. *Unit head:* Dr. Jane Schuh, Director, 701-231-7841, E-mail: jane.schuh@ndsu.edu. *Application contact:* Elizabeth Worth, Marketing, Recruitment, and Public Relations Coordinator, 701-231-8476, Fax: 701-231-6524, E-mail: elizabeth.worth@ndsu.edu.
Website: http://www.ndsu.edu/cellularmolecularbiology/

Northwestern University, The Graduate School, Interdisciplinary Biological Sciences Program (IBiS), Evanston, IL 60208. Offers biochemistry (PhD); bioengineering and biotechnology (PhD); biotechnology (PhD); cell and molecular biology (PhD); developmental and systems biology (PhD); nanotechnology (PhD); neurobiology (PhD); structural biology and biophysics (PhD). *Degree requirements:* For doctorate, thesis/dissertation, qualifying exam. *Entrance requirements:* For doctorate, GRE General Test. Additional exam requirements/recommendations for international students: Required—TOEFL (minimum score 600 paper-based). Electronic applications accepted. *Faculty research:* Biophysics/structural biology, cell/molecular biology, synthetic biology, developmental systems biology, chemical biology/nanotechnology.

The Ohio State University, Graduate School, College of Arts and Sciences, Division of Natural and Mathematical Sciences, Department of Molecular Genetics, Columbus, OH 43210. Offers cell and developmental biology (MS, PhD); genetics (MS, PhD); molecular biology (MS, PhD). *Degree requirements:* For master's, thesis; for doctorate, thesis/dissertation. *Entrance requirements:* For doctorate, GRE General Test, GRE Subject Test in biology or chemistry (recommended). Additional exam requirements/recommendations for international students: Required—TOEFL (minimum score 550 paper-based; 79 iBT), Michigan English Language Assessment Battery (minimum score 82); Recommended—IELTS (minimum score 7). Electronic applications accepted.

The Ohio State University, Graduate School, College of Arts and Sciences, Division of Natural and Mathematical Sciences, Program in Molecular, Cellular and Developmental Biology, Columbus, OH 43210. Offers MS, PhD. Terminal master's awarded for partial completion of doctoral program. *Degree requirements:* For master's, thesis; for doctorate, thesis/dissertation. *Entrance requirements:* For doctorate, GRE General Test, GRE Subject Test in any science (desired, preferably biology or chemistry, biochemistry or cell and molecular biology). Additional exam requirements/recommendations for international students: Required—TOEFL (minimum score 600 paper-based; 85 iBT); Recommended—IELTS (minimum score 8). Electronic applications accepted.

Ohio University, Graduate College, College of Arts and Sciences, Department of Biological Sciences, Athens, OH 45701-2979. Offers biological sciences (MS, PhD); cell biology and physiology (MS, PhD); ecology and evolutionary biology (MS, PhD); exercise physiology and muscle biology (MS, PhD); microbiology (MS, PhD); neuroscience (MS, PhD). Terminal master's awarded for partial completion of doctoral program. *Degree requirements:* For master's, comprehensive exam, thesis, 1 quarter of teaching experience; for doctorate, comprehensive exam, thesis/dissertation, 2 quarters of teaching experience. *Entrance requirements:* For master's, GRE General Test, names of three faculty members whose research interests most closely match the applicant's interest; for doctorate, GRE General Test, essay concerning prior training, research interest and career goals, plus names of three faculty members whose research interests most closely match the applicant's interest. Additional exam requirements/recommendations for international students: Required—TOEFL (minimum score 620 paper-based; 105 iBT) or IELTS (minimum score 7.5). Electronic applications accepted. *Faculty research:* Ecology and evolutionary biology, exercise physiology and muscle biology, neurobiology, cell biology, physiology.

Ohio University, Graduate College, College of Arts and Sciences, Interdisciplinary Graduate Program in Molecular and Cellular Biology, Athens, OH 45701-2979. Offers MS, PhD. *Degree requirements:* For master's, comprehensive exam, thesis, research proposal, teaching experience; for doctorate, comprehensive exam, thesis/dissertation, research proposal, teaching experience. *Entrance requirements:* For master's and doctorate, GRE General Test. Additional exam requirements/recommendations for international students: Required—TOEFL (minimum score 620 paper-based; 105 iBT); Recommended—TWE. Electronic applications accepted. *Faculty research:* Animal biotechnology, plant molecular biology RNA, immunology, cellular genetics, biochemistry of signal transduction, cancer research, membrane transport, bioinformatics, bioengineering, chemical biology and drug discovery, diabetes, microbiology, neuroscience.

Oregon Health & Science University, School of Medicine, Graduate Programs in Medicine, Program in Molecular and Cellular Biosciences, Cell and Developmental Biology Graduate Program, Portland, OR 97239-3098. Offers PhD. *Faculty:* 11 full-time (6 women), 38 part-time/adjunct (6 women). *Students:* 11 full-time (8 women); includes 1 minority (Asian, non-Hispanic/Latino), 2 international. Average age 28. In 2015, 7 doctorates awarded. *Degree requirements:* For doctorate, comprehensive exam, thesis/dissertation, qualifying exam. *Entrance requirements:* For doctorate, GRE General Test (minimum scores: 153 Verbal/148 Quantitative/4.5 Analytical) or MCAT. Additional exam requirements/recommendations for international students: Required—IELTS or TOEFL. *Application deadline:* For fall admission, 12/1 for domestic and international students. Application fee: $70. *Financial support:* Health care benefits, tuition waivers (full), and full tuition and stipends available. *Faculty research:* Biosynthesis, intracellular trafficking, and function of essential cellular components; signal transduction and developmental regulation of gene expression; regulation of cell proliferation, growth, and motility; mechanisms of morphogenesis and differentiation; mechanisms controlling the onset, progression, and dissemination of cancer. *Unit head:* Dr. Philip Copenhaver, Program Director, 503-494-4646, E-mail: copenhav@ohsu.edu. *Application contact:* Lola Bichler, Program Coordinator, 503-494-5824, E-mail: bichler@ohsu.edu.
Website: http://www.ohsu.edu/xd/education/schools/school-of-medicine/departments/basic-science-departments/cell-and-developmental-biology/graduate-program/CDB-

Oregon State University, College of Science, Program in Zoology, Corvallis, OR 97331. Offers behavioral ecology (MA, MS, PhD); behavioral endocrinology (MA, MS, PhD); cell biology (MA, MS, PhD); chemical ecology (MA, MS, PhD); conservation biology (MA, MS, PhD); developmental biology (MA, MS, PhD). *Faculty:* 21 full-time (9 women), 2 part-time/adjunct (1 woman). *Students:* 58 full-time (38 women), 1 part-time (0 women); includes 11 minority (1 Black or African American, non-Hispanic/Latino; 1 American Indian or Alaska Native, non-Hispanic/Latino; 7 Asian, non-Hispanic/Latino; 1 Hispanic/Latino; 1 Two or more races, non-Hispanic/Latino), 3 international. Average age 28. 75 applicants, 13% accepted, 9 enrolled. In 2015, 1 master's, 5 doctorates awarded. Terminal master's awarded for partial completion of doctoral program. *Degree requirements:* For doctorate, thesis/dissertation. *Entrance requirements:* For master's and doctorate, GRE. Additional exam requirements/recommendations for international students: Required—TOEFL (minimum score 80 iBT), IELTS (minimum score 6.5). *Application deadline:* For fall admission, 12/15 for domestic and international students. Application fee: $75 ($85 for international students). *Expenses:* Tuition, state resident: full-time $12,150; part-time $450 per credit. Tuition, nonresident: full-time $20,952; part-time $776 per credit. *Required fees:* $1572; $1443 per unit. One-time fee: $350. Tuition and fees vary according to course load, campus/location and program. *Financial support:* Fellowships, research assistantships, teaching assistantships, Federal Work-Study, and institutionally sponsored loans available. Support available to part-time students. *Faculty research:* Ecology and evolutionary biology, physiology and behavior, development and cell biology. *Unit head:* Dr. Virginia M. Weis, Professor and Chair of Integrative Biology, 541-737-4359. *Application contact:* Graduate Admissions Coordinator, 541-737-5335, E-mail: ib@science.oregonstate.edu.
Website: http://ib.oregonstate.edu/

Oregon State University, Interdisciplinary/Institutional Programs, Program in Molecular and Cellular Biology, Corvallis, OR 97331. Offers bioinformatics (PhD); biotechnology (PhD); cell biology (PhD); developmental biology (PhD); genome biology (PhD); molecular biology (PhD); molecular pathogenesis (PhD); molecular virology (PhD); plant molecular biology (PhD); structural biology (PhD). *Students:* 28 full-time (14 women), 2 part-time (1 woman); includes 4 minority (2 Asian, non-Hispanic/Latino; 2 Hispanic/Latino), 10 international. Average age 29. 104 applicants, 5% accepted, 5 enrolled. In 2015, 5 doctorates awarded. *Degree requirements:* For doctorate, thesis/dissertation, oral and written qualifying exams. *Entrance requirements:* For doctorate, GRE.

Additional exam requirements/recommendations for international students: Required—TOEFL (minimum score 80 iBT), IELTS (minimum score 6.5). *Application deadline:* For fall admission, 8/1 for domestic students, 4/1 for international students; for winter admission, 12/1 for domestic students, 7/1 for international students; for spring admission, 2/1 for domestic students, 10/1 for international students; for summer admission, 5/1 for domestic students, 1/1 for international students. Application fee: $75 ($85 for international students). *Expenses:* Tuition, state resident: full-time $12,150; part-time $450 per credit. Tuition, nonresident: full-time $20,952; part-time $776 per credit. *Required fees:* $1572; $1443 per unit. One-time fee: $350. Tuition and fees vary according to course load, campus/location and program. *Financial support:* Fellowships, career-related internships or fieldwork, Federal Work-Study, and institutionally sponsored loans available. Support available to part-time students. Financial award application deadline: 1/1. *Unit head:* Dr. Dee Denver, Director, Molecular and Cellular Biology Graduate Program, 541-737-3698. *Application contact:* Kristin Carroll, Assistant Director, 541-737-5259, E-mail: kristin.carroll@oregonstate.edu.
Website: http://www.mcb.oregonstate.edu/

Penn State Hershey Medical Center, College of Medicine, Graduate School Programs in the Biomedical Sciences, The Huck Institutes of the Life Sciences, Intercollege Graduate Program in Molecular Cellular and Integrative Biosciences, Hershey, PA 17033. Offers cell and developmental biology (PhD); immunology and infectious disease (PhD); molecular and evolutionary genetics (PhD); molecular medicine (PhD); molecular toxicology (PhD); neurobiology (PhD). *Students:* 3 full-time (2 women); includes 2 minority (both Asian, non-Hispanic/Latino). 2 applicants, 100% accepted, 2 enrolled. In 2015, 1 doctorate awarded. *Degree requirements:* For doctorate, comprehensive exam, thesis/dissertation, oral exam. *Entrance requirements:* For doctorate, GRE, minimum GPA of 3.0. Additional exam requirements/recommendations for international students: Required—TOEFL (minimum score 500 paper-based). *Application deadline:* For fall admission, 1/31 priority date for domestic students, 2/1 priority date for international students. Applications are processed on a rolling basis. Application fee: $65. Electronic applications accepted. *Financial support:* In 2015–16, research assistantships with full tuition reimbursements (averaging $26,196 per year) were awarded; fellowships with full tuition reimbursements, career-related internships or fieldwork, Federal Work-Study, scholarships/grants, health care benefits, and unspecified assistantships also available. Financial award applicants required to submit FAFSA. *Faculty research:* Vascular biology, molecular toxicology, chemical biology, immune system, pathophysiological basis of human disease. *Unit head:* Dr. Peter Hudson, Director, 814-865-6057, E-mail: pjh18@psu.edu. *Application contact:* Kathy Shuey, Administrative Assistant, 717-531-8982, Fax: 717-531-0786, E-mail: grad-hmc@psu.edu.
Website: http://www.huck.psu.edu/education/molecular-cellular-and-integrative-biosciences

Penn State University Park, Graduate School, Intercollege Graduate Programs, Program in Molecular, Cellular, and Integrative Biosciences, University Park, PA 16802. Offers molecular, cellular, and integrative biosciences (MS, PhD). *Unit head:* Dr. Regina Vasilatos-Younken, Dean, 814-865-2516, Fax: 814-863-4627. *Application contact:* Lori Stania, Director, Graduate Student Services, 814-865-1795, Fax: 814-863-4627, E-mail: l-gswww@lists.psu.edu.

Purdue University, Graduate School, College of Science, Department of Biological Sciences, West Lafayette, IN 47907. Offers biochemistry (PhD); biophysics (PhD); cell and developmental biology (PhD); ecology, evolutionary and population biology (MS, PhD), including ecology, evolutionary biology, population biology; genetics (MS, PhD); microbiology (MS, PhD); molecular biology (PhD); neurobiology (MS, PhD); plant physiology (PhD). Terminal master's awarded for partial completion of doctoral program. *Degree requirements:* For master's, thesis (for some programs); for doctorate, thesis/dissertation, seminars, teaching experience. *Entrance requirements:* For master's, GRE General Test (minimum analytical writing score of 3.5), minimum undergraduate GPA of 3.0; for doctorate, GRE General Test (minimum analytical writing score of 3.5), minimum undergraduate GPA of 3.5. Additional exam requirements/recommendations for international students: Required—TOEFL (minimum score 600 paper-based; 107 iBT for MS, 80 iBT for PhD). Electronic applications accepted.

Queen's University at Kingston, School of Graduate Studies, Faculty of Health Sciences, Department of Anatomy and Cell Biology, Kingston, ON K7L 3N6, Canada. Offers biology of reproduction (M Sc, PhD); cancer (M Sc, PhD); cardiovascular pathophysiology (M Sc, PhD); cell and molecular biology (M Sc, PhD); drug metabolism (M Sc, PhD); endocrinology (M Sc, PhD); motor control (M Sc, PhD); neural regeneration (M Sc, PhD); neurophysiology (M Sc, PhD). *Program availability:* Part-time. *Degree requirements:* For master's, thesis; for doctorate, one foreign language, comprehensive exam, thesis/dissertation. *Entrance requirements:* Additional exam requirements/recommendations for international students: Required—TOEFL. Electronic applications accepted. *Faculty research:* Human kinetics, neuroscience, reproductive biology, cardiovascular.

Quinnipiac University, College of Arts and Sciences, Program in Molecular and Cell Biology, Hamden, CT 06518-1940. Offers MS. *Program availability:* Part-time, evening/weekend. *Faculty:* 6 full-time (4 women), 3 part-time/adjunct (0 women). *Students:* 14 full-time (4 women), 20 part-time (14 women); includes 6 minority (2 Black or African American, non-Hispanic/Latino; 2 Asian, non-Hispanic/Latino; 2 Hispanic/Latino), 7 international. 49 applicants, 45% accepted, 12 enrolled. In 2015, 10 master's awarded. *Degree requirements:* For master's, thesis optional. *Entrance requirements:* For master's, bachelor's degree in biological, medical, or health sciences. Additional exam requirements/recommendations for international students: Required—TOEFL (minimum score 575 paper-based; 90 iBT), IELTS (minimum score 6.5). *Application deadline:* For fall admission, 7/30 priority date for domestic students, 4/15 priority date for international students; for spring admission, 12/15 priority date for domestic students, 9/15 priority date for international students. Applications are processed on a rolling basis. Application fee: $45. Electronic applications accepted. *Expenses:* $985 per credit tuition; $40 per credit student fee (not to exceed $360 per semester); $150 per semester technology fee part-time (fall/spring); $340 per semester technology fee full-time (fall/spring); $75 per semester technology fee (summer). *Financial support:* Career-related internships or fieldwork, Federal Work-Study, scholarships/grants, and unspecified assistantships available. Support available to part-time students. Financial award application deadline: 6/1; financial award applicants required to submit FAFSA. *Unit head:* Dr. Lise Thomas, Director, E-mail: graduate@quinnipiac.edu. *Application contact:* Office of Graduate Admissions, 800-462-1944, Fax: 203-582-3443, E-mail: graduate@quinnipiac.edu.
Website: http://www.quinnipiac.edu/gradmolecular

Rice University, Graduate Programs, Wiess School of Natural Sciences, Department of Biochemistry and Cell Biology, Houston, TX 77251-1892. Offers MA, PhD. Terminal master's awarded for partial completion of doctoral program. *Degree requirements:* For master's, thesis; for doctorate, thesis/dissertation. *Entrance requirements:* For master's and doctorate, GRE. Additional exam requirements/recommendations for international students: Required—TOEFL (minimum score 600 paper-based; 90 iBT). Electronic applications accepted. *Expenses:* Contact institution. *Faculty research:* Steroid metabolism, protein structure NMR, biophysics, cell growth and movement.

Rosalind Franklin University of Medicine and Science, School of Graduate and Postdoctoral Studies - Interdisciplinary Graduate Program in Biomedical Sciences, Department of Cell Biology and Anatomy, North Chicago, IL 60064-3095. Offers PhD, MD/PhD. Terminal master's awarded for partial completion of doctoral program. *Degree requirements:* For doctorate, comprehensive exam, thesis/dissertation, original research project. *Entrance requirements:* For doctorate, GRE General Test, minimum GPA of 3.0. Additional exam requirements/recommendations for international students: Required—TOEFL, TWE. *Faculty research:* Neuroscience, molecular biology.

Rush University, Graduate College, Division of Anatomy and Cell Biology, Chicago, IL 60612-3832. Offers MS, PhD, MD/MS, MD/PhD. Terminal master's awarded for partial completion of doctoral program. *Degree requirements:* For master's, thesis; for doctorate, comprehensive exam, thesis/dissertation, preliminary exam, dissertation proposal. *Entrance requirements:* For master's, GRE General Test, minimum GPA of 3.0, bachelor's degree in biology or chemistry (preferred), interview; for doctorate, GRE General Test, minimum GPA of 3.0, interview. Additional exam requirements/recommendations for international students: Required—TOEFL. Electronic applications accepted. *Faculty research:* Incontinence following vaginal distension, knee replacement, biomimetric materials, injured spinal motoneurons, implant fixation.

Rutgers University–Newark, Graduate School of Biomedical Sciences, Department of Cell Biology and Molecular Medicine, Newark, NJ 07107. Offers PhD. *Degree requirements:* For doctorate, thesis/dissertation, qualifying exam. *Entrance requirements:* For doctorate, GRE General Test. Additional exam requirements/recommendations for international students: Required—TOEFL. Electronic applications accepted.

Rutgers University–New Brunswick, Graduate School-New Brunswick, Programs in the Molecular Biosciences, Program in Cell and Developmental Biology, Piscataway, NJ 08854-8097. Offers MS, PhD. MS, PhD offered jointly with University of Medicine and Dentistry of New Jersey. *Program availability:* Part-time. Terminal master's awarded for partial completion of doctoral program. *Degree requirements:* For master's, thesis; for doctorate, thesis/dissertation, written qualifying exam. *Entrance requirements:* For master's, GRE General Test; for doctorate, GRE General Test, GRE Subject Test (recommended), minimum GPA of 3.0. Additional exam requirements/recommendations for international students: Required—TOEFL. Electronic applications accepted. *Faculty research:* Signal transduction and regulation of gene expression, developmental genetics, cellular biology, developmental genetics, neurobiology.

San Diego State University, Graduate and Research Affairs, College of Sciences, Department of Biology, San Diego, CA 92182. Offers biology (MA, MS), including ecology (MS), molecular biology (MS), physiology (MS), systematics/evolution (MS); cell and molecular biology (PhD); ecology (MS, PhD); microbiology (MS). Terminal master's awarded for partial completion of doctorate. *Degree requirements:* For master's, thesis; for doctorate, thesis/dissertation. *Entrance requirements:* For master's, GRE General Test, GRE Subject Test, resume or curriculum vitae, 2 letters of recommendation. Additional exam requirements/recommendations for international students: Required—TOEFL. Electronic applications accepted.

San Diego State University, Graduate and Research Affairs, College of Sciences, Molecular Biology Institute, Program in Cell and Molecular Biology, San Diego, CA 92182. Offers PhD. Program offered jointly with University of California, San Diego. *Degree requirements:* For doctorate, thesis/dissertation, oral comprehensive qualifying exam. *Entrance requirements:* For doctorate, GRE General Test, GRE Subject Test, resumé or curriculum vitae, 3 letters of recommendation. Electronic applications accepted. *Faculty research:* Structure/dynamics of protein kinesis, chromatin structure and DNA methylation membrane biochemistry, secretory protein targeting, molecular biology of cardiac myocytes.

San Francisco State University, Division of Graduate Studies, College of Science and Engineering, Department of Biology, Program in Cell and Molecular Biology, San Francisco, CA 94132-1722. Offers MS. *Application deadline:* Applications are processed on a rolling basis. *Expenses:* Tuition, state resident: full-time $6738. Tuition, nonresident: full-time $15,666. *Required fees:* $1004. *Unit head:* Dr. Diana Chu, Program Coordinator, 415-405-3487, Fax: 415-338-2295, E-mail: chud@sfsu.edu. *Application contact:* Graduate Coordinator.
Website: http://biology.sfsu.edu/programs/graduate

Sonoma State University, School of Science and Technology, Department of Biology, Rohnert Park, CA 94928. Offers biochemistry (MA); ecology (MS); environmental biology (MS); evolutionary biology (MS); functional morphology (MS); molecular and cell biology (MS); organismal biology (MS). *Program availability:* Part-time. *Degree requirements:* For master's, thesis or alternative, oral exam. *Entrance requirements:* For master's, GRE General Test, GRE Subject Test, minimum GPA of 3.0. Additional exam requirements/recommendations for international students: Required—TOEFL (minimum score 500 paper-based). *Faculty research:* Plant physiology, comparative physiology, community ecology, restoration ecology, marine ecology, conservation genetics, primate behavior, behavioral ecology, developmental biology, plant and animal systematics.

Southern Methodist University, Dedman College of Humanities and Sciences, Department of Biological Sciences, Dallas, TX 75275. Offers molecular and cellular biology (MA, MS, PhD). Terminal master's awarded for partial completion of doctoral program. *Degree requirements:* For master's, thesis (for MS), oral exam; for doctorate, thesis/dissertation, qualifying exam. *Entrance requirements:* For master's, GRE General Test (minimum score 1200), minimum GPA of 3.0; for doctorate, GRE General Test (minimum score: 1200), minimum GPA of 3.0. Additional exam requirements/recommendations for international students: Required—TOEFL (minimum score 550 paper-based). Electronic applications accepted. *Faculty research:* Free radicals and aging, protein structure, chromatin structure, signal processes, retroviral pathogenesis.

State University of New York Downstate Medical Center, School of Graduate Studies, Program in Molecular and Cellular Biology, Brooklyn, NY 11203-2098. Offers PhD, MD/PhD. Affiliation with a particular PhD degree-granting program is deferred to the second year. *Degree requirements:* For doctorate, comprehensive exam, thesis/dissertation. *Entrance requirements:* For doctorate, GRE General Test. Additional exam requirements/recommendations for international students: Recommended—TOEFL. *Faculty research:* Mechanism of gene regulation, molecular virology.

State University of New York Upstate Medical University, College of Graduate Studies, Program in Cell and Developmental Biology, Syracuse, NY 13210-2334. Offers anatomy (MS, PhD); MD/PhD. Terminal master's awarded for partial completion of doctoral program. *Degree requirements:* For master's, thesis; for doctorate, comprehensive exam, thesis/dissertation. *Entrance requirements:* For master's, GRE General Test, interview; for doctorate, GRE General Test, telephone interview. Additional exam requirements/recommendations for international students: Required—TOEFL. Electronic applications accepted. *Faculty research:* Cancer, disorders of the nervous system, infectious diseases, diabetes/metabolic disorders/cardiovascular diseases.

Stony Brook University, State University of New York, Graduate School, College of Arts and Sciences, Department of Biochemistry and Cell Biology, Biochemistry and Cell Biology Program, Stony Brook, NY 11794. Offers MS. *Program availability:* Part-time.

Cell Biology

Students: 17 full-time (6 women), 4 part-time (1 woman); includes 5 minority (1 Black or African American, non-Hispanic/Latino; 2 Asian, non-Hispanic/Latino; 2 Hispanic/Latino), 4 international. 76 applicants, 34% accepted, 14 enrolled. In 2015, 11 master's awarded. *Degree requirements:* For master's, thesis. *Entrance requirements:* For master's, three letters of recommendation, BS or BA in a life science related field with minimum B average, personal statement. Additional exam requirements/recommendations for international students: Required—TOEFL (minimum score 550 paper-based; 90 iBT). *Application deadline:* For fall admission, 4/1 for domestic and international students. Applications are processed on a rolling basis. Electronic applications accepted. *Expenses:* $12,421 full-time resident tuition and fees, $453 per credit hour; $23,761 full-time non-resident tuition and fees, $925 per credit hour. *Unit head:* Prof. Aaron Neiman, Chair, 631-632-1543, Fax: 631-632-9730, E-mail: aaron.neiman@stonybrook.edu. *Application contact:* Pam Wolfskill, Coordinator, 631-632-8585, Fax: 631-632-8575, E-mail: carol.juliano@stonybrook.edu. Website: http://www.stonybrook.edu/commcms/biochem/education/graduate/overview.html

Stony Brook University, State University of New York, Graduate School, College of Arts and Sciences, Department of Biochemistry and Cell Biology, Molecular and Cellular Biology Program, Stony Brook, NY 11794. Offers biochemistry and molecular biology (PhD); biological sciences (MA); immunology and pathology (PhD); molecular and cellular biology (PhD). *Faculty:* 22 full-time (7 women). *Students:* 66 full-time (41 women); includes 11 minority (2 Black or African American, non-Hispanic/Latino; 6 Asian, non-Hispanic/Latino; 3 Hispanic/Latino), 38 international. Average age 28. 175 applicants, 16% accepted, 8 enrolled. In 2015, 11 doctorates awarded. *Degree requirements:* For doctorate, comprehensive exam, thesis/dissertation, teaching experience. *Entrance requirements:* For doctorate, GRE General Test, GRE Subject Test. Additional exam requirements/recommendations for international students: Required—TOEFL. *Application deadline:* For fall admission, 1/15 for domestic students; for spring admission, 10/1 for domestic students. *Application fee:* $100. *Expenses:* $12,421 per year full-time resident tuition and fees, $453 per credit hour; $23,761 per year full-time non-resident tuition and fees, $925 per credit hour. *Financial support:* In 2015–16, 4 fellowships, 33 research assistantships, 8 teaching assistantships were awarded; Federal Work-Study also available. *Unit head:* Prof. Aaron Neiman, Chair, 631-632-1543, E-mail: aaron.neiman@stonybrook.edu. *Application contact:* Pam Wolfskill, Administrative Specialist/Program Administrator, 631-632-8585, Fax: 631-632-9730, E-mail: pamela.wolfskill@stonybrook.edu.

Texas Tech University Health Sciences Center, Graduate School of Biomedical Sciences, Program in Biomedical Sciences, Lubbock, TX 79430. Offers MS, PhD, MD/PhD, MS/PhD. Terminal master's awarded for partial completion of doctoral program. *Degree requirements:* For master's, comprehensive exam, thesis; for doctorate, comprehensive exam, thesis/dissertation. *Entrance requirements:* For master's and doctorate, GRE General Test, minimum GPA of 3.0. Additional exam requirements/recommendations for international students: Required—TOEFL (minimum score 550 paper-based). Electronic applications accepted. *Faculty research:* Biochemical endocrinology, neurobiology, molecular biology, reproductive biology, biology of developing systems.

Thomas Jefferson University, Jefferson College of Biomedical Sciences, MS Program in Cell and Developmental Biology, Philadelphia, PA 19107. Offers MS. *Program availability:* Part-time, evening/weekend. *Faculty:* 44 full-time (14 women), 27 part-time/adjunct (11 women). *Students:* 22 part-time (15 women); includes 3 minority (2 Black or African American, non-Hispanic/Latino; 1 Asian, non-Hispanic/Latino), 2 international. Average age 29. 13 applicants, 77% accepted, 9 enrolled. In 2015, 5 master's awarded. *Degree requirements:* For master's, thesis, clerkship. *Entrance requirements:* For master's, GRE General Test or MCAT, minimum GPA of 3.0. Additional exam requirements/recommendations for international students: Required—TOEFL, IELTS (minimum score 7). *Application deadline:* For fall admission, 8/1 priority date for domestic students, 3/1 priority date for international students; for winter admission, 12/1 priority date for domestic students, 6/1 priority date for international students; for spring admission, 4/1 priority date for domestic students. Applications are processed on a rolling basis. *Application fee:* $50. Electronic applications accepted. *Financial support:* Federal Work-Study and institutionally sponsored loans available. Support available to part-time students. Financial award application deadline: 5/1; financial award applicants required to submit FAFSA. *Faculty research:* Developmental biology, cell biology, planning and management, drug development. *Unit head:* Dr. Gerald B. Grunwald, Dean and Program Director, 215-503-4191, Fax: 215-503-6690, E-mail: gerald.grunwald@jefferson.edu. *Application contact:* Marc E. Stearns, Director of Admissions, 215-503-0155, Fax: 215-503-3433, E-mail: jgsbs-info@jefferson.edu. Website: http://www.jefferson.edu/university/biomedical-sciences/degrees-programs/master-programs/cell-developmental-biology.html

Thomas Jefferson University, Jefferson College of Biomedical Sciences, PhD Program in Cell and Developmental Biology, Philadelphia, PA 19107. Offers PhD. *Faculty:* 75 full-time (17 women). *Students:* 27 full-time (18 women); includes 3 minority (all Hispanic/Latino), 7 international. 19 applicants, 26% accepted, 3 enrolled. In 2015, 3 doctorates awarded. *Degree requirements:* For doctorate, comprehensive exam, thesis/dissertation. *Entrance requirements:* For doctorate, GRE General Test, minimum GPA of 3.2. Additional exam requirements/recommendations for international students: Required—TOEFL (minimum score 100 iBT), IELTS (minimum score 7). *Application deadline:* For fall admission, 12/15 priority date for domestic and international students. Applications are processed on a rolling basis. *Application fee:* $50. Electronic applications accepted. *Financial support:* In 2015–16, 27 fellowships with full tuition reimbursements (averaging $56,298 per year) were awarded; Federal Work-Study, institutionally sponsored loans, scholarships/grants, traineeships and stipends also available. Support available to part-time students. Financial award application deadline: 5/1; financial award applicants required to submit FAFSA. *Unit head:* Dr. Nancy J. Philp, Program Director, 215-503-7854, E-mail: nancy.philp@jefferson.edu. *Application contact:* Marc E. Stearns, Director of Admissions, 215-503-0155, Fax: 215-503-3433, E-mail: jgsbs-info@jefferson.edu. Website: http://www.jefferson.edu/university/biomedical-sciences/degrees-programs/phd-programs/cell-biology.html

Tufts University, Sackler School of Graduate Biomedical Sciences, Cell, Molecular, and Developmental Biology Program, Medford, MA 02155. Offers cancer biology (PhD); developmental and regenerative biology (PhD); molecular and cellular medicine (PhD); structural and chemical biology (PhD). *Faculty:* 45 full-time (15 women). *Students:* 36 full-time (18 women); includes 13 minority (2 Black or African American, non-Hispanic/Latino; 9 Asian, non-Hispanic/Latino; 1 Hispanic/Latino; 1 Two or more races, non-Hispanic/Latino), 4 international. Average age 28. 189 applicants, 7% accepted, 6 enrolled. In 2015, 2 doctorates awarded. Terminal master's awarded for partial completion of doctoral program. *Degree requirements:* For doctorate, comprehensive exam, thesis/dissertation. *Entrance requirements:* For doctorate, GRE General Test, 3 letters of reference. Additional exam requirements/recommendations for international students: Required—TOEFL (minimum score 600 paper-based; 100 iBT). *Application deadline:* For fall admission, 12/15 priority date for domestic and international students. Application fee: $70. Electronic applications accepted. *Expenses: Tuition, area resident:* Full-time $48,412; part-time $1210 per credit hour. *Required fees:* $806. Full-time tuition and fees vary according to degree level, program and student level. Part-time tuition and fees vary according to course load. *Financial support:* In 2015–16, 36 students received support, including 36 research assistantships with full tuition reimbursements available (averaging $32,000 per year); health care benefits also available. *Faculty research:* Reproduction and hormone action, control of gene expression, cell-matrix and cell-cell interactions, growth control and tumorigenesis, cytoskeleton and contractile proteins. *Unit head:* Dr. Ira Herman, Program Director, 617-636-2991, Fax: 617-636-0375. *Application contact:* Dr. Elizabeth Storrs, Registrar/Director of Academic Services, 617-636-6767, Fax: 617-636-0375, E-mail: sackler-school@tufts.edu. Website: http://sackler.tufts.edu/Academics/CMDB-Welcome

Tulane University, School of Medicine and School of Liberal Arts, Graduate Programs in Biomedical Sciences, Department of Structural and Cellular Biology, New Orleans, LA 70118-5669. Offers MS, PhD, MD/PhD. MS and PhD offered through the Graduate School. *Degree requirements:* For master's, one foreign language, thesis; for doctorate, 2 foreign languages, thesis/dissertation. *Entrance requirements:* For master's, GRE General Test, minimum B average in undergraduate course work; for doctorate, GRE General Test. Additional exam requirements/recommendations for international students: Required—TOEFL. Electronic applications accepted. *Expenses: Tuition, area resident:* Full-time $47,658; part-time $2648 per credit hour. *Required fees:* $1980; $44.50 per credit hour. $550 per term. Tuition and fees vary according to course load, degree level and program. *Faculty research:* Reproductive endocrinology, visual neuroscience, neural response to altered hormones.

Tulane University, School of Medicine and School of Liberal Arts, Graduate Programs in Biomedical Sciences, Interdisciplinary Graduate Program in Molecular and Cellular Biology, New Orleans, LA 70118-5669. Offers PhD, MD/PhD. PhD offered through the Graduate School. *Degree requirements:* For doctorate, thesis/dissertation. *Entrance requirements:* For doctorate, GRE General Test, GRE Subject Test. Additional exam requirements/recommendations for international students: Required—TOEFL. Electronic applications accepted. *Expenses: Tuition, area resident:* Full-time $47,658; part-time $2648 per credit hour. *Required fees:* $1980; $44.50 per credit hour. $550 per term. Tuition and fees vary according to course load, degree level and program. *Faculty research:* Developmental biology, neuroscience, virology.

Tulane University, School of Science and Engineering, Department of Cell and Molecular Biology, New Orleans, LA 70118-5669. Offers MS, PhD. Terminal master's awarded for partial completion of doctoral program. *Degree requirements:* For doctorate, thesis/dissertation. *Entrance requirements:* For master's, GRE General Test, minimum B average in undergraduate course work; for doctorate, GRE General Test. Additional exam requirements/recommendations for international students: Required—TOEFL. *Application deadline:* For fall admission, 2/1 for domestic and international students. Application fee: $45. Electronic applications accepted. *Expenses: Tuition, area resident:* Full-time $47,658; part-time $2648 per credit hour. *Required fees:* $1980; $44.50 per credit hour. $550 per term. Tuition and fees vary according to course load, degree level and program. *Financial support:* Fellowships with full tuition reimbursements, research assistantships with full tuition reimbursements, and teaching assistantships with full tuition reimbursements available. Financial award application deadline: 2/1.

Uniformed Services University of the Health Sciences, F. Edward Hebert School of Medicine, Graduate Programs in the Biomedical Sciences and Public Health, Graduate Program in Molecular and Cell Biology, Bethesda, MD 20814-4799. Offers MS, PhD. *Faculty:* 43 full-time (11 women), 3 part-time/adjunct (0 women). *Students:* 22 full-time (13 women); includes 6 minority (2 Asian, non-Hispanic/Latino; 4 Hispanic/Latino), 3 international. Average age 25. 40 applicants, 25% accepted, 6 enrolled. In 2015, 4 doctorates awarded. *Degree requirements:* For doctorate, comprehensive exam, thesis/dissertation, qualifying exam. *Entrance requirements:* For doctorate, GRE General Test, minimum GPA of 3.0. *Application deadline:* For fall admission, 12/15 priority date for domestic students. Applications are processed on a rolling basis. Application fee: $0. Electronic applications accepted. *Financial support:* In 2015–16, fellowships with full tuition reimbursements (averaging $27,000 per year) were awarded; scholarships/grants, health care benefits, and tuition waivers (full) also available. *Faculty research:* Immunology, biochemistry, cancer biology, stem cell biology. *Unit head:* Dr. Mary Lou Cutler, Director, 301-295-3453, Fax: 301-295-1996, E-mail: mary.cutler@usuhs.edu. *Application contact:* Tina Finley, Administrative Assistant, 301-295-3642, Fax: 301-295-1996, E-mail: netina.finley@usuhs.edu. Website: https://www.usuhs.edu/mcb

See Display on page 205 and Close-Up on page 223.

Universidad Central del Caribe, School of Medicine, Program in Biomedical Sciences, Bayamón, PR 00960-6032. Offers anatomy and cell biology (MA, MS); biochemistry (MS); biomedical sciences (MA); cellular and molecular biology (PhD); microbiology and immunology (MA, MS); pharmacology (MS); physiology (MS).

Université de Montréal, Faculty of Medicine, Department of Pathology and Cellular Biology, Montréal, QC H3C 3J7, Canada. Offers M Sc, PhD. Terminal master's awarded for partial completion of doctoral program. *Degree requirements:* For master's, thesis; for doctorate, thesis/dissertation, general exam. *Entrance requirements:* For master's and doctorate, proficiency in French, knowledge of English. Electronic applications accepted. *Faculty research:* Immunopathology, cardiovascular pathology, oncogenetics, cellular neurocytology, muscular dystrophy.

Université de Sherbrooke, Faculty of Medicine and Health Sciences, Graduate Programs in Medicine, Department of Anatomy and Cell Biology, Sherbrooke, QC J1H 5N4, Canada. Offers cell biology (M Sc, PhD). Terminal master's awarded for partial completion of doctoral program. *Degree requirements:* For master's, thesis; for doctorate, thesis/dissertation. Electronic applications accepted. *Faculty research:* Biology of the gut epithelium, signal transduction, gene expression and differentiation, intestinal inflammation, vascular and skeletal muscle cell biology.

Université Laval, Faculty of Medicine, Graduate Programs in Medicine, Programs in Cellular and Molecular Biology, Québec, QC G1K 7P4, Canada. Offers M Sc, PhD. Terminal master's awarded for partial completion of doctoral program. *Degree requirements:* For master's, thesis; for doctorate, comprehensive exam, thesis/dissertation. *Entrance requirements:* For master's and doctorate, knowledge of French, comprehension of written English. Electronic applications accepted. *Faculty research:* Oral bacterial metabolism, sugar transport.

University at Albany, State University of New York, College of Arts and Sciences, Department of Biological Sciences, Specialization in Molecular, Cellular, Developmental, and Neural Biology, Albany, NY 12222-0001. Offers PhD. *Degree requirements:* For doctorate, one foreign language, thesis/dissertation. *Entrance requirements:* For doctorate, GRE General Test.

University at Albany, State University of New York, School of Public Health, Department of Biomedical Sciences, Program in Structural and Cell Biology, Albany, NY 12222-0001. Offers MS, PhD. *Degree requirements:* For master's, thesis; for doctorate, thesis/dissertation. *Entrance requirements:* For master's and doctorate, GRE General Test, GRE Subject Test.

University at Buffalo, the State University of New York, Graduate School, Graduate Programs in Cancer Research and Biomedical Sciences at Roswell Park Cancer Institute, Department of Cellular and Molecular Biology at Roswell Park Cancer Institute, Buffalo, NY 14260. Offers PhD. *Faculty:* 24 full-time (2 women). *Students:* 19 full-time (11 women); includes 2 minority (1 Black or African American, non-Hispanic/Latino; 1 Hispanic/Latino), 5 international. 46 applicants, 30% accepted, 4 enrolled. In 2015, 2 doctorates awarded. *Degree requirements:* For doctorate, comprehensive exam, thesis/dissertation, oral defense of disseration. *Entrance requirements:* For doctorate, GRE General Test. Additional exam requirements/recommendations for international students: Required—TOEFL (minimum score 79 iBT). *Application deadline:* For fall admission, 1/5 priority date for domestic and international students. Application fee: $75. Electronic applications accepted. *Financial support:* In 2015–16, 19 students received support, including 19 research assistantships with full tuition reimbursements available (averaging $25,000 per year); scholarships/grants, health care benefits, and unspecified assistantships also available. Financial award application deadline: 1/5. *Faculty research:* Cancer genetics, chromatin structure and replication, regulation of transcription, human gene mapping, genetic and structural approaches to regulation of gene expression. *Unit head:* Dr. Dominic J. Smiraglia, Director of Graduate Studies, 716-845-1347, Fax: 716-845-1698, E-mail: dominic.smiraglia@roswellpark.org. *Application contact:* Dr. Norman J. Karin, Associate Dean, 716-845-2339, Fax: 716-845-8178, E-mail: norman.karin@roswellpark.edu.
Website: http://www.roswellpark.edu/education/phd-programs/cellular-molecular-biology

The University of Alabama at Birmingham, Graduate Programs in Joint Health Sciences, Cell, Molecular, and Developmental Biology Theme, Birmingham, AL 35294. Offers PhD. *Degree requirements:* For doctorate, variable foreign language requirement, comprehensive exam, thesis/dissertation. *Entrance requirements:* For doctorate, GRE General Test, interview. Additional exam requirements/recommendations for international students: Required—TOEFL (minimum score 600 paper-based). Electronic applications accepted. *Expenses:* Tuition, state resident: full-time $7340. Tuition, nonresident: full-time $16,628. Full-time tuition and fees vary according to course load and program.

University of Alberta, Faculty of Graduate Studies and Research, Department of Biological Sciences, Edmonton, AB T6G 2E1, Canada. Offers environmental biology and ecology (M Sc, PhD); microbiology and biotechnology (M Sc, PhD); molecular biology and genetics (M Sc, PhD); physiology and cell biology (M Sc, PhD); plant biology (M Sc, PhD); systematics and evolution (M Sc, PhD). Terminal master's awarded for partial completion of doctoral program. *Degree requirements:* For master's, thesis; for doctorate, thesis/dissertation. *Entrance requirements:* Additional exam requirements/recommendations for international students: Required—TOEFL.

University of Alberta, Faculty of Medicine and Dentistry and Faculty of Graduate Studies and Research, Graduate Programs in Medicine, Department of Cell Biology, Edmonton, AB T6G 2E1, Canada. Offers cell and molecular biology (M Sc, PhD). Terminal master's awarded for partial completion of doctoral program. *Degree requirements:* For master's, thesis; for doctorate, thesis/dissertation. *Entrance requirements:* For master's and doctorate, 3 letters of reference, curriculum vitae. Additional exam requirements/recommendations for international students: Required—TOEFL (minimum score 600 paper-based). *Faculty research:* Protein targeting, membrane trafficking, signal transduction, cell growth and division, cell-cell interaction and development.

The University of Arizona, College of Science, Department of Molecular and Cellular Biology, Tucson, AZ 85721. Offers molecular and cellular biology (MS, PhD). *Program availability:* Evening/weekend. Terminal master's awarded for partial completion of doctoral program. *Degree requirements:* For master's, thesis; for doctorate, thesis/dissertation. *Entrance requirements:* For master's, 3 letters of recommendation; for doctorate, 3 letters of recommendation, statement of purpose. Additional exam requirements/recommendations for international students: Required—TOEFL (minimum score 600 paper-based; 90 iBT), IELTS (minimum score 7). *Application deadline:* For fall admission, 1/1 for domestic and international students. Applications are processed on a rolling basis. Application fee: $75. Electronic applications accepted. *Financial support:* Research assistantships, teaching assistantships, career-related internships or fieldwork, scholarships/grants, health care benefits, and unspecified assistantships available. *Faculty research:* Plant molecular biology, cellular and molecular aspects of development, genetics of bacteria and lower eukaryotes. *Unit head:* Tricia Serio, Department Head, E-mail: tserio@email.arizona.edu. *Application contact:* Tricia Serio, Department Head, E-mail: tserio@email.arizona.edu.
Website: http://bmcb.biology.arizona.edu/

University of Arkansas, Graduate School, Interdisciplinary Program in Cell and Molecular Biology, Fayetteville, AR 72701-1201. Offers MS, PhD. *Students:* 33 full-time (17 women), 61 part-time (34 women); includes 6 minority (2 Black or African American, non-Hispanic/Latino; 1 American Indian or Alaska Native, non-Hispanic/Latino; 2 Asian, non-Hispanic/Latino; 1 Hispanic/Latino), 60 international. In 2015, 5 master's, 9 doctorates awarded. *Degree requirements:* For doctorate, thesis/dissertation. *Application deadline:* For fall admission, 4/1 for international students; for spring admission, 10/1 for international students. Applications are processed on a rolling basis. Application fee: $40 ($50 for international students). Electronic applications accepted. *Financial support:* In 2015–16, 31 research assistantships, 12 teaching assistantships were awarded; fellowships with tuition reimbursements also available. Financial award application deadline: 4/1; financial award applicants required to submit FAFSA. *Unit head:* Dr. Douglas Rhoads, Head, 479-575-7396, Fax: 479-575-5908, E-mail: drhoads@uark.edu. *Application contact:* Graduate Admissions, 479-575-6246, Fax: 479-575-5908, E-mail: gradinfo@uark.edu.
Website: http://www.uark.edu/depts/cemb/

The University of British Columbia, Faculty of Medicine, Department of Cellular and Physiological Sciences, Vancouver, BC V6T 1Z3, Canada. Offers M Sc, PhD. *Degree requirements:* For master's, thesis, oral defense; for doctorate, comprehensive exam, thesis/dissertation, oral defense. *Entrance requirements:* For master's, minimum overall B+ average in third- and fourth-year courses; for doctorate, minimum overall B+ average in a master's degree (or equivalent) from an approved institution with clear evidence of research ability or potential. Additional exam requirements/recommendations for international students: Required—TOEFL (minimum score 550 paper-based), IELTS (minimum score 6.5).

University of California, Berkeley, Graduate Division, College of Letters and Science, Department of Molecular and Cell Biology, Berkeley, CA 94720-1500. Offers PhD. *Degree requirements:* For doctorate, comprehensive exam, thesis/dissertation, qualifying exam, 2 semesters of teaching. *Entrance requirements:* For doctorate, GRE General Test, GRE Subject Test (recommended), minimum GPA of 3.0. Additional exam requirements/recommendations for international students: Required—TOEFL (minimum score 570 paper-based; 68 iBT), IELTS (minimum score 7). Electronic applications accepted. *Faculty research:* Biochemistry, biophysics and structural biology; cell and developmental biology; genetics, genomics and development; immunology and pathogenesis; neurobiology.

University of California, Davis, Graduate Studies, Graduate Group in Cell and Developmental Biology, Davis, CA 95616. Offers MS, PhD. *Degree requirements:* For master's, comprehensive exam (for some programs), thesis (for some programs); for doctorate, thesis/dissertation. *Entrance requirements:* For doctorate, GRE General Test, GRE Subject Test. Additional exam requirements/recommendations for international students: Required—TOEFL (minimum score 550 paper-based). Electronic applications accepted. *Faculty research:* Molecular basis of cell function and development.

University of California, Irvine, Francisco J. Ayala School of Biological Sciences, Department of Developmental and Cell Biology, Irvine, CA 92697. Offers biological sciences (MS, PhD). *Students:* 40 full-time (23 women); includes 20 minority (1 American Indian or Alaska Native, non-Hispanic/Latino; 10 Asian, non-Hispanic/Latino; 8 Hispanic/Latino; 1 Native Hawaiian or other Pacific Islander, non-Hispanic/Latino), 2 international. Average age 29. 1 applicant, 100% accepted, 1 enrolled. In 2015, 3 master's, 6 doctorates awarded. *Degree requirements:* For doctorate, thesis/dissertation. *Entrance requirements:* For master's and doctorate, GRE General Test, GRE Subject Test, minimum GPA of 3.0. Additional exam requirements/recommendations for international students: Required—TOEFL (minimum score 550 paper-based). *Application deadline:* For fall admission, 12/15 priority date for domestic and international students. Application fee: $90 ($110 for international students). Electronic applications accepted. *Financial support:* Fellowships, research assistantships with full tuition reimbursements, teaching assistantships, institutionally sponsored loans, traineeships, health care benefits, and unspecified assistantships available. Financial award application deadline: 3/1; financial award applicants required to submit FAFSA. *Faculty research:* Genetics and development, oncogene signaling pathways, gene regulation, tissue regeneration and molecular genetics. *Unit head:* Prof. Thomas F. Schilling, Chair, 949-824-4562, Fax: 949-824-1105, E-mail: dkodowd@uci.edu. *Application contact:* Prof. Aimee Edinger, Graduate Advisor, 949-824-1921, Fax: 949-824-4709, E-mail: aedinger@uci.edu.
Website: http://devcell.bio.uci.edu/

University of California, Irvine, Francisco J. Ayala School of Biological Sciences and School of Medicine, Interdisciplinary Graduate Program in Cellular and Molecular Biosciences, Irvine, CA 92697. Offers PhD. *Students:* 26 full-time (14 women); includes 11 minority (5 Asian, non-Hispanic/Latino; 3 Two or more races, non-Hispanic/Latino), 2 international. Average age 25. 322 applicants, 18% accepted, 25 enrolled. *Degree requirements:* For doctorate, thesis/dissertation, teaching assignment, preliminary exam. *Entrance requirements:* For doctorate, GRE General Test, three letters of recommendation, interview. Additional exam requirements/recommendations for international students: Required—TOEFL or IELTS. *Application deadline:* For fall admission, 12/8 for domestic and international students. Application fee: $90 ($110 for international students). Electronic applications accepted. *Expenses:* Contact institution. *Financial support:* Fellowships with full tuition reimbursements, institutionally sponsored loans, scholarships/grants, tuition waivers (full), unspecified assistantships, and stipends available. Financial award application deadline: 1/1; financial award applicants required to submit FAFSA. *Faculty research:* Cellular biochemistry; gene structure and expression; protein structure, function, and design; molecular genetics; pathogenesis and inherited disease. *Unit head:* Melanie Cocco, Director, 949-824-4487, Fax: 949-824-1965, E-mail: mcocco@uci.edu. *Application contact:* Renee Frigo, Administrator, 949-824-8145, Fax: 949-824-1965, E-mail: rfrigo@uci.edu.
Website: http://cmb.uci.edu/

University of California, Los Angeles, David Geffen School of Medicine and Graduate Division, Graduate Programs in Medicine, Department of Neurobiology, Los Angeles, CA 90095. Offers MS, PhD. Terminal master's awarded for partial completion of doctoral program. *Degree requirements:* For master's, comprehensive exam; for doctorate, thesis/dissertation, oral and written qualifying exams; 2 quarters of teaching experience. *Entrance requirements:* For doctorate, GRE General Test; GRE Subject Test, bachelor's degree; minimum undergraduate GPA of 3.0 (or its equivalent if letter grade system not used). Additional exam requirements/recommendations for international students: Required—TOEFL. Electronic applications accepted.

University of California, Los Angeles, Graduate Division, College of Letters and Science, Department of Molecular, Cell and Developmental Biology, Los Angeles, CA 90095. Offers MA, PhD. Terminal master's awarded for partial completion of doctoral program. *Degree requirements:* For master's, comprehensive exam, thesis; for doctorate, thesis/dissertation, oral and written qualifying exams; 2 quarters of teaching experience. *Entrance requirements:* For doctorate, GRE General Test. Additional exam requirements/recommendations for international students: Required—TOEFL. Electronic applications accepted.

University of California, Los Angeles, Graduate Division, College of Letters and Science and David Geffen School of Medicine, UCLA ACCESS to Programs in the Molecular, Cellular and Integrative Life Sciences, Los Angeles, CA 90095. Offers biochemistry and molecular biology (PhD); biological chemistry (PhD); cellular and molecular pathology (PhD); human genetics (PhD); microbiology, immunology, and molecular genetics (PhD); molecular biology (PhD); molecular toxicology (PhD); molecular, cellular and integrative physiology (PhD); neurobiology (PhD); oral biology (PhD); physiology (PhD). *Degree requirements:* For doctorate, thesis/dissertation, oral and written qualifying exams. *Entrance requirements:* For doctorate, GRE General Test, bachelor's degree; minimum undergraduate GPA of 3.0 (or its equivalent if letter grade system not used). Additional exam requirements/recommendations for international students: Required—TOEFL. Electronic applications accepted.

University of California, Riverside, Graduate Division, Program in Cell, Molecular, and Developmental Biology, Riverside, CA 92521-0102. Offers MS, PhD. Terminal master's awarded for partial completion of doctoral program. *Degree requirements:* For master's, thesis, oral defense of thesis; for doctorate, thesis/dissertation, oral defense of thesis, qualifying exams, 2 quarters of teaching experience. *Entrance requirements:* For master's and doctorate, GRE General Test, minimum GPA of 3.2. Additional exam requirements/recommendations for international students: Required—TOEFL (minimum score 550 paper-based; 80 iBT). *Application deadline:* For fall admission, 1/5 priority date for domestic and international students. Applications are processed on a rolling basis. Application fee: $60 ($75 for international students). Electronic applications accepted. *Expenses:* Tuition, area resident: Full-time $16,665.50; part-time $11,055.54. Tuition, state resident: full-time $16,665.50; part-time $11,055.54. Tuition, nonresident: full-time $31,768. International tuition: $31,767.50 full-time. *Required fees:* $16,665.50; $11,055.54 per quarter. $3685.18 per quarter. Tuition and fees vary according to program. *Financial support:* Fellowships with tuition reimbursements, research assistantships with tuition reimbursements, teaching assistantships with tuition reimbursements, scholarships/grants, traineeships, health care benefits, tuition waivers (partial), and unspecified assistantships available. Support available to part-time students. Financial award application deadline: 1/5.
Website: http://www.cmdb.ucr.edu/

University of California, San Francisco, Graduate Division and School of Medicine, Tetrad Graduate Program, Cell Biology Track, San Francisco, CA 94143. Offers PhD, MD/PhD. *Degree requirements:* For doctorate, thesis/dissertation. *Entrance requirements:* For doctorate, GRE General Test, GRE Subject Test. Additional exam requirements/recommendations for international students: Required—TOEFL. *Expenses:* Contact institution.

University of California, Santa Barbara, Graduate Division, College of Letters and Sciences, Division of Mathematics, Life, and Physical Sciences, Department of Molecular, Cellular, and Developmental Biology, Santa Barbara, CA 93106-9625. Offers MA, PhD, MA/PhD. *Faculty:* 35 full-time (5 women), 3 part-time/adjunct (0 women). *Students:* 55 full-time (28 women); includes 16 minority (1 Black or African American, non-Hispanic/Latino; 1 American Indian or Alaska Native, non-Hispanic/Latino; 8 Asian, non-Hispanic/Latino; 4 Hispanic/Latino; 2 Native Hawaiian or other Pacific Islander, non-Hispanic/Latino), 4 international. Average age 27. 183 applicants, 24% accepted, 23 enrolled. In 2015, 5 master's, 10 doctorates awarded. Terminal master's awarded for partial completion of doctoral program. *Degree requirements:* For master's, comprehensive exam (for some programs), thesis (for some programs); for doctorate, comprehensive exam, thesis/dissertation. *Entrance requirements:* For master's and doctorate, GRE General Test, 3 letters of recommendation, statement of purpose, personal achievements/contributions statement, resume/curriculum vitae, transcripts for post-secondary institutions attended. Additional exam requirements/recommendations for international students: Required—TOEFL (minimum score 550 paper-based; 80 iBT), IELTS (minimum score 7). *Application deadline:* For fall admission, 12/7 priority date for domestic and international students. Application fee: $90 ($110 for international students). Electronic applications accepted. *Financial support:* In 2015–16, 3 students received support, including 3 fellowships with tuition reimbursements available (averaging $22,000 per year), 40 research assistantships with tuition reimbursements available (averaging $26,250 per year), 46 teaching assistantships with partial tuition reimbursements available (averaging $17,655 per year); career-related internships or fieldwork, Federal Work-Study, institutionally sponsored loans, scholarships/grants, traineeships, health care benefits, and unspecified assistantships also available. Financial award application deadline: 3/2; financial award applicants required to submit FAFSA. *Faculty research:* Microbiology, neurobiology (including stem cell research), developmental, virology, cell biology. *Unit head:* Dr. Stephen Poole, Chair, 805-893-8122, E-mail: william.smith@lifesci.ucsb.edu. *Application contact:* Anthony Galaviz, Graduate Program Advisor, 805-893-8499, E-mail: anthony.galaviz@lifesci.ucsb.edu. Website: https://www.mcdb.ucsb.edu/grad

University of California, Santa Cruz, Division of Graduate Studies, Division of Physical and Biological Sciences, Program in Molecular, Cellular, and Developmental Biology, Santa Cruz, CA 95064. Offers MA, PhD. Terminal master's awarded for partial completion of doctoral program. *Degree requirements:* For master's, thesis; for doctorate, thesis/dissertation, qualifying exam. *Entrance requirements:* For master's and doctorate, GRE General Test, 3 letters of recommendation, interview. Additional exam requirements/recommendations for international students: Required—TOEFL (minimum score 550 paper-based; 83 iBT); Recommended—IELTS (minimum score 8). Electronic applications accepted. *Faculty research:* RNA biology, chromatin and chromosome biology, neurobiology, stem cell biology and differentiation, cell structure and function.

University of Chicago, Division of the Biological Sciences, Department of Cell and Molecular Biology, Chicago, IL 60637. Offers PhD. *Students:* 28 full-time (12 women); includes 7 minority (3 Black or African American, non-Hispanic/Latino; 2 Asian, non-Hispanic/Latino; 1 Hispanic/Latino; 1 Two or more races, non-Hispanic/Latino), 5 international. Average age 29. 85 applicants, 27% accepted, 5 enrolled. In 2015, 3 doctorates awarded. *Degree requirements:* For doctorate, thesis/dissertation, ethics class, 2 teaching assistantships. *Entrance requirements:* For doctorate, GRE General Test. Additional exam requirements/recommendations for international students: Required—TOEFL (minimum score 600 paper-based; 104 iBT), IELTS (minimum score 7). *Application deadline:* For fall admission, 12/1 for domestic and international students. Application fee: $90. Electronic applications accepted. *Financial support:* In 2015–16, 28 students received support, including fellowships (averaging $29,781 per year), research assistantships (averaging $29,781 per year); institutionally sponsored loans, scholarships/grants, traineeships, and health care benefits also available. Financial award applicants required to submit FAFSA. *Faculty research:* Gene expression, chromosome structure, animal viruses, plant molecular genetics. *Total annual research expenditures:* $8 million. *Unit head:* Dr. Richard Fehon, Chair, 773-702-5694, E-mail: rfehon@uchicago.edu. *Application contact:* Kristine Gaston, Graduate Administrative Director, 773-702-8037, Fax: 773-702-3172, E-mail: kristine@bsd.uchicago.edu. Website: http://cellmolbio.bsd.uchicago.edu/

University of Cincinnati, Graduate School, College of Medicine, Graduate Programs in Biomedical Sciences, Cancer and Cell Biology Graduate Program, Cincinnati, OH 45267. Offers PhD. *Degree requirements:* For doctorate, thesis/dissertation, qualifying exam. *Entrance requirements:* For doctorate, GRE General Test. Additional exam requirements/recommendations for international students: Required—TOEFL. Electronic applications accepted. *Faculty research:* Cancer biology, cell and molecular biology, breast cancer, pancreatic cancer, drug discovery.

University of Colorado Boulder, Graduate School, College of Arts and Sciences, Department of Molecular, Cellular, and Developmental Biology, Boulder, CO 80309. Offers cellular structure and function (MA, PhD); developmental biology (MA, PhD); molecular biology (MA, PhD). *Faculty:* 28 full-time (8 women). *Students:* 71 full-time (34 women), 1 part-time (0 women); includes 7 minority (1 Asian, non-Hispanic/Latino; 4 Hispanic/Latino; 1 Native Hawaiian or other Pacific Islander, non-Hispanic/Latino; 1 Two or more races, non-Hispanic/Latino), 7 international. Average age 27. 310 applicants, 6% accepted, 7 enrolled. In 2015, 6 doctorates awarded. Terminal master's awarded for partial completion of doctoral program. *Degree requirements:* For master's, comprehensive exam, thesis or alternative; for doctorate, comprehensive exam, thesis/dissertation. *Entrance requirements:* For master's, GRE General Test, GRE Subject Test, minimum undergraduate GPA of 3.0; for doctorate, GRE General Test, GRE Subject Test. *Application deadline:* For fall admission, 12/1 for domestic students, 12/15 for international students. Application fee: $50 ($70 for international students). Electronic applications accepted. Application fee is waived when completed online. *Financial support:* In 2015–16, 125 students received support, including 10 fellowships (averaging $5,729 per year), 53 research assistantships with tuition reimbursements available (averaging $28,304 per year), 9 teaching assistantships with tuition reimbursements available (averaging $30,852 per year); institutionally sponsored loans, scholarships/grants, health care benefits, and unspecified assistantships also available. Financial award application deadline: 2/1; financial award applicants required to submit FAFSA. *Faculty research:* Molecular biology, cellular biology, genetics, biochemistry, gene cloning, proteins. *Total annual research expenditures:* $15.4 million. *Application contact:* E-mail: mcdbgrad@colorado.edu. Website: http://mcdb.colorado.edu/graduate

University of Colorado Denver, College of Liberal Arts and Sciences, Department of Integrative and Systems Biology, Denver, CO 80217. Offers animal behavior (MS); biology (MS); cell and developmental biology (MS); ecology (MS); evolutionary biology (MS); genetics (MS); integrative and systems biology (PhD); microbiology (MS); molecular biology (MS); neurobiology (MS); plant systematics (MS). *Program availability:* Part-time. *Faculty:* 21 full-time (8 women), 3 part-time/adjunct (1 woman). *Students:* 31 full-time (19 women), 7 part-time (3 women); includes 8 minority (1 Black or African American, non-Hispanic/Latino; 1 Asian, non-Hispanic/Latino; 3 Hispanic/Latino;

3 Two or more races, non-Hispanic/Latino), 1 international. Average age 28. 34 applicants, 29% accepted, 8 enrolled. In 2015, 6 master's awarded. *Degree requirements:* For master's, comprehensive exam, thesis, 30-32 credit hours; for doctorate, comprehensive exam, thesis/dissertation. *Entrance requirements:* For master's, GRE General Test (minimum score in 50th percentile in each section), BA/BS from accredited institution awarded within the last 10 years; minimum undergraduate GPA of 3.0; prerequisite courses: 1 year each of general biology and general chemistry; 1 semester each of general genetics, general ecology, and cell biology; and a structure/function course; for doctorate, GRE, minimum undergraduate GPA of 3.2, three letters of recommendation, official transcripts from all universities and colleges attended. Additional exam requirements/recommendations for international students: Required—TOEFL (minimum score 537 paper-based; 75 iBT); Recommended—IELTS (minimum score 6.5). *Application deadline:* For fall admission, 1/15 for domestic and international students. Application fee: $50 ($75 for international students). Electronic applications accepted. *Financial support:* In 2015–16, 32 students received support. Fellowships, research assistantships, teaching assistantships, Federal Work-Study, institutionally sponsored loans, scholarships/grants, and traineeships available. Financial award application deadline: 4/1; financial award applicants required to submit FAFSA. *Faculty research:* Molecular developmental biology; quantitative ecology, biogeography, and population dynamics; environmental signaling and endocrine disruption; speciation, the evolution of reproductive isolation, and hybrid zones; evolutionary, behavioral, and conservation ecology. *Unit head:* Dr. John Swallow, Chair, 303-556-6154, E-mail: john.swallow@ucdenver.edu. *Application contact:* Dr. Michael Wunder, Graduate Advisor, 303-556-8870, E-mail: michael.wunder@ucdenver.edu. Website: http://www.ucdenver.edu/academics/colleges/CLAS/Departments/biology/Programs/MasterofScience/Pages/BiologyMasterOfScience.aspx

University of Colorado Denver, School of Medicine, Program in Cell Biology, Stem Cells, and Developmental Biology, Aurora, CO 80045. Offers cell biology, stem cells, and developmental biology (PhD); modern human anatomy (MS). *Students:* 29 full-time (13 women); includes 7 minority (1 Asian, non-Hispanic/Latino; 4 Hispanic/Latino; 2 Two or more races, non-Hispanic/Latino), 3 international. Average age 29. 42 applicants, 7% accepted, 3 enrolled. In 2015, 1 doctorate awarded. *Degree requirements:* For doctorate, comprehensive exam, thesis/dissertation, at least 30 credit hours of coursework and 30 credit hours of thesis research; laboratory rotations. *Entrance requirements:* For doctorate, GRE, minimum GPA of 3.0; 3 letters of reference; prerequisite coursework in organic chemistry, biology, biochemistry, physics and calculus; research experience (highly recommended). Additional exam requirements/recommendations for international students: Required—TOEFL (minimum score 550 paper-based; 80 iBT). *Application deadline:* For fall admission, 12/1 for domestic students, 11/1 priority date for international students. Application fee: $50 ($75 for international students). Electronic applications accepted. *Expenses:* Contact institution. *Financial support:* In 2015–16, 29 students received support. Fellowships, research assistantships, teaching assistantships, Federal Work-Study, institutionally sponsored loans, scholarships/grants, traineeships, health care benefits, and tuition waivers (full) available. Financial award application deadline: 3/15; financial award applicants required to submit FAFSA. *Faculty research:* Development and repair of the vertebrate nervous system; molecular, genetic and developmental mechanisms involved in the patterning of the early spinal cord (neural plate) during vertebrate embryogenesis; structural analysis of protein glycosylation using NMR and mass spectrometry; small RNAs and post-transcriptional gene regulation during nematode gametogenesis and early development; diabetes-mediated changes in cardiovascular gene expression and functional exercise capacity. *Total annual research expenditures:* $5.7 million. *Unit head:* Dr. Bruce Appel, Director, 303-724-3465, E-mail: bruce.appel@ucdenver.edu. *Application contact:* Kenton Owsley, Program Administrator, 303-724-3468, Fax: 303-724-3420, E-mail: kenton.owsley@ucdenver.edu. Website: http://www.ucdenver.edu/academics/colleges/medicalschool/programs/CSD/Pages/CSD.aspx

★ **University of Connecticut Health Center,** Graduate School, Graduate Program in Cell Analysis and Modeling, Farmington, CT 06030. Offers PhD. *Degree requirements:* For doctorate, comprehensive exam, thesis/dissertation. *Entrance requirements:* For doctorate, GRE General Test. Additional exam requirements/recommendations for international students: Required—TOEFL (minimum score 600 paper-based). Electronic applications accepted.

See Display on next page and Close-Up on page 225.

★ **University of Connecticut Health Center,** Graduate School, Programs in Biomedical Sciences, Graduate Program in Cell Biology, Farmington, CT 06030. Offers PhD, DMD/PhD, MD/PhD. *Degree requirements:* For doctorate, comprehensive exam, thesis/dissertation. *Entrance requirements:* For doctorate, GRE General Test. Additional exam requirements/recommendations for international students: Required—TOEFL (minimum score 600 paper-based). Electronic applications accepted. *Faculty research:* Vascular biology, computational biology, cytoskeleton and molecular motors, reproductive biology, signal transduction.

See Display on next page and Close-Up on page 227.

University of Delaware, College of Arts and Sciences, Department of Biological Sciences, Newark, DE 19716. Offers biotechnology (MS); cancer biology (MS, PhD); cell and extracellular matrix biology (MS, PhD); cell and systems physiology (MS, PhD); developmental biology (MS, PhD); ecology and evolution (MS, PhD); microbiology (MS, PhD); molecular biology and genetics (MS, PhD). Terminal master's awarded for partial completion of doctoral program. *Degree requirements:* For master's, thesis, preliminary exam; for doctorate, comprehensive exam, thesis/dissertation, preliminary exam. *Entrance requirements:* For master's and doctorate, GRE General Test. Additional exam requirements/recommendations for international students: Required—TOEFL (minimum score 600 paper-based); Recommended—TWE. Electronic applications accepted. *Faculty research:* Microorganisms, bone, cancer metastasis, developmental biology, cell biology, DNA.

University of Denver, Division of Natural Sciences and Mathematics, Department of Biological Sciences, Denver, CO 80208. Offers biology, ecology and evolution (MS, PhD); biomedical sciences (PSM); cell and molecular biology (MS, PhD). *Program availability:* Part-time. *Faculty:* 23 full-time (7 women), 2 part-time/adjunct (both women). *Students:* 8 full-time (all women), 27 part-time (21 women); includes 4 minority (2 Black or African American, non-Hispanic/Latino; 2 Hispanic/Latino), 6 international. Average age 26. 77 applicants, 38% accepted, 21 enrolled. In 2015, 6 master's, 3 doctorates awarded. Terminal master's awarded for partial completion of doctoral program. *Degree requirements:* For master's, comprehensive exam (for some programs), thesis; for doctorate, one foreign language, comprehensive exam (for some programs), thesis/dissertation. *Entrance requirements:* For master's and doctorate, GRE General Test, bachelor's degree in biology or related field, transcripts, personal statement, three letters of recommendation. Additional exam requirements/recommendations for international students: Required—TOEFL (minimum score 550 paper-based; 80 iBT). *Application deadline:* For fall admission, 1/1 priority date for domestic and international students. Applications are processed on a rolling basis. Application fee: $65. Electronic applications accepted. *Expenses:* $30,477. *Financial support:* In 2015–16, 35 students received support, including 8 research assistantships with tuition reimbursements available (averaging $15,834 per year), 23 teaching assistantships with tuition reimbursements available (averaging $17,210 per year); Federal Work-Study, institutionally sponsored loans, scholarships/grants, and unspecified assistantships also available. Support available to part-time students. Financial award application deadline: 2/15; financial award applicants required to submit FAFSA. *Faculty research:* Molecular biology, cell biology, neurobiology, ecology, molecular evolution. *Unit head:* Dr. Joseph Angleson, Associate Professor and Chair, 303-871-3463, Fax: 303-871-3471, E-mail: jangleso@du.edu. *Application contact:* Randi Flageolle, Assistant to the Chair, 303-871-3457, Fax: 303-871-3471, E-mail: rflageol@du.edu. Website: http://www.du.edu/nsm/departments/biologicalsciences

University of Florida, College of Medicine and Graduate School, Interdisciplinary Program in Biomedical Sciences, Concentration in Molecular Cell Biology, Gainesville, FL 32611. Offers PhD. *Degree requirements:* For doctorate, thesis/dissertation. *Entrance requirements:* For doctorate, GRE General Test, minimum GPA of 3.0, biochemistry before enrollment. Additional exam requirements/recommendations for international students: Required—TOEFL, IELTS. Electronic applications accepted.

University of Florida, Graduate School, College of Agricultural and Life Sciences, Department of Animal Sciences, Interdisciplinary Concentration in Animal Molecular and Cellular Biology, Gainesville, FL 32611. Offers MS, PhD. *Faculty:* 14. *Students:* 16 full-time (11 women), 1 (woman) part-time; includes 2 minority (both Hispanic/Latino), 12 international. Average age 31. 15 applicants, 20% accepted, 3 enrolled. In 2015, 1 master's, 2 doctorates awarded. *Entrance requirements:* For master's and doctorate, GRE General Test, minimum GPA of 3.0. Additional exam requirements/recommendations for international students: Required—TOEFL (minimum score 550 paper-based; 80 iBT), IELTS (minimum score 6) Application fee: $30. Electronic applications accepted. *Financial support:* In 2015–16, 1 fellowship, 11 research assistantships, 1 teaching assistantship were awarded. Financial award applicants required to submit FAFSA. *Unit head:* Geoffrey E. Dahl, PhD, Professor and Department Chair, 352-392-1981, Fax: 352-392-5595, E-mail: gdahl@ufl.edu. *Application contact:* Office of Admissions, 352-392-1365, E-mail: webrequests@admissions.ufl.edu. Website: http://www.animal.ufl.edu/amcb/

University of Florida, Graduate School, College of Agricultural and Life Sciences, Department of Microbiology and Cell Science, Gainesville, FL 32611. Offers microbiology and cell science (MS, PhD), including medical microbiology and biochemistry (MS), toxicology (PhD). *Degree requirements:* For master's, comprehensive exam, thesis (for some programs); for doctorate, comprehensive exam, thesis/dissertation. *Entrance requirements:* For master's and doctorate, GRE General Test, minimum GPA of 3.0. Additional exam requirements/recommendations for international students: Required—TOEFL (minimum score 550 paper-based; 80 iBT), IELTS (minimum score 6). Electronic applications accepted. *Faculty research:* Biomass conversion, membrane and cell wall chemistry, plant biochemistry and genetics.

University of Florida, Graduate School, College of Liberal Arts and Sciences, Department of Biology, Gainesville, FL 32611. Offers botany (MS, MST, PhD), including botany, tropical conservation and development, wetland sciences; zoology (MS, MST, PhD), including animal molecular and cellular biology (PhD), tropical conservation and development, wetland sciences, zoology. *Faculty:* 9 full-time, 9 part-time/adjunct. *Students:* 96 full-time (41 women), 6 part-time (3 women); includes 9 minority (4 Asian, non-Hispanic/Latino; 5 Hispanic/Latino), 35 international. 77 applicants, 30% accepted, 16 enrolled. In 2015, 8 master's, 15 doctorates awarded. *Degree requirements:* For master's, comprehensive exam (for some programs), thesis; for doctorate, comprehensive exam, thesis/dissertation. *Entrance requirements:* For master's and doctorate, GRE General Test, minimum GPA of 3.0. Additional exam requirements/

recommendations for international students: Required—TOEFL (minimum score 550 paper-based; 80 iBT), IELTS (minimum score 6). *Application deadline:* For fall admission, 12/1 for domestic and international students. Applications are processed on a rolling basis. Application fee: $30. Electronic applications accepted. *Financial support:* In 2015–16, 9 fellowships, 36 research assistantships, 62 teaching assistantships were awarded; unspecified assistantships also available. Financial award application deadline: 12/15; financial award applicants required to submit FAFSA. *Faculty research:* Ecology of natural populations, plant and animal genome evolution, biodiversity, plant biology, behavior. *Total annual research expenditures:* $3.6 million. *Unit head:* Marta Wayne, PhD, Professor and Chair, 352-392-9925, E-mail: mlwayne@ufl.edu. *Application contact:* William T. Barbazuk, PhD, Associate Professor/Graduate Coordinator, 352-273-8624, Fax: 352-392-3704, E-mail: bbarbazuk@ufl.edu. Website: http://www.biology.ufl.edu/

University of Georgia, Franklin College of Arts and Sciences, Department of Cellular Biology, Athens, GA 30602. Offers MS, PhD. *Degree requirements:* For master's, thesis; for doctorate, one foreign language, thesis/dissertation. *Entrance requirements:* For master's and doctorate, GRE General Test. Electronic applications accepted.

University of Guelph, Graduate Studies, College of Biological Science, Department of Molecular and Cellular Biology, Guelph, ON N1G 2W1, Canada. Offers biochemistry (M Sc, PhD); biophysics (M Sc, PhD); botany (M Sc, PhD); microbiology (M Sc, PhD); molecular biology and genetics (M Sc, PhD). *Degree requirements:* For master's, thesis, research proposal; for doctorate, comprehensive exam, thesis/dissertation, research proposal. *Entrance requirements:* For master's, minimum B-average during previous 2 years of coursework; for doctorate, minimum A-average. Additional exam requirements/recommendations for international students: Required—TOEFL (minimum score 550 paper-based), IELTS (minimum score 6.5). Electronic applications accepted. *Faculty research:* Physiology, structure, genetics, and ecology of microbes; virology and microbial technology.

University of Illinois at Chicago, College of Medicine and Graduate College, Graduate Programs in Medicine, Department of Anatomy and Cell Biology, Chicago, IL 60607. Offers MS, MD/PhD. *Faculty:* 15 full-time (6 women), 21 part-time/adjunct (12 women). *Students:* 6 full-time (4 women); includes 1 minority (Black or African American, non-Hispanic/Latino), 2 international. Average age 27. *Degree requirements:* For master's, preliminary oral examination, dissertation and oral defense. *Entrance requirements:* For master's, GRE General Test, minimum GPA of 2.75, 3 letters of recommendation. Additional exam requirements/recommendations for international students: Required—TOEFL (minimum score 550 paper-based). *Application deadline:* For fall admission, 5/15 for domestic students, 2/15 for international students. Applications are processed on a rolling basis. Application fee: $60. Electronic applications accepted. *Expenses:* Tuition, state resident: full-time $11,480; part-time $3826 per credit. Tuition, nonresident: full-time $23,720; part-time $7906 per credit. Required fees: $1333 per semester. Part-time tuition and fees vary according to course load and program. *Financial support:* Research or teaching assistantships with stipend of $24,000 per year, plus a tuition waiver available. *Faculty research:* Synapses, axonal transport, neurodegenerative diseases. *Unit head:* Prof. Scott T. Brady, Head, 312-996-3313, Fax: 312-413-0354, E-mail: stbrady@uic.edu. *Application contact:* Dr. Ernesto R. Bongarzone, Associate Professor/Director of Graduate Studies, 312-996-6791, Fax: 312-413-0354, E-mail: ebongarz@uic.edu. Website: http://www.anatomy.uic.edu/

University of Illinois at Chicago, Program in Neuroscience, Chicago, IL 60607. Offers cellular and systems neuroscience and cell biology (PhD); neuroscience (MS). *Faculty:* 1 (woman) full-time, 1 part-time/adjunct (0 women). *Students:* 17 full-time (11 women), 1 (woman) part-time; includes 4 minority (1 Asian, non-Hispanic/Latino; 2 Hispanic/Latino;

Cell Biology

1 Two or more races, non-Hispanic/Latino), 1 international. Average age 28. 64 applicants, 6% accepted, 2 enrolled. In 2015, 1 master's, 4 doctorates awarded. *Expenses:* Tuition, state resident: full-time $11,480; part-time $3826 per credit. Tuition, nonresident: full-time $23,720; part-time $7906 per credit. *Required fees:* $1333 per semester. Part-time tuition and fees vary according to course load and program. *Unit head:* Dr. John Larson, Director of Graduate Studies, 312-996-7370, Fax: 312-423-3699, E-mail: uicneuroscience@uic.edu. Website: http://www.uic.edu/depts/neurosci/

University of Illinois at Urbana–Champaign, Graduate College, College of Liberal Arts and Sciences, School of Molecular and Cellular Biology, Department of Cell and Developmental Biology, Champaign, IL 61820. Offers PhD.

The University of Iowa, Graduate College, College of Liberal Arts and Sciences, Department of Biology, Iowa City, IA 52242-1324. Offers biology (MS, PhD); cell and developmental biology (MS, PhD); evolution (MS, PhD); genetics (MS, PhD); neurobiology (MS, PhD). Terminal master's awarded for partial completion of doctoral program. *Degree requirements:* For master's, thesis optional, exam; for doctorate, comprehensive exam, thesis/dissertation. *Entrance requirements:* For master's and doctorate, GRE General Test, minimum GPA of 3.0. Additional exam requirements/recommendations for international students: Required—TOEFL (minimum score 600 paper-based; 100 iBT). Electronic applications accepted. *Faculty research:* Neurobiology, evolutionary biology, genetics, cell and developmental biology.

The University of Iowa, Graduate College, Program in Molecular and Cellular Biology, Iowa City, IA 52242-1316. Offers PhD. *Degree requirements:* For doctorate, comprehensive exam, thesis/dissertation. *Entrance requirements:* For doctorate, GRE General Test, minimum GPA of 3.0. Additional exam requirements/recommendations for international students: Required—TOEFL (minimum score 600 paper-based; 100 iBT). Electronic applications accepted. *Faculty research:* Regulation of gene expression, inherited human genetic diseases, signal transduction mechanisms, structural biology and function.

The University of Iowa, Roy J. and Lucille A. Carver College of Medicine and Graduate College, Graduate Programs in Medicine, Department of Anatomy and Cell Biology, Iowa City, IA 52242-1316. Offers PhD. *Degree requirements:* For doctorate, comprehensive exam, thesis/dissertation. *Entrance requirements:* For doctorate, GRE General Test, minimum GPA of 3.0. Additional exam requirements/recommendations for international students: Required—TOEFL (minimum score 600 paper-based; 100 iBT). Electronic applications accepted. *Faculty research:* Biology of differentiation and transformation, developmental and vascular cell biology, neurobiology.

The University of Kansas, Graduate Studies, College of Liberal Arts and Sciences, Department of Molecular Biosciences, Lawrence, KS 66044. Offers biochemistry and biophysics (MA, PhD); microbiology (MA, PhD); molecular, cellular, and developmental biology (MA, PhD). *Students:* 57 full-time (34 women), 4 part-time (1 woman); includes 9 minority (5 Asian, non-Hispanic/Latino; 2 Hispanic/Latino; 2 Two or more races, non-Hispanic/Latino), 23 international. Average age 27. 78 applicants, 46% accepted, 18 enrolled. In 2015, 3 master's, 7 doctorates awarded. Terminal master's awarded for partial completion of doctoral program. *Entrance requirements:* For master's and doctorate, GRE General Test. Additional exam requirements/recommendations for international students: Required—TOEFL or IELTS. *Application deadline:* For fall admission, 12/15 for domestic and international students. Application fee: $65 ($85 for international students). Electronic applications accepted. *Financial support:* Fellowships, research assistantships, teaching assistantships, health care benefits, and unspecified assistantships available. Financial award application deadline: 3/1. *Faculty research:* Structure and function of proteins, genetics of organism development, molecular genetics, neurophysiology, molecular virology and pathogenics, developmental biology, cell biology. *Unit head:* Susan M. Egan, Chair, 785-864-4294, E-mail: sme@ku.edu. *Application contact:* John Connolly, Graduate Admissions Contact, 785-864-4311, E-mail: jconnolly@ku.edu. Website: http://www.molecularbiosciences.ku.edu/

The University of Kansas, University of Kansas Medical Center, School of Medicine, Department of Anatomy and Cell Biology, Kansas City, KS 66160. Offers MS, PhD, MD/PhD. *Faculty:* 28 full-time (11 women), 9 part-time/adjunct (6 women). *Students:* 12 full-time (6 women), 6 international. Average age 28. In 2015, 6 doctorates awarded. Terminal master's awarded for partial completion of doctoral program. *Degree requirements:* For master's, thesis; for doctorate, comprehensive exam, thesis/dissertation. *Entrance requirements:* For master's and doctorate, GRE. Additional exam requirements/recommendations for international students: Required—TOEFL. *Application deadline:* For fall admission, 1/15 priority date for domestic students. Applications are processed on a rolling basis. Application fee: $0. Electronic applications accepted. *Financial support:* In 2015–16, 16 research assistantships with full tuition reimbursements (averaging $24,500 per year), 3 teaching assistantships with full tuition reimbursements (averaging $24,500 per year) were awarded; fellowships, institutionally sponsored loans, scholarships/grants, health care benefits, and unspecified assistantships also available. Financial award application deadline: 3/1; financial award applicants required to submit FAFSA. *Faculty research:* Development of the synapse and neuromuscular junction, pain perception and diabetic neuropathies, cardiovascular and kidney development, reproductive immunology, post-fertilization signaling events. *Total annual research expenditures:* $11 million. *Unit head:* Dr. Dale R. Abrahamson, Chairman, 913-588-0702, Fax: 913-588-2710, E-mail: dabrahamson@kumc.edu. *Application contact:* Dr. Julie A. Christianson, Assistant Professor, 913-945-6430, Fax: 913-588-5677, E-mail: jchristianson@kumc.edu. Website: http://www.kumc.edu/school-of-medicine/anatomy-and-cell-biology.html

The University of Manchester, Faculty of Life Sciences, Manchester, United Kingdom. Offers adaptive organismal biology (M Phil, PhD); animal biology (M Phil, PhD); biochemistry (M Phil, PhD); bioinformatics (M Phil, PhD); biomolecular sciences (M Phil, PhD); biotechnology (M Phil, PhD); cell biology (M Phil, PhD); cell matrix research (M Phil, PhD); channels and transporters (M Phil, PhD); developmental biology (M Phil, PhD); Egyptology (M Phil, PhD); environmental biology (M Phil, PhD); evolutionary biology (M Phil, PhD); gene expression (M Phil, PhD); genetics (M Phil, PhD); history of science, technology and medicine (M Phil, PhD); immunology (M Phil, PhD); integrative neurobiology and behavior (M Phil, PhD); membrane trafficking (M Phil, PhD); microbiology (M Phil, PhD); molecular and cellular neuroscience (M Phil, PhD); molecular biology (M Phil, PhD); molecular cancer studies (M Phil, PhD); neuroscience (M Phil, PhD); ophthalmology (M Phil, PhD); optometry (M Phil, PhD); organelle function (M Phil, PhD); pharmacology (M Phil, PhD); physiology (M Phil, PhD); plant sciences (M Phil, PhD); stem cell research (M Phil, PhD); structural biology (M Phil, PhD); systems neuroscience (M Phil, PhD); toxicology (M Phil, PhD).

University of Maryland, Baltimore, Graduate School, Graduate Program in Life Sciences, Program in Cellular and Molecular Biomedical Science, Baltimore, MD 21201. Offers MS. *Program availability:* Part-time. Electronic applications accepted. Tuition and fees vary according to program.

University of Maryland, Baltimore, Graduate School, Graduate Program in Life Sciences, Program in Molecular Medicine, Baltimore, MD 21201. Offers cancer biology (PhD); cell and molecular physiology (PhD); human genetics and genomic medicine (PhD); molecular medicine (MS); molecular toxicology and pharmacology (PhD); MD/PhD. *Degree requirements:* For doctorate, comprehensive exam, thesis/dissertation. *Entrance requirements:* For master's and doctorate, GRE. Additional exam requirements/recommendations for international students: Required—TOEFL (minimum score 600 paper-based; 100 iBT). Recommended—IELTS (minimum score 7). Electronic applications accepted. Tuition and fees vary according to program.

University of Maryland, Baltimore County, The Graduate School, College of Natural and Mathematical Sciences, Department of Biological Sciences, Program in Molecular and Cell Biology, Baltimore, MD 21250. Offers PhD. *Faculty:* 26 full-time (11 women). *Students:* 6 full-time (4 women); includes 1 minority (Hispanic/Latino), 2 international. Average age 29. 34 applicants, 9% accepted, 1 enrolled. In 2015, 2 doctorates awarded. *Degree requirements:* For doctorate, thesis/dissertation. *Entrance requirements:* For doctorate, GRE General Test, GRE Subject Test, minimum GPA of 3.0. Additional exam requirements/recommendations for international students: Required—TOEFL (minimum score 80 iBT). *Application deadline:* For fall admission, 1/1 priority date for domestic and international students. Application fee: $50. Electronic applications accepted. *Expenses:* Tuition, state resident: full-time $12,816. Tuition, nonresident: full-time $19,710. *Financial support:* In 2015–16, 7 students received support, including 3 research assistantships with full tuition reimbursements available (averaging $24,000 per year), 4 teaching assistantships with full tuition reimbursements available (averaging $24,000 per year). *Unit head:* Dr. Michelle Starz-Gaiano, Graduate Program Director, 410-455-2217, Fax: 410-455-3875, E-mail: biograd@umbc.edu. *Application contact:* Dr. Michelle Starz-Gaiano, Director, 410-455-2217, Fax: 410-455-3875, E-mail: biograd@umbc.edu. Website: http://biology.umbc.edu/grad/graduate-programs/mocb/

University of Maryland, College Park, Academic Affairs, College of Computer, Mathematical and Natural Sciences, Department of Biology, PhD Program in Biological Sciences, College Park, MD 20742. Offers behavior, ecology, evolution, and systematics (PhD); computational biology, bioinformatics and genomics (PhD); molecular and cellular biology (PhD); physiological systems (PhD). *Degree requirements:* For doctorate, comprehensive exam, thesis/dissertation, thesis work presentation in seminar. *Entrance requirements:* For doctorate, GRE General Test; GRE Subject Test in biology (recommended), academic transcripts, statement of purpose/research interests, 3 letters of recommendation. Additional exam requirements/recommendations for international students: Required—TOEFL. Electronic applications accepted.

University of Maryland, College Park, Academic Affairs, College of Computer, Mathematical and Natural Sciences, Department of Cell Biology and Molecular Genetics, Program in Cell Biology and Molecular Genetics, College Park, MD 20742. Offers MS, PhD. *Degree requirements:* For master's, thesis; for doctorate, thesis/dissertation, exams. *Faculty research:* Cytoskeletal activity, membrane biology, cell division, genetics and genomics, virology.

University of Maryland, College Park, Academic Affairs, College of Computer, Mathematical and Natural Sciences, Department of Cell Biology and Molecular Genetics, Program in Molecular and Cellular Biology, College Park, MD 20742. Offers PhD. *Program availability:* Part-time, evening/weekend. *Degree requirements:* For doctorate, thesis/dissertation, exam, public service. *Faculty research:* Monoclonal antibody production, oligonucleotide synthesis, macronolular processing, signal transduction, developmental biology.

University of Massachusetts Amherst, Graduate School, Interdisciplinary Programs, Program in Molecular and Cellular Biology, Amherst, MA 01003. Offers biological chemistry and molecular biophysics (PhD); biomedicine (PhD); cellular and developmental biology (PhD). *Program availability:* Part-time. Terminal master's awarded for partial completion of doctoral program. *Degree requirements:* For doctorate, comprehensive exam, thesis/dissertation. *Entrance requirements:* For doctorate, GRE General Test. Additional exam requirements/recommendations for international students: Required—TOEFL (minimum score 550 paper-based; 80 iBT), IELTS (minimum score 6.5). Electronic applications accepted.

University of Massachusetts Amherst, Graduate School, Interdisciplinary Programs, Program in Plant Biology, Amherst, MA 01003. Offers biochemistry and metabolism (MS, PhD); cell biology and physiology (MS, PhD); environmental, ecological and integrative biology (MS, PhD); genetics and evolution (MS, PhD). *Degree requirements:* For master's, thesis; for doctorate, 2 foreign languages, comprehensive exam, thesis/dissertation. *Entrance requirements:* For master's and doctorate, GRE General Test. Additional exam requirements/recommendations for international students: Required—TOEFL (minimum score 550 paper-based; 80 iBT), IELTS (minimum score 6.5). Electronic applications accepted.

University of Massachusetts Medical School, Graduate School of Biomedical Sciences, Worcester, MA 01655-0115. Offers biomedical sciences (PhD), including biochemistry and molecular pharmacology, bioinformatics and computational biology, cancer biology, cell biology, immunology and microbiology, interdisciplinary, neuroscience, translational science; biomedical sciences (millennium program) (PhD); clinical and population health research (PhD); clinical investigation (MS). *Faculty:* 1,339 full-time (521 women), 301 part-time/adjunct (189 women). *Students:* 363 full-time (184 women); includes 58 minority (13 Black or African American, non-Hispanic/Latino; 30 Asian, non-Hispanic/Latino; 15 Hispanic/Latino), 141 international. Average age 29. 661 applicants, 26% accepted, 51 enrolled. In 2015, 10 master's, 58 doctorates awarded. Terminal master's awarded for partial completion of doctoral program. *Degree requirements:* For master's, comprehensive exam, thesis; for doctorate, comprehensive exam, thesis/dissertation. *Entrance requirements:* For master's, MD, DVM, or PharmD; for doctorate, GRE General Test, bachelor's degree. Additional exam requirements/recommendations for international students: Required—TOEFL (minimum score 100 iBT) or IELTS (minimum score 7.5). *Application deadline:* For fall admission, 12/15 for domestic and international students; for spring admission, 5/15 for domestic students. Application fee: $80. Electronic applications accepted. *Expenses:* $6,966 resident per year; $14,182 non-resident per year. *Financial support:* In 2015–16, 383 students received support, including research assistantships with full tuition reimbursements available (averaging $30,600 per year); scholarships/grants, health care benefits, tuition waivers (full), and unspecified assistantships also available. Financial award application deadline: 5/16. *Faculty research:* RNA interference, cell/molecular/developmental biology, bioinformatics, clinical/translational research, infectious disease. *Total annual research expenditures:* $250.3 million. *Unit head:* Dr. Anthony Carruthers, Dean, 508-856-4135, E-mail: anthony.carruthers@umassmed.edu. *Application contact:* Dr. Kendall Knight, Assistant Vice Provost for Admissions, 508-856-5628, Fax: 508-856-3659, E-mail: kendall.knight@umassmed.edu. Website: http://www.umassmed.edu/gsbs/

University of Miami, Graduate School, Miller School of Medicine, Graduate Programs in Medicine, Department of Cell Biology and Anatomy, Coral Gables, FL 33124. Offers molecular cell and developmental biology (PhD); MD/PhD. *Degree requirements:* For doctorate, thesis/dissertation. *Entrance requirements:* For doctorate, GRE General Test, GRE Subject Test. Additional exam requirements/recommendations for international students: Required—TOEFL. Electronic applications accepted.

University of Michigan, Rackham Graduate School, College of Literature, Science, and the Arts, Department of Molecular, Cellular, and Developmental Biology, Ann Arbor, MI 48109. Offers MS, PhD. *Program availability:* Part-time. *Faculty:* 37 full-time (15 women). *Students:* 90 full-time (54 women), 4 part-time (3 women); includes 11 minority (4 Black or African American, non-Hispanic/Latino; 1 Asian, non-Hispanic/Latino; 6 Hispanic/Latino), 50 international. Average age 26. 106 applicants, 34% accepted, 19 enrolled. In 2015, 12 master's, 10 doctorates awarded. Terminal master's awarded for partial completion of doctoral program. *Degree requirements:* For master's, thesis (for some programs), 24 credits with at least 16 in molecular, cellular, and developmental biology and 4 in a cognate field; for doctorate, thesis/dissertation, preliminary exam, oral defense. *Entrance requirements:* For master's and doctorate, GRE General Test. Additional exam requirements/recommendations for international students: Required—TOEFL (minimum score 560 paper-based; 83 iBT). *Application deadline:* For fall admission, 1/5 for domestic and international students; for winter admission, 11/1 for domestic and international students; for spring admission, 4/1 for domestic and international students. Application fee: $75 ($90 for international students). Electronic applications accepted. *Expenses:* Contact institution. *Financial support:* In 2015–16, 67 students received support, including 23 fellowships with full tuition reimbursements available (averaging $29,025 per year), 28 research assistantships with full tuition reimbursements available (averaging $28,500 per year), 18 teaching assistantships with full tuition reimbursements available (averaging $28,500 per year); traineeships and health care benefits also available. *Faculty research:* Cell biology, microbiology, neurobiology and physiology, developmental biology and plant molecular biology. *Total annual research expenditures:* $8.2 million. *Unit head:* Dr. Robert J. Denver, Department Chair, 734-764-7476, Fax: 734-615-6337, E-mail: rdenver@umich.edu. *Application contact:* Mary Carr, Graduate Coordinator, 734-615-1635, Fax: 734-764-0884, E-mail: carrmm@umich.edu.
Website: http://www.mcdb.lsa.umich.edu

University of Michigan, Rackham Graduate School, Program in Biomedical Sciences (PIBS), Department of Cell and Developmental Biology, Ann Arbor, MI 48109. Offers PhD. *Faculty:* 37 full-time (13 women). *Students:* 21 full-time (11 women); includes 11 minority (9 Asian, non-Hispanic/Latino; 2 Hispanic/Latino). Average age 29. 57 applicants, 18% accepted, 6 enrolled. In 2015, 6 doctorates awarded. *Degree requirements:* For doctorate, thesis/dissertation, oral defense of dissertation, preliminary exam. *Entrance requirements:* For doctorate, GRE General Test, 3 letters of recommendation, research experience. Additional exam requirements/recommendations for international students: Required—TOEFL (minimum score 84 iBT). *Application deadline:* For fall admission, 12/1 for domestic and international students. Application fee: $75 ($90 for international students). Electronic applications accepted. *Financial support:* In 2015–16, fellowships (averaging $29,025 per year) were awarded; scholarships/grants, health care benefits, tuition waivers (full), and unspecified assistantships also available. Financial award application deadline: 12/1. *Faculty research:* Cell signaling, stem cells, organogenesis, cell biology, developmental genetics. *Total annual research expenditures:* $5.8 million. *Unit head:* Dr. Deborah L. Gumucio, Professor/Interim Chair, 734-647-0172, Fax: 734-763-1166, E-mail: dgumucio@umich.edu. *Application contact:* Michelle S. Melis, Director of Student Life, 734-615-6538, Fax: 734-647-7022, E-mail: msmtegan@umich.edu.
Website: http://cdb.med.umich.edu/

University of Michigan, Rackham Graduate School, Program in Biomedical Sciences (PIBS), Interdisciplinary Program in Cellular and Molecular Biology, Ann Arbor, MI 48109. Offers PhD. *Faculty:* 166 part-time/adjunct (43 women). *Students:* 59 full-time (32 women); includes 20 minority (1 Black or African American, non-Hispanic/Latino; 1 American Indian or Alaska Native, non-Hispanic/Latino; 11 Asian, non-Hispanic/Latino; 5 Hispanic/Latino; 2 Two or more races, non-Hispanic/Latino), 1 international. Average age 26. 71 applicants, 49% accepted, 7 enrolled. In 2015, 16 doctorates awarded. *Degree requirements:* For doctorate, comprehensive exam, thesis/dissertation, preliminary exam; oral defense of dissertation. *Entrance requirements:* For doctorate, GRE General Test. Additional exam requirements/recommendations for international students: Required—TOEFL (minimum score 560 paper-based; 84 iBT), IELTS (minimum score 6.5), Michigan English Language Assessment Battery. *Application deadline:* For fall admission, 12/1 for domestic students. Application fee: $75 ($90 for international students). Electronic applications accepted. *Expenses:* Contact institution. *Financial support:* In 2015–16, 59 students received support, including 17 fellowships with full tuition reimbursements available (averaging $29,025 per year), 34 research assistantships with full tuition reimbursements available (averaging $29,025 per year), 8 teaching assistantships with full tuition reimbursements available (averaging $29,025 per year); scholarships/grants, traineeships, and health care benefits also available. *Faculty research:* Cell and systems biology, cell physiology, biochemistry, genetics/gene regulation, genomics/proteomics, computational biology, microbial pathogenesis, immunology, development, aging, neurobiology, molecular mechanisms of disease, cancer biology. *Total annual research expenditures:* $20 million. *Unit head:* Dr. Robert S. Fuller, Director, 734-936-9764, Fax: 734-763-7799, E-mail: bfuller@umich.edu. *Application contact:* Margarita Bekiares, Intermediate Administrative Specialist, 734-764-5428, Fax: 734-647-7022, E-mail: cmbgrad@umich.edu.
Website: http://www.med.umich.edu/cmb/

University of Minnesota, Twin Cities Campus, Graduate School, Program in Molecular, Cellular, Developmental Biology and Genetics, Minneapolis, MN 55455-0213. Offers genetic counseling (MS); molecular, cellular, developmental biology and genetics (PhD). Terminal master's awarded for partial completion of doctoral program. *Degree requirements:* For master's, thesis optional; for doctorate, thesis/dissertation. *Entrance requirements:* For master's and doctorate, GRE General Test. Additional exam requirements/recommendations for international students: Required—TOEFL (minimum score 625 paper-based; 80 iBT). Electronic applications accepted. *Faculty research:* Membrane receptors and membrane transport, cell interactions, cytoskeleton and cell mobility, regulation of gene expression, plant cell and molecular biology.

University of Minnesota, Twin Cities Campus, Graduate School, Stem Cell Biology Graduate Program, Minneapolis, MN 55455-3007. Offers MS. *Degree requirements:* For master's, thesis. *Entrance requirements:* For master's, GRE, BS, BA, or foreign equivalent in biological sciences or related field; minimum undergraduate GPA of 3.2. Additional exam requirements/recommendations for international students: Required—TOEFL (minimum score 580 paper-based, with a minimum score of 4 in the TWE, or 94 Internet-based, with a minimum score of 22 on each of the reading and listening, 26 on the speaking, and 26 on the writing section. *Faculty research:* Stem cell and developmental biology; embryonic stem cells; iPS cells; muscle satellite cells; hematopoietic stem cells; neuronal stem cells; cardiovascular, kidney and limb development; regenerating systems.

University of Missouri–Kansas City, School of Biological Sciences, Program in Cell Biology and Biophysics, Kansas City, MO 64110-2499. Offers PhD. Offered through the School of Graduate Studies. *Faculty:* 31 full-time (9 women), 3 part-time/adjunct (2 women). *Students:* 2 full-time (both women), 7 part-time (1 woman); includes 1 minority (Hispanic/Latino), 4 international. Average age 31. 8 applicants, 25% accepted. *Degree requirements:* For doctorate, comprehensive exam, thesis/dissertation. *Entrance requirements:* For doctorate, GRE General Test, bachelor's degree in chemistry, biology

or related field; minimum GPA of 3.0. Additional exam requirements/recommendations for international students: Required—TOEFL (minimum score 550 paper-based; 80 iBT). *Application deadline:* For fall admission, 2/15 priority date for domestic and international students. Applications are processed on a rolling basis. Application fee: $45 ($50 for international students). Electronic applications accepted. *Financial support:* In 2015–16, 11 research assistantships with full tuition reimbursements (averaging $24,189 per year), 17 teaching assistantships with tuition reimbursements (averaging $15,312 per year) were awarded; fellowships with full tuition reimbursements, scholarships/grants, tuition waivers (full and partial), and unspecified assistantships also available. Financial award application deadline: 3/1; financial award applicants required to submit FAFSA. *Unit head:* Dr. Marilyn Yoder, Interim Head, 816-235-1986, E-mail: sbsgradrecruit@umkc.edu. *Application contact:* Mary Flores, Information Contact, 816-235-5247, Fax: 816-235-5158, E-mail: sbsgradrecruit@umkc.edu.
Website: http://sbs.umkc.edu/

University of Montana, Graduate School, College of Humanities and Sciences, Division of Biological Sciences, Program in Cellular, Molecular and Microbial Biology, Missoula, MT 59812-0002. Offers cellular and developmental biology (PhD); microbial evolution and ecology (PhD); microbiology and immunology (PhD); molecular biology and biochemistry (PhD). Terminal master's awarded for partial completion of doctoral program. *Degree requirements:* For doctorate, variable foreign language requirement, thesis/dissertation. *Entrance requirements:* For doctorate, GRE General Test. *Faculty research:* Ribosome structure, medical microbiology/pathogenesis, microbial ecology/environmental microbiology.

University of Nebraska Medical Center, Department of Genetics, Cell Biology and Anatomy, Omaha, NE 68198. Offers MS, PhD. *Faculty:* 22 full-time (5 women), 1 (woman) part-time/adjunct. *Students:* 41 full-time (17 women); includes 6 minority (2 Black or African American, non-Hispanic/Latino; 1 American Indian or Alaska Native, non-Hispanic/Latino; 2 Asian, non-Hispanic/Latino; 1 Hispanic/Latino), 9 international. Average age 25. 19 applicants, 32% accepted, 6 enrolled. In 2015, 14 master's, 7 doctorates awarded. Terminal master's awarded for partial completion of doctoral program. *Degree requirements:* For master's, comprehensive exam, thesis; for doctorate, comprehensive exam, thesis/dissertation. *Entrance requirements:* For master's and doctorate, GRE General Test. Additional exam requirements/recommendations for international students: Required—TOEFL (minimum score 550 paper-based; 80 iBT). *Application deadline:* For fall admission, 4/1 priority date for domestic and international students; for spring admission, 8/1 for domestic and international students; for summer admission, 1/1 for domestic and international students. Applications are processed on a rolling basis. Application fee: $45. Electronic applications accepted. *Expenses:* Tuition, state resident: full-time $7830; part-time $3915 per credit hour. Tuition, nonresident: full-time $22,410; part-time $11,205 per credit hour. *Required fees:* $521. *Financial support:* In 2015–16, 1 fellowship with full tuition reimbursement (averaging $23,100 per year), 1 research assistantship with full tuition reimbursement (averaging $24,000 per year) were awarded; scholarships/grants also available. Support available to part-time students. Financial award application deadline: 3/1; financial award applicants required to submit FAFSA. *Faculty research:* Hematology, immunology, developmental biology, genetics cancer biology, neuroscience. *Unit head:* Dr. Karen Gould, Graduate Committee Chair, 402-559-2456, E-mail: kagould@unmc.edu. *Application contact:* Bryan Katafiasa, Administrative Associate, 402-559-4031, Fax: 402-559-7328, E-mail: bkatafiasz@unmc.edu.
Website: http://www.unmc.edu/genetics

University of Nevada, Reno, Graduate School, Interdisciplinary Program in Cell and Molecular Biology, Reno, NV 89557. Offers MS, PhD. Terminal master's awarded for partial completion of doctoral program. *Degree requirements:* For master's, thesis; for doctorate, thesis/dissertation. *Entrance requirements:* For master's, GRE Subject Test (recommended), minimum GPA of 2.75; for doctorate, GRE Subject Test (recommended), minimum GPA of 3.0. Additional exam requirements/recommendations for international students: Required—TOEFL (minimum score 500 paper-based; 61 iBT), IELTS (minimum score 6). Electronic applications accepted. *Faculty research:* Cellular biology, biophysics, cancer, microbiology, insect biochemistry.

University of New Haven, Graduate School, College of Arts and Sciences, Program in Cellular and Molecular Biology, West Haven, CT 06516-1916. Offers MS, Graduate Certificate. *Program availability:* Part-time, evening/weekend. *Students:* 32 full-time (23 women), 12 part-time (7 women); includes 11 minority (7 Black or African American, non-Hispanic/Latino; 2 Asian, non-Hispanic/Latino; 2 Hispanic/Latino), 13 international. Average age 25. 61 applicants, 82% accepted, 26 enrolled. In 2015, 24 master's awarded. *Degree requirements:* For master's, thesis or alternative. *Entrance requirements:* Additional exam requirements/recommendations for international students: Required—TOEFL (minimum score 80 iBT), IELTS, PTE. *Application deadline:* For fall admission, 5/31 for international students; for winter admission, 10/15 for international students; for spring admission, 1/15 for international students. Applications are processed on a rolling basis. Application fee: $75. Electronic applications accepted. Application fee is waived when completed online. *Expenses:* Tuition, area resident: Full-time $15,282; part-time $849 per credit hour. *Required fees:* $150; $60 per term. Tuition and fees vary according to program. *Financial support:* Research assistantships with partial tuition reimbursements, teaching assistantships with partial tuition reimbursements, career-related internships or fieldwork, Federal Work-Study, scholarships/grants, and unspecified assistantships available. Support available to part-time students. Financial award application deadline: 5/1; financial award applicants required to submit FAFSA. *Unit head:* Dr. Christina Zito, Assistant Professor, 203-479-4299, E-mail: czito@newhaven.edu.
Website: http://www.newhaven.edu/4724/

University of New Mexico, Graduate Studies, Health Sciences Center, Program in Biomedical Sciences, Albuquerque, NM 87131-5196. Offers biochemistry and molecular biology (MS, PhD); cell biology and physiology (MS, PhD); molecular genetics and microbiology (MS, PhD); neuroscience (MS, PhD); pathology (MS, PhD); toxicology (MS, PhD). *Program availability:* Part-time. *Faculty:* 18 full-time (10 women), 1 part-time/adjunct (0 women). *Students:* 31 full-time (17 women), 45 part-time (26 women); includes 29 minority (1 American Indian or Alaska Native, non-Hispanic/Latino; 3 Asian, non-Hispanic/Latino; 22 Hispanic/Latino; 2 Native Hawaiian or other Pacific Islander, non-Hispanic/Latino; 1 Two or more races, non-Hispanic/Latino), 18 international. Average age 30. 98 applicants, 11% accepted, 11 enrolled. In 2015, 11 master's, 14 doctorates awarded. Terminal master's awarded for partial completion of doctoral program. *Degree requirements:* For master's, thesis; for doctorate, comprehensive exam, thesis/dissertation, qualifying exam at the end of year 1/core curriculum. *Entrance requirements:* For master's and doctorate, GRE General Test, minimum undergraduate GPA of 3.0. Additional exam requirements/recommendations for international students: Required—TOEFL. *Application deadline:* For fall admission, 3/1 priority date for domestic and international students. Applications are processed on a rolling basis. Application fee: $50. Electronic applications accepted. *Financial support:* Fellowships with tuition reimbursements, research assistantships with full tuition reimbursements, teaching assistantships, career-related internships or fieldwork, Federal Work-Study, institutionally sponsored loans, scholarships/grants, traineeships, health care benefits, and unspecified assistantships available. Financial award application deadline: 1/1;

financial award applicants required to submit FAFSA. *Faculty research:* Infectious disease/immunity, cancer biology, cardiovascular and metabolic diseases, brain and behavioral illness, environmental health. *Unit head:* Dr. Helen J. Hathaway, Program Director, 505-272-1887, Fax: 505-272-2412, E-mail: hhathaway@salud.unm.edu. *Application contact:* Mary Fenton, Admissions Coordinator, 505-272-1887, Fax: 505-272-2412, E-mail: mfenton@salud.unm.edu.

The University of North Carolina at Chapel Hill, Graduate School, College of Arts and Sciences, Department of Biology, Chapel Hill, NC 27599. Offers botany (MA, MS, PhD); cell biology, development, and physiology (MA, MS, PhD); cell motility and cytoskeleton (PhD); ecology and behavior (MA, MS, PhD); genetics and molecular biology (MA, MS, PhD); morphology, systematics, and evolution (MA, MS, PhD). Terminal master's awarded for partial completion of doctoral program. *Degree requirements:* For master's, comprehensive exam, thesis (for some programs); for doctorate, comprehensive exam, thesis/dissertation. *Entrance requirements:* For master's, GRE General Test, GRE Subject Test, 2 semesters of calculus or statistics; 2 semesters of physics, organic chemistry; 3 semesters of biology; for doctorate, GRE General Test, GRE Subject Test, 2 semesters calculus or statistics, 2 semesters physics, organic chemistry, 3 semesters of biology. Additional exam requirements/recommendations for international students: Required—TOEFL (minimum score 550 paper-based). Electronic applications accepted. *Faculty research:* Gene expression, biomechanics, yeast genetics, plant ecology, plant molecular biology.

The University of North Carolina at Chapel Hill, School of Medicine and Graduate School, Graduate Programs in Medicine, Department of Cell and Developmental Biology, Chapel Hill, NC 27599. Offers PhD. *Degree requirements:* For doctorate, comprehensive exam, thesis/dissertation. *Entrance requirements:* For doctorate, GRE General Test, GRE Subject Test. Electronic applications accepted. *Faculty research:* Cell adhesion, motility and cytoskeleton; molecular analysis of signal transduction; development biology and toxicology; reproductive biology; cell and molecular imaging.

University of North Dakota, Graduate School and Graduate School, Graduate Programs in Medicine, Department of Anatomy and Cell Biology, Grand Forks, ND 58202. Offers MS, PhD. *Degree requirements:* For master's, thesis, final exam; for doctorate, comprehensive exam, thesis/dissertation, final exam. *Entrance requirements:* For master's and doctorate, GRE General Test, minimum GPA of 3.0. Additional exam requirements/recommendations for international students: Required—TOEFL (minimum score 550 paper-based; 79 iBT), IELTS (minimum score 6.5). Electronic applications accepted. *Faculty research:* Coronary vessel, vasculogenesis, acellular glomerular and retinal microvessel membranes, ependymal cells, cardiac muscle.

University of Notre Dame, Graduate School, College of Science, Department of Biological Sciences, Notre Dame, IN 46556. Offers aquatic ecology, evolution and environmental biology (MS, PhD); cellular and molecular biology (MS, PhD); genetics (MS, PhD); physiology (MS, PhD); vector biology and parasitology (MS, PhD). Terminal master's awarded for partial completion of doctoral program. *Degree requirements:* For master's, comprehensive exam, thesis; for doctorate, comprehensive exam, thesis/dissertation, candidacy exam. *Entrance requirements:* For master's and doctorate, GRE General Test. Additional exam requirements/recommendations for international students: Required—TOEFL (minimum score 600 paper-based; 80 iBT). Electronic applications accepted. *Faculty research:* Tropical disease, molecular genetics, neurobiology, evolutionary biology, aquatic biology.

University of Oklahoma Health Sciences Center, College of Medicine and Graduate College, Graduate Programs in Medicine, Department of Cell Biology, Oklahoma City, OK 73190. Offers MS, PhD. *Degree requirements:* For master's, thesis; for doctorate, thesis/dissertation. *Entrance requirements:* For doctorate, GRE General Test, GRE Subject Test, 3 letters of recommendation. Additional exam requirements/recommendations for international students: Required—TOEFL. *Faculty research:* Neurobiology, reproductive, neuronal plasticity, extracellular matrix, neuroendocrinology.

University of Ottawa, Faculty of Graduate and Postdoctoral Studies, Faculty of Medicine, Department of Cellular and Molecular Medicine, Ottawa, ON K1H 8M5, Canada. Offers M Sc, PhD. *Degree requirements:* For master's, thesis, seminar; for doctorate, comprehensive exam, thesis/dissertation, seminar. *Entrance requirements:* For master's, honors degree or equivalent, minimum B average; for doctorate, master's degree, minimum B+ average. Electronic applications accepted. *Faculty research:* Physiology, pharmacology, growth and development.

University of Pennsylvania, Perelman School of Medicine, Biomedical Graduate Studies, Graduate Group in Cell and Molecular Biology, Philadelphia, PA 19104. Offers cancer biology (PhD); cell biology, physiology, and metabolism (PhD); developmental stem cell regenerative biology (PhD); gene therapy and vaccines (PhD); genetics and gene regulation (PhD); microbiology, virology, and parasitology (PhD); MD/PhD; VMD/PhD. *Faculty:* 317. *Students:* 339 full-time (189 women); includes 100 minority (7 Black or African American, non-Hispanic/Latino; 2 American Indian or Alaska Native, non-Hispanic/Latino; 45 Asian, non-Hispanic/Latino; 34 Hispanic/Latino; 1 Native Hawaiian or other Pacific Islander, non-Hispanic/Latino; 11 Two or more races, non-Hispanic/Latino), 52 international. 493 applicants, 22% accepted, 37 enrolled. In 2015, 51 doctorates awarded. *Degree requirements:* For doctorate, thesis/dissertation. *Entrance requirements:* For doctorate, GRE General Test. Additional exam requirements/recommendations for international students: Required—TOEFL. *Application deadline:* For fall admission, 12/1 priority date for domestic and international students. Applications are processed on a rolling basis. Application fee: $80. Electronic applications accepted. *Expenses: Tuition, area resident:* Full-time $31,068; part-time $5762 per course. *Required fees:* $3200; $336 per course. Full-time tuition and fees vary according to degree level, program and student level. Part-time tuition and fees vary according to course load, degree level and program. *Financial support:* In 2015–16, 339 students received support. Fellowships, research assistantships, scholarships/grants, traineeships, and unspecified assistantships available. *Unit head:* Dr. Daniel Kessler, Graduate Group Chair, 215-898-1478. *Application contact:* Meagan Schofer, Coordinator, 215-898-4360.
Website: http://www.med.upenn.edu/camb/

University of Pittsburgh, Dietrich School of Arts and Sciences, Department of Biological Sciences, Program in Molecular, Cellular, and Developmental Biology, Pittsburgh, PA 15260. Offers PhD. *Faculty:* 21 full-time (5 women). *Students:* 36 full-time (19 women); includes 2 minority (1 Black or African American, non-Hispanic/Latino; 1 Asian, non-Hispanic/Latino), 8 international. Average age 23. 109 applicants, 24% accepted, 7 enrolled. In 2015, 3 doctorates awarded. *Degree requirements:* For doctorate, comprehensive exam, thesis/dissertation, completion of research integrity module. *Entrance requirements:* For doctorate, GRE General Test, GRE Subject Test. Additional exam requirements/recommendations for international students: Required—TOEFL (minimum score 90 iBT). *Application deadline:* For fall admission, 1/3 priority date for domestic students, 12/9 priority date for international students. Applications are processed on a rolling basis. Application fee: $0 ($50 for international students). Electronic applications accepted. Tuition and fees vary according to program. *Financial support:* In 2015–16, 26 fellowships with full tuition reimbursements (averaging $33,193 per year), 63 research assistantships with full tuition reimbursements (averaging

$27,573 per year), 18 teaching assistantships with full tuition reimbursements (averaging $26,813 per year) were awarded; Federal Work-Study, traineeships, health care benefits, and tuition waivers (full) also available. *Unit head:* Dr. Karen M. Arndt, Professor, 412-624-6963, Fax: 412-624-4349, E-mail: arndt@pitt.edu. *Application contact:* Cathleen M. Barr, Graduate Administrator, 412-624-4268, Fax: 412-624-4349, E-mail: cbarr@pitt.edu.
Website: http://www.biology.pitt.edu

University of Pittsburgh, School of Medicine, Graduate Programs in Medicine, Cell Biology and Molecular Physiology Graduate Program, Pittsburgh, PA 15260. Offers PhD. *Faculty:* 44 full-time (9 women). *Students:* 5 full-time (4 women). Average age 28. 386 applicants, 17% accepted, 25 enrolled. In 2015, 1 doctorate awarded. *Degree requirements:* For doctorate, comprehensive exam, thesis/dissertation. *Entrance requirements:* For doctorate, GRE General Test, GRE Subject Test, minimum QPA of 3.0. Additional exam requirements/recommendations for international students: Required—TOEFL (minimum score 600 paper-based; 100 iBT), IELTS (minimum score 7). *Application deadline:* For fall admission, 12/1 priority date for domestic and international students. Application fee: $50. Electronic applications accepted. Tuition and fees vary according to program. *Financial support:* In 2015–16, 5 students received support, including 3 fellowships with full tuition reimbursements available (averaging $27,000 per year), 2 research assistantships with full tuition reimbursements available (averaging $27,000 per year), teaching assistantships with full tuition reimbursements available (averaging $27,000 per year); scholarships/grants, traineeships, and health care benefits also available. *Faculty research:* Genetic disorders of ion channels, regulation of gene expression/development, membrane traffic of proteins and lipids, reproductive biology, signal transduction in diabetes and metabolism. *Unit head:* Dr. Donna B. Stolz, Program Director, 412-383-7283, Fax: 412-648-2927, E-mail: dstolz@pitt.edu. *Application contact:* Carol Williams, Admissions and Recruiting Manager, 412-648-8957, Fax: 412-648-1077, E-mail: gradstudies@medschool.pitt.edu.
Website: http://www.gradbiomed.pitt.edu

University of Puerto Rico, Río Piedras Campus, College of Natural Sciences, Department of Biology, San Juan, PR 00931-3300. Offers ecology/systematics (MS, PhD); evolution/genetics (MS, PhD); molecular/cellular biology (MS, PhD); neuroscience (MS, PhD). *Program availability:* Part-time. *Degree requirements:* For master's, one foreign language, comprehensive exam, thesis; for doctorate, one foreign language, comprehensive exam, thesis/dissertation. *Entrance requirements:* For master's, GRE Subject Test, interview, minimum GPA of 3.0, letter of recommendation; for doctorate, GRE Subject Test, interview, master's degree, minimum GPA of 3.0, letter of recommendation. *Faculty research:* Environmental, poblational and systematic biology.

University of Rhode Island, Graduate School, College of the Environment and Life Sciences, Department of Cell and Molecular Biology, Kingston, RI 02881. Offers biochemistry (MS, PhD); clinical laboratory sciences (MS), including biotechnology, clinical laboratory science, cytopathology; microbiology (MS, PhD); molecular genetics (MS, PhD). *Program availability:* Part-time. *Faculty:* 11 full-time (4 women), 1 (woman) part-time/adjunct. *Students:* 12 full-time (6 women), 36 part-time (27 women); includes 10 minority (4 Black or African American, non-Hispanic/Latino; 3 Asian, non-Hispanic/Latino; 2 Hispanic/Latino; 1 Two or more races, non-Hispanic/Latino), 8 international. In 2015, 19 master's, 1 doctorate awarded. *Degree requirements:* For master's, comprehensive exam (for some programs), thesis optional; for doctorate, comprehensive exam, thesis/dissertation. *Entrance requirements:* For master's and doctorate, GRE, 2 letters of recommendation. Additional exam requirements/recommendations for international students: Required—TOEFL (minimum score 550 paper-based). *Application deadline:* For fall admission, 7/15 for domestic students, 2/1 for international students; for spring admission, 11/15 for domestic students, 7/15 for international students. Application fee: $65. Electronic applications accepted. *Expenses:* Tuition, state resident: full-time $11,796; part-time $655 per credit. Tuition, nonresident: full-time $24,206; part-time $1345 per credit. *Required fees:* $1546; $44 per credit. One-time fee: $155 full-time; $35 part-time. *Financial support:* In 2015–16, 3 research assistantships with tuition reimbursements (averaging $13,507 per year), 8 teaching assistantships with tuition reimbursements (averaging $13,305 per year) were awarded; traineeships also available. Financial award application deadline: 2/1; financial award applicants required to submit FAFSA. *Faculty research:* Genomics. *Total annual research expenditures:* $6.7 million. *Unit head:* Dr. Gongqing Sun, Chairperson, 401-874-5937, Fax: 401-874-2202, E-mail: gsun@mail.uri.edu. *Application contact:* Graduate Admissions, 401-874-2872, E-mail: gradadm@etal.uri.edu.
Website: http://cels.uri.edu/cmb/

University of Saskatchewan, College of Medicine, Department of Anatomy and Cell Biology, Saskatoon, SK S7N 5A2, Canada. Offers M Sc, PhD. *Degree requirements:* For master's, thesis; for doctorate, thesis/dissertation. *Entrance requirements:* Additional exam requirements/recommendations for international students: Required—TOEFL.

University of South Carolina, The Graduate School, College of Arts and Sciences, Department of Biological Sciences, Graduate Training Program in Molecular, Cellular, and Developmental Biology, Columbia, SC 29208. Offers MS, PhD. *Degree requirements:* For master's, one foreign language, thesis; for doctorate, one foreign language, thesis/dissertation. *Entrance requirements:* For master's and doctorate, GRE General Test, minimum GPA of 3.0 in science. Electronic applications accepted. *Faculty research:* Marine ecology, population and evolutionary biology, molecular biology and genetics, development.

The University of South Dakota, Graduate School, Sanford School of Medicine and Graduate School, Biomedical Sciences Graduate Program, Cellular and Molecular Biology Group, Vermillion, SD 57069-2390. Offers MS, PhD. *Students:* Average age 26. Terminal master's awarded for partial completion of doctoral program. *Degree requirements:* For master's, thesis; for doctorate, comprehensive exam, thesis/dissertation. *Entrance requirements:* For master's and doctorate, GRE General Test, GRE Subject Test, minimum GPA of 3.0. Additional exam requirements/recommendations for international students: Required—TOEFL (minimum score 550 paper-based; 80 iBT), IELTS (minimum score 6). *Application deadline:* For fall admission, 4/15 priority date for domestic students, 3/15 for international students. Applications are processed on a rolling basis. Application fee: $35. Electronic applications accepted. *Expenses:* Contact institution. *Financial support:* In 2015–16, 10 students received support. Fellowships with partial tuition reimbursements available and research assistantships with partial tuition reimbursements available available. Financial award application deadline: 4/15; financial award applicants required to submit FAFSA. *Faculty research:* Molecular aspects of protein and DNA, neurochemistry and energy transduction, gene regulation, cellular development. *Unit head:* 605-658-6322, Fax: 605-677-6381, E-mail: biomed@usd.edu.

University of Southern California, Keck School of Medicine and Graduate School, Graduate Programs in Medicine, Master of Science Program in Stem Cell Biology and Regenerative Medicine, Los Angeles, CA 90033. Offers MS. *Program availability:* Part-time. *Faculty:* 15 full-time (8 women). *Students:* 36 full-time (15 women), 2 part-time (0 women); includes 15 minority (1 Black or African American, non-Hispanic/Latino; 11 Asian, non-Hispanic/Latino; 2 Hispanic/Latino; 1 Two or more races, non-Hispanic/Latino), 5 international. Average age 25. 132 applicants, 45% accepted, 30 enrolled. In 2015, 28 master's awarded. *Entrance requirements:* For master's, GRE, MCAT, or DAT.

Additional exam requirements/recommendations for international students: Required—TOEFL (minimum score 90 iBT), IELTS (minimum score 6.5). *Application deadline:* For fall admission, 5/15 for domestic and international students. Application fee: $85. Electronic applications accepted. *Faculty research:* Developmental and stem cell biology, regeneration of pancreatic beta cells, genetic factors in neurodegenerative disease, stem cell self-renewal and differentiation, etiology of congenital cardiovascular defects. *Unit head:* Dr. Henry Sucov, Program Director, 323-442-2563, Fax: 323-442-2230, E-mail: sucov@usc.edu. *Application contact:* M. Cort Brinkerhoff, Student Services Advisor, 323-865-1266, Fax: 323-442-8067, E-mail: mcbrinke@med.usc.edu. Website: http://scrm.usc.edu/

University of Southern California, Keck School of Medicine, Program in Development, Stem Cells and Regenerative Medicine, Los Angeles, CA 90089. Offers development, stem cells and regenerative medicine (PhD). *Faculty:* 36 full-time (15 women). *Students:* 23 full-time (9 women); includes 4 minority (3 Asian, non-Hispanic/Latino; 1 Hispanic/Latino), 11 international. Average age 26. 1 applicant, 100% accepted, 1 enrolled. *Degree requirements:* For doctorate, comprehensive exam, thesis/dissertation. *Entrance requirements:* For doctorate, GRE, minimum GPA of 3.0. Additional exam requirements/recommendations for international students: Required—TOEFL (minimum score 600 paper-based; 100 iBT), IELTS (minimum score 7), PTE. *Application deadline:* For fall admission, 12/1 priority date for domestic and international students. Application fee: $85. Electronic applications accepted. *Financial support:* In 2015–16, 23 students received support, including 6 fellowships with full tuition reimbursements available (averaging $32,000 per year), 17 research assistantships with full tuition reimbursements available (averaging $32,000 per year); institutionally sponsored loans, scholarships/grants, traineeships, health care benefits, and unspecified assistantships also available. Financial award application deadline: 5/4; financial award applicants required to submit CSS PROFILE or FAFSA. *Unit head:* Dr. Gage Crump, Director, 323-442-1475, Fax: 323-442-1199, E-mail: gcrump@med.usc.edu. *Application contact:* Dr. Joyce Perez, Manager of Student Programs, 323-442-1645, Fax: 323-442-1199, E-mail: jpperez@med.usc.edu. Website: http://pibbs.usc.edu/research-and-programs/phd-programs/

University of South Florida, College of Arts and Sciences, Department of Cell Biology, Microbiology, and Molecular Biology, Tampa, FL 33620-9951. Offers biology (MS), including cell and molecular biology; cancer biology (PhD); cell and molecular biology (PhD); microbiology (MS). *Faculty:* 21 full-time (7 women). *Students:* 41 full-time (6 women), 45 part-time (2 women); includes 11 minority (1 Black or African American, non-Hispanic/Latino; 2 Asian, non-Hispanic/Latino; 5 Hispanic/Latino; 3 Two or more races, non-Hispanic/Latino), 22 international. Average age 27. 171 applicants, 14% accepted, 18 enrolled. In 2015, 22 master's, 14 doctorates awarded. *Degree requirements:* For master's, thesis or alternative; for doctorate, comprehensive exam, thesis/dissertation. *Entrance requirements:* For master's and doctorate, GRE General Test, minimum GPA of 3.0, extensive background in biology or chemistry. Additional exam requirements/recommendations for international students: Required—TOEFL (minimum score 570 paper-based; 79 iBT) or IELTS (minimum score 6.5). *Application deadline:* For fall admission, 2/1 for domestic students, 1/1 for international students. Application fee: $30. *Financial support:* Career-related internships or fieldwork, health care benefits, and unspecified assistantships available. Financial award application deadline: 4/1. *Faculty research:* Cell biology, microbiology and molecular biology: basic and applied science in bacterial pathogenesis, genome integrity and mechanisms of aging, structural and computational biology; cancer biology: immunology, cancer control, signal transduction, drug discovery, genomics. *Total annual research expenditures:* $1.9 million. *Unit head:* Dr. James Garey, Professor/Chair, 813-974-7103, Fax: 813-974-1614, E-mail: garey@usf.edu. *Application contact:* Dr. Kenneth Wright, Associate Professor of Cancer Biology, H. Lee Moffitt Cancer Center and Research Institute, 813-745-3918, Fax: 813-974-1614, E-mail: ken.wright@moffitt.org. Website: http://biology.usf.edu/cmmb/

The University of Texas at Austin, Graduate School, Institute for Cellular and Molecular Biology, Austin, TX 78712-1111. Offers PhD.

The University of Texas at Dallas, School of Natural Sciences and Mathematics, Department of Biological Sciences, Richardson, TX 75080. Offers bioinformatics and computational biology (MS); biotechnology (MS); molecular and cell biology (MS, PhD). *Program availability:* Part-time, evening/weekend. *Faculty:* 22 full-time (4 women), 1 part-time/adjunct (0 women). *Students:* 114 full-time (71 women), 13 part-time (6 women); includes 15 minority (1 Black or African American, non-Hispanic/Latino; 9 Asian, non-Hispanic/Latino; 4 Hispanic/Latino; 1 Two or more races, non-Hispanic/Latino), 90 international. Average age 27. 359 applicants, 25% accepted, 40 enrolled. In 2015, 32 master's, 4 doctorates awarded. *Degree requirements:* For master's, thesis optional; for doctorate, thesis/dissertation, publishable paper. *Entrance requirements:* For master's and doctorate, GRE (minimum combined score of 1000 on verbal and quantitative). Additional exam requirements/recommendations for international students: Required—TOEFL (minimum score 550 paper-based; 80 iBT). *Application deadline:* For fall admission, 7/15 for domestic students, 5/1 priority date for international students; for spring admission, 11/15 for domestic students, 9/1 priority date for international students. Applications are processed on a rolling basis. Application fee: $50 ($100 for international students). Electronic applications accepted. *Expenses:* Tuition, state resident: full-time $11,940; part-time $663 per semester hour. Tuition, nonresident: full-time $22,786; part-time $1266 per semester hour. Tuition and fees vary according to course load. *Financial support:* In 2015–16, 71 students received support, including 2 fellowships with partial tuition reimbursements available (averaging $350 per year), 18 research assistantships with partial tuition reimbursements available (averaging $23,800 per year), 53 teaching assistantships with partial tuition reimbursements available (averaging $17,134 per year); career-related internships or fieldwork, Federal Work-Study, institutionally sponsored loans, scholarships/grants, and unspecified assistantships also available. Support available to part-time students. Financial award application deadline: 4/30; financial award applicants required to submit FAFSA. *Faculty research:* Role of mitochondria in neurodegenerative diseases, protein-DNA interactions in site-specific recombination, eukaryotic gene expression, bio-nanotechnology, sickle cell research. *Unit head:* Dr. Stephen Spiro, Department Head, 972-883-6032, Fax: 972-883-2409, E-mail: stephen.spiro@utdallas.edu. *Application contact:* Dr. Lawrence Reitzer, Graduate Advisor, 972-883-2502, Fax: 972-883-2409, E-mail: reitzer@utdallas.edu. Website: http://www.utdallas.edu/biology/

The University of Texas at San Antonio, College of Sciences, Department of Biology, San Antonio, TX 78249-0617. Offers biology (MS); biotechnology (MS); cell and molecular biology (PhD); neurobiology (PhD). *Faculty:* 36 full-time (10 women), 1 part-time/adjunct (0 women). *Students:* 96 full-time (53 women), 60 part-time (28 women); includes 73 minority (5 Black or African American, non-Hispanic/Latino; 1 American Indian or Alaska Native, non-Hispanic/Latino; 7 Asian, non-Hispanic/Latino; 54 Hispanic/Latino; 1 Native Hawaiian or other Pacific Islander, non-Hispanic/Latino; 5 Two or more races, non-Hispanic/Latino), 28 international. Average age 28. 147 applicants, 46% accepted, 40 enrolled. In 2015, 43 master's, 8 doctorates awarded. Terminal master's awarded for partial completion of doctoral program. *Degree requirements:* For master's, comprehensive exam, thesis or alternative; for doctorate, comprehensive exam, thesis/

dissertation. *Entrance requirements:* For master's, GRE General Test, bachelor's degree with 18 credit hours in field of study or in another appropriate field of study; for doctorate, GRE General Test, 3 letters of recommendation, statement of purpose, resume. Additional exam requirements/recommendations for international students: Required—TOEFL (minimum score 500 paper-based; 100 iBT), IELTS (minimum score 5). *Application deadline:* For fall admission, 7/1 for domestic students, 4/1 for international students; for spring admission, 11/1 for domestic students, 9/1 for international students. Application fee: $45 ($80 for international students). Electronic applications accepted. *Faculty research:* Development of human and veterinary vaccines against a fungal disease, mammalian germ cells and stem cells, dopamine neuron physiology and addiction, plant biochemistry, dendritic computation and synaptic plasticity. *Unit head:* Dr. Garry Sunter, Chair, 210-458-5479, E-mail: garry.sunter@utsa.edu. *Application contact:* Rene Munguia, Jr., Senior Program Coordinator, 210-458-4642, Fax: 210-458-5658, E-mail: rene.munguia@utsa.edu. Website: http://bio.utsa.edu/

The University of Texas Health Science Center at Houston, Graduate School of Biomedical Sciences, Program in Cell and Regulatory Biology, Houston, TX 77225-0036. Offers MS, PhD, MD/PhD. Terminal master's awarded for partial completion of doctoral program. *Degree requirements:* For master's, thesis; for doctorate, thesis/dissertation. *Entrance requirements:* For master's and doctorate, GRE General Test. Additional exam requirements/recommendations for international students: Required—TOEFL. Electronic applications accepted. *Faculty research:* Pharmacology, cell biology, physiology, signal transduction, systems biology.

The University of Texas Health Science Center at San Antonio, Graduate School of Biomedical Sciences, Department of Cellular and Structural Biology, San Antonio, TX 78229-3900. Offers MS, PhD. *Degree requirements:* For master's, thesis; for doctorate, comprehensive exam, thesis/dissertation.

The University of Texas Medical Branch, Graduate School of Biomedical Sciences, Program in Biochemistry and Molecular Biology, Galveston, TX 77555. Offers biochemistry (PhD); bioinformatics (PhD); biophysics (PhD); cell biology (PhD); computational biology (PhD); structural biology (PhD). *Degree requirements:* For doctorate, thesis/dissertation. *Entrance requirements:* Additional exam requirements/recommendations for international students: Required—TOEFL (minimum score 550 paper-based). Electronic applications accepted.

The University of Texas Southwestern Medical Center, Southwestern Graduate School of Biomedical Sciences, Division of Basic Science, Program in Cell Regulation, Dallas, TX 75390. Offers PhD. *Degree requirements:* For doctorate, thesis/dissertation, qualifying exam. *Entrance requirements:* For doctorate, GRE General Test, minimum GPA of 3.0. Additional exam requirements/recommendations for international students: Required—TOEFL. Electronic applications accepted. *Faculty research:* Molecular and cellular approaches to regulatory biology, receptor-effector coupling, membrane structure, function, and assembly.

University of the Sciences, Program in Cell Biology and Biotechnology, Philadelphia, PA 19104-4495. Offers MS. *Program availability:* Part-time, evening/weekend. *Degree requirements:* For master's, thesis optional. *Entrance requirements:* For master's, GRE General Test. Additional exam requirements/recommendations for international students: Required—TOEFL, TWE. *Application deadline:* For fall admission, 5/1 for international students; for winter admission, 10/1 for international students; for spring admission, 3/1 for international students. Applications are processed on a rolling basis. Application fee: $50. *Expenses:* Contact institution. *Financial support:* Teaching assistantships with full tuition reimbursements, scholarships/grants, and tuition waivers (partial) available. Financial award application deadline: 5/1. *Unit head:* Dr. James R. McKee, Director, 215-596-8847, E-mail: j.mckee@usciences.edu. *Application contact:* Dr. James R. McKee, Director, 215-596-8847, E-mail: j.mckee@usciences.edu.

University of Toronto, School of Graduate Studies, Faculty of Arts and Science, Department of Cell and Systems Biology, Toronto, ON M5S 1A1, Canada. Offers M Sc, PhD. *Degree requirements:* For master's, thesis, thesis defense; for doctorate, thesis/dissertation, thesis defense, oral thesis examination. *Entrance requirements:* For master's, minimum B+ average in final year, B overall, 3 letters of reference. Additional exam requirements/recommendations for international students: Required—TOEFL (minimum score 580 paper-based; 93 iBT), TWE (minimum score 5). Electronic applications accepted.

University of Vermont, Graduate College, Cellular, Molecular and Biomedical Sciences Program, Burlington, VT 05405. Offers PhD. *Degree requirements:* For doctorate, thesis/dissertation. *Entrance requirements:* For doctorate, GRE General Test. Additional exam requirements/recommendations for international students: Required—TOEFL (minimum score 550 paper-based; 80 iBT). *Application deadline:* For fall admission, 12/1 priority date for domestic students, 12/1 for international students. Application fee: $65. Electronic applications accepted. *Financial support:* Fellowships, research assistantships, teaching assistantships, and career-related internships or fieldwork available. Financial award application deadline: 3/1. *Unit head:* Dr. Matthew Poynter, 802-656-9673, E-mail: cmb@uvm.edu. *Application contact:* Dr. Matthew Poynter, 802-656-9673, E-mail: cmb@uvm.edu.

University of Virginia, School of Medicine, Department of Cell Biology, Charlottesville, VA 22903. Offers PhD, MD/PhD. *Degree requirements:* For doctorate, one foreign language, thesis/dissertation. *Entrance requirements:* For doctorate, GRE General Test, GRE Subject Test (recommended), 2 letters of recommendation. Additional exam requirements/recommendations for international students: Required—TOEFL. Electronic applications accepted.

University of Washington, Graduate School, School of Medicine, Graduate Programs in Medicine, Program in Molecular and Cellular Biology, Seattle, WA 98195. Offers PhD. Offered in partnership with Fred Hutchinson Cancer Research Center, Seattle Biomedical Research Center, and Institute for Systems Biology. *Degree requirements:* For doctorate, thesis/dissertation. *Entrance requirements:* For doctorate, GRE General Test. Additional exam requirements/recommendations for international students: Required—TOEFL. Electronic applications accepted.

See Display on next page and Close-Up on page 231.

The University of Western Ontario, Faculty of Graduate Studies, Biosciences Division, Department of Anatomy and Cell Biology, London, ON N6A 5B8, Canada. Offers anatomy and cell biology (M Sc, PhD); clinical anatomy (M Sc). *Degree requirements:* For master's, thesis; for doctorate, comprehensive exam, thesis/dissertation. *Entrance requirements:* For master's, honors degree or equivalent in biological sciences; for doctorate, master's degree. Additional exam requirements/recommendations for international students: Required—TOEFL. *Faculty research:* Cell and molecular biology, developmental biology, neuroscience, immunobiology and cancer.

University of Wisconsin–La Crosse, College of Science and Health, Department of Biology, La Crosse, WI 54601-3742. Offers aquatic sciences (MS); biology (MS); cellular and molecular biology (MS); clinical microbiology (MS); microbiology (MS); nurse anesthesia (MS); physiology (MS). *Program availability:* Part-time. *Students:* 19 full-time (12 women), 50 part-time (26 women); includes 4 minority (3 Asian, non-Hispanic/

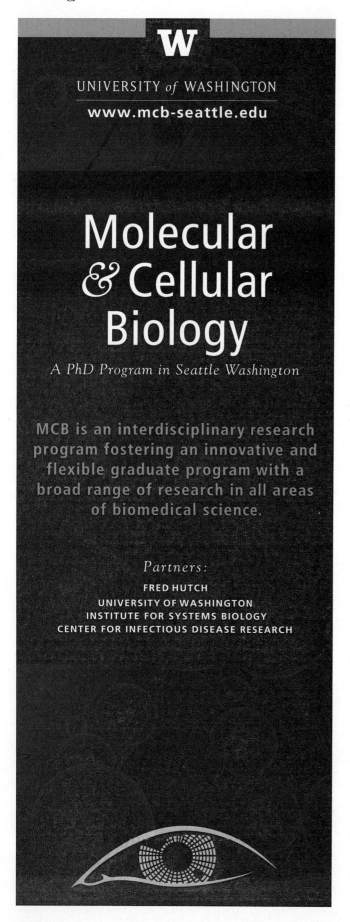

Molecular & Cellular Biology

A PhD Program in Seattle Washington

MCB is an interdisciplinary research program fostering an innovative and flexible graduate program with a broad range of research in all areas of biomedical science.

Partners:

FRED HUTCH
UNIVERSITY OF WASHINGTON
INSTITUTE FOR SYSTEMS BIOLOGY
CENTER FOR INFECTIOUS DISEASE RESEARCH

Latino; 1 Hispanic/Latino), 1 international. Average age 29. 44 applicants, 75% accepted, 27 enrolled. In 2015, 27 master's awarded. *Degree requirements:* For master's, comprehensive exam, thesis. *Entrance requirements:* For master's, GRE General Test, minimum GPA of 2.85. Additional exam requirements/recommendations for international students: Required—TOEFL (minimum score 550 paper-based; 79 iBT). *Application deadline:* For fall admission, 2/1 priority date for domestic and international students; for spring admission, 1/4 priority date for domestic and international students. Applications are processed on a rolling basis. Electronic applications accepted. *Financial support:* Research assistantships with partial tuition reimbursements, Federal Work-Study, scholarships/grants, health care benefits, and tuition waivers (partial) available. Support available to part-time students. Financial award application deadline: 3/15; financial award applicants required to submit FAFSA. *Unit head:* Dr. Mark Sandheinrich, Department Chair, 608-785-8261, E-mail: msandheinrich@uwlax.edu. *Application contact:* Brandon Schaller, Senior Graduate Student Status Examiner, 608-785-8941, E-mail: admissions@uwlax.edu.
Website: http://uwlax.edu/biology/

University of Wisconsin–Madison, Graduate School, Program in Cellular and Molecular Biology, Madison, WI 53706-1596. Offers PhD. *Degree requirements:* For doctorate, comprehensive exam, thesis/dissertation. *Entrance requirements:* For doctorate, GRE General Test, GRE Subject Test (recommended), minimum GPA of 3.0, lab experience. Additional exam requirements/recommendations for international students: Required—TOEFL (minimum score 580 paper-based; 92 iBT). Electronic applications accepted. *Expenses:* Tuition, state resident: full-time $5364. Tuition, nonresident: full-time $12,027. *Required fees:* $571. Tuition and fees vary according to campus/location, program and reciprocity agreements. *Faculty research:* Virology, cancer biology, transcriptional mechanisms, plant biology, immunology.

University of Wyoming, Graduate Program in Molecular and Cellular Life Sciences, Laramie, WY 82071. Offers PhD. *Degree requirements:* For doctorate, thesis/dissertation, four eight-week laboratory rotations, comprehensive basic practical exam, two-part qualifying exam, seminars, symposium.

Vanderbilt University, School of Medicine, Department of Cell and Developmental Biology, Nashville, TN 37240-1001. Offers MS, PhD, MD/PhD. *Faculty:* 20 full-time (6 women). *Students:* 71 full-time (46 women); includes 16 minority (4 Black or African American, non-Hispanic/Latino; 3 Asian, non-Hispanic/Latino; 6 Hispanic/Latino; 1 Native Hawaiian or other Pacific Islander, non-Hispanic/Latino; 2 Two or more races, non-Hispanic/Latino), 11 international. Average age 27. 2 applicants, 100% accepted, 3 enrolled. In 2015, 17 doctorates awarded. Terminal master's awarded for partial completion of doctoral program. *Degree requirements:* For master's, thesis or alternative; for doctorate, thesis/dissertation, preliminary, qualifying, and final exams. *Entrance requirements:* For master's, GRE General Test; for doctorate, GRE General Test, GRE Subject Test (recommended). Additional exam requirements/ recommendations for international students: Required—TOEFL (minimum score 570 paper-based; 88 iBT). *Application deadline:* For fall admission, 1/15 for domestic and international students. Application fee: $0. Electronic applications accepted. *Financial support:* Fellowships with tuition reimbursements, research assistantships with tuition reimbursements, career-related internships or fieldwork, Federal Work-Study, institutionally sponsored loans, scholarships/grants, traineeships, health care benefits, and tuition waivers (partial) available. Financial award application deadline: 1/15; financial award applicants required to submit CSS PROFILE or FAFSA. *Faculty research:* Cancer biology, cell cycle regulation, cell signaling, cytoskeletal biology, developmental biology, neurobiology, proteomics, stem cell biology, structural biology, reproductive biology, trafficking and transport, medical education and gross anatomy. *Unit head:* Dr. Steve Hann, Director of Graduate Studies, 615-322-2134, Fax: 615-343-4539, E-mail: steve.hann@vanderbilt.edu. *Application contact:* Kristi Hargrove, Coordinator, 615-322-2294, Fax: 615-343-4539, E-mail: kristi.l.hargrove@vanderbilt.edu.
Website: http://www.mc.vanderbilt.edu/cdb/

Washington State University, College of Veterinary Medicine, Program in Molecular Biosciences, Pullman, WA 99164. Offers molecular biology (PhD), including genetics, microbiology; molecular biosciences (PSM, PhD), including biochemistry (PhD), cell biology (PhD). *Program availability:* Online learning. *Faculty:* 30 full-time (12 women), 17 part-time/adjunct (5 women). *Students:* 47 full-time (26 women), 14 part-time (11 women); includes 13 minority (1 Black or African American, non-Hispanic/Latino; 1 American Indian or Alaska Native, non-Hispanic/Latino; 4 Asian, non-Hispanic/Latino; 5 Hispanic/Latino; 2 Two or more races, non-Hispanic/Latino), 1 international. Average age 28. 61 applicants, 23% accepted, 14 enrolled. In 2015, 5 master's, 8 doctorates awarded. Terminal master's awarded for partial completion of doctoral program. *Degree requirements:* For master's, thesis or alternative, oral exam; for doctorate, comprehensive exam, thesis/dissertation, oral exam, written exam. *Entrance requirements:* For master's and doctorate, GRE General Test, minimum GPA of 3.0. Additional exam requirements/recommendations for international students: Required—TOEFL (minimum score 100 iBT). *Application deadline:* For fall admission, 12/15 for domestic and international students. Application fee: $75. Electronic applications accepted. *Financial support:* In 2015–16, 5 fellowships with full tuition reimbursements (averaging $23,316 per year), 24 research assistantships with full tuition reimbursements (averaging $23,316 per year), 17 teaching assistantships with full tuition reimbursements (averaging $23,316 per year) were awarded; career-related internships or fieldwork, Federal Work-Study, traineeships, health care benefits, and unspecified assistantships also available. Financial award application deadline: 4/1; financial award applicants required to submit FAFSA. *Faculty research:* Gene regulation, signal transduction, protein export, reproductive biology, DNA repair. *Total annual research expenditures:* $5.8 million. *Unit head:* Dr. Jonathan Jones, Director, 509-335-8724, Fax: 509-335-9688, E-mail: jcr.jones@vetmed.wsu.edu. *Application contact:* Tami Breske, Coordinator, 509-335-4318, E-mail: tbreske@vetmed.wsu.edu.
Website: http://www.smb.wsu.edu

Washington University in St. Louis, Graduate School of Arts and Sciences, Division of Biology and Biomedical Sciences, Program in Molecular Cell Biology, St. Louis, MO 63130-4899. Offers PhD. *Students:* 77 full-time (34 women); includes 19 minority (5 Black or African American, non-Hispanic/Latino; 1 American Indian or Alaska Native, non-Hispanic/Latino; 9 Asian, non-Hispanic/Latino; 4 Two or more races, non-Hispanic/Latino), 17 international. 150 applicants, 19% accepted, 9 enrolled. In 2015, 22 doctorates awarded. *Degree requirements:* For doctorate, thesis/dissertation. *Entrance requirements:* For doctorate, GRE General Test, GRE Subject Test. Additional exam requirements/recommendations for international students: Required—TOEFL. *Application deadline:* For fall admission, 12/1 for domestic students. Application fee: $0. Electronic applications accepted. *Financial support:* Fellowships, research assistantships, and teaching assistantships available. Financial award application deadline: 1/15; financial award applicants required to submit CSS PROFILE. *Faculty research:* Cell adhesion, protein trafficking and organelle biogenesis, cell cycle, receptors, signal transduction, gene expression, metabolism, cytoskeleton and motility, membrane excitability, molecular basis of diseases. *Unit head:* Stacy Kiel, Coordinator, 314-362-1421. *Application contact:* Rebecca Riney, 314-747-4648, E-mail: dbbsphdadmissions@wusm.wustl.edu.

Weill Cornell Medicine, Weill Cornell Graduate School of Medical Sciences, Biochemistry, Cell and Molecular Biology Allied Program, New York, NY 10065. Offers MS, PhD. Terminal master's awarded for partial completion of doctoral program. *Degree requirements:* For master's, comprehensive exam; for doctorate, thesis/dissertation, final exam. *Entrance requirements:* For doctorate, GRE General Test, background in genetics, molecular biology, chemistry, or biochemistry. Additional exam requirements/recommendations for international students: Required—TOEFL. Electronic applications accepted. *Faculty research:* Molecular structure determination, protein structure, gene structure, stem cell biology, control of gene expression, DNA replication, chromosome maintenance, RNA biosynthesis.

Wesleyan University, Graduate Studies, Department of Biology, Middletown, CT 06459. Offers cell and developmental biology (PhD); evolution and ecology (PhD); genetics and genomics (PhD), including bioinformatics; neurobiology and behavior (PhD). *Faculty:* 14 full-time (5 women). *Students:* 26 full-time (12 women); includes 5 minority (2 Black or African American, non-Hispanic/Latino; 3 Asian, non-Hispanic/Latino), 5 international. In 2015, 3 doctorates awarded. Terminal master's awarded for partial completion of doctoral program. *Degree requirements:* For doctorate, comprehensive exam, thesis/dissertation, public seminar. *Entrance requirements:* For doctorate, GRE. Additional exam requirements/recommendations for international students: Required—TOEFL or IELTS. *Application deadline:* For fall admission, 1/15 for domestic and international students. Application fee: $0. Electronic applications accepted. *Financial support:* Stipends available. *Faculty research:* Evolution and ecology, neurobiology and behavior, cell and developmental biology, genetics, genomics and bioinformatics. *Unit head:* Dr. John Kirn, Chair/Professor, 860-685-3494, E-mail: jrkirn@wesleyan.edu. *Application contact:* Marjorie Fitzgibbons, Administrative Assistant, 860-685-2157, E-mail: mfitzgibbons@wesleyan.edu. Website: http://www.wesleyan.edu/bio/

West Virginia University, Eberly College of Arts and Sciences, Department of Biology, Morgantown, WV 26506. Offers cell and molecular biology (MS, PhD); environmental and evolutionary biology (MS, PhD); forensic biology (MS, PhD); genomic biology (MS, PhD); neurobiology (MS, PhD). Terminal master's awarded for partial completion of doctoral program. *Degree requirements:* For master's, thesis, final exam; for doctorate, thesis/dissertation, preliminary and final exams. *Entrance requirements:* For master's, GRE General Test, GRE Subject Test, minimum GPA of 3.0; for doctorate, GRE General Test, minimum GPA of 3.0. Additional exam requirements/recommendations for international students: Required—TOEFL. *Expenses:* Tuition, state resident: full-time $8568. Tuition, nonresident: full-time $22,140. Tuition and fees vary according to program. *Faculty research:* Environmental biology, genetic engineering, developmental biology, global change, biodiversity.

Yale University, Graduate School of Arts and Sciences, Department of Cell Biology, New Haven, CT 06520. Offers PhD. *Degree requirements:* For doctorate, thesis/dissertation. *Entrance requirements:* For doctorate, GRE General Test. *Expenses:* Contact institution.

Yale University, Graduate School of Arts and Sciences, Department of Molecular, Cellular, and Developmental Biology, Program in Cellular and Developmental Biology, New Haven, CT 06520. Offers PhD. *Degree requirements:* For doctorate, thesis/dissertation. *Entrance requirements:* For doctorate, GRE General Test, GRE Subject Test.

Yale University, School of Medicine and Graduate School of Arts and Sciences, Combined Program in Biological and Biomedical Sciences (BBS), Molecular Cell Biology, Genetics, and Development Track, New Haven, CT 06520. Offers PhD, MD/PhD. *Entrance requirements:* Additional exam requirements/recommendations for international students: Required—TOEFL.

Molecular Biology

Albany College of Pharmacy and Health Sciences, School of Arts and Sciences, Albany, NY 12208. Offers clinical laboratory sciences (MS); cytotechnology and molecular cytology (MS); molecular biosciences (MS). *Degree requirements:* For master's, thesis. *Entrance requirements:* For master's, GRE, minimum GPA of 3.0. Additional exam requirements/recommendations for international students: Required—TOEFL (minimum score 84 iBT). Electronic applications accepted.

Albany Medical College, Center for Cell Biology and Cancer Research, Albany, NY 12208-3479. Offers MS, PhD. *Program availability:* Part-time. Terminal master's awarded for partial completion of doctoral program. *Degree requirements:* For master's, thesis; for doctorate, comprehensive exam, thesis/dissertation. *Entrance requirements:* For master's and doctorate, GRE General Test, all transcripts, letters of recommendation. Additional exam requirements/recommendations for international students: Required—TOEFL. *Faculty research:* Cancer cell biology, tissue remodeling, signal transduction, gene regulation, cell adhesion, angiogenesis.

Albert Einstein College of Medicine, Graduate Division of Biomedical Sciences, Department of Developmental and Molecular Biology, Bronx, NY 10461. Offers PhD, MD/PhD. *Degree requirements:* For doctorate, thesis/dissertation. *Entrance requirements:* For doctorate, GRE General Test. Additional exam requirements/recommendations for international students: Required—TOEFL. *Faculty research:* DNA, RNA, and protein synthesis in prokaryotes and eukaryotes; chemical and enzymatic alteration of RNA; glycoproteins.

American University of Beirut, Graduate Programs, Faculty of Arts and Sciences, Beirut, Lebanon. Offers anthropology (MA); Arab and Middle Eastern history (PhD); Arabic language and literature (MA, PhD); archaeology (MA); biology (MS); cell and molecular biology (PhD); chemistry (MS); clinical psychology (MA); computational sciences (MS); computer science (MS); economics (MA); English language (MA); English literature (MA); environmental policy planning (MS); financial economics (MAFE); geology (MS); history (MA); mathematics (MA, MS); media studies (MA); Middle Eastern studies (MA); physics (MS); political studies (MA); psychology (MS); public administration (MA); sociology (MA); statistics (MA, MS); theoretical physics (PhD); transnational American studies (MA). *Program availability:* Part-time. *Faculty:* 114 full-time (36 women), 4 part-time/adjunct (2 women). *Students:* 258 full-time (190 women), 207 part-time (142 women). Average age 27. 241 applicants, 71% accepted, 98 enrolled. In 2015, 47 master's, 3 doctorates awarded. *Degree requirements:* For master's, one foreign language, comprehensive exam, thesis (for some programs); for doctorate, one foreign language, comprehensive exam, thesis/dissertation. *Entrance requirements:* For master's, GRE (for some MA, MS programs), letter of recommendation; for doctorate, GRE, letters of recommendation. Additional exam requirements/recommendations for international students: Required—TOEFL (minimum score 600 paper-based; 97 iBT), IELTS (minimum score 7). *Application deadline:* For fall admission, 4/1 for domestic and international students; for spring admission, 11/1 for domestic and international students. Application fee: $50. Electronic applications accepted. *Expenses: Tuition, area resident:* Full-time $16,254; part-time $903 per credit. *Required fees:* $699. Tuition and fees vary according to course load and program. *Financial support:* Research assistantships, career-related internships or fieldwork, institutionally sponsored loans, scholarships/grants, health care benefits, and unspecified assistantships available. Financial award application deadline: 2/4; financial award applicants required to submit FAFSA. *Faculty research:* Analysis and algebra; software engineering; machine learning and big data analysis; philosophy of mind and political philosophy; anthropology of art, anthropology of migration and medical anthropology; sociology of knowledge, sociology of migration, critical theory; sociology of education; hybrid solid materials; photocatalysis; human creativity. *Total annual research expenditures:* $680,360. *Unit head:* Dr. Patrick McGreevy, Dean, 961-1374374 Ext. 3800, Fax: 961-1744461, E-mail: pm07@aub.edu.lb. *Application contact:* Dr. Salim Kanaan, Director, Admissions Office, 961-1350000 Ext. 2590, Fax: 961-1750775, E-mail: sk00@aub.edu.lb. Website: http://www.aub.edu.lb/fas/

Appalachian State University, Cratis D. Williams Graduate School, Department of Biology, Boone, NC 28608. Offers cell and molecular biology (MS); general biology (MS). *Program availability:* Part-time. *Degree requirements:* For master's, comprehensive exam, thesis. *Entrance requirements:* For master's, GRE General Test, 3 letters of recommendation. Additional exam requirements/recommendations for international students: Required—TOEFL (minimum score 570 paper-based; 79 iBT), IELTS (minimum score 6.5). Electronic applications accepted. *Faculty research:* Aquatic and terrestrial ecology, animal and plant physiology, behavior and systematics, immunology and cell biology, molecular biology and microbiology.

Arizona State University at the Tempe campus, College of Liberal Arts and Sciences, School of Life Sciences, Tempe, AZ 85287-4601. Offers animal behavior (PhD); applied ethics (biomedical and health ethics) (MA); biology (MS, PhD), including biology, biology and society, complex adaptive systems science (PhD), plant biology and conservation (MS); environmental life sciences (PhD); evolutionary biology (PhD); history and philosophy of science (PhD); human and social dimensions of science and technology (PhD); microbiology (PhD); molecular and cellular biology (PhD); neuroscience (PhD). Terminal master's awarded for partial completion of doctoral program. *Degree requirements:* For master's, thesis (for some programs), interactive Program of Study (iPOS) submitted before completing 50 percent of required credit hours; for doctorate, variable foreign language requirement, comprehensive exam, thesis/dissertation, interactive Program of Study (iPOS) submitted before completing 50 percent of required credit hours. *Entrance requirements:* For master's and doctorate, GRE, minimum GPA of 3.0 or equivalent in last 2 years of work leading to bachelor's degree. Additional exam requirements/recommendations for international students: Required—TOEFL (minimum score 600 paper-based; 100 iBT). Electronic applications accepted.

Arkansas State University, Graduate School, College of Sciences and Mathematics, Program in Molecular Biosciences, State University, AR 72467. Offers molecular biosciences (MS, PhD). *Program availability:* Part-time. *Faculty:* 1 full-time (0 women). *Students:* 14 full-time (8 women), 1 part-time (0 women), 11 international. Average age 31. 16 applicants, 25% accepted, 3 enrolled. In 2015, 4 doctorates awarded. *Degree requirements:* For master's, comprehensive exam, thesis; for doctorate, comprehensive exam, thesis/dissertation. *Entrance requirements:* For master's, GRE, appropriate bachelor's degree, official transcripts, immunization records, letters of reference, autobiography; for doctorate, GRE, appropriate bachelor's or master's degree, interview, letters of recommendation, official transcripts, personal statement, immunization records. Additional exam requirements/recommendations for international students: Required—TOEFL (minimum score 550 paper-based; 79 iBT), IELTS (minimum score 6), PTE (minimum score 56). *Application deadline:* For fall admission, 2/15 for domestic and international students; for spring admission, 7/15 for domestic and international students. Applications are processed on a rolling basis. Electronic applications accepted. *Expenses:* Tuition, state resident: full-time $4572; part-time $254 per credit hour. Tuition, nonresident: full-time $9144; part-time $508 per credit hour. International tuition: $9844 full-time. *Required fees:* $1188; $66 per credit hour. $25 per term. Tuition and fees vary according to course load and program. *Financial support:* In 2015–16, 8 students received support. Fellowships, research assistantships, teaching assistantships, career-related internships or fieldwork, scholarships/grants, and unspecified assistantships available. Financial award application deadline: 7/1; financial award applicants required to submit FAFSA. *Unit head:* Dr. Malathi Srivatsan, Assistant Director of Arkansas Biosciences Institute/Director of Molecular Biosciences, 870-972-2007, Fax: 870-972-2008, E-mail: msrivatsan@astate.edu. *Application contact:* Vickey Ring, Graduate Admissions Coordinator, 870-972-2737, Fax: 870-972-3917, E-mail: vickeyring@astate.edu. Website: http://www.astate.edu/college/sciences-and-mathematics/doctoral-programs/molecular-biosciences/

Auburn University, Graduate School, Interdepartmental Programs, Auburn University, AL 36849. Offers applied economics (PhD); cell and molecular biology (PhD); real estate development (MRED); sociology and rural sociology (MA, MS), including rural sociology (MS), sociology. *Program availability:* Part-time. *Students:* 35 full-time (18 women), 44 part-time (11 women); includes 15 minority (13 Black or African American, non-Hispanic/Latino; 1 Asian, non-Hispanic/Latino; 1 Hispanic/Latino), 30 international. Average age 34. 62 applicants, 50% accepted, 24 enrolled. In 2015, 18 master's, 4 doctorates awarded. *Entrance requirements:* For master's, GRE General Test. *Application deadline:* Applications are processed on a rolling basis. Application fee: $50 ($60 for international students). Electronic applications accepted. *Expenses:* Tuition, state resident: full-time $8802; part-time $489 per credit hour. Tuition, nonresident: full-time $26,406; part-time $1467 per credit hour. *Required fees:* $808 per semester. Tuition and fees vary according to degree level and program. *Financial support:* Fellowships, research assistantships, teaching assistantships, and Federal Work-Study available. Support available to part-time students. Financial award application deadline: 3/15; financial award applicants required to submit FAFSA. *Application contact:* Dr. George Flowers, Dean of the Graduate School, 334-844-2125.

Baylor College of Medicine, Graduate School of Biomedical Sciences, Department of Biochemistry and Molecular Biology, Houston, TX 77030-3498. Offers PhD, MD/PhD. *Degree requirements:* For doctorate, thesis/dissertation, public defense. *Entrance requirements:* For doctorate, GRE General Test, GRE Subject Test (strongly

Molecular Biology

recommended), minimum GPA of 3.0. Additional exam requirements/recommendations for international students: Required—TOEFL. Electronic applications accepted. *Faculty research:* DNA repair, homologous recombination, gene therapy, trinucleotide repeat diseases, retinitis pigmentosa.

Baylor College of Medicine, Graduate School of Biomedical Sciences, Department of Molecular and Cellular Biology, Houston, TX 77030-3498. Offers PhD, MD/PhD. *Degree requirements:* For doctorate, thesis/dissertation, public defense, qualifying exam. *Entrance requirements:* For doctorate, GRE General Test, GRE Subject Test (strongly recommended), minimum GPA of 3.0. Additional exam requirements/recommendations for international students: Required—TOEFL. Electronic applications accepted. *Faculty research:* Hormone action, development, cancer, gene therapy, neurobiology.

Baylor College of Medicine, Graduate School of Biomedical Sciences, Interdepartmental Program in Cell and Molecular Biology, Houston, TX 77030-3498. Offers biochemistry (PhD); cell and molecular biology (PhD); genetics (PhD); human genetics (PhD); immunology (PhD); microbiology (PhD); virology (PhD); MD/PhD. *Degree requirements:* For doctorate, thesis/dissertation, public defense. *Entrance requirements:* For doctorate, GRE General Test, GRE Subject Test (strongly recommended), minimum GPA of 3.0. Additional exam requirements/recommendations for international students: Required—TOEFL. Electronic applications accepted. *Faculty research:* Molecular and cellular biology; cancer, aging and stem cells; genomics and proteomics; microbiome, molecular microbiology; infectious disease, immunology and translational research.

Baylor College of Medicine, Graduate School of Biomedical Sciences, Program in Developmental Biology, Houston, TX 77030-3498. Offers PhD, MD/PhD. *Degree requirements:* For doctorate, thesis/dissertation, public defense. *Entrance requirements:* For doctorate, GRE General Test, GRE Subject Test (strongly recommended), minimum GPA of 3.0. Additional exam requirements/recommendations for international students: Required—TOEFL. Electronic applications accepted. *Faculty research:* Stem cells, cancer, neurobiology, organogenesis, genetics of model organisms.

Boise State University, College of Arts and Sciences, Department of Biological Sciences, Boise, ID 83725-1515. Offers biology (MA, MS); biomolecular sciences (PhD); raptor biology (MS). *Program availability:* Part-time. *Faculty:* 26. *Students:* 51 full-time (23 women), 10 part-time (5 women); includes 7 minority (1 Black or African American, non-Hispanic/Latino; 1 American Indian or Alaska Native, non-Hispanic/Latino; 1 Asian, non-Hispanic/Latino; 3 Hispanic/Latino; 1 Native Hawaiian or other Pacific Islander, non-Hispanic/Latino), 6 international. Average age 30. 45 applicants, 27% accepted, 19 enrolled. In 2015, 13 master's awarded. *Degree requirements:* For master's, thesis. *Entrance requirements:* For master's, GRE General Test, minimum GPA of 3.0. Additional exam requirements/recommendations for international students: Required—TOEFL (minimum score 550 paper-based; 80 iBT), IELTS (minimum score 6). *Application deadline:* For fall admission, 1/15 for domestic and international students; for spring admission, 10/1 for domestic and international students. Application fee: $65 ($95 for international students). Electronic applications accepted. *Expenses:* Tuition, state resident: full-time $6058; part-time $358 per credit hour. Tuition, nonresident: full-time $20,108; part-time $608 per credit hour. *Required fees:* $2108. Tuition and fees vary according to program. *Financial support:* In 2015–16, 6 students received support, including 18 research assistantships (averaging $7,534 per year), 29 teaching assistantships (averaging $8,918 per year); institutionally sponsored loans and unspecified assistantships also available. Financial award application deadline: 1/15; financial award applicants required to submit FAFSA. *Faculty research:* Soil and stream microbial ecology, avian ecology. *Unit head:* Dr. Kevin Feris, Chair, 208-426-5498, E-mail: kevinferis@boisestate.edu. *Application contact:* Dr. Julie Heath, Graduate Coordinator, 208-426-3208, E-mail: julieheath@boisestate.edu.
Website: http://biology.boisestate.edu/graduate-programs/

Boston University, Graduate School of Arts and Sciences, Molecular Biology, Cell Biology, and Biochemistry Program (MCBB), Boston, MA 02215. Offers MA, PhD. *Students:* 32 full-time (14 women), 3 part-time (2 women); includes 10 minority (3 Black or African American, non-Hispanic/Latino; 2 Asian, non-Hispanic/Latino; 4 Hispanic/Latino; 1 Two or more races, non-Hispanic/Latino), 8 international. Average age 29. 139 applicants, 11% accepted, 3 enrolled. In 2015, 16 master's, 3 doctorates awarded. Terminal master's awarded for partial completion of doctoral program. *Degree requirements:* For master's, one foreign language, thesis (for some programs); for doctorate, one foreign language, comprehensive exam, thesis/dissertation. *Entrance requirements:* For master's and doctorate, GRE General Test, GRE Subject Test (recommended), 3 letters of recommendation, transcripts, personal statement. Additional exam requirements/recommendations for international students: Required—TOEFL (minimum score 550 paper-based; 84 iBT). *Application deadline:* For fall admission, 12/7 for domestic and international students. Application fee: $95. Electronic applications accepted. *Financial support:* In 2015–16, 30 students received support, including 2 fellowships with full tuition reimbursements available (averaging $21,000 per year), 15 research assistantships with full tuition reimbursements available (averaging $21,000 per year), 12 teaching assistantships with full tuition reimbursements available (averaging $21,000 per year); Federal Work-Study, scholarships/grants, traineeships, and health care benefits also available. Financial award application deadline: 12/7; financial award applicants required to submit FAFSA. *Unit head:* Dr. Ulla Hansen, Director, 617-353-2432, Fax: 617-353-6340, E-mail: uhansen@bu.edu. *Application contact:* Christina Honeycutt, Academic Administrator, 617-353-2432, Fax: 617-353-6340, E-mail: cjhoney@bu.edu.
Website: http://www.bu.edu/mcbb/

Boston University, School of Medicine, Division of Graduate Medical Sciences, Department of Biochemistry, Boston, MA 02118. Offers MA, PhD, MD/PhD. *Program availability:* Part-time. Terminal master's awarded for partial completion of doctoral program. *Degree requirements:* For master's, thesis or alternative; for doctorate, thesis/dissertation. *Application deadline:* For fall admission, 1/15 for domestic students; for spring admission, 10/15 for domestic students. *Unit head:* Dr. David A. Harris, Chair, 617-638-5090. *Application contact:* GMS Admissions Office, 617-638-5255, E-mail: askgms@bu.edu.
Website: http://www.bumc.bu.edu/biochemistry/

Boston University, School of Medicine, Division of Graduate Medical Sciences, Program in Cell and Molecular Biology, Boston, MA 02118. Offers PhD. *Degree requirements:* For doctorate, thesis/dissertation. *Application deadline:* For fall admission, 1/15 for domestic students; for spring admission, 10/15 for domestic students. *Financial support:* Scholarships/grants and traineeships available. Financial award applicants required to submit FAFSA. *Unit head:* Dr. Vickery Trinkaus-Randall, Director, 617-638-6099, Fax: 617-638-5337, E-mail: vickery@bu.edu. *Application contact:* GMS Admissions Office, 617-638-5255, E-mail: askgms@bu.edu.
Website: http://www.bumc.bu.edu/cmbio/

Brandeis University, Graduate School of Arts and Sciences, Program in Molecular and Cell Biology, Waltham, MA 02454-9110. Offers genetics (PhD); microbiology (PhD); molecular and cell biology (MS, PhD); molecular biology (PhD); neurobiology (PhD); quantitative biology (PhD). *Faculty:* 26 full-time (12 women), 4 part-time/adjunct (2 women). *Students:* 60 full-time (30 women); includes 5 minority (1 Black or African

American, non-Hispanic/Latino; 1 American Indian or Alaska Native, non-Hispanic/Latino; 1 Asian, non-Hispanic/Latino; 2 Hispanic/Latino), 25 international. 183 applicants, 27% accepted, 12 enrolled. In 2015, 13 master's, 7 doctorates awarded. Terminal master's awarded for partial completion of doctoral program. *Degree requirements:* For master's, thesis optional, research project, research lab, or project lab; for doctorate, comprehensive exam, thesis/dissertation, journal clubs; research seminar; colloquia; qualifying exam. *Entrance requirements:* For master's, GRE General Test, official transcript(s), resume, 2 letters of recommendation, statement of purpose; for doctorate, GRE General Test, official transcript(s), resume, 3 letters of recommendation, statement of purpose, list of previous research experience. Additional exam requirements/recommendations for international students: Required—TOEFL (minimum score 600 paper-based; 100 iBT); Recommended—IELTS (minimum score 7), TSE (minimum score 68). *Application deadline:* For fall admission, 12/15 priority date for domestic students. Application fee: $75. Electronic applications accepted. *Financial support:* In 2015–16, 35 students received support, including 16 fellowships with full tuition reimbursements available (averaging $30,500 per year), 19 research assistantships with full tuition reimbursements available (averaging $30,500 per year); scholarships/grants and tuition waivers (partial) also available. Financial award application deadline: 4/15; financial award applicants required to submit FAFSA. *Faculty research:* Molecular biology, genetics and development; structural and cell biology; neurobiology. *Unit head:* Dr. Maria Miara, Director of Graduate Studies, 781-736-2300, Fax: 781-736-3107, E-mail: scigradoffice@brandeis.edu. *Application contact:* Dr. Maryanna Aldrich, Department Administrator, 781-736-2300, Fax: 781-736-3107, E-mail: scigradoffice@brandeis.edu.
Website: http://www.brandeis.edu/gsas

Brigham Young University, Graduate Studies, College of Life Sciences, Department of Microbiology and Molecular Biology, Provo, UT 85602. Offers MS, PhD. *Faculty:* 15 full-time (3 women). *Students:* 38 full-time (18 women); includes 12 minority (6 Asian, non-Hispanic/Latino; 5 Hispanic/Latino; 1 Native Hawaiian or other Pacific Islander, non-Hispanic/Latino), 12 international. Average age 27. 22 applicants, 73% accepted, 12 enrolled. In 2015, 5 master's, 3 doctorates awarded. Terminal master's awarded for partial completion of doctoral program. *Degree requirements:* For master's, comprehensive exam, thesis; for doctorate, comprehensive exam, thesis/dissertation. *Entrance requirements:* For master's, GRE General Test, minimum GPA of 3.0 during previous 2 years; for doctorate, GRE General Test, minimum GPA of 3.0. Additional exam requirements/recommendations for international students: Required—TOEFL (minimum score 580 paper-based; 85 iBT), IELTS (minimum score 7). *Application deadline:* For fall admission, 2/1 for domestic and international students. Application fee: $50. Electronic applications accepted. *Financial support:* In 2015–16, 18 students received support, including 16 research assistantships with full tuition reimbursements available (averaging $21,000 per year), 2 teaching assistantships with tuition reimbursements available (averaging $18,000 per year); institutionally sponsored loans, scholarships/grants, health care benefits, and unspecified assistantships also available. Financial award application deadline: 2/1. *Faculty research:* Immunobiology, molecular genetics, molecular virology, cancer biology, pathogenic and environmental microbiology. Total annual research expenditures: $845,216. *Unit head:* Dr. Richard Robison, Chair, 801-422-2416, Fax: 801-422-0004, E-mail: richard_robison@byu.edu. *Application contact:* Dr. Joel Griffitts, Graduate Coordinator, 801-422-7997, Fax: 801-422-0004, E-mail: joel_griffitts@byu.edu.
Website: http://mmbio.byu.edu/

Brown University, Graduate School, Division of Biology and Medicine, Department of Molecular Biology, Cell Biology, and Biochemistry, Providence, RI 02912. Offers MA, PhD. *Program availability:* Part-time. Terminal master's awarded for partial completion of doctoral program. *Degree requirements:* For master's, thesis (for some programs); for doctorate, one foreign language, thesis/dissertation, preliminary exam. *Entrance requirements:* For master's and doctorate, GRE General Test, GRE Subject Test. Additional exam requirements/recommendations for international students: Required—TOEFL. Electronic applications accepted. *Faculty research:* Molecular genetics, gene regulation.

California Institute of Technology, Division of Biology, Program in Molecular Biology, Pasadena, CA 91125-0001. Offers PhD. *Degree requirements:* For doctorate, thesis/dissertation, qualifying exam. *Entrance requirements:* For doctorate, GRE General Test.

California State University, Sacramento, Office of Graduate Studies, College of Natural Sciences and Mathematics, Department of Biological Sciences, Sacramento, CA 95819. Offers biological conservation (MS); molecular and cellular biology (MS); stem cell (MA). *Program availability:* Part-time. *Degree requirements:* For master's, thesis, writing proficiency exam. *Entrance requirements:* For master's, GRE, bachelor's degree in biology or equivalent; minimum GPA of 3.0 in biology, 2.75 overall during last 2 years of course work. Additional exam requirements/recommendations for international students: Required—TOEFL. Electronic applications accepted.

Carnegie Mellon University, Mellon College of Science, Department of Biological Sciences, Pittsburgh, PA 15213-3891. Offers biochemistry (PhD); biophysics (PhD); cell and developmental biology (PhD); computational biology (MS, PhD); genetics (PhD); molecular biology (PhD); neuroscience (PhD); structural biology (PhD). *Degree requirements:* For doctorate, comprehensive exam, thesis/dissertation. *Entrance requirements:* For doctorate, GRE General Test, GRE Subject Test, interview. Electronic applications accepted. *Faculty research:* Genetic structure, function, and regulation; protein structure and function; biological membranes; biological spectroscopy.

Case Western Reserve University, School of Medicine and School of Graduate Studies, Graduate Programs in Medicine, Department of Molecular Biology and Microbiology, Cleveland, OH 44106-4960. Offers cellular biology (PhD); microbiology (PhD); molecular biology (PhD); molecular virology (PhD); MD/PhD. Students are admitted to an integrated Biomedical Sciences Training Program involving 11 basic science programs at Case Western Reserve University. *Degree requirements:* For doctorate, thesis/dissertation. *Entrance requirements:* For doctorate, GRE General Test, GRE Subject Test. Additional exam requirements/recommendations for international students: Required—TOEFL. Electronic applications accepted. *Expenses:* Tuition, area resident: Full-time $41,137; part-time $1714 per credit hour. *Required fees:* $32. Tuition and fees vary according to course load and program. *Faculty research:* Gene expression in eukaryotic and prokaryotic systems; microbial physiology; intracellular transport and signaling; mechanisms of oncogenesis; molecular mechanisms of RNA processing, editing, and catalysis.

Central Connecticut State University, School of Graduate Studies, School of Engineering, Science and Technology, Department of Biomolecular Sciences, New Britain, CT 06050-4010. Offers MS, Certificate. *Program availability:* Part-time, evening/weekend. *Faculty:* 9 full-time (3 women). *Students:* 28 full-time (20 women), 28 part-time (14 women); includes 21 minority (10 Black or African American, non-Hispanic/Latino; 7 Asian, non-Hispanic/Latino; 3 Hispanic/Latino; 1 Two or more races, non-Hispanic/Latino), 2 international. Average age 28. 42 applicants, 90% accepted, 29 enrolled. In 2015, 15 master's, 6 other advanced degrees awarded. *Degree requirements:* For master's, comprehensive exam, thesis or alternative; for Certificate, qualifying exam. *Entrance requirements:* For master's, minimum undergraduate GPA of 2.7, essay,

letters of recommendation; for Certificate, essay. Additional exam requirements/recommendations for international students: Required—TOEFL (minimum score 550 paper-based; 79 iBT). *Application deadline:* For fall admission, 6/1 for domestic students, 5/1 for international students; for spring admission, 11/1 for domestic and international students. Applications are processed on a rolling basis. Application fee: $50. Electronic applications accepted. *Expenses: Tuition, area resident:* Full-time $6188. Tuition, state resident: full-time $9284; part-time $577 per credit. Tuition, nonresident: full-time $17,240; part-time $592 per credit. *Required fees:* $4266; $234 per credit. *Financial support:* In 2015–16, 11 students received support, including 2 research assistantships; career-related internships or fieldwork, Federal Work-Study, scholarships/grants, and unspecified assistantships also available. Support available to part-time students. Financial award application deadline: 3/1; financial award applicants required to submit FAFSA. *Unit head:* Dr. Kathy Martin, Chair, 860-832-3560, E-mail: martink@ccsu.edu. *Application contact:* Patricia Gardner, Associate Director of Graduate Studies, 860-832-2350, Fax: 860-832-2362, E-mail: graduateadmissions@ccsu.edu.
Website: http://www.ccsu.edu/bms/

Clemson University, Graduate School, College of Science, Department of Genetics and Biochemistry, Program in Biochemistry and Molecular Biology, Clemson, SC 29634. Offers PhD. *Faculty:* 28 full-time (14 women), 1 (woman) part-time/adjunct. *Students:* 15 full-time (8 women); includes 1 minority (Asian, non-Hispanic/Latino), 7 international. Average age 29. 24 applicants, 25% accepted, 1 enrolled. In 2015, 5 doctorates awarded. *Degree requirements:* For doctorate, comprehensive exam, thesis/dissertation. *Entrance requirements:* For doctorate, GRE General Test, unofficial transcripts, letters of recommendation. Additional exam requirements/recommendations for international students: Required—TOEFL (minimum score 80 iBT), IELTS (minimum score 6.5). *Application deadline:* For fall admission, 1/1 for domestic and international students; for spring admission, 9/1 for domestic and international students. Application fee: $80 ($90 for international students). Electronic applications accepted. *Expenses:* $4,060 per semester full-time resident, $8,103 per semester full-time non-resident, $448 per credit hour part-time resident, $898 per credit hour part-time non-resident. *Financial support:* In 2015–16, 15 students received support, including 3 fellowships with partial tuition reimbursements available (averaging $3,333 per year), 5 research assistantships with partial tuition reimbursements available (averaging $21,881 per year), 9 teaching assistantships with partial tuition reimbursements available (averaging $21,044 per year); health care benefits also available. Financial award application deadline: 1/1. *Faculty research:* Cell and developmental biology, microbial pathogenesis, protein structure and function, plant biochemistry. *Unit head:* Dr. William Marcotte, Jr., Department Chair, 864-656-3586, Fax: 864-656-6879, E-mail: marcotw@clemson.edu. *Application contact:* Nicole Clark-Mount, Administrative Assistant, 864-656-6237, Fax: 864-656-6879, E-mail: hluo@clemson.edu.
Website: http://www.clemson.edu/genbiochem/graduate_programs/

Colorado State University, Interdisciplinary College, Program in Cell and Molecular Biology, Fort Collins, CO 80523-1618. Offers MS, PhD. *Students:* 31 full-time (22 women), 44 part-time (25 women); includes 8 minority (2 Black or African American, non-Hispanic/Latino; 1 Asian, non-Hispanic/Latino; 4 Hispanic/Latino; 1 Two or more races, non-Hispanic/Latino), 25 international. Average age 30. 10 applicants, 70% accepted, 7 enrolled. In 2015, 4 master's, 10 doctorates awarded. Terminal master's awarded for partial completion of doctoral program. *Degree requirements:* For master's, comprehensive exam (for some programs), thesis; for doctorate, comprehensive exam, thesis/dissertation, preliminary exam. *Entrance requirements:* For master's and doctorate, GRE General Test, GRE Subject Test in biology (strongly recommended), minimum GPA of 3.0; BA/BS in biology, biochemistry, or physics; calculus sequence; letters of recommendation; transcript; personal statement; curriculum vitae. Additional exam requirements/recommendations for international students: Required—TOEFL (minimum score 625 paper-based; 107 iBT). *Application deadline:* For fall admission, 1/1 priority date for domestic and international students. Applications are processed on a rolling basis. Application fee: $60 ($70 for international students). Electronic applications accepted. *Expenses:* Tuition, state resident: full-time $9348. Tuition, nonresident: full-time $22,916. *Required fees:* $2174; $473.72 per credit hour. $236.86 per semester. Tuition and fees vary according to course load and program. *Financial support:* In 2015–16, 10 research assistantships with full tuition reimbursements (averaging $24,065 per year), 3 teaching assistantships with full tuition reimbursements (averaging $23,328 per year) were awarded. Financial award application deadline: 1/1. *Faculty research:* Cancer biology and infectious diseases; genomics and computational biology; metabolic regulation and regulation of gene expression; neuroscience and molecular physiology; reproductive and developmental biology. *Unit head:* Dr. Howard Liber, Program Director, 970-491-0580, Fax: 970-491-2194, E-mail: howard.liber@colostate.edu. *Application contact:* Lori Williams, Program Coordinator, 970-491-0241, Fax: 970-491-2194, E-mail: lori.williams@colostate.edu.
Website: http://cmb.colostate.edu/

Columbia University, College of Physicians and Surgeons, Integrated Program in Cellular, Molecular, Structural and Genetic Studies, New York, NY 10032. Offers PhD. Terminal master's awarded for partial completion of doctoral program. *Degree requirements:* For doctorate, thesis/dissertation. *Entrance requirements:* For doctorate, GRE General Test, GRE Subject Test. Additional exam requirements/recommendations for international students: Required—TOEFL. *Expenses:* Contact institution. *Faculty research:* Transcription, macromolecular sorting, gene expression during development, cellular interaction.

Cornell University, Graduate School, Graduate Fields of Agriculture and Life Sciences, Field of Biochemistry, Molecular and Cell Biology, Ithaca, NY 14853-0001. Offers biochemistry (PhD); biophysics (PhD); cell biology (PhD); molecular biology (PhD). *Degree requirements:* For doctorate, comprehensive exam, thesis/dissertation, 2 semesters of teaching experience. *Entrance requirements:* For doctorate, GRE General Test, GRE Subject Test (biology, chemistry, physics, biochemistry, cell and molecular biology), 3 letters of recommendation. Additional exam requirements/recommendations for international students: Required—TOEFL (minimum score 600 paper-based; 77 iBT). Electronic applications accepted. *Faculty research:* Biophysics, structural biology.

Cornell University, Graduate School, Graduate Fields of Agriculture and Life Sciences and Graduate Fields of Human Ecology, Field of Nutrition, Ithaca, NY 14853-0001. Offers animal nutrition (MPS, PhD); community nutrition (MPS, PhD); human nutrition (MPS, PhD); international nutrition (MPS, PhD); molecular biochemistry (MPS, PhD). *Degree requirements:* For master's, thesis (MS), project papers (MPS); for doctorate, comprehensive exam, thesis/dissertation. *Entrance requirements:* For master's and doctorate, GRE General Test, previous course work in organic chemistry (with laboratory) and biochemistry; 2 letters of recommendation. Additional exam requirements/recommendations for international students: Required—TOEFL (minimum score 550 paper-based; 77 iBT). Electronic applications accepted. *Faculty research:* Nutritional biochemistry, experimental human and animal nutrition, international nutrition, community nutrition.

Dartmouth College, Graduate Program in Molecular and Cellular Biology, Hanover, NH 03755. Offers PhD, MBA/PhD, MD/PhD. *Faculty:* 72 full-time (19 women), 4 part-time/adjunct (1 woman). *Students:* 98 full-time (52 women); includes 17 minority (7 Asian,

non-Hispanic/Latino; 9 Hispanic/Latino; 1 Two or more races, non-Hispanic/Latino), 28 international. Average age 26. 193 applicants, 38% accepted, 30 enrolled. In 2015, 16 doctorates awarded. *Entrance requirements:* For doctorate, GRE General Test, letters of recommendation, minimum GPA of 3.0. Additional exam requirements/recommendations for international students: Required—TOEFL (minimum score paper-based 550, iBT 100) or IELTS (7.0). *Application deadline:* For fall admission, 12/1 for domestic students. Applications are processed on a rolling basis. Application fee: $75. Electronic applications accepted. *Expenses: Tuition, area resident:* Full-time $48,120. *Required fees:* $296. One-time fee: $50 full-time. *Financial support:* In 2015–16, fellowships with full tuition reimbursements (averaging $28,200 per year) were awarded; health care benefits also available. *Unit head:* Dr. Patrick J. Dolph, Chair, 603-650-1092, E-mail: mcb@dartmouth.edu. *Application contact:* Janet Cheney, Program Coordinator, 603-650-1612, Fax: 603-650-1006, E-mail: mcb@dartmouth.edu.
Website: http://dms.dartmouth.edu/mcb/

Drexel University, College of Medicine, Biomedical Graduate Programs, Interdisciplinary Program in Molecular and Cell Biology and Genetics, Philadelphia, PA 19104-2875. Offers MS, PhD, MD/PhD. Terminal master's awarded for partial completion of doctoral program. *Degree requirements:* For master's, comprehensive exam, thesis; for doctorate, thesis/dissertation, qualifying exam. *Entrance requirements:* For master's, GRE General Test, minimum GPA of 2.75; for doctorate, GRE General Test, minimum GPA of 3.0. Additional exam requirements/recommendations for international students: Required—TOEFL. Electronic applications accepted. *Faculty research:* Molecular anatomy, biochemistry, medical biotechnology, molecular pathology, microbiology and immunology.

Duke University, Graduate School, Department of Evolutionary Anthropology, Durham, NC 27708. Offers cellular and molecular biology (PhD); gross anatomy and physical anthropology (PhD), including comparative morphology of human and non-human primates, primate social behavior, vertebrate paleontology; neuroanatomy (PhD). *Degree requirements:* For doctorate, one foreign language, thesis/dissertation. *Entrance requirements:* For doctorate, GRE General Test. Additional exam requirements/recommendations for international students: Required—TOEFL (minimum score 577 paper-based; 90 iBT) or IELTS (minimum score 7). Electronic applications accepted.

Duke University, Graduate School, Program in Cell and Molecular Biology, Durham, NC 27710. Offers Certificate. Students must be enrolled in a participating PhD program (biology, cell biology, immunology, molecular genetics, neurobiology, pathology, pharmacology). *Entrance requirements:* Additional exam requirements/recommendations for international students: Required—TOEFL (minimum score 577 paper-based; 90 iBT) or IELTS (minimum score 7). Electronic applications accepted.

East Carolina University, Brody School of Medicine, Department of Biochemistry and Molecular Biology, Greenville, NC 27858-4353. Offers biochemistry and molecular biology (PhD); biomedical science (MS). *Students:* 7 full-time (4 women), 1 international. Average age 24. 15 applicants, 33% accepted, 4 enrolled. In 2015, 6 master's awarded. *Degree requirements:* For doctorate, comprehensive exam, thesis/dissertation. *Entrance requirements:* For doctorate, GRE General Test. Additional exam requirements/recommendations for international students: Required—TOEFL. *Application deadline:* For fall admission, 6/1 priority date for domestic students. Applications are processed on a rolling basis. *Financial support:* Fellowships with tuition reimbursements available. Financial award application deadline: 6/1. *Faculty research:* Gene regulation, development and differentiation, contractility and motility, macromolecular interactions, cancer. *Unit head:* Dr. Phillip H. Pekala, Chairman, 252-744-2684, Fax: 252-744-3383, E-mail: pekalap@ecu.edu.
Website: http://www.ecu.edu/cs-dhs/biochemistry/gradProgram.cfm

East Carolina University, Graduate School, Thomas Harriot College of Arts and Sciences, Department of Biology, Greenville, NC 27858-4353. Offers biology (MS); molecular biology and biotechnology (MS). *Program availability:* Part-time. *Students:* 41 full-time (22 women), 13 part-time (7 women); includes 6 minority (2 Black or African American, non-Hispanic/Latino; 2 Asian, non-Hispanic/Latino; 1 Hispanic/Latino; 1 Two or more races, non-Hispanic/Latino). Average age 26. 67 applicants, 51% accepted, 26 enrolled. In 2015, 12 master's awarded. *Degree requirements:* For master's, one foreign language, comprehensive exam, thesis. *Entrance requirements:* For master's, GRE General Test, GRE Subject Test. Additional exam requirements/recommendations for international students: Required—TOEFL. *Application deadline:* For fall admission, 6/1 priority date for domestic students; for spring admission, 10/15 for domestic students. Applications are processed on a rolling basis. Application fee: $50. *Financial support:* Fellowships with partial tuition reimbursements, research assistantships with partial tuition reimbursements, teaching assistantships with partial tuition reimbursements, career-related internships or fieldwork, Federal Work-Study, scholarships/grants, and unspecified assistantships available. Support available to part-time students. Financial award application deadline: 6/1. *Faculty research:* Biochemistry, microbiology, cell biology. *Unit head:* Dr. Jeff McKinnon, Chair, 252-328-6718, E-mail: mckinnonj@ecu.edu. *Application contact:* Dean of Graduate School, 252-328-6012, Fax: 252-328-6071, E-mail: gradschool@ecu.edu.
Website: http://www.ecu.edu/cs-cas/biology/graduate.cfm

Eastern Michigan University, Graduate School, College of Arts and Sciences, Department of Biology, Ypsilanti, MI 48197. Offers cell and molecular biology (MS); community college biology teaching (MS); ecology and organismal biology (MS); general biology (MS); water resources (MS). *Program availability:* Part-time, evening/weekend, online learning. *Faculty:* 26 full-time (8 women). *Students:* 15 full-time (9 women), 33 part-time (19 women); includes 8 minority (3 Black or African American, non-Hispanic/Latino; 2 Asian, non-Hispanic/Latino; 2 Hispanic/Latino; 1 Two or more races, non-Hispanic/Latino), 3 international. Average age 27. 47 applicants, 51% accepted, 19 enrolled. In 2015, 14 master's awarded. *Entrance requirements:* For master's, GRE General Test, GRE Subject Test. Additional exam requirements/recommendations for international students: Required—TOEFL. *Application deadline:* Applications are processed on a rolling basis. Application fee: $45. *Financial support:* Fellowships, research assistantships with full tuition reimbursements, teaching assistantships with full tuition reimbursements, career-related internships or fieldwork, Federal Work-Study, institutionally sponsored loans, scholarships/grants, tuition waivers (partial), and unspecified assistantships available. Support available to part-time students. Financial award applicants required to submit FAFSA. *Unit head:* Dr. Daniel Clemans, Department Head, 734-487-4242, Fax: 734-487-9235, E-mail: dclemans@emich.edu. *Application contact:* Dr. David Kass, Graduate Coordinator, 734-487-4242, Fax: 734-487-9235, E-mail: dkass@emich.edu.
Website: http://www.emich.edu/biology

Eastern New Mexico University, Graduate School, College of Liberal Arts and Sciences, Department of Biology, Portales, NM 88130. Offers applied ecology (MS); botany (MS); cell, molecular biology and biotechnology (MS); microbiology (MS); zoology (MS). *Program availability:* Part-time. *Degree requirements:* For master's, comprehensive exam, thesis optional. *Entrance requirements:* For master's, GRE, minimum GPA of 3.0, 2 letters of recommendation, statement of research interest, bachelor's degree related to field of study or proof of common knowledge. Additional exam requirements/recommendations for international students: Required—TOEFL

Molecular Biology

(minimum score 550 paper-based; 79 iBT), IELTS (minimum score 6). Electronic applications accepted.

Emory University, Laney Graduate School, Division of Biological and Biomedical Sciences, Program in Genetics and Molecular Biology, Atlanta, GA 30322-1100. Offers PhD. *Degree requirements:* For doctorate, comprehensive exam, thesis/dissertation. *Entrance requirements:* For doctorate, GRE General Test, minimum GPA of 3.0 in science course work (recommended). Additional exam requirements/recommendations for international students: Required—TOEFL. Electronic applications accepted. *Faculty research:* Gene regulation, genetic combination, developmental regulation.

Florida Institute of Technology, College of Science, Program in Biological Sciences, Melbourne, FL 32901-6975. Offers biological science (PhD); biotechnology (MS); cell and molecular biology (MS); ecology (MS); marine biology (MS). *Program availability:* Part-time. *Students:* 65 full-time (39 women), 10 part-time (3 women); includes 4 minority (2 Asian, non-Hispanic/Latino; 1 Two or more races, non-Hispanic/Latino), 38 international. Average age 26. 230 applicants, 24% accepted, 21 enrolled. In 2015, 23 master's, 3 doctorates awarded. *Degree requirements:* For master's, thesis (for some programs), research, seminar, internship, or summer lab; for doctorate, comprehensive exam, thesis/dissertation, dissertations seminar, publications. *Entrance requirements:* For master's, GRE General Test, 3 letters of recommendation; statement of objectives; bachelor's degree in biology, chemistry, biochemistry or equivalent; for doctorate, GRE General Test, resume, 3 letters of recommendation, minimum GPA of 3.2, statement of objectives. Additional exam requirements/recommendations for international students: Required—TOEFL (minimum score 550 paper-based; 79 iBT). *Application deadline:* For fall admission, 3/1 for domestic students, 4/1 for international students; for spring admission, 9/1 for domestic and international students. Applications are processed on a rolling basis. Electronic applications accepted. *Expenses: Tuition, area resident:* Full-time $21,690; part-time $1205 per credit hour. *Required fees:* $500. Tuition and fees vary according to degree level, campus/location and program. *Financial support:* Career-related internships or fieldwork, institutionally sponsored loans, tuition waivers (partial), unspecified assistantships, and tuition remissions available. Support available to part-time students. Financial award application deadline: 3/1; financial award applicants required to submit FAFSA. *Faculty research:* Initiation of protein synthesis in eukaryotic cells, fixation of radioactive carbon, changes in DNA molecule, endangered or threatened avian and mammalian species, hydroacoustics and feeding preference of the West Indian manatee. *Unit head:* Dr. Richard B. Aronson, Department Head, 321-674-8034, Fax: 321-674-7238, E-mail: raronson@fit.edu. *Application contact:* Cheryl A. Brown, Associate Director of Graduate Admissions, 321-674-7581, Fax: 321-723-9468, E-mail: cbrown@fit.edu.
Website: http://cos.fit.edu/biology/

Florida State University, The Graduate School, College of Arts and Sciences, Department of Biological Science, Specialization in Cell and Molecular Biology, Tallahassee, FL 32306-4295. Offers MS. *Faculty:* 25 full-time (7 women). *Students:* 62 full-time (28 women); includes 7 minority (1 Black or African American, non-Hispanic/Latino; 1 Asian, non-Hispanic/Latino; 5 Hispanic/Latino), 23 international. 113 applicants, 20% accepted, 9 enrolled. In 2015, 1 master's, 3 doctorates awarded. Terminal master's awarded for partial completion of doctoral program. *Degree requirements:* For master's, comprehensive exam, thesis, teaching experience, seminar presentation; for doctorate, comprehensive exam, thesis/dissertation, teaching experience; seminar presentation. *Entrance requirements:* For master's and doctorate, GRE General Test, minimum upper-division GPA of 3.0. Additional exam requirements/recommendations for international students: Required—TOEFL (minimum score 600 paper-based; 92 iBT). *Application deadline:* For fall admission, 12/1 for domestic and international students. Application fee: $30. Electronic applications accepted. *Expenses: Tuition, area resident:* Full-time $7263; part-time $403.50 per credit hour. Tuition, nonresident: full-time $18,087; part-time $1004.85 per credit hour. *Required fees:* $1365; $75.81 per credit hour. $20 per semester. Tuition and fees vary according to campus/location. *Financial support:* In 2015–16, 62 students received support, including 2 fellowships with full tuition reimbursements available (averaging $30,000 per year), 17 research assistantships with full tuition reimbursements available (averaging $21,500 per year), 43 teaching assistantships with full tuition reimbursements available (averaging $21,500 per year); scholarships/grants and unspecified assistantships also available. Financial award application deadline: 12/1; financial award applicants required to submit FAFSA. *Faculty research:* Molecular biology; genetics and genomics; developmental biology and gene expression; cell structure, function, and motility; cellular and organismal physiology; biophysical and structural biology. *Unit head:* Dr. Thomas A. Houpt, Professor and Associate Chair, 850-644-4907, Fax: 850-644-8447, E-mail: houpt@neuro.fsu.edu. *Application contact:* Dr. Michael B. Miller, Coordinator, Graduate Affairs, 850-644-3023, Fax: 850-644-8447, E-mail: gradinfo@bio.fsu.edu.
Website: http://www.bio.fsu.edu/cmb/

Georgetown University, Graduate School of Arts and Sciences, Department of Biochemistry and Molecular and Cellular Biology, Washington, DC 20057. Offers MS, PhD. *Degree requirements:* For doctorate, comprehensive exam, thesis/dissertation. *Entrance requirements:* For doctorate, GRE General Test. Additional exam requirements/recommendations for international students: Required—TOEFL.

Georgia State University, College of Arts and Sciences, Department of Biology, Program in Cellular and Molecular Biology and Physiology, Atlanta, GA 30302-3083. Offers bioinformatics (MS); cellular and molecular biology and physiology (MS, PhD). *Program availability:* Part-time. Terminal master's awarded for partial completion of doctoral program. *Degree requirements:* For master's, comprehensive exam (for some programs), thesis optional; for doctorate, comprehensive exam, thesis/dissertation. *Entrance requirements:* For master's and doctorate, GRE. Additional exam requirements/recommendations for international students: Required—TOEFL (minimum score 550 paper-based; 82 iBT) or IELTS (minimum score 7). *Application deadline:* For fall admission, 7/1 priority date for domestic students, 6/1 priority date for international students; for spring admission, 11/15 priority date for domestic students, 10/15 priority date for international students. Applications are processed on a rolling basis. Application fee: $50. Electronic applications accepted. *Expenses:* Tuition, state resident: full-time $6876; part-time $382 per credit hour. Tuition, nonresident: full-time $22,374; part-time $1243 per credit hour. *Required fees:* $2128; $2128 per term. $1064 per term. Part-time tuition and fees vary according to course load and program. *Financial support:* In 2015–16, fellowships with full tuition reimbursements (averaging $22,000 per year), research assistantships with full tuition reimbursements (averaging $20,000 per year) were awarded. Financial award application deadline: 12/3. *Faculty research:* Membrane transport, viral infection, molecular immunology, protein modeling, gene regulation. *Unit head:* Dr. Charles Derby, Director of Graduate Studies, 404-413-5393, Fax: 404-413-5446, E-mail: cderby@gsu.edu.
Website: http://biology.gsu.edu/

Grand Valley State University, College of Liberal Arts and Sciences, Program in Cell and Molecular Biology, Allendale, MI 49401-9403. Offers MS. *Faculty:* 9 full-time (6 women). *Students:* 25 full-time (17 women), 32 part-time (19 women); includes 4 minority (1 Black or African American, non-Hispanic/Latino; 2 Asian, non-Hispanic/Latino; 1 Hispanic/Latino), 14 international. Average age 27. 26 applicants, 85%

accepted, 22 enrolled. In 2015, 11 master's awarded. *Entrance requirements:* For master's, minimum GPA of 3.0. Application fee: $30. *Financial support:* In 2015–16, 22 students received support, including 2 fellowships (averaging $2,833 per year), 21 research assistantships with tuition reimbursements available (averaging $4,969 per year); unspecified assistantships also available. *Faculty research:* Plant cell biology, plant development, cell/signal integration. *Unit head:* Dr. Mark Staves, Associate Professor/Coordinator, 616-331-2473, E-mail: stavesm@gvsu.edu. *Application contact:* Dr. Tim Born, Coordinator, 616-331-8643, E-mail: bornt@gvsu.edu.

Harvard University, Graduate School of Arts and Sciences, Department of Molecular and Cellular Biology, Cambridge, MA 02138. Offers PhD. *Degree requirements:* For doctorate, thesis/dissertation, oral exam. *Entrance requirements:* For doctorate, GRE General Test, GRE Subject Test (recommended). Additional exam requirements/recommendations for international students: Required—TOEFL.

Harvard University, Graduate School of Arts and Sciences, Program in Chemical Biology, Cambridge, MA 02138. Offers PhD.

Hood College, Graduate School, Program in Biomedical Science, Frederick, MD 21701-8575. Offers bioinformatics (Certificate); biomedical science (MS), including biotechnology/molecular biology, microbiology/immunology/virology, regulatory compliance. *Program availability:* Part-time, evening/weekend. *Degree requirements:* For master's, comprehensive exam, thesis or alternative. *Entrance requirements:* For master's, bachelor's degree in biology; minimum GPA of 2.75; undergraduate course work in cell biology, chemistry, organic chemistry, and genetics. Additional exam requirements/recommendations for international students: Required—TOEFL (minimum score 575 paper-based; 89 iBT), IELTS (minimum score 6.5). *Application deadline:* For fall admission, 7/15 priority date for domestic students, 7/15 for international students; for spring admission, 12/1 priority date for domestic students, 12/1 for international students. Applications are processed on a rolling basis. Application fee: $35. Electronic applications accepted. Application fee is waived when completed online. *Expenses: Tuition, area resident:* Part-time $450 per credit hour. *Required fees:* $105 per term. Part-time tuition and fees vary according to degree level, campus/location and program. *Financial support:* Research assistantships with full tuition reimbursements, tuition waivers (partial), and unspecified assistantships available. Financial award applicants required to submit FAFSA.
Website: http://www.hood.edu/graduate

See Display on page 64 and Close-Up on page 109.

Howard University, College of Medicine, Department of Biochemistry and Molecular Biology, Washington, DC 20059-0002. Offers biochemistry and molecular biology (PhD); biotechnology (MS); MD/PhD. *Program availability:* Part-time. *Degree requirements:* For master's, externship; for doctorate, comprehensive exam, thesis/dissertation. *Entrance requirements:* For master's and doctorate, GRE General Test, minimum GPA of 3.0. *Faculty research:* Cellular and molecular biology of olfaction, gene regulation and expression, enzymology, NMR spectroscopy of molecular structure, hormone regulation/metabolism.

Illinois Institute of Technology, Graduate College, College of Science, Department of Biological Sciences, Chicago, IL 60616. Offers biochemistry (MS); biology (MS, PhD); cell and molecular biology (MS); microbiology (MS); molecular biochemistry and biophysics (MS, PhD). *Program availability:* Part-time, evening/weekend, online learning. Terminal master's awarded for partial completion of doctoral program. *Degree requirements:* For master's, comprehensive exam, thesis (for some programs); for doctorate, comprehensive exam, thesis/dissertation. *Entrance requirements:* For master's, GRE General Test (minimum score 300 Quantitative and Verbal, 2.5 Analytical Writing), minimum undergraduate GPA of 3.0; for doctorate, GRE General Test (minimum score 310 Quantitative and Verbal, 3.0 Analytical Writing); GRE Subject Test (strongly recommended), minimum undergraduate GPA of 3.0. Additional exam requirements/recommendations for international students: Required—TOEFL (minimum score 550 paper-based; 80 iBT). Electronic applications accepted. *Faculty research:* Macromolecular crystallography, insect immunity and basic cell biology, improvement of bacterial strains for enhanced biodesulfurization of petroleum, programmed cell death in cancer cells.

Illinois State University, Graduate School, College of Arts and Sciences, Department of Biological Sciences, Normal, IL 61790-2200. Offers animal behavior (MS); bacteriology (MS); biochemistry (MS); biological sciences (MS); biology (PhD); biophysics (MS); biotechnology (MS); botany (MS, PhD); cell biology (MS); conservation biology (MS); developmental biology (MS); ecology (MS, PhD); entomology (MS); evolutionary biology (MS); genetics (MS, PhD); immunology (MS); microbiology (MS, PhD); molecular biology (MS); molecular genetics (MS); neurobiology (MS); neuroscience (MS); parasitology (MS); physiology (MS, PhD); plant biology (MS); plant molecular biology (MS); plant sciences (MS); structural biology (MS); zoology (MS, PhD). *Program availability:* Part-time. *Degree requirements:* For master's, thesis or alternative; for doctorate, variable foreign language requirement, thesis/dissertation, 2 terms of residency. *Entrance requirements:* For master's, GRE General Test, minimum GPA of 2.6 in last 60 hours of course work; for doctorate, GRE General Test. *Application deadline:* Applications are processed on a rolling basis. Application fee: $40. *Financial support:* Research assistantships, teaching assistantships, Federal Work-Study, tuition waivers (full), and unspecified assistantships available. Financial award application deadline: 4/1. *Faculty research:* Redox balance and drug development in schistosoma mansoni, control of the growth of listeria monocytogenes at low temperature, regulation of cell expansion and microtubule function by SPR1, CRUI: physiology and fitness consequences of different life history phenotypes. *Application contact:* Steven Juliano, Graduate Coordinator, E-mail: sajulian@ilstu.edu.
Website: http://www.bio.ilstu.edu/

Indiana State University, College of Graduate and Professional Studies, College of Arts and Sciences, Department of Biology, Terre Haute, IN 47809. Offers cellular and molecular biology (PhD); ecology, systematics and evolution (PhD); life sciences (MS); physiology (PhD); science education (MS). *Degree requirements:* For master's, thesis optional; for doctorate, comprehensive exam, thesis/dissertation. *Entrance requirements:* For master's and doctorate, GRE General Test. Electronic applications accepted.

Indiana University Bloomington, University Graduate School, College of Arts and Sciences, Department of Biology, Bloomington, IN 47405. Offers biology teaching (MAT); biotechnology (MA); evolution, ecology, and behavior (MA, PhD); genetics (PhD); microbiology (MA, PhD); molecular, cellular, and developmental biology (PhD); plant sciences (MA, PhD); zoology (MA, PhD). Terminal master's awarded for partial completion of doctoral program. *Degree requirements:* For master's, thesis, oral defense; for doctorate, thesis/dissertation, oral defense. *Entrance requirements:* For master's and doctorate, GRE General Test. Additional exam requirements/recommendations for international students: Required—TOEFL (minimum score 100 iBT). Electronic applications accepted. *Faculty research:* Evolution, ecology and behavior; microbiology; molecular biology and genetics; plant biology.

Indiana University–Purdue University Indianapolis, Indiana University School of Medicine, Department of Biochemistry and Molecular Biology, Indianapolis, IN 46202.

Offers MS, PhD, MD/MS, MD/PhD. Terminal master's awarded for partial completion of doctoral program. *Degree requirements:* For master's, thesis; for doctorate, thesis/dissertation. *Entrance requirements:* For master's and doctorate, GRE General Test, GRE Subject Test (recommended), previous course work in organic chemistry. Additional exam requirements/recommendations for international students: Required—TOEFL. Electronic applications accepted. *Faculty research:* Metabolic regulation, enzymology, peptide and protein chemistry, cell biology, signal transduction.

Inter American University of Puerto Rico, Metropolitan Campus, Graduate Programs, Program in Medical Technology, San Juan, PR 00919-1293. Offers administration of clinical laboratories (MS); molecular microbiology (MS). *Accreditation:* NAACLS. *Program availability:* Part-time. *Degree requirements:* For master's, comprehensive exam. *Entrance requirements:* For master's, BS in medical technology, minimum GPA of 2.5. Electronic applications accepted.

Iowa State University of Science and Technology, Bioinformatics and Computational Biology Program, Ames, IA 50011. Offers MS, PhD. *Degree requirements:* For doctorate, thesis/dissertation. *Entrance requirements:* For master's and doctorate, GRE General Test. Additional exam requirements/recommendations for international students: Recommended—TOEFL, IELTS. Electronic applications accepted. *Faculty research:* Functional and structural genomics, genome evolution, macromolecular structure and function, mathematical biology and biological statistics, metabolic and developmental networks.

Iowa State University of Science and Technology, Program in Molecular, Cellular, and Developmental Biology, Ames, IA 50011. Offers MS, PhD. *Entrance requirements:* For master's and doctorate, GRE General Test. Additional exam requirements/recommendations for international students: Required—TOEFL (minimum score 580 paper based; 85 iBT), IELTS (minimum score 7). Electronic applications accepted.

Irell & Manella Graduate School of Biological Sciences, Graduate Program, Duarte, CA 91010. Offers brain metastatic cancer (PhD); cancer and stem cell metabolism (PhD); cancer biology (PhD); cancer biology and developmental therapeutics (PhD); cell biology (PhD); chemical biology (PhD); chromosomal break repair (PhD); diabetes and pancreatic progenitor cell biology (PhD); DNA repair and cancer biology (PhD); germline epigenetic remodeling and endocrine disruptors (PhD); hematology and hematopoietic cell transplantation (PhD); hematology and immunology (PhD); inflammation and cancer (PhD); micrornas and gene regulation in cardiovascular disease (PhD); mixed chimrism for reversal of autoimmunity (PhD); molecular and cellular biology (PhD); molecular biology and genetics (PhD); nanoparticle mediated twist1 silencing in metastatic cancer (PhD); neuro-oncology and stem cell biology (PhD); neuroscience (PhD); rna directed therapies for hiv-1 (PhD); small rna-induced transcriptional gene activation (PhD); stem cell regulation by the microenvironment (PhD); translational oncology and pharmaceutical sciences (PhD); tumor biology (PhD). *Faculty:* 70 full-time (18 women). *Students:* 75 full-time (40 women); includes 28 minority (2 Black or African American, non-Hispanic/Latino; 10 Asian, non-Hispanic/Latino; 10 Hispanic/Latino; 2 Native Hawaiian or other Pacific Islander, non-Hispanic/Latino; 4 Two or more races, non-Hispanic/Latino), 15 international. Average age 26. 197 applicants, 12% accepted, 19 enrolled. In 2015, 12 doctorates awarded. *Degree requirements:* For doctorate, comprehensive exam, thesis/dissertation, qualifying exams, two advanced courses. *Entrance requirements:* For doctorate, GRE General Test; GRE Subject Test (recommended), 2 years of course work in chemistry (general and organic); 1 year of course work each in biochemistry, general biology, and general physics; 2 semesters of course work in mathematics; significant research laboratory experience. Additional exam requirements/recommendations for international students: Required—TOEFL. *Application deadline:* For fall admission, 1/1 priority date for domestic and international students. Application fee: $0. Electronic applications accepted. Full-time tuition and fees vary according to class time, course level, course load, degree level, campus/location, program and student level. *Financial support:* In 2015–16, 12 students received support, including 35 fellowships with full tuition reimbursements available (averaging $32,000 per year); teaching assistantships, health care benefits, and tuition waivers (full) also available. Financial award applicants required to submit FAFSA. *Faculty research:* Cancer biology, diabetes, stem cell biology, neuroscience, immunology. *Unit head:* Dr. John J. Rossi, Dean, 877-715-GRAD, Fax: 626-471-3901, E-mail: gradschool@coh.org. *Application contact:* Dr. Kate Sleeth, Interim Associate Dean of Administration and Student Development, 626-218-1742, Fax: 626-471-3901, E-mail: gradschool@coh.org. Website: http://cityofhope.org/gradschool

See Display on page 66 and Close-Up on page 111.

Johns Hopkins University, Bloomberg School of Public Health, Department of Biochemistry and Molecular Biology, Baltimore, MD 21205. Offers MHS, Sc M, PhD. *Program availability:* Part-time. *Degree requirements:* For master's, thesis; for doctorate, comprehensive exam, thesis/dissertation, oral and written exams. *Entrance requirements:* For master's, MCAT or GRE, 3 letters of recommendation, curriculum vitae; for doctorate, GRE General Test, 3 letters of recommendation, curriculum vitae. Additional exam requirements/recommendations for international students: Required—TOEFL (minimum score 600 paper-based). Electronic applications accepted. *Faculty research:* DNA replication, repair, structure, carcinogenesis, protein structure, enzyme catalysts, reproductive biology.

Johns Hopkins University, National Institutes of Health Sponsored Programs, Baltimore, MD 21218. Offers biology (PhD), including biochemistry, biophysics, cell biology, developmental biology, genetic biology, molecular biology; cell, molecular, and developmental biology and biophysics (PhD). *Degree requirements:* For doctorate, comprehensive exam, thesis/dissertation. *Entrance requirements:* For doctorate, GRE General Test. Additional exam requirements/recommendations for international students: Required—TOEFL (minimum score 600 paper-based), TWE. Electronic applications accepted. *Faculty research:* Protein and nucleic acid biochemistry and biophysical chemistry, molecular biology and development.

Johns Hopkins University, School of Medicine, Graduate Programs in Medicine, Department of Pharmacology and Molecular Sciences, Baltimore, MD 21205. Offers PhD. *Degree requirements:* For doctorate, comprehensive exam, thesis/dissertation, departmental seminar. *Entrance requirements:* For doctorate, GRE General Test. Additional exam requirements/recommendations for international students: Required—TOEFL. Electronic applications accepted.

Johns Hopkins University, School of Medicine, Graduate Programs in Medicine, Predoctoral Training Program in Human Genetics, Baltimore, MD 21218. Offers PhD, MD/PhD. Terminal master's awarded for partial completion of doctoral program. *Degree requirements:* For doctorate, comprehensive exam, thesis/dissertation. *Entrance requirements:* For doctorate, GRE General Test, GRE Subject Test. Additional exam requirements/recommendations for international students: Recommended—TOEFL. Electronic applications accepted. *Faculty research:* Human, mammalian, and molecular genetics, bioinformatics, genomics.

Johns Hopkins University, School of Medicine, Graduate Programs in Medicine, Program in Biochemistry, Cellular and Molecular Biology, Baltimore, MD 21205. Offers PhD. *Degree requirements:* For doctorate, comprehensive exam, thesis/dissertation. *Entrance requirements:* For doctorate, GRE General Test. Additional exam

requirements/recommendations for international students: Required—TOEFL. Electronic applications accepted. *Faculty research:* Developmental biology, genomics/proteomics, protein targeting, signal transduction, structural biology.

Kent State University, College of Arts and Sciences, School of Biomedical Sciences, Kent, OH 44242-0001. Offers biological anthropology (PhD); cellular and molecular biology (PhD); cellular biology and structures, molecular biology and genetics; neurosciences (PhD); pharmacology (MS); physiology (PhD). *Students:* 76 full-time (46 women), 1 (woman) part-time; includes 6 minority (1 Black or African American, non-Hispanic/Latino; 2 Asian, non-Hispanic/Latino; 1 Hispanic/Latino; 2 Two or more races, non-Hispanic/Latino), 28 international. Average age 29. 223 applicants, 13% accepted, 22 enrolled. In 2015, 5 master's, 7 doctorates awarded. Terminal master's awarded for partial completion of doctoral program. *Degree requirements:* For master's, thesis; for doctorate, thesis/dissertation, candidacy exam. *Entrance requirements:* For master's and doctorate, GRE General Test, minimum GPA of 3.0, transcript, goal statement, resume, 3 letters of recommendation. Additional exam requirements/recommendations for international students: Required—TOEFL (minimum score: paper-based 525, iBT 71), Michigan English Language Assessment Battery (minimum score of 75), IELTS (minimum score of 6.0), PTE Academic (minimum score of 48), or completion of ELS level 112 Intensive Program. *Application deadline:* For fall admission, 1/1 for domestic students. Application fee: $45 ($70 for international students). Electronic applications accepted. *Expenses:* Tuition, state resident: full-time $10,864; part-time $495 per credit hour. Tuition, nonresident: full-time $18,380; part-time $837 per credit hour. *Financial support:* In 2015–16, 76 students received support. Research assistantships with full tuition reimbursements available, teaching assistantships, career-related internships or fieldwork, Federal Work-Study, and unspecified assistantships available. Financial award application deadline: 1/1. *Unit head:* Dr. Eric Mintz, Director, 330-672-2263, E-mail: emintz@kent.edu. *Application contact:* 330-672-2263, Fax: 330-672-9391, E-mail: jwearden@kent.edu.
Website: http://www.kent.edu/biomedical/

Lehigh University, College of Arts and Sciences, Department of Biological Sciences, Bethlehem, PA 18015. Offers biochemistry (PhD); cell and molecular biology (PhD); integrative biology (PhD); molecular biology (MS). *Program availability:* Part-time, 100% online. *Faculty:* 19 full-time (9 women). *Students:* 38 full-time (22 women), 21 part-time (15 women); includes 13 minority (5 Black or African American, non-Hispanic/Latino; 1 American Indian or Alaska Native, non-Hispanic/Latino; 6 Hispanic/Latino; 1 Two or more races, non-Hispanic/Latino), 5 international. Average age 27. 38 applicants, 50% accepted, 10 enrolled. In 2015, 6 master's, 1 doctorate awarded. Terminal master's awarded for partial completion of doctoral program. *Degree requirements:* For master's, thesis optional; for doctorate, comprehensive exam, thesis/dissertation. *Entrance requirements:* For doctorate, GRE General Test. Additional exam requirements/recommendations for international students: Required—TOEFL (minimum score 85 iBT). *Application deadline:* For fall admission, 12/15 for domestic and international students. Application fee: $75. *Expenses:* $1,185 per credit hour tuition (PhD); $925 per credit hour tuition (MS). *Financial support:* In 2015–16, 34 students received support, including 8 fellowships with full tuition reimbursements available (averaging $29,667 per year), 6 research assistantships with full tuition reimbursements available (averaging $27,000 per year), 19 teaching assistantships with full tuition reimbursements available (averaging $27,000 per year); scholarships/grants also available. Financial award application deadline: 12/15. *Faculty research:* Gene expression, cytoskeleton and cell structure, cell cycle and growth regulation, neuroscience, animal behavior, microbiology. Total annual research expenditures: $1.9 million. *Unit head:* Dr. Murray Itzkowitz, Chairperson, 610-758-3680, Fax: 610-758-4004, E-mail: mi00@lehigh.edu. *Application contact:* Dr. Mary Kathryn Iovine, Graduate Coordinator, 610-758-6981, Fax: 610-758-4004, E-mail: mki3@lehigh.edu.
Website: http://www.lehigh.edu/~inbios/

Lipscomb University, Program in Biomolecular Science, Nashville, TN 37204-3951. Offers MS. *Program availability:* Part-time, evening/weekend. *Faculty:* 5 full-time (3 women), 1 part-time/adjunct (0 women). *Students:* 21 full-time (9 women), 5 part-time (3 women); includes 6 minority (4 Black or African American, non-Hispanic/Latino; 1 Hispanic/Latino; 1 Two or more races, non-Hispanic/Latino). Average age 26. 75 applicants, 24% accepted, 13 enrolled. In 2015, 18 master's awarded. *Degree requirements:* For master's, capstone project. *Entrance requirements:* For master's, GRE (minimum score of 300/1000 on prior scoring system), MCAT (minimum score of 24), DAT (minimum score of 17), BS in related field, transcripts, minimum undergraduate GPA of 3.0, 2 letters of recommendation, resume. Additional exam requirements/recommendations for international students: Required—TOEFL (minimum score 570 paper-based). *Application deadline:* For fall admission, 8/1 for domestic students; for winter admission, 12/14 for domestic students; for spring admission, 5/14 for domestic students. Applications are processed on a rolling basis. Application fee: $50 ($75 for international students). Electronic applications accepted. *Expenses:* $934 per credit hour. *Financial support:* Unspecified assistantships available. Financial award applicants required to submit FAFSA. *Unit head:* Dr. Kent Gallaher, Director, 615-966-5721, E-mail: kent.gallaher@lipscomb.edu. *Application contact:* Tina Fulford, Administrative Assistant, 615-966-5330, E-mail: tina.fulford@lipscomb.edu.
Website: http://www.lipscomb.edu/biology/Graduate-Program

Louisiana State University Health Sciences Center at Shreveport, Department of Biochemistry and Molecular Biology, Shreveport, LA 71130-3932. Offers MS, PhD, MD/PhD. *Faculty:* 13 full-time (3 women). *Students:* 12 full-time (6 women), 10 international. Average age 28. 16 applicants, 31% accepted, 3 enrolled. In 2015, 1 master's, 3 doctorates awarded. *Degree requirements:* For master's, thesis; for doctorate, thesis/dissertation. *Entrance requirements:* For master's and doctorate, GRE General Test. Additional exam requirements/recommendations for international students: Required—TOEFL (minimum score 100 iBT), IELTS (minimum score 7). *Application deadline:* For fall admission, 3/15 for domestic and international students. Applications are processed on a rolling basis. Electronic applications accepted. *Expenses:* Contact institution. *Financial support:* In 2015–16, 3 fellowships (averaging $28,000 per year), 9 research assistantships (averaging $26,000 per year) were awarded. *Faculty research:* Yeast genetics, prostate cancer, cell biology, mTOR signaling, Parkinson's Disease, transcriptional mechanisms, chromatin, DNA repair and damage response, protein synthesis, neuroscience, diabetes, cell cycle regulation, tRNA synthetases, stress response, glucose transporters, transmigration and wound repair. *Unit head:* Dr. Stephan N. Witt, Interim Head, 318-675-5161, Fax: 318-675-5180. *Application contact:* April Coutee, Coordinator, 318-675-5160, Fax: 318-675-5180, E-mail: admissions-bmb@lsuhsc.edu.

Louisiana Tech University, Graduate School, College of Applied and Natural Sciences, School of Biological Sciences, Ruston, LA 71272. Offers biology (MS); molecular sciences and nanotechnology (MS). *Program availability:* Part-time. *Degree requirements:* For master's, thesis or alternative. *Entrance requirements:* For master's, GRE General Test, GRE Subject Test. *Application deadline:* For fall admission, 7/29 priority date for domestic students; for spring admission, 2/3 for domestic students. Applications are processed on a rolling basis. Application fee: $20 ($30 for international students). *Financial support:* Fellowships, research assistantships, and teaching assistantships available. Financial award application deadline: 2/1. *Faculty research:*

Genetics, animal biology, plant biology. *Unit head:* Dr. William J. Campbell, Director, 318-257-4573, Fax: 318-257-4574, E-mail: campbell@latech.edu.
Website: http://ans.latech.edu/bls.html

Loyola University Chicago, Graduate School, Integrated Program in Biomedical Sciences, Maywood, IL 60153. Offers biochemistry and molecular biology (MS, PhD); cell and molecular physiology (PhD); infectious disease and immunology (MS); integrative cell biology (PhD); medical physiology (MS); microbiology and immunology (MS, PhD); molecular pharmacology and therapeutics (MS, PhD); neuroscience (MS, PhD). *Students:* 135 full-time (65 women), 1 part-time (0 women); includes 28 minority (5 Black or African American, non-Hispanic/Latino; 15 Asian, non-Hispanic/Latino; 6 Hispanic/Latino; 2 Two or more races, non-Hispanic/Latino), 16 international. Average age 28. 442 applicants, 23% accepted, 55 enrolled. In 2015, 40 master's, 17 doctorates awarded. *Expenses: Tuition, area resident:* Full-time $18,054; part-time $9027 per credit hour. *Required fees:* $832; $284 per credit hour. Part-time tuition and fees vary according to course load, degree level and program. *Unit head:* Dr. Samuel Attoh, Dean, 773-508-3459, Fax: 773-508-2460, E-mail: sattoh@luc.edu. *Application contact:* Ron Martin, Associate Director of Enrollment Management, 312-915-8950, Fax: 312-915-8905, E-mail: gradapp@luc.edu.
Website: http://ssom.luc.edu/graduate_school/degree-programs/ipbsphd/

Marquette University, Graduate School, College of Arts and Sciences, Department of Biology, Milwaukee, WI 53201-1881. Offers cell biology (MS, PhD); developmental biology (MS, PhD); ecology (MS, PhD); epithelial physiology (MS, PhD); genetics (MS, PhD); microbiology (MS, PhD); molecular biology (MS, PhD); muscle and exercise physiology (MS, PhD); neuroscience (PhD). *Faculty:* 22 full-time (7 women), 3 part-time/adjunct (2 women). *Students:* 28 full-time (11 women), 12 part-time (4 women); includes 4 minority (1 Asian, non-Hispanic/Latino; 1 Hispanic/Latino; 2 Two or more races, non-Hispanic/Latino), 11 international. Average age 27. 72 applicants, 28% accepted, 5 enrolled. In 2015, 2 master's, 4 doctorates awarded. Terminal master's awarded for partial completion of doctoral program. *Degree requirements:* For master's, comprehensive exam, thesis, 1 year of teaching experience or equivalent; for doctorate, comprehensive exam, thesis/dissertation, 1 year of teaching experience or equivalent, qualifying exam. *Entrance requirements:* For master's and doctorate, GRE General Test, GRE Subject Test, official transcripts from all current and previous colleges/universities except Marquette, statement of professional goals and aspirations, three letters of recommendation. Additional exam requirements/recommendations for international students: Required—TOEFL (minimum score 530 paper-based). *Application deadline:* For fall admission, 12/15 for domestic and international students. Application fee: $50. Electronic applications accepted. *Financial support:* In 2015–16, 9 students received support, including 6 fellowships (averaging $1,208 per year), 4 research assistantships with full tuition reimbursements available (averaging $21,750 per year), 29 teaching assistantships with full tuition reimbursements available (averaging $21,750 per year); scholarships/grants, health care benefits, tuition waivers (full and partial), and unspecified assistantships also available. Support available to part-time students. Financial award application deadline: 2/15. *Faculty research:* Neurobiology, neuroendocrinology, epithelial physiology, neuropeptide interactions, synaptic transmission. *Total annual research expenditures:* $1.2 million. *Unit head:* Dr. Ed Blumenthal, Chair, 414-288-1748. *Application contact:* Dr. Michael Schlappi, Recruiting Contact, 414-288-1467.
Website: http://www.marquette.edu/biology/

Massachusetts Institute of Technology, School of Science, Department of Biology, Cambridge, MA 02139. Offers biochemistry (PhD); biological oceanography (PhD); biology (PhD); biophysical chemistry and molecular structure (PhD); cell biology (PhD); computational and systems biology (PhD); developmental biology (PhD); genetics (PhD); immunology (PhD); microbiology (PhD); molecular biology (PhD); neurobiology (PhD). *Faculty:* 57 full-time (14 women). *Students:* 283 full-time (137 women); includes 83 minority (3 Black or African American, non-Hispanic/Latino; 1 American Indian or Alaska Native, non-Hispanic/Latino; 38 Asian, non-Hispanic/Latino; 31 Hispanic/Latino; 10 Two or more races, non-Hispanic/Latino), 48 international. Average age 26. 673 applicants, 14% accepted, 46 enrolled. In 2015, 32 doctorates awarded. *Degree requirements:* For doctorate, comprehensive exam, thesis/dissertation, teaching assistantship during two semesters. *Entrance requirements:* For doctorate, GRE General Test. Additional exam requirements/recommendations for international students: Required—TOEFL (minimum score 577 paper-based), IELTS. *Application deadline:* For fall admission, 12/1 for domestic and international students. Application fee: $75. Electronic applications accepted. *Expenses: Tuition:* Full-time $46,400; part-time $725 per credit. One-time fee: $304 full-time. Full-time tuition and fees vary according to course load and program. *Financial support:* In 2015–16, 235 students received support, including 118 fellowships (averaging $37,500 per year), 163 research assistantships (averaging $38,900 per year), 1 teaching assistantship; Federal Work-Study, institutionally sponsored loans, scholarships/grants, traineeships, health care benefits, and unspecified assistantships also available. Support available to part-time students. Financial award application deadline: 4/15; financial award applicants required to submit FAFSA. *Faculty research:* Cellular, developmental and molecular (plant and animal) biology; biochemistry, bioengineering, biophysics and structural biology; classical and molecular genetics, stem cell and epigenetics; immunology and microbiology; cancer biology, molecular medicine, neurobiology and human disease; computational and systems biology. *Total annual research expenditures:* $42.8 million. *Unit head:* Prof. Alan Grossman, Department Head, 617-253-4701. *Application contact:* Biology Education Office, 617-253-3717, Fax: 617-258-9329, E-mail: gradbio@mit.edu.
Website: https://biology.mit.edu/

Mayo Graduate School, Graduate Programs in Biomedical Sciences, Programs in Biochemistry, Structural Biology, Cell Biology, and Genetics, Rochester, MN 55905. Offers biochemistry and structural biology (PhD); cell biology and genetics (PhD); molecular biology (PhD). *Degree requirements:* For doctorate, oral defense of dissertation, qualifying oral and written exam. *Entrance requirements:* For doctorate, GRE, 1 year of chemistry, biology, calculus, and physics. Additional exam requirements/recommendations for international students: Required—TOEFL. Electronic applications accepted. *Faculty research:* Gene structure and function, membranes and receptors/cytoskeleton, oncogenes and growth factors, protein structure and function, steroid hormonal action.

McMaster University, Faculty of Health Sciences and School of Graduate Studies, Program in Medical Sciences, Hamilton, ON L8S 4M2, Canada. Offers blood and vascular (M Sc, PhD); genetics and cancer (M Sc, PhD); immunity and infection (M Sc, PhD); metabolism and nutrition (M Sc, PhD); neurosciences and behavioral sciences (M Sc, PhD); physiology/pharmacology (M Sc, PhD); MD/PhD. *Degree requirements:* For master's, thesis; for doctorate, comprehensive exam, thesis/dissertation. *Entrance requirements:* For master's, honors B Sc, B+ average in related field; for doctorate, M Sc, minimum B+ average. Additional exam requirements/recommendations for international students: Required—TOEFL (minimum score 580 paper-based; 92 iBT).

Medical University of South Carolina, College of Graduate Studies, Department of Biochemistry and Molecular Biology, Charleston, SC 29425. Offers MS, PhD, MD/PhD. Terminal master's awarded for partial completion of doctoral program. *Degree requirements:* For master's, thesis, oral exam/thesis defense; for doctorate, thesis/dissertation, oral and written exams/dissertation defense. *Entrance requirements:* For master's, GRE General Test; for doctorate, GRE General Test, interview, minimum GPA of 3.0. Additional exam requirements/recommendations for international students: Required—TOEFL (minimum score 600 paper-based; 100 iBT). Electronic applications accepted. *Faculty research:* Lipid biochemistry, DNA replication, nucleic acids, protein structure.

Medical University of South Carolina, College of Graduate Studies, Program in Molecular and Cellular Biology and Pathobiology, Charleston, SC 29425. Offers cancer biology (PhD); cardiovascular biology (PhD); cardiovascular imaging (PhD); cell regulation (PhD); craniofacial biology (PhD); genetics and development (PhD); marine biomedicine (PhD); DMD/PhD; MD/PhD. *Degree requirements:* For doctorate, thesis/dissertation, oral and written exams. *Entrance requirements:* For doctorate, GRE General Test, interview, minimum GPA of 3.0. Additional exam requirements/recommendations for international students: Required—TOEFL (minimum score 600 paper-based; 100 iBT). Electronic applications accepted.

Michigan State University, The Graduate School, College of Agriculture and Natural Resources, MSU-DOE Plant Research Laboratory, East Lansing, MI 48824. Offers biochemistry and molecular biology (PhD); cellular and molecular biology (PhD); crop and soil sciences (PhD); genetics (PhD); microbiology and molecular genetics (PhD); plant biology (PhD); plant physiology (PhD). Offered jointly with the Department of Energy. *Degree requirements:* For doctorate, comprehensive exam, thesis/dissertation, laboratory rotation, defense of dissertation. *Entrance requirements:* For doctorate, GRE General Test, acceptance into one of the affiliated department programs; 3 letters of recommendation; bachelor's degree or equivalent in life sciences, chemistry, biochemistry, or biophysics; research experience. Electronic applications accepted. *Faculty research:* Role of hormones in the regulation of plant development and physiology, molecular mechanisms associated with signal recognition, development and application of genetic methods and materials, protein routing and function.

Michigan State University, The Graduate School, College of Natural Science and Graduate Programs in Human Medicine and Graduate Studies in Osteopathic Medicine, Department of Biochemistry and Molecular Biology, East Lansing, MI 48824. Offers biochemistry and molecular biology (MS, PhD); biochemistry and molecular biology/environmental toxicology (PhD). *Entrance requirements:* Additional exam requirements/recommendations for international students: Required—TOEFL. Electronic applications accepted.

Michigan State University, The Graduate School, College of Natural Science, Program in Cell and Molecular Biology, East Lansing, MI 48824. Offers cell and molecular biology (MS, PhD); cell and molecular biology/environmental toxicology (PhD). *Entrance requirements:* Additional exam requirements/recommendations for international students: Required—TOEFL. Electronic applications accepted.

Michigan Technological University, Graduate School, Interdisciplinary Programs, Houghton, MI 49931. Offers atmospheric sciences (PhD); biochemistry and molecular biology (PhD); computational science and engineering (PhD); data science (MS, Graduate Certificate); engineering (M Eng); environmental engineering (PhD); international profile (Graduate Certificate); nanotechnology (Graduate Certificate); sustainability (Graduate Certificate); sustainable water resources systems (Graduate Certificate). *Program availability:* Part-time. *Faculty:* 118 full-time (26 women), 12 part-time/adjunct. *Students:* 53 full-time (22 women), 10 part-time; includes 2 minority (1 Asian, non-Hispanic/Latino; 1 Two or more races, non-Hispanic/Latino), 44 international. Average age 30. 300 applicants, 19% accepted, 17 enrolled. In 2015, 3 master's, 7 doctorates, 4 other advanced degrees awarded. Terminal master's awarded for partial completion of doctoral program. *Degree requirements:* For master's, comprehensive exam (for some programs), thesis (for some programs); for doctorate, comprehensive exam, thesis/dissertation. *Entrance requirements:* For master's, doctorate, and Graduate Certificate, GRE, statement of purpose, personal statement, official transcripts, 2-3 letters of recommendation. Additional exam requirements/recommendations for international students: Required—TOEFL or IELTS. *Application deadline:* Applications are processed on a rolling basis. Electronic applications accepted. *Expenses:* Tuition, state resident: full-time $15,507; part-time $861.50 per credit. Tuition, nonresident: full-time $15,507; part-time $861.50 per credit. *Required fees:* $248; $248. Tuition and fees vary according to course load and program. *Financial support:* In 2015–16, 41 students received support, including 7 fellowships with tuition reimbursements available (averaging $14,516 per year), 16 research assistantships with tuition reimbursements available (averaging $14,516 per year), 9 teaching assistantships with tuition reimbursements available (averaging $14,516 per year); career-related internships or fieldwork, Federal Work-Study, scholarships/grants, health care benefits, unspecified assistantships, and cooperative program also available. Financial award applicants required to submit FAFSA. *Faculty research:* Big data, atmospheric sciences, bioinformatics and systems biology, molecular dynamics, environmental studies. *Unit head:* Dr. Jacqueline E. Huntoon, Provost and Vice President for Academic Affairs, 906-487-2440, Fax: 906-487-2284, E-mail: jeh@mtu.edu. *Application contact:* Carol T. Wingeron, Administrative Aide, 906-487-2328, Fax: 906-487-2284, E-mail: gradadms@mtu.edu.

Middle Tennessee State University, College of Graduate Studies, College of Basic and Applied Sciences, Interdisciplinary Program in Molecular Biosciences, Murfreesboro, TN 37132. Offers PhD. *Degree requirements:* For doctorate, comprehensive exam, thesis/dissertation. *Entrance requirements:* For doctorate, GRE. Additional exam requirements/recommendations for international students: Required—TOEFL (minimum score 525 paper-based; 71 iBT) or IELTS (minimum score 6). Electronic applications accepted.

Mississippi State University, College of Agriculture and Life Sciences, Department of Biochemistry, Molecular Biology, Entomology and Plant Pathology, Mississippi State, MS 39762. Offers agriculture life sciences (MS), including biochemistry (MS, PhD); entomology (MS, PhD), plant pathology (MS, PhD); life science (PhD), including biochemistry (MS, PhD), entomology (MS, PhD), plant pathology (MS, PhD); molecular biology (PhD). *Faculty:* 32 full-time (6 women), 2 part-time/adjunct (1 woman). *Students:* 44 full-time (20 women), 11 part-time (6 women); includes 6 minority (3 Black or African American, non-Hispanic/Latino; 1 Asian, non-Hispanic/Latino; 1 Hispanic/Latino; 1 Two or more races, non-Hispanic/Latino), 12 international. Average age 29. 35 applicants, 40% accepted, 12 enrolled. In 2015, 12 master's, 7 doctorates awarded. Terminal master's awarded for partial completion of doctoral program. *Degree requirements:* For master's, thesis (for some programs), final oral exam; for doctorate, thesis/dissertation, preliminary oral and written exam. *Entrance requirements:* For master's, GRE General Test, minimum GPA of 2.75; for doctorate, GRE. Additional exam requirements/recommendations for international students: Required—TOEFL (minimum score 500 paper-based; 61 iBT); Recommended—IELTS (minimum score 5.5). *Application deadline:* For fall admission, 7/1 for domestic students, 5/1 for international students; for spring admission, 11/1 for domestic students, 9/1 for international students. Applications are processed on a rolling basis. Application fee: $60. Electronic applications accepted. *Expenses:* Tuition, area resident: Full-time $7502; part-time $833.74 per credit hour. Tuition, nonresident: full-time $20,142; part-time $2238.24 per credit hour. *Financial support:* In 2015–16, 40 research assistantships with full tuition reimbursements (averaging $16,730 per year) were awarded; Federal Work-Study, institutionally

sponsored loans, and unspecified assistantships also available. Financial award application deadline: 4/1; financial award applicants required to submit FAFSA. *Faculty research:* Fish nutrition, plant and animal molecular biology, plant biochemistry, enzymology, lipid metabolism, chromatin, cell wall synthesis in rice, a model grass bioenergy species and the source of rice Stover residues using reverse genetic and functional genomic and proteomic approaches. *Unit head:* Dr. Jeffrey Dean, Professor and Department Head, 662-325-0643, Fax: 662-325-8664, E-mail: jd1891@msstate.edu. *Application contact:* Marina Hunt, Admissions Assistant, 662-325-5188, E-mail: mhunt@grad.msstate.edu.
Website: http://www.biochemistry.msstate.edu

Missouri State University, Graduate College, College of Health and Human Services, Department of Biomedical Sciences, Program in Cell and Molecular Biology, Springfield, MO 65897. Offers MS. *Program availability:* Part-time. *Students:* 9 full-time (5 women), 3 part-time (2 women); includes 2 minority (1 Asian, non-Hispanic/Latino; 1 Hispanic/Latino), 2 international. Average age 25. 21 applicants, 43% accepted, 7 enrolled. In 2015, 4 master's awarded. *Degree requirements:* For master's, thesis or alternative, oral and written exams. *Entrance requirements:* For master's, GRE General Test, 2 semesters of course work in organic chemistry and physics, 1 semester of course work in calculus, minimum GPA of 3.0 in last 60 hours of course work. Additional exam requirements/recommendations for international students: Required—TOEFL (minimum score 550 paper-based; 79 iBT), IELTS (minimum score 6). *Application deadline:* For fall admission, 7/20 priority date for domestic students, 5/1 for international students; for spring admission, 12/20 priority date for domestic students, 9/1 for international students. Applications are processed on a rolling basis. Application fee: $35 ($50 for international students). Electronic applications accepted. *Expenses:* Tuition, state resident: full-time $5500. Tuition, nonresident: full-time $10,108. *Required fees:* $1000. *Financial support:* In 2015–16, 11 research assistantships (averaging $8,600 per year) were awarded; career-related internships or fieldwork, Federal Work-Study, institutionally sponsored loans, scholarships/grants, and unspecified assistantships also available. Support available to part-time students. Financial award application deadline: 3/31; financial award applicants required to submit FAFSA. *Faculty research:* Extracellular matrix membrane protein, P2 nucleotide receptors, double stranded RNA viruses. *Unit head:* Dr. Scott Zimmerman, Program Director, 417-836-5478, Fax: 417-836-5588, E-mail: scottzimmerman@missouristate.edu. *Application contact:* Michael Edwards, Coordinator of Graduate Admissions, 417-836-5033, Fax: 417-836-6200, E-mail: michaeledwards@missouristate.edu.
Website: http://www.missouristate.edu/bms/CMB/

Montclair State University, The Graduate School, College of Science and Mathematics, Molecular Biology Certificate Program, Montclair, NJ 07043-1624. Offers Certificate. *Students:* 7 part-time (4 women); includes 4 minority (1 Black or African American, non-Hispanic/Latino; 1 Asian, non-Hispanic/Latino; 2 Hispanic/Latino). Average age 27. 5 applicants, 60% accepted, 2 enrolled. In 2015, 3 Certificates awarded. *Degree requirements:* For Certificate, thesis optional. Application fee: $60. *Expenses:* Tuition, state resident: part-time $553 per credit. Tuition, nonresident: part-time $854 per credit. *Required fees:* $91 per credit. Tuition and fees vary according to program. *Unit head:* Dr. Quinn Vega, Coordinator, 973-655-7178, E-mail: vegaq@mail.montclair.edu. *Application contact:* Amy Aiello, Director of Graduate Admissions and Operations, 973-655-5147, Fax: 973-655-7869, E-mail: graduate.school@montclair.edu.

Montclair State University, The Graduate School, College of Science and Mathematics, MS Program in Molecular Biology, Montclair, NJ 07043-1624. Offers MS. *Students:* 14 full-time (6 women), 23 part-time (17 women); includes 16 minority (5 Black or African American, non-Hispanic/Latino; 2 Asian, non-Hispanic/Latino; 7 Hispanic/Latino; 2 Two or more races, non-Hispanic/Latino), 4 international. Average age 29. 26 applicants, 62% accepted, 12 enrolled. In 2015, 13 master's awarded. *Degree requirements:* For master's, thesis optional. Application fee: $60. *Expenses:* Tuition, state resident: part-time $553 per credit. Tuition, nonresident: part-time $854 per credit. *Required fees:* $91 per credit. Tuition and fees vary according to program. *Unit head:* Dr. Quinn Vega, Coordinator, 973-655-7178, E-mail: vegaq@mail.montclair.edu. *Application contact:* Amy Aiello, Director of Graduate Admissions and Operations, 973-655-5147, Fax: 973-655-7869, E-mail: graduate.school@montclair.edu.

New Mexico State University, Graduate School, Program in Molecular Biology, Las Cruces, NM 88003-8001. Offers MS, PhD. *Program availability:* Part-time. *Students:* 9 full-time (7 women), 2 part-time (both women), 8 international. Average age 32. 14 applicants, 14% accepted, 2 enrolled. In 2015, 2 master's, 2 doctorates awarded. *Degree requirements:* For master's, thesis, oral seminars; for doctorate, comprehensive exam, thesis/dissertation, oral seminars. *Entrance requirements:* For master's and doctorate, GRE General Test, minimum GPA of 3.3. Additional exam requirements/recommendations for international students: Required—TOEFL (minimum score 550 paper-based; 79 iBT), IELTS (minimum score 6.5). *Application deadline:* For fall admission, 12/15 for domestic and international students; for spring admission, 10/15 for domestic and international students. Applications are processed on a rolling basis. Application fee: $40 ($50 for international students). Electronic applications accepted. *Expenses:* $274.50 per credit hour for in-state students, and all students enrolled in six or fewer credits; $839.30 per credit hour for out-of-state and international students enrolled in at least seven hours. *Financial support:* In 2015–16, 9 students received support, including 5 research assistantships (averaging $18,016 per year), 3 teaching assistantships (averaging $18,151 per year); career-related internships or fieldwork, Federal Work-Study, scholarships/grants, health care benefits, and unspecified assistantships also available. Financial award application deadline: 3/1. *Faculty research:* Emerging pathogens, plant-molecular biology and virology, molecular symbiotic interactions, cell and organismal biology, applied and environmental microbiology. *Unit head:* Dr. Charles B. Shuster, Program Head, 575-646-1325, Fax: 575-646-5665, E-mail: cshuster@nmsu.edu. *Application contact:* Nancy Treffler-McDow, Administrative Assistant, 575-646-3437, Fax: 575-646-8087, E-mail: nancyt@nmsu.edu.
Website: http://molb.research.nmsu.edu

New York Medical College, Graduate School of Basic Medical Sciences, Biochemistry and Molecular Biology - Master's Program, Valhalla, NY 10595-1691. Offers MS, MD/PhD. *Program availability:* Part-time, evening/weekend. *Degree requirements:* For master's, thesis. *Entrance requirements:* For master's, GRE General Test, MCAT, or DAT. Additional exam requirements/recommendations for international students: Required—TOEFL. Electronic applications accepted. *Expenses:* Tuition, area resident: Full-time $44,355; part-time $1025 per credit. *Required fees:* $500; $95 per year. One-time fee: $140 part-time. Tuition and fees vary according to course load and program. *Faculty research:* Expression, mechanisms of hormone action and cell signaling, enzymology, mechanisms of DNA replication and repair, cell cycle regulation, control of cell growth, molecular biology of cancer cells and the cancer process, mechanisms of nutrition and cancer prevention, molecular neurobiology and studies of neurodegenerative disorders, the aging process.

New York Medical College, Graduate School of Basic Medical Sciences, Integrated PhD Program, Valhalla, NY 10595-1691. Offers biochemistry and molecular biology (PhD); cell biology and anatomy (PhD); microbiology and immunology (PhD); pathology (PhD); pharmacology (PhD); physiology (PhD). *Degree requirements:* For doctorate, comprehensive exam, thesis/dissertation. *Entrance requirements:* For doctorate, GRE General Test. Additional exam requirements/recommendations for international students: Required—TOEFL. Electronic applications accepted. *Expenses: Tuition, area resident:* Full-time $44,355; part-time $1025 per credit. *Required fees:* $500; $95 per year. One-time fee: $140 part-time. Tuition and fees vary according to course load and program. *Faculty research:* Cardiovascular sciences, infectious diseases, neuroscience, cancer and cell signaling.

New York University, Graduate School of Arts and Science, Department of Biology, New York, NY 10012-1019. Offers biology (PhD); biomedical journalism (MS); cancer and molecular biology (PhD); computational biology (PhD); computers in biological research (MS); developmental genetics (PhD); general biology (MS); immunology and microbiology (PhD); molecular genetics (PhD); neurobiology (PhD); oral biology (MS); plant biology (PhD); recombinant DNA technology (MS); MS/MBA. *Program availability:* Part-time. Terminal master's awarded for partial completion of doctoral program. *Degree requirements:* For master's, thesis or alternative, qualifying paper; for doctorate, comprehensive exam, thesis/dissertation. *Entrance requirements:* For master's and doctorate, GRE General Test. Additional exam requirements/recommendations for international students: Required—TOEFL. *Faculty research:* Genomics, molecular and cell biology, development and molecular genetics, molecular evolution of plants and animals.

New York University, School of Medicine and Graduate School of Arts and Science, Sackler Institute of Graduate Biomedical Sciences, Program in Cellular and Molecular Biology, New York, NY 10012-1019. Offers PhD. *Degree requirements:* For doctorate, comprehensive exam, thesis/dissertation, qualifying exam. *Faculty research:* Membrane and organelle structure and biogenesis, intracellular transport and processing of proteins, cellular recognition and cell adhesion, oncogene structure and function, action of growth factors.

North Dakota State University, College of Graduate and Interdisciplinary Studies, College of Science and Mathematics, Department of Biological Sciences, Fargo, ND 58102. Offers biology (MS); botany (MS, PhD); cellular and molecular biology (PhD); genomics (PhD); zoology (MS, PhD). *Degree requirements:* For master's, thesis; for doctorate, thesis/dissertation. *Entrance requirements:* For master's and doctorate, GRE General Test. Additional exam requirements/recommendations for international students: Required—TOEFL. *Application deadline:* For fall admission, 1/15 for domestic students. Applications are processed on a rolling basis. Application fee: $35. Electronic applications accepted. *Financial support:* Fellowships with full tuition reimbursements, research assistantships with full tuition reimbursements, teaching assistantships with full tuition reimbursements, career-related internships or fieldwork, Federal Work-Study, institutionally sponsored loans, scholarships/grants, tuition waivers (full), and unspecified assistantships available. Support available to part-time students. Financial award application deadline: 4/15; financial award applicants required to submit FAFSA. *Faculty research:* Comparative endocrinology, physiology, behavioral ecology, plant cell biology, aquatic biology. *Unit head:* Dr. Wendy Reed, Head, 701-231-5921, E-mail: wendy.reed@ndsu.edu. *Application contact:* Elizabeth Worth, Marketing, Recruitment, and Public Relations Coordinator, 701-231-8476, Fax: 701-231-6524, E-mail: elizabeth.worth@ndsu.edu.
Website: http://www.ndsu.edu/biology/

North Dakota State University, College of Graduate and Interdisciplinary Studies, Interdisciplinary Program in Cellular and Molecular Biology, Fargo, ND 58102. Offers PhD. Program offered in cooperation with 11 departments in the university. *Degree requirements:* For doctorate, thesis/dissertation. *Entrance requirements:* For doctorate, GRE. Additional exam requirements/recommendations for international students: Required—TOEFL (minimum score 525 paper-based; 71 iBT). *Application deadline:* Applications are processed on a rolling basis. Application fee: $35. Electronic applications accepted. *Financial support:* Fellowships with full tuition reimbursements, research assistantships with full tuition reimbursements, teaching assistantships with full tuition reimbursements, and unspecified assistantships available. Financial award application deadline: 3/15. *Faculty research:* Plant and animal cell biology, gene regulation, molecular genetics, plant and animal virology. *Unit head:* Dr. Jane Schuh, Director, 701-231-7841, E-mail: jane.schuh@ndsu.edu. *Application contact:* Elizabeth Worth, Marketing, Recruitment, and Public Relations Coordinator, 701-231-8476, Fax: 701-231-6524, E-mail: elizabeth.worth@ndsu.edu.
Website: http://www.ndsu.edu/cellularmolecularbiology/

Northwestern University, The Graduate School, Interdisciplinary Biological Sciences Program (IBiS), Evanston, IL 60208. Offers biochemistry (PhD); bioengineering and biotechnology (PhD); biotechnology (PhD); cell and molecular biology (PhD); developmental and systems biology (PhD); nanotechnology (PhD); neurobiology (PhD); structural biology and biophysics (PhD). *Degree requirements:* For doctorate, thesis/dissertation, qualifying exam. *Entrance requirements:* For doctorate, GRE General Test. Additional exam requirements/recommendations for international students: Required—TOEFL (minimum score 600 paper-based). Electronic applications accepted. *Faculty research:* Biophysics/structural biology, cell/molecular biology, synthetic biology, developmental systems biology, chemical biology/nanotechnology.

The Ohio State University, Graduate School, College of Arts and Sciences, Division of Natural and Mathematical Sciences, Department of Molecular Genetics, Columbus, OH 43210. Offers cell and developmental biology (MS, PhD); genetics (MS, PhD); molecular biology (MS, PhD). *Degree requirements:* For master's, thesis; for doctorate, thesis/dissertation. *Entrance requirements:* For doctorate, GRE General Test, GRE Subject Test in biology or chemistry (recommended). Additional exam requirements/recommendations for international students: Required—TOEFL (minimum score 550 paper-based; 79 iBT), Michigan English Language Assessment Battery (minimum score 82); Recommended—IELTS (minimum score 7). Electronic applications accepted.

The Ohio State University, Graduate School, College of Arts and Sciences, Division of Natural and Mathematical Sciences, Program in Molecular, Cellular and Developmental Biology, Columbus, OH 43210. Offers MS, PhD. Terminal master's awarded for partial completion of doctoral program. *Degree requirements:* For master's, thesis; for doctorate, thesis/dissertation. *Entrance requirements:* For doctorate, GRE General Test, GRE Subject Test in any science (desired, preferably biology or chemistry, biochemistry or cell and molecular biology). Additional exam requirements/recommendations for international students: Required—TOEFL (minimum score 600 paper-based; 85 iBT); Recommended—IELTS (minimum score 8). Electronic applications accepted.

Ohio University, Graduate College, College of Arts and Sciences, Interdisciplinary Graduate Program in Molecular and Cellular Biology, Athens, OH 45701-2979. Offers MS, PhD. *Degree requirements:* For master's, comprehensive exam, thesis, research proposal, teaching experience; for doctorate, comprehensive exam, thesis/dissertation, research proposal, teaching experience. *Entrance requirements:* For master's and doctorate, GRE General Test. Additional exam requirements/recommendations for international students: Required—TOEFL (minimum score 620 paper-based; 105 iBT); Recommended—TWE. Electronic applications accepted. *Faculty research:* Animal biotechnology, plant molecular biology RNA, immunology, cellular genetics,

Molecular Biology

biochemistry of signal transduction, cancer research, membrane transport, bioinformatics, bioengineering, chemical biology and drug discovery, diabetes, microbiology, neuroscience.

Oklahoma State University, College of Agricultural Science and Natural Resources, Department of Biochemistry and Molecular Biology, Stillwater, OK 74078. Offers MS, PhD. *Faculty:* 18 full-time (6 women). *Students:* 5 full-time (2 women), 19 part-time (7 women); includes 4 minority (1 American Indian or Alaska Native, non-Hispanic/Latino; 1 Asian, non-Hispanic/Latino; 2 Hispanic/Latino), 12 international. Average age 29. 25 applicants, 36% accepted, 4 enrolled. In 2015, 3 master's, 5 doctorates awarded. *Degree requirements:* For master's, thesis, oral exam; for doctorate, comprehensive exam, thesis/dissertation. *Entrance requirements:* For master's and doctorate, GRE or GMAT. Additional exam requirements/recommendations for international students: Required—TOEFL (minimum score 550 paper-based; 79 iBT). *Application deadline:* For fall admission, 3/1 priority date for international students; for spring admission, 8/1 priority date for international students. Applications are processed on a rolling basis. Application fee: $40 ($75 for international students). Electronic applications accepted. *Expenses:* Tuition, state resident: full-time $3528; part-time $196 per credit hour. Tuition, nonresident: full-time $14,144; part-time $785.75 per credit hour. *Required fees:* $1895; $105.25 per credit hour. Tuition and fees vary according to campus/location. *Financial support:* In 2015–16, 23 research assistantships (averaging $19,619 per year), 2 teaching assistantships (averaging $19,722 per year) were awarded; career-related internships or fieldwork, Federal Work-Study, scholarships/grants, health care benefits, tuition waivers (partial), and unspecified assistantships also available. Support available to part-time students. Financial award application deadline: 3/1; financial award applicants required to submit FAFSA. *Unit head:* Dr. John Gustafson, Department Head, 405-744-6189, Fax: 405-744-7799, E-mail: john.gustafson@okstate.edu. *Website:* http://biochemistry.okstate.edu/

Oregon Health & Science University, School of Medicine, Graduate Programs in Medicine, Department of Environmental and Biomolecular Systems, Portland, OR 97239-3098. Offers biochemistry and molecular biology (MS, PhD); environmental science and engineering (MS, PhD). *Program availability:* Part-time. *Faculty:* 13 full-time (4 women). *Students:* 19 full-time (16 women), 2 part-time (1 woman); includes 8 minority (2 Black or African American, non-Hispanic/Latino; 3 Asian, non-Hispanic/Latino; 2 Hispanic/Latino; 1 Two or more races, non-Hispanic/Latino), 4 international. Average age 26. 42 applicants, 33% accepted, 7 enrolled. In 2015, 10 master's, 5 doctorates awarded. Terminal master's awarded for partial completion of doctoral program. *Degree requirements:* For master's, thesis (for some programs); for doctorate, comprehensive exam, thesis/dissertation, qualifying exam. *Entrance requirements:* For master's and doctorate, GRE General Test (minimum scores: 153 Verbal/148 Quantitative/4.5 Analytical) or MCAT (for some programs). Additional exam requirements/recommendations for international students: Required—TOEFL. *Application deadline:* For fall admission, 7/15 for domestic students, 5/15 for international students; for winter admission, 10/15 for domestic students, 9/15 for international students; for spring admission, 1/15 for domestic students, 12/15 for international students. Applications are processed on a rolling basis. Application fee: $70. Electronic applications accepted. *Financial support:* Health care benefits and full tuition and stipends (for PhD students) available. *Faculty research:* Metalloprotein biochemistry, molecular microbiology, environmental microbiology, environmental chemistry, biogeochemistry. *Unit head:* Dr. Bradley Tebo, Program Director, 503-346-3438, E-mail: tebob@ohsu.edu. *Application contact:* Vanessa Green, Program Coordinator, 503-346-3411, E-mail: greenva@ohsu.edu.

Oregon Health & Science University, School of Medicine, Graduate Programs in Medicine, Program in Molecular and Cellular Biosciences, Department of Biochemistry and Molecular Biology, Portland, OR 97239-3098. Offers PhD. *Faculty:* 12 full-time (3 women), 21 part-time/adjunct (3 women). *Students:* 7 full-time (3 women), 1 international. Average age 27. *Degree requirements:* For doctorate, comprehensive exam, thesis/dissertation, qualifying exam. *Entrance requirements:* For doctorate, GRE General Test (minimum scores: 153 Verbal/148 Quantitative/4.5 Analytical). Additional exam requirements/recommendations for international students: Required—TOEFL. *Application deadline:* For fall admission, 12/1 for domestic and international students. Application fee: $70. Electronic applications accepted. *Financial support:* Health care benefits, tuition waivers (full), and full tuition and stipends (for PhD students) available. *Faculty research:* Leishmania, parasites, structure and function of G proteins, cystic fibrosis, genomic instability, biology of ion channels. *Unit head:* Dr. David Farrens, Program Director, 503-494-7781, E-mail: farrensd@ohsu.edu. *Application contact:* Lola Bichler, Administrative Coordinator, 503-494-5824, E-mail: bichler@ohsu.edu. *Website:* http://www.ohsu.edu/som-biochem/

Oregon State University, Interdisciplinary/Institutional Programs, Program in Molecular and Cellular Biology, Corvallis, OR 97331. Offers bioinformatics (PhD); biotechnology (PhD); cell biology (PhD); developmental biology (PhD); genome biology (PhD); molecular biology (PhD); molecular pathogenesis (PhD); molecular virology (PhD); plant molecular biology (PhD); structural biology (PhD). *Students:* 28 full-time (14 women), 1 part-time (1 woman); includes 4 minority (2 Asian, non-Hispanic/Latino; 2 Hispanic/Latino), 10 international. Average age 29. 104 applicants, 5% accepted, 5 enrolled. In 2015, 5 doctorates awarded. *Degree requirements:* For doctorate, thesis/dissertation, oral and written qualifying exams. *Entrance requirements:* For doctorate, GRE. Additional exam requirements/recommendations for international students: Required—TOEFL (minimum score 80 iBT), IELTS (minimum score 6.5). *Application deadline:* For fall admission, 8/1 for domestic students, 4/1 for international students; for winter admission, 12/1 for domestic students, 7/1 for international students; for spring admission, 2/1 for domestic students, 10/1 for international students; for summer admission, 5/1 for domestic students, 1/1 for international students. Application fee: $75 ($85 for international students). *Expenses:* Tuition, state resident: full-time $12,150; part-time $450 per credit. Tuition, nonresident: full-time $20,952; part-time $776 per credit. *Required fees:* $1572; $1443 per unit. One-time fee: $350. Tuition and fees vary according to course load, campus/location and program. *Financial support:* Fellowships, career-related internships or fieldwork, Federal Work-Study, and institutionally sponsored loans available. Support available to part-time students. Financial award application deadline: 1/1. *Unit head:* Dr. Dee Denver, Director, Molecular and Cellular Biology Graduate Program, 541-737-3698. *Application contact:* Kristin Carroll, Assistant Director, 541-737-5259, E-mail: kristin.carroll@oregonstate.edu. *Website:* http://www.mcb.oregonstate.edu/

Pace University, Dyson College of Arts and Sciences, Program in Biochemistry and Molecular Biology, New York, NY 10038. Offers MS. *Program availability:* Part-time, evening/weekend. *Students:* 11 full-time (6 women); includes 4 minority (2 Black or African American, non-Hispanic/Latino; 2 Hispanic/Latino). Average age 24. 22 applicants, 86% accepted, 11 enrolled. *Degree requirements:* For master's, thesis. *Entrance requirements:* For master's, official transcripts, two letters of recommendation, personal statement. Additional exam requirements/recommendations for international students: Required—TOEFL (minimum score 88 iBT), IELTS (minimum score 7) or PTE (minimum score 60). *Application deadline:* For fall admission, 4/15 priority date for domestic students. Applications are processed on a rolling basis. Application fee: $70. Electronic applications accepted. *Expenses: Tuition, area resident:* Part-time $1195 per credit. *Required fees:* $260 per semester. Tuition and fees vary according to degree level, campus/location and program. *Financial support:* 3 credit scholarships for full-time students with minimum GPA of 3.5 available. Financial award application deadline: 2/15; financial award applicants required to submit FAFSA. *Unit head:* Dr. Nigel Yarlett, Director, MS in Biochemistry and Molecular Biology, 212-346-1853, E-mail: nyarlett@pace.edu. *Application contact:* Susan Ford-Goldschein, Director of Admissions, 212-346-1531, Fax: 212-346-1585, E-mail: graduateadmission@pace.edu. *Website:* http://www.pace.edu/dyson/programs/ms-biochemistry-molecular-biology-nyc

Penn State University Park, Graduate School, Eberly College of Science, Department of Biochemistry and Molecular Biology, University Park, PA 16802. Offers biochemistry, microbiology, and molecular biology (MS, PhD); biotechnology (MBIOT). *Unit head:* Dr. Douglas R. Cavener, Dean, 814-865-9591, Fax: 814-865-3634. *Application contact:* Lori Stania, Director, Graduate Student Services, 814-865-1795, Fax: 814-863-4627, E-mail: l-gswww@lists.psu.edu. *Website:* http://bmb.psu.edu/

Penn State University Park, Graduate School, Intercollege Graduate Programs, Program in Molecular, Cellular, and Integrative Biosciences, University Park, PA 16802. Offers molecular, cellular, and integrative biosciences (MS, PhD). *Unit head:* Dr. Regina Vasilatos-Younken, Dean, 814-865-2516, Fax: 814-863-4627. *Application contact:* Lori Stania, Director, Graduate Student Services, 814-865-1795, Fax: 814-863-4627, E-mail: l-gswww@lists.psu.edu.

Princeton University, Graduate School, Department of Molecular Biology, Princeton, NJ 08544-1019. Offers PhD. *Degree requirements:* For doctorate, thesis/dissertation. *Entrance requirements:* For doctorate, GRE General Test. Additional exam requirements/recommendations for international students: Required—TOEFL (minimum score 600 paper-based). Electronic applications accepted. *Faculty research:* Genetics, virology, biochemistry.

Purdue University, College of Pharmacy and Pharmacal Sciences and Graduate School, Graduate Programs in Pharmacy and Pharmacal Sciences, Department of Medicinal Chemistry and Molecular Pharmacology, West Lafayette, IN 47907. Offers biophysical and computational chemistry (PhD); cancer research (PhD); immunology and infectious disease (PhD); medicinal biochemistry and molecular biology (PhD); medicinal chemistry and chemical biology (PhD); molecular pharmacology (PhD); neuropharmacology, neurodegeneration, and neurotoxicity (PhD); systems biology and functional genomics (PhD). *Degree requirements:* For doctorate, thesis/dissertation. *Entrance requirements:* For doctorate, GRE General Test; GRE Subject Test in biology, biochemistry, and chemistry (recommended), minimum undergraduate GPA of 3.0. Additional exam requirements/recommendations for international students: Required—TOEFL (minimum score 550 paper-based; 77 iBT); Recommended—TWE. Electronic applications accepted. *Faculty research:* Drug design and development, cancer research, drug synthesis and analysis, chemical pharmacology, environmental toxicology.

Purdue University, Graduate School, College of Science, Department of Biological Sciences, West Lafayette, IN 47907. Offers biochemistry (PhD); biophysics (PhD); cell and developmental biology (PhD); ecology, evolutionary and population biology (MS, PhD), including ecology, evolutionary biology, population biology; genetics (MS, PhD); microbiology (MS, PhD); molecular biology (PhD); neurobiology (MS, PhD); plant physiology (PhD). Terminal master's awarded for partial completion of doctoral program. *Degree requirements:* For master's, thesis (for some programs); for doctorate, thesis/dissertation, seminars, teaching experience. *Entrance requirements:* For master's, GRE General Test (minimum analytical writing score of 3.5), minimum undergraduate GPA of 3.0; for doctorate, GRE General Test (minimum analytical writing score of 3.5), minimum undergraduate GPA of 3.5. Additional exam requirements/recommendations for international students: Required—TOEFL (minimum score 600 paper-based; 107 iBT for MS, 80 iBT for PhD). Electronic applications accepted.

Purdue University, Graduate School, PULSe - Purdue University Life Sciences Program, West Lafayette, IN 47907. Offers biomolecular structure and biophysics (PhD); biotechnology (PhD); chemical biology (PhD); chromatin and regulation of gene expression (PhD); integrative neuroscience (PhD); integrative plant sciences (PhD); membrane biology (PhD); microbiology (PhD); molecular evolutionary and cancer biology (PhD); molecular evolutionary genetics (PhD); molecular virology (PhD). *Entrance requirements:* For doctorate, GRE, minimum undergraduate GPA of 3.0. Additional exam requirements/recommendations for international students: Required—TOEFL (minimum score 550 paper-based; 77 iBT). Electronic applications accepted.

Queen's University at Kingston, School of Graduate Studies, Faculty of Health Sciences, Department of Anatomy and Cell Biology, Kingston, ON K7L 3N6, Canada. Offers biology of reproduction (M Sc, PhD); cancer (M Sc, PhD); cardiovascular pathophysiology (M Sc, PhD); cell and molecular biology (M Sc, PhD); drug metabolism (M Sc, PhD); endocrinology (M Sc, PhD); motor control (M Sc, PhD); neural regeneration (M Sc, PhD); neurophysiology (M Sc, PhD). *Program availability:* Part-time. *Degree requirements:* For master's, thesis; for doctorate, one foreign language, comprehensive exam, thesis/dissertation. *Entrance requirements:* Additional exam requirements/recommendations for international students: Required—TOEFL. Electronic applications accepted. *Faculty research:* Human kinetics, neuroscience, reproductive biology, cardiovascular.

Quinnipiac University, College of Arts and Sciences, Program in Molecular and Cell Biology, Hamden, CT 06518-1940. Offers MS. *Program availability:* Part-time, evening/weekend. *Faculty:* 6 full-time (4 women), 3 part-time/adjunct (0 women). *Students:* 14 full-time (4 women), 20 part-time (14 women); includes 6 minority (2 Black or African American, non-Hispanic/Latino; 2 Asian, non-Hispanic/Latino; 2 Hispanic/Latino), 7 international. 49 applicants, 45% accepted, 12 enrolled. In 2015, 10 master's awarded. *Degree requirements:* For master's, thesis optional. *Entrance requirements:* For master's, bachelor's degree in biological, medical, or health sciences. Additional exam requirements/recommendations for international students: Required—TOEFL (minimum score 575 paper-based; 90 iBT), IELTS (minimum score 6.5). *Application deadline:* For fall admission, 7/30 priority date for domestic students, 4/15 priority date for international students; for spring admission, 12/15 priority date for domestic students, 9/15 priority date for international students. Applications are processed on a rolling basis. Application fee: $45. Electronic applications accepted. *Expenses:* $985 per credit tuition; $40 per credit student fee (not to exceed $360 per semester); $150 per semester technology fee part-time (fall/spring); $340 per semester technology fee full-time (fall/spring); $75 per semester technology fee (summer). *Financial support:* Career-related internships or fieldwork, Federal Work-Study, scholarships/grants, and unspecified assistantships available. Support available to part-time students. Financial award application deadline: 6/1; financial award applicants required to submit FAFSA. *Unit head:* Dr. Lise Thomas, Director, E-mail: graduate@quinnipiac.edu. *Application contact:* Office of Graduate Admissions, 800-462-1944, Fax: 203-582-3443, E-mail: graduate@quinnipiac.edu. *Website:* http://www.quinnipiac.edu/gradmolecular

Rosalind Franklin University of Medicine and Science, School of Graduate and Postdoctoral Studies - Interdisciplinary Graduate Program in Biomedical Sciences, Department of Biochemistry and Molecular Biology, North Chicago, IL 60064-3095.

Offers PhD, MD/PhD. Terminal master's awarded for partial completion of doctoral program. *Degree requirements:* For doctorate, comprehensive exam, thesis/dissertation. *Entrance requirements:* For doctorate, GRE General Test, minimum GPA of 3.0. Additional exam requirements/recommendations for international students: Required—TOEFL, TWE. Electronic applications accepted. *Faculty research:* Structure of control enzymes, extracellular matrix, glucose metabolism, gene expression, ATP synthesis.

Rutgers University–Newark, Graduate School of Biomedical Sciences, Department of Biochemistry and Molecular Biology, Newark, NJ 07107. Offers MS, PhD. *Degree requirements:* For master's, thesis; for doctorate, thesis/dissertation, qualifying exam. *Entrance requirements:* For master's and doctorate, GRE General Test. Additional exam requirements/recommendations for international students: Required—TOEFL. Electronic applications accepted.

Rutgers University–New Brunswick, Graduate School-New Brunswick, Programs in the Molecular Biosciences, Piscataway, NJ 08854-8097. Offers biochemistry (PhD); cell and developmental biology (MS, PhD); microbiology and molecular genetics (MS, PhD), including applied microbiology, clinical microbiology (MS), clinical mircobiology (PhD), computational molecular biology (PhD), immunology, microbial biochemistry, molecular genetics, virology. MS, PhD offered jointly with University of Medicine and Dentistry of New Jersey.

Rutgers University–New Brunswick, Graduate School of Biomedical Sciences, Piscataway, NJ 08854-5635. Offers biochemistry and molecular biology (MS, PhD); biomedical engineering (MS, PhD); biomedical science (MS); cellular and molecular pharmacology (MS, PhD); clinical and translational science (PhD); environmental sciences/exposure assessment (PhD); molecular genetics, microbiology and immunology (MS, PhD); neuroscience (MS, PhD); physiology and integrative biology (MS, PhD); toxicology (PhD); MD/PhD. Terminal master's awarded for partial completion of doctoral program. *Degree requirements:* For master's, thesis (for some programs), ethics training; for doctorate, comprehensive exam, thesis/dissertation, ethics training. *Entrance requirements:* For master's, GRE General Test, MCAT, DAT; for doctorate, GRE General Test. Additional exam requirements/recommendations for international students: Required—TOEFL. Electronic applications accepted.

Saint Louis University, Graduate Education and School of Medicine, Graduate Program in Biomedical Sciences and Graduate Education, Department of Biochemistry and Molecular Biology, St. Louis, MO 63103. Offers PhD. *Degree requirements:* For doctorate, comprehensive exam, thesis/dissertation, departmental qualifying exams. *Entrance requirements:* For doctorate, GRE General Test, GRE Subject Test (optional), letters of recommendation, resume, interview. Additional exam requirements/recommendations for international students: Required—TOEFL (minimum score 525 paper-based). Electronic applications accepted. *Faculty research:* Transcription, chromatin modification and regulation of gene expression; structure/function of proteins and enzymes, including x-ray crystallography; inflammatory mediators in pathogenesis of diabetes and arteriosclerosis; cellular signaling in response to growth factors, opiates and angiogenic mediators; genomics and proteomics of Cryptococcus neoformans.

San Diego State University, Graduate and Research Affairs, College of Sciences, Department of Biology, San Diego, CA 92182. Offers biology (MA, MS), including ecology (MS), molecular biology (MS), physiology (MS), systematics/evolution (MS); cell and molecular biology (PhD); ecology (MS, PhD); microbiology (MS). Terminal master's awarded for partial completion of doctoral program. *Degree requirements:* For master's, thesis; for doctorate, thesis/dissertation. *Entrance requirements:* For master's, GRE General Test, GRE Subject Test, resume or curriculum vitae, 2 letters of recommendation. Additional exam requirements/recommendations for international students: Required—TOEFL. Electronic applications accepted.

San Diego State University, Graduate and Research Affairs, College of Sciences, Molecular Biology Institute, Program in Cell and Molecular Biology, San Diego, CA 92182. Offers PhD. Program offered jointly with University of California, San Diego. *Degree requirements:* For doctorate, thesis/dissertation, oral comprehensive qualifying exam. *Entrance requirements:* For doctorate, GRE General Test, GRE Subject Test, resumé or curriculum vitae, 3 letters of recommendation. Electronic applications accepted. *Faculty research:* Structure/dynamics of protein kinesis, chromatin structure and DNA methylation membrane biochemistry, secretory protein targeting, molecular biology of cardiac myocytes.

San Francisco State University, Division of Graduate Studies, College of Science and Engineering, Department of Biology, Program in Cell and Molecular Biology, San Francisco, CA 94132-1722. Offers MS. *Application deadline:* Applications are processed on a rolling basis. *Expenses:* Tuition, state resident: full-time $6738. Tuition, nonresident: full-time $15,666. *Required fees:* $1004. *Unit head:* Dr. Diana Chu, Program Coordinator, 415-405-3487, Fax: 415-338-2295, E-mail: chud@sfsu.edu. *Application contact:* Graduate Coordinator. Website: http://biology.sfsu.edu/programs/graduate

San Jose State University, Graduate Studies and Research, College of Science, San Jose, CA 95192-0001. Offers biological sciences (MA, MS), including molecular biology and microbiology (MS), organismal biology, conservation and ecology (MS), physiology (MS); chemistry (MA, MS); computer science (MS); cybersecurity (Certificate), cybersecurity: core technologies (Certificate); geology (MS); marine science (MS); master biotechnology (MBT); mathematics (MA, MS), including mathematics education (MA), science; meteorology (MS); physics (MS), including computational physics, modern optics, science (MA, MS); science education (MA); statistics (MS); Unix system administration (Certificate). *Program availability:* Part-time, evening/weekend. *Students:* 118 full-time (68 women), 52 part-time (25 women); includes 125 minority (5 Black or African American, non-Hispanic/Latino; 97 Asian, non-Hispanic/Latino; 23 Hispanic/Latino), 121 international. Average age 27. 1,236 applicants, 21% accepted, 171 enrolled. In 2015, 168 master's awarded. *Entrance requirements:* For master's, GRE. *Application deadline:* For fall admission, 6/29 for domestic students; for spring admission, 11/30 for domestic students. Applications are processed on a rolling basis. Application fee: $55. Electronic applications accepted. *Financial support:* Teaching assistantships, career-related internships or fieldwork, Federal Work-Study, and institutionally sponsored loans available. Support available to part-time students. Financial award applicants required to submit FAFSA. *Faculty research:* Radiochemistry/environmental analysis, health physics, radiation effects. *Unit head:* J. Michael Parrish, Dean, 408-924-4800, Fax: 408-924-4815. *Application contact:* 408-924-2480, Fax: 408-924-2477. Website: http://www.science.sjsu.edu/

Seton Hall University, College of Arts and Sciences, Department of Biological Sciences, South Orange, NJ 07079-2697. Offers biology (MS); biology/business administration (MS); microbiology (MS); molecular bioscience (PhD); molecular bioscience/neuroscience (PhD). *Program availability:* Part-time, evening/weekend. *Degree requirements:* For master's, thesis optional; for doctorate, comprehensive exam, thesis/dissertation. *Entrance requirements:* For master's, GRE or undergraduate degree (BS in biological sciences) with minimum GPA of 3.0 from accredited U.S. institution; for doctorate, GRE. Additional exam requirements/recommendations for international

students: Required—TOEFL. Electronic applications accepted. *Faculty research:* Neurobiology, genetics, immunology, molecular biology, cellular physiology, toxicology, microbiology, bioinformatics.

Simon Fraser University, Office of Graduate Studies, Faculty of Science, Department of Molecular Biology and Biochemistry, Burnaby, BC V5A 1S6, Canada. Offers bioinformatics (Graduate Diploma); molecular biology and biochemistry (M Sc, PhD). *Degree requirements:* For master's, thesis; for doctorate, thesis/dissertation; for Graduate Diploma, practicum. *Entrance requirements:* For master's, minimum GPA of 3.0 (on scale of 4.33), or 3.33 based on last 60 credits of undergraduate courses; for doctorate, minimum GPA of 3.5; for Graduate Diploma, minimum GPA of 2.5 (on scale of 4.33), or 2.67 based on the last 60 credits of undergraduate courses. Additional exam requirements/recommendations for international students: Recommended—TOEFL (minimum score 580 paper-based; 100 iBT), IELTS (minimum score 7.5), TWE (minimum score 5). Electronic applications accepted. *Faculty research:* Genomics and bioinformatics, cell and developmental biology, structural biology/biochemistry, immunology, nucleic acid function.

Sonoma State University, School of Science and Technology, Department of Biology, Rohnert Park, CA 94928. Offers biochemistry (MA); ecology (MS); environmental biology (MS); evolutionary biology (MS); functional morphology (MS); molecular and cell biology (MS); organismal biology (MS). *Program availability:* Part-time. *Degree requirements:* For master's, thesis or alternative, oral exam. *Entrance requirements:* For master's, GRE General Test, GRE Subject Test, minimum GPA of 3.0. Additional exam requirements/recommendations for international students: Required—TOEFL (minimum score 500 paper-based). *Faculty research:* Plant physiology, comparative physiology, community ecology, restoration ecology, marine ecology, conservation genetics, primate behavior, behavioral ecology, developmental biology, plant and animal systematics.

Southern Illinois University Carbondale, Graduate School, College of Science, Program in Molecular Biology, Microbiology, and Biochemistry, Carbondale, IL 62901-4701. Offers MS, PhD. *Faculty:* 16 full-time (2 women). *Students:* 38 full-time (28 women), 29 part-time (13 women); includes 5 minority (2 Black or African American, non-Hispanic/Latino; 3 Asian, non-Hispanic/Latino), 43 international. Average age 25. 83 applicants, 17% accepted, 612 enrolled. In 2015, 9 master's, 13 doctorates awarded. *Degree requirements:* For master's, thesis; for doctorate, thesis/dissertation. *Entrance requirements:* For master's, GRE, minimum GPA of 2.7; for doctorate, GRE, minimum GPA of 3.25. Additional exam requirements/recommendations for international students: Required—TOEFL. *Application deadline:* Applications are processed on a rolling basis. Application fee: $65. *Financial support:* In 2015–16, 49 students received support, including 42 research assistantships with full tuition reimbursements available, 7 teaching assistantships with full tuition reimbursements available; fellowships with full tuition reimbursements available, Federal Work-Study, and institutionally sponsored loans also available. Support available to part-time students. Financial award application deadline: 3/1. *Faculty research:* Prokaryotic gene regulation and expression; eukaryotic gene regulation; microbial, phylogenetic, and metabolic diversity; immune responses to tumors, pathogens, and autoantigens; protein folding and structure. *Unit head:* Dr. Judy Davie, Director, 618-453-5002, E-mail: jdavie@siumed.edu. *Application contact:* Donna K. Mueller, Office Manager, 618-453-8911, E-mail: mueller1@siu.edu. Website: http://mbmb.siu.edu/

Southern Methodist University, Dedman College of Humanities and Sciences, Department of Biological Sciences, Dallas, TX 75275. Offers molecular and cellular biology (MA, MS, PhD). Terminal master's awarded for partial completion of doctoral program. *Degree requirements:* For master's, thesis (for MS), oral exam; for doctorate, thesis/dissertation, qualifying exam. *Entrance requirements:* For master's, GRE General Test (minimum score 1200), minimum GPA of 3.0; for doctorate, GRE General Test (minimum score: 1200), minimum GPA of 3.0. Additional exam requirements/recommendations for international students: Required—TOEFL (minimum score 550 paper-based). Electronic applications accepted. *Faculty research:* Free radicals and aging, protein structure, chromatin structure, signal processes, retroviral pathogenesis.

State University of New York Downstate Medical Center, School of Graduate Studies, Program in Molecular and Cellular Biology, Brooklyn, NY 11203-2098. Offers PhD, MD/PhD. Affiliation with a particular PhD degree-granting program is deferred to the second year. *Degree requirements:* For doctorate, comprehensive exam, thesis/dissertation. *Entrance requirements:* For doctorate, GRE General Test. Additional exam requirements/recommendations for international students: Recommended—TOEFL. *Faculty research:* Mechanism of gene regulation, molecular virology.

State University of New York Upstate Medical University, College of Graduate Studies, Program in Biochemistry and Molecular Biology, Syracuse, NY 13210-2334. Offers biochemistry (MS); biochemistry and molecular biology (PhD); MD/PhD. Terminal master's awarded for partial completion of doctoral program. *Degree requirements:* For master's, thesis; for doctorate, comprehensive exam, thesis/dissertation. *Entrance requirements:* For master's, GRE General Test, interview; for doctorate, GRE General Test, telephone interview. Additional exam requirements/recommendations for international students: Required—TOEFL. Electronic applications accepted. *Faculty research:* Enzymology, membrane structure and functions, developmental biochemistry.

Stony Brook University, State University of New York, Graduate School, College of Arts and Sciences, Department of Biochemistry and Cell Biology, Molecular and Cellular Biology Program, Stony Brook, NY 11794. Offers biochemistry and molecular biology (PhD); biological sciences (MA); immunology and pathology (PhD); molecular and cellular biology (PhD). *Faculty:* 22 full-time (7 women). *Students:* 66 full-time (41 women); includes 11 minority (2 Black or African American, non-Hispanic/Latino; 6 Asian, non-Hispanic/Latino; 3 Hispanic/Latino), 38 international. Average age 28. 175 applicants, 16% accepted, 8 enrolled. In 2015, 11 doctorates awarded. *Degree requirements:* For doctorate, comprehensive exam, thesis/dissertation, teaching experience. *Entrance requirements:* For doctorate, GRE General Test, GRE Subject Test. Additional exam requirements/recommendations for international students: Required—TOEFL. *Application deadline:* For fall admission, 1/15 for domestic students; for spring admission, 10/1 for domestic students. Application fee: $100. *Expenses:* $12,421 per year full-time resident tuition and fees, $453 per credit hour; $23,761 per year full-time non-resident tuition and fees, $925 per credit hour. *Financial support:* In 2015–16, 4 fellowships, 33 research assistantships, 8 teaching assistantships were awarded; Federal Work-Study also available. *Unit head:* Prof. Aaron Neiman, Chair, 631-632-1543, E-mail: aaron.neiman@stonybrook.edu. *Application contact:* Pam Wolfskill, Administrative Specialist/Program Administrator, 631-632-8585, Fax: 631-632-9730, E-mail: pamela.wolfskill@stonybrook.edu.

Texas Woman's University, Graduate School, College of Arts and Sciences, Department of Biology, Denton, TX 76201. Offers biology (MS); molecular biology (PhD). *Program availability:* Part-time. Terminal master's awarded for partial completion of doctoral program. *Degree requirements:* For master's, comprehensive exam, thesis; for doctorate, comprehensive exam, thesis/dissertation, residency. *Entrance requirements:* For master's, GRE General Test (preferred minimum score 149 [425 old version] verbal, 141 [425 old version] quantitative), 3 letters of reference; letter of interest; for doctorate, GRE General Test (preferred minimum score 153 [500 old version] verbal, 144 [500 old version] quantitative), 3 letters of reference, letter of

interest. Additional exam requirements/recommendations for international students: Required—TOEFL (minimum score 550 paper-based; 79 iBT). *Application deadline:* For fall admission, 2/1 priority date for domestic students, 2/1 for international students. Applications are processed on a rolling basis. Application fee: $50 ($75 for international students). Electronic applications accepted. *Expenses:* Tuition, state resident: full-time $4380; part-time $243 per credit hour. Tuition, nonresident: full-time $11,400; part-time $633 per credit hour. *International tuition:* $11,465 full-time. *Required fees:* $1778; $99 per credit hour. *One-time fee:* $50. Tuition and fees vary according to course load and program. *Financial support:* Research assistantships, career-related internships or fieldwork, Federal Work-Study, institutionally sponsored loans, scholarships/grants, traineeships, health care benefits, and unspecified assistantships available. Support available to part-time students. Financial award application deadline: 3/1; financial award applicants required to submit FAFSA. *Faculty research:* Computational biology, protein-protein Interactions, chromatin structure and regulation, regulation of RNA synthesis, virus-host interactions, regulation of axon growth and guidance in neurons, estrogen compounds in plants, regulation of gene expression in male reproductive tissues, female gonadal hormones in the development of anxiety and depression, electron microscopy. *Unit head:* Dr. DiAnna Hynds, Interim Co-Chair, 940-898-2359, Fax: 940-898-2382, E-mail: dhynds@twu.edu. *Application contact:* Dr. Samuel Wheeler, Assistant Director of Admissions, 940-898-3188, Fax: 940-898-3081, E-mail: wheelersr@twu.edu.
Website: http://www.twu.edu/biology

Tufts University, Sackler School of Graduate Biomedical Sciences, Cell, Molecular, and Developmental Biology Program, Medford, MA 02155. Offers cancer biology (PhD); developmental and regenerative biology (PhD); molecular and cellular medicine (PhD); structural and chemical biology (PhD). *Faculty:* 45 full-time (15 women). *Students:* 36 full-time (18 women); includes 13 minority (2 Black or African American, non-Hispanic/Latino; 9 Asian, non-Hispanic/Latino; 1 Hispanic/Latino; 1 Two or more races, non-Hispanic/Latino), 4 international. Average age 28. 189 applicants, 7% accepted, 6 enrolled. In 2015, 2 doctorates awarded. Terminal master's awarded for partial completion of doctoral program. *Degree requirements:* For doctorate, comprehensive exam, thesis/dissertation. *Entrance requirements:* For doctorate, GRE General Test, 3 letters of reference. Additional exam requirements/recommendations for international students: Required—TOEFL (minimum score 600 paper-based; 100 iBT). *Application deadline:* For fall admission, 12/15 priority date for domestic and international students. Application fee: $70. Electronic applications accepted. *Expenses: Tuition, area resident:* Full-time $48,412; part-time $1210 per credit hour. *Required fees:* $806. Full-time tuition and fees vary according to degree level, program and student level. Part-time tuition and fees vary according to course load. *Financial support:* In 2015–16, 36 students received support, including 36 research assistantships with full tuition reimbursements available (averaging $32,000 per year); health care benefits also available. *Faculty research:* Reproduction and hormone action, control of gene expression, cell-matrix and cell-cell interactions, growth control and tumorigenesis, cytoskeleton and contractile proteins. *Unit head:* Dr. Ira Herman, Program Director, 617-636-2991, Fax: 617-636-0375. *Application contact:* Dr. Elizabeth Storrs, Registrar/Director of Academic Services, 617-636-6767, Fax: 617-636-0375, E-mail: sackler-school@tufts.edu.
Website: http://sackler.tufts.edu/Academics/CMDB-Welcome

Tufts University, Sackler School of Graduate Biomedical Sciences, Molecular Microbiology Program, Medford, MA 02155. Offers medically-oriented research in graduate education (PhD); molecular microbiology (PhD). *Faculty:* 17 full-time (7 women). *Students:* 29 full-time (24 women); includes 8 minority (2 Black or African American, non-Hispanic/Latino; 2 Asian, non-Hispanic/Latino; 4 Two or more races, non-Hispanic/Latino), 1 international. Average age 28. 83 applicants, 20% accepted, 5 enrolled. In 2015, 5 doctorates awarded. Terminal master's awarded for partial completion of doctoral program. *Degree requirements:* For doctorate, comprehensive exam, thesis/dissertation. *Entrance requirements:* For doctorate, GRE General Test, 3 letters of reference. Additional exam requirements/recommendations for international students: Required—TOEFL (minimum score 600 paper-based; 100 iBT), IELTS (minimum score 7). *Application deadline:* For fall admission, 12/15 priority date for domestic and international students. Application fee: $90. Electronic applications accepted. *Expenses: Tuition, area resident:* Full-time $48,412; part-time $1210 per credit hour. *Required fees:* $806. Full-time tuition and fees vary according to degree level, program and student level. Part-time tuition and fees vary according to course load. *Financial support:* In 2015–16, 29 students received support, including 29 research assistantships with full tuition reimbursements available (averaging $32,000 per year); traineeships and health care benefits also available. *Faculty research:* Mechanisms of gene regulation, interactions of microorganisms and viruses with host cells, infection response. *Unit head:* Dr. Michael Malamy, Director, 617-636-6750, Fax: 617-636-0337, E-mail: michael.malamy@tufts.edu. *Application contact:* Dr. Elizabeth Storrs, 617-636-6767, Fax: 617-636-0375, E-mail: sackler-school@tufts.edu.
Website: http://sackler.tufts.edu/Academics/Degree-Programs/Molecular-Microbiology

Tulane University, School of Medicine and School of Liberal Arts, Graduate Programs in Biomedical Sciences, Interdisciplinary Graduate Program in Molecular and Cellular Biology, New Orleans, LA 70118-5669. Offers PhD, MD/PhD. PhD offered through the Graduate School. *Degree requirements:* For doctorate, thesis/dissertation. *Entrance requirements:* For doctorate, GRE General Test, GRE Subject Test. Additional exam requirements/recommendations for international students: Required—TOEFL. Electronic applications accepted. *Expenses:* Tuition, area resident: Full-time $47,658; part-time $2648 per credit hour. *Required fees:* $1980; $44.50 per credit hour. $550 per term. Tuition and fees vary according to course load, degree level and program. *Faculty research:* Developmental biology, neuroscience, virology.

Tulane University, School of Science and Engineering, Department of Cell and Molecular Biology, New Orleans, LA 70118-5669. Offers MS, PhD. Terminal master's awarded for partial completion of doctoral program. *Degree requirements:* For doctorate, thesis/dissertation. *Entrance requirements:* For master's, GRE General Test, minimum B average in undergraduate course work; for doctorate, GRE General Test. Additional exam requirements/recommendations for international students: Required—TOEFL. *Application deadline:* For fall admission, 2/1 for domestic and international students. Application fee: $45. Electronic applications accepted. *Expenses: Tuition, area resident:* Full-time $47,658; part-time $2648 per credit hour. *Required fees:* $1980; $44.50 per credit hour. $550 per term. Tuition and fees vary according to course load, degree level and program. *Financial support:* Fellowships with full tuition reimbursements, research assistantships with full tuition reimbursements, and teaching assistantships with full tuition reimbursements available. Financial award application deadline: 2/1.

★ **Uniformed Services University of the Health Sciences,** F. Edward Hebert School of Medicine, Graduate Programs in the Biomedical Sciences and Public Health, Graduate Program in Molecular and Cell Biology, Bethesda, MD 20814-4799. Offers MS, PhD. *Faculty:* 43 full-time (11 women), 3 part-time/adjunct (0 women). *Students:* 22 full-time (13 women); includes 6 minority (2 Asian, non-Hispanic/Latino; 4 Hispanic/Latino), 3 international. Average age 25. 40 applicants, 25% accepted, 6 enrolled. In 2015, 4 doctorates awarded. *Degree requirements:* For doctorate, comprehensive exam, thesis/dissertation, qualifying exam. *Entrance requirements:* For doctorate, GRE General Test, minimum GPA of 3.0. *Application*

deadline: For fall admission, 12/15 priority date for domestic students. Applications are processed on a rolling basis. Application fee: $0. Electronic applications accepted. *Financial support:* In 2015–16, fellowships with full tuition reimbursements (averaging $27,000 per year) were awarded; scholarships/grants, health care benefits, and tuition waivers (full) also available. *Faculty research:* Immunology, biochemistry, cancer biology, stem cell biology. *Unit head:* Dr. Mary Lou Cutler, Director, 301-295-3453, Fax: 301-295-1996, E-mail: mary.cutler@usuhs.edu. *Application contact:* Tina Finley, Administrative Assistant, 301-295-3642, Fax: 301-295-1996, E-mail: netina.finley@usuhs.edu.
Website: https://www.usuhs.edu/mcb

See Display on next page and Close-Up on page 223.

Universidad Central del Caribe, School of Medicine, Program in Biomedical Sciences, Bayamón, PR 00960-6032. Offers anatomy and cell biology (MA, MS); biochemistry (MS); biomedical sciences (MA); cellular and molecular biology (PhD); microbiology and immunology (MA, MS); pharmacology (MS); physiology (MS).

Université de Montréal, Faculty of Medicine, Program in Molecular Biology, Montréal, QC H3C 3J7, Canada. Offers M Sc, PhD. Terminal master's awarded for partial completion of doctoral program. *Degree requirements:* For master's, thesis; for doctorate, thesis/dissertation, general exam. *Entrance requirements:* For master's and doctorate, proficiency in French, knowledge of English. Electronic applications accepted. *Faculty research:* Protein interactions, intracellular signaling, development and differentiation, hematopoiesis, stem cells.

Université Laval, Faculty of Medicine, Graduate Programs in Medicine, Programs in Cellular and Molecular Biology, Québec, QC G1K 7P4, Canada. Offers M Sc, PhD. Terminal master's awarded for partial completion of doctoral program. *Degree requirements:* For master's, thesis; for doctorate, comprehensive exam, thesis/dissertation. *Entrance requirements:* For master's and doctorate, knowledge of French, comprehension of written English. Electronic applications accepted. *Faculty research:* Oral bacterial metabolism, sugar transport.

University at Albany, State University of New York, College of Arts and Sciences, Department of Biological Sciences, Specialization in Molecular, Cellular, Developmental, and Neural Biology, Albany, NY 12222-0001. Offers PhD. *Degree requirements:* For doctorate, one foreign language, thesis/dissertation. *Entrance requirements:* For doctorate, GRE General Test.

University at Buffalo, the State University of New York, Graduate School, Graduate Programs in Cancer Research and Biomedical Sciences at Roswell Park Cancer Institute, Department of Cellular and Molecular Biology at Roswell Park Cancer Institute, Buffalo, NY 14260. Offers PhD. *Faculty:* 24 full-time (2 women). *Students:* 19 full-time (11 women); includes 2 minority (1 Black or African American, non-Hispanic/Latino; 1 Hispanic/Latino), 5 international. 46 applicants, 30% accepted, 4 enrolled. In 2015, 2 doctorates awarded. *Degree requirements:* For doctorate, comprehensive exam, thesis/dissertation, oral defense of dissertation. *Entrance requirements:* For doctorate, GRE General Test. Additional exam requirements/recommendations for international students: Required—TOEFL (minimum score 79 iBT). *Application deadline:* For fall admission, 1/5 priority date for domestic and international students. Application fee: $75. Electronic applications accepted. *Financial support:* In 2015–16, 19 students received support, including 19 research assistantships with full tuition reimbursements available (averaging $25,000 per year); scholarships/grants, health care benefits, and unspecified assistantships also available. Financial award application deadline: 1/5. *Faculty research:* Cancer genetics, chromatin structure and replication, regulation of transcription, human gene mapping, genetic and structural approaches to regulation of gene expression. *Unit head:* Dr. Dominic J. Smiraglia, Director of Graduate Studies, 716-845-1347, Fax: 716-845-1698, E-mail: dominic.smiraglia@roswellpark.org. *Application contact:* Dr. Norman J. Karin, Associate Dean, 716-845-2339, Fax: 716-845-8178, E-mail: norman.karin@roswellpark.edu.
Website: http://www.roswellpark.edu/education/phd-programs/cellular-molecular-biology

The University of Alabama at Birmingham, Graduate Programs in Joint Health Sciences, Cell, Molecular, and Developmental Biology Theme, Birmingham, AL 35294. Offers PhD. *Degree requirements:* For doctorate, variable foreign language requirement, comprehensive exam, thesis/dissertation. *Entrance requirements:* For doctorate, GRE General Test, interview. Additional exam requirements/recommendations for international students: Required—TOEFL (minimum score 600 paper-based). Electronic applications accepted. *Expenses:* Tuition, state resident: full-time $7340. Tuition, nonresident: full-time $16,628. Full-time tuition and fees vary according to course load and program.

University of Alberta, Faculty of Graduate Studies and Research, Department of Biological Sciences, Edmonton, AB T6G 2E1, Canada. Offers environmental biology and ecology (M Sc, PhD); microbiology and biotechnology (M Sc, PhD); molecular biology and genetics (M Sc, PhD); physiology and cell biology (M Sc, PhD); plant biology (M Sc, PhD); systematics and evolution (M Sc, PhD). Terminal master's awarded for partial completion of doctoral program. *Degree requirements:* For master's, thesis; for doctorate, thesis/dissertation. *Entrance requirements:* Additional exam requirements/recommendations for international students: Required—TOEFL.

University of Alberta, Faculty of Medicine and Dentistry and Faculty of Graduate Studies and Research, Graduate Programs in Medicine, Department of Cell Biology, Edmonton, AB T6G 2E1, Canada. Offers cell and molecular biology (M Sc, PhD). Terminal master's awarded for partial completion of doctoral program. *Degree requirements:* For master's, thesis; for doctorate, thesis/dissertation. *Entrance requirements:* For master's and doctorate, 3 letters of reference, curriculum vitae. Additional exam requirements/recommendations for international students: Required—TOEFL (minimum score 600 paper-based). *Faculty research:* Protein targeting, membrane trafficking, signal transduction, cell growth and division, cell-cell interaction and development.

The University of Arizona, College of Science, Department of Molecular and Cellular Biology, Tucson, AZ 85721. Offers molecular and cellular biology (MS, PhD). *Program availability:* Evening/weekend. Terminal master's awarded for partial completion of doctoral program. *Degree requirements:* For master's, thesis; for doctorate, thesis/dissertation. *Entrance requirements:* For master's, 3 letters of recommendation; for doctorate, 3 letters of recommendation, statement of purpose. Additional exam requirements/recommendations for international students: Required—TOEFL (minimum score 600 paper-based; 90 iBT), IELTS (minimum score 7). *Application deadline:* For fall admission, 1/1 for domestic and international students. Applications are processed on a rolling basis. Application fee: $75. Electronic applications accepted. *Financial support:* Research assistantships, teaching assistantships, career-related internships or fieldwork, scholarships/grants, health care benefits, and unspecified assistantships available. *Faculty research:* Plant molecular biology, cellular and molecular aspects of development, genetics of bacteria and lower eukaryotes. *Unit head:* Tricia Serio, Department Head, E-mail: tserio@email.arizona.edu. *Application contact:* Tricia Serio, Department Head, E-mail: tserio@email.arizona.edu.
Website: http://bmcb.biology.arizona.edu/

University of Arkansas, Graduate School, Interdisciplinary Program in Cell and Molecular Biology, Fayetteville, AR 72701-1201. Offers MS, PhD. *Students:* 33 full-time (17 women), 61 part-time (34 women); includes 6 minority (2 Black or African American, non-Hispanic/Latino; 1 American Indian or Alaska Native, non-Hispanic/Latino; 2 Asian, non-Hispanic/Latino; 1 Hispanic/Latino), 60 international. In 2015, 5 master's, 9 doctorates awarded. *Degree requirements:* For doctorate, thesis/dissertation. *Application deadline:* For fall admission, 4/1 for international students; for spring admission, 10/1 for international students. Applications are processed on a rolling basis. Application fee: $40 ($50 for international students). Electronic applications accepted. *Financial support:* In 2015–16, 31 research assistantships, 12 teaching assistantships were awarded; fellowships with tuition reimbursements also available. Financial award application deadline: 4/1; financial award applicants required to submit FAFSA. *Unit head:* Dr. Douglas Rhoads, Head, 479-575-7396, Fax: 479-575-5908, E-mail: drhoads@uark.edu. *Application contact:* Graduate Admissions, 479-575-6246, Fax: 479-575-5908, E-mail: gradinfo@uark.edu.
Website: http://www.uark.edu/depts/cemb/

University of Arkansas for Medical Sciences, Graduate School, Little Rock, AR 72205. Offers biochemistry and molecular biology (MS, PhD); bioinformatics (MS, PhD); cellular physiology and molecular biophysics (MS, PhD); clinical nutrition (MS); interdisciplinary biomedical sciences (MS, PhD, Certificate); interdisciplinary toxicology (MS); microbiology and immunology (PhD); neurobiology and developmental sciences (PhD); pharmacology (PhD); MD/PhD. Bioinformatics programs hosted jointly with the University of Arkansas at Little Rock. *Program availability:* Part-time. Terminal master's awarded for partial completion of doctoral program. *Degree requirements:* For master's, comprehensive exam (for some programs), thesis (for some programs); for doctorate, thesis/dissertation. *Entrance requirements:* For master's and doctorate, GRE. Additional exam requirements/recommendations for international students: Required—TOEFL. Electronic applications accepted. *Expenses:* Contact institution.

The University of British Columbia, Faculty of Medicine, Department of Biochemistry and Molecular Biology, Vancouver, BC V6T 1Z1, Canada. Offers M Sc, PhD. *Degree requirements:* For master's, thesis; for doctorate, comprehensive exam, thesis/dissertation. *Entrance requirements:* For master's, first class B Sc; for doctorate, master's or first class honors bachelor's degree in biochemistry. Additional exam requirements/recommendations for international students: Required—TOEFL (minimum score 625 paper-based). Electronic applications accepted. *Faculty research:* Membrane biochemistry, protein structure/function, signal transduction, biochemistry.

University of Calgary, Cumming School of Medicine and Faculty of Graduate Studies, Department of Biochemistry and Molecular Biology, Calgary, AB T2N 1N4, Canada. Offers M Sc, PhD. *Degree requirements:* For master's, thesis; for doctorate, thesis/dissertation, candidacy exam. *Entrance requirements:* For master's and doctorate, GRE General Test, minimum GPA of 3.2. Additional exam requirements/recommendations for international students: Required—TOEFL. Electronic applications accepted. *Faculty research:* Molecular and developmental genetics; molecular biology of disease; genomics, proteomics and bioinformatics; cell signaling and structure.

University of California, Berkeley, Graduate Division, College of Letters and Science, Department of Molecular and Cell Biology, Berkeley, CA 94720-1500. Offers PhD. *Degree requirements:* For doctorate, comprehensive exam, thesis/dissertation, qualifying exam, 2 semesters of teaching. *Entrance requirements:* For doctorate, GRE General Test, GRE Subject Test (recommended), minimum GPA of 3.0. Additional exam requirements/recommendations for international students: Required—TOEFL (minimum score 570 paper-based; 68 iBT), IELTS (minimum score 7). Electronic applications accepted. *Faculty research:* Biochemistry, biophysics and structural biology; cell and developmental biology; genetics, genomics and development; immunology and pathogenesis; neurobiology.

University of California, Davis, Graduate Studies, Graduate Group in Biochemistry and Molecular Biology, Davis, CA 95616. Offers MS, PhD. Terminal master's awarded for partial completion of doctoral program. *Degree requirements:* For master's, comprehensive exam (for some programs), thesis (for some programs); for doctorate, thesis/dissertation. *Entrance requirements:* For master's and doctorate, GRE General Test, GRE Subject Test. Additional exam requirements/recommendations for international students: Required—TOEFL (minimum score 550 paper-based). Electronic applications accepted. *Faculty research:* Gene expression, protein structure, molecular virology, protein synthesis, enzymology, membrane transport and structural biology.

University of California, Irvine, Francisco J. Ayala School of Biological Sciences, Department of Molecular Biology and Biochemistry, Irvine, CA 92697. Offers biological science (MS); biological sciences (PhD); biotechnology (MS); biotechnology management (MS); MD/PhD. *Students:* 43 full-time (19 women), 1 part-time (0 women); includes 16 minority (2 Black or African American, non-Hispanic/Latino; 9 Asian, non-Hispanic/Latino; 5 Hispanic/Latino), 3 international. Average age 28. In 2015, 1 master's, 16 doctorates awarded. *Degree requirements:* For doctorate, thesis/dissertation. *Entrance requirements:* For master's, GRE, minimum GPA of 3.0; for doctorate, GRE General Test, GRE Subject Test, minimum GPA of 3.0. Additional exam requirements/recommendations for international students: Required—TOEFL (minimum score 550 paper-based). *Application deadline:* For fall admission, 12/15 priority date for domestic students, 12/15 for international students. Applications are processed on a rolling basis. Application fee: $90 ($110 for international students). Electronic applications accepted. *Financial support:* Fellowships, research assistantships with full tuition reimbursements, teaching assistantships, institutionally sponsored loans, traineeships, health care benefits, and unspecified assistantships available. Financial award application deadline: 3/1; financial award applicants required to submit FAFSA. *Faculty research:* Structure and synthesis of nucleic acids and proteins, regulation, virology, biochemical genetics, gene organization. *Unit head:* Prof. Christopher Hughes, Chair, 949-824-8771, Fax: 949-824-8551, E-mail: cchughes@uci.edu. *Application contact:* Morgan Oldham, Student Affairs Assistant, 949-826-6034, Fax: 949-824-8551, E-mail: morgano@uci.edu.
Website: http://www.bio.uci.edu/

University of California, Irvine, Francisco J. Ayala School of Biological Sciences and School of Medicine, Interdisciplinary Graduate Program in Cellular and Molecular Biosciences, Irvine, CA 92697. Offers PhD. *Students:* 26 full-time (14 women); includes 11 minority (5 Asian, non-Hispanic/Latino; 3 Hispanic/Latino; 3 Two or more races, non-Hispanic/Latino), 2 international. Average age 25. 322 applicants, 18% accepted, 25 enrolled. *Degree requirements:* For doctorate, thesis/dissertation, teaching assignment, preliminary exam. *Entrance requirements:* For doctorate, GRE General Test, three letters of recommendation, interview. Additional exam requirements/recommendations for international students: Required—TOEFL or IELTS. *Application deadline:* For fall admission, 12/8 for domestic and international students. Application fee: $90 ($110 for international students). Electronic applications accepted. *Expenses:* Contact institution. *Financial support:* Fellowships with full tuition reimbursements, institutionally sponsored loans, scholarships/grants, tuition waivers (full), unspecified assistantships, and stipends available. Financial award application deadline: 1/1; financial award applicants required to submit FAFSA. *Faculty research:* Cellular biochemistry; gene structure and expression; protein structure, function, and design; molecular genetics; pathogenesis and inherited disease. *Unit head:* Melanie Cocco, Director, 949-824-4487, Fax: 949-824-1965, E-mail: mcocco@uci.edu. *Application contact:* Renee Frigo, Administrator, 949-824-8145, Fax: 949-824-1965, E-mail: rfrigo@uci.edu.
Website: http://cmb.uci.edu/

SECTION 6: CELL, MOLECULAR, AND STRUCTURAL BIOLOGY

Molecular Biology

University of California, Los Angeles, Graduate Division, College of Letters and Science, Department of Chemistry and Biochemistry, Program in Biochemistry and Molecular Biology, Los Angeles, CA 90095. Offers MS, PhD. Terminal master's awarded for partial completion of doctoral program. *Degree requirements:* For master's, comprehensive exam or thesis; for doctorate, thesis/dissertation, oral and written qualifying exams; 3 quarters of teaching experience. *Entrance requirements:* For doctorate, GRE General Test, GRE Subject Test (recommended), bachelor's degree; minimum undergraduate GPA of 3.0 (or its equivalent if letter grade system not used). Additional exam requirements/recommendations for international students: Required—TOEFL. Electronic applications accepted.

University of California, Los Angeles, Graduate Division, College of Letters and Science, Department of Molecular, Cell and Developmental Biology, Los Angeles, CA 90095. Offers MA, PhD. Terminal master's awarded for partial completion of doctoral program. *Degree requirements:* For master's, comprehensive exam, thesis; for doctorate, thesis/dissertation, oral and written qualifying exams; 2 quarters of teaching experience. *Entrance requirements:* For doctorate, GRE General Test. Additional exam requirements/recommendations for international students: Required—TOEFL. Electronic applications accepted.

University of California, Los Angeles, Graduate Division, College of Letters and Science, Program in Molecular Biology, Los Angeles, CA 90095. Offers PhD, MD/PhD. *Degree requirements:* For doctorate, thesis/dissertation, oral and written qualifying exams. *Entrance requirements:* For doctorate, GRE General Test; GRE Subject Test (biochemistry, chemistry, biology, or physics), bachelor's degree; minimum undergraduate GPA of 3.0 (or its equivalent if letter grade system not used). Additional exam requirements/recommendations for international students: Required—TOEFL. Electronic applications accepted.

University of California, Los Angeles, Graduate Division, College of Letters and Science and David Geffen School of Medicine, UCLA ACCESS to Programs in the Molecular, Cellular and Integrative Life Sciences, Los Angeles, CA 90095. Offers biochemistry and molecular biology (PhD); biological chemistry (PhD); cellular and molecular pathology (PhD); human genetics (PhD); microbiology, immunology, and molecular genetics (PhD); molecular biology (PhD); molecular toxicology (PhD); molecular, cellular and integrative physiology (PhD); neurobiology (PhD); oral biology (PhD); physiology (PhD). *Degree requirements:* For doctorate, thesis/dissertation, oral and written qualifying exams. *Entrance requirements:* For doctorate, GRE General Test, bachelor's degree; minimum undergraduate GPA of 3.0 (or its equivalent if letter grade system not used). Additional exam requirements/recommendations for international students: Required—TOEFL. Electronic applications accepted.

University of California, Riverside, Graduate Division, Department of Biochemistry and Molecular Biology, Riverside, CA 92521-0102. Offers biochemistry and molecular biology (MS, PhD). *Program availability:* Part-time. Terminal master's awarded for partial completion of doctoral program. *Degree requirements:* For master's, thesis (for some programs), comprehensive exam or thesis; for doctorate, comprehensive exam, thesis/dissertation, 2 quarters of teaching experience, written exam, oral qualifying exam. *Entrance requirements:* For master's, GRE General Test, minimum GPA of 3.0; for doctorate, GRE General Test, minimum GPA of 3.25. Additional exam requirements/recommendations for international students: Required—TOEFL (minimum score 550 paper-based; 80 iBT). *Application deadline:* For fall admission, 1/5 priority date for domestic and international students; for winter admission, 12/1 for domestic students, 7/1 for international students; for spring admission, 3/1 for domestic students, 10/1 for international students. Application fee: $80 ($100 for international students). Electronic applications accepted. *Expenses: Tuition, area resident:* Full-time $16,665.50; part-time $11,055.54. *Tuition, state resident:* full-time $16,665.50; part-time $11,055.54. *Tuition, nonresident:* full-time $31,768. *International tuition:* $31,767.50 full-time. *Required fees:* $16,665.50; $11,055.54 per quarter. $3685.18 per quarter. Tuition and fees vary according to program. *Financial support:* Fellowships with full tuition reimbursements, research assistantships with full tuition reimbursements, teaching assistantships with full tuition reimbursements, career-related internships or fieldwork, institutionally sponsored loans, and scholarships/grants available. Financial award application deadline: 1/5; financial award applicants required to submit FAFSA. *Faculty research:* Structural biology and molecular biophysics, signal transduction, plant biochemistry and molecular biology, gene expression and metabolic regulation, molecular toxicology and pathogenesis.
Website: http://www.biochemistry.ucr.edu/

University of California, Riverside, Graduate Division, Program in Cell, Molecular, and Developmental Biology, Riverside, CA 92521-0102. Offers MS, PhD. Terminal master's awarded for partial completion of doctoral program. *Degree requirements:* For master's, thesis, oral defense of thesis; for doctorate, thesis/dissertation, oral defense of thesis, qualifying exams, 2 quarters of teaching experience. *Entrance requirements:* For master's and doctorate, GRE General Test, minimum GPA of 3.2. Additional exam requirements/recommendations for international students: Required—TOEFL (minimum score 550 paper-based; 80 iBT). *Application deadline:* For fall admission, 1/5 priority date for domestic and international students. Applications are processed on a rolling basis. Application fee: $60 ($75 for international students). Electronic applications accepted. *Expenses: Tuition, area resident:* Full-time $16,665.50; part-time $11,055.54. Tuition, state resident: full-time $16,665.50; part-time $11,055.54. Tuition, nonresident: full-time $31,768. *International tuition:* $31,767.50 full-time. *Required fees:* $16,665.50; $11,055.54 per quarter. $3685.18 per quarter. Tuition and fees vary according to program. *Financial support:* Fellowships with tuition reimbursements, research assistantships with tuition reimbursements, teaching assistantships with tuition reimbursements, scholarships/grants, traineeships, health care benefits, tuition waivers (partial), and unspecified assistantships available. Support available to part-time students. Financial award application deadline: 1/5.
Website: http://www.cmdb.ucr.edu/

University of California, San Francisco, Graduate Division and School of Medicine, Tetrad Graduate Program, Biochemistry and Molecular Biology Track, San Francisco, CA 94143. Offers PhD, MD/PhD. *Degree requirements:* For doctorate, thesis/dissertation. *Entrance requirements:* For doctorate, GRE General Test, GRE Subject Test. Additional exam requirements/recommendations for international students: Required—TOEFL. *Expenses:* Contact institution. *Faculty research:* Structural biology, genetics, cell biology, cell physiology, metabolism.

University of California, Santa Barbara, Graduate Division, College of Letters and Sciences, Division of Mathematics, Life, and Physical Sciences, Department of Molecular, Cellular, and Developmental Biology, Santa Barbara, CA 93106-9625. Offers MA, PhD, MA/PhD. *Faculty:* 35 full-time (5 women), 3 part-time/adjunct (0 women). *Students:* 55 full-time (28 women); includes 16 minority (1 Black or African American, non-Hispanic/Latino; 1 American Indian or Alaska Native, non-Hispanic/Latino; 8 Asian, non-Hispanic/Latino; 4 Hispanic/Latino; 2 Native Hawaiian or other Pacific Islander, non-Hispanic/Latino), 4 international. Average age 27. 183 applicants, 24% accepted, 23 enrolled. In 2015, 5 master's, 10 doctorates awarded. Terminal master's awarded for partial completion of doctoral program. *Degree requirements:* For master's, comprehensive exam (for some programs), thesis (for some programs); for doctorate, comprehensive exam, thesis/dissertation. *Entrance requirements:* For master's and

doctorate, GRE General Test, 3 letters of recommendation, statement of purpose, personal achievements/contributions statement, resume/curriculum vitae, transcripts for post-secondary institutions attended. Additional exam requirements/recommendations for international students: Required—TOEFL (minimum score 550 paper-based; 80 iBT), IELTS (minimum score 7). *Application deadline:* For fall admission, 12/7 priority date for domestic and international students. Application fee: $90 ($110 for international students). Electronic applications accepted. *Financial support:* In 2015–16, 3 students received support, including 3 fellowships with tuition reimbursements available (averaging $22,000 per year), 40 research assistantships with tuition reimbursements available (averaging $26,250 per year), 46 teaching assistantships with partial tuition reimbursements available (averaging $17,655 per year); career-related internships or fieldwork, Federal Work-Study, institutionally sponsored loans, scholarships/grants, traineeships, health care benefits, and unspecified assistantships also available. Financial award application deadline: 3/2; financial award applicants required to submit FAFSA. *Faculty research:* Microbiology, neurobiology (including stem cell research), developmental, virology, cell biology. *Unit head:* Dr. Stephen Poole, Chair, 805-893-8122, E-mail: william.smith@lifesci.ucsb.edu. *Application contact:* Anthony Galaviz, Graduate Program Advisor, 805-893-8499, E-mail: anthony.galaviz@lifesci.ucsb.edu.
Website: https://www.mcdb.ucsb.edu/grad

University of California, Santa Barbara, Graduate Division, College of Letters and Sciences, Division of Mathematics, Life, and Physical Sciences, Interdepartmental Graduate Program in Biomolecular Science and Engineering, Santa Barbara, CA 93106-2014. Offers biochemistry and molecular biology (PhD), including biochemistry and molecular biology, biophysics and bioengineering. *Faculty:* 35 full-time (3 women), 3 part-time/adjunct (all women). *Students:* 27 full-time (9 women); includes 7 minority (5 Asian, non-Hispanic/Latino; 2 Hispanic/Latino), 1 international. Average age 26. 105 applicants, 21% accepted, 11 enrolled. In 2015, 8 doctorates awarded. Terminal master's awarded for partial completion of doctoral program. *Degree requirements:* For doctorate, thesis/dissertation. *Entrance requirements:* For doctorate, GRE General Test. Additional exam requirements/recommendations for international students: Required—TOEFL (minimum score 630 paper-based; 109 iBT), IELTS (minimum score 7). *Application deadline:* For fall admission, 12/15 for domestic and international students. Application fee: $90 ($110 for international students). Electronic applications accepted. *Financial support:* In 2015–16, 28 students received support, including 16 fellowships with tuition reimbursements available, 31 research assistantships with tuition reimbursements available, 16 teaching assistantships with tuition reimbursements available; Federal Work-Study, traineeships, health care benefits, tuition waivers (full and partial), and unspecified assistantships also available. Financial award application deadline: 12/15; financial award applicants required to submit FAFSA. *Faculty research:* Biochemistry and molecular biology, biophysics, biomaterials, bioengineering, systems biology. *Unit head:* Prof. Omar A. Saleh, Director/Professor, 805-893-8814, E-mail: saleh@engineering.ucsb.edu. *Application contact:* Lauren Baker, Graduate Program Assistant, 805-893-3011, E-mail: bmse-gradasst@lifesci.ucsb.edu.
Website: http://www.bmse.ucsb.edu/

University of California, Santa Cruz, Division of Graduate Studies, Division of Physical and Biological Sciences, Program in Molecular, Cellular, and Developmental Biology, Santa Cruz, CA 95064. Offers MA. Terminal master's awarded for partial completion of doctoral program. *Degree requirements:* For master's, thesis; for doctorate, thesis/dissertation, qualifying exam. *Entrance requirements:* For master's and doctorate, GRE General Test, 3 letters of recommendation, interview. Additional exam requirements/recommendations for international students: Required—TOEFL (minimum score 550 paper-based; 83 iBT); Recommended—IELTS (minimum score 8). Electronic applications accepted. *Faculty research:* RNA biology, chromatin and chromosome biology, neurobiology, stem cell biology and differentiation, cell structure and function.

University of Chicago, Division of the Biological Sciences, Department of Cell and Molecular Biology, Chicago, IL 60637. Offers PhD. *Students:* 28 full-time (12 women); includes 7 minority (3 Black or African American, non-Hispanic/Latino; 2 Asian, non-Hispanic/Latino; 1 Hispanic/Latino; 1 Two or more races, non-Hispanic/Latino), 5 international. Average age 29. 85 applicants, 27% accepted, 5 enrolled. In 2015, 3 doctorates awarded. *Degree requirements:* For doctorate, thesis/dissertation, ethics class, 2 teaching assistantships. *Entrance requirements:* For doctorate, GRE General Test. Additional exam requirements/recommendations for international students: Required—TOEFL (minimum score 600 paper-based; 104 iBT), IELTS (minimum score 7). *Application deadline:* For fall admission, 12/1 for domestic and international students. Application fee: $90. Electronic applications accepted. *Financial support:* In 2015–16, 28 students received support, including fellowships (averaging $29,781 per year), research assistantships (averaging $29,781 per year); institutionally sponsored loans, scholarships/grants, traineeships, and health care benefits also available. Financial award applicants required to submit FAFSA. *Faculty research:* Gene expression, chromosome structure, animal viruses, plant molecular genetics. *Total annual research expenditures:* $8 million. *Unit head:* Dr. Richard Fehon, Chair, 773-702-5694, E-mail: rfehon@uchicago.edu. *Application contact:* Kristine Gaston, Graduate Administrative Director, 773-702-8037, Fax: 773-702-3172, E-mail: kristine@bsd.uchicago.edu.
Website: http://cellmolbio.bsd.uchicago.edu/

University of Cincinnati, Graduate School, College of Medicine, Graduate Programs in Biomedical Sciences, Department of Environmental Health, Programs in Environmental Genetics and Molecular Toxicology, Cincinnati, OH 45221. Offers MS, PhD. *Degree requirements:* For doctorate, thesis/dissertation. *Entrance requirements:* For master's, GRE, minimum GPA of 3.0, 3 letters of recommendation. Additional exam requirements/recommendations for international students: Required—TOEFL (minimum score 520 paper-based).

University of Cincinnati, Graduate School, College of Medicine, Graduate Programs in Biomedical Sciences, Department of Molecular Genetics, Biochemistry and Microbiology, Cincinnati, OH 45221. Offers MS, PhD. Terminal master's awarded for partial completion of doctoral program. *Degree requirements:* For master's, thesis or alternative; for doctorate, thesis/dissertation, qualifying exam. *Entrance requirements:* For master's and doctorate, GRE General Test. Additional exam requirements/recommendations for international students: Required—TOEFL (minimum score 600 paper-based; 100 iBT), TWE. Electronic applications accepted. *Faculty research:* Cancer biology and developmental genetics, gene regulation and chromosome structure, microbiology and pathogenic mechanisms, structural biology, membrane biochemistry and signal transduction.

University of Cincinnati, Graduate School, College of Medicine, Graduate Programs in Biomedical Sciences, Department of Pediatrics, Program in Molecular and Developmental Biology, Cincinnati, OH 45221. Offers PhD. *Degree requirements:* For doctorate, thesis/dissertation, qualifying exam. *Entrance requirements:* For doctorate, GRE General Test, minimum GPA of 3.2. Additional exam requirements/recommendations for international students: Required—TOEFL (minimum score 520 paper-based). Electronic applications accepted. *Faculty research:* Cancer biology, cardiovascular biology, developmental biology, human genetics, gene therapy, genomics and bioinformatics, immunobiology, molecular medicine, neuroscience, pulmonary biology, reproductive biology, stem cell biology.

University of Colorado Boulder, Graduate School, College of Arts and Sciences, Department of Molecular, Cellular, and Developmental Biology, Boulder, CO 80309. Offers cellular structure and function (MA, PhD); developmental biology (MA, PhD); molecular biology (MA, PhD). *Faculty:* 28 full-time (8 women). *Students:* 71 full-time (34 women), 1 part-time (0 women); includes 7 minority (1 Asian, non-Hispanic/Latino; 4 Hispanic/Latino; 1 Native Hawaiian or other Pacific Islander, non-Hispanic/Latino; 1 Two or more races, non-Hispanic/Latino), 7 international. Average age 27. 310 applicants, 6% accepted, 7 enrolled. In 2015, 6 doctorates awarded. Terminal master's awarded for partial completion of doctoral program. *Degree requirements:* For master's, comprehensive exam, thesis or alternative; for doctorate, comprehensive exam, thesis/dissertation. *Entrance requirements:* For master's, GRE General Test, GRE Subject Test, minimum undergraduate GPA of 3.0; for doctorate, GRE General Test, GRE Subject Test. *Application deadline:* For fall admission, 12/1 for domestic students, 12/15 for international students. Application fee: $50 ($70 for international students). Electronic applications accepted. Application fee is waived when completed online. *Financial support:* In 2015–16, 125 students received support, including 10 fellowships (averaging $5,729 per year), 53 research assistantships with tuition reimbursements available (averaging $28,304 per year), 9 teaching assistantships with tuition reimbursements available (averaging $30,852 per year); institutionally sponsored loans, scholarships/grants, health care benefits, and unspecified assistantships also available. Financial award application deadline: 2/1; financial award applicants required to submit FAFSA. *Faculty research:* Molecular biology, cellular biology, genetics, biochemistry, gene cloning, proteins. *Total annual research expenditures:* $15.4 million. *Application contact:* E-mail: mcdbgrad@colorado.edu.
Website: http://mcdb.colorado.edu/graduate

University of Colorado Denver, College of Liberal Arts and Sciences, Department of Integrative and Systems Biology, Denver, CO 80217. Offers animal behavior (MS); biology (MS); cell and developmental biology (MS); ecology (MS); evolutionary biology (MS); genetics (MS); integrative and systems biology (PhD); microbiology (MS); molecular biology (MS); neurobiology (MS); plant systematics (MS). *Program availability:* Part-time. *Faculty:* 21 full-time (8 women), 3 part-time/adjunct (1 woman). *Students:* 31 full-time (19 women), 7 part-time (3 women); includes 8 minority (1 Black or African American, non-Hispanic/Latino; 1 Asian, non-Hispanic/Latino; 3 Hispanic/Latino; 3 Two or more races, non-Hispanic/Latino), 1 international. Average age 28. 34 applicants, 29% accepted, 8 enrolled. In 2015, 6 master's awarded. *Degree requirements:* For master's, comprehensive exam, thesis, 30-32 credit hours; for doctorate, comprehensive exam, thesis/dissertation. *Entrance requirements:* For master's, GRE General Test (minimum score in 50th percentile in each section), BA/BS from accredited institution awarded within the last 10 years; minimum undergraduate GPA of 3.0; prerequisite courses: 1 year each of general biology and general chemistry; 1 semester each of general genetics, general ecology, and cell biology; and a structure/function course; for doctorate, GRE, minimum undergraduate GPA of 3.2, three letters of recommendation, official transcripts from all universities and colleges attended. Additional exam requirements/recommendations for international students: Required—TOEFL (minimum score 537 paper-based; 75 iBT); Recommended—IELTS (minimum score 6.5). *Application deadline:* For fall admission, 1/15 for domestic and international students. Application fee: $50 ($75 for international students). Electronic applications accepted. *Financial support:* In 2015–16, 32 students received support. Fellowships, research assistantships, teaching assistantships, Federal Work-Study, institutionally sponsored loans, scholarships/grants, and traineeships available. Financial award application deadline: 4/1; financial award applicants required to submit FAFSA. *Faculty research:* Molecular developmental biology; quantitative ecology, biogeography, and population dynamics; environmental signaling and endocrine disruption; speciation, the evolution of reproductive isolation, and hybrid zones; evolutionary, behavioral, and conservation ecology. *Unit head:* Dr. John Swallow, Chair, 303-556-6154, E-mail: john.swallow@ucdenver.edu. *Application contact:* Dr. Michael Wunder, Graduate Advisor, 303-556-8870, E-mail: michael.wunder@ucdenver.edu.
Website: http://www.ucdenver.edu/academics/colleges/CLAS/Departments/biology/Programs/MasterofScience/Pages/BiologyMasterOfScience.aspx

University of Colorado Denver, School of Medicine, Program in Molecular Biology, Aurora, CO 80045. Offers biomolecular structure (PhD); molecular biology (PhD). *Students:* 43 full-time (25 women), 2 part-time (both women); includes 10 minority (1 Black or African American, non-Hispanic/Latino; 4 Asian, non-Hispanic/Latino; 4 Hispanic/Latino; 1 Two or more races, non-Hispanic/Latino), 4 international. Average age 29. 38 applicants, 16% accepted, 6 enrolled. In 2015, 4 doctorates awarded. *Degree requirements:* For doctorate, comprehensive exam, thesis/dissertation, 2 years of structured didactic courses, 2-3 years of research, laboratory work, thesis project. *Entrance requirements:* For doctorate, GRE, organic chemistry (2 semesters, including 1 semester of laboratory), biology, general physics, college-level mathematics through calculus, three letters of reference. Additional exam requirements/recommendations for international students: Required—TOEFL (minimum score 550 paper-based; 80 iBT). *Application deadline:* For fall admission, 12/1 for domestic students, 11/1 for international students. Application fee: $50 ($75 for international students). Electronic applications accepted. *Expenses:* Contact institution. *Financial support:* In 2015–16, 43 students received support. Fellowships, research assistantships, teaching assistantships, institutionally sponsored loans, scholarships/grants, traineeships, health care benefits, tuition waivers (full), and unspecified assistantships available. Financial award application deadline: 3/15; financial award applicants required to submit FAFSA. *Faculty research:* Gene transcription, RNA processing, chromosome dynamics, DNA damage and repair, chromatin assembly. *Unit head:* Dr. Mark Johnston, Chair, 303-724-3203, E-mail: mark.johnston@ucdenver.edu. *Application contact:* Sabrena Heilman, Program Administrator, 303-724-3245, E-mail: sabrena.heilman@ucdenver.edu.
Website: http://www.ucdenver.edu/academics/colleges/medicalschool/programs/Molbio/Pages/MolecularBiology.aspx

University of Colorado Denver, School of Medicine, Program in Pharmacology, Aurora, CO 80045. Offers bioinformatics (PhD); biomolecular structure (PhD); pharmacology (PhD). *Students:* 19 full-time (11 women); includes 5 minority (2 Asian, non-Hispanic/Latino; 2 Hispanic/Latino; 1 Two or more races, non-Hispanic/Latino). Average age 26. 32 applicants, 16% accepted, 5 enrolled. In 2015, 3 doctorates awarded. *Degree requirements:* For doctorate, comprehensive exam, thesis/dissertation, major seminar, 3 research rotations in the first year, 30 hours each of course work and thesis. *Entrance requirements:* For doctorate, GRE General Test, three letters of recommendation, personal statement. Additional exam requirements/recommendations for international students: Required—TOEFL (minimum score 550 paper-based; 80 iBT). *Application deadline:* For fall admission, 12/15 for domestic students, 11/15 for international students. Application fee: $50 ($75 for international students). Electronic applications accepted. *Expenses:* Contact institution. *Financial support:* In 2015–16, 23 students received support. Fellowships, research assistantships, teaching assistantships, institutionally sponsored loans, scholarships/grants, traineeships, health care benefits, tuition waivers (full), and unspecified assistantships available. Financial award application deadline: 3/15; financial award applicants required to submit FAFSA. *Faculty research:* Cancer biology, drugs of abuse, neuroscience, signal transduction, structural biology. *Total annual research expenditures:* $16.7 million. *Unit head:* Dr. Andrew Thorburn, Interim Chair, 303-724-

3290, Fax: 303-724-3663, E-mail: andrew.thorburn@ucdenver.edu. *Application contact:* Elizabeth Bowen, Graduate Program Coordinator, 303-724-3565, E-mail: elizabeth.bowen@ucdenver.edu.
Website: http://www.ucdenver.edu/academics/colleges/medicalschool/departments/Pharmacology/Pages/Pharmacology.aspx

University of Connecticut Health Center, Graduate School, Programs in Biomedical Sciences, Graduate Program in Molecular Biology and Biochemistry, Farmington, CT 06030. Offers PhD, DMD/PhD, MD/PhD. *Degree requirements:* For doctorate, comprehensive exam, thesis/dissertation. *Entrance requirements:* For doctorate, GRE General Test. Additional exam requirements/recommendations for international students: Required—TOEFL (minimum score 600 paper-based). Electronic applications accepted. *Faculty research:* Molecular biology, structural biology, protein biochemistry, microbial physiology and pathogenesis.
See Display on next page and Close-Up on page 229.

University of Delaware, College of Arts and Sciences, Department of Biological Sciences, Newark, DE 19716. Offers biotechnology (MS); cancer biology (MS, PhD); cell and extracellular matrix biology (MS, PhD); cell and systems physiology (MS, PhD); developmental biology (MS, PhD); ecology and evolution (MS, PhD); microbiology (MS, PhD); molecular biology and genetics (MS, PhD). Terminal master's awarded for partial completion of doctoral program. *Degree requirements:* For master's, thesis, preliminary exam; for doctorate, comprehensive exam, thesis/dissertation, preliminary exam. *Entrance requirements:* For master's and doctorate, GRE General Test. Additional exam requirements/recommendations for international students: Required—TOEFL (minimum score 600 paper-based); Recommended—TWE. Electronic applications accepted. *Faculty research:* Microorganisms, bone, cancer metastasis, developmental biology, cell biology, DNA.

University of Denver, Division of Natural Sciences and Mathematics, Department of Biological Sciences, Denver, CO 80208. Offers biology, ecology and evolution (MS, PhD); biomedical sciences (PSM); cell and molecular biology (MS, PhD). *Program availability:* Part-time. *Faculty:* 23 full-time (7 women), 2 part-time/adjunct (both women). *Students:* 8 full-time (all women), 27 part-time (21 women); includes 6 minority (2 Black or African American, non-Hispanic/Latino; 2 Hispanic/Latino), 6 international. Average age 26. 77 applicants, 38% accepted, 21 enrolled. In 2015, 6 master's, 3 doctorates awarded. Terminal master's awarded for partial completion of doctoral program. *Degree requirements:* For master's, comprehensive exam (for some programs), thesis; for doctorate, one foreign language, comprehensive exam (for some programs), thesis/dissertation. *Entrance requirements:* For master's and doctorate, GRE General Test, bachelor's degree in biology or related field, transcripts, personal statement, three letters of recommendation. Additional exam requirements/recommendations for international students: Required—TOEFL (minimum score 550 paper-based; 80 iBT). *Application deadline:* For fall admission, 1/1 priority date for domestic and international students. Applications are processed on a rolling basis. Application fee: $65. Electronic applications accepted. *Expenses:* $30,477. *Financial support:* In 2015–16, 35 students received support, including 8 research assistantships with tuition reimbursements available (averaging $15,834 per year), 23 teaching assistantships with tuition reimbursements available (averaging $17,210 per year); Federal Work-Study, institutionally sponsored loans, scholarships/grants, and unspecified assistantships also available. Support available to part-time students. Financial award application deadline: 2/15; financial award applicants required to submit FAFSA. *Faculty research:* Molecular biology, cell biology, neurobiology, ecology, molecular evolution. *Unit head:* Dr. Joseph Angleson, Associate Professor and Chair, 303-871-3463, Fax: 303-871-3471, E-mail: jangleso@du.edu. *Application contact:* Randi Flageolle, Assistant to the Chair, 303-871-3457, Fax: 303-871-3471, E-mail: rflageol@du.edu.
Website: http://www.du.edu/nsm/departments/biologicalsciences

University of Florida, College of Medicine and Graduate School, Interdisciplinary Program in Biomedical Sciences, Concentration in Biochemistry and Molecular Biology, Gainesville, FL 32611. Offers PhD. *Degree requirements:* For doctorate, thesis/dissertation. *Entrance requirements:* For doctorate, GRE General Test, minimum GPA of 3.0, biochemistry before enrollment. Additional exam requirements/recommendations for international students: Required—TOEFL. Electronic applications accepted. *Faculty research:* Gene expression, metabolic regulation, structural biology, enzyme mechanism, membrane transporters.

University of Florida, Graduate School, College of Agricultural and Life Sciences, Department of Animal Sciences, Interdisciplinary Concentration in Animal Molecular and Cellular Biology, Gainesville, FL 32611. Offers MS, PhD. *Faculty:* 14. *Students:* 16 full-time (11 women), 1 (woman) part-time; includes 2 minority (both Hispanic/Latino), 12 international. Average age 31. 15 applicants, 20% accepted, 3 enrolled. In 2015, 1 master's, 2 doctorates awarded. *Entrance requirements:* For master's and doctorate, GRE General Test, minimum GPA of 3.0. Additional exam requirements/recommendations for international students: Required—TOEFL (minimum score 550 paper-based; 80 iBT), IELTS (minimum score 6). Application fee: $30. Electronic applications accepted. *Financial support:* In 2015–16, 1 fellowship, 11 research assistantships, 1 teaching assistantship were awarded. Financial award applicants required to submit FAFSA. *Unit head:* Geoffrey E. Dahl, PhD, Professor and Department Chair, 352-392-1981, Fax: 352-392-5595, E-mail: gdahl@ufl.edu. *Application contact:* Office of Admissions, 352-392-1365, E-mail: webrequests@admissions.ufl.edu.
Website: http://www.animal.ufl.edu/amcb/

University of Florida, Graduate School, College of Liberal Arts and Sciences, Department of Biology, Gainesville, FL 32611. Offers botany (MS, MST, PhD), including botany, tropical conservation and development, wetland sciences; zoology (MS, MST, PhD), including animal molecular and cellular biology (PhD), tropical conservation and development, wetland sciences, zoology. *Faculty:* 9 full-time, 9 part-time/adjunct. *Students:* 96 full-time (41 women), 6 part-time (3 women); includes 9 minority (4 Asian, non-Hispanic/Latino; 5 Hispanic/Latino), 35 international. 77 applicants, 30% accepted, 16 enrolled. In 2015, 8 master's, 15 doctorates awarded. *Degree requirements:* For master's, comprehensive exam (for some programs), thesis; for doctorate, comprehensive exam, thesis/dissertation. *Entrance requirements:* For master's and doctorate, GRE General Test, minimum GPA of 3.0. Additional exam requirements/recommendations for international students: Required—TOEFL (minimum score 550 paper-based; 80 iBT), IELTS (minimum score 6). *Application deadline:* For fall admission, 12/1 for domestic and international students. Applications are processed on a rolling basis. Application fee: $30. Electronic applications accepted. *Financial support:* In 2015–16, 9 fellowships, 36 research assistantships, 62 teaching assistantships were awarded; unspecified assistantships also available. Financial award application deadline: 12/15; financial award applicants required to submit FAFSA. *Faculty research:* Ecology of natural populations, plant and animal genome evolution, biodiversity, plant biology, behavior. *Total annual research expenditures:* $3.6 million. *Unit head:* Marta Wayne, PhD, Professor and Chair, 352-392-9925, E-mail: mlwayne@ufl.edu. *Application contact:* William T. Barbazuk, PhD, Associate Professor/Graduate Coordinator, 352-273-8624, Fax: 352-392-3704, E-mail: bbarbazuk@ufl.edu.
Website: http://www.biology.ufl.edu/

Molecular Biology

University of Georgia, Franklin College of Arts and Sciences, Department of Biochemistry and Molecular Biology, Athens, GA 30602. Offers MS, PhD. *Degree requirements:* For master's, one foreign language, thesis; for doctorate, one foreign language, thesis/dissertation. *Entrance requirements:* For master's and doctorate, GRE General Test. Additional exam requirements/recommendations for international students: Required—TOEFL. Electronic applications accepted.

University of Guelph, Graduate Studies, College of Biological Science, Department of Molecular and Cellular Biology, Guelph, ON N1G 2W1, Canada. Offers biochemistry (M Sc, PhD); biophysics (M Sc, PhD); botany (M Sc, PhD); microbiology (M Sc, PhD); molecular biology and genetics (M Sc, PhD). *Degree requirements:* For master's, thesis, research proposal; for doctorate, comprehensive exam, thesis/dissertation, research proposal. *Entrance requirements:* For master's, minimum B-average during previous 2 years of coursework; for doctorate, minimum A-average. Additional exam requirements/recommendations for international students: Required—TOEFL (minimum score 550 paper-based), IELTS (minimum score 6.5). Electronic applications accepted. *Faculty research:* Physiology, structure, genetics, and ecology of microbes; virology and microbial technology.

University of Hawaii at Manoa, Graduate Division, College of Tropical Agriculture and Human Resources, Department of Molecular Biosciences and Bioengineering, Honolulu, HI 96822. Offers bioengineering (MS); molecular bioscience and bioengineering (MS); molecular biosciences and bioengineering (PhD). *Program availability:* Part-time. *Faculty:* 71 full-time (18 women), 10 part-time/adjunct (4 women). *Students:* 5 full-time (2 women), 2 part-time; includes 31 minority (16 Asian, non-Hispanic/Latino; 6 Hispanic/Latino; 1 Native Hawaiian or other Pacific Islander, non-Hispanic/Latino; 8 Two or more races, non-Hispanic/Latino), 23 international. Average age 31. 43 applicants, 70% accepted, 19 enrolled. In 2015, 14 master's, 5 doctorates awarded. *Degree requirements:* For master's, thesis optional; for doctorate, comprehensive exam, thesis/dissertation. *Entrance requirements:* For master's and doctorate, GRE General Test. Additional exam requirements/recommendations for international students: Required—TOEFL (minimum score 550 paper-based; 79 iBT), IELTS (minimum score 5). *Application deadline:* For fall admission, 5/30 for domestic students, 4/30 for international students; for spring admission, 10/30 for domestic students, 9/30 for international students. Application fee: $100. *Financial support:* In 2015–16, 11 fellowships (averaging $1,927 per year), 52 research assistantships (averaging $18,421 per year), 11 teaching assistantships (averaging $15,788 per year) were awarded; Federal Work-Study, institutionally sponsored loans, and tuition waivers (full) also available. *Faculty research:* Mechanization, agricultural systems, waste management, water management, cell culture. *Total annual research expenditures:* $1.4 million. *Unit head:* Sylvia Yuen, Interim Dean, 808-956-8234, Fax: 808-956-9105, E-mail: syuen@hawaii.edu. *Application contact:* Dulal Borthakur, Graduate Chair, 808-956-6660, Fax: 808-956-3542, E-mail: dulal@hawaii.edu.
Website: http://www.ctahr.hawaii.edu/mbbe/

University of Hawaii at Manoa, John A. Burns School of Medicine, Program in Cell and Molecular Biology, Honolulu, HI 96813. Offers MS, PhD. *Program availability:* Part-time. *Faculty:* 55 full-time (16 women), 5 part-time/adjunct (1 woman). *Students:* 32 full-time (23 women), 1 (woman) part-time; includes 20 minority (8 Asian, non-Hispanic/Latino; 4 Hispanic/Latino; 1 Native Hawaiian or other Pacific Islander, non-Hispanic/Latino; 7 Two or more races, non-Hispanic/Latino), 2 international. Average age 31. 28 applicants, 61% accepted, 11 enrolled. In 2015, 5 doctorates awarded. Terminal master's awarded for partial completion of doctoral program. *Degree requirements:* For master's, thesis optional; for doctorate, comprehensive exam, thesis/dissertation. *Entrance requirements:* For master's and doctorate, GRE General Test, minimum GPA of 3.0. Additional exam requirements/recommendations for international students: Required—TOEFL (minimum score 500 paper-based; 61 iBT), IELTS (minimum score 5).

Application deadline: For fall admission, 1/15 for domestic and international students. Applications are processed on a rolling basis. Application fee: $100. *Financial support:* In 2015–16, 19 fellowships (averaging $824 per year), 36 research assistantships (averaging $20,351 per year), 1 teaching assistantship (averaging $16,824 per year) were awarded; Federal Work-Study and institutionally sponsored loans also available. Financial award application deadline: 2/1. *Total annual research expenditures:* $2.7 million. *Unit head:* Dr. Jerris R. Hedges, Dean, 808-692-0881. *Application contact:* Marla Berry, Graduate Co-Chair, 808-692-1506, Fax: 808-692-1968, E-mail: mberry@hawaii.edu.
Website: http://www.hawaii.edu/cmb/

University of Illinois at Chicago, College of Medicine and Graduate College, Graduate Programs in Medicine, Department of Biochemistry and Molecular Genetics, Chicago, IL 60607-7128. Offers PhD, MD/PhD. *Faculty:* 31 full-time (12 women), 19 part-time/adjunct (9 women). *Students:* 22 full-time (12 women); includes 5 minority (1 Black or African American, non-Hispanic/Latino; 3 Asian, non-Hispanic/Latino; 1 Hispanic/Latino), 9 international. Average age 29. Terminal master's awarded for partial completion of doctoral program. *Degree requirements:* For doctorate, thesis/dissertation. *Entrance requirements:* For doctorate, GRE General Test. Additional exam requirements/recommendations for international students: Required—TOEFL. *Application deadline:* For fall admission, 3/1 priority date for domestic students, 2/15 for international students. Applications are processed on a rolling basis. Application fee: $60. Electronic applications accepted. *Expenses:* Tuition, state resident: full-time $11,480; part-time $3826 per credit. Tuition, nonresident: full-time $23,720; part-time $7906 per credit. *Required fees:* $1333 per semester. Part-time tuition and fees vary according to course load and program. *Financial support:* Fellowships with full tuition reimbursements, research assistantships with full tuition reimbursements, teaching assistantships with full tuition reimbursements, career-related internships or fieldwork, Federal Work-Study, institutionally sponsored loans, traineeships, tuition waivers (full), and unspecified assistantships available. Financial award application deadline: 3/1; financial award applicants required to submit FAFSA. *Faculty research:* Signal transduction, cell cycle regulation, membrane biology, regulation of gene function and development, protein and nucleic acid structure and function, cancer biology. *Unit head:* Dr. Jack Kaplan, Head, 312-355-2732, Fax: 312-413-0353, E-mail: kaplanj@uic.edu. *Application contact:* Dr. Karen Colley, Co-Director of Graduate Studies, 312-996-7756.
Website: http://www.uic.edu/com/bcmg/

The University of Iowa, Graduate College, Program in Molecular and Cellular Biology, Iowa City, IA 52242-1316. Offers PhD. *Degree requirements:* For doctorate, comprehensive exam, thesis/dissertation. *Entrance requirements:* For doctorate, GRE General Test, minimum GPA of 3.0. Additional exam requirements/recommendations for international students: Required—TOEFL (minimum score 600 paper-based; 100 iBT). Electronic applications accepted. *Faculty research:* Regulation of gene expression, inherited human genetic diseases, signal transduction mechanisms, structural biology and function.

The University of Kansas, Graduate Studies, College of Liberal Arts and Sciences, Department of Molecular Biosciences, Lawrence, KS 66044. Offers biochemistry and biophysics (MA, PhD); microbiology (MA, PhD); molecular, cellular, and developmental biology (MA, PhD). *Students:* 57 full-time (34 women), 4 part-time (1 woman); includes 9 minority (5 Asian, non-Hispanic/Latino; 2 Hispanic/Latino; 2 Two or more races, non-Hispanic/Latino), 23 international. Average age 27. 78 applicants, 46% accepted, 18 enrolled. In 2015, 3 master's, 7 doctorates awarded. Terminal master's awarded for partial completion of doctoral program. *Entrance requirements:* For master's and doctorate, GRE General Test. Additional exam requirements/recommendations for international students: Required—TOEFL or IELTS. *Application deadline:* For fall admission, 12/15 for domestic and international students. Application fee: $65 ($85 for

international students). Electronic applications accepted. *Financial support:* Fellowships, research assistantships, teaching assistantships, health care benefits, and unspecified assistantships available. Financial award application deadline: 3/1. *Faculty research:* Structure and function of proteins, genetics of organism development, molecular genetics, neurophysiology, molecular virology and pathogenics, developmental biology, cell biology. *Unit head:* Susan M. Egan, Chair, 785-864-4294, E-mail: sme@ku.edu. *Application contact:* John Connolly, Graduate Admissions Contact, 785-864-4311, E-mail: jconnolly@ku.edu.
Website: http://www.molecularbiosciences.ku.edu/

The University of Kansas, University of Kansas Medical Center, School of Medicine, Department of Biochemistry and Molecular Biology, Kansas City, KS 66160. Offers PhD, MD/PhD. *Faculty:* 22. *Students:* 7 full-time (4 women), 3 international. Average age 27. In 2015, 3 doctorates awarded. Terminal master's awarded for partial completion of doctoral program. *Degree requirements:* For doctorate, thesis/dissertation, comprehensive oral and written exam. *Entrance requirements:* For doctorate, GRE. Additional exam requirements/recommendations for international students: Required—TOEFL. *Application deadline:* For fall admission, 12/1 for domestic and international students. Applications are processed on a rolling basis. Application fee: $60. Electronic applications accepted. Application fee is waived when completed online. *Financial support:* In 2015–16, 3 research assistantships with partial tuition reimbursements, 4 teaching assistantships with partial tuition reimbursements were awarded; fellowships, traineeships, health care benefits, and unspecified assistantships also available. Financial award application deadline: 3/1; financial award applicants required to submit FAFSA. *Faculty research:* Determination of portion structure, underlying bases for interaction of proteins with their target, mapping allosteric circuiting within proteins, mechanism of action of transcription factors, renal signal transduction. *Total annual research expenditures:* $1.5 million. *Unit head:* Dr. Gerald M. Carlson, Chairman, 913-588-7005, Fax: 913-588-9896, E-mail: gcarlson@kumc.edu. *Application contact:* Dr. Liskin Swint-Kruse, Associate Professor, 913-588-0399, Fax: 913-588-9896, E-mail: lswint-kruse@kumc.edu.
Website: http://www.kumc.edu/school-of-medicine/biochemistry-and-molecular-biology.html

University of Lethbridge, School of Graduate Studies, Lethbridge, AB T1K 3M4, Canada. Offers addictions counseling (M Sc); agricultural biotechnology (M Sc); agricultural studies (M Sc, MA); anthropology (MA); archaeology (M Sc, MA); art (MA, MFA); biochemistry (M Sc); biological sciences (M Sc); biomolecular science (PhD); biosystems and biodiversity (PhD); Canadian studies (MA); chemistry (M Sc); computer science (M Sc); computer science and geographical information science (M Sc); counseling (MC); counseling psychology (M Ed); dramatic arts (MA); earth, space, and physical science (PhD); economics (MA); education (MA, PhD); educational leadership (M Ed); English (MA); environmental science (M Sc); evolution and behavior (PhD); exercise science (M Sc); French (MA); French/German (MA); French/Spanish (MA); general education (M Ed); geography (M Sc, MA); German (MA); health sciences (M Sc); individualized multidisciplinary (M Sc, MA); kinesiology (M Sc, MA); management (M Sc), including accounting, finance, human resource management and labor relations, information systems, international management, marketing, policy and strategy; mathematics (M Sc); music (M Mus, MA); Native American studies (MA); neuroscience (M Sc, PhD); new media (MA, MFA); nursing (M Sc, MN); philosophy (MA); physics (M Sc); political science (MA); psychology (M Sc, MA); religious studies (MA); sociology (MA); theatre and dramatic arts (MFA); theoretical and computational science (PhD); urban and regional studies (MA); women and gender studies (MA). *Program availability:* Part-time, evening/weekend. *Students:* 448 full-time (249 women), 110 part-time (64 women). Average age 32. 285 applicants, 36% accepted, 96 enrolled. In 2015, 154 master's, 11 doctorates awarded. *Degree requirements:* For master's, thesis (for some programs); for doctorate, comprehensive exam, thesis/dissertation. *Entrance requirements:* For master's, GMAT (for M Sc in management), bachelor's degree in related field, minimum GPA of 3.0 during previous 20 graded semester courses, 2 years' teaching or related experience (M Ed); for doctorate, master's degree, minimum graduate GPA of 3.5. Additional exam requirements/recommendations for international students: Required—TOEFL (minimum score 580 paper-based; 93 iBT). Application fee: $100 Canadian dollars ($140 Canadian dollars for international students). Electronic applications accepted. *Financial support:* Fellowships, research assistantships, teaching assistantships, scholarships/grants, health care benefits, and unspecified assistantships available. *Faculty research:* Movement and brain plasticity, gibberellin physiology, photosynthesis, carbon cycling, molecular properties of main-group ring components. *Unit head:* Kathleen Schrage, Manager, School of Graduate Studies, 403-329-2121, E-mail: schrage@uleth.ca. *Application contact:* School of Graduate Studies, 403-329-5194, E-mail: sgsinquiries@uleth.ca.
Website: http://www.uleth.ca/graduate-studies/

University of Louisville, School of Medicine, Department of Biochemistry and Molecular Biology, Louisville, KY 40292-0001. Offers MS, PhD, MD/PhD. *Students:* 24 full-time (13 women), 7 part-time (2 women); includes 3 minority (2 Black or African American, non-Hispanic/Latino; 1 Asian, non-Hispanic/Latino), 8 international. Average age 29. 39 applicants, 18% accepted, 5 enrolled. In 2015, 9 master's, 1 doctorate awarded. Terminal master's awarded for partial completion of doctoral program. *Degree requirements:* For master's, thesis; for doctorate, comprehensive exam, thesis/dissertation, one first-author publication. *Entrance requirements:* For master's and doctorate, GRE General Test (minimum score of 1000 verbal and quantitative), minimum GPA of 3.0. Additional exam requirements/recommendations for international students: Required—TOEFL. *Application deadline:* For fall admission, 4/15 for domestic and international students. Applications are processed on a rolling basis. Application fee: $60. Electronic applications accepted. *Expenses:* Tuition, state resident: full-time $11,664; part-time $649 per credit hour. Tuition, nonresident: full-time $24,274; part-time $1350 per credit hour. *Required fees:* $196. Tuition and fees vary according to program and reciprocity agreements. *Financial support:* In 2015–16, 246,603 students received support, including 12 fellowships with full tuition reimbursements available (averaging $22,000 per year), 23 research assistantships with full tuition reimbursements available (averaging $22,000 per year); teaching assistantships with tuition reimbursements available, scholarships/grants, traineeships, tuition waivers (full and partial), and unspecified assistantships also available. Financial award application deadline: 4/15. *Faculty research:* Genetic regulatory mechanisms, microRNAs, vesicular trafficking in cancer metastasis and angiogenesis, ribosome biogenesis and disease, regulation of foreign compound metabolism/lipid and steroid metabolism. *Total annual research expenditures:* $2.4 million. *Unit head:* Dr. Ronald G. Gregg, Chair, 502-852-5217, Fax: 502-852-6222, E-mail: rggreg02@gwise.louisville.edu. *Application contact:* Dr. William L. Dean, Information Contact, 502-852-5227, Fax: 502-852-6222, E-mail: wldean01@gwise.louisville.edu.

University of Maine, Graduate School, College of Natural Sciences, Forestry, and Agriculture, Department of Molecular and Biomedical Sciences, Orono, ME 04469. Offers microbiology (PhD). *Faculty:* 30 full-time (6 women), 20 part-time/adjunct (4 women). *Students:* 22 full-time (12 women); includes 2 minority (1 Asian, non-Hispanic/Latino; 1 Two or more races, non-Hispanic/Latino), 3 international. Average age 30. 40 applicants, 28% accepted, 6 enrolled. In 2015, 7 master's, 3 doctorates awarded. *Degree requirements:* For master's, thesis (for some programs); for doctorate, comprehensive exam, thesis/dissertation. *Entrance requirements:* For master's and doctorate, GRE General Test. Additional exam requirements/recommendations for international students: Required—TOEFL. *Application deadline:* For fall admission, 2/1 priority date for domestic students. Applications are processed on a rolling basis. Application fee: $65. Electronic applications accepted. *Financial support:* In 2015–16, 20 students received support, including 8 research assistantships with full tuition reimbursements available (averaging $16,800 per year), 12 teaching assistantships with full tuition reimbursements available (averaging $19,000 per year); tuition waivers (full and partial) also available. Financial award application deadline: 3/1. *Total annual research expenditures:* $242,844. *Unit head:* Dr. Robert Gundersen, Chair, 207-581-2802, Fax: 207-581-2801. *Application contact:* Scott G. Delcourt, Assistant Vice President for Graduate Studies and Senior Associate Dean, 207-581-3291, Fax: 207-581-3232, E-mail: graduate@maine.edu.
Website: http://umaine.edu/biomed/

The University of Manchester, Faculty of Life Sciences, Manchester, United Kingdom. Offers adaptive organismal biology (M Phil, PhD); animal biology (M Phil, PhD); biochemistry (M Phil, PhD); bioinformatics (M Phil, PhD); biomolecular sciences (M Phil, PhD); biotechnology (M Phil, PhD); cell biology (M Phil, PhD); cell matrix research (M Phil, PhD); channels and transporters (M Phil, PhD); developmental biology (M Phil, PhD); Egyptology (M Phil, PhD); environmental biology (M Phil, PhD); evolutionary biology (M Phil, PhD); gene expression (M Phil, PhD); genetics (M Phil, PhD); history of science, technology and medicine (M Phil, PhD); immunology (M Phil, PhD); integrative neurobiology and behavior (M Phil, PhD); membrane trafficking (M Phil, PhD); microbiology (M Phil, PhD); molecular and cellular neuroscience (M Phil, PhD); molecular biology (M Phil, PhD); molecular cancer studies (M Phil, PhD); neuroscience (M Phil, PhD); ophthalmology (M Phil, PhD); optometry (M Phil, PhD); organelle function (M Phil, PhD); pharmacology (M Phil, PhD); physiology (M Phil, PhD); plant sciences (M Phil, PhD); stem cell research (M Phil, PhD); structural biology (M Phil, PhD); systems neuroscience (M Phil, PhD); toxicology (M Phil, PhD).

The University of Manchester, School of Dentistry, Manchester, United Kingdom. Offers basic dental sciences (cancer studies) (M Phil, PhD); basic dental sciences (molecular genetics) (M Phil, PhD); basic dental sciences (stem cell biology) (M Phil, PhD); biomaterials sciences and dental technology (M Phil, PhD); dental public health/community dentistry (M Phil, PhD); dental science (clinical) (PhD); endodontology (M Phil, PhD); fixed and removable prosthodontics (M Phil, PhD); operative dentistry (M Phil, PhD); oral and maxillofacial surgery (M Phil, PhD); oral radiology (M Phil, PhD); orthodontics (M Phil, PhD); restorative dentistry (M Phil, PhD).

University of Maryland, Baltimore, Graduate School, Graduate Program in Life Sciences, Program in Biochemistry and Molecular Biology, Baltimore, MD 21201. Offers biochemistry (MS, PhD); MD/PhD. *Degree requirements:* For doctorate, comprehensive exam, thesis/dissertation. *Entrance requirements:* For doctorate, GRE General Test. Additional exam requirements/recommendations for international students: Required—TOEFL (minimum score 550 paper-based; 80 iBT); Recommended—IELTS (minimum score 7). Electronic applications accepted. Tuition and fees vary according to program. *Faculty research:* Membrane transport, hormonal regulation, protein structure, molecular virology.

University of Maryland, Baltimore, Graduate School, Graduate Program in Life Sciences, Program in Cellular and Molecular Biomedical Science, Baltimore, MD 21201. Offers MS. *Program availability:* Part-time. Electronic applications accepted. Tuition and fees vary according to program.

University of Maryland, Baltimore, Graduate School, Graduate Program in Life Sciences, Program in Molecular Medicine, Baltimore, MD 21201. Offers cancer biology (PhD); cell and molecular physiology (PhD); human genetics and genomic medicine (PhD); molecular medicine (MS); molecular toxicology and pharmacology (PhD); MD/PhD. *Degree requirements:* For doctorate, comprehensive exam, thesis/dissertation. *Entrance requirements:* For master's and doctorate, GRE. Additional exam requirements/recommendations for international students: Required—TOEFL (minimum score 600 paper-based; 100 iBT); Recommended—IELTS (minimum score 7). Electronic applications accepted. Tuition and fees vary according to program.

University of Maryland, Baltimore County, The Graduate School, College of Natural and Mathematical Sciences, Department of Biological Sciences, Program in Applied Molecular Biology, Baltimore, MD 21250. Offers MS. *Faculty:* 26 full-time (11 women). *Students:* 8 full-time (4 women), 5 part-time (3 women); includes 4 minority (3 Asian, non-Hispanic/Latino; 1 Hispanic/Latino). Average age 23. 30 applicants, 40% accepted, 10 enrolled. In 2015, 13 master's awarded. *Entrance requirements:* For master's, GRE General Test, GRE Subject Test (recommended), minimum GPA of 3.0. Additional exam requirements/recommendations for international students: Required—TOEFL (minimum score 600 paper-based; 80 iBT), IELTS (minimum score 6.5). *Application deadline:* For fall admission, 2/1 priority date for domestic and international students. Applications are processed on a rolling basis. Application fee: $50. Electronic applications accepted. *Expenses:* Tuition, state resident: full-time $12,816. Tuition, nonresident: full-time $19,710. *Financial support:* Applicants required to submit FAFSA. *Faculty research:* Structure-function of RNA, genetics and molecular biology, biological chemistry. *Unit head:* Dr. Michelle Starz-Gaiano, Director, Applied Molecular Biology Graduate Program, 410-455-2217, Fax: 410-455-3875, E-mail: biograd@umbc.edu. *Application contact:* Melody Wright, Graduate Program Coordinator, 410-455-3669, Fax: 410-455-3875, E-mail: biograd@umbc.edu.
Website: http://biology.umbc.edu/grad/graduate-programs/apmb/

University of Maryland, Baltimore County, The Graduate School, College of Natural and Mathematical Sciences, Department of Biological Sciences, Program in Molecular and Cell Biology, Baltimore, MD 21250. Offers PhD. *Faculty:* 26 full-time (11 women). *Students:* 6 full-time (4 women); includes 1 minority (Hispanic/Latino), 2 international. Average age 29. 34 applicants, 9% accepted, 1 enrolled. In 2015, 2 doctorates awarded. *Degree requirements:* For doctorate, thesis/dissertation. *Entrance requirements:* For doctorate, GRE General Test, GRE Subject Test, minimum GPA of 3.0. Additional exam requirements/recommendations for international students: Required—TOEFL (minimum score 80 iBT). *Application deadline:* For fall admission, 1/1 priority date for domestic and international students. Application fee: $50. Electronic applications accepted. *Expenses:* Tuition, state resident: full-time $12,816. Tuition, nonresident: full-time $19,710. *Financial support:* In 2015–16, 7 students received support, including 3 research assistantships with full tuition reimbursements available (averaging $24,000 per year), 4 teaching assistantships with full tuition reimbursements available (averaging $24,000 per year). *Unit head:* Dr. Michelle Starz-Gaiano, Graduate Program Director, 410-455-2217, Fax: 410-455-3875, E-mail: biograd@umbc.edu. *Application contact:* Dr. Michelle Starz-Gaiano, Director, 410-455-2217, Fax: 410-455-3875, E-mail: biograd@umbc.edu.
Website: http://biology.umbc.edu/grad/graduate-programs/mocb/

University of Maryland, College Park, Academic Affairs, College of Computer, Mathematical and Natural Sciences, Department of Biology, PhD Program in Biological Sciences, College Park, MD 20742. Offers behavior, ecology, evolution, and systematics (PhD); computational biology, bioinformatics, and genomics (PhD); molecular and cellular biology (PhD); physiological systems (PhD). *Degree requirements:* For doctorate, comprehensive exam, thesis/dissertation, thesis work presentation in seminar. *Entrance requirements:* For doctorate, GRE General Test; GRE Subject Test in biology (recommended), academic transcripts, statement of purpose/research interests, 3 letters of recommendation. Additional exam requirements/recommendations for international students: Required—TOEFL. Electronic applications accepted.

University of Maryland, College Park, Academic Affairs, College of Computer, Mathematical and Natural Sciences, Department of Cell Biology and Molecular Genetics, Program in Molecular and Cellular Biology, College Park, MD 20742. Offers PhD. *Program availability:* Part-time, evening/weekend. *Degree requirements:* For doctorate, thesis/dissertation, exam, public service. *Faculty research:* Monoclonal antibody production, oligonucleotide synthesis, macronular processing, signal transduction, developmental biology.

University of Miami, Graduate School, Miller School of Medicine, Graduate Programs in Medicine, Department of Biochemistry and Molecular Biology, Coral Gables, FL 33124. Offers PhD, MD/PhD. *Degree requirements:* For doctorate, comprehensive exam, thesis/dissertation, proposition exams. *Faculty research:* Macromolecule metabolism, molecular genetics, protein folding and 3-D structure, regulation of gene expression and enzyme function, signal transduction and developmental biology.

University of Miami, Graduate School, Miller School of Medicine, Graduate Programs in Medicine, Department of Cell Biology and Anatomy, Coral Gables, FL 33124. Offers molecular cell and developmental biology (PhD); MD/PhD. *Degree requirements:* For doctorate, thesis/dissertation. *Entrance requirements:* For doctorate, GRE General Test, GRE Subject Test. Additional exam requirements/recommendations for international students: Required—TOEFL. Electronic applications accepted.

University of Michigan, Rackham Graduate School, College of Literature, Science, and the Arts, Department of Molecular, Cellular, and Developmental Biology, Ann Arbor, MI 48109. Offers MS, PhD. *Program availability:* Part-time. *Faculty:* 37 full-time (15 women). *Students:* 90 full-time (54 women), 4 part-time (3 women); includes 11 minority (4 Black or African American, non-Hispanic/Latino; 1 Asian, non-Hispanic/Latino; 6 Hispanic/Latino), 50 international. Average age 26. 106 applicants, 34% accepted, 19 enrolled. In 2015, 12 master's, 10 doctorates awarded. Terminal master's awarded for partial completion of doctoral program. *Degree requirements:* For master's, thesis (for some programs), 24 credits with at least 16 in molecular, cellular, and developmental biology and 4 in a cognate field; for doctorate, thesis/dissertation, preliminary exam, oral defense. *Entrance requirements:* For master's and doctorate, GRE General Test. Additional exam requirements/recommendations for international students: Required—TOEFL (minimum score 560 paper-based; 83 iBT). *Application deadline:* For fall admission, 1/5 for domestic and international students; for winter admission, 11/1 for domestic and international students; for spring admission, 4/1 for domestic and international students. Application fee: $75 ($90 for international students). Electronic applications accepted. *Expenses:* Contact institution. *Financial support:* In 2015–16, 67 students received support, including 23 fellowships with full tuition reimbursements available (averaging $29,025 per year), 28 research assistantships with full tuition reimbursements available (averaging $28,500 per year), 18 teaching assistantships with full tuition reimbursements available (averaging $28,500 per year); traineeships and health care benefits also available. *Faculty research:* Cell biology, microbiology, neurobiology and physiology, developmental biology and plant molecular biology. *Total annual research expenditures:* $8.2 million. *Unit head:* Dr. Robert J. Denver, Department Chair, 734-764-7476, Fax: 734-615-6337, E-mail: rdenver@umich.edu. *Application contact:* Mary Carr, Graduate Coordinator, 734-615-1635, Fax: 734-764-0884, E-mail: carrmm@umich.edu.
Website: http://www.mcdb.lsa.umich.edu

University of Michigan, Rackham Graduate School, Program in Biomedical Sciences (PIBS), Interdisciplinary Program in Cellular and Molecular Biology, Ann Arbor, MI 48109. Offers PhD. *Faculty:* 166 part-time/adjunct (43 women). *Students:* 59 full-time (32 women); includes 20 minority (1 Black or African American, non-Hispanic/Latino; 1 American Indian or Alaska Native, non-Hispanic/Latino; 11 Asian, non-Hispanic/Latino; 5 Hispanic/Latino; 2 Two or more races, non-Hispanic/Latino), 1 international. Average age 26. 71 applicants, 49% accepted, 7 enrolled. In 2015, 16 doctorates awarded. *Degree requirements:* For doctorate, comprehensive exam, thesis/dissertation, preliminary exam; oral defense of dissertation. *Entrance requirements:* For doctorate, GRE General Test. Additional exam requirements/recommendations for international students: Required—TOEFL (minimum score 560 paper-based; 84 iBT), IELTS (minimum score 6.5), Michigan English Language Assessment Battery. *Application deadline:* For fall admission, 12/1 for domestic students. Application fee: $75 ($90 for international students). Electronic applications accepted. *Expenses:* Contact institution. *Financial support:* In 2015–16, 59 students received support, including 17 fellowships with full tuition reimbursements available (averaging $29,025 per year), 34 research assistantships with full tuition reimbursements available (averaging $29,025 per year), 8 teaching assistantships with full tuition reimbursements available (averaging $29,025 per year); scholarships/grants, traineeships, and health care benefits also available. *Faculty research:* Cell and systems biology, cell physiology, biochemistry, genetics/gene regulation, genomics/proteomics, computational biology, microbial pathogenesis, immunology, development, aging, neurobiology, molecular mechanisms of disease, cancer biology. *Total annual research expenditures:* $20 million. *Unit head:* Dr. Robert S. Fuller, Director, 734-936-9764, Fax: 734-763-7799, E-mail: bfuller@umich.edu. *Application contact:* Margarita Bekiares, Intermediate Administrative Specialist, 734-764-5428, Fax: 734-647-7022, E-mail: cmbgrad@umich.edu.
Website: http://www.med.umich.edu/cmb/

University of Minnesota, Duluth, Medical School, Department of Biochemistry, Molecular Biology and Biophysics, Duluth, MN 55812-2496. Offers biochemistry, molecular biology and biophysics (MS); biology and biophysics (PhD); social, administrative, and clinical pharmacy (MS, PhD); toxicology (MS, PhD). Terminal master's awarded for partial completion of doctoral program. *Degree requirements:* For master's, comprehensive exam, thesis; for doctorate, comprehensive exam, thesis/dissertation. *Entrance requirements:* For master's and doctorate, GRE General Test. Additional exam requirements/recommendations for international students: Required—TOEFL. Electronic applications accepted. *Faculty research:* Intestinal cancer biology; hepatotoxins and mitochondriopathies; toxicology; cell cycle regulation in stem cells; neurobiology of brain development, trace metal function and blood-brain barrier; hibernation biology.

University of Minnesota, Twin Cities Campus, Graduate School, College of Biological Sciences, Biochemistry, Molecular Biology and Biophysics Graduate Program, Minneapolis, MN 55455-0213. Offers PhD. *Degree requirements:* For doctorate, thesis/dissertation. *Entrance requirements:* For doctorate, GRE, 3 letters of recommendation, more than 1 semester of laboratory experience. Additional exam requirements/recommendations for international students: Required—TOEFL (minimum score 625 paper-based; 108 iBT with writing subsection 25 and reading subsection 25) or IELTS (minimum score 7). Electronic applications accepted. *Faculty research:* Microbial biochemistry, biotechnology, molecular biology, regulatory biochemistry, structural biology and biophysics, physical biochemistry, enzymology, physiological chemistry.

University of Minnesota, Twin Cities Campus, Graduate School, Program in Molecular, Cellular, Developmental Biology and Genetics, Minneapolis, MN 55455-0213. Offers genetic counseling (MS); molecular, cellular, developmental biology and genetics (PhD). Terminal master's awarded for partial completion of doctoral program. *Degree requirements:* For master's, thesis optional; for doctorate, thesis/dissertation. *Entrance requirements:* For master's and doctorate, GRE General Test. Additional exam requirements/recommendations for international students: Required—TOEFL (minimum score 625 paper-based; 80 iBT). Electronic applications accepted. *Faculty research:* Membrane receptors and membrane transport, cell interactions, cytoskeleton and cell mobility, regulation of gene expression, plant cell and molecular biology.

University of Missouri–Kansas City, School of Biological Sciences, Program in Molecular Biology and Biochemistry, Kansas City, MO 64110-2499. Offers PhD. Offered through the School of Graduate Studies. *Faculty:* 31 full-time (9 women), 3 part-time/adjunct (2 women). *Students:* 5 full-time (3 women), 12 part-time (3 women); includes 6 minority (1 Black or African American, non-Hispanic/Latino; 2 Asian, non-Hispanic/Latino; 2 Hispanic/Latino; 1 Two or more races, non-Hispanic/Latino), 1 international. Average age 26. 33 applicants, 33% accepted, 10 enrolled. *Degree requirements:* For doctorate, comprehensive exam, thesis/dissertation. *Entrance requirements:* For doctorate, GRE General Test, bachelor's degree in chemistry, biology, or a related discipline; minimum GPA of 3.0. Additional exam requirements/recommendations for international students: Required—TOEFL (minimum score 550 paper-based; 80 iBT). *Application deadline:* For fall admission, 2/15 priority date for domestic and international students. Application fee: $45 ($50 for international students). *Financial support:* In 2015–16, 11 research assistantships with full tuition reimbursements (averaging $24,189 per year), 17 teaching assistantships with tuition reimbursements (averaging $15,312 per year) were awarded; scholarships/grants, tuition waivers (full and partial), and unspecified assistantships also available. Financial award application deadline: 3/1; financial award applicants required to submit FAFSA. *Unit head:* Dr. Xiao-Qiang Yu, Interim Head, 816-235-6379, E-mail: yux@umkc.edu. *Application contact:* Karen Bame, Graduate Programs Officer, 816-235-2243, Fax: 816-235-5595, E-mail: bamek@umkc.edu.
Website: http://sbs.umkc.edu/

University of Montana, Graduate School, College of Humanities and Sciences, Division of Biological Sciences, Program in Cellular, Molecular and Microbial Biology, Missoula, MT 59812-0002. Offers cellular and developmental biology (PhD); microbial evolution and ecology (PhD); microbiology and immunology (PhD); molecular biology and biochemistry (PhD). Terminal master's awarded for partial completion of doctoral program. *Degree requirements:* For doctorate, variable foreign language requirement, thesis/dissertation. *Entrance requirements:* For doctorate, GRE General Test. *Faculty research:* Ribosome structure, medical microbiology/pathogenesis, microbial ecology/environmental microbiology.

University of Nebraska Medical Center, Department of Biochemistry and Molecular Biology, Omaha, NE 68198. Offers MS, PhD. *Faculty:* 32 full-time (8 women). *Students:* 42 full-time (23 women); includes 3 minority (1 Asian, non-Hispanic/Latino; 1 Hispanic/Latino; 1 Two or more races, non-Hispanic/Latino), 26 international. Average age 28. 18 applicants, 33% accepted, 6 enrolled. In 2015, 4 doctorates awarded. Terminal master's awarded for partial completion of doctoral program. *Degree requirements:* For master's, comprehensive exam, thesis; for doctorate, comprehensive exam, thesis/dissertation. *Entrance requirements:* For master's, GRE General Test; for doctorate, GRE General Test, MCAT, PCAT, DCAT. Additional exam requirements/recommendations for international students: Required—TOEFL (minimum score 550 paper-based). *Application deadline:* For fall admission, 3/1 for domestic students, 4/1 for international students; for spring admission, 8/1 for domestic and international students; for summer admission, 1/1 for domestic and international students. Application fee: $45. Electronic applications accepted. *Expenses:* Tuition, state resident: full-time $7830; part-time $3915 per credit hour. Tuition, nonresident: full-time $22,410; part-time $11,205 per credit hour. *Required fees:* $521. *Financial support:* In 2015–16, 13 students received support, including 4 fellowships with full tuition reimbursements available (averaging $23,100 per year), 7 research assistantships with full tuition reimbursements available (averaging $23,100 per year); scholarships/grants, health care benefits, and unspecified assistantships also available. Support available to part-time students. Financial award application deadline: 2/15; financial award applicants required to submit FAFSA. *Faculty research:* Recombinant DNA, cancer biology, diabetes and drug metabolism, biochemical endocrinology. *Unit head:* Dr. Paul Sorgen, Chairman, Graduate Committee, 402-559-7557, Fax: 402-559-6650, E-mail: psorgen@unmc.edu. *Application contact:* Karen Hankins, Office Associate, 402-559-4417, E-mail: karen.hankins@unmc.edu.
Website: http://www.unmc.edu/biochemistry/

University of Nevada, Reno, Graduate School, Interdisciplinary Program in Cell and Molecular Biology, Reno, NV 89557. Offers MS, PhD. Terminal master's awarded for partial completion of doctoral program. *Degree requirements:* For master's, thesis; for doctorate, thesis/dissertation. *Entrance requirements:* For master's, GRE Subject Test (recommended), minimum GPA of 2.75; for doctorate, GRE Subject Test (recommended), minimum GPA of 3.0. Additional exam requirements/recommendations for international students: Required—TOEFL (minimum score 500 paper-based; 61 iBT), IELTS (minimum score 6). Electronic applications accepted. *Faculty research:* Cellular biology, biophysics, cancer, microbiology, insect biochemistry.

University of New Haven, Graduate School, College of Arts and Sciences, Program in Cellular and Molecular Biology, West Haven, CT 06516-1916. Offers MS, Graduate Certificate. *Program availability:* Part-time, evening/weekend. *Students:* 32 full-time (23 women), 12 part-time (7 women); includes 11 minority (7 Black or African American, non-Hispanic/Latino; 2 Asian, non-Hispanic/Latino; 2 Hispanic/Latino), 13 international. Average age 25. 61 applicants, 82% accepted, 26 enrolled. In 2015, 24 master's awarded. *Degree requirements:* For master's, thesis or alternative. *Entrance requirements:* Additional exam requirements/recommendations for international students: Required—TOEFL (minimum score 80 iBT), IELTS, PTE. *Application deadline:* For fall admission, 5/31 for international students; for winter admission, 10/15 for international students; for spring admission, 1/15 for international students. Applications are processed on a rolling basis. Application fee: $75. Electronic applications accepted. Application fee is waived when completed online. *Expenses:* Tuition, area resident: Full-time $15,282; part-time $849 per credit hour. *Required fees:* $150; $60 per term. Tuition and fees vary according to program. *Financial support:* Research assistantships with partial tuition reimbursements, teaching assistantships with partial tuition reimbursements, career-related internships or fieldwork, Federal Work-Study, scholarships/grants, and unspecified assistantships available. Support available to part-time students. Financial award application deadline: 5/1; financial award applicants required to submit FAFSA. *Unit head:* Dr. Christina Zito, Assistant Professor, 203-479-4299, E-mail: czito@newhaven.edu.
Website: http://www.newhaven.edu/4724/

University of New Mexico, Graduate Studies, Health Sciences Center, Program in Biomedical Sciences, Albuquerque, NM 87131-5196. Offers biochemistry and molecular biology (MS, PhD); cell biology and physiology (MS, PhD); molecular genetics and microbiology (MS, PhD); neuroscience (MS, PhD); pathology (MS, PhD); toxicology

(MS, PhD). *Program availability:* Part-time. *Faculty:* 18 full-time (10 women), 1 part-time/adjunct (0 women). *Students:* 31 full-time (17 women), 45 part-time (26 women); includes 29 minority (1 American Indian or Alaska Native, non-Hispanic/Latino; 3 Asian, non-Hispanic/Latino; 22 Hispanic/Latino; 2 Native Hawaiian or other Pacific Islander, non-Hispanic/Latino; 1 Two or more races, non-Hispanic/Latino), 18 international. Average age 30. 98 applicants, 11% accepted, 11 enrolled. In 2015, 11 master's, 14 doctorates awarded. Terminal master's awarded for partial completion of doctoral program. *Degree requirements:* For master's, thesis; for doctorate, comprehensive exam, thesis/dissertation, qualifying exam at the end of year 1/core curriculum. *Entrance requirements:* For master's and doctorate, GRE General Test, minimum undergraduate GPA of 3.0. Additional exam requirements/recommendations for international students: Required—TOEFL. *Application deadline:* For fall admission, 3/1 priority date for domestic and international students. Applications are processed on a rolling basis. Application fee: $50. Electronic applications accepted. *Financial support:* Fellowships with tuition reimbursements, research assistantships with full tuition reimbursements, teaching assistantships, career-related internships or fieldwork, Federal Work-Study, institutionally sponsored loans, scholarships/grants, traineeships, health care benefits, and unspecified assistantships available. Financial award application deadline: 1/1; financial award applicants required to submit FAFSA. *Faculty research:* Infectious disease/immunity, cancer biology, cardiovascular and metabolic diseases, brain and behavioral illness, environmental health. *Unit head:* Dr. Helen J. Hathaway, Program Director, 505-272-1887, Fax: 505-272-2412, E-mail: hhathaway@salud.unm.edu. *Application contact:* Mary Fenton, Admissions Coordinator, 505-272-1887, Fax: 505-272-2412, E-mail: mfenton@salud.unm.edu.

The University of North Carolina at Chapel Hill, Graduate School, College of Arts and Sciences, Department of Biology, Chapel Hill, NC 27599. Offers botany (MA, MS, PhD); cell biology, development, and physiology (MA, MS, PhD); cell motility and cytoskeleton (PhD); ecology and behavior (MA, MS, PhD); genetics and molecular biology (MA, MS, PhD); morphology, systematics, and evolution (MA, MS, PhD). Terminal master's awarded for partial completion of doctoral program. *Degree requirements:* For master's, comprehensive exam, thesis (for some programs); for doctorate, comprehensive exam, thesis/dissertation. *Entrance requirements:* For master's, GRE General Test, GRE Subject Test, 2 semesters of calculus or statistics; 2 semesters of physics, organic chemistry; 3 semesters of biology; for doctorate, GRE General Test, GRE Subject Test, 2 semesters calculus or statistics, 2 semesters physics, organic chemistry, 3 semesters of biology. Additional exam requirements/recommendations for international students: Required—TOEFL (minimum score 550 paper-based). Electronic applications accepted. *Faculty research:* Gene expression, biomechanics, yeast genetics, plant ecology, plant molecular biology.

The University of North Carolina at Chapel Hill, School of Medicine and Graduate School, Graduate Programs in Medicine, Curriculum in Genetics and Molecular Biology, Chapel Hill, NC 27599. Offers MS, PhD. *Degree requirements:* For doctorate, comprehensive exam, thesis/dissertation. *Entrance requirements:* For doctorate, GRE, minimum GPA of 3.0. Additional exam requirements/recommendations for international students: Required—TOEFL. Electronic applications accepted. *Faculty research:* Telomere replication and germline immortality, experimental evolution in microorganisms, genetic vulnerabilities in tumor genomes, genetics of cell cycle control during Drosophila development, mammalian genetics.

University of North Dakota, Graduate School and Graduate School, Graduate Programs in Medicine, Department of Biochemistry and Molecular Biology, Grand Forks, ND 58202. Offers MS, PhD. *Degree requirements:* For master's, thesis, final exam; for doctorate, comprehensive exam, thesis/dissertation, final exam. *Entrance requirements:* For master's and doctorate, GRE General Test, minimum GPA of 3.0. Additional exam requirements/recommendations for international students: Required—TOEFL (minimum score 550 paper-based; 79 iBT), IELTS (minimum score 6.5). Electronic applications accepted. *Faculty research:* Glucose-6-phosphatase, guanine nucleotides, carbohydrate and lipid metabolism, cytoskeletal proteins, chromatin structure.

University of North Texas, Robert B. Toulouse School of Graduate Studies, Denton, TX 76203-5459. Offers accounting (MS, MBA, MS); applied anthropology (MA, MS); applied behavior analysis (Certificate); applied geography (MA); applied technology and performance improvement (M Ed, MS); art education (MA); art history (MA); art museum education (Certificate); arts leadership (Certificate); audiology (Au D); behavior analysis (MS); behavioral science (PhD); biochemistry and molecular biology (MS); biology (MA, MS); biomedical engineering (MS); business analysis (MS); chemistry (MS); clinical health psychology (PhD); communication studies (MA, MS); computer engineering (MS); computer science (MS); counseling (M Ed, MS), including clinical mental health counseling (MS), college and university counseling, elementary school counseling, secondary school counseling; creative writing (MA); criminal justice (MS); curriculum and instruction (M Ed); decision sciences (MBA); design (MA, MFA), including fashion design (MFA), innovation studies, interior design (MFA); early childhood studies (MS); economics (MS); educational leadership (M Ed, Ed D); educational psychology (MS, PhD), including family studies (MS), gifted and talented (MS), human development (MS), learning and cognition (MS), research, measurement and evaluation (MS); electrical engineering (MS); emergency management (MPA); engineering technology (MS); English (MA); English as a second language (MA); environmental science (MS); finance (MBA, MS); financial management (MPA); French (MA); health services management (MBA); higher education (M Ed, Ed D); history (MA, MS); hospitality management (MS); human resources management (MPA); information science (MS); information systems (PhD); information technologies (MBA); interdisciplinary studies (MA, MS); international studies (MA); international sustainable tourism (MS); jazz studies (MM); journalism (MA, MJ, Graduate Certificate), including interactive and virtual digital communication (Graduate Certificate), narrative journalism (Graduate Certificate), public relations (Graduate Certificate); kinesiology (MS); linguistics (MA); local government management (MPA); logistics (PhD); logistics and supply chain management (MBA); long-term care, senior housing, and aging services (MA); management (PhD); marketing (MBA); mathematics (MA, MS); mechanical and energy engineering (MS, PhD); music (MA), including ethnomusicology, music theory, musicology, performance; music composition (PhD); music education (MM Ed, PhD); nonprofit management (MPA); operations and supply chain management (MBA); performance (MM, DMA); philosophy (MA); political science (MA); professional and technical communication (MA); radio, television and film (MA, MFA); rehabilitation counseling (Certificate); sociology (MA); Spanish (MA); special education (M Ed); speech-language pathology (MA); strategic management (MBA); studio art (MFA); teaching (M Ed); MBA/MS. *Program availability:* Part-time, evening/weekend, online learning. Terminal master's awarded for partial completion of doctoral program. *Degree requirements:* For master's, variable foreign language requirement, comprehensive exam (for some programs), thesis (for some programs); for doctorate, variable foreign language requirement, comprehensive exam (for some programs), thesis/dissertation; for other advanced degree, variable foreign language requirement, comprehensive exam (for some programs). *Entrance requirements:* For master's and doctorate, GRE, GMAT. Additional exam requirements/recommendations for international students: Required—TOEFL (minimum score 550 paper-based; 79 iBT). Electronic applications accepted.

University of North Texas Health Science Center at Fort Worth, Graduate School of Biomedical Sciences, Fort Worth, TX 76107-2699. Offers anatomy and cell biology (MS, PhD); biochemistry and molecular biology (MS, PhD); biomedical sciences (MS, PhD); biotechnology (MS); forensic genetics (MS); integrative physiology (MS, PhD); medical science (MS); microbiology and immunology (MS, PhD); pharmacology (MS, PhD); science education (MS); DO/MS; DO/PhD. Terminal master's awarded for partial completion of doctoral program. *Degree requirements:* For master's, thesis; for doctorate, thesis/dissertation. *Entrance requirements:* For master's and doctorate, GRE General Test. Additional exam requirements/recommendations for international students: Required—TOEFL. *Expenses:* Contact institution. *Faculty research:* Alzheimer's disease, aging, eye diseases, cancer, cardiovascular disease.

University of Notre Dame, Graduate School, College of Science, Department of Biological Sciences, Notre Dame, IN 46556. Offers aquatic ecology, evolution and environmental biology (MS, PhD); cellular and molecular biology (MS, PhD); genetics (MS, PhD); physiology (MS, PhD); vector biology and parasitology (MS, PhD). Terminal master's awarded for partial completion of doctoral program. *Degree requirements:* For master's, comprehensive exam, thesis; for doctorate, comprehensive exam, thesis/dissertation, candidacy exam. *Entrance requirements:* For master's and doctorate, GRE General Test. Additional exam requirements/recommendations for international students: Required—TOEFL (minimum score 600 paper-based; 80 iBT). Electronic applications accepted. *Faculty research:* Tropical disease, molecular genetics, neurobiology, evolutionary biology, aquatic biology.

University of Oklahoma Health Sciences Center, College of Medicine and Graduate College, Graduate Programs in Medicine, Department of Biochemistry and Molecular Biology, Oklahoma City, OK 73190. Offers biochemistry (MS, PhD); molecular biology (MS, PhD). *Program availability:* Part-time. Terminal master's awarded for partial completion of doctoral program. *Degree requirements:* For master's, thesis; for doctorate, thesis/dissertation. *Entrance requirements:* For master's, GRE General Test, 2 letters of recommendation; for doctorate, GRE General Test, 3 letters of recommendation. Additional exam requirements/recommendations for international students: Required—TOEFL. *Faculty research:* Gene expression, regulation of transcription, enzyme evolution, melanogenesis, signal transduction.

University of Oregon, Graduate School, College of Arts and Sciences, Department of Biology, Eugene, OR 97403. Offers ecology and evolution (MA, MS, PhD); marine biology (MA, MS, PhD); molecular, cellular and genetic biology (PhD); neuroscience and development (PhD). Terminal master's awarded for partial completion of doctoral program. *Degree requirements:* For master's, thesis (for some programs); for doctorate, thesis/dissertation. *Entrance requirements:* For master's and doctorate, GRE General Test, minimum GPA of 3.2. Additional exam requirements/recommendations for international students: Required—TOEFL. *Faculty research:* Developmental neurobiology; evolution, population biology, and quantitative genetics; regulation of gene expression; biochemistry of marine organisms.

University of Ottawa, Faculty of Graduate and Postdoctoral Studies, Faculty of Medicine, Department of Cellular and Molecular Medicine, Ottawa, ON K1H 8M5, Canada. Offers M Sc, PhD. *Degree requirements:* For master's, thesis, seminar; for doctorate, comprehensive exam, thesis/dissertation, seminar. *Entrance requirements:* For master's, honors degree or equivalent, minimum B average; for doctorate, master's degree, minimum B+ average. Electronic applications accepted. *Faculty research:* Physiology, pharmacology, growth and development.

University of Pennsylvania, Perelman School of Medicine, Biomedical Graduate Studies, Graduate Group in Cell and Molecular Biology, Philadelphia, PA 19104. Offers cancer biology (PhD); cell biology, physiology, and metabolism (PhD); developmental stem cell regenerative biology (PhD); gene therapy and vaccines (PhD); genetics and gene regulation (PhD); microbiology, virology, and parasitology (PhD); MD/PhD; VMD/PhD. *Faculty:* 317. *Students:* 339 full-time (189 women); includes 100 minority (7 Black or African American, non-Hispanic/Latino; 2 American Indian or Alaska Native, non-Hispanic/Latino; 45 Asian, non-Hispanic/Latino; 34 Hispanic/Latino; 1 Native Hawaiian or other Pacific Islander, non-Hispanic/Latino; 11 Two or more races, non-Hispanic/Latino), 52 international. 493 applicants, 22% accepted, 37 enrolled. In 2015, 51 doctorates awarded. *Degree requirements:* For doctorate, thesis/dissertation. *Entrance requirements:* For doctorate, GRE General Test. Additional exam requirements/recommendations for international students: Required—TOEFL. *Application deadline:* For fall admission, 12/1 priority date for domestic and international students. Applications are processed on a rolling basis. Application fee: $80. Electronic applications accepted. *Expenses:* Tuition, area resident: Full-time $31,068; part-time $5762 per course. *Required fees:* $3200; $336 per course. Full-time tuition and fees vary according to degree level, program and student level. Part-time tuition and fees vary according to course load, degree level and program. *Financial support:* In 2015–16, 339 students received support. Fellowships, research assistantships, scholarships/grants, traineeships, and unspecified assistantships available. *Unit head:* Dr. Daniel Kessler, Graduate Group Chair, 215-898-1478. *Application contact:* Meagan Schofer, Coordinator, 215-898-4360.
Website: http://www.med.upenn.edu/camb/

University of Pittsburgh, Dietrich School of Arts and Sciences, Department of Biological Sciences, Program in Molecular, Cellular, and Developmental Biology, Pittsburgh, PA 15260. Offers PhD. *Students:* 36 full-time (19 women); includes 2 minority (1 Black or African American, non-Hispanic/Latino; 1 Asian, non-Hispanic/Latino), 8 international. Average age 23. 109 applicants, 24% accepted, 7 enrolled. In 2015, 3 doctorates awarded. *Degree requirements:* For doctorate, comprehensive exam, thesis/dissertation, completion of research integrity module. *Entrance requirements:* For doctorate, GRE General Test, GRE Subject Test. Additional exam requirements/recommendations for international students: Required—TOEFL (minimum score 90 iBT). *Application deadline:* For fall admission, 1/3 priority date for domestic students, 12/9 priority date for international students. Applications are processed on a rolling basis. Application fee: $0 ($50 for international students). Electronic applications accepted. Tuition and fees vary according to program. *Financial support:* In 2015–16, 26 fellowships with full tuition reimbursements (averaging $33,193 per year), 63 research assistantships with full tuition reimbursements (averaging $27,573 per year), 18 teaching assistantships with full tuition reimbursements (averaging $26,813 per year) were awarded; Federal Work-Study, traineeships, health care benefits, and tuition waivers (full) also available. *Unit head:* Dr. Karen M. Arndt, Professor, 412-624-6963, Fax: 412-624-4349, E-mail: arndt@pitt.edu. *Application contact:* Cathleen M. Barr, Graduate Administrator, 412-624-4268, Fax: 412-624-4349, E-mail: cbarr@pitt.edu.
Website: http://www.biology.pitt.edu

University of Puerto Rico, Río Piedras Campus, College of Natural Sciences, Department of Biology, San Juan, PR 00931-3300. Offers ecology/systematics (MS, PhD); evolution/genetics (MS, PhD); molecular/cellular biology (MS, PhD); neuroscience (MS, PhD). *Program availability:* Part-time. *Degree requirements:* For master's, one foreign language, comprehensive exam, thesis; for doctorate, one foreign language, comprehensive exam, thesis/dissertation. *Entrance requirements:* For master's, GRE Subject Test, interview, minimum GPA of 3.0, letter of recommendation; for doctorate,

Molecular Biology

GRE Subject Test, interview, master's degree, minimum GPA of 3.0, letter of recommendation. *Faculty research:* Environmental, poblational and systematic biology.

University of Rhode Island, Graduate School, College of the Environment and Life Sciences, Department of Cell and Molecular Biology, Kingston, RI 02881. Offers biochemistry (MS, PhD); clinical laboratory sciences (MS), including biotechnology, clinical laboratory science, cytopathology; microbiology (MS, PhD); molecular genetics (MS, PhD). *Program availability:* Part-time. *Faculty:* 11 full-time (4 women), 1 (woman) part-time/adjunct. *Students:* 12 full-time (6 women), 36 part-time (27 women); includes 10 minority (4 Black or African American, non-Hispanic/Latino; 3 Asian, non-Hispanic/Latino; 2 Hispanic/Latino; 1 Two or more races, non-Hispanic/Latino), 8 international. In 2015, 19 master's, 1 doctorate awarded. *Degree requirements:* For master's, comprehensive exam (for some programs), thesis optional; for doctorate, comprehensive exam, thesis/dissertation. *Entrance requirements:* For master's and doctorate, GRE, 2 letters of recommendation. Additional exam requirements/recommendations for international students: Required—TOEFL (minimum score 550 paper-based). *Application deadline:* For fall admission, 7/15 for domestic students, 2/1 for international students; for spring admission, 11/15 for domestic students, 7/15 for international students. Application fee: $65. Electronic applications accepted. *Expenses:* Tuition, state resident: full-time $11,796; part-time $655 per credit. Tuition, nonresident: full-time $24,206; part-time $1345 per credit. *Required fees:* $1546; $44 per credit. One-time fee: $155 full-time; $35 part-time. *Financial support:* In 2015–16, 3 research assistantships with tuition reimbursements (averaging $13,507 per year), 8 teaching assistantships with tuition reimbursements (averaging $13,305 per year) were awarded; traineeships also available. Financial award application deadline: 2/1; financial award applicants required to submit FAFSA. *Faculty research:* Genomics. *Total annual research expenditures:* $6.7 million. *Unit head:* Dr. Gongqing Sun, Chairperson, 401-874-5937, Fax: 401-874-2202, E-mail: gsun@mail.uri.edu. *Application contact:* Graduate Admissions, 401-874-2872, E-mail: gradadm@etal.uri.edu.
Website: http://cels.uri.edu/cmb/

University of Rochester, School of Medicine and Dentistry, Graduate Programs in Medicine and Dentistry, Department of Biochemistry and Biophysics, Programs in Biochemistry, Rochester, NY 14627. Offers biochemistry and molecular biology (PhD). Terminal master's awarded for partial completion of doctoral program. *Degree requirements:* For doctorate, thesis/dissertation, qualifying exam. *Entrance requirements:* For doctorate, GRE General Test. *Expenses: Tuition, area resident:* Full-time $47,450; part-time $1482 per credit hour. *Required fees:* $528. Tuition and fees vary according to program.

University of South Carolina, The Graduate School, College of Arts and Sciences, Department of Biological Sciences, Graduate Training Program in Molecular, Cellular, and Developmental Biology, Columbia, SC 29208. Offers MS, PhD. *Degree requirements:* For master's, one foreign language, thesis; for doctorate, one foreign language, thesis/dissertation. *Entrance requirements:* For master's and doctorate, GRE General Test, minimum GPA of 3.0 in science. Electronic applications accepted. *Faculty research:* Marine ecology, population and evolutionary biology, molecular biology and genetics, development.

The University of South Dakota, Graduate School, Sanford School of Medicine and Graduate School, Biomedical Sciences Graduate Program, Cellular and Molecular Biology Group, Vermillion, SD 57069-2390. Offers MS, PhD. *Students:* Average age 26. Terminal master's awarded for partial completion of doctoral program. *Degree requirements:* For master's, thesis; for doctorate, comprehensive exam, thesis/dissertation. *Entrance requirements:* For master's and doctorate, GRE General Test, GRE Subject Test, minimum GPA of 3.0. Additional exam requirements/recommendations for international students: Required—TOEFL (minimum score 550 paper-based; 80 iBT), IELTS (minimum score 6). *Application deadline:* For fall admission, 4/15 priority date for domestic students, 3/15 for international students. Applications are processed on a rolling basis. Application fee: $35. Electronic applications accepted. *Expenses:* Contact institution. *Financial support:* In 2015–16, 10 students received support. Fellowships with partial tuition reimbursements available and research assistantships with partial tuition reimbursements available available. Financial award application deadline: 4/15; financial award applicants required to submit FAFSA. *Faculty research:* Molecular aspects of protein and DNA, neurochemistry and energy transduction, gene regulation, cellular development. *Unit head:* 605-658-6322, Fax: 605-677-6381, E-mail: biomed@usd.edu.

University of Southern California, Graduate School, Dana and David Dornsife College of Letters, Arts and Sciences, Department of Biological Sciences, Program in Molecular and Computational Biology, Los Angeles, CA 90089. Offers computational biology and bioinformatics (PhD); molecular biology (PhD). *Degree requirements:* For doctorate, comprehensive exam, thesis/dissertation, qualifying examination, dissertation defense. *Entrance requirements:* For doctorate, GRE, 3 letters of recommendation, personal statement, resume, minimum GPA of 3.0. Additional exam requirements/recommendations for international students: Required—TOEFL (minimum score 600 paper-based; 100 iBT). Electronic applications accepted. *Faculty research:* Biochemistry and molecular biology; genomics; computational biology and bioinformatics; cell and developmental biology, and genetics; DNA replication and repair, and cancer biology.

University of Southern California, Keck School of Medicine and Graduate School, Graduate Programs in Medicine, Department of Biochemistry and Molecular Biology, Los Angeles, CA 90089. Offers MS. *Students:* 22 full-time (4 women). *Students:* 45 full-time (31 women); includes 6 minority (4 Asian, non-Hispanic/Latino; 2 Hispanic/Latino), 37 international. Average age 24. 76 applicants, 58% accepted, 28 enrolled. In 2015, 17 master's awarded. Terminal master's awarded for partial completion of doctoral program. *Degree requirements:* For master's, thesis. *Entrance requirements:* For master's, GRE General Test, minimum GPA of 3.0. Additional exam requirements/recommendations for international students: Required—TOEFL (minimum score 600 paper-based; 100 iBT). *Application deadline:* For fall admission, 4/15 priority date for domestic and international students. Applications are processed on a rolling basis. Application fee: $85. Electronic applications accepted. *Expenses:* Contact institution. *Financial support:* Application deadline: 5/4; applicants required to submit CSS PROFILE or FAFSA. *Faculty research:* Molecular genetics, gene expression, membrane biochemistry, metabolic regulation, cancer biology. *Total annual research expenditures:* $7.4 million. *Unit head:* Dr. Michael R. Stallcup, Chair, 323-442-1145, Fax: 323-442-1224, E-mail: stallcup@usc.edu. *Application contact:* Janet Stoeckert, Administrative Director, Basic Science Departments, 323-442-3568, Fax: 323-442-1610, E-mail: janet.stoeckert@usc.edu.
Website: http://keck.usc.edu/en/Education/Academic_Department_and_Divisions/Department_of_Biochemistry_and_Molecular_Biology.aspx

University of Southern California, Keck School of Medicine and Graduate School, Graduate Programs in Medicine, Department of Preventive Medicine, Los Angeles, CA 90089. Offers biostatistics (MS, PhD), including applied biostatistics and epidemiology (MS), biostatistics, epidemiology (MS); molecular epidemiology (MS); health behavior research (PhD); public health (MPH), including biostatistics-epidemiology, child and family health, environmental health, global health leadership, health communication, health education and promotion, public health policy. *Program availability:* Part-time. *Faculty:* 90 full-time (33 women), 11 part-time/adjunct (4 women). *Students:* 337 full-time (231 women), 36 part-time (25 women); includes 158 minority (23 Black or African American, non-Hispanic/Latino; 1 American Indian or Alaska Native, non-Hispanic/Latino; 86 Asian, non-Hispanic/Latino; 45 Hispanic/Latino; 2 Native Hawaiian or other Pacific Islander, non-Hispanic/Latino; 1 Two or more races, non-Hispanic/Latino), 111 international. Average age 28. 394 applicants, 59% accepted, 111 enrolled. In 2015, 120 master's, 14 doctorates awarded. Terminal master's awarded for partial completion of doctoral program. *Degree requirements:* For master's, thesis, practicum, final report, oral presentations; for doctorate, comprehensive exam, thesis/dissertation. *Entrance requirements:* For master's, GRE General Test, MCAT, GMAT, minimum GPA of 3.0; for doctorate, GRE General Test, minimum GPA of 3.0. Additional exam requirements/recommendations for international students: Required—TOEFL (minimum score 600 paper-based; 100 iBT). Application fee: $85. Electronic applications accepted. *Expenses:* Contact institution. *Financial support:* In 2015–16, 21 fellowships with full tuition reimbursements (averaging $32,000 per year), 43 research assistantships with tuition reimbursements (averaging $32,000 per year), 22 teaching assistantships with tuition reimbursements (averaging $32,000 per year) were awarded; career-related internships or fieldwork, Federal Work-Study, institutionally sponsored loans, scholarships/grants, traineeships, health care benefits, tuition waivers, and unspecified assistantships also available. Support available to part-time students. Financial award application deadline: 5/4; financial award applicants required to submit CSS PROFILE or FAFSA. *Unit head:* Dr. Jonthan Samet, Chair, 323-865-0803, Fax: 323-865-0103, E-mail: jsamet@usc.edu. *Application contact:* Susan Largent, Project Director, 323-852-0805, Fax: 323-852-0103, E-mail: slargent@med.usc.edu.

University of Southern California, Keck School of Medicine, Program in Molecular Structure and Signaling, Los Angeles, CA 90089. Offers molecular structure and signaling (PhD). *Faculty:* 23 full-time (6 women). *Students:* 2 full-time (1 woman). Average age 24. *Degree requirements:* For doctorate, comprehensive exam, thesis/dissertation. *Entrance requirements:* For doctorate, GRE, minimum GPA of 3.0. Additional exam requirements/recommendations for international students: Required—TOEFL (minimum score 600 paper-based; 100 iBT), IELTS (minimum score 7), PTE. *Application deadline:* For fall admission, 12/1 priority date for domestic and international students. Application fee: $85. Electronic applications accepted. *Financial support:* In 2015–16, 2 students received support, including 2 research assistantships with full tuition reimbursements available (averaging $32,000 per year); institutionally sponsored loans, scholarships/grants, traineeships, health care benefits, and unspecified assistantships also available. Financial award application deadline: 5/4; financial award applicants required to submit CSS PROFILE or FAFSA. *Unit head:* Dr. Wei Li, Director, 323-442-1475, Fax: 323-442-1199, E-mail: wli@usc.edu. *Application contact:* Dr. Joyce Perez, Manager of Student Programs, 323-442-1645, Fax: 323-442-1199, E-mail: jpperez@med.usc.edu.
Website: http://pibbs.usc.edu/research-and-programs/phd-programs/

University of Southern Maine, College of Science, Technology, and Health, Program in Applied Medical Sciences, Portland, ME 04103. Offers MS. *Program availability:* Part-time. *Degree requirements:* For master's, thesis. *Entrance requirements:* For master's, GRE General Test, minimum GPA of 3.0. Additional exam requirements/recommendations for international students: Required—TOEFL. Electronic applications accepted. *Expenses: Tuition, area resident:* Full-time $6840; part-time $380 per credit hour. Tuition, state resident: full-time $10,260; part-time $570 per credit hour. Tuition, nonresident: full-time $18,468; part-time $1026 per credit hour. *Required fees:* $830; $83 per credit hour. Tuition and fees vary according to course load and program. *Faculty research:* Cancer biology, toxicology, environmental health, epidemiology, autoimmune disease, immunology, infectious disease, virology.

University of Southern Mississippi, Graduate School, College of Science and Technology, Department of Biological Sciences, Hattiesburg, MS 39406-0001. Offers environmental biology (MS); marine biology (MS); microbiology (MS, PhD); molecular biology (MS, PhD). Terminal master's awarded for partial completion of doctoral program. *Degree requirements:* For master's, comprehensive exam, thesis; for doctorate, comprehensive exam, thesis/dissertation. *Entrance requirements:* For master's, GRE General Test, minimum GPA of 3.0 on last 60 hours; for doctorate, GRE General Test, minimum GPA of 3.5. Additional exam requirements/recommendations for international students: Required—TOEFL, IELTS.

University of South Florida, College of Arts and Sciences, Department of Cell Biology, Microbiology, and Molecular Biology, Tampa, FL 33620-9951. Offers biology (MS), including cancer biology (PhD); cell and molecular biology (PhD); microbiology (MS). *Faculty:* 21 full-time (7 women). *Students:* 41 full-time (6 women), 45 part-time (2 women); includes 11 minority (1 Black or African American, non-Hispanic/Latino; 2 Asian, non-Hispanic/Latino; 5 Hispanic/Latino; 3 Two or more races, non-Hispanic/Latino), 22 international. Average age 27. 171 applicants, 14% accepted, 18 enrolled. In 2015, 22 master's, 14 doctorates awarded. *Degree requirements:* For master's, thesis or alternative; for doctorate, comprehensive exam, thesis/dissertation. *Entrance requirements:* For master's and doctorate, GRE General Test, minimum GPA of 3.0, extensive background in biology or chemistry. Additional exam requirements/recommendations for international students: Required—TOEFL (minimum score 570 paper-based; 79 iBT) or IELTS (minimum score 6.5). *Application deadline:* For fall admission, 2/1 for domestic students, 1/1 for international students. Application fee: $30. *Financial support:* Career-related internships or fieldwork, health care benefits, and unspecified assistantships available. Financial award application deadline: 4/1. *Faculty research:* Cell biology, microbiology and molecular biology: basic and applied science in bacterial pathogenesis, genome integrity and mechanisms of aging, structural and computational biology; cancer biology: immunology, cancer control, signal transduction, drug discovery, genomics. *Total annual research expenditures:* $1.9 million. *Unit head:* Dr. James Garey, Professor/Chair, 813-974-7103, Fax: 813-974-1614, E-mail: garey@usf.edu. *Application contact:* Dr. Kenneth Wright, Associate Professor of Cancer Biology, H. Lee Moffitt Cancer Center and Research Institute, 813-745-3918, Fax: 813-974-1614, E-mail: ken.wright@moffitt.org.
Website: http://biology.usf.edu/cmmb/

The University of Texas at Austin, Graduate School, Institute for Cellular and Molecular Biology, Austin, TX 78712-1111. Offers PhD.

The University of Texas at Dallas, School of Natural Sciences and Mathematics, Department of Biological Sciences, Richardson, TX 75080. Offers bioinformatics and computational biology (MS); biotechnology (MS); molecular and cell biology (MS, PhD). *Program availability:* Part-time, evening/weekend. *Faculty:* 22 full-time (4 women), 1 part-time/adjunct (0 women). *Students:* 114 full-time (71 women), 13 part-time (6 women); includes 15 minority (1 Black or African American, non-Hispanic/Latino; 9 Asian, non-Hispanic/Latino; 4 Hispanic/Latino; 1 Two or more races, non-Hispanic/Latino), 90 international. Average age 27. 359 applicants, 25% accepted, 40 enrolled. In 2015, 32 master's, 4 doctorates awarded. *Degree requirements:* For master's, thesis optional; for doctorate, thesis/dissertation, publishable paper. *Entrance requirements:* For master's and doctorate, GRE (minimum combined score of 1000 on verbal and quantitative). Additional exam requirements/recommendations for international students: Required—TOEFL (minimum score 550 paper-based; 80 iBT). *Application deadline:* For fall admission, 7/15 for domestic students, 5/1 priority date for international students; for spring admission, 11/15 for domestic students, 9/1 priority date for international

students. Applications are processed on a rolling basis. Application fee: $50 ($100 for international students). Electronic applications accepted. *Expenses:* Tuition, state resident: full-time $11,940; part-time $663 per semester hour. Tuition, nonresident: full-time $22,786; part-time $1266 per semester hour. Tuition and fees vary according to course load. *Financial support:* In 2015–16, 71 students received support, including 2 fellowships with partial tuition reimbursements available (averaging $350 per year), 18 research assistantships with partial tuition reimbursements available (averaging $23,800 per year), 53 teaching assistantships with partial tuition reimbursements available (averaging $17,134 per year); career-related internships or fieldwork, Federal Work-Study, institutionally sponsored loans, scholarships/grants, and unspecified assistantships also available. Support available to part-time students. Financial award application deadline: 4/30; financial award applicants required to submit FAFSA. *Faculty research:* Role of mitochondria in neurodegenerative diseases, protein-DNA interactions in site-specific recombination, eukaryotic gene expression, bio-nanotechnology, sickle cell research. *Unit head:* Dr. Stephen Spiro, Department Head, 972-883-6032, Fax: 972-883-2409, E-mail: stephen.spiro@utdallas.edu. *Application contact:* Dr. Lawrence Reitzer, Graduate Advisor, 972-883-2502, Fax: 972-883-2409, E-mail: reitzer@utdallas.edu.
Website: http://www.utdallas.edu/biology/

The University of Texas at San Antonio, College of Sciences, Department of Biology, San Antonio, TX 78249-0617. Offers biology (MS); biotechnology (MS); cell and molecular biology (PhD); neurobiology (PhD). *Faculty:* 36 full-time (10 women), 1 part-time/adjunct (0 women). *Students:* 96 full-time (53 women), 60 part-time (28 women); includes 73 minority (5 Black or African American, non-Hispanic/Latino; 1 American Indian or Alaska Native, non-Hispanic/Latino; 7 Asian, non-Hispanic/Latino; 54 Hispanic/Latino; 1 Native Hawaiian or other Pacific Islander, non-Hispanic/Latino; 5 Two or more races, non-Hispanic/Latino), 28 international. Average age 28. 147 applicants, 46% accepted, 40 enrolled. In 2015, 43 master's, 8 doctorates awarded. Terminal master's awarded for partial completion of doctoral program. *Degree requirements:* For master's, comprehensive exam, thesis or alternative; for doctorate, comprehensive exam, thesis/dissertation. *Entrance requirements:* For master's, GRE General Test, bachelor's degree with 18 credit hours in field of study or in another appropriate field of study; for doctorate, GRE General Test, 3 letters of recommendation, statement of purpose, resume. Additional exam requirements/recommendations for international students: Required—TOEFL (minimum score 500 paper-based; 100 iBT), IELTS (minimum score 5). *Application deadline:* For fall admission, 7/1 for domestic students, 4/1 for international students; for spring admission, 11/1 for domestic students, 9/1 for international students. Application fee: $45 ($80 for international students). Electronic applications accepted. *Faculty research:* Development of human and veterinary vaccines against a fungal disease, mammalian germ cells and stem cells, dopamine neuron physiology and addiction, plant biochemistry, dendritic computation and synaptic plasticity. *Unit head:* Dr. Garry Sunter, Chair, 210-458-5479, E-mail: garry.sunter@utsa.edu. *Application contact:* Rene Munguia, Jr., Senior Program Coordinator, 210-458-4642, Fax: 210-458-5658, E-mail: rene.munguia@utsa.edu.
Website: http://bio.utsa.edu/

The University of Texas Health Science Center at Houston, Graduate School of Biomedical Sciences, Program in Biochemistry and Molecular Biology, Houston, TX 77225-0036. Offers MS, PhD, MD/PhD. Terminal master's awarded for partial completion of doctoral program. *Degree requirements:* For master's, thesis; for doctorate, thesis/dissertation. *Entrance requirements:* For master's and doctorate, GRE General Test. Additional exam requirements/recommendations for international students: Required—TOEFL. Electronic applications accepted. *Faculty research:* Biochemistry, membrane biology, macromolecular structure, structural biophysics, molecular models of human disease, molecular biology of the cell.

The University of Texas Health Science Center at Houston, Graduate School of Biomedical Sciences, Program in Cell and Regulatory Biology, Houston, TX 77225-0036. Offers MS, PhD, MD/PhD. Terminal master's awarded for partial completion of doctoral program. *Degree requirements:* For master's, thesis; for doctorate, thesis/dissertation. *Entrance requirements:* For master's and doctorate, GRE General Test. Additional exam requirements/recommendations for international students: Required—TOEFL. Electronic applications accepted. *Faculty research:* Pharmacology, cell biology, physiology, signal transduction, systems biology.

University of Utah, School of Medicine, Program in Molecular Biology, Salt Lake City, UT 84132. Offers PhD. *Degree requirements:* For doctorate, thesis/dissertation, preliminary exams. *Entrance requirements:* For doctorate, GRE General Test, personal statement, transcripts, letters of recommendation. Additional exam requirements/recommendations for international students: Required—TOEFL (minimum score 500 paper-based; 60 iBT). Electronic applications accepted. *Faculty research:* Biochemistry/structural biology; cancer/cell biology; genetics; developmental biology; gene expression; microbiology/immunology and neurobiology.

University of Vermont, Graduate College, Cellular, Molecular and Biomedical Sciences Program, Burlington, VT 05405. Offers PhD. *Degree requirements:* For doctorate, thesis/dissertation. *Entrance requirements:* For doctorate, GRE General Test. Additional exam requirements/recommendations for international students: Required—TOEFL (minimum score 550 paper-based; 80 iBT). *Application deadline:* For fall admission, 12/1 priority date for domestic students, 12/1 for international students. Application fee: $65. Electronic applications accepted. *Financial support:* Fellowships, research assistantships, teaching assistantships, and career-related internships or fieldwork available. Financial award application deadline: 3/1. *Unit head:* Dr. Matthew Poynter, 802-656-9673, E-mail: cmb@uvm.edu. *Application contact:* Dr. Matthew Poynter, 802-656-9673, E-mail: cmb@uvm.edu.

★ **University of Washington,** Graduate School, School of Medicine, Graduate Programs in Medicine, Program in Molecular and Cellular Biology, Seattle, WA 98195. Offers PhD. Offered in partnership with Fred Hutchinson Cancer Research Center, Seattle Biomedical Research Center, and Institute for Systems Biology. *Degree requirements:* For doctorate, thesis/dissertation. *Entrance requirements:* For doctorate, GRE General Test. Additional exam requirements/recommendations for international students: Required—TOEFL. Electronic applications accepted.

See Display on page 193 and Close-Up on page 231.

University of Wisconsin–La Crosse, College of Science and Health, Department of Biology, La Crosse, WI 54601-3742. Offers aquatic sciences (MS); biology (MS); cellular and molecular biology (MS); clinical microbiology (MS); microbiology (MS); nurse anesthesia (MS); physiology (MS). *Program availability:* Part-time. *Students:* 19 full-time (12 women), 50 part-time (26 women); includes 4 minority (3 Asian, non-Hispanic/Latino; 1 Hispanic/Latino), 1 international. Average age 29. 44 applicants, 75% accepted, 27 enrolled. In 2015, 27 master's awarded. *Degree requirements:* For master's, comprehensive exam, thesis. *Entrance requirements:* For master's, GRE General Test, minimum GPA of 2.85. Additional exam requirements/recommendations for international students: Required—TOEFL (minimum score 550 paper-based; 79 iBT). *Application deadline:* For fall admission, 2/1 priority date for domestic and international students; for spring admission, 1/4 priority date for domestic and international students.

Applications are processed on a rolling basis. Electronic applications accepted. *Financial support:* Research assistantships with partial tuition reimbursements, Federal Work-Study, scholarships/grants, health care benefits, and tuition waivers (partial) available. Support available to part-time students. Financial award application deadline: 3/15; financial award applicants required to submit FAFSA. *Unit head:* Dr. Mark Sandheinrich, Department Chair, 608-785-8261, E-mail: msandheinrich@uwlax.edu. *Application contact:* Brandon Schaller, Senior Graduate Student Status Examiner, 608-785-8941, E-mail: admissions@uwlax.edu.
Website: http://uwlax.edu/biology/

University of Wisconsin–Madison, Graduate School, Program in Cellular and Molecular Biology, Madison, WI 53706-1596. Offers PhD. *Degree requirements:* For doctorate, comprehensive exam, thesis/dissertation. *Entrance requirements:* For doctorate, GRE General Test, GRE Subject Test (recommended), minimum GPA of 3.0, lab experience. Additional exam requirements/recommendations for international students: Required—TOEFL (minimum score 580 paper-based; 92 iBT). Electronic applications accepted. *Expenses:* Tuition, state resident: full-time $5364. Tuition, nonresident: full-time $12,027. *Required fees:* $571. Tuition and fees vary according to campus/location, program and reciprocity agreements. *Faculty research:* Virology, cancer biology, transcriptional mechanisms, plant biology, immunology.

University of Wisconsin–Parkside, College of Natural and Health Sciences, Program in Applied Molecular Biology, Kenosha, WI 53141-2000. Offers MSBS. *Program availability:* Part-time. *Faculty:* 7 full-time (2 women), 1 (woman) part-time/adjunct. *Students:* 8 full-time (5 women); includes 1 minority (Asian, non-Hispanic/Latino). Average age 28. 15 applicants, 47% accepted, 4 enrolled. In 2015, 1 master's awarded. *Degree requirements:* For master's, thesis, oral exam. *Entrance requirements:* For master's, GRE General Test, minimum GPA of 3.0; course work in biology, chemistry, math, and physics. Additional exam requirements/recommendations for international students: Required—TOEFL (minimum score 525 paper-based; 71 iBT). *Application deadline:* For fall admission, 2/1 for domestic and international students; for spring admission, 9/1 for domestic and international students. Application fee: $56. Electronic applications accepted. *Financial support:* Career-related internships or fieldwork and Federal Work-Study available. Financial award application deadline: 7/1. *Faculty research:* Enzyme kinetics, bacterial stress responses, RNA stability, proteomic analysis, genomic analysis. *Unit head:* Dr. Bryan Lewis, Interim Associate Dean, 262-595-2327, Fax: 262-595-2056, E-mail: lewisb@uwp.edu. *Application contact:* Dr. Byran Lewis, Interim Associate Dean, 262-595-2327, Fax: 262-595-2056, E-mail: lewisb@uwp.edu.

University of Wyoming, College of Agriculture and Natural Resources, Department of Molecular Biology, Laramie, WY 82071. Offers MA, MS, PhD. Terminal master's awarded for partial completion of doctoral program. *Degree requirements:* For master's, comprehensive exam (for some programs), thesis; for doctorate, comprehensive exam, thesis/dissertation. *Entrance requirements:* For master's and doctorate, GRE General Test, GRE Subject Test (recommended), minimum GPA of 3.0. Additional exam requirements/recommendations for international students: Required—TOEFL. Electronic applications accepted. *Faculty research:* Protein structure/function, developmental regulation, yeast genetics, bacterial pathogenesis.

University of Wyoming, Graduate Program in Molecular and Cellular Life Sciences, Laramie, WY 82071. Offers PhD. *Degree requirements:* For doctorate, thesis/dissertation, four eight-week laboratory rotations, comprehensive basic practical exam, two-part qualifying exam, seminars, symposium.

Vanderbilt University, School of Medicine, Department of Molecular Physiology and Biophysics, Nashville, TN 37240-1001. Offers MS, PhD, MD/PhD. *Faculty:* 31 full-time (4 women). *Students:* 44 full-time (25 women); includes 7 minority (2 Black or African American, non-Hispanic/Latino; 1 Asian, non-Hispanic/Latino; 3 Hispanic/Latino; 1 Two or more races, non-Hispanic/Latino), 2 international. Average age 26. In 2015, 8 doctorates awarded. *Degree requirements:* For doctorate, comprehensive exam, thesis/dissertation, preliminary, qualifying, and final exams. *Entrance requirements:* For doctorate, GRE General Test, GRE Subject Test (recommended). Additional exam requirements/recommendations for international students: Required—TOEFL (minimum score 570 paper-based; 88 iBT). *Application deadline:* For fall admission, 1/15 for domestic and international students. Application fee: $0. Electronic applications accepted. *Financial support:* Fellowships with full tuition reimbursements, research assistantships with full tuition reimbursements, Federal Work-Study, institutionally sponsored loans, scholarships/grants, traineeships, health care benefits, and tuition waivers (partial) available. Financial award application deadline: 1/15; financial award applicants required to submit CSS PROFILE or FAFSA. *Faculty research:* Biophysics, cell signaling and gene regulation, human genetics, diabetes and obesity, neuroscience. *Unit head:* Dr. Alyssa Hasty, Director of Graduate Studies, 615-322-7000, Fax: 615-343-0490, E-mail: alyssa.hasty@vanderbilt.edu. *Application contact:* Walter B. Bieschke, Program Coordinator for Graduate Admissions, 615-342-0236, E-mail: walter.bieschke@vanderbilt.edu.
Website: http://www.mc.vanderbilt.edu/root/vumc.php?site-MPB

Virginia Commonwealth University, Medical College of Virginia-Professional Programs, School of Medicine, School of Medicine Graduate Programs, Department of Biochemistry, Richmond, VA 23284-9005. Offers biochemistry (MS, PhD); molecular biology (MS, PhD); MD/PhD. *Degree requirements:* For master's, thesis; for doctorate, thesis/dissertation, comprehensive oral and written exams. *Entrance requirements:* For master's and doctorate, GRE, MCAT or DAT. Electronic applications accepted. *Faculty research:* Molecular biology, peptide/protein chemistry, neurochemistry, enzyme mechanisms, macromolecular structure determination.

Virginia Commonwealth University, Medical College of Virginia-Professional Programs, School of Medicine, School of Medicine Graduate Programs, Department of Human and Molecular Genetics, Richmond, VA 23284-9005. Offers genetic counseling (MS); human genetics (PhD); molecular biology and genetics (MS, PhD); MD/PhD. *Degree requirements:* For master's, thesis; for doctorate, thesis/dissertation, comprehensive oral and written exams. *Entrance requirements:* For master's, GRE; for doctorate, GRE General Test. Additional exam requirements/recommendations for international students: Required—TOEFL (minimum score 600 paper-based; 100 iBT). Electronic applications accepted. *Faculty research:* Genetic epidemiology, biochemical genetics, quantitative genetics, human cytogenetics, molecular genetics.

Wake Forest University, School of Medicine and Graduate School of Arts and Sciences, Graduate Programs in Medicine, Molecular Genetics and Genomics Program, Winston-Salem, NC 27109. Offers PhD, MD/PhD. *Degree requirements:* For doctorate, thesis/dissertation. *Entrance requirements:* For doctorate, GRE General Test. Additional exam requirements/recommendations for international students: Required—TOEFL. Electronic applications accepted. *Faculty research:* Control of gene expression, molecular pathogenesis, protein biosynthesis, cell development, clinical cytogenetics.

Washington University in St. Louis, Graduate School of Arts and Sciences, Division of Biology and Biomedical Sciences, Program in Molecular Cell Biology, St. Louis, MO 63130-4899. Offers PhD. *Students:* 77 full-time (34 women); includes 19 minority (5 Black or African American, non-Hispanic/Latino; 1 American Indian or Alaska Native, non-Hispanic/Latino; 9 Asian, non-Hispanic/Latino; 4 Two or more races, non-Hispanic/

Molecular Biology

Latino), 17 international. 150 applicants, 19% accepted, 9 enrolled. In 2015, 22 doctorates awarded. *Degree requirements:* For doctorate, thesis/dissertation. *Entrance requirements:* For doctorate, GRE General Test, GRE Subject Test. Additional exam requirements/recommendations for international students: Required—TOEFL. *Application deadline:* For fall admission, 12/1 for domestic students. Application fee: $0. Electronic applications accepted. *Financial support:* Fellowships, research assistantships, and teaching assistantships available. Financial award application deadline: 1/15; financial award applicants required to submit CSS PROFILE. *Faculty research:* Cell adhesion, protein trafficking and organelle biogenesis, cell cycle, receptors, signal transduction, gene expression, metabolism, cytoskeleton and motility, membrane excitability, molecular basis of diseases. *Unit head:* Stacy Kiel, Coordinator, 314-362-1421. *Application contact:* Rebecca Riney, 314-747-4648, E-mail: dbbsphdadmissions@wusm.wustl.edu.

Wayne State University, College of Liberal Arts and Sciences, Department of Biological Sciences, Detroit, MI 48202. Offers biological sciences (MA, MS); cell development and neurobiology (PhD); evolution and organismal biology (PhD); molecular biology and biotechnology (PhD); molecular biotechnology (MS). PhD and MS programs admit for fall only. *Faculty:* 27. *Students:* 56 full-time (31 women), 8 part-time (2 women); includes 5 minority (2 Black or African American, non-Hispanic/Latino; 2 Asian, non-Hispanic/Latino; 1 Two or more races, non-Hispanic/Latino), 37 international. Average age 29. 210 applicants, 9% accepted, 7 enrolled. In 2015, 5 master's, 10 doctorates awarded. *Degree requirements:* For master's, thesis (for some programs); for doctorate, thesis/dissertation. *Entrance requirements:* For master's, GRE (for MS applicants), minimum GPA of 3.0; adequate preparation in biological sciences and supporting courses in chemistry, physics and mathematics; curriculum vitae; personal statement; three letters of recommendation (two for MA); for doctorate, GRE, curriculum vitae, statement of goals and career objectives, three letters of reference, bachelor's or master's degree in biological or other science. Additional exam requirements/recommendations for international students: Required—TOEFL (minimum score 550 paper-based; 79 iBT), TWE (minimum score 5.5), Michigan English Language Assessment Battery (minimum score 85); Recommended—IELTS (minimum score 6.5). Application fee: $0. Electronic applications accepted. *Expenses:* Tuition, state resident: full-time $14,165; part-time $590.20 per credit hour. Tuition, nonresident: full-time $30,682; part-time $1278.40 per credit hour. *Required fees:* $1688; $47.45 per credit hour. $274.60 per semester. Tuition and fees vary according to course load and program. *Financial support:* In 2015–16, 55 students received support, including 3 fellowships with tuition reimbursements available (averaging $16,000 per year), 8 research assistantships with tuition reimbursements available (averaging $19,506 per year), 45 teaching assistantships with tuition reimbursements available (averaging $19,536 per year); scholarships/grants and unspecified assistantships also available. Financial award application deadline: 3/31; financial award applicants required to submit FAFSA. *Faculty research:* Transcription and chromatin remodeling, genomic and developmental evolution, community and landscape ecology and environmental degradation, microbiology and virology, cell and neurobiology. *Total annual research expenditures:* $2.1 million. *Unit head:* Dr. David Njus, Professor and Chair, 313-577-3105, E-mail: dnjus@wayne.edu. *Application contact:* Rose Mary Priest, Graduate Secretary, 313-577-6818, E-mail: rpriest@wayne.edu. Website: http://clas.wayne.edu/Biology/

Wayne State University, School of Medicine, Office of Biomedical Graduate Programs, Department of Biochemistry and Molecular Biology, Detroit, MI 48202. Offers MS, PhD, MD/PhD. *Faculty:* 11. *Students:* 27 full-time (15 women), 2 part-time (1 woman); includes 3 minority (1 Black or African American, non-Hispanic/Latino; 2 Asian, non-Hispanic/Latino), 12 international. Average age 28. 143 applicants, 9% accepted, 9 enrolled. In 2015, 1 master's, 2 doctorates awarded. *Degree requirements:* For master's, research project; for doctorate, thesis/dissertation. *Entrance requirements:* For master's, GRE, BA or BS in biology, chemistry, or (if approved) physics or mathematics with minimum GPA of 2.6 from accredited university; three letters of recommendation; personal statement; for doctorate, GRE, BA or BS in biology, chemistry, or (if approved) physics or mathematics with minimum GPA of 3.0 from accredited university; three letters of recommendation; personal statement; copies of any abstracts or papers on which the applicant is a co-author. Additional exam requirements/recommendations for international students: Required—TOEFL (minimum score 100 iBT). *Application deadline:* For fall admission, 2/1 priority date for domestic and international students. Applications are processed on a rolling basis. Application fee: $0. Electronic applications accepted. *Expenses:* $17,645 per year resident tuition; $33,311 non-resident tuition; $735.20 per credit hour resident tuition, $1,387.95 per credit hour non-resident tuition; fees include $47.45 per credit hour student services fee and $274.60 per semester registration fee. *Financial support:* In 2015–16, 27 students received support, including 3 fellowships with tuition reimbursements available (averaging $26,909 per year), 12 research assistantships with tuition reimbursements available (averaging $26,716 per year); scholarships/grants, health care benefits, and unspecified assistantships also available. Financial award application deadline: 3/31. *Faculty research:* Structural biology, cellular metal homeostasis and drug resistance, molecular biology and cancer, molecular and cellular bioenergetics, enzymology. *Unit head:* Dr. David Evans, 313-577-1016, E-mail: drevans@med.wayne.edu. *Application contact:* Dr. Zhe Yang, PhD Program in Biochemistry and Molecular Biology Director, 313-577-1514, E-mail: zyang@med.wayne.edu. Website: http://www.biochem.med.wayne.edu/phd/

Weill Cornell Medicine, Weill Cornell Graduate School of Medical Sciences, Biochemistry, Cell and Molecular Biology Allied Program, New York, NY 10065. Offers MS, PhD. Terminal master's awarded for partial completion of doctoral program. *Degree requirements:* For master's, comprehensive exam; for doctorate, thesis/dissertation, final exam. *Entrance requirements:* For doctorate, GRE General Test, background in genetics, molecular biology, chemistry, or biochemistry. Additional exam requirements/recommendations for international students: Required—TOEFL. Electronic applications accepted. *Faculty research:* Molecular structure determination, protein structure, gene structure, stem cell biology, control of gene expression, DNA replication, chromosome maintenance, RNA biosynthesis.

Wesleyan University, Graduate Studies, Department of Molecular Biology and Biochemistry, Middletown, CT 06459. Offers biochemistry (PhD); molecular biology (PhD); molecular biophysics (PhD); molecular genetics (PhD). *Faculty:* 8 full-time (3 women), 1 (woman) part-time/adjunct. *Students:* 18 full-time (9 women); includes 4 minority (2 Asian, non-Hispanic/Latino; 1 Hispanic/Latino; 1 Two or more races, non-Hispanic/Latino), 11 international. Average age 24. 28 applicants, 14% accepted, 1 enrolled. Terminal master's awarded for partial completion of doctoral program. *Degree requirements:* For doctorate, comprehensive exam, thesis/dissertation. *Entrance requirements:* For doctorate, GRE General Test, GRE Subject Test. Additional exam requirements/recommendations for international students: Required—TOEFL. *Application deadline:* For fall admission, 1/15 for domestic and international students. Application fee: $0. Electronic applications accepted. *Financial support:* Research assistantships with full tuition reimbursements, teaching assistantships with full tuition reimbursements, and institutionally sponsored loans available. Financial award application deadline: 4/15; financial award applicants required to submit FAFSA. *Faculty research:* The olfactory system and new frontiers in genome research, chromosome structure and gene expression, gene co-regulation, crystallographic and spectroscopic analysis, DNA replication and repair. *Unit head:* Scott Holmes, Chair, 860-685-2443, E-mail: sholmes@wesleyan.edu. *Application contact:* Anika Dane, Administrative Assistant, 860-685-2404, E-mail: adane@wesleyan.edu. Website: http://www.wesleyan.edu/mbb/.

West Virginia University, Eberly College of Arts and Sciences, Department of Biology, Morgantown, WV 26506. Offers cell and molecular biology (MS, PhD); environmental and evolutionary biology (MS, PhD); forensic biology (MS, PhD); genomic biology (MS, PhD); neurobiology (MS, PhD). Terminal master's awarded for partial completion of doctoral program. *Degree requirements:* For master's, thesis, final exam; for doctorate, thesis/dissertation, preliminary and final exams. *Entrance requirements:* For master's, GRE General Test, GRE Subject Test, minimum GPA of 3.0; for doctorate, GRE General Test, minimum GPA of 3.0. Additional exam requirements/recommendations for international students: Required—TOEFL. *Expenses:* Tuition, state resident: full-time $8568. Tuition, nonresident: full-time $22,140. Tuition and fees vary according to program. *Faculty research:* Environmental biology, genetic engineering, developmental biology, global change, biodiversity.

West Virginia University, School of Medicine, Graduate Programs at the Health Sciences Center, Interdisciplinary Graduate Programs in Biomedical Sciences, Program in Biochemistry and Molecular Biology, Morgantown, WV 26506. Offers MS, PhD, MD/PhD. *Degree requirements:* For doctorate, comprehensive exam, thesis/dissertation. *Entrance requirements:* For doctorate, GRE General Test, minimum GPA of 3.0. Additional exam requirements/recommendations for international students: Required—TOEFL. Electronic applications accepted. *Expenses:* Tuition, state resident: full-time $8568. Tuition, nonresident: full-time $22,140. Tuition and fees vary according to program. *Faculty research:* Regulation of gene expression, cell survival mechanisms, signal transduction, regulation of metabolism, sensory neuroscience.

Wright State University, School of Graduate Studies, College of Science and Mathematics, Department of Biochemistry and Molecular Biology, Dayton, OH 45435. Offers MS. *Degree requirements:* For master's, thesis. *Entrance requirements:* Additional exam requirements/recommendations for international students: Required—TOEFL. *Faculty research:* Regulation of gene expression, macromolecular structural function, NMR imaging, visual biochemistry.

Yale University, Graduate School of Arts and Sciences, Department of Molecular, Cellular, and Developmental Biology, Program in Biochemistry, Molecular Biology and Chemical Biology, New Haven, CT 06520. Offers PhD. *Degree requirements:* For doctorate, thesis/dissertation. *Entrance requirements:* For doctorate, GRE General Test, GRE Subject Test.

Yale University, School of Medicine and Graduate School of Arts and Sciences, Combined Program in Biological and Biomedical Sciences (BBS), Molecular Cell Biology, Genetics, and Development Track, New Haven, CT 06520. Offers PhD, MD/PhD. *Entrance requirements:* Additional exam requirements/recommendations for international students: Required—TOEFL.

Youngstown State University, Graduate School, College of Science, Technology, Engineering and Mathematics, Department of Biological Sciences, Youngstown, OH 44555-0001. Offers environmental biology (MS); molecular biology, microbiology, and genetic (MS); physiology and anatomy (MS). *Program availability:* Part-time. *Degree requirements:* For master's, comprehensive exam, thesis, oral review. *Entrance requirements:* For master's, GRE General Test, minimum GPA of 2.7. Additional exam requirements/recommendations for international students: Required—TOEFL. *Faculty research:* Cell biology, neurophysiology, molecular biology, neurobiology, gene regulation.

Molecular Medicine

Augusta University, The Graduate School, Program in Molecular Medicine, Augusta, GA 30912. Offers PhD. *Degree requirements:* For doctorate, comprehensive exam, thesis/dissertation. *Entrance requirements:* For doctorate, GRE General Test. Additional exam requirements/recommendations for international students: Required—TOEFL (minimum score 550 paper-based; 79 iBT). *Application deadline:* For fall admission, 1/15 for domestic and international students. Application fee: $50. Electronic applications accepted. *Financial support:* Fellowships with partial tuition reimbursements, research assistantships with partial tuition reimbursements, teaching assistantships, Federal Work-Study, institutionally sponsored loans, and scholarships/grants available. Support available to part-time students. Financial award application deadline: 5/31; financial award applicants required to submit FAFSA. *Faculty research:* Developmental neurobiology, cancer, regenerative medicine, molecular chaperones, molecular immunology. *Unit head:* Dr. Lynnette McCluskey, Director, 706-721-5616, Fax: 706-721-0340, E-mail: lmccluskey@augusta.edu. *Application contact:* Angie Compton, Program Administrator, 706-721-0487, E-mail: acompton@augusta.edu. Website: http://www.augusta.edu/mcg/dnrm/molecularmedicine/

Baylor College of Medicine, Graduate School of Biomedical Sciences, Program in Translational Biology and Molecular Medicine, Houston, TX 77030-3498. Offers PhD. *Degree requirements:* For doctorate, thesis/dissertation, public defense. *Entrance requirements:* For doctorate, GRE, minimum GPA of 3.0. Additional exam requirements/recommendations for international students: Required—TOEFL. Electronic applications accepted. *Faculty research:* Molecular medicine, translational biology, human disease biology and therapy.

Boston University, School of Medicine, Division of Graduate Medical Sciences, Program in Molecular Medicine, Boston, MA 02215. Offers PhD, MD/PhD. *Degree requirements:* For doctorate, thesis/dissertation. *Application deadline:* For fall admission, 1/15 for domestic students; for spring admission, 10/15 for domestic students. *Unit head:* Dr. Matt Jones, Director, 617-638-4860, E-mail: mattj@bu.edu.

Application contact: GMS Admissions Office, 617-638-5255, E-mail: askgms@bu.edu. Website: http://www.bumc.bu.edu/gpmm

Case Western Reserve University, School of Graduate Studies, Cleveland Clinic Lerner Research Institute–Molecular Medicine PhD Program, Cleveland, OH 44106. Offers PhD. *Degree requirements:* For doctorate, comprehensive exam, thesis/dissertation, seminar. *Entrance requirements:* For doctorate, GRE, 3 letters of reference, prior research experience, interview. Additional exam requirements/recommendations for international students: Required—TOEFL (minimum score 577 paper-based; 90 iBT); Recommended—IELTS (minimum score 7). Electronic applications accepted. *Expenses: Tuition,* area resident: Full-time $41,137; part-time $1714 per credit hour. *Required fees:* $32. Tuition and fees vary according to course load and program. *Faculty research:* Cancer, cardiovascular disease, neuroscience, molecular biology, genetics.

Case Western Reserve University, School of Medicine and School of Graduate Studies, Graduate Programs in Medicine, Department of Molecular Medicine at the Lerner Research Institute, Cleveland, OH 44106. Offers PhD. *Degree requirements:* For doctorate, comprehensive exam, thesis/dissertation. *Entrance requirements:* For doctorate, GRE. Additional exam requirements/recommendations for international students: Required—TOEFL. Electronic applications accepted. *Expenses: Tuition,* area resident: Full-time $41,137; part-time $1714 per credit hour. *Required fees:* $32. Tuition and fees vary according to course load and program.

Cleveland State University, College of Graduate Studies, College of Sciences and Health Professions, Department of Chemistry, Cleveland, OH 44115. Offers analytical chemistry (MS); clinical chemistry (PhD), including cellular and molecular medicine, clinical/bioanalytical chemistry; inorganic chemistry (MS); organic chemistry (MS); physical chemistry (MS). *Program availability:* Part-time, evening/weekend. *Faculty:* 17 full-time (3 women). *Students:* 63 full-time (30 women), 25 part-time (10 women); includes 4 minority (1 Black or African American, non-Hispanic/Latino; 1 Asian, non-Hispanic/Latino; 2 Hispanic/Latino), 48 international. Average age 30. 22 applicants, 64% accepted, 12 enrolled. In 2015, 16 master's, 8 doctorates awarded. *Degree requirements:* For master's, thesis optional; for doctorate, comprehensive exam, thesis/dissertation. *Entrance requirements:* For master's and doctorate, GRE General Test. Additional exam requirements/recommendations for international students: Required—TOEFL (minimum score 550 paper-based; 78 iBT). *Application deadline:* For fall admission, 1/15 priority date for domestic and international students. Applications are processed on a rolling basis. Application fee: $30. Electronic applications accepted. *Expenses:* Tuition, state resident: full-time $9565. Tuition, nonresident: full-time $17,980. Tuition and fees vary according to program. *Financial support:* In 2015–16, 44 students received support, including 10 fellowships with full tuition reimbursements available (averaging $22,500 per year), 6 research assistantships with full tuition reimbursements available (averaging $22,500 per year), 34 teaching assistantships with full tuition reimbursements available (averaging $21,000 per year); scholarships/grants and unspecified assistantships also available. Financial award application deadline: 1/15. *Faculty research:* Bioanalytical techniques and molecular diagnostics, glycoproteomics and antithrombotic agents, drug discovery and innovation, analytical pharmacology, inflammatory disease research. *Total annual research expenditures:* $3 million. *Unit head:* Dr. David W. Ball, Chair, 216-687-2467, Fax: 216-687-9298, E-mail: d.ball@csuohio.edu. *Application contact:* Richelle P. Emery, Administrative Coordinator, 216-687-2457, Fax: 216-687-9298, E-mail: r.emery@csuohio.edu. Website: http://www.csuohio.edu/sciences/chemistry

Cornell University, Graduate School, Graduate Fields of Comparative Biomedical Sciences, Field of Comparative Biomedical Sciences, Ithaca, NY 14853-0001. Offers cellular and molecular medicine (MS, PhD); developmental and reproductive biology (MS, PhD); infectious diseases (MS, PhD); population medicine and epidemiology (MS, PhD); structural and functional biology (MS, PhD). *Degree requirements:* For master's, thesis; for doctorate, comprehensive exam, thesis/dissertation. *Entrance requirements:* For master's and doctorate, GRE General Test, 2 letters of recommendation. Additional exam requirements/recommendations for international students: Required—TOEFL (minimum score 550 paper-based; 77 iBT). Electronic applications accepted. *Faculty research:* Receptors and signal transduction, viral and bacterial infectious diseases, tumor metastasis, clinical sciences/nutritional disease, developmental/neurological disorders.

Dartmouth College, Program in Experimental and Molecular Medicine, Hanover, NH 03755. Offers MBA/PhD, MD/PhD. *Faculty:* 29 full-time (10 women), 11 part-time/adjunct (3 women). *Students:* 52 full-time (31 women); includes 6 minority (4 Asian, non-Hispanic/Latino; 2 Hispanic/Latino), 8 international. Average age 26. 127 applicants, 15% accepted, 10 enrolled. *Entrance requirements:* Additional exam requirements/recommendations for international students: Required—TOEFL (minimum score 620 paper-based; 105 iBT). *Application deadline:* For fall admission, 1/1 for domestic and international students. Application fee: $75. Electronic applications accepted. *Expenses: Tuition,* area resident: Full-time $48,120. *Required fees:* $296. One-time fee: $50 full-time. *Financial support:* In 2015–16, fellowships with full tuition reimbursements (averaging $28,200 per year) were awarded; health care benefits also available. *Faculty research:* Biomedical physiology and immunotherapy, cancer biology and molecular therapeutics, molecular pharmacology toxicology and experimental therapeutics, neuroscience. *Unit head:* Dr. Michael Spinella, Director, 603-650-4933, Fax: 603-650-4932. *Application contact:* Gail L. Paige, Program Coordinator, 603-650-4933, Fax: 603-650-4932, E-mail: molecular.medicine@dartmouth.edu. Website: http://geiselmed.dartmouth.edu/pemm/

Drexel University, College of Medicine, Biomedical Graduate Programs, Molecular Medicine Program, Philadelphia, PA 19104-2875. Offers MS.

Elmezzi Graduate School of Molecular Medicine, Graduate Program, Manhasset, NY 11030. Offers PhD. *Faculty:* 41 full-time (13 women). *Students:* 8 full-time (2 women), 7 international. *Degree requirements:* For doctorate, comprehensive exam, thesis/dissertation. *Entrance requirements:* For doctorate, MD or equivalent. *Application deadline:* Applications are processed on a rolling basis. Application fee: $25. *Financial support:* In 2015–16, 8 students received support. Fellowships with full tuition reimbursements available, health care benefits, and tuition waivers (full) available. *Faculty research:* Cardiopulmonary disease, cancer, inflammation, genetics of complex disorders, cytokine biology. *Unit head:* Dr. Bettie M. Steinberg, Chief Scientific Officer, 516-562-1159, Fax: 516-562-1022, E-mail: bsteinbe@lij.edu. *Application contact:* Emilia C. Hristis, Education Coordinator, 516-562-3405, Fax: 516-562-1022, E-mail: ehristis@nshs.edu. Website: http://www.feinsteininstitute.org/education/the-elmezzi-graduate-school-of-molecular-medicine/

The George Washington University, Columbian College of Arts and Sciences, Institute for Biomedical Sciences, Program in Molecular Medicine, Washington, DC 20037. Offers molecular and cellular oncology (PhD); neurosciences (PhD); pharmacology and physiology (PhD). *Students:* 7 full-time (5 women), 12 part-time (10 women); includes 3 minority (1 Black or African American, non-Hispanic/Latino; 1 Hispanic/Latino; 1 Hispanic/Latino), 4 international. Average age 29. In 2015, 2 doctorates awarded. *Degree requirements:* For doctorate, comprehensive exam, thesis/

dissertation, general exams. *Entrance requirements:* For doctorate, GRE General Test, interview, minimum GPA of 3.0. Additional exam requirements/recommendations for international students: Required—TOEFL (minimum score 600 paper-based). *Application deadline:* For fall admission, 12/15 priority date for domestic and international students. Applications are processed on a rolling basis. Application fee: $75. Electronic applications accepted. *Financial support:* In 2015–16, 10 students received support. Fellowships with tuition reimbursements available, Federal Work-Study, institutionally sponsored loans, and tuition waivers available. Financial award application deadline: 2/1. *Unit head:* Dr. Norman Lee, Director, 202-994-2114, E-mail: beb@gwu.edu. *Application contact:* 202-994-2179, Fax: 202-994-0967, E-mail: gwibs@gwu.edu. Website: http://smhs.gwu.edu/ibs/program/introduction-molecular-medicine-program

Hofstra University, School of Medicine, Hempstead, NY 11549. Offers medicine (MD); molecular basis of medicine (PhD); MD/PhD. *Accreditation:* LCME/AMA. *Faculty:* 12 full-time (6 women), 9 part-time/adjunct (5 women). *Students:* 277 full-time (130 women); includes 104 minority (14 Black or African American, non-Hispanic/Latino; 50 Asian, non-Hispanic/Latino; 30 Hispanic/Latino; 2 Native Hawaiian or other Pacific Islander, non-Hispanic/Latino; 8 Two or more races, non-Hispanic/Latino), 1 international. Average age 25. 6,199 applicants, 4% accepted, 99 enrolled. *Entrance requirements:* For doctorate, MCAT. Additional exam requirements/recommendations for international students: Required—TOEFL (minimum score 600 paper-based; 100 iBT). *Application deadline:* For fall admission, 12/1 priority date for domestic students. Application fee: $100. Electronic applications accepted. *Expenses:* Contact institution. *Financial support:* In 2015–16, 239 students received support, including 222 fellowships with tuition reimbursements available (averaging $23,020 per year); research assistantships with tuition reimbursements available, Federal Work-Study, institutionally sponsored loans, scholarships/grants, and tuition waivers (full and partial) also available. Support available to part-time students. Financial award applicants required to submit FAFSA. *Faculty research:* Pathogenesis of sepsis, pathogenesis of autoimmune disease, pathogenesis of schizophrenia and movement disorders, population health, healthcare quality and effectiveness. *Unit head:* Dr. Veronica Catanese, Vice Dean, 516-463-7517, Fax: 516-463-7543, E-mail: medvmc@hofstra.edu. *Application contact:* Sunil Samuel, Assistant Vice President of Admissions, 516-463-4723, Fax: 516-463-4664. Website: http://medicine.hofstra.edu/index.html

Johns Hopkins University, School of Medicine, Graduate Programs in Medicine, Graduate Program in Cellular and Molecular Medicine, Baltimore, MD 21218. Offers PhD. *Degree requirements:* For doctorate, comprehensive exam, thesis/dissertation, oral exam. *Entrance requirements:* For doctorate, GRE. Additional exam requirements/recommendations for international students: Required—TOEFL. Electronic applications accepted. *Faculty research:* Cellular and molecular basis of disease.

Penn State Hershey Medical Center, College of Medicine, Graduate School Programs in the Biomedical Sciences, The Huck Institutes of the Life Sciences, Intercollege Graduate Program in Molecular Cellular and Integrative Biosciences, Hershey, PA 17033. Offers cell and developmental biology (PhD); immunology and infectious disease (PhD); molecular and evolutionary genetics (PhD); molecular medicine (PhD); molecular toxicology (PhD); neurobiology (PhD). *Students:* 3 full-time (2 women); includes 2 minority (both Asian, non-Hispanic/Latino). 2 applicants, 100% accepted, 2 enrolled. In 2015, 1 doctorate awarded. *Degree requirements:* For doctorate, comprehensive exam, thesis/dissertation, oral exam. *Entrance requirements:* For doctorate, GRE, minimum GPA of 3.0. Additional exam requirements/recommendations for international students: Required—TOEFL (minimum score 500 paper-based). *Application deadline:* For fall admission, 1/31 priority date for domestic students, 2/1 priority date for international students. Applications are processed on a rolling basis. Application fee: $65. Electronic applications accepted. *Financial support:* In 2015–16, research assistantships with full tuition reimbursements (averaging $26,196 per year) were awarded; fellowships with full tuition reimbursements, career-related internships or fieldwork, Federal Work-Study, scholarships/grants, health care benefits, and unspecified assistantships also available. Financial award applicants required to submit FAFSA. *Faculty research:* Vascular biology, molecular toxicology, chemical biology, immune system, pathophysiological basis of human disease. *Unit head:* Dr. Peter Hudson, Director, 814-865-6057, E-mail: pjh18@psu.edu. *Application contact:* Kathy Shuey, Administrative Assistant, 717-531-8982, Fax: 717-531-0786, E-mail: grad-hmc@psu.edu. Website: http://www.huck.psu.edu/education/molecular-cellular-and-integrative-biosciences

Queen's University at Kingston, School of Graduate Studies, Faculty of Health Sciences, Department of Pathology and Molecular Medicine, Kingston, ON K7L 3N6, Canada. Offers M Sc, PhD. *Program availability:* Part-time. *Degree requirements:* For master's, thesis; for doctorate, comprehensive exam, thesis/dissertation. *Entrance requirements:* Additional exam requirements/recommendations for international students: Required—TOEFL. *Faculty research:* Immunopathology, cancer biology, immunology and metastases, cell differentiation, blood coagulation.

Rutgers University–Newark, Graduate School of Biomedical Sciences, Department of Cell Biology and Molecular Medicine, Newark, NJ 07107. Offers PhD. *Degree requirements:* For doctorate, thesis/dissertation, qualifying exam. *Entrance requirements:* For doctorate, GRE General Test. Additional exam requirements/recommendations for international students: Required—TOEFL. Electronic applications accepted.

Tufts University, Sackler School of Graduate Biomedical Sciences, Cell, Molecular, and Developmental Biology Program, Medford, MA 02155. Offers cancer biology (PhD); developmental and regenerative biology (PhD); molecular and cellular medicine (PhD); structural and chemical biology (PhD). *Faculty:* 45 full-time (15 women). *Students:* 36 full-time (18 women); includes 13 minority (2 Black or African American, non-Hispanic/Latino; 9 Asian, non-Hispanic/Latino; 1 Hispanic/Latino; 1 Two or more races, non-Hispanic/Latino), 4 international. Average age 28. 189 applicants, 7% accepted, 6 enrolled. In 2015, 2 doctorates awarded. Terminal master's awarded for partial completion of doctoral program. *Degree requirements:* For doctorate, comprehensive exam, thesis/dissertation. *Entrance requirements:* For doctorate, GRE General Test, 3 letters of reference. Additional exam requirements/recommendations for international students: Required—TOEFL (minimum score 600 paper-based; 100 iBT). *Application deadline:* For fall admission, 12/15 priority date for domestic and international students. Application fee: $70. Electronic applications accepted. *Expenses: Tuition,* area resident: Full-time $48,412; part-time $1210 per credit hour. *Required fees:* $806. Full-time tuition and fees vary according to degree level, program and student level. Part-time tuition and fees vary according to course load. *Financial support:* In 2015–16, 36 students received support, including 36 research assistantships with full tuition reimbursements available (averaging $32,000 per year); health care benefits also available. *Faculty research:* Reproduction and hormone action, control of gene expression, cell-matrix and cell-cell interactions, growth control and tumorigenesis, cytoskeleton and contractile proteins. *Unit head:* Dr. Ira Herman, Program Director, 617-636-2991, Fax: 617-636-0375. *Application contact:* Dr. Elizabeth Storrs, Registrar/Director of Academic Services, 617-636-6767, Fax: 617-636-0375, E-mail: sackler-school@tufts.edu. Website: http://sackler.tufts.edu/Academics/CMDB-Welcome

Molecular Medicine

The University of Alabama at Birmingham, Graduate Programs in Joint Health Sciences, Pathobiology and Molecular Medicine Theme, Birmingham, AL 35294. Offers PhD. *Students:* 46 full-time (20 women), 1 (woman) part-time; includes 9 minority (5 Black or African American, non-Hispanic/Latino; 1 Asian, non-Hispanic/Latino; 3 Hispanic/Latino), 9 international. Average age 27. *Degree requirements:* For doctorate, comprehensive exam, thesis/dissertation. *Entrance requirements:* For doctorate, GRE (minimum combined verbal/quantitative score of 300 new test or 1100 old test), baccalaureate degree in natural or physical sciences, research experience, interview, reference letters. Additional exam requirements/recommendations for international students: Required—TOEFL (minimum score 600 paper-based; 100 iBT). *Application deadline:* For fall admission, 12/15 priority date for domestic students, 1/15 for international students. Applications are processed on a rolling basis. Application fee: $0 ($60 for international students). Electronic applications accepted. *Expenses:* Tuition, state resident: full-time $7340. Tuition, nonresident: full-time $16,628. Full-time tuition and fees vary according to course load and program. *Financial support:* Fellowships with tuition reimbursements and competitive annual stipends, health insurance, and fully-paid tuition and fees available. *Faculty research:* Molecular basis of disease, AIDS vaccine development and T-cell biology of HIV infection and pathogenesis of AIDS; metabolic bone disease and cellular signaling and death; extracellular matrix control of normal and cancerous cell movement and growth; mechanisms of neuronal cell death and neoplasia; tumor invasion, tumor markers, and cancer genetics; bacterial and mycotic infections; mechanisms of insulin and growth hormone action. *Unit head:* Dr. Yabing Chen, Director, 205-996-6293, E-mail: yabingchen@uabmc.edu. *Application contact:* Director of Graduate School Operations, Fax: 205-934-8413, E-mail: gradschool@uab.edu.
Website: http://www.uab.edu/gbs/pathobiology/

The University of Arizona, College of Medicine, Department of Cellular and Molecular Medicine, Tucson, AZ 85721. Offers MS, PhD. *Degree requirements:* For doctorate, comprehensive exam. *Entrance requirements:* Additional exam requirements/recommendations for international students: Required—TOEFL, IELTS. *Application deadline:* For fall admission, 6/18 for domestic students; for spring admission, 11/15 for domestic students. Applications are processed on a rolling basis. Application fee: $75. Electronic applications accepted. *Financial support:* Research assistantships available. *Faculty research:* Heart and vascular development, neural development, cellular toxicology, immunobiology, cell biology and cancer biology. *Unit head:* Dr. Carol Gregorio, Head, 520-626-3184, E-mail: gregorio@email.arizona.edu. *Application contact:* Dr. Carol Gregorio, Head, 520-626-3184, E-mail: gregorio@email.arizona.edu.
Website: http://cmm.arizona.edu/

University of Cincinnati, Graduate School, College of Medicine, Graduate Programs in Biomedical Sciences, Program in Pathobiology and Molecular Medicine, Cincinnati, OH 45221. Offers pathology (PhD), including anatomic pathology, laboratory medicine, pathobiology and molecular medicine. *Degree requirements:* For doctorate, thesis/dissertation, qualifying exam. *Entrance requirements:* For doctorate, GRE General Test. Additional exam requirements/recommendations for international students: Required—TOEFL (minimum score 620 paper-based). Electronic applications accepted. *Faculty research:* Cardiovascular and lipid disorders, digestive and kidney disease, endocrine and metabolic disorders, hematological and oncogenic, immunology and infectious disease.

University of Maryland, Baltimore, Graduate School, Graduate Program in Life Sciences, Program in Molecular Medicine, Baltimore, MD 21201. Offers cancer biology (PhD); cell and molecular physiology (PhD); human genetics and genomic medicine (PhD); molecular medicine (MS); molecular toxicology and pharmacology (PhD); MD/PhD. *Degree requirements:* For doctorate, comprehensive exam, thesis/dissertation. *Entrance requirements:* For master's and doctorate, GRE. Additional exam requirements/recommendations for international students: Required—TOEFL (minimum score 600 paper-based; 100 iBT); Recommended—IELTS (minimum score 7). Electronic applications accepted. Tuition and fees vary according to program.

University of South Florida, Morsani College of Medicine and College of Graduate Studies, Graduate Programs in Medical Sciences, Tampa, FL 33620-9951. Offers advanced athletic training (MS); athletic training (MS); bioinformatics and computational biology (MSBCB); biotechnology (MSB); health informatics (MSHI); medical sciences (MSMS, PhD), including aging and neuroscience (MSMS), allergy, immunology and infectious disease (PhD), anatomy, athletic training (MSMS), clinical and translational research, health informatics (MSMS), health science (MSMS), interdisciplinary medical sciences (MSMS), medical microbiology and immunology (MSMS), metabolic and nutritional medicine (MSMS), molecular medicine, molecular pharmacology and physiology (PhD), neurology (PhD), pathology and laboratory medicine (PhD), pharmacology and therapeutics (PhD), physiology and biophysics (PhD), women's health (MSMS). *Students:* 510 full-time (261 women), 318 part-time (208 women); includes 360 minority (108 Black or African American, non-Hispanic/Latino; 3 American Indian or Alaska Native, non-Hispanic/Latino; 101 Asian, non-Hispanic/Latino; 124 Hispanic/Latino; 1 Native Hawaiian or other Pacific Islander, non-Hispanic/Latino; 23 Two or more races, non-Hispanic/Latino), 52 international. Average age 26. 6,567 applicants, 13% accepted, 469 enrolled. In 2015, 216 master's awarded. Terminal master's awarded for partial completion of doctoral program. *Degree requirements:* For master's, comprehensive exam, thesis; for doctorate, comprehensive exam, thesis/dissertation. *Entrance requirements:* For master's, GRE General Test or GMAT, bachelor's degree or equivalent from regionally-accredited university with minimum GPA of 3.0 in upper-division sciences coursework; prerequisites in general biology, general chemistry, general physics, organic chemistry, quantitative analysis, and integral and differential calculus; for doctorate, GRE General Test, bachelor's degree from regionally-accredited university with minimum GPA of 3.0 in upper-division sciences coursework; 3 letters of recommendation; personal interview; 1-2 page personal statement; prerequisites in biology, chemistry, physics, organic chemistry, quantitative analysis, and integral/differential calculus. Additional exam requirements/

recommendations for international students: Required—TOEFL (minimum score 550 paper-based; 79 iBT) or IELTS (minimum score 6.5). *Application deadline:* For fall admission, 2/15 for domestic students, 1/2 for international students. Application fee: $30. *Expenses:* Contact institution. *Faculty research:* Anatomy, biochemistry, cancer biology, cardiovascular disease, cell biology, immunology, microbiology, molecular biology, neuroscience, pharmacology, physiology. *Unit head:* Dr. Michael Barber, Professor/Associate Dean for Graduate and Postdoctoral Affairs, 813-974-9908, Fax: 813-974-4317, E-mail: mbarber@health.usf.edu. *Application contact:* Dr. Eric Bennett, Graduate Director, PhD Program in Medical Sciences, 813-974-1545, Fax: 813-974-4317, E-mail: esbennet@health.usf.edu.
Website: http://health.usf.edu/nocms/medicine/graduatestudies/

The University of Texas Health Science Center at San Antonio, Graduate School of Biomedical Sciences, Department of Molecular Medicine, San Antonio, TX 78245-3207. Offers MS, PhD. Terminal master's awarded for partial completion of doctoral program. *Degree requirements:* For master's, comprehensive exam, thesis; for doctorate, comprehensive exam, thesis/dissertation.

University of Washington, Graduate School, School of Public Health, Department of Global Health, Graduate Program in Pathobiology, Seattle, WA 98195. Offers PhD. *Degree requirements:* For doctorate, comprehensive exam, thesis/dissertation, published paper from thesis work. *Entrance requirements:* For doctorate, GRE General Test, minimum GPA of 3.0. Additional exam requirements/recommendations for international students: Required—TOEFL, IELTS. Electronic applications accepted. *Expenses:* Contact institution. *Faculty research:* Malaria, immunological response to mycobacteria infections, HIV-cell interaction and the development of an anti-HIV vaccine, regulation of intercellular communication via gap junctions, genetic and nutritional regulation of proteins involved in lipid transport.

Wake Forest University, School of Medicine and Graduate School of Arts and Sciences, Graduate Programs in Medicine, Molecular Genetics and Genomics Program, Winston-Salem, NC 27109. Offers PhD, MD/PhD. *Degree requirements:* For doctorate, thesis/dissertation. *Entrance requirements:* For doctorate, GRE General Test. Additional exam requirements/recommendations for international students: Required—TOEFL. Electronic applications accepted. *Faculty research:* Control of gene expression, molecular pathogenesis, protein biosynthesis, cell development, clinical cytogenetics.

Wake Forest University, School of Medicine and Graduate School of Arts and Sciences, Graduate Programs in Medicine, Program in Molecular Medicine, Winston-Salem, NC 27109. Offers MS, PhD, MD/PhD. *Degree requirements:* For master's, thesis; for doctorate, thesis/dissertation. *Entrance requirements:* For master's and doctorate, GRE General Test. Additional exam requirements/recommendations for international students: Required—TOEFL. Electronic applications accepted. *Faculty research:* Human biology and disease, scientific basis of medicine, cellular and molecular mechanisms of health and disease.

Wayne State University, School of Medicine, Office of Biomedical Graduate Programs, Detroit, MI 48202. Offers anatomy and cell biology (PhD); basic medical sciences (MS); biochemistry and molecular biology (MS); cancer biology (MS, PhD); clinical and translational science (Graduate Certificate); family medicine and public health sciences (MPH, Graduate Certificate), including public health practice; genetic counseling (MS); immunology and microbiology (MS, PhD); medical physics (MS, PhD, Graduate Certificate); medical research (MS); molecular medicine and genomics (MS, PhD), including molecular genetics and genomics; pathology (PhD); pharmacology (MS, PhD); physiology (MS, PhD), including physiology, reproductive sciences (PhD); psychiatry and behavioral neurosciences (PhD), including translational neuroscience; MD/MPH; MD/PhD; MPH/MA. *Program availability:* Part-time, evening/weekend. *Students:* 277 full-time (143 women), 84 part-time (41 women); includes 92 minority (13 Black or African American, non-Hispanic/Latino; 54 Asian, non-Hispanic/Latino; 15 Hispanic/Latino; 10 Two or more races, non-Hispanic/Latino), 67 international. Average age 27. 1,053 applicants, 20% accepted, 141 enrolled. In 2015, 69 master's, 26 doctorates, 13 other advanced degrees awarded. Terminal master's awarded for partial completion of doctoral program. *Degree requirements:* For master's, thesis (for some programs); for doctorate, thesis/dissertation. *Entrance requirements:* For master's, doctorate, and Graduate Certificate, GRE. Additional exam requirements/recommendations for international students: Required—TOEFL (minimum score 550 paper-based; 100 iBT), Michigan English Language Assessment Battery (minimum score 85); Recommended—IELTS (minimum score 6.5), TWE (minimum score 5.5). *Application deadline:* For fall admission, 2/1 for domestic and international students. Application fee: $0. Electronic applications accepted. *Expenses:* $17,645 per year resident tuition, $33,311 non-resident tuition; $735.20 per credit hour resident tuition, $1,387.95 per credit hour non-resident tuition; fees include $47.45 per credit hour student services fee and $274.60 per semester registration fee. *Financial support:* In 2015–16, 186 students received support, including 64 fellowships with full tuition reimbursements available (averaging $25,445 per year), 103 research assistantships with full tuition reimbursements available (averaging $26,275 per year); Federal Work-Study, scholarships/grants, traineeships, health care benefits, and unspecified assistantships also available. Support available to part-time students. Financial award application deadline: 3/31. *Faculty research:* Cancer biology, neurosciences, vision sciences, molecular biology, pathology, physiology, pharmacology, public health, medical physics. *Unit head:* Dr. Stanley R. Terlecky, Associate Dean of Graduate Programs, 313-577-1455, Fax: 313-577-8796, E-mail: gradprogs@med.wayne.edu.
Website: http://gradprograms.med.wayne.edu/

Yale University, School of Medicine and Graduate School of Arts and Sciences, Combined Program in Biological and Biomedical Sciences (BBS), Pharmacological Sciences and Molecular Medicine Track, New Haven, CT 06520. Offers PhD, MD/PhD. *Degree requirements:* For doctorate, thesis/dissertation. *Entrance requirements:* For doctorate, GRE General Test. Additional exam requirements/recommendations for international students: Required—TOEFL. Electronic applications accepted.

Structural Biology

Baylor College of Medicine, Graduate School of Biomedical Sciences, Program in Structural and Computational Biology and Molecular Biophysics, Houston, TX 77030-3498. Offers PhD, MD/PhD. MD/PhD offered jointly with Rice University and University of Houston. *Degree requirements:* For doctorate, thesis/dissertation, public defense. *Entrance requirements:* For doctorate, GRE General Test, GRE Subject Test (strongly recommended), minimum GPA of 3.0. Additional exam requirements/recommendations for international students: Required—TOEFL. Electronic applications accepted. *Faculty research:* Computational biology, structural biology, biophysics.

Carnegie Mellon University, Mellon College of Science, Department of Biological Sciences, Pittsburgh, PA 15213-3891. Offers biochemistry (PhD); biophysics (PhD); cell and developmental biology (PhD); computational biology (MS, PhD); genetics (PhD); molecular biology (PhD); neuroscience (PhD); structural biology (PhD). *Degree requirements:* For doctorate, comprehensive exam, thesis/dissertation. *Entrance requirements:* For doctorate, GRE General Test, GRE Subject Test, interview. Electronic applications accepted. *Faculty research:* Genetic structure, function, and regulation; protein structure and function; biological membranes; biological spectroscopy.

Carnegie Mellon University, Mellon College of Science, Joint Pitt + CMU Molecular Biophysics and Structural Biology Graduate Program, Pittsburgh, PA 15213-3891. Offers PhD. Program offered jointly with University of Pittsburgh. *Degree requirements:* For doctorate, comprehensive exam, thesis/dissertation. *Entrance requirements:* For doctorate, GRE General Test. Additional exam requirements/recommendations for international students: Required—TOEFL (minimum score 600 paper-based; 100 iBT), IELTS (minimum score 7). Electronic applications accepted. *Faculty research:* Structural biology, protein dynamics and folding, computational biophysics, molecular informatics, membrane biophysics and ion channels, NMR, x-ray crystallography cryaelectron microscopy.

Columbia University, College of Physicians and Surgeons, Integrated Program in Cellular, Molecular, Structural and Genetic Studies, New York, NY 10032. Offers PhD. Terminal master's awarded for partial completion of doctoral program. *Degree requirements:* For doctorate, thesis/dissertation. *Entrance requirements:* For doctorate, GRE General Test, GRE Subject Test. Additional exam requirements/recommendations for international students: Required—TOEFL. *Expenses:* Contact institution. *Faculty research:* Transcription, macromolecular sorting, gene expression during development, cellular interaction.

Cornell University, Graduate School, Graduate Fields of Comparative Biomedical Sciences, Field of Comparative Biomedical Sciences, Ithaca, NY 14853-0001. Offers cellular and molecular medicine (MS, PhD); developmental and reproductive biology (MS, PhD); infectious diseases (MS, PhD); population medicine and epidemiology (MS, PhD); structural and functional biology (MS, PhD). *Degree requirements:* For master's, thesis; for doctorate, comprehensive exam, thesis/dissertation. *Entrance requirements:* For master's and doctorate, GRE General Test, 2 letters of recommendation. Additional exam requirements/recommendations for international students: Required—TOEFL (minimum score 550 paper-based; 77 iBT). Electronic applications accepted. *Faculty research:* Receptors and signal transduction, viral and bacterial infectious diseases, tumor metastasis, clinical sciences/nutritional disease, developmental/neurological disorders.

Duke University, Graduate School, University Program in Structural Biology and Biophysics, Durham, NC 27710. Offers Certificate. Students must be enrolled in a participating PhD program (biochemistry, cell biology, chemistry, molecular genetics, neurobiology, pharmacology). *Entrance requirements:* For degree, GRE General Test. Additional exam requirements/recommendations for international students: Required—TOEFL (minimum score 577 paper-based; 90 iBT) or IELTS (minimum score 7).

Florida State University, The Graduate School, College of Arts and Sciences, Department of Biological Science, Specialization in Structural Biology, Tallahassee, FL 32306-4295. Offers MS, PhD. *Faculty:* 12 full-time (4 women). *Students:* 22 full-time (12 women); includes 3 minority (1 Black or African American, non-Hispanic/Latino; 2 Hispanic/Latino), 5 international. In 2015, 1 doctorate awarded. Terminal master's awarded for partial completion of doctoral program. *Degree requirements:* For master's, comprehensive exam, thesis, teaching experience, seminar presentation; for doctorate, comprehensive exam, thesis/dissertation, teaching experience, seminar presentation. *Entrance requirements:* For master's and doctorate, GRE General Test, minimum upper-division GPA of 3.0. Additional exam requirements/recommendations for international students: Required—TOEFL (minimum score 600 paper-based; 92 iBT). *Application deadline:* For fall admission, 12/1 for domestic and international students. Application fee: $30. Electronic applications accepted. *Expenses: Tuition, area resident:* Full-time $7263; part-time $403.50 per credit hour. Tuition, nonresident: full-time $18,087; part-time $1004.85 per credit hour. *Required fees:* $1365; $75.81 per credit hour. $20 per semester. Tuition and fees vary according to campus/location. *Financial support:* In 2015–16, 22 students received support, including 1 fellowship (averaging $23,000 per year), 7 research assistantships with full tuition reimbursements available (averaging $21,500 per year), 14 teaching assistantships with full tuition reimbursements available (averaging $21,500 per year); traineeships and unspecified assistantships also available. Financial award application deadline: 12/1; financial award applicants required to submit FAFSA. *Faculty research:* Molecular genetics, signal transduction and regulation of gene expression, cell and molecular biology of the cytoskeleton, olfactory signal transduction, ion channel structure-function, neuromodulation, 3-D electron microscopy and x-ray crystallography of protein complexes involved in mRNA and sulfur metabolism, olfaction, synaptic physiology and plasticity, ion channel modulation, biomechanics of cardiac and skeletal muscle, magnetic resonance of proteins. *Unit head:* Dr. Thomas A. Houpt, Professor and Associate Chair, 850-644-4907, Fax: 850-644-8447, E-mail: houpt@neuro.fsu.edu. *Application contact:* Dr. Michael B. Miller, Coordinator, Graduate Affairs, 850-644-3023, Fax: 850-644-9829, E-mail: gradinfo@bio.fsu.edu.
Website: http://www.bio.fsu.edu/

Florida State University, The Graduate School, College of Arts and Sciences, Program in Molecular Biophysics, Tallahassee, FL 32306. Offers molecular biophysics (PhD); structural biology and computational biophysics (PhD). *Faculty:* 34 full-time (7 women). *Students:* 19 full-time (5 women); includes 2 minority (both Hispanic/Latino), 8 international. Average age 29. 14 applicants, 36% accepted, 2 enrolled. In 2015, 5 doctorates awarded. *Degree requirements:* For doctorate, comprehensive exam, thesis/dissertation, teaching 1 term in professor's major department. *Entrance requirements:* For doctorate, GRE General Test. Additional exam requirements/recommendations for international students: Required—TOEFL (minimum score 600 paper-based; 90 iBT). *Application deadline:* For fall admission, 12/15 for domestic and international students. Application fee: $30. Electronic applications accepted. *Expenses: Tuition, area resident:* Full-time $7263; part-time $403.50 per credit hour. Tuition, nonresident: full-time $18,087; part-time $1004.85 per credit hour. *Required fees:* $1365; $75.81 per credit hour. $20 per semester. Tuition and fees vary according to campus/location. *Financial support:* In 2015–16, 23 students received support, including 1 fellowship with tuition reimbursement available (averaging $34,200 per year), 20 research assistantships with tuition reimbursements available (averaging $24,200 per year), 2 teaching assistantships with tuition reimbursements available (averaging $24,200 per year); scholarships/grants, health care benefits, and unspecified assistantships also available. *Faculty research:* Protein and nucleic acid structure and function, membrane protein structure, computational biophysics, 3-D image reconstruction. *Total annual research expenditures:* $2.3 million. *Unit head:* Dr. Hong Li, Director, 850-644-6785, Fax: 850-644-7244, E-mail: hli4@fsu.edu. *Application contact:* Katie Mikusak, Academic Coordinator, Graduate Programs, 850-644-1012, Fax: 850-644-7244, E-mail: kmikusak@chem.fsu.edu.
Website: http://www.biophysics.fsu.edu/graduate-program

Harvard University, Graduate School of Arts and Sciences, Department of Systems Biology, Cambridge, MA 02138. Offers PhD. *Degree requirements:* For doctorate, thesis/dissertation, lab rotation, qualifying examination. *Entrance requirements:* For doctorate, GRE. Additional exam requirements/recommendations for international students: Required—TOEFL. Electronic applications accepted.

Illinois State University, Graduate School, College of Arts and Sciences, Department of Biological Sciences, Normal, IL 61790-2200. Offers animal behavior (MS); bacteriology (MS); biochemistry (MS); biological sciences (MS); biology (PhD); biophysics (MS); biotechnology (MS); botany (MS, PhD); cell biology (MS); conservation biology (MS); developmental biology (MS); ecology (MS, PhD); entomology (MS); evolutionary biology (MS); genetics (MS, PhD); immunology (MS); microbiology (MS, PhD); molecular biology (MS); molecular genetics (MS); neurobiology (MS); neuroscience (MS); parasitology (MS); physiology (MS, PhD); plant biology (MS); plant molecular biology (MS); plant sciences (MS); structural biology (MS); zoology (MS, PhD). *Program availability:* Part-time. *Degree requirements:* For master's, thesis or alternative; for doctorate, variable foreign language requirement, thesis/dissertation, 2 terms of residency. *Entrance requirements:* For master's, GRE General Test, minimum GPA of 2.6 in last 60 hours of course work; for doctorate, GRE General Test. *Application deadline:* Applications are processed on a rolling basis. Application fee: $40. *Financial support:* Research assistantships, teaching assistantships, Federal Work-Study, tuition waivers (full), and unspecified assistantships available. Financial award application deadline: 4/1. *Faculty research:* Redoc balance and drug development in schistosoma mansoni, control of the growth of listeria monocytogenes at low temperature, regulation of cell expansion and microtubule function by SPRI, CRUI: physiology and fitness consequences of different life history phenotypes. *Application contact:* Steven Juliano, Graduate Coordinator, E-mail: sajulian@ilstu.edu.
Website: http://www.bio.ilstu.edu

Iowa State University of Science and Technology, Bioinformatics and Computational Biology Program, Ames, IA 50011. Offers MS, PhD. *Degree requirements:* For doctorate, thesis/dissertation. *Entrance requirements:* For master's and doctorate, GRE General Test. Additional exam requirements/recommendations for international students: Recommended—TOEFL, IELTS. Electronic applications accepted. *Faculty research:* Functional and structural genomics, genome evolution, macromolecular structure and function, mathematical biology and biological statistics, metabolic and developmental networks.

Massachusetts Institute of Technology, School of Science, Department of Biology, Cambridge, MA 02139. Offers biochemistry (PhD); biological oceanography (PhD); biology (PhD); biophysical chemistry and molecular structure (PhD); cell biology (PhD); computational and systems biology (PhD); developmental biology (PhD); genetics (PhD); immunology (PhD); microbiology (PhD); molecular biology (PhD); neurobiology (PhD). *Faculty:* 57 full-time (14 women). *Students:* 283 full-time (137 women); includes 83 minority (3 Black or African American, non-Hispanic/Latino; 1 American Indian or Alaska Native, non-Hispanic/Latino; 38 Asian, non-Hispanic/Latino; 31 Hispanic/Latino; 10 Two or more races, non-Hispanic/Latino), 48 international. Average age 26. 673 applicants, 14% accepted, 46 enrolled. In 2015, 32 doctorates awarded. *Degree requirements:* For doctorate, comprehensive exam, thesis/dissertation, teaching assistantship during two semesters. *Entrance requirements:* For doctorate, GRE General Test. Additional exam requirements/recommendations for international students: Required—TOEFL (minimum score 577 paper-based), IELTS. *Application deadline:* For fall admission, 12/1 for domestic and international students. Application fee: $75. Electronic applications accepted. *Expenses: Tuition:* Full-time $46,400; part-time $725 per credit. One-time fee: $304 full-time. Full-time tuition and fees vary according to course load and program. *Financial support:* In 2015–16, 235 students received support, including 118 fellowships (averaging $37,500 per year), 163 research assistantships (averaging $38,900 per year), 1 teaching assistantship; Federal Work-Study, institutionally sponsored loans, scholarships/grants, traineeships, health care benefits, and unspecified assistantships also available. Support available to part-time students. Financial award application deadline: 4/15; financial award applicants required to submit FAFSA. *Faculty research:* Cellular, developmental and molecular (plant and animal) biology; biochemistry, bioengineering, biophysics and structural biology; classical and molecular genetics, stem cell and epigenetics; immunology and microbiology; cancer biology, molecular medicine, neurobiology and human disease; computational and systems biology. *Total annual research expenditures:* $42.8 million. *Unit head:* Prof. Alan Grossman, Department Head, 617-253-4701. *Application contact:* Biology Education Office, 617-253-3717, Fax: 617-258-9329, E-mail: gradbio@mit.edu.
Website: https://biology.mit.edu/

Mayo Graduate School, Graduate Programs in Biomedical Sciences, Programs in Biochemistry, Structural Biology, Cell Biology, and Genetics, Rochester, MN 55905. Offers biochemistry and structural biology (PhD); cell biology and genetics (PhD); molecular biology (PhD). *Degree requirements:* For doctorate, oral defense of dissertation, qualifying oral and written exam. *Entrance requirements:* For doctorate, GRE, 1 year of chemistry, biology, calculus, and physics. Additional exam requirements/recommendations for international students: Required—TOEFL. Electronic applications accepted. *Faculty research:* Gene structure and function, membranes and receptors/cytoskeleton, oncogenes and growth factors, protein structure and function, steroid hormonal action.

Michigan State University, The Graduate School, College of Natural Science, Quantitative Biology Program, East Lansing, MI 48824. Offers PhD.

New York University, School of Medicine and Graduate School of Arts and Science, Sackler Institute of Graduate Biomedical Sciences, New York, NY 10010. Offers biomedical imaging (PhD); biomedical informatics (PhD); cellular and molecular biology (PhD); computational biology (PhD); developmental genetics (PhD); genome integrity (PhD); immunology and inflammation (PhD); microbiology (PhD); molecular biophysics (PhD); molecular oncology and tumor immunology (PhD), including immunology, molecular oncology; molecular pharmacology (PhD); neuroscience and physiology (PhD); pathobiology and translational medicine (PhD); stem cell biology (PhD); MD/PhD. *Degree requirements:* For doctorate, comprehensive exam, thesis/dissertation, qualifying exam. *Entrance requirements:* For doctorate, GRE General Test. Additional exam requirements/recommendations for international students: Required—TOEFL. Electronic applications accepted. *Expenses:* Contact institution.

Northwestern University, The Graduate School, Interdisciplinary Biological Sciences Program (IBiS), Evanston, IL 60208. Offers biochemistry (PhD); bioengineering and biotechnology (PhD); biotechnology (PhD); cell and molecular biology (PhD); developmental and systems biology (PhD); nanotechnology (PhD); neurobiology (PhD); structural biology and biophysics (PhD). *Degree requirements:* For doctorate, thesis/dissertation, qualifying exam. *Entrance requirements:* For doctorate, GRE General Test. Additional exam requirements/recommendations for international students: Required—TOEFL (minimum score 600 paper-based). Electronic applications accepted. *Faculty research:* Biophysics/structural biology, cell/molecular biology, synthetic biology, developmental systems biology, chemical biology/nanotechnology.

Oregon State University, Interdisciplinary/Institutional Programs, Program in Molecular and Cellular Biology, Corvallis, OR 97331. Offers bioinformatics (PhD); biotechnology (PhD); cell biology (PhD); developmental biology (PhD); genome biology (PhD); molecular biology (PhD); molecular pathogenesis (PhD); molecular virology (PhD); plant molecular biology (PhD); structural biology (PhD). *Students:* 28 full-time (14 women), 2 part-time (1 woman); includes 4 minority (2 Asian, non-Hispanic/Latino; 2 Hispanic/Latino), 10 international. Average age 29. 104 applicants, 5% accepted, 5 enrolled. In 2015, 5 doctorates awarded. *Degree requirements:* For doctorate, thesis/dissertation,

oral and written qualifying exams. *Entrance requirements:* For doctorate, GRE. Additional exam requirements/recommendations for international students: Required—TOEFL (minimum score 80 iBT), IELTS (minimum score 6.5). *Application deadline:* For fall admission, 8/1 for domestic students, 4/1 for international students; for winter admission, 12/1 for domestic students, 7/1 for international students; for spring admission, 2/1 for domestic students, 10/1 for international students; for summer admission, 5/1 for domestic students, 1/1 for international students. Application fee: $75 ($85 for international students). *Expenses:* Tuition, state resident: full-time $12,150; part-time $450 per credit. Tuition, nonresident: full-time $20,952; part-time $776 per credit. *Required fees:* $1572; $1443 per unit. One-time fee: $350. Tuition and fees vary according to course load, campus/location and program. *Financial support:* Fellowships, career-related internships or fieldwork, Federal Work-Study, and institutionally sponsored loans available. Support available to part-time students. Financial award application deadline: 1/1. *Unit head:* Dr. Dee Denver, Director, Molecular and Cellular Biology Graduate Program, 541-737-3698. *Application contact:* Kristin Carroll, Assistant Director, 541-737-5259, E-mail: kristin.carroll@oregonstate.edu.
Website: http://www.mcb.oregonstate.edu/

Stanford University, School of Medicine, Graduate Programs in Medicine, Department of Structural Biology, Stanford, CA 94305-9991. Offers PhD. *Degree requirements:* For doctorate, thesis/dissertation. *Entrance requirements:* For doctorate, GRE General Test, GRE Subject Test. Additional exam requirements/recommendations for international students: Required—TOEFL. Electronic applications accepted. *Expenses:* Tuition, area resident: Full-time $45,729. *Required fees:* $591.

Stony Brook University, State University of New York, Graduate School, College of Arts and Sciences, Department of Biochemistry and Cell Biology, Program in Biochemistry and Structural Biology, Stony Brook, NY 11794. Offers PhD. *Students:* 32 full-time (14 women); includes 5 minority (1 Black or African American, non-Hispanic/Latino; 1 Asian, non-Hispanic/Latino; 2 Hispanic/Latino; 1 Native Hawaiian or other Pacific Islander, non-Hispanic/Latino), 15 international. Average age 27. 49 applicants, 33% accepted, 4 enrolled. In 2015, 5 doctorates awarded. *Entrance requirements:* For doctorate, GRE. Additional exam requirements/recommendations for international students: Required—TOEFL (minimum score 90 iBT). *Application deadline:* For fall admission, 1/15 for domestic students; for spring admission, 10/1 for domestic students. Application fee: $100. *Expenses:* $12,421 per year full-time resident tuition and fees, $453 per credit hour; $23,761 per year full-time non-resident tuition and fees, $925 per credit hour. *Financial support:* In 2015–16, 2 fellowships, 18 research assistantships, 8 teaching assistantships were awarded. *Unit head:* Prof. Robert Haltiwanger, Chair, 631-632-7336, Fax: 631-632-9730, E-mail: robert.haltiwanger@stonybrook.edu. *Application contact:* Joann DeLucia-Conlon, Graduate Program Assistant, 631-632-8613, Fax: 631-632-8575, E-mail: joann.delucia-conlon@stonybrook.edu.
Website: http://www.stonybrook.edu/commcms/biochem/education/graduate/overview.html

Syracuse University, College of Arts and Sciences, Ph.D. Program in Structural Biology, Biochemistry and Biophysics, Syracuse, NY 13244. Offers structural biology, biochemistry, and biophysics (PhD). *Students:* Average age 28. *Degree requirements:* For doctorate, comprehensive exam, thesis/dissertation. *Entrance requirements:* For doctorate, GRE General Test, GRE Subject Test, three letters of recommendation, resume, personal statement, transcripts. Additional exam requirements/recommendations for international students: Required—TOEFL (minimum score 100 iBT). *Application deadline:* For fall admission, 12/15 priority date for domestic and international students. Application fee: $75. Electronic applications accepted. *Expenses: Tuition, area resident:* Full-time $25,974; part-time $1443 per credit hour. *Required fees:* $802; $50 per course. Tuition and fees vary according to course load and program. *Financial support:* Fellowships with full tuition reimbursements, research assistantships with tuition reimbursements, teaching assistantships with tuition reimbursements, scholarships/grants, and tuition waivers available. Financial award application deadline: 1/1. *Faculty research:* Biochemistry, genetic engineering, biomolecular modeling, methods for computerized simulation of molecules, ethical conduct of science. *Unit head:* Prof. Liviu Movileanu, Associate Professor, Physics, 315-443-9154, Fax: 315-443-2012, E-mail: lmovilea@syr.edu. *Application contact:* Patty Whitmore, Academic Program Coordinator, 315-443-5958, E-mail: pawhitmo@syr.edu.
Website: http://sb3.syr.edu/

Tufts University, Sackler School of Graduate Biomedical Sciences, Cell, Molecular, and Developmental Biology Program, Medford, MA 02155. Offers cancer biology (PhD); developmental and regenerative biology (PhD); molecular and cellular medicine (PhD); structural and chemical biology (PhD). *Faculty:* 45 full-time (15 women). *Students:* 36 full-time (18 women); includes 13 minority (2 Black or African American, non-Hispanic/Latino; 9 Asian, non-Hispanic/Latino; 1 Hispanic/Latino; 1 Two or more races, non-Hispanic/Latino), 4 international. Average age 28. 189 applicants, 7% accepted, 6 enrolled. In 2015, 2 doctorates awarded. Terminal master's awarded for partial completion of doctoral program. *Degree requirements:* For doctorate, comprehensive exam, thesis/dissertation. *Entrance requirements:* For doctorate, GRE General Test, 3 letters of reference. Additional exam requirements/recommendations for international students: Required—TOEFL (minimum score 600 paper-based; 100 iBT). *Application deadline:* For fall admission, 12/15 priority date for domestic and international students. Application fee: $70. Electronic applications accepted. *Expenses: Tuition, area resident:* Full-time $48,412; part-time $1210 per credit hour. *Required fees:* $806. Full-time tuition and fees vary according to degree level, program and student level. Part-time tuition and fees vary according to course load. *Financial support:* In 2015–16, 36 students received support, including 36 research assistantships with full tuition reimbursements available (averaging $32,000 per year); health care benefits also available. *Faculty research:* Reproduction and hormone action, control of gene expression, cell-matrix and cell-cell interactions, growth control and tumorigenesis, cytoskeleton and contractile proteins. *Unit head:* Dr. Ira Herman, Program Director, 617-636-2991, Fax: 617-636-0375. *Application contact:* Dr. Elizabeth Storrs, Registrar/Director of Academic Services, 617-636-6767, Fax: 617-636-0375, E-mail: sackler-school@tufts.edu.
Website: http://sackler.tufts.edu/Academics/CMDB-Welcome

Tulane University, School of Medicine and School of Liberal Arts, Graduate Programs in Biomedical Sciences, Department of Structural and Cellular Biology, New Orleans, LA 70118-5669. Offers MS, PhD, MD/PhD. MS and PhD offered through the Graduate School. *Degree requirements:* For master's, one foreign language, thesis; for doctorate, 2 foreign languages, thesis/dissertation. *Entrance requirements:* For master's, GRE General Test, minimum B average in undergraduate course work; for doctorate, GRE General Test. Additional exam requirements/recommendations for international students: Required—TOEFL. Electronic applications accepted. *Expenses: Tuition, area resident:* Full-time $47,658; part-time $2648 per credit hour. *Required fees:* $1980; $44.50 per credit hour. $550 per term. Tuition and fees vary according to course load, degree level and program. *Faculty research:* Reproductive endocrinology, visual neuroscience, neural response to altered hormones.

University at Albany, State University of New York, School of Public Health, Department of Biomedical Sciences, Program in Structural and Cell Biology, Albany, NY 12222-0001. Offers MS, PhD. *Degree requirements:* For master's, thesis; for doctorate,

thesis/dissertation. *Entrance requirements:* For master's and doctorate, GRE General Test, GRE Subject Test.

University at Buffalo, the State University of New York, Graduate School, School of Medicine and Biomedical Sciences, Graduate Programs in Medicine and Biomedical Sciences, Department of Structural Biology, Buffalo, NY 14260. Offers MS, PhD. *Faculty:* 1 full-time (0 women), 6 part-time/adjunct (1 woman). *Students:* 4 full-time (0 women). Average age 27. In 2015, 1 master's awarded. *Degree requirements:* For master's, comprehensive exam, thesis; for doctorate, comprehensive exam, thesis/dissertation. *Entrance requirements:* For master's, BS or BA in science, engineering, or math; for doctorate, GRE General Test, BS or BA in science, engineering, or math. Additional exam requirements/recommendations for international students: Required—TOEFL (minimum score 600 paper-based; 100 iBT). *Application deadline:* For fall admission, 2/1 priority date for domestic and international students. Applications are processed on a rolling basis. Application fee: $50. Electronic applications accepted. *Financial support:* In 2015–16, 8 research assistantships (averaging $24,000 per year) were awarded; Federal Work-Study, scholarships/grants, traineeships, and unspecified assistantships also available. Financial award application deadline: 2/1; financial award applicants required to submit FAFSA. *Faculty research:* Biomacromolecular structure and function at the level of three-dimensional atomic architecture. *Total annual research expenditures:* $4.5 million. *Unit head:* Dr. Michael Malkowski, Chair/Professor, 716-898-8624, Fax: 716-898-8660, E-mail: malkowski@hwi.buffalo.edu. *Application contact:* Elizabeth A. White, Administrative Director, 716-829-3399, Fax: 716-829-2437, E-mail: bethw@buffalo.edu.
Website: http://www.hwi.buffalo.edu/graduate_studies/graduate_studies.html

The University of Alabama at Birmingham, Graduate Programs in Joint Health Sciences, Biochemistry, Structural and Stem Cell Biology Program, Birmingham, AL 35294-0024. Offers PhD. *Students:* 34 full-time (11 women); includes 7 minority (4 Black or African American, non-Hispanic/Latino; 2 Hispanic/Latino; 1 Two or more races, non-Hispanic/Latino), 5 international. Average age 26. *Degree requirements:* For doctorate, comprehensive exam, thesis/dissertation. *Entrance requirements:* For doctorate, GRE (minimum combined verbal/quantitative score of 300, 1100 on old exam), interview, letters of recommendation, minimum GPA of 3.0, research experience. Additional exam requirements/recommendations for international students: Required—TOEFL (minimum score 600 paper-based; 100 iBT). *Application deadline:* For fall admission, 12/1 priority date for domestic students, 1/15 for international students. Application fee: $0 ($60 for international students). Electronic applications accepted. *Expenses:* Tuition, state resident: full-time $7340. Tuition, nonresident: full-time $16,628. Full-time tuition and fees vary according to course load and program. *Financial support:* In 2015–16, fellowships with full tuition reimbursements (averaging $29,000 per year) were awarded. *Faculty research:* Enzymology, chromatin structure, gene expression, cell signaling, protein structure. *Unit head:* Dr. Thomas Ryan, Program Director, 205-996-2175, E-mail: tryan@uab.edu. *Application contact:* Holly Hebard, Director of Student and Academic Services, 205-996-5696, E-mail: hghebard@uab.edu.
Website: http://www.uab.edu/gbs/bssb/

The University of Manchester, Faculty of Life Sciences, Manchester, United Kingdom. Offers adaptive organismal biology (M Phil, PhD); animal biology (M Phil, PhD); biochemistry (M Phil, PhD); bioinformatics (M Phil, PhD); biomolecular sciences (M Phil, PhD); biotechnology (M Phil, PhD); cell biology (M Phil, PhD); cell matrix research (M Phil, PhD); channels and transporters (M Phil, PhD); developmental biology (M Phil, PhD); Egyptology (M Phil, PhD); environmental biology (M Phil, PhD); evolutionary biology (M Phil, PhD); gene expression (M Phil, PhD); genetics (M Phil, PhD); history of science, technology and medicine (M Phil, PhD); immunology (M Phil, PhD); integrative neurobiology and behavior (M Phil, PhD); membrane trafficking (M Phil, PhD); microbiology (M Phil, PhD); molecular and cellular neuroscience (M Phil, PhD); molecular biology (M Phil, PhD); molecular cancer studies (M Phil, PhD); neuroscience (M Phil, PhD); ophthalmology (M Phil, PhD); optometry (M Phil, PhD); organelle function (M Phil, PhD); pharmacology (M Phil, PhD); physiology (M Phil, PhD); plant sciences (M Phil, PhD); stem cell research (M Phil, PhD); structural biology (M Phil, PhD); systems neuroscience (M Phil, PhD); toxicology (M Phil, PhD).

University of Minnesota, Twin Cities Campus, Graduate School, College of Biological Sciences, Biochemistry, Molecular Biology and Biophysics Graduate Program, Minneapolis, MN 55455-0213. Offers PhD. *Degree requirements:* For doctorate, thesis/dissertation. *Entrance requirements:* For doctorate, GRE, 3 letters of recommendation, more than 1 semester of laboratory experience. Additional exam requirements/recommendations for international students: Required—TOEFL (minimum score 625 paper-based; 108 iBT with writing subsection 25 and reading subsection 25) or IELTS (minimum score 7). Electronic applications accepted. *Faculty research:* Microbial biochemistry, biotechnology, molecular biology, regulatory biochemistry, structural biology and biophysics, physical biochemistry, enzymology, physiological chemistry.

University of Pittsburgh, School of Medicine and Dietrich School of Arts and Sciences, Molecular Biophysics and Structural Biology Graduate Program, Pittsburgh, PA 15260. Offers PhD. PhD jointly offered with Carnegie Mellon University. *Faculty:* 51 full-time (13 women). *Students:* 10 full-time (6 women); includes 1 minority (Hispanic/Latino), 2 international. Average age 26. 46 applicants, 22% accepted. In 2015, 4 doctorates awarded. *Degree requirements:* For doctorate, comprehensive exam, thesis/dissertation. *Entrance requirements:* For doctorate, GRE General Test. Additional exam requirements/recommendations for international students: Required—TOEFL (minimum score 600 paper-based; 100 iBT), IELTS (minimum score 7). *Application deadline:* For fall admission, 12/1 priority date for domestic and international students. Application fee: $50. Electronic applications accepted. Tuition and fees vary according to program. *Financial support:* In 2015–16, 10 students received support, including 2 fellowships with full tuition reimbursements available (averaging $27,000 per year), 8 research assistantships with full tuition reimbursements available (averaging $27,000 per year); teaching assistantships, scholarships/grants, traineeships, and health care benefits also available. *Faculty research:* Structural biology, protein dynamics and folding, computational biophysics, molecular informatics, membrane biophysics and ion channels, x-ray crystallography cryaelectron microscopy. *Unit head:* Dr. James Conway, Director, 412-648-8957, Fax: 412-648-1077, E-mail: mbsbinfo@medschool.pitt.edu. *Application contact:* Lauren Zielinski, Student Affairs Specialist, 412-383-7866, E-mail: mbsbinfo@medschool.pitt.edu.
Website: http://www.mbsb.pitt.edu

University of Rochester, School of Medicine and Dentistry, Graduate Programs in Medicine and Dentistry, Department of Biochemistry and Biophysics, Programs in Biophysics, Rochester, NY 14627. Offers biophysics, structural and computational biology (PhD). Terminal master's awarded for partial completion of doctoral program. *Degree requirements:* For doctorate, thesis/dissertation, qualifying exam. *Entrance requirements:* For doctorate, GRE General Test. *Expenses: Tuition, area resident:* Full-time $47,450; part-time $1482 per credit hour. *Required fees:* $528. Tuition and fees vary according to program.

The University of Texas Health Science Center at San Antonio, Graduate School of Biomedical Sciences, Department of Cellular and Structural Biology, San Antonio, TX 78229-3900. Offers MS, PhD. *Degree requirements:* For master's, thesis; for doctorate, comprehensive exam, thesis/dissertation.

The University of Texas Medical Branch, Graduate School of Biomedical Sciences, Program in Biochemistry and Molecular Biology, Galveston, TX 77555. Offers biochemistry (PhD); bioinformatics (PhD); biophysics (PhD); cell biology (PhD); computational biology (PhD); structural biology (PhD). *Degree requirements:* For doctorate, thesis/dissertation. *Entrance requirements:* Additional exam requirements/recommendations for international students: Required—TOEFL (minimum score 550 paper-based). Electronic applications accepted.

University of Washington, Graduate School, School of Medicine, Graduate Programs in Medicine, Department of Biological Structure, Seattle, WA 98195. Offers PhD. *Degree requirements:* For doctorate, thesis/dissertation. *Faculty research:* Cellular and developmental biology, experimental immunology and hematology, molecular structure and molecular biology, neurobiology, x-rays.

Weill Cornell Medicine, Weill Cornell Graduate School of Medical Sciences, Biochemistry, Cell and Molecular Biology Allied Program, New York, NY 10065. Offers MS, PhD. Terminal master's awarded for partial completion of doctoral program. *Degree requirements:* For master's, comprehensive exam; for doctorate, thesis/dissertation, final exam. *Entrance requirements:* For doctorate, GRE General Test, background in genetics, molecular biology, chemistry, or biochemistry. Additional exam requirements/recommendations for international students: Required—TOEFL. Electronic applications accepted. *Faculty research:* Molecular structure determination, protein structure, gene structure, stem cell biology, control of gene expression, DNA replication, chromosome maintenance, RNA biosynthesis.

GERSTNER SLOAN KETTERING GRADUATE SCHOOL OF BIOMEDICAL SCIENCES

Ph.D. in Cancer Biology Program

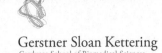

Gerstner Sloan Kettering
Graduate School of Biomedical Sciences

 For more information, visit http://petersons.to/sloanketteringcancerbiology

Program of Study

The Louis V. Gerstner, Jr. Graduate School of Biomedical Sciences, Memorial Sloan Kettering Cancer Center offers a doctoral program that trains laboratory scientists to work in research areas directly applicable to human disease and, in particular, cancer.

The unique curriculum integrates Memorial Sloan Kettering's basic science and clinical arms to maximize the potential of future basic scientists to improve human health.

During the first year, students complete a core course that introduces recent findings in relevant topics through didactic lecture and discussion of research papers. A separate course in quantitative and computational biology is offered in the spring semester. Students will also complete three 5-week laboratory rotations, with each one culminating in an oral presentation of their findings; three visits with clinicians; course work in logic and critical analysis; and two semesters of the President's Research Seminar Series Journal Club, which introduces students to the published works of world-renowned speakers.

After completing the didactic portion of their education in the first year, students focus full time on thesis research. Students are expected to present a written and oral thesis proposal by March 31 of the second year. Continuing throughout their graduate programs, students take part in the Current Topics Journal Club, along with the Graduate Student Seminar, in which students present their own research.

Students also have the opportunity to select a clinical mentor who directs the student in participating in hospital-based academic activities such as grand rounds and conferences with pathology and disease management teams.

Research Facilities

Memorial Sloan Kettering's research space totals approximately 575,000 square feet, with many cutting-edge laboratories and facilities housed within the Rockefeller Research Laboratories building and the Zuckerman Research Center, a building with open, spacious floors designed to encourage collaboration.

There are dozens of research core facilities that serve both basic and clinical research needs, offering state-of-the-art instruments and technical staff support to graduate students. The Memorial Sloan Kettering Cancer Center library subscribes to a full range of science, medical, and healthcare resources. Students have access to an array of published literature, with the majority of these titles available electronically. The library's website provides access to an extensive collection of resources, including an online catalog, databases, electronic books, and electronic journals.

Financial Aid

All matriculated students receive a fellowship package that includes an annual stipend ($37,530 for 2016–17); a first-year allowance to be used for books, journals, and other school expenses; a scholarship that covers the full cost of tuition and fees; comprehensive medical, dental, and vision insurance; a laptop computer; relocation costs (up to $500); and paid membership in the New York Academy of Sciences.

Eligible students may also apply for independent funding from agencies such as the National Institutes of Health and the National Science Foundation. Recipients of one of these fellowships receive an additional stipend of $5,000 per year during the award period from the school; this is in addition to any supplement necessary to bring the stipend to the common level. Travel awards are given to students who present a poster or a short talk at a scientific meeting.

Living and Housing Costs

Affordable housing in proximity to the research buildings is provided to all Gerstner Sloan Kettering students. Housing units are located in family-oriented neighborhoods on or near Manhattan's Upper East Side. Students who have spouses or significant others can apply for family units. The housing contract runs for the student's duration of study and is automatically renewed each year based on academic progress.

Student Group

Currently there are 68 full-time students (27 women, 41 men), with 15 percent minority and 40 percent international. Applicants are expected to hold an undergraduate degree from an accredited institution and have significant basic science research experience. College-level coursework in the following areas is required: biology, chemistry, physics, organic chemistry, mathematics, and biochemistry.

Student Outcomes

Graduates of the program are expected to enter into careers as researchers, scientists, and educators in excellent laboratories, hospitals, medical schools, and research institutions throughout the country and around the world.

Location

The campus is located on Manhattan's Upper East Side, home to some of New York City's best shopping and dining. Several world-famous museums are within walking distance, and Central Park is a few blocks away. New York also offers theater, live music, outdoor recreation, and cultural attractions such as the Metropolitan Museum of Art, all accessible by public transportation.

The Faculty

Information regarding the faculty members is available online at: http://www.sloankettering.edu/research/faculty.

Gerstner Sloan Kettering Graduate School of Biomedical Sciences

The Graduate School

The Louis V. Gerstner, Jr. Graduate School of Biomedical Sciences, Memorial Sloan Kettering Cancer Center, offers the next generation of basic scientists an intensive Ph.D. program to study the biological sciences through the lens of cancer.

The Gerstner Sloan Kettering Graduate School of Biomedical Sciences is accredited by the New York State Board of Regents and the Commissioner of Education, located at 89 Washington Avenue, Albany, New York 12234; phone: 518-474-3852.

Applying

Prospective students must submit the online application, official transcripts from all colleges previously attended, three letters of recommendation from advisers and/or research mentors, and official GRE scores. Official scores for the Test of English as a Foreign Language (TOEFL) exams are required for applicants who do not speak English as their first language (can be waived for those who earned their undergraduate degrees in the United States). An in-person interview is requested from those applicants being seriously considered for admission, but the requirement may be waived if geographical constraints are overwhelming and may be substituted with video interviews. There is currently no application fee. The deadline to apply is December 1, and interviews take place the following January.

Correspondence and Information

Gerstner Sloan Kettering Graduate School of Biomedical
    Sciences
1275 York Avenue, Box 441
New York, New York 10065
Phone: 646-888-6639
Fax: 646-422-2351
E-mail: gradstudies@sloankettering.edu
Website: http://www.sloankettering.edu

The school is located on Manhattan's Upper East Side, in the heart of a thriving biomedical research community.

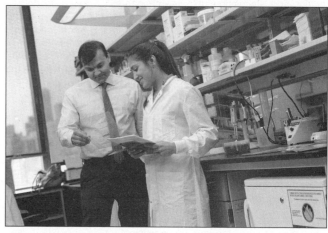

The Louis V. Gerstner, Jr. Graduate School of Biomedical Sciences, Memorial Sloan Kettering Cancer Center offers a doctoral program that trains laboratory scientists to work in research areas directly applicable to human disease, and in particular, cancer.

UNIFORMED SERVICES UNIVERSITY OF THE HEALTH SCIENCES

F. Edward Hébert School of Medicine
Graduate Program in Molecular and Cell Biology

 For more information, visit http://petersons.to/uniformedserviceshealthsciences

Program of Study

The program of study is designed for full-time students who wish to obtain a Ph.D. degree in the area of molecular and cell biology. This interdepartmental graduate program, which includes faculty members from both basic and clinical departments, offers research expertise in a wide range of areas, including bacteriology, immunology, genetics, biochemistry, regulation of gene expression, and cancer biology. The program includes core courses in molecular and cell biology that provide necessary knowledge for modern biomedical research, as well as advanced electives in areas of faculty expertise. The first-year curriculum includes courses in biochemistry, cell biology, experimental methodology, genetics, and immunology. During the first summer, students participate in laboratory rotations in two laboratories of their choice, leading to the choice of a mentor for their doctoral research. The second-year curriculum offers advanced elective courses in a variety of disciplines, including biochemistry, cell biology, immunology, molecular endocrinology, and virology, and marks the transition from classwork to original laboratory research. Throughout their graduate experience, students participate in journal clubs designed to foster interaction across disciplines and to develop the critical skills needed for data presentation and analysis. A year-round seminar series brings renowned scientists to the Uniformed Services University of the Health Sciences (USUHS) to share their results and to meet with students and faculty members. Students may also take advantage of seminars hosted by other programs and departments as well as those presented at the National Institutes of Health. Completion of the research project and preparation and successful defense of a written dissertation leads to the degree of Doctor of Philosophy.

Research Facilities

The University possesses outstanding facilities for research in molecular and cell biology. Well-equipped laboratories and extramurally funded faculty members provide an outstanding environment in which to pursue state-of-the-art research. Shared equipment in a modern biomedical instrumentation core facility includes oligonucleotide and peptide synthesizers and sequencers; a variety of imaging equipment, including laser confocal and electron microscopes; fluorescent-activated cell sorters; and an ACAS workstation. A recently added proteomics facility contains both MADLI-TOF and ESI tandem mass spectrometers. All offices, laboratories, and the Learning Resource Center are equipped with high-speed Internet connectivity and have access to an extensive online journal collection.

Financial Aid

USUHS provides an attractive package of financial support that is administered as a federal salary. This salary is available on a competitive basis to all civilian graduate students. Salaries are made on an annual basis and are renewable for up to three years. For the 2016–17 academic year, salaries for graduate students are $43,400. In addition to this base support, health insurance and transit benefits are provided if needed.

Cost of Study

Graduate students are **not** required to pay tuition. Civilian graduate students do **not** incur any obligation to the United States government for service after completion of their graduate training programs. Active-duty military personnel incur an obligation for additional military service by Department of Defense regulations that govern sponsored graduate education. Students are required to maintain health insurance.

Living and Housing Costs

The University does not have housing for graduate students. However, there is an abundant supply of rental housing in the area. Living costs in the greater Washington, D.C., area are comparable to those of other East Coast metropolitan areas.

Student Group

The first graduate students in the interdisciplinary Graduate Program in Molecular and Cell Biology at USUHS were admitted in 1995. Over the last decade, the Graduate Program in Molecular and Cell Biology has grown significantly; 25 students are currently enrolled. Forty Ph.D. degrees in molecular and cell biology have been awarded over the past fifteen years.

Location

Metropolitan Washington has a population of about 5 million residents in the District of Columbia and the surrounding areas of Maryland and Virginia. The region is a center of education and research and is home to five major universities, four medical schools, the National Library of Medicine and the National Institutes of Health (next to the USUHS campus), Walter Reed National Military Medical Center, the Armed Forces Institute of Pathology, the Library of Congress, the Smithsonian Institution, the National Bureau of Standards, and many other private and government research centers. Many cultural advantages of the area include the theater, a major symphony orchestra, major-league sports, and world-famous museums. The Metro subway system has a station near campus and provides a convenient connection from the University to museums and cultural attractions of downtown Washington. The University is within easy distance of three major airports: Baltimore Washington International, Reagan International, and Dulles International. Both Reagan and Dulles International airports are accessible from the University via metro subway. For outdoor activities, the Blue Ridge Mountains, the Chesapeake Bay, and the Atlantic coast beaches are all within a few hours' drive.

The University

USUHS is located just outside Washington, D.C., in Bethesda, Maryland. The campus is situated on an attractive, wooded site at the Walter Reed National Military Medical Center and is close to several major federal health research facilities. Through various affiliation agreements, these institutes provide additional resources to enhance the educational experience of graduate students at USUHS.

Applying

Both civilians and military personnel are eligible to apply for graduate study at USUHS. Before matriculation, each applicant must complete a baccalaureate degree that includes college-level courses in biology, inorganic chemistry, mathematics, organic chemistry, and physics. Advanced courses in biology, chemistry, or related fields, such as biochemistry, cell biology, genetics, immunology, microbiology, molecular biology, and physical chemistry, are desirable but not essential. Each applicant must complete an online application and have sent to USU complete academic transcripts of postsecondary education, GRE scores (in addition to the aptitude sections, one advanced examination is recommended), three letters of recommendation from individuals familiar with the academic achievements or research experience of the applicant, and a personal statement expressing the applicant's career objectives. Active-duty military personnel must obtain the approval and sponsorship of their parent military department in addition to acceptance from USUHS. USUHS subscribes fully to the policy of equal educational opportunity and selects students on a competitive basis without regard to race, sex, creed, or national origin. Students may apply online at https://registrar.usuhs.edu or https://www.usuhs.edu/graded/prospectivestudents. Completed applications must be received before December 1 for matriculation in August. Applications received between December 2 and June 1 may be considered if space is available.

Correspondence and Information

For an application and information about the molecular and cell biology program:

Dr. Mary Lou Cutler, Director
Graduate Program in Molecular and Cell Biology
Uniformed Services University of the Health Sciences
4301 Jones Bridge Road
Bethesda, Maryland 20814
United States
Phone: 301-295-3642
Fax: 301-295-1996
E-mail: mary.cutler@usuhs.edu
Website: http://www.usuhs.mil/mcb/

Tina Finley

Administrative Officer
Uniformed Services University of the Health Sciences
4301 Jones Bridge Road
Bethesda, Maryland 20814
United States
Phone: 301-295-3642
E-mail: netina.finley@usuhs.edu

THE FACULTY AND THEIR RESEARCH

Regina C. Armstrong, Professor; Ph.D., North Carolina at Chapel Hill, 1987. Cellular and molecular mechanisms of neural stem/progenitor cell development and regeneration in demyelinating diseases and brain injury models.
Roopa Biswas, Assistant Professor, Ph.D. Ohio State, 1997. Mechanisms of regulation of inflammation; https://www.usuhs.edu/apg/faculty.

Uniformed Services University of the Health Sciences

Jorge Blanco, Adjunct Assistant Professor; Ph.D., Buenos Aires, 1991. Receptor characterization and susceptibility of cotton rats to avian and 2009 pandemic influenza strains. *J. Virol.* 87(4):2036–45, 2013.

Christopher C. Broder, Professor and Director; Ph.D., Florida, 1989. Virus-host cell interactions, vaccines, and therapeutics; Henipaviruses; Filoviruses; Australian bat lyssavirus.

Teodor Brumeanu, Professor; M.D., Carol Davila (Romania), 1978. Medicine.

Rolf Bünger, Professor; M.D./Ph.D., Munich, 1979. Cellular, molecular, and metabolic mechanisms of heart and brain circulation and resuscitation at various levels of organization: intact animal/isolated perfused organs/subcellular compartments of cytosol and mitochondria. *NMR Biomed.*, doi: 10.1002/nbm.1717; *Exp. Biol. Med. 234(12):1395–416, 2009; in Recent Research Developments in Physiology, Vol. 4, ed. S. G. Pandalai, 2006; Exerc. Sport Sci. Rev.* 32(4):174–9, 2004.

Barrington G. Burnett, Assistant Professor; Ph.D., Pennsylvania, 2005. The ubiquitin-proteasome system in neuronal maintenance and neurodegeneration.

Thomas P. Conrads, Professor, Ph.D., Ohio State, 1999. Discovery and validation of genomic, proteomic, and small molecule biomarkers and surrogates for enhanced cancer patient management through improved early detection, patient stratification, and monitoring for therapeutic efficacy, outcome, and recurrence.

Rachel Cox, Assistant Professor, Ph.D., North Carolina at Chapel Hill, 1998. Mitochondrial dynamics and inheritance during development. *Disease Models & Mechanisms* 2(9/10):490–9, 2009.

Mary Lou Cutler, Professor and Director; Ph.D., Hahnemann, 1980. Role of molecules that suppress transformation by the Ras oncogene; Ras signal transduction and human carcinogenesis. *Eur. J. Cell Biol.* 87:721–34, 2008; *J. Cell. Physiol.* 214:38–46, 2007; *BMC Cell Biol.* 7:34, 2006; *Exp. Cell Res.* 306:168–79, 2005.

Clifton Dalgard, Assistant Professor; Ph.D., Uniformed Services University of the Health Sciences, 2005. *Front. Mol. Neurosci.* 5:6, 2012.

Michael Daly, Professor; Ph.D., London, 1988. Pathology.

Thomas N. Darling, Professor; M.D./Ph.D., Duke, 1990. mTOR signaling pathway in skin regeneration and disease. *JAMA Dermatol.* 150:1095–101, 2014; *Hum. Mol. Genet.* 23:2023–9, 2014; *J. Investig. Dermatol.* 134:538–40, 2014; *J. Investig. Dermatol.* 134:543–6, 2014.

Stephen Davies, Assistant Professor; Ph.D., Cornell. Microbiology.

Regina Day, Associate Professor; Ph.D., Tufts, 1995. Mechanisms of normal tissue repair and mechanisms of fibrotic remodeling, especially radiation. *Mol. Biol. Cell* 21:4240–50, 2010; *Mol. Biol. Cell* 24:2088–07, 2013; *Mol. Pharmacol.* 85:898–908, 2014.

Saibal Dey, Associate Professor; Ph.D., Wayne State (Michigan), 1995. Allosteric modulation of the human multidrug transporter P-glycoprotein (MDR1 or ABCB1), which confers multidrug resistance in cancer cells and alters bioavailability of many anticancer and antimicrobial agents. *J. Biol. Chem.* 281(16):10699–777, 2006; *Biochemistry* 45:2739–51, 2006; *J. Biol. Chem.* 278(20):18132–9, 2003.

Martin Doughty, Associate Professor, Department of Anatomy, Physiology, and Genetics; Ph.D. Optimizing induced pluripotent stem cells (iPSCs) for cell replacement therapy to treat traumatic brain injury (TBI); identifying transcriptional programs that function in cerebellar neurogenesis and pattern formation.

Yang Du, Assistant Professor; Ph.D., Texas Tech, 2000. Leukemia development mechanisms. *Nat. Genet.* 45:942–6, 2013; *Blood* 119:6099–108, 2012.

Teresa M. Dunn, Professor; Ph.D., Brandeis, 1984. Sphingolipid synthesis and function. *J. Biol. Chem.* 277:11481–8, 2002 and 277:10194–200, 2002; *Mol. Cell Biol.* 21:109–25, 2001; *Methods Enzymol.* 312:317–30, 2000.

Gabriela S. Dveksler, Professor; Ph.D., Uniformed Services University of the Health Sciences, 1991. *J. Biol. Chem.* 286(9):7577–86, 2011; *Biol. Reprod.* 83(1):27–35, 2010.

Ying-Hong Feng, Associate Professor; Ph.D., Oxford, 1993. Pharmacology.

Thomas P. Flagg, Ph.D., Assistant Professor, Maryland, Baltimore, 2001. Cardiac ATP-sensitive potassium channel structure and function.

Zygmund Galdzicki, Assistant Professor, Ph.D., Wroclaw (Poland), 1982. Molecular and electrophysiological approach to understanding mental retardation in trisomy 21/Down syndrome.

Chou Zen Giam, Professor; Ph.D., UConn Health Center, 1983. Human T-lymphotropic viruses and Kaposi's sarcoma herpes virus; cellular senescence; cell-cycle control, I-kappa B kinases, protein ubiquitylation, cell transformation; viral oncogenesis; HTLV-1 pathogenesis; HTLV-1 latency and reactivation; transcriptional regulation. *PLoS Pathogens* 10:e1004040, 2014; *J. Virol.* 88:3496–504, 2014; *Oncogene* doi: 10.1038/onc.2013.567, 2014; *PLoS Pathogens* 7:e1002025, 2011.

David A. Grahame, Professor; Ph.D., Ohio State, 1984. Metalloenzyme structure and function in bacteria and archaea. *Biochemistry* 52:1705–16, 2013; *J. Biol. Chem.* 285(20):15450–63, 2010.

Philip M. Grimley, Professor; M.D., Albany Medical College, 1961. Population studies relevant to the pathogenesis and molecular biology of ovarian and mammary epithelial cancers.

David Horowitz, Associate Professor; Ph.D., Harvard, 1986. Biochemistry of pre-mRNA splicing.

Ann E. Jerse, Associate Professor; Ph.D., Maryland, Baltimore, 1991. Estradiol-treated female mice as surrogate hosts for *Neisseria gonorrhoeae* genital-tract infections. *Front. Microbio.* 2:107, 2011, doi: 10.3389/fmicb.2011.00107.

Sharon L. Juliano, Professor; Ph.D., Pennsylvania, 1982. Mechanisms of development and plasticity in the cerebral cortex, with particular emphasis on the migration of neurons into the cortical plate; factors maintaining the function and morphology of radial glia and Cajal-Retzius cells.

Jason Lees, Assistant Professor; Ph.D., Iowa, 2004. T cell trafficking and lesion development in neuroinflammation.

Joseph Mattapallil, Associate Professor; Ph.D., California, Davis, 1997. Molecular and cellular mechanisms of viral pathogenesis using nonhuman primate models. *Curr. HIV Res.* 2014; *Plos One* 9(5):e98060; *J. Virol.* 87(12):7093–101, 2013; *PLos One* 8(3):e59758, 2013; *Clin. Dev. Immunol.* 2013:852418, 2013; *J. Virol.* 86(2):1069–78, 2012; *AIDS Res. Hum. Retroviruses* 27(7):763–75, 2011; *Mucosal Immunol.* 2(5):439–49, 2009; *J. Immunol.* 182(3):1439–48, 2009; *J. Virol.* 82(22):11467–71, 2008; *Nature* 434(7037):1093–7, 2005.

Anthony T. Maurelli, Professor; Ph.D., Alabama at Birmingham, 1983. Molecular genetics of bacterial pathogens; molecular biology and pathogenesis of the intracellular pathogens *Shigella* and *Chlamydia. Nature* 506:507–10, 2014; *BMC Genom.* 11:272, 2010; *mBio* 2:e00051–11, 2011.

Ernest Maynard, Assistant Professor; Ph.D., Texas A&M, 2001. Zinc binding to the HCCH motif of HIV-1 virion infectivity factor induces a conformational change that mediates protein-protein interactions. *Proc. Natl. Acad. Sci. U.S.A.* 103:18475–80, 2006.

Joseph T. McCabe, Professor and Vice Chair; Ph.D., CUNY Graduate Center, 1983. Diazoxide, as a postconditioning and delayed preconditioner trigger, increases HSP25 and HSP70 in the central nervous system following combined cerebral stroke and hemorrhagic shock. *J. Neurotrauma* 24(3):532–46. 2007.

D. Scott Merrell, Professor; Ph.D., Tufts, 2001. *H. pylori*, gene regulation; gastric cancer; role of the microbiome in health and disease; https://www.usuhs.edu/mic/faculty. *Infect. Immun.* 83(2):802–11, 2015.

Eleanor S. Metcalf, Professor; Ph.D., Pennsylvania, 1976. *J. Immun.*, in press; *Infect. Immun.* 80:441–9, 2012.

Alexandra C. Miller, Assistant Professor; Ph.D., SUNY, 1986. Low dose radiation and heavy metal exposure induced late effects: mechanisms and prevention. Development of models to study radiation late effects. *Rev. Environ. Health* 29(3):25–34, 2013.

Edward Mitre, Assistant Professor; M.D., Johns Hopkins, 1995. Immune modulation by parasitic helminthes; www.usuhs.mil/mic/mitre.html.

Alison D. O'Brien, Professor and Chair; Ph.D., Ohio State, 1976. The role of *E. coli* shiga toxins in the pathogenesis of hemorrhagic colitis and the hemolytic uremic syndrome; the role of toxins in the pathogenesis of *E. coli*–mediated urinary-tract infections; development of vaccines and therapeutics against *Bacillus anthracis. Proc. Natl. Acad. Sci. USA* 110(23):E2126–33, 2013.

Galina Petukhova, Associate Professor, Ph.D., Shemyakin & Ovchinnikov Institute of Bioorganic Chemistry, Moscow, 1994. Molecular mechanisms of genetic recombination in mammals. *Nature* 472:375–78, 2011.

Harvey Pollard, Professor and Chair; Ph.D., 1969, M.D., 1973, Chicago. Differential regulation of inflammation by inflammatory mediators in cystic fibrosis lung epithelial cells. *J. Interferon Cytokine Res.* 33:121–9, 2013.

Gerald Quinnan, Professor; M.D., Saint Louis, 1973. Understanding the significance of mutations in the envelope gene of HIV in determining the resistance of virus to neutralization; induction of neutralizing antibody responses using novel HIV-1 envelope glycoproteins and methods of administration with the goal of inducing protection against infection; attempting to understand the factors that limit B cell responses to neutralization epitopes on HIV envelope glycoproteins.

Brian C. Schaefer, Associate Professor; Ph.D., Harvard, 1995. Mechanisms of leukocyte activation, particularly regulation of cytoplasmic signals to NF-kappaB; role of immune response in cancer, traumatic brain injury, and neurotropic viral infections; imaging, biochemical, and cellular approaches to elucidate signal transduction mechanisms. *Science Signaling* 7:ra45, 2014; *Immunity* 36:947–58, 2012; *Front. Neurol.* 3:155, 2012.

Michael Shamblott, Assistant Professor; Ph.D., Johns Hopkins, 2001. Human stem cells and regenerative medicine; development of new tools for bioinformatic research. *Proc. Natl. Acad. Sci. U.S.A.* 98:113–8, 2001.

Frank Shewmaker, Assistant Professor; Ph.D., Tulane. Prions, amyloid, and protein aggregation, especially in relation to neurodegenerative disease.

Vijay K. Singh, Professor, Ph.D. Mechanism of action of radiation injury and advanced development of radiation countermeasures. *Cytokine* 71:22–37, 2015; *Health Phys.* 108:607–30, 2015; *Brain Res.* 1600:42–58, 2015; *Expet. Opin. Biol. Ther.* 15:465–71, 2015; *PLos One* 9:e114078, 2014.

Clifford M. Snapper, Professor; M.D., Albany Medical College, 1981. In vivo regulation of protein- and polysaccharide-specific humoral immunity to extracellular bacteria and development of antibacterial and antiviral vaccines. *Vaccine* 31(30):3039–45, 2013.

Andrew Snow, Assistant Professor; Ph.D., Stanford, 2005. Molecular control of human lymphocyte homeostasis via antigen receptor signaling and apoptosis; dysregulation of lymphocyte homeostasis in XLP and BENTA disease. *J. Clin. Immunol.* 35(1) 32–46, 2015; *J. Immunol.* 192(9):4202–9, 2014; *J. Exp. Med.* 209(12):2247–61, 2012; *J. Clin. Investig.* 119(10):2976–89, 2009.

Shiv Srivastava, Professor and Co-Director, Center for Prostate Disease Research, Department of Surgery; Ph.D., Indian Institute of Technology (New Delhi), 1980. Molecular genetics of human cancer; prostate cancer. *Clin. Chem.* 51:102–12, 2005; *Oncogene* 23:605–11, 2004; *Cancer Res.* 63:4299–304, 2003.

Tharun Sundaresan, Associate Professor; Ph.D., Centre for Cellular and Molecular Biology (India), 1995. Mechanism of eukaryotic mRNA decay, with particular focus on the role of Lsm1-7-Pat1 complex. *RNA* 20:1465–75, 2014; *Int. Rev. Cell Mol. Biol.* 272:149–89, 2009.

Viqar Syed, Associate Professor, Ph.D., Karolinska Institute, Stockholm. Understanding the process of carcinogenesis and developing novel therapeutic strategies for cancer prevention. *J. Cell. Biochem.* 116:1797–1805, 2015; *Mol. Carcinog.* 54:368–78, 2015; *Canc. Prev. Res.* 7:1045–55, 2014.

Aviva Symes, Associate Professor; Ph.D., University College (London), 1990. Neuroinflammation, neurogenesis, and therapeutics after traumatic brain injury. *J. Neurochem.* 129:155–68, 2014; *Front. Neurol.* doi: 10.3389/fneur.2014.00082, 2014; *PLOS one* 10.1371/journal.pone.0059250, 2013.

Charles S. Via, Professor; M.D., Virginia, 1973. The role of T cells in lupus and in graft-versus-host disease. *J. Immunol.* 190(9):4562–72, 2013.

Shuishu Wang, Assistant Professor; Ph.D., Purdue, 1999. Structural and functional studies of potential drug target proteins from *Mycobacterium tuberculosis* by X-ray crystallography and biochemical techniques.

T. John Wu, Professor; Ph.D., Texas A&M, 1991. Molecular and cellular neuroendocrinology of reproduction and stress. *Mol. Cell. Endocrinol.* (in press); *Endocrine* 49(2):470–8, 2015; *New Engl. J. Med.* 371:2363–74, 2014; *Mol. Endocrinol.* 28:80–98, 2014; *Endocrinology* 154:4726–36, 2013.

Xin Xiang, Professor; Ph.D., University of Medicine and Dentistry of New Jersey, 1991. HookA is a novel dynein-early endosome linker critical for cargo movement in vivo. *J. Cell Biol.* 204:1009–26, 2014.

UCONN HEALTH

Graduate Program in Cell Analysis and Modeling

 For more information, visit http://petersons.to/uconnhealth_cellanalysis

Program of Study

UConn Health's quantitative cell biology research has grown into the area in cell analysis and modeling (CAM). Faculty members associated with this area explore complex biological systems using computational cell biology, optical imaging, and other quantitative approaches to analyze processes in living cells. The program is designed to train students from diverse disciplinary backgrounds in the cutting-edge research techniques that comprise the interdisciplinary research of modern cell biology. Students are provided with rigorous cross-training in areas of mathematical, physical, and computational sciences and biology. CAM students take courses, attend seminars, and work on interdisciplinary research projects to broaden and strengthen their abilities to conduct quantitative cell biology research.

The Cell Analysis and Modeling area of concentration is based within the Richard D. Berlin Center for Cell Analysis and Modeling (CCAM) at UConn Health. Established in 1994, CCAM has emerged as a center that promotes the application of physics, chemistry, and computation to cell biology. The environment of CCAM is designed to promote interdisciplinary interactions and its cadre of physical scientists are supported and valued in a way that is unique for a medical school. CAM is also the home of the virtual cell modeling and simulation software project (http://vcell.org).

The CAM program is particularly strong in the following areas of research: cell modeling (data-driven analysis and simulation, virtual microscopy, modeling cell migration, modularity and multistate complexes, molecular flux in cellular spaces, stochastic modeling and discrete particles); biophysics (biological signaling platforms, single molecule and particle tracking, cytoskeletal dynamics, and morphogenesis); optical imaging (fluorescent correlation spectroscopy, optical probe development, nonlinear optical microscopy single-molecule imaging); cell biology (cellular tissues and development, RNA trafficking, signal transduction, molecular medicine).

Research Facilities

The program is situated at UConn Health in Farmington. This complex provides excellent physical facilities for research in both basic and clinical sciences, a computer center, and the Lyman Maynard Stowe Library. The program provides research facilities and guidance for graduate and postdoctoral work in cell biology—particularly membrane and surface function, membrane protein synthesis and turnover, cytoskeleton structure and function, stimulus-response coupling, gene expression and regulation, vascular biology, fertilization, bone biology, molecular medicine, early development, signal transduction, angiogenesis, computer modeling, and tumor biology. Facilities for training in cell culture, electron microscopy, electrophysiology, fluorescence spectroscopy, molecular biology, molecular modeling, fluorescence imaging, and intravital microscopy are available.

Financial Aid

Support for doctoral students engaged in full-time degree programs at UConn Health is provided on a competitive basis. Graduate research assistantships for 2016–17 provide a stipend of $29,000 per year, which includes a waiver of tuition/most University fees for the fall and spring semesters and the option of participating in a student health insurance plan. While financial aid is offered competitively, the UConn Health makes every possible effort to address the financial needs of all students during their period of training.

Cost of Study

For 2016–17, tuition is $14,310 per year for full-time students who are Connecticut residents and $35,346 per year for full-time students who are out-of-state residents. General University fees are added to the cost of tuition for students who do not receive a tuition waiver. These costs are usually met by traineeships or research assistantships for doctoral students.

Living and Housing Costs

There is a wide range of affordable housing options in the greater Hartford area within easy commuting distance of the campus, including an extensive complex that is adjacent to UConn Health. Costs range from $700 to $1,000 per month for a one-bedroom unit; 2 or more students sharing an apartment usually pay less. University housing is not available at on campus.

Student Group

The total number of Ph.D. students at UConn Health is approximately 150, while the medical and dental schools combined currently enroll 130 students per class.

Location

UConn Health is located in the historic town of Farmington, Connecticut. Set in the beautiful New England countryside on a hill overlooking the Farmington Valley, it is close to ski areas, hiking trails, and facilities for boating, fishing, and swimming. Connecticut's capital city of Hartford, 7 miles east of Farmington, is the center of an urban region of approximately 800,000 people. The beaches of the Long Island Sound are about 50 minutes away to the south, and the beautiful Berkshires are a short drive to the northwest. New York City and Boston can be reached within 2½ hours by car. Hartford is the home of the acclaimed Hartford Stage Company, TheatreWorks, the Hartford Symphony and Chamber orchestras, two ballet companies, an opera company, the Wadsworth Athenaeum (the oldest public art museum in the nation), the Mark Twain house, the Hartford Civic Center, and many other interesting cultural and recreational facilities. The area is also home to several branches of the University of Connecticut, Trinity College, and the University of Hartford, which includes the Hartt School of Music. Bradley International Airport (about 30 minutes from campus) serves the Hartford/Springfield area with frequent airline connections to major cities in this country and abroad. Frequent bus and rail service is also available from Hartford.

The UConn Health Campus

The 200-acre UConn Health campus at Farmington houses a division of the University of Connecticut Graduate School, as well as the Schools of Medicine and Dental Medicine. The campus also includes the John Dempsey Hospital, associated clinics, and extensive medical research facilities, all in a centralized facility with more than 1 million square feet of floor space. The Academic Research Building, built in 1999, is an impressive eleven-story structure providing 170,000 square feet of laboratory space and renovations are underway in the main Laboratory building, converting existing lab space to state-of-the-art open lab areas. In addition, The Jackson Laboratory for Genomic Medicine opened its 189,000-square-foot facility on the UConn Health Campus in fall 2014. The faculty at the center includes more than 260 full-time members. The institution has a strong commitment to graduate study within an environment that promotes social and intellectual interaction among the various educational programs. Graduate students are represented on various administrative committees concerned with curricular affairs, and the Graduate Student Organization (GSO) represents graduate students' needs and concerns to the faculty and administration, in addition to fostering social contact among graduate students in UConn Health.

Applying

Applications for admission should be submitted via the online application system and should be filed together with transcripts, three letters of recommendation, a personal statement, and recent results from the General Test of the Graduate Record Examinations. International students must take the Test of English as a Foreign Language (TOEFL) to satisfy Graduate School requirements. The deadline for completed applications and receipt of all supplemental materials is **December 1**. Please note that GRE and TOEFL exams taken after the due date will not be accepted for consideration for admission. In accordance with the laws of the state of Connecticut and of the United States, UConn Health Center does not discriminate against any person in its educational and employment activities on the grounds of race, color, creed, national origin, sex, age, or physical disability.

Correspondence and Information

Graduate Admissions Office
Ph.D. in Biomedical Science Program
UConn Health
263 Farmington Ave., MC 3906
Farmington, Connecticut 06030-3906
United States
Phone: 860-679-4509
E-mail: BiomedSciAdmissions@uchc.edu
Website: http://health.uconn.edu/graduate-school/academics/
        programs/ph-d-biomedical-science
        http://www.ccam.uchc.edu

THE FACULTY AND THEIR RESEARCH

Michael Blinov, Assistant Professor of Genetics and Developmental Biology; Ph.D., Weizmann Institute (Israel). Computational biology: modeling of signal transcription systems and protein-DNA interactions; bioinformatics: data mining and visualization; developing software tools and mathematical methods for rule-based modeling of signal transduction systems.

John H. Carson, Professor of Molecular, Microbial and Structural Biology; Ph.D., MIT. RNA transport in cells of the nervous system.

Ann E. Cowan, Professor of Molecular, Microbial, and Structural Biology; Deputy Director, Center for Biomedical Imaging Technology; Ph.D., Colorado. Research encompassing several areas of mammalian sperm development.

Reinhard Laubenbacher, Professor of Cell Biology; Ph.D., Northwestern. Development of mathematical algorithms and their application to problems in systems biology, in particular the modeling and simulation of molecular networks. An application area of particular interest is cancer systems biology, especially the role of iron metabolism in breast cancer.

Leslie M. Loew, Professor of Cell Biology and of Computer Science and Engineering; Ph.D., Cornell. Morphological determinants of cell physiology; image-based computational models of cellular biology; spatial variations of cell membrane electrophysiology; new optical methods for probing living cells.

Bruce J. Mayer, Professor of Genetics and Developmental Biology; Ph.D., Rockefeller. Mechanisms of signal transduction.

William A. Mohler, Ph.D., Stanford. Associate Professor of Genetics and Developmental Biology. Developmental cell fusion; *C. elegans* genetics; multidimensional imaging of developmental and cell biological processes.

Ion I. Moraru, Associate Professor of Cell Biology; M.D., Ph.D., Carol Davila (Romania). Understanding signal transduction mechanisms, in particular those related to calcium and phosphoinositides.

Vladimir Rodionov, Professor of Cell Biology; Ph.D., Moscow, 1980. Molecular mechanisms of intracellular transport; organization of microtubule cytoskeleton.

Boris Slepchenko, Associate Professor of Cell Biology.

Paola Vera-Licona, Assistant Professor of Cell Biology; Ph.D., Virginia Tech. Computational systems biology of cancer; reverse-engineering of biological networks; network theory; development and application of algorithms for mathematical modeling and analysis of biological networks; discovery and development of combinations of targeted therapies.

Yi Wu, Assistant Professor of Genetics and Developmental Biology; Ph.D., Northwestern. Developing quantitative imaging tools that are capable of revealing dynamics of cellular signaling at high spatial and temporal resolution (biosensors) or that enable optical control of signaling proteins at precise times and subcellular locations (optogenetics).

Ji Yu, Associate Professor of Genetics and Developmental Biology; Ph.D., Texas at Austin. Optical imaging technology; regulation mechanisms in dendritic RNA translation; cytoskeletal dynamics.

UCONN HEALTH
Graduate Program in Cell Biology

 For more information, visit http://petersons.to/uconnhealth_cellbiology

Program of Study

The Cell Biology Area of Concentration (CB AoC) at the University of Connecticut Health Center offers training leading to a Ph.D. in Biomedical Sciences. Faculty members in the CB AoC are engaged in cutting-edge research in a wide range of topics related to the molecular and cellular basis of biology and disease, and are from multiple departments and research centers, including but not limited to the Department of Cell Biology, Center for Vascular Biology, Calhoun Cardiology Center, and Department of Molecular Medicine. First-year students will take core courses and participate in Cell Biology Journal Club. An equally important activity in the first year is laboratory rotations, which offer students opportunities to acquaint themselves with research activities in different laboratories, and identify a major thesis adviser. In the second year, while students continue to take some advanced elective courses, the main emphasis shifts towards research and preparation for general examination. Individual students should form advisory committees, and complete general examination before the end of their second year. From third year on, students will continue to participate in Cell Biology Journal Club and focus on their thesis research with the aim of completing their thesis before the end of the fifth year. Through rigorous course and research training, the CB AoC prepares students for successful careers in academic research, biotech industry, and education.

Research Facilities

The program is situated at the modern UConn Health campus in Farmington. This complex provides excellent physical facilities for research in both basic and clinical sciences, a computer center, and the Lyman Maynard Stowe Library. The program provides research facilities and guidance for graduate and postdoctoral work in cell biology—particularly membrane and surface function, membrane protein synthesis and turnover, cytoskeleton structure and function, stimulus-response coupling, gene expression and regulation, vascular biology, fertilization, bone biology, molecular medicine, early development, signal transduction, angiogenesis, computer modeling, and tumor biology. Facilities for training in cell culture, electron microscopy, electrophysiology, fluorescence spectroscopy, molecular biology, molecular modeling, fluorescence imaging, and intravital microscopy are available.

Financial Aid

Support for doctoral students engaged in full-time degree programs at UConn Health is provided on a competitive basis. Graduate research assistantships for 2016–17 provide a stipend of $29,000 per year, which includes a waiver of tuition/most University fees for the fall and spring semesters and the option of participating in a student health insurance plan. While financial aid is offered competitively, UConn Health makes every possible effort to address the financial needs of all students during their period of training.

Cost of Study

For 2016–17, tuition is $14,310 per year for full-time students who are Connecticut residents and $35,346 per year for full-time students who are out-of-state residents. General University fees are added to the cost of tuition for students who do not receive a tuition waiver. These costs are usually met by traineeships or research assistantships for doctoral students.

Living and Housing Costs

There is a wide range of affordable housing options in the greater Hartford area within easy commuting distance of the campus, including an extensive complex that is adjacent to the UConn Health. Costs range from $700 to $1,000 per month for a one-bedroom unit; 2 or more students sharing an apartment usually pay less. University housing is not available on campus.

Student Group

Currently, approximately 10 students are pursuing doctoral studies in the program. The total number of Ph.D. students at UConn Health is approximately 150, while the medical and dental schools combined currently enroll 130 students per class.

Location

UConn Health is located in the historic town of Farmington, Connecticut. Set in the beautiful New England countryside on a hill overlooking the Farmington Valley, it is close to ski areas, hiking trails, and facilities for boating, fishing, and swimming. Connecticut's capital city of Hartford, 7 miles east of Farmington, is the center of an urban region of approximately 800,000 people. The beaches of the Long Island Sound are about 50 minutes away to the south, and the beautiful Berkshires are a short drive to the northwest. New York City and Boston can be reached within 2½ hours by car. Hartford is the home of the acclaimed Hartford Stage Company, TheatreWorks, the Hartford Symphony and Chamber orchestras, two ballet companies, an opera company, the Wadsworth Atheneaum (the oldest public art museum in the nation), the Mark Twain house, the Hartford Civic Center, and many other interesting cultural and recreational facilities. The area is also home to several branches of the University of Connecticut, Trinity College, and the University of Hartford, which includes the Hartt School of Music. Bradley International Airport (about 30 minutes from campus) serves the Hartford/Springfield area with frequent airline connections to major cities in this country and abroad. Frequent bus and rail service is also available from Hartford.

The UConn Health Campus

The 200-acre UConn Health campus at Farmington houses a division of the University of Connecticut Graduate School, as well as the Schools of Medicine and Dental Medicine. The campus also includes the John Dempsey Hospital, associated clinics, and extensive medical research facilities, all in a centralized facility with more than 1 million square feet of floor space. The Academic Research Building, built in 1999, is an impressive eleven-story structure providing 170,000 square feet of laboratory space and renovations are underway in the main Laboratory building, converting existing lab space into state-of-the-art open lab areas. In addition, The Jackson Laboratory for Genomic Medicine opened its 189,000-square-foot facility on the UConn Health Campus in fall 2014. The faculty includes more than 260 full-time members. The institution has a strong commitment to graduate study within an environment that promotes social and intellectual interaction among the various educational programs. Graduate students are represented on various administrative committees concerned with curricular affairs, and the Graduate Student Organization (GSO) represents graduate students' needs and concerns to the faculty and administration, in addition to fostering social contact among graduate students at UConn Health.

Applying

Applications for admission should be submitted via the online application system and should be filed together with transcripts, three letters of recommendation, a personal statement, and recent results from the General Test of the Graduate Record Examinations. International students must take the Test of English as a Foreign Language (TOEFL) to satisfy Graduate School requirements. The deadline for completed applications and receipt of all supplemental materials is **December 1**. Please note that GRE and TOEFL exams taken after the due date will not be accepted for consideration for admission. In accordance with the laws of the state of Connecticut and of the United States, UConn Health does not discriminate against any person in its educational and employment activities on the grounds of race, color, creed, national origin, sex, age, or physical disability.

Correspondence and Information

Graduate Admissions Office
Ph.D. in Biomedical Science Program
UConn Health
263 Farmington Ave., MC 3906
Farmington, Connecticut 06030-3906
United States
Phone: 860-679-4509
E-mail: BiomedSciAdmissions@uchc.edu
Website: http://health.uconn.edu/graduate-school/academics/programs/
ph-d-biomedical-science

THE FACULTY AND THEIR RESEARCH

Andrew Arnold, Professor and Director, Center for Molecular Medicine; M.D., Harvard. Structure and function of the cyclin D1 oncogene and cell-cycle regulator; molecular genetics and biology of endocrine tumors; inherited endocrine neoplastic diseases.

UConn Health

Stefan Brocke, Associate Professor of Immunology; M.D., Freie Universistaet Berlin School of Medicine. Cellular and molecular mechanisms of brain injury in inflammatory and inflammation-associated disorders of the central nervous system.

Ernesto Canalis, Professor of Orthopaedic Surgery and Medicine; M.D., Universidad Peruana Cayetano Heredia. Skeletal growth factors; insulin-like growth factors; hormonal action in bone, mechanisms of glucocorticoid action in bone; anabolic agents and osteoporosis.

Kevin P. Claffey, Professor of Cell Biology and Center for Vascular Biology; Ph.D., Boston University. Angiogenesis in human cancer progression and metastasis; vascular endothelial growth factor (VEGF) expression; hypoxia-mediated gene regulation.

Robert B. Clark, Professor of Medicine, Division of Rheumatic Diseases; M.D., Stanford. Basic T-lymphocyte biology, especially as it relates to autoimmune diseases, such as multiple sclerosis and rheumatoid arthritis; molecular biology and structure of the T-cell antigen receptor; T-cell function; T-cell activation.

Ann Cowan, Professor of Biochemistry and Deputy Director of the Center for Biomedical Imaging Technology; Ph.D., Colorado. Mammalian sperm development.

Anne Delany, Associate Professor of Medicine; Ph.D., Dartmouth. Function and regulation of the noncollagen matrix protein osteonectin/SPARC in bone; regulation of osteoblast gene expression by microRNAs; exploring how the extracellular matrix regulates gene expression in bone-metastatic prostate carcinoma.

Kimberly Dodge-Kafka, Associate Professor of Cell Biology, Center for Cardiology and Cardiovascular Research; Ph.D., Texas–Houston Health Science Center. Molecular mechanism of signaling pathways in the heart.

David I. Dorsky, Associate Professor of Medicine; M.D./Ph.D., Harvard. The structure and function of herpesvirus DNA polymerases and their roles in viral DNA replication.

Paul Epstein, Associate Professor of Cell Biology; Ph.D., Yeshiva (Einstein). Signal transduction in relation to leukemia and breast cancer; purification and cloning of cyclic nucleotide phosphodiesterases.

Alan Fein, Professor of Cell Biology; Ph.D., Johns Hopkins. Molecular basis of visual excitation and adaptation; signal transduction and calcium homeostasis in platelets.

Guo-Hua Fong, Associate Professor of Cell Biology and Center for Vascular Biology; Ph.D., Illinois. Cardiovascular biology.

David Han, Associate Professor of Cell Biology and Center for Vascular Biology; Ph.D., George Washington. Proteomic analysis of complex protein mixtures.

Marc Hansen, Professor of Medicine; Ph.D., Cincinnati. Analysis of genes involved in the development of the bone tumor osteosarcoma.

J. Travis Hinson, Assistant Professor of Cardiology and Genetics; M.D., Harvard. Human iPS disease modeling of cardiovascular disorders; functional genomics; regenerative medicine related to the heart; CRISPR/CAS9 genomewide screens in iPS-cell assays.

Marja Hurley, Professor of Medicine; M.D., Connecticut Health Center. Molecular mechanisms by which members of the fibroblast growth factor (FGFs) and fibroblast growth factor receptor (FGFR) families (produced by osteoblasts, osteoclasts, and stromal cells) regulate bone development, remodeling, and disorders of bone: Fgf2 knockout and Fgf2 transgenic mice are utilized in loss and gain of function experiments to elucidate the role of FGF-2 in disorders of bone, including osteoporosis.

Laurinda A. Jaffe, Professor of Cell Biology; Ph.D., UCLA. Physiology of fertilization, in particular the mechanisms by which membrane potential regulates sperm-egg fusion; transduction mechanisms coupling sperm-egg interaction to egg exocytosis; opening of ion channels in the egg membrane.

Reinhard Laubenbacher, Professor of Cell Biology; Ph.D., Northwestern. Development of mathematical algorithms and their application to problems in systems biology, in particular the modeling and simulation of molecular networks. An application area of particular interest is cancer systems biology, especially the role of iron metabolism in breast cancer.

Eric S. Levine, Professor of Neuroscience; Ph.D., Princeton. Synaptic physiology and plasticity; roles of nerve growth factors and endogenous cannabinoids in hippocampus and cortex.

Bruce Liang, Professor of Cardiopulmonary Medicine; M.D., Harvard. Signal transduction; cardiac and vascular cell biology; receptors; G proteins; transgenic mice.

Leslie M. Loew, Professor of Cell Biology and Director, Center for Cell Analysis and Modeling; Ph.D., Cornell. Spectroscopic methods for measuring spatial and temporal variations in membrane potential; electric field effects on cell membranes; membrane pores induced by toxins and antibiotics.

Nilanjana Maulik, Associate Professor of Surgery; Ph.D., Calcutta. Molecular and cellular signaling during myocardial ischemia and reperfusion.

Lisa Mehlmann, Assistant Professor of Cell Biology; Ph.D., Kent State. Cell signaling events that regulate oocyte maturation and fertilization; maintenance of oocyte meiotic arrest by G-protein receptors; hormonal regulation of oocyte maturation.

Joel Pachter, Professor of Cell Biology; Ph.D., NYU. Elucidating the mechanisms by which leukocytes and pathogens invade the central nervous system.

John J. Peluso, Professor of Cell Biology and Obstetrics and Gynecology; Ph.D., West Virginia. Cell and molecular mechanisms involving the regulating ovarian cell mitosis and apoptosis; cell-cell interaction as a regulator of ovarian cell function; identification and characterization of a putative membrane receptor for progesterone.

Carol C. Pilbeam, Professor of Medicine; M.D./Ph.D., Yale. Regulation and function of prostaglandins in bone; transcriptional regulation of cyclooxygenase-2; role of cytokines and estrogen in bone physiology and osteoporosis.

Vladimir Rodionov, Professor of Cell Biology; Ph.D., Moscow. Dynamics of cytoskeleton; self-organization of microtubule arrays; regulation of the activity of microtubule motors.

Annabelle Rodriguez-Oquendo, Professor of Cell Biology; M.D., New Jersey Medical School. Genetic link between healthy HDL cholesterol, heart disease, and infertility in women.

Daniel Rosenberg, Professor of Medicine; Ph.D., Michigan. Molecular genetics of colorectal cancer; signaling pathways in the development of tumors; toxicogenomics.

Archana Sanjay, Assistant Professor of Orthopaedic Surgery, School of Medicine; Ph.D. Regulation of bone remodeling; examining signaling pathways that regulate osteoblast and osteoclast differentiation and function.

Linda H. Shapiro, Associate Professor of Cell Biology and Center for Vascular Biology; Ph.D., Michigan. Regulation and function of CD 13/aminopeptidase N in angiogenic vasculature and early myeloid cells; control of tumor and myocardial angiogenesis by peptidases; inflammatory regulation of angiogenesis.

Henry Smilowitz, Associate Professor of Cell Biology; Ph.D., MIT. Preclinical experimental therapeutics of cancer using glioma, intracerebral melanoma, as well as breast, head, and neck, and bladder cancer models. Gold nanoparticles as radiation enhancers (with an emphasis on glioma); gold and iron nanoparticles for hyperthermia and hyperthermia mediated radiation enhancement (with an emphasis on head and neck cancer); combination of radiation therapy and immunotherapy for intracerebral tumors.

Mark R. Terasaki, Associate Professor of Cell Biology; Ph.D., Berkeley. Structure and function of the endoplasmic reticulum; confocal microscopy.

Paola Vera-Licona, Assistant Professor of Cell Biology; Ph.D., Virginia Tech. Computational systems biology of cancer; reverse-engineering of biological networks; network theory, development, and application of algorithms for mathematical modeling and analysis of biological networks; discovery and development of combinations of targeted therapies.

Zhao-Wen Wang, Associate Professor of Neuroscience. Cellular and molecular mechanisms of neurotransmitter release; potassium and calcium channel function; synaptic localization of potassium channels.

James Watras, Associate Professor of Medicine; Ph.D., Washington State. The mechanisms by which the sarcoplasmic reticulum regulates intracellular calcium concentration in vascular smooth muscle.

Bruce A. White, Professor of Cell Biology; Ph.D., Berkeley. Regulation of prolactin gene expression by Ca and calmodulin in rat pituitary tumor cells; examination of nuclear DNA-binding proteins, nuclear calmodulin-binding proteins, and nuclear Ca-calmodulin-dependent protein kinase activity.

George Y. Wu, Professor of Medicine; M.D./Ph.D., Yeshiva (Einstein). Receptor-mediated endocytosis of glycoproteins; drug delivery by endocytic targeting; targeted gene delivery and expression.

Siu-Pok Yee, Assistant Professor of Genetics and Genome Sciences; Ph.D., McMaster. Molecular biology; mouse genetics; mouse developmental biology.

Lixia Yue, Associate Professor of Cell Biology and Center for Cardiovascular Research; Ph.D., McGill. TRP channels and Ca^{2+} signaling mechanisms in cardiac remodeling.

UCONN HEALTH

Graduate Program in Molecular Biology and Biochemistry

 For more information, visit http://petersons.to/uconnhealth_molecularbio

Program of Study

The Graduate Program in Molecular Biology and Biochemistry (MBB) uniquely bridges modern molecular biology, microbiology, biochemistry, cell biology, and structural biology, leading to a Ph.D. in the biomedical sciences. From cancer to host-pathogen interactions, students study the proteins and pathways involved with an eye toward improving disease diagnosis, prevention and treatment.

MBB students are affiliated with the Department of Molecular Biology and Biophysics, which provides a rigorous, yet supportive community of faculty, students, and staff to guide them through the Ph.D. degree process.

The primary goal of the MBB graduate program is to train students for the broad range of careers available in biomedical science. Whether the graduate pursues a career in academic research, biomedical industry, teaching, government, or any of the other careers now available to Ph.D.s in biomedical science, they have been prepared with a solid base of knowledge, critical thinking skills, and the confidence in their abilities to be successful. Graduates are expected to have demonstrated a high degree of competence in research, as judged by publications in first-rank journals. They will have developed essential skills in identifying important research problems, planning appropriate experimental approaches, and effectively communicating their research results and their significance both orally and in written form. The success of our students in these areas is exemplified by the number of first-author publications in quality scientific journals and awards received both internally at UConn Health and from national and international conferences and societies.

Categories of faculty research include microbiology and infectious diseases, structural biology and biophysics, computational and modeling, cellular pathways, and cancer biology.

Research Facilities

In addition to the general facilities of UConn Health, the program offers complete physical research facilities. There is research equipment, as well as expertise, for all areas of genetic, biochemical, molecular, cellular, and biophysical investigation. The department houses the UConn Health NMR Structural Biology Facility (http://structbio.uchc.edu), which includes a 400-MHz NMR spectrometer and cryoprobe-equipped 500- and 600-MHz NMR spectrometers, as well as a circular dichroism spectropolarimeter, isothermal titration calorimeter, and multi-angle laser light scattering facilities. An 800-MHz NMR spectrometer and X-ray crystallography facilities are planned. The department also houses the UConn Health Structural Biology Computational Facility, which includes a bank of Mac and Linux desktop computers connected to ultrafast servers with the latest structural biology software. Facilities are also available for electron and confocal laser scanning microscopy, low-light-level imaging microscopy (in the state-of-the-art Center for Cell Analysis and Modeling), protein purification and sequencing, cell culture, monoclonal antibody production, DNA oligonucleotide and peptide synthesis and sequencing, and gene silencing using RNAi.

Financial Aid

Support for doctoral students engaged in full-time degree programs at UConn Health is provided on a competitive basis. Graduate research assistantships for 2016–17 provide a stipend of $29,000 per year, which includes a waiver of tuition/most University fees for the fall and spring semesters and the option of participating in a student health insurance plan. While financial aid is offered competitively, UConn Health makes every possible effort to address the financial needs of all students during their period of training.

Cost of Study

For 2016–17, tuition is $14,310 per year for full-time students who are Connecticut residents and $35,346 per year for full-time out-of-state residents. General University fees are added to the cost of tuition for students who do not receive a tuition waiver. These costs are usually met by traineeships or research assistantships for doctoral students.

Living and Housing Costs

There is a wide range of affordable housing options in the greater Hartford area within easy commuting distance of the campus, including an extensive complex that is adjacent to UConn Health. Costs range from $700 to $1,000 per month for a one-bedroom unit; 2 or more students sharing an apartment usually pay less. University housing is not available on campus.

Student Group

There are approximately 15 graduate students in the molecular biology and biochemistry program. There are approximately 150 graduate students in Ph.D. programs on the UConn Health campus, and the total enrollment is about 1,000.

Location

UConn Health is located in the historic town of Farmington, Connecticut. Set in the beautiful New England countryside on a hill overlooking the Farmington Valley, it is close to ski areas, hiking trails, and facilities for boating, fishing, and swimming. Connecticut's capital city of Hartford, 7 miles east of Farmington, is the center of an urban region of approximately 800,000 people. The beaches of the Long Island Sound are about 50 minutes away to the south, and the beautiful Berkshires are a short drive to the northwest. New York City and Boston can be reached within 2½ hours by car. Hartford is the home of the acclaimed Hartford Stage Company, TheatreWorks, the Hartford Symphony and Chamber orchestras, two ballet companies, an opera company, the Wadsworth Athenaeum (the oldest public art museum in the nation), the Mark Twain house, the Hartford Civic Center, and many other interesting cultural and recreational facilities. The area is also home to several branches of the University of Connecticut, Trinity College, and the University of Hartford, which includes the Hartt School of Music. Bradley International Airport (about 30 minutes from campus) serves the Hartford/Springfield area with frequent airline connections to major cities in this country and abroad. Frequent bus and rail service is also available from Hartford.

UConn Health

The UConn Health Campus

The 200-acre UConn Health campus at Farmington houses a division of the University of Connecticut Graduate School, as well as the Schools of Medicine and Dental Medicine. The campus also includes the John Dempsey Hospital, associated clinics, and extensive medical research facilities, all in a centralized facility with more than 1 million square feet of floor space. The Academic Research Building, built in 1999, is an impressive eleven-story structure providing 170,000 square feet of laboratory space and renovations are underway in the main Laboratory building, converting existing lab space to state-of-the-art open lab areas. In addition, The Jackson Laboratory for Genomic Medicine opened its 189,000-square-foot facility on the UConn Health Campus in fall 2014. The faculty includes more than 260 full-time members. The institution has a strong commitment to graduate study within an environment that promotes social and intellectual interaction among the various educational programs. Graduate students are represented on various administrative committees concerned with curricular affairs, and the Graduate Student Organization (GSO) represents graduate students' needs and concerns to the faculty and administration, in addition to fostering social contact among graduate students.

Applying

Applications for admission should be submitted via the online application system and should be filed together with transcripts, three letters of recommendation, a personal statement, and recent results from the General Test of the Graduate Record Examinations. International students must take the Test of English as a Foreign Language (TOEFL) to satisfy Graduate School requirements. The deadline for completed applications and receipt of all supplemental materials is **December 1**. Please note that GRE and TOEFL exams taken after the due date will not be accepted for consideration for admission. In accordance with the laws of the state of Connecticut and of the United States, UConn Health does not discriminate against any person in its educational and employment activities on the grounds of race, color, creed, national origin, sex, age, or physical disability.

Correspondence and Information

Graduate Admissions Office
Ph.D. in Biomedical Science Program
UConn Health
263 Farmington Ave., MC 3906
Farmington, Connecticut 06030-3906
United States
Phone: 860-679-4509
E-mail: BiomedSciAdmissions@uchc.edu
Website: http://health.uconn.edu/graduate-school/academics/programs/
ph-d-biomedical-science

THE FACULTY AND THEIR RESEARCH

Irina Besonova, Assistant Professor of Molecular, Microbial, and Structural Biology; Ph.D., Toronto. Structural and biochemical characterization of proteins and protein complexes of p53 pathway, especially, proteins responsible for maintenance of an appropriate level of p53 in the cell.

Melissa Caimano, Assistant Professor; Ph.D., Alabama at Birmingham. Regulatory pathways and molecular mechanisms underlying mammalian host adaptation and maintenance of Borrelia burgdorferi within its natural enzootic cycle.

Gordon G. Carmichael, Professor; Ph.D., Harvard. Regulation of viral gene expression and function.

John H. Carson, Professor; Ph.D., MIT. RNA transport in cells of the nervous system.

Ann Cowan, Professor; Ph.D., Colorado at Boulder. Plasma membrane proteins in sperm.

Asis Das, Professor; Ph.D., Calcutta. Gene control in bacterial adaptive response.

Kimberly Dodge-Kafka, Associate Professor of Cell Biology/Center for Cardiology and Cardiovascular Research; Ph.D., Texas Health Science Center at Houston, 1999. Molecular mechanism of signaling pathways in the heart.

Betty Eipper, Professor; Ph.D., Harvard. Biosynthesis and secretion of peptides by neurons and endocrine cells.

Michael Gryk, Associate Professor; Ph.D., Stanford. Three-dimensional structure and function of proteins involved in DNA repair.

Bing Hao, Assistant Professor of Molecular, Microbial, and Structural Biology; Ph.D., Ohio State. Understanding how the cell cycle is regulated by ubiquitin-mediated proteolysis using X-ray crystallography as a primary tool.

Christopher Heinen, Associate Professor of Medicine; Ph.D., Cincinnati. Biochemical and cellular defects of the DNA mismatch repair pathway during tumorigenesis.

Jeffrey Hoch, Professor; Ph.D., Harvard. Biophysical chemistry of proteins.

Stephen M. King, Professor; Ph.D., University College, London. Structure and function of microtubule-based molecular motor proteins.

Lawrence A. Klobutcher, Professor and Associate Dean of the Graduate School; Ph.D., Yale. DNA rearrangement, programmed translational frameshifting, and phagocytosis in ciliated protozoa.

Dmitry Korzhnev, Assistant Professor, Molecular, Microbial, and Structural Biology; Ph.D., Moscow Institute of Physics and Technology. Liquid-state nuclear magnetic resonance (NMR) studies of structure and dynamics of proteins and their assemblies; multiprotein complexes involved in DNA replication and repair; protein folding.

Mark Maciejewski, Associate Professor; Ph.D., Ohio State. Enzymes of DNA replication, repair, and recombination.

Adam Schuyler, Assistant Professor of Molecular Biology and Biophysics; Ph.D., Johns Hopkins. Computational modeling of molecular dynamics and allosteric activation, nonuniform sampling techniques for multidimensional NMR experiments.

Peter Setlow, Professor; Ph.D., Brandeis. Biochemistry of bacterial spore germination.

Aziz Taghbalout, Assistant Professor of Molecular, Microbial, and Structural Biology; Ph.D., Hassan II University (Morocco). Understanding the molecular organization of the RNA degradosome, a multiprotein complex that plays essential role in the normal RNA degradation and processing in *Escherichia coli*.

Suzy V. Torti, Professor of Molecular, Microbial, and Structural Biology; Ph.D., Tufts.

Sandra K. Weller, Professor and Department Head; Ph.D., Wisconsin. Mechanisms of DNA replication and DNA encapsidation in herpes simplex virus; virus-host interactions.

UNIVERSITY OF WASHINGTON/ FRED HUTCHINSON CANCER RESEARCH CENTER

Molecular and Cellular Biology Program

UNIVERSITY *of* WASHINGTON

FRED HUTCH
CURES START HERE™

 For more information, visit http://petersons.to/uwashingtonmolecularcellbiology

Program of Study

The University of Washington (UW) and the Fred Hutchinson Cancer Research Center (Fred Hutch) offer a Ph.D. program in molecular and cellular biology. More than 200 faculty members participate in the program and are located on the UW campus in the Departments of Biochemistry, Biological Structure, Biology, Environmental Health, Genome Sciences, Immunology, Microbiology, Global Health, Pathology, Pharmacology, and Physiology and Biophysics, as well as on the Fred Hutch campus, primarily in the Division of Basic Sciences and the Division of Human Biology, but also incorporating the Divisions of Clinical Research, Public Health Sciences, and Vaccines & Infectious Diseases. Recently, the Institute for Systems Biology (ISB), the Benaroya Research Institute (BRI), and the Center for Infectious Disease Research (CIDR, formerly Seattle BioMed) have joined the Molecular and Cellular Biology (MCB) program.

The goals of MCB are to give a sound background in molecular and cellular biology and to provide access to the research expertise of all faculty members and laboratories working in this area. The program includes keystone courses in a student's area of interest, advanced elective courses in molecular and cellular biology, a literature review course, one quarter of grant writing, three or more lab rotations, two quarters of teaching experience, and a series of informal workshops and seminars. Emphasis is placed on critical evaluation of the literature, exposure to current research methods, and creative thinking through independent research. Students are expected to begin active research in the first year during lab rotations and to choose a permanent thesis adviser at the end of the first year.

Research Facilities

The laboratories of participating faculty members are well equipped with the latest in research equipment and are funded by external support. The program uses the research facilities of the individual UW departments, Fred Hutch, ISB, BRI, and CIDR. The School of Medicine is housed in the Health Sciences Center and the South Lake Union research hub (SLU). The University Hospital and the College of Arts and Sciences are in nearby buildings. Fred Hutch is located near UW, in South Lake Union on a modern, spectacular 15-acre campus that focuses on technology and sustainability. The ISB, BRI, and CIDR are within easy commuting distance. Some of the other facilities available are two Howard Hughes Medical Institute research units, the Markey Molecular Medicine Center, animal quarters, shared major instrument facilities, oligonucleotide and peptide synthesis facilities, a marine biology station at Friday Harbor in the San Juan Islands, and an extensive Health Sciences Library.

Financial Aid

The program offers a salary of approximately $34,416 annually. Students with satisfactory academic progress can anticipate funding that includes tuition and health insurance for the duration of their studies.

Cost of Study

Tuition, salary, and medical, dental, and vision benefits are funded for the duration of the program for students in good academic standing.

Living and Housing Costs

The University has a wide variety of housing available for single students, married students, and students with families. The University Housing Office (phone: 206-543-4059) can provide further information. Private accommodations may be found within easy walking or biking distance.

Student Group

At UW, approximately 2,500 full-time faculty members serve a student population of 54,000 that is drawn from all over the United States and other countries. An average of 20 new students are admitted to the program each year. There are approximately 500 graduate students in the biological sciences at UW.

Student Outcomes

MCB received degree-granting status in 1994. The majority of students, upon earning Ph.D. degrees, secure postdoctoral research positions.

Location

Seattle enjoys a moderate climate, with an abundance of outdoor recreation options in the lakes, mountains, rivers, and parks that surround the area. Hiking, camping, skiing, and biking are popular activities. The city offers many cultural and educational advantages, including theater, museums, symphony, and films, while the waterfront is home to a large marketplace, galleries, and fresh seafood restaurants. The UW, Fred Hutch, and other participating institutes are all located within easy distance of each other, and near downtown.

The University

The University of Washington is located in a residential section of Seattle near the downtown area. It is bordered by two lakes and is one of the largest and most scenic institutions of higher education in the country. The University is a research-intensive institution, regularly ranking first overall among public universities in externally funded research programs. It is recognized for graduate instruction of high quality, offering more than ninety graduate and professional programs that enroll more than 12,000 graduate students on campus. Fred Hutch's state-of-the-art research laboratories are located near Lake Union just north of downtown Seattle, a short shuttle ride from the UW and affiliated institutions. Celebrating its 40th anniversary in 2015, it is the largest independent cancer research center in the country, with more than 200 faculty spread throughout five scientific divisions. Fred Hutch is also home to 3 Nobel Laureates, as well as many award-winning faculty members.

Applying

Applicants must have completed a baccalaureate or advanced degree by the time of matriculation; degrees emphasizing biology, physical or natural sciences, and mathematics are preferred. It is advisable to take the GRE (the General Test) by August 1 so that scores can be recorded before the deadline (code for MCB is 0206, code for UW is 4854, on the GRE registration form). New students enter the graduate program in the autumn quarter. The deadline for completion of applications is currently December 1 of the academic year preceding entrance. Students must apply via the online application available at the MCB Program website (https://www.grad.uw.edu/applForAdmiss).

Correspondence and Information

Graduate Program Specialist
Molecular and Cellular Biology Program, Box 357275
University of Washington
Seattle, Washington 98195-7275
United States
Phone: 206-685-3155
Fax: 206-685-8174
E-mail: mcb@uw.edu
Website: http://www.mcb-seattle.edu

THE FACULTY AND THEIR RESEARCH

UNIVERSITY OF WASHINGTON

Cancer Biology
Charles Asbury, Trisha Davis, Maitreya Dunham, Douglas Fowler, Richard Gardner, Philip Greenberg, Liangcai Gu, Barry Gumbiner, Suzanne Hoppins, Brian Iritani, Michael Lagunoff, Lawrence Loeb, Nancy Maizels, Raymond Monnat, Shao-En Ong, Junko Oshima, Bradley Preston, Rosa Ana Risques, Hannele Ruohola-Baker, Andrew Scharenberg, Daniel Stetson, Judit Villen, Alejandro Wolf-Yadlin.

Cell Signaling and Cell/Environment Interactions
Michael Ailion, John Aitchison, Charles Asbury, Sandra Bajjalieh, Joseph Beavo, Celeste Berg, Karol Bomsztyk, Karin Bornfeldt, Mark Bothwell, Susan Brockerhoff, Steven Carlson, William Catterall, Sharon Doty, Elaine Faustman, Stanley Froehner, Richard Gardner, Sharona Gordon, E. Peter Greenberg, Ted Gross, Christoph Grundner, Barry Gumbiner, Chris Hague, Suzanne Hoppins, James Hurley, Takato Imaizumi, Matthew Kaeberlein, David Kimelman, Michael Laflamme, John Leigh, Jaisri Lingappa, Qinghang Liu, Dustin Maly, Stanley McKnight, Alex Merz, Dana Miller, Neil Nathanson, Jennifer Nemhauser, Andrew Oberst, Leo Pallanck, Alexander Paredez, David Parichy, Marilyn Parsons, Christine Queitsch, David Raible, Hannele Ruohola-Baker, John Scott, Daniel Stetson, Daniel Storm, Rong Tian, Keiko Torii, Judit Villen, Alejandro Wolf-Yadlin, Zhengui Xia, Zipora Yablonka-Reuveni, William Zagotta.

Developmental Biology, Stem Cells, and Aging
Chris Amemiya, David Beier, Celeste Berg, Mark Bothwell, Steven Carlson, Jeffrey Chamberlain, Michael Chin, Vincenzo Cirulli, John Clark, Mark Cooper, Michael Cunningham, Ajay Dhaka, Christine Disteche, Barry

University of Washington/Fred Hutchinson Cancer Research Center

Gumbiner, Marshall Horwitz, Matthew Kaeberlein, David Kimelman, Young Kwon, Michael Laflamme, Michael MacCoss, Alex Merz, Dana Miller, William Moody, Randall Moon, Charles Murry, Jennifer Nemhauser, Leo Pallanck, David Parichy, Jay Parrish, Daniel Promislow, Peter Rabinovitch, David Raible, Thomas Reh, Hannele Ruohola-Baker, Billie Swalla, Keiko Torii, Judit Villen, Barbara Wakimoto, Robert Waterston, Andrea E. Willis, Zhengui Xia, Zipora Yablonka-Reuveni.

Gene Expression, Cell Cycle, and Chromosome Biology
John Aitchison, Charles Asbury, Nitin Baliga, Karol Bomsztyk, Eliot Brenowitz, Bonita Brewer, Roger Bumgarner, Daniel Campbell, Trisha Davis, Christine Disteche, Maitreya Dunham, Elaine Faustman, Takato Imaizumi, Nancy Maizels, Stanley McKinight, Houra Merrikh, Dana Miller, Raymond Monnat, James Mullins, Peter Myler, Shao-En Ong, Alexander Paredez, Hannele Ruohola-Baker, Keiko Torii, Edith Wang, Robert Waterston, Linda Wordeman, Zipora Yablonka-Reuveni.

Genetics, Genomics, and Evolution
Michael Ailion, Chris Amemiya, Nitin Baliga, Celeste Berg, Elhanan Borenstein, Bonita Brewer, Roger Bumgarner, Peter Byers, Jeffrey Chamberlain, Michael Cunningham, Christine Disteche, Aimee Dudley, Maitreya Dunham, Elaine Faustman, Stanley Fields, Douglas Fowler, Clement Furlong, Richard Gardner, Marshall Horwitz, Matthew Kaeberlein, Benjamin Kerr, Mary-Claire King, Young Kwon, John Leigh, Lawrence Loeb, Nancy Maizels, Houra Merrikh, Dana Miller, Raymond Monnat, James Mullins, Peter Myler, Shao-En Ong, Junko Oshima, Leo Pallanck, Alexander Paredez, David Parichy, Jay Parrish, Bradley Preston, Daniel Promislow, Christine Queitsch, David Raible, Lalita Ramakrishnan, Jay Shendure, David Sherman, Ilya Shmulevich, Daniel Stetson, Kenneth Stuart, Billie Swalla, Bruce Tempel, Rong Tian, Keiko Torii, Barbara Wakimoto, Robert Waterston, Andrea E. Wills, Zipora Yablonka-Reuveni.

Microbiology, Infection, and Immunity
Alan Aderem, John Aitchison, Nitin Baliga, Elhanan Borenstein, Roger Bumgarner, Daniel Campbell, James Champoux, Edward Clark, Brad Cookson, Ian Nicholas Crispe, Keith Elkon, Ferric Fang, Pamela Fink, Michael Gale, Joan Goverman, E. Peter Greenberg, Philip Greenberg, Christoph Grundner, Liangcai Gu, Jessica Hamerman, Caroline Harwood, Lucas Hoffmann, Michael Katze, Nichole Klatt, Michael Lagunoff, Kelly Lee, Jaisri Lingappa, Jennifer Lund, Houra Merrikh, Alex Merz, Samuel Miller, Joseph Mougous, James Mullins, Peter Myler, Andrew Oberst, Matthew Parsek, Marilyn Parsons, Lakshmi Rajgopal, Lalita Ramakrishnan, David Rawlings, Marilyn Roberts, Andrew Scharenberg, Jay Shendure, David Sherman, Pradeep Singh, Jason Smith, Joseph Smith, Kelly Smith, Donald Sodora, Leonidas Stamatatos, Daniel Stetson, Kenneth Stuart, Naeha Subramanian, Justin Taylor, Wendy Thomas, Beth Traxler, Kevin Urdahl, Wesley Van Voorhis, Joshua Woodward, Tuofu Zhu, Steven Ziegler.

Molecular Structure and Computational Biology
John Aitchison, Charles Asbury, David Baker, Elhanan Borenstein, James Champoux, Douglas Fowler, Sharona Gordon, Liangcai Gu, Rachel Klevit, Justin Kollman, Kelly Lee, Michael MacCoss, Raymond Monnat, James Mullins, Peter Myler, Shao-En Ong, Ram Samudrala, Ilya Shmulevich, Wendy Thomas, Gabriele Varani, Edith Wang, Liguo Wang, Wenqing Xu, William Zagotta, Ning Zheng.

Neuroscience
Michael Ailion, Sandra Bajjalieh, Andres Barria, Joseph Beavo, Olivia Bermingham-McDonogh, Mark Bothwell, Eliot Brenowitz, Susan Brockerhoff, Steven Carlson, Jeffrey Chamberlain, Charles Chavkin, Horacio de la Iglesia, Ajay Dhaka, Sharona Gordon, Robert Hevner, Bertil Hille, James Hurley, Matthew Kaeberlein, Brian Kraemer, Stanley McKnight, William Moody, Neil Nathanson, John Neumaier, Leo Pallanck, Richard Palmiter, Jay Parrish, Paul Phillips, Nicholas Poolos, David Raible, Thomas Reh, Fred Rieke, Robert Steiner, Nephi Stella, Daniel Storm, Bruce Tempel, Rachel Wong, Zhengui Xia, William Zagotta.

FRED HUTCHINSON CANCER RESEARCH CENTER

Cancer Biology
Antonio Bedalov, Slobodan Beronja, Jason Bielas, Robert Bradley, Kevin Cheung, Bruce Clurman, Denise Galloway, Cyrus Ghajar, William Grady, Philip Greenberg, David Hockenbery, Andrew Hsieh, Christopher Kemp, Hans-Peter Kiem, Paul Lampe, David MacPherson, Peter Nelson, Patrick Paddison, Susan Parkhurst, Amanda Paulovich, Peggy Porter, Martin Prlic, Nina Salama, Julian Simon, Toshiyasu Taniguchi, Stephen Tapscott, Valeri Vasioukhin, Edus Warren.

Cell Signaling and Cell/Environment Interactions
Jihong Bai, Linda Breeden, Kevin Cheung, Jonathan Cooper, Cyrus Ghajar, David Hockenbery, Andrew Hsieh, Paul Lampe, Susan Parkhurst, Amanda Paulovich, Mark Roth, Wenying Shou, Valera Vasioukhin.

Developmental Biology, Stem Cells, and Aging
Jihong Bai, Jonathan Cooper, Cyrus Ghajar, Hans-Peter Kiem, Cecilia Moens, Patrick Paddison, Susan Parkhurst, James Priess, Akiko Shimamura, Valera Vasioukhin.

Gene Expression, Cell Cycle, and Chromosome Biology
Antonio Bedalov, Susan Biggins, Linda Breeden, Bruce Clurman, Adam Geballe, Mark Groudine, Steven Hahn, Steven Henikoff, David MacPherson, Harmit Malik, Susan Parkhurst, Amanda Paulovich, Arvind "Rasi" Subramaniam, Mark Roth, Gerald Smith, Stephen Tapscott, Toshio Tsukiyama.

Genetics, Genomics, and Evolution
Antonio Bedalov, Trevor Bedford, Jesse Bloom, Robert Bradley, Roger Brent, Michael Emerman, Adam Geballe, Steven Henikoff, David MacPherson, Harmit Malik, J. Lee Nelson, Peter Nelson, Amanda Paulovich, Katie Peichel, Wenying Shou, Gerald Smith, Arvind "Rasi" Subramaniam, Edus Warren.

Microbiology, Infection, and Immunity
Trevor Bedford, Jesse Bloom, Michael Emerman, Denise Galloway, Adam Geballe, Keith Jerome, Hans-Peter Kiem, Harmit Malik, Julie Overbaugh, Martin Prlic, Stanley Riddell, Nina Salama, Wenying Shou, Roland Strong, Edus Warren.

Molecular Structure and Computational Biology
Trevor Bedford, Jesse Bloom, Steven Hahn, Andrew Hsieh, Wenying Shou, Barry Stoddard, Roland Strong, Arvind "Rasi" Subramaniam, Edus Warren.

Neuroscience
Jihong Bai, Linda Buck, Cecilia Moens, James Olson, Valera Vasioukhin.

Section 7
Computational, Systems, and Translational Biology

This section contains a directory of institutions offering graduate work in computational, systems, and translational biology, followed by in in-depth entry prepared by an institution that chose to submit a detailed program description. Additional information about programs listed in the directory may be obtained by writing directly to the dean of a graduate school or chair of a department at the address given in the directory.

CONTENTS

Computational Biology

Albert Einstein College of Medicine, Graduate Division of Biomedical Sciences, Systems and Computational Biology Program, Bronx, NY 10461. Offers PhD.

Baylor College of Medicine, Graduate School of Biomedical Sciences, Program in Structural and Computational Biology and Molecular Biophysics, Houston, TX 77030-3498. Offers PhD, MD/PhD. MD/PhD offered jointly with Rice University and University of Houston. *Degree requirements:* For doctorate, thesis/dissertation, public defense. *Entrance requirements:* For doctorate, GRE General Test, GRE Subject Test (strongly recommended), minimum GPA of 3.0. Additional exam requirements/recommendations for international students: Required—TOEFL. Electronic applications accepted. *Faculty research:* Computational biology, structural biology, biophysics.

Carnegie Mellon University, Joint CMU-Pitt PhD Program in Computational Biology, Pittsburgh, PA 15213-3891. Offers PhD.

Carnegie Mellon University, Mellon College of Science, Department of Biological Sciences, Program in Computational Biology, Pittsburgh, PA 15213-3891. Offers MS. *Entrance requirements:* For master's, GRE General Test, GRE Subject Test, interview.

Claremont Graduate University, Graduate Programs, Institute of Mathematical Sciences, Claremont, CA 91711-6160. Offers computational and systems biology (PhD); computational mathematics and numerical analysis (MA, MS); computational science (PhD); engineering and industrial applied mathematics (PhD); mathematics (PhD); operations research and statistics (MA, MS); physical applied mathematics (MA, MS); pure mathematics (MA, MS); scientific computing (MA, MS); systems and control theory (MA, MS). *Program availability:* Part-time. *Faculty:* 6 full-time (1 woman), 2 part-time/adjunct (0 women). *Students:* 74 full-time (19 women), 35 part-time (12 women); includes 23 minority (2 Black or African American, non-Hispanic/Latino; 12 Asian, non-Hispanic/Latino; 8 Hispanic/Latino; 1 Two or more races, non-Hispanic/Latino), 51 international. Average age 30. In 2015, 25 master's, 10 doctorates awarded. Terminal master's awarded for partial completion of doctoral program. *Entrance requirements:* For master's and doctorate, GRE General Test. Additional exam requirements/recommendations for international students: Required—TOEFL (minimum score 75 iBT). *Application deadline:* For fall admission, 2/1 priority date for domestic and international students. Applications are processed on a rolling basis. Application fee: $80. Electronic applications accepted. *Expenses: Tuition, area resident:* Full-time $43,032; part-time $1793 per unit. *Required fees:* $600; $300 per semester. $300 per semester. Tuition and fees vary according to course load and program. *Financial support:* Fellowships, research assistantships, Federal Work-Study, institutionally sponsored loans, scholarships/grants, and tuition waivers (full and partial) available. Support available to part-time students. Financial award application deadline: 2/15; financial award applicants required to submit FAFSA. *Unit head:* Ali Nadim, Director, 909-607-9413, E-mail: ali.nadim@cgu.edu. *Application contact:* Jake Campbell, Assistant Director of Admissions, 909-607-3024, E-mail: jake.campbell@cgu.edu. Website: http://www.cgu.edu/pages/168.asp

The College of William and Mary, Faculty of Arts and Sciences, Department of Applied Science, Williamsburg, VA 23187-8795. Offers accelerator science (PhD); applied mathematics (PhD); applied mechanics (PhD); applied robotics (PhD); applied science (MS); atmospheric and environmental science (PhD); computational neuroscience (PhD); interface, thin film and surface science (PhD); lasers and optics (PhD); magnetic resonance (PhD); materials science and engineering (PhD); mathematical and computational biology (PhD); medical imaging (PhD); nanotechnology (PhD); neuroscience (PhD); non-destructive evaluation (PhD); polymer chemistry (PhD); remote sensing (PhD). *Program availability:* Part-time. *Faculty:* 7 full-time (1 woman), 1 part-time/adjunct (0 women). *Students:* 26 full-time (9 women), 3 part-time (1 woman); includes 5 minority (2 Black or African American, non-Hispanic/Latino; 1 Asian, non-Hispanic/Latino; 2 Hispanic/Latino), 12 international. Average age 28. 34 applicants, 46% accepted, 6 enrolled. In 2015, 2 master's, 6 doctorates awarded. Terminal master's awarded for partial completion of doctoral program. *Degree requirements:* For master's, comprehensive exam, thesis; for doctorate, comprehensive exam, thesis/dissertation, 4 core courses. *Entrance requirements:* For master's and doctorate, GRE General Test, GRE Subject Test. Additional exam requirements/recommendations for international students: Required—TOEFL, TWE. *Application deadline:* For fall admission, 2/3 priority date for domestic students, 2/3 for international students; for spring admission, 10/15 priority date for domestic students, 10/14 for international students. Applications are processed on a rolling basis. Application fee: $45. Electronic applications accepted. *Expenses:* $6,550 per semester; $13,100 per year. *Financial support:* Fellowships, research assistantships, teaching assistantships, Federal Work-Study, health care benefits, tuition waivers (full), and unspecified assistantships available. Financial award application deadline: 4/15; financial award applicants required to submit FAFSA. *Faculty research:* Computational biology, non-destructive evaluation, neurophysiology, lasers and optics. *Total annual research expenditures:* $1.7 million. *Unit head:* Dr. Christopher Del Negro, Chair, 757-221-7808, Fax: 757-221-2050, E-mail: cadeln@wm.edu. *Application contact:* Lianne Rios Ashburne, Graduate Program Coordinator, 757-221-2563, Fax: 757-221-2050, E-mail: lrashburne@wm.edu. Website: http://www.wm.edu/as/appliedscience

Cornell University, Graduate School, Graduate Fields of Agriculture and Life Sciences, Field of Computational Biology, Ithaca, NY 14853-0001. Offers computational behavioral biology (PhD); computational biology (PhD); computational cell biology (PhD); computational ecology (PhD); computational genetics (PhD); computational macromolecular biology (PhD); computational organismal biology (PhD). *Degree requirements:* For doctorate, comprehensive exam, thesis/dissertation, 2 semesters of teaching experience. *Entrance requirements:* For doctorate, GRE General Test, GRE Subject Test (biology), 2 letters of recommendation. Additional exam requirements/recommendations for international students: Required—TOEFL (minimum score 550 paper-based; 77 iBT). Electronic applications accepted. *Faculty research:* Computational behavioral biology, computational biology, computational cell biology, computational ecology, computational genetics, computational macromolecular biology, computational organismal biology.

Duke University, Graduate School, Department of Computational Biology and Bioinformatics, Durham, NC 27708. Offers PhD, Certificate. *Degree requirements:* For doctorate, thesis/dissertation. *Entrance requirements:* For doctorate, GRE General Test. Additional exam requirements/recommendations for international students: Required—TOEFL (minimum score 577 paper-based; 90 iBT) or IELTS (minimum score 7). Electronic applications accepted.

Florida State University, The Graduate School, College of Arts and Sciences, Program in Molecular Biophysics, Tallahassee, FL 32306. Offers molecular biophysics (PhD); structural biology and computational biophysics (PhD). *Faculty:* 34 full-time (7 women). *Students:* 19 full-time (5 women); includes 2 minority (both Hispanic/Latino), 8 international. Average age 29. 14 applicants, 36% accepted, 2 enrolled. In 2015, 5 doctorates awarded. *Degree requirements:* For doctorate, comprehensive exam, thesis/dissertation, teaching 1 term in professor's major department. *Entrance requirements:* For doctorate, GRE General Test. Additional exam requirements/recommendations for international students: Required—TOEFL (minimum score 600 paper-based; 90 iBT). *Application deadline:* For fall admission, 12/15 for domestic and international students. Application fee: $30. Electronic applications accepted. *Expenses: Tuition, area resident:* Full-time $7263; part-time $403.50 per credit hour. Tuition, nonresident: full-time $18,087; part-time $1004.85 per credit hour. *Required fees:* $1365; $75.81 per credit hour. $20 per semester. Tuition and fees vary according to campus/location. *Financial support:* In 2015–16, 23 students received support, including 1 fellowship with tuition reimbursement available (averaging $34,200 per year), 20 research assistantships with tuition reimbursements available (averaging $24,200 per year), 2 teaching assistantships with tuition reimbursements available (averaging $24,200 per year); scholarships/grants, health care benefits, and unspecified assistantships also available. *Faculty research:* Protein and nucleic acid structure and function, membrane protein structure, computational biophysics, 3-D image reconstruction. *Total annual research expenditures:* $2.3 million. *Unit head:* Dr. Hong Li, Director, 850-644-6785, Fax: 850-644-7244, E-mail: hli4@fsu.edu. *Application contact:* Katie Mikusak, Academic Coordinator, Graduate Programs, 850-644-1012, Fax: 850-644-7244, E-mail: kmikusak@chem.fsu.edu.
Website: http://www.biophysics.fsu.edu/graduate-program

Harvard University, Harvard T.H. Chan School of Public Health, Master of Science Program in Computational Biology and Quantitative Genetics, Cambridge, MA 02138. Offers SM. Offered jointly by the Department of Biostatistics and the Department of Epidemiology. *Faculty:* 2 full-time (0 women). *Students:* 25 full-time (15 women); includes 7 minority (all Asian, non-Hispanic/Latino), 16 international. Average age 25. 28 applicants, 79% accepted, 12 enrolled. *Entrance requirements:* For master's, GRE. Additional exam requirements/recommendations for international students: Recommended—TOEFL (minimum score 600 paper-based; 100 iBT), IELTS (minimum score 7). *Application deadline:* For fall admission, 12/15 for domestic and international students. Application fee: $120. Electronic applications accepted. Application fee is waived when completed online. *Financial support:* Application deadline: 2/15; applicants required to submit FAFSA. *Unit head:* Dr. John Quackenbush, Director, 617-582-8163. *Application contact:* Vincent W. James, Director of Admissions, 617-432-1031, Fax: 617-432-7080, E-mail: admissions@hsph.harvard.edu.
Website: http://www.hsph.harvard.edu/sm-computational-biology/

Iowa State University of Science and Technology, Bioinformatics and Computational Biology Program, Ames, IA 50011. Offers MS, PhD. *Degree requirements:* For doctorate, thesis/dissertation. *Entrance requirements:* For master's and doctorate, GRE General Test. Additional exam requirements/recommendations for international students: Recommended—TOEFL, IELTS. Electronic applications accepted. *Faculty research:* Functional and structural genomics, genome evolution, macromolecular structure and function, mathematical biology and biological statistics, metabolic and developmental networks.

Massachusetts Institute of Technology, School of Engineering and School of Science, Program in Computational and Systems Biology, Cambridge, MA 02139-4307. Offers PhD. *Degree requirements:* For doctorate, comprehensive exam, thesis/dissertation, teaching assistantship during one semester; training in the ethical conduct of research. *Entrance requirements:* For doctorate, GRE General Test. Additional exam requirements/recommendations for international students: Required—TOEFL (minimum score 600 paper-based; 95 iBT), IELTS (minimum score 6). Electronic applications accepted. *Expenses: Tuition:* Full-time $46,400; part-time $725 per credit. One-time fee: $304 full-time. Full-time tuition and fees vary according to course load and program. *Faculty research:* Computational biology and bioinformatics, biological design and synthetic biology, gene and protein networks, systems biology of cancer, nanobiology and microsystems.

Massachusetts Institute of Technology, School of Science, Department of Biology, Cambridge, MA 02139. Offers biochemistry (PhD); biological oceanography (PhD); biology (PhD); biophysical chemistry and molecular structure (PhD); cell biology (PhD); computational and systems biology (PhD); developmental biology (PhD); genetics (PhD); immunology (PhD); microbiology (PhD); molecular biology (PhD); neurobiology (PhD). *Faculty:* 57 full-time (14 women). *Students:* 283 full-time (137 women); includes 83 minority (3 Black or African American, non-Hispanic/Latino; 1 American Indian or Alaska Native, non-Hispanic/Latino; 38 Asian, non-Hispanic/Latino; 31 Hispanic/Latino; 10 Two or more races, non-Hispanic/Latino), 48 international. Average age 26. 673 applicants, 14% accepted, 46 enrolled. In 2015, 32 doctorates awarded. *Degree requirements:* For doctorate, comprehensive exam, thesis/dissertation, teaching assistantship during two semesters. *Entrance requirements:* For doctorate, GRE General Test. Additional exam requirements/recommendations for international students: Required—TOEFL (minimum score 577 paper-based), IELTS. *Application deadline:* For fall admission, 12/1 for domestic and international students. Application fee: $75. Electronic applications accepted. *Expenses: Tuition:* Full-time $46,400; part-time $725 per credit. One-time fee: $304 full-time. Full-time tuition and fees vary according to course load and program. *Financial support:* In 2015–16, 235 students received support, including 118 fellowships (averaging $37,500 per year), 163 research assistantships (averaging $38,900 per year), 1 teaching assistantship; Federal Work-Study, institutionally sponsored loans, scholarships/grants, traineeships, health care benefits, and unspecified assistantships also available. Support available to part-time students. Financial award application deadline: 4/15; financial award applicants required to submit FAFSA. *Faculty research:* Cellular, developmental and molecular (plant and animal) biology; biochemistry, bioengineering, biophysics and structural biology; classical and molecular genetics, stem cell and epigenetics; immunology and microbiology; cancer biology, molecular medicine, neurobiology and human disease; computational and systems biology. *Total annual research expenditures:* $42.8 million. *Unit head:* Prof. Alan Grossman, Department Head, 617-253-4701. *Application contact:* Biology Education Office, 617-253-3717, Fax: 617-258-9329, E-mail: gradbio@mit.edu. Website: https://biology.mit.edu

New Jersey Institute of Technology, College of Science and Liberal Arts, Newark, NJ 07102. Offers applied mathematics (MS); applied physics (M Sc, PhD); applied statistics (MS, Certificate); biology (MS, PhD); biostatistics (MS); chemistry (MS, PhD); computational biology (MS); environmental science (MS, PhD); history (MA, MAT); materials science and engineering (MS, PhD); mathematical and computational finance (MS); mathematics science (PhD); pharmaceutical chemistry (MS); practice of technical communications (Certificate); professional and technical communications (MS). *Program availability:* Part-time, evening/weekend. *Faculty:* 153 full-time (35 women), 100 part-time/adjunct (40 women). *Students:* 212 full-time (82 women), 94 part-time (37 women); includes 72 minority (22 Black or African American, non-Hispanic/Latino; 25

Asian, non-Hispanic/Latino; 19 Hispanic/Latino; 6 Two or more races, non-Hispanic/Latino), 164 international. Average age 29. 519 applicants, 62% accepted, 104 enrolled. In 2015, 98 master's, 21 doctorates, 3 other advanced degrees awarded. Terminal master's awarded for partial completion of doctoral program. *Degree requirements:* For master's, thesis optional; for doctorate, thesis/dissertation. *Entrance requirements:* For master's, GRE General Test; for doctorate, GRE General Test, minimum graduate GPA of 3.5. Additional exam requirements/recommendations for international students: Required—TOEFL (minimum score 550 paper-based; 79 iBT). *Application deadline:* For fall admission, 6/1 priority date for domestic students, 5/1 priority date for international students; for spring admission, 11/15 priority date for domestic and international students. Applications are processed on a rolling basis. Application fee: $75. Electronic applications accepted. *Expenses:* $28,800 per year non-resident full-time. *Financial support:* In 2015–16, 56 research assistantships with full tuition reimbursements (averaging $17,711 per year), 52 teaching assistantships with full tuition reimbursements (averaging $17,914 per year) were awarded; fellowships with full tuition reimbursements also available. Financial award application deadline: 1/15. *Total annual research expenditures:* $23.1 million. *Unit head:* Dr. Kevin Belfield, Dean, 973-596-3676, Fax: 973-565-0586, E-mail: kevin.d.belfield@njit.edu. *Application contact:* Stephen Eck, Director of Admissions, 973-596-3300, Fax: 973-596-3461, E-mail: admissions@njit.edu.
Website: http://csla.njit.edu/

New York University, Graduate School of Arts and Science, Department of Biology, Program in Computational Biology, New York, NY 10012-1019. Offers PhD. *Entrance requirements:* For doctorate, GRE. Additional exam requirements/recommendations for international students: Required—TOEFL.

New York University, School of Medicine and Graduate School of Arts and Science, Sackler Institute of Graduate Biomedical Sciences, Program in Computational Biology, New York, NY 10012-1019. Offers PhD. *Faculty research:* Protein engineering, cheminformatics and rational drug design; bioinformatics; computational methods to analyze the transcriptional regulation of the mammalian cell cycle.

Princeton University, Graduate School, Department of Molecular Biology, Princeton, NJ 08544-1019. Offers PhD. *Degree requirements:* For doctorate, thesis/dissertation. *Entrance requirements:* For doctorate, GRE General Test. Additional exam requirements/recommendations for international students: Required—TOEFL (minimum score 600 paper-based). Electronic applications accepted. *Faculty research:* Genetics, virology, biochemistry.

Rutgers University–Camden, Graduate School of Arts and Sciences, Program in Computational and Integrative Biology, Camden, NJ 08102-1401. Offers MS, PhD. *Degree requirements:* For doctorate, original research, oral defense. *Entrance requirements:* For master's and doctorate, GRE General Test; GRE Subject Test (recommended), transcripts, personal statement, three letters of recommendation. Additional exam requirements/recommendations for international students: Required—TOEFL. Electronic applications accepted.

Rutgers University–Newark, Graduate School, Program in Computational Biology, Newark, NJ 07102. Offers MS. Program offered jointly with New Jersey Institute of Technology. *Entrance requirements:* For master's, GRE, minimum undergraduate B average. Additional exam requirements/recommendations for international students: Required—TOEFL.

Rutgers University–New Brunswick, Graduate School-New Brunswick, BioMaPS Institute for Quantitative Biology, Piscataway, NJ 08854-8097. Offers computational biology and molecular biophysics (PhD). *Degree requirements:* For doctorate, comprehensive exam, thesis/dissertation. *Entrance requirements:* For doctorate, GRE. Additional exam requirements/recommendations for international students: Required—TOEFL. Electronic applications accepted. *Faculty research:* Structural biology, systems biology, bioinformatics, translational medicine, genomics.

University of California, Irvine, Francisco J. Ayala School of Biological Sciences, Program in Mathematical, Computational and Systems Biology, Irvine, CA 92697. Offers PhD. *Students:* 13 full-time (3 women); includes 6 minority (3 Asian, non-Hispanic/Latino; 2 Hispanic/Latino; 1 Two or more races, non-Hispanic/Latino), 1 international. Average age 24. 77 applicants, 32% accepted, 8 enrolled. Application fee: $90 ($110 for international students). *Unit head:* Prof. John Lowengrub, Director, 949-824-8456, Fax: 949-824-7993, E-mail: jlowengr@uci.edu. *Application contact:* Aracely Dean, Assistant Administrative Analyst, 949-824-4120, Fax: 949-824-6444, E-mail: mcsb@uci.edu.
Website: http://mcsb.bio.uci.edu/

University of Colorado Denver, College of Liberal Arts and Sciences, Department of Mathematical and Statistical Sciences, Denver, CO 80217. Offers applied mathematics (MS, PhD), including applied mathematics, applied probability (MS) applied statistics (MS), computational biology, computational mathematics (PhD), discrete mathematics, finite geometry (PhD), mathematics education (PhD), mathematics of engineering and science (MS), numerical analysis, operations research (MS), optimization and operations research (PhD), probability (PhD), statistics (PhD). *Program availability:* Part-time. *Faculty:* 18 full-time (4 women), 5 part-time/adjunct (0 women). *Students:* 48 full-time (16 women), 15 part-time (6 women); includes 7 minority (1 Black or African American, non-Hispanic/Latino; 2 Asian, non-Hispanic/Latino; 3 Hispanic/Latino; 1 Two or more races, non-Hispanic/Latino), 12 international. Average age 32. 105 applicants, 70% accepted, 21 enrolled. In 2015, 10 master's, 3 doctorates awarded. *Degree requirements:* For master's, comprehensive exam, thesis optional, 30 hours of course work with minimum GPA of 3.0; for doctorate, comprehensive exam, thesis/dissertation, 42 hours of course work with minimum GPA of 3.25. *Entrance requirements:* For master's, GRE General Test; GRE Subject Test in math (recommended), 30 hours of course work in mathematics (24 of which must be upper-division mathematics), bachelor's degree with minimum GPA of 3.0; for doctorate, GRE General Test; GRE Subject Test in math (recommended), 30 hours of course work in mathematics (24 of which must be upper-division mathematics), master's degree with minimum GPA of 3.25. Additional exam requirements/recommendations for international students: Required—TOEFL (minimum score 537 paper-based; 75 iBT); Recommended—IELTS (minimum score 6.5). *Application deadline:* For fall admission, 4/1 for domestic and international students; for spring admission, 10/1 for domestic and international students; for summer admission, 4/1 for domestic and international students. Application fee: $50 ($75 for international students). Electronic applications accepted. *Financial support:* In 2015–16, 46 students received support. Fellowships with partial tuition reimbursements available, research assistantships with full tuition reimbursements available, teaching assistantships with full tuition reimbursements available, Federal Work-Study, institutionally sponsored loans, scholarships/grants, and traineeships available. Financial award application deadline: 4/1; financial award applicants required to submit FAFSA. *Faculty research:* Computational mathematics, computational biology, discrete mathematics and geometry, probability and statistics, optimization. *Unit head:* Dr. Michael Ferrara, Graduate Chair, 303-315-1705, E-mail: michael.ferrara@ucdenver.edu. *Application contact:* Julie Blunck, Program Assistant, 303-315-1743, E-mail: julie.blunck@ucdenver.edu.
Website: http://www.ucdenver.edu/academics/colleges/CLAS/Departments/math/Pages/MathStats.aspx

University of Colorado Denver, School of Medicine, Program in Computational Bioscience, Aurora, CO 80045-0511. Offers PhD. *Program availability:* Part-time. *Students:* 13 full-time (6 women), 3 part-time (1 woman); includes 3 minority (1 Hispanic/Latino; 2 Two or more races, non-Hispanic/Latino), 2 international. Average age 29. 25 applicants, 16% accepted, 4 enrolled. In 2015, 2 doctorates awarded. *Degree requirements:* For doctorate, comprehensive exam, thesis/dissertation, minimum of 30 semester credit hours of course work and 30 semester hours of dissertation research. *Entrance requirements:* For doctorate, GRE General Test, GRE Subject Test in computer science (recommended), demonstrated adequate computational and biological backgrounds, interviews. Additional exam requirements/recommendations for international students: Required—TOEFL (minimum score 550 paper-based; 80 iBT). *Application deadline:* For fall admission, 12/1 for domestic students, 11/1 for international students. Application fee: $50 ($75 for international students). Electronic applications accepted. *Expenses:* Contact institution. *Financial support:* In 2015–16, 16 students received support. Fellowships, research assistantships, teaching assistantships, Federal Work-Study, institutionally sponsored loans, scholarships/grants, traineeships, health care benefits, tuition waivers (full), and unspecified assistantships available. Financial award application deadline: 4/1; financial award applicants required to submit FAFSA. *Faculty research:* Physical simulations of biological macromolecules and their dynamics, gene expression array analysis and interpretation of expression data, natural language processing in the biomedical literature, metabolic and signaling pathway analysis, evolutionary reconstruction and disease gene finding. *Unit head:* Dr. Larry Hunter, Director, 303-724-3574, E-mail: larry.hunter@ucdenver.edu. *Application contact:* Elizabeth Wethington, Administrative Coordinator, 303-724-7280, Fax: 303-724-6881, E-mail: elizabeth.wethington@ucdenver.edu.
Website: http://compbio.ucdenver.edu/

University of Idaho, College of Graduate Studies, College of Science, Program in Bioinformatics and Computational Biology, Moscow, ID 83844-3051. Offers MS, PhD. *Faculty:* 16 full-time. *Students:* 19 full-time, 4 part-time. Average age 30. *Entrance requirements:* For master's, GRE, minimum GPA of 2.8. Additional exam requirements/recommendations for international students: Required—TOEFL. *Application deadline:* For fall admission, 8/1 for domestic students; for spring admission, 12/15 for domestic students. Applications are processed on a rolling basis. Application fee: $60. Electronic applications accepted. *Expenses:* Tuition, state resident: full-time $6205; part-time $399 per credit hour. Tuition, nonresident: full-time $20,209; part-time $1177 per credit hour. *Required fees:* $2017; $58 per credit hour. Full-time tuition and fees vary according to course load and reciprocity agreements. *Financial support:* Applicants required to submit FAFSA. *Unit head:* Dr. Eva Top, Director, 208-885-6010, E-mail: bcb@uidaho.edu. *Application contact:* Sean Scoggin, Graduate Recruitment Coordinator, 208-885-4723, Fax: 208-885-4406, E-mail: graduateadmissions@uidaho.edu.
Website: http://www.uidaho.edu/cogs/bcb

University of Illinois at Urbana–Champaign, Graduate College, College of Liberal Arts and Sciences, School of Molecular and Cellular Biology, Center for Biophysics and Computational Biology, Champaign, IL 61820. Offers MS, PhD.

The University of Iowa, Graduate College, Program in Informatics, Iowa City, IA 52242-1316. Offers bioinformatics (MS, PhD); bioinformatics and computational biology (Certificate); geoinformatics (MS, PhD, Certificate); health informatics (MS, PhD, Certificate); information science (MS, PhD, Certificate). *Degree requirements:* For master's, thesis optional; for doctorate, comprehensive exam, thesis/dissertation. *Entrance requirements:* For master's and doctorate, GRE General Test, minimum GPA of 3.0. Additional exam requirements/recommendations for international students: Required—TOEFL (minimum score 550 paper-based; 81 iBT). Electronic applications accepted.

The University of Kansas, Graduate Studies, College of Liberal Arts and Sciences, Department of Computational Biology, Lawrence, KS 66047. Offers PhD. *Students:* 21 full-time (8 women); includes 2 minority (both Asian, non-Hispanic/Latino), 12 international. Average age 29. 20 applicants, 55% accepted, 6 enrolled. In 2015, 2 doctorates awarded. *Entrance requirements:* For doctorate, bachelor's or master's degree in natural sciences, mathematics, engineering, or another relevant field. Additional exam requirements/recommendations for international students: Required—TOEFL. *Application deadline:* For fall admission, 12/15 for domestic and international students. Application fee: $65 ($85 for international students). Electronic applications accepted. *Faculty research:* Life sciences, computational modeling tools, community-wide activities in bioinformatics, education for the new generation of researchers. *Unit head:* Illya Vakser, Director, 785-864-1057, E-mail: vakser@ku.edu. *Application contact:* Debbie Douglass-Metsker, Office Manager, 785-864-1057, E-mail: douglass@ku.edu.
Website: http://www.bioinformatics.ku.edu/

University of Maryland, College Park, Academic Affairs, College of Computer, Mathematical and Natural Sciences, Department of Biology, PhD Program in Biological Sciences, College Park, MD 20742. Offers behavior, ecology, evolution, and systematics (PhD); computational biology, bioinformatics, and genomics (PhD); molecular and cellular biology (PhD); physiological systems (PhD). *Degree requirements:* For doctorate, comprehensive exam, thesis/dissertation, thesis work presentation in seminar. *Entrance requirements:* For doctorate, GRE General Test; GRE Subject Test in biology (recommended), academic transcripts, statement of purpose/research interests, 3 letters of recommendation. Additional exam requirements/recommendations for international students: Required—TOEFL. Electronic applications accepted.

University of Massachusetts Medical School, Graduate School of Biomedical Sciences, Worcester, MA 01655-0115. Offers biomedical sciences (PhD), including biochemistry and molecular pharmacology, bioinformatics and computational biology, cancer biology, cell biology, immunology and microbiology, interdisciplinary, neuroscience, translational science; biomedical sciences (millennium program) (PhD); clinical and population health research (PhD); clinical investigation (MS). *Faculty:* 1,339 full-time (521 women), 301 part-time/adjunct (189 women). *Students:* 363 full-time (184 women); includes 58 minority (13 Black or African American, non-Hispanic/Latino; 30 Asian, non-Hispanic/Latino; 15 Hispanic/Latino), 141 international. Average age 29. 661 applicants, 26% accepted, 51 enrolled. In 2015, 10 master's, 58 doctorates awarded. Terminal master's awarded for partial completion of doctoral program. *Degree requirements:* For master's, comprehensive exam, thesis; for doctorate, comprehensive exam, thesis/dissertation. *Entrance requirements:* For master's, MD, PhD, DVM, or PharmD; for doctorate, GRE General Test, bachelor's degree. Additional exam requirements/recommendations for international students: Required—TOEFL (minimum score 100 iBT) or IELTS (minimum score 7.5). *Application deadline:* For fall admission, 12/15 for domestic and international students; for spring admission, 5/15 for domestic students. Application fee: $80. Electronic applications accepted. *Expenses:* $6,966 resident per year; $14,182 non-resident per year. *Financial support:* In 2015–16, 383 students received support, including research assistantships with full tuition reimbursements available (averaging $30,600 per year); scholarships/grants, health care benefits, tuition waivers (full), and unspecified assistantships also available. Financial award application deadline: 5/16. *Faculty research:* RNA interference, cell/molecular/developmental biology, bioinformatics, clinical/translational research,

Computational Biology

infectious disease. *Total annual research expenditures:* $250.3 million. *Unit head:* Dr. Anthony Carruthers, Dean, 508-856-4135, E-mail: anthony.carruthers@umassmed.edu. *Application contact:* Dr. Kendall Knight, Assistant Vice Provost for Admissions, 508-856-5628, Fax: 508-856-3659, E-mail: kendall.knight@umassmed.edu.
Website: http://www.umassmed.edu/gsbs/

The University of North Carolina at Chapel Hill, School of Medicine and Graduate School, Graduate Programs in Medicine, Curriculum in Bioinformatics and Computational Biology, Chapel Hill, NC 27599. Offers PhD. *Degree requirements:* For doctorate, comprehensive exam, thesis/dissertation. *Entrance requirements:* For doctorate, GRE, minimum GPA of 3.0. Additional exam requirements/recommendations for international students: Required—TOEFL. Electronic applications accepted. *Faculty research:* Protein folding, design and evolution and molecular biophysics of disease; mathematical modeling of signaling pathways and regulatory networks; bioinformatics, medical informatics, user interface design; statistical genetics and genetic epidemiology datamining, classification and clustering analysis of gene-expression data.

University of Pennsylvania, Perelman School of Medicine, Biomedical Graduate Studies, Graduate Group in Genomics and Computational Biology, Philadelphia, PA 19104. Offers PhD, MD/PhD, VMD/PhD. *Faculty:* 78. *Students:* 40 full-time (15 women); includes 10 minority (7 Asian, non-Hispanic/Latino; 1 Hispanic/Latino; 2 Two or more races, non-Hispanic/Latino), 10 international. 127 applicants, 17% accepted, 11 enrolled. In 2015, 5 doctorates awarded. *Degree requirements:* For doctorate, thesis/dissertation. *Entrance requirements:* For doctorate, GRE. Additional exam requirements/recommendations for international students: Required—TOEFL. *Application deadline:* For fall admission, 12/1 priority date for domestic students, 12/1 for international students. Applications are processed on a rolling basis. Application fee: $80. Electronic applications accepted. *Expenses: Tuition, area resident:* Full-time $31,068; part-time $5762 per course. *Required fees:* $3200; $336 per course. Full-time tuition and fees vary according to degree level, program and student level. Part-time tuition and fees vary according to course load, degree level and program. *Financial support:* In 2015–16, 40 students received support. Fellowships, research assistantships, scholarships/grants, traineeships, and unspecified assistantships available. *Unit head:* Dr. Li-San Wang, Chairperson, 215-746-7015. *Application contact:* Maureen Kirsch, Graduate Coordinator, 215-746-2807.
Website: http://www.med.upenn.edu/gcb/

University of Pittsburgh, School of Medicine, Graduate Programs in Medicine, Computational Biology Program, Pittsburgh, PA 15260. Offers PhD. Program jointly offered with Carnegie Mellon University. *Faculty:* 21 full-time (4 women), 68 part-time/adjunct (16 women). *Students:* 24 full-time (10 women); includes 2 minority (both Hispanic/Latino), 11 international. Average age 28. 141 applicants, 26% accepted, 11 enrolled. In 2015, 12 doctorates awarded. Terminal master's awarded for partial completion of doctoral program. *Degree requirements:* For doctorate, comprehensive exam, thesis/dissertation, ethics training service as course assistant, seminar. *Entrance requirements:* For doctorate, GRE Subject Test (recommended), GRE General Test, 3 letters of recommendation, resume. Additional exam requirements/recommendations for international students: Required—TOEFL (minimum score 600 paper-based; 100 iBT), IELTS (minimum score 7). *Application deadline:* For fall admission, 12/15 priority date for domestic and international students. Application fee: $75. Electronic applications accepted. Tuition and fees vary according to program. *Financial support:* In 2015–16, 24 students received support, including 7 fellowships with full tuition reimbursements available (averaging $27,000 per year), 17 research assistantships with full tuition reimbursements available (averaging $27,000 per year); teaching assistantships, scholarships/grants, traineeships, and health care benefits also available. *Faculty research:* Computational structural biology, computational genomics, cellular and systems modeling, bioimage informatics, mathematical biology. *Total annual research expenditures:* $6.3 million. *Unit head:* Dr. Daniel M. Zuckerman, Director, 412-648-3335, Fax: 412-648-3163, E-mail: ddmmzz@pitt.edu. *Application contact:* Kelly Gentille, Educational Programs Administrator, 412-648-8107, Fax: 412-648-3163, E-mail: kmg120@pitt.edu.
Website: http://www.compbio.pitt.edu/

University of Rochester, School of Medicine and Dentistry, Graduate Programs in Medicine and Dentistry, Department of Biochemistry and Biophysics, Programs in Biophysics, Rochester, NY 14627. Offers biophysics, structural and computational biology (PhD). Terminal master's awarded for partial completion of doctoral program. *Degree requirements:* For doctorate, thesis/dissertation, qualifying exam. *Entrance requirements:* For doctorate, GRE General Test. *Expenses: Tuition, area resident:* Full-time $47,450; part-time $1482 per credit hour. *Required fees:* $528. Tuition and fees vary according to program.

University of Southern California, Graduate School, Dana and David Dornsife College of Letters, Arts and Sciences, Department of Biological Sciences, Program in Molecular and Computational Biology, Los Angeles, CA 90089. Offers computational biology and bioinformatics (PhD); molecular biology (PhD). *Degree requirements:* For doctorate, comprehensive exam, thesis/dissertation, qualifying examination, dissertation defense. *Entrance requirements:* For doctorate, GRE, 3 letters of recommendation, personal statement, resume, minimum GPA of 3.0. Additional exam requirements/recommendations for international students: Required—TOEFL (minimum score 600 paper-based; 100 iBT). Electronic applications accepted. *Faculty research:* Biochemistry and molecular biology; genomics; computational biology and bioinformatics; cell and developmental biology, and genetics; DNA replication and repair, and cancer biology.

University of South Florida, Morsani College of Medicine and College of Graduate Studies, Graduate Programs in Medical Sciences, Tampa, FL 33620-9951. Offers advanced athletic training (MS); athletic training (MS); bioinformatics and computational biology (MSBCB); biotechnology (MSB); health informatics (MSHI); medical sciences (MSMS, PhD), including aging and neuroscience (MSMS), allergy, immunology and infectious disease (PhD), anatomy, athletic training (MSMS), clinical and translational research, health informatics (MSMS), health science (MSMS), interdisciplinary medical sciences (MSMS), medical microbiology and immunology (MSMS), metabolic and nutritional medicine (MSMS), molecular medicine, molecular pharmacology and physiology (PhD), neurology (PhD), pathology and laboratory medicine (PhD), pharmacology and therapeutics (PhD), physiology and biophysics (PhD), women's health (MSMS). *Students:* 510 full-time (261 women), 318 part-time (208 women); includes 360 minority (108 Black or African American, non-Hispanic/Latino; 3 American Indian or Alaska Native, non-Hispanic/Latino; 101 Asian, non-Hispanic/Latino; 124 Hispanic/Latino; 1 Native Hawaiian or other Pacific Islander, non-Hispanic/Latino, 23 Two or more races, non-Hispanic/Latino), 52 international. Average age 26. 6,567 applicants, 13% accepted, 469 enrolled. In 2015, 216 master's awarded. Terminal master's awarded for partial completion of doctoral program. *Degree requirements:* For master's, comprehensive exam, thesis; for doctorate, comprehensive exam, thesis/dissertation. *Entrance requirements:* For master's, GRE General Test or GMAT, bachelor's degree or equivalent from regionally-accredited university with minimum GPA of 3.0 in upper-division sciences coursework; prerequisites in general biology, general chemistry, general physics, organic chemistry, quantitative analysis, and integral and differential calculus; for doctorate, GRE General Test, bachelor's degree from regionally-accredited university with minimum GPA of 3.0 in upper-division sciences

coursework; 3 letters of recommendation; personal interview; 1-2 page personal statement; prerequisites in biology, chemistry, physics, organic chemistry, quantitative analysis, and integral/differential calculus. Additional exam requirements/recommendations for international students: Required—TOEFL (minimum score 550 paper-based; 79 iBT) or IELTS (minimum score 6.5). *Application deadline:* For fall admission, 2/15 for domestic students, 1/2 for international students. Application fee: $30. *Expenses:* Contact institution. *Faculty research:* Anatomy, biochemistry, cancer biology, cardiovascular disease, cell biology, immunology, microbiology, molecular biology, neuroscience, pharmacology, physiology. *Unit head:* Dr. Michael Barber, Professor/Associate Dean for Graduate and Postdoctoral Affairs, 813-974-9908, Fax: 813-974-4317, E-mail: mbarber@health.usf.edu. *Application contact:* Dr. Eric Bennett, Graduate Director, PhD Program in Medical Sciences, 813-974-1545, Fax: 813-974-4317, E-mail: esbennet@health.usf.edu.
Website: http://health.usf.edu/nocms/medicine/graduatestudies/

The University of Texas Medical Branch, Graduate School of Biomedical Sciences, Program in Biochemistry and Molecular Biology, Galveston, TX 77555. Offers biochemistry (PhD); bioinformatics (PhD); biophysics (PhD); cell biology (PhD); computational biology (PhD); structural biology (PhD). *Degree requirements:* For doctorate, thesis/dissertation. *Entrance requirements:* Additional exam requirements/recommendations for international students: Required—TOEFL (minimum score 550 paper-based). Electronic applications accepted.

University of Wyoming, Graduate Program in Molecular and Cellular Life Sciences, Laramie, WY 82071. Offers PhD. *Degree requirements:* For doctorate, thesis/dissertation, four eight-week laboratory rotations, comprehensive basic practical exam, two-part qualifying exam, seminars, symposium.

Washington University in St. Louis, Graduate School of Arts and Sciences, Division of Biology and Biomedical Sciences, Program in Computational and Systems Biology, St. Louis, MO 63130-4899. Offers PhD. *Students:* 37 full-time (11 women); includes 11 minority (7 Asian, non-Hispanic/Latino; 4 Two or more races, non-Hispanic/Latino), 13 international. 71 applicants, 27% accepted, 5 enrolled. In 2015, 3 doctorates awarded. *Degree requirements:* For doctorate, thesis/dissertation. *Entrance requirements:* For doctorate, GRE General Test, GRE Subject Test. Additional exam requirements/recommendations for international students: Required—TOEFL. *Application deadline:* For fall admission, 12/1 for domestic students. Application fee: $0. Electronic applications accepted. *Financial support:* Fellowships, research assistantships, and teaching assistantships available. Financial award application deadline: 1/15. *Faculty research:* Systems biology, genomics, sequence analysis, regulatory networks, synthetic biology, metagenomics, metabolomics, proteomics, epigenomics, transcriptomics, lipidomics, single cell dynamics, high-throughput technology development, applied math and mathematical models of biological processes, computational biology, comparative genomics, personalized medicine, genome engineering, machine learning, big data science, next generation sequencing and its applications, bioinformatics. *Unit head:* Melanie Puhar, Coordinator, 314-362-2763, E-mail: puharm@dbbs.wustl.edu. *Application contact:* Jenny Larner, Admissions and Recruitment Coordinator, 800-852-9074, E-mail: admissions@dbbs.wustl.edu.
Website: http://dbbs.wustl.edu/divprograms/compbio/Pages/default.aspx

Wayne State University, College of Engineering, Department of Computer Science, Detroit, MI 48202. Offers computer science (MS, PhD), including bioinformatics (PhD), computational biology (PhD), computer science (PhD); scientific computing (Graduate Certificate). *Faculty:* 22. *Students:* 134 full-time (41 women), 55 part-time (21 women); includes 12 minority (2 Black or African American, non-Hispanic/Latino; 8 Asian, non-Hispanic/Latino; 1 Hispanic/Latino; 1 Two or more races, non-Hispanic/Latino), 154 international. Average age 27. 534 applicants, 36% accepted, 50 enrolled. In 2015, 70 master's, 10 doctorates awarded. *Degree requirements:* For master's, thesis (for some programs); for doctorate, thesis/dissertation. *Entrance requirements:* For master's, GRE, minimum GPA of 3.0, three letters of recommendation, adequate preparation in computer science and mathematics courses, personal statement; for doctorate, GRE, minimum GPA of 3.3 in most recent degree; three letters of recommendation; personal statement; adequate preparation in computer science and mathematics courses. Additional exam requirements/recommendations for international students: Required—TOEFL (minimum score 550 paper-based; 79 iBT), TWE (minimum score 5.5), Michigan English Language Assessment Battery (minimum score 85); Recommended—IELTS (minimum score 6.5). *Application deadline:* For fall admission, 6/1 priority date for domestic students, 5/1 priority date for international students; for winter admission, 10/1 priority date for domestic students, 9/1 priority date for international students; for spring admission, 2/1 priority date for domestic students, 1/2 priority date for international students. Applications are processed on a rolling basis. Application fee: $0. Electronic applications accepted. *Expenses:* $16,444 annual resident tuition, $32,915 non-resident tuition; $685 per credit hour resident tuition, $1,371.45 per credit hour non-resident tuition; fees include $47.45 per credit hour student services fee and $274.60 per semester registration fee. *Financial support:* In 2015–16, 80 students received support, including 5 fellowships with tuition reimbursements available (averaging $16,000 per year), 29 research assistantships with tuition reimbursements available (averaging $20,065 per year), 33 teaching assistantships with tuition reimbursements available (averaging $19,058 per year); scholarships/grants, health care benefits, and unspecified assistantships also available. Financial award application deadline: 3/31; financial award applicants required to submit FAFSA. *Faculty research:* Software engineering, databases, bioinformatics, artificial intelligence, networking, distributed and parallel computing, security, graphics, visualizations. *Total annual research expenditures:* $1.8 million. *Unit head:* Dr. Loren Schwiebert, Interim Chair, 313-577-5474, E-mail: loren@cs.wayne.edu. *Application contact:* Nathan Fisher, Graduate Program Director, E-mail: csgradadvisor@cs.wayne.edu.
Website: http://engineering.wayne.edu/cs/

Weill Cornell Medicine, Weill Cornell Graduate School of Medical Sciences, Cornell/Weill Cornell/Sloan Kettering Tri-Institutional PhD Program in Computational Biology and Medicine, New York, NY 10065. Offers PhD. Terminal master's awarded for partial completion of doctoral program. *Degree requirements:* For doctorate, comprehensive exam, thesis/dissertation. *Entrance requirements:* For doctorate, GRE General Test, three letters of recommendation. Additional exam requirements/recommendations for international students: Required—TOEFL. Electronic applications accepted. *Faculty research:* Computational genomics and gene regulation, quantitative and systems biology, cancer biology and genomics, structural biology and biophysics, computational neuroscience.

Worcester Polytechnic Institute, Graduate Studies and Research, Program in Bioinformatics and Computational Biology, Worcester, MA 01609-2280. Offers MS, PhD. *Program availability:* Evening/weekend. *Students:* 8 full-time (4 women), 2 international. 14 applicants, 86% accepted, 5 enrolled. In 2015, 2 master's awarded. *Entrance requirements:* For master's and doctorate, GRE, 3 letters of recommendation, statement of purpose. Additional exam requirements/recommendations for international students: Required—TOEFL (minimum score 563 paper-based; 84 iBT), IELTS (minimum score 7). *Application deadline:* For fall admission, 1/1 priority date for domestic and international students; for spring admission, 10/1 priority date for domestic and international students. Applications are processed on a rolling basis. Application

fee: $70. Electronic applications accepted. *Financial support:* Research assistantships, teaching assistantships, and career-related internships or fieldwork available. Financial award application deadline: 1/1; financial award applicants required to submit FAFSA. *Unit head:* Elizabeth Ryder, Professor, 508-831-5543, Fax: 508-831-5936, E-mail: ryder@wpi.edu. *Application contact:* Jenny McGarty, Administrative Assistant, 508-831-5543, Fax: 508-831-5936, E-mail: jrmcgourty@wpi.edu.
Website: http://www.wpi.edu/academics/bcb

Yale University, School of Medicine and Graduate School of Arts and Sciences, Combined Program in Biological and Biomedical Sciences (BBS), Computational Biology and Bioinformatics Track, New Haven, CT 06520. Offers PhD, MD/PhD. *Entrance requirements:* Additional exam requirements/recommendations for international students: Required—TOEFL.

Systems Biology

Albert Einstein College of Medicine, Graduate Division of Biomedical Sciences, Systems and Computational Biology Program, Bronx, NY 10461. Offers PhD.

The George Washington University, Columbian College of Arts and Sciences, Institute for Biomedical Sciences, Program in Biochemistry and Systems Biology, Washington, DC 20037. Offers PhD. *Students:* 5 full-time (2 women), 8 part-time (3 women); includes 5 minority (3 Asian, non-Hispanic/Latino; 1 Hispanic/Latino; 1 Two or more races, non-Hispanic/Latino), 3 international. Average age 32. Terminal master's awarded for partial completion of doctoral program. *Degree requirements:* For doctorate, thesis/dissertation, general exam. *Entrance requirements:* For doctorate, GRE General Test, interview, minimum GPA of 3.0. Additional exam requirements/recommendations for international students: Required—TOEFL (minimum score 600 paper-based). *Application deadline:* For fall admission, 12/15 priority date for domestic and international students; for spring admission, 10/1 priority date for domestic and international students. Applications are processed on a rolling basis. Application fee: $75. Electronic applications accepted. *Financial support:* In 2015–16, 3 students received support. Fellowships, Federal Work-Study, institutionally sponsored loans, and tuition waivers available. Financial award application deadline: 2/1. *Unit head:* Dr. Eric Hoffman, Director, 202-476-6029, E-mail: ehoffman@cnmcresearch.org. *Application contact:* Information Contact, 202-994-7120, Fax: 202-994-6100, E-mail: genetics@gwu.edu.
Website: http://smhs.gwu.edu/

Harvard University, Graduate School of Arts and Sciences, Department of Systems Biology, Cambridge, MA 02138. Offers PhD. *Degree requirements:* For doctorate, thesis/dissertation, lab rotation, qualifying examination. *Entrance requirements:* For doctorate, GRE. Additional exam requirements/recommendations for international students: Required—TOEFL. Electronic applications accepted.

Massachusetts Institute of Technology, School of Engineering and School of Science, Program in Computational and Systems Biology, Cambridge, MA 02139-4307. Offers PhD. *Degree requirements:* For doctorate, comprehensive exam, thesis/dissertation, teaching assistantship during one semester; training in the ethical conduct of research. *Entrance requirements:* For doctorate, GRE General Test. Additional exam requirements/recommendations for international students: Required—TOEFL (minimum score 600 paper-based; 95 iBT), IELTS (minimum score 6). Electronic applications accepted. *Expenses: Tuition:* Full-time $46,400; part-time $725 per credit. One-time fee: $304 full-time. Full-time tuition and fees vary according to course load and program. *Faculty research:* Computational biology and bioinformatics, biological design and synthetic biology, gene and protein networks, systems biology of cancer, nanobiology and microsystems.

Michigan State University, The Graduate School, College of Natural Science, Quantitative Biology Program, East Lansing, MI 48824. Offers PhD.

Northwestern University, The Graduate School, Interdisciplinary Biological Sciences Program (IBiS), Evanston, IL 60208. Offers biochemistry (PhD); bioengineering and biotechnology (PhD); biotechnology (PhD); cell and molecular biology (PhD); developmental and systems biology (PhD); nanotechnology (PhD); neurobiology (PhD); structural biology and biophysics (PhD). *Degree requirements:* For doctorate, thesis/dissertation, qualifying exam. *Entrance requirements:* For doctorate, GRE General Test. Additional exam requirements/recommendations for international students: Required—TOEFL (minimum score 600 paper-based). Electronic applications accepted. *Faculty research:* Biophysics/structural biology, cell/molecular biology, synthetic biology, developmental systems biology, chemical biology/nanotechnology.

Purdue University, College of Pharmacy and Pharmacal Sciences and Graduate School, Graduate Programs in Pharmacy and Pharmacal Sciences, Department of Medicinal Chemistry and Molecular Pharmacology, West Lafayette, IN 47907. Offers biophysical and computational chemistry (PhD); cancer research (PhD); immunology and infectious disease (PhD); medicinal biochemistry and molecular biology (PhD); medicinal chemistry and chemical biology (PhD); molecular pharmacology (PhD); neuropharmacology, neurodegeneration, and neurotoxicity (PhD); systems biology and functional genomics (PhD). *Degree requirements:* For doctorate, thesis/dissertation. *Entrance requirements:* For doctorate, GRE General Test; GRE Subject Test in biology, biochemistry, and chemistry (recommended), minimum undergraduate GPA of 3.0. Additional exam requirements/recommendations for international students: Required—TOEFL (minimum score 550 paper-based; 77 iBT); Recommended—TWE. Electronic applications accepted. *Faculty research:* Drug design and development, cancer research, drug synthesis and analysis, chemical pharmacology, environmental toxicology.

Rutgers University–New Brunswick, Graduate School-New Brunswick, BioMaPS Institute for Quantitative Biology, Piscataway, NJ 08854-8097. Offers computational biology and molecular biophysics (PhD). *Degree requirements:* For doctorate, comprehensive exam, thesis/dissertation. *Entrance requirements:* For doctorate, GRE. Additional exam requirements/recommendations for international students: Required—TOEFL. Electronic applications accepted. *Faculty research:* Structural biology, systems biology, bioinformatics, translational medicine, genomics.

Stanford University, School of Medicine, Graduate Programs in Medicine, Department of Chemical and Systems Biology, Stanford, CA 94305-9991. Offers PhD. *Degree requirements:* For doctorate, thesis/dissertation, qualifying examination. *Entrance requirements:* For doctorate, GRE General Test, GRE Subject Test. Additional exam requirements/recommendations for international students: Required—TOEFL. Electronic applications accepted. *Expenses: Tuition, area resident:* Full-time $45,729. *Required fees:* $591. *Faculty research:* Action of drugs such as epinephrine, cell differentiation and development, microsomal enzymes, neuropeptide gene expression.

University of California, Irvine, Francisco J. Ayala School of Biological Sciences, Program in Mathematical, Computational and Systems Biology, Irvine, CA 92697. Offers PhD. *Students:* 13 full-time (3 women); includes 6 minority (3 Asian, non-Hispanic/Latino; 2 Hispanic/Latino; 1 Two or more races, non-Hispanic/Latino), 1 international. Average age 24. 77 applicants, 32% accepted, 8 enrolled. Application fee: $90 ($110 for international students). *Unit head:* Prof. John Lowengrub, Director, 949-824-8456, Fax: 949-824-7993, E-mail: jlowengr@uci.edu. *Application contact:* Aracely Dean, Assistant Administrative Analyst, 949-824-4120, Fax: 949-824-6444, E-mail: mcsb@uci.edu.
Website: http://mcsb.bio.uci.edu/

University of California, Merced, Graduate Division, School of Natural Sciences, Merced, CA 95343. Offers applied mathematics (MS, PhD); chemistry and chemical biology (MS, PhD); physics (MS, PhD); quantitative and systems biology (MS, PhD). *Faculty:* 63 full-time (25 women). *Students:* 156 full-time (64 women); includes 58 minority (3 Black or African American, non-Hispanic/Latino; 23 Asian, non-Hispanic/Latino; 22 Hispanic/Latino; 1 Native Hawaiian or other Pacific Islander, non-Hispanic/Latino; 9 Two or more races, non-Hispanic/Latino), 37 international. Average age 27. 199 applicants, 57% accepted, 45 enrolled. In 2015, 12 master's, 11 doctorates awarded. Terminal master's awarded for partial completion of doctoral program. *Degree requirements:* For master's, variable foreign language requirement, comprehensive exam, thesis or alternative; for doctorate, variable foreign language requirement, comprehensive exam, thesis/dissertation. *Entrance requirements:* For master's and doctorate, GRE. Additional exam requirements/recommendations for international students: Required—TOEFL (minimum score 550 paper-based; 80 iBT); Recommended—IELTS (minimum score 7). *Application deadline:* For fall admission, 1/15 for domestic and international students. Application fee: $90 ($110 for international students). Electronic applications accepted. *Expenses:* $11,220 per year resident tuition, $15,102 per year non-resident tuition. *Financial support:* In 2015–16, 151 students received support, including 12 fellowships with full tuition reimbursements available (averaging $23,614 per year), 37 research assistantships with full tuition reimbursements available (averaging $18,842 per year), 127 teaching assistantships with full tuition reimbursements available (averaging $18,538 per year); scholarships/grants, traineeships, and health care benefits also available. Financial award application deadline: 1/15. *Faculty research:* Computational science, soft matter physics, neurobiology, genomics, biochemistry. *Total annual research expenditures:* $5.3 million. *Unit head:* Dr. Juan C. Meza, Dean, 209-228-4487, Fax: 209-228-4060, E-mail: jcmeza@ucmerced.edu. *Application contact:* Tsu Ya, Director of Graduate Admissions and Academic Services, 209-228-4521, Fax: 209-228-6906, E-mail: tya@ucmerced.edu.

★ **University of California, San Diego,** Graduate Division, Program in Bioinformatics and Systems Biology, La Jolla, CA 92093. Offers biomedical informatics (PhD). *Students:* 62 full-time (16 women), 2 part-time (0 women); includes 19 minority (1 Black or African American, non-Hispanic/Latino; 18 Asian, non-Hispanic/Latino), 13 international. 217 applicants, 13% accepted, 11 enrolled. In 2015, 11 doctorates awarded. *Degree requirements:* For doctorate, comprehensive exam, thesis/dissertation. *Entrance requirements:* For doctorate, GRE General Test. Additional exam requirements/recommendations for international students: Required—TOEFL (minimum score 550 paper-based; 80 iBT), IELTS (minimum score 7). *Application deadline:* For fall admission, 12/14 for domestic students. Application fee: $90 ($110 for international students). Electronic applications accepted. *Expenses: Tuition,* state resident: full-time $11,220. *Tuition, nonresident:* full-time $26,322. *Required fees:* $1800. *Financial support:* Fellowships, research assistantships, teaching assistantships, scholarships/grants, and traineeships available. Financial award applicants required to submit FAFSA. *Faculty research:* Quantitative foundations of computational biology, structural bioinformatics and systems pharmacology, proteomics and metabolomics, epigenomics and gene expression control, genetic and molecular networks. *Unit head:* Vineet Bafna, Chair, 858-822-4978, E-mail: vbafna@ucsd.edu. *Application contact:* Begum Asena, Graduate Coordinator, 858-822-4948, E-mail: bioinfo@ucsd.edu.
Website: http://bioinformatics.ucsd.edu/

See Display on next page and Close-Up on page 241.

University of Chicago, Division of the Biological Sciences, Committee on Genetics, Genomics and Systems Biology, Chicago, IL 60637. Offers PhD. *Students:* 27 full-time (11 women); includes 7 minority (1 Black or African American, non-Hispanic/Latino; 4 Asian, non-Hispanic/Latino; 1 Hispanic/Latino; 1 Native Hawaiian or other Pacific Islander, non-Hispanic/Latino), 6 international. Average age 28. 71 applicants, 18% accepted, 4 enrolled. In 2015, 4 doctorates awarded. *Degree requirements:* For doctorate, thesis/dissertation, ethics class, 2 teaching assistantships. *Entrance requirements:* For doctorate, GRE General Test. Additional exam requirements/recommendations for international students: Required—TOEFL (minimum score 600 paper-based; 104 iBT), IELTS (minimum score 7). *Application deadline:* For fall admission, 12/1 for domestic and international students. Application fee: $90. Electronic applications accepted. *Financial support:* In 2015–16, 21 students received support, including fellowships with tuition reimbursements available (averaging $29,781 per year), research assistantships with tuition reimbursements available (averaging $29,781 per year); institutionally sponsored loans, scholarships/grants, traineeships, and health care benefits also available. Financial award applicants required to submit FAFSA. *Faculty research:* Molecular genetics, developmental genetics, population genetics, human genetics. *Application contact:* Sue Levison, Administrator, 773-702-2464, Fax: 773-702-3172, E-mail: committee-on-genetics@uchicago.edu.
Website: http://cg.bsd.uchicago.edu/

University of Pittsburgh, School of Medicine, Graduate Programs in Medicine, Computational Biology Program, Pittsburgh, PA 15260. Offers PhD. Program jointly offered with Carnegie Mellon University. *Faculty:* 21 full-time (4 women), 68 part-time/adjunct (16 women). *Students:* 24 full-time (10 women); includes 2 minority (both Hispanic/Latino), 11 international. Average age 28. 141 applicants, 26% accepted, 11 enrolled. In 2015, 12 doctorates awarded. Terminal master's awarded for partial completion of doctoral program. *Degree requirements:* For doctorate, comprehensive exam, thesis/dissertation, ethics training service as course assistant, seminar. *Entrance requirements:* For doctorate, GRE Subject Test (recommended), GRE General Test, 3 letters of recommendation, resume. Additional exam requirements/recommendations for international students: Required—TOEFL (minimum score 600 paper-based; 100 iBT),

Systems Biology

IELTS (minimum score 7). *Application deadline:* For fall admission, 12/15 priority date for domestic and international students. Application fee: $75. Electronic applications accepted. Tuition and fees vary according to program. *Financial support:* In 2015–16, 24 students received support, including 7 fellowships with full tuition reimbursements available (averaging $27,000 per year), 17 research assistantships with full tuition reimbursements available (averaging $27,000 per year); teaching assistantships, scholarships/grants, traineeships, and health care benefits also available. *Faculty research:* Computational structural biology, computational genomics, cellular and systems modeling, bioimage informatics, mathematical biology. *Total annual research expenditures:* $6.3 million. *Unit head:* Dr. Daniel M. Zuckerman, Director, 412-648-3335, Fax: 412-648-3163, E-mail: ddmmzz@pitt.edu. *Application contact:* Kelly Gentille, Educational Programs Administrator, 412-648-8107, Fax: 412-648-3163, E-mail: kmg120@pitt.edu.
Website: http://www.compbio.pitt.edu/

University of Pittsburgh, School of Medicine and Dietrich School of Arts and Sciences, integrative Systems Biology Graduate Program, Pittsburgh, PA 15260. Offers PhD. *Faculty:* 48 full-time (8 women). *Students:* 8 full-time (3 women); includes 5 minority (all Black or African American, non-Hispanic/Latino), 2 international. Average age 24. 39 applicants, 10% accepted, 4 enrolled. In 2015, 2 doctorates awarded. *Degree requirements:* For doctorate, comprehensive exam, thesis/dissertation. *Entrance requirements:* For doctorate, GRE, minimum GPA of 3.7, 3 letters of reference. Additional exam requirements/recommendations for international students: Required—TOEFL (minimum score 650 paper-based; 114 iBT), IELTS (minimum score 7.5). *Application deadline:* For fall admission, 1/1 priority date for domestic and international students. Application fee: $50. Electronic applications accepted. Tuition and fees vary according to program. *Financial support:* In 2015–16, 8 students received support, including fellowships with full tuition reimbursements available (averaging $27,000 per year), 8 research assistantships with full tuition reimbursements available (averaging $27,000 per year); teaching assistantships, scholarships/grants, traineeships, and health care benefits also available. *Faculty research:* Cellular, molecular, developmental biology; genomics; proteomics and gene function. *Unit head:* Dr. Neil Hukriede, Program Director, 412-648-9918, E-mail: hukriede@pitt.edu. *Application contact:* Shari Murphy, Program Coordinator, 412-692-9907, E-mail: sas101@pitt.edu.
Website: http://www.pimb.pitt.edu

University of Toronto, School of Graduate Studies, Faculty of Arts and Science, Department of Cell and Systems Biology, Toronto, ON M5S 1A1, Canada. Offers M Sc, PhD. *Degree requirements:* For master's, thesis, thesis defense; for doctorate, thesis/dissertation, thesis defense, oral thesis examination. *Entrance requirements:* For master's, minimum B+ average in final year, B overall, 3 letters of reference. Additional exam requirements/recommendations for international students: Required—TOEFL

(minimum score 580 paper-based; 93 iBT), TWE (minimum score 5). Electronic applications accepted.

Virginia Commonwealth University, Graduate School, School of Life Sciences, Doctoral Program in Integrative Life Sciences, Richmond, VA 23284-9005. Offers PhD. *Entrance requirements:* For doctorate, GRE, minimum GPA of 60 credits of undergraduate work or in graduate degree, 3 letters of recommendation. Additional exam requirements/recommendations for international students: Required—TOEFL (minimum score 600 paper-based; 100 iBT). Electronic applications accepted.

Washington University in St. Louis, Graduate School of Arts and Sciences, Division of Biology and Biomedical Sciences, Program in Computational and Systems Biology, St. Louis, MO 63130-4899. Offers PhD. *Students:* 37 full-time (11 women); includes 11 minority (7 Asian, non-Hispanic/Latino; 4 Two or more races, non-Hispanic/Latino), 13 international. 71 applicants, 27% accepted, 5 enrolled. In 2015, 3 doctorates awarded. *Degree requirements:* For doctorate, thesis/dissertation. *Entrance requirements:* For doctorate, GRE General Test, GRE Subject Test. Additional exam requirements/recommendations for international students: Required—TOEFL. *Application deadline:* For fall admission, 12/1 for domestic students. Application fee: $0. Electronic applications accepted. *Financial support:* Fellowships, research assistantships, and teaching assistantships available. Financial award application deadline: 1/15. *Faculty research:* Systems biology, genomics, sequence analysis, regulatory networks, synthetic biology, metagenomics, metabolomics, proteomics, epigenomics, transcriptomics, lipidomics, single cell dynamics, high-throughput technology development, applied math and mathematical models of biological processes, computational biology, comparative genomics, personalized medicine, genome engineering, machine learning, big data science, next generation sequencing and its applications, bioinformatics. *Unit head:* Melanie Puhar, Coordinator, 314-362-2763, E-mail: puharm@dbbs.wustl.edu. *Application contact:* Jenny Lawler, Admissions and Recruitment Coordinator, 800-852-9074, E-mail: admissions@dbbs.wustl.edu.
Website: http://dbbs.wustl.edu/divprograms/compbio/Pages/default.aspx

Weill Cornell Medicine, Weill Cornell Graduate School of Medical Sciences, Physiology, Biophysics and Systems Biology Program, New York, NY 10065. Offers MS, PhD. Terminal master's awarded for partial completion of doctoral program. *Degree requirements:* For master's, comprehensive exam; for doctorate, thesis/dissertation, final exam. *Entrance requirements:* For doctorate, GRE General Test, introductory courses in biology, inorganic and organic chemistry, physics, and mathematics. Additional exam requirements/recommendations for international students: Required—TOEFL. *Faculty research:* Receptor-mediated regulation of cell function, molecular properties of channels or receptors, bioinformatics, mathematical modeling.

Translational Biology

Baylor College of Medicine, Graduate School of Biomedical Sciences, Program in Translational Biology and Molecular Medicine, Houston, TX 77030-3498. Offers PhD. *Degree requirements:* For doctorate, thesis/dissertation, public defense. *Entrance requirements:* For doctorate, GRE, minimum GPA of 3.0. Additional exam requirements/ recommendations for international students: Required—TOEFL. Electronic applications accepted. *Faculty research:* Molecular medicine, translational biology, human disease biology and therapy.

Cedars-Sinai Medical Center, Graduate Program in Biomedical Sciences and Translational Medicine, Los Angeles, CA 90048. Offers PhD. *Degree requirements:* For doctorate, comprehensive exam, thesis/dissertation. *Entrance requirements:* For doctorate, GRE, 3 letters of recommendation. Additional exam requirements/recommendations for international students: Required—TOEFL (minimum score 550 paper-based; 80 iBT), IELTS (minimum score 6.5). Electronic applications accepted. *Faculty research:* Immunology and infection, neuroscience, cardiovascular science, cancer, human genetics.

Rutgers University–New Brunswick, Graduate School of Biomedical Sciences, Program in Clinical and Translational Science, Piscataway, NJ 08854-8097. Offers MS. *Program availability:* Part-time. *Degree requirements:* For master's, thesis.

University of California, Irvine, School of Medicine, Program in Biomedical and Translational Science, Irvine, CA 92697. Offers MS. *Students:* 12 full-time (8 women), 1 part-time (0 women); includes 6 minority (1 Black or African American, non-Hispanic/Latino; 2 Asian, non-Hispanic/Latino; 3 Hispanic/Latino), 3 international. Average age 28. 38 applicants, 50% accepted, 11 enrolled. In 2015, 11 master's awarded. *Entrance requirements:* For master's, curriculum vitae. *Application deadline:* For fall admission, 1/15 priority date for domestic students. Application fee: $90 ($110 for international students). *Unit head:* Dr. Sherrie Kaplan, Director, 949-824-0095. Website: http://www.som.uci.edu/bats/education/ms-degree.asp

The University of Iowa, Graduate College, Program in Translational Biomedicine, Iowa City, IA 52242-1316. Offers MS, PhD. Terminal master's awarded for partial completion of doctoral program. *Degree requirements:* For master's, comprehensive exam; for doctorate, comprehensive exam, thesis/dissertation. *Entrance requirements:* For master's and doctorate, minimum GPA of 3.0. Additional exam requirements/recommendations for international students: Required—TOEFL (minimum score 550 paper-based; 81 iBT). Electronic applications accepted.

University of Massachusetts Medical School, Graduate School of Biomedical Sciences, Worcester, MA 01655-0115. Offers biomedical sciences (PhD), including biochemistry and molecular pharmacology, bioinformatics and computational biology, cancer biology, cell biology, immunology and microbiology, interdisciplinary, neuroscience, translational science; biomedical sciences (millennium program) (PhD); clinical and population health research (PhD); clinical investigation (MS). *Faculty:* 1,339 full-time (521 women), 301 part-time/adjunct (189 women). *Students:* 363 full-time (184 women); includes 58 minority (13 Black or African American, non-Hispanic/Latino; 30 Asian, non-Hispanic/Latino; 15 Hispanic/Latino), 141 international. Average age 29. 661 applicants, 26% accepted, 51 enrolled. In 2015, 10 master's, 58 doctorates awarded. Terminal master's awarded for partial completion of doctoral program. *Degree requirements:* For master's, comprehensive exam, thesis; for doctorate, comprehensive exam, thesis/dissertation. *Entrance requirements:* For master's, MD, PhD, DVM, or PharmD; for doctorate, GRE General Test, bachelor's degree. Additional exam requirements/recommendations for international students: Required—TOEFL (minimum score 100 iBT) or IELTS (minimum score 7.5). *Application deadline:* For fall admission, 12/15 for domestic and international students; for spring admission, 5/15 for domestic students. Application fee: $80. Electronic applications accepted. *Expenses:* $6,966 resident per year; $14,182 non-resident per year. *Financial support:* In 2015–16, 383 students received support, including research assistantships with full tuition reimbursements available (averaging $30,600 per year); scholarships/grants, health care benefits, tuition waivers (full), and unspecified assistantships also available. Financial award application deadline: 5/16. *Faculty research:* RNA interference, cell/molecular/developmental biology, bioinformatics, clinical/translational research, infectious disease. *Total annual research expenditures:* $250.3 million. *Unit head:* Dr. Anthony Carruthers, Dean, 508-856-4135, E-mail: anthony.carruthers@umassmed.edu. *Application contact:* Dr. Kendall Knight, Assistant Vice Provost for Admissions, 508-856-5628, Fax: 508-856-3659, E-mail: kendall.knight@umassmed.edu. Website: http://www.umassmed.edu/gsbs/

The University of Texas at San Antonio, Joint PhD Program in Translational Science, San Antonio, TX 78249-0617. Offers PhD. Program offered in partnership with The University of Texas Health Science Center at San Antonio, The University of Texas at Austin, and The University of Texas Health Science Center at Houston. *Program availability:* Part-time. *Degree requirements:* For doctorate, comprehensive exam, thesis/dissertation. *Entrance requirements:* For doctorate, GRE General Test, official transcripts, copy of U.S. medical license/certificate, criminal background check, resume or curriculum vitae, 3 letters of recommendation, statement of purpose. Additional exam requirements/recommendations for international students: Required—TOEFL (minimum score 565 paper-based; 86 iBT), IELTS (minimum score 6.5). *Application deadline:* For fall admission, 11/1 for domestic and international students. Application fee: $45 ($80 for international students). Electronic applications accepted. *Expenses:* Contact institution. *Financial support:* In 2015–16, 1 student received support, including 3 research assistantships (averaging $26,000 per year), 3 teaching assistantships (averaging $34,000 per year); scholarships/grants and unspecified assistantships also available. *Faculty research:* Community-acquired methicillin-resistant staphylococcus (CA-MRSA); epigenetic changes in cancer genomes; occupational injury and prevention; addiction science; inflammation, tissue injury, and regeneration. *Unit head:* Dr. Michael J. Lichtenstein, Program Director, 210-567-4304, Fax: 210-564-4301, E-mail: lichtenstei@uthscsa.edu. *Application contact:* Susan Stappenbeck, Senior Project Coordinator, 210-567-4304, Fax: 210-567-4301, E-mail: stappenbeck@uthscsa.edu.

UNIVERSITY OF CALIFORNIA, SAN DIEGO

Bioinformatics and Systems Biology Program

UC San Diego
Bioinformatics and Systems Biology

 For more information, visit http://petersons.to/uc-sandiego_bioinformatics

Program of Study

There is an enormous need for trained professionals who are experts in biology, biomedicine, and computing. The Bioinformatics and Systems Biology Graduate Program at University of California, San Diego (UCSD), founded in 2001 by Professor Shankar Subramaniam, addresses this need. It includes five schools and divisions on the UC San Diego campus: the Jacobs School of Engineering (bioengineering, computer science and engineering, and nanoengineering), the Division of Biological Sciences (molecular biology, cell and developmental biology, neurobiology, ecology/behavior/evolution), the Division of Physical Sciences (chemistry and biochemistry, physics, and mathematics), the School of Medicine, and the Skaggs School of Pharmacy and Pharmaceutical Sciences. The graduate program is supported by the respective schools, divisions, and departments as well as by a substantial NIH Training Grant and more than fifty associated faculty.

The Bioinformatics and Systems Biology Graduate Program is organized around two disciplinary tracks that have distinct, yet overlapping, faculty and curricular requirements: Bioinformatics and Systems Biology (BISB) and Biomedical Informatics (BMI). Students indicate their interest in one track, but are able to request a switch at any time during their study. For each track there are four required core courses (generally completed within the first year) and 16 units to be chosen from a list of elective fields to be completed within the first two years. The core curriculum ensures that every student within the program has the same knowledge basis in key areas of bioinformatics, systems biology, and biomedical informatics. The electives are intended to provide students with in-depth courses related to their own research interests.

In addition, students must also take the colloquium for their track; one of two ethics courses; the Research Rotation requirement; research units with their dissertation advisor after joining a lab; and two quarters as a teaching assistant.

Research Facilities

UC San Diego recently ranked fifth in the nation for annual federal research and development spending. The University excels in both traditional scholarly disciplines and fields that cross these disciplines, such as neuroscience, nanoscience, and climate science.

UC San Diego researchers consistently earn international acclaim. They include Nobel and Pulitzer prize winners, members of the National Academies, and recipients of MacArthur Foundation "genius grants."

The Jacobs School of Engineering ranks seventh in the nation and 23rd in the world according to a *U.S. News & World Report* best global universities ranking, published October 2015. With $162 million in federal, state, and industry research support in FY15, the Jacobs School of Engineering ranks ninth in the nation for research expenditures per faculty member (*U.S. News & World Report*, published March 2016), reflecting UC San Diego's leadership as a research university.

The UC San Diego Library, ranked among the nation's top public academic libraries, plays a critical role in advancing and supporting the university's research, teaching, patient care, and public service missions. The world-renowned research for which UC San Diego is known starts at the UC San Diego Library, which provides the foundation of knowledge needed to advance cutting-edge discoveries in a wide range of disciplines.

Financial Aid

All U.S. citizens and residents admitted into the Ph.D. program are supported by a financial support package to cover tuition and fees (determined by the Graduate Division), as well as a stipend (set by the program; $32,000 as of October 1, 2016) that covers living expenses, so long as they are in good academic standing with university and program requirements.

Living and Housing costs

UCSD has several options for on-campus living; additional details are available on the Associated Rental Community Housing (ARCH) website, http://hdh.ucsd.edu/arch/pages/. Those looking for off-campus housing can find more information at http://offcampushousing.ucsd.edu/.

Student Group

The University's diverse student population is drawn from the best and brightest worldwide. With over 500 student organizations, there is something for everyone. The Graduate Bioinformatics Council (GBIC) represents the students of the Bioinformatics and System Biology Ph.D. program.

Student Outcomes

There is enormous demand from academia, industry, and government for trained professionals in bioinformatics and biomedical informatics. A report from the Working Group on Data and Informatics to the NIH Advisory Committee to the Director recognized the shortage of biomedical scientists with appropriate computing expertise and called for strong NIH support of cross-disciplinary education and training. Academic institutions in health sciences, the healthcare industry, and government institutions are seeking highly skilled individuals who can manage and analyze large amounts of data, and who can connect discoveries at different biological scales (from molecular to individual to population levels).

Location

The university's main campus is located near the Pacific Ocean on 1,200 acres of coastal woodland in La Jolla, California. About a 25-minute drive to downtown, and hour trip to Tijuana, Mexico, UCSD is not far from any fun destination.

The University

The University of California, San Diego is a student-centered, research-focused, service-oriented public institution that provides opportunity for all. Recognized as one of the top 15 research universities worldwide, a culture of collaboration sparks discoveries that advance society and drive economic impact. UCSD is home to over 500 student organizations, and six colleges. UCSD sponsors 23 intercollegiate men's and women's sports at the NCAA Division II level. The Tritons compete primarily in California Collegiate Athletic Association, widely regarded as the premiere conference for D-II athletics.

Applying

Admission review will be on a competitive basis based on the applicants' undergraduate track record, Graduate Record Examination General Test (GRE) scores, and other scholastic achievements. Special attention will be given to the quantitative and analytical section scores of the GRE and the formal education in quantitative methods. The applications will be screened and evaluated by the Admissions Committee with input from program faculty. Applicants must apply online at https://gradapply.ucsd.edu/ and must submit a completed UC San Diego Application for Graduate Admission.

Correspondence and Information

Begum Asena
Bioinformatics and Systems Biology Graduate Coordinator
Powell-Focht Bioengineering Hall
University of California, San Diego
9500 Gilman Drive MC 0419
La Jolla, California 92093-0419
United States
Phone: 858-822-4948
E-mail: bioinfo@ucsd.edu
Website: http://bioinformatics.ucsd.edu

THE FACULTY AND THEIR RESEARCH

Bioinformatics and Systems Biology Research Areas
Ruben Abagyan, Professor, School of Pharmacy.
Vineet Bafna, Professor, Computer Science and Engineering, Graduate and Undergraduate, Program Director Bioinformatics.
Nuno Bandeira, Assistant Professor, Computer Science and Engineering.
Vikas Bansal, Assistant Professor, Pediatrics.
Steve Briggs, Professor, Biological Sciences.
Hannah Carter, Assistant Professor of Medicine, School of Medicine.
Pieter Dorrestein, Assistant Professor, School of Pharmacy.
Joseph Ecker, Professor, Biological Sciences.
Charles Elkan, Professor, Computer Science and Engineering.
Ronald M. Evans, Professor and Director, Salk Institute for Biological Studies.
Kelly Frazer, Professor, Pediatrics.
Yoav Freund, Professor, Computer Science and Engineering.
Terry Gaasterland, Professor and Director of Scripps Genome Center, Marine Biology Research Division.
Kyle Gaulton, Assistant Professor, Pediatrics.
Michael Gilson, Professor, School of Pharmacy.
Christopher Glass, Professor, Cellular and Molecular Medicine.
Joseph Gleeson, Professor/HHMI Investigator, Neurosciences (School of Medicine).
Lawrence Goldstein, Professor, Cellular and Molecular Medicine.
Nan Hao, Assistant Professor, Biological Sciences.
Jeff Hasty, Associate Professor, Biological Sciences.

University of California, San Diego

Michael Holst, Professor, Mathematics.
Vivian Hook, Professor, School of Pharmacy.
Xiaohua Huang, Assistant Professor, Bioengineering.
Terence Hwa, Professor, Physics Professor, Biological Sciences.
Lilia Iakoucheva, Associate Professor, Psychiatry.
Trey Ideker, Professor, School of Medicine.
Suckjoon Jun, Assistant Professor, Physics Assistant Professor, Biological Sciences.
Amy Kiger, Assistant Professor, Biological Sciences.
Rob Knight, Professor, Pediatrics.
Richard Kolodner, Professor, School of Medicine.
Julie Law, Assistant Professor, Salk Institute for Biological Studies.
Nathan E. Lewis, Assistant Professor, Pediatrics.
Prashant Mali, Assistant Professor, Bioengineering.
Andrew McCammon, Professor, Chemistry and Biochemistry.
Andrew McCulloch, Professor, Bioengineering.
Graham McVicker, Assistant Professor, Salk Institute for Biological Studies.
Jill Mesirov, Professor, School of Medicine Associate Vice Chancellor, Computational Health Sciences, Professor of Medicine, Division of Medical Genetics.
Christian Metallo, Assistant Professor, Bioengineering.
Siavash Mirarab, Assistant Professor, Electrical and Computer Engineering.
Eran Mukamel, Assistant Professor, Cognitive Science.
Saket Navlakha, Assistant Professor, Salk Institute for Biological Studies.
Lucila Ohno-Machado, Professor, Division of Biomedical Informatics.
Bernhard Palsson, Professor, Bioengineering.
Pavel Pevzner, Professor and Ronald R Taylor Chair, Computer Science and Engineering.
Anjana Rao, Adjunct Professor, Pharmacology.
Bing Ren, Professor, Cellular and Molecular Medicine Graduate Program Associate Director, Bioinformatics.
Doug Richman, Professor, Pathology.
Scott Rifkin, Assistant Professor, Biological Sciences.
Michael Rosenfeld, Professor, School of Medicine.
Debashis Sahoo, Assistant Professor, Pediatrics.
Nicholas Schork, Professor, Scripps Research Institute.
Julian Schroeder, Professor, Biological Sciences.
Dorothy Sears, Associate Professor, School of Medicine.
Jonathan Sebat, Chief, Beyster Center for Molecular Genomics of Neuropsychiatric Diseases; Associate Professor of Psychiatry and Cellular & Molecular Medicine, Cellular and Molecular Medicine.
Shankar Subramaniam, Professor, Bioengineering.
Gurol Suel, Associate Professor, Biological Sciences.
Palmer Taylor, Professor and Dean, School of Pharmacy.
Susan Taylor, Professor, Chemistry and Biochemistry.
Glenn Tesler Associate Professor, Mathematics.
Roger Tsien, Professor, Pharmacology.
Inder Verma, Adjunct Professor, Biological Sciences.
Yingxiao (Peter) Wang, Associate Professor, Bioengineering.
Wei Wang, Professor, Chemistry and Biochemistry.
Joel Wertheim, Assistant Professor of Medicine, Division of Infectious Diseases, School of Medicine.
Ruth Williams, Professor, Mathematics.
Christopher Woelk, Assistant Professor; Dir., Genomics Core, CFAR, School of Medicine.
Roy Wollman, Assistant Professor, Chemistry and Biochemistry.
Ronghui (Lily) Xu, Professor, Mathematics.
Gene Yeo, Professor, Cellular and Molecular Medicine.
Kun Zhang, Associate Professor, Bioengineering.
Sheng Zhong, Associate Professor, Bioengineering.

Biomedical Informatics Research Areas

Predictive Modeling and Personalized Medicine
Olivier Harismendy
Chun-Nan Hsu
Lucila Ohno-Machado
Gene Yeo

Privacy Technology, Data Sharing, and Big Data Analytics
Charles Elkan
Yoav Freundm
Lucila Ohno-Machado
Staal Vinterbo
Gene Yeo
Data Models and Knowledge Representation
Chun-Nan Hsu
Hyeon-eui Kim

Decision Support Systems
Robert El-Kareh

Biomedical Natural Language Processing
Charles ElkanChun-Nan Hsu

Bioinformatics Applications in Human Disease
Olivier Harismendy
Lilia Iakoucheva
Dorothy Sears
Christopher Woelk
Gene Yeo, Professor
Jason Young, Assistant Professor

Section 8
Ecology, Environmental Biology, and Evolutionary Biology

This section contains a directory of institutions offering graduate work in ecology, environmental biology, and evolutionary biology. Additional information about programs listed in the directory may be obtained by writing directly to the dean of a graduate school or chair of a department at the address given in the directory.

For programs offering related work, see also in this book *Biological and Biomedical Sciences; Botany and Plant Biology; Entomology; Genetics, Developmental Biology, and Reproductive Biology; Microbiological Sciences; Pharmacology and Toxicology; Public Health;* and *Zoology.* In the other guides in this series:

Graduate Programs in the Humanities, Arts & Social Sciences
See *Sociology, Anthropology, and Archaeology*
Graduate Programs in the Physical Sciences, Mathematics, Agricultural Sciences, the Environment & Natural Resources
See *Agricultural and Food Sciences, Geosciences, Marine Sciences and Oceanography,* and *Mathematical Sciences*
Graduate Programs in Engineering & Applied Sciences
See *Civil and Environmental Engineering, Management of Engineering and Technology,* and *Ocean Engineering*

CONTENTS

Program Directories

Conservation Biology

Antioch University New England, Graduate School, Department of Environmental Studies, Program in Conservation Biology, Keene, NH 03431-3552. Offers MS. *Degree requirements:* For master's, thesis or project. *Entrance requirements:* For master's, resume, 3 letters of recommendation. Additional exam requirements/recommendations for international students: Required—TOEFL (minimum score 550 paper-based). Electronic applications accepted.

Arizona State University at the Tempe campus, College of Liberal Arts and Sciences, School of Life Sciences, Tempe, AZ 85287-4601. Offers animal behavior (PhD); applied ethics (biomedical and health ethics) (MA); biology (MS, PhD), including biology, biology and society, complex adaptive systems science (PhD), plant biology and conservation (MS); environmental life sciences (PhD); evolutionary biology (PhD); history and philosophy of science (PhD); human and social dimensions of science and technology (PhD); microbiology (PhD); molecular and cellular biology (PhD); neuroscience (PhD). Terminal master's awarded for partial completion of doctoral program. *Degree requirements:* For master's, thesis (for some programs), interactive Program of Study (iPOS) submitted before completing 50 percent of required credit hours; for doctorate, variable foreign language requirement, comprehensive exam, thesis/dissertation, interactive Program of Study (iPOS) submitted before completing 50 percent of required credit hours. *Entrance requirements:* For master's and doctorate, GRE, minimum GPA of 3.0 or equivalent in last 2 years of work leading to bachelor's degree. Additional exam requirements/recommendations for international students: Required—TOEFL (minimum score 600 paper-based; 100 iBT). Electronic applications accepted.

California State University, Sacramento, Office of Graduate Studies, College of Natural Sciences and Mathematics, Department of Biological Sciences, Sacramento, CA 95819. Offers biological conservation (MS); molecular and cellular biology (MS); stem cell (MS). *Program availability:* Part-time. *Degree requirements:* For master's, thesis, writing proficiency exam. *Entrance requirements:* For master's, GRE, bachelor's degree in biology or equivalent; minimum GPA of 3.0 in biology, 2.75 overall during last 2 years of course work. Additional exam requirements/recommendations for international students: Required—TOEFL. Electronic applications accepted.

California State University, Stanislaus, College of Natural Sciences, Program in Ecology and Sustainability (MS), Turlock, CA 95382. Offers ecological conservation (MS); ecological economics (MS). *Program availability:* Part-time. *Degree requirements:* For master's, thesis. *Entrance requirements:* For master's, GRE, minimum GPA of 3.0, 3 letters of recommendation, personal statement. Additional exam requirements/recommendations for international students: Required—TOEFL (minimum score 550 paper-based). Electronic applications accepted.

Central Michigan University, College of Graduate Studies, College of Science and Technology, Department of Biology, Mount Pleasant, MI 48859. Offers biology (MS); conservation biology (MS). *Program availability:* Part-time. *Degree requirements:* For master's, thesis or alternative. *Entrance requirements:* For master's, GRE, bachelor's degree with a major in biological science, minimum GPA of 3.0. Electronic applications accepted. *Faculty research:* Conservation biology, morphology and taxonomy of aquatic plants, molecular biology and genetics, microbials and invertebrate ecology, vertebrates.

Colorado State University, Warner College of Natural Resources, Department of Fish, Wildlife, and Conservation Biology, Fort Collins, CO 80523-1474. Offers MFWCB, MS, PhD. *Program availability:* Part-time, blended/hybrid learning. *Faculty:* 12 full-time (2 women), 3 part-time/adjunct (1 woman). *Students:* 8 full-time (5 women), 18 part-time (6 women); includes 2 minority (1 Hispanic/Latino; 1 Two or more races, non-Hispanic/Latino). Average age 29. 5 applicants, 20% accepted, 1 enrolled. In 2015, 7 master's, 2 doctorates awarded. Terminal master's awarded for partial completion of doctoral program. *Degree requirements:* For master's, comprehensive exam, thesis; for doctorate, comprehensive exam, thesis/dissertation. *Entrance requirements:* For master's, GRE General Test (minimum 70th percentile), minimum GPA of 3.0, BA or BS in related field, letters of recommendation, resume, transcripts; for doctorate, GRE General Test (minimum 70th percentile), minimum GPA of 3.0, MS in related field, letters of recommendation, resume, transcripts. Additional exam requirements/recommendations for international students: Required—TOEFL (minimum score 550 paper-based; 80 iBT), IELTS (minimum score 6.5). *Application deadline:* For fall admission, 2/1 for domestic and international students. Applications are processed on a rolling basis. Application fee: $60 ($70 for international students). Electronic applications accepted. *Expenses:* Tuition, state resident: full-time $9348. Tuition, nonresident: full-time $22,916. *Required fees:* $2174; $473.72 per credit hour. $236.86 per semester. Tuition and fees vary according to course load and program. *Financial support:* In 2015–16, 26 students received support, including 8 fellowships with tuition reimbursements available (averaging $49,625 per year), 8 research assistantships with tuition reimbursements available (averaging $25,168 per year), 6 teaching assistantships with tuition reimbursements available (averaging $14,123 per year); career-related internships or fieldwork, scholarships/grants, tuition waivers (full and partial), and unspecified assistantships also available. Financial award application deadline: 2/15; financial award applicants required to submit FAFSA. *Faculty research:* Quantitative, spatio-temporal ecological methods applied to management; behavioral ecology; aquatic, avian, wildlife ecology; management and protection of biodiverse populations; fish ecology, physiology, dynamics. *Total annual research expenditures:* $3.4 million. *Unit head:* Dr. Kenneth R. Wilson, Professor/Department Head, 970-491-5020, Fax: 970-491-5091, E-mail: kenneth.wilson@colostate.edu. *Application contact:* Joyce Pratt, Assistant to Department Head, 970-491-5020, Fax: 970-491-5091, E-mail: joyce.pratt@colostate.edu.
Website: http://warnercnr.colostate.edu/fwcb-home/

Columbia University, Graduate School of Arts and Sciences, New York, NY 10027. Offers African-American studies (MA); American studies (MA); anthropology (MA, PhD); art history and archaeology (MA, PhD); astronomy (PhD); biological sciences (PhD); biotechnology (MA); chemical physics (PhD); chemistry (PhD); classical studies (MA, PhD); classics (MA, PhD); climate and society (MA); conservation biology (MA); earth and environmental sciences (PhD); East Asia: regional studies (MA); East Asian languages and cultures (MA, PhD); ecology, evolution and environmental biology (MA), including conservation biology; ecology, evolution, and environmental biology (PhD), including ecology and evolutionary biology, evolutionary primatology; economics (MA, PhD); English and comparative literature (MA, PhD); French and Romance philology (MA, PhD); Germanic languages (MA, PhD); global French studies (MA); global thought (MA); Hispanic cultural studies (MA); history (PhD); history and literature (MA); human rights studies (MA); Islamic studies (MA); Italian (MA, PhD); Japanese pedagogy (MA); Jewish studies (MA); Latin America and the Caribbean: regional studies (MA); Latin American and Iberian cultures (PhD); mathematics (MA, PhD), including finance (MA); medieval and Renaissance studies (MA); Middle Eastern, South Asian, and African studies (MA, PhD); modern art: critical and curatorial studies (MA); modern European

studies (MA); museum anthropology (MA); music (DMA, PhD); oral history (MA); philosophical foundations of physics (MA); philosophy (MA, PhD); physics (PhD); political science (MA, PhD); psychology (PhD); quantitative methods in the social sciences (MA); religion (MA, PhD); Russia, Eurasia and East Europe: regional studies (MA); Russian translation (MA); Slavic cultures (MA); Slavic languages (MA, PhD); sociology (MA, PhD); South Asian studies (MA); statistics (MA, PhD); theatre (PhD). Dual-degree programs require admission to both Graduate School of Arts and Sciences and another Columbia school. *Program availability:* Part-time. *Students:* 3,030 full-time, 235 part-time; includes 861 minority (88 Black or African American, non-Hispanic/Latino; 5 American Indian or Alaska Native, non-Hispanic/Latino; 517 Asian, non-Hispanic/Latino; 159 Hispanic/Latino; 4 Native Hawaiian or other Pacific Islander, non-Hispanic/Latino; 88 Two or more races, non-Hispanic/Latino), 1,697 international. 13,288 applicants, 21% accepted, 1162 enrolled. In 2015, 1,061 master's, 553 doctorates awarded. Terminal master's awarded for partial completion of doctoral program. *Degree requirements:* For master's, variable foreign language requirement, comprehensive exam (for some programs), thesis (for some programs); for doctorate, variable foreign language requirement, comprehensive exam (for some programs), thesis/dissertation. *Entrance requirements:* For master's and doctorate, GRE General Test, GRE Subject Test (for some programs). Additional exam requirements/recommendations for international students: Required—TOEFL, IELTS. Application fee: $105. Electronic applications accepted. *Financial support:* Fellowships, research assistantships, teaching assistantships, career-related internships or fieldwork, Federal Work-Study, institutionally sponsored loans, scholarships/grants, traineeships, health care benefits, tuition waivers, and unspecified assistantships available. Support available to part-time students. Financial award application deadline: 12/15. *Unit head:* Carlos J. Alonso, Dean of the Graduate School of Arts and Sciences, 212-854-5177. *Application contact:* GSAS Office of Admissions, 212-854-8903, E-mail: gsas-admissions@columbia.edu.
Website: http://gsas.columbia.edu/

Cornell University, Graduate School, Graduate Fields of Agriculture and Life Sciences, Field of Natural Resources, Ithaca, NY 14853-0001. Offers community-based natural resources management (MS, PhD); conservation biology (MS, PhD); ecosystem biology and biogeochemistry (MPS, MS, PhD); environmental management (MPS); fishery and aquatic science (MPS, MS, PhD); forest science (MPS, MS, PhD); human dimensions of natural resources management (MPS, MS, PhD); policy and institutional analysis (MS, PhD); program development and evaluation (MPS, MS, PhD); quantitative ecology (MS, PhD); wildlife science (MPS, MS, PhD). *Degree requirements:* For master's, thesis (MS), project paper (MPS); for doctorate, comprehensive exam, thesis/dissertation. *Entrance requirements:* For master's and doctorate, GRE General Test, 2 letters of recommendation. Additional exam requirements/recommendations for international students: Required—TOEFL (minimum score 550 paper-based; 77 iBT). Electronic applications accepted. *Faculty research:* Ecosystem-level dynamics, systems modeling, conservation biology/management, resource management's human dimensions, biogeochemistry.

Florida Institute of Technology, College of Science, Program in Conservation Technology, Melbourne, FL 32901-6975. Offers MS. *Program availability:* Part-time. *Students:* 3 full-time (all women), 5 part-time (4 women). Average age 25. 6 applicants, 50% accepted. In 2015, 1 master's awarded. *Degree requirements:* For master's, 30 credit hours. *Entrance requirements:* For master's, GRE General Test, 3 letters of recommendation, statement of objectives. Additional exam requirements/recommendations for international students: Required—TOEFL (minimum score 550 paper-based; 79 iBT). *Application deadline:* Applications are processed on a rolling basis. Electronic applications accepted. *Expenses: Tuition, area resident:* Full-time $21,690; part-time $1205 per credit hour. *Required fees:* $500. Tuition and fees vary according to degree level, campus/location and program. *Financial support:* Applicants required to submit FAFSA. *Unit head:* Dr. Richard B. Aronson, Department Head, 321-674-8034, Fax: 321-674-7238, E-mail: raronson@fit.edu. *Application contact:* Cheryl A. Brown, Associate Director of Graduate Admissions, 321-674-7581, Fax: 321-723-9468, E-mail: cbrown@fit.edu.
Website: http://www.fit.edu/programs/

Fordham University, Graduate School of Arts and Sciences, Department of Biological Sciences, New York, NY 10458. Offers biological sciences (MS, PhD); conservation biology (Graduate Certificate). *Program availability:* Part-time, evening/weekend. *Faculty:* 18 full-time (2 women). *Students:* 43 full-time (20 women), 10 part-time (8 women); includes 3 minority (1 Black or African American, non-Hispanic/Latino; 2 Asian, non-Hispanic/Latino), 13 international. Average age 29. 123 applicants, 24% accepted, 13 enrolled. In 2015, 8 master's, 3 doctorates, 4 other advanced degrees awarded. Terminal master's awarded for partial completion of doctoral program. *Degree requirements:* For master's, one foreign language, comprehensive exam, thesis optional; for doctorate, one foreign language, comprehensive exam, thesis/dissertation. *Entrance requirements:* For master's and doctorate, GRE General Test, GRE Subject Test (recommended). Additional exam requirements/recommendations for international students: Required—TOEFL (minimum score 550 paper-based). *Application deadline:* For fall admission, 1/4 priority date for domestic students; for spring admission, 11/1 for domestic students. Application fee: $70. Electronic applications accepted. *Financial support:* In 2015–16, 28 students received support, including 4 fellowships with tuition reimbursements available (averaging $31,000 per year), 42 teaching assistantships with tuition reimbursements available (averaging $29,270 per year); Federal Work-Study, institutionally sponsored loans, scholarships/grants, tuition waivers (full and partial), and unspecified assistantships also available. Support available to part-time students. Financial award application deadline: 1/4; financial award applicants required to submit FAFSA. *Faculty research:* Avian ecology, behavioral ecology, and conservation biology; plant, community and ecosystem responses to invasive organisms; neurobiology and ion channel disorders; biochemical, physiological and morphological basis of pattern formation; behavioral, physiological and biochemical adaptations of mammals to extreme environments; evolutionary ecology, functional morphology and ichthyology; genotypic response to biogeographic and anthropogenic factors; community-based sustainable resource use. *Total annual research expenditures:* $1.5 million. *Unit head:* Dr. James Lewis, Chair, 718-817-3642, Fax: 718-817-3645, E-mail: jdlewis@fordham.edu. *Application contact:* Bernadette Valentino-Morrison, Director of Graduate Admissions, 718-817-4419, Fax: 718-817-3566, E-mail: valentinomor@fordham.edu.

Frostburg State University, Graduate School, College of Liberal Arts and Sciences, Department of Biology, Program in Applied Ecology and Conservation Biology, Frostburg, MD 21532-1099. Offers MS. *Degree requirements:* For master's, thesis. *Entrance requirements:* For master's, GRE General Test, resume. Additional exam requirements/recommendations for international students: Required—TOEFL. Electronic applications accepted. *Faculty research:* Forest ecology, microbiology of man-made wetlands, invertebrate zoology and entomology, wildlife and carnivore ecology, aquatic pollution ecology.

Illinois State University, Graduate School, College of Arts and Sciences, Department of Biological Sciences, Normal, IL 61790-2200. Offers animal behavior (MS); bacteriology (MS); biochemistry (MS); biological sciences (MS); biology (PhD); biophysics (MS); biotechnology (MS); botany (MS, PhD); cell biology (MS); conservation biology (MS); developmental biology (MS); ecology (MS, PhD); entomology (MS); evolutionary biology (MS); genetics (MS, PhD); immunology (MS); microbiology (MS, PhD); molecular biology (MS); molecular genetics (MS); neurobiology (MS); neuroscience (MS); parasitology (MS); physiology (MS, PhD); plant biology (MS); plant molecular biology (MS); plant sciences (MS); structural biology (MS); zoology (MS, PhD). *Program availability:* Part-time. *Degree requirements:* For master's, thesis or alternative; for doctorate, variable foreign language requirement, thesis/dissertation, 2 terms of residency. *Entrance requirements:* For master's, GRE General Test, minimum GPA of 2.6 in last 60 hours of course work; for doctorate, GRE General Test. *Application deadline:* Applications are processed on a rolling basis. Application fee: $40. *Financial support:* Research assistantships, teaching assistantships, Federal Work-Study, tuition waivers (full), and unspecified assistantships available. Financial award application deadline: 4/1. *Faculty research:* Redoc balance and drug development in schistosoma mansoni, control of the growth of listeria monocytogenes at low temperature, regulation of cell expansion and microtubule function by SPRI, CRUI: physiology and fitness consequences of different life history phenotypes. *Application contact:* Steven Juliano, Graduate Coordinator, E-mail: sajulian@ilstu.edu.
Website: http://www.bio.ilstu.edu/

Oregon State University, College of Science, Program in Zoology, Corvallis, OR 97331. Offers behavioral ecology (MA, MS, PhD); behavioral endocrinology (MA, MS, PhD); cell biology (MA, MS, PhD); chemical ecology (MA, MS, PhD); conservation biology (MA, MS, PhD); developmental biology (MA, MS, PhD). *Faculty:* 21 full-time (9 women), 2 part-time/adjunct (1 woman). *Students:* 58 full-time (38 women), 1 part-time (0 women); includes 11 minority (1 Black or African American, non-Hispanic/Latino; 1 American Indian or Alaska Native, non-Hispanic/Latino; 7 Asian, non-Hispanic/Latino; 1 Hispanic/Latino; 1 Two or more races, non-Hispanic/Latino), 3 international. Average age 28. 75 applicants, 13% accepted, 9 enrolled. In 2015, 1 master's, 5 doctorates awarded. Terminal master's awarded for partial completion of doctoral program. *Degree requirements:* For doctorate, thesis/dissertation. *Entrance requirements:* For master's and doctorate, GRE. Additional exam requirements/recommendations for international students: Required—TOEFL (minimum score 80 iBT), IELTS (minimum score 6.5). *Application deadline:* For fall admission, 12/15 for domestic and international students. Application fee: $75 ($85 for international students). *Expenses:* Tuition, state resident: full-time $12,150; part-time $450 per credit. Tuition, nonresident: full-time $20,952; part-time $776 per credit. *Required fees:* $1572; $1443 per unit. One-time fee: $350. Tuition and fees vary according to course load, campus/location and program. *Financial support:* Fellowships, research assistantships, teaching assistantships, Federal Work-Study, and institutionally sponsored loans available. Support available to part-time students. *Faculty research:* Ecology and evolutionary biology, physiology and behavior, development and cell biology. *Unit head:* Dr. Virginia M. Weis, Professor and Chair of Integrative Biology, 541-737-4359. *Application contact:* Graduate Admissions Coordinator, 541-737-5335, E-mail: ib@science.oregonstate.edu.
Website: http://ib.oregonstate.edu/

State University of New York College of Environmental Science and Forestry, Department of Environmental and Forest Biology, Syracuse, NY 13210-2779. Offers applied ecology (MPS); chemical ecology (MPS, MS, PhD); conservation biology (MPS, MS, PhD); ecology (MPS, MS, PhD); entomology (MPS, MS, PhD); environmental interpretation (MPS, MS, PhD); environmental physiology (MPS, MS, PhD); fish and wildlife biology and management (MPS, MS, PhD); forest pathology and mycology (MPS, MS, PhD); plant biotechnology (MPS); plant science and biotechnology (MPS, MS, PhD). *Faculty:* 29 full-time (9 women), 4 part-time/adjunct (3 women). *Students:* 81 full-time (47 women), 57 part-time (24 women); includes 9 minority (1 Black or African American, non-Hispanic/Latino; 2 American Indian or Alaska Native, non-Hispanic/Latino; 1 Asian, non-Hispanic/Latino; 3 Hispanic/Latino; 2 Two or more races, non-Hispanic/Latino), 15 international. Average age 28. 47 applicants, 49% accepted, 15 enrolled. In 2015, 15 master's, 7 doctorates awarded. *Degree requirements:* For master's, thesis (for some programs), capstone seminar; for doctorate, comprehensive exam, thesis/dissertation, capstone seminar. *Entrance requirements:* For master's and doctorate, GRE General Test, minimum GPA of 3.0. Additional exam requirements/recommendations for international students: Required—TOEFL (minimum score 550 paper-based; 80 iBT), IELTS (minimum score 6). *Application deadline:* For fall admission, 2/1 priority date for domestic and international students; for spring admission, 11/1 priority date for domestic and international students. Applications are processed on a rolling basis. Application fee: $60. *Expenses:* Tuition, state resident: full-time $10,870; part-time $453 per credit. Tuition, nonresident: full-time $22,210; part-time $925 per credit. *Required fees:* $1075; $89.22 per credit. *Financial support:* In 2015–16, 4 fellowships with tuition reimbursements, 36 research assistantships with tuition reimbursements, 39 teaching assistantships with tuition reimbursements (averaging $11,490 per year) were awarded; Federal Work-Study, institutionally sponsored loans, scholarships/grants, health care benefits, and unspecified assistantships also available. Financial award application deadline: 6/30. *Faculty research:* Ecology, conservation biology, fish and wildlife biology and management, plant science, entomology. *Total annual research expenditures:* $4.1 million. *Unit head:* Dr. Donald J. Leopold, Chair, 315-470-6760, Fax: 315-470-6934, E-mail: djleopold@esf.edu. *Application contact:* Dr. Danilo D. Fernando, Director, Graduate Program/Associate Professor, 315-470-6746, Fax: 315-470-6934, E-mail: dfernando@esf.edu.
Website: http://www.esf.edu/efb/grad/default.asp

Texas State University, The Graduate College, College of Science and Engineering, Program in Population and Conservation Biology, San Marcos, TX 78666. Offers MS. *Faculty:* 5 full-time (2 women). *Students:* 17 full-time (11 women), 2 part-time (1 woman); includes 3 minority (all Hispanic/Latino), 1 international. Average age 28. 13 applicants, 69% accepted, 8 enrolled. In 2015, 4 master's awarded. *Degree requirements:* For master's, comprehensive exam, thesis. *Entrance requirements:* For master's, GRE (minimum recommended score in at least the 50th percentile on both the verbal and quantitative portions), baccalaureate degree in biology or related discipline from regionally-accredited university with minimum GPA of 3.0 on last 60 undergraduate semester hours, statement of purpose, current curriculum vitae, 3 letters of recommendation, intent to mentor letter from faculty member of Biology Department. Additional exam requirements/recommendations for international students: Required—TOEFL (minimum score 550 paper-based; 78 iBT). *Application deadline:* For fall admission, 2/1 priority date for domestic and international students; for spring admission, 10/15 for domestic students, 10/1 for international students; for summer admission, 4/15 for domestic students, 3/15 for international students. Applications are processed on a rolling basis. Application fee: $40 ($90 for international students). Electronic applications accepted. *Expenses:* $3,615 in-state tuition (for 12 semester credit hours/1 full-time semester), $974 in-state fees. *Financial support:* In 2015–16, 11 students received support, including 1 research assistantship (averaging $15,300 per year), 15 teaching assistantships (averaging $12,664 per year); Federal Work-Study,

institutionally sponsored loans, scholarships/grants, health care benefits, and unspecified assistantships also available. Support available to part-time students. Financial award application deadline: 3/1; financial award applicants required to submit FAFSA. *Faculty research:* Assessing and minimizing wildlife collisions on public roads; fire ant management in roadway construction; mitigation for potential impacts to endangered Houston toad; Houston toad response to ongoing habitat restoration; understanding the potential of urban impacts on the Jollyville Salamander; red ant control; migratory bird documentation/assessment. *Total annual research expenditures:* $1.1 million. *Unit head:* Dr. Noland Martin, Graduate Advisor, 512-245-3317, E-mail: nm14@txstate.edu. *Application contact:* Dr. Andrea Golato, Dean of the Graduate School, 512-245-2581, Fax: 512-245-8365, E-mail: jw02@swt.edu.
Website: http://www.bio.txstate.edu/Graduate-Programs/pop-and-con-biology.html

Tropical Agriculture Research and Higher Education Center, Graduate School, Turrialba, Costa Rica. Offers agribusiness management (MS); agroforestry systems (PhD); development practices (MS); ecological agriculture (MS); environmental socioeconomics (MS); forestry in tropical and subtropical zones (PhD); integrated watershed management (MS); international sustainable tourism (MS); management and conservation of tropical rainforests and biodiversity (MS); tropical agriculture (PhD); tropical agroforestry (MS). *Entrance requirements:* For master's, GRE, 2 years of related professional experience, letters of recommendation; for doctorate, GRE, 4 letters of recommendation, letter of support from employing organization, master's degree in agronomy, biological sciences, forestry, natural resources or related field. Additional exam requirements/recommendations for international students: Required—TOEFL (minimum score 550 paper-based). Electronic applications accepted. *Faculty research:* Biodiversity in fragmented landscapes, ecosystem management, integrated pest management, environmental livestock production, biotechnology carbon balances in diverse land uses.

University at Albany, State University of New York, College of Arts and Sciences, Department of Biological Sciences, Program in Biodiversity, Conservation, and Policy, Albany, NY 12222-0001. Offers MS. *Degree requirements:* For master's, one foreign language. *Entrance requirements:* For master's, GRE General Test. *Faculty research:* Aquatic ecology, plant community ecology, biodiversity and public policy, restoration ecology, coastal and estuarine science.

University of Alberta, Faculty of Graduate Studies and Research, Department of Renewable Resources, Edmonton, AB T6G 2E1, Canada. Offers agroforestry (M Ag, M Sc, MF); conservation biology (M Sc, PhD); forest biology and management (M Sc, PhD); land reclamation and remediation (M Sc, PhD); protected areas and wildlands management (M Sc, PhD); soil science (M Ag, M Sc, PhD); water and land resources (M Ag, M Sc, PhD); wildlife ecology and management (M Sc, PhD); MBA/M Ag; MBA/MF. *Program availability:* Part-time. *Degree requirements:* For master's, thesis (for some programs); for doctorate, comprehensive exam, thesis/dissertation. *Entrance requirements:* For master's, minimum 2 years of relevant professional experiences, minimum GPA of 3.0; for doctorate, minimum GPA of 3.0. Additional exam requirements/recommendations for international students: Required—TOEFL (minimum score 550 paper-based). Electronic applications accepted. *Faculty research:* Natural and managed landscapes.

University of Central Florida, College of Sciences, Department of Biology, Orlando, FL 32816. Offers conservation biology (MS, PhD, Certificate). *Program availability:* Part-time, evening/weekend. *Faculty:* 25 full-time (11 women), 3 part-time/adjunct (0 women). *Students:* 49 full-time (27 women), 12 part-time (7 women); includes 4 minority (1 Asian, non-Hispanic/Latino; 3 Hispanic/Latino), 5 international. Average age 28. 63 applicants, 43% accepted, 16 enrolled. In 2015, 13 master's, 3 doctorates, 1 other advanced degree awarded. *Degree requirements:* For master's, comprehensive exam, thesis or alternative, field exam. *Entrance requirements:* For master's, GRE General Test, minimum GPA of 3.0 in last 60 hours. Additional exam requirements/recommendations for international students: Required—TOEFL. *Application deadline:* For fall admission, 3/1 priority date for domestic students; for spring admission, 10/15 for domestic students. Application fee: $30. Electronic applications accepted. *Expenses:* Tuition, state resident: part-time $288.16 per credit hour. Tuition, nonresident: part-time $1071.31 per credit hour. *Financial support:* In 2015–16, 46 students received support, including 13 fellowships with partial tuition reimbursements available (averaging $5,800 per year), 12 research assistantships with partial tuition reimbursements available (averaging $7,200 per year), 41 teaching assistantships with partial tuition reimbursements available (averaging $10,200 per year); career-related internships or fieldwork, Federal Work-Study, institutionally sponsored loans, tuition waivers (partial), and unspecified assistantships also available. Financial award application deadline: 3/1; financial award applicants required to submit FAFSA. *Unit head:* Dr. Graham Worthy, Chair, 407-823-2141, Fax: 407-823-5769, E-mail: graham.worthy@ucf.edu. *Application contact:* Associate Director, Admissions and Student Services, 407-823-2766, Fax: 407-823-6442, E-mail: gradadmissions@ucf.edu.
Website: http://biology.cos.ucf.edu/

University of Hawaii at Hilo, Program in Tropical Conservation Biology and Environmental Science, Hilo, HI 96720-4091. Offers MS. *Entrance requirements:* Additional exam requirements/recommendations for international students: Required—TOEFL, IELTS. Electronic applications accepted.

University of Illinois at Urbana–Champaign, Graduate College, College of Liberal Arts and Sciences, School of Integrative Biology, Program in Ecology, Evolution and Conservation Biology, Champaign, IL 61820. Offers MS, PhD.

University of Maryland, College Park, Academic Affairs, College of Computer, Mathematical and Natural Sciences, Department of Biology, Program in Sustainable Development and Conservation Biology, College Park, MD 20742. Offers MS. *Program availability:* Part-time, evening/weekend. *Degree requirements:* For master's, internship, scholarly paper. *Entrance requirements:* For master's, GRE General Test, minimum GPA of 3.0, 3 letters of recommendation. Electronic applications accepted. *Faculty research:* Biodiversity, global change, conservation.

University of Minnesota, Twin Cities Campus, Graduate School, College of Food, Agricultural and Natural Resource Sciences, Program in Conservation Biology, Minneapolis, MN 55455-0213. Offers MS, PhD. *Program availability:* Part-time. Terminal master's awarded for partial completion of doctoral program. *Degree requirements:* For master's, comprehensive exam, thesis; for doctorate, comprehensive exam, thesis/dissertation. *Entrance requirements:* For master's and doctorate, GRE, advanced ecology course. Additional exam requirements/recommendations for international students: Required—TOEFL (minimum score 550 paper-based; 79 iBT), IELTS (minimum score 6.5). Electronic applications accepted. *Faculty research:* Wildlife conservation, fisheries and aquatic biology, invasive species, human dimensions, GIS, restoration ecology.

University of Missouri, Office of Research and Graduate Studies, College of Agriculture, Food and Natural Resources, Department of Agricultural and Applied Economics, Columbia, MO 65211. Offers agricultural economics (MS, PhD); conservation biology (Graduate Certificate). *Degree requirements:* For doctorate, comprehensive exam, thesis/dissertation. *Entrance requirements:* For master's and doctorate, GRE General Test, minimum GPA of 3.0. Additional exam requirements/

Conservation Biology

recommendations for international students: Required—TOEFL (minimum score 550 paper-based; 80 iBT). *Application deadline:* For fall admission, 2/15 priority date for domestic students, 2/15 for international students; for winter admission, 9/15 for domestic and international students. Applications are processed on a rolling basis. Application fee: $55 ($75 for international students). Electronic applications accepted. *Financial support:* Fellowships, research assistantships with tuition reimbursements, teaching assistantships with tuition reimbursements, Federal Work-Study, institutionally sponsored loans, scholarships/grants, health care benefits, and unspecified assistantships available. Financial award application deadline: 3/1; financial award applicants required to submit FAFSA. *Faculty research:* Agribusiness management, contracting and strategy; collective action and cooperative theory; econometrics and price analysis; entrepreneurship; environmental and natural resource economics; food, biofuel and agricultural policy and regulation; international development; regional economics and rural development policy; science policy and innovation; sustainable agriculture and applied ethics.
Website: http://dass.missouri.edu/agecon/grad/

University of Missouri, Office of Research and Graduate Studies, College of Agriculture, Food and Natural Resources, School of Natural Resources, Department of Fisheries and Wildlife Sciences, Columbia, MO 65211. Offers conservation biology (Certificate); fisheries and wildlife (MS, PhD). *Degree requirements:* For doctorate, thesis/dissertation. *Entrance requirements:* For master's and doctorate, GRE General Test, minimum GPA of 3.0. Additional exam requirements/recommendations for international students: Required—TOEFL (minimum score 550 paper-based; 79 iBT). *Application deadline:* Applications are processed on a rolling basis. Application fee: $55 ($75 for international students). Electronic applications accepted. *Financial support:* Fellowships, research assistantships, teaching assistantships, institutionally sponsored loans, and scholarships/grants available.
Website: http://www.snr.missouri.edu/fw/academics/graduate-program.php

University of Nevada, Reno, Graduate School, Interdisciplinary Program in Ecology, Evolution, and Conservation Biology, Reno, NV 89557. Offers PhD. Offered through the College of Arts and Science, the M. C. Fleischmann College of Agriculture, and the Desert Research Institute. *Degree requirements:* For doctorate, thesis/dissertation. *Entrance requirements:* For doctorate, GRE General Test, GRE Subject Test, minimum GPA of 3.0. Additional exam requirements/recommendations for international students: Required—TOEFL (minimum score 500 paper-based; 61 iBT), IELTS (minimum score 6). Electronic applications accepted. *Faculty research:* Population biology, behavioral

ecology, plant response to climate change, conservation of endangered species, restoration of natural ecosystems.

University of New Hampshire, Graduate School, College of Life Sciences and Agriculture, Department of Natural Resources and the Environment, Durham, NH 03824. Offers environmental conservation (MS); environmental economics (MS); forestry (MS); natural resources (MS); resource administration and management (MS); soil and water resource management (MS); wildlife and conservation biology (MS). *Program availability:* Part-time. *Degree requirements:* For master's, thesis or alternative. *Entrance requirements:* For master's, GRE General Test. Additional exam requirements/recommendations for international students: Required—TOEFL (minimum score 550 paper-based; 80 iBT). *Application deadline:* For fall admission, 6/1 for domestic students, 4/1 for international students; for spring admission, 12/1 for domestic students. Applications are processed on a rolling basis. Application fee: $65. Electronic applications accepted. *Expenses:* Tuition, state resident: full-time $13,840; part-time $770 per credit hour. Tuition, nonresident: full-time $27,130; part-time $1175 per credit hour. *Required fees:* $2080; $1040. Tuition and fees vary according to degree level and program. *Financial support:* Fellowships, research assistantships, teaching assistantships, career-related internships or fieldwork, Federal Work-Study, scholarships/grants, and tuition waivers (full and partial) available. Support available to part-time students. Financial award application deadline: 2/15. *Unit head:* Pete Pekins, Chair, 603-862-1017, E-mail: natural.resources@unh.edu. *Application contact:* Wendy Rose, Administrative Assistant, 603-862-3933, E-mail: natural.resources@unh.edu.
Website: http://www.colsa.unh.edu/nren

University of Wisconsin–Madison, Graduate School, Gaylord Nelson Institute for Environmental Studies, Environmental Conservation Program, Madison, WI 53706-1380. Offers MS. *Degree requirements:* For master's, thesis or alternative, spring/summer leadership (internship) experience. *Entrance requirements:* Additional exam requirements/recommendations for international students: Required—TOEFL (minimum score 550 paper-based; 80 iBT). Electronic applications accepted. *Expenses:* Tuition, state resident: full-time $5364. Tuition, nonresident: full-time $12,027. *Required fees:* $571. Tuition and fees vary according to campus/location, program and reciprocity agreements. *Faculty research:* Ornithology, forestry, sociology, rural sociology, plant ecology, biodiversity, sustainability, sustainable development, conservation biology.

University of Wisconsin–Stout, Graduate School, College of Science, Technology, Engineering and Mathematics, Program in Conservation Biology, Menomonie, WI 54751. Offers PSM. *Program availability:* Online learning.

Ecology

Baylor University, Graduate School, College of Arts and Sciences, The Institute of Ecological, Earth and Environmental Sciences, Waco, TX 76798. Offers PhD. *Degree requirements:* For doctorate, variable foreign language requirement, comprehensive exam, thesis/dissertation or alternative. *Entrance requirements:* For doctorate, GRE. Additional exam requirements/recommendations for international students: Required—TOEFL (minimum score 550 paper-based; 80 iBT); Recommended—IELTS (minimum score 6.5). Electronic applications accepted. *Faculty research:* Ecosystem processes, environmental toxicology and risk assessment, biogeochemical cycling, chemical fate and transport, conservation management.

Brown University, Graduate School, Division of Biology and Medicine, Department of Ecology and Evolutionary Biology, Providence, RI 02912. Offers PhD. *Degree requirements:* For doctorate, thesis/dissertation, preliminary exam. *Entrance requirements:* For doctorate, GRE General Test, GRE Subject Test. Additional exam requirements/recommendations for international students: Required—TOEFL. Electronic applications accepted. *Faculty research:* Marine ecology, behavioral ecology, population genetics, evolutionary morphology, plant ecology.

California Institute of Integral Studies, School of Consciousness and Transformation, San Francisco, CA 94103. Offers anthropology and social change (MA, PhD); Asian philosophies and cultures (MA, PhD); creative inquiry/interdisciplinary arts (MFA); East-West psychology (MA, PhD); integral and transpersonal psychology (PhD); philosophy and religion (MA, PhD), including ecology, spirituality, and religion, philosophy, cosmology, and consciousness, women's spirituality (PhD); theater and performance making (MFA); transformative leadership (MA); transformative studies (PhD); women, gender, spirituality and social justice (MA); writing and consciousness (MFA). *Program availability:* Part-time, evening/weekend, 100% online, blended/hybrid learning. *Students:* 386 full-time (263 women), 111 part-time (80 women); includes 127 minority (31 Black or African American, non-Hispanic/Latino; 3 American Indian or Alaska Native, non-Hispanic/Latino; 18 Asian, non-Hispanic/Latino; 43 Hispanic/Latino; 2 Native Hawaiian or other Pacific Islander, non-Hispanic/Latino; 30 Two or more races, non-Hispanic/Latino), 39 international. Average age 38. 188 applicants, 91% accepted, 107 enrolled. In 2015, 75 master's, 41 doctorates awarded. Terminal master's awarded for partial completion of doctoral program. *Degree requirements:* For master's, thesis optional; for doctorate, comprehensive exam, thesis/dissertation, 1 foreign language (for Asian philosophies and cultures). *Entrance requirements:* For master's, minimum GPA of 3.0, letters of recommendation, writing sample; for doctorate, master's degree, minimum GPA of 3.0, letters of recommendation, writing sample. Additional exam requirements/recommendations for international students: Required—TOEFL. *Application deadline:* For fall admission, 2/1 priority date for domestic and international students; for spring admission, 10/15 priority date for domestic and international students. Applications are processed on a rolling basis. Application fee: $65. Electronic applications accepted. *Financial support:* Research assistantships, teaching assistantships, career-related internships or fieldwork, Federal Work-Study, and scholarships/grants available. Support available to part-time students. Financial award application deadline: 4/15; financial award applicants required to submit FAFSA. *Faculty research:* Ecology and sustainability, philosophy and religion, East-West psychology, integrative health, social and cultural anthropology, transformative leadership. *Application contact:* Ellen Durst, Interim Director of Admissions, 415-575-6100, Fax: 415-575-1268, E-mail: admissions@ciis.edu.
Website: http://www.ciis.edu/

California State University, Stanislaus, College of Natural Sciences, Program in Ecology and Sustainability (MS), Turlock, CA 95382. Offers ecological conservation (MS); ecological economics (MS). *Program availability:* Part-time. *Degree requirements:* For master's, thesis. *Entrance requirements:* For master's, GRE, minimum GPA of 3.0, 3 letters of recommendation, personal statement. Additional exam requirements/recommendations for international students: Required—TOEFL (minimum score 550 paper-based). Electronic applications accepted.

Clemson University, Graduate School, College of Science, Department of Biological Sciences, Program in Biological Sciences, Clemson, SC 29634. Offers MS, PhD. *Program availability:* Part-time. *Faculty:* 9 full-time (2 women). *Students:* 31 full-time (20 women); includes 1 minority (Two or more races, non-Hispanic/Latino), 8 international. Average age 28. 45 applicants, 31% accepted, 6 enrolled. In 2015, 1 master's, 5 doctorates awarded. *Degree requirements:* For master's, thesis; for doctorate, comprehensive exam, thesis/dissertation. *Entrance requirements:* For master's and doctorate, GRE General Test, unofficial transcripts, letters of recommendation. Additional exam requirements/recommendations for international students: Required—TOEFL (minimum score 100 iBT), IELTS (minimum score 7.5), PTE (minimum score 7). *Application deadline:* For fall admission, 1/5 for domestic and international students. Application fee: $80 ($90 for international students). Electronic applications accepted. *Expenses:* $4,060 per semester full-time resident, $8,103 per semester full-time non-resident, $448 per credit hour part-time resident, $898 per credit hour part-time non-resident. *Financial support:* In 2015–16, 31 students received support, including 1 fellowship with partial tuition reimbursement available (averaging $5,000 per year), 2 research assistantships with partial tuition reimbursements available (averaging $21,600 per year), 29 teaching assistantships with partial tuition reimbursements available (averaging $26,656 per year); career-related internships or fieldwork and health care benefits also available. Financial award application deadline: 1/5. *Faculty research:* Cell and developmental biology, evolutionary biology, ecology, molecular biology. *Unit head:* Dr. Robert Cohen, Department Chair, 864-656-1112, Fax: 864-656-0435, E-mail: rscohen@clemson.edu. *Application contact:* Jay Lyn Martin, Student Services Program Coordinator, 864-656-3587, Fax: 864-656-0435, E-mail: jaylyn@clemson.edu.
Website: http://www.clemson.edu/cafls/departments/biosci/

Colorado State University, Interdisciplinary College, Graduate Degree Program in Ecology, Fort Collins, CO 80523-1401. Offers MS, PhD. *Program availability:* Part-time. *Students:* 43 full-time (27 women), 108 part-time (57 women); includes 12 minority (2 Black or African American, non-Hispanic/Latino; 4 Asian, non-Hispanic/Latino; 5 Hispanic/Latino; 1 Two or more races, non-Hispanic/Latino), 16 international. Average age 32. 72 applicants, 24% accepted, 16 enrolled. In 2015, 19 master's, 20 doctorates awarded. Terminal master's awarded for partial completion of doctoral program. *Degree requirements:* For master's, comprehensive exam, thesis (for some programs), project paper; for doctorate, comprehensive exam, thesis/dissertation. *Entrance requirements:* For master's and doctorate, GRE General Test, minimum GPA of 3.0, BA/BS in related field, 3 letters of recommendation, personal statement, confirmation from a CSU ecology faculty advisor. Additional exam requirements/recommendations for international students: Required—TOEFL (minimum score 550 paper-based; 80 iBT). *Application deadline:* For fall admission, 1/1 priority date for domestic students, 1/1 for international students; for spring admission, 11/1 priority date for domestic students, 11/1 for international students. Applications are processed on a rolling basis. Application fee: $60 ($70 for international students). Electronic applications accepted. *Expenses:* Tuition, state resident: full-time $9348. Tuition, nonresident: full-time $22,916. *Required fees:* $2174; $473.72 per credit hour. $236.86 per semester. Tuition and fees vary according to course load and program. *Financial support:* In 2015–16, 8 fellowships (averaging $47,076 per year), 18 research assistantships with partial tuition reimbursements (averaging $22,742 per year) were awarded; teaching assistantships with partial tuition reimbursements and scholarships/grants also available. Financial award application deadline: 1/1; financial award applicants required to submit FAFSA. *Faculty research:* Physiology, dynamics of species population, interacting species in communities, energy and material flux in ecosystems, landscape determinants of ecological organization. *Unit head:* Dr. N. Leroy Poff, Director, 970-491-4373, E-mail: nleroy.poff@colostate.edu. *Application contact:* Sara Rose, Program Coordinator, 970-491-4373, E-mail: sara.rose@colostate.edu.
Website: http://www.ecology.colostate.edu/

Columbia University, Graduate School of Arts and Sciences, New York, NY 10027. Offers African-American studies (MA); American studies (MA); anthropology (MA, PhD);

art history and archaeology (MA, PhD); astronomy (PhD); biological sciences (PhD); biotechnology (MA); chemical physics (PhD); chemistry (PhD); classical studies (MA, PhD); classics (MA, PhD); climate and society (MA); conservation biology (MA); earth and environmental sciences (PhD); East Asia: regional studies (MA); East Asian languages and cultures (MA, PhD); ecology, evolution and environmental biology (MA), including conservation biology; ecology, evolution, and environmental biology (PhD), including ecology and evolutionary biology, evolutionary primatology; economics (MA, PhD); English and comparative literature (MA, PhD); French and Romance philology (MA, PhD); Germanic languages (MA, PhD); global French studies (MA); global thought (MA); Hispanic cultural studies (MA); history (PhD); history and literature (MA); human rights studies (MA); Islamic studies (MA); Italian (MA, PhD); Japanese pedagogy (MA); Jewish studies (MA); Latin America and the Caribbean: regional studies (MA); Latin American and Iberian cultures (PhD); mathematics (MA, PhD), including finance (MA); medieval and Renaissance studies (MA); Middle Eastern, South Asian, and African studies (MA, PhD); modern art: critical and curatorial studies (MA); modern European studies (MA); museum anthropology (MA); music (DMA, PhD); oral history (MA); philosophical foundations of physics (MA); philosophy (MA, PhD); physics (PhD); political science (MA, PhD); psychology (PhD); quantitative methods in the social sciences (MA); religion (MA, PhD); Russia, Eurasia and East Europe: regional studies (MA); Russian translation (MA); Slavic cultures (MA); Slavic languages (MA, PhD); sociology (MA, PhD); South Asian studies (MA); statistics (MA, PhD); theatre (PhD). Dual-degree programs require admission to both Graduate School of Arts and Sciences and another Columbia school. *Program availability:* Part-time. *Students:* 3,030 full-time, 235 part-time; includes 861 minority (88 Black or African American, non-Hispanic/Latino; 5 American Indian or Alaska Native, non-Hispanic/Latino; 517 Asian, non-Hispanic/Latino; 159 Hispanic/Latino; 4 Native Hawaiian or other Pacific Islander, non-Hispanic/Latino; 88 Two or more races, non-Hispanic/Latino), 1,697 international. 13,288 applicants, 21% accepted, 1162 enrolled. In 2015, 1,061 master's, 553 doctorates awarded. Terminal master's awarded for partial completion of doctoral program. *Degree requirements:* For master's, variable foreign language requirement, comprehensive exam (for some programs), thesis (for some programs); for doctorate, variable foreign language requirement, comprehensive exam (for some programs), thesis/dissertation. *Entrance requirements:* For master's and doctorate, GRE General Test, GRE Subject Test (for some programs). Additional exam requirements/recommendations for international students: Required—TOEFL, IELTS. Application fee: $105. Electronic applications accepted. *Financial support:* Fellowships, research assistantships, teaching assistantships, career-related internships or fieldwork, Federal Work-Study, institutionally sponsored loans, scholarships/grants, traineeships, health care benefits, tuition waivers, and unspecified assistantships available. Support available to part-time students. Financial award application deadline: 12/15. *Unit head:* Carlos J. Alonso, Dean of the Graduate School of Arts and Sciences, 212-854-5177. *Application contact:* GSAS Office of Admissions, 212-854-8903, E-mail: gsas-admissions@columbia.edu. Website: http://gsas.columbia.edu/

Cornell University, Graduate School, Graduate Fields of Agriculture and Life Sciences, Field of Computational Biology, Ithaca, NY 14853-0001. Offers computational behavioral biology (PhD); computational biology (PhD); computational cell biology (PhD); computational ecology (PhD); computational genetics (PhD); computational macromolecular biology (PhD); computational organismal biology (PhD). *Degree requirements:* For doctorate, comprehensive exam, thesis/dissertation, 2 semesters of teaching experience. *Entrance requirements:* For doctorate, GRE General Test, GRE Subject Test (biology), 2 letters of recommendation. Additional exam requirements/recommendations for international students: Required—TOEFL (minimum score 550 paper-based; 77 iBT). Electronic applications accepted. *Faculty research:* Computational behavioral biology, computational biology, computational cell biology, computational ecology, computational genetics, computational macromolecular biology, computational organismal biology.

Cornell University, Graduate School, Graduate Fields of Agriculture and Life Sciences, Field of Ecology and Evolutionary Biology, Ithaca, NY 14853-0001. Offers ecology (PhD), including animal ecology, applied ecology, biogeochemistry, community and ecosystem ecology, limnology, oceanography, physiological ecology, plant ecology, population ecology, theoretical ecology, vertebrate zoology; evolutionary biology (PhD), including ecological genetics, paleobiology, population biology, systematics. *Degree requirements:* For doctorate, comprehensive exam, thesis/dissertation, 2 semesters of teaching experience. *Entrance requirements:* For doctorate, GRE General Test, GRE Subject Test (biology), 2 letters of recommendation. Additional exam requirements/recommendations for international students: Required—TOEFL (minimum score 550 paper-based; 77 iBT). Electronic applications accepted. *Faculty research:* Population and organismal biology, population and evolutionary genetics, systematics and macroevolution, biochemistry, conservation biology.

Cornell University, Graduate School, Graduate Fields of Agriculture and Life Sciences, Field of Horticulture, Ithaca, NY 14853-0001. Offers breeding of horticultural crops (MPS); horticultural crop management systems (MPS); human-plant interactions (MPS, PhD); physiology and ecology of horticultural crops (MPS, MS, PhD). *Degree requirements:* For master's, thesis (MS); for doctorate, comprehensive exam, thesis/dissertation. *Entrance requirements:* For master's and doctorate, GRE General Test, 3 letters of recommendation. Additional exam requirements/recommendations for international students: Required—TOEFL (minimum score 550 paper-based; 77 iBT). Electronic applications accepted. *Faculty research:* Plant selection/plant materials, greenhouse management, greenhouse crop production, urban landscape management, turfgrass management.

Cornell University, Graduate School, Graduate Fields of Agriculture and Life Sciences, Field of Natural Resources, Ithaca, NY 14853-0001. Offers community-based natural resources management (MS, PhD); conservation biology (MS, PhD); ecosystem biology and biogeochemistry (MPS, MS, PhD); environmental management (MPS); fishery and aquatic science (MPS, MS, PhD); forest science (MPS, MS, PhD); human dimensions of natural resources management (MPS, MS, PhD); policy and institutional analysis (MS, PhD); program development and evaluation (MPS, MS, PhD); quantitative ecology (MS, PhD); wildlife science (MPS, MS, PhD). *Degree requirements:* For master's, thesis (MS), project paper (MPS); for doctorate, comprehensive exam, thesis/dissertation. *Entrance requirements:* For master's and doctorate, GRE General Test, 2 letters of recommendation. Additional exam requirements/recommendations for international students: Required—TOEFL (minimum score 550 paper-based; 77 iBT). Electronic applications accepted. *Faculty research:* Ecosystem-level dynamics, systems modeling, conservation biology/management, resource management's human dimensions, biogeochemistry.

Cornell University, Graduate School, Graduate Fields of Agriculture and Life Sciences, Field of Zoology and Wildlife Conservation, Ithaca, NY 14853-0001. Offers animal cytology (PhD); comparative and functional anatomy (PhD); developmental biology (PhD); ecology (PhD); histology (PhD); wildlife conservation (PhD). *Degree requirements:* For doctorate, comprehensive exam, thesis/dissertation, 2 semesters of teaching experience. *Entrance requirements:* For doctorate, GRE General Test, GRE Subject Test (biology), 2 letters of recommendation. Additional exam requirements/recommendations for international students: Required—TOEFL (minimum score 550

paper-based; 77 iBT). Electronic applications accepted. *Faculty research:* Organismal biology, functional morphology, biomechanics, comparative vertebrate anatomy, comparative invertebrate anatomy, paleontology.

Dalhousie University, Faculty of Agriculture, Halifax, NS B3H 4R2, Canada. Offers agriculture (M Sc), including air quality, animal behavior, animal molecular genetics, animal nutrition, animal technology, aquaculture, botany, crop management, crop physiology, ecology, environmental microbiology, food science, horticulture, nutrient management, pest management, physiology, plant biotechnology, plant pathology, soil chemistry, soil fertility, waste management and composting, water quality. *Program availability:* Part-time. *Degree requirements:* For master's, thesis, ATC Exam Teaching Assistantship. *Entrance requirements:* For master's, honors B Sc, minimum GPA of 3.0. Additional exam requirements/recommendations for international students: Required—TOEFL (minimum score 580 paper-based; 92 iBT), IELTS, Michigan English Language Assessment Battery, CanTEST, CAEL. *Faculty research:* Bio-product development, organic agriculture, nutrient management, air and water quality, agricultural biotechnology.

Dartmouth College, Arts and Sciences Graduate Programs, Program in Ecology and Evolutionary Biology, Hanover, NH 03755. Offers PhD. *Faculty:* 8 full-time (4 women). *Students:* 28 full-time (18 women); includes 3 minority (1 American Indian or Alaska Native, non-Hispanic/Latino; 1 Asian, non-Hispanic/Latino; 1 Two or more races, non-Hispanic/Latino), 4 international. Average age 29. 35 applicants, 26% accepted, 7 enrolled. In 2015, 10 doctorates awarded. *Entrance requirements:* For doctorate, GRE General Test, GRE Subject Test in biology (highly recommended). Additional exam requirements/recommendations for international students: Required—TOEFL. *Application deadline:* For fall admission, 12/1 for domestic students. Electronic applications accepted. *Expenses: Tuition,* area resident: Full-time $48,120. *Required fees:* $296. One-time fee: $50 full-time. *Financial support:* Fellowships with full tuition reimbursements, research assistantships with full tuition reimbursements, teaching assistantships with full tuition reimbursements, institutionally sponsored loans, traineeships, and unspecified assistantships available. Financial award applicants required to submit FAFSA. *Unit head:* Dr. Mathew Ayres, 603-646-2788. *Application contact:* Amy Layne, 603-646-3847, Fax: 603-646-3488. Website: http://sites.dartmouth.edu/EEES/

Duke University, Graduate School, Department of Ecology, Durham, NC 27708-0329. Offers PhD, Certificate. *Degree requirements:* For doctorate, thesis/dissertation. *Entrance requirements:* For doctorate, GRE General Test. Additional exam requirements/recommendations for international students: Required—TOEFL (minimum score 577 paper-based; 90 iBT) or IELTS (minimum score 7). Electronic applications accepted.

Eastern Kentucky University, The Graduate School, College of Arts and Sciences, Department of Biological Sciences, Richmond, KY 40475-3102. Offers biological sciences (MS); ecology (MS). *Program availability:* Part-time. *Degree requirements:* For master's, thesis. *Entrance requirements:* For master's, GRE General Test, minimum GPA of 2.5. *Faculty research:* Systematics, ecology, and biodiversity; animal behavior; protein structure and molecular genetics; biomonitoring and aquatic toxicology; pathogenesis of microbes and parasites.

Eastern Michigan University, Graduate School, College of Arts and Sciences, Department of Biology, Ypsilanti, MI 48197. Offers cell and molecular biology (MS); community college biology teaching (MS); ecology and organismal biology (MS); general biology (MS); water resources (MS). *Program availability:* Part-time, evening/weekend, online learning. *Faculty:* 26 full-time (8 women). *Students:* 15 full-time (9 women), 33 part-time (19 women); includes 8 minority (3 Black or African American, non-Hispanic/Latino; 2 Asian, non-Hispanic/Latino; 2 Hispanic/Latino; 1 Two or more races, non-Hispanic/Latino), 3 international. Average age 27. 47 applicants, 51% accepted, 19 enrolled. In 2015, 14 master's awarded. *Entrance requirements:* For master's, GRE General Test, GRE Subject Test. Additional exam requirements/recommendations for international students: Required—TOEFL. *Application deadline:* Applications are processed on a rolling basis. Application fee: $45. *Financial support:* Fellowships, research assistantships with full tuition reimbursements, teaching assistantships with full tuition reimbursements, career-related internships or fieldwork, Federal Work-Study, institutionally sponsored loans, scholarships/grants, tuition waivers (partial), and unspecified assistantships available. Support available to part-time students. Financial award applicants required to submit FAFSA. *Unit head:* Dr. Daniel Clemans, Department Head, 734-487-4242, Fax: 734-487-9235, E-mail: dclemans@emich.edu. *Application contact:* Dr. David Kass, Graduate Coordinator, 734-487-4242, Fax: 734-487-9235, E-mail: dkass@emich.edu. Website: http://www.emich.edu/biology

Eastern New Mexico University, Graduate School, College of Liberal Arts and Sciences, Department of Biology, Portales, NM 88130. Offers applied ecology (MS); botany (MS); cell, molecular biology and biotechnology (MS); microbiology (MS); zoology (MS). *Program availability:* Part-time. *Degree requirements:* For master's, comprehensive exam, thesis optional. *Entrance requirements:* For master's, GRE, minimum GPA of 3.0, 2 letters of recommendation, statement of research interest, bachelor's degree related to field of study or proof of common knowledge. Additional exam requirements/recommendations for international students: Required—TOEFL (minimum score 550 paper-based; 79 iBT), IELTS (minimum score 6). Electronic applications accepted.

Emory University, Laney Graduate School, Division of Biological and Biomedical Sciences, Program in Population Biology, Ecology and Evolution, Atlanta, GA 30322-1100. Offers PhD. *Degree requirements:* For doctorate, comprehensive exam, thesis/dissertation. *Entrance requirements:* For doctorate, GRE General Test, minimum GPA of 3.0 in science course work (recommended). Additional exam requirements/recommendations for international students: Required—TOEFL. Electronic applications accepted. *Faculty research:* Evolution of microbes, infectious disease, the immune system, genetic disease in humans, evolution of behavior.

Florida Institute of Technology, College of Science, Program in Biological Sciences, Melbourne, FL 32901-6975. Offers biological science (PhD); biotechnology (MS); cell and molecular biology (MS); ecology (MS); marine biology (MS). *Program availability:* Part-time. *Students:* 65 full-time (39 women), 10 part-time (3 women); includes 4 minority (2 Asian, non-Hispanic/Latino; 1 Hispanic/Latino; 1 Two or more races, non-Hispanic/Latino), 38 international. Average age 26. 230 applicants, 24% accepted, 21 enrolled. In 2015, 23 master's, 3 doctorates awarded. *Degree requirements:* For master's, thesis (for some programs), research, seminar, internship, or summer lab; for doctorate, comprehensive exam, thesis/dissertation, dissertations seminar, publications. *Entrance requirements:* For master's, GRE General Test, 3 letters of recommendation; statement of objectives; bachelor's degree in biology, chemistry, biochemistry or equivalent; for doctorate, GRE General Test, resume, 3 letters of recommendation, minimum GPA of 3.2, statement of objectives. Additional exam requirements/recommendations for international students: Required—TOEFL (minimum score 550 paper-based; 79 iBT). *Application deadline:* For fall admission, 3/1 for domestic students, 4/1 for international students; for spring admission, 9/1 for domestic and international students. Applications are processed on a rolling basis. Electronic

Ecology

applications accepted. *Expenses: Tuition, area resident:* Full-time $21,690; part-time $1205 per credit hour. *Required fees:* $500. Tuition and fees vary according to degree level, campus/location and program. *Financial support:* Career-related internships or fieldwork, institutionally sponsored loans, tuition waivers (partial), unspecified assistantships, and tuition remissions available. Support available to part-time students. Financial award application deadline: 3/1; financial award applicants required to submit FAFSA. *Faculty research:* Initiation of protein synthesis in eukaryotic cells, fixation of radioactive carbon, changes in DNA molecule, endangered or threatened avian and mammalian species, hydroacoustics and feeding preference of the West Indian manatee. *Unit head:* Dr. Richard B. Aronson, Department Head, 321-674-8034, Fax: 321-674-7238, E-mail: raronson@fit.edu. *Application contact:* Cheryl A. Brown, Associate Director of Graduate Admissions, 321-674-7581, Fax: 321-723-9468, E-mail: cbrown@fit.edu.
Website: http://cos.fit.edu/biology/

Florida State University, The Graduate School, College of Arts and Sciences, Department of Biological Science, Specialization in Ecology and Evolutionary Biology, Tallahassee, FL 32306-4295. Offers MS, PhD. *Faculty:* 21 full-time (7 women). *Students:* 56 full-time (27 women); includes 4 minority (1 Black or African American, non-Hispanic/Latino; 3 Hispanic/Latino), 5 international. 120 applicants, 13% accepted, 9 enrolled. In 2015, 2 master's, 3 doctorates awarded. Terminal master's awarded for partial completion of doctoral program. *Degree requirements:* For master's, comprehensive exam, thesis, teaching experience, seminar presentation; for doctorate, comprehensive exam, thesis/dissertation, teaching experience; seminar presentation. *Entrance requirements:* For master's and doctorate, GRE General Test, minimum upper-division GPA of 3.0. Additional exam requirements/recommendations for international students: Required—TOEFL (minimum score 600 paper-based; 92 iBT). *Application deadline:* For fall admission, 12/1 for domestic and international students. Application fee: $30. Electronic applications accepted. *Expenses: Tuition, area resident:* Full-time $7263; part-time $403.50 per credit hour. Tuition, nonresident: full-time $18,087; part-time $1004.85 per credit hour. *Required fees:* $1365; $75.81 per credit hour. $20 per semester. Tuition and fees vary according to campus/location. *Financial support:* In 2015–16, 55 students received support, including 4 fellowships with tuition reimbursements available (averaging $30,000 per year), 20 research assistantships with full tuition reimbursements available (averaging $21,500 per year), 31 teaching assistantships with full tuition reimbursements available (averaging $21,500 per year); scholarships/grants and unspecified assistantships also available. Financial award application deadline: 12/1; financial award applicants required to submit FAFSA. *Faculty research:* Ecology and conservation biology; evolution; marine biology; phylogeny and systematics; theoretical, computational and mathematical biology. *Unit head:* Dr. Thomas A. Houpt, Professor and Associate Chair, 850-644-4907, Fax: 850-644-8447, E-mail: houpt@neuro.fsu.edu. *Application contact:* Dr. Michael B. Miller, Coordinator, Graduate Affairs, 850-644-3023, Fax: 850-644-9829, E-mail: gradinfo@bio.fsu.edu.
Website: http://www.bio.fsu.edu/

Frostburg State University, Graduate School, College of Liberal Arts and Sciences, Department of Biology, Program in Applied Ecology and Conservation Biology, Frostburg, MD 21532-1099. Offers MS. *Degree requirements:* For master's, thesis. *Entrance requirements:* For master's, GRE General Test, resume. Additional exam requirements/recommendations for international students: Required—TOEFL. Electronic applications accepted. *Faculty research:* Forest ecology, microbiology of man-made wetlands, invertebrate zoology and entomology, wildlife and carnivore ecology, aquatic pollution ecology.

George Mason University, College of Science, Department of Environmental Science and Policy, Fairfax, VA 22030. Offers aquatic ecology (MS). *Faculty:* 20 full-time (10 women), 6 part-time/adjunct (0 women). *Students:* 58 full-time (37 women), 73 part-time (49 women); includes 21 minority (8 Black or African American, non-Hispanic/Latino; 7 Asian, non-Hispanic/Latino; 5 Hispanic/Latino; 1 Native Hawaiian or other Pacific Islander, non-Hispanic/Latino), 9 international. Average age 35. 40 applicants, 70% accepted, 14 enrolled. In 2015, 22 master's, 13 doctorates awarded. *Degree requirements:* For doctorate, comprehensive exam, thesis/dissertation, internship; seminar. *Entrance requirements:* For master's, GRE, bachelor's degree with minimum GPA of 3.0 in related field; 3 letters of recommendation; expanded goals statement; 2 official copies of transcripts; for doctorate, GRE, bachelor's degree with minimum GPA of 3.0; 3 letters of recommendation; current resume; expanded goals statement; 2 official copies of transcripts. Additional exam requirements/recommendations for international students: Required—TOEFL (minimum score 575 paper-based; 88 iBT), IELTS (minimum score 6.5), PTE (minimum score 59). Application fee: $75 ($80 for international students). Electronic applications accepted. *Financial support:* In 2015–16, 54 students received support, including 6 fellowships (averaging $7,149 per year), 13 research assistantships with tuition reimbursements available (averaging $15,186 per year), 36 teaching assistantships with tuition reimbursements available (averaging $14,546 per year); career-related internships or fieldwork, Federal Work-Study, scholarships/grants, unspecified assistantships, and health care benefits (for full-time research or teaching assistantship recipients) also available. Support available to part-time students. Financial award application deadline: 3/1; financial award applicants required to submit FAFSA. *Faculty research:* Wetland ecosystems, comparative physiology, systematics, molecular phylogenetics, conservation genetics, estuarine and oceanic systems, biodiversity of fungi, environmental and resource management, human ecology. *Total annual research expenditures:* $751,706. *Unit head:* Dr. Robert B. Jonas, Chair, 703-993-7590, Fax: 703-993-1066, E-mail: rjonas@gmu.edu. *Application contact:* Sharon Bloomquist, Graduate Program Coordinator, 703-993-3187, Fax: 703-993-1066, E-mail: sbloomqu@gmu.edu.
Website: http://esp.gmu.edu/

Illinois State University, Graduate School, College of Arts and Sciences, Department of Biological Sciences, Normal, IL 61790-2200. Offers animal behavior (MS); bacteriology (MS); biochemistry (MS); biological sciences (MS); biology (PhD); biophysics (MS); biotechnology (MS); botany (MS, PhD); cell biology (MS); conservation biology (MS); developmental biology (MS); ecology (MS, PhD); entomology (MS); evolutionary biology (MS); genetics (MS, PhD); immunology (MS); microbiology (MS, PhD); molecular biology (MS); molecular genetics (MS); neurobiology (MS); neuroscience (MS); parasitology (MS); physiology (MS, PhD); plant biology (MS); plant molecular biology (MS); plant sciences (MS); structural biology (MS); zoology (MS, PhD). *Program availability:* Part-time. *Degree requirements:* For master's, thesis or alternative; for doctorate, variable foreign language requirement, thesis/dissertation, 2 terms of residency. *Entrance requirements:* For master's, GRE General Test, minimum GPA of 2.6 in last 60 hours of course work; for doctorate, GRE General Test. *Application deadline:* Applications are processed on a rolling basis. Application fee: $40. *Financial support:* Research assistantships, teaching assistantships, Federal Work-Study, tuition waivers (full), and unspecified assistantships available. Financial award application deadline: 4/1. *Faculty research:* Redox balance and drug development in schistosoma mansoni, control of the growth of listeria monocytogenes at low temperature, regulation of cell expansion and microtubule function by SPR1, CRUI: physiology and fitness consequences of different life history phenotypes. *Application contact:* Steven Juliano, Graduate Coordinator, E-mail: sajulian@ilstu.edu.
Website: http://www.bio.ilstu.edu/

Indiana State University, College of Graduate and Professional Studies, College of Arts and Sciences, Department of Biology, Terre Haute, IN 47809. Offers cellular and molecular biology (PhD); ecology, systematics and evolution (PhD); life sciences (MS); physiology (PhD); science education (MS). *Degree requirements:* For master's, thesis optional; for doctorate, comprehensive exam, thesis/dissertation. *Entrance requirements:* For master's and doctorate, GRE General Test. Electronic applications accepted.

Indiana University Bloomington, School of Public and Environmental Affairs, Environmental Science Programs, Bloomington, IN 47405. Offers applied ecology (MSES); energy (MSES); environmental chemistry, toxicology, and risk assessment (MSES); environmental science (PhD); hazardous materials management (Certificate); specialized environmental science (MSES); water resources (MSES); JD/MSES; MSES/MA; MSES/MPA; MSES/MS. *Program availability:* Part-time. Terminal master's awarded for partial completion of doctoral program. *Degree requirements:* For master's, capstone or thesis; internship; for doctorate, comprehensive exam, thesis/dissertation. *Entrance requirements:* For master's, GRE General Test or GMAT, official transcripts, 3 letters of recommendation, resume, personal statement; for doctorate, GRE General Test or LSAT, official transcripts, 3 letters of recommendation, resume or curriculum vitae, statement of purpose. Additional exam requirements/recommendations for international students: Required—TOEFL (minimum score 600 paper-based; 96 iBT); Recommended—IELTS (minimum score 7). Electronic applications accepted. *Faculty research:* Applied ecology, bio-geochemistry, toxicology, wetlands ecology, environmental microbiology, forest ecology, environmental chemistry.

Indiana University Bloomington, University Graduate School, College of Arts and Sciences, Department of Biology, Bloomington, IN 47405. Offers biology teaching (MAT); biotechnology (MA); evolution, ecology, and behavior (MA, PhD); genetics (PhD); microbiology (MA, PhD); molecular, cellular, and developmental biology (PhD); plant sciences (MA, PhD); zoology (MA, PhD). Terminal master's awarded for partial completion of doctoral program. *Degree requirements:* For master's, thesis, oral defense; for doctorate, thesis/dissertation, oral defense. *Entrance requirements:* For master's and doctorate, GRE General Test. Additional exam requirements/recommendations for international students: Required—TOEFL (minimum score 100 iBT). Electronic applications accepted. *Faculty research:* Evolution, ecology and behavior; microbiology; molecular biology and genetics; plant biology.

Inter American University of Puerto Rico, Bayamón Campus, Graduate School, Bayamón, PR 00957. Offers biology (MS), including environmental sciences and ecology, molecular biotechnology; human resources (MBA). *Program availability:* Part-time, evening/weekend. *Faculty:* 14 full-time (3 women), 5 part-time/adjunct (3 women). *Students:* 6 full-time (4 women), 117 part-time (68 women); includes 122 minority (1 Asian, non-Hispanic/Latino; 121 Hispanic/Latino). *Degree requirements:* For master's, comprehensive exam, research project. *Entrance requirements:* For master's, EXADEP, GRE General Test, letters of recommendation. *Application deadline:* For fall admission, 7/1 for domestic students, 5/1 priority date for international students; for winter admission, 11/15 priority date for domestic and international students; for spring admission, 2/15 priority date for domestic and international students. Application fee: $31. *Expenses: Tuition, area resident:* Part-time $207 per credit. *Required fees:* $328 per semester. *Unit head:* Prof. Juan F. Martinez, Chancellor, 787-279-1200 Ext. 2295, Fax: 787-279-2205, E-mail: jmartinez@bayamon.inter.edu. *Application contact:* Hector Vargas, Interim Director of Admissions, 787-279-1912 Ext. 2017, Fax: 787-279-2205, E-mail: hvargas@bayamon.inter.edu.

Iowa State University of Science and Technology, Program in Ecology and Evolutionary Biology, Ames, IA 50011. Offers MS, PhD. *Degree requirements:* For master's, thesis or alternative; for doctorate, thesis/dissertation. *Entrance requirements:* For master's and doctorate, GRE General Test. Additional exam requirements/recommendations for international students: Required—TOEFL (minimum score 550 paper-based; 79 iBT), IELTS (minimum score 6.5). Electronic applications accepted. *Faculty research:* Landscape ecology, aquatic and method ecology, physiological ecology, population genetics and evolution, systematics.

Kent State University, College of Arts and Sciences, Department of Biological Sciences, Kent, OH 44242-0001. Offers biological sciences (MS, PhD), including ecology, physiology. *Program availability:* Part-time. *Faculty:* 37 full-time (12 women). *Students:* 52 full-time (33 women), 15 part-time (9 women); includes 7 minority (3 Black or African American, non-Hispanic/Latino; 2 Asian, non-Hispanic/Latino; 2 Two or more races, non-Hispanic/Latino), 20 international. Average age 30. 142 applicants, 27% accepted, 24 enrolled. In 2015, 15 master's, 9 doctorates awarded. *Degree requirements:* For master's, thesis (for some programs); for doctorate, thesis/dissertation. *Entrance requirements:* For master's and doctorate, GRE General Test, minimum GPA of 3.0, transcript, resume, statement of purpose, 3 letters of recommendation. Additional exam requirements/recommendations for international students: Required—TOEFL (minimum score: paper-based 525, iBT 71), Michigan English Language Assessment Battery (minimum score of 75), IELTS (minimum score of 6.0), PTE Academic (minimum score of 48), or completion of ELS level 112 Intensive Program. *Application deadline:* For fall admission, 12/15 for domestic students, 12/5 for international students; for spring admission, 11/29 for domestic and international students. Application fee: $45 ($70 for international students). Electronic applications accepted. *Expenses:* Tuition, state resident: full-time $10,864; part-time $495 per credit hour. Tuition, nonresident: full-time $18,380; part-time $837 per credit hour. *Financial support:* Research assistantships with full tuition reimbursements, teaching assistantships with full tuition reimbursements, career-related internships or fieldwork, Federal Work-Study, scholarships/grants, and unspecified assistantships available. Financial award application deadline: 2/1. *Unit head:* Dr. James L. Blank, Dean, 330-672-2650, E-mail: jblank@kent.edu. *Application contact:* Dr. Heather K. Caldwell, Associate Professor and Graduate Coordinator, 330-672-3636, E-mail: hcaldwel@kent.edu.
Website: http://www.kent.edu/biology/

Laurentian University, School of Graduate Studies and Research, Programme in Biology, Sudbury, ON P3E 2C6, Canada. Offers biology (M Sc); boreal ecology (PhD). *Program availability:* Part-time. *Degree requirements:* For master's, thesis. *Entrance requirements:* For master's, honors degree with second class or better. *Faculty research:* Recovery of acid-stressed lakes, effects of climate change, origin and maintenance of biocomplexity, radionuclide dynamics, cytogenetic studies of plants.

Lesley University, Graduate School of Education, Cambridge, MA 02138-2790. Offers arts, community, and education (M Ed); autism studies (Certificate); curriculum and instruction (M Ed); early childhood education (M Ed); ecological teaching and learning (MS); educational studies (PhD), including adult learning, educational leadership, individually designed; elementary education (M Ed); emergent technologies for educators (Certificate); ESLArts: language learning through the arts (M Ed); high school education (M Ed); individually designed (M Ed); integrated teaching through the arts (M Ed); literacy for K-8 classroom teachers (M Ed); mathematics education (M Ed); middle school education (M Ed); moderate disabilities (M Ed); online learning (Certificate); reading (CAGS); science in education (M Ed); severe disabilities (M Ed); special needs (CAGS); specialist teacher of reading (M Ed); teacher of visual art (M Ed); technology in education (M Ed, CAGS). *Accreditation:* Teacher Education Accreditation

Council. *Program availability:* Part-time, evening/weekend, online learning. *Degree requirements:* For master's, practicum; for doctorate, thesis/dissertation. *Entrance requirements:* For master's, Massachusetts Tests for Educator Licensure (MTEL), transcripts, statement of purpose, recommendations; interview (for special education); for doctorate, GRE General Test, transcripts, statement of purpose, recommendations, interview, master's degree, resume; for other advanced degree, interview, master's degree. Additional exam requirements/recommendations for international students: Required—TOEFL (minimum score 550 paper-based; 80 iBT). Electronic applications accepted. *Faculty research:* Assessment in literacy, mathematics and science; autism spectrum disorders; instructional technology and online learning; multicultural education and English language learners.

Marquette University, Graduate School, College of Arts and Sciences, Department of Biology, Milwaukee, WI 53201-1881. Offers cell biology (MS, PhD); developmental biology (MS, PhD); ecology (MS, PhD); epithelial physiology (MS, PhD); genetics (MS, PhD); microbiology (MS, PhD); molecular biology (MS, PhD); muscle and exercise physiology (MS, PhD); neuroscience (PhD). *Faculty:* 22 full-time (7 women), 3 part-time/adjunct (2 women). *Students:* 28 full-time (11 women), 12 part-time (4 women); includes 4 minority (1 Asian, non-Hispanic/Latino; 1 Hispanic/Latino; 2 Two or more races, non-Hispanic/Latino), 11 international. Average age 27. 72 applicants, 28% accepted, 5 enrolled. In 2015, 2 master's, 4 doctorates awarded. Terminal master's awarded for partial completion of doctoral program. *Degree requirements:* For master's, comprehensive exam, thesis, 1 year of teaching experience or equivalent; for doctorate, thesis/dissertation, 1 year of teaching experience or equivalent, qualifying exam. *Entrance requirements:* For master's and doctorate, GRE General Test, GRE Subject Test, official transcripts from all current and previous colleges/universities except Marquette, statement of professional goals and aspirations, three letters of recommendation. Additional exam requirements/recommendations for international students: Required—TOEFL (minimum score 530 paper-based). *Application deadline:* For fall admission, 12/15 for domestic and international students. Application fee: $50. Electronic applications accepted. *Financial support:* In 2015–16, 39 students received support, including 6 fellowships (averaging $1,208 per year), 4 research assistantships with full tuition reimbursements available (averaging $21,750 per year), 29 teaching assistantships with full tuition reimbursements available (averaging $21,750 per year); scholarships/grants, health care benefits, tuition waivers (full and partial), and unspecified assistantships also available. Support available to part-time students. Financial award application deadline: 2/15. *Faculty research:* Neurobiology, neuroendocrinology, epithelial physiology, neuropeptide interactions, synaptic transmission. *Total annual research expenditures:* $1.2 million. *Unit head:* Dr. Ed Blumenthal, Chair, 414-288-1748. *Application contact:* Dr. Michael Schlappi, Recruiting Contact, 414-288-1467.
Website: http://www.marquette.edu/biology/

Michigan State University, The Graduate School, College of Natural Science, Interdepartmental Program in Ecology, Evolutionary Biology and Behavior, East Lansing, MI 48824. Offers PhD. *Entrance requirements:* Additional exam requirements/recommendations for international students: Required—TOEFL. Electronic applications accepted.

Michigan Technological University, Graduate School, School of Forest Resources and Environmental Science, Houghton, MI 49931. Offers applied ecology (MS); forest ecology and management (MS); forest molecular genetics and biotechnology (MS, PhD); forest science (PhD); forestry (MF, MS); geographic information science (MGIS). *Accreditation:* SAF. *Program availability:* Part-time. *Faculty:* 41 full-time (11 women), 52 part-time/adjunct (18 women). *Students:* 58 full-time (24 women), 23 part-time (6 women); includes 2 minority (both Two or more races, non-Hispanic/Latino), 19 international. Average age 31. 92 applicants, 51% accepted, 32 enrolled. In 2015, 16 master's, 5 doctorates awarded. Terminal master's awarded for partial completion of doctoral program. *Degree requirements:* For master's, thesis (for some programs), comprehensive exam (for non-research degrees); for doctorate, comprehensive exam, thesis/dissertation. *Entrance requirements:* For master's and doctorate, GRE, statement of purpose, personal statement, official transcripts, 3 letters of recommendation, resume/curriculum vitae. Additional exam requirements/recommendations for international students: Required—TOEFL (recommended score 79 iBT) or IELTS. *Application deadline:* Applications are processed on a rolling basis. Electronic applications accepted. *Expenses:* Tuition, state resident: full-time $15,507; part-time $861.50 per credit. Tuition, nonresident: full-time $15,507; part-time $861.50 per credit. *Required fees:* $248; $248. Tuition and fees vary according to course load and program. *Financial support:* In 2015–16, 51 students received support, including 6 fellowships with tuition reimbursements available (averaging $14,516 per year), 17 research assistantships with tuition reimbursements available (averaging $14,516 per year), 6 teaching assistantships with tuition reimbursements available (averaging $14,516 per year); career-related internships or fieldwork, Federal Work-Study, scholarships/grants, health care benefits, unspecified assistantships, and cooperative program also available. Financial award applicants required to submit FAFSA. *Faculty research:* Forest ecology and management, forest molecular genetics and biotechnology, forest biomaterials, restoration ecology, wildlife ecology and management. *Total annual research expenditures:* $3.7 million. *Unit head:* Dr. Terry Sharik, Dean, 906-487-2352, Fax: 906-487-2915, E-mail: tlsharik@mtu.edu. *Application contact:* Dr. Andrew J. Storer, Associate Dean, 906-487-3470, Fax: 906-487-2915, E-mail: storer@mtu.edu.
Website: http://www.mtu.edu/forest/

Montana State University, The Graduate School, College of Letters and Science, Department of Ecology, Bozeman, MT 59717. Offers ecological and environmental statistics (MS); ecology and environmental sciences (PhD); fish and wildlife biology (PhD); fish and wildlife management (MS). *Program availability:* Part-time. *Degree requirements:* For master's, comprehensive exam, thesis (for some programs); for doctorate, comprehensive exam, thesis/dissertation. *Entrance requirements:* For master's and doctorate, GRE, minimum GPA of 3.0, letters of recommendation, essay. Additional exam requirements/recommendations for international students: Required—TOEFL (minimum score 550 paper-based). Electronic applications accepted. *Faculty research:* Community ecology, population ecology, land-use effects, management and conservation, environmental modeling.

Montclair State University, The Graduate School, College of Science and Mathematics, Program in Biology, Montclair, NJ 07043-1624. Offers biological science/education (MS); biology (MS); ecology and evolution (MS); physiology (MS). *Students:* 10 full-time (7 women), 35 part-time (27 women); includes 9 minority (6 Asian, non-Hispanic/Latino; 2 Hispanic/Latino; 1 Two or more races, non-Hispanic/Latino). Average age 28. 23 applicants, 57% accepted, 12 enrolled. In 2015, 18 master's awarded. *Expenses:* Tuition, state resident: part-time $553 per credit. Tuition, nonresident: part-time $854 per credit. *Required fees:* $91 per credit. Tuition and fees vary according to program. *Unit head:* Dr. Liza C. Hazard, Chairperson, 973-655-4397, E-mail: hazardl@mail.montclair.edu. *Application contact:* Amy Aiello, Director of Graduate Admissions and Operations, 973-655-5147, Fax: 973-655-7869, E-mail: graduate.school@montclair.edu.

North Dakota State University, College of Graduate and Interdisciplinary Studies, Interdisciplinary Program in Environmental and Conservation Sciences, Fargo, ND 58102. Offers MS, PhD. *Degree requirements:* For master's, comprehensive exam, thesis. *Entrance requirements:* Additional exam requirements/recommendations for international students: Required—TOEFL (minimum score 550 paper-based; 79 iBT). *Application deadline:* For fall admission, 5/1 for international students; for spring admission, 8/1 for international students. Application fee: $35. *Unit head:* Eakalak Khan, Director, 701-231-7717, Fax: 701-231-6185, E-mail: eakalak.khan@ndsu.edu. *Application contact:* Madonna Fitzgerald, Academic Assistant, 701-231-6456, E-mail: madonna.fitzgerald@ndsu.edu.
Website: http://www.ndsu.edu/ecs/

Northeastern University, College of Science, Boston, MA 02115-5096. Offers applied mathematics (MS); bioinformatics (MS); biology (PhD); biotechnology (MS); chemistry (MS, PhD); ecology, evolution, and marine biology (PhD); marine biology (MS); mathematics (MS, PhD); network science (PhD); operations research (MSOR); physics (MS, PhD); psychology (PhD). *Program availability:* Part-time. *Faculty:* 216 full-time (70 women), 62 part-time/adjunct (20 women). *Students:* 517 full-time (252 women), 80 part-time (39 women). In 2015, 94 master's, 46 doctorates awarded. Terminal master's awarded for partial completion of doctoral program. *Degree requirements:* For master's, comprehensive exam (for some programs), thesis; for doctorate, comprehensive exam (for some programs), thesis/dissertation. *Entrance requirements:* For master's, GRE General Test. *Application deadline:* Applications are processed on a rolling basis. Application fee: $75. Electronic applications accepted. *Expenses:* $1,325 per credit; $1,170 per credit (for marine biology). *Financial support:* Fellowships with tuition reimbursements, research assistantships with tuition reimbursements, teaching assistantships with tuition reimbursements, career-related internships or fieldwork, scholarships/grants, health care benefits, tuition waivers (full and partial), and unspecified assistantships available. Support available to part-time students. Financial award applicants required to submit FAFSA. *Unit head:* Dr. Jonathan Tilly, Interim Dean. *Application contact:* Graduate Student Services, 617-373-4275, E-mail: gradcos@neu.edu.
Website: http://www.northeastern.edu/cos/

The Ohio State University, Graduate School, College of Arts and Sciences, Division of Natural and Mathematical Sciences, Department of Evolution, Ecology, and Organismal Biology, Columbus, OH 43210. Offers MS, PhD. *Faculty:* 25. *Students:* 55 full-time (21 women), 1 (woman) part-time. Average age 29. In 2015, 5 master's, 7 doctorates awarded. *Degree requirements:* For master's, thesis optional; for doctorate, thesis/dissertation. *Entrance requirements:* For master's and doctorate, GRE General Test. Additional exam requirements/recommendations for international students: Required—TOEFL (minimum score 550 paper-based; 79 iBT), Michigan English Language Assessment Battery (minimum score 86); Recommended—IELTS (minimum score 7). *Application deadline:* For fall admission, 12/1 priority date for domestic students, 11/30 priority date for international students. Applications are processed on a rolling basis. Application fee: $60 ($70 for international students). Electronic applications accepted. *Financial support:* Fellowships with tuition reimbursements, research assistantships with tuition reimbursements, teaching assistantships with tuition reimbursements, Federal Work-Study, and institutionally sponsored loans available. Support available to part-time students. *Unit head:* Dr. Elizabeth Marschall, Chair, 614-292-8767, E-mail: marschall.2@osu.edu. *Application contact:* Graduate and Professional Admissions, 614-292-9444, Fax: 614-292-3895, E-mail: gpadmissions@osu.edu.
Website: http://eeob.osu.edu/

The Ohio State University, Graduate School, College of Food, Agricultural, and Environmental Sciences, School of Environment and Natural Resources, Columbus, OH 43210. Offers ecological restoration (MS, PhD); ecosystem science (MS, PhD); environment and natural resources (MENR); environmental social sciences (MS, PhD); fisheries and wildlife science (MS, PhD); forest science (MS, PhD); rural sociology (MS, PhD); soil science (MS, PhD). *Faculty:* 38. *Students:* 90 full-time (58 women), 5 part-time (2 women); includes 12 minority (3 Black or African American, non-Hispanic/Latino; 7 Hispanic/Latino; 2 Two or more races, non-Hispanic/Latino), 6 international. Average age 28. In 2015, 22 master's, 4 doctorates awarded. *Degree requirements:* For master's, thesis; for doctorate, thesis/dissertation. *Entrance requirements:* For master's and doctorate, GRE. Additional exam requirements/recommendations for international students: Required—TOEFL (minimum score 550 paper-based; 79 iBT), Michigan English Language Assessment Battery (minimum score 82); Recommended—IELTS (minimum score 7). *Application deadline:* For fall admission, 1/1 priority date for domestic students, 12/15 priority date for international students; for spring admission, 11/1 for domestic students, 9/15 for international students. Applications are processed on a rolling basis. Application fee: $60 ($70 for international students). Electronic applications accepted. *Financial support:* Fellowships with tuition reimbursements, research assistantships with tuition reimbursements, teaching assistantships with tuition reimbursements, health care benefits, and unspecified assistantships available. *Unit head:* Dr. Jeff S. Sharp, Director, 614-292-9410, E-mail: sharp.123@osu.edu. *Application contact:* Graduate and Professional Admissions, 614-292-9444, Fax: 614-292-3895, E-mail: gpadmissions@osu.edu.
Website: http://senr.osu.edu/

Ohio University, Graduate College, College of Arts and Sciences, Department of Biological Sciences, Athens, OH 45701-2979. Offers biological sciences (MS, PhD); cell biology and physiology (MS, PhD); ecology and evolutionary biology (MS, PhD); exercise physiology and muscle biology (MS, PhD); microbiology (MS, PhD); neuroscience (MS, PhD). Terminal master's awarded for partial completion of doctoral program. *Degree requirements:* For master's, comprehensive exam, thesis, 1 quarter of teaching experience; for doctorate, comprehensive exam, thesis/dissertation, 2 quarters of teaching experience. *Entrance requirements:* For master's, GRE General Test, names of three faculty members whose research interests most closely match the applicant's interest; for doctorate, GRE General Test, essay concerning prior training, research interest and career goals, plus names of three faculty members whose research interests/recommendations most closely match the applicant's interest. Additional exam requirements/recommendations for international students: Required—TOEFL (minimum score 620 paper-based; 105 iBT) or IELTS (minimum score 7.5). Electronic applications accepted. *Faculty research:* Ecology and evolutionary biology, exercise physiology and muscle biology, neurobiology, cell biology, physiology.

Oklahoma State University, College of Arts and Sciences, Department of Plant Biology, Ecology, and Evolution, Stillwater, OK 74078. Offers botany (MS); environmental science (MS, PhD); plant science (PhD). *Faculty:* 14 full-time (5 women). *Students:* 8 part-time (3 women); includes 4 minority (1 Asian, non-Hispanic/Latino; 1 Hispanic/Latino; 2 Two or more races, non-Hispanic/Latino). Average age 32. 3 applicants, 67% accepted. In 2015, 3 master's awarded. *Degree requirements:* For master's, thesis; for doctorate, comprehensive exam, thesis/dissertation. *Entrance requirements:* For master's and doctorate, GRE or GMAT. Additional exam requirements/recommendations for international students: Required—TOEFL (minimum score 550 paper-based; 79 iBT). *Application deadline:* For fall admission, 3/1 priority date for international students; for spring admission, 8/1 priority date for international students. Applications are processed on a rolling basis. Application fee: $40 ($75 for international students). Electronic applications accepted. *Expenses:* Tuition, state resident: full-time $3528; part-time $196 per credit hour. Tuition, nonresident: full-time

Ecology

$14,144; part-time $785.75 per credit hour. *Required fees:* $1895; $105.25 per credit hour. Tuition and fees vary according to campus/location. *Financial support:* In 2015–16, 1 research assistantship (averaging $18,504 per year), 12 teaching assistantships (averaging $20,754 per year) were awarded; career-related internships or fieldwork, Federal Work-Study, scholarships/grants, health care benefits, tuition waivers (partial), and unspecified assistantships also available. Support available to part-time students. Financial award application deadline: 3/1; financial award applicants required to submit FAFSA. *Faculty research:* Ethnobotany, developmental genetics of arabidopsis, biological roles of plasmodesmata, community ecology and biodiversity, nutrient cycling in grassland ecosystems. *Unit head:* Dr. Linda Watson, Department Head, 405-744-5559, Fax: 405-744-7074, E-mail: linda.watson10@okstate.edu. Website: http://plantbio.okstate.edu

Old Dominion University, College of Sciences, Program in Ecological Sciences, Norfolk, VA 23529. Offers PhD. *Faculty:* 13 full-time (3 women), 41 part-time/adjunct (7 women). *Students:* 9 full-time (5 women), 11 part-time (7 women), 2 international. Average age 31. 17 applicants, 24% accepted, 4 enrolled. In 2015, 3 doctorates awarded. *Degree requirements:* For doctorate, one foreign language, comprehensive exam, thesis/dissertation. *Entrance requirements:* For doctorate, GRE General Test, 3 letters of recommendation. Additional exam requirements/recommendations for international students: Required—TOEFL (minimum score 550 paper-based; 79 iBT). *Application deadline:* For fall admission, 2/1 priority date for domestic and international students. Applications are processed on a rolling basis. Application fee: $50. Electronic applications accepted. *Expenses:* Tuition, state resident: full-time $11,136; part-time $464 per credit hour. Tuition, nonresident: full-time $27,840; part-time $1160 per credit hour. *Required fees:* $64 per semester. Tuition and fees vary according to campus/location, program and reciprocity agreements. *Financial support:* In 2015–16, 3 fellowships with full tuition reimbursements (averaging $17,000 per year), 4 research assistantships with full tuition reimbursements (averaging $15,750 per year), 9 teaching assistantships with full tuition reimbursements (averaging $15,000 per year) were awarded; scholarships/grants also available. Financial award application deadline: 2/15; financial award applicants required to submit FAFSA. *Faculty research:* Marine ecology, physiological ecology, systematics and speciation, ecological and evolutionary processes, molecular genetics. *Total annual research expenditures:* $2 million. *Unit head:* Dr. Holly Gaff, Graduate Program Director, 757-683-6903, Fax: 757-683-5283, E-mail: hgaff@odu.edu. *Application contact:* William Heffelfinger, Director of Graduate Admissions, 757-683-5554, Fax: 757-683-3255, E-mail: gradadmit@odu.edu. Website: http://www.odu.edu/academics/programs/doctoral/ecological-sciences

Oregon State University, Interdisciplinary/Institutional Programs, Program in Environmental Sciences, Corvallis, OR 97331. Offers biogeochemistry (MS, PhD); ecology (MS, PhD); environmental education (MS, PhD); environmental sciences (PSM); natural resources (MS, PhD); quantitative analysis (MS, PhD); social science (MS, PhD); water resources (MS, PhD). *Program availability:* Part-time. *Students:* 17 full-time (12 women), 12 part-time (6 women); includes 7 minority (1 Black or African American, non-Hispanic/Latino; 2 Asian, non-Hispanic/Latino; 2 Hispanic/Latino; 2 Two or more races, non-Hispanic/Latino), 3 international. Average age 34. 42 applicants, 19% accepted, 3 enrolled. In 2015, 6 master's, 4 doctorates awarded. *Entrance requirements:* For master's and doctorate, GRE. Additional exam requirements/recommendations for international students: Required—TOEFL (minimum score 80 iBT), IELTS (minimum score 6.5). *Application deadline:* For fall admission, 1/15 for domestic students. Application fee: $75 ($85 for international students). *Expenses:* Contact institution. *Unit head:* Dr. Carolyn Fonyo Boggess, Interim Director, E-mail: carolyn.fonyo@oregonstate.edu. Website: http://envsci.science.oregonstate.edu/

Penn State University Park, Graduate School, Intercollege Graduate Programs, Intercollege Graduate Program in Ecology, University Park, PA 16802. Offers ecology (MS, PhD). *Unit head:* Dr. Regina Vasilatos-Younken, Dean, 814-865-2516, Fax: 814-863-4627. *Application contact:* Lori Stania, Director, Graduate Student Services, 814-865-1795, Fax: 814-863-4627, E-mail: l-gswww@lists.psu.edu.

Princeton University, Graduate School, Department of Ecology and Evolutionary Biology, Princeton, NJ 08544-1019. Offers PhD. *Degree requirements:* For doctorate, thesis/dissertation. *Entrance requirements:* For doctorate, GRE General Test, GRE Subject Test. Additional exam requirements/recommendations for international students: Required—TOEFL (minimum score 600 paper-based). Electronic applications accepted.

Purdue University, College of Engineering, Division of Environmental and Ecological Engineering, West Lafayette, IN 47907. Offers MS, PhD.

Purdue University, Graduate School, College of Agriculture, Department of Forestry and Natural Resources, West Lafayette, IN 47907. Offers fisheries and aquatic sciences (MS, MSF, PhD); forest biology (MS, MSF, PhD); natural resource social science (MS, PhD); natural resources social science (MSF); quantitative ecology (MS, MSF, PhD); wildlife science (MS, MSF, PhD); wood products and wood products manufacturing (MS, MSF, PhD). *Degree requirements:* For master's, thesis; for doctorate, thesis/dissertation. *Entrance requirements:* For master's and doctorate, GRE General Test (minimum score: verbal 50th percentile; quantitative 50th percentile; analytical writing 4.0), minimum undergraduate GPA of 3.2 or equivalent. Additional exam requirements/recommendations for international students: Required—TOEFL (minimum score 550 paper-based; 77 iBT). Electronic applications accepted. *Faculty research:* Wildlife management, forest management, forest ecology, forest soils, limnology.

Purdue University, Graduate School, College of Science, Department of Biological Sciences, West Lafayette, IN 47907. Offers biochemistry (PhD); biophysics (PhD); cell and developmental biology (PhD); ecology, evolutionary and population biology (MS, PhD), including ecology, evolutionary biology, population biology; genetics (MS, PhD); microbiology (MS, PhD); molecular biology (PhD); neurobiology (MS, PhD); plant physiology (PhD). Terminal master's awarded for partial completion of doctoral program. *Degree requirements:* For master's, thesis (for some programs); for doctorate, thesis/dissertation, seminars, teaching experience. *Entrance requirements:* For master's, GRE General Test (minimum analytical writing score of 3.5), minimum undergraduate GPA of 3.0; for doctorate, GRE General Test (minimum analytical writing score of 3.5), minimum undergraduate GPA of 3.5. Additional exam requirements/recommendations for international students: Required—TOEFL (minimum score 600 paper-based; 107 iBT for MS, 80 iBT for PhD). Electronic applications accepted.

Purdue University, Graduate School, Interdisciplinary Graduate Program in Ecological Sciences and Engineering, West Lafayette, IN 47907. Offers MS, PhD. *Degree requirements:* For master's, thesis optional; for doctorate, thesis/dissertation, written and oral preliminary exam. *Entrance requirements:* For master's and doctorate, GRE (minimum old score Verbal and Quantitative combined 1200, Analytical writing 4.0; new score 300/4.0), previous research or environmental project experience; minimum GPA of 3.3. Additional exam requirements/recommendations for international students: Required—TOEFL (minimum score 550 paper-based; 77 iBT), IELTS (minimum score 6.5); Recommended—TWE. Electronic applications accepted.

Rice University, Graduate Programs, Wiess School of Natural Sciences, Department of Ecology and Evolutionary Biology, Houston, TX 77251-1892. Offers MA, MS, PhD.

Terminal master's awarded for partial completion of doctoral program. *Degree requirements:* For master's, comprehensive exam (for some programs), thesis (for some programs); for doctorate, comprehensive exam, thesis/dissertation. *Entrance requirements:* For master's and doctorate, GRE General Test, GRE Subject Test. Additional exam requirements/recommendations for international students: Required—TOEFL (minimum score 600 paper-based; 90 iBT). Electronic applications accepted. *Faculty research:* Trace gas emissions, wetlands, biology, community ecology of forests and grasslands, conservation biology specialization.

Rutgers University–New Brunswick, Graduate School-New Brunswick, Program in Ecology and Evolution, Piscataway, NJ 08854-8097. Offers MS, PhD. *Program availability:* Part-time. Terminal master's awarded for partial completion of doctoral program. *Degree requirements:* For master's, comprehensive exam; for doctorate, comprehensive exam, thesis/dissertation. *Entrance requirements:* For master's and doctorate, GRE General Test, minimum GPA of 3.0. Additional exam requirements/recommendations for international students: Required—TOEFL (minimum score 550 paper-based). Electronic applications accepted. *Faculty research:* Population and community ecology, population genetics, evolutionary biology, conservation biology, ecosystem ecology.

San Diego State University, Graduate and Research Affairs, College of Sciences, Department of Biology, Program in Ecology, San Diego, CA 92182. Offers MS, PhD. PhD offered jointly with University of California, Davis. *Degree requirements:* For master's, thesis; for doctorate, thesis/dissertation. *Entrance requirements:* For master's, GRE General Test, resumé or curriculum vitae, 2 letters of recommendation; for doctorate, GRE General Test, GRE Subject Test, resume or curriculum vitae, 3 letters of recommendation. Electronic applications accepted. *Faculty research:* Conservation and restoration ecology, coastal and marine ecology, global change and ecosystem ecology.

San Francisco State University, Division of Graduate Studies, College of Science and Engineering, Department of Biology, Program in Ecology, Evolution, and Conservation Biology, San Francisco, CA 94132-1722. Offers MS. *Application deadline:* Applications are processed on a rolling basis. *Expenses:* Tuition, state resident: full-time $6738. Tuition, nonresident: full-time $15,666. *Required fees:* $1004. *Unit head:* Dr. Andrew Zink, Acting Coordinator, 415-405-2761, Fax: 415-338-2295, E-mail: zink@sfsu.edu. Website: http://biology.sfsu.edu/graduate/ecology-evolution-and-conservation-biology-eecb-0

San Jose State University, Graduate Studies and Research, College of Science, San Jose, CA 95192-0001. Offers biological sciences (MA, MS), including molecular biology and microbiology (MS); organismal biology, conservation and ecology (MS), physiology (MS); chemistry (MA, MS); computer science (MS); cybersecurity (Certificate); cybersecurity: core technologies (Certificate); geology (MS); marine science (MS); master biotechnology (MBT); mathematics (MA, MS), including mathematics education (MA), science; meteorology (MS); physics (MS), including computational physics, modern optics, science (MA, MS); science education (MS); statistics (MS); Unix system administration (Certificate). *Program availability:* Part-time, evening/weekend. *Students:* 118 full-time (68 women), 52 part-time (25 women); includes 125 minority (5 Black or African American, non-Hispanic/Latino; 97 Asian, non-Hispanic/Latino; 23 Hispanic/Latino), 121 international. Average age 27. 1,236 applicants, 21% accepted, 171 enrolled. In 2015, 168 master's awarded. *Entrance requirements:* For master's, GRE. *Application deadline:* For fall admission, 6/29 for domestic students; for spring admission, 11/30 for domestic students. Applications are processed on a rolling basis. Application fee: $55. Electronic applications accepted. *Financial support:* Teaching assistantships, career-related internships or fieldwork, Federal Work-Study, and institutionally sponsored loans available. Support available to part-time students. Financial award applicants required to submit FAFSA. *Faculty research:* Radiochemistry/environmental analysis, health physics, radiation effects. *Unit head:* J. Michael Parrish, Dean, 408-924-4800, Fax: 408-924-4815. *Application contact:* 408-924-2480, Fax: 408-924-2477. Website: http://www.science.sjsu.edu/

Sonoma State University, School of Science and Technology, Department of Biology, Rohnert Park, CA 94928. Offers biochemistry (MA); ecology (MS); environmental biology (MS); evolutionary biology (MS); functional morphology (MS); molecular and cell biology (MS); organismal biology (MS). *Program availability:* Part-time. *Degree requirements:* For master's, thesis or alternative, oral exam. *Entrance requirements:* For master's, GRE General Test, GRE Subject Test, minimum GPA of 3.0. Additional exam requirements/recommendations for international students: Required—TOEFL (minimum score 500 paper-based). *Faculty research:* Plant physiology, comparative physiology, community ecology, restoration ecology, marine ecology, conservation genetics, primate behavior, behavioral ecology, developmental biology, plant and animal systematics.

Stanford University, School of Humanities and Sciences, Department of Anthropology, Stanford, CA 94305-9991. Offers anthropology (MA); archaeology (PhD); culture and society (PhD); ecology and environment (PhD). Terminal master's awarded for partial completion of doctoral program. *Degree requirements:* For master's, thesis; for doctorate, one foreign language, thesis/dissertation. *Entrance requirements:* For master's and doctorate, GRE General Test. Additional exam requirements/recommendations for international students: Required—TOEFL. Electronic applications accepted. *Expenses: Tuition, area resident:* Full-time $45,729. *Required fees:* $591.

State University of New York College of Environmental Science and Forestry, Department of Environmental and Forest Biology, Syracuse, NY 13210-2779. Offers applied ecology (MPS); chemical ecology (MPS, MS, PhD); conservation biology (MPS, MS, PhD); ecology (MPS, MS, PhD); entomology (MPS, MS, PhD); environmental interpretation (MPS, MS, PhD); environmental physiology (MPS, MS, PhD); fish and wildlife biology and management (MPS, MS, PhD); forest pathology and mycology (MPS, MS, PhD); plant biotechnology (MPS); plant science and biotechnology (MPS, MS, PhD). *Faculty:* 29 full-time (9 women), 4 part-time/adjunct (3 women). *Students:* 81 full-time (47 women), 57 part-time (24 women); includes 9 minority (1 Black or African American, non-Hispanic/Latino; 2 American Indian or Alaska Native, non-Hispanic/Latino; 1 Asian, non-Hispanic/Latino; 3 Hispanic/Latino; 2 Two or more races, non-Hispanic/Latino), 15 international. Average age 28. 47 applicants, 49% accepted, 15 enrolled. In 2015, 15 master's, 7 doctorates awarded. *Degree requirements:* For master's, thesis (for some programs), capstone seminar; for doctorate, comprehensive exam, thesis/dissertation, capstone seminar. *Entrance requirements:* For master's and doctorate, GRE General Test, minimum GPA of 3.0. Additional exam requirements/recommendations for international students: Required—TOEFL (minimum score 550 paper-based; 80 iBT), IELTS (minimum score 6). *Application deadline:* For fall admission, 2/1 priority date for domestic and international students; for spring admission, 11/1 priority date for domestic and international students. Applications are processed on a rolling basis. Application fee: $60. *Expenses:* Tuition, state resident: full-time $10,870; part-time $453 per credit. Tuition, nonresident: full-time $22,210; part-time $925 per credit. *Required fees:* $1075; $89.22 per credit. *Financial support:* In 2015–16, 4 fellowships with tuition reimbursements, 36 research assistantships with tuition reimbursements, 39 teaching assistantships with tuition reimbursements (averaging $11,490 per year) were awarded; Federal Work-Study, institutionally sponsored loans, scholarships/grants, health care benefits, and unspecified assistantships also available. Financial award application deadline: 6/30. *Faculty* *research:* Ecology, conservation biology, fish and wildlife biology and management, plant science, entomology. *Total annual research expenditures:* $4.1 million. *Unit head:* Dr. Donald J. Leopold, Chair, 315-470-6760, Fax: 315-470-6934, E-mail: djleopold@esf.edu. *Application contact:* Dr. Danilo D. Fernando, Director, Graduate Program/Associate Professor, 315-470-6746, Fax: 315-470-6934, E-mail: dfernando@esf.edu. Website: http://www.esf.edu/efb/grad/default.asp

State University of New York College of Environmental Science and Forestry, Department of Forest and Natural Resources Management, Syracuse, NY 13210-2779. Offers ecology and ecosystems (MPS, MS, PhD); economics, governance and human dimensions (MPS, MS, PhD); forest and natural resources management (MPS, MS, PhD); monitoring, analysis and modeling (MPS, MS, PhD). *Accreditation:* SAF. *Faculty:* 34 full-time (9 women), 7 part-time/adjunct (0 women). *Students:* 40 full-time (24 women), 5 part-time (0 women); includes 6 minority (2 American Indian or Alaska Native, non-Hispanic/Latino; 1 Asian, non-Hispanic/Latino; 2 Hispanic/Latino; 1 Two or more races, non-Hispanic/Latino), 10 international. 41 applicants, 68% accepted, 16 enrolled. *Degree requirements:* For master's, thesis (for some programs); for doctorate, comprehensive exam, thesis/dissertation. *Entrance requirements:* For master's and doctorate, GRE General Test, minimum GPA of 3.0. Additional exam requirements/recommendations for international students: Required—TOEFL (minimum score 550 paper-based; 80 iBT), IELTS (minimum score 6). *Application deadline:* For fall admission, 2/1 priority date for domestic and international students; for spring admission, 11/1 priority date for domestic and international students. Applications are processed on a rolling basis. Application fee: $60. *Expenses:* Tuition, state resident: full-time $10,870; part-time $453 per credit. Tuition, nonresident: full-time $22,210; part-time $925 per credit. *Required fees:* $1075; $89.22 per credit. *Financial support:* Fellowships with tuition reimbursements, research assistantships with tuition reimbursements, teaching assistantships with tuition reimbursements, career-related internships or fieldwork, Federal Work-Study, institutionally sponsored loans, scholarships/grants, health care benefits, and unspecified assistantships available. Financial award application deadline: 6/30; financial award applicants required to submit FAFSA. *Faculty research:* Silviculture recreation management, tree improvement, operations management, economics. *Unit head:* Dr. David Newman, Chair, 315-470-6534, Fax: 315-470-6535. *Application contact:* Scott Shannon, Dean, Instruction and Graduate Studies, 315-470-6599, Fax: 315-470-6978, E-mail: esfgrad@esf.edu. Website: http://www.esf.edu/fnrm/

Stony Brook University, State University of New York, Graduate School, College of Arts and Sciences, Department of Ecology and Evolution, Stony Brook, NY 11794. Offers applied ecology (MA); ecology and evolution (PhD). *Faculty:* 18 full-time (6 women). *Students:* 51 full-time (30 women), 1 part-time (0 women); includes 2 minority (1 Asian, non-Hispanic/Latino; 1 Hispanic/Latino), 12 international. Average age 26. 34 applicants, 68% accepted, 5 enrolled. In 2015, 9 doctorates awarded. *Degree requirements:* For doctorate, one foreign language, comprehensive exam, thesis/dissertation, teaching experience. *Entrance requirements:* For doctorate, GRE General Test, GRE Subject Test. Additional exam requirements/recommendations for international students: Required—TOEFL. *Application deadline:* For fall admission, 1/15 for domestic students; for spring admission, 10/1 for domestic students. Application fee: $100. *Expenses:* $12,421 full-time resident tuition and fees, $453 per credit hour; $23,761 full-time nonresident tuition and fees, $925 per credit hour. *Financial support:* In 2015–16, 7 research assistantships, 25 teaching assistantships were awarded; fellowships and Federal Work-Study also available. *Faculty research:* Ecology, ecology and population, evolution, biodiversity, environmental conservation. *Total annual research expenditures:* $1.3 million. *Unit head:* Dr. Robert W. Thacker, Chair, 631-632-8590, Fax: 631-632-7626, E-mail: robert.thacker@stonybrook.edu. *Application contact:* Melissa Cohen, Coordinator, 631-246-8604, Fax: 631-632-7626, E-mail: melissa.j.cohen@stonybrook.edu. Website: http://life.bio.sunysb.edu/ee/

Tulane University, School of Science and Engineering, Department of Ecology and Evolutionary Biology, New Orleans, LA 70118-5669. Offers MS, PhD. Terminal master's awarded for partial completion of doctoral program. *Degree requirements:* For master's, thesis or alternative; for doctorate, thesis/dissertation. *Entrance requirements:* For master's, GRE General Test, minimum B average in undergraduate course work; for doctorate, GRE General Test. Additional exam requirements/recommendations for international students: Required—TOEFL. *Application deadline:* For fall admission, 2/1 for domestic and international students. Application fee: $45. Electronic applications accepted. *Expenses:* Tuition, area resident: Full-time $47,658; part-time $2648 per credit hour. *Required fees:* $1980; $44.50 per credit hour. $550 per term. Tuition and fees vary according to course load, degree level and program. *Financial support:* Fellowships with full tuition reimbursements, research assistantships with full tuition reimbursements, teaching assistantships with full tuition reimbursements, and career-related internships or fieldwork available. Financial award application deadline: 2/1. *Faculty research:* Ichthyology, plant systematics, crustacean endocrinology, ecotoxicology, ornithology.

Universidad Nacional Pedro Henriquez Urena, Graduate School, Santo Domingo, Dominican Republic. Offers agricultural diversity (MS), including horticultural/fruit production, tropical animal production; conservation of monuments and cultural assets (M Arch); ecology and environment (MS); environmental engineering (MEE); international relations (MA); natural resource management (MS); political science (MA); project optimization (MPM); project feasibility (MPM); project management (MPM); sanitation engineering (ME); science for teachers (MS); tropical Caribbean architecture (M Arch).

University at Albany, State University of New York, College of Arts and Sciences, Department of Biological Sciences, Program in Ecology and Evolutionary Biology, Albany, NY 12222-0001. Offers PhD. *Degree requirements:* For doctorate, one foreign language, thesis/dissertation. *Entrance requirements:* For doctorate, GRE General Test.

University at Buffalo, the State University of New York, Graduate School, College of Arts and Sciences, Program in Evolution, Ecology and Behavior, Buffalo, NY 14260. Offers MS, PhD, Certificate. *Faculty:* 16 full-time (7 women), 5 part-time/adjunct (2 women). *Students:* 17 full-time (11 women), 4 international. Average age 25. 27 applicants, 74% accepted, 5 enrolled. In 2015, 2 master's awarded. Terminal master's awarded for partial completion of doctoral program. *Degree requirements:* For master's, project; for doctorate, comprehensive exam, thesis/dissertation. *Entrance requirements:* For master's, GRE, minimum undergraduate GPA of 3.0; for doctorate, GRE, minimum GPA of 3.0. Additional exam requirements/recommendations for international students: Required—TOEFL (minimum score 550 paper-based; 79 iBT). *Application deadline:* For fall admission, 1/15 priority date for domestic and international students. Applications are processed on a rolling basis. Application fee: $75. Electronic applications accepted. *Financial support:* In 2015–16, 3 fellowships with full tuition reimbursements (averaging $24,600 per year), 5 research assistantships with full tuition reimbursements (averaging $24,000 per year), 3 teaching assistantships with full tuition reimbursements (averaging $17,000 per year) were awarded; Federal Work-Study, scholarships/grants, health care benefits, and unspecified assistantships also available. Financial award application deadline: 1/15; financial award applicants required to submit FAFSA. *Faculty research:* Coral reef ecology, evolution and ecology of aquatic invertebrates, animal communication, paleobiology, primate behavior. *Unit head:* Dr. Katharina Dittmar De La Cruz, Program Director, 716-645-4912, E-mail: ub-evb@buffalo.edu. *Application contact:* Joseph C. Syracuse, Graduate Enrollment Manager, 716-645-2711, Fax: 716-645-3888, E-mail: jcs32@buffalo.edu. Website: http://www.evolutionecologybehavior.buffalo.edu/

University at Buffalo, the State University of New York, Graduate School, School of Architecture and Planning, Department of Architecture, Buffalo, NY 14214. Offers architecture (M Arch); ecological practices (MS Arch); historic preservation and urban design (MS Arch); inclusive design (MS Arch); real estate development (MS Arch); situated technology (MS Arch); M Arch/MBA; M Arch/MFA; M Arch/MUP. *Faculty:* 28 full-time (9 women), 16 part-time/adjunct (8 women). *Students:* 128 full-time (54 women), 12 part-time (4 women); includes 17 minority (3 Black or African American, non-Hispanic/Latino; 5 Asian, non-Hispanic/Latino; 5 Hispanic/Latino; 4 Two or more races, non-Hispanic/Latino), 33 international. Average age 26. 296 applicants, 29% accepted, 63 enrolled. In 2015, 44 master's awarded. *Degree requirements:* For master's, thesis or alternative, project. *Entrance requirements:* For master's, GRE, portfolio, 3 letters of recommendation, transcripts, 500-word personal statement. Additional exam requirements/recommendations for international students: Required—TOEFL (minimum score 79 iBT), IELTS (minimum score 6.5). *Application deadline:* For fall admission, 1/1 priority date for domestic and international students. Application fee: $75. Electronic applications accepted. *Expenses:* $15,284 resident full-time; $24,505 nonresident full-time. *Financial support:* In 2015–16, 6 fellowships with full tuition reimbursements (averaging $22,000 per year), 10 research assistantships with tuition reimbursements (averaging $7,515 per year), 29 teaching assistantships with partial tuition reimbursements (averaging $4,865 per year) were awarded; career-related internships or fieldwork, Federal Work-Study, scholarships/grants, health care benefits, and unspecified assistantships also available. Financial award application deadline: 3/1; financial award applicants required to submit FAFSA. *Faculty research:* Ecological practices, inclusive design, material culture, situated technologies, urban design. *Total annual research expenditures:* $3.4 million. *Unit head:* Prof. Omar Khan, Chair, 716-829-3483 Ext. 105, Fax: 716-829-3256, E-mail: omar.khan@buffalo.edu. *Application contact:* Debra Eggebrecht, Assistant to the Chair, 716-829-3486 Ext. 105, Fax: 716-829-3256, E-mail: dle2@buffalo.edu. Website: http://www.ap.buffalo.edu/architecture/

University of Alberta, Faculty of Graduate Studies and Research, Department of Biological Sciences, Edmonton, AB T6G 2E1, Canada. Offers environmental biology and ecology (M Sc, PhD); microbiology and biotechnology (M Sc, PhD); molecular biology and genetics (M Sc, PhD); physiology and cell biology (M Sc, PhD); plant biology (M Sc, PhD); systematics and evolution (M Sc, PhD). Terminal master's awarded for partial completion of doctoral program. *Degree requirements:* For master's, thesis; for doctorate, thesis/dissertation. *Entrance requirements:* Additional exam requirements/recommendations for international students: Required—TOEFL.

The University of Arizona, College of Science, Department of Ecology and Evolutionary Biology, Tucson, AZ 85721. Offers MS, PhD. Terminal master's awarded for partial completion of doctoral program. *Degree requirements:* For master's, thesis optional; for doctorate, one foreign language, comprehensive exam, thesis/dissertation. *Entrance requirements:* For master's, GRE General Test, GRE Subject Test, statement of purpose, curriculum vitae, 3 letters of recommendation; for doctorate, GRE General Test, GRE Subject Test, curriculum vitae, 3 letters of recommendation. Additional exam requirements/recommendations for international students: Required—TOEFL (minimum score 550 paper-based; 79 iBT). *Application deadline:* For fall admission, 12/1 for domestic students, 12/8 for international students. Application fee: $75. *Financial support:* Research assistantships, teaching assistantships, career-related internships or fieldwork, scholarships/grants, health care benefits, and unspecified assistantships available. *Faculty research:* Biological diversity, evolutionary history, evolutionary mechanisms, community structure. *Unit head:* Dr. Michael Worobey, Head, E-mail: worobey@email.arizona.edu. *Application contact:* Dr. Michael Worobey, Head, E-mail: worobey@email.arizona.edu. Website: http://eebweb.arizona.edu/

University of California, Davis, Graduate Studies, Graduate Group in Ecology, Davis, CA 95616. Offers MS, PhD. PhD offered jointly with San Diego State University. *Degree requirements:* For master's, comprehensive exam (for some programs), thesis (for some programs); for doctorate, thesis/dissertation. *Entrance requirements:* For master's and doctorate, GRE General Test. Additional exam requirements/recommendations for international students: Required—TOEFL (minimum score 550 paper-based). Electronic applications accepted. *Faculty research:* Agricultural conservation, physiological restoration, environmental policy, ecotoxicology.

University of California, Irvine, Francisco J. Ayala School of Biological Sciences, Department of Ecology and Evolutionary Biology, Irvine, CA 92697. Offers biological sciences (MS, PhD). *Students:* 61 full-time (32 women); includes 21 minority (4 Asian, non-Hispanic/Latino; 11 Hispanic/Latino; 6 Two or more races, non-Hispanic/Latino), 2 international. Average age 28. 64 applicants, 19% accepted, 10 enrolled. In 2015, 8 master's, 8 doctorates awarded. *Degree requirements:* For master's, thesis; for doctorate, thesis/dissertation. *Entrance requirements:* For master's and doctorate, GRE General Test, GRE Subject Test, minimum GPA of 3.0. Additional exam requirements/recommendations for international students: Required—TOEFL (minimum score 550 paper-based). *Application deadline:* For fall admission, 1/15 priority date for domestic students, 1/15 for international students. Applications are processed on a rolling basis. Application fee: $90 ($110 for international students). Electronic applications accepted. *Financial support:* Fellowships, research assistantships with full tuition reimbursements, teaching assistantships, career-related internships or fieldwork, institutionally sponsored loans, traineeships, health care benefits, and unspecified assistantships available. Financial award application deadline: 3/1; financial award applicants required to submit FAFSA. *Faculty research:* Ecological energetics, quantitative genetics, life history evolution, plant-herbivore and plant-pollinator interactions, molecular evolution. *Unit head:* Laurence D. Mueller, Professor/Department Chair, 949-824-4744, Fax: 949-824-2181, E-mail: ldmueller@uci.edu. *Application contact:* Pam McDonald, Student Affairs Coordinator, 949-824-4743, Fax: 949-824-2181, E-mail: pmcdonal@uci.edu. Website: http://ecoevo.bio.uci.edu/

University of California, Los Angeles, Graduate Division, College of Letters and Science, Department of Ecology and Evolutionary Biology, Los Angeles, CA 90095. Offers MA, PhD. Terminal master's awarded for partial completion of doctoral program. *Degree requirements:* For master's, comprehensive exam or thesis; for doctorate, thesis/dissertation, oral and written qualifying exams; 3 quarters of teaching experience. *Entrance requirements:* For master's and doctorate, GRE General Test, GRE Subject Test (biology), bachelor's degree; minimum undergraduate GPA of 3.0 (or its equivalent if letter grade system not used). Additional exam requirements/recommendations for international students: Required—TOEFL. Electronic applications accepted.

University of California, Santa Barbara, Graduate Division, College of Letters and Sciences, Division of Mathematics, Life, and Physical Sciences, Department of Ecology, Evolution, and Marine Biology, Santa Barbara, CA 93106-9620. Offers MA, PhD, MA/PhD. *Faculty:* 33 full-time (8 women). *Students:* 69 full-time (44 women); includes 15 minority (2 Black or African American, non-Hispanic/Latino; 5 Asian, non-Hispanic/

Ecology

Latino; 6 Hispanic/Latino; 2 Native Hawaiian or other Pacific Islander, non-Hispanic/Latino), 3 international. Average age 29. 157 applicants, 14% accepted, 17 enrolled. In 2015, 7 master's, 8 doctorates awarded. *Degree requirements:* For master's, comprehensive exam (for some programs), thesis (for some programs); for doctorate, comprehensive exam, thesis/dissertation. *Entrance requirements:* For master's and doctorate, GRE General Test. Additional exam requirements/recommendations for international students: Required—TOEFL (minimum score 550 paper-based; 80 iBT), IELTS. *Application deadline:* For fall admission, 12/15 for domestic and international students. Application fee: $90 ($110 for international students). Electronic applications accepted. *Financial support:* In 2015–16, 50 students received support, including 55 fellowships with tuition reimbursements available (averaging $10,812 per year), 24 research assistantships with tuition reimbursements available (averaging $8,441 per year), 97 teaching assistantships with partial tuition reimbursements available (averaging $9,346 per year); Federal Work-Study, scholarships/grants, traineeships, health care benefits, and tuition waivers (full and partial) also available. Financial award application deadline: 12/15; financial award applicants required to submit FAFSA. *Faculty research:* Community ecology, evolution, marine biology, population genetics, stream ecology. *Unit head:* Dr. Craig Carlson, Chair, 805-893-2415, Fax: 805-893-5885, E-mail: eembchair@lifesci.ucsb.edu. *Application contact:* Melanie Fujii, Student Affairs Officer, 805-893-2979, Fax: 805-893-5885, E-mail: eemb-info@lifesci.ucsb.edu. Website: http://www.lifesci.ucsb.edu/EEMB/index.html

University of California, Santa Cruz, Division of Graduate Studies, Division of Physical and Biological Sciences, Department of Ecology and Evolutionary Biology, Santa Cruz, CA 95064. Offers MA, PhD. *Degree requirements:* For master's, thesis; for doctorate, comprehensive exam, thesis/dissertation. *Entrance requirements:* For master's and doctorate, GRE General Test, GRE Subject Test, 3 letters of recommendation. Additional exam requirements/recommendations for international students: Required—TOEFL (minimum score 550 paper-based; 83 iBT); Recommended—IELTS (minimum score 8). Electronic applications accepted. *Faculty research:* Population and community ecology, evolutionary biology, physiology and behavior (marine and terrestrial), systematics and biodiversity.

University of Chicago, Division of the Biological Sciences, Department of Ecology and Evolution, Chicago, IL 60637. Offers PhD. *Students:* 31 full-time (16 women); includes 2 minority (both Asian, non-Hispanic/Latino), 8 international. Average age 28. 52 applicants, 17% accepted, 5 enrolled. In 2015, 3 doctorates awarded. *Degree requirements:* For doctorate, thesis/dissertation, ethics class, 2 teaching assistantships. *Entrance requirements:* For doctorate, GRE General Test. Additional exam requirements/recommendations for international students: Required—TOEFL (minimum score 600 paper-based; 104 iBT), IELTS (minimum score 7). *Application deadline:* For fall admission, 12/1 for domestic and international students. Application fee: $90. Electronic applications accepted. *Financial support:* In 2015–16, 22 students received support, including fellowships with tuition reimbursements available (averaging $29,781 per year), research assistantships with tuition reimbursements available (averaging $29,781 per year); institutionally sponsored loans, scholarships/grants, traineeships, and health care benefits also available. Financial award applicants required to submit FAFSA. *Faculty research:* Population genetics, molecular evolution, behavior. *Unit head:* Dr. Joy Bergelson, Chair, 773-702-3855, Fax: 773-702-9740, E-mail: j-bergelson@uchicago.edu. Website: http://pondside.uchicago.edu/ee/

University of Colorado Boulder, Graduate School, College of Arts and Sciences, Department of Ecology and Evolutionary Biology, Boulder, CO 80309. Offers animal behavior (MA); biology (MA, PhD); environmental biology (MA, PhD); evolutionary biology (MA, PhD); neurobiology (MA); population biology (MA); population genetics (PhD). *Faculty:* 31 full-time (12 women). *Students:* 67 full-time (31 women), 3 part-time (1 woman); includes 8 minority (1 Asian, non-Hispanic/Latino; 3 Hispanic/Latino; 4 Two or more races, non-Hispanic/Latino), 4 international. Average age 30. 119 applicants, 11% accepted, 13 enrolled. In 2015, 10 master's, 14 doctorates awarded. Terminal master's awarded for partial completion of doctoral program. *Degree requirements:* For master's, comprehensive exam, thesis or alternative; for doctorate, comprehensive exam, thesis/dissertation. *Entrance requirements:* For master's, GRE General Test, GRE Subject Test, minimum undergraduate GPA of 3.0; for doctorate, GRE General Test, GRE Subject Test. *Application deadline:* For fall admission, 12/31 for domestic students, 12/1 for international students. Application fee: $50 ($70 for international students). Electronic applications accepted. Application fee is waived when completed online. *Financial support:* In 2015–16, 138 students received support, including 14 fellowships (averaging $7,260 per year), 12 research assistantships with tuition reimbursements available (averaging $31,833 per year), 47 teaching assistantships with tuition reimbursements available (averaging $33,448 per year); institutionally sponsored loans, scholarships/grants, health care benefits, and unspecified assistantships also available. Financial award applicants required to submit FAFSA. *Faculty research:* Ecology, botany, evolutionary biology, biological sciences, conservation biology. *Total annual research expenditures:* $6.3 million. *Application contact:* E-mail: ebiograd@colorado.edu. Website: http://ebio.colorado.edu

University of Colorado Denver, College of Liberal Arts and Sciences, Department of Geography and Environmental Sciences, Denver, CO 80217. Offers environmental sciences (MS), including air quality, ecosystems, environmental health, environmental science education, geospatial analysis, urban agriculture, water quality. *Program availability:* Part-time, evening/weekend. *Faculty:* 12 full-time (4 women), 2 part-time/adjunct (1 woman). *Students:* 46 full-time (26 women), 12 part-time (5 women); includes 11 minority (1 Black or African American, non-Hispanic/Latino; 1 Asian, non-Hispanic/Latino; 6 Hispanic/Latino; 3 Two or more races, non-Hispanic/Latino), 3 international. Average age 30. 75 applicants, 61% accepted, 24 enrolled. In 2015, 11 master's awarded. *Degree requirements:* For master's, thesis or alternative, 30 credits including 21 of core requirements and 9 of environmental science electives. *Entrance requirements:* For master's, GRE General Test, BA in one of the natural/physical sciences or engineering (or equivalent background); prerequisite coursework in calculus and physics (one semester each), general chemistry with lab and general biology with lab (two semesters each); three letters of recommendation. Additional exam requirements/recommendations for international students: Required—TOEFL (minimum score 537 paper-based; 75 iBT); Recommended—IELTS (minimum score 6.5). *Application deadline:* For fall admission, 1/20 for domestic and international students; for spring admission, 10/1 for domestic and international students. Application fee: $50 ($75 for international students). Electronic applications accepted. *Financial support:* In 2015–16, 8 students received support. Fellowships, research assistantships, teaching assistantships, Federal Work-Study, institutionally sponsored loans, scholarships/grants, and traineeships available. Financial award application deadline: 4/1; financial award applicants required to submit FAFSA. *Faculty research:* Air quality, environmental health, ecosystems, hazardous waste, water quality, geo-spatial analysis and environmental science education. *Unit head:* Anne Chinn, Director of MS in Environmental Sciences Program, 303-556-3958, E-mail: ges@ucdenver.edu. *Application contact:* Sue Eddleman, Program Assistant, 303-352-3698, E-mail: sue.eddleman@ucdenver.edu.

Website: http://www.ucdenver.edu/academics/colleges/CLAS/Departments/ges/Programs/MasterofScience/Pages/MasterofScience.aspx

University of Colorado Denver, College of Liberal Arts and Sciences, Department of Integrative and Systems Biology, Denver, CO 80217. Offers animal behavior (MS); biology (MS); cell and developmental biology (MS); ecology (MS); evolutionary biology (MS); genetics (MS); integrative and systems biology (PhD); microbiology (MS); molecular biology (MS); neurobiology (MS); plant systematics (MS). *Program availability:* Part-time. *Faculty:* 21 full-time (8 women), 3 part-time/adjunct (1 woman). *Students:* 31 full-time (19 women), 7 part-time (3 women); includes 8 minority (1 Black or African American, non-Hispanic/Latino; 1 Asian, non-Hispanic/Latino; 3 Hispanic/Latino; 3 Two or more races, non-Hispanic/Latino), 1 international. Average age 28. 34 applicants, 29% accepted, 8 enrolled. In 2015, 6 master's awarded. *Degree requirements:* For master's, comprehensive exam, thesis, 30-32 credit hours; for doctorate, comprehensive exam, thesis/dissertation. *Entrance requirements:* For master's, GRE General Test (minimum score in 50th percentile in each section), BA/BS from accredited institution awarded within the last 10 years; minimum undergraduate GPA of 3.0; prerequisite courses: 1 year each of general biology and general chemistry; 1 semester each of general genetics, general ecology, and cell biology; and a structure/function course; for doctorate, GRE, minimum undergraduate GPA of 3.2, three letters of recommendation, official transcripts from all universities and colleges attended. Additional exam requirements/recommendations for international students: Required—TOEFL (minimum score 537 paper-based; 75 iBT); Recommended—IELTS (minimum score 6.5). *Application deadline:* For fall admission, 1/15 for domestic and international students. Application fee: $50 ($75 for international students). Electronic applications accepted. *Financial support:* In 2015–16, 32 students received support. Fellowships, research assistantships, teaching assistantships, Federal Work-Study, institutionally sponsored loans, scholarships/grants, and traineeships available. Financial award application deadline: 4/1; financial award applicants required to submit FAFSA. *Faculty research:* Molecular developmental biology; quantitative ecology, biogeography, and population dynamics; environmental signaling and endocrine disruption; speciation, the evolution of reproductive isolation, and hybrid zones; evolutionary, behavioral, and conservation ecology. *Unit head:* Dr. John Swallow, Chair, 303-556-6154, E-mail: john.swallow@ucdenver.edu. *Application contact:* Dr. Michael Wunder, Graduate Advisor, 303-556-8870, E-mail: michael.wunder@ucdenver.edu. Website: http://www.ucdenver.edu/academics/colleges/CLAS/Departments/biology/Programs/MasterofScience/Pages/BiologyMasterOfScience.aspx

University of Connecticut, Graduate School, College of Liberal Arts and Sciences, Department of Psychology, Storrs, CT 06269. Offers behavioral neuroscience (PhD); biopsychology (PhD); clinical psychology (MA, PhD); cognition and instruction (PhD); developmental psychology (MA, PhD); ecological psychology (PhD); experimental psychology (PhD); general psychology (MA, PhD); industrial/organizational psychology (PhD); language and cognition (PhD); neuroscience (PhD); social psychology (MA, PhD). *Accreditation:* APA. Terminal master's awarded for partial completion of doctoral program. *Degree requirements:* For master's, comprehensive exam; for doctorate, thesis/dissertation. *Entrance requirements:* For master's and doctorate, GRE General Test, GRE Subject Test. Additional exam requirements/recommendations for international students: Required—TOEFL (minimum score 550 paper-based). *Application deadline:* For fall admission, 2/1 priority date for domestic and international students; for spring admission, 11/1 for domestic students, 10/1 for international students. Applications are processed on a rolling basis. Application fee: $55. Electronic applications accepted. *Financial support:* Fellowships, research assistantships with full tuition reimbursements, teaching assistantships with full tuition reimbursements, career-related internships or fieldwork, Federal Work-Study, scholarships/grants, health care benefits, and unspecified assistantships available. Financial award application deadline: 2/1; financial award applicants required to submit FAFSA. Website: http://www.psychology.uconn.edu/

University of Delaware, College of Agriculture and Natural Resources, Department of Entomology and Wildlife Ecology, Newark, DE 19716. Offers entomology and applied ecology (MS, PhD), including avian ecology, evolution and taxonomy, insect biological control, insect ecology and behavior (MS), insect genetics, pest management, plant-insect interactions, wildlife ecology and management. *Program availability:* Part-time. *Degree requirements:* For master's, comprehensive exam, thesis, oral exam, seminar; for doctorate, comprehensive exam, thesis/dissertation, qualifying exam, seminar. *Entrance requirements:* For master's, GRE General Test, minimum GPA of 3.0 in field, 2.8 overall; for doctorate, GRE General Test, GRE Subject Test (biology), minimum GPA of 3.0 in field, 2.8 overall. Additional exam requirements/recommendations for international students: Required—TOEFL. Electronic applications accepted. *Faculty research:* Ecology and evolution of plant-insect interactions, ecology of wildlife conservation management, habitat restoration, biological control, applied ecosystem management.

University of Delaware, College of Arts and Sciences, Department of Biological Sciences, Newark, DE 19716. Offers biotechnology (MS); cancer biology (MS, PhD); cell and extracellular matrix biology (MS, PhD); cell and systems physiology (MS, PhD); developmental biology (MS, PhD); ecology and evolution (MS, PhD); microbiology (MS, PhD); molecular biology and genetics (MS, PhD). Terminal master's awarded for partial completion of doctoral program. *Degree requirements:* For master's, thesis, preliminary exam; for doctorate, comprehensive exam, thesis/dissertation, preliminary exam. *Entrance requirements:* For master's and doctorate, GRE General Test. Additional exam requirements/recommendations for international students: Required—TOEFL (minimum score 600 paper-based); Recommended—TWE. Electronic applications accepted. *Faculty research:* Microorganisms, bone, cancer metastasis, developmental biology, cell biology, DNA.

University of Denver, Division of Natural Sciences and Mathematics, Department of Biological Sciences, Denver, CO 80208. Offers biology, ecology and evolution (MS, PhD); biomedical sciences (PSM); cell and molecular biology (MS, PhD). *Program availability:* Part-time. *Faculty:* 23 full-time (7 women), 2 part-time/adjunct (both women). *Students:* 8 full-time (all women), 27 part-time (21 women); includes 4 minority (2 Black or African American, non-Hispanic/Latino; 2 Hispanic/Latino), 6 international. Average age 26. 77 applicants, 38% accepted, 21 enrolled. In 2015, 6 master's, 3 doctorates awarded. Terminal master's awarded for partial completion of doctoral program. *Degree requirements:* For master's, comprehensive exam (for some programs), thesis; for doctorate, one foreign language, comprehensive exam (for some programs), thesis/dissertation. *Entrance requirements:* For master's and doctorate, GRE General Test, bachelor's degree in biology or related field, transcripts, personal statement, three letters of recommendation. Additional exam requirements/recommendations for international students: Required—TOEFL (minimum score 550 paper-based; 80 iBT). *Application deadline:* For fall admission, 1/1 priority date for domestic and international students. Applications are processed on a rolling basis. Application fee: $65. Electronic applications accepted. *Expenses:* $30,477. *Financial support:* In 2015–16, 35 students received support, including 8 research assistantships with tuition reimbursements available (averaging $15,834 per year), 23 teaching assistantships with tuition reimbursements available (averaging $17,210 per year); Federal Work-Study, institutionally sponsored loans, scholarships/grants, and unspecified assistantships also

available. Support available to part-time students. Financial award application deadline: 2/15; financial award applicants required to submit FAFSA. *Faculty research:* Molecular biology, cell biology, neurobiology, ecology, molecular evolution. *Unit head:* Dr. Joseph Angleson, Associate Professor and Chair, 303-871-3463, Fax: 303-871-3471, E-mail: jangleso@du.edu. *Application contact:* Randi Flageolle, Assistant to the Chair, 303-871-3457, Fax: 303-871-3471, E-mail: rflageol@du.edu.
Website: http://www.du.edu/nsm/departments/biologicalsciences

University of Florida, Graduate School, College of Agricultural and Life Sciences, Department of Wildlife Ecology and Conservation, Gainesville, FL 32611. Offers environmental education and communications (Certificate); wildlife ecology and conservation (MS, PhD), including geographic information systems, tropical conservation and development, wetland sciences. *Faculty:* 58. *Students:* Average age 32. 33 applicants, 30% accepted, 9 enrolled. In 2015, 15 master's, 4 doctorates awarded. *Degree requirements:* For master's, comprehensive exam, thesis optional; for doctorate, comprehensive exam, thesis/dissertation. *Entrance requirements:* For master's and doctorate, GRE General Test (minimum 34th percentile for Quantitative), minimum GPA of 3.3. Additional exam requirements/recommendations for international students: Required—TOEFL (minimum score 550 paper-based; 80 iBT), IELTS (minimum score 6). *Application deadline:* For fall admission, 12/15 priority date for domestic students, 12/15 for international students; for spring admission, 12/1 for domestic students. Applications are processed on a rolling basis. Application fee: $30. Electronic applications accepted. *Financial support:* In 2015–16, 4 fellowships, 36 research assistantships, 11 teaching assistantships were awarded; institutionally sponsored loans also available. Financial award applicants required to submit FAFSA. *Faculty research:* Conservation biology, spatial ecology, wildlife conservation and management, wetlands ecology and conservation, human dimensions in wildlife conservation. *Total annual research expenditures:* $4.8 million. *Unit head:* Eric C. Hellgren, PhD, Professor and Department Chair, 352-846-0552, E-mail: hellgren@ufl.edu. *Application contact:* Katie Sieving, PhD, Professor and Graduate Coordinator, 352-846-0569, Fax: 352-846-0841, E-mail: chucao@ufl.edu.
Website: http://www.wec.ufl.edu/

University of Florida, Graduate School, School of Natural Resources and Environment, Gainesville, FL 32611. Offers interdisciplinary ecology (MS, PhD). *Faculty:* 265. *Students:* 93 full-time (57 women), 12 part-time (8 women); includes 11 minority (3 Black or African American, non-Hispanic/Latino; 1 American Indian or Alaska Native, non-Hispanic/Latino; 2 Asian, non-Hispanic/Latino; 5 Hispanic/Latino), 32 international. Average age 32. 42 applicants, 62% accepted, 24 enrolled. In 2015, 9 master's, 13 doctorates awarded. *Degree requirements:* For master's, comprehensive exam, thesis; for doctorate, comprehensive exam, thesis/dissertation. *Entrance requirements:* For master's and doctorate, GRE General Test, minimum GPA of 3.0. Additional exam requirements/recommendations for international students: Required—TOEFL (minimum score 550 paper-based; 80 iBT), IELTS (minimum score 6). *Application deadline:* For fall admission, 2/1 priority date for domestic students, 2/1 for international students. Applications are processed on a rolling basis. Application fee: $30. Electronic applications accepted. *Financial support:* Applicants required to submit FAFSA. *Faculty research:* Natural sciences, social sciences, sustainability studies, research design and methods. *Total annual research expenditures:* $11,475. *Unit head:* Dr. Thomas K. Frazer, Director, 352-392-9230, Fax: 352-392-9748, E-mail: frazer@ufl.edu. *Application contact:* Office of Graduate Admissions, 352-392-1365, E-mail: webrequests@admissions.ufl.edu.
Website: http://www.snre.ufl.edu/

University of Georgia, School of Ecology, Athens, GA 30602. Offers conservation ecology and sustainable development (MS); ecology (MS, PhD). *Degree requirements:* For master's, thesis; for doctorate, one foreign language, thesis/dissertation. *Entrance requirements:* For master's and doctorate, GRE General Test. Electronic applications accepted.

University of Guelph, Graduate Studies, College of Biological Science, Department of Integrative Biology, Botany and Zoology, Guelph, ON N1G 2W1, Canada. Offers botany (M Sc, PhD); zoology (M Sc, PhD). *Program availability:* Part-time. *Degree requirements:* For master's, thesis, research proposal; for doctorate, thesis/dissertation, research proposal, qualifying exam. *Entrance requirements:* For master's, minimum B average during previous 2 years of course work. Additional exam requirements/recommendations for international students: Required—TOEFL (minimum score 550 paper-based), IELTS (minimum score 6.5). Electronic applications accepted. *Faculty research:* Aquatic science, environmental physiology, parasitology, wildlife biology, management.

University of Illinois at Urbana–Champaign, Graduate College, College of Liberal Arts and Sciences, School of Integrative Biology, Department of Animal Biology, Champaign, IL 61820. Offers animal biology (ecology, ethology and evolution) (MS, PhD).

University of Illinois at Urbana–Champaign, Graduate College, College of Liberal Arts and Sciences, School of Integrative Biology, Program in Ecology, Evolution and Conservation Biology, Champaign, IL 61820. Offers MS, PhD.

The University of Kansas, Graduate Studies, College of Liberal Arts and Sciences, Department of Ecology and Evolutionary Biology, Lawrence, KS 66045. Offers botany (MA, PhD); ecology and evolutionary biology (MA, PhD); entomology (MA, PhD). *Students:* 69 full-time (35 women), 1 part-time (0 women); includes 8 minority (1 Black or African American, non-Hispanic/Latino; 1 Asian, non-Hispanic/Latino; 4 Native Hawaiian or other Pacific Islander, non-Hispanic/Latino; 2 Two or more races, non-Hispanic/Latino), 22 international. Average age 28. 66 applicants, 39% accepted, 20 enrolled. In 2015, 3 master's, 5 doctorates awarded. Terminal master's awarded for partial completion of doctoral program. *Degree requirements:* For master's, comprehensive exam, thesis (for some programs), 30-36 credits, thesis presentation; for doctorate, comprehensive exam, thesis/dissertation, residency, responsible scholarship and research skills, final exam, dissertation defense. *Entrance requirements:* For master's, GRE General Test, bachelor's degree with minimum undergraduate GPA of 3.0; for doctorate, GRE General Test, bachelor's degree; minimum undergraduate/graduate GPA of 3.0. Additional exam requirements/recommendations for international students: Required—TOEFL or IELTS. *Application deadline:* For fall admission, 12/1 for domestic and international students; for spring admission, 9/15 for domestic and international students. Application fee: $65 ($85 for international students). Electronic applications accepted. *Financial support:* Fellowships, research assistantships, teaching assistantships, scholarships/grants, traineeships, health care benefits, and unspecified assistantships available. Financial award application deadline: 12/1. *Faculty research:* Ecology and global change, diversity and macroevolution, evolutionary mechanisms, systematics/phylogenetics, biogeography. *Unit head:* Dr. Christopher H. Haufler, Chair, 785-864-3255, E-mail: vulgare@ku.edu. *Application contact:* Aagje Ashe, Graduate Coordinator, 785-864-2362, Fax: 785-864-5860, E-mail: a4ashe@ku.edu.
Website: http://eeb.ku.edu/

University of Maine, Graduate School, College of Natural Sciences, Forestry, and Agriculture, School of Biology and Ecology, Orono, ME 04469. Offers biological sciences (PhD); botany and plant pathology (MS); ecology and environmental science (MS, PhD); entomology (MS); plant science (PhD); zoology (MS, PhD). *Program availability:* Part-time. *Faculty:* 24 full-time (12 women), 34 part-time/adjunct (13 women). *Students:* 64 full-time (36 women), 1 part-time (0 women); includes 4 minority (1 American Indian or Alaska Native, non-Hispanic/Latino; 1 Asian, non-Hispanic/Latino; 1 Hispanic/Latino; 1 Two or more races, non-Hispanic/Latino), 8 international. Average age 29. 52 applicants, 25% accepted, 11 enrolled. In 2015, 7 master's, 8 doctorates awarded. Terminal master's awarded for partial completion of doctoral program. *Degree requirements:* For master's, thesis (for some programs); for doctorate, comprehensive exam, thesis/dissertation. *Entrance requirements:* For master's and doctorate, GRE General Test. Additional exam requirements/recommendations for international students: Required—TOEFL. *Application deadline:* For fall admission, 2/1 priority date for domestic students. Applications are processed on a rolling basis. Application fee: $65. Electronic applications accepted. *Financial support:* In 2015–16, 14 students received support, including 6 research assistantships with full tuition reimbursements available (averaging $14,600 per year), 8 teaching assistantships with full tuition reimbursements available (averaging $14,600 per year); career-related internships or fieldwork, Federal Work-Study, institutionally sponsored loans, and tuition waivers (full and partial) also available. Financial award application deadline: 3/1. *Faculty research:* Ecology and evolution (aquatic, terrestrial, paleo); development and genetics; biomedical research; ecophysiology and stress; invasion ecology and pest management. *Total annual research expenditures:* $3.2 million. *Unit head:* Dr. Andrei Aloykhin, Director, 207-581-2977, Fax: 207-581-2537. *Application contact:* Scott G. Delcourt, Assistant Vice President for Graduate Studies and Senior Associate Dean, 207-581-3291, Fax: 207-581-3232, E-mail: graduate@maine.edu.
Website: http://sbe.umaine.edu/

The University of Manchester, Faculty of Life Sciences, Manchester, United Kingdom. Offers adaptive organismal biology (M Phil, PhD); animal biology (M Phil, PhD); biochemistry (M Phil, PhD); bioinformatics (M Phil, PhD); biomolecular sciences (M Phil, PhD); biotechnology (M Phil, PhD); cell biology (M Phil, PhD); cell matrix research (M Phil, PhD); channels and transporters (M Phil, PhD); developmental biology (M Phil, PhD); Egyptology (M Phil, PhD); environmental biology (M Phil, PhD); evolutionary biology (M Phil, PhD); gene expression (M Phil, PhD); genetics (M Phil, PhD); history of science, technology and medicine (M Phil, PhD); immunology (M Phil, PhD); integrative neurobiology and behavior (M Phil, PhD); membrane trafficking (M Phil, PhD); microbiology (M Phil, PhD); molecular and cellular neuroscience (M Phil, PhD); molecular biology (M Phil, PhD); molecular cancer studies (M Phil, PhD); neuroscience (M Phil, PhD); ophthalmology (M Phil, PhD); optometry (M Phil, PhD); organelle function (M Phil, PhD); pharmacology (M Phil, PhD); physiology (M Phil, PhD); plant sciences (M Phil, PhD); stem cell research (M Phil, PhD); structural biology (M Phil, PhD); systems neuroscience (M Phil, PhD); toxicology (M Phil, PhD).

University of Manitoba, Faculty of Graduate Studies, Faculty of Science, Department of Biological Sciences, Winnipeg, MB R3T 2N2, Canada. Offers botany (M Sc, PhD); ecology (M Sc, PhD); zoology (M Sc, PhD).

University of Maryland, College Park, Academic Affairs, College of Computer, Mathematical and Natural Sciences, Department of Biology, Behavior, Ecology, Evolution, and Systematics Program, College Park, MD 20742. Offers MS, PhD. *Degree requirements:* For master's, thesis, oral defense, seminar; for doctorate, thesis/dissertation, exam, 4 seminars. *Entrance requirements:* For master's and doctorate, GRE General Test, GRE Subject Test (biology), 3 letters of recommendation. Additional exam requirements/recommendations for international students: Required—TOEFL. *Faculty research:* Animal behavior, biostatistics, ecology, evolution, neurothology.

University of Maryland, College Park, Academic Affairs, College of Computer, Mathematical and Natural Sciences, Department of Biology, PhD Program in Biological Sciences, College Park, MD 20742. Offers behavior, ecology, evolution, and systematics (PhD); computational biology, bioinformatics, and genomics (PhD); molecular and cellular biology (PhD); physiological systems (PhD). *Degree requirements:* For doctorate, comprehensive exam, thesis/dissertation, thesis work presentation in seminar. *Entrance requirements:* For doctorate, GRE General Test; GRE Subject Test in biology (recommended), academic transcripts, statement of purpose/research interests, 3 letters of recommendation. Additional exam requirements/recommendations for international students: Required—TOEFL. Electronic applications accepted.

University of Michigan, Rackham Graduate School, College of Literature, Science, and the Arts, Department of Ecology and Evolutionary Biology, Ann Arbor, MI 48109. Offers MS, PhD. *Program availability:* Part-time. *Faculty:* 57 full-time (22 women). *Students:* 72 full-time (36 women); includes 28 minority (2 Black or African American, non-Hispanic/Latino; 1 American Indian or Alaska Native, non-Hispanic/Latino; 5 Asian, non-Hispanic/Latino; 13 Hispanic/Latino; 1 Native Hawaiian or other Pacific Islander, non-Hispanic/Latino; 6 Two or more races, non-Hispanic/Latino), 13 international. Average age 28. 143 applicants, 22% accepted, 14 enrolled. In 2015, 9 master's, 7 doctorates awarded. Terminal master's awarded for partial completion of doctoral program. *Degree requirements:* For master's, thesis (for some programs), two seminars; for doctorate, comprehensive exam, thesis/dissertation, 2 semesters of teaching. *Entrance requirements:* For master's and doctorate, GRE. Additional exam requirements/recommendations for international students: Required—TOEFL (minimum score 84 iBT). *Application deadline:* For fall admission, 12/1 priority date for domestic and international students; for winter admission, 10/15 priority date for domestic and international students. Applications are processed on a rolling basis. Application fee: $65 ($75 for international students). Electronic applications accepted. *Financial support:* In 2015–16, 67 students received support, including 30 fellowships with full tuition reimbursements available (averaging $26,350 per year), 11 research assistantships with full tuition reimbursements available (averaging $26,350 per year), 37 teaching assistantships with full tuition reimbursements available (averaging $26,350 per year); scholarships/grants, traineeships, health care benefits, and unspecified assistantships also available. Financial award applicants required to submit FAFSA. *Faculty research:* Population and community ecology, ecosystem ecology and biogeochemistry, global change biology, biogeography and paleobiology, evolution of behavior, evolutionary genetics, phylogenetic and phylogeography, ecology and evolution of infectious disease. *Total annual research expenditures:* $5.1 million. *Unit head:* Diarmaid O Foighil, Chair, 734-615-4912, Fax: 734-763-0544. *Application contact:* Cynthia Carl, Graduate Program Coordinator, 734-615-7338, Fax: 734-763-0544, E-mail: eeb.gradcoord@umich.edu.
Website: http://www.lsa.umich.edu/eeb/

University of Michigan, School of Natural Resources and Environment, Program in Natural Resources and Environment, Ann Arbor, MI 48109. Offers behavior, education and communication (MS); conservation ecology (MS); environmental informatics (MS); environmental justice (MS); environmental policy and planning (MS); natural resources and environment (PhD); sustainable systems (MS); MS/JD; MS/MBA; MS/MPP; MS/MSE; MUP/MS. *Students:* 342 full-time (184 women). Average age 27. Terminal master's awarded for partial completion of doctoral program. *Degree requirements:* For master's, practicum or group project; for doctorate, comprehensive exam, thesis/dissertation, oral defense of dissertation, preliminary exam. *Entrance requirements:* For master's, GRE General Test; for doctorate, GRE General Test, master's degree.

Ecology

Additional exam requirements/recommendations for international students: Required—TOEFL (minimum score 560 paper-based; 84 iBT). *Application deadline:* For fall admission, 4/30 for domestic and international students. Application fee: $75 ($90 for international students). Electronic applications accepted. *Financial support:* Application deadline: 1/6; applicants required to submit FAFSA. *Unit head:* Dr. Marie Lynn Miranda, Interim Dean, 734-764-2550, Fax: 734-763-8965, E-mail: danbrown@umich.edu. *Application contact:* Sondra R. Auerbach, Director of Academic Programs, 734-764-6453, Fax: 734-936-2195, E-mail: sshowen@umich.edu.
Website: http://www.snre.umich.edu/

University of Minnesota, Twin Cities Campus, Graduate School, College of Biological Sciences, Department of Ecology, Evolution, and Behavior, St. Paul, MN 55418. Offers MS, PhD. Terminal master's awarded for partial completion of doctoral program. *Degree requirements:* For master's, comprehensive exam, thesis or projects; for doctorate, comprehensive exam, thesis/dissertation. *Entrance requirements:* For master's and doctorate, GRE General Test, minimum GPA of 3.0. Additional exam requirements/recommendations for international students: Required—TOEFL (minimum score 550 paper-based; 79 iBT), Michigan English Language Assessment Battery. Electronic applications accepted. *Faculty research:* Behavioral ecology, community ecology, community genetics, ecosystem and global change, evolution and systematics.

University of Missouri, Office of Research and Graduate Studies, College of Arts and Science, Division of Biological Sciences, Columbia, MO 65211. Offers evolutionary biology and ecology (MA, PhD). Terminal master's awarded for partial completion of doctoral program. *Degree requirements:* For master's, thesis; for doctorate, comprehensive exam, thesis/dissertation. *Entrance requirements:* For master's and doctorate, GRE General Test (minimum score 1200 verbal and quantitative), minimum GPA of 3.0. Additional exam requirements/recommendations for international students: Required—TOEFL (minimum score 600 paper-based; 100 iBT). *Application deadline:* For fall admission, 12/15 priority date for domestic and international students. Applications are processed on a rolling basis. Application fee: $55 ($75 for international students). Electronic applications accepted. *Financial support:* Fellowships with full tuition reimbursements, research assistantships with full tuition reimbursements, teaching assistantships with full tuition reimbursements, institutionally sponsored loans, traineeships, health care benefits, and unspecified assistantships available. Website: http://biology.missouri.edu/graduate-studies/

University of Montana, Graduate School, College of Forestry and Conservation, Missoula, MT 59812-0002. Offers fish and wildlife biology (PhD); forest and conservation sciences (PhD); forestry (MS); recreation management (MS); resource conservation (MS); systems ecology (MS, PhD); wildlife biology (MS). *Degree requirements:* For doctorate, thesis/dissertation. *Entrance requirements:* For master's and doctorate, GRE General Test. Additional exam requirements/recommendations for international students: Required—TOEFL (minimum score 575 paper-based).

University of Montana, Graduate School, College of Humanities and Sciences, Division of Biological Sciences, Interdisciplinary Program in Systems Ecology, Missoula, MT 59812-0002. Offers MS, PhD.

University of Montana, Graduate School, College of Humanities and Sciences, Division of Biological Sciences, Program in Organismal Biology and Ecology, Missoula, MT 59812-0002. Offers MS, PhD. Terminal master's awarded for partial completion of doctoral program. *Degree requirements:* For master's, one foreign language, thesis; for doctorate, 2 foreign languages, thesis/dissertation. *Entrance requirements:* For master's and doctorate, GRE General Test. *Faculty research:* Conservation biology, ecology and behavior, evolutionary genetics, avian biology.

University of Nevada, Reno, Graduate School, Interdisciplinary Program in Ecology, Evolution, and Conservation Biology, Reno, NV 89557. Offers PhD. Offered through the College of Arts and Science, the M. C. Fleischmann College of Agriculture, and the Desert Research Institute. *Degree requirements:* For doctorate, thesis/dissertation. *Entrance requirements:* For doctorate, GRE General Test, GRE Subject Test, minimum GPA of 3.0. Additional exam requirements/recommendations for international students: Required—TOEFL (minimum score 500 paper-based; 61 iBT), IELTS (minimum score 6). Electronic applications accepted. *Faculty research:* Population biology, behavioral ecology, plant response to climate change, conservation of endangered species, restoration of natural ecosystems.

University of New Haven, Graduate School, College of Arts and Sciences, Program in Environmental Science, West Haven, CT 06516-1916. Offers environmental ecology (MS); environmental education (MS); environmental geoscience (MS); environmental health and management (MS); environmental science (MS); geographical information systems (MS, Graduate Certificate). *Program availability:* Part-time, evening/weekend. *Students:* 20 full-time (10 women), 6 part-time (5 women); includes 2 minority (1 Black or African American, non-Hispanic/Latino; 1 Hispanic/Latino), 5 international. Average age 26. 25 applicants, 88% accepted, 13 enrolled. In 2015, 19 master's awarded. *Degree requirements:* For master's, thesis optional, research project. *Entrance requirements:* Additional exam requirements/recommendations for international students: Required—TOEFL (minimum score 80 iBT), IELTS, PTE. *Application deadline:* For fall admission, 5/31 for international students; for winter admission, 10/15 for international students; for spring admission, 1/15 for international students. Applications are processed on a rolling basis. Application fee: $75. Electronic applications accepted. Application fee is waived when completed online. *Expenses: Tuition,* area resident: Full-time $15,282; part-time $849 per credit hour. *Required fees:* $150; $60 per term. Tuition and fees vary according to program. *Financial support:* Research assistantships with partial tuition reimbursements, teaching assistantships with partial tuition reimbursements, career-related internships or fieldwork, Federal Work-Study, scholarships/grants, and unspecified assistantships available. Support available to part-time students. Financial award applicants required to submit FAFSA. *Unit head:* Dr. Roman Zajac, Coordinator, 203-932-7114, E-mail: rzajac@newhaven.edu. *Application contact:* Michelle Mason, Director of Graduate Enrollment, 203-932-7067, E-mail: mmason@newhaven.edu. Website: http://www.newhaven.edu/4728/

The University of North Carolina at Chapel Hill, Graduate School, College of Arts and Sciences, Curriculum in Ecology, Chapel Hill, NC 27599. Offers MA, MS, PhD. *Degree requirements:* For master's, comprehensive exam, thesis (for some programs), oral defense of thesis; for doctorate, comprehensive exam, thesis/dissertation, oral exams, oral defense of dissertation. *Entrance requirements:* For master's and doctorate, GRE General Test. Additional exam requirements/recommendations for international students: Required—TOEFL (minimum score 550 paper-based). Electronic applications accepted. *Faculty research:* Community and population ecology and ecosystems, human ecology, landscape ecology, conservation ecology, marine ecology.

The University of North Carolina at Chapel Hill, Graduate School, College of Arts and Sciences, Department of Biology, Chapel Hill, NC 27599. Offers botany (MA, MS, PhD); cell biology, development, and physiology (MA, MS, PhD); cell motility and cytoskeleton (PhD); ecology and behavior (MA, MS, PhD); genetics and molecular biology (MA, MS, PhD); morphology, systematics, and evolution (MA, MS, PhD). Terminal master's awarded for partial completion of doctoral program. *Degree requirements:* For master's, comprehensive exam, thesis (for some programs); for doctorate, comprehensive exam, thesis/dissertation. *Entrance requirements:* For master's, GRE General Test, GRE

Subject Test, 2 semesters of calculus or statistics; 2 semesters of physics, organic chemistry; 3 semesters of biology; for doctorate, GRE General Test, GRE Subject Test, 2 semesters calculus or statistics, 2 semesters physics, organic chemistry, 3 semesters of biology. Additional exam requirements/recommendations for international students: Required—TOEFL (minimum score 550 paper-based). Electronic applications accepted. *Faculty research:* Gene expression, biomechanics, yeast genetics, plant ecology, plant molecular biology.

University of North Dakota, Graduate School, College of Arts and Sciences, Department of Biology, Grand Forks, ND 58202. Offers botany (MS, PhD); ecology (MS, PhD); entomology (MS, PhD); environmental biology (MS, PhD); fisheries/wildlife (MS, PhD); genetics (MS, PhD); zoology (MS, PhD). Terminal master's awarded for partial completion of doctoral program. *Degree requirements:* For master's, thesis, final exam; for doctorate, comprehensive exam, thesis/dissertation, final exam. *Entrance requirements:* For master's, GRE General Test, GRE Subject Test, minimum GPA of 3.0; for doctorate, GRE General Test, GRE Subject Test, minimum GPA of 3.5. Additional exam requirements/recommendations for international students: Required—TOEFL (minimum score 550 paper-based; 79 iBT), IELTS (minimum score 6.5). Electronic applications accepted. *Faculty research:* Population biology, wildlife ecology, RNA processing, hormonal control of behavior.

University of Notre Dame, Graduate School, College of Science, Department of Biological Sciences, Notre Dame, IN 46556. Offers aquatic ecology, evolution and environmental biology (MS, PhD); cellular and molecular biology (MS, PhD); genetics (MS, PhD); physiology (MS, PhD); vector biology and parasitology (MS, PhD). Terminal master's awarded for partial completion of doctoral program. *Degree requirements:* For master's, comprehensive exam, thesis; for doctorate, comprehensive exam, thesis/dissertation, candidacy exam. *Entrance requirements:* For master's and doctorate, GRE General Test. Additional exam requirements/recommendations for international students: Required—TOEFL (minimum score 600 paper-based; 80 iBT). Electronic applications accepted. *Faculty research:* Tropical disease, molecular genetics, neurobiology, evolutionary biology, aquatic biology.

University of Oklahoma, College of Arts and Sciences, Department of Biology, Program in Ecology and Evolutionary Biology, Norman, OK 73019. Offers PhD. *Students:* 16 full-time (8 women), 9 part-time (7 women); includes 1 minority (Hispanic/Latino), 1 international. Average age 28. 18 applicants, 39% accepted, 7 enrolled. In 2015, 5 degrees awarded. *Degree requirements:* For doctorate, comprehensive exam, thesis/dissertation, course in biostatistics; 2 semesters as a teaching assistant. *Entrance requirements:* For doctorate, GRE General Test, transcripts, 3 letters of recommendation, personal statement, CV. Additional exam requirements/recommendations for international students: Required—TOEFL (minimum score 79 iBT) or IELTS (minimum score 6.5). *Application deadline:* For fall admission, 12/15 for domestic and international students. Application fee: $50 ($100 for international students). Electronic applications accepted. *Expenses:* Tuition, state resident: full-time $4577; part-time $190.70 per credit hour. Tuition, nonresident: full-time $17,758; part-time $739.90 per credit hour. *Required fees:* $3060; $115.70 per credit hour. $141.50 per semester. *Financial support:* In 2015–16, 23 students received support. Fellowships, research assistantships with full tuition reimbursements available, teaching assistantships with full tuition reimbursements available, scholarships/grants, health care benefits, unspecified assistantships, and assistantships (with tuition waivers and health insurance), supplementary scholarship funding available. Financial award application deadline: 6/1; financial award applicants required to submit FAFSA. *Faculty research:* Geographical ecology, global change biology, evolutionary biology, phylogenetics, ecosystem ecology. *Unit head:* Dr. Michael Kaspari, Professor, 405-325-3371, Fax: 405-325-6202, E-mail: mkaspari@ou.edu. *Application contact:* Dianna Wilson, Academic Counselor, 405-325-9139, Fax: 405-325-6202, E-mail: biologygrad@ou.edu.
Website: http://www.ou.edu/eeb

University of Oklahoma, College of Arts and Sciences, Department of Microbiology and Plant Biology, Program in Ecology and Evolutionary Biology, Norman, OK 73019. Offers PhD. *Students:* 8 full-time (3 women), 2 part-time (1 woman), 9 international. Average age 27. 4 applicants, 75% accepted, 3 enrolled. In 2015, 1 doctorate awarded. *Entrance requirements:* Additional exam requirements/recommendations for international students: Required—TOEFL (minimum score 79 iBT) or IELTS (minimum score 6.5). *Application deadline:* For fall admission, 4/1 for domestic and international students; for spring admission, 9/1 for domestic and international students. Application fee: $50 ($100 for international students). Electronic applications accepted. *Expenses:* Tuition, state resident: full-time $4577; part-time $190.70 per credit hour. Tuition, nonresident: full-time $17,758; part-time $739.90 per credit hour. *Required fees:* $3060; $115.70 per credit hour. $141.50 per semester. *Financial support:* In 2015–16, 10 students received support. Scholarships/grants, health care benefits, tuition waivers (partial), and unspecified assistantships available. Financial award application deadline: 6/1; financial award applicants required to submit FAFSA. *Faculty research:* Geographical ecology, global change biology, evolutionary biology, phylogenetics, ecosystem ecology. *Unit head:* Dr. Michael Kaspari, Professor/Director of EEB Graduate Program, 405-325-4321, Fax: 405-325-7619, E-mail: mkaspari@ou.edu. *Application contact:* Adell Hopper, Staff Assistant, 405-325-4321, Fax: 405-325-7619, E-mail: ahopper@ou.edu.
Website: http://mpbio.ou.edu/

University of Oregon, Graduate School, College of Arts and Sciences, Department of Biology, Eugene, OR 97403. Offers ecology and evolution (MA, MS, PhD); marine biology (MA, MS, PhD); molecular, cellular and genetic biology (PhD); neuroscience and development (PhD). Terminal master's awarded for partial completion of doctoral program. *Degree requirements:* For master's, thesis (for some programs); for doctorate, thesis/dissertation. *Entrance requirements:* For master's and doctorate, GRE General Test, minimum GPA of 3.2. Additional exam requirements/recommendations for international students: Required—TOEFL. *Faculty research:* Developmental neurobiology; evolution, population biology, and quantitative genetics; regulation of gene expression; biochemistry of marine organisms.

University of Pittsburgh, Dietrich School of Arts and Sciences, Department of Biological Sciences, Program in Ecology and Evolution, Pittsburgh, PA 15260. Offers PhD. *Faculty:* 5 full-time (2 women). *Students:* 15 full-time (10 women); includes 1 minority (Hispanic/Latino), 2 international. Average age 23. 27 applicants, 22% accepted, 3 enrolled. In 2015, 4 doctorates awarded. *Degree requirements:* For doctorate, comprehensive exam, thesis/dissertation, completion of research integrity module. *Entrance requirements:* For doctorate, GRE General Test, GRE Subject Test. Additional exam requirements/recommendations for international students: Required—TOEFL (minimum score 90 iBT). *Application deadline:* For fall admission, 1/3 priority date for domestic students, 12/9 priority date for international students. Applications are processed on a rolling basis. Application fee: $0 ($50 for international students). Electronic applications accepted. Tuition and fees vary according to program. *Financial support:* In 2015–16, 15 fellowships with full tuition reimbursements (averaging $33,193 per year), 13 research assistantships with full tuition reimbursements (averaging $27,645 per year), 15 teaching assistantships with full tuition reimbursements (averaging $26,850 per year) were awarded; Federal Work-Study, traineeships, health

care benefits, and tuition waivers (full) also available. *Unit head:* Dr. Karen M. Arndt, Professor, 412-624-6963, Fax: 412-624-4349, E-mail: arndt@pitt.edu. *Application contact:* Cathleen M. Barr, Graduate Administrator, 412-624-4268, Fax: 412-624-4349, E-mail: cbarr@pitt.edu.
Website: http://www.biology.pitt.edu

University of Puerto Rico, Río Piedras Campus, College of Natural Sciences, Department of Biology, San Juan, PR 00931-3300. Offers ecology/systematics (MS, PhD); evolution/genetics (MS, PhD); molecular/cellular biology (MS, PhD); neuroscience (MS, PhD). *Program availability:* Part-time. *Degree requirements:* For master's, one foreign language, comprehensive exam, thesis; for doctorate, one foreign language, comprehensive exam, thesis/dissertation. *Entrance requirements:* For master's, GRE Subject Test, interview, minimum GPA of 3.0, letter of recommendation; for doctorate, GRE Subject Test, interview, master's degree, minimum GPA of 3.0, letter of recommendation. *Faculty research:* Environmental, poblational and systematic biology.

University of South Carolina, The Graduate School, College of Arts and Sciences, Department of Biological Sciences, Graduate Training Program in Ecology, Evolution, and Organismal Biology, Columbia, SC 29208. Offers MS, PhD. *Degree requirements:* For master's, one foreign language, comprehensive exam, thesis; for doctorate, one foreign language, comprehensive exam, thesis/dissertation. *Entrance requirements:* For master's and doctorate, GRE General Test, minimum GPA of 3.0 in science. Additional exam requirements/recommendations for international students: Required—TOEFL (minimum score 570 paper-based). Electronic applications accepted.

University of South Florida, College of Arts and Sciences, Department of Integrative Biology, Tampa, FL 33620-9951. Offers biology (MS), including ecology and evolution (MS, PhD), environmental and ecological microbiology (MS, PhD), physiology and morphology (MS, PhD); integrative biology (PhD), including ecology and evolution (MS, PhD), environmental and ecological microbiology (MS, PhD), physiology and morphology (MS, PhD). *Program availability:* Part-time. *Faculty:* 14 full-time (6 women). *Students:* 48 full-time (30 women), 6 part-time (3 women); includes 10 minority (1 American Indian or Alaska Native, non-Hispanic/Latino; 1 Asian, non-Hispanic/Latino; 7 Hispanic/Latino; 1 Two or more races, non-Hispanic/Latino), 3 international. Average age 30. 43 applicants, 37% accepted, 12 enrolled. In 2015, 8 master's, 3 doctorates awarded. *Degree requirements:* For master's, comprehensive exam, thesis (for some programs); for doctorate, comprehensive exam, thesis/dissertation. *Entrance requirements:* For master's and doctorate, GRE General Test, minimum GPA of 3.0 in last 60 hours of BS. Additional exam requirements/recommendations for international students: Required—TOEFL (minimum score 570 paper-based; 88 iBT). *Application deadline:* For fall admission, 2/15 priority date for domestic students, 1/2 for international students; for spring admission, 8/1 for domestic students, 6/1 for international students. Application fee: $30. Electronic applications accepted. *Financial support:* Research assistantships, teaching assistantships, and unspecified assistantships available. Financial award application deadline: 6/30; financial award applicants required to submit FAFSA. *Faculty research:* Marine ecology, ecosystem responses to urbanization, biomechanical and physiological mechanisms of animal movement, population biology and conservation, microbial ecology and public health microbiology, natural diversity of parasites and herbivores; ecosystems, vertebrates, disturbance ecology, functional and ecological morphology of feeding in fishes, rare amphibians and reptiles, genomics in ecological experiments, ecotoxicology, global carbon cycle, plant-animal interactions. *Total annual research expenditures:* $1.3 million. *Unit head:* Dr. Valerie Harwood, Professor and Chair, 813-974-1524, Fax: 813-974-3263, E-mail: vharwood@usf.edu. *Application contact:* Dr. Lynn Martin, Associate Professor and Graduate Program Director, 813-974-0157, Fax: 813-974-3263, E-mail: lbmartin@usf.edu.
Website: http://biology.usf.edu/ib/grad/

The University of Tennessee, Graduate School, College of Arts and Sciences, Department of Ecology and Evolutionary Biology, Knoxville, TN 37996. Offers behavior (MS, PhD); ecology (MS, PhD); evolutionary biology (MS, PhD). *Program availability:* Part-time. *Degree requirements:* For master's, thesis; for doctorate, thesis/dissertation. *Entrance requirements:* For master's and doctorate, GRE General Test, minimum GPA of 2.7. Additional exam requirements/recommendations for international students: Required—TOEFL. Electronic applications accepted.

The University of Tennessee, Graduate School, College of Arts and Sciences, Department of Mathematics, Knoxville, TN 37996. Offers applied mathematics (MS); mathematical ecology (PhD); mathematics (M Math, MS, PhD). *Program availability:* Part-time. *Degree requirements:* For master's, thesis or alternative; for doctorate, one foreign language, thesis/dissertation. *Entrance requirements:* For master's and doctorate, minimum GPA of 2.7. Additional exam requirements/recommendations for international students: Required—TOEFL. Electronic applications accepted.

The University of Texas at Austin, Graduate School, College of Natural Sciences, School of Biological Sciences, Program in Ecology, Evolution and Behavior, Austin, TX 78712-1111. Offers PhD. *Entrance requirements:* For doctorate, GRE General Test. Additional exam requirements/recommendations for international students: Required—TOEFL. Electronic applications accepted.

The University of Toledo, College of Graduate Studies, College of Natural Sciences and Mathematics, Department of Environmental Sciences, Toledo, OH 43606-3390. Offers biology (MS, PhD), including ecology; geology (MS), including earth surface processes. *Program availability:* Part-time. *Degree requirements:* For master's, thesis or alternative. *Entrance requirements:* For master's, GRE General Test, minimum cumulative point-hour ratio of 2.7 for all previous academic work, three letters of recommendation, statement of purpose, transcripts from all prior institutions attended. Additional exam requirements/recommendations for international students: Required—TOEFL (minimum score 550 paper-based; 80 iBT). Electronic applications accepted. *Faculty research:* Environmental geochemistry, geophysics, petrology and mineralogy, paleontology, geohydrology.

University of Toronto, School of Graduate Studies, Faculty of Arts and Science, Department of Ecology and Evolutionary Biology, Toronto, ON M5S 1A1, Canada. Offers M Sc, PhD. *Degree requirements:* For master's, thesis, thesis defense; for doctorate, thesis/dissertation, thesis defense. *Entrance requirements:* For master's, minimum B average in last 2 years; knowledge of physics, chemistry, and biology. Additional exam requirements/recommendations for international students: Required—TOEFL (minimum score 580 paper-based; 93 iBT), TWE (minimum score 5). Electronic applications accepted.

University of Washington, Graduate School, College of the Environment, School of Environmental and Forest Resources, Seattle, WA 98195. Offers bioresource science and engineering (MS, PhD); environmental horticulture (MEH); forest ecology (MS, PhD); forest management (MFR); forest soils (MS, PhD); restoration ecology (MS, PhD); restoration ecology and environmental horticulture (MS, PhD); social sciences (MS, PhD); sustainable resource management (MS, PhD); wildlife science (MS, PhD); MFR/MAIS; MPA/MS. *Accreditation:* SAF. *Program availability:* Part-time. *Degree requirements:* For master's, thesis; for doctorate, comprehensive exam, thesis/dissertation. *Entrance requirements:* For master's and doctorate, GRE, minimum GPA of 3.0. Additional exam requirements/recommendations for international students: Required—TOEFL. Electronic applications accepted. *Faculty research:* Ecosystem analysis, silviculture and forest protection, paper

science and engineering, environmental horticulture and urban forestry, natural resource policy and economics, restoration ecology and environment horticulture, conservation, human dimensions, wildlife, bioresource science and engineering.

University of Wisconsin–Madison, Graduate School, College of Agricultural and Life Sciences, Agroecology Program, Madison, WI 53706-1380. Offers MS. *Degree requirements:* For master's, thesis (for some programs). *Entrance requirements:* For master's, GRE. Additional exam requirements/recommendations for international students: Required—TOEFL (minimum score 580 paper-based; 92 iBT), IELTS (minimum score 7). Electronic applications accepted. *Expenses:* Tuition, state resident: full-time $5364. Tuition, nonresident: full-time $12,027. *Required fees:* $571. Tuition and fees vary according to campus/location, program and reciprocity agreements. *Faculty research:* Multifunctional landscape, socio-ecological systems, participatory solutions to environmental problems.

University of Wyoming, Program in Ecology, Laramie, WY 82071. Offers MS, PhD. *Entrance requirements:* For master's and doctorate, GRE.

Utah State University, School of Graduate Studies, College of Natural Resources, Department of Environment and Society, Logan, UT 84322. Offers bioregional planning (MS); geography (MA, MS); human dimensions of ecosystem science and management (MS, PhD); recreation resource management (MS, PhD). *Degree requirements:* For master's, comprehensive exam, thesis (for some programs). *Entrance requirements:* For master's and doctorate, GRE General Test, minimum GPA of 3.0. Additional exam requirements/recommendations for international students: Required—TOEFL. Electronic applications accepted. *Faculty research:* Geographic information systems/ geographic and environmental education, bioregional planning, natural resource and environmental policy, outdoor recreation and tourism, natural resource and environmental management.

Utah State University, School of Graduate Studies, College of Natural Resources, Department of Watershed Sciences, Logan, UT 84322. Offers ecology (MS, PhD); fisheries biology (MS, PhD); watershed science (MS, PhD). *Degree requirements:* For master's, thesis (for some programs); for doctorate, thesis/dissertation. *Entrance requirements:* For master's and doctorate, GRE General Test, minimum GPA of 3.2. Additional exam requirements/recommendations for international students: Required—TOEFL. Electronic applications accepted. *Faculty research:* Behavior, population ecology, habitat, conservation biology, restoration, aquatic ecology, fisheries management, fluvial geomorphology, remote sensing, conservation biology.

Utah State University, School of Graduate Studies, College of Natural Resources, Department of Wildland Resources, Logan, UT 84322. Offers ecology (MS, PhD); forestry (MS, PhD); range science (MS, PhD); wildlife biology (MS, PhD). *Program availability:* Part-time. *Degree requirements:* For master's, thesis; for doctorate, comprehensive exam, thesis/dissertation. *Entrance requirements:* For master's and doctorate, GRE General Test, minimum GPA of 3.0. Additional exam requirements/ recommendations for international students: Required—TOEFL. *Faculty research:* Range plant ecophysiology, plant community ecology, ruminant nutrition, population ecology.

Utah State University, School of Graduate Studies, College of Science, Department of Biology, Logan, UT 84322. Offers biology (MS, PhD); ecology (MS, PhD). *Program availability:* Part-time. *Degree requirements:* For master's, thesis; for doctorate, thesis/ dissertation. *Entrance requirements:* For master's and doctorate, GRE General Test, minimum GPA of 3.0. Additional exam requirements/recommendations for international students: Required—TOEFL (minimum score 575 paper-based). *Faculty research:* Plant, insect, microbial, and animal biology.

Washington University in St. Louis, Graduate School of Arts and Sciences, Division of Biology and Biomedical Sciences, Program in Evolution, Ecology and Population Biology, St. Louis, MO 63130-4899. Offers ecology (PhD). *Students:* 26 full-time (15 women); includes 3 minority (1 Black or African American, non-Hispanic/Latino; 1 Asian, non-Hispanic/Latino; 1 Two or more races, non-Hispanic/Latino), 2 international. 27 applicants, 37% accepted, 5 enrolled. In 2015, 3 doctorates awarded. *Degree requirements:* For doctorate, thesis/dissertation. *Entrance requirements:* For doctorate, GRE General Test, GRE Subject Test. Additional exam requirements/recommendations for international students: Required—TOEFL. *Application deadline:* For fall admission, 12/1 for domestic students. Application fee: $0. Electronic applications accepted. *Financial support:* Fellowships, research assistantships, and teaching assistantships available. Financial award application deadline: 1/15. *Faculty research:* Population ecology, community ecology, plant and animal evolution; microbial evolution, evolution of behavior, phylogenetics, systematics, theoretical and experimental population genetics. *Unit head:* Stacia Burd, Coordinator, 314-362-3364. *Application contact:* Rebecca Riney, 314-747-4648, E-mail: dbbsphdadmissions@wusm.wustl.edu.

Wesleyan University, Graduate Studies, Department of Biology, Middletown, CT 06459. Offers cell and developmental biology (PhD); evolution and ecology (PhD); genetics and genomics (PhD), including bioinformatics; neurobiology and behavior (PhD). *Faculty:* 14 full-time (5 women). *Students:* 26 full-time (12 women); includes 5 minority (2 Black or African American, non-Hispanic/Latino; 3 Asian, non-Hispanic/ Latino) 5 international. In 2015, 3 doctorates awarded. Terminal master's awarded for partial completion of doctoral program. *Degree requirements:* For doctorate, comprehensive exam, thesis/dissertation, public seminar. *Entrance requirements:* For doctorate, GRE. Additional exam requirements/recommendations for international students: Required—TOEFL or IELTS. *Application deadline:* For fall admission, 1/15 for domestic and international students. Application fee: $0. Electronic applications accepted. *Financial support:* Stipends available. *Faculty research:* Evolution and ecology, neurobiology and behavior, cell and developmental biology, genetics, genomics and bioinformatics. *Unit head:* Dr. John Kirn, Chair/Professor, 860-685-3494, E-mail: jrkirn@wesleyan.edu. *Application contact:* Marjorie Fitzgibbons, Administrative Assistant, 860-685-2157, E-mail: mfitzgibbons@wesleyan.edu.
Website: http://www.wesleyan.edu/bio/

Western Illinois University, School of Graduate Studies, College of Arts and Sciences, Program in Environmental Science: Large River Ecosystems, Macomb, IL 61455-1390. Offers PhD. *Students:* 1 full-time (0 women), 2 part-time (both women). Average age 35. 3 applicants, 33% accepted, 1 enrolled. *Degree requirements:* For doctorate, thesis/ dissertation. *Entrance requirements:* For doctorate, GRE, three letters of recommendation, official transcripts, statement of research intent, curriculum vitae. Additional exam requirements/recommendations for international students: Required— TOEFL. *Application deadline:* Applications are processed on a rolling basis. Application fee: $30. *Financial support:* In 2015–16, 1 student received support, including 1 research assistantship with full tuition reimbursement available (averaging $7,544 per year). *Unit head:* Dr. Roger Viadero, Director, Institute for Environmental Sciences, 309-298-2040. *Application contact:* Dr. Nancy Parsons, Associate Provost and Director of Graduate Studies, 309-298-1806, Fax: 309-298-2345, E-mail: grad-office@wiu.edu.
Website: http://wiu.edu/graduate_studies/programs_of_study/environsci_profile.php

Yale University, Graduate School of Arts and Sciences, Department of Ecology and Evolutionary Biology, New Haven, CT 06520. Offers PhD. *Entrance requirements:* For doctorate, GRE General Test, GRE Subject Test (biology).

Environmental Biology

Baylor University, Graduate School, College of Arts and Sciences, Department of Biology, Waco, TX 76798. Offers biology (MA, MS, PhD); environmental biology (MS); limnology (MS). *Program availability:* Part-time. *Degree requirements:* For master's, thesis (for some programs); for doctorate, thesis/dissertation. *Entrance requirements:* For master's and doctorate, GRE General Test. Additional exam requirements/recommendations for international students: Required—TOEFL. *Faculty research:* Terrestrial ecology, aquatic ecology, genetics.

Chatham University, Program in Biology, Pittsburgh, PA 15232-2826. Offers environmental biology (MS); human biology (MS). *Program availability:* Part-time. *Faculty:* 1 (woman) full-time, 1 (woman) part-time/adjunct. *Students:* 52 full-time (33 women), 11 part-time (7 women); includes 20 minority (11 Black or African American, non-Hispanic/Latino; 4 Asian, non-Hispanic/Latino; 5 Hispanic/Latino), 7 international. Average age 25. 149 applicants, 66% accepted, 42 enrolled. In 2015, 35 master's awarded. *Degree requirements:* For master's, thesis optional. *Entrance requirements:* For master's, 3 letters of recommendation. Additional exam requirements/recommendations for international students: Required—TOEFL (minimum score 600 paper-based; 100 iBT), IELTS (minimum score 7), TWE. *Application deadline:* For fall admission, 4/1 priority date for domestic and international students; for spring admission, 11/1 priority date for domestic students, 10/1 priority date for international students. Applications are processed on a rolling basis. Application fee: $45. Electronic applications accepted. Application fee is waived when completed online. *Expenses: Tuition, area resident:* Full-time $15,786; part-time $877 per credit hour. *Required fees:* $468; $26 per credit hour. *Financial support:* Applicants required to submit FAFSA. *Faculty research:* Molecular evolution of iron homeostasis, characteristics of soil bacterial communities, gene flow through seed movement, role of gonadotropins in spermatogonial proliferation, phosphatid/linositol metabolism in epithelial cells. *Unit head:* Dr. Lisa Lambert, Director, 412-365-1217, E-mail: lambert@chatham.edu. *Application contact:* Ashlee Bartko, Senior Assistant Director of Graduate Admission, 412-365-1115, Fax: 412-365-1609, E-mail: gradadmissions@chatham.edu. Website: http://www.chatham.edu/departments/sciences/graduate/biology

Dalhousie University, Faculty of Agriculture, Halifax, NS B3H 4R2, Canada. Offers agriculture (M Sc), including air quality, animal behavior, animal molecular genetics, animal nutrition, animal technology, aquaculture, botany, crop management, crop physiology, ecology, environmental microbiology, food science, horticulture, nutrient management, pest management, physiology, plant biotechnology, plant pathology, soil chemistry, soil fertility, waste management and composting, water quality. *Program availability:* Part-time. *Degree requirements:* For master's, thesis, ATC Exam Teaching Assistantship. *Entrance requirements:* For master's, honors B Sc, minimum GPA of 3.0. Additional exam requirements/recommendations for international students: Required—TOEFL (minimum score 580 paper-based; 92 iBT), IELTS, Michigan English Language Assessment Battery, CanTEST, CAEL. *Faculty research:* Bio-product development, organic agriculture, nutrient management, air and water quality, agricultural biotechnology.

Emporia State University, Department of Biological Sciences, Emporia, KS 66801-5415. Offers botany (MS); environmental biology (MS); general biology (MS); microbial and cellular biology (MS); zoology (MS). *Program availability:* Part-time. *Faculty:* 14 full-time (3 women), 1 part-time/adjunct (0 women). *Students:* 26 full-time (13 women), 15 part-time (7 women); includes 1 minority (Two or more races, non-Hispanic/Latino), 24 international. 16 applicants, 100% accepted, 11 enrolled. In 2015, 17 master's awarded. *Degree requirements:* For master's, comprehensive exam or thesis. *Entrance requirements:* For master's, GRE, appropriate undergraduate degree, interview, letters of reference. Additional exam requirements/recommendations for international students: Required—TOEFL (minimum score 520 paper-based; 68 iBT). *Application deadline:* For fall admission, 8/15 priority date for domestic students. Applications are processed on a rolling basis. Application fee: $30 ($75 for international students). Electronic applications accepted. *Expenses:* Tuition, state resident: full-time $5640; part-time $235 per credit hour. Tuition, nonresident: full-time $17,544; part-time $731 per credit hour. *Required fees:* $1848; $77 per credit hour. *Financial support:* In 2015–16, 7 research assistantships with full tuition reimbursements (averaging $7,344 per year), 12 teaching assistantships with full tuition reimbursements (averaging $7,844 per year) were awarded; career-related internships or fieldwork, Federal Work-Study, institutionally sponsored loans, health care benefits, and unspecified assistantships also available. Financial award application deadline: 3/15; financial award applicants required to submit FAFSA. *Faculty research:* Fisheries, range, and wildlife management; aquatic, plant, grassland, vertebrate, and invertebrate ecology; mammalian and plant systematics, taxonomy, and evolution; immunology, virology, and molecular biology. *Unit head:* Dr. Yixin Eric Yang, Chair, 620-341-5311, Fax: 620-341-5608, E-mail: yyang@emporia.edu. Website: http://www.emporia.edu/info/degrees-courses/grad/biology

Georgia State University, College of Arts and Sciences, Department of Biology, Program in Applied and Environmental Microbiology, Atlanta, GA 30302-3083. Offers applied and environmental microbiology (MS, PhD); bioinformatics (MS). *Program availability:* Part-time. Terminal master's awarded for partial completion of doctoral program. *Degree requirements:* For master's, comprehensive exam (for some programs), thesis optional; for doctorate, comprehensive exam, thesis/dissertation. *Entrance requirements:* For master's and doctorate, GRE. Additional exam requirements/recommendations for international students: Required—TOEFL (minimum score 550 paper-based; 82 iBT) or IELTS (minimum score 7). *Application deadline:* For fall admission, 7/1 priority date for domestic students, 6/1 priority date for international students; for spring admission, 11/15 priority date for domestic students, 10/15 priority date for international students. Applications are processed on a rolling basis. Application fee: $50. Electronic applications accepted. *Expenses:* Tuition, state resident: full-time $6876; part-time $382 per credit hour. Tuition, nonresident: full-time $22,374; part-time $1243 per credit hour. *Required fees:* $2128; $2128 per term. $1064 per term. Part-time tuition and fees vary according to course load and program. *Financial support:* In 2015–16, fellowships with full tuition reimbursements (averaging $22,000 per year), research assistantships with full tuition reimbursements (averaging $20,000 per year) were awarded. Financial award application deadline: 12/3. *Faculty research:* Bioremediation, biofilms, indoor air quality control, environmental toxicology, product biosynthesis. *Unit head:* Dr. Charles Derby, Director of Graduate Studies, 404-413-5393, Fax: 404-413-5446, E-mail: cderby@gsu.edu. Website: http://biology.gsu.edu/

Governors State University, College of Arts and Sciences, Program in Environmental Biology, University Park, IL 60484. Offers MS. *Program availability:* Part-time, evening/weekend. *Degree requirements:* For master's, thesis or alternative. *Faculty research:* Animal physiology, cell biology, animal behavior, plant physiology, plant populations.

Hampton University, School of Science, Department of Biological Sciences, Hampton, VA 23668. Offers biology (MS); environmental science (MS); medical science (MS). *Program availability:* Part-time. *Degree requirements:* For master's, comprehensive exam (for some programs), thesis optional. *Entrance requirements:* For master's, GRE General Test. Additional exam requirements/recommendations for international students: Required—TOEFL (minimum score 525 paper-based) or IELTS (6.5). Electronic applications accepted. *Expenses: Tuition, area resident:* Full-time $10,263; part-time $522 per credit hour. *Required fees:* $35. Tuition and fees vary according to course load and program. *Faculty research:* Molecular mechanisms responsible for initiation, promotion, and progression of breast, colon, prostate, thyroid, and skin cancers; isolation and characterization of bacteria in natural and contaminated environments and study of probable uses in biocontrol, diabetes, and hypertension.

Hood College, Graduate School, Program in Environmental Biology, Frederick, MD 21701-8575. Offers MS. *Program availability:* Part-time, evening/weekend. *Degree requirements:* For master's, thesis or alternative. *Entrance requirements:* For master's, minimum GPA of 2.75, 1 year of undergraduate biology and chemistry, 1 semester of mathematics. Additional exam requirements/recommendations for international students: Required—TOEFL (minimum score 575 paper-based; 89 iBT), IELTS (minimum score 6.5). *Application deadline:* For fall admission, 7/15 priority date for domestic students, 7/15 for international students; for spring admission, 12/1 priority date for domestic students, 12/1 for international students. Applications are processed on a rolling basis. Application fee: $35. Electronic applications accepted. Application fee is waived when completed online. *Expenses: Tuition, area resident:* Part-time $450 per credit hour. *Required fees:* $105 per term. Part-time tuition and fees vary according to degree level, campus/location and program. *Financial support:* Tuition waivers (partial) and unspecified assistantships available. Financial award applicants required to submit FAFSA. Website: http://www.hood.edu/graduate

Massachusetts Institute of Technology, School of Engineering, Department of Civil and Environmental Engineering, Cambridge, MA 02139. Offers biological oceanography (PhD, Sc D); chemical oceanography (PhD, Sc D); civil and environmental systems (M Eng, SM, PhD, Sc D); civil engineering (PhD, Sc D, CE); coastal engineering (PhD, Sc D); construction engineering and management (PhD, Sc D); environmental biology (PhD, Sc D); environmental chemistry (PhD, Sc D); environmental engineering (PhD, Sc D); environmental fluid mechanics (PhD, Sc D); geotechnical and geoenvironmental engineering (PhD, Sc D); hydrology (PhD, Sc D); information technology (PhD, Sc D); oceanographic engineering (PhD, Sc D); structures and materials (PhD, Sc D); transportation (PhD, Sc D); SM/MBA. *Faculty:* 27 full-time (5 women). *Students:* 183 full-time (59 women); includes 19 minority (1 Black or African American, non-Hispanic/Latino; 7 Asian, non-Hispanic/Latino; 8 Hispanic/Latino; 3 Two or more races, non-Hispanic/Latino), 106 international. Average age 27. 513 applicants, 20% accepted, 56 enrolled. In 2015, 77 master's, 18 doctorates, 1 other advanced degree awarded. *Degree requirements:* For master's, thesis; for doctorate, comprehensive exam, thesis/dissertation; for CE, comprehensive exam, thesis. *Entrance requirements:* For master's, doctorate, and CE, GRE General Test. Additional exam requirements/recommendations for international students: Required—TOEFL (minimum score 577 paper-based; 100 iBT), IELTS (minimum score 7). *Application deadline:* For fall admission, 12/15 for domestic and international students. Application fee: $75. Electronic applications accepted. *Expenses: Tuition:* Full-time $46,400; part-time $725 per credit. One-time fee: $304 full-time. Full-time tuition and fees vary according to course load and program. *Financial support:* In 2015–16, 150 students received support, including 38 fellowships (averaging $38,000 per year), 111 research assistantships (averaging $35,100 per year), 9 teaching assistantships (averaging $39,900 per year); Federal Work-Study, institutionally sponsored loans, scholarships/grants, traineeships, health care benefits, and unspecified assistantships also available. Support available to part-time students. Financial award application deadline: 4/15; financial award applicants required to submit FAFSA. *Faculty research:* Environmental chemistry, environmental fluid mechanics and coastal engineering, environmental microbiology, geotechnical engineering and geomechanics, hydrology and hydroclimatology, infrastructure systems, mechanics of materials and structures, transportation systems. *Total annual research expenditures:* $24.8 million. *Unit head:* Prof. Markus Buehler, Department Head, 617-253-7101. *Application contact:* Graduate Admissions Coordinator, 617-253-7119, E-mail: cee-admissions@mit.edu. Website: http://cee.mit.edu/

Missouri University of Science and Technology, Graduate School, Department of Biological Sciences, Rolla, MO 65409. Offers applied and environmental biology (MS). *Faculty:* 10 full-time (3 women). *Students:* 10 full-time (6 women), 6 part-time (5 women); includes 1 minority (Hispanic/Latino), 6 international. Average age 28. 19 applicants, 68% accepted, 7 enrolled. In 2015, 8 master's awarded. *Entrance requirements:* For master's, GRE (minimum score 600 quantitative, 4 writing). Additional exam requirements/recommendations for international students: Required—TOEFL (minimum score 570 paper-based). Application fee: $50. *Expenses:* Tuition, state resident: full-time $10,536. Tuition, nonresident: full-time $27,015. Full-time tuition and fees vary according to course load. *Financial support:* In 2015–16, 6 research assistantships (averaging $1,810 per year), 1 teaching assistantship (averaging $1,814 per year) were awarded; institutionally sponsored loans and unspecified assistantships also available. *Total annual research expenditures:* $306,173. *Unit head:* Dr. Robert Aronstam, Chair, 573-341-4819, Fax: 573-341-4821, E-mail: aronstam@mst.edu. *Application contact:* Debbie Schwertz, Admissions Coordinator, 573-341-6013, Fax: 573-341-6271, E-mail: schwertz@mst.edu. Website: http://biosci.mst.edu/

Morgan State University, School of Graduate Studies, School of Computer, Mathematical, and Natural Sciences, Department of Biology, Program in Bioenvironmental Science, Baltimore, MD 21251. Offers PhD. *Degree requirements:* For doctorate, comprehensive exam, thesis/dissertation, oral defense of dissertation. *Entrance requirements:* For doctorate, GRE General Test, GRE Subject Test (biology, chemistry, or related science), bachelor's or master's degree in biology, chemistry, physics or related field; minimum GPA of 3.0. Additional exam requirements/recommendations for international students: Required—TOEFL (minimum score 550 paper-based).

Nicholls State University, Graduate Studies, College of Arts and Sciences, Department of Biological Sciences, Thibodaux, LA 70310. Offers marine and environmental biology (MS). *Program availability:* Part-time. *Degree requirements:* For master's, comprehensive exam, thesis. *Entrance requirements:* For master's, GRE. Additional exam requirements/recommendations for international students: Required—TOEFL (minimum score 600 paper-based). *Application deadline:* For fall admission, 6/17 priority date for domestic and international students; for spring admission, 11/15

priority date for domestic and international students. Application fee: $20 ($30 for international students). *Financial support:* Research assistantships, teaching assistantships with tuition reimbursements, career-related internships or fieldwork, and scholarships/grants available. *Faculty research:* Bioremediation, ecology, public health, biotechnology, physiology.
Website: http://www.nicholls.edu/biol/

Ohio University, Graduate College, College of Arts and Sciences, Department of Environmental and Plant Biology, Athens, OH 45701-2979. Offers MS, PhD. *Program availability:* Part-time. *Degree requirements:* For master's, thesis, 2 terms of teaching experience; for doctorate, comprehensive exam, thesis/dissertation, 2 terms of teaching experience. *Entrance requirements:* For master's, GRE General Test, minimum GPA of 3.0; for doctorate, GRE General Test, minimum GPA of 3.2. Additional exam requirements/recommendations for international students: Required—TOEFL (minimum score 620 paper-based; 105 iBT) or IELTS (minimum score 7.5). Electronic applications accepted. *Faculty research:* Eastern deciduous forest ecology, evolutionary developmental plant biology, phylogenetic systematics, plant cell wall biotechnology.

Regis University, Regis College, Denver, CO 80221-1099. Offers biomedical sciences (MS); development practice (MA); environmental biology (MS). *Accreditation:* Teacher Education Accreditation Council. *Program availability:* Part-time. *Faculty:* 2 full-time (1 woman), 22 part-time/adjunct (12 women). *Students:* 60 full-time (38 women), 11 part-time (8 women); includes 13 minority (4 Asian, non-Hispanic/Latino; 7 Hispanic/Latino; 2 Two or more races, non-Hispanic/Latino), 2 international. Average age 27. 390 applicants, 71% accepted, 45 enrolled. In 2015, 29 master's awarded. *Degree requirements:* For master's, thesis (for some programs), capstone presentation. *Entrance requirements:* For master's, official transcript reflecting baccalaureate degree awarded from U.S.-based regionally-accredited college or university. Additional exam requirements/recommendations for international students: Required—TOEFL (minimum score 550 paper-based; 82 iBT). *Application deadline:* For fall admission, 5/15 priority date for domestic students, 4/1 priority date for international students; for spring admission, 12/15 priority date for domestic students. Applications are processed on a rolling basis. Application fee: $75. Electronic applications accepted. *Expenses:* Contact institution. *Financial support:* Federal Work-Study and scholarships/grants available. Financial award application deadline: 4/15; financial award applicants required to submit FAFSA. *Unit head:* Dr. Thomas Bowie, Academic Dean. *Application contact:* Sarah Engel, Director of Admissions, 303-458-4900, Fax: 303-964-5534, E-mail: ruadmissions@regis.edu.
Website: http://www.regis.edu/RC.aspx

Rutgers University–New Brunswick, Graduate School-New Brunswick, Department of Environmental Sciences, Piscataway, NJ 08854-8097. Offers air pollution and resources (MS, PhD); aquatic biology (MS, PhD); aquatic chemistry (MS, PhD); atmospheric science (MS, PhD); chemistry and physics of aerosol and hydrosol systems (MS, PhD); environmental chemistry (MS, PhD); environmental microbiology (MS, PhD); environmental toxicology (PhD); exposure assessment (PhD); fate and effects of pollutants (MS, PhD); pollution prevention and control (MS, PhD); water and wastewater treatment (MS, PhD); water resources (MS, PhD). Terminal master's awarded for partial completion of doctoral program. *Degree requirements:* For master's, comprehensive exam, thesis or alternative, oral final exam; for doctorate, comprehensive exam, thesis/dissertation, thesis defense, qualifying exam. *Entrance requirements:* For master's and doctorate, GRE General Test. Additional exam requirements/recommendations for international students: Required—TOEFL. Electronic applications accepted. *Faculty research:* Biological waste treatment; contaminant fate and transport; air, soil and water quality.

Sonoma State University, School of Science and Technology, Department of Biology, Rohnert Park, CA 94928. Offers biochemistry (MA); ecology (MS); environmental biology (MS); evolutionary biology (MS); functional morphology (MS); molecular and cell biology (MS); organismal biology (MS). *Program availability:* Part-time. *Degree requirements:* For master's, thesis or alternative, oral exam. *Entrance requirements:* For master's, GRE General Test, GRE Subject Test, minimum GPA of 3.0. Additional exam requirements/recommendations for international students: Required—TOEFL (minimum score 500 paper-based). *Faculty research:* Plant physiology, comparative physiology, community ecology, restoration ecology, marine ecology, conservation genetics, primate behavior, behavioral ecology, developmental biology, plant and animal systematics.

State University of New York College of Environmental Science and Forestry, Department of Environmental and Forest Biology, Syracuse, NY 13210-2779. Offers applied ecology (MPS); chemical ecology (MPS, MS, PhD); conservation biology (MPS, MS, PhD); ecology (MPS, MS, PhD); entomology (MPS, MS, PhD); environmental interpretation (MPS, MS, PhD); environmental physiology (MPS, MS, PhD); fish and wildlife biology and management (MPS, MS, PhD); forest pathology and mycology (MPS, MS, PhD); plant biotechnology (MPS); plant science and biotechnology (MPS, MS, PhD). *Faculty:* 29 full-time (9 women), 4 part-time/adjunct (3 women). *Students:* 81 full-time (47 women), 57 part-time (24 women); includes 16 minority (1 Black or African American, non-Hispanic/Latino; 2 American Indian or Alaska Native, non-Hispanic/Latino; 1 Asian, non-Hispanic/Latino; 3 Hispanic/Latino; 2 Two or more races, non-Hispanic/Latino), 15 international. Average age 28. 47 applicants, 49% accepted, 15 enrolled. In 2015, 15 master's, 7 doctorates awarded. *Degree requirements:* For master's, thesis (for some programs), capstone seminar; for doctorate, comprehensive exam, thesis/dissertation, capstone seminar. *Entrance requirements:* For master's and doctorate, GRE General Test, minimum GPA of 3.0. Additional exam requirements/recommendations for international students: Required—TOEFL (minimum score 550 paper-based; 80 iBT), IELTS (minimum score 6). *Application deadline:* For fall admission, 2/1 priority date for domestic and international students; for spring admission, 11/1 priority date for domestic and international students. Applications are processed on a rolling basis. Application fee: $60. *Expenses:* Tuition, state resident: full-time $10,870; part-time $453 per credit. Tuition, nonresident: full-time $22,210; part-time $925 per credit. *Required fees:* $1075; $89.22 per credit. *Financial support:* In 2015–16, 4 fellowships with tuition reimbursements, 36 research assistantships with tuition reimbursements, 39 teaching assistantships with tuition reimbursements (averaging $11,490 per year) were awarded; Federal Work-Study, institutionally sponsored loans, scholarships/grants, health care benefits, and unspecified assistantships also available. Financial award application deadline: 6/30. *Faculty research:* Ecology, conservation biology, fish and wildlife biology and management, plant science, entomology. *Total annual research expenditures:* $4.1 million. *Unit head:* Dr. Donald J. Leopold, Chair, 315-470-6760, Fax: 315-470-6934, E-mail: djleopold@esf.edu. *Application contact:* Dr. Danilo D. Fernando, Director, Graduate Program/Associate Professor, 315-470-6746, Fax: 315-470-6934, E-mail: dfernando@esf.edu.
Website: http://www.esf.edu/efb/grad/default.asp

Universidad del Turabo, Graduate Programs, Programs in Science and Technology, Gurabo, PR 00778-3030. Offers environmental analysis (MSE), including environmental chemistry; environmental management (MSE), including pollution management; environmental science (D Sc), including environmental biology. *Entrance requirements:* For master's, GRE, EXADEP, interview.

University of Alberta, Faculty of Graduate Studies and Research, Department of Biological Sciences, Edmonton, AB T6G 2E1, Canada. Offers environmental biology

and ecology (M Sc, PhD); microbiology and biotechnology (M Sc, PhD); molecular biology and genetics (M Sc, PhD); physiology and cell biology (M Sc, PhD); plant biology (M Sc, PhD); systematics and evolution (M Sc, PhD). Terminal master's awarded for partial completion of doctoral program. *Degree requirements:* For master's, thesis; for doctorate, thesis/dissertation. *Entrance requirements:* Additional exam requirements/recommendations for international students: Required—TOEFL.

University of California, Santa Cruz, Division of Graduate Studies, Division of Physical and Biological Sciences, Environmental Toxicology Department, Santa Cruz, CA 95064. Offers MS, PhD. Terminal master's awarded for partial completion of doctoral program. *Degree requirements:* For master's, comprehensive exam, thesis; for doctorate, thesis/dissertation, qualifying exams. *Entrance requirements:* For master's and doctorate, GRE. Additional exam requirements/recommendations for international students: Required—TOEFL (minimum score 550 paper-based; 83 iBT); Recommended—IELTS (minimum score 8). Electronic applications accepted. *Faculty research:* Molecular mechanisms of reactive DNA methylation toxicity, anthropogenic perturbations of biogeochemical cycles, anaerobic microbiology and biotransformation of pollutants and toxic metals, organismal responses and therapeutic treatment of toxins, microbiology, molecular genetics, genomics.

University of Guelph, Graduate Studies, Ontario Agricultural College, Department of Environmental Biology, Guelph, ON N1G 2W1, Canada. Offers entomology (M Sc, PhD); environmental microbiology and biotechnology (M Sc, PhD); environmental toxicology (M Sc, PhD); plant and forest systems (M Sc, PhD); plant pathology (M Sc, PhD). *Program availability:* Part-time. *Degree requirements:* For master's, thesis; for doctorate, comprehensive exam, thesis/dissertation. *Entrance requirements:* For master's, minimum 75% average during previous 2 years of course work; for doctorate, minimum 75% average. Additional exam requirements/recommendations for international students. Required—TOEFL or IELTS. Electronic applications accepted. *Faculty research:* Entomology, environmental microbiology and biotechnology, environmental toxicology, forest ecology, plant pathology.

University of Louisiana at Lafayette, College of Sciences, Department of Biology, Lafayette, LA 70504. Offers biology (MS); environmental and evolutionary biology (PhD). Terminal master's awarded for partial completion of doctoral program. *Degree requirements:* For master's, thesis; for doctorate, 2 foreign languages, comprehensive exam, thesis/dissertation. *Entrance requirements:* For master's, GRE General Test, minimum GPA of 2.75; for doctorate, GRE General Test, GRE Subject Test, minimum GPA of 3.0. Additional exam requirements/recommendations for international students: Required—TOEFL (minimum score 550 paper-based). Electronic applications accepted. *Faculty research:* Structure and ultrastructure, system biology, ecology, processes, environmental physiology.

University of Louisville, Graduate School, College of Arts and Sciences, Department of Biology, Louisville, KY 40292-0001. Offers biology (MS); environmental biology (PhD). *Program availability:* Part-time. *Students:* 52 full-time (29 women), 2 part-time (0 women); includes 4 minority (1 Black or African American, non-Hispanic/Latino; 1 Asian, non-Hispanic/Latino; 1 Hispanic/Latino; 1 Two or more races, non-Hispanic/Latino), 11 international. Average age 29. 35 applicants, 54% accepted, 15 enrolled. In 2015, 3 master's, 1 doctorate awarded. Terminal master's awarded for partial completion of doctoral program. *Degree requirements:* For master's, comprehensive exam, thesis (for some programs); for doctorate, comprehensive exam, thesis/dissertation. *Entrance requirements:* For master's, GRE, MCAT, or DAT; for doctorate, GRE. Additional exam requirements/recommendations for international students: Required—TOEFL (minimum score 550 paper-based, 83 iBT) or IELTS (6.5). *Application deadline:* For fall admission, 1/31 priority date for domestic and international students; for spring admission, 12/1 for domestic and international students; for summer admission, 4/15 for domestic and international students. Applications are processed on a rolling basis. Application fee: $60. *Expenses:* Tuition, state resident: full-time $11,664; part-time $649 per credit hour. Tuition, nonresident: full-time $24,274; part-time $1350 per credit hour. *Required fees:* $196. Tuition and fees vary according to program and reciprocity agreements. *Financial support:* In 2015–16, 415,878 students received support, including 2 fellowships with full tuition reimbursements available (averaging $22,000 per year), 2 research assistantships with full tuition reimbursements available (averaging $22,000 per year), 24 teaching assistantships with full tuition reimbursements available (averaging $22,000 per year); Federal Work-Study and unspecified assistantships also available. Financial award application deadline: 1/31. *Faculty research:* Molecular, microbiology, ecology, animal behavior, evolution. *Total annual research expenditures:* $717,917. *Unit head:* Dr. Ronald Fell, Chair, 502-852-6771, Fax: 502-852-0725, E-mail: rdfell@louisville.edu. *Application contact:* Libby Leggett, Director, Graduate Admissions, 502-852-3101, Fax: 502-852-6536, E-mail: gradadm@louisville.edu.
Website: http://louisville.edu/biology

The University of Manchester, Faculty of Life Sciences, Manchester, United Kingdom. Offers adaptive organismal biology (M Phil, PhD); animal biology (M Phil, PhD); biochemistry (M Phil, PhD); bioinformatics (M Phil, PhD); biomolecular sciences (M Phil, PhD); biotechnology (M Phil, PhD); cell biology (M Phil, PhD); cell matrix research (M Phil, PhD); channels and transporters (M Phil, PhD); developmental biology (M Phil, PhD); Egyptology (M Phil, PhD); environmental biology (M Phil, PhD); evolutionary biology (M Phil, PhD); gene expression (M Phil, PhD); genetics (M Phil, PhD); history of science, technology and medicine (M Phil, PhD); immunology (M Phil, PhD); integrative neurobiology and behavior (M Phil, PhD); membrane trafficking (M Phil, PhD); microbiology (M Phil, PhD); molecular and cellular neuroscience (M Phil, PhD); molecular biology (M Phil, PhD); molecular cancer studies (M Phil, PhD); neuroscience (M Phil, PhD); ophthalmology (M Phil, PhD); optometry (M Phil, PhD); organelle function (M Phil, PhD); pharmacology (M Phil, PhD); physiology (M Phil, PhD); plant sciences (M Phil, PhD); stem cell research (M Phil, PhD); structural biology (M Phil, PhD); systems neuroscience (M Phil, PhD); toxicology (M Phil, PhD).

University of Massachusetts Amherst, Graduate School, College of Natural Sciences, Department of Environmental Conservation, Amherst, MA 01003. Offers building systems (MS, PhD); environmental policy and human dimensions (MS, PhD); forest resources (MS, PhD); sustainability science (MS); water, wetlands and watersheds (MS, PhD); wildlife and fisheries conservation (MS, PhD). *Program availability:* Part-time. Terminal master's awarded for partial completion of doctoral program. *Degree requirements:* For master's, thesis or alternative; for doctorate, comprehensive exam, thesis/dissertation. *Entrance requirements:* For master's and doctorate, GRE General Test. Additional exam requirements/recommendations for international students: Required—TOEFL (minimum score 550 paper-based; 80 iBT), IELTS (minimum score 6.5). Electronic applications accepted.

University of North Dakota, Graduate School, College of Arts and Sciences, Department of Biology, Grand Forks, ND 58202. Offers botany (MS, PhD); ecology (MS, PhD); entomology (MS, PhD); environmental biology (MS, PhD); fisheries/wildlife (MS, PhD); genetics (MS, PhD); zoology (MS, PhD). Terminal master's awarded for partial completion of doctoral program. *Degree requirements:* For master's, thesis, final exam; for doctorate, comprehensive exam, thesis/dissertation, final exam. *Entrance requirements:* For master's, GRE General Test, GRE Subject Test, minimum GPA of 3.0; for doctorate, GRE General Test, GRE Subject Test, minimum GPA of 3.5.

Environmental Biology

Additional exam requirements/recommendations for international students: Required—TOEFL (minimum score 550 paper-based; 79 iBT), IELTS (minimum score 6.5). Electronic applications accepted. *Faculty research:* Population biology, wildlife ecology, RNA processing, hormonal control of behavior.

University of Southern California, Graduate School, Dana and David Dornsife College of Letters, Arts and Sciences, Department of Biological Sciences, Program in Marine Biology and Biological Oceanography, Los Angeles, CA 90089. Offers marine and environmental biology (MS); marine biology and biological oceanography (PhD). Terminal master's awarded for partial completion of doctoral program. *Degree requirements:* For master's, research paper; for doctorate, comprehensive exam, thesis/dissertation, qualifying examination, dissertation defense. *Entrance requirements:* For master's and doctorate, GRE, 3 letters of recommendation, personal statement, resume, minimum GPA of 3.0. Additional exam requirements/recommendations for international students: Required—TOEFL (minimum score 600 paper-based; 100 iBT). Electronic applications accepted. *Faculty research:* Microbial ecology, biogeochemistry, and geobiology; biodiversity and molecular ecology; integrative organismal biology; conservation biology; marine genomics.

University of Southern Mississippi, Graduate School, College of Science and Technology, Department of Biological Sciences, Hattiesburg, MS 39406-0001. Offers environmental biology (MS); marine biology (MS); microbiology (MS, PhD); molecular biology (MS, PhD). Terminal master's awarded for partial completion of doctoral program. *Degree requirements:* For master's, comprehensive exam, thesis; for doctorate, comprehensive exam, thesis/dissertation. *Entrance requirements:* For master's, GRE General Test, minimum GPA of 3.0 on last 60 hours; for doctorate, GRE General Test, minimum GPA of 3.5. Additional exam requirements/recommendations for international students: Required—TOEFL, IELTS.

University of South Florida, College of Arts and Sciences, Department of Integrative Biology, Tampa, FL 33620-9951. Offers biology (MS), including ecology and evolution (MS, PhD), environmental and ecological microbiology (MS, PhD), physiology and morphology (MS, PhD); integrative biology (PhD), including ecology and evolution (MS, PhD), environmental and ecological microbiology (MS, PhD), physiology and morphology (MS, PhD). *Program availability:* Part-time. *Faculty:* 14 full-time (6 women). *Students:* 48 full-time (30 women), 6 part-time (3 women); includes 10 minority (1 American Indian or Alaska Native, non-Hispanic/Latino; 1 Asian, non-Hispanic/Latino; 7 Hispanic/Latino; 1 Two or more races, non-Hispanic/Latino), 3 international. Average age 30. 43 applicants, 37% accepted, 12 enrolled. In 2015, 8 master's, 3 doctorates awarded. *Degree requirements:* For master's, comprehensive exam, thesis (for some programs); for doctorate, comprehensive exam, thesis/dissertation. *Entrance requirements:* For master's and doctorate, GRE General Test, minimum GPA of 3.0 in last 60 hours of BS. Additional exam requirements/recommendations for international students: Required—TOEFL (minimum score 570 paper-based; 88 iBT). *Application deadline:* For fall admission, 2/15 priority date for domestic students, 1/2 for international students; for spring admission, 8/1 for domestic students, 6/1 for international students. Application fee: $30. Electronic applications accepted. *Financial support:* Research assistantships, teaching assistantships, and unspecified assistantships available. Financial award application deadline: 6/30; financial award applicants required to submit FAFSA. *Faculty research:* Marine ecology, ecosystem responses to urbanization, biomechanical and physiological mechanisms of animal movement, population biology and conservation, microbial ecology and public health microbiology, natural diversity of parasites and herbivores; ecosystems, vertebrates, disturbance ecology, functional and ecological morphology of feeding in fishes, rare amphibians and reptiles, genomics in ecological experiments, ecotoxicology, global carbon cycle, plant-animal interactions. *Total annual research expenditures:* $1.3 million. *Unit head:* Dr. Valerie Harwood, Professor and Chair, 813-974-1524, Fax: 813-974-3263, E-mail: vharwood@usf.edu. *Application contact:* Dr. Lynn Martin, Associate Professor and Graduate Program Director, 813-974-0157, Fax: 813-974-3263, E-mail: lbmartin@usf.edu.
Website: http://biology.usf.edu/ib/grad/

University of West Florida, College of Science and Engineering, School of Allied Health and Life Sciences, Department of Biology, Pensacola, FL 32514-5750. Offers biological chemistry (MS); biology (MS); biology education (MST); biotechnology (MS); coastal zone studies (MS); environmental biology (MS). *Degree requirements:* For master's, thesis. *Entrance requirements:* For master's, GRE (minimum score: verbal 450, quantitative 550), official transcripts; BS in biology or related field; letter of interest; relevant past experience; three letters of recommendation from individuals who can

evaluate applicant's academic ability. Additional exam requirements/recommendations for international students: Required—TOEFL (minimum score 550 paper-based).

University of Wisconsin–Madison, School of Medicine and Public Health, Molecular and Environmental Toxicology Graduate Program, Madison, WI 53706. Offers MS, PhD. Terminal master's awarded for partial completion of doctoral program. *Expenses:* Tuition, state resident: full-time $5364. Tuition, nonresident: full-time $12,027. *Required fees:* $571. Tuition and fees vary according to campus/location, program and reciprocity agreements.
Website: http://www.med.wisc.edu/metc/

Washington University in St. Louis, Graduate School of Arts and Sciences, Division of Biology and Biomedical Sciences, St. Louis, MO 63130-4899. Offers biochemistry (PhD); computational and molecular biophysics (PhD); computational and systems biology (PhD); developmental, regenerative, and stem cell biology (PhD); evolution, ecology and population biology (PhD), including ecology, environmental biology, evolutionary biology, genetics; human and statistical genetics (PhD); immunology (PhD); molecular cell biology (PhD); molecular genetics and genomics (PhD); molecular microbiology and microbial pathogenesis (PhD); neurosciences (PhD); plant and microbial biosciences (PhD); MD/PhD. *Students:* 542 full-time (246 women); includes 106 minority (27 Black or African American, non-Hispanic/Latino; 5 American Indian or Alaska Native, non-Hispanic/Latino; 60 Asian, non-Hispanic/Latino; 11 Hispanic/Latino; 3 Two or more races, non-Hispanic/Latino), 115 international. 1,085 applicants, 21% accepted, 77 enrolled. In 2015, 87 doctorates awarded. *Degree requirements:* For doctorate, thesis/dissertation. *Entrance requirements:* For doctorate, GRE General Test, GRE Subject Test. Additional exam requirements/recommendations for international students: Required—TOEFL. *Application deadline:* For fall admission, 12/1 for domestic students. Application fee: $0. Electronic applications accepted. *Financial support:* Fellowships, research assistantships, and tuition waivers (full) available. Financial award application deadline: 1/15. *Unit head:* Dr. John Russell, Associate Dean, 314-747-0840. *Application contact:* Rebecca Riney, 314-474-4648, E-mail: dbbsphdadmissions@wusm.wustl.edu.
Website: http://dbbs.wustl.edu/

West Virginia University, Davis College of Agriculture, Forestry and Consumer Sciences, Division of Plant and Soil Sciences, Morgantown, WV 26506. Offers agricultural sciences (PhD), including animal and food sciences, plant and soil sciences; agronomy (MS); entomology (MS); environmental microbiology (MS); horticulture (MS); plant pathology (MS). *Degree requirements:* For master's, thesis. *Entrance requirements:* For master's, GRE, minimum GPA of 2.5. Additional exam requirements/recommendations for international students: Required—TOEFL. *Expenses:* Tuition, state resident: full-time $8568. Tuition, nonresident: full-time $22,140. Tuition and fees vary according to program. *Faculty research:* Water quality, reclamation of disturbed land, crop production, pest control, environmental protection.

West Virginia University, Eberly College of Arts and Sciences, Department of Biology, Morgantown, WV 26506. Offers cell and molecular biology (MS, PhD); environmental and evolutionary biology (MS, PhD); forensic biology (MS, PhD); genomic biology (MS, PhD); neurobiology (MS, PhD). Terminal master's awarded for partial completion of doctoral program. *Degree requirements:* For master's, thesis, final exam; for doctorate, thesis/dissertation, preliminary and final exams. *Entrance requirements:* For master's, GRE General Test, GRE Subject Test, minimum GPA of 3.0; for doctorate, GRE General Test, minimum GPA of 3.0. Additional exam requirements/recommendations for international students: Required—TOEFL. *Expenses:* Tuition, state resident: full-time $8568. Tuition, nonresident: full-time $22,140. Tuition and fees vary according to program. *Faculty research:* Environmental biology, genetic engineering, developmental biology, global change, biodiversity.

Youngstown State University, Graduate School, College of Science, Technology, Engineering and Mathematics, Department of Biological Sciences, Youngstown, OH 44555-0001. Offers environmental biology (MS); molecular biology, microbiology, and genetic (MS); physiology and anatomy (MS). *Program availability:* Part-time. *Degree requirements:* For master's, comprehensive exam, thesis, oral review. *Entrance requirements:* For master's, GRE General Test, minimum GPA of 2.7. Additional exam requirements/recommendations for international students: Required—TOEFL. *Faculty research:* Cell biology, neurophysiology, molecular biology, neurobiology, gene regulation.

Evolutionary Biology

Arizona State University at the Tempe campus, College of Liberal Arts and Sciences, School of Life Sciences, Tempe, AZ 85287-4601. Offers animal behavior (PhD); applied ethics (biomedical and health ethics) (MA); biology (MS, PhD), including biology, biology and society, complex adaptive systems science (PhD), plant biology and conservation (MS); environmental life sciences (PhD); evolutionary biology (PhD); history and philosophy of science (PhD); human and social dimensions of science and technology (PhD); microbiology (PhD); molecular and cellular biology (PhD); neuroscience (PhD). Terminal master's awarded for partial completion of doctoral program. *Degree requirements:* For master's, thesis (for some programs), interactive Program of Study (iPOS) submitted before completing 50 percent of required credit hours; for doctorate, variable foreign language requirement, comprehensive exam, thesis/dissertation, interactive Program of Study (iPOS) submitted before completing 50 percent of required credit hours. *Entrance requirements:* For master's and doctorate, GRE, minimum GPA of 3.0 or equivalent in last 2 years of work leading to bachelor's degree. Additional exam requirements/recommendations for international students: Required—TOEFL (minimum score 600 paper-based; 100 iBT). Electronic applications accepted.

Brown University, Graduate School, Division of Biology and Medicine, Department of Ecology and Evolutionary Biology, Providence, RI 02912. Offers PhD. *Degree requirements:* For doctorate, thesis/dissertation, preliminary exam. *Entrance requirements:* For doctorate, GRE General Test, GRE Subject Test. Additional exam requirements/recommendations for international students: Required—TOEFL. Electronic applications accepted. *Faculty research:* Marine ecology, behavioral ecology, population genetics, evolutionary morphology, plant ecology.

Clemson University, Graduate School, College of Science, Department of Biological Sciences, Program in Biological Sciences, Clemson, SC 29634. Offers MS, PhD. *Program availability:* Part-time. *Faculty:* 9 full-time (2 women). *Students:* 31 full-time (20 women); includes 1 minority (Two or more races, non-Hispanic/Latino), 8 international. Average age 28. 45 applicants, 31% accepted, 6 enrolled. In 2015, 1 master's, 5 doctorates awarded. *Degree requirements:* For master's, thesis; for doctorate,

comprehensive exam, thesis/dissertation. *Entrance requirements:* For master's and doctorate, GRE General Test, unofficial transcripts, letters of recommendation. Additional exam requirements/recommendations for international students: Required—TOEFL (minimum score 100 iBT), IELTS (minimum score 7.5), PTE (minimum score 7). *Application deadline:* For fall admission, 1/5 for domestic and international students. Application fee: $80 ($90 for international students). Electronic applications accepted. *Expenses:* $4,060 per semester full-time resident, $8,103 per semester full-time non-resident, $448 per credit hour part-time resident, $898 per credit hour part-time non-resident. *Financial support:* In 2015–16, 31 students received support, including 1 fellowship with partial tuition reimbursement available (averaging $5,000 per year), 2 research assistantships with partial tuition reimbursements available (averaging $21,600 per year), 29 teaching assistantships with partial tuition reimbursements available (averaging $26,656 per year); career-related internships or fieldwork and health care benefits also available. Financial award application deadline: 1/5. *Faculty research:* Cell and developmental biology, evolutionary biology, ecology, molecular biology. *Unit head:* Dr. Robert Cohen, Department Chair, 864-656-1112, Fax: 864-656-0435, E-mail: rscohen@clemson.edu. *Application contact:* Jay Lyn Martin, Student Services Program Coordinator, 864-656-3587, Fax: 864-656-0435, E-mail: jaylyn@clemson.edu.
Website: http://www.clemson.edu/cafls/departments/biosci/

Columbia University, Graduate School of Arts and Sciences, New York, NY 10027. Offers African-American studies (MA); American studies (MA); anthropology (MA, PhD); art history and archaeology (MA, PhD); astronomy (PhD); biological sciences (PhD); biotechnology (MA); chemical physics (PhD); chemistry (PhD); classical studies (MA, PhD); classics (MA, PhD); climate and society (MA); conservation biology (MA); earth and environmental sciences (PhD); East Asia: regional studies (MA); East Asian languages and cultures (MA, PhD); ecology, evolution and environmental biology (MA), including conservation biology; ecology, evolution, and environmental biology (PhD), including ecology and evolutionary biology, evolutionary primatology; economics (MA, PhD); English and comparative literature (MA, PhD); French and Romance philology

(MA, PhD); Germanic languages (MA, PhD); global French studies (MA); global thought (MA); Hispanic cultural studies (MA); history (PhD); history and literature (MA); human rights studies (MA); Islamic studies (MA); Italian (MA, PhD); Japanese pedagogy (MA); Jewish studies (MA); Latin America and the Caribbean: regional studies (MA); Latin American and Iberian cultures (PhD); mathematics (MA, PhD), including finance (MA); medieval and Renaissance studies (MA); Middle Eastern, South Asian, and African studies (MA, PhD); modern art: critical and curatorial studies (MA); modern European studies (MA); museum anthropology (MA); music (DMA, PhD); oral history (MA); philosophical foundations of physics (MA); philosophy (MA, PhD); physics (PhD); political science (MA, PhD); psychology (PhD); quantitative methods in the social sciences (MA); religion (MA, PhD); Russia, Eurasia and East Europe: regional studies (MA); Russian translation (MA); Slavic cultures (MA); Slavic languages (MA, PhD); sociology (MA, PhD); South Asian studies (MA); statistics (MA, PhD); theatre (PhD). Dual-degree programs require admission to both Graduate School of Arts and Sciences and another Columbia school. *Program availability:* Part-time. *Students:* 3,030 full-time, 235 part-time; includes 861 minority (88 Black or African American, non-Hispanic/Latino; 5 American Indian or Alaska Native, non-Hispanic/Latino; 517 Asian, non-Hispanic/Latino; 159 Hispanic/Latino; 4 Native Hawaiian or other Pacific Islander, non-Hispanic/Latino; 88 Two or more races, non-Hispanic/Latino), 1,697 international. 13,288 applicants, 21% accepted, 1162 enrolled. In 2015, 1,061 master's, 553 doctorates awarded. Terminal master's awarded for partial completion of doctoral program. *Degree requirements:* For master's, variable foreign language requirement, comprehensive exam (for some programs), thesis (for some programs); for doctorate, variable foreign language requirement, comprehensive exam (for some programs), thesis/dissertation. *Entrance requirements:* For master's and doctorate, GRE General Test, GRE Subject Test (for some programs). Additional exam requirements/recommendations for international students: Required—TOEFL, IELTS. Application fee: $105. Electronic applications accepted. *Financial support:* Fellowships, research assistantships, teaching assistantships, career-related internships or fieldwork, Federal Work-Study, institutionally sponsored loans, scholarships/grants, traineeships, health care benefits, tuition waivers, and unspecified assistantships available. Support available to part-time students. Financial award application deadline: 12/15. *Unit head:* Carlos J. Alonso, Dean of the Graduate School of Arts and Sciences, 212-854-5177. *Application contact:* GSAS Office of Admissions, 212-854-8903, E-mail: gsas-admissions@columbia.edu.
Website: http://gsas.columbia.edu/

Cornell University, Graduate School, Graduate Fields of Agriculture and Life Sciences, Field of Ecology and Evolutionary Biology, Ithaca, NY 14853-0001. Offers ecology (PhD), including animal ecology, applied ecology, biogeochemistry, community and ecosystem ecology, limnology, oceanography, physiological ecology, plant ecology, population ecology, theoretical ecology, vertebrate zoology; evolutionary biology (PhD), including ecological genetics, paleobiology, population biology, systematics. *Degree requirements:* For doctorate, comprehensive exam, thesis/dissertation, 2 semesters of teaching experience. *Entrance requirements:* For doctorate, GRE General Test, GRE Subject Test (biology), 2 letters of recommendation. Additional exam requirements/recommendations for international students: Required—TOEFL (minimum score 550 paper-based; 77 iBT). Electronic applications accepted. *Faculty research:* Population and organismal biology, population and evolutionary genetics, systematics and macroevolution, biochemistry, conservation biology.

Dartmouth College, Arts and Sciences Graduate Programs, Program in Ecology and Evolutionary Biology, Hanover, NH 03755. Offers PhD. *Faculty:* 8 full-time (4 women). *Students:* 28 full-time (18 women); includes 3 minority (1 American Indian or Alaska Native, non-Hispanic/Latino; 1 Asian, non-Hispanic/Latino; 1 Two or more races, non-Hispanic/Latino), 4 international. Average age 29. 35 applicants, 26% accepted, 7 enrolled. In 2015, 10 doctorates awarded. *Entrance requirements:* For doctorate, GRE General Test, GRE Subject Test in biology (highly recommended). Additional exam requirements/recommendations for international students: Required—TOEFL. *Application deadline:* For fall admission, 12/1 for domestic students. Electronic applications accepted. *Expenses:* Tuition, area resident: Full-time $48,120. *Required fees:* $296. One-time fee: $50 full-time. *Financial support:* Fellowships with full tuition reimbursements, research assistantships with full tuition reimbursements, teaching assistantships with full tuition reimbursements, institutionally sponsored loans, traineeships, and unspecified assistantships available. Financial award applicants required to submit FAFSA. *Unit head:* Dr. Mathew Ayres, 603-646-2788. *Application contact:* Amy Layne, 603-646-3847, Fax: 603-646-3488.
Website: http://sites.dartmouth.edu/EEES/

Emory University, Laney Graduate School, Division of Biological and Biomedical Sciences, Program in Population Biology, Ecology and Evolution, Atlanta, GA 30322-1100. Offers PhD. *Degree requirements:* For doctorate, comprehensive exam, thesis/dissertation. *Entrance requirements:* For doctorate, GRE General Test, minimum GPA of 3.0 in science course work (recommended). Additional exam requirements/recommendations for international students: Required—TOEFL. Electronic applications accepted. *Faculty research:* Evolution of microbes, infectious disease, the immune system, genetic disease in humans, evolution of behavior.

Florida State University, The Graduate School, College of Arts and Sciences, Department of Biological Science, Specialization in Ecology and Evolutionary Biology, Tallahassee, FL 32306-4295. Offers MS, PhD. *Faculty:* 21 full-time (7 women). *Students:* 56 full-time (27 women); includes 4 minority (1 Black or African American, non-Hispanic/Latino; 3 Hispanic/Latino), 5 international. 120 applicants, 13% accepted, 9 enrolled. In 2015, 2 master's, 3 doctorates awarded. Terminal master's awarded for partial completion of doctoral program. *Degree requirements:* For master's, comprehensive exam, thesis, teaching experience, seminar presentation; for doctorate, comprehensive exam, thesis/dissertation, teaching experience, seminar presentation. *Entrance requirements:* For master's and doctorate, GRE General Test, minimum upper-division GPA of 3.0. Additional exam requirements/recommendations for international students: Required—TOEFL (minimum score 600 paper-based; 92 iBT). *Application deadline:* For fall admission, 12/1 for domestic and international students. Application fee: $30. Electronic applications accepted. *Expenses: Tuition, area resident:* Full-time $7263; part-time $403.50 per credit hour. *Tuition, nonresident:* full-time $18,087; part-time $1004.85 per credit hour. *Required fees:* $1365; $75.81 per credit hour. $20 per semester. Tuition and fees vary according to campus/location. *Financial support:* In 2015–16, 55 students received support, including 4 fellowships with tuition reimbursements available (averaging $30,000 per year), 20 research assistantships with full tuition reimbursements available (averaging $21,500 per year), 31 teaching assistantships with full tuition reimbursements available (averaging $21,500 per year); scholarships/grants and unspecified assistantships also available. Financial award application deadline: 12/1; financial award applicants required to submit FAFSA. *Faculty research:* Ecology and conservation biology; evolution; marine biology; phylogeny and systematics; theoretical, computational and mathematical biology. *Unit head:* Dr. Thomas A. Houpt, Professor and Associate Chair, 850-644-4907, Fax: 850-644-8447, E-mail: houpt@neuro.fsu.edu. *Application contact:* Dr. Michael B. Miller, Coordinator, Graduate Affairs, 850-644-3023, Fax: 850-644-9829, E-mail: gradinfo@bio.fsu.edu.
Website: http://www.bio.fsu.edu/

Harvard University, Graduate School of Arts and Sciences, Department of Organismic and Evolutionary Biology, Cambridge, MA 02138. Offers biology (PhD). *Degree requirements:* For doctorate, 2 foreign languages, public presentation of thesis research, exam. *Entrance requirements:* For doctorate, GRE General Test, GRE Subject Test (recommended), 7 courses in biology, chemistry, physics, mathematics, computer science, or geology. Additional exam requirements/recommendations for international students: Required—TOEFL.

Illinois State University, Graduate School, College of Arts and Sciences, Department of Biological Sciences, Normal, IL 61790-2200. Offers animal behavior (MS); bacteriology (MS); biochemistry (MS); biological sciences (MS); biology (PhD); biophysics (MS); biotechnology (MS); botany (MS, PhD); cell biology (MS); conservation biology (MS); developmental biology (MS); ecology (MS, PhD); entomology (MS); evolutionary biology (MS); genetics (MS, PhD); immunology (MS); microbiology (MS, PhD); molecular biology (MS); molecular genetics (MS); neurobiology (MS); neuroscience (MS); parasitology (MS); physiology (MS, PhD); plant biology (MS); plant molecular biology (MS); plant sciences (MS); structural biology (MS); zoology (MS, PhD). *Program availability:* Part-time. *Degree requirements:* For master's, thesis or alternative; for doctorate, variable foreign language requirement, thesis/dissertation, 2 terms of residency. *Entrance requirements:* For master's, GRE General Test, minimum GPA of 2.6 in last 60 hours of course work; for doctorate, GRE General Test. *Application deadline:* Applications are processed on a rolling basis. Application fee: $40. *Financial support:* Research assistantships, teaching assistantships, Federal Work-Study, tuition waivers (full), and unspecified assistantships available. Financial award application deadline: 4/1. *Faculty research:* Redoc balance and drug development in schistosoma mansoni, control of the growth of listeria monocytogenes at low temperature, regulation of cell expansion and microtubule function by SPRI, CRUI: physiology and fitness consequences of different life history phenotypes. *Application contact:* Steven Juliano, Graduate Coordinator, E-mail: sajulian@ilstu.edu.
Website: http://www.bio.ilstu.edu/

Indiana State University, College of Graduate and Professional Studies, College of Arts and Sciences, Department of Biology, Terre Haute, IN 47809. Offers cellular and molecular biology (PhD); ecology, systematics and evolution (PhD); life sciences (MS); physiology (PhD); science education (MS). *Degree requirements:* For master's, thesis optional; for doctorate, comprehensive exam, thesis/dissertation. *Entrance requirements:* For master's and doctorate, GRE General Test. Electronic applications accepted.

Indiana University Bloomington, University Graduate School, College of Arts and Sciences, Department of Biology, Bloomington, IN 47405. Offers biology teaching (MAT); biotechnology (MA); evolution, ecology, and behavior (MA, PhD); genetics (PhD); microbiology (MA, PhD); molecular, cellular, and developmental biology (PhD); plant sciences (MA, PhD); zoology (MA, PhD). Terminal master's awarded for partial completion of doctoral program. *Degree requirements:* For master's, thesis, oral defense; for doctorate, thesis/dissertation, oral defense. *Entrance requirements:* For master's and doctorate, GRE General Test. Additional exam requirements/recommendations for international students: Required—TOEFL (minimum score 100 iBT). Electronic applications accepted. *Faculty research:* Evolution, ecology and behavior; microbiology; molecular biology and genetics; plant biology.

Iowa State University of Science and Technology, Program in Ecology and Evolutionary Biology, Ames, IA 50011. Offers MS, PhD. *Degree requirements:* For master's, thesis or alternative; for doctorate, thesis/dissertation. *Entrance requirements:* For master's and doctorate, GRE General Test. Additional exam requirements/recommendations for international students: Required—TOEFL (minimum score 550 paper-based; 79 iBT), IELTS (minimum score 6.5). Electronic applications accepted. *Faculty research:* Landscape ecology, aquatic and method ecology, physiological ecology, population genetics and evolution, systematics.

Johns Hopkins University, School of Medicine, Graduate Programs in Medicine, Center for Functional Anatomy and Evolution, Baltimore, MD 21218. Offers PhD. *Degree requirements:* For doctorate, comprehensive exam, thesis/dissertation, oral exams. *Entrance requirements:* For doctorate, GRE. Additional exam requirements/recommendations for international students: Required—TOEFL. *Faculty research:* Vertebrate evolution, functional anatomy, primate evolution, vertebrate paleobiology, vertebrate morphology.

Michigan State University, The Graduate School, College of Natural Science, Interdepartmental Program in Ecology, Evolutionary Biology and Behavior, East Lansing, MI 48824. Offers PhD. *Entrance requirements:* Additional exam requirements/recommendations for international students: Required—TOEFL. Electronic applications accepted.

Montclair State University, The Graduate School, College of Science and Mathematics, Program in Biology, Montclair, NJ 07043-1624. Offers biological science/education (MS); biology (MS); ecology and evolution (MS); physiology (MS). *Students:* 10 full-time (7 women), 35 part-time (27 women); includes 9 minority (6 Asian, non-Hispanic/Latino; 2 Hispanic/Latino; 1 Two or more races, non-Hispanic/Latino). Average age 28. 23 applicants, 57% accepted, 12 enrolled. In 2015, 18 master's awarded. *Expenses:* Tuition, state resident: part-time $553 per credit. Tuition, nonresident: part-time $854 per credit. *Required fees:* $91 per credit. Tuition and fees vary according to program. *Unit head:* Dr. Liza C. Hazard, Chairperson, 973-655-4397, E-mail: hazardl@mail.montclair.edu. *Application contact:* Amy Aiello, Director of Graduate Admissions and Operations, 973-655-5147, Fax: 973-655-7869, E-mail: graduate.school@montclair.edu.

Northeastern University, College of Science, Boston, MA 02115-5096. Offers applied mathematics (MS); bioinformatics (MS); biology (PhD); biotechnology (MS); chemistry (MS, PhD); ecology, evolution, and marine biology (PhD); marine biology (MS); mathematics (MS, PhD); network science (PhD); operations research (MSOR); physics (MS, PhD); psychology (PhD). *Program availability:* Part-time. *Faculty:* 216 full-time (70 women), 62 part-time/adjunct (20 women). *Students:* 517 full-time (252 women), 80 part-time (39 women). In 2015, 94 master's, 46 doctorates awarded. Terminal master's awarded for partial completion of doctoral program. *Degree requirements:* For master's, comprehensive exam (for some programs), thesis; for doctorate, comprehensive exam (for some programs), thesis/dissertation. *Entrance requirements:* For master's, GRE General Test. *Application deadline:* Applications are processed on a rolling basis. Application fee: $75. Electronic applications accepted. *Expenses:* $1,325 per credit; $1,170 per credit for marine biology). *Financial support:* Fellowships with tuition reimbursements, research assistantships with tuition reimbursements, teaching assistantships with tuition reimbursements, career-related internships or fieldwork, scholarships/grants, health care benefits, tuition waivers (full and partial), and unspecified assistantships available. Support available to part-time students. Financial award applicants required to submit FAFSA. *Unit head:* Dr. Jonathan Tilly, Interim Dean. *Application contact:* Graduate Student Services, 617-373-4275, E-mail: gradcos@neu.edu.
Website: http://www.northeastern.edu/cos/

The Ohio State University, Graduate School, College of Arts and Sciences, Division of Natural and Mathematical Sciences, Department of Evolution, Ecology, and Organismal

Evolutionary Biology

Biology, Columbus, OH 43210. Offers MS, PhD. *Faculty:* 25. *Students:* 55 full-time (21 women), 1 (woman) part-time. Average age 29. In 2015, 5 master's, 7 doctorates awarded. *Degree requirements:* For master's, thesis optional; for doctorate, thesis/dissertation. *Entrance requirements:* For master's and doctorate, GRE General Test. Additional exam requirements/recommendations for international students: Required—TOEFL (minimum score 550 paper-based; 79 iBT), Michigan English Language Assessment Battery (minimum score 86); Recommended—IELTS (minimum score 7). *Application deadline:* For fall admission, 12/1 priority date for domestic students, 11/30 priority date for international students. Applications are processed on a rolling basis. Application fee: $60 ($70 for international students). Electronic applications accepted. *Financial support:* Fellowships with tuition reimbursements, research assistantships with tuition reimbursements, teaching assistantships with tuition reimbursements, Federal Work-Study, and institutionally sponsored loans available. Support available to part-time students. *Unit head:* Dr. Elizabeth Marschall, Chair, 614-292-8767, E-mail: marschall.2@osu.edu. *Application contact:* Graduate and Professional Admissions, 614-292-9444, Fax: 614-292-3895, E-mail: gpadmissions@osu.edu. Website: http://eeob.osu.edu/

Ohio University, Graduate College, College of Arts and Sciences, Department of Biological Sciences, Athens, OH 45701-2979. Offers biological sciences (MS, PhD); cell biology and physiology (MS, PhD); ecology and evolutionary biology (MS, PhD); exercise physiology and muscle biology (MS, PhD); microbiology (MS, PhD); neuroscience (MS, PhD). Terminal master's awarded for partial completion of doctoral program. *Degree requirements:* For master's, comprehensive exam, thesis, 1 quarter of teaching experience; for doctorate, comprehensive exam, thesis/dissertation, 2 quarters of teaching experience. *Entrance requirements:* For master's, GRE General Test, names of three faculty members whose research interests most closely match the applicant's interest; for doctorate, GRE General Test, essay concerning prior training, research interest and career goals, plus names of three faculty members whose research interests most closely match the applicant's interest. Additional exam requirements/recommendations for international students: Required—TOEFL (minimum score 620 paper-based; 105 iBT) or IELTS (minimum score 7.5). Electronic applications accepted. *Faculty research:* Ecology and evolutionary biology, exercise physiology and muscle biology, neurobiology, cell biology, physiology.

Oklahoma State University, College of Arts and Sciences, Department of Plant Biology, Ecology, and Evolution, Stillwater, OK 74078. Offers botany (MS); environmental science (MS, PhD); plant science (PhD). *Faculty:* 14 full-time (5 women). *Students:* 8 part-time (3 women); includes 4 minority (1 Asian, non-Hispanic/Latino; 1 Hispanic/Latino; 2 Two or more races, non-Hispanic/Latino). Average age 32. 3 applicants, 67% accepted. In 2015, 3 master's awarded. *Degree requirements:* For master's, thesis; for doctorate, comprehensive exam, thesis/dissertation. *Entrance requirements:* For master's and doctorate, GRE or GMAT. Additional exam requirements/recommendations for international students: Required—TOEFL (minimum score 550 paper-based; 79 iBT). *Application deadline:* For fall admission, 3/1 priority date for international students; for spring admission, 8/1 priority date for international students. Applications are processed on a rolling basis. Application fee: $40 ($75 for international students). Electronic applications accepted. *Expenses:* Tuition, state resident: full-time $3528; part-time $196 per credit hour. Tuition, nonresident: full-time $14,144; part-time $785.75 per credit hour. *Required fees:* $1895; $105.25 per credit hour. Tuition and fees vary according to campus/location. *Financial support:* In 2015–16, 1 research assistantship (averaging $18,504 per year), 12 teaching assistantships (averaging $20,754 per year) were awarded; career-related internships or fieldwork, Federal Work-Study, scholarships/grants, health care benefits, tuition waivers (partial), and unspecified assistantships also available. Support available to part-time students. Financial award application deadline: 3/1; financial award applicants required to submit FAFSA. *Faculty research:* Ethnobotany, developmental genetics of arabidopsis, biological roles of plasmodesmata, community ecology and biodiversity, nutrient cycling in grassland ecosystems. *Unit head:* Dr. Linda Watson, Department Head, 405-744-5559, Fax: 405-744-7074, E-mail: linda.watson10@okstate.edu. Website: http://plantbio.okstate.edu

Princeton University, Graduate School, Department of Ecology and Evolutionary Biology, Princeton, NJ 08544-1019. Offers PhD. *Degree requirements:* For doctorate, thesis/dissertation. *Entrance requirements:* For doctorate, GRE General Test, GRE Subject Test. Additional exam requirements/recommendations for international students: Required—TOEFL (minimum score 600 paper-based). Electronic applications accepted.

Purdue University, Graduate School, College of Science, Department of Biological Sciences, West Lafayette, IN 47907. Offers biochemistry (PhD); biophysics (PhD); cell and developmental biology (PhD); ecology, evolutionary and population biology (MS, PhD), including ecology, evolutionary biology, population biology; genetics (MS, PhD); microbiology (MS, PhD); molecular biology (PhD); neurobiology (MS, PhD); plant physiology (PhD). Terminal master's awarded for partial completion of doctoral program. *Degree requirements:* For master's, thesis (for some programs); for doctorate, thesis/dissertation, seminars, teaching experience. *Entrance requirements:* For master's, GRE General Test (minimum analytical writing score of 3.5), minimum undergraduate GPA of 3.0; for doctorate, GRE General Test (minimum analytical writing score of 3.5), minimum undergraduate GPA of 3.5. Additional exam requirements/recommendations for international students: Required—TOEFL (minimum score 600 paper-based; 107 iBT for MS, 80 iBT for PhD). Electronic applications accepted.

Purdue University, Graduate School, PULSe - Purdue University Life Sciences Program, West Lafayette, IN 47907. Offers biomolecular structure and biophysics (PhD); biotechnology (PhD); chemical biology (PhD); chromatin and regulation of gene expression (PhD); integrative neuroscience (PhD); integrative plant sciences (PhD); membrane biology (PhD); microbiology (PhD); molecular evolutionary and cancer biology (PhD); molecular evolutionary genetics (PhD); molecular virology (PhD). *Entrance requirements:* For doctorate, GRE, minimum undergraduate GPA of 3.0. Additional exam requirements/recommendations for international students: Required—TOEFL (minimum score 550 paper-based; 77 iBT). Electronic applications accepted.

Rice University, Graduate Programs, Wiess School of Natural Sciences, Department of Ecology and Evolutionary Biology, Houston, TX 77251-1892. Offers MA, MS, PhD. Terminal master's awarded for partial completion of doctoral program. *Degree requirements:* For master's, comprehensive exam (for some programs), thesis (for some programs); for doctorate, comprehensive exam, thesis/dissertation. *Entrance requirements:* For master's and doctorate, GRE General Test, GRE Subject Test. Additional exam requirements/recommendations for international students: Required—TOEFL (minimum score 600 paper-based; 90 iBT). Electronic applications accepted. *Faculty research:* Trace gas emissions, wetlands, biology, community ecology of forests and grasslands, conservation biology specialization.

Rutgers University–New Brunswick, Graduate School-New Brunswick, Program in Ecology and Evolution, Piscataway, NJ 08854-8097. Offers MS, PhD. *Program availability:* Part-time. Terminal master's awarded for partial completion of doctoral program. *Degree requirements:* For master's, comprehensive exam; for doctorate, comprehensive exam, thesis/dissertation. *Entrance requirements:* For master's and doctorate, GRE General Test, minimum GPA of 3.0. Additional exam requirements/

recommendations for international students: Required—TOEFL (minimum score 550 paper-based). Electronic applications accepted. *Faculty research:* Population and community ecology, population genetics, evolutionary biology, conservation biology, ecosystem ecology.

Rutgers University–New Brunswick, Graduate School-New Brunswick, Program in Plant Biology, Piscataway, NJ 08854-8097. Offers horticulture and plant technology (MS, PhD); molecular and cellular biology (MS, PhD); organismal and population biology (MS, PhD); plant pathology (MS, PhD). *Program availability:* Part-time. Terminal master's awarded for partial completion of doctoral program. *Degree requirements:* For master's, comprehensive exam, thesis or alternative; for doctorate, comprehensive exam, thesis/dissertation. *Entrance requirements:* For master's and doctorate, GRE General Test, GRE Subject Test (recommended). Additional exam requirements/recommendations for international students: Required—TOEFL (minimum score 600 paper-based). Electronic applications accepted. *Faculty research:* Molecular biology and biochemistry of plants, plant development and genomics, plant protection, plant improvement, plant management of horticultural and field crops.

Sonoma State University, School of Science and Technology, Department of Biology, Rohnert Park, CA 94928. Offers biochemistry (MA); ecology (MS); environmental biology (MS); evolutionary biology (MS); functional morphology (MS); molecular and cell biology (MS); organismal biology (MS). *Program availability:* Part-time. *Degree requirements:* For master's, thesis or alternative, oral exam. *Entrance requirements:* For master's, GRE General Test, GRE Subject Test, minimum GPA of 3.0. Additional exam requirements/recommendations for international students: Required—TOEFL (minimum score 500 paper-based). *Faculty research:* Plant physiology, comparative physiology, community ecology, restoration ecology, marine ecology, conservation genetics, primate behavior, behavioral ecology, developmental biology, plant and animal systematics.

Stony Brook University, State University of New York, Graduate School, College of Arts and Sciences, Department of Ecology and Evolution, Stony Brook, NY 11794. Offers applied ecology (MA); ecology and evolution (PhD). *Faculty:* 18 full-time (6 women). *Students:* 51 full-time (30 women), 1 part-time (0 women); includes 2 minority (1 Asian, non-Hispanic/Latino; 1 Hispanic/Latino), 12 international. Average age 26. 34 applicants, 68% accepted, 5 enrolled. In 2015, 9 doctorates awarded. *Degree requirements:* For doctorate, one foreign language, comprehensive exam, thesis/dissertation, teaching experience. *Entrance requirements:* For doctorate, GRE General Test, GRE Subject Test. Additional exam requirements/recommendations for international students: Required—TOEFL. *Application deadline:* For fall admission, 1/15 for domestic students; for spring admission, 10/1 for domestic students. Application fee: $100. *Expenses:* $12,421 full-time resident tuition and fees, $453 per credit hour; $23,761 full-time nonresident tuition and fees, $925 per credit hour. *Financial support:* In 2015–16, 7 research assistantships, 25 teaching assistantships were awarded; fellowships and Federal Work-Study also available. *Faculty research:* Ecology, ecology and population, evolution, biodiversity, environmental conservation. *Total annual research expenditures:* $1.3 million. *Unit head:* Dr. Robert W. Thacker, Chair, 631-632-8590, Fax: 631-632-7626, E-mail: robert.thacker@stonybrook.edu. *Application contact:* Melissa Cohen, Coordinator, 631-246-8604, Fax: 631-632-7626, E-mail: melissa.j.cohen@stonybrook.edu. Website: http://life.bio.sunysb.edu/ee/

Tulane University, School of Science and Engineering, Department of Ecology and Evolutionary Biology, New Orleans, LA 70118-5669. Offers MS, PhD. Terminal master's awarded for partial completion of doctoral program. *Degree requirements:* For master's, thesis or alternative; for doctorate, thesis/dissertation. *Entrance requirements:* For master's, GRE General Test, minimum B average in undergraduate course work; for doctorate, GRE General Test. Additional exam requirements/recommendations for international students: Required—TOEFL. *Application deadline:* For fall admission, 2/1 for domestic and international students. Application fee: $45. Electronic applications accepted. *Expenses: Tuition, area resident:* Full-time $47,658; part-time $2648 per credit hour. *Required fees:* $1980; $44.50 per credit hour. $550 per term. Tuition and fees vary according to course load, degree level and program. *Financial support:* Fellowships with full tuition reimbursements, research assistantships with full tuition reimbursements, teaching assistantships with full tuition reimbursements, and career-related internships or fieldwork available. Financial award application deadline: 2/1. *Faculty research:* Ichthyology, plant systematics, crustacean endocrinology, ecotoxicology, ornithology.

University at Albany, State University of New York, College of Arts and Sciences, Department of Biological Sciences, Program in Ecology and Evolutionary Biology, Albany, NY 12222-0001. Offers PhD. *Degree requirements:* For doctorate, one foreign language, thesis/dissertation. *Entrance requirements:* For doctorate, GRE General Test.

University at Buffalo, the State University of New York, Graduate School, College of Arts and Sciences, Program in Evolution, Ecology and Behavior, Buffalo, NY 14260. Offers MS, PhD, Certificate. *Faculty:* 16 full-time (7 women), 5 part-time/adjunct (2 women). *Students:* 17 full-time (11 women), 4 international. Average age 25. 27 applicants, 74% accepted, 5 enrolled. In 2015, 2 master's awarded. Terminal master's awarded for partial completion of doctoral program. *Degree requirements:* For master's, project; for doctorate, comprehensive exam, thesis/dissertation. *Entrance requirements:* For master's, GRE, minimum undergraduate GPA of 3.0; for doctorate, GRE, minimum GPA of 3.0. Additional exam requirements/recommendations for international students: Required—TOEFL (minimum score 550 paper-based; 79 iBT). *Application deadline:* For fall admission, 1/15 priority date for domestic and international students. Applications are processed on a rolling basis. Application fee: $75. Electronic applications accepted. *Financial support:* In 2015–16, 3 fellowships with full tuition reimbursements (averaging $24,600 per year), 5 research assistantships with full tuition reimbursements (averaging $24,000 per year), 3 teaching assistantships with full tuition reimbursements (averaging $17,000 per year) were awarded; Federal Work-Study, scholarships/grants, health care benefits, and unspecified assistantships also available. Financial award application deadline: 1/15; financial award applicants required to submit FAFSA. *Faculty research:* Coral reef ecology, evolution and ecology of aquatic invertebrates, animal communication, paleobiology, primate behavior. *Unit head:* Dr. Katharina Dittmar De La Cruz, Program Director, 716-645-4912, E-mail: ub-evb@buffalo.edu. *Application contact:* Joseph C. Syracuse, Graduate Enrollment Manager, 716-645-2711, Fax: 716-645-3888, E-mail: jcs32@buffalo.edu. Website: http://www.evolutionecologybehavior.buffalo.edu/

University of Alberta, Faculty of Graduate Studies and Research, Department of Biological Sciences, Edmonton, AB T6G 2E1, Canada. Offers environmental biology and ecology (M Sc, PhD); microbiology and biotechnology (M Sc, PhD); molecular biology and genetics (M Sc, PhD); physiology and cell biology (M Sc, PhD); plant biology (M Sc, PhD); systematics and evolution (M Sc, PhD). Terminal master's awarded for partial completion of doctoral program. *Degree requirements:* For master's, thesis; for doctorate, thesis/dissertation. *Entrance requirements:* Additional exam requirements/recommendations for international students: Required—TOEFL.

The University of Arizona, College of Science, Department of Ecology and Evolutionary Biology, Tucson, AZ 85721. Offers MS, PhD. Terminal master's awarded for partial completion of doctoral program. *Degree requirements:* For master's, thesis

optional; for doctorate, one foreign language, comprehensive exam, thesis/dissertation. *Entrance requirements:* For master's, GRE General Test, GRE Subject Test, statement of purpose, curriculum vitae, 3 letters of recommendation; for doctorate, GRE General Test, GRE Subject Test, curriculum vitae, 3 letters of recommendation. Additional exam requirements/recommendations for international students: Required—TOEFL (minimum score 550 paper-based; 79 iBT). *Application deadline:* For fall admission, 12/1 for domestic students, 12/8 for international students. Application fee: $75. *Financial support:* Research assistantships, teaching assistantships, career-related internships or fieldwork, scholarships/grants, health care benefits, and unspecified assistantships available. *Faculty research:* Biological diversity, evolutionary history, evolutionary mechanisms, community structure. *Unit head:* Dr. Michael Worobey, Head, E-mail: worobey@email.arizona.edu. *Application contact:* Dr. Michael Worobey, Head, E-mail: worobey@email.arizona.edu.
Website: http://eebweb.arizona.edu/

University of California, Davis, Graduate Studies, Graduate Group in Population Biology, Davis, CA 95616. Offers PhD. *Degree requirements:* For doctorate, thesis/dissertation. *Entrance requirements:* For doctorate, GRE General Test, GRE Subject Test. Additional exam requirements/recommendations for international students: Required—TOEFL (minimum score 550 paper-based). Electronic applications accepted. *Faculty research:* Population ecology, population genetics, systematics, evolution, community ecology.

University of California, Irvine, Francisco J. Ayala School of Biological Sciences, Department of Ecology and Evolutionary Biology, Irvine, CA 92697. Offers biological sciences (MS, PhD). *Students:* 61 full-time (32 women); includes 21 minority (4 Asian, non-Hispanic/Latino; 11 Hispanic/Latino; 6 Two or more races, non-Hispanic/Latino), 2 international. Average age 28. 64 applicants, 19% accepted, 10 enrolled. In 2015, 8 master's, 8 doctorates awarded. *Degree requirements:* For master's, thesis; for doctorate, thesis/dissertation. *Entrance requirements:* For master's and doctorate, GRE General Test, GRE Subject Test, minimum GPA of 3.0. Additional exam requirements/recommendations for international students: Required—TOEFL (minimum score 550 paper-based). *Application deadline:* For fall admission, 1/15 priority date for domestic students, 1/15 for international students. Applications are processed on a rolling basis. Application fee: $90 ($110 for international students). Electronic applications accepted. *Financial support:* Fellowships, research assistantships with full tuition reimbursements, teaching assistantships, career-related internships or fieldwork, institutionally sponsored loans, traineeships, health care benefits, and unspecified assistantships available. Financial award application deadline: 3/1; financial award applicants required to submit FAFSA. *Faculty research:* Ecological energetics, quantitative genetics, life history evolution, plant-herbivore and plant-pollinator interactions, molecular evolution. *Unit head:* Laurence D. Mueller, Professor/Department Chair, 949-824-4744, Fax: 949-824-2181, E-mail: ldmuelle@uci.edu. *Application contact:* Pam McDonald, Student Affairs Coordinator, 949-824-4743, Fax: 949-824-2181, E-mail: pmcdonal@uci.edu.
Website: http://ecoevo.bio.uci.edu/

University of California, Los Angeles, Graduate Division, College of Letters and Science, Department of Ecology and Evolutionary Biology, Los Angeles, CA 90095. Offers MA, PhD. Terminal master's awarded for partial completion of doctoral program. *Degree requirements:* For master's, comprehensive exam or thesis; for doctorate, thesis/dissertation, oral and written qualifying exams; 3 quarters of teaching experience. *Entrance requirements:* For master's and doctorate, GRE General Test, GRE Subject Test (biology), bachelor's degree; minimum undergraduate GPA of 3.0 (or its equivalent if letter grade system not used). Additional exam requirements/recommendations for international students: Required—TOEFL. Electronic applications accepted.

University of California, Riverside, Graduate Division, Department of Biology, Riverside, CA 92521-0102. Offers evolution, ecology and organismal biology (MS, PhD). Terminal master's awarded for partial completion of doctoral program. *Degree requirements:* For master's, thesis, oral defense of thesis; for doctorate, thesis/dissertation, 3 quarters of teaching experience, qualifying exams. *Entrance requirements:* For master's and doctorate, GRE General Test, minimum GPA of 3.2. Additional exam requirements/recommendations for international students: Required—TOEFL (minimum score 550 paper-based, 80 iBT) or IELTS. Electronic applications accepted. *Expenses: Tuition, area resident:* Full-time $16,665.50; part-time $11,055.54. Tuition, state resident: full-time $16,665.50; part-time $11,055.54. Tuition, nonresident: full-time $31,768. *International tuition:* $31,767.50 full-time. *Required fees:* $16,665.50; $11,055.54 per quarter. $3685.18 per quarter. Tuition and fees vary according to program. *Faculty research:* Ecology, evolutionary biology, physiology, quantitative genetics, conservation biology.

University of California, Santa Barbara, Graduate Division, College of Letters and Sciences, Division of Mathematics, Life, and Physical Sciences, Department of Ecology, Evolution, and Marine Biology, Santa Barbara, CA 93106-9620. Offers MA, PhD, MA/PhD. *Faculty:* 33 full-time (8 women). *Students:* 69 full-time (44 women); includes 15 minority (2 Black or African American, non-Hispanic/Latino; 5 Asian, non-Hispanic/Latino; 6 Hispanic/Latino; 2 Native Hawaiian or other Pacific Islander, non-Hispanic/Latino), 3 international. Average age 29. 157 applicants, 14% accepted, 17 enrolled. In 2015, 7 master's, 8 doctorates awarded. *Degree requirements:* For master's, comprehensive exam (for some programs), thesis (for some programs); for doctorate, comprehensive exam, thesis/dissertation. *Entrance requirements:* For master's and doctorate, GRE General Test. Additional exam requirements/recommendations for international students: Required—TOEFL (minimum score 550 paper-based; 80 iBT), IELTS. *Application deadline:* For fall admission, 12/15 for domestic and international students. Application fee: $90 ($110 for international students). Electronic applications accepted. *Financial support:* In 2015–16, 50 students received support, including 55 fellowships with tuition reimbursements available (averaging $10,812 per year), 24 research assistantships with tuition reimbursements available (averaging $8,441 per year), 97 teaching assistantships with partial tuition reimbursements available (averaging $9,346 per year); Federal Work-Study, scholarships/grants, traineeships, health care benefits, and tuition waivers (full and partial) also available. Financial award application deadline: 12/15; financial award applicants required to submit FAFSA. *Faculty research:* Community ecology, evolution, marine biology, population genetics, stream ecology. *Unit head:* Dr. Craig Carlson, Chair, 805-893-2415, Fax: 805-893-5885, E-mail: eembchair@lifesci.ucsb.edu. *Application contact:* Melanie Fujii, Student Affairs Officer, 805-893-2979, Fax: 805-893-5885, E-mail: eemb-info@lifesci.ucsb.edu.
Website: http://www.lifesci.ucsb.edu/EEMB/index.html

University of California, Santa Cruz, Division of Graduate Studies, Division of Physical and Biological Sciences, Department of Ecology and Evolutionary Biology, Santa Cruz, CA 95064. Offers MA, PhD. *Degree requirements:* For master's, thesis; for doctorate, comprehensive exam, thesis/dissertation. *Entrance requirements:* For master's and doctorate, GRE General Test, GRE Subject Test, 3 letters of recommendation. Additional exam requirements/recommendations for international students: Required—TOEFL (minimum score 550 paper-based; 83 iBT); Recommended—IELTS (minimum score 8). Electronic applications accepted. *Faculty research:* Population and community ecology, evolutionary biology, physiology and behavior (marine and terrestrial), systematics and biodiversity.

University of Chicago, Division of the Biological Sciences, Committee on Evolutionary Biology, Chicago, IL 60637. Offers PhD. *Students:* 28 full-time (14 women); includes 10 minority (2 Black or African American, non-Hispanic/Latino; 1 Asian, non-Hispanic/Latino; 7 Hispanic/Latino), 2 international. Average age 29. 44 applicants, 20% accepted, 4 enrolled. In 2015, 7 doctorates awarded. Terminal master's awarded for partial completion of doctoral program. *Degree requirements:* For doctorate, thesis/dissertation, ethics class, 2 teaching assistantships. *Entrance requirements:* For doctorate, GRE General Test. Additional exam requirements/recommendations for international students: Required—TOEFL (minimum score 600 paper-based; 104 iBT), IELTS (minimum score 7). *Application deadline:* For fall admission, 12/1 for domestic and international students. Application fee: $90. Electronic applications accepted. *Financial support:* In 2015–16, 29 students received support, including fellowships with tuition reimbursements available (averaging $29,781 per year), research assistantships (averaging $29,781 per year); institutionally sponsored loans, scholarships/grants, traineeships, and health care benefits also available. Financial award applicants required to submit FAFSA. *Faculty research:* Systematics and evolutionary theory, genetics, functional morphology and physiology, behavior, ecology and biogeography. *Unit head:* Dr. Michael Coates, Chairman, 773-834-8417, Fax: 773-702-4699, E-mail: mcoates@uchicago.edu. *Application contact:* Carolyn Johnson, Graduate Administrative Director, 773-702-9474, Fax: 773-702-4699, E-mail: csjohnso@uchicago.edu.
Website: http://evbio.uchicago.edu/

University of Colorado Boulder, Graduate School, College of Arts and Sciences, Department of Ecology and Evolutionary Biology, Boulder, CO 80309. Offers animal behavior (MA); biology (MA, PhD); environmental biology (MA, PhD); evolutionary biology (MA, PhD); neurobiology (MA); population biology (MA); population genetics (PhD). *Faculty:* 31 full-time (11 women). *Students:* 67 full-time (31 women), 3 part-time (1 woman); includes 8 minority (1 Asian, non-Hispanic/Latino; 3 Hispanic/Latino; 4 Two or more races, non-Hispanic/Latino), 4 international. Average age 30. 119 applicants, 11% accepted, 13 enrolled. In 2015, 10 master's, 14 doctorates awarded. Terminal master's awarded for partial completion of doctoral program. *Degree requirements:* For master's, comprehensive exam, thesis or alternative; for doctorate, comprehensive exam, thesis/dissertation. *Entrance requirements:* For master's, GRE General Test, GRE Subject Test, minimum undergraduate GPA of 3.0; for doctorate, GRE General Test, GRE Subject Test. *Application deadline:* For fall admission, 12/31 for domestic students, 12/1 for international students. Application fee: $50 ($70 for international students). Electronic applications accepted. Application fee is waived when completed online. *Financial support:* In 2015–16, 138 students received support, including 14 fellowships (averaging $7,260 per year), 12 research assistantships with tuition reimbursements available (averaging $31,833 per year), 47 teaching assistantships with tuition reimbursements available (averaging $33,448 per year); institutionally sponsored loans, scholarships/grants, health care benefits, and unspecified assistantships also available. Financial award applicants required to submit FAFSA. *Faculty research:* Ecology, botany, evolutionary biology, biological sciences, conservation biology. *Total annual research expenditures:* $6.3 million. *Application contact:* E-mail: ebiograd@colorado.edu.
Website: http://ebio.colorado.edu

University of Colorado Denver, College of Liberal Arts and Sciences, Department of Integrative and Systems Biology, Denver, CO 80217. Offers animal behavior (MS); biology (MS); cell and developmental biology (MS); ecology (MS); evolutionary biology (MS); genetics (MS); integrative and systems biology (PhD); microbiology (MS); molecular biology (MS); neurobiology (MS); plant systematics (MS). *Program availability:* Part-time. *Faculty:* 21 full-time (8 women), 3 part-time/adjunct (1 woman). *Students:* 31 full-time (19 women), 7 part-time (3 women); includes 8 minority (1 Black or African American, non-Hispanic/Latino; 1 Asian, non-Hispanic/Latino; 3 Hispanic/Latino; 3 Two or more races, non-Hispanic/Latino), 1 international. Average age 28. 34 applicants, 29% accepted, 8 enrolled. In 2015, 6 master's awarded. *Degree requirements:* For master's, comprehensive exam, thesis, 30-32 credit hours; for doctorate, comprehensive exam, thesis/dissertation. *Entrance requirements:* For master's, GRE General Test (minimum score in 50th percentile in each section), BA/BS from accredited institution awarded within the last 10 years; minimum undergraduate GPA of 3.0; prerequisite courses: 1 year each of general biology and general chemistry; 1 semester each of general genetics, general ecology, and cell biology; and a structure/function course; for doctorate, GRE, minimum undergraduate GPA of 3.2, three letters of recommendation, official transcripts from all universities and colleges attended. Additional exam requirements/recommendations for international students: Required—TOEFL (minimum score 537 paper-based; 75 iBT); Recommended—IELTS (minimum score 6.5). *Application deadline:* For fall admission, 1/15 for domestic and international students. Application fee: $50 ($75 for international students). Electronic applications accepted. *Financial support:* In 2015–16, 32 students received support. Fellowships, research assistantships, teaching assistantships, Federal Work-Study, institutionally sponsored loans, scholarships/grants, and traineeships available. Financial award application deadline: 4/1; financial award applicants required to submit FAFSA. *Faculty research:* Molecular developmental biology; quantitative ecology, biogeography, and population dynamics; environmental signaling and endocrine disruption; speciation, the evolution of reproductive isolation, and hybrid zones; evolutionary, behavioral, and conservation ecology. *Unit head:* Dr. John Swallow, Chair, 303-556-6154, E-mail: john.swallow@ucdenver.edu. *Application contact:* Dr. Michael Wunder, Graduate Advisor, 303-556-8870, E-mail: michael.wunder@ucdenver.edu.
Website: http://www.ucdenver.edu/academics/colleges/CLAS/Departments/biology/Programs/MasterofScience/Pages/BiologyMasterOfScience.aspx

University of Delaware, College of Arts and Sciences, Department of Biological Sciences, Newark, DE 19716. Offers biotechnology (MS); cancer biology (MS, PhD); cell and extracellular matrix biology (MS, PhD); cell and systems physiology (MS, PhD); developmental biology (MS, PhD); ecology and evolution (MS, PhD); microbiology (MS, PhD); molecular biology and genetics (MS, PhD). Terminal master's awarded for partial completion of doctoral program. *Degree requirements:* For master's, thesis, preliminary exam; for doctorate, comprehensive exam, thesis/dissertation, preliminary exam. *Entrance requirements:* For master's and doctorate, GRE General Test. Additional exam requirements/recommendations for international students: Required—TOEFL (minimum score 600 paper-based); Recommended—TWE. Electronic applications accepted. *Faculty research:* Microorganisms, bone, cancer metastasis, developmental biology, cell biology, DNA.

University of Denver, Division of Natural Sciences and Mathematics, Department of Biological Sciences, Denver, CO 80208. Offers biology, ecology and evolution (MS, PhD); biomedical sciences (PSM); cell and molecular biology (MS, PhD). *Program availability:* Part-time. *Faculty:* 23 full-time (7 women), 2 part-time/adjunct (both women). *Students:* 8 full-time (all women), 27 part-time (21 women); includes 4 minority (2 Black or African American, non-Hispanic/Latino; 2 Hispanic/Latino), 6 international. Average age 26. 77 applicants, 38% accepted, 21 enrolled. In 2015, 6 master's, 3 doctorates awarded. Terminal master's awarded for partial completion of doctoral program. *Degree requirements:* For master's, comprehensive exam (for some programs), thesis; for doctorate, one foreign language, comprehensive exam (for some programs), thesis/dissertation. *Entrance requirements:* For master's and doctorate, GRE General Test,

Evolutionary Biology

bachelor's degree in biology or related field, transcripts, personal statement, three letters of recommendation. Additional exam requirements/recommendations for international students: Required—TOEFL (minimum score 550 paper-based; 80 iBT). *Application deadline:* For fall admission, 1/1 priority date for domestic and international students. Applications are processed on a rolling basis. Application fee: $65. Electronic applications accepted. *Expenses:* $30,477. *Financial support:* In 2015–16, 35 students received support, including 8 research assistantships with tuition reimbursements available (averaging $15,834 per year), 23 teaching assistantships with tuition reimbursements available (averaging $17,210 per year); Federal Work-Study, institutionally sponsored loans, scholarships/grants, and unspecified assistantships also available. Support available to part-time students. Financial award application deadline: 2/15; financial award applicants required to submit FAFSA. *Faculty research:* Molecular biology, cell biology, neurobiology, ecology, molecular evolution. *Unit head:* Dr. Joseph Angleson, Associate Professor and Chair, 303-871-3463, Fax: 303-871-3471, E-mail: jangleso@du.edu. *Application contact:* Randi Flageolle, Assistant to the Chair, 303-871-3457, Fax: 303-871-3471, E-mail: rflageol@du.edu.
Website: http://www.du.edu/nsm/departments/biologicalsciences

University of Guelph, Graduate Studies, College of Biological Science, Department of Integrative Biology, Botany and Zoology, Guelph, ON N1G 2W1, Canada. Offers biology (M Sc, PhD); zoology (M Sc, PhD). *Program availability:* Part-time. *Degree requirements:* For master's, thesis, research proposal; for doctorate, thesis/dissertation, research proposal, qualifying exam. *Entrance requirements:* For master's, minimum B average during previous 2 years of course work. Additional exam requirements/recommendations for international students: Required—TOEFL (minimum score 550 paper-based), IELTS (minimum score 6.5). Electronic applications accepted. *Faculty research:* Aquatic science, environmental physiology, parasitology, wildlife biology, management.

University of Illinois at Urbana–Champaign, Graduate College, College of Liberal Arts and Sciences, School of Integrative Biology, Department of Animal Biology, Champaign, IL 61820. Offers animal biology (ecology, ethology and evolution) (MS, PhD).

University of Illinois at Urbana–Champaign, Graduate College, College of Liberal Arts and Sciences, School of Integrative Biology, Program in Ecology, Evolution and Conservation Biology, Champaign, IL 61820. Offers MS, PhD.

The University of Iowa, Graduate College, College of Liberal Arts and Sciences, Department of Biology, Iowa City, IA 52242-1324. Offers biology (MS, PhD); cell and developmental biology (MS, PhD); evolution (MS, PhD); genetics (MS, PhD); neurobiology (MS, PhD). Terminal master's awarded for partial completion of doctoral program. *Degree requirements:* For master's, thesis optional, exam; for doctorate, comprehensive exam, thesis/dissertation. *Entrance requirements:* For master's and doctorate, GRE General Test, minimum GPA of 3.0. Additional exam requirements/recommendations for international students: Required—TOEFL (minimum score 600 paper-based; 100 iBT). Electronic applications accepted. *Faculty research:* Neurobiology, evolutionary biology, genetics, cell and developmental biology.

The University of Kansas, Graduate Studies, College of Liberal Arts and Sciences, Department of Ecology and Evolutionary Biology, Lawrence, KS 66045. Offers botany (MA, PhD); ecology and evolutionary biology (MA, PhD); entomology (MA, PhD). *Students:* 69 full-time (35 women), 1 part-time (0 women); includes 8 minority (1 Black or African American, non-Hispanic/Latino; 1 Asian, non-Hispanic/Latino; 4 Native Hawaiian or other Pacific Islander, non-Hispanic/Latino; 2 Two or more races, non-Hispanic/Latino), 22 international. Average age 28. 66 applicants, 39% accepted, 20 enrolled. In 2015, 3 master's, 5 doctorates awarded. Terminal master's awarded for partial completion of doctoral program. *Degree requirements:* For master's, comprehensive exam, thesis (for some programs), 30-36 credits, thesis presentation; for doctorate, comprehensive exam, thesis/dissertation, residency, responsible scholarship and research skills, final exam, dissertation defense. *Entrance requirements:* For master's, GRE General Test, bachelor's degree with minimum undergraduate GPA of 3.0; for doctorate, GRE General Test, bachelor's degree; minimum undergraduate/graduate GPA of 3.0. Additional exam requirements/recommendations for international students: Required—TOEFL or IELTS. *Application deadline:* For fall admission, 12/1 for domestic and international students; for spring admission, 9/15 for domestic and international students. Application fee: $65 ($85 for international students). Electronic applications accepted. *Financial support:* Fellowships, research assistantships, teaching assistantships, scholarships/grants, traineeships, health care benefits, and unspecified assistantships available. Financial award application deadline: 12/1. *Faculty research:* Ecology and global change, diversity and macroevolution, evolutionary mechanisms, systematics/phylogenetics, biogeography. *Unit head:* Dr. Christopher H. Haufler, Chair, 785-864-3255, E-mail: vulgare@ku.edu. *Application contact:* Aagje Ashe, Graduate Coordinator, 785-864-2362, Fax: 785-864-5860, E-mail: a4ashe@ku.edu.
Website: http://eeb.ku.edu/

University of Louisiana at Lafayette, College of Sciences, Department of Biology, Lafayette, LA 70504. Offers biology (MS); environmental and evolutionary biology (PhD). Terminal master's awarded for partial completion of doctoral program. *Degree requirements:* For master's, thesis; for doctorate, 2 foreign languages, comprehensive exam, thesis/dissertation. *Entrance requirements:* For master's, GRE General Test, minimum GPA of 2.75; for doctorate, GRE General Test, GRE Subject Test, minimum GPA of 3.0. Additional exam requirements/recommendations for international students: Required—TOEFL (minimum score 550 paper-based). Electronic applications accepted. *Faculty research:* Structure and ultrastructure, system biology, ecology, processes, environmental physiology.

The University of Manchester, Faculty of Life Sciences, Manchester, United Kingdom. Offers adaptive organismal biology (M Phil, PhD); animal biology (M Phil, PhD); biochemistry (M Phil, PhD); bioinformatics (M Phil, PhD); biomolecular sciences (M Phil, PhD); biotechnology (M Phil, PhD); cell biology (M Phil, PhD); cell matrix research (M Phil, PhD); channels and transporters (M Phil, PhD); developmental biology (M Phil, PhD); Egyptology (M Phil, PhD); environmental biology (M Phil, PhD); evolutionary biology (M Phil, PhD); gene expression (M Phil, PhD); genetics (M Phil, PhD); history of science, technology and medicine (M Phil, PhD); immunology (M Phil, PhD); integrative neurobiology and behavior (M Phil, PhD); membrane trafficking (M Phil, PhD); microbiology (M Phil, PhD); molecular and cellular neuroscience (M Phil, PhD); molecular biology (M Phil, PhD); molecular cancer studies (M Phil, PhD); neuroscience (M Phil, PhD); ophthalmology (M Phil, PhD); optometry (M Phil, PhD); organelle function (M Phil, PhD); pharmacology (M Phil, PhD); physiology (M Phil, PhD); plant sciences (M Phil, PhD); stem cell research (M Phil, PhD); structural biology (M Phil, PhD); systems neuroscience (M Phil, PhD); toxicology (M Phil, PhD).

University of Maryland, College Park, Academic Affairs, College of Computer, Mathematical and Natural Sciences, Department of Biology, Behavior, Ecology, Evolution, and Systematics Program, College Park, MD 20742. Offers MS, PhD. *Degree requirements:* For master's, thesis, oral defense, seminar; for doctorate, thesis/dissertation, exam, 4 seminars. *Entrance requirements:* For master's and doctorate, GRE General Test, GRE Subject Test (biology), 3 letters of recommendation. Additional

exam requirements/recommendations for international students: Required—TOEFL. *Faculty research:* Animal behavior, biostatistics, ecology, evolution, neurothology.

University of Maryland, College Park, Academic Affairs, College of Computer, Mathematical and Natural Sciences, Department of Biology, PhD Program in Biological Sciences, College Park, MD 20742. Offers behavior, ecology, evolution, and systematics (PhD); computational biology, bioinformatics, and genomics (PhD); molecular and cellular biology (PhD); physiological systems (PhD). *Degree requirements:* For doctorate, comprehensive exam, thesis/dissertation, thesis work presentation in seminar. *Entrance requirements:* For doctorate, GRE General Test; GRE Subject Test in biology (recommended), academic transcripts, statement of purpose/research interests, 3 letters of recommendation. Additional exam requirements/recommendations for international students: Required—TOEFL. Electronic applications accepted.

University of Massachusetts Amherst, Graduate School, Interdisciplinary Programs, Program in Organismic and Evolutionary Biology, Amherst, MA 01003. Offers MS, PhD. *Program availability:* Part-time. Terminal master's awarded for partial completion of doctoral program. *Degree requirements:* For master's, thesis or alternative; for doctorate, comprehensive exam, thesis/dissertation. *Entrance requirements:* For master's and doctorate, GRE General Test, 3 letters of recommendation. Additional exam requirements/recommendations for international students: Required—TOEFL (minimum score 550 paper-based; 80 iBT), IELTS (minimum score 6.5). Electronic applications accepted.

University of Massachusetts Amherst, Graduate School, Interdisciplinary Programs, Program in Plant Biology, Amherst, MA 01003. Offers biochemistry and metabolism (MS, PhD); cell biology and physiology (MS, PhD); environmental, ecological and integrative biology (MS, PhD); genetics and evolution (MS, PhD). *Degree requirements:* For master's, thesis; for doctorate, 2 foreign languages, comprehensive exam, thesis/dissertation. *Entrance requirements:* For master's and doctorate, GRE General Test. Additional exam requirements/recommendations for international students: Required—TOEFL (minimum score 550 paper-based; 80 iBT), IELTS (minimum score 6.5). Electronic applications accepted.

University of Miami, Graduate School, College of Arts and Sciences, Department of Biology, Coral Gables, FL 33124. Offers biology (MS, PhD); genetics and evolution (MS, PhD). Terminal master's awarded for partial completion of doctoral program. *Degree requirements:* For master's, comprehensive exam (for some programs), thesis (for some programs); for doctorate, thesis/dissertation, oral and written qualifying exam. *Entrance requirements:* For master's, GRE General Test, 3 letters of recommendation, research papers; for doctorate, GRE General Test, 3 letters of recommendation, research papers, sponsor letter. Additional exam requirements/recommendations for international students: Required—TOEFL (minimum score 550 paper-based; 59 iBT). Electronic applications accepted. *Faculty research:* Neuroscience to ethology; plants, vertebrates and mycorrhizae; phylogenies, life histories and species interactions; molecular biology, gene expression and populations; cells, auditory neurons and vertebrate locomotion.

University of Michigan, Rackham Graduate School, College of Literature, Science, and the Arts, Department of Ecology and Evolutionary Biology, Ann Arbor, MI 48109. Offers MS, PhD. *Program availability:* Part-time. *Faculty:* 57 full-time (22 women). *Students:* 72 full-time (36 women); includes 28 minority (2 Black or African American, non-Hispanic/Latino; 1 American Indian or Alaska Native, non-Hispanic/Latino; 5 Asian, non-Hispanic/Latino; 13 Hispanic/Latino; 1 Native Hawaiian or other Pacific Islander, non-Hispanic/Latino; 6 Two or more races, non-Hispanic/Latino), 13 international. Average age 28. 143 applicants, 22% accepted, 14 enrolled. In 2015, 9 master's, 7 doctorates awarded. Terminal master's awarded for partial completion of doctoral program. *Degree requirements:* For master's, thesis (for some programs), two seminars; for doctorate, comprehensive exam, thesis/dissertation, 2 semesters of teaching. *Entrance requirements:* For master's and doctorate, GRE. Additional exam requirements/recommendations for international students: Required—TOEFL (minimum score 84 iBT). *Application deadline:* For fall admission, 12/1 priority date for domestic and international students; for winter admission, 10/15 priority date for domestic and international students. Applications are processed on a rolling basis. Application fee: $65 ($75 for international students). Electronic applications accepted. *Financial support:* In 2015–16, 67 students received support, including 30 fellowships with full tuition reimbursements available (averaging $26,350 per year), 11 research assistantships with full tuition reimbursements available (averaging $26,350 per year), 37 teaching assistantships with full tuition reimbursements available (averaging $26,350 per year); scholarships/grants, traineeships, health care benefits, and unspecified assistantships also available. Financial award applicants required to submit FAFSA. *Faculty research:* Population and community ecology, ecosystem ecology and biogeochemistry, global change biology, biogeography and paleobiology, evolution of behavior, evolutionary genetics, phylogenetic and phylogeography, ecology and evolution of infectious disease. *Total annual research expenditures:* $5.1 million. *Unit head:* Diarmaid O Foighil, Chair, 734-615-4912, Fax: 734-763-0544. *Application contact:* Cynthia Carl, Graduate Program Coordinator, 734-615-7338, Fax: 734-763-0544, E-mail: eeb.gradcoord@umich.edu.
Website: http://www.lsa.umich.edu/eeb/

University of Minnesota, Twin Cities Campus, Graduate School, College of Biological Sciences, Department of Ecology, Evolution, and Behavior, St. Paul, MN 55418. Offers MS, PhD. Terminal master's awarded for partial completion of doctoral program. *Degree requirements:* For master's, comprehensive exam, thesis or projects; for doctorate, comprehensive exam, thesis/dissertation. *Entrance requirements:* For master's and doctorate, GRE General Test, minimum GPA of 3.0. Additional exam requirements/recommendations for international students: Required—TOEFL (minimum score 550 paper-based; 79 iBT), Michigan English Language Assessment Battery. Electronic applications accepted. *Faculty research:* Behavioral ecology, community ecology, community genetics, ecosystem and global change, evolution and systematics.

University of Missouri, Office of Research and Graduate Studies, College of Arts and Science, Division of Biological Sciences, Columbia, MO 65211. Offers evolutionary biology and ecology (MA, PhD). Terminal master's awarded for partial completion of doctoral program. *Degree requirements:* For master's, thesis; for doctorate, comprehensive exam, thesis/dissertation. *Entrance requirements:* For master's and doctorate, GRE General Test (minimum score 1200 verbal and quantitative), minimum GPA of 3.0. Additional exam requirements/recommendations for international students: Required—TOEFL (minimum score 600 paper-based; 100 iBT). *Application deadline:* For fall admission, 12/15 priority date for domestic and international students. Applications are processed on a rolling basis. Application fee: $55 ($75 for international students). Electronic applications accepted. *Financial support:* Fellowships with full tuition reimbursements, research assistantships with full tuition reimbursements, teaching assistantships with full tuition reimbursements, institutionally sponsored loans, traineeships, health care benefits, and unspecified assistantships available.
Website: http://biology.missouri.edu/graduate-studies/

University of Nevada, Reno, Graduate School, Interdisciplinary Program in Ecology, Evolution, and Conservation Biology, Reno, NV 89557. Offers PhD. Offered through the College of Arts and Science, the M. C. Fleischmann College of Agriculture, and the

Desert Research Institute. *Degree requirements:* For doctorate, thesis/dissertation. *Entrance requirements:* For doctorate, GRE General Test, GRE Subject Test, minimum GPA of 3.0. Additional exam requirements/recommendations for international students: Required—TOEFL (minimum score 500 paper-based; 61 iBT), IELTS (minimum score 6). Electronic applications accepted. *Faculty research:* Population biology, behavioral ecology, plant response to climate change, conservation of endangered species, restoration of natural ecosystems.

University of New Hampshire, Graduate School, College of Life Sciences and Agriculture, Department of Molecular, Cellular and Biomedical Sciences, Program in Molecular and Evolutionary Systems Biology, Durham, NH 03824. Offers PhD. *Program availability:* Part-time. *Students:* 1 part-time. *Degree requirements:* For doctorate, comprehensive exam, thesis/dissertation. *Entrance requirements:* For doctorate, GRE General Test. Additional exam requirements/recommendations for international students: Required—TOEFL (minimum score 550 paper-based; 80 iBT). *Application deadline:* For fall admission, 1/15 priority date for domestic and international students. Application fee: $65. Electronic applications accepted. *Expenses:* Tuition, state resident: full-time $13,840; part-time $770 per credit hour. Tuition, nonresident: full-time $27,130; part-time $1175 per credit hour. *Required fees:* $2080; $1040. Tuition and fees vary according to degree level and program. *Financial support:* Research assistantships, Federal Work-Study, scholarships/grants, and tuition waivers (full and partial) available. Support available to part-time students. *Unit head:* Dr. W. Kelley Thomas, Director, 603-862-2470. *Application contact:* Dovev L. Levine, Admissions Officer, 603-862-3000, Fax: 603-862-0275, E-mail: grad.school@unh.edu. Website: http://colsa.unh.edu/mcbs/mesb/mesb-phd

The University of North Carolina at Chapel Hill, Graduate School, College of Arts and Sciences, Department of Biology, Chapel Hill, NC 27500. Offers botany (MA, MS, PhD); cell biology, development, and physiology (MA, MS, PhD); cell motility and cytoskeleton (PhD); ecology and behavior (MA, MS, PhD); genetics and molecular biology (MA, MS, PhD); morphology, systematics, and evolution (MA, MS, PhD). Terminal master's awarded for partial completion of doctoral program. *Degree requirements:* For master's, comprehensive exam, thesis (for some programs); for doctorate, comprehensive exam, thesis/dissertation. *Entrance requirements:* For master's, GRE General Test, GRE Subject Test, 2 semesters of calculus or statistics; 2 semesters of physics, organic chemistry; 3 semesters of biology; for doctorate, GRE General Test, GRE Subject Test, 2 semesters calculus or statistics, 2 semesters physics, organic chemistry, 3 semesters of biology. Additional exam requirements/recommendations for international students: Required—TOEFL (minimum score 550 paper-based). Electronic applications accepted. *Faculty research:* Gene expression, biomechanics, yeast genetics, plant ecology, plant molecular biology.

University of Notre Dame, Graduate School, College of Science, Department of Biological Sciences, Notre Dame, IN 46556. Offers aquatic ecology, evolution and environmental biology (MS, PhD); cellular and molecular biology (MS, PhD); genetics (MS, PhD); physiology (MS, PhD); vector biology and parasitology (MS, PhD). Terminal master's awarded for partial completion of doctoral program. *Degree requirements:* For master's, comprehensive exam, thesis; for doctorate, comprehensive exam, thesis/dissertation, candidacy exam. *Entrance requirements:* For master's and doctorate, GRE General Test. Additional exam requirements/recommendations for international students: Required—TOEFL (minimum score 600 paper-based; 80 iBT). Electronic applications accepted. *Faculty research:* Tropical disease, molecular genetics, neurobiology, evolutionary biology, aquatic biology.

University of Oklahoma, College of Arts and Sciences, Department of Biology, Program in Ecology and Evolutionary Biology, Norman, OK 73019. Offers PhD. *Students:* 16 full-time (8 women), 9 part-time (7 women); includes 1 minority (Hispanic/Latino), 1 international. Average age 28. 18 applicants, 39% accepted, 7 enrolled. In 2015, 5 degrees awarded. *Degree requirements:* For doctorate, comprehensive exam, thesis/dissertation, course in biostatistics; 2 semesters as a teaching assistant. *Entrance requirements:* For doctorate, GRE General Test, transcripts, 3 letters of recommendation, personal statement, CV. Additional exam requirements/recommendations for international students: Required—TOEFL (minimum score 79 iBT) or IELTS (minimum score 6.5). *Application deadline:* For fall admission, 12/15 for domestic and international students. Application fee: $50 ($100 for international students). Electronic applications accepted. *Expenses:* Tuition, state resident: full-time $4577; part-time $190.70 per credit hour. Tuition, nonresident: full-time $17,758; part-time $739.90 per credit hour. *Required fees:* $3060; $115.70 per credit hour. $141.50 per semester. *Financial support:* In 2015–16, 23 students received support. Fellowships, research assistantships with full tuition reimbursements available, teaching assistantships with full tuition reimbursements available, scholarships/grants, health care benefits, unspecified assistantships, and assistantships (with tuition waivers and health insurance), supplementary scholarship funding available. Financial award application deadline: 6/1; financial award applicants required to submit FAFSA. *Faculty research:* Geographical ecology, global change biology, evolutionary biology, phylogenetics, ecosystem ecology. *Unit head:* Dr. Michael Kaspari, Professor, 405-325-3371, Fax: 405-325-6202, E-mail: mkaspari@ou.edu. *Application contact:* Dianna Wilson, Academic Counselor, 405-325-9139, Fax: 405-325-6202, E-mail: biologygrad@ou.edu.
Website: http://www.ou.edu/eeb

University of Oklahoma, College of Arts and Sciences, Department of Microbiology and Plant Biology, Program in Ecology and Evolutionary Biology, Norman, OK 73019. Offers PhD. *Students:* 8 full-time (3 women), 2 part-time (1 woman), 9 international. Average age 27. 4 applicants, 75% accepted, 3 enrolled. In 2015, 1 doctorate awarded. *Entrance requirements:* Additional exam requirements/recommendations for international students: Required—TOEFL (minimum score 79 iBT) or IELTS (minimum score 6.5). *Application deadline:* For fall admission, 4/1 for domestic and international students; for spring admission, 9/1 for domestic and international students. Application fee: $50 ($100 for international students). Electronic applications accepted. *Expenses:* Tuition, state resident: full-time $4577; part-time $190.70 per credit hour. Tuition, nonresident: full-time $17,758; part-time $739.90 per credit hour. *Required fees:* $3060; $115.70 per credit hour. $141.50 per semester. *Financial support:* In 2015–16, 10 students received support. Scholarships/grants, health care benefits, tuition waivers (partial), and unspecified assistantships available. Financial award application deadline: 6/1; financial award applicants required to submit FAFSA. *Faculty research:* Geographical ecology, global change biology, evolutionary biology, phylogenetics, ecosystem ecology. *Unit head:* Dr. Michael Kaspari, Professor/Director of EEB Graduate Program, 405-325-4321, Fax: 405-325-7619, E-mail: mkaspari@ou.edu. *Application contact:* Adell Hopper, Staff Assistant, 405-325-4321, Fax: 405-325-7619, E-mail: ahopper@ou.edu.
Website: http://mpbio.ou.edu/

University of Oregon, Graduate School, College of Arts and Sciences, Department of Biology, Eugene, OR 97403. Offers ecology and evolution (MA, MS, PhD); marine biology (MA, MS, PhD); molecular, cellular and genetic biology (PhD); neuroscience and development (PhD). Terminal master's awarded for partial completion of doctoral program. *Degree requirements:* For master's, thesis (for some programs); for doctorate, thesis/dissertation. *Entrance requirements:* For master's and doctorate, GRE General

Test, minimum GPA of 3.2. Additional exam requirements/recommendations for international students: Required—TOEFL. *Faculty research:* Developmental neurobiology; evolution, population biology, and quantitative genetics; regulation of gene expression; biochemistry of marine organisms.

University of Pittsburgh, Dietrich School of Arts and Sciences, Department of Biological Sciences, Program in Ecology and Evolution, Pittsburgh, PA 15260. Offers PhD. *Faculty:* 5 full-time (2 women). *Students:* 15 full-time (10 women); includes 1 minority (Hispanic/Latino), 2 international. Average age 23. 27 applicants, 22% accepted, 3 enrolled. In 2015, 4 doctorates awarded. *Degree requirements:* For doctorate, comprehensive exam, thesis/dissertation, completion of research integrity module. *Entrance requirements:* For doctorate, GRE General Test, GRE Subject Test. Additional exam requirements/recommendations for international students: Required—TOEFL (minimum score 90 iBT). *Application deadline:* For fall admission, 1/3 priority date for domestic students, 12/9 priority date for international students. Applications are processed on a rolling basis. Application fee: $0 ($50 for international students). Electronic applications accepted. Tuition and fees vary according to program. *Financial support:* In 2015–16, 15 fellowships with full tuition reimbursements (averaging $33,193 per year), 13 research assistantships with full tuition reimbursements (averaging $27,645 per year), 15 teaching assistantships with full tuition reimbursements (averaging $26,850 per year) were awarded; Federal Work-Study, traineeships, health care benefits, and tuition waivers (full) also available. *Unit head:* Dr. Karen M. Arndt, Professor, 412-624-6963, Fax: 412-624-4349, E-mail: arndt@pitt.edu. *Application contact:* Cathleen M. Barr, Graduate Administrator, 412-624-4268, Fax: 412-624-4349, E-mail: cbarr@pitt.edu.
Website: http://www.biology.pitt.edu

University of Puerto Rico, Río Piedras Campus, College of Natural Sciences, Department of Biology, San Juan, PR 00931-3300. Offers ecology/systematics (MS, PhD); evolution/genetics (MS, PhD); molecular/cellular biology (MS, PhD); neuroscience (MS, PhD). *Program availability:* Part-time. *Degree requirements:* For master's, one foreign language, comprehensive exam, thesis; for doctorate, one foreign language, comprehensive exam, thesis/dissertation. *Entrance requirements:* For master's, GRE Subject Test, interview, minimum GPA of 3.0, letter of recommendation; for doctorate, GRE Subject Test, interview, master's degree, minimum GPA of 3.0, letter of recommendation. *Faculty research:* Environmental, poblational and systematic biology.

University of South Carolina, The Graduate School, College of Arts and Sciences, Department of Biological Sciences, Graduate Training Program in Ecology, Evolution, and Organismal Biology, Columbia, SC 29208. Offers MS, PhD. *Degree requirements:* For master's, one foreign language, comprehensive exam, thesis; for doctorate, one foreign language, comprehensive exam, thesis/dissertation. *Entrance requirements:* For master's and doctorate, GRE General Test, minimum GPA of 3.0 in science. Additional exam requirements/recommendations for international students: Required—TOEFL (minimum score 570 paper-based). Electronic applications accepted.

University of Southern California, Graduate School, Dana and David Dornsife College of Letters, Arts and Sciences, Department of Biological Sciences, Program in Integrative and Evolutionary Biology, Los Angeles, CA 90089. Offers PhD. M.S. in Biology is a terminal degree only. Terminal master's awarded for partial completion of doctoral program. *Degree requirements:* For doctorate, comprehensive exam, thesis/dissertation, qualifying examination, dissertation defense. *Entrance requirements:* For doctorate, GRE, 3 letters of recommendation, personal statement, resume, minimum GPA of 3.0. Additional exam requirements/recommendations for international students: Required—TOEFL (minimum score 600 paper-based; 100 iBT). Electronic applications accepted. *Faculty research:* Organisms and their interaction with the environment, evolution and life history, integration of the control and dynamics of physiological processes, biomechanics and rehabilitation engineering, primate behavior and ecology.

University of South Florida, College of Arts and Sciences, Department of Integrative Biology, Tampa, FL 33620-9951. Offers biology (MS), including ecology and evolution (MS, PhD), environmental and ecological microbiology (MS, PhD), physiology and morphology (MS, PhD); integrative biology (PhD), including ecology and evolution (MS, PhD), environmental and ecological microbiology (MS, PhD), physiology and morphology (MS, PhD). *Program availability:* Part-time. *Faculty:* 14 full-time (6 women). *Students:* 48 full-time (30 women), 6 part-time (3 women); includes 10 minority (1 American Indian or Alaska Native, non-Hispanic/Latino; 1 Asian, non-Hispanic/Latino; 7 Hispanic/Latino; 1 Two or more races, non-Hispanic/Latino), 3 international. Average age 30. 43 applicants, 37% accepted, 12 enrolled. In 2015, 8 master's, 3 doctorates awarded. *Degree requirements:* For master's, comprehensive exam, thesis (for some programs); for doctorate, comprehensive exam, thesis/dissertation. *Entrance requirements:* For master's and doctorate, GRE General Test, minimum GPA of 3.0 in last 60 hours of BS. Additional exam requirements/recommendations for international students: Required—TOEFL (minimum score 570 paper-based; 88 iBT). *Application deadline:* For fall admission, 2/15 priority date for domestic students, 1/2 for international students; for spring admission, 8/1 for domestic students, 6/1 for international students. Application fee: $30. Electronic applications accepted. *Financial support:* Research assistantships, teaching assistantships, and unspecified assistantships available. Financial award application deadline: 6/30; financial award applicants required to submit FAFSA. *Faculty research:* Marine ecology, ecosystem responses to urbanization, biomechanical and physiological mechanisms of animal movement, population biology and conservation, microbial ecology and public health microbiology, natural diversity of parasites and herbivores; ecosystems, vertebrates, disturbance ecology, functional and ecological morphology of feeding in fishes, rare amphibians and reptiles, genomics in ecological experiments, ecotoxicology, global carbon cycle, plant-animal interactions. *Total annual research expenditures:* $1.3 million. *Unit head:* Dr. Valerie Harwood, Professor and Chair, 813-974-1524, Fax: 813-974-3263, E-mail: vharwood@usf.edu. *Application contact:* Dr. Lynn Martin, Associate Professor and Graduate Program Director, 813-974-0157, Fax: 813-974-3263, E-mail: lbmartin@usf.edu.
Website: http://biology.usf.edu/ib/grad/

The University of Tennessee, Graduate School, College of Arts and Sciences, Department of Ecology and Evolutionary Biology, Knoxville, TN 37996. Offers behavior (MS, PhD); ecology (MS, PhD); evolutionary biology (MS, PhD). *Program availability:* Part-time. *Degree requirements:* For master's, thesis; for doctorate, thesis/dissertation. *Entrance requirements:* For master's and doctorate, GRE General Test, minimum GPA of 2.7. Additional exam requirements/recommendations for international students: Required—TOEFL. Electronic applications accepted.

The University of Texas at Austin, Graduate School, College of Natural Sciences, School of Biological Sciences, Program in Ecology, Evolution and Behavior, Austin, TX 78712-1111. Offers PhD. *Entrance requirements:* For doctorate, GRE General Test. Additional exam requirements/recommendations for international students: Required—TOEFL. Electronic applications accepted.

University of Toronto, School of Graduate Studies, Faculty of Arts and Science, Department of Ecology and Evolutionary Biology, Toronto, ON M5S 1A1, Canada. Offers M Sc, PhD. *Degree requirements:* For master's, thesis, thesis defense; for doctorate, thesis/dissertation, thesis defense. *Entrance requirements:* For master's, minimum B average in last 2 years; knowledge of physics, chemistry, and biology.

Evolutionary Biology

Additional exam requirements/recommendations for international students: Required—TOEFL (minimum score 580 paper-based; 93 iBT), TWE (minimum score 5). Electronic applications accepted.

Washington University in St. Louis, Graduate School of Arts and Sciences, Division of Biology and Biomedical Sciences, Program in Evolution, Ecology and Population Biology, St. Louis, MO 63130-4899. Offers ecology (PhD). *Students:* 26 full-time (15 women); includes 3 minority (1 Black or African American, non-Hispanic/Latino; 1 Asian, non-Hispanic/Latino; 1 Two or more races, non-Hispanic/Latino), 2 international. 27 applicants, 37% accepted, 5 enrolled. In 2015, 3 doctorates awarded. *Degree requirements:* For doctorate, thesis/dissertation. *Entrance requirements:* For doctorate, GRE General Test, GRE Subject Test. Additional exam requirements/recommendations for international students: Required—TOEFL. *Application deadline:* For fall admission, 12/1 for domestic students. Application fee: $0. Electronic applications accepted. *Financial support:* Fellowships, research assistantships, and teaching assistantships available. Financial award application deadline: 1/15. *Faculty research:* Population ecology, community ecology, plant and animal evolution; microbial evolution, evolution of behavior, phylogenetics, systematics, theoretical and experimental population genetics. *Unit head:* Stacia Burd, Coordinator, 314-362-3364. *Application contact:* Rebecca Riney, 314-747-4648, E-mail: dbbsphdadmissions@wusm.wustl.edu.

Wayne State University, College of Liberal Arts and Sciences, Department of Biological Sciences, Detroit, MI 48202. Offers biological sciences (MA, MS); cell development and neurobiology (PhD); evolution and organismal biology (PhD); molecular biology and biotechnology (PhD); molecular biotechnology (MS). PhD and MS programs admit for fall only. *Faculty:* 27. *Students:* 56 full-time (31 women), 8 part-time (2 women); includes 5 minority (2 Black or African American, non-Hispanic/Latino; 2 Asian, non-Hispanic/Latino; 1 Two or more races, non-Hispanic/Latino), 37 international. Average age 29. 210 applicants, 9% accepted, 7 enrolled. In 2015, 5 master's, 10 doctorates awarded. *Degree requirements:* For master's, thesis (for some programs); for doctorate, thesis/dissertation. *Entrance requirements:* For master's, GRE (for MS applicants), minimum GPA of 3.0; adequate preparation in biological sciences and supporting courses in chemistry, physics and mathematics; curriculum vitae; personal statement; three letters of recommendation (two for MA); for doctorate, GRE, curriculum vitae, statement of goals and career objectives, three letters of reference, bachelor's or master's degree in biological or other science. Additional exam requirements/recommendations for international students: Required—TOEFL (minimum score 550 paper-based; 79 iBT), TWE (minimum score 5.5), Michigan English Language Assessment Battery (minimum score 85); Recommended—IELTS (minimum score 6.5). Application fee: $0. Electronic applications accepted. *Expenses:* Tuition, state resident: full-time $14,165; part-time $590.20 per credit hour. Tuition, nonresident: full-time $30,682; part-time $1278.40 per credit hour. *Required fees:* $1688; $47.45 per credit hour. $274.60 per semester. Tuition and fees vary according to course load and program. *Financial support:* In 2015–16, 55 students received support, including 3 fellowships with tuition reimbursements available (averaging $16,000 per year), 8 research assistantships with tuition reimbursements available (averaging $19,506 per year), 45 teaching assistantships with tuition reimbursements available (averaging $19,536 per year); scholarships/grants and unspecified assistantships also available. Financial award application deadline: 3/31; financial award applicants required to submit FAFSA. *Faculty research:* Transcription and chromatin remodeling, genomic and developmental evolution, community and landscape ecology and environmental degradation, microbiology and virology, cell and neurobiology. *Total annual research expenditures:* $2.1 million. *Unit head:* Dr. David Njus, Professor and Chair, 313-577-3105, E-mail: dnjus@wayne.edu. *Application contact:* Rose Mary Priest, Graduate Secretary, 313-577-6818, E-mail: rpriest@wayne.edu. Website: http://clas.wayne.edu/Biology/

Wesleyan University, Graduate Studies, Department of Biology, Middletown, CT 06459. Offers cell and developmental biology (PhD); evolution and ecology (PhD); genetics and genomics (PhD), including bioinformatics; neurobiology and behavior (PhD). *Faculty:* 14 full-time (5 women). *Students:* 26 full-time (12 women); includes 5 minority (2 Black or African American, non-Hispanic/Latino; 3 Asian, non-Hispanic/Latino), 5 international. In 2015, 3 doctorates awarded. Terminal master's awarded for partial completion of doctoral program. *Degree requirements:* For doctorate, comprehensive exam, thesis/dissertation, public seminar. *Entrance requirements:* For doctorate, GRE. Additional exam requirements/recommendations for international students: Required—TOEFL or IELTS. *Application deadline:* For fall admission, 1/15 for domestic and international students. Application fee: $0. Electronic applications accepted. *Financial support:* Stipends available. *Faculty research:* Evolution and ecology, neurobiology and behavior, cell and developmental biology, genetics, genomics and bioinformatics. *Unit head:* Dr. John Kirn, Chair/Professor, 860-685-3494, E-mail: jrkirn@wesleyan.edu. *Application contact:* Marjorie Fitzgibbons, Administrative Assistant, 860-685-2157, E-mail: mfitzgibbons@wesleyan.edu. Website: http://www.wesleyan.edu/bio/

West Virginia University, Eberly College of Arts and Sciences, Department of Biology, Morgantown, WV 26506. Offers cell and molecular biology (MS, PhD); environmental and evolutionary biology (MS, PhD); forensic biology (MS, PhD); genomic biology (MS, PhD); neurobiology (MS, PhD). Terminal master's awarded for partial completion of doctoral program. *Degree requirements:* For master's, thesis, final exam; for doctorate, thesis/dissertation, preliminary and final exams. *Entrance requirements:* For master's, GRE General Test, GRE Subject Test, minimum GPA of 3.0; for doctorate, GRE General Test, minimum GPA of 3.0. Additional exam requirements/recommendations for international students: Required—TOEFL. *Expenses:* Tuition, state resident: full-time $8568. Tuition, nonresident: full-time $22,140. Tuition and fees vary according to program. *Faculty research:* Environmental biology, genetic engineering, developmental biology, global change, biodiversity.

Yale University, Graduate School of Arts and Sciences, Department of Ecology and Evolutionary Biology, New Haven, CT 06520. Offers PhD. *Entrance requirements:* For doctorate, GRE General Test, GRE Subject Test (biology).

Section 9
Entomology

This section contains a directory of institutions offering graduate work in entomology. Additional information about programs listed in the directory may be obtained by writing directly to the dean of a graduate school or chair of a department at the address given in the directory.

For programs offering related work, see also in this book *Biochemistry; Biological and Biomedical Sciences; Botany and Plant Biology; Ecology, Environmental Biology, and Evolutionary Biology; Genetics, Developmental Biology, and Reproductive Biology; Microbiological Sciences; Physiology;* and *Zoology.* In the other guides in this series:

Graduate Programs in the Humanities, Arts & Social Sciences
See *Economics (Agricultural Economics and Agribusiness)*
Graduate Programs in the Physical Sciences, Mathematics, Agricultural Sciences, the Environment & Natural Resources
See *Agricultural and Food Sciences* and *Environmental Sciences and Management*
Graduate Programs in Engineering & Applied Sciences
See *Agricultural Engineering* and *Bioengineering*

CONTENTS

Entomology

Auburn University, Graduate School, College of Agriculture, Department of Entomology and Plant Pathology, Auburn University, AL 36849. Offers entomology (M Ag, MS, PhD); plant pathology (M Ag, MS, PhD). *Program availability:* Part-time. *Faculty:* 16 full-time (6 women). *Students:* 27 full-time (15 women), 10 part-time (1 woman); includes 2 minority (1 Black or African American, non-Hispanic/Latino; 1 Hispanic/Latino), 23 international. Average age 26. 28 applicants, 50% accepted, 13 enrolled. In 2015, 3 master's, 3 doctorates awarded. *Degree requirements:* For master's, thesis (for some programs); for doctorate, one foreign language, thesis/dissertation. *Entrance requirements:* For master's, GRE General Test; for doctorate, GRE General Test, GRE Subject Test, master's degree with thesis. *Application deadline:* Applications are processed on a rolling basis. Application fee: $50 ($60 for international students). Electronic applications accepted. *Expenses:* Tuition, state resident: full-time $8802; part-time $489 per credit hour. Tuition, nonresident: full-time $26,406; part-time $1467 per credit hour. *Required fees:* $808 per semester. Tuition and fees vary according to degree level and program. *Financial support:* Research assistantships, teaching assistantships, and Federal Work-Study available. Support available to part-time students. Financial award application deadline: 3/15; financial award applicants required to submit FAFSA. *Faculty research:* Pest management, biological control, systematics, medical entomology. *Unit head:* Dr. Nannan Liu, Chair, 334-844-4266. *Application contact:* Dr. George Flowers, Dean of the Graduate School, 334-844-2125.

Clemson University, Graduate School, College of Agriculture, Forestry and Life Sciences, Department of Plant and Environmental Sciences, Program in Entomology, Clemson, SC 29634. Offers MS, PhD. *Program availability:* Part-time. *Faculty:* 9 full-time (1 woman). *Students:* 9 full-time (4 women), 3 part-time (2 women); includes 1 minority (Black or African American, non-Hispanic/Latino), 4 international. Average age 25. 14 applicants, 57% accepted, 5 enrolled. In 2015, 3 doctorates awarded. *Degree requirements:* For master's, thesis, peer-reviewed manuscript submission; conference presentation; for doctorate, comprehensive exam, thesis/dissertation, peer-reviewed manuscript submission; conference presentation. *Entrance requirements:* For master's and doctorate, GRE General Test, unofficial transcripts, letters of recommendation. Additional exam requirements/recommendations for international students: Required—TOEFL (minimum score 550 paper-based; 80 iBT), IELTS (minimum score 6.5). *Application deadline:* For fall admission, 4/15 priority date for domestic and international students; for spring admission, 9/15 priority date for domestic and international students. Applications are processed on a rolling basis. Application fee: $80 ($90 for international students). Electronic applications accepted. *Expenses:* $4,060 per semester full-time resident, $8,103 per semester full-time non-resident, $448 per credit hour part-time resident, $898 per credit hour part-time non-resident. *Financial support:* In 2015–16, 10 students received support, including 10 research assistantships with partial tuition reimbursements available (averaging $19,300 per year); career-related internships or fieldwork and health care benefits also available. Financial award application deadline: 4/15. *Faculty research:* Biodiversity, urban entomology, agricultural entomology. *Unit head:* Dr. Patricia Zungoli, Department Head, 864-656-5041, Fax: 864-656-4960, E-mail: pzngl@clemson.edu. *Application contact:* Dr. Matthew Turnbull, Graduate Program Coordinator, 864-656-4964, E-mail: turnbul@clemson.edu. Website: http://www.clemson.edu/cafls/departments/entomology/index.html

Colorado State University, College of Agricultural Sciences, Department of Bioagricultural Sciences and Pest Management, Fort Collins, CO 80523-1177. Offers entomology (MS, PhD); pest management (MS); plant pathology and weed science (MS, PhD). *Program availability:* Part-time, evening/weekend. *Faculty:* 18 full-time (6 women), 5 part-time/adjunct (2 women). *Students:* 22 full-time (12 women), 13 part-time (7 women); includes 2 minority (both Two or more races, non-Hispanic/Latino), 8 international. Average age 28. 15 applicants, 100% accepted, 13 enrolled. In 2015, 3 master's, 4 doctorates awarded. *Degree requirements:* For master's, comprehensive exam, thesis; for doctorate, comprehensive exam, thesis/dissertation. *Entrance requirements:* For master's and doctorate, GRE General Test, minimum GPA of 3.0, letters of recommendation, essay, transcripts. Additional exam requirements/recommendations for international students: Required—TOEFL (minimum score 550 paper-based; 80 iBT), IELTS (minimum score 6.5). *Application deadline:* For fall admission, 1/15 priority date for domestic and international students; for spring admission, 9/1 priority date for domestic and international students. Applications are processed on a rolling basis. Application fee: $60 ($70 for international students). Electronic applications accepted. *Expenses:* Tuition, state resident: full-time $9348. Tuition, nonresident: full-time $22,916. *Required fees:* $2174; $473.72 per credit hour. $236.86 per semester. Tuition and fees vary according to course load and program. *Financial support:* In 2015–16, 4 fellowships with full tuition reimbursements (averaging $39,950 per year), 20 research assistantships with full tuition reimbursements (averaging $20,192 per year), 8 teaching assistantships with full tuition reimbursements (averaging $16,403 per year) were awarded. Financial award application deadline: 1/15. *Faculty research:* Genomics and molecular biology, ecology and biodiversity, biology and management of invasive species, integrated pest management. *Total annual research expenditures:* $3.3 million. *Unit head:* Dr. Louis Bjostad, Department Head, 970-491-3612, Fax: 970-491-3862, E-mail: louis.bjostad@colostate.edu. *Application contact:* Janet Dill, Graduate Coordinator, 970-491-0402, Fax: 970-491-3862, E-mail: janet.dill@colostate.edu. Website: http://bspm.agsci.colostate.edu/

Cornell University, Graduate School, Graduate Fields of Agriculture and Life Sciences, Field of Entomology, Ithaca, NY 14853-0001. Offers acarology (MS, PhD); apiculture (MS, PhD); applied entomology (MS, PhD); aquatic entomology (MS, PhD); biological control (MS, PhD); insect behavior (MS, PhD); insect biochemistry (MS, PhD); insect ecology (MS, PhD); insect genetics (MS, PhD); insect morphology (MS, PhD); insect pathology (MS, PhD); insect physiology (MS, PhD); insect systematics (MS, PhD); insect toxicology and insecticide chemistry (MS, PhD); integrated pest management (MS, PhD); medical and veterinary entomology (MS, PhD). *Degree requirements:* For master's, thesis; for doctorate, comprehensive exam, thesis/dissertation. *Entrance requirements:* For master's and doctorate, GRE General Test, GRE Subject Test (biology), 3 letters of recommendation. Additional exam requirements/recommendations for international students: Required—TOEFL (minimum score 550 paper-based; 77 iBT). Electronic applications accepted. *Faculty research:* Systematics and biodiversity, integrated pest management, pathology and biological control, toxicology and physiology, ecology and behavior.

Illinois State University, Graduate School, College of Arts and Sciences, Department of Biological Sciences, Normal, IL 61790-2200. Offers animal behavior (MS); bacteriology (MS); biochemistry (MS); biological sciences (MS); biology (PhD); biophysics (MS); biotechnology (MS); botany (MS, PhD); cell biology (MS); conservation biology (MS); developmental biology (MS); ecology (MS, PhD); entomology (MS); evolutionary biology (MS); genetics (MS, PhD); immunology (MS); microbiology (MS,

PhD); molecular biology (MS); molecular genetics (MS); neurobiology (MS); neuroscience (MS); parasitology (MS); physiology (MS, PhD); plant biology (MS); plant molecular biology (MS); plant sciences (MS); structural biology (MS); zoology (MS, PhD). *Program availability:* Part-time. *Degree requirements:* For master's, thesis or alternative; for doctorate, variable foreign language requirement, thesis/dissertation, 2 terms of residency. *Entrance requirements:* For master's, GRE General Test, minimum GPA of 2.6 in last 60 hours of course work; for doctorate, GRE General Test. *Application deadline:* Applications are processed on a rolling basis. Application fee: $40. *Financial support:* Research assistantships, teaching assistantships, Federal Work-Study, tuition waivers (full), and unspecified assistantships available. Financial award application deadline: 4/1. *Faculty research:* Redoc balance and drug development in schistosoma mansoni, control of the growth of listeria monocytogenes at low temperature, regulation of cell expansion and microtubule function by SPRI, CRUI: physiology and fitness consequences of different life history phenotypes. *Application contact:* Steven Juliano, Graduate Coordinator, E-mail: sajulian@ilstu.edu. Website: http://www.bio.ilstu.edu/

Iowa State University of Science and Technology, Department of Entomology, Ames, IA 50011. Offers MS, PhD. *Degree requirements:* For master's, thesis; for doctorate, thesis/dissertation. *Entrance requirements:* For master's and doctorate, GRE General Test, GRE Subject Test (biology). Additional exam requirements/recommendations for international students: Required—TOEFL (minimum score 550 paper-based; 79 iBT), IELTS (minimum score 6.5). Electronic applications accepted.

Kansas State University, Graduate School, College of Agriculture, Department of Entomology, Manhattan, KS 66506. Offers MS, PhD. *Degree requirements:* For master's, thesis, oral exam; for doctorate, comprehensive exam, thesis/dissertation, written and oral exams. *Entrance requirements:* Additional exam requirements/recommendations for international students: Required—TOEFL (minimum score 550 paper-based; 79 iBT). Electronic applications accepted. *Faculty research:* Molecular genetics, biologically-based pest management, host plant resistance, ecological genomics, stored product entomology.

Louisiana State University and Agricultural & Mechanical College, Graduate School, College of Agriculture, Department of Entomology, Baton Rouge, LA 70803. Offers MS, PhD.

McGill University, Faculty of Graduate and Postdoctoral Studies, Faculty of Agricultural and Environmental Sciences, Department of Natural Resource Sciences, Montréal, QC H3A 2T5, Canada. Offers entomology (M Sc, PhD); environmental assessment (M Sc); forest science (M Sc, PhD); microbiology (M Sc, PhD); micrometeorology (M Sc, PhD); neotropical environment (M Sc, PhD); soil science (M Sc, PhD); wildlife biology (M Sc, PhD).

Michigan State University, The Graduate School, College of Agriculture and Natural Resources and College of Natural Science, Department of Entomology, East Lansing, MI 48824. Offers entomology (MS, PhD); integrated pest management (MS). *Entrance requirements:* Additional exam requirements/recommendations for international students: Required—TOEFL (minimum score 550 paper-based), Michigan State University ELT (minimum score 85), Michigan English Language Assessment Battery (minimum score 83). Electronic applications accepted.

Mississippi State University, College of Agriculture and Life Sciences, Department of Biochemistry, Molecular Biology, Entomology and Plant Pathology, Mississippi State, MS 39762. Offers agriculture life sciences (MS), including biochemistry (MS, PhD), entomology (MS, PhD), plant pathology (MS, PhD); life science (PhD), including biochemistry (MS, PhD), entomology (MS, PhD), plant pathology (MS, PhD); molecular biology (PhD). *Faculty:* 32 full-time (6 women), 2 part-time/adjunct (1 woman). *Students:* 44 full-time (20 women), 11 part-time (6 women); includes 6 minority (3 Black or African American, non-Hispanic/Latino; 1 Asian, non-Hispanic/Latino; 1 Hispanic/Latino; 1 Two or more races, non-Hispanic/Latino), 12 international. Average age 29. 35 applicants, 40% accepted, 12 enrolled. In 2015, 12 master's, 7 doctorates awarded. Terminal master's awarded for partial completion of doctoral program. *Degree requirements:* For master's, thesis (for some programs), final oral exam; for doctorate, thesis/dissertation, preliminary oral and written exam. *Entrance requirements:* For master's, GRE General Test, minimum GPA of 2.75; for doctorate, GRE. Additional exam requirements/recommendations for international students: Required—TOEFL (minimum score 500 paper-based; 61 iBT); Recommended—IELTS (minimum score 5.5). *Application deadline:* For fall admission, 7/1 for domestic students, 5/1 for international students; for spring admission, 11/1 for domestic students, 9/1 for international students. Applications are processed on a rolling basis. Application fee: $60. Electronic applications accepted. *Expenses: Tuition, area resident:* Full-time $7502; part-time $833.74 per credit hour. Tuition, nonresident: full-time $20,142; part-time $2238.24 per credit hour. *Financial support:* In 2015–16, 40 research assistantships with full tuition reimbursements (averaging $16,730 per year) were awarded; Federal Work-Study, institutionally sponsored loans, and unspecified assistantships also available. Financial award application deadline: 4/1; financial award applicants required to submit FAFSA. *Faculty research:* Fish nutrition, plant and animal molecular biology, plant biochemistry, enzymology, lipid metabolism, chromatin, cell wall synthesis in rice, a model grass bioenergy species and the source of rice Stover residues using reverse genetic and functional genomic and proteomic approaches. *Unit head:* Dr. Jeffrey Dean, Professor and Department Head, 662-325-0643, Fax: 662-325-8664, E-mail: jd1891@msstate.edu. *Application contact:* Marina Hunt, Admissions Assistant, 662-325-5188, E-mail: mhunt@grad.msstate.edu. Website: http://www.biochemistry.msstate.edu

New Mexico State University, College of Agricultural, Consumer and Environmental Sciences, Department of Entomology, Plant Pathology and Weed Science, Las Cruces, NM 88003-8001. Offers MS. *Program availability:* Part-time. *Faculty:* 10 full-time (1 woman). *Students:* 8 full-time (3 women), 3 part-time (all women); includes 3 minority (1 American Indian or Alaska Native, non-Hispanic/Latino; 2 Hispanic/Latino), 4 international. Average age 29. 4 applicants, 75% accepted, 3 enrolled. In 2015, 6 master's awarded. *Degree requirements:* For master's, comprehensive exam, thesis. *Entrance requirements:* For master's, GRE General Test. Additional exam requirements/recommendations for international students: Required—TOEFL (minimum score 550 paper-based; 79 iBT), IELTS (minimum score 6.5). *Application deadline:* For fall admission, 7/1 priority date for domestic students; for spring admission, 11/1 priority date for domestic students. Applications are processed on a rolling basis. Application fee: $40 ($50 for international students). Electronic applications accepted. *Expenses:* $274.50 per credit hour for in-state students, and all students enrolled in six or fewer credits; $839.30 per credit hour for out-of-state and international students enrolled in at least seven hours. *Financial support:* In 2015–16, 10 students received support, including 6 research assistantships (averaging $21,962 per year), 3 teaching

assistantships (averaging $16,022 per year); career-related internships or fieldwork, Federal Work-Study, scholarships/grants, traineeships, health care benefits, and unspecified assistantships also available. Support available to part-time students. Financial award application deadline: 3/1. *Faculty research:* Entomology, nematology, plant pathology, weed science. *Total annual research expenditures:* $2.3 million. *Unit head:* Dr. Gerald K. Sims, Department Head, 575-646-3225, Fax: 575-646-8087, E-mail: gksims@nmsu.edu. *Application contact:* Belinda Williams, 575-646-3225, Fax: 575-646-8087.
Website: http://eppws.nmsu.edu/

North Carolina State University, Graduate School, College of Agriculture and Life Sciences, Department of Entomology, Raleigh, NC 27695. Offers MS, PhD. Terminal master's awarded for partial completion of doctoral program. *Degree requirements:* For master's, thesis (for some programs); for doctorate, thesis/dissertation. *Entrance requirements:* For master's and doctorate, GRE General Test. Electronic applications accepted. *Faculty research:* Physiology, biocontrol, ecology, forest entomology, apiculture.

North Dakota State University, College of Graduate and Interdisciplinary Studies, College of Agriculture, Food Systems, and Natural Resources, Department of Entomology, Fargo, ND 58102. Offers entomology (MS, PhD). *Program availability:* Part-time. *Degree requirements:* For master's, thesis; for doctorate, comprehensive exam, thesis/dissertation. *Entrance requirements:* For master's and doctorate, minimum GPA of 3.0. Additional exam requirements/recommendations for international students: Required—TOEFL (minimum score 550 paper-based; 79 iBT). *Application deadline:* For fall admission, 5/1 for international students; for winter admission, 8/1 for international students. Application fee: $35. Electronic applications accepted. *Financial support:* Research assistantships with full tuition reimbursements, Federal Work-Study, institutionally sponsored loans, and unspecified assistantships available. Financial award application deadline: 4/15. *Faculty research:* Insect systematics, conservation biology, integrated pest management, insect behavior, insect biology. *Unit head:* Jason Harmon, Program Leader, 701-231-5083, Fax: 701-231-8557, E-mail: jason.harmon@ndsu.edu. *Application contact:* Jason Harmon, Program Leader, 701-231-5083, Fax: 701-231-8557, E-mail: jason.harmon@ndsu.edu.
Website: http://www.ndsu.edu/entomology/

The Ohio State University, Graduate School, College of Food, Agricultural, and Environmental Sciences, Department of Entomology, Columbus, OH 43210. Offers MPHM, MS, PhD. MPHM offered jointly with Department of Plant Pathology. *Faculty:* 13. *Students:* 23 full-time (11 women); includes 2 minority (1 Black or African American, non-Hispanic/Latino; 1 Hispanic/Latino), 6 international. Average age 27. In 2015, 3 master's, 6 doctorates awarded. *Degree requirements:* For master's, variable foreign language requirement, thesis optional; for doctorate, variable foreign language requirement, thesis/dissertation. *Entrance requirements:* For master's and doctorate, GRE General Test. Additional exam requirements/recommendations for international students: Required—TOEFL (minimum score 550 paper-based; 79 iBT), Michigan English Language Assessment Battery (minimum score 82); Recommended—IELTS (minimum score 7). *Application deadline:* For fall admission, 12/15 priority date for domestic students, 11/30 priority date for international students; for spring admission, 12/12 for domestic students, 11/10 for international students; for summer admission, 4/10 for domestic students, 3/13 for international students. Applications are processed on a rolling basis. Application fee: $60 ($70 for international students). Electronic applications accepted. *Financial support:* Fellowships with tuition reimbursements, research assistantships with tuition reimbursements, teaching assistantships with tuition reimbursements, Federal Work-Study, and institutionally sponsored loans available. Support available to part-time students. *Faculty research:* Acarology, insect systematics, soil ecology, integrated pest management, chemical ecology. *Unit head:* Dr. Carol Anelli, Professor and Interim Chair, 614-292-9325, E-mail: anelli.7@osu.edu. *Application contact:* Graduate and Professional Admissions, 614-292-9444, Fax: 614-292-3895, E-mail: gpadmissions@osu.edu.
Website: http://entomology.osu.edu/

Oklahoma State University, College of Agricultural Science and Natural Resources, Department of Entomology and Plant Pathology, Stillwater, OK 74078. Offers entomology (PhD); entomology and plant pathology (MS); plant pathology (PhD). *Faculty:* 29 full-time (10 women), 1 part-time/adjunct (0 women). *Students:* 6 full-time (2 women), 33 part-time (20 women); includes 3 minority (1 American Indian or Alaska Native, non-Hispanic/Latino; 2 Two or more races, non-Hispanic/Latino), 14 international. Average age 30. 13 applicants, 62% accepted, 4 enrolled. In 2015, 10 master's, 1 doctorate awarded. *Degree requirements:* For master's, thesis or alternative; for doctorate, comprehensive exam, thesis/dissertation. *Entrance requirements:* For master's and doctorate, GRE or GMAT. Additional exam requirements/recommendations for international students: Required—TOEFL (minimum score 550 paper-based; 79 iBT). *Application deadline:* For fall admission, 3/1 priority date for international students; for spring admission, 8/1 priority date for international students. Applications are processed on a rolling basis. Application fee: $40 ($75 for international students). Electronic applications accepted. *Expenses:* Tuition, state resident: full-time $3528; part-time $196 per credit hour. Tuition, nonresident: full-time $14,144; part-time $785.75 per credit hour. *Required fees:* $1895; $105.25 per credit hour. Tuition and fees vary according to campus/location. *Financial support:* In 2015–16, 30 research assistantships (averaging $18,582 per year), 2 teaching assistantships (averaging $17,046 per year) were awarded; career-related internships or fieldwork, Federal Work-Study, scholarships/grants, health care benefits, tuition waivers (partial), and unspecified assistantships also available. Support available to part-time students. Financial award application deadline: 3/1; financial award applicants required to submit FAFSA. *Unit head:* Dr. Phillip Mulder, Jr., Department Head, 405-744-5527, Fax: 405-744-6039, E-mail: phil.mulder@okstate.edu. *Application contact:* Dr. Bob Hunger, Graduate Coordinator, 405-744-9958, Fax: 405-744-6039, E-mail: bob.hunger@okstate.edu.
Website: http://entoplp.okstate.edu/

Penn State University Park, Graduate School, College of Agricultural Sciences, Department of Entomology, University Park, PA 16802. Offers entomology (MS, PhD). *Unit head:* Dr. Richard T. Roush, Dean, 814-865-2541, Fax: 814-865-3103. *Application contact:* Lori Stania, Director, Graduate Student Services, 814-865-1795, Fax: 814-863-4627, E-mail: l-gswww@lists.psu.edu.
Website: http://ento.psu.edu/

Purdue University, Graduate School, College of Agriculture, Department of Entomology, West Lafayette, IN 47907. Offers MS, PhD. *Program availability:* Part-time. *Degree requirements:* For master's, thesis (for some programs), seminar; for doctorate, thesis/dissertation, seminar. *Entrance requirements:* For master's, GRE General Test, minimum undergraduate GPA of 3.0 or equivalent; for doctorate, GRE, minimum undergraduate GPA of 3.0 or equivalent; master's degree (highly recommended). Additional exam requirements/recommendations for international students: Required—TOEFL (minimum score 550 paper-based; 77 iBT). Electronic applications accepted. *Faculty research:* Insect biochemistry, nematology, aquatic diptera, behavioral ecology, insect physiology.

Rutgers University–New Brunswick, Graduate School-New Brunswick, Program in Entomology, Piscataway, NJ 08854-8097. Offers MS, PhD. *Degree requirements:* For master's, thesis or alternative; for doctorate, thesis/dissertation. *Entrance requirements:* For master's and doctorate, GRE General Test, GRE Subject Test (recommended). Additional exam requirements/recommendations for international students: Required—TOEFL. Electronic applications accepted. *Faculty research:* Insect toxicology, biolorial control, pathology, IPM and ecology, insect systematics.

Simon Fraser University, Office of Graduate Studies, Faculty of Science, Department of Biological Sciences, Burnaby, BC V5A 1S6, Canada. Offers bioinformatics (Graduate Diploma); biological sciences (M Sc, PhD); environmental toxicology (MET); pest management (MPM). *Degree requirements:* For master's, thesis; for doctorate, thesis/dissertation, candidacy exam; for Graduate Diploma, practicum. *Entrance requirements:* For master's, minimum GPA of 3.0 (on scale of 4.33), or 3.33 based on last 60 credits of undergraduate courses; for doctorate, minimum GPA of 3.5 (on scale of 4.33); for Graduate Diploma, minimum GPA of 2.5 (on scale of 4.33), or 2.67 based on the last 60 credits of undergraduate courses. Additional exam requirements/recommendations for international students: Recommended—TOEFL (minimum score 580 paper-based; 93 iBT), IELTS (minimum score 7), TWE (minimum score 5). Electronic applications accepted. *Faculty research:* Cell biology, wildlife ecology, environmental and evolutionary physiology, environmental toxicology, pest management.

State University of New York College of Environmental Science and Forestry, Department of Environmental and Forest Biology, Syracuse, NY 13210-2779. Offers applied ecology (MPS); chemical ecology (MPS, MS, PhD); conservation biology (MPS, MS, PhD); ecology (MPS, MS, PhD); entomology (MPS, MS, PhD); environmental interpretation (MPS, MS, PhD); environmental physiology (MPS, MS, PhD); fish and wildlife biology and management (MPS, MS, PhD); forest pathology and mycology (MPS, MS, PhD); plant biotechnology (MPS); plant science and biotechnology (MPS, MS, PhD). *Faculty:* 29 full-time (9 women), 4 part-time/adjunct (3 women). *Students:* 81 full-time (47 women), 57 part-time (24 women); includes 9 minority (1 Black or African American, non-Hispanic/Latino; 2 American Indian or Alaska Native, non-Hispanic/Latino; 1 Asian, non-Hispanic/Latino; 3 Hispanic/Latino; 2 Two or more races, non-Hispanic/Latino), 15 international. Average age 28. 47 applicants, 49% accepted, 15 enrolled. In 2015, 15 master's, 7 doctorates awarded. *Degree requirements:* For master's, thesis (for some programs), capstone seminar; for doctorate, comprehensive exam, thesis/dissertation, capstone seminar. *Entrance requirements:* For master's and doctorate, GRE General Test, minimum GPA of 3.0. Additional exam requirements/recommendations for international students: Required—TOEFL (minimum score 550 paper-based; 80 iBT), IELTS (minimum score 6). *Application deadline:* For fall admission, 2/1 priority date for domestic and international students; for spring admission, 11/1 priority date for domestic and international students. Applications are processed on a rolling basis. Application fee: $60. *Expenses:* Tuition, state resident: full-time $10,870; part-time $453 per credit. Tuition, nonresident: full-time $22,210; part-time $925 per credit. *Required fees:* $1075; $89.22 per credit. *Financial support:* In 2015–16, 4 fellowships with tuition reimbursements, 36 research assistantships with tuition reimbursements, 39 teaching assistantships with tuition reimbursements (averaging $11,490 per year) were awarded; Federal Work-Study, institutionally sponsored loans, scholarships/grants, health care benefits, and unspecified assistantships also available. Financial award application deadline: 6/30. *Faculty research:* Ecology, conservation biology, fish and wildlife biology and management, plant science, entomology. *Total annual research expenditures:* $4.1 million. *Unit head:* Dr. Donald J. Leopold, Chair, 315-470-6760, Fax: 315-470-6934, E-mail: djleopold@esf.edu. *Application contact:* Dr. Danilo D. Fernando, Director, Graduate Program/Associate Professor, 315-470-6746, Fax: 315-470-6934, E-mail: dfernando@esf.edu.
Website: http://www.esf.edu/efb/grad/default.asp

Texas A&M University, College of Agriculture and Life Sciences, Department of Entomology, College Station, TX 77843. Offers MS, PhD. *Faculty:* 25. *Students:* 60 full-time (28 women), 14 part-time (5 women); includes 17 minority (2 Black or African American, non-Hispanic/Latino; 4 Asian, non-Hispanic/Latino; 10 Hispanic/Latino; 1 Two or more races, non-Hispanic/Latino), 16 international. Average age 29. 34 applicants, 71% accepted, 16 enrolled. In 2015, 11 master's, 10 doctorates awarded. *Degree requirements:* For master's, comprehensive exam, thesis (for some programs); for doctorate, comprehensive exam, thesis/dissertation. *Entrance requirements:* For master's and doctorate, GRE General Test. Additional exam requirements/recommendations for international students: Required—TOEFL (minimum score 550 paper-based; 80 iBT), IELTS (minimum score 6), PTE (minimum score 53). *Application deadline:* For fall admission, 2/1 priority date for domestic students; for spring admission, 10/1 for domestic students. Applications are processed on a rolling basis. Application fee: $50 ($90 for international students). Electronic applications accepted. *Expenses:* Contact institution. *Financial support:* In 2015–16, 65 students received support, including 12 fellowships with tuition reimbursements available (averaging $14,063 per year), 26 research assistantships with tuition reimbursements available (averaging $7,800 per year), 24 teaching assistantships with tuition reimbursements available (averaging $7,517 per year); career-related internships or fieldwork, institutionally sponsored loans, scholarships/grants, traineeships, health care benefits, tuition waivers (full and partial), and unspecified assistantships also available. Support available to part-time students. Financial award application deadline: 3/15; financial award applicants required to submit FAFSA. *Faculty research:* Biology, biological control, integrated pest management, systematics, host plant resistance. *Unit head:* Dr. David Ragsdale, Head, 979-845-2510, Fax: 979-845-6305, E-mail: dragsdale@tamu.edu. *Application contact:* Rebecca Hapes, Senior Academic Advisor II, 979-845-9733, E-mail: rhapes@tamu.edu.
Website: http://entomology.tamu.edu

The University of Arizona, Graduate Interdisciplinary Programs, Graduate Interdisciplinary Program in Entomology and Insect Science, Tucson, AZ 85721. Offers MS, PhD. *Program availability:* Part-time. *Degree requirements:* For master's, thesis; for doctorate, comprehensive exam, thesis/dissertation. *Entrance requirements:* For master's, GRE General Test, GRE Subject Test, minimum GPA of 3.0, 3 letters of recommendation; for doctorate, GRE General Test, GRE Subject Test, minimum GPA of 3.0, 3 letters of recommendation, statement of purpose. Additional exam requirements/recommendations for international students: Required—TOEFL (minimum score 550 paper-based). *Application deadline:* For fall admission, 1/1 for domestic students, 12/1 for international students. Applications are processed on a rolling basis. Application fee: $75. *Financial support:* Fellowships, research assistantships, teaching assistantships, Federal Work-Study, institutionally sponsored loans, scholarships/grants, health care benefits, tuition waivers (full and partial), and unspecified assistantships available. Financial award application deadline: 3/1. *Faculty research:* Toxicology and physiology, plant/insect relations, vector biology, insect pest management, chemical ecology. *Unit head:* Dr. Molly E. Hunter, Professor and Head, 520-621-0847, Fax: 520-621-1150, E-mail: mhunter@ag.arizona.edu. *Application contact:* Rachel Mattull, Graduate Coordinator, 520-621-1151, Fax: 520-621-1150, E-mail: aliciag@email.arizona.edu.
Website: http://insects.arizona.edu/

University of Arkansas, Graduate School, Dale Bumpers College of Agricultural, Food and Life Sciences, Department of Entomology, Fayetteville, AR 72701-1201. Offers MS,

Entomology

PhD. *Students:* 1 full-time (0 women), 18 part-time (8 women); includes 1 minority (Hispanic/Latino), 3 international. In 2015, 3 master's, 3 doctorates awarded. *Degree requirements:* For master's, thesis; for doctorate, one foreign language, thesis/dissertation. *Entrance requirements:* For master's, GRE, minimum GPA of 3.0; for doctorate, GRE, minimum GPA of 3.25. *Application deadline:* For fall admission, 4/1 for international students; for spring admission, 10/1 for international students. Applications are processed on a rolling basis. Application fee: $40 ($50 for international students). Electronic applications accepted. *Financial support:* In 2015–16, 19 research assistantships were awarded; fellowships with tuition reimbursements, teaching assistantships, career-related internships or fieldwork, and Federal Work-Study also available. Support available to part-time students. Financial award application deadline: 4/1; financial award applicants required to submit FAFSA. *Faculty research:* Integrated pest management, insect virology, insect taxonomy. *Unit head:* Dr. Robert Wiedenmann, Chair, 479-575-6628, E-mail: rwieden@uark.edu. *Application contact:* Graduate Admissions, 479-575-6246, Fax: 479-575-5908, E-mail: gradinfo@uark.edu. Website: http://entomology.uark.edu/

University of California, Davis, Graduate Studies, Graduate Group in Integrated Pest Management, Davis, CA 95616. Offers MS. *Degree requirements:* For master's, comprehensive exam (for some programs), thesis (for some programs). *Entrance requirements:* For master's, GRE General Test, GRE Subject Test (biology), minimum GPA of 3.0. Additional exam requirements/recommendations for international students: Required—TOEFL (minimum score 550 paper-based). Electronic applications accepted.

University of California, Davis, Graduate Studies, Program in Entomology, Davis, CA 95616. Offers MS, PhD. Terminal master's awarded for partial completion of doctoral program. *Degree requirements:* For master's, comprehensive exam (for some programs), thesis (for some programs); for doctorate, thesis/dissertation. *Entrance requirements:* For master's and doctorate, GRE General Test, GRE Subject Test (biology). Additional exam requirements/recommendations for international students: Required—TOEFL (minimum score 550 paper-based). Electronic applications accepted. *Faculty research:* Bee biology, biological control, systematics, medical/veterinary entomology, pest management.

University of California, Riverside, Graduate Division, Department of Entomology, Riverside, CA 92521-0102. Offers entomology (MS, PhD). *Program availability:* Part-time. Terminal master's awarded for partial completion of doctoral program. *Degree requirements:* For master's, thesis; for doctorate, thesis/dissertation, qualifying exams. *Entrance requirements:* For master's and doctorate, GRE General Test, minimum GPA of 3.2. Additional exam requirements/recommendations for international students: Required—TOEFL (minimum score 550 paper-based; 80 iBT) or IELTS. *Application deadline:* For fall admission, 5/1 for domestic students, 2/1 for international students; for winter admission, 9/1 for domestic students, 7/1 for international students; for spring admission, 12/1 for domestic students, 10/1 for international students. Applications are processed on a rolling basis. Application fee: $80 ($100 for international students). Electronic applications accepted. *Expenses: Tuition, area resident:* Full-time $16,665.50; part-time $11,055.54. Tuition, state resident: full-time $16,665.50; part-time $11,055.54. Tuition, nonresident: full-time $31,768. *International tuition:* $31,767.50 full-time. *Required fees:* $16,665.50; $11,055.54 per quarter. $3685.18 per quarter. Tuition and fees vary according to program. *Financial support:* Fellowships with tuition reimbursements, research assistantships with tuition reimbursements, teaching assistantships with tuition reimbursements, career-related internships or fieldwork, Federal Work-Study, institutionally sponsored loans, and tuition waivers (full and partial) available. Financial award application deadline: 1/5; financial award applicants required to submit FAFSA. *Faculty research:* Agricultural, urban, medical, and veterinary entomology; biological control; chemical ecology; insect pathogens; novel toxicants. Website: http://www.entomology.ucr.edu/

University of Delaware, College of Agriculture and Natural Resources, Department of Entomology and Wildlife Ecology, Newark, DE 19716. Offers entomology and applied ecology (MS, PhD), including avian ecology, evolution and taxonomy, insect biological control, insect ecology and behavior (MS), insect genetics, pest management, plant-insect interactions, wildlife ecology and management. *Program availability:* Part-time. *Degree requirements:* For master's, comprehensive exam, thesis, oral exam, seminar; for doctorate, comprehensive exam, thesis/dissertation, qualifying exam, seminar. *Entrance requirements:* For master's, GRE General Test, minimum GPA of 3.0 in field, 2.8 overall; for doctorate, GRE General Test, GRE Subject Test (biology), minimum GPA of 3.0 in field, 2.8 overall. Additional exam requirements/recommendations for international students: Required—TOEFL. Electronic applications accepted. *Faculty research:* Ecology and evolution of plant-insect interactions, ecology of wildlife conservation management, habitat restoration, biological control, applied ecosystem management.

University of Georgia, College of Agricultural and Environmental Sciences, Department of Entomology, Athens, GA 30602. Offers entomology (MS, PhD); plant protection and pest management (MPPPM). *Degree requirements:* For master's, thesis (MS); for doctorate, one foreign language, thesis/dissertation. *Entrance requirements:* For master's and doctorate, GRE General Test. Electronic applications accepted. *Faculty research:* Apiculture, acarology, aquatic and soil biology, ecology, systematics.

University of Guelph, Graduate Studies, Ontario Agricultural College, Department of Environmental Biology, Guelph, ON N1G 2W1, Canada. Offers entomology (M Sc, PhD); environmental microbiology and biotechnology (M Sc, PhD); environmental toxicology (M Sc, PhD); plant and forest systems (M Sc, PhD); plant pathology (M Sc, PhD). *Program availability:* Part-time. *Degree requirements:* For master's, thesis; for doctorate, comprehensive exam, thesis/dissertation. *Entrance requirements:* For master's, minimum 75% average during previous 2 years of course work; for doctorate, minimum 75% average. Additional exam requirements/recommendations for international students: Required—TOEFL or IELTS. Electronic applications accepted. *Faculty research:* Entomology, environmental microbiology and biotechnology, environmental toxicology, forest ecology, plant pathology.

University of Hawaii at Manoa, Graduate Division, College of Tropical Agriculture and Human Resources, Department of Plant and Environmental Protection Sciences, Program in Entomology, Honolulu, HI 96822. Offers MS, PhD. *Program availability:* Part-time. *Faculty:* 14 full-time (3 women), 2 part-time/adjunct (1 woman). *Students:* 14 full-time (4 women), 3 part-time (1 woman); includes 10 minority (5 Asian, non-Hispanic/Latino; 1 Hispanic/Latino; 4 Two or more races, non-Hispanic/Latino), 3 international. Average age 32. 14 applicants, 36% accepted, 4 enrolled. *Degree requirements:* For master's, thesis optional; for doctorate, comprehensive exam, thesis/dissertation. *Entrance requirements:* For master's and doctorate, GRE General Test, GRE Subject Test (biology). Additional exam requirements/recommendations for international students: Required—TOEFL (minimum score 500 paper-based; 61 iBT), IELTS (minimum score 5). *Application deadline:* For fall admission, 3/1 for domestic and international students; for spring admission, 10/1 for domestic and international students. Application fee: $100. *Financial support:* In 2015–16, 5 fellowships (averaging $1,148 per year), 16 research assistantships (averaging $19,580 per year) were awarded; tuition waivers (full) also available. *Faculty research:* Integrated pest management, biological control, urban entomology, medical/forensic entomology resistance. *Total annual research expenditures:* $200,000. *Unit head:* Dr. J. Kenneth

Grace, Chair, 808-956-7076, Fax: 808-956-2428. *Application contact:* Mark Wright, Graduate Chair, 808-956-6747, Fax: 808-956-2458, E-mail: markwrig@hawaii.edu. Website: http://www.ctahr.hawaii.edu/peps/academic/graduate_ento.htm

University of Idaho, College of Graduate Studies, College of Agricultural and Life Sciences, Department of Plant, Soil, and Entomological Sciences, Moscow, ID 83844-2339. Offers entomology (MS, PhD); plant science (MS, PhD); soil and land resources (MS, PhD). *Faculty:* 30 full-time. *Students:* 28 full-time (9 women), 19 part-time (9 women). Average age 32. In 2015, 5 master's, 2 doctorates awarded. *Degree requirements:* For doctorate, thesis/dissertation. *Entrance requirements:* For master's and doctorate, GRE General Test, minimum GPA of 3.0. *Application deadline:* For fall admission, 7/1 for domestic students; for spring admission, 11/1 for domestic students. Applications are processed on a rolling basis. Application fee: $60. Electronic applications accepted. *Expenses:* Tuition, state resident: full-time $6205; part-time $399 per credit hour. Tuition, nonresident: full-time $20,209; part-time $1177 per credit hour. *Required fees:* $2017; $58 per credit hour. Full-time tuition and fees vary according to course load and reciprocity agreements. *Financial support:* Research assistantships and teaching assistantships available. Financial award applicants required to submit FAFSA. *Faculty research:* Entomological sciences, crop and weed science, horticultural science, soil and land resources. *Unit head:* Dr. Paul McDaniel, Department Head, 208-885-6274, Fax: 208-885-7760, E-mail: pses@uidaho.edu. *Application contact:* Sean Scoggin, Graduate Recruitment Coordinator, 208-885-4001, Fax: 208-885-4406, E-mail: graduateadmissions@uidaho.edu. Website: http://www.uidaho.edu/cals/pses/

University of Illinois at Urbana–Champaign, Graduate College, College of Liberal Arts and Sciences, School of Integrative Biology, Department of Entomology, Champaign, IL 61820. Offers MS, PhD. Terminal master's awarded for partial completion of doctoral program.

The University of Kansas, Graduate Studies, College of Liberal Arts and Sciences, Department of Ecology and Evolutionary Biology, Lawrence, KS 66045. Offers botany (MA, PhD); ecology and evolutionary biology (MA, PhD); entomology (MA, PhD). *Students:* 69 full-time (35 women), 1 part-time (0 women); includes 8 minority (1 Black or African American, non-Hispanic/Latino; 1 Asian, non-Hispanic/Latino; 4 Native Hawaiian or other Pacific Islander, non-Hispanic/Latino; 2 Two or more races, non-Hispanic/Latino), 22 international. Average age 28. 66 applicants, 39% accepted, 20 enrolled. In 2015, 3 master's, 5 doctorates awarded. Terminal master's awarded for partial completion of doctoral program. *Degree requirements:* For master's, comprehensive exam, thesis (for some programs), 30-36 credits, thesis presentation; for doctorate, comprehensive exam, thesis/dissertation, residency, responsible scholarship and research skills, final exam, dissertation defense. *Entrance requirements:* For master's, GRE General Test, bachelor's degree with minimum undergraduate GPA of 3.0; for doctorate, GRE General Test, bachelor's degree; minimum undergraduate/graduate GPA of 3.0. Additional exam requirements/recommendations for international students: Required—TOEFL or IELTS. *Application deadline:* For fall admission, 12/1 for domestic and international students; for spring admission, 9/15 for domestic and international students. Application fee: $65 ($85 for international students). Electronic applications accepted. *Financial support:* Fellowships, research assistantships, teaching assistantships, scholarships/grants, traineeships, health care benefits, and unspecified assistantships available. Financial award application deadline: 12/1. *Faculty research:* Ecology and global change, diversity and macroevolution, evolutionary mechanisms, systematics/phylogenetics, biogeography. *Unit head:* Dr. Christopher H. Haufler, Chair, 785-864-3255, E-mail: vulgare@ku.edu. *Application contact:* Aagje Ashe, Graduate Coordinator, 785-864-2362, Fax: 785-864-5860, E-mail: a4ashe@ku.edu. Website: http://eeb.ku.edu/

University of Kentucky, Graduate School, College of Agriculture, Food and Environment, Program in Entomology, Lexington, KY 40506-0032. Offers MS, PhD. *Degree requirements:* For master's, comprehensive exam, thesis optional; for doctorate, comprehensive exam, thesis/dissertation. *Entrance requirements:* For master's, GRE General Test, minimum undergraduate GPA of 2.75; for doctorate, GRE General Test, minimum graduate GPA of 3.0. Additional exam requirements/recommendations for international students: Required—TOEFL (minimum score 550 paper-based). Electronic applications accepted. *Faculty research:* Applied entomology, behavior, insect biology and ecology, biological control, insect physiology and molecular biology.

University of Maine, Graduate School, College of Natural Sciences, Forestry, and Agriculture, School of Biology and Ecology, Orono, ME 04469. Offers biological sciences (PhD); botany and plant pathology (MS); ecology and environmental science (MS, PhD); entomology (MS); plant science (PhD); zoology (MS, PhD). *Program availability:* Part-time. *Faculty:* 24 full-time (12 women), 34 part-time/adjunct (13 women). *Students:* 64 full-time (36 women), 1 part-time (0 women); includes 4 minority (1 American Indian or Alaska Native, non-Hispanic/Latino; 1 Asian, non-Hispanic/Latino; 1 Hispanic/Latino; 1 Two or more races, non-Hispanic/Latino), 8 international. Average age 29. 52 applicants, 25% accepted, 11 enrolled. In 2015, 7 master's, 8 doctorates awarded. Terminal master's awarded for partial completion of doctoral program. *Degree requirements:* For master's, thesis (for some programs); for doctorate, comprehensive exam, thesis/dissertation. *Entrance requirements:* For master's and doctorate, GRE General Test. Additional exam requirements/recommendations for international students: Required—TOEFL. *Application deadline:* For fall admission, 2/1 priority date for domestic students. Applications are processed on a rolling basis. Application fee: $65. Electronic applications accepted. *Financial support:* In 2015–16, 14 students received support, including 6 research assistantships with full tuition reimbursements available (averaging $14,600 per year), 8 teaching assistantships with full tuition reimbursements available (averaging $14,600 per year); career-related internships or fieldwork, Federal Work-Study, institutionally sponsored loans, and tuition waivers (full and partial) also available. Financial award application deadline: 3/1. *Faculty research:* Ecology and evolution (aquatic, terrestrial, paleo); development and genetics; biomedical research; ecophysiology and stress; invasion ecology and pest management. *Total annual research expenditures:* $3.2 million. *Unit head:* Dr. Andrei Aloykhin, Director, 207-581-2977, Fax: 207-581-2537. *Application contact:* Scott G. Delcourt, Assistant Vice President for Graduate Studies and Senior Associate Dean, 207-581-3291, Fax: 207-581-3232, E-mail: graduate@maine.edu. Website: http://sbe.umaine.edu/

University of Manitoba, Faculty of Graduate Studies, Faculty of Agricultural and Food Sciences, Department of Entomology, Winnipeg, MB R3T 2N2, Canada. Offers M Sc, PhD. *Degree requirements:* For master's, thesis; for doctorate, one foreign language, thesis/dissertation.

University of Maryland, College Park, Academic Affairs, College of Computer, Mathematical and Natural Sciences, Department of Entomology, College Park, MD 20742. Offers MS, PhD. *Program availability:* Part-time, evening/weekend. Terminal master's awarded for partial completion of doctoral program. *Degree requirements:* For master's, thesis; for doctorate, thesis/dissertation, oral qualifying exam. *Entrance requirements:* For master's and doctorate, GRE General Test, minimum GPA of 3.0, 3 letters of recommendation. Electronic applications accepted. *Faculty research:* Pest management, biosystematics, physiology and morphology, toxicology.

University of Minnesota, Twin Cities Campus, Graduate School, College of Food, Agricultural and Natural Resource Sciences, Entomology Graduate Program, Saint Paul, MN 55108. Offers MS, PhD. *Program availability:* Part-time. Terminal master's awarded for partial completion of doctoral program. *Degree requirements:* For master's, comprehensive exam, thesis; for doctorate, comprehensive exam, thesis/dissertation. *Entrance requirements:* For master's, GRE, minimum undergraduate GPA of 3.0; for doctorate, GRE, minimum undergraduate GPA of 3.0, graduate 3.5. Additional exam requirements/recommendations for international students: Required—TOEFL (minimum score 550 paper-based; 79 iBT), IELTS (minimum score 6.5). Electronic applications accepted. *Faculty research:* Behavior, ecology, molecular genetics, physiology, systematics and taxonomy.

University of Missouri, Office of Research and Graduate Studies, College of Agriculture, Food and Natural Resources, Division of Plant Insect Microbial Sciences, Columbia, MO 65211. Offers crop, soil and pest management (MS, PhD); entomology (MS, PhD); horticulture (MS, PhD); plant biology and genetics (MS, PhD); plant stress biology (MS, PhD). Terminal master's awarded for partial completion of doctoral program. *Degree requirements:* For master's, thesis; for doctorate, comprehensive exam, thesis/dissertation. *Entrance requirements:* For master's and doctorate, GRE General Test, minimum GPA of 3.0; bachelor's degree from accredited college. Additional exam requirements/recommendations for international students: Required—TOEFL (minimum score 500 paper-based; 61 iBT), IELTS (minimum score 5.5). *Application deadline:* For fall admission, 1/15 priority date for domestic students, 1/15 for international students. Applications are processed on a rolling basis. Application fee: $65 ($90 for international students). Electronic applications accepted. *Financial support:* Fellowships with tuition reimbursements, research assistantships with tuition reimbursements, teaching assistantships with tuition reimbursements, institutionally sponsored loans, scholarships/grants, health care benefits, and unspecified assistantships available. Support available to part-time students. *Faculty research:* Crop, soil and pest management; entomology; horticulture; plant biology and genetics; plant microbiology and pathology.
Website: http://plantsci.missouri.edu/graduate/

University of Nebraska–Lincoln, Graduate College, College of Agricultural Sciences and Natural Resources, Department of Entomology, Lincoln, NE 68588. Offers MS, PhD. *Program availability:* Online learning. *Degree requirements:* For master's, thesis optional; for doctorate, comprehensive exam, thesis/dissertation. *Entrance requirements:* For master's and doctorate, GRE General Test. Additional exam requirements/recommendations for international students: Required—TOEFL (minimum score 550 paper-based). Electronic applications accepted. *Faculty research:* Ecology and behavior, insect-plant interactions, integrated pest management, genetics, urban entomology.

University of North Dakota, Graduate School, College of Arts and Sciences, Department of Biology, Grand Forks, ND 58202. Offers botany (MS, PhD); ecology (MS, PhD); entomology (MS, PhD); environmental biology (MS, PhD); fisheries/wildlife (MS, PhD); genetics (MS, PhD); zoology (MS, PhD). Terminal master's awarded for partial completion of doctoral program. *Degree requirements:* For master's, thesis, final exam; for doctorate, comprehensive exam, thesis/dissertation, final exam. *Entrance requirements:* For master's, GRE General Test, GRE Subject Test, minimum GPA of 3.0; for doctorate, GRE General Test, GRE Subject Test, minimum GPA of 3.5. Additional exam requirements/recommendations for international students: Required—TOEFL (minimum score 550 paper-based; 79 iBT), IELTS (minimum score 6.5). Electronic applications accepted. *Faculty research:* Population biology, wildlife ecology, RNA processing, hormonal control of behavior.

The University of Tennessee, Graduate School, College of Agricultural Sciences and Natural Resources, Department of Entomology and Plant Pathology, Knoxville, TN 37996. Offers entomology (MS, PhD); integrated pest management and bioactive natural products (PhD); plant pathology (MS, PhD). *Program availability:* Part-time. *Degree requirements:* For master's, thesis, seminar. *Entrance requirements:* For master's, GRE General Test, minimum GPA of 2.7, 3 reference letters, letter of intent; for doctorate, GRE General Test, minimum GPA of 2.7, 3 reference letters, letter of intent, proposed dissertation research. Additional exam requirements/recommendations for international students: Required—TOEFL. Electronic applications accepted.

University of Wisconsin–Madison, Graduate School, College of Agricultural and Life Sciences, Department of Entomology, Madison, WI 53706-1380. Offers MS, PhD. *Degree requirements:* For master's, thesis; for doctorate, thesis/dissertation. *Entrance requirements:* For master's and doctorate, GRE General Test, minimum GPA of 3.0. Additional exam requirements/recommendations for international students: Required—TOEFL. Electronic applications accepted. *Expenses:* Tuition, state resident: full-time $5364. Tuition, nonresident: full-time $12,027. *Required fees:* $571. Tuition and fees vary according to campus/location, program and reciprocity agreements. *Faculty research:* Ecology, biocontrol, molecular.

University of Wyoming, College of Agriculture and Natural Resources, Department of Renewable Resources, Program in Entomology, Laramie, WY 82071. Offers MS, PhD. *Degree requirements:* For master's, thesis; for doctorate, thesis/dissertation. *Entrance requirements:* For master's and doctorate, GRE General Test, minimum GPA of 3.0. Additional exam requirements/recommendations for international students: Required—TOEFL. Electronic applications accepted. *Faculty research:* Insect pest management, taxonomy, biocontrol of weeds, forest insects, insects affecting humans and animals.

Virginia Polytechnic Institute and State University, Graduate School, College of Agriculture and Life Sciences, Blacksburg, VA 24061. Offers agricultural and applied economics (MS); agricultural and life sciences (MS); animal and poultry science (MS, PhD); crop and soil environmental sciences (MS, PhD); dairy science (MS); entomology (PhD); horticulture (MS, PhD); human nutrition, foods and exercise (MS, PhD); life sciences (MS, PhD); plant pathology, physiology and weed science (PhD). *Degree requirements:* For master's, comprehensive exam (for some programs), thesis (for some programs); for doctorate, comprehensive exam (for some programs), thesis/dissertation (for some programs). *Entrance requirements:* For master's and doctorate, GRE/GMAT (may vary by department). Additional exam requirements/recommendations for international students: Required—TOEFL (minimum score 550 paper-based). Electronic applications accepted.

Washington State University, College of Agricultural, Human, and Natural Resource Sciences, Department of Entomology, Pullman, WA 99164. Offers MS, PhD. Programs offered at the Pullman campus. Terminal master's awarded for partial completion of doctoral program. *Degree requirements:* For master's, comprehensive exam, thesis, oral exam; for doctorate, comprehensive exam, thesis/dissertation, oral exam, written exam. *Entrance requirements:* For master's, GRE General Test, GRE Subject Test in advanced biology (recommended), undergraduate degree in biology, ecology or related area; minimum GPA of 3.0; 3 letters of recommendation; for doctorate, GRE General Test, MS in entomology, biology, ecology or related area; minimum GPA of 3.0; 3 letters of recommendation. Additional exam requirements/recommendations for international students: Required—TOEFL (minimum score 550 paper-based), IELTS. Electronic applications accepted. *Faculty research:* Apiculture, biological control of arthropods, integrated pest management, ecology, physiology and systematics of insects.

West Virginia University, Davis College of Agriculture, Forestry and Consumer Sciences, Division of Plant and Soil Sciences, Morgantown, WV 26506. Offers agricultural sciences (PhD), including animal and food sciences, plant and soil sciences; agronomy (MS); entomology (MS); environmental microbiology (MS); horticulture (MS); plant pathology (MS). *Degree requirements:* For master's, thesis. *Entrance requirements:* For master's, GRE, minimum GPA of 2.5. Additional exam requirements/recommendations for international students: Required—TOEFL. *Expenses:* Tuition, state resident: full-time $8568. Tuition, nonresident: full-time $22,140. Tuition and fees vary according to program. *Faculty research:* Water quality, reclamation of disturbed land, crop production, pest control, environmental protection.

Section 10
Genetics, Developmental Biology, and Reproductive Biology

This section contains a directory of institutions offering graduate work in genetics, developmental biology, and reproductive biology, followed by an in-depth entry submitted by an institution that chose to prepare a detailed program description. Additional information about programs listed in the directory but not augmented by an in-depth entry may be obtained by writing directly to the dean of a graduate school or chair of a department at the address given in the directory.

For programs offering related work, see also all other sections of this book. In the other guides in this series:

Graduate Programs in the Physical Sciences, Mathematics, Agricultural Sciences, the Environment & Natural Resources

See *Agricultural and Food Sciences, Chemistry,* and *Environmental Sciences and Management*

Graduate Programs in Engineering & Applied Sciences

See *Agricultural Engineering and Bioengineering* and *Biomedical Engineering and Biotechnology*

CONTENTS

Program Directories

Displays and Close-Ups

See also:

Developmental Biology

Albert Einstein College of Medicine, Graduate Division of Biomedical Sciences, Department of Anatomy and Structural Biology, Bronx, NY 10461. Offers anatomy (PhD); cell and developmental biology (PhD); MD/PhD. *Degree requirements:* For doctorate, thesis/dissertation. *Entrance requirements:* For doctorate, GRE General Test. Additional exam requirements/recommendations for international students: Required—TOEFL. Electronic applications accepted. *Faculty research:* Cell motility, cell membranes and membrane-cytoskeletal interactions as applied to processing of pancreatic hormones, mechanisms of secretion.

Albert Einstein College of Medicine, Graduate Division of Biomedical Sciences, Department of Developmental and Molecular Biology, Bronx, NY 10461. Offers PhD, MD/PhD. *Degree requirements:* For doctorate, thesis/dissertation. *Entrance requirements:* For doctorate, GRE General Test. Additional exam requirements/recommendations for international students: Required—TOEFL. *Faculty research:* DNA, RNA, and protein synthesis in prokaryotes and eukaryotes; chemical and enzymatic alteration of RNA; glycoproteins.

Baylor College of Medicine, Graduate School of Biomedical Sciences, Program in Developmental Biology, Houston, TX 77030-3498. Offers PhD, MD/PhD. *Degree requirements:* For doctorate, thesis/dissertation, public defense. *Entrance requirements:* For doctorate, GRE General Test, GRE Subject Test (strongly recommended), minimum GPA of 3.0. Additional exam requirements/recommendations for international students: Required—TOEFL. Electronic applications accepted. *Faculty research:* Stem cells, cancer, neurobiology, organogenesis, genetics of model organisms.

Brigham Young University, Graduate Studies, College of Life Sciences, Department of Physiology and Developmental Biology, Provo, UT 84602. Offers neuroscience (MS, PhD); physiology and developmental biology (MS, PhD). *Program availability:* Part-time. *Faculty:* 20 full-time (1 woman), 4 part-time/adjunct (3 women). *Students:* 33 full-time (20 women); includes 6 minority (1 American Indian or Alaska Native, non-Hispanic/Latino; 3 Asian, non-Hispanic/Latino; 1 Hispanic/Latino; 1 Two or more races, non-Hispanic/Latino). Average age 29. 17 applicants, 29% accepted, 5 enrolled. In 2015, 6 master's, 3 doctorates awarded. Terminal master's awarded for partial completion of doctoral program. *Degree requirements:* For master's, thesis, oral exam; for doctorate, comprehensive exam, thesis/dissertation. *Entrance requirements:* For master's, GRE General Test, minimum GPA of 3.0 during previous 2 years; for doctorate, GRE General Test, minimum GPA of 3.0 overall. Additional exam requirements/recommendations for international students: Required—TOEFL (minimum score 580 paper-based; 85 iBT); Recommended—IELTS. *Application deadline:* For fall admission, 2/1 priority date for domestic and international students; for winter admission, 9/10 priority date for domestic and international students. Application fee: $50. Electronic applications accepted. *Financial support:* In 2015–16, 37 students received support, including 2 fellowships with partial tuition reimbursements available (averaging $7,100 per year), 17 research assistantships with full tuition reimbursements available (averaging $15,500 per year), 18 teaching assistantships with partial tuition reimbursements available (averaging $14,900 per year); career-related internships or fieldwork, institutionally sponsored loans, scholarships/grants, tuition waivers (full and partial), unspecified assistantships, and tuition awards also available. Financial award application deadline: 2/1. *Faculty research:* Sex differentiation of the brain, exercise physiology, developmental biology, membrane biophysics, neuroscience, heart differentiation/birth defects. *Total annual research expenditures:* $747,261. *Unit head:* Dr. Dixon J. Woodbury, Chair, 801-422-7562, Fax: 801-422-0004, E-mail: dixon_woodbury@byu.edu. *Application contact:* Connie L. Provost, Graduate Program Administrator, 801-422-3706, Fax: 801-422-0004, E-mail: connie_provost@byu.edu.
Website: http://pdbio.byu.edu

California Institute of Technology, Division of Biology, Program in Developmental Biology, Pasadena, CA 91125-0001. Offers PhD. *Degree requirements:* For doctorate, thesis/dissertation, qualifying exam. *Entrance requirements:* For doctorate, GRE General Test.

California State University, Sacramento, Office of Graduate Studies, College of Natural Sciences and Mathematics, Department of Biological Sciences, Sacramento, CA 95819. Offers biological conservation (MS); molecular and cellular biology (MS); stem cell (MA). *Program availability:* Part-time. *Degree requirements:* For master's, thesis, writing proficiency exam. *Entrance requirements:* For master's, GRE, bachelor's degree in biology or equivalent; minimum GPA of 3.0 in biology, 2.75 overall during last 2 years of course work. Additional exam requirements/recommendations for international students: Required—TOEFL. Electronic applications accepted.

Carnegie Mellon University, Mellon College of Science, Department of Biological Sciences, Pittsburgh, PA 15213-3891. Offers biochemistry (PhD); biophysics (PhD); cell and developmental biology (PhD); computational biology (MS, PhD); genetics (PhD); molecular biology (PhD); neuroscience (PhD); structural biology (PhD). *Degree requirements:* For doctorate, comprehensive exam, thesis/dissertation. *Entrance requirements:* For doctorate, GRE General Test, GRE Subject Test, interview. Electronic applications accepted. *Faculty research:* Genetic structure, function, and regulation; protein structure and function; biological membranes; biological spectroscopy.

Columbia University, College of Physicians and Surgeons, Department of Genetics and Development, New York, NY 10032. Offers genetics (M Phil, MA, PhD); MD/PhD. Only candidates for the PhD are admitted. Terminal master's awarded for partial completion of doctoral program. *Degree requirements:* For doctorate, thesis/dissertation. *Entrance requirements:* For master's and doctorate, GRE General Test. Additional exam requirements/recommendations for international students: Required—TOEFL. *Faculty research:* Mammalian cell differentiation and meiosis, developmental genetics, yeast and human genetics, chromosome structure, molecular and cellular biology.

Cornell University, Graduate School, Graduate Fields of Agriculture and Life Sciences, Field of Genetics, Genomics and Development, Ithaca, NY 14853-0001. Offers developmental biology (PhD); genetics (PhD); genomics (PhD). *Degree requirements:* For doctorate, comprehensive exam, thesis/dissertation, 2 semesters of teaching experience. *Entrance requirements:* For doctorate, GRE General Test, GRE Subject Test in biology or biochemistry (recommended), 2 letters of recommendation. Additional exam requirements/recommendations for international students: Required—TOEFL (minimum score 550 paper-based; 77 iBT). Electronic applications accepted. *Faculty research:* Molecular and general genetics, developmental biology and developmental genetics, evolution and population genetics, plant genetics, microbial genetics.

Cornell University, Graduate School, Graduate Fields of Agriculture and Life Sciences, Field of Zoology and Wildlife Conservation, Ithaca, NY 14853-0001. Offers animal cytology (PhD); comparative and functional anatomy (PhD); developmental biology (PhD); ecology (PhD); histology (PhD); wildlife conservation (PhD). *Degree requirements:* For doctorate, comprehensive exam, thesis/dissertation, 2 semesters of teaching experience. *Entrance requirements:* For doctorate, GRE General Test, GRE Subject Test (biology), 2 letters of recommendation. Additional exam requirements/recommendations for international students: Required—TOEFL (minimum score 550 paper-based; 77 iBT). Electronic applications accepted. *Faculty research:* Organismal biology, functional morphology, biomechanics, comparative vertebrate anatomy, comparative invertebrate anatomy, paleontology.

Cornell University, Graduate School, Graduate Fields of Comparative Biomedical Sciences, Field of Comparative Biomedical Sciences, Ithaca, NY 14853-0001. Offers cellular and molecular medicine (MS, PhD); developmental and reproductive biology (MS, PhD); infectious diseases (MS, PhD); population medicine and epidemiology (MS, PhD); structural and functional biology (MS, PhD). *Degree requirements:* For master's, thesis; for doctorate, comprehensive exam, thesis/dissertation. *Entrance requirements:* For master's and doctorate, GRE General Test, 2 letters of recommendation. Additional exam requirements/recommendations for international students: Required—TOEFL (minimum score 550 paper-based; 77 iBT). Electronic applications accepted. *Faculty research:* Receptors and signal transduction, viral and bacterial infectious diseases, tumor metastasis, clinical sciences/nutritional disease, developmental/neurological disorders.

Duke University, Graduate School, Program in Developmental and Stem Cell Biology, Durham, NC 27710. Offers Certificate. *Entrance requirements:* For degree, GRE General Test. Additional exam requirements/recommendations for international students: Required—TOEFL (minimum score 577 paper-based; 90 iBT) or IELTS (minimum score 7).

Emory University, Laney Graduate School, Division of Biological and Biomedical Sciences, Program in Biochemistry, Cell and Developmental Biology, Atlanta, GA 30322. Offers PhD. *Degree requirements:* For doctorate, comprehensive exam, thesis/dissertation. *Entrance requirements:* For doctorate, GRE General Test, minimum GPA of 3.0 in science course work (recommended). Additional exam requirements/recommendations for international students: Required—TOEFL. Electronic applications accepted. *Faculty research:* Signal transduction, molecular biology, enzymes and cofactors, receptor and ion channel function, membrane biology.

Illinois State University, Graduate School, College of Arts and Sciences, Department of Biological Sciences, Normal, IL 61790-2200. Offers animal behavior (MS); bacteriology (MS); biochemistry (MS); biological sciences (MS); biology (PhD); biophysics (MS); biotechnology (MS); botany (MS, PhD); cell biology (MS); conservation biology (MS); developmental biology (MS); ecology (MS, PhD); entomology (MS); evolutionary biology (MS); genetics (MS, PhD); immunology (MS); microbiology (MS, PhD); molecular biology (MS); molecular genetics (MS); neurobiology (MS); neuroscience (MS); parasitology (MS); physiology (MS, PhD); plant biology (MS); plant molecular biology (MS); plant sciences (MS); structural biology (MS); zoology (MS, PhD). *Program availability:* Part-time. *Degree requirements:* For master's, thesis or alternative; for doctorate, variable foreign language requirement, thesis/dissertation, 2 terms of residency. *Entrance requirements:* For master's, GRE General Test, minimum GPA of 2.6 in last 60 hours of course work; for doctorate, GRE General Test. *Application deadline:* Applications are processed on a rolling basis. Application fee: $40. *Financial support:* Research assistantships, teaching assistantships, Federal Work-Study, tuition waivers (full), and unspecified assistantships available. Financial award application deadline: 4/1. *Faculty research:* Redoc balance and drug development in schistosoma mansoni, control of the growth of listeria monocytogenes at low temperature, regulation of cell expansion and microtubule function by SPRI, CRUI: physiology and fitness consequences of different life history phenotypes. *Application contact:* Steven Juliano, Graduate Coordinator, E-mail: sajulian@ilstu.edu.
Website: http://www.bio.ilstu.edu/

Iowa State University of Science and Technology, Program in Molecular, Cellular, and Developmental Biology, Ames, IA 50011. Offers MS, PhD. *Entrance requirements:* For master's and doctorate, GRE General Test. Additional exam requirements/recommendations for international students: Required—TOEFL (minimum score 580 paper-based; 85 iBT), IELTS (minimum score 7). Electronic applications accepted.

Irell & Manella Graduate School of Biological Sciences, Graduate Program, Duarte, CA 91010. Offers brain metastatic cancer (PhD); cancer and stem cell metabolism (PhD); cancer biology (PhD); cancer biology and developmental therapeutics (PhD); cell biology (PhD); chemical biology (PhD); chromosomal break repair (PhD); diabetes and pancreatic progenitor cell biology (PhD); DNA repair and cancer biology (PhD); germline epigenetic remodeling and endocrine disruptors (PhD); hematology and hematopoietic cell transplantation (PhD); hematology and immunology (PhD); inflammation and cancer (PhD); micrornas and gene regulation in cardiovascular disease (PhD); mixed chimrism for reversal of autoimmunity (PhD); molecular and cellular biology (PhD); molecular biology and genetics (PhD); nanoparticle mediated twist1 silencing in metastatic cancer (PhD); neuro-oncology and stem cell biology (PhD); neuroscience (PhD); rna directed therapies for hiv-1 (PhD); small rna-induced transcriptional gene activation (PhD); stem cell regulation by the microenvironment (PhD); translational oncology and pharmaceutical sciences (PhD); tumor biology (PhD). *Faculty:* 70 full-time (18 women). *Students:* 75 full-time (40 women); includes 28 minority (2 Black or African American, non-Hispanic/Latino; 10 Asian, non-Hispanic/Latino; 10 Hispanic/Latino; 2 Native Hawaiian or other Pacific Islander, non-Hispanic/Latino; 4 Two or more races, non-Hispanic/Latino), 15 international. Average age 26. 197 applicants, 12% accepted, 19 enrolled. In 2015, 12 doctorates awarded. *Degree requirements:* For doctorate, comprehensive exam, thesis/dissertation, qualifying exams, two advanced courses. *Entrance requirements:* For doctorate, GRE General Test; GRE Subject Test (recommended), 2 years of course work in chemistry (general and organic); 1 year of course work each in biochemistry, general biology, and general physics; 2 semesters of course work in mathematics; significant research laboratory experience. Additional exam requirements/recommendations for international students: Required—TOEFL. *Application deadline:* For fall admission, 1/1 priority date for domestic and international students. Application fee: $0. Electronic applications accepted. Full-time tuition and fees vary according to class time, course level, course load, degree level, campus/location, program and student level. *Financial support:* In 2015–16, 12 students received support, including 35 fellowships with full tuition reimbursements available (averaging $32,000 per year); teaching assistantships, health care benefits, and tuition waivers (full) also available. Financial award applicants required to submit FAFSA. *Faculty research:* Cancer biology, diabetes, stem cell biology, neuroscience, immunology. *Unit head:* Dr. John J. Rossi, Dean, 877-715-GRAD, Fax: 626-471-3901, E-mail: gradschool@coh.org. *Application contact:* Dr. Kate Sleeth, Interim Associate Dean of Administration and

Student Development, 626-218-1742, Fax: 626-471-3901, E-mail: gradschool@coh.org. Website: http://cityofhope.org/gradschool

See Display on page 66 and Close-Up on page 111.

Johns Hopkins University, National Institutes of Health Sponsored Programs, Baltimore, MD 21218. Offers biology (PhD), including biochemistry, biophysics, cell biology, developmental biology, genetic biology, molecular biology; cell, molecular, and developmental biology and biophysics (PhD). *Degree requirements:* For doctorate, comprehensive exam, thesis/dissertation. *Entrance requirements:* For doctorate, GRE General Test. Additional exam requirements/recommendations for international students: Required—TOEFL (minimum score 600 paper-based), TWE. Electronic applications accepted. *Faculty research:* Protein and nucleic acid biochemistry and biophysical chemistry, molecular biology and development.

Louisiana State University Health Sciences Center, School of Graduate Studies in New Orleans, Department of Cell Biology and Anatomy, New Orleans, LA 70112-2223. Offers cell biology and anatomy (PhD), including clinical anatomy, development, cell, and neurobiology; MD/PhD. *Faculty:* 17 full-time (2 women). *Students:* 5 full-time (2 women), 1 international. 2 applicants, 100% accepted, 2 enrolled. *Degree requirements:* For doctorate, comprehensive exam, thesis/dissertation. *Entrance requirements:* For doctorate, GRE General Test, minimum undergraduate GPA of 3.0. Additional exam requirements/recommendations for international students: Recommended—TOEFL, IELTS. *Application deadline:* For fall admission, 3/1 priority date for domestic students, 3/1 for international students. Applications are processed on a rolling basis. Application fee: $30. *Financial support:* In 2015–16, 6 students received support. Unspecified assistantships available. Financial award application deadline: 4/1. *Faculty research:* Visual system organization, neural development, plasticity of sensory systems, information processing through the nervous system, visuomotor integration. *Total annual research expenditures:* $900,000. *Unit head:* Dr. Samuel McClugage, Head, 504-568-4011, Fax: 504-568-2165, E-mail: smcclu@lsuhsc.edu. *Application contact:* Dr. R. John Cork, Graduate Coordinator and Professor, 504-568-7177, E-mail: jcork@lsuhsc.edu.
Website: http://www.medschool.lsuhsc.edu/cell_biology/

Marquette University, Graduate School, College of Arts and Sciences, Department of Biology, Milwaukee, WI 53201-1881. Offers cell biology (MS, PhD); developmental biology (MS, PhD); ecology (MS, PhD); epithelial physiology (MS, PhD); genetics (MS, PhD); microbiology (MS, PhD); molecular biology (MS, PhD); muscle and exercise physiology (MS, PhD); neuroscience (PhD). *Faculty:* 22 full-time (7 women), 3 part-time/adjunct (2 women). *Students:* 28 full-time (11 women), 12 part-time (4 women); includes 4 minority (1 Asian, non-Hispanic/Latino; 1 Hispanic/Latino; 2 Two or more races, non-Hispanic/Latino), 11 international. Average age 27. 72 applicants, 28% accepted, 5 enrolled. In 2015, 2 master's, 4 doctorates awarded. Terminal master's awarded for partial completion of doctoral program. *Degree requirements:* For master's, comprehensive exam, thesis, 1 year of teaching experience or equivalent; for doctorate, thesis/dissertation, 1 year of teaching experience or equivalent, qualifying exam. *Entrance requirements:* For master's and doctorate, GRE General Test, GRE Subject Test, official transcripts from all current and previous colleges/universities except Marquette, statement of professional goals and aspirations, three letters of recommendation. Additional exam requirements/recommendations for international students: Required—TOEFL (minimum score 530 paper-based). *Application deadline:* For fall admission, 12/15 for domestic and international students. Application fee: $50. Electronic applications accepted. *Financial support:* In 2015–16, 39 students received support, including 6 fellowships (averaging $1,208 per year), 4 research assistantships with full tuition reimbursements available (averaging $21,750 per year), 29 teaching assistantships with full tuition reimbursements available (averaging $21,750 per year); scholarships/grants, health care benefits, tuition waivers (full and partial), and unspecified assistantships also available. Support available to part-time students. Financial award application deadline: 2/15. *Faculty research:* Neurobiology, neuroendocrinology, epithelial physiology, neuropeptide interactions, synaptic transmission. *Total annual research expenditures:* $1.2 million. *Unit head:* Dr. Ed Blumenthal, Chair, 414-288-1748. *Application contact:* Dr. Michael Schlappi, Recruiting Contact, 414-288-1467.
Website: http://www.marquette.edu/biology/

Massachusetts Institute of Technology, School of Science, Department of Biology, Cambridge, MA 02139. Offers biochemistry (PhD); biological oceanography (PhD); biology (PhD); biophysical chemistry and molecular structure (PhD); cell biology (PhD); computational and systems biology (PhD); developmental biology (PhD); genetics (PhD); immunology (PhD); microbiology (PhD); molecular biology (PhD); neurobiology (PhD). *Faculty:* 57 full-time (14 women). *Students:* 283 full-time (137 women); includes 83 minority (3 Black or African American, non-Hispanic/Latino; 1 American Indian or Alaska Native, non-Hispanic/Latino; 38 Asian, non-Hispanic/Latino; 31 Hispanic/Latino; 10 Two or more races, non-Hispanic/Latino), 48 international. Average age 26. 673 applicants, 14% accepted, 46 enrolled. In 2015, 32 doctorates awarded. *Degree requirements:* For doctorate, comprehensive exam, thesis/dissertation, teaching assistantship during two semesters. *Entrance requirements:* For doctorate, GRE General Test. Additional exam requirements/recommendations for international students: Required—TOEFL (minimum score 577 paper-based), IELTS. *Application deadline:* For fall admission, 12/1 for domestic and international students. Application fee: $75. Electronic applications accepted. *Expenses: Tuition:* Full-time $46,400; part-time $725 per credit. One-time fee: $304 full-time. Full-time tuition and fees vary according to course load and program. *Financial support:* In 2015–16, 235 students received support, including 118 fellowships (averaging $37,500 per year), 163 research assistantships (averaging $38,900 per year), 1 teaching assistantship; Federal Work-Study, institutionally sponsored loans, scholarships/grants, traineeships, health care benefits, and unspecified assistantships also available. Support available to part-time students. Financial award application deadline: 4/15; financial award applicants required to submit FAFSA. *Faculty research:* Cellular, developmental and molecular (plant and animal) biology; biochemistry, bioengineering, biophysics and structural biology; classical and molecular genetics, stem cell and epigenetics; immunology and microbiology; cancer biology, molecular medicine, neurobiology and human disease; computational and systems biology. *Total annual research expenditures:* $42.8 million. *Unit head:* Prof. Alan Grossman, Department Head, 617-253-4701. *Application contact:* Biology Education Office, 617-253-3717, Fax: 617-258-9329, E-mail: gradbio@mit.edu.
Website: https://biology.mit.edu/

Medical University of South Carolina, College of Graduate Studies, Program in Molecular and Cellular Biology and Pathobiology, Charleston, SC 29425. Offers cancer biology (PhD); cardiovascular biology (PhD); cardiovascular imaging (PhD); cell regulation (PhD); craniofacial biology (PhD); genetics and development (PhD); marine biomedicine (PhD); DMD/PhD; MD/PhD. *Degree requirements:* For doctorate, thesis/dissertation, oral and written exams. *Entrance requirements:* For doctorate, GRE General Test, interview, minimum GPA of 3.0. Additional exam requirements/recommendations for international students: Required—TOEFL (minimum score 600 paper-based; 100 iBT). Electronic applications accepted.

New York University, Graduate School of Arts and Science, Department of Biology, New York, NY 10012-1019. Offers biology (PhD); biomedical journalism (MS); cancer and molecular biology (PhD); computational biology (PhD); computers in biological research (MS); developmental genetics (PhD); general biology (MS); immunology and microbiology (PhD); molecular genetics (PhD); neurobiology (PhD); oral biology (MS); plant biology (PhD); recombinant DNA technology (MS); MS/MBA. *Program availability:* Part-time. Terminal master's awarded for partial completion of doctoral program. *Degree requirements:* For master's, thesis or alternative, qualifying paper; for doctorate, comprehensive exam, thesis/dissertation. *Entrance requirements:* For master's and doctorate, GRE General Test. Additional exam requirements/recommendations for international students: Required—TOEFL. *Faculty research:* Genomics, molecular and cell biology, development and molecular genetics, molecular evolution of plants and animals.

New York University, School of Medicine and Graduate School of Arts and Science, Sackler Institute of Graduate Biomedical Sciences, Program in Developmental Genetics, New York, NY 10012-1019. Offers PhD, MD/PhD. *Degree requirements:* For doctorate, comprehensive exam, thesis/dissertation, qualifying exam. *Faculty research:* Developmental genetics of germline proliferation in C. elegans, maternal/fetal immune interactions, signaling mechanisms of neuromuscular synapses formation in mice.

New York University, School of Medicine and Graduate School of Arts and Science, Sackler Institute of Graduate Biomedical Sciences, Program in Stem Cell Biology, New York, NY 10012-1019. Offers PhD, MD/PhD. *Degree requirements:* For doctorate, comprehensive exam, thesis/dissertation, qualifying exam. *Faculty research:* Stem cell self-renewal in Drosophila, electrophysiology of cardiac stem cells, developmental and physiological control of stem cells.

Northwestern University, The Graduate School, Interdisciplinary Biological Sciences Program (IBiS), Evanston, IL 60208. Offers biochemistry (PhD); bioengineering and biotechnology (PhD); biotechnology (PhD); cell and molecular biology (PhD); developmental and systems biology (PhD); nanotechnology (PhD); neurobiology (PhD); structural biology and biophysics (PhD). *Degree requirements:* For doctorate, thesis/ dissertation, qualifying exam. *Entrance requirements:* For doctorate, GRE General Test. Additional exam requirements/recommendations for international students: Required—TOEFL (minimum score 600 paper-based). Electronic applications accepted. *Faculty research:* Biophysics/structural biology, cell/molecular biology, synthetic biology, developmental systems biology, chemical biology/nanotechnology.

The Ohio State University, Graduate School, College of Arts and Sciences, Division of Natural and Mathematical Sciences, Department of Molecular Genetics, Columbus, OH 43210. Offers cell and developmental biology (MS, PhD); genetics (MS, PhD); molecular biology (MS, PhD). *Degree requirements:* For master's, thesis; for doctorate, thesis/dissertation. *Entrance requirements:* For doctorate, GRE General Test, GRE Subject Test in biology or chemistry (recommended). Additional exam requirements/recommendations for international students: Required—TOEFL (minimum score 550 paper-based; 79 iBT), Michigan English Language Assessment Battery (minimum score 82); Recommended—IELTS (minimum score 7). Electronic applications accepted.

The Ohio State University, Graduate School, College of Arts and Sciences, Division of Natural and Mathematical Sciences, Program in Molecular, Cellular and Developmental Biology, Columbus, OH 43210. Offers MS, PhD. Terminal master's awarded for partial completion of doctoral program. *Degree requirements:* For master's, thesis; for doctorate, thesis/dissertation. *Entrance requirements:* For doctorate, GRE General Test, GRE Subject Test in any science (desired, preferably biology or chemistry, biochemistry or cell and molecular biology). Additional exam requirements/ recommendations for international students: Required—TOEFL (minimum score 600 paper-based; 85 iBT); Recommended—IELTS (minimum score 8). Electronic applications accepted.

Oregon Health & Science University, School of Medicine, Graduate Programs in Medicine, Program in Molecular and Cellular Biosciences, Cell and Developmental Biology Graduate Program, Portland, OR 97239-3098. Offers PhD. *Faculty:* 11 full-time (6 women), 38 part-time/adjunct (6 women). *Students:* 11 full-time (8 women); includes 1 minority (Asian, non-Hispanic/Latino), 2 international. Average age 28. In 2015, 7 doctorates awarded. *Degree requirements:* For doctorate, comprehensive exam, thesis/ dissertation, qualifying exam. *Entrance requirements:* For doctorate, GRE General Test (minimum scores: 153 Verbal/148 Quantitative/4.5 Analytical) or MCAT. Additional exam requirements/recommendations for international students: Required—IELTS or TOEFL. *Application deadline:* For fall admission, 12/1 for domestic and international students. Application fee: $70. *Financial support:* Health care benefits, tuition waivers (full), and full tuition and stipends available. *Faculty research:* Biosynthesis, intracellular trafficking, and function of essential cellular components; signal transduction and developmental regulation of gene expression; regulation of cell proliferation, growth, and motility; mechanisms of morphogenesis and differentiation; mechanisms controlling the onset, progression, and dissemination of cancer. *Unit head:* Dr. Philip Copenhaver, Program Director, 503-494-4646, E-mail: copenhav@ohsu.edu. *Application contact:* Lola Bichler, Program Coordinator, 503-494-5824, E-mail: bichler@ohsu.edu.
Website: http://www.ohsu.edu/xd/education/schools/school-of-medicine/departments/basic-science-departments/cell-and-developmental-biology/graduate-program/CDB-

Oregon State University, College of Science, Program in Zoology, Corvallis, OR 97331. Offers behavioral ecology (MA, MS, PhD); behavioral endocrinology (MA, MS, PhD); cell biology (MA, MS, PhD); chemical ecology (MA, MS, PhD); conservation biology (MA, MS, PhD); developmental biology (MA, MS, PhD). *Faculty:* 21 full-time (9 women), 2 part-time/adjunct (1 woman). *Students:* 58 full-time (38 women), 1 part-time (0 women); includes 11 minority (1 Black or African American, non-Hispanic/Latino; 1 American Indian or Alaska Native, non-Hispanic/Latino; 7 Asian, non-Hispanic/Latino; 1 Hispanic/Latino; 1 Two or more races, non-Hispanic/Latino), 3 international. Average age 28. 75 applicants, 13% accepted, 9 enrolled. In 2015, 1 master's, 5 doctorates awarded. Terminal master's awarded for partial completion of doctoral program. *Degree requirements:* For doctorate, thesis/dissertation. *Entrance requirements:* For master's and doctorate, GRE. Additional exam requirements/recommendations for international students: Required—TOEFL (minimum score 80 iBT), IELTS (minimum score 6.5). *Application deadline:* For fall admission, 12/15 for domestic and international students. Application fee: $75 ($85 for international students). *Expenses: Tuition,* state resident: full-time $12,150; part-time $450 per credit. Tuition, nonresident: full-time $20,952; part-time $776 per credit. *Required fees:* $1572; $1443 per unit. One-time fee: $350. Tuition and fees vary according to course load, campus/location and program. *Financial support:* Fellowships, research assistantships, teaching assistantships, Federal Work-Study, and institutionally sponsored loans available. Support available to part-time students. *Faculty research:* Ecology and evolutionary biology, physiology and behavior, development and cell biology. *Unit head:* Dr. Virginia M. Weis, Professor and Chair of Integrative Biology, 541-737-4359. *Application contact:* Graduate Admissions Coordinator, 541-737-5335, E-mail: ib@science.oregonstate.edu.
Website: http://ib.oregonstate.edu/

Oregon State University, Interdisciplinary/Institutional Programs, Program in Molecular and Cellular Biology, Corvallis, OR 97331. Offers bioinformatics (PhD); biotechnology (PhD); cell biology (PhD); developmental biology (PhD); genome biology (PhD);

Developmental Biology

molecular biology (PhD); molecular pathogenesis (PhD); molecular virology (PhD); plant molecular biology (PhD); structural biology (PhD). *Students:* 28 full-time (14 women), 2 part-time (1 woman); includes 4 minority (2 Asian, non-Hispanic/Latino; 2 Hispanic/Latino), 10 international. Average age 29. 104 applicants, 5% accepted, 5 enrolled. In 2015, 5 doctorates awarded. *Degree requirements:* For doctorate, thesis/dissertation, oral and written qualifying exams. *Entrance requirements:* For doctorate, GRE. Additional exam requirements/recommendations for international students: Required—TOEFL (minimum score 80 iBT), IELTS (minimum score 6.5). *Application deadline:* For fall admission, 8/1 for domestic students, 4/1 for international students; for winter admission, 12/1 for domestic students, 7/1 for international students; for spring admission, 2/1 for domestic students, 10/1 for international students; for summer admission, 5/1 for domestic students, 1/1 for international students. Application fee: $75 ($85 for international students). *Expenses:* Tuition, state resident: full-time $12,150; part-time $450 per credit. Tuition, nonresident: full-time $20,952; part-time $776 per credit. *Required fees:* $1572; $1443 per unit. One-time fee: $350. Tuition and fees vary according to course load, campus/location and program. *Financial support:* Fellowships, career-related internships or fieldwork, Federal Work-Study, and institutionally sponsored loans available. Support available to part-time students. Financial award application deadline: 1/1. *Unit head:* Dr. Dee Denver, Director, Molecular and Cellular Biology Graduate Program, 541-737-3698. *Application contact:* Kristin Carroll, Assistant Director, 541-737-5259, E-mail: kristin.carroll@oregonstate.edu.
Website: http://www.mcb.oregonstate.edu/

Penn State Hershey Medical Center, College of Medicine, Graduate School Programs in the Biomedical Sciences, The Huck Institutes of the Life Sciences, Intercollege Graduate Program in Molecular Cellular and Integrative Biosciences, Hershey, PA 17033. Offers cell and developmental biology (PhD); immunology and infectious disease (PhD); molecular and evolutionary genetics (PhD); molecular medicine (PhD); molecular toxicology (PhD); neurobiology (PhD). *Students:* 3 full-time (2 women); includes 2 minority (both Asian, non-Hispanic/Latino). 2 applicants, 100% accepted, 2 enrolled. In 2015, 1 doctorate awarded. *Degree requirements:* For doctorate, comprehensive exam, thesis/dissertation, oral exam. *Entrance requirements:* For doctorate, GRE, minimum GPA of 3.0. Additional exam requirements/recommendations for international students: Required—TOEFL (minimum score 500 paper-based). *Application deadline:* For fall admission, 1/31 priority date for domestic students, 2/1 priority date for international students. Applications are processed on a rolling basis. Application fee: $65. Electronic applications accepted. *Financial support:* In 2015–16, research assistantships with full tuition reimbursements (averaging $26,196 per year) were awarded; fellowships with full tuition reimbursements, career-related internships or fieldwork, Federal Work-Study, scholarships/grants, health care benefits, and unspecified assistantships also available. Financial award applicants required to submit FAFSA. *Faculty research:* Vascular biology, molecular toxicology, chemical biology, immune system, pathophysiological basis of human disease. *Unit head:* Dr. Peter Hudson, Director, 814-865-6057, E-mail: pjh18@psu.edu. *Application contact:* Kathy Shuey, Administrative Assistant, 717-531-8982, Fax: 717-531-0786, E-mail: grad-hmc@psu.edu.
Website: http://www.huck.psu.edu/education/molecular-cellular-and-integrative-biosciences

Purdue University, Graduate School, College of Science, Department of Biological Sciences, West Lafayette, IN 47907. Offers biochemistry (PhD); biophysics (PhD); cell and developmental biology (PhD); ecology, evolutionary and population biology (MS, PhD), including ecology, evolutionary biology, population biology; genetics (MS, PhD); microbiology (MS, PhD); molecular biology (PhD); neurobiology (MS, PhD); plant physiology (PhD). Terminal master's awarded for partial completion of doctoral program. *Degree requirements:* For master's, thesis (for some programs); for doctorate, thesis/dissertation, seminars, teaching experience. *Entrance requirements:* For master's, GRE General Test (minimum analytical writing score of 3.5), minimum undergraduate GPA of 3.0; for doctorate, GRE General Test (minimum analytical writing score of 3.5), minimum undergraduate GPA of 3.5. Additional exam requirements/recommendations for international students: Required—TOEFL (minimum score 600 paper-based; 107 iBT for MS, 80 iBT for PhD). Electronic applications accepted.

Rutgers University–Newark, Graduate School of Biomedical Sciences, Newark, NJ 07107. Offers biodefense (Certificate); biomedical engineering (PhD); biomedical sciences (multidisciplinary) (PhD); cellular biology, neuroscience and physiology (PhD), including neuroscience, physiology, biophysics, cardiovascular biology, molecular pharmacology, stem cell biology; infection, immunity and inflammation (PhD), including immunology, infectious disease, microbiology, oral biology; molecular biology, genetics and cancer (PhD), including biochemistry, molecular genetics, cancer biology, radiation biology, bioinformatics; neuroscience (Certificate); pharmacological sciences (Certificate); stem cell (Certificate); DMD/PhD; MD/PhD. PhD in biomedical engineering offered jointly with New Jersey Institute of Technology. *Program availability:* Part-time, evening/weekend. Terminal master's awarded for partial completion of doctoral program. *Degree requirements:* For doctorate, thesis/dissertation, qualifying exam. *Entrance requirements:* For doctorate, GRE General Test. Additional exam requirements/recommendations for international students: Required—TOEFL. Electronic applications accepted.

Rutgers University–New Brunswick, Graduate School-New Brunswick, Programs in the Molecular Biosciences, Program in Cell and Developmental Biology, Piscataway, NJ 08854-8097. Offers MS, PhD. MS, PhD offered jointly with University of Medicine and Dentistry of New Jersey. *Program availability:* Part-time. Terminal master's awarded for partial completion of doctoral program. *Degree requirements:* For master's, thesis; for doctorate, thesis/dissertation, written qualifying exam. *Entrance requirements:* For master's, GRE General Test; for doctorate, GRE General Test, GRE Subject Test (recommended), minimum GPA of 3.0. Additional exam requirements/recommendations for international students: Required—TOEFL. Electronic applications accepted. *Faculty research:* Signal transduction and regulation of gene expression, developmental biology, cellular biology, developmental genetics, neurobiology.

San Francisco State University, Division of Graduate Studies, College of Science and Engineering, Department of Biology, Professional Science Master's Program, San Francisco, CA 94132-1722. Offers biotechnology (PSM); stem cell science (PSM). *Expenses:* Tuition, state resident: full-time $6738. Tuition, nonresident: full-time $15,666. *Required fees:* $1004. *Unit head:* Dr. Lily Chen, Director, 415-338-6763, Fax: 415-338-2295, E-mail: lilychen@sfsu.edu. *Application contact:* Dr. Linda H. Chen, Associate Director and Program Coordinator, 415-338-1696, Fax: 415-338-2295, E-mail: psm@sfsu.edu.
Website: http://psm.sfsu.edu/

Stanford University, School of Medicine, Graduate Programs in Medicine, Department of Developmental Biology, Stanford, CA 94305-9991. Offers MS, PhD. *Degree requirements:* For doctorate, thesis/dissertation, qualifying examination. *Entrance requirements:* For doctorate, GRE General Test, GRE Subject Test. Additional exam requirements/recommendations for international students: Required—TOEFL. Electronic applications accepted. *Expenses:* Tuition, area resident: Full-time $45,729. *Required fees:* $591. *Faculty research:* Mammalian embryology; developmental

genetics with particular emphasis on microbial systems; &ITDictyostelium&RO, &ITDrosophila&RO, the nematode, and the mouse.

Stony Brook University, State University of New York, Graduate School, College of Arts and Sciences, Department of Biochemistry and Cell Biology, Stony Brook, NY 11794. Offers biochemistry and cell biology (MS); biochemistry and structural biology (PhD); molecular and cellular biology (MA, PhD), including biochemistry and molecular biology (PhD), biological sciences (MA), cellular and developmental biology (PhD), immunology and pathology (PhD), molecular and cellular biology (PhD). *Faculty:* 22 full-time (7 women). *Students:* 115 full-time (61 women), 4 part-time (1 woman); includes 21 minority (4 Black or African American, non-Hispanic/Latino; 9 Asian, non-Hispanic/Latino; 7 Hispanic/Latino; 1 Native Hawaiian or other Pacific Islander, non-Hispanic/Latino), 57 international. Average age 27. 300 applicants, 23% accepted, 26 enrolled. In 2015, 11 master's, 16 doctorates awarded. *Degree requirements:* For doctorate, comprehensive exam, thesis/dissertation, teaching experience. *Entrance requirements:* For doctorate, GRE General Test, GRE Subject Test. Additional exam requirements/recommendations for international students: Required—TOEFL. *Application deadline:* For fall admission, 1/15 for domestic students; for spring admission, 10/15 for domestic students. Application fee: $100. *Expenses:* $12,421 full-time resident tuition and fees, $453 per credit hour; $23,761 full-time nonresident tuition and fees, $925 per credit hour. *Financial support:* In 2015–16, 6 fellowships, 51 research assistantships, 16 teaching assistantships were awarded; Federal Work-Study also available. *Faculty research:* Bioimaging, cell signaling, cell biology, biochemistry, pathogenesis. *Total annual research expenditures:* $6.6 million. *Unit head:* Prof. Aaron Neiman, Chair, 631-632-1543, Fax: 631-632-8575, E-mail: aaron.neiman@stonybrook.edu. *Application contact:* Pam Wolfskill, Coordinator, 631-632-8585, Fax: 631-632-8575, E-mail: pamela.wolfskill@stonybrook.edu.
Website: http://www.sunysb.edu/biochem

Thomas Jefferson University, Jefferson College of Biomedical Sciences, MS Program in Cell and Developmental Biology, Philadelphia, PA 19107. Offers MS. *Program availability:* Part-time, evening/weekend. *Faculty:* 44 full-time (14 women), 27 part-time/adjunct (11 women). *Students:* 22 part-time (15 women); includes 3 minority (2 Black or African American, non-Hispanic/Latino; 1 Asian, non-Hispanic/Latino), 2 international. Average age 29. 13 applicants, 77% accepted, 9 enrolled. In 2015, 5 master's awarded. *Degree requirements:* For master's, thesis, clerkship. *Entrance requirements:* For master's, GRE General Test or MCAT, minimum GPA of 3.0. Additional exam requirements/recommendations for international students: Required—TOEFL, IELTS (minimum score 7). *Application deadline:* For fall admission, 8/1 priority date for domestic students, 3/1 priority date for international students; for winter admission, 12/1 priority date for domestic students, 6/1 priority date for international students; for spring admission, 4/1 priority date for domestic students. Applications are processed on a rolling basis. Application fee: $50. Electronic applications accepted. *Financial support:* Federal Work-Study and institutionally sponsored loans available. Support available to part-time students. Financial award application deadline: 5/1; financial award applicants required to submit FAFSA. *Faculty research:* Developmental biology, cell biology, planning and management, drug development. *Unit head:* Dr. Gerald B. Grunwald, Dean and Program Director, 215-503-4191, Fax: 215-503-6690, E-mail: gerald.grunwald@jefferson.edu. *Application contact:* Marc E. Stearns, Director of Admissions, 215-503-0155, Fax: 215-503-3433, E-mail: jgsbs-info@jefferson.edu.
Website: http://www.jefferson.edu/university/biomedical-sciences/degrees-programs/master-programs/cell-developmental-biology.html

Thomas Jefferson University, Jefferson College of Biomedical Sciences, PhD Program in Cell and Developmental Biology, Philadelphia, PA 19107. Offers PhD. *Faculty:* 75 full-time (17 women). *Students:* 27 full-time (18 women); includes 3 minority (all Hispanic/Latino), 7 international. 19 applicants, 26% accepted, 3 enrolled. In 2015, 3 doctorates awarded. *Degree requirements:* For doctorate, comprehensive exam, thesis/dissertation. *Entrance requirements:* For doctorate, GRE General Test, minimum GPA of 3.2. Additional exam requirements/recommendations for international students: Required—TOEFL (minimum score 100 iBT), IELTS (minimum score 7). *Application deadline:* For fall admission, 12/15 priority date for domestic and international students. Applications are processed on a rolling basis. Application fee: $50. Electronic applications accepted. *Financial support:* In 2015–16, 27 fellowships with full tuition reimbursements (averaging $56,298 per year) were awarded; Federal Work-Study, institutionally sponsored loans, scholarships/grants, traineeships, and stipends also available. Support available to part-time students. Financial award application deadline: 5/1; financial award applicants required to submit FAFSA. *Unit head:* Dr. Nancy J. Philp, Program Director, 215-503-7854, E-mail: nancy.philp@jefferson.edu. *Application contact:* Marc E. Stearns, Director of Admissions, 215-503-0155, Fax: 215-503-3433, E-mail: jgsbs-info@jefferson.edu.
Website: http://www.jefferson.edu/university/biomedical-sciences/degrees-programs/phd-programs/cell-biology.html

Tufts University, Sackler School of Graduate Biomedical Sciences, Cell, Molecular, and Developmental Biology Program, Medford, MA 02155. Offers cancer biology (PhD); developmental and regenerative biology (PhD); molecular and cellular medicine (PhD); structural and chemical biology (PhD). *Faculty:* 45 full-time (15 women). *Students:* 36 full-time (18 women); includes 13 minority (2 Black or African American, non-Hispanic/Latino; 9 Asian, non-Hispanic/Latino; 1 Hispanic/Latino; 1 Two or more races, non-Hispanic/Latino), 4 international. Average age 28. 189 applicants, 7% accepted, 6 enrolled. In 2015, 2 doctorates awarded. Terminal master's awarded for partial completion of doctoral program. *Degree requirements:* For doctorate, comprehensive exam, thesis/dissertation. *Entrance requirements:* For doctorate, GRE General Test, 3 letters of reference. Additional exam requirements/recommendations for international students: Required—TOEFL (minimum score 600 paper-based; 100 iBT). *Application deadline:* For fall admission, 12/15 priority date for domestic and international students. Application fee: $70. Electronic applications accepted. *Expenses:* Tuition, area resident: Full-time $48,412; part-time $1210 per credit hour. *Required fees:* $806. Full-time tuition and fees vary according to degree level, program and student level. Part-time tuition and fees vary according to course load. *Financial support:* In 2015–16, 36 students received support, including 36 research assistantships with full tuition reimbursements available (averaging $32,000 per year); health care benefits also available. *Faculty research:* Reproduction and hormone action, control of gene expression, cell-matrix and cell-cell interactions, growth control and tumorigenesis, cytoskeleton and contractile proteins. *Unit head:* Dr. Ira Herman, Program Director, 617-636-2991, Fax: 617-636-0375. *Application contact:* Dr. Elizabeth Storrs, Registrar/Director of Academic Services, 617-636-6767, Fax: 617-636-0375, E-mail: sackler-school@tufts.edu.
Website: http://sackler.tufts.edu/Academics/CMDB-Welcome

University at Albany, State University of New York, College of Arts and Sciences, Department of Biological Sciences, Specialization in Molecular, Cellular, Developmental, and Neural Biology, Albany, NY 12222-0001. Offers PhD. *Degree requirements:* For doctorate, one foreign language, thesis/dissertation. *Entrance requirements:* For doctorate, GRE General Test.

The University of Alabama at Birmingham, Graduate Programs in Joint Health Sciences, Cell, Molecular, and Developmental Biology Theme, Birmingham, AL 35294. Offers PhD. *Degree requirements:* For doctorate, variable foreign language requirement, comprehensive exam, thesis/dissertation. *Entrance requirements:* For doctorate, GRE General Test, interview. Additional exam requirements/recommendations for international students: Required—TOEFL (minimum score 600 paper-based). Electronic applications accepted. *Expenses:* Tuition, state resident: full-time $7340. Tuition, nonresident: full-time $16,628. Full-time tuition and fees vary according to course load and program.

The University of British Columbia, Faculty of Medicine, Department of Cellular and Physiological Sciences, Vancouver, BC V6T 1Z3, Canada. Offers M Sc, PhD. *Degree requirements:* For master's, thesis, oral defense; for doctorate, comprehensive exam, thesis/dissertation, oral defense. *Entrance requirements:* For master's, minimum overall B+ average in third- and fourth-year courses; for doctorate, minimum overall B+ average in a master's degree (or equivalent) from an approved institution with clear evidence of research ability or potential. Additional exam requirements/recommendations for international students: Required—TOEFL (minimum score 550 paper-based), IELTS (minimum score 6.5).

University of California, Davis, Graduate Studies, Graduate Group in Cell and Developmental Biology, Davis, CA 95616. Offers MS, PhD. *Degree requirements:* For master's, comprehensive exam (for some programs), thesis (for some programs); for doctorate, thesis/dissertation. *Entrance requirements:* For doctorate, GRE General Test, GRE Subject Test. Additional exam requirements/recommendations for international students: Required—TOEFL (minimum score 550 paper-based). Electronic applications accepted. *Faculty research:* Molecular basis of cell function and development.

University of California, Irvine, Francisco J. Ayala School of Biological Sciences, Department of Developmental and Cell Biology, Irvine, CA 92697. Offers biological sciences (MS, PhD). *Students:* 40 full-time (23 women); includes 20 minority (1 American Indian or Alaska Native, non-Hispanic/Latino; 10 Asian, non-Hispanic/Latino; 8 Hispanic/Latino; 1 Native Hawaiian or other Pacific Islander, non-Hispanic/Latino), 2 international. Average age 29. 1 applicant, 100% accepted, 1 enrolled. In 2015, 3 master's, 6 doctorates awarded. *Degree requirements:* For doctorate, thesis/ dissertation. *Entrance requirements:* For master's and doctorate, GRE General Test, GRE Subject Test, minimum GPA of 3.0. Additional exam requirements/ recommendations for international students: Required—TOEFL (minimum score 550 paper-based). *Application deadline:* For fall admission, 12/15 priority date for domestic and international students. Application fee: $90 ($110 for international students). Electronic applications accepted. *Financial support:* Fellowships, research assistantships with full tuition reimbursements, teaching assistantships, institutionally sponsored loans, traineeships, health care benefits, and unspecified assistantships available. Financial award application deadline: 3/1; financial award applicants required to submit FAFSA. *Faculty research:* Genetics and development, oncogene signaling pathways, gene regulation, tissue regeneration and molecular genetics. *Unit head:* Prof. Thomas F. Schilling, Chair, 949-824-4562, Fax: 949-824-1105, E-mail: dkodowd@ uci.edu. *Application contact:* Prof. Aimee Edinger, Graduate Advisor, 949-824-1921, Fax: 949-824-4709, E-mail: aedinger@uci.edu.
Website: http://devcellbio.uci.edu/

University of California, Los Angeles, Graduate Division, College of Letters and Science, Department of Molecular, Cell and Developmental Biology, Los Angeles, CA 90095. Offers MA, PhD. Terminal master's awarded for partial completion of doctoral program. *Degree requirements:* For master's, comprehensive exam, thesis; for doctorate, thesis/dissertation, oral and written qualifying exams; 2 quarters of teaching experience. *Entrance requirements:* For doctorate, GRE General Test. Additional exam requirements/recommendations for international students: Required—TOEFL. Electronic applications accepted.

University of California, Riverside, Graduate Division, Program in Cell, Molecular, and Developmental Biology, Riverside, CA 92521-0102. Offers MS, PhD. Terminal master's awarded for partial completion of doctoral program. *Degree requirements:* For master's, thesis, oral defense of thesis; for doctorate, thesis/dissertation, oral defense of thesis, qualifying exams, 2 quarters of teaching experience. *Entrance requirements:* For master's and doctorate, GRE General Test, minimum GPA of 3.2. Additional exam requirements/recommendations for international students: Required—TOEFL (minimum score 550 paper-based; 80 iBT). *Application deadline:* For fall admission, 1/5 priority date for domestic and international students. Applications are processed on a rolling basis. Application fee: $60 ($75 for international students). Electronic applications accepted. *Expenses: Tuition, area resident:* full-time $16,665.50; part-time $11,055.54. Tuition, state resident: full-time $16,665.50; part-time $11,055.54. Tuition, nonresident: full-time $31,768. *International tuition:* $31,767.50 full-time. *Required fees:* $16,665.50; $11,055.54 per quarter. $3685.18 per quarter. Tuition and fees vary according to program. *Financial support:* Fellowships with tuition reimbursements, research assistantships with tuition reimbursements, teaching assistantships with tuition reimbursements, scholarships/grants, traineeships, health care benefits, tuition waivers (partial), and unspecified assistantships available. Support available to part-time students. Financial award application deadline: 1/5.
Website: http://www.cmdb.ucr.edu/

University of California, San Francisco, Graduate Division and School of Medicine, Tetrad Graduate Program, San Francisco, CA 94143. Offers biochemistry and molecular biology (PhD); cell biology (PhD); developmental biology (PhD); genetics (PhD); MD/PhD. *Degree requirements:* For doctorate, thesis/dissertation. *Entrance requirements:* For doctorate, GRE General Test, GRE Subject Test. Additional exam requirements/recommendations for international students: Required—TOEFL. *Expenses:* Contact institution.

University of California, Santa Barbara, Graduate Division, College of Letters and Sciences, Division of Mathematics, Life, and Physical Sciences, Department of Molecular, Cellular, and Developmental Biology, Santa Barbara, CA 93106-9625. Offers MA, PhD, MA/PhD. *Faculty:* 35 full-time (5 women), 3 part-time/adjunct (0 women). *Students:* 55 full-time (28 women); includes 16 minority (1 Black or African American, non-Hispanic/Latino; 1 American Indian or Alaska Native, non-Hispanic/Latino; 8 Asian, non-Hispanic/Latino; 4 Hispanic/Latino; 2 Native Hawaiian or other Pacific Islander, non-Hispanic/Latino), 4 international. Average age 27. 183 applicants, 24% accepted, 23 enrolled. In 2015, 5 master's, 10 doctorates awarded. Terminal master's awarded for partial completion of doctoral program. *Degree requirements:* For master's, comprehensive exam (for some programs), thesis (for some programs); for doctorate, comprehensive exam, thesis/dissertation. *Entrance requirements:* For master's and doctorate, GRE General Test, 3 letters of recommendation, statement of purpose, personal achievements/contributions statement, resume/curriculum vitae, transcripts for post-secondary institutions attended. Additional exam requirements/recommendations for international students: Required—TOEFL (minimum score 550 paper-based; 80 iBT), IELTS (minimum score 7). *Application deadline:* For fall admission, 12/7 priority date for domestic and international students. Application fee: $90 ($110 for international students). Electronic applications accepted. *Financial support:* In 2015–16, 3 students received support, including 3 fellowships with tuition reimbursements available (averaging $22,000 per year), 40 research assistantships with tuition reimbursements available (averaging $26,250 per year), 46 teaching assistantships with partial tuition reimbursements available (averaging $17,655 per year); career-related internships or fieldwork, Federal Work-Study, institutionally sponsored loans, scholarships/grants,

traineeships, health care benefits, and unspecified assistantships also available. Financial award application deadline: 3/2; financial award applicants required to submit FAFSA. *Faculty research:* Microbiology, neurobiology (including stem cell research), developmental, virology, cell biology. *Unit head:* Dr. Stephen Poole, Chair, 805-893-8122, E-mail: william.smith@lifesci.ucsb.edu. *Application contact:* Anthony Galaviz, Graduate Program Advisor, 805-893-8499, E-mail: anthony.galaviz@lifesci.ucsb.edu.
Website: https://www.mcdb.ucsb.edu/grad

University of California, Santa Cruz, Division of Graduate Studies, Division of Physical and Biological Sciences, Program in Molecular, Cellular, and Developmental Biology, Santa Cruz, CA 95064. Offers MA, PhD. Terminal master's awarded for partial completion of doctoral program. *Degree requirements:* For master's, thesis; for doctorate, thesis/dissertation, qualifying exam. *Entrance requirements:* For master's and doctorate, GRE General Test, 3 letters of recommendation, interview. Additional exam requirements/recommendations for international students: Required—TOEFL (minimum score 550 paper-based; 83 iBT); Recommended—IELTS (minimum score 8). Electronic applications accepted. *Faculty research:* RNA biology, chromatin and chromosome biology, neurobiology, stem cell biology and differentiation, cell structure and function.

University of Chicago, Division of the Biological Sciences, Committee on Development, Regeneration, and Stem Cell Biology, Chicago, IL 60637-1513. Offers PhD. *Students:* 22 full-time (10 women); includes 8 minority (4 Asian, non-Hispanic/Latino; 3 Hispanic/Latino; 1 Two or more races, non-Hispanic/Latino), 5 international. Average age 28. 49 applicants, 20% accepted, 3 enrolled. In 2015, 2 doctorates awarded. *Degree requirements:* For doctorate, thesis/dissertation, ethics class, 2 teaching assistantships. *Entrance requirements:* For doctorate, GRE General Test. Additional exam requirements/recommendations for international students: Required—TOEFL (minimum score 600 paper-based; 104 iBT), IELTS (minimum score 7). *Application deadline:* For fall admission, 12/1 for domestic and international students. Application fee: $90. Electronic applications accepted. *Financial support:* In 2015–16, 16 students received support, including fellowships with full tuition reimbursements available (averaging $29,781 per year), research assistantships with full tuition reimbursements available (averaging $29,781 per year); institutionally sponsored loans, scholarships/grants, traineeships, and health care benefits also available. Financial award applicants required to submit FAFSA. *Faculty research:* Epidermal differentiation, neural lineages, pattern formation. *Unit head:* Dr. Edwin Ferguson, Chair. *Application contact:* Kristine Gaston, Graduate Administrative Director, 773-702-8037, Fax: 773-702-3172, E-mail: kristine@bsd.uchicago.edu.
Website: http://devbio.bsd.uchicago.edu/

University of Cincinnati, Graduate School, College of Medicine, Graduate Programs in Biomedical Sciences, Department of Pediatrics, Program in Molecular and Developmental Biology, Cincinnati, OH 45221. Offers PhD. *Degree requirements:* For doctorate, thesis/dissertation, qualifying exam. *Entrance requirements:* For doctorate, GRE General Test, minimum GPA of 3.2. Additional exam requirements/ recommendations for international students: Required—TOEFL (minimum score 520 paper-based). Electronic applications accepted. *Faculty research:* Cancer biology, cardiovascular biology, developmental biology, human genetics, gene therapy, genomics and bioinformatics, immunobiology, molecular medicine, neuroscience, pulmonary biology, reproductive biology, stem cell biology.

University of Colorado Boulder, Graduate School, College of Arts and Sciences, Department of Molecular, Cellular, and Developmental Biology, Boulder, CO 80309. Offers cellular structure and function (MA, PhD); developmental biology (MA, PhD); molecular biology (MA, PhD). *Faculty:* 28 full-time (8 women). *Students:* 71 full-time (34 women), 1 part-time (0 women); includes 7 minority (1 Asian, non-Hispanic/Latino; 4 Hispanic/Latino; 1 Native Hawaiian or other Pacific Islander, non-Hispanic/Latino; 1 Two or more races, non-Hispanic/Latino), 7 international. Average age 27. 310 applicants, 6% accepted, 7 enrolled. In 2015, 6 doctorates awarded. Terminal master's awarded for partial completion of doctoral program. *Degree requirements:* For master's, comprehensive exam, thesis or alternative; for doctorate, comprehensive exam, thesis/ dissertation. *Entrance requirements:* For master's, GRE General Test, GRE Subject Test, minimum undergraduate GPA of 3.0; for doctorate, GRE General Test, GRE Subject Test. *Application deadline:* For fall admission, 12/1 for domestic students, 12/15 for international students. Application fee: $50 ($70 for international students). Electronic applications accepted. Application fee is waived when completed online. *Financial support:* In 2015–16, 125 students received support, including 10 fellowships (averaging $5,729 per year), 53 research assistantships with tuition reimbursements available (averaging $28,304 per year), 9 teaching assistantships with tuition reimbursements available (averaging $30,852 per year); institutionally sponsored loans, scholarships/grants, health care benefits, and unspecified assistantships also available. Financial award application deadline: 2/1; financial award applicants required to submit FAFSA. *Faculty research:* Molecular biology, cellular biology, genetics, biochemistry, gene cloning, proteins. *Total annual research expenditures:* $15.4 million. *Application contact:* E-mail: mcdbgrad@colorado.edu.
Website: http://mcdb.colorado.edu/graduate

University of Colorado Denver, College of Liberal Arts and Sciences, Department of Integrative and Systems Biology, Denver, CO 80217. Offers animal behavior (MS); biology (MS); cell and developmental biology (MS); ecology (MS); evolutionary biology (MS); genetics (MS); integrative and systems biology (PhD); microbiology (MS); molecular biology (MS); neurobiology (MS); plant systematics (MS). *Program availability:* Part-time. *Faculty:* 21 full-time (8 women), 3 part-time/adjunct (1 woman). *Students:* 31 full-time (19 women), 7 part-time (3 women); includes 8 minority (1 Black or African American, non-Hispanic/Latino; 1 Asian, non-Hispanic/Latino; 3 Hispanic/Latino; 3 Two or more races, non-Hispanic/Latino), 1 international. Average age 28. 34 applicants, 29% accepted, 8 enrolled. In 2015, 6 master's awarded. *Degree requirements:* For master's, comprehensive exam, thesis, 30-32 credit hours; for doctorate, comprehensive exam, thesis/dissertation. *Entrance requirements:* For master's, GRE General Test (minimum score in 50th percentile in each section), BA/BS from accredited institution awarded within the last 10 years; minimum undergraduate GPA of 3.0; prerequisite courses: 1 year each of general biology and general chemistry; 1 semester each of general genetics, general ecology, and cell biology; and a structure/ function course; for doctorate, GRE, minimum undergraduate GPA of 3.2, three letters of recommendation, official transcripts from all universities and colleges attended. Additional exam requirements/recommendations for international students: Required— TOEFL (minimum score 537 paper-based; 75 iBT); Recommended—IELTS (minimum score 6.5). *Application deadline:* For fall admission, 1/15 for domestic and international students. Application fee: $50 ($75 for international students). Electronic applications accepted. *Financial support:* In 2015–16, 32 students received support. Fellowships, research assistantships, teaching assistantships, Federal Work-Study, institutionally sponsored loans, scholarships/grants, and traineeships available. Financial award application deadline: 4/1; financial award applicants required to submit FAFSA. *Faculty research:* Molecular developmental biology; quantitative ecology, biogeography, and population dynamics; environmental signaling and endocrine disruption; speciation, the evolution of reproductive isolation, and hybrid zones; evolutionary, behavioral, and conservation ecology. *Unit head:* Dr. John Swallow, Chair, 303-556-6154, E-mail: john.swallow@ucdenver.edu. *Application contact:* Dr. Michael Wunder, Graduate

Developmental Biology

Advisor, 303-556-8870, E-mail: michael.wunder@ucdenver.edu. Website: http://www.ucdenver.edu/academics/colleges/CLAS/Departments/biology/Programs/MasterofScience/Pages/BiologyMasterOfScience.aspx

University of Colorado Denver, School of Medicine, Program in Cell Biology, Stem Cells, and Developmental Biology, Aurora, CO 80045. Offers cell biology, stem cells, and developmental biology (PhD); modern human anatomy (MS). *Students:* 29 full-time (13 women); includes 7 minority (1 Asian, non-Hispanic/Latino; 4 Hispanic/Latino; 2 Two or more races, non-Hispanic/Latino), 3 international. Average age 29. 42 applicants, 7% accepted, 3 enrolled. In 2015, 1 doctorate awarded. *Degree requirements:* For doctorate, comprehensive exam, thesis/dissertation, at least 30 credit hours of coursework and 30 credit hours of thesis research; laboratory rotations. *Entrance requirements:* For doctorate, GRE, minimum GPA of 3.0; 3 letters of reference; prerequisite coursework in organic chemistry, biology, biochemistry, physics and calculus; research experience (highly recommended). Additional exam requirements/recommendations for international students: Required—TOEFL (minimum score 550 paper-based; 80 iBT). *Application deadline:* For fall admission, 12/1 for domestic students, 11/1 priority date for international students. Application fee: $50 ($75 for international students). Electronic applications accepted. *Expenses:* Contact institution. *Financial support:* In 2015–16, 29 students received support. Fellowships, research assistantships, teaching assistantships, Federal Work-Study, institutionally sponsored loans, scholarships/grants, traineeships, health care benefits, and tuition waivers (full) available. Financial award application deadline: 3/15; financial award applicants required to submit FAFSA. *Faculty research:* Development and repair of the vertebrate nervous system; molecular, genetic and developmental mechanisms involved in the patterning of the early spinal cord (neural plate) during vertebrate embryogenesis; structural analysis of protein glycosylation using NMR and mass spectrometry; small RNAs and post-transcriptional gene regulation during nematode gametogenesis and early development; diabetes-mediated changes in cardiovascular gene expression and functional exercise capacity. *Total annual research expenditures:* $5.7 million. *Unit head:* Dr. Bruce Appel, Director, 303-724-3465, E-mail: bruce.appel@ucdenver.edu. *Application contact:* Kenton Owsley, Program Administrator, 303-724-3468, Fax: 303-724-3420, E-mail: kenton.owsley@ucdenver.edu.
Website: http://www.ucdenver.edu/academics/colleges/medicalschool/programs/CSD/Pages/CSD.aspx

★ **University of Connecticut Health Center,** Graduate School, Programs in Biomedical Sciences, Program in Genetics and Developmental Biology, Farmington, CT 06030. Offers PhD, DMD/PhD, MD/PhD. *Degree requirements:* For doctorate, comprehensive exam, thesis/dissertation. *Entrance requirements:* For doctorate, GRE General Test, GRE Subject Test. Additional exam requirements/recommendations for international students: Required—TOEFL (minimum score 600 paper-based). Electronic applications accepted. *Faculty research:* Developmental biology, genomic imprinting, RNA biology, RNA alternative splicing, human embryonic stem cells.
See Display on page 283 and Close-Up on page 295.

University of Delaware, College of Arts and Sciences, Department of Biological Sciences, Newark, DE 19716. Offers biotechnology (MS); cancer biology (MS, PhD); cell and extracellular matrix biology (MS, PhD); cell and systems physiology (MS, PhD); developmental biology (MS, PhD); ecology and evolution (MS, PhD); microbiology (MS, PhD); molecular biology and genetics (MS, PhD). Terminal master's awarded for partial completion of doctoral program. *Degree requirements:* For master's, thesis, preliminary exam; for doctorate, comprehensive exam, thesis/dissertation, preliminary exam. *Entrance requirements:* For master's and doctorate, GRE General Test. Additional exam requirements/recommendations for international students: Required—TOEFL (minimum score 600 paper-based); Recommended—TWE. Electronic applications accepted. *Faculty research:* Microorganisms, bone, cancer metastasis, developmental biology, cell biology, DNA.

University of Hawaii at Manoa, John A. Burns School of Medicine, Program in Developmental and Reproductive Biology, Honolulu, HI 96813. Offers MS, PhD. *Program availability:* Part-time. *Faculty:* 24 full-time (7 women). *Students:* 11 full-time (5 women), 3 part-time (1 woman); includes 9 minority (7 Asian, non-Hispanic/Latino; 2 Two or more races, non-Hispanic/Latino), 2 international. 19 applicants, 32% accepted, 2 enrolled. In 2015, 1 master's, 1 doctorate awarded. *Degree requirements:* For doctorate, thesis/dissertation. *Entrance requirements:* For doctorate, GRE General Test, GRE Subject Test. Additional exam requirements/recommendations for international students: Recommended—TOEFL (minimum score 560 paper-based), IELTS (minimum score 5). *Application deadline:* For fall admission, 3/1 for domestic and international students. Application fee: $100. *Financial support:* In 2015–16, 2 fellowships (averaging $4,577 per year), 10 research assistantships (averaging $16,328 per year) were awarded; teaching assistantships also available. *Faculty research:* Biology of gametes and fertilization, reproductive endocrinology. *Total annual research expenditures:* $5.4 million. *Unit head:* Dr. Yusuke Marikawa, Chair, 808-692-1411.
Website: http://www2.jabsom.hawaii.edu/Grad_DRB/

University of Illinois at Urbana–Champaign, Graduate College, College of Liberal Arts and Sciences, School of Molecular and Cellular Biology, Department of Cell and Developmental Biology, Champaign, IL 61820. Offers PhD.

The University of Kansas, Graduate Studies, College of Liberal Arts and Sciences, Department of Molecular Biosciences, Lawrence, KS 66044. Offers biochemistry and biophysics (MA, PhD); microbiology (MA, PhD); molecular, cellular, and developmental biology (MA, PhD). *Students:* 57 full-time (34 women), 4 part-time (1 woman); includes 9 minority (5 Asian, non-Hispanic/Latino; 2 Hispanic/Latino; 2 Two or more races, non-Hispanic/Latino), 23 international. Average age 27. 78 applicants, 46% accepted, 18 enrolled. In 2015, 3 master's, 7 doctorates awarded. Terminal master's awarded for partial completion of doctoral program. *Entrance requirements:* For master's and doctorate, GRE General Test. Additional exam requirements/recommendations for international students: Required—TOEFL or IELTS. *Application deadline:* For fall admission, 12/15 for domestic and international students. Application fee: $65 ($85 for international students). Electronic applications accepted. *Financial support:* Fellowships, research assistantships, teaching assistantships, health care benefits, and unspecified assistantships available. Financial award application deadline: 3/1. *Faculty research:* Structure and function of proteins, genetics of organism development, molecular genetics, neurophysiology, molecular virology and pathogenics, developmental biology, cell biology. *Unit head:* Susan M. Egan, Chair, 785-864-4294, E-mail: sme@ku.edu. *Application contact:* John Connolly, Graduate Admissions Contact, 785-864-4311, E-mail: jconnolly@ku.edu.
Website: http://www.molecularbiosciences.ku.edu/

The University of Manchester, Faculty of Life Sciences, Manchester, United Kingdom. Offers adaptive organismal biology (M Phil, PhD); animal biology (M Phil, PhD); biochemistry (M Phil, PhD); bioinformatics (M Phil, PhD); biomolecular sciences (M Phil, PhD); biotechnology (M Phil, PhD); cell biology (M Phil, PhD); cell matrix research (M Phil, PhD); channels and transporters (M Phil, PhD); developmental biology (M Phil, PhD); Egyptology (M Phil, PhD); environmental biology (M Phil, PhD); evolutionary biology (M Phil, PhD); gene expression (M Phil, PhD); genetics (M Phil, PhD); history of

science, technology and medicine (M Phil, PhD); immunology (M Phil, PhD); integrative neurobiology and behavior (M Phil, PhD); membrane trafficking (M Phil, PhD); microbiology (M Phil, PhD); molecular and cellular neuroscience (M Phil, PhD); molecular biology (M Phil, PhD); molecular cancer studies (M Phil, PhD); neuroscience (M Phil, PhD); ophthalmology (M Phil, PhD); optometry (M Phil, PhD); organelle function (M Phil, PhD); pharmacology (M Phil, PhD); physiology (M Phil, PhD); plant sciences (M Phil, PhD); stem cell research (M Phil, PhD); structural biology (M Phil, PhD); systems neuroscience (M Phil, PhD); toxicology (M Phil, PhD).

The University of Manchester, School of Dentistry, Manchester, United Kingdom. Offers basic dental sciences (cancer studies) (M Phil, PhD); basic dental sciences (molecular genetics) (M Phil, PhD); basic dental sciences (stem cell biology) (M Phil, PhD); biomaterials sciences and dental technology (M Phil, PhD); dental public health/community dentistry (M Phil, PhD); dental science (clinical) (PhD); endodontology (M Phil, PhD); fixed and removable prosthodontics (M Phil, PhD); operative dentistry (M Phil, PhD); oral and maxillofacial surgery (M Phil, PhD); oral radiology (M Phil, PhD); orthodontics (M Phil, PhD); restorative dentistry (M Phil, PhD).

University of Massachusetts Amherst, Graduate School, Interdisciplinary Programs, Program in Molecular and Cellular Biology, Amherst, MA 01003. Offers biological chemistry and molecular biophysics (PhD); biomedicine (PhD); cellular and developmental biology (PhD). *Program availability:* Part-time. Terminal master's awarded for partial completion of doctoral program. *Degree requirements:* For doctorate, comprehensive exam, thesis/dissertation. *Entrance requirements:* For doctorate, GRE General Test. Additional exam requirements/recommendations for international students: Required—TOEFL (minimum score 550 paper-based; 80 iBT), IELTS (minimum score 6.5). Electronic applications accepted.

University of Miami, Graduate School, Miller School of Medicine, Graduate Programs in Medicine, Department of Cell Biology and Anatomy, Coral Gables, FL 33124. Offers molecular cell and developmental biology (PhD); MD/PhD. *Degree requirements:* For doctorate, thesis/dissertation. *Entrance requirements:* For doctorate, GRE General Test, GRE Subject Test. Additional exam requirements/recommendations for international students: Required—TOEFL. Electronic applications accepted.

University of Michigan, Rackham Graduate School, College of Literature, Science, and the Arts, Department of Molecular, Cellular, and Developmental Biology, Ann Arbor, MI 48109. Offers MS, PhD. *Program availability:* Part-time. *Faculty:* 37 full-time (15 women). *Students:* 90 full-time (54 women), 4 part-time (3 women); includes 11 minority (4 Black or African American, non-Hispanic/Latino; 1 Asian, non-Hispanic/Latino; 6 Hispanic/Latino), 50 international. Average age 26. 106 applicants, 34% accepted, 19 enrolled. In 2015, 12 master's, 10 doctorates awarded. Terminal master's awarded for partial completion of doctoral program. *Degree requirements:* For master's, thesis (for some programs), 24 credits with at least 16 in molecular, cellular, and developmental biology and 4 in a cognate field; for doctorate, thesis/dissertation, preliminary exam, oral defense. *Entrance requirements:* For master's and doctorate, GRE General Test. Additional exam requirements/recommendations for international students: Required—TOEFL (minimum score 560 paper-based; 83 iBT). *Application deadline:* For fall admission, 1/5 for domestic and international students; for winter admission, 11/1 for domestic and international students; for spring admission, 4/1 for domestic and international students. Application fee: $75 ($90 for international students). Electronic applications accepted. *Expenses:* Contact institution. *Financial support:* In 2015–16, 67 students received support, including 23 fellowships with full tuition reimbursements available (averaging $29,025 per year), 28 research assistantships with full tuition reimbursements available (averaging $28,500 per year), 18 teaching assistantships with full tuition reimbursements available (averaging $28,500 per year); traineeships and health care benefits also available. *Faculty research:* Cell biology, microbiology, neurobiology and physiology, developmental biology and plant molecular biology. *Total annual research expenditures:* $8.2 million. *Unit head:* Dr. Robert J. Denver, Department Chair, 734-764-7476, Fax: 734-615-6337, E-mail: rdenver@umich.edu. *Application contact:* Mary Carr, Graduate Coordinator, 734-615-1635, Fax: 734-764-0884, E-mail: carrmm@umich.edu.
Website: http://www.mcdb.lsa.umich.edu

University of Michigan, Rackham Graduate School, Program in Biomedical Sciences (PIBS), Department of Cell and Developmental Biology, Ann Arbor, MI 48109. Offers PhD. *Faculty:* 37 full-time (13 women). *Students:* 21 full-time (11 women); includes 11 minority (9 Asian, non-Hispanic/Latino; 2 Hispanic/Latino). Average age 29. 57 applicants, 18% accepted, 6 enrolled. In 2015, 6 doctorates awarded. *Degree requirements:* For doctorate, thesis/dissertation, oral defense of dissertation, preliminary exam. *Entrance requirements:* For doctorate, GRE General Test, 3 letters of recommendation, research experience. Additional exam requirements/recommendations for international students: Required—TOEFL (minimum score 84 iBT). *Application deadline:* For fall admission, 12/1 for domestic and international students. Application fee: $75 ($90 for international students). Electronic applications accepted. *Financial support:* In 2015–16, fellowships (averaging $29,025 per year) were awarded; scholarships/grants, health care benefits, tuition waivers (full), and unspecified assistantships also available. Financial award application deadline: 12/1. *Faculty research:* Cell signaling, stem cells, organogenesis, cell biology, developmental genetics. *Total annual research expenditures:* $5.8 million. *Unit head:* Dr. Deborah L. Gumucio, Professor/Interim Chair, 734-647-0172, Fax: 734-763-1166, E-mail: dgumucio@umich.edu. *Application contact:* Michelle S. Melis, Director of Student Life, 734-615-6538, Fax: 734-647-7022, E-mail: msmtegan@umich.edu.
Website: http://cdb.med.umich.edu/

University of Minnesota, Twin Cities Campus, Graduate School, Program in Molecular, Cellular, Developmental Biology and Genetics, Minneapolis, MN 55455-0213. Offers genetic counseling (MS); molecular, cellular, developmental biology and genetics (PhD). Terminal master's awarded for partial completion of doctoral program. *Degree requirements:* For master's, thesis optional; for doctorate, thesis/dissertation. *Entrance requirements:* For master's and doctorate, GRE General Test. Additional exam requirements/recommendations for international students: Required—TOEFL (minimum score 625 paper-based; 80 iBT). Electronic applications accepted. *Faculty research:* Membrane receptors and membrane transport, cell interactions, cytoskeleton and cell mobility, regulation of gene expression, plant cell and molecular biology.

University of Minnesota, Twin Cities Campus, Graduate School, Stem Cell Biology Graduate Program, Minneapolis, MN 55455-3007. Offers MS. *Degree requirements:* For master's, thesis. *Entrance requirements:* For master's, GRE, BS, BA, or foreign equivalent in biological sciences or related field; minimum undergraduate GPA of 3.2. Additional exam requirements/recommendations for international students: Required—TOEFL (minimum score 580 paper-based, with a minimum score of 4 in the TWE, or 94 Internet-based, with a minimum score of 22 on each of the reading and listening, 26 on the speaking, and 26 on the writing section. *Faculty research:* Stem cell and developmental biology; embryonic stem cells; iPS cells; muscle satellite cells; hematopoietic stem cells; neuronal stem cells; cardiovascular, kidney and limb development; regenerating systems.

University of Montana, Graduate School, College of Humanities and Sciences, Division of Biological Sciences, Program in Cellular, Molecular and Microbial Biology,

Missoula, MT 59812-0002. Offers cellular and developmental biology (PhD); microbial evolution and ecology (PhD); microbiology and immunology (PhD); molecular biology and biochemistry (PhD). Terminal master's awarded for partial completion of doctoral program. *Degree requirements:* For doctorate, variable foreign language requirement, thesis/dissertation. *Entrance requirements:* For doctorate, GRE General Test. *Faculty research:* Ribosome structure, medical microbiology/pathogenesis, microbial ecology/environmental microbiology.

The University of North Carolina at Chapel Hill, Graduate School, College of Arts and Sciences, Department of Biology, Chapel Hill, NC 27599. Offers botany (MA, MS, PhD); cell biology, development, and physiology (MA, MS, PhD); cell motility and cytoskeleton (PhD); ecology and behavior (MA, MS, PhD); genetics and molecular biology (MA, MS, PhD); morphology, systematics, and evolution (MA, MS, PhD). Terminal master's awarded for partial completion of doctoral program. *Degree requirements:* For master's, comprehensive exam, thesis (for some programs); for doctorate, comprehensive exam, thesis/dissertation. *Entrance requirements:* For master's, GRE General Test, GRE Subject Test, 2 semesters of calculus or statistics; 2 semesters of physics, organic chemistry; 3 semesters of biology; for doctorate, GRE General Test, GRE Subject Test, 2 semesters calculus or statistics, 2 semesters physics, organic chemistry, 3 semesters of biology. Additional exam requirements/recommendations for international students: Required—TOEFL (minimum score 550 paper-based). Electronic applications accepted. *Faculty research:* Gene expression, biomechanics, yeast genetics, plant ecology, plant molecular biology.

The University of North Carolina at Chapel Hill, School of Medicine and Graduate School, Graduate Programs in Medicine, Department of Cell and Developmental Biology, Chapel Hill, NC 27599. Offers PhD. *Degree requirements:* For doctorate, comprehensive exam, thesis/dissertation. *Entrance requirements:* For doctorate, GRE General Test, GRE Subject Test. Electronic applications accepted. *Faculty research:* Cell adhesion, motility and cytoskeleton; molecular analysis of signal transduction; development biology and toxicology; reproductive biology; cell and molecular imaging.

University of Pennsylvania, Perelman School of Medicine, Biomedical Graduate Studies, Graduate Group in Cell and Molecular Biology, Philadelphia, PA 19104. Offers cancer biology (PhD); cell biology, physiology, and metabolism (PhD); developmental stem cell regenerative biology (PhD); gene therapy and vaccines (PhD); genetics and gene regulation (PhD); microbiology, virology, and parasitology (PhD); MD/PhD; VMD/PhD. *Faculty:* 317. *Students:* 339 full-time (189 women); includes 100 minority (7 Black or African American, non-Hispanic/Latino; 2 American Indian or Alaska Native, non-Hispanic/Latino; 45 Asian, non-Hispanic/Latino; 34 Hispanic/Latino; 1 Native Hawaiian or other Pacific Islander, non-Hispanic/Latino; 11 Two or more races, non-Hispanic/Latino), 52 international. 493 applicants, 22% accepted, 37 enrolled. In 2015, 51 doctorates awarded. *Degree requirements:* For doctorate, thesis/dissertation. *Entrance requirements:* For doctorate, GRE General Test. Additional exam requirements/recommendations for international students: Required—TOEFL. *Application deadline:* For fall admission, 12/1 priority date for domestic and international students. Applications are processed on a rolling basis. Application fee: $80. Electronic applications accepted. *Expenses: Tuition, area resident:* Full-time $31,068; part-time $5762 per course. *Required fees:* $3200; $336 per course. Full-time tuition and fees vary according to degree level, program and student level. Part-time tuition and fees vary according to course load, degree level and program. *Financial support:* In 2015–16, 339 students received support. Fellowships, research assistantships, scholarships/grants, traineeships, and unspecified assistantships available. *Unit head:* Dr. Daniel Kessler, Graduate Group Chair, 215-898-1478. *Application contact:* Meagan Schofer, Coordinator, 215-898-4360.
Website: http://www.med.upenn.edu/camb/

University of Pittsburgh, Dietrich School of Arts and Sciences, Department of Biological Sciences, Program in Molecular, Cellular, and Developmental Biology, Pittsburgh, PA 15260. Offers PhD. *Faculty:* 21 full-time (5 women). *Students:* 36 full-time (19 women); includes 2 minority (1 Black or African American, non-Hispanic/Latino; 1 Asian, non-Hispanic/Latino), 8 international. Average age 23. 109 applicants, 24% accepted, 7 enrolled. In 2015, 3 doctorates awarded. *Degree requirements:* For doctorate, comprehensive exam, thesis/dissertation, completion of research integrity module. *Entrance requirements:* For doctorate, GRE General Test, GRE Subject Test. Additional exam requirements/recommendations for international students: Required—TOEFL (minimum score 90 iBT). *Application deadline:* For fall admission, 1/3 priority date for domestic students, 12/9 priority date for international students. Applications are processed on a rolling basis. Application fee: $0 ($50 for international students). Electronic applications accepted. Tuition and fees vary according to program. *Financial support:* In 2015–16, 26 fellowships with full tuition reimbursements (averaging $33,193 per year), 63 research assistantships with full tuition reimbursements (averaging $27,573 per year), 18 teaching assistantships with full tuition reimbursements (averaging $26,813 per year) were awarded; Federal Work-Study, traineeships, health care benefits, and tuition waivers (full) also available. *Unit head:* Dr. Karen M. Arndt, Professor, 412-624-6963, Fax: 412-624-4349, E-mail: arndt@pitt.edu. *Application contact:* Cathleen M. Barr, Graduate Administrator, 412-624-4268, Fax: 412-624-4349, E-mail: cbarr@pitt.edu.
Website: http://www.biology.pitt.edu

University of Pittsburgh, School of Medicine, Graduate Programs in Medicine, Molecular Genetics and Developmental Biology Graduate Program, Pittsburgh, PA 15260. Offers PhD. *Faculty:* 56 full-time (16 women). *Students:* 11 full-time (9 women); includes 5 minority (1 Black or African American, non-Hispanic/Latino; 4 Asian, non-Hispanic/Latino). Average age 29. 386 applicants, 17% accepted, 25 enrolled. In 2015, 3 doctorates awarded. *Degree requirements:* For doctorate, comprehensive exam, thesis/dissertation. *Entrance requirements:* For doctorate, GRE General Test, GRE Subject Test, minimum QPA of 3.0. Additional exam requirements/recommendations for international students: Required—TOEFL (minimum score 600 paper-based; 100 iBT), IELTS (minimum score 7). *Application deadline:* For fall admission, 12/1 priority date for domestic and international students. Application fee: $50. Electronic applications accepted. Tuition and fees vary according to program. *Financial support:* In 2015–16, 11 students received support, including 2 fellowships with full tuition reimbursements available (averaging $27,000 per year), 9 research assistantships with full tuition reimbursements available (averaging $27,000 per year), teaching assistantships with full tuition reimbursements available (averaging $27,000 per year); scholarships/grants, traineeships, and health care benefits also available. *Faculty research:* Developmental and stem cell biology, DNA replication and repair, gene regulation and signal transduction, oncogenes and tumor suppressor genes, protein structure and molecular dynamics. *Unit head:* Dr. Kyle E. Orwig, Graduate Program Director, 412-641-2460, Fax: 412-641-3899, E-mail: korwig@mwri.magee.edu. *Application contact:* Carol Williams, Admissions and Recruiting Manager, 412-648-8957, Fax: 412-648-1077, E-mail: gradstudies@medschool.pitt.edu.
Website: http://www.gradbiomed.pitt.edu/

University of South Carolina, The Graduate School, College of Arts and Sciences, Department of Biological Sciences, Graduate Training Program in Molecular, Cellular, and Developmental Biology, Columbia, SC 29208. Offers MS, PhD. *Degree requirements:* For master's, one foreign language, thesis; for doctorate, one foreign language, thesis/dissertation. *Entrance requirements:* For master's and doctorate, GRE General Test, minimum GPA of 3.0 in science. Electronic applications accepted. *Faculty research:* Marine ecology, population and evolutionary biology, molecular biology and genetics, development.

University of Southern California, Keck School of Medicine, Program in Development, Stem Cells and Regenerative Medicine, Los Angeles, CA 90089. Offers development, stem cells and regenerative medicine (PhD). *Faculty:* 36 full-time (15 women). *Students:* 23 full-time (9 women); includes 4 minority (3 Asian, non-Hispanic/Latino; 1 Hispanic/Latino), 11 international. Average age 26. 1 applicant, 100% accepted, 1 enrolled. *Degree requirements:* For doctorate, comprehensive exam, thesis/dissertation. *Entrance requirements:* For doctorate, GRE, minimum GPA of 3.0. Additional exam requirements/recommendations for international students: Required—TOEFL (minimum score 600 paper-based; 100 iBT), IELTS (minimum score 7), PTE. *Application deadline:* For fall admission, 12/1 priority date for domestic and international students. Application fee: $85. Electronic applications accepted. *Financial support:* In 2015–16, 23 students received support, including 6 fellowships with full tuition reimbursements available (averaging $32,000 per year), 17 research assistantships with full tuition reimbursements available (averaging $32,000 per year); institutionally sponsored loans, scholarships/grants, traineeships, health care benefits, and unspecified assistantships also available. Financial award application deadline: 5/4; financial award applicants required to submit CSS PROFILE or FAFSA. *Unit head:* Dr. Gage Crump, Director, 323-442-1475, Fax: 323-442-1199, E-mail: gcrump@med.usc.edu. *Application contact:* Dr. Joyce Perez, Manager of Student Programs, 323-442-1645, Fax: 323-442-1199, E-mail: jpperez@med.usc.edu.
Website: http://pibbs.usc.edu/research-and-programs/phd-programs/

The University of Texas Health Science Center at Houston, Graduate School of Biomedical Sciences, Program in Genes and Development, Houston, TX 77225-0036. Offers MS, PhD, MD/PhD. Terminal master's awarded for partial completion of doctoral program. *Degree requirements:* For master's, thesis; for doctorate, thesis/dissertation. *Entrance requirements:* For master's and doctorate, GRE General Test. Additional exam requirements/recommendations for international students: Required—TOEFL. Electronic applications accepted. *Faculty research:* Developmental biology, genetics, cell biology, structural biology, cancer.

The University of Texas Southwestern Medical Center, Southwestern Graduate School of Biomedical Sciences, Division of Basic Science, Program in Genetics and Development, Dallas, TX 75390. Offers PhD. *Degree requirements:* For doctorate, thesis/dissertation, qualifying exam. *Entrance requirements:* For doctorate, GRE General Test, minimum GPA of 3.0. Additional exam requirements/recommendations for international students: Required—TOEFL. Electronic applications accepted. *Faculty research:* Human molecular genetics, chromosome structure, gene regulation, molecular biology, gene expression.

Vanderbilt University, School of Medicine, Department of Cell and Developmental Biology, Nashville, TN 37240-1001. Offers MS, PhD, MD/PhD. *Faculty:* 20 full-time (6 women). *Students:* 71 full-time (46 women); includes 16 minority (4 Black or African American, non-Hispanic/Latino; 3 Asian, non-Hispanic/Latino; 6 Hispanic/Latino; 1 Native Hawaiian or other Pacific Islander, non-Hispanic/Latino; 2 Two or more races, non-Hispanic/Latino), 11 international. Average age 27. 2 applicants, 100% accepted, 3 enrolled. In 2015, 17 doctorates awarded. Terminal master's awarded for partial completion of doctoral program. *Degree requirements:* For master's, thesis or alternative; for doctorate, thesis/dissertation, preliminary, qualifying, and final exams. *Entrance requirements:* For master's, GRE General Test; for doctorate, GRE General Test, GRE Subject Test (recommended). Additional exam requirements/recommendations for international students: Required—TOEFL (minimum score 570 paper-based; 88 iBT). *Application deadline:* For fall admission, 1/15 for domestic and international students. Application fee: $0. Electronic applications accepted. *Financial support:* Fellowships with tuition reimbursements, research assistantships with tuition reimbursements, career-related internships or fieldwork, Federal Work-Study, institutionally sponsored loans, scholarships/grants, traineeships, health care benefits, and tuition waivers (partial) available. Financial award application deadline: 1/15; financial award applicants required to submit CSS PROFILE or FAFSA. *Faculty research:* Cancer biology, cell cycle regulation, cell signaling, cytoskeletal biology, developmental biology, neurobiology, proteomics, stem cell biology, structural biology, reproductive biology, trafficking and transport, medical education and gross anatomy. *Unit head:* Dr. Steve Hann, Director of Graduate Studies, 615-322-2134, Fax: 615-343-4539, E-mail: steve.hann@vanderbilt.edu. *Application contact:* Kristi Hargrove, Coordinator, 615-322-2294, Fax: 615-343-4539, E-mail: kristi.l.hargrove@vanderbilt.edu.
Website: http://www.mc.vanderbilt.edu/cdb/

Washington University in St. Louis, Graduate School of Arts and Sciences, Division of Biology and Biomedical Sciences, Program in Developmental, Regenerative, and Stem Cell Biology, St. Louis, MO 63130-4899. Offers PhD. *Students:* 31 full-time (17 women); includes 7 minority (2 Black or African American, non-Hispanic/Latino; 3 Asian, non-Hispanic/Latino; 2 Hispanic/Latino), 6 international. 85 applicants, 25% accepted, 5 enrolled. In 2015, 5 doctorates awarded. *Degree requirements:* For doctorate, thesis/dissertation. *Entrance requirements:* For doctorate, GRE General Test, GRE Subject Test. Additional exam requirements/recommendations for international students: Required—TOEFL. *Application deadline:* For fall admission, 12/1 for domestic students. Application fee: $0. Electronic applications accepted. *Financial support:* Fellowships, research assistantships, and teaching assistantships available. Financial award application deadline: 1/15. *Faculty research:* Development, stem cell biology, regenerative biology, cell reprogramming, cell biology, genetics, cell signaling, the biology of cancer, epigenetics, circadian rhythms, systems biology. *Unit head:* Sally Vogt, Coordinator, 314-362-7189, E-mail: vogts@wustl.edu. *Application contact:* Rebecca Riney, 314-747-4648, E-mail: dbbsphdadmissions@wusm.wustl.edu.
Website: http://dbbs.wustl.edu/divprograms/devbio/Pages/default.aspx

Wesleyan University, Graduate Studies, Department of Biology, Middletown, CT 06459. Offers cell and developmental biology (PhD); evolution and ecology (PhD); genetics and genomics (PhD), including bioinformatics; neurobiology and behavior (PhD). *Faculty:* 14 full-time (5 women). *Students:* 26 full-time (12 women); includes 5 minority (2 Black or African American, non-Hispanic/Latino; 3 Asian, non-Hispanic/Latino), 5 international. In 2015, 3 doctorates awarded. Terminal master's awarded for partial completion of doctoral program. *Degree requirements:* For doctorate, comprehensive exam, thesis/dissertation, public seminar. *Entrance requirements:* For doctorate, GRE. Additional exam requirements/recommendations for international students: Required—TOEFL or IELTS. *Application deadline:* For fall admission, 1/15 for domestic and international students. Application fee: $0. Electronic applications accepted. *Financial support:* Stipends available. *Faculty research:* Evolution and ecology, neurobiology and behavior, cell and developmental biology, genetics, genomics and bioinformatics. *Unit head:* Dr. John Kirn, Chair/Professor, 860-685-3494, E-mail: jrkirn@wesleyan.edu. *Application contact:* Marjorie Fitzgibbons, Administrative Assistant, 860-685-2157, E-mail: mfitzgibbons@wesleyan.edu.
Website: http://www.wesleyan.edu/bio/

Developmental Biology

West Virginia University, Davis College of Agriculture, Forestry and Consumer Sciences, Interdisciplinary Program in Genetics and Developmental Biology, Morgantown, WV 26506. Offers animal breeding (MS, PhD); biochemical and molecular genetics (MS, PhD); cytogenetics (MS, PhD); descriptive embryology (MS, PhD); developmental genetics (MS); experimental morphogenesis/teratology (MS); human genetics (MS, PhD); immunogenetics (MS, PhD); life cycles of animals and plants (MS, PhD); molecular aspects of development (MS, PhD); mutagenesis (MS, PhD); oncology (MS, PhD); plant genetics (MS, PhD); population and quantitative genetics (MS, PhD); regeneration (MS, PhD); teratology (PhD); toxicology (MS, PhD). *Degree requirements:* For master's, thesis; for doctorate, comprehensive exam, thesis/dissertation. *Entrance requirements:* For master's, GRE or MCAT, minimum GPA of 2.75. Additional exam requirements/recommendations for international students: Required—TOEFL. *Expenses:* Tuition, state resident: full-time $8568. Tuition, nonresident: full-time $22,140. Tuition and fees vary according to program.

Yale University, Graduate School of Arts and Sciences, Department of Molecular, Cellular, and Developmental Biology, New Haven, CT 06520. Offers biochemistry, molecular biology and chemical biology (PhD); cellular and developmental biology (PhD); genetics (PhD); neurobiology (PhD); plant sciences (PhD). *Degree requirements:* For doctorate, thesis/dissertation. *Entrance requirements:* For doctorate, GRE General Test, GRE Subject Test.

Genetics

Albert Einstein College of Medicine, Graduate Division of Biomedical Sciences, Department of Genetics, Bronx, NY 10461. Offers computational genetics (PhD); molecular genetics (PhD); translational genetics (PhD); MD/PhD. *Degree requirements:* For doctorate, thesis/dissertation. *Entrance requirements:* For doctorate, GRE General Test. Additional exam requirements/recommendations for international students: Required—TOEFL. *Faculty research:* Neurologic genetics in &ITDrosophila&RO, biochemical genetics of yeast, developmental genetics in the mouse.

American University of Beirut, Graduate Programs, Faculty of Medicine, Beirut, Lebanon. Offers anatomy, cell biology and human morphology (MS); biochemistry and medical genetics (MS); biomedical sciences (PhD); experimental pathology, immunology and microbiology (MS); medicine (MD); neuroscience (MS); pharmacology and toxicology (MS). *Program availability:* Part-time. *Faculty:* 302 full-time (95 women), 64 part-time/adjunct (11 women). *Students:* 381 full-time (173 women), 61 part-time (51 women). Average age 23. In 2015, 14 master's awarded. *Degree requirements:* For master's, one foreign language, comprehensive exam, thesis (for some programs); for doctorate, one foreign language, comprehensive exam, thesis/dissertation. *Entrance requirements:* For master's, letter of recommendation; for doctorate, MCAT, bachelor's degree. Additional exam requirements/recommendations for international students: Required—TOEFL (minimum score 600 paper-based; 100 iBT), IELTS (minimum score 7.5). *Application deadline:* For fall admission, 4/30 for domestic and international students; for spring admission, 11/1 for domestic and international students. Application fee: $50. Electronic applications accepted. *Expenses: Tuition, area resident:* Full-time $16,254; part-time $903 per credit. *Required fees:* $699. Tuition and fees vary according to course load and program. *Financial support:* In 2015–16, 273 students received support, including 45 teaching assistantships (averaging $9,000 per year); career-related internships or fieldwork, institutionally sponsored loans, scholarships/grants, health care benefits, and unspecified assistantships also available. Financial award application deadline: 2/2. *Faculty research:* Cancer research (targeted therapy, mechanisms of leukemogenesis, tumor cell extravasation and metastasis, cancer stem cells), stem cell research (regenerative medicine, drug discovery), genetic research (neurogenetics, hereditary cardiomyopathy, hemoglobinopathies, pharmacogenomics, proteomics), neuroscience research (pain, neurodegenerative disorder), metabolism (inflammation and metabolism, metabolic disorder, diabetes mellitus); vascular and renal biology, signal transduction. *Total annual research expenditures:* $2.6 million. *Unit head:* Dr. Mohamed Sayegh, Dean, 961-1350000 Ext. 4700, Fax: 961-1744464, E-mail: msayegh@aub.edu.lb. *Application contact:* Dr. Salim Kanaan, Director, Admissions Office, 961-1350000 Ext. 2594, Fax: 961-1750775, E-mail: sk00@aub.edu.lb. Website: http://www.aub.edu.lb/fm/fm_home/Pages/index.aspx

Baylor College of Medicine, Graduate School of Biomedical Sciences, Department of Molecular and Human Genetics, Houston, TX 77030-3498. Offers PhD, MD/PhD. *Degree requirements:* For doctorate, thesis/dissertation, public defense. *Entrance requirements:* For doctorate, GRE General Test, GRE Subject Test (strongly recommended), minimum GPA of 3.0. Additional exam requirements/recommendations for international students: Required—TOEFL. Electronic applications accepted. *Faculty research:* Human genetics, genome biology, epigenetics, gene therapy, model organisms.

Baylor College of Medicine, Graduate School of Biomedical Sciences, Interdepartmental Program in Cell and Molecular Biology, Houston, TX 77030-3498. Offers biochemistry (PhD); cell and molecular biology (PhD); genetics (PhD); human genetics (PhD); immunology (PhD); microbiology (PhD); virology (PhD); MD/PhD. *Degree requirements:* For doctorate, thesis/dissertation, public defense. *Entrance requirements:* For doctorate, GRE General Test, GRE Subject Test (strongly recommended), minimum GPA of 3.0. Additional exam requirements/recommendations for international students: Required—TOEFL. Electronic applications accepted. *Faculty research:* Molecular and cellular biology; cancer, aging and stem cells; genomics and proteomics; microbiome, molecular microbiology; infectious disease, immunology and translational research.

Baylor College of Medicine, Graduate School of Biomedical Sciences, Program in Developmental Biology, Houston, TX 77030-3498. Offers PhD, MD/PhD. *Degree requirements:* For doctorate, thesis/dissertation, public defense. *Entrance requirements:* For doctorate, GRE General Test, GRE Subject Test (strongly recommended), minimum GPA of 3.0. Additional exam requirements/recommendations for international students: Required—TOEFL. Electronic applications accepted. *Faculty research:* Stem cells, cancer, neurobiology, organogenesis, genetics of model organisms.

Baylor College of Medicine, Graduate School of Biomedical Sciences, Program in Translational Biology and Molecular Medicine, Houston, TX 77030-3498. Offers PhD. *Degree requirements:* For doctorate, thesis/dissertation, public defense. *Entrance requirements:* For doctorate, GRE, minimum GPA of 3.0. Additional exam requirements/recommendations for international students: Required—TOEFL. Electronic applications accepted. *Faculty research:* Molecular medicine, translational biology, human disease biology and therapy.

Boston University, School of Medicine, Division of Graduate Medical Sciences, Program in Genetics and Genomics, Boston, MA 02215. Offers PhD. *Degree requirements:* For doctorate, thesis/dissertation. *Application deadline:* For fall admission, 1/15 for domestic students; for spring admission, 10/15 for domestic students. *Unit head:* Dr. Shoumita Dasgupta, Associate Professor and Director of Graduate Studies, 617-414-1580, E-mail: dasgupta@bu.edu. *Application contact:* GMS Admissions Office, 617-638-5255, E-mail: askgms@bu.edu. Website: http://www.bumc.bu.edu/gpgg/graduate-program/

Brandeis University, Graduate School of Arts and Sciences, Program in Molecular and Cell Biology, Waltham, MA 02454-9110. Offers genetics (PhD); microbiology (PhD); molecular and cell biology (MS, PhD); molecular biology (PhD); neurobiology (PhD); quantitative biology (PhD). *Faculty:* 26 full-time (12 women), 4 part-time/adjunct (2 women). *Students:* 60 full-time (30 women); includes 5 minority (1 Black or African American, non-Hispanic/Latino; 1 American Indian or Alaska Native, non-Hispanic/Latino; 1 Asian, non-Hispanic/Latino; 2 Hispanic/Latino), 25 international. 183 applicants, 27% accepted, 12 enrolled. In 2015, 13 master's, 7 doctorates awarded. Terminal master's awarded for partial completion of doctoral program. *Degree requirements:* For master's, thesis optional, research project, research lab, or project lab; for doctorate, comprehensive exam, thesis/dissertation, journal clubs; research seminar; colloquia; qualifying exam. *Entrance requirements:* For master's, GRE General Test, official transcript(s), resume, 2 letters of recommendation, statement of purpose; for doctorate, GRE General Test, official transcript(s), resume, 3 letters of recommendation, statement of purpose, list of previous research experience. Additional exam requirements/recommendations for international students: Required—TOEFL (minimum score 600 paper-based; 100 iBT); Recommended—IELTS (minimum score 7), TSE (minimum score 68). *Application deadline:* For fall admission, 12/15 priority date for domestic students. Application fee: $75. Electronic applications accepted. *Financial support:* In 2015–16, 35 students received support, including 16 fellowships with full tuition reimbursements available (averaging $30,500 per year), 19 research assistantships with full tuition reimbursements available (averaging $30,500 per year); scholarships/grants and tuition waivers (partial) also available. Financial award application deadline: 4/15; financial award applicants required to submit FAFSA. *Faculty research:* Molecular biology, genetics and development; structural and cell biology; neurobiology. *Unit head:* Dr. Maria Miara, Director of Graduate Studies, 781-736-2300, Fax: 781-736-3107, E-mail: scigradoffice@brandeis.edu. *Application contact:* Dr. Maryanna Aldrich, Department Administrator, 781-736-2300, Fax: 781-736-3107, E-mail: scigradoffice@brandeis.edu.
Website: http://www.brandeis.edu/gsas

California Institute of Technology, Division of Biology, Program in Genetics, Pasadena, CA 91125-0001. Offers PhD. *Degree requirements:* For doctorate, thesis/dissertation, qualifying exam. *Entrance requirements:* For doctorate, GRE General Test.

Carnegie Mellon University, Mellon College of Science, Department of Biological Sciences, Pittsburgh, PA 15213-3891. Offers biochemistry (PhD); biophysics (PhD); cell and developmental biology (PhD); computational biology (MS, PhD); genetics (PhD); molecular biology (PhD); neuroscience (PhD); structural biology (PhD). *Degree requirements:* For doctorate, comprehensive exam, thesis/dissertation. *Entrance requirements:* For doctorate, GRE General Test, GRE Subject Test, interview. Electronic applications accepted. *Faculty research:* Genetic structure, function, and regulation; protein structure and function; biological membranes; biological spectroscopy.

Case Western Reserve University, School of Medicine and School of Graduate Studies, Graduate Programs in Medicine, Department of Genetics and Genome Sciences, Program in Human, Molecular, and Developmental Genetics and Genomics, Cleveland, OH 44106. Offers PhD, MD/PhD. *Degree requirements:* For doctorate, comprehensive exam, thesis/dissertation. *Entrance requirements:* For doctorate, GRE General Test, GRE Subject Test. Additional exam requirements/recommendations for international students: Required—TOEFL. *Expenses: Tuition, area resident:* Full-time $41,137; part-time $1714 per credit hour. *Required fees:* $32. Tuition and fees vary according to course load and program. *Faculty research:* Regulation of gene expression, molecular control of development, genomics.

Clemson University, Graduate School, College of Behavioral, Social and Health Sciences, School of Nursing, Clemson, SC 29634-0743. Offers healthcare genetics (PhD); nursing (MS). *Accreditation:* AACN. *Program availability:* Part-time. *Faculty:* 30 full-time (28 women), 2 part-time/adjunct (both women). *Students:* 33 full-time (29 women), 76 part-time (65 women); includes 10 minority (3 Black or African American, non-Hispanic/Latino; 1 American Indian or Alaska Native, non-Hispanic/Latino; 2 Hispanic/Latino; 4 Two or more races, non-Hispanic/Latino), 6 international. Average age 39. 20 applicants, 85% accepted, 13 enrolled. In 2015, 40 master's, 1 doctorate awarded. *Degree requirements:* For master's, comprehensive exam, thesis or alternative; for doctorate, comprehensive exam, thesis/dissertation. *Entrance requirements:* For master's, GRE General Test, South Carolina RN license, unofficial transcripts, resume, letters of recommendation; for doctorate, GRE General Test, unofficial transcripts, MS/MA thesis or publications, curriculum vitae, statement of career goals, letters of recommendation. Additional exam requirements/recommendations for international students: Required—TOEFL (minimum score 80 iBT), IELTS (minimum score 6.5). *Application deadline:* For fall admission, 3/1 priority date for domestic and international students; for spring admission, 10/1 priority date for domestic and international students. Application fee: $80 ($90 for international students). Electronic applications accepted. *Expenses:* $5,349 per semester full-time resident, $10,683 per semester full-time non-resident, $663 per credit hour part-time resident, $1,327 per credit hour part-time non-resident. *Financial support:* In 2015–16, 37 students received support, including 4 fellowships with partial tuition reimbursements available (averaging $6,848 per year), 2 research assistantships with partial tuition reimbursements available (averaging $8,874 per year), 26 teaching assistantships with partial tuition reimbursements available (averaging $6,877 per year); career-related internships or fieldwork, health care benefits, and unspecified assistantships also available. Financial award application deadline: 3/1. *Faculty research:* Breast cancer, healthcare, genetics, international healthcare, educational innovation and technology. *Total annual research expenditures:* $503,531. *Unit head:* Dr. Rosanne Pruitt, Director and Associate College Dean, 864-656-7622, Fax: 864-656-5488, E-mail: prosan@clemson.edu. *Application contact:* Dr. Stephanie Davis, Graduate Studies Coordinator, 864-656-2588, Fax: 864-

656-5488, E-mail: stephad@clemson.edu.
Website: http://www.clemson.edu/nursing/

Clemson University, Graduate School, College of Science, Department of Genetics and Biochemistry, Program in Genetics, Clemson, SC 29634. Offers PhD. *Faculty:* 28 full-time (14 women), 1 (woman) part-time/adjunct. *Students:* 13 full-time (6 women), 1 (woman) part-time; includes 1 minority (Hispanic/Latino), 5 international. Average age 27. 20 applicants, 30% accepted, 3 enrolled. In 2015, 3 doctorates awarded. *Degree requirements:* For doctorate, comprehensive exam, thesis/dissertation. *Entrance requirements:* For doctorate, GRE General Test, unofficial transcripts, letters of recommendation. Additional exam requirements/recommendations for international students: Required—TOEFL (minimum score 80 iBT), IELTS (minimum score 6.5). *Application deadline:* For fall admission, 1/1 for domestic and international students; for spring admission, 9/1 for domestic and international students. Application fee: $80 ($90 for international students). Electronic applications accepted. *Expenses:* $4,060 per semester full-time resident, $8,103 per semester full-time non-resident, $448 per credit hour part-time resident, $898 per credit hour part-time non-resident. *Financial support:* In 2015–16, 14 students received support, including 7 fellowships with partial tuition reimbursements available (averaging $4,707 per year), 9 research assistantships with partial tuition reimbursements available (averaging $21,571 per year), 4 teaching assistantships with partial tuition reimbursements available (averaging $21,391 per year); health care benefits also available. Financial award application deadline: 1/1. *Faculty research:* Animal genetics, genomics, bioinformatics, population genetics. *Unit head:* Dr. William Marcotte, Jr., Department Chair, 864-656-3586, Fax: 864-656-6879, E-mail: marcotw@clemson.edu. *Application contact:* Nicole Clark-Mount, Administrative Assistant, 864-656-6237, Fax: 864-656-6879, E-mail: nicolec@clemson.edu. Website: http://www.clemson.edu/genbiochem/graduate_programs/

Columbia University, College of Physicians and Surgeons, Department of Genetics and Development, New York, NY 10032. Offers genetics (M Phil, MA, PhD); MD/PhD. Only candidates for the PhD are admitted. Terminal master's awarded for partial completion of doctoral program. *Degree requirements:* For doctorate, thesis/dissertation. *Entrance requirements:* For master's and doctorate, GRE General Test. Additional exam requirements/recommendations for international students: Required—TOEFL. *Faculty research:* Mammalian cell differentiation and meiosis, developmental genetics, yeast and human genetics, chromosome structure, molecular and cellular biology.

Columbia University, College of Physicians and Surgeons, Integrated Program in Cellular, Molecular, Structural and Genetic Studies, New York, NY 10032. Offers PhD. Terminal master's awarded for partial completion of doctoral program. *Degree requirements:* For doctorate, thesis/dissertation. *Entrance requirements:* For doctorate, GRE General Test, GRE Subject Test. Additional exam requirements/recommendations for international students: Required—TOEFL. *Expenses:* Contact institution. *Faculty research:* Transcription, macromolecular sorting, gene expression during development, cellular interaction.

Cornell University, Graduate School, Graduate Fields of Agriculture and Life Sciences, Field of Computational Biology, Ithaca, NY 14853-0001. Offers computational behavioral biology (PhD); computational biology (PhD); computational cell biology (PhD); computational ecology (PhD); computational genetics (PhD); computational macromolecular biology (PhD); computational organismal biology (PhD). *Degree requirements:* For doctorate, comprehensive exam, thesis/dissertation, 2 semesters of teaching experience. *Entrance requirements:* For doctorate, GRE General Test, GRE Subject Test (biology), 2 letters of recommendation. Additional exam requirements/recommendations for international students: Required—TOEFL (minimum score 550 paper-based; 77 iBT). Electronic applications accepted. *Faculty research:* Computational behavioral biology, computational biology, computational cell biology, computational ecology, computational genetics, computational macromolecular biology, computational organismal biology.

Cornell University, Graduate School, Graduate Fields of Agriculture and Life Sciences, Field of Genetics, Genomics and Development, Ithaca, NY 14853-0001. Offers developmental biology (PhD); genetics (PhD); genomics (PhD). *Degree requirements:* For doctorate, comprehensive exam, thesis/dissertation, 2 semesters of teaching experience. *Entrance requirements:* For doctorate, GRE General Test, GRE Subject Test in biology or biochemistry (recommended), 2 letters of recommendation. Additional exam requirements/recommendations for international students: Required—TOEFL (minimum score 550 paper-based; 77 iBT). Electronic applications accepted. *Faculty research:* Molecular and general genetics, developmental biology and developmental genetics, evolution and population genetics, plant genetics, microbial genetics.

Dartmouth College, Graduate Program in Molecular and Cellular Biology, Department of Genetics, Hanover, NH 03755. Offers PhD, MBA/PhD, MD/PhD. *Faculty:* 7 full-time (1 woman), 1 part-time/adjunct (0 women). *Students:* 30 full-time (16 women); includes 8 minority (5 Asian, non-Hispanic/Latino; 3 Hispanic/Latino), 13 international. Average age 27. In 2015, 8 doctorates awarded. *Entrance requirements:* For doctorate, GRE General Test, letters of recommendation, minimum GPA of 3.0. Additional exam requirements/recommendations for international students: Required—TOEFL (minimum score paper-based 550, iBT 100) or IELTS (7.0). *Application deadline:* For fall admission, 12/1 for domestic students. Application fee: $75. Electronic applications accepted. *Expenses:* Tuition, area resident: Full-time $48,120. *Required fees:* $296. One-time fee: $50 full-time. *Financial support:* In 2015–16, fellowships with full tuition reimbursements (averaging $28,200 per year) were awarded; health care benefits also available. *Unit head:* Dr. Jay C. Dunlap, Chair and Professor, 603-650-1108, E-mail: genetics@dartmouth.edu. *Application contact:* Janet Cheney, Program Coordinator, 603-650-1612, Fax: 603-650-1006, E-mail: mcb@dartmouth.edu. Website: http://www.dartmouth.edu/~genetics/

Drexel University, College of Medicine, Biomedical Graduate Programs, Interdisciplinary Program in Molecular and Cell Biology and Genetics, Philadelphia, PA 19104-2875. Offers MS, PhD, MD/PhD. Terminal master's awarded for partial completion of doctoral program. *Degree requirements:* For master's, comprehensive exam, thesis; for doctorate, thesis/dissertation, qualifying exam. *Entrance requirements:* For master's, GRE General Test, minimum GPA of 2.75; for doctorate, GRE General Test, minimum GPA of 3.0. Additional exam requirements/recommendations for international students: Required—TOEFL. Electronic applications accepted. *Faculty research:* Molecular anatomy, biochemistry, medical biotechnology, molecular pathology, microbiology and immunology.

Duke University, Graduate School, Department of Biochemistry, Durham, NC 27710. Offers crystallography of macromolecules (PhD); enzyme mechanisms (PhD); lipid biochemistry (PhD); membrane structure and function (PhD); molecular genetics (PhD); neurochemistry (PhD); nucleic acid structure and function (PhD); protein structure and function (PhD). *Degree requirements:* For doctorate, thesis/dissertation. *Entrance requirements:* For doctorate, GRE General Test, GRE Subject Test (recommended). Additional exam requirements/recommendations for international students: Required—TOEFL (minimum score 577 paper-based; 90 iBT) or IELTS (minimum score 7). Electronic applications accepted.

Duke University, Graduate School, University Program in Genetics and Genomics, Durham, NC 27710. Offers PhD. *Degree requirements:* For doctorate, variable foreign language requirement, thesis/dissertation. *Entrance requirements:* For doctorate, GRE General Test. Additional exam requirements/recommendations for international students: Required—TOEFL (minimum score 577 paper-based; 90 iBT) or IELTS (minimum score 7).

Emory University, Laney Graduate School, Division of Biological and Biomedical Sciences, Program in Genetics and Molecular Biology, Atlanta, GA 30322-1100. Offers PhD. *Degree requirements:* For doctorate, comprehensive exam, thesis/dissertation. *Entrance requirements:* For doctorate, GRE General Test, minimum GPA of 3.0 in science course work (recommended). Additional exam requirements/recommendations for international students: Required—TOEFL. Electronic applications accepted. *Faculty research:* Gene regulation, genetic combination, developmental regulation.

Harvard University, Graduate School of Arts and Sciences, Division of Medical Sciences, Boston, MA 02115. Offers biological chemistry and molecular pharmacology (PhD); cell biology (PhD); genetics (PhD); microbiology and molecular genetics (PhD); pathology (PhD), including experimental pathology. *Degree requirements:* For doctorate, thesis/dissertation. *Entrance requirements:* For doctorate, GRE General Test, GRE Subject Test. Additional exam requirements/recommendations for international students: Required—TOEFL.

Illinois State University, Graduate School, College of Arts and Sciences, Department of Biological Sciences, Normal, IL 61790-2200. Offers animal behavior (MS); bacteriology (MS); biochemistry (MS); biological sciences (MS); biology (PhD); biophysics (MS); biotechnology (MS); botany (MS, PhD); cell biology (MS); conservation biology (MS); developmental biology (MS); ecology (MS, PhD); entomology (MS); evolutionary biology (MS); genetics (MS, PhD); immunology (MS); microbiology (MS, PhD); molecular biology (MS); molecular genetics (MS); neurobiology (MS); neuroscience (MS); parasitology (MS); physiology (MS, PhD); plant biology (MS); plant molecular biology (MS); plant sciences (MS); structural biology (MS); zoology (MS, PhD). *Program availability:* Part-time. *Degree requirements:* For master's, thesis or alternative; for doctorate, variable foreign language requirement, thesis/dissertation, 2 terms of residency. *Entrance requirements:* For master's, GRE General Test, minimum GPA of 2.6 in last 60 hours of course work; for doctorate, GRE General Test. *Application deadline:* Applications are processed on a rolling basis. Application fee: $40. *Financial support:* Research assistantships, teaching assistantships, Federal Work-Study, tuition waivers (full), and unspecified assistantships available. Financial award application deadline: 4/1. *Faculty research:* Redox balance and drug development in schistosoma mansoni, control of the growth of listeria monocytogenes at low temperature, regulation of cell expansion and microtubule function by SPRI, CRUI: physiology and fitness consequences of different life history phenotypes. *Application contact:* Steven Juliano, Graduate Coordinator, E-mail: sajulian@ilstu.edu. Website: http://www.bio.ilstu.edu/

Indiana University Bloomington, University Graduate School, College of Arts and Sciences, Department of Biology, Bloomington, IN 47405. Offers biology teaching (MAT); biotechnology (MA); evolution, ecology, and behavior (MA, PhD); genetics (PhD); microbiology (MA); molecular, cellular, and developmental biology (PhD); plant sciences (MA, PhD); zoology (MA, PhD). Terminal master's awarded for partial completion of doctoral program. *Degree requirements:* For master's, thesis, oral defense; for doctorate, thesis/dissertation, oral defense. *Entrance requirements:* For master's and doctorate, GRE General Test. Additional exam requirements/recommendations for international students: Required—TOEFL (minimum score 100 iBT). Electronic applications accepted. *Faculty research:* Evolution, ecology and behavior; microbiology; molecular biology and genetics; plant biology.

Iowa State University of Science and Technology, Bioinformatics and Computational Biology Program, Ames, IA 50011. Offers MS, PhD. *Degree requirements:* For doctorate, thesis/dissertation. *Entrance requirements:* For master's and doctorate, GRE General Test. Additional exam requirements/recommendations for international students: Recommended—TOEFL, IELTS. Electronic applications accepted. *Faculty research:* Functional and structural genomics, genome evolution, macromolecular structure and function, mathematical biology and biological statistics, metabolic and developmental networks.

Iowa State University of Science and Technology, Program in Genetics, Ames, IA 50011. Offers MS, PhD. *Entrance requirements:* For master's and doctorate, GRE General Test. Additional exam requirements/recommendations for international students: Required—TOEFL (minimum score 550 paper-based; 79 iBT), IELTS (minimum score 6.5). Electronic applications accepted.

Irell & Manella Graduate School of Biological Sciences, Graduate Program, Duarte, CA 91010. Offers brain metastatic cancer (PhD); cancer and stem cell metabolism (PhD); cancer biology (PhD); cancer biology and developmental therapeutics (PhD); cell biology (PhD); chemical biology (PhD); chromosomal break repair (PhD); diabetes and pancreatic progenitor cell biology (PhD); DNA repair and cancer biology (PhD); germline epigenetic remodeling and endocrine disruptors (PhD); hematology and hematopoietic cell transplantation (PhD); hematology and immunology (PhD); inflammation and cancer (PhD); micrornas and gene regulation in cardiovascular disease (PhD); mixed chimrism for reversal of autoimmunity (PhD); molecular and cellular biology (PhD); molecular biology and genetics (PhD); nanoparticle mediated twist1 silencing in metastatic cancer (PhD); neuro-oncology and stem cell biology (PhD); neuroscience (PhD); rna directed therapies for hiv-1 (PhD); small rna-induced transcriptional gene activation (PhD); stem cell regulation by the microenvironment (PhD); translational oncology and pharmaceutical sciences (PhD); tumor biology (PhD). *Faculty:* 70 full-time (18 women). *Students:* 75 full-time (40 women); includes 28 minority (2 Black or African American, non-Hispanic/Latino; 10 Asian, non-Hispanic/Latino; 10 Hispanic/Latino; 2 Native Hawaiian or other Pacific Islander, non-Hispanic/Latino; 4 Two or more races, non-Hispanic/Latino), 15 international. Average age 26. 197 applicants, 12% accepted, 19 enrolled. In 2015, 12 doctorates awarded. *Degree requirements:* For doctorate, comprehensive exam, thesis/dissertation, qualifying exams, two advanced courses. *Entrance requirements:* For doctorate, GRE General Test; GRE Subject Test (recommended), 2 years of course work in chemistry (general and organic); 1 year of course work each in biochemistry, general biology, and general physics; 2 semesters of course work in mathematics; significant research laboratory experience. Additional exam requirements/recommendations for international students: Required—TOEFL. *Application deadline:* For fall admission, 1/1 priority date for domestic and international students. Application fee: $0. Electronic applications accepted. Full-time tuition and fees vary according to class time, course level, course load, degree level, campus/location, program and student level. *Financial support:* In 2015–16, 12 students received support, including 35 fellowships with full tuition reimbursements available (averaging $32,000 per year); teaching assistantships, health care benefits, and tuition waivers (full) also available. Financial award applicants required to submit FAFSA. *Faculty research:* Cancer biology, diabetes, stem cell biology, neuroscience, immunology. *Unit head:* Dr. John J. Rossi, Dean, 877-715-GRAD, Fax: 626-471-3901, E-mail: gradschool@coh.org. *Application contact:* Dr. Kate Sleeth, Interim Associate Dean of Administration and Student Development, 626-218-1742, Fax: 626-471-3901, E-mail: gradschool@coh.org. Website: http://cityofhope.org/gradschool

See Display on page 66 and Close-Up on page 111.

Genetics

Johns Hopkins University, Bloomberg School of Public Health, Department of Epidemiology, Baltimore, MD 21205. Offers cancer etiology and prevention (MHS, Sc M, PhD, Sc D); cardiovascular diseases (MHS, Sc M, PhD, Sc D); clinical epidemiology (MHS, Sc M, PhD, Sc D); clinical trials (PhD, Sc D); epidemiology (MHS, Sc M, Dr PH, PhD, Sc D); epidemiology of aging (MHS, Sc M, PhD, Sc D); genetic epidemiology (MHS, Sc M, PhD, Sc D); infectious disease epidemiology (MHS, Sc M, PhD, Sc D); occupational and environmental epidemiology (MHS, Sc M, PhD, Sc D). *Program availability:* Part-time. *Degree requirements:* For master's, comprehensive exam, thesis, 1-year full-time residency; for doctorate, comprehensive exam, thesis/dissertation, 2 years' full-time residency, oral and written exams, student teaching. *Entrance requirements:* For master's, GRE General Test or MCAT, 3 letters of recommendation, curriculum vitae; for doctorate, GRE General Test, minimum 1 year of work experience, 3 letters of recommendation, curriculum vitae, academic records from all schools. Additional exam requirements/recommendations for international students: Required—TOEFL (minimum score 600 paper-based; 100 iBT); Recommended—IELTS (minimum score 7.5), TWE. Electronic applications accepted. *Faculty research:* Cancer and congenital malformations, nutritional epidemiology, AIDS, tuberculosis, cardiovascular disease, risk assessment.

Johns Hopkins University, National Institutes of Health Sponsored Programs, Baltimore, MD 21218. Offers biology (PhD), including biochemistry, biophysics, cell biology, developmental biology, genetic biology, molecular biology; cell, molecular, and developmental biology and biophysics (PhD). *Degree requirements:* For doctorate, comprehensive exam, thesis/dissertation. *Entrance requirements:* For doctorate, GRE General Test. Additional exam requirements/recommendations for international students: Required—TOEFL (minimum score 600 paper-based), TWE. Electronic applications accepted. *Faculty research:* Protein and nucleic acid biochemistry and biophysical chemistry, molecular biology and development.

Kansas State University, Graduate School, College of Agriculture, Department of Plant Pathology, Manhattan, KS 66506. Offers genetics (MS, PhD); plant pathology (MS, PhD). Terminal master's awarded for partial completion of doctoral program. *Degree requirements:* For master's, thesis, oral exam; for doctorate, thesis/dissertation, preliminary exams. *Entrance requirements:* For master's and doctorate, minimum undergraduate GPA of 3.0. Additional exam requirements/recommendations for international students: Required—TOEFL (minimum score 550 paper-based; 79 iBT). Electronic applications accepted. *Faculty research:* Applied microbiology, microbial genetics, microbial ecology/epidemiology, integrated pest management, plant genetics/genomics/molecular biology.

Kent State University, College of Arts and Sciences, School of Biomedical Sciences, Kent, OH 44242-0001. Offers biological anthropology (PhD); cellular and molecular biology (PhD), including cellular biology and structures, molecular biology and genetics; neurosciences (PhD); pharmacology (MS); physiology (PhD). *Students:* 76 full-time (46 women), 1 (woman) part-time; includes 6 minority (1 Black or African American, non-Hispanic/Latino; 2 Asian, non-Hispanic/Latino; 1 Hispanic/Latino; 2 Two or more races, non-Hispanic/Latino), 28 international. Average age 29. 223 applicants, 13% accepted, 22 enrolled. In 2015, 5 master's, 7 doctorates awarded. Terminal master's awarded for partial completion of doctoral program. *Degree requirements:* For master's, thesis; for doctorate, thesis/dissertation, candidacy exam. *Entrance requirements:* For master's and doctorate, GRE General Test, minimum GPA of 3.0, transcript, goal statement, resume, 3 letters of recommendation. Additional exam requirements/recommendations for international students: Required—TOEFL (minimum score: paper-based 525, iBT 71), Michigan English Language Assessment Battery (minimum score of 75), IELTS (minimum score of 6.0), PTE Academic (minimum score of 48), or completion of ELS level 112 Intensive Program. *Application deadline:* For fall admission, 1/1 for domestic students. Application fee: $45 ($70 for international students). Electronic applications accepted. *Expenses:* Tuition, state resident: full-time $10,864; part-time $495 per credit hour. Tuition, nonresident: full-time $18,380; part-time $837 per credit hour. *Financial support:* In 2015–16, 76 students received support. Research assistantships with full tuition reimbursements available, teaching assistantships, career-related internships or fieldwork, Federal Work-Study, and unspecified assistantships available. Financial award application deadline: 1/1. *Unit head:* Dr. Eric Mintz, Director, 330-672-2263, E-mail: emintz@kent.edu. *Application contact:* 330-672-2263, Fax: 330-672-9391, E-mail: jwearden@kent.edu.
Website: http://www.kent.edu/biomedical/

Marquette University, Graduate School, College of Arts and Sciences, Department of Biology, Milwaukee, WI 53201-1881. Offers cell biology (MS, PhD); developmental biology (MS, PhD); ecology (MS, PhD); epithelial physiology (MS, PhD); genetics (MS, PhD); microbiology (MS, PhD); molecular biology (MS, PhD); muscle and exercise physiology (MS, PhD); neuroscience (PhD). *Faculty:* 22 full-time (7 women), 3 part-time/adjunct (2 women). *Students:* 28 full-time (11 women), 12 part-time (4 women); includes 4 minority (1 Asian, non-Hispanic/Latino; 1 Hispanic/Latino; 2 Two or more races, non-Hispanic/Latino), 11 international. Average age 27. 72 applicants, 28% accepted, 5 enrolled. In 2015, 2 master's, 4 doctorates awarded. Terminal master's awarded for partial completion of doctoral program. *Degree requirements:* For master's, comprehensive exam, thesis, 1 year of teaching experience or equivalent; for doctorate, thesis/dissertation, 1 year of teaching experience or equivalent, qualifying exam. *Entrance requirements:* For master's and doctorate, GRE General Test, GRE Subject Test, official transcripts from all current and previous colleges/universities except Marquette, statement of professional goals and aspirations, three letters of recommendation. Additional exam requirements/recommendations for international students: Required—TOEFL (minimum score 530 paper-based). *Application deadline:* For fall admission, 12/15 for domestic and international students. Application fee: $50. Electronic applications accepted. *Financial support:* In 2015–16, 39 students received support, including 6 fellowships (averaging $1,208 per year), 4 research assistantships with full tuition reimbursements available (averaging $21,750 per year), 29 teaching assistantships with full tuition reimbursements available (averaging $21,750 per year); scholarships/grants, health care benefits, tuition waivers (full and partial), and unspecified assistantships also available. Support available to part-time students. Financial award application deadline: 2/15. *Faculty research:* Neurobiology, neuroendocrinology, epithelial physiology, neuropeptide interactions, synaptic transmission. *Total annual research expenditures:* $1.2 million. *Unit head:* Dr. Ed Blumenthal, Chair, 414-288-1748. *Application contact:* Dr. Michael Schlappi, Recruiting Contact, 414-288-1467.
Website: http://www.marquette.edu/biology/

Massachusetts Institute of Technology, School of Science, Department of Biology, Cambridge, MA 02139. Offers biochemistry (PhD); biological oceanography (PhD); biology (PhD); biophysical chemistry and molecular structure (PhD); cell biology (PhD); computational and systems biology (PhD); developmental biology (PhD); genetics (PhD); immunology (PhD); microbiology (PhD); molecular biology (PhD); neurobiology (PhD). *Faculty:* 57 full-time (14 women). *Students:* 283 full-time (137 women); includes 83 minority (3 Black or African American, non-Hispanic/Latino; 1 American Indian or Alaska Native, non-Hispanic/Latino; 38 Asian, non-Hispanic/Latino; 31 Hispanic/Latino; 10 Two or more races, non-Hispanic/Latino), 48 international. Average age 26. 673 applicants, 14% accepted, 46 enrolled. In 2015, 32 doctorates awarded. *Degree*

requirements: For doctorate, comprehensive exam, thesis/dissertation, teaching assistantship during two semesters. *Entrance requirements:* For doctorate, GRE General Test. Additional exam requirements/recommendations for international students: Required—TOEFL (minimum score 577 paper-based), IELTS. *Application deadline:* For fall admission, 12/1 for domestic and international students. Application fee: $75. Electronic applications accepted. *Expenses:* Tuition: Full-time $46,400; part-time $725 per credit. One-time fee: $304 full-time. Full-time tuition and fees vary according to course load and program. *Financial support:* In 2015–16, 235 students received support, including 118 fellowships (averaging $37,500 per year), 163 research assistantships (averaging $38,900 per year), 1 teaching assistantship; Federal Work-Study, institutionally sponsored loans, scholarships/grants, traineeships, health care benefits, and unspecified assistantships also available. Support available to part-time students. Financial award application deadline: 4/15; financial award applicants required to submit FAFSA. *Faculty research:* Cellular, developmental and molecular (plant and animal) biology; biochemistry, bioengineering, biophysics and structural biology; classical and molecular genetics, stem cell and epigenetics; immunology and microbiology; cancer biology, molecular medicine, neurobiology and human disease; computational and systems biology. *Total annual research expenditures:* $42.8 million. *Unit head:* Prof. Alan Grossman, Department Head, 617-253-4701. *Application contact:* Biology Education Office, 617-253-3717, Fax: 617-258-9329, E-mail: gradbio@mit.edu. Website: https://biology.mit.edu/

Mayo Graduate School, Graduate Programs in Biomedical Sciences, Program in Virology and Gene Therapy, Rochester, MN 55905. Offers PhD.

Mayo Graduate School, Graduate Programs in Biomedical Sciences, Programs in Biochemistry, Structural Biology, Cell Biology, and Genetics, Rochester, MN 55905. Offers biochemistry and structural biology (PhD); cell biology and genetics (PhD); molecular biology (PhD). *Degree requirements:* For doctorate, oral defense of dissertation, qualifying oral and written exam. *Entrance requirements:* For doctorate, GRE, 1 year of chemistry, biology, calculus, and physics. Additional exam requirements/recommendations for international students: Required—TOEFL. Electronic applications accepted. *Faculty research:* Gene structure and function, membranes and receptors/cytoskeleton, oncogenes and growth factors, protein structure and function, steroid hormonal action.

McMaster University, Faculty of Health Sciences and School of Graduate Studies, Program in Medical Sciences, Genetics and Cancer Area, Hamilton, ON L8S 4M2, Canada. Offers M Sc, PhD, MD/PhD. *Degree requirements:* For master's, thesis; for doctorate, comprehensive exam, thesis/dissertation. *Entrance requirements:* For master's, honors B Sc, B+ average in related field; for doctorate, M Sc, minimum B+ average, students with proven research experience and an A average may be admitted with a B Sc degree. Additional exam requirements/recommendations for international students: Required—TOEFL (minimum score 580 paper-based; 92 iBT).

Medical University of South Carolina, College of Graduate Studies, Program in Molecular and Cellular Biology and Pathobiology, Charleston, SC 29425. Offers cancer biology (PhD); cardiovascular biology (PhD); cardiovascular imaging (PhD); cell regulation (PhD); craniofacial biology (PhD); genetics and development (PhD); marine biomedicine (PhD); DMD/PhD; MD/PhD. *Degree requirements:* For doctorate, thesis/dissertation, oral and written exams. *Entrance requirements:* For doctorate, GRE General Test, interview, minimum GPA of 3.0. Additional exam requirements/recommendations for international students: Required—TOEFL (minimum score 600 paper-based; 100 iBT). Electronic applications accepted.

Michigan State University, College of Veterinary Medicine and The Graduate School, Graduate Programs in Veterinary Medicine and College of Natural Science and Graduate Programs in Human Medicine, Department of Microbiology and Molecular Genetics, East Lansing, MI 48824. Offers industrial microbiology (MS, PhD); microbiology (MS, PhD); microbiology and molecular genetics (MS, PhD); microbiology–environmental toxicology (PhD). *Entrance requirements:* For master's, GRE General Test. Additional exam requirements/recommendations for international students: Required—TOEFL (minimum score 550 paper-based), Michigan State University ELT (minimum score 85), Michigan English Language Assessment Battery (minimum score 83). Electronic applications accepted.

Michigan State University, The Graduate School, College of Agriculture and Natural Resources, MSU-DOE Plant Research Laboratory, East Lansing, MI 48824. Offers biochemistry and molecular biology (PhD); cellular and molecular biology (PhD); crop and soil sciences (PhD); genetics (PhD); microbiology and molecular genetics (PhD); plant biology (PhD); plant physiology (PhD). Offered jointly with the Department of Energy. *Degree requirements:* For doctorate, comprehensive exam, thesis/dissertation, laboratory rotation, defense of dissertation. *Entrance requirements:* For doctorate, GRE General Test, acceptance into one of the affiliated department programs; 3 letters of recommendation; bachelor's degree or equivalent in life sciences, chemistry, biochemistry, or biophysics; research experience. Electronic applications accepted. *Faculty research:* Role of hormones in the regulation of plant development and physiology, molecular mechanisms associated with signal recognition, development and application of genetic methods and materials, protein routing and function.

Michigan State University, The Graduate School, College of Natural Science, Program in Genetics, East Lansing, MI 48824. Offers genetics (MS, PhD); genetics–environmental toxicology (PhD). *Entrance requirements:* Additional exam requirements/recommendations for international students: Required—TOEFL. Electronic applications accepted.

Mississippi State University, College of Agriculture and Life Sciences, Department of Animal Dairy Sciences, Mississippi State, MS 39762. Offers agricultural life sciences (MS), including animal physiology (MS, PhD), genetics (MS, PhD); agricultural science (PhD), including animal dairy sciences, animal nutrition (MS, PhD); agriculture (MS), including animal nutrition (MS, PhD), animal science; life sciences (PhD), including animal physiology (MS, PhD), genetics (MS, PhD). *Faculty:* 18 full-time (6 women). *Students:* 15 full-time (10 women), 10 part-time (4 women); includes 1 minority (Black or African American, non-Hispanic/Latino), 7 international. Average age 28. 27 applicants, 44% accepted, 9 enrolled. In 2015, 7 master's, 2 doctorates awarded. *Degree requirements:* For master's, comprehensive exam (for some programs), thesis, written proposal of intended research area; for doctorate, comprehensive exam, thesis/dissertation, written proposal of intended research area. *Entrance requirements:* For master's, GRE General Test, minimum GPA of 3.0; for doctorate, GRE General Test. Additional exam requirements/recommendations for international students: Required—TOEFL (minimum score 575 paper-based; 84 iBT), IELTS (minimum score 7). *Application deadline:* For fall admission, 7/1 for domestic students, 5/1 for international students; for spring admission, 11/1 for domestic students, 9/1 for international students. Applications are processed on a rolling basis. Application fee: $60. Electronic applications accepted. *Expenses:* Tuition, area resident: Full-time $7502; part-time $833.74 per credit hour. Tuition, nonresident: full-time $20,142; part-time $2238.24 per credit hour. *Financial support:* In 2015–16, 10 research assistantships (averaging $13,661 per year) were awarded; Federal Work-Study, institutionally sponsored loans, and unspecified assistantships also available. Financial award application deadline: 4/1; financial award applicants required to submit FAFSA. *Faculty research:* Ecology and population dynamics, physiology, biochemistry and behavior, systematics. *Unit head:* Dr. John Blanton, Department Head, 662-325-2935, Fax: 662-325-8873, E-mail: jblanton@ads.msstate.edu. *Application contact:* Marina Hunt, Admissions Assistant, 662-325-5188, E-mail: mhunt@grad.msstate.edu. Website: http://www.ads.msstate.edu/

New York University, Graduate School of Arts and Science, Department of Biology, New York, NY 10012-1019. Offers biology (PhD); biomedical journalism (MS); cancer and molecular biology (PhD); computational biology (PhD); computers in biological research (MS); developmental genetics (PhD); general biology (MS); immunology and microbiology (PhD); molecular genetics (PhD); neurobiology (PhD); oral biology (MS); plant biology (PhD); recombinant DNA technology (MS); MS/MBA. *Program availability:* Part-time. Terminal master's awarded for partial completion of doctoral program. *Degree requirements:* For master's, thesis or alternative, qualifying paper; for doctorate, comprehensive exam, thesis/dissertation. *Entrance requirements:* For master's and doctorate, GRE General Test. Additional exam requirements/recommendations for international students: Required—TOEFL. *Faculty research:* Genomics, molecular and cell biology, development and molecular genetics, molecular evolution of plants and animals.

North Carolina State University, Graduate School, College of Agriculture and Life Sciences, Department of Genetics, Raleigh, NC 27695. Offers MG, MS, PhD. Terminal master's awarded for partial completion of doctoral program. *Degree requirements:* For master's, thesis (for some programs); for doctorate, thesis/dissertation. *Entrance requirements:* For master's and doctorate, GRE General Test, minimum GPA of 3.0. Electronic applications accepted. *Faculty research:* Population and quantitative genetics, plant molecular genetics, developmental genetics.

The Ohio State University, Graduate School, College of Arts and Sciences, Division of Natural and Mathematical Sciences, Department of Molecular Genetics, Columbus, OH 43210. Offers cell and developmental biology (MS, PhD); genetics (MS, PhD); molecular biology (MS, PhD). *Degree requirements:* For master's, thesis; for doctorate, thesis/dissertation. *Entrance requirements:* For doctorate, GRE General Test, GRE Subject Test in biology or chemistry (recommended). Additional exam requirements/recommendations for international students: Required—TOEFL (minimum score 550 paper-based; 79 iBT), Michigan English Language Assessment Battery (minimum score 82); Recommended—IELTS (minimum score 7). Electronic applications accepted.

Oregon Health & Science University, School of Medicine, Graduate Programs in Medicine, Program in Molecular and Cellular Biosciences, Department of Molecular and Medical Genetics, Portland, OR 97239-3098. Offers PhD. *Faculty:* 15 full-time (6 women), 30 part-time/adjunct (12 women). *Students:* 9 full-time (6 women); includes 2 minority (1 Black or African American, non-Hispanic/Latino; 1 Hispanic/Latino), 1 international. Average age 27. Terminal master's awarded for partial completion of doctoral program. *Degree requirements:* For doctorate, comprehensive exam, thesis/dissertation. *Entrance requirements:* For doctorate, GRE General Test (minimum scores: 153 Verbal/148 Quantitative/4.5 Analytical) or MCAT (for some programs). Additional exam requirements/recommendations for international students: Required—IELTS or TOEFL. *Application deadline:* For fall admission, 12/1 for domestic and international students. Application fee: $70. Electronic applications accepted. *Financial support:* Health care benefits and full tuition and stipends (for PhD students) available. *Faculty research:* Human molecular genetics and cytogenetics, neurogenomics, epigenetics/epigenomics, cancer genetics, biochemical genetics, gene therapy. *Unit head:* Dr. Mike Liskay, Program Director, 503-494-3475, E-mail: liskaym@oshsu.edu. *Application contact:* Brandi Colbert, Program Coordinator, 503-418-9457, E-mail: colbertb@ohsu.edu. Website: http://www.ohsu.edu/xd/education/schools/school-of-medicine/departments/basic-science-departments/molecular-and-medical-genetics/index.cfm

Purdue University, Graduate School, College of Science, Department of Biological Sciences, West Lafayette, IN 47907. Offers biochemistry (PhD); biophysics (PhD); cell and developmental biology (PhD); ecology, evolutionary and population biology (MS, PhD), including ecology, evolutionary biology, population biology; genetics (MS, PhD); microbiology (MS, PhD); molecular biology (PhD); neurobiology (MS, PhD); plant physiology (PhD). Terminal master's awarded for partial completion of doctoral program. *Degree requirements:* For master's, thesis (for some programs); for doctorate, thesis/dissertation, seminars, teaching experience. *Entrance requirements:* For master's, GRE General Test (minimum analytical writing score of 3.5), minimum undergraduate GPA of 3.0; for doctorate, GRE General Test (minimum analytical writing of 3.5), minimum undergraduate GPA of 3.5. Additional exam requirements/recommendations for international students: Required—TOEFL (minimum score 600 paper-based; 107 iBT for MS, 80 iBT for PhD). Electronic applications accepted.

Purdue University, Graduate School, PULSe - Purdue University Life Sciences Program, West Lafayette, IN 47907. Offers biomolecular structure and biophysics (PhD); biotechnology (PhD); chemical biology (PhD); chromatin and regulation of gene expression (PhD); integrative neuroscience (PhD); integrative plant sciences (PhD); membrane biology (PhD); microbiology (PhD); molecular evolutionary and cancer biology (PhD); molecular evolutionary genetics (PhD); molecular virology (PhD). *Entrance requirements:* For doctorate, GRE, minimum undergraduate GPA of 3.0. Additional exam requirements/recommendations for international students: Required—TOEFL (minimum score 550 paper-based; 77 iBT). Electronic applications accepted.

Rutgers University–New Brunswick, Graduate School-New Brunswick, Programs in the Molecular Biosciences, Piscataway, NJ 08854-8097. Offers biochemistry (PhD); cell and developmental biology (MS, PhD); microbiology and molecular genetics (MS, PhD), including applied microbiology, clinical microbiology (MS), clinical mircobiology (PhD), computational molecular biology (PhD), immunology, microbial biochemistry, molecular genetics, virology. MS, PhD offered jointly with University of Medicine and Dentistry of New Jersey.

Stanford University, School of Medicine, Graduate Programs in Medicine, Department of Genetics, Stanford, CA 94305-9991. Offers genetics (PhD). *Degree requirements:* For doctorate, thesis/dissertation, qualifying examination, teaching requirement. *Entrance requirements:* For doctorate, GRE General Test, GRE Subject Test. Additional exam requirements/recommendations for international students: Required—TOEFL. Electronic applications accepted. *Expenses: Tuition, area resident:* Full-time $45,729. *Required fees:* $591. *Faculty research:* Molecular biology of DNA replication in human cells, analysis of existing and search for new DNA polymorphisms in humans, molecular genetics of prokaryotic and eukaryotic genetic elements, proteins in DNA replication.

Stony Brook University, State University of New York, Graduate School, College of Arts and Sciences, Graduate Program in Genetics, Stony Brook, NY 11794. Offers PhD. *Students:* 34 full-time (16 women), 1 (woman) part-time; includes 7 minority (3 Asian, non-Hispanic/Latino; 3 Hispanic/Latino; 1 Two or more races, non-Hispanic/Latino), 11 international. Average age 27. 97 applicants, 23% accepted, 9 enrolled. In 2015, 6 doctorates awarded. *Degree requirements:* For doctorate, comprehensive exam, thesis/dissertation, teaching experience. *Entrance requirements:* For doctorate, GRE General Test, GRE Subject Test. Additional exam requirements/recommendations for international students: Required—TOEFL (minimum score 90 iBT). *Application deadline:* For fall admission, 1/15 for domestic students; for spring admission, 10/1 for domestic

students. Application fee: $100. *Expenses:* $12,421 full-time resident tuition and fees, $453 per credit hour; $23,761 full-time nonresident tuition and fees, $925 per credit hour. *Financial support:* In 2015–16, 6 fellowships, 14 research assistantships, 4 teaching assistantships were awarded; Federal Work-Study also available. *Faculty research:* Gene structure, gene regulation, genetics. *Unit head:* Dr. Jorge Benach, Dean, 631-632-4225, Fax: 631-632-9797, E-mail: jorge.benach@stonybrook.edu. *Application contact:* Kathryn Bell, Coordinator, 631-632-8812, Fax: 631-632-4294, E-mail: kathryn.bell@stonybrook.edu. Website: http://life.bio.sunysb.edu/gen/

Thomas Jefferson University, Jefferson College of Biomedical Sciences, PhD Program in Genetics, Genomics and Cancer Biology, Philadelphia, PA 19107. Offers PhD. *Faculty:* 48 full-time (16 women), 4 part-time/adjunct (3 women). *Students:* 21 full-time (12 women); includes 3 minority (1 Asian, non-Hispanic/Latino; 2 Hispanic/Latino), 3 international. 46 applicants, 11% accepted, 6 enrolled. In 2015, 1 doctorate awarded. *Degree requirements:* For doctorate, comprehensive exam, thesis/dissertation. *Entrance requirements:* For doctorate, GRE General Test, minimum GPA of 3.2. Additional exam requirements/recommendations for international students: Required—TOEFL, IELTS (minimum score 7). *Application deadline:* For fall admission, 12/15 priority date for domestic and international students. Applications are processed on a rolling basis. Application fee: $50. Electronic applications accepted. *Financial support:* In 2015–16, 21 students received support, including 21 fellowships with full tuition reimbursements available (averaging $56,298 per year); Federal Work-Study, institutionally sponsored loans, scholarships/grants, traineeships, and stipends also available. Support available to part-time students. Financial award application deadline: 5/1; financial award applicants required to submit FAFSA. *Faculty research:* Functional genomics, cancer susceptibility, cell cycle, regulation oncogenes and tumor suppressor genes, genetics of neoplastic disease. *Unit head:* Dr. Lucia Languino, Program Director, 215-503-3442, E-mail: lucia.languino@jefferson.edu. *Application contact:* Marc E. Stearns, Director of Admissions, 215-503-0155, Fax: 215-503-3433, E-mail: jgsbs-info@jefferson.edu. Website: http://www.jefferson.edu/university/biomedical-sciences/degrees-programs/phd-programs/genetics.html

Tufts University, Sackler School of Graduate Biomedical Sciences, Genetics Program, Medford, MA 02155. Offers genetics (PhD); mammalian genetics at jax (PhD). *Faculty:* 64 full-time (19 women). *Students:* 27 full-time (16 women); includes 5 minority (3 Asian, non-Hispanic/Latino; 1 Hispanic/Latino; 1 Two or more races, non-Hispanic/Latino), 4 international. Average age 28. 55 applicants, 20% accepted, 6 enrolled. In 2015, 5 doctorates awarded. Terminal master's awarded for partial completion of doctoral program. *Degree requirements:* For doctorate, comprehensive exam, thesis/dissertation. *Entrance requirements:* For doctorate, GRE General Test, 3 letters of reference. Additional exam requirements/recommendations for international students: Required—TOEFL (minimum score 600 paper-based; 100 iBT). *Application deadline:* For fall admission, 12/15 priority date for domestic and international students. Application fee: $90. Electronic applications accepted. *Expenses: Tuition, area resident:* Full-time $48,412; part-time $1210 per credit hour. *Required fees:* $806. Full-time tuition and fees vary according to degree level, program and student level. Part-time tuition and fees vary according to course load. *Financial support:* In 2015–16, 26 students received support, including 26 research assistantships with full tuition reimbursements available (averaging $32,000 per year); health care benefits also available. *Faculty research:* Cancer genetics, developmental and neurogenetics, microbial and yeast genetics, the genetics of bacterial and viral pathogens, Drosophila genetics, human genetics and gene discovery. *Unit head:* Dr. Rajendra Kumar-Singh, Program Director, 617-636-6836. *Application contact:* Dr. Elizabeth Storrs, 617-636-6767, Fax: 617-636-0375. Website: http://sackler.tufts.edu/Academics/Degree-Programs/PhD-Programs/Genetics

Université de Montréal, Faculty of Medicine, Program in Medical Genetics, Montréal, QC H3C 3J7, Canada. Offers DESS.

Université du Québec à Chicoutimi, Graduate Programs, Program in Experimental Medicine, Chicoutimi, QC G7H 2B1, Canada. Offers genetics (M Sc). *Degree requirements:* For master's, thesis. *Entrance requirements:* For master's, appropriate bachelor's degree, proficiency in French.

University at Buffalo, the State University of New York, Graduate School, School of Medicine and Biomedical Sciences, Graduate Programs in Medicine and Biomedical Sciences, Program in Genetics, Genomics and Bioinformatics, Buffalo, NY 14203. Offers MS, PhD. *Faculty:* 60 full-time (17 women). *Students:* 4 full-time (1 woman); includes 2 minority (both Asian, non-Hispanic/Latino), 1 international. Average age 28. 13 applicants, 69% accepted, 1 enrolled. In 2015, 1 master's awarded. Terminal master's awarded for partial completion of doctoral program. *Degree requirements:* For master's, thesis or alternative; for doctorate, thesis/dissertation. *Entrance requirements:* For master's and doctorate, GRE. Additional exam requirements/recommendations for international students: Required—TOEFL (minimum score 100 iBT). *Application deadline:* For fall admission, 3/1 for domestic and international students. Application fee: $85. Electronic applications accepted. *Expenses:* $10,870 tuition per year in-state; $22,210 tuition per year out-of-state. *Financial support:* Support by faculty mentor available. *Faculty research:* Human and medical genetics and genomics, developmental genomics and genetics, microbial genetics and pathogenesis, bioinformatics. *Unit head:* Dr. Richard Gronostajski, Director, 716-829-3471, Fax: 716-849-6655, E-mail: rgron@buffalo.edu. *Application contact:* Greg Korosec, Program Administrator, 716-881-8209, Fax: 716-849-6655, E-mail: korosec@buffalo.edu. Website: http://medicine.buffalo.edu/education/ggb.html

The University of Alabama at Birmingham, Graduate Programs in Joint Health Sciences, Genetics, Genomics and Bioinformatics Theme, Birmingham, AL 35294. Offers PhD. *Degree requirements:* For doctorate, comprehensive exam, thesis/dissertation. *Entrance requirements:* For doctorate, GRE General Test, interview, previous research experience. Additional exam requirements/recommendations for international students: Required—TOEFL. Electronic applications accepted. *Expenses:* Tuition, state resident: full-time $7340. Tuition, nonresident: full-time $16,628. Full-time tuition and fees vary according to course load and program.

University of Alberta, Faculty of Graduate Studies and Research, Department of Biological Sciences, Edmonton, AB T6G 2E1, Canada. Offers environmental biology and ecology (M Sc, PhD); microbiology and biotechnology (M Sc, PhD); molecular biology and genetics (M Sc, PhD); physiology and cell biology (M Sc, PhD); plant biology (M Sc, PhD); systematics and evolution (M Sc, PhD). Terminal master's awarded for partial completion of doctoral program. *Degree requirements:* For master's, thesis; for doctorate, thesis/dissertation. *Entrance requirements:* Additional exam requirements/recommendations for international students: Required—TOEFL.

University of Alberta, Faculty of Medicine and Dentistry and Faculty of Graduate Studies and Research, Graduate Programs in Medicine, Department of Medical Genetics, Edmonton, AB T6G 2E1, Canada. Offers M Sc, PhD. *Degree requirements:* For master's, comprehensive exam, thesis; for doctorate, comprehensive exam, thesis/dissertation. *Entrance requirements:* For master's and doctorate, minimum GPA of 3.2. *Faculty research:* Clinical and molecular cytogenetics, ocular genetics, Prader-Willi syndrome, genomic instability, developmental genetics.

Genetics

The University of Arizona, Graduate Interdisciplinary Programs, Graduate Interdisciplinary Program in Genetics, Tucson, AZ 85719. Offers MS, PhD. Terminal master's awarded for partial completion of doctoral program. *Degree requirements:* For master's, thesis; for doctorate, one foreign language, comprehensive exam, thesis/dissertation. *Entrance requirements:* For master's, GRE General Test, 3 letters of recommendation; for doctorate, GRE General Test, statement of purpose, 3 letters of recommendation. Additional exam requirements/recommendations for international students: Required—TOEFL (minimum score 550 paper-based; 79 iBT). *Application deadline:* For fall admission, 6/1 for domestic students, 12/1 for international students. Applications are processed on a rolling basis. Application fee: $75. Electronic applications accepted. *Financial support:* Career-related internships or fieldwork, scholarships/grants, health care benefits, and unspecified assistantships available. *Faculty research:* Cancer research; DNA repair; plant and animal cytogenetics; molecular, population, and ecological genetics. *Unit head:* Dr. Melanie Culver, Chair, 520-626-1452, Fax: 520-626-5097, E-mail: mculver@email.arizona.edu. *Application contact:* Angela Nelson, Program Coordinator, 520-626-1452, Fax: 520-626-5097, E-mail: cora@email.arizona.edu.
Website: http://www.genetics.arizona.edu/

The University of British Columbia, Faculty of Medicine, Department of Medical Genetics, Medical Genetics Graduate Program, Vancouver, BC V6T 1Z1, Canada. Offers M Sc, PhD. *Degree requirements:* For master's, thesis, 18 credits of coursework; for doctorate, comprehensive exam, thesis/dissertation, 18 credits of coursework. Electronic applications accepted.

The University of British Columbia, Genetics Graduate Program, Vancouver, BC V6T 1Z1, Canada. Offers M Sc, PhD. *Degree requirements:* For master's, comprehensive exam, thesis, thesis defense; for doctorate, comprehensive exam, thesis/dissertation, qualifying exam, oral and written comprehensive exams. *Entrance requirements:* Additional exam requirements/recommendations for international students: Required—TOEFL (minimum score 600 paper-based; 100 iBT). *Faculty research:* Prokaryote and eukaryote genetics.

University of Calgary, Cumming School of Medicine and Faculty of Graduate Studies, Medical Science Graduate Program, Calgary, AB T2N 1N4, Canada. Offers cancer biology (M Sc, PhD); critical care medicine (M Sc, PhD); joint injury and arthritis (M Sc, PhD); molecular and medical genetics (M Sc, PhD); mountain medicine and high altitude physiology (M Sc, PhD); pathologists' assistant (M Sc, PhD). *Degree requirements:* For master's, thesis; for doctorate, thesis/dissertation, candidacy exam. *Entrance requirements:* For master's, minimum undergraduate GPA of 3.2; for doctorate, minimum graduate GPA of 3.2. Additional exam requirements/recommendations for international students: Required—TOEFL (minimum score 600 paper-based). Electronic applications accepted. *Faculty research:* Cancer biology, immunology, joint injury and arthritis, medical education, population genomics.

University of California, Davis, Graduate Studies, Graduate Group in Genetics, Davis, CA 95616. Offers MS, PhD. Terminal master's awarded for partial completion of doctoral program. *Degree requirements:* For master's, comprehensive exam (for some programs), thesis (for some programs); for doctorate, thesis/dissertation. *Entrance requirements:* For master's and doctorate, GRE General Test, GRE Subject Test. Additional exam requirements/recommendations for international students: Required—TOEFL (minimum score 550 paper-based). Electronic applications accepted. *Faculty research:* Molecular, quantitative, and developmental genetics; cytogenetics; plant breeding.

University of California, Irvine, Francisco J. Ayala School of Biological Sciences and School of Medicine, Interdisciplinary Graduate Program in Cellular and Molecular Biosciences, Irvine, CA 92697. Offers PhD. *Students:* 26 full-time (14 women); includes 11 minority (5 Asian, non-Hispanic/Latino; 3 Hispanic/Latino; 3 Two or more races, non-Hispanic/Latino), 2 international. Average age 25. 322 applicants, 18% accepted, 25 enrolled. *Degree requirements:* For doctorate, thesis/dissertation, teaching assignment, preliminary exam. *Entrance requirements:* For doctorate, GRE General Test, three letters of recommendation, interview. Additional exam requirements/recommendations for international students: Required—TOEFL or IELTS. *Application deadline:* For fall admission, 12/8 for domestic and international students. Application fee: $90 ($110 for international students). Electronic applications accepted. *Expenses:* Contact institution. *Financial support:* Fellowships with full tuition reimbursements, institutionally sponsored loans, scholarships/grants, tuition waivers (full), unspecified assistantships, and stipends available. Financial award application deadline: 1/1; financial award applicants required to submit FAFSA. *Faculty research:* Cellular biochemistry; gene structure and expression; protein structure, function, and design; molecular genetics; pathogenesis and inherited disease. *Unit head:* Melanie Cocco, Director, 949-824-4487, Fax: 949-824-1965, E-mail: mcocco@uci.edu. *Application contact:* Renee Frigo, Administrator, 949-824-8145, Fax: 949-824-1965, E-mail: rfrigo@uci.edu.
Website: http://cmb.uci.edu/

University of California, Riverside, Graduate Division, Graduate Program in Genetics, Genomics, and Bioinformatics, Riverside, CA 92521-0102. Offers genomics and bioinformatics (PhD). *Degree requirements:* For doctorate, thesis/dissertation, qualifying exams, teaching experience. *Entrance requirements:* For doctorate, GRE General Test, minimum GPA of 3.2. Additional exam requirements/recommendations for international students: Required—TOEFL (minimum score 550 paper-based; 80 iBT). *Application deadline:* For fall admission, 12/1 priority date for domestic students, 1/1 priority date for international students; for winter admission, 9/1 for domestic students, 7/1 for international students; for spring admission, 12/1 for domestic students, 10/1 for international students. Applications are processed on a rolling basis. Application fee: $85 ($100 for international students). Electronic applications accepted. *Expenses:* Tuition, area resident: Full-time $16,665.50; part-time $11,055.54. Tuition, state resident: full-time $16,665.50; part-time $11,055.54. Tuition, nonresident: full-time $31,768. International tuition: $31,767.50 full-time. *Required fees:* $16,665.50; $11,055.54 per quarter. $3685.18 per quarter. Tuition and fees vary according to program. *Financial support:* Fellowships with tuition reimbursements, research assistantships with tuition reimbursements, teaching assistantships with tuition reimbursements, career-related internships or fieldwork, Federal Work-Study, institutionally sponsored loans, and tuition waivers (full and partial) available. *Faculty research:* Molecular genetics, evolution and population genetics, genomics and bioinformatics.
Website: http://ggb.ucr.edu/

University of California, San Francisco, Graduate Division and School of Medicine, Tetrad Graduate Program, Genetics Track, San Francisco, CA 94143. Offers PhD, MD/PhD. *Degree requirements:* For doctorate, thesis/dissertation. *Entrance requirements:* For doctorate, GRE General Test, GRE Subject Test. Additional exam requirements/recommendations for international students: Required—TOEFL. *Expenses:* Contact institution. *Faculty research:* Gene expression; chromosome structure and mechanics; medical, somatic cell, and radiation genetics.

University of Chicago, Division of the Biological Sciences, Committee on Genetics, Genomics and Systems Biology, Chicago, IL 60637. Offers PhD. *Students:* 27 full-time (11 women); includes 7 minority (1 Black or African American, non-Hispanic/Latino; 4

Asian, non-Hispanic/Latino; 1 Hispanic/Latino; 1 Native Hawaiian or other Pacific Islander, non-Hispanic/Latino), 6 international. Average age 28. 71 applicants, 18% accepted, 4 enrolled. In 2015, 4 doctorates awarded. *Degree requirements:* For doctorate, thesis/dissertation, ethics class, 2 teaching assistantships. *Entrance requirements:* For doctorate, GRE General Test. Additional exam requirements/recommendations for international students: Required—TOEFL (minimum score 600 paper-based; 104 iBT), IELTS (minimum score 7). *Application deadline:* For fall admission, 12/1 for domestic and international students. Application fee: $90. Electronic applications accepted. *Financial support:* In 2015–16, 21 students received support, including fellowships with tuition reimbursements available (averaging $29,781 per year), research assistantships with tuition reimbursements available (averaging $29,781 per year); institutionally sponsored loans, scholarships/grants, traineeships, and health care benefits also available. Financial award applicants required to submit FAFSA. *Faculty research:* Molecular genetics, developmental genetics, population genetics, human genetics. *Application contact:* Sue Levison, Administrator, 773-702-2464, Fax: 773-702-3172, E-mail: committee-on-genetics@uchicago.edu.
Website: http://cg.bsd.uchicago.edu/

University of Colorado Boulder, Graduate School, College of Arts and Sciences, Department of Ecology and Evolutionary Biology, Boulder, CO 80309. Offers animal behavior (MA); biology (MA, PhD); environmental biology (MA, PhD); evolutionary biology (MA, PhD); neurobiology (MA); population biology (MA); population genetics (PhD). *Faculty:* 31 full-time (12 women). *Students:* 67 full-time (31 women), 3 part-time (1 woman); includes 8 minority (1 Asian, non-Hispanic/Latino; 3 Hispanic/Latino; 4 Two or more races, non-Hispanic/Latino), 4 international. Average age 30. 119 applicants, 11% accepted, 13 enrolled. In 2015, 10 master's, 14 doctorates awarded. Terminal master's awarded for partial completion of doctoral program. *Degree requirements:* For master's, comprehensive exam, thesis or alternative; for doctorate, comprehensive exam, thesis/dissertation. *Entrance requirements:* For master's, GRE General Test, GRE Subject Test, minimum undergraduate GPA of 3.0; for doctorate, GRE General Test, GRE Subject Test. *Application deadline:* For fall admission, 12/31 for domestic students, 12/1 for international students. Application fee: $50 ($70 for international students). Electronic applications accepted. Application fee is waived when completed online. *Financial support:* In 2015–16, 138 students received support, including 14 fellowships (averaging $7,260 per year), 12 research assistantships with tuition reimbursements available (averaging $31,833 per year), 47 teaching assistantships with tuition reimbursements available (averaging $33,448 per year); institutionally sponsored loans, scholarships/grants, health care benefits, and unspecified assistantships also available. Financial award applicants required to submit FAFSA. *Faculty research:* Ecology, botany, evolutionary biology, biological sciences, conservation biology. *Total annual research expenditures:* $6.3 million. *Application contact:* E-mail: ebiograd@colorado.edu.
Website: http://ebio.colorado.edu

University of Colorado Denver, College of Liberal Arts and Sciences, Department of Integrative and Systems Biology, Denver, CO 80217. Offers animal behavior (MS); biology (MS); cell and developmental biology (MS); ecology (MS); evolutionary biology (MS); genetics (MS); integrative and systems biology (MS); microbiology (MS); molecular biology (MS); neurobiology (MS); plant systematics (MS). *Program availability:* Part-time. *Faculty:* 21 full-time (8 women), 3 part-time/adjunct (1 woman). *Students:* 31 full-time (19 women), 7 part-time (3 women); includes 8 minority (1 Black or African American, non-Hispanic/Latino; 1 Asian, non-Hispanic/Latino; 3 Hispanic/Latino; 3 Two or more races, non-Hispanic/Latino), 1 international. Average age 28. 34 applicants, 29% accepted, 8 enrolled. In 2015, 6 master's awarded. *Degree requirements:* For master's, comprehensive exam, thesis, 30-32 credit hours; for doctorate, comprehensive exam, thesis/dissertation. *Entrance requirements:* For master's, GRE General Test (minimum score in 50th percentile in each section), BA/BS from accredited institution awarded within the last 10 years; minimum undergraduate GPA of 3.0; prerequisite courses: 1 year each of general biology and general chemistry; 1 semester each of general genetics, general ecology, and cell biology; and a structure/function course; for doctorate, GRE, minimum undergraduate GPA of 3.2, three letters of recommendation, official transcripts from all universities and colleges attended. Additional exam requirements/recommendations for international students: Required—TOEFL (minimum score 537 paper-based; 75 iBT); Recommended—IELTS (minimum score 6.5). *Application deadline:* For fall admission, 1/15 for domestic and international students. Application fee: $50 ($75 for international students). Electronic applications accepted. *Financial support:* In 2015–16, 32 students received support. Fellowships, research assistantships, teaching assistantships, Federal Work-Study, institutionally sponsored loans, scholarships/grants, and traineeships available. Financial award application deadline: 4/1; financial award applicants required to submit FAFSA. *Faculty research:* Molecular developmental biology; quantitative ecology, biogeography, and population dynamics; environmental signaling and endocrine disruption; speciation, the evolution of reproductive isolation, and hybrid zones; evolutionary, behavioral, and conservation ecology. *Unit head:* Dr. John Swallow, Chair, 303-556-6154, E-mail: john.swallow@ucdenver.edu. *Application contact:* Dr. Michael Wunder, Graduate Advisor, 303-556-8870, E-mail: michael.wunder@ucdenver.edu.
Website: http://www.ucdenver.edu/academics/colleges/CLAS/Departments/biology/Programs/MasterofScience/Pages/BiologyMasterOfScience.aspx

University of Colorado Denver, School of Medicine, Program in Human Medical Genetics and Genomics, Aurora, CO 80045. Offers PhD. *Students:* 16 full-time (14 women); includes 4 minority (1 Black or African American, non-Hispanic/Latino; 3 Hispanic/Latino). Average age 27. 43 applicants, 7% accepted, 2 enrolled. In 2015, 3 doctorates awarded. *Degree requirements:* For doctorate, comprehensive exam, thesis/dissertation, at least 30 semester hours in course work (rotations and research courses taken prior to the completion of the comprehensive examination) and 30 semester hours of thesis/didactic credits prior to defending. *Entrance requirements:* For doctorate, GRE General Test (minimum combined score of 1205), minimum GPA of 3.0, 4 letters of recommendation; prerequisite courses in biology, chemistry (general and organic), physics, genetics, calculus, and statistics (recommended). Additional exam requirements/recommendations for international students: Required—TOEFL (minimum score 570 paper-based; 80 iBT). *Application deadline:* For fall admission, 12/1 for domestic students, 1/1 priority date for international students. Application fee: $50 ($75 for international students). Electronic applications accepted. *Expenses:* Contact institution. *Financial support:* In 2015–16, 15 students received support. Fellowships, research assistantships, teaching assistantships, Federal Work-Study, institutionally sponsored loans, scholarships/grants, traineeships, health care benefits, and unspecified assistantships available. Financial award application deadline: 3/15; financial award applicants required to submit FAFSA. *Faculty research:* Mapping, discovery, and function of disease genes affecting skin and craniofacial development and autoimmunity; genetics of colon cancer; clinical proteomics; biochemical markers of disease, including cancer; modeling human genetic diseases with patient-derived induced pluripotent stem cells; cell cycle control of DNA replication and mutagenesis in yeast and human cancer cells; mechanisms of cancer chemoprevention. *Unit head:* Dr. Richard A. Spritz, Director, 303-724-3107, E-mail: richard.spritz@ucdenver.edu. *Application contact:* Maia Evans, Program Administrator, 303-724-3102, Fax: 303-724-3100, E-mail: adama.evans@ucdenver.edu.

Website: http://www.ucdenver.edu/academics/colleges/medicalschool/programs/HumanMedicalGenetics/Pages/Genetics.aspx

University of Connecticut Health Center, Graduate School, Programs in Biomedical Sciences, Program in Genetics and Developmental Biology, Farmington, CT 06030. Offers PhD, DMD/PhD, MD/PhD. *Degree requirements:* For doctorate, comprehensive exam, thesis/dissertation. *Entrance requirements:* For doctorate, GRE General Test, GRE Subject Test. Additional exam requirements/recommendations for international students: Required—TOEFL (minimum score 600 paper-based). Electronic applications accepted. *Faculty research:* Developmental biology, genomic imprinting, RNA biology, RNA alternative splicing, human embryonic stem cells.

See Display below and Close-Up on page 295.

University of Delaware, College of Arts and Sciences, Department of Biological Sciences, Newark, DE 19716. Offers biotechnology (MS); cancer biology (MS, PhD); cell and extracellular matrix biology (MS, PhD); cell and systems physiology (MS, PhD); developmental biology (MS, PhD); ecology and evolution (MS, PhD); microbiology (MS, PhD); molecular biology and genetics (MS, PhD). Terminal master's awarded for partial completion of doctoral program. *Degree requirements:* For master's, thesis, preliminary exam; for doctorate, comprehensive exam, thesis/dissertation, preliminary exam. *Entrance requirements:* For master's and doctorate, GRE General Test. Additional exam requirements/recommendations for international students: Required—TOEFL (minimum score 600 paper-based); Recommended—TWE. Electronic applications accepted. *Faculty research:* Microorganisms, bone, cancer metastasis, developmental biology, cell biology, DNA.

University of Florida, College of Medicine and Graduate School, Interdisciplinary Program in Biomedical Sciences, Concentration in Genetics, Gainesville, FL 32611. Offers PhD. *Degree requirements:* For doctorate, thesis/dissertation. *Entrance requirements:* For doctorate, GRE General Test, minimum GPA of 3.0, biochemistry before enrollment. Additional exam requirements/recommendations for international students: Required—TOEFL, IELTS. Electronic applications accepted.

University of Georgia, College of Agricultural and Environmental Sciences, Institute of Plant Breeding, Genetics and Genomics, Athens, GA 30602. Offers MS, PhD.

University of Georgia, Franklin College of Arts and Sciences, Department of Genetics, Athens, GA 30602. Offers MS, PhD. Terminal master's awarded for partial completion of doctoral program. *Degree requirements:* For master's, thesis; for doctorate, comprehensive exam, thesis/dissertation. *Entrance requirements:* For master's and doctorate, GRE General Test. Additional exam requirements/recommendations for international students: Required—TOEFL. Electronic applications accepted.

University of Hawaii at Manoa, John A. Burns School of Medicine, Program in Cell and Molecular Biology, Honolulu, HI 96813. Offers MS, PhD. *Program availability:* Part-time. *Faculty:* 55 full-time (16 women), 5 part-time/adjunct (1 woman). *Students:* 32 full-time (23 women), 1 (woman) part-time; includes 20 minority (8 Asian, non-Hispanic/Latino; 4 Hispanic/Latino; 1 Native Hawaiian or other Pacific Islander, non-Hispanic/Latino; 7 Two or more races, non-Hispanic/Latino), 2 international. Average age 31. 28 applicants, 61% accepted, 11 enrolled. In 2015, 5 doctorates awarded. Terminal master's awarded for partial completion of doctoral program. *Degree requirements:* For master's, thesis optional; for doctorate, comprehensive exam, thesis/dissertation. *Entrance requirements:* For master's and doctorate, GRE General Test, minimum GPA of 3.0. Additional exam requirements/recommendations for international students: Required—TOEFL (minimum score 500 paper-based; 61 iBT), IELTS (minimum score 5). *Application deadline:* For fall admission, 1/15 for domestic and international students. Applications are processed on a rolling basis. Application fee: $100. *Financial support:*

In 2015–16, 19 fellowships (averaging $824 per year), 36 research assistantships (averaging $20,351 per year), 1 teaching assistantship (averaging $16,824 per year) were awarded; Federal Work-Study and institutionally sponsored loans also available. Financial award application deadline: 2/1. *Total annual research expenditures:* $2.7 million. *Unit head:* Dr. Jerris R. Hedges, Dean, 808-692-0881. *Application contact:* Marla Berry, Graduate Co-Chair, 808-692-1506, Fax: 808-692-1968, E-mail: mberry@hawaii.edu.
Website: http://www.hawaii.edu/cmb/

University of Illinois at Chicago, College of Medicine and Graduate College, Graduate Programs in Medicine, Department of Biochemistry and Molecular Genetics, Chicago, IL 60607-7128. Offers PhD, MD/PhD. *Faculty:* 31 full-time (12 women), 19 part-time/adjunct (9 women). *Students:* 22 full-time (12 women); includes 5 minority (1 Black or African American, non-Hispanic/Latino; 3 Asian, non-Hispanic/Latino; 1 Hispanic/Latino), 9 international. Average age 29. Terminal master's awarded for partial completion of doctoral program. *Degree requirements:* For doctorate, thesis/dissertation. *Entrance requirements:* For doctorate, GRE General Test. Additional exam requirements/recommendations for international students: Required—TOEFL. *Application deadline:* For fall admission, 3/1 priority date for domestic students, 2/15 for international students. Applications are processed on a rolling basis. Application fee: $60. Electronic applications accepted. *Expenses:* Tuition, state resident: full-time $11,480; part-time $3826 per credit. Tuition, nonresident: full-time $23,720; part-time $7906 per credit. *Required fees:* $1333 per semester. Part-time tuition and fees vary according to course load and program. *Financial support:* Fellowships with full tuition reimbursements, research assistantships with full tuition reimbursements, teaching assistantships with full tuition reimbursements, career-related internships or fieldwork, Federal Work-Study, institutionally sponsored loans, traineeships, tuition waivers (full), and unspecified assistantships available. Financial award application deadline: 3/1; financial award applicants required to submit FAFSA. *Faculty research:* Signal transduction, cell cycle regulation, membrane biology, regulation of gene function and development, protein and nucleic acid structure and function, cancer biology. *Unit head:* Dr. Jack Kaplan, Head, 312-355-2732, Fax: 312-413-0353, E-mail: kaplanj@uic.edu. *Application contact:* Dr. Karen Colley, Co-Director of Graduate Studies, 312-996-7756. Website: http://www.uic.edu/com/bcmg/

The University of Iowa, Graduate College, College of Liberal Arts and Sciences, Department of Biology, Iowa City, IA 52242-1324. Offers biology (MS, PhD); cell and developmental biology (MS, PhD); evolution (MS, PhD); genetics (MS, PhD); neurobiology (MS, PhD). Terminal master's awarded for partial completion of doctoral program. *Degree requirements:* For master's, thesis optional, exam; for doctorate, comprehensive exam, thesis/dissertation. *Entrance requirements:* For master's and doctorate, GRE General Test, minimum GPA of 3.0. Additional exam requirements/recommendations for international students: Required—TOEFL (minimum score 600 paper-based; 100 iBT). Electronic applications accepted. *Faculty research:* Neurobiology, evolutionary biology, genetics, cell and developmental biology.

The University of Iowa, Graduate College, Program in Genetics, Iowa City, IA 52242-1316. Offers PhD. *Degree requirements:* For doctorate, comprehensive exam, thesis/dissertation. *Entrance requirements:* For doctorate, GRE General Test, minimum GPA of 3.0. Additional exam requirements/recommendations for international students: Required—TOEFL (minimum score 600 paper-based; 100 iBT). Electronic applications accepted. *Expenses:* Contact institution. *Faculty research:* Developmental genetics, eukaryotic gene expression, human genetics, molecular and biochemical genetics, evolutionary genetics.

The University of Iowa, Roy J. and Lucille A. Carver College of Medicine and Graduate College, Graduate Programs in Medicine, Department of Microbiology, Iowa City, IA

52242-1316. Offers general microbiology and microbial physiology (MS, PhD); immunology (MS, PhD); microbial genetics (MS, PhD); pathogenic bacteriology (MS, PhD); virology (MS, PhD). *Degree requirements:* For master's, thesis; for doctorate, comprehensive exam, thesis/dissertation. *Entrance requirements:* For master's and doctorate, GRE General Test. Additional exam requirements/recommendations for international students: Required—TOEFL (minimum score 600 paper-based). Electronic applications accepted. *Faculty research:* Gene regulation, processing and transport of HIV, retroviral pathogenesis, biodegradation, biofilm.

The University of Manchester, Faculty of Life Sciences, Manchester, United Kingdom. Offers adaptive organismal biology (M Phil, PhD); animal biology (M Phil, PhD); biochemistry (M Phil, PhD); bioinformatics (M Phil, PhD); biomolecular sciences (M Phil, PhD); biotechnology (M Phil, PhD); cell biology (M Phil, PhD); cell matrix research (M Phil, PhD); channels and transporters (M Phil, PhD); developmental biology (M Phil, PhD); Egyptology (M Phil, PhD); environmental biology (M Phil, PhD); evolutionary biology (M Phil, PhD); gene expression (M Phil, PhD); genetics (M Phil, PhD); history of science, technology and medicine (M Phil, PhD); immunology (M Phil, PhD); integrative neurobiology and behavior (M Phil, PhD); membrane trafficking (M Phil, PhD); microbiology (M Phil, PhD); molecular and cellular neuroscience (M Phil, PhD); molecular biology (M Phil, PhD); molecular cancer studies (M Phil, PhD); neuroscience (M Phil, PhD); ophthalmology (M Phil, PhD); optometry (M Phil, PhD); organelle function (M Phil, PhD); pharmacology (M Phil, PhD); physiology (M Phil, PhD); plant sciences (M Phil, PhD); stem cell research (M Phil, PhD); structural biology (M Phil, PhD); systems neuroscience (M Phil, PhD); toxicology (M Phil, PhD).

University of Massachusetts Amherst, Graduate School, Interdisciplinary Programs, Program in Plant Biology, Amherst, MA 01003. Offers biochemistry and metabolism (MS, PhD); cell biology and physiology (MS, PhD); environmental, ecological and integrative biology (MS, PhD); genetics and evolution (MS, PhD). *Degree requirements:* For master's, thesis; for doctorate, 2 foreign languages, comprehensive exam, thesis/dissertation. *Entrance requirements:* For master's and doctorate, GRE General Test. Additional exam requirements/recommendations for international students: Required—TOEFL (minimum score 550 paper-based; 80 iBT), IELTS (minimum score 6.5). Electronic applications accepted.

University of Miami, Graduate School, College of Arts and Sciences, Department of Biology, Coral Gables, FL 33124. Offers biology (MS, PhD); genetics and evolution (MS, PhD). Terminal master's awarded for partial completion of doctoral program. *Degree requirements:* For master's, comprehensive exam (for some programs), thesis (for some programs); for doctorate, thesis/dissertation, oral and written qualifying exam. *Entrance requirements:* For master's, GRE General Test, 3 letters of recommendation, research papers; for doctorate, GRE General Test, 3 letters of recommendation, research papers, sponsor letter. Additional exam requirements/recommendations for international students: Required—TOEFL (minimum score 550 paper-based; 59 iBT). Electronic applications accepted. *Faculty research:* Neuroscience to ethology; plants, vertebrates and mycorrhizae; phylogenies, life histories and species interactions; molecular biology, gene expression and populations; cells, auditory neurons and vertebrate locomotion.

University of Minnesota, Twin Cities Campus, Graduate School, Program in Molecular, Cellular, Developmental Biology and Genetics, Minneapolis, MN 55455-0213. Offers genetic counseling (MS); molecular, cellular, developmental biology and genetics (PhD). Terminal master's awarded for partial completion of doctoral program. *Degree requirements:* For master's, thesis optional; for doctorate, thesis/dissertation. *Entrance requirements:* For master's and doctorate, GRE General Test. Additional exam requirements/recommendations for international students: Required—TOEFL (minimum score 625 paper-based; 80 iBT). Electronic applications accepted. *Faculty research:* Membrane receptors and membrane transport, cell interactions, cytoskeleton and cell mobility, regulation of gene expression, plant cell and molecular biology.

University of Missouri, Office of Research and Graduate Studies, Genetics Area Program, Columbia, MO 65211. Offers PhD. *Degree requirements:* For doctorate, comprehensive exam, thesis/dissertation. *Entrance requirements:* For doctorate, GRE General Test, minimum GPA of 3.0. Additional exam requirements/recommendations for international students: Required—TOEFL (minimum score 580 paper-based; 92 iBT). *Application deadline:* For fall admission, 1/15 priority date for domestic students, 1/15 for international students. Applications are processed on a rolling basis. Application fee: $55 ($75 for international students). Electronic applications accepted. *Financial support:* Fellowships with tuition reimbursements, research assistantships with tuition reimbursements, teaching assistantships with tuition reimbursements, institutionally sponsored loans, scholarships/grants, traineeships, health care benefits, and unspecified assistantships available. Support available to part-time students. Website: http://www.gap.missouri.edu/

University of Nebraska Medical Center, Department of Genetics, Cell Biology and Anatomy, Omaha, NE 68198. Offers MS, PhD. *Faculty:* 22 full-time (5 women), 1 (woman) part-time/adjunct. *Students:* 41 full-time (17 women); includes 6 minority (2 Black or African American, non-Hispanic/Latino; 1 American Indian or Alaska Native, non-Hispanic/Latino; 2 Asian, non-Hispanic/Latino; 1 Hispanic/Latino), 9 international. Average age 25. 19 applicants, 32% accepted, 6 enrolled. In 2015, 14 master's, 7 doctorates awarded. Terminal master's awarded for partial completion of doctoral program. *Degree requirements:* For master's, comprehensive exam, thesis; for doctorate, comprehensive exam, thesis/dissertation. *Entrance requirements:* For master's and doctorate, GRE General Test. Additional exam requirements/recommendations for international students: Required—TOEFL (minimum score 550 paper-based; 80 iBT). *Application deadline:* For fall admission, 4/1 priority date for domestic and international students; for spring admission, 8/1 for domestic and international students; for summer admission, 1/1 for domestic and international students. Applications are processed on a rolling basis. Application fee: $45. Electronic applications accepted. *Expenses:* Tuition, state resident: full-time $7830; part-time $3915 per credit hour. Tuition, nonresident: full-time $22,410; part-time $11,205 per credit hour. Required fees: $521. *Financial support:* In 2015–16, 1 fellowship with full tuition reimbursement (averaging $23,100 per year), 1 research assistantship with full tuition reimbursement (averaging $24,000 per year) were awarded; scholarships/grants also available. Support available to part-time students. Financial award application deadline: 3/1; financial award applicants required to submit FAFSA. *Faculty research:* Hematology, immunology, developmental biology, genetics cancer biology, neuroscience. *Unit head:* Dr. Karen Gould, Graduate Committee Chair, 402-559-2456, E-mail: kagould@unmc.edu. *Application contact:* Bryan Katafiasz, Administrative Associate, 402-559-4031, Fax: 402-559-7328, E-mail: bkatafiasz@unmc.edu. Website: http://www.unmc.edu/genetics/

University of Nebraska Medical Center, Medical Sciences Interdepartmental Area, Omaha, NE 68198. Offers genetics, cell biology and anatomy (MS); internal medicine (MS). *Program availability:* Part-time. *Faculty:* 195 full-time, 20 part-time/adjunct. *Students:* 49 full-time (28 women), 40 part-time (27 women); includes 10 minority (1 Black or African American, non-Hispanic/Latino; 6 Asian, non-Hispanic/Latino; 3 Hispanic/Latino), 16 international. Average age 32. 46 applicants, 41% accepted, 19 enrolled. In 2015, 12 master's, 17 doctorates awarded. Terminal master's awarded for partial completion of doctoral program. *Degree requirements:* For master's, comprehensive exam, thesis; for doctorate, comprehensive exam, thesis/dissertation.

Entrance requirements: For master's, GRE General Test; for doctorate, GRE General Test, MCAT or DCAT. Additional exam requirements/recommendations for international students: Required—TOEFL (minimum score 550 paper-based; 80 iBT). *Application deadline:* For fall admission, 4/1 for domestic and international students; for spring admission, 8/1 for domestic and international students; for summer admission, 1/1 for domestic and international students. Applications are processed on a rolling basis. Application fee: $45. Electronic applications accepted. *Expenses:* Tuition, state resident: full-time $7830; part-time $3915 per credit hour. Tuition, nonresident: full-time $22,410; part-time $11,205 per credit hour. Required fees: $521. *Financial support:* In 2015–16, 3 fellowships with full tuition reimbursements (averaging $23,100 per year), 4 research assistantships with full tuition reimbursements (averaging $23,100 per year) were awarded; teaching assistantships and scholarships/grants also available. Support available to part-time students. Financial award application deadline: 2/15; financial award applicants required to submit FAFSA. *Faculty research:* Molecular genetics, oral biology, veterinary pathology, newborn medicine, immunology, clinical research. *Unit head:* Dr. Laura Bilek, Graduate Committee Chair, 402-559-6923, E-mail: lbilek@unmc.edu.
Website: http://www.unmc.edu/gradstudies/programs/msia/

University of New Hampshire, Graduate School, College of Life Sciences and Agriculture, Department of Molecular, Cellular and Biomedical Sciences, Program in Genetics, Durham, NH 03824. Offers MS, PhD. *Program availability:* Part-time. *Degree requirements:* For master's, thesis; for doctorate, thesis/dissertation. *Entrance requirements:* For master's and doctorate, GRE General Test, GRE Subject Test. Additional exam requirements/recommendations for international students: Required—TOEFL (minimum score 550 paper-based; 80 iBT). *Application deadline:* For fall admission, 6/1 priority date for domestic students, 4/1 for international students; for spring admission, 12/1 for domestic students. Applications are processed on a rolling basis. Application fee: $65. Electronic applications accepted. *Expenses:* Tuition, state resident: full-time $13,840; part-time $770 per credit hour. Tuition, nonresident: full-time $27,130; part-time $1175 per credit hour. Required fees: $2080; $1040. Tuition and fees vary according to degree level and program. *Financial support:* Fellowships, research assistantships, teaching assistantships, career-related internships or fieldwork, Federal Work-Study, and scholarships/grants available. Support available to part-time students. Financial award application deadline: 2/15. *Unit head:* Dr. Subhash C. Minocha, Director, 603-862-3840. *Application contact:* Flora Joyal, Administrative Assistant, 603-862-2250, E-mail: genetics.dept@unh.edu.
Website: http://colsa.unh.edu/mcbs/genetics-graduate-programs/

University of New Mexico, Graduate Studies, Health Sciences Center, Program in Biomedical Sciences, Albuquerque, NM 87131-5196. Offers biochemistry and molecular biology (MS, PhD); cell biology and physiology (MS, PhD); molecular genetics and microbiology (MS, PhD); neuroscience (MS, PhD); pathology (MS, PhD); toxicology (MS, PhD). *Program availability:* Part-time. *Faculty:* 18 full-time (10 women), 1 part-time/adjunct (0 women). *Students:* 31 full-time (17 women), 45 part-time (26 women); includes 29 minority (1 American Indian or Alaska Native, non-Hispanic/Latino; 3 Asian, non-Hispanic/Latino; 22 Hispanic/Latino; 2 Native Hawaiian or other Pacific Islander, non-Hispanic/Latino; 1 Two or more races, non-Hispanic/Latino), 18 international. Average age 30. 98 applicants, 11% accepted, 11 enrolled. In 2015, 11 master's, 14 doctorates awarded. Terminal master's awarded for partial completion of doctoral program. *Degree requirements:* For master's, thesis; for doctorate, comprehensive exam, thesis/dissertation, qualifying exam at the end of year 1/core curriculum. *Entrance requirements:* For master's and doctorate, GRE General Test, minimum undergraduate GPA of 3.0. Additional exam requirements/recommendations for international students: Required—TOEFL. *Application deadline:* For fall admission, 3/1 priority date for domestic and international students. Applications are processed on a rolling basis. Application fee: $50. Electronic applications accepted. *Financial support:* Fellowships with tuition reimbursements, research assistantships with full tuition reimbursements, teaching assistantships, career-related internships or fieldwork, Federal Work-Study, institutionally sponsored loans, scholarships/grants, traineeships, health care benefits, and unspecified assistantships available. Financial award application deadline: 1/1; financial award applicants required to submit FAFSA. *Faculty research:* Infectious disease/immunity, cancer biology, cardiovascular and metabolic diseases, brain and behavioral illness, environmental health. *Unit head:* Dr. Helen J. Hathaway, Program Director, 505-272-1887, Fax: 505-272-2412, E-mail: hhathaway@salud.unm.edu. *Application contact:* Mary Fenton, Admissions Coordinator, 505-272-1887, Fax: 505-272-2412, E-mail: mfenton@salud.unm.edu.

The University of North Carolina at Chapel Hill, Graduate School, College of Arts and Sciences, Department of Biology, Chapel Hill, NC 27599. Offers botany (MA, MS, PhD); cell biology, development, and physiology (MA, MS, PhD); cell motility and cytoskeleton (PhD); ecology and behavior (MA, MS, PhD); genetics and molecular biology (MA, MS, PhD); morphology, systematics, and evolution (MA, MS, PhD). Terminal master's awarded for partial completion of doctoral program. *Degree requirements:* For master's, comprehensive exam, thesis (for some programs); for doctorate, comprehensive exam, thesis/dissertation. *Entrance requirements:* For master's, GRE General Test, GRE Subject Test, 2 semesters of calculus or statistics; 2 semesters of physics, organic chemistry; 3 semesters of biology; for doctorate, GRE General Test, GRE Subject Test, 2 semesters calculus or statistics, 2 semesters physics, organic chemistry, 3 semesters of biology. Additional exam requirements/recommendations for international students: Required—TOEFL (minimum score 550 paper-based). Electronic applications accepted. *Faculty research:* Gene expression, biomechanics, yeast genetics, plant ecology, plant molecular biology.

The University of North Carolina at Chapel Hill, School of Medicine and Graduate School, Graduate Programs in Medicine, Curriculum in Genetics and Molecular Biology, Chapel Hill, NC 27599. Offers MS, PhD. *Degree requirements:* For doctorate, comprehensive exam, thesis/dissertation. *Entrance requirements:* For doctorate, GRE, minimum GPA of 3.0. Additional exam requirements/recommendations for international students: Required—TOEFL. Electronic applications accepted. *Faculty research:* Telomere replication and germline immortality, experimental evolution in microorganisms, genetic vulnerabilities in tumor genomes, genetics of cell cycle control during Drosophila development, mammalian genetics.

University of North Dakota, Graduate School, College of Arts and Sciences, Department of Biology, Grand Forks, ND 58202. Offers botany (MS, PhD); ecology (MS, PhD); entomology (MS, PhD); environmental biology (MS, PhD); fisheries/wildlife (MS, PhD); genetics (MS, PhD); zoology (MS, PhD). Terminal master's awarded for partial completion of doctoral program. *Degree requirements:* For master's, thesis, final exam; for doctorate, comprehensive exam, thesis/dissertation, final exam. *Entrance requirements:* For master's, GRE General Test, GRE Subject Test, minimum GPA of 3.0; for doctorate, GRE General Test, GRE Subject Test, minimum GPA of 3.5. Additional exam requirements/recommendations for international students: Required—TOEFL (minimum score 550 paper-based; 79 iBT), IELTS (minimum score 6.5). Electronic applications accepted. *Faculty research:* Population biology, wildlife ecology, RNA processing, hormonal control of behavior.

University of North Texas Health Science Center at Fort Worth, Graduate School of Biomedical Sciences, Fort Worth, TX 76107-2699. Offers anatomy and cell biology (MS,

PhD); biochemistry and molecular biology (MS, PhD); biomedical sciences (MS, PhD); biotechnology (MS); forensic genetics (MS); integrative physiology (MS, PhD); medical science (MS); microbiology and immunology (MS, PhD); pharmacology (MS, PhD); science education (MS); DO/MS; DO/PhD. Terminal master's awarded for partial completion of doctoral program. *Degree requirements:* For master's, thesis; for doctorate, thesis/dissertation. *Entrance requirements:* For master's and doctorate, GRE General Test. Additional exam requirements/recommendations for international students: Required—TOEFL. *Expenses:* Contact institution. *Faculty research:* Alzheimer's disease, aging, eye diseases, cancer, cardiovascular disease.

University of Notre Dame, Graduate School, College of Science, Department of Biological Sciences, Notre Dame, IN 46556. Offers aquatic ecology, evolution and environmental biology (MS, PhD); cellular and molecular biology (MS, PhD); genetics (MS, PhD); physiology (MS, PhD); vector biology and parasitology (MS, PhD). Terminal master's awarded for partial completion of doctoral program. *Degree requirements:* For master's, comprehensive exam, thesis; for doctorate, comprehensive exam, thesis/ dissertation, candidacy exam. *Entrance requirements:* For master's and doctorate, GRE General Test. Additional exam requirements/recommendations for international students: Required—TOEFL (minimum score 600 paper-based; 80 iBT). Electronic applications accepted. *Faculty research:* Tropical disease, molecular genetics, neurobiology, evolutionary biology, aquatic biology.

University of Oregon, Graduate School, College of Arts and Sciences, Department of Biology, Eugene, OR 97403. Offers ecology and evolution (MA, MS, PhD); marine biology (MA, MS, PhD); molecular, cellular and genetic biology (PhD); neuroscience and development (PhD). Terminal master's awarded for partial completion of doctoral program. *Degree requirements:* For master's, thesis (for some programs); for doctorate, thesis/dissertation. *Entrance requirements:* For master's and doctorate, GRE General Test, minimum GPA of 3.2. Additional exam requirements/recommendations for international students: Required—TOEFL. *Faculty research:* Developmental neurobiology; evolution, population biology, and quantitative genetics; regulation of gene expression; biochemistry of marine organisms.

University of Pennsylvania, Perelman School of Medicine, Biomedical Graduate Studies, Graduate Group in Cell and Molecular Biology, Philadelphia, PA 19104. Offers cancer biology (PhD); cell biology, physiology, and metabolism (PhD); developmental stem cell regenerative biology (PhD); gene therapy and vaccines (PhD); genetics and gene regulation (PhD); microbiology, virology, and parasitology (PhD); MD/PhD; VMD/ PhD. *Faculty:* 317. *Students:* 339 full-time (189 women); includes 100 minority (7 Black or African American, non-Hispanic/Latino; 2 American Indian or Alaska Native, non-Hispanic/Latino; 45 Asian, non-Hispanic/Latino; 34 Hispanic/Latino; 1 Native Hawaiian or other Pacific Islander, non-Hispanic/Latino; 11 Two or more races, non-Hispanic/ Latino), 52 international. 493 applicants, 22% accepted, 37 enrolled. In 2015, 51 doctorates awarded. *Degree requirements:* For doctorate, thesis/dissertation. *Entrance requirements:* For doctorate, GRE General Test. Additional exam requirements/ recommendations for international students: Required—TOEFL. *Application deadline:* For fall admission, 12/1 priority date for domestic and international students. Applications are processed on a rolling basis. Application fee: $80. Electronic applications accepted. *Expenses:* Tuition, area resident: Full-time $31,068; part-time $5762 per course. *Required fees:* $3200; $336 per course. Full-time tuition and fees vary according to degree level, program and student level. Part-time tuition and fees vary according to course load, degree level and program. *Financial support:* In 2015–16, 339 students received support. Fellowships, research assistantships, scholarships/ grants, traineeships, and unspecified assistantships available. *Unit head:* Dr. Daniel Kessler, Graduate Group Chair, 215-898-1478. *Application contact:* Meagan Schofer, Coordinator, 215-898-4360.
Website: http://www.med.upenn.edu/camb/

University of Puerto Rico, Río Piedras Campus, College of Natural Sciences, Department of Biology, San Juan, PR 00931-3300. Offers ecology/systematics (MS, PhD); evolution/genetics (MS, PhD); molecular/cellular biology (MS, PhD); neuroscience (MS, PhD). *Program availability:* Part-time. *Degree requirements:* For master's, one foreign language, comprehensive exam, thesis; for doctorate, one foreign language, comprehensive exam, thesis/dissertation. *Entrance requirements:* For master's, GRE Subject Test, interview, minimum GPA of 3.0, letter of recommendation; for doctorate, GRE Subject Test, interview, master's degree, minimum GPA of 3.0, letter of recommendation. *Faculty research:* Environmental, poblational and systematic biology.

University of Rochester, School of Medicine and Dentistry, Graduate Programs in Medicine and Dentistry, Department of Biomedical Genetics, Rochester, NY 14627. Offers genetics, genomics and development (PhD). *Degree requirements:* For doctorate, thesis/dissertation, qualifying exam. *Entrance requirements:* For doctorate, GRE General Test. *Expenses:* Tuition, area resident: Full-time $47,450; part-time $1482 per credit hour. *Required fees:* $528. Tuition and fees vary according to program.

The University of Tennessee, Graduate School, College of Arts and Sciences, Program in Life Sciences, Knoxville, TN 37996. Offers genome science and technology (MS, PhD); plant physiology and genetics (MS, PhD). *Degree requirements:* For doctorate, one foreign language, thesis/dissertation. *Entrance requirements:* For master's and doctorate, GRE General Test, minimum GPA of 2.7. Additional exam requirements/recommendations for international students: Required—TOEFL. Electronic applications accepted.

The University of Texas Health Science Center at Houston, Graduate School of Biomedical Sciences, Program in Genes and Development, Houston, TX 77225-0036. Offers MS, PhD, MD/PhD. Terminal master's awarded for partial completion of doctoral program. *Degree requirements:* For master's, thesis; for doctorate, thesis/dissertation. *Entrance requirements:* For master's and doctorate, GRE General Test. Additional exam requirements/recommendations for international students: Required—TOEFL. Electronic applications accepted. *Faculty research:* Developmental biology, genetics, cell biology, structural biology, cancer.

The University of Texas MD Anderson Cancer Center, School of Health Professions, Houston, TX 77030. Offers diagnostic genetics (MS). *Degree requirements:* For master's, successful defense of a written applied research project. *Entrance requirements:* For master's, bachelor's degree, minimum GPA of 3.0, clinical certification, three reference letters, personal interview. Additional exam requirements/ recommendations for international students: Required—TOEFL.

The University of Texas Medical Branch, Graduate School of Biomedical Sciences, Program in Biochemistry and Molecular Biology, Galveston, TX 77555. Offers biochemistry (PhD); bioinformatics (PhD); biophysics (PhD); cell biology (PhD); computational biology (PhD); structural biology (PhD). *Degree requirements:* For doctorate, thesis/dissertation. *Entrance requirements:* Additional exam requirements/ recommendations for international students: Required—TOEFL (minimum score 550 paper-based). Electronic applications accepted.

The University of Texas Southwestern Medical Center, Southwestern Graduate School of Biomedical Sciences, Division of Basic Science, Program in Genetics and Development, Dallas, TX 75390. Offers PhD. *Degree requirements:* For doctorate, thesis/dissertation, qualifying exam. *Entrance requirements:* For doctorate, GRE General Test, minimum GPA of 3.0. Additional exam requirements/recommendations for

international students: Required—TOEFL. Electronic applications accepted. *Faculty research:* Human molecular genetics, chromosome structure, gene regulation, molecular biology, gene expression.

University of Washington, Graduate School, School of Public Health, Institute for Public Health Genetics, Seattle, WA 98195. Offers genetic epidemiology (MS); public health genetics (MPH, PhD); MPH/JD. *Program availability:* Part-time. Terminal master's awarded for partial completion of doctoral program. *Degree requirements:* For master's, thesis, practicum (MPH); for doctorate, comprehensive exam, thesis/dissertation. *Entrance requirements:* For master's, GRE General Test, experience in health sciences, bachelor's degree in related field and course in human genetics (preferred); minimum GPA of 3.0; for doctorate, GRE General Test, experience in health sciences and master's degree in related field (preferred); coursework in human genetics, minimum GPA of 3.0. Additional exam requirements/recommendations for international students: Required—TOEFL (minimum score 580 paper-based; 92 iBT). Electronic applications accepted. *Expenses:* Contact institution. *Faculty research:* Genetic epidemiology; ethical, legal, social issues of genetics; ecogenetics; health policy.

University of Wisconsin–Madison, Graduate School, College of Agricultural and Life Sciences and Graduate Programs in Medicine, Department of Genetics, Madison, WI 53706-1380. Offers genetic counseling (MS); genetics (PhD). *Degree requirements:* For doctorate, thesis/dissertation. *Expenses:* Tuition, state resident: full-time $5364. Tuition, nonresident: full-time $12,027. *Required fees:* $571. Tuition and fees vary according to campus/location, program and reciprocity agreements.

University of Wyoming, Graduate Program in Molecular and Cellular Life Sciences, Laramie, WY 82071. Offers PhD. *Degree requirements:* For doctorate, thesis/ dissertation, four eight-week laboratory rotations, comprehensive basic practical exam, two-part qualifying exam, seminars, symposium.

Van Andel Institute Graduate School, PhD Program, Grand Rapids, MI 49503. Offers cell and molecular genetics (PhD). *Faculty:* 33 full-time (9 women). *Students:* 22 full-time (13 women); includes 3 minority (1 Black or African American, non-Hispanic/Latino; 2 Asian, non-Hispanic/Latino). Average age 24. 38 applicants, 24% accepted, 7 enrolled. In 2015, 3 degrees awarded. *Median time to degree:* Of those who began their doctoral program in fall 2007, 77% received their degree in 8 years or less. *Degree requirements:* For doctorate, comprehensive exam, thesis/dissertation. *Entrance requirements:* For doctorate, GRE or MCAT, personal statement, 3 letters of recommendation, official transcripts from all institutions attended, sample of scientific writing (research paper). Additional exam requirements/recommendations for international students: Required— TOEFL. *Application deadline:* For fall admission, 1/5 for domestic and international students. Applications are processed on a rolling basis. Application fee: $0. Electronic applications accepted. *Expenses:* Tuition, area resident: Full-time $25,000; part-time $835 per credit. *Financial support:* In 2015–16, 22 students received support, including 22 fellowships; health care benefits also available. *Faculty research:* Epigenetics, neurodegenerative science, cancer and cell biology. *Unit head:* Steve Triezenberg, President and Dean, 616-234-5708, Fax: 616-234-5709, E-mail: steve.triezenberg@ vai.org.

Virginia Commonwealth University, Medical College of Virginia-Professional Programs, School of Medicine, School of Medicine Graduate Programs, Department of Human and Molecular Genetics, Richmond, VA 23284-9005. Offers genetic counseling (MS); human genetics (PhD); molecular biology and genetics (MS, PhD); MD/PhD. *Degree requirements:* For master's, thesis; for doctorate, thesis/dissertation, comprehensive oral and written exams. *Entrance requirements:* For master's, GRE; for doctorate, GRE General Test. Additional exam requirements/recommendations for international students: Required—TOEFL (minimum score 600 paper-based; 100 iBT). Electronic applications accepted. *Faculty research:* Genetic epidemiology, biochemical genetics, quantitative genetics, human cytogenetics, molecular genetics.

Virginia Polytechnic Institute and State University, Graduate School, Intercollege, Blacksburg, VA 24061. Offers genetics, bioinformatics and computational biology (PhD); information technology (MIT); macromolecular science and engineering (MS, PhD). *Degree requirements:* For master's, comprehensive exam (for some programs), thesis (for some programs); for doctorate, comprehensive exam (for some programs), thesis/ dissertation (for some programs). *Entrance requirements:* For master's and doctorate, GRE/GMAT (may vary by department). Additional exam requirements/recommendations for international students: Required—TOEFL (minimum score 550 paper-based). Electronic applications accepted.

Washington State University, College of Veterinary Medicine, Program in Molecular Biosciences, Pullman, WA 99164. Offers molecular biology (PhD), including genetics, microbiology; molecular biosciences (PSM, PhD), including biochemistry (PhD), cell biology (PhD). *Program availability:* Online learning. *Faculty:* 30 full-time (12 women), 17 part-time/adjunct (5 women). *Students:* 47 full-time (26 women), 14 part-time (11 women); includes 13 minority (1 Black or African American, non-Hispanic/Latino; 1 American Indian or Alaska Native, non-Hispanic/Latino; 4 Asian, non-Hispanic/Latino; 5 Hispanic/Latino; 2 Two or more races, non-Hispanic/Latino), 1 international. Average age 28. 61 applicants, 23% accepted, 14 enrolled. In 2015, 5 master's, 8 doctorates awarded. Terminal master's awarded for partial completion of doctoral program. *Degree requirements:* For master's, thesis or alternative, oral exam; for doctorate, comprehensive exam, thesis/dissertation, oral exam, written exam. *Entrance requirements:* For master's and doctorate, GRE General Test, minimum GPA of 3.0. Additional exam requirements/recommendations for international students: Required— TOEFL (minimum score 100 iBT). *Application deadline:* For fall admission, 12/15 for domestic and international students. Application fee: $75. Electronic applications accepted. *Financial support:* In 2015–16, 5 fellowships with full tuition reimbursements (averaging $23,316 per year), 24 research assistantships with full tuition reimbursements (averaging $23,316 per year), 17 teaching assistantships with full tuition reimbursements (averaging $23,316 per year) were awarded; career-related internships or fieldwork, Federal Work-Study, traineeships, health care benefits, and unspecified assistantships also available. Financial award application deadline: 4/1; financial award applicants required to submit FAFSA. *Faculty research:* Gene regulation, signal transduction, protein export, reproductive biology, DNA repair. *Total annual research expenditures:* $5.8 million. *Unit head:* Dr. Jonathan Jones, Director, 509-335-8724, Fax: 509-335-9688, E-mail: jcr.jones@vetmed.wsu.edu. *Application contact:* Tami Breske, Coordinator, 509-335-4318, E-mail: tbreske@vetmed.wsu.edu.
Website: http://www.smb.wsu.edu

Washington University in St. Louis, Graduate School of Arts and Sciences, Division of Biology and Biomedical Sciences, St. Louis, MO 63130-4899. Offers biochemistry (PhD); computational and molecular biophysics (PhD); computational and systems biology (PhD); developmental, regenerative, and stem cell biology (PhD); evolution, ecology and population biology (PhD), including ecology, environmental biology, evolutionary biology, genetics; human and statistical genetics (PhD); immunology (PhD); molecular cell biology (PhD); molecular genetics and genomics (PhD); molecular microbiology and microbial pathogenesis (PhD); neurosciences (PhD); plant and microbial biosciences (PhD); MD/PhD. *Students:* 542 full-time (246 women); includes 106 minority (27 Black or African American, non-Hispanic/Latino; 5 American Indian or Alaska Native, non-Hispanic/Latino; 60 Asian, non-Hispanic/Latino; 11 Hispanic/Latino;

Genetics

3 Two or more races, non-Hispanic/Latino), 115 international. 1,085 applicants, 21% accepted, 77 enrolled. In 2015, 87 doctorates awarded. *Degree requirements:* For doctorate, thesis/dissertation. *Entrance requirements:* For doctorate, GRE General Test, GRE Subject Test. Additional exam requirements/recommendations for international students: Required—TOEFL. *Application deadline:* For fall admission, 12/1 for domestic students. Application fee: $0. Electronic applications accepted. *Financial support:* Fellowships, research assistantships, and tuition waivers (full) available. Financial award application deadline: 1/15. *Unit head:* Dr. John Russell, Associate Dean, 314-747-0840. *Application contact:* Rebecca Riney, 314-474-4648, E-mail: dbbsphdadmissions@wusm.wustl.edu.
Website: http://dbbs.wustl.edu/

Washington University in St. Louis, School of Medicine, Program in Clinical Investigation, St. Louis, MO 63130-4899. Offers clinical investigation (MS), including bioethics, entrepreneurship, genetics/genomics, translational medicine. *Program availability:* Part-time, evening/weekend. *Faculty:* 61 full-time (14 women), 2 part-time/adjunct (both women). *Students:* 15 full-time (5 women), 39 part-time (19 women); includes 15 minority (3 Black or African American, non-Hispanic/Latino; 8 Asian, non-Hispanic/Latino; 2 Hispanic/Latino; 2 Two or more races, non-Hispanic/Latino), 3 international. Average age 32. 34 applicants, 65% accepted, 22 enrolled. In 2015, 35 master's awarded. *Degree requirements:* For master's, thesis. *Entrance requirements:* For master's, doctoral-level degree or in process of obtaining doctoral-level degree. *Application deadline:* For fall admission, 5/15 for domestic students; for spring admission, 10/15 for domestic students. Application fee: $0. Electronic applications accepted. *Financial support:* In 2015–16, 4 students received support. Tuition waivers (partial) available. Financial award application deadline: 12/12. *Faculty research:* Anesthesiology, infectious diseases, neurology, obstetrics and gynecology, orthopedic surgery. *Unit head:* Dr. David Warren, Associate Professor of Medicine, 314-454-8225, Fax: 314-454-8279, E-mail: dwarren@wustl.edu. *Application contact:* Suzie Fragale, Curriculum and Evaluation Coordinator, 314-454-8936, Fax: 314-454-8279, E-mail: fragale@wustl.edu.
Website: http://crtc.wustl.edu/

Wesleyan University, Graduate Studies, Department of Biology, Middletown, CT 06459. Offers cell and developmental biology (PhD); evolution and ecology (PhD); genetics and genomics (PhD), including bioinformatics; neurobiology and behavior (PhD). *Faculty:* 14 full-time (5 women). *Students:* 26 full-time (12 women); includes 5 minority (2 Black or African American, non-Hispanic/Latino; 3 Asian, non-Hispanic/Latino), 5 international. In 2015, 3 doctorates awarded. Terminal master's awarded for partial completion of doctoral program. *Degree requirements:* For doctorate, comprehensive exam, thesis/dissertation, public seminar. *Entrance requirements:* For doctorate, GRE. Additional exam requirements/recommendations for international students: Required—TOEFL or IELTS. *Application deadline:* For fall admission, 1/15 for domestic and international students. Application fee: $0. Electronic applications accepted. *Financial support:* Stipends available. *Faculty research:* Evolution and ecology, neurobiology and behavior, cell and developmental biology, genetics, genomics and bioinformatics. *Unit head:* Dr. John Kirn, Chair/Professor, 860-685-3494, E-mail: jrkirn@wesleyan.edu. *Application contact:* Marjorie Fitzgibbons, Administrative Assistant, 860-685-2157, E-mail: mfitzgibbons@wesleyan.edu.
Website: http://www.wesleyan.edu/bio/

West Virginia University, Davis College of Agriculture, Forestry and Consumer Sciences, Interdisciplinary Program in Genetics and Developmental Biology, Morgantown, WV 26506. Offers animal breeding (MS, PhD); biochemical and molecular genetics (MS, PhD); cytogenetics (MS, PhD); descriptive embryology (MS, PhD); developmental genetics (MS); experimental morphogenesis/teratology (MS); human genetics (MS, PhD); immunogenetics (MS, PhD); life cycles of animals and plants (MS, PhD); molecular aspects of development (MS, PhD); mutagenesis (MS, PhD); oncology (MS, PhD); plant genetics (MS, PhD); population and quantitative genetics (MS, PhD); regeneration (MS, PhD); teratology (PhD); toxicology (MS, PhD). *Degree requirements:* For master's, thesis; for doctorate, comprehensive exam, thesis/dissertation. *Entrance requirements:* For master's, GRE or MCAT, minimum GPA of 2.75. Additional exam requirements/recommendations for international students: Required—TOEFL. *Expenses:* Tuition, state resident: full-time $8568. Tuition, nonresident: full-time $22,140. Tuition and fees vary according to program.

Yale University, Graduate School of Arts and Sciences, Department of Genetics, New Haven, CT 06520. Offers PhD, MD/PhD. *Degree requirements:* For doctorate, thesis/dissertation. *Entrance requirements:* For doctorate, GRE General Test, GRE Subject Test.

Yale University, Graduate School of Arts and Sciences, Department of Molecular, Cellular, and Developmental Biology, Program in Genetics, New Haven, CT 06520. Offers PhD. *Degree requirements:* For doctorate, thesis/dissertation. *Entrance requirements:* For doctorate, GRE General Test, GRE Subject Test.

Yale University, School of Medicine and Graduate School of Arts and Sciences, Combined Program in Biological and Biomedical Sciences (BBS), Molecular Cell Biology, Genetics, and Development Track, New Haven, CT 06520. Offers PhD, MD/PhD. *Entrance requirements:* Additional exam requirements/recommendations for international students: Required—TOEFL.

Genomic Sciences

Albert Einstein College of Medicine, Graduate Division of Biomedical Sciences, Department of Genetics, Bronx, NY 10461. Offers computational genetics (PhD); molecular genetics (PhD); translational genetics (PhD); MD/PhD. *Degree requirements:* For doctorate, thesis/dissertation. *Entrance requirements:* For doctorate, GRE General Test. Additional exam requirements/recommendations for international students: Required—TOEFL. *Faculty research:* Neurologic genetics in &ITDrosophila&RO, biochemical genetics of yeast, developmental genetics in the mouse.

Augusta University, The Graduate School, Program in Genomic Medicine, Augusta, GA 30912. Offers MS, PhD. *Faculty:* 1 full-time. *Degree requirements:* For doctorate, comprehensive exam, thesis/dissertation. *Entrance requirements:* For doctorate, GRE General Test. Additional exam requirements/recommendations for international students: Required—TOEFL (minimum score 550 paper-based; 79 iBT). *Application deadline:* For fall admission, 1/15 for domestic and international students. Application fee: $50. Electronic applications accepted. *Financial support:* Research assistantships with partial tuition reimbursements, Federal Work-Study, institutionally sponsored loans, and scholarships/grants available. Support available to part-time students. Financial award application deadline: 5/31; financial award applicants required to submit FAFSA. *Faculty research:* Genetic and genomic basis of diseases (diabetes, cancer, autoimmunity), development of diagnostic markers, bioinformatics, computational biology. *Unit head:* Dr. Jin-Xiong She, Director, Center for Biotechnology and Genomic Medicine, 706-721-3540, E-mail: jshe@augusta.edu.
Website: http://www.cbgm.gru.edu/GraduateProgram.aspx

Black Hills State University, Graduate Studies, Program in Integrative Genomics, Spearfish, SD 57799. Offers MS. *Entrance requirements:* Additional exam requirements/recommendations for international students: Required—TOEFL (minimum score 500 paper-based; 60 iBT).

Boston University, School of Medicine, Division of Graduate Medical Sciences, Program in Genetics and Genomics, Boston, MA 02215. Offers PhD. *Degree requirements:* For doctorate, thesis/dissertation. *Application deadline:* For fall admission, 1/15 for domestic students; for spring admission, 10/15 for domestic students. *Unit head:* Dr. Shoumita Dasgupta, Associate Professor and Director of Graduate Studies, 617-414-1580, E-mail: dasgupta@bu.edu. *Application contact:* GMS Admissions Office, 617-638-5255, E-mail: askgms@bu.edu.
Website: http://www.bumc.bu.edu/gpgg/graduate-program/

Case Western Reserve University, School of Medicine and School of Graduate Studies, Graduate Programs in Medicine, Department of Genetics and Genome Sciences, Program in Human, Molecular, and Developmental Genetics and Genomics, Cleveland, OH 44106. Offers MS, MD/PhD. *Degree requirements:* For doctorate, comprehensive exam, thesis/dissertation. *Entrance requirements:* For doctorate, GRE General Test, GRE Subject Test. Additional exam requirements/recommendations for international students: Required—TOEFL. *Expenses:* Tuition, area resident: Full-time $41,137; part-time $1714 per credit hour. *Required fees:* $32. Tuition and fees vary according to course load and program. *Faculty research:* Regulation of gene expression, molecular control of development, genomics.

Concordia University, School of Graduate Studies, Faculty of Arts and Science, Department of Biology, Montréal, QC H3G 1M8, Canada. Offers biology (M Sc, PhD); biotechnology and genomics (Diploma). *Degree requirements:* For master's, thesis; for doctorate, thesis/dissertation, pedagogical training. *Entrance requirements:* For master's, honors degree in biology; for doctorate, M Sc in life science. *Application deadline:* For fall admission, 1/15 priority date for domestic students; for winter admission, 8/31 for domestic students. Application fee: $50. Tuition and fees vary according to course load, degree level and program. *Faculty research:* Cell biology, animal physiology, ecology, microbiology/molecular biology, plant physiology/biochemistry and biotechnology. *Unit head:* Patrick Gulick, Chair, 514-848-2424 Ext. 3407, Fax: 514-848-2881. *Application contact:* Selvadurai Dayanandan, Graduate Program Director, 514-848-2424 Ext. 3414, Fax: 514-848-2881.
Website: http://www.concordia.ca/artsci/biology.html

Cornell University, Graduate School, Graduate Fields of Agriculture and Life Sciences, Field of Genetics, Genomics and Development, Ithaca, NY 14853-0001. Offers developmental biology (PhD); genetics (PhD); genomics (PhD). *Degree requirements:* For doctorate, comprehensive exam, thesis/dissertation, 2 semesters of teaching experience. *Entrance requirements:* For doctorate, GRE General Test, GRE Subject Test in biology or biochemistry (recommended), 2 letters of recommendation. Additional exam requirements/recommendations for international students: Required—TOEFL (minimum score 550 paper-based; 77 iBT). Electronic applications accepted. *Faculty research:* Molecular and general genetics, developmental biology and developmental genetics, evolution and population genetics, plant genetics, microbial genetics.

Duke University, Graduate School, University Program in Genetics and Genomics, Durham, NC 27710. Offers PhD. *Degree requirements:* For doctorate, variable foreign language requirement, thesis/dissertation. *Entrance requirements:* For doctorate, GRE General Test. Additional exam requirements/recommendations for international students: Required—TOEFL (minimum score 577 paper-based; 90 iBT) or IELTS (minimum score 7).

Harvard University, Graduate School of Arts and Sciences, Department of Systems Biology, Cambridge, MA 02138. Offers PhD. *Degree requirements:* For doctorate, thesis/dissertation, lab rotation, qualifying examination. *Entrance requirements:* For doctorate, GRE. Additional exam requirements/recommendations for international students: Required—TOEFL. Electronic applications accepted.

Massachusetts Institute of Technology, School of Engineering, Harvard-MIT Health Sciences and Technology Program, Cambridge, MA 02139. Offers health sciences and technology (SM, PhD, Sc D), including bioastronautics (PhD, Sc D), bioinformatics and integrative genomics (PhD, Sc D), medical engineering and medical physics (PhD, Sc D), speech and hearing bioscience and technology (PhD, Sc D). *Faculty:* 125 full-time (20 women). *Students:* 271 full-time (111 women), 15 part-time (4 women); includes 79 minority (2 Black or African American, non-Hispanic/Latino; 1 American Indian or Alaska Native, non-Hispanic/Latino; 61 Asian, non-Hispanic/Latino; 12 Hispanic/Latino; 3 Two or more races, non-Hispanic/Latino), 51 international. Average age 26. 265 applicants, 11% accepted, 21 enrolled. In 2015, 3 master's, 25 doctorates awarded. Terminal master's awarded for partial completion of doctoral program. *Degree requirements:* For master's, thesis; for doctorate, comprehensive exam, thesis/dissertation. *Entrance requirements:* For doctorate, GRE General Test (for medical engineering and medical physics). Additional exam requirements/recommendations for international students: Required—TOEFL (minimum score 600 paper-based; 100 iBT), IELTS (minimum score 7). *Application deadline:* For fall admission, 12/15 for domestic and international students. Application fee: $75. Electronic applications accepted. *Expenses: Tuition:* Full-time $46,400; part-time $725 per credit. One-time fee: $304 full-time. Full-time tuition and fees vary according to course load and program. *Financial support:* In 2015–16, 128 students received support, including 57 fellowships (averaging $38,200 per year), 52 research assistantships (averaging $34,200 per year), 1 teaching assistantship (averaging $19,500 per year); Federal Work-Study, institutionally sponsored loans, scholarships/grants, traineeships, health care benefits, and unspecified assistantships also available. Support available to part-time students. Financial award application deadline: 4/15; financial award applicants required to submit FAFSA. *Faculty research:* Signal processing, biomedical imaging, drug delivery, medical devices, medical diagnostics, regenerative biomedical technologies. *Unit head:* Emery N. Brown, Director, 617-452-4091. *Application contact:* 617-253-3609, Fax: 617-253-6692, E-mail: hst-phd-admissions@mit.edu.
Website: http://hst.mit.edu/

New York University, School of Medicine and Graduate School of Arts and Science, Sackler Institute of Graduate Biomedical Sciences, New York, NY 10010. Offers biomedical imaging (PhD); biomedical informatics (PhD); cellular and molecular biology (PhD); computational biology (PhD); developmental genetics (PhD); genome integrity (PhD); immunology and inflammation (PhD); microbiology (PhD); molecular biophysics (PhD); molecular oncology and tumor immunology (PhD), including immunology, molecular oncology; molecular pharmacology (PhD); neuroscience and physiology (PhD); pathobiology and translational medicine (PhD); stem cell biology (PhD); MD/PhD. *Degree requirements:* For doctorate, comprehensive exam, thesis/dissertation, qualifying exam. *Entrance requirements:* For doctorate, GRE General Test. Additional exam requirements/recommendations for international students: Required—TOEFL. Electronic applications accepted. *Expenses:* Contact institution.

North Carolina State University, Graduate School, College of Agriculture and Life Sciences, Graduate Program in Genomic Sciences, Raleigh, NC 27695. Offers MS, PhD.

North Carolina State University, Graduate School, College of Agriculture and Life Sciences, Program in Functional Genomics, Raleigh, NC 27695. Offers MFG, MS, PhD. *Degree requirements:* For master's, thesis (for some programs); for doctorate, thesis/dissertation. *Entrance requirements:* For master's and doctorate, GRE, minimum B average. Additional exam requirements/recommendations for international students: Required—TOEFL. Electronic applications accepted. *Faculty research:* Genome structure, genome expression, molecular evolution, nucleic acid structure/function, proteomics.

North Dakota State University, College of Graduate and Interdisciplinary Studies, College of Science and Mathematics, Department of Biological Sciences, Fargo, ND 58102. Offers biology (MS); botany (MS, PhD); cellular and molecular biology (PhD); genomics (PhD); zoology (MS, PhD). *Degree requirements:* For master's, thesis; for doctorate, thesis/dissertation. *Entrance requirements:* For master's and doctorate, GRE General Test. Additional exam requirements/recommendations for international students: Required—TOEFL. *Application deadline:* For fall admission, 1/15 for domestic students. Applications are processed on a rolling basis. Application fee: $35. Electronic applications accepted. *Financial support:* Fellowships with full tuition reimbursements, research assistantships with full tuition reimbursements, teaching assistantships with full tuition reimbursements, career-related internships or fieldwork, Federal Work-Study, institutionally sponsored loans, scholarships/grants, tuition waivers (full), and unspecified assistantships available. Support available to part-time students. Financial award application deadline: 4/15; financial award applicants required to submit FAFSA. *Faculty research:* Comparative endocrinology, physiology, behavioral ecology, plant cell biology, aquatic biology. *Unit head:* Dr. Wendy Reed, Head, 701-231-5921, E-mail: wendy.reed@ndsu.edu. *Application contact:* Elizabeth Worth, Marketing, Recruitment, and Public Relations Coordinator, 701-231-8476, Fax: 701-231-6524, E-mail: elizabeth.worth@ndsu.edu.
Website: http://www.ndsu.edu/biology/

North Dakota State University, College of Graduate and Interdisciplinary Studies, Interdisciplinary Program in Genomics and Bioinformatics, Fargo, ND 58102. Offers MS, PhD. *Program availability:* Part-time. *Degree requirements:* For master's, thesis; for doctorate, comprehensive exam, thesis/dissertation. *Entrance requirements:* For master's and doctorate, minimum GPA of 3.0. Additional exam requirements/recommendations for international students: Required—TOEFL (minimum score 525 paper-based; 71 iBT). *Application deadline:* For fall admission, 5/1 for international students; for spring admission, 8/1 for international students. Applications are processed on a rolling basis. Application fee: $35. Electronic applications accepted. *Financial support:* Research assistantships with full tuition reimbursements and unspecified assistantships available. *Faculty research:* Genome evolution, genome mapping, genome expression, bioinformatics, data mining. *Unit head:* Dr. Phillip E. McClean, Director, 701-231-8443, Fax: 701-231-8474. *Application contact:* Elizabeth Worth, Marketing, Recruitment, and Public Relations Coordinator, 701-231-8476, Fax: 701-231-6524, E-mail: elizabeth.worth@ndsu.edu.

Oregon State University, College of Science, Program in Microbiology, Corvallis, OR 97331. Offers environmental microbiology (MA, MS, PhD); food microbiology (MA, MS, PhD); genomics (MA, MS, PhD); immunology (MA, MS, PhD); microbial ecology (MA, MS, PhD); microbial evolution (MA, MS, PhD); parasitology (MA, MS, PhD); pathogenic microbiology (MA, MS, PhD); virology (MA). *Program availability:* Part-time. *Faculty:* 14 full-time (5 women), 1 part-time/adjunct (0 women). *Students:* 32 full-time (12 women); includes 5 minority (4 Asian, non-Hispanic/Latino; 1 Two or more races, non-Hispanic/Latino), 2 international. Average age 28. 79 applicants, 10% accepted, 4 enrolled. In 2015, 3 master's, 4 doctorates awarded. Terminal master's awarded for partial completion of doctoral program. *Degree requirements:* For master's, thesis; for doctorate, one foreign language, thesis/dissertation. *Entrance requirements:* For master's and doctorate, GRE. Additional exam requirements/recommendations for international students: Required—TOEFL (minimum score 600 paper-based; 100 iBT). *Application deadline:* For fall admission, 8/1 for domestic students, 4/1 for international students; for winter admission, 12/1 for domestic students, 7/1 for international students; for spring admission, 2/1 for domestic students, 10/1 for international students; for summer admission, 5/1 for domestic students, 1/1 for international students. Application fee: $75 ($85 for international students). *Expenses:* Tuition, state resident: full-time $12,150; part-time $450 per credit. Tuition, nonresident: full-time $20,952; part-time $776 per credit. *Required fees:* $1572; $1443 per unit. One-time fee: $350. Tuition and fees vary according to course load, campus/location and program. *Financial support:* Fellowships, research assistantships, and teaching assistantships available. Financial award application deadline: 1/15. *Faculty research:* Genetics, physiology, biotechnology, pathogenic microbiology, plant virology. *Unit head:* Dr. Jerri Bartholomew, Professor and Department Head, 541-737-1856. *Application contact:* Mary Fulton, Microbiology Advisor, 541-737-1833, E-mail: mary.fulton@oregonstate.edu.
Website: http://microbiology.science.oregonstate.edu/

Purdue University, College of Pharmacy and Pharmacal Sciences and Graduate School, Graduate Programs in Pharmacy and Pharmacal Sciences, Department of Medicinal Chemistry and Molecular Pharmacology, West Lafayette, IN 47907. Offers biophysical and computational chemistry (PhD); cancer research (PhD); immunology and infectious disease (PhD); medicinal biochemistry and molecular biology (PhD); medicinal chemistry and chemical biology (PhD); molecular pharmacology (PhD); neuropharmacology, neurodegeneration, and neurotoxicity (PhD); systems biology and functional genomics (PhD). *Degree requirements:* For doctorate, thesis/dissertation. *Entrance requirements:* For doctorate, GRE General Test; GRE Subject Test in biology, biochemistry, and chemistry (recommended), minimum undergraduate GPA of 3.0. Additional exam requirements/recommendations for international students: Required—TOEFL (minimum score 550 paper-based; 77 iBT); Recommended—TWE. Electronic applications accepted. *Faculty research:* Drug design and development, cancer research, drug synthesis and analysis, chemical pharmacology, environmental toxicology.

Thomas Jefferson University, Jefferson College of Biomedical Sciences, PhD Program in Genetics, Genomics and Cancer Biology, Philadelphia, PA 19107. Offers

PhD. *Faculty:* 48 full-time (16 women), 4 part-time/adjunct (3 women). *Students:* 21 full-time (12 women); includes 3 minority (1 Asian, non-Hispanic/Latino; 2 Hispanic/Latino), 3 international. 46 applicants, 11% accepted, 4 enrolled. In 2015, 1 doctorate awarded. *Degree requirements:* For doctorate, comprehensive exam, thesis/dissertation. *Entrance requirements:* For doctorate, GRE General Test, minimum GPA of 3.2. Additional exam requirements/recommendations for international students: Required—TOEFL, IELTS (minimum score 7). *Application deadline:* For fall admission, 12/15 priority date for domestic and international students. Applications are processed on a rolling basis. Application fee: $50. Electronic applications accepted. *Financial support:* In 2015–16, 21 students received support, including 21 fellowships with full tuition reimbursements available (averaging $56,298 per year); Federal Work-Study, institutionally sponsored loans, scholarships/grants, traineeships, and stipends also available. Support available to part-time students. Financial award application deadline: 5/1; financial award applicants required to submit FAFSA. *Faculty research:* Functional genomics, cancer susceptibility, cell cycle, regulation oncogenes and tumor suppressor genes, genetics of neoplastic disease. *Unit head:* Dr. Lucia Languino, Program Director, 215-503-3442, E-mail: lucia.languino@jefferson.edu. *Application contact:* Marc E. Stearns, Director of Admissions, 215-503-0155, Fax: 215-503-3433, E-mail: jgsbs-info@jefferson.edu.
Website: http://www.jefferson.edu/university/biomedical-sciences/degrees-programs/phd-programs/genetics.html

University at Buffalo, the State University of New York, Graduate School, School of Medicine and Biomedical Sciences, Graduate Programs in Medicine and Biomedical Sciences, Program in Genetics, Genomics and Bioinformatics, Buffalo, NY 14203. Offers MS, PhD. *Faculty:* 60 full-time (17 women). *Students:* 4 full-time (1 woman); includes 2 minority (both Asian, non-Hispanic/Latino), 1 international. Average age 28. 13 applicants, 69% accepted, 1 enrolled. In 2015, 1 master's awarded. Terminal master's awarded for partial completion of doctoral program. *Degree requirements:* For master's, thesis or alternative; for doctorate, thesis/dissertation. *Entrance requirements:* For master's and doctorate, GRE. Additional exam requirements/recommendations for international students: Required—TOEFL (minimum score 100 iBT). *Application deadline:* For fall admission, 3/1 for domestic and international students. Application fee: $85. Electronic applications accepted. *Expenses:* $10,870 tuition per year in-state; $22,210 tuition per year out-of-state. *Financial support:* Support by faculty mentor available. *Faculty research:* Human and medical genetics and genomics, developmental genomics and genetics, microbial genetics and pathogenesis, bioinformatics. *Unit head:* Dr. Richard Gronostajski, Director, 716-829-3471, Fax: 716-849-6655, E-mail: rgron@buffalo.edu. *Application contact:* Greg Korosec, Program Administrator, 716-881-8209, Fax: 716-849-6655, E-mail: korosec@buffalo.edu.
Website: http://medicine.buffalo.edu/education/ggb.html

The University of Alabama at Birmingham, Graduate Programs in Joint Health Sciences, Genetics, Genomics and Bioinformatics Theme, Birmingham, AL 35294. Offers PhD. *Degree requirements:* For doctorate, comprehensive exam, thesis/dissertation. *Entrance requirements:* For doctorate, GRE General Test, interview, previous research experience. Additional exam requirements/recommendations for international students: Required—TOEFL. Electronic applications accepted. *Expenses:* Tuition, state resident: full-time $7340. Tuition, nonresident: full-time $16,628. Full-time tuition and fees vary according to course load and program.

University of California, Riverside, Graduate Division, Graduate Program in Genetics, Genomics, and Bioinformatics, Riverside, CA 92521-0102. Offers genomics and bioinformatics (PhD). *Degree requirements:* For doctorate, thesis/dissertation, qualifying exams, teaching experience. *Entrance requirements:* For doctorate, GRE General Test, minimum GPA of 3.2. Additional exam requirements/recommendations for international students: Required—TOEFL (minimum score 550 paper-based; 80 iBT). *Application deadline:* For fall admission, 12/1 priority date for domestic students, 1/1 priority date for international students; for winter admission, 9/1 for domestic students, 7/1 for international students; for spring admission, 12/1 for domestic students, 10/1 for international students. Applications are processed on a rolling basis. Application fee: $85 ($100 for international students). Electronic applications accepted. *Expenses:* Tuition, area resident: Full-time $16,665.50; part-time $11,055.54. Tuition, state resident: full-time $16,665.50; part-time $11,055.54. Tuition, nonresident: full-time $31,768. *International tuition:* $31,767.50 full-time. *Required fees:* $16,665.50; $11,055.54 per quarter. $3685.18 per quarter. Tuition and fees vary according to program. *Financial support:* Fellowships with tuition reimbursements, research assistantships with tuition reimbursements, teaching assistantships with tuition reimbursements, career-related internships or fieldwork, Federal Work-Study, institutionally sponsored loans, and tuition waivers (full and partial) available. *Faculty research:* Molecular genetics, evolution and population genetics, genomics and bioinformatics.
Website: http://ggb.ucr.edu/

University of California, San Francisco, School of Pharmacy and Graduate Division, Pharmaceutical Sciences and Pharmacogenomics Program, San Francisco, CA 94158-0775. Offers PhD. *Degree requirements:* For doctorate, comprehensive exam, thesis/dissertation. *Entrance requirements:* For doctorate, GRE General Test, bachelor's degree, 3 letters of recommendation, personal statement. Additional exam requirements/recommendations for international students: Required—TOEFL. Electronic applications accepted. *Faculty research:* Drug development sciences, molecular pharmacology, therapeutic bioengineering, pharmacogenomics and functional genomics, quantitative and systems pharmacology, computational genomics.
See Display on page 926 and Close-Up on page 937.

University of Chicago, Division of the Biological Sciences, Committee on Genetics, Genomics and Systems Biology, Chicago, IL 60637. Offers PhD. *Students:* 27 full-time (11 women); includes 7 minority (1 Black or African American, non-Hispanic/Latino; 4 Asian, non-Hispanic/Latino; 1 Hispanic/Latino; 1 Native Hawaiian or other Pacific Islander, non-Hispanic/Latino), 6 international. Average age 28. 71 applicants, 18% accepted, 4 enrolled. In 2015, 4 doctorates awarded. *Degree requirements:* For doctorate, thesis/dissertation, ethics class, 2 teaching assistantships. *Entrance requirements:* For doctorate, GRE General Test. Additional exam requirements/recommendations for international students: Required—TOEFL (minimum score 600 paper-based; 104 iBT), IELTS (minimum score 7). *Application deadline:* For fall admission, 12/1 for domestic and international students. Application fee: $90. Electronic applications accepted. *Financial support:* In 2015–16, 21 students received support, including fellowships with tuition reimbursements available (averaging $29,781 per year), research assistantships with tuition reimbursements available (averaging $29,781 per year); institutionally sponsored loans, scholarships/grants, traineeships, and health care benefits also available. Financial award applicants required to submit FAFSA. *Faculty research:* Molecular genetics, developmental genetics, population genetics, human genetics. *Application contact:* Sue Levison, Administrator, 773-702-2464, Fax: 773-702-3172, E-mail: committee-on-genetics@uchicago.edu.
Website: http://cg.bsd.uchicago.edu/

University of Cincinnati, Graduate School, College of Medicine, Graduate Programs in Biomedical Sciences, Department of Environmental Health, Programs in Environmental

Genomic Sciences

Genetics and Molecular Toxicology, Cincinnati, OH 45221. Offers MS, PhD. *Degree requirements:* For doctorate, thesis/dissertation. *Entrance requirements:* For master's, GRE, minimum GPA of 3.0, 3 letters of recommendation. Additional exam requirements/recommendations for international students: Required—TOEFL (minimum score 520 paper-based).

University of Connecticut, Graduate School, College of Liberal Arts and Sciences, Department of Molecular and Cell Biology, Field of Applied Genomics, Storrs, CT 06269. Offers MS. *Degree requirements:* For master's, comprehensive exam. *Entrance requirements:* For master's, GRE General Test, GRE Subject Test. Additional exam requirements/recommendations for international students: Required—TOEFL (minimum score 550 paper-based). *Application deadline:* For fall admission, 2/1 priority date for domestic and international students; for spring admission, 11/1 for domestic students, 10/1 for international students. Applications are processed on a rolling basis. Application fee: $55. Electronic applications accepted. *Financial support:* Fellowships, research assistantships with full tuition reimbursements, teaching assistantships with full tuition reimbursements, Federal Work-Study, scholarships/grants, health care benefits, and unspecified assistantships available. Financial award application deadline: 2/1; financial award applicants required to submit FAFSA. Website: http://www.mcb.uconn.edu/

University of Georgia, College of Agricultural and Environmental Sciences, Institute of Plant Breeding, Genetics and Genomics, Athens, GA 30602. Offers MS, PhD.

University of Maryland, Baltimore, School of Medicine, Department of Epidemiology and Public Health, Baltimore, MD 21201. Offers biostatistics (MS); clinical research (MS); epidemiology and preventive medicine (MPH, MS, PhD); gerontology (PhD); human genetics and genomic medicine (MS, PhD); molecular epidemiology (MS, PhD); toxicology (MS, PhD); JD/MS; MD/PhD; MS/PhD. *Accreditation:* CEPH. *Program availability:* Part-time. *Students:* 73 full-time (58 women), 56 part-time (32 women); includes 45 minority (23 Black or African American, non-Hispanic/Latino; 12 Asian, non-Hispanic/Latino; 5 Hispanic/Latino; 5 Two or more races, non-Hispanic/Latino), 17 international. Average age 31. In 2015, 34 master's, 17 doctorates awarded. *Degree requirements:* For doctorate, comprehensive exam, thesis/dissertation. *Entrance requirements:* For master's and doctorate, GRE General Test. Additional exam requirements/recommendations for international students: Required—TOEFL (minimum score 550 paper-based; 80 iBT); Recommended—IELTS (minimum score 7). *Application deadline:* For fall admission, 1/15 for domestic and international students. Application fee: $75. Electronic applications accepted. *Expenses:* Contact institution. *Financial support:* In 2015–16, research assistantships with partial tuition reimbursements (averaging $26,000 per year) were awarded; fellowships, Federal Work-Study, scholarships/grants, and unspecified assistantships also available. Financial award application deadline: 3/1; financial award applicants required to submit FAFSA. *Unit head:* Dr. Laura Hungerford, Program Director, 410-706-8492, Fax: 410-706-4225. *Application contact:* Jessica Kelley, Program Coordinator, 410-706-8492, Fax: 410-706-4225, E-mail: jkelley@som.umaryland.edu. Website: http://lifesciences.umaryland.edu/epidemiology/

University of Maryland, College Park, Academic Affairs, College of Computer, Mathematical and Natural Sciences, Department of Biology, PhD Program in Biological Sciences, College Park, MD 20742. Offers behavior, ecology, evolution, and systematics (PhD); computational biology, bioinformatics, and genomics (PhD); molecular and cellular biology (PhD); physiological systems (PhD). *Degree requirements:* For doctorate, comprehensive exam, thesis/dissertation, thesis work presentation in seminar. *Entrance requirements:* For doctorate, GRE General Test; GRE Subject Test in biology (recommended), academic transcripts, statement of purpose/research interests, 3 letters of recommendation. Additional exam requirements/recommendations for international students: Required—TOEFL. Electronic applications accepted.

University of Pennsylvania, Perelman School of Medicine, Biomedical Graduate Studies, Graduate Group in Genomics and Computational Biology, Philadelphia, PA 19104. Offers MD, MD/PhD, VMD/PhD. *Faculty:* 78. *Students:* 40 full-time (15 women); includes 10 minority (7 Asian, non-Hispanic/Latino; 1 Hispanic/Latino; 2 Two or more races, non-Hispanic/Latino), 10 international. 127 applicants, 17% accepted, 11 enrolled. In 2015, 5 doctorates awarded. *Degree requirements:* For doctorate, thesis/dissertation. *Entrance requirements:* For doctorate, GRE. Additional exam requirements/recommendations for international students: Required—TOEFL. *Application deadline:* For fall admission, 12/1 priority date for domestic students, 12/1 for international students. Applications are processed on a rolling basis. Application fee: $80. Electronic applications accepted. *Expenses:* Tuition, area resident: Full-time $31,068; part-time $5762 per course. *Required fees:* $3200; $336 per course. Full-time tuition and fees vary according to degree level, program and student level. Part-time tuition and fees vary according to course load, degree level and program. *Financial support:* In 2015–16, 40 students received support. Fellowships, research assistantships, scholarships/grants, traineeships, and unspecified assistantships available. *Unit head:* Dr. Li-San Wang, Chairperson, 215-746-7015. *Application contact:* Maureen Kirsch, Graduate Coordinator, 215-746-2807. Website: http://www.med.upenn.edu/gcb/

University of Rochester, School of Medicine and Dentistry, Graduate Programs in Medicine and Dentistry, Department of Biomedical Genetics, Rochester, NY 14627. Offers genetics, genomics and development (PhD). *Degree requirements:* For doctorate, thesis/dissertation, qualifying exam. *Entrance requirements:* For doctorate, GRE General Test. *Expenses:* Tuition, area resident: Full-time $47,450; part-time $1482 per credit hour. *Required fees:* $528. Tuition and fees vary according to program.

University of Southern California, Keck School of Medicine, Program in Cancer Biology and Genomics, Los Angeles, CA 90089. Offers cancer biology and genomics (PhD). *Faculty:* 43 full-time (10 women). *Students:* 15 full-time (11 women); includes 5 minority (4 Asian, non-Hispanic/Latino; 1 Hispanic/Latino), 8 international. Average age 28. 3 applicants, 100% accepted, 3 enrolled. *Degree requirements:* For doctorate, comprehensive exam, thesis/dissertation. *Entrance requirements:* For doctorate, GRE, minimum GPA of 3.0. Additional exam requirements/recommendations for international students: Required—TOEFL (minimum score 600 paper-based; 100 iBT), IELTS (minimum score 7), PTE. *Application deadline:* For fall admission, 12/1 priority date for domestic and international students. Application fee: $85. Electronic applications accepted. *Financial support:* In 2015–16, 15 students received support, including 2 fellowships with full tuition reimbursements available (averaging $32,000 per year), 13 research assistantships with full tuition reimbursements available (averaging $32,000 per year); institutionally sponsored loans, scholarships/grants, traineeships, health care benefits, and unspecified assistantships also available. Financial award application deadline: 5/4; financial award applicants required to submit CSS PROFILE or FAFSA. *Unit head:* Dr. Baruch Frenkel, Director, 323-442-1475, Fax: 323-442-1199, E-mail: frenkel@med.usc.edu. *Application contact:* Dr. Joyce Perez, Manager of Student Programs, 323-442-1645, Fax: 323-442-1199, E-mail: jpperez@med.usc.edu. Website: http://pibbs.usc.edu/research-and-programs/phd-programs/

The University of Tennessee, Graduate School, College of Arts and Sciences, Program in Life Sciences, Knoxville, TN 37996. Offers genome science and technology

(MS, PhD); plant physiology and genetics (MS, PhD). *Degree requirements:* For doctorate, one foreign language, thesis/dissertation. *Entrance requirements:* For master's and doctorate, GRE General Test, minimum GPA of 2.7. Additional exam requirements/recommendations for international students: Required—TOEFL. Electronic applications accepted.

The University of Tennessee–Oak Ridge National Laboratory, Graduate Program in Genome Science and Technology, Knoxville, TN 37966. Offers life sciences (MS, PhD). *Degree requirements:* For master's, thesis; for doctorate, comprehensive exam, thesis/dissertation. *Entrance requirements:* For master's and doctorate, GRE General Test. Additional exam requirements/recommendations for international students: Required—TOEFL. Electronic applications accepted. *Faculty research:* Genetics/genomics, structural biology/proteomics, computational biology/bioinformatics, bioanalytical technologies.

The University of Toledo, College of Graduate Studies, College of Medicine and Life Sciences, Interdepartmental Programs, Toledo, OH 43606-3390. Offers bioinformatics and proteomics/genomics (MSBS); biomarkers and bioinformatics (Certificate); biomarkers and diagnostics (PSM); human donation sciences (MSBS); medical sciences (MSBS); MD/MSBS. *Degree requirements:* For master's, thesis or alternative. *Entrance requirements:* For master's, GRE, minimum undergraduate GPA of 3.0, three letters of recommendation, statement of purpose, transcripts from all prior institutions attended, resume; for Certificate, minimum undergraduate GPA of 3.0, three letters of recommendation, statement of purpose, transcripts from all prior institutions attended, resume. Additional exam requirements/recommendations for international students: Required—TOEFL (minimum score 550 paper-based; 80 iBT). Electronic applications accepted.

University of Washington, Graduate School, School of Medicine, Graduate Programs in Medicine, Department of Genome Sciences, Seattle, WA 98195. Offers PhD. *Degree requirements:* For doctorate, thesis/dissertation, general exam. *Entrance requirements:* For doctorate, GRE General Test, minimum GPA of 3.0. Additional exam requirements/recommendations for international students: Required—TOEFL. Electronic applications accepted. *Faculty research:* Model organism genetics, human and medical genetics, genomics and proteomics, computational biology.

Wake Forest University, School of Medicine and Graduate School of Arts and Sciences, Graduate Programs in Medicine, Molecular Genetics and Genomics Program, Winston-Salem, NC 27109. Offers PhD, MD/PhD. *Degree requirements:* For doctorate, thesis/dissertation. *Entrance requirements:* For doctorate, GRE General Test. Additional exam requirements/recommendations for international students: Required—TOEFL. Electronic applications accepted. *Faculty research:* Control of gene expression, molecular pathogenesis, protein biosynthesis, cell development, clinical cytogenetics.

Washington University in St. Louis, School of Medicine, Program in Clinical Investigation, St. Louis, MO 63130-4899. Offers clinical investigation (MS), including bioethics, entrepreneurship, genetics/genomics, translational medicine. *Program availability:* Part-time, evening/weekend. *Faculty:* 61 full-time (14 women), 2 part-time/adjunct (both women). *Students:* 15 full-time (5 women), 39 part-time (19 women); includes 15 minority (3 Black or African American, non-Hispanic/Latino; 8 Asian, non-Hispanic/Latino; 2 Hispanic/Latino; 2 Two or more races, non-Hispanic/Latino), 3 international. Average age 32. 34 applicants, 65% accepted, 22 enrolled. In 2015, 35 master's awarded. *Degree requirements:* For master's, thesis. *Entrance requirements:* For master's, doctoral-level degree or in process of obtaining doctoral-level degree. *Application deadline:* For fall admission, 5/15 for domestic students; for spring admission, 10/15 for domestic students. Application fee: $0. Electronic applications accepted. *Financial support:* In 2015–16, 4 students received support. Tuition waivers (partial) available. Financial award application deadline: 12/12. *Faculty research:* Anesthesiology, infectious diseases, neurology, obstetrics and gynecology, orthopedic surgery. *Unit head:* Dr. David Warren, Associate Professor of Medicine, 314-454-8225, Fax: 314-454-8279, E-mail: dwarren@wustl.edu. *Application contact:* Suzie Fragale, Curriculum and Evaluation Coordinator, 314-454-8936, Fax: 314-454-8279, E-mail: fragale@wustl.edu. Website: http://crtc.wustl.edu/

Wayne State University, School of Medicine, Office of Biomedical Graduate Programs, Program in Molecular Genetics and Genomics, Detroit, MI 48201. Offers MS, PhD, MD/PhD. *Faculty:* 20. *Students:* 13 full-time (7 women), 2 part-time (both women); includes 2 minority (both Asian, non-Hispanic/Latino), 3 international. Average age 27. 39 applicants, 15% accepted, 5 enrolled. In 2015, 4 doctorates awarded. Terminal master's awarded for partial completion of doctoral program. *Degree requirements:* For master's, thesis; for doctorate, thesis/dissertation. *Entrance requirements:* For master's and doctorate, GRE General Test, GRE Subject Test (chemistry or biology), minimum GPA of 3.0, strong background in one of the chemical or biological sciences, three letters of recommendation, personal statement, interview. Additional exam requirements/recommendations for international students: Required—TOEFL, Michigan English Language Assessment Battery (minimum score 85); Recommended—IELTS, TWE. *Application deadline:* For fall admission, 1/31 priority date for domestic and international students. Application fee: $0. Electronic applications accepted. *Expenses:* $17,645 per year resident tuition, $33,311 non-resident tuition; $735.20 per credit hour resident tuition, $1,387.95 per credit hour non-resident tuition; fees include $47.45 per credit hour student services fee and $274.60 per semester registration fee. *Financial support:* In 2015–16, 15 students received support, including 3 fellowships with tuition reimbursements available (averaging $26,377 per year), 12 research assistantships with tuition reimbursements available (averaging $26,716 per year); scholarships/grants and unspecified assistantships also available. Financial award application deadline: 3/31; financial award applicants required to submit FAFSA. *Faculty research:* Human gene mapping, genome organization and sequencing, gene regulation, molecular evolution. *Unit head:* Dr. Gregory Kapatos, Director, 313-577-5965, E-mail: gkapato@med.wayne.edu. *Application contact:* 313-577-5523, Fax: 313-577-5218, E-mail: info@genetics.wayne.edu. Website: http://genetics.wayne.edu/

Wesleyan University, Graduate Studies, Department of Biology, Middletown, CT 06459. Offers cell and developmental biology (PhD); evolution and ecology (PhD); genetics and genomics (PhD), including bioinformatics; neurobiology and behavior (PhD). *Faculty:* 14 full-time (5 women). *Students:* 26 full-time (12 women); includes 5 minority (2 Black or African American, non-Hispanic/Latino; 3 Asian, non-Hispanic/Latino), 5 international. In 2015, 3 doctorates awarded. Terminal master's awarded for partial completion of doctoral program. *Degree requirements:* For doctorate, comprehensive exam, thesis/dissertation, public seminar. *Entrance requirements:* For doctorate, GRE. Additional exam requirements/recommendations for international students: Required—TOEFL or IELTS. *Application deadline:* For fall admission, 1/15 for domestic and international students. Application fee: $0. Electronic applications accepted. *Financial support:* Stipends available. *Faculty research:* Evolution and ecology, neurobiology and behavior, cell and developmental biology, genetics, genomics and bioinformatics. *Unit head:* Dr. John Kirn, Chair/Professor, 860-685-3494, E-mail: jrkirn@wesleyan.edu. *Application contact:* Marjorie Fitzgibbons, Administrative Assistant, 860-685-2157, E-mail: mfitzgibbons@wesleyan.edu. Website: http://www.wesleyan.edu/bio/

West Virginia University, Eberly College of Arts and Sciences, Department of Biology, Morgantown, WV 26506. Offers cell and molecular biology (MS, PhD); environmental and evolutionary biology (MS, PhD); forensic biology (MS, PhD); genomic biology (MS, PhD); neurobiology (MS, PhD). Terminal master's awarded for partial completion of doctoral program. *Degree requirements:* For master's, thesis, final exam; for doctorate, thesis/dissertation, preliminary and final exams. *Entrance requirements:* For master's, GRE General Test, GRE Subject Test, minimum GPA of 3.0; for doctorate, GRE General Test, minimum GPA of 3.0. Additional exam requirements/recommendations for international students: Required—TOEFL. *Expenses:* Tuition, state resident: full-time $8568. Tuition, nonresident: full-time $22,140. Tuition and fees vary according to program. *Faculty research:* Environmental biology, genetic engineering, developmental biology, global change, biodiversity.

Yale University, School of Medicine and Graduate School of Arts and Sciences, Combined Program in Biological and Biomedical Sciences (BBS), Computational Biology and Bioinformatics Track, New Haven, CT 06520. Offers PhD, MD/PhD. *Entrance requirements:* Additional exam requirements/recommendations for international students: Required—TOEFL.

Human Genetics

Baylor College of Medicine, Graduate School of Biomedical Sciences, Department of Molecular and Human Genetics, Houston, TX 77030-3498. Offers PhD, MD/PhD. *Degree requirements:* For doctorate, thesis/dissertation, public defense. *Entrance requirements:* For doctorate, GRE General Test, GRE Subject Test (strongly recommended), minimum GPA of 3.0. Additional exam requirements/recommendations for international students: Required—TOEFL. Electronic applications accepted. *Faculty research:* Human genetics, genome biology, epigenetics, gene therapy, model organisms.

Baylor College of Medicine, Graduate School of Biomedical Sciences, Interdepartmental Program in Cell and Molecular Biology, Houston, TX 77030-3498. Offers biochemistry (PhD); cell and molecular biology (PhD); genetics (PhD); human genetics (PhD); immunology (PhD); microbiology (PhD); virology (PhD); MD/PhD. *Degree requirements:* For doctorate, thesis/dissertation, public defense. *Entrance requirements:* For doctorate, GRE General Test, GRE Subject Test (strongly recommended), minimum GPA of 3.0. Additional exam requirements/recommendations for international students: Required—TOEFL. Electronic applications accepted. *Faculty research:* Molecular and cellular biology; cancer, aging and stem cells; genomics and proteomics; microbiome, molecular microbiology; infectious disease, immunology and translational research.

Case Western Reserve University, School of Medicine and School of Graduate Studies, Graduate Programs in Medicine, Department of Genetics and Genome Sciences, Program in Human, Molecular, and Developmental Genetics and Genomics, Cleveland, OH 44106. Offers PhD, MD/PhD. *Degree requirements:* For doctorate, comprehensive exam, thesis/dissertation. *Entrance requirements:* For doctorate, GRE General Test, GRE Subject Test. Additional exam requirements/recommendations for international students: Required—TOEFL. *Expenses: Tuition, area resident:* Full-time $41,137; part-time $1714 per credit hour. *Required fees:* $32. Tuition and fees vary according to course load and program. *Faculty research:* Regulation of gene expression, molecular control of development, genomics.

Emory University, School of Medicine, Programs in Allied Health Professions, Genetic Counseling Training Program, Atlanta, GA 30322. Offers MM Sc. *Degree requirements:* For master's, thesis, capstone project. *Entrance requirements:* For master's, GRE General Test, minimum GPA of 3.0; prerequisites: genetics, statistics, psychology, and biochemistry. Additional exam requirements/recommendations for international students: Required—TOEFL. *Faculty research:* Cancer genetics, lysosomal storage disease, carrier screening, public health genomics, genetic counseling, psychology, molecular genetics.

Johns Hopkins University, School of Medicine, Graduate Programs in Medicine, Predoctoral Training Program in Human Genetics, Baltimore, MD 21218. Offers PhD, MD/PhD. Terminal master's awarded for partial completion of doctoral program. *Degree requirements:* For doctorate, comprehensive exam, thesis/dissertation. *Entrance requirements:* For doctorate, GRE General Test, GRE Subject Test. Additional exam requirements/recommendations for international students: Recommended—TOEFL. Electronic applications accepted. *Faculty research:* Human, mammalian, and molecular genetics, bioinformatics, genomics.

Louisiana State University Health Sciences Center, School of Graduate Studies in New Orleans, Department of Human Genetics, New Orleans, LA 70112-2223. Offers PhD, MD/PhD. *Faculty:* 10 full-time (4 women). *Students:* 7 full-time (5 women); includes 3 minority (1 Black or African American, non-Hispanic/Latino; 2 Asian, non-Hispanic/Latino). Average age 26. 8 applicants. In 2015, 4 doctorates awarded. Terminal master's awarded for partial completion of doctoral program. *Degree requirements:* For doctorate, comprehensive exam, thesis/dissertation. *Entrance requirements:* For doctorate, GRE General Test. Additional exam requirements/recommendations for international students: Recommended—TOEFL, IELTS. *Application deadline:* For fall admission, 4/1 priority date for domestic students, 4/1 for international students. Applications are processed on a rolling basis. Application fee: $30. *Financial support:* Unspecified assistantships available. Financial award application deadline: 4/1. *Faculty research:* Genetic epidemiology, segregation and linkage analysis, gene mapping. *Unit head:* Dr. Lucio Miele, Professor and Head, 504-568-6150. *Application contact:* Dr. Diptasri Mandal, Graduate Coordinator, 504-568-6156, Fax: 504-568-8500, E-mail: dmanda@lsuhsc.edu.
Website: http://www.medschool.lsuhsc.edu/genetics/

McGill University, Faculty of Graduate and Postdoctoral Studies, Faculty of Medicine, Department of Human Genetics, Montréal, QC H3A 2T5, Canada. Offers genetic counseling (M Sc); human genetics (M Sc, PhD).

Memorial University of Newfoundland, Faculty of Medicine and School of Graduate Studies, Graduate Programs in Medicine, Division of Human Genetics, St. John's, NL A1C 5S7, Canada. Offers M Sc, PhD, MD/PhD. *Program availability:* Part-time. *Degree requirements:* For master's, thesis; for doctorate, comprehensive exam, thesis/dissertation, oral defense of thesis. *Entrance requirements:* For master's, MD or B Sc; for doctorate, MD or M Sc. Additional exam requirements/recommendations for international students: Required—TOEFL. *Expenses: Tuition, area resident:* Full-time $2199 Canadian dollars. *International tuition:* $2859 Canadian dollars full-time. *Faculty research:* Cancer genetics, gene mapping, medical genetics, birth defects, population genetics.

Sarah Lawrence College, Graduate Studies, Joan H. Marks Graduate Program in Human Genetics, Bronxville, NY 10708-5999. Offers MS. *Program availability:* Part-time. *Degree requirements:* For master's, thesis, fieldwork. *Entrance requirements:* For master's, previous course work in biology, chemistry, developmental biology, genetics, probability and statistics. Additional exam requirements/recommendations for international students: Required—TOEFL (minimum score 600 paper-based). Electronic applications accepted. *Expenses:* Contact institution.

Tulane University, School of Medicine and School of Liberal Arts, Graduate Programs in Biomedical Sciences, Program in Human Genetics, New Orleans, LA 70118-5669. Offers MS. MS and PhD offered through the Graduate School. *Degree requirements:* For master's, thesis. *Entrance requirements:* For master's, GRE, MCAT. Additional exam requirements/recommendations for international students: Required—TOEFL. *Application deadline:* For fall admission, 2/1 for domestic and international students. Application fee: $45. Electronic applications accepted. *Expenses: Tuition, area resident:* Full-time $47,658; part-time $2648 per credit hour. *Required fees:* $1980; $44.50 per credit hour. $550 per term. Tuition and fees vary according to course load, degree level and program. *Financial support:* Fellowships with full tuition reimbursements and research assistantships with full tuition reimbursements available. Financial award application deadline: 2/1. *Faculty research:* Inborn errors of metabolism, DNA methylation, gene therapy.

University of California, Los Angeles, David Geffen School of Medicine and Graduate Division, Graduate Programs in Medicine, Department of Human Genetics, Los Angeles, CA 90095. Offers MS, PhD. *Degree requirements:* For master's, thesis; for doctorate, thesis/dissertation, written and oral qualifying examination; 2 quarters of teaching experience. *Entrance requirements:* For master's and doctorate, GRE General Test; GRE Subject Test (recommended); bachelor's degree; minimum undergraduate GPA of 3.0 (or its equivalent if letter grade system not used). Additional exam requirements/recommendations for international students: Required—TOEFL. Electronic applications accepted.

University of California, Los Angeles, Graduate Division, College of Letters and Science and David Geffen School of Medicine, UCLA ACCESS to Programs in the Molecular, Cellular and Integrative Life Sciences, Los Angeles, CA 90095. Offers biochemistry and molecular biology (PhD); biological chemistry (PhD); cellular and molecular pathology (PhD); human genetics (PhD); microbiology, immunology, and molecular genetics (PhD); molecular biology (PhD); molecular toxicology (PhD); molecular, cellular and integrative physiology (PhD); neurobiology (PhD); oral biology (PhD); physiology (PhD). *Degree requirements:* For doctorate, thesis/dissertation, oral and written qualifying exams. *Entrance requirements:* For doctorate, GRE General Test, bachelor's degree; minimum undergraduate GPA of 3.0 (or its equivalent if letter grade system not used). Additional exam requirements/recommendations for international students: Required—TOEFL. Electronic applications accepted.

University of Chicago, Division of the Biological Sciences, Department of Human Genetics, Chicago, IL 60637. Offers PhD. *Students:* 25 full-time (12 women); includes 4 minority (1 Black or African American, non-Hispanic/Latino; 2 Asian, non-Hispanic/Latino; 1 Hispanic/Latino), 6 international. Average age 28. 58 applicants, 28% accepted, 10 enrolled. In 2015, 3 doctorates awarded. *Degree requirements:* For doctorate, thesis/dissertation, ethics class, 2 teaching assistantships. *Entrance requirements:* For doctorate, GRE General Test. Additional exam requirements/recommendations for international students: Required—TOEFL (minimum score 600 paper-based; 104 iBT), IELTS (minimum score 7). *Application deadline:* For fall admission, 12/1 for domestic and international students. Application fee: $90. Electronic applications accepted. *Financial support:* In 2015–16, 21 students received support, including fellowships with tuition reimbursements available (averaging $29,781 per year), research assistantships with tuition reimbursements available (averaging $29,781 per year); institutionally sponsored loans, scholarships/grants, traineeships, and health care benefits also available. Financial award applicants required to submit FAFSA. *Unit head:* Dr. Carole Ober, Chair, 773-834-0735, Fax: 773-834-0505. *Application contact:* Justin Shelton, Graduate Administrative Director, 773-834-8073, Fax: 773-702-3172, E-mail: jshelton@bsd.uchicago.edu.
Website: http://genes.bsd.uchicago.edu/

University of Manitoba, Faculty of Medicine and Faculty of Graduate Studies, Graduate Programs in Medicine, Department of Biochemistry and Medical Genetics, Winnipeg, MB R3T 2N2, Canada. Offers M Sc, PhD. Terminal master's awarded for partial completion of doctoral program. *Degree requirements:* For master's, thesis; for doctorate, thesis/dissertation. *Faculty research:* Cancer, gene expression, membrane lipids, metabolic control, genetic diseases.

University of Maryland, Baltimore, School of Medicine, Department of Epidemiology and Public Health, Baltimore, MD 21201. Offers biostatistics (MS); clinical research (MS); epidemiology and preventive medicine (MPH, MS, PhD); gerontology (PhD); human genetics and genomic medicine (MS, PhD); molecular epidemiology (MS, PhD); toxicology (MS, PhD); JD/MS; MD/PhD; MS/PhD. *Accreditation:* CEPH. *Program availability:* Part-time. *Students:* 73 full-time (58 women), 56 part-time (32 women); includes 45 minority (23 Black or African American, non-Hispanic/Latino; 12 Asian, non-Hispanic/Latino; 5 Hispanic/Latino; 5 Two or more races, non-Hispanic/Latino), 17 international. Average age 31. In 2015, 34 master's, 17 doctorates awarded. *Degree requirements:* For doctorate, comprehensive exam, thesis/dissertation. *Entrance requirements:* For master's and doctorate, GRE General Test. Additional exam requirements/recommendations for international students: Required—TOEFL (minimum score 550 paper-based; 80 iBT); Recommended—IELTS (minimum score 7). *Application deadline:* For fall admission, 1/15 for domestic and international students. Application fee: $75. Electronic applications accepted. *Expenses:* Contact institution. *Financial support:* In 2015–16, research assistantships with partial tuition reimbursements (averaging $26,000 per year) were awarded; fellowships, Federal Work-Study, scholarships/grants, and unspecified assistantships also available. Financial award application deadline: 3/1; financial award applicants required to submit FAFSA. *Unit head:* Dr. Laura Hungerford, Program Director, 410-706-8492, Fax: 410-706-4225. *Application contact:* Jessica Kelley, Program Coordinator, 410-706-8492, Fax: 410-706-4225, E-mail: jkelley@som.umaryland.edu.
Website: http://lifesciences.umaryland.edu/epidemiology/

University of Michigan, Rackham Graduate School, Program in Biomedical Sciences (PIBS), Department of Human Genetics, Ann Arbor, MI 48109-5618. Offers genetic

Human Genetics

counseling (MS); human genetics (MS, PhD). *Faculty:* 35 full-time (16 women). *Students:* 42 full-time (28 women); includes 8 minority (5 Asian, non-Hispanic/Latino; 1 Hispanic/Latino; 2 Two or more races, non-Hispanic/Latino), 6 international. Average age 27. 234 applicants, 18% accepted, 16 enrolled. In 2015, 8 master's, 4 doctorates awarded. Terminal master's awarded for partial completion of doctoral program. *Degree requirements:* For master's, research project; for doctorate, thesis/dissertation, oral preliminary exam, oral defense of dissertation. *Entrance requirements:* For master's, GRE General Test, bachelor's degree; 3 letters of recommendation; advocacy experience (for the MS in genetic counseling); for doctorate, GRE General Test, bachelor's degree; 3 letters of recommendation. Additional exam requirements/recommendations for international students: Required—TOEFL (minimum score 84 iBT). Application fee: $75 ($90 for international students). Electronic applications accepted. *Expenses:* Contact institution. *Financial support:* In 2015–16, 37 students received support, including 24 fellowships with tuition reimbursements available, 6 research assistantships with full tuition reimbursements available (averaging $29,025 per year), 7 teaching assistantships with full tuition reimbursements available (averaging $29,025 per year); Federal Work-Study, scholarships/grants, traineeships, and health care benefits also available. Financial award application deadline: 4/30; financial award applicants required to submit FAFSA. *Faculty research:* Molecular and developmental genetics, genetics of Mendelian and complex human disease, genome biology, statistical and population genetics, epigenetics. *Total annual research expenditures:* $7.1 million. *Unit head:* Sherry Cogswell, Chief Department Administrator, 734-764-6361, Fax: 734-763-3784, E-mail: shercogs@umich.edu. *Application contact:* Karen L. Grahl, Student Services Coordinator, 734-764-5490, Fax: 734-763-3784, E-mail: kgrahl@umich.edu.
Website: http://www.hg.med.umich.edu/

University of Pennsylvania, Perelman School of Medicine, Center for Clinical Epidemiology and Biostatistics, Philadelphia, PA 19104. Offers clinical epidemiology (MSCE), including bioethics, clinical trials, human genetics, patient centered outcome research, pharmacoepidemiology. *Accreditation:* CEPH. *Program availability:* Part-time. *Faculty:* 97 full-time (47 women), 90 part-time/adjunct (27 women). *Students:* 94 full-time (63 women), 2 part-time (1 woman); includes 34 minority (6 Black or African American, non-Hispanic/Latino; 17 Asian, non-Hispanic/Latino; 11 Hispanic/Latino). Average age 35. 40 applicants, 95% accepted, 33 enrolled. In 2015, 36 master's awarded. *Degree requirements:* For master's, comprehensive exam, thesis. *Entrance requirements:* For master's, GRE General Test or MCAT, advanced degree, clinical experience. Additional exam requirements/recommendations for international students: Required—TOEFL. *Application deadline:* For fall admission, 12/1 priority date for domestic students, 12/1 for international students. Application fee: $0. *Expenses:* Contact institution. *Financial support:* In 2015–16, 60 students received support, including 65 fellowships with tuition reimbursements available (averaging $45,500 per year); career-related internships or fieldwork, scholarships/grants, health care benefits, and unspecified assistantships also available. Financial award application deadline: 12/1. *Faculty research:* Health services research, pharmacoepidemiology, women's health, cancer epidemiology, genetic epidemiology. *Total annual research expenditures:* $38.7 million. *Unit head:* Dr. Harold I. Feldman, Director, 215-573-0901, E-mail: hfeldman@mail.med.upenn.edu. *Application contact:* Jennifer Kuklinski, Program Coordinator, 215-573-2382, E-mail: jkuklins@mail.med.upenn.edu.
Website: http://www.cceb.upenn.edu/

University of Pittsburgh, Graduate School of Public Health, Department of Human Genetics, Pittsburgh, PA 15261. Offers genetic counseling (MS); human genetics (MS, PhD); public health genetics (MPH, Certificate); MD/PhD; MS/MPH. *Faculty:* 18 full-time (8 women), 42 part-time/adjunct (36 women). *Students:* 43 full-time (28 women), 29 part-time (23 women); includes 14 minority (2 Black or African American, non-Hispanic/Latino; 4 Asian, non-Hispanic/Latino; 5 Hispanic/Latino; 3 Two or more races, non-Hispanic/Latino), 14 international. Average age 27. 143 applicants, 42% accepted, 20 enrolled. In 2015, 18 master's, 4 doctorates awarded. *Degree requirements:* For master's, comprehensive exam, thesis; for doctorate, comprehensive exam, thesis/dissertation, qualifying examination. *Entrance requirements:* For master's and doctorate, GRE General Test (above the 70th percentile for the verbal and quantitative tests), previous course work in biochemistry and behavioral or social sciences (recommended); bachelor's degree in a discipline related to the biological or behavioral sciences from accredited college or university with minimum GPA of 3.0, introductory courses in genetics and calculus. Additional exam requirements/recommendations for international students: Required—TOEFL (minimum score 550 paper-based, 80 iBT) or IELTS (minimum score 6.5). *Application deadline:* For fall admission, 1/15 priority date for domestic and international students; for spring admission, 10/15 priority date for domestic students, 8/1 priority date for international students. Applications are processed on a rolling basis. Application fee: $120. Electronic applications accepted. *Expenses:* $12,464 per term full-time in-state, $20,502 per term full-time out-of-state; $1,016 per credit part-time in-state, $1,680 per credit part-time out-of-state. *Financial support:* In 2015–16, 25 students received support, including 1 fellowship (averaging $20,902 per year), 24 research assistantships (averaging $17,186 per year); scholarships/grants, traineeships, and health care benefits also available. Financial award application deadline: 4/15; financial award applicants required to submit CSS PROFILE or FAFSA. *Faculty research:* Atherosclerotic cardiovascular disease, Alzheimer's disease, statistical genetics, chromosomal instability, gene mapping. *Total annual research expenditures:* $3.1 million. *Unit head:* Dr. Dietrich A. Stephan, Chair, 412-648-3353, Fax: 412-624-3020, E-mail: dstephan@pitt.edu. *Application contact:* Noel C. Harrie, Student Services Coordinator, 412-624-3066, Fax: 412-624-3020, E-mail: nce1@pitt.edu.
Website: http://www.publichealth.pitt.edu/human-genetics

The University of Texas Health Science Center at Houston, Graduate School of Biomedical Sciences, Program in Human and Molecular Genetics, Houston, TX 77225-0036. Offers MS, PhD, MD/PhD. Terminal master's awarded for partial completion of

doctoral program. *Degree requirements:* For master's, thesis; for doctorate, thesis/dissertation. *Entrance requirements:* For master's and doctorate, GRE General Test. Additional exam requirements/recommendations for international students: Required—TOEFL. Electronic applications accepted. *Faculty research:* Computational genomics, cancer genetics, complex disease genetics, medical genetics.

University of Utah, School of Medicine and Graduate School, Graduate Programs in Medicine, Department of Human Genetics, Salt Lake City, UT 84112-1107. Offers MS, PhD. Terminal master's awarded for partial completion of doctoral program. *Degree requirements:* For master's, comprehensive exam, thesis optional; for doctorate, comprehensive exam, thesis/dissertation. Electronic applications accepted. *Faculty research:* RNA metabolism, drosophilia genetics, mouse genetics, protein synthesis.

Vanderbilt University, Program in Human Genetics, Nashville, TN 37240-1001. Offers PhD, MD/PhD. *Faculty:* 27 full-time (5 women). *Students:* 13 full-time (7 women); includes 2 minority (1 American Indian or Alaska Native, non-Hispanic/Latino; 1 Hispanic/Latino). Average age 29. In 2015, 7 doctorates awarded. *Degree requirements:* For doctorate, comprehensive exam, thesis/dissertation. *Entrance requirements:* For doctorate, GRE General Test. Additional exam requirements/recommendations for international students: Required—TOEFL (minimum score 570 paper-based; 88 iBT). *Application deadline:* For fall admission, 1/15 for domestic and international students. Application fee: $0. Electronic applications accepted. *Financial support:* Fellowships with tuition reimbursements, research assistantships with tuition reimbursements, Federal Work-Study, institutionally sponsored loans, traineeships, and health care benefits available. Financial award application deadline: 1/15; financial award applicants required to submit CSS PROFILE or FAFSA. *Faculty research:* Disease gene discovery, computational genomics, translational genetics. *Unit head:* Dr. David Samuels, Director of Graduate Studies, 615-343-8555, Fax: 615-322-1453, E-mail: david.c.samuels@vanderbilt.edu. *Application contact:* Walter B. Bieschke, Program Coordinator for Graduate Admissions, 615-342-0236, E-mail: vandygrad@vanderbilt.edu.
Website: https://medschool.vanderbilt.edu/igp/human-genetics

Virginia Commonwealth University, Medical College of Virginia-Professional Programs, School of Medicine, School of Medicine Graduate Programs, Department of Human and Molecular Genetics, Richmond, VA 23284-9005. Offers genetic counseling (MS); human genetics (PhD); molecular biology and genetics (MS, PhD); MD/PhD. *Degree requirements:* For master's, thesis; for doctorate, thesis/dissertation, comprehensive oral and written exams. *Entrance requirements:* For master's, GRE; for doctorate, GRE General Test. Additional exam requirements/recommendations for international students: Required—TOEFL (minimum score 600 paper-based; 100 iBT). Electronic applications accepted. *Faculty research:* Genetic epidemiology, biochemical genetics, quantitative genetics, human cytogenetics, molecular genetics.

Virginia Commonwealth University, Program in Pre-Medical Basic Health Sciences, Richmond, VA 23284-9005. Offers anatomy (CBHS); biochemistry (CBHS); human genetics (CBHS); microbiology (CBHS); pharmacology (CBHS); physiology (CBHS). *Entrance requirements:* For degree, GRE, MCAT or DAT, course work in organic chemistry, minimum undergraduate GPA of 2.8. Additional exam requirements/recommendations for international students: Required—TOEFL (minimum score 600 paper-based). Electronic applications accepted.

Wake Forest University, School of Medicine and Graduate School of Arts and Sciences, Graduate Programs in Medicine, Molecular Genetics and Genomics Program, Winston-Salem, NC 27109. Offers PhD, MD/PhD. *Degree requirements:* For doctorate, thesis/dissertation. *Entrance requirements:* For doctorate, GRE General Test. Additional exam requirements/recommendations for international students: Required—TOEFL. Electronic applications accepted. *Faculty research:* Control of gene expression, molecular pathogenesis, protein biosynthesis, cell development, clinical cytogenetics.

Washington University in St. Louis, Graduate School of Arts and Sciences, Division of Biology and Biomedical Sciences, Program in Human and Statistical Genetics, St. Louis, MO 63130-4899. Offers PhD. *Students:* 19 full-time (11 women); includes 4 minority (1 Black or African American, non-Hispanic/Latino; 1 Asian, non-Hispanic/Latino; 2 Hispanic/Latino), 6 international. 28 applicants, 29% accepted, 3 enrolled. In 2015, 5 doctorates awarded. *Degree requirements:* For doctorate, thesis/dissertation. *Entrance requirements:* For doctorate, GRE General Test, GRE Subject Test. Additional exam requirements/recommendations for international students: Required—TOEFL. *Application deadline:* For fall admission, 12/1 for domestic students. Application fee: $0. Electronic applications accepted. *Financial support:* Fellowships, research assistantships, and teaching assistantships available. *Faculty research:* Human genetics, statistical genetics, functional genomics, molecular genetics, Mendelian disease, complex disease, human disease models, systems biology. *Unit head:* Jeanne Silvestrini, Coordinator, 314-362-4806. *Application contact:* Rebecca Riney, E-mail: dbbsphdadmissions@wusm.wustl.edu.
Website: http://dbbs.wustl.edu/divprograms/hsg/Pages/default.aspx

West Virginia University, Davis College of Agriculture, Forestry and Consumer Sciences, Interdisciplinary Program in Genetics and Developmental Biology, Morgantown, WV 26506. Offers animal breeding (MS, PhD); biochemical and molecular genetics (MS, PhD); cytogenetics (MS, PhD); descriptive embryology (MS, PhD); developmental genetics (MS); experimental morphogenesis/teratology (MS); human genetics (MS, PhD); immunogenetics (MS, PhD); life cycles of animals and plants (MS, PhD); molecular aspects of development (MS, PhD); mutagenesis (MS, PhD); oncology (MS, PhD); plant genetics (MS, PhD); population and quantitative genetics (MS, PhD); regeneration (MS, PhD); teratology (PhD); toxicology (MS, PhD). *Degree requirements:* For master's, thesis; for doctorate, comprehensive exam, thesis/dissertation. *Entrance requirements:* For master's, GRE or MCAT, minimum GPA of 2.75. Additional exam requirements/recommendations for international students: Required—TOEFL. *Expenses:* Tuition, state resident: full-time $8568. Tuition, nonresident: full-time $22,140. Tuition and fees vary according to program.

Molecular Genetics

Albert Einstein College of Medicine, Graduate Division of Biomedical Sciences, Department of Genetics, Bronx, NY 10461. Offers computational genetics (PhD); molecular genetics (PhD); translational genetics (PhD); MD/PhD. *Degree requirements:* For doctorate, thesis/dissertation. *Entrance requirements:* For doctorate, GRE General Test. Additional exam requirements/recommendations for international students: Required—TOEFL. *Faculty research:* Neurologic genetics in &ITDrosophila&RO, biochemical genetics of yeast, developmental genetics in the mouse.

Duke University, Graduate School, Department of Molecular Genetics and Microbiology, Durham, NC 27710. Offers PhD. *Degree requirements:* For doctorate, thesis/dissertation. *Entrance requirements:* For doctorate, GRE General Test, GRE Subject Test in biology, chemistry, or biochemistry, cell and molecular biology (recommended). Additional exam requirements/recommendations for international students: Required—TOEFL (minimum score 577 paper-based; 90 iBT) or IELTS (minimum score 7). Electronic applications accepted.

Emory University, Laney Graduate School, Division of Biological and Biomedical Sciences, Program in Microbiology and Molecular Genetics, Atlanta, GA 30322-1100. Offers PhD. *Degree requirements:* For doctorate, comprehensive exam, thesis/dissertation. *Entrance requirements:* For doctorate, GRE General Test, minimum GPA of 3.0 in science course work (recommended). Additional exam requirements/recommendations for international students: Required—TOEFL. Electronic applications accepted. *Faculty research:* Bacterial genetics and physiology, microbial development, molecular biology of viruses and bacterial pathogens, DNA recombination.

Georgia State University, College of Arts and Sciences, Department of Biology, Program in Molecular Genetics and Biochemistry, Atlanta, GA 30302-3083. Offers bioinformatics (MS); molecular genetics and biochemistry (MS, PhD). *Program availability:* Part-time. Terminal master's awarded for partial completion of doctoral program. *Degree requirements:* For master's, comprehensive exam (for some programs), thesis optional; for doctorate, comprehensive exam, thesis/dissertation. *Entrance requirements:* For master's and doctorate, GRE. Additional exam requirements/recommendations for international students: Required—TOEFL (minimum score 550 paper-based; 82 iBT) or IELTS (minimum score 7). *Application deadline:* For fall admission, 7/1 priority date for domestic students, 6/1 priority date for international students; for spring admission, 11/15 priority date for domestic students, 10/15 priority date for international students. Applications are processed on a rolling basis. Application fee: $50. Electronic applications accepted. *Expenses:* Tuition, state resident: full-time $6876; part-time $382 per credit hour. Tuition, nonresident: full-time $22,374; part-time $1243 per credit hour. *Required fees:* $2128; $2128 per term. $1064 per term. Part-time tuition and fees vary according to course load and program. *Financial support:* In 2015–16, fellowships with full tuition reimbursements (averaging $22,000 per year), research assistantships with full tuition reimbursements (averaging $20,000 per year) were awarded. Financial award application deadline: 12/3. *Faculty research:* Gene regulation, microbial pathogenesis, molecular transport, protein modeling, viral pathogenesis. *Unit head:* Dr. Charles Derby, Director of Graduate Studies, 404-413-5393, Fax: 404-413-5446, E-mail: cderby@gsu.edu. Website: http://biology.gsu.edu/

Harvard University, Graduate School of Arts and Sciences, Division of Medical Sciences, Boston, MA 02115. Offers biological chemistry and molecular pharmacology (PhD); cell biology (PhD); genetics (PhD); microbiology and molecular genetics (PhD); pathology (PhD), including experimental pathology. *Degree requirements:* For doctorate, thesis/dissertation. *Entrance requirements:* For doctorate, GRE General Test, GRE Subject Test. Additional exam requirements/recommendations for international students: Required—TOEFL.

Illinois State University, Graduate School, College of Arts and Sciences, Department of Biological Sciences, Normal, IL 61790-2200. Offers animal behavior (MS); bacteriology (MS); biochemistry (MS); biological sciences (MS); biology (PhD); biophysics (MS); biotechnology (MS); botany (MS, PhD); cell biology (MS); conservation biology (MS); developmental biology (MS); ecology (MS, PhD); entomology (MS); evolutionary biology (MS); genetics (MS, PhD); immunology (MS); microbiology (MS, PhD); molecular biology (MS); molecular genetics (MS); neurobiology (MS); neuroscience (MS); parasitology (MS); physiology (MS, PhD); plant biology (MS); plant molecular biology (MS); plant sciences (MS); structural biology (MS); zoology (MS, PhD). *Program availability:* Part-time. *Degree requirements:* For master's, thesis or alternative; for doctorate, variable foreign language requirement, thesis/dissertation, 2 terms of residency. *Entrance requirements:* For master's, GRE General Test, minimum GPA of 2.6 in last 60 hours of course work; for doctorate, GRE General Test. *Application deadline:* Applications are processed on a rolling basis. Application fee: $40. *Financial support:* Research assistantships, teaching assistantships, Federal Work-Study, tuition waivers (full), and unspecified assistantships available. Financial award application deadline: 4/1. *Faculty research:* Redox balance and drug development in schistosoma mansoni, control of the growth of listeria monocytogenes at low temperature, regulation of cell expansion and microtubule function by SPRI, CRUI: physiology and fitness consequences of different life history phenotypes. *Application contact:* Steven Juliano, Graduate Coordinator, E-mail: sajulian@ilstu.edu. Website: http://www.bio.ilstu.edu/

Indiana University–Purdue University Indianapolis, Indiana University School of Medicine, Department of Medical and Molecular Genetics, Indianapolis, IN 46202-5251. Offers genetic counseling (MS); medical and molecular genetics (MS, PhD); MD/MS; MD/PhD. *Program availability:* Part-time. Terminal master's awarded for partial completion of doctoral program. *Degree requirements:* For master's, thesis optional; for doctorate, thesis/dissertation, research ethics. *Entrance requirements:* For master's and doctorate, GRE General Test, minimum GPA of 3.0. Additional exam requirements/recommendations for international students: Required—TOEFL, IELTS. *Faculty research:* Twins, human gene mapping, chromosomes and malignancy, clinical genetics.

Iowa State University of Science and Technology, Program in Animal Breeding and Genetics, Ames, IA 50011. Offers animal breeding and genetics (MS); immunogenetics (PhD); molecular genetics (PhD); quantitative genetics (PhD). *Entrance requirements:* For master's and doctorate, GRE. Additional exam requirements/recommendations for international students: Required—TOEFL (minimum score 550 paper-based; 80 iBT), IELTS (minimum score 6.5). Electronic applications accepted.

Medical College of Wisconsin, Graduate School of Biomedical Sciences, Department of Microbiology and Molecular Genetics, Milwaukee, WI 53226-0509. Offers MS, PhD, MD/PhD. *Degree requirements:* For doctorate, comprehensive exam, thesis/dissertation. *Entrance requirements:* For master's and doctorate, GRE, official transcripts, three letters of recommendation. Additional exam requirements/recommendations for international students: Required—TOEFL. *Faculty research:* Virology, immunology, bacterial toxins, regulation of gene expression.

Michigan State University, College of Human Medicine and The Graduate School, Graduate Programs in Human Medicine, East Lansing, MI 48824. Offers biochemistry and molecular biology (MS, PhD); epidemiology (MS, PhD); microbiology (MS); microbiology and molecular genetics (PhD); pharmacology and toxicology (MS, PhD); physiology (MS, PhD); public health (MPH). *Entrance requirements:* Additional exam requirements/recommendations for international students: Required—TOEFL.

Michigan State University, College of Osteopathic Medicine and The Graduate School, Graduate Studies in Osteopathic Medicine, East Lansing, MI 48824. Offers biochemistry and molecular biology (MS, PhD); microbiology (MS); microbiology and molecular genetics (PhD); pharmacology and toxicology (MS, PhD), including integrative pharmacology (MS), pharmacology and toxicology, pharmacology and toxicology-environmental toxicology (PhD); physiology (MS, PhD).

New York University, Graduate School of Arts and Science, Department of Biology, New York, NY 10012-1019. Offers biology (PhD); biomedical journalism (MS); cancer and molecular biology (PhD); computational biology (PhD); computers in biological research (MS); developmental genetics (PhD); general biology (MS); immunology and microbiology (PhD); molecular genetics (PhD); neurobiology (PhD); oral biology (MS); plant biology (PhD); recombinant DNA technology (MS); MS/MBA. *Program availability:* Part-time. Terminal master's awarded for partial completion of doctoral program. *Degree*

requirements: For master's, thesis or alternative, qualifying paper; for doctorate, comprehensive exam, thesis/dissertation. *Entrance requirements:* For master's and doctorate, GRE General Test. Additional exam requirements/recommendations for international students: Required—TOEFL. *Faculty research:* Genomics, molecular and cell biology, development and molecular genetics, molecular evolution of plants and animals.

Northern Michigan University, Office of Graduate Education and Research, College of Health Sciences and Professional Studies, School of Clinical Sciences, Marquette, MI 49855-5301. Offers clinical molecular genetics (MS). *Program availability:* Part-time. *Degree requirements:* For master's, thesis or project to be presented as a seminar at the conclusion of the program. *Entrance requirements:* For master's, minimum undergraduate GPA of 3.0; bachelor's degree in clinical laboratory science or biology; laboratory experience; statement of intent that includes lab skills and experiences along with reason for pursuing this degree; 3 letters of recommendation (instructors or professional references). Additional exam requirements/recommendations for international students: Required—TOEFL (minimum score 550 paper-based; 79 iBT), IELTS (minimum score 6.5). Electronic applications accepted.

The Ohio State University, Graduate School, College of Arts and Sciences, Division of Natural and Mathematical Sciences, Department of Molecular Genetics, Columbus, OH 43210. Offers cell and developmental biology (MS, PhD); genetics (MS, PhD); molecular biology (MS, PhD). *Degree requirements:* For master's, thesis; for doctorate, thesis/dissertation. *Entrance requirements:* For doctorate, GRE General Test, GRE Subject Test in biology or chemistry (recommended). Additional exam requirements/recommendations for international students: Required—TOEFL (minimum score 550 paper-based; 79 iBT), Michigan English Language Assessment Battery (minimum score 82); Recommended—IELTS (minimum score 7). Electronic applications accepted.

Oklahoma State University, College of Arts and Sciences, Department of Microbiology and Molecular Genetics, Stillwater, OK 74078. Offers MS, PhD. *Faculty:* 19 full-time (5 women), 1 part-time/adjunct (0 women). *Students:* 12 full-time (6 women), 21 part-time (14 women); includes 9 minority (2 American Indian or Alaska Native, non-Hispanic/Latino; 2 Asian, non-Hispanic/Latino; 2 Hispanic/Latino; 3 Two or more races, non-Hispanic/Latino), 13 international. Average age 29. 44 applicants, 23% accepted, 9 enrolled. In 2015, 7 master's, 2 doctorates awarded. *Degree requirements:* For master's, thesis; for doctorate, comprehensive exam, thesis/dissertation. *Entrance requirements:* For master's and doctorate, GRE General Test. Additional exam requirements/recommendations for international students: Required—TOEFL (minimum score 550 paper-based; 79 iBT). *Application deadline:* For fall admission, 3/1 priority date for international students; for spring admission, 8/1 priority date for international students. Applications are processed on a rolling basis. Application fee: $40 ($75 for international students). Electronic applications accepted. *Expenses:* Tuition, state resident: full-time $3528; part-time $196 per credit hour. Tuition, nonresident: full-time $14,144; part-time $785.75 per credit hour. *Required fees:* $1895; $105.25 per credit hour. Tuition and fees vary according to campus/location. *Financial support:* In 2015–16, 12 research assistantships (averaging $17,445 per year), 14 teaching assistantships (averaging $18,093 per year) were awarded; career-related internships or fieldwork, Federal Work-Study, scholarships/grants, health care benefits, tuition waivers (partial), and unspecified assistantships also available. Support available to part-time students. Financial award application deadline: 3/1; financial award applicants required to submit FAFSA. *Faculty research:* Bioinformatics, genomics-genetics, virology, environmental microbiology, development-molecular mechanisms. *Unit head:* Dr. Tyrrell Conway, Professor and Department Head, 405-744-6243, Fax: 405-744-6790, E-mail: tconway@okstate.edu. *Application contact:* Dr. Wouter Hoff, Graduate Program Coordinator, 405-744-6243, Fax: 405-744-6790, E-mail: wouter.hoff@okstate.edu. Website: http://microbiology.okstate.edu

Penn State Hershey Medical Center, College of Medicine, Graduate School Programs in the Biomedical Sciences, Graduate Program in Biomedical Sciences, Hershey, PA 17033. Offers biochemistry and molecular genetics (MS, PhD); biomedical sciences (MS, PhD); translational therapeutics (MS, PhD); virology and immunology (MS, PhD); MD/PhD; PhD/MBA. *Students:* 79 full-time (43 women); includes 27 minority (7 Black or African American, non-Hispanic/Latino; 15 Asian, non-Hispanic/Latino; 4 Hispanic/Latino; 1 Native Hawaiian or other Pacific Islander, non-Hispanic/Latino), 17 international. 275 applicants, 16% accepted, 17 enrolled. Terminal master's awarded for partial completion of doctoral program. *Degree requirements:* For master's, thesis (for some programs); for doctorate, comprehensive exam, thesis/dissertation, candidacy exam. *Entrance requirements:* For doctorate, GRE General Test. Additional exam requirements/recommendations for international students: Required—TOEFL (minimum score 550 paper-based; 81 iBT). *Application deadline:* For fall admission, 1/1 for domestic and international students. Applications are processed on a rolling basis. Application fee: $65. Electronic applications accepted. *Expenses:* Contact institution. *Financial support:* In 2015–16, 79 students received support, including 79 research assistantships with full tuition reimbursements available (averaging $26,196 per year); fellowships, scholarships/grants, health care benefits, and unspecified assistantships also available. *Unit head:* Dr. Ralph L. Keil, Chair, 717-531-8595, Fax: 717-531-0786, E-mail: rlk9@psu.edu. *Application contact:* Kristin E. Smith, Director of Graduate Admissions, 717-531-1045, Fax: 717-531-0786, E-mail: kec17@psu.edu. Website: http://med.psu.edu/bms

Penn State Hershey Medical Center, College of Medicine, Graduate School Programs in the Biomedical Sciences, The Huck Institutes of the Life Sciences, Intercollege Graduate Program in Molecular Cellular and Integrative Biosciences, Hershey, PA 17033. Offers cell and developmental biology (PhD); immunology and infectious disease (PhD); molecular and evolutionary genetics (PhD); molecular medicine (PhD); molecular toxicology (PhD); neurobiology (PhD). *Students:* 3 full-time (2 women); includes 2 minority (both Asian, non-Hispanic/Latino). 2 applicants, 100% accepted, 2 enrolled. In 2015, 1 doctorate awarded. *Degree requirements:* For doctorate, comprehensive exam, thesis/dissertation, oral exam. *Entrance requirements:* For doctorate, GRE, minimum GPA of 3.0. Additional exam requirements/recommendations for international students: Required—TOEFL (minimum score 500 paper-based). *Application deadline:* For fall admission, 1/31 priority date for domestic students, 2/1 priority date for international students. Applications are processed on a rolling basis. Application fee: $65. Electronic applications accepted. *Financial support:* In 2015–16, research assistantships with full tuition reimbursements (averaging $26,196 per year) were awarded; fellowships with full tuition reimbursements, career-related internships or fieldwork, Federal Work-Study, scholarships/grants, health care benefits, and unspecified assistantships also available. Financial award applicants required to submit FAFSA. *Faculty research:* Vascular biology, molecular toxicology, chemical biology, immune system, pathophysiological basis of human disease. *Unit head:* Dr. Peter Hudson, Director, 814-865-6057, E-mail: pjh18@psu.edu. *Application contact:* Kathy Shuey, Administrative Assistant, 717-531-8982, Fax: 717-531-0786, E-mail: grad-hmc@psu.edu. Website: http://www.huck.psu.edu/education/molecular-cellular-and-integrative-biosciences

Rutgers University–Newark, Graduate School of Biomedical Sciences, Department of Microbiology and Molecular Genetics, Newark, NJ 07107. Offers PhD. *Degree requirements:* For doctorate, thesis/dissertation, qualifying exam. *Entrance*

requirements: For doctorate, GRE General Test. Additional exam requirements/recommendations for international students: Required—TOEFL. Electronic applications accepted. *Faculty research:* Molecular genetics of yeast, mutagenesis and carcinogenesis of DNA, bacterial protein synthesis, mammalian cell genetics, adenovirus gene expression.

Rutgers University–New Brunswick, Graduate School-New Brunswick, Programs in the Molecular Biosciences, Piscataway, NJ 08854-8097. Offers biochemistry (PhD); cell and developmental biology (MS, PhD); microbiology and molecular genetics (MS, PhD), including applied microbiology, clinical microbiology (MS), clinical mircobiology (PhD), computational molecular biology (PhD), immunology, microbial biochemistry, molecular genetics, virology. MS, PhD offered jointly with University of Medicine and Dentistry of New Jersey.

Rutgers University–New Brunswick, Graduate School of Biomedical Sciences, Program in Microbiology and Molecular Genetics, Piscataway, NJ 08854-5635. Offers MS, PhD, MD/PhD. Terminal master's awarded for partial completion of doctoral program. *Degree requirements:* For master's, thesis, qualifying exam; for doctorate, thesis/dissertation, qualifying exam. *Entrance requirements:* For master's and doctorate, GRE General Test. Additional exam requirements/recommendations for international students: Required—TOEFL. Electronic applications accepted. *Faculty research:* Interferon, receptors, retrovirus evolution, Arbo virus/host cell interactions.

Stony Brook University, State University of New York, Stony Brook Medicine, School of Medicine and Graduate School, Graduate Programs in Medicine, Department of Molecular Genetics and Microbiology, Stony Brook, NY 11794. Offers PhD. *Faculty:* 16 full-time (4 women), 2 part-time/adjunct (1 woman). *Students:* 25 full-time (8 women); includes 7 minority (5 Asian, non-Hispanic/Latino; 2 Hispanic/Latino), 6 international. Average age 27. 49 applicants, 18% accepted, 4 enrolled. In 2015, 1 doctorate awarded. *Degree requirements:* For doctorate, comprehensive exam, thesis/dissertation. *Entrance requirements:* For doctorate, GRE General Test, GRE Subject Test, undergraduate training in biochemistry, genetics, and cell biology; recommendations; personal statement. Additional exam requirements/recommendations for international students: Required—TOEFL (minimum score 550 paper-based; 90 iBT). *Application deadline:* For fall admission, 1/15 for domestic students; for spring admission, 10/1 for domestic students. Application fee: $100. *Expenses:* $12,421 per year full-time resident tuition and fees, $453 per credit hour; $23,761 per year full-time non-resident tuition and fees, $925 per credit hour. *Financial support:* In 2015–16, 6 fellowships, 14 research assistantships, 4 teaching assistantships were awarded; Federal Work-Study also available. Financial award application deadline: 3/15. *Faculty research:* Bioimaging, infectious diseases or agents, pathogenesis, viral studies (virology), genetics. *Total annual research expenditures:* $19.7 million. *Unit head:* Dr. David G. Thanassi, Interim Chair, 631-632-4549, Fax: 631-632-9797, E-mail: david.thanassi@stonybrook.edu. *Application contact:* Kathryn Bell, Program Administrator, 631-632-8812, Fax: 631-632-9797, E-mail: kathryn.bell@stonybrook.edu.
Website: http://www.mgm.stonybrook.edu/index.shtml

University of Calgary, Cumming School of Medicine and Faculty of Graduate Studies, Medical Science Graduate Program, Calgary, AB T2N 1N4, Canada. Offers cancer biology (M Sc, PhD); critical care medicine (M Sc, PhD); joint injury and arthritis (M Sc, PhD); molecular and medical genetics (M Sc, PhD); mountain medicine and high altitude physiology (M Sc, PhD); pathologists' assistant (M Sc, PhD). *Degree requirements:* For master's, thesis; for doctorate, thesis/dissertation, candidacy exam. *Entrance requirements:* For master's, minimum undergraduate GPA of 3.2; for doctorate, minimum graduate GPA of 3.2. Additional exam requirements/recommendations for international students: Required—TOEFL (minimum score 600 paper-based). Electronic applications accepted. *Faculty research:* Cancer biology, immunology, joint injury and arthritis, medical education, population genomics.

University of California, Irvine, School of Medicine and Francisco J. Ayala School of Biological Sciences, Department of Microbiology and Molecular Genetics, Irvine, CA 92697. Offers biological sciences (MS, PhD); MD/PhD. *Students:* 19 full-time (11 women), 1 (woman) part-time; includes 9 minority (1 Black or African American, non-Hispanic/Latino; 1 American Indian or Alaska Native, non-Hispanic/Latino; 3 Asian, non-Hispanic/Latino; 4 Hispanic/Latino), 1 international. Average age 29. In 2015, 1 master's, 4 doctorates awarded. *Degree requirements:* For doctorate, thesis/dissertation. *Entrance requirements:* For doctorate, GRE General Test, GRE Subject Test, minimum GPA of 3.0. Additional exam requirements/recommendations for international students: Required—TOEFL (minimum score 550 paper-based). *Application deadline:* For fall admission, 12/15 priority date for domestic students, 12/15 for international students. Application fee: $90 ($110 for international students). Electronic applications accepted. *Financial support:* Fellowships, research assistantships with full tuition reimbursements, teaching assistantships, institutionally sponsored loans, traineeships, health care benefits, and unspecified assistantships available. Financial award applicants required to submit FAFSA. *Faculty research:* Molecular biology and genetics of viruses, bacteria, and yeast; immune response; molecular biology of cultured animal cells; genetic basis of cancer; genetics and physiology of infectious agents. *Unit head:* Rozanne M. Sandri-Goldin, Chair, 949-824-7570, Fax: 949-824-8598, E-mail: rmsandri@uci.edu. *Application contact:* Janet Horwitz, Graduate Student Coordinator, 949-824-7669, E-mail: horwitz@uci.edu.
Website: http://www.microbiology.uci.edu/graduate-students.asp

University of California, Los Angeles, David Geffen School of Medicine and Graduate Division, Graduate Programs in Medicine, Department of Microbiology, Immunology and Molecular Genetics, Los Angeles, CA 90095. Offers MS, PhD. *Degree requirements:* For master's, thesis; for doctorate, thesis/dissertation, oral and written qualifying exams; 2 quarters of teaching experience. *Entrance requirements:* For master's and doctorate, GRE General Test, bachelor's degree; minimum undergraduate GPA of 3.0 (or its equivalent if letter grade system not used). Additional exam requirements/recommendations for international students: Required—TOEFL. Electronic applications accepted.

University of Cincinnati, Graduate School, College of Medicine, Graduate Programs in Biomedical Sciences, Department of Molecular Genetics, Biochemistry and Microbiology, Cincinnati, OH 45221. Offers MS, PhD. Terminal master's awarded for partial completion of doctoral program. *Degree requirements:* For master's, thesis or alternative; for doctorate, thesis/dissertation, qualifying exam. *Entrance requirements:* For master's and doctorate, GRE General Test. Additional exam requirements/recommendations for international students: Required—TOEFL (minimum score 600 paper-based; 100 iBT), TWE. Electronic applications accepted. *Faculty research:* Cancer biology and developmental genetics, gene regulation and chromosome structure, microbiology and pathogenic mechanisms, structural biology, membrane biochemistry and signal transduction.

University of Colorado Denver, School of Medicine, Biochemistry Program, Aurora, CO 80045. Offers biochemistry (PhD); biochemistry and molecular genetics (PhD). *Students:* 14 full-time (4 women); includes 3 minority (2 Asian, non-Hispanic/Latino; 1 Hispanic/Latino). Average age 28. 24 applicants, 17% accepted, 4 enrolled. In 2015, 2 doctorates awarded. *Degree requirements:* For doctorate, comprehensive exam, thesis/dissertation, 30 credit hours each of coursework and thesis research. *Entrance requirements:* For doctorate, GRE, minimum of three letters of recommendation from qualified referees.

Additional exam requirements/recommendations for international students: Required—TOEFL (minimum score 550 paper-based; 80 iBT). *Application deadline:* For fall admission, 12/1 for domestic students. Applications are processed on a rolling basis. Application fee: $50 ($75 for international students). Electronic applications accepted. *Expenses:* Contact institution. *Financial support:* In 2015–16, 14 students received support. Fellowships, research assistantships, teaching assistantships, Federal Work-Study, institutionally sponsored loans, scholarships/grants, traineeships, health care benefits, tuition waivers (full), and unspecified assistantships available. Financial award application deadline: 3/15; financial award applicants required to submit FAFSA. *Faculty research:* DNA damage, cancer and neurodegeneration, molecular mechanisms of pro-MRNA splicing, yeast RNA polymerases, DNA replication. *Total annual research expenditures:* $8.6 million. *Unit head:* Dr. Mark Johnston, Professor and Chair, 303-724-3203, Fax: 303-724-3215, E-mail: mark.johnston@ucdenver.edu. *Application contact:* Sue Brozowski, Department Contact, 303-724-3202, Fax: 303-724-3215, E-mail: sue.brozowski@ucdenver.edu.
Website: http://www.ucdenver.edu/academics/colleges/medicalschool/departments/biochemistry/Pages/Home.aspx

University of Florida, College of Medicine, Department of Molecular Genetics and Microbiology, Gainesville, FL 32610-0266. Offers MS. Terminal master's awarded for partial completion of doctoral program. *Degree requirements:* For master's, thesis. *Entrance requirements:* For master's, GRE General Test, minimum GPA of 3.0. Additional exam requirements/recommendations for international students: Required—TOEFL, IELTS. Electronic applications accepted.

University of Guelph, Graduate Studies, College of Biological Science, Department of Molecular and Cellular Biology, Guelph, ON N1G 2W1, Canada. Offers biochemistry (M Sc, PhD); biophysics (M Sc, PhD); botany (M Sc, PhD); microbiology (M Sc, PhD); molecular biology and genetics (M Sc, PhD). *Degree requirements:* For master's, thesis, research proposal; for doctorate, comprehensive exam, thesis/dissertation, research proposal. *Entrance requirements:* For master's, minimum B-average during previous 2 years of coursework; for doctorate, minimum A-average. Additional exam requirements/recommendations for international students: Required—TOEFL (minimum score 550 paper-based), IELTS (minimum score 6.5). Electronic applications accepted. *Faculty research:* Physiology, structure, genetics, and ecology of microbes; virology and microbial technology.

University of Illinois at Chicago, College of Medicine and Graduate College, Graduate Programs in Medicine, Department of Biochemistry and Molecular Genetics, Chicago, IL 60607-7128. Offers MS, MD/PhD. *Faculty:* 31 full-time (12 women), 19 part-time/adjunct (9 women). *Students:* 22 full-time (12 women); includes 5 minority (1 Black or African American, non-Hispanic/Latino; 3 Asian, non-Hispanic/Latino; 1 Hispanic/Latino), 9 international. Average age 29. Terminal master's awarded for partial completion of doctoral program. *Degree requirements:* For doctorate, thesis/dissertation. *Entrance requirements:* For doctorate, GRE General Test. Additional exam requirements/recommendations for international students: Required—TOEFL. *Application deadline:* For fall admission, 3/1 priority date for domestic students, 2/15 for international students. Applications are processed on a rolling basis. Application fee: $60. Electronic applications accepted. *Expenses:* Tuition, state resident: full-time $11,480; part-time $3826 per credit. Tuition, nonresident: full-time $23,720; part-time $7906 per credit. *Required fees:* $1333 per semester. Part-time tuition and fees vary according to course load and program. *Financial support:* Fellowships with full tuition reimbursements, research assistantships with full tuition reimbursements, teaching assistantships with full tuition reimbursements, career-related internships or fieldwork, Federal Work-Study, institutionally sponsored loans, traineeships, tuition waivers (full), and unspecified assistantships available. Financial award application deadline: 3/1; financial award applicants required to submit FAFSA. *Faculty research:* Signal transduction, cell cycle regulation, membrane biology, regulation of gene function and development, protein and nucleic acid structure and function, cancer biology. *Unit head:* Dr. Jack Kaplan, Head, 312-355-2732, Fax: 312-413-0353, E-mail: kaplanj@uic.edu. *Application contact:* Dr. Karen Colley, Co-Director of Graduate Studies, 312-996-7756.
Website: http://www.uic.edu/com/bcmg/

The University of Manchester, Faculty of Life Sciences, Manchester, United Kingdom. Offers adaptive organismal biology (M Phil, PhD); animal biology (M Phil, PhD); biochemistry (M Phil, PhD); bioinformatics (M Phil, PhD); biomolecular sciences (M Phil, PhD); biotechnology (M Phil, PhD); cell biology (M Phil, PhD); cell matrix research (M Phil, PhD); channels and transporters (M Phil, PhD); developmental biology (M Phil, PhD); Egyptology (M Phil, PhD); environmental biology (M Phil, PhD); evolutionary biology (M Phil, PhD); gene expression (M Phil, PhD); genetics (M Phil, PhD); history of science, technology and medicine (M Phil, PhD); immunology (M Phil, PhD); integrative neurobiology and behavior (M Phil, PhD); membrane trafficking (M Phil, PhD); microbiology (M Phil, PhD); molecular and cellular neuroscience (M Phil, PhD); molecular biology (M Phil, PhD); molecular cancer studies (M Phil, PhD); neuroscience (M Phil, PhD); ophthalmology (M Phil, PhD); optometry (M Phil, PhD); organelle function (M Phil, PhD); pharmacology (M Phil, PhD); physiology (M Phil, PhD); plant sciences (M Phil, PhD); stem cell research (M Phil, PhD); structural biology (M Phil, PhD); systems neuroscience (M Phil, PhD); toxicology (M Phil, PhD).

University of Maryland, College Park, Academic Affairs, College of Computer, Mathematical and Natural Sciences, Department of Cell Biology and Molecular Genetics, Program in Cell Biology and Molecular Genetics, College Park, MD 20742. Offers MS, PhD. *Degree requirements:* For master's, thesis; for doctorate, thesis/dissertation, exams. *Faculty research:* Cytoskeletal activity, membrane biology, cell division, genetics and genomics, virology.

University of Pittsburgh, School of Medicine, Graduate Programs in Medicine, Molecular Genetics and Developmental Biology Graduate Program, Pittsburgh, PA 15260. Offers PhD. *Faculty:* 56 full-time (16 women). *Students:* 11 full-time (9 women); includes 5 minority (1 Black or African American, non-Hispanic/Latino; 4 Asian, non-Hispanic/Latino). Average age 29. 386 applicants, 17% accepted, 25 enrolled. In 2015, 3 doctorates awarded. *Degree requirements:* For doctorate, comprehensive exam, thesis/dissertation. *Entrance requirements:* For doctorate, GRE General Test, GRE Subject Test, minimum QPA of 3.0. Additional exam requirements/recommendations for international students: Required—TOEFL (minimum score 600 paper-based; 100 iBT), IELTS (minimum score 7). *Application deadline:* For fall admission, 12/1 priority date for domestic and international students. Application fee: $50. Electronic applications accepted. Tuition and fees vary according to program. *Financial support:* In 2015–16, 11 students received support, including 2 fellowships with full tuition reimbursements available (averaging $27,000 per year), 9 research assistantships with full tuition reimbursements available (averaging $27,000 per year), teaching assistantships with full tuition reimbursements available (averaging $27,000 per year); scholarships/grants, traineeships, and health care benefits also available. *Faculty research:* Developmental and stem cell biology, DNA replication and repair, gene regulation and signal transduction, oncogenes and tumor suppressor genes, protein structure and molecular dynamics. *Unit head:* Dr. Kyle E. Orwig, Graduate Program Director, 412-641-2460, Fax: 412-641-3899, E-mail: korwig@mwri.magee.edu. *Application contact:* Carol Williams, Admissions and Recruiting Manager, 412-648-8957, Fax: 412-648-1077, E-mail: gradstudies@medschool.pitt.edu.
Website: http://www.gradbiomed.pitt.edu/

University of Rhode Island, Graduate School, College of the Environment and Life Sciences, Department of Cell and Molecular Biology, Kingston, RI 02881. Offers biochemistry (MS, PhD); clinical laboratory sciences (MS), including biotechnology, clinical laboratory science, cytopathology; microbiology (MS, PhD); molecular genetics (MS, PhD). *Program availability:* Part-time. *Faculty:* 11 full-time (4 women), 1 (woman) part-time/adjunct. *Students:* 12 full-time (6 women), 36 part-time (27 women); includes 10 minority (4 Black or African American, non-Hispanic/Latino; 3 Asian, non-Hispanic/Latino; 2 Hispanic/Latino; 1 Two or more races, non-Hispanic/Latino), 8 international. In 2015, 19 master's, 1 doctorate awarded. *Degree requirements:* For master's, comprehensive exam (for some programs), thesis optional; for doctorate, comprehensive exam, thesis/dissertation. *Entrance requirements:* For master's and doctorate, GRE, 2 letters of recommendation. Additional exam requirements/recommendations for international students: Required—TOEFL (minimum score 550 paper-based). *Application deadline:* For fall admission, 7/15 for domestic students, 2/1 for international students; for spring admission, 11/15 for domestic students, 7/15 for international students. Application fee: $65. Electronic applications accepted. *Expenses:* Tuition, state resident: full-time $11,796; part-time $655 per credit. Tuition, nonresident: full-time $24,206; part-time $1345 per credit. *Required fees:* $1546; $44 per credit. One-time fee: $155 full-time; $35 part-time. *Financial support:* In 2015–16, 3 research assistantships with tuition reimbursements (averaging $13,507 per year), 8 teaching assistantships with tuition reimbursements (averaging $13,305 per year) were awarded; traineeships also available. Financial award application deadline: 2/1; financial award applicants required to submit FAFSA. *Faculty research:* Genomics. *Total annual research expenditures:* $6.7 million. *Unit head:* Dr. Gongqing Sun, Chairperson, 401-874-5937, Fax: 401-874-2202, E-mail: gsun@mail.uri.edu. *Application contact:* Graduate Admissions, 401-874-2872, E-mail: gradadm@etal.uri.edu.
Website: http://cels.uri.edu/cmb/

The University of Texas Health Science Center at Houston, Graduate School of Biomedical Sciences, Program in Human and Molecular Genetics, Houston, TX 77225-0036. Offers MS, PhD, MD/PhD. Terminal master's awarded for partial completion of doctoral program. *Degree requirements:* For master's, thesis; for doctorate, thesis/dissertation. *Entrance requirements:* For master's and doctorate, GRE General Test. Additional exam requirements/recommendations for international students: Required—TOEFL. Electronic applications accepted. *Faculty research:* Computational genomics, cancer genetics, complex disease genetics, medical genetics.

The University of Texas Health Science Center at Houston, Graduate School of Biomedical Sciences, Program in Microbiology and Molecular Genetics, Houston, TX 77225-0036. Offers MS, PhD, MD/PhD. Terminal master's awarded for partial completion of doctoral program. *Degree requirements:* For master's, thesis; for doctorate, thesis/dissertation. *Entrance requirements:* For master's and doctorate, GRE General Test. Additional exam requirements/recommendations for international students: Required—TOEFL. Electronic applications accepted. *Faculty research:* Disease causation, environmental signaling, gene regulation, cell growth and division, cell structure and architecture.

University of Toronto, Faculty of Medicine, Department of Molecular Genetics, Toronto, ON M5S 1A1, Canada. Offers genetic counseling (M Sc); molecular genetics (M Sc, PhD). *Degree requirements:* For master's, thesis; for doctorate, thesis/dissertation. *Entrance requirements:* For master's, B Sc or equivalent; for doctorate, M Sc or equivalent, minimum B+ average. Additional exam requirements/recommendations for international students: Required—TOEFL, IELTS (minimum score 7), Michigan English Language Assessment Battery (minimum score 85), or COPE (minimum score 4). Electronic applications accepted. *Faculty research:* Structural biology, developmental genetics, molecular medicine, genetic counseling.

University of Virginia, School of Medicine, Department of Biochemistry and Molecular Genetics, Charlottesville, VA 22903. Offers biochemistry (PhD); MD/PhD. *Degree requirements:* For doctorate, thesis/dissertation, written research proposal and defense. *Entrance requirements:* For doctorate, GRE General Test, 3 letters of recommendation. Additional exam requirements/recommendations for international students: Recommended—TOEFL (minimum score 630 paper-based; 90 iBT). Electronic applications accepted.

Van Andel Institute Graduate School, PhD Program, Grand Rapids, MI 49503. Offers cell and molecular genetics (PhD). *Faculty:* 33 full-time (9 women). *Students:* 22 full-time (13 women); includes 3 minority (1 Black or African American, non-Hispanic/Latino; 2 Asian, non-Hispanic/Latino). Average age 24. 38 applicants, 24% accepted, 7 enrolled. In 2015, 3 degrees awarded. *Median time to degree:* Of those who began their doctoral program in fall 2007, 77% received their degree in 8 years or less. *Degree requirements:* For doctorate, comprehensive exam, thesis/dissertation. *Entrance requirements:* For doctorate, GRE or MCAT, personal statement, 3 letters of recommendation, official transcripts from all institutions attended, sample of scientific writing (research paper). Additional exam requirements/recommendations for international students: Required—TOEFL. *Application deadline:* For fall admission, 1/5 for domestic and international students. Applications are processed on a rolling basis. Application fee: $0. Electronic applications accepted. *Expenses:* Tuition, area resident: Full-time $25,000; part-time $835 per credit. *Financial support:* In 2015–16, 22 students received support, including 22 fellowships; health care benefits also available. *Faculty research:* Epigenetics, neurodegenerative science, cancer and cell biology. *Unit head:* Steve Triezeberg, President and Dean, 616-234-5708, Fax: 616-234-5709, E-mail: steve.triezenberg@vai.org.

Wake Forest University, School of Medicine and Graduate School of Arts and Sciences, Graduate Programs in Medicine, Molecular Genetics and Genomics Program, Winston-Salem, NC 27109. Offers PhD, MD/PhD. *Degree requirements:* For doctorate, thesis/dissertation. *Entrance requirements:* For doctorate, GRE General Test. Additional exam requirements/recommendations for international students: Required—TOEFL. Electronic applications accepted. *Faculty research:* Control of gene expression, molecular pathogenesis, protein biosynthesis, cell development, clinical cytogenetics.

Washington University in St. Louis, Graduate School of Arts and Sciences, Division of Biology and Biomedical Sciences, Program in Molecular Genetics and Genomics, St. Louis, MO 63130-4899. Offers PhD. *Students:* 77 full-time (36 women); includes 19 minority (5 Black or African American, non-Hispanic/Latino; 1 American Indian or Alaska Native, non-Hispanic/Latino; 7 Asian, non-Hispanic/Latino; 2 Hispanic/Latino; 4 Two or more races, non-Hispanic/Latino), 12 international. 107 applicants, 20% accepted, 9 enrolled. In 2015, 9 doctorates awarded. *Degree requirements:* For doctorate, thesis/dissertation. *Entrance requirements:* For doctorate, GRE General Test, GRE Subject Test. Additional exam requirements/recommendations for international students: Required—TOEFL. *Application deadline:* For fall admission, 12/1 for domestic students. Application fee: $0. Electronic applications accepted. *Financial support:* Fellowships, research assistantships, and teaching assistantships available. Financial award application deadline: 1/15. *Faculty research:* Genetics, genetic basis of disease, genomics, epigenetics, genetic engineering, genome editing, model organism genetics, development, cell biology, molecular biology, complex traits, bioinformatics, systems biology. *Unit head:* Melanie Relich, Coordinator, 314-362-2763. *Application contact:* Rebecca Riney, 314-747-4648, E-mail: dbbsphdadmissions@wusm.wustl.edu.
Website: http://dbbs.wustl.edu/divprograms/genetics/Pages/default.aspx

Wayne State University, School of Medicine, Office of Biomedical Graduate Programs, Detroit, MI 48202. Offers anatomy and cell biology (PhD); basic medical sciences (MS); biochemistry and molecular biology (MS); cancer biology (MS, PhD); clinical and translational science (Graduate Certificate); family medicine and public health sciences (MPH, Graduate Certificate), including public health practice; genetic counseling (MS); immunology and microbiology (MS, PhD); medical physics (MS, PhD, Graduate Certificate); medical research (MS); molecular medicine and genomics (MS, PhD), including molecular genetics and genomics; pathology (PhD); pharmacology (MS, PhD); physiology (MS, PhD), including physiology, reproductive sciences (PhD); psychiatry and behavioral neurosciences (PhD), including translational neuroscience; MD/MPH; MD/PhD; MPH/MA. *Program availability:* Part-time, evening/weekend. *Students:* 277 full-time (143 women), 84 part-time (41 women); includes 92 minority (13 Black or African American, non-Hispanic/Latino; 54 Asian, non-Hispanic/Latino; 15 Hispanic/Latino; 10 Two or more races, non-Hispanic/Latino), 67 international. Average age 27. 1,053 applicants, 20% accepted, 141 enrolled. In 2015, 69 master's, 26 doctorates, 13 other advanced degrees awarded. Terminal master's awarded for partial completion of doctoral program. *Degree requirements:* For master's, thesis (for some programs); for doctorate, thesis/dissertation. *Entrance requirements:* For master's, doctorate, and Graduate Certificate, GRE. Additional exam requirements/recommendations for international students: Required—TOEFL (minimum score 550 paper-based; 100 iBT), Michigan English Language Assessment Battery (minimum score 85); Recommended—IELTS (minimum score 6.5), TWE (minimum score 5.5). *Application deadline:* For fall admission, 2/1 for domestic and international students. Application fee: $0. Electronic applications accepted. *Expenses:* $17,645 per year resident tuition, $33,311 non-resident tuition; $735.20 per credit hour resident tuition, $1,387.95 per credit hour non-resident tuition; fees include $47.45 per credit hour student services fee and $274.60 per semester registration fee. *Financial support:* In 2015–16, 186 students received support, including 64 fellowships with full tuition reimbursements available (averaging $25,445 per year), 103 research assistantships with full tuition reimbursements available (averaging $26,275 per year); Federal Work-Study, scholarships/grants, traineeships, health care benefits, and unspecified assistantships also available. Support available to part-time students. Financial award application deadline: 3/31. *Faculty research:* Cancer biology, neurosciences, vision sciences, molecular biology, pathology, physiology, pharmacology, public health, medical physics. *Unit head:* Dr. Stanley R. Terlecky, Associate Dean of Graduate Programs, 313-577-1455, Fax: 313-577-8796, E-mail: gradprogs@med.wayne.edu.
Website: http://gradprograms.med.wayne.edu/

Wesleyan University, Graduate Studies, Department of Molecular Biology and Biochemistry, Middletown, CT 06459. Offers biochemistry (PhD); molecular biology (PhD); molecular biophysics (PhD); molecular genetics (PhD). *Faculty:* 8 full-time (3 women), 1 (woman) part-time/adjunct. *Students:* 18 full-time (9 women); includes 4 minority (2 Asian, non-Hispanic/Latino; 1 Hispanic/Latino; 1 Two or more races, non-Hispanic/Latino), 11 international. Average age 24. 28 applicants, 14% accepted, 1 enrolled. Terminal master's awarded for partial completion of doctoral program. *Degree requirements:* For doctorate, comprehensive exam, thesis/dissertation. *Entrance requirements:* For doctorate, GRE General Test, GRE Subject Test. Additional exam requirements/recommendations for international students: Required—TOEFL. *Application deadline:* For fall admission, 1/15 for domestic and international students. Application fee: $0. Electronic applications accepted. *Financial support:* Research assistantships with full tuition reimbursements, teaching assistantships with full tuition reimbursements, and institutionally sponsored loans available. Financial award application deadline: 4/15; financial award applicants required to submit FAFSA. *Faculty research:* The olfactory system and new frontiers in genome research, chromosome structure and gene expression, gene co-regulation, crystallographic and spectroscopic analysis, DNA replication and repair. *Unit head:* Scott Holmes, Chair, 860-685-2443, E-mail: sholmes@wesleyan.edu. *Application contact:* Anika Dane, Administrative Assistant, 860-685-2404, E-mail: adane@wesleyan.edu.
Website: http://www.wesleyan.edu/mbb/

Reproductive Biology

Cornell University, Graduate School, Graduate Fields of Comparative Biomedical Sciences, Field of Comparative Biomedical Sciences, Ithaca, NY 14853-0001. Offers cellular and molecular medicine (MS, PhD); developmental and reproductive biology (MS, PhD); infectious diseases (MS, PhD); population medicine and epidemiology (MS, PhD); structural and functional biology (MS, PhD). *Degree requirements:* For master's, thesis; for doctorate, comprehensive exam, thesis/dissertation. *Entrance requirements:* For master's and doctorate, GRE General Test, 2 letters of recommendation. Additional exam requirements/recommendations for international students: Required—TOEFL (minimum score 550 paper-based; 77 iBT). Electronic applications accepted. *Faculty research:* Receptors and signal transduction, viral and bacterial infectious diseases, tumor metastasis, clinical sciences/nutritional disease, developmental/neurological disorders.

Eastern Virginia Medical School, Master's Program in Clinical Embryology and Andrology, Norfolk, VA 23501-1980. Offers MS. *Program availability:* Online learning. *Entrance requirements:* Additional exam requirements/recommendations for international students: Required—TOEFL (minimum score 550 paper-based; 80 iBT). Electronic applications accepted. *Expenses:* Contact institution.

Queen's University at Kingston, School of Graduate Studies, Faculty of Health Sciences, Department of Anatomy and Cell Biology, Kingston, ON K7L 3N6, Canada. Offers biology of reproduction (M Sc, PhD); cancer (M Sc, PhD); cardiovascular pathophysiology (M Sc, PhD); cell and molecular biology (M Sc, PhD); drug metabolism (M Sc, PhD); endocrinology (M Sc, PhD); motor control (M Sc, PhD); neural regeneration (M Sc, PhD); neurophysiology (M Sc, PhD). *Program availability:* Part-

Reproductive Biology

time. *Degree requirements:* For master's, thesis; for doctorate, one foreign language, comprehensive exam, thesis/dissertation. *Entrance requirements:* Additional exam requirements/recommendations for international students: Required—TOEFL. Electronic applications accepted. *Faculty research:* Human kinetics, neuroscience, reproductive biology, cardiovascular.

Rutgers University–New Brunswick, Graduate School-New Brunswick, Program in Endocrinology and Animal Biosciences, Piscataway, NJ 08854-8097. Offers MS, PhD. Terminal master's awarded for partial completion of doctoral program. *Degree requirements:* For master's, thesis; for doctorate, comprehensive exam, thesis/dissertation. *Entrance requirements:* For master's and doctorate, GRE General Test. Additional exam requirements/recommendations for international students: Required—TOEFL. Electronic applications accepted. *Faculty research:* Comparative and behavioral endocrinology, epigenetic regulation of the endocrine system, exercise physiology and immunology, fetal and neonatal developmental programming, mammary gland biology and breast cancer, neuroendocrinology and alcohol studies, reproductive and developmental toxicology.

Tufts University, Cummings School of Veterinary Medicine, North Grafton, MA 01536. Offers animals and public policy (MS); biomedical sciences (PhD), including digestive diseases, infectious diseases, neuroscience and reproductive biology, pathology; conservation medicine (MS); veterinary medicine (DVM); DVM/MPH; DVM/MS. *Accreditation:* AVMA (one or more programs are accredited). *Degree requirements:* For master's, thesis (for some programs); for doctorate, comprehensive exam, thesis/dissertation (for some programs). *Entrance requirements:* For master's and doctorate, GRE General Test. Additional exam requirements/recommendations for international students: Required—TOEFL or IELTS. Electronic applications accepted. *Expenses:* Contact institution. *Faculty research:* Oncology, veterinary ethics, international veterinary medicine, veterinary genomics, pathogenesis of Clostridium difficile, wildlife fertility control.

The University of British Columbia, Faculty of Medicine, Department of Obstetrics and Gynecology, Program in Reproductive and Developmental Sciences, Vancouver, BC V6H 3N1, Canada. Offers M Sc, PhD. *Program availability:* Part-time. Terminal master's awarded for partial completion of doctoral program. *Degree requirements:* For master's, thesis; for doctorate, thesis/dissertation. *Entrance requirements:* For master's, B Sc or equivalent, MD, DVM, DDS; for doctorate, B Sc with first class honors, M Sc, MD, DVM, DDS. Additional exam requirements/recommendations for international students: Required—TOEFL (minimum score 580 paper-based; 80 iBT), IELTS (minimum score 7). Electronic applications accepted. *Faculty research:* Reproductive and placental endocrinology; immunology of reproductive, fertilization, and embryonic development; perinatal metabolism; neonatal development.

University of Hawaii at Manoa, John A. Burns School of Medicine, Program in Developmental and Reproductive Biology, Honolulu, HI 96813. Offers MS, PhD. *Program availability:* Part-time. *Faculty:* 24 full-time (7 women). *Students:* 11 full-time (5 women), 3 part-time (1 woman); includes 9 minority (7 Asian, non-Hispanic/Latino; 2 Two or more races, non-Hispanic/Latino), 2 international. 19 applicants, 32% accepted, 2 enrolled. In 2015, 1 master's, 1 doctorate awarded. *Degree requirements:* For doctorate, thesis/dissertation. *Entrance requirements:* For doctorate, GRE General Test, GRE Subject Test. Additional exam requirements/recommendations for international students: Recommended—TOEFL (minimum score 560 paper-based), IELTS (minimum score 5). *Application deadline:* For fall admission, 3/1 for domestic and international students. Application fee: $100. *Financial support:* In 2015–16, 2 fellowships (averaging $4,577 per year), 10 research assistantships (averaging $16,328 per year) were awarded; teaching assistantships also available. *Faculty research:* Biology of gametes and fertilization, reproductive endocrinology. *Total annual research expenditures:* $5.4 million. *Unit head:* Dr. Yusuke Marikawa, Chair, 808-692-1411. Website: http://www2.jabsom.hawaii.edu/Grad_DRB/

University of Saskatchewan, College of Medicine, Department of Obstetrics, Gynecology and Reproductive Services, Saskatoon, SK S7N 5A2, Canada. Offers M Sc, PhD. *Degree requirements:* For master's, thesis; for doctorate, thesis/dissertation. *Entrance requirements:* Additional exam requirements/recommendations for international students: Required—TOEFL.

University of Wyoming, College of Agriculture and Natural Resources, Department of Animal Sciences, Program in Reproductive Biology, Laramie, WY 82071. Offers MS, PhD. *Degree requirements:* For master's, thesis; for doctorate, thesis/dissertation. *Entrance requirements:* For master's, GRE General Test, minimum GPA of 3.0; for doctorate, GRE General Test, minimum GPA of 3.0 or MS degree. Additional exam requirements/recommendations for international students: Required—TOEFL. *Faculty research:* Fetal programming, chemical suppression, ovaria function, genetics.

West Virginia University, Davis College of Agriculture, Forestry and Consumer Sciences, Interdisciplinary Program in Genetics and Developmental Biology, Morgantown, WV 26506. Offers animal breeding (MS, PhD); biochemical and molecular genetics (MS, PhD); cytogenetics (MS, PhD); descriptive embryology (MS, PhD); developmental genetics (MS); experimental morphogenesis/teratology (MS); human genetics (MS, PhD); immunogenetics (MS, PhD); life cycles of animals and plants (MS, PhD); molecular aspects of development (MS, PhD); mutagenesis (MS, PhD); oncology (MS, PhD); plant genetics (MS, PhD); population and quantitative genetics (MS, PhD); regeneration (MS, PhD); teratology (PhD); toxicology (MS, PhD). *Degree requirements:* For master's, thesis; for doctorate, comprehensive exam, thesis/dissertation. *Entrance requirements:* For master's, GRE or MCAT, minimum GPA of 2.75. Additional exam requirements/recommendations for international students: Required—TOEFL. *Expenses:* Tuition, state resident: full-time $8568. Tuition, nonresident: full-time $22,140. Tuition and fees vary according to program.

Teratology

West Virginia University, Davis College of Agriculture, Forestry and Consumer Sciences, Interdisciplinary Program in Genetics and Developmental Biology, Morgantown, WV 26506. Offers animal breeding (MS, PhD); biochemical and molecular genetics (MS, PhD); cytogenetics (MS, PhD); descriptive embryology (MS, PhD); developmental genetics (MS); experimental morphogenesis/teratology (MS); human genetics (MS, PhD); immunogenetics (MS, PhD); life cycles of animals and plants (MS, PhD); molecular aspects of development (MS, PhD); mutagenesis (MS, PhD); oncology (MS, PhD); plant genetics (MS, PhD); population and quantitative genetics (MS, PhD); regeneration (MS, PhD); teratology (PhD); toxicology (MS, PhD). *Degree requirements:* For master's, thesis; for doctorate, comprehensive exam, thesis/dissertation. *Entrance requirements:* For master's, GRE or MCAT, minimum GPA of 2.75. Additional exam requirements/recommendations for international students: Required—TOEFL. *Expenses:* Tuition, state resident: full-time $8568. Tuition, nonresident: full-time $22,140. Tuition and fees vary according to program.

UCONN HEALTH
Graduate Program in Genetics and Developmental Biology

 For more information, visit http://petersons.to/uconnhealth_genetics

Program of Study

The Genetics and Developmental Biology graduate program provides students with fundamental interdisciplinary training in modern molecular genetics and developmental biology, emphasizing cellular and molecular aspects as well as tissue interactions. It prepares students to compete for job opportunities in traditional medical and dental school departments as well as a productive research career in either academia or industry. Faculty members are from several basic science and clinical departments and study a wide range of organisms including yeast, worms, fruit flies, mice, and humans.

Areas of research include the mapping and cloning of human genes responsible for disease, RNA processing (including RNA editing, alternative splicing, antisense regulation, and RNA interference), the molecular mechanisms of aging, signal transduction pathways, microbial pathogenesis, developmental neurobiology, cell differentiation, musculoskeletal development, morphogenesis and pattern formation, reproductive biology, and endocrinology.

Research Facilities

The Department of Genetics and Developmental Biology is the academic home of the genetics and developmental biology graduate program which houses equipment and facilities for mouse transgenics, ES cell manipulation, DNA microarrays, nucleic acid sequencing, fluorescence microscopy, and digital imaging. Students also have ready access to first-rate flow cytometry and confocal microscopy facilities. Other institutional resources include a computer center and the Lyman Maynard Stowe Library which contains approximately 200,000 volumes and subscribes to more than 1,700 current periodicals. Students of the program therefore have an excellent opportunity for research and training in cutting-edge areas of genetics and developmental biology.

Financial Aid

Support for doctoral students engaged in full-time degree programs at UConn Health is provided on a competitive basis. Graduate research assistantships for 2016–17 provide a stipend of $29,000 per year, which includes a waiver of tuition/most University fees for the fall and spring semesters and the option of participating in a student health insurance plan. While financial aid is offered competitively, UConn Health makes every possible effort to address the financial needs of all students during their period of training.

Cost of Study

For 2016–17, tuition is $14,310 per year for full-time students who are Connecticut residents and $35,346 per year for full-time out-of-state residents. General University fees are added to the cost of tuition for students who do not receive a tuition waiver. These costs are usually met by traineeships or research assistantships for doctoral students.

Living and Housing Costs

There is a wide range of affordable housing options in the greater Hartford area within easy commuting distance of the campus, including an extensive complex that is adjacent to UConn Health. Costs range from $700 to $1,000 per month for a one-bedroom unit; 2 or more students sharing an apartment usually pay less. University housing is not available on campus.

Student Group

At UConn Health, there are about 500 students in the Schools of Medicine and Dental Medicine, 150 Ph.D. students, and 50 postdoctoral fellows. There are no restrictions on the admission of out-of-state graduate students.

Location

UConn Health is located in the historic town of Farmington, Connecticut. Set in the beautiful New England countryside on a hill overlooking the Farmington Valley, it is close to ski areas, hiking trails, and facilities for boating, fishing, and swimming. Connecticut's capital city of Hartford, 7 miles east of Farmington, is the center of an urban region of approximately 800,000 people. The beaches of the Long Island Sound are about 50 minutes away to the south, and the beautiful Berkshires are a short drive to the northwest. New York City and Boston can be reached within 2½ hours by car. Hartford

is the home of the acclaimed Hartford Stage Company, TheatreWorks, the Hartford Symphony and Chamber orchestras, two ballet companies, an opera company, the Wadsworth Athenaeum (the oldest public art museum in the nation), the Mark Twain house, the Hartford Civic Center, and many other interesting cultural and recreational facilities. The area is also home to several branches of the University of Connecticut, Trinity College, and the University of Hartford, which includes the Hartt School of Music. Bradley International Airport (about 30 minutes from campus) serves the Hartford/Springfield area with frequent airline connections to major cities in this country and abroad. Frequent bus and rail service is also available from Hartford.

The UConn Health Campus

The 200-acre UConn Health campus at Farmington houses a division of the University of Connecticut Graduate School, as well as the Schools of Medicine and Dental Medicine. The campus also includes the John Dempsey Hospital, associated clinics, and extensive medical research facilities, all in a centralized facility with more than 1 million square feet of floor space. The Academic Research Building, built in 1999, is an impressive eleven-story structure providing 170,000 square feet of laboratory space and renovations are underway in the main Laboratory building, converting existing lab space to state-of-the-art open lab areas. In addition, The Jackson Laboratory for Genomic Medicine opened its 189,000-square-foot facility on the UConn Health Campus in fall 2014. The faculty includes more than 260 full-time members. The institution has a strong commitment to graduate study within an environment that promotes social and intellectual interaction among the various educational programs. Graduate students are represented on various administrative committees concerned with curricular affairs, and the Graduate Student Organization (GSO) represents graduate students' needs and concerns to the faculty and administration, in addition to fostering social contact among graduate students at UConn Health.

Applying

Applications for admission should be submitted via the online application system and should be filed together with transcripts, three letters of recommendation, a personal statement, and recent results from the General Test of the Graduate Record Examinations. International students must take the Test of English as a Foreign Language (TOEFL) to satisfy Graduate School requirements. The deadline for completed applications and receipt of all supplemental materials is **December 1**. Please note that GRE and TOEFL exams taken after the due date will not be accepted for consideration for admission. In accordance with the laws of the state of Connecticut and of the United States, UConn Health does not discriminate against any person in its educational and employment activities on the grounds of race, color, creed, national origin, sex, age, or physical disability.

Correspondence and Information

Graduate Admissions Office
Ph.D. in Biomedical Science Program
UConn Health
263 Farmington Ave., MC 3906
Farmington, Connecticut 06030-3906
United States
Phone: 860-679-4509
E-mail: BiomedSciAdmissions@uchc.edu
Website: http://health.uconn.edu/graduate-school/academics/
      programs/ph-d-biomedical-science

THE FACULTY AND THEIR RESEARCH

Hector Leonardo Aguila, Ph.D., Associate Professor of Immunology. Hematopoiesis and bone marrow microenvironment; lymphoid cell development; stem cell biology.

Andrew Arnold, M.D., Professor of Medicine and Murray-Heilig Chair in Molecular Medicine. Molecular genetic underpinnings of tumors of the endocrine glands; role of the cyclin D1 oncogene.

Michael Blinov, Ph.D., Assistant Professor of Genetics and Developmental Biology. Modeling of signal transcription systems and protein-DNA interactions; bioinformatics: data mining and visualization; developing software tools and mathematical methods for rule-based modeling of signal transduction systems.

Gordon Carmichael, Ph.D., Professor of Genetics and Developmental Biology. Regulation of gene expression in eukaryotes.

Stormy J. Chamberlain, Ph.D., Assistant Professor of Genetics and Developmental Biology. Human induced pluripotent stem (iPS) cell models to study 15q11-q13 imprinting disorders.

Albert Cheng, Assistant Professor of Genetics and Developmental Biology; Ph.D., MIT. Engineering and applying artificial DNA and RNA binding proteins to study the genome, epigenome and transcriptome.

Jeffrey Chuang, Ph.D., Associate Professor, Genetics and Developmental Biology. Computational biology and bioinformatics; genomics, gene regulation, molecular evolution, and metabolomics; post-transcriptional regulation and cancer genomics.

Kevin Claffey, Ph.D., Assistant Professor of Cell Biology. Angiogenesis in cancer progression and metastasis; vascular endothelial growth factor (VEGF) expression; hypoxia-mediated gene regulation.

Soheil (Sam) Dadras, M.D., Ph.D., Associate Professor of Dermatology, and Genetics and Developmental Biology, Discovery of small RNAs (including microRNA) as novel biomarkers in human melanoma progression and metastasis using next generation sequencing.

Asis Das, Ph.D., Professor of Microbiology. Basic genetic and biomechanical mechanisms that govern the elongation-termination and decision in transcription.

Caroline N. Dealy, Ph.D., Associate Professor of Anatomy. Roles of various growth factors and signaling molecules, particularly IGF-I and insulin, in the regulation of chick limb development.

Paul Epstein, Ph.D., Associate Professor of Pharmacology. Receptor signal transduction, second messengers, and protein phosphorylation in control of cell growth and regulation; purification and regulation of cyclic nucleotide phosphodiesterases; role of calmodulin in mediating Ca^{2+}-dependent cell processes.

Guo-Hua Fong, Ph.D., Associate Professor of Cell Biology. Developmental biology of the vascular system, VEGF-A receptor signal transduction, embryonic stem cells, and gene knock-out in mice.

Brenton R. Graveley, Ph.D., Professor of Genetics and Developmental Biology. Regulation of alternative splicing in the mammalian nervous system and mechanisms of alternative splicing.

Arthur Günzl, Ph.D., Professor, Center for Microbial Pathogenesis. Transcription and antigenic variation in the mammalian parasite *Trypanosoma brucei.*

Marc Hansen, Ph.D., Professor of Medicine. Molecular genetics of osteosarcoma and related bone diseases.

Laura Haynes, Ph.D., Professor of Immunology. Rochester. Influence of aging on CD4 T cell function and how this impacts responses to infection and vaccination.

J. Travis Hinson, Assistant Professor of Cardiology and Genetics; M.D., Harvard. Human iPS disease modeling of cardiovascular disorders; functional genomics; regenerative medicine related to the heart; CRISPR/CAS9 genomewide screens in iPS-cell assays.

Laurinda Jaffe, Ph.D., Professor of Cell Biology. Physiology of fertilization.

Barbara Kream, Ph.D., Professor of Medicine. Hormonal regulation of collagen gene expression in bone.

George Kuchel, M.D., Professor of Medicine. Role of hormones and cytokines in geriatric disability. Pathogenesis of impaired detrusor contractility and urinary retention. Molecular mechanisms of bladder muscle survival.

Marc Lalande, Ph.D., Professor of Genetics and Developmental Biology. Genomic imprinting; Angelman syndrome; mechanism of tissue-specific silencing of the Angelman ubiquitin ligase in mouse and human.

James Li, Ph.D., Assistant Professor of Genetics and Developmental Biology. Identifying the molecular mechanisms underlying formation of the mammalian cerebellum.

Alexander Lichtler, Ph.D., Associate Professor of Pediatrics. Regulation of collagen gene transcription; retrovirus vectors; role of homeobox genes in limb development.

Edison T. Liu, M.D., Professor, President and CEO of The Jackson Laboratory.

Bruce Mayer, Ph.D., Professor of Genetics and Developmental Biology. Biologically relevant Nck-interacting proteins.

Mina Mina, D.M.D., Ph.D., Associate Professor of Pediatric Dentistry. Characterization of genetic and epigenetic influences involved in pattern formation and skeletogenesis of the chick mandible and mouse tooth germ.

William Mohler, Ph.D., Associate Professor of Genetics and Developmental Biology. Molecular and cellular mechanisms of cell fusion.

Julia Oh, Assistant Professor of Genetics and Developmental Biology; Ph.D., Stanford. Potential of the human microbiome—the diverse bacteria, fungi, and viruses that inhabit our bodies—to deliver treatments for infectious and other diseases.

Zhengqing Ouyang, Ph.D., Assistant Professor of Genetics and Developmental Biology. Development and application of statistical and computational methodologies in the area of regulatory genomics;

chromatin structure; lncRNA; epigenomics and epitranscriptomics; regulatory network.

John Peluso, Ph.D., Professor of Cell Biology. Control of ovarian follicle growth steroidogenesis in vitro; proto-oncogene expression and ovarian follicular growth.

Carol C. Pilbeam, Ph.D., M.D., Professor of Medicine; Mechanisms of regulation of bone formation and resorption.

Stefan Pinter, Assistant Professor of Genetics and Genomic Science; Ph.D., Princeton. How chromosome topology, non-coding (nc)RNA and chromatin modifiers orchestrate gene expression.

Justin D. Radolf, M.D., Professor of Medicine and Genetics and Developmental Biology. Molecular pathogenesis and immunobiology of spirochetal infections.

Blanka Rogina, Ph.D., Associate Professor of Genetics and Developmental Biology. Molecular mechanism underlying aging process in *Drosophila melanogaster.*

Daniel W. Rosenberg, Ph.D., Professor of Medicine. Molecular genetics of colorectal cancer; signaling pathways in the development of tumors; toxicogenomics.

Edward F. Rossomando, D.D.S., Ph.D., Professor of BioStructure and Function. Control of gene expression in tumor and nontumor cell lines in response to stimulation by monokines; coding, transmission, and processing of environmental signals in normal and abnormal development.

Yijun Ruan, Ph.D., Professor of Genetics and Developmental Biology. Elucidating the structures and dynamics of all functional DNA elements in complex genomes through DNA sequencing analysis of genetic variations in genomes and transcriptomes.

Archana Sanjay, Ph.D., Assistant Professor of Orthopaedic Surgery, School of Medicine. Regulation of bone remodeling; examining signaling pathways that regulate osteoblast and osteoclast differentiation and function.

Mansoor Sarfarazi, Ph.D., Professor of Surgery. Positional mapping and mutation analysis of human genetic disorders; primary open angle glaucoma; primary congenital glaucoma; synpolydactyly; dyslexia; mitral valve prolapse and ascending aortic aneurysm.

Duygu Ucar, Ph.D., Assistant Professor of Genetics. Developing computational models to take advantage of existing datasets to study the dynamics and mechanisms of transcriptional gene regulation and propose testable hypotheses.

Zhao-Wen Wang, Ph.D., Associate Professor of Neuroscience. Function and regulation of potassium channels and gap junctions; mechanisms of synaptic transmission.

George Weinstock, Ph.D., Associate Director for Microbial Genomics [Professor], The Jackson Laboratory for Genomic Medicine.

Bruce White, Ph.D., Professor of Physiology. Control of prolactin gene expression at pretranslational level in GH3 cells; control of aromatase gene expression in ovarian and testicular tissues.

Adam Williams, Ph.D., Assistant Professor of Genetics. The role of non-coding RNAs in regulating gene expression relating to immune cell function, in particular, CD4+ T cells.

George Y. Wu, M.D., Ph.D., Professor of Medicine; Chief, Hepatology Section, Herman Lopata Chair in Hepatitis Research. Targeted delivery of biological substances specifically to liver cells; novel Inhibitors of hepatitis C viral (HCV) replication; animal models of HCV.

Yi Wu, Assistant Professor of Genetics and Developmental Biology. Developing quantitative imaging tools capable of revealing dynamics of cellular signaling at high spatial and temporal resolution (biosensors), or that enable optical control of signaling proteins at precise times and subcellular locations (optogenetics).

Erin Young, Ph.D., Assistant Professor of Genetics and Developmental Biology. The understanding of gene x environment interactions on pain outcomes, with a particular focus on stress and injury/inflammation as environmental factors.

Ji Yu, Ph.D., Associate Professor of Genetics and Developmental Biology; Optical imaging technology; regulation mechanisms in dendritic RNA translation; cytoskeletal dynamics.

Section 11
Marine Biology

This section contains a directory of institutions offering graduate work in marine biology. Additional information about programs listed in the directory may be obtained by writing directly to the dean of a graduate school or chair of a department at the address given in the directory.

For programs offering related work, see also in this book *Biological and Biomedical Sciences* and *Zoology*. In another guide in this series:

Graduate Programs in the Physical Sciences, Mathematics, Agricultural Sciences, the Environment & Natural Resources

See *Marine Sciences and Oceanography*

CONTENTS

Program Directory

Marine Biology

College of Charleston, Graduate School, School of Sciences and Mathematics, Program in Marine Biology, Charleston, SC 29412. Offers MS. *Degree requirements:* For master's, comprehensive exam, thesis. *Entrance requirements:* For master's, GRE General Test, 3 letters of recommendation. Additional exam requirements/recommendations for international students: Required—TOEFL (minimum score 81 iBT). Electronic applications accepted. *Faculty research:* Ecology, environmental physiology, marine genomics, bioinformatics, toxicology, cell biology, population biology, fisheries science, animal physiology, biodiversity, estuarine ecology, evolution and systematics, microbial processes, plant physiology, immunology.

Florida Institute of Technology, College of Science, Program in Biological Sciences, Melbourne, FL 32901-6975. Offers biological science (PhD); biotechnology (MS); cell and molecular biology (MS); ecology (MS); marine biology (MS). *Program availability:* Part-time. *Students:* 65 full-time (39 women), 10 part-time (3 women); includes 4 minority (2 Asian, non-Hispanic/Latino; 1 Hispanic/Latino; 1 Two or more races, non-Hispanic/Latino), 38 international. Average age 26. 230 applicants, 24% accepted, 21 enrolled. In 2015, 23 master's, 3 doctorates awarded. *Degree requirements:* For master's, thesis (for some programs), research, seminar, internship, or summer lab; for doctorate, comprehensive exam, thesis/dissertation, dissertations seminar, publications. *Entrance requirements:* For master's, GRE General Test, 3 letters of recommendation; statement of objectives; bachelor's degree in biology, chemistry, biochemistry or equivalent; for doctorate, GRE General Test, resume, 3 letters of recommendation, minimum GPA of 3.2, statement of objectives. Additional exam requirements/recommendations for international students: Required—TOEFL (minimum score 550 paper-based; 79 iBT). *Application deadline:* For fall admission, 3/1 for domestic students, 4/1 for international students; for spring admission, 9/1 for domestic and international students. Applications are processed on a rolling basis. Electronic applications accepted. *Expenses:* Tuition, area resident: Full-time $21,690; part-time $1205 per credit hour. *Required fees:* $500. Tuition and fees vary according to degree level, campus/location and program. *Financial support:* Career-related internships or fieldwork, institutionally sponsored loans, tuition waivers (partial), unspecified assistantships, and tuition remissions available. Support available to part-time students. Financial award application deadline: 3/1; financial award applicants required to submit FAFSA. *Faculty research:* Initiation of protein synthesis in eukaryotic cells, fixation of radioactive carbon, changes in DNA molecule, endangered or threatened avian and mammalian species, hydroacoustics and feeding preference of the West Indian manatee. *Unit head:* Dr. Richard B. Aronson, Department Head, 321-674-8034, Fax: 321-674-7238, E-mail: raronson@fit.edu. *Application contact:* Cheryl A. Brown, Associate Director of Graduate Admissions, 321-674-7581, Fax: 321-723-9468, E-mail: cbrown@fit.edu.
Website: http://cos.fit.edu/biology/

Montclair State University, The Graduate School, College of Science and Mathematics, Program in Marine Biology and Coastal Sciences, Montclair, NJ 07043-1624. Offers MS. *Students:* 14 full-time (6 women), 23 part-time (17 women); includes 16 minority (5 Black or African American, non-Hispanic/Latino; 2 Asian, non-Hispanic/Latino; 7 Hispanic/Latino; 2 Two or more races, non-Hispanic/Latino), 4 international. Average age 29. 33 applicants, 67% accepted, 12 enrolled. In 2015, 13 master's awarded. *Degree requirements:* For master's, thesis. *Expenses:* Tuition, state resident: part-time $553 per credit. Tuition, nonresident: part-time $854 per credit. *Required fees:* $91 per credit. Tuition and fees vary according to program. *Unit head:* Dr. Paul Bologna, Coordinator, 973-655-4112, E-mail: bolognap@mail.montclair.edu. *Application contact:* Amy Aiello, Director of Graduate Admissions and Operations, 973-655-5147, Fax: 973-655-7869, E-mail: graduate.school@montclair.edu.

Nicholls State University, Graduate Studies, College of Arts and Sciences, Department of Biological Sciences, Thibodaux, LA 70310. Offers marine and environmental biology (MS). *Program availability:* Part-time. *Degree requirements:* For master's, comprehensive exam, thesis. *Entrance requirements:* For master's, GRE. Additional exam requirements/recommendations for international students: Required—TOEFL (minimum score 600 paper-based). *Application deadline:* For fall admission, 6/17 priority date for domestic and international students; for spring admission, 11/15 priority date for domestic and international students. Application fee: $20 ($30 for international students). *Financial support:* Research assistantships, teaching assistantships with tuition reimbursements, career-related internships or fieldwork, and scholarships/grants available. *Faculty research:* Bioremediation, ecology, public health, biotechnology, physiology.
Website: http://www.nicholls.edu/biol/

Northeastern University, College of Science, Boston, MA 02115-5096. Offers applied mathematics (MS); bioinformatics (MS); biology (PhD); biotechnology (MS); chemistry (MS, PhD); ecology, evolution, and marine biology (PhD); marine biology (MS); mathematics (MS, PhD); network science (PhD); operations research (MSOR); physics (MS, PhD); psychology (PhD). *Program availability:* Part-time. *Faculty:* 216 full-time (70 women), 62 part-time/adjunct (20 women). *Students:* 517 full-time (252 women), 80 part-time (39 women). In 2015, 94 master's, 46 doctorates awarded. Terminal master's awarded for partial completion of doctoral program. *Degree requirements:* For master's, comprehensive exam (for some programs), thesis; for doctorate, comprehensive exam (for some programs), thesis/dissertation. *Entrance requirements:* For master's, GRE General Test. *Application deadline:* Applications are processed on a rolling basis. Application fee: $75. Electronic applications accepted. *Expenses:* $1,325 per credit; $1,170 per credit (for marine biology). *Financial support:* Fellowships with tuition reimbursements, research assistantships with tuition reimbursements, teaching assistantships with tuition reimbursements, career-related internships or fieldwork, scholarships/grants, health care benefits, tuition waivers (full and partial), and unspecified assistantships available. Support available to part-time students. Financial award applicants required to submit FAFSA. *Unit head:* Dr. Jonathan Tilly, Interim Dean. *Application contact:* Graduate Student Services, 617-373-4275, E-mail: gradcos@neu.edu.
Website: http://www.northeastern.edu/cos/

Nova Southeastern University, Halmos College of Natural Sciences and Oceanography, Fort Lauderdale, FL 33314-7796. Offers biological sciences (MS); coastal studies (Certificate); coastal zone management (MS); marine and coastal climate change (Certificate); marine and coastal studies (MA); marine biology (MS); marine biology and oceanography (PhD), including marine biology, oceanography; marine environmental sciences (MS). *Program availability:* Part-time, evening/weekend, 100% online, blended/hybrid learning. *Faculty:* 17 full-time (3 women), 22 part-time/adjunct (11 women). *Students:* 100 full-time (57 women), 114 part-time (76 women); includes 32 minority (6 Black or African American, non-Hispanic/Latino; 1 American Indian or Alaska Native, non-Hispanic/Latino; 6 Asian, non-Hispanic/Latino; 10 Hispanic/Latino; 9 Two or more races, non-Hispanic/Latino), 5 international. Average age 30. 85

applicants, 60% accepted, 39 enrolled. In 2015, 47 master's, 2 doctorates, 9 other advanced degrees awarded. *Degree requirements:* For master's, thesis; for doctorate, comprehensive exam, thesis/dissertation, departmental qualifying exam. *Entrance requirements:* For master's, GRE General Test, 3 letters of recommendation, BS/BA in natural science (for marine biology program), BS/BA in biology (for biological sciences program), minor in the natural sciences or equivalent (for coastal zone management and marine environmental sciences); for doctorate, GRE General Test, master's degree. Additional exam requirements/recommendations for international students: Required—TOEFL (minimum score 550 paper-based). *Application deadline:* Applications are processed on a rolling basis. Application fee: $50. Electronic applications accepted. *Expenses:* $34,749 per year (for PhD); $3,738 per course (for MS and Graduate Certificate). *Financial support:* In 2015–16, 157 students received support, including 14 fellowships with tuition reimbursements available (averaging $25,000 per year), 42 research assistantships with tuition reimbursements available (averaging $19,000 per year); teaching assistantships, career-related internships or fieldwork, Federal Work-Study, scholarships/grants, health care benefits, tuition waivers (full and partial), and unspecified assistantships also available. Support available to part-time students. Financial award application deadline: 4/15; financial award applicants required to submit FAFSA. *Faculty research:* Physical oceanography, biological oceanography, molecular and microbiology, ecology and evolution, coral reefs. *Total annual research expenditures:* $5 million. *Unit head:* Dr. Richard Dodge, Dean, 954-262-3600, Fax: 954-262-4020, E-mail: dodge@nsu.nova.edu. *Application contact:* Dr. Bernhard Riegl, Chair, Department of Marine and Environmental Sciences, 954-262-3600, Fax: 954-262-4020, E-mail: rieglb@nova.edu.
Website: http://cnso.nova.edu

Princeton University, Graduate School, Department of Geosciences, Princeton, NJ 08544-1019. Offers atmospheric and oceanic sciences (PhD); geosciences (PhD); ocean sciences and marine biology (PhD). *Degree requirements:* For doctorate, one foreign language, thesis/dissertation. *Entrance requirements:* For doctorate, GRE General Test. Additional exam requirements/recommendations for international students: Required—TOEFL (minimum score 600 paper-based). Electronic applications accepted. *Faculty research:* Biogeochemistry, climate science, earth history, regional geology and tectonics, solid–earth geophysics.

Rutgers University–New Brunswick, Graduate School-New Brunswick, Department of Environmental Sciences, Piscataway, NJ 08854-8097. Offers air pollution and resources (MS, PhD); aquatic biology (MS, PhD); aquatic chemistry (MS, PhD); atmospheric science (MS, PhD); chemistry and physics of aerosol and hydrosol systems (MS, PhD); environmental chemistry (MS, PhD); environmental microbiology (MS, PhD); environmental toxicology (PhD); exposure assessment (PhD); fate and effects of pollutants (MS, PhD); pollution prevention and control (MS, PhD); water and wastewater treatment (MS, PhD); water resources (MS, PhD). Terminal master's awarded for partial completion of doctoral program. *Degree requirements:* For master's, comprehensive exam, thesis or alternative, oral final exam; for doctorate, comprehensive exam, thesis/dissertation, thesis defense, qualifying exam. *Entrance requirements:* For master's and doctorate, GRE General Test. Additional exam requirements/recommendations for international students: Required—TOEFL. Electronic applications accepted. *Faculty research:* Biological waste treatment; contaminant fate and transport; air, soil and water quality.

San Francisco State University, Division of Graduate Studies, College of Science and Engineering, Department of Biology, Program in Marine Biology, San Francisco, CA 94132-1722. Offers MS. *Expenses:* Tuition, state resident: full-time $6738. Tuition, nonresident: full-time $15,666. *Required fees:* $1004. *Unit head:* Dr. Karen Crow, Program Coordinator, 415-405-2760, Fax: 415-338-2295, E-mail: crow@sfsu.edu. *Application contact:* Graduate Coordinator.
Website: http://biology.sfsu.edu/graduate/marine_biology

Texas A&M University at Galveston, Department of Marine Biology, Galveston, TX 77553-1675. Offers MS, PhD. *Faculty:* 18 full-time (5 women). *Students:* 45 full-time (31 women), 9 part-time (4 women); includes 5 minority (1 Black or African American, non-Hispanic/Latino; 1 Asian, non-Hispanic/Latino; 2 Hispanic/Latino; 1 Two or more races, non-Hispanic/Latino), 9 international. Average age 29. 42 applicants, 55% accepted, 16 enrolled. In 2015, 3 master's, 3 doctorates awarded. Terminal master's awarded for partial completion of doctoral program. *Degree requirements:* For master's, comprehensive exam (for some programs), thesis (for some programs); for doctorate, comprehensive exam, thesis/dissertation. *Entrance requirements:* For master's and doctorate, GRE. Additional exam requirements/recommendations for international students: Required—TOEFL (minimum score 550 paper-based; 80 iBT), IELTS (minimum score 6). *Application deadline:* For fall admission, 5/15 for domestic students, 5/1 for international students; for spring admission, 10/15 for domestic students, 10/1 for international students. Application fee: $50. Electronic applications accepted. *Expenses:* Contact institution. *Financial support:* In 2015–16, 44 students received support, including 15 research assistantships (averaging $7,603 per year), 25 teaching assistantships (averaging $7,045 per year); scholarships/grants, health care benefits, and unspecified assistantships also available. Financial award application deadline: 3/1; financial award applicants required to submit FAFSA. *Faculty research:* Fisheries, coastal and wetland ecologies, phytoplankton, marine mammals, seafood safety, marine invertebrates and marine biospeleology. *Unit head:* Dr. John Schwarz, Professor/Chair of Marine Biology Interdisciplinary Program, 409-740-4428, E-mail: schwarzj@tamug.edu. *Application contact:* Nicole Kinslow, Director of Graduate Studies, 409-740-4937, Fax: 409-740-4754, E-mail: kinslown@tamug.edu.
Website: http://www.tamug.edu/marb/index.html

Texas State University, The Graduate College, College of Science and Engineering, Program in Aquatic Resources, San Marcos, TX 78666. Offers MS, PhD. *Faculty:* 9 full-time (2 women). *Students:* 38 full-time (19 women), 13 part-time (6 women); includes 8 minority (2 Black or African American, non-Hispanic/Latino; 2 Asian, non-Hispanic/Latino; 4 Hispanic/Latino), 11 international. Average age 32. 19 applicants, 74% accepted, 12 enrolled. In 2015, 3 master's, 6 doctorates awarded. *Degree requirements:* For master's, comprehensive exam, thesis, 3 seminars. *Entrance requirements:* For master's, GRE General Test (minimum recommended score in at least the 50th percentile on both the verbal and quantitative portions), baccalaureate degree in biology or related discipline from regionally-accredited university with minimum GPA of 3.0 on last 60 undergraduate semester hours; for doctorate, GRE (recommended score in at least the 60th percentile on both the verbal and quantitative portions), baccalaureate degree from regionally-accredited university; master's degree in biology, chemistry, engineering, geology, or related natural science field with minimum GPA of 3.25 on all completed graduate work. Additional exam requirements/recommendations for international students: Required—TOEFL (minimum score 550 paper-based; 78 iBT). *Application deadline:* For fall admission, 1/15 priority date for domestic and international

students; for spring admission, 8/15 for domestic students, 8/1 for international students; for summer admission, 4/15 for domestic students, 3/15 for international students. Applications are processed on a rolling basis. Application fee: $40 ($90 for international students). Electronic applications accepted. *Expenses:* $3,615 in-state tuition (for 12 semester credit hours/1 full-time semester); $974 in-state fees. *Financial support:* In 2015–16, 17 students received support, including 15 research assistantships (averaging $18,045 per year), 29 teaching assistantships (averaging $20,870 per year); Federal Work-Study, institutionally sponsored loans, scholarships/grants, health care benefits, and unspecified assistantships also available. Support available to part-time students. Financial award application deadline: 3/1; financial award applicants required to submit FAFSA. *Faculty research:* Data synthesis/assessment to determine future status of plants; possible role of invasive Herpestes Javanicus in sustaining cattle fever tick; occupancy, distribution, and abundance of black rails along Texas Gulf Coast, population genetic structure of ixodes scapularis and disease transmission, instream flow studies for Guadalupe, San Antonio, Mission and Aransas Rivers. *Total annual research expenditures:* $300,139. *Unit head:* Dr. Michael Clay Green, PhD Advisor, 512-245-8037, Fax: 512-245-8713, E-mail: mg54@txstate.edu. *Application contact:* Dr. Andrea Golato, Dean of the Graduate School, 512-245-2581, Fax: 512-245-8365, E-mail: jw02@swt.edu.
Website: http://www.bio.txstate.edu/

University of Alaska Fairbanks, School of Fisheries and Ocean Sciences, Program in Marine Sciences and Limnology, Fairbanks, AK 99775-7220. Offers marine biology (MS, PhD); oceanography (MS, PhD). *Program availability:* Part-time. *Faculty:* 4 full-time (1 woman). *Students:* 31 full-time (20 women), 10 part-time (7 women); includes 6 minority (1 Asian, non-Hispanic/Latino; 4 Hispanic/Latino; 1 Two or more races, non-Hispanic/Latino), 8 international. Average age 31. 26 applicants, 46% accepted, 12 enrolled. In 2015, 10 master's, 3 doctorates awarded. *Median time to degree:* Of those who began their doctoral program in fall 2007, 100% received their degree in 8 years or less. *Degree requirements:* For master's, comprehensive exam, oral defense of thesis; for doctorate, comprehensive exam, thesis/dissertation, oral defense of dissertation. *Entrance requirements:* For master's, GRE General Test, bachelor's degree from accredited institution with minimum cumulative undergraduate and major GPA of 3.0; for doctorate, GRE General Test, minimum cumulative GPA of 3.0. Additional exam requirements/recommendations for international students: Required—TOEFL (minimum score 550 paper-based; 79 iBT), IELTS (minimum score 6.5). *Application deadline:* For fall admission, 5/1 for domestic students, 4/1 for international students; for spring admission, 9/15 for domestic students, 8/15 for international students. Applications are processed on a rolling basis. Application fee: $60. Electronic applications accepted. *Expenses:* Tuition, state resident: full-time $7614; part-time $423 per credit. Tuition, nonresident: full-time $15,552; part-time $864 per credit. *Required fees:* $38 per credit. $187 per semester. Tuition and fees vary according to course level, course load, program and reciprocity agreements. *Financial support:* In 2015–16, 29 research assistantships with full tuition reimbursements (averaging $14,427 per year), 5 teaching assistantships with full tuition reimbursements (averaging $7,083 per year) were awarded; fellowships with full tuition reimbursements, career-related internships or fieldwork, Federal Work-Study, scholarships/grants, health care benefits, and unspecified assistantships also available. Support available to part-time students. Financial award application deadline: 7/1; financial award applicants required to submit FAFSA. *Total annual research expenditures:* $24.1 million. *Unit head:* Katrin Iken, Co-Chair, 907-474-7289, Fax: 907-474-5863, E-mail: info@sfos.uaf.edu. *Application contact:* Mary Kreta, Director of Admissions, 907-474-7500, Fax: 907-474-7097, E-mail: admissions@alaska.edu.
Website: http://www.uaf.edu/sfos/academics/graduate/

University of California, San Diego, Graduate Division, Scripps Institution of Oceanography, La Jolla, CA 92093. Offers climate science and policy (MAS); earth sciences (MS, PhD); geophysics (PhD); marine biodiversity and conservation (MAS); marine biology (MS, PhD); oceanography (MS, PhD). PhD in geophysics is offered jointly with San Diego State University. *Students:* 262 full-time (137 women), 11 part-time (1 woman); includes 51 minority (11 Black or African American, non-Hispanic/Latino; 3 American Indian or Alaska Native, non-Hispanic/Latino; 21 Asian, non-Hispanic/Latino; 16 Hispanic/Latino), 56 international. 332 applicants, 24% accepted, 47 enrolled. In 2015, 38 master's, 28 doctorates awarded. Terminal master's awarded for partial completion of doctoral program. *Degree requirements:* For master's, comprehensive exam (for some programs), thesis (for some programs); for doctorate, comprehensive exam, thesis/dissertation. *Entrance requirements:* For master's and doctorate, GRE General Test, GRE Subject Test (encouraged for ocean biosciences applicants), minimum GPA of 3.0. Additional exam requirements/recommendations for international students: Required—TOEFL (minimum score 550 paper-based; 80 iBT), IELTS (minimum score 7). *Application deadline:* For fall admission, 12/10 for domestic students. Application fee: $90 ($110 for international students). Electronic applications accepted. *Expenses:* Tuition, state resident: full-time $11,220. Tuition, nonresident: full-time $26,322. *Required fees:* $1800. *Financial support:* Fellowships, research assistantships, teaching assistantships, scholarships/grants, traineeships, and unspecified assistantships available. Financial award applicants required to submit FAFSA. *Faculty research:* Biodiversity and conservation, earth and planetary chemistry, alternative energy, global environmental monitoring, air-sea boundary, tectonic margins and the interactions between systems and environments. *Unit head:* Brian Palenik, Chair, 858-534-7505, E-mail: bpalenik@ucsd.edu. *Application contact:* Gilbert Bretado, Graduate Coordinator, 858-534-1694, E-mail: siodept@sio.ucsd.edu.
Website: https://scripps.ucsd.edu/education

University of California, Santa Barbara, Graduate Division, College of Letters and Sciences, Division of Mathematics, Life, and Physical Sciences, Department of Ecology, Evolution, and Marine Biology, Santa Barbara, CA 93106-9620. Offers MA, PhD, MA/PhD. *Faculty:* 33 full-time (8 women). *Students:* 69 full-time (44 women); includes 15 minority (2 Black or African American, non-Hispanic/Latino; 5 Asian, non-Hispanic/Latino; 6 Hispanic/Latino; 2 Native Hawaiian or other Pacific Islander, non-Hispanic/Latino), 3 international. Average age 29. 157 applicants, 14% accepted, 17 enrolled. In 2015, 7 master's, 8 doctorates awarded. *Degree requirements:* For master's, comprehensive exam (for some programs), thesis (for some programs); for doctorate, comprehensive exam, thesis/dissertation. *Entrance requirements:* For master's and doctorate, GRE General Test. Additional exam requirements/recommendations for international students: Required—TOEFL (minimum score 550 paper-based; 80 iBT), IELTS. *Application deadline:* For fall admission, 12/15 for domestic and international students. Application fee: $90 ($110 for international students). Electronic applications accepted. *Financial support:* In 2015–16, 50 students received support, including 55 fellowships with tuition reimbursements available (averaging $10,812 per year), 24 research assistantships with tuition reimbursements available (averaging $8,441 per year), 97 teaching assistantships with partial tuition reimbursements available (averaging $9,346 per year); Federal Work-Study, scholarships/grants, traineeships, health care benefits, and tuition waivers (full and partial) also available. Financial award application deadline: 12/15; financial award applicants required to submit FAFSA. *Faculty research:* Community ecology, evolution, marine biology, population genetics, stream ecology. *Unit head:* Dr. Craig Carlson, Chair, 805-893-2415, Fax: 805-893-5885, E-mail: eembchair@lifesci.ucsb.edu. *Application contact:* Melanie Fujii, Student Affairs

Officer, 805-893-2979, Fax: 805-893-5885, E-mail: eemb-info@lifesci.ucsb.edu.
Website: http://www.lifesci.ucsb.edu/EEMB/index.html

University of Colorado Boulder, Graduate School, College of Arts and Sciences, Department of Ecology and Evolutionary Biology, Boulder, CO 80309. Offers animal behavior (MA); biology (MA, PhD); environmental biology (MA, PhD); evolutionary biology (MA, PhD); neurobiology (MA); population biology (MA); population genetics (PhD). *Faculty:* 31 full-time (12 women). *Students:* 67 full-time (31 women), 3 part-time (1 woman); includes 6 minority (1 Asian, non-Hispanic/Latino; 3 Hispanic/Latino; 4 Two or more races, non-Hispanic/Latino), 4 international. Average age 30. 119 applicants, 11% accepted, 13 enrolled. In 2015, 10 master's, 14 doctorates awarded. Terminal master's awarded for partial completion of doctoral program. *Degree requirements:* For master's, comprehensive exam, thesis or alternative; for doctorate, comprehensive exam, thesis/dissertation. *Entrance requirements:* For master's, GRE General Test, GRE Subject Test, minimum undergraduate GPA of 3.0; for doctorate, GRE General Test, GRE Subject Test. *Application deadline:* For fall admission, 12/31 for domestic students, 12/1 for international students. Application fee: $50 ($70 for international students). Electronic applications accepted. Application fee is waived when completed online. *Financial support:* In 2015–16, 138 students received support, including 14 fellowships (averaging $7,260 per year), 12 research assistantships with tuition reimbursements available (averaging $31,833 per year), 47 teaching assistantships with tuition reimbursements available (averaging $33,448 per year); institutionally sponsored loans, scholarships/grants, health care benefits, and unspecified assistantships also available. Financial award applicants required to submit FAFSA. *Faculty research:* Ecology, botany, evolutionary biology, biological sciences, conservation biology. *Total annual research expenditures:* $6.3 million. *Application contact:* E-mail: ebiograd@colorado.edu.
Website: http://ebio.colorado.edu

University of Guam, Office of Graduate Studies, College of Natural and Applied Sciences, Program in Biology, Mangilao, GU 96923. Offers tropical marine biology (MS). *Degree requirements:* For master's, comprehensive exam, thesis. *Entrance requirements:* For master's, GRE General Test, GRE Subject Test. Additional exam requirements/recommendations for international students: Required—TOEFL. *Faculty research:* Maintenance and ecology of coral reefs.

University of Hawaii at Hilo, Program in Tropical Conservation Biology and Environmental Science, Hilo, HI 96720-4091. Offers MS. *Entrance requirements:* Additional exam requirements/recommendations for international students: Required—TOEFL, IELTS. Electronic applications accepted.

University of Hawaii at Manoa, Graduate Division, School of Ocean and Earth Science and Technology, Program in Marine Biology, Honolulu, HI 96822. Offers MS, PhD. Offered in conjunction with the College of Natural Sciences. *Students:* 57 full-time (37 women), 6 part-time (3 women); includes 17 minority (6 Asian, non-Hispanic/Latino; 1 Hispanic/Latino; 10 Two or more races, non-Hispanic/Latino), 5 international. 82 applicants, 21% accepted, 12 enrolled. *Degree requirements:* For master's, thesis, research project; for doctorate, thesis/dissertation, research project. *Entrance requirements:* For master's and doctorate, GRE. Additional exam requirements/recommendations for international students: Required—TOEFL. Application fee: $100. *Expenses:* Contact institution. *Financial support:* Research assistantships, teaching assistantships, tuition waivers, and unspecified assistantships available. *Faculty research:* Ecology, ichthyology, behavior of marine animals, developmental biology. *Unit head:* Brian Taylor, Dean, 808-956-6182, E-mail: taylorb@hawaii.edu. *Application contact:* Graduate Division, 808-956-8544.
Website: http://www.hawaii.edu/marine_biology/

University of Maine, Graduate School, College of Natural Sciences, Forestry, and Agriculture, School of Marine Sciences, Orono, ME 04469. Offers marine bio-resources (MS, PhD); marine biology (MS, PhD); marine policy (MS); oceanography (MS, PhD). *Program availability:* Part-time. *Faculty:* 26 full-time (9 women), 11 part-time/adjunct (0 women). *Students:* 57 full-time (38 women); includes 2 minority (1 American Indian or Alaska Native, non-Hispanic/Latino; 1 Asian, non-Hispanic/Latino), 8 international. Average age 28. 95 applicants, 19% accepted, 16 enrolled. In 2015, 9 master's, 5 doctorates awarded. *Degree requirements:* For master's, thesis; for doctorate, comprehensive exam, thesis/dissertation. *Entrance requirements:* For master's and doctorate, GRE General Test. Additional exam requirements/recommendations for international students: Required—TOEFL (minimum score 550 paper-based; 79 iBT). *Application deadline:* Applications are processed on a rolling basis. Application fee: $65. Electronic applications accepted. *Financial support:* In 2015–16, 54 students received support, including 2 fellowships (averaging $22,400 per year), 41 research assistantships with tuition reimbursements available (averaging $14,600 per year), 10 teaching assistantships with tuition reimbursements available (averaging $14,600 per year); career-related internships or fieldwork, Federal Work-Study, and tuition waivers (full and partial) also available. Support available to part-time students. Financial award application deadline: 3/1. *Faculty research:* Oceanography, marine biology, marine policy, aquaculture and fisheries. *Total annual research expenditures:* $12 million. *Unit head:* Dr. Fei Chai, Director, 207-581-3321, Fax: 207-581-4388. *Application contact:* Scott L. Delcourt, Assistant Vice President for Graduate Studies and Senior Associate Dean, 207-581-3291, Fax: 207-581-3232, E-mail: graduate@maine.edu.
Website: http://www.umaine.edu/marine/

University of Massachusetts Dartmouth, Graduate School, College of Arts and Sciences, Department of Biology, North Dartmouth, MA 02747-2300. Offers biology (MS); marine biology (MS). *Program availability:* Part-time. *Faculty:* 19 full-time (8 women), 2 part-time/adjunct (both women). *Students:* 11 full-time (8 women), 9 part-time (6 women); includes 2 minority (1 Hispanic/Latino; 1 Two or more races, non-Hispanic/Latino). Average age 26. 20 applicants, 65% accepted, 6 enrolled. In 2015, 5 master's awarded. *Degree requirements:* For master's, thesis. *Entrance requirements:* For master's, GRE, statement of purpose (minimum of 300 words), resume, official transcripts, 3 letters of recommendation. Additional exam requirements/recommendations for international students: Required—TOEFL (minimum score 533 paper-based; 72 iBT). *Application deadline:* For fall admission, 2/15 priority date for domestic students, 1/15 priority date for international students. Applications are processed on a rolling basis. Application fee: $60. Electronic applications accepted. *Expenses:* Tuition, state resident: full-time $2071; part-time $86.29 per credit. Tuition, nonresident: full-time $8099; part-time $337.46 per credit. *Required fees:* $18,074; $762.08 per credit. Tuition and fees vary according to course load and reciprocity agreements. *Financial support:* In 2015–16, 1 research assistantship (averaging $16,000 per year), 8 teaching assistantships (averaging $16,000 per year) were awarded; career-related internships or fieldwork and unspecified assistantships also available. Support available to part-time students. Financial award application deadline: 3/1; financial award applicants required to submit FAFSA. *Faculty research:* Shark biology, marine mammal biology, domestication of fish, cell body, fish biology. *Total annual research expenditures:* $1.9 million. *Unit head:* Whitney Hable, Graduate Program Director, 508-999-8206, E-mail: whable@umassd.edu. *Application contact:* Steven Briggs, Director of Recruitment and Marketing for Graduate Studies, 508-999-8604, Fax: 508-999-8183, E-mail: graduate@umassd.edu.
Website: http://www.umassd.edu/cas/biology/

Marine Biology

University of Miami, Graduate School, Rosenstiel School of Marine and Atmospheric Science, Division of Marine Biology and Fisheries, Coral Gables, FL 33124. Offers MA, MS, PhD. Terminal master's awarded for partial completion of doctoral program. *Degree requirements:* For master's, comprehensive exam, thesis; for doctorate, comprehensive exam, thesis/dissertation. *Entrance requirements:* For master's and doctorate, GRE General Test. Additional exam requirements/recommendations for international students: Required—TOEFL (minimum score 550 paper-based). Electronic applications accepted. *Faculty research:* Biochemistry, physiology, plankton, coral, biology.

University of New Hampshire, Graduate School, School of Marine Science and Ocean Engineering, Durham, NH 03824. Offers marine biology (MS, PhD); ocean engineering (MS, PhD); ocean mapping (MS, Postbaccalaureate Certificate); oceanography (MS, PhD). *Degree requirements:* For master's, thesis. *Entrance requirements:* Additional exam requirements/recommendations for international students: Required—TOEFL (minimum score 550 paper-based; 80 iBT). *Application deadline:* For fall admission, 4/1 priority date for domestic students; for spring admission, 12/1 for domestic students. Applications are processed on a rolling basis. Electronic applications accepted. *Expenses:* Tuition, state resident: full-time $13,840; part-time $770 per credit hour. Tuition, nonresident: full-time $27,130; part-time $1175 per credit hour. *Required fees:* $2080; $1040. Tuition and fees vary according to degree level and program. *Financial support:* Fellowships, research assistantships, teaching assistantships, Federal Work-Study, scholarships/grants, and tuition waivers (full and partial) available. Support available to part-time students. Financial award application deadline: 2/15. *Unit head:* Dr. Kenneth Baldwin, Chairperson, 603-862-1898. *Application contact:* Abby Pagan-Allis, Administrative Assistant, 603-862-3433, E-mail: ocean.engineering@unh.edu.
Website: http://www.marine.unh.edu/oe

The University of North Carolina Wilmington, College of Arts and Sciences, Department of Biology and Marine Biology, Wilmington, NC 28403-3297. Offers biology (MS); marine biology (MS, PhD). *Program availability:* Part-time. *Faculty:* 38 full-time (11 women). *Students:* 2 full-time (1 woman), 65 part-time (36 women); includes 10 minority (1 Black or African American, non-Hispanic/Latino; 2 Asian, non-Hispanic/Latino; 6 Hispanic/Latino; 1 Two or more races, non-Hispanic/Latino), 4 international. Average age 31. 89 applicants, 17 enrolled. In 2015, 14 master's, 1 doctorate awarded. *Degree requirements:* For master's, comprehensive exam, thesis; for doctorate, comprehensive exam, thesis/dissertation. *Entrance requirements:* For master's, GRE General Test, minimum B average in undergraduate work, 3 recommendations, resume, statement of interest, bachelor's degree in field of biology; for doctorate, GRE General Test, minimum B average in undergraduate and graduate work, resume, summary of MS thesis research, master's degree, statement of interest. Additional exam requirements/recommendations for international students: Required—TOEFL (minimum score 79 iBT), IELTS (minimum score 6.5). *Application deadline:* For fall admission, 6/15 for domestic students; for spring admission, 11/30 for domestic students. Applications are processed on a rolling basis. Application fee: $60. Electronic applications accepted. *Expenses:* $8,854 in-state full-time per year; $20,945 out-of-state full-time per year. *Financial support:* Research assistantships with tuition reimbursements, teaching assistantships with tuition reimbursements, and scholarships/grants available. Support available to part-time students. Financial award application deadline: 3/15; financial award applicants required to submit FAFSA. *Faculty research:* Ecology, physiology, cell and molecular biology, systematics, biomechanics. *Unit head:* Dr. Chris Finelli, Chair, 910-962-3487, E-mail: finellic@uncw.edu. *Application contact:* Dr. Stephen Kinsey, Graduate Coordinator, 910-962-7398, Fax: 910-962-4066, E-mail: kinseys@uncw.edu. Website: http://www.uncw.edu/bio/graduate.html

University of Oregon, Graduate School, College of Arts and Sciences, Department of Biology, Eugene, OR 97403. Offers ecology and evolution (MA, MS, PhD); marine biology (MA, MS, PhD); molecular, cellular and genetic biology (PhD); neuroscience and development (PhD). Terminal master's awarded for partial completion of doctoral program. *Degree requirements:* For master's, thesis (for some programs); for doctorate,

thesis/dissertation. *Entrance requirements:* For master's and doctorate, GRE General Test, minimum GPA of 3.2. Additional exam requirements/recommendations for international students: Required—TOEFL. *Faculty research:* Developmental neurobiology; evolution, population biology, and quantitative genetics; regulation of gene expression; biochemistry of marine organisms.

University of Southern California, Graduate School, Dana and David Dornsife College of Letters, Arts and Sciences, Department of Biological Sciences, Program in Marine Biology and Biological Oceanography, Los Angeles, CA 90089. Offers marine and environmental biology (MS); marine biology and biological oceanography (PhD). Terminal master's awarded for partial completion of doctoral program. *Degree requirements:* For master's, research paper; for doctorate, comprehensive exam, thesis/dissertation, qualifying examination, dissertation defense. *Entrance requirements:* For master's and doctorate, GRE, 3 letters of recommendation, personal statement, resume, minimum GPA of 3.0. Additional exam requirements/recommendations for international students: Required—TOEFL (minimum score 600 paper-based; 100 iBT). Electronic applications accepted. *Faculty research:* Microbial ecology, biogeochemistry, and geobiology; biodiversity and molecular ecology; integrative organismal biology; conservation biology; marine genomics.

University of Southern Mississippi, Graduate School, College of Science and Technology, Department of Biological Sciences, Hattiesburg, MS 39406-0001. Offers environmental biology (MS); marine biology (MS); microbiology (MS, PhD); molecular biology (MS, PhD). Terminal master's awarded for partial completion of doctoral program. *Degree requirements:* For master's, comprehensive exam, thesis; for doctorate, comprehensive exam, thesis/dissertation. *Entrance requirements:* For master's, GRE General Test, minimum GPA of 3.0 on last 60 hours; for doctorate, GRE General Test, minimum GPA of 3.5. Additional exam requirements/recommendations for international students: Required—TOEFL, IELTS.

Western Illinois University, School of Graduate Studies, College of Arts and Sciences, Department of Biological Sciences, Macomb, IL 61455-1390. Offers biological sciences (MS); environmental geographic information systems (Certificate); zoo and aquarium studies (Certificate). *Program availability:* Part-time. *Students:* 57 full-time (40 women), 32 part-time (23 women); includes 5 minority (2 Black or African American, non-Hispanic/Latino; 1 Hispanic/Latino; 2 Two or more races, non-Hispanic/Latino), 25 international. Average age 28. 56 applicants, 84% accepted, 30 enrolled. In 2015, 15 master's, 11 other advanced degrees awarded. *Degree requirements:* For master's, thesis or alternative. *Entrance requirements:* Additional exam requirements/recommendations for international students: Required—TOEFL (minimum score 550 paper-based; 80 iBT); Recommended—IELTS. *Application deadline:* Applications are processed on a rolling basis. Application fee: $30. Electronic applications accepted. *Financial support:* In 2015–16, 15 research assistantships with full tuition reimbursements (averaging $7,544 per year), 15 teaching assistantships with full tuition reimbursements (averaging $8,688 per year) were awarded; unspecified assistantships also available. Financial award applicants required to submit FAFSA. *Unit head:* Dr. Charles Lydeard, Chairperson, 309-298-1546. *Application contact:* Dr. Nancy Parsons, Associate Provost and Director of Graduate Studies, 309-298-1806, Fax: 309-298-2345, E-mail: grad-office@wiu.edu.
Website: http://wiu.edu/biology

Woods Hole Oceanographic Institution, MIT/WHOI Joint Program in Oceanography/Applied Ocean Science and Engineering, Woods Hole, MA 02543-1541. Offers applied ocean science and engineering (PhD); biological oceanography (PhD); chemical oceanography (PhD); marine geology and geophysics (PhD); physical oceanography (PhD). Program offered jointly with Massachusetts Institute of Technology. *Degree requirements:* For doctorate, thesis/dissertation. *Entrance requirements:* For doctorate, GRE General Test, GRE Subject Test. Additional exam requirements/recommendations for international students: Required—TOEFL. Electronic applications accepted.

Section 12
Microbiological Sciences

This section contains a directory of institutions offering graduate work in microbiological sciences, followed by in-depth entries submitted by institutions that chose to prepare detailed program descriptions. Additional information about programs listed in the directory but not augmented by an in-depth entry may be obtained by writing directly to the dean of a graduate school or chair of a department at the address given in the directory.

For programs offering related work, see also in this book *Allied Health; Biochemistry; Biological and Biomedical Sciences; Botany and Plant Biology; Cell, Molecular, and Structural Biology; Dentistry and Dental Sciences; Ecology, Environmental Biology, and Evolutionary Biology; Entomology; Genetics, Developmental Biology, and Reproductive Biology; Parasitology; Pathology and Pathobiology; Pharmacy and Pharmaceutical Sciences; Public Health; Physiology; Veterinary Medicine and Sciences;* and *Zoology.* In the other guides in this series:

Graduate Programs in the Physical Sciences, Mathematics, Agricultural Sciences, the Environment & Natural Resources

See *Agricultural and Food Sciences* and *Chemistry*

Graduate Programs in Engineering & Applied Sciences

See *Agricultural Engineering and Bioengineering* and *Biomedical Engineering and Biotechnology*

CONTENTS

Program Directories

Displays and Close-Ups

See also:

Bacteriology

Illinois State University, Graduate School, College of Arts and Sciences, Department of Biological Sciences, Normal, IL 61790-2200. Offers animal behavior (MS); bacteriology (MS); biochemistry (MS); biological sciences (MS); biology (PhD); biophysics (MS); biotechnology (MS); botany (MS, PhD); cell biology (MS); conservation biology (MS); developmental biology (MS); ecology (MS, PhD); entomology (MS); evolutionary biology (MS); genetics (MS, PhD); immunology (MS); microbiology (MS, PhD); molecular biology (MS); molecular genetics (MS); neurobiology (MS); neuroscience (MS); parasitology (MS); physiology (MS, PhD); plant biology (MS); plant molecular biology (MS); plant sciences (MS); structural biology (MS); zoology (MS, PhD). *Program availability:* Part-time. *Degree requirements:* For master's, thesis or alternative; for doctorate, variable foreign language requirement, thesis/dissertation, 2 terms of residency. *Entrance requirements:* For master's, GRE General Test, minimum GPA of 2.6 in last 60 hours of course work; for doctorate, GRE General Test. *Application deadline:* Applications are processed on a rolling basis. Application fee: $40. *Financial support:* Research assistantships, teaching assistantships, Federal Work-Study, tuition waivers (full), and unspecified assistantships available. Financial award application deadline: 4/1. *Faculty research:* Redoc balance and drug development in schistosoma mansoni, control of the growth of listeria monocytogenes at low temperature, regulation of cell expansion and microtubule function by SPRI, CRUI: physiology and fitness consequences of different life history phenotypes. *Application contact:* Steven Juliano, Graduate Coordinator, E-mail: sajulian@ilstu.edu. Website: http://www.bio.ilstu.edu/

The University of Iowa, Roy J. and Lucille A. Carver College of Medicine and Graduate College, Graduate Programs in Medicine, Department of Microbiology, Iowa City, IA 52242-1316. Offers general microbiology and microbial physiology (MS, PhD); immunology (MS, PhD); microbial genetics (MS, PhD); pathogenic bacteriology (MS, PhD); virology (MS, PhD). *Degree requirements:* For master's, thesis; for doctorate, comprehensive exam, thesis/dissertation. *Entrance requirements:* For master's and doctorate, GRE General Test. Additional exam requirements/recommendations for international students: Required—TOEFL (minimum score 600 paper-based). Electronic applications accepted. *Faculty research:* Gene regulation, processing and transport of HIV, retroviral pathogenesis, biodegradation, biofilm.

University of Prince Edward Island, Atlantic Veterinary College, Graduate Program in Veterinary Medicine, Charlottetown, PE C1A 4P3, Canada. Offers anatomy (M Sc, PhD); bacteriology (M Sc, PhD); clinical pharmacology (M Sc, PhD); clinical sciences (M Sc, PhD); epidemiology (M Sc, PhD), including reproduction; fish health (M Sc, PhD); food animal nutrition (M Sc, PhD); immunology (M Sc, PhD); microanatomy (M Sc, PhD); parasitology (M Sc, PhD); pathology (M Sc, PhD); pharmacology (M Sc, PhD); physiology (M Sc, PhD); toxicology (M Sc, PhD); veterinary science (M Vet Sc); virology (M Sc, PhD). *Program availability:* Part-time. *Degree requirements:* For master's, thesis; for doctorate, thesis/dissertation. *Entrance requirements:* For master's, DVM, B Sc honors degree, or equivalent; for doctorate, M Sc. Additional exam requirements/recommendations for international students: Required—TOEFL (minimum score 550 paper-based; 80 iBT). *Expenses:* Contact institution. *Faculty research:* Animal health management, infectious diseases, fin fish and shellfish health, basic biomedical sciences, ecosystem health.

The University of Texas Medical Branch, Graduate School of Biomedical Sciences, Program in Emerging and Tropical Infectious Diseases, Galveston, TX 77555. Offers PhD, MD/PhD. *Degree requirements:* For doctorate, thesis/dissertation. *Entrance requirements:* For doctorate, GRE General Test. *Faculty research:* Emerging diseases, tropical diseases, parasitology, vitology and bacteriology.

University of Washington, Graduate School, School of Public Health, Department of Global Health, Graduate Program in Pathobiology, Seattle, WA 98195. Offers PhD. *Degree requirements:* For doctorate, comprehensive exam, thesis/dissertation, published paper from thesis work. *Entrance requirements:* For doctorate, GRE General Test, minimum GPA of 3.0. Additional exam requirements/recommendations for international students: Required—TOEFL, IELTS. Electronic applications accepted. *Expenses:* Contact institution. *Faculty research:* Malaria, immunological response to mycobacteria infections, HIV-cell interaction and the development of an anti-HIV vaccine, regulation of intercellular communication via gap junctions, genetic and nutritional regulation of proteins involved in lipid transport.

University of Wisconsin–Madison, Graduate School, College of Agricultural and Life Sciences, Department of Bacteriology, Madison, WI 53706-1380. Offers MS. *Program availability:* Part-time. *Entrance requirements:* Additional exam requirements/recommendations for international students: Required—TOEFL. Electronic applications accepted. *Expenses:* Tuition, state resident: full-time $5364. Tuition, nonresident: full-time $12,027. *Required fees:* $571. Tuition and fees vary according to campus/location, program and reciprocity agreements. *Faculty research:* Microbial physiology, gene regulation, microbial ecology, plant-microbe interactions, symbiosis.

Immunology

Albany Medical College, Center for Immunology and Microbial Disease, Albany, NY 12208-3479. Offers MS, PhD. *Program availability:* Part-time. Terminal master's awarded for partial completion of doctoral program. *Degree requirements:* For master's, thesis; for doctorate, comprehensive exam, thesis/dissertation, oral qualifying exam, written preliminary exam, 1 published paper-peer review. *Entrance requirements:* For master's, GRE General Test, all transcripts, letters of recommendation; for doctorate, GRE General Test, letters of recommendation. Additional exam requirements/recommendations for international students: Required—TOEFL. *Faculty research:* Microbial and viral pathogenesis, cancer development and cell transformation, biochemical and genetic mechanisms responsible for human disease.

Albert Einstein College of Medicine, Graduate Division of Biomedical Sciences, Department of Microbiology and Immunology, Bronx, NY 10461. Offers PhD, MD/PhD. *Degree requirements:* For doctorate, thesis/dissertation. *Entrance requirements:* For doctorate, GRE General Test. Additional exam requirements/recommendations for international students: Required—TOEFL. *Faculty research:* Nature of histocompatibility antigens, lymphoid cell receptors, regulation of immune responses and mechanisms of resistance to infection.

American University of Beirut, Graduate Programs, Faculty of Medicine, Beirut, Lebanon. Offers anatomy, cell biology and human morphology (MS); biochemistry and medical genetics (MS); biomedical sciences (PhD); experimental pathology, immunology and microbiology (MS); medicine (MD); neuroscience (MS); pharmacology and toxicology (MS). *Program availability:* Part-time. *Faculty:* 302 full-time (95 women), 64 part-time/adjunct (11 women). *Students:* 381 full-time (173 women), 61 part-time (51 women). Average age 23. In 2015, 14 master's awarded. *Degree requirements:* For master's, one foreign language, comprehensive exam, thesis (for some programs); for doctorate, one foreign language, comprehensive exam, thesis/dissertation. *Entrance requirements:* For master's, letter of recommendation; for doctorate, MCAT, bachelor's degree. Additional exam requirements/recommendations for international students: Required—TOEFL (minimum score 600 paper-based; 100 iBT), IELTS (minimum score 7.5). *Application deadline:* For fall admission, 4/30 for domestic and international students; for spring admission, 11/1 for domestic and international students. Application fee: $50. Electronic applications accepted. *Expenses: Tuition, area resident:* Full-time $16,254; part-time $903 per credit. *Required fees:* $699. Tuition and fees vary according to course load and program. *Financial support:* In 2015–16, 273 students received support, including 45 teaching assistantships (averaging $9,000 per year); career-related internships or fieldwork, institutionally sponsored loans, scholarships/grants, health care benefits, and unspecified assistantships also available. Financial award application deadline: 2/2. *Faculty research:* Cancer research (targeted therapy, mechanisms of leukemogenesis, tumor cell extravasation and metastasis, cancer stem cells), stem cell research (regenerative medicine, drug discovery), genetic research (neurogenetics, hereditary cardiomyopathy, hemoglobinopathies, pharmacogenomics, proteomics), neuroscience research (pain, nourodegenerative disorder), metabolism (inflammation and metabolism, metabolic disorder, diabetes mellitus), vascular and renal biology, signal transduction. *Total annual research expenditures:* $2.6 million. *Unit head:* Dr. Mohamed Sayegh, Dean, 961-1350000 Ext. 4700, Fax: 961-1744464, E-mail: msayegh@aub.edu.lb. *Application contact:* Dr. Salim Kanaan, Director, Admissions Office, 961-1350000 Ext. 2594, Fax: 961-1750775, E-mail: sk00@aub.edu.lb. Website: http://www.aub.edu.lb/fm/fm_home/Pages/index.aspx

Baylor College of Medicine, Graduate School of Biomedical Sciences, Department of Immunology, Houston, TX 77030-3498. Offers PhD, MD/PhD. *Degree requirements:* For doctorate, thesis/dissertation, public defense. *Entrance requirements:* For doctorate, GRE General Test, GRE Subject Test (strongly recommended), minimum GPA of 3.0. Additional exam requirements/recommendations for international students: Required—TOEFL. Electronic applications accepted. *Faculty research:* MHC expression, inflammation and allergy, germinal center biology, HIV pathogenesis, immune responses to gene therapy.

Baylor College of Medicine, Graduate School of Biomedical Sciences, Interdepartmental Program in Cell and Molecular Biology, Houston, TX 77030-3498. Offers biochemistry (PhD); cell and molecular biology (PhD); genetics (PhD); human genetics (PhD); immunology (PhD); microbiology (PhD); virology (PhD); MD/PhD. *Degree requirements:* For doctorate, thesis/dissertation, public defense. *Entrance requirements:* For doctorate, GRE General Test, GRE Subject Test (strongly recommended), minimum GPA of 3.0. Additional exam requirements/recommendations for international students: Required—TOEFL. Electronic applications accepted. *Faculty research:* Molecular and cellular biology; cancer, aging and stem cells; genomics and proteomics; microbiome, molecular microbiology; infectious disease, immunology and translational research.

Boston University, School of Medicine, Division of Graduate Medical Sciences, Immunology Training Program, Boston, MA 02215. Offers PhD, MD/PhD. *Degree requirements:* For doctorate, thesis/dissertation. *Application deadline:* For fall admission, 1/15 for domestic students; for spring admission, 10/15 for domestic students. *Unit head:* Dr. David Sherr, Director, 617-638-6464, Fax: 617-638-5254. *Application contact:* GMS Admissions Office, 617-638-5255, E-mail: askgms@bu.edu. Website: http://www.bumc.bu.edu/immunology/

California Institute of Technology, Division of Biology, Program in Immunology, Pasadena, CA 91125-0001. Offers PhD. *Degree requirements:* For doctorate, thesis/dissertation, qualifying exam. *Entrance requirements:* For doctorate, GRE General Test.

Case Western Reserve University, School of Medicine and School of Graduate Studies, Graduate Programs in Medicine, Programs in Molecular and Cellular Basis of Disease/Pathology, Immunology Training Program, Cleveland, OH 44106. Offers MS, PhD, MD/PhD. *Degree requirements:* For doctorate, comprehensive exam, thesis/dissertation. *Entrance requirements:* For doctorate, GRE General Test, GRE Subject Test. Additional exam requirements/recommendations for international students: Required—TOEFL (minimum score 550 paper-based). Electronic applications accepted. *Expenses: Tuition, area resident:* Full-time $41,137; part-time $1714 per credit hour. *Required fees:* $32. Tuition and fees vary according to course load and program. *Faculty research:* Immunology, immunopathology, immunochemistry, infectious diseases.

Colorado State University, College of Veterinary Medicine and Biomedical Sciences, Department of Microbiology, Immunology and Pathology, Fort Collins, CO 80523. Offers microbiology (MS, PhD); pathology (PhD). *Faculty:* 75 full-time (35 women), 10 part-time/adjunct (6 women). *Students:* 81 full-time (60 women), 28 part-time (18 women); includes 21 minority (2 American Indian or Alaska Native, non-Hispanic/Latino; 3 Asian, non-Hispanic/Latino; 13 Hispanic/Latino; 3 Two or more races, non-Hispanic/Latino), 8 international. Average age 29. 133 applicants, 38% accepted, 47 enrolled. In 2015, 47 master's, 7 doctorates awarded. *Degree requirements:* For master's, comprehensive exam, thesis; for doctorate, comprehensive exam, thesis/dissertation. *Entrance requirements:* For master's, GRE General Test, minimum GPA of 3.0, BA/BS in biomedical field, resume, transcripts, personal statement, 3 letters of recommendation; for doctorate, GRE General Test, minimum GPA of 3.0, BA/BS in biomedical field, resume, personal statement, transcripts, 3 letters of recommendation. Additional exam requirements/recommendations for international students: Required—TOEFL (minimum score 550 paper-based; 80 iBT); Recommended—IELTS (minimum score 6.5), TWE,

TSE. *Application deadline:* For fall admission, 12/15 priority date for domestic and international students. Application fee: $60 ($70 for international students). Electronic applications accepted. *Expenses:* Contact institution. *Financial support:* In 2015–16, 82 students received support, including 33 fellowships with full tuition reimbursements available (averaging $39,971 per year), 29 research assistantships with full tuition reimbursements available (averaging $21,981 per year), 2 teaching assistantships with full tuition reimbursements available (averaging $17,190 per year); scholarships/grants, traineeships, and unspecified assistantships also available. Financial award applicants required to submit FAFSA. *Faculty research:* Prions, tuberculosis, vector-borne diseases, rna biology, host-pathogen interactions. *Total annual research expenditures:* $21.5 million. *Unit head:* Dr. Gregg A. Dean, Department Head, 970-491-6144, E-mail: gregg.dean@colostate.edu. *Application contact:* Heidi Runge, Academic Support Coordinator for Graduate Studies, 970-491-1630, Fax: 970-491-0603, E-mail: heidi.runge@colostate.edu.
Website: http://csu-cvmbs.colostate.edu/academics/mip/graduate/Pages/microbiology-immunology-professional-masters.aspx

Cornell University, Graduate School, Graduate Fields of Comparative Biomedical Sciences, Field of Immunology, Ithaca, NY 14853-0001. Offers cellular immunology (MS, PhD); immunochemistry (MS, PhD); immunogenetics (MS, PhD); immunopathology (MS, PhD); infection and immunity (MS, PhD). Terminal master's awarded for partial completion of doctoral program. *Degree requirements:* For master's, thesis; for doctorate, comprehensive exam, thesis/dissertation. *Entrance requirements:* For master's and doctorate, GRE General Test, 2 letters of recommendation. Additional exam requirements/recommendations for international students: Required—TOEFL (minimum score 550 paper-based; 77 iBT). Electronic applications accepted. *Faculty research:* Avian immunology, mucosal immunity, anti-parasite and anti-viral immunity, neutrophil function, reproductive immunology.

Creighton University, School of Medicine and Graduate School, Graduate Programs in Medicine, Omaha, NE 68178-0001. Offers biomedical sciences (MS, PhD); clinical anatomy (MS); medical microbiology and immunology (MS, PhD); pharmacology (MS, PhD), including pharmaceutical sciences (MS); pharmacology; MD/PhD; Pharm D/MS. Terminal master's awarded for partial completion of doctoral program. *Degree requirements:* For master's, thesis; for doctorate, thesis/dissertation. *Entrance requirements:* For master's and doctorate, GRE General Test. Additional exam requirements/recommendations for international students: Required—TOEFL (minimum score 550 paper-based; 80 iBT). Electronic applications accepted. *Expenses:* Contact institution. *Faculty research:* Molecular biology and gene transfection, infectious disease, antimicrobial agents and chemotherapy, virology, pharmacological secretion.

Dalhousie University, Faculty of Medicine, Department of Microbiology and Immunology, Halifax, NS B3H 4R2, Canada. Offers M Sc, PhD. *Degree requirements:* For master's, thesis; for doctorate, comprehensive exam, thesis/dissertation. *Entrance requirements:* For master's, GRE General Test, honors B Sc; for doctorate, GRE General Test, honors B Sc in microbiology, M Sc in discipline or transfer after 1 year in master's program. Additional exam requirements/recommendations for international students: Required—1 of 5 approved tests: TOEFL, IELTS, CANTEST, CAEL, Michigan English Language Assessment Battery. Electronic applications accepted. *Faculty research:* Virology, molecular genetics, pathogenesis, bacteriology, immunology.

Dartmouth College, Graduate Program in Molecular and Cellular Biology, Department of Microbiology and Immunology, Program in Immunology, Hanover, NH 03755. Offers PhD, MBA/PhD, MD/PhD. *Entrance requirements:* For doctorate, GRE, letters of recommendation. Additional exam requirements/recommendations for international students: Required—TOEFL (minimum score paper-based 550, iBT 100) or IELTS (7.0). *Application deadline:* For fall admission, 12/1 for domestic students. Application fee: $75. Electronic applications accepted. *Expenses: Tuition, area resident:* Full-time $48,120. *Required fees:* $296. One-time fee: $50 full-time. *Financial support:* In 2015–16, fellowships with full tuition reimbursements (averaging $28,200 per year) were awarded; health care benefits also available. *Faculty research:* Tumor immunotherapy, cell and molecular biology of connective tissue degradation in rheumatoid arthritis and cancer, immunology and immunotherapy of tumors of the central nervous system, transcriptional regulation of hematopoiesis and leukemia, bacterial pathogenesis. *Unit head:* Dr. William R. Green, Chair, 603-650-4919, Fax: 603-650-6223, E-mail: immunology@dartmouth.edu. *Application contact:* Marcia L. Ingalls, Administrative Assistant, 603-650-4919, Fax: 603-650-6223, E-mail: immunology@dartmouth.edu.
Website: https://geiselmed.dartmouth.edu/immuno/

Drexel University, College of Medicine, Biomedical Graduate Programs, Program in Microbiology and Immunology, Philadelphia, PA 19104-2875. Offers MS, PhD, MD/PhD. Terminal master's awarded for partial completion of doctoral program. *Degree requirements:* For master's, comprehensive exam, thesis; for doctorate, thesis/dissertation, qualifying exam. *Entrance requirements:* For master's, GRE General Test, minimum GPA of 2.75; for doctorate, GRE General Test, minimum GPA of 3.0. Additional exam requirements/recommendations for international students: Required—TOEFL. Electronic applications accepted. *Faculty research:* Immunology of malarial parasites, virology, bacteriology, molecular biology, parasitology.

Duke University, Graduate School, Department of Immunology, Durham, NC 27710. Offers PhD. *Degree requirements:* For doctorate, thesis/dissertation. *Entrance requirements:* For doctorate, GRE General Test, GRE Subject Test in biology or biochemistry, cell and molecular biology (strongly recommended). Additional exam requirements/recommendations for international students: Required—TOEFL (minimum score 577 paper-based; 90 iBT) or IELTS (minimum score 7). Electronic applications accepted.

East Carolina University, Brody School of Medicine, Department of Microbiology and Immunology, Greenville, NC 27858-4353. Offers MS, MD, PhD. *Students:* 15 full-time (8 women); includes 1 minority (Asian, non-Hispanic/Latino), 5 international. Average age 28. 19 applicants, 26% accepted, 5 enrolled. In 2015, 3 doctorates awarded. *Degree requirements:* For doctorate, comprehensive exam, thesis/dissertation. *Entrance requirements:* For doctorate, GRE General Test. Additional exam requirements/recommendations for international students: Required—TOEFL. *Application deadline:* For fall admission, 4/15 priority date for domestic students. Applications are processed on a rolling basis. Application fee: $50. *Financial support:* Fellowships with tuition reimbursements available. Financial award application deadline: 6/1. *Faculty research:* Molecular virology, genetics of bacteria, yeast and somatic cells, bacterial physiology and metabolism, bioterrorism. *Unit head:* Dr. Charles J. Smith, Chair, 252-744-2700, Fax: 252-744-3104, E-mail: smithcha@ecu.edu. *Application contact:* Jamaal Peele, Program Director, 252-744-2701, E-mail: peelej@ecu.edu.
Website: http://www.ecu.edu/cs-dhs/microbiology/guidelines.cfm

Emory University, Laney Graduate School, Division of Biological and Biomedical Sciences, Program in Immunology and Molecular Pathogenesis, Atlanta, GA 30322-1100. Offers PhD. *Degree requirements:* For doctorate, comprehensive exam, thesis/dissertation. *Entrance requirements:* For doctorate, GRE General Test, minimum GPA of 3.0 in science course work (recommended). Additional exam requirements/recommendations for international students: Required—TOEFL. Electronic applications

accepted. *Faculty research:* Transplantation immunology, autoimmunity, microbial pathogenesis.

Georgetown University, Graduate School of Arts and Sciences, Department of Microbiology and Immunology, Washington, DC 20057. Offers biohazardous threat agents and emerging infectious diseases (MS); biomedical science policy and advocacy (MS); general microbiology and immunology (MS); global infectious diseases (PhD); microbiology and immunology (PhD). *Program availability:* Part-time. *Degree requirements:* For master's, 30 credit hours of coursework; for doctorate, comprehensive exam, thesis/dissertation. *Entrance requirements:* For master's, GRE General Test, 3 letters of reference, bachelor's degree in related field; for doctorate, GRE General Test, 3 letters of reference, MS/BS in related field. Additional exam requirements/recommendations for international students: Required—TOEFL (minimum score 505 paper-based). Electronic applications accepted. *Faculty research:* Pathogenesis and basic biology of the fungus Candida albicans, molecular biology of viral immunopathological mechanisms in Multiple Sclerosis.

The George Washington University, Columbian College of Arts and Sciences, Institute for Biomedical Sciences, Program in Microbiology and Immunology, Washington, DC 20037. Offers PhD. *Faculty:* 13 full-time (2 women). *Students:* 2 full-time (1 woman), 15 part-time (10 women); includes 6 minority (1 Black or African American, non-Hispanic/Latino; 1 American Indian or Alaska Native, non-Hispanic/Latino; 2 Asian, non-Hispanic/Latino; 1 Hispanic/Latino; 1 Two or more races, non-Hispanic/Latino), 3 international. Average age 30. In 2015, 5 doctorates awarded. *Degree requirements:* For doctorate, thesis/dissertation. *Entrance requirements:* For doctorate, GRE General Test, minimum GPA of 3.0. Additional exam requirements/recommendations for international students: Required—TOEFL (minimum score 600 paper-based). *Application deadline:* For fall admission, 12/15 priority date for domestic and international students. Applications are processed on a rolling basis. Application fee: $75. Electronic applications accepted. *Financial support:* In 2015–16, 10 students received support. Fellowships with tuition reimbursements available and tuition waivers available. *Unit head:* Dr. David Leitenberg, Director, 202-994-9475, Fax: 202-994-2913, E-mail: dleit@gwu.edu. *Application contact:* Information Contact, 202-994-3532, Fax: 202-994-2913, E-mail: mtmjxl@gwumc.edu.
Website: http://smhs.gwu.edu/microbiology/

Hood College, Graduate School, Program in Biomedical Science, Frederick, MD 21701-8575. Offers bioinformatics (Certificate); biomedical science (MS), including biotechnology/molecular biology, microbiology/immunology/virology, regulatory compliance. *Program availability:* Part-time, evening/weekend. *Degree requirements:* For master's, comprehensive exam, thesis or alternative. *Entrance requirements:* For master's, bachelor's degree in biology; minimum GPA of 2.75; undergraduate course work in cell biology, chemistry, organic chemistry, and genetics. Additional exam requirements/recommendations for international students: Required—TOEFL (minimum score 575 paper-based; 89 iBT), IELTS (minimum score 6.5). *Application deadline:* For fall admission, 7/15 priority date for domestic students, 7/15 for international students; for spring admission, 12/1 priority date for domestic students, 12/1 for international students. Applications are processed on a rolling basis. Application fee: $35. Electronic applications accepted. Application fee is waived when completed online. *Expenses: Tuition, area resident:* Part-time $450 per credit hour. *Required fees:* $105 per term. Part-time tuition and fees vary according to degree level, campus/location and program. *Financial support:* Research assistantships with full tuition reimbursements, tuition waivers (partial), and unspecified assistantships available. Financial award applicants required to submit FAFSA.
Website: http://www.hood.edu/graduate

See Display on page 64 and Close-Up on page 109.

Illinois State University, Graduate School, College of Arts and Sciences, Department of Biological Sciences, Normal, IL 61790-2200. Offers animal behavior (MS); bacteriology (MS); biochemistry (MS); biological sciences (MS); biology (PhD); biophysics (MS); biotechnology (MS); botany (MS, PhD); cell biology (MS); conservation biology (MS); developmental biology (MS); ecology (MS, PhD); entomology (MS); evolutionary biology (MS); genetics (MS, PhD); immunology (MS); microbiology (MS, PhD); molecular biology (MS); molecular genetics (MS); neurobiology (MS); neuroscience (MS); parasitology (MS); physiology (MS, PhD); plant biology (MS); plant molecular biology (MS); plant sciences (MS); structural biology (MS); zoology (MS, PhD). *Program availability:* Part-time. *Degree requirements:* For master's, thesis or alternative; for doctorate, variable foreign language requirement, thesis/dissertation, 2 terms of residency. *Entrance requirements:* For master's, GRE General Test, minimum GPA of 2.6 in last 60 hours of course work; for doctorate, GRE General Test. *Application deadline:* Applications are processed on a rolling basis. Application fee: $40. *Financial support:* Research assistantships, teaching assistantships, Federal Work-Study, tuition waivers (full), and unspecified assistantships available. Financial award application deadline: 4/1. *Faculty research:* Redoc balance and drug development in schistosoma mansoni, control of the growth of listeria monocytogenes at low temperature, regulation of cell expansion and microtubule function by SPRI, CRUI: physiology and fitness consequences of different life history phenotypes. *Application contact:* Steven Juliano, Graduate Coordinator, E-mail: sajulian@ilstu.edu.
Website: http://www.bio.ilstu.edu/

Indiana University–Purdue University Indianapolis, Indiana University School of Medicine, Department of Microbiology and Immunology, Indianapolis, IN 46202. Offers MS, PhD, MD/MS, MD/PhD. Terminal master's awarded for partial completion of doctoral program. *Degree requirements:* For master's, thesis; for doctorate, thesis/dissertation. *Entrance requirements:* For master's and doctorate, GRE General Test, previous course work in calculus, cell biology, chemistry, genetics, physics, and biochemistry. *Faculty research:* Host-parasite interactions, molecular biology, cellular and molecular immunology and hematology, viral and bacterial pathogenesis, cancer research.

Iowa State University of Science and Technology, Program in Immunobiology, Ames, IA 50011. Offers MS, PhD. *Entrance requirements:* For master's and doctorate, GRE General Test, resume. Additional exam requirements/recommendations for international students: Required—TOEFL (minimum score 600 paper-based; 85 iBT), IELTS (minimum score 7). Electronic applications accepted. *Faculty research:* Immunogenetics, cellular and molecular immunology, infectious disease, neuroimmunology.

Irell & Manella Graduate School of Biological Sciences, Graduate Program, Duarte, CA 91010. Offers brain metastatic cancer (PhD); cancer and stem cell metabolism (PhD); cancer biology (PhD); cancer biology and developmental therapeutics (PhD); cell biology (PhD); chemical biology (PhD); chromosomal break repair (PhD); diabetes and pancreatic progenitor cell biology (PhD); DNA repair and cancer biology (PhD); germline epigenetic remodeling and endocrine disruptors (PhD); hematology and hematopoietic cell transplantation (PhD); hematology and immunology (PhD); inflammation and cancer (PhD); micrornas and gene regulation in cardiovascular disease (PhD); mixed chimrism for reversal of autoimmunity (PhD); molecular and cellular biology (PhD); molecular biology and genetics (PhD); nanoparticle mediated twist1 silencing in metastatic cancer (PhD); neuro-oncology and stem cell biology (PhD); neuroscience (PhD); rna directed therapies for hiv-1 (PhD); small rna-induced transcriptional gene activation (PhD); stem cell regulation by the microenvironment (PhD); translational oncology and pharmaceutical sciences (PhD); tumor biology (PhD). *Faculty:* 70 full-time (18 women). *Students:* 75 full-time (40 women); includes 28 minority (2 Black or African American, non-Hispanic/Latino; 10 Asian, non-Hispanic/Latino; 10 Hispanic/Latino; 2 Native Hawaiian or other Pacific Islander, non-Hispanic/Latino; 4 Two or more races, non-Hispanic/Latino), 15 international. Average age 26. 197 applicants, 12% accepted, 19 enrolled. In 2015, 12 doctorates awarded. *Degree requirements:* For doctorate, comprehensive exam, thesis/dissertation, qualifying exams, two advanced courses. *Entrance requirements:* For doctorate, GRE General Test; GRE Subject Test (recommended), 2 years of course work in chemistry (general and organic); 1 year of course work each in biochemistry, general biology, and general physics; 2 semesters of course work in mathematics; significant research laboratory experience. Additional exam requirements/recommendations for international students: Required—TOEFL. *Application deadline:* For fall admission, 1/1 priority date for domestic and international students. Application fee: $0. Electronic applications accepted. Full-time tuition and fees vary according to class time, course level, course load, degree level, campus/location, program and student level. *Financial support:* In 2015–16, 12 students received support, including 35 fellowships with full tuition reimbursements available (averaging $32,000 per year); teaching assistantships, health care benefits, and tuition waivers (full) also available. Financial award applicants required to submit FAFSA. *Faculty research:* Cancer biology, diabetes, stem cell biology, neuroscience, immunology. *Unit head:* Dr. John J. Rossi, Dean, 877-715-GRAD, Fax: 626-471-3901, E-mail: gradschool@coh.org. *Application contact:* Dr. Kate Sleeth, Interim Associate Dean of Administration and Student Development, 626-218-1742, Fax: 626-471-3901, E-mail: gradschool@coh.org. Website: http://cityofhope.org/gradschool

See Display on page 66 and Close-Up on page 111.

Johns Hopkins University, Bloomberg School of Public Health, W. Harry Feinstone Department of Molecular Microbiology and Immunology, Baltimore, MD 21218. Offers MHS, Sc M, PhD. *Faculty:* 41 full-time (10 women), 10 part-time/adjunct (1 woman). *Students:* 95 full-time (52 women), 2 part-time (1 woman); includes 23 minority (3 Black or African American, non-Hispanic/Latino; 13 Asian, non-Hispanic/Latino; 5 Hispanic/Latino; 2 Two or more races, non-Hispanic/Latino), 25 international. Average age 26. 192 applicants, 47% accepted, 37 enrolled. In 2015, 34 master's, 7 doctorates awarded. Terminal master's awarded for partial completion of doctoral program. *Degree requirements:* For master's, comprehensive exam, thesis (for some programs), essay, written exams; for doctorate, comprehensive exam, thesis/dissertation, 1-year full-time residency, oral and written exams. *Entrance requirements:* For master's, GRE General Test or MCAT, 3 letters of recommendation, curriculum vitae; for doctorate, GRE General Test, 3 letters of recommendation, transcripts, curriculum vitae. Additional exam requirements/recommendations for international students: Required—TOEFL (minimum score 600 paper-based). *Application deadline:* For fall admission, 1/2 priority date for domestic and international students. Applications are processed on a rolling basis. Application fee: $45. Electronic applications accepted. *Financial support:* Fellowships with tuition reimbursements, research assistantships with tuition reimbursements, Federal Work-Study, institutionally sponsored loans, scholarships/grants, and stipends available. Financial award application deadline: 3/15; financial award applicants required to submit FAFSA. *Faculty research:* Immunology, virology, bacteriology, parasitology, vector biology, disease ecology, pathogenesis of infectious disease, immune responses to infectious agents, vector-borne and tropical diseases, biochemistry and molecular biology of infectious agents, population genetics of insect vectors, genetic regulation and immune responses in insect vectors, vaccine development, hormonal effects on pathogenesis and immune responses. *Total annual research expenditures:* $14.5 million. *Unit head:* Dr. Arturo Casadevall, Chair, 410-955-3459, Fax: 410-955-0105, E-mail: acasade1@jhu.edu. *Application contact:* Gail O'Connor, Academic Program Administrator, 410-614-4232, Fax: 410-955-0105, E-mail: goconnor@jhsph.edu.
Website: http://www.jhsph.edu/dept/MMI/

Johns Hopkins University, School of Medicine, Graduate Programs in Medicine, Immunology Training Program, Baltimore, MD 21218. Offers PhD. *Degree requirements:* For doctorate, comprehensive exam, thesis/dissertation, oral exam, final thesis seminar. *Entrance requirements:* For doctorate, GRE General Test, 2 letters of recommendation. Additional exam requirements/recommendations for international students: Required—TOEFL (minimum score 550 paper-based). Electronic applications accepted. *Faculty research:* HIV immunity, tumor immunity, major histocompatibility complex, transplantation, genetics of antibodies and T-cell receptors; immune response to infectious agents; antigen recognition; immune regulation; autoimmune diseases; immune cell signaling.

London Metropolitan University, Graduate Programs, London, United Kingdom. Offers applied psychology (M Sc); architecture (MA); biomedical science (M Sc); blood science (M Sc); cancer pharmacology (M Sc); computer networking and cyber security (M Sc); computing and information systems (M Sc); conference interpreting (MA); counter-terrorism studies (M Sc); creative, digital and professional writing (MA); crime, violence and prevention (M Sc); criminology (M Sc); curating contemporary art (MA); data analytics (M Sc); digital media (MA); early childhood studies (MA); education (MA, Ed D); financial services law, regulation and compliance (LL M); food science (M Sc); forensic psychology (M Sc); health and social care management and policy (M Sc); human nutrition (M Sc); human resource management (MA); human rights and international conflict (MA); information technology (M Sc); intelligence and security studies (M Sc); international oil, gas and energy law (LL M); international relations (MA); interpreting (MA); learning and teaching in higher education (MA); legal practice (LL M); media and entertainment law (LL M); organizational and consumer psychology (M Sc); psychological therapy (M Sc); psychology of mental health (M Sc); public health (M Sc); public policy and management (MPA); security studies (M Sc); social work (M Sc); spatial planning and urban design (MA); sports therapy (M Sc); supporting older children and young people with dyslexia (MA); teaching languages (MA), including Arabic, English; translation (MA); woman and child abuse (MA).

Louisiana State University Health Sciences Center, School of Graduate Studies in New Orleans, Department of Microbiology, Immunology, and Parasitology, New Orleans, LA 70112-1393. Offers microbiology and immunology (PhD); MD/PhD. *Faculty:* 22 full-time (5 women). *Students:* 18 full-time (10 women); includes 3 minority (2 Black or African American, non-Hispanic/Latino; 1 Hispanic/Latino), 4 international. Average age 26. 14 applicants, 21% accepted, 1 enrolled. In 2015, 3 doctorates awarded. *Degree requirements:* For doctorate, comprehensive exam, thesis/dissertation, preliminary exam, qualifying exam. *Entrance requirements:* For doctorate, GRE General Test. Additional exam requirements/recommendations for international students: Recommended—TOEFL, IELTS. *Application deadline:* For fall admission, 4/1 for domestic and international students. Applications are processed on a rolling basis. Application fee: $30. *Financial support:* Unspecified assistantships available. Financial award application deadline: 4/15. *Faculty research:* Microbial physiology, animal virology, vaccine development, AIDS drug studies, pathogenic mechanisms, molecular immunology. *Unit head:* Dr. Alistair Ramsay, Professor and Head, 504-568-4062, Fax: 504-568-2918, E-mail: aramsa@lsuhsc.edu. *Application contact:* Dr. Angela Amedee,

Associate Professor, 504-568-5608, Fax: 504-568-2918, E-mail: aamede@lsuhsc.edu. Website: http://www.medschool.lsuhsc.edu/microbiology/

Louisiana State University Health Sciences Center at Shreveport, Department of Microbiology and Immunology, Shreveport, LA 71130-3932. Offers MS, PhD, MD/PhD. *Faculty:* 13 full-time (3 women). *Students:* 17 full-time (9 women), 2 international. Average age 27. 9 applicants, 100% accepted, 7 enrolled. In 2015, 5 master's, 5 doctorates awarded. Terminal master's awarded for partial completion of doctoral program. *Degree requirements:* For master's, comprehensive exam, thesis; for doctorate, comprehensive exam, thesis/dissertation, research proposal. *Entrance requirements:* For master's and doctorate, GRE General Test. Additional exam requirements/recommendations for international students: Required—TOEFL. *Application deadline:* For fall admission, 1/31 for domestic and international students. Application fee: $0. Electronic applications accepted. *Expenses:* $6,467.25 resident tuition; $15,872 non-resident tuition; $410.50 student fees. *Financial support:* In 2015–16, 20 students received support, including 20 fellowships with full tuition reimbursements available (averaging $26,000 per year); institutionally sponsored loans, scholarships/grants, and tuition waivers (for all full-time PhD students) also available. Financial award application deadline: 1/31. *Faculty research:* Infectious disease, molecular bacteriology, pathogenesis, molecular virology and immunology. *Unit head:* Dr. Dennis J. O'Callaghan, Head, 318-675-5750, Fax: 318-675-5764. *Application contact:* Marti Glass, Administrative Coordinator, 318-675-7851 Ext. 4781, Fax: 318-675-5764, E-mail: mglass@lsuhsc.edu.
Website: http://www.lsuhscmicrobiology.com

Loyola University Chicago, Graduate School, Integrated Program in Biomedical Sciences, Maywood, IL 60153. Offers biochemistry and molecular biology (MS, PhD); cell and molecular physiology (PhD); infectious disease and immunology (MS); integrative cell biology (PhD); medical physiology (MS); microbiology and immunology (MS, PhD); molecular pharmacology and therapeutics (MS, PhD); neuroscience (MS, PhD). *Students:* 135 full-time (65 women), 1 part-time (0 women); includes 28 minority (5 Black or African American, non-Hispanic/Latino; 15 Asian, non-Hispanic/Latino; 6 Hispanic/Latino; 2 Two or more races, non-Hispanic/Latino), 16 international. Average age 28. 442 applicants, 23% accepted, 55 enrolled. In 2015, 40 master's, 17 doctorates awarded. *Expenses:* Tuition, area resident: Full-time $18,054; part-time $9027 per credit hour. Required fees: $832; $284 per credit hour. Part-time tuition and fees vary according to course load, degree level and program. *Unit head:* Dr. Samuel Attoh, Dean, 773-508-3459, Fax: 773-508-2460, E-mail: sattoh@luc.edu. *Application contact:* Ron Martin, Associate Director of Enrollment Management, 312-915-8950, Fax: 312-915-8905, E-mail: gradapp@luc.edu.
Website: http://ssom.luc.edu/graduate_school/degree-programs/ipbsphd/

Massachusetts Institute of Technology, School of Science, Department of Biology, Cambridge, MA 02139. Offers biochemistry (PhD); biological oceanography (PhD); biology (PhD); biophysical chemistry and molecular structure (PhD); cell biology (PhD); computational and systems biology (PhD); developmental biology (PhD); genetics (PhD); immunology (PhD); microbiology (PhD); molecular biology (PhD); neurobiology (PhD). *Faculty:* 57 full-time (14 women). *Students:* 283 full-time (137 women); includes 83 minority (3 Black or African American, non-Hispanic/Latino; 1 American Indian or Alaska Native, non-Hispanic/Latino; 38 Asian, non-Hispanic/Latino; 31 Hispanic/Latino; 10 Two or more races, non-Hispanic/Latino), 48 international. Average age 26. 673 applicants, 14% accepted, 46 enrolled. In 2015, 32 doctorates awarded. *Degree requirements:* For doctorate, comprehensive exam, thesis/dissertation, teaching assistantship during two semesters. *Entrance requirements:* For doctorate, GRE General Test. Additional exam requirements/recommendations for international students: Required—TOEFL (minimum score 577 paper-based), IELTS. *Application deadline:* For fall admission, 12/1 for domestic and international students. Application fee: $75. Electronic applications accepted. *Expenses:* Tuition: Full-time $46,400; part-time $725 per credit. One-time fee: $304 full-time. Full-time tuition and fees vary according to course load and program. *Financial support:* In 2015–16, 235 students received support, including 118 fellowships (averaging $37,500 per year), 163 research assistantships (averaging $38,900 per year), 1 teaching assistantship; Federal Work-Study, institutionally sponsored loans, scholarships/grants, traineeships, health care benefits, and unspecified assistantships also available. Support available to part-time students. Financial award application deadline: 4/15; financial award applicants required to submit FAFSA. *Faculty research:* Cellular, developmental and molecular (plant and animal) biology; biochemistry, bioengineering, biophysics and structural biology; classical and molecular genetics, stem cell and epigenetics; immunology and microbiology; cancer biology, molecular medicine, neurobiology and human disease; computational and systems biology. *Total annual research expenditures:* $42.8 million. *Unit head:* Prof. Alan Grossman, Department Head, 617-253-4701. *Application contact:* Biology Education Office, 617-253-3717, Fax: 617-258-9329, E-mail: gradbio@mit.edu. Website: https://biology.mit.edu/

Mayo Graduate School, Graduate Programs in Biomedical Sciences, Program in Immunology, Rochester, MN 55905. Offers PhD. *Degree requirements:* For doctorate, oral defense of dissertation, qualifying oral and written exam. *Entrance requirements:* For doctorate, GRE, 1 year of chemistry, biology, calculus, and physics. Additional exam requirements/recommendations for international students: Required—TOEFL. Electronic applications accepted. *Faculty research:* Immunogenetics, autoimmunity, receptor signal transduction, T lymphocyte activation, transplantation.

McGill University, Faculty of Graduate and Postdoctoral Studies, Faculty of Medicine, Department of Microbiology and Immunology, Montréal, QC H3A 2T5, Canada. Offers M Sc, M Sc A, PhD.

McMaster University, Faculty of Health Sciences and School of Graduate Studies, Program in Medical Sciences, Immunity and Infection Area, Hamilton, ON L8S 4M2, Canada. Offers M Sc, PhD, MD/PhD. *Degree requirements:* For master's, thesis; for doctorate, comprehensive exam, thesis/dissertation. *Entrance requirements:* For master's, honors B Sc, B+ average in related field; for doctorate, M Sc, minimum B+ average, students with proven research experience and an A average may be admitted with a B Sc degree. Additional exam requirements/recommendations for international students: Required—TOEFL (minimum score 580 paper-based; 92 iBT).

Medical University of South Carolina, College of Graduate Studies, Department of Microbiology and Immunology, Charleston, SC 29425. Offers MS, PhD, DMD/PhD, MD/PhD. Terminal master's awarded for partial completion of doctoral program. *Degree requirements:* For master's, thesis; for doctorate, thesis/dissertation, oral and written exams. *Entrance requirements:* For master's, GRE General Test, MCAT, or DAT, minimum GPA of 3.0; for doctorate, GRE General Test, interview, minimum GPA of 3.0, research experience. Additional exam requirements/recommendations for international students: Required—TOEFL (minimum score 600 paper-based; 100 iBT). Electronic applications accepted. *Faculty research:* Innate and adaptive immunology, gene therapy/vector development, vaccinology, proteomics of biowarfare agents, bacterial and fungal pathogenesis.

Meharry Medical College, School of Graduate Studies, Program in Biomedical Sciences, Microbiology and Immunology Emphasis, Nashville, TN 37208-9989. Offers PhD, MD/PhD. *Degree requirements:* For doctorate, comprehensive exam, thesis/

dissertation. *Entrance requirements:* For doctorate, GRE General Test, GRE Subject Test, undergraduate degree in related science. *Application deadline:* For fall admission, 6/1 for domestic students. Applications are processed on a rolling basis. Application fee: $65. *Financial support:* Fellowships, research assistantships, and Federal Work-Study available. Financial award application deadline: 4/15. *Faculty research:* Microbial and bacterial pathogenesis, viral transcription, immune response to viruses and parasites.

Memorial University of Newfoundland, Faculty of Medicine and School of Graduate Studies, Graduate Programs in Medicine, Division of Biomedical Sciences, St. John's, NL A1C 5S7, Canada. Offers cancer (M Sc, PhD); cardiovascular (M Sc, PhD); immunology (M Sc, PhD); neuroscience (M Sc, PhD). *Program availability:* Part-time. *Degree requirements:* For master's, thesis; for doctorate, comprehensive exam, thesis/dissertation, oral defense of thesis. *Entrance requirements:* For master's, MD or B Sc; for doctorate, MD or M Sc. Additional exam requirements/recommendations for international students: Required—TOEFL. *Expenses: Tuition, area resident:* Full-time $2199 Canadian dollars. *International tuition:* $2859 Canadian dollars full-time. *Faculty research:* Neuroscience, immunology, cardiovascular, and cancer.

Montana State University, The Graduate School, College of Agriculture, Department of Immunology and Infectious Diseases, Bozeman, MT 59717. Offers MS, PhD. *Program availability:* Part-time. *Degree requirements:* For master's, comprehensive exam; for doctorate, comprehensive exam, thesis/dissertation. *Entrance requirements:* For master's and doctorate, GRE General Test. Additional exam requirements/recommendations for international students: Required—TOEFL (minimum score 550 paper-based). Electronic applications accepted. *Faculty research:* Immunology, mechanisms of infectious disease pathogenesis, mechanisms of host defense, lymphocyte development, host-pathogen interactions.

New York Medical College, Graduate School of Basic Medical Sciences, Integrated PhD Program, Valhalla, NY 10595-1691. Offers biochemistry and molecular biology (PhD); cell biology and anatomy (PhD); microbiology and immunology (PhD); pathology (PhD); pharmacology (PhD); physiology (PhD). *Degree requirements:* For doctorate, comprehensive exam, thesis/dissertation. *Entrance requirements:* For doctorate, GRE General Test. Additional exam requirements/recommendations for international students: Required—TOEFL. Electronic applications accepted. *Expenses: Tuition, area resident:* Full-time $44,355; part-time $1025 per credit. *Required fees:* $500; $95 per year. One-time fee: $140 part-time. Tuition and fees vary according to course load and program. *Faculty research:* Cardiovascular sciences, infectious diseases, neuroscience, cancer and cell signaling.

New York Medical College, Graduate School of Basic Medical Sciences, Microbiology and Immunology - Master's Program, Valhalla, NY 10595-1691. Offers MS, MD/PhD. *Program availability:* Part-time, evening/weekend. *Degree requirements:* For master's, thesis. *Entrance requirements:* For master's, GRE General Test, MCAT, or DAT. Additional exam requirements/recommendations for international students: Required—TOEFL. Electronic applications accepted. *Expenses: Tuition, area resident:* Full-time $44,355; part-time $1025 per credit. *Required fees:* $500; $95 per year. One-time fee: $140 part-time. Tuition and fees vary according to course load and program. *Faculty research:* Tumor cells, cancer vaccines, the role of stem cells in cancer, bacterial genetics pathogenesis of infectious disease and function of influenza virus antigens, molecular virology, and the biochemistry and genetics of emerging pathogens.

New York University, Graduate School of Arts and Science, Department of Biology, New York, NY 10012-1019. Offers biology (PhD); biomedical journalism (MS); cancer and molecular biology (PhD); computational biology (PhD); computers in biological research (MS); developmental genetics (PhD); general biology (PhD); immunology and microbiology (PhD); molecular genetics (PhD); neurobiology (PhD); oral biology (MS); plant biology (PhD); recombinant DNA technology (MS); MS/MBA. *Program availability:* Part-time. Terminal master's awarded for partial completion of doctoral program. *Degree requirements:* For master's, thesis or alternative, qualifying paper; for doctorate, comprehensive exam, thesis/dissertation. *Entrance requirements:* For master's and doctorate, GRE General Test. Additional exam requirements/recommendations for international students: Required—TOEFL. *Faculty research:* Genomics, molecular and cell biology, development and molecular genetics, molecular evolution of plants and animals.

New York University, School of Medicine and Graduate School of Arts and Science, Sackler Institute of Graduate Biomedical Sciences, Program in Immunology and Inflammation, New York, NY 10012-1019. Offers PhD, MD/PhD. *Degree requirements:* For doctorate, comprehensive exam, thesis/dissertation, qualifying exam. *Faculty research:* Molecular regulation of hematopoietic stem cell differentiation, immunological synapse and immunotherapy, adenosine as a regulator of inflammation.

New York University, School of Medicine and Graduate School of Arts and Science, Sackler Institute of Graduate Biomedical Sciences, Program in Molecular Oncology and Tumor Immunology, New York, NY 10012-1019. Offers immunology (PhD); molecular oncology (PhD). *Degree requirements:* For doctorate, one foreign language, comprehensive exam, thesis/dissertation, qualifying exam. *Faculty research:* Stem cells, immunology, genome instability, DNA damage checkpoints.

North Carolina State University, Graduate School, College of Agriculture and Life Sciences and College of Veterinary Medicine, Program in Immunology, Raleigh, NC 27695. Offers MS, PhD. *Degree requirements:* For master's, thesis; for doctorate, thesis/dissertation. *Entrance requirements:* For master's and doctorate, GRE General Test. Additional exam requirements/recommendations for international students: Required—TOEFL (minimum score 550 paper-based). Electronic applications accepted. *Faculty research:* Immunogenetics, immunopathology, immunotoxicology, immunoparasitology, molecular and infectious disease immunology.

Oregon Health & Science University, School of Medicine, Graduate Programs in Medicine, Program in Molecular and Cellular Biosciences, Department of Molecular Microbiology and Immunology, Portland, OR 97239-3098. Offers PhD. *Faculty:* 28 full-time (8 women), 21 part-time/adjunct (6 women). *Students:* 17 full-time (12 women); includes 5 minority (2 Asian, non-Hispanic/Latino; 3 Two or more races, non-Hispanic/Latino), 3 international. Average age 30. Terminal master's awarded for partial completion of doctoral program. *Degree requirements:* For doctorate, comprehensive exam, thesis/dissertation, qualifying exam. *Entrance requirements:* For doctorate, GRE General Test (minimum scores: 153 Verbal/148 Quantitative/4.5 Analytical) or MCAT (for some programs). Additional exam requirements/recommendations for international students: Required—IELTS or TOEFL. *Application deadline:* For fall admission, 12/1 for domestic and international students. Application fee: $70. Electronic applications accepted. *Financial support:* Health care benefits and full tuition and stipends available. *Faculty research:* Molecular biology of bacterial and viral pathogens, cellular and humoral immunology, molecular biology of microbes. *Unit head:* Dr. Eric Barklis, Program Director, 503-494-7768, E-mail: mmi@ohsu.edu. *Application contact:* Brandi Colbert, Program Coordinator, 503-418-9457, E-mail: colbertb@ohsu.edu. Website: http://www.ohsu.edu/microbiology

Oregon State University, College of Science, Program in Microbiology, Corvallis, OR 97331. Offers environmental microbiology (MA, MS, PhD); food microbiology (MA, MS, PhD); genomics (MA, MS, PhD); immunology (MA, MS, PhD); microbial ecology (MA, MS, PhD); microbial evolution (MA, MS, PhD); parasitology (MA, MS, PhD); pathogenic microbiology (MA, MS, PhD); virology (MA). *Program availability:* Part-time. *Faculty:* 14 full-time (5 women), 1 part-time/adjunct (0 women). *Students:* 32 full-time (12 women); includes 5 minority (4 Asian, non-Hispanic/Latino; 1 Two or more races, non-Hispanic/Latino), 2 international. Average age 28. 79 applicants, 10% accepted, 4 enrolled. In 2015, 3 master's, 4 doctorates awarded. Terminal master's awarded for partial completion of doctoral program. *Degree requirements:* For master's, thesis; for doctorate, one foreign language, thesis/dissertation. *Entrance requirements:* For master's and doctorate, GRE. Additional exam requirements/recommendations for international students: Required—TOEFL (minimum score 600 paper-based; 100 iBT). *Application deadline:* For fall admission, 8/1 for domestic students, 4/1 for international students; for winter admission, 12/1 for domestic students, 7/1 for international students; for spring admission, 2/1 for domestic students, 10/1 for international students; for summer admission, 5/1 for domestic students, 1/1 for international students. Application fee: $75 ($85 for international students). *Expenses: Tuition,* state resident: full-time $12,150; part-time $450 per credit. Tuition, nonresident: full-time $20,952; part-time $776 per credit. *Required fees:* $1572; $1443 per unit. One-time fee: $350. Tuition and fees vary according to course load, campus/location and program. *Financial support:* Fellowships, research assistantships, and teaching assistantships available. Financial award application deadline: 1/15. *Faculty research:* Genetics, physiology, biotechnology, pathogenic microbiology, plant virology. *Unit head:* Dr. Jerri Bartholomew, Professor and Department Head, 541-737-1856. *Application contact:* Mary Fulton, Microbiology Advisor, 541-737-1833, E-mail: mary.fulton@oregonstate.edu.
Website: http://microbiology.science.oregonstate.edu/

Penn State Hershey Medical Center, College of Medicine, Graduate School Programs in the Biomedical Sciences, Graduate Program in Biomedical Sciences, Hershey, PA 17033. Offers biochemistry and molecular genetics (MS, PhD); biomedical sciences (MS, PhD); translational therapeutics (MS, PhD); virology and immunology (MS, PhD); MD/PhD; PhD/MBA. *Students:* 79 full-time (43 women); includes 27 minority (7 Black or African American, non-Hispanic/Latino; 15 Asian, non-Hispanic/Latino; 4 Hispanic/Latino; 1 Native Hawaiian or other Pacific Islander, non-Hispanic/Latino), 17 international. 275 applicants, 16% accepted, 17 enrolled. Terminal master's awarded for partial completion of doctoral program. *Degree requirements:* For master's, thesis (for some programs); for doctorate, comprehensive exam, thesis/dissertation, candidacy exam. *Entrance requirements:* For doctorate, GRE General Test. Additional exam requirements/recommendations for international students: Required—TOEFL (minimum score 550 paper-based; 81 iBT). *Application deadline:* For fall admission, 1/1 for domestic and international students. Applications are processed on a rolling basis. Application fee: $65. Electronic applications accepted. *Expenses:* Contact institution. *Financial support:* In 2015–16, 79 students received support, including 79 research assistantships with full tuition reimbursements available (averaging $26,196 per year); fellowships, scholarships/grants, health care benefits, and unspecified assistantships also available. *Unit head:* Dr. Ralph L. Keil, Chair, 717-531-8595, Fax: 717-531-0786, E-mail: rlk9@psu.edu. *Application contact:* Kristin E. Smith, Director of Graduate Admissions, 717-531-1045, Fax: 717-531-0786, E-mail: kec17@psu.edu.
Website: http://med.psu.edu/bms

Penn State Hershey Medical Center, College of Medicine, Graduate School Programs in the Biomedical Sciences, The Huck Institutes of the Life Sciences, Intercollege Graduate Program in Molecular Cellular and Integrative Biosciences, Hershey, PA 17033. Offers cell and developmental biology (PhD); immunology and infectious disease (PhD); molecular and evolutionary genetics (PhD); molecular medicine (PhD); molecular toxicology (PhD); neurobiology (PhD). *Students:* 3 full-time (2 women); includes 2 minority (both Asian, non-Hispanic/Latino). 2 applicants, 100% accepted, 2 enrolled. In 2015, 1 doctorate awarded. *Degree requirements:* For doctorate, comprehensive exam, thesis/dissertation, oral exam. *Entrance requirements:* For doctorate, GRE, minimum GPA of 3.0. Additional exam requirements/recommendations for international students: Required—TOEFL (minimum score 500 paper-based). *Application deadline:* For fall admission, 1/31 priority date for domestic students, 2/1 priority date for international students. Applications are processed on a rolling basis. Application fee: $65. Electronic applications accepted. *Financial support:* In 2015–16, research assistantships with full tuition reimbursements (averaging $26,196 per year) were awarded; fellowships with full tuition reimbursements, career-related internships or fieldwork, Federal Work-Study, scholarships/grants, health care benefits, and unspecified assistantships also available. Financial award applicants required to submit FAFSA. *Faculty research:* Vascular biology, molecular toxicology, chemical biology, immune system, pathophysiological basis of human disease. *Unit head:* Dr. Peter Hudson, Director, 814-865-6057, E-mail: pjh18@psu.edu. *Application contact:* Kathy Shuey, Administrative Assistant, 717-531-8982, Fax: 717-531-0786, E-mail: grad-hmc@psu.edu.
Website: http://www.huck.psu.edu/education/molecular-cellular-and-integrative-biosciences

Purdue University, College of Pharmacy and Pharmacal Sciences and Graduate School, Graduate Programs in Pharmacy and Pharmacal Sciences, Department of Medicinal Chemistry and Molecular Pharmacology, West Lafayette, IN 47907. Offers biophysical and computational chemistry (PhD); cancer research (PhD); immunology and infectious disease (PhD); medicinal biochemistry and molecular biology (PhD); medicinal chemistry and chemical biology (PhD); molecular pharmacology (PhD); neuropharmacology, neurodegeneration, and neurotoxicity (PhD); systems biology and functional genomics (PhD). *Degree requirements:* For doctorate, thesis/dissertation. *Entrance requirements:* For doctorate, GRE General Test; GRE Subject Test in biology, biochemistry, and chemistry (recommended), minimum undergraduate GPA of 3.0. Additional exam requirements/recommendations for international students: Required—TOEFL (minimum score 550 paper-based; 77 iBT); Recommended—TWE. Electronic applications accepted. *Faculty research:* Drug design and development, cancer research, drug synthesis and analysis, chemical pharmacology, environmental toxicology.

Purdue University, School of Veterinary Medicine and Graduate School, Graduate Programs in Veterinary Medicine, Department of Comparative Pathobiology, West Lafayette, IN 47907-2027. Offers comparative epidemiology and public health (MS); comparative epidemiology and public heath (PhD); comparative microbiology and immunology (MS, PhD); comparative pathobiology (MS, PhD); interdisciplinary studies (PhD), including microbial pathogenesis, molecular signaling and cancer biology, molecular virology; lab animal medicine (MS); veterinary anatomic pathology (MS); veterinary clinical pathology (MS). Terminal master's awarded for partial completion of doctoral program. *Degree requirements:* For master's, thesis (for some programs); for doctorate, thesis/dissertation. *Entrance requirements:* For master's and doctorate, GRE General Test. Additional exam requirements/recommendations for international students: Required—TOEFL (minimum score 575 paper-based), IELTS (minimum score 6.5), TWE (minimum score 4). Electronic applications accepted.

Queen's University at Kingston, School of Graduate Studies, Faculty of Health Sciences, Department of Microbiology and Immunology, Kingston, ON K7L 3N6, Canada. Offers M Sc, PhD. *Program availability:* Part-time. *Degree requirements:* For master's, thesis; for doctorate, comprehensive exam, thesis/dissertation. *Entrance requirements:* For master's and doctorate, minimum B+ average. Additional exam

Immunology

requirements/recommendations for international students: Required—TOEFL (minimum score 600 paper-based). Electronic applications accepted. *Faculty research:* Bacteriology, virology, immunology, education in microbiology and immunology, microbial pathogenesis.

Rosalind Franklin University of Medicine and Science, School of Graduate and Postdoctoral Studies - Interdisciplinary Graduate Program in Biomedical Sciences, Department of Microbiology and Immunology, North Chicago, IL 60064-3095. Offers PhD, MD/PhD. Terminal master's awarded for partial completion of doctoral program. *Degree requirements:* For doctorate, comprehensive exam, thesis/dissertation. *Entrance requirements:* For doctorate, GRE General Test. Additional exam requirements/recommendations for international students: Required—TOEFL, TWE. *Faculty research:* Molecular biology, parasitology, virology.

Rush University, Graduate College, Division of Immunology and Microbiology, Program in Immunology/Microbiology, Chicago, IL 60612-3832. Offers immunology (MS, PhD); virology (MS, PhD); MD/PhD. *Program availability:* Part-time. Terminal master's awarded for partial completion of doctoral program. *Degree requirements:* For master's, thesis; for doctorate, thesis/dissertation, comprehensive preliminary exam. *Entrance requirements:* For master's, GRE General Test; for doctorate, GRE General Test, interview, minimum GPA of 3.0. Additional exam requirements/recommendations for international students: Required—TOEFL. Electronic applications accepted. *Faculty research:* Human genetics, autoimmunity, tumor biology, complement, HIV immunopathology genesis.

Rutgers University–Newark, Graduate School of Biomedical Sciences, Program in Molecular Pathology and Immunology, Newark, NJ 07107. Offers PhD. *Entrance requirements:* Additional exam requirements/recommendations for international students: Required—TOEFL. Electronic applications accepted.

Rutgers University–New Brunswick, Graduate School-New Brunswick, Programs in the Molecular Biosciences, Piscataway, NJ 08854-8097. Offers biochemistry (PhD); cell and developmental biology (MS, PhD); microbiology and molecular genetics (MS, PhD), including applied microbiology, clinical microbiology (MS), clinical mircobiology (PhD), computational molecular biology (PhD); immunology, microbial biochemistry, molecular genetics, virology. MS, PhD offered jointly with University of Medicine and Dentistry of New Jersey.

Saint Louis University, Graduate Education and School of Medicine, Graduate Program in Biomedical Sciences, Department of Molecular Microbiology and Immunology, St. Louis, MO 63103. Offers PhD. *Degree requirements:* For doctorate, comprehensive exam, thesis/dissertation, qualifying exams. *Entrance requirements:* For doctorate, GRE General Test (GRE Subject Test optional), letters of recommendation, resume, interview. Additional exam requirements/recommendations for international students: Required—TOEFL (minimum score 525 paper-based). Electronic applications accepted. *Faculty research:* Pathogenesis of hepatitis C virus, herperviruses, pox viruses, rheumatoid arthritis, antiviral drugs and vaccines in biodefense, cancer gene therapy, virology and immunology.

⭐ **Stanford University,** School of Medicine, Graduate Programs in Medicine, Department of Microbiology and Immunology, Stanford, CA 94305-9991. Offers PhD. *Degree requirements:* For doctorate, comprehensive exam, thesis/dissertation, 2 quarter teaching assistantship. *Entrance requirements:* For doctorate, GRE General Test, GRE Subject Test (biology or biochemistry). Additional exam requirements/recommendations for international students: Required—TOEFL. Electronic applications accepted. *Expenses: Tuition, area resident:* Full-time $45,729. *Required fees:* $591. *Faculty research:* Molecular pathogenesis of bacteria viruses and parasites, immune system function, autoimmunity, molecular biology.

See Close-Up on page 331.

State University of New York Upstate Medical University, College of Graduate Studies, Program in Microbiology and Immunology, Syracuse, NY 13210-2334. Offers microbiology (MS); microbiology and immunology (PhD); MD/PhD. Terminal master's awarded for partial completion of doctoral program. *Degree requirements:* For master's, thesis; for doctorate, comprehensive exam, thesis/dissertation. *Entrance requirements:* For master's, GRE General Test, interview; for doctorate, GRE General Test, telephone interview. Additional exam requirements/recommendations for international students: Required—TOEFL. Electronic applications accepted. *Faculty research:* Cancer, disorders of the nervous system, infectious diseases, diabetes/metabolic disorders/cardiovascular diseases.

Stony Brook University, State University of New York, Graduate School, College of Arts and Sciences, Department of Biochemistry and Cell Biology, Molecular and Cellular Biology Program, Stony Brook, NY 11794. Offers biochemistry and molecular biology (PhD); biological sciences (MA); immunology and pathology (PhD); molecular and cellular biology (PhD). *Faculty:* 22 full-time (7 women). *Students:* 66 full-time (41 women); includes 11 minority (2 Black or African American, non-Hispanic/Latino; 6 Asian, non-Hispanic/Latino; 3 Hispanic/Latino), 38 international. Average age 28. 175 applicants, 16% accepted, 8 enrolled. In 2015, 11 doctorates awarded. *Degree requirements:* For doctorate, comprehensive exam, thesis/dissertation, teaching experience. *Entrance requirements:* For doctorate, GRE General Test, GRE Subject Test. Additional exam requirements/recommendations for international students: Required—TOEFL. *Application deadline:* For fall admission, 1/15 for domestic students; for spring admission, 10/1 for domestic students. Application fee: $100. *Expenses:* $12,421 per year full-time resident tuition and fees, $453 per credit hour; $23,761 per year full-time non-resident tuition and fees, $925 per credit hour. *Financial support:* In 2015–16, 4 fellowships, 33 research assistantships, 8 teaching assistantships were awarded; Federal Work-Study also available. *Unit head:* Prof. Aaron Neiman, Chair, 631-632-1543, E-mail: aaron.neiman@stonybrook.edu. *Application contact:* Pam Wolfskill, Administrative Specialist/Program Administrator, 631-632-8585, Fax: 631-632-9730, E-mail: pamela.wolfskill@stonybrook.edu.

Thomas Jefferson University, Jefferson College of Biomedical Sciences, PhD Program in Immunology and Microbial Pathogenesis, Philadelphia, PA 19107. Offers PhD. *Faculty:* 35 full-time (5 women), 1 part-time/adjunct (0 women). *Students:* 16 full-time (9 women); includes 4 minority (3 Asian, non-Hispanic/Latino; 1 Hispanic/Latino), 1 international. Average age 28. 35 applicants, 9% accepted, 2 enrolled. In 2015, 6 doctorates awarded. *Degree requirements:* For doctorate, comprehensive exam, thesis/dissertation. *Entrance requirements:* For doctorate, GRE General Test, minimum GPA of 3.2. Additional exam requirements/recommendations for international students: Required—TOEFL, IELTS (minimum score 7). *Application deadline:* For fall admission, 12/15 priority date for domestic and international students. Applications are processed on a rolling basis. Application fee: $50. Electronic applications accepted. *Financial support:* In 2015–16, 16 students received support, including 16 fellowships with full tuition reimbursements available (averaging $56,298 per year); Federal Work-Study, institutionally sponsored loans, scholarships/grants, traineeships, and stipends also available. Support available to part-time students. Financial award application deadline: 5/1; financial award applicants required to submit FAFSA. *Unit head:* Dr. Matthias J. Schnell, Program Director, 215-503-4634, Fax: 215-503-5393, E-mail: matthias.schnell@jefferson.edu. *Application contact:* Marc E. Stearns, Director of

Admissions, 215-503-0155, Fax: 215-503-3433, E-mail: jgsbs-info@jefferson.edu. Website: http://www.jefferson.edu/university/biomedical-sciences/degrees-programs/phd-programs/immunology.html

Tufts University, Sackler School of Graduate Biomedical Sciences, Immunology Program, Medford, MA 02155. Offers PhD. *Faculty:* 25 full-time (8 women). *Students:* 25 full-time (11 women); includes 7 minority (2 Black or African American, non-Hispanic/Latino; 2 Asian, non-Hispanic/Latino; 2 Hispanic/Latino; 1 Two or more races, non-Hispanic/Latino), 2 international. Average age 30. 59 applicants, 8% accepted, 4 enrolled. In 2015, 5 doctorates awarded. Terminal master's awarded for partial completion of doctoral program. *Degree requirements:* For doctorate, comprehensive exam, thesis/dissertation. *Entrance requirements:* For doctorate, GRE General Test, 3 letters of reference. Additional exam requirements/recommendations for international students: Required—TOEFL (minimum score 600 paper-based; 100 iBT). *Application deadline:* For fall admission, 12/15 priority date for domestic and international students. Application fee: $90. Electronic applications accepted. *Expenses: Tuition, area resident:* Full-time $48,412; part-time $1210 per credit hour. *Required fees:* $806. Full-time tuition and fees vary according to degree level, program and student level. Part-time tuition and fees vary according to course load. *Financial support:* In 2015–16, 24 students received support, including 24 research assistantships with full tuition reimbursements available (averaging $32,000 per year); traineeships also available. *Faculty research:* Genetic regulation of the ontogeny and activation of lymphocytes, mechanisms of antigen-receptor gene rearrangement, biology and molecular biology of negative selection (tolerance) of B and T cells, activation signal pathways, gene expression and the biochemistry of apoptosis. *Unit head:* Dr. Brigitte Huber, Director, 617-636-6836, Fax: 617-636-2990. *Application contact:* Dr. Elizabeth Storrs, 617-636-6767, Fax: 617-636-0375, E-mail: sackler-school@tufts.edu.
Website: http://sackler.tufts.edu/Academics/Degree-Programs/Immunology

Tulane University, School of Medicine and School of Liberal Arts, Graduate Programs in Biomedical Sciences, Department of Microbiology and Immunology, New Orleans, LA 70118-5669. Offers MS. MS and PhD offered through the Graduate School. *Degree requirements:* For master's, thesis. *Entrance requirements:* For master's, GRE General Test, minimum B average in undergraduate course work. Additional exam requirements/recommendations for international students: Required—TOEFL. *Application deadline:* For fall admission, 2/1 for domestic and international students. Application fee: $45. Electronic applications accepted. *Expenses: Tuition, area resident:* Full-time $47,658; part-time $2648 per credit hour. *Required fees:* $1980; $44.50 per credit hour. $550 per term. Tuition and fees vary according to course load, degree level and program. *Financial support:* Fellowships with full tuition reimbursements, research assistantships with full tuition reimbursements, career-related internships or fieldwork, Federal Work-Study, and institutionally sponsored loans available. Financial award application deadline: 2/1. *Faculty research:* Vaccine development, viral pathogenesis, molecular virology, bacterial pathogenesis, fungal pathogenesis.

⭐ **Uniformed Services University of the Health Sciences,** F. Edward Hebert School of Medicine, Graduate Programs in the Biomedical Sciences and Public Health, Graduate Program in Emerging Infectious Diseases, Bethesda, MD 20814-4799. Offers PhD. *Faculty:* 35 full-time (5 women), 17 part-time/adjunct (6 women). *Students:* 26 full-time (20 women); includes 2 minority (1 Black or African American, non-Hispanic/Latino; 1 Asian, non-Hispanic/Latino), 2 international. Average age 25. 53 applicants, 13% accepted, 5 enrolled. In 2015, 10 doctorates awarded. *Degree requirements:* For doctorate, comprehensive exam, thesis/dissertation, qualifying exam. *Entrance requirements:* For doctorate, GRE General Test. *Application deadline:* For fall admission, 12/15 priority date for domestic students. Applications are processed on a rolling basis. Application fee: $0. Electronic applications accepted. *Financial support:* In 2015–16, fellowships with full tuition reimbursements (averaging $43,000 per year) were awarded; scholarships/grants, health care benefits, and tuition waivers (full) also available. *Faculty research:* Pathogenesis, host response, and epidemiology of infectious diseases. *Unit head:* Dr. Christopher Broder, Director, 301-295-3401, E-mail: christopher.broder@usuhs.edu. *Application contact:* Patricia Grant, Program Administrative Specialist, 301-295-3400, Fax: 301-295-3773, E-mail: patricia.grant@usuhs.edu.
Website: http://www.usuhs.mil/eid

See Display on page 313 and Close-Up on page 333.

Universidad Central del Caribe, School of Medicine, Program in Biomedical Sciences, Bayamón, PR 00960-6032. Offers anatomy and cell biology (MA, MS); biochemistry (MS); biomedical sciences (MA); cellular and molecular biology (PhD); microbiology and immunology (MA, MS); pharmacology (MS); physiology (MS).

Université de Montréal, Faculty of Medicine, Department of Microbiology and Immunology, Montréal, QC H3C 3J7, Canada. Offers M Sc, PhD. Programs offered jointly with Faculty of Veterinary Medicine and Université du Québec, Institut Armand-Frappier. Terminal master's awarded for partial completion of doctoral program. *Degree requirements:* For master's, thesis; for doctorate, thesis/dissertation, general exam. *Entrance requirements:* For master's and doctorate, proficiency in French, knowledge of English. Electronic applications accepted.

Université de Montréal, Faculty of Veterinary Medicine, Program in Virology and Immunology, Montréal, QC H3C 3J7, Canada. Offers PhD. Program offered jointly with Université du Québec, Institut Armand-Frappier. *Degree requirements:* For doctorate, thesis/dissertation, general exam. *Entrance requirements:* For doctorate, proficiency in French, knowledge of English. Electronic applications accepted.

Université de Sherbrooke, Faculty of Medicine and Health Sciences, Graduate Programs in Medicine, Program in Immunology, Sherbrooke, QC J1H 5N4, Canada. Offers M Sc, PhD. Electronic applications accepted. *Faculty research:* Cytokine receptor signal transduction, lipid mediators and inflammation, TGFbeta convertases.

Université du Québec, Institut National de la Recherche Scientifique, Graduate Programs, Research Center–INRS–Institut Armand-Frappier, Laval, QC H7V 1B7, Canada. Offers applied microbiology (M Sc); biology (PhD); experimental health sciences (M Sc); virology and immunology (M Sc, PhD). *Program availability:* Part-time. *Degree requirements:* For master's, thesis; for doctorate, thesis/dissertation. *Entrance requirements:* For master's, appropriate bachelor's degree, proficiency in French; for doctorate, appropriate master's degree, proficiency in French. Electronic applications accepted. *Faculty research:* Immunity, infection and cancer; toxicology and environmental biotechnology; molecular pharmacochemistry.

Université Laval, Faculty of Medicine, Graduate Programs in Medicine, Programs in Microbiology-Immunology, Québec, QC G1K 7P4, Canada. Offers M Sc, PhD. Terminal master's awarded for partial completion of doctoral program. *Degree requirements:* For master's, thesis; for doctorate, comprehensive exam, thesis/dissertation. *Entrance requirements:* For master's and doctorate, knowledge of French, comprehension of written English. Electronic applications accepted.

University at Albany, State University of New York, School of Public Health, Department of Biomedical Sciences, Program in Immunology and Infectious Diseases, Albany, NY 12222-0001. Offers MS, PhD. *Degree requirements:* For master's, thesis; for doctorate, thesis/dissertation. *Entrance requirements:* For master's and doctorate, GRE General Test, GRE Subject Test.

University at Buffalo, the State University of New York, Graduate School, Graduate Programs in Cancer Research and Biomedical Sciences at Roswell Park Cancer Institute, Department of Immunology at Roswell Park Cancer Institute, Buffalo, NY 14260. Offers PhD. *Faculty:* 23 full-time (8 women). *Students:* 24 full-time (16 women); includes 4 minority (2 Black or African American, non-Hispanic/Latino; 1 Asian, non-Hispanic/Latino; 1 Two or more races, non-Hispanic/Latino), 5 international. 25 applicants, 24% accepted, 2 enrolled. In 2015, 3 doctorates awarded. *Degree requirements:* For doctorate, comprehensive exam, thesis/dissertation, oral defense of dissertation. *Entrance requirements:* For doctorate, GRE General Test. Additional exam requirements/recommendations for international students: Required—TOEFL (minimum score 79 iBT). *Application deadline:* For fall admission, 1/5 priority date for domestic and international students. Application fee: $75. Electronic applications accepted. *Financial support:* In 2015–16, 23 students received support, including 23 research assistantships with full tuition reimbursements available (averaging $25,000 per year); scholarships/grants, health care benefits, and unspecified assistantships also available. Financial award application deadline: 1/5. *Faculty research:* Immunochemistry, immunobiology, molecular immunology, hybridoma studies, recombinant DNA studies. *Unit head:* Dr. Kelvin Lee, Chair, 716-845-4106, Fax: 716-845-2993, E-mail: kelvin.lee@roswellpark.org. *Application contact:* Dr. Norman J. Karin, Associate Dean, 716-845-4630, Fax: 716-845-8178, E-mail: norman.karin@roswellpark.edu.
Website: http://www.roswellpark.edu/education/phd-programs/immunology

University at Buffalo, the State University of New York, Graduate School, School of Medicine and Biomedical Sciences, Graduate Programs in Medicine and Biomedical Sciences, Department of Microbiology and Immunology, Buffalo, NY 14214-3000. Offers MA, PhD. *Faculty:* 18 full-time (5 women). *Students:* 19 full-time (10 women); includes 5 minority (1 Black or African American, non-Hispanic/Latino; 4 Asian, non-Hispanic/Latino). Average age 27. 16 applicants, 19% accepted. In 2015, 1 master's, 6 doctorates awarded. *Degree requirements:* For master's, comprehensive exam; for doctorate, thesis/dissertation, departmental qualifying exam. *Entrance requirements:* For master's and doctorate, GRE General Test, 3 letters of recommendation. Additional exam requirements/recommendations for international students: Required—TOEFL (minimum score 100 iBT). *Application deadline:* For fall admission, 4/1 priority date for domestic and international students. Applications are processed on a rolling basis. Application fee: $85. Electronic applications accepted. *Financial support:* In 2015–16, 6 fellowships with tuition reimbursements (averaging $28,000 per year), 8 research assistantships with tuition reimbursements (averaging $27,000 per year) were awarded; traineeships and unspecified assistantships also available. Financial award application deadline: 2/1; financial award applicants required to submit FAFSA. *Faculty research:* Bacteriology, immunology, parasitology, virology, mycology. Total annual research expenditures: $5 million. *Unit head:* Dr. James Bangs, Chair/Professor, 716-829-2907, Fax: 716-829-2158. *Application contact:* Dr. John Panepinto, Director of Graduate Studies, 716-829-2176, Fax: 716-829-2158.
Website: http://www.smbs.buffalo.edu/microb/

University of Alberta, Faculty of Medicine and Dentistry and Faculty of Graduate Studies and Research, Graduate Programs in Medicine, Department of Medical Microbiology and Immunology, Edmonton, AB T6G 2E1, Canada. Offers M Sc, PhD. Terminal master's awarded for partial completion of doctoral program. *Degree requirements:* For master's, thesis; for doctorate, thesis/dissertation. *Entrance requirements:* For master's and doctorate, minimum GPA of 3.3. Additional exam requirements/recommendations for international students: Required—TOEFL (minimum score 600 paper-based; 96 iBT). *Faculty research:* Cellular and reproductive immunology, microbial pathogenesis, mechanisms of antibiotic resistance, molecular biology of mammalian viruses, antiviral chemotherapy.

The University of Arizona, College of Medicine, Department of Immunobiology, Tucson, AZ 85721. Offers PhD. *Degree requirements:* For doctorate, thesis/dissertation. *Entrance requirements:* For doctorate, GRE General Test, minimum GPA of 3.0. *Application deadline:* For fall admission, 3/1 priority date for domestic students; for spring admission, 9/1 for domestic students. Application fee: $75. *Financial support:* Fellowships, research assistantships, teaching assistantships, institutionally sponsored loans, and tuition waivers (full) available. Financial award application deadline: 4/30. *Faculty research:* Environmental and pathogenic microbiology, molecular biology. *Unit head:* Dr. Janko Nikolich-Zugich, Head, 520-626-6065, Fax: 520-626-2100, E-mail: nikolich@email.arizona.edu. *Application contact:* Tammy Rippberger, Senior business Manager, 520-626-6888, E-mail: trippberger@email.arizona.edu.
Website: http://immunobiology.arizona.edu/

University of Arkansas for Medical Sciences, Graduate School, Little Rock, AR 72205. Offers biochemistry and molecular biology (MS, PhD); bioinformatics (MS, PhD); cellular physiology and molecular biophysics (MS, PhD); clinical nutrition (MS); interdisciplinary biomedical sciences (MS, PhD, Certificate); interdisciplinary toxicology (MS); microbiology and immunology (PhD); neurobiology and developmental sciences (PhD); pharmacology (PhD); MD/PhD. Bioinformatics programs hosted jointly with the University of Arkansas at Little Rock. *Program availability:* Part-time. Terminal master's awarded for partial completion of doctoral program. *Degree requirements:* For master's, comprehensive exam (for some programs), thesis (for some programs); for doctorate, thesis/dissertation. *Entrance requirements:* For master's and doctorate, GRE. Additional exam requirements/recommendations for international students: Required—TOEFL. Electronic applications accepted. *Expenses:* Contact institution.

The University of British Columbia, Faculty of Science, Department of Microbiology and Immunology, Vancouver, BC V6T 1Z1, Canada. Offers M Sc, PhD. *Degree requirements:* For master's, thesis; for doctorate, comprehensive exam, thesis/dissertation. *Entrance requirements:* For master's and doctorate, GRE General Test. Additional exam requirements/recommendations for international students: Required—TOEFL (minimum score 590 paper-based). Electronic applications accepted. *Faculty research:* Bacterial genetics, metabolism, pathogenic bacteriology, virology.

University of Calgary, Cumming School of Medicine and Faculty of Graduate Studies, Department of Microbiology, Immunology and Infectious Diseases, Calgary, AB T2N 1N4, Canada. Offers M Sc, PhD. *Degree requirements:* For master's, thesis, oral thesis exam; for doctorate, thesis/dissertation, candidacy exam, oral thesis exam. *Entrance requirements:* For master's and doctorate, minimum GPA of 3.2. Additional exam requirements/recommendations for international students: Required—TOEFL (minimum score 580 paper-based). Electronic applications accepted. *Faculty research:* Bacteriology, virology, parasitology, immunology.

University of California, Berkeley, Graduate Division, School of Public Health, Group in Infectious Diseases and Immunity, Berkeley, CA 94720-1500. Offers PhD. *Entrance requirements:* For doctorate, GRE General Test, minimum GPA of 3.0, 3 letters of recommendation.

University of California, Davis, Graduate Studies, Graduate Group in Immunology, Davis, CA 95616. Offers MS, PhD. Terminal master's awarded for partial completion of doctoral program. *Degree requirements:* For master's, comprehensive exam (for some programs), thesis (for some programs); for doctorate, thesis/dissertation. *Entrance requirements:* For master's and doctorate, GRE General Test. Additional exam requirements/recommendations for international students: Required—TOEFL (minimum score 550 paper-based). Electronic applications accepted. *Faculty research:* Immune regulation in autoimmunity, immunopathology, immunotoxicology, tumor immunology, avian immunology.

University of California, Los Angeles, David Geffen School of Medicine and Graduate Division, Graduate Programs in Medicine, Department of Microbiology, Immunology and Molecular Genetics, Los Angeles, CA 90095. Offers MS, PhD. *Degree requirements:* For master's, thesis; for doctorate, thesis/dissertation, oral and written qualifying exams; 2 quarters of teaching experience. *Entrance requirements:* For master's and doctorate, GRE General Test, bachelor's degree; minimum undergraduate GPA of 3.0 (or its equivalent if letter grade system not used). Additional exam requirements/recommendations for international students: Required—TOEFL. Electronic applications accepted.

University of California, Los Angeles, Graduate Division, College of Letters and Science and David Geffen School of Medicine, UCLA ACCESS to Programs in the Molecular, Cellular and Integrative Life Sciences, Los Angeles, CA 90095. Offers biochemistry and molecular biology (PhD); biological chemistry (PhD); cellular and molecular pathology (PhD); human genetics (PhD); microbiology, immunology, and molecular genetics (PhD); molecular biology (PhD); molecular toxicology (PhD); molecular, cellular and integrative physiology (PhD); neurobiology (PhD); oral biology (PhD); physiology (PhD). *Degree requirements:* For doctorate, thesis/dissertation, oral and written qualifying exams. *Entrance requirements:* For doctorate, GRE General Test, bachelor's degree; minimum undergraduate GPA of 3.0 (or its equivalent if letter grade system not used). Additional exam requirements/recommendations for international students: Required—TOEFL. Electronic applications accepted.

University of Chicago, Division of the Biological Sciences, Committee on Immunology, Chicago, IL 60637. Offers PhD. *Students:* 32 full-time (14 women); includes 7 minority (2 Black or African American, non-Hispanic/Latino; 4 Asian, non-Hispanic/Latino; 1 Hispanic/Latino), 4 international. Average age 28. 87 applicants, 22% accepted, 5 enrolled. In 2015, 6 doctorates awarded. *Degree requirements:* For doctorate, thesis/dissertation, ethics class, 2 teaching assistantships. *Entrance requirements:* For doctorate, GRE General Test. Additional exam requirements/recommendations for international students: Required—TOEFL (minimum score 600 paper-based; 104 iBT), IELTS (minimum score 7). *Application deadline:* For fall admission, 12/1 for domestic and international students. Application fee: $90. Electronic applications accepted. *Financial support:* In 2015–16, 27 students received support, including 10 fellowships with full tuition reimbursements available (averaging $29,781 per year), 16 research assistantships with full tuition reimbursements available (averaging $29,781 per year); institutionally sponsored loans, scholarships/grants, traineeships, and health care benefits also available. Financial award applicants required to submit FAFSA. *Faculty research:* Molecular immunology, transplantation, autoimmunology, neuroimmunology, tumor immunology. Total annual research expenditures: $15 million. *Unit head:* Dr. Alexander Chervonsky, Interim Chairman, 773-702-1371, Fax: 773-834-5251.
Website: http://biomedsciences.uchicago.edu/page/committee-immunology-0

University of Cincinnati, Graduate School, College of Medicine, Graduate Programs in Biomedical Sciences, Department of Pediatrics, Cincinnati, OH 45221. Offers immunobiology (PhD); molecular and developmental biology (PhD). *Degree requirements:* For doctorate, thesis/dissertation, qualifying exam. *Entrance requirements:* For doctorate, GRE General Test, minimum GPA of 3.0. Additional exam requirements/recommendations for international students: Required—TOEFL (minimum score 600 paper-based; 100 iBT). Electronic applications accepted. *Faculty research:* Pulmonary biology, molecular cardiovascular, developmental biology, cancer biology, genetics.

University of Cincinnati, Graduate School, College of Medicine, Graduate Programs in Biomedical Sciences, Immunology Graduate Program, Cincinnati, OH 45229. Offers MS, PhD. *Program availability:* Part-time. *Degree requirements:* For master's, seminar, thesis with oral defense; for doctorate, seminar, dissertation with oral defense, written and oral candidacy exams. *Entrance requirements:* For master's, GRE, bachelor's degree in biology-related field or bachelor's degree in any field and work experience in biology-related field; for doctorate, GRE, bachelor's degree in biology-related field. Additional exam requirements/recommendations for international students: Required—TOEFL (minimum score 100 iBT). Electronic applications accepted. *Faculty research:* Allergy and asthma, cancer, organ transplantation, immunodeficiences: Lupus and AIDS, diabetes.

University of Colorado Denver, School of Medicine, Integrated Department of Immunology, Aurora, CO 80206. Offers PhD. *Students:* 40 full-time (21 women), 1 (woman) part-time; includes 8 minority (1 Black or African American, non-Hispanic/Latino; 1 American Indian or Alaska Native, non-Hispanic/Latino; 3 Asian, non-Hispanic/Latino; 3 Hispanic/Latino), 1 international. Average age 28. 61 applicants, 5% accepted, 3 enrolled. In 2015, 6 doctorates awarded. *Degree requirements:* For doctorate, thesis/dissertation, 30 credit hours of formal course work, three laboratory rotations, oral comprehensive examination, 30 credit hours of dissertation research, final defense of the dissertation. *Entrance requirements:* For doctorate, GRE, letters of recommendation, statement of purpose, interview. Additional exam requirements/recommendations for international students: Required—TOEFL (minimum score 550 paper-based; 89 iBT). *Application deadline:* For fall admission, 12/1 for domestic students, 11/1 for international students. Application fee: $50 ($75 for international students). Electronic applications accepted. *Expenses:* Contact institution. *Financial support:* In 2015–16, 41 students received support. Fellowships with full tuition reimbursements available, research assistantships, teaching assistantships, Federal Work-Study, institutionally sponsored loans, scholarships/grants, traineeships, health care benefits, tuition waivers (full), and unspecified assistantships available. Financial award application deadline: 3/15; financial award applicants required to submit FAFSA. *Faculty research:* Gene regulation, immune signaling, apoptosis, stem cells, vaccines. *Unit head:* Dr. John Cambier, Professor/Chairman, 303-724-8663, E-mail: john.cambier@ucdenver.edu. *Application contact:* Elizabeth Wethington, LEAD Program Administrator, 303-724-7280, E-mail: elizabeth.wethington@ucdenver.edu.
Website: http://www.ucdenver.edu/academics/colleges/medicalschool/departments/ImmunologyMicrobiology/gradprogram/immugradprog/Pages/ImmuGradHome.aspx

University of Colorado Denver, School of Medicine, Program in Microbiology, Aurora, CO 80045. Offers microbiology (PhD); microbiology and immunology (PhD). *Students:* 16 full-time (7 women); includes 1 minority (Hispanic/Latino), 1 international. Average age 27. 57 applicants, 4% accepted, 2 enrolled. In 2015, 3 doctorates awarded. *Degree requirements:* For doctorate, comprehensive exam, thesis/dissertation, 3 lab rotations; 30 credit hours of coursework. *Entrance requirements:* For doctorate, GRE, three letters of reference, two copies of official transcripts, minimum GPA of 3.0. Additional exam requirements/recommendations for international students: Required—TOEFL (minimum score 550 paper-based; 80 iBT). *Application deadline:* For fall admission, 12/1 for domestic students, 11/1 for international students. Application fee: $50 ($75 for international students). Electronic applications accepted. *Expenses:* Contact institution. *Financial support:* In 2015–16, 17 students received support. Fellowships with tuition reimbursements available, research assistantships, teaching assistantships,

Immunology

institutionally sponsored loans, scholarships/grants, traineeships, health care benefits, and tuition waivers (full) available. Financial award application deadline: 3/15; financial award applicants required to submit FAFSA. *Faculty research:* Molecular mechanisms of picornavirus replication, mechanisms of papovavirus assembly, human immune response in multiple sclerosis. *Total annual research expenditures:* $5.9 million. *Unit head:* Dr. John Cambier, Chair, 303-724-8663, E-mail: john.cambier@ucdenver.edu. *Application contact:* Elizabeth Wethington, Program Administrator, 303-724-7280, E-mail: elizabeth.wethington@ucdenver.edu.
Website: http://www.ucdenver.edu/academics/colleges/medicalschool/departments/ImmunologyMicrobiology/Pages/welcome.aspx

University of Connecticut Health Center, Graduate School, Programs in Biomedical Sciences, Graduate Program in Immunology, Farmington, CT 06030. Offers PhD, DMD/PhD, MD/PhD. *Degree requirements:* For doctorate, comprehensive exam, thesis/dissertation. *Entrance requirements:* For doctorate, GRE General Test. Additional exam requirements/recommendations for international students: Required—TOEFL (minimum score 600 paper-based). Electronic applications accepted. *Faculty research:* Developmental immunology, T-cell immunity, lymphoid cell development, tolerance and tumor immunity, leukocyte chemotaxis.

See Display below and Close-Up on page 335.

University of Florida, College of Medicine and Graduate School, Interdisciplinary Program in Biomedical Sciences, Concentration in Immunology and Microbiology, Gainesville, FL 32611. Offers PhD. *Degree requirements:* For doctorate, thesis/dissertation. *Entrance requirements:* For doctorate, GRE General Test, minimum GPA of 3.0, biochemistry before enrollment. Additional exam requirements/recommendations for international students: Required—TOEFL. Electronic applications accepted.

University of Guelph, Ontario Veterinary College and Graduate Studies, Graduate Programs in Veterinary Sciences, Department of Pathobiology, Guelph, ON N1G 2W1, Canada. Offers anatomic pathology (DV Sc, Diploma); clinical pathology (Diploma); comparative pathology (M Sc, PhD); immunology (M Sc, PhD); laboratory animal science (DV Sc); pathology (M Sc, PhD, Diploma); veterinary infectious diseases (M Sc, PhD); zoo animal/wildlife medicine (DV Sc). *Degree requirements:* For master's, thesis; for doctorate, thesis/dissertation. *Entrance requirements:* For master's, DVM with B average or an honours degree in biological sciences; for doctorate, DVM or MSC degree, minimum B+ average. Additional exam requirements/recommendations for international students: Required—TOEFL (minimum score 550 paper-based). *Faculty research:* Pathogenesis; diseases of animals, wildlife, fish, and laboratory animals; parasitology; immunology; veterinary infectious diseases; laboratory animal science.

University of Illinois at Chicago, College of Medicine and Graduate College, Graduate Programs in Medicine, Department of Microbiology and Immunology, Chicago, IL 60607-7128. Offers PhD, MD/PhD. *Faculty:* 18 full-time (5 women), 10 part-time/adjunct (6 women). *Students:* 10 full-time (6 women); includes 2 minority (1 Hispanic/Latino; 1 Two or more races, non-Hispanic/Latino), 4 international. Average age 29. *Degree requirements:* For doctorate, thesis/dissertation. *Entrance requirements:* For doctorate, GRE General Test, minimum GPA of 2.75. Additional exam requirements/recommendations for international students: Required—TOEFL. *Application deadline:* For fall admission, 3/1 priority date for domestic students, 2/15 priority date for international students. Application fee: $60. *Expenses:* Tuition, state resident: full-time $11,480; part-time $3826 per credit. Tuition, nonresident: full-time $23,720; part-time $7906 per credit. *Required fees:* $1333 per semester. Part-time tuition and fees vary according to course load and program. *Financial support:* In 2015–16, 5 fellowships with full tuition reimbursements were awarded; research assistantships with full tuition reimbursements, teaching assistantships with full tuition reimbursements, Federal Work-Study, scholarships/grants, traineeships, tuition waivers (full), and unspecified

assistantships also available. Financial award application deadline: 3/1; financial award applicants required to submit FAFSA. *Faculty research:* Class I major histocompatibility complex molecules; proteins such as azurin with the immunoglobulin folds; T cell immunobiology relevant to disease pathogenesis, immunotherapeutics and vaccines for HIV/AIDS, tuberculosis, AIDS-related tuberculosis, and malaria, plague and smallpox; intracellular bacterial pathogen Listeria monocytogenes; virus infection. *Unit head:* Prof. Bellur S. Prabhakar, Department Head, 312-996-4915, Fax: 312-996-6415, E-mail: bprabkhar@uic.edu. *Application contact:* Mia Johnson, Admissions and Records Officer, 312-996-9477, Fax: 312-996-6415, E-mail: mimi@uic.edu.
Website: http://www.uic.edu/depts/mcmi/index.htm

The University of Iowa, Graduate College, Program in Immunology, Iowa City, IA 52242-1316. Offers PhD. *Degree requirements:* For doctorate, comprehensive exam, thesis/dissertation. *Entrance requirements:* For doctorate, GRE General Test, minimum GPA of 3.0. Additional exam requirements/recommendations for international students: Required—TOEFL (minimum score 600 paper-based; 100 iBT). Electronic applications accepted.

The University of Iowa, Roy J. and Lucille A. Carver College of Medicine and Graduate College, Graduate Programs in Medicine, Department of Microbiology, Iowa City, IA 52242-1316. Offers general microbiology and microbial physiology (MS, PhD); immunology (MS, PhD); microbial genetics (MS, PhD); pathogenic bacteriology (MS, PhD); virology (MS, PhD). *Degree requirements:* For master's, thesis; for doctorate, comprehensive exam, thesis/dissertation. *Entrance requirements:* For master's and doctorate, GRE General Test. Additional exam requirements/recommendations for international students: Required—TOEFL (minimum score 600 paper-based). Electronic applications accepted. *Faculty research:* Gene regulation, processing and transport of HIV, retroviral pathogenesis, biodegradation, biofilm.

University of Kentucky, Graduate School, Graduate School Programs from the College of Medicine, Program in Microbiology and Immunology, Lexington, KY 40506-0032. Offers PhD. *Degree requirements:* For doctorate, comprehensive exam, thesis/dissertation. *Entrance requirements:* For doctorate, GRE General Test, minimum undergraduate GPA of 2.75. Additional exam requirements/recommendations for international students: Required—TOEFL (minimum score 550 paper-based). Electronic applications accepted.

University of Louisville, School of Medicine, Department of Microbiology and Immunology, Louisville, KY 40292-0001. Offers MS, PhD, MD/PhD. *Program availability:* Part-time. *Students:* 38 full-time (20 women); includes 4 minority (1 Black or African American, non-Hispanic/Latino; 2 Hispanic/Latino; 1 Two or more races, non-Hispanic/Latino), 12 international. Average age 29. 55 applicants, 15% accepted, 7 enrolled. In 2015, 3 master's, 3 doctorates awarded. Terminal master's awarded for partial completion of doctoral program. *Median time to degree:* Of those who began their doctoral program in fall 2007, 100% received their degree in 8 years or less. *Degree requirements:* For master's, comprehensive exam, thesis or alternative; for doctorate, comprehensive exam, thesis/dissertation. *Entrance requirements:* For master's and doctorate, GRE General Test (minimum score of 300 verbal and quantitative), minimum GPA of 3.0; 1 year of course work in biology and organic chemistry; 1 semester of course work in introductory calculus and biochemistry. Additional exam requirements/recommendations for international students: Required—TOEFL (minimum score 550 paper-based; 79 iBT), IELTS (minimum score 6.5). *Application deadline:* For fall admission, 3/1 priority date for domestic and international students. Applications are processed on a rolling basis. Application fee: $60. Electronic applications accepted. *Expenses:* Tuition, state resident: full-time $11,664; part-time $649 per credit hour. Tuition, nonresident: full-time $24,274; part-time $1350 per credit hour. *Required fees:* $196. Tuition and fees vary according to program and reciprocity agreements. *Financial*

support: In 2015–16, 12 fellowships with full tuition reimbursements (averaging $25,500 per year), 15 research assistantships with full tuition reimbursements (averaging $25,500 per year) were awarded; health care benefits also available. Financial award application deadline: 3/1. *Faculty research:* Biodefense/emerging infectious diseases; autoimmune disease and basic immune mechanisms; bacterial and viral pathogenesis; vaccines; tumor immunity. *Total annual research expenditures:* $373,681. *Unit head:* Dr. Nejat Egilmez, Chair, 502-852-5351, Fax: 502-852-7531, E-mail: nejat.egilmez@louisville.edu. *Application contact:* Carolyn Burton, Graduate Program Coordinator, 502-852-6208, Fax: 502-852-7531, E-mail: cmburt01@louisville.edu.
Website: http://louisville.edu/medicine/departments/microbiology

The University of Manchester, Faculty of Life Sciences, Manchester, United Kingdom. Offers adaptive organismal biology (M Phil, PhD); animal biology (M Phil, PhD); biochemistry (M Phil, PhD); bioinformatics (M Phil, PhD); biomolecular sciences (M Phil, PhD); biotechnology (M Phil, PhD); cell biology (M Phil, PhD); cell matrix research (M Phil, PhD); channels and transporters (M Phil, PhD); developmental biology (M Phil, PhD); Egyptology (M Phil, PhD); environmental biology (M Phil, PhD); evolutionary biology (M Phil, PhD); gene expression (M Phil, PhD); genetics (M Phil, PhD); history of science, technology and medicine (M Phil, PhD); immunology (M Phil, PhD); integrative neurobiology and behavior (M Phil, PhD); membrane trafficking (M Phil, PhD); microbiology (M Phil, PhD); molecular and cellular neuroscience (M Phil, PhD); molecular biology (M Phil, PhD); molecular cancer studies (M Phil, PhD); neuroscience (M Phil, PhD); ophthalmology (M Phil, PhD); optometry (M Phil, PhD); organelle function (M Phil, PhD); pharmacology (M Phil, PhD); physiology (M Phil, PhD); plant sciences (M Phil, PhD); stem cell research (M Phil, PhD); structural biology (M Phil, PhD); systems neuroscience (M Phil, PhD); toxicology (M Phil, PhD).

University of Manitoba, Faculty of Medicine and Faculty of Graduate Studies, Graduate Programs in Medicine, Department of Immunology, Winnipeg, MB R3T 2N2, Canada. Offers M Sc, PhD. Terminal master's awarded for partial completion of doctoral program. *Degree requirements:* For master's, thesis; for doctorate, one foreign language, thesis/dissertation. *Faculty research:* Immediate hypersensitivity, regulation of the immune response, natural immunity, cytokines, inflammation.

University of Maryland, Baltimore, Graduate School, Graduate Program in Life Sciences, Program in Molecular Microbiology and Immunology, Baltimore, MD 21201. Offers PhD, MD/PhD. *Degree requirements:* For doctorate, comprehensive exam, thesis/dissertation. *Entrance requirements:* For doctorate, GRE. Additional exam requirements/recommendations for international students: Required—TOEFL (minimum score 550 paper-based; 80 iBT); Recommended—IELTS (minimum score 7). Electronic applications accepted. Tuition and fees vary according to program.

University of Massachusetts Medical School, Graduate School of Biomedical Sciences, Worcester, MA 01655-0115. Offers biomedical sciences (PhD), including biochemistry and molecular pharmacology, bioinformatics and computational biology, cancer biology, cell biology, immunology and microbiology, interdisciplinary, neuroscience, translational science; biomedical sciences (millennium program) (PhD); clinical and population health research (PhD); clinical investigation (MS). *Faculty:* 1,339 full-time (521 women), 301 part-time/adjunct (189 women). *Students:* 363 full-time (184 women); includes 58 minority (13 Black or African American, non-Hispanic/Latino; 30 Asian, non-Hispanic/Latino; 15 Hispanic/Latino), 141 international. Average age 29. 661 applicants, 26% accepted, 51 enrolled. In 2015, 10 master's, 58 doctorates awarded. Terminal master's awarded for partial completion of doctoral program. *Degree requirements:* For master's, comprehensive exam, thesis; for doctorate, comprehensive exam, thesis/dissertation. *Entrance requirements:* For master's, MD, PhD, DVM, or PharmD; for doctorate, GRE General Test, bachelor's degree. Additional exam requirements/recommendations for international students: Required—TOEFL (minimum score 100 iBT) or IELTS (minimum score 7.5). *Application deadline:* For fall admission, 12/15 for domestic and international students; for spring admission, 5/15 for domestic students. Application fee: $80. Electronic applications accepted. *Expenses:* $6,966 resident per year; $14,182 non-resident per year. *Financial support:* In 2015–16, 383 students received support, including research assistantships with full tuition reimbursements available (averaging $30,600 per year); scholarships/grants, health care benefits, tuition waivers (full), and unspecified assistantships also available. Financial award application deadline: 5/16. *Faculty research:* RNA interference, cell/molecular/developmental biology, bioinformatics, clinical/translational research, infectious disease. *Total annual research expenditures:* $250.3 million. *Unit head:* Dr. Anthony Carruthers, Dean, 508-856-4135, E-mail: anthony.carruthers@umassmed.edu. *Application contact:* Dr. Kendall Knight, Assistant Vice Provost for Admissions, 508-856-5628, Fax: 508-856-3659, E-mail: kendall.knight@umassmed.edu.
Website: http://www.umassmed.edu/gsbs/

University of Miami, Graduate School, Miller School of Medicine, Graduate Programs in Medicine, Department of Microbiology and Immunology, Coral Gables, FL 33124. Offers PhD, MD/PhD. *Degree requirements:* For doctorate, thesis/dissertation, oral and written qualifying exams. *Entrance requirements:* For doctorate, GRE General Test. Additional exam requirements/recommendations for international students: Required—TOEFL. Electronic applications accepted. *Faculty research:* Cellular and molecular immunology, molecular and pathogenic virology, pathogenic bacteriology and gene therapy of cancer.

University of Michigan, Rackham Graduate School, Program in Biomedical Sciences (PIBS), Department of Microbiology and Immunology, Ann Arbor, MI 48109. Offers MS, PhD. *Program availability:* Part-time. *Faculty:* 25 full-time (13 women), 13 part-time/adjunct (4 women). *Students:* 46 full-time (24 women); includes 8 minority (1 Black or African American, non-Hispanic/Latino; 1 American Indian or Alaska Native, non-Hispanic/Latino; 3 Asian, non-Hispanic/Latino; 3 Hispanic/Latino), 3 international. Average age 27. 128 applicants, 10% accepted, 6 enrolled. In 2015, 5 master's, 11 doctorates awarded. Terminal master's awarded for partial completion of doctoral program. *Degree requirements:* For master's, thesis optional; for doctorate, comprehensive exam, thesis/dissertation, oral defense of dissertation, preliminary exam. *Entrance requirements:* For master's and doctorate, GRE General Test. Additional exam requirements/recommendations for international students: Required—TOEFL (minimum score 600 paper-based; 84 iBT), TWE. *Application deadline:* For fall admission, 12/1 for domestic and international students. Application fee: $75. Electronic applications accepted. *Financial support:* In 2015–16, 15 fellowships with full tuition reimbursements (averaging $28,500 per year), 20 research assistantships with full tuition reimbursements (averaging $28,500 per year) were awarded; health care benefits and tuition waivers (full) also available. Financial award application deadline: 2/1. *Faculty research:* Mechanisms by which viruses, bacteria, fungi, and parasites elicit pathogenesis in the infected host; viral pathogens; bacterial pathogens; eukaryotic pathogens; innate immunity; adaptive immunity cell biology of infection. *Total annual research expenditures:* $10.2 million. *Unit head:* Dr. Harry L. T. Mobley, Chair, 734-764-1466, Fax: 734-764-3562, E-mail: hmobley@umich.edu. *Application contact:* Heidi Thompson, Senior Student Administrative Assistant, 734-763-3532, Fax: 734-764-3562, E-mail: heiditho@umich.edu.
Website: http://www.med.umich.edu/microbio/

University of Michigan, Rackham Graduate School, Program in Biomedical Sciences (PIBS), Program in Immunology, Ann Arbor, MI 48109-0619. Offers PhD. *Faculty:* 57

full-time (16 women). *Students:* 24 full-time (12 women); all minorities (2 Black or African American, non-Hispanic/Latino; 12 American Indian or Alaska Native, non-Hispanic/Latino; 4 Asian, non-Hispanic/Latino; 5 Hispanic/Latino; 1 Native Hawaiian or other Pacific Islander, non-Hispanic/Latino). Average age 28. 28 applicants, 32% accepted, 4 enrolled. In 2015, 6 doctorates awarded. *Degree requirements:* For doctorate, thesis/dissertation, oral defense of dissertation, preliminary exam. *Entrance requirements:* For doctorate, GRE General Test, 3 letters of recommendation, research experience, personal statement. Additional exam requirements/recommendations for international students: Required—TOEFL (minimum score 84 iBT). *Application deadline:* For fall admission, 12/1 for domestic students. Application fee: $75. Electronic applications accepted. *Expenses:* Contact institution. *Financial support:* In 2015–16, 24 students received support, including 15 fellowships with full tuition reimbursements available (averaging $29,025 per year), 9 research assistantships with full tuition reimbursements available (averaging $29,025 per year); scholarships/grants, health care benefits, tuition waivers (full), and unspecified assistantships also available. Financial award application deadline: 12/1. *Faculty research:* Cytokine networks, T and B cell activation, autoimmunity, antigen processing/ presentation, cell signaling. *Unit head:* Dr. Bethany Moore, Director, 734-647-8378, Fax: 734-615-2331, E-mail: bmoore@umich.edu. *Application contact:* Michelle S. Melis, Director of Student Life, 734-615-6538, Fax: 734-647-7022, E-mail: msmtegan@umich.edu.
Website: http://www.med.umich.edu/immprog/

University of Minnesota, Duluth, Medical School, Microbiology, Immunology and Molecular Pathobiology Section, Duluth, MN 55812-2496. Offers MS, PhD. MS, PhD offered jointly with University of Minnesota, Twin Cities Campus. Terminal master's awarded for partial completion of doctoral program. *Degree requirements:* For master's, thesis, final oral exam; for doctorate, thesis/dissertation, final exam, oral and written preliminary exams. *Entrance requirements:* For master's and doctorate, GRE General Test. Additional exam requirements/recommendations for international students: Required—TOEFL. *Faculty research:* Immunomodulation, molecular diagnosis of rabies, cytokines, cancer immunology, cytomegalovirus infection.

University of Minnesota, Twin Cities Campus, Graduate School, PhD Program in Microbiology, Immunology and Cancer Biology, Minneapolis, MN 55455-0213. Offers PhD. *Degree requirements:* For doctorate, thesis/dissertation. *Entrance requirements:* For doctorate, GRE General Test. Additional exam requirements/recommendations for international students: Required—TOEFL (minimum score 600 paper-based). Electronic applications accepted. *Faculty research:* Virology, microbiology, cancer biology, immunology.

University of Missouri, School of Medicine and Office of Research and Graduate Studies, Graduate Programs in Medicine, Department of Molecular Microbiology and Immunology, Columbia, MO 65211. Offers PhD. Terminal master's awarded for partial completion of doctoral program. *Degree requirements:* For doctorate, thesis/dissertation. *Entrance requirements:* For doctorate, GRE General Test, minimum GPA of 3.0. Additional exam requirements/recommendations for international students: Required—TOEFL (minimum score 580 paper-based; 92 iBT). *Application deadline:* For fall admission, 1/15 priority date for domestic and international students. Application fee: $55 ($75 for international students). Electronic applications accepted. *Financial support:* Fellowships, research assistantships, teaching assistantships, institutionally sponsored loans, scholarships/grants, traineeships, health care benefits, and unspecified assistantships available. Support available to part-time students. Financial award application deadline: 3/1.
Website: http://medicine.missouri.edu/education/phd.html

University of Montana, Graduate School, College of Humanities and Sciences, Division of Biological Sciences, Program in Cellular, Molecular and Microbial Biology, Missoula, MT 59812-0002. Offers cellular and developmental biology (PhD); microbial evolution and ecology (PhD); microbiology and immunology (PhD); molecular biology and biochemistry (PhD). Terminal master's awarded for partial completion of doctoral program. *Degree requirements:* For doctorate, variable foreign language requirement, thesis/dissertation. *Entrance requirements:* For doctorate, GRE General Test. *Faculty research:* Ribosome structure, medical microbiology/pathogenesis, microbial ecology/environmental microbiology.

The University of North Carolina at Chapel Hill, School of Medicine and Graduate School, Graduate Programs in Medicine, Department of Microbiology and Immunology, Chapel Hill, NC 27599-7290. Offers immunology (MS, PhD); microbiology (MS, PhD). Terminal master's awarded for partial completion of doctoral program. *Degree requirements:* For master's, comprehensive exam, thesis; for doctorate, comprehensive exam, thesis/dissertation. *Entrance requirements:* For master's and doctorate, GRE General Test, minimum GPA of 3.0. Electronic applications accepted. *Faculty research:* HIV pathogenesis, immune response, t-cell mediated autoimmunity, alpha-viruses, bacterial chemotaxis, francisella tularensis, pertussis, Mycobacterium tuberculosis, Burkholderia, Dengue virus.

University of North Dakota, Graduate School and Graduate School, Graduate Programs in Medicine, Department of Microbiology and Immunology, Grand Forks, ND 58202. Offers MS, PhD. *Degree requirements:* For master's, comprehensive exam, thesis or alternative; for doctorate, comprehensive exam, thesis/dissertation, final examination. *Entrance requirements:* For master's and doctorate, GRE General Test, minimum GPA of 3.0. Additional exam requirements/recommendations for international students: Required—TOEFL (minimum score 550 paper-based; 79 iBT), IELTS (minimum score 6.5). Electronic applications accepted. *Faculty research:* Genetic and immunological aspects of a murine model of human multiple sclerosis, termination of DNA replication, cell division in bacteria, yersinia pestis.

University of North Texas Health Science Center at Fort Worth, Graduate School of Biomedical Sciences, Fort Worth, TX 76107-2699. Offers anatomy and cell biology (MS, PhD); biochemistry and molecular biology (MS, PhD); biomedical sciences (MS, PhD); biotechnology (MS); forensic genetics (MS); integrative physiology (MS, PhD); medical science (MS); microbiology and immunology (MS, PhD); pharmacology (MS, PhD); science education (MS); DO/MS; DO/PhD. Terminal master's awarded for partial completion of doctoral program. *Degree requirements:* For master's, thesis; for doctorate, thesis/dissertation. *Entrance requirements:* For master's and doctorate, GRE General Test. Additional exam requirements/recommendations for international students: Required—TOEFL. *Expenses:* Contact institution. *Faculty research:* Alzheimer's disease, aging, eye diseases, cancer, cardiovascular disease.

University of Oklahoma Health Sciences Center, College of Medicine and Graduate College, Graduate Programs in Medicine, Department of Microbiology and Immunology, Oklahoma City, OK 73190. Offers immunology (MS, PhD); microbiology (MS, PhD). *Program availability:* Part-time. Terminal master's awarded for partial completion of doctoral program. *Degree requirements:* For master's, thesis or alternative; for doctorate, one foreign language, thesis/dissertation. *Entrance requirements:* For doctorate, GRE General Test, 3 letters of recommendation. Additional exam requirements/recommendations for international students: Required—TOEFL. *Faculty research:* Molecular genetics, pathogenesis, streptococcal infections, gram-positive virulence, monoclonal antibodies.

University of Ottawa, Faculty of Graduate and Postdoctoral Studies, Faculty of Medicine, Department of Biochemistry, Microbiology and Immunology, Ottawa, ON K1N 6N5, Canada. Offers biochemistry (M Sc, PhD); microbiology and immunology (M Sc, PhD). *Degree requirements:* For master's, thesis; for doctorate, comprehensive exam, thesis/dissertation, seminar. *Entrance requirements:* For master's, honors degree or equivalent, minimum B average; for doctorate, master's degree, minimum B+ average. Electronic applications accepted. *Faculty research:* General biochemistry, molecular biology, microbiology, host biology, nutrition and metabolism.

University of Pennsylvania, Perelman School of Medicine, Biomedical Graduate Studies, Graduate Group in Immunology, Philadelphia, PA 19104. Offers PhD, MD/PhD, VMD/PhD. *Faculty:* 113. *Students:* 55 full-time (23 women); includes 21 minority (1 Black or African American, non-Hispanic/Latino; 1 American Indian or Alaska Native, non-Hispanic/Latino; 13 Asian, non-Hispanic/Latino; 1 Hispanic/Latino; 5 Two or more races, non-Hispanic/Latino), 4 international. 123 applicants, 19% accepted, 9 enrolled. In 2015, 11 doctorates awarded. *Degree requirements:* For doctorate, thesis/dissertation, 2 preliminary exams. *Entrance requirements:* For doctorate, GRE General Test, undergraduate major in natural or physical science. Additional exam requirements/recommendations for international students: Required—TOEFL. *Application deadline:* For fall admission, 12/1 for domestic and international students. Applications are processed on a rolling basis. Application fee: $80. Electronic applications accepted. *Expenses: Tuition, area resident:* Full-time $31,068; part-time $5762 per course. *Required fees:* $3200; $336 per course. Full-time tuition and fees vary according to degree level, program and student level. Part-time tuition and fees vary according to course load, degree level and program. *Financial support:* In 2015–16, 55 students received support. Fellowships, research assistantships, scholarships/grants, traineeships, and unspecified assistantships available. *Faculty research:* Immunoglobulin structure and function, cell surface receptors, lymphocyte functional transplantation immunology, cellular immunology, molecular biology of immunoglobulins. *Unit head:* Dr. David Allman, Chair, 215-746-5547. *Application contact:* Mary Taylor, Graduate Coordinator, 215-573-4394.
Website: http://www.med.upenn.edu/immun

University of Pittsburgh, School of Medicine, Graduate Programs in Medicine, Immunology Graduate Program, Pittsburgh, PA 15260. Offers PhD. *Faculty:* 58 full-time (19 women). *Students:* 28 full-time (16 women); includes 15 minority (1 Black or African American, non-Hispanic/Latino; 10 Asian, non-Hispanic/Latino; 2 Hispanic/Latino; 2 Two or more races, non-Hispanic/Latino). Average age 29. 386 applicants, 17% accepted, 25 enrolled. In 2015, 4 doctorates awarded. *Degree requirements:* For doctorate, comprehensive exam, thesis/dissertation. *Entrance requirements:* For doctorate, GRE General Test, GRE Subject Test, minimum QPA of 3.0. Additional exam requirements/recommendations for international students: Required—TOEFL (minimum score 600 paper-based; 100 iBT), IELTS (minimum score 7). *Application deadline:* For fall admission, 12/1 priority date for domestic and international students. Application fee: $50. Electronic applications accepted. Tuition and fees vary according to program. *Financial support:* In 2015–16, 28 students received support, including 13 fellowships with full tuition reimbursements available (averaging $27,000 per year), 15 research assistantships with full tuition reimbursements available (averaging $27,000 per year); teaching assistantships, scholarships/grants, traineeships, and health care benefits also available. *Faculty research:* Human T-cell biology, opportunistic infections associated with AIDS, autoimmunity, immunoglobin gene expression, tumor immunology. *Unit head:* Dr. Robert Binder, Program Director, 412-383-7722, E-mail: rjb42@pitt.edu. *Application contact:* Carol Williams, Admissions and Recruiting Manager, 412-648-8957, Fax: 412-648-1007, E-mail: gradstudies@medschool.pitt.edu.
Website: http://www.gradbiomed.pitt.edu

University of Prince Edward Island, Atlantic Veterinary College, Graduate Program in Veterinary Medicine, Charlottetown, PE C1A 4P3, Canada. Offers anatomy (M Sc, PhD); bacteriology (M Sc, PhD); clinical pharmacology (M Sc, PhD); clinical sciences (M Sc, PhD); epidemiology (M Sc, PhD), including reproduction; fish health (M Sc, PhD); food animal nutrition (M Sc, PhD); immunology (M Sc, PhD); microanatomy (M Sc, PhD); parasitology (M Sc, PhD); pathology (M Sc, PhD); pharmacology (M Sc, PhD); physiology (M Sc, PhD); toxicology (M Sc, PhD); veterinary science (M Vet Sc); virology (M Sc, PhD). *Program availability:* Part-time. *Degree requirements:* For master's, thesis; for doctorate, thesis/dissertation. *Entrance requirements:* For master's, DVM, B Sc honors degree, or equivalent; for doctorate, M Sc. Additional exam requirements/recommendations for international students: Required—TOEFL (minimum score 550 paper-based; 80 iBT). *Expenses:* Contact institution. *Faculty research:* Animal health management, infectious diseases, fin fish and shellfish health, basic biomedical sciences, ecosystem health.

University of Rochester, School of Medicine and Dentistry, Graduate Programs in Medicine and Dentistry, Department of Microbiology and Immunology, Program in Microbiology and Immunology, Rochester, NY 14627. Offers MS, PhD. *Expenses: Tuition, area resident:* Full-time $47,450; part-time $1482 per credit hour. *Required fees:* $528. Tuition and fees vary according to program.

University of Saskatchewan, College of Medicine, Department of Microbiology and Immunology, Saskatoon, SK S7N 5A2, Canada. Offers M Sc, PhD. *Degree requirements:* For master's, thesis; for doctorate, thesis/dissertation. *Entrance requirements:* Additional exam requirements/recommendations for international students: Required—TOEFL.

The University of South Dakota, Graduate School, Sanford School of Medicine and Graduate School, Biomedical Sciences Graduate Program, Molecular Microbiology and Immunology Group, Vermillion, SD 57069-2390. Offers MS, PhD. Terminal master's awarded for partial completion of doctoral program. *Degree requirements:* For master's, thesis; for doctorate, comprehensive exam, thesis/dissertation. *Entrance requirements:* For master's and doctorate, GRE General Test, minimum GPA of 3.0. Additional exam requirements/recommendations for international students: Required—TOEFL (minimum score 550 paper-based; 80 iBT), IELTS (minimum score 6). *Application deadline:* For fall admission, 4/15 priority date for domestic students, 3/15 for international students. Applications are processed on a rolling basis. Application fee: $35. Electronic applications accepted. *Expenses:* Contact institution. *Financial support:* In 2015–16, 6 students received support. Fellowships with partial tuition reimbursements available, research assistantships with partial tuition reimbursements available, and unspecified assistantships available. Financial award application deadline: 4/15; financial award applicants required to submit FAFSA. *Faculty research:* Structure-function membranes, plasmids, immunology, virology, pathogenesis. *Total annual research expenditures:* $325,000. *Unit head:* 605-658-6322, Fax: 605-677-6381, E-mail: biomed@usd.edu.

University of Southern California, Keck School of Medicine and Graduate School, Graduate Programs in Medicine, Department of Molecular Microbiology and Immunology, Los Angeles, CA 90033. Offers MS. *Program availability:* Part-time. *Faculty:* 23 full-time (5 women), 1 (woman) part-time/adjunct. *Students:* 16 full-time (10 women); includes 2 minority (both Asian, non-Hispanic/Latino), 12 international. Average age 24. 34 applicants, 65% accepted, 6 enrolled. In 2015, 16 degrees awarded. *Degree requirements:* For master's, comprehensive exam (for some programs), thesis optional. *Entrance requirements:* For master's, GRE General Test, minimum GPA of 3.0. Additional exam requirements/recommendations for international students: Required—

TOEFL (minimum score 100 iBT), IELTS. *Application deadline:* For fall admission, 6/1 for domestic students, 5/1 for international students; for spring admission, 11/1 for domestic students, 10/1 for international students. Applications are processed on a rolling basis. Application fee: $85. Electronic applications accepted. *Expenses:* Contact institution. *Financial support:* Federal Work-Study, institutionally sponsored loans, and scholarships/grants available. Financial award application deadline: 3/2; financial award applicants required to submit FAFSA. *Faculty research:* Animal virology, microbial genetics, molecular and cellular immunology, cellular differentiation control of protein synthesis, HIV. *Unit head:* Dr. Axel H. Schonthal, Associate Professor/Program Chairman, 323-442-1730, Fax: 323-442-1721, E-mail: schontha@usc.edu. *Application contact:* Silvina V. Campos, Administrative Assistant II, 323-442-1713, Fax: 323-442-1721, E-mail: scampos@usc.edu.
Website: http://keck.usc.edu/molecular-microbiology-and-immunology/

University of Southern Maine, College of Science, Technology, and Health, Program in Applied Medical Sciences, Portland, ME 04103. Offers MS. *Program availability:* Part-time. *Degree requirements:* For master's, thesis. *Entrance requirements:* For master's, GRE General Test, minimum GPA of 3.0. Additional exam requirements/recommendations for international students: Required—TOEFL. Electronic applications accepted. *Expenses: Tuition, area resident:* Full-time $6840; part-time $380 per credit hour. Tuition, state resident: full-time $10,260; part-time $570 per credit hour. Tuition, nonresident: full-time $18,468; part-time $1026 per credit hour. *Required fees:* $830; $83 per credit hour. Tuition and fees vary according to course load and program. *Faculty research:* Cancer biology, toxicology, environmental health, epidemiology, autoimmune disease, immunology, infectious disease, virology.

University of South Florida, Morsani College of Medicine and College of Graduate Studies, Graduate Programs in Medical Sciences, Tampa, FL 33620-9951. Offers advanced athletic training (MS); athletic training (MS); bioinformatics and computational biology (MSBCB); biotechnology (MSB); health informatics (MSHI); medical sciences (MSMS, PhD), including aging and neuroscience (MSMS), allergy, immunology and infectious disease (PhD), anatomy, athletic training (MSMS), clinical and translational research, health informatics (MSMS), health science (MSMS), interdisciplinary medical sciences (MSMS), medical microbiology and immunology (MSMS), metabolic and nutritional medicine (MSMS), molecular medicine, molecular pharmacology and physiology (PhD), neurology (PhD), pathology and laboratory medicine (PhD), pharmacology and therapeutics (PhD), physiology and biophysics (PhD), women's health (MSMS). *Students:* 510 full-time (261 women), 318 part-time (208 women); includes 360 minority (108 Black or African American, non-Hispanic/Latino; 3 American Indian or Alaska Native, non-Hispanic/Latino; 101 Asian, non-Hispanic/Latino; 124 Hispanic/Latino; 1 Native Hawaiian or other Pacific Islander, non-Hispanic/Latino; 23 Two or more races, non-Hispanic/Latino), 52 international. Average age 26. 6,567 applicants, 13% accepted, 469 enrolled. In 2015, 216 master's awarded. Terminal master's awarded for partial completion of doctoral program. *Degree requirements:* For master's, comprehensive exam, thesis; for doctorate, comprehensive exam, thesis/dissertation. *Entrance requirements:* For master's, GRE General Test or GMAT, bachelor's degree or equivalent from regionally-accredited university with minimum GPA of 3.0 in upper-division sciences coursework; prerequisites in general biology, general chemistry, general physics, organic chemistry, quantitative analysis, and integral and differential calculus; for doctorate, GRE General Test, bachelor's degree from regionally-accredited university with minimum GPA of 3.0 in upper-division sciences coursework; 3 letters of recommendation; personal interview; 1-2 page personal statement; prerequisites in biology, chemistry, physics, organic chemistry, quantitative analysis, and integral/differential calculus. Additional exam requirements/recommendations for international students: Required—TOEFL (minimum score 550 paper-based; 79 iBT) or IELTS (minimum score 6.5). *Application deadline:* For fall admission, 2/15 for domestic students, 1/2 for international students. Application fee: $30. *Expenses:* Contact institution. *Faculty research:* Anatomy, biochemistry, cancer biology, cardiovascular disease, cell biology, immunology, microbiology, molecular biology, neuroscience, pharmacology, physiology. *Unit head:* Dr. Michael Barber, Professor/Associate Dean for Graduate and Postdoctoral Affairs, 813-974-9908, Fax: 813-974-4317, E-mail: mbarber@health.usf.edu. *Application contact:* Dr. Eric Bennett, Graduate Director, PhD Program in Medical Sciences, 813-974-1545, Fax: 813-974-4317, E-mail: esbennet@health.usf.edu.
Website: http://health.usf.edu/nocms/medicine/graduatestudies/

The University of Texas Health Science Center at Houston, Graduate School of Biomedical Sciences, Program in Immunology, Houston, TX 77225-0036. Offers MS, PhD, MD/PhD. Terminal master's awarded for partial completion of doctoral program. *Degree requirements:* For master's, thesis; for doctorate, thesis/dissertation. *Entrance requirements:* For master's and doctorate, GRE General Test. Additional exam requirements/recommendations for international students: Required—TOEFL. Electronic applications accepted. *Faculty research:* Cancer immunology, molecular immunology, immune cell signaling, immune disease, immune system development.

The University of Texas Health Science Center at San Antonio, Graduate School of Biomedical Sciences, Department of Microbiology and Immunology, San Antonio, TX 78229-3900. Offers MS, PhD. *Degree requirements:* For master's, thesis; for doctorate, comprehensive exam, thesis/dissertation.

The University of Texas Medical Branch, Graduate School of Biomedical Sciences, Program in Microbiology and Immunology, Galveston, TX 77555. Offers MS, PhD. Terminal master's awarded for partial completion of doctoral program. *Degree requirements:* For master's, thesis or alternative; for doctorate, thesis/dissertation. *Entrance requirements:* For doctorate, GRE General Test, minimum GPA of 3.0. Additional exam requirements/recommendations for international students: Required—TOEFL (minimum score 550 paper-based). Electronic applications accepted.

The University of Texas Southwestern Medical Center, Southwestern Graduate School of Biomedical Sciences, Division of Basic Science, Program in Immunology, Dallas, TX 75390. Offers PhD. *Degree requirements:* For doctorate, thesis/dissertation, qualifying exam. *Entrance requirements:* For doctorate, GRE General Test, minimum GPA of 3.0. Additional exam requirements/recommendations for international students: Required—TOEFL. Electronic applications accepted. *Faculty research:* Antibody diversity and idiotype, cytotoxic effector mechanisms, natural killer cells, biology of immunoglobulins, oncogenes.

The University of Toledo, College of Graduate Studies, College of Medicine and Life Sciences, Department of Medical Microbiology and Immunology, Toledo, OH 43606-3390. Offers infection, immunity, and transplantation (MSBS, PhD); MD/MSBS; MD/PhD. Terminal master's awarded for partial completion of doctoral program. *Degree requirements:* For master's, thesis, qualifying exam; for doctorate, thesis/dissertation, qualifying exam. *Entrance requirements:* For master's and doctorate, GRE, minimum undergraduate GPA of 3.0, three letters of recommendation, statement of purpose, transcripts from all prior institutions attended, resume. Additional exam requirements/recommendations for international students: Required—TOEFL (minimum score 550 paper-based; 80 iBT). Electronic applications accepted.

University of Toronto, Faculty of Medicine, Department of Immunology, Toronto, ON M5S 1A1, Canada. Offers M Sc, PhD, MD/PhD. *Degree requirements:* For master's, thesis, thesis defense; for doctorate, thesis/dissertation, thesis defense. *Entrance requirements:* For master's, resume, 3 letters of reference. Additional exam requirements/recommendations for international students: Required—TOEFL (minimum score 580 paper-based; 93 iBT), TWE (minimum score 5). Electronic applications accepted.

University of Washington, Graduate School, School of Medicine, Graduate Programs in Medicine, Department of Immunology, Seattle, WA 98109-8059. Offers PhD. *Degree requirements:* For doctorate, thesis/dissertation, 1st-authored paper, accepted for publication. *Entrance requirements:* For doctorate, GRE General Test, BA or BS in related field. Additional exam requirements/recommendations for international students: Required—TOEFL (minimum score 600 paper-based; 100 iBT). Electronic applications accepted. *Faculty research:* Molecular and cellular immunology, regulation of lymphocyte differentiation and responses, genetics of immune recognition genetics and pathogenesis of autoimmune diseases, signal transduction.

The University of Western Ontario, Faculty of Graduate Studies, Biosciences Division, Department of Microbiology and Immunology, London, ON N6A 5B8, Canada. Offers M Sc, PhD. *Degree requirements:* For master's, thesis, oral and written exam; for doctorate, thesis/dissertation, oral and written exam. *Entrance requirements:* For master's, honors degree or equivalent in microbiology, immunology, or other biological science; minimum B average; for doctorate, M Sc in microbiology and immunology. Additional exam requirements/recommendations for international students: Required—TOEFL. *Faculty research:* Virology, molecular pathogenesis, cellular immunology, molecular biology.

University of Wisconsin–Milwaukee, Graduate School, College of Health Sciences, Program in Biomedical Sciences, Milwaukee, WI 53211. Offers cancer (MS); immunology (MS); microbiology (MS); neurodegenerative disease (MS); pharmacology and toxicology (MS); photobiomodulation (MS). *Accreditation:* NAACLS. *Program availability:* Part-time. *Faculty:* 8 full-time (4 women). *Students:* 8 full-time (7 women), 3 part-time (1 woman); includes 1 minority (Two or more races, non-Hispanic/Latino), 2 international. Average age 29. 42 applicants, 14% accepted, 4 enrolled. In 2015, 7 master's awarded. *Degree requirements:* For master's, thesis. *Entrance requirements:* For master's, GRE General Test. Additional exam requirements/recommendations for international students: Required—TOEFL (minimum score 550 paper-based; 79 iBT), IELTS (minimum score 6.5). *Application deadline:* For fall admission, 1/1 priority date for domestic students; for spring admission, 9/1 for domestic students. Applications are processed on a rolling basis. Application fee: $56 ($96 for international students). *Financial support:* In 2015–16, 6 teaching assistantships were awarded; fellowships, research assistantships, career-related internships or fieldwork, and unspecified assistantships also available. Support available to part-time students. Financial award application deadline: 4/15. *Unit head:* Raymond Fleming, Representative, 414-229-3980, E-mail: mundo@uwm.edu. *Application contact:* Roger O. Smith, General Information Contact, 414-229-6697, Fax: 414-229-6697, E-mail: smithro@uwm.edu. Website: http://www4.uwm.edu/chs/academics/biomedical_sciences/bms_masters/

Vanderbilt University, School of Medicine, Department of Microbiology and Immunology, Nashville, TN 37240-1001. Offers MS, PhD, MD/PhD. *Faculty:* 39 full-time (13 women). *Students:* 61 full-time (36 women); includes 10 minority (3 Black or African American, non-Hispanic/Latino; 1 American Indian or Alaska Native, non-Hispanic/Latino; 2 Asian, non-Hispanic/Latino; 2 Hispanic/Latino; 2 Two or more races, non-Hispanic/Latino), 8 international. Average age 27. In 2015, 2 master's, 6 doctorates awarded. Terminal master's awarded for partial completion of doctoral program. *Degree requirements:* For master's, thesis; for doctorate, thesis/dissertation, final and qualifying exams. *Entrance requirements:* For master's and doctorate, GRE General Test, GRE Subject Test (recommended). Additional exam requirements/recommendations for international students: Required—TOEFL (minimum score 570 paper-based; 88 iBT). *Application deadline:* For fall admission, 1/15 for domestic and international students. Application fee: $0. Electronic applications accepted. *Financial support:* Fellowships with full tuition reimbursements, research assistantships with full tuition reimbursements, Federal Work-Study, institutionally sponsored loans, scholarships/grants, traineeships, health care benefits, and tuition waivers (partial) available. Financial award application deadline: 1/15; financial award applicants required to submit CSS PROFILE or FAFSA. *Faculty research:* Cellular and molecular microbiology, viruses, genes, cancer, molecular pathogenesis of microbial diseases, immunobiology. *Unit head:* Dr. Christopher Aiken, Director of Graduate Studies, 615-322-2087, Fax: 615-322-5551, E-mail: chris.aiken@vanderbilt.edu. *Application contact:* Walter B. Bieschke, Program Coordinator for Graduate Admissions, 615-342-0236, E-mail: walter.bieschke@vanderbilt.edu.
Website: http://www.mc.vanderbilt.edu/root/vumc.php?site-vmcpathology

Virginia Commonwealth University, Medical College of Virginia-Professional Programs, School of Medicine, School of Medicine Graduate Programs, Department of Microbiology and Immunology, Richmond, VA 23284-9005. Offers microbiology and immunology (MS, PhD); MD/PhD. *Degree requirements:* For master's, thesis; for doctorate, thesis/dissertation, comprehensive oral and written exams. *Entrance requirements:* For master's and doctorate, GRE General Test or MCAT. Additional exam requirements/recommendations for international students: Required—TOEFL (minimum score 600 paper-based; 100 iBT). Electronic applications accepted. *Faculty research:* Microbial physiology and genetics, molecular biology, crystallography of biological molecules, antibiotics and chemotherapy, membrane transport.

Wake Forest University, School of Medicine and Graduate School of Arts and Sciences, Graduate Programs in Medicine, Department of Microbiology and Immunology, Winston-Salem, NC 27109. Offers PhD, MD/PhD. *Degree requirements:* For doctorate, thesis/dissertation. *Entrance requirements:* For doctorate, GRE General Test. Additional exam requirements/recommendations for international students: Required—TOEFL. Electronic applications accepted. *Faculty research:* Molecular immunology, bacterial pathogenesis and molecular genetics, viral pathogenesis, regulation of mRNA metabolism, leukocyte biology.

Washington State University, College of Veterinary Medicine, Paul G. Allen School for Global Animal Health, Pullman, WA 99164. Offers immunology and infectious diseases (MS, PhD). *Program availability:* Part-time. *Faculty:* 14 full-time (4 women), 13 part-time/adjunct (6 women). *Students:* 20 full-time (9 women); includes 2 minority (1 Black or African American, non-Hispanic/Latino; 1 Native Hawaiian or other Pacific Islander, non-Hispanic/Latino). Average age 30. 2 applicants, 100% accepted, 2 enrolled. In 2015, 1 doctorate awarded. Terminal master's awarded for partial completion of doctoral program. *Degree requirements:* For master's, thesis, 30 credits of course work; for doctorate, thesis/dissertation, 15 credits of course work. *Entrance requirements:* Additional exam requirements/recommendations for international students: Required—TOEFL (minimum score 550 paper-based; 80 iBT), IELTS (7.0), or Michigan English Language Assessment Battery. *Application deadline:* For fall admission, 1/10 priority date for domestic and international students; for spring admission, 7/1 priority date for domestic and international students. Application fee: $75. Electronic applications accepted. *Financial support:* In 2015–16, 13 students received support, including 2 fellowships with full tuition reimbursements available (averaging $7,000 per year), 10 research assistantships with full tuition reimbursements available (averaging $23,544 per year), 1 teaching assistantship (averaging $21,738 per year); scholarships/grants

and health care benefits also available. Financial award application deadline: 1/1; financial award applicants required to submit FAFSA. *Faculty research:* Immunology, infectious disease, virology, disease surveillance, vaccine development. *Total annual research expenditures:* $6.8 million. *Unit head:* Dr. Guy H. Palmer, Director, Paul G. Allen School for Global Animal Health, 509-335-5861, Fax: 509-335-6328, E-mail: gpalmer@vetmed.wsu.edu. *Application contact:* Jill Griffin, Administrative Manager, 509-335-5861, Fax: 509-335-6328, E-mail: griffinj@vetmed.wsu.edu.
Website: http://globalhealth.wsu.edu/

Washington State University, College of Veterinary Medicine, Program in Immunology and Infectious Diseases, Pullman, WA 99164. Offers veterinary science (MS, PhD). *Faculty:* 22 full-time (7 women), 43 part-time/adjunct (19 women). *Students:* 39 full-time (26 women); includes 5 minority (2 Black or African American, non-Hispanic/Latino; 1 Asian, non-Hispanic/Latino; 2 Hispanic/Latino), 14 international. Average age 31. 47 applicants, 11% accepted, 5 enrolled. In 2015, 1 master's, 8 doctorates awarded. Terminal master's awarded for partial completion of doctoral program. *Degree requirements:* For master's, thesis, oral exam; for doctorate, thesis/dissertation, oral exam. *Entrance requirements:* For master's and doctorate, minimum GPA of 3.0. Additional exam requirements/recommendations for international students: Required—TOEFL (minimum score 550 paper-based; 80 iBT). *Application deadline:* Applications are processed on a rolling basis. Application fee: $75. Electronic applications accepted. *Financial support:* In 2015–16, 17 fellowships, 20 research assistantships, 2 teaching assistantships were awarded; institutionally sponsored loans, scholarships/grants, traineeships, health care benefits, and unspecified assistantships also available. Financial award application deadline: 3/1. *Faculty research:* Microbial pathogenesis, veterinary and wildlife parasitology, laboratory animal pathology, immune responses to infectious diseases. *Unit head:* Dr. Michele E. Hardy, Chair, 509-335-6030, Fax: 509-335-8529, E-mail: mhardy@votmed.wsu.edu. *Application contact:* Sue Zumwalt, Graduate Coordinator, 509-335-6027, Fax: 509-335-8529, E-mail: szumwalt@vetmed.wsu.edu.
Website: http://vmp.vetmed.wsu.edu/graduate-programs/master-phd

Washington University in St. Louis, Graduate School of Arts and Sciences, Division of Biology and Biomedical Sciences, Program in Immunology, St. Louis, MO 63130-4899. Offers PhD. *Students:* 66 full-time (27 women); includes 24 minority (2 Black or African American, non-Hispanic/Latino; 1 American Indian or Alaska Native, non-Hispanic/Latino; 17 Asian, non-Hispanic/Latino; 2 Hispanic/Latino; 2 Two or more races, non-Hispanic/Latino), 15 international. 92 applicants, 18% accepted, 6 enrolled. In 2015, 14 doctorates awarded. *Degree requirements:* For doctorate, thesis/dissertation. *Entrance requirements:* For doctorate, GRE General Test, GRE Subject Test. Additional exam requirements/recommendations for international students: Required—TOEFL. *Application deadline:* For fall admission, 12/1 priority date for domestic students. Application fee: $0. Electronic applications accepted. *Financial support:* Fellowships, research assistantships, and teaching assistantships available. Financial award application deadline: 1/15. *Faculty research:* Cellular immunology, molecular immunology, lineage development, autoimmunity, cancer immunotherapy, transcription factors, epigenomics, mucosal immunity, innate immunity, bacterial, viral, and parasite immunity, immune evasion, antigen processing and presentation, dendritic cells, T cell signaling, antigen receptor diversification. *Unit head:* Melanie Relich, Coordinator, 314-362-2763. *Application contact:* Rebecca Riney, 314-747-4648, E-mail: dbbsphdadmissions@wusm.wustl.edu.

Wayne State University, School of Medicine, Office of Biomedical Graduate Programs, Department of Immunology and Microbiology, Detroit, MI 48202. Offers MS, PhD, MD/PhD. *Faculty:* 11. *Students:* 8 full-time (3 women), 1 part-time (0 women); includes 4 minority (1 Black or African American, non-Hispanic/Latino; 1 Asian, non-Hispanic/Latino; 1 Hispanic/Latino; 1 Two or more races, non-Hispanic/Latino). Average age 29. 94 applicants, 5% accepted, 4 enrolled. In 2015, 2 master's, 3 doctorates awarded. *Degree requirements:* For master's, thesis; for doctorate, thesis/dissertation. *Entrance requirements:* For master's and doctorate, GRE, minimum GPA of 3.0 in BS in biology or related scientific discipline, three letters of recommendation, statement of purpose. Additional exam requirements/recommendations for international students: Required—TOEFL (minimum score 100 iBT). *Application deadline:* For fall admission, 2/1 priority date for domestic and international students. Application fee: $0. Electronic applications accepted. *Expenses:* $17,645 annual resident tuition, $33,311 non-resident tuition; $735.20 per credit hour resident tuition, $1,387.95 per credit hour non-resident tuition; fees include $47.45 per credit hour student services fee and $274.60 per semester registration fee. *Financial support:* In 2015–16, 8 students received support, including 2 fellowships with tuition reimbursements available (averaging $26,614 per year), 5 research assistantships with tuition reimbursements available (averaging $26,716 per year); scholarships/grants, health care benefits, and unspecified assistantships also available. Financial award application deadline: 3/31. *Faculty research:* Viral replication and pathogenesis, bacterial pathogenesis, mucosal immunity, autoimmune diseases. *Unit head:* Dr. T.R. Reddy, Department Graduate Officer, 313-577-1591, Fax: 313-577-1155, E-mail: trreddy@med.wayne.edu.
Website: http://www.immunomicro.med.wayne.edu/gradprogram.php

Weill Cornell Medicine, Weill Cornell Graduate School of Medical Sciences, Immunology and Microbial Pathogenesis Program, New York, NY 10065. Offers immunology (MS, PhD), including immunology, microbiology, pathology. Terminal master's awarded for partial completion of doctoral program. *Degree requirements:* For master's, comprehensive exam; for doctorate, thesis/dissertation, final exam. *Entrance requirements:* For doctorate, GRE General Test, laboratory research experience, course work in biological sciences. Additional exam requirements/recommendations for international students: Required—TOEFL. Electronic applications accepted. *Faculty research:* Microbial immunity, tumor immunology, lymphocyte and leukocyte biology, auto immunity, stem cell/bone marrow transplantation.

West Virginia University, Davis College of Agriculture, Forestry and Consumer Sciences, Interdisciplinary Program in Genetics and Developmental Biology, Morgantown, WV 26506. Offers animal breeding (MS, PhD); biochemical and molecular genetics (MS, PhD); cytogenetics (MS, PhD); descriptive embryology (MS, PhD); developmental genetics (MS); experimental morphogenesis/teratology (MS); human genetics (MS, PhD); immunogenetics (MS, PhD); life cycles of animals and plants (MS, PhD); molecular aspects of development (MS, PhD); mutagenesis (MS, PhD); oncology (MS, PhD); plant genetics (MS, PhD); population and quantitative genetics (MS, PhD); regeneration (MS, PhD); teratology (PhD); toxicology (MS, PhD). *Degree requirements:* For master's, thesis; for doctorate, comprehensive exam, thesis/dissertation. *Entrance requirements:* For master's, GRE or MCAT, minimum GPA of 2.75. Additional exam requirements/recommendations for international students: Required—TOEFL. *Expenses:* Tuition, state resident: full-time $8568. Tuition, nonresident: full-time $22,140. Tuition and fees vary according to program.

West Virginia University, School of Medicine, Graduate Programs at the Health Sciences Center, Interdisciplinary Graduate Programs in Biomedical Sciences, Program in Immunology and Microbial Pathogenesis, Morgantown, WV 26506. Offers MS, PhD, MD/PhD. *Degree requirements:* For doctorate, comprehensive exam, thesis/dissertation. *Entrance requirements:* For doctorate, GRE General Test, minimum GPA of 3.0. Additional exam requirements/recommendations for international students:

Required—TOEFL. Electronic applications accepted. *Expenses:* Tuition, state resident: full-time $8568. Tuition, nonresident: full-time $22,140. Tuition and fees vary according to program. *Faculty research:* Regulation of signal transduction in immune responses, immune responses in bacterial and viral diseases, peptide and DNA vaccines for contraception, inflammatory bowel disease, physiology of pathogenic microbes.

Wright State University, School of Graduate Studies, College of Science and Mathematics, Program in Microbiology and Immunology, Dayton, OH 45435. Offers MS. *Program availability:* Part-time. *Degree requirements:* For master's, thesis. *Entrance requirements:* Additional exam requirements/recommendations for international students: Required—TOEFL. *Faculty research:* Reproductive immunology, viral pathogenesis, virus-host cell interactions.

Yale University, Graduate School of Arts and Sciences, Department of Immunobiology, New Haven, CT 06520. Offers PhD. *Degree requirements:* For doctorate, thesis/dissertation. *Entrance requirements:* For doctorate, GRE General Test.

Yale University, School of Medicine and Graduate School of Arts and Sciences, Combined Program in Biological and Biomedical Sciences (BBS), Immunology Track, New Haven, CT 06520. Offers PhD, MD/PhD. *Degree requirements:* For doctorate, thesis/dissertation. *Entrance requirements:* For doctorate, GRE General Test. Additional exam requirements/recommendations for international students: Required—TOEFL. Electronic applications accepted.

Infectious Diseases

Cornell University, Graduate School, Graduate Fields of Comparative Biomedical Sciences, Field of Comparative Biomedical Sciences, Ithaca, NY 14853-0001. Offers cellular and molecular medicine (MS, PhD); developmental and reproductive biology (MS, PhD); infectious diseases (MS, PhD); population medicine and epidemiology (MS, PhD); structural and functional biology (MS, PhD). *Degree requirements:* For master's, thesis; for doctorate, comprehensive exam, thesis/dissertation. *Entrance requirements:* For master's and doctorate, GRE General Test, 2 letters of recommendation. Additional exam requirements/recommendations for international students: Required—TOEFL (minimum score 550 paper-based; 77 iBT). Electronic applications accepted. *Faculty research:* Receptors and signal transduction, viral and bacterial infectious diseases, tumor metastasis, clinical sciences/nutritional disease, developmental/neurological disorders.

Georgetown University, Graduate School of Arts and Sciences, Department of Microbiology and Immunology, Washington, DC 20057. Offers biohazardous threat agents and emerging infectious diseases (MS); biomedical science policy and advocacy (MS); general microbiology and immunology (MS); global infectious diseases (PhD); microbiology and immunology (PhD). *Program availability:* Part-time. *Degree requirements:* For master's, 30 credit hours of coursework; for doctorate, comprehensive exam, thesis/dissertation. *Entrance requirements:* For master's, GRE General Test, 3 letters of reference, bachelor's degree in related field; for doctorate, GRE General Test, 3 letters of reference, MS/BS in related field. Additional exam requirements/recommendations for international students: Required—TOEFL (minimum score 505 paper-based). Electronic applications accepted. *Faculty research:* Pathogenesis and basic biology of the fungus Candida albicans, molecular biology of viral immunopathological mechanisms in Multiple Sclerosis.

The George Washington University, Milken Institute School of Public Health, Department of Epidemiology and Biostatistics, Washington, DC 20052. Offers biostatistics (MPH); epidemiology (MPH); microbiology and emerging infectious diseases (MSPH). *Faculty:* 30 full-time (20 women), 9 part-time/adjunct (7 women). *Students:* 65 full-time (49 women), 70 part-time (54 women); includes 40 minority (12 Black or African American, non-Hispanic/Latino; 15 Asian, non-Hispanic/Latino; 8 Hispanic/Latino; 5 Two or more races, non-Hispanic/Latino), 12 international. Average age 29. 493 applicants, 55% accepted, 47 enrolled. In 2015, 56 master's awarded. *Degree requirements:* For master's, case study or special project. *Entrance requirements:* For master's, GMAT, GRE General Test, or MCAT. Additional exam requirements/recommendations for international students: Required—TOEFL. *Application deadline:* For fall admission, 4/15 priority date for domestic students, 4/15 for international students; for spring admission, 11/1 for domestic and international students. Applications are processed on a rolling basis. Application fee: $75. *Financial support:* In 2015–16, 6 students received support. Tuition waivers available. Financial award application deadline: 2/15. *Unit head:* Dr. Alan E. Greenberg, Chair, 202-994-0612, E-mail: aeg1@gwu.edu. *Application contact:* Jane Smith, Director of Admissions, 202-994-0248, Fax: 202-994-1860, E-mail: sphhsinfo@gwumc.edu.

The George Washington University, School of Medicine and Health Sciences, Health Sciences Programs, Washington, DC 20052. Offers clinical practice management (MSHS); clinical research administration (MSHS); emergency services management (MSHS); end-of-life care (MSHS); immunohematology (MSHS); immunohematology and biotechnology (MSHS); physical therapy (DPT); physician assistant (MSHS). *Program availability:* Online learning. *Faculty:* 22 full-time (17 women), 13 part-time/adjunct (10 women). *Students:* 277 full-time (198 women), 249 part-time (182 women); includes 159 minority (54 Black or African American, non-Hispanic/Latino; 2 American Indian or Alaska Native, non-Hispanic/Latino; 53 Asian, non-Hispanic/Latino; 40 Hispanic/Latino; 3 Native Hawaiian or other Pacific Islander, non-Hispanic/Latino; 7 Two or more races, non-Hispanic/Latino), 13 international. Average age 33. 1,905 applicants, 19% accepted, 197 enrolled. In 2015, 146 master's, 35 doctorates, 5 other advanced degrees awarded. *Entrance requirements:* Additional exam requirements/recommendations for international students: Required—TOEFL (minimum score 550 paper-based). *Application deadline:* Applications are processed on a rolling basis. Application fee: $75. *Expenses:* Contact institution. *Unit head:* Jean E. Johnson, Senior Associate Dean, 202-994-3725, E-mail: jejohns@gwu.edu. *Application contact:* Joke Ogundiran, Director of Admission, 202-994-1668, Fax: 202-994-0870, E-mail: jokeogun@gwu.edu.

Johns Hopkins University, Bloomberg School of Public Health, Department of Epidemiology, Baltimore, MD 21205. Offers cancer etiology and prevention (MHS, Sc M, PhD, Sc D); cardiovascular disease (MHS, Sc M, PhD, Sc D); clinical epidemiology (MHS, Sc M, PhD, Sc D); clinical trials (PhD, Sc D); epidemiology (MHS, Sc M, Dr PH, PhD, Sc D); epidemiology of aging (MHS, Sc M, PhD, Sc D); genetic epidemiology (MHS, Sc M, PhD, Sc D); infectious disease epidemiology (MHS, Sc M, PhD, Sc D); occupational and environmental epidemiology (MHS, Sc M, PhD, Sc D). *Program availability:* Part-time. *Degree requirements:* For master's, comprehensive exam, thesis, 1-year full-time residency; for doctorate, comprehensive exam, thesis/dissertation, 2 years' full-time residency, oral and written exams, student teaching. *Entrance requirements:* For master's, GRE General Test or MCAT, 3 letters of recommendation, curriculum vitae; for doctorate, GRE General Test, minimum 1 year of work experience, 3 letters of recommendation, curriculum vitae, academic records from all schools. Additional exam requirements/recommendations for international students: Required—TOEFL (minimum score 600 paper-based; 100 iBT); Recommended—IELTS (minimum score 7.5), TWE. Electronic applications accepted. *Faculty research:* Cancer and congenital malformations, nutritional epidemiology, AIDS, tuberculosis, cardiovascular disease, risk assessment.

Long Island University–LIU Post, School of Health Professions and Nursing, Brookville, NY 11548-1300. Offers biomedical sciences (MS), including applied laboratory medicine, cancer biology, medical and molecular immunology, microbiology/

infectious diseases; cardiovascular perfusion (MS); dietetic internship (Advanced Certificate); family nurse practitioner (MS); forensic social work (Advanced Certificate); nursing education (MS); social work (MSW). *Program availability:* Part-time, evening/weekend, blended/hybrid learning. *Faculty:* 16 full-time (14 women), 46 part-time/adjunct (33 women). *Students:* 190 full-time (139 women), 181 part-time (157 women); includes 141 minority (51 Black or African American, non-Hispanic/Latino; 46 Asian, non-Hispanic/Latino; 41 Hispanic/Latino; 3 Two or more races, non-Hispanic/Latino), 47 international. Average age 36. 422 applicants, 64% accepted, 141 enrolled. In 2015, 96 master's, 28 other advanced degrees awarded. *Degree requirements:* For master's, comprehensive exam (for some programs), thesis (for some programs). *Entrance requirements:* Additional exam requirements/recommendations for international students: Required—TOEFL, IELTS. *Application deadline:* Applications are processed on a rolling basis. Application fee: $50. Electronic applications accepted. *Expenses:* $1,155 per credit, $934 per term full-time university fee, $442 per term part-time university fee. *Financial support:* In 2015–16, 6 research assistantships with partial tuition reimbursements were awarded; career-related internships or fieldwork, Federal Work-Study, institutionally sponsored loans, tuition waivers (partial), and unspecified assistantships also available. Support available to part-time students. Financial award application deadline: 2/15; financial award applicants required to submit FAFSA. *Faculty research:* Breast cancer, childhood obesity, dietary beverage consumption, emotional distress, histone modification, interprofessional practice, interstitial cystitis, lung cancer, pancreatic cancer, pediatric pain management, post-traumatic growth, poverty, renal nutrition, social ethics, yeast and bacterial drug resistance. *Total annual research expenditures:* $15,000. *Unit head:* Dr. Stacy Gropack, Acting Dean, 516-299-2486, Fax: 516-299-2527, E-mail: post-shpn@liu.edu. *Application contact:* Carol Zerah, Director of Graduate and International Admissions, 516-299-2900 Ext. 3952, Fax: 516-299-2137, E-mail: post-enroll@liu.edu.
Website: http://liu.edu/post/health

Loyola University Chicago, Graduate School, Integrated Program in Biomedical Sciences, Maywood, IL 60153. Offers biochemistry and molecular biology (MS, PhD); cell and molecular physiology (PhD); infectious disease and immunology (MS); integrative cell biology (PhD); medical physiology (MS); microbiology and immunology (MS, PhD); molecular pharmacology and therapeutics (MS, PhD); neuroscience (MS, PhD). *Students:* 135 full-time (65 women), 1 part-time (0 women); includes 28 minority (5 Black or African American, non-Hispanic/Latino; 15 Asian, non-Hispanic/Latino; 6 Hispanic/Latino; 2 Two or more races, non-Hispanic/Latino), 16 international. Average age 28. 442 applicants, 23% accepted, 55 enrolled. In 2015, 40 master's, 17 doctorates awarded. *Expenses: Tuition, area resident:* Full-time $18,054; part-time $9027 per credit hour. *Required fees:* $832; $284 per credit hour. Part-time tuition and fees vary according to course load, degree level and program. *Unit head:* Dr. Samuel Attoh, Dean, 773-508-3459, Fax: 773-508-2460, E-mail: sattoh@luc.edu. *Application contact:* Ron Martin, Associate Director of Enrollment Management, 312-915-8950, Fax: 312-915-8905, E-mail: gradapp@luc.edu.
Website: http://ssom.luc.edu/graduate_school/degree-programs/ipbsphd/

Montana State University, The Graduate School, College of Agriculture, Department of Immunology and Infectious Diseases, Bozeman, MT 59717. Offers MS, PhD. *Program availability:* Part-time. *Degree requirements:* For master's, comprehensive exam; for doctorate, comprehensive exam, thesis/dissertation. *Entrance requirements:* For master's and doctorate, GRE General Test. Additional exam requirements/recommendations for international students: Required—TOEFL (minimum score 550 paper-based). Electronic applications accepted. *Faculty research:* Immunology, mechanisms of infectious disease pathogenesis, mechanisms of host defense, lymphocyte development, host-pathogen interactions.

North Carolina State University, College of Veterinary Medicine, Program in Comparative Biomedical Sciences, Raleigh, NC 27695. Offers cell biology (MS, PhD); infectious disease (MS, PhD); pathology (MS, PhD); pharmacology (MS, PhD); population medicine (MS, PhD). *Program availability:* Part-time. *Degree requirements:* For master's, thesis; for doctorate, thesis/dissertation. *Entrance requirements:* For master's and doctorate, GRE General Test. Additional exam requirements/recommendations for international students: Required—TOEFL (minimum score 550 paper-based). Electronic applications accepted. *Expenses:* Contact institution. *Faculty research:* Infectious diseases, cell biology, pharmacology and toxicology, genomics, pathology and population medicine.

Penn State Hershey Medical Center, College of Medicine, Graduate School Programs in the Biomedical Sciences, The Huck Institutes of the Life Sciences, Intercollege Graduate Program in Molecular Cellular and Integrative Biosciences, Hershey, PA 17033. Offers cell and developmental biology (PhD); immunology and infectious disease (PhD); molecular and evolutionary genetics (PhD); molecular medicine (PhD); molecular toxicology (PhD); neurobiology (PhD). *Students:* 3 full-time (2 women); includes 2 minority (both Asian, non-Hispanic/Latino). 2 applicants, 100% accepted, 2 enrolled. In 2015, 1 doctorate awarded. *Degree requirements:* For doctorate, comprehensive exam, thesis/dissertation, oral exam. *Entrance requirements:* For doctorate, GRE, minimum GPA of 3.0. Additional exam requirements/recommendations for international students: Required—TOEFL (minimum score 500 paper-based). *Application deadline:* For fall admission, 1/31 priority date for domestic students, 2/1 priority date for international students. Applications are processed on a rolling basis. Application fee: $65. Electronic applications accepted. *Financial support:* In 2015–16, research assistantships with full tuition reimbursements (averaging $26,196 per year) were awarded; fellowships with full tuition reimbursements, career-related internships or fieldwork, Federal Work-Study, scholarships/grants, health care benefits, and unspecified assistantships also available. Financial award applicants required to submit FAFSA. *Faculty research:* Vascular biology, molecular toxicology, chemical biology, immune system, pathophysiological

basis of human disease. *Unit head:* Dr. Peter Hudson, Director, 814-865-6057, E-mail: pjh18@psu.edu. *Application contact:* Kathy Shuey, Administrative Assistant, 717-531-8982, Fax: 717-531-0786, E-mail: grad-hmc@psu.edu.
Website: http://www.huck.psu.edu/education/molecular-cellular-and-integrative-biosciences

Rutgers University–Newark, Graduate School of Biomedical Sciences, Newark, NJ 07107. Offers biodefense (Certificate); biomedical engineering (PhD); biomedical sciences (multidisciplinary) (PhD); cellular biology, neuroscience and physiology (PhD), including neuroscience, physiology, biophysics, cardiovascular biology, molecular pharmacology, stem cell biology; infection, immunity and inflammation (PhD), including immunology, infectious disease, microbiology, oral biology; molecular biology, genetics and cancer (PhD), including biochemistry, molecular genetics, cancer biology, radiation biology, bioinformatics; neuroscience (Certificate); pharmacological sciences (Certificate); stem cell (Certificate); DMD/PhD; MD/PhD. PhD in biomedical engineering offered jointly with New Jersey Institute of Technology. *Program availability:* Part-time, evening/weekend. Terminal master's awarded for partial completion of doctoral program. *Degree requirements:* For doctorate, thesis/dissertation, qualifying exam. *Entrance requirements:* For doctorate, GRE General Test. Additional exam requirements/recommendations for international students: Required—TOEFL. Electronic applications accepted.

Thomas Jefferson University, Jefferson College of Biomedical Sciences, Certificate Program in Infectious Disease Control, Philadelphia, PA 19107. Offers Certificate. *Program availability:* Part-time. *Students:* 7 part-time (4 women); includes 2 minority (both Black or African American, non-Hispanic/Latino). Average age 27. 13 applicants, 85% accepted, 8 enrolled. In 2015, 2 Certificates awarded. *Entrance requirements:* For degree, GRE General Test (recommended). Additional exam requirements/recommendations for international students: Required—TOEFL, IELTS (minimum score 7). *Application deadline:* For fall admission, 8/1 priority date for domestic students, 3/1 priority date for international students; for winter admission, 12/1 priority date for domestic students, 6/1 priority date for international students; for spring admission, 4/1 priority date for domestic students. Applications are processed on a rolling basis. Application fee: $50. *Financial support:* Federal Work-Study and institutionally sponsored loans available. Support available to part-time students. Financial award application deadline: 5/1; financial award applicants required to submit FAFSA. *Unit head:* Dr. James P. McGettigan, Program Director, 215-503-4629, Fax: 215-503-5393. *Application contact:* Marc E. Stearns, Director of Admissions, 215-503-0155, Fax: 215-503-3433, E-mail: jgsbs-info@jefferson.edu.
Website: http://www.jefferson.edu/university/biomedical-sciences/degrees-programs/graduate-certificate.html

Thomas Jefferson University, Jefferson College of Biomedical Sciences, Graduate Certificate Programs, Philadelphia, PA 19107. Offers clinical research and trials: implementation (Certificate); clinical research: operations (Certificate); human clinical investigation: theory (Certificate). *Program availability:* Part-time. *Faculty:* 44 full-time (14 women), 27 part-time/adjunct (11 women). *Students:* 7 part-time (6 women); includes 1 minority (Black or African American, non-Hispanic/Latino), 1 international. Average age 36. 4 applicants, 100% accepted, 4 enrolled. In 2015, 1 Certificate awarded. *Entrance requirements:* For degree, GRE General Test (recommended). Additional exam requirements/recommendations for international students: Required—TOEFL, IELTS (minimum score 7). *Application deadline:* For fall admission, 8/1 priority date for domestic students, 3/1 priority date for international students; for winter admission, 12/1 priority date for domestic students, 6/1 priority date for international students; for spring admission, 4/1 priority date for domestic students. Applications are processed on a rolling basis. Application fee: $50. *Financial support:* Federal Work-Study and institutionally sponsored loans available. Support available to part-time

students. Financial award application deadline: 5/1; financial award applicants required to submit FAFSA. *Faculty research:* Epidemiology, clinical research, statistics, planning and management, disease control. *Unit head:* Dr. Dennis M. Gross, Associate Dean, 215-503-0156, Fax: 215-503-3433, E-mail: dennis.gross@jefferson.edu. *Application contact:* Marc E. Stearns, Director of Admissions, 215-503-0155, Fax: 215-503-3433, E-mail: jgsbs-info@jefferson.edu.
Website: http://www.jefferson.edu/university/biomedical-sciences/degrees-programs/graduate-certificate.html

Tufts University, Cummings School of Veterinary Medicine, North Grafton, MA 01536. Offers animals and public policy (MS); biomedical sciences (PhD), including digestive diseases, infectious diseases, neuroscience and reproductive biology, pathology; conservation medicine (MS); veterinary medicine (DVM); DVM/MPH; DVM/MS. *Accreditation:* AVMA (one or more programs are accredited). *Degree requirements:* For master's, thesis (for some programs); for doctorate, comprehensive exam, thesis/dissertation (for some programs). *Entrance requirements:* For master's and doctorate, GRE General Test. Additional exam requirements/recommendations for international students: Required—TOEFL or IELTS. Electronic applications accepted. *Expenses:* Contact institution. *Faculty research:* Oncology, veterinary ethics, international veterinary medicine, veterinary genomics, pathogenesis of Clostridium difficile, wildlife fertility control.

 Uniformed Services University of the Health Sciences, F. Edward Hebert School of Medicine, Graduate Programs in the Biomedical Sciences and Public Health, Graduate Program in Emerging Infectious Diseases, Bethesda, MD 20814-4799. Offers PhD. *Faculty:* 35 full-time (5 women), 17 part-time/adjunct (6 women). *Students:* 26 full-time (20 women); includes 2 minority (1 Black or African American, non-Hispanic/Latino; 1 Asian, non-Hispanic/Latino), 2 international. Average age 25. 53 applicants, 13% accepted, 5 enrolled. In 2015, 10 doctorates awarded. *Degree requirements:* For doctorate, comprehensive exam, thesis/dissertation, qualifying exam. *Entrance requirements:* For doctorate, GRE General Test. *Application deadline:* For fall admission, 12/15 priority date for domestic students. Applications are processed on a rolling basis. Application fee: $0. Electronic applications accepted. *Financial support:* In 2015–16, fellowships with full tuition reimbursements (averaging $43,000 per year) were awarded; scholarships/grants, health care benefits, and tuition waivers (full) also available. *Faculty research:* Pathogenesis, host response, and epidemiology of infectious diseases. *Unit head:* Dr. Christopher Broder, Director, 301-295-3401, E-mail: christopher.broder@usuhs.edu. *Application contact:* Patricia Grant, Program Administrative Specialist, 301-295-3400, Fax: 301-295-3773, E-mail: patricia.grant@usuhs.edu.
Website: http://www.usuhs.mil/eid

See Display below and Close-Up on page 333.

Université Laval, Faculty of Medicine, Post-Professional Programs in Medical Studies, Québec, QC G1K 7P4, Canada. Offers anatomy–pathology (DESS); anesthesiology (DESS); cardiology (DESS); care of older people (Diploma); clinical research (DESS); community health (DESS); dermatology (DESS); diagnostic radiology (DESS); emergency medicine (Diploma); family medicine (DESS); general surgery (DESS); geriatrics (DESS); hematology (DESS); internal medicine (DESS); maternal and fetal medicine (Diploma); medical biochemistry (DESS); medical microbiology and infectious diseases (DESS); medical oncology (DESS); nephrology (DESS); neurology (DESS); neurosurgery (DESS); obstetrics and gynecology (DESS); ophthalmology (DESS); orthopedic surgery (DESS); oto-rhino-laryngology (DESS); palliative medicine (Diploma); pediatrics (DESS); plastic surgery (DESS); psychiatry (DESS); pulmonary medicine (DESS); radiology–oncology (DESS); thoracic surgery (DESS); urology (DESS). *Degree requirements:* For other advanced degree, comprehensive exam.

Infectious Diseases

Entrance requirements: For degree, knowledge of French. Electronic applications accepted.

University of Calgary, Cumming School of Medicine and Faculty of Graduate Studies, Department of Microbiology, Immunology and Infectious Diseases, Calgary, AB T2N 1N4, Canada. Offers M Sc, PhD. *Degree requirements:* For master's, thesis, oral thesis exam; for doctorate, thesis/dissertation, candidacy exam, oral thesis exam. *Entrance requirements:* For master's and doctorate, minimum GPA of 3.2. Additional exam requirements/recommendations for international students: Required—TOEFL (minimum score 580 paper-based). Electronic applications accepted. *Faculty research:* Bacteriology, virology, parasitology, immunology.

University of California, Berkeley, Graduate Division, School of Public Health, Group in Epidemiology, Berkeley, CA 94720-1500. Offers epidemiology (MS, PhD); infectious diseases (MPH, PhD). *Accreditation:* CEPH (one or more programs are accredited). *Degree requirements:* For master's, comprehensive exam; for doctorate, thesis/ dissertation, oral and written exam. *Entrance requirements:* For master's, GRE General Test, minimum GPA of 3.0; MD, DDS, DVM, or PhD in biomedical science (MPH); for doctorate, GRE General Test, minimum GPA of 3.0.

University of California, Berkeley, Graduate Division, School of Public Health, Group in Infectious Diseases and Immunity, Berkeley, CA 94720-1500. Offers PhD. *Entrance requirements:* For doctorate, GRE General Test, minimum GPA of 3.0, 3 letters of recommendation.

Université of Georgia, College of Veterinary Medicine, Department of Infectious Diseases, Athens, GA 30602. Offers MS, PhD. *Degree requirements:* For master's, thesis; for doctorate, one foreign language, thesis/dissertation. *Entrance requirements:* For master's and doctorate, GRE General Test. Electronic applications accepted.

University of Guelph, Ontario Veterinary College and Graduate Studies, Graduate Programs in Veterinary Sciences, Department of Pathobiology, Guelph, ON N1G 2W1, Canada. Offers anatomic pathology (DV Sc, Diploma); clinical pathology (Diploma); comparative pathology (M Sc, PhD); immunology (M Sc, PhD); laboratory animal science (DV Sc); pathology (M Sc, PhD, Diploma); veterinary infectious diseases (M Sc, PhD); zoo animal/wildlife medicine (DV Sc). *Degree requirements:* For master's, thesis; for doctorate, thesis/dissertation. *Entrance requirements:* For master's, DVM with B average or an honours degree in biological sciences; for doctorate, DVM or MSC degree, minimum B+ average. Additional exam requirements/recommendations for international students: Required—TOEFL (minimum score 550 paper-based). *Faculty research:* Pathogenesis; diseases of animals, wildlife, fish, and laboratory animals; parasitology; immunology; veterinary infectious diseases; laboratory animal science.

University of Minnesota, Twin Cities Campus, School of Public Health, Division of Environmental Health Sciences, Area in Environmental Infectious Diseases, Minneapolis, MN 55455-0213. Offers MPH, MS, PhD. *Degree requirements:* For doctorate, thesis/dissertation. *Entrance requirements:* For master's and doctorate, GRE General Test. Electronic applications accepted.

University of Pittsburgh, Graduate School of Public Health, Department of Infectious Diseases and Microbiology, Pittsburgh, PA 15261. Offers infectious disease management, intervention, and community practice (MPH); infectious disease pathogenesis, eradication, and laboratory practice (MPH); infectious diseases and microbiology (MS, PhD). *Program availability:* Part-time. *Faculty:* 19 full-time (5 women), 5 part-time/adjunct (2 women). *Students:* 67 full-time (47 women), 14 part-time (10 women); includes 19 minority (5 Black or African American, non-Hispanic/Latino; 5 Asian, non-Hispanic/Latino; 7 Hispanic/Latino; 2 Two or more races, non-Hispanic/ Latino), 11 international. Average age 26. 178 applicants, 65% accepted, 39 enrolled. In 2015, 15 master's, 3 doctorates awarded. *Degree requirements:* For master's, comprehensive exam (for some programs), thesis; for doctorate, comprehensive exam, thesis/dissertation, preliminary exam, dissertation approval. *Entrance requirements:* For master's and doctorate, GRE General Test, MCAT, DAT, or GMAT. Additional exam requirements/recommendations for international students: Required—TOEFL (minimum score 550 paper-based, 80 iBT) or IELTS (minimum score 6.5). *Application deadline:* For fall admission, 1/15 priority date for domestic and international students. Applications are processed on a rolling basis. Application fee: $120. Electronic applications accepted. *Expenses:* $12,464 per semester in-state, $20,502 per semester out-of-state; $450 fees. *Financial support:* In 2015–16, 19 students received support, including 6 fellowships (averaging $19,210 per year), 13 research assistantships (averaging $16,556 per year); scholarships/grants, traineeships, health care benefits, and unspecified assistantships also available. Financial award applicants required to submit FAFSA. *Faculty research:* HIV, complications of antiretroviral therapy, Hepatitis C, emerging infections, clinical and molecular epidemiology, genetic basis of innate immune response, HIV prevention and care, AIDS education and training. *Total annual research expenditures:* $10.8 million. *Unit head:* Dr. Charles R. Rinaldo, Chair, 412-624-3928, Fax: 412-624-4953, E-mail: rinaldo@pitt.edu. *Application contact:* Meredith Mavero, Student Services Coordinator, 412-624-3331, Fax: 412-383-8926, E-mail: mlm72@pitt.edu.
Website: http://www.idm.pitt.edu/

The University of Texas Medical Branch, Graduate School of Biomedical Sciences, Program in Emerging and Tropical Infectious Diseases, Galveston, TX 77555. Offers PhD, MD/PhD. *Degree requirements:* For doctorate, thesis/dissertation. *Entrance requirements:* For doctorate, GRE General Test. *Faculty research:* Emerging diseases, tropical diseases, parasitology, vitology and bacteriology.

Yale University, School of Medicine and Graduate School of Arts and Sciences, Combined Program in Biological and Biomedical Sciences (BBS), Microbiology Track, New Haven, CT 06520. Offers PhD, MD/PhD. *Degree requirements:* For doctorate, thesis/dissertation. *Entrance requirements:* For doctorate, GRE General Test, GRE Subject Test. Additional exam requirements/recommendations for international students: Required—TOEFL. Electronic applications accepted.

Medical Microbiology

Creighton University, School of Medicine and Graduate School, Graduate Programs in Medicine, Omaha, NE 68178-0001. Offers biomedical sciences (MS, PhD); clinical anatomy (MS); medical microbiology and immunology (MS, PhD); pharmacology (MS, PhD), including pharmaceutical sciences (MS), pharmacology; MD/PhD; Pharm D/MS. Terminal master's awarded for partial completion of doctoral program. *Degree requirements:* For master's, thesis; for doctorate, thesis/dissertation. *Entrance requirements:* For master's and doctorate, GRE General Test. Additional exam requirements/recommendations for international students: Required—TOEFL (minimum score 550 paper-based; 80 iBT). Electronic applications accepted. *Expenses:* Contact institution. *Faculty research:* Molecular biology and gene transfection, infectious disease, antimicrobial agents and chemotherapy, virology, pharmacological secretion.

Idaho State University, Office of Graduate Studies, College of Science and Engineering, Department of Biological Sciences, Pocatello, ID 83209-8007. Offers biology (MNS, MS, DA, PhD); clinical laboratory science (MS); microbiology (MS). *Accreditation:* NAACLS. *Program availability:* Part-time. *Degree requirements:* For master's, comprehensive exam, thesis; for doctorate, comprehensive exam, thesis/ dissertation, 9 credits of internship (for DA). *Entrance requirements:* For master's, GRE General Test, minimum GPA of 3.0 in all upper division classes; for doctorate, GRE General Test, GRE Subject Test (biology), diagnostic exam (DA), minimum GPA of 3.0 in all upper division classes. Additional exam requirements/recommendations for international students: Required—TOEFL (minimum score 550 paper-based; 80 iBT). Electronic applications accepted. *Faculty research:* Ecology, plant and animal physiology, plant and animal developmental biology, immunology, molecular biology, bioinfomatics.

Rutgers University–New Brunswick, Graduate School-New Brunswick, Programs in the Molecular Biosciences, Piscataway, NJ 08854-8097. Offers biochemistry (PhD); cell and developmental biology (MS, PhD); microbiology and molecular genetics (MS, PhD), including applied microbiology, clinical microbiology (MS), clinical mircobiology (PhD), computational molecular biology (PhD), immunology, microbial biochemistry, molecular genetics, virology. MS, PhD offered jointly with University of Medicine and Dentistry of New Jersey.

Université du Québec, Institut National de la Recherche Scientifique, Graduate Programs, Research Center–INRS–Institut Armand-Frappier, Laval, QC H7V 1B7, Canada. Offers applied microbiology (M Sc); biology (PhD); experimental health sciences (M Sc); virology and immunology (M Sc, PhD). *Program availability:* Part-time. *Degree requirements:* For master's, thesis; for doctorate, thesis/dissertation. *Entrance requirements:* For master's, appropriate bachelor's degree, proficiency in French; for doctorate, appropriate master's degree, proficiency in French. Electronic applications accepted. *Faculty research:* Immunity, infection and cancer; toxicology and environmental biotechnology; molecular pharmacochemistry.

University of Alberta, Faculty of Medicine and Dentistry and Faculty of Graduate Studies and Research, Graduate Programs in Medicine, Department of Medical Microbiology and Immunology, Edmonton, AB T6G 2E1, Canada. Offers M Sc, PhD. Terminal master's awarded for partial completion of doctoral program. *Degree requirements:* For master's, thesis; for doctorate, thesis/dissertation. *Entrance requirements:* For master's and doctorate, minimum GPA of 3.3. Additional exam requirements/recommendations for international students: Required—TOEFL (minimum score 600 paper-based; 96 iBT). *Faculty research:* Cellular and reproductive immunology, microbial pathogenesis, mechanisms of antibiotic resistance, molecular biology of mammalian viruses, antiviral chemotherapy.

University of Hawaii at Manoa, John A. Burns School of Medicine and Graduate Division, Graduate Programs in Biomedical Sciences, Department of Tropical Medicine, Medical Microbiology and Pharmacology, Honolulu, HI 96822. Offers tropical medicine (MS, PhD). *Program availability:* Part-time. *Faculty:* 27 full-time (11 women), 1 part-time/ adjunct (0 women). *Students:* 20 full-time (12 women), 1 part-time; includes 12 minority (6 Asian, non-Hispanic/Latino; 3 Hispanic/Latino; 3 Two or more races, non-Hispanic/ Latino), 6 international. Average age 33. 16 applicants, 25% accepted, 4 enrolled. In 2015, 2 master's, 1 doctorate awarded. Terminal master's awarded for partial completion of doctoral program. *Degree requirements:* For master's, thesis optional; for doctorate, comprehensive exam, thesis/dissertation. *Entrance requirements:* For master's and doctorate, GRE General Test. Additional exam requirements/ recommendations for international students: Required—TOEFL (minimum score 580 paper-based; 92 iBT), IELTS (minimum score 5). *Application deadline:* For fall admission, 1/15 for domestic and international students; for spring admission, 9/1 for domestic and international students. Application fee: $100. *Financial support:* In 2015–16, 6 fellowships (averaging $1,583 per year), 15 research assistantships (averaging $20,967 per year) were awarded; teaching assistantships and tuition waivers (full) also available. *Faculty research:* Immunological studies of dengue, malaria, Kawasaki's disease, lupus erythematosus, rheumatoid disease. *Total annual research expenditures:* $2.4 million. *Unit head:* Dr. Jerris R. Hedges, Dean, 808-692-0881. *Application contact:* Sandra Chang, Graduate Chair, 808-692-1617, Fax: 808-692-1979, E-mail: sandrac@ hawaii.edu.

University of Manitoba, Faculty of Medicine and Faculty of Graduate Studies, Graduate Programs in Medicine, Department of Medical Microbiology, Winnipeg, MB R3T 2N2, Canada. Offers M Sc, PhD. *Program availability:* Part-time. Terminal master's awarded for partial completion of doctoral program. *Degree requirements:* For master's, thesis; for doctorate, one foreign language, thesis/dissertation. *Entrance requirements:* For master's and doctorate, minimum GPA of 3.0. Electronic applications accepted. *Faculty research:* HIV, bacterial adhesion, sexually transmitted diseases, virus structure/ function and assembly.

University of Minnesota, Duluth, Medical School, Microbiology, Immunology and Molecular Pathobiology Section, Duluth, MN 55812-2496. Offers MS, PhD. MS, PhD offered jointly with University of Minnesota, Twin Cities Campus. Terminal master's awarded for partial completion of doctoral program. *Degree requirements:* For master's, thesis, final oral exam; for doctorate, thesis/dissertation, final exam, oral and written preliminary exams. *Entrance requirements:* For master's and doctorate, GRE General Test. Additional exam requirements/recommendations for international students: Required—TOEFL. *Faculty research:* Immunomodulation, molecular diagnosis of rabies, cytokines, cancer immunology, cytomegalovirus infection.

University of Southern California, Keck School of Medicine, Program in Medical Biology, Los Angeles, CA 90089. Offers medical biology (PhD). *Faculty:* 46 full-time (13 women). *Students:* 15 full-time (10 women); includes 5 minority (4 Asian, non-Hispanic/ Latino; 1 Hispanic/Latino), 3 international. Average age 26. 3 applicants, 100% accepted, 3 enrolled. *Degree requirements:* For doctorate, comprehensive exam, thesis/ dissertation. *Entrance requirements:* For doctorate, GRE, minimum GPA of 3.0. Additional exam requirements/recommendations for international students: Required— TOEFL (minimum score 600 paper-based; 100 iBT), IELTS (minimum score 7), PTE.

Application deadline: For fall admission, 12/1 priority date for domestic and international students. Application fee: $85. Electronic applications accepted. *Financial support:* In 2015–16, 15 students received support, including 2 fellowships with full tuition reimbursements available (averaging $32,000 per year), 13 research assistantships with full tuition reimbursements available (averaging $32,000 per year); institutionally sponsored loans, scholarships/grants, traineeships, health care benefits, and unspecified assistantships also available. Financial award application deadline: 5/4; financial award applicants required to submit CSS PROFILE or FAFSA. *Unit head:* Dr. Martin Kast, Director, 323-442-1645, Fax: 323-442-1199, E-mail: mkast@usc.edu. *Application contact:* Dr. Joyce Perez, Manager of Student Programs, 323-442-1645, Fax: 323-442-1199, E-mail: jpperez@med.usc.edu.
Website: http://pibbs.usc.edu/research-and-programs/phd-programs/

University of South Florida, Morsani College of Medicine and College of Graduate Studies, Graduate Programs in Medical Sciences, Tampa, FL 33620-9951. Offers advanced athletic training (MS); athletic training (MS); bioinformatics and computational biology (MSBCB); biotechnology (MSB); health informatics (MSHI); medical sciences (MSMS, PhD), including aging and neuroscience (MSMS), allergy, immunology and infectious disease (PhD), anatomy, athletic training (MSMS), clinical and translational research, health informatics (MSMS), health science (MSMS), interdisciplinary medical sciences (MSMS), medical microbiology and immunology (MSMS), metabolic and nutritional medicine (MSMS), molecular medicine, molecular pharmacology and physiology (PhD), neurology (PhD), pathology and laboratory medicine (PhD), pharmacology and therapeutics (PhD), physiology and biophysics (PhD), women's health (MSMS). *Students:* 510 full-time (261 women), 318 part-time (208 women); includes 360 minority (108 Black or African American, non-Hispanic/Latino; 3 American Indian or Alaska Native, non-Hispanic/Latino; 101 Asian, non-Hispanic/Latino; 124 Hispanic/Latino; 1 Native Hawaiian or other Pacific Islander, non-Hispanic/Latino; 23 Two or more races, non-Hispanic/Latino; 52 international. Average age 26. 6,567 applicants, 13% accepted, 469 enrolled. In 2015, 216 master's awarded. Terminal master's awarded for partial completion of doctoral program. *Degree requirements:* For master's, comprehensive exam, thesis; for doctorate, comprehensive exam, thesis/dissertation. *Entrance requirements:* For master's, GRE General Test or GMAT, bachelor's degree or equivalent from regionally-accredited university with minimum GPA of 3.0 in upper-division sciences coursework; prerequisites in general biology, general chemistry, general physics, organic chemistry, quantitative analysis, and integral and differential calculus; for doctorate, GRE General Test, bachelor's degree from regionally-accredited university with minimum GPA of 3.0 in upper-division sciences coursework; 3 letters of recommendation; personal interview; 1-2 page personal statement; prerequisites in biology, chemistry, physics, organic chemistry, quantitative analysis, and integral/differential calculus. Additional exam requirements/

recommendations for international students: Required—TOEFL (minimum score 550 paper-based; 79 iBT) or IELTS (minimum score 6.5). *Application deadline:* For fall admission, 2/15 for domestic students, 1/2 for international students. Application fee: $30. *Expenses:* Contact institution. *Faculty research:* Anatomy, biochemistry, cancer biology, cardiovascular disease, cell biology, immunology, microbiology, molecular biology, neuroscience, pharmacology, physiology. *Unit head:* Dr. Michael Barber, Professor/Associate Dean for Graduate and Postdoctoral Affairs, 813-974-9908, Fax: 813-974-4317, E-mail: mbarber@health.usf.edu. *Application contact:* Dr. Eric Bennett, Graduate Director, PhD Program in Medical Sciences, 813-974-1545, Fax: 813-974-4317, E-mail: esbennet@health.usf.edu.
Website: http://health.usf.edu/nocms/medicine/graduatestudies/

University of Wisconsin–La Crosse, College of Science and Health, Department of Biology, La Crosse, WI 54601-3742. Offers aquatic sciences (MS); biology (MS); cellular and molecular biology (MS); clinical microbiology (MS); microbiology (MS); nurse anesthesia (MS); physiology (MS). *Program availability:* Part-time. *Students:* 19 full-time (12 women), 50 part-time (26 women); includes 4 minority (3 Asian, non-Hispanic/Latino; 1 Hispanic/Latino), 1 international. Average age 29. 44 applicants, 75% accepted, 27 enrolled. In 2015, 27 master's awarded. *Degree requirements:* For master's, comprehensive exam, thesis. *Entrance requirements:* For master's, GRE General Test, minimum GPA of 2.85. Additional exam requirements/recommendations for international students: Required—TOEFL (minimum score 550 paper-based; 79 iBT). *Application deadline:* For fall admission, 2/1 priority date for domestic and international students; for spring admission, 1/4 priority date for domestic and international students. Applications are processed on a rolling basis. Electronic applications accepted. *Financial support:* Research assistantships with partial tuition reimbursements, Federal Work-Study, scholarships/grants, health care benefits, and tuition waivers (partial) available. Support available to part-time students. Financial award application deadline: 3/15; financial award applicants required to submit FAFSA. *Unit head:* Dr. Mark Sandheinrich, Department Chair, 608-785-8261, E-mail: msandheinrich@uwlax.edu. *Application contact:* Brandon Schaller, Senior Graduate Student Status Examiner, 608-785-8941, E-mail: admissions@uwlax.edu.
Website: http://uwlax.edu/biology/

University of Wisconsin–Madison, School of Medicine and Public Health and College of Agricultural and Life Sciences, Microbiology Doctoral Training Program, Madison, WI 53706. Offers PhD. *Expenses:* Tuition, state resident: full-time $5364. Tuition, nonresident: full-time $12,027. *Required fees:* $571. Tuition and fees vary according to campus/location, program and reciprocity agreements.
Website: http://www.microbiology.wisc.edu/

Microbiology

Albany Medical College, Center for Immunology and Microbial Disease, Albany, NY 12208-3479. Offers MS, PhD. *Program availability:* Part-time. Terminal master's awarded for partial completion of doctoral program. *Degree requirements:* For master's, thesis; for doctorate, comprehensive exam, thesis/dissertation, oral qualifying exam, written preliminary exam, 1 published paper-peer review. *Entrance requirements:* For master's, GRE General Test, all transcripts, letters of recommendation; for doctorate, GRE General Test, letters of recommendation. Additional exam requirements/recommendations for international students: Required—TOEFL. *Faculty research:* Microbial and viral pathogenesis, cancer development and cell transformation, biochemical and genetic mechanisms responsible for human disease.

Albert Einstein College of Medicine, Graduate Division of Biomedical Sciences, Department of Microbiology and Immunology, Bronx, NY 10461. Offers PhD, MD/PhD. *Degree requirements:* For doctorate, thesis/dissertation. *Entrance requirements:* For doctorate, GRE General Test. Additional exam requirements/recommendations for international students: Required—TOEFL. *Faculty research:* Nature of histocompatibility antigens, lymphoid cell receptors, regulation of immune responses and mechanisms of resistance to infection.

American University of Beirut, Graduate Programs, Faculty of Medicine, Beirut, Lebanon. Offers anatomy, cell biology and human morphology (MS); biochemistry and medical genetics (MS); biomedical sciences (PhD); experimental pathology, immunology and microbiology (MS); medicine (MD); neuroscience (MS); pharmacology and toxicology (MS). *Program availability:* Part-time. *Faculty:* 302 full-time (95 women), 64 part-time/adjunct (11 women). *Students:* 381 full-time (173 women), 61 part-time (51 women). Average age 23. In 2015, 14 master's awarded. *Degree requirements:* For master's, one foreign language, comprehensive exam, thesis (for some programs); for doctorate, one foreign language, comprehensive exam, thesis/dissertation. *Entrance requirements:* For master's, letter of recommendation; for doctorate, MCAT, bachelor's degree. Additional exam requirements/recommendations for international students: Required—TOEFL (minimum score 600 paper-based; 100 iBT), IELTS (minimum score 7.5). *Application deadline:* For fall admission, 4/30 for domestic and international students; for spring admission, 11/1 for domestic and international students. Application fee: $50. Electronic applications accepted. *Expenses:* Tuition, area resident: Full-time $16,254; part-time $903 per credit. *Required fees:* $699. Tuition and fees vary according to course load and program. *Financial support:* In 2015–16, 273 students received support, including 45 teaching assistantships (averaging $9,000 per year); career-related internships or fieldwork, institutionally sponsored loans, scholarships/grants, health care benefits, and unspecified assistantships also available. Financial award application deadline: 2/2. *Faculty research:* Cancer research (targeted therapy, mechanisms of leukemogenesis, tumor cell extravasation and metastasis, cancer stem cells), stem cell research (regenerative medicine, drug discovery), genetic research (neurogenetics, hereditary cardiomyopathy, hemoglobinopathies, pharmacogenomics, proteomics), neuroscience research (pain, neurodegenerative disorder), metabolism (inflammation and metabolism, metabolic disorder, diabetes mellitus), vascular and renal biology, signal transduction. *Total annual research expenditures:* $2.6 million. *Unit head:* Dr. Mohamed Sayegh, Dean, 961-1350000 Ext. 4700, Fax: 961-1744464, E-mail: msayegh@aub.edu.lb. *Application contact:* Dr. Salim Kanaan, Director, Admissions Office, 961-1350000 Ext. 2594, Fax: 961-1750775, E-mail: sk00@aub.edu.lb.
Website: http://www.aub.edu.lb/fm/fm_home/Pages/index.aspx

Arizona State University at the Tempe campus, College of Liberal Arts and Sciences, School of Life Sciences, Tempe, AZ 85287-4601. Offers animal behavior (PhD); applied ethics (biomedical and health ethics) (MA); biology (MS, PhD), including biology, biology and society, complex adaptive systems science (PhD); plant biology and conservation (MS); environmental life sciences (PhD); evolutionary biology (PhD); history and

philosophy of science (PhD); human and social dimensions of science and technology (PhD); microbiology (PhD); molecular and cellular biology (PhD); neuroscience (PhD). Terminal master's awarded for partial completion of doctoral program. *Degree requirements:* For master's, thesis (for some programs), interactive Program of Study (iPOS) submitted before completing 50 percent of required credit hours; for doctorate, variable foreign language requirement, comprehensive exam, thesis/dissertation, interactive Program of Study (iPOS) submitted before completing 50 percent of required credit hours. *Entrance requirements:* For master's and doctorate, GRE, minimum GPA of 3.0 or equivalent in last 2 years of work leading to bachelor's degree. Additional exam requirements/recommendations for international students: Required—TOEFL (minimum score 600 paper-based; 100 iBT). Electronic applications accepted.

Baylor College of Medicine, Graduate School of Biomedical Sciences, Department of Molecular Virology and Microbiology, Houston, TX 77030-3498. Offers PhD, MD/PhD. *Degree requirements:* For doctorate, thesis/dissertation, public defense. *Entrance requirements:* For doctorate, GRE General Test, GRE Subject Test (strongly recommended), minimum GPA of 3.0. Additional exam requirements/recommendations for international students: Required—TOEFL. Electronic applications accepted. *Faculty research:* Microbiology, viral molecular biology, bacterial molecular biology, microbial pathogenesis, microbial genomics.

Baylor College of Medicine, Graduate School of Biomedical Sciences, Interdepartmental Program in Cell and Molecular Biology, Houston, TX 77030-3498. Offers biochemistry (PhD); cell and molecular biology (PhD); genetics (PhD); human genetics (PhD); immunology (PhD); microbiology (PhD); virology (PhD); MD/PhD. *Degree requirements:* For doctorate, thesis/dissertation, public defense. *Entrance requirements:* For doctorate, GRE General Test, GRE Subject Test (strongly recommended), minimum GPA of 3.0. Additional exam requirements/recommendations for international students: Required—TOEFL. Electronic applications accepted. *Faculty research:* Molecular and cellular biology; cancer, aging and stem cells; genomics and proteomics; microbiome, molecular microbiology; infectious disease, immunology and translational research.

Brandeis University, Graduate School of Arts and Sciences, Program in Molecular and Cell Biology, Waltham, MA 02454-9110. Offers genetics (PhD); microbiology (PhD); molecular and cell biology (MS, PhD); molecular biology (PhD); neurobiology (PhD); quantitative biology (PhD). *Faculty:* 26 full-time (12 women), 4 part-time/adjunct (2 women). *Students:* 60 full-time (30 women); includes 5 minority (1 Black or African American, non-Hispanic/Latino; 1 American Indian or Alaska Native, non-Hispanic/Latino; 1 Asian, non-Hispanic/Latino; 2 Hispanic/Latino), 25 international. 183 applicants, 27% accepted, 12 enrolled. In 2015, 13 master's, 7 doctorates awarded. Terminal master's awarded for partial completion of doctoral program. *Degree requirements:* For master's, thesis optional, research project, research lab, or project lab; for doctorate, comprehensive exam, thesis/dissertation, journal clubs; research seminar; colloquia; qualifying exam. *Entrance requirements:* For master's, GRE General Test, official transcript(s), resume, 2 letters of recommendation, statement of purpose; for doctorate, GRE General Test, official transcript(s), resume, 3 letters of recommendation, statement of purpose, list of previous research experience. Additional exam requirements/recommendations for international students: Required—TOEFL (minimum score 600 paper-based; 100 iBT); Recommended—IELTS (minimum score 7), TSE (minimum score 68). *Application deadline:* For fall admission, 12/15 priority date for domestic students. Application fee: $75. Electronic applications accepted. *Financial support:* In 2015–16, 35 students received support, including 16 fellowships with full tuition reimbursements available (averaging $30,500 per year), 19 research assistantships with full tuition reimbursements available (averaging $30,500 per year); scholarships/grants and tuition waivers (partial) also available. Financial award

Microbiology

application deadline: 4/15; financial award applicants required to submit FAFSA. *Faculty research:* Molecular biology, genetics and development; structural and cell biology; neurobiology. *Unit head:* Dr. Maria Miara, Director of Graduate Studies, 781-736-2300, Fax: 781-736-3107, E-mail: scigradoffice@brandeis.edu. *Application contact:* Dr. Maryanna Aldrich, Department Administrator, 781-736-2300, Fax: 781-736-3107, E-mail: scigradoffice@brandeis.edu.
Website: http://www.brandeis.edu/gsas

Brigham Young University, Graduate Studies, College of Life Sciences, Department of Microbiology and Molecular Biology, Provo, UT 85602. Offers MS, PhD. *Faculty:* 15 full-time (3 women). *Students:* 38 full-time (18 women); includes 12 minority (6 Asian, non-Hispanic/Latino; 5 Hispanic/Latino; 1 Native Hawaiian or other Pacific Islander, non-Hispanic/Latino), 12 international. Average age 27. 22 applicants, 73% accepted, 12 enrolled. In 2015, 5 master's, 3 doctorates awarded. Terminal master's awarded for partial completion of doctoral program. *Degree requirements:* For master's, comprehensive exam, thesis; for doctorate, comprehensive exam, thesis/dissertation. *Entrance requirements:* For master's, GRE General Test, minimum GPA of 3.0 during previous 2 years; for doctorate, GRE General Test, minimum GPA of 3.0. Additional exam requirements/recommendations for international students: Required—TOEFL (minimum score 580 paper-based; 85 iBT), IELTS (minimum score 7). *Application deadline:* For fall admission, 2/1 for domestic and international students. Application fee: $50. Electronic applications accepted. *Financial support:* In 2015–16, 18 students received support, including 16 research assistantships with full tuition reimbursements available (averaging $21,000 per year), 2 teaching assistantships with tuition reimbursements available (averaging $18,000 per year); institutionally sponsored loans, scholarships/grants, health care benefits, and unspecified assistantships also available. Financial award application deadline: 2/1. *Faculty research:* Immunobiology, molecular genetics, molecular virology, cancer biology, pathogenic and environmental microbiology. *Total annual research expenditures:* $845,216. *Unit head:* Dr. Richard Robison, Chair, 801-422-2416, Fax: 801-422-0004, E-mail: richard_robison@byu.edu. *Application contact:* Dr. Joel Griffitts, Graduate Coordinator, 801-422-7997, Fax: 801-422-0004, E-mail: joel_griffitts@byu.edu. Website: http://mmbio.byu.edu/

California State University, Long Beach, Graduate Studies, College of Natural Sciences and Mathematics, Department of Biological Sciences, Long Beach, CA 90840. Offers biology (MS); microbiology (MS). *Program availability:* Part-time. *Entrance requirements:* For master's, GRE Subject Test, minimum GPA of 3.0. Electronic applications accepted.

Case Western Reserve University, School of Medicine and School of Graduate Studies, Graduate Programs in Medicine, Department of Molecular Biology and Microbiology, Cleveland, OH 44106-4960. Offers cellular biology (PhD); microbiology (PhD); molecular biology (PhD); molecular virology (PhD); MD/PhD. Students are admitted to an integrated Biomedical Sciences Training Program involving 11 basic science programs at Case Western Reserve University. *Degree requirements:* For doctorate, thesis/dissertation. *Entrance requirements:* For doctorate, GRE General Test, GRE Subject Test. Additional exam requirements/recommendations for international students: Required—TOEFL. Electronic applications accepted. *Expenses: Tuition, area resident:* Full-time $41,137; part-time $1714 per credit hour. *Required fees:* $32. Tuition and fees vary according to course load and program. *Faculty research:* Gene expression in eukaryotic and prokaryotic systems; microbial physiology; intracellular transport and signaling; mechanisms of oncogenesis; molecular mechanisms of RNA processing, editing, and catalysis.

The Catholic University of America, School of Arts and Sciences, Department of Biology, Washington, DC 20064. Offers biotechnology (MS); cell and microbial biology (MS, PhD), including cell biology; clinical laboratory science (MS, PhD); MSLS/MS. *Program availability:* Part-time. *Faculty:* 9 full-time (4 women), 7 part-time/adjunct (1 woman). *Students:* 29 full-time (18 women), 36 part-time (22 women); includes 8 minority (3 Black or African American, non-Hispanic/Latino; 2 Asian, non-Hispanic/Latino; 1 Hispanic/Latino; 2 Two or more races, non-Hispanic/Latino), 44 international. Average age 30. 68 applicants, 38% accepted, 13 enrolled. In 2015, 21 master's, 1 doctorate awarded. *Degree requirements:* For master's and doctorate, comprehensive exam. *Entrance requirements:* For master's and doctorate, GRE General Test, GRE Subject Test, statement of purpose, official copies of academic transcripts, three letters of recommendation. Additional exam requirements/recommendations for international students: Required—TOEFL (minimum score 550 paper-based; 80 iBT). *Application deadline:* For fall admission, 7/15 priority date for domestic students, 7/1 for international students; for spring admission, 11/15 priority date for domestic students, 11/1 for international students. Applications are processed on a rolling basis. Application fee: $55. Electronic applications accepted. *Expenses:* $20,700 per semester full-time tuition, $200 per semester full-time fees; $1,650 per credit hour part-time tuition, $145 per semester part-time fees. *Financial support:* Fellowships, research assistantships, teaching assistantships, Federal Work-Study, scholarships/grants, tuition waivers (full and partial), and unspecified assistantships available. Financial award application deadline: 2/1; financial award applicants required to submit FAFSA. *Faculty research:* Virus structure and assembly, hepatic and epithelial cell biology, drug resistance and genome stabilization in yeast, biophysics of ion-conductive nanostructures, eukaryotic gene regulation, cancer and vaccine research. *Total annual research expenditures:* $2.2 million. *Unit head:* Dr. Venigalla Rao, Chair, 202-319-5271, Fax: 202-319-5721, E-mail: rao@cua.edu. *Application contact:* Director of Graduate Admissions, 202-319-5057, Fax: 202-319-6533, E-mail: cua-admissions@cua.edu.
Website: http://biology.cua.edu/

Clemson University, Graduate School, College of Science, Department of Biological Sciences, Program in Microbiology, Clemson, SC 29634. Offers MS, PhD. *Faculty:* 10 full-time (4 women). *Students:* 18 full-time (7 women), 2 part-time (1 woman), 9 international. Average age 28. 33 applicants, 15% accepted, 6 enrolled. In 2015, 5 master's, 1 doctorate awarded. *Degree requirements:* For master's, thesis; for doctorate, comprehensive exam, thesis/dissertation. *Entrance requirements:* For master's, GRE General Test, unofficial transcripts, letters of recommendation; for doctorate, GRE General Test, unofficial transcripts, letters of recommendation. Additional exam requirements/recommendations for international students: Required—TOEFL (minimum score 100 iBT), IELTS (minimum score 7.5), PTE (minimum score 72). *Application deadline:* For fall admission, 1/5 for domestic and international students. Application fee: $80 ($90 for international students). Electronic applications accepted. *Expenses:* $4,060 per semester full-time resident, $8,103 per semester full-time non-resident, $448 per credit hour part-time resident, $898 per credit hour part-time non-resident. *Financial support:* In 2015–16, 18 students received support, including 2 research assistantships with partial tuition reimbursements available (averaging $19,500 per year), 16 teaching assistantships with partial tuition reimbursements available (averaging $19,969 per year); career-related internships or fieldwork and health care benefits also available. Financial award application deadline: 1/5. *Faculty research:* Anaerobic microbiology, microbiology and ecology of soil and aquatic systems, microbial genetics, biofilms, nanotechnology. *Unit head:* Dr. Robert Cohen, Department Chair, 864-656-1112, E-mail: rscohen@clemson.edu. *Application contact:* Jay Lyn Martin, Student Services Program Coordinator, 864-656-3587, Fax: 864-656-0435, E-mail: jaylyn@clemson.edu.
Website: http://www.clemson.edu/cafls/departments/biosci/graduates/index.html

Colorado State University, College of Veterinary Medicine and Biomedical Sciences, Department of Microbiology, Immunology and Pathology, Fort Collins, CO 80523. Offers microbiology (MS, PhD); pathology (PhD). *Faculty:* 75 full-time (35 women), 10 part-time/adjunct (6 women). *Students:* 81 full-time (60 women), 28 part-time (18 women); includes 21 minority (2 American Indian or Alaska Native, non-Hispanic/Latino; 3 Asian, non-Hispanic/Latino; 13 Hispanic/Latino; 3 Two or more races, non-Hispanic/Latino), 8 international. Average age 29. 133 applicants, 38% accepted, 47 enrolled. In 2015, 47 master's, 7 doctorates awarded. *Degree requirements:* For master's, comprehensive exam, thesis; for doctorate, comprehensive exam, thesis/dissertation. *Entrance requirements:* For master's, GRE General Test, minimum GPA of 3.0, BA/BS in biomedical field, resume, transcripts, personal statement, 3 letters of recommendation; for doctorate, GRE General Test, minimum GPA of 3.0, BA/BS in biomedical field, resume, personal statement, transcripts, 3 letters of recommendation. Additional exam requirements/recommendations for international students: Required—TOEFL (minimum score 550 paper-based; 80 iBT); Recommended—IELTS (minimum score 6.5), TWE, TSE. *Application deadline:* For fall admission, 12/15 priority date for domestic and international students. Application fee: $60 ($70 for international students). Electronic applications accepted. *Expenses:* Contact institution. *Financial support:* In 2015–16, 82 students received support, including 33 fellowships with full tuition reimbursements available (averaging $39,971 per year), 29 research assistantships with full tuition reimbursements available (averaging $21,981 per year), 2 teaching assistantships with full tuition reimbursements available (averaging $17,190 per year); scholarships/grants, traineeships, and unspecified assistantships also available. Financial award applicants required to submit FAFSA. *Faculty research:* Prions, tuberculosis, vector-borne diseases, rna biology, host-pathogen interactions. *Total annual research expenditures:* $21.5 million. *Unit head:* Dr. Gregg A. Dean, Department Head, 970-491-6144, E-mail: gregg.dean@colostate.edu. *Application contact:* Heidi Runge, Academic Support Coordinator for Graduate Studies, 970-491-1630, Fax: 970-491-0603, E-mail: heidi.runge@colostate.edu.
Website: http://csu-cvmbs.colostate.edu/academics/mip/graduate/Pages/microbiology-immunology-professional-masters.aspx

Columbia University, College of Physicians and Surgeons, Department of Microbiology, New York, NY 10032. Offers biomedical sciences (M Phil, MA, PhD); MD/PhD. Only candidates for the PhD are admitted. Terminal master's awarded for partial completion of doctoral program. *Degree requirements:* For doctorate, thesis/dissertation. *Entrance requirements:* For master's, GRE General Test; for doctorate, GRE. Additional exam requirements/recommendations for international students: Required—TOEFL. *Faculty research:* Prokaryotic molecular biology, immunology, virology, yeast molecular genetics, regulation of gene expression.

Cornell University, Graduate School, Graduate Fields of Agriculture and Life Sciences, Field of Microbiology, Ithaca, NY 14853-0001. Offers PhD. *Degree requirements:* For doctorate, comprehensive exam, thesis/dissertation, 2 semesters of teaching experience. *Entrance requirements:* For doctorate, GRE General Test, 3 letters of recommendation. Additional exam requirements/recommendations for international students: Required—TOEFL (minimum score 550 paper-based; 77 iBT). Electronic applications accepted. *Faculty research:* Microbial diversity, molecular biology, biotechnology, microbial ecology, phytobacteriology.

Dalhousie University, Faculty of Medicine, Department of Microbiology and Immunology, Halifax, NS B3H 4R2, Canada. Offers M Sc, PhD. *Degree requirements:* For master's, thesis; for doctorate, comprehensive exam, thesis/dissertation. *Entrance requirements:* For master's, GRE General Test, honors B Sc; for doctorate, GRE General Test, honors B Sc in microbiology, M Sc in discipline or transfer after 1 year in master's program. Additional exam requirements/recommendations for international students: Required—1 of 5 approved tests: TOEFL, IELTS, CANTEST, CAEL, Michigan English Language Assessment Battery. Electronic applications accepted. *Faculty research:* Virology, molecular genetics, pathogenesis, bacteriology, immunology.

Dartmouth College, Graduate Program in Molecular and Cellular Biology, Department of Microbiology and Immunology, Program in Immunology, Hanover, NH 03755. Offers PhD, MBA/PhD, MD/PhD. *Entrance requirements:* For doctorate, GRE, letters of recommendation. Additional exam requirements/recommendations for international students: Required—TOEFL (minimum score paper-based 550, iBT 100) or IELTS (7.0). *Application deadline:* For fall admission, 12/1 for domestic students. Application fee: $75. Electronic applications accepted. *Expenses: Tuition, area resident:* Full-time $48,120. *Required fees:* $296. One-time fee: $50 full-time. *Financial support:* In 2015–16, fellowships with full tuition reimbursements (averaging $28,200 per year) were awarded; health care benefits also available. *Faculty research:* Tumor immunotherapy, cell and molecular biology of connective tissue degradation in rheumatoid arthritis and cancer, immunology and immunotherapy of tumors of the central nervous system, transcriptional regulation of hematopoiesis and leukemia, bacterial pathogenesis. *Unit head:* Dr. William R. Green, Chair, 603-650-4919, Fax: 603-650-6223, E-mail: immunology@dartmouth.edu. *Application contact:* Marcia L. Ingalls, Administrative Assistant, 603-650-4919, Fax: 603-650-6223, E-mail: immunology@dartmouth.edu.
Website: https://geiselmed.dartmouth.edu/immuno/

Dartmouth College, Graduate Program in Molecular and Cellular Biology, Department of Microbiology and Immunology, Program in Molecular Pathogenesis, Hanover, NH 03755. Offers microbiology and immunology (PhD); MBA/PhD; MD/PhD. *Entrance requirements:* Additional exam requirements/recommendations for international students: Required—TOEFL (minimum score paper-based 550, iBT 100) or IELTS (7.0). *Application deadline:* For fall admission, 12/1 for domestic students. Application fee: $75. Electronic applications accepted. *Expenses: Tuition, area resident:* Full-time $48,120. *Required fees:* $296. One-time fee: $50 full-time. *Financial support:* In 2015–16, fellowships with full tuition reimbursements (averaging $28,200 per year) were awarded; health care benefits also available. *Unit head:* Dr. William R. Green, Chair, 603-650-8607, Fax: 603-650-6223. *Application contact:* Janet Cheney, Program Administrator, 608-650-1612, Fax: 608-650-6223.
Website: https://www.dartmouth.edu/~m2p2/

Drexel University, College of Medicine, Biomedical Graduate Programs, Program in Microbiology and Immunology, Philadelphia, PA 19104-2875. Offers MS, PhD, MD/PhD. Terminal master's awarded for partial completion of doctoral program. *Degree requirements:* For master's, comprehensive exam, thesis; for doctorate, thesis/dissertation, qualifying exam. *Entrance requirements:* For master's, GRE General Test, minimum GPA of 2.75; for doctorate, GRE General Test, minimum GPA of 3.0. Additional exam requirements/recommendations for international students: Required—TOEFL. Electronic applications accepted. *Faculty research:* Immunology of malarial parasites, virology, bacteriology, molecular biology, parasitology.

Duke University, Graduate School, Department of Molecular Genetics and Microbiology, Durham, NC 27710. Offers PhD. *Degree requirements:* For doctorate, thesis/dissertation. *Entrance requirements:* For doctorate, GRE General Test, GRE Subject Test in biology, chemistry, or biochemistry, cell and molecular biology (recommended). Additional exam requirements/recommendations for international students: Required—TOEFL (minimum score 577 paper-based; 90 iBT) or IELTS (minimum score 7). Electronic applications accepted.

East Carolina University, Brody School of Medicine, Department of Microbiology and Immunology, Greenville, NC 27858-4353. Offers MS, MD, PhD. *Students:* 15 full-time (8 women); includes 1 minority (Asian, non-Hispanic/Latino), 5 international. Average age 28. 19 applicants, 26% accepted, 5 enrolled. In 2015, 3 doctorates awarded. *Degree requirements:* For doctorate, comprehensive exam, thesis/dissertation. *Entrance requirements:* For doctorate, GRE General Test. Additional exam requirements/recommendations for international students: Required—TOEFL. *Application deadline:* For fall admission, 4/15 priority date for domestic students. Applications are processed on a rolling basis. Application fee: $50. *Financial support:* Fellowships with tuition reimbursements available. Financial award application deadline: 6/1. *Faculty research:* Molecular virology, genetics of bacteria, yeast and somatic cells, bacterial physiology and metabolism, bioterrorism. *Unit head:* Dr. Charles J. Smith, Chair, 252-744-2700, Fax: 252-744-3104, E-mail: smithcha@ecu.edu. *Application contact:* Jamaal Peele, Program Director, 252-744-2701, E-mail: peelej@ecu.edu.
Website: http://www.ecu.edu/cs-dhs/microbiology/guidelines.cfm

Eastern New Mexico University, Graduate School, College of Liberal Arts and Sciences, Department of Biology, Portales, NM 88130. Offers applied ecology (MS); botany (MS); cell, molecular biology and biotechnology (MS); microbiology (MS); zoology (MS). *Program availability:* Part-time. *Degree requirements:* For master's, comprehensive exam, thesis optional. *Entrance requirements:* For master's, GRE, minimum GPA of 3.0, 2 letters of recommendation, statement of research interest, bachelor's degree related to field of study or proof of common knowledge. Additional exam requirements/recommendations for international students: Required—TOEFL (minimum score 550 paper-based; 79 iBT), IELTS (minimum score 6). Electronic applications accepted.

East Tennessee State University, James H. Quillon College of Medicine, Department of Biomedical Sciences, Johnson City, TN 37614. Offers anatomy (PhD); biochemistry (PhD); microbiology (PhD); pharmaceutical sciences (PhD); pharmacology (PhD); physiology (PhD); quantitative biosciences (PhD). *Faculty:* 30 full-time (6 women). *Students:* 35 full-time (17 women), 2 part-time (1 woman); includes 13 minority (9 Black or African American, non-Hispanic/Latino; 4 Asian, non-Hispanic/Latino), 13 international. Average age 29. 53 applicants, 17% accepted, 8 enrolled. In 2015, 8 doctorates awarded. *Degree requirements:* For doctorate, thesis/dissertation, comprehensive qualifying exam. *Entrance requirements:* For doctorate, GRE General Test, GRE Subject Test, 3 letters of recommendation. Additional exam requirements/recommendations for international students: Required—TOEFL (minimum score 550 paper-based; 79 iBT). *Application deadline:* For fall admission, 3/15 priority date for domestic students, 3/1 priority date for international students. Application fee: $35 ($45 for international students). Electronic applications accepted. *Expenses:* Contact institution. *Financial support:* In 2015–16, 30 students received support, including 27 research assistantships with full tuition reimbursements available (averaging $20,000 per year); career-related internships or fieldwork, institutionally sponsored loans, scholarships/grants, and unspecified assistantships also available. Financial award application deadline: 7/1; financial award applicants required to submit FAFSA. *Faculty research:* Cardiovascular, infectious disease, neurosciences, cancer, immunology. *Unit head:* Dr. Mitchell E. Robinson, Associate Dean/Program Director, 423-439-2031, Fax: 423-439-2140, E-mail: robinson@etsu.edu. *Application contact:* Shella Bennett, Graduate Specialist, 423-439-4708, Fax: 423-439-5624, E-mail: bennetsg@etsu.edu.
Website: http://www.etsu.edu/com/dbms/

Emory University, Laney Graduate School, Division of Biological and Biomedical Sciences, Program in Microbiology and Molecular Genetics, Atlanta, GA 30322-1100. Offers PhD. *Degree requirements:* For doctorate, comprehensive exam, thesis/dissertation. *Entrance requirements:* For doctorate, GRE General Test, minimum GPA of 3.0 in science course work (recommended). Additional exam requirements/recommendations for international students: Required—TOEFL. Electronic applications accepted. *Faculty research:* Bacterial genetics and physiology, microbial development, molecular biology of viruses and bacterial pathogens, DNA recombination.

Emporia State University, Department of Biological Sciences, Emporia, KS 66801-5415. Offers botany (MS); environmental biology (MS); general biology (MS); microbial and cellular biology (MS); zoology (MS). *Program availability:* Part-time. *Faculty:* 14 full-time (3 women), 1 part-time/adjunct (0 women). *Students:* 26 full-time (13 women), 15 part-time (7 women); includes 1 minority (Two or more races, non-Hispanic/Latino), 24 international. 16 applicants, 100% accepted, 11 enrolled. In 2015, 17 master's awarded. *Degree requirements:* For master's, comprehensive exam or thesis. *Entrance requirements:* For master's, GRE, appropriate undergraduate degree, interview, letters of reference. Additional exam requirements/recommendations for international students: Required—TOEFL (minimum score 520 paper-based; 68 iBT). *Application deadline:* For fall admission, 8/15 priority date for domestic students. Applications are processed on a rolling basis. Application fee: $30 ($75 for international students). Electronic applications accepted. *Expenses:* Tuition, state resident: full-time $5640; part-time $235 per credit hour. Tuition, nonresident: full-time $17,544; part-time $731 per credit hour. *Required fees:* $1848; $77 per credit hour. *Financial support:* In 2015–16, 7 research assistantships with full tuition reimbursements (averaging $7,344 per year), 12 teaching assistantships with full tuition reimbursements (averaging $7,844 per year) were awarded; career-related internships or fieldwork, Federal Work-Study, institutionally sponsored loans, health care benefits, and unspecified assistantships also available. Financial award application deadline: 3/15; financial award applicants required to submit FAFSA. *Faculty research:* Fisheries, range, and wildlife management; aquatic, plant, grassland, vertebrate, and invertebrate ecology; mammalian and plant systematics, taxonomy, and evolution; immunology, virology, and molecular biology. *Unit head:* Dr. Yixin Eric Yang, Chair, 620-341-5311, Fax: 620-341-5608, E-mail: yyang@emporia.edu.
Website: http://www.emporia.edu/info/degrees-courses/grad/biology

Georgetown University, Graduate School of Arts and Sciences, Department of Microbiology and Immunology, Washington, DC 20057. Offers biohazardous threat agents and emerging infectious diseases (MS); biomedical science policy and advocacy (MS); general microbiology and immunology (MS); global infectious diseases (PhD); microbiology and immunology (PhD). *Program availability:* Part-time. *Degree requirements:* For master's, 30 credit hours of coursework; for doctorate, comprehensive exam, thesis/dissertation. *Entrance requirements:* For master's, GRE General Test, 3 letters of reference, bachelor's degree in related field; for doctorate, GRE General Test, 3 letters of reference, MS/BS in related field. Additional exam requirements/recommendations for international students: Required—TOEFL (minimum score 505 paper-based). Electronic applications accepted. *Faculty research:* Pathogenesis and basic biology of the fungus Candida albicans, molecular biology of viral immunopathological mechanisms in Multiple Sclerosis.

The George Washington University, Columbian College of Arts and Sciences, Institute for Biomedical Sciences, Program in Microbiology and Immunology, Washington, DC 20037. Offers PhD. *Faculty:* 13 full-time (2 women). *Students:* 2 full-time (1 woman), 15 part-time (10 women); includes 6 minority (1 Black or African American, non-Hispanic/Latino; 1 American Indian or Alaska Native, non-Hispanic/Latino; 2 Asian, non-Hispanic/Latino; 1 Hispanic/Latino; 1 Two or more races, non-Hispanic/Latino), 3 international. Average age 30. In 2015, 5 doctorates awarded. *Degree requirements:* For doctorate, thesis/dissertation. *Entrance requirements:* For

doctorate, GRE General Test, minimum GPA of 3.0. Additional exam requirements/recommendations for international students: Required—TOEFL (minimum score 600 paper-based). *Application deadline:* For fall admission, 12/15 priority date for domestic and international students. Applications are processed on a rolling basis. Application fee: $75. Electronic applications accepted. *Financial support:* In 2015–16, 10 students received support. Fellowships with tuition reimbursements available and tuition waivers available. *Unit head:* Dr. David Leitenberg, Director, 202-994-9475, Fax: 202-994-2913, E-mail: dleit@gwu.edu. *Application contact:* Information Contact, 202-994-3532, Fax: 202-994-2913, E-mail: mtmjxl@gwumc.edu.
Website: http://smhs.gwu.edu/microbiology/

The George Washington University, Milken Institute School of Public Health, Department of Epidemiology and Biostatistics, Washington, DC 20052. Offers biostatistics (MPH); epidemiology (MPH); microbiology and emerging infectious diseases (MSPH). *Faculty:* 30 full-time (20 women), 9 part-time/adjunct (7 women). *Students:* 65 full-time (49 women), 70 part-time (54 women); includes 40 minority (12 Black or African American, non-Hispanic/Latino; 15 Asian, non-Hispanic/Latino; 8 Hispanic/Latino; 5 Two or more races, non-Hispanic/Latino), 12 international. Average age 29. 493 applicants, 55% accepted, 47 enrolled. In 2015, 56 master's awarded. *Degree requirements:* For master's, case study or special project. *Entrance requirements:* For master's, GMAT, GRE General Test, or MCAT. Additional exam requirements/recommendations for international students: Required—TOEFL. *Application deadline:* For fall admission, 4/15 priority date for domestic students, 4/15 for international students; for spring admission, 11/1 for domestic and international students. Applications are processed on a rolling basis. Application fee: $75. *Financial support:* In 2015–16, 6 students received support. Tuition waivers available. Financial award application deadline: 2/15. *Unit head:* Dr. Alan E. Greenberg, Chair, 202-994-0612, E-mail: aeg1@gwu.edu. *Application contact:* Jane Smith, Director of Admissions, 202-994-0248, Fax: 202-994-1860, E-mail: sphhsinfo@gwumc.edu.

The George Washington University, School of Medicine and Health Sciences, Health Sciences Programs, Washington, DC 20052. Offers clinical practice management (MSHS); clinical research administration (MSHS); emergency services management (MSHS); end-of-life care (MSHS); immunohematology (MSHS); immunohematology and biotechnology (MSHS); physical therapy (DPT); physician assistant (MSHS). *Program availability:* Online learning. *Faculty:* 22 full-time (17 women), 13 part-time/adjunct (10 women). *Students:* 277 full-time (198 women), 249 part-time (182 women); includes 159 minority (54 Black or African American, non-Hispanic/Latino; 2 American Indian or Alaska Native, non-Hispanic/Latino; 53 Asian, non-Hispanic/Latino; 40 Hispanic/Latino; 3 Native Hawaiian or other Pacific Islander, non-Hispanic/Latino; 7 Two or more races, non-Hispanic/Latino), 13 international. Average age 33. 1,905 applicants, 19% accepted, 197 enrolled. In 2015, 146 master's, 35 doctorates, 5 other advanced degrees awarded. *Entrance requirements:* Additional exam requirements/recommendations for international students: Required—TOEFL (minimum score 550 paper-based). *Application deadline:* Applications are processed on a rolling basis. Application fee: $75. *Expenses:* Contact institution. *Unit head:* Jean E. Johnson, Senior Associate Dean, 202-994-3725, E-mail: jejohns@gwu.edu. *Application contact:* Joke Ogundiran, Director of Admission, 202-994-1668, Fax: 202-994-0870, E-mail: jokeogun@gwu.edu.

Georgia State University, College of Arts and Sciences, Department of Biology, Program in Applied and Environmental Microbiology, Atlanta, GA 30302-3083. Offers applied and environmental microbiology (MS, PhD); bioinformatics (MS). *Program availability:* Part-time. Terminal master's awarded for partial completion of doctoral program. *Degree requirements:* For master's, comprehensive exam (for some programs), thesis optional; for doctorate, comprehensive exam, thesis/dissertation. *Entrance requirements:* For master's and doctorate, GRE. Additional exam requirements/recommendations for international students: Required—TOEFL (minimum score 550 paper-based; 82 iBT) or IELTS (minimum score 7). *Application deadline:* For fall admission, 7/1 priority date for domestic students, 6/1 priority date for international students; for spring admission, 11/15 priority date for domestic students, 10/15 priority date for international students. Applications are processed on a rolling basis. Application fee: $50. Electronic applications accepted. *Expenses:* Tuition, state resident: full-time $6876; part-time $382 per credit hour. Tuition, nonresident: full-time $22,374; part-time $1243 per credit hour. *Required fees:* $2128; $2128 per term. $1064 per term. Part-time tuition and fees vary according to course load and program. *Financial support:* In 2015–16, fellowships with full tuition reimbursements (averaging $22,000 per year), research assistantships with full tuition reimbursements (averaging $20,000 per year) were awarded. Financial award application deadline: 12/3. *Faculty research:* Bioremediation, biofilms, indoor air quality control, environmental toxicology, product biosynthesis. *Unit head:* Dr. Charles Derby, Director of Graduate Studies, 404-413-5393, Fax: 404-413-5446, E-mail: cderby@gsu.edu.
Website: http://biology.gsu.edu/

Harvard University, Graduate School of Arts and Sciences, Division of Medical Sciences, Boston, MA 02115. Offers biological chemistry and molecular pharmacology (PhD); cell biology (PhD); genetics (PhD); microbiology and molecular genetics (PhD); pathology (PhD), including experimental pathology. *Degree requirements:* For doctorate, thesis/dissertation. *Entrance requirements:* For doctorate, GRE General Test, GRE Subject Test. Additional exam requirements/recommendations for international students: Required—TOEFL.

Hood College, Graduate School, Program in Biomedical Science, Frederick, MD 21701-8575. Offers bioinformatics (Certificate); biomedical science (MS), including biotechnology/molecular biology, microbiology/immunology/virology, regulatory compliance. *Program availability:* Part-time, evening/weekend. *Degree requirements:* For master's, comprehensive exam, thesis or alternative. *Entrance requirements:* For master's, bachelor's degree in biology; minimum GPA of 2.75; undergraduate course work in cell biology, chemistry, organic chemistry, and genetics. Additional exam requirements/recommendations for international students: Required—TOEFL (minimum score 575 paper-based; 89 iBT), IELTS (minimum score 6.5). *Application deadline:* For fall admission, 7/15 priority date for domestic students, 7/15 for international students; for spring admission, 12/1 priority date for domestic students, 12/1 for international students. Applications are processed on a rolling basis. Application fee: $35. Electronic applications accepted. Application fee is waived when completed online. *Expenses:* Tuition, area resident: Part-time $450 per credit hour. *Required fees:* $105 per term. Part-time tuition and fees vary according to degree level, campus/location and program. *Financial support:* Research assistantships with full tuition reimbursements, tuition waivers (partial), and unspecified assistantships available. Financial award applicants required to submit FAFSA.
Website: http://www.hood.edu/graduate

See Display on page 64 and Close-Up on page 109.

Howard University, College of Medicine, Department of Microbiology, Washington, DC 20059-0002. Offers PhD. *Degree requirements:* For doctorate, one foreign language, comprehensive exam, thesis/dissertation, qualifying exam, teaching experience. *Entrance requirements:* For doctorate, GRE General Test, minimum GPA of 3.0 in sciences. Additional exam requirements/recommendations for international students: Required—TOEFL. *Faculty research:* Immunology, molecular and cellular microbiology,

Microbiology

microbial genetics, microbial physiology, pathogenic bacteriology, medical mycology, medical parasitology, virology.

Idaho State University, Office of Graduate Studies, College of Science and Engineering, Department of Biological Sciences, Pocatello, ID 83209-8007. Offers biology (MNS, MS, DA, PhD); clinical laboratory science (MS); microbiology (MS). *Accreditation:* NAACLS. *Program availability:* Part-time. *Degree requirements:* For master's, comprehensive exam, thesis; for doctorate, comprehensive exam, thesis/dissertation, 9 credits of internship (for DA). *Entrance requirements:* For master's, GRE General Test, minimum GPA of 3.0 in all upper division classes; for doctorate, GRE General Test, GRE Subject Test (biology), diagnostic exam (DA), minimum GPA of 3.0 in all upper division classes. Additional exam requirements/recommendations for international students: Required—TOEFL (minimum score 550 paper-based; 80 iBT). Electronic applications accepted. *Faculty research:* Ecology, plant and animal physiology, plant and animal developmental biology, immunology, molecular biology, bioinfomatics.

Illinois Institute of Technology, Graduate College, College of Science, Department of Biological Sciences, Chicago, IL 60616. Offers biochemistry (MS); biology (MS, PhD); cell and molecular biology (MS); microbiology (MS); molecular biochemistry and biophysics (MS, PhD). *Program availability:* Part-time, evening/weekend, online learning. Terminal master's awarded for partial completion of doctoral program. *Degree requirements:* For master's, comprehensive exam, thesis (for some programs); for doctorate, comprehensive exam, thesis/dissertation. *Entrance requirements:* For master's, GRE General Test (minimum score 300 Quantitative and Verbal, 2.5 Analytical Writing), minimum undergraduate GPA of 3.0; for doctorate, GRE General Test (minimum score 310 Quantitative and Verbal, 3.0 Analytical Writing); GRE Subject Test (strongly recommended), minimum undergraduate GPA of 3.0. Additional exam requirements/recommendations for international students: Required—TOEFL (minimum score 550 paper-based; 80 iBT). Electronic applications accepted. *Faculty research:* Macromolecular crystallography, insect immunity and basic cell biology, improvement of bacterial strains for enhanced biodesulfurization of petroleum, programmed cell death in cancer cells.

Illinois State University, Graduate School, College of Arts and Sciences, Department of Biological Sciences, Normal, IL 61790-2200. Offers animal behavior (MS); bacteriology (MS); biochemistry (MS); biological sciences (MS); biology (PhD); biophysics (MS); biotechnology (MS); botany (MS, PhD); cell biology (MS); conservation biology (MS); developmental biology (MS); ecology (MS, PhD); entomology (MS); evolutionary biology (MS); genetics (MS, PhD); immunology (MS); microbiology (MS, PhD); molecular biology (MS); molecular genetics (MS); neurobiology (MS); neuroscience (MS); parasitology (MS); physiology (MS, PhD); plant biology (MS); plant molecular biology (MS); plant sciences (MS); structural biology (MS); zoology (MS, PhD). *Program availability:* Part-time. *Degree requirements:* For master's, thesis or alternative; for doctorate, variable foreign language requirement, thesis/dissertation, 2 terms of residency. *Entrance requirements:* For master's, GRE General Test, minimum GPA of 2.6 in last 60 hours of course work; for doctorate, GRE General Test. *Application deadline:* Applications are processed on a rolling basis. Application fee: $40. *Financial support:* Research assistantships, teaching assistantships, Federal Work-Study, tuition waivers (full), and unspecified assistantships available. Financial award application deadline: 4/1. *Faculty research:* Redoc balance and drug development in schistosoma mansoni, control of the growth of listeria monocytogenes at low temperature, regulation of cell expansion and microtubule function by SPRI, CRUI: physiology and fitness consequences of different life history phenotypes. *Application contact:* Steven Juliano, Graduate Coordinator, E-mail: sajulian@ilstu.edu.
Website: http://www.bio.ilstu.edu/

Indiana University Bloomington, University Graduate School, College of Arts and Sciences, Department of Biology, Bloomington, IN 47405. Offers biology teaching (MAT); biotechnology (MA); evolution, ecology, and behavior (MA, PhD); genetics (PhD); microbiology (MA, PhD); molecular, cellular, and developmental biology (PhD); plant sciences (MA, PhD); zoology (MA, PhD). Terminal master's awarded for partial completion of doctoral program. *Degree requirements:* For master's, thesis, oral defense; for doctorate, thesis/dissertation, oral defense. *Entrance requirements:* For master's and doctorate, GRE General Test. Additional exam requirements/recommendations for international students: Required—TOEFL (minimum score 100 iBT). Electronic applications accepted. *Faculty research:* Evolution, ecology and behavior; microbiology; molecular biology and genetics; plant biology.

Indiana University–Purdue University Indianapolis, Indiana University School of Medicine, Department of Microbiology and Immunology, Indianapolis, IN 46202. Offers MS, PhD, MD/MS, MD/PhD. Terminal master's awarded for partial completion of doctoral program. *Degree requirements:* For master's, thesis; for doctorate, thesis/dissertation. *Entrance requirements:* For master's and doctorate, GRE General Test, previous course work in calculus, cell biology, chemistry, genetics, physics, and biochemistry. *Faculty research:* Host-parasite interactions, molecular biology, cellular and molecular immunology and hematology, viral and bacterial pathogenesis, cancer research.

Inter American University of Puerto Rico, Metropolitan Campus, Graduate Programs, Program in Medical Technology, San Juan, PR 00919-1293. Offers administration of clinical laboratories (MS); molecular microbiology (MS). *Accreditation:* NAACLS. *Program availability:* Part-time. *Degree requirements:* For master's, comprehensive exam. *Entrance requirements:* For master's, BS in medical technology, minimum GPA of 2.5. Electronic applications accepted.

Iowa State University of Science and Technology, Department of Veterinary Microbiology and Preventive Medicine, Ames, IA 50011. Offers veterinary microbiology (MS, PhD). *Entrance requirements:* For master's and doctorate, GRE General Test. Additional exam requirements/recommendations for international students: Required—TOEFL (minimum score 550 paper-based; 79 iBT), IELTS (minimum score 6.5). Electronic applications accepted. *Faculty research:* Bacteriology, immunology, virology, public health and food safety.

Iowa State University of Science and Technology, Program in Microbiology, Ames, IA 50011. Offers MS, PhD. *Entrance requirements:* For master's and doctorate, GRE General Test. Additional exam requirements/recommendations for international students: Required—TOEFL (minimum score 550 paper-based; 79 iBT), IELTS (minimum score 6.5). Electronic applications accepted.

Johns Hopkins University, Bloomberg School of Public Health, W. Harry Feinstone Department of Molecular Microbiology and Immunology, Baltimore, MD 21218. Offers MHS, Sc M, PhD. *Faculty:* 41 full-time (10 women), 10 part-time/adjunct (1 woman). *Students:* 95 full-time (52 women), 2 part-time (1 woman); includes 23 minority (3 Black or African American, non-Hispanic/Latino; 13 Asian, non-Hispanic/Latino; 5 Hispanic/Latino; 2 Two or more races, non-Hispanic/Latino), 25 international. Average age 26. 192 applicants, 47% accepted, 37 enrolled. In 2015, 34 master's, 7 doctorates awarded. Terminal master's awarded for partial completion of doctoral program. *Degree requirements:* For master's, comprehensive exam, thesis (for some programs), essay, written exams; for doctorate, comprehensive exam, thesis/dissertation, 1-year full-time residency, oral and written exams. *Entrance requirements:* For master's, GRE General Test or MCAT, 3 letters of recommendation, curriculum vitae; for doctorate, GRE General Test, 3 letters of recommendation, transcripts, curriculum vitae. Additional exam requirements/recommendations for international students: Required—TOEFL (minimum score 600 paper-based). *Application deadline:* For fall admission, 1/2 priority date for domestic and international students. Applications are processed on a rolling basis. Application fee: $45. Electronic applications accepted. *Financial support:* Fellowships with tuition reimbursements, research assistantships with tuition reimbursements, Federal Work-Study, institutionally sponsored loans, scholarships/grants, and stipends available. Financial award application deadline: 3/15; financial award applicants required to submit FAFSA. *Faculty research:* Immunology, virology, bacteriology, parasitology, vector biology, disease ecology, pathogenesis of infectious disease, immune responses to infectious agents, vector-borne and tropical diseases, biochemistry and molecular biology of infectious agents, population genetics of insect vectors, genetic regulation and immune responses in insect vectors, vaccine development, hormonal effects on pathogenesis and immune responses. *Total annual research expenditures:* $14.5 million. *Unit head:* Dr. Arturo Casadevall, Chair, 410-955-3459, Fax: 410-955-0105, E-mail: acasade1@jhu.edu. *Application contact:* Gail O'Connor, Academic Program Administrator, 410-614-4232, Fax: 410-955-0105, E-mail: goconnor@jhsph.edu.
Website: http://www.jhsph.edu/dept/MMI/

Loma Linda University, School of Medicine, Programs in Biochemistry and Microbiology, Loma Linda, CA 92350. Offers biochemistry (MS, PhD); microbiology (PhD). *Program availability:* Part-time. *Degree requirements:* For master's, thesis or alternative; for doctorate, thesis/dissertation. *Entrance requirements:* For master's and doctorate, GRE General Test. Additional exam requirements/recommendations for international students: Required—TOEFL (minimum score 550 paper-based). *Application deadline:* For fall admission, 7/1 for domestic students. Applications are processed on a rolling basis. Application fee: $60. *Financial support:* Tuition waivers (full and partial) available. Support available to part-time students. *Faculty research:* Physical chemistry of macromolecules, biochemistry of endocrine system, biochemical mechanism of bone volume regulation. *Unit head:* Dr. Hansel Fletcher, Vice Chair, 909-558-8497. *Application contact:* Admissions Office, 909-651-5029, Fax: 909-558-4879, E-mail: admissions.app@llu.edu.

Long Island University–LIU Post, School of Health Professions and Nursing, Brookville, NY 11548-1300. Offers biomedical sciences (MS), including applied laboratory medicine, cancer biology, medical and molecular immunology, microbiology/infectious diseases; cardiovascular perfusion (MS); dietetic internship (Advanced Certificate); family nurse practitioner (MS); forensic social work (Advanced Certificate); nursing education (MS); social work (MSW). *Program availability:* Part-time, evening/weekend, blended/hybrid learning. *Faculty:* 16 full-time (14 women), 46 part-time/adjunct (33 women). *Students:* 190 full-time (139 women), 181 part-time (157 women); includes 141 minority (51 Black or African American, non-Hispanic/Latino; 46 Asian, non-Hispanic/Latino; 41 Hispanic/Latino; 3 Two or more races, non-Hispanic/Latino), 47 international. Average age 36. 422 applicants, 64% accepted, 141 enrolled. In 2015, 96 master's, 28 other advanced degrees awarded. *Degree requirements:* For master's, comprehensive exam (for some programs), thesis (for some programs). *Entrance requirements:* Additional exam requirements/recommendations for international students: Required—TOEFL, IELTS. *Application deadline:* Applications are processed on a rolling basis. Application fee: $50. Electronic applications accepted. *Expenses:* $1,155 per credit, $934 per term full-time university fee, $442 per term part-time university fee. *Financial support:* In 2015–16, 6 research assistantships with partial tuition reimbursements were awarded; career-related internships or fieldwork, Federal Work-Study, institutionally sponsored loans, tuition waivers (partial), and unspecified assistantships also available. Support available to part-time students. Financial award application deadline: 2/15; financial award applicants required to submit FAFSA. *Faculty research:* Breast cancer, childhood obesity, dietary beverage consumption, emotional distress, histone modification, interprofessional practice, interstitial cystitis, lung cancer, pancreatic cancer, pediatric pain management, post-traumatic growth, poverty, renal nutrition, social ethics, yeast and bacterial drug resistance. *Total annual research expenditures:* $15,000. *Unit head:* Dr. Stacy Gropack, Acting Dean, 516-299-2486, Fax: 516-299-2527, E-mail: post-shpn@liu.edu. *Application contact:* Carol Zerah, Director of Graduate and International Admissions, 516-299-2900 Ext. 3952, Fax: 516-299-2137, E-mail: post-enroll@liu.edu.
Website: http://liu.edu/post/health

Louisiana State University Health Sciences Center, School of Graduate Studies in New Orleans, Department of Microbiology, Immunology, and Parasitology, New Orleans, LA 70112-1393. Offers microbiology and immunology (PhD); MD/PhD. *Faculty:* 22 full-time (5 women). *Students:* 18 full-time (10 women); includes 3 minority (2 Black or African American, non-Hispanic/Latino; 1 Hispanic/Latino), 4 international. Average age 26. 14 applicants, 21% accepted, 1 enrolled. In 2015, 3 doctorates awarded. *Degree requirements:* For doctorate, comprehensive exam, thesis/dissertation, preliminary exam, qualifying exam. *Entrance requirements:* For doctorate, GRE General Test. Additional exam requirements/recommendations for international students: Recommended—TOEFL, IELTS. *Application deadline:* For fall admission, 4/1 for domestic and international students. Applications are processed on a rolling basis. Application fee: $30. *Financial support:* Unspecified assistantships available. Financial award application deadline: 4/15. *Faculty research:* Microbial physiology, animal virology, vaccine development, AIDS drug studies, pathogenic mechanisms, molecular immunology. *Unit head:* Dr. Alistair Ramsay, Professor and Head, 504-568-4062, Fax: 504-568-2918, E-mail: aramsa@lsuhsc.edu. *Application contact:* Dr. Angela Amedee, Associate Professor, 504-568-5608, Fax: 504-568-2918, E-mail: aamede@lsuhsc.edu.
Website: http://www.medschool.lsuhsc.edu/microbiology/

Louisiana State University Health Sciences Center at Shreveport, Department of Microbiology and Immunology, Shreveport, LA 71130-3932. Offers MS, PhD, MD/PhD. *Faculty:* 13 full-time (3 women). *Students:* 17 full-time (9 women), 2 international. Average age 27. 9 applicants, 100% accepted, 7 enrolled. In 2015, 5 master's, 5 doctorates awarded. Terminal master's awarded for partial completion of doctoral program. *Degree requirements:* For master's, comprehensive exam, thesis; for doctorate, comprehensive exam, thesis/dissertation, research proposal. *Entrance requirements:* For master's and doctorate, GRE General Test. Additional exam requirements/recommendations for international students: Required—TOEFL. *Application deadline:* For fall admission, 1/31 for domestic and international students. Application fee: $0. Electronic applications accepted. *Expenses:* $6,467.25 resident tuition; $15,872 non-resident tuition; $410.50 student fees. *Financial support:* In 2015–16, 20 students received support, including 20 fellowships with full tuition reimbursements available (averaging $26,000 per year); institutionally sponsored loans, scholarships/grants, and tuition waivers (for all full-time PhD students) also available. Financial award application deadline: 1/31. *Faculty research:* Infectious disease, molecular bacteriology, pathogenesis, molecular virology and immunology. *Unit head:* Dr. Dennis J. O'Callaghan, Head, 318-675-5750, Fax: 318-675-5764. *Application contact:* Marti Glass, Administrative Coordinator, 318-675-7851 Ext. 4781, Fax: 318-675-5764, E-mail: mglass@lsuhsc.edu.
Website: http://www.lsuhscmicrobiology.com

Loyola University Chicago, Graduate School, Integrated Program in Biomedical Sciences, Maywood, IL 60153. Offers biochemistry and molecular biology (MS, PhD); cell and molecular physiology (PhD); infectious disease and immunology (MS); integrative cell biology (PhD); medical physiology (MS); microbiology and immunology (MS, PhD); molecular pharmacology and therapeutics (MS, PhD); neuroscience (MS, PhD). *Students:* 135 full-time (65 women), 1 part-time (0 women); includes 28 minority (5 Black or African American, non-Hispanic/Latino; 15 Asian, non-Hispanic/Latino; 6 Hispanic/Latino; 2 Two or more races, non-Hispanic/Latino), 16 international. Average age 28. 442 applicants, 23% accepted, 55 enrolled. In 2015, 40 master's, 17 doctorates awarded. *Expenses: Tuition, area resident:* Full-time $18,054; part-time $9027 per credit hour. *Required fees:* $832; $284 per credit hour. Part-time tuition and fees vary according to course load, degree level and program. *Unit head:* Dr. Samuel Attoh, Dean, 773-508-3459, Fax: 773-508-2460, E-mail: sattoh@luc.edu. *Application contact:* Ron Martin, Associate Director of Enrollment Management, 312-915-8950, Fax: 312-915-8905, E-mail: gradapp@luc.edu.
Website: http://ssom.luc.edu/graduate_school/degree-programs/ipbsphd/

Marquette University, Graduate School, College of Arts and Sciences, Department of Biology, Milwaukee, WI 53201-1881. Offers cell biology (MS, PhD); developmental biology (MS, PhD); ecology (MS, PhD); epithelial physiology (MS, PhD); genetics (MS, PhD); microbiology (MS, PhD); molecular biology (MS, PhD); muscle and exercise physiology (MS, PhD); neuroscience (PhD). *Faculty:* 22 full-time (7 women), 3 part-time/adjunct (2 women). *Students:* 28 full-time (11 women), 12 part-time (4 women); includes 4 minority (1 Asian, non-Hispanic/Latino; 1 Hispanic/Latino; 2 Two or more races, non-Hispanic/Latino), 11 international. Average age 27. 72 applicants, 28% accepted, 5 enrolled. In 2015, 2 master's, 4 doctorates awarded. Terminal master's awarded for partial completion of doctoral program. *Degree requirements:* For master's, comprehensive exam, thesis, 1 year of teaching experience or equivalent; for doctorate, thesis/dissertation, 1 year of teaching experience or equivalent, qualifying exam. *Entrance requirements:* For master's and doctorate, GRE General Test, GRE Subject Test, official transcripts from all current and previous colleges/universities except Marquette, statement of professional goals and aspirations, three letters of recommendation. Additional exam requirements/recommendations for international students: Required—TOEFL (minimum score 530 paper-based). *Application deadline:* For fall admission, 12/15 for domestic and international students. Application fee: $50. Electronic applications accepted. *Financial support:* In 2015–16, 39 students received support, including 6 fellowships (averaging $1,208 per year), 4 research assistantships with full tuition reimbursements available (averaging $21,750 per year), 29 teaching assistantships with full tuition reimbursements available (averaging $21,750 per year); scholarships/grants, health care benefits, tuition waivers (full and partial), and unspecified assistantships also available. Support available to part-time students. Financial award application deadline: 2/15. *Faculty research:* Neurobiology, neuroendocrinology, epithelial physiology, neuropeptide interactions, synaptic transmission. *Total annual research expenditures:* $1.2 million. *Unit head:* Dr. Ed Blumenthal, Chair, 414-288-1748. *Application contact:* Dr. Michael Schlappi, Recruiting Contact, 414-288-1467.
Website: http://www.marquette.edu/biology/

Massachusetts Institute of Technology, School of Science, Department of Biology, Cambridge, MA 02139. Offers biochemistry (PhD); biological oceanography (PhD); biology (PhD); biophysical chemistry and molecular structure (PhD); cell biology (PhD); computational and systems biology (PhD); developmental biology (PhD); genetics (PhD); immunology (PhD); microbiology (PhD); molecular biology (PhD); neurobiology (PhD). *Faculty:* 57 full-time (14 women). *Students:* 283 full-time (137 women); includes 83 minority (3 Black or African American, non-Hispanic/Latino; 1 American Indian or Alaska Native, non-Hispanic/Latino; 38 Asian, non-Hispanic/Latino; 31 Hispanic/Latino; 10 Two or more races, non-Hispanic/Latino), 48 international. Average age 26. 673 applicants, 14% accepted, 46 enrolled. In 2015, 32 doctorates awarded. *Degree requirements:* For doctorate, comprehensive exam, thesis/dissertation, teaching assistantship during two semesters. *Entrance requirements:* For doctorate, GRE General Test. Additional exam requirements/recommendations for international students: Required—TOEFL (minimum score 577 paper-based), IELTS. *Application deadline:* For fall admission, 12/1 for domestic and international students. Application fee: $75. Electronic applications accepted. *Expenses: Tuition:* Full-time $46,400; part-time $725 per credit. One-time fee: $304 full-time. Full-time tuition and fees vary according to course load and program. *Financial support:* In 2015–16, 235 students received support, including 118 fellowships (averaging $37,500 per year), 163 research assistantships (averaging $38,900 per year), 1 teaching assistantship; Federal Work-Study, institutionally sponsored loans, scholarships/grants, traineeships, health care benefits, and unspecified assistantships also available. Support available to part-time students. Financial award application deadline: 4/15; financial award applicants required to submit FAFSA. *Faculty research:* Cellular, developmental and molecular (plant and animal) biology; biochemistry, bioengineering, biophysics and structural biology; classical and molecular genetics, stem cell and epigenetics; immunology and microbiology; cancer biology, molecular medicine, neurobiology and human disease; computational and systems biology. *Total annual research expenditures:* $42.8 million. *Unit head:* Prof. Alan Grossman, Department Head, 617-253-4701. *Application contact:* Biology Education Office, 617-253-3717, Fax: 617-258-9329, E-mail: gradbio@mit.edu.
Website: https://biology.mit.edu/

McGill University, Faculty of Graduate and Postdoctoral Studies, Faculty of Agricultural and Environmental Sciences, Department of Natural Resource Sciences, Montréal, QC H3A 2T5, Canada. Offers entomology (M Sc, PhD); environmental assessment (M Sc); forest science (M Sc, PhD); microbiology (M Sc, PhD); micrometeorology (M Sc, PhD); neotropical environment (M Sc, PhD); soil science (M Sc, PhD); wildlife biology (M Sc, PhD).

McGill University, Faculty of Graduate and Postdoctoral Studies, Faculty of Medicine, Department of Microbiology and Immunology, Montréal, QC H3A 2T5, Canada. Offers M Sc, M Sc A, PhD.

Medical College of Wisconsin, Graduate School of Biomedical Sciences, Department of Microbiology and Molecular Genetics, Milwaukee, WI 53226-0509. Offers MS, PhD, MD/PhD. *Degree requirements:* For doctorate, comprehensive exam, thesis/dissertation. *Entrance requirements:* For master's and doctorate, GRE, official transcripts, three letters of recommendation. Additional exam requirements/recommendations for international students: Required—TOEFL. *Faculty research:* Virology, immunology, bacterial toxins, regulation of gene expression.

Medical University of South Carolina, College of Graduate Studies, Department of Microbiology and Immunology, Charleston, SC 29425. Offers MS, PhD, DMD/PhD, MD/PhD. Terminal master's awarded for partial completion of doctoral program. *Degree requirements:* For master's, thesis; for doctorate, thesis/dissertation, oral and written exams. *Entrance requirements:* For master's, GRE General Test, MCAT, or DAT, minimum GPA of 3.0; for doctorate, GRE General Test, interview, minimum GPA of 3.0, research experience. Additional exam requirements/recommendations for international students: Required—TOEFL (minimum score 600 paper-based; 100 iBT). Electronic applications accepted. *Faculty research:* Inmate and adaptive immunology, gene

therapy/vector development, vaccinology, proteomics of biowarfare agents, bacterial and fungal pathogenesis.

Meharry Medical College, School of Graduate Studies, Program in Biomedical Sciences, Microbiology and Immunology Emphasis, Nashville, TN 37208-9989. Offers PhD, MD/PhD. *Degree requirements:* For doctorate, comprehensive exam, thesis/dissertation. *Entrance requirements:* For doctorate, GRE General Test, GRE Subject Test, undergraduate degree in related science. *Application deadline:* For fall admission, 6/1 for domestic students. Applications are processed on a rolling basis. Application fee: $65. *Financial support:* Fellowships, research assistantships, and Federal Work-Study available. Financial award application deadline: 4/15. *Faculty research:* Microbial and bacterial pathogenesis, viral transcription, immune response to viruses and parasites.

Miami University, College of Arts and Science, Department of Microbiology, Oxford, OH 45056. Offers MS, PhD. *Students:* 22 full-time (15 women), 1 part-time (0 women); includes 3 minority (1 Black or African American, non-Hispanic/Latino; 1 Asian, non-Hispanic/Latino; 1 Hispanic/Latino), 4 international. Average age 27. In 2015, 4 master's, 4 doctorates awarded. *Entrance requirements:* For master's and doctorate, GRE General Test, brief statement of research interests and career objectives; three letters of recommendation. Additional exam requirements/recommendations for international students: Recommended—TOEFL (minimum score 80 iBT), IELTS (minimum score 6.5), TSE (minimum score 54). *Application deadline:* For fall admission, 1/15 for domestic and international students. Application fee: $50. Electronic applications accepted. *Expenses:* Tuition, state resident: full-time $12,888; part-time $537 per credit hour. Tuition, nonresident: full-time $29,022; part-time $1209 per credit hour. *Required fees:* $530; $24 per credit hour. $30 per semester. Part-time tuition and fees vary according to course load and program. *Financial support:* Application deadline: 1/15; applicants required to submit FAFSA. *Unit head:* Dr. Louis A. Actis, Chair, 513-529-5424, E-mail: actisla@miamioh.edu. *Application contact:* Dr. Mitchell Balish, Associate Professor and Director of Graduate Studies, 513-529-0167, E-mail: balishmf@miamioh.edu.
Website: http://www.miamioh.edu/microbiology

Michigan State University, College of Human Medicine and The Graduate School, Graduate Programs in Human Medicine, East Lansing, MI 48824. Offers biochemistry and molecular biology (MS, PhD); epidemiology (MS, PhD); microbiology (MS); microbiology and molecular genetics (PhD); pharmacology and toxicology (MS, PhD); physiology (MS, PhD); public health (MPH). *Entrance requirements:* Additional exam requirements/recommendations for international students: Required—TOEFL.

Michigan State University, College of Osteopathic Medicine and The Graduate School, Graduate Studies in Osteopathic Medicine, East Lansing, MI 48824. Offers biochemistry and molecular biology (MS, PhD); microbiology (MS); microbiology and molecular genetics (PhD); pharmacology and toxicology (MS, PhD), including integrative pharmacology (MS), pharmacology and toxicology, pharmacology and toxicology-environmental toxicology (PhD); physiology (MS, PhD).

Michigan State University, College of Veterinary Medicine and The Graduate School, Graduate Programs in Veterinary Medicine and College of Natural Science and Graduate Programs in Human Medicine, Department of Microbiology and Molecular Genetics, East Lansing, MI 48824. Offers industrial microbiology (MS, PhD); microbiology (MS, PhD); microbiology and molecular genetics (PhD); microbiology—environmental toxicology (PhD). *Entrance requirements:* For master's, GRE General Test. Additional exam requirements/recommendations for international students: Required—TOEFL (minimum score 550 paper-based), Michigan State University ELT (minimum score 85), Michigan English Language Assessment Battery (minimum score 83). Electronic applications accepted.

Michigan State University, The Graduate School, College of Agriculture and Natural Resources, MSU-DOE Plant Research Laboratory, East Lansing, MI 48824. Offers biochemistry and molecular biology (PhD); cellular and molecular biology (PhD); crop and soil sciences (PhD); genetics (PhD); microbiology and molecular genetics (PhD); plant biology (PhD); plant physiology (PhD). Offered jointly with the Department of Energy. *Degree requirements:* For doctorate, comprehensive exam, thesis/dissertation, laboratory rotation, defense of dissertation. *Entrance requirements:* For doctorate, GRE General Test, acceptance into one of the affiliated department programs; 3 letters of recommendation; bachelor's degree or equivalent in life sciences, chemistry, biochemistry, or biophysics; research experience. Electronic applications accepted. *Faculty research:* Role of hormones in the regulation of plant development and physiology, molecular mechanisms associated with signal recognition, development and application of genetic methods and materials, protein routing and function.

Montana State University, The Graduate School, College of Letters and Science, Department of Microbiology, Bozeman, MT 59717. Offers MS, PhD. *Program availability:* Part-time. *Degree requirements:* For master's, comprehensive exam; for doctorate, comprehensive exam, thesis/dissertation. *Entrance requirements:* For master's and doctorate, GRE General Test. Additional exam requirements/recommendations for international students: Required—TOEFL (minimum score 550 paper-based). Electronic applications accepted. *Faculty research:* Medical microbiology, environmental microbiology, biofilms, immunology, molecular biology and bioinformatics.

New York Medical College, Graduate School of Basic Medical Sciences, Integrated PhD Program, Valhalla, NY 10595-1691. Offers biochemistry and molecular biology (PhD); cell biology and anatomy (PhD); microbiology and immunology (PhD); pathology (PhD); pharmacology (PhD); physiology (PhD). *Degree requirements:* For doctorate, comprehensive exam, thesis/dissertation. *Entrance requirements:* For doctorate, GRE General Test. Additional exam requirements/recommendations for international students: Required—TOEFL. Electronic applications accepted. *Expenses: Tuition, area resident:* Full-time $44,355; part-time $1025 per credit. *Required fees:* $500; $95 per year. One-time fee: $140 full-time. Tuition and fees vary according to course load and program. *Faculty research:* Cardiovascular sciences, infectious diseases, neuroscience, cancer and cell signaling.

New York Medical College, Graduate School of Basic Medical Sciences, Microbiology and Immunology - Master's Program, Valhalla, NY 10595-1691. Offers MS, MD/PhD. *Program availability:* Part-time, evening/weekend. *Degree requirements:* For master's, thesis. *Entrance requirements:* For master's, GRE General Test, MCAT, or DAT. Additional exam requirements/recommendations for international students: Required—TOEFL. Electronic applications accepted. *Expenses: Tuition, area resident:* Full-time $44,355; part-time $1025 per credit. *Required fees:* $500; $95 per year. One-time fee: $140 part-time. Tuition and fees vary according to course load and program. *Faculty research:* Tumor cells, cancer vaccines, the role of stem cells in cancer, bacterial genetics pathogenesis of infectious disease and function of influenza virus antigens, molecular virology, and the biochemistry and genetics of emerging pathogens.

New York University, Graduate School of Arts and Science, Department of Biology, New York, NY 10012-1019. Offers biology (PhD); biomedical journalism (MS); cancer and molecular biology (PhD); computational biology (PhD); computers in biological research (MS); developmental genetics (PhD); general biology (MS); immunology and microbiology (PhD); molecular genetics (PhD); neurobiology (PhD); oral biology (MS); plant biology (PhD); recombinant DNA technology (MS); MS/MBA. *Program availability:*

Microbiology

Part-time. Terminal master's awarded for partial completion of doctoral program. *Degree requirements:* For master's, thesis or alternative, qualifying paper; for doctorate, comprehensive exam, thesis/dissertation. *Entrance requirements:* For master's and doctorate, GRE General Test. Additional exam requirements/recommendations for international students: Required—TOEFL. *Faculty research:* Genomics, molecular and cell biology, development and molecular genetics, molecular evolution of plants and animals.

New York University, School of Medicine and Graduate School of Arts and Science, Sackler Institute of Graduate Biomedical Sciences, Program in Microbiology, New York, NY 10012-1019. Offers PhD. *Degree requirements:* For doctorate, one foreign language, comprehensive exam, thesis/dissertation, qualifying exam. *Faculty research:* Microbiology, parasitology, and genetics; virology.

North Carolina State University, Graduate School, College of Agriculture and Life Sciences, Department of Microbiology, Program in Microbiology, Raleigh, NC 27695. Offers MS, PhD. *Degree requirements:* For master's, thesis (for some programs); for doctorate, thesis/dissertation. *Entrance requirements:* For master's and doctorate, GRE. Electronic applications accepted.

North Dakota State University, College of Graduate and Interdisciplinary Studies, College of Agriculture, Food Systems, and Natural Resources, Department of Microbiological Sciences, Fargo, ND 58102. Offers microbiology (MS); molecular pathogenesis (PhD). *Program availability:* Part-time. *Degree requirements:* For master's, thesis; for doctorate, thesis/dissertation, oral and written preliminary exams. *Entrance requirements:* For master's and doctorate, GRE. Additional exam requirements/recommendations for international students: Required—TOEFL (minimum score 525 paper-based; 71 iBT). *Application deadline:* For fall admission, 2/15 priority date for domestic students. Applications are processed on a rolling basis. Application fee: $35. *Financial support:* Fellowships with full tuition reimbursements, research assistantships with full tuition reimbursements, teaching assistantships with full tuition reimbursements, Federal Work-Study, and institutionally sponsored loans available. Financial award application deadline: 4/15. *Faculty research:* Bacterial gene regulation, antibiotic resistance, molecular virology, mechanisms of bacterial pathogenesis, immunology of animals. *Unit head:* John McEvoy, Interim Head, 701-231-8530, E-mail: john.mcevoy@ndsu.edu. *Application contact:* Eugene Berry, Associate Professor, 701-231-7520, Fax: 701-231-7514, E-mail: eugene.berry@ndsu.edu.
Website: http://www.ndsu.edu/micro/

The Ohio State University, Graduate School, College of Arts and Sciences, Division of Natural and Mathematical Sciences, Department of Microbiology, Columbus, OH 43210. Offers MS, PhD. Terminal master's awarded for partial completion of doctoral program. *Degree requirements:* For master's, thesis optional; for doctorate, thesis/dissertation. *Entrance requirements:* For doctorate, GRE General Test. Additional exam requirements/recommendations for international students: Required—TOEFL (minimum score 600 paper-based; 100 iBT), Michigan English Language Assessment Battery (minimum score 82); Recommended—IELTS (minimum score 8). Electronic applications accepted.

Ohio University, Graduate College, College of Arts and Sciences, Department of Biological Sciences, Athens, OH 45701-2979. Offers biological sciences (MS, PhD); cell biology and physiology (MS, PhD); ecology and evolutionary biology (MS, PhD); exercise physiology and muscle biology (MS, PhD); microbiology (MS, PhD); neuroscience (MS, PhD). Terminal master's awarded for partial completion of doctoral program. *Degree requirements:* For master's, comprehensive exam, thesis, 1 quarter of teaching experience; for doctorate, comprehensive exam, thesis/dissertation, 2 quarters of teaching experience. *Entrance requirements:* For master's, GRE General Test, names of three faculty members whose research interests most closely match the applicant's interest; for doctorate, GRE General Test, essay concerning prior training, research interest and career goals, plus names of three faculty members whose research interests most closely match the applicant's interest. Additional exam requirements/recommendations for international students: Required—TOEFL (minimum score 620 paper-based; 105 iBT) or IELTS (minimum score 7.5). Electronic applications accepted. *Faculty research:* Ecology and evolutionary biology, exercise physiology and muscle biology, neurobiology, cell biology, physiology.

Oklahoma State University, College of Arts and Sciences, Department of Microbiology and Molecular Genetics, Stillwater, OK 74078. Offers MS, PhD. *Faculty:* 19 full-time (5 women), 1 part-time/adjunct (0 women). *Students:* 12 full-time (6 women), 21 part-time (14 women); includes 9 minority (2 American Indian or Alaska Native, non-Hispanic/Latino; 2 Asian, non-Hispanic/Latino; 2 Hispanic/Latino; 3 Two or more races, non-Hispanic/Latino), 13 international. Average age 29. 44 applicants, 23% accepted, 9 enrolled. In 2015, 7 master's, 2 doctorates awarded. *Degree requirements:* For master's, thesis; for doctorate, comprehensive exam, thesis/dissertation. *Entrance requirements:* For master's and doctorate, GRE General Test. Additional exam requirements/recommendations for international students: Required—TOEFL (minimum score 550 paper-based; 79 iBT). *Application deadline:* For fall admission, 3/1 priority date for international students; for spring admission, 8/1 priority date for international students. Applications are processed on a rolling basis. Application fee: $40 ($75 for international students). Electronic applications accepted. *Expenses:* Tuition, state resident: full-time $3528; part-time $196 per credit hour. Tuition, nonresident: full-time $14,144; part-time $785.75 per credit hour. *Required fees:* $1895; $105.25 per credit hour. Tuition and fees vary according to campus/location. *Financial support:* In 2015–16, 12 research assistantships (averaging $17,445 per year), 14 teaching assistantships (averaging $18,093 per year) were awarded; career-related internships or fieldwork, Federal Work-Study, scholarships/grants, health care benefits, tuition waivers (partial), and unspecified assistantships also available. Support available to part-time students. Financial award application deadline: 3/1; financial aid applicants required to submit FAFSA. *Faculty research:* Bioinformatics, genomics-genetics, virology, environmental microbiology, development-molecular mechanisms. *Unit head:* Dr. Tyrrell Conway, Professor and Department Head, 405-744-6243, Fax: 405-744-6790, E-mail: tconway@okstate.edu. *Application contact:* Dr. Wouter Hoff, Graduate Program Coordinator, 405-744-6243, Fax: 405-744-6790, E-mail: wouter.hoff@okstate.edu.
Website: http://microbiology.okstate.edu

Oregon Health & Science University, School of Medicine, Graduate Programs in Medicine, Program in Molecular and Cellular Biosciences, Department of Molecular Microbiology and Immunology, Portland, OR 97239-3098. Offers PhD. *Faculty:* 28 full-time (8 women), 21 part-time/adjunct (6 women). *Students:* 17 full-time (12 women); includes 5 minority (2 Asian, non-Hispanic/Latino; 3 Two or more races, non-Hispanic/Latino), 3 international. Average age 30. Terminal master's awarded for partial completion of doctoral program. *Degree requirements:* For doctorate, comprehensive exam, thesis/dissertation, qualifying exam. *Entrance requirements:* For doctorate, GRE General Test (minimum scores: 153 Verbal/148 Quantitative/4.5 Analytical) or MCAT (for some programs). Additional exam requirements/recommendations for international students: Required—IELTS or TOEFL. *Application deadline:* For fall admission, 12/1 for domestic and international students. Application fee: $70. Electronic applications accepted. *Financial support:* Health care benefits and full tuition and stipends available. *Faculty research:* Molecular biology of bacterial and viral pathogens, cellular and humoral immunology, molecular biology of microbes. *Unit head:* Dr. Eric Barklis, Program Director, 503-494-7768, E-mail: mmi@ohsu.edu. *Application contact:* Brandi Colbert, Program Coordinator, 503-418-9457, E-mail: colbertb@ohsu.edu.
Website: http://www.ohsu.edu/microbiology

Oregon State University, College of Science, Program in Microbiology, Corvallis, OR 97331. Offers environmental microbiology (MA, MS, PhD); food microbiology (MA, MS, PhD); genomics (MA, MS, PhD); immunology (MA, MS, PhD); microbial ecology (MA, MS, PhD); microbial evolution (MA, MS, PhD); parasitology (MA, MS, PhD); pathogenic microbiology (MA, MS, PhD); virology (MA). *Program availability:* Part-time. *Faculty:* 14 full-time (5 women), 1 part-time/adjunct (0 women). *Students:* 32 full-time (12 women); includes 5 minority (4 Asian, non-Hispanic/Latino; 1 Two or more races, non-Hispanic/Latino), 2 international. Average age 28. 79 applicants, 10% accepted, 4 enrolled. In 2015, 3 master's, 4 doctorates awarded. Terminal master's awarded for partial completion of doctoral program. *Degree requirements:* For master's, thesis; for doctorate, one foreign language, thesis/dissertation. *Entrance requirements:* For master's and doctorate, GRE. Additional exam requirements/recommendations for international students: Required—TOEFL (minimum score 600 paper-based; 100 iBT). *Application deadline:* For fall admission, 8/1 for domestic students, 4/1 for international students; for winter admission, 12/1 for domestic students, 7/1 for international students; for spring admission, 2/1 for domestic students, 10/1 for international students; for summer admission, 5/1 for domestic students, 1/1 for international students. Application fee: $75 ($85 for international students). *Expenses:* Tuition, state resident: full-time $12,150; part-time $450 per credit. Tuition, nonresident: full-time $20,952; part-time $776 per credit. *Required fees:* $1572; $1443 per unit. One-time fee: $350. Tuition and fees vary according to course load, campus/location and program. *Financial support:* Fellowships, research assistantships, and teaching assistantships available. Financial award application deadline: 1/15. *Faculty research:* Genetics, physiology, biotechnology, pathogenic microbiology, plant virology. *Unit head:* Dr. Jerri Bartholomew, Professor and Department Head, 541-737-1856. *Application contact:* Mary Fulton, Microbiology Advisor, 541-737-1833, E-mail: mary.fulton@oregonstate.edu.
Website: http://microbiology.science.oregonstate.edu/

Penn State University Park, Graduate School, Eberly College of Science, Department of Biochemistry and Molecular Biology, University Park, PA 16802. Offers biochemistry, microbiology, and molecular biology (MS, PhD); biotechnology (MBIOT). *Unit head:* Dr. Douglas R. Cavener, Dean, 814-865-9591, Fax: 814-865-3634. *Application contact:* Lori Stania, Director, Graduate Student Services, 814-865-1795, Fax: 814-863-4627, E-mail: l-gswww@lists.psu.edu.
Website: http://bmb.psu.edu/

Purdue University, Graduate School, College of Science, Department of Biological Sciences, West Lafayette, IN 47907. Offers biochemistry (PhD); biophysics (PhD); cell and developmental biology (PhD); ecology, evolutionary and population biology (MS, PhD), including ecology, evolutionary biology, population biology; genetics (MS, PhD); microbiology (MS, PhD); molecular biology (PhD); neurobiology (MS, PhD); plant physiology (PhD). Terminal master's awarded for partial completion of doctoral program. *Degree requirements:* For master's, thesis (for some programs); for doctorate, thesis/dissertation, seminars, teaching experience. *Entrance requirements:* For master's, GRE General Test (minimum analytical writing score of 3.5), minimum undergraduate GPA of 3.0; for doctorate, GRE General Test (minimum analytical writing score of 3.5), minimum undergraduate GPA of 3.5. Additional exam requirements/recommendations for international students: Required—TOEFL (minimum score 600 paper-based; 107 iBT for MS, 80 iBT for PhD). Electronic applications accepted.

Purdue University, Graduate School, PULSe - Purdue University Life Sciences Program, West Lafayette, IN 47907. Offers biomolecular structure and biophysics (PhD); biotechnology (PhD); chemical biology (PhD); chromatin and regulation of gene expression (PhD); integrative neuroscience (PhD); integrative plant sciences (PhD); membrane biology (PhD); microbiology (PhD); molecular evolutionary and cancer biology (PhD); molecular evolutionary genetics (PhD); molecular virology (PhD). *Entrance requirements:* For doctorate, GRE, minimum undergraduate GPA of 3.0. Additional exam requirements/recommendations for international students: Required—TOEFL (minimum score 550 paper-based; 77 iBT). Electronic applications accepted.

Purdue University, School of Veterinary Medicine and Graduate School, Graduate Programs in Veterinary Medicine, Department of Comparative Pathobiology, West Lafayette, IN 47907-2027. Offers comparative epidemiology and public health (MS); comparative epidemiology and public heath (PhD); comparative microbiology and immunology (MS, PhD); comparative pathobiology (MS, PhD); interdisciplinary studies (PhD), including microbial pathogenesis, molecular signaling and cancer biology, molecular virology; lab animal medicine (MS); veterinary anatomic pathology (MS); veterinary clinical pathology (MS). Terminal master's awarded for partial completion of doctoral program. *Degree requirements:* For master's, thesis (for some programs); for doctorate, thesis/dissertation. *Entrance requirements:* For master's and doctorate, GRE General Test. Additional exam requirements/recommendations for international students: Required—TOEFL (minimum score 575 paper-based), IELTS (minimum score 6.5), TWE (minimum score 4). Electronic applications accepted.

Queen's University at Kingston, School of Graduate Studies, Faculty of Health Sciences, Department of Microbiology and Immunology, Kingston, ON K7L 3N6, Canada. Offers M Sc, PhD. *Program availability:* Part-time. *Degree requirements:* For master's, thesis; for doctorate, comprehensive exam, thesis/dissertation. *Entrance requirements:* For master's and doctorate, minimum B+ average. Additional exam requirements/recommendations for international students: Required—TOEFL (minimum score 600 paper-based). Electronic applications accepted. *Faculty research:* Bacteriology, virology, immunology, education in microbiology and immunology, microbial pathogenesis.

Rosalind Franklin University of Medicine and Science, School of Graduate and Postdoctoral Studies - Interdisciplinary Graduate Program in Biomedical Sciences, Department of Microbiology and Immunology, North Chicago, IL 60064-3095. Offers PhD, MD/PhD. Terminal master's awarded for partial completion of doctoral program. *Degree requirements:* For doctorate, comprehensive exam, thesis/dissertation. *Entrance requirements:* For doctorate, GRE General Test. Additional exam requirements/recommendations for international students: Required—TOEFL, TWE. *Faculty research:* Molecular biology, parasitology, virology.

Rush University, Graduate College, Division of Immunology and Microbiology, Chicago, IL 60612-3832. Offers microbiology (PhD); virology (MS, PhD), including immunology, virology; MD/PhD. *Degree requirements:* For doctorate, thesis/dissertation, comprehensive preliminary exam. *Entrance requirements:* For doctorate, GRE General Test, interview, minimum GPA of 3.0. Additional exam requirements/recommendations for international students: Required—TOEFL. *Faculty research:* Immune interactions of cells and membranes, HIV immunopathogenesis, autoimmunity, tumor biology.

Rutgers University–Newark, Graduate School of Biomedical Sciences, Department of Microbiology and Molecular Genetics, Newark, NJ 07107. Offers PhD. *Degree requirements:* For doctorate, thesis/dissertation, qualifying exam. *Entrance requirements:* For doctorate, GRE General Test. Additional exam requirements/recommendations for international students: Required—TOEFL. Electronic applications accepted. *Faculty research:* Molecular genetics of yeast, mutagenesis and carcinogenesis of DNA, bacterial protein synthesis, mammalian cell genetics, adenovirus gene expression.

Rutgers University–New Brunswick, Graduate School-New Brunswick, Programs in the Molecular Biosciences, Piscataway, NJ 08854-8097. Offers biochemistry (PhD); cell and developmental biology (MS, PhD); microbiology and molecular genetics (MS, PhD), including applied microbiology, clinical microbiology (MS), clinical mircobiology (PhD), computational molecular biology (PhD), immunology, microbial biochemistry, molecular genetics, virology. MS, PhD offered jointly with University of Medicine and Dentistry of New Jersey.

Rutgers University–New Brunswick, Graduate School of Biomedical Sciences, Program in Microbiology and Molecular Genetics, Piscataway, NJ 08854-5635. Offers MS, PhD, MD/PhD. Terminal master's awarded for partial completion of doctoral program. *Degree requirements:* For master's, thesis, qualifying exam; for doctorate, thesis/dissertation, qualifying exam. *Entrance requirements:* For master's and doctorate, GRE General Test. Additional exam requirements/recommendations for international students: Required—TOEFL. Electronic applications accepted. *Faculty research:* Interferon, receptors, retrovirus evolution, Arbo virus/host cell interactions.

Saint Louis University, Graduate Education and School of Medicine, Graduate Program in Biomedical Sciences, Department of Molecular Microbiology and Immunology, St. Louis, MO 63103. Offers PhD. *Degree requirements:* For doctorate, comprehensive exam, thesis/dissertation, qualifying exams. *Entrance requirements:* For doctorate, GRE General Test (GRE Subject Test optional), letters of recommendation, resume, interview. Additional exam requirements/recommendations for international students: Required—TOEFL (minimum score 525 paper-based). Electronic applications accepted. *Faculty research:* Pathogenesis of hepatitis C virus, herperviruses, pox viruses, rheumatoid arthritis, antiviral drugs and vaccines in biodefense, cancer gene therapy, virology and immunology.

San Diego State University, Graduate and Research Affairs, College of Sciences, Department of Biology, Program in Microbiology, San Diego, CA 92182. Offers MS. *Degree requirements:* For master's, thesis, oral exam. *Entrance requirements:* For master's, GRE General Test, GRE Subject Test, resume or curriculum vitae, 2 letters of recommendation. Additional exam requirements/recommendations for international students: Required—TOEFL. Electronic applications accepted.

San Francisco State University, Division of Graduate Studies, College of Science and Engineering, Department of Biology, Program in Microbiology, San Francisco, CA 94132-1722. Offers MS. *Application deadline:* Applications are processed on a rolling basis. *Expenses:* Tuition, state resident: full-time $6738. Tuition, nonresident: full-time $15,666. *Required fees:* $1004. *Unit head:* Dr. Diana Chu, Program Coordinator, 415-405-3487, Fax: 415-338-2295, E-mail: chud@sfsu.edu.
Website: http://biology.sfsu.edu/graduate/microbiology

Seton Hall University, College of Arts and Sciences, Department of Biological Sciences, South Orange, NJ 07079-2697. Offers biology (MS); biology/business administration (MS); microbiology (MS); molecular bioscience (PhD); molecular bioscience/neuroscience (PhD). *Program availability:* Part-time, evening/weekend. *Degree requirements:* For master's, thesis optional; for doctorate, comprehensive exam, thesis/dissertation. *Entrance requirements:* For master's, GRE or undergraduate degree (BS in biological sciences) with minimum GPA of 3.0 from accredited U.S. institution; for doctorate, GRE. Additional exam requirements/recommendations for international students: Required—TOEFL. Electronic applications accepted. *Faculty research:* Neurobiology, genetics, immunology, molecular biology, cellular physiology, toxicology, microbiology, bioinformatics.

South Dakota State University, Graduate School, College of Agriculture and Biological Sciences, Department of Biology and Microbiology, Brookings, SD 57007. Offers biological sciences (MS, PhD). *Program availability:* Part-time. *Degree requirements:* For master's, thesis (for some programs), oral exam; for doctorate, comprehensive exam, thesis/dissertation, oral exam. *Entrance requirements:* For master's and doctorate, GRE General Test. Additional exam requirements/recommendations for international students: Required—TOEFL (minimum score 600 paper-based; 100 iBT). *Faculty research:* Ecosystem ecology; plant, animal and microbial genomics; animal infectious disease, microbial bioproducts.

Southern Illinois University Carbondale, Graduate School, College of Science, Program in Molecular Biology, Microbiology, and Biochemistry, Carbondale, IL 62901-4701. Offers MS, PhD. *Faculty:* 16 full-time (2 women). *Students:* 38 full-time (28 women), 29 part-time (13 women); includes 5 minority (2 Black or African American, non-Hispanic/Latino; 3 Asian, non-Hispanic/Latino), 43 international. Average age 25. 83 applicants, 17% accepted, 612 enrolled. In 2015, 9 master's, 13 doctorates awarded. *Degree requirements:* For master's, thesis; for doctorate, thesis/dissertation. *Entrance requirements:* For master's, GRE, minimum GPA of 2.7; for doctorate, GRE, minimum GPA of 3.25. Additional exam requirements/recommendations for international students: Required—TOEFL. *Application deadline:* Applications are processed on a rolling basis. Application fee: $65. *Financial support:* In 2015–16, 49 students received support, including 42 research assistantships with full tuition reimbursements available, 7 teaching assistantships with full tuition reimbursements available; fellowships with full tuition reimbursements available, Federal Work-Study, and institutionally sponsored loans also available. Support available to part-time students. Financial award application deadline: 3/1. *Faculty research:* Prokaryotic gene regulation and expression; eukaryotic gene regulation; microbial, phylogenetic, and metabolic diversity; immune responses to tumors, pathogens, and autoantigens; protein folding and structure. *Unit head:* Dr. Judy Davie, Director, 618-453-5002, E-mail: jdavie@siumed.edu. *Application contact:* Donna K. Mueller, Office Manager, 618-453-8911, E-mail: mueller1@siu.edu.
Website: http://mbmb.siu.edu/

Southwestern Oklahoma State University, College of Professional and Graduate Studies, School of Behavioral Sciences and Education, Specialization in Health Sciences and Microbiology, Weatherford, OK 73096-3098. Offers M Ed.

⭐ **Stanford University,** School of Medicine, Graduate Programs in Medicine, Department of Microbiology and Immunology, Stanford, CA 94305-9991. Offers PhD. *Degree requirements:* For doctorate, comprehensive exam, thesis/dissertation, 2 quarter teaching assistantship. *Entrance requirements:* For doctorate, GRE General Test, GRE Subject Test (biology or biochemistry). Additional exam requirements/recommendations for international students: Required—TOEFL. Electronic applications accepted. *Expenses:* Tuition, area resident: Full-time $45,729. *Required fees:* $591. *Faculty research:* Molecular pathogenesis of bacteria viruses and parasites, immune system function, autoimmunity, molecular biology.

See Close-Up on page 331.

State University of New York Upstate Medical University, College of Graduate Studies, Program in Microbiology and Immunology, Syracuse, NY 13210-2334. Offers microbiology (MS); microbiology and immunology (PhD); MD/PhD. Terminal master's awarded for partial completion of doctoral program. *Degree requirements:* For master's, thesis; for doctorate, comprehensive exam, thesis/dissertation. *Entrance requirements:* For master's, GRE General Test, interview; for doctorate, GRE General Test, telephone interview. Additional exam requirements/recommendations for international students: Required—TOEFL. Electronic applications accepted. *Faculty research:* Cancer, disorders of the nervous system, infectious diseases, diabetes/metabolic disorders/cardiovascular diseases.

Stony Brook University, State University of New York, Stony Brook Medicine, School of Medicine and Graduate School, Graduate Programs in Medicine, Department of Molecular Genetics and Microbiology, Stony Brook, NY 11794. Offers PhD. *Faculty:* 16 full-time (4 women), 2 part-time/adjunct (1 woman). *Students:* 25 full-time (8 women); includes 7 minority (5 Asian, non-Hispanic/Latino; 2 Hispanic/Latino), 6 international. Average age 27. 49 applicants, 18% accepted, 4 enrolled. In 2015, 1 doctorate awarded. *Degree requirements:* For doctorate, comprehensive exam, thesis/dissertation. *Entrance requirements:* For doctorate, GRE General Test, GRE Subject Test, undergraduate training in biochemistry, genetics, and cell biology; recommendations; personal statement. Additional exam requirements/recommendations for international students: Required—TOEFL (minimum score 550 paper-based; 90 iBT). *Application deadline:* For fall admission, 1/15 for domestic students; for spring admission, 10/1 for domestic students. Application fee: $100. *Expenses:* $12,421 per year full-time resident tuition and fees, $453 per credit hour; $23,761 per year full-time non-resident tuition and fees, $925 per credit hour. *Financial support:* In 2015–16, 6 fellowships, 14 research assistantships, 4 teaching assistantships were awarded; Federal Work-Study also available. Financial award application deadline: 3/15. *Faculty research:* Bioimaging, infectious diseases or agents, pathogenesis, viral studies (virology), genetics. *Total annual research expenditures:* $19.7 million. *Unit head:* Dr. David G. Thanassi, Interim Chair, 631-632-4549, Fax: 631-632-9797, E-mail: david.thanassi@stonybrook.edu. *Application contact:* Kathryn Bell, Program Administrator, 631-632-8812, Fax: 631-632-9797, E-mail: kathryn.bell@stonybrook.edu.
Website: http://www.mgm.stonybrook.edu/index.shtml

Texas A&M University, College of Science, Department of Biology, College Station, TX 77843. Offers biology (MS, PhD); microbiology (MS, PhD). *Faculty:* 37. *Students:* 97 full-time (58 women), 4 part-time (2 women); includes 13 minority (2 Black or African American, non-Hispanic/Latino; 1 American Indian or Alaska Native, non-Hispanic/Latino; 2 Asian, non-Hispanic/Latino; 7 Hispanic/Latino; 1 Two or more races, non-Hispanic/Latino), 52 international. Average age 28. 97 applicants, 24% accepted, 12 enrolled. In 2015, 3 master's, 7 doctorates awarded. *Degree requirements:* For master's, thesis or alternative; for doctorate, comprehensive exam, thesis/dissertation. *Entrance requirements:* For master's and doctorate, GRE General Test. Additional exam requirements/recommendations for international students: Required—TOEFL. *Application deadline:* For fall admission, 1/15 for domestic students. Applications are processed on a rolling basis. Application fee: $50 ($90 for international students). Electronic applications accepted. *Expenses:* Contact institution. *Financial support:* In 2015–16, 102 students received support, including 7 fellowships with tuition reimbursements available (averaging $23,990 per year), 29 research assistantships with tuition reimbursements available (averaging $8,464 per year), 63 teaching assistantships with tuition reimbursements available (averaging $8,222 per year); career-related internships or fieldwork, institutionally sponsored loans, scholarships/grants, traineeships, health care benefits, tuition waivers (full and partial), and unspecified assistantships also available. Support available to part-time students. Financial award application deadline: 4/1; financial award applicants required to submit FAFSA. *Faculty research:* Biological clocks, cell, molecular and developmental biology, ecology and evolutionary biology, genetics and genomics, microbiology. *Unit head:* Dr. Tom McKnight, Department Head, 979-845-3896, Fax: 979-845-2891, E-mail: mcknight@bio.tamu.edu. *Application contact:* Dr. Arne Lekven, Graduate Advisor, 979-458-3461, Fax: 979-845-2891, E-mail: alekven@bio.tamu.edu.
Website: http://www.bio.tamu.edu/index.html

Texas Tech University, Graduate School, College of Arts and Sciences, Department of Biological Sciences, Lubbock, TX 79409-3131. Offers biology (MS, PhD); environmental sustainability and natural resources management (PSM); microbiology (MS); zoology (MS, PhD). *Program availability:* Part-time, blended/hybrid learning. *Faculty:* 41 full-time (12 women), 2 part-time/adjunct (1 woman). *Students:* 94 full-time (51 women), 5 part-time (3 women); includes 6 minority (1 American Indian or Alaska Native, non-Hispanic/Latino; 1 Asian, non-Hispanic/Latino; 3 Hispanic/Latino; 1 Two or more races, non-Hispanic/Latino), 53 international. Average age 29. 92 applicants, 39% accepted, 21 enrolled. In 2015, 7 master's, 9 doctorates awarded. *Degree requirements:* For master's, thesis or alternative; for doctorate, thesis/dissertation. *Entrance requirements:* For master's and doctorate, GRE General Test. Additional exam requirements/recommendations for international students: Required—TOEFL (minimum score 550 paper-based; 79 iBT). *Application deadline:* For fall admission, 6/1 priority date for domestic students, 1/15 priority date for international students; for spring admission, 9/1 priority date for domestic students, 6/15 priority date for international students. Applications are processed on a rolling basis. Application fee: $60. Electronic applications accepted. *Expenses:* Tuition, state resident: full-time $6477; part-time $269.89 per credit hour. Tuition, nonresident: full-time $15,837; part-time $659.89 per credit hour. *Required fees:* $2751; $36.50 per credit hour. $937.50 per semester. Tuition and fees vary according to course level. *Financial support:* In 2015–16, 98 students received support, including 79 fellowships (averaging $1,515 per year), 36 research assistantships (averaging $6,272 per year), 98 teaching assistantships (averaging $13,936 per year). Financial award application deadline: 4/15; financial award applicants required to submit FAFSA. *Faculty research:* Biodiversity, genomics and evolution, climate change in arid ecosystems, plant biology and biotechnology, animal communication and behavior, zoonotic and emerging diseases. *Total annual research expenditures:* $1.4 million. *Unit head:* Dr. Ron Chesser, Chair, 806-834-0121, Fax: 806-742-2963, E-mail: ron.chesser@ttu.edu. *Application contact:* Dr. Lou Densmore, Graduate Adviser, 806-834-6479, Fax: 806-742-2963, E-mail: lou.densmore@ttu.edu.
Website: http://www.depts.ttu.edu/biology/

Thomas Jefferson University, Jefferson College of Biomedical Sciences, MS Program in Microbiology, Philadelphia, PA 19107. Offers MS. *Program availability:* Part-time, evening/weekend. *Faculty:* 44 full-time (14 women), 27 part-time/adjunct (11 women). *Students:* 26 part-time (16 women); includes 5 minority (2 Black or African American, non-Hispanic/Latino; 2 Asian, non-Hispanic/Latino; 1 Hispanic/Latino). Average age 29. 25 applicants, 68% accepted, 12 enrolled. In 2015, 19 master's awarded. *Degree requirements:* For master's, thesis, clerkship. *Entrance requirements:* For master's, GRE General Test or MCAT, minimum GPA of 3.0. Additional exam requirements/recommendations for international students: Required—TOEFL, IELTS (minimum score 7). *Application deadline:* For fall admission, 8/1 priority date for domestic students, 3/1 priority date for international students; for winter admission, 12/1 priority date for domestic students, 6/1 priority date for international students; for spring admission, 4/1 priority date for domestic students. Applications are processed on a rolling basis. Application fee: $50. Electronic applications accepted. *Financial support:* Federal Work-Study and institutionally sponsored loans available. Support available to part-time students. Financial award application deadline: 5/1; financial award applicants required to submit FAFSA. *Faculty research:* Vaccinology, epidemiology, planning and management, microbiology. *Unit head:* Dr. James P. McGettigan, Program Director, 215-503-4629, Fax: 215-503-5393, E-mail: james.mcgettigan@jefferson.edu. *Application contact:* Marc E. Stearns, Director of Admissions, 215-503-0155, Fax: 215-

Microbiology

503-3433, E-mail: jgsbs-info@jefferson.edu.
Website: http://www.jefferson.edu/university/biomedical-sciences/degrees-programs/master-programs/microbiology.html

Thomas Jefferson University, Jefferson College of Biomedical Sciences, PhD Program in Immunology and Microbial Pathogenesis, Philadelphia, PA 19107. Offers PhD. *Faculty:* 35 full-time (5 women), 1 part-time/adjunct (0 women). *Students:* 16 full-time (9 women); includes 4 minority (3 Asian, non-Hispanic/Latino; 1 Hispanic/Latino), 1 international. Average age 28. 35 applicants, 9% accepted, 2 enrolled. In 2015, 6 doctorates awarded. *Degree requirements:* For doctorate, comprehensive exam, thesis/dissertation. *Entrance requirements:* For doctorate, GRE General Test, minimum GPA of 3.2. Additional exam requirements/recommendations for international students: Required—TOEFL, IELTS (minimum score 7). *Application deadline:* For fall admission, 12/15 priority date for domestic and international students. Applications are processed on a rolling basis. Application fee: $50. Electronic applications accepted. *Financial support:* In 2015–16, 16 students received support, including 16 fellowships with full tuition reimbursements available (averaging $56,298 per year); Federal Work-Study, institutionally sponsored loans, scholarships/grants, traineeships and stipends also available. Support available to part-time students. Financial award application deadline: 5/1; financial award applicants required to submit FAFSA. *Unit head:* Dr. Matthias J. Schnell, Program Director, 215-503-4634, Fax: 215-503-5393, E-mail: matthias.schnell@jefferson.edu. *Application contact:* Marc E. Stearns, Director of Admissions, 215-503-0155, Fax: 215-503-3433, E-mail: jgsbs-info@jefferson.edu. Website: http://www.jefferson.edu/university/biomedical-sciences/degrees-programs/phd-programs/immunology.html

Tufts University, Sackler School of Graduate Biomedical Sciences, Molecular Microbiology Program, Medford, MA 02155. Offers medically-oriented research in graduate education (PhD); molecular microbiology (PhD). *Faculty:* 17 full-time (7 women). *Students:* 29 full-time (24 women); includes 8 minority (2 Black or African American, non-Hispanic/Latino; 2 Asian, non-Hispanic/Latino; 4 Two or more races, non-Hispanic/Latino), 1 international. Average age 28. 83 applicants, 20% accepted, 5 enrolled. In 2015, 5 doctorates awarded. Terminal master's awarded for partial completion of doctoral program. *Degree requirements:* For doctorate, comprehensive exam, thesis/dissertation. *Entrance requirements:* For doctorate, GRE General Test, 3 letters of reference. Additional exam requirements/recommendations for international students: Required—TOEFL (minimum score 600 paper-based; 100 iBT), IELTS (minimum score 7). *Application deadline:* For fall admission, 12/15 priority date for domestic and international students. Application fee: $90. Electronic applications accepted. *Expenses: Tuition, area resident:* Full-time $48,412; part-time $1210 per credit hour. *Required fees:* $806. Full-time tuition and fees vary according to degree level, program and student level. Part-time tuition and fees vary according to course load. *Financial support:* In 2015–16, 29 students received support, including 29 research assistantships with full tuition reimbursements available (averaging $32,000 per year); traineeships and health care benefits also available. *Faculty research:* Mechanisms of gene regulation, interactions of microorganisms and viruses with host cells, infection response. *Unit head:* Dr. Michael Malamy, Director, 617-636-6750, Fax: 617-636-0337, E-mail: michael.malamy@tufts.edu. *Application contact:* Dr. Elizabeth Storrs, 617-636-6767, Fax: 617-636-0375, E-mail: sackler-school@tufts.edu. Website: http://sackler.tufts.edu/Academics/Degree-Programs/Molecular-Microbiology

Tulane University, School of Medicine and School of Liberal Arts, Graduate Programs in Biomedical Sciences, Department of Microbiology and Immunology, New Orleans, LA 70118-5669. Offers MS. MS and PhD offered through the Graduate School. *Degree requirements:* For master's, thesis. *Entrance requirements:* For master's, GRE General Test, minimum B average in undergraduate course work. Additional exam requirements/recommendations for international students: Required—TOEFL. *Application deadline:* For fall admission, 2/1 for domestic and international students. Application fee: $45. Electronic applications accepted. *Expenses: Tuition, area resident:* Full-time $47,658; part-time $2648 per credit hour. *Required fees:* $1980; $44.50 per credit hour. $550 per term. Tuition and fees vary according to course load, degree level and program. *Financial support:* Fellowships with full tuition reimbursements, research assistantships with full tuition reimbursements, career-related internships or fieldwork, Federal Work-Study, and institutionally sponsored loans available. Financial award application deadline: 2/1. *Faculty research:* Vaccine development, viral pathogenesis, molecular virology, bacterial pathogenesis, fungal pathogenesis.

Universidad Central del Caribe, School of Medicine, Program in Biomedical Sciences, Bayamón, PR 00960-6032. Offers anatomy and cell biology (MA, MS); biochemistry (MS); biomedical sciences (MA); cellular and molecular biology (PhD); microbiology and immunology (MA, MS); pharmacology (MS); physiology (MS).

Université de Montréal, Faculty of Medicine, Department of Microbiology and Immunology, Montréal, QC H3C 3J7, Canada. Offers M Sc, PhD. Programs offered jointly with Faculty of Veterinary Medicine and Université du Québec, Institut Armand-Frappier. Terminal master's awarded for partial completion of doctoral program. *Degree requirements:* For master's, thesis; for doctorate, thesis/dissertation, general exam. *Entrance requirements:* For master's and doctorate, proficiency in French, knowledge of English. Electronic applications accepted.

Université de Sherbrooke, Faculty of Medicine and Health Sciences, Graduate Programs in Medicine, Program in Microbiology, Sherbrooke, QC J1H 5N4, Canada. Offers M Sc, PhD. Terminal master's awarded for partial completion of doctoral program. *Degree requirements:* For master's, thesis; for doctorate, thesis/dissertation. Electronic applications accepted. *Faculty research:* Oncogenes, alternative splicing mechanisms, genomics, telomerase, DNA repair, Clostridium difficile, Campylobacter jejuni.

Université du Québec, Institut National de la Recherche Scientifique, Graduate Programs, Research Center–INRS–Institut Armand-Frappier, Laval, QC H7V 1B7, Canada. Offers applied microbiology (M Sc); biology (PhD); experimental health sciences (M Sc); virology and immunology (M Sc, PhD). *Program availability:* Part-time. *Degree requirements:* For master's, thesis; for doctorate, thesis/dissertation. *Entrance requirements:* For master's, appropriate bachelor's degree, proficiency in French; for doctorate, appropriate master's degree, proficiency in French. Electronic applications accepted. *Faculty research:* Immunity, infection and cancer; toxicology and environmental biotechnology; molecular pharmacochemistry.

Université Laval, Faculty of Agricultural and Food Sciences, Program in Agricultural Microbiology, Québec, QC G1K 7P4, Canada. Offers agricultural microbiology (M Sc); agro-food microbiology (PhD). Terminal master's awarded for partial completion of doctoral program. *Degree requirements:* For master's, thesis; for doctorate, comprehensive exam, thesis/dissertation. *Entrance requirements:* For master's and doctorate, knowledge of French and English. Electronic applications accepted.

Université Laval, Faculty of Medicine, Graduate Programs in Medicine, Programs in Microbiology-Immunology, Québec, QC G1K 7P4, Canada. Offers M Sc, PhD. Terminal master's awarded for partial completion of doctoral program. *Degree requirements:* For master's, thesis; for doctorate, comprehensive exam, thesis/dissertation. *Entrance requirements:* For master's and doctorate, knowledge of French, comprehension of written English. Electronic applications accepted.

Université Laval, Faculty of Sciences and Engineering, Department of Biochemistry and Microbiology, Programs in Microbiology, Québec, QC G1K 7P4, Canada. Offers M Sc, PhD. Terminal master's awarded for partial completion of doctoral program. *Degree requirements:* For master's, thesis; for doctorate, comprehensive exam, thesis/dissertation. *Entrance requirements:* For master's and doctorate, knowledge of French, comprehension of written English. Electronic applications accepted.

University at Buffalo, the State University of New York, Graduate School, School of Medicine and Biomedical Sciences, Graduate Programs in Medicine and Biomedical Sciences, Department of Microbiology and Immunology, Buffalo, NY 14214-3000. Offers MA, PhD. *Faculty:* 18 full-time (5 women). *Students:* 19 full-time (10 women); includes 5 minority (1 Black or African American, non-Hispanic/Latino; 4 Asian, non-Hispanic/Latino). Average age 27. 16 applicants, 19% accepted. In 2015, 1 master's, 6 doctorates awarded. *Degree requirements:* For master's, comprehensive exam; for doctorate, thesis/dissertation, departmental qualifying exam. *Entrance requirements:* For master's and doctorate, GRE General Test, 3 letters of recommendation. Additional exam requirements/recommendations for international students: Required—TOEFL (minimum score 100 iBT). *Application deadline:* For fall admission, 4/1 priority date for domestic and international students. Applications are processed on a rolling basis. Application fee: $85. Electronic applications accepted. *Financial support:* In 2015–16, 6 fellowships with tuition reimbursements (averaging $28,000 per year), 8 research assistantships with tuition reimbursements (averaging $27,000 per year) were awarded; traineeships and unspecified assistantships also available. Financial award application deadline: 2/1; financial award applicants required to submit FAFSA. *Faculty research:* Bacteriology, immunology, parasitology, virology, mycology. Total annual research expenditures: $5 million. *Unit head:* Dr. James Bangs, Chair/Professor, 716-829-2907, Fax: 716-829-2158. *Application contact:* Dr. John Panepinto, Director of Graduate Studies, 716-829-2176, Fax: 716-829-2158.
Website: http://www.smbs.buffalo.edu/microb/

The University of Alabama at Birmingham, Graduate Programs in Joint Health Sciences, Microbiology Theme, Birmingham, AL 35294-2182. Offers PhD. *Faculty:* 67 full-time (15 women). *Students:* 36 full-time (17 women); includes 21 minority (5 Black or African American, non-Hispanic/Latino; 13 Asian, non-Hispanic/Latino; 3 Hispanic/Latino), 7 international. Average age 27. In 2015, 4 doctorates awarded. *Degree requirements:* For doctorate, comprehensive exam, thesis/dissertation. *Entrance requirements:* For doctorate, GRE (minimum combined verbal/quantitative score of 300), minimum GPA of 3.0; interview; strong background in biology, chemistry, and/or mathematics. Additional exam requirements/recommendations for international students: Required—TOEFL (minimum score 100 iBT). *Application deadline:* For fall admission, 12/1 priority date for domestic students, 1/15 for international students. Application fee: $0 ($60 for international students). Electronic applications accepted. *Expenses:* Contact institution. *Financial support:* In 2015–16, 36 students received support. Fellowships, traineeships, and competitive annual stipends, health insurance, and fully-paid tuition and fees available. *Faculty research:* Streptococcus pneumoniae capsular polysaccharides, genetics, and pathogenesis; protective and pathogenic CD4 T cell responses; anti-viral immunity; immunological memory; microbiome, bacteria and host interactions, structural biology and glycobiology; the role of oxidative stress on autoimmune Type 1 diabetes. *Unit head:* Dr. Janet Yother, Program Director, 205-934-9531, Fax: 205-996-6749, E-mail: jyother@uab.edu. *Application contact:* Susan Noblitt Banks, Director of Graduate School Operations, 205-934-8227, Fax: 205-934-8413, E-mail: gradschool@uab.edu.
Website: http://www.uab.edu/gbs/microbiology/

University of Alberta, Faculty of Graduate Studies and Research, Department of Biological Sciences, Edmonton, AB T6G 2E1, Canada. Offers environmental biology and ecology (M Sc, PhD); microbiology and biotechnology (M Sc, PhD); molecular biology and genetics (M Sc, PhD); physiology and cell biology (M Sc, PhD); plant biology (M Sc, PhD); systematics and evolution (M Sc, PhD). Terminal master's awarded for partial completion of doctoral program. *Degree requirements:* For master's, thesis; for doctorate, thesis/dissertation. *Entrance requirements:* Additional exam requirements/recommendations for international students: Required—TOEFL.

The University of Arizona, College of Medicine, Department of Immunobiology, Tucson, AZ 85721. Offers PhD. *Degree requirements:* For doctorate, thesis/dissertation. *Entrance requirements:* For doctorate, GRE General Test, minimum GPA of 3.0. *Application deadline:* For fall admission, 3/1 priority date for domestic students; for spring admission, 9/1 for domestic students. Application fee: $75. *Financial support:* Fellowships, research assistantships, teaching assistantships, institutionally sponsored loans, and tuition waivers (full) available. Financial award application deadline: 4/30. *Faculty research:* Environmental and pathogenic microbiology, molecular biology. *Unit head:* Dr. Janko Nikolich-Zugich, Head, 520-626-6065, Fax: 520-626-2100, E-mail: nikolich@email.arizona.edu. *Application contact:* Tammy Rippberger, Senior business Manager, 520-626-6888, E-mail: trippberger@email.arizona.edu.
Website: http://immunobiology.arizona.edu/

University of Arkansas for Medical Sciences, Graduate School, Little Rock, AR 72205. Offers biochemistry and molecular biology (MS, PhD); bioinformatics (MS, PhD); cellular physiology and molecular biophysics (MS, PhD); clinical nutrition (MS); interdisciplinary biomedical sciences (MS, PhD, Certificate); interdisciplinary toxicology (MS); microbiology and immunology (PhD); neurobiology and developmental sciences (PhD); pharmacology (PhD); MD/PhD. Bioinformatics programs hosted jointly with the University of Arkansas at Little Rock. *Program availability:* Part-time. Terminal master's awarded for partial completion of doctoral program. *Degree requirements:* For master's, comprehensive exam (for some programs), thesis (for some programs); for doctorate, thesis/dissertation. *Entrance requirements:* For master's and doctorate, GRE. Additional exam requirements/recommendations for international students: Required—TOEFL. Electronic applications accepted. *Expenses:* Contact institution.

The University of British Columbia, Faculty of Science, Department of Microbiology and Immunology, Vancouver, BC V6T 1Z1, Canada. Offers M Sc, PhD. *Degree requirements:* For master's, thesis; for doctorate, comprehensive exam, thesis/dissertation. *Entrance requirements:* For master's and doctorate, GRE General Test. Additional exam requirements/recommendations for international students: Required—TOEFL (minimum score 590 paper-based). Electronic applications accepted. *Faculty research:* Bacterial genetics, metabolism, pathogenic bacteriology, virology.

University of Calgary, Cumming School of Medicine and Faculty of Graduate Studies, Department of Microbiology, Immunology and Infectious Diseases, Calgary, AB T2N 1N4, Canada. Offers M Sc, PhD. *Degree requirements:* For master's, thesis, oral thesis exam; for doctorate, thesis/dissertation, candidacy exam, oral thesis exam. *Entrance requirements:* For master's and doctorate, minimum GPA of 3.2. Additional exam requirements/recommendations for international students: Required—TOEFL (minimum score 580 paper-based). Electronic applications accepted. *Faculty research:* Bacteriology, virology, parasitology, immunology.

University of California, Berkeley, Graduate Division, College of Natural Resources, Group in Microbiology, Berkeley, CA 94720-1500. Offers PhD. *Degree requirements:* For doctorate, thesis/dissertation. *Entrance requirements:* For doctorate, GRE General Test, minimum GPA of 3.0, 3 letters of recommendation.

University of California, Davis, Graduate Studies, Graduate Group in Microbiology, Davis, CA 95616. Offers MS, PhD. Terminal master's awarded for partial completion of doctoral program. *Degree requirements:* For master's, thesis; for doctorate, thesis/dissertation. *Entrance requirements:* For master's and doctorate, GRE General Test, minimum GPA of 3.0. Additional exam requirements/recommendations for international students: Required—TOEFL (minimum score 550 paper-based). Electronic applications accepted. *Faculty research:* Microbial physiology and genetics, microbial molecular and cellular biology, microbial ecology, microbial pathogenesis and immunology, urology.

University of California, Irvine, School of Medicine and Francisco J. Ayala School of Biological Sciences, Department of Microbiology and Molecular Genetics, Irvine, CA 92697. Offers biological sciences (MS, PhD); MD/PhD. *Students:* 19 full-time (11 women), 1 (woman) part-time; includes 9 minority (1 Black or African American, non-Hispanic/Latino; 1 American Indian or Alaska Native, non-Hispanic/Latino; 3 Asian, non-Hispanic/Latino; 4 Hispanic/Latino), 1 international. Average age 29. In 2015, 1 master's, 4 doctorates awarded. *Degree requirements:* For doctorate, thesis/dissertation. *Entrance requirements:* For doctorate, GRE General Test, GRE Subject Test, minimum GPA of 3.0. Additional exam requirements/recommendations for international students: Required—TOEFL (minimum score 550 paper-based). *Application deadline:* For fall admission, 12/15 priority date for domestic students, 12/15 for international students. Application fee: $90 ($110 for international students). Electronic applications accepted. *Financial support:* Fellowships, research assistantships with full tuition reimbursements, teaching assistantships, institutionally sponsored loans, traineeships, health care benefits, and unspecified assistantships available. Financial award applicants required to submit FAFSA. *Faculty research:* Molecular biology and genetics of viruses, bacteria, and yeast; immune response; molecular biology of cultured animal cells; genetic basis of cancer; genetics and physiology of infectious agents. *Unit head:* Rozanne M. Sandri-Goldin, Chair, 949-824-7570, Fax: 949-824-8598, E-mail: rmsandri@uci.edu. *Application contact:* Janet Horwitz, Graduate Student Coordinator, 949-824-7669, E-mail: horwitz@uci.edu. Website: http://www.microbiology.uci.edu/graduate-students.asp

University of California, Los Angeles, David Geffen School of Medicine and Graduate Division, Graduate Programs in Medicine, Department of Microbiology, Immunology and Molecular Genetics, Los Angeles, CA 90095. Offers MS, PhD. *Degree requirements:* For master's, thesis; for doctorate, thesis/dissertation, oral and written qualifying exams; 2 quarters of teaching experience. *Entrance requirements:* For master's and doctorate, GRE General Test, bachelor's degree; minimum undergraduate GPA of 3.0 (or its equivalent if letter grade system not used). Additional exam requirements/recommendations for international students: Required—TOEFL. Electronic applications accepted.

University of California, Riverside, Graduate Division, Program in Microbiology, Riverside, CA 92521-0102. Offers MS, PhD. *Program availability:* Part-time. Terminal master's awarded for partial completion of doctoral program. *Degree requirements:* For master's, thesis; for doctorate, thesis/dissertation, qualifying exams. *Entrance requirements:* For master's and doctorate, GRE General Test, minimum GPA of 3.2. Additional exam requirements/recommendations for international students: Required—TOEFL (minimum score 550 paper-based; 80 iBT). Electronic applications accepted. *Expenses:* Tuition, area resident: Full-time $16,665.50; part-time $11,055.54. Tuition, state resident: full-time $16,665.50; part-time $11,055.54. Tuition, nonresident: full-time $31,768. *International tuition:* $31,767.50 full-time. *Required fees:* $16,665.50; $11,055.54 per quarter. $3685.18 per quarter. Tuition and fees vary according to program. *Faculty research:* Host-pathogen interactions; environmental microbiology; bioremediation; molecular microbiology; microbial genetics, physiology, and pathogenesis.

University of Chicago, Division of the Biological Sciences, Committee on Microbiology, Chicago, IL 60637. Offers PhD. *Students:* 18 full-time (7 women); includes 5 minority (1 Black or African American, non-Hispanic/Latino; 2 Hispanic/Latino; 2 Two or more races, non-Hispanic/Latino), 2 international. Average age 27. 71 applicants, 23% accepted, 4 enrolled. In 2015, 2 doctorates awarded. *Degree requirements:* For doctorate, thesis/dissertation, ethics class, 2 teaching assistantships. *Entrance requirements:* For doctorate, GRE General Test. Additional exam requirements/recommendations for international students: Required—TOEFL (minimum score 600 paper-based; 104 iBT), IELTS (minimum score 7). *Application deadline:* For fall admission, 12/1 for domestic and international students. Application fee: $90. Electronic applications accepted. *Financial support:* In 2015–16, 18 students received support, including fellowships with full tuition reimbursements available (averaging $29,781 per year), research assistantships with full tuition reimbursements available (averaging $29,781 per year); institutionally sponsored loans, scholarships/grants, traineeships, and health care benefits also available. Financial award application deadline: 1/5; financial award applicants required to submit FAFSA. *Faculty research:* Molecular genetics, herpes virus, adipoviruses, Picarna viruses, ENS viruses. *Unit head:* Dr. Olaf Schneewind, Chairman, 773-834-9060, Fax: 773-834-8150. *Application contact:* Emily Traw, Administrator, 773-834-3550, Fax: 773-834-7473, E-mail: etraw@bsd.uchicago.edu. Website: http://biomed.bsd.uchicago.edu/common/programs/microbiology/microbiology.html

University of Cincinnati, Graduate School, College of Medicine, Graduate Programs in Biomedical Sciences, Department of Molecular Genetics, Biochemistry and Microbiology, Cincinnati, OH 45221. Offers MS, PhD. Terminal master's awarded for partial completion of doctoral program. *Degree requirements:* For master's, thesis or alternative; for doctorate, thesis/dissertation, qualifying exam. *Entrance requirements:* For master's and doctorate, GRE General Test. Additional exam requirements/recommendations for international students: Required—TOEFL (minimum score 600 paper-based; 100 iBT), TWE. Electronic applications accepted. *Faculty research:* Cancer biology and developmental genetics, gene regulation and chromosome structure, microbiology and pathogenic mechanisms, structural biology, membrane biochemistry and signal transduction.

University of Colorado Boulder, Graduate School, College of Arts and Sciences, Department of Ecology and Evolutionary Biology, Boulder, CO 80309. Offers animal behavior (MA); biology (MA, PhD); environmental biology (MA, PhD); evolutionary biology (MA, PhD); neurobiology (MA); population biology (MA); population genetics (PhD). *Faculty:* 31 full-time (12 women). *Students:* 67 full-time (31 women), 3 part-time (1 woman); includes 8 minority (1 Asian, non-Hispanic/Latino; 3 Hispanic/Latino; 4 Two or more races, non-Hispanic/Latino), 4 international. Average age 30. 119 applicants, 11% accepted, 13 enrolled. In 2015, 10 master's, 14 doctorates awarded. Terminal master's awarded for partial completion of doctoral program. *Degree requirements:* For master's, comprehensive exam, thesis or alternative; for doctorate, comprehensive exam, thesis/dissertation. *Entrance requirements:* For master's, GRE General Test, GRE Subject Test, minimum undergraduate GPA of 3.0; for doctorate, GRE General Test, GRE Subject Test. *Application deadline:* For fall admission, 12/31 for domestic students, 12/1 for international students. Application fee: $50 ($70 for international students). Electronic applications accepted. Application fee is waived when completed online. *Financial support:* In 2015–16, 138 students received support, including 14 fellowships (averaging $7,260 per year), 12 research assistantships with tuition reimbursements available (averaging $31,833 per year), 47 teaching assistantships with tuition reimbursements available (averaging $33,448 per year); institutionally sponsored loans, scholarships/grants, health care benefits, and unspecified assistantships also available. Financial award applicants required to submit FAFSA. *Faculty research:* Ecology, botany, evolutionary biology, biological sciences, conservation biology. *Total annual research expenditures:* $6.3 million. *Application contact:* E-mail: ebiograd@colorado.edu. Website: http://ebio.colorado.edu

University of Colorado Denver, College of Liberal Arts and Sciences, Department of Integrative and Systems Biology, Denver, CO 80217. Offers animal behavior (MS); biology (MS); cell and developmental biology (MS); ecology (MS); evolutionary biology (MS); genetics (MS); integrative and systems biology (PhD); microbiology (MS); molecular biology (MS); neurobiology (MS); plant systematics (MS). *Program availability:* Part-time. *Faculty:* 21 full-time (8 women), 3 part-time/adjunct (1 woman). *Students:* 31 full-time (19 women), 7 part-time (3 women); includes 8 minority (1 Black or African American, non-Hispanic/Latino; 1 Asian, non-Hispanic/Latino; 3 Hispanic/Latino; 3 Two or more races, non-Hispanic/Latino), 1 international. Average age 28. 34 applicants, 29% accepted, 8 enrolled. In 2015, 6 master's awarded. *Degree requirements:* For master's, comprehensive exam, thesis, 30-32 credit hours; for doctorate, comprehensive exam, thesis/dissertation. *Entrance requirements:* For master's, GRE General Test (minimum score in 50th percentile in each section), BA/BS from accredited institution awarded within the last 10 years; minimum undergraduate GPA of 3.0; prerequisite courses: 1 year each of general biology and general chemistry; 1 semester each of general genetics, general ecology, and cell biology; and a structure/function course; for doctorate, GRE, minimum undergraduate GPA of 3.2, three letters of recommendation, official transcripts from all universities and colleges attended. Additional exam requirements/recommendations for international students: Required—TOEFL (minimum score 537 paper-based; 75 iBT); Recommended—IELTS (minimum score 6.5). *Application deadline:* For fall admission, 1/15 for domestic and international students. Application fee: $50 ($75 for international students). Electronic applications accepted. *Financial support:* In 2015–16, 32 students received support. Fellowships, research assistantships, teaching assistantships, Federal Work-Study, institutionally sponsored loans, scholarships/grants, and traineeships available. Financial award application deadline: 4/1; financial award applicants required to submit FAFSA. *Faculty research:* Molecular developmental biology; quantitative ecology, biogeography, and population dynamics; environmental signaling and endocrine disruption; speciation, the evolution of reproductive isolation, and hybrid zones; evolutionary, behavioral, and conservation ecology. *Unit head:* Dr. John Swallow, Chair, 303-556-6154, E-mail: john.swallow@ucdenver.edu. *Application contact:* Dr. Michael Wunder, Graduate Advisor, 303-556-8870, E-mail: michael.wunder@ucdenver.edu. Website: http://www.ucdenver.edu/academics/colleges/CLAS/Departments/biology/Programs/MasterofScience/Pages/BiologyMasterOfScience.aspx

University of Colorado Denver, School of Medicine, Program in Microbiology, Aurora, CO 80045. Offers microbiology (PhD); microbiology and immunology (PhD). *Students:* 16 full-time (7 women); includes 1 minority (Hispanic/Latino), 1 international. Average age 27. 57 applicants, 4% accepted, 2 enrolled. In 2015, 3 doctorates awarded. *Degree requirements:* For doctorate, comprehensive exam, thesis/dissertation, 3 lab rotations; 30 credit hours of coursework. *Entrance requirements:* For doctorate, GRE, three letters of reference, two copies of official transcripts, minimum GPA of 3.0. Additional exam requirements/recommendations for international students: Required—TOEFL (minimum score 550 paper-based; 80 iBT). *Application deadline:* For fall admission, 12/1 for domestic students, 11/1 for international students. Application fee: $50 ($75 for international students). Electronic applications accepted. *Expenses:* Contact institution. *Financial support:* In 2015–16, 17 students received support. Fellowships with tuition reimbursements available, research assistantships, teaching assistantships, institutionally sponsored loans, scholarships/grants, traineeships, health care benefits, and tuition waivers (full) available. Financial award application deadline: 3/15; financial award applicants required to submit FAFSA. *Faculty research:* Molecular mechanisms of picornavirus replication, mechanisms of papovavirus assembly, human immune response in multiple sclerosis. *Total annual research expenditures:* $5.9 million. *Unit head:* Dr. John Cambier, Chair, 303-724-8663, E-mail: john.cambier@ucdenver.edu. *Application contact:* Elizabeth Wethington, Program Administrator, 303-724-7280, E-mail: elizabeth.wethington@ucdenver.edu. Website: http://www.ucdenver.edu/academics/colleges/medicalschool/departments/ImmunologyMicrobiology/Pages/welcome.aspx

University of Delaware, College of Arts and Sciences, Department of Biological Sciences, Newark, DE 19716. Offers biotechnology (MS); cancer biology (MS, PhD); cell and extracellular matrix biology (MS, PhD); cell and systems physiology (MS, PhD); developmental biology (MS, PhD); ecology and evolution (MS, PhD); microbiology (MS, PhD); molecular biology and genetics (MS, PhD). Terminal master's awarded for partial completion of doctoral program. *Degree requirements:* For master's, thesis, preliminary exam; for doctorate, comprehensive exam, thesis/dissertation, preliminary exam. *Entrance requirements:* For master's and doctorate, GRE General Test. Additional exam requirements/recommendations for international students: Required—TOEFL (minimum score 600 paper-based); Recommended—TWE. Electronic applications accepted. *Faculty research:* Microorganisms, bone, cancer metastasis, developmental biology, cell biology, DNA.

University of Florida, College of Medicine, Department of Molecular Genetics and Microbiology, Gainesville, FL 32610-0266. Offers MS. Terminal master's awarded for partial completion of doctoral program. *Degree requirements:* For master's, thesis. *Entrance requirements:* For master's, GRE General Test, minimum GPA of 3.0. Additional exam requirements/recommendations for international students: Required—TOEFL, IELTS. Electronic applications accepted.

University of Florida, College of Medicine and Graduate School, Interdisciplinary Program in Biomedical Sciences, Concentration in Immunology and Microbiology, Gainesville, FL 32611. Offers PhD. *Degree requirements:* For doctorate, thesis/dissertation. *Entrance requirements:* For doctorate, GRE General Test, minimum GPA of 3.0, biochemistry before enrollment. Additional exam requirements/recommendations for international students: Required—TOEFL. Electronic applications accepted.

University of Florida, Graduate School, College of Agricultural and Life Sciences, Department of Microbiology and Cell Science, Gainesville, FL 32611. Offers microbiology and cell science (MS, PhD), including medical microbiology and biochemistry (MS), toxicology (PhD). *Degree requirements:* For master's, comprehensive exam, thesis (for some programs); for doctorate, comprehensive exam, thesis/dissertation. *Entrance requirements:* For master's and doctorate, GRE General Test, minimum GPA of 3.0. Additional exam requirements/recommendations for international students: Required—TOEFL (minimum score 550 paper-based; 80 iBT), IELTS (minimum score 6). Electronic applications accepted. *Faculty research:* Biomass conversion, membrane and cell wall chemistry, plant biochemistry and genetics.

University of Georgia, Franklin College of Arts and Sciences, Department of Microbiology, Athens, GA 30602. Offers MS, PhD. *Degree requirements:* For master's, thesis; for doctorate, one foreign language, thesis/dissertation. *Entrance requirements:* For master's and doctorate, GRE General Test. Additional exam requirements/

Microbiology

recommendations for international students: Required—TOEFL (minimum score 550 paper-based). Electronic applications accepted.

University of Guelph, Graduate Studies, College of Biological Science, Department of Molecular and Cellular Biology, Guelph, ON N1G 2W1, Canada. Offers biochemistry (M Sc, PhD); biophysics (M Sc, PhD); botany (M Sc, PhD); microbiology (M Sc, PhD); molecular biology and genetics (M Sc, PhD). *Degree requirements:* For master's, thesis, research proposal; for doctorate, comprehensive exam, thesis/dissertation, research proposal. *Entrance requirements:* For master's, minimum B-average during previous 2 years of coursework; for doctorate, minimum A-average. Additional exam requirements/recommendations for international students: Required—TOEFL (minimum score 550 paper-based), IELTS (minimum score 6.5). Electronic applications accepted. *Faculty research:* Physiology, structure, genetics, and ecology of microbes; virology and microbial technology.

University of Hawaii at Manoa, Graduate Division, College of Natural Sciences, Department of Microbiology, Honolulu, HI 96822. Offers MS, PhD. *Program availability:* Part-time. *Faculty:* 25 full-time (6 women), 2 part-time/adjunct (1 woman). *Students:* 18 full-time (11 women), 17 part-time (11 women); includes 5 minority (5 Asian, non-Hispanic/Latino; 2 Hispanic/Latino), 4 international. Average age 30. 12 applicants, 17% accepted, 2 enrolled. In 2015, 4 master's, 5 doctorates awarded. *Degree requirements:* For master's, thesis optional; for doctorate, comprehensive exam, thesis/dissertation. *Entrance requirements:* For master's and doctorate, GRE General Test. Additional exam requirements/recommendations for international students: Required—TOEFL (minimum score 580 paper-based; 92 iBT), IELTS (minimum score 5). *Application deadline:* For fall admission, 2/1 for domestic and international students; for spring admission, 8/1 for domestic and international students. Application fee: $100. *Financial support:* In 2015–16, 1 fellowship (averaging $2,000 per year), 15 research assistantships (averaging $18,180 per year), 12 teaching assistantships (averaging $16,086 per year) were awarded. *Faculty research:* Virology, immunology, microbial physiology, medical microbiology, bacterial genetics. *Total annual research expenditures:* $852,000. *Unit head:* William Ditto, Dean, 808-956-6451, E-mail: wditto@hawaii.edu. *Application contact:* Dr. Paul Q. Patek, Chairperson, 808-956-7025, Fax: 808-956-5339, E-mail: patek@hawaii.edu.
Website: http://www.hawaii.edu/microbiology/

University of Idaho, College of Graduate Studies, College of Science, Department of Biological Sciences, Moscow, ID 83844-3051. Offers biology (MS, PhD); microbiology, molecular biology and biochemistry (PhD); neuroscience (MS, PhD). *Faculty:* 18 full-time. *Students:* 25 full-time, 2 part-time. Average age 29. In 2015, 5 doctorates awarded. *Degree requirements:* For doctorate, one foreign language, thesis/dissertation. *Entrance requirements:* For master's, GRE, minimum GPA of 2.8; for doctorate, GRE, minimum undergraduate GPA of 2.8, 3.0 graduate. Additional exam requirements/recommendations for international students: Required—TOEFL. *Application deadline:* For fall admission, 8/1 for domestic students; for spring admission, 12/15 for domestic students. Applications are processed on a rolling basis. Application fee: $60. Electronic applications accepted. *Expenses:* Tuition, state resident: full-time $6205; part-time $399 per credit hour. Tuition, nonresident: full-time $20,209; part-time $1177 per credit hour. *Required fees:* $2017; $58 per credit hour. Full-time tuition and fees vary according to course load and reciprocity agreements. *Financial support:* Research assistantships and teaching assistantships available. Financial award applicants required to submit FAFSA. *Faculty research:* Animal behavior development, germ cell development, evolutionary biology, fish reproductive biology, molecular mechanisms. *Unit head:* Dr. James J. Nagler, Interim Department Chair, 208-885-6280, E-mail: biosci@uidaho.edu. *Application contact:* Sean Scoggin, Graduate Recruitment Coordinator, 208-885-4723, Fax: 208-885-4406, E-mail: graduateadmissions@uidaho.edu.
Website: http://www.uidaho.edu/sci/biology

University of Illinois at Chicago, College of Medicine and Graduate College, Graduate Programs in Medicine, Department of Microbiology and Immunology, Chicago, IL 60607-7128. Offers PhD, MD/PhD. *Faculty:* 18 full-time (5 women), 10 part-time/adjunct (6 women). *Students:* 10 full-time (6 women); includes 2 minority (1 Hispanic/Latino; 1 Two or more races, non-Hispanic/Latino), 4 international. Average age 29. *Degree requirements:* For doctorate, thesis/dissertation. *Entrance requirements:* For doctorate, GRE General Test, minimum GPA of 2.75. Additional exam requirements/recommendations for international students: Required—TOEFL. *Application deadline:* For fall admission, 3/1 priority date for domestic students, 2/15 priority date for international students. Application fee: $60. *Expenses:* Tuition, state resident: full-time $11,480; part-time $3826 per credit. Tuition, nonresident: full-time $23,720; part-time $7906 per credit. *Required fees:* $1333 per semester. Part-time tuition and fees vary according to course load and program. *Financial support:* In 2015–16, 5 fellowships with full tuition reimbursements were awarded; research assistantships with full tuition reimbursements, teaching assistantships with full tuition reimbursements, Federal Work-Study, scholarships/grants, traineeships, tuition waivers (full), and unspecified assistantships also available. Financial award application deadline: 3/1; financial award applicants required to submit FAFSA. *Faculty research:* Class I major histocompatibility complex molecules; proteins such as azurin with the immunoglobulin folds; T cell immunobiology relevant to disease pathogenesis, immunotherapeutics and vaccines for HIV/AIDS, tuberculosis, AIDS-related tuberculosis, and malaria, plague and smallpox; intracellular bacterial pathogen Listeria monocytogenes; virus infection. *Unit head:* Prof. Bellur S. Prabhakar, Department Head, 312-996-4915, Fax: 312-996-6415, E-mail: bprabkhar@uic.edu. *Application contact:* Mia Johnson, Admissions and Records Officer, 312-996-9477, Fax: 312-996-6415, E-mail: mimi@uic.edu.
Website: http://www.uic.edu/depts/mcmi/index.htm

University of Illinois at Urbana–Champaign, Graduate College, College of Liberal Arts and Sciences, School of Molecular and Cellular Biology, Department of Microbiology, Champaign, IL 61820. Offers MS, PhD.

The University of Iowa, Roy J. and Lucille A. Carver College of Medicine and Graduate College, Graduate Programs in Medicine, Department of Microbiology, Iowa City, IA 52242-1316. Offers general microbiology and microbial physiology (MS, PhD); immunology (MS, PhD); microbial genetics (MS, PhD); pathogenic bacteriology (MS, PhD); virology (MS, PhD). *Degree requirements:* For master's, thesis; for doctorate, comprehensive exam, thesis/dissertation. *Entrance requirements:* For master's and doctorate, GRE General Test. Additional exam requirements/recommendations for international students: Required—TOEFL (minimum score 600 paper-based). Electronic applications accepted. *Faculty research:* Gene regulation, processing and transport of HIV, retroviral pathogenesis, biodegradation, biofilm.

The University of Kansas, Graduate Studies, College of Liberal Arts and Sciences, Department of Molecular Biosciences, Lawrence, KS 66044. Offers biochemistry and biophysics (MA, PhD); microbiology (MA, PhD); molecular, cellular, and developmental biology (MA, PhD). *Students:* 57 full-time (34 women), 4 part-time (1 woman); includes 9 minority (5 Asian, non-Hispanic/Latino; 2 Hispanic/Latino; 2 Two or more races, non-Hispanic/Latino), 23 international. Average age 27. 78 applicants, 46% accepted, 18 enrolled. In 2015, 3 master's, 7 doctorates awarded. Terminal master's awarded for partial completion of doctoral program. *Entrance requirements:* For master's and doctorate, GRE General Test. Additional exam requirements/recommendations for international students: Required—TOEFL or IELTS. *Application deadline:* For fall

admission, 12/15 for domestic and international students. Application fee: $65 ($85 for international students). Electronic applications accepted. *Financial support:* Fellowships, research assistantships, teaching assistantships, health care benefits, and unspecified assistantships available. Financial award application deadline: 3/1. *Faculty research:* Structure and function of proteins, genetics of organism development, molecular genetics, neurophysiology, molecular virology and pathogenics, developmental biology, cell biology. *Unit head:* Susan M. Egan, Chair, 785-864-4294, E-mail: sme@ku.edu. *Application contact:* John Connolly, Graduate Admissions Contact, 785-864-4311, E-mail: jconnolly@ku.edu.
Website: http://www.molecularbiosciences.ku.edu/

The University of Kansas, University of Kansas Medical Center, School of Medicine, Department of Microbiology, Molecular Genetics and Immunology, Kansas City, KS 66160. Offers MS, PhD, MD/PhD. *Faculty:* 13. *Students:* 11 full-time (5 women), 1 part-time (0 women); includes 2 minority (1 Hispanic/Latino; 1 Two or more races, non-Hispanic/Latino), 4 international. Average age 29. In 2015, 1 doctorate awarded. Terminal master's awarded for partial completion of doctoral program. *Degree requirements:* For master's, thesis; for doctorate, comprehensive exam, thesis/dissertation, research skills. *Entrance requirements:* For master's and doctorate, GRE General Test, B Sc. Additional exam requirements/recommendations for international students: Required—TOEFL or IELTS. *Application deadline:* For fall admission, 3/1 priority date for domestic and international students. Applications are processed on a rolling basis. Application fee: $60. Electronic applications accepted. *Financial support:* Research assistantships with full tuition reimbursements, teaching assistantships with full tuition reimbursements, and unspecified assistantships available. Financial award application deadline: 3/1; financial award applicants required to submit FAFSA. *Faculty research:* Immunology, infectious disease, virology, molecular genetics, bacteriology. *Total annual research expenditures:* $4 million. *Unit head:* Dr. Michael Parmely, Professor/Chair, 913-588-7053, Fax: 913-588-7295, E-mail: mparmely@kumc.edu. *Application contact:* Dr. Jianming Qiu, Microbiology Graduate Program Director, 913-588-4329, Fax: 913-588-7295, E-mail: jqiu@kumc.edu.
Website: http://www.kumc.edu/school-of-medicine/microbiology-molecular-genetics-and-immunology.html

University of Kentucky, Graduate School, Graduate School Programs from the College of Medicine, Program in Microbiology and Immunology, Lexington, KY 40506-0032. Offers PhD. *Degree requirements:* For doctorate, comprehensive exam, thesis/dissertation. *Entrance requirements:* For doctorate, GRE General Test, minimum undergraduate GPA of 2.75. Additional exam requirements/recommendations for international students: Required—TOEFL (minimum score 550 paper-based). Electronic applications accepted.

University of Louisville, School of Medicine, Department of Microbiology and Immunology, Louisville, KY 40292-0001. Offers MS, PhD, MD/PhD. *Program availability:* Part-time. *Students:* 38 full-time (20 women); includes 4 minority (1 Black or African American, non-Hispanic/Latino; 2 Hispanic/Latino; 1 Two or more races, non-Hispanic/Latino), 12 international. Average age 29. 55 applicants, 15% accepted, 7 enrolled. In 2015, 3 master's, 3 doctorates awarded. Terminal master's awarded for partial completion of doctoral program. *Median time to degree:* Of those who began their doctoral program in fall 2007, 100% received their degree in 8 years or less. *Degree requirements:* For master's, comprehensive exam, thesis or alternative; for doctorate, comprehensive exam, thesis/dissertation. *Entrance requirements:* For master's and doctorate, GRE General Test (minimum score of 300 verbal and quantitative), minimum GPA of 3.0; 1 year of course work in biology and organic chemistry; 1 semester of course work in introductory calculus and biochemistry. Additional exam requirements/recommendations for international students: Required—TOEFL (minimum score 550 paper-based; 79 iBT), IELTS (minimum score 6.5). *Application deadline:* For fall admission, 3/1 priority date for domestic and international students. Applications are processed on a rolling basis. Application fee: $60. Electronic applications accepted. *Expenses:* Tuition, state resident: full-time $11,664; part-time $649 per credit hour. Tuition, nonresident: full-time $24,274; part-time $1350 per credit hour. *Required fees:* $196. Tuition and fees vary according to program and reciprocity agreements. *Financial support:* In 2015–16, 12 fellowships with full tuition reimbursements (averaging $25,500 per year), 15 research assistantships with full tuition reimbursements (averaging $25,500 per year) were awarded; health care benefits also available. Financial award application deadline: 3/1. *Faculty research:* Biodefense/emerging infectious diseases; autoimmune disease and basic immune mechanisms; bacterial and viral pathogenesis; vaccines; tumor immunity. *Total annual research expenditures:* $373,681. *Unit head:* Dr. Nejat Egilmez, Chair, 502-852-5351, Fax: 502-852-7531, E-mail: nejat.egilmez@louisville.edu. *Application contact:* Carolyn Burton, Graduate Program Coordinator, 502-852-6208, Fax: 502-852-7531, E-mail: cmburt01@louisville.edu.
Website: http://louisville.edu/medicine/departments/microbiology

University of Maine, Graduate School, College of Natural Sciences, Forestry, and Agriculture, Department of Molecular and Biomedical Sciences, Orono, ME 04469. Offers microbiology (PhD). *Faculty:* 30 full-time (6 women), 20 part-time/adjunct (4 women). *Students:* 22 full-time (12 women); includes 2 minority (1 Asian, non-Hispanic/Latino; 1 Two or more races, non-Hispanic/Latino), 3 international. Average age 30. 40 applicants, 28% accepted, 6 enrolled. In 2015, 7 master's, 3 doctorates awarded. *Degree requirements:* For master's, thesis (for some programs); for doctorate, comprehensive exam, thesis/dissertation. *Entrance requirements:* For master's and doctorate, GRE General Test. Additional exam requirements/recommendations for international students: Required—TOEFL. *Application deadline:* For fall admission, 2/1 priority date for domestic students. Applications are processed on a rolling basis. Application fee: $65. Electronic applications accepted. *Financial support:* In 2015–16, 20 students received support, including 8 research assistantships with full tuition reimbursements available (averaging $16,800 per year), 12 teaching assistantships with full tuition reimbursements available (averaging $19,000 per year); tuition waivers (full and partial) also available. Financial award application deadline: 3/1. *Total annual research expenditures:* $242,844. *Unit head:* Dr. Robert Gundersen, Chair, 207-581-2802, Fax: 207-581-2801. *Application contact:* Scott G. Delcourt, Assistant Vice President for Graduate Studies and Senior Associate Dean, 207-581-3291, Fax: 207-581-3232, E-mail: graduate@maine.edu.
Website: http://umaine.edu/biomed/

The University of Manchester, Faculty of Life Sciences, Manchester, United Kingdom. Offers adaptive organismal biology (M Phil, PhD); animal biology (M Phil, PhD); biochemistry (M Phil, PhD); bioinformatics (M Phil, PhD); biomolecular sciences (M Phil, PhD); biotechnology (M Phil, PhD); cell biology (M Phil, PhD); cell matrix research (M Phil, PhD); channels and transporters (M Phil, PhD); developmental biology (M Phil, PhD); Egyptology (M Phil, PhD); environmental biology (M Phil, PhD); evolutionary biology (M Phil, PhD); gene expression (M Phil, PhD); genetics (M Phil, PhD); history of science, technology and medicine (M Phil, PhD); immunology (M Phil, PhD); integrative neurobiology and behavior (M Phil, PhD); membrane trafficking (M Phil, PhD); microbiology (M Phil, PhD); molecular and cellular neuroscience (M Phil, PhD); molecular biology (M Phil, PhD); molecular cancer studies (M Phil, PhD); neuroscience (M Phil, PhD); ophthalmology (M Phil, PhD); optometry (M Phil, PhD); organelle function (M Phil, PhD); pharmacology (M Phil, PhD); physiology (M Phil, PhD); plant sciences

(M Phil, PhD); stem cell research (M Phil, PhD); structural biology (M Phil, PhD); systems neuroscience (M Phil, PhD); toxicology (M Phil, PhD).

University of Manitoba, Faculty of Graduate Studies, Faculty of Science, Department of Microbiology, Winnipeg, MB R3T 2N2, Canada. Offers M Sc, PhD. *Degree requirements:* For master's, thesis; for doctorate, one foreign language, thesis/dissertation.

University of Maryland, Baltimore, Graduate School, Graduate Program in Life Sciences, Program in Molecular Microbiology and Immunology, Baltimore, MD 21201. Offers PhD, MD/PhD. *Degree requirements:* For doctorate, comprehensive exam, thesis/dissertation. *Entrance requirements:* For doctorate, GRE. Additional exam requirements/recommendations for international students: Required—TOEFL (minimum score 550 paper-based; 80 iBT); Recommended—IELTS (minimum score 7). Electronic applications accepted. Tuition and fees vary according to program.

University of Massachusetts Amherst, Graduate School, College of Natural Sciences, Department of Microbiology, Amherst, MA 01003. Offers MS, PhD. *Program availability:* Part-time. Terminal master's awarded for partial completion of doctoral program. *Degree requirements:* For master's, thesis or alternative; for doctorate, comprehensive exam, thesis/dissertation. *Entrance requirements:* For master's and doctorate, GRE General Test. Additional exam requirements/recommendations for international students: Required—TOEFL (minimum score 550 paper-based; 80 iBT), IELTS (minimum score 6.5). Electronic applications accepted. *Faculty research:* Microbial physiology, genetics, immunology, parasitology, pathogenic bacteriology.

See Display below and Close-Up on page 337.

University of Massachusetts Medical School, Graduate School of Biomedical Sciences, Worcester, MA 01655-0115. Offers biomedical sciences (PhD), including biochemistry and molecular pharmacology, bioinformatics and computational biology, cancer biology, cell biology, immunology and microbiology, interdisciplinary, neuroscience, translational science; biomedical sciences (millennium program) (PhD); clinical and population health research (PhD); clinical investigation (MS). *Faculty:* 1,339 full-time (521 women), 301 part-time/adjunct (189 women). *Students:* 363 full-time (184 women); includes 58 minority (13 Black or African American, non-Hispanic/Latino; 30 Asian, non-Hispanic/Latino; 15 Hispanic/Latino), 141 international. Average age 29. 661 applicants, 26% accepted, 51 enrolled. In 2015, 10 master's, 58 doctorates awarded. Terminal master's awarded for partial completion of doctoral program. *Degree requirements:* For master's, comprehensive exam, thesis; for doctorate, comprehensive exam, thesis/dissertation. *Entrance requirements:* For master's, MD, PhD, DVM, or PharmD; for doctorate, GRE General Test, bachelor's degree. Additional exam requirements/recommendations for international students: Required—TOEFL (minimum score 100 iBT) or IELTS (minimum score 7.5). *Application deadline:* For fall admission, 12/15 for domestic and international students; for spring admission, 5/15 for domestic students. Application fee: $80. Electronic applications accepted. *Expenses:* $6,966 resident per year; $14,182 non-resident per year. *Financial support:* In 2015–16, 383 students received support, including research assistantships with full tuition reimbursements available (averaging $30,600 per year); scholarships/grants, health care benefits, tuition waivers (full), and unspecified assistantships also available. Financial award application deadline: 5/16. *Faculty research:* RNA interference, cell/molecular/developmental biology, bioinformatics, clinical/translational research, infectious disease. *Total annual research expenditures:* $250.3 million. *Unit head:* Dr. Anthony Carruthers, Dean, 508-856-4135, E-mail: anthony.carruthers@umassmed.edu. *Application contact:* Dr. Kendall Knight, Assistant Vice Provost for Admissions, 508-856-5628, Fax: 508-856-3659, E-mail: kendall.knight@umassmed.edu.
Website: http://www.umassmed.edu/gsbs/

University of Miami, Graduate School, Miller School of Medicine, Graduate Programs in Medicine, Department of Microbiology and Immunology, Coral Gables, FL 33124. Offers PhD, MD/PhD. *Degree requirements:* For doctorate, thesis/dissertation, oral and written qualifying exams. *Entrance requirements:* For doctorate, GRE General Test. Additional exam requirements/recommendations for international students: Required—TOEFL. Electronic applications accepted. *Faculty research:* Cellular and molecular immunology, molecular and pathogenic virology, pathogenic bacteriology and gene therapy of cancer.

University of Michigan, Rackham Graduate School, Program in Biomedical Sciences (PIBS), Department of Microbiology and Immunology, Ann Arbor, MI 48109. Offers MS, PhD. *Program availability:* Part-time. *Faculty:* 25 full-time (13 women), 13 part-time/adjunct (4 women). *Students:* 46 full-time (24 women); includes 8 minority (1 Black or African American, non-Hispanic/Latino; 1 American Indian or Alaska Native, non-Hispanic/Latino; 3 Asian, non-Hispanic/Latino; 3 Hispanic/Latino), 3 international. Average age 27. 128 applicants, 10% accepted, 6 enrolled. In 2015, 5 master's, 11 doctorates awarded. Terminal master's awarded for partial completion of doctoral program. *Degree requirements:* For master's, thesis optional; for doctorate, comprehensive exam, thesis/dissertation, oral defense of dissertation, preliminary exam. *Entrance requirements:* For master's and doctorate, GRE General Test. Additional exam requirements/recommendations for international students: Required—TOEFL (minimum score 600 paper-based; 84 iBT), TWE. *Application deadline:* For fall admission, 12/1 for domestic and international students. Application fee: $75. Electronic applications accepted. *Financial support:* In 2015–16, 15 fellowships with full tuition reimbursements (averaging $28,500 per year), 20 research assistantships with full tuition reimbursements (averaging $28,500 per year) were awarded; health care benefits and tuition waivers (full) also available. Financial award application deadline: 2/1. *Faculty research:* Mechanisms by which viruses, bacteria, fungi, and parasites elicit pathogenesis in the infected host; viral pathogens, bacterial pathogens; eukaryotic pathogens; innate immunity; adaptive immunity cell biology of infection. *Total annual research expenditures:* $10.2 million. *Unit head:* Dr. Harry L. T. Mobley, Chair, 734-764-1466, Fax: 734-764-3562, E-mail: hmobley@umich.edu. *Application contact:* Heidi Thompson, Senior Student Administrative Assistant, 734-763-3532, Fax: 734-764-3562, E-mail: heiditho@umich.edu.
Website: http://www.med.umich.edu/microbio/

University of Minnesota, Twin Cities Campus, Graduate School, PhD Program in Microbiology, Immunology and Cancer Biology, Minneapolis, MN 55455-0213. Offers PhD. *Degree requirements:* For doctorate, thesis/dissertation. *Entrance requirements:* For doctorate, GRE General Test. Additional exam requirements/recommendations for international students: Required—TOEFL (minimum score 600 paper-based). Electronic applications accepted. *Faculty research:* Virology, microbiology, cancer biology, immunology.

University of Mississippi Medical Center, School of Graduate Studies in the Health Sciences, Department of Microbiology, Jackson, MS 39216-4505. Offers PhD, MD/PhD. *Degree requirements:* For doctorate, comprehensive exam, thesis/dissertation, first authored publication. *Entrance requirements:* For doctorate, GRE General Test (minimum score of 300), minimum GPA of 3.0. Additional exam requirements/recommendations for international students: Recommended—TOEFL (minimum score 550 paper-based; 79 iBT), IELTS (minimum score 6.5), TSE (minimum score 53). Electronic applications accepted. *Faculty research:* Host-pathogen interaction, microbial population genetics, immunology, virology, parasitology.

University of Missouri, School of Medicine and Office of Research and Graduate Studies, Graduate Programs in Medicine, Department of Molecular Microbiology and Immunology, Columbia, MO 65211. Offers PhD. Terminal master's awarded for partial

Microbiology

completion of doctoral program. *Degree requirements:* For doctorate, thesis/dissertation. *Entrance requirements:* For doctorate, GRE General Test, minimum GPA of 3.0. Additional exam requirements/recommendations for international students: Required—TOEFL (minimum score 580 paper-based; 92 iBT). *Application deadline:* For fall admission, 1/15 priority date for domestic and international students. Application fee: $55 ($75 for international students). Electronic applications accepted. *Financial support:* Fellowships, research assistantships, teaching assistantships, institutionally sponsored loans, scholarships/grants, traineeships, health care benefits, and unspecified assistantships available. Support available to part-time students. Financial award application deadline: 3/1.
Website: http://medicine.missouri.edu/education/phd.html

University of Montana, Graduate School, College of Humanities and Sciences, Division of Biological Sciences, Program in Cellular, Molecular and Microbial Biology, Missoula, MT 59812-0002. Offers cellular and developmental biology (PhD); microbial evolution and ecology (PhD); microbiology and immunology (PhD); molecular biology and biochemistry (PhD). Terminal master's awarded for partial completion of doctoral program. *Degree requirements:* For doctorate, variable foreign language requirement, thesis/dissertation. *Entrance requirements:* For doctorate, GRE General Test. *Faculty research:* Ribosome structure, medical microbiology/pathogenesis, microbial ecology/environmental microbiology.

University of Nebraska Medical Center, Department of Pathology and Microbiology, Omaha, NE 68198. Offers MS, PhD. *Program availability:* Part-time. *Faculty:* 53 full-time (17 women), 4 part-time/adjunct (2 women). *Students:* 37 full-time (22 women), 2 part-time (1 woman); includes 2 minority (1 Asian, non-Hispanic/Latino; 1 Hispanic/Latino), 22 international. Average age 27. 36 applicants, 17% accepted, 6 enrolled. In 2015, 4 master's, 10 doctorates awarded. Terminal master's awarded for partial completion of doctoral program. *Degree requirements:* For master's, comprehensive exam, thesis; for doctorate, comprehensive exam, thesis/dissertation. *Entrance requirements:* For master's, previous course work in biology, chemistry, mathematics, and physics; for doctorate, GRE General Test, previous course work in biology, chemistry, mathematics, and physics. Additional exam requirements/recommendations for international students: Required—TOEFL (minimum score 550 paper-based; 90 iBT). *Application deadline:* For fall admission, 3/1 for domestic and international students; for spring admission, 10/1 for domestic and international students; for summer admission, 3/1 for domestic and international students. Applications are processed on a rolling basis. Application fee: $45. Electronic applications accepted. *Expenses:* Tuition, state resident: full-time $7830; part-time $3915 per credit hour. Tuition, nonresident: full-time $22,410; part-time $11,205 per credit hour. *Required fees:* $521. *Financial support:* In 2015–16, 7 students received support, including 1 fellowship with full tuition reimbursement available (averaging $23,100 per year), 3 research assistantships with full tuition reimbursements available (averaging $23,100 per year); scholarships/grants also available. Support available to part-time students. Financial award application deadline: 2/15; financial award applicants required to submit FAFSA. *Faculty research:* Carcinogenesis, cancer biology, immunobiology, molecular virology, molecular genetics. *Unit head:* Dr. Rakesh K. Singh, Chair, Graduate Committee, 402-559-9949, Fax: 402-559-5900, E-mail: rsingh@unmc.edu. *Application contact:* Tuire Cechin, Office Associate, 402-559-4042, Fax: 402-559-5900, E-mail: tcechin@unmc.edu.
Website: http://www.unmc.edu/pathology/

University of New Hampshire, Graduate School, College of Life Sciences and Agriculture, Department of Molecular, Cellular and Biomedical Sciences, Program in Microbiology, Durham, NH 03824. Offers MS, PhD. *Program availability:* Part-time. Terminal master's awarded for partial completion of doctoral program. *Degree requirements:* For master's, thesis; for doctorate, thesis/dissertation. *Entrance requirements:* For master's and doctorate, GRE General Test. Additional exam requirements/recommendations for international students: Required—TOEFL (minimum score 550 paper-based; 80 iBT). *Application deadline:* For fall admission, 1/15 priority date for domestic students, 1/15 for international students; for spring admission, 11/1 for domestic students. Applications are processed on a rolling basis. Application fee: $65. Electronic applications accepted. *Expenses:* Tuition, state resident: full-time $13,840; part-time $770 per credit hour. Tuition, nonresident: full-time $27,130; part-time $1175 per credit hour. *Required fees:* $2080; $1040. Tuition and fees vary according to degree level and program. *Financial support:* Fellowships, research assistantships, teaching assistantships, career-related internships or fieldwork, Federal Work-Study, scholarships/grants, and tuition waivers (full and partial) available. Support available to part-time students. Financial award application deadline: 2/15. *Faculty research:* Bacterial host-parasite interactions, immunology, microbial structures, bacterial and bacteriophage genetics, virology. *Unit head:* Dr. W. Kelley Thomas, Director, 603-862-2470. *Application contact:* Flora Joyal, Administrative Assistant, 603-862-4095, E-mail: flora.joyal@unh.edu.
Website: http://colsa.unh.edu/mcbs/microbiology/microbiology-ms

University of New Mexico, Graduate Studies, Health Sciences Center, Program in Biomedical Sciences, Albuquerque, NM 87131-5196. Offers biochemistry and molecular biology (MS, PhD); cell biology and physiology (MS, PhD); molecular genetics and microbiology (MS, PhD); neuroscience (MS, PhD); pathology (MS, PhD); toxicology (MS, PhD). *Program availability:* Part-time. *Faculty:* 18 full-time (10 women), 1 part-time/adjunct (0 women). *Students:* 31 full-time (17 women), 45 part-time (26 women); includes 29 minority (1 American Indian or Alaska Native, non-Hispanic/Latino; 3 Asian, non-Hispanic/Latino; 22 Hispanic/Latino; 2 Native Hawaiian or other Pacific Islander, non-Hispanic/Latino; 1 Two or more races, non-Hispanic/Latino), 18 international. Average age 30. 98 applicants, 11% accepted, 11 enrolled. In 2015, 11 master's, 14 doctorates awarded. Terminal master's awarded for partial completion of doctoral program. *Degree requirements:* For master's, thesis; for doctorate, comprehensive exam, thesis/dissertation, qualifying exam at the end of year 1/core curriculum. *Entrance requirements:* For master's and doctorate, GRE General Test, minimum undergraduate GPA of 3.0. Additional exam requirements/recommendations for international students: Required—TOEFL. *Application deadline:* For fall admission, 3/1 priority date for domestic and international students. Applications are processed on a rolling basis. Application fee: $50. Electronic applications accepted. *Financial support:* Fellowships with tuition reimbursements, research assistantships with full tuition reimbursements, teaching assistantships, career-related internships or fieldwork, Federal Work-Study, institutionally sponsored loans, scholarships/grants, traineeships, health care benefits, and unspecified assistantships available. Financial award application deadline: 1/1; financial award applicants required to submit FAFSA. *Faculty research:* Infectious disease/immunity, cancer biology, cardiovascular and metabolic diseases, brain and behavioral illness, environmental health. *Unit head:* Dr. Helen J. Hathaway, Program Director, 505-272-1887, Fax: 505-272-2412, E-mail: hhathaway@salud.unm.edu. *Application contact:* Mary Fenton, Admissions Coordinator, 505-272-1887, Fax: 505-272-2412, E-mail: mfenton@salud.unm.edu.

The University of North Carolina at Chapel Hill, School of Medicine and Graduate School, Graduate Programs in Medicine, Department of Microbiology and Immunology, Chapel Hill, NC 27599-7290. Offers immunology (MS, PhD); microbiology (MS, PhD). Terminal master's awarded for partial completion of doctoral program. *Degree requirements:* For master's, comprehensive exam, thesis; for doctorate, comprehensive

exam, thesis/dissertation. *Entrance requirements:* For master's and doctorate, GRE General Test, minimum GPA of 3.0. Electronic applications accepted. *Faculty research:* HIV pathogenesis, immune response, t-cell mediated autoimmunity, alpha-viruses, bacterial chemotaxis, francisella tularensis, pertussis, Mycobacterium tuberculosis, Burkholderia, Dengue virus.

University of North Dakota, Graduate School and Graduate School, Graduate Programs in Medicine, Department of Microbiology and Immunology, Grand Forks, ND 58202. Offers MS, PhD. *Degree requirements:* For master's, comprehensive exam, thesis or alternative; for doctorate, comprehensive exam, thesis/dissertation, final examination. *Entrance requirements:* For master's and doctorate, GRE General Test, minimum GPA of 3.0. Additional exam requirements/recommendations for international students: Required—TOEFL (minimum score 550 paper-based; 79 iBT), IELTS (minimum score 6.5). Electronic applications accepted. *Faculty research:* Genetic and immunological aspects of a murine model of human multiple sclerosis, termination of DNA replication, cell division in bacteria, yersinia pestis.

University of North Texas Health Science Center at Fort Worth, Graduate School of Biomedical Sciences, Fort Worth, TX 76107-2699. Offers anatomy and cell biology (MS, PhD); biochemistry and molecular biology (MS, PhD); biomedical sciences (MS, PhD); biotechnology (MS); forensic genetics (MS); integrative physiology (MS, PhD); medical science (MS); microbiology and immunology (MS, PhD); pharmacology (MS, PhD); science education (MS); DO/MS; DO/PhD. Terminal master's awarded for partial completion of doctoral program. *Degree requirements:* For master's, thesis; for doctorate, thesis/dissertation. *Entrance requirements:* For master's and doctorate, GRE General Test. Additional exam requirements/recommendations for international students: Required—TOEFL. *Expenses:* Contact institution. *Faculty research:* Alzheimer's disease, aging, eye diseases, cancer, cardiovascular disease.

University of Oklahoma, College of Arts and Sciences, Department of Microbiology and Plant Biology, Program in Microbiology, Norman, OK 73019. Offers MS, PhD. *Students:* 21 full-time (13 women), 22 part-time (7 women); includes 10 minority (2 Black or African American, non-Hispanic/Latino; 1 American Indian or Alaska Native, non-Hispanic/Latino; 3 Asian, non-Hispanic/Latino; 1 Hispanic/Latino; 3 Two or more races, non-Hispanic/Latino), 16 international. Average age 28. 15 applicants, 40% accepted, 6 enrolled. In 2015, 5 master's, 4 doctorates awarded. Terminal master's awarded for partial completion of doctoral program. *Degree requirements:* For master's, thesis; for doctorate, comprehensive exam, thesis/dissertation. *Entrance requirements:* For master's and doctorate, GRE, 3 recommendation letters, letter of intent, bachelor's degree. Additional exam requirements/recommendations for international students: Required—TOEFL (minimum score 80 iBT). *Application deadline:* For fall admission, 3/1 for domestic students, 4/1 for international students; for spring admission, 9/1 for domestic and international students; for summer admission, 9/1 for domestic and international students. Application fee: $50 ($100 for international students). Electronic applications accepted. *Expenses:* Tuition, state resident: full-time $4577; part-time $190.70 per credit hour. Tuition, nonresident: full-time $17,758; part-time $739.90 per credit hour. *Required fees:* $3060; $115.70 per credit hour. $141.50 per semester. *Financial support:* In 2015–16, 36 students received support. Research assistantships with full tuition reimbursements available, teaching assistantships with full tuition reimbursements available, Federal Work-Study, institutionally sponsored loans, scholarships/grants, health care benefits, and unspecified assistantships available. Support available to part-time students. Financial award application deadline: 6/1; financial award applicants required to submit FAFSA. *Faculty research:* Anaerobic microbiology, biodegradation and bioremediation, environmental microbiology and genomics, microbial genetics and molecular biology, microbial stress responses. *Unit head:* Dr. Anne K. Dunn, Interim Department Chair/Associate Professor of Microbiology, 405-325-4321, Fax: 405-325-7619, E-mail: akdunn@ou.edu. *Application contact:* Adell Hopper, Staff Assistant, 405-325-4322, Fax: 405-325-7619, E-mail: ahopper@ou.edu.
Website: http://mpbio.ou.edu/

University of Oklahoma Health Sciences Center, College of Medicine and Graduate College, Graduate Programs in Medicine, Department of Microbiology and Immunology, Oklahoma City, OK 73190. Offers immunology (MS, PhD); microbiology (MS, PhD). *Program availability:* Part-time. Terminal master's awarded for partial completion of doctoral program. *Degree requirements:* For master's, thesis or alternative; for doctorate, one foreign language, thesis/dissertation. *Entrance requirements:* For doctorate, GRE General Test, 3 letters of recommendation. Additional exam requirements/recommendations for international students: Required—TOEFL. *Faculty research:* Molecular genetics, pathogenesis, streptococcal infections, gram-positive virulence, monoclonal antibodies.

University of Ottawa, Faculty of Graduate and Postdoctoral Studies, Faculty of Medicine, Department of Biochemistry, Microbiology and Immunology, Ottawa, ON K1N 6N5, Canada. Offers biochemistry (M Sc, PhD); microbiology and immunology (M Sc, PhD). *Degree requirements:* For master's, thesis; for doctorate, comprehensive exam, thesis/dissertation, seminar. *Entrance requirements:* For master's, honors degree or equivalent, minimum B average; for doctorate, master's degree, minimum B+ average. Electronic applications accepted. *Faculty research:* General biochemistry, molecular biology, microbiology, host biology, nutrition and metabolism.

University of Pennsylvania, Perelman School of Medicine, Biomedical Graduate Studies, Graduate Group in Cell and Molecular Biology, Philadelphia, PA 19104. Offers cancer biology (PhD); cell biology, physiology, and metabolism (PhD); developmental stem cell regenerative biology (PhD); gene therapy and vaccines (PhD); genetics and gene regulation (PhD); microbiology, virology, and parasitology (PhD); MD/PhD; VMD/PhD. *Faculty:* 317. *Students:* 339 full-time (189 women); includes 100 minority (7 Black or African American, non-Hispanic/Latino; 2 American Indian or Alaska Native, non-Hispanic/Latino; 45 Asian, non-Hispanic/Latino; 34 Hispanic/Latino; 1 Native Hawaiian or other Pacific Islander, non-Hispanic/Latino; 11 Two or more races, non-Hispanic/Latino), 52 international. 493 applicants, 22% accepted, 37 enrolled. In 2015, 51 doctorates awarded. *Degree requirements:* For doctorate, thesis/dissertation. *Entrance requirements:* For doctorate, GRE General Test. Additional exam requirements/recommendations for international students: Required—TOEFL. *Application deadline:* For fall admission, 12/1 priority date for domestic and international students. Applications are processed on a rolling basis. Application fee: $80. Electronic applications accepted. *Expenses:* Tuition, area resident: Full-time $31,068; part-time $5762 per course. *Required fees:* $3200; $336 per course. Full-time tuition and fees vary according to degree level, program and student level. Part-time tuition and fees vary according to course load, degree level and program. *Financial support:* In 2015–16, 339 students received support. Fellowships, research assistantships, scholarships/grants, traineeships, and unspecified assistantships available. *Unit head:* Dr. Daniel Kessler, Graduate Group Chair, 215-898-1478. *Application contact:* Meagan Schofer, Coordinator, 215-898-4360.
Website: http://www.med.upenn.edu/camb/

University of Pittsburgh, Graduate School of Public Health, Department of Infectious Diseases and Microbiology, Pittsburgh, PA 15261. Offers infectious disease management, intervention, and community practice (MPH); infectious disease pathogenesis, eradication, and laboratory practice (MPH); infectious diseases and microbiology (MS, PhD). *Program availability:* Part-time. *Faculty:* 19 full-time (5 women),

5 part-time/adjunct (2 women). *Students:* 67 full-time (47 women), 14 part-time (10 women); includes 19 minority (5 Black or African American, non-Hispanic/Latino; 5 Asian, non-Hispanic/Latino; 7 Hispanic/Latino; 2 Two or more races, non-Hispanic/Latino), 11 international. Average age 26. 178 applicants, 65% accepted, 39 enrolled. In 2015, 15 master's, 3 doctorates awarded. *Degree requirements:* For master's, comprehensive exam (for some programs), thesis; for doctorate, comprehensive exam, thesis/dissertation, preliminary exam, dissertation approval. *Entrance requirements:* For master's and doctorate, GRE General Test, MCAT, DAT, or GMAT. Additional exam requirements/recommendations for international students: Required—TOEFL (minimum score 550 paper-based, 80 iBT) or IELTS (minimum score 6.5). *Application deadline:* For fall admission, 1/15 priority date for domestic and international students. Applications are processed on a rolling basis. Application fee: $120. Electronic applications accepted. *Expenses:* $12,464 per semester in-state, $20,502 per semester out-of-state; $450 fees. *Financial support:* In 2015–16, 19 students received support, including 6 fellowships (averaging $19,210 per year), 13 research assistantships (averaging $16,556 per year); scholarships/grants, traineeships, health care benefits, and unspecified assistantships also available. Financial award applicants required to submit FAFSA. *Faculty research:* HIV, complications of antiretroviral therapy, Hepatitis C, emerging infections, clinical and molecular epidemiology, genetic basis of innate immune response, HIV prevention and care, AIDS education and training. *Total annual research expenditures:* $10.8 million. *Unit head:* Dr. Charles R. Rinaldo, Chair, 412-624-3928, Fax: 412-624-4953, E-mail: rinaldo@pitt.edu. *Application contact:* Meredith Mavero, Student Services Coordinator, 412-624-3331, Fax: 412-383-8926, E-mail: mlm72@pitt.edu.
Website: http://www.idm.pitt.edu/

University of Pittsburgh, School of Medicine, Graduate Programs in Medicine, Molecular Virology and Microbiology Graduate Program, Pittsburgh, PA 15260. Offers PhD. *Faculty:* 47 full-time (14 women). *Students:* 24 full-time (9 women); includes 7 minority (1 Black or African American, non-Hispanic/Latino; 5 Asian, non-Hispanic/Latino; 1 Hispanic/Latino). Average age 28. 386 applicants, 17% accepted, 25 enrolled. In 2015, 7 doctorates awarded. *Degree requirements:* For doctorate, comprehensive exam, thesis/dissertation. *Entrance requirements:* For doctorate, GRE General Test, GRE Subject Test, minimum QPA of 3.0. Additional exam requirements/recommendations for international students: Required—TOEFL (minimum score 600 paper-based; 100 iBT), IELTS (minimum score 7). *Application deadline:* For fall admission, 12/1 priority date for domestic and international students. Application fee: $50. Electronic applications accepted. Tuition and fees vary according to program. *Financial support:* In 2015–16, 24 students received support, including 8 fellowships with full tuition reimbursements available (averaging $27,000 per year), 14 research assistantships with full tuition reimbursements available (averaging $27,000 per year), 2 teaching assistantships with full tuition reimbursements available (averaging $27,000 per year); scholarships/grants, traineeships, and health care benefits also available. *Faculty research:* Host-pathogen interactions, persistent microbial infections, microbial genetics and gene expression, microbial pathogenesis, anti-bacterial therapeutics. *Unit head:* Dr. Carolyn Coyne, Graduate Program Director, 412-383-5149, Fax: 412-624-1401, E-mail: ndeluca@pitt.edu. *Application contact:* Carol Williams, Admissions and Recruiting Manager, 412-648-8957, Fax: 412-648-1077, E-mail: gradstudies@medschool.pitt.edu.
Website: http://www.gradbiomed.pitt.edu

University of Puerto Rico, Medical Sciences Campus, School of Medicine, Biomedical Sciences Graduate Program, Department of Microbiology and Medical Zoology, San Juan, PR 00936-5067. Offers MS, PhD. *Degree requirements:* For master's, one foreign language, thesis; for doctorate, one foreign language, comprehensive exam, thesis/dissertation. *Entrance requirements:* For master's and doctorate, GRE General Test, GRE Subject Test, interview, minimum GPA of 3.0, 3 letters of recommendation. *Faculty research:* Molecular and general parasitology, immunology, development of viral vaccines and antiviral agents, antibiotic resistance, bacteriology.

University of Rhode Island, Graduate School, College of the Environment and Life Sciences, Department of Cell and Molecular Biology, Kingston, RI 02881. Offers biochemistry (MS, PhD); clinical laboratory sciences (MS), including biotechnology, clinical laboratory science, cytopathology; microbiology (MS, PhD); molecular genetics (MS, PhD). *Program availability:* Part-time. *Faculty:* 11 full-time (4 women), 1 (woman) part-time/adjunct. *Students:* 12 full-time (6 women), 36 part-time (27 women); includes 10 minority (4 Black or African American, non-Hispanic/Latino; 3 Asian, non-Hispanic/Latino; 2 Hispanic/Latino; 1 Two or more races, non-Hispanic/Latino), 8 international. In 2015, 19 master's, 1 doctorate awarded. *Degree requirements:* For master's, comprehensive exam (for some programs), thesis optional; for doctorate, comprehensive exam, thesis/dissertation. *Entrance requirements:* For master's and doctorate, GRE, 2 letters of recommendation. Additional exam requirements/recommendations for international students: Required—TOEFL (minimum score 550 paper-based). *Application deadline:* For fall admission, 7/15 for domestic students, 2/1 for international students; for spring admission, 11/15 for domestic students, 7/15 for international students. Application fee: $65. Electronic applications accepted. *Expenses:* Tuition, state resident: full-time $11,796; part-time $655 per credit. Tuition, nonresident: full-time $24,206; part-time $1345 per credit. *Required fees:* $1546; $44 per credit. One-time fee: $155 full-time; $35 part-time. *Financial support:* In 2015–16, 3 research assistantships with tuition reimbursements (averaging $13,507 per year), 8 teaching assistantships with tuition reimbursements (averaging $13,305 per year) were awarded; traineeships also available. Financial award application deadline: 2/1; financial award applicants required to submit FAFSA. *Faculty research:* Genomics. *Total annual research expenditures:* $6.7 million. *Unit head:* Dr. Gongqing Sun, Chairperson, 401-874-5937, Fax: 401-874-2202, E-mail: gsun@mail.uri.edu. *Application contact:* Graduate Admissions, 401-874-2872, E-mail: gradadm@etal.uri.edu.
Website: http://cels.uri.edu/cmb/

University of Rochester, School of Medicine and Dentistry, Graduate Programs in Medicine and Dentistry, Department of Microbiology and Immunology, Program in Medical Microbiology, Rochester, NY 14627. Offers MS, PhD. *Expenses:* Tuition, area resident: Full-time $47,450; part-time $1482 per credit hour. *Required fees:* $528. Tuition and fees vary according to program.

University of Rochester, School of Medicine and Dentistry, Graduate Programs in Medicine and Dentistry, Department of Microbiology and Immunology, Program in Microbiology and Immunology, Rochester, NY 14627. Offers MS, PhD. *Expenses:* Tuition, area resident: Full-time $47,450; part-time $1482 per credit hour. *Required fees:* $528. Tuition and fees vary according to program.

University of Saskatchewan, College of Medicine, Department of Microbiology and Immunology, Saskatoon, SK S7N 5A2, Canada. Offers M Sc, PhD. *Degree requirements:* For master's, thesis; for doctorate, thesis/dissertation. *Entrance requirements:* Additional exam requirements/recommendations for international students: Required—TOEFL.

University of Saskatchewan, Western College of Veterinary Medicine and College of Graduate Studies and Research, Graduate Programs in Veterinary Medicine, Department of Veterinary Microbiology, Saskatoon, SK S7N 5A2, Canada. Offers M Sc,

M Vet Sc, PhD. *Degree requirements:* For master's, thesis; for doctorate, comprehensive exam (for some programs), thesis/dissertation. *Entrance requirements:* Additional exam requirements/recommendations for international students: Required—TOEFL (minimum score 80 iBT) or IELTS (minimum score 6.5). Electronic applications accepted. *Faculty research:* Immunology, vaccinology, epidemiology, virology, parasitology.

The University of South Dakota, Graduate School, Sanford School of Medicine and Graduate School, Biomedical Sciences Graduate Program, Molecular Microbiology and Immunology Group, Vermillion, SD 57069-2390. Offers MS, PhD. Terminal master's awarded for partial completion of doctoral program. *Degree requirements:* For master's, thesis; for doctorate, comprehensive exam, thesis/dissertation. *Entrance requirements:* For master's and doctorate, GRE General Test, minimum GPA of 3.0. Additional exam requirements/recommendations for international students: Required—TOEFL (minimum score 550 paper-based; 80 iBT), IELTS (minimum score 6). *Application deadline:* For fall admission, 4/15 priority date for domestic students, 3/15 for international students. Applications are processed on a rolling basis. Application fee: $35. Electronic applications accepted. *Expenses:* Contact institution. *Financial support:* In 2015–16, 6 students received support. Fellowships with partial tuition reimbursements available, research assistantships with partial tuition reimbursements available, and unspecified assistantships available. Financial award application deadline: 4/15; financial award applicants required to submit FAFSA. *Faculty research:* Structure-function membranes, plasmids, immunology, virology, pathogenesis. *Total annual research expenditures:* $325,000. *Unit head:* 605-658-6322, Fax: 605-677-6381, E-mail: biomed@usd.edu.

University of Southern California, Keck School of Medicine and Graduate School, Graduate Programs in Medicine, Department of Molecular Microbiology and Immunology, Los Angeles, CA 90033. Offers MS. *Program availability:* Part-time. *Faculty:* 23 full-time (5 women), 1 (woman) part-time/adjunct. *Students:* 16 full-time (10 women); includes 2 minority (both Asian, non-Hispanic/Latino), 12 international. Average age 24. 34 applicants, 65% accepted, 6 enrolled. In 2015, 16 degrees awarded. *Degree requirements:* For master's, comprehensive exam (for some programs), thesis optional. *Entrance requirements:* For master's, GRE General Test, minimum GPA of 3.0. Additional exam requirements/recommendations for international students: Required—TOEFL (minimum score 100 iBT), IELTS. *Application deadline:* For fall admission, 6/1 for domestic students, 5/1 for international students; for spring admission, 11/1 for domestic students, 10/1 for international students. Applications are processed on a rolling basis. Application fee: $85. Electronic applications accepted. *Expenses:* Contact institution. *Financial support:* Federal Work-Study, institutionally sponsored loans, and scholarships/grants available. Financial award application deadline: 3/2; financial award applicants required to submit FAFSA. *Faculty research:* Animal virology, microbial genetics, molecular and cellular immunology, cellular differentiation control of protein synthesis, HIV. *Unit head:* Dr. Axel H. Schonthal, Associate Professor/Program Chairman, 323-442-1730, Fax: 323-442-1721, E-mail: schonthal@usc.edu. *Application contact:* Silvina V. Campos, Administrative Assistant II, 323-442-1713, Fax: 323-442-1721, E-mail: scampos@usc.edu.
Website: http://keck.usc.edu/molecular-microbiology-and-immunology/

University of Southern Mississippi, Graduate School, College of Science and Technology, Department of Biological Sciences, Hattiesburg, MS 39406-0001. Offers environmental biology (MS); marine biology (MS); microbiology (MS, PhD); molecular biology (MS, PhD). Terminal master's awarded for partial completion of doctoral program. *Degree requirements:* For master's, comprehensive exam, thesis; for doctorate, comprehensive exam, thesis/dissertation. *Entrance requirements:* For master's, GRE General Test, minimum GPA of 3.0 on last 60 hours; for doctorate, GRE General Test, minimum GPA of 3.5. Additional exam requirements/recommendations for international students: Required—TOEFL, IELTS.

University of South Florida, College of Arts and Sciences, Department of Cell Biology, Microbiology, and Molecular Biology, Tampa, FL 33620-9951. Offers biology (MS), including cell and molecular biology; cancer biology (PhD); cell and molecular biology (PhD); microbiology (MS). *Faculty:* 21 full-time (7 women). *Students:* 41 full-time (6 women), 45 part-time (2 women); includes 11 minority (1 Black or African American, non-Hispanic/Latino; 2 Asian, non-Hispanic/Latino; 5 Hispanic/Latino; 3 Two or more races, non-Hispanic/Latino), 22 international. Average age 27. 171 applicants, 14% accepted, 18 enrolled. In 2015, 22 master's, 14 doctorates awarded. *Degree requirements:* For master's, thesis or alternative; for doctorate, comprehensive exam, thesis/dissertation. *Entrance requirements:* For master's and doctorate, GRE General Test, minimum GPA of 3.0, extensive background in biology or chemistry. Additional exam requirements/recommendations for international students: Required—TOEFL (minimum score 570 paper-based; 79 iBT) or IELTS (minimum score 6.5). *Application deadline:* For fall admission, 2/1 for domestic students, 1/1 for international students. Application fee: $30. *Financial support:* Career-related internships or fieldwork, health care benefits, and unspecified assistantships available. Financial award application deadline: 4/1. *Faculty research:* Cell biology, microbiology and molecular biology: basic and applied science in bacterial pathogenesis, genome integrity and mechanisms of aging, structural and computational biology; cancer biology: immunology, cancer control, signal transduction, drug discovery, genomics. *Total annual research expenditures:* $1.9 million. *Unit head:* Dr. James Garey, Professor/Chair, 813-974-7103, Fax: 813-974-1614, E-mail: garey@usf.edu. *Application contact:* Dr. Kenneth Wright, Associate Professor of Cancer Biology, H. Lee Moffitt Cancer Center and Research Institute, 813-745-3918, Fax: 813-974-1614, E-mail: ken.wright@moffitt.org.
Website: http://biology.usf.edu/cmmb/

University of South Florida, College of Arts and Sciences, Department of Integrative Biology, Tampa, FL 33620-9951. Offers biology (MS), including ecology and evolution (MS, PhD), environmental and ecological microbiology (MS, PhD), physiology and morphology (MS, PhD); integrative biology (PhD), including ecology and evolution (MS, PhD), environmental and ecological microbiology (MS, PhD), physiology and morphology (MS, PhD). *Program availability:* Part-time. *Faculty:* 14 full-time (6 women). *Students:* 48 full-time (30 women), 6 part-time (3 women); includes 10 minority (1 American Indian or Alaska Native, non-Hispanic/Latino; 1 Asian, non-Hispanic/Latino; 7 Hispanic/Latino; 1 Two or more races, non-Hispanic/Latino), 3 international. Average age 30. 43 applicants, 37% accepted, 12 enrolled. In 2015, 8 master's, 3 doctorates awarded. *Degree requirements:* For master's, comprehensive exam, thesis (for some programs); for doctorate, comprehensive exam, thesis/dissertation. *Entrance requirements:* For master's and doctorate, GRE General Test, minimum GPA of 3.0 in last 60 hours of BS. Additional exam requirements/recommendations for international students: Required—TOEFL (minimum score 570 paper-based; 88 iBT). *Application deadline:* For fall admission, 2/15 priority date for domestic students, 1/2 for international students; for spring admission, 8/1 for domestic students, 6/1 for international students. Application fee: $30. Electronic applications accepted. *Financial support:* Research assistantships, teaching assistantships, and unspecified assistantships available. Financial award application deadline: 6/30; financial award applicants required to submit FAFSA. *Faculty research:* Marine ecology, ecosystem responses to urbanization, biomechanical and physiological mechanisms of animal movement, population biology and conservation, microbial ecology and public health microbiology, natural diversity of parasites and herbivores; ecosystems, vertebrates, disturbance ecology, functional and

Microbiology

ecological morphology of feeding in fishes, rare amphibians and reptiles, genomics in ecological experiments, ecotoxicology, global carbon cycle, plant-animal interactions. *Total annual research expenditures:* $1.3 million. *Unit head:* Dr. Valerie Harwood, Professor and Chair, 813-974-1524, Fax: 813-974-3263, E-mail: vharwood@usf.edu. *Application contact:* Dr. Lynn Martin, Associate Professor and Graduate Program Director, 813-974-0157, Fax: 813-974-3263, E-mail: lbmartin@usf.edu. Website: http://biology.usf.edu/ib/grad/

The University of Tennessee, Graduate School, College of Arts and Sciences, Department of Microbiology, Knoxville, TN 37996. Offers MS, PhD. *Program availability:* Part-time. *Degree requirements:* For master's, thesis; for doctorate, thesis/dissertation. *Entrance requirements:* For master's and doctorate, GRE General Test, minimum GPA of 2.7. Additional exam requirements/recommendations for international students: Required—TOEFL. Electronic applications accepted.

The University of Texas at Austin, Graduate School, College of Natural Sciences, School of Biological Sciences, Program in Microbiology, Austin, TX 78712-1111. Offers PhD. *Entrance requirements:* For doctorate, GRE General Test. Electronic applications accepted.

The University of Texas Health Science Center at Houston, Graduate School of Biomedical Sciences, Program in Microbiology and Molecular Genetics, Houston, TX 77225-0036. Offers MS, PhD, MD/PhD. Terminal master's awarded for partial completion of doctoral program. *Degree requirements:* For master's, thesis; for doctorate, thesis/dissertation. *Entrance requirements:* For master's and doctorate, GRE General Test. Additional exam requirements/recommendations for international students: Required—TOEFL. Electronic applications accepted. *Faculty research:* Disease causation, environmental signaling, gene regulation, cell growth and division, cell structure and architecture.

The University of Texas Health Science Center at San Antonio, Graduate School of Biomedical Sciences, Department of Microbiology and Immunology, San Antonio, TX 78229-3900. Offers MS, PhD. *Degree requirements:* For master's, thesis; for doctorate, comprehensive exam, thesis/dissertation.

The University of Texas Medical Branch, Graduate School of Biomedical Sciences, Program in Microbiology and Immunology, Galveston, TX 77555. Offers MS, PhD. Terminal master's awarded for partial completion of doctoral program. *Degree requirements:* For master's, thesis or alternative; for doctorate, thesis/dissertation. *Entrance requirements:* For doctorate, GRE General Test, minimum GPA of 3.0. Additional exam requirements/recommendations for international students: Required—TOEFL (minimum score 550 paper-based). Electronic applications accepted.

The University of Texas Southwestern Medical Center, Southwestern Graduate School of Biomedical Sciences, Division of Basic Science, Program in Molecular Microbiology, Dallas, TX 75390. Offers PhD. *Degree requirements:* For doctorate, thesis/dissertation, oral and written exams. *Entrance requirements:* For doctorate, GRE General Test, minimum GPA of 3.0. Additional exam requirements/recommendations for international students: Required—TOEFL. Electronic applications accepted. *Faculty research:* Cell and molecular immunology, molecular pathogenesis of infectious disease, virology.

University of Victoria, Faculty of Graduate Studies, Faculty of Science, Department of Biochemistry and Microbiology, Victoria, BC V8W 2Y2, Canada. Offers biochemistry (M Sc, PhD); microbiology (M Sc, PhD). *Degree requirements:* For master's, thesis, seminar; for doctorate, thesis/dissertation, seminar, candidacy exam. *Entrance requirements:* For master's, GRE General Test, minimum B+ average; for doctorate, GRE General Test, minimum B+ average, M Sc. Additional exam requirements/recommendations for international students: Required—TOEFL (minimum score 600 paper-based). Electronic applications accepted. *Faculty research:* Molecular pathogenesis, prokaryotic, eukaryotic, macromolecular interactions, microbial surfaces, virology, molecular genetics.

University of Virginia, School of Medicine, Department of Microbiology, Immunology, and Cancer Biology, Charlottesville, VA 22903. Offers PhD, MD/PhD. *Degree requirements:* For doctorate, thesis/dissertation. *Entrance requirements:* For doctorate, GRE General Test, 2 or more letters of recommendation. Additional exam requirements/recommendations for international students: Required—TOEFL (minimum score 600 paper-based; 90 iBT). Electronic applications accepted. *Faculty research:* Virology, membrane biology and molecular genetics.

University of Washington, Graduate School, School of Medicine, Graduate Programs in Medicine, Department of Microbiology, Seattle, WA 98195. Offers PhD. *Degree requirements:* For doctorate, thesis/dissertation. *Entrance requirements:* For doctorate, GRE General Test, GRE Subject Test (recommended). Electronic applications accepted. *Faculty research:* Bacterial genetics and physiology, mechanisms of bacterial and viral pathogenesis, bacterial-plant interaction.

The University of Western Ontario, Faculty of Graduate Studies, Biosciences Division, Department of Microbiology and Immunology, London, ON N6A 5B8, Canada. Offers M Sc, PhD. *Degree requirements:* For master's, thesis, oral and written exam; for doctorate, thesis/dissertation, oral and written exam. *Entrance requirements:* For master's, honors degree or equivalent in microbiology, immunology, or other biological science; minimum B average; for doctorate, M Sc in microbiology and immunology. Additional exam requirements/recommendations for international students: Required—TOEFL. *Faculty research:* Virology, molecular pathogenesis, cellular immunology, molecular biology.

University of Wisconsin–La Crosse, College of Science and Health, Department of Biology, La Crosse, WI 54601-3742. Offers aquatic sciences (MS); biology (MS); cellular and molecular biology (MS); clinical microbiology (MS); microbiology (MS); nurse anesthesia (MS); physiology (MS). *Program availability:* Part-time. *Students:* 19 full-time (12 women), 50 part-time (26 women); includes 4 minority (3 Asian, non-Hispanic/Latino; 1 Hispanic/Latino), 1 international. Average age 29. 44 applicants, 75% accepted, 27 enrolled. In 2015, 27 master's awarded. *Degree requirements:* For master's, comprehensive exam, thesis. *Entrance requirements:* For master's, GRE General Test, minimum GPA of 2.85. Additional exam requirements/recommendations for international students: Required—TOEFL (minimum score 550 paper-based; 79 iBT). *Application deadline:* For fall admission, 2/1 priority date for domestic and international students; for spring admission, 1/4 priority date for domestic and international students. Applications are processed on a rolling basis. Electronic applications accepted. *Financial support:* Research assistantships with partial tuition reimbursements, Federal Work-Study, scholarships/grants, health care benefits, and tuition waivers (partial) available. Support available to part-time students. Financial award application deadline: 3/15; financial award applicants required to submit FAFSA. *Unit head:* Dr. Mark Sandheinrich, Department Chair, 608-785-8261, E-mail: msandheinrich@uwlax.edu. *Application contact:* Brandon Schaller, Senior Graduate Student Status Examiner, 608-785-8941, E-mail: admissions@uwlax.edu. Website: http://uwlax.edu/biology/

University of Wisconsin–Madison, School of Medicine and Public Health and College of Agricultural and Life Sciences, Microbiology Doctoral Training Program, Madison, WI 53706. Offers PhD. *Expenses:* Tuition, state resident: full-time $5364. Tuition, nonresident: full-time $12,027. *Required fees:* $571. Tuition and fees vary according to campus/location, program and reciprocity agreements. Website: http://www.microbiology.wisc.edu/

University of Wisconsin–Milwaukee, Graduate School, College of Health Sciences, Program in Biomedical Sciences, Milwaukee, WI 53211. Offers cancer (MS); immunology (MS); microbiology (MS); neurodegenerative disease (MS); pharmacology and toxicology (MS); photobiomodulation (MS). *Accreditation:* NAACLS. *Program availability:* Part-time. *Faculty:* 8 full-time (4 women). *Students:* 8 full-time (7 women), 3 part-time (1 woman); includes 1 minority (Two or more races, non-Hispanic/Latino), 2 international. Average age 29. 42 applicants, 14% accepted, 4 enrolled. In 2015, 7 master's awarded. *Degree requirements:* For master's, thesis. *Entrance requirements:* For master's, GRE General Test. Additional exam requirements/recommendations for international students: Required—TOEFL (minimum score 550 paper-based; 79 iBT), IELTS (minimum score 6.5). *Application deadline:* For fall admission, 1/1 priority date for domestic students; for spring admission, 9/1 for domestic students. Applications are processed on a rolling basis. Application fee: $56 ($96 for international students). *Financial support:* In 2015–16, 6 teaching assistantships were awarded; fellowships, research assistantships, career-related internships or fieldwork, and unspecified assistantships also available. Support available to part-time students. Financial award application deadline: 4/15. *Unit head:* Raymond Fleming, Representative, 414-229-3980, E-mail: mundo@uwm.edu. *Application contact:* Roger O. Smith, General Information Contact, 414-229-6697, Fax: 414-229-6697, E-mail: smithro@uwm.edu. Website: http://www4.uwm.edu/chs/academics/biomedical_sciences/bms_masters/

University of Wisconsin–Oshkosh, Graduate Studies, College of Letters and Science, Department of Biology and Microbiology, Oshkosh, WI 54901. Offers biology (MS), including botany, microbiology, zoology. *Degree requirements:* For master's, comprehensive exam, thesis. *Entrance requirements:* For master's, GRE General Test, minimum GPA of 3.0, BS in biology. Additional exam requirements/recommendations for international students: Required—TOEFL (minimum score 550 paper-based; 79 iBT). Electronic applications accepted.

University of Wyoming, Graduate Program in Molecular and Cellular Life Sciences, Laramie, WY 82071. Offers PhD. *Degree requirements:* For doctorate, thesis/dissertation, four eight-week laboratory rotations, comprehensive basic practical exam, two-part qualifying exam, seminars, symposium.

Vanderbilt University, School of Medicine, Department of Microbiology and Immunology, Nashville, TN 37240-1001. Offers MS, PhD, MD/PhD. *Faculty:* 39 full-time (13 women). *Students:* 61 full-time (36 women); includes 10 minority (3 Black or African American, non-Hispanic/Latino; 1 American Indian or Alaska Native, non-Hispanic/Latino; 2 Asian, non-Hispanic/Latino; 2 Hispanic/Latino; 2 Two or more races, non-Hispanic/Latino), 8 international. Average age 27. In 2015, 2 master's, 6 doctorates awarded. Terminal master's awarded for partial completion of doctoral program. *Degree requirements:* For master's, thesis; for doctorate, thesis/dissertation, final and qualifying exams. *Entrance requirements:* For master's and doctorate, GRE General Test, GRE Subject Test (recommended). Additional exam requirements/recommendations for international students: Required—TOEFL (minimum score 570 paper-based; 88 iBT). *Application deadline:* For fall admission, 1/15 for domestic and international students. Application fee: $0. Electronic applications accepted. *Financial support:* Fellowships with full tuition reimbursements, research assistantships with full tuition reimbursements, Federal Work-Study, institutionally sponsored loans, scholarships/grants, traineeships, health care benefits, and tuition waivers (partial) available. Financial award application deadline: 1/15; financial award applicants required to submit CSS PROFILE or FAFSA. *Faculty research:* Cellular and molecular microbiology, viruses, genes, cancer, molecular pathogenesis of microbial diseases, immunobiology. *Unit head:* Dr. Christopher Aiken, Director of Graduate Studies, 615-322-2087, Fax: 615-322-5551, E-mail: chris.aiken@vanderbilt.edu. *Application contact:* Walter B. Bieschke, Program Coordinator for Graduate Admissions, 615-342-0236, E-mail: walter.bieschke@vanderbilt.edu. Website: http://www.mc.vanderbilt.edu/root/vumc.php?site-vmcpathology

Virginia Commonwealth University, Medical College of Virginia-Professional Programs, School of Medicine, School of Medicine Graduate Programs, Department of Microbiology and Immunology, Richmond, VA 23284-9005. Offers microbiology and immunology (MS, PhD); MD/PhD. *Degree requirements:* For master's, thesis; for doctorate, thesis/dissertation, comprehensive oral and written exams. *Entrance requirements:* For master's and doctorate, GRE General Test or MCAT. Additional exam requirements/recommendations for international students: Required—TOEFL (minimum score 600 paper-based; 100 iBT). Electronic applications accepted. *Faculty research:* Microbial physiology and genetics, molecular biology, crystallography of biological molecules, antibiotics and chemotherapy, membrane transport.

Virginia Commonwealth University, Program in Pre-Medical Basic Health Sciences, Richmond, VA 23284-9005. Offers anatomy (CBHS); biochemistry (CBHS); human genetics (CBHS); microbiology (CBHS); pharmacology (CBHS); physiology (CBHS). *Entrance requirements:* For degree, GRE, MCAT or DAT, course work in organic chemistry, minimum undergraduate GPA of 2.8. Additional exam requirements/recommendations for international students: Required—TOEFL (minimum score 600 paper-based). Electronic applications accepted.

Wagner College, Division of Graduate Studies, Program in Microbiology, Staten Island, NY 10301-4495. Offers MS. *Program availability:* Part-time, evening/weekend. *Degree requirements:* For master's, comprehensive exam or thesis. *Entrance requirements:* For master's, minimum GPA of 2.6, proficiency in statistics, undergraduate major in biological science or chemistry, undergraduate microbiology course, 16 credits of chemistry including organic chemistry with lab. Additional exam requirements/recommendations for international students: Required—TOEFL (minimum score 550 paper-based; 79 iBT). *Faculty research:* Listeria monocytogenes pathogenesis, plant extracts as anti-microbial agents, neuroimmunology.

Wake Forest University, School of Medicine and Graduate School of Arts and Sciences, Graduate Programs in Medicine, Department of Microbiology and Immunology, Winston-Salem, NC 27109. Offers PhD, MD/PhD. *Degree requirements:* For doctorate, thesis/dissertation. *Entrance requirements:* For doctorate, GRE General Test. Additional exam requirements/recommendations for international students: Required—TOEFL. Electronic applications accepted. *Faculty research:* Molecular immunology, bacterial pathogenesis and molecular genetics, viral pathogenesis, regulation of mRNA metabolism, leukocyte biology.

Washington State University, College of Veterinary Medicine, Program in Molecular Biosciences, Pullman, WA 99164. Offers molecular biology (PhD), including genetics, microbiology; molecular biosciences (PSM, PhD), including biochemistry (PhD), cell biology (PhD). *Program availability:* Online learning. *Faculty:* 30 full-time (12 women), 17 part-time/adjunct (5 women). *Students:* 47 full-time (26 women), 14 part-time (11 women); includes 13 minority (1 Black or African American, non-Hispanic/Latino; 1 American Indian or Alaska Native, non-Hispanic/Latino; 4 Asian, non-Hispanic/Latino; 5 Hispanic/Latino; 2 Two or more races, non-Hispanic/Latino), 1 international. Average age 28. 61 applicants, 23% accepted, 14 enrolled. In 2015, 5 master's, 8 doctorates awarded. Terminal master's awarded for partial completion of doctoral program. *Degree* *requirements:* For master's, thesis or alternative, oral exam; for doctorate, comprehensive exam, thesis/dissertation, oral exam, written exam. *Entrance requirements:* For master's and doctorate, GRE General Test, minimum GPA of 3.0. Additional exam requirements/recommendations for international students: Required—TOEFL (minimum score 100 iBT). *Application deadline:* For fall admission, 12/15 for domestic and international students. Application fee: $75. Electronic applications accepted. *Financial support:* In 2015–16, 5 fellowships with full tuition reimbursements (averaging $23,316 per year), 24 research assistantships with full tuition reimbursements (averaging $23,316 per year), 17 teaching assistantships with full tuition reimbursements (averaging $23,316 per year) were awarded; career-related internships or fieldwork, Federal Work-Study, traineeships, health care benefits, and unspecified assistantships also available. Financial award application deadline: 4/1; financial award applicants required to submit FAFSA. *Faculty research:* Gene regulation, signal transduction, protein export, reproductive biology, DNA repair. *Total annual research expenditures:* $5.8 million. *Unit head:* Dr. Jonathan Jones, Director, 509-335-8724, Fax: 509-335-9688, E-mail: jcr.jones@vetmed.wsu.edu. *Application contact:* Tami Breske, Coordinator, 509-335-4318, E-mail: tbreske@vetmed.wsu.edu. Website: http://www.smb.wsu.edu

Washington University in St. Louis, Graduate School of Arts and Sciences, Division of Biology and Biomedical Sciences, Program in Molecular Microbiology and Microbial Pathogenesis, St. Louis, MO 63130-4899. Offers PhD. *Students:* 47 full-time (24 women); includes 10 minority (3 Black or African American, non-Hispanic/Latino; 1 American Indian or Alaska Native, non-Hispanic/Latino; 4 Asian, non-Hispanic/Latino; 1 Hispanic/Latino; 1 Two or more races, non-Hispanic/Latino), 8 international. 136 applicants, 15% accepted, 7 enrolled. *Degree requirements:* For doctorate, thesis/dissertation. *Entrance requirements:* For doctorate, GRE General Test, GRE Subject Test. Additional exam requirements/recommendations for international students: Required—TOEFL. *Application deadline:* For fall admission, 12/1 for domestic students. Application fee: $0. Electronic applications accepted. *Financial support:* Fellowships, research assistantships, and teaching assistantships available. Financial award application deadline: 1/15. *Faculty research:* Host-pathogen interactions, cellular microbiology, molecular microbiology, microbial pathogenesis, pathogen discovery, emerging infectious diseases, microbial physiology and biochemistry, comparative genomics, gene expression and regulation, microbiome and host interactions, virology, bacteriology, mycology, parasitology. *Unit head:* Jeanne Silvestrini, Coordinator, 314-362-4806. *Application contact:* Rebecca Riney, 314-747-4648, E-mail: dbbsphdadmissions@wusm.wustl.edu.

Wayne State University, School of Medicine, Office of Biomedical Graduate Programs, Department of Immunology and Microbiology, Detroit, MI 48202. Offers MS, PhD, MD/PhD. *Faculty:* 11. *Students:* 8 full-time (3 women), 1 part-time (0 women); includes 4 minority (1 Black or African American, non-Hispanic/Latino; 1 Asian, non-Hispanic/Latino; 1 Hispanic/Latino; 1 Two or more races, non-Hispanic/Latino). Average age 29. 94 applicants, 5% accepted, 4 enrolled. In 2015, 2 master's, 3 doctorates awarded. *Degree requirements:* For master's, thesis; for doctorate, thesis/dissertation. *Entrance requirements:* For master's and doctorate, GRE, minimum GPA of 3.0 in BS in biology or related scientific discipline, three letters of recommendation, statement of purpose. Additional exam requirements/recommendations for international students: Required—

TOEFL (minimum score 100 iBT). *Application deadline:* For fall admission, 2/1 priority date for domestic and international students. Application fee: $0. Electronic applications accepted. *Expenses:* $17,645 annual resident tuition, $33,311 non-resident tuition; $735.20 per credit hour resident tuition, $1,387.95 per credit hour non-resident tuition; fees include $47.45 per credit hour student services fee and $274.60 per semester registration fee. *Financial support:* In 2015–16, 8 students received support, including 2 fellowships with tuition reimbursements available (averaging $26,614 per year), 5 research assistantships with tuition reimbursements available (averaging $26,716 per year); scholarships/grants, health care benefits, and unspecified assistantships also available. Financial award application deadline: 3/31. *Faculty research:* Viral replication and pathogenesis, bacterial pathogenesis, mucosal immunity, autoimmune diseases. *Unit head:* Dr. T.R. Reddy, Department Graduate Officer, 313-577-1591, Fax: 313-577-1155, E-mail: trreddy@med.wayne.edu. Website: http://www.immunomicro.med.wayne.edu/gradprogram.php

West Virginia University, School of Medicine, Graduate Programs at the Health Sciences Center, Interdisciplinary Graduate Programs in Biomedical Sciences, Program in Immunology and Microbial Pathogenesis, Morgantown, WV 26506. Offers MS, PhD, MD/PhD. *Degree requirements:* For doctorate, comprehensive exam, thesis/dissertation. *Entrance requirements:* For doctorate, GRE General Test, minimum GPA of 3.0. Additional exam requirements/recommendations for international students: Required—TOEFL. Electronic applications accepted. *Expenses:* Tuition, state resident: full-time $8568. Tuition, nonresident: full-time $22,140. Tuition and fees vary according to program. *Faculty research:* Regulation of signal transduction in immune responses, immune responses in bacterial and viral diseases, peptide and DNA vaccines for contraception, inflammatory bowel disease, physiology of pathogenic microbes.

Wright State University, School of Graduate Studies, College of Science and Mathematics, Program in Microbiology and Immunology, Dayton, OH 45435. Offers MS. *Program availability:* Part-time. *Degree requirements:* For master's, thesis. *Entrance requirements:* Additional exam requirements/recommendations for international students: Required—TOEFL. *Faculty research:* Reproductive immunology, viral pathogenesis, virus-host cell interactions.

Yale University, School of Medicine and Graduate School of Arts and Sciences, Combined Program in Biological and Biomedical Sciences (BBS), Microbiology Track, New Haven, CT 06520. Offers PhD, MD/PhD. *Degree requirements:* For doctorate, thesis/dissertation. *Entrance requirements:* For doctorate, GRE General Test, GRE Subject Test. Additional exam requirements/recommendations for international students: Required—TOEFL. Electronic applications accepted.

Youngstown State University, Graduate School, College of Science, Technology, Engineering and Mathematics, Department of Biological Sciences, Youngstown, OH 44555-0001. Offers environmental biology (MS); molecular biology, microbiology, and genetic (MS); physiology and anatomy (MS). *Program availability:* Part-time. *Degree requirements:* For master's, comprehensive exam, thesis, oral review. *Entrance requirements:* For master's, GRE General Test, minimum GPA of 2.7. Additional exam requirements/recommendations for international students: Required—TOEFL. *Faculty research:* Cell biology, neurophysiology, molecular biology, neurobiology, gene regulation.

Virology

Baylor College of Medicine, Graduate School of Biomedical Sciences, Department of Molecular Virology and Microbiology, Houston, TX 77030-3498. Offers PhD, MD/PhD. *Degree requirements:* For doctorate, thesis/dissertation, public defense. *Entrance requirements:* For doctorate, GRE General Test, GRE Subject Test (strongly recommended), minimum GPA of 3.0. Additional exam requirements/recommendations for international students: Required—TOEFL. Electronic applications accepted. *Faculty research:* Microbiology, viral molecular biology, bacterial molecular biology, microbial pathogenesis, microbial genomics.

Baylor College of Medicine, Graduate School of Biomedical Sciences, Interdepartmental Program in Cell and Molecular Biology, Houston, TX 77030-3498. Offers biochemistry (PhD); cell and molecular biology (PhD); genetics (PhD); human genetics (PhD); immunology (PhD); microbiology (PhD); virology (PhD); MD/PhD. *Degree requirements:* For doctorate, thesis/dissertation, public defense. *Entrance requirements:* For doctorate, GRE General Test, GRE Subject Test (strongly recommended), minimum GPA of 3.0. Additional exam requirements/recommendations for international students: Required—TOEFL. Electronic applications accepted. *Faculty research:* Molecular and cellular biology; cancer, aging and stem cells; genomics and proteomics; microbiome, molecular microbiology; infectious disease, immunology and translational research.

Case Western Reserve University, School of Medicine and School of Graduate Studies, Graduate Programs in Medicine, Department of Molecular Biology and Microbiology, Program in Molecular Virology, Cleveland, OH 44106. Offers PhD. *Entrance requirements:* Additional exam requirements/recommendations for international students: Required—TOEFL (minimum score 550 paper-based). *Expenses: Tuition, area resident:* Full-time $41,137; part-time $1714 per credit hour. *Required fees:* $32. Tuition and fees vary according to course load and program.

Mayo Graduate School, Graduate Programs in Biomedical Sciences, Program in Virology and Gene Therapy, Rochester, MN 55905. Offers PhD.

McMaster University, Faculty of Health Sciences and School of Graduate Studies, Program in Medical Sciences, Hamilton, ON L8S 4M2, Canada. Offers blood and vascular (M Sc, PhD); genetics and cancer (M Sc, PhD); immunity and infection (M Sc, PhD); metabolism and nutrition (M Sc, PhD); neurosciences and behavioral sciences (M Sc, PhD); physiology/pharmacology (M Sc, PhD); MD/PhD. *Degree requirements:* For master's, thesis; for doctorate, comprehensive exam, thesis/dissertation. *Entrance requirements:* For master's, honors B Sc, B+ average in related field; for doctorate, M Sc, minimum B+ average. Additional exam requirements/recommendations for international students: Required—TOEFL (minimum score 580 paper-based; 92 iBT).

Oregon State University, College of Science, Program in Microbiology, Corvallis, OR 97331. Offers environmental microbiology (MA, MS, PhD); food microbiology (MA, MS, PhD); genomics (MA, MS, PhD); immunology (MA, MS, PhD); microbial ecology (MA, MS, PhD); microbial evolution (MA, MS, PhD); parasitology (MA, MS, PhD); pathogenic microbiology (MA, MS, PhD); virology (MA). *Program availability:* Part-time. *Faculty:* 14 full-time (5 women), 1 part-time/adjunct (0 women). *Students:* 32 full-time (12 women); includes 5 minority (4 Asian, non-Hispanic/Latino; 1 Two or more races, non-Hispanic/Latino), 2 international. Average age 28. 79 applicants, 10% accepted, 4 enrolled. In 2015, 3 master's, 4 doctorates awarded. Terminal master's awarded for partial completion of

doctoral program. *Degree requirements:* For master's, thesis; for doctorate, one foreign language, thesis/dissertation. *Entrance requirements:* For master's and doctorate, GRE. Additional exam requirements/recommendations for international students: Required—TOEFL (minimum score 600 paper-based; 100 iBT). *Application deadline:* For fall admission, 8/1 for domestic students, 4/1 for international students; for winter admission, 12/1 for domestic students, 7/1 for international students; for spring admission, 2/1 for domestic students, 10/1 for international students; for summer admission, 5/1 for domestic students, 1/1 for international students. Application fee: $75 ($85 for international students). *Expenses:* Tuition, state resident: full-time $12,150; part-time $450 per credit. Tuition, nonresident: full-time $20,952; part-time $776 per credit. *Required fees:* $1572; $1443 per unit. One-time fee: $350. Tuition and fees vary according to course load, campus/location and program. *Financial support:* Fellowships, research assistantships, and teaching assistantships available. Financial award application deadline: 1/15. *Faculty research:* Genetics, physiology, biotechnology, pathogenic microbiology, plant virology. *Unit head:* Dr. Jerri Bartholomew, Professor and Department Head, 541-737-1856. *Application contact:* Mary Fulton, Microbiology Advisor, 541-737-1833, E-mail: mary.fulton@oregonstate.edu. Website: http://microbiology.science.oregonstate.edu/

Oregon State University, Interdisciplinary/Institutional Programs, Program in Molecular and Cellular Biology, Corvallis, OR 97331. Offers bioinformatics (PhD); biotechnology (PhD); cell biology (PhD); developmental biology (PhD); genome biology (PhD); molecular biology (PhD); molecular pathogenesis (PhD); molecular virology (PhD); plant molecular biology (PhD); structural biology (PhD). *Students:* 28 full-time (14 women), 2 part-time (1 woman); includes 4 minority (2 Asian, non-Hispanic/Latino; 2 Hispanic/Latino), 10 international. Average age 29. 104 applicants, 5% accepted, 5 enrolled. In 2015, 5 doctorates awarded. *Degree requirements:* For doctorate, thesis/dissertation, oral and written qualifying exams. *Entrance requirements:* For doctorate, GRE. Additional exam requirements/recommendations for international students: Required—TOEFL (minimum score 80 iBT), IELTS (minimum score 6.5). *Application deadline:* For fall admission, 8/1 for domestic students, 4/1 for international students; for winter admission, 12/1 for domestic students, 7/1 for international students; for spring admission, 2/1 for domestic students, 10/1 for international students; for summer admission, 5/1 for domestic students, 1/1 for international students. Application fee: $75 ($85 for international students). *Expenses:* Tuition, state resident: full-time $12,150; part-time $450 per credit. Tuition, nonresident: full-time $20,952; part-time $776 per credit. *Required fees:* $1572; $1443 per unit. One-time fee: $350. Tuition and fees vary according to course load, campus/location and program. *Financial support:* Fellowships, career-related internships or fieldwork, Federal Work-Study, and institutionally sponsored loans available. Support available to part-time students. Financial award application deadline: 1/1. *Unit head:* Dr. Dee Denver, Director, Molecular and Cellular Biology Graduate Program, 541-737-3698. *Application contact:* Kristin Carroll, Assistant Director, 541-737-5259, E-mail: kristin.carroll@oregonstate.edu. Website: http://www.mcb.oregonstate.edu/

Penn State Hershey Medical Center, College of Medicine, Graduate School Programs in the Biomedical Sciences, Graduate Program in Biomedical Sciences, Hershey, PA 17033. Offers biochemistry and molecular genetics (MS, PhD); biomedical sciences

Virology

(MS, PhD); translational therapeutics (MS, PhD); virology and immunology (MS, PhD); MD/PhD; PhD/MBA. *Students:* 79 full-time (43 women); includes 27 minority (7 Black or African American, non-Hispanic/Latino; 15 Asian, non-Hispanic/Latino; 4 Hispanic/Latino; 1 Native Hawaiian or other Pacific Islander, non-Hispanic/Latino), 17 international. 275 applicants, 16% accepted, 17 enrolled. Terminal master's awarded for partial completion of doctoral program. *Degree requirements:* For master's, thesis (for some programs); for doctorate, comprehensive exam, thesis/dissertation, candidacy exam. *Entrance requirements:* For doctorate, GRE General Test. Additional exam requirements/recommendations for international students: Required—TOEFL (minimum score 550 paper-based; 81 iBT). *Application deadline:* For fall admission, 1/1 for domestic and international students. Applications are processed on a rolling basis. Application fee: $65. Electronic applications accepted. *Expenses:* Contact institution. *Financial support:* In 2015–16, 79 students received support, including 79 research assistantships with full tuition reimbursements available (averaging $26,196 per year); fellowships, scholarships/grants, health care benefits, and unspecified assistantships also available. *Unit head:* Dr. Ralph L. Keil, Chair, 717-531-8595, Fax: 717-531-0786, E-mail: rlk9@psu.edu. *Application contact:* Kristin E. Smith, Director of Graduate Admissions, 717-531-1045, Fax: 717-531-0786, E-mail: kec17@psu.edu. Website: http://med.psu.edu/bms

Purdue University, Graduate School, PULSe - Purdue University Life Sciences Program, West Lafayette, IN 47907. Offers biomolecular structure and biophysics (PhD); biotechnology (PhD); chemical biology (PhD); chromatin and regulation of gene expression (PhD); integrative neuroscience (PhD); integrative plant sciences (PhD); membrane biology (PhD); microbiology (PhD); molecular evolutionary and cancer biology (PhD); molecular evolutionary genetics (PhD); molecular virology (PhD). *Entrance requirements:* For doctorate, GRE, minimum undergraduate GPA of 3.0. Additional exam requirements/recommendations for international students: Required—TOEFL (minimum score 550 paper-based; 77 iBT). Electronic applications accepted.

Purdue University, School of Veterinary Medicine and Graduate School, Graduate Programs in Veterinary Medicine, Department of Comparative Pathobiology, West Lafayette, IN 47907-2027. Offers comparative epidemiology and public health (MS); comparative epidemiology and public heath (PhD); comparative microbiology and immunology (MS, PhD); comparative pathobiology (MS, PhD); interdisciplinary studies (PhD), including microbial pathogenesis, molecular signaling and cancer biology, molecular virology; lab animal medicine (MS); veterinary anatomic pathology (MS); veterinary clinical pathology (MS). Terminal master's awarded for partial completion of doctoral program. *Degree requirements:* For master's, thesis (for some programs); for doctorate, thesis/dissertation. *Entrance requirements:* For master's and doctorate, GRE General Test. Additional exam requirements/recommendations for international students: Required—TOEFL (minimum score 575 paper-based), IELTS (minimum score 6.5), TWE (minimum score 4). Electronic applications accepted.

Rush University, Graduate College, Division of Immunology and Microbiology, Program in Immunology/Microbiology, Chicago, IL 60612-3832. Offers immunology (MS, PhD); virology (MS, PhD); MD/PhD. *Program availability:* Part-time. Terminal master's awarded for partial completion of doctoral program. *Degree requirements:* For master's, thesis; for doctorate, thesis/dissertation, comprehensive preliminary exam. *Entrance requirements:* For master's, GRE General Test; for doctorate, GRE General Test, interview, minimum GPA of 3.0. Additional exam requirements/recommendations for international students: Required—TOEFL. Electronic applications accepted. *Faculty research:* Human genetics, autoimmunity, tumor biology, complement, HIV immunopathology genesis.

Rutgers University–New Brunswick, Graduate School-New Brunswick, Programs in the Molecular Biosciences, Piscataway, NJ 08854-8097. Offers biochemistry (PhD); cell and developmental biology (MS, PhD); microbiology and molecular genetics (MS, PhD), including applied microbiology, clinical microbiology (MS), clinical mircobiology (PhD), computational molecular biology (PhD), immunology, microbial biochemistry, molecular genetics, virology. MS, PhD offered jointly with University of Medicine and Dentistry of New Jersey.

Université de Montréal, Faculty of Veterinary Medicine, Program in Virology and Immunology, Montréal, QC H3C 3J7, Canada. Offers PhD. Program offered jointly with Université du Québec, Institut Armand-Frappier. *Degree requirements:* For doctorate, thesis/dissertation, general exam. *Entrance requirements:* For doctorate, proficiency in French, knowledge of English. Electronic applications accepted.

Université du Québec, Institut National de la Recherche Scientifique, Graduate Programs, Research Center–INRS–Institut Armand-Frappier, Laval, QC H7V 1B7, Canada. Offers applied microbiology (M Sc); biology (PhD); experimental health sciences (M Sc); virology and immunology (M Sc, PhD). *Program availability:* Part-time. *Degree requirements:* For master's, thesis; for doctorate, thesis/dissertation. *Entrance requirements:* For master's, appropriate bachelor's degree, proficiency in French; for doctorate, appropriate master's degree, proficiency in French. Electronic applications accepted. *Faculty research:* Immunity, infection and cancer; toxicology and environmental biotechnology; molecular pharmacochemistry.

The University of Iowa, Roy J. and Lucille A. Carver College of Medicine and Graduate College, Graduate Programs in Medicine, Department of Microbiology, Iowa City, IA 52242-1316. Offers general microbiology and microbial physiology (MS, PhD); immunology (MS, PhD); microbial genetics (MS, PhD); pathogenic bacteriology (MS, PhD); virology (MS, PhD). *Degree requirements:* For master's, thesis; for doctorate, comprehensive exam, thesis/dissertation. *Entrance requirements:* For master's and doctorate, GRE General Test. Additional exam requirements/recommendations for international students: Required—TOEFL (minimum score 600 paper-based). Electronic applications accepted. *Faculty research:* Gene regulation, processing and transport of HIV, retroviral pathogenesis, biodegradation, biofilm.

University of Minnesota, Twin Cities Campus, Graduate School, PhD Program in Microbiology, Immunology and Cancer Biology, Minneapolis, MN 55455-0213. Offers PhD. *Degree requirements:* For doctorate, thesis/dissertation. *Entrance requirements:*

For doctorate, GRE General Test. Additional exam requirements/recommendations for international students: Required—TOEFL (minimum score 600 paper-based). Electronic applications accepted. *Faculty research:* Virology, microbiology, cancer biology, immunology.

University of Pennsylvania, Perelman School of Medicine, Biomedical Graduate Studies, Graduate Group in Cell and Molecular Biology, Philadelphia, PA 19104. Offers cancer biology (PhD); cell biology, physiology, and metabolism (PhD); developmental stem cell regenerative biology (PhD); gene therapy and vaccines (PhD); genetics and gene regulation (PhD); microbiology, virology, and parasitology (PhD); MD/PhD; VMD/PhD. *Faculty:* 317. *Students:* 339 full-time (189 women); includes 100 minority (7 Black or African American, non-Hispanic/Latino; 2 American Indian or Alaska Native, non-Hispanic/Latino; 45 Asian, non-Hispanic/Latino; 34 Hispanic/Latino; 1 Native Hawaiian or other Pacific Islander, non-Hispanic/Latino; 11 Two or more races, non-Hispanic/Latino), 52 international. 493 applicants, 22% accepted, 37 enrolled. In 2015, 51 doctorates awarded. *Degree requirements:* For doctorate, thesis/dissertation. *Entrance requirements:* For doctorate, GRE General Test. Additional exam requirements/recommendations for international students: Required—TOEFL. *Application deadline:* For fall admission, 12/1 priority date for domestic and international students. Applications are processed on a rolling basis. Application fee: $80. Electronic applications accepted. *Expenses: Tuition, area resident:* Full-time $31,068; part-time $5762 per course. *Required fees:* $3200; $336 per course. Full-time tuition and fees vary according to degree level, program and student level. Part-time tuition and fees vary according to course load, degree level and program. *Financial support:* In 2015–16, 339 students received support. Fellowships, research assistantships, scholarships/grants, traineeships, and unspecified assistantships available. *Unit head:* Dr. Daniel Kessler, Graduate Group Chair, 215-898-1478. *Application contact:* Meagan Schofer, Coordinator, 215-898-4360.
Website: http://www.med.upenn.edu/camb/

University of Pittsburgh, School of Medicine, Graduate Programs in Medicine, Molecular Virology and Microbiology Graduate Program, Pittsburgh, PA 15260. Offers PhD. *Faculty:* 47 full-time (14 women). *Students:* 24 full-time (9 women); includes 7 minority (1 Black or African American, non-Hispanic/Latino; 5 Asian, non-Hispanic/Latino; 1 Hispanic/Latino). Average age 28. 386 applicants, 17% accepted, 25 enrolled. In 2015, 7 doctorates awarded. *Degree requirements:* For doctorate, comprehensive exam, thesis/dissertation. *Entrance requirements:* For doctorate, GRE General Test, GRE Subject Test, minimum QPA of 3.0. Additional exam requirements/recommendations for international students: Required—TOEFL (minimum score 600 paper-based; 100 iBT), IELTS (minimum score 7). *Application deadline:* For fall admission, 12/1 priority date for domestic and international students. Application fee: $50. Electronic applications accepted. Tuition and fees vary according to program. *Financial support:* In 2015–16, 24 students received support, including 8 fellowships with full tuition reimbursements available (averaging $27,000 per year), 14 research assistantships with full tuition reimbursements available (averaging $27,000 per year), 2 teaching assistantships with full tuition reimbursements available (averaging $27,000 per year); scholarships/grants, traineeships, and health care benefits also available. *Faculty research:* Host-pathogen interactions, persistent microbial infections, microbial genetics and gene expression, microbial pathogenesis, anti-bacterial therapeutics. *Unit head:* Dr. Carolyn Coyne, Graduate Program Director, 412-383-5149, Fax: 412-624-1401, E-mail: ndeluca@pitt.edu. *Application contact:* Carol Williams, Admissions and Recruiting Manager, 412-648-8957, Fax: 412-648-1077, E-mail: gradstudies@medschool.pitt.edu.
Website: http://www.gradbiomed.pitt.edu

University of Prince Edward Island, Atlantic Veterinary College, Graduate Program in Veterinary Medicine, Charlottetown, PE C1A 4P3, Canada. Offers anatomy (M Sc, PhD); bacteriology (M Sc, PhD); clinical pharmacology (M Sc, PhD); clinical sciences (M Sc, PhD); epidemiology (M Sc, PhD), including reproduction; fish health (M Sc, PhD); food animal nutrition (M Sc, PhD); immunology (M Sc, PhD); microanatomy (M Sc, PhD); parasitology (M Sc, PhD); pathology (M Sc, PhD); pharmacology (M Sc, PhD); physiology (M Sc, PhD); toxicology (M Sc, PhD); veterinary science (M Vet Sc); virology (M Sc, PhD). *Program availability:* Part-time. *Degree requirements:* For master's, thesis; for doctorate, thesis/dissertation. *Entrance requirements:* For master's, DVM, B Sc honors degree, or equivalent; for doctorate, M Sc. Additional exam requirements/recommendations for international students: Required—TOEFL (minimum score 550 paper-based; 80 iBT). *Expenses:* Contact institution. *Faculty research:* Animal health management, infectious diseases, fin fish and shellfish health, basic biomedical sciences, ecosystem health.

The University of Texas Health Science Center at Houston, Graduate School of Biomedical Sciences, Program in Virology and Gene Therapy, Houston, TX 77225-0036. Offers MS, PhD; MD/PhD. Terminal master's awarded for partial completion of doctoral program. *Degree requirements:* For master's, thesis; for doctorate, thesis/dissertation. *Entrance requirements:* For master's and doctorate, GRE General Test. Additional exam requirements/recommendations for international students: Required—TOEFL. Electronic applications accepted. *Faculty research:* Viruses, infectious diseases, vaccines, gene therapy, cancer.

The University of Texas Medical Branch, Graduate School of Biomedical Sciences, Program in Emerging and Tropical Infectious Diseases, Galveston, TX 77555. Offers PhD, MD/PhD. *Degree requirements:* For doctorate, thesis/dissertation. *Entrance requirements:* For doctorate, GRE General Test. *Faculty research:* Emerging diseases, tropical diseases, parasitology, vitology and bacteriology.

Yale University, School of Medicine and Graduate School of Arts and Sciences, Combined Program in Biological and Biomedical Sciences (BBS), Microbiology Track, New Haven, CT 06520. Offers PhD, MD/PhD. *Degree requirements:* For doctorate, thesis/dissertation. *Entrance requirements:* For doctorate, GRE General Test, GRE Subject Test. Additional exam requirements/recommendations for international students: Required—TOEFL. Electronic applications accepted.

STANFORD UNIVERSITY

Ph.D. Program in Immunology

 For more information, visit http://petersons.to/stanford_immunology

Program of Study

The mission of the interdisciplinary Ph.D. Program in Immunology is to provide cutting-edge training in research and teaching leading to the Ph.D., graduating productive and innovative young scientists prepared for successful careers in immunology and related disciplines. The Ph.D. Program in Immunology is part of a community called "Stanford Immunology" of over 800 individuals, all of whom share a common passion for research and learning. The Ph.D. is offered in two tracks: Molecular, Cellular, and Translational Immunology (MCT) and Computational and Systems Immunology (CSI). Both tracks share a common curriculum, and after the first year, immunology graduate students in the CSI track continue taking bioinformatics courses. Courses are taught by expert faculty and emphasize current research and critical thinking. The Program provides teaching opportunities in undergraduate and graduate courses; an annual scientific conference, a seminar series featuring outstanding immunologists from across the country; and training in writing research papers and proposals, public speaking, data presentation, and the responsible conduct of research. Incoming first-year graduate students participate in a week-long "Immunology Startup," which prepares them for research at the bench and a general overview of important first principles and fundamental concepts in immunology.

The 76 faculty members in the Ph.D. Program in Immunology have a broad spectrum of expertise and represent some of the most outstanding scientists in their respective areas. The research interests of the faculty cover the major areas of modern immunology, including cellular, molecular, clinical, and structural immunology, and many aspects of the function of the immune system in each of these areas. Research includes studies of the development and function of T- and B- lymphocytes, natural killer cells, regulatory T cells, macrophages, dendritic cells, and the specific tissues and organs that contribute to host defenses. Faculty members also have made significant discoveries and contributions in clinical immunological research, such as cancer immunotherapies, transplantation, and microbiome studies. Students seeking admission to the Ph.D. Program in Immunology typically have an undergraduate major in biological sciences, but majors from other areas are acceptable if the applicants have sufficient coursework in biology, chemistry, general physics, and mathematics. Applications are evaluated by the Immunology Graduate Program committee based upon the following: GRE scores; grades; evidence of research experience; letters of recommendation, including letters from research sponsor(s); and commitment to a career in biomedical research. The GRE Subject test is not required. Applicants should plan on taking the GRE at least one month prior to the application deadline of December 1 to ensure that official scores are available when applications are evaluated. Interested Stanford medical students are welcome to apply to the program and should also submit a formal application by December 1.

For more information regarding the Ph.D. Program in Immunology, please refer to: http://med.stanford.edu/immunol.

Research Facilities

Students in the Ph.D. Program in Immunology benefit from outstanding facilities and resources provided by Stanford University and its schools, particularly the School of Medicine. The extraordinary level of investment of the University and school in the research environment—new buildings, centers and institutes, shared instrumentation facilities, and other research resources—has played a large role in building an outstanding faculty in immunology and other biomedical sciences. The laboratories of the 62 of the 76 immunology program faculty are located primarily in the School of Medicine; the proximity of the immunology labs fosters interactions and collaborations among the research groups. Rooms for classes, seminars, conferences, and meetings; a student fitness center, study commons, a café, and School of Medicine offices are in the Li Ka Shing Center for Learning and Knowledge, located among the research buildings previously mentioned. In addition, Biology, Bioengineering, Chemistry, Computer Science, and other Engineering departments are also right across Campus Drive from the School of Medicine, fostering cross-disciplinary interactions.

Financial Aid

All graduate students in the Ph.D. Program in Immunology are guaranteed support in the form of tuition, health insurance, and a living stipend. The level of this support is set annually and is generally the same (after tax) for all students regardless of the source of their support. The support used for a graduate student's tuition and stipend can be derived from a variety of sources including governmental grants; contracts and fellowships; private, industrial, and philanthropic sources; and University funds. Students will be informed of the initial source of their funding when they arrive at Stanford and are informed of changes as they occur.

Some students are supported by fellowships that require that they devote full time to study (usually 10–15 units of research or courses per quarter).

Living and Housing

About 64 percent of graduate students eligible for housing live in university-provided housing designed for single students, couples without children, and students with children. New graduate students are guaranteed housing their first year at Stanford when they apply by the spring deadline.

Location

Located 35 miles south of San Francisco and 20 miles north of San Jose, Stanford University is in the heart of Northern California's dynamic Silicon Valley, home to Yahoo!, Google, Hewlett-Packard, and many other cutting-edge companies that were started by and continue to be led by Stanford alumni and faculty.

Stanford University

To the west of the University's 8,180-acre campus are the Santa Cruz Mountains and Pacific Ocean, and to the east San Francisco Bay. Known as The Peninsula, the area is rich in natural beauty, culture, and entertainment.

Although the University is virtually a community unto itself, it calls the City of Palo Alto home. Downtown Palo Alto is a short walk from campus and includes many attractions, as well as many shops and restaurants.

The University

Stanford University is one of the world's leading teaching and research universities. Since its opening in 1891, Stanford has been dedicated to finding solutions to big challenges and to preparing students for leadership in a complex world.

Stanford Medicine's strength lies in interdisciplinary scholarship, dedicated faculty, and a culture of innovation that sets the training ground for the next generation of biomedical leaders and pioneers.

The Faculty

There are 76 faculty members; approximately 58 graduate students; more than 400 post-doctoral fellows; approximately 55 research, administrative, and support staff; and approximately 50 undergraduate and medical students working in labs.

Applying

Applications are made to the Office of Graduate Admissions for admission and financial support for the autumn quarter. The department requires the results of the General Test of the Graduate Record Examinations (GRE). It is strongly advised that the GRE be taken before October so that scores will be available when applications are evaluated. Applicants will be considered without regard to race, color, creed, religion, sex, marital status, age, physical handicap, or national origin. The Ph.D. Program in Immunology at Stanford University School of Medicine is committed to increasing its training of underrepresented minority groups.

Additional information, including application deadlines and the online application, can be found online at http://biosciences.stanford. edu/prospective/how-to-apply/index.html.

Correspondence and Information

Maureen Panganiba
Student Services Officer II and Program Manager
Ph.D. Program in Immunology
Stanford University School of Medicine
1215 Welch Road, Modular B, Room 55
Stanford, California 94305-5244
United States
Phone: 650-725-5076
E-mail: mopan@stanford.edu
Website: http://med.stanford.edu/immunol

UNIFORMED SERVICES UNIVERSITY OF THE HEALTH SCIENCES

F. Edward Hébert School of Medicine
Graduate Program in Emerging Infectious Diseases

 For more information, visit http://petersons.to/uniformedserviceshealthsciences

Program of Study

One of the missions of the Uniformed Services University of the Health Sciences (USUHS) is to provide both civilians and military students with high-quality training leading to advanced degrees in the biomedical sciences. The Graduate Program in Emerging Infectious Diseases (EID) is designed for applicants who wish to pursue an interdisciplinary program of study leading to the Ph.D. degree and was created for students who are primarily interested in the pathogenesis, host response, and epidemiology of infectious diseases. No M.S. degree program is currently offered. A broadly based core program of formal training is combined with an intensive laboratory research experience in the different disciplines encompassed by the field of infectious diseases. Courses are taught by an interdisciplinary EID faculty who hold primary appointments in the Departments of Microbiology and Immunology, Pathology, Preventive Medicine and Biometrics, Pediatrics, and Medicine. Research training emphasizes modern methods in molecular biology and cell biology, as well as interdisciplinary approaches.

During the first two years, all students are required to complete a series of broadly based core courses and laboratory rotations. Students also select one of two academic tracks in which to focus the remainder of their course work. The two tracks are Microbiology and Immunology, and Preventive Medicine and Biometrics. Advanced course work is required in each academic track. In addition, each student selects a faculty member with whom he or she would like to carry out a thesis research project. By the end of the second year, the student must complete all requirements for advancement to candidacy for the Ph.D. degree, which includes satisfactory completion of formal course work and passage of the qualifying examination. After advancement to candidacy, the student must complete an original research project and prepare and defend a written dissertation under the supervision of his or her faculty adviser and an advisory committee.

Research Facilities

Each academic department of the University is provided with laboratories for the support of a variety of research projects. Laboratories are available in most areas of study that encompass the interdisciplinary field of emerging infectious diseases, including both basic and medical aspects of bacteriology, bacterial genetics, virology, cellular and molecular immunology, parasitology, pathogenic mechanisms of disease, pathology of infectious disease, and epidemiology of infectious diseases. Resources available to students within the University include real-time PCR, microarray spotters and readers, EPICS, FACSAria and LSRII cell sorters and analyzers, Luminex 100 analyzer, automated oligonucleotide and peptide synthesizers and sequencing, MALDI-TOF Mass Spectrometer, high-resolution electron microscopes, confocal microscopes, a certified central animal facility, and state-of-the-art computer facilities. In addition, a BSL-3 biohazard containment laboratory suite is available. The library/learning resources center houses more than 521,000 bound volumes, subscribes to nearly 3,000 journals (print and online), and maintains 100 IBM and Macintosh personal computers for use by students, faculty members, and staff members. Biostatisticians serve as a resource for students and faculty members.

Financial Aid

USUHS provides an attractive package of financial support that is administered as a federal salary. This support is available on a competitive basis to all civilian graduate students. Awards are made on an annual basis and are renewable for up to three years. For the 2016–17 academic year, financial support for graduate students is $43,400. In addition to this base support, health insurance and transit benefits are provided, if needed.

Cost of Study

Graduate students in the Emerging Infectious Diseases Program are not required to pay tuition or fees. Civilian students do not incur obligations to the United States government for service after completion of their graduate training programs.

Living and Housing Costs

There is a reasonable supply of affordable rental housing in the area. The University does not have housing for graduate students. Living costs in the greater Washington, D.C., area are comparable to those of other East Coast metropolitan areas.

Student Group

The first full-time graduate students were admitted to the EID program in 2000. There are currently 30 full-time students enrolled in the EID graduate program. The University also has Ph.D. programs in departmentally based basic biomedical sciences, as well as interdisciplinary graduate programs in molecular and cell biology and in neurosciences.

Student Outcomes

Graduates hold faculty, research associate, postdoctoral, science policy, and other positions in universities, medical schools, government, and industrial research institutions. Since 2005, 61 Ph.D.'s have been awarded.

Location

The greater Washington metropolitan area has a population of about 3 million that includes the District of Columbia and the surrounding areas of Maryland and Virginia. The region is a center of education and research and is home to five major universities, four medical schools, and numerous other internationally recognized private and government research centers. In addition, multiple cultural advantages exist in the area and include theaters, a major symphony orchestra, major-league sports, and world-famous museums. The Metro subway system has a station adjacent to the campus and provides a convenient connection from the University to cultural attractions and activities in downtown Washington. The international community in Washington is the source of many diverse cuisines and international cultural events. For a wide variety of outdoor activities, the Blue Ridge Mountains, Chesapeake Bay, and Atlantic coast beaches are all within a 1- to 3-hour drive. Many national and local parks serve the area for weekend hikes, bicycling, and picnics.

The University

USUHS is located just outside Washington, D.C., in Bethesda, Maryland. The campus is situated in an attractive, park-like setting on the grounds of the Walter Reed National Military Medical Center (WRNMMC) and across the street from the National Institutes of Health (NIH). Wooded areas with jogging and biking trails surround the University. NIH and other research institutes in the area provide additional resources to enhance the education experience of graduate students at USUHS. Students can visit the USUHS website at http://www.usuhs.edu/eid.

Uniformed Services University of the Health Sciences

Applying

The Admissions Committee, in consultation with other faculty members, evaluates applications to the program. Each applicant must complete the online application form and have academic transcripts of postsecondary education, and results of the Graduate Record Examinations sent. No GRE Subject Test is required. In addition, three letters of recommendation from individuals familiar with the academic achievements and/or research experience of the applicant are required, as well as a personal statement that expresses the applicant's career objectives. USUHS subscribes fully to the policy of equal educational opportunity and selects students on a competitive basis without regard to race, color, gender, creed, or national origin. Prospective students may apply at https://registrar. usuhs.edu. Completed applications should be received on or before December 1.

Both civilians and military personnel are eligible to apply. Prior to acceptance, each applicant must complete a baccalaureate degree that includes required courses in mathematics, biology, physics, and chemistry (inorganic, organic, and biochemistry). Advanced-level courses in microbiology, molecular biology, genetics, and cell biology are very strongly recommended. All students are expected to have a reasonable level of computer literacy. Active-duty military applicants must obtain the approval and sponsorship of their parent military service, in addition to acceptance into the EID graduate program.

Correspondence and Information

Dr. Christopher C. Broder, Director
Graduate Program in Emerging Infectious Diseases
Uniformed Services University
4301 Jones Bridge Road
Bethesda, Maryland 20814-4755
United States
Phone: 301-295-5749
Fax: 301-295-9861
E-mail: christopher.broder@usuhs.edu
Website: http://www.usuhs.edu/eid

Patricia Sinclair
Administrative Officer
Graduate Program in Emerging Infectious Diseases
Uniformed Services University
4301 Jones Bridge Road
Bethesda, Maryland 20814-4755
United States
Phone: 301-295-3400
Fax: 301-295-9861
E-mail: patricia.sinclair@usuhs.edu

THE FACULTY

The interdisciplinary graduate programs at USUHS are superimposed on the departmental structure. Therefore, all faculty members in the interdisciplinary Graduate Program in Emerging Infectious Diseases (EID) have primary appointments in either a basic science or a clinical department and secondary appointments in EID. The faculty is derived primarily from the Departments of Microbiology and Immunology, Pathology, Preventive Medicine and Biometrics, Pediatrics, and Medicine. Thus, the faculty in EID includes the experts in infectious diseases, regardless of department. For additional information, students should visit the USUHS Academic Department website at http://www.usuhs.mil/academic.html. To address e-mail to specific faculty members at USUHS, students should use the first name, a period, the last name, and @usuhs.edu as the address; for example, to send e-mail to John Doe, the address would be john.doe@usuhs.edu.

Naomi E. Aronson, M.D.; Professor, Medicine.
Kimberly A. Bishop-Lilly, Ph.D.; Adjunct Assistant Professor, Navy Medical Research Center.
Christopher C. Broder, Ph.D.; Professor, Microbiology and Immunology.
Timothy H. Burgess, M.D., M.P.H.; Assistant Professor, Medicine.
Drusilla L. Burns, Ph.D.; Adjunct Assistant Professor, CBER, FDA.
David F. Cruess, Ph.D.; Professor, Preventive Medicine and Biometrics.
Stephen J. Davies, Ph.D.; Associate Professor, Microbiology and Immunology.
Saibal Dey, Ph.D.; Adjunct Assistant Professor, Biochemistry.
Michael W. Ellis, M.D.; Assistant Professor, Medicine.
Chou-Zen Giam, Ph.D.; Professor, Microbiology and Immunology.
Scott W. Gordon, Ph.D.; Adjunct Assistant Professor, Preventive Medicine and Biometrics.
Patricia Guerry, Ph.D.; Assistant Professor, Immunology, NMRC.
Val G. Hemming, M.D.; Professor, Pediatrics.
Ann E. Jerse, Ph.D.; Professor, Microbiology and Immunology.
Barbara Knollman-Ritschel, M.D.; Professor, Pathology.
Philip R. Krause, M.D.; Assistant Professor, CBER, FDA.
Larry W. Laughlin, M.D., Ph.D.; Professor, Preventive Medicine and Biometrics.
Radha K. Maheshwari, Ph.D.; Professor, Pathology.
Joseph Mattapallil, Ph.D.; Associate Professor, Microbiology and Immunology.
D. Scotty Merrell, Ph.D.; Professor, Microbiology and Immunology.
Nelson L. Michael, M.D., Ph.D.; Adjunct Assistant Professor, Medicine.
Edward Mitre, M.D.; Associate Professor, Microbiology and Immunology.
Alison D. O'Brien, Ph.D.; Professor, Microbiology and Immunology.
Christian F. Ockenhouse, M.D., Ph.D.; Adjunct Assistant Professor, Infectious Diseases, WRAIR.
Martin G. Ottolini, M.D.; Associate Professor, Pediatrics.
Julie A. Pavlin, M.D., Ph.D.; Associate Professor, Preventive Medicine and Biometrics.
Allen L. Richards, Ph.D.; Professor, Preventive Medicine and Biometrics.
Capt. Stephen J. Savarino, M.D.; Adjunct Assistant Professor, Infectious Diseases, NMRC.
Brian C. Schaefer, Ph.D.; Associate Professor, Microbiology and Immunology.
Connie S. Schmaljohn, Ph.D.; Adjunct Assistant Professor, USAMRIID.
David W. Scott, Ph.D.; Professor, Medicine.
Frank P. Shewmaker, Ph.D.; Assistant Professor, Pharmacology.
Clifford M. Snapper, M.D.; Professor, Pathology.
Andrew L. Snow, Ph.D.; Assistant Professor, Pharmacology.
V. Ann Stewart, D.V.M., Ph.D.; Professor, Preventive Medicine and Biometrics.
J. Thomas Stocker, M.D.; Professor, Pathology.
Terrill L. Tops, M.D., Assistant Professor, Pathology.
Charles Via, M.D.; Assistant Professor, Pathology.
Shuishu Wang, Ph.D.; Assistant Professor, Biochemistry.
Lt. Col. Glenn W. Wortmann, M.D.; Adjunct Assistant Professor. Infectious Diseases, WRAIR.
Shuenn-Jue L. Wu, Ph.D.; Adjunct Associate Professor, Immunology, NMRC.
Pengfei Zhang, Ph.D.; Research Associate Professor, Preventive Medicine and Biometrics.

UCONN HEALTH
Graduate Program in Immunology

 For more information, visit http://petersons.to/uconnhealth_immunology

Program of Study

The UConn Health Graduate Program in Immunology focuses on educating and training students to become independent investigators and educators who will contribute to expanding knowledge in the areas of basic and/or applied immunology. This goal will be achieved by course work, research seminars, laboratory experience, presentations, experimental work, and review of the literature of immunology. In addition to basic and advanced immunology courses, the student is given a strong foundation in basic biomedical sciences through the core curriculum in genetics, molecular biology, and cell biology. Research laboratory training aims to provide a foundation in modern laboratory technique and concentrates on hypothesis-based analysis of projects. The program will develop the student's ability to conceive and solve experimental problems, critically evaluate data, and communicate information in order to become productive members of a community of scientists that increases understanding and application of the basic principles of immunity to the treatment and prevention of disease.

The immunology graduate program emphasizes several areas, including:

- Molecular immunology; mechanisms of antigen presentation; T cell receptor genetics, major histocompatibility complex genetics, and function; cytokines and cytokine receptors; tumor antigens.
- Cellular immunology; biochemical mechanisms and biological aspects of signal transduction of lymphocytes and granulocytes; requirements for thymic and extrathymic T cell development; cytokines in B and T cell development; immunotherapy of tumors and infectious disease; immunoparasitology including parasite genetics and immune recognition of parasite antigens; mechanisms of inflammation.
- Organ-based immunology; immune effector mechanisms of the intestine; lymphocyte interactions in the lung; immune regulation of the eye.
- Autoimmunity; animal models of autoimmune disease; effector mechanisms in human autoimmunity.

Research Facilities

The Graduate Program in Immunology is interdepartmental, and therefore provides a broad base of training possibilities as well as ample shared facilities. State-of-the-art equipment is available in individual laboratories for analysis of molecular and cellular parameters of immune system structure and function. In addition, UConn Health–supported facilities provide equipment and expertise in areas of advanced data acquisition and analysis. These facilities include the Center for Cell Analysis and Modeling, the Fluorescence Flow Cytometry Facility, the Gene Targeting and Transgenic Facility, the Molecular Core Facility, the Microarray Facility, the Gregory P. Mullen Structural Biology Facility, and the Electron Microscopy Facility. The Lyman Maynard Stowe Library is well equipped with extensive journal and book holdings and rapid electronic access to database searching, Internet, and library holdings. A computer center is also housed in the library for student use and training.

Financial Aid

Support for doctoral students engaged in full-time degree programs at UConn Health is provided on a competitive basis. Graduate research assistantships for 2016–17 provide a stipend of $29,000 per year, which includes a waiver of tuition/most University fees for the fall and spring semesters and the option of participating in a student health insurance plan. While financial aid is offered competitively, UConn Health makes every possible effort to address the financial needs of all students.

Cost of Study

For 2016–17, tuition is $14,310 per year for full-time students who are Connecticut residents and $35,346 per year for full-time out-of-state residents. General University fees are added to the cost of tuition for students who do not receive a tuition waiver. These costs are usually met by traineeships or research assistantships for doctoral students.

Living and Housing Costs

There is a wide range of affordable housing options in the greater Hartford area within easy commuting distance of the campus, including an extensive complex that is adjacent to UConn Health. Costs range from $700 to $1,000 per month for a one-bedroom unit; 2 or more students sharing an apartment usually pay less. University housing is not available.

Student Group

At present, there are approximately 15 students in the Graduate Program in Immunology. There are 150 students in the various Ph.D. programs on the UConn Health campus.

Student Outcomes

Graduates have traditionally been accepted into high-quality laboratories for postdoctoral training. Following their training, graduates have accepted a wide range of positions in research in universities, colleges, research institutes, and industry, including the biotechnology sector.

Location

UConn Health is located in the historic town of Farmington, Connecticut. Set in the beautiful New England countryside on a hill overlooking the Farmington Valley, it is close to ski areas, hiking trails, and facilities for boating, fishing, and swimming. Connecticut's capital city of Hartford, 7 miles east of Farmington, is the center of an urban region of approximately 800,000 people. The beaches of the Long Island Sound are about 50 minutes away to the south, and the beautiful Berkshires are a short drive to the northwest. New York City and Boston can be reached within 2½ hours by car. Hartford is the home of the acclaimed Hartford Stage Company, TheatreWorks, the Hartford Symphony and Chamber orchestras, two ballet companies, an opera company, the Wadsworth Athenaeum (the oldest public art museum in the nation), the Mark Twain house, the Hartford Civic Center, and many other interesting cultural and recreational facilities. The area is also home to several branches of the University of Connecticut, Trinity College, and the University of Hartford, which includes the Hartt School of Music. Bradley International Airport (about 30 minutes from campus) serves the Hartford/Springfield area with frequent airline connections to major cities in this country and abroad. Frequent bus and rail service is also available from Hartford.

UConn Health

The UConn Health Campus

The 200-acre UConn Health campus at Farmington houses a division of the University of Connecticut Graduate School, as well as the Schools of Medicine and Dental Medicine. The campus also includes the John Dempsey Hospital, associated clinics, and extensive medical research facilities, all in a centralized facility with more than 1 million square feet of floor space. The Academic Research Building, built in 1999, is an impressive eleven-story structure providing 170,000 square feet of laboratory space and renovations are underway in the main laboratory building, converting existing lab space to state-of-the-art open lab areas. In addition, the Jackson Laboratory for Genomic Medicine opened its 189,000-square-foot facility on the UConn Health Campus in fall 2014. The faculty includes more than 260 full-time members. The institution has a strong commitment to graduate study within an environment that promotes social and intellectual interaction among the various educational programs. Graduate students are represented on various administrative committees concerned with curricular affairs, and the Graduate Student Organization (GSO) represents graduate students' needs and concerns to the faculty and administration, in addition to fostering social contact among graduate students at UConn Health.

Applying

Applications for admission should be submitted via the online application system and should be filed together with transcripts, three letters of recommendation, a personal statement, and recent results from the General Test of the Graduate Record Examinations. International students must take the Test of English as a Foreign Language (TOEFL) to satisfy Graduate School requirements. The deadline for completed applications and receipt of all supplemental materials is **December 1**. Please note that GRE and TOEFL exams taken after the due date will not be accepted for consideration for admission. In accordance with the laws of the state of Connecticut and of the United States, UConn Health does not discriminate against any person in its educational and employment activities on the grounds of race, color, creed, national origin, sex, age, or physical disability.

Correspondence and Information

Graduate Admissions Office
Ph.D. in Biomedical Science Program
UConn Health
263 Farmington Ave., MC 3906
Farmington, Connecticut 06030-3906
United States
Phone: 860-679-4509
E-mail: BiomedSciAdmissions@uchc.edu
Website:
  http://health.uconn.edu/graduate-school/academics/programs/ph-d-biomedical-science

THE FACULTY AND THEIR RESEARCH

Adam J. Adler, Professor of Immunology; Ph.D., Columbia. Mechanisms of T-cell tolerance induction to peripheral self- and tumor-antigens; immunological properties of prostate cancer.

Hector L. Aguila, Associate Professor of Immunology; Ph.D., Yeshiva (Einstein). Hematopoiesis and bone marrow microenvironment; lymphoid cell development; stem cell biology.

Jacques Banchereau, Professor of Immunology; Ph.D., University of Paris. Systems biology (omics) of the human immune response in health and diseases.

Linda Cauley, Assistant Professor of Immunology; D.Phil., Oxford. T-cell memory and respiratory virus infections.

Robert B. Clark, Professor of Immunology; M.D., Stanford. Autoimmunity; immune regulation; regulatory T cells.

Laura Haynes, Professor of Immunology, Ph.D., Rochester. Influence of aging on CD4 T-cell function and how this impacts responses to infection and vaccination.

Kamal Khanna, Assistant Professor of Immunology, Ph.D., Pittsburgh. Identifying the factors and the role they play in controlling the anatomy of a primary and secondary immune response in the hopes of explicating the underlying mechanisms that guide the complex movement of T cells during infection and recall responses in lymphoid and non-lymphoid tissues.

Joseph A. Lorenzo, Professor of Medicine; M.D., SUNY Downstate Medical Center. Relationships between bone-absorbing osteoclasts and immune cells.

Andrei Medvedev, Associate Professor of Immunology; Ph.D., Gabrichevsky Institute of Epidemiology and Microbiology (Moscow). How distorted control of TLR signaling underlies immune pathologies.

Lynn Puddington, Associate Professor of Immunology; Ph.D., Wake Forest. Allergic asthma; neonatal immunity and tolerance; developmental immunology.

Justin D. Radolf, Professor of Medicine and Center for Microbial Pathogenesis; M.D., California, San Francisco. Molecular pathogenesis and immunobiology of spirochetal infections.

Vijay Rathinam, Assistant Professor of Immunology; Ph.D., Michigan State. Immunologic basis of infectious and inflammatory diseases.

Juan C. Salazar, Professor of Pediatrics; M.D., Universidad Javeriana (Bogatá, Columbia). Analysis of the immunologic interactions between syphilis and HIV and the pathogenesis of spirochetal diseases including Lyme disease.

Pramod K. Srivastava, Professor of Medicine; Ph.D., Hyderabad (India). Heat shock proteins as peptide chaperones; roles in antigen presentation and applications in immunotherapy of cancer, infectious diseases, and autoimmune disorders.

Derya Unutmaz, Professor of Immunology; M.D., Mamara University Medical School. Decoding the functional and differentiation programs of different human T-lymphocyte subsets; developing various approaches towards development of T-cells for cancer immunotherapy, HIV infection, and regeneration during aging; mapping the immune profiles in cancer, HIV, and other inflammatory diseases to translate this knowledge as potential diagnostics.

Anthony T. Vella, Professor of Immunology; Ph.D., Cornell. T-cell immunity; costimulation; adjuvants and cytokines.

Kepeng Wang, Assistant Professor of Immunology; Ph.D., Hong Kong University of Science and Technology. Understanding the role of IL-17 in the development, immune regulation, and treatment of colorectal cancer.

Richard A. Zeff, Professor of Immunology; Ph.D., Rush. Major histocompatibility complex; antigen processing and presentation.

Beiyan Zhou, Associate Professor of Immunology; Ph.D., Northwestern. Understanding the systemic network governed by epigenetic factors in immune cell development and function in obesity; incorporating animal models and omics-technologies to address the critical questions in the field, including mechanisms underlying histone modification factors and non-coding RNAs In modulating tissue specific stem cell features and immune cell interactions within the host tissue niche.

UNIVERSITY OF MASSACHUSETTS AMHERST

Department of Microbiology

 For more information, visit http://petersons.to/umassmicrobiology

Programs of Study

The Department of Microbiology at the University of Massachusetts Amherst (UMass) offers programs of graduate study leading to the M.S. and Ph.D. degrees in microbiology. Postdoctoral training is also available. Courses covering various areas in the field of microbiology are offered by the Departmental faculty members, listed in the Faculty and Their Research section.

In the Ph.D. program, formal course work is completed during the first two years. From the start, a large portion of a student's time is dedicated to research. Students actively participate in ongoing research during two 1-semester rotations and then select dissertation problems from the wide spectrum of research areas pursued by the faculty. The following research fields are represented: microbial physiology, genetics, immunology, parasitology, pathogenic bacteriology, molecular biology, microbial ecology, and environmental microbiology. In the second year, Ph.D. candidates must pass a comprehensive preliminary examination. Degree requirements are completed by submission and defense of a dissertation. There is no foreign language requirement. Completion of the Ph.D. program generally takes four years beyond the bachelor's degree.

Research Facilities

The Department of Microbiology occupies space in the Morrill Science Center, Life Science Laboratories, and Fernald Hall. Laboratories are spacious and well equipped for research and teaching. State-of-the-art equipment necessary for investigation into all aspects of microbiology is available within the Department. The Department's facilities include tissue- and cell-culture laboratories, animal quarters, and various instrument rooms containing preparative and analytical ultracentrifuges, scintillation counters, fermentors, anaerobic chambers, equipment for chromatographic and electrophoretic procedures, photography, and other standard laboratory procedures. Centralized facilities provide state-of-the-art equipment and expertise to support research projects, such as the Light Microscopy Core, Genomics Resource Laboratory, Mass Spectrometry Facility and Flow Cytometry. A full list of core facilities can be found at http://www.umass.edu/ials/core-facilities.

Financial Aid

Financial aid is available in the form of University fellowships and teaching assistantships. Research assistantships are available for advanced graduate students. All assistantships include a waiver of tuition.

Cost of Study

In academic year 2016–17, annual tuition for in-state residents is $1,905 per credit; nonresident tuition is $3,627 per credit. Full-time students register for at least 9 credits per semester. The mandatory fees and tuition assessed for full-time graduate students (9 credits) is $7,457 per semester for in-state residents and $14,556 for nonresidents. Tuition is waived with eligible graduate assistantships. Tuition and fees are subject to change. More information is available in the Bursar's Office fee schedule online at http://www.umass.edu/bursar.

Living and Housing Costs

Graduate student housing is available in several twelve-month campus residence halls through University Housing Services. The University owns and manages unfurnished apartments of various sizes for family housing on or near the campus. Off-campus housing is available; rents vary widely and depend on factors such as size and location. A free bus system connects UMass with all neighboring communities.

Student Group

The Department has approximately 40 graduate and 225 undergraduate students as well as 10 postdoctoral fellows. Enrollment at the Amherst campus is about 29,000, including 6,500 graduate students.

Microbiology graduate students have the option of participating in activities sponsored by the Microbiology Graduate Student Group (MGSG). The group is open to all students pursuing a master's or doctoral degree from the Department of Microbiology at UMass Amherst. The purpose of this organization is (1) fostering student involvement in and communication within the Microbiology program at the University of Massachusetts Amherst, (2) creating an environment for student researchers to present their work and engage in scientific discourse, (3) encouraging participation in scientific conferences, (4) increasing the number of visiting speakers, and (5) promoting student participation in local, state and national American Society for Microbiology activities.

Location

The 1,450-acre campus of the University provides a rich cultural environment in a rural setting. Amherst is situated in the picturesque Pioneer Valley in historic western Massachusetts. The area is renowned for its natural beauty. Green open land framed by the outline of the Holyoke Range, clear streams, country roads, forests, grazing cattle, and shade trees are characteristic of the region. A broad spectrum of cultural activities and extensive recreational facilities are available within the University and at four neighboring colleges—Smith, Amherst, Mount Holyoke, and Hampshire. Opportunities for outdoor winter sports are exceptional. Amherst is 90 miles west of Boston and 175 miles north of New York City, and Cape Cod is a 3½-hour drive away.

The University

The University of Massachusetts is the state university of the Commonwealth of Massachusetts and is the flagship campus of the five-campus UMass system. Departments affiliated with the ten colleges and schools of the University offer a variety of graduate degrees through the Graduate School. The Amherst campus consists of approximately 150 buildings, including the twenty-eight-story W. E. B. DuBois Library, which is the largest at a state-supported institution in New England. The library features more than 5.8 million items and is home to a state-of-the-art learning commons equipped with computer workstations and high-speed network access.

Applying

The secure online application is available on the University of Massachusetts Graduate School website: http://www.umass.edu/gradschool. Prospective students are required to take the Graduate Record Examination. Applications for admission should be received by the Graduate Admissions Office by December 1 for September enrollment. Applications received after this date are considered only if space is available.

Correspondence and Information

Graduate Program Director
Department of Microbiology
Morrill IV, N416
639 North Pleasant Street
University of Massachusetts Amherst
Amherst, Massachusetts 01003-9298
United States
Phone: 413-545-2051
Fax: 413-545-1578
E-mail: microbio-dept@microbio.umass.edu
Website: http://www.micro.umass.edu

THE FACULTY AND THEIR RESEARCH

S. J. Sandler, Professor and Department Head; Ph.D., Berkeley. Molecular genetics of recombination; DNA replication and DNA repair in bacteria. *Mol. Microbiol.* 57:1074, 2005; *Mol. Microbiol.* 53:1343, 2004.

C. L. Baldwin, Adjunct Professor; Ph.D., Cornell. Cellular responses to bacterial and protozoan pathogens of humans and livestock including *Brucella, Leptospira, Mycobacteria,* and *Theileria. J. Immunol,* 192:6, 2014; *Plos One.* 10.1371/journal.pone.0089357; *BMC Genet.* 13:86.

J. P. Burand, Professor; Ph.D., Washington State. Biology and molecular biology of insect pathogenic viruses, particularly nonoccluded insect viruses and bee viruses, with emphasis on virus-host interactions that affect the virulence and persistence of these viruses in insects. *Viruses*

University of Massachusetts Amherst

4:28–61, 2012; *J. Invertebr. Pathol.* 108:217–9, 2011; *Appl. Environ. Micro.* 75:7862–5, 2009; *Virol. Sin.* 24:428–35, 2009; *Arch. Virol.* 154:909–18, 2009.

P. Chien, Adjunct Assistant Professor; Ph.D., California, San Francisco. Protein degradation during bacterial cell-cycle progression. *Proc. Natl. Acad. Sci. Unit. States Am.* Nov 5:110(45):18138–43, 2013; *Cell* 154:623–36, 2013. *Mol. Microbiol.* 88(6):1083–92, 2013; *Mol. Microbiol.* 87(6):1277–89, 2013; *Mol. Cell* 43(4):550–60, 2013; *Structure* 20(7):1223–32, 2012.

K. M. DeAngelis, Assistant Professor; Ph.D., Berkeley. Microbial ecology of carbon cycling in soils; microbial feedbacks to climate change; lignocellulosic biofuels. *Front. Microbiol.* 6:480, 2015; *Front. Microbiol.* 6:104, 2015; *Soil Biol. Biochem.* 66:60–8, 2013.

S. Goodwin, Dean, College of Natural Sciences; Ph.D., Wisconsin.

K. L. Griffith, Assistant Professor; Ph.D., Maryland. Cell-cell signaling in bacteria; development of tools for studying regulatory networks. *J. Mol. Bio.* 381:261–75, 2008; *Mol. Microbiol.* 70:1012–25, 2008.

J. F. Holden, Professor; Ph.D., Washington (Seattle). Physiology of hyperthermophilic archaea; geomicrobiology; hydrothermal vents; agricultural waste remediation and bioenergy using thermophiles. *Front. Microbiol.* 7:167, 2016; *G-cubed* 17:300–23, 2016; *Environ. Microbiol. Rep.* 8:196–200, 2016.

M. M. Klingbeil, Associate Professor and Graduate Program Director; Ph.D., Toledo. Molecular and biochemical parasitology, replication and repair of mitochondrial DNA (kinetoplast DNA) and nuclear DNA replication initiation in African trypanosomes. *Trends Parasitol.* [Epub ahead of print], 2016; *PLos One* 10:e0130998, 2015; *MBio* 6:e02425–14, 2015; *Mol. Microbiol.* 87:196–210, 2013; *Eukaryot. Cell* 11:844–55, 2012; *Mol. Biochem. Parasitol.* 175:68–75, 2011; *Mol. Microbiol.* 75:1414–25, 2010; *Mol. Cell* 5:398–400, 2009; *Eukaryot. Cell* 7:2141–6, 2008; *Science* 309:409–15, 2005; *Proc. Natl. Acad. Sci. U.S.A.* 101:4333–4, 2004; *J. Biol. Chem.* 278:49095–101, 2003; *Mol. Cell* 10:175–86, 2002.

J. M. Lopes, Professor and Associate Dean; Ph.D., South Carolina. Regulation of gene expression in eukaryotes. *Genes, Genomes & Genomics* 4:761–7, 2014; *J. Mol. Biol.* 425:457–65, 2013; *Mol. Microbiol.* 83:395–407, 2012.

D. R. Lovley, Distinguished University Professor; Ph.D., Michigan State. Physiology, ecology, and evolution of novel anaerobic microorganisms; microbe-electrode interactions with a focus on novel bioenergy solutions and environmental sensors; interspecies electron exchange; microbial nanowires; anaerobic bioremediation. *Nature Nanotechnology* 9:1012–17, 2014: *Curr. Opin. Biotechnol.* 24:385–90, 2013; *Nature Nanotechnology* 6:573–9, 2011; *Adv. Microb. Physiol.* 59:1–100, 2011; *Science* 330:1413–5, 2010; *Nature* 435:1098–101, 2005; *Science* 295:483–5, 2002.

Y. S. Morita, Assistant Professor; Ph.D., Johns Hopkins. Biosynthesis of lipids and glycans and the pathogenesis of mycobacterial diseases. *Proc. Natl. Acad. Sci. Unit. States Am.* 113:5400–5, 2016; *mBio* 4:e00472–512, 2013; *J. Biol. Chem.* 285:16643–50, 2010; *J. Biol. Chem.* 285:13326–36, 2010.

K. Nüsslein, Professor; Ph.D., Michigan State. Microbial ecology of terrestrial and aquatic environments; relating the stress of environmental influences to community structure and function, with emphasis on understanding interactions among bacterial communities. *Appl. Soil Ecol.* 107:48–56, 2016; *Front. Microbiol.* 6:1057 & 6:779, 2015; *Soil Biol. Biochem.* 80:1–8; *The ISME Journal* 8:1548–50, 2014; *Mol. Ecol.* 23:2988–99, 2014; *Appl. Environ. Microbiol.* 80:281–8, 2014; *PNAS* 110:988–93, 2013; *Appl. Microbio. Biotechnol.*, 2013, doi: 10.1007/s00253-013-4963-1; *Front. Extr. Microbiol.* 3:175, 2012; *Bioresource Technology* 123:207–13, 2012; *Appl. Microbiol. Biotechnol.* 2:6, 2012; *Biointerfaces* 87(1):109–15, 2011; *Water Res.* 44:4970–9, 2010; *Curr. Opin. Biotechnol.* 21:339–45, 2010; *Geomicrobiology* 26:9–20, 2009; *Geology* 36:139–42, 2008.

S. T. Petsch, Adjunct Associate Professor; Ph.D., Yale. Transport, transformation, and biodegradation of natural organic matter in sediments, soils, and sedimentary rocks. *Geology,* 36:139–42, 2008; *Appl. Environ. Microbiol.* 73:4171–9, 2007; *Geochim. Cosmochim. Acta* 71:4233–50, 2007; *SEPM* 5:5–9, 2007; *Am. J. Sci.* 306:575–615, 2006; *Palaeogeogr. Palaeoclim. Palaeoecol.* 219:157–70, 2005; *Gas Technol. Inst.* GRI-05/0023, 2004; *Am. J. Sci.* 304:234–49, 2004; *Org. Geochem.* 34:731–43, 2003.

S. M. Rich, Professor; Ph.D. California, Irvine. Population genetics and evolution of vectorborne and zoonotic diseases. *Proc. Natl. Acad. Sci. Unit. States Am.* 106:14902–7; *Emerg. Infect. Dis.* 15:585–7; *Gene* 304:65–75; *Proc. Natl. Acad. Sci. Unit. States Am.* 98:15038–43; *J. Clin. Microbiol.* 39:494–7; *Proc. Natl. Acad. Sci. Unit. States Am.* 95:4425–30; *Proc. Natl. Acad. Sci. Unit. States Am.* 94:13040–45; *Insect Mol. Biol.* 6:123–9; *Proc. Natl. Acad. Sci. Unit. States Am.* 92:6284–8.

D. A. Sela, Adjunct Assistant Professor; Ph.D., California, Davis. Breast milk interactions with the infant microbiome; nutritional microbiology; comparative microbial genomics. *Evolution, Medicine, and Public Health* PMID: 25835022, 2015; *Am. J. Clin. Nutr.* PMID:24452239, 2014; *Appl. Environ. Microbiol.* PMID:22138995, 2013; *J. Biol. Chem.* PMID:21288901, 2011; *Trends Microbiol.* PMID:20409714, 2010; *Proc. Natl. Acad. Sci. Unit. States Am.* PMID:19033196, 2008.

M. Sloan Siegrist, Assistant Professor; Ph.D., Harvard School of Public Health. Mycobacterial cell envelope; mechanisms by which *Mycobacterium* tuberculosis adapts to the host environment; bacterial cell wall engineering for basic and translational applications. *Cell Reports,* PMID: 25892235, 2015; *FEMS Microbiol. Rev.,* PMID: 25725012, 2014; *Proc. Natl. Acad. Sci. Unit. States Am.,* PMID: 25049412, 2014; *mBio,* PMID: 24803520, 2014; *Proc. Natl. Acad. Sci. Unit. States Am.,* PMID: 24706769, 2014; *ACS Chemical Biology,* PMID: 23240806, 2013; *J. Am. Chem. Soc.,* PMID: 22978752, 2012; *Proc. Natl. Acad. Sci. Unit. States Am.,* PMID: 19846780, 2009.

D. Wang, Adjunct Assistant Professor; Ph.D., Duke. Mechanisms of intracellular symbiosis between eukaryotic legume hosts and nitrogen-fixing bacteria. *Mol. Plant* 4(4):581, 2011; *Science* 327(5969):1126, 2010; *Current Biology* 17(20):1784, 2007.

W. Webley, Associate Professor and Director of Pre-Medical/Pre-Dental Advising; Ph.D., Massachusetts. Immunology and pathogenic bacteriology; understanding the role and mechanism of *Chlamydia* involvement in chronic severe asthma; design and development of a novel multi-subunit vaccine display/delivery system for *Chlamydia;* design of a point-of-care diagnostic test for Chlamydia infections in farm animals. *PLos One* 8(12), 2013; *Biology of AIDS,* 2nd edition, Kendall/Hunt Publishing; *Vaccine* 30(41):5942–8, 2012; *Plos One* 7(4), 2012; *Resp. Res.* 13(1):32, 2012; *Eur. Respir. J.* 38(4)994–5, 2011; *Respirology* 16(7):1081–7, 2011; *Pediatr. Infect. Dis. J.,* 29(12):1093–8, 2010; *Eur. Respir. J.,* 33:1–8, 2009; *Biology of AIDS,* 2nd ed., Dubuque, Iowa: Kendall/Hunt Publishing Company, 2008; *CHEST* 134(suppl.), 2008; *CHEST* 132(4):607, 2007; *J. Clin. Apheresis* 3, 2006; *BMC Infect. Dis.* 6:23, 2006; *Am. J. Respir. Crit. Care Med.* 171(10):1083–8, 2005; *BMC Infect. Dis.* 4(1):23, 2004 (with Stuart and Norkin); *Curr. Microbiol.* 49(1):13–21, 2004; *Am. J. Respir. Crit. Care Med.* 169(7):A586, 2004; *J. Clin. Apheresis* 18(2), 2003; *Exp. Cell Res.* 287(1):67–78, 2003.

H. Xiao, Adjunct Associate Professor; Ph.D., Wisconsin–Madison. Cancer preventive dietary components; diet-based strategy for cancer prevention; interaction between dietary components and human microbiome; enhancement of biological activity of dietary components by combination regimen; food processing, and nanotechnology.

Section 13
Neuroscience and Neurobiology

This section contains a directory of institutions offering graduate work in neuroscience and neurobiology, followed by in-depth entries submitted by institutions that chose to prepare detailed program descriptions. Additional information about programs listed in the directory but not augmented by an in-depth entry may be obtained by writing directly to the dean of a graduate school or chair of a department at the address given in the directory.

For programs offering related work, see also in this book *Anatomy; Biochemistry; Biological and Biomedical Sciences; Biophysics; Cell, Molecular, and Structural Biology; Genetics, Developmental Biology, and Reproductive Biology; Optometry and Vision Sciences; Pathology and Pathobiology; Pharmacology and Toxicology; Physiology;* and *Zoology.* In another guide in this series:

Graduate Programs in the Humanities, Arts & Social Sciences
See Psychology and Counseling

CONTENTS

Program Directories

Displays and Close-Ups

See also:

Biopsychology

Adler University, Programs in Psychology, Chicago, IL 60602. Offers advanced Adlerian psychotherapy (Certificate); art therapy (MA); clinical mental health counseling (MA); clinical neuropsychology (Certificate); clinical psychology (Psy D); community psychology (MA); counseling and organizational psychology (MA); counseling psychology (MA); counselor education and supervision (PhD); couple and family therapy (DCFT); criminology (MA); emergency management leadership (MA); forensic psychology (MA); marriage and family counseling (MA); marriage and family therapy (Certificate); military psychology (MA); nonprofit management (MA); organizational psychology (MA); police psychology (MA); public policy and administration (MA); rehabilitation counseling (MA); sport and health psychology (MA); substance abuse counseling (Certificate; Psy D/Certificate; Psy D/MACAT; Psy D/MACP; Psy D/MAMFC; Psy D/MASAC. *Accreditation:* APA. *Program availability:* Part-time, evening/weekend, online learning. Terminal master's awarded for partial completion of doctoral program. *Degree requirements:* For master's, thesis or alternative, oral exam, practicum; for doctorate, thesis/dissertation, clinical exam, internship, oral exam, practicum, written qualifying exam. *Entrance requirements:* For master's, 12 semester hours in psychology, minimum GPA of 3.0; for doctorate, 18 semester hours in psychology, minimum GPA of 3.25; for Certificate, appropriate master's or doctoral degree. Additional exam requirements/recommendations for international students: Required—TOEFL (minimum score 550 paper-based; 79 iBT). Electronic applications accepted.

American University, College of Arts and Sciences, Department of Psychology, Washington, DC 22016-8062. Offers addiction and addictive behavior (Certificate); behavior, cognition, and neuroscience (PhD); clinical psychology (PhD); psychobiology of healing (Certificate); psychology (MA). *Accreditation:* APA. *Program availability:* Part-time. *Faculty:* 22 full-time (8 women), 8 part-time/adjunct (5 women). *Students:* 88 full-time (67 women), 19 part-time (17 women); includes 20 minority (5 Black or African American, non-Hispanic/Latino; 5 Asian, non-Hispanic/Latino; 6 Hispanic/Latino; 4 Two or more races, non-Hispanic/Latino), 7 international. Average age 28. 564 applicants, 13% accepted, 30 enrolled. In 2015, 15 master's, 19 doctorates awarded. *Degree requirements:* For master's, comprehensive exam, thesis or alternative; for doctorate, comprehensive exam, thesis/dissertation. *Entrance requirements:* For master's, GRE General Test, GRE Subject Test, statement of purpose, transcripts, 2 letters of recommendation; for doctorate, GRE General Test, GRE Subject Test, 3 letters of recommendation, statement of purpose, transcripts, resume. Additional exam requirements/recommendations for international students: Required—TOEFL (minimum score 100 iBT), IELTS (minimum score 7), PTE (minimum score 68). Application fee: $55. *Expenses:* Tuition, area resident: Full-time $27,468; part-time $1526 per credit hour. *Required fees:* $430. Tuition and fees vary according to course level and program. *Financial support:* Application deadline: 2/1. *Unit head:* Dr. David Haaga, Department Chair, 202-885-1718, Fax: 202-885-1023, E-mail: ahrens@american.edu. *Application contact:* Kathy Clowery, Associate Director, Graduate Admission, 202-885-3620, Fax: 202-885-1344, E-mail: clowery@american.edu.
Website: http://www.american.edu/CAS/Psychology/

Argosy University, Atlanta, Georgia School of Professional Psychology, Atlanta, GA 30328. Offers clinical psychology (MA, Psy D, Postdoctoral Respecialization Certificate), including child and family psychology (Psy D), general adult clinical (Psy D), health psychology (Psy D), neuropsychology/geropsychology (Psy D); community counseling (MA), including marriage and family therapy; counselor education and supervision (Ed D); forensic psychology (MA); industrial organizational psychology (MA); marriage and family therapy (Certificate); sport-exercise psychology (MA). *Accreditation:* APA.

Argosy University, Twin Cities, Minnesota School of Professional Psychology, Eagan, MN 55121. Offers clinical psychology (MA, Psy D), including child and family psychology (Psy D), forensic psychology (Psy D), health and neuropsychology (Psy D), trauma (Psy D); forensic counseling (Post-Graduate Certificate); forensic psychology (MA); industrial organizational psychology (MA); marriage and family therapy (MA, DMFT), including forensic counseling (MA). *Accreditation:* AAMFT; AAMFT/COAMFTE; APA.

Binghamton University, State University of New York, Graduate School, School of Arts and Sciences, Department of Psychology, Specialization in Behavioral Neuroscience, Binghamton, NY 13902-6000. Offers PhD. *Program availability:* Part-time. *Students:* 12 full-time (8 women), 12 part-time (8 women); includes 6 minority (2 Black or African American, non-Hispanic/Latino; 4 Asian, non-Hispanic/Latino). Average age 27. 31 applicants, 35% accepted, 5 enrolled. In 2015, 2 doctorates awarded. Terminal master's awarded for partial completion of doctoral program. *Degree requirements:* For doctorate, thesis/dissertation. *Entrance requirements:* For doctorate, GRE General Test. Additional exam requirements/recommendations for international students: Required—TOEFL (minimum score 550 paper-based; 80 iBT). *Application deadline:* For fall admission, 12/15 priority date for domestic and international students. Application fee: $75. Electronic applications accepted. *Financial support:* In 2015–16, 23 students received support, including 3 research assistantships with full tuition reimbursements available (averaging $18,500 per year), 15 teaching assistantships with full tuition reimbursements available (averaging $18,500 per year); career-related internships or fieldwork, Federal Work-Study, institutionally sponsored loans, scholarships/grants, health care benefits, tuition waivers (full and partial), and unspecified assistantships also available. Financial award applicants required to submit FAFSA. *Unit head:* Dr. Lisa Savage, Program Coordinator, 607-777-4383, E-mail: lsavage@binghamton.edu. *Application contact:* Kishan Zuber, Recruiting and Admissions Coordinator, 607-777-2151, Fax: 607-777-2501, E-mail: kzuber@binghamton.edu.

Boston University, School of Medicine, Division of Graduate Medical Sciences, Program in Mental Health Counseling and Behavioral Medicine, Boston, MA 02215. Offers MA. *Faculty research:* HIV/AIDS, trauma, behavioral medicine (obesity, breast cancer), neurosciences, autism, serious mental illness, sports psychology. *Unit head:* Dr. Stephen Brady, Director, 617-414-2320, Fax: 617-414-2323, E-mail: sbrady@bu.edu. *Application contact:* GMS Admissions Office, 617-638-5255, E-mail: askgms@bu.edu.
Website: http://www.bumc.bu.edu/mhbm/

Carnegie Mellon University, Dietrich College of Humanities and Social Sciences, Department of Psychology, Area of Cognitive Neuroscience, Pittsburgh, PA 15213-3891. Offers PhD. *Degree requirements:* For doctorate, comprehensive exam, thesis/dissertation. *Entrance requirements:* For doctorate, GRE General Test. Additional exam requirements/recommendations for international students: Required—TOEFL.

Connecticut College, Department of Psychology, New London, CT 06320. Offers behavioral medicine/health psychology (MA); clinical psychology (MA); neuroscience/psychobiology (MA); social/personality psychology (MA). *Program availability:* Part-time. *Degree requirements:* For master's, thesis. *Entrance requirements:* For master's, GRE

General Test, statistics course. Additional exam requirements/recommendations for international students: Required—TOEFL (minimum score 600 paper-based).

Cornell University, Graduate School, Graduate Fields of Arts and Sciences, Field of Psychology, Ithaca, NY 14853-0001. Offers biopsychology (PhD); human experimental psychology (PhD); personality and social psychology (PhD). *Degree requirements:* For doctorate, comprehensive exam, thesis/dissertation, 2 semesters of teaching experience. *Entrance requirements:* For doctorate, GRE General Test, 3 letters of recommendation. Additional exam requirements/recommendations for international students: Required—TOEFL (minimum score 550 paper-based; 77 iBT). Electronic applications accepted. *Faculty research:* Sensory and perceptual systems, social cognition, cognitive development, quantitative and computational modeling, behavioral neuroscience.

Drexel University, College of Arts and Sciences, Department of Psychology, Philadelphia, PA 19104-2875. Offers clinical psychology (PhD), including clinical psychology, forensic psychology, health psychology, neuropsychology; law-psychology (PhD); psychology (MS); JD/PhD. *Accreditation:* APA (one or more programs are accredited). *Degree requirements:* For doctorate, thesis/dissertation, internship. *Entrance requirements:* For doctorate, GRE General Test. Additional exam requirements/recommendations for international students: Required—TOEFL. Electronic applications accepted. *Expenses:* Contact institution. *Faculty research:* Neurosciences, rehabilitation psychology, cognitive science, neurological assessment.

Duke University, Graduate School, Department of Psychology and Neuroscience, Durham, NC 27708. Offers biological psychology (PhD); clinical psychology (PhD); cognitive psychology (PhD); developmental psychology (PhD); experimental psychology (PhD); health psychology (PhD); human social development (PhD); JD/MA. *Accreditation:* APA (one or more programs are accredited). *Degree requirements:* For doctorate, thesis/dissertation. *Entrance requirements:* For doctorate, GRE General Test. Additional exam requirements/recommendations for international students: Required—TOEFL (minimum score 577 paper-based; 90 iBT) or IELTS (minimum score 7). Electronic applications accepted.

The Graduate Center, City University of New York, Graduate Studies, Program in Psychology, New York, NY 10016-4039. Offers basic applied neurocognition (PhD); biopsychology (PhD); clinical psychology (PhD); developmental psychology (PhD); environmental psychology (PhD); experimental psychology (PhD); industrial psychology (PhD); learning processes (PhD); neuropsychology (PhD); psychology (PhD); social personality (PhD). *Degree requirements:* For doctorate, one foreign language, thesis/dissertation. *Entrance requirements:* For doctorate, GRE General Test. Additional exam requirements/recommendations for international students: Required—TOEFL. Electronic applications accepted.

Harvard University, Graduate School of Arts and Sciences, Department of Psychology, Cambridge, MA 02138. Offers psychology (PhD), including behavior and decision analysis, cognition, developmental psychology, experimental psychology, personality, psychobiology, psychopathology; social psychology (PhD). *Accreditation:* APA. *Degree requirements:* For doctorate, thesis/dissertation, general exams. *Entrance requirements:* For doctorate, GRE General Test. Additional exam requirements/recommendations for international students: Required—TOEFL.

Howard University, Graduate School, Department of Psychology, Washington, DC 20059-0002. Offers clinical psychology (PhD); developmental psychology (PhD); experimental psychology (PhD); neuropsychology (PhD); personality psychology (PhD); psychology (MS); social psychology (PhD). *Accreditation:* APA (one or more programs are accredited). *Program availability:* Part-time. *Degree requirements:* For master's, thesis; for doctorate, comprehensive exam, thesis/dissertation, qualifying exam. *Entrance requirements:* For master's, GRE General Test, minimum GPA of 2.5, bachelor's degree in psychology or related field; for doctorate, GRE General Test, minimum GPA of 3.0. *Faculty research:* Personality and psychophysiology, educational and social development of African-American children, child and adult psychopathology.

Indiana University–Purdue University Indianapolis, School of Science, Department of Psychology, Indianapolis, IN 46202-3275. Offers clinical psychology (MS); industrial/organizational psychology (MS); psychobiology of addictions (PhD). *Accreditation:* APA (one or more programs are accredited). Terminal master's awarded for partial completion of doctoral program. *Degree requirements:* For master's, thesis; for doctorate, thesis/dissertation. *Entrance requirements:* For master's, GRE General Test, minimum undergraduate GPA of 3.0; for doctorate, GRE General Test, GRE Subject Test (clinical psychology), minimum undergraduate GPA of 3.2. Additional exam requirements/recommendations for international students: Required—TOEFL (minimum score 567 paper-based; 86 iBT), IELTS (minimum score 6.5). Electronic applications accepted. *Faculty research:* Severe mental illness, health psychology, neurological research, alcoholism and psychopathology, functional activities within organizations.

Louisiana State University and Agricultural & Mechanical College, Graduate School, College of Humanities and Social Sciences, Department of Psychology, Baton Rouge, LA 70803. Offers biological psychology (MA, PhD); clinical psychology (MA, PhD); cognitive psychology (MA, PhD); developmental psychology (MA, PhD); school psychology (MA, PhD). *Accreditation:* APA (one or more programs are accredited).

Memorial University of Newfoundland, School of Graduate Studies, Interdisciplinary Program in Cognitive and Behavioral Ecology, St. John's, NL A1C 5S7, Canada. Offers M Sc, PhD. *Degree requirements:* For master's, thesis, public lecture; for doctorate, comprehensive exam, thesis/dissertation, oral defense of dissertation. *Entrance requirements:* For master's, honors degree (minimum 2nd class standing) in related field; for doctorate, master's degree. *Application deadline:* For fall admission, 1/31 priority date for domestic students, 1/31 for international students. Applications are processed on a rolling basis. Application fee: $50 Canadian dollars ($100 Canadian dollars for international students). Electronic applications accepted. *Expenses:* Tuition, area resident: Full-time $2199 Canadian dollars. *International tuition:* $2859 Canadian dollars full-time. *Financial support:* Fellowships, research assistantships, and teaching assistantships available. *Faculty research:* Seabird feeding ecology, marine mammal and seabird energetics, systems of fish, seabird/seal/fisheries interaction. *Unit head:* Dr. Mark Abrams, Dean, 709-864-8153, Fax: 709-864-3316. *Application contact:* Gail Kenny, Secretary, 709-864-8154, Fax: 709-864-3316, E-mail: gkenny@mun.ca.

Northwestern University, The Graduate School, Judd A. and Marjorie Weinberg College of Arts and Sciences, Department of Psychology, Evanston, IL 60208. Offers brain, behavior and cognition (PhD); clinical psychology (PhD); cognitive psychology (PhD); personality psychology (PhD); social psychology (PhD); JD/PhD. Admissions and degrees offered through The Graduate School. *Accreditation:* APA (one or more programs are accredited). *Program availability:* Part-time. *Degree requirements:* For doctorate, thesis/dissertation. *Entrance requirements:* For doctorate, GRE General Test,

GRE Subject Test. Additional exam requirements/recommendations for international students: Required—TOEFL. Electronic applications accepted. *Faculty research:* Memory and higher order cognition, anxiety and depression, effectiveness of psychotherapy, social cognition, molecular basis of memory.

Northwestern University, The Graduate School and Feinberg School of Medicine, Program in Clinical Psychology, Evanston, IL 60208. Offers clinical psychology (PhD), including clinical neuropsychology. Admissions and degree offered through The Graduate School. *Accreditation:* APA. *Degree requirements:* For doctorate, thesis/dissertation, clinical internship. *Entrance requirements:* For doctorate, GRE General Test, GRE Subject Test, minimum GPA of 3.2, course work in psychology. Additional exam requirements/recommendations for international students: Required—TOEFL. *Faculty research:* Cancer and cardiovascular risk reduction, evaluation of mental health services and policy, neuropsychological assessment, outcome of psychotherapy, cognitive therapy, pediatric and clinical child psychology.

Oregon Health & Science University, School of Medicine, Graduate Programs in Medicine, Department of Behavioral Neuroscience, Portland, OR 97239-3098. Offers PhD. *Faculty:* 21 full-time (7 women), 25 part-time/adjunct (9 women). *Students:* 28 full-time (18 women); includes 11 minority (1 Black or African American, non-Hispanic/Latino; 2 Asian, non-Hispanic/Latino; 8 Hispanic/Latino). Average age 28. 75 applicants, 13% accepted, 6 enrolled. In 2015, 6 doctorates awarded. Terminal master's awarded for partial completion of doctoral program. *Degree requirements:* For doctorate, comprehensive exam, thesis/dissertation, qualifying exam. *Entrance requirements:* For doctorate, GRE General Test (minimum scores: 153 Verbal/148 Quantitative/4.5 Analytical), undergraduate coursework in biopsychology and other basic science areas. Additional exam requirements/recommendations for international students: Required—IELTS or TOEFL. *Application deadline:* For fall admission, 12/1 for domestic and international students. Application fee: $70. Electronic applications accepted. *Financial support:* Fellowships, research assistantships, health care benefits, tuition waivers (full), and stipends (for PhD students) available. *Faculty research:* Behavioral neuroscience, behavioral genomics, biological basis of drug and alcohol abuse, cognitive neuroscience, neuropharmacology and neuroendocrinology. *Unit head:* Dr. Suzanne Mitchell, Program Director, 503-494-1650, E-mail: mitchesu@ohsu.edu. *Application contact:* Kris Thomason, Graduate Program Manager, 503-494-8464, E-mail: thomason@ohsu.edu.
Website: http://www.ohsu.edu/som-BehNeuro/

Palo Alto University, PGSP-Stanford Psy D Consortium Program, Palo Alto, CA 94304. Offers Psy D. Program offered jointly with Stanford University. *Accreditation:* APA. *Degree requirements:* For doctorate, comprehensive exam, thesis/dissertation, 2000-hour clinical internship. *Entrance requirements:* For doctorate, GRE General Test (minimum overall score 1200); GRE Subject Test in psychology (highly recommended), undergraduate degree in psychology or related area with minimum GPA of 3.3. Additional exam requirements/recommendations for international students: Required—TOEFL, IELTS. Electronic applications accepted. *Expenses:* Contact institution.

Penn State University Park, Graduate School, College of Health and Human Development, Department of Biobehavioral Health, University Park, PA 16802. Offers biobehavioral health (MS, PhD). *Unit head:* Dr. Ann C. Crouter, Dean, 814-865-1420, Fax: 814-865-3282. *Application contact:* Lori Stania, Director, Graduate Student Services, 814-865-1795, Fax: 814-863-4627, E-mail: l-gswww@lists.psu.edu.
Website: http://bbh.hhdev.psu.edu/

Philadelphia College of Osteopathic Medicine, Graduate and Professional Programs, Department of Psychology, Philadelphia, PA 19131-1694. Offers applied behavior analysis (Certificate); clinical health psychology (Post-Doctoral Certificate); clinical neuropsychology (Post-Doctoral Certificate); clinical psychology (Psy D); mental health counseling (MS); organizational development and leadership (MS); psychology (Certificate); school psychology (MS, Psy D, Ed S). *Accreditation:* APA. Terminal master's awarded for partial completion of doctoral program. *Degree requirements:* For master's, comprehensive exam (for some programs), thesis (for some programs); for doctorate, comprehensive exam, thesis/dissertation. *Entrance requirements:* For master's, GRE or MAT, minimum GPA of 3.0; bachelor's degree from regionally-accredited college or university; for doctorate, PRAXIS II (for Psy D in school psychology), minimum undergraduate GPA of 3.0; for other advanced degree, GRE (for Ed S). Additional exam requirements/recommendations for international students: Required—TOEFL (minimum score 79 iBT). Electronic applications accepted. *Faculty research:* Adult and childhood anxiety and ADHD; coping with chronic illness; primary care psychology/integrated health care; applied behavior analysis; psychological, educational, and neuropsychological assessment.

Rutgers University–Newark, Graduate School, Program in Psychology, Newark, NJ 07102. Offers cognitive neuroscience (PhD); cognitive science (PhD); perception (PhD); psychobiology (PhD); social cognition (PhD). *Degree requirements:* For doctorate, comprehensive exam, thesis/dissertation. *Entrance requirements:* For doctorate, GRE General Test, GRE Subject Test, minimum undergraduate B average. Electronic applications accepted. *Faculty research:* Visual perception (luminance, motion), neuroendocrine mechanisms in behavior (reproduction, pain), attachment theory, connectionist modeling of cognition.

Rutgers University–New Brunswick, Graduate School-New Brunswick, Program in Psychology, Piscataway, NJ 08854-8097. Offers behavioral neuroscience (PhD); clinical psychology (PhD); cognitive psychology (PhD); interdisciplinary health psychology (PhD); social psychology (PhD). *Accreditation:* APA. *Degree requirements:* For doctorate, comprehensive exam, thesis/dissertation. *Entrance requirements:* For doctorate, GRE General Test, 3 letters of recommendation. Additional exam requirements/recommendations for international students: Required—TOEFL (minimum score 577 paper-based). Electronic applications accepted. *Faculty research:* Learning and memory, behavioral ecology, hormones and behavior, psychopharmacology, anxiety disorders.

The University of British Columbia, Faculty of Arts and Faculty of Graduate Studies, Department of Psychology, Vancouver, BC V6T 1Z4, Canada. Offers behavioral neuroscience (MA, PhD); clinical psychology (MA, PhD); cognitive science (MA, PhD); developmental psychology (MA, PhD); health psychology (MA, PhD); quantitative methods (MA, PhD); social/personality psychology (MA, PhD). *Accreditation:* APA (one or more programs are accredited). Terminal master's awarded for partial completion of doctoral program. *Degree requirements:* For master's, thesis; for doctorate, comprehensive exam, thesis/dissertation. *Entrance requirements:* For master's and doctorate, GRE General Test. Additional exam requirements/recommendations for international students: Required—TOEFL (minimum score 550 paper-based; 80 iBT). Electronic applications accepted. *Faculty research:* Clinical, developmental, social/personality, cognition, behavioral neuroscience.

University of Connecticut, Graduate School, College of Liberal Arts and Sciences, Department of Psychology, Storrs, CT 06269. Offers behavioral neuroscience (PhD); biopsychology (PhD); clinical psychology (MA, PhD); cognition and instruction (PhD); developmental psychology (MA, PhD); ecological psychology (PhD); experimental psychology (PhD); general psychology (MA, PhD); industrial/organizational psychology (PhD); language and cognition (PhD); neuroscience (PhD); social psychology (MA,

PhD). *Accreditation:* APA. Terminal master's awarded for partial completion of doctoral program. *Degree requirements:* For master's, comprehensive exam; for doctorate, thesis/dissertation. *Entrance requirements:* For master's and doctorate, GRE General Test, GRE Subject Test. Additional exam requirements/recommendations for international students: Required—TOEFL (minimum score 550 paper-based). *Application deadline:* For fall admission, 2/1 priority date for domestic and international students; for spring admission, 11/1 for domestic students, 10/1 for international students. Applications are processed on a rolling basis. Application fee: $55. Electronic applications accepted. *Financial support:* Fellowships, research assistantships with full tuition reimbursements, teaching assistantships with full tuition reimbursements, career-related internships or fieldwork, Federal Work-Study, scholarships/grants, health care benefits, and unspecified assistantships available. Financial award application deadline: 2/1; financial award applicants required to submit FAFSA.
Website: http://www.psychology.uconn.edu/

University of Michigan, Rackham Graduate School, College of Literature, Science, and the Arts, Department of Psychology, Ann Arbor, MI 48109. Offers biopsychology (PhD); clinical science (PhD); cognition and cognitive neuroscience (PhD); developmental psychology (PhD); personality and social contexts (PhD); social psychology (PhD). *Accreditation:* APA. *Faculty:* 57 full-time (27 women), 31 part-time/adjunct (17 women). *Students:* 120 full-time (86 women); includes 59 minority (13 Black or African American, non-Hispanic/Latino; 2 American Indian or Alaska Native, non-Hispanic/Latino; 14 Asian, non-Hispanic/Latino; 25 Hispanic/Latino; 5 Two or more races, non-Hispanic/Latino), 10 international. Average age 27. 687 applicants, 7% accepted, 25 enrolled. In 2015, 20 doctorates awarded. *Degree requirements:* For doctorate, comprehensive exam, thesis/dissertation, oral defense of dissertation, preliminary exam. *Entrance requirements:* For doctorate, GRE General Test. Additional exam requirements/recommendations for international students: Required—TOEFL. *Application deadline:* For fall admission, 12/1 for domestic and international students. Application fee: $75 ($90 for international students). Electronic applications accepted. *Financial support:* In 2015–16, 46 fellowships with full tuition reimbursements (averaging $19,800 per year), 86 teaching assistantships with full tuition reimbursements (averaging $24,750 per year) were awarded; career-related internships or fieldwork and health care benefits also available. Financial award application deadline: 4/15. *Unit head:* Prof. Patricia Reuter-Lorenz, Department Chair, 734-764-7429. *Application contact:* Tina Griffith, Psychology Student Academic Affairs, 734-764-2580, Fax: 734-615-7584, E-mail: psych.saa@umich.edu.
Website: http://www.lsa.umich.edu/psych/

University of Minnesota, Twin Cities Campus, Graduate School, College of Liberal Arts, Department of Psychology, Program in Cognitive and Biological Psychology, Minneapolis, MN 55455-0213. Offers PhD. *Degree requirements:* For doctorate, comprehensive exam, thesis/dissertation. *Entrance requirements:* For doctorate, GRE General Test, GRE Subject Test (recommended), 12 credits of upper-level psychology courses, including a course in statistics or psychological measurement. Additional exam requirements/recommendations for international students: Required—TOEFL (minimum score 550 paper-based; 79 iBT).

University of Nebraska–Lincoln, Graduate College, College of Arts and Sciences, Department of Psychology, Lincoln, NE 68588. Offers biopsychology (PhD); clinical psychology (PhD); cognitive psychology (PhD); developmental psychology (PhD); psychology (MA); social/personality psychology (PhD); JD/MA; JD/PhD. *Accreditation:* APA (one or more programs are accredited). *Degree requirements:* For master's, thesis optional; for doctorate, comprehensive exam, thesis/dissertation. *Entrance requirements:* For master's and doctorate, GRE General Test. Additional exam requirements/recommendations for international students: Required—TOEFL (minimum score 550 paper-based). Electronic applications accepted. *Faculty research:* Law and psychology, rural mental health, chronic mental illness, neuropsychology, child clinical psychology.

The University of North Carolina at Chapel Hill, Graduate School, College of Arts and Sciences, Department of Psychology, Chapel Hill, NC 27599-3270. Offers behavioral neuroscience psychology (PhD); clinical psychology (PhD); cognitive psychology (PhD); developmental psychology (PhD); quantitative psychology (PhD); social psychology (PhD). *Accreditation:* APA. *Degree requirements:* For doctorate, comprehensive exam, thesis/dissertation. *Entrance requirements:* For doctorate, GRE General Test, minimum GPA of 3.0. Additional exam requirements/recommendations for international students: Required—TOEFL (minimum score 550 paper-based; 79 iBT), IELTS (minimum score 7). Electronic applications accepted. *Faculty research:* Expressed emotion, cognitive development, social cognitive neuroscience, human memory personality.

University of Oklahoma Health Sciences Center, College of Medicine and Graduate College, Graduate Programs in Medicine, Department of Psychiatry and Behavioral Sciences, Oklahoma City, OK 73190. Offers biological psychology (MS, PhD). *Degree requirements:* For master's, thesis; for doctorate, thesis/dissertation. *Entrance requirements:* For doctorate, GRE General Test, 3 letters of recommendation. Additional exam requirements/recommendations for international students: Required—TOEFL. *Faculty research:* Behavioral neuroscience, human neuropsychology, psychophysiology, behavioral medicine, health psychology.

University of Oregon, Graduate School, College of Arts and Sciences, Department of Psychology, Eugene, OR 97403. Offers clinical psychology (PhD); cognitive psychology (MA, MS, PhD); developmental psychology (MA, MS, PhD); physiological psychology (MA, MS, PhD); psychology (MA, MS, PhD); social/personality psychology (MA, MS, PhD). *Accreditation:* APA (one or more programs are accredited). Terminal master's awarded for partial completion of doctoral program. *Degree requirements:* For doctorate, thesis/dissertation. *Entrance requirements:* For master's, GRE General Test, minimum GPA of 3.0; for doctorate, GRE General Test. Additional exam requirements/recommendations for international students: Required—TOEFL.

The University of Texas at Austin, Graduate School, The Institute for Neuroscience, Austin, TX 78712-1111. Offers PhD, MD/PhD. Terminal master's awarded for partial completion of doctoral program. *Degree requirements:* For doctorate, thesis/dissertation. *Entrance requirements:* For doctorate, GRE. Electronic applications accepted. *Faculty research:* Cellular/molecular biology, neurobiology, pharmacology, behavioral neuroscience.

University of Windsor, Faculty of Graduate Studies, Faculty of Arts and Social Sciences, Department of Psychology, Windsor, ON N9B 3P4, Canada. Offers adult clinical (MA, PhD); applied social psychology (MA, PhD); child clinical (MA, PhD); clinical neuropsychology (MA, PhD). *Accreditation:* APA (one or more programs are accredited). *Degree requirements:* For master's, thesis; for doctorate, comprehensive exam, thesis/dissertation. *Entrance requirements:* For master's, GRE General Test, GRE Subject Test in psychology, minimum B average; for doctorate, GRE General Test, GRE Subject Test in psychology, master's degree. Additional exam requirements/recommendations for international students: Required—TOEFL (minimum score 600 paper-based). Electronic applications accepted. *Faculty research:* Gambling, suicidology, emotional competence, psychotherapy and trauma.

University of Wisconsin–Madison, Graduate School, College of Letters and Science, Department of Psychology, Program in Biology of Brain and Behavior, Madison, WI

Biopsychology

53706-1380. Offers PhD. *Degree requirements:* For doctorate, comprehensive exam, thesis/dissertation. *Entrance requirements:* For doctorate, GRE General Test, minimum undergraduate GPA of 3.0. Additional exam requirements/recommendations for international students: Required—TOEFL. Electronic applications accepted. *Expenses:* Tuition, state resident: full-time $5364. Tuition, nonresident: full-time $12,027. *Required fees:* $571. Tuition and fees vary according to campus/location, program and reciprocity agreements.

Virginia Commonwealth University, Graduate School, College of Humanities and Sciences, Department of Psychology, Program in General Psychology, Richmond, VA 23284-9005. Offers biopsychology (PhD); developmental psychology (PhD); social psychology (PhD). *Degree requirements:* For doctorate, thesis/dissertation. *Entrance requirements:* For doctorate, GRE General Test. Additional exam requirements/recommendations for international students: Required—TOEFL (minimum score 600 paper-based; 100 iBT); Recommended—IELTS (minimum score 6.5). Electronic applications accepted. *Faculty research:* Biopsychology, developmental and social psychology.

Wayne State University, School of Medicine, Office of Biomedical Graduate Programs, Department of Psychiatry and Behavioral Neurosciences, Detroit, MI 48202. Offers translational neuroscience (PhD). *Faculty:* 28. *Students:* 12 full-time (6 women); includes 3 minority (2 Asian, non-Hispanic/Latino; 1 Two or more races, non-Hispanic/Latino), 1 international. Average age 27. 20 applicants, 15% accepted, 2 enrolled. In

2015, 2 doctorates awarded. *Degree requirements:* For doctorate, thesis/dissertation. *Entrance requirements:* For doctorate, GRE, minimum undergraduate GPA of 3.0, bachelor's degree from accredited institution, coursework in biological sciences and other scientific disciplines, personal statement, three letters of recommendation, curriculum vitae. Additional exam requirements/recommendations for international students: Required—TOEFL (minimum score 600 paper-based; 100 iBT). *Application deadline:* For fall admission, 12/15 for domestic and international students. Application fee: $0. Electronic applications accepted. *Expenses:* $17,645 per year resident tuition, $33,311 per year non-resident tuition; $735.20 per credit hour resident tuition, $1,387.95 per credit hour non-resident tuition; fees include $47.45 per credit hour student services fee and $274.60 per semester registration fee. *Financial support:* In 2015–16, 12 students received support, including 2 fellowships with tuition reimbursements available (averaging $27,057 per year), 10 research assistantships with tuition reimbursements available (averaging $26,951 per year); scholarships/grants, health care benefits, and unspecified assistantships also available. Financial award application deadline: 3/31. *Faculty research:* Substance abuse, brain imaging, schizophrenia, child psychopathy, child development, neurobiology of monoamine systems. *Unit head:* Dr. Jeffrey Stanley, Graduate Program Director, 313-577-9090, E-mail: jstanley@med.wayne.edu. *Application contact:* 313-577-1841, E-mail: tnp@med.wayne.edu.
Website: http://psychiatry.med.wayne.edu/

Neurobiology

Albert Einstein College of Medicine, Graduate Division of Biomedical Sciences, Department of Neuroscience, Bronx, NY 10461. Offers PhD, MD/PhD. *Degree requirements:* For doctorate, thesis/dissertation. *Entrance requirements:* For doctorate, GRE General Test. Additional exam requirements/recommendations for international students: Required—TOEFL. *Faculty research:* Structure-function relations at chemical and electrical synapses, mechanisms of electrogenesis, analysis of neuronal subsystems.

Boston University, School of Medicine, Division of Graduate Medical Sciences, Department of Anatomy and Neurobiology, Boston, MA 02118. Offers MA, PhD, MD/PhD. *Program availability:* Part-time. Terminal master's awarded for partial completion of doctoral program. *Degree requirements:* For master's, thesis; for doctorate, thesis/dissertation. *Application deadline:* For fall admission, 1/15 for domestic students; for spring admission, 10/15 for domestic students. *Unit head:* Dr. Mark Moss, Chairman, 617-638-4200, Fax: 617-638-4216. *Application contact:* GMS Admissions Office, 617-638-5255, E-mail: askgms@bu.edu.
Website: http://www.bumc.bu.edu/anatneuro/

Brandeis University, Graduate School of Arts and Sciences, Program in Molecular and Cell Biology, Waltham, MA 02454-9110. Offers genetics (PhD); microbiology (PhD); molecular and cell biology (MS, PhD); molecular biology (PhD); neurobiology (PhD); quantitative biology (PhD). *Faculty:* 26 full-time (12 women), 4 part-time/adjunct (2 women). *Students:* 60 full-time (30 women); includes 5 minority (1 Black or African American, non-Hispanic/Latino; 1 American Indian or Alaska Native, non-Hispanic/Latino; 1 Asian, non-Hispanic/Latino; 2 Hispanic/Latino), 25 international. 183 applicants, 27% accepted, 12 enrolled. In 2015, 13 master's, 7 doctorates awarded. Terminal master's awarded for partial completion of doctoral program. *Degree requirements:* For master's, thesis optional, research project, research lab, or project lab; for doctorate, comprehensive exam, thesis/dissertation, journal clubs; research seminar; colloquia; qualifying exam. *Entrance requirements:* For master's, GRE General Test, official transcript(s), resume, 2 letters of recommendation, statement of purpose; for doctorate, GRE General Test, official transcript(s), resume, 3 letters of recommendation, statement of purpose, list of previous research experience. Additional exam requirements/recommendations for international students: Required—TOEFL (minimum score 600 paper-based; 100 iBT); Recommended—IELTS (minimum score 7), TSE (minimum score 68). *Application deadline:* For fall admission, 12/15 priority date for domestic students. Application fee: $75. Electronic applications accepted. *Financial support:* In 2015–16, 35 students received support, including 16 fellowships with full tuition reimbursements available (averaging $30,500 per year), 19 research assistantships with full tuition reimbursements available (averaging $30,500 per year); scholarships/grants and tuition waivers (partial) also available. Financial award application deadline: 4/15; financial award applicants required to submit FAFSA. *Faculty research:* Molecular biology, genetics and development; structural and cell biology; neurobiology. *Unit head:* Dr. Maria Miara, Director of Graduate Studies, 781-736-2300, Fax: 781-736-3107, E-mail: scigradoffice@brandeis.edu. *Application contact:* Dr. Maryanna Aldrich, Department Administrator, 781-736-2300, Fax: 781-736-3107, E-mail: scigradoffice@brandeis.edu.
Website: http://www.brandeis.edu/gsas

California Institute of Technology, Division of Biology, Program in Neurobiology, Pasadena, CA 91125-0001. Offers PhD. *Degree requirements:* For doctorate, thesis/dissertation, qualifying exam. *Entrance requirements:* For doctorate, GRE General Test.

Carnegie Mellon University, Mellon College of Science, Department of Biological Sciences, Pittsburgh, PA 15213-3891. Offers biochemistry (PhD); biophysics (PhD); cell and developmental biology (PhD); computational biology (MS, PhD); genetics (PhD); molecular biology (PhD); neuroscience (PhD); structural biology (PhD). *Degree requirements:* For doctorate, comprehensive exam, thesis/dissertation. *Entrance requirements:* For doctorate, GRE General Test, GRE Subject Test, interview. Electronic applications accepted. *Faculty research:* Genetic structure, function, and regulation; protein structure and function; biological membranes; biological spectroscopy.

Columbia University, College of Physicians and Surgeons, Program in Neurobiology and Behavior, New York, NY 10032. Offers PhD. Only candidates for the PhD are admitted. *Degree requirements:* For doctorate, thesis/dissertation. *Entrance requirements:* For doctorate, GRE General Test. Additional exam requirements/recommendations for international students: Required—TOEFL. *Expenses:* Contact institution. *Faculty research:* Cellular and molecular mechanisms of neural development, neuropathology, neuropharmacology.

Cornell University, Graduate School, Graduate Fields of Agriculture and Life Sciences, Field of Neurobiology and Behavior, Ithaca, NY 14853-0001. Offers behavioral biology (PhD), including behavioral ecology, chemical ecology, ethology, neuroethology, sociobiology; neurobiology (PhD), including cellular and molecular neurobiology, neuroanatomy, neurochemistry, neuropharmacology, neurophysiology, sensory physiology. *Degree requirements:* For doctorate, comprehensive exam, thesis/

dissertation, 1 year of teaching experience, seminar presentation. *Entrance requirements:* For doctorate, GRE General Test, GRE Subject Test (biology), 3 letters of recommendation. Additional exam requirements/recommendations for international students: Required—TOEFL (minimum score 550 paper-based; 77 iBT). Electronic applications accepted. *Faculty research:* Cellular neurobiology and neuropharmacology, integrative neurobiology, social behavior, chemical ecology, neuroethology.

Dalhousie University, Faculty of Graduate Studies and Faculty of Medicine, Graduate Programs in Medicine, Department of Anatomy and Neurobiology, Halifax, NS B3H 4R2, Canada. Offers M Sc, PhD. *Degree requirements:* For master's, thesis; for doctorate, thesis/dissertation. *Entrance requirements:* For master's and doctorate, GRE (recommended), minimum A- average. Additional exam requirements/recommendations for international students: Required—1 of 5 approved tests: TOEFL, IELTS, CANTEST, CAEL, Michigan English Language Assessment Battery. Electronic applications accepted. *Faculty research:* Neuroscience histology, cell biology, neuroendocrinology, evolutionary biology.

Duke University, Graduate School, Department of Evolutionary Anthropology, Durham, NC 27708. Offers cellular and molecular biology (PhD); gross anatomy and physical anthropology (PhD), including comparative morphology of human and non-human primates, primate social behavior, vertebrate paleontology; neuroanatomy (PhD). *Degree requirements:* For doctorate, one foreign language, thesis/dissertation. *Entrance requirements:* For doctorate, GRE General Test. Additional exam requirements/recommendations for international students: Required—TOEFL (minimum score 577 paper-based; 90 iBT) or IELTS (minimum score 7). Electronic applications accepted.

Duke University, Graduate School, Department of Neurobiology, Durham, NC 27710. Offers PhD. *Degree requirements:* For doctorate, variable foreign language requirement, thesis/dissertation. *Entrance requirements:* For doctorate, GRE General Test. Additional exam requirements/recommendations for international students: Required—TOEFL (minimum score 577 paper-based; 90 iBT) or IELTS (minimum score 7). Electronic applications accepted.

Georgia State University, College of Arts and Sciences, Department of Biology, Program in Neurobiology and Behavior, Atlanta, GA 30302-3083. Offers bioinformatics (MS); neurobiology and behavior (MS, PhD). *Program availability:* Part-time. Terminal master's awarded for partial completion of doctoral program. *Degree requirements:* For master's, comprehensive exam (for some programs), thesis optional; for doctorate, comprehensive exam, thesis/dissertation. *Entrance requirements:* For master's and doctorate, GRE. Additional exam requirements/recommendations for international students: Required—TOEFL (minimum score 550 paper-based; 82 iBT) or IELTS (minimum score 7). *Application deadline:* For fall admission, 7/1 priority date for domestic students, 6/1 priority date for international students; for spring admission, 11/15 priority date for domestic students, 10/15 priority date for international students. Applications are processed on a rolling basis. Application fee: $50. Electronic applications accepted. *Expenses:* Tuition, state resident: full-time $6876; part-time $382 per credit hour. Tuition, nonresident: full-time $22,374; part-time $1243 per credit hour. *Required fees:* $2128; $2128 per term. $1064 per term. Part-time tuition and fees vary according to course load and program. *Financial support:* In 2015–16, fellowships with full tuition reimbursements (averaging $22,000 per year), research assistantships with full tuition reimbursements (averaging $20,000 per year) were awarded. Financial award application deadline: 12/3. *Faculty research:* Behavior, Circadian and Circa-annual rhythms, developmental genetics, neuroendocrinology, cytoskeletal dynamics. *Unit head:* Dr. Charles Derby, Director of Graduate Studies, 404-413-5393, Fax: 404-413-5446, E-mail: cderby@gsu.edu.
Website: http://biology.gsu.edu/

Harvard University, Graduate School of Arts and Sciences, Program in Neuroscience, Boston, MA 02115. Offers neurobiology (PhD). *Degree requirements:* For doctorate, thesis/dissertation, qualifying exam. *Entrance requirements:* For doctorate, GRE General Test, GRE Subject Test. Additional exam requirements/recommendations for international students: Required—TOEFL. *Faculty research:* Relationship between diseases of the nervous system and basic science.

Illinois State University, Graduate School, College of Arts and Sciences, Department of Biological Sciences, Normal, IL 61790-2200. Offers animal behavior (MS); bacteriology (MS); biochemistry (MS); biological sciences (MS); biology (PhD); biophysics (MS); biotechnology (MS); botany (MS, PhD); cell biology (MS); conservation biology (MS); developmental biology (MS); ecology (MS, PhD); entomology (MS); evolutionary biology (MS); genetics (MS, PhD); immunology (MS); microbiology (MS, PhD); molecular biology (MS); molecular genetics (MS); neurobiology (MS); neuroscience (MS); parasitology (MS); physiology (MS, PhD); plant biology (MS); plant molecular biology (MS); plant sciences (MS); structural biology (MS); zoology (MS, PhD). *Program availability:* Part-time. *Degree requirements:* For master's, thesis or alternative; for doctorate, variable foreign language requirement, thesis/dissertation, 2 terms of residency. *Entrance requirements:* For master's, GRE General Test, minimum GPA of 2.6 in last 60 hours of course work; for doctorate, GRE General Test. *Application*

deadline: Applications are processed on a rolling basis. Application fee: $40. *Financial support:* Research assistantships, teaching assistantships, Federal Work-Study, tuition waivers (full), and unspecified assistantships available. Financial award application deadline: 4/1. *Faculty research:* Redoc balance and drug development in schistosoma mansoni, control of the growth of listeria monocytogenes at low temperature, regulation of cell expansion and microtubule function by SPRI, CRUI: physiology and fitness consequences of different life history phenotypes. *Application contact:* Steven Juliano, Graduate Coordinator, E-mail: sajulian@ilstu.edu.
Website: http://www.bio.ilstu.edu/

Indiana University–Purdue University Indianapolis, Indiana University School of Medicine, Stark Neurosciences Research Institute, Indianapolis, IN 46202. Offers PhD. *Degree requirements:* For doctorate, thesis/dissertation. *Entrance requirements:* For doctorate, GRE General Test, previous course work in calculus, organic chemistry, and physics. *Faculty research:* Neurobiology from molecular level to complex behavioral interactions.

Louisiana State University Health Sciences Center, School of Graduate Studies in New Orleans, Department of Cell Biology and Anatomy, New Orleans, LA 70112-2223. Offers cell biology and anatomy (PhD), including clinical anatomy, development, cell, and neurobiology; MD/PhD. *Faculty:* 17 full-time (2 women). *Students:* 5 full-time (2 women), 1 international. 2 applicants, 100% accepted, 2 enrolled. *Degree requirements:* For doctorate, comprehensive exam, thesis/dissertation. *Entrance requirements:* For doctorate, GRE General Test, minimum undergraduate GPA of 3.0. Additional exam requirements/recommendations for international students: Recommended—TOEFL, IELTS. *Application deadline:* For fall admission, 3/1 priority date for domestic students, 3/1 for international students. Applications are processed on a rolling basis. Application fee: $30. *Financial support:* In 2015–16, 6 students received support. Unspecified assistantships available. Financial award application deadline: 4/1. *Faculty research:* Visual system organization, neural development, plasticity of sensory systems, information processing through the nervous system, visuomotor integration. *Total annual research expenditures:* $900,000. *Unit head:* Dr. Samuel McClugage, Head, 504-568-4011, Fax: 504-568-2165, E-mail: smcclu@lsuhsc.edu. *Application contact:* Dr. R. John Cork, Graduate Coordinator and Professor, 504-568-7177, E-mail: jcork@lsuhsc.edu.
Website: http://www.medschool.lsuhsc.edu/cell_biology/

Massachusetts Institute of Technology, School of Science, Department of Biology, Cambridge, MA 02139. Offers biochemistry (PhD); biological oceanography (PhD); biology (PhD); biophysical chemistry and molecular structure (PhD); cell biology (PhD); computational and systems biology (PhD); developmental biology (PhD); genetics (PhD); immunology (PhD); microbiology (PhD); molecular biology (PhD); neurobiology (PhD). *Faculty:* 57 full-time (14 women). *Students:* 283 full-time (137 women); includes 83 minority (3 Black or African American, non-Hispanic/Latino; 1 American Indian or Alaska Native, non-Hispanic/Latino; 38 Asian, non-Hispanic/Latino; 31 Hispanic/Latino; 10 Two or more races, non-Hispanic/Latino), 48 international. Average age 26. 673 applicants, 14% accepted, 46 enrolled. In 2015, 32 doctorates awarded. *Degree requirements:* For doctorate, comprehensive exam, thesis/dissertation, teaching assistantship during two semesters. *Entrance requirements:* For doctorate, GRE General Test. Additional exam requirements/recommendations for international students: Required—TOEFL (minimum score 577 paper-based), IELTS. *Application deadline:* For fall admission, 12/1 for domestic and international students. Application fee: $75. Electronic applications accepted. *Expenses: Tuition:* Full-time $46,400; part-time $725 per credit. One-time fee: $304 full-time. Full-time tuition and fees vary according to course load and program. *Financial support:* In 2015–16, 235 students received support, including 118 fellowships (averaging $37,500 per year), 163 research assistantships (averaging $38,900 per year), 1 teaching assistantship; Federal Work-Study, institutionally sponsored loans, scholarships/grants, traineeships, health care benefits, and unspecified assistantships also available. Support available to part-time students. Financial award application deadline: 4/15; financial award applicants required to submit FAFSA. *Faculty research:* Cellular, developmental and molecular (plant and animal) biology; biochemistry, bioengineering, biophysics and structural biology; classical and molecular genetics, stem cell and epigenetics; immunology and microbiology; cancer biology, molecular medicine, neurobiology and human disease; computational and systems biology. *Total annual research expenditures:* $42.8 million. *Unit head:* Prof. Alan Grossman, Department Head, 617-253-4701. *Application contact:* Biology Education Office, 617-253-3717, Fax: 617-258-9329, E-mail: gradbio@mit.edu.
Website: https://biology.mit.edu/

New York University, Graduate School of Arts and Science, Department of Biology, New York, NY 10012-1019. Offers biology (PhD); biomedical journalism (MS); cancer and molecular biology (PhD); computational biology (PhD); computers in biological research (MS); developmental genetics (PhD); general biology (MS); immunology and microbiology (PhD); molecular genetics (PhD); neurobiology (PhD); oral biology (MS); plant biology (PhD); recombinant DNA technology (MS); MS/MBA. *Program availability:* Part-time. Terminal master's awarded for partial completion of doctoral program. *Degree requirements:* For master's, thesis or alternative, qualifying paper; for doctorate, comprehensive exam, thesis/dissertation. *Entrance requirements:* For master's and doctorate, GRE General Test. Additional exam requirements/recommendations for international students: Required—TOEFL. *Faculty research:* Genomics, molecular and cell biology, development and molecular genetics, molecular evolution of plants and animals.

Northwestern University, The Graduate School, Interdisciplinary Biological Sciences Program (IBiS), Evanston, IL 60208. Offers biochemistry (PhD); bioengineering and biotechnology (PhD); biotechnology (PhD); cell and molecular biology (PhD); developmental and systems biology (PhD); nanotechnology (PhD); neurobiology (PhD); structural biology and biophysics (PhD). *Degree requirements:* For doctorate, thesis/dissertation, qualifying exam. *Entrance requirements:* For doctorate, GRE General Test. Additional exam requirements/recommendations for international students: Required—TOEFL (minimum score 600 paper-based). Electronic applications accepted. *Faculty research:* Biophysics/structural biology, cell/molecular biology, synthetic biology, developmental systems biology, chemical biology/nanotechnology.

Northwestern University, The Graduate School, Judd A. and Marjorie Weinberg College of Arts and Sciences, Department of Neurobiology, Evanston, IL 60208. Offers neurobiology and physiology (MS). Admissions and degrees offered through The Graduate School. *Program availability:* Part-time. *Degree requirements:* For master's, thesis. *Entrance requirements:* For master's, GRE General Test and MCAT (strongly recommended). Additional exam requirements/recommendations for international students: Required—TOEFL. Electronic applications accepted. *Expenses:* Contact institution. *Faculty research:* Sensory neurobiology and neuroendocrinology, reproductive biology, vision physiology and psychophysics, cell and developmental biology.

Penn State Hershey Medical Center, College of Medicine, Graduate School Programs in the Biomedical Sciences, The Huck Institutes of the Life Sciences, Intercollege Graduate Program in Molecular Cellular and Integrative Biosciences, Hershey, PA 17033. Offers cell and developmental biology (PhD); immunology and infectious disease (PhD); molecular and evolutionary genetics (PhD); molecular medicine (PhD); molecular

toxicology (PhD); neurobiology (PhD). *Students:* 3 full-time (2 women); includes 2 minority (both Asian, non-Hispanic/Latino). 2 applicants, 100% accepted, 2 enrolled. In 2015, 1 doctorate awarded. *Degree requirements:* For doctorate, comprehensive exam, thesis/dissertation, oral exam. *Entrance requirements:* For doctorate, GRE, minimum GPA of 3.0. Additional exam requirements/recommendations for international students: Required—TOEFL (minimum score 500 paper-based). *Application deadline:* For fall admission, 1/31 priority date for domestic students, 2/1 priority date for international students. Applications are processed on a rolling basis. Application fee: $65. Electronic applications accepted. *Financial support:* In 2015–16, research assistantships with full tuition reimbursements (averaging $26,196 per year) were awarded; fellowships with full tuition reimbursements, career-related internships or fieldwork, Federal Work-Study, scholarships/grants, health care benefits, and unspecified assistantships also available. Financial award applicants required to submit FAFSA. *Faculty research:* Vascular biology, molecular toxicology, chemical biology, immune system, pathophysiological basis of human disease. *Unit head:* Dr. Peter Hudson, Director, 814-865-6057, E-mail: pjh18@psu.edu. *Application contact:* Kathy Shuey, Administrative Assistant, 717-531-8982, Fax: 717-531-0786, E-mail: grad-hmc@psu.edu.
Website: http://www.huck.psu.edu/education/molecular-cellular-and-integrative-biosciences

Purdue University, Graduate School, College of Science, Department of Biological Sciences, West Lafayette, IN 47907. Offers biochemistry (PhD); biophysics (PhD); cell and developmental biology (PhD); ecology, evolutionary and population biology (MS, PhD), including ecology, evolutionary biology, population biology; genetics (MS, PhD); microbiology (MS, PhD); molecular biology (PhD); neurobiology (MS, PhD); plant physiology (PhD). Terminal master's awarded for partial completion of doctoral program. *Degree requirements:* For master's, thesis (for some programs); for doctorate, thesis/dissertation, seminars, teaching experience. *Entrance requirements:* For master's, GRE General Test (minimum analytical writing score of 3.5), minimum undergraduate GPA of 3.0; for doctorate, GRE General Test (minimum analytical writing score of 3.5), minimum undergraduate GPA of 3.5. Additional exam requirements/recommendations for international students: Required—TOEFL (minimum score 600 paper-based; 107 iBT for MS, 80 iBT for PhD). Electronic applications accepted.

Queen's University at Kingston, School of Graduate Studies, Faculty of Health Sciences, Department of Anatomy and Cell Biology, Kingston, ON K7L 3N6, Canada. Offers biology of reproduction (M Sc, PhD); cancer (M Sc, PhD); cardiovascular pathophysiology (M Sc, PhD); cell and molecular biology (M Sc, PhD); drug metabolism (M Sc, PhD); endocrinology (M Sc, PhD); motor control (M Sc, PhD); neural regeneration (M Sc, PhD); neurophysiology (M Sc, PhD). *Program availability:* Part-time. *Degree requirements:* For master's, thesis; for doctorate, one foreign language, comprehensive exam, thesis/dissertation. *Entrance requirements:* Additional exam requirements/recommendations for international students: Required—TOEFL. Electronic applications accepted. *Faculty research:* Human kinetics, neuroscience, reproductive biology, cardiovascular.

Université Laval, Faculty of Medicine, Graduate Programs in Medicine, Programs in Neurobiology, Québec, QC G1K 7P4, Canada. Offers M Sc, PhD. Terminal master's awarded for partial completion of doctoral program. *Degree requirements:* For master's, thesis; for doctorate, comprehensive exam, thesis/dissertation. *Entrance requirements:* For master's and doctorate, knowledge of French and English. Electronic applications accepted.

University at Albany, State University of New York, College of Arts and Sciences, Department of Biological Sciences, Specialization in Molecular, Cellular, Developmental, and Neural Biology, Albany, NY 12222-0001. Offers PhD. *Degree requirements:* For doctorate, one foreign language, thesis/dissertation. *Entrance requirements:* For doctorate, GRE General Test.

The University of Alabama at Birmingham, Graduate Programs in Joint Health Sciences, Neurobiology Program, Birmingham, AL 35294. Offers PhD. *Degree requirements:* For doctorate, comprehensive exam, thesis/dissertation. *Entrance requirements:* For doctorate, GRE or MCAT, interview. Additional exam requirements/recommendations for international students: Required—TOEFL. Electronic applications accepted. *Expenses:* Tuition, state resident: full-time $7340. Tuition, nonresident: full-time $16,628. Full-time tuition and fees vary according to course load and program.

University of Arkansas for Medical Sciences, Graduate School, Little Rock, AR 72205. Offers biochemistry and molecular biology (MS, PhD); bioinformatics (MS, PhD); cellular physiology and molecular biophysics (MS, PhD); clinical nutrition (MS); interdisciplinary biomedical sciences (MS, PhD, Certificate); interdisciplinary toxicology (MS); microbiology and immunology (MS, PhD); neurobiology and developmental sciences (PhD); pharmacology (PhD); MD/PhD. Bioinformatics programs hosted jointly with the University of Arkansas at Little Rock. *Program availability:* Part-time. Terminal master's awarded for partial completion of doctoral program. *Degree requirements:* For master's, comprehensive exam (for some programs), thesis (for some programs); for doctorate, thesis/dissertation. *Entrance requirements:* For master's and doctorate, GRE. Additional exam requirements/recommendations for international students: Required—TOEFL. Electronic applications accepted. *Expenses:* Contact institution.

University of California, Irvine, Francisco J. Ayala School of Biological Sciences, Department of Neurobiology and Behavior, Irvine, CA 92697. Offers biological sciences (MS, PhD); MD/PhD. *Students:* 35 full-time (20 women); includes 15 minority (2 Black or African American, non-Hispanic/Latino; 8 Asian, non-Hispanic/Latino; 5 Hispanic/Latino). Average age 28. In 2015, 5 master's, 6 doctorates awarded. *Degree requirements:* For doctorate, thesis/dissertation. *Entrance requirements:* For master's and doctorate, GRE General Test, GRE Subject Test, minimum GPA of 3.0. Additional exam requirements/recommendations for international students: Required—TOEFL (minimum score 550 paper-based). *Application deadline:* For fall admission, 1/15 priority date for domestic students, 1/15 for international students. Applications are processed on a rolling basis. Application fee: $90 ($110 for international students). Electronic applications accepted. *Financial support:* Fellowships, research assistantships with full tuition reimbursements, teaching assistantships, institutionally sponsored loans, traineeships, health care benefits, and unspecified assistantships available. Financial award application deadline: 3/1; financial award applicants required to submit FAFSA. *Faculty research:* Synaptic processes, neurophysiology, neuroendocrinology, neuroanatomy, molecular neurobiology. *Unit head:* Marcelo A. Wood, Chair, 949-824-6114, Fax: 949-824-2447, E-mail: mwood@uci.edu. *Application contact:* Sally Dabiri, Department Administrator, 949-824-4727, Fax: 949-824-2447, E-mail: sfdabiri@uci.edu.
Website: http://neurobiology.uci.edu/

University of California, Irvine, School of Medicine and Francisco J. Ayala School of Biological Sciences, Department of Anatomy and Neurobiology, Irvine, CA 92697. Offers biological sciences (MS, PhD); MD/PhD. *Faculty:* 26 full-time (13 women), 2 part-time/adjunct (1 woman). *Students:* 19 full-time (12 women), 2 part-time (both women); includes 8 minority (all Asian, non-Hispanic/Latino), 3 international. Average age 28. In 2015, 1 master's, 5 doctorates awarded. *Degree requirements:* For doctorate, thesis/dissertation. *Entrance requirements:* For master's and doctorate, GRE General Test, GRE Subject Test. Additional exam requirements/recommendations for international students: Required—TOEFL (minimum score 550 paper-based). *Application deadline:*

Neurobiology

For fall admission, 1/15 priority date for domestic students, 1/15 for international students. Applications are processed on a rolling basis. Application fee: $90 ($110 for international students). Electronic applications accepted. *Financial support:* Fellowships, research assistantships with full tuition reimbursements, teaching assistantships, institutionally sponsored loans, traineeships, health care benefits, and unspecified assistantships available. Financial award application deadline: 3/1; financial award applicants required to submit FAFSA. *Faculty research:* Neurotransmitter immunocytochemistry, intracellular physiology, molecular neurobiology, forebrain organization and development, structure and function of sensory and motor systems. *Unit head:* Prof. Christine Gall, Interim Chair, 949-824-8652, Fax: 949-824-1255, E-mail: cmgall@uci.edu. *Application contact:* David Lyon, Director of Graduate Studies, 949-824-0447, E-mail: dclyon@uci.edu.

University of California, Los Angeles, David Geffen School of Medicine and Graduate Division, Graduate Programs in Medicine, Department of Neurobiology, Los Angeles, CA 90095. Offers MS, PhD. Terminal master's awarded for partial completion of doctoral program. *Degree requirements:* For master's, comprehensive exam; for doctorate, thesis/dissertation, oral and written qualifying exams; 2 quarters of teaching experience. *Entrance requirements:* For doctorate, GRE General Test; GRE Subject Test, bachelor's degree; minimum undergraduate GPA of 3.0 (or its equivalent if letter grade system not used). Additional exam requirements/recommendations for international students: Required—TOEFL. Electronic applications accepted.

University of California, Los Angeles, Graduate Division, College of Letters and Science and David Geffen School of Medicine, UCLA ACCESS to Programs in the Molecular, Cellular and Integrative Life Sciences, Los Angeles, CA 90095. Offers biochemistry and molecular biology (PhD); biological chemistry (PhD); cellular and molecular pathology (PhD); human genetics (PhD); microbiology, immunology, and molecular genetics (PhD); molecular biology (PhD); molecular toxicology (PhD); molecular, cellular and integrative physiology (PhD); neurobiology (PhD); oral biology (PhD); physiology (PhD). *Degree requirements:* For doctorate, thesis/dissertation, oral and written qualifying exams. *Entrance requirements:* For doctorate, GRE General Test, bachelor's degree; minimum undergraduate GPA of 3.0 (or its equivalent if letter grade system not used). Additional exam requirements/recommendations for international students: Required—TOEFL. Electronic applications accepted.

University of Chicago, Division of the Biological Sciences, Committee on Neurobiology, Chicago, IL 60637. Offers PhD. *Faculty:* 45 full-time (14 women). *Students:* 27 full-time (15 women); includes 6 minority (2 Black or African American, non-Hispanic/Latino; 4 Asian, non-Hispanic/Latino; 2 Hispanic/Latino), 3 international. 151 applicants, 13% accepted, 7 enrolled. *Degree requirements:* For doctorate, thesis/dissertation, ethics class, 2 teaching assistantships. *Entrance requirements:* For doctorate, GRE General Test. Additional exam requirements/recommendations for international students: Required—TOEFL (minimum score 600 paper-based; 104 iBT), IELTS (minimum score 7). *Application deadline:* For fall admission, 12/1 for domestic and international students. Application fee: $90. Electronic applications accepted. *Financial support:* In 2015–16, 27 students received support, including fellowships with tuition reimbursements available (averaging $29,781 per year), research assistantships with tuition reimbursements available (averaging $29,781 per year); institutionally sponsored loans, scholarships/grants, traineeships, and health care benefits also available. Financial award applicants required to submit FAFSA. *Faculty research:* Immunogenetic aspects of neurologic disease. *Unit head:* Murry Sherman, Chair, E-mail: neurobiology@chicago.edu. Website: http://neuroscience.uchicago.edu/?p-neuro/neurobio

University of Colorado Boulder, Graduate School, College of Arts and Sciences, Department of Ecology and Evolutionary Biology, Boulder, CO 80309. Offers animal behavior (MA); biology (MA, PhD); environmental biology (MA, PhD); evolutionary biology (MA, PhD); neurobiology (MA); population biology (MA, PhD); population genetics (PhD). *Faculty:* 31 full-time (12 women). *Students:* 67 full-time (31 women), 3 part-time (1 woman); includes 8 minority (1 Asian, non-Hispanic/Latino; 3 Hispanic/Latino; 4 Two or more races, non-Hispanic/Latino), 4 international. Average age 30. 119 applicants, 11% accepted, 13 enrolled. In 2015, 10 master's, 14 doctorates awarded. Terminal master's awarded for partial completion of doctoral program. *Degree requirements:* For master's, comprehensive exam, thesis or alternative; for doctorate, comprehensive exam, thesis/dissertation. *Entrance requirements:* For master's, GRE General Test, GRE Subject Test, minimum undergraduate GPA of 3.0; for doctorate, GRE General Test, GRE Subject Test. *Application deadline:* For fall admission, 12/31 for domestic students, 12/1 for international students. Application fee: $50 ($70 for international students). Electronic applications accepted. Application fee is waived when completed online. *Financial support:* In 2015–16, 138 students received support, including 14 fellowships (averaging $7,260 per year), 12 research assistantships with tuition reimbursements available (averaging $31,833 per year), 47 teaching assistantships with tuition reimbursements available (averaging $33,448 per year); institutionally sponsored loans, scholarships/grants, health care benefits, and unspecified assistantships also available. Financial award applicants required to submit FAFSA. *Faculty research:* Ecology, botany, evolutionary biology, biological sciences, conservation biology. *Total annual research expenditures:* $6.3 million. *Application contact:* E-mail: ebiograd@colorado.edu. Website: http://ebio.colorado.edu

University of Colorado Denver, College of Liberal Arts and Sciences, Department of Integrative and Systems Biology, Denver, CO 80217. Offers animal behavior (MS); biology (MS); cell and developmental biology (MS); ecology (MS); evolutionary biology (MS); genetics (MS); integrative and systems biology (PhD); microbiology (MS); molecular biology (MS); neurobiology (MS); plant systematics (MS). *Program availability:* Part-time. *Faculty:* 21 full-time (8 women), 3 part-time/adjunct (1 woman). *Students:* 31 full-time (19 women), 7 part-time (3 women); includes 8 minority (1 Black or African American, non-Hispanic/Latino; 1 Asian, non-Hispanic/Latino; 3 Hispanic/Latino; 3 Two or more races, non-Hispanic/Latino), 1 international. Average age 28. 34 applicants, 29% accepted, 8 enrolled. In 2015, 6 master's awarded. *Degree requirements:* For master's, comprehensive exam, thesis, 30-32 credit hours; for doctorate, comprehensive exam, thesis/dissertation. *Entrance requirements:* For master's, GRE General Test (minimum score in 50th percentile in each section), BA/BS from accredited institution awarded within the last 10 years; minimum undergraduate GPA of 3.0; prerequisite courses: 1 year each of general biology and general chemistry; 1 semester each of general genetics, general ecology, and cell biology; and a structure/function course; for doctorate, GRE, minimum undergraduate GPA of 3.2, three letters of recommendation, official transcripts from all universities and colleges attended. Additional exam requirements/recommendations for international students: Required—TOEFL (minimum score 537 paper-based; 75 iBT); Recommended—IELTS (minimum score 6.5). *Application deadline:* For fall admission, 1/15 for domestic and international students. Application fee: $50 ($75 for international students). Electronic applications accepted. *Financial support:* In 2015–16, 32 students received support. Fellowships, research assistantships, teaching assistantships, Federal Work-Study, institutionally sponsored loans, scholarships/grants, and traineeships available. Financial award application deadline: 4/1; financial award applicants required to submit FAFSA. *Faculty research:* Molecular developmental biology; quantitative ecology, biogeography, and population dynamics; environmental signaling and endocrine disruption; speciation, the evolution of reproductive isolation, and hybrid zones; evolutionary, behavioral, and conservation ecology. *Unit head:* Dr. John Swallow, Chair, 303-556-6154, E-mail: john.swallow@ucdenver.edu. *Application contact:* Dr. Michael Wunder, Graduate Advisor, 303-556-8870, E-mail: michael.wunder@ucdenver.edu. Website: http://www.ucdenver.edu/academics/colleges/CLAS/Departments/biology/Programs/MasterofScience/Pages/BiologyMasterOfScience.aspx

University of Connecticut, Graduate School, College of Liberal Arts and Sciences, Department of Physiology and Neurobiology, Storrs, CT 06269. Offers comparative physiology (MS, PhD). Terminal master's awarded for partial completion of doctoral program. *Degree requirements:* For master's, comprehensive exam; for doctorate, thesis/dissertation. *Entrance requirements:* For master's and doctorate, GRE General Test, GRE Subject Test. Additional exam requirements/recommendations for international students: Required—TOEFL (minimum score 550 paper-based). *Application deadline:* For fall admission, 2/1 priority date for domestic and international students; for spring admission, 11/1 for domestic students, 10/1 for international students. Applications are processed on a rolling basis. Application fee: $55. Electronic applications accepted. *Financial support:* Fellowships, research assistantships with full tuition reimbursements, teaching assistantships with full tuition reimbursements, Federal Work-Study, scholarships/grants, health care benefits, tuition waivers (full), and unspecified assistantships available. Financial award application deadline: 2/1. Website: http://www.pnb.uconn.edu/

See Display on page 428 and Close-Up on page 435.

The University of Iowa, Graduate College, College of Liberal Arts and Sciences, Department of Biology, Iowa City, IA 52242-1324. Offers biology (MS, PhD); cell and developmental biology (MS, PhD); evolution (MS, PhD); genetics (MS, PhD); neurobiology (MS, PhD). Terminal master's awarded for partial completion of doctoral program. *Degree requirements:* For master's, thesis optional, exam; for doctorate, comprehensive exam, thesis/dissertation. *Entrance requirements:* For master's and doctorate, GRE General Test, minimum GPA of 3.0. Additional exam requirements/recommendations for international students: Required—TOEFL (minimum score 600 paper-based; 100 iBT). Electronic applications accepted. *Faculty research:* Neurobiology, evolutionary biology, genetics, cell and developmental biology.

University of Kentucky, Graduate School, Graduate School Programs from the College of Medicine, Program in Anatomy and Neurobiology, Lexington, KY 40506-0032. Offers PhD. *Degree requirements:* For doctorate, comprehensive exam, thesis/dissertation. *Entrance requirements:* For doctorate, GRE General Test, minimum undergraduate GPA of 2.75. Additional exam requirements/recommendations for international students: Required—TOEFL (minimum score 550 paper-based). Electronic applications accepted. *Faculty research:* Neuroendocrinology, developmental neurobiology, neurotrophic substances, neural plasticity and trauma, neurobiology of aging.

University of Louisville, School of Medicine, Department of Anatomical Sciences and Neurobiology, Louisville, KY 40292-0001. Offers MS, PhD. *Students:* 21 full-time (10 women), 7 part-time (4 women); includes 5 minority (2 Hispanic/Latino; 3 Two or more races, non-Hispanic/Latino), 2 international. Average age 28. 43 applicants, 23% accepted, 7 enrolled. In 2015, 1 master's, 2 doctorates awarded. Terminal master's awarded for partial completion of doctoral program. *Degree requirements:* For master's, thesis; for doctorate, comprehensive exam, thesis/dissertation. *Entrance requirements:* For master's and doctorate, GRE General Test (minimum score of 1000 verbal and quantitative), minimum GPA of 3.0. Additional exam requirements/recommendations for international students: Required—TOEFL. *Application deadline:* For fall admission, 1/15 priority date for domestic students; for spring admission, 4/15 priority date for domestic and international students. Applications are processed on a rolling basis. Application fee: $60. Electronic applications accepted. *Expenses:* Tuition, state resident: full-time $11,664; part-time $649 per credit hour. Tuition, nonresident: full-time $24,274; part-time $1350 per credit hour. *Required fees:* $196. Tuition and fees vary according to program and reciprocity agreements. *Financial support:* In 2015–16, 235,179 students received support. Fellowships with full tuition reimbursements available, research assistantships with full tuition reimbursements available, health care benefits, and unspecified assistantships available. Financial award application deadline: 4/15. *Faculty research:* Human adult neural stem cells, development and plasticity of the nervous system, organization of the dorsal thalamus, electrophysiology/neuroanatomy of central neurons mediating control of reproductive and pelvic organs, normal neural mechanisms and plasticity following injury and/or chronic pain, differentiation and regeneration of motor neurons and oligodendrocytes. *Total annual research expenditures:* $3.5 million. *Unit head:* Dr. William Guido, Chair, 502-852-6227, Fax: 502-852-6228, E-mail: w0guid01@gwise.louisville.edu. *Application contact:* Dr. Charles Hubscher, Director of Graduate Studies, 502-852-3058, Fax: 502-852-6228, E-mail: chhub01@louisville.edu. Website: http://louisville.edu/medicine/departments/anatomy

The University of Manchester, Faculty of Life Sciences, Manchester, United Kingdom. Offers adaptive organismal biology (M Phil, PhD); animal biology (M Phil, PhD); biochemistry (M Phil, PhD); bioinformatics (M Phil, PhD); biomolecular sciences (M Phil, PhD); biotechnology (M Phil, PhD); cell biology (M Phil, PhD); cell matrix research (M Phil, PhD); channels and transporters (M Phil, PhD); developmental biology (M Phil, PhD); Egyptology (M Phil, PhD); environmental biology (M Phil, PhD); evolutionary biology (M Phil, PhD); gene expression (M Phil, PhD); genetics (M Phil, PhD); history of science, technology and medicine (M Phil, PhD); immunology (M Phil, PhD); integrative neurobiology and behavior (M Phil, PhD); membrane trafficking (M Phil, PhD); microbiology (M Phil, PhD); molecular and cellular neuroscience (M Phil, PhD); molecular biology (M Phil, PhD); molecular cancer studies (M Phil, PhD); neuroscience (M Phil, PhD); ophthalmology (M Phil, PhD); optometry (M Phil, PhD); organelle function (M Phil, PhD); pharmacology (M Phil, PhD); physiology (M Phil, PhD); plant sciences (M Phil, PhD); stem cell research (M Phil, PhD); structural biology (M Phil, PhD); systems neuroscience (M Phil, PhD); toxicology (M Phil, PhD).

University of Maryland, Baltimore, Graduate School, Graduate Program in Life Sciences, Program in Neuroscience, Baltimore, MD 21201. Offers PhD, MD/PhD. *Program availability:* Part-time. *Degree requirements:* For doctorate, comprehensive exam, thesis/dissertation. *Entrance requirements:* For doctorate, GRE General Test, minimum GPA of 3.0. Additional exam requirements/recommendations for international students: Required—TOEFL (minimum score 550 paper-based; 80 iBT), Recommended—IELTS (minimum score 7). Electronic applications accepted. Tuition and fees vary according to program. *Faculty research:* Molecular, biochemical, and cellular pharmacology; membrane biophysics; synaptology; developmental neurobiology.

University of Minnesota, Twin Cities Campus, Graduate School, Graduate Program in Neuroscience, Minneapolis, MN 55455-0213. Offers MS, PhD. Terminal master's awarded for partial completion of doctoral program. *Degree requirements:* For master's, thesis; for doctorate, thesis/dissertation. *Entrance requirements:* For doctorate, GRE. Additional exam requirements/recommendations for international students: Required—TOEFL. Electronic applications accepted. *Faculty research:* Cellular and molecular neuroscience, behavioral neuroscience, developmental neuroscience, neurodegenerative diseases, pain, addiction, motor control.

The University of North Carolina at Chapel Hill, School of Medicine and Graduate School, Graduate Programs in Medicine, Curriculum in Neurobiology, Chapel Hill, NC 27599. Offers PhD. *Degree requirements:* For doctorate, comprehensive exam, thesis/dissertation. *Entrance requirements:* For doctorate, GRE General Test, minimum GPA of 3.0. Electronic applications accepted.

University of Oklahoma, College of Arts and Sciences, Department of Biology and School of Aerospace and Mechanical Engineering and Department of Chemistry and Biochemistry, Program in Cellular and Behavioral Neurobiology, Norman, OK 73019. Offers PhD. *Students:* 1 (woman) full-time, 1 part-time (0 women), both international. Average age 26. 4 applicants. In 2015, 2 doctorates awarded. *Degree requirements:* For doctorate, comprehensive exam, thesis/dissertation, neurobiology, current topics in neurobiology, and biostatistics courses; 2-3 lab rotations. *Entrance requirements:* For doctorate, GRE General Test, transcripts, 3 letters of recommendation, personal statement. Additional exam requirements/recommendations for international students: Required—TOEFL (minimum score 79 iBT) or IELTS (minimum score 6.5). *Application deadline:* For fall admission, 12/15 for domestic and international students. Application fee: $50 ($100 for international students). Electronic applications accepted. *Expenses:* Tuition, state resident: full-time $4577; part-time $190.70 per credit hour. Tuition, nonresident: full-time $17,758; part-time $739.90 per credit hour. *Required fees:* $3060; $115.70 per credit hour. $141.50 per semester. *Financial support:* In 2015–16, 1 student received support. Fellowships, research assistantships with full tuition reimbursements available, teaching assistantships with full tuition reimbursements available, scholarships/grants, health care benefits, and unspecified assistantships available. Financial award application deadline: 6/1; financial award applicants required to submit FAFSA. *Faculty research:* Behavioral neurobiology, cellular neurobiology, molecular neurobiology, developmental neurobiology, cell signaling. *Unit head:* Dr. Ari Berkowitz, Director, Graduate Program, 405-325-3492, Fax: 405-325-6202, E-mail: ari@ou.edu.
Website: http://www.ou.edu/cbn

University of Pittsburgh, Dietrich School of Arts and Sciences and School of Medicine, Center for Neuroscience, Pittsburgh, PA 15260. Offers neurobiology (PhD); neuroscience (PhD). Program held jointly with School of Medicine. *Faculty:* 108 full-time (38 women). *Students:* 78 full-time (37 women); includes 13 minority (1 American Indian or Alaska Native, non-Hispanic/Latino; 8 Asian, non-Hispanic/Latino; 4 Hispanic/Latino), 9 international. Average age 25. 182 applicants, 22% accepted, 15 enrolled. In 2015, 13 doctorates awarded. *Degree requirements:* For doctorate, comprehensive exam, thesis/ dissertation. *Entrance requirements:* For doctorate, GRE, interview. Additional exam requirements/recommendations for international students: Required—TOEFL (minimum score 600 paper-based; 100 iBT). *Application deadline:* For fall admission, 12/1 priority date for domestic and international students. Application fee: $50. Electronic applications accepted. Tuition and fees vary according to program. *Financial support:* In 2015–16, 69 students received support, including 32 fellowships with full tuition reimbursements available (averaging $27,000 per year), 23 research assistantships with full tuition reimbursements available (averaging $27,000 per year), 5 teaching assistantships with full tuition reimbursements available (averaging $27,000 per year); traineeships, health care benefits, and tuition waivers (full) also available. Financial award application deadline: 12/1. *Faculty research:* Behavioral/systems/cognitive, cell and molecular, development/plasticity/repair, neurobiology of disease. *Unit head:* Dr. Alan Sved, Co-Director, 412-624-6996, Fax: 412-624-9198, E-mail: sved@pitt.edu. *Application contact:* Missy Deasy, Graduate Program Administrator, 412-383-7582, Fax: 412-624-9198, E-mail: deasym@pitt.edu.
Website: http://cnup.neurobio.pitt.edu/

University of Rochester, School of Medicine and Dentistry, Graduate Programs in Medicine and Dentistry, Department of Neurobiology and Anatomy, Programs in Neurobiology and Anatomy, Rochester, NY 14627. Offers PhD, MD/MS. *Degree requirements:* For doctorate, thesis/dissertation, qualifying exam. *Entrance requirements:* For doctorate, GRE General Test. *Expenses: Tuition,* area resident: Full-time $47,450; part-time $1482 per credit hour. *Required fees:* $528. Tuition and fees vary according to program.

University of Southern California, Graduate School, Dana and David Dornsife College of Letters, Arts and Sciences, Department of Biological Sciences, Program in Neurobiology, Los Angeles, CA 90089. Offers PhD. M.S. is terminal degree only. Terminal master's awarded for partial completion of doctoral program. *Degree requirements:* For doctorate, comprehensive exam, thesis/dissertation, qualifying examination, dissertation defense. *Entrance requirements:* For doctorate, GRE, 3 letters of recommendation, personal statement, resume, minimum GPA of 3.0. Additional exam requirements/recommendations for international students: Required—TOEFL (minimum score 600 paper-based; 100 iBT). Electronic applications accepted. *Faculty research:* Neural basis of emotion and motivation, learning and memory, cell biology and physiology of neuronal signaling, sensory processing, development and aging.

The University of Texas at Austin, Graduate School, The Institute for Neuroscience, Austin, TX 78712-1111. Offers PhD, MD/PhD. Terminal master's awarded for partial completion of doctoral program. *Degree requirements:* For doctorate, thesis/ dissertation. *Entrance requirements:* For doctorate, GRE. Electronic applications accepted. *Faculty research:* Cellular/molecular biology, neurobiology, pharmacology, behavioral neuroscience.

The University of Texas at San Antonio, College of Sciences, Department of Biology, San Antonio, TX 78249-0617. Offers biology (MS); biotechnology (MS); cell and molecular biology (PhD); neurobiology (PhD). *Faculty:* 36 full-time (10 women), 1 part-time/adjunct (0 women). *Students:* 96 full-time (53 women), 60 part-time (28 women); includes 73 minority (5 Black or African American, non-Hispanic/Latino; 1 American Indian or Alaska Native, non-Hispanic/Latino; 7 Asian, non-Hispanic/Latino; 54 Hispanic/ Latino; 1 Native Hawaiian or other Pacific Islander, non-Hispanic/Latino; 5 Two or more races, non-Hispanic/Latino), 28 international. Average age 28. 147 applicants, 46% accepted, 40 enrolled. In 2015, 43 master's, 8 doctorates awarded. Terminal master's awarded for partial completion of doctoral program. *Degree requirements:* For master's, comprehensive exam, thesis or alternative; for doctorate, comprehensive exam, thesis/ dissertation. *Entrance requirements:* For master's, GRE General Test, bachelor's degree with 18 credit hours in field of study or in another appropriate field of study; for doctorate, GRE General Test, 3 letters of recommendation, statement of purpose, resume. Additional exam requirements/recommendations for international students: Required—TOEFL (minimum score 500 paper-based; 100 iBT), IELTS (minimum score 5). *Application deadline:* For fall admission, 7/1 for domestic students, 4/1 for international students; for spring admission, 11/1 for domestic students, 9/1 for international students. Application fee: $45 ($80 for international students). Electronic applications accepted. *Faculty research:* Development of human and veterinary vaccines against a fungal disease, mammalian germ cells and stem cells, dopamine neuron physiology and addiction, plant biochemistry, dendritic computation and synaptic plasticity. *Unit head:* Dr. Garry Sunter, Chair, 210-458-5479, E-mail: garry.sunter@ utsa.edu. *Application contact:* Rene Munguia, Jr., Senior Program Coordinator, 210-458-4642, Fax: 210-458-5658, E-mail: rene.munguia@utsa.edu.
Website: http://bio.utsa.edu/

University of Utah, School of Medicine and Graduate School, Graduate Programs in Medicine, Department of Neurobiology and Anatomy, Salt Lake City, UT 84112-1107. Offers PhD. *Program availability:* Part-time. Terminal master's awarded for partial completion of doctoral program. *Degree requirements:* For doctorate, comprehensive exam, thesis/dissertation. *Entrance requirements:* For doctorate, GRE General Test. Additional exam requirements/recommendations for international students: Required— TOEFL. *Faculty research:* Neuroscience, neuroanatomy, developmental neurobiology, neurogenetics.

University of Washington, Graduate School, School of Medicine, Graduate Programs in Medicine, Graduate Program in Neurobiology and Behavior, Seattle, WA 98195. Offers PhD. *Degree requirements:* For doctorate, thesis/dissertation. *Entrance requirements:* For doctorate, GRE. Additional exam requirements/recommendations for international students: Required—TOEFL. Electronic applications accepted. *Faculty research:* Motor, sensory systems, neuroplasticity, animal behavior, neuroendocrinology, computational neuroscience.

Virginia Commonwealth University, Medical College of Virginia-Professional Programs, School of Medicine, School of Medicine Graduate Programs, Department of Anatomy and Neurobiology, Program in Anatomy and Neurobiology, Richmond, VA 23284-9005. Offers PhD. *Accreditation:* APTA. *Degree requirements:* For doctorate, thesis/dissertation. *Entrance requirements:* For doctorate, GRE, MCAT or DAT. Electronic applications accepted.

Wake Forest University, School of Medicine and Graduate School of Arts and Sciences, Graduate Programs in Medicine, Department of Neurobiology and Anatomy, Winston-Salem, NC 27109. Offers PhD, MD/PhD. *Degree requirements:* For doctorate, thesis/dissertation. *Entrance requirements:* For doctorate, GRE General Test. Additional exam requirements/recommendations for international students: Required—TOEFL. Electronic applications accepted. *Faculty research:* Sensory neurobiology, reproductive endocrinology, regulatory processes in cell biology.

Wayne State University, College of Liberal Arts and Sciences, Department of Biological Sciences, Detroit, MI 48202. Offers biological sciences (MA, MS); cell development and neurobiology (PhD); evolution and organismal biology (PhD); molecular biology and biotechnology (PhD); molecular biotechnology (MS). PhD and MS programs admit for fall only. *Faculty:* 27. *Students:* 56 full-time (31 women), 8 part-time (2 women); includes 5 minority (2 Black or African American, non-Hispanic/Latino; 2 Asian, non-Hispanic/Latino; 1 Two or more races, non-Hispanic/Latino), 37 international. Average age 29. 210 applicants, 9% accepted, 7 enrolled. In 2015, 5 master's, 10 doctorates awarded. *Degree requirements:* For master's, thesis (for some programs); for doctorate, thesis/dissertation. *Entrance requirements:* For master's, GRE (for MS applicants), minimum GPA of 3.0; adequate preparation in biological sciences and supporting courses in chemistry, physics and mathematics; curriculum vitae; personal statement; three letters of recommendation (two for MA); for doctorate, GRE, curriculum vitae, statement of goals and career objectives, three letters of reference, bachelor's or master's degree in biological or other science. Additional exam requirements/ recommendations for international students: Required—TOEFL (minimum score 550 paper-based; 79 iBT), TWE (minimum score 5.5), Michigan English Language Assessment Battery (minimum score 85); Recommended—IELTS (minimum score 6.5). Application fee: $0. Electronic applications accepted. *Expenses:* Tuition, state resident: full-time $14,165; part-time $590.20 per credit hour. Tuition, nonresident: full-time $30,682; part-time $1278.40 per credit hour. *Required fees:* $1688; $47.45 per credit hour. $274.60 per semester. Tuition and fees vary according to course load and program. *Financial support:* In 2015–16, 55 students received support, including 3 fellowships with tuition reimbursements available (averaging $16,000 per year), 8 research assistantships with tuition reimbursements available (averaging $19,506 per year), 45 teaching assistantships with tuition reimbursements available (averaging $19,536 per year); scholarships/grants and unspecified assistantships also available. Financial award application deadline: 3/31; financial award applicants required to submit FAFSA. *Faculty research:* Transcription and chromatin remodeling, genomic and developmental evolution, community and landscape ecology and environmental degradation, microbiology and virology, cell and neurobiology. *Total annual research expenditures:* $2.1 million. *Unit head:* Dr. David Njus, Professor and Chair, 313-577-3105, E-mail: dnjus@wayne.edu. *Application contact:* Rose Mary Priest, Graduate Secretary, 313-577-6818, E-mail: rpriest@wayne.edu.
Website: http://clas.wayne.edu/Biology/

Wesleyan University, Graduate Studies, Department of Biology, Middletown, CT 06459. Offers cell and developmental biology (PhD); evolution and ecology (PhD); genetics and genomics (PhD), including bioinformatics; neurobiology and behavior (PhD). *Faculty:* 14 full-time (5 women). *Students:* 26 full-time (12 women); includes 5 minority (2 Black or African American, non-Hispanic/Latino; 3 Asian, non-Hispanic/ Latino), 5 international. In 2015, 3 doctorates awarded. Terminal master's awarded for partial completion of doctoral program. *Degree requirements:* For doctorate, comprehensive exam, thesis/dissertation, public seminar. *Entrance requirements:* For doctorate, GRE. Additional exam requirements/recommendations for international students: Required—TOEFL or IELTS. *Application deadline:* For fall admission, 1/15 for domestic and international students. Application fee: $0. Electronic applications accepted. *Financial support:* Stipends available. *Faculty research:* Evolution and ecology, neurobiology and behavior, cell and developmental biology, genetics, genomics and bioinformatics. *Unit head:* Dr. John Kirn, Chair/Professor, 860-685-3494, E-mail: jrkirn@wesleyan.edu. *Application contact:* Marjorie Fitzgibbons, Administrative Assistant, 860-685-2157, E-mail: mfitzgibbons@wesleyan.edu.
Website: http://www.wesleyan.edu/bio/

West Virginia University, Eberly College of Arts and Sciences, Department of Biology, Morgantown, WV 26506. Offers cell and molecular biology (MS, PhD); environmental and evolutionary biology (MS, PhD); forensic biology (MS, PhD); genomic biology (MS, PhD); neurobiology (MS, PhD). Terminal master's awarded for partial completion of doctoral program. *Degree requirements:* For master's, thesis, final exam; for doctorate, thesis/dissertation, preliminary and final exams. *Entrance requirements:* For master's, GRE General Test, GRE Subject Test, minimum GPA of 3.0; for doctorate, GRE General Test, minimum GPA of 3.0. Additional exam requirements/recommendations for international students: Required—TOEFL. *Expenses:* Tuition, state resident: full-time $8568. Tuition, nonresident: full-time $22,140. Tuition and fees vary according to program. *Faculty research:* Environmental biology, genetic engineering, developmental biology, global change, biodiversity.

Yale University, Graduate School of Arts and Sciences, Department of Molecular, Cellular, and Developmental Biology, Program in Neurobiology, New Haven, CT 06520. Offers PhD. *Degree requirements:* For doctorate, thesis/dissertation. *Entrance requirements:* For doctorate, GRE General Test, GRE Subject Test.

Yale University, School of Medicine and Graduate School of Arts and Sciences, Combined Program in Biological and Biomedical Sciences (BBS), Department of Neurobiology, New Haven, CT 06520. Offers PhD. *Degree requirements:* For doctorate, thesis/dissertation. *Entrance requirements:* For doctorate, GRE General Test, GRE Subject Test.

Neuroscience

Albany Medical College, Center for Neuropharmacology and Neuroscience, Albany, NY 12208-3479. Offers MS, PhD. Terminal master's awarded for partial completion of doctoral program. *Degree requirements:* For master's, thesis; for doctorate, comprehensive exam, thesis/dissertation. *Entrance requirements:* For master's, GRE General Test, all transcripts, letters of recommendation; for doctorate, GRE General Test, letters of recommendation. Additional exam requirements/recommendations for international students: Required—TOEFL. *Faculty research:* Molecular and cellular neuroscience, neuronal development, addiction.

Alliant International University–San Diego, Shirley M. Hufstedler School of Education, Educational Psychology Programs, San Diego, CA 92131-1799. Offers educational psychology (Psy D); pupil personnel services (Credential); school neuropsychology (Certificate); school psychology (MA); school-based mental health (Certificate). *Program availability:* Part-time. *Degree requirements:* For doctorate, comprehensive exam, thesis/dissertation, internship. *Entrance requirements:* For master's, minimum GPA of 2.5, letters of recommendation; for doctorate, minimum GPA of 3.0, letters of recommendation. Additional exam requirements/recommendations for international students: Required—TOEFL (minimum score 550 paper-based; 80 iBT), TWE (minimum score 5). Electronic applications accepted. *Faculty research:* School-based mental health, pupil personnel services, childhood mood, school-based assessment.

American University, College of Arts and Sciences, Department of Psychology, Washington, DC 22016-8062. Offers addiction and addictive behavior (Certificate); behavior, cognition, and neuroscience (PhD); clinical psychology (PhD); psychobiology of healing (Certificate); psychology (MA). *Accreditation:* APA. *Program availability:* Part-time. *Faculty:* 22 full-time (8 women), 8 part-time/adjunct (5 women). *Students:* 88 full-time (67 women), 19 part-time (17 women); includes 20 minority (5 Black or African American, non-Hispanic/Latino; 5 Asian, non-Hispanic/Latino; 6 Hispanic/Latino; 4 Two or more races, non-Hispanic/Latino), 7 international. Average age 28. 564 applicants, 13% accepted, 30 enrolled. In 2015, 15 master's, 19 doctorates awarded. *Degree requirements:* For master's, comprehensive exam, thesis or alternative; for doctorate, comprehensive exam, thesis/dissertation. *Entrance requirements:* For master's, GRE General Test, GRE Subject Test, statement of purpose, transcripts, 2 letters of recommendation; for doctorate, GRE General Test, GRE Subject Test, 3 letters of recommendation, statement of purpose, transcripts, resume. Additional exam requirements/recommendations for international students: Required—TOEFL (minimum score 100 iBT), IELTS (minimum score 7), PTE (minimum score 68). Application fee: $55. *Expenses: Tuition,* area resident: Full-time $27,468; part-time $1526 per credit hour. *Required fees:* $430. Tuition and fees vary according to course level and program. *Financial support:* Application deadline: 2/1. *Unit head:* Dr. David Haaga, Department Chair, 202-885-1718, Fax: 202-885-1023, E-mail: ahrens@american.edu. *Application contact:* Kathy Clowery, Associate Director, Graduate Admission, 202-885-3620, Fax: 202-885-1344, E-mail: clowery@american.edu. Website: http://www.american.edu/CAS/Psychology/

American University of Beirut, Graduate Programs, Faculty of Medicine, Beirut, Lebanon. Offers anatomy, cell biology and human morphology (MS); biochemistry and medical genetics (MS); biomedical sciences (PhD); experimental pathology, immunology and microbiology (MS); medicine (MD); neuroscience (MS); pharmacology and toxicology (MS). *Program availability:* Part-time. *Faculty:* 302 full-time (95 women), 64 part-time/adjunct (11 women). *Students:* 381 full-time (173 women), 61 part-time (51 women). Average age 23. In 2015, 14 master's awarded. *Degree requirements:* For master's, one foreign language, comprehensive exam, thesis (for some programs); for doctorate, one foreign language, comprehensive exam, thesis/dissertation. *Entrance requirements:* For master's, letter of recommendation; for doctorate, MCAT, bachelor's degree. Additional exam requirements/recommendations for international students: Required—TOEFL (minimum score 600 paper-based; 100 iBT), IELTS (minimum score 7.5). *Application deadline:* For fall admission, 4/30 for domestic and international students; for spring admission, 11/1 for domestic and international students. Application fee: $50. Electronic applications accepted. *Expenses: Tuition,* area resident: Full-time $16,254; part-time $903 per credit. *Required fees:* $699. Tuition and fees vary according to course load and program. *Financial support:* In 2015–16, 273 students received support, including 45 teaching assistantships (averaging $9,000 per year); career-related internships or fieldwork, institutionally sponsored loans, scholarships/grants, health care benefits, and unspecified assistantships also available. Financial award application deadline: 2/2. *Faculty research:* Cancer research (targeted therapy, mechanisms of leukemogenesis, tumor cell extravasation and metastasis, cancer stem cells), stem cell research (regenerative medicine, drug discovery), genetic research (neurogenetics, hereditary cardiomyopathy, hemoglobinopathies, pharmacogenomics, proteomics), neuroscience research (pain, neurodegenerative disorder), metabolism (inflammation and metabolism, metabolic disorder, diabetes mellitus), vascular and renal biology, signal transduction. *Total annual research expenditures:* $2.6 million. *Unit head:* Dr. Mohamed Sayegh, Dean, 961-1350000 Ext. 4700, Fax: 961-1744464, E-mail: msayegh@aub.edu.lb. *Application contact:* Dr. Salim Kanaan, Director, Admissions Office, 961-1350000 Ext. 2594, Fax: 961-1750775, E-mail: sk00@aub.edu.lb. Website: http://www.aub.edu.lb/fm/fm_home/Pages/index.aspx

Argosy University, Chicago, Illinois School of Professional Psychology, Doctoral Program in Clinical Psychology, Chicago, IL 60601. Offers child and adolescent psychology (Psy D); client-centered and experiential psychotherapies (Psy D); diversity and multicultural psychology (Psy D); family psychology (Psy D); forensic psychology (Psy D); health psychology (Psy D); neuropsychology (Psy D); organizational consulting (Psy D); psychoanalytic psychology (Psy D); psychology and spirituality (Psy D). *Accreditation:* APA.

Argosy University, Phoenix, Arizona School of Professional Psychology, Program in Clinical Psychology, Phoenix, AZ 85021. Offers clinical psychology (MA); neuropsychology (Psy D); sports-exercise psychology (Psy D). *Accreditation:* APA (one or more programs are accredited).

Argosy University, Phoenix, Arizona School of Professional Psychology, Program in Neuropsychology, Phoenix, AZ 85021. Offers Psy D.

Argosy University, Tampa, Florida School of Professional Psychology, Program in Clinical Psychology, Tampa, FL 33607. Offers clinical psychology (MA, Psy D), including child and adolescent psychology (Psy D), geropsychology (Psy D), marriage/couples and family therapy (Psy D), neuropsychology (Psy D). *Accreditation:* APA.

Arizona State University at the Tempe campus, College of Liberal Arts and Sciences, Department of Psychology, Tempe, AZ 85287-1104. Offers applied behavior analysis (MS); behavioral neuroscience (PhD); clinical psychology (PhD); cognitive science (PhD); developmental psychology (PhD); quantitative psychology (PhD); social psychology (PhD). *Accreditation:* APA. *Degree requirements:* For doctorate,

comprehensive exam, thesis/dissertation, interactive Program of Study (iPOS) submitted before completing 50 percent of required credit hours. *Entrance requirements:* For doctorate, GRE General Test, GRE Subject Test, minimum GPA of 3.0 or equivalent in last 2 years of work leading to bachelor's degree. Additional exam requirements/recommendations for international students: Required—TOEFL, IELTS, or PTE. Electronic applications accepted.

Arizona State University at the Tempe campus, College of Liberal Arts and Sciences, School of Life Sciences, Tempe, AZ 85287-4601. Offers animal behavior (PhD); applied ethics (biomedical and health ethics) (MA); biology (MS, PhD), including biology, biology and society, complex adaptive systems science (PhD), plant biology and conservation (MS); environmental life sciences (PhD); evolutionary biology (PhD); history and philosophy of science (PhD); human and social dimensions of science and technology (PhD); microbiology (PhD); molecular and cellular biology (PhD); neuroscience (PhD). Terminal master's awarded for partial completion of doctoral program. *Degree requirements:* For master's, thesis (for some programs), interactive Program of Study (iPOS) submitted before completing 50 percent of required credit hours; for doctorate, variable foreign language requirement, comprehensive exam, thesis/dissertation, interactive Program of Study (iPOS) submitted before completing 50 percent of required credit hours. *Entrance requirements:* For master's and doctorate, GRE, minimum GPA of 3.0 or equivalent in last 2 years of work leading to bachelor's degree. Additional exam requirements/recommendations for international students: Required—TOEFL (minimum score 600 paper-based; 100 iBT). Electronic applications accepted.

Arizona State University at the Tempe campus, Graduate College, Interdisciplinary Graduate Program in Neuroscience, Tempe, AZ 85287-1003. Offers PhD. Terminal master's awarded for partial completion of doctoral program. *Degree requirements:* For doctorate, comprehensive exam, thesis/dissertation, All students must submit an interactive Program of Study (iPOS) before completing 50 percent of the credit hours required for their degree program. A student is not eligible to apply for the Foreign Language Examination (if appl), comprehensive exams, dissertation proposal/ prospectus or dissertation defense (if appl) without an approved iPOS. *Entrance requirements:* For doctorate, GRE, GPA of 3.0 or better in the last 2 years of work leading to the bachelor's degree, 3 letters of recommendation, statement of research interests and goals, CV or resume, and the completed Interdisciplinary Neuroscience Academic Record form. Additional exam requirements/recommendations for international students: Required—TOEFL (minimum score 550 paper-based; 80 iBT), IELTS (minimum score 6.5). Electronic applications accepted.

Augusta University, The Graduate School, Program in Neuroscience, Augusta, GA 30912. Offers PhD. *Degree requirements:* For doctorate, comprehensive exam, thesis/ dissertation. *Entrance requirements:* For doctorate, GRE General Test. Additional exam requirements/recommendations for international students: Required—TOEFL (minimum score 550 paper-based; 79 iBT). *Application deadline:* For fall admission, 1/15 for domestic and international students. Application fee: $50. Electronic applications accepted. *Financial support:* Research assistantships with partial tuition reimbursements and Federal Work-Study available. Support available to part-time students. Financial award application deadline: 5/31. *Faculty research:* Learning and memory, neuronal migration, synapse formation, regeneration, developmental neurobiology, neurodegeneration and neural repair. *Unit head:* Dr. Darrell Brann, Director, 706-721-7779, Fax: 706-721-8685, E-mail: dbrann@augusta.edu. *Application contact:* Angie Compton, Coordinator, 706-721-0487, E-mail: acompton@augusta.edu. Website: http://www.augusta.edu/mcg/dnrm/neuroscience/

Ball State University, Graduate School, Teachers College, Department of Educational Psychology, Muncie, IN 47306. Offers educational psychology (MA, MS), including educational psychology (MA, MS, PhD); educational psychology (PhD), including educational psychology (MA, MS, PhD); gifted and talented education (Certificate); human development and learning (Certificate); instructional design and assessment (Certificate); neuropsychology (Certificate); quantitative psychology (MS); response to intervention (Certificate); school psychology (MA, PhD), including school psychology (MA, PhD, Ed S); school psychology (Ed S), including school psychology (MA, PhD, Ed S). *Program availability:* 100% online. *Faculty:* 18 full-time (11 women), 3 part-time/ adjunct (all women). *Students:* 60 full-time (46 women), 86 part-time (64 women); includes 23 minority (10 Black or African American, non-Hispanic/Latino; 1 American Indian or Alaska Native, non-Hispanic/Latino; 3 Asian, non-Hispanic/Latino; 3 Hispanic/ Latino; 1 Native Hawaiian or other Pacific Islander, non-Hispanic/Latino; 5 Two or more races, non-Hispanic/Latino), 2 international. Average age 31. 70 applicants, 59% accepted, 36 enrolled. In 2015, 23 master's, 5 doctorates, 19 other advanced degrees awarded. *Degree requirements:* For doctorate, thesis/dissertation; for other advanced degree, thesis. *Entrance requirements:* For master's, GRE General Test, minimum baccalaureate GPA of 2.75 or 3.0 in latter half of baccalauareate, professional goals and self-assessment; for doctorate, GRE General Test, minimum graduate GPA of 3.2; for other advanced degree, GRE General Test. Additional exam requirements/ recommendations for international students: Required—TOEFL (minimum score 550 paper-based; 79 iBT), IELTS (minimum score 6.5). *Application deadline:* Applications are processed on a rolling basis. Application fee: $60. Electronic applications accepted. *Expenses: Tuition,* area resident: Full-time $6948; part-time $2316 per semester. Tuition, state resident: full-time $10,422; part-time $3474 per semester. Tuition, nonresident: full-time $19,062; part-time $6354 per semester. *Required fees:* $651 per semester. Tuition and fees vary according to campus/location, program and reciprocity agreements. *Financial support:* In 2015–16, 39 students received support, including 27 research assistantships with partial tuition reimbursements available (averaging $11,922 per year), 5 teaching assistantships with partial tuition reimbursements available (averaging $10,715 per year); unspecified assistantships also available. Financial award application deadline: 3/1; financial award applicants required to submit FAFSA. *Unit head:* Dr. Sharon Paulson, Chairperson, 765-285-8500, Fax: 765-285-5455, E-mail: spaulson@bsu.edu. *Application contact:* Dr. Jerrell Cassady, Director, Master's and Graduate Programs, 765-285-8522, Fax: 765-285-5455, E-mail: jccassady@bsu.edu. Website: http://www.bsu.edu/edpsych

Baylor College of Medicine, Graduate School of Biomedical Sciences, Department of Neuroscience, Houston, TX 77030-3498. Offers PhD, MD/PhD. *Degree requirements:* For doctorate, thesis/dissertation, public defense. *Entrance requirements:* For doctorate, GRE General Test, GRE Subject Test (strongly recommended), minimum GPA of 3.0. Additional exam requirements/recommendations for international students: Required—TOEFL. Electronic applications accepted. *Faculty research:* Neurodegenerative, neurodevelopment, neurophysiology, addiction, learning and memory.

Baylor College of Medicine, Graduate School of Biomedical Sciences, Program in Developmental Biology, Houston, TX 77030-3498. Offers PhD, MD/PhD. *Degree requirements:* For doctorate, thesis/dissertation, public defense. *Entrance requirements:*

For doctorate, GRE General Test, GRE Subject Test (strongly recommended), minimum GPA of 3.0. Additional exam requirements/recommendations for international students: Required—TOEFL. Electronic applications accepted. *Faculty research:* Stem cells, cancer, neurobiology, organogenesis, genetics of model organisms.

Boston University, School of Medicine, Division of Graduate Medical Sciences, Graduate Program for Neuroscience, Boston, MA 02215. Offers PhD, MD/PhD. *Degree requirements:* For doctorate, thesis/dissertation. *Unit head:* Dr. Shelley Russek, Director, 617-638-4319, E-mail: srussek@bu.edu. *Application contact:* GMS Admissions Office, 617-638-5255, E-mail: askgms@bu.edu.
Website: http://www.bu.edu/neuro/graduate/

Boston University, School of Medicine, Division of Graduate Medical Sciences, Program in Behavioral Neuroscience, Boston, MA 02215. Offers PhD, MD/PhD. *Program availability:* Part-time. *Degree requirements:* For doctorate, thesis/dissertation. *Application deadline:* For fall admission, 1/15 for domestic students; for spring admission, 10/15 for domestic students. *Financial support:* Federal Work-Study, scholarships/grants, and traineeships available. *Unit head:* Dr. Carol Palumbo, Director, 617-638-5255, E-mail: cpalumbo@bu.edu. *Application contact:* GMS Admissions Office, 617-638-5255, E-mail: askgms@bu.edu.
Website: http://www.bumc.bu.edu/busm-bns/

Brandeis University, Graduate School of Arts and Sciences, Department of Psychology, Waltham, MA 02454-9110. Offers brain, body and behavior (PhD); cognitive neuroscience (PhD); general psychology (MA); social/developmental psychology (PhD). *Program availability:* Part-time. *Faculty:* 15 full-time (7 women), 3 part-time/adjunct (2 women). *Students:* 36 full-time (27 women), 1 (woman) part-time; includes 7 minority (1 Black or African American, non-Hispanic/Latino; 1 Asian, non-Hispanic/Latino; 3 Hispanic/Latino; 2 Two or more races, non-Hispanic/Latino), 7 international. 183 applicants, 13% accepted, 12 enrolled. In 2015, 13 master's, 3 doctorates awarded. Terminal master's awarded for partial completion of doctoral program. *Degree requirements:* For master's, thesis or alternative; for doctorate, thesis/dissertation, research reports. *Entrance requirements:* For master's and doctorate, GRE General Test; GRE Subject Test (recommended), 3 letters of recommendation, statement of purpose, transcript(s), resume. Additional exam requirements/recommendations for international students: Required—TOEFL (minimum score 600 paper-based; 100 iBT); Recommended—IELTS (minimum score 7), TSE (minimum score 68). *Application deadline:* For fall admission, 1/15 priority date for domestic and international students. Application fee: $75. Electronic applications accepted. *Financial support:* In 2015–16, 47 students received support, including 23 fellowships with full tuition reimbursements available (averaging $22,000 per year), 24 teaching assistantships with partial tuition reimbursements available (averaging $3,200 per year); Federal Work-Study, scholarships/grants, health care benefits, and tuition waivers (full and partial) also available. Support available to part-time students. Financial award application deadline: 4/15; financial award applicants required to submit FAFSA. *Faculty research:* Brain, body, and behavior across the lifespan; face perception and nonverbal communication; learning and memory; motor control and spatial orientation; neurophysiology of learning and decision making; personality and cognition in adulthood and old age; social, cultural and affective neuroscience; social relations and health physiology; speech comprehension and memory; taste physiology and psychophysics; visual perception. *Unit head:* Prof. Paul DiZio, Department Chair, 781-736-3300, Fax: 781-736-3291, E-mail: dizio@brandeis.edu. *Application contact:* Phil Gnatowski, Department Administrator, 781-736-3302, Fax: 781-736-3291, E-mail: gnat@brandeis.edu.
Website: http://www.brandeis.edu/departments/psych/

Brandeis University, Graduate School of Arts and Sciences, Program in Neuroscience, Waltham, MA 02454-9110. Offers neuroscience (MS, PhD); quantitative biology (PhD). *Faculty:* 21 full-time (9 women). *Students:* 58 full-time (24 women), 1 (woman) part-time; includes 14 minority (1 Black or African American, non-Hispanic/Latino; 1 American Indian or Alaska Native, non-Hispanic/Latino; 6 Asian, non-Hispanic/Latino; 6 Hispanic/Latino), 9 international. 192 applicants, 23% accepted, 15 enrolled. In 2015, 10 master's, 6 doctorates awarded. Terminal master's awarded for partial completion of doctoral program. *Degree requirements:* For master's, thesis optional, research project; for doctorate, comprehensive exam, thesis/dissertation, qualifying exams, teaching experience, journal club, research seminars. *Entrance requirements:* For master's, GRE General Test, official transcript(s), statement of purpose, resume, 2 letters of recommendation; for doctorate, GRE General Test, official transcript(s), statement of purpose, resume, 3 letters of recommendation, listing of previous research experience. Additional exam requirements/recommendations for international students: Required—TOEFL (minimum score 600 paper-based; 100 iBT); Recommended—IELTS (minimum score 7), TSE (minimum score 68). *Application deadline:* For fall admission, 12/15 priority date for domestic students. Application fee: $75. Electronic applications accepted. *Financial support:* In 2015–16, 49 students received support, including 32 fellowships with full tuition reimbursements available (averaging $30,500 per year), 17 research assistantships with full tuition reimbursements available (averaging $30,500 per year); Federal Work-Study, scholarships/grants, health care benefits, and tuition waivers (full and partial) also available. Financial award application deadline: 4/15; financial award applicants required to submit FAFSA. *Faculty research:* Behavioral/cognitive neuroscience, cellular and molecular neuroscience, computational neuroscience and systems neuroscience, and developmental neuroscience. *Unit head:* Dr. Don Katz, Director of Graduate Studies, 781-736-3100, Fax: 781-736-3107, E-mail: dbkatz@brandeis.edu. *Application contact:* Dr. Maryanna Aldrich, Department Administrator, 781-736-2300, Fax: 781-736-3107, E-mail: scigradoffice@brandeis.edu.
Website: http://www.brandeis.edu/gsas

Brigham Young University, Graduate Studies, College of Life Sciences, Department of Physiology and Developmental Biology, Provo, UT 84602. Offers neuroscience (MS, PhD); physiology and developmental biology (MS, PhD). *Program availability:* Part-time. *Faculty:* 20 full-time (1 woman), 4 part-time/adjunct (3 women). *Students:* 33 full-time (20 women); includes 6 minority (1 American Indian or Alaska Native, non-Hispanic/Latino; 3 Asian, non-Hispanic/Latino; 1 Hispanic/Latino; 1 Two or more races, non-Hispanic/Latino). Average age 29. 17 applicants, 29% accepted, 5 enrolled. In 2015, 6 master's, 3 doctorates awarded. Terminal master's awarded for partial completion of doctoral program. *Degree requirements:* For master's, thesis, oral exam; for doctorate, comprehensive exam, thesis/dissertation. *Entrance requirements:* For master's, GRE General Test, minimum GPA of 3.0 during previous 2 years; for doctorate, GRE General Test, minimum GPA of 3.0 overall. Additional exam requirements/recommendations for international students: Required—TOEFL (minimum score 580 paper-based; 85 iBT); Recommended—IELTS. *Application deadline:* For fall admission, 2/1 priority date for domestic and international students; for winter admission, 9/10 priority date for domestic and international students. Application fee: $50. Electronic applications accepted. *Financial support:* In 2015–16, 37 students received support, including 2 fellowships with partial tuition reimbursements available (averaging $7,100 per year), 17 research assistantships with full tuition reimbursements available (averaging $15,500 per year), 18 teaching assistantships with partial tuition reimbursements available (averaging $14,900 per year); career-related internships or fieldwork, institutionally sponsored loans, scholarships/grants, tuition waivers (full and partial), unspecified assistantships,

and tuition awards also available. Financial award application deadline: 2/1. *Faculty research:* Sex differentiation of the brain, exercise physiology, developmental biology, membrane biophysics, neuroscience, heart differentiation/birth defects. *Total annual research expenditures:* $747,261. *Unit head:* Dr. Dixon J. Woodbury, Chair, 801-422-7562, Fax: 801-422-0004, E-mail: dixon_woodbury@byu.edu. *Application contact:* Connie L. Provost, Graduate Program Administrator, 801-422-3706, Fax: 801-422-0004, E-mail: connie_provost@byu.edu.
Website: http://pdbio.byu.edu

Brock University, Faculty of Graduate Studies, Faculty of Social Sciences, Program in Psychology, St. Catharines, ON L2S 3A1, Canada. Offers behavioral neuroscience (MA, PhD); life span development (MA, PhD); social personality (MA, PhD). *Program availability:* Part-time. *Degree requirements:* For master's, thesis; for doctorate, thesis/dissertation. *Entrance requirements:* For master's, GRE, honors degree; for doctorate, GRE, master's degree. Additional exam requirements/recommendations for international students: Required—TOEFL (minimum score 550 paper-based; 80 iBT), IELTS (minimum score 6.5), TWE (minimum score 4). Electronic applications accepted. *Faculty research:* Social personality, behavioral neuroscience, life-span development.

Brown University, Graduate School, Division of Biology and Medicine, Department of Neuroscience, Providence, RI 02912. Offers PhD. *Degree requirements:* For doctorate, thesis/dissertation, preliminary exam. *Entrance requirements:* For doctorate, GRE General Test, GRE Subject Test. Additional exam requirements/recommendations for international students: Required—TOEFL. Electronic applications accepted. *Faculty research:* Neurophysiology, systems neuroscience, membrane biophysics, neuropharmacology, sensory systems.

Brown University, National Institutes of Health Sponsored Programs, Providence, RI 02912. Offers neuroscience (PhD).

California Institute of Technology, Division of Engineering and Applied Science, Option in Computation and Neural Systems, Pasadena, CA 91125-0001. Offers MS, PhD. Terminal master's awarded for partial completion of doctoral program. *Degree requirements:* For doctorate, thesis/dissertation, qualifying exam. *Entrance requirements:* For doctorate, GRE General Test. *Faculty research:* Biological and artificial computational devices, modeling of sensory processes and learning, theory of collective computation.

Carleton University, Faculty of Graduate Studies, Faculty of Arts and Social Sciences, Department of Psychology, Ottawa, ON K1S 5B6, Canada. Offers neuroscience (M Sc); psychology (MA, PhD). *Program availability:* Part-time. *Degree requirements:* For master's, thesis; for doctorate, comprehensive exam, thesis/dissertation. *Entrance requirements:* For master's, honors degree; for doctorate, GRE, master's degree. Additional exam requirements/recommendations for international students: Required—TOEFL. *Faculty research:* Behavioral neuroscience, social and personality psychology, cognitive/perception, developmental psychology, computer user research and evaluation, forensic psychology, health psychology.

Carnegie Mellon University, Center for the Neural Basis of Cognition, Pittsburgh, PA 15213-3891. Offers PhD.

Case Western Reserve University, School of Medicine and School of Graduate Studies, Graduate Programs in Medicine, Department of Neurosciences, Cleveland, OH 44106. Offers neuroscience (PhD); MD/PhD. Terminal master's awarded for partial completion of doctoral program. *Degree requirements:* For doctorate, thesis/dissertation. *Entrance requirements:* For doctorate, GRE General Test, 3 letters of recommendation. Additional exam requirements/recommendations for international students: Required—TOEFL (minimum score 90 iBT). Electronic applications accepted. *Expenses:* Tuition, area resident: Full-time $41,137; part-time $1714 per credit hour. *Required fees:* $32. Tuition and fees vary according to course load and program. *Faculty research:* Neurotropic factors, synapse formation, regeneration, determination of cell fate, cellular neuroscience.

Central Michigan University, College of Graduate Studies, College of Humanities and Social and Behavioral Sciences, Department of Psychology, Program in Neuroscience, Mount Pleasant, MI 48859. Offers MS, PhD. *Degree requirements:* For master's, comprehensive exam, thesis or alternative; for doctorate, thesis/dissertation. *Entrance requirements:* For master's and doctorate, GRE. Electronic applications accepted.

College of Staten Island of the City University of New York, Graduate Programs, Division of Science and Technology, Program in Neuroscience and Developmental Disabilities, Staten Island, NY 10314-6600. Offers MS. *Program availability:* Part-time, evening/weekend. *Faculty:* 4 full-time, 3 part-time/adjunct. *Students:* 4 full-time, 17 part-time. Average age 29. 32 applicants, 56% accepted, 15 enrolled. In 2015, 9 master's awarded. Terminal master's awarded for partial completion of doctoral program. *Degree requirements:* For master's, thesis, oral preliminary exam, thesis defense. *Entrance requirements:* For master's, three letters of recommendation; minimum GPA of 3.0 in undergraduate biology, mathematics, psychology or other science; interview. Additional exam requirements/recommendations for international students: Required—TOEFL (minimum score 550 paper-based; 79 iBT), IELTS (minimum score 6.5). *Application deadline:* For fall admission, 4/22 priority date for international students; for spring admission, 11/19 priority date for international students. Applications are processed on a rolling basis. Application fee: $125. Electronic applications accepted. *Expenses:* Tuition, state resident: Full-time $10,130; part-time $425 per credit. Tuition, nonresident: full-time $18,720; part-time $780 per credit. *Required fees:* $181.10 per semester. Tuition and fees vary according to program. *Financial support:* Applicants required to submit FAFSA. *Unit head:* Dr. Alejandra Alonso, Graduate Program Coordinator, 718-982-4153, Fax: 718-982-3953, E-mail: alejandra.alonso@csi.cuny.edu. *Application contact:* Sasha Spence, Associate Director for Graduate Admissions, 718-982-2019, Fax: 718-982-2500, E-mail: sasha.spence@csi.cuny.edu.
Website: http://www.csi.cuny.edu/catalog/graduate/master-of-science-in-neuroscience-and-developmental-disabilities-ms.htm

The College of William and Mary, Faculty of Arts and Sciences, Department of Applied Science, Williamsburg, VA 23187-8795. Offers accelerator science (PhD); applied mathematics (PhD); applied mechanics (PhD); applied robotics (PhD); applied science (MS); atmospheric and environmental science (PhD); computational neuroscience (PhD); interface, thin film and surface science (PhD); lasers and optics (PhD); magnetic resonance (PhD); materials science and engineering (PhD); mathematical and computational biology (PhD); medical imaging (PhD); nanotechnology (PhD); neuroscience (PhD); non-destructive evaluation (PhD); polymer chemistry (PhD); remote sensing (PhD). *Program availability:* Part-time. *Faculty:* 7 full-time (1 woman), 1 part-time/adjunct (0 women). *Students:* 26 full-time (9 women), 3 part-time (1 woman); includes 5 minority (2 Black or African American, non-Hispanic/Latino; 1 Asian, non-Hispanic/Latino; 2 Hispanic/Latino), 12 international. Average age 28. 24 applicants, 46% accepted, 6 enrolled. In 2015, 2 master's, 6 doctorates awarded. Terminal master's awarded for partial completion of doctoral program. *Degree requirements:* For master's, comprehensive exam, thesis; for doctorate, comprehensive exam, thesis/dissertation, 4 core courses. *Entrance requirements:* For master's and doctorate, GRE General Test, GRE Subject Test. Additional exam requirements/recommendations for international students: Required—TOEFL, TWE. *Application deadline:* For fall admission, 2/3 priority date for domestic students, 2/3 for international students; for spring admission, 10/15

Neuroscience

priority date for domestic students, 10/14 for international students. Applications are processed on a rolling basis. Application fee: $45. Electronic applications accepted. *Expenses:* $6,550 per semester; $13,100 per year. *Financial support:* Fellowships, research assistantships, teaching assistantships, Federal Work-Study, health care benefits, tuition waivers (full), and unspecified assistantships available. Financial award application deadline: 4/15; financial award applicants required to submit FAFSA. *Faculty research:* Computational biology, non-destructive evaluation, neurophysiology, lasers and optics. *Total annual research expenditures:* $1.7 million. *Unit head:* Dr. Christopher Del Negro, Chair, 757-221-7808, Fax: 757-221-2050, E-mail: cadeln@wm.edu. *Application contact:* Lianne Rios Ashburne, Graduate Program Coordinator, 757-221-2563, Fax: 757-221-2050, E-mail: lrashburne@wm.edu.
Website: http://www.wm.edu/as/appliedscience

Colorado State University, Interdisciplinary College, Program in Molecular, Cellular and Integrative Neurosciences, Fort Collins, CO 80523-1617. Offers PhD. *Students:* 3 full-time (2 women). Average age 26. 36 applicants, 8% accepted, 3 enrolled. *Degree requirements:* For doctorate, comprehensive exam, thesis/dissertation. *Entrance requirements:* For doctorate, GRE, minimum GPA of 3.0. Additional exam requirements/recommendations for international students: Required—TOEFL (minimum score 630 paper-based; 109 iBT). *Application deadline:* For fall admission, 12/15 priority date for domestic and international students. Application fee: $60 ($70 for international students). Electronic applications accepted. *Expenses:* Tuition, state resident: full-time $9348. Tuition, nonresident: full-time $22,916. *Required fees:* $2174; $473.72 per credit hour. $236.86 per semester. Tuition and fees vary according to course load and program. *Financial support:* In 2015–16, 3 research assistantships with partial tuition reimbursements (averaging $19,392 per year) were awarded; fellowships, teaching assistantships with partial tuition reimbursements, scholarships/grants, and unspecified assistantships also available. Financial award application deadline: 12/15; financial award applicants required to submit FAFSA. *Faculty research:* Ion channels synapse plasticity; neurophysiology and neuroimaging; sensory biology and perception; neurological and neurodegenerative disorders; computational biology and modeling. *Unit head:* Dr. Noreen E. Reist, Director, 970-491-0425, Fax: 970-491-7907, E-mail: noreen.reist@colostate.edu. *Application contact:* Nancy Graham, Administrative Assistant, 970-491-0425, Fax: 970-491-7907, E-mail: nancy.graham@colostate.edu.
Website: http://mcin.colostate.edu/

Connecticut College, Department of Psychology, New London, CT 06320. Offers behavioral medicine/health psychology (MA); clinical psychology (MA); neuroscience/psychobiology (MA); social/personality psychology (MA). *Program availability:* Part-time. *Degree requirements:* For master's, thesis. *Entrance requirements:* For master's, GRE General Test, statistics course. Additional exam requirements/recommendations for international students: Required—TOEFL (minimum score 600 paper-based).

Dalhousie University, Faculty of Graduate Studies, Neuroscience Institute, Halifax, NS B3H 4H7, Canada. Offers M Sc, PhD. *Degree requirements:* For doctorate, thesis/dissertation. *Entrance requirements:* For master's and doctorate, 4 year honors degree or equivalent, minimum A- average. Additional exam requirements/recommendations for international students: Required—1 of 5 approved tests: TOEFL, IELTS, CANTEST, CAEL, Michigan English Language Assessment Battery. Electronic applications accepted. *Faculty research:* Molecular, cellular, systems, behavioral and clinical neuroscience.

Dalhousie University, Faculty of Science, Department of Psychology, Halifax, NS B3H 4R2, Canada. Offers clinical psychology (PhD); psychology (M Sc, PhD); psychology/neuroscience (M Sc, PhD). *Degree requirements:* For master's, thesis; for doctorate, thesis/dissertation. *Entrance requirements:* For doctorate, GRE General Test. Additional exam requirements/recommendations for international students: Required—TOEFL, IELTS, CANTEST, CAEL, or Michigan English Language Assessment Battery. Electronic applications accepted. *Faculty research:* Physiological psychology, psychology of learning, learning and behavior, forensic clinical health psychology, development perception and cognition.

Dartmouth College, Arts and Sciences Graduate Programs, Department of Psychological and Brain Sciences, Hanover, NH 03755. Offers cognitive neuroscience (PhD); psychology (PhD). *Faculty:* 26 full-time (7 women), 3 part-time/adjunct (1 woman). *Students:* 39 full-time (19 women); includes 5 minority (1 American Indian or Alaska Native, non-Hispanic/Latino; 2 Asian, non-Hispanic/Latino; 2 Hispanic/Latino), 14 international. Average age 27. 129 applicants, 12% accepted, 9 enrolled. In 2015, 5 doctorates awarded. *Degree requirements:* For doctorate, thesis/dissertation. *Entrance requirements:* For doctorate, GRE General Test, GRE Subject Test. Additional exam requirements/recommendations for international students: Required—TOEFL. *Application deadline:* For fall admission, 11/30 for domestic students. Application fee: $50. Electronic applications accepted. *Expenses:* Tuition, area resident: Full-time $48,120. *Required fees:* $296. One-time fee: $50 full-time. *Faculty research:* Behavioral neuroscience, cognitive neuroscience, cognitive science, social/personality psychology. *Unit head:* Dr. David Bucci, Chair, 603-646-3439, Fax: 603-646-1419. *Application contact:* Julia Abraham, Department Administrator, 603-646-2744, E-mail: julia.s.abraham@dartmouth.edu.
Website: http://www.dartmouth.edu/~psych/graduate/

Delaware State University, Graduate Programs, Department of Biological Sciences, Dover, DE 19901-2277. Offers biological sciences (MA, MS); biology education (MS); molecular and cellular neuroscience (MS); neuroscience (PhD). *Program availability:* Part-time, evening/weekend. *Degree requirements:* For master's, thesis (for some programs). *Entrance requirements:* For master's, GRE, minimum GPA of 3.0 in major, 2.75 overall. Additional exam requirements/recommendations for international students: Required—TOEFL (minimum score 550 paper-based). Electronic applications accepted. *Faculty research:* Cell biology, immunology, microbiology, genetics, ecology.

Drexel University, College of Arts and Sciences, Department of Psychology, Clinical Psychology Program, Philadelphia, PA 19104-2875. Offers clinical psychology (PhD); forensic psychology (PhD); health psychology (PhD); neuropsychology (PhD). *Accreditation:* APA. Terminal master's awarded for partial completion of doctoral program. *Degree requirements:* For doctorate, thesis/dissertation, qualifying exam. *Entrance requirements:* For doctorate, GRE General Test, GRE Subject Test, minimum GPA of 3.0. Electronic applications accepted. *Expenses:* Contact institution. *Faculty research:* Cognitive behavioral therapy, stress and coping, eating disorders, substance abuse, developmental disabilities.

Drexel University, College of Medicine, Biomedical Graduate Programs, Program in Neuroscience, Philadelphia, PA 19104-2875. Offers MS, PhD, MD/PhD. *Degree requirements:* For doctorate, thesis/dissertation, qualifying exam. *Entrance requirements:* For doctorate, GRE General Test, or MCAT, minimum GPA of 2.75. Additional exam requirements/recommendations for international students: Required—TOEFL. Electronic applications accepted. *Faculty research:* Central monoamine systems, drugs of abuse, anatomy/physiology of sensory systems, neurodegenerative disorders and recovery of function, neuromodulation and synaptic plasticity.

Duke University, Graduate School, Cognitive Neuroscience Admitting Program, Durham, NC 27708. Offers PhD, Certificate. PhD offered through one of the participating departments: Neurobiology, Psychology and Neuroscience, Biomedical Engineering,

Computer Science, Evolutionary Anthropology, or Philosophy. *Degree requirements:* For doctorate, thesis/dissertation. *Entrance requirements:* For doctorate, GRE General Test. Additional exam requirements/recommendations for international students: Required—TOEFL (minimum score 577 paper-based; 90 iBT) or IELTS (minimum score 7). Electronic applications accepted.

Emory University, Laney Graduate School, Department of Psychology, Atlanta, GA 30322-1100. Offers clinical psychology (PhD); cognition and development (PhD); neuroscience and animal behavior (PhD). *Accreditation:* APA. *Degree requirements:* For doctorate, comprehensive exam, thesis/dissertation. *Entrance requirements:* For doctorate, GRE General Test, minimum GPA of 3.25. Additional exam requirements/recommendations for international students: Required—TOEFL. Electronic applications accepted. *Faculty research:* Neuroscience and animal behavior; adult and child psychopathology, cognition development assessment.

Emory University, Laney Graduate School, Division of Biological and Biomedical Sciences, Program in Neuroscience, Atlanta, GA 30322-1100. Offers PhD. *Degree requirements:* For doctorate, comprehensive exam, thesis/dissertation. *Entrance requirements:* For doctorate, GRE General Test, minimum GPA of 3.0 in science course work (recommended). Additional exam requirements/recommendations for international students: Required—TOEFL. Electronic applications accepted. *Faculty research:* Cell and molecular biology, development, behavior, neurodegenerative disease.

Fielding Graduate University, Graduate Programs, School of Psychology, Santa Barbara, CA 93105-3814. Offers clinical psychology (PhD, Graduate Certificate), including forensic psychology (PhD), health psychology (PhD), neuropsychology (PhD), parent-infant mental health (PhD), violence prevention and control (PhD); clinical psychology respecialization (Post-Doctoral Certificate); media psychology (MA, PhD, Graduate Certificate), including forensic psychology (PhD); neuropsychology (Post-Doctoral Certificate). *Accreditation:* APA. *Program availability:* Part-time, 100% online, blended/hybrid learning. *Faculty:* 32 full-time (21 women), 42 part-time/adjunct (19 women). *Students:* 521 full-time (380 women), 75 part-time (55 women); includes 189 minority (76 Black or African American, non-Hispanic/Latino; 4 American Indian or Alaska Native, non-Hispanic/Latino; 19 Asian, non-Hispanic/Latino; 64 Hispanic/Latino; 1 Native Hawaiian or other Pacific Islander, non-Hispanic/Latino; 25 Two or more races, non-Hispanic/Latino), 4 international. Average age 41. 278 applicants, 61% accepted, 130 enrolled. In 2015, 19 master's, 63 doctorates, 38 other advanced degrees awarded. Terminal master's awarded for partial completion of doctoral program. *Degree requirements:* For master's, thesis or alternative, capstone project; for doctorate, comprehensive exam, thesis/dissertation. *Entrance requirements:* For master's, BA from regionally-accredited institution or equivalent, minimum GPA of 2.5; for doctorate, BA or MA from regionally-accredited institution or equivalent, writing sample, minimum GPA of 3.0. *Application deadline:* For fall admission, 1/24 for domestic and international students; for spring admission, 11/1 for domestic and international students; for summer admission, 3/1 for domestic and international students. Application fee: $75. Electronic applications accepted. *Expenses:* Tuition, area resident: Full-time $26,640; part-time $720 per credit. Tuition and fees vary according to course load, degree level and program. *Financial support:* In 2015–16, 82 students received support, including 11 teaching assistantships (averaging $1,600 per year); scholarships/grants also available. Support available to part-time students. Financial award applicants required to submit FAFSA. *Unit head:* Dr. Gerald Porter, Provost and Senior Vice President, 805-898-2940, E-mail: gporter@fielding.edu. *Application contact:* Enrollment Coordinator, 800-340-1099 Ext. 4098, Fax: 805-687-9793, E-mail: psyadmission@fielding.edu.
Website: http://www.fielding.edu/our-programs/school-of-psychology/

Florida Atlantic University, Charles E. Schmidt College of Science, Center for Complex Systems and Brain Sciences, Boca Raton, FL 33431-0991. Offers PhD. *Degree requirements:* For doctorate, thesis/dissertation. *Entrance requirements:* For doctorate, GRE General Test, minimum GPA of 3.0 in last 60 hours of undergraduate course work. Additional exam requirements/recommendations for international students: Required—TOEFL (minimum score 500 paper-based; 61 iBT), IELTS (minimum score 6). *Application deadline:* For fall admission, 1/15 priority date for domestic and international students. Application fee: $30. *Expenses:* Tuition, area resident: Full-time $7392; part-time $369.82 per credit hour. Tuition, state resident: full-time $7392; part-time $369.82 per credit hour. Tuition, nonresident: full-time $19,432; part-time $1024.81 per credit hour. *Financial support:* Fellowships with full tuition reimbursements, research assistantships with partial tuition reimbursements, teaching assistantships with partial tuition reimbursements, Federal Work-Study, and traineeships available. *Faculty research:* Motor behavior, speech perception, nonlinear dynamics and fractals, behavioral neuroscience, cellular and molecular neuroscience.
Website: http://www.ccs.fau.edu/

Florida International University, College of Arts, Sciences, and Education, Department of Psychology, Miami, FL 33199. Offers behavioral analysis (MS); clinical science (PhD); cognitive neuroscience (PhD); counseling psychology (MS); developmental science (PhD); legal psychology (PhD); organizational psychology (MS, PhD). Program has fall admissions only. *Program availability:* Part-time, evening/weekend. *Faculty:* 44 full-time (26 women), 40 part-time/adjunct (30 women). *Students:* 136 full-time (106 women), 14 part-time (7 women); includes 86 minority (6 Black or African American, non-Hispanic/Latino; 4 Asian, non-Hispanic/Latino; 76 Hispanic/Latino), 3 international. Average age 27. 257 applicants, 26% accepted, 53 enrolled. In 2015, 62 master's, 21 doctorates awarded. Terminal master's awarded for partial completion of doctoral program. *Degree requirements:* For master's, thesis; for doctorate, comprehensive exam, thesis/dissertation. *Entrance requirements:* For master's, GRE General Test, minimum GPA of 3.0, resume, 3 letters of recommendation; for doctorate, GRE General Test, 3 letters of recommendation, resume, letter of intent, two writing samples, minimum GPA of 3.0. Additional exam requirements/recommendations for international students: Required—TOEFL (minimum score 550 paper-based; 80 iBT). *Application deadline:* For fall admission, 12/15 for domestic and international students. Application fee: $30. Electronic applications accepted. *Expenses:* Tuition, state resident: full-time $10,708; part-time $455.64 per credit hour. Tuition, nonresident: full-time $23,816; part-time $1001.69 per credit hour. *Required fees:* $390; $195 per semester. Tuition and fees vary according to program. *Financial support:* Institutionally sponsored loans and scholarships/grants available. Financial award application deadline: 3/1. *Faculty research:* Legal psychology, organizational and industrial psychology, child behavior psychology. *Unit head:* Dr. William Pelham, Chair, 305-348-3002, Fax: 305-348-3646, E-mail: wpelham@fiu.edu. *Application contact:* Lara Wilson, Senior Secretary, 305-348-2881, Fax: 305-348-3879, E-mail: lara.wilson@fiu.edu.

Florida State University, College of Medicine, Department of Biomedical Sciences, Tallahassee, FL 32306-4300. Offers biomedical sciences (PhD); neuroscience (PhD). *Faculty:* 33 full-time (11 women). *Students:* 33 full-time (22 women); includes 10 minority (2 Black or African American, non-Hispanic/Latino; 3 Asian, non-Hispanic/Latino; 5 Hispanic/Latino). Average age 27. 67 applicants, 15% accepted, 8 enrolled. In 2015, 8 doctorates awarded. *Degree requirements:* For doctorate, comprehensive exam, thesis/dissertation. *Entrance requirements:* For doctorate, GRE. Additional exam requirements/recommendations for international students: Required—TOEFL (minimum score 550 paper-based; 80 iBT). *Application deadline:* For fall admission, 12/15 for domestic and international students. Application fee: $30. *Expenses:* Contact institution. *Financial support:* In 2015–16, 25,000 students received support, including 33 research assistantships with full tuition reimbursements available (averaging $25,000 per year). Financial award application deadline: 1/15; financial award applicants required to submit FAFSA. *Faculty research:* Development, neuroscience, the molecular basis of human disease. *Unit head:* Dr. Richard S. Nowakowski, Professor/Chair, 850-644-7963, Fax: 850-644-5781, E-mail: richard.nowakowski@med.fsu.edu. *Application contact:* Christina Rene' Goswick-Childers, Academic Program Specialist, 850-645-6420, Fax: 850-644-5781, E-mail: cgoswick-childers@med.fsu.edu.

Florida State University, The Graduate School, College of Arts and Sciences, Department of Biological Science, Tallahassee, FL 32306-4295. Offers cell and molecular biology (MS, PhD); ecology and evolutionary biology (MS, PhD); neuroscience (MS, PhD); plant biology (MS, PhD); science teaching (MST), including community college science teaching; structural biology (MS, PhD). *Faculty:* 45 full-time (14 women). *Students:* 106 full-time (53 women); includes 13 minority (3 Black or African American, non-Hispanic/Latino; 1 Asian, non-Hispanic/Latino; 9 Hispanic/Latino), 27 international. Average age 28. 191 applicants, 18% accepted, 16 enrolled. In 2015, 4 master's, 12 doctorates awarded. Terminal master's awarded for partial completion of doctoral program. *Degree requirements:* For master's, comprehensive exam, thesis, teaching experience, seminar presentations; for doctorate, comprehensive exam, thesis/dissertation, teaching experience; seminar presentations. *Entrance requirements:* For master's and doctorate, GRE General Test, minimum upper-division GPA of 3.0. Additional exam requirements/recommendations for international students: Required—TOEFL (minimum score 600 paper-based; 92 iBT). *Application deadline:* For fall admission, 12/1 for domestic and international students. Application fee: $30. Electronic applications accepted. *Expenses: Tuition, area resident:* Full-time $7263; part-time $403.50 per credit hour. Tuition, nonresident: full-time $18,087; part time $1004.85 per credit hour. *Required fees:* $1365; $75.81 per credit hour. $20 per semester. Tuition and fees vary according to campus/location. *Financial support:* In 2015–16, 113 students received support, including 8 fellowships with full tuition reimbursements available (averaging $30,000 per year), 29 research assistantships with full tuition reimbursements available (averaging $21,500 per year), 76 teaching assistantships with full tuition reimbursements available (averaging $21,500 per year); scholarships/grants, traineeships, and unspecified assistantships also available. Financial award application deadline: 12/1; financial award applicants required to submit FAFSA. *Faculty research:* Cell and molecular biology and genetics, ecology and evolutionary biology, plant science, structural biology. *Unit head:* Dr. Thomas A. Houpt, Professor and Associate Chair, 850-644-4906, Fax: 850-644-4907, E-mail: houpt@neuro.fsu.edu. *Application contact:* Dr. Michael B. Miller, Academic Program Specialist, 850-644-3023, Fax: 850-644-9829, E-mail: gradinfo@bio.fsu.edu.
Website: http://www.bio.fsu.edu/

Florida State University, The Graduate School, College of Arts and Sciences, Department of Psychology, Interdisciplinary Program in Neuroscience, Tallahassee, FL 32306. Offers PhD. *Faculty:* 10 full-time (4 women). *Students:* 19 full-time (9 women), 3 part-time (2 women); includes 5 minority (2 Black or African American, non-Hispanic/Latino; 1 Asian, non-Hispanic/Latino; 2 Hispanic/Latino), 1 international. Average age 26. 37 applicants, 19% accepted, 4 enrolled. In 2015, 3 doctorates awarded. *Degree requirements:* For doctorate, thesis/dissertation, preliminary exam. *Entrance requirements:* For doctorate, GRE General Test (suggested minimum score above 60th percentile on both verbal and quantitative sections), minimum GPA of 3.0, research experience, letters of recommendation. Additional exam requirements/ recommendations for international students: Required—TOEFL (minimum score 550 paper-based; 80 iBT). *Application deadline:* For fall admission, 12/1 for domestic and international students. Application fee: $30. Electronic applications accepted. *Expenses:* $8,622 resident full-time per year; $19,980 non-resident full-time per year. *Financial support:* In 2015–16, 16 students received support, including 10 fellowships with full tuition reimbursements available (averaging $22,000 per year), 6 research assistantships with full tuition reimbursements available (averaging $22,000 per year), 6 teaching assistantships with full tuition reimbursements available (averaging $22,815 per year); Federal Work-Study, institutionally sponsored loans, scholarships/grants, traineeships, health care benefits, and unspecified assistantships also available. Financial award application deadline: 12/1; financial award applicants required to submit FAFSA. *Faculty research:* Sensory processes, neural development and plasticity, circadian rhythms, behavioral and molecular genetics, hormonal control of behavior. *Total annual research expenditures:* $2.3 million. *Unit head:* Dr. Frank Johnson, Director, 850-644-8566, Fax: 850-645-0349, E-mail: johnson@psy.fsu.edu. *Application contact:* Cherie P. Miller, Graduate Program Associate, 850-644-2499, Fax: 850-644-7739, E-mail: grad-info@psy.fsu.edu.
Website: http://www.neuro.fsu.edu

Gallaudet University, The Graduate School, Washington, DC 20002-3625. Offers American Sign Language/English bilingual early childhood deaf education: birth to 5 (Certificate); audiology (Au D); clinical psychology (PhD); deaf and hard of hearing infants, toddlers, and their families (Certificate); deaf education (MA, Ed S); deaf history (Certificate); deaf studies (Certificate); educating deaf students with disabilities (Certificate); education: teacher preparation (MA), including deaf education, early childhood education and deaf education, elementary education and deaf education, secondary education and deaf education; educational neuroscience (PhD); hearing, speech and language sciences (MS, PhD); international development (MA); interpretation (MA, PhD), including combined interpreting practice and research (MA), interpreting research (MA); linguistics (MA, PhD); mental health counseling (MA); peer mentoring (Certificate); public administration (MPA); school counseling (MA); school psychology (Psy S); sign language teaching (MA); social work (MSW); speech-language pathology (MS). *Program availability:* Part-time. *Students:* 295 full-time (229 women), 149 part-time (104 women); includes 127 minority (32 Black or African American, non-Hispanic/Latino; 2 American Indian or Alaska Native, non-Hispanic/Latino; 14 Asian, non-Hispanic/Latino; 35 Hispanic/Latino; 44 Two or more races, non-Hispanic/Latino), 26 international. Average age 31. 598 applicants, 47% accepted, 158 enrolled. In 2015, 140 master's, 17 doctorates, 8 other advanced degrees awarded. Terminal master's awarded for partial completion of doctoral program. *Degree requirements:* For master's, comprehensive exam (for some programs), thesis optional; for doctorate, comprehensive exam, thesis/dissertation. *Entrance requirements:* For master's and doctorate, GRE General Test or MAT, letters of recommendation, interviews, goals statement, American Sign Language proficiency interview, written English competency. Additional exam requirements/recommendations for international students: Required—TOEFL. *Application deadline:* For fall admission, 2/15 for domestic students. Applications are processed on a rolling basis. Application fee: $75. Electronic applications accepted. *Expenses: Tuition, area resident:* Full-time $16,596; part-time $922 per credit hour. *International tuition:* $33,192 full-time. *Required fees:* $3047; $263 per semester. *Financial support:* In 2015–16, 229 students received support. Fellowships, research assistantships, teaching assistantships, career-related internships or fieldwork, Federal Work-Study, scholarships/grants, tuition waivers (partial), and unspecified assistantships available. Support available to part-time students. Financial award application deadline: 7/1; financial award applicants required to submit FAFSA. *Faculty research:* Signing math dictionaries, telecommunications

access, cancer genetics, linguistics, visual language and visual learning, integrated quantum materials, deaf legal discourse, advance recruitment and retention in geosciences. *Unit head:* Dr. Gaurav Mathur, Dean, Graduate School and Continuing Studies, 202-250-2380, Fax: 202-651-5027, E-mail: gaurav.mathur@gallaudet.edu. *Application contact:* Wednesday Luria, Coordinator of Prospective Graduate Student Services, 202-651-5400, Fax: 202-651-5295, E-mail: graduate.school@gallaudet.edu.
Website: http://www.gallaudet.edu/x26696.xml

George Mason University, College of Humanities and Social Sciences, Department of Psychology, Fairfax, VA 22030. Offers applied developmental psychology (Certificate); cognitive and behavioral neuroscience (MA); industrial/organizational psychology (PhD). *Accreditation:* APA. *Faculty:* 41 full-time (21 women), 17 part-time/adjunct (14 women). *Students:* 179 full-time (121 women), 46 part-time (24 women); includes 41 minority (8 Black or African American, non-Hispanic/Latino; 7 Asian, non-Hispanic/Latino; 19 Hispanic/Latino; 1 Native Hawaiian or other Pacific Islander, non-Hispanic/Latino; 6 Two or more races, non-Hispanic/Latino), 9 international. Average age 27. 814 applicants, 18% accepted, 72 enrolled. In 2015, 57 master's, 19 doctorates, 6 other advanced degrees awarded. *Degree requirements:* For master's, comprehensive exam, thesis (for biopsychology); for doctorate, comprehensive exam, thesis/dissertation, 2nd-year project. *Entrance requirements:* For master's, GRE, 2 official transcripts; goals statement; 15 undergraduate credits in concentration for which the applicant is applying; for doctorate, GRE, 3 letters of recommendation; resume; goals statement; minimum GPA of 3.0 overall for last 60 undergraduate credits, 3.25 in psychology courses; 15 undergraduate credits in concentration for which the applicant is applying; 2 official transcripts; for Certificate, GRE, 2 official transcripts; expanded goals statement; 3 letters of recommendation. Additional exam requirements/recommendations for international students: Required—TOEFL (minimum score 575 paper-based; 88 iBT), IELTS (minimum score 6.5), PTE (minimum score 59). Application fee: $75 ($80 for international students). Electronic applications accepted. *Financial support:* In 2015–16, 130 students received support, including 8 fellowships (averaging $10,437 per year), 65 research assistantships with tuition reimbursements available (averaging $11,768 per year), 76 teaching assistantships with tuition reimbursements available (averaging $6,537 per year); career-related internships or fieldwork, Federal Work-Study, scholarships/grants, tuition waivers (partial), unspecified assistantships, and health care benefits (for full-time research or teaching assistantship recipients) also available. Support available to part-time students. Financial award application deadline: 3/1; financial award applicants required to submit FAFSA. *Faculty research:* Applied developmental psychology, biopsychology, clinical psychology, human factors/applied cognition psychology, industrial/organizational psychology, school psychology. *Total annual research expenditures:* $5.6 million. *Unit head:* Reeshad Dalal, Department Chair, 703-993-9487, Fax: 703-993-1359, E-mail: rdalal@gmu.edu. *Application contact:* Debbie McCain Wesley, Graduate Program Coordinator, 703-993-1548, Fax: 703-993-1359, E-mail: dwesley@gmu.edu.
Website: http://psychology.gmu.edu

George Mason University, College of Science, Program in Neuroscience, Fairfax, VA 22030. Offers MAIS, PhD. *Faculty:* 27 full-time (9 women), 1 part-time/adjunct (0 women). *Students:* 13 full-time (4 women), 3 part-time (2 women); includes 2 minority (1 Asian, non-Hispanic/Latino; 1 Hispanic/Latino), 5 international. Average age 35. 16 applicants, 44% accepted. In 2015, 6 doctorates awarded. *Degree requirements:* For doctorate, comprehensive exam, thesis/dissertation, at least one publication in a refereed journal (print or press). *Entrance requirements:* For doctorate, GRE, bachelor's degree in related field with minimum GPA of 3.25; expanded goals statement; 2 copies of official transcripts; 3 letters of recommendation. Additional exam requirements/ recommendations for international students: Required—TOEFL (minimum score 575 paper-based; 88 iBT), IELTS (minimum score 6.5), PTE (minimum score 59). Application fee: $75 ($80 for international students). Electronic applications accepted. *Financial support:* In 2015–16, 18 students received support, including 4 fellowships (averaging $13,324 per year), 12 research assistantships with tuition reimbursements available (averaging $18,372 per year), 2 teaching assistantships with tuition reimbursements available (averaging $12,938 per year); career-related internships or fieldwork, Federal Work-Study, scholarships/grants, unspecified assistantships, and health care benefits (for full-time research or teaching assistantship recipients) also available. Support available to part-time students. Financial award application deadline: 3/1; financial award applicants required to submit FAFSA. *Faculty research:* Complexity of the human brain; research in behavior, anatomy, physiology, biochemistry; computational modeling, informatics. *Unit head:* James L. Olds, Director, 703-292-8254, Fax: 703-993-4325, E-mail: jolds@gmu.edu. *Application contact:* Avrama L. Blackwell, Director of PhD Program, 703-993-4381, Fax: 703-993-4325, E-mail: avrama@gmu.edu.
Website: http://neuroscience.gmu.edu/

Georgetown University, Graduate School of Arts and Sciences, Interdisciplinary Program in Neuroscience, Washington, DC 20057. Offers PhD, MD/PhD. *Degree requirements:* For doctorate, thesis/dissertation. *Entrance requirements:* For doctorate, GRE General Test. Additional exam requirements/recommendations for international students: Required—TOEFL.

Georgia State University, College of Arts and Sciences, Department of Psychology, Atlanta, GA 30302-3083. Offers clinical (PhD); cognitive sciences (PhD); community (PhD); developmental (PhD); neuropsychology and behavioral neuroscience (PhD). *Accreditation:* APA. *Faculty:* 17 full-time (16 women). *Students:* 116 full-time (94 women), 3 part-time (2 women); includes 29 minority (9 Black or African American, non-Hispanic/Latino; 11 Asian, non-Hispanic/Latino; 4 Hispanic/Latino; 5 Two or more races, non-Hispanic/Latino), 10 international. Average age 28. 513 applicants, 7% accepted, 20 enrolled. In 2015, 7 degrees awarded. *Degree requirements:* For doctorate, comprehensive exam, thesis/dissertation, residency year (for clinical only). *Entrance requirements:* For doctorate, GRE. Additional exam requirements/recommendations for international students: Required—TOEFL (minimum score 550 paper-based; 80 iBT). *Application deadline:* For fall admission, 12/1 for domestic and international students. Application fee: $50. Electronic applications accepted. *Expenses:* Tuition, state resident: full-time $6876; part-time $382 per credit hour. Tuition, nonresident: full-time $22,374; part-time $1243 per credit hour. *Required fees:* $2128; $2128 per term. $1064 per term. Part-time tuition and fees vary according to course load and program. *Financial support:* In 2015–16, fellowships with full tuition reimbursements (averaging $19,282 per year), research assistantships with full tuition reimbursements (averaging $5,173 per year), teaching assistantships with full tuition reimbursements (averaging $6,389 per year) were awarded; scholarships/grants, traineeships, health care benefits, and unspecified assistantships also available. Financial award applicants required to submit FAFSA. *Faculty research:* Clinical psychology, developmental psychology, community psychology, neuropsychology and behavioral neuroscience, cognitive sciences. *Unit head:* Dr. Lisa Armistead, Chair, 404-413-6205, Fax: 404-413-6207, E-mail: lparmistead@gsu.edu. *Application contact:* Dr. Lindsey Cohen, Director of Graduate Studies, 404-413-6263, Fax: 404-413-6207, E-mail: llcohen@gsu.edu.

Georgia State University, College of Arts and Sciences, Neuroscience Institute, Atlanta, GA 30302-3083. Offers PhD. *Faculty:* 18 full-time (7 women). *Students:* 51 full-time (27 women); includes 9 minority (1 Black or African American, non-Hispanic/Latino;

2 Asian, non-Hispanic/Latino; 2 Hispanic/Latino; 2 Native Hawaiian or other Pacific Islander, non-Hispanic/Latino; 2 Two or more races, non-Hispanic/Latino; 9 international. Average age 29. 53 applicants, 30% accepted, 11 enrolled. In 2015, 10 doctorates awarded. Terminal master's awarded for partial completion of doctoral program. *Degree requirements:* For doctorate, comprehensive exam, thesis/dissertation. *Entrance requirements:* For doctorate, GRE. Additional exam requirements/recommendations for international students: Required—TOEFL. *Application deadline:* For fall admission, 12/10 for domestic and international students. Application fee: $50. Electronic applications accepted. *Expenses:* Tuition, state resident: full-time $6876; part-time $382 per credit hour. Tuition, nonresident: full-time $22,374; part-time $1243 per credit hour. *Required fees:* $2128; $2128 per term. $1064 per term. Part-time tuition and fees vary according to course load and program. *Financial support:* In 2015–16, fellowships (averaging $22,000 per year), research assistantships (averaging $22,000 per year) were awarded. Financial award applicants required to submit FAFSA. *Faculty research:* Neuroendocrinology; computational neuroscience; brain plasticity; neuromodulation of social behavior; neurobiology of learning and memory, drugs of abuse, and motor and sensory systems. *Unit head:* Prof. Walter Wilczynski, Director, 404-413-6307, E-mail: wwilczynski@gsu.edu. *Application contact:* Dr. Laura L. Carruth, Director of Graduate Studies, 404-413-5340, E-mail: lcarruth@gsu.edu.
Website: http://www.neuroscience.gsu.edu/

The Graduate Center, City University of New York, Graduate Studies, Program in Psychology, New York, NY 10016-4039. Offers basic applied neurocognition (PhD); biopsychology (PhD); clinical psychology (PhD); developmental psychology (PhD); environmental psychology (PhD); experimental psychology (PhD); industrial psychology (PhD); learning processes (PhD); neuropsychology (PhD); psychology (PhD); social personality (PhD). *Degree requirements:* For doctorate, one foreign language, thesis/dissertation. *Entrance requirements:* For doctorate, GRE General Test. Additional exam requirements/recommendations for international students: Required—TOEFL. Electronic applications accepted.

Harvard University, Graduate School of Arts and Sciences, Program in Neuroscience, Boston, MA 02115. Offers neurobiology (PhD). *Degree requirements:* For doctorate, thesis/dissertation, qualifying exam. *Entrance requirements:* For doctorate, GRE General Test, GRE Subject Test. Additional exam requirements/recommendations for international students: Required—TOEFL. *Faculty research:* Relationship between diseases of the nervous system and basic science.

Icahn School of Medicine at Mount Sinai, Graduate School of Biomedical Sciences, New York, NY 10029-6504. Offers biomedical sciences (MS, PhD); clinical research education (MS, PhD); community medicine (MPH); genetic counseling (MS); neurosciences (PhD); MD/PhD. Terminal master's awarded for partial completion of doctoral program. *Degree requirements:* For master's, thesis; for doctorate, comprehensive exam, thesis/dissertation. *Entrance requirements:* For master's, GRE General Test; for doctorate, GRE General Test, GRE Subject Test, 3 years of college pre-med course work. Additional exam requirements/recommendations for international students: Required—TOEFL. Electronic applications accepted. *Faculty research:* Cancer, genetics and genomics, immunology, neuroscience, developmental and stem cell biology, translational research.

Illinois State University, Graduate School, College of Arts and Sciences, Department of Biological Sciences, Normal, IL 61790-2200. Offers animal behavior (MS); bacteriology (MS); biochemistry (MS); biological sciences (MS); biology (PhD); biophysics (MS); biotechnology (MS); botany (MS, PhD); cell biology (MS); conservation biology (MS); developmental biology (MS); ecology (MS, PhD); entomology (MS); evolutionary biology (MS); genetics (MS, PhD); immunology (MS); microbiology (MS, PhD); molecular biology (MS); molecular genetics (MS); neurobiology (MS); neuroscience (MS); parasitology (MS); physiology (MS, PhD); plant biology (MS); plant molecular biology (MS); plant sciences (MS); structural biology (MS); zoology (MS, PhD). *Program availability:* Part-time. *Degree requirements:* For master's, thesis or alternative; for doctorate, variable foreign language requirement, thesis/dissertation, 2 terms of residency. *Entrance requirements:* For master's, GRE General Test, minimum GPA of 2.6 in last 60 hours of course work; for doctorate, GRE General Test. *Application deadline:* Applications are processed on a rolling basis. Application fee: $40. *Financial support:* Research assistantships, teaching assistantships, Federal Work-Study, tuition waivers (full), and unspecified assistantships available. Financial award application deadline: 4/1. *Faculty research:* Redoc balance and drug development in schistosoma mansoni, control of the growth of listeria monocytogenes at low temperature, regulation of cell expansion and microtubule function by SPRI, CRUI: physiology and fitness consequences of different life history phenotypes. *Application contact:* Steven Juliano, Graduate Coordinator, E-mail: sajulian@ilstu.edu.
Website: http://www.bio.ilstu.edu/

Immaculata University, College of Graduate Studies, Department of Psychology, Immaculata, PA 19345. Offers clinical mental health counseling (MA); clinical psychology (Psy D); forensic psychology (Graduate Certificate); integrative psychotherapy (Graduate Certificate); neuropsychology (Graduate Certificate); psychodynamic psychotherapy (Graduate Certificate); psychological testing (Graduate Certificate); school counseling (MA, Graduate Certificate); school psychology (MA). *Accreditation:* APA. *Program availability:* Part-time, evening/weekend. Terminal master's awarded for partial completion of doctoral program. *Degree requirements:* For master's, comprehensive exam, thesis optional; for doctorate, comprehensive exam, thesis/dissertation. *Entrance requirements:* For master's, GRE General Test or MAT, minimum GPA of 3.0; for doctorate, GRE General Test or MAT, minimum GPA of 3.5. Additional exam requirements/recommendations for international students: Required—TOEFL, IELTS. Electronic applications accepted. *Faculty research:* Supervision ethics, psychology of teaching, gender.

Indiana University Bloomington, University Graduate School, College of Arts and Sciences, Department of Psychological and Brain Sciences, Bloomington, IN 47405. Offers clinical science (PhD); cognitive neuroscience (PhD); cognitive psychology (PhD); developmental psychology (PhD); methods of behavior (PhD); molecular systems neuroscience (PhD); social psychology (PhD). *Accreditation:* APA. *Degree requirements:* For doctorate, comprehensive exam, 90 credit hours, 2 advanced statistics/methods courses, 2 written research projects, the teaching of psychology course, teaching 1 semester of undergraduate methods course, qualifying examination, minor or a second major, first-year research seminar course, dissertation defense, written dissertation. *Entrance requirements:* For doctorate, GRE. Additional exam requirements/recommendations for international students: Required—TOEFL (minimum score 550 paper-based; 79 iBT). Electronic applications accepted. *Faculty research:* Clinical science, cognitive neuroscience, cognitive psychology, developmental psychology, mechanisms of behavior, molecular and systems neuroscience, social psychology.

Indiana University Bloomington, University Graduate School, College of Arts and Sciences, Program in Neuroscience, Bloomington, IN 47405. Offers PhD. *Degree requirements:* For doctorate, comprehensive exam, thesis/dissertation, qualifying exam. *Entrance requirements:* For doctorate, GRE, bachelor's degree. Additional exam requirements/recommendations for international students: Required—TOEFL.

Electronic applications accepted. *Faculty research:* Cellular and molecular neuroscience, cognitive neuroscience, developmental neuroscience, disorders of the nervous system, sensory and motor processes.

Iowa State University of Science and Technology, Program in Neuroscience, Ames, IA 50011. Offers MS, PhD. *Degree requirements:* For master's, thesis; for doctorate, thesis/dissertation. *Entrance requirements:* For master's and doctorate, GRE General Test, resume. Additional exam requirements/recommendations for international students: Required—TOEFL (minimum score 580 paper-based; 85 iBT), IELTS (minimum score 7). Electronic applications accepted. *Faculty research:* Behavioral pharmacology and immunology, developmental neurobiology, neuroendocrinology, neuroregulatory mechanisms at the cellular level, signal transduction in neurons.

Irell & Manella Graduate School of Biological Sciences, Graduate Program, Duarte, CA 91010. Offers brain metastatic cancer (PhD); cancer and stem cell metabolism (PhD); cancer biology (PhD); cancer biology and developmental therapeutics (PhD); cell biology (PhD); chemical biology (PhD); chromosomal break repair (PhD); diabetes and pancreatic progenitor cell biology (PhD); DNA repair and cancer biology (PhD); germline epigenetic remodeling and endocrine disruptors (PhD); hematology and hematopoietic cell transplantation (PhD); hematology and immunology (PhD); inflammation and cancer (PhD); micrornas and gene regulation in cardiovascular disease (PhD); mixed chimrism for reversal of autoimmunity (PhD); molecular and cellular biology (PhD); molecular biology and genetics (PhD); nanoparticle mediated twist1 silencing in metastatic cancer (PhD); neuro-oncology and stem cell biology (PhD); neuroscience (PhD); rna directed therapies for hiv-1 (PhD); small rna-induced transcriptional gene activation (PhD); stem cell regulation by the microenvironment (PhD); translational oncology and pharmaceutical sciences (PhD); tumor biology (PhD). *Faculty:* 70 full-time (18 women). *Students:* 75 full-time (40 women); includes 28 minority (2 Black or African American, non-Hispanic/Latino; 10 Asian, non-Hispanic/Latino; 10 Hispanic/Latino; 2 Native Hawaiian or other Pacific Islander, non-Hispanic/Latino; 4 Two or more races, non-Hispanic/Latino), 15 international. Average age 26. 197 applicants, 12% accepted, 19 enrolled. In 2015, 12 doctorates awarded. *Degree requirements:* For doctorate, comprehensive exam, thesis/dissertation, qualifying exams, two advanced courses. *Entrance requirements:* For doctorate, GRE General Test; GRE Subject Test (recommended), 2 years of course work in chemistry (general and organic); 1 year of course work each in biochemistry, general biology, and general physics; 2 semesters of course work in mathematics; significant research laboratory experience. Additional exam requirements/recommendations for international students: Required—TOEFL. *Application deadline:* For fall admission, 1/1 priority date for domestic and international students. Application fee: $0. Electronic applications accepted. Full-time tuition and fees vary according to class time, course level, course load, degree level, campus/location, program and student level. *Financial support:* In 2015–16, 12 students received support, including 35 fellowships with full tuition reimbursements available (averaging $32,000 per year); teaching assistantships, health care benefits, and tuition waivers (full) also available. Financial award applicants required to submit FAFSA. *Faculty research:* Cancer biology, diabetes, stem cell biology, neuroscience, immunology. *Unit head:* Dr. John J. Rossi, Dean, 877-715-GRAD, Fax: 626-471-3901, E-mail: gradschool@coh.org. *Application contact:* Dr. Kate Sleeth, Interim Associate Dean of Administration and Student Development, 626-218-1742, Fax: 626-471-3901, E-mail: gradschool@coh.org. Website: http://cityofhope.org/gradschool

See Display on page 66 and Close-Up on page 111.

Johns Hopkins University, School of Medicine, Graduate Programs in Medicine, Neuroscience Training Program, Baltimore, MD 21218. Offers PhD. *Degree requirements:* For doctorate, comprehensive exam, thesis/dissertation, thesis defense. *Entrance requirements:* For doctorate, GRE General Test, bachelor's degree in science or mathematics. Additional exam requirements/recommendations for international students: Required—TOEFL. Electronic applications accepted. *Faculty research:* Neurophysiology, neurochemistry, neuroanatomy, pharmacology, development.

Kent State University, College of Arts and Sciences, School of Biomedical Sciences, Kent, OH 44242-0001. Offers biological anthropology (PhD); cellular and molecular biology (PhD), including cellular biology and structures, molecular biology and genetics; neurosciences (PhD); pharmacology (MS); physiology (PhD). *Students:* 76 full-time (46 women), 1 (woman) part-time; includes 6 minority (1 Black or African American, non-Hispanic/Latino; 2 Asian, non-Hispanic/Latino; 1 Hispanic/Latino; 2 Two or more races, non-Hispanic/Latino), 28 international. Average age 29. 223 applicants, 13% accepted, 22 enrolled. In 2015, 5 master's, 7 doctorates awarded. Terminal master's awarded for partial completion of doctoral program. *Degree requirements:* For master's, thesis; for doctorate, thesis/dissertation, candidacy exam. *Entrance requirements:* For master's and doctorate, GRE General Test, minimum GPA of 3.0, transcript, goal statement, resume, 3 letters of recommendation. Additional exam requirements/recommendations for international students: Required—TOEFL (minimum score: paper-based 525, iBT 71), Michigan English Language Assessment Battery (minimum score of 75), IELTS (minimum score of 6.0), PTE Academic (minimum score of 48), or completion of ELS level 112 Intensive Program. *Application deadline:* For fall admission, 1/1 for domestic students. Application fee: $45 ($70 for international students). Electronic applications accepted. *Expenses:* Tuition, state resident: full-time $10,864; part-time $495 per credit hour. Tuition, nonresident: full-time $18,380; part-time $837 per credit hour. *Financial support:* In 2015–16, 76 students received support. Research assistantships with full tuition reimbursements available, teaching assistantships, career-related internships or fieldwork, Federal Work-Study, and unspecified assistantships available. Financial award application deadline: 1/1. *Unit head:* Dr. Eric Mintz, Director, 330-672-2263, E-mail: emintz@kent.edu. *Application contact:* 330-672-2263, Fax: 330-672-9391, E-mail: jwearden@kent.edu.
Website: http://www.kent.edu/biomedical/

Louisiana State University Health Sciences Center, School of Graduate Studies in New Orleans, Interdisciplinary Neuroscience Graduate Program, New Orleans, LA 70112-2223. Offers PhD, MD/PhD. *Faculty:* 16 full-time (5 women). *Students:* 5 full-time (1 woman); includes 1 minority (Hispanic/Latino), 4 international. Average age 26. 12 applicants, 17% accepted, 1 enrolled. In 2015, 5 doctorates awarded. *Degree requirements:* For doctorate, comprehensive exam, thesis/dissertation. *Entrance requirements:* For doctorate, GRE General Test, previous course work in chemistry, mathematics, physics, and computer science. Additional exam requirements/recommendations for international students: Recommended—TOEFL, IELTS. *Application deadline:* For fall admission, 4/1 for domestic and international students. Applications are processed on a rolling basis. Application fee: $30. *Financial support:* Unspecified assistantships available. Financial award application deadline: 8/1. *Faculty research:* Visual system, second messengers, drugs and behavior, signal transduction, plasticity and development. *Unit head:* Dr. Nicolas G. Bazan, Department Head, 504-599-0831, Fax: 504-568-5801. *Application contact:* Dr. Hamilton Farris, Graduate Coordinator, 504-568-4027, Fax: 504-599-0685, E-mail: hfarri@lsuhsc.edu.
Website: http://www.medschool.lsuhsc.edu/neuroscience/grad_program/

Loyola University Chicago, Graduate School, Integrated Program in Biomedical Sciences, Maywood, IL 60153. Offers biochemistry and molecular biology (MS, PhD); cell and molecular physiology (PhD); infectious disease and immunology (MS);

integrative cell biology (PhD); medical physiology (MS); microbiology and immunology (MS, PhD); molecular pharmacology and therapeutics (MS, PhD); neuroscience (MS, PhD). *Students:* 135 full-time (65 women), 1 part-time (0 women); includes 28 minority (5 Black or African American, non-Hispanic/Latino; 15 Asian, non-Hispanic/Latino; 6 Hispanic/Latino; 2 Two or more races, non-Hispanic/Latino), 16 international. Average age 28. 442 applicants, 23% accepted, 55 enrolled. In 2015, 40 master's, 17 doctorates awarded. *Expenses: Tuition, area resident:* Full-time $18,054; part-time $9027 per credit hour. *Required fees:* $832; $284 per credit hour. Part-time tuition and fees vary according to course load, degree level and program. *Unit head:* Dr. Samuel Attoh, Dean, 773-508-3459, Fax: 773-508-2460, E-mail: sattoh@luc.edu. *Application contact:* Ron Martin, Associate Director of Enrollment Management, 312-915-8950, Fax: 312-915-8905, E-mail: gradapp@luc.edu.
Website: http://ssom.luc.edu/graduate_school/degree-programs/ipbsphd/

Marquette University, Graduate School, College of Arts and Sciences, Department of Biology, Milwaukee, WI 53201-1881. Offers cell biology (MS, PhD); developmental biology (MS, PhD); ecology (MS, PhD); epithelial physiology (MS, PhD); genetics (MS, PhD); microbiology (MS, PhD); molecular biology (MS, PhD); muscle and exercise physiology (MS, PhD); neuroscience (PhD). *Faculty:* 22 full-time (7 women), 3 part-time/adjunct (2 women). *Students:* 28 full-time (11 women), 12 part-time (4 women); includes 4 minority (1 Asian, non-Hispanic/Latino; 1 Hispanic/Latino; 2 Two or more races, non-Hispanic/Latino), 11 international. Average age 27. 72 applicants, 28% accepted, 5 enrolled. In 2015, 2 master's, 4 doctorates awarded. Terminal master's awarded for partial completion of doctoral program. *Degree requirements:* For master's, comprehensive exam, thesis, 1 year of teaching experience or equivalent; for doctorate, thesis/dissertation, 1 year of teaching experience or equivalent, qualifying exam. *Entrance requirements:* For master's and doctorate, GRE General Test, GRE Subject Test, official transcripts from all current and previous colleges/universities except Marquette, statement of professional goals and aspirations, three letters of recommendation. Additional exam requirements/recommendations for international students: Required—TOEFL (minimum score 530 paper-based). *Application deadline:* For fall admission, 12/15 for domestic and international students. Application fee: $50. Electronic applications accepted. *Financial support:* In 2015–16, 39 students received support, including 6 fellowships (averaging $1,208 per year), 4 research assistantships with full tuition reimbursements available (averaging $21,750 per year), 29 teaching assistantships with full tuition reimbursements available (averaging $21,750 per year); scholarships/grants, health care benefits, tuition waivers (full and partial), and unspecified assistantships also available. Support available to part-time students. Financial award application deadline: 2/15. *Faculty research:* Neurobiology, neuroendocrinology, epithelial physiology, neuropeptide interactions, synaptic transmission. *Total annual research expenditures:* $1.2 million. *Unit head:* Dr. Ed Blumenthal, Chair, 414-288-1748. *Application contact:* Dr. Michael Schlappi, Recruiting Contact, 414-288-1467.
Website: http://www.marquette.edu/biology/

Massachusetts Institute of Technology, School of Science, Department of Brain and Cognitive Sciences, Cambridge, MA 02139. Offers cognitive science (PhD); neuroscience (PhD). *Faculty:* 36 full-time (14 women), 1 (woman) part-time/adjunct. *Students:* 107 full-time (35 women); includes 20 minority (3 Black or African American, non-Hispanic/Latino; 6 Asian, non-Hispanic/Latino; 8 Hispanic/Latino; 3 Two or more races, non-Hispanic/Latino), 37 international. Average age 28. 463 applicants, 9% accepted, 16 enrolled. In 2015, 11 doctorates awarded. *Degree requirements:* For doctorate, comprehensive exam, thesis/dissertation. *Entrance requirements:* For doctorate, GRE General Test. Additional exam requirements/recommendations for international students: Required—TOEFL (minimum score 577 paper-based; 90 iBT), IELTS (minimum score 7). *Application deadline:* For fall admission, 12/1 for domestic and international students. Application fee: $75. Electronic applications accepted. *Expenses: Tuition:* Full-time $46,400; part-time $725 per credit. One-time fee: $304 full-time. Full-time tuition and fees vary according to course load and program. *Financial support:* In 2015–16, 95 students received support, including 54 fellowships (averaging $39,200 per year), 47 research assistantships (averaging $43,900 per year), 6 teaching assistantships (averaging $39,600 per year); Federal Work-Study, institutionally sponsored loans, scholarships/grants, traineeships, health care benefits, and unspecified assistantships also available. Support available to part-time students. Financial award application deadline: 4/15; financial award applicants required to submit FAFSA. *Faculty research:* Vision, audition, and other perceptual systems: physiology and computation; learning, memory, and executive control: molecular and systems approaches; sensorimotor systems: physiology and computation; neural and cognitive development and plasticity; language and high-level cognition: learning, acquisition, and computation. *Total annual research expenditures:* $34.1 million. *Unit head:* Prof. James Dicarlo, Head, 617-253-5748, Fax: 617-258-9126, E-mail: bcs-info@mit.edu. *Application contact:* Academic Office, 617-253-7403, Fax: 617-253-9767, E-mail: bcs-admissions@mit.edu.
Website: http://bcs.mit.edu/

Mayo Graduate School, Graduate Programs in Biomedical Sciences, Program in Molecular Neuroscience, Rochester, MN 55905. Offers PhD. Program also offered in Jacksonville, FL. *Degree requirements:* For doctorate, oral defense of dissertation, qualifying oral and written exam. *Entrance requirements:* For doctorate, GRE, 1 year of chemistry, biology, calculus, and physics. Additional exam requirements/recommendations for international students: Required—TOEFL. Electronic applications accepted. *Faculty research:* Cholinergic receptor/Alzheimer's; molecular biology, channels, receptors, and mental disease; neuronal cytoskeleton; growth factors; gene regulation.

McGill University, Faculty of Graduate and Postdoctoral Studies, Faculty of Medicine, Department of Neurology and Neurosurgery, Montréal, QC H3A 2T5, Canada. Offers M Sc, PhD.

McMaster University, Faculty of Health Sciences and School of Graduate Studies, Program in Medical Sciences, Neurosciences and Behavioral Sciences Area, Hamilton, ON L8S 4M2, Canada. Offers M Sc, PhD, MD/PhD. *Degree requirements:* For master's, thesis; for doctorate, comprehensive exam, thesis/dissertation. *Entrance requirements:* For master's, honors B Sc, B+ average in related field; for doctorate, M Sc, minimum B+ average, students with proven research experience and an A average may be admitted with a B Sc degree. Additional exam requirements/recommendations for international students: Required—TOEFL (minimum score 580 paper-based).

Medical College of Wisconsin, Graduate School of Biomedical Sciences, Neuroscience Doctoral Program, Milwaukee, WI 53226-0509. Offers PhD, MD/PhD. *Degree requirements:* For doctorate, comprehensive exam, thesis/dissertation. *Entrance requirements:* For doctorate, GRE, official transcripts, three letters of recommendation. Additional exam requirements/recommendations for international students: Required—TOEFL. *Faculty research:* Neurobiology, development, neuroscience, teratology.

Medical University of South Carolina, College of Graduate Studies, Department of Neurosciences, Charleston, SC 29425. Offers MS, PhD, DMD/PhD, MD/PhD. Terminal master's awarded for partial completion of doctoral program. *Degree requirements:* For master's, thesis; for doctorate, thesis/dissertation, oral and written exams. *Entrance*

requirements: For master's, GRE General Test; for doctorate, GRE General Test, interview, minimum GPA of 3.0. Additional exam requirements/recommendations for international students: Required—TOEFL (minimum score 600 paper-based; 100 iBT). Electronic applications accepted. *Faculty research:* Addiction, aging, movement disorders, membrane physiology, neurotransmission and behavior.

Meharry Medical College, School of Graduate Studies, Program in Biomedical Sciences, Neuroscience Emphasis, Nashville, TN 37208-9989. Offers PhD, MD/PhD. *Degree requirements:* For doctorate, comprehensive exam, thesis/dissertation. *Entrance requirements:* For doctorate, GRE. *Application deadline:* For fall admission, 6/1 for domestic students. Applications are processed on a rolling basis. Application fee: $65. *Financial support:* Fellowships and institutionally sponsored loans available. Financial award application deadline: 4/15; financial award applicants required to submit FAFSA. *Faculty research:* Neurochemistry, pain, smooth muscle tone, HP axis and peptides neural plasticity.

Memorial University of Newfoundland, Faculty of Medicine and School of Graduate Studies, Graduate Programs in Medicine, Division of Biomedical Sciences, St. John's, NL A1C 5S7, Canada. Offers cancer (M Sc, PhD); cardiovascular (M Sc, PhD); immunology (M Sc, PhD); neuroscience (M Sc, PhD). *Program availability:* Part-time. *Degree requirements:* For master's, thesis; for doctorate, comprehensive exam, thesis/dissertation, oral defense of thesis. *Entrance requirements:* For master's, MD or B Sc; for doctorate, MD or M Sc. Additional exam requirements/recommendations for international students: Required—TOEFL. *Expenses: Tuition, area resident:* Full-time $2199 Canadian dollars. *International tuition:* $2859 Canadian dollars full-time. *Faculty research:* Neuroscience, immunology, cardiovascular, and cancer.

Michigan State University, The Graduate School, College of Natural Science, Program in Neuroscience, East Lansing, MI 48824. Offers MS, PhD. *Entrance requirements:* Additional exam requirements/recommendations for international students: Required—TOEFL. Electronic applications accepted.

Montana State University, The Graduate School, College of Letters and Science, Department of Cell Biology and Neuroscience, Bozeman, MT 59717. Offers biological sciences (PhD); neuroscience (MS, PhD). *Program availability:* Part-time. *Degree requirements:* For master's, comprehensive exam; for doctorate, comprehensive exam, thesis/dissertation. *Entrance requirements:* For master's and doctorate, GRE General Test. Additional exam requirements/recommendations for international students: Required—TOEFL (minimum score 550 paper-based). Electronic applications accepted. *Faculty research:* Development of the nervous system, neuronal mechanisms of visual perception, ion channel biophysics, mechanisms of sensory coding, neuroinformatics.

New York University, Graduate School of Arts and Science, Center for Neural Science, New York, NY 10012-1019. Offers PhD. *Degree requirements:* For doctorate, one foreign language, thesis/dissertation. *Entrance requirements:* For doctorate, GRE, interview. Additional exam requirements/recommendations for international students: Required—TOEFL. *Faculty research:* Systems and integrative neuroscience; combining biology, cognition, computation, and theory.

New York University, School of Medicine and Graduate School of Arts and Science, Sackler Institute of Graduate Biomedical Sciences, Program in Neuroscience and Physiology, New York, NY 10012-1019. Offers PhD. *Degree requirements:* For doctorate, one foreign language, comprehensive exam, thesis/dissertation, qualifying exam. *Faculty research:* Rhythms in neural networks, genetic basis of neural circuit formation and function, behavior and memory formation in mouse models of neurodevelopmental disorders.

Northwestern University, Feinberg School of Medicine, Department of Physical Therapy and Human Movement Sciences, Chicago, IL 60611-2814. Offers neuroscience (PhD), including movement and rehabilitation science; physical therapy (DPT); DPT/PhD. *Accreditation:* APTA. *Faculty:* 30 full-time, 26 part-time/adjunct. *Students:* 281 full-time (208 women); includes 56 minority (8 Black or African American, non-Hispanic/Latino; 1 American Indian or Alaska Native, non-Hispanic/Latino; 32 Asian, non-Hispanic/Latino; 12 Hispanic/Latino; 1 Native Hawaiian or other Pacific Islander, non-Hispanic/Latino; 2 Two or more races, non-Hispanic/Latino). Average age 25. 556 applicants, 34% accepted, 93 enrolled. *Degree requirements:* For doctorate, synthesis research project. *Entrance requirements:* For doctorate, GRE General Test (for DPT), baccalaureate degree with minimum GPA of 3.0 in required course work (DPT). Additional exam requirements/recommendations for international students: Required—TOEFL (minimum score 600 paper-based; 100 iBT). *Application deadline:* For fall admission, 10/3 for domestic and international students. Applications are processed on a rolling basis. Application fee: $50. Electronic applications accepted. *Expenses:* Contact institution. *Financial support:* Institutionally sponsored loans and scholarships/grants available. Financial award application deadline: 3/1; financial award applicants required to submit FAFSA. *Faculty research:* Motor control, robotics, neuromuscular imaging, student performance (academic/professional), clinical outcomes. *Unit head:* Dr. Julius P. A. Dewald, Professor and Chair, 312-908-8160, Fax: 312-908-0741. *Application contact:* Dr. Jane Sullivan, Associate Professor/Assistant Chair for Recruitment and Admissions, 312-908-8160, Fax: 312-908-0741, E-mail: dpt-admissions@northwestern.edu.
Website: http://www.feinberg.northwestern.edu/sites/pthms/

Northwestern University, The Graduate School, Interdepartmental Neuroscience Program, Evanston, IL 60208. Offers PhD. Admissions and degree offered through The Graduate School. *Degree requirements:* For doctorate, thesis/dissertation. *Entrance requirements:* For doctorate, GRE General Test. Additional exam requirements/recommendations for international students: Required—TOEFL. *Faculty research:* Circadian rhythms, synaptic neurotransmissions, cognitive neuroscience, sensory/motor systems, cell biology and structure/function, neurobiology of disease.

The Ohio State University, Graduate School, College of Arts and Sciences, Division of Natural and Mathematical Sciences, Neuroscience Graduate Studies Program, Columbus, OH 43210. Offers PhD. *Degree requirements:* For doctorate, comprehensive exam, thesis/dissertation. *Entrance requirements:* For doctorate, GRE General Test, GRE Subject Test in biology, psychology, biochemistry, or cell and molecular biology (recommended). Additional exam requirements/recommendations for international students: Required—TOEFL (minimum score 600 paper-based; 100 iBT); Recommended—IELTS (minimum score 8). Electronic applications accepted. *Faculty research:* Neurotrauma and disease, behavioral neuroscience, systems neuroscience, stress and neuroimmunology, molecular and cellular neuroscience.

The Ohio State University, Graduate School, College of Arts and Sciences, Division of Social and Behavioral Sciences, Department of Psychology, Columbus, OH 43210. Offers behavioral neuroscience (PhD); clinical psychology (PhD); cognitive psychology (PhD); developmental psychology (PhD); intellectual and developmental disabilities psychology (PhD); quantitative psychology (PhD); social psychology (PhD). *Accreditation:* APA. *Faculty:* 57. *Students:* 154 full-time (88 women); includes 27 minority (5 Black or African American, non-Hispanic/Latino; 2 American Indian or Alaska Native, non-Hispanic/Latino; 8 Asian, non-Hispanic/Latino; 10 Hispanic/Latino; 2 Two or more races, non-Hispanic/Latino), 29 international. Average age 27. In 2015, 22 doctorates awarded. *Degree requirements:* For doctorate, thesis/dissertation. *Entrance requirements:* For doctorate, GRE General Test. Additional exam requirements/

Neuroscience

recommendations for international students: Required—TOEFL (minimum score 600 paper-based; 100 iBT); Recommended—IELTS (minimum score 8). *Application deadline:* For fall admission, 12/1 for domestic and international students. Applications are processed on a rolling basis. Application fee: $60 ($70 for international students). Electronic applications accepted. *Financial support:* Fellowships with tuition reimbursements, research assistantships with tuition reimbursements, and teaching assistantships with tuition reimbursements available. *Unit head:* Dr. John Bruno, Chair, 614-292-3038, E-mail: bruno.1@osu.edu. *Application contact:* Graduate and Professional Admissions, 614-292-9444, Fax: 614-292-3895, E-mail: gpadmissions@osu.edu.
Website: http://www.psy.ohio-state.edu/

Ohio University, Graduate College, College of Arts and Sciences, Department of Biological Sciences, Athens, OH 45701-2979. Offers biological sciences (MS, PhD); cell biology and physiology (MS, PhD); ecology and evolutionary biology (MS, PhD); exercise physiology and muscle biology (MS, PhD); microbiology (MS, PhD); neuroscience (MS, PhD). Terminal master's awarded for partial completion of doctoral program. *Degree requirements:* For master's, comprehensive exam, thesis, 1 quarter of teaching experience; for doctorate, comprehensive exam, thesis/dissertation, 2 quarters of teaching experience. *Entrance requirements:* For master's, GRE General Test, names of three faculty members whose research interests most closely match the applicant's interest; for doctorate, GRE General Test, essay concerning prior training, research interest and career goals, plus names of three faculty members whose research interests most closely match the applicant's interest. Additional exam requirements/recommendations for international students: Required—TOEFL (minimum score 620 paper-based; 105 iBT) or IELTS (minimum score 7.5). Electronic applications accepted. *Faculty research:* Ecology and evolutionary biology, exercise physiology and muscle biology, neurobiology, cell biology, physiology.

Oregon Health & Science University, School of Medicine, Graduate Programs in Medicine, Department of Behavioral Neuroscience, Portland, OR 97239-3098. Offers PhD. *Faculty:* 21 full-time (7 women), 25 part-time/adjunct (9 women). *Students:* 28 full-time (18 women); includes 11 minority (1 Black or African American, non-Hispanic/Latino; 2 Asian, non-Hispanic/Latino; 8 Hispanic/Latino). Average age 28. 75 applicants, 13% accepted, 6 enrolled. In 2015, 6 doctorates awarded. Terminal master's awarded for partial completion of doctoral program. *Degree requirements:* For doctorate, comprehensive exam, thesis/dissertation, qualifying exam. *Entrance requirements:* For doctorate, GRE General Test (minimum scores: 153 Verbal/148 Quantitative/4.5 Analytical), undergraduate coursework in biopsychology and other basic science areas. Additional exam requirements/recommendations for international students: Required—IELTS or TOEFL. *Application deadline:* For fall admission, 12/1 for domestic and international students. Application fee: $70. Electronic applications accepted. *Financial support:* Fellowships, research assistantships, health care benefits, tuition waivers (full), and stipends (for PhD students) available. *Faculty research:* Behavioral neuroscience, behavioral genomics, biological basis of drug and alcohol abuse, cognitive neuroscience, neuropharmacology and neuroendocrinology. *Unit head:* Dr. Suzanne Mitchell, Program Director, 503-494-1650, E-mail: mitchesu@ohsu.edu. *Application contact:* Kris Thomason, Graduate Program Manager, 503-494-8464, E-mail: thomason@ohsu.edu.
Website: http://www.ohsu.edu/som-BehNeuro/

Oregon Health & Science University, School of Medicine, Graduate Programs in Medicine, Neuroscience Graduate Program, Portland, OR 97239-3098. Offers PhD. *Faculty:* 44 full-time (13 women), 105 part-time/adjunct (34 women). *Students:* 44 full-time (22 women); includes 5 minority (2 Asian, non-Hispanic/Latino; 2 Hispanic/Latino; 1 Two or more races, non-Hispanic/Latino), 3 international. Average age 28. 105 applicants, 19% accepted, 6 enrolled. Terminal master's awarded for partial completion of doctoral program. *Degree requirements:* For doctorate, comprehensive exam, thesis/dissertation, qualifying exam. *Entrance requirements:* For doctorate, GRE General Test (minimum scores: 153 Verbal/148 Quantitative/4.5 Analytical) or MCAT (for some programs). Additional exam requirements/recommendations for international students: Required—IELTS or TOEFL. *Application deadline:* For fall admission, 12/1 for domestic and international students. Application fee: $70. Electronic applications accepted. *Financial support:* Health care benefits and full tuition and stipends (for PhD students) available. *Faculty research:* Development, neurobiology of disease, molecular, systems, behavioral, cellular, biophysics of channels and transporters, gene regulation, neuronal signaling, synapses and circuits, sensory systems, neuroendocrinology, neurobiology of disease. *Unit head:* Dr. Gary Westbrook, Program Director, 503-494-6932, E-mail: ngp@ohsu.edu. *Application contact:* Liz Lawson-Weber, Program Coordinator, 503-494-6932, E-mail: ngp@ohsu.edu.
Website: http://www.ohsu.edu/ngp

Penn State Hershey Medical Center, College of Medicine, Graduate School Programs in the Biomedical Sciences, The Huck Institutes of the Life Sciences, Intercollege Graduate Program in Neuroscience, Hershey, PA 17033. Offers MS, PhD, MD/PhD. *Students:* 20 full-time (11 women); includes 1 minority (Black or African American, non-Hispanic/Latino), 3 international. 32 applicants, 16% accepted, 4 enrolled. Terminal master's awarded for partial completion of doctoral program. *Degree requirements:* For master's, thesis or alternative; for doctorate, comprehensive exam, thesis/dissertation, oral exam. *Entrance requirements:* For master's, GRE General Test; for doctorate, GRE General Test, minimum GPA of 3.0. Additional exam requirements/recommendations for international students: Required—TOEFL (minimum score 500 paper-based). *Application deadline:* For fall admission, 12/31 for domestic and international students. Applications are processed on a rolling basis. Application fee: $65. Electronic applications accepted. *Financial support:* In 2015–16, research assistantships with full tuition reimbursements (averaging $26,196 per year) were awarded; fellowships with full tuition reimbursements, career-related internships or fieldwork, institutionally sponsored loans, scholarships/grants, health care benefits, and unspecified assistantships also available. Financial award applicants required to submit FAFSA. *Faculty research:* Behavioral neuroscience, growth factors and neuropeptides, molecular neurobiology and neurogenetics, neuronal aging and brain metabolism, neuronal and glial development. *Unit head:* Dr. Colin Barnstable, Program Director, 717-531-8982, Fax: 717-531-0786, E-mail: neuro-grad-hmc@psu.edu. *Application contact:* Kathy Shuey, Program Assistant, 717-531-8982, Fax: 717-531-0786, E-mail: neuro-grad-hmc@psu.edu.
Website: http://www2.med.psu.edu/neurograd/

Princeton University, Graduate School, Department of Psychology, Princeton, NJ 08544 1019. Offers neuroscience (PhD); psychology (PhD). *Degree requirements:* For doctorate, thesis/dissertation. *Entrance requirements:* For doctorate, GRE General Test, GRE Subject Test. Additional exam requirements/recommendations for international students: Required—TOEFL (minimum score 550 paper-based). Electronic applications accepted.

Princeton University, Princeton Neuroscience Institute, Princeton, NJ 08544-1019. Offers PhD. Electronic applications accepted.

Purdue University, College of Pharmacy and Pharmacal Sciences and Graduate School, Graduate Programs in Pharmacy and Pharmacal Sciences, Department of Medicinal Chemistry and Molecular Pharmacology, West Lafayette, IN 47907. Offers

biophysical and computational chemistry (PhD); cancer research (PhD); immunology and infectious disease (PhD); medicinal biochemistry and molecular biology (PhD); medicinal chemistry and chemical biology (PhD); molecular pharmacology (PhD); neuropharmacology, neurodegeneration, and neurotoxicity (PhD); systems biology and functional genomics (PhD). *Degree requirements:* For doctorate, thesis/dissertation. *Entrance requirements:* For doctorate, GRE General Test; GRE Subject Test in biology, biochemistry, and chemistry (recommended), minimum undergraduate GPA of 3.0. Additional exam requirements/recommendations for international students: Required—TOEFL (minimum score 550 paper-based; 77 iBT); Recommended—TWE. Electronic applications accepted. *Faculty research:* Drug design and development, cancer research, drug synthesis and analysis, chemical pharmacology, environmental toxicology.

Purdue University, Graduate School, College of Health and Human Sciences, Department of Psychological Sciences, West Lafayette, IN 47907. Offers behavioral neuroscience (PhD); clinical psychology (PhD); cognitive psychology (PhD); industrial/organizational psychology (PhD); mathematical and computational cognitive science (PhD). *Accreditation:* APA. Terminal master's awarded for partial completion of doctoral program. *Degree requirements:* For doctorate, thesis/dissertation. *Entrance requirements:* For doctorate, GRE General Test, minimum undergraduate GPA of 3.0 or equivalent. Additional exam requirements/recommendations for international students: Required—TOEFL (minimum score 550 paper-based; 77 iBT); Recommended—TWE. Electronic applications accepted. *Faculty research:* Career development of women in science, development of friendships during childhood and adolescence, social competence, human information processing.

Purdue University, Graduate School, PULSe - Purdue University Life Sciences Program, West Lafayette, IN 47907. Offers biomolecular structure and biophysics (PhD); biotechnology (PhD); chemical biology (PhD); chromatin and regulation of gene expression (PhD); integrative neuroscience (PhD); integrative plant sciences (PhD); membrane biology (PhD); microbiology (PhD); molecular evolutionary and cancer biology (PhD); molecular evolutionary genetics (PhD); molecular virology (PhD). *Entrance requirements:* For doctorate, GRE, minimum undergraduate GPA of 3.0. Additional exam requirements/recommendations for international students: Required—TOEFL (minimum score 550 paper-based; 77 iBT). Electronic applications accepted.

Queens College of the City University of New York, Mathematics and Natural Sciences Division, Department of Psychology, Flushing, NY 11367-1597. Offers applied behavior analysis (MA, AC); behavioral neuroscience (MA); psychology (MA). *Program availability:* Part-time. *Faculty:* 29 full-time (17 women), 58 part-time/adjunct (44 women). *Students:* 9 full-time (6 women), 111 part-time (92 women); includes 41 minority (10 Black or African American, non-Hispanic/Latino; 1 American Indian or Alaska Native, non-Hispanic/Latino; 7 Asian, non-Hispanic/Latino; 23 Hispanic/Latino), 2 international. Average age 28. 173 applicants, 51% accepted, 59 enrolled. In 2015, 20 master's awarded. *Degree requirements:* For master's, comprehensive exam, thesis or alternative. *Entrance requirements:* For master's, minimum GPA of 3.0. Additional exam requirements/recommendations for international students: Required—TOEFL, IELTS. *Application deadline:* For fall admission, 4/1 for domestic students; for spring admission, 11/1 for domestic students. Applications are processed on a rolling basis. Application fee: $125. Electronic applications accepted. *Expenses:* Tuition, state resident: full-time $5065; part-time $425 per credit. Tuition, nonresident: part-time $780 per credit. *Required fees:* $522. Part-time tuition and fees vary according to course load and program. *Financial support:* Career-related internships or fieldwork, institutionally sponsored loans, and unspecified assistantships available. Financial award application deadline: 4/1; financial award applicants required to submit FAFSA. *Unit head:* Dr. Jeffery Halperin, Acting Chair, 718-997-3200, E-mail: jeffery.halperin@qc.cuny.edu.

Queen's University at Kingston, School of Graduate Studies, Faculty of Health Sciences, Department of Anatomy and Cell Biology, Kingston, ON K7L 3N6, Canada. Offers biology of reproduction (M Sc, PhD); cancer (M Sc, PhD); cardiovascular pathophysiology (M Sc, PhD); cell and molecular biology (M Sc, PhD); drug metabolism (M Sc, PhD); endocrinology (M Sc, PhD); motor control (M Sc, PhD); neural regeneration (M Sc, PhD); neurophysiology (M Sc, PhD). *Program availability:* Part-time. *Degree requirements:* For master's, thesis; for doctorate, one foreign language, comprehensive exam, thesis/dissertation. *Entrance requirements:* Additional exam requirements/recommendations for international students: Required—TOEFL. Electronic applications accepted. *Faculty research:* Human kinetics, neuroscience, reproductive biology, cardiovascular.

Rosalind Franklin University of Medicine and Science, School of Graduate and Postdoctoral Studies - Interdisciplinary Graduate Program in Biomedical Sciences, Department of Neuroscience, North Chicago, IL 60064-3095. Offers PhD, MD/PhD. *Degree requirements:* For doctorate, comprehensive exam, thesis/dissertation, original research project. *Entrance requirements:* For doctorate, GRE General Test. Additional exam requirements/recommendations for international students: Required—TOEFL, TWE.

Rush University, Graduate College, Division of Neuroscience, Chicago, IL 60612-3832. Offers MS, PhD. Terminal master's awarded for partial completion of doctoral program. *Degree requirements:* For master's, thesis; for doctorate, thesis/dissertation. *Entrance requirements:* For master's and doctorate, GRE General Test. Additional exam requirements/recommendations for international students: Required—TOEFL. Electronic applications accepted. *Faculty research:* Neurodegenerative disorders, neurobiology of memory, aging, pathology and genetics of Alzheimer's disease.

Rutgers University–Newark, Graduate School of Biomedical Sciences, Program in Integrative Neuroscience, Newark, NJ 07107. Offers PhD. Program offered jointly with Rutgers, The State University of New Jersey, New Brunswick. *Degree requirements:* For doctorate, thesis/dissertation, qualifying exam. *Entrance requirements:* For doctorate, GRE General Test, minimum GPA of 3.5. Additional exam requirements/recommendations for international students: Required—TOEFL. Electronic applications accepted.

Rutgers University–Newark, Graduate School, Program in Psychology, Newark, NJ 07102. Offers cognitive neuroscience (PhD); cognitive science (PhD); perception (PhD); psychobiology (PhD); social cognition (PhD). *Degree requirements:* For doctorate, comprehensive exam, thesis/dissertation. *Entrance requirements:* For doctorate, GRE General Test, GRE Subject Test, minimum undergraduate B average. Electronic applications accepted. *Faculty research:* Visual perception (luminance, motion), neuroendocrine mechanisms in behavior (reproduction, pain), attachment theory, connectionist modeling of cognition.

Rutgers University–New Brunswick, Graduate School-New Brunswick, Program in Endocrinology and Animal Biosciences, Piscataway, NJ 08854-8097. Offers MS, PhD. Terminal master's awarded for partial completion of doctoral program. *Degree requirements:* For master's, thesis; for doctorate, comprehensive exam, thesis/dissertation. *Entrance requirements:* For master's and doctorate, GRE General Test. Additional exam requirements/recommendations for international students: Required—TOEFL. Electronic applications accepted. *Faculty research:* Comparative and behavioral endocrinology, epigenetic regulation of the endocrine system, exercise physiology and immunology, fetal and neonatal developmental programming, mammary gland biology and breast cancer, neuroendocrinology and alcohol studies, reproductive and developmental toxicology.

Rutgers University–New Brunswick, Graduate School of Biomedical Sciences, Program in Neuroscience, Piscataway, NJ 08854-5635. Offers MS, PhD, MD/PhD. *Degree requirements:* For master's, thesis, qualifying exam; for doctorate, thesis/dissertation, qualifying exam. *Entrance requirements:* Additional exam requirements/recommendations for international students: Required—TOEFL. Electronic applications accepted.

Seton Hall University, College of Arts and Sciences, Department of Biological Sciences, South Orange, NJ 07079-2697. Offers biology (MS); biology/business administration (MS); microbiology (MS); molecular bioscience (PhD); molecular bioscience/neuroscience (PhD). *Program availability:* Part-time, evening/weekend. *Degree requirements:* For master's, thesis optional; for doctorate, comprehensive exam, thesis/dissertation. *Entrance requirements:* For master's, GRE or undergraduate degree (BS in biological sciences) with minimum GPA of 3.0 from accredited U.S. institution; for doctorate, GRE. Additional exam requirements/recommendations for international students: Required—TOEFL. Electronic applications accepted. *Faculty research:* Neurobiology, genetics, immunology, molecular biology, cellular physiology, toxicology, microbiology, bioinformatics.

State University of New York Downstate Medical Center, School of Graduate Studies, Program in Neural and Behavioral Science, Brooklyn, NY 11203-2098. Offers PhD, MD/PhD. *Degree requirements:* For doctorate, comprehensive exam, thesis/dissertation. *Entrance requirements:* For doctorate, GRE. Additional exam requirements/recommendations for international students: Recommended—TOEFL. *Faculty research:* Molecular neuroscience, cellular neuroscience, systems neuroscience, behavioral neuroscience, behavior.

State University of New York Upstate Medical University, College of Graduate Studies, Program in Neuroscience, Syracuse, NY 13210-2334. Offers PhD. *Degree requirements:* For doctorate, comprehensive exam, thesis/dissertation. *Entrance requirements:* For doctorate, GRE General Test, telephone interview. Additional exam requirements/recommendations for international students: Required—TOEFL. Electronic applications accepted. *Faculty research:* Cancer, disorders of the nervous system, infectious diseases, diabetes/metabolic disorders/cardiovascular diseases.

Stony Brook University, State University of New York, Graduate School, College of Arts and Sciences, Department of Neurobiology and Behavior, Stony Brook, NY 11794. Offers neuroscience (MS, PhD). *Faculty:* 17 full-time (4 women), 2 part-time/adjunct (0 women). *Students:* 32 full-time (15 women); includes 10 minority (3 Black or African American, non-Hispanic/Latino; 2 Asian, non-Hispanic/Latino; 3 Hispanic/Latino; 2 Two or more races, non-Hispanic/Latino), 8 international. Average age 28. 97 applicants, 12% accepted, 4 enrolled. In 2015, 6 doctorates awarded. *Degree requirements:* For doctorate, comprehensive exam, thesis/dissertation, teaching experience. *Entrance requirements:* For doctorate, GRE General Test, GRE Subject Test, minimum GPA of 3.0. Additional exam requirements/recommendations for international students: Required—TOEFL (minimum score 90 iBT). *Application deadline:* For fall admission, 1/15 for domestic students; for spring admission, 10/1 for domestic students. Application fee: $100. *Expenses:* $12,421 full-time resident tuition and fees, $453 per credit hour; $23,761 full-time nonresident tuition and fees, $925 per credit hour. *Financial support:* In 2015–16, 7 fellowships, 9 research assistantships, 8 teaching assistantships were awarded; Federal Work-Study also available. *Faculty research:* Cerebral cortex, neurobiology, neurodegenerative diseases, brain, brain disorders, ion channels, synaptic transmission, neocortex, cell signaling, cerebral cortex. *Total annual research expenditures:* $4.5 million. *Unit head:* Dr. Lorna Role, Director, PhD Program, 631-632-8616, Fax: 631-632-6661, E-mail: lorna.role@stonybrook.edu. *Application contact:* Odalis Hernandez, Coordinator, 631-632-8078, Fax: 631-632-6661, E-mail: odalis.hernandez@stonybrook.edu.
Website: http://medicine.stonybrookmedicine.edu/neurobiology/

Stony Brook University, State University of New York, Graduate School, College of Arts and Sciences, Department of Psychology, Program in Integrative Neuroscience, Stony Brook, NY 11794. Offers PhD. *Students:* 14 full-time (10 women); includes 1 minority (Black or African American, non-Hispanic/Latino), 2 international. Average age 28. 26 applicants, 15% accepted, 3 enrolled. In 2015, 2 doctorates awarded. *Degree requirements:* For doctorate, thesis/dissertation. *Entrance requirements:* For doctorate, GRE General Test, GRE Subject Test. Additional exam requirements/recommendations for international students: Required—TOEFL (minimum score 90 iBT). *Application deadline:* For fall admission, 1/15 for domestic students; for spring admission, 10/1 for domestic students. Application fee: $100. *Expenses:* $12,421 per year full-time resident tuition and fees, $453 per credit hour; $23,761 per year full-time non-resident tuition and fees, $925 per credit hour. *Financial support:* In 2015–16, 13 teaching assistantships were awarded. *Unit head:* Dr. Arthur Samuel, Chair, 631-632-7808, Fax: 631-632-7876, E-mail: arthur.samuel@stonybrook.edu. *Application contact:* Marilynn Wollmuth, Coordinator, 631-632-7855, Fax: 631-632-7876, E-mail: marilyn.wollmuth@stonybrook.edu.
Website: http://www.stonybrook.edu/commcms/psychology/integrative_neuroscience/overview.html

Syracuse University, College of Arts and Sciences, Programs in Biology, Syracuse, NY 13244. Offers biology (MS, PhD), including biology (MS), neuroscience (PhD). *Program availability:* Part-time. *Students:* Average age 26. In 2015, 2 master's, 3 doctorates awarded. Terminal master's awarded for partial completion of doctoral program. *Degree requirements:* For master's, thesis; for doctorate, thesis/dissertation. *Entrance requirements:* For master's and doctorate, GRE General Test, GRE Subject Test (recommended), BS or BA, at least a minimal background in both physical and biological sciences, three letters of recommendation, personal statement, transcripts. Additional exam requirements/recommendations for international students: Required—TOEFL (minimum score 100 iBT). *Application deadline:* For fall admission, 12/15 priority date for domestic and international students. Application fee: $75. Electronic applications accepted. *Expenses: Tuition, area resident:* Full-time $25,974; part-time $1443 per credit hour. *Required fees:* $802; $50 per course. Tuition and fees vary according to course load and program. *Financial support:* Fellowships with full tuition reimbursements, research assistantships with tuition reimbursements, teaching assistantships with tuition reimbursements, and scholarships/grants available. Financial award application deadline: 1/1; financial award applicants required to submit FAFSA. *Faculty research:* Cell signaling, plant ecosystem ecology, aquatic ecology, genetics and molecular biology of color vision, ion transport by cell membranes. *Unit head:* Dr. Steve Dorus, Graduate Program Director, 315-443-7091, E-mail: biology@syr.edu. *Application contact:* Lynn Fall, Graduate Program Administrator, 315-443-9154, E-mail: biology@syr.edu.
Website: http://biology.syr.edu/

Teachers College, Columbia University, Department of Biobehavioral Sciences, New York, NY 10027-6696. Offers applied exercise physiology (Ed M, MA, Ed D); communication sciences and disorders (MS, Ed D, PhD); kinesiology (PhD); motor learning and control (Ed M, MA); motor learning/movement science (Ed D); neuroscience and education (MS); physical education (MA, Ed D). *Program availability:* Part-time, evening/weekend. *Students:* 121 full-time (103 women), 218 part-time (171 women); includes 157 minority (30 Black or African American, non-Hispanic/Latino; 58 Asian, non-Hispanic/Latino; 63 Hispanic/Latino; 6 Two or more races, non-Hispanic/Latino), 6 international. *Expenses: Tuition, area resident:* Part-time $1454 per credit. *Required fees:* $428 per semester. One-time fee: $475 full-time. Full-time tuition and fees vary according to course load. *Financial support:* Fellowships, teaching assistantships, career-related internships or fieldwork, Federal Work-Study, institutionally sponsored loans, traineeships, and tuition waivers (full and partial) available. Support available to part-time students. *Unit head:* Prof. Carol Garber, Chair, E-mail: garber@tc.columbia.edu. *Application contact:* David Estrella, Director of Admissions, E-mail: estrella@tc.columbia.edu.
Website: http://www.tc.columbia.edu/biobehavioral-sciences/

Texas Christian University, College of Science and Engineering, Department of Psychology, Fort Worth, TX 76129. Offers developmental trauma (MS); experimental psychology (MS, PhD), including behavioral neuroscience (MS), cognition (MS), learning (MS), social (MS). *Faculty:* 12 full-time (5 women), 2 part-time/adjunct (1 woman). *Students:* 26 full-time (17 women), 1 part-time; includes 2 minority (1 Hispanic/Latino; 1 Two or more races, non-Hispanic/Latino), 2 international. Average age 26. 35 applicants, 29% accepted, 9 enrolled. In 2015, 8 master's, 7 doctorates awarded. Terminal master's awarded for partial completion of doctoral program. *Degree requirements:* For master's, thesis; for doctorate, thesis/dissertation. *Entrance requirements:* For doctorate, GRE General Test. Additional exam requirements/recommendations for international students: Required—TOEFL. *Application deadline:* For fall admission, 2/1 for domestic and international students. Application fee: $60 ($0 for international students). Electronic applications accepted. *Expenses:* $27,000. *Financial support:* In 2015–16, 23 students received support, including 23 teaching assistantships with full tuition reimbursements available (averaging $19,750 per year); scholarships/grants also available. Financial award application deadline: 2/1; financial award applicants required to submit FAFSA. *Faculty research:* Neuroscience, human and animal learning, cognition, development, experimental social psychology. *Unit head:* Dr. Mauricio Papini, Chair, 817-257-7410, Fax: 817-257-7681, E-mail: m.papini@tcu.edu. *Application contact:* Cindy Hayes, Administrative Assistant, 817-257-7410, Fax: 817-257-7681, E-mail: c.hayes@tcu.edu.
Website: http://www.psy.tcu.edu/gradpro.html

Thomas Jefferson University, Jefferson College of Biomedical Sciences, PhD Program in Neuroscience, Philadelphia, PA 19107. Offers PhD. Offered jointly with the Farber Institute for Neuroscience. *Faculty:* 37 full-time (12 women). *Students:* 24 full-time (7 women); includes 3 minority (1 Black or African American, non-Hispanic/Latino; 2 Asian, non-Hispanic/Latino), 3 international. Average age 27. 40 applicants, 5% accepted, 2 enrolled. In 2015, 4 doctorates awarded. *Degree requirements:* For doctorate, comprehensive exam, thesis/dissertation. *Entrance requirements:* For doctorate, GRE General Test, strong background in the sciences, interview, previous research experience. Additional exam requirements/recommendations for international students: Required—TOEFL, IELTS (minimum score 7). *Application deadline:* For fall admission, 12/15 priority date for domestic and international students. Applications are processed on a rolling basis. Application fee: $50. Electronic applications accepted. *Financial support:* In 2015–16, 24 students received support, including 24 fellowships with full tuition reimbursements available (averaging $56,298 per year); institutionally sponsored loans, scholarships/grants, and stipends also available. Financial award application deadline: 5/1; financial award applicants required to submit FAFSA. *Unit head:* Dr. Melanie Elliott, Program Director, 215-955-3776, Fax: 215-503-9871, E-mail: melanie.elliott@jefferson.edu. *Application contact:* Marc E. Stearns, Director of Admissions and Recruitment, 215-503-4400, Fax: 215-503-3433, E-mail: jgsbs-info@jefferson.edu.
Website: http://www.jefferson.edu/university/biomedical-sciences/degrees-programs/phd-programs/neuroscience.html

Tufts University, Cummings School of Veterinary Medicine, North Grafton, MA 01536. Offers animals and public policy (MS); biomedical sciences (PhD), including digestive diseases, infectious diseases, neuroscience and reproductive biology, pathology; conservation medicine (MS); veterinary medicine (DVM); DVM/MPH; DVM/MS. *Accreditation:* AVMA (one or more programs are accredited). *Degree requirements:* For master's, thesis (for some programs); for doctorate, comprehensive exam, thesis/dissertation (for some programs). *Entrance requirements:* For master's and doctorate, GRE General Test. Additional exam requirements/recommendations for international students: Required—TOEFL or IELTS. Electronic applications accepted. *Expenses:* Contact institution. *Faculty research:* Oncology, veterinary ethics, international veterinary medicine, veterinary genomics, pathogenesis of Clostridium difficile, wildlife fertility control.

Tufts University, Sackler School of Graduate Biomedical Sciences, Neuroscience Program, Medford, MA 02155. Offers PhD. *Faculty:* 32 full-time (14 women). *Students:* 30 full-time (19 women); includes 8 minority (6 Black or African American, non-Hispanic/Latino; 5 Asian, non-Hispanic/Latino; 1 Hispanic/Latino; 1 Two or more races, non-Hispanic/Latino), 1 international. Average age 28. 113 applicants, 4% accepted, 2 enrolled. In 2015, 3 doctorates awarded. Terminal master's awarded for partial completion of doctoral program. *Degree requirements:* For doctorate, comprehensive exam, thesis/dissertation. *Entrance requirements:* For doctorate, GRE General Test, 3 letters of reference. Additional exam requirements/recommendations for international students: Required—TOEFL (minimum score 600 paper-based; 100 iBT). *Application deadline:* For fall admission, 12/15 priority date for domestic and international students. Application fee: $90. Electronic applications accepted. *Expenses: Tuition, area resident:* Full-time $48,412; part-time $1210 per credit hour. *Required fees:* $806. Full-time tuition and fees vary according to degree level, program and student level. Part-time tuition and fees vary according to course load. *Financial support:* In 2015–16, 30 students received support, including 30 research assistantships with full tuition reimbursements available (averaging $32,000 per year); health care benefits also available. *Faculty research:* Molecular, cellular, and systems analyses of synapses and circuits and their implications for neurological disease. *Unit head:* Dr. F. Rob Jackson, Director, 617-636-3796, E-mail: rob.jackson@tufts.edu. *Application contact:* Dr. Elizabeth Storrs, 617-636-6767, Fax: 617-636-0375, E-mail: sackler-school@tufts.edu.
Website: http://sackler.tufts.edu/Academics/Degree-Programs/Neuroscience

Tulane University, School of Medicine and School of Liberal Arts, Graduate Programs in Biomedical Sciences, Program in Neuroscience, New Orleans, LA 70118-5669. Offers MS, PhD, MD/PhD. MS and PhD offered through the Graduate School. *Degree requirements:* For doctorate, thesis/dissertation, qualifying exam. *Entrance requirements:* For doctorate, GRE General Test. Additional exam requirements/recommendations for international students: Required—TOEFL. Electronic applications accepted. *Expenses: Tuition, area resident:* Full-time $47,658; part-time $2648 per credit hour. *Required fees:* $1980; $44.50 per credit hour. $550 per term. Tuition and fees vary according to course load, degree level and program. *Faculty research:* Neuroendocrinology, ion channels, neuropeptides.

Tulane University, School of Science and Engineering, Neuroscience Program, New Orleans, LA 70118-5669. Offers MS, PhD. *Expenses: Tuition, area resident:* Full-time $47,658; part-time $2648 per credit hour. *Required fees:* $1980; $44.50 per credit hour.

$550 per term. Tuition and fees vary according to course load, degree level and program.

Uniformed Services University of the Health Sciences, F. Edward Hebert School of Medicine, Graduate Programs in the Biomedical Sciences and Public Health, Graduate Program in Neuroscience, Bethesda, MD 20814-4799. Offers PhD. *Faculty:* 54 full-time (18 women), 2 part-time/adjunct (1 woman). *Students:* 30 full-time (15 women); includes 7 minority (2 Black or African American, non-Hispanic/Latino; 5 Asian, non-Hispanic/Latino), 5 international. Average age 25. 34 applicants, 24% accepted, 5 enrolled. In 2015, 3 doctorates awarded. *Degree requirements:* For doctorate, comprehensive exam, thesis/dissertation, qualifying exams. *Entrance requirements:* For doctorate, GRE General Test, minimum GPA of 3.0; course work in biology, general chemistry, organic chemistry. *Application deadline:* For fall admission, 12/15 priority date for domestic students. Applications are processed on a rolling basis. Application fee: $0. Electronic applications accepted. *Financial support:* In 2015–16, fellowships with full tuition reimbursements (averaging $27,000 per year) were awarded; scholarships/grants, health care benefits, and tuition waivers (full) also available. *Faculty research:* Neuronal development and plasticity, molecular neurobiology, environmental adaptations, stress and injury. *Unit head:* Dr. Sharon Juliano, Director, 301-295-3673, Fax: 301-295-1996, E-mail: sharon.juliano@usuhs.edu. *Application contact:* Tina Finley, Administrative Assistant, 301-295-3642, Fax: 301-295-1996, E-mail: netina.finley@usuhs.edu.
Website: http://www.usuhs.edu/nes

See Display below and Close-Up on page 363.

Universidad de Iberoamerica, Graduate School, San Jose, Costa Rica. Offers clinical neuropsychology (PhD); clinical psychology (M Psych); educational psychology (M Psych); forensic psychology (M Psych); hospital management (MHA); intensive care nursing (MN); medicine (MD).

Université de Montréal, Faculty of Medicine, Department of Physiology, Program in Neurological Sciences, Montréal, QC H3C 3J7, Canada. Offers M Sc, PhD. Terminal master's awarded for partial completion of doctoral program. *Degree requirements:* For master's, thesis; for doctorate, thesis/dissertation, general exam. *Entrance requirements:* For master's and doctorate, proficiency in French, knowledge of English. Electronic applications accepted.

University at Albany, State University of New York, College of Arts and Sciences, Department of Psychology, Albany, NY 12222-0001. Offers behavioral neuroscience (PhD); clinical psychology (PhD); cognitive psychology (PhD); industrial/organizational psychology (MA, PhD); social-personality psychology (PhD). *Accreditation:* APA (one or more programs are accredited). *Degree requirements:* For doctorate, thesis/dissertation. *Entrance requirements:* For doctorate, GRE General Test, GRE Subject Test. Additional exam requirements/recommendations for international students: Required—TOEFL (minimum score 550 paper-based). Electronic applications accepted.

University at Albany, State University of New York, School of Public Health, Department of Biomedical Sciences, Program in Neuroscience, Albany, NY 12222-0001. Offers MS, PhD. *Degree requirements:* For master's, thesis; for doctorate, thesis/dissertation. *Entrance requirements:* For master's and doctorate, GRE General Test, GRE Subject Test.

University at Buffalo, the State University of New York, Graduate School, School of Medicine and Biomedical Sciences, Graduate Programs in Medicine and Biomedical Sciences, Neuroscience Program, Buffalo, NY 14260. Offers neuroscience (MS, PhD). *Faculty:* 88 full-time (24 women), 1 part-time/adjunct. *Students:* 36 full-time (17 women); includes 7 minority (3 Black or African American, non-Hispanic/Latino; 3 Asian, non-Hispanic/Latino; 1 Hispanic/Latino), 10 international. Average age 25. 34 applicants, 44% accepted, 6 enrolled. In 2015, 5 master's, 3 doctorates awarded. Terminal master's awarded for partial completion of doctoral program. *Degree requirements:* For master's, thesis (for some programs); for doctorate, comprehensive exam, thesis/dissertation. *Entrance requirements:* For master's, GRE General Test, 3 letters of recommendation, transcripts. Additional exam requirements/recommendations for international students: Required—TOEFL (minimum score 100 iBT), GRE. *Application deadline:* For fall admission, 7/15 priority date for domestic and international students. Applications are processed on a rolling basis. Application fee: $75. Electronic applications accepted. *Expenses:* Contact institution. *Financial support:* In 2015–16, 21 students received support, including 21 research assistantships with full tuition reimbursements available (averaging $26,000 per year); health care benefits also available. Financial award application deadline: 9/1. *Faculty research:* Neural degeneration and regeneration, synapse formation and elimination, glial cell biology, sensory systems, ion channels and receptors. *Total annual research expenditures:* $6 million. *Unit head:* Dr. Malcolm Slaughter, Professor, 716-829-3240, E-mail: mslaught@buffalo.edu. *Application contact:* Kristen Kahi, Program Administrator, 716-829-2419, E-mail: kkms@buffalo.edu. Website: http://wings.buffalo.edu/neuroscience/

The University of Alabama at Birmingham, College of Arts and Sciences, Program in Psychology, Birmingham, AL 35294. Offers behavioral neuroscience (PhD); lifespan developmental psychology (PhD); medical/clinical psychology (PhD); psychology (MA). *Accreditation:* APA (one or more programs are accredited). *Entrance requirements:* For master's and doctorate, GRE General Test, letters of recommendation. Electronic applications accepted. *Expenses:* Tuition, state resident: full-time $7340. Tuition, nonresident: full-time $16,628. Full-time tuition and fees vary according to course load and program. *Faculty research:* Biological basis of behavior structure, function of the nervous system.

University of Alaska Fairbanks, College of Natural Sciences and Mathematics, Department of Chemistry and Biochemistry, Fairbanks, AK 99775-6160. Offers biochemistry and neuroscience (PhD); chemistry (MA, MS), including chemistry (MS); environmental chemistry (PhD). *Program availability:* Part-time. *Faculty:* 10 full-time (3 women), 4 part-time (2 women); includes 3 minority (1 Asian, non-Hispanic/Latino; 2 Two or more races, non-Hispanic/Latino), 9 international. Average age 29. 27 applicants, 30% accepted, 7 enrolled. In 2015, 4 master's, 1 doctorate awarded. *Degree requirements:* For master's, comprehensive exam, thesis (for some programs), oral defense of project or thesis; for doctorate, comprehensive exam, thesis/dissertation, oral defense of dissertation. *Entrance requirements:* For master's, GRE General Test (for MS), bachelor's degree from accredited institution with minimum cumulative undergraduate and major GPA of 3.0; for doctorate, GRE General Test, minimum cumulative GPA of 3.0. Additional exam requirements/recommendations for international students: Required—TOEFL (minimum score 550 paper-based; 79 iBT), TWE. *Application deadline:* For fall admission, 6/1 for domestic students, 3/1 for international students; for spring admission, 10/15 for domestic students, 9/1 for international students. Applications are processed on a rolling basis. Application fee: $60. Electronic applications accepted. *Expenses:* Tuition, state resident: full-time $7614; part-time $423 per credit. Tuition, nonresident: full-time $15,552; part-time $864 per credit. *Required fees:* $38 per credit. $187 per semester. Tuition and fees vary according to course level, course load, program and reciprocity agreements. *Financial support:* In 2015–16, 14 research assistantships with full tuition reimbursements (averaging $16,421 per year), 14 teaching assistantships with full tuition reimbursements (averaging $17,322 per year) were awarded; fellowships with full tuition reimbursements, Federal Work-Study, scholarships/grants, health care benefits, and unspecified assistantships also available. Support available to part-time students. Financial award application deadline: 7/1; financial award applicants required to submit FAFSA. *Faculty research:* Atmospheric aerosols, cold adaptation, hibernation and

neuroprotection, liganogated ion channels, arctic contaminants. *Unit head:* Bill Simpson, Department Chair, 907-474-5510, Fax: 907-474-5640, E-mail: uaf-chem-biochem@alaska.edu. *Application contact:* Mary Kreta, Director of Admissions, 907-474-7500, Fax: 907-474-7097, E-mail: admissions@uaf.edu.
Website: http://www.uaf.edu/chem

University of Alberta, Faculty of Medicine and Dentistry and Faculty of Graduate Studies and Research, Graduate Programs in Medicine, Centre for Neuroscience, Edmonton, AB T6G 2E1, Canada. Offers M Sc, PhD. Terminal master's awarded for partial completion of doctoral program. *Degree requirements:* For master's, thesis; for doctorate, thesis/dissertation. *Entrance requirements:* For master's and doctorate, minimum GPA of 3.3. Additional exam requirements/recommendations for international students: Required—TOEFL (minimum score 600 paper-based). Electronic applications accepted. *Faculty research:* Sensory and motor mechanisms, neural growth and regeneration, molecular neurobiology, synaptic mechanisms, behavioral and psychiatric neuroscience.

The University of Arizona, Graduate Interdisciplinary Programs, Graduate Interdisciplinary Program in Neuroscience, Tucson, AZ 85719. Offers PhD. *Degree requirements:* For doctorate, thesis/dissertation. *Entrance requirements:* For doctorate, GRE (minimum score 1100), minimum GPA of 3.5, 3 letters of recommendation. Additional exam requirements/recommendations for international students: Required—TOEFL (minimum score 550 paper-based; 79 iBT). *Application deadline:* For fall admission, 12/1 for domestic and international students. Application fee: $75. Electronic applications accepted. *Financial support:* Research assistantships, teaching assistantships, health care benefits, tuition waivers (full), and unspecified assistantships available. Financial award application deadline: 12/1. *Faculty research:* Cognitive neuroscience, developmental neurobiology, speech and hearing, motor control, insect neurobiology. *Unit head:* Dr. Alan Nighorn, Director, 520-621-1343, Fax: 520-621-8282, E-mail: nighorn@neurobio.arizona.edu. *Application contact:* Kristen Grabo, Graduate Coordinator, 520-621-8380, Fax: 520-626-2618, E-mail: nrsc@u.arizona.edu.
Website: http://www.neuroscience.arizona.edu/

The University of British Columbia, Faculty of Arts and Faculty of Graduate Studies, Department of Psychology, Vancouver, BC V6T 1Z4, Canada. Offers behavioral neuroscience (MA, PhD); clinical psychology (MA, PhD); cognitive science (MA, PhD); developmental psychology (MA, PhD); health psychology (MA, PhD); quantitative methods (MA, PhD); social/personality psychology (MA, PhD). *Accreditation:* APA (one or more programs are accredited). Terminal master's awarded for partial completion of doctoral program. *Degree requirements:* For master's, thesis; for doctorate, comprehensive exam, thesis/dissertation. *Entrance requirements:* For master's and doctorate, GRE General Test. Additional exam requirements/recommendations for international students: Required—TOEFL (minimum score 550 paper-based; 80 iBT). Electronic applications accepted. *Faculty research:* Clinical, developmental, social/personality, cognition, behavioral neuroscience.

University of Calgary, Cumming School of Medicine and Faculty of Graduate Studies, Department of Neuroscience, Calgary, AB T2N 1N4, Canada. Offers M Sc, PhD. *Degree requirements:* For master's, thesis, oral thesis exam; for doctorate, thesis/dissertation, candidacy exam, oral thesis exam. *Entrance requirements:* For master's and doctorate, minimum GPA of 3.2 during previous 2 years. Additional exam requirements/recommendations for international students: Required—TOEFL (minimum score 580 paper-based). Electronic applications accepted. *Faculty research:* Cellular pharmacology and neurotoxicology, developmental neurobiology, molecular basis of neurodegenerative diseases, neural systems, ion channels.

University of California, Berkeley, Graduate Division, Neuroscience Graduate Program, Berkeley, CA 94720-3370. Offers PhD. *Degree requirements:* For doctorate, qualifying exam, teaching, research thesis/dissertation. *Entrance requirements:* For doctorate, GRE General Test, minimum GPA of 3.0, 3 letters of recommendation, at least one year of laboratory experience. Additional exam requirements/recommendations for international students: Required—TOEFL or IELTS. Electronic applications accepted. *Faculty research:* Analysis of ion channels, signal transduction mechanisms, and gene regulation; development of neurons, synapses, and circuits; synapse function and plasticity; mechanisms of sensory processing; principles of function of cerebral cortex; neural basis for learning, attention, and sleep; neural basis for human emotion, language, motor control, and other high-level cognitive processes.

University of California, Davis, Graduate Studies, Graduate Group in Neuroscience, Davis, CA 95616. Offers PhD. *Degree requirements:* For doctorate, thesis/dissertation. *Entrance requirements:* For doctorate, GRE General Test, GRE Subject Test. Additional exam requirements/recommendations for international students: Required—TOEFL (minimum score 550 paper-based). Electronic applications accepted. *Faculty research:* Neuroethology, cognitive neurosciences, cortical neurophysics, cellular and molecular neurobiology.

University of California, Irvine, Francisco J. Ayala School of Biological Sciences, Interdepartmental Neuroscience Program, Irvine, CA 92697. Offers PhD. *Students:* 12 full-time (7 women); includes 4 minority (1 Asian, non-Hispanic/Latino; 2 Hispanic/Latino; 1 Two or more races, non-Hispanic/Latino), 2 international. Average age 24. 179 applicants, 15% accepted, 12 enrolled. *Application deadline:* For fall admission, 12/2 for domestic students. Application fee: $90 ($110 for international students). Electronic applications accepted. *Unit head:* Prof. Karina S. Cramer, Director, 949-824-4211, Fax: 949-824-2447, E-mail: cramerk@uci.edu. *Application contact:* Gary R. Roman, Program Administrator, 949-824-6226, Fax: 949-824-4150, E-mail: gary.roman@uci.edu.
Website: http://www.inp.uci.edu/

University of California, Los Angeles, David Geffen School of Medicine and Graduate Division, Graduate Programs in Medicine, Interdepartmental Program in Neuroscience, Los Angeles, CA 90095. Offers PhD. *Degree requirements:* For doctorate, thesis/dissertation, oral and written qualifying exams; 1 quarter of teaching experience. *Entrance requirements:* For doctorate, GRE General Test or MCAT, bachelor's degree; minimum undergraduate GPA of 3.0 (or its equivalent if letter grade system not used). Additional exam requirements/recommendations for international students: Required—TOEFL. Electronic applications accepted.

University of California, Riverside, Graduate Division, Program in Neuroscience, Riverside, CA 92521. Offers PhD. *Degree requirements:* For doctorate, comprehensive exam, thesis/dissertation, 2 quarters of teaching experience, qualifying exams. *Entrance requirements:* For doctorate, GRE General Test, minimum GPA of 3.25. Additional exam requirements/recommendations for international students: Required—TOEFL (minimum score 550 paper-based; 80 iBT); Recommended—IELTS. *Application deadline:* For fall admission, 1/5 priority date for domestic and international students. Application fee: $80 ($100 for international students). Electronic applications accepted. *Expenses:* Tuition, area resident: Full-time $16,665.50; part-time $11,055.54. Tuition, state resident: full-time $16,665.50; part-time $11,055.54. Tuition, nonresident: full-time $31,768. International tuition: $31,767.50 full-time. Required fees: $16,665.50; $11,055.54 per quarter. $3685.18 per quarter. Tuition and fees vary according to program. *Financial support:* Fellowships with full tuition reimbursements, research assistantships with full tuition reimbursements, teaching assistantships with full tuition reimbursements, institutionally sponsored loans, scholarships/grants, health care benefits, and tuition

waivers available. Financial award application deadline: 1/5; financial award applicants required to submit FAFSA. *Faculty research:* Cellular and molecular neuroscience, development and plasticity, systems neuroscience and behavior, computational neuroscience, cognitive neuroscience, medical neuroscience. *Unit head:* Dr. Michael Adams, Director, 951-827-4180, Fax: 951-827-3087, E-mail: michael.adams@ucr.edu. *Application contact:* Perla Fabelo.
Website: http://www.neuro.ucr.edu/

University of California, San Diego, School of Medicine and Graduate Division, Program in Neurosciences, La Jolla, CA 92093. Offers PhD. *Students:* 95 full-time (45 women); includes 34 minority (3 Black or African American, non-Hispanic/Latino; 2 American Indian or Alaska Native, non-Hispanic/Latino; 18 Asian, non-Hispanic/Latino; 11 Hispanic/Latino), 7 international. 585 applicants, 8% accepted, 16 enrolled. In 2015, 7 doctorates awarded. *Degree requirements:* For doctorate, comprehensive exam, thesis/dissertation, 1-quarter teaching assistantship. *Entrance requirements:* For doctorate, GRE General Test. Additional exam requirements/recommendations for international students: Required—TOEFL (minimum score 550 paper-based; 80 iBT), IELTS (minimum score 7). *Application deadline:* For fall admission, 12/1 for domestic students. Application fee: $90 ($110 for international students). Electronic applications accepted. *Expenses:* Tuition, state resident: full-time $11,220. Tuition, nonresident: full-time $26,322. Required fees: $1800. *Financial support:* Fellowships, research assistantships, teaching assistantships, scholarships/grants, traineeships, unspecified assistantships, and readerships available. Financial award application deadline: 1/1; financial award applicants required to submit FAFSA. *Faculty research:* Cellular and developmental; biochemistry and molecular; cognitive, behavioral and psychopharmacology; clinical; computational; systems. *Unit head:* Timothy Gentner, Chair, 858-822-6763, E-mail: tgentner@ucsd.edu. *Application contact:* Erin Gilbert, Graduate Coordinator, 858-534-3377, E-mail: neurograd@ucsd.edu.
Website: http://neurograd.ucsd.edu

University of California, San Francisco, Graduate Division, Program in Neuroscience, San Francisco, CA 94143. Offers PhD. *Degree requirements:* For doctorate, thesis/dissertation. *Entrance requirements:* For doctorate, GRE General Test or MCAT, official transcripts, two letters of recommendation. Additional exam requirements/recommendations for international students: Required—TOEFL. Electronic applications accepted. *Faculty research:* Molecular neurobiology, synaptic plasticity, mechanisms of motor learning.

University of California, Santa Barbara, Graduate Division, College of Letters and Sciences, Division of Mathematics, Life, and Physical Sciences, Interdepartmental Graduate Program in Dynamical Neuroscience, Santa Barbara, CA 93106-2014. Offers PhD. *Faculty:* 13 full-time (1 woman). *Students:* 6 full-time (3 women); includes 1 minority (American Indian or Alaska Native, non-Hispanic/Latino), 2 international. Average age 24. 17 applicants, 12% accepted, 2 enrolled. *Degree requirements:* For doctorate, comprehensive exam, thesis/dissertation. *Entrance requirements:* Additional exam requirements/recommendations for international students: Required—TOEFL. *Application deadline:* For winter admission, 1/5 for domestic and international students. Application fee: $90 ($110 for international students). Electronic applications accepted. *Financial support:* In 2015–16, 4 students received support, including fellowships (averaging $60,000 per year), research assistantships (averaging $25,000 per year). Financial award applicants required to submit FAFSA. *Faculty research:* Computational neuroscience, network science, computational vision, neuro imaging, signal processing. *Unit head:* Prof. Barry Giesbrecht, Department Chair, 805-893-7909, E-mail: giesbrecht@psych.ucsb.edu. *Application contact:* Graduate Admissions Coordinator, 805-893-2104, Fax: 805-893-8259, E-mail: gradadmissions@graddiv.ucsb.edu.
Website: http://www.dyns.ucsb.edu

University of Chicago, Division of the Biological Sciences, Committee on Computational Neuroscience, Chicago, IL 60637-1513. Offers PhD. *Students:* 26 full-time (4 women); includes 3 minority (1 Black or African American, non-Hispanic/Latino; 2 Asian, non-Hispanic/Latino), 6 international. Average age 28. 55 applicants, 27% accepted, 5 enrolled. In 2015, 3 doctorates awarded. *Degree requirements:* For doctorate, thesis/dissertation, ethics class, 2 teaching assistantships. *Entrance requirements:* For doctorate, GRE General Test. Additional exam requirements/recommendations for international students: Required—TOEFL (minimum score 600 paper-based; 104 iBT), IELTS (minimum score 7). *Application deadline:* For fall admission, 12/1 for domestic and international students. Application fee: $90. Electronic applications accepted. *Financial support:* In 2015–16, 21 students received support, including fellowships with tuition reimbursements available (averaging $29,781 per year), research assistantships with tuition reimbursements available (averaging $29,781 per year); institutionally sponsored loans, scholarships/grants, traineeships, and health care benefits also available. Financial award applicants required to submit FAFSA.
Website: http://neuroscience.uchicago.edu/?p-neuro/cns

University of Cincinnati, Graduate School, Interdisciplinary PhD Study Program in Neuroscience, Cincinnati, OH 45221. Offers PhD. *Degree requirements:* For doctorate, thesis/dissertation, qualifying exam. *Entrance requirements:* For doctorate, GRE General Test. Additional exam requirements/recommendations for international students: Required—TOEFL. Electronic applications accepted. *Faculty research:* Developmental neurobiology, membrane and channel biophysics, molecular neurobiology, neuroendocrinology, neuronal cell biology.

University of Colorado Denver, School of Medicine, Program in Neuroscience, Aurora, CO 80045. Offers PhD. *Students:* 33 full-time (16 women); includes 6 minority (2 Black or African American, non-Hispanic/Latino; 3 Hispanic/Latino; 1 Two or more races, non-Hispanic/Latino). Average age 28. 66 applicants, 8% accepted, 5 enrolled. In 2015, 6 doctorates awarded. *Degree requirements:* For doctorate, comprehensive exam, thesis/dissertation, structured class schedule each year paired with lab rotations. *Entrance requirements:* For doctorate, GRE, baccalaureate degree in a biological science, chemistry, physics or engineering (recommended); minimum GPA of 3.2. Additional exam requirements/recommendations for international students: Required—TOEFL (minimum score 550 paper-based; 80 iBT). *Application deadline:* For fall admission, 12/1 for domestic students, 11/1 priority date for international students. Application fee: $50 ($75 for international students). Electronic applications accepted. *Expenses:* Contact institution. *Financial support:* In 2015–16, 33 students received support. Fellowships, research assistantships, teaching assistantships, Federal Work-Study, institutionally sponsored loans, scholarships/grants, traineeships, health care benefits, tuition waivers (full), and unspecified assistantships available. Financial award application deadline: 3/15; financial award applicants required to submit FAFSA. *Faculty research:* Neurobiology of olfaction, ion channels, schizophrenia, spinal cord regeneration, neurotransplantation. *Unit head:* Dr. Wendy Macklin, Professor and Chair, 303-724-3426, Fax: 303-724-3420, E-mail: wendy.macklin@ucdenver.edu. *Application contact:* Deanne Sylvester, Program Administrator, 303-724-3120, Fax: 303-724-3121, E-mail: deanne.sylvester@ucdenver.edu.
Website: http://www.ucdenver.edu/academics/colleges/medicalschool/programs/Neuroscience/Pages/Neuroscience.aspx

University of Connecticut, Graduate School, College of Liberal Arts and Sciences, Department of Psychology, Storrs, CT 06269. Offers behavioral neuroscience (PhD); biopsychology (PhD); clinical psychology (MA, PhD); cognition and instruction (PhD);

Neuroscience

developmental psychology (MA, PhD); ecological psychology (PhD); experimental psychology (PhD); general psychology (MA, PhD); industrial/organizational psychology (PhD); language and cognition (PhD); neuroscience (PhD); social psychology (MA, PhD). *Accreditation:* APA. Terminal master's awarded for partial completion of doctoral program. *Degree requirements:* For master's, comprehensive exam; for doctorate, thesis/dissertation. *Entrance requirements:* For master's and doctorate, GRE General Test, GRE Subject Test. Additional exam requirements/recommendations for international students: Required—TOEFL (minimum score 550 paper-based). *Application deadline:* For fall admission, 2/1 priority date for domestic and international students; for spring admission, 11/1 for domestic students, 10/1 for international students. Applications are processed on a rolling basis. Application fee: $55. Electronic applications accepted. *Financial support:* Fellowships, research assistantships with full tuition reimbursements, teaching assistantships with full tuition reimbursements, career-related internships or fieldwork, Federal Work-Study, scholarships/grants, health care benefits, and unspecified assistantships available. Financial award application deadline: 2/1; financial award applicants required to submit FAFSA.
Website: http://www.psychology.uconn.edu/

University of Connecticut Health Center, Graduate School, Programs in Biomedical Sciences, Program in Neuroscience, Farmington, CT 06030. Offers PhD, DMD/PhD, MD/PhD. *Degree requirements:* For doctorate, comprehensive exam, thesis/dissertation. *Entrance requirements:* For doctorate, GRE General Test, interview (recommended). Additional exam requirements/recommendations for international students: Required—TOEFL (minimum score 600 paper-based). Electronic applications accepted. *Faculty research:* Molecular and systems neuroscience, neuroanatomy, neurophysiology, neurochemistry, neuropathology.

See Display below and Close-Up on page 365.

University of Delaware, College of Arts and Sciences, Department of Psychology, Newark, DE 19716. Offers behavioral neuroscience (PhD); clinical psychology (PhD); cognitive psychology (PhD); social psychology (PhD). *Accreditation:* APA. *Degree requirements:* For doctorate, thesis/dissertation. *Entrance requirements:* For doctorate, GRE General Test. Additional exam requirements/recommendations for international students: Required—TOEFL (minimum score 600 paper-based). Electronic applications accepted. *Faculty research:* Emotion development, neural and cognitive aspects of memory, neural control of feeding, intergroup relations, social cognition and communication.

University of Florida, College of Medicine and Graduate School, Interdisciplinary Program in Biomedical Sciences, Concentration in Neuroscience, Gainesville, FL 32611. Offers PhD. *Degree requirements:* For doctorate, thesis/dissertation. *Entrance requirements:* For doctorate, GRE General Test, minimum GPA of 3.0, biochemistry before enrollment. Additional exam requirements/recommendations for international students: Required—TOEFL. Electronic applications accepted. *Faculty research:* Neural injury and repair, neurophysiology, neurotoxicology, cellular and molecular neurobiology, neuroimmunology and endocrinology.

University of Georgia, Biomedical and Health Sciences Institute, Athens, GA 30602. Offers neuroscience (PhD). *Entrance requirements:* For doctorate, GRE, official transcripts, 3 letters of recommendation, statement of interest. Additional exam requirements/recommendations for international students: Required—TOEFL.

University of Guelph, Ontario Veterinary College and Graduate Studies, Graduate Programs in Veterinary Sciences, Department of Biomedical Sciences, Guelph, ON N1G 2W1, Canada. Offers morphology (M Sc, DV Sc, PhD); neuroscience (M Sc, DV Sc, PhD); pharmacology (M Sc, DV Sc, PhD); physiology (M Sc, DV Sc, PhD); toxicology (M Sc, DV Sc, PhD). *Program availability:* Part-time. *Degree requirements:*

For master's, thesis; for doctorate, comprehensive exam, thesis/dissertation. *Entrance requirements:* For master's, honors B Sc, minimum 75% average in last 20 courses; for doctorate, M Sc with thesis from accredited institution. Additional exam requirements/recommendations for international students: Required—TOEFL (minimum score 550 paper-based; 89 iBT). Electronic applications accepted. *Faculty research:* Cellular morphology; endocrine, vascular and reproductive physiology; clinical pharmacology; veterinary toxicology; developmental biology, neuroscience.

University of Guelph, Ontario Veterinary College and Graduate Studies, Graduate Programs in Veterinary Sciences, Department of Clinical Studies, Guelph, ON N1G 2W1, Canada. Offers anesthesiology (M Sc, DV Sc); cardiology (DV Sc, Diploma); clinical studies (Diploma); dermatology (M Sc); diagnostic imaging (M Sc, DV Sc); emergency/critical care (M Sc, DV Sc, Diploma); medicine (M Sc, DV Sc); neurology (M Sc, DV Sc); ophthalmology (M Sc, DV Sc); surgery (M Sc, DV Sc). *Degree requirements:* For master's, thesis; for doctorate, comprehensive exam, thesis/dissertation. *Entrance requirements:* Additional exam requirements/recommendations for international students: Required—TOEFL (minimum score 550 paper-based), IELTS (minimum score 6.5). Electronic applications accepted. *Faculty research:* Orthopedics, respirology, oncology, exercise physiology, cardiology.

University of Hartford, College of Arts and Sciences, Department of Biology, Program in Neuroscience, West Hartford, CT 06117-1599. Offers MS. *Program availability:* Part-time, evening/weekend. *Degree requirements:* For master's, comprehensive exam, thesis optional, oral exams. *Entrance requirements:* For master's, GRE General Test, GRE Subject Test, MCAT. Additional exam requirements/recommendations for international students: Required—TOEFL (minimum score 550 paper-based). Electronic applications accepted. *Faculty research:* Neurobiology of aging, central actions of neural steroids, neuroendocrine control of reproduction, retinopathies in sharks, plasticity in the central nervous system.

University of Idaho, College of Graduate Studies, College of Science, Department of Biological Sciences, Program in Neuroscience, Moscow, ID 83844. Offers MS, PhD. *Faculty:* 4 full-time. *Students:* 5 full-time. Average age 28. *Entrance requirements:* Additional exam requirements/recommendations for international students: Required—TOEFL. *Application deadline:* For fall admission, 2/15 for domestic students. Applications are processed on a rolling basis. Application fee: $60. Electronic applications accepted. *Expenses:* Tuition, state resident: full-time $6205; part-time $399 per credit hour. Tuition, nonresident: full-time $20,209; part-time $1177 per credit hour. *Required fees:* $2017; $58 per credit hour. Full-time tuition and fees vary according to course load and reciprocity. *Financial support:* Applicants required to submit FAFSA. *Unit head:* Dr. Steffen Werner, Director, 208-885-6010, Fax: 208-885-6198, E-mail: neuro@uidaho.edu. *Application contact:* Sean Scoggin, Graduate Recruitment Coordinator, 208-885-4723, Fax: 208-885-4406, E-mail: gadms@uidaho.edu.

University of Illinois at Chicago, Program in Neuroscience, Chicago, IL 60607. Offers cellular and systems neuroscience and cell biology (PhD); neuroscience (MS). *Faculty:* 1 (woman) full-time, 1 part-time/adjunct (0 women). *Students:* 17 full-time (11 women), 1 (woman) part-time; includes 4 minority (1 Asian, non-Hispanic/Latino; 2 Hispanic/Latino; 1 Two or more races, non-Hispanic/Latino), 1 international. Average age 28. 64 applicants, 6% accepted, 2 enrolled. In 2015, 1 master's, 4 doctorates awarded. *Expenses:* Tuition, state resident: full-time $11,480; part-time $3826 per credit. Tuition, nonresident: full-time $23,720; part-time $7906 per credit. *Required fees:* $1333 per semester. Part-time tuition and fees vary according to course load and program. *Unit head:* Dr. John Larson, Director of Graduate Studies, 312-996-7370, Fax: 312-423-3699, E-mail: uicneuroscience@uic.edu.
Website: http://www.uic.edu/depts/neurosci/

University of Illinois at Urbana–Champaign, Graduate College, College of Liberal Arts and Sciences, School of Molecular and Cellular Biology, Neuroscience Program, Champaign, IL 61820. Offers PhD.

The University of Iowa, Graduate College, Program in Neuroscience, Iowa City, IA 52242-1316. Offers PhD. *Degree requirements:* For doctorate, comprehensive exam, thesis/dissertation. *Entrance requirements:* For doctorate, GRE General Test, minimum GPA of 3.0. Additional exam requirements/recommendations for international students: Required—TOEFL (minimum score 600 paper-based; 100 iBT). Electronic applications accepted. *Faculty research:* Molecular, cellular, and developmental systems; behavioral neurosciences.

The University of Kansas, Graduate Studies, School of Pharmacy, Department of Pharmacology and Toxicology, Lawrence, KS 66045. Offers neurosciences (MS, PhD); pharmacology and toxicology (MS, PhD). *Students:* 34 full-time (19 women); includes 3 minority (1 Asian, non-Hispanic/Latino; 2 Hispanic/Latino), 15 international. Average age 25. 88 applicants, 14% accepted, 8 enrolled. In 2015, 5 doctorates awarded. Terminal master's awarded for partial completion of doctoral program. *Entrance requirements:* For master's and doctorate, GRE General Test, bachelor's degree in related field, 3 letters of recommendation, resume or curriculum vitae, official transcripts, 1-2 page personal statement. Additional exam requirements/recommendations for international students: Required—TOEFL. *Application deadline:* For fall admission, 1/1 priority date for domestic students, 1/15 priority date for international students. Application fee: $65 ($85 for international students). Electronic applications accepted. *Financial support:* Fellowships, research assistantships, and teaching assistantships available. Financial award application deadline: 2/1. *Faculty research:* Molecular neurobiology, gene regulation, neurotransmitter receptors, drug metabolism. *Unit head:* Nancy Muma, Chair, 785-864-4002, E-mail: nmuma@ku.edu. *Application contact:* Sheila Stice, Graduate Admissions Contact, 785-864-4002, E-mail: sstice@ku.edu.
Website: http://pharmtox.ku.edu/

The University of Kansas, Graduate Studies, School of Pharmacy, Program in Neurosciences, Lawrence, KS 66045. Offers MS, PhD. *Students:* 11 full-time (4 women); includes 2 minority (both Hispanic/Latino). Average age 26. 35 applicants, 9% accepted, 2 enrolled. In 2015, 3 doctorates awarded. *Entrance requirements:* For master's, GRE, BA or BS in neuroscience or a related study, three letters of recommendation, personal statement, minimum GPA of 3.0; for doctorate, GRE. Additional exam requirements/recommendations for international students: Required—TOEFL. *Application deadline:* For fall admission, 1/15 priority date for domestic and international students. Application fee: $65 ($85 for international students). Electronic applications accepted. *Financial support:* Fellowships, research assistantships, and teaching assistantships available. Financial award application deadline: 1/15. *Unit head:* Ruth Anne Atchley, Chair, 785-864-4131, E-mail: ratchley@ku.edu. *Application contact:* Susan D. Wakefield, Program Assistant, 785-864-7339, Fax: 785-864-5738, E-mail: swakefield@ku.edu.
Website: http://www.neuroscience.ku.edu/

The University of Kansas, University of Kansas Medical Center, School of Medicine, Neuroscience Graduate Program, Kansas City, KS 66160. Offers PhD, MD/PhD. *Students:* 7 full-time (3 women); includes 1 minority (Hispanic/Latino). Average age 26. In 2015, 2 doctorates awarded. Terminal master's awarded for partial completion of doctoral program. *Degree requirements:* For doctorate, comprehensive exam, thesis/dissertation. *Entrance requirements:* For doctorate, GRE. Additional exam requirements/recommendations for international students: Required—TOEFL or IELTS. Application fee: $60. Application fee is waived when completed online. *Financial support:* Fellowships with partial tuition reimbursements, research assistantships with full tuition reimbursements, and teaching assistantships with full tuition reimbursements available. Financial award application deadline: 3/1; financial award applicants required to submit FAFSA. *Unit head:* Dr. Doug Wright, Professor, Department of Anatomy and Cell Biology, 913-588-2713, Fax: 913-588-2710, E-mail: dwright@kumc.edu. *Application contact:* Marcia Jones, Director of Graduate Studies, 913-588-1238, Fax: 913-588-5242, E-mail: mjones@kumc.edu.
Website: http://www.kumc.edu/school-of-medicine/neuroscience.html

University of Lethbridge, School of Graduate Studies, Lethbridge, AB T1K 3M4, Canada. Offers addictions counseling (M Sc); agricultural biotechnology (M Sc); agricultural studies (M Sc, MA); anthropology (MA); archaeology (M Sc, MA); art (MA, MFA); biochemistry (M Sc); biological sciences (M Sc); biomolecular science (PhD); biosystems and biodiversity (PhD); Canadian studies (MA); chemistry (M Sc); computer science (M Sc); computer science and geographical information science (M Sc); counseling (MC); counseling psychology (M Ed); dramatic arts (MA); earth, space, and physical science (PhD); economics (MA); education (MA, PhD); educational leadership (M Ed); English (MA); environmental science (M Sc); evolution and behavior (PhD); exercise science (M Sc); French (MA); French/German (MA); French/Spanish (MA); general education (M Ed); geography (M Sc, MA); German (MA); health sciences (M Sc); individualized multidisciplinary (M Sc, MA); kinesiology (M Sc, MA); management (M Sc), including accounting, finance, human resource management and labor relations, information systems, international management, marketing, policy and strategy; mathematics (M Sc); music (M Mus, MA); Native American studies (MA); neuroscience (M Sc, PhD); new media (MA, MFA); nursing (M Sc, MN); philosophy (MA); physics (M Sc); political science (MA); psychology (M Sc, MA); religious studies (MA); sociology (MA); theatre and dramatic arts (MFA); theoretical and computational science (PhD); urban and regional studies (MA); women and gender studies (MA). *Program availability:* Part-time, evening/weekend. *Students:* 448 full-time (249 women), 110 part-time (64 women). Average age 32. 285 applicants, 36% accepted, 96 enrolled. In 2015, 154 master's, 11 doctorates awarded. *Degree requirements:* For master's, thesis (for some programs); for doctorate, comprehensive exam, thesis/dissertation. *Entrance requirements:* For master's, GMAT (for M Sc in management), bachelor's degree in related field, minimum GPA of 3.0 during previous 20 graded semester courses, 2 years' teaching or related experience (M Ed); for doctorate, master's degree, minimum graduate GPA of 3.5. Additional exam requirements/recommendations for international students: Required—TOEFL (minimum score 580 paper-based; 93 iBT). Application fee: $100 Canadian dollars ($140 Canadian dollars for international students). Electronic applications accepted. *Financial support:* Fellowships, research assistantships, teaching assistantships, scholarships/grants, health care benefits, and unspecified assistantships available. *Faculty research:* Movement and brain plasticity, gibberellin physiology, photosynthesis, carbon cycling, molecular properties of main-group ring components. *Unit head:* Kathleen Schrage, Manager, School of Graduate Studies, 403-329-2121, E-mail: schrage@uleth.ca. *Application contact:* School of Graduate Studies, 403-329-5194, E-mail: sgsinquiries@uleth.ca.
Website: http://www.uleth.ca/graduate-studies/

The University of Manchester, Faculty of Life Sciences, Manchester, United Kingdom. Offers adaptive organismal biology (M Phil, PhD); animal biology (M Phil, PhD); biochemistry (M Phil, PhD); bioinformatics (M Phil, PhD); biomolecular sciences (M Phil, PhD); biotechnology (M Phil, PhD); cell biology (M Phil, PhD); cell matrix research (M Phil, PhD); channels and transporters (M Phil, PhD); developmental biology (M Phil, PhD); Egyptology (M Phil, PhD); environmental biology (M Phil, PhD); evolutionary biology (M Phil, PhD); gene expression (M Phil, PhD); genetics (M Phil, PhD); history of

science, technology and medicine (M Phil, PhD); immunology (M Phil, PhD); integrative neurobiology and behavior (M Phil, PhD); membrane trafficking (M Phil, PhD); microbiology (M Phil, PhD); molecular and cellular neuroscience (M Phil, PhD); molecular biology (M Phil, PhD); molecular cancer studies (M Phil, PhD); neuroscience (M Phil, PhD); ophthalmology (M Phil, PhD); optometry (M Phil, PhD); organelle function (M Phil, PhD); pharmacology (M Phil, PhD); physiology (M Phil, PhD); plant sciences (M Phil, PhD); stem cell research (M Phil, PhD); structural biology (M Phil, PhD); systems neuroscience (M Phil, PhD); toxicology (M Phil, PhD).

University of Maryland, Baltimore, Graduate School, Graduate Program in Life Sciences, Program in Neuroscience, Baltimore, MD 21201. Offers PhD, MD/PhD. *Program availability:* Part-time. *Degree requirements:* For doctorate, comprehensive exam, thesis/dissertation. *Entrance requirements:* For doctorate, GRE General Test, minimum GPA of 3.0. Additional exam requirements/recommendations for international students: Required—TOEFL (minimum score 550 paper-based; 80 iBT); Recommended—IELTS (minimum score 7). Electronic applications accepted. Tuition and fees vary according to program. *Faculty research:* Molecular, biochemical, and cellular pharmacology; membrane biophysics; synaptology; developmental neurobiology.

University of Maryland, Baltimore County, The Graduate School, College of Natural and Mathematical Sciences, Department of Biological Sciences, Program in Neuroscience and Cognitive Sciences, Baltimore, MD 21250. Offers PhD. *Faculty:* 6 full-time (3 women). *Students:* 1 (woman) full-time; minority (Black or African American, non-Hispanic/Latino). Average age 24. 11 applicants, 9% accepted, 1 enrolled. In 2015, 1 doctorate awarded. *Degree requirements:* For doctorate, thesis/dissertation. *Entrance requirements:* For doctorate, GRE General Test, minimum GPA of 3.0. Additional exam requirements/recommendations for international students: Required—TOEFL (minimum score 80 iBT). *Application deadline:* For fall admission, 1/1 priority date for domestic and international students. Application fee: $50. Electronic applications accepted. *Expenses:* Tuition, state resident: full-time $12,816. Tuition, nonresident: full-time $19,710. *Financial support:* In 2015–16, 2 students received support, including 2 fellowships with full tuition reimbursements available (averaging $23,000 per year); health care benefits also available. *Unit head:* Dr. Michelle Starz-Gaiano, Graduate Program Director, 410-455-2217, Fax: 410-455-3875, E-mail: biograd@umbc.edu. *Application contact:* Dr. Michelle Starz-Gaiano, Director, 410-455-2217, Fax: 410-455-3875, E-mail: biograd@umbc.edu.
Website: http://biology.umbc.edu

University of Maryland, College Park, Academic Affairs, College of Behavioral and Social Sciences, Department of Hearing and Speech Sciences, College Park, MD 20742. Offers audiology (MA, AuD); hearing and speech sciences (Au D); language pathology (MA, PhD); neuroscience (PhD); speech (MA, PhD). *Accreditation:* ASHA (one or more programs are accredited). *Degree requirements:* For master's, thesis optional; for doctorate, thesis/dissertation, written and oral exams. *Entrance requirements:* For master's, GRE General Test, minimum GPA of 3.5, 3 letters of recommendation; for doctorate, GRE General Test, minimum GPA of 3.5. Additional exam requirements/recommendations for international students: Required—TOEFL. Electronic applications accepted. *Faculty research:* Speech perception, language acquisition, bilingualism, hearing loss.

University of Maryland, College Park, Academic Affairs, College of Behavioral and Social Sciences, Program in Neurosciences and Cognitive Sciences, College Park, MD 20742. Offers PhD. *Degree requirements:* For doctorate, comprehensive exam, thesis/dissertation. *Entrance requirements:* For doctorate, GRE General Test, 3 letters of recommendation. Additional exam requirements/recommendations for international students: Required—TOEFL. Electronic applications accepted. *Faculty research:* Molecular neurobiology, cognition, neural and behavioral systems language, memory, human development.

University of Massachusetts Amherst, Graduate School, Interdisciplinary Programs, Program in Neuroscience and Behavior, Amherst, MA 01003. Offers animal behavior and learning (PhD); molecular and cellular neuroscience (PhD); neural and behavioral development (PhD); neuroendocrinology (PhD); neuroscience and behavior (MS); sensorimotor, cognitive, and computational neuroscience (PhD). Terminal master's awarded for partial completion of doctoral program. *Degree requirements:* For master's, thesis or alternative; for doctorate, comprehensive exam, thesis/dissertation. *Entrance requirements:* For master's, GRE General Test; for doctorate, GRE General Test; GRE Subect Test in psychology, biology, or mathematics (recommended). Additional exam requirements/recommendations for international students: Required—TOEFL (minimum score 550 paper-based; 80 iBT), IELTS (minimum score 6.5). Electronic applications accepted.

University of Massachusetts Medical School, Graduate School of Biomedical Sciences, Worcester, MA 01655-0115. Offers biomedical sciences (PhD), including biochemistry and molecular pharmacology, bioinformatics and computational biology, cancer biology, cell biology, immunology and microbiology, interdisciplinary, neuroscience, translational science; biomedical sciences (millennium program) (PhD); clinical and population health research (PhD); clinical investigation (MS). *Faculty:* 1,339 full-time (521 women), 301 part-time/adjunct (189 women). *Students:* 363 full-time (184 women); includes 58 minority (13 Black or African American, non-Hispanic/Latino; 30 Asian, non-Hispanic/Latino; 15 Hispanic/Latino), 141 international. Average age 29. 661 applicants, 26% accepted, 51 enrolled. In 2015, 10 master's, 58 doctorates awarded. Terminal master's awarded for partial completion of doctoral program. *Degree requirements:* For master's, comprehensive exam, thesis; for doctorate, comprehensive exam, thesis/dissertation. *Entrance requirements:* For master's, MD, PhD, DVM, or PharmD; for doctorate, GRE General Test, bachelor's degree. Additional exam requirements/recommendations for international students: Required—TOEFL (minimum score 100 iBT) or IELTS (minimum score 7.5). *Application deadline:* For fall admission, 12/15 for domestic and international students; for spring admission, 5/15 for domestic students. Application fee: $80. Electronic applications accepted. *Expenses:* $6,966 resident per year; $14,182 non-resident per year. *Financial support:* In 2015–16, 383 students received support, including research assistantships with full tuition reimbursements available (averaging $30,600 per year); scholarships/grants, health care benefits, tuition waivers (full), and unspecified assistantships also available. Financial award application deadline: 5/16. *Faculty research:* RNA interference, cell/molecular/developmental biology, bioinformatics, clinical/translational research, infectious disease. *Total annual research expenditures:* $250.3 million. *Unit head:* Dr. Anthony Carruthers, Dean, 508-856-4135, E-mail: anthony.carruthers@umassmed.edu. *Application contact:* Dr. Kendall Knight, Assistant Vice Provost for Admissions, 508-856-5628, Fax: 508-856-3659, E-mail: kendall.knight@umassmed.edu.
Website: http://www.umassmed.edu/gsbs/

University of Miami, Graduate School, College of Arts and Sciences, Department of Psychology, Coral Gables, FL 33124. Offers adult clinical (PhD); behavioral neuroscience (PhD); child clinical (PhD); developmental psychology (PhD); health clinical (PhD); psychology (MS). *Accreditation:* APA (one or more programs are accredited). *Degree requirements:* For doctorate, comprehensive exam, thesis/dissertation. *Entrance requirements:* For doctorate, GRE General Test, minimum GPA of 3.5. Additional exam requirements/recommendations for international students:

Neuroscience

Required—TOEFL. Electronic applications accepted. *Faculty research:* Behavioral factors in cardiovascular disease and cancer adult psychopathology, developmental disabilities, social and emotional development, mechanisms of coping.

University of Miami, Graduate School, Miller School of Medicine, Graduate Programs in Medicine, Neuroscience Program, Coral Gables, FL 33124. Offers PhD, MD/PhD. *Degree requirements:* For doctorate, thesis/dissertation, qualifying exam. *Entrance requirements:* For doctorate, GRE General Test. Additional exam requirements/recommendations for international students: Required—TOEFL (minimum score 550 paper-based). Electronic applications accepted. *Faculty research:* Cellular and molecular biology, transduction, nerve regeneration and embryonic development, membrane biophysics.

University of Michigan, Rackham Graduate School, College of Literature, Science, and the Arts, Department of Psychology, Ann Arbor, MI 48109. Offers biopsychology (PhD); clinical science (PhD); cognition and cognitive neuroscience (PhD); developmental psychology (PhD); personality and social contexts (PhD); social psychology (PhD). *Accreditation:* APA. *Faculty:* 57 full-time (27 women), 31 part-time/adjunct (17 women). *Students:* 120 full-time (86 women); includes 59 minority (13 Black or African American, non-Hispanic/Latino; 2 American Indian or Alaska Native, non-Hispanic/Latino; 14 Asian, non-Hispanic/Latino; 25 Hispanic/Latino; 5 Two or more races, non-Hispanic/Latino), 10 international. Average age 27. 687 applicants, 7% accepted, 25 enrolled. In 2015, 20 doctorates awarded. *Degree requirements:* For doctorate, comprehensive exam, thesis/dissertation, oral defense of dissertation, preliminary exam. *Entrance requirements:* For doctorate, GRE General Test. Additional exam requirements/recommendations for international students: Required—TOEFL. *Application deadline:* For fall admission, 12/1 for domestic and international students. Application fee: $75 ($90 for international students). Electronic applications accepted. *Financial support:* In 2015–16, 46 fellowships with full tuition reimbursements (averaging $19,800 per year), 86 teaching assistantships with full tuition reimbursements (averaging $24,750 per year) were awarded; career-related internships or fieldwork and health care benefits also available. Financial award application deadline: 4/15. *Unit head:* Prof. Patricia Reuter-Lorenz, Department Chair, 734-764-7429. *Application contact:* Tina Griffith, Psychology Student Academic Affairs, 734-764-2580, Fax: 734-615-7584, E-mail: psych.saa@umich.edu.
Website: http://www.lsa.umich.edu/psych/

University of Michigan, Rackham Graduate School, Program in Biomedical Sciences (PIBS), Neuroscience Graduate Program, Ann Arbor, MI 48109. Offers PhD. *Faculty:* 130 full-time (38 women). *Students:* 55 full-time (31 women); includes 18 minority (4 Black or African American, non-Hispanic/Latino; 1 American Indian or Alaska Native, non-Hispanic/Latino; 4 Asian, non-Hispanic/Latino; 9 Hispanic/Latino), 2 international. Average age 27. 138 applicants, 14% accepted, 8 enrolled. In 2015, 23 doctorates awarded. *Degree requirements:* For doctorate, thesis/dissertation, oral defense of dissertation, preliminary exam. *Entrance requirements:* For doctorate, GRE General Test, 3 letters of recommendation, research experience. Additional exam requirements/recommendations for international students: Required—TOEFL (minimum score 84 iBT). *Application deadline:* For fall admission, 12/1 for domestic and international students. Application fee: $75 ($90 for international students). Electronic applications accepted. *Financial support:* In 2015–16, 55 students received support, including 55 fellowships with full tuition reimbursements available (averaging $29,025 per year); scholarships/grants, health care benefits, tuition waivers (full), and unspecified assistantships also available. Financial award application deadline: 12/1. *Faculty research:* Developmental neurobiology, cellular and molecular neurobiology, cognitive neuroscience, sensory neuroscience, behavioral neuroscience. *Unit head:* Dr. Edward Stuenkel, Director, 734-763-9638, Fax: 734-647-0717, E-mail: esterm@umich.edu. *Application contact:* Rachel A. Harbach, Student Services Administrator, 734-763-9638, Fax: 734-647-0717, E-mail: rachelfk@umich.edu.
Website: http://neuroscience.med.umich.edu/

University of Michigan–Flint, School of Health Professions and Studies, Program in Physical Therapy, Flint, MI 48502-1950. Offers geriatrics (DPT, PhD, Certificate); neurology (DPT, PhD, Certificate); orthopedics (DPT, PhD, Certificate); pediatrics (DPT, PhD, Certificate); physical therapy (DPT). *Accreditation:* APTA. *Program availability:* Part-time. *Faculty:* 15 full-time (11 women), 6 part-time/adjunct (3 women). *Students:* 190 full-time (109 women), 41 part-time (28 women); includes 25 minority (1 Black or African American, non-Hispanic/Latino; 1 American Indian or Alaska Native, non-Hispanic/Latino; 13 Asian, non-Hispanic/Latino; 7 Hispanic/Latino; 3 Two or more races, non-Hispanic/Latino), 20 international. Average age 27. 531 applicants, 30% accepted, 70 enrolled. In 2015, 79 doctorates, 1 other advanced degree awarded. *Degree requirements:* For doctorate, comprehensive exam, thesis/dissertation or alternative. *Entrance requirements:* For doctorate, GRE (minimum Verbal score between 340-480; Quantitative 370-710); for Certificate, physical therapy degree from accredited institution; current physical therapy license in the United States or Canada; minimum overall GPA of 3.0 in the physical therapy degree; current CPR certification. Additional exam requirements/recommendations for international students: Required—TOEFL (minimum score 560 paper-based; 84 iBT), IELTS (minimum score 6.5). *Application deadline:* For fall admission, 5/1 for domestic students, 2/1 for international students; for winter admission, 7/31 for domestic students, 4/1 for international students; for spring admission, 3/1 for domestic students, 12/1 for international students. Application fee: $55. Electronic applications accepted. *Expenses:* Contact institution. *Financial support:* Federal Work-Study, scholarships/grants, and unspecified assistantships available. Support available to part-time students. Financial award application deadline: 3/1; financial award applicants required to submit FAFSA. *Faculty research:* Cumulative trauma disorders, oncology rehabilitation, neurological rehabilitation, musculoskeletal rehabilitation, cardiopulmonary rehabilitation. *Unit head:* Dr. Amy Yorke, Admissions Chair, 810-762-3373, E-mail: amyorke@umflint.edu. *Application contact:* Crystal Quaderer, Administrative Assistant, 810-762-3373, Fax: 810-766-6668, E-mail: quaderer@umflint.edu.
Website: https://www.umflint.edu/pt/pt_career

University of Minnesota, Twin Cities Campus, Graduate School, Graduate Program in Neuroscience, Minneapolis, MN 55455-0213. Offers MS, PhD. Terminal master's awarded for partial completion of doctoral program. *Degree requirements:* For master's, thesis; for doctorate, thesis/dissertation. *Entrance requirements:* For doctorate, GRE. Additional exam requirements/recommendations for international students: Required—TOEFL. Electronic applications accepted. *Faculty research:* Cellular and molecular neuroscience, behavioral neuroscience, developmental neuroscience, neurodegenerative diseases, pain, addiction, motor control.

University of Mississippi Medical Center, School of Graduate Studies in the Health Sciences, Program in Neuroscience, Jackson, MS 39216-4505. Offers PhD. *Degree requirements:* For doctorate, comprehensive exam, thesis/dissertation, 1st authored publication. *Entrance requirements:* For doctorate, GRE, BA, BS. Additional exam requirements/recommendations for international students: Required—TOEFL (minimum score 550 paper-based, 79 iBT), IELTS (minimum score 6.5), or PTE (minimum score 53). Electronic applications accepted. *Faculty research:* Neuroendocrinology, drugs of abuse, psychiatric neuroscience, sensory neuroscience, circadian rhythms.

University of Missouri, Office of Research and Graduate Studies, Interdisciplinary Neuroscience Program, Columbia, MO 65211. Offers MS, PhD, Graduate Certificate. *Entrance requirements:* For master's and doctorate, GRE (minimum score: Verbal and Quantitative 1200), bachelor's degree or its equivalent. Additional exam requirements/recommendations for international students: Required—TOEFL (minimum score 600 paper-based; 100 iBT). *Application deadline:* For fall admission, 1/15 priority date for domestic and international students. Application fee: $55 ($75 for international students). Electronic applications accepted. *Financial support:* Scholarships/grants, health care benefits, and unspecified assistantships available. Support available to part-time students.
Website: http://neuroscience.missouri.edu/graduate-studies/

University of Missouri–St. Louis, College of Arts and Sciences, Department of Psychological Sciences, St. Louis, MO 63121. Offers behavioral neuroscience (MA, PhD); clinical psychology (PhD); clinical psychology respecialization (Certificate); industrial/organizational psychology (MA, PhD); trauma studies (Certificate). *Accreditation:* APA (one or more programs are accredited). *Program availability:* Evening/weekend. *Faculty:* 1 full-time (0 women). *Students:* 62 full-time (41 women), 18 part-time (12 women); includes 10 minority (4 Black or African American, non-Hispanic/Latino; 1 American Indian or Alaska Native, non-Hispanic/Latino; 1 Asian, non-Hispanic/Latino; 4 Hispanic/Latino), 3 international. Average age 27. 226 applicants, 11% accepted, 21 enrolled. Terminal master's awarded for partial completion of doctoral program. *Degree requirements:* For master's, thesis; for doctorate, thesis/dissertation. *Entrance requirements:* For master's, GRE General Test, 3 letters of recommendation; for doctorate, GRE General Test, GRE Subject Test, 3 letters of recommendation. Additional exam requirements/recommendations for international students: Required—TOEFL (minimum score 550 paper-based; 79 iBT), IELTS (minimum score 6.5). *Application deadline:* For fall admission, 12/15 for domestic and international students. Application fee: $50 ($40 for international students). Electronic applications accepted. *Financial support:* Fellowships with full tuition reimbursements, research assistantships with tuition reimbursements, and teaching assistantships with tuition reimbursements available. Financial award applicants required to submit FAFSA. *Faculty research:* Bereavement and loss, neuroscience, post-traumatic stress disorder, conflict and negotiation, social psychology. *Unit head:* Michael G. Griffin, Chair, 314-516-5391, Fax: 314-516-5392, E-mail: michael_griffin@umsl.edu. *Application contact:* 314-516-5458, Fax: 314-516-6996, E-mail: gradadm@umsl.edu.
Website: http://www.umsl.edu/divisions/artscience/psychology/

University of Montana, Graduate School, College of Health Professions and Biomedical Sciences, Skaggs School of Pharmacy, Department of Biomedical and Pharmaceutical Sciences, Missoula, MT 59812-0002. Offers biomedical sciences (PhD); medicinal chemistry (MS, PhD); molecular and cellular toxicology (MS, PhD); neuroscience (PhD); pharmaceutical sciences (MS). *Accreditation:* ACPE. *Degree requirements:* For master's, oral defense of thesis; for doctorate, research dissertation defense. *Entrance requirements:* For master's and doctorate, GRE General Test. Additional exam requirements/recommendations for international students: Required—TOEFL (minimum score 540 paper-based). Electronic applications accepted. *Faculty research:* Cardiovascular pharmacology, medicinal chemistry, neurosciences, environmental toxicology, pharmacogenetics, cancer.

University of Nebraska Medical Center, Department of Pharmacology and Experimental Neuroscience, Omaha, NE 68198. Offers PhD. *Faculty:* 26 full-time (8 women), 2 part-time/adjunct (0 women). *Students:* 33 full-time (12 women), 2 part-time (0 women); includes 2 minority (1 Black or African American, non-Hispanic/Latino; 1 Two or more races, non-Hispanic/Latino), 14 international. Average age 27. 22 applicants. In 2015, 8 doctorates awarded. Terminal master's awarded for partial completion of doctoral program. *Degree requirements:* For doctorate, comprehensive exam, thesis/dissertation. *Entrance requirements:* For doctorate, GRE General Test. Additional exam requirements/recommendations for international students: Required—TOEFL (minimum score 550 paper-based; 80 iBT). *Application deadline:* For fall admission, 4/1 for domestic and international students. Applications are processed on a rolling basis. Application fee: $45. Electronic applications accepted. *Expenses:* Tuition, state resident: full-time $7830; part-time $3915 per credit hour. Tuition, nonresident: full-time $22,410; part-time $11,205 per credit hour. *Required fees:* $521. *Financial support:* In 2015–16, 8 students received support, including 2 fellowships with full tuition reimbursements available (averaging $24,000 per year), 3 research assistantships with full tuition reimbursements available (averaging $24,000 per year); scholarships/grants, health care benefits, and unspecified assistantships also available. Financial award application deadline: 2/15. *Faculty research:* Neuropharmacology, molecular pharmacology, toxicology, molecular biology, neuroscience. *Unit head:* Dr. Keshore Bidasee, Chair, Graduate Studies, 402-559-9018, Fax: 402-559-7495, E-mail: kbidasee@unmc.edu. *Application contact:* Leticia Tran, Office Assistant, 402-559-4044, E-mail: leticia.tran@unmc.edu.
Website: http://www.unmc.edu/pharmacology/

University of New Mexico, Graduate Studies, College of Arts and Sciences, Program in Psychology, Albuquerque, NM 87131-2039. Offers behavioral neuroscience (PhD); clinical psychology (PhD); cognitive neuroimaging (PhD); developmental psychology (PhD); evolution (PhD); health psychology (PhD); quantitative methodology (PhD). *Accreditation:* APA. *Faculty:* 18 full-time (8 women), 2 part-time/adjunct (1 woman). *Students:* 53 full-time (33 women), 23 part-time (13 women); includes 19 minority (2 Black or African American, non-Hispanic/Latino; 2 American Indian or Alaska Native, non-Hispanic/Latino; 2 Asian, non-Hispanic/Latino; 11 Hispanic/Latino; 2 Two or more races, non-Hispanic/Latino), 2 international. Average age 31. 135 applicants, 10% accepted, 13 enrolled. In 2015, 10 doctorates awarded. *Degree requirements:* For doctorate, comprehensive exam, thesis/dissertation. *Entrance requirements:* For doctorate, GRE General Test, GRE Subject Test (psychology), minimum GPA of 3.0. Additional exam requirements/recommendations for international students: Required—TOEFL (minimum score 550 paper-based; 79 iBT), IELTS (minimum score 6.5). *Application deadline:* For fall admission, 12/15 priority date for domestic and international students. Applications are processed on a rolling basis. Application fee: $50. Electronic applications accepted. *Financial support:* Fellowships, research assistantships with tuition reimbursements, teaching assistantships with tuition reimbursements, career-related internships or fieldwork, Federal Work-Study, institutionally sponsored loans, scholarships/grants, health care benefits, tuition waivers (partial), and unspecified assistantships available. Financial award application deadline: 3/1; financial award applicants required to submit FAFSA. *Faculty research:* Addiction, cognition, brain and behavior, developmental, evolutionary, functioning neuroimaging, health psychology, learning and memory, neuroscience. *Total annual research expenditures:* $727,970. *Unit head:* Dr. Jane Ellen Smith, Department Chair, 505-277-4121, Fax: 505-277-1394. *Application contact:* Rikk Murphy, Graduate Program Coordinator, 505-277-5009, Fax: 505-277-1394, E-mail: advising@unm.edu.
Website: http://psych.unm.edu

University of New Mexico, Graduate Studies, Health Sciences Center, Program in Biomedical Sciences, Albuquerque, NM 87131-5196. Offers biochemistry and molecular biology (MS, PhD); cell biology and physiology (MS, PhD); molecular genetics and microbiology (MS, PhD); neuroscience (MS, PhD); pathology (MS, PhD); toxicology

(MS, PhD). *Program availability:* Part-time. *Faculty:* 18 full-time (10 women), 1 part-time/adjunct (0 women). *Students:* 31 full-time (17 women), 45 part-time (26 women); includes 29 minority (1 American Indian or Alaska Native, non-Hispanic/Latino; 3 Asian, non-Hispanic/Latino; 22 Hispanic/Latino; 2 Native Hawaiian or other Pacific Islander, non-Hispanic/Latino; 1 Two or more races, non-Hispanic/Latino), 18 international. Average age 30. 98 applicants, 11% accepted, 11 enrolled. In 2015, 11 master's, 14 doctorates awarded. Terminal master's awarded for partial completion of doctoral program. *Degree requirements:* For master's, thesis; for doctorate, comprehensive exam, thesis/dissertation, qualifying exam at the end of year 1/core curriculum. *Entrance requirements:* For master's and doctorate, GRE General Test, minimum undergraduate GPA of 3.0. Additional exam requirements/recommendations for international students: Required—TOEFL. *Application deadline:* For fall admission, 3/1 priority date for domestic and international students. Applications are processed on a rolling basis. Application fee: $50. Electronic applications accepted. *Financial support:* Fellowships with tuition reimbursements, research assistantships with full tuition reimbursements, teaching assistantships, career-related internships or fieldwork, Federal Work-Study, institutionally sponsored loans, scholarships/grants, traineeships, health care benefits, and unspecified assistantships available. Financial award application deadline: 1/1; financial award applicants required to submit FAFSA. *Faculty research:* Infectious disease/immunity, cancer biology, cardiovascular and metabolic diseases, brain and behavioral illness, environmental health. *Unit head:* Dr. Helen J. Hathaway, Program Director, 505-272-1887, Fax: 505-272-2412, E-mail: hhathaway@salud.unm.edu. *Application contact:* Mary Fenton, Admissions Coordinator, 505-272-1887, Fax: 505-272-2412, E-mail: mfenton@salud.unm.edu.

The University of North Carolina at Chapel Hill, Graduate School, College of Arts and Sciences, Department of Psychology, Chapel Hill, NC 27599-3270. Offers behavioral neuroscience psychology (PhD); clinical psychology (PhD); cognitive psychology (PhD); developmental psychology (PhD); quantitative psychology (PhD); social psychology (PhD). *Accreditation:* APA. *Degree requirements:* For doctorate, comprehensive exam, thesis/dissertation. *Entrance requirements:* For doctorate, GRE General Test, minimum GPA of 3.0. Additional exam requirements/recommendations for international students: Required—TOEFL (minimum score 550 paper-based; 79 iBT), IELTS (minimum score 7). Electronic applications accepted. *Faculty research:* Expressed emotion, cognitive development, social cognitive neuroscience, human memory personality.

University of Oklahoma Health Sciences Center, College of Medicine and Graduate College, Graduate Programs in Medicine, Department of Neuroscience, Oklahoma City, OK 73190. Offers MS, PhD. *Degree requirements:* For doctorate, thesis/dissertation. *Entrance requirements:* For master's and doctorate, GRE General Test, 3 letters of recommendation. Additional exam requirements/recommendations for international students: Required—TOEFL.

University of Oregon, Graduate School, College of Arts and Sciences, Department of Biology, Eugene, OR 97403. Offers ecology and evolution (MA, MS, PhD); marine biology (MA, MS, PhD); molecular, cellular and genetic biology (PhD); neuroscience and development (PhD). Terminal master's awarded for partial completion of doctoral program. *Degree requirements:* For master's, thesis (for some programs); for doctorate, thesis/dissertation. *Entrance requirements:* For master's and doctorate, GRE General Test, minimum GPA of 3.2. Additional exam requirements/recommendations for international students: Required—TOEFL. *Faculty research:* Developmental neurobiology; evolution, population biology, and quantitative genetics; regulation of gene expression; biochemistry of marine organisms.

University of Pennsylvania, Perelman School of Medicine, Biomedical Graduate Studies, Graduate Group in Neuroscience, Philadelphia, PA 19104. Offers PhD, MD/PhD, VMD/PhD. *Faculty:* 143. *Students:* 110 full-time (64 women); includes 35 minority (3 Black or African American, non-Hispanic/Latino; 19 Asian, non-Hispanic/Latino; 12 Hispanic/Latino; 1 Two or more races, non-Hispanic/Latino), 6 international. 263 applicants, 17% accepted, 10 enrolled. In 2015, 21 doctorates awarded. *Degree requirements:* For doctorate, thesis/dissertation. *Entrance requirements:* For doctorate, GRE General Test. Additional exam requirements/recommendations for international students: Required—TOEFL. *Application deadline:* For fall admission, 12/1 for domestic and international students. Application fee: $80. *Expenses:* Tuition, area resident: Full-time $31,068; part-time $5762 per course. *Required fees:* $3200; $336 per course. Full-time tuition and fees vary according to degree level, program and student level. Part-time tuition and fees vary according to course load, degree level and program. *Financial support:* In 2015–16, 110 students received support. Fellowships, research assistantships, teaching assistantships, scholarships/grants, traineeships, and unspecified assistantships available. *Faculty research:* Molecular and cellular neuroscience, behavioral neuroscience, developmental neuroscience, systems neuroscience and neurophysiology, neurochemistry. *Unit head:* Dr. Joshua Gold, Chair, 215-746-0028. *Application contact:* Christine Clay, Coordinator, 215-898-8048. Website: http://www.med.upenn.edu/ngg

University of Pittsburgh, Dietrich School of Arts and Sciences and School of Medicine, Center for Neuroscience, Pittsburgh, PA 15260. Offers neurobiology (PhD); neuroscience (PhD). Program held jointly with School of Medicine. *Faculty:* 108 full-time (38 women). *Students:* 78 full-time (37 women); includes 13 minority (1 American Indian or Alaska Native, non-Hispanic/Latino; 8 Asian, non-Hispanic/Latino; 4 Hispanic/Latino), 9 international. Average age 25. 182 applicants, 22% accepted, 15 enrolled. In 2015, 13 doctorates awarded. *Degree requirements:* For doctorate, comprehensive exam, thesis/dissertation. *Entrance requirements:* For doctorate, GRE, interview. Additional exam requirements/recommendations for international students: Required—TOEFL (minimum score 600 paper-based; 100 iBT). *Application deadline:* For fall admission, 12/1 priority date for domestic and international students. Application fee: $50. Electronic applications accepted. Tuition and fees vary according to program. *Financial support:* In 2015–16, 69 students received support, including 32 fellowships with full tuition reimbursements available (averaging $27,000 per year), 33 research assistantships with full tuition reimbursements available (averaging $27,000 per year), 5 teaching assistantships with full tuition reimbursements available (averaging $27,000 per year); traineeships, health care benefits, and tuition waivers (full) also available. Financial award application deadline: 12/1. *Faculty research:* Behavioral/systems/cognitive, cell and molecular, development/plasticity/repair, neurobiology of disease. *Unit head:* Dr. Alan Sved, Co-Director, 412-624-6996, Fax: 412-624-9198, E-mail: sved@pitt.edu. *Application contact:* Missy Deasy, Graduate Program Administrator, 412-383-7582, Fax: 412-624-9198, E-mail: deasym@pitt.edu. Website: http://cnup.neurobio.pitt.edu/

University of Puerto Rico, Río Piedras Campus, College of Natural Sciences, Department of Biology, San Juan, PR 00931-3300. Offers ecology/systematics (MS, PhD); evolution/genetics (MS, PhD); molecular/cellular biology (MS, PhD); neuroscience (MS, PhD). *Program availability:* Part-time. *Degree requirements:* For master's, one foreign language, comprehensive exam, thesis; for doctorate, one foreign language, comprehensive exam, thesis/dissertation. *Entrance requirements:* For master's, GRE Subject Test, interview, minimum GPA of 3.0, letter of recommendation; for doctorate, GRE Subject Test, interview, master's degree, minimum GPA of 3.0, letter of recommendation. *Faculty research:* Environmental, poblational and systematic biology.

University of Rochester, School of Medicine and Dentistry, Graduate Programs in Medicine and Dentistry, Department of Neurobiology and Anatomy, Interdepartmental Programs in Neuroscience, Rochester, NY 14627. Offers PhD. Terminal master's awarded for partial completion of doctoral program. *Degree requirements:* For doctorate, one foreign language, thesis/dissertation, qualifying exam. *Entrance requirements:* For doctorate, GRE General Test. *Expenses:* Tuition, area resident: Full-time $47,450; part-time $1482 per credit hour. *Required fees:* $528. Tuition and fees vary according to program.

The University of South Dakota, Graduate School, Sanford School of Medicine and Graduate School, Biomedical Sciences Graduate Program, Program in Neuroscience, Vermillion, SD 57069-2390. Offers MS, PhD. Terminal master's awarded for partial completion of doctoral program. *Degree requirements:* For master's, thesis; for doctorate, comprehensive exam, thesis/dissertation. *Entrance requirements:* For master's and doctorate, GRE General Test, minimum GPA of 3.0. Additional exam requirements/recommendations for international students: Required—TOEFL (minimum score 550 paper-based; 80 iBT), IELTS (minimum score 6). *Application deadline:* For fall admission, 4/15 for domestic students, 3/15 for international students. Applications are processed on a rolling basis. Application fee: $35. Electronic applications accepted. *Expenses:* Contact institution. *Financial support:* Fellowships with partial tuition reimbursements, research assistantships with partial tuition reimbursements, and unspecified assistantships available. Financial award application deadline: 4/15; financial award applicants required to submit FAFSA. *Faculty research:* Central nervous system learning, neural plasticity, respiratory control. *Unit head:* 605-658-6322, Fax: 605-677-6381, E-mail: biomed@usd.edu.

University of Southern California, Graduate School, Dana and David Dornsife College of Letters, Arts and Sciences, Program in Neuroscience, Los Angeles, CA 90089. Offers MS, PhD. M.S. degree is terminal degree only. Terminal master's awarded for partial completion of doctoral program. *Degree requirements:* For master's, research paper; for doctorate, comprehensive exam, thesis/dissertation, qualifying examination, dissertation defense. *Entrance requirements:* For doctorate, GRE, 3 letters of recommendation, personal statement, resume. Additional exam requirements/recommendations for international students: Required—TOEFL (minimum score 600 paper-based; 100 iBT). Electronic applications accepted. *Faculty research:* Cellular and molecular neurobiology, behavioral and systems neurobiology, cognitive neuroscience, computation neuroscience and neural engineering, neuroscience of aging.

University of South Florida, College of Arts and Sciences, Department of Psychology, Tampa, FL 33620-9951. Offers psychology (PhD), including clinical psychology, cognitive and neural sciences, industrial-organizational psychology. *Accreditation:* APA. *Faculty:* 34 full-time (15 women), 1 part-time/adjunct (0 women). *Students:* 93 full-time (65 women), 19 part-time (12 women); includes 20 minority (2 Black or African American, non-Hispanic/Latino; 7 Asian, non-Hispanic/Latino; 7 Hispanic/Latino; 4 Two or more races, non-Hispanic/Latino), 11 international. Average age 29. 493 applicants, 4% accepted, 16 enrolled. In 2015, 16 doctorates awarded. *Degree requirements:* For doctorate, comprehensive exam, thesis/dissertation, internship. *Entrance requirements:* For doctorate, GRE General Test, minimum upper-division GPA of 3.4, three letters of recommendation, personal goals statement. Additional exam requirements/recommendations for international students: Required—TOEFL (minimum score 550 paper-based; 79 iBT) or IELTS (minimum score 6.5). *Application deadline:* For fall admission, 12/1 for domestic and international students. Application fee: $30. Electronic applications accepted. *Expenses:* Contact institution. *Financial support:* In 2015–16, 75 students received support, including 18 research assistantships with tuition reimbursements available (averaging $14,727 per year), 57 teaching assistantships with tuition reimbursements available (averaging $14,543 per year); tuition waivers (partial) and unspecified assistantships also available. Financial award applicants required to submit FAFSA. *Faculty research:* Clinical, cognitive, neuroscience, social, and industrial/organizational. *Total annual research expenditures:* $1.3 million. *Unit head:* Dr. Toru Shimizu, Chairperson, 813-974-0352, Fax: 813-974-4617, E-mail: shimizu@usf.edu. *Application contact:* Dr. Joseph Vandello, Associate Professor and Graduate Program Director, 813-974-0362, Fax: 813-974-4617, E-mail: vandello@usf.edu. Website: http://psychology.usf.edu/

University of South Florida, Innovative Education, Tampa, FL 33620-9951. Offers adult, career and higher education (Graduate Certificate), including college teaching, leadership in developing human resources, leadership in higher education; Africana studies (Graduate Certificate), including diasporas and health disparities, genocide and human rights; aging studies (Graduate Certificate), including gerontology; art research (Graduate Certificate), including museum studies; business foundations (Graduate Certificate); chemical and biomedical engineering (Graduate Certificate), including materials science and engineering, water, health and sustainability; child and family studies (Graduate Certificate), including positive behavior support; civil and industrial engineering (Graduate Certificate), including transportation systems analysis; community and family health (Graduate Certificate), including maternal and child health, social marketing and public health, violence and injury: prevention and intervention, women's health; criminology (Graduate Certificate), including criminal justice administration; educational measurement and research (Graduate Certificate), including evaluation; English (Graduate Certificate), including comparative literary studies, creative writing, professional and technical communication; entrepreneurship (Graduate Certificate); environmental health (Graduate Certificate), including safety management; epidemiology and biostatistics (Graduate Certificate), including applied biostatistics, biostatistics, concepts and tools of epidemiology, epidemiology, epidemiology of infectious diseases; geography, environment and planning (Graduate Certificate), including community development, environmental policy and management, geographical information systems; geology (Graduate Certificate), including hydrogeology; global health (Graduate Certificate), including disaster management, global health and Latin American and Caribbean studies, global health practice, humanitarian assistance, infection control; government and international affairs (Graduate Certificate), including Cuban studies, globalization studies; health policy and management (Graduate Certificate), including health management and leadership, public health policy and programs; hearing specialist: early intervention (Graduate Certificate); industrial and management systems engineering (Graduate Certificate), including systems engineering, technology management; information studies (Graduate Certificate), including school library media specialist; information systems/decision sciences (Graduate Certificate), including analytics and business intelligence; instructional technology (Graduate Certificate), including distance education, Florida digital/virtual educator, instructional design, multimedia design, Web design; internal medicine, bioethics and medical humanities (Graduate Certificate), including biomedical ethics; Latin American and Caribbean studies (Graduate Certificate); mass communications (Graduate Certificate), including multimedia journalism; mathematics and statistics (Graduate Certificate), including mathematics; medicine (Graduate Certificate), including aging and neuroscience, bioinformatics, biotechnology, brain fitness and memory management, clinical investigation, health informatics, health sciences, integrative weight management, intellectual property, medicine and gender, metabolic and nutritional medicine, metabolic cardiology, pharmacy sciences; national and competitive intelligence (Graduate Certificate); psychological and social foundations (Graduate Certificate), including career counseling, college teaching, diversity in

Neuroscience

education, mental health counseling, school counseling; public affairs (Graduate Certificate), including nonprofit management, public management, research administration; public health (Graduate Certificate), including environmental health, health equity, public health generalist, translational research in adolescent behavioral health; public health practices (Graduate Certificate), including planning for healthy communities; rehabilitation and mental health counseling (Graduate Certificate), including integrative mental health care, marriage and family therapy, rehabilitation technology; secondary education (Graduate Certificate), including ESOL, foreign language education: culture and content, foreign language education: professional; social work (Graduate Certificate), including geriatric social work/clinical gerontology; special education (Graduate Certificate), including autism spectrum disorder, disabilities education: severe/profound; world languages (Graduate Certificate), including teaching English as a second language (TESL) or foreign language. *Unit head:* Kathy Barnes, Interdisciplinary Programs Coordinator, 813-974-8031, Fax: 813-974-7061, E-mail: barnesk@usf.edu. *Application contact:* Karen Tylinski, Metro Initiatives, 813-974-9943, Fax: 813-974-7061, E-mail: ktylinsk@usf.edu.
Website: http://www.usf.edu/innovative-education/

University of South Florida, Morsani College of Medicine and College of Graduate Studies, Graduate Programs in Medical Sciences, Tampa, FL 33620-9951. Offers advanced athletic training (MS); athletic training (MS); bioinformatics and computational biology (MSBCB); biotechnology (MSB); health informatics (MSHI); medical sciences (MSMS, PhD), including aging and neuroscience (MSMS), allergy, immunology and infectious disease (PhD), anatomy, athletic training (MSMS), clinical and translational research, health informatics (MSMS), health science (MSMS), interdisciplinary medical sciences (MSMS), medical microbiology and immunology (MSMS), metabolic and nutritional medicine (MSMS), molecular medicine, molecular pharmacology and physiology (PhD), neurology (PhD), pathology and laboratory medicine (PhD), pharmacology and therapeutics (PhD), physiology and biophysics (PhD), women's health (MSMS). *Students:* 510 full-time (261 women), 318 part-time (208 women); includes 360 minority (108 Black or African American, non-Hispanic/Latino; 3 American Indian or Alaska Native, non-Hispanic/Latino; 101 Asian, non-Hispanic/Latino; 124 Hispanic/Latino; 1 Native Hawaiian or other Pacific Islander, non-Hispanic/Latino; 23 Two or more races, non-Hispanic/Latino), 52 international. Average age 26. 6,567 applicants, 13% accepted, 469 enrolled. In 2015, 216 master's awarded. Terminal master's awarded for partial completion of doctoral program. *Degree requirements:* For master's, comprehensive exam, thesis; for doctorate, comprehensive exam, thesis/dissertation. *Entrance requirements:* For master's, GRE General Test or GMAT, bachelor's degree or equivalent from regionally-accredited university with minimum GPA of 3.0 in upper-division sciences coursework; prerequisites in general biology, general chemistry, general physics, organic chemistry, quantitative analysis, and integral and differential calculus; for doctorate, GRE General Test, bachelor's degree from regionally-accredited university with minimum GPA of 3.0 in upper-division sciences coursework; 3 letters of recommendation; personal interview; 1-2 page personal statement; prerequisites in biology, chemistry, physics, organic chemistry, quantitative analysis, and integral/differential calculus. Additional exam requirements/recommendations for international students: Required—TOEFL (minimum score 550 paper-based; 79 iBT) or IELTS (minimum score 6.5). *Application deadline:* For fall admission, 2/15 for domestic students, 1/2 for international students. Application fee: $30. *Expenses:* Contact institution. *Faculty research:* Anatomy, biochemistry, cancer biology, cardiovascular disease, cell biology, immunology, microbiology, molecular biology, neuroscience, pharmacology, physiology. *Unit head:* Dr. Michael Barber, Professor/Associate Dean for Graduate and Postdoctoral Affairs, 813-974-9908, Fax: 813-974-4317, E-mail: mbarber@health.usf.edu. *Application contact:* Dr. Eric Bennett, Graduate Director, PhD Program in Medical Sciences, 813-974-1545, Fax: 813-974-4317, E-mail: esbennet@health.usf.edu.
Website: http://health.usf.edu/nocms/medicine/graduatestudies/

The University of Texas at Austin, Graduate School, College of Liberal Arts, Department of Psychology, Austin, TX 78712-1111. Offers behavioral neuroscience (PhD); clinical psychology (PhD); cognitive systems (PhD); developmental psychology (PhD); individual differences and evolutionary psychology (PhD); perceptual systems (PhD); social psychology (PhD). *Accreditation:* APA. *Degree requirements:* For doctorate, thesis/dissertation. *Entrance requirements:* For doctorate, GRE General Test. Electronic applications accepted. *Faculty research:* Behavioral neuroscience, sensory neuroscience, evolutionary psychology, cognitive processes in psychopathology, cognitive processes and their development.

The University of Texas at Austin, Graduate School, The Institute for Neuroscience, Austin, TX 78712-1111. Offers PhD, MD/PhD. Terminal master's awarded for partial completion of doctoral program. *Degree requirements:* For doctorate, thesis/dissertation. *Entrance requirements:* For doctorate, GRE. Electronic applications accepted. *Faculty research:* Cellular/molecular biology, neurobiology, pharmacology, behavioral neuroscience.

The University of Texas at Dallas, School of Behavioral and Brain Sciences, Program in Cognition and Neuroscience, Richardson, TX 75080. Offers applied cognition and neuroscience (MS); cognition and neuroscience (PhD). *Program availability:* Part-time, evening/weekend. *Faculty:* 31 full-time (12 women), 2 part-time/adjunct (1 woman). *Students:* 174 full-time (101 women), 32 part-time (26 women); includes 62 minority (8 Black or African American, non-Hispanic/Latino; 1 American Indian or Alaska Native, non-Hispanic/Latino; 21 Asian, non-Hispanic/Latino; 25 Hispanic/Latino; 7 Two or more races, non-Hispanic/Latino), 37 international. Average age 29. 174 applicants, 47% accepted, 65 enrolled. In 2015, 59 master's, 8 doctorates awarded. *Degree requirements:* For master's, internship; for doctorate, thesis/dissertation. *Entrance requirements:* For master's and doctorate, GRE General Test, minimum GPA of 3.0 in upper-level coursework in field. Additional exam requirements/recommendations for international students: Required—TOEFL (minimum score 550 paper-based). *Application deadline:* For fall admission, 7/15 for domestic students, 5/1 priority date for international students; for spring admission, 11/15 for domestic students, 9/1 priority date for international students. Applications are processed on a rolling basis. Application fee: $50 ($100 for international students). Electronic applications accepted. *Expenses:* Tuition, state resident: full-time $11,940; part-time $663 per semester hour. Tuition, nonresident: full-time $22,786; part-time $1266 per semester hour. Tuition and fees vary according to course load. *Financial support:* In 2015–16, 155 students received support, including 27 research assistantships with partial tuition reimbursements available (averaging $26,645 per year), 39 teaching assistantships with partial tuition reimbursements available (averaging $18,216 per year); fellowships, career-related internships or fieldwork, Federal Work-Study, institutionally sponsored loans, scholarships/grants, and unspecified assistantships also available. Support available to part-time students. Financial award application deadline: 4/30; financial award applicants required to submit FAFSA. *Faculty research:* Neural plasticity, neuroimaging, face recognition, cognitive and neurobiological mechanisms of human memory, treatment interventions for semantic memory retrieval problems. *Unit head:* Dr. Christa McIntyre Rodriguez, Program Head, 972-883-2235, Fax: 972-883-2491, E-mail: christa.mcintyre@utdallas.edu. *Application contact:* Dr. Theodore Price, Assistant Program Head, 972-883-4311, Fax: 972-883-2491, E-mail: cogneurophd@utdallas.edu.
Website: http://bbs.utdallas.edu/cogneuro/

The University of Texas Health Science Center at Houston, Graduate School of Biomedical Sciences, Program in Neuroscience, Houston, TX 77225-0036. Offers MS, PhD, MD/PhD. Terminal master's awarded for partial completion of doctoral program. *Degree requirements:* For master's, thesis; for doctorate, thesis/dissertation. *Entrance requirements:* For master's and doctorate, GRE General Test. Additional exam requirements/recommendations for international students: Required—TOEFL. Electronic applications accepted. *Faculty research:* Behavior, cognitive, computational, neuroimaging, substance abuse.

The University of Texas Health Science Center at San Antonio, Graduate School of Biomedical Sciences, Department of Pharmacology, San Antonio, TX 78229-3900. Offers neuroscience (PhD). *Degree requirements:* For doctorate, comprehensive exam, thesis/dissertation.

The University of Texas Medical Branch, Graduate School of Biomedical Sciences, Program in Neuroscience, Galveston, TX 77555. Offers PhD. *Degree requirements:* For doctorate, thesis/dissertation. *Entrance requirements:* For doctorate, GRE General Test. Additional exam requirements/recommendations for international students: Required—TOEFL (minimum score 550 paper-based). Electronic applications accepted.

The University of Texas Southwestern Medical Center, Southwestern Graduate School of Biomedical Sciences, Division of Basic Science, Program in Neuroscience, Dallas, TX 75390. Offers PhD. *Degree requirements:* For doctorate, thesis/dissertation, qualifying exam. *Entrance requirements:* For doctorate, GRE General Test, minimum GPA of 3.0. Additional exam requirements/recommendations for international students: Required—TOEFL. Electronic applications accepted. *Faculty research:* Ion channels, sensory transduction, membrane excitability and biophysics, synaptic transmission, developmental neurogenetics.

The University of Toledo, College of Graduate Studies, College of Medicine and Life Sciences, Department of Neurosciences, Toledo, OH 43606-3390. Offers MSBS, PhD, MD/MSBS, MD/PhD. Terminal master's awarded for partial completion of doctoral program. *Degree requirements:* For master's, thesis, qualifying exam; for doctorate, thesis/dissertation, qualifying exam. *Entrance requirements:* For master's and doctorate, GRE, minimum undergraduate GPA of 3.0, three letters of recommendation, statement of purpose, transcripts from all prior institutions attended, resume. Additional exam requirements/recommendations for international students: Required—TOEFL (minimum score 550 paper-based; 80 iBT). Electronic applications accepted.

University of Utah, School of Medicine and Graduate School, Graduate Programs in Medicine, Program in Neuroscience, Salt Lake City, UT 84112-1107. Offers PhD. *Degree requirements:* For doctorate, thesis/dissertation. *Entrance requirements:* For doctorate, GRE General Test, minimum GPA of 3.0. Additional exam requirements/recommendations for international students: Required—TOEFL (minimum score 500 paper-based); Recommended—TWE (minimum score 6). Electronic applications accepted. *Faculty research:* Brain and behavioral neuroscience, cellular neuroscience, molecular neuroscience, neurobiology of disease, developmental neuroscience.

University of Vermont, College of Medicine and Graduate College, Graduate Programs in Medicine, Graduate Program in Neuroscience, Burlington, VT 05405. Offers PhD. *Degree requirements:* For doctorate, thesis/dissertation. *Entrance requirements:* For doctorate, GRE General Test. Additional exam requirements/recommendations for international students: Required—TOEFL (minimum score 550 paper-based; 80 iBT). *Application deadline:* For fall admission, 12/1 priority date for domestic students, 12/1 for international students. Application fee: $65. Electronic applications accepted. *Financial support:* Research assistantships and teaching assistantships available. Financial award application deadline: 3/1. *Unit head:* Dr. Anthony Morielli, 802-656-2230, E-mail: anthony.morielli@uvm.edu. *Application contact:* Dr. Anthony Morielli, 802-656-2230, E-mail: anthony.morielli@uvm.edu.

University of Virginia, School of Medicine, Department of Neuroscience, Charlottesville, VA 22903. Offers PhD, MD/PhD. *Degree requirements:* For doctorate, thesis/dissertation. *Entrance requirements:* For doctorate, GRE General Test, 2 letters of recommendation. Additional exam requirements/recommendations for international students: Required—TOEFL. Electronic applications accepted.

The University of Western Ontario, Faculty of Graduate Studies, Biosciences Division, Department of Clinical Neurological Sciences, London, ON N6A 5B8, Canada. Offers M Sc, PhD. Terminal master's awarded for partial completion of doctoral program. *Degree requirements:* For master's, thesis; for doctorate, thesis/dissertation. *Entrance requirements:* For master's, honors degree or equivalent, minimum B+ average; for doctorate, master's degree, minimum B+ average. *Faculty research:* Behavioral neuroscience, neural regeneration and degeneration, visual development, human motor function.

University of Wisconsin–Madison, Graduate School, College of Letters and Science, Department of Psychology, Program in Cognitive Neurosciences, Madison, WI 53706-1380. Offers PhD. *Degree requirements:* For doctorate, comprehensive exam, thesis/dissertation. *Entrance requirements:* For doctorate, GRE General Test, minimum undergraduate GPA of 3.0. Additional exam requirements/recommendations for international students: Required—TOEFL. Electronic applications accepted. *Expenses:* Tuition, state resident: full-time $5364. Tuition, nonresident: full-time $12,027. *Required fees:* $571. Tuition and fees vary according to campus/location, program and reciprocity agreements.

Virginia Commonwealth University, Medical College of Virginia-Professional Programs, School of Medicine, Graduate Program in Neuroscience, Richmond, VA 23284-9005. Offers PhD. Program offered with Departments of Anatomy, Biochemistry and Molecular Biophysics, Pharmacology and Toxicology, and Physiology. *Entrance requirements:* For doctorate, GRE or MCAT. Additional exam requirements/recommendations for international students: Required—TOEFL (minimum score 600 paper-based; 100 iBT). Electronic applications accepted.

Virginia Commonwealth University, Medical College of Virginia-Professional Programs, School of Medicine, School of Medicine Graduate Programs, Department of Anatomy and Neurobiology, Richmond, VA 23284-9005. Offers anatomy (MS); anatomy and neurobiology (PhD); neurobiology (MS); neuroscience (MS); MD/PhD. *Degree requirements:* For master's, thesis; for doctorate, thesis/dissertation, comprehensive oral and written exams. *Entrance requirements:* For master's and doctorate, GRE, MCAT or DAT. Electronic applications accepted.

Virginia Commonwealth University, Medical College of Virginia-Professional Programs, School of Medicine, School of Medicine Graduate Programs, Department of Pharmacology and Toxicology, Richmond, VA 23284-9005. Offers neuroscience (PhD); pharmacology (Certificate); pharmacology and toxicology (MS, PhD); MD/PhD. Terminal master's awarded for partial completion of doctoral program. *Degree requirements:* For master's, thesis; for doctorate, thesis/dissertation, comprehensive oral and written exams. *Entrance requirements:* For master's and doctorate, GRE or MCAT. Additional exam requirements/recommendations for international students: Required—TOEFL (minimum score 600 paper-based; 100 iBT). Electronic applications accepted. *Faculty research:* Drug abuse, drug metabolism, pharmacodynamics, peptide synthesis, receptor mechanisms.

Wake Forest University, School of Medicine and Graduate School of Arts and Sciences, Graduate Programs in Medicine, Interdisciplinary Program in Neuroscience, Winston-Salem, NC 27109. Offers PhD, MD/PhD. *Degree requirements:* For doctorate, thesis/dissertation. *Entrance requirements:* For doctorate, GRE General Test. Additional exam requirements/recommendations for international students: Required—TOEFL. Electronic applications accepted. *Faculty research:* Neurobiology of substance abuse, learning and memory, aging, sensory neurobiology, nervous system development.

Washington State University, College of Veterinary Medicine, Program in Neuroscience, Pullman, WA 99164-6520. Offers MS, PhD. *Program availability:* Part-time. *Faculty:* 54 full-time (15 women). *Students:* 28 full-time (14 women); includes 4 minority (all Asian, non-Hispanic/Latino), 3 international. Average age 29. 43 applicants, 23% accepted, 2 enrolled. In 2015, 3 doctorates awarded. Terminal master's awarded for partial completion of doctoral program. *Degree requirements:* For master's, thesis, written exam; for doctorate, thesis/dissertation, written exam, oral exam. *Entrance requirements:* For master's and doctorate, GRE General Test, minimum GPA of 3.0. Additional exam requirements/recommendations for international students: Required—TOEFL (minimum score 550 paper-based; 100 iBT). *Application deadline:* For fall admission, 12/15 priority date for domestic and international students. Applications are processed on a rolling basis. Application fee: $75. Electronic applications accepted. *Financial support:* In 2015–16, 25 students received support, including 10 research assistantships with full tuition reimbursements available (averaging $23,319 per year), 16 teaching assistantships with full tuition reimbursements available (averaging $23,319 per year); fellowships, scholarships/grants, health care benefits, and unspecified assistantships also available. Financial award application deadline: 1/31. *Faculty research:* Addiction, sleep and performance, body weight and energy balance, emotion and well being, learning and memory, reproduction, vision, movement. *Total annual research expenditures:* $4.7 million. *Unit head:* Dr. Steve Simasko, Chair, 509-335-6624, Fax: 509-335-4650, E-mail: simasko@vetmed.wsu.edu. *Application contact:* Becky Morton, Department Manager, 509-335-6621, Fax: 509-335-4650, E-mail: grad.neuro@vetmed.wsu.edu.
Website: http://ipn.vetmed.wsu.edu/neuroscience/graduate

Washington University in St. Louis, Graduate School of Arts and Sciences, Department of Philosophy, Program in Philosophy-Neuroscience-Psychology, St. Louis, MO 63130-4899. Offers PhD. *Students:* 20 full-time (9 women); includes 1 minority (Asian, non-Hispanic/Latino), 4 international. 45 applicants, 22% accepted, 4 enrolled. In 2015, 1 doctorate awarded. *Degree requirements:* For doctorate, thesis/dissertation. *Entrance requirements:* For doctorate, GRE General Test, sample of written work. Additional exam requirements/recommendations for international students: Required—TOEFL. *Application deadline:* For fall admission, 12/31 for domestic students. Application fee: $45. Electronic applications accepted. *Financial support:* Fellowships, teaching assistantships, and tuition waivers (full and partial) available. Financial award application deadline: 1/15. *Faculty research:* Philosophy of mind and language with a special emphasis on the philosophical dimensions of psychology, neuroscience, and linguistics. *Unit head:* Dr. Kit Wellman, Chair, 314-935-6670. *Application contact:* Bridget Coleman, Director of Admissions, 314-935-6880, Fax: 314-935-4887.
Website: http://pnp.artsci.wustl.edu/

Washington University in St. Louis, Graduate School of Arts and Sciences, Division of Biology and Biomedical Sciences, Program in Neurosciences, St. Louis, MO 63130-4899. Offers PhD. *Students:* 90 full-time (43 women); includes 15 minority (2 Black or African American, non-Hispanic/Latino; 1 American Indian or Alaska Native, non-Hispanic/Latino; 7 Asian, non-Hispanic/Latino; 2 Hispanic/Latino; 3 Two or more races, non-Hispanic/Latino), 20 international. 229 applicants, 17% accepted, 16 enrolled. In 2015, 14 doctorates awarded. *Degree requirements:* For doctorate, thesis/dissertation. *Entrance requirements:* For doctorate, GRE General Test, GRE Subject Test. Additional exam requirements/recommendations for international students: Required—TOEFL. *Application deadline:* For fall admission, 12/1 for domestic students. Application fee: $0. Electronic applications accepted. *Financial support:* Fellowships, research assistantships, and teaching assistantships available. Financial award application deadline: 1/15. *Faculty research:* Neurobiology, neurology, functional imaging, behavior, cognition, computational neuroscience, electrophysiology, sensory systems, motor systems, neuroglia, neuronal development, learning, memory, language, synaptic plasticity, mind, consciousness, neurodegeneration, diseases of the nervous system, neuronal injury, clinical neuroscience, motor control, biological rhythms, connectivity mapping. *Unit head:* Sally Vogt, Coordinator, 314-362-7189. *Application contact:* Rebecca Riney, 314-747-4648, E-mail: dbbsphdadmissions@wusm.wustl.edu.

Wayne State University, College of Liberal Arts and Sciences, Department of Psychology, Detroit, MI 48202. Offers behavioral and cognitive neuroscience (PhD); clinical psychology (PhD); cognitive, developmental and social psychology (PhD); industrial/organizational psychology (MA, PhD); social psychology (PhD). Doctoral programs admit for fall only. *Accreditation:* APA (one or more programs are accredited). *Faculty:* 37 full-time (13 women), 8 part-time/adjunct (4 women). *Students:* 103 full-time (67 women), 36 part-time (20 women); includes 22 minority (5 Black or African American, non-Hispanic/Latino; 3 Asian, non-Hispanic/Latino; 8 Hispanic/Latino; 6 Two or more races, non-Hispanic/Latino), 9 international. Average age 28. 443 applicants, 11% accepted, 23 enrolled. In 2015, 24 master's, 16 doctorates awarded. Terminal master's awarded for partial completion of doctoral program. *Degree requirements:* For master's, thesis (for some programs); for doctorate, thesis/dissertation, training assignments. *Entrance requirements:* For master's, GRE General Test, minimum undergraduate upper-division cumulative GPA of 3.0, courses in introductory psychology and statistics, two letters of recommendation, professional statement; for doctorate, GRE General Test, bachelor's, master's, or other advanced degree; at least twelve credits in psychology with minimum GPA of 3.0; courses in laboratory psychology and statistical methods in psychology; at least three letters of recommendation; statement of purpose. Additional exam requirements/recommendations for international students: Required—TOEFL (minimum score 550 paper-based; 79 iBT), TWE (minimum score 5.5), Michigan English Language Assessment Battery (minimum score 85); Recommended—IELTS (minimum score 6.5). Application fee: $0. Electronic applications accepted. *Expenses:* Tuition, state resident: full-time $14,165; part-time $590.20 per credit hour. Tuition, nonresident: full-time $30,682; part-time $1278.40 per credit hour. *Required fees:* $1688; $47.45 per credit hour. $274.60 per semester. Tuition and fees vary according to course load and program. *Financial support:* In 2015–16, 93 students received support, including 15 fellowships with tuition reimbursements available (averaging $14,792 per year), 12 research assistantships with tuition reimbursements available (averaging $18,558 per year), 48 teaching assistantships with tuition reimbursements available (averaging $17,427 per year); scholarships/grants, health care benefits, and unspecified assistantships also available. Financial award application deadline: 3/31; financial award applicants required to submit FAFSA. *Faculty research:* Neuroscience, including functional cognitive imaging, neural physiology, behavioral pharmacology, and neurobehavioral teratology; cognitive and neurochemical processes associated with aging, drug addiction and neurological disorders to studies of the neural circuits that underlie learning, emotion, and weight regulation; the life-long developmental plasticity of the neurobiological processes of behavior; neuropsychology; child clinical psychology; health psychology; community psychology. *Total annual research expenditures:* $1.7 million. *Unit head:* Boris Baltes, PhD, Chair/Professor, 313-577-2803, E-mail: b.baltes@wayne.edu. *Application contact:* Alia Allen, Academic Services Officer, 313-577-2823, E-mail: aallen@wayne.edu.
Website: http://clas.wayne.edu/psychology/

Wayne State University, School of Medicine, Office of Biomedical Graduate Programs, Department of Psychiatry and Behavioral Neurosciences, Detroit, MI 48202. Offers translational neuroscience (PhD). *Faculty:* 28. *Students:* 12 full-time (6 women); includes 3 minority (2 Asian, non-Hispanic/Latino; 1 Two or more races, non-Hispanic/Latino), 1 international. Average age 27. 20 applicants, 15% accepted, 2 enrolled. In 2015, 2 doctorates awarded. *Degree requirements:* For doctorate, thesis/dissertation. *Entrance requirements:* For doctorate, GRE, minimum undergraduate GPA of 3.0, bachelor's degree from accredited institution, coursework in biological sciences and other scientific disciplines, personal statement, three letters of recommendation, curriculum vitae. Additional exam requirements/recommendations for international students: Required—TOEFL (minimum score 600 paper-based; 100 iBT). *Application deadline:* For fall admission, 12/15 for domestic and international students. Application fee: $0. Electronic applications accepted. *Expenses:* $17,645 per year resident tuition, $33,311 per year non-resident tuition; $735.20 per credit hour resident tuition, $1,387.95 per credit hour non-resident tuition; fees include $47.45 per credit hour student services fee and $274.60 per semester registration fee. *Financial support:* In 2015–16, 12 students received support, including 2 fellowships with tuition reimbursements available (averaging $27,057 per year), 10 research assistantships with tuition reimbursements available (averaging $26,951 per year); scholarships/grants, health care benefits, and unspecified assistantships also available. Financial award application deadline: 3/31. *Faculty research:* Substance abuse, brain imaging, schizophrenia, child psychopathy, child development, neurobiology of monoamine systems. *Unit head:* Dr. Jeffrey Stanley, Graduate Program Director, 313-577-9090, E-mail: jstanley@med.wayne.edu. *Application contact:* 313-577-1841, E-mail: tnp@med.wayne.edu.
Website: http://psychiatry.med.wayne.edu/

Weill Cornell Medicine, Weill Cornell Graduate School of Medical Sciences, Neuroscience Program, New York, NY 10065. Offers MS, PhD. Terminal master's awarded for partial completion of doctoral program. *Degree requirements:* For master's, comprehensive exam; for doctorate, thesis/dissertation, final exam. *Entrance requirements:* For doctorate, GRE General Test, undergraduate training in biology, organic chemistry, physics, and mathematics. Additional exam requirements/recommendations for international students: Required—TOEFL. Electronic applications accepted. *Faculty research:* Neural disease, synaptic transmission, developmental neurobiology and regeneration, vision and computational and systems neuroscience, neuropharmacology.

West Virginia University, School of Medicine, Graduate Programs at the Health Sciences Center, Interdisciplinary Graduate Programs in Biomedical Sciences, Program in Neuroscience, Morgantown, WV 26506. Offers PhD, MD/PhD. *Degree requirements:* For doctorate, comprehensive exam, thesis/dissertation. *Entrance requirements:* For doctorate, GRE General Test, minimum GPA of 3.0. Additional exam requirements/recommendations for international students: Required—TOEFL. Electronic applications accepted. *Expenses:* Tuition, state resident: full-time $8568. Tuition, nonresident: full-time $22,140. Tuition and fees vary according to program. *Faculty research:* Sensory neuroscience, cognitive neuroscience, neural injury, homeostasis, behavioral neuroscience.

Wilfrid Laurier University, Faculty of Graduate and Postdoctoral Studies, Faculty of Science, Department of Psychology, Waterloo, ON N2L 3C5, Canada. Offers behavioral neuroscience (M Sc, PhD); cognitive neuroscience (M Sc, PhD); community psychology (MA, PhD); social and developmental psychology (MA, PhD). *Program availability:* Part-time. *Degree requirements:* For master's, thesis; for doctorate, thesis/dissertation. *Entrance requirements:* For master's, GRE General Test, honors BA or the equivalent in psychology, minimum B average in undergraduate course work; for doctorate, GRE General Test, master's degree, minimum A- average. Additional exam requirements/recommendations for international students: Required—TOEFL (minimum score 89 iBT). Electronic applications accepted. *Faculty research:* Brain and cognition, community psychology, social and developmental psychology.

Yale University, Graduate School of Arts and Sciences, Department of Psychology, New Haven, CT 06520. Offers behavioral neuroscience (PhD); clinical psychology (PhD); cognitive psychology (PhD); developmental psychology (PhD); social/personality psychology (PhD). *Accreditation:* APA. *Degree requirements:* For doctorate, thesis/dissertation. *Entrance requirements:* For doctorate, GRE General Test.

Yale University, Graduate School of Arts and Sciences, Interdepartmental Neuroscience Program, New Haven, CT 06520. Offers PhD. *Degree requirements:* For doctorate, thesis/dissertation. *Entrance requirements:* For doctorate, GRE General Test. *Expenses:* Contact institution.

Yale University, School of Medicine and Graduate School of Arts and Sciences, Combined Program in Biological and Biomedical Sciences (BBS), Neuroscience Track, New Haven, CT 06520. Offers PhD, MD/PhD. *Degree requirements:* For doctorate, thesis/dissertation. *Entrance requirements:* For doctorate, GRE General Test. Additional exam requirements/recommendations for international students: Required—TOEFL. Electronic applications accepted.

UNIFORMED SERVICES UNIVERSITY OF THE HEALTH SCIENCES

F. Edward Hébert School of Medicine
Graduate Program in Neuroscience

 For more information, visit http://petersons.to/uniformedserviceshealthsciences

Program of Study

The Uniformed Services University of the Health Sciences (USUHS) offers the Graduate Program in Neuroscience, a broadly based interdisciplinary program leading to the Ph.D. degree in neuroscience. Courses and research training are provided by the neuroscience faculty members, who hold primary appointments in the Departments of Anatomy, Physiology, and Genetics; Biochemistry; Medical and Clinical Psychology; Microbiology and Immunology; Neurology; Pathology; Pediatrics; Pharmacology; and Psychiatry at the University. The program permits considerable flexibility in the choice of courses and research areas; training programs are tailored to meet the individual requirements of each student. The program is designed for students with strong undergraduate training in the physical sciences, biology, or psychology who wish to pursue a professional career in neuroscience research. Integrated instruction in the development, structure, function, and pathology of the nervous system and its interaction with the environment is provided. Students in the program conduct their research under the direction of neuroscience faculty members in laboratories that are located in the medical school. During the first year of study, students begin formal course work. Each student is required to take laboratory training rotations in the research laboratories of program faculty members. By the end of the first year, students select a research area and a faculty thesis adviser. During the second year, students complete requirements for advancement to candidacy, including required course work and passage of the qualifying examination. After advancement to candidacy, each student develops an original research project and prepares and defends a written dissertation under the guidance of his or her faculty adviser and advisory committee.

Research Facilities

Each academic department at the University is provided with laboratories for the support of a variety of research projects. Neuroscience research laboratories available to students are suitable for research in most areas of neuroscience, including behavioral studies, electrophysiology, molecular and cellular neurobiology, neuroanatomy, neurochemistry, neuropathology, neuropharmacology, and neurophysiology. High-resolution electron microscopes, confocal microscopes, two photon microscopes, deconvolution wide-field fluorescence microscopes, a central resource facility providing custom synthesis of oligonucleotides and peptides and DNA sequencing, RNA sequencing, centralized animal facilities, computer support, a medical library, and a learning resources center are available within the University.

Financial Aid

USUHS provides an attractive package of financial support that is administered as a federal salary. This support is available on a competitive basis to all civilian graduate students. Awards are made on an annual basis and are renewable for up to three years. For the 2016–17 academic year, financial support for graduate students is $43,400. In addition to this base support, health insurance and transit benefits are provided if needed.

Cost of Study

Graduate students in the neuroscience program are not required to pay tuition or fees. Civilian students incur no obligation to the United States government for service after completion of their graduate training program. Students are required to carry health insurance.

Living and Housing Costs

There is a reasonable supply of affordable rental housing in the area. The University does not have housing for graduate students. Students are responsible for making their own arrangements for accommodations. Costs in the Washington, D.C., area are comparable to those in other major metropolitan areas.

Student Group

The neuroscience graduate program is an active and growing graduate program; approximately 31 students are enrolled. The Uniformed Services University (USU) also has Ph.D. programs in departmentally based basic biomedical sciences, as well as interdisciplinary graduate programs in molecular and cell biology and in emerging infectious diseases. In addition to the graduate and medical programs in the medical school, the nursing school has graduate programs for nurse practitioners and nurse anesthetists.

Student Outcomes

Graduates hold faculty, research associate, postdoctoral, science policy, and other positions in universities, medical schools, government, and industrial research institutions. Forty Ph.D.'s have been awarded since 1998. Currently 3 USU neuroscience graduates hold faculty positions within the Neuroscience Graduate Program.

Location

Metropolitan Washington has a population of about 5 million residents in the District of Columbia and the surrounding areas of Maryland and Virginia. The region is a center of education and research and is home to five major universities, four medical schools, the National Library of Medicine and the National Institutes of Health (next to the USUHS campus), Walter Reed National Military Medical Center, the Armed Forces Institute of Pathology, the Library of Congress, the Smithsonian Institution, the National Bureau of Standards, and many other private and government research centers. Many cultural advantages of the area include the theater, a major symphony orchestra, major league sports, and world-famous museums. The Metro subway system has a station near campus and provides a convenient connection from the University to museums and cultural attractions of downtown Washington. The University is within an easy distance of three major airports, Baltimore Washington International, Reagan International, and Dulles International. Both Reagan and Dulles International airports are accessible from the campus via Metro subway. For outdoor activities, the Blue Ridge Mountains, the Chesapeake Bay, and the Atlantic coast beaches are all within a few hours of driving distance.

The University

The University was established by Congress in 1972 to provide a comprehensive education in medicine to those who demonstrate potential for careers as Medical Corps officers in the uniformed services. Graduate programs in the basic medical sciences are offered to both civilian and military students and are an essential part of the academic environment at the University. The University is located in proximity to major research facilities, including the National Institutes of Health (NIH), the National Library of Medicine, Walter Reed Army Medical Center at the National Naval Medical Center, the Armed Forces Institute of Pathology, the National Institute of Standards and Technology, and numerous biotechnology companies.

Uniformed Services University subscribes fully to the policy of equal educational opportunity and accepts students on a competitive basis without regard to race, color, sex, age, or creed.

Applying

Civilian applicants are accepted as full-time students only. Each applicant must have a bachelor's degree from an accredited academic institution. A strong background in science with courses in several of the following disciplines—biochemistry, biology, chemistry, mathematics, physics, physiology, and psychology—is desirable. Applicants must arrange for official transcripts of all prior college-level courses taken and their GRE scores (taken within the last two years) to be sent to the Office of Graduate Education. Students may elect to submit scores obtained in one or more GRE Subject Tests (from the subject areas listed above) in support of their application, but this is not required. Applicants must also arrange for letters of recommendation from 3 people who are familiar with their academic work to be sent to the University. For full consideration and evaluation for stipend support, completed applications should be received before December 1 for matriculation in late August. Late applications are evaluated on a space-available basis. There is no application fee. Students may complete an application at https://registrar.usuhs.edu..

Correspondence and Information

For information about the neuroscience program:

Sharon L. Juliano, Ph.D.
Director, Graduate Program in Neuroscience
Uniformed Services University
4301 Jones Bridge Road
Bethesda, Maryland 20814-4799
United States
Phone: 301-295-3642
Fax: 301-295-1996
E-mail: sharon.juliano@usuhs.edu
Website: http://www.usuhs.mil/nes/index.html

Tina Finley
Administrative Officer
Uniformed Services University
4301 Jones Bridge Road
Bethesda, Maryland 20814-4799
United States
Phone: 301-295-3642
E-mail: netina.finley@usuhs.edu

Uniformed Services University of the Health Sciences

THE FACULTY AND THEIR RESEARCH

Denes V. Agoston, M.D., Ph.D., Professor, Department of Anatomy, Physiology, and Genetics. The pathology of traumatic brain injury (TBI); molecular and imaging biomarkers for diagnosis and prognosis of chronic TBI.

Juanita Anders, Ph.D., Professor, Department of Anatomy, Physiology, and Genetics. Innovative therapies for neuronal regeneration of injured central and peripheral nervous systems; light-cellular interaction.

Regina Armstrong, Ph.D., Professor, Department of Anatomy, Physiology, and Genetics, and Director, Center for Neuroscience and Regenerative Medicine. Cellular and molecular mechanisms of neural stem/progenitor cell development and regeneration in demyelinating diseases and brain injury models.

David Benedek, M.D., Professor, Department of Psychiatry.

Diane E. Borst, Ph.D., Research Assistant Professor, Department of Anatomy, Physiology, and Genetics. Molecular mechanisms of retinal gene regulation and function.

Maria F. Braga, D.D.S., Ph.D., Professor, Department of Anatomy, Physiology, and Genetics. Cellular and molecular mechanisms regulating neuronal excitability in the amygdala; pathophysiology of anxiety disorders and epilepsy.

Barrington G. Burnett, Ph.D., Assistant Professor, Department of Anatomy, Physiology, and Genetics. The ubiquitin-proteasome system in neuronal maintenance and neurodegeneration.

Howard Bryant, Ph.D., Associate Professor, Department of Anatomy, Physiology, and Genetics. Electrophysiology of vascular smooth muscle.

Kimberly Byrnes, Ph.D., Associate Professor, Department of Anatomy, Physiology, and Genetics. Microglial and macrophage-based chronic inflammation after traumatic brain and spinal cord injury; noninvasive imaging of post-injury metabolic and inflammatory events.

Kwang Choi, Ph.D., Assistant Professor, Department of Psychiatry. Translational research on posttraumatic stress and substance use disorders using intravenous drug self-administration, Pavlovian fear conditioning, and PET brain imaging in rodents.

Jeffrey Cole, Ph.D., Assistant Professor, Department of Neurology. Translational research on traumatic brain injury, focusing on branched chain amino acids and metabolomics.

De-Maw Chuang, Ph.D., Adjunct Professor, Department of Psychiatry. Molecular and cellular of actions of mood stabilizers: neuroprotection against excitotoxicity-related neurodegeneration.

Thomas Côté, Ph.D., Associate Professor, Department of Pharmacology. Mu opioid receptor interaction with GTP-binding proteins and RGS proteins.

Brian Cox, Ph.D., Professor, Department of Pharmacology. Opiate drugs, endogenous opioids, neuropeptides; mechanisms underlying synaptic plasticity, drug tolerance and dependence, and responses to brain injury.

Clifton Dalgard, Ph.D., Assistant Professor, Department of Anatomy, Physiology, and Genetics. Molecular mechanisms of damage-associated inflammation.

Patricia A. Deuster, Ph.D., M.P.H., Professor, Department of Military and Emergency Medicine. Mechanisms of neuroendocrine and immune activation with stress.

Martin Doughty, Ph.D., Associate Professor, Department of Anatomy, Physiology, and Genetics. Optimizing induced pluripotent stem cells (iPSCs) for cell replacement therapy to treat traumatic brain injury (TBI); identifying transcriptional programs that function in cerebellar neurogenesis and pattern formation.

Ying-Hong Feng, Associate Professor, M.D., Ph.D. Angiotensin receptor and signal transduction.

Zygmunt Galdzicki, Ph.D., Professor, Department of Anatomy, Physiology, and Genetics. Molecular and electrophysiological approach to understand mental retardation in Down syndrome; neuroepigenetics and role of stress and brain trauma in neurodegenerative disorders

Neil Grunberg, Ph.D., Professor, Department of Medical and Clinical Psychology. Nicotine and tobacco; drug abuse; stress; traumatic brain injury; PTSD.

David Jacobowitz, Ph.D., Professor, Department of Anatomy, Physiology, and Genetics. Gene and protein discovery in the diseased and developing brain.

Sharon Juliano, Ph.D., Professor, Department of Anatomy, Physiology, and Genetics. Mechanisms of development and plasticity in the cerebral cortex, with particular emphasis on the migration of neurons into the cortical plate and factors maintaining the function and morphology of radial glia and Cajal-Retzius cells; assessing architectural reorganization in the neocortex after traumatic brain injury.

Fabio Leonessa, M.D., Research Assistant Professor, Department of Neurology. Pathobiology and biomarkers of blast-related neurotrauma.

He Li, M.D., Ph.D., Associate Professor, Department of Psychiatry. Neurobiological basis of post-traumatic stress disorder: synaptic plasticity and neuronal signaling in the amygdala circuitry.

Geoffrey Ling, M.D., Ph.D., Professor, Departments of Anesthesiology, Neurology, and Surgery. Novel therapeutics and diagnostic tools for traumatic brain injury and hemorrhagic shock; mechanisms of cellular injury and edema formation in traumatic brain injury.

Ann M. Marini, Ph.D., M.D., Professor, Department of Neurology. Molecular and cellular mechanisms of intrinsic survival pathways to protect against neurodegenerative disorders.

Joseph McCabe, Ph.D., Professor and Vice Chair, Department of Anatomy, Physiology, and Genetics. Traumatic brain injury and modeling; neuroprotection.

David Mears, Ph.D., Associate Professor, Department of Anatomy, Physiology, and Genetics. Electrophysiology and calcium signaling in neuroendocrine cells.

Chantal Moratz, Ph.D, Assistant Professor, Department of Medicine. Mechanisms of inflammation regulation in systemic lupus erythematosus, neuroinflammation in mild traumatic brain injury.

Gregory Mueller, Ph.D., Professor, Department of Anatomy, Physiology, and Genetics. Neuroimmunology; brain autoantibodies; brain injury biomarkers and the proteomics of brain injury.

Aryan Namboodiri, Ph.D., Associate Professor, Department of Anatomy, Physiology, and Genetics. Neurobiology of N-acetylaspartate (NAA); pathogenesis and treatment of Canavan disease and intranasal brain delivery of neuroprotectants.

Fereshteh Nugent, Ph.D., Assistant Professor, Department of Pharmacology. Synaptic plasticity and drug addiction.

Paul Pasquina, M.D., Chairman, Department of Physical Medicine and Rehabilitation, and Director, Center for Rehabilitation Sciences Research. Clinical studies on advanced prosthetics, neurorehabilitation, traumatic brain injury, and pain management.

Harvey B. Pollard, M.D., Ph.D., Professor and Chair, Department of Anatomy, Physiology, and Genetics. Molecular biology of secretory processes.

Sylvie Poluch, Ph.D., Research Assistant Professor, Department of Anatomy, Physiology, and Genetics. Development of the cerebral cortex.

Brian Schaefer, Ph.D., Associate Professor, Department of Microbiology and Immunology. Mechanisms of leukocyte activation, particularly regulation of cytoplasmic signals to NF-kappaB; development of therapeutic approaches for neurotropic viral infections; role of inflammation in traumatic brain injury.

Jeremy T. Smyth, Ph.D., Assistant Professor, Department of Anatomy, Physiology, and Genetics. Physiology of the endoplasmic reticulum in developmental and neurodegenerative processes; intracellular calcium signaling; Drosophila developmental genetics.

Aviva Symes, Ph.D., Professor, Department of Pharmacology. Glial response to traumatic brain and spinal cord injury; mechanism of cytokine action in the CNS after injury.

Jack W. Tsao, M.D., Ph.D., Professor, Departments of Neurology and Physical Medicine and Rehabilitation. Clinical studies on phantom limb pain and traumatic brain injury; basic science studies on cellular and developmental mechanisms governing nerve degeneration.

Robert J. Ursano, M.D., Professor and Chairman, Department of Psychiatry, and Director, Center for the Study of Traumatic Stress. Posttraumatic stress disorder.

Gary H. Wynn, M.D., Associate Professor, Department of Psychiatry. Neurobiology and clinical treatment of trauma-related disorders.

T. John Wu, Ph.D., Associate Professor, Department of Obstetrics and Gynecology. Neuroendocrine regulation of reproduction and stress.

Lei Zhang, M.D., Associate Professor, Department of Psychiatry. PTSD and biomarkers.

Yumin Zhang, M.D., Ph.D., Associate Professor, Department of Anatomy, Physiology, and Genetics. Cellular and molecular mechanisms of oligodendroglial and neuronal toxicity.

UCONN HEALTH
Graduate Program in Neuroscience

UCONN
HEALTH

 For more information, visit http://petersons.to/uconnhealth_neuroscience

Program of Study

The neuroscience graduate program at UConn Health is committed to fostering an interdisciplinary training environment for students towards understanding the normal function and disorders of the nervous system. Special emphasis is placed upon preparing students for a research and teaching career in both academic and industrial settings.

The interdepartmental nature of the program offers comprehensive conceptual and experimental training in molecular, systems, and behavioral neuroscience. The faculty of the neuroscience program engages in research that involves cellular, molecular, and developmental neurobiology, neuroanatomy, neurophysiology, neurochemistry, neuroendocrinology, neuropharmacology, neuroimaging, and neuropathology. Specific examples of research topics include:

- Cellular and molecular bases of synaptic neurotransmission, including the structure and function of ligand-gated neurotransmitter receptors and voltage-sensitive ion channels
- Genetic and epigenetic regulation of membrane biogenesis in neurons and glia
- Electrophysiology of excitable tissue
- Development of the autonomic nervous system
- Development of neural tissue and of the neural crest
- Stimulus coding, synaptic organization, and development of sensory systems
- Structure and function of auditory and gustatory systems
- Computational neuroscience
- Degeneration, regeneration, plasticity, and transplantation
- fMRI research/functional mapping of normal and diseased brain
- Neurobiology of degenerative disorders, notably Huntington's Disease
- Alzheimer's Disease, multiple sclerosis, deafness, and loss of hearing

Research Facilities

Because of the interdepartmental format, the students have access to all of the facilities of modern biomedical research at UConn Health, including those in clinical and basic science departments. Most of the neuroscience faculty members are housed in the same building on adjoining floors, providing for a congenial atmosphere of informal scientific exchange and collaborations between laboratories. The Center for Cell Analysis and Modeling (CCAM) has state-of-the-art facilities for confocal and two-photon microscopy and image analysis and is available to members of the Program in Neuroscience. The Lyman Maynard Stowe Library has an extensive collection of periodicals and monographs as well as subscriptions to journals of current interest in the field of neuroscience.

Financial Aid

Support for doctoral students engaged in full-time degree programs at UConn Health is provided on a competitive basis. Graduate research assistantships for 2016–17 provide a stipend of $29,000 per year, which includes a waiver of tuition/most University fees for the fall and spring semesters and the option of participating in a student health insurance plan. While financial aid is offered competitively, UConn Health makes every possible effort to address the financial needs of all students.

Cost of Study

For 2016–17, tuition is $14,310 per year for full-time students who are Connecticut residents and $35,346 per year for full-time students who are out-of-state residents. General University fees are added to the cost of tuition for students who do not receive a tuition waiver. These costs are usually met by traineeships or research assistantships for doctoral students.

Living and Housing Costs

There is a wide range of affordable housing options in the greater Hartford area within easy commuting distance of the campus, including an extensive complex that is adjacent to UConn Health. Costs range from $700 to $1,000 per month for a one-bedroom unit; 2 or more students sharing an apartment usually pay less. University housing is not available.

Student Group

Twelve students are registered in the Ph.D. program in the Neuroscience Program (including combined-degree students). The total number of master's and Ph.D. students at UConn Health is approximately 400, and there are about 125 medical and dental students per class.

Location

UConn Health is located in the historic town of Farmington, Connecticut. Set in the beautiful New England countryside on a hill overlooking the Farmington Valley, it is close to ski areas, hiking trails, and facilities for boating, fishing, and swimming. Connecticut's capital city of Hartford, 7 miles east of Farmington, is the center of an urban region of approximately 800,000 people. The beaches of the Long Island Sound are about 50 minutes away to the south, and the beautiful Berkshires are a short drive to the northwest. New York City and Boston can be reached within 2½ hours by car. Hartford is the home of the acclaimed Hartford Stage Company, TheatreWorks, the Hartford Symphony and Chamber orchestras, two ballet companies, an opera company, the Wadsworth Athenaeum (the oldest public art museum in the nation), the Mark Twain house, the Hartford Civic Center, and many other interesting cultural and recreational facilities. The area is also home to several branches of the University of Connecticut, Trinity College, and the University of Hartford, which includes the Hartt School of Music. Bradley International Airport (about 30 minutes from campus) serves the Hartford/Springfield area with frequent airline connections to major cities in this country and abroad. Frequent bus and rail service is also available from Hartford.

The UConn Health Campus

The 200-acre UConn Health campus at Farmington houses a division of the University of Connecticut Graduate School, as well as the School of Medicine and Dental Medicine. The campus also includes the John Dempsey Hospital, associated clinics, and extensive medical research facilities, all in a centralized facility with more than 1 million square feet of floor space. The Academic Research Building, built in 1999, is an impressive eleven-story structure providing 170,000 square feet of laboratory space and renovations are underway in the main Laboratory building, converting existing lab space to state-of-the-art open lab areas. In addition, the Jackson Laboratory for Genomic Medicine opened its 189,000-square-foot facility on the UConn Health Campus in fall 2014. The faculty includes more than 260 full-time members. The institution has a strong commitment to graduate study within an environment that promotes social and intellectual interaction among the various educational programs. Graduate students are represented on various administrative committees concerned with curricular affairs, and the Graduate Student Organization (GSO) represents graduate students' needs and concerns to the faculty and administration, in addition to fostering social contact among graduate students at UConn Health.

Applying

Applications for admission should be submitted via the online application system and should be filed together with transcripts, three letters of recommendation, a personal statement, and recent results from the General Test of the Graduate Record Examinations. International students must take the Test of English as a Foreign Language (TOEFL) to satisfy Graduate School requirements. The deadline for completed applications and receipt of all supplemental materials is **December 1**. Please note that GRE and TOEFL exams taken after the due date will not be accepted for consideration for admission. Applicants should have had undergraduate instruction in chemistry and biology. In accordance with the laws of the state of Connecticut and of the United States, UConn Health does not discriminate against any person in its educational and employment activities on the grounds of race, color, creed, national origin, sex, age, or physical disability.

Correspondence and Information

Graduate Admissions Office
Ph.D. in Biomedical Science Program
UConn Health
263 Farmington Ave., MC 3906
Farmington, Connecticut 06030-3906
United States
Phone: 860-679-4509
E-mail: BiomedSciAdmissions@uchc.edu
Website: http://health.uconn.edu/graduate-school/academics/
         programs/ph-d-biomedical-science

THE FACULTY AND THEIR RESEARCH

Srdjan Antic, Associate Professor of Neuroscience; M.D., Belgrade. Dendritic integration of synaptic inputs; dopaminergic modulation of dendritic excitability.

Rashmi Bansal, Professor of Neuroscience; Ph.D., Central Drug Research Institute. Developmental, cellular, and molecular biology of oligodendrocytes; growth-factor regulation of development and function and its relationship to neurodegenerative disease, including multiple sclerosis.

Elisa Barbarese, Professor of Neuroscience and Neurology; Ph.D. McGill. Molecular and cellular biology of neural cells, with emphasis on RNA trafficking.

Kyle Baumbauer, Assistant Professor of Neuroscience; Ph.D., Kent State. Neurons responsible for transmitting sensory information to the central nervous system; the primary afferents.

Leslie R. Bernstein, Professor of Neuroscience; Ph.D., Illinois. Behavioral neuroscience: psychoacoustics, binaural hearing.

John H. Carson, Professor of Molecular, Microbial, and Structural Biology; Ph.D., MIT. Molecular and developmental neurobiology; myelination; intracellular RNA trafficking.

Jonathan Covault, Professor of Psychiatry; M.D., Ph.D., Iowa. Genetic correlates of alcohol use disorders; role of neuroactive steroids in the effects of alcohol.

Stephen Crocker, Assistant Professor of Neuroscience; Ph.D., Ottawa. Brain injury and repair in neurodegenerative diseases, with a focus on neuroinflammation; myelin injury; neural stem cell differentiation; signal transduction; glia; matrix metalloproteinases and their tissue inhibitors.

Betty Eipper, Professor of Neuroscience; Ph.D., Harvard. Cell biology, biochemistry, and physiology of peptide synthesis, storage, and secretion in neurons and endocrine cells.

Marion E. Frank, Professor of BioStructure and Function and Director, Connecticut Chemosensory Clinical Research Center; Ph.D., Brown. Gustatory neurophysiology, neuroanatomy, behavior, and disorders; chemosensory information processing; clinical testing of oral chemosensory function in humans.

Duck O. Kim, Professor of Neuroscience and Biological Engineering Program; D.Sc., Washington (St. Louis). Neurobiology and biophysics of the auditory system; computational neuroscience of single neurons and neural systems; experimental otolaryngology; biomedical engineering.

Shigeyuki Kuwada, Professor of Neuroscience; Ph.D., Cincinnati. Neurophysiology and anatomy of mammalian auditory system; principles of binaural signal processing, electrical audiometry in infants.

Eric S. Levine, Professor of Neuroscience; Ph.D., Princeton. Synapse plasticity and role of neuromodulators in brain development and learning, focusing on neurotrophins and endocannabinoids.

James Li, Associate Professor of Genetics and Developmental Biology; Ph.D., Texas. Development of the central nervous system, with an emphasis on the cellular and molecular mechanisms underlying formation of the mammalian cerebellum.

Leslie Loew, Professor of Cell Biology; Ph.D., Cornell. Morphological determinants of cell physiology; image-based computational models of cellular biology; spatial variations of cell membrane electrophysiology; new optical methods for probing living cells.

Xin-Ming Ma, Assistant Professor of Neuroscience; Ph.D., Beijing. Synaptogenesis and spine plasticity in hippocampal neurons; estrogen hormones and synaptic plasticity; stress and neuronal plasticity.

Richard Mains, Professor and Chair of Neuroscience; Ph.D., Harvard. Pituitary; neuronal tissue culture; peptides, vesicles; enzymes; drug abuse; development.

Royce Mohan, Associate Professor of Neuroscience; Ph.D., Ohio State. Chemical genetic approaches in corneal angiogenesis, fibrosis, and retinal gliosis.

Douglas L. Oliver, Professor of Neuroscience and Biomedical Engineering; Ph.D., Duke. Synaptic organization; parallel information processing in CNS; role of ionic currents, channel expression in information processing; neurocytology, morphology, cellular physiology of CNS sensory systems; biology of hearing and deafness.

Joel S. Pachter, Professor of Cell Biology; Ph.D., NYU. Mechanisms regulating pathogenesis of CNS infectious/inflammatory disease.

Zhaowen Wang, Associate Professor of Neuroscience; Ph.D., Michigan State. Molecular mechanisms of synaptic transmission, focusing on neurotransmitter release and mechanisms of potassium channel localization, using *C. elegans* as a model organism.

Ji Yu, Associate Professor of Genetics and Developmental Biology; Ph.D., Texas. Optical imaging technology; regulatory mechanisms in dendritic RNA translation; cytoskeletal dynamics.

Nada Zecevic, Professor of Neuroscience; M.D., Ph.D., Belgrade. Cellular and molecular aspects of CNS development; primate cerebral cortex; oligodendrocyte progenitors, stem cells, microglia; multiple sclerosis.

Section 14
Nutrition

This section contains a directory of institutions offering graduate work in nutrition, followed by an in-depth entry submitted by an institution that chose to prepare a detailed program description. Additional information about programs listed in the directory but not augmented by an in-depth entry may be obtained by writing directly to the dean of a graduate school or chair of a department at the address given in the directory.

For programs offering related work, see also in this book *Allied Health, Biochemistry, Biological and Biomedical Sciences, Botany and Plant Biology, Microbiological Sciences, Pathology and Pathobiology, Pharmacology and Toxicology, Physiology, Public Health,* and *Veterinary Medicine and Sciences*. In the other guides in this series:

Graduate Programs in the Humanities, Arts & Social Sciences

See *Economics (Agricultural Economics and Agribusiness)* and *Family and Consumer Sciences*

Graduate Programs in the Physical Sciences, Mathematics, Agricultural Sciences, the Environment & Natural Resources

See *Agricultural and Food Sciences* and *Chemistry*

Graduate Programs in Engineering & Applied Sciences

See *Agricultural Engineering and Bioengineering* and *Biomedical Engineering and Biotechnology*

CONTENTS

Nutrition

Abilene Christian University, Graduate School, College of Education and Human Services, Department of Kinesiology and Nutrition, Abilene, TX 79699-9100. Offers dietetic internship (Certificate). *Faculty:* 2 part-time/adjunct (both women). *Students:* 12 full-time (11 women); includes 2 minority (1 Black or African American, non-Hispanic/Latino; 1 Two or more races, non-Hispanic/Latino), 1 international. 27 applicants, 44% accepted, 12 enrolled. In 2015, 9 Certificates awarded. *Entrance requirements:* Additional exam requirements/recommendations for international students: Required—TOEFL (minimum score 550 paper-based; 90 iBT), IELTS (minimum score 6.5), PTE. Application fee: $50. *Expenses:* $1,133 per credit hour. *Financial support:* In 2015–16, 1 student received support. Application deadline: 4/1; applicants required to submit FAFSA. *Unit head:* Sheila Jones, Chair, 325-674-2089, E-mail: joness@acu.edu. *Application contact:* Kay Williams, Program Director, 254-744-3707, E-mail: jkw14a@acu.edu.

Adelphi University, College of Nursing and Public Health, Garden City, NY 11530. Offers adult health nurse (MS); health information technology (Advanced Certificate); nurse practitioner in adult health nursing (Certificate); nursing (PhD); nursing administration (MS, Certificate); nutrition (MS); public health (MPH). *Accreditation:* AACN. *Program availability:* Part-time, evening/weekend. *Degree requirements:* For master's, thesis or alternative. *Entrance requirements:* For master's, BSN, clinical experience, 1 course in basic statistics, minimum GPA of 3.0, 2 letters of recommendation, resume or curriculum vitae; for doctorate, GRE, licensure as RN in New York, professional writing sample (scholarly writing), 3 letters of recommendation, resume or curriculum vitae; for other advanced degree, MSN. Additional exam requirements/recommendations for international students: Required—TOEFL (minimum score 550 paper-based; 80 iBT). Electronic applications accepted. *Faculty research:* Social practices in healthcare, bereavement, family grief, historiography, gerontology.

Alabama Agricultural and Mechanical University, School of Graduate Studies, College of Agricultural, Life and Natural Sciences, Department of Family and Consumer Sciences, Huntsville, AL 35811. Offers apparel, merchandising and design (MS); family and consumer sciences (MS); human development and family studies (MS); nutrition and hospitality management (MS). *Program availability:* Part-time, evening/weekend. *Degree requirements:* For master's, comprehensive exam, thesis optional. *Entrance requirements:* For master's, GRE General Test. Additional exam requirements/recommendations for international students: Required—TOEFL (minimum score 500 paper-based; 61 iBT). Electronic applications accepted. *Faculty research:* Food biotechnology, nutrition, food microbiology, food engineering, food chemistry.

American College of Healthcare Sciences, Graduate Programs, Portland, OR 97239-3719. Offers aromatherapy (Graduate Certificate); complementary alternative medicine (MS, Graduate Certificate); herbal medicine (Graduate Certificate); nutrition (Graduate Certificate). *Program availability:* Part-time, evening/weekend, online learning. *Degree requirements:* For master's, capstone project. *Entrance requirements:* For master's, interview, letters of recommendation, essay.

American University, College of Arts and Sciences, Department of Health Studies, Program in Nutrition Education, Washington, DC 20016-8001. Offers MS, Certificate. *Program availability:* Online only, 100% online. *Students:* 64 part-time (58 women); includes 7 minority (2 Black or African American, non-Hispanic/Latino; 2 American Indian or Alaska Native, non-Hispanic/Latino; 3 Hispanic/Latino), 2 international. Average age 30. 59 applicants, 93% accepted, 38 enrolled. *Entrance requirements:* For master's, GRE; for Certificate, statement of purpose, transcripts, resume. Additional exam requirements/recommendations for international students: Required—TOEFL (minimum score 100 iBT), IELTS (minimum score 7), PTE (minimum score 68). Application fee: $55. *Expenses: Tuition, area resident:* Full-time $27,468; part-time $1526 per credit hour. *Required fees:* $430. Tuition and fees vary according to course level and program. *Unit head:* Anastasia Snelling, Department Chair, Health Studies, 202-885-6278, Fax: 202-885-1187, E-mail: stacey@american.edu. *Application contact:* Kathleen Clowery, Associate Director, Graduate Enrollment Management, 202-885-3620, Fax: 202-885-1344, E-mail: clowery@american.edu.
Website: http://www.american.edu/cas/seth/nutrition-education-ms.cfm

American University of Beirut, Graduate Programs, Faculty of Agricultural and Food Sciences, Beirut, Lebanon. Offers agricultural economics (MS); animal sciences (MS); ecosystem management (MSES); food technology (MS); irrigation (MS); nutrition (MS); plant protection (MS); plant science (MS); poultry science (MS); rural community development (MS). *Program availability:* Part-time. *Faculty:* 19 full-time (4 women). *Students:* 13 full-time (5 women), 55 part-time (41 women). Average age 26. 93 applicants, 52% accepted, 25 enrolled. In 2015, 27 master's awarded. *Degree requirements:* For master's, one foreign language, comprehensive exam, thesis (for some programs). *Entrance requirements:* Additional exam requirements/recommendations for international students: Required—TOEFL (minimum score 600 paper-based; 100 iBT), IELTS (minimum score 7.5). *Application deadline:* For fall admission, 2/10 for domestic and international students; for spring admission, 11/2 for domestic and international students. Application fee: $50. Electronic applications accepted. *Expenses: Tuition, area resident:* Full-time $16,254; part-time $903 per credit. *Required fees:* $699. Tuition and fees vary according to course load and program. *Financial support:* In 2015–16, 1 research assistantship with partial tuition reimbursement (averaging $1,800 per year), 48 teaching assistantships with tuition reimbursements (averaging $1,400 per year) were awarded; scholarships/grants, health care benefits, and unspecified assistantships also available. Financial award application deadline: 2/2. *Faculty research:* Developing skills in the field of integrated energy planning in med landscaper; profiling refugee households in Lebanon; Improving the nutrition of Syrian refugees and host communities though garden walls; monitoring and evaluation of salt iodization in Lebanon; mother and child cohorts: towards curbing the epidemic of non-communicable diseases in Qatar and Lebanon. *Total annual research expenditures:* $852,730. *Unit head:* Prof. Nahla Hwalla, Dean, 961-1343002 Ext. 4400, Fax: 961-1744460, E-mail: nahla@aub.edu.lb. *Application contact:* Dr. Rabih Talhouk, Director, Graduate Council, 961-1350000 Ext. 4386, Fax: 961-1374374, E-mail: graduate.council@aub.edu.lb.
Website: http://www.aub.edu.lb/fafs/fafs_home/Pages/index.aspx

Andrews University, School of Health Professions, Department of Nutrition, Berrien Springs, MI 49104. Offers nutrition (MS); nutrition and dietetics (Certificate); public health (MPH). *Program availability:* Part-time. *Faculty:* 1 (woman) full-time, 7 part-time/adjunct (2 women). *Students:* 19 full-time (18 women), 22 part-time (19 women); includes 15 minority (5 Black or African American, non-Hispanic/Latino; 2 Asian, non-Hispanic/Latino; 7 Hispanic/Latino; 1 Two or more races, non-Hispanic/Latino), 4 international. Average age 31. 50 applicants, 50% accepted, 25 enrolled. In 2015, 1 master's, 11 other advanced degrees awarded. *Entrance requirements:* For master's, GRE. Additional exam requirements/recommendations for international students: Required—TOEFL (minimum score 550 paper-based). *Application deadline:* Applications are processed on a rolling basis. Application fee: $40. *Faculty research:* Exercise education. *Unit head:* Dr. Sherine Brown-Fraser, Chairperson, 269-471-3370. *Application contact:* Monica Wringer, Supervisor of Graduate Admission, 800-253-2874, Fax: 269-471-6321, E-mail: graduate@andrews.edu.
Website: http://www.andrews.edu/shp/nutrition/

Appalachian State University, Cratis D. Williams Graduate School, Department of Nutrition and Health Care Management, Boone, NC 28608. Offers nutrition (MS). *Program availability:* Part-time. Electronic applications accepted. *Faculty research:* Food antioxidants and nutrition.

Arizona State University at the Tempe campus, College of Health Solutions, School of Nutrition and Health Promotion, Tempe, AZ 85287. Offers clinical exercise physiology (MS); exercise and wellness (MS); nutrition (MS), including dietetics, human nutrition; obesity prevention and management (MS); physical activity, nutrition and wellness (PhD).

Auburn University, Graduate School, College of Human Sciences, Department of Nutrition and Food Science, Auburn University, AL 36849. Offers global hospitality and retailing (Graduate Certificate); nutrition (MS, PhD). *Program availability:* Part-time. *Faculty:* 14 full-time (6 women). *Students:* 38 full-time (33 women), 36 part-time (21 women); includes 11 minority (4 Black or African American, non-Hispanic/Latino; 1 American Indian or Alaska Native, non-Hispanic/Latino; 1 Asian, non-Hispanic/Latino; 3 Hispanic/Latino; 2 Two or more races, non-Hispanic/Latino), 22 international. Average age 30. 73 applicants, 64% accepted, 33 enrolled. In 2015, 7 master's, 5 doctorates awarded. *Degree requirements:* For master's, thesis (for some programs); for doctorate, thesis/dissertation. *Entrance requirements:* For master's and doctorate, GRE General Test. *Application deadline:* Applications are processed on a rolling basis. Application fee: $50 ($60 for international students). Electronic applications accepted. *Expenses:* Tuition, state resident: full-time $8802; part-time $489 per credit hour. Tuition, nonresident: full-time $26,406; part-time $1467 per credit hour. *Required fees:* $808 per semester. Tuition and fees vary according to degree level and program. *Financial support:* Research assistantships, teaching assistantships, career-related internships or fieldwork, and Federal Work-Study available. Support available to part-time students. Financial award application deadline: 3/15; financial award applicants required to submit FAFSA. *Faculty research:* Food quality and safety, diet, food supply, physical activity in maintenance of health, prevention of selected chronic disease states. *Unit head:* Dr. Martin O'Neill, Head, 334-844-3266. *Application contact:* Dr. George Flowers, Dean of the Graduate School, 334-844-2125.
Website: http://www.humsci.auburn.edu/ndhm/grad.php

Ball State University, Graduate School, College of Applied Sciences and Technology, Department of Family and Consumer Sciences, Muncie, IN 47306. Offers family and consumer science (MS), including apparel design (MA, MS), fashion merchandising (MA, MS), interior design (MA, MS), residential property management (MA, MS); family and consumer sciences (MA), including apparel design (MA, MS), fashion merchandising (MA, MS), interior design (MA, MS), residential property management (MA, MS); nutrition and dietetics (MA, MS). *Program availability:* Part-time, evening/weekend, 100% online. *Faculty:* 8 full-time (7 women), 3 part-time/adjunct (all women). *Students:* 34 full-time (33 women), 40 part-time (35 women); includes 4 minority (1 Black or African American, non-Hispanic/Latino; 2 Asian, non-Hispanic/Latino; 1 Hispanic/Latino), 7 international. Average age 25. 63 applicants, 32% accepted, 18 enrolled. In 2015, 24 master's awarded. *Degree requirements:* For master's, thesis or alternative. *Entrance requirements:* For master's, letter of intent, resume, two letters of recommendation, portfolio (for interior design option). Additional exam requirements/recommendations for international students: Required—TOEFL (minimum score 550 paper-based; 79 iBT), IELTS (minimum score 6.5). *Application deadline:* For fall admission, 2/15 for domestic students; for spring admission, 9/25 for domestic students. Applications are processed on a rolling basis. Application fee: $60. Electronic applications accepted. *Expenses: Tuition, area resident:* Full-time $6948; part-time $2316 per semester. Tuition, state resident: full-time $10,422; part-time $3474 per semester. Tuition, nonresident: full-time $19,062; part-time $6354 per semester. *Required fees:* $651 per semester. Tuition and fees vary according to campus/location, program and reciprocity agreements. *Financial support:* In 2015–16, 8 students received support, including 7 research assistantships with partial tuition reimbursements available (averaging $12,288 per year); unspecified assistantships also available. Financial award application deadline: 3/1; financial award applicants required to submit FAFSA. *Faculty research:* Maternal and infant nutrition, nutrition education. *Unit head:* Dr. Sotiris Hji-Avgoustis, Chairperson, 765-285-5922, Fax: 765-285-2314, E-mail: shjiavgousti@bsu.edu. *Application contact:* Dr. Scott Hall, Assistant Chairperson, 765-285-5943, Fax: 765-285-2314, E-mail: sshall@bsu.edu.
Website: http://www.bsu.edu/fcs/

Bastyr University, School of Natural Health Arts and Sciences, Kenmore, WA 98028-4966. Offers counseling psychology (MA); holistic landscape design (Certificate); midwifery (MS); nutrition (MS); nutrition and clinical health psychology (MS). *Accreditation:* AND. *Program availability:* Part-time. *Degree requirements:* For master's, thesis optional. *Entrance requirements:* For master's, 1-2 years' basic sciences course work (depending on program). Additional exam requirements/recommendations for international students: Required—TOEFL (minimum score 550 paper-based; 79 iBT). *Faculty research:* Whole-food nutrition for type 2 diabetes; meditation in end-of-life care; stress management; Qi Gong, Tai Chi and yoga for older adults; Echinacea and immunology.

Baylor University, Graduate School, Military Programs, Program in Nutrition, Waco, TX 76798. Offers MS. *Faculty:* 7 full-time (6 women), 6 part-time/adjunct (all women). *Students:* 19 full-time (14 women), 4 part-time (all women); includes 3 minority (1 Black or African American, non-Hispanic/Latino; 1 Hispanic/Latino; 1 Two or more races, non-Hispanic/Latino). Average age 26. 25 applicants, 48% accepted, 12 enrolled. In 2015, 11 master's awarded. *Degree requirements:* For master's, comprehensive exam, thesis. *Entrance requirements:* For master's, GRE. *Application deadline:* Applications are processed on a rolling basis. Electronic applications accepted. *Faculty research:* Weight control, critical care nutrition, breast feeding, intuitive eating. *Unit head:* Col. LesLee Funderburk, Graduate Program Director, 210-221-6274, Fax: 210-221-7363, E-mail: leslee.k.funderburk.mil@mail.mil. *Application contact:* Sgt. Doshka Bbowens, Administrative Assistant, 210-295-6274, E-mail: bowensdoshka@gmail.com.
Website: http://www.baylor.edu/graduate/nutrition/

Baylor University, Graduate School, Robbins College of Health and Human Sciences, Department of Family and Consumer Sciences, Waco, TX 76798. Offers nutrition sciences (MS).

Benedictine University, Graduate Programs, Program in Nutrition and Wellness, Lisle, IL 60532. Offers MS. *Entrance requirements:* Additional exam requirements/recommendations for international students: Required—TOEFL (minimum score 550 paper-based). Electronic applications accepted. *Faculty research:* Community and corporate wellness risk assessment, health behavior change, self-efficacy, evaluation of health program impact and effectiveness.

Benedictine University, Graduate Programs, Program in Public Health, Lisle, IL 60532. Offers administration of health care institutions (MPH); dietetics (MPH); disaster management (MPH); health education (MPH); health information systems (MPH); MBA/MPH; MPH/MS. *Accreditation:* CEPH. *Program availability:* Part-time, evening/weekend, online learning. *Entrance requirements:* For master's, MAT, GRE, or GMAT. Additional exam requirements/recommendations for international students: Required—TOEFL (minimum score 550 paper-based).

Boston University, College of Health and Rehabilitation Sciences: Sargent College, Department of Health Sciences, Program in Nutrition, Boston, MA 02215. Offers MS. *Faculty:* 10 full-time (9 women), 5 part-time/adjunct (3 women). *Students:* 47 full-time (45 women), 1 (woman) part-time; includes 9 minority (1 Black or African American, non-Hispanic/Latino; 6 Asian, non-Hispanic/Latino; 1 Hispanic/Latino; 1 Two or more races, non-Hispanic/Latino), 1 international. Average age 25. 136 applicants, 23% accepted, 17 enrolled. In 2015, 15 master's awarded. *Entrance requirements:* For master's, GRE General Test, minimum GPA of 3.0. Additional exam requirements/recommendations for international students: Required—TOEFL (minimum score 550 paper-based; 84 iBT). *Application deadline:* For fall admission, 2/15 priority date for domestic and international students; for spring admission, 10/1 for domestic and international students. Applications are processed on a rolling basis. Application fee: $80. Electronic applications accepted. *Expenses:* $1,537 per credit. *Financial support:* In 2015–16, 31 students received support, including 4 teaching assistantships (averaging $2,500 per year); career-related internships or fieldwork, Federal Work-Study, institutionally sponsored loans, and scholarships/grants also available. Financial award application deadline: 2/15; financial award applicants required to submit FAFSA. *Faculty research:* Metabolism, health promotion, obesity, epidemiology. *Unit head:* Dr. Paula Quatromoni, Chair, 617-353-5797, Fax: 617-353-7567, E-mail: paulaq@bu.edu. *Application contact:* Sharon Sankey, Assistant Dean, Student Services, 617-353-2713, Fax: 617-353-7500, E-mail: ssankey@bu.edu.

Boston University, School of Medicine, Division of Graduate Medical Sciences, Nutrition and Metabolism, Boston, MA 02215. Offers MA, PhD. *Degree requirements:* For master's, thesis; for doctorate, thesis/dissertation. *Application deadline:* For fall admission, 1/15 for domestic students; for spring admission, 10/15 for domestic students. *Unit head:* Dr. Susan K. Fried, Director, 617-638-8088, E-mail: llmoore@bu.edu. *Application contact:* Dr. Lynn Moore, GMS Admissions Office, 617-638-5255, E-mail: askgms@bu.edu.
Website: http://www.bumc.bu.edu/gms/nutrition-metabolism/

Bowling Green State University, Graduate College, College of Education and Human Development, School of Family and Consumer Sciences, Bowling Green, OH 43403. Offers food and nutrition (MFCS); human development and family studies (MFCS). *Program availability:* Part-time. *Degree requirements:* For master's, thesis. *Entrance requirements:* For master's, GRE General Test, minimum GPA of 3.0. Additional exam requirements/recommendations for international students: Required—TOEFL. Electronic applications accepted. *Faculty research:* Public health, wellness, social issues and policies, ethnic foods, nutrition and aging.

Brigham Young University, Graduate Studies, College of Life Sciences, Department of Nutrition, Dietetics and Food Science, Provo, UT 84602. Offers food science (MS); nutrition (MS). *Faculty:* 12 full-time (5 women). *Students:* 16 full-time (8 women); includes 1 minority (Asian, non-Hispanic/Latino). Average age 24. 12 applicants, 50% accepted, 6 enrolled. In 2015, 2 master's awarded. *Degree requirements:* For master's, comprehensive exam, thesis. *Entrance requirements:* For master's, GRE General Test. Additional exam requirements/recommendations for international students: Required—TOEFL; Recommended—TSE. *Application deadline:* For fall admission, 2/1 priority date for domestic and international students; for winter admission, 6/30 priority date for domestic and international students. Application fee: $50. Electronic applications accepted. *Financial support:* In 2015–16, 6 students received support, including 6 research assistantships (averaging $20,325 per year), 6 teaching assistantships (averaging $20,325 per year); career-related internships or fieldwork, institutionally sponsored loans, and scholarships/grants also available. Financial award application deadline: 4/1. *Faculty research:* Dairy foods, lipid oxidation, food processes, magnesium and selenium nutrition, nutrient effect on gene expression. *Total annual research expenditures:* $326,945. *Unit head:* Dr. Michael L. Dunn, Chair, 801-422-6670, Fax: 801-422-0258, E-mail: michael_dunn@byu.edu. *Application contact:* Dr. Susan Fullmer, Graduate Coordinator, 801-422-3349, Fax: 801-422-0258, E-mail: susan_fullmer@byu.edu.
Website: http://ndfs.byu.edu/

Brooklyn College of the City University of New York, School of Natural and Behavioral Sciences, Department of Health and Nutrition Sciences, Program in Nutrition, Brooklyn, NY 11210-2889. Offers MS. *Program availability:* Part-time. *Degree requirements:* For master's, thesis or comprehensive exam. *Entrance requirements:* For master's, 18 credits in health-related areas, 2 letters of recommendation, essay. Additional exam requirements/recommendations for international students: Required—TOEFL. Electronic applications accepted. *Faculty research:* Medical ethics, AIDS, history of public health, diet restriction, palliative care, risk reduction/disease prevention, metabolism, diabetes.

California State Polytechnic University, Pomona, Program in Agriculture, Pomona, CA 91768-2557. Offers agricultural science (MS); nutrition and food science (MS). *Program availability:* Part-time. *Students:* 13 full-time (9 women), 23 part-time (15 women); includes 16 minority (3 Black or African American, non-Hispanic/Latino; 4 Asian, non-Hispanic/Latino; 9 Hispanic/Latino), 3 international. Average age 28. 64 applicants, 42% accepted, 13 enrolled. In 2015, 12 master's awarded. *Degree requirements:* For master's, thesis or alternative. *Application deadline:* For fall admission, 5/1 priority date for domestic students; for winter admission, 10/15 priority date for domestic students; for spring admission, 1/2 priority date for domestic students. Applications are processed on a rolling basis. Application fee: $55. Electronic applications accepted. *Expenses:* Tuition, state resident: full-time $6738. Tuition, nonresident: full-time $13,434. *Required fees:* $1504. Tuition and fees vary according to course load, degree level and program. *Financial support:* Career-related internships or fieldwork, Federal Work-Study, and institutionally sponsored loans available. Support available to part-time students. Financial award application deadline: 3/2; financial award applicants required to submit FAFSA. *Faculty research:* Equine nutrition, physiology, and reproduction; leadership development; bioartificial pancreas; plant science; ruminant and human nutrition. *Unit head:* Dr. Harmit Singh, Director of Research and Graduate Studies, 909-869-3023, Fax: 909-869-5078, E-mail: harmitsingh@cpp.edu.
Website: http://www.cpp.edu/~agri/agmasters/index.shtml

California State University, Chico, Office of Graduate Studies, College of Natural Sciences, Department of Nutrition and Food Science, Chico, CA 95929-0722. Offers general nutritional science (MS); nutrition education (MS). *Program availability:* Part-time. *Degree requirements:* For master's, thesis, professional paper, or oral defense. *Entrance requirements:* For master's, GRE General Test, two letters of recommendation, statement of purpose, resume. Additional exam requirements/recommendations for international students: Required—TOEFL (minimum score 550 paper-based; 80 iBT), IELTS (minimum score 6.5), PTE (minimum score 59). *Application deadline:* For fall admission, 3/1 priority date for domestic students, 3/1 for international students; for spring admission, 9/15 priority date for domestic students, 9/15 for international students. Application fee: $55. Electronic applications accepted. *Expenses: Tuition, area resident:* Full-time $4146; part-time $2730. *Financial support:* Teaching assistantships, career-related internships or fieldwork, and scholarships/grants available. Financial award application deadline: 3/1; financial award applicants required to submit FAFSA. *Unit head:* Dr. Katie Silliman, Chair, 530-898-6245, Fax: 530-898-5586, E-mail: ksilliman@csuchico.edu. *Application contact:* Judy L. Rice, Graduate Admissions Coordinator, 530-898-5416, Fax: 530-898-3342, E-mail: jlrice@csuchico.edu.
Website: http://www.csuchico.edu/nfsc/

California State University, Long Beach, Graduate Studies, College of Health and Human Services, Department of Family and Consumer Sciences, Master of Science in Nutritional Science Program, Long Beach, CA 90840. Offers food science (MS); hospitality foodservice and hotel management (MS); nutritional science (MS). *Program availability:* Part-time. *Degree requirements:* For master's, thesis, oral presentation of thesis or directed project. *Entrance requirements:* For master's, GRE, minimum GPA of 2.5 in last 60 units. Electronic applications accepted. *Faculty research:* Protein and water-soluble vitamins, sensory evaluation of foods, mineral deficiencies in humans, child nutrition, minerals and blood pressure.

California State University, Long Beach, Graduate Studies, College of Health and Human Services, Department of Kinesiology, Long Beach, CA 90840. Offers adapted physical education (MA); coaching and student athlete development (MA); exercise physiology and nutrition (MS); exercise science (MS); individualized studies (MA); kinesiology (MA); pedagogical studies (MA); sport and exercise psychology (MS); sport management (MA); sports medicine and injury studies (MS). *Program availability:* Part-time. *Degree requirements:* For master's, oral and written comprehensive exams or thesis. *Entrance requirements:* For master's, GRE General Test, minimum GPA of 2.75 during previous 2 years of course work. Electronic applications accepted. *Faculty research:* Pulmonary functioning, feedback and practice structure, strength training, history and politics of sports, special population research issues.

California State University, Los Angeles, Graduate Studies, College of Health and Human Services, Department of Kinesiology and Nutritional Sciences, Los Angeles, CA 90032-8530. Offers nutritional science (MS); physical education and kinesiology (MA). *Accreditation:* AND. *Program availability:* Part-time, evening/weekend. *Degree requirements:* For master's, comprehensive exam, project or thesis. *Entrance requirements:* For master's, minimum GPA of 2.75. Additional exam requirements/recommendations for international students: Required—TOEFL (minimum score 500 paper-based). *Application deadline:* For fall admission, 5/1 for domestic and international students. Applications are processed on a rolling basis. Application fee: $55. *Financial support:* Federal Work-Study available. Support available to part-time students. Financial award application deadline: 3/1.
Website: http://www.calstatela.edu/dept/pe/

Canisius College, Graduate Division, School of Education and Human Services, Office of Professional Studies, Buffalo, NY 14208-1098. Offers applied nutrition (MS, Certificate); community and school health (MS); health and human performance (MS); health information technology (MS); respiratory care (MS). *Program availability:* Part-time, evening/weekend, 100% online, blended/hybrid learning. *Faculty:* 1 full-time (0 women), 11 part-time/adjunct (7 women). *Students:* 23 full-time (14 women), 79 part-time (58 women); includes 13 minority (7 Black or African American, non-Hispanic/Latino; 1 American Indian or Alaska Native, non-Hispanic/Latino; 3 Asian, non-Hispanic/Latino; 2 Hispanic/Latino), 4 international. Average age 35. 62 applicants, 81% accepted, 32 enrolled. In 2015, 37 master's awarded. *Entrance requirements:* For master's, GRE (recommended), bachelor's degree transcript, two letters of recommendation, current licensure (for applied nutrition), minimum GPA of 2.7, current resume. Additional exam requirements/recommendations for international students: Required—TOEFL (minimum score 550 paper-based, 80 iBT), IELTS (minimum score 6.5), or CAEL (minimum score 70). *Application deadline:* Applications are processed on a rolling basis. Application fee: $25. Electronic applications accepted. Application fee is waived when completed online. *Expenses:* $780 per credit hour; $644 per year full-time fees. *Financial support:* Career-related internships or fieldwork, Federal Work-Study, scholarships/grants, tuition waivers (partial), and unspecified assistantships available. Support available to part-time students. Financial award application deadline: 4/30; financial award applicants required to submit FAFSA. *Faculty research:* Nutrition, community and school health; community and health; health and human performance applied; nutrition and respiratory care. *Unit head:* Sandy McKenna, Director, Professional Studies, 716-888-8296, E-mail: mckekkas@canisius.edu. *Application contact:* Kathleen B. Davis, Vice President of Enrollment Management, 716-888-2500, Fax: 716-888-3195, E-mail: daviskb@canisius.edu.
Website: http://www.canisius.edu/graduate/

Case Western Reserve University, School of Medicine and School of Graduate Studies, Graduate Programs in Medicine, Department of Nutrition, Cleveland, OH 44106-4954. Offers dietetics (MS); nutrition (MS, PhD), including molecular nutrition (PhD), nutrition and biochemistry (PhD); public health nutrition (MS). *Program availability:* Part-time. Terminal master's awarded for partial completion of doctoral program. *Degree requirements:* For master's, thesis (for some programs); for doctorate, thesis/dissertation. *Entrance requirements:* For master's, GRE General Test; for doctorate, GRE General Test, GRE Subject Test. Additional exam requirements/recommendations for international students: Required—TOEFL. *Expenses: Tuition, area resident:* Full-time $41,137; part-time $1714 per credit hour. *Required fees:* $32. Tuition and fees vary according to course load and program. *Faculty research:* Fatty acid metabolism, application of gene therapy to nutritional problems, dietary intake methodology, nutrition and physical fitness, metabolism during infancy and pregnancy.

Cedar Crest College, Dietetic Internship Certificate Program, Allentown, PA 18104-6196. Offers Graduate Certificate. *Program availability:* Part-time, evening/weekend, blended/hybrid learning. *Faculty:* 1 (woman) full-time, 2 part-time/adjunct (1 woman). *Students:* 26 part-time (24 women); includes 1 minority (Hispanic/Latino). Average age 26. In 2015, 23 Graduate Certificates awarded. *Entrance requirements:* For degree, two semesters of medical nutrition therapy coursework completed no more than four years prior to application; one biochemistry course completed no more than five years prior to application. *Application deadline:* Applications are processed on a rolling basis. Electronic applications accepted. *Expenses:* Contact institution. *Unit head:* Kati Fosselius, Director, 610-606-4666 Ext. 3445, E-mail: kdfossel@cedarcrest.edu. *Application contact:* Mary Ellen Hickes, Director of School of Adult and Graduate

Nutrition

Education, 610-437-4471, E-mail: sage@cedarcrest.edu.
Website: http://sage.cedarcrest.edu/graduate/dietetic-internship/

Central Michigan University, Central Michigan University Global Campus, Program in Health Administration, Mount Pleasant, MI 48859. Offers health administration (DHA); international health (Certificate); nutrition and dietetics (MS). *Program availability:* Part-time, evening/weekend, online learning. Electronic applications accepted.

Central Michigan University, College of Graduate Studies, College of Education and Human Services, Department of Human Environmental Studies, Mount Pleasant, MI 48859. Offers apparel product development and merchandising technology (MS); gerontology (Graduate Certificate); human development and family studies (MA); nutrition and dietetics (MS). *Program availability:* Part-time, evening/weekend. *Degree requirements:* For master's, thesis or alternative. Electronic applications accepted. *Faculty research:* Human growth and development, family studies and human sexuality, human nutrition and dietetics, apparel and textile retailing, computer-aided design for apparel.

Central Washington University, Graduate Studies and Research, College of Education and Professional Studies, Department of Nutrition, Exercise and Health Services, Ellensburg, WA 98926. Offers exercise science (MS); nutrition (MS). *Program availability:* Part-time. *Degree requirements:* For master's, thesis or alternative. *Entrance requirements:* For master's, GRE, minimum GPA of 3.0; writing sample (for exercise students). Additional exam requirements/recommendations for international students: Required—TOEFL (minimum score 550 paper-based; 79 iBT). Electronic applications accepted.

Chapman University, Schmid College of Science and Technology, Food Science Program, Orange, CA 92866. Offers MS, MS/MBA. *Program availability:* Part-time, evening/weekend. *Faculty:* 4 full-time (3 women), 8 part-time/adjunct (6 women). *Students:* 12 full-time (9 women), 31 part-time (22 women); includes 12 minority (1 Black or African American, non-Hispanic/Latino; 10 Asian, non-Hispanic/Latino; 1 Hispanic/Latino), 10 international. Average age 26. 38 applicants, 71% accepted, 19 enrolled. In 2015, 22 master's awarded. *Degree requirements:* For master's, thesis or alternative. *Entrance requirements:* For master's, GRE or GMAT. Additional exam requirements/recommendations for international students: Required—TOEFL (minimum score 550 paper-based; 80 iBT). *Application deadline:* For fall admission, 5/1 priority date for domestic students. Applications are processed on a rolling basis. Application fee: $60. Electronic applications accepted. *Expenses:* $940 per unit. *Financial support:* Fellowships, research assistantships, teaching assistantships, Federal Work-Study, and scholarships/grants available. Financial award applicants required to submit FAFSA. *Unit head:* Dr. Anuradha Prakash, Program Director, 714-744-7895, E-mail: prakash@chapman.edu. *Application contact:* Monica Chen, Graduate Admission Counselor, 714-289-3590, E-mail: mchen@chapman.edu.

Clemson University, Graduate School, College of Agriculture, Forestry and Life Sciences, Department of Food, Nutrition and Packaging Sciences, Program in Food, Nutrition and Culinary Sciences, Clemson, SC 29634-0316. Offers MS. *Program availability:* Part-time. *Faculty:* 19 full-time (8 women). *Students:* 18 full-time (14 women), 3 part-time (all women); includes 3 minority (2 Black or African American, non-Hispanic/Latino; 1 Hispanic/Latino), 4 international. Average age 25. 42 applicants, 17% accepted, 5 enrolled. In 2015, 20 master's awarded. *Degree requirements:* For master's, thesis. *Entrance requirements:* For master's, GRE General Test, unofficial transcripts, letters of recommendation. Additional exam requirements/recommendations for international students: Required—TOEFL (minimum score 80 iBT), IELTS (minimum score 6.5). *Application deadline:* For fall admission, 6/1 for domestic students, 4/15 for international students; for spring admission, 9/15 for international students. Applications are processed on a rolling basis. Application fee: $80 ($90 for international students). Electronic applications accepted. *Expenses:* $4,060 per semester full-time resident, $8,103 per semester full-time non-resident, $448 per credit hour part-time resident, $898 per credit hour part-time non-resident. *Financial support:* In 2015–16, 16 students received support, including 8 research assistantships with partial tuition reimbursements available (averaging $12,450 per year), 7 teaching assistantships with partial tuition reimbursements available (averaging $14,142 per year); health care benefits and unspecified assistantships also available. Financial award application deadline: 2/15. *Unit head:* Dr. E. Jeffery Rhodehamel, Department Chair, 864-656-1211, Fax: 864-656-0331, E-mail: jrhode@clemson.edu. *Application contact:* Dr. Paul Dawson, Graduate Coordinator, 864-656-1138, E-mail: pdawson@clemson.edu.
Website: http://www.clemson.edu/cafls/departments/fnps/graduate/

College of Saint Elizabeth, Department of Foods and Nutrition, Morristown, NJ 07960. Offers dietetic internship (Certificate); dietetics verification (Certificate); nutrition (MS); sports nutrition and wellness (Certificate). *Accreditation:* AND. *Program availability:* Part-time, blended/hybrid learning. *Faculty:* 1 (woman) full-time, 2 part-time/adjunct (both women). *Students:* 35 full-time (34 women), 32 part-time (31 women); includes 11 minority (2 Black or African American, non-Hispanic/Latino; 5 Asian, non-Hispanic/Latino; 3 Hispanic/Latino; 1 Two or more races, non-Hispanic/Latino). Average age 28. 45 applicants, 73% accepted, 29 enrolled. In 2015, 7 master's awarded. *Degree requirements:* For master's, thesis. *Entrance requirements:* For master's, GRE, GMAT, minimum cumulative undergraduate GPA of 3.0. Additional exam requirements/recommendations for international students: Required—TOEFL (minimum score 550 paper-based; 79 iBT), IELTS (minimum score 6.5). *Application deadline:* For fall admission, 5/1 for international students. Applications are processed on a rolling basis. Application fee: $35. Electronic applications accepted. Application fee is waived when completed online. *Expenses:* Contact institution. *Financial support:* Career-related internships or fieldwork, scholarships/grants, and unspecified assistantships available. Financial award applicants required to submit FAFSA. *Faculty research:* Medical nutrition intervention, public policy, hunger and food security, osteoporosis, nutrition and exercise. *Unit head:* Dr. Marie Boyle, Program Chair, 973-290-4127, Fax: 973-290-4167, E-mail: mboyle01@cse.edu. *Application contact:* Scolavino Marie, Admissions Director of Graduate and Continuing Studies, 973-290-4413, Fax: 973-290-4710, E-mail: apply@cse.edu.
Website: http://www.cse.edu/academics/prof-studies/foods-and-nutrition/

Colorado State University, College of Health and Human Sciences, Department of Food Science and Human Nutrition, Fort Collins, CO 80523-1571. Offers MS, PhD. *Accreditation:* AND. *Program availability:* Part-time, 100% online, blended/hybrid learning. *Faculty:* 18 full-time (11 women). *Students:* 40 full-time (31 women), 54 part-time (48 women); includes 11 minority (1 American Indian or Alaska Native, non-Hispanic/Latino; 2 Asian, non-Hispanic/Latino; 5 Hispanic/Latino; 3 Two or more races, non-Hispanic/Latino), 1 international. Average age 32. 124 applicants, 36% accepted, 29 enrolled. In 2015, 24 master's, 5 doctorates awarded. Terminal master's awarded for partial completion of doctoral program. *Degree requirements:* For master's, thesis; for doctorate, thesis/dissertation. *Entrance requirements:* For master's, GRE (minimum 50th percentile), minimum GPA of 3.0 overall and in science classes, transcripts, three letters of recommendation, statement of purpose, resume; for doctorate, GRE (minimum 50th percentile), minimum GPA of 3.0, transcripts, three letters of recommendation, statement of purpose, resume. Additional exam requirements/recommendations for international students: Required—TOEFL (minimum score 550 paper-based; 80 iBT), IELTS (minimum score 6.5). *Application deadline:* For fall admission, 2/1 priority date for

domestic and international students. Application fee: $60 ($70 for international students). Electronic applications accepted. *Expenses:* $545 per credit hour tuition for online program. *Financial support:* In 2015–16, 21 students received support, including 1 fellowship with partial tuition reimbursement available (averaging $34,848 per year), 13 research assistantships with partial tuition reimbursements available (averaging $13,608 per year), 11 teaching assistantships with partial tuition reimbursements available (averaging $11,815 per year); Federal Work-Study, scholarships/grants, and unspecified assistantships also available. Financial award application deadline: 2/1; financial award applicants required to submit FAFSA. *Faculty research:* Community nutrition, bioactive compounds, nutrition and obesity, nutrition and health disparities, fatty acids and obesity-related disorders. *Total annual research expenditures:* $1.7 million. *Unit head:* Dr. Michael Pagliassotti, Professor and Department Head, 970-491-1390, Fax: 970-491-3875, E-mail: michael.pagliassotti@colostate.edu. *Application contact:* Paula Coleman, Administrative Assistant, 970-491-3819, Fax: 970-491-3875, E-mail: paula.coleman@colostate.edu.
Website: http://www.fshn.chhs.colostate.edu/

Colorado State University, College of Health and Human Sciences, Department of Health and Exercise Science, Fort Collins, CO 80523-1582. Offers exercise science and nutrition (MS); health and exercise science (MS); human bioenergetics (PhD). *Program availability:* Part-time. *Faculty:* 5 full-time (2 women). *Students:* 25 full-time (10 women), 11 part-time (6 women); includes 3 minority (all Hispanic/Latino). Average age 28. 65 applicants, 11% accepted, 7 enrolled. In 2015, 10 master's, 2 doctorates awarded. *Degree requirements:* For master's, thesis; for doctorate, comprehensive exam, thesis/dissertation, mentored teaching experience. *Entrance requirements:* For master's, GRE, minimum overall GPA of 3.0, personal statement; for doctorate, GRE, minimum overall GPA of 3.0, three letters of recommendation, letter of interest. Additional exam requirements/recommendations for international students: Required—TOEFL (minimum score 550 paper-based; 79 iBT). *Application deadline:* For fall admission, 1/31 priority date for domestic and international students; for spring admission, 9/30 priority date for domestic and international students. Application fee: $60 ($70 for international students). Electronic applications accepted. *Expenses:* Tuition, state resident: full-time $9348. Tuition, nonresident: full-time $22,916. *Required fees:* $2174; $473.72 per credit hour. $236.86 per semester. Tuition and fees vary according to course load and program. *Financial support:* In 2015–16, 16 students received support, including 1 fellowship with full tuition reimbursement available (averaging $48,192 per year), 5 research assistantships with full tuition reimbursements available (averaging $12,540 per year), 14 teaching assistantships with full tuition reimbursements available (averaging $15,697 per year); career-related internships or fieldwork and unspecified assistantships also available. Financial award application deadline: 1/31. *Faculty research:* Gerontology, neurophysiology, cardiovascular physiology, cell and molecular biology, energy balance and metabolism. *Total annual research expenditures:* $1.1 million. *Unit head:* Dr. Barry Braun, Professor and Department Head, 970-491-7875, Fax: 970-491-0445, E-mail: barry.braun@colostate.edu. *Application contact:* Dr. Matthew Hickey, Professor and Director, Graduate Program, 970-491-5727, Fax: 970-491-0445, E-mail: matthew.hickey@colostate.edu.
Website: http://www.hes.chhs.colostate.edu/

Columbia University, College of Physicians and Surgeons, Institute of Human Nutrition, MS Program in Nutrition, New York, NY 10032. Offers MS, MPH/MS. *Program availability:* Part-time. *Faculty:* 11 full-time (9 women). *Students:* 80 full-time (40 women), 2 part-time (1 woman); includes 28 minority (5 Black or African American, non-Hispanic/Latino; 21 Asian, non-Hispanic/Latino; 2 Hispanic/Latino), 1 international. Average age 23. 200 applicants, 63% accepted, 75 enrolled. In 2015, 85 master's awarded. *Degree requirements:* For master's, thesis. *Entrance requirements:* For master's, GRE General Test, MCAT. Additional exam requirements/recommendations for international students: Required—TOEFL; Recommended—IELTS. *Application deadline:* For fall and spring admission, 7/15 priority date for domestic and international students. Applications are processed on a rolling basis. Application fee: $95. Electronic applications accepted. *Financial support:* In 2015–16, 46 students received support. Federal Work-Study, institutionally sponsored loans, and traineeships available. Support available to part-time students. Financial award application deadline: 7/15; financial award applicants required to submit FAFSA. *Unit head:* Dr. Richard J. Deckelbaum, Director, 212-305-4808, Fax: 212-305-3079, E-mail: nutrition@columbia.edu. *Application contact:* Dr. Sharon R. Akabas, Director, MS Program in Human Nutrition, 212-305-4808, Fax: 212-305-3079, E-mail: sa109@columbia.edu.
Website: http://cumc.columbia.edu/dept/ihn/

Columbia University, College of Physicians and Surgeons, Institute of Human Nutrition and Graduate School of Arts and Sciences at the College of Physicians and Surgeons, PhD Program in Nutrition, New York, NY 10032. Offers PhD. *Degree requirements:* For doctorate, thesis/dissertation. *Entrance requirements:* For doctorate, GRE General Test. Additional exam requirements/recommendations for international students: Required—TOEFL. *Faculty research:* Growth and development, nutrition and metabolism.

Cornell University, Graduate School, Graduate Fields of Agriculture and Life Sciences, Field of Global Development, Ithaca, NY 14853-0001. Offers development policy (MPS); international agriculture and development (MPS); international development (MPS); international nutrition (MPS); international planning (MPS); international population (MPS); science and technology policy (MPS). *Degree requirements:* For master's, project paper. *Entrance requirements:* For master's, GRE General Test (recommended), 2 years of development experience, 2 letters of recommendation. Additional exam requirements/recommendations for international students: Required—TOEFL (minimum score 550 paper-based; 77 iBT). Electronic applications accepted.

Cornell University, Graduate School, Graduate Fields of Agriculture and Life Sciences and Graduate Fields of Human Ecology, Field of Nutrition, Ithaca, NY 14853-0001. Offers animal nutrition (MPS, PhD); community nutrition (MPS, PhD); human nutrition (MPS, PhD); international nutrition (MPS, PhD); molecular biochemistry (MPS, PhD). *Degree requirements:* For master's, thesis (MS), project papers (MPS); for doctorate, comprehensive exam, thesis/dissertation. *Entrance requirements:* For master's and doctorate, GRE General Test, previous course work in organic chemistry (with laboratory) and biochemistry; 2 letters of recommendation. Additional exam requirements/recommendations for international students: Required—TOEFL (minimum score 550 paper-based; 77 iBT). Electronic applications accepted. *Faculty research:* Nutritional biochemistry, experimental human and animal nutrition, international nutrition, community nutrition.

Drexel University, College of Arts and Sciences, Department of Biology, Program in Human Nutrition, Philadelphia, PA 19104-2875. Offers MS. *Accreditation:* AND. *Program availability:* Part-time. Terminal master's awarded for partial completion of doctoral program. *Degree requirements:* For master's, thesis. *Entrance requirements:* For master's, GRE General Test. Additional exam requirements/recommendations for international students: Required—TOEFL. Electronic applications accepted. *Faculty research:* Metabolism of lipids, W-3 fatty acids, obesity, diabetes and heart disease, mineral metabolism.

D'Youville College, Department of Dietetics, Buffalo, NY 14201-1084. Offers MS. Five-year program begins at freshman entry. *Accreditation:* AND. *Students:* 92 full-time (82 women), 16 part-time (15 women); includes 13 minority (4 Black or African American, non-Hispanic/Latino; 4 Asian, non-Hispanic/Latino; 1 Hispanic/Latino; 4 Two or more races, non-Hispanic/Latino), 10 international. Average age 24. 69 applicants, 90% accepted, 31 enrolled. In 2015, 22 master's awarded. *Degree requirements:* For master's, thesis. *Entrance requirements:* Additional exam requirements/ recommendations for international students: Required—TOEFL (minimum score 500 paper-based). *Application deadline:* For fall admission, 5/1 priority date for international students; for spring admission, 9/1 priority date for international students. Applications are processed on a rolling basis. Electronic applications accepted. *Expenses: Tuition, area resident:* Full-time $21,120; part-time $880 per credit hour. *Required fees:* $235; $96. One-time fee: $100. *Faculty research:* Nutrition education, clinical nutrition, herbal supplements, obesity. *Unit head:* Dr. Charlotte Baumgart, Chair, 716-829-7752, Fax: 716-829-8137. *Application contact:* Dr. Steven Smith, Director of Admissions, 716-829-7600, Fax: 716-829-7900, E-mail: admissons@dyc.edu.

East Carolina University, Graduate School, College of Allied Health Sciences, Department of Nutrition Science, Greenville, NC 27858-4353. Offers MS. *Program availability:* Part-time. *Students:* 16 full-time (13 women), 19 part-time (17 women); includes 4 minority (all Black or African American, non-Hispanic/Latino). Average age 27. 31 applicants, 90% accepted, 28 enrolled. In 2015, 7 master's awarded. *Degree requirements:* For master's, comprehensive exam, thesis optional. *Entrance requirements:* For master's, GRE. Additional exam requirements/recommendations for international students: Required—TOEFL. *Application deadline:* For fall admission, 6/1 priority date for domestic students. Applications are processed on a rolling basis. Application fee: $50. *Financial support:* Fellowships, teaching assistantships with partial tuition reimbursements, Federal Work-Study, institutionally sponsored loans, scholarships/grants, and unspecified assistantships available. Support available to part-time students. Financial award application deadline: 6/1. *Faculty research:* Lifecycle nutrition, nutrition and disease, nutrition for fish species, food service management. *Unit head:* Dr. Melani Duffrin, Interim Chair, 252-328-5698, E-mail: duffrinm@ecu.edu. *Application contact:* Dean of Graduate School, 252-328-6012, Fax: 252-328-6071, E-mail: gradschool@ecu.edu.
Website: http://www.ecu.edu/nutr/

Eastern Illinois University, Graduate School, Lumpkin College of Business and Applied Sciences, School of Family and Consumer Sciences, Program in Nutrition and Dietetics, Charleston, IL 61920. Offers MS. *Program availability:* Part-time, evening/ weekend. *Degree requirements:* For master's, comprehensive exam (for some programs), thesis (for some programs). *Entrance requirements:* For master's, GMAT or GRE. Additional exam requirements/recommendations for international students: Required—TOEFL (minimum score 500 paper-based; 61 iBT), IELTS (minimum score 6). Electronic applications accepted.

Eastern Kentucky University, The Graduate School, College of Health Sciences, Department of Family and Consumer Sciences, Richmond, KY 40475-3102. Offers community nutrition (MS). *Program availability:* Part-time. *Entrance requirements:* For master's, GRE General Test, minimum GPA of 2.5.

Eastern Michigan University, Graduate School, College of Health and Human Services, School of Health Sciences, Programs in Dietetics and Human Nutrition, Ypsilanti, MI 48197. Offers dietetics (MS); human nutrition (MS). *Accreditation:* AND. *Program availability:* Part-time, evening/weekend, online learning. *Students:* 42 full-time (39 women), 35 part-time (30 women); includes 13 minority (4 Black or African American, non-Hispanic/Latino; 5 Asian, non-Hispanic/Latino; 4 Hispanic/Latino), 3 international. Average age 34. 50 applicants, 52% accepted. In 2015, 34 master's awarded. *Entrance requirements:* Additional exam requirements/recommendations for international students: Required—TOEFL. *Application deadline:* Applications are processed on a rolling basis. Application fee: $45. *Financial support:* Fellowships, research assistantships with full tuition reimbursements, teaching assistantships with full tuition reimbursements, career-related internships or fieldwork, Federal Work-Study, institutionally sponsored loans, scholarships/grants, tuition waivers (partial), and unspecified assistantships available. Support available to part-time students. Financial award applicants required to submit FAFSA. *Application contact:* Lydia Kret, Program Director, 734-487-7862, Fax: 734-487-4095, E-mail: lydia.kret@emich.edu.

East Tennessee State University, School of Graduate Studies, College of Clinical and Rehabilitative Health Sciences, Department of Allied Health Science, Johnson City, TN 37614. Offers allied health (MSAH); clinical nutrition (MS). *Program availability:* Part-time, online learning. *Faculty:* 13 full-time (9 women). *Students:* 23 full-time (22 women), 22 part-time (18 women); includes 1 minority (Asian, non-Hispanic/Latino). Average age 31. 52 applicants, 31% accepted, 16 enrolled. In 2015, 15 master's awarded. *Degree requirements:* For master's, comprehensive exam, thesis or advanced practice seminar (for MSAH); internship (for MS). *Entrance requirements:* For master's, GRE General Test, professional license in allied health discipline, minimum GPA of 2.75, and three professional letters of recommendation (for MSAH); bachelor's degree from an undergraduate didactic program in dietetics with minimum GPA of 3.0 in DPD coursework and three letters of recommendation (for MS). Additional exam requirements/recommendations for international students: Required—TOEFL (minimum score 550 paper-based; 79 iBT). *Application deadline:* For fall admission, 2/15 for domestic and international students; for spring admission, 11/1 for domestic students, 9/30 for international students. Application fee: $35 ($45 for international students). Electronic applications accepted. *Financial support:* In 2015–16, 18 students received support, including 14 research assistantships with partial tuition reimbursements available (averaging $3,000 per year), 4 teaching assistantships with partial tuition reimbursements available (averaging $3,000 per year); career-related internships or fieldwork, institutionally sponsored loans, scholarships/grants, and unspecified assistantships also available. Financial award application deadline: 7/1; financial award applicants required to submit FAFSA. *Faculty research:* Recruitment and retention of allied health professionals, relationship between APACHEE II scores and the need for a tracheotomy, health care workers, patient care, occupational stress, radiofrequency lesioning, absorption of lipophilic compounds, Vitamin D status in college-age students, childhood and adolescence obesity, nutrition education/interventions. *Unit head:* Dr. Ester Verhovsek, Chair, 423-547-4900, Fax: 423-439-4921, E-mail: verhovse@etsu.edu. *Application contact:* Mary Duncan, Graduate Specialist, 423-439-4302, Fax: 423-439-5624, E-mail: duncanm@etsu.edu.
Website: http://www.etsu.edu/crhs/alliedhealth/

Emory University, Laney Graduate School, Division of Biological and Biomedical Sciences, Program in Nutrition and Health Sciences, Atlanta, GA 30322-1100. Offers PhD. *Degree requirements:* For doctorate, comprehensive exam, thesis/dissertation. *Entrance requirements:* For doctorate, GRE General Test, minimum GPA of 3.0 in science course work (recommended). Additional exam requirements/recommendations for international students: Required—TOEFL. Electronic applications accepted. *Faculty research:* Biochemistry, molecular and cell biology, clinical nutrition, community and preventive health, nutritional epidemiology.

Emory University, Rollins School of Public Health, Hubert Department of Global Health, Atlanta, GA 30322-1100. Offers global health (MPH); public nutrition (MSPH). *Accreditation:* CEPH. *Degree requirements:* For master's, thesis, practicum. *Entrance requirements:* For master's, GRE General Test. Additional exam requirements/

recommendations for international students: Required—TOEFL (minimum score 550 paper-based; 80 iBT). Electronic applications accepted.

Florida International University, Robert Stempel College of Public Health and Social Work, Department of Dietetics and Nutrition, Miami, FL 33199. Offers MS, PhD. *Program availability:* Part-time. *Faculty:* 11 full-time (10 women), 8 part-time/adjunct (all women). *Students:* 59 full-time (52 women), 40 part-time (36 women); includes 56 minority (5 Black or African American, non-Hispanic/Latino; 6 Asian, non-Hispanic/Latino; 44 Hispanic/Latino; 1 Two or more races, non-Hispanic/Latino), 16 international. Average age 29. 80 applicants, 34% accepted, 17 enrolled. In 2015, 36 master's, 5 doctorates awarded. *Degree requirements:* For master's, thesis; for doctorate, comprehensive exam, thesis/dissertation. *Entrance requirements:* For master's, minimum GPA of 3.0; for doctorate, GRE General Test, minimum GPA of 3.0, resume, letters of recommendation, faculty sponsor. Additional exam requirements/ recommendations for international students: Required—TOEFL (minimum score 550 paper-based; 80 iBT). *Application deadline:* For fall admission, 6/1 for domestic students, 4/1 for international students; for spring admission, 10/1 for domestic students, 9/1 for international students. Applications are processed on a rolling basis. Application fee: $30. Electronic applications accepted. *Expenses:* Tuition, state resident: full-time $10,708; part-time $455.64 per credit hour. Tuition, nonresident: full-time $23,816; part-time $1001.69 per credit hour. *Required fees:* $390; $195 per semester. Tuition and fees vary according to program. *Financial support:* Career-related internships or fieldwork, Federal Work-Study, institutionally sponsored loans, and scholarships/grants available. Financial award application deadline: 3/1; financial award applicants required to submit FAFSA. *Faculty research:* Clinical nutrition, cultural food habits, pediatric nutrition, diabetes, dietetic education. *Unit head:* Dr. Fatma Huffman, Chair, 305-348-3788, Fax: 305-348-1996, E-mail: huffmanf@fiu.edu. *Application contact:* Nanett Rojas, Manager, Admissions Operations, 305-348-7464, Fax: 305-348-7441, E-mail: gradadm@fiu.edu.

Florida State University, The Graduate School, College of Human Sciences, Department of Nutrition, Food and Exercise Sciences, Tallahassee, FL 32306-1493. Offers exercise physiology (MS, PhD); nutrition and food science (MS, PhD), including clinical nutrition (MS), food science, human nutrition (PhD), nutrition education and health promotion (MS), nutrition science (MS); sports nutrition (MS); sports sciences (MS). *Program availability:* Part-time. *Faculty:* 20 full-time (9 women). *Students:* 89 full-time (51 women), 5 part-time (3 women); includes 12 minority (2 Black or African American, non-Hispanic/Latino; 1 Asian, non-Hispanic/Latino; 4 Hispanic/Latino; 5 Two or more races, non-Hispanic/Latino), 17 international. Average age 28. 185 applicants, 40% accepted, 31 enrolled. In 2015, 38 master's, 3 doctorates awarded. *Degree requirements:* For master's, comprehensive exam (for some programs), thesis optional; for doctorate, thesis/dissertation. *Entrance requirements:* For master's, GRE General Test, minimum upper-division GPA of 3.0; for doctorate, GRE General Test, minimum upper-division GPA of 3.0, MS. Additional exam requirements/recommendations for international students: Required—TOEFL (minimum score 550 paper-based; 80 iBT). *Application deadline:* For fall admission, 4/1 for domestic and international students; for spring admission, 10/1 for domestic and international students. Applications are processed on a rolling basis. Application fee: $30. Electronic applications accepted. *Expenses: Tuition, area resident:* Full-time $7263; part-time $403.50 per credit hour. Tuition, nonresident: full-time $18,087; part-time $1004.85 per credit hour. *Required fees:* $1365; $75.81 per credit hour. $20 per semester. Tuition and fees vary according to campus/location. *Financial support:* In 2015–16, 48 students received support, including 20 research assistantships with full tuition reimbursements available (averaging $5,975 per year), 37 teaching assistantships with full tuition reimbursements available (averaging $9,477 per year); career-related internships or fieldwork, Federal Work-Study, institutionally sponsored loans, scholarships/grants, and unspecified assistantships also available. Financial award application deadline: 2/1; financial award applicants required to submit FAFSA. *Faculty research:* Body composition, functional food, chronic disease and aging response; food safety, food allergy, and safety/quality detection methods; sports nutrition, energy and human performance; strength training, functional performance, cardiovascular physiology, sarcopenia. *Total annual research expenditures:* $543,728. *Unit head:* Dr. Robert J. Moffatt, Professor/Interim Chair, 850-644-1520, Fax: 850-645-5000, E-mail: rmoffatt@fsu.edu. *Application contact:* Ann R. Smith, Office Administrator, 850-644-1828, Fax: 850-645-5000, E-mail: asmith@fsu.edu.
Website: http://www.chs.fsu.edu/Departments/Nutrition-Food-Exercise-Sciences

Framingham State University, Continuing Education, Programs in Food and Nutrition, Coordinated Program in Dietetics, Framingham, MA 01701-9101. Offers MS.

Framingham State University, Continuing Education, Programs in Food and Nutrition, Food Science and Nutrition Science Program, Framingham, MA 01701-9101. Offers MS. *Program availability:* Part-time, evening/weekend. *Entrance requirements:* For master's, GRE General Test.

Framingham State University, Continuing Education, Programs in Food and Nutrition, Program in Human Nutrition: Education and Media Technologies, Framingham, MA 01701-9101. Offers MS.

George Mason University, College of Health and Human Services, Department of Nutrition and Food Studies, Fairfax, VA 22030. Offers MS. *Faculty:* 4 full-time (all women), 8 part-time/adjunct (all women). *Students:* 17 full-time (12 women), 31 part-time (29 women); includes 8 minority (3 Black or African American, non-Hispanic/Latino; 3 Asian, non-Hispanic/Latino; 2 Hispanic/Latino), 2 international. Average age 33. 25 applicants, 60% accepted, 10 enrolled. In 2015, 11 master's awarded. *Degree requirements:* For master's, comprehensive exam, thesis optional. *Entrance requirements:* For master's, resume, 3 letters of recommendation, expanded goal statement. Additional exam requirements/recommendations for international students: Required—TOEFL (minimum score 575 paper-based; 88 iBT), IELTS (minimum score 6.5), PTE (minimum score 59). *Application deadline:* For fall admission, 4/1 for domestic and international students; for spring admission, 11/1 for domestic and international students. Application fee: $75 ($80 for international students). Electronic applications accepted. *Financial support:* In 2015–16, 4 research assistantships with tuition reimbursements (averaging $13,250 per year) were awarded; career-related internships or fieldwork, Federal Work-Study, and health care benefits (for full-time research or teaching assistantship recipients) also available. Support available to part-time students. Financial award applicants required to submit FAFSA. *Total annual research expenditures:* $6,845. *Application contact:* Joe Wilson, Manager, Department of Food and Nutrition, 703-993-9709, Fax: 703-993-2193, E-mail: jwilso25@gmu.edu.
Website: https://chhs.gmu.edu/nfs/

Georgia Southern University, Jack N. Averitt College of Graduate Studies, College of Health and Human Sciences, School of Health and Kinesiology, Dietetic Internship Program, Statesboro, GA 30458. Offers Certificate. *Students:* 20 full-time (16 women); includes 3 minority (2 Asian, non-Hispanic/Latino; 1 Hispanic/Latino). Average age 24. 60 applicants, 33% accepted. *Degree requirements:* For Certificate, 1,200 hours of supervised practice experiences. *Entrance requirements:* Additional exam requirements/recommendations for international students: Required—TOEFL (minimum score 550 paper-based; 80 iBT), IELTS (minimum score 6). *Application deadline:* For fall admission, 1/16 for domestic students. Application fee: $50. Electronic applications accepted. *Expenses:* Tuition, state resident: full-time $7236; part-time $277 per

Nutrition

semester hour. Tuition, nonresident: full-time $27,118; part-time $1105 per semester hour. *Required fees:* $2092. *Financial support:* Application deadline: 4/20; applicants required to submit FAFSA. *Faculty research:* Community and school nutrition, energy balance, medical nutrition. *Unit head:* Dr. Donna O. Burnett, Director, 912-478-2123, E-mail: dburnett@georgiasouthern.edu.
Website: http://chhs.georgiasouthern.edu/hk/graduate/dietetic-internship/

Georgia State University, Byrdine F. Lewis School of Nursing, Division of Nutrition, Atlanta, GA 30302-3083. Offers MS. *Accreditation:* AND. *Program availability:* Part-time. *Faculty:* 7 full-time (4 women). *Students:* 34 full-time (29 women), 3 part-time (all women); includes 5 minority (3 Asian, non-Hispanic/Latino; 2 Two or more races, non-Hispanic/Latino), 1 international. Average age 29. 49 applicants, 37% accepted, 12 enrolled. In 2015, 23 master's awarded. *Degree requirements:* For master's, portfolio or thesis. *Entrance requirements:* For master's, GRE, prerequisite courses in inorganic chemistry (1 semester), organic chemistry (1 semester), and human anatomy and physiology (2 semesters); transcripts; resume; statement of goals; letters of recommendation. Additional exam requirements/recommendations for international students: Required—TOEFL (minimum score 550 paper-based; 80 iBT). *Application deadline:* For fall admission, 5/15 for domestic and international students; for spring admission, 10/1 for domestic and international students. Application fee: $50. Electronic applications accepted. *Expenses:* Tuition, state resident: full-time $6876; part-time $382 per credit hour. Tuition, nonresident: full-time $22,374; part-time $1243 per credit hour. *Required fees:* $2128; $2128 per term. $1064 per term. Part-time tuition and fees vary according to course load and program. *Financial support:* In 2015–16, research assistantships with tuition reimbursements (averaging $1,647 per year), teaching assistantships with full tuition reimbursements (averaging $2,666 per year) were awarded. Financial award application deadline: 4/1. *Faculty research:* Energy balance and body composition, nutrition and HIV in Kenya, lipid peroxidation, energy requirements in obese children, diet and incidence of type I diabetes. *Unit head:* Dr. Anita Nucci, Department Head, 404-413-1234, Fax: 404-413-1228.
Website: http://nutrition.gsu.edu/

Harvard University, Harvard T.H. Chan School of Public Health, Department of Nutrition, Boston, MA 02115-6096. Offers nutrition (SD); nutritional epidemiology (SD); public health nutrition (SD). *Faculty:* 28 full-time (10 women), 16 part-time/adjunct (6 women). *Students:* 22 full-time (13 women), 3 part-time (2 women); includes 6 minority (1 Black or African American, non-Hispanic/Latino; 1 Asian, non-Hispanic/Latino; 1 Hispanic/Latino; 3 Two or more races, non-Hispanic/Latino), 11 international. Average age 30. 46 applicants, 11% accepted, 5 enrolled. In 2015, 8 doctorates awarded. *Degree requirements:* For doctorate, thesis/dissertation, qualifying exam. *Entrance requirements:* For doctorate, GRE. Additional exam requirements/recommendations for international students: Recommended—TOEFL (minimum score 600 paper-based; 100 iBT), IELTS (minimum score 7). *Application deadline:* For fall admission, 12/15 for domestic and international students. Application fee: $120. Electronic applications accepted. *Financial support:* Fellowships, research assistantships, teaching assistantships, Federal Work-Study, scholarships/grants, traineeships, and unspecified assistantships available. Support available to part-time students. Financial award application deadline: 2/15; financial award applicants required to submit FAFSA. *Faculty research:* Dietary and genetic factors affecting heart diseases in humans; interactions among nutrition, immunity, and infection; role of diet and lifestyle in preventing macrovascular complications in diabetics. *Unit head:* Dr. Walter Willett, Chair, 617-432-1333, Fax: 617-432-2435, E-mail: walter.willett@channing.harvard.edu. *Application contact:* Vincent W. James, Director of Admissions, 617-432-1031, Fax: 617-432-7080, E-mail: admissions@hsph.harvard.edu.
Website: http://www.hsph.harvard.edu/nutrition/

Howard University, Graduate School, Department of Nutritional Sciences, Washington, DC 20059-0002. Offers nutrition (MS, PhD). *Program availability:* Part-time, evening/weekend. *Degree requirements:* For master's, comprehensive exam, thesis; for doctorate, comprehensive exam, thesis/dissertation. *Entrance requirements:* For master's and doctorate, minimum GPA of 3.0, general chemistry, organic chemistry, biochemistry, nutrition. Additional exam requirements/recommendations for international students: Required—TOEFL. Electronic applications accepted. *Faculty research:* Dietary fiber, phytate, trace minerals, cardio-vascular diseases, overweight/obesity.

Hunter College of the City University of New York, Graduate School, Schools of the Health Professions, School of Health Sciences, Programs in Urban Public Health, Program in Nutrition, New York, NY 10065-5085. Offers MPH. *Accreditation:* AND. *Program availability:* Part-time, evening/weekend. *Students:* 4 full-time (all women), 47 part-time (27 women); includes 9 minority (1 Black or African American, non-Hispanic/Latino; 4 Asian, non-Hispanic/Latino; 4 Hispanic/Latino), 6 international. Average age 28. 83 applicants, 48% accepted, 27 enrolled. In 2015, 21 master's awarded. *Degree requirements:* For master's, comprehensive exam, thesis and essay, internship. *Entrance requirements:* For master's, GRE General Test, previous course work in calculus and statistics. Additional exam requirements/recommendations for international students: Required—TOEFL. *Application deadline:* For fall admission, 4/1 for domestic students; for spring admission, 11/1 for domestic students. *Financial support:* In 2015–16, 6 fellowships were awarded; career-related internships or fieldwork, Federal Work-Study, institutionally sponsored loans, and tuition waivers (partial) also available. Support available to part-time students. *Unit head:* Prof. Krusheed Navder, Program Director, 212-396-7775, Fax: 212-481-5260, E-mail: knavder@hunter.cuny.edu. *Application contact:* Milena Solo, Director of Graduate Admissions, 212-772-4288, E-mail: milena.solo@hunter.cuny.edu.
Website: http://cuny.edu/site/sph/hunter-college/a-programs/graduate/nutrition/nutrition-msdpd.html

Huntington College of Health Sciences, Program in Nutrition, Knoxville, TN 37918. Offers clinical nutrition (DHS); nutrition (MS); personalized option (DHS). *Program availability:* Part-time, evening/weekend, online learning. *Degree requirements:* For doctorate, comprehensive exam, thesis/dissertation. *Entrance requirements:* For master's, bachelor's degree, essay, resume/curriculum vitae; for doctorate, master's degree, essay, references, interview, resume/curriculum vitae. Additional exam requirements/recommendations for international students: Required—TOEFL (minimum score 550 paper-based; 80 iBT); Recommended—IELTS. Electronic applications accepted.

Idaho State University, Office of Graduate Studies, Kasiska College of Health Professions, Department of Health and Nutrition Sciences, Pocatello, ID 83209-8109. Offers dietetics (Certificate); health education (MHE); public health (MPH). *Program availability:* Part-time. *Degree requirements:* For master's, comprehensive exam, internship, thesis or project. *Entrance requirements:* For master's, GRE General Test or GPA greater than 3.5, minimum GPA of 3.0 for upper division classes, 2 letters of recommendation. Additional exam requirements/recommendations for international students: Required—TOEFL (minimum score 600 paper-based). Electronic applications accepted. *Faculty research:* Epidemiology, environmental health, nutrition and aging, dietetics.

Immaculata University, College of Graduate Studies, Program in Nutrition Education, Immaculata, PA 19345. Offers nutrition education for the registered dietitian (MA); nutrition education with dietetic internship (MA); nutrition education with wellness

promotion (MA). *Program availability:* Part-time, evening/weekend. *Degree requirements:* For master's, comprehensive exam, thesis optional. *Entrance requirements:* For master's, GRE or MAT, minimum GPA of 3.0. Additional exam requirements/recommendations for international students: Required—TOEFL. Electronic applications accepted. *Faculty research:* Sports nutrition, pediatric nutrition, changes in food consumption patterns in weight loss, nutritional counseling.

Indiana University Bloomington, School of Public Health, Department of Applied Health Science, Bloomington, IN 47405. Offers behavioral, social, and community health (MPH); family health (MPH); health behavior (PhD); nutrition science (MS); professional health education (MPH); public health administration (MPH); safety management (MS); school and college health education (MS). *Accreditation:* CEPH (one or more programs are accredited). *Degree requirements:* For master's, thesis optional; for doctorate, comprehensive exam, thesis/dissertation. *Entrance requirements:* For master's, GRE (for MS in nutrition science), 3 recommendations; for doctorate, GRE, 3 recommendations. Additional exam requirements/recommendations for international students: Required—TOEFL (minimum score 550 paper-based; 80 iBT). Electronic applications accepted. *Faculty research:* Cancer education, HIV/AIDS and drug education, public health, parent-child interactions, safety education, obesity, public health policy, public health administration, school health, health education, human development, nutrition, human sexuality, chronic disease, early childhood health.

Indiana University of Pennsylvania, School of Graduate Studies and Research, College of Health and Human Services, Department of Food and Nutrition, Indiana, PA 15705-1087. Offers MS. *Program availability:* Part-time, online learning. *Faculty:* 5 full-time (all women). *Students:* 6 full-time (all women), 35 part-time (33 women); includes 1 minority (Black or African American, non-Hispanic/Latino). Average age 25. 33 applicants, 70% accepted, 20 enrolled. In 2015, 7 master's awarded. *Degree requirements:* For master's, thesis optional. *Entrance requirements:* For master's, GRE General Test, 2 letters of recommendation. Additional exam requirements/recommendations for international students: Required—TOEFL (minimum score 540 paper-based). *Application deadline:* Applications are processed on a rolling basis. Application fee: $50. Electronic applications accepted. *Financial support:* In 2015–16, 5 research assistantships with tuition reimbursements (averaging $4,664 per year) were awarded; fellowships with partial tuition reimbursements and Federal Work-Study also available. Support available to part-time students. Financial award application deadline: 4/15; financial award applicants required to submit FAFSA. *Unit head:* Dr. Rita M. Johnson, Chairperson, 724-357-4440, E-mail: rita.johnson@iup.edu. *Application contact:* Dr. Stephanie Taylor-Davis, Graduate Coordinator, 724-357-7733, E-mail: stdavis@iup.edu.

Indiana University–Purdue University Indianapolis, School of Health and Rehabilitation Sciences, Indianapolis, IN 46202-5119. Offers health and rehabilitation sciences (PhD); health sciences (MS); nutrition and dietetics (MS); occupational therapy (MS); physical therapy (DPT); physician assistant (MPAS). *Program availability:* Part-time, evening/weekend. *Degree requirements:* For master's, thesis (for some programs). *Entrance requirements:* For master's, GRE General Test, minimum GPA of 3.0 (for MS in health sciences, nutrition and dietetics), 3.2 (for MS in occupational therapy), 3.0 cumulative and prerequisite math/science (for MPAS); for doctorate, GRE, minimum cumulative and prerequisite math/science GPA of 3.2. Additional exam requirements/recommendations for international students: Required—TOEFL (minimum score 550 paper-based; 79 iBT), IELTS (minimum score 6.5), PTE (minimum score 54). Electronic applications accepted. *Expenses:* Contact institution. *Faculty research:* Function and mobility across the lifespan, pediatric nutrition, driving and mobility rehabilitation, neurorehabilitation and biomechanics, rehabilitation and integrative therapy.

Instituto Tecnologico de Santo Domingo, Graduate School, Area of Health Sciences, Santo Domingo, Dominican Republic. Offers bioethics (M Bioethics); clinical bioethics (Certificate); clinical nutrition (Certificate); comprehensive health and the adolescent (Certificate); comrehensive adloescent health (MS); health and social security (M Mgmt).

Iowa State University of Science and Technology, Program in Diet and Exercise, Ames, IA 50011. Offers MS. *Entrance requirements:* For master's, GRE, minimum GPA of 3.5, 3 letters of recommendation. Additional exam requirements/recommendations for international students: Required—TOEFL (minimum score 550 paper-based; 79 iBT), IELTS (minimum score 6.5). Electronic applications accepted.

Iowa State University of Science and Technology, Program in Nutritional Sciences, Ames, IA 50011. Offers MS, PhD. *Entrance requirements:* For master's and doctorate, GRE General Test. Additional exam requirements/recommendations for international students: Required—TOEFL (minimum score 550 paper-based; 79 iBT), IELTS (minimum score 6.5). Electronic applications accepted.

James Madison University, The Graduate School, College of Health and Behavioral Sciences, Program in Health Sciences, Harrisonburg, VA 22807. Offers nutrition and physical activity (MS). *Program availability:* Part-time. *Students:* 9 full-time (6 women), 1 (woman) part-time; includes 2 minority (1 Asian, non-Hispanic/Latino; 1 Hispanic/Latino), 1 international. Average age 30. 9 applicants, 78% accepted, 5 enrolled. In 2015, 5 master's awarded. Application fee: $55. Electronic applications accepted. *Financial support:* In 2015–16, 6 students received support. Federal Work-Study, unspecified assistantships, and assistantships (averaging $7530), athletic assistantships (averaging $8837) available. Financial award application deadline: 3/1; financial award applicants required to submit FAFSA. *Unit head:* Dr. Allen Lewis, Department Head, 540-568-6510, E-mail: lewis6an@jmu.edu. *Application contact:* Lynette D. Michael, Director of Graduate Admissions, 540-568-6131 Ext. 6395, Fax: 540-568-7860, E-mail: michaeld@jmu.edu.
Website: http://www.healthsci.jmu.edu/index.html

James Madison University, The Graduate School, College of Health and Behavioral Sciences, Program in Kinesiology, Harrisonburg, VA 22807. Offers clinical exercise physiology (MS); exercise physiology (MS); kinesiology (MAT, MS); nutrition and exercise (MS); physical and health education (MAT); sport and recreation leadership (MS). *Program availability:* Part-time, evening/weekend. *Faculty:* 9 full-time (3 women), 2 part-time/adjunct (1 woman). *Students:* 64 full-time (32 women), 7 part-time (3 women); includes 6 minority (2 Black or African American, non-Hispanic/Latino; 1 Asian, non-Hispanic/Latino; 3 Two or more races, non-Hispanic/Latino), 1 international. Average age 30. 140 applicants, 70% accepted, 44 enrolled. In 2015, 43 master's awarded. Application fee: $55. Electronic applications accepted. *Financial support:* In 2015–16, 44 students received support, including 14 teaching assistantships with full tuition reimbursements available (averaging $8,837 per year); Federal Work-Study, unspecified assistantships, and athletic assistantships (averaging $8837); service assistantships (averaging $7530), assistantships (averaging $7530) also available. Financial award application deadline: 3/1; financial award applicants required to submit FAFSA. *Unit head:* Dr. Christopher J. Womack, Department Head, 540-568-6145, E-mail: womackcx@jmu.edu. *Application contact:* Lynette D. Michael, Director of Graduate Admissions, 540-568-6131 Ext. 6395, Fax: 540-568-7860, E-mail: michaeld@jmu.edu.
Website: http://www.jmu.edu/kinesiology/

Johns Hopkins University, Bloomberg School of Public Health, Department of International Health, Baltimore, MD 21205. Offers global disease epidemiology and control (MHS, PhD); health systems (MHS, PhD); human nutrition (MHS, PhD); international health (MSPH, Dr PH); registered dietician (MSPH); social and behavioral interventions (MHS, PhD). *Degree requirements:* For master's, comprehensive exam, thesis (for some programs), 1-year full-time residency, 4-9 month internship; for doctorate, comprehensive exam, thesis/dissertation or alternative, 1.5 years' full-time residency, oral and written exams. *Entrance requirements:* For master's, GRE General Test or MCAT, 3 letters of recommendation, resume; for doctorate, GRE General Test or MCAT, 3 letters of recommendation, resume, transcripts. Additional exam requirements/recommendations for international students: Required—TOEFL (minimum score 600 paper-based; 100 iBT); Recommended—IELTS (minimum score 7). Electronic applications accepted. *Faculty research:* Nutrition, infectious diseases, health systems, health economics, humanitarian emergencies.

Kansas State University, Graduate School, College of Human Ecology, Department of Human Nutrition, Manhattan, KS 66506. Offers human nutrition (MS, PhD); nutritional sciences (PhD); public health nutrition (PhD); public health physical activity (PhD); sensory analysis and consumer behavior (PhD). *Program availability:* Part-time. *Degree requirements:* For master's, thesis or alternative, residency; for doctorate, thesis/dissertation, residency. *Entrance requirements:* For master's, GRE General Test, minimum undergraduate GPA of 3.0; for doctorate, GRE General Test, minimum graduate GPA of 3.0. Additional exam requirements/recommendations for international students: Required—TOEFL (minimum score 550 paper-based; 79 iBT), IELTS (minimum score 6.5). Electronic applications accepted. *Faculty research:* Cancer and immunology, obesity, sensory analysis and consumer behavior, nutrient metabolism, clinical and community interventions.

Kent State University, College of Education, Health and Human Services, School of Health Sciences, Program in Nutrition, Kent, OH 44242-0001. Offers MS. *Degree requirements:* For master's, thesis optional. *Entrance requirements:* For master's, 3 letters of reference, goals statement, minimum GPA of 3.0. Additional exam requirements/recommendations for international students: Required—TOEFL (minimum score 550 paper-based; 80 iBT). *Expenses:* Tuition, state resident: full-time $10,864; part-time $495 per credit hour. Tuition, nonresident: full-time $18,380; part-time $837 per credit hour.

Lehman College of the City University of New York, School of Natural and Social Sciences, Department of Health Sciences, Program in Nutrition, Bronx, NY 10468-1589. Offers clinical nutrition (MS); community nutrition (MS); dietetic internship (MS). *Degree requirements:* For master's, thesis or alternative.

Liberty University, School of Health Sciences, Lynchburg, VA 24515. Offers biomedical sciences (MS); global health (MPH); health promotion (MPH); healthcare management (Certificate); nutrition (MPH). *Program availability:* Part-time, online learning. *Students:* 435 full-time (342 women), 609 part-time (489 women); includes 301 minority (238 Black or African American, non-Hispanic/Latino; 6 American Indian or Alaska Native, non-Hispanic/Latino; 25 Asian, non-Hispanic/Latino; 12 Hispanic/Latino; 1 Native Hawaiian or other Pacific Islander, non-Hispanic/Latino; 19 Two or more races, non-Hispanic/Latino), 71 international. Average age 33. 1,433 applicants, 43% accepted, 295 enrolled. In 2015, 50 master's, 8 other advanced degrees awarded. *Degree requirements:* For master's, thesis (for some programs). *Entrance requirements:* Additional exam requirements/recommendations for international students: Required—TOEFL (minimum score 600 paper-based; 100 iBT). Application fee: $50. *Unit head:* Dr. Ralph Linstra, Dean. *Application contact:* Jay Bridge, Director of Admissions, 800-424-9595, Fax: 800-628-7977, E-mail: gradadmissions@liberty.edu.

Life University, Graduate Programs, Marietta, GA 30060-2903. Offers athletic training (MAT); chiropractic sport science (MS); clinical nutrition (MS); nutrition and sport science (MS), including chiropractic sport science; sport coaching (MS), including exercise sport science; sport injury management (MS), including nutrition and sport science; sports health science (MS). *Program availability:* Part-time, 100% online, blended/hybrid learning. *Faculty:* 6 full-time (1 woman), 7 part-time/adjunct (2 women). *Students:* 100 full-time (60 women), 107 part-time (68 women); includes 104 minority (88 Black or African American, non-Hispanic/Latino; 2 American Indian or Alaska Native, non-Hispanic/Latino; 6 Asian, non-Hispanic/Latino; 8 Hispanic/Latino), 8 international. Average age 30. *Degree requirements:* For master's, comprehensive exam (for some programs), thesis optional. *Entrance requirements:* For master's, GRE General Test, minimum GPA of 3.0, 3 letters of recommendation, curriculum vitae. Additional exam requirements/recommendations for international students: Required—TOEFL (minimum score 500 paper-based). *Application deadline:* For fall admission, 4/1 priority date for domestic and international students; for winter admission, 12/1 priority date for domestic and international students; for spring admission, 3/1 priority date for domestic and international students. Applications are processed on a rolling basis. Application fee: $50. Electronic applications accepted. *Expenses:* Contact institution. *Financial support:* Career-related internships or fieldwork, Federal Work-Study, and tuition waivers (full and partial) available. Support available to part-time students. Financial award application deadline: 9/1; financial award applicants required to submit FAFSA. *Unit head:* Dr. Jana Holwick, Dean of Graduate and Undergraduate Studies, 678-331-4407, Fax: 770-426-2699, E-mail: jana.holwick@life.edu. *Application contact:* Robyn Stanley, Director of Enrollment, 770-426-2889, E-mail: robin.stanley@life.edu.
Website: http://www.life.edu/enrollment/admissions/graduate-admissions

Lipscomb University, Program in Exercise and Nutrition Science, Nashville, TN 37204-3951. Offers MS. *Program availability:* Part-time, evening/weekend. *Faculty:* 4 full-time (3 women), 3 part-time/adjunct (1 woman). *Students:* 11 full-time (6 women), 37 part-time (21 women); includes 7 minority (3 Black or African American, non-Hispanic/Latino; 1 Asian, non-Hispanic/Latino; 3 Hispanic/Latino), 1 international. Average age 28. In 2015, 21 master's awarded. *Degree requirements:* For master's, comprehensive exam (for some programs), thesis optional. *Entrance requirements:* For master's, GRE (minimum score of 800), minimum GPA of 2.75 on all undergraduate work; 2 letters of recommendation; resume. Additional exam requirements/recommendations for international students: Required—TOEFL (minimum score 570 paper-based; 80 iBT). *Application deadline:* For fall admission, 6/1 for domestic students; for spring admission, 12/1 for domestic students. Applications are processed on a rolling basis. Application fee: $50 ($75 for international students). Electronic applications accepted. *Expenses:* $930 per credit hour. *Financial support:* Unspecified assistantships available. Financial award applicants required to submit FAFSA. *Unit head:* Dr. Karen Robichaud, Director, 615-966-5602, E-mail: karen.robichaud@lipscomb.edu. *Application contact:* Julie Lillicrap, Administrative Assistant, 615-966-5700, E-mail: julie.lillicrap@lipscomb.edu.
Website: http://www.lipscomb.edu/kinesiology/graduate-programs

Logan University, College of Health Sciences, Chesterfield, MO 63017. Offers health informatics (MS); health professionals education (DHPE); nutrition and human performance (MS); sports science and rehabilitation (MS). *Program availability:* Part-time, 100% online, blended/hybrid learning. *Faculty:* 3 full-time (2 women), 14 part-time/adjunct (5 women). *Students:* 19 full-time (15 women), 96 part-time (60 women); includes 12 minority (6 Black or African American, non-Hispanic/Latino; 1 Asian, non-Hispanic/Latino; 4 Hispanic/Latino; 1 Two or more races, non-Hispanic/Latino). Average age 31. 74 applicants, 85% accepted, 63 enrolled. In 2015, 95 master's awarded.

Entrance requirements: For master's, minimum GPA of 2.5. Additional exam requirements/recommendations for international students: Required—TOEFL (minimum score 500 paper-based; 79 iBT); Recommended—IELTS (minimum score 6.5). *Application deadline:* Applications are processed on a rolling basis. Application fee: $50. Electronic applications accepted. *Expenses:* Contact institution. *Financial support:* In 2015–16, 4 students received support. Federal Work-Study and scholarships/grants available. Support available to part-time students. Financial award applicants required to submit FAFSA. *Faculty research:* Ankle injury prevention in high school athletes, low back pain in college football players, short arc banding and low back pain, the effects of enzymes on inflammatory blood markers, gait analysis in high school and college athletes. *Unit head:* Dr. Sherri Cole, Dean, College of Health Sciences, 636-227-2100 Ext. 2702, Fax: 636-207-2418, E-mail: sherri.cole@logan.edu. *Application contact:* Jordan LaMarca, Assistant Director of Admissions, 636-227-2100 Ext. 1973, Fax: 636-207-2425, E-mail: admissions@logan.edu.
Website: http://www.logan.edu

Loma Linda University, School of Public Health, Programs in Nutrition, Loma Linda, CA 92350. Offers public health nutrition (MPH, Dr PH). *Accreditation:* AND. *Degree requirements:* For doctorate, thesis/dissertation. *Entrance requirements:* For doctorate, GRE General Test. Additional exam requirements/recommendations for international students: Required—Michigan English Language Assessment Battery or TOEFL. *Application deadline:* Applications are processed on a rolling basis. Application fee: $100. *Expenses:* $880 per unit. *Financial support:* Application deadline: 5/15. *Faculty research:* Sports nutrition in minorities, dietary determinance of chronic disease, protein adequacy in vegetarian diets, relationship of dietary intake to hormone level. *Unit head:* Ella Haddad, Director, 909-824-4598, Fax: 909-824-4087, E-mail: ehaddad@llu.edu. *Application contact:* Wendy Genovez, Assistant Dean of Admissions and Records, 909-824-4694, Fax: 909-824-4087, E-mail: wgenovez@llu.edu.

London Metropolitan University, Graduate Programs, London, United Kingdom. Offers applied psychology (M Sc); architecture (MA); biomedical science (M Sc); blood science (M Sc); cancer pharmacology (M Sc); computer networking and cyber security (M Sc); computing and information systems (M Sc); conference interpreting (MA); counter-terrorism studies (M Sc); creative, digital and professional writing (MA); crime, violence and prevention (M Sc); criminology (M Sc); curating contemporary art (MA); data analytics (M Sc); digital media (MA); early childhood studies (MA); education (MA, Ed D); financial services law, regulation and compliance (LL M); food science (M Sc); forensic psychology (M Sc); health and social care management and policy (M Sc); human nutrition (M Sc); human resource management (MA); human rights and international conflict (MA); information technology (M Sc); intelligence and security studies (M Sc); international oil, gas and energy law (LL M); international relations (MA); interpreting (MA); learning and teaching in higher education (MA); legal practice (LL M); media and entertainment law (LL M); organizational and consumer psychology (M Sc); psychological therapy (M Sc); psychology of mental health (M Sc); public health (M Sc); public policy and management (MPA); security studies (M Sc); social work (M Sc); spatial planning and urban design (MA); sports therapy (M Sc); supporting older children and young people with dyslexia (MA); teaching languages (MA), including Arabic, English; translation (MA); woman and child abuse (MA).

Long Island University–LIU Post, School of Health Professions and Nursing, Brookville, NY 11548-1300. Offers biomedical sciences (MS), including applied laboratory medicine, cancer biology, medical and molecular immunology, microbiology/infectious diseases; cardiovascular perfusion (MS); dietetic internship (Advanced Certificate); family nurse practitioner (MS); forensic social work (Advanced Certificate); nursing education (MS); social work (MSW). *Program availability:* Part-time, evening/weekend, blended/hybrid learning. *Faculty:* 16 full-time (14 women), 46 part-time/adjunct (33 women). *Students:* 190 full-time (139 women), 181 part-time (157 women); includes 141 minority (51 Black or African American, non-Hispanic/Latino; 46 Asian, non-Hispanic/Latino; 41 Hispanic/Latino; 3 Two or more races, non-Hispanic/Latino), 47 international. Average age 36. 422 applicants, 64% accepted, 141 enrolled. In 2015, 96 master's, 28 other advanced degrees awarded. *Degree requirements:* For master's, comprehensive exam (for some programs), thesis (for some programs). *Entrance requirements:* Additional exam requirements/recommendations for international students: Required—TOEFL, IELTS. *Application deadline:* Applications are processed on a rolling basis. Application fee: $50. Electronic applications accepted. *Expenses:* $1,155 per credit, $934 per term full-time university fee, $442 per term part-time university fee. *Financial support:* In 2015–16, 6 research assistantships with partial tuition reimbursements were awarded; career-related internships or fieldwork, Federal Work-Study, institutionally sponsored loans, tuition waivers (partial), and unspecified assistantships also available. Support available to part-time students. Financial award application deadline: 2/15; financial award applicants required to submit FAFSA. *Faculty research:* Breast cancer, childhood obesity, dietary beverage consumption, emotional distress, histone modification, interprofessional practice, interstitial cystitis, lung cancer, pancreatic cancer, pediatric pain management, post-traumatic growth, poverty, renal nutrition, social ethics, yeast and bacterial drug resistance. *Total annual research expenditures:* $15,000. *Unit head:* Dr. Stacy Gropack, Acting Dean, 516-299-2486, Fax: 516-299-2527, E-mail: post-shpn@liu.edu. *Application contact:* Carol Zerah, Director of Graduate and International Admissions, 516-299-2900 Ext. 3952, Fax: 516-299-2137, E-mail: post-enroll@liu.edu.
Website: http://liu.edu/post/health

Louisiana Tech University, Graduate School, College of Applied and Natural Sciences, School of Human Ecology, Ruston, LA 71272. Offers nutrition and dietetics (MS). *Program availability:* Part-time. *Degree requirements:* For master's, thesis or alternative, Registered Dietician Exam eligibility. *Entrance requirements:* For master's, GRE General Test. *Application deadline:* For fall admission, 7/29 priority date for domestic students; for spring admission, 2/3 for domestic students. Applications are processed on a rolling basis. Application fee: $20 ($30 for international students). *Financial support:* Fellowships, research assistantships, career-related internships or fieldwork, and Federal Work-Study available. Financial award application deadline: 2/1. *Unit head:* Dr. Amy Yates, Director, 318-257-3727, Fax: 318-257-4014.
Website: http://ans.latech.edu/human-ecology.html

Loyola University Chicago, Graduate School, Marcella Niehoff School of Nursing, Maywood, IL 60153. Offers adult gerontology acute care clinical nurse specialist (MSN), including emergency care (MSN, Certificate); adult gerontology acute care nurse practitioner (MSN), including oncology (MSN, Certificate); adult gerontology clinical nurse specialist (MSN), including oncology (MSN, Certificate); adult gerontology nursing (Certificate), including oncology (MSN, Certificate); adult nurse practitioner (Certificate); dietetics (MS); family nurse practitioner (MSN, Certificate), including emergency care; informatics (MSN); leadership (DNP), including healthcare quality using education in safety and technology, infection prevention; nursing science (PhD); women's health nurse practitioner (MSN); women's health nursing (Certificate). *Accreditation:* AACN. *Program availability:* Part-time, blended/hybrid learning. *Faculty:* 27 full-time (25 women), 12 part-time/adjunct (10 women). *Students:* 174 full-time (161 women), 232 part-time (221 women); includes 95 minority (19 Black or African American, non-Hispanic/Latino; 2 American Indian or Alaska Native, non-Hispanic/Latino; 38 Asian, non-Hispanic/Latino; 28 Hispanic/Latino; 2 Native Hawaiian or other Pacific Islander,

Nutrition

non-Hispanic/Latino; 6 Two or more races, non-Hispanic/Latino), 3 international. Average age 35. 209 applicants, 52% accepted, 83 enrolled. In 2015, 78 master's, 10 doctorates, 17 other advanced degrees awarded. *Degree requirements:* For master's, comprehensive exam; for doctorate, thesis/dissertation, qualifying examination (for PhD); capstone project (for DNP). *Entrance requirements:* For master's, BSN, minimum nursing GPA of 3.0, Illinois RN license, 3 letters of recommendation, 1000 hours of experience in area of specialty prior to starting clinical rotations, personal statement; for doctorate, GRE General Test (for PhD), BSN or MSN, minimum GPA of 3.0, professional nursing license, 3 letters of recommendation, personal statement. Additional exam requirements/recommendations for international students: Required—TOEFL (minimum score 550 paper-based; 79 iBT), IELTS (minimum score 6.5). *Application deadline:* For fall admission, 6/1 priority date for domestic and international students; for spring admission, 11/15 priority date for domestic and international students; for summer admission, 3/15 priority date for domestic and international students. Applications are processed on a rolling basis. Application fee: $50. Electronic applications accepted. Application fee is waived when completed online. *Expenses:* $1,081 per credit hour. *Financial support:* In 2015–16, 10 students received support, including 3 research assistantships with full tuition reimbursements available (averaging $18,000 per year), 1 teaching assistantship with full tuition reimbursement available (averaging $18,000 per year); scholarships/grants, unspecified assistantships, and nurse faculty loan program also available. Financial award application deadline: 5/1; financial award applicants required to submit FAFSA. *Faculty research:* Epigenetics and social determinants of health, women's health, vitamin D, interprofessional education, prevention and self-management of chronic disease. *Total annual research expenditures:* $649,606. *Unit head:* Dr. Vicky Keough, Dean, 708-216-5448, Fax: 708-216-9555, E-mail: vkeough@luc.edu. *Application contact:* Toni Topalova, Enrollment Advisor, 708-216-3751, Fax: 708-216-9555, E-mail: atopalova@luc.edu. Website: http://www.luc.edu/nursing/

Marshall University, Academic Affairs Division, College of Health Professions, Department of Dietetics, Huntington, WV 25755. Offers MS. *Students:* 17 full-time (16 women), 2 part-time (both women); includes 3 minority (1 Asian, non-Hispanic/Latino; 1 Hispanic/Latino; 1 Two or more races, non-Hispanic/Latino). Average age 26. In 2015, 11 master's awarded. *Unit head:* Dr. Kelli Williams, Chairperson, 304-696-4336, E-mail: williamsk@marshall.edu. *Application contact:* Information Contact, 304-746-1900, Fax: 304-746-1902, E-mail: services@marshall.edu.

Marywood University, Academic Affairs, College of Health and Human Services, Department of Nutrition and Dietetics, Program in Dietetic Internship, Scranton, PA 18509-1598. Offers Certificate. *Program availability:* Online learning. Electronic applications accepted.

Marywood University, Academic Affairs, College of Health and Human Services, Department of Nutrition and Dietetics, Program in Nutrition, Scranton, PA 18509-1598. Offers MS. *Program availability:* Part-time. Electronic applications accepted.

Marywood University, Academic Affairs, College of Health and Human Services, Department of Nutrition and Dietetics, Program in Sports Nutrition and Exercise Science, Scranton, PA 18509-1598. Offers MS. *Program availability:* Part-time. Electronic applications accepted.

McGill University, Faculty of Graduate and Postdoctoral Studies, Faculty of Agricultural and Environmental Sciences, School of Dietetics and Human Nutrition, Montréal, QC H3A 2T5, Canada. Offers dietetics (M Sc A, Graduate Diploma); human nutrition (M Sc, M Sc A, PhD).

McMaster University, Faculty of Health Sciences and School of Graduate Studies, Program in Medical Sciences, Metabolism and Nutrition Area, Hamilton, ON L8S 4M2, Canada. Offers M Sc, PhD, MD/PhD. *Degree requirements:* For master's, thesis; for doctorate, comprehensive exam, thesis/dissertation. *Entrance requirements:* For master's, honors B Sc, B+ average in related field; for doctorate, M Sc, minimum B+ average, students with proven research experience and an A average may be admitted with a B Sc degree. Additional exam requirements/recommendations for international students: Required—TOEFL (minimum score 580 paper-based; 92 iBT).

McNeese State University, Doré School of Graduate Studies, Burton College of Education, Department of Health and Human Performance, Lake Charles, LA 70609. Offers exercise physiology (MS); health promotion (MS); nutrition and wellness (MS). *Accreditation:* NCATE. *Program availability:* Evening/weekend. *Entrance requirements:* For master's, GRE, undergraduate major or minor in health and human performance or related field of study.

Meredith College, Nutrition, Health and Human Performance Department, Raleigh, NC 27607-5298. Offers dietetic internship (Postbaccalaureate Certificate); nutrition (MS). *Faculty:* 4 full-time (3 women), 6 part-time/adjunct (all women). *Students:* 75 full-time (71 women), 35 part-time (33 women); includes 7 minority (4 Black or African American, non-Hispanic/Latino; 1 American Indian or Alaska Native, non-Hispanic/Latino; 1 Asian, non-Hispanic/Latino; 1 Hispanic/Latino), 2 international. Average age 27. 252 applicants, 31% accepted, 72 enrolled. In 2015, 18 master's, 27 other advanced degrees awarded. *Degree requirements:* For master's, thesis optional. *Entrance requirements:* For master's, GRE, recommendations, interview. Additional exam requirements/recommendations for international students: Required—TOEFL. *Application deadline:* For fall admission, 7/1 priority date for domestic and international students; for spring admission, 11/1 priority date for domestic and international students. Applications are processed on a rolling basis. Application fee: $50. Electronic applications accepted. *Expenses:* Contact institution. *Financial support:* Application deadline: 2/15; applicants required to submit FAFSA. *Unit head:* Dr. Judy Peel, Head, 919-760-8014, E-mail: peeljudy@meredith.edu. *Application contact:* Dr. William H. Landis, Director, 919-760-2355, Fax: 919-760-2819, E-mail: landish@meredith.edu.

Michigan State University, The Graduate School, College of Agriculture and Natural Resources and College of Natural Science, Department of Food Science and Human Nutrition, East Lansing, MI 48824. Offers food science (MS, PhD); food science - environmental toxicology (PhD); human nutrition (MS, PhD); human nutrition-environmental toxicology (PhD). *Entrance requirements:* Additional exam requirements/recommendations for international students: Required—TOEFL (minimum score 550 paper-based), Michigan State University ELT (minimum score 85), Michigan English Language Assessment Battery (minimum score 83). Electronic applications accepted.

Mississippi State University, College of Agriculture and Life Sciences, Department of Food Science, Nutrition and Health Promotion, Mississippi State, MS 39762. Offers food science and technology (MS); food science and technology (PhD); health promotion (MS); nutrition (MS, PhD). *Program availability:* Online learning. *Faculty:* 18 full-time (6 women), 2 part-time/adjunct (one woman). *Students:* 55 full-time (40 women), 40 part-time (33 women); includes 25 minority (16 Black or African American, non-Hispanic/Latino; 2 Asian, non-Hispanic/Latino; 6 Hispanic/Latino; 1 Two or more races, non-Hispanic/Latino), 25 international. Average age 28. 105 applicants, 47% accepted, 29 enrolled. In 2015, 27 master's, 6 doctorates awarded. *Degree requirements:* For master's, comprehensive exam, thesis; for doctorate, comprehensive exam, thesis/ dissertation. *Entrance requirements:* For master's, GRE General Test, minimum GPA of 2.75; for doctorate, GRE General Test, minimum GPA of 2.75 undergraduate, 3.0 graduate. Additional exam requirements/recommendations for international students:

Required—TOEFL (minimum score 550 paper-based; 79 iBT); Recommended—IELTS (minimum score 6.5). *Application deadline:* For fall admission, 7/1 for domestic students, 5/1 for international students; for spring admission, 11/1 for domestic students, 9/1 for international students. Applications are processed on a rolling basis. Application fee: $60. Electronic applications accepted. *Expenses: Tuition, area resident:* Full-time $7502; part-time $833.74 per credit hour. Tuition, nonresident: full-time $20,142; part-time $2238.24 per credit hour. *Financial support:* In 2015–16, 17 research assistantships with full tuition reimbursements (averaging $15,465 per year), 4 teaching assistantships with full tuition reimbursements (averaging $11,861 per year) were awarded; Federal Work-Study, institutionally sponsored loans, scholarships/grants, and unspecified assistantships also available. Financial award application deadline: 4/1; financial award applicants required to submit FAFSA. *Faculty research:* Food preservation, food chemistry, food safety, food processing, product development. *Unit head:* Dr. Will Evans, Professor and Head, 662-325-5055, Fax: 662-325-8728, E-mail: mwe59@msstate.edu. *Application contact:* Marina Hunt, Admissions Assistant, 662-325-5188, E-mail: mhunt@grad.msstate.edu. Website: http://www.fsnhp.msstate.edu

Missouri State University, Graduate College, College of Health and Human Services, Department of Biomedical Sciences, Springfield, MO 65897. Offers cell and molecular biology (MS); dietetic internship (Certificate); nurse anesthesia (DNAP). *Accreditation:* AANA/CANAEP (one or more programs are accredited). *Program availability:* Part-time. *Faculty:* 15 full-time (6 women), 17 part-time/adjunct (8 women). *Students:* 64 full-time (39 women), 27 part-time (21 women); includes 10 minority (4 Black or African American, non-Hispanic/Latino; 2 American Indian or Alaska Native, non-Hispanic/ Latino; 2 Asian, non-Hispanic/Latino; 2 Hispanic/Latino), 2 international. Average age 29. 55 applicants, 29% accepted, 14 enrolled. In 2015, 25 master's, 1 other advanced degree awarded. *Degree requirements:* For master's, thesis or alternative, oral exam. *Entrance requirements:* For master's, GRE, minimum GPA of 3.0. Additional exam requirements/recommendations for international students: Required—TOEFL (minimum score 550 paper-based; 79 iBT), IELTS (minimum score 6). *Application deadline:* For fall admission, 7/20 for domestic students, 5/1 for international students; for spring admission, 12/20 for domestic students, 9/1 for international students. Application fee: $35 ($50 for international students). Electronic applications accepted. *Expenses:* Tuition, state resident: full-time $5500. Tuition, nonresident: full-time $10,108. *Required fees:* $1000. *Financial support:* In 2015–16, 11 teaching assistantships with full tuition reimbursements (averaging $8,450 per year) were awarded; Federal Work-Study, institutionally sponsored loans, scholarships/grants, and unspecified assistantships also available. Financial award application deadline: 3/31; financial award applicants required to submit FAFSA. *Unit head:* Dr. Collette Witkowski, Department Head, 417-836-5603, Fax: 417-836-5588, E-mail: biomedicalsciences@missouristate.edu. *Application contact:* Michael Edwards, Coordinator of Graduate Admissions, 417-836-5330, Fax: 417-836-6200, E-mail: michaeledwards@missouristate.edu. Website: http://www.missouristate.edu/bms/

Montclair State University, The Graduate School, College of Education and Human Services, American Dietetics Certificate Program, Montclair, NJ 07043-1624. Offers Postbaccalaureate Certificate. *Program availability:* Part-time, evening/weekend. *Students:* 5 full-time (4 women), 4 part-time (3 women); includes 3 minority (1 Asian, non-Hispanic/Latino; 2 Hispanic/Latino). Average age 27. In 2015, 8 Postbaccalaureate Certificates awarded. *Entrance requirements:* Additional exam requirements/ recommendations for international students: Required—TOEFL (minimum score 65 iBT), IELTS. *Application deadline:* Applications are processed on a rolling basis. Application fee: $60. Electronic applications accepted. *Expenses:* Tuition, state resident: part-time $553 per credit. Tuition, nonresident: part-time $854 per credit. *Required fees:* $91 per credit. Tuition and fees vary according to program. *Financial support:* Federal Work-Study, scholarships/grants, and unspecified assistantships available. Support available to part-time students. Financial award application deadline: 3/1; financial award applicants required to submit FAFSA. *Unit head:* Dr. Eva Goldfarb, Chairperson, 973-655-4154. *Application contact:* Amy Aiello, Director of Graduate Admissions and Operations, 973-655-5147, Fax: 973-655-7869, E-mail: graduate.school@montclair.edu.

Montclair State University, The Graduate School, College of Education and Human Services, Nutrition and Exercise Science Certificate Program, Montclair, NJ 07043-1624. Offers Certificate. *Students:* 3 full-time (all women), 2 part-time (both women); includes 2 minority (1 Asian, non-Hispanic/Latino; 1 Two or more races, non-Hispanic/ Latino). Average age 27. 4 applicants, 75% accepted, 2 enrolled. In 2015, 1 Certificate awarded. *Application deadline:* Applications are processed on a rolling basis. Application fee: $60. Electronic applications accepted. *Expenses:* Tuition, state resident: part-time $553 per credit. Tuition, nonresident: part-time $854 per credit. *Required fees:* $91 per credit. Tuition and fees vary according to program. *Financial support:* Federal Work-Study and scholarships/grants available. Support available to part-time students. *Unit head:* Dr. Susana Juniu, Chairperson, 973-655-7093. *Application contact:* Amy Aiello, Executive Director of The Graduate School, 973-655-5147, Fax: 973-655-7869, E-mail: graduate.school@montclair.edu. Website: http://www.montclair.edu/catalog/view_requirements.php?CurriculumID-3081

Montclair State University, The Graduate School, College of Education and Human Services, Program in Nutrition and Food Science, Montclair, NJ 07043-1624. Offers MS. *Program availability:* Part-time, evening/weekend. *Students:* 33 full-time (27 women), 48 part-time (36 women); includes 18 minority (5 Black or African American, non-Hispanic/ Latino; 3 Asian, non-Hispanic/Latino; 8 Hispanic/Latino; 1 Native Hawaiian or other Pacific Islander, non-Hispanic/Latino; 1 Two or more races, non-Hispanic/Latino), 6 international. Average age 29. 38 applicants, 76% accepted, 22 enrolled. In 2015, 32 master's awarded. *Degree requirements:* For master's, comprehensive exam, thesis or alternative. *Entrance requirements:* For master's, GRE General Test, essay, 2 letters of recommendation. Additional exam requirements/recommendations for international students: Required—TOEFL (minimum score 83 iBT), IELTS (minimum score 6.5). *Application deadline:* Applications are processed on a rolling basis. Application fee: $60. Electronic applications accepted. *Expenses:* Tuition, state resident: part-time $553 per credit. Tuition, nonresident: part-time $854 per credit. *Required fees:* $91 per credit. Tuition and fees vary according to program. *Financial support:* In 2015–16, 8 research assistantships with full tuition reimbursements (averaging $7,000 per year), 1 teaching assistantship with partial tuition reimbursement (averaging $7,000 per year) were awarded; Federal Work-Study, scholarships/grants, and unspecified assistantships also available. Support available to part-time students. Financial award application deadline: 3/1; financial award applicants required to submit FAFSA. *Unit head:* Dr. Eva Goldfarb, Chairperson, 973-655-4154. *Application contact:* Amy Aiello, Executive Director of The Graduate School, 973-655-5147, Fax: 973-655-7869, E-mail: graduate.school@ montclair.edu. Website: http://www.montclair.edu/graduate/programs-of-study/nutrition-and-food-science/

Mount Mary University, Graduate Division, Program in Dietetics, Milwaukee, WI 53222-4597. Offers administrative dietetics (MS); clinical dietetics (MS); nutrition education (MS). *Program availability:* Part-time, evening/weekend. *Faculty:* 2 full-time (both women), 3 part-time/adjunct (2 women). *Students:* 11 full-time (10 women), 16

part-time (all women); includes 2 minority (both Hispanic/Latino). Average age 32. 97 applicants, 16% accepted, 12 enrolled. In 2015, 10 master's awarded. *Degree requirements:* For master's, thesis or alternative. *Entrance requirements:* For master's, minimum GPA of 2.75, completion of ADA and DPD requirements. Additional exam requirements/recommendations for international students: Required—TOEFL (minimum score 550 paper-based; 80 iBT); Recommended—IELTS (minimum score 6.5). *Application deadline:* For fall admission, 8/1 for domestic and international students; for spring admission, 12/1 for domestic and international students. Applications are processed on a rolling basis. Application fee: $45. Electronic applications accepted. *Expenses:* $625 per credit. *Financial support:* Career-related internships or fieldwork and Federal Work-Study available. Support available to part-time students. Financial award application deadline: 5/1; financial award applicants required to submit FAFSA. *Unit head:* Tara LaRowe, Director, 414-930-3292, E-mail: larowet@mtmary.edu. *Application contact:* Kirk Heller de Messer, Director, Graduate Admissions, 414-930-3221, E-mail: hellerk@mtmary.edu.
Website: http://www.mtmary.edu/majors-programs/graduate/dietetics/index.html

Mount Saint Vincent University, Graduate Programs, Department of Applied Human Nutrition, Halifax, NS B3M 2J6, Canada. Offers M Sc AHN, MAHN. *Program availability:* Part-time, evening/weekend. *Degree requirements:* For master's, thesis (for some programs). *Entrance requirements:* For master's, bachelor's degree in related field, minimum GPA of 3.0, professional experience. Electronic applications accepted.

New Mexico State University, College of Agricultural, Consumer and Environmental Sciences, Department of Family and Consumer Sciences, Las Cruces, NM 88003. Offers family and child science (MS); family and consumer science education (MS); food science and technology (MS); human nutrition and dietetic science (MS); marriage and family therapy (MS). *Program availability:* Part-time. *Faculty:* 11 full-time (9 women), 1 (woman) part-time/adjunct. *Students:* 31 full-time (26 women), 6 part-time (3 women); includes 16 minority (1 Black or African American, non-Hispanic/Latino; 1 Asian, non-Hispanic/Latino; 14 Hispanic/Latino), 2 international. Average age 27. 16 applicants, 75% accepted, 11 enrolled. In 2015, 15 master's awarded. *Degree requirements:* For master's, comprehensive exam (for some programs), thesis (for some programs), oral exam. *Entrance requirements:* For master's, GRE, 3 letters of reference, resume, letter of interest. Additional exam requirements/recommendations for international students: Required—TOEFL (minimum score 550 paper-based; 79 iBT), IELTS (minimum score 6.5). *Application deadline:* For fall admission, 3/1 priority date for domestic and international students; for spring admission, 11/30 for domestic and international students. Applications are processed on a rolling basis. Application fee: $40 ($50 for international students). Electronic applications accepted. *Expenses:* $274.50 per credit hour for in-state students, and all students enrolled in six or fewer credits; $839.30 per credit hour for out-of-state and international students enrolled in at least seven hours. *Financial support:* In 2015–16, 28 students received support, including 2 fellowships (averaging $4,088 per year), 9 teaching assistantships (averaging $13,666 per year); career-related internships or fieldwork, Federal Work-Study, scholarships/grants, traineeships, health care benefits, and unspecified assistantships also available. Support available to part-time students. Financial award application deadline: 3/1. *Faculty research:* Food product analysis, childhood obesity, couple relationship education, military families, Latino college students. *Total annual research expenditures:* $476,012. *Unit head:* Dr. Esther Lynn Devall, Department Head, 575-646-1161, Fax: 575-646-1889, E-mail: edevall@nmsu.edu. *Application contact:* Dr. Margaret Ann Bock, Graduate Program Contact, 575-646-3936, Fax: 575-646-1889, E-mail: marbock@nmsu.edu.
Website: http://aces.nmsu.edu/academics/fcs

New York Chiropractic College, Program in Applied Clinical Nutrition, Seneca Falls, NY 13148-0800. Offers MS. *Program availability:* Part-time, evening/weekend. *Entrance requirements:* For master's, minimum GPA of 2.5, transcripts, writing sample. Additional exam requirements/recommendations for international students: Recommended—TOEFL. Electronic applications accepted.

New York Institute of Technology, School of Health Professions, Department of Interdisciplinary Health Sciences, Old Westbury, NY 11568-8000. Offers clinical nutrition (MS). *Program availability:* Part-time, evening/weekend, online only, 100% online. *Faculty:* 1 (woman) full-time, 12 part-time/adjunct (10 women). *Students:* 5 full-time (4 women), 23 part-time (20 women); includes 11 minority (5 Black or African American, non-Hispanic/Latino; 4 Asian, non-Hispanic/Latino; 1 Hispanic/Latino; 1 Two or more races, non-Hispanic/Latino). Average age 33. 22 applicants, 68% accepted, 9 enrolled. In 2015, 14 master's awarded. *Degree requirements:* For master's, comprehensive exam, thesis. *Entrance requirements:* For master's, minimum undergraduate GPA of 2.85, satisfactory preparation in science courses. Additional exam requirements/recommendations for international students: Required—TOEFL (minimum score 550 paper-based; 79 iBT), IELTS (minimum score 6). *Application deadline:* For fall admission, 7/1 for international students; for spring admission, 12/1 for international students. Applications are processed on a rolling basis. Application fee: $50. Electronic applications accepted. *Expenses: Tuition, area resident:* Full-time $20,790; part-time $1155 per credit. *Required fees:* $95; $75 per credit. Full-time tuition and fees vary according to degree level, campus/location and program. Part-time tuition and fees vary according to course load and campus/location. *Financial support:* Research assistantships with partial tuition reimbursements, career-related internships or fieldwork, scholarships/grants, health care benefits, tuition waivers (full and partial), and unspecified assistantships available. Support available to part-time students. Financial award application deadline: 3/1; financial award applicants required to submit FAFSA. *Faculty research:* Diabetes prevention and treatment, college students' health behavior, online education in health sciences, health policy, wellness in underserved populations. *Unit head:* Dr. Mindy Haar, Director, 516-686-3818, Fax: 516-686-3795, E-mail: mhaar@nyit.edu. *Application contact:* Alice Dolitsky, Director, Graduate Admissions, 516-686-7520, Fax: 516-686-1116, E-mail: nyitgrad@nyit.edu.
Website: http://www.nyit.edu/degrees/clinical_nutrition

New York University, College of Global Public Health, New York, NY 10003. Offers biological basis of public health (PhD); community and international health (MPH); global health leadership (MPH); health systems and health services research (PhD); population and community health (PhD); public health nutrition (MPH); social and behavioral sciences (MPH); socio-behavioral health (PhD). *Program availability:* Part-time, online learning. *Degree requirements:* For master's, thesis (for some programs); for doctorate, thesis/dissertation. *Entrance requirements:* For master's and doctorate, GRE. Additional exam requirements/recommendations for international students: Required—TOEFL. Electronic applications accepted.

New York University, Steinhardt School of Culture, Education, and Human Development, Department of Nutrition, Food Studies, and Public Health, Programs in Nutrition and Dietetics, New York, NY 10003. Offers clinical nutrition (MS); nutrition and dietetics (MS, PhD), including food and nutrition (MS); rehabilitation sciences (PhD). *Program availability:* Part-time. *Degree requirements:* For master's, thesis (for some programs); for doctorate, thesis/dissertation. *Entrance requirements:* For doctorate, GRE General Test, interview. Additional exam requirements/recommendations for international students: Required—TOEFL (minimum score 100 iBT). Electronic applications accepted. *Faculty research:* Nutrition and race, childhood obesity and other

eating disorders, nutritional epidemiology, nutrition policy, nutrition and health promotion.

North Carolina Agricultural and Technical State University, School of Graduate Studies, School of Agriculture and Environmental Sciences, Department of Family and Consumer Sciences, Greensboro, NC 27411. Offers child development early education and family studies (MAT); family and consumer sciences (MAT); food and nutrition (MS). *Program availability:* Part-time, evening/weekend. *Degree requirements:* For master's, comprehensive exam, thesis or alternative, qualifying exam. *Entrance requirements:* For master's, GRE General Test, minimum GPA of 2.6.

North Carolina State University, Graduate School, College of Agriculture and Life Sciences and College of Veterinary Medicine, Program in Nutrition, Raleigh, NC 27695. Offers MN, MS, PhD. *Program availability:* Part-time. *Degree requirements:* For master's, thesis (for some programs); for doctorate, thesis/dissertation. *Entrance requirements:* For master's and doctorate, GRE General Test. Additional exam requirements/recommendations for international students: Required—TOEFL (minimum score 550 paper-based). Electronic applications accepted. *Faculty research:* Effects of food/feed ingredients and components on health and growth, community nutrition, waste management and reduction, experimental animal nutrition.

North Dakota State University, College of Graduate and Interdisciplinary Studies, College of Human Development and Education, Department of Health, Nutrition, and Exercise Sciences, Fargo, ND 58102. Offers athletic training (MAT, MS); dietetics (MS); exercise science and nutrition (PhD); exercise/nutrition science (MS); health promotion (MPH); leadership in physical education and sport (MS). *Program availability:* Part-time, evening/weekend, online learning. *Degree requirements:* For master's, thesis (for some programs). *Entrance requirements:* For master's, minimum GPA of 3.0. Additional exam requirements/recommendations for international students: Required—TOEFL (minimum score 525 paper-based; 71 iBT). *Application deadline:* For fall admission, 3/1 priority date for domestic and international students. Applications are processed on a rolling basis. Application fee: $35. Electronic applications accepted. *Financial support:* Teaching assistantships with full tuition reimbursements available. Financial award application deadline: 3/31. *Faculty research:* Biomechanics, sport specialization, recreation, nutrition, athletic training. *Unit head:* Dr. Yeong Rhee, Head, 701-231-7476, Fax: 701-231-8872, E-mail: yeong.rhee@ndsu.edu. *Application contact:* Nancy Moberg, Academic Assistant, 701-231-7474, Fax: 701-231-6524.
Website: http://www.ndsu.edu/hnes/

Northeastern University, College of Professional Studies, Boston, MA 02115-5096. Offers applied nutrition (MS); college athletics administration (MSL); commerce and economic development (MS); corporate and organizational communication (MS); criminal justice (MS); digital media (MPS); elearning and instructional design (M Ed); elementary education (MAT); geographic information technology (MPS); global studies and international relations (MS); higher education administration (M Ed); homeland security (MA); human services (MS); informatics (MPS); leadership (MS); learning analytics (M Ed); learning and instruction (M Ed); nonprofit management (MS); professional sports administration (MSL); project management (MS); regulatory affairs for drugs, biologics, and medical devices (MS); respiratory care leadership (MS); special education (M Ed); technical communication (MS). *Program availability:* Part-time, evening/weekend, 100% online, blended/hybrid learning. *Faculty:* 72 full-time (44 women), 865 part-time/adjunct (380 women). *Students:* 4,930 part-time (3,046 women). In 2015, 1,310 master's awarded. *Application deadline:* Applications are processed on a rolling basis. Application fee: $0. Electronic applications accepted. *Expenses:* Contact institution. *Financial support:* Applicants required to submit FAFSA. *Unit head:* Dr. John LaBrie, Dean/Vice President for Professional Education.
Website: http://www.cps.neu.edu/

Northern Illinois University, Graduate School, College of Health and Human Sciences, School of Family, Consumer and Nutrition Sciences, De Kalb, IL 60115-2854. Offers applied family and child studies (MS); nutrition and dietetics (MS). *Accreditation:* AAMFT/COAMFTE. *Program availability:* Part-time. *Faculty:* 16 full-time (14 women), 2 part-time/adjunct (1 woman). *Students:* 53 full-time (50 women), 16 part-time (all women); includes 11 minority (2 Black or African American, non-Hispanic/Latino; 1 Asian, non-Hispanic/Latino; 5 Hispanic/Latino; 3 Two or more races, non-Hispanic/Latino), 2 international. Average age 27. 80 applicants, 46% accepted, 20 enrolled. In 2015, 29 master's awarded. *Degree requirements:* For master's, comprehensive exam, internship, thesis (for nutrition and dietetics). *Entrance requirements:* For master's, GRE General Test, minimum GPA of 2.75. Additional exam requirements/recommendations for international students: Required—TOEFL (minimum score 550 paper-based). *Application deadline:* For fall admission, 6/1 for domestic students, 5/1 for international students; for spring admission, 11/1 for domestic students, 10/1 for international students. Applications are processed on a rolling basis. Application fee: $40. Electronic applications accepted. *Financial support:* In 2015–16, 8 research assistantships with full tuition reimbursements, 35 teaching assistantships with full tuition reimbursements were awarded; fellowships with full tuition reimbursements, career-related internships or fieldwork, Federal Work-Study, scholarships/grants, tuition waivers (full), and staff assistantships also available. Support available to part-time students. Financial award applicants required to submit FAFSA. *Faculty research:* Preliminary child development, hospitality administration in Asia, sports nutrition, eating disorders. *Unit head:* Dr. Thomas Pavkov, Chair, 815-753-6342, Fax: 815-753-1321, E-mail: tpavkov@niu.edu. *Application contact:* Graduate School Office, 815-753-0395, E-mail: gradsch@niu.edu.
Website: http://www.fcns.niu.edu/

The Ohio State University, Graduate School, College of Education and Human Ecology, Department of Human Sciences, Columbus, OH 43210. Offers consumer sciences (MS, PhD); human development and family science (PhD); human nutrition (MS, PhD); kinesiology (MA, PhD). *Program availability:* Part-time. *Faculty:* 52. *Students:* 115 full-time (69 women), 11 part-time (9 women); includes 22 minority (9 Black or African American, non-Hispanic/Latino; 1 American Indian or Alaska Native, non-Hispanic/Latino; 1 Asian, non-Hispanic/Latino; 7 Hispanic/Latino; 4 Two or more races, non-Hispanic/Latino), 30 international. Average age 28. In 2015, 33 master's, 15 doctorates awarded. *Degree requirements:* For master's, thesis optional; for doctorate, thesis/dissertation. *Entrance requirements:* For master's and doctorate, GRE. Additional exam requirements/recommendations for international students: Required—TOEFL (minimum score 550 paper-based; 79 iBT), Michigan English Language Assessment Battery (minimum score 82); Recommended—IELTS (minimum score 7). *Application deadline:* For fall admission, 12/1 priority date for domestic and international students. Applications are processed on a rolling basis. Application fee: $60 ($70 for international students). Electronic applications accepted. *Financial support:* Fellowships with tuition reimbursements, research assistantships with tuition reimbursements, teaching assistantships with tuition reimbursements, Federal Work-Study, and institutionally sponsored loans available. Support available to part-time students. *Unit head:* Dr. Carl M. Maresh, Chair, E-mail: maresh.15@osu.edu. *Application contact:* Graduate and Professional Admissions, 614-292-9444, Fax: 614-292-3895, E-mail: gpadmissions@osu.edu.
Website: http://ehe.osu.edu/human-sciences/

The Ohio State University, Graduate School, College of Education and Human Ecology, Human Nutrition Program, Columbus, OH 43210. Offers PhD. Offered jointly

Nutrition

with College of Food, Agricultural, and Environmental Sciences, College of Medicine, and College of Veterinary Medicine. *Faculty:* 43. *Students:* 32 full-time (21 women); includes 4 minority (2 Asian, non-Hispanic/Latino; 2 Hispanic/Latino), 7 international. Average age 27. In 2015, 3 doctorates awarded. *Degree requirements:* For doctorate, thesis/dissertation. *Entrance requirements:* For doctorate, GRE. Additional exam requirements/recommendations for international students: Required—TOEFL (minimum score 600 paper-based; 100 iBT). Recommended—IELTS (minimum score 8). *Application deadline:* For fall admission, 12/1 priority date for domestic and international students. Applications are processed on a rolling basis. Application fee: $60 ($70 for international students). Electronic applications accepted. *Financial support:* Applicants required to submit FAFSA. *Unit head:* Dr. Jeffrey L. Firkins, Director, 614-292-9957, E-mail: osun@osu.edu. *Application contact:* Graduate and Professional Admissions, 614-292-9444, Fax: 614-292-3895, E-mail: gpadmissions@osu.edu.
Website: http://osun.osu.edu/

Ohio University, Graduate College, College of Health Sciences and Professions, School of Applied Health Sciences and Wellness, Program in Food and Nutrition, Athens, OH 45701-2979. Offers human and consumer sciences (MS).

Oklahoma State University, College of Human Sciences, Department of Nutritional Sciences, Stillwater, OK 74078. Offers MS, PhD. *Program availability:* Online learning. *Faculty:* 22 full-time (17 women), 2 part-time/adjunct (both women). *Students:* 40 full-time (31 women), 35 part-time (30 women); includes 13 minority (3 Black or African American, non-Hispanic/Latino; 2 American Indian or Alaska Native, non-Hispanic/Latino; 3 Asian, non-Hispanic/Latino; 2 Hispanic/Latino; 3 Two or more races, non-Hispanic/Latino), 14 international. Average age 29. 46 applicants, 74% accepted, 25 enrolled. In 2015, 20 master's, 5 doctorates awarded. *Degree requirements:* For master's, thesis (for some programs); for doctorate, comprehensive exam, thesis/dissertation. *Entrance requirements:* For master's and doctorate, GRE or GMAT. Additional exam requirements/recommendations for international students: Required—TOEFL (minimum score 550 paper-based; 79 iBT). *Application deadline:* For fall admission, 3/1 priority date for international students; for spring admission, 8/1 priority date for international students. Applications are processed on a rolling basis. Application fee: $40 ($75 for international students). Electronic applications accepted. *Expenses:* Tuition, state resident: full-time $3528; part-time $196 per credit hour. Tuition, nonresident: full-time $14,144; part-time $785.75 per credit hour. *Required fees:* $1895; $105.25 per credit hour. Tuition and fees vary according to campus/location. *Financial support:* In 2015–16, 24 research assistantships (averaging $13,618 per year), 15 teaching assistantships (averaging $10,989 per year) were awarded; career-related internships or fieldwork, Federal Work-Study, scholarships/grants, health care benefits, tuition waivers (partial), and unspecified assistantships also available. Support available to part-time students. Financial award application deadline: 3/1; financial award applicants required to submit FAFSA. *Faculty research:* Nutritional sciences, micronutrients and chronic disease, phytochemicals, nutrition education, osteoporosis, food service administration. *Unit head:* Dr. Nancy M. Betts, Department Head, 405-744-5040, Fax: 405-744-1357, E-mail: nancy.betts@okstate.edu. *Application contact:* Dr. Gail Gates, Graduate Coordinator, 405-744-3845, Fax: 405-744-1357, E-mail: gail.gates@okstate.edu.
Website: http://humansciences.okstate.edu/nsci/

Oregon Health & Science University, School of Medicine, Graduate Programs in Medicine, Program in Clinical Nutrition, Portland, OR 97239-3098. Offers dietetics (Certificate); human nutrition (MS). *Program availability:* Part-time. *Faculty:* 7 part-time/adjunct (all women). *Students:* 28 full-time (27 women); includes 4 minority (1 American Indian or Alaska Native, non-Hispanic/Latino; 3 Hispanic/Latino). Average age 27. 75 applicants, 24% accepted, 18 enrolled. *Degree requirements:* For master's, thesis optional. *Entrance requirements:* For master's, GRE General Test (minimum scores: 153 Verbal/148 Quantitative/4.5 Analytical). *Application deadline:* For fall admission, 1/1 for domestic students. Application fee: $120. *Faculty research:* Inborn errors of metabolism, weight loss/weight regulation, body composition/energy expenditure, nutritional epidemiology, medical nutrition therapy. *Unit head:* Dr. Diane Stadler, Program Director. *Application contact:* Alexis Young, 503-494-7596, E-mail: gphn@ohsu.edu.

Oregon State University, College of Public Health and Human Sciences, Program in Nutrition, Corvallis, OR 97331. Offers MS, PhD. *Program availability:* Part-time. *Faculty:* 8 full-time (5 women), 1 (woman) part-time/adjunct. *Students:* 10 full-time (9 women); includes 2 minority (1 Asian, non-Hispanic/Latino; 1 Hispanic/Latino), 2 international. Average age 27. 10 applicants, 10% accepted, 1 enrolled. In 2015, 1 master's, 1 doctorate awarded. *Degree requirements:* For master's, thesis; for doctorate, thesis/dissertation. *Entrance requirements:* For master's and doctorate, GRE, minimum GPA of 3.0 in last 90 hours of course work. Additional exam requirements/recommendations for international students: Required—TOEFL (minimum score 80 iBT), IELTS (minimum score 6.5). *Application deadline:* For fall admission, 12/1 for domestic and international students. Applications are processed on a rolling basis. *Expenses:* Tuition, state resident: full-time $12,150; part-time $450 per credit. Tuition, nonresident: full-time $20,952; part-time $776 per credit. *Required fees:* $1572; $1443 per unit. One-time fee: $350. Tuition and fees vary according to course load, campus/location and program. *Financial support:* Fellowships, research assistantships, teaching assistantships, career-related internships or fieldwork, Federal Work-Study, and institutionally sponsored loans available. Support available to part-time students. Financial award application deadline: 12/1. *Faculty research:* Human metabolic studies, trace minerals, food science, food management. *Unit head:* Dr. Donald B. Jump, Professor and Director, Nutrition Graduate Program, 541-737-4007. *Application contact:* Debi Rothermund, Nutrition Advisor, 541-737-3324, Fax: 541-737-6914, E-mail: debi.rothermund@oregonstate.edu.
Website: http://health.oregonstate.edu/degrees/graduate/nutrition

[Pennsylvania State] University Park, Graduate School, College of Health and Human [Development], Department of Nutritional Sciences, University Park, PA 16802. Offers [nutritional scien]ce (MS, PhD). *Unit head:* Dr. Ann C. Crouter, Dean, 814-865-1420, Fax: [814-865-59]2. *Application contact:* Lori Stania, Director, Graduate Student Services, [814-863-2911], Fax: 814-863-4627, E-mail: l-gswww@lists.psu.edu.
Website: http://nutrition.hhd.psu.edu/

[Purdue] University, Graduate School, College of Health and Human Sciences, [Departm]ent of Nutrition Science, West Lafayette, IN 47907. Offers animal health (MS, [PhD); bi]ochemical and molecular nutrition (MS, PhD); growth and development (MS, [PhD); h]uman and clinical nutrition (MS, PhD); public health and education (MS, PhD). *Degree requirements:* For master's, thesis; for doctorate, thesis/dissertation. *Entrance requirements:* For master's and doctorate, GRE General Test (minimum scores in verbal and quantitative areas of 1000 or 300 on new scoring), minimum undergraduate GPA of 3.0 or equivalent. Additional exam requirements/recommendations for international students: Required—TOEFL (minimum score 600 paper-based; 77 iBT). Electronic applications accepted. *Faculty research:* Nutrient requirements, nutrient metabolism, nutrition and disease prevention.

Queens College of the City University of New York, Mathematics and Natural Sciences Division, Department of Family, Nutrition and Exercise Sciences, Flushing, NY 11367-1597. Offers exercise science specialist (MS); family and consumer science (K-12) (AC);

family and consumer science/teacher (K-12) (MS Ed); nutrition and exercise science (MS); nutrition specialist (MS); physical education (K-12) (AC); physical education/teaching curriculum (pre K-12) (MS Ed). *Program availability:* Part-time, evening/weekend. *Faculty:* 14 full-time (13 women), 53 part-time/adjunct (37 women). *Students:* 25 full-time (10 women), 142 part-time (87 women); includes 54 minority (28 Black or African American, non-Hispanic/Latino; 12 Asian, non-Hispanic/Latino; 14 Hispanic/Latino), 16 international. Average age 31. 102 applicants, 66% accepted, 54 enrolled. In 2015, 16 master's, 7 other advanced degrees awarded. *Degree requirements:* For master's, research project. *Entrance requirements:* For master's, minimum GPA of 3.0. Additional exam requirements/recommendations for international students: Required—TOEFL, IELTS. *Application deadline:* For fall admission, 4/1 for domestic students; for spring admission, 11/1 for domestic students. Applications are processed on a rolling basis. Application fee: $125. Electronic applications accepted. *Expenses:* Tuition, state resident: $5065; part-time $425 per credit. Tuition, nonresident: part-time $780 per credit. *Required fees:* $522. Part-time tuition and fees vary according to course load and program. *Financial support:* Career-related internships or fieldwork and unspecified assistantships available. Financial award application deadline: 4/1; financial award applicants required to submit FAFSA. *Unit head:* Dr. Michael Toner, Chairperson, 718-997-4168, E-mail: michael.toner@qc.cuny.edu.

Rosalind Franklin University of Medicine and Science, College of Health Professions, Department of Nutrition, North Chicago, IL 60064-3095. Offers clinical nutrition (MS); health promotion and wellness (MS); nutrition education (MS). *Program availability:* Part-time, evening/weekend, online learning. *Degree requirements:* For master's, thesis optional, portfolio. *Entrance requirements:* For master's, minimum GPA of 2.75, registered dietitian (RD), professional certificate or license. Additional exam requirements/recommendations for international students: Required—TOEFL. *Expenses:* Contact institution. *Faculty research:* Nutrition education, distance learning, computer-based graduate education, childhood obesity, nutrition medical education.

Rush University, College of Health Sciences, Department of Clinical Nutrition, Chicago, IL 60612. Offers MS. *Program availability:* Part-time. *Degree requirements:* For master's, thesis. *Entrance requirements:* For master's, GRE General Test, minimum GPA of 3.0, course work in statistics, undergraduate didactic program approved by the American Dietetic Association. Additional exam requirements/recommendations for international students: Required—TOEFL. *Application deadline:* For winter admission, 2/15 for domestic and international students. Application fee: $40. Electronic applications accepted. *Financial support:* Career-related internships or fieldwork, Federal Work-Study, institutionally sponsored loans, scholarships/grants, and stipends available. Support available to part-time students. Financial award applicants required to submit FAFSA. *Faculty research:* Food service management, chronic disease prevention/treatment, obesity, Alzheimer's. *Unit head:* Dr. Kathryn S. Keim, Interim Chair, 312-942-5926, Fax: 312-942-5203.
Website: http://www.rushu.rush.edu/nutrition/

Rutgers University–Newark, School of Health Related Professions, Department of Nutritional Sciences, Dietetic Internship Program, Newark, NJ 07102. Offers Certificate. *Program availability:* Online learning. *Entrance requirements:* For degree, bachelor's degree in dietetics, nutrition, or related field; interview; minimum GPA of 2.9. Additional exam requirements/recommendations for international students: Required—TOEFL (minimum score 500 paper-based; 79 iBT). Electronic applications accepted.

Rutgers University–Newark, School of Health Related Professions, Department of Nutritional Sciences, Program in Clinical Nutrition, Newark, NJ 07102. Offers MS, DCN. *Program availability:* Part-time, evening/weekend, online learning. *Entrance requirements:* For master's, statement of career goals, minimum GPA of 3.2, proof of registered dietician status, interview, transcript of highest degree, bachelor's degree, 1 reference letter; for doctorate, minimum GPA of 3.4, transcript of highest degree, statement of career goals, interview, master's degree, 1 reference letter. Additional exam requirements/recommendations for international students: Required—TOEFL (minimum score 500 paper-based; 79 iBT). Electronic applications accepted.

Rutgers University–New Brunswick, Graduate School-New Brunswick, Program in Nutritional Sciences, Piscataway, NJ 08854-8097. Offers MS, PhD. *Program availability:* Part-time. Terminal master's awarded for partial completion of doctoral program. *Degree requirements:* For master's, thesis; for doctorate, thesis/dissertation, written qualifying exam. *Entrance requirements:* For master's and doctorate, GRE General Test, 3 letters of recommendation. Additional exam requirements/recommendations for international students: Required—TOEFL (minimum score 560 paper-based; 83 iBT). Electronic applications accepted. *Faculty research:* Nutrition and gene expression, nutrition and disease (obesity, diabetes, cancer, osteoporosis, alcohol), community nutrition and nutrition education, cellular lipid transport and metabolism.

Sacred Heart University, Graduate Programs, College of Health Professions, Department of Exercise Science, Fairfield, CT 06825. Offers exercise science and nutrition (MS). *Program availability:* Part-time, evening/weekend. *Faculty:* 6 full-time (3 women). *Students:* 29 full-time (18 women), 1 part-time (0 women); includes 3 minority (2 Hispanic/Latino; 1 Two or more races, non-Hispanic/Latino). Average age 25. 53 applicants, 68% accepted, 14 enrolled. In 2015, 12 master's awarded. *Entrance requirements:* For master's, bachelor's degree in related major, minimum GPA of 3.0, anatomy and physiology (with labs), exercise physiology, nutrition, statistics or health/exercise-specific research methods course, kinesiology (preferred). Additional exam requirements/recommendations for international students: Required—PTE; Recommended—TOEFL (minimum score 570 paper-based; 80 iBT), IELTS (minimum score 6.5). *Application deadline:* Applications are processed on a rolling basis. Application fee: $75. Electronic applications accepted. *Expenses:* Tuition, area resident: Part-time $654 per credit hour. *Financial support:* Unspecified assistantships available. Financial award applicants required to submit FAFSA. *Unit head:* Dr. Kevin Chui, Associate Professor/Chair, Physical Therapy and Human Movement, 203-371-7976, E-mail: chuik@sacredheart.edu. *Application contact:* William Sweeney, Director of Graduate Admissions, 203-396-4827, E-mail: sweeneyw@sacredheart.edu.
Website: http://www.sacredheart.edu/academics/collegeofhealthprofessions/academicprograms/exercisescience/masterofscienceinexercisesciencenutrition/

Sage Graduate School, School of Health Sciences, Program in Nutrition, Troy, NY 12180-4115. Offers applied nutrition (MS); dietetic internship (Certificate); nutrition (Certificate). *Program availability:* Part-time, evening/weekend, 100% online. *Faculty:* 4 full-time (all women), 1 (woman) part-time/adjunct. *Students:* 71 full-time (66 women), 27 part-time (26 women); includes 10 minority (1 Black or African American, non-Hispanic/Latino; 3 Asian, non-Hispanic/Latino; 2 Hispanic/Latino; 4 Two or more races, non-Hispanic/Latino). Average age 27. 202 applicants, 31% accepted, 50 enrolled. In 2015, 13 master's, 24 other advanced degrees awarded. *Entrance requirements:* For master's, minimum GPA of 3.0, resume, 2 letters of recommendation, interview with director. Additional exam requirements/recommendations for international students: Required—TOEFL (minimum score 550 paper-based). *Application deadline:* Applications are processed on a rolling basis. Application fee: $40. Electronic applications accepted. *Expenses: Tuition, area resident:* Full-time $12,240; part-time $680 per credit hour. Tuition and fees vary according to degree level and program. *Financial support:* Fellowships, research assistantships, Federal Work-Study, scholarships/grants, and unspecified assistantships available. Support available to part-time students. Financial award applicants required to submit FAFSA. *Unit head:* Dr. Theresa Hand, Dean, School of Health Sciences, 518-244-2264, Fax: 518-244-4571, E-mail: handt@sage.edu. *Application contact:* Rayane AbuSabha, Program Director, Nutrition, 518-935-3214, E-mail: abusar@sage.edu.

Saint Louis University, Graduate Education, Doisy College of Health Sciences and Graduate Education, Department of Nutrition and Dietetics, St. Louis, MO 63103. Offers medical dietetics (MS); nutrition and physical performance (MS). *Program availability:* Part-time. *Degree requirements:* For master's, comprehensive exam (for some programs). *Entrance requirements:* For master's, GRE General Test, letters of recommendation, resume, interview. Additional exam requirements/recommendations for international students: Required—TOEFL (minimum score 525 paper-based). Electronic applications accepted. *Faculty research:* Sustainable food systems, nutrition education, public health nutrition, culinary nutrition and physical performance.

See Display below and Close-Up on page 387.

Sam Houston State University, College of Health Sciences, Department of Family and Consumer Sciences, Huntsville, TX 77341. Offers dietetics (MS); family and consumer sciences (MS). *Program availability:* Part-time, evening/weekend. *Degree requirements:* For master's, comprehensive exam, thesis optional, internship. *Entrance requirements:* For master's, GRE General Test, letters of recommendation, personal statement, writing sample. Additional exam requirements/recommendations for international students: Required—TOEFL (minimum score 550 paper-based; 79 iBT), IELTS (minimum score 6.5). Electronic applications accepted.

San Diego State University, Graduate and Research Affairs, College of Health and Human Services, School of Exercise and Nutritional Sciences, Program in Nutritional Sciences, San Diego, CA 92182. Offers MS, MS/MS. *Degree requirements:* For master's, thesis. *Entrance requirements:* For master's, GRE General Test, 2 letters of reference. Additional exam requirements/recommendations for international students: Required—TOEFL. Electronic applications accepted.

San Jose State University, Graduate Studies and Research, College of Applied Sciences and Arts, San Jose, CA 95192-0001. Offers big data (Certificate); California library media teacher services (Credential); collaborative response to family violence (Certificate); justice studies (MS); kinesiology (MA), including applied sciences and arts (MA, MS), athletic training, exercise physiology, sport management, sport studies; library and information science (MLIS, Certificate); mass communication (MA); master of social work (MSW); nutritional science (MS); occupational therapy (MS); public health (MPH); pupil personnel services (Credential); recreation (MS), including applied sciences and arts (MA, MS), international tourism; Spanish language counseling (Certificate); strategic management of digital assets and services (Certificate). *Program availability:* Part-time, evening/weekend. *Students:* 219 full-time (155 women), 140 part-time (103 women); includes 472 minority (38 Black or African American, non-Hispanic/Latino; 2 American Indian or Alaska Native, non-Hispanic/Latino; 190 Asian, non-Hispanic/Latino; 238 Hispanic/Latino; 4 Native Hawaiian or other Pacific Islander, non-Hispanic/Latino), 28 international. Average age 31. 1,404 applicants, 37% accepted, 360 enrolled. In 2015, 850 master's awarded. *Application deadline:* For fall admission, 6/29 for domestic students; for spring admission, 11/30 for domestic students. Applications are processed on a rolling basis. Application fee: $55. Electronic applications accepted. *Financial support:* Career-related internships or fieldwork, Federal Work-Study, institutionally sponsored loans, and scholarships/grants available. Support available to part-time students. Financial award application deadline: 6/15; financial award applicants required to submit FAFSA. *Unit head:* Dr. Mary Schutten, Dean, 408-924-2900, Fax: 408-924-2901, E-mail: mary.schutten@sjsu.edu. *Application contact:* 408-924-2480, Fax: 408-924-2477.
Website: http://www.sjsu.edu/casa/

Saybrook University, School of Mind-Body Medicine, San Francisco, CA 94111-1920. Offers MS, PhD, Certificate. *Entrance requirements:* Additional exam requirements/recommendations for international students: Required—TOEFL (minimum score 580 paper-based; 93 iBT). Electronic applications accepted.

Simmons College, School of Nursing and Health Sciences, Boston, MA 02115. Offers didactic dietetics (Certificate); dietetic internship (Certificate); health education profession (PhD); health professions education (CAGS); nursing (MS), including family nurse practitioner; nursing practice (DNP); nutrition and health promotion (MS); physical therapy (DPT); sports nutrition (Certificate). *Program availability:* Part-time, blended/hybrid learning. *Faculty:* 21 full-time (17 women), 171 part-time/adjunct (157 women). *Students:* 333 full-time (305 women), 889 part-time (813 women); includes 250 minority (88 Black or African American, non-Hispanic/Latino; 3 American Indian or Alaska Native, non-Hispanic/Latino; 65 Asian, non-Hispanic/Latino; 67 Hispanic/Latino; 2 Native Hawaiian or other Pacific Islander, non-Hispanic/Latino; 25 Two or more races, non-Hispanic/Latino), 9 international. Average age 33. 846 applicants, 66% accepted, 441 enrolled. In 2015, 70 master's, 45 doctorates awarded. *Entrance requirements:* For doctorate, GRE. Additional exam requirements/recommendations for international students: Required—TOEFL (minimum score 570 paper-based; 88 iBT). *Application deadline:* For fall admission, 6/1 for international students. Application fee: $50. Electronic applications accepted. *Expenses:* Contact institution. *Financial support:* In 2015–16, 12 research assistantships (averaging $6,000 per year) were awarded; scholarships/grants and unspecified assistantships also available. *Unit head:* Dr. Judy Beal, Dean, 617-521-2139. *Application contact:* Brett DiMarzo, Director of Graduate Admission, 617-521-2651, Fax: 617-521-3137, E-mail: brett.dimarzo@simmons.edu. Website: http://www.simmons.edu/snhs/

South Carolina State University, College of Graduate and Professional Studies, Department of Family and Consumer Sciences, Orangeburg, SC 29117-0001. Offers individual and family development (MS); nutritional sciences (MS). *Program availability:* Part-time, evening/weekend. *Faculty:* 4 full-time (all women). *Students:* 3 full-time (2 women), 10 part-time (all women); all minorities (all Black or African American, non-Hispanic/Latino). Average age 31. 6 applicants, 83% accepted, 2 enrolled. *Degree requirements:* For master's, comprehensive exam, thesis optional, departmental qualifying exam. *Entrance requirements:* For master's, GRE, MAT, or NTE, minimum GPA of 2.7. *Application deadline:* For fall admission, 6/15 priority date for domestic students, 6/15 for international students; for spring admission, 11/1 for domestic and international students. Applications are processed on a rolling basis. Application fee: $25. Electronic applications accepted. *Expenses:* Tuition, state resident: full-time $8906; part-time $495 per credit hour. Tuition, nonresident: full-time $18,674; part-time $1037 per credit hour. *Required fees:* $2497; $66 per credit hour. *Financial support:* Fellowships, Federal Work-Study, and scholarships/grants available. Financial award application deadline: 6/1. *Unit head:* Dr. Ethel G. Jones, Chair, Department of Family and Consumer Sciences, 803-536-8958, Fax: 803-533-3268, E-mail: egjones@scsu.edu. *Application contact:* Curtis Foskey, Coordinator of Graduate Admission, 803-536-8419, Fax: 803-536-8812, E-mail: cfoskey@scsu.edu.

South Dakota State University, Graduate School, College of Education and Human Sciences, Department of Health and Nutritional Sciences, Brookings, SD 57007. Offers athletic training (MS); dietetics (MS); nutrition and exercise sciences (MS, PhD); sport and recreation studies (MS). *Program availability:* Part-time. *Degree requirements:* For master's, comprehensive exam (for some programs), thesis (for some programs), oral exam. *Entrance requirements:* Additional exam requirements/recommendations for international students: Required—TOEFL (minimum score 525 paper-based). *Faculty research:* Food chemistry, bone density, functional food, nutrition education, nutrition biochemistry.

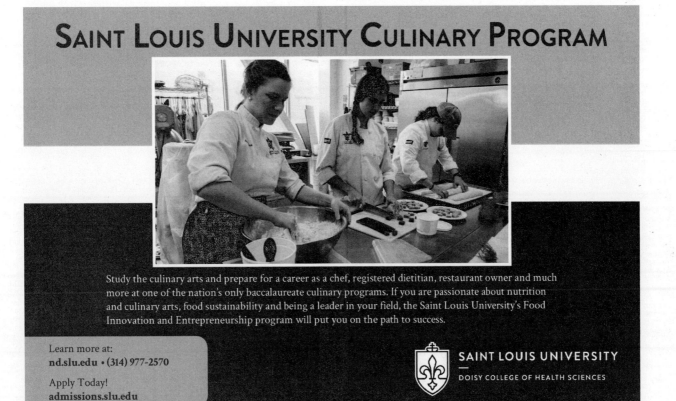

Nutrition

Southeast Missouri State University, School of Graduate Studies, Department of Health, Human Performance and Recreation, Cape Girardeau, MO 63701-4799. Offers nutrition and exercise science (MS). *Program availability:* Part-time. *Faculty:* 8 full-time (2 women), 2 part-time/adjunct (1 woman). *Students:* 22 full-time (11 women), 17 part-time (12 women); includes 2 minority (1 Black or African American, non-Hispanic/Latino; 1 Hispanic/Latino), 20 international. Average age 25. 22 applicants, 82% accepted, 15 enrolled. In 2015, 7 master's awarded. *Degree requirements:* For master's, comprehensive exam, thesis optional. *Entrance requirements:* For master's, GRE General Test (minimum combined score of 950). Additional exam requirements/recommendations for international students: Required—TOEFL (minimum score 550 paper-based; 79 iBT), IELTS (minimum score 6), PTE (minimum score 53). *Application deadline:* For fall admission, 8/1 for domestic students, 5/1 for international students; for spring admission, 11/21 for domestic students, 10/1 for international students; for summer admission, 5/15 for domestic students. Applications are processed on a rolling basis. Application fee: $30 ($40 for international students). Electronic applications accepted. *Expenses:* Tuition, state resident: part-time $260.80 per credit hour. Tuition, nonresident: part-time $486.80 per credit hour. *Required fees:* $33.70 per credit hour. *Financial support:* In 2015–16, 19 students received support, including 5 teaching assistantships with full tuition reimbursements available (averaging $8,467 per year); career-related internships or fieldwork, Federal Work-Study, scholarships/grants, traineeships, tuition waivers (full), and unspecified assistantships also available. Financial award application deadline: 6/30; financial award applicants required to submit FAFSA. *Faculty research:* Body composition assessment techniques, serum lipid adaptations with physical activity in smokers, professional attitudes of pre-service teachers, high intensity training with clinical populations. *Unit head:* Dr. Joe Pujol, Professor and Chairperson, 573-651-2664, Fax: 573-651-5150, E-mail: jpujol@semo.edu. *Application contact:* Dr. Jeremy Barnes, Professor/Graduate Coordinator, 573-651-2197, Fax: 573-651-5150, E-mail: jbarnes@semo.edu.
Website: http://www.semo.edu/health/

Southern Illinois University Carbondale, Graduate School, College of Agriculture, Department of Animal Science, Food and Nutrition, Program in Food and Nutrition, Carbondale, IL 62901-4701. Offers MS. *Faculty:* 12 full-time (4 women). *Students:* 17 full-time (13 women), 6 part-time (5 women); includes 2 minority (both Black or African American, non-Hispanic/Latino), 3 international. Average age 29. 28 applicants, 29% accepted, 8 enrolled. In 2015, 9 master's awarded. *Degree requirements:* For master's, thesis or alternative. *Entrance requirements:* For master's, GRE, minimum GPA of 2.7. Additional exam requirements/recommendations for international students: Required—TOEFL (minimum score 550 paper-based; 80 iBT). *Application deadline:* For fall admission, 1/1 for domestic students. Application fee: $65. Electronic applications accepted. *Financial support:* In 2015–16, 12 students received support, including 1 fellowship with full tuition reimbursement available, 3 research assistantships with full tuition reimbursements available, 8 teaching assistantships with full tuition reimbursements available; career-related internships or fieldwork, Federal Work-Study, institutionally sponsored loans, and tuition waivers (full) also available. Support available to part-time students. *Faculty research:* Public health nutrition, nutrition physiology, soybean utilization, nutrition education. *Unit head:* Dr. William Banz, Chair, 618-453-1763, E-mail: banz@siu.edu. *Application contact:* Terry Richardson, Office Support Specialist, 618-453-1762, E-mail: cerebus@siu.edu.
Website: http://coas.siu.edu/academics/departments/animal-science-food-nutrition/index.html

State University of New York College at Oneonta, Graduate Education, Department of Human Ecology, Oneonta, NY 13820-4015. Offers nutrition and dietetics (MS). *Program availability:* Online learning.

Stony Brook University, State University of New York, Stony Brook Medicine, School of Medicine and Graduate School, Graduate Programs in Medicine, Department of Family Medicine, Stony Brook, NY 11794. Offers nutrition (MS, Advanced Certificate). *Program availability:* Online learning. *Faculty:* 15 full-time (6 women), 6 part-time/adjunct (3 women). *Students:* 4 full-time (all women), 56 part-time (51 women); includes 6 minority (4 Asian, non-Hispanic/Latino; 1 Hispanic/Latino; 1 Two or more races, non-Hispanic/Latino), 1 international. Average age 29. 59 applicants, 66% accepted, 29 enrolled. In 2015, 2 master's, 1 other advanced degree awarded. *Entrance requirements:* For master's, baccalaureate degree with minimum preferred GPA of 3.0; physiology (laboratory not required) and statistics; for Advanced Certificate, physiology (laboratory not required). Additional exam requirements/recommendations for international students: Required—TOEFL. *Application deadline:* For fall admission, 7/1 for domestic students; for winter admission, 7/1 for domestic students; for spring admission, 12/1 for domestic students; for summer admission, 4/1 for domestic students. Application fee: $100. Electronic applications accepted. *Expenses:* $12,421 per year full-time resident tuition and fees; $453 per credit hour; $23,761 per year full-time out-of-state tuition and fees; $925 per credit hour. *Faculty research:* Family medicine, health of underserved populations, medical education, minority health, obstetrics or gynecology. *Total annual research expenditures:* $1.1 million. *Unit head:* Dr. Josephine Connolly-Schoonen, Executive Director, 631-444-2132, E-mail: josephine.connolly-schoonen@stonybrookmedicine.edu. *Application contact:* Sharon Schmidt, Staff Associate, 631-638-2132, E-mail: sharon.schmidt@stonybrookmedicine.edu.
Website: http://medicine.stonybrookmedicine.edu/gradnutrition

Syracuse University, David B. Falk College of Sport and Human Dynamics, Programs in Nutrition Science, Syracuse, NY 13244. Offers MA, MS. *Accreditation:* AND. *Program availability:* Part-time. *Students:* Average age 28. In 2015, 17 degrees awarded. *Degree requirements:* For master's, comprehensive exam, thesis. *Entrance requirements:* For master's, GRE General Test, personal statement, resume, official transcripts, three letters of recommendation. Additional exam requirements/recommendations for international students: Required—TOEFL (minimum score 100 iBT). *Application deadline:* For fall admission, 2/15 priority date for domestic and international students; for spring admission, 11/1 priority date for domestic and international students. Application fee: $75. Electronic applications accepted. *Expenses:* Tuition, area resident: Full-time $25,974; part-time $1443 per credit hour. *Required fees:* $802; $50 per course. Tuition and fees vary according to course load and program. *Financial support:* Fellowships with full tuition reimbursements, research assistantships with tuition reimbursements, teaching assistantships with tuition reimbursements, career-related internships or fieldwork, and tuition waivers available. Financial award application deadline: 1/1; financial award applicants required to submit FAFSA. *Faculty research:* Vegetarianism, cultural food practices, consequences of global nutrition transition, food and agricultural policy. *Unit head:* Dr. Sudha Raj, Program Director, 315-443-2556, E-mail: sraj@syr.edu. *Application contact:* Felicia Otero, Information Contact, 315-443-5555, E-mail: falk@syr.edu.
Website: http://falk.syr.edu/NutritionScienceDietetics/Default.aspx

Teachers College, Columbia University, Department of Health and Behavior Studies, New York, NY 10027-6696. Offers applied behavior analysis (MA, PhD); applied educational psychology: school psychology (Ed M, PhD); behavioral nutrition (PhD), including nutrition (Ed D, PhD); community health education (MS); community nutrition education (Ed M), including community nutrition education; education of deaf and hard

of hearing (MA, PhD); health education (MA, Ed D); hearing impairment (Ed D); intellectual disability/autism (MA, Ed D, PhD); nursing education (Advanced Certificate); nutrition and education (MS); nutrition and exercise physiology (MS); nutrition and public health (MS); nutrition education (Ed D), including nutrition (Ed D, PhD); physical disabilities (Ed D); reading specialist (MA); severe or multiple disabilities (MA); special education (Ed M, MA, Ed D); teaching of sign language (MA). *Program availability:* Part-time, evening/weekend. *Students:* 186 full-time (168 women), 362 part-time (319 women); includes 199 minority (50 Black or African American, non-Hispanic/Latino; 1 American Indian or Alaska Native, non-Hispanic/Latino; 73 Asian, non-Hispanic/Latino; 59 Hispanic/Latino; 1 Native Hawaiian or other Pacific Islander, non-Hispanic/Latino; 15 Two or more races, non-Hispanic/Latino), 13 international. Terminal master's awarded for partial completion of doctoral program. *Expenses: Tuition, area resident:* Part-time $1454 per credit. *Required fees:* $428 per semester. One-time fee: $475 full-time. Full-time tuition and fees vary according to course load. *Unit head:* Prof. Stephen T. Peverly, Chair, 212-678-3964, Fax: 212-678-8259, E-mail: stp4@columbia.edu. *Application contact:* David Estrella, Director of Admission, 212-678-3305, E-mail: estrella@tc.columbia.edu.
Website: http://www.tc.columbia.edu/health-and-behavior-studies/

Texas A&M University, College of Agriculture and Life Sciences, Department of Nutrition and Food Science, College Station, TX 77843. Offers food science and technology (M Agr); nutrition (MS, PhD). *Students:* 56 full-time (42 women), 10 part-time (5 women); includes 11 minority (3 Asian, non-Hispanic/Latino; 7 Hispanic/Latino; 1 Two or more races, non-Hispanic/Latino), 17 international. Average age 27. 149 applicants, 13% accepted, 13 enrolled. In 2015, 12 master's, 1 doctorate awarded. *Degree requirements:* For master's, thesis; for doctorate, thesis/dissertation. *Entrance requirements:* For master's and doctorate, GRE General Test. Additional exam requirements/recommendations for international students: Required—TOEFL (minimum score 550 paper-based; 80 iBT), IELTS (minimum score 6), PTE (minimum score 53). *Application deadline:* For fall admission, 12/1 priority date for domestic students, 12/1 for international students; for spring admission, 8/1 for domestic and international students; for summer admission, 12/1 priority date for domestic students, 12/1 for international students. Applications are processed on a rolling basis. Application fee: $50 ($90 for international students). Electronic applications accepted. *Expenses:* Contact institution. *Financial support:* In 2015–16, 56 students received support, including 5 fellowships with tuition reimbursements available (averaging $6,964 per year), 21 research assistantships with tuition reimbursements available (averaging $5,592 per year), 16 teaching assistantships with tuition reimbursements available (averaging $5,260 per year); career-related internships or fieldwork, institutionally sponsored loans, scholarships/grants, traineeships, health care benefits, tuition waivers (full and partial), and unspecified assistantships also available. Support available to part-time students. Financial award application deadline: 3/15; financial award applicants required to submit FAFSA. *Faculty research:* Food safety, microbiology, product development. *Unit head:* Dr. Boon Chew, Department Head, 979-862-6655, E-mail: boon.chew@tamu.edu. *Application contact:* Graduate Admissions, 979-845-1044, E-mail: admissions@tamu.edu.
Website: http://nfs.tamu.edu

Texas State University, The Graduate College, College of Applied Arts, School of Family and Consumer Sciences, San Marcos, TX 78666. Offers family and child studies (MS); human nutrition (MS); merchandising and consumer studies (MS). *Program availability:* Part-time. *Faculty:* 18 full-time (14 women), 5 part-time/adjunct (all women). *Students:* 87 full-time (76 women), 46 part-time (37 women); includes 38 minority (6 Black or African American, non-Hispanic/Latino; 3 Asian, non-Hispanic/Latino; 21 Hispanic/Latino; 8 Two or more races, non-Hispanic/Latino), 12 international. Average age 27. 119 applicants, 57% accepted, 43 enrolled. In 2015, 47 master's awarded. *Degree requirements:* For master's, comprehensive exam, thesis (for some programs). *Entrance requirements:* For master's, GRE General Test (preferred), baccalaureate degree from regionally-accredited institution with minimum GPA of 3.0 in last 60 hours of course work. Additional exam requirements/recommendations for international students: Required—TOEFL (minimum score 550 paper-based; 78 iBT). *Application deadline:* For fall admission, 3/1 priority date for domestic students, 3/1 for international students; for spring admission, 10/15 priority date for domestic students, 10/1 for international students. Applications are processed on a rolling basis. Application fee: $40 ($90 for international students). Electronic applications accepted. *Expenses:* $3,615 in-state tuition (for 12 semester credit hour/1 full-time semester), $974 in-state fees. *Financial support:* In 2015–16, 54 students received support, including 21 research assistantships (averaging $11,981 per year), 20 teaching assistantships (averaging $12,253 per year). Financial award application deadline: 4/1; financial award applicants required to submit FAFSA. *Faculty research:* Investigating use of mobile technology for nutrition and breastfeeding education, WIC mobile App data analysis, influence of prosynbiotic on cardiometabolic in the obese, Mexican origin student success, academic identity and its role in predicting postsecondary achievement. *Total annual research expenditures:* $174,517. *Unit head:* Dr. Rodney C. Runyan, Director, 512-245-2155, Fax: 512-245-3829, E-mail: rcr56@txstate.edu. *Application contact:* Dr. Andrea Golato, Dean of the Graduate College, 512-245-2581, Fax: 512-245-8365, E-mail: gradcollege@txstate.edu.
Website: http://www.fcs.txstate.edu/

Texas Tech University, Graduate School, College of Human Sciences, Department of Nutritional Sciences, Lubbock, TX 79409. Offers MS, PhD. *Program availability:* Part-time, online learning. *Faculty:* 17 full-time (11 women), 4 part-time/adjunct (all women). *Students:* 62 full-time (47 women), 9 part-time (all women); includes 7 minority (1 Black or African American, non-Hispanic/Latino; 1 Asian, non-Hispanic/Latino; 3 Hispanic/Latino; 2 Two or more races, non-Hispanic/Latino), 26 international. Average age 27. 54 applicants, 63% accepted, 29 enrolled. In 2015, 15 master's, 6 doctorates awarded. Terminal master's awarded for partial completion of doctoral program. *Degree requirements:* For master's, comprehensive exam (for some programs), thesis (for some programs); for doctorate, thesis/dissertation, qualifying exams. *Entrance requirements:* For master's, GRE, minimum undergraduate cumulative GPA of 3.0; for doctorate, GRE, minimum undergraduate or graduate cumulative GPA of 3.0. Additional exam requirements/recommendations for international students: Required—TOEFL (minimum score 550 paper-based, 79 iBT) or IELTS (6.5). *Application deadline:* For fall admission, 6/1 priority date for domestic students, 1/15 priority date for international students; for spring admission, 9/1 priority date for domestic students, 6/15 priority date for international students. Applications are processed on a rolling basis. Application fee: $60. Electronic applications accepted. *Expenses:* Tuition, state resident: full-time $6477; part-time $269.89 per credit hour. Tuition, nonresident: full-time $15,837; part-time $659.89 per credit hour. *Required fees:* $2751; $36.50 per credit hour. $937.50 per semester. Tuition and fees vary according to course level. *Financial support:* In 2015–16, 63 students received support, including 59 fellowships (averaging $5,176 per year), 24 research assistantships (averaging $9,839 per year), 22 teaching assistantships (averaging $10,902 per year); Federal Work-Study, scholarships/grants, and unspecified assistantships also available. Financial award application deadline: 1/15; financial award applicants required to submit FAFSA. *Faculty research:* Obesity and chronic diseases, clinical and cellular lipid metabolism, community nutrition education, domestic and international food security. *Total annual research expenditures:* $371,255.

Unit head: Dr. Nikhil Dhurandhar, Chair, 806-742-5270, Fax: 806-742-2926, E-mail: nikhil.dhurandhar@ttu.edu. *Application contact:* Dr. Debra Reed, Graduate Program Director, 806-834-6629, Fax: 806-742-2926, E-mail: debra.reed@ttu.edu.
Website: http://www.depts.ttu.edu/hs/ns/

Texas Woman's University, Graduate School, College of Health Sciences, Department of Nutrition and Food Sciences, Program in Exercise and Sports Nutrition, Denton, TX 76201. Offers MS. *Program availability:* Part-time. *Degree requirements:* For master's, comprehensive exam, thesis optional. *Entrance requirements:* For master's, GRE General Test (preferred minimum score 153 [500 old version] Verbal, 140 [400 old version] Quantitative), 9 hours each of chemistry, nutrition, and kinesiology; 3 hours of human physiology; minimum GPA of 3.0 in last 60 hours; resume; 2 letters of recommendation. Additional exam requirements/recommendations for international students: Required—TOEFL (minimum score 550 paper-based; 79 iBT). *Application deadline:* For fall admission, 6/15 for domestic students; for spring admission, 10/1 for domestic students; for summer admission, 4/1 for domestic students. Applications are processed on a rolling basis. Application fee: $50 ($75 for international students). Electronic applications accepted. *Expenses:* Tuition, state resident: full-time $4380; part-time $243 per credit hour. Tuition, nonresident: full-time $11,400; part-time $633 per credit hour. *International tuition:* $11,465 full-time. *Required fees:* $1778; $99 per credit hour. $283 per semester. One-time fee: $50. Tuition and fees vary according to course load and program. *Financial support:* Research assistantships, teaching assistantships, career-related internships or fieldwork, Federal Work-Study, institutionally sponsored loans, scholarships/grants, traineeships, health care benefits, and unspecified assistantships available. Support available to part-time students. Financial award application deadline: 3/1; financial award applicants required to submit FAFSA. *Faculty research:* Metabolism of lipoproteins, bone metabolism, osteoporosis, adult and childhood obesity. *Unit head:* Dr. Nancy DiMarco, Director, 940-898-2785, Fax: 940-898-2634, E-mail: nutrfdsci@twu.edu. *Application contact:* Dr. Samuel Wheeler, Assistant Director of Admissions, 940-898-3188, Fax: 940-898-3081, E-mail: wheelersr@twu.edu.
Website: http://www.twu.edu/nutrition-food-sciences/

Tufts University, The Gerald J. and Dorothy R. Friedman School of Nutrition Science and Policy, Boston, MA 02111. Offers agriculture, food and environment (MS, PhD); biochemical and molecular nutrition (PhD); dietetic internship (MS); food policy and applied nutrition (MS, PhD); humanitarian assistance (MAHA); nutrition (MS, PhD); nutrition communication (MS); nutritional epidemiology (MS, PhD). *Program availability:* Part-time. *Degree requirements:* For doctorate, comprehensive exam, thesis/ dissertation. *Entrance requirements:* For master's and doctorate, GRE General Test. Additional exam requirements/recommendations for international students: Required— TOEFL. Electronic applications accepted. *Expenses:* Contact institution. *Faculty research:* Nutritional biochemistry and metabolism, cell and molecular biochemistry, epidemiology, policy/planning, applied nutrition.

Tufts University, School of Medicine, Public Health and Professional Degree Programs, Boston, MA 02111. Offers biomedical sciences (MS); health communication (MS, Certificate); pain research, education and policy (MS, Certificate); physician assistant (MS); public health (MPH, Dr PH), including behavioral science (MPH), biostatistics (MPH), epidemiology (MPH), health communication (MPH), health services (MPH), management and policy (MPH), nutrition (MPH); DMD/MPH; DVM/MPH; JD/ MPH; MD/MPH; MMS/MPH; MS/MBA; MS/MPH. MS programs offered jointly with Emerson College. *Accreditation:* CEPH (one or more programs are accredited). *Program availability:* Part-time, evening/weekend. *Faculty:* 78 full-time (29 women), 42 part-time/adjunct (20 women). *Students:* 457 full-time (266 women), 61 part-time (46 women); includes 187 minority (21 Black or African American, non-Hispanic/Latino; 107 Asian, non-Hispanic/Latino; 37 Hispanic/Latino; 22 Two or more races, non-Hispanic/ Latino), 24 international. Average age 27. 1,599 applicants, 48% accepted, 222 enrolled. In 2015, 219 master's awarded. *Degree requirements:* For master's, thesis (for some programs); for doctorate, thesis/dissertation. *Entrance requirements:* For master's, GRE General Test, MCAT, or GMAT; for doctorate, GRE General Test or MCAT. Additional exam requirements/recommendations for international students: Required—TOEFL (minimum score 100 iBT). *Application deadline:* For fall admission, 1/15 priority date for domestic students, 12/15 priority date for international students; for spring admission, 10/25 priority date for domestic and international students. Applications are processed on a rolling basis. Application fee: $70. Electronic applications accepted. *Expenses:* Contact institution. *Financial support:* In 2015–16, 12 students received support, including 1 fellowship (averaging $3,000 per year), 50 research assistantships (averaging $1,000 per year), 65 teaching assistantships (averaging $2,000 per year); Federal Work-Study and scholarships/grants also available. Support available to part-time students. Financial award application deadline: 2/19; financial award applicants required to submit FAFSA. *Faculty research:* Environmental and occupational health, nutrition, epidemiology, health communication, biostatics, obesity/chronic disease, health policy and health care delivery, global health, health inequality and social determinants of health. *Unit head:* Dr. Aviva Must, Dean, 617-636-0935, Fax: 617-636-0898, E-mail: aviva.must@tufts.edu. *Application contact:* Emily Keily, Director of Admissions, 617-636-0935, Fax: 617-636-0898, E-mail: med-phpd@tufts.edu.
Website: http://publichealth.tufts.edu

Tuskegee University, Graduate Programs, College of Agriculture, Environment and Nutrition Sciences, Department of Food and Nutritional Sciences, Tuskegee, AL 36088. Offers MS. *Degree requirements:* For master's, thesis. *Entrance requirements:* For master's, GRE General Test. Additional exam requirements/recommendations for international students: Required—TOEFL (minimum score 500 paper-based).

Université de Moncton, School of Food Science, Nutrition and Family Studies, Moncton, NB E1A 3E9, Canada. Offers foods/nutrition (M Sc). *Program availability:* Part-time. *Degree requirements:* For master's, one foreign language, thesis. *Entrance requirements:* For master's, previous course work in statistics. Electronic applications accepted. *Faculty research:* Clinic nutrition (anemia, elderly, osteoporosis), applied nutrition, metabolic activities of lactic bacteria, solubility of low density lipoproteins, bile acids.

Université de Montréal, Faculty of Medicine, Department of Nutrition, Montréal, QC H3C 3J7, Canada. Offers M Sc, PhD, DESS. Terminal master's awarded for partial completion of doctoral program. *Degree requirements:* For master's, thesis; for doctorate, thesis/dissertation, general exam. *Entrance requirements:* For master's, MD, B Sc in nutrition or equivalent, proficiency in French; for doctorate, M Sc in nutrition or equivalent, proficiency in French. Electronic applications accepted. *Faculty research:* Nutritional aspects of diabetes, obesity, anorexia nervosa, lipid metabolism, hepatic function.

Université Laval, Faculty of Agricultural and Food Sciences, Department of Food Sciences and Nutrition, Programs in Nutrition, Québec, QC G1K 7P4, Canada. Offers M Sc, PhD. Terminal master's awarded for partial completion of doctoral program. *Degree requirements:* For master's, thesis; for doctorate, comprehensive exam, thesis/ dissertation. *Entrance requirements:* For master's and doctorate, knowledge of French and English. Electronic applications accepted.

University at Buffalo, the State University of New York, Graduate School, School of Public Health and Health Professions, Department of Exercise and Nutrition Sciences, Buffalo, NY 14260. Offers exercise science (MS, PhD); nutrition (MS, Advanced Certificate). *Program availability:* Part-time. *Faculty:* 16 full-time (6 women), 6 part-time/ adjunct (3 women). *Students:* 76 full-time (52 women), 6 part-time (5 women); includes 3 minority (all Asian, non-Hispanic/Latino), 15 international. Average age 24. 123 applicants, 58% accepted, 52 enrolled. In 2015, 31 master's, 1 doctorate, 18 other advanced degrees awarded. *Degree requirements:* For master's, comprehensive exam or thesis; for doctorate, comprehensive exam, thesis/dissertation. *Entrance requirements:* For master's, doctorate, and Advanced Certificate, GRE General Test, minimum GPA of 3.0. Additional exam requirements/recommendations for international students: Required—TOEFL (minimum score 550 paper-based; 79 iBT), IELTS (minimum score 6.5). *Application deadline:* For fall admission, 4/1 for domestic students, 3/1 for international students; for spring admission, 8/15 for international students. Applications are processed on a rolling basis. Application fee: $50. Electronic applications accepted. *Financial support:* In 2015–16, 14 students received support, including 1 research assistantship with full tuition reimbursement available (averaging $15,000 per year), 11 teaching assistantships with tuition reimbursements available (averaging $6,980 per year); tuition waivers (full) and Fulbright scholarship also available. Financial award application deadline: 3/15; financial award applicants required to submit FAFSA. *Faculty research:* Cardiovascular disease-diet and exercise, respiratory control and muscle function, plasticity of connective and neural tissue, exercise nutrition, diet and cancer. *Unit head:* Dr. David Hostler, Chair, 716-829-6756, Fax: 716-829-2428, E-mail: dhostler@buffalo.edu. *Application contact:* Dr. Jennifer Temple, Director of Graduate Studies, 716-829-5593, Fax: 716-829-2428, E-mail: jltemple@buffalo.edu.
Website: http://sphhp.buffalo.edu/exercise-and-nutrition-sciences.html

The University of Alabama, Graduate School, College of Human Environmental Sciences, Department of Human Nutrition and Hospitality Management, Tuscaloosa, AL 35487. Offers MSHES. *Program availability:* Part-time, online only, 100% online. *Faculty:* 13 full-time (11 women), 1 (woman) part-time/adjunct. *Students:* 20 full-time (all women), 85 part-time (82 women); includes 6 minority (2 Black or African American, non-Hispanic/Latino; 5 Hispanic/Latino; 2 Two or more races, non-Hispanic/Latino), 1 international. Average age 31. 65 applicants, 65% accepted, 30 enrolled. In 2015, 36 master's awarded. *Degree requirements:* For master's, comprehensive exam, thesis optional. *Entrance requirements:* For master's, minimum GPA of 3.0. Additional exam requirements/recommendations for international students: Required—TOEFL, IELTS. *Application deadline:* For fall admission, 6/1 for domestic students; for spring admission, 11/1 for domestic students; for summer admission, 4/1 for domestic students. Applications are processed on a rolling basis. Application fee: $50 ($60 for international students). Electronic applications accepted. *Expenses:* Tuition, state resident: full-time $10,170. Tuition, nonresident: full-time $25,950. *Financial support:* In 2015–16, 4 students received support, including 2 research assistantships (averaging $8,100 per year), 4 teaching assistantships (averaging $8,100 per year); career-related internships or fieldwork also available. Financial award application deadline: 3/15. *Faculty research:* Maternal and child nutrition, childhood obesity, community nutrition interventions, geriatric nutrition, family eating patterns, food chemistry, phytochemicals, dietary antioxidants. *Unit head:* Dr. Jeannine C. Lawrence, Chair/Associate Professor, 205-348-6252, Fax: 205-348-2982, E-mail: jlawrence@ches.ua.edu. *Application contact:* Patrick D. Fuller, Admissions Officer, 205-348-5923, Fax: 205-348-0400, E-mail: patrick.d.fuller@ua.edu.
Website: http://www.nhm.ches.ua.edu/

The University of Alabama at Birmingham, School of Health Professions, Program in Nutrition Sciences, Birmingham, AL 35294. Offers MS, PhD. Terminal master's awarded for partial completion of doctoral program. *Degree requirements:* For master's, thesis optional; for doctorate, thesis/dissertation. *Entrance requirements:* For master's, GRE or MAT, letters of recommendation; for doctorate, GRE. Additional exam requirements/ recommendations for international students: Required—TOEFL. *Expenses:* Tuition, state resident: full-time $7340. Tuition, nonresident: full-time $16,628. Full-time tuition and fees vary according to course load and program. *Faculty research:* Energy metabolism, obesity, body composition, cancer prevention, bone metabolism, diabetes.

The University of Arizona, College of Agriculture and Life Sciences, Department of Nutritional Sciences, Tucson, AZ 85721. Offers MS, PhD. *Entrance requirements:* For master's, GRE, minimum GPA of 3.0, 2 letters of recommendation; for doctorate, GRE, minimum GPA of 3.0, 2 letters of recommendation, statement of purpose. Additional exam requirements/recommendations for international students: Required—TOEFL (minimum score 550 paper-based; 79 iBT). *Application deadline:* For fall admission, 12/ 15 for domestic and international students. Applications are processed on a rolling basis. Application fee: $75. Electronic applications accepted. *Financial support:* Fellowships, research assistantships, teaching assistantships, scholarships/grants, health care benefits, tuition waivers (full and partial), and unspecified assistantships available. *Faculty research:* Bioactive compounds, nutrients and lifestyle: relationships to cancer; metabolic and behavior factors Influencing body composition; diabetes, obesity, musculoskeletal and cardiovascular diseases. *Unit head:* Dr. Scott Going, Department Head, E-mail: going@email.arizona.edu.

University of Arkansas for Medical Sciences, Graduate School, Little Rock, AR 72205. Offers biochemistry and molecular biology (MS, PhD); bioinformatics (MS, PhD); cellular physiology and molecular biophysics (MS, PhD); clinical nutrition (MS); interdisciplinary biomedical sciences (MS, PhD, Certificate); interdisciplinary toxicology (MS); microbiology and immunology (PhD); neurobiology and developmental sciences (PhD); pharmacology (PhD); MD/PhD. Bioinformatics programs hosted jointly with the University of Arkansas at Little Rock. *Program availability:* Part-time. Terminal master's awarded for partial completion of doctoral program. *Degree requirements:* For master's, comprehensive exam (for some programs), thesis (for some programs); for doctorate, thesis/dissertation. *Entrance requirements:* For master's and doctorate, GRE. Additional exam requirements/recommendations for international students: Required—TOEFL. Electronic applications accepted. *Expenses:* Contact institution.

University of Bridgeport, Nutrition Institute, Bridgeport, CT 06604. Offers human nutrition (MS). *Program availability:* Part-time, evening/weekend, online learning. *Degree requirements:* For master's, thesis, research project. *Entrance requirements:* For master's, previous course work in anatomy, biochemistry, organic chemistry, or physiology. Additional exam requirements/recommendations for international students: Recommended—TOEFL (minimum score 550 paper-based; 80 iBT), IELTS (minimum score 6.5). *Application deadline:* For fall admission, 8/1 priority date for domestic and international students; for spring admission, 12/1 priority date for domestic and international students. Applications are processed on a rolling basis. Application fee: $50. Electronic applications accepted. *Expenses:* Contact institution. *Financial support:* Available to part-time students. Application deadline: 6/1; applicants required to submit FAFSA.

The University of British Columbia, Faculty of Land and Food Systems, Human Nutrition Program, Vancouver, BC V6T 1Z1, Canada. Offers M Sc, PhD. *Program availability:* Part-time. Terminal master's awarded for partial completion of doctoral program. *Degree requirements:* For master's, thesis; for doctorate, comprehensive

Nutrition

exam, thesis/dissertation. *Entrance requirements:* Additional exam requirements/recommendations for international students: Required—TOEFL (minimum score 577 paper-based; 90 iBT), IELTS (minimum score 6.5). Electronic applications accepted. *Faculty research:* Basic nutrition, clinical nutrition, community nutrition, women's health, pediatric nutrition.

University of California, Berkeley, Graduate Division, College of Natural Resources, Group in Molecular and Biochemical Nutrition, Berkeley, CA 94720-1500. Offers PhD. *Degree requirements:* For doctorate, thesis/dissertation, qualifying exam. *Entrance requirements:* For doctorate, GRE General Test, minimum GPA of 3.0, 3 letters of recommendation. Additional exam requirements/recommendations for international students: Required—TOEFL. Electronic applications accepted. *Faculty research:* Regulation of metabolism; nutritional genomics and nutrient-gene interactions; transport, metabolism and function of minerals; carcinogenesis and dietary anti-carcinogens.

University of California, Davis, Graduate Studies, Graduate Group in Nutritional Biology, Davis, CA 95616. Offers MS, PhD. *Degree requirements:* For master's, thesis; for doctorate, thesis/dissertation. *Entrance requirements:* For master's and doctorate, GRE General Test, minimum GPA of 3.0. Additional exam requirements/recommendations for international students: Required—TOEFL (minimum score 550 paper-based). Electronic applications accepted. *Faculty research:* Human/animal nutrition.

University of California, Davis, Graduate Studies, Program in Maternal and Child Nutrition, Davis, CA 95616. Offers MAS. *Degree requirements:* For master's, comprehensive exam. *Entrance requirements:* Additional exam requirements/recommendations for international students: Required—TOEFL (minimum score 550 paper-based).

University of Central Oklahoma, The Jackson College of Graduate Studies, College of Education and Professional Studies, Department of Human Environmental Sciences, Edmond, OK 73034-5209. Offers family and child studies (MS), including family life education, infant/child specialist, marriage and family therapy; nutrition-food management (MS). *Program availability:* Part-time. *Degree requirements:* For master's, comprehensive exam (for some programs), thesis (for some programs). *Entrance requirements:* For master's, GRE, essay, physical, CPR and First Aid training. Additional exam requirements/recommendations for international students: Required—TOEFL (minimum score 550 paper-based; 79 iBT), IELTS (minimum score 6.5). Electronic applications accepted.

University of Chicago, Division of the Biological Sciences, Committee on Molecular Metabolism and Nutrition, Chicago, IL 60637. Offers PhD. *Faculty:* 43. *Students:* 15 full-time (9 women); includes 6 minority (2 Asian, non-Hispanic/Latino; 4 Hispanic/Latino; 1 international. Average age 29. 30 applicants, 23% accepted, 2 enrolled. In 2015, 5 doctorates awarded. *Degree requirements:* For doctorate, thesis/dissertation, ethics class, 2 teaching assistantships. *Entrance requirements:* For doctorate, GRE General Test. Additional exam requirements/recommendations for international students: Required—TOEFL (minimum score 600 paper-based; 104 iBT), IELTS (minimum score 7). *Application deadline:* For fall admission, 12/1 for domestic and international students. Application fee: $90. Electronic applications accepted. *Financial support:* In 2015–16, 11 students received support, including fellowships with full tuition reimbursements available (averaging $29,781 per year), research assistantships with full tuition reimbursements available (averaging $29,781 per year); institutionally sponsored loans, scholarships/grants, traineeships, and health care benefits also available. Financial award applicants required to submit FAFSA. *Faculty research:* Regulation of lipoprotein metabolism, cellular vitamin metabolism, obesity and body composition, adipocyte differentiation. *Unit head:* Dr. Christopher J. Rhodes, Chairman, 773-702-8128, Fax: 773-834-0851. Website: http://biomedsciences.uchicago.edu/page/molecular-metabolism-and-nutrition

University of Cincinnati, Graduate School, College of Allied Health Sciences, Department of Nutritional Sciences, Cincinnati, OH 45221. Offers MS. *Program availability:* Part-time. *Degree requirements:* For master's, thesis. *Entrance requirements:* For master's, GRE General Test. Additional exam requirements/recommendations for international students: Required—TOEFL (minimum score 550 paper-based). Electronic applications accepted. *Faculty research:* Phytochemicals-osteoarthritis, pediatric hypertension and hypercholesterol, cancer prevention/Type II diabetes.

University of Connecticut, Graduate School, College of Agriculture, Health and Natural Resources, Department of Nutritional Sciences, Storrs, CT 06269. Offers MS, PhD. Terminal master's awarded for partial completion of doctoral program. *Degree requirements:* For master's, comprehensive exam, thesis; for doctorate, thesis/dissertation. *Entrance requirements:* For master's and doctorate, GRE General Test. Additional exam requirements/recommendations for international students: Required—TOEFL (minimum score 550 paper-based). *Application deadline:* For fall admission, 2/1 priority date for domestic and international students; for spring admission, 11/1 for domestic students, 10/1 for international students. Applications are processed on a rolling basis. Application fee: $55. Electronic applications accepted. *Financial support:* Fellowships, research assistantships with full tuition reimbursements, teaching assistantships with full tuition reimbursements, Federal Work-Study, scholarships/grants, health care benefits, and unspecified assistantships available. Financial award application deadline: 2/1; financial award applicants required to submit FAFSA. Website: http://www.canr.uconn.edu/nutsci/nutsci/

University of Delaware, College of Health Sciences, Department of Behavioral Health and Nutrition, Newark, DE 19716. Offers health promotion (MS); human nutrition (MS). *Program availability:* Part-time. *Degree requirements:* For master's, thesis. *Entrance requirements:* For master's, GRE General Test, interview, minimum GPA of 3.0. Additional exam requirements/recommendations for international students: Required—TOEFL (minimum score 550 paper-based). Electronic applications accepted. *Faculty research:* Sport biomechanics, rehabilitation biomechanics, vascular dynamics.

University of Florida, Graduate School, College of Agricultural and Life Sciences, Department of Food Science and Human Nutrition, Gainesville, FL 32611. Offers food science (PhD), including toxicology; food science and human nutrition (MS), including nutritional sciences; nutritional sciences (MS, PhD), including clinical and translational science (PhD). *Faculty:* 13 full-time, 1 part-time/adjunct. *Students:* 43 full-time (32 women), 4 part-time (1 woman); includes 6 minority (3 Black or African American, non-Hispanic/Latino; 2 Asian, non-Hispanic/Latino; 2 Hispanic/Latino), 27 international. Average age 27. 150 applicants, 23% accepted, 23 enrolled. In 2015, 22 master's awarded. *Degree requirements:* For master's, thesis optional; for doctorate, thesis/dissertation. *Entrance requirements:* For master's and doctorate, GRE General Test, minimum GPA of 3.0. Additional exam requirements/recommendations for international students: Required—TOEFL. *Application deadline:* For fall admission, 6/1 priority date for domestic students. Applications are processed on a rolling basis. Application fee: $30. Electronic applications accepted. *Financial support:* In 2015–16, 2 fellowships, 16 research assistantships, 23 teaching assistantships were awarded; career-related internships or fieldwork also available. Financial award applicants required to submit FAFSA. *Faculty research:* Pesticide research, nutritional biochemistry and microbiology, food safety and toxicology assessment and dietetics, food chemistry. *Total annual research expenditures:* $7.5 million. *Unit head:* Susan S. Percival, PhD, Chair and Professor, 352-392-1991 Ext. 202, Fax: 352-392-1991, E-mail: percival@ufl.edu. Website: http://fshn.ifas.ufl.edu/

University of Georgia, College of Family and Consumer Sciences, Department of Foods and Nutrition, Athens, GA 30602. Offers MFCS, MS, PhD. *Degree requirements:* For master's, thesis (MS); for doctorate, thesis/dissertation. *Entrance requirements:* For master's, GRE General Test, minimum GPA of 3.0, course work in biochemistry and physiology; for doctorate, GRE General Test, master's degree, minimum GPA of 3.0. Electronic applications accepted.

University of Guelph, Graduate Studies, College of Biological Science, Department of Human Health and Nutritional Sciences, Guelph, ON N1G 2W1, Canada. Offers nutritional sciences (M Sc, PhD). *Program availability:* Part-time. *Degree requirements:* For master's, thesis (for some programs); for doctorate, comprehensive exam, thesis/dissertation. *Entrance requirements:* For master's, minimum B-average during previous 2 years of coursework; for doctorate, minimum A-average. Additional exam requirements/recommendations for international students: Required—TOEFL (minimum score 550 paper-based). Electronic applications accepted. *Faculty research:* Nutrition and biochemistry, exercise metabolism and physiology, toxicology, gene expression, biomechanics and ergonomics.

University of Guelph, Graduate Studies, College of Social and Applied Human Sciences, Department of Family Relations and Applied Nutrition, Guelph, ON N1G 2W1, Canada. Offers applied nutrition (MAN); family relations and human development (M Sc, PhD), including applied human nutrition, couple and family therapy (M Sc), family relations and human development. *Accreditation:* AAMFT/COAMFTE (one or more programs are accredited). *Program availability:* Part-time. *Degree requirements:* For master's, thesis (for some programs); for doctorate, comprehensive exam, thesis/dissertation. *Entrance requirements:* For master's, minimum B+ average; for doctorate, master's degree in family relations and human development or related field with a minimum B+ average or master's degree in applied human nutrition. Additional exam requirements/recommendations for international students: Required—TOEFL (minimum score 600 paper-based). Electronic applications accepted. *Faculty research:* Child and adolescent development, social gerontology, family roles and relations, couple and family therapy, applied human nutrition.

University of Hawaii at Manoa, Graduate Division, College of Tropical Agriculture and Human Resources, Department of Human Nutrition, Food and Animal Sciences, Program in Nutrition, Honolulu, HI 96822. Offers PhD. *Program availability:* Part-time. *Faculty:* 26 full-time (11 women), 2 part-time/adjunct (1 woman). *Students:* 4 full-time (2 women), 1 part-time; includes 1 minority (Asian, non-Hispanic/Latino), 2 international. Average age 30. 6 applicants, 67% accepted, 1 enrolled. *Degree requirements:* For doctorate, comprehensive exam, thesis/dissertation. *Entrance requirements:* For doctorate, GRE General Test. Additional exam requirements/recommendations for international students: Required—TOEFL (minimum score 580 paper-based; 92 iBT), IELTS (minimum score 5). *Application deadline:* For fall admission, 2/1 for domestic and international students; for spring admission, 9/1 for domestic and international students. Application fee: $100. *Financial support:* In 2015–16, 3 students received support, including 1 fellowship (averaging $500 per year), 2 research assistantships (averaging $17,511 per year). *Unit head:* Douglas Vincent, Chair, 808-956-8393, E-mail: vincent@hawaii.edu. *Application contact:* Dr. Michael Dunn, Graduate Chair, 808-956-8523, Fax: 808-956-4024, E-mail: mdunn@hawaii.edu.

University of Hawaii at Manoa, Graduate Division, College of Tropical Agriculture and Human Resources, Department of Human Nutrition, Food and Animal Sciences, Program in Nutritional Sciences, Honolulu, HI 96822. Offers MS, PhD. *Program availability:* Part-time. *Faculty:* 26 full-time (11 women), 2 part-time/adjunct (1 woman). *Students:* 3 full-time (2 women), 1 part-time; includes 3 minority (1 Asian, non-Hispanic/Latino; 2 Two or more races, non-Hispanic/Latino). Average age 30. 4 applicants, 75% accepted, 1 enrolled. In 2015, 3 master's awarded. *Degree requirements:* For master's, thesis optional; for doctorate, comprehensive exam, thesis/dissertation. *Entrance requirements:* For master's and doctorate, GRE General Test. Additional exam requirements/recommendations for international students: Required—TOEFL (minimum score 580 paper-based; 92 iBT), IELTS (minimum score 5). *Application deadline:* For fall admission, 2/1 for domestic and international students; for spring admission, 9/1 for domestic and international students. Application fee: $100. *Financial support:* In 2015–16, 4 fellowships (averaging $5,125 per year), 9 research assistantships (averaging $16,193 per year) were awarded; teaching assistantships and tuition waivers (full) also available. Financial award application deadline: 3/1. *Faculty research:* Nutritional biochemistry, human nutrition, nutrition education, international nutrition, nutritional epidemiology. *Total annual research expenditures:* $1 million. *Unit head:* Douglas Vincent, Chair, 808-956-8393, E-mail: vincent@hawaii.edu. *Application contact:* Dr. Michael Dunn, Graduate Chairperson, 808-956-8523, Fax: 808-956-4024, E-mail: mdunn@hawaii.edu. Website: http://www.ctahr.hawaii.edu/hnfas/academics.html

University of Houston, College of Liberal Arts and Social Sciences, Department of Health and Human Performance, Houston, TX 77204. Offers exercise science (MS); human nutrition (MS); human space exploration sciences (MS); kinesiology (PhD); physical education (M Ed). *Accreditation:* NCATE (one or more programs are accredited). *Program availability:* Part-time, evening/weekend. *Degree requirements:* For master's, comprehensive exam (for some programs), thesis (for some programs); for doctorate, comprehensive exam, thesis/dissertation, qualifying exam, candidacy paper. *Entrance requirements:* For master's, GRE (minimum 35th percentile on each section), minimum cumulative GPA of 3.0; for doctorate, GRE (minimum 35th percentile on each section), minimum cumulative GPA of 3.3. Additional exam requirements/recommendations for international students: Required—TOEFL (minimum score 550 paper-based; 79 iBT). Electronic applications accepted. *Faculty research:* Biomechanics, exercise physiology, obesity, nutrition, space exploration science.

University of Illinois at Chicago, College of Applied Health Sciences, Program in Nutrition, Chicago, IL 60607-7128. Offers MS, PhD. *Accreditation:* AND. *Students:* 97 full-time (83 women), 9 part-time (8 women); includes 23 minority (8 Black or African American, non-Hispanic/Latino; 5 Asian, non-Hispanic/Latino; 7 Hispanic/Latino; 3 Two or more races, non-Hispanic/Latino), 15 international. Average age 30. *Degree requirements:* For master's, thesis; for doctorate, thesis/dissertation. *Entrance requirements:* For master's and doctorate, GRE General Test, minimum GPA of 2.75. Additional exam requirements/recommendations for international students: Required—TOEFL. *Application deadline:* For fall admission, 12/13 priority date for domestic and international students. Application fee: $60 ($50 for international students). Electronic applications accepted. *Expenses:* Contact institution. *Financial support:* Fellowships with full tuition reimbursements, research assistantships with full tuition reimbursements, teaching assistantships with full tuition reimbursements, career-related internships or fieldwork, Federal Work-Study, institutionally sponsored loans, traineeships, tuition waivers (full), and unspecified assistantships available. Financial award application deadline: 3/1; financial award applicants required to submit FAFSA. *Faculty research:* Nutrition for the elderly, inborn errors of metabolism, nutrition and cancer, lipid metabolism, dietary fat markers. *Unit head:* Prof. Giamila Fantuzzi, Director of Graduate Studies, 312-413-5398, Fax: 312-355-1713, E-mail: giamila@uic.edu. *Application contact:* Receptionist, 312-413-2550, E-mail: gradcoll@uic.edu. Website: http://www.ahs.uic.edu/kn/academics/msncp/

University of Illinois at Urbana–Champaign, Graduate College, College of Agricultural, Consumer and Environmental Sciences, Department of Food Science and Human Nutrition, Champaign, IL 61820. Offers food science (MS); food science and human nutrition (MS, PhD), including professional science (MS); human nutrition (MS). *Program availability:* Part-time, online learning.

University of Illinois at Urbana–Champaign, Graduate College, College of Agricultural, Consumer and Environmental Sciences, Division of Nutritional Sciences, Champaign, IL 61820. Offers MS, PhD, PhD/MPH.

The University of Kansas, University of Kansas Medical Center, School of Health Professions, Department of Dietetics and Nutrition, Kansas City, KS 66160. Offers dietetic internship (Graduate Certificate); dietetics and integrative medicine (Graduate Certificate); dietetics and nutrition (MS); medical nutrition science (PhD). *Program availability:* Part-time, online learning. *Faculty:* 22. *Students:* 40 full-time (37 women), 16 part-time (14 women); includes 2 minority (both Two or more races, non-Hispanic/Latino), 3 international. Average age 28. 66 applicants, 36% accepted, 22 enrolled. In 2015, 16 master's, 2 doctorates, 12 other advanced degrees awarded. *Degree requirements:* For master's, comprehensive exam, thesis, oral exam; for doctorate, comprehensive exam, thesis/dissertation, oral exam. *Entrance requirements:* For master's, GRE, prerequisite courses in nutrition, biochemistry, and physiology; for doctorate, GRE; for Graduate Certificate, GRE, minimum cumulative GPA of 3.0. Additional exam requirements/recommendations for international students: Required—TOEFL. *Application deadline:* For fall admission, 7/1 for domestic students, 6/1 for international students; for winter admission, 12/1 for domestic students, 11/1 for international students; for spring admission, 11/1 for domestic students, 10/1 for international students; for summer admission, 4/1 for domestic students, 3/1 for international students. Applications are processed on a rolling basis. Application fee: $60. Electronic applications accepted. *Expenses:* Contact institution. *Financial support:* In 2015–16, 12 students received support. Fellowships, research assistantships with full tuition reimbursements available, teaching assistantships with full tuition reimbursements available, career-related internships or fieldwork, Federal Work-Study, institutionally sponsored loans, scholarships/grants, traineeships, tuition waivers, and unspecified assistantships available. Support available to part-time students. Financial award application deadline: 3/1; financial award applicants required to submit FAFSA. *Faculty research:* Obesity prevention and treatment, omega-3 fatty acids impact on infant development and immunity, vitamin D and bone metabolism in osteosarcoma cells, cancer prevention and recovery maternal diet intake and weight gain impact on infant body composition and development. *Total annual research expenditures:* $1.8 million. *Unit head:* Dr. Debra Kay Sullivan, Chairperson, 913-588-5357, Fax: 913-588-8946, E-mail: dsulliva@kumc.edu. *Application contact:* Dr. Heather Gibbs, Graduate Director, 913-945-9138.
Website: http://www.kumc.edu/school-of-health-professions/dietetics-and-nutrition.html

University of Kentucky, Graduate School, College of Agriculture, Food and Environment, Program in Hospitality and Dietetics Administration, Lexington, KY 40506-0032. Offers MS. *Degree requirements:* For master's, comprehensive exam, thesis optional. *Entrance requirements:* For master's, GRE General Test, minimum undergraduate GPA of 2.75. Additional exam requirements/recommendations for international students: Required—TOEFL (minimum score 550 paper-based). Electronic applications accepted.

University of Kentucky, Graduate School, College of Health Sciences, Program in Nutritional Sciences, Lexington, KY 40506-0032. Offers MSNS, PhD. *Degree requirements:* For doctorate, comprehensive exam, thesis/dissertation. *Entrance requirements:* For master's, GRE General Test, minimum undergraduate GPA of 2.75; for doctorate, GRE General Test, minimum graduate GPA of 3.0. Additional exam requirements/recommendations for international students: Required—TOEFL (minimum score 550 paper-based). Electronic applications accepted. *Faculty research:* Nutrition and AIDS, nutrition and alcoholism, nutrition and cardiovascular disease, nutrition and cancer, nutrition and diabetes.

University of Maine, Graduate School, College of Natural Sciences, Forestry, and Agriculture, School of Food and Agriculture, Orono, ME 04469. Offers animal sciences (MPS, MS); food and human nutrition (PhD); food science and human nutrition (MS); horticulture (MS); plant science (PhD). *Program availability:* Part-time. *Faculty:* 30 full-time (15 women). *Students:* 50 full-time (29 women), 2 part-time (both women); includes 3 minority (2 American Indian or Alaska Native, non-Hispanic/Latino; 1 Asian, non-Hispanic/Latino), 15 international. Average age 28. 81 applicants, 48% accepted, 20 enrolled. In 2015, 18 master's, 3 doctorates, 3 other advanced degrees awarded. *Degree requirements:* For master's, thesis (for some programs); for doctorate, comprehensive exam, thesis/dissertation. *Entrance requirements:* For master's and doctorate, GRE General Test. Additional exam requirements/recommendations for international students: Required—TOEFL. *Application deadline:* For fall admission, 2/1 priority date for domestic students. Applications are processed on a rolling basis. Application fee: $65. Electronic applications accepted. *Financial support:* In 2015–16, 36 students received support, including 1 fellowship (averaging $20,000 per year), 25 research assistantships with full tuition reimbursements available (averaging $14,600 per year), 7 teaching assistantships with full tuition reimbursements available (averaging $14,600 per year); Federal Work-Study, institutionally sponsored loans, and tuition waivers (full and partial) also available. Financial award application deadline: 3/1. *Faculty research:* Nutrition education for adults and children, food processing, food safety, sustainable crop and soil management, animal health and nutrition. *Total annual research expenditures:* $1.9 million. *Unit head:* Dr. Sue Erich, Chair, 207-581-2947, Fax: 207-581-2770. *Application contact:* Scott G. Delcourt, Assistant Vice President for Graduate Studies and Senior Associate Dean, 207-581-3291, Fax: 207-581-3232, E-mail: graduate@maine.edu.
Website: http://umaine.edu/foodandagriculture

University of Manitoba, Faculty of Graduate Studies, Faculty of Agricultural and Food Sciences, Department of Food Science, Winnipeg, MB R3T 2N2, Canada. Offers food and nutritional sciences (PhD); food science (M Sc); foods and nutrition (M Sc). *Degree requirements:* For master's, thesis.

University of Manitoba, Faculty of Graduate Studies, Faculty of Human Ecology, Department of Human Nutritional Sciences, Winnipeg, MB R3T 2N2, Canada. Offers M Sc. *Degree requirements:* For master's, thesis.

University of Maryland, College Park, Academic Affairs, College of Agriculture and Natural Resources, Department of Nutrition and Food Science, Program in Nutrition, College Park, MD 20742. Offers MS, PhD. *Degree requirements:* For master's, thesis; for doctorate, comprehensive exam, thesis/dissertation, candidacy exam. *Entrance requirements:* For master's, GRE General Test, minimum GPA of 3.0, 3 letters of recommendation; for doctorate, GRE General Test, minimum GPA of 3.0. Additional exam requirements/recommendations for international students: Required—TOEFL. Electronic applications accepted. *Faculty research:* Nutrition education, carbohydrates and physical activity.

University of Massachusetts Amherst, Graduate School, School of Public Health and Health Sciences, Department of Nutrition, Amherst, MA 01003. Offers community nutrition (MS); nutrition (MPH); nutrition science (MS). *Program availability:* Part-time, evening/weekend, online learning. Terminal master's awarded for partial completion of doctoral program. *Degree requirements:* For master's, thesis or alternative. *Entrance requirements:* For master's, GRE General Test. Additional exam requirements/recommendations for international students: Required—TOEFL (minimum score 550 paper-based; 80 iBT), IELTS (minimum score 6.5). Electronic applications accepted.

University of Massachusetts Amherst, Graduate School, School of Public Health and Health Sciences, Department of Public Health, Amherst, MA 01003. Offers biostatistics (MPH, MS, PhD); community health education (MPH, MS, PhD); environmental health sciences (MPH, MS, PhD); epidemiology (MPH, MS, PhD); health policy and management (MPH, MS, PhD); nutrition (MPH, PhD); public health practice (MPH); MPH/MPPA. *Accreditation:* CEPH (one or more programs are accredited). *Program availability:* Part-time, evening/weekend, online learning. Terminal master's awarded for partial completion of doctoral program. *Degree requirements:* For master's, thesis (for some programs); for doctorate, comprehensive exam, thesis/dissertation. *Entrance requirements:* For master's and doctorate, GRE General Test. Additional exam requirements/recommendations for international students: Required—TOEFL (minimum score 550 paper-based; 80 iBT), IELTS (minimum score 6.5). Electronic applications accepted.

University of Miami, Graduate School, School of Education and Human Development, Department of Kinesiology and Sport Sciences, Program in Nutrition for Health and Human Performance, Coral Gables, FL 33124. Offers MS Ed. *Degree requirements:* For master's, comprehensive examination or research project. *Entrance requirements:* For master's, GRE. Additional exam requirements/recommendations for international students: Required—TOEFL (minimum score 550 paper-based; 80 iBT).

University of Michigan, School of Public Health, Department of Nutritional Sciences, Ann Arbor, MI 48109. Offers dietetics (MPH); nutrition sciences (MPH, MS, PhD). *Faculty:* 7 full-time (5 women), 4 part-time/adjunct (all women). *Students:* 68 full-time (62 women); includes 12 minority (1 Black or African American, non-Hispanic/Latino; 8 Asian, non-Hispanic/Latino; 2 Hispanic/Latino; 1 Two or more races, non-Hispanic/Latino), 6 international. Average age 26. 97 applicants, 90% accepted, 39 enrolled. In 2015, 21 master's, 2 doctorates awarded. *Entrance requirements:* For master's, GRE, MCAT; for doctorate, GRE. Additional exam requirements/recommendations for international students: Required—TOEFL (minimum score 100 iBT). *Application deadline:* For fall admission, 12/15 priority date for domestic students, 1/15 for international students. Applications are processed on a rolling basis. Application fee: $75. Electronic applications accepted. *Financial support:* Fellowships, research assistantships, teaching assistantships, career-related internships or fieldwork, Federal Work-Study, institutionally sponsored loans, scholarships/grants, traineeships, health care benefits, and unspecified assistantships available. *Unit head:* Dr. Karen E. Peterson, Chair, 734-647-1923, Fax: 734-936-7283, E-mail: karenep@umich.edu. *Application contact:* Susan Aaronson, Program Coordinator, 734-763-3860, E-mail: susaaaro@umich.edu.
Website: http://sph.umich.edu/ns/

University of Minnesota, Twin Cities Campus, Graduate School, College of Food, Agricultural and Natural Resource Sciences, Program in Nutrition, Saint Paul, MN 55108. Offers MS, PhD. *Program availability:* Part-time. *Faculty:* 20 full-time (10 women), 20 part-time/adjunct (15 women). *Students:* 40 full-time (29 women), 3 part-time (all women); includes 3 minority (2 American Indian or Alaska Native, non-Hispanic/Latino; 1 Native Hawaiian or other Pacific Islander, non-Hispanic/Latino), 12 international. Average age 25. 41 applicants, 22% accepted, 9 enrolled. In 2015, 10 master's, 8 doctorates awarded. Terminal master's awarded for partial completion of doctoral program. *Degree requirements:* For master's, comprehensive exam, thesis; for doctorate, comprehensive exam, thesis/dissertation. *Entrance requirements:* For master's, GRE General Test, previous course work in general chemistry, organic chemistry, physiology, biology, biochemistry, and statistics; minimum GPA of 3.0 (preferred); for doctorate, GRE General Test, previous course work in general chemistry, organic chemistry, biology, physiology, biochemistry, and statistics; minimum GPA of 3.0 (preferred). Additional exam requirements/recommendations for international students: Required—TOEFL (minimum score 550 paper-based; 79 iBT), IELTS (minimum score 6.5). *Application deadline:* Applications are processed on a rolling basis. Application fee: $75 ($95 for international students). Electronic applications accepted. *Financial support:* In 2015–16, fellowships with full tuition reimbursements (averaging $40,000 per year), research assistantships with tuition reimbursements (averaging $40,000 per year), teaching assistantships with tuition reimbursements (averaging $40,000 per year) were awarded; career-related internships or fieldwork, tuition waivers (full and partial), and unspecified assistantships also available. Support available to part-time students. *Faculty research:* Diet and chronic disease: from basic biological and molecular biology approaches to a public health/intervention/ epidemiology perspective. *Total annual research expenditures:* $3 million. *Unit head:* Dr. Marla Reicks, Director of Graduate Studies, 612-624-4735, Fax: 612-625-5272, E-mail: mreicks@umn.edu. *Application contact:* Nancy L. Toedt, Program Coordinator, 612-624-6753, Fax: 612-625-5272, E-mail: sviker@umn.edu.
Website: http://fscn.cfans.umn.edu/graduate-programs/nutrition

University of Minnesota, Twin Cities Campus, School of Public Health, Major in Public Health Nutrition, Minneapolis, MN 55455-0213. Offers MPH. *Accreditation:* AND. *Program availability:* Part-time. *Degree requirements:* For master's, fieldwork, project. *Entrance requirements:* For master's, GRE General Test. Additional exam requirements/recommendations for international students: Required—TOEFL. Electronic applications accepted. *Expenses:* Contact institution. *Faculty research:* Nutrition and pregnancy outcomes, nutrition and women's health, child growth and nutrition, child and adolescent nutrition and eating behaviors, obesity and eating disorder prevention.

University of Mississippi, Graduate School, School of Applied Sciences, University, MS 38677. Offers communicative disorders (MS); criminal justice (MCJ); exercise science (MS); food and nutrition services (MS); health and kinesiology (PhD); health promotion (MS); park and recreation management (MA); social work (MSW). *Faculty:* 65 full-time (36 women), 32 part-time/adjunct (23 women). *Students:* 192 full-time (148 women), 43 part-time (23 women); includes 47 minority (37 Black or African American, non-Hispanic/Latino; 2 Asian, non-Hispanic/Latino; 7 Hispanic/Latino; 1 Two or more races, non-Hispanic/Latino), 12 international. In 2015, 99 master's, 3 doctorates awarded. *Entrance requirements:* For master's, GRE General Test, minimum GPA of 3.0. Additional exam requirements/recommendations for international students: Required—TOEFL. *Application deadline:* For fall admission, 4/1 for domestic students; for spring admission, 10/1 for domestic students. Applications are processed on a rolling basis. Application fee: $40. Electronic applications accepted. *Financial support:* Scholarships/grants available. Financial award application deadline: 3/1; financial award applicants required to submit FAFSA. *Unit head:* Dr. Velmer Stanley Burton, Dean, 662-915-1081, Fax: 662-915-5717, E-mail: applsci@olemiss.edu. *Application contact:* Dr. Christy M. Wyandt, Associate Dean of Graduate School, 662-915-7474, Fax: 662-915-7577, E-mail: cwyandt@olemiss.edu.

University of Missouri, Office of Research and Graduate Studies, College of Human Environmental Sciences, Department of Nutrition and Exercise Physiology, Columbia, MO 65211. Offers exercise physiology (MS); nutrition sciences (MS). *Degree requirements:* For doctorate, thesis/dissertation. *Entrance requirements:* For master's

Nutrition

and doctorate, GRE General Test, minimum GPA of 3.0. Additional exam requirements/ recommendations for international students: Required—TOEFL (minimum score 500 paper-based; 61 iBT). *Application deadline:* For fall admission, 12/31 priority date for domestic and international students. Applications are processed on a rolling basis. Application fee: $55 ($75 for international students). Electronic applications accepted. *Financial support:* Fellowships with tuition reimbursements, research assistantships with tuition reimbursements, teaching assistantships with tuition reimbursements, institutionally sponsored loans, scholarships/grants, health care benefits, and unspecified assistantships available. Support available to part-time students. Website: http://ns.missouri.edu/

University of Nebraska–Lincoln, Graduate College, College of Agricultural Sciences and Natural Resources, Interdepartmental Area of Nutrition, Lincoln, NE 68588. Offers MS, PhD. *Degree requirements:* For master's, thesis optional; for doctorate, comprehensive exam, thesis/dissertation. *Entrance requirements:* For master's and doctorate, GRE General Test. Additional exam requirements/recommendations for international students: Required—TOEFL (minimum score 550 paper-based). Electronic applications accepted. *Faculty research:* Human nutrition and metabolism, animal nutrition and metabolism, biochemistry, community and clinical nutrition.

University of Nebraska–Lincoln, Graduate College, College of Education and Human Sciences, Department of Nutrition and Health Sciences, Lincoln, NE 68588. Offers community nutrition and health promotion (MS); nutrition (MS, PhD); nutrition and exercise (MS); nutrition and health sciences (MS, PhD). *Degree requirements:* For master's, thesis optional. *Entrance requirements:* For master's, GRE General Test. Additional exam requirements/recommendations for international students: Required—TOEFL (minimum score 550 paper-based). Electronic applications accepted. *Faculty research:* Foods/food service administration, community nutrition science, diet-health relationships.

University of Nebraska Medical Center, School of Allied Health Professions and College of Medicine, UNMC Dietetic Internship Program (Medical Nutrition Education Division), Omaha, NE 68198. Offers Certificate. *Entrance requirements:* Additional exam requirements/recommendations for international students: Required—TOEFL. *Expenses:* Tuition, state resident: full-time $7830; part-time $3915 per credit hour. Tuition, nonresident: full-time $22,410; part-time $11,205 per credit hour. *Required fees:* $521. *Faculty research:* Nutrition intervention outcomes.

University of Nevada, Las Vegas, Graduate College, School of Allied Health Sciences, Department of Kinesiology and Nutrition Sciences, Las Vegas, NV 89154-3034. Offers exercise physiology (MS); kinesiology (PhD). *Program availability:* Part-time. *Faculty:* 11 full-time (5 women), 1 part-time/adjunct. *Students:* 42 full-time (24 women), 14 part-time (3 women); includes 10 minority (1 Black or African American, non-Hispanic/Latino; 3 Asian, non-Hispanic/Latino; 3 Hispanic/Latino; 3 Two or more races, non-Hispanic/Latino), 3 international. Average age 28. 37 applicants, 68% accepted, 15 enrolled. In 2015, 23 master's, 1 doctorate awarded. *Degree requirements:* For master's, thesis (for some programs), professional paper; for doctorate, comprehensive exam, thesis/dissertation. *Entrance requirements:* For master's, GRE General Test; for doctorate, GRE General Test (minimum 70th percentile on the Verbal section). Additional exam requirements/recommendations for international students: Required—TOEFL (minimum score 550 paper-based; 80 iBT), IELTS (minimum score 7). *Application deadline:* For fall admission, 6/15 for domestic students, 5/1 for international students; for spring admission, 11/15 for domestic students, 10/1 for international students. Application fee: $60 ($95 for international students). Electronic applications accepted. *Expenses:* $264 per credit state resident full-time and part-time; $6,955 per semester, $264 per credit nonresident full-time; $555 per credit nonresident part-time. *Financial support:* In 2015–16, 26 students received support, including 11 research assistantships with partial tuition reimbursements available (averaging $11,727 per year), 15 teaching assistantships with partial tuition reimbursements available (averaging $10,933 per year); institutionally sponsored loans, scholarships/grants, health care benefits, and unspecified assistantships also available. Financial award application deadline: 3/1. *Faculty research:* Biomechanics of gait, factors in motor skill acquisition and performance, nutritional supplements and performance, lipoprotein chemistry, body composition methods. *Total annual research expenditures:* $56,220. *Unit head:* John Mercer, Chair/Professor, 702-895-4672, Fax: 702-895-1500, E-mail: john.mercer@unlv.edu. *Application contact:* Graduate College Admissions Evaluator, 702-895-3367, Fax: 702-895-4180, E-mail: gradadmissions@unlv.edu. Website: http://kinesiology.unlv.edu/

University of Nevada, Reno, Graduate School, College of Agriculture, Biotechnology and Natural Resources, Department of Nutrition, Reno, NV 89557. Offers MS. *Degree requirements:* For master's, thesis optional. *Entrance requirements:* For master's, GRE, minimum GPA of 2.75. Additional exam requirements/recommendations for international students: Required—TOEFL (minimum score 500 paper-based; 61 iBT), IELTS (minimum score 6). Electronic applications accepted. *Faculty research:* Nutritional education, food technology, therapeutic human nutrition, human nutritional requirements, diet and disease.

University of New Hampshire, Graduate School, College of Life Sciences and Agriculture, Department of Molecular, Cellular and Biomedical Sciences, Program in Animal and Nutritional Sciences, Durham, NH 03824. Offers PhD. *Program availability:* Part-time. *Entrance requirements:* For doctorate, GRE. Additional exam requirements/recommendations for international students: Required—TOEFL (minimum score 550 paper-based; 80 iBT). *Application deadline:* For fall admission, 6/1 priority date for domestic students, 4/1 priority date for international students; for spring admission, 12/1 for domestic students. Applications are processed on a rolling basis. Application fee: $65. Electronic applications accepted. *Expenses:* Tuition, state resident: full-time $13,840; part-time $770 per credit hour. Tuition, nonresident: full-time $27,130; part-time $1175 per credit hour. *Required fees:* $2080; $1040. Tuition and fees vary according to degree level and program. *Financial support:* Fellowships, research assistantships, teaching assistantships, scholarships/grants, traineeships, and unspecified assistantships available. Support available to part-time students. *Unit head:* Dr. Andre Brito, Director, 603-862-1341. *Application contact:* Flora Joyal, Administrative Assistant, 603-862-4095, E-mail: ansc.grad.program.info@unh.edu.

University of New Hampshire, Graduate School, College of Life Sciences and Agriculture, Department of Molecular, Cellular and Biomedical Sciences, Program in Nutritional Sciences, Durham, NH 03824. Offers MS. *Program availability:* Part-time. *Degree requirements:* For master's, thesis. *Entrance requirements:* Additional exam requirements/recommendations for international students: Required—TOEFL (minimum score 550 paper-based; 80 iBT). *Application deadline:* For fall admission, 4/1 priority date for domestic students, 4/1 for international students; for spring admission, 12/1 for domestic students. Applications are processed on a rolling basis. Application fee: $65. Electronic applications accepted. *Expenses:* Tuition, state resident: full-time $13,840; part-time $770 per credit hour. Tuition, nonresident: full-time $27,130; part-time $1175 per credit hour. *Required fees:* $2080; $1040. Tuition and fees vary according to degree level and program. *Financial support:* Fellowships, research assistantships, teaching assistantships, career-related internships or fieldwork, Federal Work-Study, and scholarships/grants available. Support available to part-time students. Financial award application deadline: 2/15. *Unit head:* Dr. Andre Brito, Director, 603-862-1341.

Application contact: Flora Joyal, Administrative Assistant, 603-862-4095, E-mail: flora.joyal@unh.edu.

University of New Haven, Graduate School, College of Arts and Sciences, Program in Human Nutrition, West Haven, CT 06516-1916. Offers human nutrition (MS); nutritional genomics (MS, Graduate Certificate). *Program availability:* Part-time, evening/weekend. *Students:* 5 full-time (4 women), 11 part-time (9 women); includes 2 minority (1 Black or African American, non-Hispanic/Latino; 1 Two or more races, non-Hispanic/Latino), 2 international. Average age 32. 19 applicants, 89% accepted, 7 enrolled. In 2015, 9 master's, 1 other advanced degree awarded. *Degree requirements:* For master's, internship. *Entrance requirements:* Additional exam requirements/recommendations for international students: Required—TOEFL (minimum score 80 iBT), IELTS, PTE. *Application deadline:* For fall admission, 5/31 for international students; for winter admission, 10/15 for international students; for spring admission, 1/15 for international students. Applications are processed on a rolling basis. Application fee: $75. Electronic applications accepted. Application fee is waived when completed online. *Expenses:* Tuition, area resident: Full-time $15,282; part-time $849 per credit hour. *Required fees:* $150; $60 per term. Tuition and fees vary according to program. *Financial support:* Research assistantships with partial tuition reimbursements, teaching assistantships with partial tuition reimbursements, career-related internships or fieldwork, Federal Work-Study, scholarships/grants, tuition waivers, and unspecified assistantships available. Support available to part-time students. Financial award applicants required to submit FAFSA. *Unit head:* Dr. Rosa A. Mo, Chair, 203-932-7040, E-mail: rmo@newhaven.edu. *Application contact:* Michelle Mason, Director of Graduate Enrollment, 203-932-7067, E-mail: mmason@newhaven.edu. Website: http://www.newhaven.edu/4729/

University of New Mexico, Graduate Studies, College of Education, Program in Nutrition, Albuquerque, NM 87131. Offers MS. *Program availability:* Part-time. *Faculty:* 5 full-time (all women). *Students:* 12 full-time (10 women), 11 part-time (10 women); includes 8 minority (all Hispanic/Latino), 1 international. Average age 34. 16 applicants, 44% accepted, 5 enrolled. In 2015, 5 master's awarded. *Degree requirements:* For master's, comprehensive exam or thesis. *Entrance requirements:* For master's, GRE. Additional exam requirements/recommendations for international students: Required—TOEFL. *Application deadline:* For fall admission, 2/1 priority date for domestic students, 2/1 for international students; for spring admission, 11/1 priority date for domestic students, 11/1 for international students. Application fee: $50. Electronic applications accepted. *Financial support:* Teaching assistantships and unspecified assistantships available. Financial award application deadline: 3/1; financial award applicants required to submit FAFSA. *Faculty research:* Nutritional needs of children, obesity prevention, phytochemicals, international nutrition. *Unit head:* Dr. Carole Conn, Graduate Coordinator, 505-277-8185, Fax: 505-277-8361, E-mail: cconn@unm.edu. *Application contact:* Cynthia Salas, Program Office, 505-277-4535, Fax: 505-277-8361, E-mail: casalas@unm.edu. Website: http://coe.unm.edu/departments-programs/ifce/nutrition/

The University of North Carolina at Chapel Hill, Graduate School, Gillings School of Global Public Health, Department of Nutrition, Chapel Hill, NC 27599. Offers nutrition (MPH, PhD); nutritional biochemistry (MS). *Accreditation:* AND. *Faculty:* 37 full-time. *Students:* 125 full-time (105 women); includes 28 minority (8 Black or African American, non-Hispanic/Latino; 5 Asian, non-Hispanic/Latino; 7 Hispanic/Latino; 8 Two or more races, non-Hispanic/Latino), 14 international. Average age 26. 200 applicants, 30% accepted, 37 enrolled. *Degree requirements:* For master's, comprehensive exam, thesis, major paper; for doctorate, comprehensive exam, thesis/dissertation. *Entrance requirements:* For master's and doctorate, GRE General Test, minimum GPA of 3.0 (recommended). Additional exam requirements/recommendations for international students: Required—TOEFL. *Application deadline:* For fall admission, 12/10 priority date for domestic students, 12/15 priority date for international students; for spring admission, 10/15 for domestic students. Applications are processed on a rolling basis. Application fee: $85. Electronic applications accepted. *Financial support:* Fellowships with tuition reimbursements, research assistantships with tuition reimbursements, teaching assistantships with tuition reimbursements, career-related internships or fieldwork, Federal Work-Study, institutionally sponsored loans, scholarships/grants, traineeships, health care benefits, and unspecified assistantships available. Financial award application deadline: 3/1; financial award applicants required to submit FAFSA. *Faculty research:* Nutrition policy, management and leadership development, lipid and carbohydrate metabolism, dietary trends and determinants, transmembrane signal transduction and carcinogenesis, maternal and child nutrition. *Unit head:* Dr. Elizabeth Mayer-Davis, Chair, 919-966-7218, E-mail: beth_mayer-davis@unc.edu. *Application contact:* Joanne O. Lee, Student Services Manager, 919-966-7212, Fax: 919-966-7216, E-mail: joanne_lee@unc.edu. Website: http://www2.sph.unc.edu/nutr/

The University of North Carolina at Greensboro, Graduate School, School of Health and Human Sciences, Department of Nutrition, Greensboro, NC 27412-5001. Offers MS, PhD. *Degree requirements:* For master's, thesis; for doctorate, thesis/dissertation. *Entrance requirements:* For master's and doctorate, GRE General Test. Additional exam requirements/recommendations for international students: Required—TOEFL. Electronic applications accepted.

University of North Florida, Brooks College of Health, Department of Nutrition and Dietetics, Jacksonville, FL 32224. Offers MSH. *Program availability:* Part-time. *Faculty:* 7 full-time (6 women), 1 (woman) part-time/adjunct. *Students:* 29 full-time (26 women), 13 part-time (11 women); includes 6 minority (4 Black or African American, non-Hispanic/Latino; 1 Asian, non-Hispanic/Latino; 1 Hispanic/Latino). Average age 27. 37 applicants, 49% accepted, 16 enrolled. In 2015, 16 master's awarded. *Entrance requirements:* For master's, GRE General Test, minimum GPA of 3.0 in last 60 hours. Additional exam requirements/recommendations for international students: Required—TOEFL (minimum score 500 paper-based; 61 iBT). *Application deadline:* For fall admission, 7/1 for domestic students, 5/1 for international students; for spring admission, 11/1 for domestic students, 10/1 for international students. Application fee: $30. Electronic applications accepted. *Expenses:* Tuition, state resident: part-time $408.10 per credit hour. Tuition, nonresident: part-time $932.61 per credit hour. *Required fees:* $111.81 per credit hour. Tuition and fees vary according to course load, campus/location and program. *Financial support:* In 2015–16, 15 students received support, including 2 research assistantships (averaging $624 per year), 1 teaching assistantship (averaging $1,500 per year); career-related internships or fieldwork, Federal Work-Study, scholarships/grants, and tuition waivers (partial) also available. Financial award application deadline: 4/1; financial award applicants required to submit FAFSA. *Total annual research expenditures:* $3,347. *Unit head:* Dr. Judy Rodriguez, Chair, 904-620-1298, E-mail: jrodrigu@unf.edu. *Application contact:* Dr. Catherine Christie, Program Director, 904-620-1423, Fax: 904-620-1942, E-mail: c.christie@unf.edu. Website: http://www.unf.edu/brooks/nutrition

University of Oklahoma Health Sciences Center, Graduate College, College of Allied Health, Department of Nutritional Sciences, Oklahoma City, OK 73190. Offers MS. *Accreditation:* AND. *Degree requirements:* For master's, comprehensive exam, thesis optional. *Entrance requirements:* For master's, GRE General Test, interview, 3 letters of reference. Additional exam requirements/recommendations for international students: Required—TOEFL (minimum score 550 paper-based).

University of Pittsburgh, School of Health and Rehabilitation Sciences, Coordinated Master's in Nutrition and Dietetics Program, Pittsburgh, PA 15260. Offers MS. *Accreditation:* AND. *Program availability:* Part-time. *Faculty:* 6 full-time (all women), 2 part-time/adjunct (both women). *Students:* 35 full-time (32 women); includes 3 minority (1 Asian, non-Hispanic/Latino; 2 Hispanic/Latino), 1 international. Average age 26. 26 applicants, 77% accepted, 17 enrolled. In 2015, 18 master's awarded. *Entrance requirements:* For master's, GRE, volunteer experience. Additional exam requirements/ recommendations for international students: Required—TOEFL (minimum score 550 paper-based; 80 iBT), IELTS (minimum score 6.5). *Application deadline:* For fall admission, 3/15 for domestic students, 3/1 for international students. Applications are processed on a rolling basis. Application fee: $50. Electronic applications accepted. *Expenses:* Contact institution. *Financial support:* In 2015–16, 1 student received support. Scholarships/grants available. *Faculty research:* Targeted approaches to weight control, pediatric obesity treatment, effect of tart cherry juice on muscles. *Total annual research expenditures:* $32,194. *Unit head:* Dr. Kevin Conley, Department Chair/ Associate Professor, 412-383-6737, Fax: 412-383-6527, E-mail: kconley@pitt.edu. *Application contact:* Jessica Maguire, Director of Admissions, 412-383-6557, Fax: 412-383-6535, E-mail: maguire@pitt.edu.
Website: http://www.shrs.pitt.edu/ndms/

University of Puerto Rico, Medical Sciences Campus, Graduate School of Public Health, Department of Human Development, Program in Nutrition, San Juan, PR 00936-5067. Offers MS. *Program availability:* Part-time. *Degree requirements:* For master's, thesis. *Entrance requirements:* For master's, GRE, previous course work in algebra, biochemistry, biology, chemistry, and social sciences.

University of Puerto Rico, Medical Sciences Campus, School of Health Professions, Program in Dietetics Internship, San Juan, PR 00936-5067. Offers Certificate. *Degree requirements:* For Certificate, one foreign language, clinical practice. *Entrance requirements:* For degree, minimum GPA of 2.5, interview, participation in the computer matching process by the American Dietetic Association.

University of Puerto Rico, Medical Sciences Campus, School of Medicine, Biomedical Sciences Graduate Program, Department of Biochemistry, San Juan, PR 00936-5067. Offers MS, PhD. *Degree requirements:* For master's, thesis; for doctorate, comprehensive exam, thesis/dissertation. *Entrance requirements:* For master's and doctorate, GRE General Test, GRE Subject Test, interview, minimum GPA of 3.0. Electronic applications accepted. *Faculty research:* Genetics, cell and molecular biology, cancer biology, protein structure/function, glycosilation of proteins.

University of Puerto Rico, Río Piedras Campus, College of Education, Program in Family Ecology and Nutrition, San Juan, PR 00931-3300. Offers M Ed. *Program availability:* Part-time. *Degree requirements:* For master's, thesis. *Entrance requirements:* For master's, PAEG or GRE, minimum GPA of 3.0, letter of recommendation.

University of Rhode Island, Graduate School, College of the Environment and Life Sciences, Department of Nutrition and Food Sciences, Kingston, RI 02881. Offers dietetic internship (MS); nutrition (MS, PhD). *Program availability:* Part-time. *Faculty:* 6 full-time (5 women), 2 part-time/adjunct (1 woman). *Students:* 11 full-time (7 women), 9 part-time (all women); includes 4 minority (2 Asian, non-Hispanic/Latino; 1 Hispanic/ Latino; 1 Two or more races, non-Hispanic/Latino). In 2015, 5 master's awarded. *Degree requirements:* For master's, comprehensive exam (for some programs), thesis optional; for doctorate, thesis/dissertation. *Entrance requirements:* For master's, GRE, 2 letters of recommendation (3 for MS in dietetic internship); for doctorate, GRE, 2 letters of recommendation. Additional exam requirements/recommendations for international students: Required—TOEFL (minimum score 550 paper-based). *Application deadline:* For fall admission, 2/15 for domestic students, 2/1 for international students; for spring admission, 11/15 for domestic students, 7/15 for international students. Application fee: $65. Electronic applications accepted. *Expenses:* Tuition, state resident: full-time $11,796; part-time $655 per credit. Tuition, nonresident: full-time $24,206; part-time $1345 per credit. *Required fees:* $1546; $44 per credit. One-time fee: $155 full-time; $35 part-time. *Financial support:* In 2015–16, 2 research assistantships with tuition reimbursements (averaging $11,883 per year), 1 teaching assistantship (averaging $7,922 per year) were awarded. Financial award application deadline: 2/15; financial award applicants required to submit FAFSA. *Faculty research:* Food safety and quality, marine resource utilization, nutrition in underserved populations, eating behavior, lipid metabolism. *Total annual research expenditures:* $1.6 million. *Unit head:* Dr. Cathy English, Chair, 401-874-5689, Fax: 401-874-5974, E-mail: cathy@uri.edu. *Application contact:* Graduate Admissions, 401-874-2872, E-mail: gradadm@etal.uri.edu.
Website: http://cels.uri.edu/nfs/

University of Saint Joseph, Department of Nutrition and Dietetics, West Hartford, CT 06117-2700. Offers nutrition (MS). *Program availability:* Part-time, evening/weekend, online learning. *Entrance requirements:* For master's, 2 letters of recommendation, letter of intent. *Application deadline:* Applications are processed on a rolling basis. Application fee: $50. Electronic applications accepted. Application fee is waived when completed online. *Financial support:* Career-related internships or fieldwork and unspecified assistantships available. Support available to part-time students. Financial award applicants required to submit FAFSA.
Website: http://www.usj.edu/academics/schools/school-of-health-natural-sciences/nutrition-dietetics/

University of Southern Mississippi, Graduate School, College of Health, Department of Nutrition and Food Systems, Hattiesburg, MS 39406-0001. Offers nutrition (MS, PhD). *Program availability:* Part-time. *Degree requirements:* For master's, comprehensive exam, thesis (for some programs); for doctorate, comprehensive exam, thesis/ dissertation. *Entrance requirements:* For master's, GRE General Test, minimum GPA of 2.75 on last 60 hours; for doctorate, GRE General Test, minimum GPA of 3.5. Additional exam requirements/recommendations for international students: Required—TOEFL, IELTS.

University of South Florida, Innovative Education, Tampa, FL 33620-9951. Offers adult, career and higher education (Graduate Certificate), including college teaching, leadership in developing human resources, leadership in higher education; Africana studies (Graduate Certificate), including diasporas and health disparities, genocide and human rights; aging studies (Graduate Certificate), including gerontology; art research (Graduate Certificate), including museum studies; business foundations (Graduate Certificate); chemical and biomedical engineering (Graduate Certificate), including materials science and engineering, water, health and sustainability; child and family studies (Graduate Certificate), including positive behavior support; civil and industrial engineering (Graduate Certificate), including transportation systems analysis; community and family health (Graduate Certificate), including maternal and child health, social marketing and public health, violence and injury: prevention and intervention, women's health; criminology (Graduate Certificate), including criminal justice administration; educational measurement and research (Graduate Certificate), including evaluation; English (Graduate Certificate), including comparative literary studies, creative writing, professional and technical communication; entrepreneurship (Graduate Certificate); environmental health (Graduate Certificate), including safety management; epidemiology and biostatistics (Graduate Certificate), including applied biostatistics, biostatistics, concepts and tools of epidemiology, epidemiology, epidemiology of infectious diseases; geography, environment and planning (Graduate Certificate), including community development, environmental policy and management, geographical information systems; geology (Graduate Certificate), including hydrogeology; global health (Graduate Certificate), including disaster management, global health and Latin American and Caribbean studies, global health practice, humanitarian assistance, infection control; government and international affairs (Graduate Certificate), including Cuban studies, globalization studies; health policy and management (Graduate Certificate), including health management and leadership, public health policy and programs; hearing specialist: early intervention (Graduate Certificate); industrial and management systems engineering (Graduate Certificate), including systems engineering, technology management; information studies (Graduate Certificate), including school library media specialist; information systems/decision sciences (Graduate Certificate), including analytics and business intelligence; instructional technology (Graduate Certificate), including distance education, Florida digital/virtual educator, instructional design, multimedia design, Web design; internal medicine, bioethics and medical humanities (Graduate Certificate), including biomedical ethics; Latin American and Caribbean studies (Graduate Certificate); mass communications (Graduate Certificate), including multimedia journalism; mathematics and statistics (Graduate Certificate), including mathematics; medicine (Graduate Certificate), including aging and neuroscience, bioinformatics, biotechnology, brain fitness and memory management, clinical investigation, health informatics, health sciences, integrative weight management, intellectual property, medicine and gender, metabolic and nutritional medicine, metabolic cardiology, pharmacy sciences; national and competitive intelligence (Graduate Certificate); psychological and social foundations (Graduate Certificate), including career counseling, college teaching, diversity in education, mental health counseling, school counseling; public affairs (Graduate Certificate), including nonprofit management, public management, research administration; public health (Graduate Certificate), including environmental health, health equity, public health generalist, translational research in adolescent behavioral health; public health practices (Graduate Certificate), including planning for healthy communities; rehabilitation and mental health counseling (Graduate Certificate), including integrative mental health care, marriage and family therapy, rehabilitation technology; secondary education (Graduate Certificate), including ESOL, foreign language education: culture and content, foreign language education: professional; social work (Graduate Certificate), including geriatric social work/clinical gerontology; special education (Graduate Certificate), including autism spectrum disorder, disabilities education: severe/profound; world languages (Graduate Certificate), including teaching English as a second language (TESL) or foreign language. *Unit head:* Kathy Barnes, Interdisciplinary Programs Coordinator, 813-974-8031, Fax: 813-974-7061, E-mail: barnesk@usf.edu. *Application contact:* Karen Tylinski, Metro Initiatives, 813-974-9943, Fax: 813-974-7061, E-mail: ktylinsk@usf.edu.
Website: http://www.usf.edu/innovative-education/

University of South Florida, Morsani College of Medicine and College of Graduate Studies, Graduate Programs in Medical Sciences, Tampa, FL 33620-9951. Offers advanced athletic training (MS); athletic training (MS); bioinformatics and computational biology (MSBCB); biotechnology (MSB); health informatics (MSHI); medical sciences (MSMS, PhD), including aging and neuroscience (MSMS), allergy, immunology and infectious disease (PhD), anatomy, athletic training (MSMS), clinical and translational research, health informatics (MSMS), health science (MSMS), interdisciplinary medical sciences (MSMS), medical microbiology and immunology (MSMS), metabolic and nutritional medicine (MSMS), molecular medicine, molecular pharmacology and physiology (PhD), neurology (PhD), pathology and laboratory medicine (PhD), pharmacology and therapeutics (PhD), physiology and biophysics (PhD), women's health (MSMS). *Students:* 510 full-time (261 women), 318 part-time (208 women); includes 360 minority (108 Black or African American, non-Hispanic/Latino; 3 American Indian or Alaska Native, non-Hispanic/Latino; 101 Asian, non-Hispanic/Latino; 124 Hispanic/Latino; 1 Native Hawaiian or other Pacific Islander, non-Hispanic/Latino; 23 Two or more races, non-Hispanic/Latino), 52 international. Average age 26. 6,567 applicants, 13% accepted, 469 enrolled. In 2015, 216 master's awarded. Terminal master's awarded for partial completion of doctoral program. *Degree requirements:* For master's, comprehensive exam, thesis; for doctorate, comprehensive exam, thesis/ dissertation. *Entrance requirements:* For master's, GRE General Test or GMAT, bachelor's degree or equivalent from regionally-accredited university with minimum GPA of 3.0 in upper-division sciences coursework; prerequisites in general biology, general chemistry, general physics, organic chemistry, quantitative analysis, and integral and differential calculus; for doctorate, GRE General Test, bachelor's degree from regionally-accredited university with minimum GPA of 3.0 in upper-division sciences coursework; 3 letters of recommendation; personal interview; 1-2 page personal statement; prerequisites in biology, chemistry, physics, organic chemistry, quantitative analysis, and integral/differential calculus. Additional exam requirements/ recommendations for international students: Required—TOEFL (minimum score 550 paper-based; 79 iBT) or IELTS (minimum score 6.5). *Application deadline:* For fall admission, 2/15 for domestic students, 1/2 for international students. Application fee: $30. *Expenses:* Contact institution. *Faculty research:* Anatomy, biochemistry, cancer biology, cardiovascular disease, cell biology, immunology, microbiology, molecular biology, neuroscience, pharmacology, physiology. *Unit head:* Dr. Michael Barber, Professor/Associate Dean for Graduate and Postdoctoral Affairs, 813-974-9908, Fax: 813-974-4317, E-mail: mbarber@health.usf.edu. *Application contact:* Dr. Eric Bennett, Graduate Director, PhD Program in Medical Sciences, 813-974-1545, Fax: 813-974-4317, E-mail: esbennet@health.usf.edu.
Website: http://health.usf.edu/nocms/medicine/graduatestudies/

The University of Tampa, Program in Exercise and Nutrition Science, Tampa, FL 33606-1490. Offers MS. *Program availability:* Part-time, evening/weekend. *Faculty:* 6 full-time (3 women). *Students:* 47 full-time (17 women), 5 part-time (2 women); includes 2 minority (both Black or African American, non-Hispanic/Latino), 3 international. Average age 25. 185 applicants, 40% accepted, 42 enrolled. *Degree requirements:* For master's, comprehensive exam, practicum. *Entrance requirements:* For master's, GMAT or GRE, bachelor's degree in a related field. Additional exam requirements/ recommendations for international students: Required—TOEFL (minimum score 577 paper-based; 90 iBT), IELTS (minimum score 7.5). *Application deadline:* Applications are processed on a rolling basis. Application fee: $40. Electronic applications accepted. *Expenses:* $573 per credit tuition, $80 per term fees. *Financial support:* In 2015–16, 5 students received support. Career-related internships or fieldwork, scholarships/grants, and unspecified assistantships available. Financial award applicants required to submit FAFSA. *Application contact:* Chanelle Cox, Staff Assistant, Admissions for Graduate and Continuing Studies, 813-253-6249, E-mail: ccox@ut.edu.
Website: http://www.ut.edu/msexercisenutrition/

The University of Tennessee, Graduate School, College of Education, Health and Human Sciences, Department of Nutrition, Knoxville, TN 37996. Offers nutrition (MS), including nutrition science, public health nutrition; MS/MPH. *Program availability:* Part-time. *Degree requirements:* For master's, thesis or alternative. *Entrance requirements:*

Nutrition

For master's, GRE General Test, minimum GPA of 2.7. Additional exam requirements/recommendations for international students: Required—TOEFL. Electronic applications accepted.

The University of Tennessee at Martin, Graduate Programs, College of Agriculture and Applied Sciences, Department of Family and Consumer Sciences, Martin, TN 38238. Offers dietetics (MSFCS); general family and consumer sciences (MSFCS). *Program availability:* Part-time, 100% online. *Faculty:* 8. *Students:* 1 (woman) full-time, 42 part-time (38 women); includes 13 minority (9 Black or African American, non-Hispanic/Latino; 3 Hispanic/Latino; 1 Two or more races, non-Hispanic/Latino). Average age 28. 74 applicants, 74% accepted, 24 enrolled. In 2015, 9 master's awarded. *Degree requirements:* For master's, comprehensive exam, thesis optional. *Entrance requirements:* For master's, GRE General Test, minimum GPA of 2.5. Additional exam requirements/recommendations for international students: Required—TOEFL (minimum score 525 paper-based; 71 iBT). *Application deadline:* For fall admission, 7/27 priority date for domestic and international students; for spring admission, 12/17 priority date for domestic and international students; for summer admission, 5/10 priority date for domestic and international students. Applications are processed on a rolling basis. Application fee: $30 ($130 for international students). Electronic applications accepted. *Expenses:* Tuition, state resident: full-time $8254; part-time $459 per credit hour. Tuition, nonresident: full-time $22,198; part-time $1234 per credit hour. *Required fees:* $79 per credit hour. Part-time tuition and fees vary according to course load and campus/location. *Financial support:* In 2015–16, 7 students received support, including 1 research assistantship (averaging $7,540 per year), 6 teaching assistantships with full tuition reimbursements available (averaging $7,518 per year); scholarships/grants and unspecified assistantships also available. Financial award application deadline: 2/1; financial award applicants required to submit FAFSA. *Faculty research:* Children with developmental disabilities, regional food product development and marketing, parent education. *Unit head:* Dr. Lisa LeBleu, Coordinator, 731-881-7116, Fax: 731-881-7106, E-mail: llebleu@utm.edu. *Application contact:* Jolene L. Cunningham, Student Services Specialist, 731-881-7012, Fax: 731-881-7499, E-mail: jcunningham@utm.edu. Website: http://www.utm.edu/departments/caas/fcs/index.php

The University of Texas at Austin, Graduate School, College of Natural Sciences, School of Human Ecology, Program in Nutritional Sciences, Austin, TX 78712-1111. Offers nutrition (MA); nutritional sciences (PhD). *Degree requirements:* For master's, thesis; for doctorate, thesis/dissertation. *Entrance requirements:* For master's and doctorate, GRE General Test. Additional exam requirements/recommendations for international students: Required—TOEFL. Electronic applications accepted. *Faculty research:* Nutritional biochemistry, nutrient health assessment, obesity, nutrition education, molecular/cellular aspects of nutrient functions.

The University of Texas Southwestern Medical Center, Southwestern School of Health Professions, Clinical Nutrition Program, Dallas, TX 75390. Offers MCN. *Accreditation:* AND.

University of the District of Columbia, College of Agriculture, Urban Sustainability and Environmental Sciences, Program in Nutrition and Dietetics, Washington, DC 20008-1175. Offers MS. *Degree requirements:* For master's, thesis. *Entrance requirements:* For master's, GRE, 3 letters of recommendation, personal interview. *Application deadline:* For fall admission, 4/15 for domestic students. Application fee: $50. Website: http://www.udc.edu/nutrition/ms_program.htm

University of the Incarnate Word, School of Graduate Studies and Research, H-E-B School of Business and Administration, Programs in Administration, San Antonio, TX 78209-6397. Offers adult education (MAA); communication arts (MAA); nutrition (MAA); organizational development (MAA); sports management (MAA). *Program availability:* Part-time, evening/weekend, online learning. *Faculty:* 13 full-time (5 women), 14 part-time/adjunct (5 women). *Students:* 16 full-time (8 women), 27 part-time (14 women); includes 20 minority (19 Hispanic/Latino; 1 Two or more races, non-Hispanic/Latino), 12 international. Average age 30. 25 applicants, 100% accepted, 11 enrolled. In 2015, 33 master's awarded. *Degree requirements:* For master's, capstone. *Entrance requirements:* For master's, GRE, GMAT, undergraduate degree, minimum GPA of 2.5. Additional exam requirements/recommendations for international students: Required—TOEFL (minimum score 560 paper-based; 83 iBT). *Application deadline:* Applications are processed on a rolling basis. Application fee: $20. Electronic applications accepted. *Expenses:* Tuition, area resident: Part-time $885 per credit hour. *Required fees:* $40 per credit hour. Tuition and fees vary according to course load, degree level, campus/location, program and student level. *Financial support:* Federal Work-Study, scholarships/grants, tuition waivers, and unspecified assistantships available. Financial award applicants required to submit FAFSA. *Unit head:* Dr. Mark Teachout, Programs Director, 210-829-3177, Fax: 210-805-3564, E-mail: teachout@uiwtx.edu. *Application contact:* Johnny Garcia, Graduate Admissions Counselor, 210-829-3554, Fax: 210-829-3921, E-mail: admis@uiwtx.edu. Website: http://www.uiw.edu/maa/

University of the Incarnate Word, School of Graduate Studies and Research, School of Mathematics, Science, and Engineering, Program in Nutrition, San Antonio, TX 78209-6397. Offers administration (MS); nutrition education and health promotion (MS). *Program availability:* Part-time, evening/weekend. *Faculty:* 8 full-time (4 women), 1 (woman) part-time/adjunct. *Students:* 8 full-time (all women), 22 part-time (19 women); includes 18 minority (1 Asian, non-Hispanic/Latino; 17 Hispanic/Latino), 1 international. Average age 26. 46 applicants, 89% accepted, 14 enrolled. In 2015, 5 master's awarded. *Degree requirements:* For master's, comprehensive exam, thesis or alternative. *Entrance requirements:* For master's, two letters of recommendation. Additional exam requirements/recommendations for international students: Required—TOEFL (minimum score 560 paper-based; 83 iBT). *Application deadline:* Applications are processed on a rolling basis. Application fee: $20. Electronic applications accepted. *Expenses:* Tuition, area resident: Part-time $885 per credit hour. *Required fees:* $40 per credit hour. Tuition and fees vary according to course load, degree level, campus/location, program and student level. *Financial support:* In 2015–16, research assistantships (averaging $5,000 per year) were awarded; Federal Work-Study and scholarships/grants also available. Financial award applicants required to submit FAFSA. *Faculty research:* Nutrition. *Unit head:* Dr. Beth Senne-Duff, Associate Professor, 210-829-3165, Fax: 210-829-3153, E-mail: beths@uiwtx.edu. *Application contact:* Johnny Garcia, Assistant Director of Graduate Admissions, 210-805-3554, Fax: 210-829-3921, E-mail: admis@uiwtx.edu. Website: http://www.uiw.edu/nutrition/nutrition3.htm

The University of Toledo, College of Graduate Studies, College of Medicine and Life Sciences, Department of Public Health and Preventative Medicine, Toledo, OH 43606-3390. Offers biostatistics and epidemiology (Certificate); contemporary gerontological practice (Certificate); environmental and occupational health and safety (MPH); epidemiology (Certificate); global public health (Certificate); health promotion and education (MPH); industrial hygiene (MSOH); medical and health science teaching and learning (Certificate); occupational health (Certificate); public health administration (MPH); public health and emergency response (Certificate); public health epidemiology (MPH); public health nutrition (MPH); MD/MPH. *Program availability:* Part-time, evening/weekend. *Degree requirements:* For master's, thesis or alternative. *Entrance requirements:* For master's, GRE, minimum undergraduate GPA of 3.0, three letters of

recommendation, statement of purpose, transcripts from all prior institutions attended, resume; for Certificate, minimum undergraduate GPA of 3.0, three letters of recommendation, statement of purpose, transcripts from all prior institutions attended, resume. Additional exam requirements/recommendations for international students: Required—TOEFL (minimum score 550 paper-based; 80 iBT), IELTS (minimum score 6.5). Electronic applications accepted.

University of Toronto, Faculty of Medicine, Department of Nutritional Sciences, Toronto, ON M5S 1A1, Canada. Offers M Sc, PhD. *Program availability:* Part-time. *Degree requirements:* For master's, thesis, oral thesis defense; for doctorate, comprehensive exam, thesis/dissertation, departmental examination, oral examination. *Entrance requirements:* For master's, minimum B average, background in nutrition or an area of biological or health sciences, 2 letters of reference; for doctorate, minimum B+ average in final 2 years, background in nutrition or an area of biological or health sciences, 2 letters of reference. Additional exam requirements/recommendations for international students: Required—TOEFL (minimum score 580 paper-based), TWE (minimum score 5), IELTS (minimum score 7), Michigan English Language Assessment Battery (minimum score 85), or COPE (minimum score 4). Electronic applications accepted.

University of Toronto, School of Graduate Studies, Department of Public Health Sciences, Toronto, ON M5S 1A1, Canada. Offers biostatistics (M Sc, PhD); community health (M Sc); community nutrition (MPH), including nutrition and dietetics; epidemiology (MPH, PhD); family and community medicine (MPH); occupational and environmental health (MPH); social and behavioral health science (PhD); social and behavioral health sciences (MPH), including health promotion. *Accreditation:* CAHME (one or more programs are accredited); CEPH (one or more programs are accredited). *Program availability:* Part-time. *Degree requirements:* For master's, thesis (for some programs), practicum; for doctorate, comprehensive exam, thesis/dissertation, oral thesis defense. *Entrance requirements:* For master's, 2 letters of reference, relevant professional/research experience, minimum B average in final year; for doctorate, 2 letters of reference, relevant professional/research experience, minimum B+ average. Additional exam requirements/recommendations for international students: Required—TOEFL (minimum score 580 paper-based; 93 iBT), TWE (minimum score 5). Electronic applications accepted. *Expenses:* Contact institution.

University of Utah, Graduate School, College of Health, Division of Nutrition, Salt Lake City, UT 84112. Offers nutrition and integrative physiology (MS, PhD), including integrative physiology (MS), nutrition (MS). *Accreditation:* AND. *Program availability:* 100% online. *Faculty:* 4 full-time (2 women), 12 part-time/adjunct (10 women). *Students:* 36 full-time (29 women), 6 part-time (5 women); includes 3 minority (1 American Indian or Alaska Native, non-Hispanic/Latino; 1 Native Hawaiian or other Pacific Islander, non-Hispanic/Latino; 1 Two or more races, non-Hispanic/Latino), 1 international. Average age 27. 65 applicants, 26% accepted, 17 enrolled. In 2015, 17 master's awarded. Terminal master's awarded for partial completion of doctoral program. *Degree requirements:* For master's, comprehensive exam, thesis; for doctorate, thesis/dissertation. *Entrance requirements:* For master's, GRE General Test, minimum undergraduate GPA of 3.0; for doctorate, GRE General Test. Additional exam requirements/recommendations for international students: Required—TOEFL (minimum score 500 paper-based). *Application deadline:* For fall and winter admission, 2/15 for domestic and international students. Application fee: $55 ($65 for international students). Electronic applications accepted. *Expenses:* Contact institution. *Financial support:* In 2015–16, 22 students received support, including 2 research assistantships with partial tuition reimbursements available (averaging $7,250 per year), 10 teaching assistantships with partial tuition reimbursements available (averaging $7,250 per year); career-related internships or fieldwork, scholarships/grants, and unspecified assistantships also available. Financial award application deadline: 2/15; financial award applicants required to submit FAFSA. *Faculty research:* Cholesterol metabolism, sport nutrition education, metabolic and critical care, cardiovascular nutrition, wilderness nutrition, pediatric nutrition. *Total annual research expenditures:* $120,000. *Unit head:* Dr. Julie Metos, Director, 801-587-3024, Fax: 801-585-3874, E-mail: julie.metos@hsc.utah.edu. *Application contact:* Jean Zancanella, Academic Adviser, 801-581-5280, Fax: 801-585-3874, E-mail: jean.zancanella@health.utah.edu. Website: http://www.health.utah.edu/fdnu/

University of Vermont, Graduate College, College of Agriculture and Life Sciences, Department of Nutrition and Food Sciences, Burlington, VT 05405. Offers dietetics (MSD); nutritional sciences (MS). *Accreditation:* AND. *Degree requirements:* For master's, thesis. *Entrance requirements:* For master's, GRE General Test. Additional exam requirements/recommendations for international students: Required—TOEFL (minimum score 550 paper-based; 80 iBT). *Application deadline:* For fall admission, 2/15 priority date for domestic students, 2/15 for international students; for spring admission, 11/15 for domestic students. Applications are processed on a rolling basis. Application fee: $65. Electronic applications accepted. *Financial support:* Research assistantships available. Financial award application deadline: 3/1. *Unit head:* Dr. Stephen Pintauro, 802-656-3374, E-mail: stephen.pintauro@uvm.edu. *Application contact:* Dr. Stephen Pintauro, 802-656-3374, E-mail: stephen.pintauro@uvm.edu.

University of Vermont, Graduate College, College of Agriculture and Life Sciences, Program in Animal, Nutrition and Food Sciences, Burlington, VT 05405. Offers PhD. *Degree requirements:* For doctorate, one foreign language, thesis/dissertation. *Entrance requirements:* For doctorate, GRE General Test. Additional exam requirements/recommendations for international students: Required—TOEFL (minimum score 550 paper-based; 80 iBT). *Application deadline:* For fall admission, 4/1 priority date for domestic students, 4/1 for international students. Applications are processed on a rolling basis. Application fee: $65. Electronic applications accepted. *Financial support:* Application deadline: 3/1. *Application contact:* Dr. David Kerr, Coordinator, 802-656-2070, E-mail: stephen.pintauro@uvm.edu.

University of Washington, Graduate School, School of Public Health, Nutritional Sciences Program, Seattle, WA 98195. Offers MPH, MS, PhD. *Accreditation:* AND. *Program availability:* Part-time. Terminal master's awarded for partial completion of doctoral program. *Degree requirements:* For master's, thesis, practicum (MPH); for doctorate, thesis/dissertation. *Entrance requirements:* For master's, GRE General Test; for doctorate, GRE General Test, master's degree, minimum GPA of 3.0. Additional exam requirements/recommendations for international students: Required—TOEFL (minimum score 580 paper-based; 92 iBT), IELTS (minimum score 7). Electronic applications accepted. *Expenses:* Contact institution. *Faculty research:* Dietary behavior, dietary supplements, obesity, clinical nutrition, addictive behaviors.

University of Wisconsin–Madison, Graduate School, College of Agricultural and Life Sciences, Department of Nutritional Sciences, Madison, WI 53706. Offers MS, PhD. Terminal master's awarded for partial completion of doctoral program. *Degree requirements:* For master's, thesis or research report; for doctorate, comprehensive exam, thesis/dissertation. *Entrance requirements:* For master's and doctorate, GRE General Test. Additional exam requirements/recommendations for international students: Required—TOEFL (minimum score 550 paper-based; 80 iBT). Electronic applications accepted. *Expenses:* Tuition, state resident: full-time $5364. Tuition, nonresident: full-time $12,027. *Required fees:* $571. Tuition and fees vary according to campus/location, program and reciprocity agreements. *Faculty research:* Human and animal nutrition, nutrition epidemiology, nutrition education, biochemical and molecular nutrition.

University of Wisconsin–Stevens Point, College of Professional Studies, School of Health Promotion and Human Development, Program in Nutritional Sciences, Stevens Point, WI 54481-3897. Offers MS. *Program availability:* Part-time. *Degree requirements:* For master's, thesis or alternative. *Entrance requirements:* For master's, minimum GPA of 2.75.

University of Wisconsin–Stout, Graduate School, College of Education, Health and Human Sciences, Program in Food and Nutritional Sciences, Menomonie, WI 54751. Offers MS. *Program availability:* Part-time. *Degree requirements:* For master's, thesis. *Entrance requirements:* For master's, minimum GPA of 3.0. Additional exam requirements/recommendations for international students: Required—TOEFL (minimum score 500 paper-based; 61 iBT). Electronic applications accepted. *Faculty research:* Disease states and nutrition, childhood obesity, nutraceuticals, food safety, nanotechnology.

University of Wyoming, College of Agriculture and Natural Resources, Department of Animal Sciences, Program in Food Science and Human Nutrition, Laramie, WY 82071. Offers MS. *Degree requirements:* For master's, thesis. *Entrance requirements:* For master's, GRE General Test, minimum GPA of 3.0. Additional exam requirements/ recommendations for international students: Required—TOEFL (minimum score 525 paper-based). Electronic applications accepted. *Faculty research:* Protein and lipid metabolism, food microbiology, food safety, meat science.

Utah State University, School of Graduate Studies, College of Agriculture, Department of Nutrition, Dietetics, and Food Sciences, Logan, UT 84322. Offers dietetic administration (MDA); nutrition and food sciences (MS, PhD). *Program availability:* Online learning. *Degree requirements:* For master's, thesis; for doctorate, comprehensive exam, thesis/dissertation, teaching experience. *Entrance requirements:* For master's, GRE General Test, minimum GPA of 3.0, course work in chemistry, biochemistry, physics, math, bacteriology, physiology; for doctorate, GRE General Test, minimum GPA of 3.2, course work in chemistry, MS or manuscript in referred journal. Additional exam requirements/recommendations for international students: Required— TOEFL (minimum score 550 paper-based). Electronic applications accepted. *Faculty research:* Mineral balance, meat microbiology and nitrate interactions, milk ultrafiltration, lactic culture, milk coagulation.

Virginia Polytechnic Institute and State University, Graduate School, College of Agriculture and Life Sciences, Blacksburg, VA 24061. Offers agricultural and applied economics (MS); agricultural and life sciences (MS); animal and poultry science (MS, PhD); crop and soil environmental sciences (MS, PhD); dairy science (MS); entomology (PhD); horticulture (MS, PhD); human nutrition, foods and exercise (MS, PhD); life sciences (MS, PhD); plant pathology, physiology and weed science (PhD). *Degree requirements:* For master's, comprehensive exam (for some programs), thesis (for some programs); for doctorate, comprehensive exam (for some programs), thesis/dissertation (for some programs). *Entrance requirements:* For master's and doctorate, GRE/GMAT (may vary by department). Additional exam requirements/recommendations for international students: Required—TOEFL (minimum score 550 paper-based). Electronic applications accepted.

Washington State University, College of Pharmacy, Nutrition and Exercise Physiology Program, Pullman, WA 99164. Offers MS. Programs offered at the Spokane campus. *Accreditation:* AND. *Degree requirements:* For master's, internship. *Entrance requirements:* For master's, BS in nutrition and exercise physiology, exercise science, human nutrition, or related degree; interview.

Wayne State University, College of Liberal Arts and Sciences, Department of Nutrition and Food Science, Detroit, MI 48202. Offers dietetics (Postbaccalaureate Certificate); food science (PhD); nutrition (PhD); nutrition and food science (MA, MS). Postbaccalaureate Certificate program admits only in Fall with April 1 application deadline. *Faculty:* 10 full-time (7 women), 6 part-time/adjunct (3 women). *Students:* 31 full-time (23 women), 10 part-time (all women); includes 4 minority (2 Asian, non-Hispanic/Latino; 1 Hispanic/Latino; 1 Two or more races, non-Hispanic/Latino), 23 international. Average age 29. 95 applicants, 31% accepted, 13 enrolled. In 2015, 12 master's, 4 doctorates awarded. *Degree requirements:* For master's, thesis (for some programs), essay (for MA); for doctorate, thesis/dissertation. *Entrance requirements:* For

master's, GRE General Test, two letters of recommendation; minimum GPA of 3.0; basic courses in nutrition and food science; courses in human nutrition and metabolism, food chemistry, introductory microbiology, anatomy and physiology, and organic chemistry (for MS); for doctorate, GRE, MS in nutrition and/or food science or in a cognate science with a minimum GPA of 3.5; three letters of recommendation; personal statement; interview (live or web-based); for Postbaccalaureate Certificate, bachelor's degree. Additional exam requirements/recommendations for international students: Required—TOEFL (minimum score 550 paper-based; 79 iBT), TWE (minimum score 5.5), Michigan English Language Assessment Battery (minimum score 85); Recommended—IELTS (minimum score 6.5). *Application deadline:* For fall admission, 2/1 priority date for domestic and international students. Application fee: $0. Electronic applications accepted. *Expenses:* Tuition, state resident: full-time $14,165; part-time $590.20 per credit hour. Tuition, nonresident: full-time $30,682; part-time $1278.40 per credit hour. *Required fees:* $1688; $47.45 per credit hour. $274.60 per semester. Tuition and fees vary according to course load and program. *Financial support:* In 2015–16, 17 students received support, including 1 fellowship with tuition reimbursement available (averaging $16,000 per year), 1 research assistantship with tuition reimbursement available (averaging $22,000 per year), 9 teaching assistantships with tuition reimbursements available (averaging $18,801 per year); scholarships/grants, health care benefits, and unspecified assistantships also available. Financial award application deadline: 3/31; financial award applicants required to submit FAFSA. *Faculty research:* Nutrition cancer; mechanisms by which aging increases cancer risk; nutrition and exercise, nutrition, cancer and metabolomics; diet-induced obesity and diabetes; cholesterol and lipoprotein metabolism; dietetics; food microbiology, antimicrobial resistance, microbial detection; food and nutraceutical chemistry. *Total annual research expenditures:* $1 million. *Unit head:* Dr. Ahmad R. Heydari, Professor and Chair, 313-577-2500, E-mail: ahmad.heydari@wayne.edu. *Application contact:* Dr. Pramod Khosla, Graduate Director, 313-577-0448, Fax. 313-577-8010, E-mail: nfsgradprogram@wayne.edu.
Website: http://clas.wayne.edu/nfs/

West Virginia University, Davis College of Agriculture, Forestry and Consumer Sciences, Division of Animal and Nutritional Sciences, Program in Animal and Nutritional Sciences, Morgantown, WV 26506. Offers breeding (MS); food sciences (MS); nutrition (MS); physiology (MS); production management (MS); reproduction (MS). *Program availability:* Part-time. *Degree requirements:* For master's, thesis, oral and written exams. *Entrance requirements:* For master's, GRE, minimum GPA of 3.0. Additional exam requirements/recommendations for international students: Required—TOEFL. *Expenses:* Tuition, state resident: full-time $8568. Tuition, nonresident: full-time $22,140. Tuition and fees vary according to program. *Faculty research:* Animal nutrition, reproductive physiology, food science.

Winthrop University, College of Arts and Sciences, Department of Human Nutrition, Rock Hill, SC 29733. Offers dietics (Certificate); human nutrition (MS). *Program availability:* Part-time. *Faculty:* 2 full-time, 5 part-time/adjunct. *Students:* 43 full-time (38 women), 27 part-time (25 women); includes 9 minority (6 Black or African American, non-Hispanic/Latino; 1 Asian, non-Hispanic/Latino; 1 Hispanic/Latino; 1 Two or more races, non-Hispanic/Latino), 2 international. Average age 27. In 2015, 20 master's, 16 other advanced degrees awarded. *Degree requirements:* For master's, thesis. *Entrance requirements:* For master's, GRE General Test, PRAXIS, or MAT, interview, minimum GPA of 3.0. Additional exam requirements/recommendations for international students: Required—TOEFL (minimum score 550 paper-based; 79 iBT), IELTS (minimum score 6). *Application deadline:* For fall admission, 7/15 priority date for domestic students; for spring admission, 12/1 for domestic students. Applications are processed on a rolling basis. Application fee: $50. Electronic applications accepted. *Expenses: Tuition, area resident:* Part-time $579 per credit hour. Tuition, state resident: full-time $13,828. Tuition, nonresident: full-time $26,638; part-time $1114 per credit hour. *Financial support:* Research assistantships with full tuition reimbursements, career-related internships or fieldwork, Federal Work-Study, scholarships/grants, and unspecified assistantships available. Support available to part-time students. Financial award application deadline: 2/1. *Unit head:* Dr. Wanda Koszewski, Chair, 803-323-4520, E-mail: humannutrition@winthrop.edu. *Application contact:* 800-411-7041, Fax: 803-323-2292, E-mail: gradschool@winthrop.edu.

SAINT LOUIS UNIVERSITY
Department of Nutrition and Dietetics

 For more information, visit http://petersons.to/slu_nutrition-dietetics

Programs of Study

The Department of Nutrition and Dietetics at Saint Louis University is committed to education, research, and service. It cultivates competent, compassionate, and ethical dietetic professionals and prepares them for leadership roles in administration, teaching, and the expansion of knowledge in nutrition and dietetics. The department offers a Master of Science (M.S.) in Nutrition and Dietetics program with five concentrations. These programs can be completed on a full- or part-time basis, and most classes are held in the late afternoons and evenings.

The **M.S. in Nutrition and Dietetics, Nutrition and Physical Performance** was created for professionals with baccalaureate degrees in allied health fields. It consists of 30 or more semester hours of course work, depending on students' educational backgrounds and experience. Its curriculum focuses on cardiovascular fitness, health promotion, nutrition, physiology, and prevention.

The **M.S. in Nutrition and Dietetics, Medical Dietetics** is a 31-semester hour program designed for professionals with baccalaureate degrees in allied health fields. Course work focuses on administration, counseling, and education as they relate to nutrition care.

The **M.S. in Nutrition and Dietetics, Culinary Entrepreneurship** is ideal for professionals who have baccalaureate degrees in nutrition and experience in the culinary field. It includes 30 or more semester hours of course work, depending on students' educational backgrounds and experience. Its curriculum emphasizes entrepreneurship, finance, marketing, nutrition, organizational management, and sustainable food systems.

The **M.S. in Nutrition and Dietetics, Food Innovation and Entrepreneurship** is designed for individuals who aren't registered dietitians and have backgrounds in culinary arts. It includes 30 or more semester hours of course work, depending on students' educational backgrounds and experience. Its curriculum has three phases that focus on sustainability: business, culinary arts, and nutrition. Coursework integrates culinary practice and business subjects with nutrition to foster innovative business planning, entrepreneurship, and product development.

Dual M.S. in Nutrition and Dietetics and Public Health: This program prepares nutrition specialists for positions in public health and voluntary agencies as well as educational and healthcare settings. The program's curriculum trains students to design, coordinate, implement, and evaluate nutrition intervention programs related to public health. It has 54 semester hours of course work including a comprehensive oral exam and a capstone, practicum research project.

Research Opportunities

With nearly 40 research centers and institutes, Saint Louis University is a hub for medical and scholarly research. *U.S. News & World Report* ranked it among the leading research universities in the nation.

Faculty members work alongside graduate and undergraduate students to promote vigorous and innovative intellectual inquiry. Researchers team up with local and global leaders to alleviate hunger, ignorance, injustice, and poverty; provide compassionate healthcare to those in need; and improve and maintain quality of life for all people.

Faculty members in the Department of Nutrition and Dietetics conduct research in many areas including cardiovascular nutrition, community nutrition, culinary arts, geriatric nutrition, sports nutrition, sustainable food systems, and women's health and fitness.

The Faculty

Faculty members in the Department of Nutrition and Dietetics are excellent teachers who use progressive curricular methods. They are also highly-regarded practitioners and researchers who expand knowledge and practice concerning nutrition and dietetics. Three faculty members, Daniel Brewer, Kathleen Kress, and Edward Weiss, exemplify the department's goal to demonstrate innovation, conduct relevant research, and model academic excellence.

Chef and instructor Daniel Brewer, M.S., RDN manages the department's local farmer/producer network including product development, procurement, and processing. He has 15 years of experience working in the food and beverage industry, and he currently owns a business that produces small batch tofu for grocers and restaurants.

Professor Kathleen Kress, M.S., RD, LD joined the University in 1995. Her career experience includes positions as the district support dietitian/patient services manager at Marriot Management Services and clinical dietitian at St. Joseph Health Center and Sarah Bush Lincoln Center.

Professor Edward Weiss has postdoctoral training in exercise physiology, geriatrics, and nutrition. His primary research interests include cardiovascular disease and diabetes prevention, exercise and nutrition for weight loss, and slowing primary aging. He has received grants from the National Institutes of Health for the past 16 years, and he has published 50 research papers.

Financial Aid

Graduate students at Saint Louis University may qualify for graduate assistantships, graduate teaching assistantships, or graduate research assistantships. These positions provide tuition scholarships, extended library privileges, and health insurance.

Graduate students who demonstrate outstanding academic achievement and potential to succeed may receive fellowships like the Dissertation Fellowship, Diversity Fellowship, and Presidential Fellowship. Students in serious need of financial assistance may qualify for tuition scholarships.

Students may also qualify for the federal Direct Unsubsidized or Graduate Plus loan. In addition, they can pursue loans from private lenders, seek fellowships and scholarships from external sources, and enroll in the university's monthly payment plan.

Cost of Study

Graduate tuition for the 2016–17 academic year is $1,075 per credit hour.

Living and Housing Costs

The University provides graduate student housing at The Flats and Robert May Hall. Room and board rates for a full-year contract (fall, spring, and summer terms) range from $9,940 to $13,540 in 2016–17. Information regarding graduate student housing is available at http://www.slu.edu/housing.

Saint Louis University

Student Life

Saint Louis University's inclusive and supportive community helps students develop their minds, bodies, hearts, and spirits. It has more than 35 club sports, 150 chartered student organizations, 25 fraternities and sororities, and numerous service opportunities. It also offers a variety of events including concerts, dances, Division 1 NCAA athletics, guest speakers, heritage month activities, and theatre productions. Resources include the following:

- Campus Ministry
- Campus Recreation
- Center for Service and Community Engagement
- Cross Cultural Center
- Interfaith Sacred Space
- Leadership Opportunities
- Student Health Center
- Student Success Center

Location

Saint Louis University is located in St. Louis, Missouri. It also has a campus in Madrid, Spain.

St. Louis is one of the Midwest's most historic and charming cities. Live music venues, performing arts, museums, nightlife, outdoor adventures, professional sports teams, restaurants, and shopping are just some of the activities that this vibrant city offers. Attractions include the Challenger Learning Center–St. Louis, the Contemporary Art Museum of St. Louis, Forest Park, Gateway Archway, the Missouri History Museum, the Saint Louis Zoo, Six Flags St. Louis, and the St. Louis Cardinals baseball team.

The University

Established in 1818, Saint Louis University is one of the oldest and most esteemed Catholic universities in the United States. It adheres to the Jesuit traditions of educating the whole person and maintaining an enduring commitment to faith and service. Its goal is to cultivate compassionate professionals and leaders who make the world a better place. To this end, it offers approximately 13,000 students 90-plus undergraduate programs; nearly 100 graduate programs; and a variety of leadership, spiritual, and service opportunities.

Saint Louis University receives national recognition for academic excellence. *U.S. News & World Report* ranked 21 of its graduate and undergraduate programs within the top 100 in the nation.

In addition to providing excellent academics, compassionate healthcare, and ground-breaking research, the University contributes more than $715 million to the St. Louis metropolitan area annually and supports 6,800 jobs in the region.

Admission Requirements and Applying

Applicants to the Department of Nutrition and Dietetics gradual programs are required to submit a complete transcript of grades from all undergraduate institutions attended, three letters of recommendation, GRE scores, a resume, a professional goal statement, and an application fee ($55 for domestic applicants, $65 for international applicants). In addition, international applicants must provide a completed Declaration of Financial Support packet with all accompanying documents and TOEFL or IELTS scores. An on-campus or telephone interview is also desired as part of the application process.

A committee reviews each application, looking for factors such as an above-average GPA, high GRE scores, TOEFL scores (for international applicants), and overall fit with programs.

Online application deadlines for the fall term are July 1 (domestic), May 1 (international); for the spring term, November 1 (domestic), October 1 (international); and for the summer term, April 1.

Correspondence and Information

Department of Nutrition and Dietetics
Allied Health Professions Building
Saint Louis University
3437 Caroline St., Room 3096
St. Louis, Missouri 63104-1111
United States
Phone: 314-977-2570
E-mail: dchs@slu.edu
Website: http://www.slu.edu/nutrition-and-dietetics-ms

Section 15
Parasitology

This section contains a directory of institutions offering graduate work in parasitology. Additional information about programs listed in the directory may be obtained by writing directly to the dean of a graduate school or chair of a department at the address given in the directory.

For programs offering related work, see also in this book *Allied Health, Biological and Biomedical Sciences, Microbiological Sciences,* and *Public Health.*

CONTENTS

Program Directory

Parasitology

Illinois State University, Graduate School, College of Arts and Sciences, Department of Biological Sciences, Normal, IL 61790-2200. Offers animal behavior (MS); bacteriology (MS); biochemistry (MS); biological sciences (MS); biology (PhD); biophysics (MS); biotechnology (MS); botany (MS, PhD); cell biology (MS); conservation biology (MS); developmental biology (MS); ecology (MS, PhD); entomology (MS); evolutionary biology (MS); genetics (MS, PhD); immunology (MS); microbiology (MS, PhD); molecular biology (MS); molecular genetics (MS); neurobiology (MS); neuroscience (MS); parasitology (MS); physiology (MS, PhD); plant biology (MS); plant molecular biology (MS); plant sciences (MS); structural biology (MS); zoology (MS, PhD). *Program availability:* Part-time. *Degree requirements:* For master's, thesis or alternative; for doctorate, variable foreign language requirement, thesis/dissertation, 2 terms of residency. *Entrance requirements:* For master's, GRE General Test, minimum GPA of 2.6 in last 60 hours of course work; for doctorate, GRE General Test. *Application deadline:* Applications are processed on a rolling basis. Application fee: $40. *Financial support:* Research assistantships, teaching assistantships, Federal Work-Study, tuition waivers (full), and unspecified assistantships available. Financial award application deadline: 4/1. *Faculty research:* Redoc balance and drug development in schistosoma mansoni, control of the growth of listeria monocytogenes at low temperature, regulation of cell expansion and microtubule function by SPRI, CRUI: physiology and fitness consequences of different life history phenotypes. *Application contact:* Steven Juliano, Graduate Coordinator, E-mail: sajulian@ilstu.edu.
Website: http://www.bio.ilstu.edu/

Louisiana State University Health Sciences Center, School of Graduate Studies in New Orleans, Department of Microbiology, Immunology, and Parasitology, New Orleans, LA 70112-1393. Offers microbiology and immunology (PhD); MD/PhD. *Faculty:* 22 full-time (5 women). *Students:* 18 full-time (10 women); includes 3 minority (2 Black or African American, non-Hispanic/Latino; 1 Hispanic/Latino), 4 international. Average age 26. 14 applicants, 21% accepted, 1 enrolled. In 2015, 3 doctorates awarded. *Degree requirements:* For doctorate, comprehensive exam, thesis/dissertation, preliminary exam, qualifying exam. *Entrance requirements:* For doctorate, GRE General Test. Additional exam requirements/recommendations for international students: Recommended—TOEFL, IELTS. *Application deadline:* For fall admission, 4/1 for domestic and international students. Applications are processed on a rolling basis. Application fee: $30. *Financial support:* Unspecified assistantships available. Financial award application deadline: 4/15. *Faculty research:* Microbial physiology, animal virology, vaccine development, AIDS drug studies, pathogenic mechanisms, molecular immunology. *Unit head:* Dr. Alistair Ramsay, Professor and Head, 504-568-4062, Fax: 504-568-2918, E-mail: aramsa@lsuhsc.edu. *Application contact:* Dr. Angela Amedee, Associate Professor, 504-568-5608, Fax: 504-568-2918, E-mail: aamede@lsuhsc.edu.
Website: http://www.medschool.lsuhsc.edu/microbiology/

McGill University, Faculty of Graduate and Postdoctoral Studies, Faculty of Agricultural and Environmental Sciences, Institute of Parasitology, Montréal, QC H3A 2T5, Canada. Offers biotechnology (M Sc A, Certificate); parasitology (M Sc, PhD).

Oregon State University, College of Science, Program in Microbiology, Corvallis, OR 97331. Offers environmental microbiology (MA, MS, PhD); food microbiology (MA, MS, PhD); genomics (MA, MS, PhD); immunology (MA, MS, PhD); microbial ecology (MA, MS, PhD); microbial evolution (MA, MS, PhD); parasitology (MA, MS, PhD); pathogenic microbiology (MA, MS, PhD); virology (MA). *Program availability:* Part-time. *Faculty:* 14 full-time (5 women), 1 part-time/adjunct (0 women). *Students:* 32 full-time (12 women); includes 5 minority (4 Asian, non-Hispanic/Latino; 1 Two or more races, non-Hispanic/Latino), 2 international. Average age 28. 79 applicants, 10% accepted, 4 enrolled. In 2015, 3 master's, 4 doctorates awarded. Terminal master's awarded for partial completion of doctoral program. *Degree requirements:* For master's, thesis; for doctorate, one foreign language, thesis/dissertation. *Entrance requirements:* For master's and doctorate, GRE. Additional exam requirements/recommendations for international students: Required—TOEFL (minimum score 600 paper-based; 100 iBT). *Application deadline:* For fall admission, 8/1 for domestic and international students; for winter admission, 12/1 for domestic students, 7/1 for international students; for spring admission, 2/1 for domestic students, 10/1 for international students; for summer admission, 5/1 for domestic students, 1/1 for international students. Application fee: $75 ($85 for international students). *Expenses:* Tuition, state resident: full-time $12,150; part-time $450 per credit. Tuition, nonresident: full-time $20,952; part-time $776 per credit. *Required fees:* $1572; $1443 per unit. One-time fee: $350. Tuition and fees vary according to course load, campus/location and program. *Financial support:* Fellowships, research assistantships, and teaching assistantships available. Financial award application deadline: 1/15. *Faculty research:* Genetics, physiology, biotechnology, pathogenic microbiology, plant virology. *Unit head:* Dr. Jerri Bartholomew, Professor and Department Head, 541-737-1856. *Application contact:* Mary Fulton, Microbiology Advisor, 541-737-1833, E-mail: mary.fulton@oregonstate.edu.
Website: http://microbiology.science.oregonstate.edu/

Tulane University, School of Public Health and Tropical Medicine, Department of Tropical Medicine, New Orleans, LA 70118-5669. Offers clinical tropical medicine and travelers health (Diploma); parasitology (PhD); public health (MSPH); public health and tropical medicine (MPHTM); MD/MPHTM. PhD offered through the Graduate School. *Degree requirements:* For master's, thesis; for doctorate, comprehensive exam, thesis/dissertation. *Entrance requirements:* For master's, GRE General Test, minimum B average in undergraduate course work; for doctorate, GRE General Test. Additional exam requirements/recommendations for international students: Required—TOEFL. *Application deadline:* For fall admission, 2/1 for domestic and international students. *Expenses:* Tuition, area resident: Full-time $47,658; part-time $2648 per credit hour. *Required fees:* $1980; $44.50 per credit hour. $550 per term. Tuition and fees vary according to course load, degree level and program. *Financial support:* Fellowships with full tuition reimbursements and research assistantships with full tuition reimbursements available. Financial award application deadline: 2/1.

University of Notre Dame, Graduate School, College of Science, Department of Biological Sciences, Notre Dame, IN 46556. Offers aquatic ecology, evolution and environmental biology (MS, PhD); cellular and molecular biology (MS, PhD); genetics (MS, PhD); physiology (MS, PhD); vector biology and parasitology (MS, PhD). Terminal master's awarded for partial completion of doctoral program. *Degree requirements:* For master's, comprehensive exam, thesis; for doctorate, comprehensive exam, thesis/dissertation, candidacy exam. *Entrance requirements:* For master's and doctorate, GRE General Test. Additional exam requirements/recommendations for international students: Required—TOEFL (minimum score 600 paper-based; 80 iBT). Electronic applications accepted. *Faculty research:* Tropical disease, molecular genetics, neurobiology, evolutionary biology, aquatic biology.

University of Prince Edward Island, Atlantic Veterinary College, Graduate Program in Veterinary Medicine, Charlottetown, PE C1A 4P3, Canada. Offers anatomy (M Sc, PhD); bacteriology (M Sc, PhD); clinical pharmacology (M Sc, PhD); clinical sciences (M Sc, PhD); epidemiology (M Sc, PhD), including reproduction; fish health (M Sc, PhD); food animal nutrition (M Sc, PhD); immunology (M Sc, PhD); microanatomy (M Sc, PhD); parasitology (M Sc, PhD); pathology (M Sc, PhD); pharmacology (M Sc, PhD); physiology (M Sc, PhD); toxicology (M Sc, PhD); veterinary science (M Vet Sc); virology (M Sc, PhD). *Program availability:* Part-time. *Degree requirements:* For master's, thesis; for doctorate, thesis/dissertation. *Entrance requirements:* For master's, DVM, B Sc honors degree, or equivalent; for doctorate, M Sc. Additional exam requirements/recommendations for international students: Required—TOEFL (minimum score 550 paper-based; 80 iBT). *Expenses:* Contact institution. *Faculty research:* Animal health management, infectious diseases, fin fish and shellfish health, basic biomedical sciences, ecosystem health.

University of Washington, Graduate School, School of Public Health, Department of Global Health, Graduate Program in Pathobiology, Seattle, WA 98195. Offers PhD. *Degree requirements:* For doctorate, comprehensive exam, thesis/dissertation, published paper from thesis work. *Entrance requirements:* For doctorate, GRE General Test, minimum GPA of 3.0. Additional exam requirements/recommendations for international students: Required—TOEFL, IELTS. Electronic applications accepted. *Expenses:* Contact institution. *Faculty research:* Malaria, immunological response to mycobacteria infections, HIV-cell interaction and the development of an anti-HIV vaccine, regulation of intercellular communication via gap junctions, genetic and nutritional regulation of proteins involved in lipid transport.

Section 16
Pathology and Pathobiology

This section contains a directory of institutions offering graduate work in pathology and pathobiology. Additional information about programs listed in the directory may be obtained by writing directly to the dean of a graduate school or chair of a department at the address given in the directory.

For programs offering related work, see also in this book *Allied Health; Anatomy; Biochemistry; Biological and Biomedical Sciences; Cell, Molecular, and Structural Biology; Genetics, Developmental Biology, and Reproductive Biology; Microbiological Sciences; Pharmacology and Toxicology; Physiology, Public Health,* and *Veterinary Medicine and Sciences.*

CONTENTS

Program Directories

Molecular Pathogenesis

Dartmouth College, Graduate Program in Molecular and Cellular Biology, Department of Microbiology and Immunology, Program in Molecular Pathogenesis, Hanover, NH 03755. Offers microbiology and immunology (PhD); MBA/PhD; MD/PhD. *Entrance requirements:* Additional exam requirements/recommendations for international students: Required—TOEFL (minimum score paper-based 550, iBT 100) or IELTS (7.0). *Application deadline:* For fall admission, 12/1 for domestic students. Application fee: $75. Electronic applications accepted. *Expenses: Tuition, area resident:* Full-time $48,120. *Required fees:* $296. One-time fee: $50 full-time. *Financial support:* In 2015–16, fellowships with full tuition reimbursements (averaging $28,200 per year) were awarded; health care benefits also available. *Unit head:* Dr. William R. Green, Chair, 603-650-8607, Fax: 603-650-6223. *Application contact:* Janet Cheney, Program Administrator, 608-650-1612, Fax: 608-650-6223.
Website: https://www.dartmouth.edu/~m2p2/

Emory University, Laney Graduate School, Division of Biological and Biomedical Sciences, Program in Immunology and Molecular Pathogenesis, Atlanta, GA 30322-1100. Offers PhD. *Degree requirements:* For doctorate, comprehensive exam, thesis/dissertation. *Entrance requirements:* For doctorate, GRE General Test, minimum GPA of 3.0 in science course work (recommended). Additional exam requirements/recommendations for international students: Required—TOEFL. Electronic applications accepted. *Faculty research:* Transplantation immunology, autoimmunity, microbial pathogenesis.

North Dakota State University, College of Graduate and Interdisciplinary Studies, College of Agriculture, Food Systems, and Natural Resources, Department of Microbiological Sciences, Fargo, ND 58102. Offers microbiology (MS); molecular pathogenesis (PhD). *Program availability:* Part-time. *Degree requirements:* For master's, thesis; for doctorate, thesis/dissertation, oral and written preliminary exams. *Entrance requirements:* For master's and doctorate, GRE. Additional exam requirements/recommendations for international students: Required—TOEFL (minimum score 525 paper-based; 71 iBT). *Application deadline:* For fall admission, 2/15 priority date for domestic students. Applications are processed on a rolling basis. Application fee: $35. *Financial support:* Fellowships with full tuition reimbursements, research assistantships with full tuition reimbursements, teaching assistantships with full tuition reimbursements, Federal Work-Study, and institutionally sponsored loans available. Financial award application deadline: 4/15. *Faculty research:* Bacterial gene regulation, antibiotic resistance, molecular virology, mechanisms of bacterial pathogenesis, immunology of animals. *Unit head:* John McEvoy, Interim Head, 701-231-8530, E-mail: john.mcevoy@ndsu.edu. *Application contact:* Eugene Berry, Associate Professor, 701-231-7520, Fax: 701-231-7514, E-mail: eugene.berry@ndsu.edu.
Website: http://www.ndsu.edu/micro/

Oregon State University, Interdisciplinary/Institutional Programs, Program in Molecular and Cellular Biology, Corvallis, OR 97331. Offers bioinformatics (PhD); biotechnology (PhD); cell biology (PhD); developmental biology (PhD); genome biology (PhD); molecular biology (PhD); molecular pathogenesis (PhD); molecular virology (PhD); plant molecular biology (PhD); structural biology (PhD). *Students:* 28 full-time (14 women), 2 part-time (1 woman); includes 4 minority (2 Asian, non-Hispanic/Latino; 2 Hispanic/Latino), 10 international. Average age 29. 104 applicants, 5% accepted, 5 enrolled. In 2015, 5 doctorates awarded. *Degree requirements:* For doctorate, thesis/dissertation, oral and written qualifying exams. *Entrance requirements:* For doctorate, GRE. Additional exam requirements/recommendations for international students: Required—TOEFL (minimum score 80 iBT), IELTS (minimum score 6.5). *Application deadline:* For fall admission, 8/1 for domestic students, 4/1 for international students; for winter admission, 12/1 for domestic students, 7/1 for international students; for spring admission, 2/1 for domestic students, 10/1 for international students; for summer admission, 5/1 for domestic students, 1/1 for international students. Application fee: $75 ($85 for international students). *Expenses: Tuition,* state resident: full-time $12,150; part-time $450 per credit. Tuition, nonresident: full-time $20,952; part-time $776 per credit. *Required fees:* $1572; $1443 per unit. One-time fee: $350. Tuition and fees vary according to course load, campus/location and program. *Financial support:* Fellowships, career-related internships or fieldwork, Federal Work-Study, and institutionally sponsored loans available. Support available to part-time students. Financial award application deadline: 1/1. *Unit head:* Dr. Dee Denver, Director, Molecular and Cellular Biology Graduate Program, 541-737-3698. *Application contact:* Kristin Carroll, Assistant Director, 541-737-5259, E-mail: kristin.carroll@oregonstate.edu.
Website: http://www.mcb.oregonstate.edu/

Washington University in St. Louis, Graduate School of Arts and Sciences, Division of Biology and Biomedical Sciences, Program in Molecular Microbiology and Microbial Pathogenesis, St. Louis, MO 63130-4899. Offers PhD. *Students:* 47 full-time (24 women); includes 10 minority (3 Black or African American, non-Hispanic/Latino; 1 American Indian or Alaska Native, non-Hispanic/Latino; 4 Asian, non-Hispanic/Latino; 1 Hispanic/Latino; 1 Two or more races, non-Hispanic/Latino), 8 international. 136 applicants, 15% accepted, 7 enrolled. *Degree requirements:* For doctorate, thesis/dissertation. *Entrance requirements:* For doctorate, GRE General Test, GRE Subject Test. Additional exam requirements/recommendations for international students: Required—TOEFL. *Application deadline:* For fall admission, 12/1 for domestic students. Application fee: $0. Electronic applications accepted. *Financial support:* Fellowships, research assistantships, and teaching assistantships available. Financial award application deadline: 1/15. *Faculty research:* Host-pathogen interactions, cellular microbiology, molecular microbiology, microbial pathogenesis, pathogen discovery, emerging infectious diseases, microbial physiology and biochemistry, comparative genomics, gene expression and regulation, microbiome and host interactions, virology, bacteriology, mycology, parasitology. *Unit head:* Jeanne Silvestrini, Coordinator, 314-362-4806. *Application contact:* Rebecca Riney, 314-747-4648, E-mail: dbbsphdadmissions@wusm.wustl.edu.

Molecular Pathology

Rutgers University–Newark, Graduate School of Biomedical Sciences, Program in Molecular Pathology and Immunology, Newark, NJ 07107. Offers PhD. *Entrance requirements:* Additional exam requirements/recommendations for international students: Required—TOEFL. Electronic applications accepted.

Texas Tech University Health Sciences Center, School of Health Professions, Program in Molecular Pathology, Lubbock, TX 79430. Offers MS. *Faculty:* 10 full-time (8 women). *Students:* 21 full-time (13 women); includes 11 minority (2 Black or African American, non-Hispanic/Latino; 2 Asian, non-Hispanic/Latino; 7 Hispanic/Latino). Average age 25. 42 applicants, 52% accepted, 22 enrolled. In 2015, 23 master's awarded. *Entrance requirements:* Additional exam requirements/recommendations for international students: Required—TOEFL (minimum score 550 paper-based; 79 iBT), IELTS. *Application deadline:* For spring admission, 2/1 priority date for domestic students. Applications are processed on a rolling basis. Application fee: $40. Electronic applications accepted. *Expenses:* $25,678.40 non-resident; $11,248.40 resident. *Financial support:* Career-related internships or fieldwork, institutionally sponsored loans, and scholarships/grants available. Financial award application deadline: 9/1; financial award applicants required to submit FAFSA. *Unit head:* Dr. Ericka Hendrix, Program Director, 806-743-3257, Fax: 806-743-4470, E-mail: ericka.hendrix@ttuhsc.edu. *Application contact:* Lindsay Johnson, Associate Dean for Admissions and Student Affairs, 806-743-3220, Fax: 806-743-2994, E-mail: lindsay.johnson@ttuhsc.edu.
Website: http://www.ttuhsc.edu/shp/msmp/

University of Michigan, Rackham Graduate School, Program in Biomedical Sciences (PIBS), Program in Molecular and Cellular Pathology, Ann Arbor, MI 48109-2800. Offers PhD. *Faculty:* 35 full-time (10 women). *Students:* 25 full-time (16 women); includes 8 minority (1 Black or African American, non-Hispanic/Latino; 3 Asian, non-Hispanic/Latino; 3 Hispanic/Latino; 1 Two or more races, non-Hispanic/Latino), 5 international. Average age 29. 56 applicants, 16% accepted, 3 enrolled. In 2015, 4 doctorates awarded. *Degree requirements:* For doctorate, comprehensive exam, thesis/dissertation, preliminary exam; oral defense of dissertation. *Entrance requirements:* For doctorate, GRE General Test, 3 letters of recommendation, research experience, personal statement. Additional exam requirements/recommendations for international students: Required—TOEFL (minimum score 84 iBT). *Application deadline:* For fall admission, 12/1 for domestic and international students. Application fee: $90 ($90 for international students). Electronic applications accepted. *Financial support:* In 2015–16, 8 fellowships with full tuition reimbursements (averaging $29,025 per year), 17 research assistantships with full tuition reimbursements (averaging $29,025 per year) were awarded; scholarships/grants, traineeships, health care benefits, and unspecified assistantships also available. Financial award applicants required to submit FAFSA. *Faculty research:* Cancer biology, stem cell and developmental biology, immunopathology and inflammatory disease, epigenetics and gene regulation, cell death and regulation. *Total annual research expenditures:* $19.1 million. *Unit head:* Dr. Zaneta Nikolovska-Coleska, Associate Professor of Pathology/Director, 734-763-0846, Fax: 734-936-7361, E-mail: pathgradprog@med.umich.edu. *Application contact:* Jim Musgrave, Recruiting Coordinator, 734-615-1660, Fax: 734-647-7022, E-mail: jdmusg@umich.edu.
Website: http://www.pathology.med.umich.edu/

University of Pittsburgh, School of Medicine, Graduate Programs in Medicine, Cellular and Molecular Pathology Graduate Program, Pittsburgh, PA 15260. Offers PhD. *Faculty:* 77 full-time (24 women). *Students:* 28 full-time (15 women); includes 7 minority (6 Asian, non-Hispanic/Latino; 1 Two or more races, non-Hispanic/Latino). Average age 27. 386 applicants, 17% accepted, 25 enrolled. In 2015, 4 doctorates awarded. *Degree requirements:* For doctorate, comprehensive exam, thesis/dissertation. *Entrance requirements:* For doctorate, GRE General Test, GRE Subject Test, minimum QPA of 3.0. Additional exam requirements/recommendations for international students: Required—TOEFL (minimum score 600 paper-based; 100 iBT), IELTS (minimum score 7). *Application deadline:* For fall admission, 12/1 priority date for domestic and international students. Application fee: $50. Electronic applications accepted. Tuition and fees vary according to program. *Financial support:* In 2015–16, 28 students received support, including 9 fellowships with full tuition reimbursements available (averaging $27,000 per year), 18 research assistantships with full tuition reimbursements available (averaging $27,000 per year), 1 teaching assistantship with full tuition reimbursement available (averaging $27,000 per year); scholarships/grants, traineeships, and health care benefits also available. *Faculty research:* Liver growth and differentiation, pathogenesis of neurodegeneration, cancer research. *Unit head:* Dr. Wendy Mars, Graduate Program Director, 412-648-9690, Fax: 412-648-9846, E-mail: wmars@pitt.edu. *Application contact:* Carol Williams, Admissions and Recruiting Manager, 412-648-8957, Fax: 412-648-1077, E-mail: gradstudies@medschool.pitt.edu.
Website: http://www.gradbiomed.pitt.edu

The University of Texas Health Science Center at Houston, Graduate School of Biomedical Sciences, Program in Molecular Pathology, Houston, TX 77225-0036. Offers MS, PhD, MD/PhD. Terminal master's awarded for partial completion of doctoral program. *Degree requirements:* For master's, thesis; for doctorate, thesis/dissertation. *Entrance requirements:* For master's and doctorate, GRE General Test. Additional exam requirements/recommendations for international students: Required—TOEFL. Electronic applications accepted. *Faculty research:* Infectious disease, carcinogenesis, structural biology, cell biology.

University of Wisconsin–Madison, School of Medicine and Public Health, Cellular and Molecular Pathology Graduate Program, Madison, WI 53705. Offers PhD. *Accreditation:* NAACLS. *Expenses:* Tuition, state resident: full-time $5364. Tuition, nonresident: full-time $12,027. *Required fees:* $571. Tuition and fees vary according to campus/location, program and reciprocity agreements.
Website: http://www.cmp.wisc.edu/

Yale University, School of Medicine and Graduate School of Arts and Sciences, Combined Program in Biological and Biomedical Sciences (BBS), Pharmacological Sciences and Molecular Medicine Track, New Haven, CT 06520. Offers PhD, MD/PhD. *Degree requirements:* For doctorate, thesis/dissertation. *Entrance requirements:* For doctorate, GRE General Test. Additional exam requirements/recommendations for international students: Required—TOEFL. Electronic applications accepted.

Pathobiology

Auburn University, College of Veterinary Medicine and Graduate School, Graduate Programs in Veterinary Medicine, Auburn University, AL 36849. Offers biomedical sciences (MS, PhD), including anatomy, physiology and pharmacology (MS), biomedical sciences (PhD), clinical sciences (MS), large animal surgery and medicine (MS), pathobiology (MS), radiology (MS), small animal surgery and medicine (MS); DVM/MS. *Program availability:* Part-time. *Faculty:* 97 full-time (40 women), 4 part-time/adjunct (2 women). *Students:* 19 full-time (11 women), 54 part-time (34 women); includes 10 minority (2 Black or African American, non-Hispanic/Latino; 2 American Indian or Alaska Native, non-Hispanic/Latino; 2 Asian, non-Hispanic/Latino; 4 Hispanic/Latino), 23 international. Average age 31. 39 applicants, 59% accepted, 14 enrolled. In 2015, 12 master's, 6 doctorates awarded. *Degree requirements:* For master's, thesis/dissertation. *Entrance requirements:* For master's, GRE General Test; for doctorate, GRE General Test, GRE Subject Test. *Application deadline:* Applications are processed on a rolling basis. Application fee: $50 ($60 for international students). Electronic applications accepted. *Expenses:* Tuition, state resident: full-time $8802; part-time $489 per credit hour. Tuition, nonresident: full-time $26,406; part-time $1467 per credit hour. *Required fees:* $808 per semester. Tuition and fees vary according to degree level and program. *Financial support:* Research assistantships, teaching assistantships, and Federal Work-Study available. Support available to part-time students. Financial award application deadline: 3/15; financial award applicants required to submit FAFSA. *Unit head:* Dr. Calvin Johnson, Acting Dean, 334-844-2650. *Application contact:* Dr. George Flowers, Dean of the Graduate School, 334-844-2125.

Brown University, Graduate School, Division of Biology and Medicine, Department of Pathology and Laboratory Medicine, Providence, RI 02912. Offers Sc M, PhD, MD/PhD. Terminal master's awarded for partial completion of doctoral program. *Degree requirements:* For doctorate, thesis/dissertation, preliminary exam. *Entrance requirements:* For master's and doctorate, GRE General Test, GRE Subject Test. Additional exam requirements/recommendations for international students: Required—TOEFL. Electronic applications accepted. *Faculty research:* Environmental pathology, carcinogenesis, immunopathology, signal transduction, innate immunity.

Columbia University, College of Physicians and Surgeons, Department of Pathology, New York, NY 10032. Offers pathobiology (M Phil, MA, PhD); MD/PhD. Only candidates for the PhD are admitted. Terminal master's awarded for partial completion of doctoral program. *Degree requirements:* For doctorate, thesis/dissertation. *Entrance requirements:* For master's and doctorate, GRE General Test. Additional exam requirements/recommendations for international students: Required—TOEFL. *Faculty research:* Virology, molecular biology, cell biology, neurobiology, immunology.

Drexel University, College of Medicine, Biomedical Graduate Programs, Interdisciplinary Program in Molecular Pathobiology, Philadelphia, PA 19104-2875. Offers MS, PhD, MD/PhD. *Degree requirements:* For doctorate, comprehensive exam, thesis/dissertation, qualifying exams. *Entrance requirements:* For doctorate, GRE General Test, minimum GPA of 3.0. Additional exam requirements/recommendations for international students: Required—TOEFL. Electronic applications accepted. *Faculty research:* Cell and molecular immunology, tumor immunology, molecular genetics, immunopathology, immunology of aging.

Johns Hopkins University, School of Medicine, Graduate Programs in Medicine, Department of Pathology, Baltimore, MD 21218. Offers pathobiology (PhD). *Degree requirements:* For doctorate, thesis/dissertation, qualifying oral exam. *Entrance requirements:* For doctorate, GRE General Test, previous course work with laboratory in organic and inorganic chemistry, general biology, calculus; interview. Additional exam requirements/recommendations for international students: Required—TOEFL. Electronic applications accepted. *Faculty research:* Role of mutant proteins in Alzheimer's disease, nuclear protein function in breast and prostate cancer, medically important fungi, glycoproteins in HIV pathogenesis.

Kansas State University, Graduate School, College of Veterinary Medicine, Department of Diagnostic Medicine/Pathobiology, Manhattan, KS 66506. Offers biomedical science (MS); diagnostic medicine/pathobiology (PhD). Terminal master's awarded for partial completion of doctoral program. *Degree requirements:* For doctorate, thesis/dissertation. *Entrance requirements:* For master's and doctorate, interviews. Additional exam requirements/recommendations for international students: Required—TOEFL (minimum score 550 paper-based). Electronic applications accepted. *Faculty research:* Infectious disease of animals, food safety and security, epidemiology and public health, toxicology, pathology.

Medical University of South Carolina, College of Graduate Studies, Program in Molecular and Cellular Biology and Pathobiology, Charleston, SC 29425. Offers cancer biology (PhD); cardiovascular biology (PhD); cardiovascular imaging (PhD); cell regulation (PhD); craniofacial biology (PhD); genetics and development (PhD); marine biomedicine (PhD); DMD/PhD; MD/PhD. *Degree requirements:* For doctorate, thesis/dissertation, oral and written exams. *Entrance requirements:* For doctorate, GRE General Test, interview, minimum GPA of 3.0. Additional exam requirements/recommendations for international students: Required—TOEFL (minimum score 600 paper-based; 100 iBT). Electronic applications accepted.

Michigan State University, College of Veterinary Medicine and The Graduate School, Graduate Programs in Veterinary Medicine, Department of Pathobiology and Diagnostic Investigation, East Lansing, MI 48824. Offers pathology (MS, PhD); pathology–environmental toxicology (PhD). *Entrance requirements:* Additional exam requirements/recommendations for international students: Required—TOEFL. Electronic applications accepted.

New York University, School of Medicine and Graduate School of Arts and Science, Sackler Institute of Graduate Biomedical Sciences, Program in Pathobiology and Translational Medicine, New York, NY 10012-1019. Offers PhD, MD/PhD. *Degree requirements:* For doctorate, comprehensive exam, thesis/dissertation, qualifying exam. *Faculty research:* Identification of new targets for treatment in melanoma and pre-clinical drug testing, respiratory syncytial virus and pediatric infectious diseases, immunotherapy of cancer.

Penn State University Park, Graduate School, College of Agricultural Sciences, Department of Veterinary and Biomedical Sciences, University Park, PA 16802. Offers pathobiology (MS, PhD). *Unit head:* Dr. Richard T. Roush, Dean, 814-865-2541, Fax: 814-865-3103. *Application contact:* Lori Stania, Director, Graduate Student Services, 814-865-1795, Fax: 814-863-4627, E-mail: l-gswww@lists.psu.edu. Website: http://vbs.psu.edu/

Purdue University, School of Veterinary Medicine and Graduate School, Graduate Programs in Veterinary Medicine, Department of Comparative Pathobiology, West Lafayette, IN 47907-2027. Offers comparative epidemiology and public health (MS); comparative epidemiology and public heath (PhD); comparative microbiology and

immunology (MS, PhD); comparative pathobiology (MS, PhD); interdisciplinary studies (PhD), including microbial pathogenesis, molecular signaling and cancer biology, molecular virology; lab animal medicine (MS); veterinary anatomic pathology (MS); veterinary clinical pathology (MS). Terminal master's awarded for partial completion of doctoral program. *Degree requirements:* For master's, thesis (for some programs); for doctorate, thesis/dissertation. *Entrance requirements:* For master's and doctorate, GRE General Test. Additional exam requirements/recommendations for international students: Required—TOEFL (minimum score 575 paper-based), IELTS (minimum score 6.5), TWE (minimum score 4). Electronic applications accepted.

The University of Alabama at Birmingham, Graduate Programs in Joint Health Sciences, Pathobiology and Molecular Medicine Theme, Birmingham, AL 35294. Offers PhD. *Students:* 46 full-time (20 women), 1 (woman) part-time; includes 9 minority (5 Black or African American, non-Hispanic/Latino; 1 Asian, non-Hispanic/Latino; 3 Hispanic/Latino), 9 international. Average age 27. *Degree requirements:* For doctorate, comprehensive exam, thesis/dissertation. *Entrance requirements:* For doctorate, GRE (minimum combined verbal/quantitative score of 300 new test or 1100 old test), baccalaureate degree in natural or physical sciences, research experience, interview, reference letters. Additional exam requirements/recommendations for international students: Required—TOEFL (minimum score 600 paper-based; 100 iBT). *Application deadline:* For fall admission, 12/15 priority date for domestic students, 1/15 for international students. Applications are processed on a rolling basis. Application fee: $0 ($60 for international students). Electronic applications accepted. *Expenses:* Tuition, state resident: full-time $7340. Tuition, nonresident: full-time $16,628. Full-time tuition and fees vary according to course load and program. *Financial support:* Fellowships with tuition reimbursements and competitive annual stipends, health insurance, and fully-paid tuition and fees available. *Faculty research:* Molecular basis of disease, AIDS vaccine development and T-cell biology of HIV infection and pathogenesis of AIDS; metabolic bone disease and cellular signaling and death; extracellular matrix control of normal and cancerous cell movement and growth; mechanisms of neuronal cell death and neoplasia; tumor invasion, tumor markers, and cancer genetics; bacterial and mycotic infections; mechanisms of insulin and growth hormone action. *Unit head:* Dr. Yabing Chen, Director, 205-996-6293, E-mail: yabingchen@uabmc.edu. *Application contact:* Director of Graduate School Operations, Fax: 205-934-8413, E-mail: gradschool@uab.edu.
Website: http://www.uab.edu/gbs/pathobiology/

University of Cincinnati, Graduate School, College of Medicine, Graduate Programs in Biomedical Sciences, Program in Pathobiology and Molecular Medicine, Cincinnati, OH 45221. Offers pathology (PhD), including anatomic pathology, laboratory medicine, pathobiology and molecular medicine. *Degree requirements:* For doctorate, thesis/dissertation, qualifying exam. *Entrance requirements:* For doctorate, GRE General Test. Additional exam requirements/recommendations for international students: Required—TOEFL (minimum score 620 paper-based). Electronic applications accepted. *Faculty research:* Cardiovascular and lipid disorders, digestive and kidney disease, endocrine and metabolic disorders, hematologic and oncogenic, immunology and infectious disease.

University of Connecticut, Graduate School, College of Agriculture, Health and Natural Resources, Department of Pathobiology and Veterinary Science, Storrs, CT 06269. Offers pathobiology (MS, PhD). Terminal master's awarded for partial completion of doctoral program. *Degree requirements:* For master's, comprehensive exam; for doctorate, thesis/dissertation. *Entrance requirements:* For master's and doctorate, GRE General Test, GRE Subject Test. Additional exam requirements/recommendations for international students: Required—TOEFL (minimum score 550 paper-based). *Application deadline:* For fall admission, 2/1 priority date for domestic and international students; for spring admission, 11/1 for domestic students, 10/1 for international students. Applications are processed on a rolling basis. Application fee: $55. Electronic applications accepted. *Financial support:* Fellowships, research assistantships with full tuition reimbursements, teaching assistantships with full tuition reimbursements, Federal Work-Study, scholarships/grants, health care benefits, and unspecified assistantships available. Financial award application deadline: 2/1; financial award applicants required to submit FAFSA.
Website: http://patho.uconn.edu/

University of Illinois at Urbana–Champaign, College of Veterinary Medicine, Department of Pathobiology, Urbana, IL 61802. Offers MS, PhD, DVM/PhD. Terminal master's awarded for partial completion of doctoral program. *Degree requirements:* For doctorate, thesis/dissertation.

University of Missouri, College of Veterinary Medicine and Office of Research and Graduate Studies, Graduate Programs in Veterinary Medicine, Department of Veterinary Pathobiology, Columbia, MO 65211. Offers comparative medicine (MS); pathobiology (MS, PhD). *Degree requirements:* For master's, thesis; for doctorate, 2 foreign languages, thesis/dissertation. *Entrance requirements:* For master's and doctorate, GRE General Test, minimum GPA of 3.0. Additional exam requirements/recommendations for international students: Required—TOEFL (minimum score 500 paper-based; 61 iBT). *Application deadline:* For fall admission, 1/15 for domestic students; for spring admission, 9/1 for domestic students. Application fee: $65 ($90 for international students). Electronic applications accepted. *Financial support:* Research assistantships with full tuition reimbursements, teaching assistantships with full tuition reimbursements, institutionally sponsored loans, scholarships/grants, traineeships, health care benefits, and unspecified assistantships available. Support available to part-time students. *Faculty research:* Bacteriology, cell biology, clinical pathology, comparative medicine, cytoskeletal regulation, gene expression and control, gene therapy, immunology, infectious disease, inflammatory diseases, microbiology, microscopy, molecular diagnostics, molecular genetics and genomic analysis.
Website: http://vpbio.missouri.edu/

University of Toronto, Faculty of Medicine, Department of Laboratory Medicine and Pathobiology, Toronto, ON M5S 1A1, Canada. Offers M Sc, PhD. *Degree requirements:* For master's, thesis; for doctorate, thesis/dissertation, oral defense of thesis. *Entrance requirements:* For master's, minimum B+ average in final 2 years, research experience, 2 letters of recommendation, resume, interview; for doctorate, minimum A- average, 2 letters of recommendation, research experience, resume, interview. Additional exam requirements/recommendations for international students: Required—TOEFL (minimum score 600 paper-based), TWE (minimum score 5, or IELTS (minimum score 7). Electronic applications accepted.

University of Washington, Graduate School, School of Public Health, Department of Global Health, Graduate Program in Pathobiology, Seattle, WA 98195. Offers PhD. *Degree requirements:* For doctorate, comprehensive exam, thesis/dissertation, published paper from thesis work. *Entrance requirements:* For doctorate, GRE General

Pathobiology

Test, minimum GPA of 3.0. Additional exam requirements/recommendations for international students: Required—TOEFL, IELTS. Electronic applications accepted. *Expenses:* Contact institution. *Faculty research:* Malaria, immunological response to mycobacteria infections, HIV-cell interaction and the development of an anti-HIV vaccine, regulation of intercellular communication via gap junctions, genetic and nutritional regulation of proteins involved in lipid transport.

University of Wyoming, College of Agriculture and Natural Resources, Department of Veterinary Sciences, Laramie, WY 82071. Offers pathobiology (MS). *Degree requirements:* For master's, thesis. *Entrance requirements:* For master's, GRE General Test, minimum GPA of 3.0. Additional exam requirements/recommendations for international students: Required—TOEFL. *Faculty research:* Infectious diseases, pathology, toxicology, immunology, microbiology.

Wake Forest University, School of Medicine and Graduate School of Arts and Sciences, Graduate Programs in Medicine, Program in Molecular and Cellular Pathobiology, Winston-Salem, NC 27109. Offers MS, PhD, MD/PhD. *Degree requirements:* For master's, thesis; for doctorate, thesis/dissertation. *Entrance requirements:* For master's and doctorate, GRE General Test. Additional exam requirements/recommendations for international students: Required—TOEFL. Electronic applications accepted. *Faculty research:* Atherosclerosis, lipoproteins, arterial wall metabolism.

Yale University, School of Medicine and Graduate School of Arts and Sciences, Combined Program in Biological and Biomedical Sciences (BBS), Pharmacological Sciences and Molecular Medicine Track, New Haven, CT 06520. Offers PhD, MD/PhD. *Degree requirements:* For doctorate, thesis/dissertation. *Entrance requirements:* For doctorate, GRE General Test. Additional exam requirements/recommendations for international students: Required—TOEFL. Electronic applications accepted.

Pathology

Albert Einstein College of Medicine, Graduate Division of Biomedical Sciences, Department of Pathology, Bronx, NY 10467. Offers PhD, MD/PhD. *Degree requirements:* For doctorate, thesis/dissertation. *Entrance requirements:* For doctorate, GRE General Test. Additional exam requirements/recommendations for international students: Required—TOEFL. *Faculty research:* Clinical and disease-related research at tissue, cellular, and subcellular levels; biochemistry and morphology of enzyme and lysosome disorders.

Baylor College of Medicine, Graduate School of Biomedical Sciences, Program in Developmental Biology, Houston, TX 77030-3498. Offers PhD, MD/PhD. *Degree requirements:* For doctorate, thesis/dissertation, public defense. *Entrance requirements:* For doctorate, GRE General Test, GRE Subject Test (strongly recommended), minimum GPA of 3.0. Additional exam requirements/recommendations for international students: Required—TOEFL. Electronic applications accepted. *Faculty research:* Stem cells, cancer, neurobiology, organogenesis, genetics of model organisms.

Boston University, School of Medicine, Division of Graduate Medical Sciences, Department of Pathology and Laboratory Medicine, Boston, MA 02118. Offers PhD, MD/PhD. *Program availability:* Part-time. *Degree requirements:* For doctorate, thesis/dissertation. *Entrance requirements:* Additional exam requirements/recommendations for international students: Required—TOEFL. *Application deadline:* For fall admission, 1/15 for domestic students; for spring admission, 10/15 for domestic students. *Financial support:* Scholarships/grants and traineeships available. Financial award applicants required to submit FAFSA. *Unit head:* Dr. Daniel G. Remick, Chairman, 617-414-7043, E-mail: remickd@bu.edu. *Application contact:* GMS Admissions Office, 617-638-5255, E-mail: askgms@bu.edu.
Website: http://www.bumc.bu.edu/busm-pathology/

Case Western Reserve University, School of Medicine and School of Graduate Studies, Graduate Programs in Medicine, Programs in Molecular and Cellular Basis of Disease/Pathology, Cleveland, OH 44106. Offers cancer biology (PhD); cell biology (MS, PhD); immunology (MS, PhD); pathology (MS, PhD). Terminal master's awarded for partial completion of doctoral program. *Degree requirements:* For master's, thesis; for doctorate, thesis/dissertation. *Entrance requirements:* For master's and doctorate, GRE General Test, GRE Subject Test. Additional exam requirements/recommendations for international students: Required—TOEFL (minimum score 550 paper-based). Electronic applications accepted. *Expenses:* Tuition, area resident: Full-time $41,137; part-time $1714 per credit hour. *Required fees:* $32. Tuition and fees vary according to course load and program. *Faculty research:* Neurobiology, molecular biology, cancer biology, biomaterials, biocompatibility.

Colorado State University, College of Veterinary Medicine and Biomedical Sciences, Department of Microbiology, Immunology and Pathology, Fort Collins, CO 80523. Offers microbiology (MS, PhD). *Faculty:* 75 full-time (35 women), 10 part-time/adjunct (6 women). *Students:* 81 full-time (60 women), 28 part-time (18 women); includes 21 minority (2 American Indian or Alaska Native, non-Hispanic/Latino; 3 Asian, non-Hispanic/Latino; 13 Hispanic/Latino; 3 Two or more races, non-Hispanic/Latino), 8 international. Average age 29. 133 applicants, 38% accepted, 47 enrolled. In 2015, 47 master's, 7 doctorates awarded. *Degree requirements:* For master's, comprehensive exam, thesis; for doctorate, comprehensive exam, thesis/dissertation. *Entrance requirements:* For master's, GRE General Test, minimum GPA of 3.0, BA/BS in biomedical field, resume, transcripts, personal statement, 3 letters of recommendation; for doctorate, GRE General Test, minimum GPA of 3.0, BA/BS in biomedical field, resume, personal statement, transcripts, 3 letters of recommendation. Additional exam requirements/recommendations for international students: Required—TOEFL (minimum score 550 paper-based; 80 iBT); Recommended—IELTS (minimum score 6.5), TWE, TSE. *Application deadline:* For fall admission, 12/15 priority date for domestic and international students. Application fee: $60 ($70 for international students). Electronic applications accepted. *Expenses:* Contact institution. *Financial support:* In 2015–16, 82 students received support, including 33 fellowships with full tuition reimbursements available (averaging $39,971 per year), 29 research assistantships with full tuition reimbursements available (averaging $21,981 per year), 2 teaching assistantships with full tuition reimbursements available (averaging $17,190 per year); scholarships/grants, traineeships, and unspecified assistantships also available. Financial award applicants required to submit FAFSA. *Faculty research:* Prions, tuberculosis, vector-borne diseases, rna biology, host-pathogen interactions. *Total annual research expenditures:* $21.5 million. *Unit head:* Dr. Gregg A. Dean, Department Head, 970-491-6144, E-mail: gregg.dean@colostate.edu. *Application contact:* Heidi Runge, Academic Support Coordinator for Graduate Studies, 970-491-1630, Fax: 970-491-0603, E-mail: heidi.runge@colostate.edu.
Website: http://csu-cvmbs.colostate.edu/academics/mip/graduate/Pages/microbiology-immunology-professional-masters.aspx

Columbia University, College of Physicians and Surgeons, Department of Pathology, New York, NY 10032. Offers pathobiology (M Phil, MA, PhD); MD/PhD. Only candidates for the PhD are admitted. Terminal master's awarded for partial completion of doctoral program. *Degree requirements:* For doctorate, thesis/dissertation. *Entrance requirements:* For master's and doctorate, GRE General Test. Additional exam requirements/recommendations for international students: Required—TOEFL. *Faculty research:* Virology, molecular biology, cell biology, neurobiology, immunology.

Dalhousie University, Faculty of Graduate Studies and Faculty of Medicine, Graduate Programs in Medicine, Department of Pathology, Halifax, NS B3H 4R2, Canada. Offers M Sc, PhD. *Degree requirements:* For master's, oral defense of thesis. *Entrance*

requirements: Additional exam requirements/recommendations for international students: Required—1 of 5 approved tests: TOEFL, IELTS, CANTEST, CAEL, Michigan English Language Assessment Battery. Electronic applications accepted. *Faculty research:* Tumor immunology, molecular oncology, clinical chemistry, hematology, molecular genetics/oncology.

Duke University, Graduate School, Department of Pathology, Durham, NC 27710. Offers PhD. *Accreditation:* NAACLS. *Degree requirements:* For doctorate, thesis/dissertation. *Entrance requirements:* For doctorate, GRE General Test, GRE Subject Test (recommended). Additional exam requirements/recommendations for international students: Required—TOEFL (minimum score 577 paper-based; 90 iBT) or IELTS (minimum score 7). Electronic applications accepted.

Duke University, School of Medicine, Pathologists' Assistant Program, Durham, NC 27710. Offers MHS. *Accreditation:* NAACLS. *Faculty:* 1 (woman) full-time, 45 part-time/adjunct (23 women). *Students:* 16 full-time (all women). Average age 26. 41 applicants, 22% accepted, 8 enrolled. In 2015, 8 master's awarded. *Degree requirements:* For master's, comprehensive exam. *Entrance requirements:* For master's, GRE. Additional exam requirements/recommendations for international students: Required—TOEFL. *Application deadline:* For fall admission, 1/15 for domestic students. Application fee: $55. *Financial support:* Application deadline: 5/1; applicants required to submit FAFSA. *Unit head:* Dr. Rex C. Bentley, Program Director, 919-684-6423, Fax: 919-681-7634, E-mail: bentl003@mc.duke.edu. *Application contact:* Pamela Vollmer, Associate Director, 919-684-2159, Fax: 919-684-8693, E-mail: pamela.vollmer@duke.edu.
Website: http://pathology.duke.edu/academic-programs/pathologists-assistant-program

Harvard University, Graduate School of Arts and Sciences, Division of Medical Sciences, Boston, MA 02115. Offers biological chemistry and molecular pharmacology (PhD); cell biology (PhD); genetics (PhD); microbiology and molecular genetics (PhD); pathology (PhD), including experimental pathology. *Degree requirements:* For doctorate, thesis/dissertation. *Entrance requirements:* For doctorate, GRE General Test, GRE Subject Test. Additional exam requirements/recommendations for international students: Required—TOEFL.

Indiana University–Purdue University Indianapolis, Indiana University School of Medicine, Department of Pathology and Laboratory Medicine, Indianapolis, IN 46202. Offers MS, PhD, MD/PhD. *Degree requirements:* For master's, thesis; for doctorate, thesis/dissertation. *Entrance requirements:* For master's and doctorate, GRE General Test. Additional exam requirements/recommendations for international students: Required—TOEFL. *Faculty research:* Intestinal microecology and anaerobes, molecular pathogenesis of infectious diseases, AIDS, pneumocystis, sports medicine toxicology, neuropathology of aging.

Iowa State University of Science and Technology, Department of Veterinary Pathology, Ames, IA 50011. Offers MS, PhD. *Entrance requirements:* For master's and doctorate, GRE General Test. Additional exam requirements/recommendations for international students: Recommended—TOEFL (minimum score 550 paper-based; 79 iBT), IELTS (minimum score 6.5). Electronic applications accepted.

Johns Hopkins University, School of Medicine, Graduate Programs in Medicine, Department of Pathology, Baltimore, MD 21218. Offers pathobiology (PhD). *Degree requirements:* For doctorate, thesis/dissertation, qualifying oral exam. *Entrance requirements:* For doctorate, GRE General Test, previous course work with laboratory in organic and inorganic chemistry, general biology, calculus; interview. Additional exam requirements/recommendations for international students: Required—TOEFL. Electronic applications accepted. *Faculty research:* Role of mutant proteins in Alzheimer's disease, nuclear protein function in breast and prostate cancer, medically important fungi, glycoproteins in HIV pathogenesis.

Loma Linda University, School of Medicine, Programs in Pathology and Human Anatomy, Loma Linda, CA 92350. Offers human anatomy (PhD); pathology (PhD). *Program availability:* Part-time. Terminal master's awarded for partial completion of doctoral program. *Degree requirements:* For doctorate, 2 foreign languages, thesis/dissertation. *Entrance requirements:* For doctorate, GRE General Test. Additional exam requirements/recommendations for international students: Required—TOEFL (minimum score 550 paper-based). *Application deadline:* For fall admission, 7/1 for domestic students. Applications are processed on a rolling basis. Application fee: $60. *Financial support:* Tuition waivers (full and partial) available. Support available to part-time students. *Faculty research:* Neuroendocrine system, histochemistry and image analysis, effect of age and diabetes on PNS, electron microscopy, histology. *Application contact:* Admissions Office, 909-651-5029, Fax: 909-558-4879, E-mail: admissions.app@llu.edu.

McGill University, Faculty of Graduate and Postdoctoral Studies, Faculty of Medicine, Department of Pathology, Montréal, QC H3A 2T5, Canada. Offers M Sc, PhD.

Medical University of South Carolina, College of Graduate Studies, Department of Pathology and Laboratory Medicine, Charleston, SC 29425. Offers MS, PhD, DMD/PhD, MD/PhD. Terminal master's awarded for partial completion of doctoral program. *Degree requirements:* For master's, thesis; for doctorate, thesis/dissertation, oral and written exams. *Entrance requirements:* For master's, GRE General Test; for doctorate, GRE General Test, interview, minimum GPA of 3.0. Additional exam requirements/recommendations for international students: Required—TOEFL (minimum score 600 paper-based; 100 iBT). Electronic applications accepted. *Faculty research:* Neurobiology of hearing loss; inner ear ion homeostasis; cancer biology, genetics and stem cell biology; cellular defense mechanisms.

Michigan State University, College of Veterinary Medicine and The Graduate School, Graduate Programs in Veterinary Medicine, Department of Pathobiology and Diagnostic Investigation, East Lansing, MI 48824. Offers pathology (MS, PhD); pathology-environmental toxicology (PhD). *Entrance requirements:* Additional exam requirements/recommendations for international students: Required—TOEFL. Electronic applications accepted.

New York Medical College, Graduate School of Basic Medical Sciences, Integrated PhD Program, Valhalla, NY 10595-1691. Offers biochemistry and molecular biology (PhD); cell biology and anatomy (PhD); microbiology and immunology (PhD); pathology (PhD); pharmacology (PhD); physiology (PhD). *Degree requirements:* For doctorate, comprehensive exam, thesis/dissertation. *Entrance requirements:* For doctorate, GRE General Test. Additional exam requirements/recommendations for international students: Required—TOEFL. Electronic applications accepted. *Expenses: Tuition, area resident:* Full-time $44,355; part-time $1025 per credit. *Required fees:* $500; $95 per year. One-time fee: $140 part-time. Tuition and fees vary according to course load and program. *Faculty research:* Cardiovascular sciences, infectious diseases, neuroscience, cancer and cell signaling.

New York Medical College, Graduate School of Basic Medical Sciences, Pathology - Master's Program, Valhalla, NY 10595-1691. Offers MS, PhD, MD/PhD. *Program availability:* Part-time, evening/weekend. *Degree requirements:* For master's, thesis. *Entrance requirements:* For master's, GRE General Test, MCAT, or DAT. Additional exam requirements/recommendations for international students: Required—TOEFL. Electronic applications accepted. *Expenses: Tuition, area resident:* Full-time $44,355; part-time $1025 per credit. *Required fees:* $500; $95 per year. One-time fee: $140 part-time. Tuition and fees vary according to course load and program. *Faculty research:* Examination of the underlying mechanisms involved in biochemical toxicology, cancer cell biology, cell-cycle regulation and apoptosis, chemical carcinogenesis and tissue engineering.

North Carolina State University, College of Veterinary Medicine, Program in Comparative Biomedical Sciences, Raleigh, NC 27695. Offers cell biology (MS, PhD); infectious disease (MS, PhD); pathology (MS, PhD); pharmacology (MS, PhD); population medicine (MS, PhD). *Program availability:* Part-time. *Degree requirements:* For master's, thesis; for doctorate, thesis/dissertation. *Entrance requirements:* For master's and doctorate, GRE General Test. Additional exam requirements/recommendations for international students: Required—TOEFL (minimum score 550 paper-based). Electronic applications accepted. *Expenses:* Contact institution. *Faculty research:* Infectious diseases, cell biology, pharmacology and toxicology, genomics, pathology and population medicine.

North Dakota State University, College of Graduate and Interdisciplinary Studies, College of Agriculture, Food Systems, and Natural Resources, Department of Microbiological Sciences, Fargo, ND 58102. Offers microbiology (MS); molecular pathogenesis (PhD). *Program availability:* Part-time. *Degree requirements:* For master's, thesis; for doctorate, thesis/dissertation, oral and written preliminary exams. *Entrance requirements:* For master's and doctorate, GRE. Additional exam requirements/recommendations for international students: Required—TOEFL (minimum score 525 paper-based; 71 iBT). *Application deadline:* For fall admission, 2/15 priority date for domestic students. Applications are processed on a rolling basis. Application fee: $35. *Financial support:* Fellowships with full tuition reimbursements, research assistantships with full tuition reimbursements, teaching assistantships with full tuition reimbursements, Federal Work-Study, and institutionally sponsored loans available. Financial award application deadline: 4/15. *Faculty research:* Bacterial gene regulation, antibiotic resistance, molecular virology, mechanisms of bacterial pathogenesis, immunology of animals. *Unit head:* John McEvoy, Interim Head, 701-231-8530, E-mail: john.mcevoy@ndsu.edu. *Application contact:* Eugene Berry, Associate Professor, 701-231-7520, Fax: 701-231-7514, E-mail: eugene.berry@ndsu.edu. Website: http://www.ndsu.edu/micro/

Purdue University, School of Veterinary Medicine and Graduate School, Graduate Programs in Veterinary Medicine, Department of Comparative Pathobiology, West Lafayette, IN 47907-2027. Offers comparative epidemiology and public health (MS); comparative epidemiology and public heath (PhD); comparative microbiology and immunology (MS, PhD); comparative pathobiology (MS, PhD); interdisciplinary studies (PhD), including microbial pathogenesis, molecular signaling and cancer biology, molecular virology; lab animal medicine (MS); veterinary anatomic pathology (MS); veterinary clinical pathology (MS). Terminal master's awarded for partial completion of doctoral program. *Degree requirements:* For master's, thesis (for some programs); for doctorate, thesis/dissertation. *Entrance requirements:* For master's and doctorate, GRE General Test. Additional exam requirements/recommendations for international students: Required—TOEFL (minimum score 575 paper-based), IELTS (minimum score 6.5), TWE (minimum score 4). Electronic applications accepted.

Queen's University at Kingston, School of Graduate Studies, Faculty of Health Sciences, Department of Pathology and Molecular Medicine, Kingston, ON K7L 3N6, Canada. Offers M Sc, PhD. *Program availability:* Part-time. *Degree requirements:* For master's, thesis; for doctorate, comprehensive exam, thesis/dissertation. *Entrance requirements:* Additional exam requirements/recommendations for international students: Required—TOEFL. *Faculty research:* Immunopathology, cancer biology, immunology and metastases, cell differentiation, blood coagulation.

Quinnipiac University, School of Health Sciences, Program for Pathologists' Assistant, Hamden, CT 06518-1940. Offers MHS. *Accreditation:* NAACLS. *Faculty:* 3 full-time (0 women), 3 part-time/adjunct (0 women). *Students:* 45 full-time (32 women); includes 3 minority (1 Black or African American, non-Hispanic/Latino; 2 Hispanic/Latino), 1 international. 111 applicants, 26% accepted, 24 enrolled. In 2015, 22 master's awarded. *Degree requirements:* For master's, residency. *Entrance requirements:* For master's, interview, coursework in biological and health sciences, minimum GPA of 3.0. *Application deadline:* For summer admission, 9/1 for domestic students. Applications are processed on a rolling basis. Application fee: $45. Electronic applications accepted. *Expenses:* $985 per credit; $360 per semester student fee; $340 per semester (fall/spring) technology and lab fee; $75 per semester summer technology and lab fee. *Financial support:* Scholarships/grants and unspecified assistantships available. Financial award application deadline: 5/1; financial award applicants required to submit FAFSA. *Faculty research:* ACL injury mechanism and running injuries and performance; transcriptional activators upstream stimulatory factor (USF); identification of novel antimicrobials; vaccines, formites and opportunistic pathogens; molecular biology of the Lyme Disease agent, Borrelia burgdorferi; molecular and microscopic techniques in host-pathogen interactions; non-invasive vascular biology, external pneumatic compression, sports performance. *Unit head:* Robert Cottrell, Program Director, 203-582-8672, E-mail: paadmissions@quinnipiac.edu. *Application contact:* Office of Graduate Admissions, 800-462-1944, Fax: 203-582-3443, E-mail: paadmissions@quinnipiac.edu.
Website: http://www.quinnipiac.edu/gradpathologists

Rosalind Franklin University of Medicine and Science, College of Health Professions, Pathologists' Assistant Department, North Chicago, IL 60064-3095. Offers MS. *Accreditation:* NAACLS. *Entrance requirements:* For master's, bachelor's degree

from an accredited college or university, minimum cumulative GPA of 3.0. Additional exam requirements/recommendations for international students: Required—TOEFL. *Faculty research:* Adaptation of ACGME/ADASP pathology resident training competencies to pathologists' assistant clinical education, utilization of structural portfolios in pathologists' assistant clinical education.

Rutgers University–Newark, Graduate School of Biomedical Sciences, Program in Molecular Pathology and Immunology, Newark, NJ 07107. Offers PhD. *Entrance requirements:* Additional exam requirements/recommendations for international students: Required—TOEFL. Electronic applications accepted.

Saint Louis University, Graduate Education and School of Medicine, Graduate Program in Biomedical Sciences and Graduate Education, Department of Pathology, St. Louis, MO 63103. Offers PhD. *Degree requirements:* For doctorate, comprehensive exam, thesis/dissertation, oral and written preliminary exams, oral defense of dissertation. *Entrance requirements:* For doctorate, GRE General Test (GRE Subject Test optional), letters of recommendation, resume, interview. Additional exam requirements/recommendations for international students: Required—TOEFL (minimum 525 paper-based). Electronic applications accepted. *Faculty research:* Cancer research, hepatitis C virology, cell imaging, liver disease.

Stony Brook University, State University of New York, Graduate School, College of Arts and Sciences, Department of Biochemistry and Cell Biology, Molecular and Cellular Biology Program, Stony Brook, NY 11794. Offers biochemistry and molecular biology (PhD); biological sciences (MA); immunology and pathology (PhD); molecular and cellular biology (PhD). *Faculty:* 22 full-time (7 women). *Students:* 66 full-time (41 women); includes 11 minority (2 Black or African American, non-Hispanic/Latino; 6 Asian, non-Hispanic/Latino; 3 Hispanic/Latino), 38 international. Average age 28. 175 applicants, 16% accepted, 8 enrolled. In 2015, 11 doctorates awarded. *Degree requirements:* For doctorate, comprehensive exam, thesis/dissertation, teaching experience. *Entrance requirements:* For doctorate, GRE General Test, GRE Subject Test. Additional exam requirements/recommendations for international students: Required—TOEFL. *Application deadline:* For fall admission, 1/15 for domestic students; for spring admission, 10/1 for domestic students. Application fee: $100. *Expenses:* $12,421 per year full-time resident tuition and fees; $453 per credit hour; $23,761 per year full-time non-resident tuition and fees; $925 per credit hour. *Financial support:* In 2015–16, 4 fellowships, 33 research assistantships, 8 teaching assistantships were awarded; Federal Work-Study also available. *Unit head:* Prof. Aaron Neiman, Chair, 631-632-1543, E-mail: aaron.neiman@stonybrook.edu. *Application contact:* Pam Wolfskill, Administrative Specialist/Program Administrator, 631-632-8585, Fax: 631-632-9730, E-mail: pamela.wolfskill@stonybrook.edu.

Tufts University, Cummings School of Veterinary Medicine, North Grafton, MA 01536. Offers animals and public policy (MS); biomedical sciences (PhD), including digestive diseases, infectious diseases, neuroscience and reproductive biology, pathology; conservation medicine (MS); veterinary medicine (DVM); DVM/MPH; DVM/MS. *Accreditation:* AVMA (one or more programs are accredited). *Degree requirements:* For master's, thesis (for some programs); for doctorate, comprehensive exam, thesis/dissertation (for some programs). *Entrance requirements:* For master's and doctorate, GRE General Test. Additional exam requirements/recommendations for international students: Required—TOEFL or IELTS. Electronic applications accepted. *Expenses:* Contact institution. *Faculty research:* Oncology, veterinary ethics, international veterinary medicine, veterinary genomics, pathogenesis of Clostridium difficile, wildlife fertility control.

Université de Montréal, Faculty of Medicine, Department of Pathology and Cellular Biology, Montréal, QC H3C 3J7, Canada. Offers M Sc, PhD. Terminal master's awarded for partial completion of doctoral program. *Degree requirements:* For master's, thesis; for doctorate, thesis/dissertation, general exam. *Entrance requirements:* For master's and doctorate, proficiency in French, knowledge of English. Electronic applications accepted. *Faculty research:* Immunopathology, cardiovascular pathology, oncogenetics, cellular neurocytology, muscular dystrophy.

Université Laval, Faculty of Medicine, Post-Professional Programs in Medical Studies, Québec, QC G1K 7P4, Canada. Offers anatomy–pathology (DESS); anesthesiology (DESS); cardiology (DESS); care of older people (Diploma); clinical research (DESS); community health (DESS); dermatology (DESS); diagnostic radiology (DESS); emergency medicine (Diploma); family medicine (DESS); general surgery (DESS); geriatrics (DESS); hematology (DESS); internal medicine (DESS); maternal and fetal medicine (Diploma); medical biochemistry (DESS); medical microbiology and infectious diseases (DESS); medical oncology (DESS); nephrology (DESS); neurology (DESS); neurosurgery (DESS); obstetrics and gynecology (DESS); ophthalmology (DESS); orthopedic surgery (DESS); oto-rhino-laryngology (DESS); palliative medicine (Diploma); pediatrics (DESS); plastic surgery (DESS); psychiatry (DESS); pulmonary medicine (DESS); radiology–oncology (DESS); thoracic surgery (DESS); urology (DESS). *Degree requirements:* For other advanced degree, comprehensive exam. *Entrance requirements:* For degree, knowledge of French. Electronic applications accepted.

University at Buffalo, the State University of New York, Graduate School, Graduate Programs in Cancer Research and Biomedical Sciences at Roswell Park Cancer Institute, Department of Cancer Pathology and Prevention at Roswell Park Cancer Institute, Buffalo, NY 14263-0001. Offers PhD. *Faculty:* 31 full-time (16 women). *Students:* 13 full-time (6 women), 6 international. 25 applicants, 16% accepted, 4 enrolled. In 2015, 3 doctorates awarded. *Degree requirements:* For doctorate, comprehensive exam, thesis/dissertation, oral defense of dissertation. *Entrance requirements:* For doctorate, GRE General Test. Additional exam requirements/recommendations for international students: Required—TOEFL (minimum score 79 iBT). *Application deadline:* For fall admission, 1/5 priority date for domestic and international students. Application fee: $75. Electronic applications accepted. *Financial support:* In 2015–16, 11 students received support, including 13 research assistantships with full tuition reimbursements available (averaging $25,000 per year); scholarships/grants, health care benefits, and unspecified assistantships also available. Financial award application deadline: 1/5. *Faculty research:* Molecular pathology of cancer, chemoprevention of cancer, genomic instability, molecular diagnosis and prognosis of cancer, molecular epidemiology. *Unit head:* Dr. Kirsten Moysich, Chairman, 716-845-8004, Fax: 716-845-1126, E-mail: kirsten.moysich@roswellpark.org. *Application contact:* Dr. Norman J. Karin, Associate Dean, 716-845-2339, Fax: 716-845-8178, E-mail: norman.karin@roswellpark.edu.
Website: http://www.roswellpark.edu/education/phd-programs/cancer-pathology-and-prevention

University at Buffalo, the State University of New York, Graduate School, School of Medicine and Biomedical Sciences, Graduate Programs in Medicine and Biomedical Sciences, Department of Pathology and Anatomical Sciences, Buffalo, NY 14214. Offers anatomical sciences (MA, PhD); pathology (MA, PhD). *Program availability:* Part-time. *Faculty:* 17 full-time (6 women). *Students:* 9 full-time (3 women); includes 1 minority (Asian, non-Hispanic/Latino), 1 international. Average age 29. 14 applicants, 14% accepted, 2 enrolled. In 2015, 2 master's, 1 doctorate awarded. *Degree requirements:* For master's, thesis; for doctorate, comprehensive exam, thesis/

dissertation. *Entrance requirements:* For master's and doctorate, GRE, MCAT, or DAT, 3 letters of recommendation. Additional exam requirements/recommendations for international students: Required—TOEFL (minimum score 600 paper-based; 100 iBT). *Application deadline:* For fall admission, 5/1 priority date for domestic students, 3/1 priority date for international students. Application fee: $85. *Financial support:* In 2015–16, 2 students received support, including 1 research assistantship with full tuition reimbursement available (averaging $24,900 per year), 1 teaching assistantship with full tuition reimbursement available (averaging $24,900 per year); health care benefits also available. Financial award application deadline: 2/1; financial award applicants required to submit FAFSA. *Faculty research:* Immunopathology-immunobiology, experimental hypertension, neuromuscular disease, molecular pathology, cell motility and cytoskeleton. *Unit head:* Dr. John E. Tomaszewski, Department Chair, 716-829-2846, Fax: 716-829-2911, E-mail: johntoma@buffalo.edu. *Application contact:* Graduate Program Coordinator, 716-829-2846, Fax: 716-829-2911, E-mail: ubpathad@buffalo.edu.
Website: http://wings.buffalo.edu/smbs/path/

University of Alberta, Faculty of Medicine and Dentistry and Faculty of Graduate Studies and Research, Graduate Programs in Medicine, Department of Laboratory Medicine and Pathology, Edmonton, AB T6G 2E1, Canada. Offers medical sciences (M Sc, PhD). *Program availability:* Part-time. Terminal master's awarded for partial completion of doctoral program. *Degree requirements:* For master's, thesis; for doctorate, thesis/dissertation, candidacy exam. *Entrance requirements:* For master's and doctorate, 3 letters of recommendation, minimum GPA of 3.0. Additional exam requirements/recommendations for international students: Required—TOEFL. *Faculty research:* Transplantation, renal pathology, molecular mechanisms of diseases, cryobiology, immunodiagnostics, informatics/cyber medicine, neuroimmunology, microbiology.

The University of British Columbia, Faculty of Medicine, Department of Pathology and Laboratory Medicine, Vancouver, BC V5Z 1M9, Canada. Offers experimental pathology (M Sc, PhD). *Degree requirements:* For master's, thesis; for doctorate, comprehensive exam, thesis/dissertation, internal oral defense. *Entrance requirements:* For master's, GRE, upper-level course work in biochemistry and physiology; for doctorate, GRE. Additional exam requirements/recommendations for international students: Required—TOEFL (minimum score 550 paper-based), IELTS (minimum score 6.5). Electronic applications accepted. *Faculty research:* Molecular biology of disease processes, cancer, hematopathology, atherosclerosis, pulmonary and cardiovascular pathophysiology.

University of Calgary, Cumming School of Medicine and Faculty of Graduate Studies, Medical Science Graduate Program, Calgary, AB T2N 1N4, Canada. Offers cancer biology (M Sc, PhD); critical care medicine (M Sc, PhD); joint injury and arthritis (M Sc, PhD); molecular and medical genetics (M Sc, PhD); mountain medicine and high altitude physiology (M Sc, PhD); pathologists' assistant (M Sc, PhD). *Degree requirements:* For master's, thesis; for doctorate, thesis/dissertation, candidacy exam. *Entrance requirements:* For master's, minimum undergraduate GPA of 3.2; for doctorate, minimum graduate GPA of 3.2. Additional exam requirements/recommendations for international students: Required—TOEFL (minimum score 600 paper-based). Electronic applications accepted. *Faculty research:* Cancer biology, immunology, joint injury and arthritis, medical education, population genomics.

University of California, Davis, Graduate Studies, Graduate Group in Comparative Pathology, Davis, CA 95616. Offers MS, PhD. *Accreditation:* NAACLS. Terminal master's awarded for partial completion of doctoral program. *Degree requirements:* For master's, comprehensive exam (for some programs), thesis (for some programs); for doctorate, thesis/dissertation. *Entrance requirements:* For master's and doctorate, GRE General Test. Additional exam requirements/recommendations for international students: Required—TOEFL (minimum score 550 paper-based). Electronic applications accepted. *Faculty research:* Immunopathology, toxicological and environmental pathology, reproductive pathology, pathology of infectious diseases.

University of California, Irvine, School of Medicine, Department of Pathology and Laboratory Medicine, Irvine, CA 92697. Offers experimental pathology (PhD). *Accreditation:* NAACLS. *Students:* 6 full-time (2 women); includes 3 minority (all Hispanic/Latino), 1 international. Average age 30. In 2015, 1 doctorate awarded. Application fee: $90 ($110 for international students). *Unit head:* Dr. Edwin S. Monuki, Chair, 949-824-9604, Fax: 949-824-2160, E-mail: emonuki@uci.edu. *Application contact:* Stefani Ching, Graduate Student Coordinator, 949-824-5367, E-mail: shching@uci.edu.
Website: http://www.pathology.uci.edu/

University of California, Los Angeles, David Geffen School of Medicine and Graduate Division, Graduate Programs in Medicine, Program in Cellular and Molecular Pathology, Los Angeles, CA 90095. Offers MS, PhD. Terminal master's awarded for partial completion of doctoral program. *Degree requirements:* For master's, thesis; for doctorate, thesis/dissertation, written and oral qualifying examinations; 2 quarters of teaching experience. *Entrance requirements:* For doctorate, GRE General Test, bachelor's degree; minimum undergraduate GPA of 3.0 (or its equivalent if letter grade system not used). Additional exam requirements/recommendations for international students: Required—TOEFL. Electronic applications accepted.

University of California, Los Angeles, David Geffen School of Medicine and Graduate Division, Graduate Programs in Medicine, Program in Experimental Pathology, Los Angeles, CA 90095. Offers MS, PhD. *Degree requirements:* For doctorate, thesis/dissertation, oral and written qualifying exams. *Entrance requirements:* For master's, GRE General Test; for doctorate, GRE General Test, previous course work in physical chemistry and physics.

University of California, Los Angeles, Graduate Division, College of Letters and Science and David Geffen School of Medicine, UCLA ACCESS to Programs in the Molecular, Cellular and Integrative Life Sciences, Los Angeles, CA 90095. Offers biochemistry and molecular biology (PhD); biological chemistry (PhD); cellular and molecular pathology (PhD); human genetics (PhD); microbiology, immunology, and molecular genetics (PhD); molecular biology (PhD); molecular toxicology (PhD); molecular, cellular and integrative physiology (PhD); neurobiology (PhD); oral biology (PhD); physiology (PhD). *Degree requirements:* For doctorate, thesis/dissertation, oral and written qualifying exams. *Entrance requirements:* For doctorate, GRE General Test, bachelor's degree; minimum undergraduate GPA of 3.0 (or its equivalent if letter grade system not used). Additional exam requirements/recommendations for international students: Required—TOEFL. Electronic applications accepted.

University of Cincinnati, Graduate School, College of Medicine, Graduate Programs in Biomedical Sciences, Program in Pathobiology and Molecular Medicine, Cincinnati, OH 45211. Offers pathology (PhD), including anatomic pathology, laboratory medicine, pathobiology and molecular medicine. *Degree requirements:* For doctorate, thesis/dissertation, qualifying exam. *Entrance requirements:* For doctorate, GRE General Test. Additional exam requirements/recommendations for international students: Required—TOEFL (minimum score 620 paper-based). Electronic applications accepted. *Faculty research:* Cardiovascular and lipid disorders, digestive and kidney disease, endocrine

and metabolic disorders, hematologic and oncogenic, immunology and infectious disease.

University of Georgia, College of Veterinary Medicine, Department of Pathology, Athens, GA 30602. Offers MS, PhD. *Degree requirements:* For master's, thesis; for doctorate, one foreign language, thesis/dissertation. *Entrance requirements:* For master's and doctorate, GRE General Test. Electronic applications accepted.

University of Guelph, Ontario Veterinary College and Graduate Studies, Graduate Programs in Veterinary Sciences, Department of Pathobiology, Guelph, ON N1G 2W1, Canada. Offers anatomic pathology (DV Sc, Diploma); clinical pathology (Diploma); comparative pathology (M Sc, PhD); immunology (M Sc, PhD); laboratory animal science (DV Sc); pathology (M Sc, PhD, Diploma); veterinary infectious diseases (M Sc, PhD); zoo animal/wildlife medicine (DV Sc). *Degree requirements:* For master's, thesis; for doctorate, thesis/dissertation. *Entrance requirements:* For master's, DVM with B average or an honours degree in biological sciences; for doctorate, DVM or MSC degree, minimum B+ average. Additional exam requirements/recommendations for international students: Required—TOEFL (minimum score 550 paper-based). *Faculty research:* Pathogenesis; diseases of animals, wildlife, fish, and laboratory animals; parasitology; immunology; veterinary infectious diseases; laboratory animal science.

The University of Iowa, Roy J. and Lucille A. Carver College of Medicine and Graduate College, Graduate Programs in Medicine, Department of Pathology, Iowa City, IA 52242-1316. Offers MS. *Degree requirements:* For master's, thesis. *Entrance requirements:* For master's, GRE, minimum GPA of 3.0. Additional exam requirements/recommendations for international students: Required—TOEFL. Electronic applications accepted. *Faculty research:* Oncology, microbiology, vascular biology, immunology, neuroscience, virology, signaling and cell death.

The University of Kansas, University of Kansas Medical Center, School of Medicine, Department of Pathology and Laboratory Medicine, Kansas City, KS 66160. Offers PhD, MD/PhD. *Faculty:* 29. *Students:* 15 full-time (9 women), 1 (woman) part-time; includes 1 minority (Hispanic/Latino), 11 international. Average age 30. In 2015, 2 doctorates awarded. Terminal master's awarded for partial completion of doctoral program. *Degree requirements:* For doctorate, one foreign language, comprehensive exam, thesis/dissertation. *Entrance requirements:* For doctorate, GRE, curriculum vitae, statement of research and career interests, official transcripts for all undergraduate and graduate coursework, 3 reference letters. Additional exam requirements/recommendations for international students: Required—TOEFL (preferred) or IELTS. *Application deadline:* For fall admission, 1/15 priority date for domestic and international students. Applications are processed on a rolling basis. Application fee: $60. *Financial support:* In 2015–16, 1 student received support. Fellowships, research assistantships with full tuition reimbursements available, teaching assistantships with tuition reimbursements available, Federal Work-Study, scholarships/grants, traineeships, tuition waivers (full), and unspecified assistantships available. Financial award application deadline: 3/1; financial award applicants required to submit FAFSA. *Faculty research:* Cancer biology, developmental biology and cell differentiation, stem cell biology, microbial and viral pathogenesis. *Total annual research expenditures:* $7.1 million. *Unit head:* Dr. Soumen Paul, Director, Pathology Graduate Program, 913-588-7236, Fax: 913-588-5242, E-mail: spaul2@kumc.edu.
Website: http://www.kumc.edu/school-of-medicine/pathology.html

University of Manitoba, Faculty of Medicine and Faculty of Graduate Studies, Graduate Programs in Medicine, Department of Pathology, Winnipeg, MB R3E 3P5, Canada. Offers M Sc. *Degree requirements:* For master's, thesis. *Entrance requirements:* For master's, B Sc honours degree. Additional exam requirements/recommendations for international students: Required—TOEFL (minimum score 550 paper-based; 80 iBT), IELTS (minimum score 6.5). *Faculty research:* Experimental hydrocephalus; brain development; stroke; developmental neurobiology; myelination in Rett Syndrome; glial migration during cortical development; growth factors and breast cancer; transgenic models of breast cancer; molecular genetics and cancer diagnosis; graft-vs-host disease; biology of natural killer cells; transplantation immunology.

University of Maryland, Baltimore, School of Medicine, Department of Pathology, Baltimore, MD 21201. Offers pathologists' assistant (MS). *Accreditation:* NAACLS. *Students:* 21 full-time (17 women); includes 4 minority (3 Asian, non-Hispanic/Latino; 1 Hispanic/Latino). Average age 25. 81 applicants, 78% accepted, 10 enrolled. In 2015, 10 master's awarded. *Entrance requirements:* For master's, GRE General Test. Additional exam requirements/recommendations for international students: Required—TOEFL (minimum score 600 paper-based; 100 iBT); Recommended—IELTS (minimum score 8). *Application deadline:* For fall admission, 2/1 for domestic and international students. Application fee: $75. Electronic applications accepted. *Expenses:* Contact institution. *Financial support:* Application deadline: 3/1; applicants required to submit FAFSA. *Unit head:* Dr. Rudy Castellani, Program Director, 410-328-5555, Fax: 410-706-8414, E-mail: rcastellani@som.umaryland.edu. *Application contact:* Carlen Miller, Associate Program Director, 410-328-5555, Fax: 410-706-8414, E-mail: cmiller@som.umaryland.edu.
Website: http://medschool.umaryland.edu/pathology/pa/default.asp

University of Michigan, Rackham Graduate School, Program in Biomedical Sciences (PIBS), Program in Molecular and Cellular Pathology, Ann Arbor, MI 48109-2800. Offers PhD. *Faculty:* 35 full-time (10 women). *Students:* 25 full-time (16 women); includes 8 minority (1 Black or African American, non-Hispanic/Latino; 3 Asian, non-Hispanic/Latino; 3 Hispanic/Latino; 1 Two or more races, non-Hispanic/Latino), 5 international. Average age 29. 56 applicants, 16% accepted, 3 enrolled. In 2015, 4 doctorates awarded. *Degree requirements:* For doctorate, comprehensive exam, thesis/dissertation, preliminary exam; oral defense of dissertation. *Entrance requirements:* For doctorate, GRE General Test, 3 letters of recommendation, research experience, personal statement. Additional exam requirements/recommendations for international students: Required—TOEFL (minimum score 84 iBT). *Application deadline:* For fall admission, 12/1 for domestic and international students. Application fee: $75 ($90 for international students). Electronic applications accepted. *Financial support:* In 2015–16, 8 fellowships with full tuition reimbursements (averaging $29,025 per year), 17 research assistantships with full tuition reimbursements (averaging $29,025 per year) were awarded; scholarships/grants, traineeships, health care benefits, and unspecified assistantships also available. Financial award applicants required to submit FAFSA. *Faculty research:* Cancer biology, stem cell and developmental biology, immunopathology and inflammatory disease, epigenetics and gene regulation, cell death and regulation. *Total annual research expenditures:* $19.1 million. *Unit head:* Dr. Zaneta Nikolovska-Coleska, Associate Professor of Pathology/Director, 734-763-0846, Fax: 734-936-7361, E-mail: pathgradprog@med.umich.edu. *Application contact:* Jim Musgrave, Recruiting Coordinator, 734-615-1660, Fax: 734-647-7022, E-mail: jdmusg@umich.edu.
Website: http://www.pathology.med.umich.edu/

University of Mississippi Medical Center, School of Graduate Studies in the Health Sciences, Department of Pathology, Jackson, MS 39216-4505. Offers PhD, MD/PhD. *Degree requirements:* For doctorate, thesis/dissertation, first authored publication in peer-reviewed journal. *Entrance requirements:* For doctorate, GRE General Test, GRE Subject Test, minimum GPA of 3.0. Additional exam requirements/recommendations for international students: Required—TOEFL. *Faculty research:* Toll-like receptor expression and function in metastatic breast cancer patients, innate immunity, circulating tumor cells, natural killer cells, pro-inflammatory T cell transcriptional profile during progression of HIV-1 infection, renal allografts hinges on microvascular endothelium response, immunoregulatory gene expression affecting regulatory cells.

University of Missouri, School of Medicine and Office of Research and Graduate Studies, Graduate Programs in Medicine, Department of Pathology and Anatomical Sciences, Columbia, MO 65211. Offers MS. *Entrance requirements:* For master's, GRE (minimum Verbal and Analytical score of 1250), letters of recommendation, minimum GPA of 3.5. Additional exam requirements/recommendations for international students: Required—TOEFL. Application fee: $55 ($75 for international students). Electronic applications accepted.
Website: http://pathology-anatomy.missouri.edu/

University of Nebraska Medical Center, Department of Pathology and Microbiology, Omaha, NE 68198. Offers MS, PhD. *Program availability:* Part-time. *Faculty:* 53 full-time (17 women), 4 part-time/adjunct (2 women). *Students:* 37 full-time (22 women), 2 part-time (1 woman); includes 2 minority (1 Asian, non-Hispanic/Latino; 1 Hispanic/Latino), 22 international. Average age 27. 36 applicants, 17% accepted, 6 enrolled. In 2015, 4 master's, 10 doctorates awarded. Terminal master's awarded for partial completion of doctoral program. *Degree requirements:* For master's, comprehensive exam, thesis; for doctorate, comprehensive exam, thesis/dissertation. *Entrance requirements:* For master's, previous course work in biology, chemistry, mathematics, and physics; for doctorate, GRE General Test, previous course work in biology, chemistry, mathematics, and physics. Additional exam requirements/recommendations for international students: Required—TOEFL (minimum score 550 paper-based; 90 iBT). *Application deadline:* For fall admission, 3/1 for domestic and international students; for spring admission, 10/1 for domestic and international students; for summer admission, 3/1 for domestic and international students. Applications are processed on a rolling basis. Application fee: $45. Electronic applications accepted. *Expenses:* Tuition, state resident: full-time $7830; part-time $3915 per credit hour. Tuition, nonresident: full-time $22,410; part-time $11,205 per credit hour. *Required fees:* $521. *Financial support:* In 2015–16, 7 students received support, including 1 fellowship with full tuition reimbursement available (averaging $23,100 per year), 3 research assistantships with full tuition reimbursements available (averaging $23,100 per year); scholarships/grants also available. Support available to part-time students. Financial award application deadline: 2/15; financial award applicants required to submit FAFSA. *Faculty research:* Carcinogenesis, cancer biology, immunobiology, molecular virology, molecular genetics. *Unit head:* Dr. Rakesh K. Singh, Chair, Graduate Committee, 402-559-9949, Fax: 402-559-5900, E-mail: rsingh@unmc.edu. *Application contact:* Tuire Cechin, Office Associate, 402-559-4042, Fax: 402-559-5900, E-mail: tcechin@unmc.edu.
Website: http://www.unmc.edu/pathology/

University of New Mexico, Graduate Studies, Health Sciences Center, Program in Biomedical Sciences, Albuquerque, NM 87131-5196. Offers biochemistry and molecular biology (MS, PhD); cell biology and physiology (MS, PhD); molecular genetics and microbiology (MS, PhD); neuroscience (MS, PhD); pathology (MS, PhD); toxicology (MS, PhD). *Program availability:* Part-time. *Faculty:* 18 full-time (10 women), 1 part-time/adjunct (0 women). *Students:* 31 full-time (17 women), 45 part-time (26 women); includes 29 minority (1 American Indian or Alaska Native, non-Hispanic/Latino; 3 Asian, non-Hispanic/Latino; 22 Hispanic/Latino; 2 Native Hawaiian or other Pacific Islander, non-Hispanic/Latino; 1 Two or more races, non-Hispanic/Latino), 18 international. Average age 30. 98 applicants, 11% accepted, 11 enrolled. In 2015, 11 master's, 14 doctorates awarded. Terminal master's awarded for partial completion of doctoral program. *Degree requirements:* For master's, thesis; for doctorate, comprehensive exam, thesis/dissertation, qualifying exam at the end of year 1/core curriculum. *Entrance requirements:* For master's and doctorate, GRE General Test, minimum undergraduate GPA of 3.0. Additional exam requirements/recommendations for international students: Required—TOEFL. *Application deadline:* For fall admission, 3/1 priority date for domestic and international students. Applications are processed on a rolling basis. Application fee: $50. Electronic applications accepted. *Financial support:* Fellowships with tuition reimbursements, research assistantships with full tuition reimbursements, teaching assistantships, career-related internships or fieldwork, Federal Work-Study, institutionally sponsored loans, scholarships/grants, traineeships, health care benefits, and unspecified assistantships available. Financial award application deadline: 1/1; financial award applicants required to submit FAFSA. *Faculty research:* Infectious disease/immunity, cancer biology, cardiovascular and metabolic diseases, brain and behavioral illness, environmental health. *Unit head:* Dr. Helen J. Hathaway, Program Director, 505-272-1887, Fax: 505-272-2412, E-mail: hhathaway@salud.unm.edu. *Application contact:* Mary Fenton, Admissions Coordinator, 505-272-1887, Fax: 505-272-2412, E-mail: mfenton@salud.unm.edu.

The University of North Carolina at Chapel Hill, School of Medicine and Graduate School, Graduate Programs in Medicine, Department of Pathology and Laboratory Medicine, Chapel Hill, NC 27599-7525. Offers experimental pathology (PhD). *Accreditation:* NAACLS. *Degree requirements:* For doctorate, comprehensive exam, thesis/dissertation, oral exam, proposal defense. *Entrance requirements:* For doctorate, GRE General Test. Additional exam requirements/recommendations for international students: Required—TOEFL (minimum score 550 paper-based). Electronic applications accepted. *Faculty research:* Carcinogenesis, mutagenesis and cancer biology; molecular biology, genetics and animal models of human disease; cardiovascular biology, hemostasis, and thrombosis; immunology and infectious disease; progenitor cell research.

University of Oklahoma Health Sciences Center, College of Medicine and Graduate College, Graduate Programs in Medicine, Department of Pathology, Oklahoma City, OK 73190. Offers PhD. *Degree requirements:* For doctorate, thesis/dissertation. *Entrance requirements:* For doctorate, GRE General Test, 3 letters of recommendation. Additional exam requirements/recommendations for international students: Required—TOEFL. *Faculty research:* Molecular pathology, tissue response in disease, anatomic pathology, immunopathology, histocytochemistry.

University of Pittsburgh, School of Medicine, Graduate Programs in Medicine, Cellular and Molecular Pathology Graduate Program, Pittsburgh, PA 15260. Offers PhD. *Faculty:* 77 full-time (24 women). *Students:* 28 full-time (15 women); includes 7 minority (6 Asian, non-Hispanic/Latino; 1 Two or more races, non-Hispanic/Latino). Average age 27. 386 applicants, 17% accepted, 25 enrolled. In 2015, 4 doctorates awarded. *Degree requirements:* For doctorate, comprehensive exam, thesis/dissertation. *Entrance requirements:* For doctorate, GRE General Test, GRE Subject Test, minimum QPA of 3.0. Additional exam requirements/recommendations for international students: Required—TOEFL (minimum score 600 paper-based; 100 iBT), IELTS (minimum score 7). *Application deadline:* For fall admission, 12/1 priority date for domestic and international students. Application fee: $50. Electronic applications accepted. Tuition and fees vary according to program. *Financial support:* In 2015–16, 28 students received support, including 9 fellowships with full tuition reimbursements available (averaging $27,000 per year), 18 research assistantships with full tuition reimbursements available (averaging $27,000 per year), 1 teaching assistantship with full tuition reimbursement available (averaging $27,000 per year); scholarships/grants,

traineeships, and health care benefits also available. *Faculty research:* Liver growth and differentiation, pathogenesis of neurodegeneration, cancer research. *Unit head:* Dr. Wendy Mars, Graduate Program Director, 412-648-9690, Fax: 412-648-9846, E-mail: wmars@pitt.edu. *Application contact:* Carol Williams, Admissions and Recruiting Manager, 412-648-8957, Fax: 412-648-1077, E-mail: gradstudies@medschool.pitt.edu. Website: http://www.gradbiomed.pitt.edu

University of Prince Edward Island, Atlantic Veterinary College, Graduate Program in Veterinary Medicine, Charlottetown, PE C1A 4P3, Canada. Offers anatomy (M Sc, PhD); bacteriology (M Sc, PhD); clinical pharmacology (M Sc, PhD); clinical sciences (M Sc, PhD); epidemiology (M Sc, PhD), including reproduction; fish health (M Sc, PhD); food animal nutrition (M Sc, PhD); immunology (M Sc, PhD); microanatomy (M Sc, PhD); parasitology (M Sc, PhD); pathology (M Sc, PhD); pharmacology (M Sc, PhD); physiology (M Sc, PhD); toxicology (M Sc, PhD); veterinary science (M Vet Sc); virology (M Sc, PhD). *Program availability:* Part-time. *Degree requirements:* For master's, thesis; for doctorate, thesis/dissertation. *Entrance requirements:* For master's, DVM, B Sc honors degree, or equivalent; for doctorate, M Sc. Additional exam requirements/recommendations for international students: Required—TOEFL (minimum score 550 paper-based; 80 iBT). *Expenses:* Contact institution. *Faculty research:* Animal health management, infectious diseases, fin fish and shellfish health, basic biomedical sciences, ecosystem health.

University of Rochester, School of Medicine and Dentistry, Graduate Programs in Medicine and Dentistry, Department of Pathology and Laboratory Medicine, Rochester, NY 14627. Offers pathology (PhD). *Degree requirements:* For doctorate, variable foreign language requirement, thesis/dissertation, qualifying exam. *Entrance requirements:* For doctorate, GRE General Test, GRE Subject Test. *Expenses:* Tuition, area resident: Full-time $47,450; part-time $1482 per credit hour. *Required fees:* $528. Tuition and fees vary according to program.

University of Saskatchewan, College of Medicine, Department of Pathology, Saskatoon, SK S7N 5A2, Canada. Offers M Sc, PhD. *Degree requirements:* For master's, thesis; for doctorate, thesis/dissertation. *Entrance requirements:* Additional exam requirements/recommendations for international students: Required—TOEFL.

University of Saskatchewan, Western College of Veterinary Medicine and College of Graduate Studies and Research, Graduate Programs in Veterinary Medicine, Department of Veterinary Pathology, Saskatoon, SK S7N 5A2, Canada. Offers M Sc, M Vet Sc, PhD. *Degree requirements:* For master's, thesis; for doctorate, comprehensive exam (for some programs), thesis/dissertation. *Entrance requirements:* Additional exam requirements/recommendations for international students: Required—TOEFL or IELTS (minimum score 6.5). Electronic applications accepted. *Faculty research:* Thyroid, oncology, immunology/infectious diseases, vaccinology.

University of Southern California, Keck School of Medicine and Graduate School, Graduate Programs in Medicine, Department of Pathology, Los Angeles, CA 90089-9092. Offers experimental and molecular pathology (MS). *Faculty:* 32 full-time (4 women), 1 part-time/adjunct (0 women). *Students:* 9 full-time (3 women); includes 4 minority (3 Asian, non-Hispanic/Latino; 1 Hispanic/Latino), 3 international. Average age 28. 11 applicants, 55% accepted, 3 enrolled. In 2015, 7 master's awarded. *Degree requirements:* For master's, experiment-based thesis or theory-based scholarly review. *Entrance requirements:* For master's, GRE General Test, minimum GPA of 3.0. Additional exam requirements/recommendations for international students: Required—TOEFL (minimum score 600 paper-based; 100 iBT). *Application deadline:* For fall admission, 6/15 for domestic students, 6/15 priority date for international students; for spring admission, 12/1 for domestic students, 12/1 priority date for international students. Application fee: $85. Electronic applications accepted. *Expenses:* $1,666 per credit hour. *Financial support:* In 2015–16, 21 students received support, including 1 research assistantship (averaging $32,000 per year); Federal Work-Study, institutionally sponsored loans, scholarships/grants, health care benefits, and unspecified assistantships also available. Financial award application deadline: 5/4. *Faculty research:* Cellular and molecular biology of cancer; chemical carcinogenesis; virology; stem cell and developmental pathology; liver and pulmonary diseases; circulatory, endocrine, and neurodegenerative diseases. *Total annual research expenditures:* $8.9 million. *Unit head:* Dr. Michael E. Selsted, Chair, 323-442-1180, Fax: 323-442-3049, E-mail: selsted@usc.edu. *Application contact:* Lisa A. Doumak, Student Services Assistant, 323-442-1168, Fax: 323-442-3049, E-mail: doumak@usc.edu.
Website: http://www.usc.edu/hsc/medicine/pathology/

University of South Florida, Morsani College of Medicine and College of Graduate Studies, Graduate Programs in Medical Sciences, Tampa, FL 33620-9951. Offers advanced athletic training (MS); athletic training (MS); bioinformatics and computational biology (MSBCB); biotechnology (MSB); health informatics (MSHI); medical sciences (MSMS, PhD), including aging and neuroscience (MSMS), allergy, immunology and infectious disease (PhD), anatomy, athletic training (MSMS), clinical and translational research, health informatics (MSMS), health science (MSMS), interdisciplinary medical sciences (MSMS), medical microbiology and immunology (MSMS), metabolic and nutritional medicine (MSMS), molecular medicine, molecular pharmacology and physiology (PhD), neurology (PhD), pathology and laboratory medicine (PhD), pharmacology and therapeutics (PhD), physiology and biophysics (PhD), women's health (MSMS). *Students:* 510 full-time (261 women), 318 part-time (208 women); includes 360 minority (108 Black or African American, non-Hispanic/Latino; 3 American Indian or Alaska Native, non-Hispanic/Latino; 101 Asian, non-Hispanic/Latino; 124 Hispanic/Latino; 1 Native Hawaiian or other Pacific Islander, non-Hispanic/Latino; 23 Two or more races, non-Hispanic/Latino), 52 international. Average age 26. 6,567 applicants, 13% accepted, 469 enrolled. In 2015, 216 master's awarded. Terminal master's awarded for partial completion of doctoral program. *Degree requirements:* For master's, comprehensive exam, thesis; for doctorate, comprehensive exam, thesis/dissertation. *Entrance requirements:* For master's, GRE General Test or GMAT, bachelor's degree or equivalent from regionally-accredited university with minimum GPA of 3.0 in upper-division sciences coursework; prerequisites in general biology, general chemistry, general physics, organic chemistry, quantitative analysis, and integral and differential calculus; for doctorate, GRE General Test, bachelor's degree from regionally-accredited university with minimum GPA of 3.0 in upper-division sciences coursework; 3 letters of recommendation; personal interview; 1-2 page personal statement; prerequisites in biology, chemistry, physics, organic chemistry, quantitative analysis, and integral/differential calculus. Additional exam requirements/recommendations for international students: Required—TOEFL (minimum score 550 paper-based; 79 iBT) or IELTS (minimum score 6.5). *Application deadline:* For fall admission, 2/15 for domestic students, 1/2 for international students. Application fee: $30. *Expenses:* Contact institution. *Faculty research:* Anatomy, biochemistry, cancer biology, cardiovascular disease, cell biology, immunology, microbiology, molecular biology, neuroscience, pharmacology, physiology. *Unit head:* Dr. Michael Barber, Professor/Associate Dean for Graduate and Postdoctoral Affairs, 813-974-9908, Fax: 813-974-4317, E-mail: mbarber@health.usf.edu. *Application contact:* Dr. Eric Bennett, Graduate Director, PhD Program in Medical Sciences, 813-974-1545, Fax: 813-974-4317, E-mail: esbennet@health.usf.edu.
Website: http://health.usf.edu/nocms/medicine/graduatestudies/

Pathology

The University of Tennessee Health Science Center, College of Health Professions, Memphis, TN 38163-0002. Offers audiology (MS, Au D); clinical laboratory science (MSCLS); cytopathology practice (MCP); health informatics and information management (MHIIM); occupational therapy (MOT); physical therapy (DPT, ScDPT); physician assistant (MMS); speech-language pathology (MS). *Accreditation:* AOTA; APTA. *Program availability:* Part-time, evening/weekend, online learning. Terminal master's awarded for partial completion of doctoral program. *Degree requirements:* For master's, comprehensive exam, thesis; for doctorate, comprehensive exam, residency. *Entrance requirements:* For master's, GRE (MOT, MSCLS), minimum GPA of 3.0, 3 letters of reference, national accreditation (MSCLS), GRE if GPA is less than 3.0 (MCP); for doctorate, GRE. Additional exam requirements/recommendations for international students: Required—TOEFL (minimum score 550 paper-based; 80 iBT). Electronic applications accepted. *Expenses:* Contact institution. *Faculty research:* Gait deviation, muscular dystrophy and strength, hemophilia and exercise, pediatric neurology, self-efficacy.

The University of Texas Medical Branch, Graduate School of Biomedical Sciences, Program in Experimental Pathology, Galveston, TX 77555. Offers PhD. *Degree requirements:* For doctorate, thesis/dissertation. *Entrance requirements:* For doctorate, GRE General Test. Additional exam requirements/recommendations for international students: Required—TOEFL (minimum score 550 paper-based). Electronic applications accepted.

The University of Toledo, College of Graduate Studies, College of Medicine and Life Sciences, Department of Pathology, Toledo, OH 43606-3390. Offers pathology (Certificate); pathology assistant (MSBS). *Entrance requirements:* For degree, second-year medical student in good academic standing with recommendation by UT Medical School. Electronic applications accepted.

University of Utah, School of Medicine and Graduate School, Graduate Programs in Medicine, Department of Pathology, Salt Lake City, UT 84112-1107. Offers experimental pathology (PhD); laboratory medicine and biomedical science (MS). PhD offered after acceptance into the combined Program in Molecular Biology. *Degree requirements:* For doctorate, comprehensive exam, thesis/dissertation. *Entrance requirements:* For doctorate, GRE, minimum GPA of 3.0. *Faculty research:* Immunology, cell biology, signal transduction, gene regulation, receptor biology.

University of Vermont, College of Medicine and Graduate College, Graduate Programs in Medicine, Department of Pathology, Burlington, VT 05405. Offers MS. *Degree requirements:* For master's, thesis. *Entrance requirements:* For master's, GRE General Test. Additional exam requirements/recommendations for international students: Required—TOEFL (minimum score 550 paper-based; 80 iBT). *Application deadline:* For fall admission, 3/1 priority date for domestic students; 3/1 for international students. Applications are processed on a rolling basis. Application fee: $65. Electronic applications accepted. *Financial support:* Fellowships, research assistantships, and traineeships available. Financial award application deadline: 3/1. *Unit head:* Dr. Tamara Williams, E-mail: tamara.williams@uvm.edu. *Application contact:* Dr. Tamara Williams, E-mail: tamara.williams@uvm.edu.

University of Virginia, School of Medicine, Program in Experimental Pathology, Charlottesville, VA 22903. Offers PhD. *Degree requirements:* For doctorate, thesis/dissertation, oral defense of thesis. *Entrance requirements:* For doctorate, GRE General Test; GRE Subject Test (recommended), 2 letters of recommendation. Additional exam requirements/recommendations for international students: Required—TOEFL.

University of Washington, Graduate School, School of Medicine, Graduate Programs in Medicine, Department of Pathology, Seattle, WA 98195. Offers experimental and molecular pathology (PhD). *Degree requirements:* For doctorate, thesis/dissertation. *Entrance requirements:* For doctorate, GRE General Test. *Faculty research:* Viral oncogenesis, aging, mutagenesis and repair, extracellular matrix biology, vascular biology.

The University of Western Ontario, Faculty of Graduate Studies, Biosciences Division, Department of Pathology, London, ON N6A 5B8, Canada. Offers M Sc, PhD. *Degree requirements:* For master's, thesis; for doctorate, comprehensive exam, thesis/dissertation. *Entrance requirements:* For master's and doctorate, minimum B+ average, honors degree. Additional exam requirements/recommendations for international students: Required—TOEFL. *Faculty research:* Heavy metal toxicology, transplant pathology, immunopathology, immunological cancers, neurochemistry, aging and dementia, cancer pathology.

University of Wisconsin–Madison, School of Medicine and Public Health, Cellular and Molecular Pathology Graduate Program, Madison, WI 53705. Offers PhD. *Accreditation:* NAACLS. *Expenses:* Tuition, state resident: full-time $5364. Tuition, nonresident: full-time $12,027. *Required fees:* $571. Tuition and fees vary according to campus/location, program and reciprocity agreements. Website: http://www.cmp.wisc.edu/

Vanderbilt University, School of Medicine, Department of Pathology, Nashville, TN 37240-1001. Offers PhD, MD/PhD. *Faculty:* 39 full-time (13 women). *Students:* 10 full-time (6 women); includes 2 minority (1 Black or African American, non-Hispanic/Latino; 1 Asian, non-Hispanic/Latino), 2 international. Average age 29. In 2015, 8 doctorates awarded. *Degree requirements:* For doctorate, thesis/dissertation, qualifying and final exams. *Entrance requirements:* For doctorate, GRE General Test. Additional exam requirements/recommendations for international students: Required—TOEFL (minimum score 570 paper-based; 88 iBT). *Application deadline:* 1/15 for domestic and international students. Application fee: $0. Electronic applications accepted. *Financial support:* Fellowships with full tuition reimbursements, research assistantships with full tuition reimbursements, Federal Work-Study, institutionally sponsored loans, traineeships, health care benefits, and tuition waivers (partial) available. Financial award application deadline: 1/15; financial award applicants required to submit CSS PROFILE or FAFSA. *Faculty research:* Vascular biology and biochemistry, tumor pathology, the immune response, inflammation and repair, the biology of the extracellular matrix in response to disease processes, the pathogenesis of infectious agents, the regulation of gene expression in disease. *Unit head:* Lorie Franklin, Administrative Assistant/Assistant Director of Graduate Studies, 615-343-8324, Fax: 615-322-0576, E-mail: lorie.franklin@vanderbilt.edu. *Application contact:* Walter B. Bieschke, Program Coordinator for Graduate Admissions, 615-342-0236, E-mail: vandygrad@vanderbilt.edu. Website: http://www.mc.vanderbilt.edu/root/vumc.php?site-vmcpathology

Virginia Commonwealth University, Medical College of Virginia-Professional Programs, School of Medicine, School of Medicine Graduate Programs, Department of Pathology, Richmond, VA 23284-9005. Offers PhD, MD/PhD. *Program availability:* Part-time. Terminal master's awarded for partial completion of doctoral program. *Degree requirements:* For doctorate, thesis/dissertation, comprehensive oral and written exams. *Entrance requirements:* For doctorate, GRE General Test, MCAT. *Faculty research:* Biochemical and clinical applications of enzyme and protein immobilization, clinical enzymology.

Wayne State University, School of Medicine, Office of Biomedical Graduate Programs, Department of Pathology, Detroit, MI 48202. Offers PhD. *Accreditation:* NAACLS. *Faculty:* 18. *Students:* 4 full-time (3 women). Average age 26. 28 applicants, 4% accepted, 1 enrolled. *Degree requirements:* For doctorate, thesis/dissertation. *Entrance requirements:* For doctorate, GRE General Test, personal statement, three letters of recommendation, minimum undergraduate GPA of 3.0. Additional exam requirements/recommendations for international students: Required—TOEFL (minimum score 100 iBT). *Application deadline:* For fall admission, 2/1 priority date for domestic and international students. Application fee: $0. Electronic applications accepted. *Expenses:* $17,645 annual resident tuition, $33,311 non-resident tuition; $735.20 per credit hour resident tuition, $1,387.95 per credit hour non-resident tuition; fees include $47.45 per credit hour student services fee and $274.60 per semester registration fee. *Financial support:* In 2015–16, 4 students received support, including 1 fellowship with tuition reimbursement available (averaging $26,614 per year), 3 research assistantships with tuition reimbursements available (averaging $26,716 per year); scholarships/grants, health care benefits, and unspecified assistantships also available. Financial award application deadline: 3/31. *Faculty research:* Cancer, tumor microenvironment, metalloproteases, metabolism, diabetes and obesity. *Unit head:* Dr. Todd Leff, Program Director, 313-577-3006, E-mail: tleff@med.wayne.edu. Website: http://pathology.med.wayne.edu/grad_program.php

Yale University, Graduate School of Arts and Sciences, Department of Experimental Pathology, New Haven, CT 06520. Offers MS, PhD. *Degree requirements:* For doctorate, thesis/dissertation, qualifying exam. *Entrance requirements:* For doctorate, GRE General Test.

Yale University, School of Medicine and Graduate School of Arts and Sciences, Combined Program in Biological and Biomedical Sciences (BBS), Pharmacological Sciences and Molecular Medicine Track, New Haven, CT 06520. Offers PhD, MD/PhD. *Degree requirements:* For doctorate, thesis/dissertation. *Entrance requirements:* For doctorate, GRE General Test. Additional exam requirements/recommendations for international students: Required—TOEFL. Electronic applications accepted.

Section 17
Pharmacology and Toxicology

This section contains a directory of institutions offering graduate work in pharmacology and toxicology. Additional information about programs listed in the directory but not augmented by an in-depth entry may be obtained by writing directly to the dean of a graduate school or chair of a department at the address given in the directory.

For programs offering related work, see also in this book *Biochemistry; Biological and Biomedical Sciences; Cell, Molecular, and Structural Biology; Ecology, Environmental Biology, and Evolutionary Biology; Genetics, Developmental Biology, and Reproductive Biology; Neuroscience and Neurobiology; Nutrition; Pathology and Pathobiology; Pharmacy and Pharmaceutical Sciences; Physiology; Public Health;* and *Veterinary Medicine and Sciences.* In the other guides in this series:

Graduate Programs in the Humanities, Arts & Social Sciences
See *Psychology and Counseling*

Graduate Programs in the Physical Sciences, Mathematics, Agricultural Sciences, the Environment & Natural Resources
See *Chemistry* and *Environmental Sciences and Management*

Graduate Programs in Engineering & Applied Sciences
See *Chemical Engineering* and *Civil and Environmental Engineering*

CONTENTS

Program Directories

Displays and Close-Ups

See:

Molecular Pharmacology

Albert Einstein College of Medicine, Graduate Division of Biomedical Sciences, Department of Molecular Pharmacology, Bronx, NY 10461. Offers PhD, MD/PhD. *Degree requirements:* For doctorate, thesis/dissertation. *Entrance requirements:* For doctorate, GRE General Test. Additional exam requirements/recommendations for international students: Required—TOEFL. *Faculty research:* Effects of drugs on macromolecules, enzyme systems, cell morphology and function.

Brown University, Graduate School, Division of Biology and Medicine, Department of Molecular Pharmacology, Physiology and Biotechnology, Providence, RI 02912. Offers biomedical engineering (Sc M, PhD); biotechnology (PhD); molecular pharmacology and physiology (PhD); MD/PhD. *Degree requirements:* For doctorate, thesis/dissertation, preliminary exam. *Entrance requirements:* For master's and doctorate, GRE General Test, GRE Subject Test. Additional exam requirements/recommendations for international students: Required—TOEFL. Electronic applications accepted. *Faculty research:* Structural biology, antiplatelet drugs, nicotinic receptor structure/function.

Harvard University, Graduate School of Arts and Sciences, Division of Medical Sciences, Boston, MA 02115. Offers biological chemistry and molecular pharmacology (PhD); cell biology (PhD); genetics (PhD); microbiology and molecular genetics (PhD); pathology (PhD), including experimental pathology. *Degree requirements:* For doctorate, thesis/dissertation. *Entrance requirements:* For doctorate, GRE General Test, GRE Subject Test. Additional exam requirements/recommendations for international students: Required—TOEFL.

Loyola University Chicago, Graduate School, Integrated Program in Biomedical Sciences, Maywood, IL 60153. Offers biochemistry and molecular biology (MS, PhD); cell and molecular physiology (PhD); infectious disease and immunology (MS); integrative cell biology (PhD); medical physiology (MS); microbiology and immunology (MS, PhD); molecular pharmacology and therapeutics (MS, PhD); neuroscience (MS, PhD). *Students:* 135 full-time (65 women), 1 part-time (0 women); includes 28 minority (5 Black or African American, non-Hispanic/Latino; 15 Asian, non-Hispanic/Latino; 6 Hispanic/Latino; 2 Two or more races, non-Hispanic/Latino), 16 international. Average age 28. 442 applicants, 23% accepted, 55 enrolled. In 2015, 40 master's, 17 doctorates awarded. *Expenses: Tuition,* area resident: Full-time $18,054; part-time $9027 per credit hour. *Required fees:* $832; $284 per credit hour. Part-time tuition and fees vary according to course load, degree level and program. *Unit head:* Dr. Samuel Attoh, Dean, 773-508-3459, Fax: 773-508-2460, E-mail: sattoh@luc.edu. *Application contact:* Ron Martin, Associate Director of Enrollment Management, 312-915-8950, Fax: 312-915-8905, E-mail: gradapp@luc.edu.
Website: http://ssom.luc.edu/graduate_school/degree-programs/ipbsphd/

Mayo Graduate School, Graduate Programs in Biomedical Sciences, Program in Molecular Pharmacology and Experimental Therapeutics, Rochester, MN 55905. Offers PhD. *Degree requirements:* For doctorate, oral defense of dissertation, qualifying oral and written exam. *Entrance requirements:* For doctorate, GRE, 1 year of chemistry, biology, calculus, and physics. Additional exam requirements/recommendations for international students: Required—TOEFL. Electronic applications accepted. *Faculty research:* Patch clamping, G-proteins, pharmacogenetics, receptor-induced transcriptional events, cholinesterase biology.

Medical University of South Carolina, College of Graduate Studies, Program in Cell and Molecular Pharmacology and Experimental Therapeutics, Charleston, SC 29425. Offers MS, PhD, DMD/PhD, MD/PhD. Terminal master's awarded for partial completion of doctoral program. *Degree requirements:* For master's, thesis; for doctorate, comprehensive exam, thesis/dissertation, oral and written exams. *Entrance requirements:* For master's, GRE General Test; for doctorate, GRE General Test, interview, minimum GPA of 3.0. Additional exam requirements/recommendations for international students: Required—TOEFL (minimum score 600 paper-based; 100 iBT). Electronic applications accepted. *Faculty research:* Cancer drug discovery and development, growth factor receptor signaling, regulation of G-protein signaling, redox signal transduction, proteomics and mass spectrometry.

New York University, School of Medicine and Graduate School of Arts and Science, Sackler Institute of Graduate Biomedical Sciences, Program in Molecular Pharmacology, New York, NY 10012-1019. Offers PhD. *Degree requirements:* For doctorate, comprehensive exam, thesis/dissertation, qualifying exam. *Faculty research:* Pharmacology and neurobiology, neuropeptides, receptor biochemistry, cytoskeleton, endocrinology.

Purdue University, College of Pharmacy and Pharmacal Sciences and Graduate School, Graduate Programs in Pharmacy and Pharmacal Sciences, Department of Medicinal Chemistry and Molecular Pharmacology, West Lafayette, IN 47907. Offers biophysical and computational chemistry (PhD); cancer research (PhD); immunology and infectious disease (PhD); medicinal biochemistry and molecular biology (PhD); medicinal chemistry and chemical biology (PhD); molecular pharmacology (PhD); neuropharmacology, neurodegeneration, and neurotoxicity (PhD); systems biology and functional genomics (PhD). *Degree requirements:* For doctorate, thesis/dissertation. *Entrance requirements:* For doctorate, GRE General Test; GRE Subject Test in biology, biochemistry, and chemistry (recommended), minimum undergraduate GPA of 3.0. Additional exam requirements/recommendations for international students: Required—TOEFL (minimum score 550 paper-based; 77 iBT); Recommended—TWE. Electronic applications accepted. *Faculty research:* Drug design and development, cancer research, drug synthesis and analysis, chemical pharmacology, environmental toxicology.

Rosalind Franklin University of Medicine and Science, School of Graduate and Postdoctoral Studies - Interdisciplinary Graduate Program in Biomedical Sciences, Department of Cellular and Molecular Pharmacology, North Chicago, IL 60064-3095. Offers MS, PhD, MD/PhD. Terminal master's awarded for partial completion of doctoral program. *Degree requirements:* For master's, comprehensive exam, thesis; for doctorate, comprehensive exam, thesis/dissertation. *Entrance requirements:* For master's and doctorate, GRE General Test. Additional exam requirements/recommendations for international students: Required—TOEFL, TWE. Electronic applications accepted. *Faculty research:* Control of gene expression in higher organisms, molecular mechanism of action of growth factors and hormones, hormonal regulation in brain neuropsychopharmacology.

Rutgers University–New Brunswick, Graduate School of Biomedical Sciences, Program in Cellular and Molecular Pharmacology, Piscataway, NJ 08854-5635. Offers MS, PhD, MD/PhD. *Degree requirements:* For master's, thesis, qualifying exam; for doctorate, thesis/dissertation, qualifying exam. *Entrance requirements:* Additional exam requirements/recommendations for international students: Required—TOEFL. Electronic applications accepted.

Thomas Jefferson University, Jefferson College of Biomedical Sciences, PhD Program in Biochemistry and Molecular Pharmacology, Philadelphia, PA 19107. Offers PhD. *Faculty:* 68 full-time (19 women), 1 (woman) part-time/adjunct. *Students:* 36 full-time (23 women); includes 9 minority (1 Black or African American, non-Hispanic/Latino; 8 Asian, non-Hispanic/Latino), 10 international. 25 applicants, 36% accepted, 6 enrolled. In 2015, 4 doctorates awarded. *Degree requirements:* For doctorate, comprehensive exam, thesis/dissertation. *Entrance requirements:* For doctorate, GRE General Test or MCAT, minimum GPA of 3.2. Additional exam requirements/recommendations for international students: Required—TOEFL, IELTS (minimum score 7). *Application deadline:* For fall admission, 12/15 priority date for domestic and international students. Applications are processed on a rolling basis. Application fee: $50. Electronic applications accepted. *Financial support:* In 2015–16, 36 students received support, including 36 fellowships with full tuition reimbursements available (averaging $56,298 per year); Federal Work-Study, institutionally sponsored loans, scholarships/grants, traineeships, and stipends also available. Financial award application deadline: 5/1; financial award applicants required to submit FAFSA. *Faculty research:* Signal transduction and molecular genetics, translational biochemistry, human mitochondrial genetics, molecular biology of protein-RNA interaction, mammalian mitochondrial biogenesis and function. *Unit head:* Dr. Michael J. Root, MD, Program Director, 215-503-4564, Fax: 215-923-2117, E-mail: michael.root@jefferson.edu. *Application contact:* Marc E. Stearns, Director of Admissions, 215-503-0155, Fax: 215-503-3433, E-mail: jgsbs-info@jefferson.edu.
Website: http://www.jefferson.edu/university/biomedical-sciences/degrees-programs/phd-programs/biochemistry-pharmacology.html

University at Buffalo, the State University of New York, Graduate School, Graduate Programs in Cancer Research and Biomedical Sciences at Roswell Park Cancer Institute, Department of Molecular Pharmacology and Cancer Therapeutics at Roswell Park Cancer Institute, Buffalo, NY 14260. Offers PhD. *Faculty:* 19 full-time (6 women). *Students:* 18 full-time (11 women); includes 3 minority (2 Hispanic/Latino; 1 Native Hawaiian or other Pacific Islander, non-Hispanic/Latino), 3 international. 26 applicants, 23% accepted, 5 enrolled. In 2015, 2 doctorates awarded. *Degree requirements:* For doctorate, comprehensive exam, thesis/dissertation, oral defense of disseration. *Entrance requirements:* For doctorate, GRE General Test. Additional exam requirements/recommendations for international students: Required—TOEFL (minimum score 79 iBT). *Application deadline:* For fall admission, 1/5 priority date for domestic and international students. Application fee: $75. Electronic applications accepted. *Financial support:* In 2015–16, 18 students received support, including 18 research assistantships with full tuition reimbursements available (averaging $25,000 per year); scholarships/grants, health care benefits, and unspecified assistantships also available. Financial award application deadline: 1/5. *Faculty research:* Cell cycle regulation, apoptosis, signal transduction, k+s signaling pathway, drug development. *Unit head:* Dr. Barbara Foster, Director of Graduate Studies, 716-845-1260, Fax: 716-845-1258, E-mail: barbara.foster@roswellpark.org. *Application contact:* Dr. Norman J. Karin, Associate Dean, 716-845-2339, Fax: 716-845-8178, E-mail: norman.karin@roswellpark.edu.
Website: http://www.roswellpark.edu/education/phd-programs/molecular-pharmacology-cancer-therapeutics

University of Massachusetts Medical School, Graduate School of Biomedical Sciences, Worcester, MA 01655-0115. Offers biomedical sciences (PhD), including biochemistry and molecular pharmacology, bioinformatics and computational biology, cancer biology, cell biology, immunology and microbiology, interdisciplinary, neuroscience, translational science; biomedical sciences (millennium program) (PhD); clinical and population health research (PhD); clinical investigation (MS). *Faculty:* 1,339 full-time (521 women), 301 part-time/adjunct (189 women). *Students:* 363 full-time (184 women); includes 58 minority (13 Black or African American, non-Hispanic/Latino; 30 Asian, non-Hispanic/Latino; 15 Hispanic/Latino), 141 international. Average age 29. 661 applicants, 26% accepted, 51 enrolled. In 2015, 10 master's, 58 doctorates awarded. Terminal master's awarded for partial completion of doctoral program. *Degree requirements:* For master's, comprehensive exam, thesis; for doctorate, comprehensive exam, thesis/dissertation. *Entrance requirements:* For master's, MD, PhD, DVM, or PharmD; for doctorate, GRE General Test, bachelor's degree. Additional exam requirements/recommendations for international students: Required—TOEFL (minimum score 100 iBT) or IELTS (minimum score 7.5). *Application deadline:* For fall admission, 12/15 for domestic and international students; for spring admission, 5/15 for domestic students. Application fee: $80. Electronic applications accepted. *Expenses:* $6,966 resident per year; $14,182 non-resident per year. *Financial support:* In 2015–16, 383 students received support, including research assistantships with full tuition reimbursements available (averaging $30,600 per year); scholarships/grants, health care benefits, tuition waivers (full), and unspecified assistantships also available. Financial award application deadline: 5/16. *Faculty research:* RNA interference, cell/molecular/developmental biology, bioinformatics, clinical/translational research, infectious disease. *Total annual research expenditures:* $250.3 million. *Unit head:* Dr. Anthony Carruthers, Dean, 508-856-4135, E-mail: anthony.carruthers@umassmed.edu. *Application contact:* Dr. Kendall Knight, Assistant Vice Provost for Admissions, 508-856-5628, Fax: 508-856-3659, E-mail: kendall.knight@umassmed.edu.
Website: http://www.umassmed.edu/gsbs/

University of Nevada, Reno, Graduate School, Interdisciplinary Program in Cellular and Molecular Pharmacology and Physiology, Reno, NV 89557. Offers PhD. *Degree requirements:* For doctorate, one foreign language, thesis/dissertation. *Entrance requirements:* For doctorate, GRE General Test or MCAT, minimum GPA of 3.0. Additional exam requirements/recommendations for international students: Required—TOEFL (minimum score 500 paper-based; 61 iBT), IELTS (minimum score 6). Electronic applications accepted. *Faculty research:* Neuropharmacology, toxicology, cardiovascular pharmacology, neuromuscular pharmacology.

University of Pittsburgh, School of Medicine, Graduate Programs in Medicine, Molecular Pharmacology Graduate Program, Pittsburgh, PA 15260. Offers PhD. *Faculty:* 62 full-time (10 women). *Students:* 26 full-time (13 women); includes 11 minority (4 Black or African American, non-Hispanic/Latino; 4 Asian, non-Hispanic/Latino; 1 Hispanic/Latino; 2 Two or more races, non-Hispanic/Latino). Average age 27. 386 applicants, 17% accepted, 25 enrolled. In 2015, 5 doctorates awarded. *Degree requirements:* For doctorate, comprehensive exam, thesis/dissertation. *Entrance requirements:* For doctorate, GRE General Test, GRE Subject Test, minimum QPA of 3.0. Additional exam requirements/recommendations for international students: Required—TOEFL (minimum score 600 paper-based; 100 iBT), IELTS (minimum score 7). *Application deadline:* For fall admission, 1/1 priority date for domestic and international students. Application fee: $50. Electronic applications accepted. Tuition and fees vary according to program. *Financial support:* In 2015–16, 26 students

received support, including 15 fellowships with full tuition reimbursements available (averaging $27,000 per year), 11 research assistantships with full tuition reimbursements available (averaging $27,000 per year); teaching assistantships, scholarships/grants, traineeships, and health care benefits also available. *Faculty research:* Drug discovery, signal transduction, cancer therapeutics, neuropharmacology, cardiovascular and renal pharmacology. *Unit head:* Dr. Patrick Pagano, Graduate Program Director, 412-383-6505, Fax: 412-648-9009, E-mail: pagano@pitt.edu. *Application contact:* Carol Williams, Admissions and Recruiting Manager, 412-648-8957, Fax: 412-648-1007, E-mail: gradstudies@medschool.pitt.edu.
Website: http://www.gradbiomed.pitt.edu/

University of Southern California, Graduate School, School of Pharmacy, Graduate Programs in Molecular Pharmacology and Toxicology, Los Angeles, CA 90033. Offers pharmacology and pharmaceutical sciences (MS, PhD). Terminal master's awarded for partial completion of doctoral program. *Degree requirements:* For master's, comprehensive exam, thesis, 24 units of formal course work, excluding research and seminar courses; for doctorate, comprehensive exam, thesis/dissertation, 24 units of formal course work, excluding research and seminar courses. *Entrance requirements:* For master's and doctorate, GRE. Additional exam requirements/recommendations for international students: Required—TOEFL (minimum score 603 paper-based; 100 iBT). Electronic applications accepted. *Expenses:* Contact institution. *Faculty research:* Degenerative diseases, toxicology of drugs.

University of South Florida, Morsani College of Medicine and College of Graduate Studies, Graduate Programs in Medical Sciences, Tampa, FL 33620-9951. Offers advanced athletic training (MS); athletic training (MS); bioinformatics and computational biology (MSBCB); biotechnology (MSB); health informatics (MSHI); medical sciences (MGMS, PhD), including aging and neuroscience (MSMS), allergy, immunology and infectious disease (PhD), anatomy, athletic training (MSMS), clinical and translational research, health informatics (MSMS), health science (MSMS), interdisciplinary medical sciences (MSMS), medical microbiology and immunology (MSMS), metabolic and nutritional medicine (MSMS), molecular medicine, molecular pharmacology and

physiology (PhD), neurology (PhD), pathology and laboratory medicine (PhD), pharmacology and therapeutics (PhD), physiology and biophysics (PhD), women's health (MSMS). *Students:* 510 full-time (261 women), 318 part-time (208 women); includes 360 minority (108 Black or African American, non-Hispanic/Latino; 3 American Indian or Alaska Native, non-Hispanic/Latino; 101 Asian, non-Hispanic/Latino; 124 Hispanic/Latino; 1 Native Hawaiian or other Pacific Islander, non-Hispanic/Latino; 23 Two or more races, non-Hispanic/Latino), 52 international. Average age 26. 6,567 applicants, 13% accepted, 469 enrolled. In 2015, 216 master's awarded. Terminal master's awarded for partial completion of doctoral program. *Degree requirements:* For master's, comprehensive exam, thesis; for doctorate, comprehensive exam, thesis/dissertation. *Entrance requirements:* For master's, GRE General Test or GMAT, bachelor's degree or equivalent from regionally-accredited university with minimum GPA of 3.0 in upper-division sciences coursework; prerequisites in general biology, general chemistry, general physics, organic chemistry, quantitative analysis, and integral and differential calculus; for doctorate, GRE General Test, bachelor's degree from regionally-accredited university with minimum GPA of 3.0 in upper-division sciences coursework; 3 letters of recommendation; personal interview; 1-2 page personal statement; prerequisites in biology, chemistry, physics, organic chemistry, quantitative analysis, and integral/differential calculus. Additional exam requirements/recommendations for international students: Required—TOEFL (minimum score 550 paper-based; 79 iBT) or IELTS (minimum score 6.5). *Application deadline:* For fall admission, 2/15 for domestic students, 1/2 for international students. Application fee: $30. *Expenses:* Contact institution. *Faculty research:* Anatomy, biochemistry, cancer biology, cardiovascular disease, cell biology, immunology, microbiology, molecular biology, neuroscience, pharmacology, physiology. *Unit head:* Dr. Michael Barber, Professor/Associate Dean for Graduate and Postdoctoral Affairs, 813-974-9908, Fax: 813-974-4317, E-mail: mbarber@health.usf.edu. *Application contact:* Dr. Eric Bennett, Graduate Director, PhD Program in Medical Sciences, 813-974-1545, Fax: 813-974-4317, E-mail: esbennet@health.usf.edu.
Website: http://health.usf.edu/nocms/medicine/graduatestudies/

Molecular Toxicology

Massachusetts Institute of Technology, School of Science, Department of Biology, Cambridge, MA 02139. Offers biochemistry (PhD); biological oceanography (PhD); biology (PhD); biophysical chemistry and molecular structure (PhD); cell biology (PhD); computational and systems biology (PhD); developmental biology (PhD); genetics (PhD); immunology (PhD); microbiology (PhD); molecular biology (PhD); neurobiology (PhD). *Faculty:* 57 full-time (14 women). *Students:* 283 full-time (137 women); includes 83 minority (3 Black or African American, non-Hispanic/Latino; 1 American Indian or Alaska Native, non-Hispanic/Latino; 38 Asian, non-Hispanic/Latino; 31 Hispanic/Latino; 10 Two or more races, non-Hispanic/Latino), 48 international. Average age 26. 673 applicants, 14% accepted, 46 enrolled. In 2015, 32 doctorates awarded. *Degree requirements:* For doctorate, comprehensive exam, thesis/dissertation, teaching assistantship during two semesters. *Entrance requirements:* For doctorate, GRE General Test. Additional exam requirements/recommendations for international students: Required—TOEFL (minimum score 577 paper-based), IELTS. *Application deadline:* For fall admission, 12/1 for domestic and international students. Application fee: $75. Electronic applications accepted. *Expenses: Tuition:* Full-time $46,400; part-time $725 per credit. One-time fee: $304 full-time. Full-time tuition and fees vary according to course load and program. *Financial support:* In 2015–16, 235 students received support, including 118 fellowships (averaging $37,500 per year), 163 research assistantships (averaging $38,900 per year), 1 teaching assistantship; Federal Work-Study, institutionally sponsored loans, scholarships/grants, traineeships, health care benefits, and unspecified assistantships also available. Support available to part-time students. Financial award application deadline: 4/15; financial award applicants required to submit FAFSA. *Faculty research:* Cellular, developmental and molecular (plant and animal) biology; biochemistry, bioengineering, biophysics and structural biology; classical and molecular genetics, stem cell and epigenetics; immunology and microbiology; cancer biology, molecular medicine, neurobiology and human disease; computational and systems biology. Total annual research expenditures: $42.8 million. *Unit head:* Prof. Alan Grossman, Department Head, 617-253-4701. *Application contact:* Biology Education Office, 617-253-3717, Fax: 617-258-9329, E-mail: gradbio@mit.edu.
Website: https://biology.mit.edu/

New York University, Graduate School of Arts and Science, Department of Environmental Medicine, New York, NY 10012-1019. Offers environmental health sciences (MS, PhD), including biostatistics (PhD), environmental hygiene (MS), epidemiology (PhD), ergonomics and biomechanics (PhD), exposure assessment and health effects (PhD), molecular toxicology/carcinogenesis (PhD), toxicology (PhD). *Program availability:* Part-time. Terminal master's awarded for partial completion of doctoral program. *Degree requirements:* For master's, thesis or alternative; for doctorate, one foreign language, thesis/dissertation, oral and written exams. *Entrance requirements:* For master's and doctorate, GRE General Test, minimum GPA of 3.0; bachelor's degree in biological, physical, or engineering science. Additional exam requirements/recommendations for international students: Required—TOEFL.
See Close-Up on page 851.

North Carolina State University, Graduate School, College of Agriculture and Life Sciences and College of Veterinary Medicine, Department of Environmental and Molecular Toxicology, Raleigh, NC 27695. Offers M Tox, MS, PhD. Terminal master's

awarded for partial completion of doctoral program. *Degree requirements:* For master's, thesis (for some programs); for doctorate, thesis/dissertation. *Entrance requirements:* For master's and doctorate, GRE General Test, minimum GPA of 3.0. Electronic applications accepted. *Faculty research:* Chemical fate, carcinogenesis, developmental and endocrine toxicity, xenobiotic metabolism, signal transduction.

Penn State Hershey Medical Center, College of Medicine, Graduate School Programs in the Biomedical Sciences, The Huck Institutes of the Life Sciences, Intercollege Graduate Program in Molecular Cellular and Integrative Biosciences, Hershey, PA 17033. Offers cell and developmental biology (PhD); immunology and infectious disease (PhD); molecular and evolutionary genetics (PhD); molecular medicine (PhD); molecular toxicology (PhD); neurobiology (PhD). *Students:* 3 full-time (2 women); includes 2 minority (both Asian, non-Hispanic/Latino). 2 applicants, 100% accepted, 2 enrolled. In 2015, 1 doctorate awarded. *Degree requirements:* For doctorate, comprehensive exam, thesis/dissertation, oral exam. *Entrance requirements:* For doctorate, GRE, minimum GPA of 3.0. Additional exam requirements/recommendations for international students: Required—TOEFL (minimum score 500 paper-based). *Application deadline:* For fall admission, 1/31 priority date for domestic students, 2/1 priority date for international students. Applications are processed on a rolling basis. Application fee: $65. Electronic applications accepted. *Financial support:* In 2015–16, research assistantships with full tuition reimbursements (averaging $26,196 per year) were awarded; fellowships with full tuition reimbursements, career-related internships or fieldwork, Federal Work-Study, scholarships/grants, health care benefits, and unspecified assistantships also available. Financial award applicants required to submit FAFSA. *Faculty research:* Vascular biology, molecular toxicology, chemical biology, immune system, pathophysiological basis of human disease. *Unit head:* Dr. Peter Hudson, Director, 814-865-6057, E-mail: pjh18@psu.edu. *Application contact:* Kathy Shuey, Administrative Assistant, 717-531-8982, Fax: 717-531-0786, E-mail: grad-hmc@psu.edu.
Website: http://www.huck.psu.edu/education/molecular-cellular-and-integrative-biosciences

University of California, Berkeley, Graduate Division, College of Natural Resources, Group in Molecular Toxicology, Berkeley, CA 94720-1500. Offers PhD. *Entrance requirements:* For doctorate, GRE General Test, 3 letters of recommendation.

University of California, Los Angeles, Graduate Division, School of Public Health, Department of Environmental Health Sciences, Interdepartmental Program in Molecular Toxicology, Los Angeles, CA 90095. Offers PhD. *Degree requirements:* For doctorate, thesis/dissertation, oral and written qualifying exams. *Entrance requirements:* For doctorate, GRE General Test. Electronic applications accepted.

University of Cincinnati, Graduate School, College of Medicine, Graduate Programs in Biomedical Sciences, Department of Environmental Health, Programs in Environmental Genetics and Molecular Toxicology, Cincinnati, OH 45221. Offers MS, PhD. *Degree requirements:* For doctorate, thesis/dissertation. *Entrance requirements:* For master's, GRE, minimum GPA of 3.0, 3 letters of recommendation. Additional exam requirements/recommendations for international students: Required—TOEFL (minimum score 520 paper-based).

Pharmacology

Albany College of Pharmacy and Health Sciences, School of Pharmacy and Pharmaceutical Sciences, Albany, NY 12208. Offers health outcomes research (MS); pharmaceutical sciences (MS), including pharmaceutics, pharmacology; pharmacy (Pharm D). *Accreditation:* ACPE. *Degree requirements:* For master's, thesis; for doctorate, practice experience. *Entrance requirements:* For master's, GRE, minimum GPA of 3.0; for doctorate, PCAT, minimum GPA of 2.5. Additional exam requirements/

recommendations for international students: Required—TOEFL (minimum score 84 iBT). Electronic applications accepted. *Faculty research:* Therapeutic use of drugs, pharmacokinetics, drug delivery and design.

Albany Medical College, Center for Neuropharmacology and Neuroscience, Albany, NY 12208-3479. Offers MS, PhD. Terminal master's awarded for partial completion of doctoral program. *Degree requirements:* For master's, thesis; for doctorate,

Pharmacology

comprehensive exam, thesis/dissertation. *Entrance requirements:* For master's, GRE General Test, all transcripts, letters of recommendation; for doctorate, GRE General Test, letters of recommendation. Additional exam requirements/recommendations for international students: Required—TOEFL. *Faculty research:* Molecular and cellular neuroscience, neuronal development, addiction.

Alliant International University–San Francisco, California School of Professional Psychology, Program in Psychopharmacology, San Francisco, CA 94133-1221. Offers Post-Doctoral MS. *Program availability:* Part-time, online learning. *Entrance requirements:* For master's, doctorate in clinical psychology. Additional exam requirements/recommendations for international students: Required—TOEFL (minimum score 550 paper-based; 80 iBT), TWE (minimum score 5). Electronic applications accepted.

American University of Beirut, Graduate Programs, Faculty of Medicine, Beirut, Lebanon. Offers anatomy, cell biology and human morphology (MS); biochemistry and medical genetics (MS); biomedical sciences (PhD); experimental pathology, immunology and microbiology (MS); medicine (MD); neuroscience (MS); pharmacology and toxicology (MS). *Program availability:* Part-time. *Faculty* 302 full-time (95 women), 64 part-time/adjunct (11 women). *Students:* 381 full-time (173 women), 61 part-time (51 women). Average age 23. In 2015, 14 master's awarded. *Degree requirements:* For master's, one foreign language, comprehensive exam, thesis (for some programs); for doctorate, one foreign language, comprehensive exam, thesis/dissertation. *Entrance requirements:* For master's, letter of recommendation; for doctorate, MCAT, bachelor's degree. Additional exam requirements/recommendations for international students: Required—TOEFL (minimum score 600 paper-based; 100 iBT), IELTS (minimum score 7.5). *Application deadline:* For fall admission, 4/30 for domestic and international students; for spring admission, 11/1 for domestic and international students. Application fee: $50. Electronic applications accepted. *Expenses: Tuition, area resident:* Full-time $16,254; part-time $903 per credit. *Required fees:* $699. Tuition and fees vary according to course load and program. *Financial support:* In 2015–16, 273 students received support, including 45 teaching assistantships (averaging $9,000 per year); career-related internships or fieldwork, institutionally sponsored loans, scholarships/grants, health care benefits, and unspecified assistantships also available. Financial award application deadline: 2/2. *Faculty research:* Cancer research (targeted therapy, mechanisms of leukemogenesis, tumor cell extravasation and metastasis, cancer stem cells), stem cell research (regenerative medicine, drug discovery), genetic research (neurogenetics, hereditary cardiomyopathy, hemoglobinopathies, pharmacogenomics, proteomics), neuroscience research (pain, neurodegenerative disorder), metabolism (inflammation and metabolism, metabolic disorder, diabetes mellitus), vascular and renal biology, signal transduction. *Total annual research expenditures:* $2.6 million. *Unit head:* Dr. Mohamed Sayegh, Dean, 961-1350000 Ext. 4700, Fax: 961-1744464, E-mail: msayegh@aub.edu.lb. *Application contact:* Dr. Salim Kanaan, Director, Admissions Office, 961-1350000 Ext. 2594, Fax: 961-1750775, E-mail: sk00@aub.edu.lb. Website: http://www.aub.edu.lb/fm/fm_home/Pages/index.aspx

Argosy University, Hawai`i, Hawai'i School of Professional Psychology, Program in Psychopharmacology, Honolulu, HI 96813. Offers MS, Certificate.

Auburn University, College of Veterinary Medicine and Graduate School, Graduate Programs in Veterinary Medicine, Auburn University, AL 36849. Offers biomedical sciences (MS, PhD), including anatomy, physiology and pharmacology (MS); biomedical sciences (PhD); clinical sciences (MS); large animal surgery and medicine (MS); pathobiology (MS); radiology (MS); small animal surgery and medicine (MS); DVM/MS. *Program availability:* Part-time. *Faculty:* 97 full-time (40 women), 4 part-time/adjunct (2 women). *Students:* 19 full-time (11 women), 54 part-time (34 women); includes 10 minority (2 Black or African American, non-Hispanic/Latino; 2 American Indian or Alaska Native, non-Hispanic/Latino; 2 Asian, non-Hispanic/Latino; 4 Hispanic/Latino), 23 international. Average age 31. 39 applicants, 59% accepted, 14 enrolled. In 2015, 12 master's, 6 doctorates awarded. *Degree requirements:* For doctorate, thesis/dissertation. *Entrance requirements:* For master's, GRE General Test; for doctorate, GRE General Test, GRE Subject Test. *Application deadline:* Applications are processed on a rolling basis. Application fee: $50 ($60 for international students). Electronic applications accepted. *Expenses:* Tuition, state resident: full-time $8802; part-time $489 per credit hour. Tuition, nonresident: full-time $26,406; part-time $1467 per credit hour. *Required fees:* $808 per semester. Tuition and fees vary according to degree level and program. *Financial support:* Research assistantships, teaching assistantships, and Federal Work-Study available. Support available to part-time students. Financial award application deadline: 3/15; financial award applicants required to submit FAFSA. *Unit head:* Dr. Calvin Johnson, Acting Dean, 334-844-2650. *Application contact:* Dr. George Flowers, Dean of the Graduate School, 334-844-2125.

Augusta University, The Graduate School, Program in Pharmacology, Augusta, GA 30912. Offers PhD. *Degree requirements:* For doctorate, comprehensive exam, thesis/dissertation. *Entrance requirements:* For doctorate, GRE General Test. Additional exam requirements/recommendations for international students: Required—TOEFL (minimum score 550 paper-based; 79 iBT). *Application deadline:* For fall admission, 1/15 for domestic and international students. Application fee: $50. Electronic applications accepted. *Financial support:* Fellowships with partial tuition reimbursements, research assistantships with partial tuition reimbursements, Federal Work-Study, institutionally sponsored loans, and scholarships/grants available. Support available to part-time students. Financial award application deadline: 5/31; financial award applicants required to submit FAFSA. *Faculty research:* Protein signaling, neural development, cardiovascular pharmacology, endothelial cell function, neuropharmacology. *Unit head:* Dr. John A. Johnson, Director, 706-721-4173, Fax: 706-721-6059, E-mail: jjohnson@augusta.edu.
Website: http://www.augusta.edu/mcg/phmtox/phtx_graduate.php

Baylor College of Medicine, Graduate School of Biomedical Sciences, Department of Pharmacology, Houston, TX 77030-3498. Offers PhD, MD/PhD. *Degree requirements:* For doctorate, thesis/dissertation, public defense. *Entrance requirements:* For doctorate, GRE General Test, GRE Subject Test (strongly recommended), minimum GPA of 3.0. Additional exam requirements/recommendations for international students: Required—TOEFL. Electronic applications accepted. *Faculty research:* Drug discovery, antibiotics, antitumor, computational drug design, signal transduction complex.

Boston University, School of Medicine, Division of Graduate Medical Sciences, Department of Pharmacology and Experimental Therapeutics, Boston, MA 02118. Offers MA, PhD, MD/PhD. Terminal master's awarded for partial completion of doctoral program. *Degree requirements:* For master's, thesis; for doctorate, thesis/dissertation. *Application deadline:* For fall admission, 1/15 for domestic students; for spring admission, 10/15 for domestic students. *Unit head:* Dr. David H. Farb, Chairman, 617-638-4300, Fax: 617-638-4329, E-mail: dfarb@bu.edu. *Application contact:* GMS Admissions Office, 617-638-5255, E-mail: askgms@bu.edu.
Website: http://www.bumc.bu.edu/busm-pm/

Boston University, School of Medicine, Division of Graduate Medical Sciences, Program in Clinical Investigation, Boston, MA 02215. Offers MA. *Degree requirements:* For master's, thesis. *Application deadline:* For spring admission, 10/15 for domestic students. *Unit head:* Dr. Susan S. Fish, Director, 617-638-7715, E-mail: sfish@bu.edu.

Application contact: Stacey Hess Pino, GMS Admissions Office, 617-638-5255, E-mail: askgms@bu.edu.
Website: http://www.bumc.bu.edu/gms/maci/

Case Western Reserve University, School of Medicine and School of Graduate Studies, Graduate Programs in Medicine, Department of Pharmacology, Cleveland, OH 44106. Offers PhD, MD/PhD. Terminal master's awarded for partial completion of doctoral program. *Degree requirements:* For doctorate, comprehensive exam, thesis/dissertation. *Entrance requirements:* For doctorate, GRE General Test or MCAT. Additional exam requirements/recommendations for international students: Required—TOEFL (minimum score 577 paper-based; 90 iBT). Electronic applications accepted. *Expenses: Tuition, area resident:* Full-time $41,137; part-time $1714 per credit hour. *Required fees:* $32. Tuition and fees vary according to course load and program. *Faculty research:* Neuroendocrine pharmacology, translational therapeutics, cancer therapeutics, molecular pharmacology and cell regulation, membrane and structural biology and pharmacology.

Columbia University, College of Physicians and Surgeons, Department of Pharmacology, New York, NY 10032. Offers pharmacology (M Phil, MA, PhD); pharmacology-toxicology (M Phil, MA, PhD); MD/PhD. Only candidates for the PhD are admitted. Terminal master's awarded for partial completion of doctoral program. *Degree requirements:* For master's and doctorate, thesis/dissertation. *Entrance requirements:* For master's and doctorate, GRE General Test. Additional exam requirements/recommendations for international students: Required—TOEFL. *Faculty research:* Cardiovascular pharmacology, receptor pharmacology, neuropharmacology, membrane biophysics, eicosanoids.

Cornell University, Graduate School, Graduate Fields of Comparative Biomedical Sciences, Field of Pharmacology, Ithaca, NY 14853-0001. Offers MS, PhD. *Degree requirements:* For master's, thesis; for doctorate, comprehensive exam, thesis/dissertation. *Entrance requirements:* For master's and doctorate, GRE General Test, 3 letters of recommendation. Additional exam requirements/recommendations for international students: Required—TOEFL (minimum score 550 paper-based; 77 iBT). Electronic applications accepted. *Faculty research:* Signal transduction, ion channels, calcium signaling, G proteins, cancer cell biology.

Creighton University, School of Medicine and Graduate School, Graduate Programs in Medicine, Department of Pharmacology, Omaha, NE 68178-0001. Offers pharmaceutical sciences (MS); pharmacology (MS, PhD); Pharm D/MS. Terminal master's awarded for partial completion of doctoral program. *Degree requirements:* For master's, comprehensive exam, thesis; for doctorate, comprehensive exam, thesis/dissertation, oral and written preliminary exams. *Entrance requirements:* For master's and doctorate, GRE General Test, minimum GPA of 3.0, undergraduate degree in sciences. Additional exam requirements/recommendations for international students: Required—TOEFL. Electronic applications accepted. *Expenses: Tuition, area resident:* Full-time $14,400; part-time $800 per credit hour. *Required fees:* $158 per semester. Tuition and fees vary according to course load, campus/location, program, reciprocity agreements and student's religious affiliation. *Faculty research:* Pharmacology secretion, cardiovascular-renal pharmacology, adrenergic receptors, signal transduction, genetic regulation of receptors.

Dalhousie University, Faculty of Graduate Studies and Faculty of Medicine, Graduate Programs in Medicine, Department of Pharmacology, Halifax, NS B3H 4R2, Canada. Offers M Sc, PhD. *Degree requirements:* For master's, thesis; for doctorate, comprehensive exam, thesis/dissertation. *Entrance requirements:* Additional exam requirements/recommendations for international students: Required—1 of 5 approved tests: TOEFL, IELTS, CANTEST, CAEL, Michigan English Language Assessment Battery. Electronic applications accepted. *Faculty research:* Electrophysiology and neurochemistry; endocrinology, immunology and cancer research; molecular biology; cardiovascular and autonomic; drug biotransformation and metabolism; ocular pharmacology.

Drexel University, College of Medicine, Biomedical Graduate Programs, Pharmacology and Physiology Program, Philadelphia, PA 19104-2875. Offers MS, PhD, MD/PhD. *Program availability:* Part-time. Terminal master's awarded for partial completion of doctoral program. *Degree requirements:* For master's, comprehensive exam; for doctorate, thesis/dissertation, qualifying exam. *Entrance requirements:* For master's, GRE General Test, minimum GPA of 2.75; for doctorate, GRE General Test, minimum GPA of 3.0. Additional exam requirements/recommendations for international students: Required—TOEFL. Electronic applications accepted. *Faculty research:* Cardiovascular pharmacology, drugs of abuse, neurotransmitter mechanisms.

Duke University, Graduate School, Department of Pharmacology and Cancer Biology, Durham, NC 27710. Offers pharmacology (PhD). *Faculty:* 50 full-time. *Students:* 51 full-time (20 women). Average age 23. 68 applicants, 15% accepted, 6 enrolled. In 2015, 8 doctorates awarded. *Degree requirements:* For doctorate, thesis/dissertation. *Entrance requirements:* For doctorate, GRE General Test, minimum GPA of 3.0. Additional exam requirements/recommendations for international students: Required—TOEFL or IELTS. *Application deadline:* For fall admission, 12/1 priority date for domestic and international students. Application fee: $80. Electronic applications accepted. *Financial support:* In 2015–16, 10 fellowships with tuition reimbursements (averaging $29,420 per year), 52 research assistantships with tuition reimbursements (averaging $29,860 per year) were awarded; scholarships/grants, traineeships, health care benefits, and unspecified assistantships also available. Financial award application deadline: 12/1. *Faculty research:* Developmental pharmacology, neuropharmacology, molecular pharmacology, toxicology, cell growth and metabolism. *Unit head:* Dr. David MacAlpine, Director of Graduate Studies, 919-681-6077, E-mail: david.macalpine@duke.edu. *Application contact:* Jamie Baize-Smith, Assistant Director of Graduate Studies, 919-613-8600, Fax: 919-681-7139, E-mail: baize@duke.edu.
Website: http://pharmacology.mc.duke.edu/

Duquesne University, Mylan School of Pharmacy, Graduate School of Pharmaceutical Sciences, Program in Pharmacology, Pittsburgh, PA 15282-0001. Offers MS, PhD. *Faculty:* 6 full-time (4 women). *Students:* 14 full-time (8 women), 6 international. Average age 27. 30 applicants, 10% accepted, 2 enrolled. In 2015, 1 master's awarded. *Degree requirements:* For master's, thesis; for doctorate, comprehensive exam, thesis/dissertation. *Entrance requirements:* For master's and doctorate, GRE General Test. Additional exam requirements/recommendations for international students: Required—TOEFL (minimum score 100 iBT). *Application deadline:* For fall admission, 2/1 priority date for domestic and international students; for spring admission, 10/1 priority date for domestic and international students. Applications are processed on a rolling basis. Application fee: $50. Electronic applications accepted. Application fee is waived when completed online. *Expenses:* $1,432 per credit. *Financial support:* In 2015–16, 14 students received support, including 1 research assistantship with full tuition reimbursement available, 13 teaching assistantships with full tuition reimbursements available. *Unit head:* Dr. Christopher K. Surratt, Head, 412-396-5007. *Application contact:* Information Contact, 412-396-1172, E-mail: gsps-adm@duq.edu.
Website: http://www.duq.edu/academics/schools/pharmacy/graduate-school-of-pharmaceutical-sciences

East Carolina University, Brody School of Medicine, Department of Pharmacology and Toxicology, Greenville, NC 27858-4353. Offers PhD, MD/PhD. *Students:* 18 full-time (7 women), 1 (woman) part-time; includes 6 minority (3 Black or African American, non-Hispanic/Latino; 1 Asian, non-Hispanic/Latino; 1 Hispanic/Latino; 1 Two or more races, non-Hispanic/Latino), 4 international. Average age 29. 6 applicants, 33% accepted, 2 enrolled. In 2015, 2 doctorates awarded. *Degree requirements:* For doctorate, comprehensive exam, thesis/dissertation. *Entrance requirements:* For doctorate, GRE General Test, GRE Subject Test. Additional exam requirements/recommendations for international students: Required—TOEFL. *Application deadline:* For fall admission, 6/15 priority date for domestic students. Applications are processed on a rolling basis. Application fee: $50. *Financial support:* Fellowships with full tuition reimbursements available. Financial award application deadline: 6/1. *Faculty research:* GNS/behavioral pharmacology, cardiovascular pharmacology, cell signaling and second messenger, effects of calcium channel blockers. *Unit head:* Dr. David A. Taylor, Chairman, 252-744-2734, Fax: 252-744-3203, E-mail: taylorda@ecu.edu. *Application contact:* Contact Center, 252-744-1020.
Website: http://www.ecu.edu/cs-dhs/pharmacology/Graduate-Program09.cfm

East Tennessee State University, James H. Quillen College of Medicine, Department of Biomedical Sciences, Johnson City, TN 37614. Offers anatomy (PhD); biochemistry (PhD); microbiology (PhD); pharmaceutical sciences (PhD); pharmacology (PhD); physiology (PhD); quantitative biosciences (PhD). *Faculty:* 30 full-time (6 women). *Students:* 35 full-time (17 women), 2 part-time (1 woman); includes 13 minority (9 Black or African American, non-Hispanic/Latino; 4 Asian, non-Hispanic/Latino), 13 international. Average age 29. 53 applicants, 17% accepted, 8 enrolled. In 2015, 8 doctorates awarded. *Degree requirements:* For doctorate, thesis/dissertation, comprehensive qualifying exam. *Entrance requirements:* For doctorate, GRE General Test, GRE Subject Test, 3 letters of recommendation. Additional exam requirements/recommendations for international students: Required—TOEFL (minimum score 550 paper-based; 79 iBT). *Application deadline:* For fall admission, 3/15 priority date for domestic students, 3/1 priority date for international students. Application fee: $35 ($45 for international students). Electronic applications accepted. *Expenses:* Contact institution. *Financial support:* In 2015–16, 30 students received support, including 27 research assistantships with full tuition reimbursements available (averaging $20,000 per year); career-related internships or fieldwork, institutionally sponsored loans, scholarships/grants, and unspecified assistantships also available. Financial award application deadline: 7/1; financial award applicants required to submit FAFSA. *Faculty research:* Cardiovascular, infectious disease, neurosciences, cancer, immunology. *Unit head:* Dr. Mitchell E. Robinson, Associate Dean/Program Director, 423-439-2031, Fax: 423-439-2140, E-mail: robinson@etsu.edu. *Application contact:* Shella Bennett, Graduate Specialist, 423-439-4708, Fax: 423-439-5624, E-mail: bennetsg@etsu.edu.
Website: http://www.etsu.edu/com/dbms/

Emory University, Laney Graduate School, Division of Biological and Biomedical Sciences, Program in Molecular and Systems Pharmacology, Atlanta, GA 30322-1100. Offers PhD. *Degree requirements:* For doctorate, comprehensive exam, thesis/dissertation. *Entrance requirements:* For doctorate, GRE General Test, minimum GPA of 3.0 in science course work (recommended). Additional exam requirements/recommendations for international students: Required—TOEFL. Electronic applications accepted. *Faculty research:* Transmembrane signaling, neuropharmacology, neurophysiology and neurodegeneration, metabolism and molecular toxicology, cell and developmental biology.

Fairleigh Dickinson University, College at Florham, Silberman College of Business, Program in Pharmaceutical Studies, Madison, NJ 07940-1099. Offers MBA, Certificate.

Florida Agricultural and Mechanical University, Division of Graduate Studies, Research, and Continuing Education, College of Pharmacy and Pharmaceutical Sciences, Graduate Programs in Pharmaceutical Sciences, Tallahassee, FL 32307-3200. Offers environmental toxicology (PhD); health outcomes research and pharmacoeconomics (PhD); medicinal chemistry (MS, PhD); pharmaceutics (MS, PhD); pharmacology/toxicology (MS, PhD); pharmacy administration (MS). *Accreditation:* CEPH. *Degree requirements:* For master's, comprehensive exam, thesis, publishable paper; for doctorate, comprehensive exam, thesis/dissertation, publishable paper. *Entrance requirements:* For master's and doctorate, GRE General Test, minimum GPA of 3.0 in last 60 hours. Additional exam requirements/recommendations for international students: Required—TOEFL. *Faculty research:* Anticancer agents, anti-inflammatory drugs, chronopharmacology, neuroendocrinology, microbiology.

Georgetown University, Graduate School of Arts and Sciences, Department of Pharmacology and Physiology, Washington, DC 20057. Offers pharmacology (MS, PhD); physiology (MS); MD/PhD. *Degree requirements:* For doctorate, comprehensive exam, thesis/dissertation. *Entrance requirements:* For doctorate, GRE General Test, previous course work in biology and chemistry. Additional exam requirements/recommendations for international students: Required—TOEFL. *Faculty research:* Neuropharmacology, techniques in biochemistry and tissue culture.

Howard University, College of Medicine, Department of Pharmacology, Washington, DC 20059-0002. Offers MS, PhD, MD/PhD. *Program availability:* Part-time. *Degree requirements:* For master's, comprehensive exam, thesis; for doctorate, one foreign language, comprehensive exam, thesis/dissertation, qualifying exam. *Entrance requirements:* For master's, GRE General Test, minimum GPA of 3.2, BS in chemistry, biology, pharmacy, psychology or related field; for doctorate, GRE General Test, minimum graduate GPA of 3.2. Additional exam requirements/recommendations for international students: Recommended—TOEFL. *Faculty research:* Biochemical pharmacology, molecular pharmacology, neuropharmacology, drug metabolism, cancer research.

Idaho State University, Office of Graduate Studies, College of Pharmacy, Department of Biomedical and Pharmaceutical Sciences, Pocatello, ID 83209-8334. Offers biopharmaceutical analysis (PhD); drug delivery (PhD); medicinal chemistry (PhD); pharmaceutical sciences (MS); pharmacology (PhD). *Program availability:* Part-time. *Degree requirements:* For master's, one foreign language, comprehensive exam, thesis, thesis research, classes in speech and technical writing; for doctorate, comprehensive exam, thesis/dissertation, written and oral exams, classes in speech and technical writing. *Entrance requirements:* For master's, GRE General Test, minimum GPA of 3.0, 3 letters of recommendation; for doctorate, GRE General Test, BS in pharmacy or related field, minimum GPA of 3.0, 3 letters of recommendation. Additional exam requirements/recommendations for international students: Required—TOEFL (minimum score 550 paper-based; 80 iBT). Electronic applications accepted. *Expenses:* Contact institution. *Faculty research:* Metabolic toxicity of heavy metals, neuroendocrine pharmacology, cardiovascular pharmacology, cancer biology, immunopharmacology.

Indiana University–Purdue University Indianapolis, Indiana University School of Medicine, Department of Pharmacology and Toxicology, Indianapolis, IN 46202. Offers pharmacology (MS, PhD); toxicology (MS, PhD); MD/PhD. Terminal master's awarded for partial completion of doctoral program. *Degree requirements:* For master's, thesis; for doctorate, thesis/dissertation. *Entrance requirements:* For master's and doctorate, GRE General Test, GRE Subject Test, minimum GPA of 3.0. *Faculty research:* Neuropharmacology, cardiovascular biopharmacology, chemotherapy, oncogenesis.

Johns Hopkins University, School of Medicine, Graduate Programs in Medicine, Department of Pharmacology and Molecular Sciences, Baltimore, MD 21205. Offers PhD. *Degree requirements:* For doctorate, comprehensive exam, thesis/dissertation, departmental seminar. *Entrance requirements:* For doctorate, GRE General Test. Additional exam requirements/recommendations for international students: Required—TOEFL. Electronic applications accepted.

Kent State University, College of Arts and Sciences, School of Biomedical Sciences, Kent, OH 44242-0001. Offers biological anthropology (PhD); cellular and molecular biology (PhD), including cellular biology and structures, molecular biology and genetics; neurosciences (PhD); pharmacology (MS); physiology (PhD). *Students:* 76 full-time (46 women), 1 (woman) part-time; includes 6 minority (1 Black or African American, non-Hispanic/Latino; 2 Asian, non-Hispanic/Latino; 1 Hispanic/Latino; 2 Two or more races, non-Hispanic/Latino), 28 international. Average age 29. 223 applicants, 13% accepted, 22 enrolled. In 2015, 5 master's, 7 doctorates awarded. Terminal master's awarded for partial completion of doctoral program. *Degree requirements:* For master's, thesis; for doctorate, thesis/dissertation, candidacy exam. *Entrance requirements:* For master's and doctorate, GRE General Test, minimum GPA of 3.0, transcript, goal statement, resume, 3 letters of recommendation. Additional exam requirements/recommendations for international students: Required—TOEFL (minimum score: paper-based 525, iBT 71), Michigan English Language Assessment Battery (minimum score of 75), IELTS (minimum score of 6.0), PTE Academic (minimum score of 48), or completion of ELS level 112 Intensive Program. *Application deadline:* For fall admission, 1/1 for domestic students. Application fee: $45 ($70 for international students). Electronic applications accepted. *Expenses:* Tuition, state resident: full-time $10,864; part-time $495 per credit hour. Tuition, nonresident: full-time $18,380; part-time $837 per credit hour. *Financial support:* In 2015–16, 76 students received support. Research assistantships with full tuition reimbursements available, teaching assistantships, career-related internships or fieldwork, Federal Work-Study, and unspecified assistantships available. Financial award application deadline: 1/1. *Unit head:* Dr. Eric Mintz, Director, 330-672-2263, E-mail: emintz@kent.edu. *Application contact:* 330-672-2263, Fax: 330-672-9391, E-mail: jwearden@kent.edu.
Website: http://www.kent.edu/biomedical/

Loma Linda University, School of Medicine, Programs in Physiology and Pharmacology, Loma Linda, CA 92350. Offers pharmacology (PhD); physiology (PhD). *Program availability:* Part-time. *Degree requirements:* For doctorate, 2 foreign languages, thesis/dissertation. *Entrance requirements:* For doctorate, GRE General Test. *Application deadline:* Applications are processed on a rolling basis. Application fee: $40. *Financial support:* Tuition waivers (full and partial) available. Support available to part-time students. *Faculty research:* Drug metabolism, biochemical pharmacology, structure and function of cell membranes, neuropharmacology. *Unit head:* Dr. John Buchholz, Vice Chair, 909-558-7026. *Application contact:* Admissions Office, 909-651-5029, Fax: 909-558-4879, E-mail: admissions.app@llu.edu.

London Metropolitan University, Graduate Programs, London, United Kingdom. Offers applied psychology (M Sc); architecture (MA); biomedical science (M Sc); blood science (M Sc); cancer pharmacology (M Sc); computer networking and cyber security (M Sc); computing and information systems (M Sc); conference interpreting (MA); counter-terrorism studies (M Sc); creative, digital and professional writing (MA); crime, violence and prevention (M Sc); criminology (M Sc); curating contemporary art (MA); data analytics (M Sc); digital media (MA); early childhood studies (MA); education (MA, Ed D); financial services law, regulation and compliance (LL M); food science (M Sc); forensic psychology (M Sc); health and social care management and policy (M Sc); human nutrition (M Sc); human resource management (MA); human rights and international conflict (MA); information technology (M Sc); intelligence and security studies (M Sc); international oil, gas and energy law (LL M); international relations (MA); interpreting (MA); learning and teaching in higher education (MA); legal practice (LL M); media and entertainment law (LL M); organizational and consumer psychology (M Sc); psychological therapy (M Sc); psychology of mental health (M Sc); public health (M Sc); public policy and management (MPA); security studies (M Sc); social work (M Sc); spatial planning and urban design (MA); sports therapy (M Sc); supporting older children and young people with dyslexia (MA); teaching languages (MA), including Arabic, English; translation (MA); woman and child abuse (MA).

Long Island University–LIU Brooklyn, Arnold and Marie Schwartz College of Pharmacy and Health Sciences, Brooklyn, NY 11201-8423. Offers drug regulatory affairs (MS); pharmaceutics (MS, PhD), including cosmetic science (MS), industrial pharmacy (MS); pharmacology and toxicology (MS); pharmacy (Pharm D). *Accreditation:* ACPE. *Program availability:* Part-time. *Faculty:* 49 full-time (25 women), 20 part-time/adjunct (9 women). *Students:* 579 full-time (346 women), 29 part-time (14 women); includes 191 minority (24 Black or African American, non-Hispanic/Latino; 1 American Indian or Alaska Native, non-Hispanic/Latino; 144 Asian, non-Hispanic/Latino; 19 Hispanic/Latino; 3 Two or more races, non-Hispanic/Latino), 193 international. Average age 27. 350 applicants, 63% accepted, 65 enrolled. In 2015, 114 master's, 206 doctorates awarded. *Degree requirements:* For master's, comprehensive exam (for some programs), thesis optional; for doctorate, comprehensive exam, thesis/dissertation. *Entrance requirements:* For master's and doctorate, GRE, minimum GPA of 3.0. Additional exam requirements/recommendations for international students: Required—TOEFL (minimum score 550 paper-based; 79 iBT), IELTS (minimum score 6.5). *Application deadline:* Applications are processed on a rolling basis. Application fee: $50. Electronic applications accepted. *Expenses:* Contact institution. *Financial support:* In 2015–16, 185 students received support, including 6 fellowships with full tuition reimbursements available (averaging $12,800 per year), 28 teaching assistantships with full tuition reimbursements available (averaging $6,000 per year); Federal Work-Study, institutionally sponsored loans, and scholarships/grants also available. Support available to part-time students. Financial award application deadline: 2/15; financial award applicants required to submit FAFSA. *Faculty research:* Pharmaceutics, pharmacodynamics, pharmacology, pharmacometrics, pharmacotherapeutics. *Unit head:* Dr. John M. Pezzuto, Dean, 718-488-1004, Fax: 718-488-0628, E-mail: john.pezzuto@liu.edu. *Application contact:* Dr. Anait Levinson, Associate Dean of Research and Graduate Studies, 718-246-6323, E-mail: anait.levenson@liu.edu.
Website: http://liu.edu/Pharmacy

Louisiana State University Health Sciences Center, School of Graduate Studies in New Orleans, Department of Pharmacology and Experimental Therapeutics, New Orleans, LA 70112-2223. Offers PhD, MD/PhD. *Faculty:* 21 full-time (4 women). *Students:* 18 full-time (10 women); includes 3 minority (2 Black or African American, non-Hispanic/Latino; 1 Hispanic/Latino), 4 international. Average age 25. 9 applicants, 11% accepted, 1 enrolled. In 2015, 6 doctorates awarded. *Degree requirements:* For doctorate, comprehensive exam, thesis/dissertation. *Entrance requirements:* For doctorate, GRE General Test. Additional exam requirements/recommendations for international students: Recommended—TOEFL, IELTS. *Application deadline:* For fall admission, 4/1 for domestic and international students. Applications are processed on a rolling basis. Application fee: $30. *Financial support:* Unspecified assistantships available. Financial award application deadline: 2/15. *Faculty research:* Neuropharmacology, gastrointestinal pharmacology, drug metabolism, behavioral pharmacology, cardiovascular pharmacology. *Unit head:* Dr. Kurt Varner, Professor/

Pharmacology

Head, 504-568-4740, Fax: 504-568-2361, E-mail: kvarne@lsuhsc.edu. *Application contact:* Dr. Andrew Catling, Graduate Coordinator and Professor, 504-568-2222, E-mail: acatli@lsuhsc.edu.
Website: http://www.medschool.lsumc.edu/pharmacology/

Louisiana State University Health Sciences Center at Shreveport, Department of Pharmacology, Toxicology and Neuroscience, Shreveport, LA 71130-3932. Offers pharmacology (PhD); MD/PhD. *Faculty:* 10 full-time (2 women), 5 part-time/adjunct (3 women). *Students:* 15 full-time (11 women); includes 2 minority (1 Black or African American, non-Hispanic/Latino; 1 Asian, non-Hispanic/Latino), 2 international. Average age 25. 16 applicants, 25% accepted, 4 enrolled. In 2015, 1 master's, 1 doctorate awarded. Terminal master's awarded for partial completion of doctoral program. *Degree requirements:* For master's, thesis; for doctorate, thesis/dissertation. *Entrance requirements:* For master's, GRE General Test; for doctorate, GRE General Test, minimum GPA of 3.0. Additional exam requirements/recommendations for international students: Required—TOEFL (minimum score 550 paper-based). *Application deadline:* For fall admission, 2/1 priority date for domestic students, 2/1 for international students. Application fee: $0. *Financial support:* In 2015–16, 3 fellowships with full tuition reimbursements (averaging $28,000 per year), 9 research assistantships with full tuition reimbursements (averaging $24,000 per year) were awarded; institutionally sponsored loans also available. Financial award application deadline: 5/1. *Faculty research:* Behavioral, cardiovascular, clinical, and gastrointestinal pharmacology; neuropharmacology; psychopharmacology; drug abuse; pharmacokinetics; neuroendocrinology, psychoneuroimmunology, and stress; toxicology. *Unit head:* Dr. Nicholas E. Goeders, Head, 318-675-7850, Fax: 318-675-7857, E-mail: ngoede@lsuhsc.edu. *Application contact:* Ty E. Martinez, Academic Coordinator, 318-675-7851, Fax: 318-675-7857, E-mail: tmoren@lsuhsc.edu.
Website: http://lsuhscshreveport.edu/departments/BasicScience/pharmacologytoxicologyandneuroscience/index

McGill University, Faculty of Graduate and Postdoctoral Studies, Faculty of Medicine, Department of Pharmacology and Therapeutics, Montréal, QC H3A 2T5, Canada. Offers M Sc, PhD.

McMaster University, Faculty of Health Sciences and School of Graduate Studies, Program in Medical Sciences, Physiology/Pharmacology Area, Hamilton, ON L8S 4M2, Canada. Offers M Sc, PhD, MD/PhD. *Degree requirements:* For master's, thesis; for doctorate, comprehensive exam, thesis/dissertation. *Entrance requirements:* For master's, honors B Sc, B+ average in related field; for doctorate, M Sc, minimum B+ average, students with proven research experience and an A average may be admitted with a B Sc degree. Additional exam requirements/recommendations for international students: Required—TOEFL (minimum score 580 paper-based; 92 iBT).

MCPHS University, Graduate Studies, Program in Pharmacology, Boston, MA 02115-5896. Offers MS, PhD. *Accreditation:* ACPE (one or more programs are accredited). Terminal master's awarded for partial completion of doctoral program. *Degree requirements:* For master's, oral defense of thesis; for doctorate, one foreign language, oral defense of dissertation, qualifying exam. *Entrance requirements:* For master's and doctorate, GRE General Test, minimum QPA of 3.0. Additional exam requirements/recommendations for international students: Required—TOEFL (minimum score 550 paper-based; 79 iBT). *Faculty research:* Neuropharmacology, cardiovascular pharmacology, nutritional pharmacology, pulmonary physiology, drug metabolism.

Medical College of Wisconsin, Graduate School of Biomedical Sciences, Department of Pharmacology and Toxicology, Milwaukee, WI 53226-0509. Offers PhD, MD/PhD. *Degree requirements:* For doctorate, comprehensive exam, thesis/dissertation, oral and written qualifying exams. *Entrance requirements:* For doctorate, GRE, official transcripts, three letters of recommendation. Additional exam requirements/recommendations for international students: Required—TOEFL. Electronic applications accepted. *Faculty research:* Cardiovascular physiology and pharmacology, drugs of abuse, environmental and aquatic toxicology, central nervous system and biochemical pharmacology, signal transduction.

Meharry Medical College, School of Graduate Studies, Program in Biomedical Sciences, Pharmacology Emphasis, Nashville, TN 37208-9989. Offers PhD, MD/PhD. *Degree requirements:* For doctorate, comprehensive exam, thesis/dissertation. *Entrance requirements:* For doctorate, GRE. *Application deadline:* For fall admission, 6/1 for domestic students. Applications are processed on a rolling basis. Application fee: $65. *Financial support:* Fellowships, research assistantships, teaching assistantships, Federal Work-Study, institutionally sponsored loans, and tuition waivers (full) available. Support available to part-time students. Financial award application deadline: 4/15.

Michigan State University, College of Human Medicine and The Graduate School, Graduate Programs in Human Medicine, East Lansing, MI 48824. Offers biochemistry and molecular biology (MS, PhD); epidemiology (MS, PhD); microbiology (MS); microbiology and molecular genetics (PhD); pharmacology and toxicology (MS, PhD); physiology (MS, PhD); public health (MPH). *Entrance requirements:* Additional exam requirements/recommendations for international students: Required—TOEFL.

Michigan State University, College of Osteopathic Medicine and The Graduate School, Graduate Studies in Osteopathic Medicine and Graduate Programs in Human Medicine and Graduate Programs in Veterinary Medicine, Department of Pharmacology and Toxicology, East Lansing, MI 48824. Offers integrative pharmacology (MS); pharmacology and toxicology (MS, PhD); pharmacology and toxicology-environmental toxicology (PhD). *Entrance requirements:* Additional exam requirements/recommendations for international students: Required—TOEFL (minimum score 600 paper-based). Electronic applications accepted.

Michigan State University, College of Veterinary Medicine and The Graduate School, Graduate Programs in Veterinary Medicine, East Lansing, MI 48824. Offers comparative medicine and integrative biology (MS, PhD), including comparative medicine and integrative biology, comparative medicine and integrative biology–environmental toxicology (PhD); food safety and toxicology (MS), including food safety; integrative toxicology (PhD), including animal science–environmental toxicology, biochemistry and molecular biology–environmental toxicology, chemistry–environmental toxicology, crop and soil sciences–environmental toxicology, environmental engineering–environmental toxicology, environmental geosciences–environmental toxicology, fisheries and wildlife–environmental toxicology, food science–environmental toxicology, forestry–environmental toxicology, genetics–environmental toxicology, human nutrition–environmental toxicology, microbiology–environmental toxicology, pharmacology and toxicology–environmental toxicology, zoology–environmental toxicology; large animal clinical sciences (MS, PhD); microbiology and molecular genetics (MS, PhD), including industrial microbiology, microbiology, microbiology and molecular genetics, microbiology–environmental toxicology (PhD); pathobiology and diagnostic investigation (MS, PhD), including pathology, pathology–environmental toxicology (PhD); pharmacology and toxicology (MS, PhD); pharmacology and toxicology–environmental toxicology (PhD); physiology (MS, PhD); small animal clinical sciences (MS). Electronic applications accepted. *Faculty research:* Molecular genetics, food safety/toxicology, comparative orthopedics, airway disease, population medicine.

Montclair State University, The Graduate School, College of Science and Mathematics, Program in Pharmaceutical Biochemistry, Montclair, NJ 07043-1624.

Offers MS. *Program availability:* Part-time, evening/weekend. *Students:* 6 full-time (5 women), 2 part-time (0 women); includes 2 minority (1 Black or African American, non-Hispanic/Latino; 1 Hispanic/Latino), 4 international. Average age 24. 8 applicants, 63% accepted, 4 enrolled. *Entrance requirements:* For master's, GRE General Test, 24 undergraduate credits in chemistry, 2 letters of recommendation, essay. *Application deadline:* Applications are processed on a rolling basis. Application fee: $60. Electronic applications accepted. *Expenses:* Tuition, state resident: part-time $553 per credit. Tuition, nonresident: part-time $854 per credit. *Required fees:* $91 per credit. Tuition and fees vary according to program. *Financial support:* Federal Work-Study, scholarships/grants, and unspecified assistantships available. Support available to part-time students. Financial award application deadline: 3/1. *Faculty research:* Enzyme kinetics, enzyme expression, pharmaceutical biochemistry, medicinal chemistry, biophysical chemistry. *Unit head:* Dr. Marc Kasner, Chair, 973-655-6864. *Application contact:* Amy Aiello, Executive Director of The Graduate School, 973-655-5147, E-mail: graduate.school@montclair.edu.
Website: http://www.montclair.edu/graduate/programs-of-study/pharmaceutical-biochemistry/

New Jersey Institute of Technology, Newark College of Engineering, Newark, NJ 07102. Offers biomedical engineering (MS, PhD); chemical engineering (MS, PhD); computer engineering (MS, PhD); electrical engineering (MS, PhD); engineering management (MS); environmental engineering (PhD); healthcare systems management (MS); industrial engineering (MS, PhD); Internet engineering (MS); manufacturing engineering (MS); mechanical engineering (MS, PhD); occupational safety and health engineering (MS); pharmaceutical bioprocessing (MS); pharmaceutical engineering (MS); pharmaceutical systems management (MS); power and energy systems (MS); telecommunications (MS); transportation (MS, PhD). *Program availability:* Part-time, evening/weekend. *Faculty:* 139 full-time (22 women), 152 part-time/adjunct (18 women). *Students:* 946 full-time (226 women), 580 part-time (122 women); includes 397 minority (93 Black or African American, non-Hispanic/Latino; 136 Asian, non-Hispanic/Latino; 145 Hispanic/Latino; 23 Two or more races, non-Hispanic/Latino), 808 international. Average age 28. 3,111 applicants, 62% accepted, 591 enrolled. In 2015, 570 master's, 31 doctorates awarded. Terminal master's awarded for partial completion of doctoral program. *Degree requirements:* For master's, thesis optional; for doctorate, thesis/dissertation. *Entrance requirements:* For master's, GRE General Test; for doctorate, GRE General Test, minimum graduate GPA of 3.5. Additional exam requirements/recommendations for international students: Required—TOEFL (minimum score 550 paper-based; 79 iBT). *Application deadline:* For fall admission, 6/1 priority date for domestic students, 5/1 priority date for international students; for spring admission, 11/15 priority date for domestic and international students. Applications are processed on a rolling basis. Application fee: $75. Electronic applications accepted. *Expenses:* $28,800 per year non-resident full-time. *Financial support:* In 2015–16, fellowships with partial tuition reimbursements (averaging $3,900 per year), 68 research assistantships with partial tuition reimbursements (averaging $18,120 per year), 68 teaching assistantships with partial tuition reimbursements (averaging $13,325 per year) were awarded. Financial award application deadline: 1/15. *Total annual research expenditures:* $41.3 million. *Unit head:* Dr. Moshe Kam, Dean, 973-596-5534, E-mail: moshe.kam@njit.edu. *Application contact:* Stephen Eck, Director of Admissions, 973-596-3300, Fax: 973-596-3461, E-mail: admissions@njit.edu.
Website: http://engineering.njit.edu/

New York Medical College, Graduate School of Basic Medical Sciences, Integrated PhD Program, Valhalla, NY 10595-1691. Offers biochemistry and molecular biology (PhD); cell biology and anatomy (PhD); microbiology and immunology (PhD); pathology (PhD); pharmacology (PhD); physiology (PhD). *Degree requirements:* For doctorate, comprehensive exam, thesis/dissertation. *Entrance requirements:* For doctorate, GRE General Test. Additional exam requirements/recommendations for international students: Required—TOEFL. Electronic applications accepted. *Expenses: Tuition, area resident:* Full-time $44,355; part-time $1025 per credit. *Required fees:* $500; $95 per year. One-time fee: $140 part-time. Tuition and fees vary according to course load and program. *Faculty research:* Cardiovascular sciences, infectious diseases, neuroscience, cancer and cell signaling.

New York Medical College, Graduate School of Basic Medical Sciences, Pharmacology - Master's Program, Valhalla, NY 10595-1691. Offers MS, MD/PhD. *Program availability:* Part-time, evening/weekend. *Degree requirements:* For master's, thesis. *Entrance requirements:* For master's, GRE General Test, MCAT, or DAT. Additional exam requirements/recommendations for international students: Required—TOEFL. Electronic applications accepted. *Expenses: Tuition, area resident:* Full-time $44,355; part-time $1025 per credit. *Required fees:* $500; $95 per year. One-time fee: $140 part-time. Tuition and fees vary according to course load and program. *Faculty research:* Investigation into the therapeutic and pathophysiologic role of bioactive lipids (eicosanoids) in cancer, ophthalmology, and cardiovascular diseases including hypertension, kidney disease, stroke, diabetes, atherosclerosis and inflammatory conditions; cytochrome P-450 function and control; patch-clamp analysis of ion transport; the roles of vasoactive hormones and inflammatory cytokines in hypertension, end-organ damage and cardiovascular function.

North Carolina State University, College of Veterinary Medicine, Program in Comparative Biomedical Sciences, Raleigh, NC 27695. Offers cell biology (MS, PhD); infectious disease (MS, PhD); pathology (MS, PhD); pharmacology (MS, PhD); population medicine (MS, PhD). *Program availability:* Part-time. *Degree requirements:* For master's, thesis; for doctorate, thesis/dissertation. *Entrance requirements:* For master's and doctorate, GRE General Test. Additional exam requirements/recommendations for international students: Required—TOEFL (minimum score 550 paper-based). Electronic applications accepted. *Expenses:* Contact institution. *Faculty research:* Infectious diseases, cell biology, pharmacology and toxicology, genomics, pathology and population medicine.

Northeastern University, Bouvé College of Health Sciences, Boston, MA 02115-5096. Offers applied behavior analysis (MS, CAGS); audiology (Au D); biomedical nanotechnology (MS); college student development and counseling (MS, CAGS); counseling psychology (MS, CAGS); exercise science (MS); health informatics (MS); medicinal chemistry (MS); nurse anesthesia (DNP, CAGS); nursing (MS, PhD, CAGS), including administration (MS), adult-gerontology acute care nurse practitioner (MS, CAGS), adult-gerontology primary care nurse practitioner (MS, CAGS), anesthesia (MS), family nurse practitioner (MS, CAGS), neonatal nurse practitioner (MS, CAGS), pediatric nurse practitioner (MS, CAGS), psychiatric mental health nurse practitioner (MS, CAGS); nursing practice (DNP); personal health informatics (PhD); pharmaceutical sciences (MS, PhD), including interdisciplinary concentration, pharmaceutics and drug delivery systems; pharmacology (MS); pharmacy (Pharm D); physical therapy (Postbaccalaureate Certificate); physician assistant (MS); population health (PhD); school psychology (MS, PhD, CAGS); speech-language pathology (MS); urban health (MPH); MS/MBA. *Accreditation:* ACPE (one or more programs are accredited). *Program availability:* Part-time, evening/weekend, online learning. *Faculty:* 194 full-time (120 women), 169 part-time/adjunct (136 women). *Students:* 1,416 full-time (1,049 women), 310 part-time (248 women). In 2015, 374 master's, 313 doctorates, 37 other advanced degrees awarded. *Degree requirements:* For doctorate, thesis/dissertation (for some

programs); for other advanced degree, comprehensive exam. Application fee: $75. Electronic applications accepted. *Expenses:* Contact institution. *Financial support:* Applicants required to submit FAFSA. *Unit head:* John R. Reynolds, Professor and Interim Dean, 617-373-3323, Fax: 617-373-3030. *Application contact:* Molly Schnabel, Senior Director of Graduate Affairs, 617-373-2708, Fax: 617-373-4701, E-mail: bouvegrad@neu.edu.
Website: http://www.northeastern.edu/bouve/

The Ohio State University, College of Pharmacy, Columbus, OH 43210. Offers MS, PhD, Pharm D, Pharm D/MBA, Pharm D/MPH, Pharm D/PhD. *Accreditation:* ACPE (one or more programs are accredited). *Faculty:* 50. *Students:* 574 full-time (315 women); includes 142 minority (26 Black or African American, non-Hispanic/Latino; 1 American Indian or Alaska Native, non-Hispanic/Latino; 93 Asian, non-Hispanic/Latino; 17 Hispanic/Latino; 1 Native Hawaiian or other Pacific Islander, non-Hispanic/Latino; 4 Two or more races, non-Hispanic/Latino), 53 international. Average age 25. In 2015, 17 master's, 132 doctorates awarded. Terminal master's awarded for partial completion of doctoral program. *Degree requirements:* For doctorate, comprehensive exam (for some programs), thesis/dissertation (for some programs). *Entrance requirements:* For master's, GRE General Test, minimum GPA of 3.0; for doctorate, GRE General Test; PCAT (for PharmD), minimum GPA of 3.0. Additional exam requirements/recommendations for international students: Required—TOEFL (minimum score 600 paper-based, 100 iBT) for MS and PhD; TOEFL (minimum score 577 paper-based; 90 iBT), Michigan English Language Assessment Battery (minimum score 84), IELTS (minimum score 7.5) for PharmD. *Application deadline:* For fall admission, 12/15 for domestic and international students. Application fee: $60 ($70 for international students). Electronic applications accepted. *Expenses:* Contact institution. *Financial support:* Fellowships with full tuition reimbursements, research assistantships with full tuition reimbursements, teaching assistantships with full tuition reimbursements, career-related internships or fieldwork, Federal Work-Study, institutionally sponsored loans, scholarships/grants, and traineeships available. *Unit head:* Dr. Henry J. Mann, Dean and Professor, 614-292-5711, Fax: 614-292-2588, E-mail: mann.414@osu.edu. *Application contact:* Dr. Henry J. Mann, Dean and Professor, 614-292-5711, Fax: 614-292-2588, E-mail: mann.414@osu.edu.
Website: http://www.pharmacy.osu.edu

Oregon Health & Science University, School of Medicine, Graduate Programs in Medicine, Program in Molecular and Cellular Biosciences, Department of Physiology and Pharmacology, Portland, OR 97239-3098. Offers PhD. *Faculty:* 15 full-time (5 women), 20 part-time/adjunct (7 women). *Students:* 9 full-time (6 women); includes 1 minority (Hispanic/Latino). Average age 27. *Degree requirements:* For doctorate, comprehensive exam, thesis/dissertation. *Entrance requirements:* For doctorate, GRE General Test (minimum scores: 153 Verbal/148 Quantitative/4.5 Analytical) or MCAT (for some programs). Additional exam requirements/recommendations for international students: Required—IELTS or TOEFL. *Application deadline:* For fall admission, 12/1 for domestic and international students. Application fee: $70. Electronic applications accepted. *Financial support:* Full tuition and stipends available. *Faculty research:* Ion conduction and gating in K+ channels, autonomic neuron plasticity, neurotransmitter/receptor expression, fetal/neonatal pharmacology, molecular pharmacology. *Unit head:* Dr. Robert Duvoisin, Program Director, 503-418-2665, E-mail: duvoisin@ohsu.edu. *Application contact:* Nermina Radaslic, Program Coordinator, 503-418-9462, E-mail: radaslic@ohsu.edu.

Oregon State University, College of Pharmacy, Program in Pharmaceutical Sciences, Corvallis, OR 97331. Offers medicinal chemistry (MS, PhD); natural products chemistry (MS, PhD); pharmaceutics (MS, PhD); pharmacoeconomics (MS, PhD); pharmacokinetics (MS, PhD); pharmacology (MS, PhD); toxicology (MS, PhD). *Program availability:* Part-time. *Faculty:* 30 full-time (15 women). *Students:* 29 full-time (10 women); includes 2 minority (1 Asian, non-Hispanic/Latino; 1 Hispanic/Latino), 16 international. Average age 29. 79 applicants, 10% accepted, 5 enrolled. In 2015, 4 doctorates awarded. *Entrance requirements:* For master's and doctorate, GRE. Additional exam requirements/recommendations for international students: Required—TOEFL (minimum score 80 iBT), IELTS (minimum score 6.5). *Application deadline:* For fall admission, 1/1 for domestic students. Application fee: $75 ($85 for international students). *Expenses:* Tuition, state resident: full-time $12,150; part-time $450 per credit. Tuition, nonresident: full-time $20,952; part-time $776 per credit. *Required fees:* $1572; $1443 per unit. One-time fee: $350. Tuition and fees vary according to course load, campus/location and program. *Unit head:* Dr. Mark Zabriskie, Dean and Professor, 541-737-5781, E-mail: mark.zabriskie@oregonstate.edu. *Application contact:* Debra Peters, Pharmacy Advisor, 541-737-8743, E-mail: debra.peters@oregonstate.edu.
Website: http://pharmacy.oregonstate.edu/

Purdue University, College of Pharmacy and Pharmacal Sciences and Graduate School, Graduate Programs in Pharmacy and Pharmacal Sciences, Department of Medicinal Chemistry and Molecular Pharmacology, West Lafayette, IN 47907. Offers biophysical and computational chemistry (PhD); cancer research (PhD); immunology and infectious disease (PhD); medicinal biochemistry and molecular biology (PhD); medicinal chemistry and chemical biology (PhD); molecular pharmacology (PhD); neuropharmacology, neurodegeneration, and neurotoxicity (PhD); systems biology and functional genomics (PhD). *Degree requirements:* For doctorate, thesis/dissertation. *Entrance requirements:* For doctorate, GRE General Test; GRE Subject Test in biology, biochemistry, and chemistry (recommended), minimum undergraduate GPA of 3.0. Additional exam requirements/recommendations for international students: Required—TOEFL (minimum score 550 paper-based; 77 iBT); Recommended—TWE. Electronic applications accepted. *Faculty research:* Drug design and development, cancer research, drug synthesis and analysis, chemical pharmacology, environmental toxicology.

Purdue University, School of Veterinary Medicine and Graduate School, Graduate Programs in Veterinary Medicine, Department of Basic Medical Sciences, West Lafayette, IN 47907. Offers anatomy (MS, PhD); pharmacology (MS, PhD); physiology (MS, PhD). *Program availability:* Part-time. Terminal master's awarded for partial completion of doctoral program. *Degree requirements:* For master's, thesis; for doctorate, thesis/dissertation. *Entrance requirements:* For master's and doctorate, GRE General Test. Additional exam requirements/recommendations for international students: Required—TOEFL. Electronic applications accepted. *Faculty research:* Development and regeneration, tissue injury and shock, biomedical engineering, ovarian function, bone and cartilage biology, cell and molecular biology.

Queen's University at Kingston, School of Graduate Studies, Faculty of Health Sciences, Department of Pharmacology and Toxicology, Kingston, ON K7L 3N6, Canada. Offers M Sc, PhD. *Degree requirements:* For master's, thesis; for doctorate, comprehensive exam, thesis/dissertation. *Entrance requirements:* For master's, minimum 2nd class standing, honors bachelor of science degree (life sciences, health sciences, or equivalent); for doctorate, masters of science degree or outstanding performance in honors bachelor of science program. Additional exam requirements/recommendations for international students: Required—TOEFL (minimum score 600 paper-based). Electronic applications accepted. *Faculty research:* Biochemical toxicology, cardiovascular pharmacology and neuropharmacology.

Rush University, Graduate College, Division of Pharmacology, Chicago, IL 60612-3832. Offers clinical research (MS); pharmacology (MS, PhD); MD/PhD. Terminal master's awarded for partial completion of doctoral program. *Degree requirements:* For master's, thesis; for doctorate, thesis/dissertation. *Entrance requirements:* For master's and doctorate, GRE General Test, interview. Additional exam requirements/recommendations for international students: Required—TOEFL (minimum score 550 paper-based). *Faculty research:* Dopamine neurobiology and Parkinson's disease; cardiac electrophysiology and clinical pharmacology; neutrophil motility, apoptosis, and adhesion; angiogenesis; pulmonary vascular physiology.

Rutgers University–Newark, Graduate School of Biomedical Sciences, Department of Pharmacology and Physiology, Newark, NJ 07107. Offers PhD. *Degree requirements:* For doctorate, thesis/dissertation, qualifying exam. *Entrance requirements:* For doctorate, GRE General Test. Additional exam requirements/recommendations for international students: Required—TOEFL. Electronic applications accepted.

Saint Louis University, Graduate Education and School of Medicine, Graduate Program in Biomedical Sciences and Graduate Education, Department of Pharmacological and Physiological Science, St. Louis, MO 63103. Offers PhD. *Degree requirements:* For doctorate, comprehensive exam, thesis/dissertation, departmental qualifying exams. *Entrance requirements:* For doctorate, GRE General Test (GRE Subject Test optional), letters of recommendation, resume, interview. Additional exam requirements/recommendations for international students: Required—TOEFL (minimum score 525 paper-based). Electronic applications accepted. *Faculty research:* Molecular endocrinology, neuropharmacology, cardiovascular science, drug abuse, neurotransmitter and hormonal signaling mechanisms.

Southern Illinois University Carbondale, Graduate School, Graduate Programs in Medicine, Program in Pharmacology, Springfield, IL 62794-9629. Offers MS, PhD. *Faculty:* 13 full-time (1 woman). *Students:* 3 full-time (2 women), 9 part-time (6 women); includes 1 minority (Asian, non-Hispanic/Latino), 7 international. Average age 30. 23 applicants, 17% accepted, 2 enrolled. In 2015, 5 doctorates awarded. *Degree requirements:* For master's, thesis; for doctorate, thesis/dissertation. *Entrance requirements:* For master's, GRE, minimum GPA of 3.0; for doctorate, GRE, minimum GPA of 3.25. Additional exam requirements/recommendations for international students: Required—TOEFL. *Application deadline:* For fall admission, 2/1 for domestic students. Applications are processed on a rolling basis. Application fee: $65. *Financial support:* In 2015–16, 12 students received support, including 12 research assistantships with full tuition reimbursements available; fellowships with full tuition reimbursements available, teaching assistantships, tuition waivers (full), and unspecified assistantships also available. *Faculty research:* Autonomic nervous system pharmacology, biochemical pharmacology, neuropharmacology, toxicology, cardiovascular pharmacology. *Unit head:* Dr. Carl L. Faingold, Chairman, 217-545-2185, Fax: 217-524-0145, E-mail: cfaingold@siumed.edu. *Application contact:* Linda Moss, Secretary, 217-545-2875, E-mail: lmoss@siumed.edu.
Website: http://www.siumed.edu/pharm/home.html

State University of New York Upstate Medical University, College of Graduate Studies, Program in Pharmacology, Syracuse, NY 13210-2334. Offers PhD, MD/PhD. Terminal master's awarded for partial completion of doctoral program. *Degree requirements:* For doctorate, comprehensive exam, thesis/dissertation. *Entrance requirements:* For doctorate, GRE General Test, telephone interview. Additional exam requirements/recommendations for international students: Required—TOEFL. Electronic applications accepted. *Faculty research:* Cancer, disorders of the nervous system, infectious diseases, diabetes/metabolic disorders/cardiovascular diseases.

Stony Brook University, State University of New York, Stony Brook Medicine, School of Medicine and Graduate School, Graduate Programs in Medicine, Department of Pharmacological Sciences, Graduate Program in Molecular and Cellular Pharmacology, Stony Brook, NY 11794. Offers PhD. *Faculty:* 19 full-time (4 women). *Students:* 48 full-time (22 women), 2 part-time (1 woman); includes 16 minority (6 Black or African American, non-Hispanic/Latino; 6 Asian, non-Hispanic/Latino; 4 Hispanic/Latino), 7 international. Average age 26. 56 applicants, 18% accepted, 5 enrolled. In 2015, 5 doctorates awarded. *Degree requirements:* For doctorate, thesis/dissertation, departmental qualifying exam. *Entrance requirements:* For doctorate, GRE General Test. Additional exam requirements/recommendations for international students: Required—TOEFL. *Application deadline:* For fall admission, 1/15 priority date for domestic students; for spring admission, 10/1 for domestic students. Applications are processed on a rolling basis. Application fee: $100. Electronic applications accepted. *Expenses:* $12,421 full-time resident tuition and fees, $453 per credit hour; $23,761 full-time nonresident tuition and fees, $925 per credit hour. *Financial support:* In 2015–16, 17 fellowships, 16 research assistantships were awarded; teaching assistantships and Federal Work-Study also available. Financial award application deadline: 3/15; financial award applicants required to submit FAFSA. *Faculty research:* Bioimaging, pharmacology, DNA repair, DNA replication, cancer or carcinogenesis. *Total annual research expenditures:* $4.4 million. *Unit head:* Dr. Michael A. Frohman, Chair, 631-444-3050, Fax: 631-444-3218, E-mail: michael.frohman@stonybrook.edu. *Application contact:* Odalis Hernandez, Coordinator, 631-444-3057, Fax: 631-444-3218, E-mail: odalis.hernandez@stonybrook.edu.
Website: http://www.pharm.stonybrook.edu/about-graduate-program

Thomas Jefferson University, Jefferson College of Biomedical Sciences, MS Program in Pharmacology, Philadelphia, PA 19107. Offers MS. *Program availability:* Part-time, evening/weekend. *Faculty:* 44 full-time (14 women), 27 part-time/adjunct (11 women). *Students:* 31 part-time (10 women); includes 4 minority (2 Black or African American, non-Hispanic/Latino; 1 Asian, non-Hispanic/Latino; 1 Hispanic/Latino), 5 international. Average age 30. 15 applicants, 93% accepted, 9 enrolled. In 2015, 5 master's awarded. *Degree requirements:* For master's, thesis, clerkship. *Entrance requirements:* For master's, GRE General Test or MCAT, minimum GPA of 3.0. Additional exam requirements/recommendations for international students: Required—TOEFL, IELTS (minimum score 7). *Application deadline:* For fall admission, 8/1 priority date for domestic students, 3/1 priority date for international students; for winter admission, 12/1 priority date for domestic students, 6/1 priority date for international students; for spring admission, 4/1 priority date for domestic students. Applications are processed on a rolling basis. Application fee: $50. Electronic applications accepted. *Financial support:* Federal Work-Study and institutionally sponsored loans available. Support available to part-time students. Financial award application deadline: 5/1; financial award applicants required to submit FAFSA. *Faculty research:* Pharmacology, drug development, planning and management, biostatistics. *Unit head:* Dr. Carol L. Beck, Associate Dean/Program Director, 215-503-6539, Fax: 215-503-3433, E-mail: carol.beck@jefferson.edu. *Application contact:* Marc E. Stearns, Director of Admissions, 215-503-0155, Fax: 215-503-3433, E-mail: jgsbs-info@jefferson.edu.
Website: http://www.jefferson.edu/university/biomedical-sciences/degrees-programs/master-programs/pharmacology.html

Tufts University, Sackler School of Graduate Biomedical Sciences, Pharmacology and Experimental Therapeutics Program, Medford, MA 02155. Offers pharmacology and drug development (MS); pharmacology and experimental therapeutics (PhD). *Faculty:* 22 full-time (5 women). *Students:* 35 full-time (24 women); includes 6 minority (2 Black or African American, non-Hispanic/Latino; 3 Asian, non-Hispanic/Latino; 1 Hispanic/

Pharmacology

Latino), 17 international. Average age 28. 90 applicants, 22% accepted, 12 enrolled. In 2015, 4 master's, 2 doctorates awarded. Terminal master's awarded for partial completion of doctoral program. *Degree requirements:* For master's, thesis; for doctorate, comprehensive exam, thesis/dissertation. *Entrance requirements:* For master's and doctorate, GRE General Test, 3 letters of reference. Additional exam requirements/recommendations for international students: Required—TOEFL (minimum score 600 paper-based; 100 iBT). *Application deadline:* For fall admission, 12/15 priority date for domestic and international students. Application fee: $90. Electronic applications accepted. *Expenses:* $45,960 per year (MS); $31,626 per year (PhD). *Financial support:* In 2015–16, 10 students received support, including 10 research assistantships with full tuition reimbursements available (averaging $32,000 per year); health care benefits also available. *Faculty research:* Biochemical mechanisms of narcotic addiction, clinical psychopharmacology, pharmacokinetics, neurotransmitter receptors, neuropeptides. *Unit head:* Dr. Emmanuel Pothos, Director, 617-636-6940, E-mail: emmanuel.pothos@tufts.edu. *Application contact:* Dr. Elizabeth Storrs, 617-636-6767, Fax: 617-636-0375, E-mail: sackler-school@tufts.edu.
Website: http://sackler.tufts.edu/Academics/Degree-Programs/PhD-Programs/Pharmacology-and-Experimental-Therapeutics

Tulane University, School of Medicine and School of Liberal Arts, Graduate Programs in Biomedical Sciences, Department of Pharmacology, New Orleans, LA 70118-5669. Offers MS. MS and PhD offered through the Graduate School. *Degree requirements:* For master's, one foreign language, thesis. *Entrance requirements:* For master's, GRE General Test, minimum B average in undergraduate course work. Additional exam requirements/recommendations for international students: Required—TOEFL. *Application deadline:* For fall admission, 2/1 for domestic and international students. Application fee: $45. Electronic applications accepted. *Expenses: Tuition, area resident:* Full-time $47,658; part-time $2648 per credit hour. *Required fees:* $1980; $44.50 per credit hour. $550 per term. Tuition and fees vary according to course load, degree level and program. *Financial support:* Fellowships with full tuition reimbursements and research assistantships with full tuition reimbursements available. Financial award application deadline: 2/1.

Universidad Central del Caribe, School of Medicine, Program in Biomedical Sciences, Bayamón, PR 00960-6032. Offers anatomy and cell biology (MA, MS); biochemistry (MS); biomedical sciences (MA); cellular and molecular biology (PhD); microbiology and immunology (MA, MS); pharmacology (MS); physiology (MS).

Université de Montréal, Faculty of Medicine, Department of Pharmacology, Montréal, QC H3C 3J7, Canada. Offers M Sc, PhD. Terminal master's awarded for partial completion of doctoral program. *Degree requirements:* For master's, thesis; for doctorate, thesis/dissertation, general exam. *Entrance requirements:* For master's, proficiency in French, knowledge of English; for doctorate, master's degree, proficiency in French. Electronic applications accepted. *Faculty research:* Molecular, clinical, and cardiovascular pharmacology; pharmacokinetics; mechanisms of drug interactions and toxicity; neuropharmacology and receptology.

Université de Sherbrooke, Faculty of Medicine and Health Sciences, Graduate Programs in Medicine, Department of Pharmacology, Sherbrooke, QC J1H 5N4, Canada. Offers M Sc, PhD. Terminal master's awarded for partial completion of doctoral program. *Degree requirements:* For master's, thesis; for doctorate, thesis/dissertation. Electronic applications accepted. *Faculty research:* Pharmacology of peptide hormones, pharmacology of lipid mediators, protein-protein interactions, medicinal pharmacology.

University at Buffalo, the State University of New York, Graduate School, School of Medicine and Biomedical Sciences, Graduate Programs in Medicine and Biomedical Sciences, Department of Pharmacology and Toxicology, Buffalo, NY 14221. Offers pharmacology (MS, PhD); MD/PhD. *Faculty:* 21 full-time (3 women). *Students:* 25 full-time (14 women); includes 9 minority (3 Black or African American, non-Hispanic/Latino; 1 American Indian or Alaska Native, non-Hispanic/Latino; 2 Asian, non-Hispanic/Latino; 3 Hispanic/Latino), 5 international. Average age 26. 67 applicants, 24% accepted, 10 enrolled. In 2015, 11 master's, 5 doctorates awarded. Terminal master's awarded for partial completion of doctoral program. *Degree requirements:* For master's, thesis; for doctorate, thesis/dissertation. *Entrance requirements:* For master's and doctorate, GRE General Test, 3 letters of recommendation. Additional exam requirements/recommendations for international students: Required—TOEFL (minimum score 79 iBT). *Application deadline:* For fall admission, 2/14 priority date for domestic and international students. Applications are processed on a rolling basis. Application fee: $85. Electronic applications accepted. *Financial support:* In 2015–16, 3 students received support, including 19 research assistantships with full tuition reimbursements available (averaging $27,000 per year); fellowships, teaching assistantships, Federal Work-Study, scholarships/grants, health care benefits, and unspecified assistantships also available. Financial award application deadline: 2/14; financial award applicants required to submit FAFSA. *Faculty research:* Neuropharmacology, toxicology, signal transduction, molecular pharmacology, behavioral pharmacology. *Total annual research expenditures:* $9.4 million. *Unit head:* Dr. Margarita L. Dubocovich, Professor/Chair, 716-829-3048, Fax: 716-829-2801, E-mail: mdubo@buffalo.edu. *Application contact:* Linda M. LeRoy, Admissions Assistant, 716-829-2800, Fax: 716-829-2801, E-mail: pmygrad@buffalo.edu.
Website: http://medicine.buffalo.edu/pharmtox

The University of Alabama at Birmingham, Graduate Programs in Joint Health Sciences, Program in Pharmacology and Toxicology, Birmingham, AL 35294. Offers PhD. *Degree requirements:* For doctorate, thesis/dissertation. *Entrance requirements:* For doctorate, GRE General Test; GRE Subject Test (recommended), interview. Additional exam requirements/recommendations for international students: Required—TOEFL, TWE. Electronic applications accepted. *Expenses:* Contact institution. *Faculty research:* Anticancer and antiviral chemotherapy, with emphasis on drugs used in the management of AIDS and related opportunistic infections; metabolism and biliary excretion of drugs (and metabolites) as well as the mechanisms of drug toxicity.

University of Alberta, Faculty of Graduate Studies and Research, Department of Pharmacology, Edmonton, AB T6G 2E1, Canada. Offers M Sc, PhD. Terminal master's awarded for partial completion of doctoral program. *Degree requirements:* For master's, thesis; for doctorate, thesis/dissertation. *Entrance requirements:* For master's, B Sc, minimum GPA of 3.3; for doctorate, M Sc in pharmacology or closely related field, honors B Sc in pharmacology. *Faculty research:* Cardiovascular pharmacology, neuropharmacology, cancer pharmacology, molecular pharmacology, toxicology.

The University of Arizona, College of Pharmacy, Department of Pharmacology and Toxicology, Graduate Program in Medical Pharmacology, Tucson, AZ 85721. Offers medical pharmacology (PhD); perfusion science (MS). *Degree requirements:* For master's, thesis; for doctorate, comprehensive exam, thesis/dissertation. *Entrance requirements:* For master's, GRE General Test, 3 letters of recommendation; for doctorate, GRE General Test, personal statement, 3 letters of recommendation. Additional exam requirements/recommendations for international students: Required—TOEFL (minimum score 550 paper-based; 79 iBT). *Application deadline:* For fall admission, 1/1 for domestic and international students. Applications are processed on a rolling basis. Application fee: $75. Electronic applications accepted. *Financial support:* Research assistantships, institutionally sponsored loans, and tuition waivers (partial) available. Financial award applicants required to submit FAFSA. *Faculty research:*

Immunopharmacology, pharmacogenetics, pharmacogenomics, clinical pharmacology, ocularpharmacology and neuropharmacology. *Unit head:* Todd W. Vanderah, Director, 520-626-7801, Fax: 520-626-2204. *Application contact:* Anabel T. Moreno, Coordinator, 520-626-7218, Fax: 520-626-2204.
Website: http://www.pharmacology.arizona.edu/

University of Arkansas for Medical Sciences, Graduate School, Little Rock, AR 72205. Offers biochemistry and molecular biology (MS, PhD); bioinformatics (MS, PhD); cellular physiology and molecular biophysics (MS, PhD); clinical nutrition (MS); interdisciplinary biomedical sciences (MS, PhD, Certificate); interdisciplinary toxicology (MS); microbiology and immunology (PhD); neurobiology and developmental sciences (PhD); pharmacology (PhD); MD/PhD. Bioinformatics programs hosted jointly with the University of Arkansas at Little Rock. *Program availability:* Part-time. Terminal master's awarded for partial completion of doctoral program. *Degree requirements:* For master's, comprehensive exam (for some programs), thesis (for some programs); for doctorate, thesis/dissertation. *Entrance requirements:* For master's and doctorate, GRE. Additional exam requirements/recommendations for international students: Required—TOEFL. Electronic applications accepted. *Expenses:* Contact institution.

The University of British Columbia, Faculty of Medicine, Department of Anesthesiology, Pharmacology and Therapeutics, Vancouver, BC V6T 1Z3, Canada. Offers M Sc, PhD. Terminal master's awarded for partial completion of doctoral program. *Degree requirements:* For master's, thesis; for doctorate, comprehensive exam, thesis/dissertation. *Entrance requirements:* For master's, MD or appropriate bachelor's degree; for doctorate, MD or M Sc. Additional exam requirements/recommendations for international students: Required—TOEFL (minimum score 600 paper-based; 100 iBT). Electronic applications accepted. *Faculty research:* Cellular, biochemical, autonomic, and cardiovascular pharmacology; neuropharmacology and pulmonary pharmacology.

University of California, Davis, Graduate Studies, Graduate Group in Pharmacology and Toxicology, Davis, CA 95616. Offers MS, PhD. Terminal master's awarded for partial completion of doctoral program. *Degree requirements:* For master's, comprehensive exam or thesis; for doctorate, thesis/dissertation, qualifying exam. *Entrance requirements:* For master's and doctorate, GRE General Test, minimum GPA of 3.0, course work in biochemistry and/or physiology. Additional exam requirements/recommendations for international students: Required—TOEFL (minimum score 550 paper-based). Electronic applications accepted. *Faculty research:* Respiratory, neurochemical, molecular, genetic, and ecological toxicology.

University of California, Los Angeles, David Geffen School of Medicine and Graduate Division, Graduate Programs in Medicine, Department of Molecular and Medical Pharmacology, Los Angeles, CA 90095. Offers MS, PhD. *Degree requirements:* For master's, thesis; for doctorate, thesis/dissertation, written and oral qualifying exams; 2 quarters of teaching experience. *Entrance requirements:* For doctorate, GRE General Test, bachelor's degree; minimum undergraduate GPA of 3.0 (or its equivalent if letter grade system not used). Additional exam requirements/recommendations for international students: Required—TOEFL. Electronic applications accepted.

University of California, San Francisco, School of Pharmacy and Graduate Division, Pharmaceutical Sciences and Pharmacogenomics Program, San Francisco, CA 94158-0775. Offers PhD. *Degree requirements:* For doctorate, comprehensive exam, thesis/dissertation. *Entrance requirements:* For doctorate, GRE General Test, bachelor's degree, 3 letters of recommendation, personal statement. Additional exam requirements/recommendations for international students: Required—TOEFL. Electronic applications accepted. *Faculty research:* Drug development sciences, molecular pharmacology, therapeutic bioengineering, pharmacogenomics and functional genomics, quantitative and systems pharmacology, computational genomics.
See Display on page 926 and Close-Up on page 937.

University of Cincinnati, Graduate School, College of Medicine, Graduate Programs in Biomedical Sciences, Department of Pharmacology and Cell Biophysics, Cincinnati, OH 45221. Offers cell biophysics (PhD); pharmacology (PhD). *Degree requirements:* For doctorate, thesis/dissertation, qualifying exam. *Entrance requirements:* For doctorate, GRE General Test. Additional exam requirements/recommendations for international students: Required—TOEFL. Electronic applications accepted. *Faculty research:* Lipoprotein research, enzyme regulation, electrophysiology, gene actuation.

University of Colorado Denver, School of Medicine, Program in Pharmacology, Aurora, CO 80045. Offers bioinformatics (PhD); biomolecular structure (PhD); pharmacology (PhD). *Students:* 19 full-time (11 women); includes 5 minority (2 Asian, non-Hispanic/Latino; 2 Hispanic/Latino; 1 Two or more races, non-Hispanic/Latino). Average age 26. 32 applicants, 16% accepted, 5 enrolled. In 2015, 3 doctorates awarded. *Degree requirements:* For doctorate, comprehensive exam, thesis/dissertation, major seminar, 3 research rotations in the first year, 30 hours each of course work and thesis. *Entrance requirements:* For doctorate, GRE General Test, three letters of recommendation, personal statement. Additional exam requirements/recommendations for international students: Required—TOEFL (minimum score 550 paper-based; 80 iBT). *Application deadline:* For fall admission, 12/15 for domestic students, 11/15 for international students. Application fee: $50 ($75 for international students). Electronic applications accepted. *Expenses:* Contact institution. *Financial support:* In 2015–16, 23 students received support. Fellowships, research assistantships, teaching assistantships, institutionally sponsored loans, scholarships/grants, traineeships, health care benefits, tuition waivers (full), and unspecified assistantships available. Financial award application deadline: 3/15; financial award applicants required to submit FAFSA. *Faculty research:* Cancer biology, drugs of abuse, neuroscience, signal transduction, structural biology. *Total annual research expenditures:* $16.7 million. *Unit head:* Dr. Andrew Thorburn, Interim Chair, 303-724-3290, Fax: 303-724-3663, E-mail: andrew.thorburn@ucdenver.edu. *Application contact:* Elizabeth Bowen, Graduate Program Coordinator, 303-724-3565, E-mail: elizabeth.bowen@ucdenver.edu.
Website: http://www.ucdenver.edu/academics/colleges/medicalschool/departments/Pharmacology/Pages/Pharmacology.aspx

University of Connecticut, Graduate School, School of Pharmacy, Department of Pharmaceutical Sciences, Graduate Program in Pharmacology and Toxicology, Storrs, CT 06269. Offers pharmacology (MS, PhD); toxicology (MS, PhD). Terminal master's awarded for partial completion of doctoral program. *Degree requirements:* For master's, comprehensive exam, thesis; for doctorate, thesis/dissertation. *Entrance requirements:* For master's and doctorate, GRE General Test. Additional exam requirements/recommendations for international students: Required—TOEFL (minimum score 550 paper-based). *Application deadline:* For fall admission, 2/1 priority date for domestic and international students; for spring admission, 11/1 for domestic students, 10/1 for international students. Applications are processed on a rolling basis. Application fee: $55. Electronic applications accepted. *Financial support:* Fellowships, research assistantships with full tuition reimbursements, teaching assistantships with full tuition reimbursements, career-related internships or fieldwork, Federal Work-Study, scholarships/grants, traineeships, health care benefits, and unspecified assistantships available. Financial award application deadline: 2/1; financial award applicants required to submit FAFSA.
Website: http://www.pharmacy.uconn.edu/

University of Florida, College of Medicine and Graduate School, Interdisciplinary Program in Biomedical Sciences, Concentration in Physiology and Pharmacology, Gainesville, FL 32611. Offers PhD. *Degree requirements:* For doctorate, thesis/dissertation. *Entrance requirements:* For doctorate, GRE General Test, minimum GPA of 3.0, biochemistry before enrollment. Electronic applications accepted.

University of Florida, Graduate School, College of Pharmacy and Graduate School, Graduate Programs in Pharmacy, Department of Pharmacodynamics, Gainesville, FL 32611. Offers MSP, PhD, Pharm D/PhD. *Faculty:* 2 full-time. *Students:* 12 full-time (5 women), 7 international. Average age 29. In 2015, 1 master's, 1 doctorate awarded. *Degree requirements:* For doctorate, comprehensive exam, thesis/dissertation. *Entrance requirements:* For master's and doctorate, GRE General Test, minimum GPA of 3.0. Additional exam requirements/recommendations for international students: Required—TOEFL (minimum score 550 paper-based; 80 iBT), IELTS (minimum score 6). *Application deadline:* For fall admission, 2/15 priority date for domestic students, 2/15 for international students. Applications are processed on a rolling basis. Electronic applications accepted. *Financial support:* In 2015–16, 1 fellowship, 2 research assistantships, 9 teaching assistantships were awarded; institutionally sponsored loans and unspecified assistantships also available. Support available to part-time students. Financial award application deadline: 2/15; financial award applicants required to submit FAFSA. *Faculty research:* Neurological mechanisms involved in addiction, stress, and body fluid homeostasis; cellular and molecular neurobiology of epilepsy, age-related cognitive decline, and Parkinson's Disease; hypertension and cardiac hypertrophy; stress hormone effects on fetal and neonatal development. *Total annual research expenditures:* $1.3 million. *Unit head:* Maureen Keller-Wood, PhD, Professor and Chair, 352-273-7687, Fax: 352-273-7705, E-mail: kellerwd@cop.ufl.edu. *Application contact:* Charles J. Frazier, PhD, Associate Professor and Graduate Coordinator, 352-273-7686, Fax: 352-273-7705, E-mail: frazier@cop.ufl.edu.
Website: http://pharmacy.ufl.edu/pd/

University of Georgia, College of Veterinary Medicine, Department of Physiology and Pharmacology, Athens, GA 30602. Offers pharmacology (MS, PhD); physiology (MS, PhD). *Degree requirements:* For master's, thesis; for doctorate, one foreign language, thesis/dissertation. *Entrance requirements:* For master's and doctorate, GRE General Test. Electronic applications accepted.

University of Guelph, Ontario Veterinary College and Graduate Studies, Graduate Programs in Veterinary Sciences, Department of Biomedical Sciences, Guelph, ON N1G 2W1, Canada. Offers morphology (M Sc, DV Sc, PhD); neuroscience (M Sc, DV Sc, PhD); pharmacology (M Sc, DV Sc, PhD); physiology (M Sc, DV Sc, PhD); toxicology (M Sc, DV Sc, PhD). *Program availability:* Part-time. *Degree requirements:* For master's, thesis; for doctorate, comprehensive exam, thesis/dissertation. *Entrance requirements:* For master's, honors B Sc, minimum 75% average in last 20 courses; for doctorate, M Sc with thesis from accredited institution. Additional exam requirements/recommendations for international students: Required—TOEFL (minimum score 550 paper-based; 89 iBT). Electronic applications accepted. *Faculty research:* Cellular morphology; endocrine, vascular and reproductive physiology; clinical pharmacology; veterinary toxicology; developmental biology, neuroscience.

University of Hawaii at Hilo, Program in Clinical Psychopharmacology, Hilo, HI 96720-4091. Offers MS. *Entrance requirements:* Additional exam requirements/recommendations for international students: Required—TOEFL, IELTS. Electronic applications accepted.

University of Houston, College of Pharmacy, Houston, TX 77204. Offers pharmaceutics (MSPHR, PhD); pharmacology (MSPHR, PhD); pharmacy (Pharm D); pharmacy administration (MSPHR, PhD). *Accreditation:* ACPE. *Program availability:* Part-time. Terminal master's awarded for partial completion of doctoral program. *Entrance requirements:* For doctorate, PCAT (for Pharm D). Additional exam requirements/recommendations for international students: Required—TOEFL. Electronic applications accepted. *Faculty research:* Drug screening and design, cardiovascular pharmacology, infectious disease, asthma research, herbal medicine.

University of Illinois at Chicago, College of Medicine and Graduate College, Graduate Programs in Medicine, Department of Pharmacology, Chicago, IL 60612. Offers PhD, MD/PhD. *Faculty:* 45 full-time (10 women), 25 part-time/adjunct (12 women). *Students:* 25 full-time (15 women), 1 part-time (0 women); includes 7 minority (1 Black or African American, non-Hispanic/Latino; 2 Asian, non-Hispanic/Latino; 3 Hispanic/Latino; 1 Two or more races, non-Hispanic/Latino), 7 international. Average age 28. *Degree requirements:* For doctorate, thesis/dissertation. *Entrance requirements:* For doctorate, GRE General Test. Additional exam requirements/recommendations for international students: Required—TOEFL. *Application deadline:* For fall admission, 1/15 priority date for domestic students, 2/15 for international students. Application fee: $60. *Expenses:* Tuition, state resident: full-time $11,480; part-time $3826 per credit. Tuition, nonresident: full-time $23,720; part-time $7906 per credit. *Required fees:* $1333 per semester. Part-time tuition and fees vary according to course load and program. *Financial support:* In 2015–16, 4 fellowships with full tuition reimbursements were awarded; research assistantships with full tuition reimbursements, tuition waivers (full), and unspecified assistantships also available. *Faculty research:* Cardiovascular and lung biology, cell signaling, molecular pharmacology of G-proteins, immunopharmacology, molecular and cellular basis of inflammation, neuroscience. *Unit head:* Prof. Asrar B. Malik, Department Head, 312-996-7635, Fax: 312-996-1225, E-mail: abmalik@uic.edu. *Application contact:* Jackie Perry, Graduate College Receptionist, 312-413-2550, Fax: 312-413-0185, E-mail: gradcoll@uic.edu.
Website: http://mcph.uic.edu/home

The University of Iowa, Roy J. and Lucille A. Carver College of Medicine and Graduate College, Graduate Programs in Medicine, Department of Pharmacology, Iowa City, IA 52242-1316. Offers MS, PhD. Terminal master's awarded for partial completion of doctoral program. *Degree requirements:* For master's, thesis. *Entrance requirements:* For master's, GRE General Test. Additional exam requirements/recommendations for international students: Required—TOEFL (minimum score 600 paper-based). Electronic applications accepted. *Faculty research:* Cancer and cell cycle, hormones and growth factors, nervous system function and dysfunction, receptors and signal transduction, stroke and hypertension.

The University of Kansas, Graduate Studies, School of Pharmacy, Department of Pharmacology and Toxicology, Program in Pharmacology and Toxicology, Lawrence, KS 66045. Offers MS, PhD. *Students:* 23 full-time (15 women); includes 1 minority (Asian, non-Hispanic/Latino), 15 international. Average age 25. 53 applicants, 17% accepted, 6 enrolled. In 2015, 2 doctorates awarded. Terminal master's awarded for partial completion of doctoral program. *Entrance requirements:* For master's, GRE, bachelor's degree in related field, 3 letters of recommendation, resume or curriculum vitae, official transcripts, 1-2 page personal statement; for doctorate, GRE (minimum score: 600 verbal, 600 quantitative, 4.5 analytical), bachelor's degree in related field, 3 letters of recommendation, resume or curriculum vitae, official transcripts, 1-2 page personal statement. Additional exam requirements/recommendations for international students: Required—TOEFL (minimum score 600 paper-based; 100 iBT). *Application deadline:* For fall admission, 1/15 for domestic students, 2/1 for international students. Application fee: $65 ($85 for international students). Electronic applications accepted.

Financial support: Fellowships and research assistantships available. Financial award application deadline: 2/1. *Faculty research:* Neurodegeneration, diabetes, neurological disorders, neuropharmacology, drug metabolism. *Unit head:* Nancy Muma, Chair, 785-864-4002, Fax: 785-864-5219, E-mail: nmuma@ku.edu. *Application contact:* Sheila Stice, Graduate Admissions Contact, 785-864-4002, E-mail: sstice@ku.edu.
Website: http://www.pharmtox.pharm.ku.edu

The University of Kansas, University of Kansas Medical Center, School of Medicine, Department of Pharmacology, Toxicology and Therapeutics, Kansas City, KS 66160. Offers pharmacology (PhD); toxicology (PhD); MD/PhD. *Faculty:* 18. *Students:* 24 full-time (12 women); includes 2 minority (1 Black or African American, non-Hispanic/Latino; 1 Two or more races, non-Hispanic/Latino), 17 international. Average age 29. In 2015, 7 doctorates awarded. Terminal master's awarded for partial completion of doctoral program. *Degree requirements:* For doctorate, one foreign language, comprehensive exam, thesis/dissertation. *Entrance requirements:* For doctorate, GRE General Test. Additional exam requirements/recommendations for international students: Required—TOEFL. *Application deadline:* For fall admission, 12/1 priority date for domestic and international students. Applications are processed on a rolling basis. Application fee: $60. Electronic applications accepted. Application fee is waived when completed online. *Financial support:* Fellowships with full tuition reimbursements, research assistantships with full tuition reimbursements, teaching assistantships with full tuition reimbursements, Federal Work-Study, scholarships/grants, traineeships, and unspecified assistantships available. Support available to part-time students. Financial award application deadline: 3/1; financial award applicants required to submit FAFSA. *Faculty research:* Liver nuclear receptors, hepatobiliary transporters, pharmacogenomics, estrogen-induced carcinogenesis, neuropharmacology of pain and depression. *Total annual research expenditures:* $5.5 million. *Unit head:* Dr. Hartmut Jaeschke, Professor and Chair, 913-588-7500, Fax: 913-588-7501, E-mail: hjaeschke@kumc.edu. *Application contact:* Dr Bruno Hagenbuch, Chair, Departmental Graduate Committee, 913-588-7500, Fax: 913-588-7501, E-mail: bhagenbuch@kumc.edu.
Website: http://www.kumc.edu/school-of-medicine/pharmacology-toxicology-and-therapeutics.html

University of Kentucky, Graduate School, Graduate School Programs from the College of Medicine, Program in Molecular and Biomedical Pharmacology, Lexington, KY 40506-0032. Offers PhD, MD/PhD. *Degree requirements:* For doctorate, comprehensive exam, thesis/dissertation. *Entrance requirements:* For doctorate, GRE General Test, minimum undergraduate GPA of 2.75, graduate 3.0. Additional exam requirements/recommendations for international students: Required—TOEFL (minimum score 550 paper-based). Electronic applications accepted.

University of Louisville, School of Medicine, Department of Pharmacology and Toxicology, Louisville, KY 40292-0001. Offers MS, PhD, MD/PhD. *Students:* 43 full-time (21 women), 5 part-time (all women); includes 5 minority (3 Black or African American, non-Hispanic/Latino; 1 Asian, non-Hispanic/Latino; 1 Two or more races, non-Hispanic/Latino), 12 international. Average age 28. 49 applicants, 27% accepted, 13 enrolled. In 2015, 1 master's awarded. Terminal master's awarded for partial completion of doctoral program. *Degree requirements:* For master's, thesis; for doctorate, comprehensive exam, thesis/dissertation. *Entrance requirements:* For master's and doctorate, GRE General Test (minimum score of 1000 verbal and quantitative), minimum GPA of 3.0. Additional exam requirements/recommendations for international students: Required—TOEFL. *Application deadline:* For fall admission, 1/15 priority date for domestic and international students. Applications are processed on a rolling basis. Application fee: $60. Electronic applications accepted. *Expenses:* Tuition, state resident: full-time $11,664; part-time $649 per credit hour. Tuition, nonresident: full-time $24,274; part-time $1350 per credit hour. *Required fees:* $196. Tuition and fees vary according to program and reciprocity agreements. *Financial support:* In 2015–16, 394,161 students received support. Fellowships with full tuition reimbursements available and research assistantships with full tuition reimbursements available available. Financial award application deadline: 4/15. *Faculty research:* Molecular pharmacogenetics; epidemiology; functional genomics; genetic predisposition to chemical carcinogenesis and drug toxicity; mechanisms of oxidative stress; alcohol-induced hepatitis, pancreatitis, and hepatocellular carcinoma; molecular and cardiac toxicology; molecular biology and genetics of DNA damage and repair in humans; mechanisms of chemo resistance; arsenic toxicity and cell cycle disruption; molecular pharmacology of novel G protein-coupled receptors. *Total annual research expenditures:* $3.5 million. *Unit head:* Dr. David W. Hein, Chair, 502-852-5141, Fax: 502-852-7868, E-mail: dhein@louisville.edu. *Application contact:* Heddy R. Rubin, Information Contact, 502-852-5741, Fax: 502-852-7868, E-mail: hrrubi01@gwise.louisville.edu.
Website: http://louisville.edu/medicine/departments/pharmacology

The University of Manchester, Faculty of Life Sciences, Manchester, United Kingdom. Offers adaptive organismal biology (M Phil, PhD); animal biology (M Phil, PhD); biochemistry (M Phil, PhD); bioinformatics (M Phil, PhD); biomolecular sciences (M Phil, PhD); biotechnology (M Phil, PhD); cell biology (M Phil, PhD); cell matrix research (M Phil, PhD); channels and transporters (M Phil, PhD); developmental biology (M Phil, PhD); Egyptology (M Phil, PhD); environmental biology (M Phil, PhD); evolutionary biology (M Phil, PhD); gene expression (M Phil, PhD); genetics (M Phil, PhD); history of science, technology and medicine (M Phil, PhD); immunology (M Phil, PhD); integrative neurobiology and behavior (M Phil, PhD); membrane trafficking (M Phil, PhD); microbiology (M Phil, PhD); molecular and cellular neuroscience (M Phil, PhD); molecular biology (M Phil, PhD); molecular cancer studies (M Phil, PhD); neuroscience (M Phil, PhD); ophthalmology (M Phil, PhD); optometry (M Phil, PhD); organelle function (M Phil, PhD); pharmacology (M Phil, PhD); physiology (M Phil, PhD); plant sciences (M Phil, PhD); stem cell research (M Phil, PhD); structural biology (M Phil, PhD); systems neuroscience (M Phil, PhD); toxicology (M Phil, PhD).

University of Manitoba, Faculty of Medicine and Faculty of Graduate Studies, Graduate Programs in Medicine, Department of Pharmacology and Therapeutics, Winnipeg, MB R3T 2N2, Canada. Offers M Sc, PhD. *Program availability:* Part-time. Terminal master's awarded for partial completion of doctoral program. *Degree requirements:* For master's, thesis; for doctorate, thesis/dissertation. *Entrance requirements:* For master's and doctorate, GRE. Additional exam requirements/recommendations for international students: Required—TOEFL. *Faculty research:* Clinical pharmacology; neuropharmacology; cardiac, hepatic, and renal pharmacology.

University of Maryland, Baltimore, Graduate School, Graduate Program in Life Sciences, Program in Molecular Medicine, Baltimore, MD 21201. Offers cancer biology (PhD); cell and molecular physiology (PhD); human genetics and genomic medicine (PhD); molecular medicine (MS); molecular toxicology and pharmacology (PhD); MD/PhD. *Degree requirements:* For doctorate, comprehensive exam, thesis/dissertation. *Entrance requirements:* For master's and doctorate, GRE. Additional exam requirements/recommendations for international students: Required—TOEFL (minimum score 600 paper-based; 100 iBT); Recommended—IELTS (minimum score 7). Electronic applications accepted. Tuition and fees vary according to program.

University of Maryland, Baltimore, Graduate School, Graduate Programs in Pharmacy, Program in Pharmacometrics, Baltimore, MD 21201. Offers MS. Tuition and fees vary according to program.

Pharmacology

University of Miami, Graduate School, Miller School of Medicine, Graduate Programs in Medicine, Department of Molecular and Cellular Pharmacology, Coral Gables, FL 33124. Offers PhD, MD/PhD. *Degree requirements:* For doctorate, thesis/dissertation, dissertation defense, laboratory rotations, qualifying exam. *Entrance requirements:* For doctorate, GRE General Test. Additional exam requirements/recommendations for international students: Required—TOEFL (minimum score 550 paper-based). *Faculty research:* Membrane and cardiovascular pharmacology, muscle contraction, hormone action signal transduction, nuclear transport.

University of Michigan, Rackham Graduate School, Program in Biomedical Sciences (PIBS), Department of Pharmacology, Ann Arbor, MI 48109-5632. Offers MS, PhD. *Faculty:* 17 full-time (6 women). *Students:* 23 full-time (12 women); includes 1 minority (Asian, non-Hispanic/Latino), 3 international. Average age 27. 48 applicants, 35% accepted, 2 enrolled. In 2015, 8 master's, 6 doctorates awarded. Terminal master's awarded for partial completion of doctoral program. *Degree requirements:* For master's, thesis, oral presentation; for doctorate, thesis/dissertation, oral preliminary exam, oral defense of dissertation. *Entrance requirements:* For master's, 3 letters of recommendation, research experience, all undergraduate transcripts; for doctorate, GRE General Test, 3 letters of recommendation, research experience, all undergraduate transcripts. Additional exam requirements/recommendations for international students: Required—TOEFL (minimum score 560 paper-based; 84 iBT). *Application deadline:* For fall admission, 12/1 for domestic and international students. Applications are processed on a rolling basis. Application fee: $75 ($90 for international students). Electronic applications accepted. *Expenses:* Contact institution. *Financial support:* In 2015–16, 23 students received support, including 16 fellowships with full tuition reimbursements available (averaging $29,025 per year), 7 research assistantships with full tuition reimbursements available (averaging $29,025 per year); scholarships/grants, traineeships, health care benefits, and unspecified assistantships also available. Financial award application deadline: 12/1. *Faculty research:* Signal transduction, addiction research, cancer pharmacology, drug metabolism and pharmacogenetics. *Total annual research expenditures:* $5.1 million. *Unit head:* Dr. Lori L. Isom, Professor/Chair of Pharmacology, 734-764-8166, Fax: 734-763-4450, E-mail: lisom@umich.edu. *Application contact:* Jim Musgrave, Director of Graduate Admissions and Recruitment, 734-615-1581, Fax: 734-647-7022, E-mail: jdmusg@umich.edu. Website: https://medicine.umich.edu/pharmacology

University of Minnesota, Duluth, Medical School, Program in Pharmacology, Duluth, MN 55812-2496. Offers MS, PhD. MS, PhD offered jointly with University of Minnesota, Twin Cities Campus. Terminal master's awarded for partial completion of doctoral program. *Degree requirements:* For master's, thesis, final oral exam; for doctorate, thesis/dissertation, final oral exam, oral and written preliminary exams. *Entrance requirements:* For master's and doctorate, GRE General Test. Additional exam requirements/recommendations for international students: Required—TOEFL. *Faculty research:* Drug addiction, alcohol and hypertension, neurotransmission, allergic airway disease, auditory neuroscience.

University of Minnesota, Twin Cities Campus, College of Pharmacy and Graduate School, Graduate Programs in Pharmacy, Graduate Program in Experimental and Clinical Pharmacology, Minneapolis, MN 55455-0213. Offers MS, PhD. *Degree requirements:* For doctorate, thesis/dissertation.

University of Minnesota, Twin Cities Campus, Medical School, Department of Pharmacology, Minneapolis, MN 55455. Offers MS, PhD. Terminal master's awarded for partial completion of doctoral program. *Degree requirements:* For master's, thesis (for some programs); for doctorate, thesis/dissertation. *Entrance requirements:* For master's and doctorate, GRE General Test. Additional exam requirements/recommendations for international students: Required—TOEFL (minimum score 603 paper-based; 100 iBT). Electronic applications accepted. *Faculty research:* Molecular pharmacology, cancer chemotherapy, neuropharmacology, biochemical pharmacology, behavioral pharmacology.

University of Mississippi Medical Center, School of Graduate Studies in the Health Sciences, Department of Pharmacology and Toxicology, Jackson, MS 39216-4505. Offers PhD. *Degree requirements:* For doctorate, comprehensive exam, thesis/dissertation, first authored publication. *Entrance requirements:* For doctorate, GRE General Test, minimum GPA of 3.0. Additional exam requirements/recommendations for international students: Required—TOEFL (minimum score 550 paper-based, 79 iBT), IELTS or PTE. Electronic applications accepted. *Faculty research:* Renal and cardiovascular pharmacology, genetic basis of cardio-renal diseases, diabetes, obesity, metabolic diseases, cancer chemotherapy.

University of Missouri, School of Medicine and Office of Research and Graduate Studies, Graduate Programs in Medicine, Department of Medical Pharmacology and Physiology, Columbia, MO 65211. Offers MS, PhD. *Degree requirements:* For master's, thesis; for doctorate, thesis/dissertation. *Entrance requirements:* For master's and doctorate, GRE General Test, minimum GPA of 3.0. Additional exam requirements/recommendations for international students: Required—TOEFL (minimum score 500 paper-based; 61 iBT). *Application deadline:* For fall admission, 1/10 priority date for domestic and international students; for winter admission, 10/10 priority date for domestic and international students. Applications are processed on a rolling basis. Application fee: $55 ($75 for international students). Electronic applications accepted. *Financial support:* Fellowships, research assistantships, teaching assistantships, institutionally sponsored loans, scholarships/grants, health care benefits, and unspecified assistantships available. Support available to part-time students. Website: http://mpp.missouri.edu/

University of Missouri–Kansas City, School of Pharmacy, Kansas City, MO 64110-2499. Offers pharmaceutical sciences (PhD); pharmacology and toxicology (PhD); pharmacy (Pharm D). PhD offered through School of Graduate Studies. *Accreditation:* ACPE (one or more programs are accredited). *Program availability:* Online learning. *Faculty:* 49 full-time (26 women), 6 part-time/adjunct (2 women). *Students:* 447 full-time (276 women); includes 103 minority (24 Black or African American, non-Hispanic/Latino; 1 American Indian or Alaska Native, non-Hispanic/Latino; 53 Asian, non-Hispanic/Latino; 12 Hispanic/Latino; 13 Two or more races, non-Hispanic/Latino), 2 international. Average age 25. 414 applicants, 33% accepted, 133 enrolled. In 2015, 125 doctorates awarded. *Degree requirements:* For doctorate, comprehensive exam (for some programs), thesis/dissertation (for some programs). *Entrance requirements:* For doctorate, PCAT (for Pharm D). Additional exam requirements/recommendations for international students: Required—TOEFL (minimum score 550 paper-based; 80 iBT). *Application deadline:* For fall admission, 3/1 for domestic and international students. Applications are processed on a rolling basis. Application fee: $45 ($50 for international students). Electronic applications accepted. *Expenses:* Contact institution. *Financial support:* In 2015–16, 4 fellowships (averaging $40,082 per year), 14 research assistantships with tuition reimbursements (averaging $13,117 per year), 26 teaching assistantships with full tuition reimbursements (averaging $14,724 per year) were awarded; career-related internships or fieldwork, Federal Work-Study, institutionally sponsored loans, tuition waivers (full and partial), and unspecified assistantships also available. Financial award application deadline: 3/1; financial award applicants required to submit FAFSA. *Faculty research:* Bio-organic and medicinal chemistry, drug delivery, pharmaceutics, molecular neurobiology, neurology. *Unit head:* Dr. Russell B. Melchert,

Dean, 816-235-1609, Fax: 816-235-5190, E-mail: melchertr@umkc.edu. *Application contact:* Shelly M. Janasz, Director, Student Services, 816-235-2400, Fax: 816-235-5190, E-mail: janaszs@umkc.edu.
Website: http://pharmacy.umkc.edu/

University of Nebraska Medical Center, Department of Pharmacology and Experimental Neuroscience, Omaha, NE 68198. Offers PhD. *Faculty:* 26 full-time (8 women), 2 part-time/adjunct (0 women). *Students:* 33 full-time (12 women), 2 part-time (0 women); includes 2 minority (1 Black or African American, non-Hispanic/Latino; 1 Two or more races, non-Hispanic/Latino), 14 international. Average age 27. 22 applicants. In 2015, 8 doctorates awarded. Terminal master's awarded for partial completion of doctoral program. *Degree requirements:* For doctorate, comprehensive exam, thesis/dissertation. *Entrance requirements:* For doctorate, GRE General Test. Additional exam requirements/recommendations for international students: Required—TOEFL (minimum score 550 paper-based; 80 iBT). *Application deadline:* For fall admission, 4/1 for domestic and international students. Applications are processed on a rolling basis. Application fee: $45. Electronic applications accepted. *Expenses:* Tuition, state resident: full-time $7830; part-time $3915 per credit hour. Tuition, nonresident: full-time $22,410; part-time $11,205 per credit hour. *Required fees:* $521. *Financial support:* In 2015–16, 8 students received support, including 2 fellowships with full tuition reimbursements available (averaging $24,000 per year), 3 research assistantships with full tuition reimbursements available (averaging $24,000 per year); scholarships/grants, health care benefits, and unspecified assistantships also available. Financial award application deadline: 2/15. *Faculty research:* Neuropharmacology, molecular pharmacology, toxicology, molecular biology, neuroscience. *Unit head:* Dr. Keshore Bidasee, Chair, Graduate Studies, 402-559-9018, Fax: 402-559-7495, E-mail: kbidasee@unmc.edu. *Application contact:* Leticia Tran, Office Assistant, 402-559-4044, E-mail: leticia.tran@unmc.edu.
Website: http://www.unmc.edu/pharmacology/

The University of North Carolina at Chapel Hill, School of Medicine and Graduate School, Graduate Programs in Medicine, Department of Pharmacology, Chapel Hill, NC 27599-7365. Offers PhD. *Degree requirements:* For doctorate, comprehensive exam, thesis/dissertation. *Entrance requirements:* For doctorate, GRE General Test, minimum GPA of 3.0. Additional exam requirements/recommendations for international students: Required—TOEFL. Electronic applications accepted. *Faculty research:* Signal transduction, cell adhesion, receptors, ion channels.

University of North Dakota, Graduate School and Graduate School, Graduate Programs in Medicine, Department of Pharmacology, Physiology, and Therapeutics, Grand Forks, ND 58202. Offers pharmacology (MS, PhD); physiology (MS, PhD). *Degree requirements:* For master's, comprehensive exam, thesis; for doctorate, thesis/dissertation, written and oral exams. *Entrance requirements:* For master's, GRE General Test or MCAT, minimum GPA of 3.0; for doctorate, GRE General Test, minimum GPA of 3.5. Additional exam requirements/recommendations for international students: Required—TOEFL (minimum score 550 paper-based; 79 iBT), IELTS (minimum score 6.5). Electronic applications accepted.

University of North Texas Health Science Center at Fort Worth, Graduate School of Biomedical Sciences, Fort Worth, TX 76107-2699. Offers anatomy and cell biology (MS, PhD); biochemistry and molecular biology (MS, PhD); biomedical sciences (MS, PhD); biotechnology (MS); forensic genetics (MS); integrative physiology (MS, PhD); medical science (MS); microbiology and immunology (MS, PhD); pharmacology (MS, PhD); science education (MS); DO/MS; DO/PhD. Terminal master's awarded for partial completion of doctoral program. *Degree requirements:* For master's, thesis; for doctorate, thesis/dissertation. *Entrance requirements:* For master's and doctorate, GRE General Test. Additional exam requirements/recommendations for international students: Required—TOEFL. *Expenses:* Contact institution. *Faculty research:* Alzheimer's disease, aging, eye diseases, cancer, cardiovascular disease.

University of Pennsylvania, Perelman School of Medicine, Biomedical Graduate Studies, Graduate Group in Pharmacology, Philadelphia, PA 19104. Offers PhD, MD/PhD, VMD/PhD. *Faculty:* 99. *Students:* 60 full-time (34 women); includes 24 minority (7 Black or African American, non-Hispanic/Latino; 15 Asian, non-Hispanic/Latino; 1 Hispanic/Latino; 1 Native Hawaiian or other Pacific Islander, non-Hispanic/Latino), 5 international. 73 applicants, 23% accepted, 11 enrolled. In 2015, 13 doctorates awarded. *Degree requirements:* For doctorate, thesis/dissertation. *Entrance requirements:* For doctorate, GRE General Test, previous course work in physical or natural science. Additional exam requirements/recommendations for international students: Required—TOEFL. *Application deadline:* For fall admission, 12/1 priority date for domestic and international students. Applications are processed on a rolling basis. Application fee: $80. Electronic applications accepted. *Expenses: Tuition, area resident:* Full-time $31,068; part-time $5762 per course. *Required fees:* $3200; $336 per course. Full-time tuition and fees vary according to degree level, program and student level. Part-time tuition and fees vary according to course load, degree level and program. *Financial support:* In 2015–16, 60 students received support. Fellowships, research assistantships, scholarships/grants, traineeships, and unspecified assistantships available. *Faculty research:* Properties and regulation of receptors for biogenic amines, molecular aspects of transduction, mechanisms of biosynthesis, biological mechanisms of depression, developmental events in the nervous system. *Unit head:* Dr. Julie Blendy, Chair, 215-898-0730. *Application contact:* Sarah Squire, Coordinator, 215-898-1790.
Website: http://www.med.upenn.edu/ggps

University of Prince Edward Island, Atlantic Veterinary College, Graduate Program in Veterinary Medicine, Charlottetown, PE C1A 4P3, Canada. Offers anatomy (M Sc, PhD); bacteriology (M Sc, PhD); clinical pharmacology (M Sc, PhD); clinical sciences (M Sc, PhD); epidemiology (M Sc, PhD), including reproduction; fish health (M Sc, PhD); food animal nutrition (M Sc, PhD); immunology (M Sc, PhD); microanatomy (M Sc, PhD); parasitology (M Sc, PhD); pathology (M Sc, PhD); pharmacology (M Sc, PhD); physiology (M Sc, PhD); toxicology (M Sc, PhD); veterinary science (M Vet Sci); virology (M Sc, PhD). *Program availability:* Part-time. *Degree requirements:* For master's, thesis; for doctorate, thesis/dissertation. *Entrance requirements:* For master's, DVM, B Sc honors degree, or equivalent; for doctorate, M Sc. Additional exam requirements/recommendations for international students: Required—TOEFL (minimum score 550 paper-based; 80 iBT). *Expenses:* Contact institution. *Faculty research:* Animal health management, infectious diseases, fin fish and shellfish health, basic biomedical sciences, ecosystem health.

University of Puerto Rico, Medical Sciences Campus, School of Medicine, Biomedical Sciences Graduate Program, Department of Pharmacology and Toxicology, San Juan, PR 00936-5067. Offers MS, PhD. *Degree requirements:* For master's, one foreign language, thesis; for doctorate, one foreign language, comprehensive exam, thesis/dissertation. *Entrance requirements:* For master's and doctorate, GRE General Test, GRE Subject Test, interview, minimum GPA of 3.0, 3 letters of recommendation. Electronic applications accepted. *Faculty research:* Cardiovascular, central nervous system, and endocrine pharmacology; anti-cancer drugs; sodium pump; mitochondrial DNA repair; Huntington's disease.

University of Rhode Island, Graduate School, College of Pharmacy, Department of Biomedical and Pharmaceutical Sciences, Kingston, RI 02881. Offers medicinal

chemistry and pharmacognosy (MS, PhD); pharmaceutics and pharmacokinetics (MS, PhD); pharmacology and toxicology (MS, PhD). *Program availability:* Part-time. *Faculty:* 15 full-time (4 women), 4 part-time/adjunct (2 women). *Students:* 39 full-time (14 women), 10 part-time (3 women); includes 3 minority (1 Black or African American, non-Hispanic/Latino; 2 Asian, non-Hispanic/Latino), 24 international. In 2015, 4 master's, 10 doctorates awarded. *Entrance requirements:* For master's and doctorate, GRE (minimum old/new format scores: Verbal 350/143; Quantitative 550/146; Analytical 3.0), 2 letters of recommendation. Additional exam requirements/recommendations for international students: Required—TOEFL (minimum score 550 paper-based). *Application deadline:* For fall admission, 7/15 for domestic students, 2/1 for international students. Application fee: $65. Electronic applications accepted. *Expenses:* Tuition, state resident: full-time $11,796; part-time $655 per credit. Tuition, nonresident: full-time $24,206; part-time $1345 per credit. *Required fees:* $1546; $44 per credit. One-time fee: $155 full-time; $35 part-time. *Financial support:* In 2015–16, 6 research assistantships with tuition reimbursements (averaging $14,828 per year), 18 teaching assistantships with tuition reimbursements (averaging $14,851 per year) were awarded. Financial award application deadline: 2/1; financial award applicants required to submit FAFSA. *Faculty research:* Chemical carcinogenesis with a major emphasis on the structural and synthetic aspects of DNA-adduct formation, drug-drug/herb interaction, drug-genetic interaction, signaling of nuclear receptors, transcriptional regulation, oncogenesis. *Total annual research expenditures:* $5.8 million. *Unit head:* Dr. Bingfang Yan, Chair, 401-874-5032, Fax: 401-874-2181, E-mail: byan@uri.edu. *Application contact:* Graduate Admissions, 401-874-2872, E-mail: gradadm@etal.uri.edu.
Website: http://www.uri.edu/pharmacy/departments/bps/index.shtml

University of Rochester, School of Medicine and Dentistry, Graduate Programs in Medicine and Dentistry, Department of Pharmacology and Physiology, Programs in Pharmacology, Rochester, NY 14627. Offers MS, PhD. Terminal master's awarded for partial completion of doctoral program. *Degree requirements:* For master's, thesis; for doctorate, thesis/dissertation, qualifying exam. *Entrance requirements:* For master's and doctorate, GRE General Test. *Expenses: Tuition, area resident:* Full-time $47,450; part-time $1482 per credit hour. *Required fees:* $528. Tuition and fees vary according to program.

University of Saskatchewan, College of Medicine, Department of Pharmacology, Saskatoon, SK S7N 5A2, Canada. Offers M Sc, PhD. *Degree requirements:* For master's, thesis; for doctorate, thesis/dissertation. *Entrance requirements:* Additional exam requirements/recommendations for international students: Required—TOEFL. *Faculty research:* Neuropharmacology, mechanisms of action of anticancer drugs, clinical pharmacology, cardiovascular pharmacology, toxicology: alcohol-related changes in fetal brain development.

The University of South Dakota, Graduate School, Sanford School of Medicine and Graduate School, Biomedical Sciences Graduate Program, Physiology and Pharmacology Group, Vermillion, SD 57069-2390. Offers MS, PhD. *Students:* Average age 25. In 2015, 1 master's, 3 doctorates awarded. Terminal master's awarded for partial completion of doctoral program. *Degree requirements:* For master's, thesis; for doctorate, comprehensive exam, thesis/dissertation. *Entrance requirements:* For master's and doctorate, GRE General Test, minimum GPA of 3.0. Additional exam requirements/recommendations for international students: Required—TOEFL (minimum score 550 paper-based; 80 iBT), IELTS (minimum score 6). *Application deadline:* For fall admission, 4/15 priority date for domestic students, 3/15 for international students. Applications are processed on a rolling basis. Application fee: $35. Electronic applications accepted. *Expenses:* Contact institution. *Financial support:* In 2015–16, 12 students received support. Fellowships with partial tuition reimbursements available, research assistantships with partial tuition reimbursements available, scholarships/grants, and unspecified assistantships available. Financial award application deadline: 4/15; financial award applicants required to submit FAFSA. *Faculty research:* Pulmonary physiology and pharmacology, drug abuse, reproduction, signal transduction, cardiovascular physiology and pharmacology. *Unit head:* 605-658-632, Fax: 605-677-6381, E-mail: biomed@usd.edu.

University of South Florida, Morsani College of Medicine and College of Graduate Studies, Graduate Programs in Medical Sciences, Tampa, FL 33620-9951. Offers advanced athletic training (MS); athletic training (MS); bioinformatics and computational biology (MSBCB); biotechnology (MSB); health informatics (MSHI); medical sciences (MSMS, PhD), including aging and neuroscience (MSMS), allergy, immunology and infectious disease (PhD), anatomy, athletic training (MSMS), clinical and translational research, health informatics (MSMS), health science (MSMS), interdisciplinary medical sciences (MSMS), medical microbiology and immunology (MSMS), metabolic and nutritional medicine (MSMS), molecular medicine, molecular pharmacology and physiology (PhD), neurology (PhD), pathology and laboratory medicine (PhD), pharmacology and therapeutics (PhD), physiology and biophysics (PhD), women's health (MSMS). *Students:* 510 full-time (261 women), 318 part-time (208 women); includes 360 minority (108 Black or African American, non-Hispanic/Latino; 3 American Indian or Alaska Native, non-Hispanic/Latino; 101 Asian, non-Hispanic/Latino; 124 Hispanic/Latino; 1 Native Hawaiian or other Pacific Islander, non-Hispanic/Latino; 23 Two or more races, non-Hispanic/Latino), 52 international. Average age 26. 6,567 applicants, 13% accepted, 469 enrolled. In 2015, 216 master's awarded. Terminal master's awarded for partial completion of doctoral program. *Degree requirements:* For master's, comprehensive exam, thesis; for doctorate, comprehensive exam, thesis/dissertation. *Entrance requirements:* For master's, GRE General Test or GMAT, bachelor's degree or equivalent from regionally-accredited university with minimum GPA of 3.0 in upper-division sciences coursework; prerequisites in general biology, general chemistry, general physics, organic chemistry, quantitative analysis, and integral and differential calculus; for doctorate, GRE General Test, bachelor's degree from regionally-accredited university with minimum GPA of 3.0 in upper-division sciences coursework; 3 letters of recommendation; personal interview; 1-2 page personal statement; prerequisites in biology, chemistry, physics, organic chemistry, quantitative analysis, and integral/differential calculus. Additional exam requirements/recommendations for international students: Required—TOEFL (minimum score 550 paper-based; 79 iBT) or IELTS (minimum score 6.5). *Application deadline:* For fall admission, 2/15 for domestic students, 1/2 for international students. Application fee: $30. *Expenses:* Contact institution. *Faculty research:* Anatomy, biochemistry, cancer biology, cardiovascular disease, cell biology, immunology, microbiology, molecular biology, neuroscience, pharmacology, physiology. *Unit head:* Dr. Michael Barber, Professor/Associate Dean for Graduate and Postdoctoral Affairs, 813-974-9908, Fax: 813-974-4317, E-mail: mbarber@health.usf.edu. *Application contact:* Dr. Eric Bennett, Graduate Director, PhD Program in Medical Sciences, 813-974-1545, Fax: 813-974-4317, E-mail: esbennet@health.usf.edu.
Website: http://health.usf.edu/nocms/medicine/graduatestudies/

The University of Tennessee Health Science Center, College of Graduate Health Sciences, Memphis, TN 38163-0002. Offers biomedical engineering (MS, PhD); biomedical sciences (PhD); dental sciences (MDS); epidemiology (MS); health outcomes and policy research (PhD); laboratory research and management (MS); nursing science (PhD); pharmaceutical sciences (PhD); pharmacology (MS); speech and hearing science (PhD); DDS/PhD; DNP/PhD; MD/PhD; Pharm D/PhD. Terminal

master's awarded for partial completion of doctoral program. *Degree requirements:* For master's, comprehensive exam, thesis; for doctorate, comprehensive exam, thesis/dissertation, oral and written preliminary and comprehensive exams. *Entrance requirements:* For master's and doctorate, GRE General Test, minimum GPA of 3.0. Additional exam requirements/recommendations for international students: Required—TOEFL (minimum score 79 iBT); Recommended—IELTS (minimum score 6.5). Electronic applications accepted.

The University of Texas at Austin, Graduate School, College of Pharmacy, Graduate Programs in Pharmacy, Austin, TX 78712-1111. Offers health outcomes and pharmacy practice (PhD); health outcomes and pharmacy practice (MS); medicinal chemistry (PhD); pharmaceutics (PhD); pharmacology and toxicology (PhD); pharmacotherapy (MS, PhD); translational science (PhD). PhD in translational science offered jointly with The University of Texas Health Science Center at San Antonio and The University of Texas at San Antonio. *Degree requirements:* For master's, thesis; for doctorate, thesis/dissertation. *Entrance requirements:* For master's and doctorate, GRE General Test. Electronic applications accepted. *Faculty research:* Synthetic medical chemistry, synthetic molecular biology, bio-organic chemistry, pharmacoeconomics, pharmacy practice.

The University of Texas Health Science Center at San Antonio, Graduate School of Biomedical Sciences, Department of Pharmacology, San Antonio, TX 78229-3900. Offers neuroscience (PhD). *Degree requirements:* For doctorate, comprehensive exam, thesis/dissertation.

The University of Texas Medical Branch, Graduate School of Biomedical Sciences, Program in Pharmacology and Toxicology, Galveston, TX 77555. Offers pharmacology (MS); pharmacology and toxicology (PhD). *Degree requirements:* For master's, thesis or alternative; for doctorate, thesis/dissertation. *Entrance requirements:* For master's and doctorate, GRE General Test. Additional exam requirements/recommendations for international students: Required—TOEFL (minimum score 550 paper-based).

University of the Sciences, Program in Chemistry, Biochemistry and Pharmacognosy, Philadelphia, PA 19104-4495. Offers biochemistry (MS, PhD); chemistry (MS, PhD); pharmacognosy (MS, PhD). *Program availability:* Part-time. *Degree requirements:* For master's, thesis, qualifying exams; for doctorate, comprehensive exam, thesis/dissertation, qualifying exams. *Entrance requirements:* For master's and doctorate, GRE General Test, GRE Subject Test. Additional exam requirements/recommendations for international students: Required—TOEFL, TWE. *Application deadline:* For fall admission, 5/1 for international students; for winter admission, 10/1 for international students; for spring admission, 3/1 for international students. Applications are processed on a rolling basis. Application fee: $50. *Expenses:* Contact institution. *Financial support:* Fellowships with full tuition reimbursements, research assistantships with full tuition reimbursements, teaching assistantships with full tuition reimbursements, institutionally sponsored loans, scholarships/grants, and tuition waivers (full) available. Financial award application deadline: 5/1. *Unit head:* Dr. James R. McKee, Director, 215-596-8847, E-mail: j.mckee@usciences.edu. *Application contact:* Dr. James R. McKee, Director, 215-596-8847, E-mail: j.mckee@usciences.edu.

University of the Sciences, Program in Pharmacology and Toxicology, Philadelphia, PA 19104-4495. Offers pharmacology (MS, PhD); toxicology (MS, PhD). Terminal master's awarded for partial completion of doctoral program. *Degree requirements:* For master's, thesis; for doctorate, comprehensive exam, thesis/dissertation. *Entrance requirements:* For master's and doctorate, GRE General Test. Additional exam requirements/recommendations for international students: Required—TOEFL, TWE. *Application deadline:* For fall admission, 5/1 for international students; for winter admission, 10/1 for international students; for spring admission, 3/1 for international students. Applications are processed on a rolling basis. Application fee: $50. *Expenses:* Contact institution. *Financial support:* Teaching assistantships with tuition reimbursements, institutionally sponsored loans, and tuition waivers (partial) available. Financial award application deadline: 5/1. *Unit head:* Dr. Bin Chen, Director, 215-596-7481, E-mail: b.chen@usciences.edu. *Application contact:* Dr. Bin Chen, Director, 215-596-7481, E-mail: b.chen@usciences.edu.

The University of Toledo, College of Graduate Studies, College of Pharmacy and Pharmaceutical Sciences, Program in Experimental Therapeutics, Toledo, OH 43606-3390. Offers PhD. *Entrance requirements:* For doctorate, GRE, bachelors degree in chemistry, biology, pharmaceutical sciences, pharmacy or a related discipline. Additional exam requirements/recommendations for international students: Required—TOEFL.

The University of Toledo, College of Graduate Studies, College of Pharmacy and Pharmaceutical Sciences, Program in Pharmaceutical Sciences, Toledo, OH 43606-3390. Offers administrative pharmacy (MSPS); industrial pharmacy (MSPS); pharmacology toxicology (MSPS). *Degree requirements:* For master's, thesis. *Entrance requirements:* For master's, GRE General Test. Additional exam requirements/recommendations for international students: Required—TOEFL (minimum score 550 paper-based; 80 iBT). Electronic applications accepted.

University of Toronto, Faculty of Medicine, Department of Pharmacology and Toxicology, Toronto, ON M5S 1A1, Canada. Offers pharmacology (M Sc, PhD). *Program availability:* Part-time. *Degree requirements:* For master's, thesis; for doctorate, thesis/dissertation. *Entrance requirements:* For master's, B Sc or equivalent; background in pharmacology, biochemistry, and physiology; minimum B+ earned in at least 4 senior level classes; for doctorate, minimum B+ average. Additional exam requirements/recommendations for international students: Required—TOEFL (minimum score 580 paper-based; 93 iBT), TWE (minimum score 5). Electronic applications accepted.

University of Utah, Graduate School, College of Pharmacy, Department of Pharmacology and Toxicology, Salt Lake City, UT 84112. Offers PhD. *Faculty:* 16 full-time (5 women), 11 part-time/adjunct (4 women). *Students:* 9 full-time (5 women), 3 international. Average age 29. In 2015, 1 doctorate awarded. Terminal master's awarded for partial completion of doctoral program. *Degree requirements:* For doctorate, comprehensive exam, thesis/dissertation, final exam. *Entrance requirements:* For doctorate, GRE General Test, BS in biology, chemistry, or neuroscience. *Application deadline:* For fall admission, 12/15 for domestic and international students. Application fee: $0. Electronic applications accepted. *Expenses:* $1,356.08 per credit hour. *Financial support:* In 2015–16, 9 students received support, including 9 research assistantships with full tuition reimbursements available (averaging $25,000 per year); health care benefits and tuition waivers (full) also available. Financial award application deadline: 1/15. *Faculty research:* Neuropharmacology of anti-seizure drugs and drugs of abuse, drug metabolism, signal transduction pathways and oncogenic processes, drug analyses in biological samples, natural products drug discovery. *Unit head:* Dr. Karen Wilcox, Department Chair, 801-581-6287, Fax: 801-585-5111, E-mail: karen.wilcox@hsc.utah.edu. *Application contact:* Linda Wright, Program Assistant, 801-581-6281, Fax: 801-585-5111, E-mail: linda.wright@utah.edu.
Website: http://www.pharmacy.utah.edu/pharmtox/

University of Vermont, College of Medicine and Graduate College, Graduate Programs in Medicine, Department of Pharmacology, Burlington, VT 05405. Offers MS, PhD. *Degree requirements:* For master's, thesis; for doctorate, thesis/dissertation.

Pharmacology

Entrance requirements: For master's and doctorate, GRE General Test. Additional exam requirements/recommendations for international students: Required—TOEFL (minimum score 550 paper-based; 80 iBT). *Application deadline:* For fall admission, 1/15 priority date for domestic students, 1/15 for international students. Applications are processed on a rolling basis. Application fee: $65. Electronic applications accepted. *Financial support:* Fellowships, research assistantships, and teaching assistantships available. Financial award application deadline: 3/1. *Faculty research:* Cardiovascular drugs, anticancer drugs. *Unit head:* Dr. Anthony Morielli, 802-656-2500, E-mail: anthony.morielli@uvm.edu. *Application contact:* Dr. Anthony Morielli, 802-656-2500, E-mail: anthony.morielli@uvm.edu.

University of Virginia, School of Medicine, Department of Pharmacology, Charlottesville, VA 22903. Offers PhD, MD/PhD. *Degree requirements:* For doctorate, thesis/dissertation. *Entrance requirements:* For doctorate, GRE General Test, GRE Subject Test (recommended), 2 letters of recommendation. Additional exam requirements/recommendations for international students: Required—TOEFL. Electronic applications accepted.

University of Washington, Graduate School, School of Medicine, Graduate Programs in Medicine, Department of Pharmacology, Seattle, WA 98195. Offers PhD. *Degree requirements:* For doctorate, thesis/dissertation. *Entrance requirements:* For doctorate, GRE General Test, minimum GPA of 3.0. *Faculty research:* Neuroscience, cell physiology, molecular biology, regulation of metabolism, signal transduction.

University of Wisconsin–Madison, School of Medicine and Public Health, Molecular and Cellular Pharmacology Graduate Training Program, Madison, WI 53705. Offers PhD. *Faculty:* 70 full-time (20 women). *Students:* 33 full-time (17 women); includes 8 minority (1 Black or African American, non-Hispanic/Latino; 5 Asian, non-Hispanic/Latino; 1 Hispanic/Latino; 1 Native Hawaiian or other Pacific Islander, non-Hispanic/Latino), 6 international. Average age 26. 89 applicants, 15% accepted, 3 enrolled. In 2015, 4 doctorates awarded. *Degree requirements:* For doctorate, comprehensive exam, thesis/dissertation. *Entrance requirements:* For doctorate, GRE. Additional exam requirements/recommendations for international students: Required—TOEFL (minimum score 580 paper-based; 92 iBT). *Application deadline:* For fall admission, 12/1 priority date for domestic and international students. Applications are processed on a rolling basis. Application fee: $56. Electronic applications accepted. *Expenses:* Tuition, state resident: full-time $5364. Tuition, nonresident: full-time $12,027. *Required fees:* $571. Tuition and fees vary according to campus/location, program and reciprocity agreements. *Financial support:* In 2015–16, 33 students received support, including 4 fellowships with full tuition reimbursements available (averaging $25,000 per year), 29 research assistantships with full tuition reimbursements available (averaging $25,000 per year), teaching assistantships with full tuition reimbursements available (averaging $24,500 per year); scholarships/grants, traineeships, health care benefits, and unspecified assistantships also available. *Faculty research:* Protein kinases, signaling pathways, neurotransmitters, molecular recognition, receptors and transporters. *Unit head:* Dr. Anjon Audhya, Director, 608-262-3761, E-mail: audhya@wisc.edu. *Application contact:* Kristin Cooper, Program Coordinator, 608-262-9826, E-mail: kgcooper@wisc.edu.
Website: http://molpharm.wisc.edu/

University of Wisconsin–Milwaukee, Graduate School, College of Health Sciences, Program in Biomedical Sciences, Milwaukee, WI 53211. Offers cancer (MS); immunology (MS); microbiology (MS); neurodegenerative disease (MS); pharmacology and toxicology (MS); photobiomodulation (MS). *Accreditation:* NAACLS. *Program availability:* Part-time. *Faculty:* 8 full-time (4 women). *Students:* 8 full-time (7 women), 3 part-time (1 woman); includes 1 minority (Two or more races, non-Hispanic/Latino), 2 international. Average age 29. 42 applicants, 14% accepted, 4 enrolled. In 2015, 7 master's awarded. *Degree requirements:* For master's, thesis. *Entrance requirements:* For master's, GRE General Test. Additional exam requirements/recommendations for international students: Required—TOEFL (minimum score 550 paper-based; 79 iBT), IELTS (minimum score 6.5). *Application deadline:* For fall admission, 1/1 priority date for domestic students; for spring admission, 9/1 for domestic students. Applications are processed on a rolling basis. Application fee: $56 ($96 for international students). *Financial support:* In 2015–16, 6 teaching assistantships were awarded; fellowships, research assistantships, career-related internships or fieldwork, and unspecified assistantships also available. Support available to part-time students. Financial award application deadline: 4/15. *Unit head:* Raymond Fleming, Representative, 414-229-3980, E-mail: mundo@uwm.edu. *Application contact:* Roger O. Smith, General Information Contact, 414-229-6697, Fax: 414-229-6697, E-mail: smithro@uwm.edu.
Website: http://www4.uwm.edu/chs/academics/biomedical_sciences/bms_masters/

Vanderbilt University, School of Medicine, Department of Pharmacology, Nashville, TN 37240-1001. Offers PhD, MD/PhD. *Faculty:* 25 full-time (8 women). *Students:* 49 full-time (27 women); includes 10 minority (1 Black or African American, non-Hispanic/Latino; 3 Asian, non-Hispanic/Latino; 3 Hispanic/Latino; 3 Two or more races, non-Hispanic/Latino), 5 international. Average age 28. 3 applicants, 100% accepted, 3 enrolled. In 2015, 10 doctorates awarded. *Degree requirements:* For doctorate, comprehensive exam, thesis/dissertation, preliminary, qualifying, and final exams. *Entrance requirements:* For doctorate, GRE General Test, GRE Subject Test (recommended). Additional exam requirements/recommendations for international students: Required—TOEFL (minimum score 570 paper-based; 88 iBT). *Application deadline:* For fall admission, 1/15 for domestic and international students. Application fee: $0. Electronic applications accepted. *Financial support:* Fellowships with full tuition reimbursements, research assistantships with full tuition reimbursements, Federal Work-Study, institutionally sponsored loans, scholarships/grants, traineeships, health care benefits, and tuition waivers (partial) available. Financial award application deadline: 1/15; financial award applicants required to submit CSS PROFILE or FAFSA. *Faculty research:* Molecular pharmacology, neuropharmacology, drug disposition and toxicology, genetic mechanics, cell regulation. *Unit head:* Dr. Christine Konradi, Director of Graduate Studies, 615-322-2207, Fax: 615-936-3910, E-mail: christine.konradi@vanderbilt.edu. *Application contact:* Karen Gieg, Coordinator, 615-322-1182, E-mail: karen.gieg@vanderbilt.edu.
Website: http://medschool.vanderbilt.edu/pharmacology/

Virginia Commonwealth University, Medical College of Virginia-Professional Programs, School of Medicine, School of Medicine Graduate Programs, Department of Pharmacology and Toxicology, Richmond, VA 23284-9005. Offers pharmacology (PhD); pharmacology (Certificate); pharmacology and toxicology (MS, PhD); MD/PhD. Terminal master's awarded for partial completion of doctoral program. *Degree requirements:* For master's, thesis; for doctorate, thesis/dissertation, comprehensive oral and written exams. *Entrance requirements:* For master's and doctorate, GRE or MCAT. Additional exam requirements/recommendations for international students: Required—TOEFL (minimum score 600 paper-based; 100 iBT). Electronic applications accepted. *Faculty research:* Drug abuse, drug metabolism, pharmacodynamics, peptide synthesis, receptor mechanisms.

Virginia Commonwealth University, Program in Pre-Medical Basic Health Sciences, Richmond, VA 23284-9005. Offers anatomy (CBHS); biochemistry (CBHS); human genetics (CBHS); microbiology (CBHS); pharmacology (CBHS); physiology (CBHS). *Entrance requirements:* For degree, GRE, MCAT or DAT, course work in organic chemistry, minimum undergraduate GPA of 2.8. Additional exam requirements/recommendations for international students: Required—TOEFL (minimum score 600 paper-based). Electronic applications accepted.

Wake Forest University, School of Medicine and Graduate School of Arts and Sciences, Graduate Programs in Medicine, Program in Physiology and Pharmacology, Winston-Salem, NC 27109. Offers pharmacology (PhD); physiology (PhD); MD/PhD. *Degree requirements:* For doctorate, thesis/dissertation. *Entrance requirements:* For doctorate, GRE General Test. Additional exam requirements/recommendations for international students: Required—TOEFL. Electronic applications accepted. *Faculty research:* Aging, substance abuse, cardiovascular control, endocrine systems, toxicology.

Wayne State University, School of Medicine, Office of Biomedical Graduate Programs, Department of Pharmacology, Detroit, MI 48202. Offers MS, PhD, MD/PhD. *Faculty:* 23. *Students:* 11 full-time (8 women); includes 3 minority (1 Asian, non-Hispanic/Latino; 2 Hispanic/Latino), 4 international. Average age 27. 50 applicants, 4% accepted, 2 enrolled. In 2015, 1 doctorate awarded. Terminal master's awarded for partial completion of doctoral program. *Degree requirements:* For master's, thesis; for doctorate, thesis/dissertation. *Entrance requirements:* For master's and doctorate, GRE General Test, minimum undergraduate GPA of 3.0 for upper-division course work, personal statement, three letters of recommendation, background in chemical or biological sciences. Additional exam requirements/recommendations for international students: Required—TOEFL (minimum score 100 iBT). *Application deadline:* For fall admission, 2/1 priority date for domestic and international students. Applications are processed on a rolling basis. Application fee: $0. Electronic applications accepted. *Expenses:* $17,645 per year resident tuition, $33,311 non-resident tuition; $735.20 per credit hour resident tuition, $1,387.95 per credit hour non-resident tuition; fees include $47.45 per credit hour student services fee and $274.60 per semester registration fee. *Financial support:* In 2015–16, 11 students received support, including 2 fellowships with tuition reimbursements available (averaging $26,614 per year), 9 research assistantships with tuition reimbursements available (averaging $27,064 per year); teaching assistantships, scholarships/grants, health care benefits, and unspecified assistantships also available. *Faculty research:* Molecular and cellular biology of cancer and anti-cancer therapies; molecular and cellular biology of protein trafficking, signal transduction and aging; environmental toxicology and drug metabolism; functional cellular and in vivo imaging; neuroscience. *Unit head:* Dr. Roy McCauley, Graduate Program Director, 313-577-6737, E-mail: rmccaul@med.wayne.edu.
Website: http://www.med.wayne.edu/pharmacology/index.asp

Weill Cornell Medicine, Weill Cornell Graduate School of Medical Sciences, Pharmacology Program, New York, NY 10065. Offers MS, PhD. Terminal master's awarded for partial completion of doctoral program. *Degree requirements:* For master's, comprehensive exam; for doctorate, thesis/dissertation, final exam. *Entrance requirements:* For doctorate, GRE General Test, previous course work in natural and/or health sciences. Additional exam requirements/recommendations for international students: Required—TOEFL. *Faculty research:* Understanding how drugs and chemicals modify biological systems; using and developing new drugs to treat diseases, such as cancer, diabetes, atherosclerosis, epilepsy, anxiety disorders, Alzheimer's disease, and autism.

West Virginia University, School of Medicine, Graduate Programs at the Health Sciences Center, Interdisciplinary Graduate Programs in Biomedical Sciences, Program in Pharmaceutical and Pharmacological Sciences, Morgantown, WV 26506. Offers MS, PhD, MD/PhD. *Degree requirements:* For doctorate, comprehensive exam, thesis/dissertation. *Entrance requirements:* For doctorate, GRE General Test, minimum GPA of 3.0. Additional exam requirements/recommendations for international students: Required—TOEFL. Electronic applications accepted. *Expenses:* Tuition, state resident: full-time $8568. Tuition, nonresident: full-time $22,140. Tuition and fees vary according to program. *Faculty research:* Medicinal chemistry, pharmacokinetics, nano-pharmaceutics, polymer-based drug delivery, molecular therapeutics.

Wright State University, School of Medicine, Program in Pharmacology and Toxicology, Dayton, OH 45435. Offers MS. *Degree requirements:* For master's, thesis optional.

Yale University, School of Medicine and Graduate School of Arts and Sciences, Combined Program in Biological and Biomedical Sciences (BBS), Department of Pharmacology, New Haven, CT 06520. Offers PhD. *Degree requirements:* For doctorate, thesis/dissertation. *Entrance requirements:* For doctorate, GRE General Test. Additional exam requirements/recommendations for international students: Required—TOEFL. *Expenses:* Contact institution.

Yale University, School of Medicine and Graduate School of Arts and Sciences, Combined Program in Biological and Biomedical Sciences (BBS), Pharmacological Sciences and Molecular Medicine Track, New Haven, CT 06520. Offers PhD, MD/PhD. *Degree requirements:* For doctorate, thesis/dissertation. *Entrance requirements:* For doctorate, GRE General Test. Additional exam requirements/recommendations for international students: Required—TOEFL. Electronic applications accepted.

Toxicology

American University of Beirut, Graduate Programs, Faculty of Medicine, Beirut, Lebanon. Offers anatomy, cell biology and human morphology (MS); biochemistry and medical genetics (MS); biomedical sciences (PhD); experimental pathology, immunology and microbiology (MS); medicine (MD); neuroscience (MS); pharmacology and toxicology (MS). *Program availability:* Part-time. *Faculty:* 302 full-time (95 women), 64 part-time/adjunct (11 women). *Students:* 381 full-time (173 women), 61 part-time (51 women). Average age 23. In 2015, 14 master's awarded. *Degree requirements:* For master's, one foreign language, comprehensive exam, thesis (for some programs); for doctorate, one foreign language, comprehensive exam, thesis/dissertation. *Entrance requirements:* For master's, letter of recommendation; for doctorate, MCAT, bachelor's degree. Additional exam requirements/recommendations for international students: Required—TOEFL (minimum score 600 paper-based; 100 iBT), IELTS (minimum score

7.5). *Application deadline:* For fall admission, 4/30 for domestic and international students; for spring admission, 11/1 for domestic and international students. Application fee: $50. Electronic applications accepted. *Expenses: Tuition, area resident:* Full-time $16,254; part-time $903 per credit. *Required fees:* $699. Tuition and fees vary according to course load and program. *Financial support:* In 2015–16, 273 students received support, including 45 teaching assistantships (averaging $9,000 per year); career-related internships or fieldwork, institutionally sponsored loans, scholarships/grants, health care benefits, and unspecified assistantships also available. Financial award application deadline: 2/2. *Faculty research:* Cancer research (targeted therapy, mechanisms of leukemogenesis, tumor cell extravasation and metastasis, cancer stem cells), stem cell research (regenerative medicine, drug discovery), genetic research (neurogenetics, hereditary cardiomyopathy, hemoglobinopathies, pharmacogenomics, proteomics), neuroscience research (pain, neurodegenerative disorder), metabolism (inflammation and metabolism, metabolic disorder, diabetes mellitus), vascular and renal biology, signal transduction. *Total annual research expenditures:* $2.6 million. *Unit head:* Dr. Mohamed Sayegh, Dean, 961-1350000 Ext. 4700, Fax: 961-1744464, E-mail: msayegh@aub.edu.lb. *Application contact:* Dr. Salim Kanaan, Director, Admissions Office, 961-1350000 Ext. 2594, Fax: 961-1750775, E-mail: sk00@aub.edu.lb. Website: http://www.aub.edu.lb/fm/fm_home/Pages/index.aspx

Colorado State University, College of Veterinary Medicine and Biomedical Sciences, Department of Environmental and Radiological Health Sciences, Fort Collins, CO 80523-1681. Offers environmental health (MS, PhD); radiological health sciences (MS, PhD); toxicology (MS, PhD). *Program availability:* Part-time. *Faculty:* 31 full-time (13 women), 6 part-time/adjunct (3 women). *Students:* 100 full-time (48 women), 40 part-time (21 women); includes 20 minority (2 Black or African American, non-Hispanic/Latino; 1 American Indian or Alaska Native, non-Hispanic/Latino; 4 Asian, non-Hispanic/Latino; 12 Hispanic/Latino; 1 Two or more races, non-Hispanic/Latino), 9 international Average age 29. 117 applicants, 83% accepted, 69 enrolled. In 2015, 35 master's, 5 doctorates awarded. Terminal master's awarded for partial completion of doctoral program. *Degree requirements:* For master's, comprehensive exam (for some programs), thesis (for some programs); for doctorate, comprehensive exam, thesis/dissertation. *Entrance requirements:* For master's, GRE, minimum GPA of 3.0; for doctorate, GRE, minimum GPA of 3.0, MS or proof of research. Additional exam requirements/recommendations for international students: Recommended—TOEFL (minimum score 550 paper-based; 80 iBT), IELTS (minimum score 6.5). *Application deadline:* For fall admission, 7/1 for domestic students, 5/1 for international students; for spring admission, 7/1 for domestic students, 5/1 for international students. Applications are processed on a rolling basis. Application fee: $60 ($70 for international students). Electronic applications accepted. *Expenses:* Contact institution. *Financial support:* In 2015–16, 4 students received support, including 16 fellowships with full tuition reimbursements available (averaging $48,116 per year), 21 research assistantships with full tuition reimbursements available (averaging $21,807 per year), 3 teaching assistantships with full tuition reimbursements available (averaging $13,680 per year); scholarships/grants, traineeships, unspecified assistantships, and hourly employment positions also available. Financial award application deadline: 2/1. *Faculty research:* Chromosomes and telomeres in cancer and other human disease states, ambient environmental exposures, radiation physics and dosimetry, cellular toxicity, noise exposure assessment. *Total annual research expenditures:* $8.4 million. *Unit head:* Dr. Jac A. Nickoloff, Professor/Department Head, 970-491-6674, Fax: 970-491-0623, E-mail: j.nickoloff@colostate.edu. *Application contact:* Jeanne A. Brockway, Graduate Program Coordinator, 970-491-5003, Fax: 970-491-2940, E-mail: jeanne.brockway@colostate.edu. Website: http://csu-cvmbs.colostate.edu/academics/erhs/Pages/graduate-studies.aspx

Columbia University, College of Physicians and Surgeons, Department of Pharmacology, New York, NY 10032. Offers pharmacology (M Phil, MA, PhD); pharmacology-toxicology (M Phil, MA, PhD); MD/PhD. Only candidates for the PhD are admitted. Terminal master's awarded for partial completion of doctoral program. *Degree requirements:* For doctorate, thesis/dissertation. *Entrance requirements:* For master's and doctorate, GRE General Test. Additional exam requirements/recommendations for international students: Required—TOEFL. *Faculty research:* Cardiovascular pharmacology, receptor pharmacology, neuropharmacology, membrane biophysics, eicosanoids.

Cornell University, Graduate School, Graduate Fields of Agriculture and Life Sciences, Field of Environmental Toxicology, Ithaca, NY 14853-0001. Offers cellular and molecular toxicology (MS, PhD); ecotoxicology and environmental chemistry (MS, PhD); nutritional and food toxicology (MS, PhD); risk assessment, management and public policy (MS, PhD). *Degree requirements:* For master's, thesis; for doctorate, comprehensive exam, thesis/dissertation. *Entrance requirements:* For master's and doctorate, GRE General Test, GRE Subject Test (biology or chemistry recommended), 2 letters of recommendation. Additional exam requirements/recommendations for international students: Required—TOEFL (minimum score 600 paper-based; 77 iBT). Electronic applications accepted. *Faculty research:* Cellular and molecular toxicology, cancer toxicology, bioremediation, ecotoxicology, nutritional and food toxicology, reproductive toxicology.

Duke University, Graduate School, Integrated Toxicology and Environmental Health Program, Durham, NC 27708. Offers Certificate. *Entrance requirements:* Additional exam requirements/recommendations for international students: Required—TOEFL (minimum score 577 paper-based; 90 iBT) or IELTS (minimum score 7). Electronic applications accepted.

Florida Agricultural and Mechanical University, Division of Graduate Studies, Research, and Continuing Education, College of Pharmacy and Pharmaceutical Sciences, Graduate Programs in Pharmaceutical Sciences, Tallahassee, FL 32307-3200. Offers environmental toxicology (PhD); health outcomes research and pharmacoeconomics (PhD); medicinal chemistry (MS, PhD); pharmaceutics (MS, PhD); pharmacology/toxicology (MS, PhD); pharmacy administration (MS). *Accreditation:* CEPH. *Degree requirements:* For master's, comprehensive exam, thesis, publishable paper; for doctorate, comprehensive exam, thesis/dissertation, publishable paper. *Entrance requirements:* For master's and doctorate, GRE General Test, minimum GPA of 3.0 in last 60 hours. Additional exam requirements/recommendations for international students: Required—TOEFL. *Faculty research:* Anticancer agents, anti-inflammatory drugs, chronopharmacology, neuroendocrinology, microbiology.

The George Washington University, Columbian College of Arts and Sciences, Department of Forensic Sciences, Washington, DC 20052. Offers crime scene investigation (MFS); forensic chemistry (MFS); forensic molecular biology (MFS); forensic toxicology (MFS); high-technology crime investigation (MS); security management (MFS). MFS programs in high-technology crime investigation and in security management offered in Arlington, VA. *Program availability:* Part-time, evening/weekend. *Faculty:* 10 full-time (1 woman), 17 part-time/adjunct (4 women). *Students:* 64 full-time (48 women), 38 part-time (26 women); includes 34 minority (14 Black or African American, non-Hispanic/Latino; 1 American Indian or Alaska Native, non-Hispanic/Latino; 12 Asian, non-Hispanic/Latino; 6 Hispanic/Latino; 1 Two or more races, non-Hispanic/Latino), 4 international. Average age 27. 153 applicants, 71% accepted, 54 enrolled. In 2015, 42 master's, 4 other advanced degrees awarded. *Degree*

requirements: For master's, comprehensive exam. *Entrance requirements:* For master's, GRE General Test, minimum GPA of 3.0. Additional exam requirements/recommendations for international students: Required—TOEFL (minimum score 550 paper-based; 80 iBT). *Application deadline:* For fall admission, 1/16 priority date for international students; for spring admission, 10/1 priority date for domestic students, 9/1 priority date for international students. Applications are processed on a rolling basis. Application fee: $75. Electronic applications accepted. *Financial support:* In 2015–16, 19 students received support. Fellowships with partial tuition reimbursements available, Federal Work-Study, and tuition waivers available. *Unit head:* Dr. Victor Weedn, Chair, 202-994-6977, E-mail: vweedn@gwu.edu. *Application contact:* 202-994-6210, Fax: 202-994-6213, E-mail: askccas@gwu.edu. Website: http://forensicsciences.columbian.gwu.edu/

Indiana University Bloomington, School of Public and Environmental Affairs, Environmental Science Programs, Bloomington, IN 47405. Offers applied ecology (MSES); energy (MSES); environmental chemistry, toxicology, and risk assessment (MSES); environmental science (PhD); hazardous materials management (Certificate); specialized environmental science (MSES); water resources (MSES); JD/MSES; MSES/MA; MSES/MPA; MSES/MS. *Program availability:* Part-time. Terminal master's awarded for partial completion of doctoral program. *Degree requirements:* For master's, capstone or thesis; internship; for doctorate, comprehensive exam, thesis/dissertation. *Entrance requirements:* For master's, GRE General Test or GMAT, official transcripts, 3 letters of recommendation, resume, personal statement; for doctorate, GRE General Test or LSAT, official transcripts, 3 letters of recommendation, resume or curriculum vitae, statement of purpose. Additional exam requirements/recommendations for international students: Required—TOEFL (minimum score 600 paper-based; 96 iBT); Recommended—IELTS (minimum score 7). Electronic applications accepted. *Faculty research:* Applied ecology, bio-geochemistry, toxicology, wetlands ecology, environmental microbiology, forest ecology, environmental chemistry.

Indiana University–Purdue University Indianapolis, Indiana University School of Medicine, Department of Pharmacology and Toxicology, Indianapolis, IN 46202. Offers pharmacology (MS, PhD); toxicology (MS, PhD); MD/PhD. Terminal master's awarded for partial completion of doctoral program. *Degree requirements:* For master's, thesis; for doctorate, thesis/dissertation. *Entrance requirements:* For master's and doctorate, GRE General Test, GRE Subject Test, minimum GPA of 3.0. *Faculty research:* Neuropharmacology, cardiovascular biopharmacology, chemotherapy, oncogenesis.

Iowa State University of Science and Technology, Program in Toxicology, Ames, IA 50011. Offers MS, PhD. *Entrance requirements:* For master's and doctorate, GRE General Test. Additional exam requirements/recommendations for international students: Required—TOEFL (minimum score 550 paper-based; 79 iBT), IELTS (minimum score 6.5). Electronic applications accepted.

Johns Hopkins University, Bloomberg School of Public Health, Department of Environmental Health Sciences, Baltimore, MD 21218. Offers environmental health engineering (PhD); environmental health sciences (MHS, Dr PH); occupational and environmental health (PhD); physiology (PhD); toxicology (PhD). *Program availability:* Online learning. *Degree requirements:* For master's, essay, presentation; for doctorate, comprehensive exam, thesis/dissertation, 1-year full-time residency, oral and written exams. *Entrance requirements:* For master's, GRE General Test or MCAT, 3 letters of recommendation, transcripts; for doctorate, GRE General Test or MCAT, 3 letters of recommendation. Additional exam requirements/recommendations for international students: Required—TOEFL (minimum score 600 paper-based). Electronic applications accepted. *Faculty research:* Chemical carcinogenesis/toxicology, lung disease, occupational and environmental health, nuclear imaging, molecular epidemiology.

Long Island University–LIU Brooklyn, Arnold and Marie Schwartz College of Pharmacy and Health Sciences, Brooklyn, NY 11201-8423. Offers drug regulatory affairs (MS); pharmaceutics (MS, PhD), including cosmetic science (MS), industrial pharmacy (MS); pharmacology and toxicology (MS); pharmacy (Pharm D). *Accreditation:* ACPE. *Program availability:* Part-time. *Faculty:* 49 full-time (25 women), 20 part-time/adjunct (9 women). *Students:* 579 full-time (346 women), 29 part-time (14 women); includes 191 minority (24 Black or African American, non-Hispanic/Latino; 1 American Indian or Alaska Native, non-Hispanic/Latino; 144 Asian, non-Hispanic/Latino; 19 Hispanic/Latino; 3 Two or more races, non-Hispanic/Latino), 193 international. Average age 27. 350 applicants, 63% accepted, 65 enrolled. In 2015, 114 master's, 206 doctorates awarded. *Degree requirements:* For master's, comprehensive exam (for some programs), thesis optional; for doctorate, comprehensive exam, thesis/dissertation. *Entrance requirements:* For master's and doctorate, GRE, minimum GPA of 3.0. Additional exam requirements/recommendations for international students: Required—TOEFL (minimum score 550 paper-based; 79 iBT), IELTS (minimum score 6.5). *Application deadline:* Applications are processed on a rolling basis. Application fee: $50. Electronic applications accepted. *Expenses:* Contact institution. *Financial support:* In 2015–16, 185 students received support, including 6 fellowships with full tuition reimbursements available (averaging $12,800 per year), 28 teaching assistantships with full tuition reimbursements available (averaging $6,000 per year); Federal Work-Study, institutionally sponsored loans, and scholarships/grants also available. Support available to part-time students. Financial award application deadline: 2/15; financial award applicants required to submit FAFSA. *Faculty research:* Pharmaceutics, pharmacodynamics, pharmacology, pharmacometrics, pharmacotherapeutics. *Unit head:* Dr. John M. Pezzuto, Dean, 718-488-1004, Fax: 718-488-0628, E-mail: john.pezzuto@liu.edu. *Application contact:* Dr. Anait Levinsont, Associate Dean of Research and Graduate Studies, 718-246-6323, E-mail: anait.levenson@liu.edu. Website: http://liu.edu/Pharmacy

Louisiana State University and Agricultural & Mechanical College, Graduate School, School of the Coast and Environment, Department of Environmental Sciences, Baton Rouge, LA 70803. Offers environmental planning and management (MS); environmental science (PhD); environmental toxicology (MS).

Massachusetts Institute of Technology, School of Engineering, Department of Biological Engineering, Cambridge, MA 02139. Offers applied biosciences (PhD, Sc D); bioengineering (PhD, Sc D); biological engineering (PhD, Sc D); biomedical engineering (M Eng); toxicology (SM); SM/MBA. *Faculty:* 34 full-time (5 women). *Students:* 137 full-time (56 women); includes 49 minority (3 Black or African American, non-Hispanic/Latino; 35 Asian, non-Hispanic/Latino; 5 Hispanic/Latino; 6 Two or more races, non-Hispanic/Latino), 27 international. Average age 26. 470 applicants, 7% accepted, 18 enrolled. In 2015, 1 master's, 14 doctorates awarded. Terminal master's awarded for partial completion of doctoral program. *Degree requirements:* For master's, thesis; for doctorate, comprehensive exam, thesis/dissertation. *Entrance requirements:* For master's and doctorate, GRE General Test. Additional exam requirements/recommendations for international students: Required—IELTS (minimum score 7). *Application deadline:* For fall admission, 12/15 for domestic and international students. Application fee: $75. Electronic applications accepted. *Expenses: Tuition:* Full-time $46,400; part-time $725 per credit. One-time fee: $304 full-time. Full-time tuition and fees vary according to course load and program. *Financial support:* In 2015–16, 127 students received support, including 59 fellowships (averaging $42,700 per year), 74 research assistantships (averaging $39,700 per year), 2 teaching assistantships (averaging $38,300 per year); Federal Work-Study, institutionally sponsored loans,

Toxicology

scholarships/grants, traineeships, health care benefits, and unspecified assistantships also available. Support available to part-time students. Financial award application deadline: 4/15; financial award applicants required to submit FAFSA. *Faculty research:* Biomaterials; biophysics; cell and tissue engineering; computational modeling of biological and physiological systems; discovery and delivery of molecular therapeutics; new tools for genomics; functional genomics, proteomics and glycomics; macromolecular biochemistry and biophysics; molecular, cell and tissue biomechanics; synthetic biology; systems biology. *Total annual research expenditures:* $48.5 million. *Unit head:* Prof. Douglas A. Lauffenburger, Department Head, 617-452-4086. *Application contact:* Graduate Admissions, 617-253-1712, Fax: 617-253-5208, E-mail: be-acad@mit.edu.
Website: http://web.mit.edu/be/

Medical College of Wisconsin, Graduate School of Biomedical Sciences, Department of Pharmacology and Toxicology, Milwaukee, WI 53226-0509. Offers PhD, MD/PhD. *Degree requirements:* For doctorate, comprehensive exam, thesis/dissertation, oral and written qualifying exams. *Entrance requirements:* For doctorate, GRE, official transcripts, three letters of recommendation. Additional exam requirements/recommendations for international students: Required—TOEFL. Electronic applications accepted. *Faculty research:* Cardiovascular physiology and pharmacology, drugs of abuse, environmental and aquatic toxicology, central nervous system and biochemical pharmacology, signal transduction.

Medical University of South Carolina, College of Graduate Studies, Department of Pharmaceutical and Biomedical Sciences, Charleston, SC 29425. Offers cell injury and repair (PhD); drug discovery (PhD); medicinal chemistry (PhD); toxicology (PhD); DMD/PhD; MD/PhD; Pharm D/PhD. *Degree requirements:* For doctorate, thesis/dissertation, oral and written exams, teaching and research seminar. *Entrance requirements:* For doctorate, GRE General Test, interview, minimum GPA of 3.0. Additional exam requirements/recommendations for international students: Required—TOEFL (minimum score 600 paper-based; 100 iBT). Electronic applications accepted. *Faculty research:* Drug discovery, toxicology, metabolomics, cell stress and injury.

Michigan State University, College of Human Medicine and The Graduate School, Graduate Programs in Human Medicine, East Lansing, MI 48824. Offers biochemistry and molecular biology (MS, PhD); epidemiology (MS, PhD); microbiology (MS); microbiology and molecular genetics (PhD); pharmacology and toxicology (MS, PhD); physiology (MS, PhD); public health (MPH). *Entrance requirements:* Additional exam requirements/recommendations for international students: Required—TOEFL.

Michigan State University, College of Osteopathic Medicine and The Graduate School, Graduate Studies in Osteopathic Medicine and Graduate Programs in Human Medicine and Graduate Programs in Veterinary Medicine, Department of Pharmacology and Toxicology, East Lansing, MI 48824. Offers integrative pharmacology (MS); pharmacology and toxicology (MS, PhD); pharmacology and toxicology-environmental toxicology (PhD). *Entrance requirements:* Additional exam requirements/recommendations for international students: Required—TOEFL (minimum score 600 paper-based). Electronic applications accepted.

Michigan State University, College of Veterinary Medicine and The Graduate School, Graduate Programs in Veterinary Medicine, Center for Integrative Toxicology, East Lansing, MI 48824. Offers animal science–environmental toxicology (PhD); biochemistry and molecular biology–environmental toxicology (PhD); chemistry–environmental toxicology (PhD); crop and soil sciences–environmental toxicology (PhD); environmental engineering–environmental toxicology (PhD); environmental geosciences–environmental toxicology (PhD); fisheries and wildlife–environmental toxicology (PhD); food science–environmental toxicology (PhD); forestry–environmental toxicology (PhD); genetics–environmental toxicology (PhD); human nutrition–environmental toxicology (PhD); microbiology–environmental toxicology (PhD); pharmacology and toxicology–environmental toxicology (PhD); zoology–environmental toxicology (PhD). *Entrance requirements:* Additional exam requirements/recommendations for international students: Required—TOEFL (minimum score 550 paper-based), Michigan State University ELT (minimum score 85), Michigan English Language Assessment Battery (minimum score 83). Electronic applications accepted. *Faculty research:* Environmental risk assessment, toxicogenomics, phytoremediation, storage and disposal of hazardous waste, environmental regulation.

Michigan State University, College of Veterinary Medicine and The Graduate School, Graduate Programs in Veterinary Medicine and College of Natural Science and Graduate Programs in Human Medicine, Department of Microbiology and Molecular Genetics, East Lansing, MI 48824. Offers industrial microbiology (MS, PhD); microbiology (MS, PhD); microbiology and molecular genetics (MS, PhD); microbiology–environmental toxicology (PhD). *Entrance requirements:* For master's, GRE General Test. Additional exam requirements/recommendations for international students: Required—TOEFL (minimum score 550 paper-based), Michigan State University ELT (minimum score 85), Michigan English Language Assessment Battery (minimum score 83). Electronic applications accepted.

Michigan State University, The Graduate School, College of Agriculture and Natural Resources, Department of Animal Science, East Lansing, MI 48824. Offers animal science (MS, PhD); animal science-environmental toxicology (PhD). *Entrance requirements:* Additional exam requirements/recommendations for international students: Required—TOEFL (minimum score 550 paper-based), Michigan State University ELT (minimum score 85), Michigan English Language Assessment Battery (minimum score 83). Electronic applications accepted.

Michigan State University, The Graduate School, College of Agriculture and Natural Resources, Department of Crop and Soil Sciences, East Lansing, MI 48824. Offers crop and soil sciences (MS, PhD); crop and soil sciences-environmental toxicology (PhD); plant breeding and genetics-crop and soil sciences (MS); plant breeding, genetics and biotechnology-crop and soil sciences (PhD). *Entrance requirements:* Additional exam requirements/recommendations for international students: Required—TOEFL (minimum score 550 paper-based), Michigan State University ELT (minimum score 85), Michigan Michigan English Language Assessment Battery (minimum score 83). Electronic applications accepted.

Michigan State University, The Graduate School, College of Agriculture and Natural Resources and College of Natural Science, Department of Food Science and Human Nutrition, East Lansing, MI 48824. Offers food science (MS, PhD); food science - environmental toxicology (PhD); human nutrition (MS, PhD); human nutrition-onvironmental toxicology (PhD). *Entrance requirements:* Additional exam requirements/recommendations for international students: Required—TOEFL (minimum score 550 paper-based), Michigan State University ELT (minimum score 85), Michigan English Language Assessment Battery (minimum score 83). Electronic applications accepted.

Michigan State University, The Graduate School, College of Engineering, Department of Civil and Environmental Engineering, East Lansing, MI 48824. Offers civil engineering (MS, PhD); environmental engineering (MS, PhD); environmental engineering-environmental toxicology (PhD). *Program availability:* Part-time. *Entrance requirements:* Additional exam requirements/recommendations for international students: Required—TOEFL. Electronic applications accepted.

Michigan State University, The Graduate School, College of Natural Science and Graduate Programs in Human Medicine and Graduate Studies in Osteopathic Medicine, Department of Biochemistry and Molecular Biology, East Lansing, MI 48824. Offers biochemistry and molecular biology (MS, PhD); biochemistry and molecular biology/environmental toxicology (PhD). *Entrance requirements:* Additional exam requirements/recommendations for international students: Required—TOEFL. Electronic applications accepted.

Michigan State University, The Graduate School, College of Natural Science, Department of Chemistry, East Lansing, MI 48824. Offers chemical physics (PhD); chemistry (MS, PhD); chemistry-environmental toxicology (PhD); computational chemistry (MS). *Entrance requirements:* Additional exam requirements/recommendations for international students: Required—TOEFL. Electronic applications accepted. *Faculty research:* Analytical chemistry, inorganic and organic chemistry, nuclear chemistry, physical chemistry, theoretical and computational chemistry.

Michigan State University, The Graduate School, College of Natural Science, Department of Geological Sciences, East Lansing, MI 48824. Offers environmental geosciences (MS, PhD); environmental geosciences-environmental toxicology (PhD); geological sciences (MS, PhD). *Degree requirements:* For master's, thesis (for those without prior thesis work); for doctorate, thesis/dissertation. *Entrance requirements:* For master's, GRE General Test, minimum GPA of 3.0, course work in geoscience, 3 letters of recommendation; for doctorate, GRE General Test, 3 letters of recommendation. Additional exam requirements/recommendations for international students: Required—TOEFL (minimum score 550 paper-based), Michigan State University ELT (minimum score 85), Michigan English Language Assessment Battery (minimum score 83). Electronic applications accepted. *Faculty research:* Water in the environment, global and biological change, crystal dynamics.

Michigan State University, The Graduate School, College of Natural Science, Program in Genetics, East Lansing, MI 48824. Offers genetics (MS, PhD); genetics–environmental toxicology (PhD). *Entrance requirements:* Additional exam requirements/recommendations for international students: Required—TOEFL. Electronic applications accepted.

New York University, Graduate School of Arts and Science, Department of Environmental Medicine, New York, NY 10012-1019. Offers environmental health sciences (MS, PhD), including biostatistics (PhD), environmental hygiene (MS), epidemiology (PhD), ergonomics and biomechanics (PhD), exposure assessment and health effects (PhD), molecular toxicology/carcinogenesis (PhD), toxicology. *Program availability:* Part-time. Terminal master's awarded for partial completion of doctoral program. *Degree requirements:* For master's, thesis or alternative; for doctorate, one foreign language, thesis/dissertation, oral and written exams. *Entrance requirements:* For master's and doctorate, GRE General Test, minimum GPA of 3.0; bachelor's degree in biological, physical, or engineering science. Additional exam requirements/recommendations for international students: Required—TOEFL.

See Close-Up on page 851.

North Carolina State University, Graduate School, College of Agriculture and Life Sciences and College of Veterinary Medicine, Department of Environmental and Molecular Toxicology, Raleigh, NC 27695. Offers M Tox, MS, PhD. Terminal master's awarded for partial completion of doctoral program. *Degree requirements:* For master's, thesis (for some programs); for doctorate, thesis/dissertation. *Entrance requirements:* For master's and doctorate, GRE General Test, minimum GPA of 3.0. Electronic applications accepted. *Faculty research:* Chemical fate, carcinogenesis, developmental and endocrine toxicity, xenobiotic metabolism, signal transduction.

Oklahoma State University Center for Health Sciences, Graduate Program in Forensic Sciences, Tulsa, OK 74107-1898. Offers forensic sciences (MS), including arson and explosives investigation, forensic biology/DNA, forensic document examination, forensic pathology/death scene investigations, forensic psychology, forensic science administration, forensic toxicology/trace evidence. *Program availability:* Part-time, evening/weekend, 100% online, blended/hybrid learning. *Faculty:* 3 full-time (0 women), 15 part-time/adjunct (5 women). *Students:* 10 full-time (7 women), 51 part-time (13 women); includes 6 minority (2 American Indian or Alaska Native, non-Hispanic/Latino; 2 Hispanic/Latino; 1 Native Hawaiian or other Pacific Islander, non-Hispanic/Latino; 1 Two or more races, non-Hispanic/Latino). Average age 31. 63 applicants, 89% accepted, 49 enrolled. In 2015, 6 master's awarded. *Degree requirements:* For master's, comprehensive exam, thesis (for some programs), thesis or creative component. *Entrance requirements:* For master's, GRE (for thesis tracks); GRE or MAT (for options in arson and explosives investigation, forensic science administration, and forensic document examination), professional experience (for options in arson and explosives investigation, forensic science administration and forensic document examination). Additional exam requirements/recommendations for international students: Required—TOEFL (minimum score 100 iBT) or IELTS (minimum score 7.0). *Application deadline:* For fall admission, 3/1 priority date for domestic students, 3/1 for international students; for spring admission, 10/1 priority date for domestic students, 10/1 for international students; for summer admission, 7/1 priority date for domestic students, 7/1 for international students. Applications are processed on a rolling basis. Application fee: $50 ($75 for international students). Electronic applications accepted. *Financial support:* In 2015–16, 16 students received support, including 8 research assistantships (averaging $12,000 per year); career-related internships or fieldwork, Federal Work-Study, health care benefits, tuition waivers (partial), and unspecified assistantships also available. Financial award application deadline: 4/1; financial award applicants required to submit FAFSA. *Faculty research:* Studies on the variability in chromosomal DNA; development/enhancement of accessory methods useful for forensic DNA typing; forensic chemistry in the areas of controlled substances, explosives, and technology; research on explosives and IEDs (non-chemistry); therapeutic jurisprudence, issues involving inmates and their families, institutional stress suicide. *Total annual research expenditures:* $58,000. *Unit head:* Dr. Robert W. Allen, Director, 918-561-1292, Fax: 918-561-8794, E-mail: robert.w.allen@okstate.edu. *Application contact:* Cathy Newsome, Coordinator, 918-561-1108, Fax: 918-561-8414, E-mail: cathy.newsome@okstate.edu.
Website: http://www.healthsciences.okstate.edu/forensic/index.cfm

Oregon State University, College of Agricultural Sciences, Program in Toxicology, Corvallis, OR 97331. Offers M Ag, MS, PhD. *Faculty:* 12 full-time (4 women). *Students:* 25 full-time (13 women), 1 (woman) part-time; includes 4 minority (1 Asian, non-Hispanic/Latino; 1 Hispanic/Latino; 2 Two or more races, non-Hispanic/Latino), 1 international. Average age 26. 34 applicants, 24% accepted, 8 enrolled. In 2015, 2 doctorates awarded. *Degree requirements:* For master's, thesis; for doctorate, thesis/dissertation. *Entrance requirements:* For master's and doctorate, GRE, bachelor's degree in chemistry or biological sciences, minimum GPA of 3.0 in last 90 hours of course work. Additional exam requirements/recommendations for international students: Required—TOEFL (minimum score 80 iBT), IELTS (minimum score 6.5). *Application deadline:* For fall admission, 12/31 for domestic students. Application fee: $75 ($85 for international students). *Expenses:* Tuition, state resident: full-time $12,150; part-time $450 per credit. Tuition, nonresident: full-time $20,952; part-time $776 per credit. *Required fees:* $1572; $1443 per unit. One-time fee: $350. Tuition and fees vary

according to course load, campus/location and program. *Financial support:* Fellowships, research assistantships, Federal Work-Study, and institutionally sponsored loans available. Support available to part-time students. Financial award application deadline: 12/31. *Faculty research:* Biochemical mechanisms for toxicology; analytical, comparative, aquatic, and food toxicology; aquaculture of salmonids; immunotoxicology; fish toxicology. *Unit head:* Dr. Craig Marcus, Department Head, 541-737-1808, E-mail: craig.marcus@oregonstate.edu. *Application contact:* Mary Mucia, Toxicology Advisor, 541-737-9079, E-mail: mary.mucia@oregonstate.edu.
Website: http://emt.oregonstate.edu/prospectivegrads

Oregon State University, College of Pharmacy, Program in Pharmaceutical Sciences, Corvallis, OR 97331. Offers medicinal chemistry (MS, PhD); natural products chemistry (MS, PhD); pharmaceutics (MS, PhD); pharmacoeconomics (MS, PhD); pharmacokinetics (MS, PhD); pharmacology (MS, PhD); toxicology (MS, PhD). *Program availability:* Part-time. *Faculty:* 30 full-time (15 women). *Students:* 29 full-time (10 women); includes 2 minority (1 Asian, non-Hispanic/Latino; 1 Hispanic/Latino), 16 international. Average age 29. 79 applicants, 10% accepted, 5 enrolled. In 2015, 4 doctorates awarded. *Entrance requirements:* For master's and doctorate, GRE. Additional exam requirements/recommendations for international students: Required—TOEFL (minimum score 80 iBT), IELTS (minimum score 6.5). *Application deadline:* For fall admission, 1/1 for domestic students. Application fee: $75 ($85 for international students). *Expenses:* Tuition, state resident: full-time $12,150; part-time $450 per credit. Tuition, nonresident: full-time $20,952; part-time $776 per credit. *Required fees:* $1572; $1443 per unit. One-time fee: $350. Tuition and fees vary according to course load, campus/location and program. *Unit head:* Dr. Mark Zabriskie, Dean and Professor, 541-737-5781, E-mail: mark.zabriskie@oregonstate.edu. *Application contact:* Debra Peters, Pharmacy Advisor, 541-737-8743, E-mail: debra.peters@oregonstate.edu.
Website: http://pharmacy.oregonstate.edu/

Purdue University, Graduate School, College of Health and Human Sciences, School of Health Sciences, West Lafayette, IN 47907. Offers health physics (MS, PhD); medical physics (MS, PhD); occupational and environmental health science (MS, PhD), including aerosol deposition and lung disease, ergonomics, exposure and risk assessment, indoor air quality and bioaerosols (PhD), liver/lung toxicology; radiation biology (PhD); toxicology (PhD); MS/PhD. *Program availability:* Part-time. *Degree requirements:* For master's, thesis optional; for doctorate, one foreign language, thesis/dissertation. *Entrance requirements:* For master's and doctorate, GRE General Test, minimum undergraduate GPA of 3.0 or equivalent. Additional exam requirements/recommendations for international students: Required—TOEFL (minimum score 550 paper-based; 77 iBT); Recommended—TWE. Electronic applications accepted. *Faculty research:* Environmental toxicology, industrial hygiene, radiation dosimetry.

Queen's University at Kingston, School of Graduate Studies, Faculty of Health Sciences, Department of Pharmacology and Toxicology, Kingston, ON K7L 3N6, Canada. Offers M Sc, PhD. *Degree requirements:* For master's, thesis; for doctorate, comprehensive exam, thesis/dissertation. *Entrance requirements:* For master's, minimum 2nd class standing, honors bachelor of science degree (life sciences, health sciences, or equivalent); for doctorate, masters of science degree or outstanding performance in honors bachelor of science program. Additional exam requirements/recommendations for international students: Required—TOEFL (minimum score 600 paper-based). Electronic applications accepted. *Faculty research:* Biochemical toxicology, cardiovascular pharmacology and neuropharmacology.

Rutgers University–New Brunswick, Graduate School-New Brunswick, Department of Environmental Sciences, Piscataway, NJ 08854-8097. Offers air pollution and resources (MS, PhD); aquatic biology (MS, PhD); aquatic chemistry (MS, PhD); atmospheric science (MS, PhD); chemistry and physics of aerosol and hydrosol systems (MS, PhD); environmental chemistry (MS, PhD); environmental microbiology (MS, PhD); environmental toxicology (PhD); exposure assessment (PhD); fate and effects of pollutants (MS, PhD); pollution prevention and control (MS, PhD); water and wastewater treatment (MS, PhD); water resources (MS, PhD). Terminal master's awarded for partial completion of doctoral program. *Degree requirements:* For master's, comprehensive exam, thesis or alternative, oral final exam; for doctorate, comprehensive exam, thesis/dissertation, thesis defense, qualifying exam. *Entrance requirements:* For master's and doctorate, GRE General Test. Additional exam requirements/recommendations for international students: Required—TOEFL. Electronic applications accepted. *Faculty research:* Biological waste treatment; contaminant fate and transport; air, soil and water quality.

Rutgers University–New Brunswick, Graduate School-New Brunswick, Joint Program in Toxicology, Piscataway, NJ 08854-8097. Offers environmental toxicology (MS, PhD); industrial-occupational toxicology (MS, PhD); nutritional toxicology (MS, PhD); pharmaceutical toxicology (MS, PhD). MS, PhD offered jointly with University of Medicine and Dentistry of New Jersey. *Degree requirements:* For master's, thesis; for doctorate, comprehensive exam, thesis/dissertation, qualifying exams (written and oral). *Entrance requirements:* For master's and doctorate, GRE General Test. Additional exam requirements/recommendations for international students: Required—TOEFL. Electronic applications accepted. *Faculty research:* Neurotoxicants, immunotoxicology, carcinogenesis and chemoprevention, molecular toxicology, xenobiotic metabolism.

Rutgers University–New Brunswick, Graduate School of Biomedical Sciences, Piscataway, NJ 08854-5635. Offers biochemistry and molecular biology (MS, PhD); biomedical engineering (MS, PhD); biomedical science (MS); cellular and molecular pharmacology (MS, PhD); clinical and translational science (MS); environmental sciences/exposure assessment (PhD); molecular genetics, microbiology and immunology (MS, PhD); neuroscience (MS, PhD); physiology and integrative biology (MS, PhD); toxicology (MS, PhD); MD/PhD. Terminal master's awarded for partial completion of doctoral program. *Degree requirements:* For master's, thesis (for some programs), ethics training; for doctorate, comprehensive exam, thesis/dissertation, ethics training. *Entrance requirements:* For master's, GRE General Test, MCAT, DAT; for doctorate, GRE General Test. Additional exam requirements/recommendations for international students: Required—TOEFL. Electronic applications accepted.

St. John's University, College of Pharmacy and Health Sciences, Graduate Programs in Pharmaceutical Sciences, Program in Toxicology, Queens, NY 11439. Offers MS. *Program availability:* Part-time, evening/weekend. *Degree requirements:* For master's, comprehensive exam, thesis optional, one-year residency. *Entrance requirements:* For master's, GRE General Test, minimum GPA of 3.0, 2 letters of recommendation, bachelor's degree in related area. Additional exam requirements/recommendations for international students: Required—TOEFL (minimum score 600 paper-based; 100 iBT), IELTS (minimum score 7). Electronic applications accepted. *Expenses:* Contact institution. *Faculty research:* Neurotoxicology, renal toxicology, toxicology of metals, regulatory toxicology.

San Diego State University, Graduate and Research Affairs, College of Health and Human Services, Graduate School of Public Health, San Diego, CA 92182. Offers environmental health (MPH); epidemiology (MPH, PhD), including biostatistics (MPH); global emergency preparedness and response (MS); global health (PhD); health behavior (PhD); health promotion (MPH); health services administration (MPH); toxicology (MS); MPH/MA; MSW/MPH. *Accreditation:* CAHME (one or more programs

are accredited); CEPH (one or more programs are accredited). *Program availability:* Part-time. *Degree requirements:* For master's, comprehensive exam (for some programs), thesis (for some programs); for doctorate, thesis/dissertation. *Entrance requirements:* For master's, GMAT (MPH in health services administration), GRE General Test; for doctorate, GRE General Test. Additional exam requirements/recommendations for international students: Required—TOEFL. *Faculty research:* Evaluation of tobacco, AIDS prevalence and prevention, mammography, infant death project, Alzheimer's in elderly Chinese.

Simon Fraser University, Office of Graduate Studies, Faculty of Science, Department of Biological Sciences, Burnaby, BC V5A 1S6, Canada. Offers bioinformatics (Graduate Diploma); biological sciences (M Sc, PhD); environmental toxicology (MET); pest management (MPM). *Degree requirements:* For master's, thesis; for doctorate, thesis/dissertation, candidacy exam; for Graduate Diploma, practicum. *Entrance requirements:* For master's, minimum GPA of 3.0 (on scale of 4.33), or 3.33 based on last 60 credits of undergraduate courses; for doctorate, minimum GPA of 3.5 (on scale of 4.33); for Graduate Diploma, minimum GPA of 2.5 (on scale of 4.33), or 2.67 based on the last 60 credits of undergraduate courses. Additional exam requirements/recommendations for international students: Recommended—TOEFL (minimum score 580 paper-based; 93 iBT), IELTS (minimum score 7), TWE (minimum score 5). Electronic applications accepted. *Faculty research:* Cell biology, wildlife ecology, environmental and evolutionary physiology, environmental toxicology, pest management.

Syracuse University, College of Arts and Sciences, Programs in Forensic Science, Syracuse, NY 13244. Offers firearm and tool mark examination (CAS); forensic science (MS), including advanced, biology, biomedical forensic sciences, crime scene investigation, forensic anthropology, general, impressions evidence, jurisprudence, linguistics, medicolegal death investigation, national security science, nuclear forensics, psychiatry and behavioral science, regulatory science, toxicology; medicolegal death investigation (CAS); MS/JD. *Program availability:* Part-time. *Students:* Average age 25. In 2015, 15 master's awarded. *Degree requirements:* For master's, internship. *Entrance requirements:* For master's, GRE General Test, personal statement, three letters of recommendation, transcripts, telephone interview. Additional exam requirements/recommendations for international students: Required—TOEFL (minimum score 100 iBT). *Application deadline:* For fall admission, 2/15 priority date for domestic and international students; for summer admission, 2/15 for domestic students, 2/16 priority date for international students. Applications are processed on a rolling basis. Application fee: $75. Electronic applications accepted. *Expenses: Tuition, area resident:* Full-time $25,974; part-time $1443 per credit hour. *Required fees:* $802; $50 per course. Tuition and fees vary according to course load and program. *Financial support:* Fellowships with full tuition reimbursements, research assistantships, teaching assistantships, and scholarships/grants available. Financial award application deadline: 1/1; financial award applicants required to submit FAFSA. *Faculty research:* Chemical analysis, molecular genetics, forensic biochemical analysis, forensic entomology, human osteology. *Unit head:* Dr. Michael M. Sponsler, Director of Curricular Programs for the Forensic and National Security Sciences Institute, 315-443-4347, E-mail: sponsler@syr.edu. *Application contact:* Cassidy Perreault, Administrative Specialist, 315-443-2875, E-mail: forensics@syr.edu.
Website: http://forensics.syr.edu/index.html

Texas Southern University, School of Science and Technology, Program in Environmental Toxicology, Houston, TX 77004-4584. Offers MS, PhD. *Program availability:* Part-time. *Degree requirements:* For master's, thesis; for doctorate, thesis/dissertation. *Entrance requirements:* For master's, minimum GPA of 2.75; for doctorate, GRE, minimum GPA of 2.75. Electronic applications accepted. *Expenses:* Contact institution. *Faculty research:* Air quality, water quality, soil remediation, computer modeling.

Texas Tech University, Graduate School, College of Arts and Sciences, Department of Environmental Toxicology, Lubbock, TX 79409. Offers MS, PhD, JD/MS, MBA/MS. *Program availability:* Part-time. *Faculty:* 12 full-time (2 women). *Students:* 37 full-time (23 women), 1 (woman) part-time; includes 8 minority (3 Black or African American, non-Hispanic/Latino; 2 Hispanic/Latino; 3 Two or more races, non-Hispanic/Latino), 10 international. Average age 30. 32 applicants, 53% accepted, 11 enrolled. In 2015, 10 master's, 7 doctorates awarded. Terminal master's awarded for partial completion of doctoral program. *Degree requirements:* For master's, thesis; for doctorate, comprehensive exam, thesis/dissertation. *Entrance requirements:* For master's and doctorate, GRE. Additional exam requirements/recommendations for international students: Required—TOEFL (minimum score 550 paper-based; 79 iBT); Recommended—IELTS (minimum score 6.5), TSE (minimum score 60). *Application deadline:* For fall admission, 6/1 priority date for domestic students, 1/15 priority date for international students; for spring admission, 9/1 priority date for domestic students, 6/15 priority date for international students. Applications are processed on a rolling basis. Application fee: $60. Electronic applications accepted. *Expenses:* Tuition, state resident: full-time $6477; part-time $269.89 per credit hour. Tuition, nonresident: full-time $15,837; part-time $659.89 per credit hour. *Required fees:* $2751; $36.50 per credit hour. $937.50 per semester. Tuition and fees vary according to course level. *Financial support:* In 2015–16, 49 students received support, including 40 fellowships (averaging $2,617 per year), 48 research assistantships (averaging $12,456 per year), 2 teaching assistantships (averaging $13,050 per year); Federal Work-Study, institutionally sponsored loans, scholarships/grants, and health care benefits also available. Financial award application deadline: 4/15; financial award applicants required to submit FAFSA. *Faculty research:* Wildlife toxicology; molecular epidemiology and genomics; endangered species toxicology; reproductive, molecular, and developmental toxicology; environmental chemistry. *Total annual research expenditures:* $1.4 million. *Unit head:* Dr. Todd Anderson, Chair, 806-834-1587, Fax: 806-885-2132, E-mail: todd.anderson@ttu.edu. *Application contact:* Dr. Jaclyn Canas-Carrell, Graduate Officer, 806-834-6217, E-mail: jaclyn.e.canas@ttu.edu.
Website: http://www.tiehh.ttu.edu/

Thomas Jefferson University, Jefferson College of Biomedical Sciences, MS Program in Forensic Toxicology, Philadelphia, PA 19107. Offers MS. *Program availability:* Part-time, evening/weekend. *Students:* 4 part-time (2 women); includes 1 minority (Hispanic/Latino). Average age 27. 8 applicants, 75% accepted, 5 enrolled. *Degree requirements:* For master's, thesis, clerkship. *Entrance requirements:* For master's, GRE General Test or MCAT, minimum GPA of 3.0. Additional exam requirements/recommendations for international students: Required—TOEFL, IELTS (minimum score 7). *Application deadline:* For fall admission, 8/1 priority date for domestic students, 3/1 priority date for international students. Applications are processed on a rolling basis. Application fee: $50. Electronic applications accepted. *Financial support:* Federal Work-Study and institutionally sponsored loans available. Support available to part-time students. Financial award application deadline: 5/1; financial award applicants required to submit FAFSA. *Unit head:* Marc E. Stearns, Director of Admissions, 215-503-0155, Fax: 215-503-3433, E-mail: jgsbs-info@jefferson.edu. *Application contact:* Marc E. Stearns, Director of Admissions, 215-503-0155, Fax: 215-503-3433, E-mail: jgsbs-info@jefferson.edu.
Website: http://www.jefferson.edu/university/biomedical-sciences/degrees-programs/master-programs/forensic-toxicology.html

Toxicology

Université de Montréal, Faculty of Medicine, Program in Toxicology and Risk Analysis, Montréal, QC H3C 3J7, Canada. Offers DESS. Electronic applications accepted.

University at Albany, State University of New York, School of Public Health, Department of Environmental Health Sciences, Albany, NY 12222-0001. Offers environmental and occupational health (MS, PhD); environmental chemistry (MS, PhD); toxicology (MS, PhD). *Degree requirements:* For master's, thesis; for doctorate, comprehensive exam, thesis/dissertation. *Entrance requirements:* For master's and doctorate, GRE General Test, GRE Subject Test, 3 letters of reference. Additional exam requirements/recommendations for international students: Required—TOEFL (minimum score 600 paper-based). Electronic applications accepted. *Faculty research:* Xenobiotic metabolism, neurotoxicity of halogenated hydrocarbons, pharmac/toxicogenomics, environmental analytical chemistry.

University at Buffalo, the State University of New York, Graduate School, School of Medicine and Biomedical Sciences, Graduate Programs in Medicine and Biomedical Sciences, Department of Pharmacology and Toxicology, Buffalo, NY 14221. Offers pharmacology (MS, PhD); MD/PhD. *Faculty:* 21 full-time (3 women). *Students:* 25 full-time (14 women); includes 9 minority (3 Black or African American, non-Hispanic/Latino; 1 American Indian or Alaska Native, non-Hispanic/Latino; 2 Asian, non-Hispanic/Latino; 3 Hispanic/Latino), 5 international. Average age 25. 67 applicants, 24% accepted, 10 enrolled. In 2015, 11 master's, 5 doctorates awarded. Terminal master's awarded for partial completion of doctoral program. *Degree requirements:* For master's, thesis; for doctorate, thesis/dissertation. *Entrance requirements:* For master's and doctorate, GRE General Test, 3 letters of recommendation. Additional exam requirements/ recommendations for international students: Required—TOEFL (minimum score 79 iBT). *Application deadline:* For fall admission, 2/14 priority date for domestic and international students. Applications are processed on a rolling basis. Application fee: $85. Electronic applications accepted. *Financial support:* In 2015–16, 3 students received support, including 19 research assistantships with full tuition reimbursements available (averaging $27,000 per year); fellowships, teaching assistantships, Federal Work-Study, scholarships/grants, health care benefits, and unspecified assistantships also available. Financial award application deadline: 2/14; financial award applicants required to submit FAFSA. *Faculty research:* Neuropharmacology, toxicology, signal transduction, molecular pharmacology, behavioral pharmacology. *Total annual research expenditures:* $9.4 million. *Unit head:* Dr. Margarita L. Dubocovich, Professor/Chair, 716-829-3048, Fax: 716-829-2801, E-mail: mdubo@buffalo.edu. *Application contact:* Linda M. LeRoy, Admissions Assistant, 716-829-2800, Fax: 716-829-2801, E-mail: pmygrad@buffalo.edu.
Website: http://medicine.buffalo.edu/pharmtox

The University of Alabama at Birmingham, Graduate Programs in Joint Health Sciences, Program in Pharmacology and Toxicology, Birmingham, AL 35294. Offers PhD. *Degree requirements:* For doctorate, thesis/dissertation. *Entrance requirements:* For doctorate, GRE General Test; GRE Subject Test (recommended), interview. Additional exam requirements/recommendations for international students: Required— TOEFL, TWE. Electronic applications accepted. *Expenses:* Contact institution. *Faculty research:* Anticancer and antiviral chemotherapy, with emphasis on drugs used in the management of AIDS and related opportunistic infections; metabolism and biliary excretion of drugs (and metabolites) as well as the mechanisms of drug toxicity.

The University of Alabama at Birmingham, School of Public Health, Program in Public Health, Birmingham, AL 35294. Offers applied epidemiology (MSPH); pharmacoepidemiology (MSPH); biostatistics (MPH); clinical and translational science (MSPH); environmental health (MPH); environmental health and toxicology (MSPH); epidemiology (MPH); general theory and practice (MPH); health behavior (MPH); health care organization (MPH); health policy quantitative policy analysis (MPH); industrial hygiene (MPH, MSPH); maternal and child health policy (Dr PH); maternal and child health policy and leadership (MPH); occupational health and safety (MPH); outcomes research (MSPH, Dr PH); public health (PhD); public health management (Dr PH); public health preparedness management (MPH). *Accreditation:* CEPH. *Program availability:* Part-time, online learning. *Degree requirements:* For doctorate, comprehensive exam, thesis/dissertation. *Entrance requirements:* For master's and doctorate, GRE. Additional exam requirements/recommendations for international students: Recommended—TOEFL (minimum score 550 paper-based; 79 iBT), IELTS (minimum score 6.5). Electronic applications accepted. *Expenses:* Tuition, state resident: full-time $7340. Tuition, nonresident: full-time $16,628. Full-time tuition and fees vary according to course load and program.

University of Arkansas for Medical Sciences, Graduate School, Little Rock, AR 72205. Offers biochemistry and molecular biology (MS, PhD); bioinformatics (MS, PhD); cellular physiology and molecular biophysics (MS, PhD); clinical nutrition (MS); interdisciplinary biomedical sciences (MS, PhD, Certificate); interdisciplinary toxicology (MS); microbiology and immunology (PhD); neurobiology and developmental sciences (PhD); pharmacology (PhD); MD/PhD. Bioinformatics programs hosted jointly with the University of Arkansas at Little Rock. *Program availability:* Part-time. Terminal master's awarded for partial completion of doctoral program. *Degree requirements:* For master's, comprehensive exam (for some programs), thesis (for some programs); for doctorate, thesis/dissertation. *Entrance requirements:* For master's and doctorate, GRE. Additional exam requirements/recommendations for international students: Required—TOEFL. Electronic applications accepted. *Expenses:* Contact institution.

University of California, Davis, Graduate Studies, Graduate Group in Pharmacology and Toxicology, Davis, CA 95616. Offers MS, PhD. Terminal master's awarded for partial completion of doctoral program. *Degree requirements:* For master's, comprehensive exam or thesis; for doctorate, thesis/dissertation, qualifying exam. *Entrance requirements:* For master's and doctorate, GRE General Test, minimum GPA of 3.0, course work in biochemistry and/or physiology. Additional exam requirements/ recommendations for international students: Required—TOEFL (minimum score 550 paper-based). Electronic applications accepted. *Faculty research:* Respiratory, neurochemical, molecular, genetic, and ecological toxicology.

University of California, Irvine, School of Medicine, Program in Environmental Health Sciences, Irvine, CA 92697. Offers environmental health sciences (MS); environmental toxicology (PhD); exposure sciences and risk assessment (PhD). *Students:* 11 full-time (6 women); includes 2 minority (1 Asian, non-Hispanic/Latino; 1 Two or more races, non-Hispanic/Latino), 1 international. Average age 32. 15 applicants, 40% accepted, 5 enrolled. In 2015, 1 master's awarded. Terminal master's awarded for partial completion of doctoral program. *Degree requirements:* For master's, comprehensive exam; for doctorate, comprehensive exam, thesis/dissertation. *Entrance requirements:* For master's and doctorate, GRE General Test, GRE Subject Test, minimum GPA of 3.0. Additional exam requirements/recommendations for international students: Required— TOEFL (minimum score 550 paper-based). *Application deadline:* For fall admission, 1/ 15 for domestic students. Applications are processed on a rolling basis. Application fee: $90 ($110 for international students). Electronic applications accepted. *Financial support:* Fellowships, research assistantships with full tuition reimbursements, teaching assistantships, institutionally sponsored loans, traineeships, health care benefits, and unspecified assistantships available. Financial award application deadline: 2/1; financial award applicants required to submit FAFSA. *Faculty research:* Inhalation/ pulmonary toxicology, environmental carcinogenesis, biochemical neurotoxicology,

toxicokinetics, chemical pathology. *Unit head:* Dr. Ulrike Luderer, Director, 949-824-8848, E-mail: uluderer@uci.edu. *Application contact:* Armando Villalpando, Student Affairs Officer, 949-824-8848, E-mail: afvillal@uci.edu.
Website: http://www.medicine.uci.edu/occupational/graduate.asp

University of California, Los Angeles, Graduate Division, College of Letters and Science and David Geffen School of Medicine, UCLA ACCESS to Programs in the Molecular, Cellular and Integrative Life Sciences, Los Angeles, CA 90095. Offers biochemistry and molecular biology (PhD); biological chemistry (PhD); cellular and molecular pathology (PhD); human genetics (PhD); microbiology, immunology, and molecular genetics (PhD); molecular biology (PhD); molecular toxicology (PhD); molecular, cellular and integrative physiology (PhD); neurobiology (PhD); oral biology (PhD); physiology (PhD). *Degree requirements:* For doctorate, thesis/dissertation, oral and written qualifying exams. *Entrance requirements:* For doctorate, GRE General Test, bachelor's degree; minimum undergraduate GPA of 3.0 (or its equivalent if letter grade system not used). Additional exam requirements/recommendations for international students: Required—TOEFL. Electronic applications accepted.

University of California, Riverside, Graduate Division, Program in Environmental Toxicology, Riverside, CA 92521-0102. Offers MS, PhD. Terminal master's awarded for partial completion of doctoral program. *Degree requirements:* For master's, thesis; for doctorate, comprehensive exam, thesis/dissertation, preliminary written exam, oral qualifying exam. *Entrance requirements:* For master's and doctorate, GRE General Test, minimum GPA of 3.25. Additional exam requirements/recommendations for international students: Required—TOEFL (minimum score 550 paper-based; 80 iBT). *Application deadline:* For fall admission, 1/5 priority date for domestic students, 1/5 for international students; for winter admission, 12/1 for domestic students, 7/1 for international students; for spring admission, 3/1 for domestic students, 10/1 for international students. Application fee: $80 ($100 for international students). Electronic applications accepted. *Expenses: Tuition, area resident:* Full-time $16,665.50; part-time $11,055.54. Tuition, state resident: full-time $16,665.50; part-time $11,055.54. Tuition, nonresident: full-time $31,768. *International tuition:* $31,767.50 full-time. *Required fees:* $16,665.50; $11,055.54 per quarter. $3685.18 per quarter. Tuition and fees vary according to program. *Financial support:* Fellowships with full tuition reimbursements, research assistantships with full tuition reimbursements, teaching assistantships with full tuition reimbursements, career-related internships or fieldwork, institutionally sponsored loans, scholarships/grants, health care benefits, and unspecified assistantships available. Financial award application deadline: 1/5; financial award applicants required to submit FAFSA. *Faculty research:* Cellular/molecular toxicology, atmospheric chemistry, bioremediation, carcinogenesis, mechanism of toxicity.
Website: http://www.etox.ucr.edu/

University of California, Santa Cruz, Division of Graduate Studies, Division of Physical and Biological Sciences, Environmental Toxicology Department, Santa Cruz, CA 95064. Offers MS, PhD. Terminal master's awarded for partial completion of doctoral program. *Degree requirements:* For master's, comprehensive exam, thesis; for doctorate, thesis/ dissertation, qualifying exams. *Entrance requirements:* For master's and doctorate, GRE. Additional exam requirements/recommendations for international students: Required—TOEFL (minimum score 550 paper-based; 83 iBT); Recommended—IELTS (minimum score 8). Electronic applications accepted. *Faculty research:* Molecular mechanisms of reactive DNA methylation toxicity, anthropogenic perturbations of biogeochemical cycles, anaerobic microbiology and biotransformation of pollutants and toxic metals, organismal responses and therapeutic treatment of toxins, microbiology, molecular genetics, genomics.

University of Colorado Denver, School of Pharmacy, Program in Toxicology, Aurora, CO 80045. Offers PhD. *Students:* 21 full-time (12 women); includes 5 minority (1 Black or African American, non-Hispanic/Latino; 1 Asian, non-Hispanic/Latino; 3 Hispanic/ Latino), 9 international. Average age 28. 14 applicants, 21% accepted, 3 enrolled. In 2015, 2 doctorates awarded. *Degree requirements:* For doctorate, comprehensive exam, thesis/dissertation, 60 credit hours (30 in upper-level course work and 30 in thesis research hours). *Entrance requirements:* For doctorate, GRE, minimum undergraduate GPA of 3.0; prior coursework in general chemistry, organic chemistry, calculus, biology, and physics. Additional exam requirements/recommendations for international students: Required—TOEFL (minimum score 550 paper-based; 80 iBT). *Application deadline:* For fall admission, 1/15 for domestic students, 12/15 for international students. Application fee: $50 ($75 for international students). Electronic applications accepted. *Expenses:* Contact institution. *Financial support:* In 2015–16, 19 students received support. Fellowships, research assistantships, teaching assistantships, Federal Work-Study, institutionally sponsored loans, scholarships/grants, traineeships, and unspecified assistantships available. Financial award application deadline: 3/15; financial award applicants required to submit FAFSA. *Faculty research:* Regulation of apoptotic cell death; cancer chemoprevention; innate immunity and hepatotoxicity; role of chronic inflammation in cancer; Parkinson's disease, epilepsy and oxidative stress. *Unit head:* Dr. David Ross, Chair/Professor of Toxicology, 303-724-7265, Fax: 303-724-7266, E-mail: david.ross@ucdenver.edu. *Application contact:* Jackie Milowski, Information Contact, 303-724-7263, E-mail: jackie.milowski@ucdenver.edu.
Website: http://www.ucdenver.edu/academics/colleges/pharmacy/AcademicPrograms/PhDPrograms/PhDToxicology/Pages/PhDToxicology.aspx

University of Connecticut, Graduate School, School of Pharmacy, Department of Pharmaceutical Sciences, Graduate Program in Pharmacology and Toxicology, Storrs, CT 06269. Offers pharmacology (MS, PhD); toxicology (MS, PhD). Terminal master's awarded for partial completion of doctoral program. *Degree requirements:* For master's, comprehensive exam, thesis; for doctorate, thesis/dissertation. *Entrance requirements:* For master's and doctorate, GRE General Test. Additional exam requirements/ recommendations for international students: Required—TOEFL (minimum score 550 paper-based). *Application deadline:* For fall admission, 2/1 priority date for domestic and international students; for spring admission, 11/1 for domestic students, 10/1 for international students. Applications are processed on a rolling basis. Application fee: $55. Electronic applications accepted. *Financial support:* Fellowships, research assistantships with full tuition reimbursements, teaching assistantships with full tuition reimbursements, career-related internships or fieldwork, Federal Work-Study, scholarships/grants, traineeships, health care benefits, and unspecified assistantships available. Financial award application deadline: 2/1; financial award applicants required to submit FAFSA.
Website: http://www.pharmacy.uconn.edu/

University of Florida, College of Veterinary Medicine, Graduate Program in Veterinary Medical Sciences, Gainesville, FL 32611. Offers forensic toxicology (Certificate); veterinary medical sciences (MS, PhD), including forensic toxicology (MS). *Program availability:* Online learning. Terminal master's awarded for partial completion of doctoral program. *Degree requirements:* For master's, thesis; for doctorate, thesis/dissertation. *Entrance requirements:* For master's and doctorate, GRE General Test, minimum GPA of 3.0. Additional exam requirements/recommendations for international students: Required—TOEFL (minimum score 550 paper-based). Electronic applications accepted. *Expenses:* Contact institution.

University of Florida, Graduate School, College of Pharmacy, Programs in Forensic Science, Gainesville, FL 32611. Offers clinical toxicology (Certificate); drug chemistry

(Certificate); environmental forensics (Certificate); forensic death investigation (Certificate); forensic DNA and serology (MSP, Certificate); forensic drug chemistry (MSP); forensic science (MSP); forensic toxicology (Certificate). *Program availability:* Part-time, evening/weekend, online learning. *Degree requirements:* For master's, comprehensive exam. *Entrance requirements:* For master's, GRE General Test, minimum GPA of 3.0. Additional exam requirements/recommendations for international students: Required—TOEFL (minimum score 550 paper-based; 80 iBT), IELTS (minimum score 6).

University of Guelph, Graduate Studies, Ontario Agricultural College, Department of Environmental Biology, Guelph, ON N1G 2W1, Canada. Offers entomology (M Sc, PhD); environmental microbiology and biotechnology (M Sc, PhD); environmental toxicology (M Sc, PhD); plant and forest systems (M Sc, PhD); plant pathology (M Sc, PhD). *Program availability:* Part-time. *Degree requirements:* For master's, thesis; for doctorate, comprehensive exam, thesis/dissertation. *Entrance requirements:* For master's, minimum 75% average during previous 2 years of course work; for doctorate, minimum 75% average. Additional exam requirements/recommendations for international students: Required—TOEFL or IELTS. Electronic applications accepted. *Faculty research:* Entomology, environmental microbiology and biotechnology, environmental toxicology, forest ecology, plant pathology.

University of Guelph, Ontario Veterinary College and Graduate Studies, Graduate Programs in Veterinary Sciences, Department of Biomedical Sciences, Guelph, ON N1G 2W1, Canada. Offers morphology (M Sc, DV Sc, PhD); neuroscience (M Sc, DV Sc, PhD); pharmacology (M Sc, DV Sc, PhD); physiology (M Sc, DV Sc, PhD); toxicology (M Sc, DV Sc, PhD). *Program availability:* Part-time. *Degree requirements:* For master's, thesis; for doctorate, comprehensive exam, thesis/dissertation. *Entrance requirements:* For master's, honors B Sc, minimum 75% average in last 20 courses; for doctorate, M Sc with thesis from accredited institution. Additional exam requirements/ recommendations for international students: Required—TOEFL (minimum score 550 paper-based; 89 iBT). Electronic applications accepted. *Faculty research:* Cellular morphology; endocrine, vascular and reproductive physiology; clinical pharmacology; veterinary toxicology; developmental biology, neuroscience.

University of Guelph, Ontario Veterinary College, Interdepartmental Program in Toxicology, Guelph, ON N1G 2W1, Canada. Offers M Sc, PhD. *Program availability:* Part-time. *Degree requirements:* For master's, thesis (for some programs); for doctorate, comprehensive exam, thesis/dissertation. *Entrance requirements:* For master's, B Sc; for doctorate, M Sc. Additional exam requirements/recommendations for international students: Required—TOEFL (minimum score 550 paper-based; 89 iBT).

University of Illinois at Chicago, College of Pharmacy and Graduate College, Graduate Programs in Pharmacy, Program in Forensic Science, Chicago, IL 60607-7128. Offers MS. *Faculty:* 15 full-time (4 women), 10 part-time/adjunct (2 women). *Students:* 5 full-time (all women); includes 1 minority (Hispanic/Latino). Average age 30. *Degree requirements:* For master's, thesis. *Entrance requirements:* For master's, GRE General Test. Additional exam requirements/recommendations for international students: Required—TOEFL. *Application deadline:* For fall admission, 1/1 for domestic students, 2/15 for international students. Application fee: $60. *Expenses:* Tuition, state resident: full-time $11,480; part-time $3826 per credit. Tuition, nonresident: full-time $23,720; part-time $7906 per credit. *Required fees:* $1333 per semester. Part-time tuition and fees vary according to course load and program. *Financial support:* Fellowships with full tuition reimbursements, research assistantships with full tuition reimbursements, teaching assistantships with full tuition reimbursements, career-related internships or fieldwork, Federal Work-Study, institutionally sponsored loans, and tuition waivers (full) available. Financial award application deadline: 2/1; financial award applicants required to submit FAFSA. *Faculty research:* Interpretation of physical evidence, utilization of physical evidence, analytical toxicology of controlled substances, automated fingerprint systems, dye and ink characterizations. *Unit head:* Prof. Albert Karl Larsen, Director, Forensic Science Graduate Studies, 312-996-2250, E-mail: forensicdgs@uic.edu. *Application contact:* Jackie Perry, Graduate College Receptionist, 312-413-2550, Fax: 312-413-0185, E-mail: gradcoll@uic.edu.
Website: http://www.uic.edu/pharmacy/depts/Forensic_Science/

The University of Iowa, Graduate College, Program in Human Toxicology, Iowa City, IA 52242-1316. Offers MS, PhD. *Degree requirements:* For master's, thesis; for doctorate, comprehensive exam, thesis/dissertation. *Entrance requirements:* For master's and doctorate, GRE General Test, minimum GPA of 3.0. Additional exam requirements/recommendations for international students: Required—TOEFL (minimum score 600 paper-based; 100 iBT). Electronic applications accepted.

The University of Kansas, Graduate Studies, School of Pharmacy, Department of Pharmacology and Toxicology, Program in Pharmacology and Toxicology, Lawrence, KS 66045. Offers MS, PhD. *Students:* 23 full-time (15 women); includes 1 minority (Asian, non-Hispanic/Latino), 15 international. Average age 25. 53 applicants, 17% accepted, 6 enrolled. In 2015, 2 doctorates awarded. Terminal master's awarded for partial completion of doctoral program. *Entrance requirements:* For master's, GRE, bachelor's degree in related field, 3 letters of recommendation, resume or curriculum vitae, official transcripts, 1-2 page personal statement; for doctorate, GRE (minimum score: 600 verbal, 600 quantitative, 4.5 analytical), bachelor's degree in related field, 3 letters of recommendation, resume or curriculum vitae, official transcripts, 1-2 page personal statement. Additional exam requirements/recommendations for international students: Required—TOEFL (minimum score 600 paper-based; 100 iBT). *Application deadline:* For fall admission, 1/15 for domestic students, 2/1 for international students. Application fee: $65 ($85 for international students). Electronic applications accepted. *Financial support:* Fellowships and research assistantships available. Financial award application deadline: 2/1. *Faculty research:* Neurodegeneration, diabetes, neurological disorders, neuropharmacology, drug metabolism. *Unit head:* Nancy Muma, Chair, 785-864-4002, Fax: 785-864-5219, E-mail: nmuma@ku.edu. *Application contact:* Sheila Stice, Graduate Admissions Contact, 785-864-4002, E-mail: sstice@ku.edu.
Website: http://www.pharmtox.pharm.ku.edu

The University of Kansas, University of Kansas Medical Center, School of Medicine, Department of Pharmacology, Toxicology and Therapeutics, Kansas City, KS 66160. Offers pharmacology (PhD); toxicology (PhD); MD/PhD. *Faculty:* 18. *Students:* 24 full-time (12 women); includes 2 minority (1 Black or African American, non-Hispanic/Latino; 1 Two or more races, non-Hispanic/Latino), 17 international. Average age 29. In 2015, 7 doctorates awarded. Terminal master's awarded for partial completion of doctoral program. *Degree requirements:* For doctorate, one foreign language, comprehensive exam, thesis/dissertation. *Entrance requirements:* For doctorate, GRE General Test. Additional exam requirements/recommendations for international students: Required—TOEFL. *Application deadline:* For fall admission, 12/1 priority date for domestic and international students. Applications are processed on a rolling basis. Application fee: $60. Electronic applications accepted. Application fee is waived when completed online. *Financial support:* Fellowships with full tuition reimbursements, research assistantships with full tuition reimbursements, teaching assistantships with full tuition reimbursements, Federal Work-Study, scholarships/grants, traineeships, and unspecified assistantships available. Support available to part-time students. Financial award application deadline: 3/1; financial award applicants required to submit FAFSA. *Faculty research:* Liver

nuclear receptors, hepatobiliary transporters, pharmacogenomics, estrogen-induced carcinogenesis, neuropharmacology of pain and depression. *Total annual research expenditures:* $5.5 million. *Unit head:* Dr. Hartmut Jaeschke, Professor and Chair, 913-588-7500, Fax: 913-588-7501, E-mail: hjaeschke@kumc.edu. *Application contact:* Dr. Bruno Hagenbuch, Chair, Departmental Graduate Committee, 913-588-7500, Fax: 913-588-7501, E-mail: bhagenbuch@kumc.edu.
Website: http://www.kumc.edu/school-of-medicine/pharmacology-toxicology-and-therapeutics.html

University of Kentucky, Graduate School, Graduate School Programs from the College of Medicine, Program in Toxicology, Lexington, KY 40506-0032. Offers MS, PhD. Terminal master's awarded for partial completion of doctoral program. *Degree requirements:* For master's, comprehensive exam, thesis optional; for doctorate, comprehensive exam, thesis/dissertation. *Entrance requirements:* For master's, GRE General Test, minimum undergraduate GPA of 2.75; for doctorate, GRE General Test, minimum graduate GPA of 3.0. Additional exam requirements/recommendations for international students: Required—TOEFL (minimum score 550 paper-based). Electronic applications accepted. *Faculty research:* Chemical carcinogenesis, immunotoxicology, neurotoxicology, metabolism and disposition, gene regulation.

University of Louisiana at Monroe, Graduate School, College of Health and Pharmaceutical Sciences, School of Pharmacy, Monroe, LA 71209-0001. Offers pharmacy (PhD, Pharm D); toxicology (PhD). *Accreditation:* ACPE. *Degree requirements:* For doctorate, comprehensive exam, thesis/dissertation. *Entrance requirements:* For doctorate, GRE General Test, minimum undergraduate GPA of 2.5. Additional exam requirements/recommendations for international students: Required—TOEFL (minimum score 500 paper-based; 61 iBT). Electronic applications accepted.

University of Louisville, School of Medicine, Department of Pharmacology and Toxicology, Louisville, KY 40292-0001. Offers MS, PhD, MD/PhD. *Students:* 43 full-time (21 women), 5 part-time (all women); includes 5 minority (3 Black or African American, non-Hispanic/Latino; 1 Asian, non-Hispanic/Latino; 1 Two or more races, non-Hispanic/Latino), 12 international. Average age 28. 49 applicants, 27% accepted, 13 enrolled. In 2015, 1 master's awarded. Terminal master's awarded for partial completion of doctoral program. *Degree requirements:* For master's, thesis; for doctorate, comprehensive exam, thesis/dissertation. *Entrance requirements:* For master's and doctorate, GRE General Test (minimum score of 1000 verbal and quantitative), minimum GPA of 3.0. Additional exam requirements/recommendations for international students: Required—TOEFL. *Application deadline:* For fall admission, 1/15 priority date for domestic and international students. Applications are processed on a rolling basis. Application fee: $60. Electronic applications accepted. *Expenses:* Tuition, state resident: full-time $11,664; part-time $649 per credit hour. Tuition, nonresident: full-time $24,274; part-time $1350 per credit hour. *Required fees:* $196. Tuition and fees vary according to program and reciprocity agreements. *Financial support:* In 2015–16, 394,161 students received support. Fellowships with full tuition reimbursements available and research assistantships with full tuition reimbursements available available. Financial award application deadline: 4/15. *Faculty research:* Molecular pharmacogenetics; epidemiology; functional genomics; genetic predisposition to chemical carcinogenesis and drug toxicity; mechanisms of oxidative stress; alcohol-induced hepatitis, pancreatitis, and hepatocellular carcinoma; molecular and cardiac toxicology; molecular biology and genetics of DNA damage and repair in humans; mechanisms of chemo resistance; arsenic toxicity and cell cycle disruption; molecular pharmacology of novel G protein-coupled receptors. *Total annual research expenditures:* $3.5 million. *Unit head:* Dr. David W. Hein, Chair, 502-852-5141, Fax: 502-852-7868, E-mail: dhein@louisville.edu. *Application contact:* Heddy R. Rubin, Information Contact, 502-852-5741, Fax: 502-852-7868, E-mail: hrrubi01@gwise.louisville.edu.
Website: http://louisville.edu/medicine/departments/pharmacology

The University of Manchester, Faculty of Life Sciences, Manchester, United Kingdom. Offers adaptive organismal biology (M Phil, PhD); animal biology (M Phil, PhD); biochemistry (M Phil, PhD); bioinformatics (M Phil, PhD); biomolecular sciences (M Phil, PhD); biotechnology (M Phil, PhD); cell biology (M Phil, PhD); cell matrix research (M Phil, PhD); channels and transporters (M Phil, PhD); developmental biology (M Phil, PhD); Egyptology (M Phil, PhD); environmental biology (M Phil, PhD); evolutionary biology (M Phil, PhD); gene expression (M Phil, PhD); genetics (M Phil, PhD); history of science, technology and medicine (M Phil, PhD); immunology (M Phil, PhD); integrative neurobiology and behavior (M Phil, PhD); membrane trafficking (M Phil, PhD); microbiology (M Phil, PhD); molecular and cellular neuroscience (M Phil, PhD); molecular biology (M Phil, PhD); molecular cancer studies (M Phil, PhD); neuroscience (M Phil, PhD); ophthalmology (M Phil, PhD); optometry (M Phil, PhD); organelle function (M Phil, PhD); pharmacology (M Phil, PhD); physiology (M Phil, PhD); plant sciences (M Phil, PhD); stem cell research (M Phil, PhD); structural biology (M Phil, PhD); systems neuroscience (M Phil, PhD); toxicology (M Phil, PhD).

University of Maryland, Baltimore, Graduate School, Graduate Program in Life Sciences, Program in Toxicology, Baltimore, MD 21201. Offers MS, PhD, MD/MS, MD/PhD. *Program availability:* Part-time. *Degree requirements:* For doctorate, comprehensive exam, thesis/dissertation. *Entrance requirements:* For master's and doctorate, GRE General Test, GRE Subject Test, minimum GPA of 3.0. Additional exam requirements/recommendations for international students: Required—TOEFL (minimum score 550 paper-based; 80 iBT); Recommended—IELTS (minimum score 7). Electronic applications accepted. Tuition and fees vary according to program.

University of Maryland, Baltimore, School of Medicine, Department of Epidemiology and Public Health, Baltimore, MD 21201. Offers biostatistics (MS); clinical research (MS); epidemiology and preventive medicine (MPH, MS, PhD); gerontology (PhD); human genetics and genomic medicine (MS, PhD); molecular epidemiology (MS, PhD); toxicology (MS, PhD); JD/MS; MD/PhD; MS/PhD. *Accreditation:* CEPH. *Program availability:* Part-time. *Students:* 73 full-time (58 women), 56 part-time (32 women); includes 45 minority (23 Black or African American, non-Hispanic/Latino; 12 Asian, non-Hispanic/Latino; 5 Hispanic/Latino; 5 Two or more races, non-Hispanic/Latino), 17 international. Average age 31. In 2015, 34 master's, 17 doctorates awarded. *Degree requirements:* For doctorate, comprehensive exam, thesis/dissertation. *Entrance requirements:* For master's and doctorate, GRE General Test. Additional exam requirements/recommendations for international students: Required—TOEFL (minimum score 550 paper-based; 80 iBT); Recommended—IELTS (minimum score 7). *Application deadline:* For fall admission, 1/15 for domestic and international students. Application fee: $75. Electronic applications accepted. *Expenses:* Contact institution. *Financial support:* In 2015–16, research assistantships with partial tuition reimbursements (averaging $26,000 per year) were awarded; fellowships, Federal Work-Study, scholarships/grants, and unspecified assistantships also available. Financial award application deadline: 3/1; financial award applicants required to submit FAFSA. *Unit head:* Dr. Laura Hungerford, Program Director, 410-706-8492, Fax: 410-706-4225. *Application contact:* Jessica Kelley, Program Coordinator, 410-706-8492, Fax: 410-706-4225, E-mail: jkelley@som.umaryland.edu.
Website: http://lifesciences.umaryland.edu/epidemiology/

University of Maryland Eastern Shore, Graduate Programs, Department of Natural Sciences, Program in Toxicology, Princess Anne, MD 21853-1299. Offers MS, PhD.

Toxicology

University of Michigan, School of Public Health, Department of Environmental Health Sciences, Ann Arbor, MI 48109. Offers environmental health sciences (MS, PhD); environmental quality and health (MPH); industrial hygiene (MPH, MS); occupational and environmental epidemiology (MPH); toxicology (MPH, MS, PhD). *Accreditation:* CEPH (one or more programs are accredited). *Program availability:* Part-time. *Faculty:* 22 full-time (7 women), 28 part-time/adjunct (9 women). *Students:* 76 full-time (53 women), 3 part-time (all women); includes 13 minority (4 Black or African American, non-Hispanic/Latino; 5 Asian, non-Hispanic/Latino; 2 Hispanic/Latino; 2 Two or more races, non-Hispanic/Latino; 12 international. Average age 27. 263 applicants, 39% accepted, 39 enrolled. In 2015, 50 master's, 8 doctorates awarded. Terminal master's awarded for partial completion of doctoral program. *Degree requirements:* For master's, thesis (for some programs); for doctorate, thesis/dissertation, preliminary exam, oral defense of dissertation. *Entrance requirements:* For master's and doctorate, GRE General Test and/or MCAT. Additional exam requirements/recommendations for international students: Required—TOEFL (minimum score 100 iBT). *Application deadline:* For fall admission, 12/15 priority date for domestic students, 1/15 for international students. Applications are processed on a rolling basis. Application fee: $75. Electronic applications accepted. *Financial support:* Fellowships, research assistantships, teaching assistantships, career-related internships or fieldwork, Federal Work-Study, institutionally sponsored loans, scholarships/grants, traineeships, health care benefits, and unspecified assistantships available. Financial award application deadline: 12/15. *Faculty research:* Toxicology, occupational hygiene, environmental exposure sciences, environmental epidemiology. *Unit head:* Dr. Craig Harris, Chair, 734-939-3397, E-mail: charris@umich.edu. *Application contact:* Susan Crawford, Student Administrative Coordinator, 734-764-3018, E-mail: sph.inquiries@umich.edu. Website: http://www.sph.umich.edu/ehs/

University of Minnesota, Duluth, Graduate School, Program in Toxicology, Duluth, MN 55812-2496. Offers MS, PhD. MS, PhD offered jointly with University of Minnesota, Twin Cities Campus. Terminal master's awarded for partial completion of doctoral program. *Degree requirements:* For master's, thesis; for doctorate, comprehensive exam, thesis/dissertation, written and oral preliminary and final exams. *Entrance requirements:* For master's and doctorate, GRE General Test, BS in basic science; full year each of biology, chemistry, and physics; mathematics coursework through calculus. Additional exam requirements/recommendations for international students: Required—TOEFL (minimum score 550 paper-based; 79 iBT). Electronic applications accepted. *Faculty research:* Structure activity correlations, neurotoxicity, aquatic toxicology, biochemical mechanisms, immunotoxicology.

University of Minnesota, Duluth, Medical School, Department of Biochemistry, Molecular Biology and Biophysics, Duluth, MN 55812-2496. Offers biochemistry, molecular biology and biophysics (MS); biology and biophysics (PhD); social, administrative, and clinical pharmacy (MS, PhD); toxicology (MS, PhD). Terminal master's awarded for partial completion of doctoral program. *Degree requirements:* For master's, comprehensive exam, thesis; for doctorate, comprehensive exam, thesis/dissertation. *Entrance requirements:* For master's and doctorate, GRE General Test. Additional exam requirements/recommendations for international students: Required—TOEFL. Electronic applications accepted. *Faculty research:* Intestinal cancer biology; hepatotoxins and mitochondriopathies; toxicology; cell cycle regulation in stem cells; neurobiology of brain development, trace metal function and blood-brain barrier; hibernation biology.

University of Minnesota, Twin Cities Campus, School of Public Health, Division of Environmental Health Sciences, Area in Environmental Toxicology, Minneapolis, MN 55455-0213. Offers MPH, MS, PhD. *Degree requirements:* For doctorate, thesis/dissertation. *Entrance requirements:* For master's and doctorate, GRE General Test. Electronic applications accepted.

University of Mississippi Medical Center, School of Graduate Studies in the Health Sciences, Department of Pharmacology and Toxicology, Jackson, MS 39216-4505. Offers PhD. *Degree requirements:* For doctorate, comprehensive exam, thesis/dissertation, first authored publication. *Entrance requirements:* For doctorate, GRE General Test, minimum GPA of 3.0. Additional exam requirements/recommendations for international students: Required—TOEFL (minimum score 550 paper-based, 79 iBT), IELTS or PTE. Electronic applications accepted. *Faculty research:* Renal and cardiovascular pharmacology, genetic basis of cardio-renal diseases, diabetes, obesity, metabolic diseases, cancer chemotherapy.

University of Missouri–Kansas City, School of Pharmacy, Kansas City, MO 64110-2499. Offers pharmaceutical sciences (PhD); pharmacology and toxicology (PhD); pharmacy (Pharm D). PhD offered through School of Graduate Studies. *Accreditation:* ACPE (one or more programs are accredited). *Program availability:* Online learning. *Faculty:* 49 full-time (26 women), 6 part-time/adjunct (2 women). *Students:* 447 full-time (276 women); includes 103 minority (24 Black or African American, non-Hispanic/Latino; 1 American Indian or Alaska Native, non-Hispanic/Latino; 53 Asian, non-Hispanic/Latino; 12 Hispanic/Latino; 13 Two or more races, non-Hispanic/Latino), 2 international. Average age 25. 414 applicants, 33% accepted, 133 enrolled. In 2015, 125 doctorates awarded. *Degree requirements:* For doctorate, comprehensive exam (for some programs), thesis/dissertation (for some programs). *Entrance requirements:* For doctorate, PCAT (for Pharm D). Additional exam requirements/recommendations for international students: Required—TOEFL (minimum score 550 paper-based; 80 iBT). *Application deadline:* For fall admission, 3/1 for domestic and international students. Applications are processed on a rolling basis. Application fee: $45 ($50 for international students). Electronic applications accepted. *Expenses:* Contact institution. *Financial support:* In 2015–16, 4 fellowships (averaging $40,082 per year), 14 research assistantships with tuition reimbursements (averaging $13,117 per year), 26 teaching assistantships with full tuition reimbursements (averaging $14,724 per year) were awarded; career-related internships or fieldwork, Federal Work-Study, institutionally sponsored loans, tuition waivers (full and partial), and unspecified assistantships also available. Financial award application deadline: 3/1; financial award applicants required to submit FAFSA. *Faculty research:* Bio-organic and medicinal chemistry, drug delivery, pharmaceutics, molecular neurobiology, neurology. *Unit head:* Dr. Russell B. Melchert, Dean, 816-235-1609, Fax: 816-235-5190, E-mail: melchertr@umkc.edu. *Application contact:* Shelly M. Janasz, Director, Student Services, 816-235-2400, Fax: 816-235-5190, E-mail: janaszs@umkc.edu. Website: http://pharmacy.umkc.edu/

University of Montana, Graduate School, College of Health Professions and Biomedical Sciences, Skaggs School of Pharmacy, Department of Biomedical and Pharmaceutical Sciences, Missoula, MT 59812-0002. Offers biomedical sciences (PhD); medicinal chemistry (MS, PhD); molecular and cellular toxicology (MS, PhD); neuroscience (PhD); pharmaceutical sciences (MS). *Accreditation:* ACPE. *Degree requirements:* For master's, oral defense of thesis; for doctorate, research dissertation defense. *Entrance requirements:* For master's and doctorate, GRE General Test. Additional exam requirements/recommendations for international students: Required—TOEFL (minimum score 540 paper-based). Electronic applications accepted. *Faculty research:* Cardiovascular pharmacology, medicinal chemistry, neurosciences, environmental toxicology, pharmacogenetics, cancer.

University of Nebraska–Lincoln, Graduate College, Interdepartmental Area of Environmental Health, Occupational Health and Toxicology, Lincoln, NE 68588. Offers MS, PhD. MS, PhD offered jointly with University of Nebraska Medical Center. *Entrance requirements:* Additional exam requirements/recommendations for international students: Required—TOEFL (minimum score 550 paper-based). Electronic applications accepted.

University of Nebraska Medical Center, Program in Environmental Health, Occupational Health and Toxicology, Omaha, NE 68198. Offers PhD. *Faculty:* 9 full-time (1 woman). *Students:* 4 full-time (1 woman), 2 part-time (1 woman); includes 1 minority (Asian, non-Hispanic/Latino), 2 international. Average age 40. 7 applicants, 57% accepted, 4 enrolled. In 2015, 3 doctorates awarded. *Degree requirements:* For doctorate, comprehensive exam (for some programs), thesis/dissertation. *Entrance requirements:* For doctorate, GRE General Test, BS in chemistry, biology, biochemistry or related area. Additional exam requirements/recommendations for international students: Required—TOEFL (minimum score 550 paper-based; 80 iBT). *Application deadline:* For fall admission, 4/1 for domestic and international students; for spring admission, 8/1 for domestic and international students; for summer admission, 1/1 for domestic and international students. Applications are processed on a rolling basis. Application fee: $45. Electronic applications accepted. *Expenses:* Tuition, state resident: full-time $7830; part-time $3915 per credit hour. Tuition, nonresident: full-time $22,410; part-time $11,205 per credit hour. *Required fees:* $521. *Financial support:* In 2015–16, fellowships with full tuition reimbursements (averaging $23,100 per year), 1 research assistantship with full tuition reimbursement (averaging $23,100 per year) was awarded; teaching assistantships and scholarships/grants also available. Support available to part-time students. Financial award application deadline: 2/15; financial award applicants required to submit FAFSA. *Faculty research:* Mechanisms of carcinogenesis, alcohol and metal toxicity, DNA damage, human molecular genetics, agrochemicals in soil and water. *Unit head:* Dr. Chandran Achutan, Associate Professor, 402-559-8599, E-mail: cachutan@unmc.edu. *Application contact:* Sherry Cherek, Coordinator, 402-559-8924, Fax: 402-559-8068, E-mail: scherek@unmc.edu. Website: http://www.unmc.edu/publichealth/programs/phdprograms/phdenviromental.html

University of New Mexico, Graduate Studies, Health Sciences Center, Program in Biomedical Sciences, Albuquerque, NM 87131-5196. Offers biochemistry and molecular biology (MS, PhD); cell biology and physiology (MS, PhD); molecular genetics and microbiology (MS, PhD); neuroscience (MS, PhD); pathology (MS, PhD); toxicology (MS, PhD). *Program availability:* Part-time. *Faculty:* 18 full-time (10 women), 1 part-time/adjunct (1 woman). *Students:* 31 full-time (17 women), 45 part-time (26 women); includes 29 minority (1 American Indian or Alaska Native, non-Hispanic/Latino; 3 Asian, non-Hispanic/Latino; 22 Hispanic/Latino; 2 Native Hawaiian or other Pacific Islander, non-Hispanic/Latino; 1 Two or more races, non-Hispanic/Latino), 18 international. Average age 30. 98 applicants, 11% accepted, 11 enrolled. In 2015, 11 master's, 14 doctorates awarded. Terminal master's awarded for partial completion of doctoral program. *Degree requirements:* For master's, thesis; for doctorate, comprehensive exam, thesis/dissertation, qualifying exam at the end of year 1/core curriculum. *Entrance requirements:* For master's and doctorate, GRE General Test, minimum undergraduate GPA of 3.0. Additional exam requirements/recommendations for international students: Required—TOEFL. *Application deadline:* For fall admission, 3/1 priority date for domestic and international students. Applications are processed on a rolling basis. Application fee: $50. Electronic applications accepted. *Financial support:* Fellowships with tuition reimbursements, research assistantships with full tuition reimbursements, teaching assistantships, career-related internships or fieldwork, Federal Work-Study, institutionally sponsored loans, scholarships/grants, traineeships, health care benefits, and unspecified assistantships available. Financial award application deadline: 1/1; financial award applicants required to submit FAFSA. *Faculty research:* Infectious disease/immunity, cancer biology, cardiovascular and metabolic diseases, brain and behavioral illness, environmental health. *Unit head:* Dr. Helen J. Hathaway, Program Director, 505-272-1887, Fax: 505-272-2412, E-mail: hhathaway@salud.unm.edu. *Application contact:* Mary Fenton, Admissions Coordinator, 505-272-1887, Fax: 505-272-2412, E-mail: mfenton@salud.unm.edu.

The University of North Carolina at Chapel Hill, School of Medicine, Curriculum in Toxicology, Chapel Hill, NC 27599. Offers MS, PhD. Terminal master's awarded for partial completion of doctoral program. *Degree requirements:* For master's, comprehensive exam, thesis; for doctorate, comprehensive exam, thesis/dissertation. *Entrance requirements:* For doctorate, GRE General Test. Electronic applications accepted. *Faculty research:* Molecular and cellular toxicology, carcinogenesis, neurotoxicology, pulmonary toxicology, developmental toxicology.

University of Prince Edward Island, Atlantic Veterinary College, Graduate Program in Veterinary Medicine, Charlottetown, PE C1A 4P3, Canada. Offers anatomy (M Sc, PhD); bacteriology (M Sc, PhD); clinical pharmacology (M Sc, PhD); clinical sciences (M Sc, PhD); epidemiology (M Sc, PhD), including reproduction; fish health (M Sc, PhD); food animal nutrition (M Sc, PhD); immunology (M Sc, PhD); microanatomy (M Sc, PhD); parasitology (M Sc, PhD); pathology (M Sc, PhD); pharmacology (M Sc, PhD); physiology (M Sc, PhD); toxicology (M Sc, PhD); veterinary science (M Vet Sc); virology (M Sc, PhD). *Program availability:* Part-time. *Degree requirements:* For master's, thesis; for doctorate, thesis/dissertation. *Entrance requirements:* For master's, DVM, B Sc honors degree, or equivalent; for doctorate, M Sc. Additional exam requirements/recommendations for international students: Required—TOEFL (minimum score 550 paper-based; 80 iBT). *Expenses:* Contact institution. *Faculty research:* Animal health management, infectious diseases, fin fish and shellfish health, basic biomedical sciences, ecosystem health.

University of Puerto Rico, Medical Sciences Campus, School of Medicine, Biomedical Sciences Graduate Program, Department of Pharmacology and Toxicology, San Juan, PR 00936-5067. Offers MS, PhD. *Degree requirements:* For master's, one foreign language, thesis; for doctorate, one foreign language, comprehensive exam, thesis/dissertation. *Entrance requirements:* For master's and doctorate, GRE General Test, GRE Subject Test, interview, minimum GPA of 3.0, 3 letters of recommendation. Electronic applications accepted. *Faculty research:* Cardiovascular, central nervous system, and endocrine pharmacology; anti-cancer drugs; sodium pump; mitochondrial DNA repair; Huntington's disease.

University of Rhode Island, Graduate School, College of Pharmacy, Department of Biomedical and Pharmaceutical Sciences, Kingston, RI 02881. Offers medicinal chemistry and pharmacognosy (MS, PhD); pharmaceutics and pharmacokinetics (MS, PhD); pharmacology and toxicology (MS, PhD). *Program availability:* Part-time. *Faculty:* 15 full-time (4 women), 4 part-time/adjunct (2 women). *Students:* 39 full-time (14 women), 10 part-time (3 women); includes 3 minority (1 Black or African American, non-Hispanic/Latino; 2 Asian, non-Hispanic/Latino), 24 international. In 2015, 4 master's, 10 doctorates awarded. *Entrance requirements:* For master's and doctorate, GRE (minimum old/new format scores: Verbal 350/143; Quantitative 550/146; Analytical 3.0), 2 letters of recommendation. Additional exam requirements/recommendations for international students: Required—TOEFL (minimum score 550 paper-based). *Application deadline:* For fall admission, 7/15 for domestic students, 2/1 for international students. Application fee: $65. Electronic applications accepted. *Expenses:* Tuition,

state resident: full-time $11,796; part-time $655 per credit. Tuition, nonresident: full-time $24,206; part-time $1345 per credit. *Required fees:* $1546; $44 per credit. One-time fee: $155 full-time; $35 part-time. *Financial support:* In 2015–16, 6 research assistantships with tuition reimbursements (averaging $14,828 per year), 18 teaching assistantships with tuition reimbursements (averaging $14,851 per year) were awarded. Financial award application deadline: 2/1; financial award applicants required to submit FAFSA. *Faculty research:* Chemical carcinogenesis with a major emphasis on the structural and synthetic aspects of DNA-adduct formation, drug-drug/herb interaction, drug-genetic interaction, signaling of nuclear receptors, transcriptional regulation, oncogenesis. *Total annual research expenditures:* $5.8 million. *Unit head:* Dr. Bingfang Yan, Chair, 401-874-5032, Fax: 401-874-2181, E-mail: byan@uri.edu. *Application contact:* Graduate Admissions, 401-874-2872, E-mail: gradadm@etal.uri.edu.
Website: http://www.uri.edu/pharmacy/departments/bps/index.shtml

University of Rochester, School of Medicine and Dentistry, Graduate Programs in Medicine and Dentistry, Department of Environmental Medicine, Programs in Toxicology, Rochester, NY 14627. Offers PhD. *Degree requirements:* For doctorate, thesis/dissertation, qualifying exam. *Entrance requirements:* For doctorate, GRE General Test. *Expenses: Tuition, area resident:* Full-time $47,450; part-time $1482 per credit hour. *Required fees:* $528. Tuition and fees vary according to program.

University of Saskatchewan, College of Graduate Studies and Research, Toxicology Centre, Saskatoon, SK S7N 5A2, Canada. Offers M Sc, PhD, Diploma. *Degree requirements:* For master's, thesis; for doctorate, thesis/dissertation. *Entrance requirements:* Additional exam requirements/recommendations for international students: Required—TOEFL.

University of South Alabama, Graduate School, Program in Environmental Toxicology, Mobile, AL 36688. Offers MS. *Faculty:* 1 full-time (0 women). *Students:* 5 full-time (4 women), 4 part-time (3 women); includes 2 minority (both Black or African American, non-Hispanic/Latino). Average age 26. 12 applicants, 25% accepted, 2 enrolled. In 2015, 5 master's awarded. *Degree requirements:* For master's, comprehensive exam, research project or thesis. *Entrance requirements:* For master's, GRE, BA/BS in related discipline, minimum undergraduate GPA of 3.0. Additional exam requirements/recommendations for international students: Required—TOEFL (minimum score 525 paper-based; 71 iBT). *Application deadline:* For fall admission, 7/15 for domestic students, 6/15 for international students; for spring admission, 12/1 for domestic students, 11/1 for international students. Application fee: $35. Electronic applications accepted. *Expenses: Tuition, state resident:* full-time $9480; part-time $395 per credit hour. Tuition, nonresident: full-time $18,960; part-time $790 per credit hour. *Financial support:* Fellowships, research assistantships, teaching assistantships, career-related internships or fieldwork, Federal Work-Study, institutionally sponsored loans, scholarships/grants, and unspecified assistantships available. Support available to part-time students. Financial award application deadline: 5/31; financial award applicants required to submit FAFSA. *Unit head:* Dr. B. Keith Harrison, Dean and Senior Vice President for Academic Affairs, 251-460-6310, E-mail: gradschool@southalabam.edu. *Application contact:* Dr. David Forbes, Chair, Chemistry, 251-460-6181, E-mail: dforbes@southalabama.edu.
Website: http://www.southalabama.edu/graduatemajors/etox/index.html

University of Southern California, Graduate School, School of Pharmacy, Graduate Programs in Molecular Pharmacology and Toxicology, Los Angeles, CA 90033. Offers pharmacology and pharmaceutical sciences (MS, PhD). Terminal master's awarded for partial completion of doctoral program. *Degree requirements:* For master's, comprehensive exam, thesis, 24 units of formal course work, excluding research and seminar courses; for doctorate, comprehensive exam, thesis/dissertation, 24 units of formal course work, excluding research and seminar courses. *Entrance requirements:* For master's and doctorate, GRE. Additional exam requirements/recommendations for international students: Required—TOEFL (minimum score 603 paper-based; 100 iBT). Electronic applications accepted. *Expenses:* Contact institution. *Faculty research:* Degenerative diseases, toxicology of drugs.

The University of Texas at Austin, Graduate School, College of Pharmacy, Graduate Programs in Pharmacy, Austin, TX 78712-1111. Offers health outcomes and pharmacy practice (PhD); health outcomes and pharmacy practice (MS); medicinal chemistry (PhD); pharmaceutics (PhD); pharmacology and toxicology (PhD); pharmacotherapy (MS, PhD); translational science (PhD). PhD in translational science offered jointly with The University of Texas Health Science Center at San Antonio and The University of Texas at San Antonio. *Degree requirements:* For master's, thesis; for doctorate, thesis/dissertation. *Entrance requirements:* For master's and doctorate, GRE General Test. Electronic applications accepted. *Faculty research:* Synthetic medical chemistry, synthetic molecular biology, bio-organic chemistry, pharmacoeconomics, pharmacy practice.

The University of Texas Health Science Center at San Antonio, Graduate School of Biomedical Sciences, Program in Toxicology, San Antonio, TX 78229-3900. Offers MS.

The University of Texas Medical Branch, Graduate School of Biomedical Sciences, Program in Pharmacology and Toxicology, Galveston, TX 77555. Offers pharmacology (MS); pharmacology and toxicology (PhD). *Degree requirements:* For master's, thesis or alternative; for doctorate, thesis/dissertation. *Entrance requirements:* For master's and doctorate, GRE General Test. Additional exam requirements/recommendations for international students: Required—TOEFL (minimum score 550 paper-based).

University of the Sciences, Program in Pharmacology and Toxicology, Philadelphia, PA 19104-4495. Offers pharmacology (MS, PhD); toxicology (MS, PhD). Terminal master's awarded for partial completion of doctoral program. *Degree requirements:* For master's, thesis; for doctorate, comprehensive exam, thesis/dissertation. *Entrance requirements:* For master's and doctorate, GRE General Test. Additional exam requirements/recommendations for international students: Required—TOEFL, TWE. *Application deadline:* For fall admission, 5/1 for international students; for winter admission, 10/1 for international students; for spring admission, 3/1 for international students. Applications are processed on a rolling basis. Application fee: $50. *Expenses:* Contact institution. *Financial support:* Teaching assistantships with tuition reimbursements, institutionally sponsored loans, and tuition waivers (partial) available. Financial award application deadline: 5/1. *Unit head:* Dr. Bin Chen, Director, 215-596-7481, E-mail: b.chen@usciences.edu. *Application contact:* Dr. Bin Chen, Director, 215-596-7481, E-mail: b.chen@usciences.edu.

University of Utah, Graduate School, College of Pharmacy, Department of Pharmacology and Toxicology, Salt Lake City, UT 84112. Offers PhD. *Faculty:* 16 full-time (5 women), 11 part-time/adjunct (4 women). *Students:* 9 full-time (5 women), 3 international. Average age 29. In 2015, 1 doctorate awarded. Terminal master's awarded for partial completion of doctoral program. *Degree requirements:* For doctorate, comprehensive exam, thesis/dissertation, final exam. *Entrance requirements:* For doctorate, GRE General Test, BS in biology, chemistry, or neuroscience. *Application deadline:* For fall admission, 12/15 for domestic and international students. Application fee: $0. Electronic applications accepted. *Expenses:* $1,356.08 per credit hour. *Financial support:* In 2015–16, 9 students received support, including 9 research assistantships with full tuition reimbursements available (averaging $25,000 per year); health care benefits and tuition waivers (full) also available. Financial award application

deadline: 1/15. *Faculty research:* Neuropharmacology of anti-seizure drugs and drugs of abuse, drug metabolism, signal transduction pathways and oncogenic processes, drug analyses in biological samples, natural products drug discovery. *Unit head:* Dr. Karen Wilcox, Department Chair, 801-581-6287, Fax: 801-585-5111, E-mail: karen.wilcox@hsc.utah.edu. *Application contact:* Linda Wright, Program Assistant, 801-581-6281, Fax: 801-585-5111, E-mail: linda.wright@utah.edu.
Website: http://www.pharmacy.utah.edu/pharmtox/

University of Washington, Graduate School, School of Public Health, Department of Environmental and Occupational Health Sciences, Seattle, WA 98195. Offers environmental and occupational health (MPH); environmental and occupational hygiene (PhD); environmental health (MS); occupational and environmental exposure sciences (MS); occupational and environmental medicine (MPH); toxicology (MS, PhD); MPH/MPA; MS/MPA. *Program availability:* Part-time. Terminal master's awarded for partial completion of doctoral program. *Degree requirements:* For master's, comprehensive exam, thesis (for some programs), project or thesis; for doctorate, comprehensive exam, thesis/dissertation. *Entrance requirements:* For master's, GRE General Test, one year each of physics, general chemistry, and biology; two quarters of organic chemistry; one quarter of calculus; for doctorate, GRE General Test, minimum GPA of 3.0, prerequisite course work in biology, chemistry, physics, calculus. Additional exam requirements/recommendations for international students: Required—TOEFL (minimum score 580 paper-based; 92 iBT). Electronic applications accepted. *Expenses:* Contact institution. *Faculty research:* Developmental and behavioral toxicology, biochemical toxicology, exposure assessment, hazardous waste, industrial chemistry.

University of Wisconsin–Madison, School of Medicine and Public Health, Molecular and Environmental Toxicology Graduate Program, Madison, WI 53706. Offers MS, PhD. Terminal master's awarded for partial completion of doctoral program. *Expenses:* Tuition, state resident: full-time $5564. Tuition, nonresident: full-time $12,027. *Required fees:* $571. Tuition and fees vary according to campus/location, program and reciprocity agreements.
Website: http://www.med.wisc.edu/metc/

University of Wisconsin–Milwaukee, Graduate School, College of Health Sciences, Program in Biomedical Sciences, Milwaukee, WI 53211. Offers cancer (MS); immunology (MS); microbiology (MS); neurodegenerative disease (MS); pharmacology and toxicology (MS); photobiomodulation (MS). *Accreditation:* NAACLS. *Program availability:* Part-time. *Faculty:* 8 full-time (4 women). *Students:* 8 full-time (7 women), 3 part-time (1 woman); includes 1 minority (Two or more races, non-Hispanic/Latino), 2 international. Average age 29. 42 applicants, 14% accepted, 4 enrolled. In 2015, 7 master's awarded. *Degree requirements:* For master's, thesis. *Entrance requirements:* For master's, GRE General Test. Additional exam requirements/recommendations for international students: Required—TOEFL (minimum score 550 paper-based; 79 iBT), IELTS (minimum score 6.5). *Application deadline:* For fall admission, 1/1 priority date for domestic students; for spring admission, 9/1 for domestic students. Applications are processed on a rolling basis. Application fee: $56 ($96 for international students). *Financial support:* In 2015–16, 6 teaching assistantships were awarded; fellowships, research assistantships, career-related internships or fieldwork, and unspecified assistantships also available. Support available to part-time students. Financial award application deadline: 4/15. *Unit head:* Raymond Fleming, Representative, 414-229-3980, E-mail: mundo@uwm.edu. *Application contact:* Roger O. Smith, General Information Contact, 414-229-6697, Fax: 414-229-6697, E-mail: smithro@uwm.edu.
Website: http://www4.uwm.edu/chs/academics/biomedical_sciences/bms_masters/

Utah State University, School of Graduate Studies, College of Agriculture, Program in Toxicology, Logan, UT 84322. Offers MS, PhD. Terminal master's awarded for partial completion of doctoral program. *Degree requirements:* For master's, thesis; for doctorate, thesis/dissertation. *Entrance requirements:* For master's and doctorate, GRE General Test, minimum GPA of 3.0. Additional exam requirements/recommendations for international students: Required—TOEFL. *Faculty research:* Free-radical mechanisms, toxicity of iron, carcinogenesis of natural compounds, molecular mechanisms of retinoid toxicity, aflatoxins.

Virginia Commonwealth University, Graduate School, College of Humanities and Sciences, Department of Forensic Science, Richmond, VA 23284-9005. Offers forensic biology (MS); forensic chemistry/drugs and toxicology (MS); forensic chemistry/trace (MS); forensic physical evidence (MS). *Program availability:* Part-time. *Entrance requirements:* For master's, GRE General Test, bachelor's degree in a natural science discipline, including forensic science, or a degree with equivalent work. Additional exam requirements/recommendations for international students: Required—TOEFL (minimum score 600 paper-based; 100 iBT) or IELTS (minimum score 6.5). Electronic applications accepted.

Virginia Commonwealth University, Medical College of Virginia-Professional Programs, School of Medicine, School of Medicine Graduate Programs, Department of Pharmacology and Toxicology, Richmond, VA 23284-9005. Offers neuroscience (PhD); pharmacology (Certificate); pharmacology and toxicology (MS, PhD); MD/PhD. Terminal master's awarded for partial completion of doctoral program. *Degree requirements:* For master's, thesis; for doctorate, thesis/dissertation, comprehensive oral and written exams. *Entrance requirements:* For master's and doctorate, GRE or MCAT. Additional exam requirements/recommendations for international students: Required—TOEFL (minimum score 600 paper-based; 100 iBT). Electronic applications accepted. *Faculty research:* Drug abuse, drug metabolism, pharmacodynamics, peptide synthesis, receptor mechanisms.

Wayne State University, Eugene Applebaum College of Pharmacy and Health Sciences, Department of Pharmaceutical Sciences, Detroit, MI 48202. Offers medicinal chemistry (MS, PhD); pharmaceutics (MS, PhD), including medicinal chemistry (PhD); pharmacology/toxicology (MS, PhD). *Accreditation:* ACPE (one or more programs are accredited). *Faculty:* 17 full-time (3 women). *Students:* 26 full-time (14 women), 3 part-time (1 woman); includes 3 minority (1 Black or African American, non-Hispanic/Latino; 1 American Indian or Alaska Native, non-Hispanic/Latino; 1 Asian, non-Hispanic/Latino), 23 international. Average age 26. 184 applicants, 15% accepted, 10 enrolled. In 2015, 9 master's, 102 doctorates awarded. *Degree requirements:* For master's, thesis; for doctorate, thesis/dissertation. *Entrance requirements:* For master's, GRE General Test, bachelor's degree; adequate background in biology, physics, calculus, and chemistry; three letters of recommendation; personal statement; for doctorate, GRE General Test, bachelor's or master's degree in one of the behavioral, biological, pharmaceutical or physical sciences; three letters of recommendation. Additional exam requirements/recommendations for international students: Required—TOEFL (minimum score 550 paper-based; 79 iBT), Michigan English Language Assessment Battery (minimum score 85); Recommended—IELTS (minimum score 6.5), TWE (minimum score 5.5). *Application deadline:* For fall admission, 12/1 priority date for domestic and international students. Applications are processed on a rolling basis. Application fee: $0. Electronic applications accepted. *Expenses:* $16,104 per year resident tuition, $32,401 non-resident tuition; $671 per credit hour resident tuition, $1,350.05 per credit hour non-resident tuition; fees include $47.45 per credit hour student services fee and $274.60 per semester registration fee. *Financial support:* In 2015–16, 15 students received support, including 2 fellowships with tuition reimbursements available (averaging $24,179 per year), 10 research assistantships with full tuition reimbursements available (averaging

Toxicology

$24,595 per year); teaching assistantships, scholarships/grants, health care benefits, and unspecified assistantships also available. Financial award application deadline: 3/31; financial award applicants required to submit FAFSA. *Faculty research:* Design of new anthracyclines, genetic and epigenetic effects of extracellular inducers, cellular injury and cell death, drug metabolism and nutrition, anti-infective agents, carcinogenesis, diabetes research, theragnostic nanomedicines, neurotoxicity, drug discovery, insulin resistance. *Unit head:* Dr. George Corcoran, Chair and Professor, 313-577-1737, E-mail: corcoran@wayne.edu. *Application contact:* 313-577-5415, Fax: 313-577-2033, E-mail: pscgrad@wayne.edu.
Website: http://cphs.wayne.edu/sciences/index.php

West Virginia University, Davis College of Agriculture, Forestry and Consumer Sciences, Interdisciplinary Program in Genetics and Developmental Biology, Morgantown, WV 26506. Offers animal breeding (MS, PhD); biochemical and molecular genetics (MS, PhD); cytogenetics (MS, PhD); descriptive embryology (MS, PhD); developmental genetics (MS); experimental morphogenesis/teratology (MS); human genetics (MS, PhD); immunogenetics (MS, PhD); life cycles of animals and plants (MS, PhD); molecular aspects of development (MS, PhD); mutagenesis (MS, PhD); oncology (MS, PhD); plant genetics (MS, PhD); population and quantitative genetics (MS, PhD); regeneration (MS, PhD); teratology (PhD); toxicology (MS, PhD). *Degree requirements:* For master's, thesis; for doctorate, comprehensive exam, thesis/dissertation. *Entrance requirements:* For master's, GRE or MCAT, minimum GPA of 2.75. Additional exam requirements/recommendations for international students: Required—TOEFL. *Expenses:* Tuition, state resident: full-time $8568. Tuition, nonresident: full-time $22,140. Tuition and fees vary according to program.

West Virginia University, School of Pharmacy, Program in Pharmaceutical and Pharmacological Sciences, Morgantown, WV 26506. Offers administrative pharmacy (PhD); behavioral pharmacy (MS, PhD); biopharmaceutics/pharmacokinetics (MS, PhD); industrial pharmacy (MS); medicinal chemistry (MS, PhD); pharmaceutical chemistry (MS, PhD); pharmaceutics (MS, PhD); pharmacology and toxicology (MS); pharmacy (MS); pharmacy administration (MS). *Program availability:* Part-time. Terminal master's awarded for partial completion of doctoral program. *Degree requirements:* For master's, thesis; for doctorate, one foreign language, comprehensive exam, thesis/dissertation. *Entrance requirements:* For master's and doctorate, GRE General Test, minimum GPA of 2.75. Additional exam requirements/recommendations for international students: Required—TOEFL; Recommended—TWE. Electronic applications accepted. *Expenses:* Contact institution. *Faculty research:* Pharmaceutics, medicinal chemistry, biopharmaceutics/pharmacokinetics, health outcomes research.

Wright State University, School of Medicine, Program in Pharmacology and Toxicology, Dayton, OH 45435. Offers MS. *Degree requirements:* For master's, thesis optional.

Section 18
Physiology

This section contains a directory of institutions offering graduate work in physiology, followed by an in-depth entry submitted by an institution that chose to prepare a detailed program description. Additional information about programs listed in the directory but not augmented by an in-depth entry may be obtained by writing directly to the dean of a graduate school or chair of a department at the address given in the directory.

For programs offering related work, see also all other sections in this book. In the other guides in this series:

Graduate Programs in the Physical Sciences, Mathematics, Agricultural Sciences, the Environment & Natural Resources

See *Agricultural and Food Sciences, Chemistry,* and *Marine Sciences and Oceanography*

Graduate Programs in Engineering & Applied Sciences

See *Agricultural Engineering and Bioengineering, Biomedical Engineering and Biotechnology, Electrical and Computer Engineering,* and *Mechanical Engineering and Mechanics*

CONTENTS

Program Directories

Displays and Close-Ups

See also:

Cardiovascular Sciences

Albany Medical College, Center for Cardiovascular Sciences, Albany, NY 12208-3479. Offers MS, PhD. *Program availability:* Part-time. Terminal master's awarded for partial completion of doctoral program. *Degree requirements:* For master's, thesis; for doctorate, comprehensive exam, thesis/dissertation, candidacy exam, written preliminary exam, 1 published paper-peer review. *Entrance requirements:* For master's, GRE General Test, letters of recommendation; for doctorate, GRE General Test, all transcripts, letters of recommendation. Additional exam requirements/recommendations for international students: Required—TOEFL. *Faculty research:* Vascular smooth muscle, endothelial cell biology, molecular and genetic bases underlying cardiac disease, reactive oxygen and nitrogen species biology, fatty acid trafficking and fatty acid mediated transcription control.

Augusta University, The Graduate School, Program in Vascular Biology, Augusta, GA 30912. Offers PhD. *Degree requirements:* For doctorate, comprehensive exam, thesis/dissertation. *Entrance requirements:* For doctorate, GRE General Test. Additional exam requirements/recommendations for international students: Required—TOEFL (minimum score 550 paper-based; 79 iBT). *Application deadline:* For fall admission, 1/15 for domestic and international students. Application fee: $50. Electronic applications accepted. *Financial support:* Fellowships with partial tuition reimbursements, research assistantships with partial tuition reimbursements, Federal Work-Study, institutionally sponsored loans, scholarships/grants, and traineeships available. Support available to part-time students. Financial award application deadline: 5/31. *Faculty research:* Hypertension and renal disease, diabetes and obesity, peripheral vascular disease, acute lung injury, signal transduction. *Unit head:* Dr. David J. Fulton, Director, Vascular Biology Center, 706-721-6338, Fax: 706-721-9799, E-mail: dfulton@augusta.edu. *Application contact:* Kari Martin, Graduate Program Coordinator, 706-721-6338, E-mail: kmartin@augusta.edu.
Website: http://www.augusta.edu/centers/vbc/grad_prog.php

Baylor College of Medicine, Graduate School of Biomedical Sciences, Department of Molecular Physiology and Biophysics, Houston, TX 77030-3498. Offers cardiovascular sciences (PhD); molecular physiology and biophysics (PhD); MD/PhD. *Degree requirements:* For doctorate, thesis/dissertation, public defense. *Entrance requirements:* For doctorate, GRE General Test, GRE Subject Test (strongly recommended), minimum GPA of 3.0. Additional exam requirements/recommendations for international students: Required—TOEFL. Electronic applications accepted. *Faculty research:* Cardiovascular disease; skeletal muscle disease (myasthenia gravis, muscular dystrophy, malignant hyperthermia, central core disease); cancer; Alzheimer's disease; developmental diseases of the nervous system, eye and heart; diabetes; motor neuron disease (amyotrophic lateral sclerosis and spinal muscular atrophy); asthma; autoimmune diseases.

Geneva College, Master of Science in Cardiovascular Science Program, Beaver Falls, PA 15010-3599. Offers MS. *Faculty:* 1 full-time (0 women), 2 part-time/adjunct (1 woman). *Students:* 3 full-time (0 women), 1 international. Average age 28. In 2015, 1 master's awarded. *Degree requirements:* For master's, six semesters (includes 2 summers), RCIS and RCES registry exams. *Entrance requirements:* For master's, GRE, BS in biology or related field, minimum undergraduate GPA of 3.0, two letters of reference, one-day orientation at the cardiac catheterization labs at INOVA Heart and Vascular Institute campus. Additional exam requirements/recommendations for international students: Required—TOEFL. *Application deadline:* For fall admission, 5/30 for domestic students. Applications are processed on a rolling basis. Electronic applications accepted. *Expenses:* Contact institution. *Financial support:* Application deadline: 8/1; applicants required to submit FAFSA. *Unit head:* Dr. David A. Essig, Program Coordinator, 724-847-6900, E-mail: dessig@geneva.edu.
Website: http://www.geneva.edu/object/cvt

Johns Hopkins University, Bloomberg School of Public Health, Department of Epidemiology, Baltimore, MD 21205. Offers cancer etiology and prevention (MHS, Sc M, PhD, Sc D); cardiovascular diseases (MHS, Sc M, PhD, Sc D); clinical epidemiology (MHS, Sc M, PhD, Sc D); clinical trials (PhD, Sc D); epidemiology (MHS, Sc M, Dr PH, PhD, Sc D); epidemiology of aging (MHS, Sc M, PhD, Sc D); genetic epidemiology (MHS, Sc M, PhD, Sc D); infectious disease epidemiology (MHS, Sc M, PhD, Sc D); occupational and environmental epidemiology (MHS, Sc M, PhD, Sc D). *Program availability:* Part-time. *Degree requirements:* For master's, comprehensive exam, thesis, 1-year full-time residency; for doctorate, comprehensive exam, thesis/dissertation, 2 years' full-time residency, oral and written exams, student teaching. *Entrance requirements:* For master's, GRE General Test or MCAT, 3 letters of recommendation, curriculum vitae; for doctorate, GRE General Test, minimum 1 year of work experience, 3 letters of recommendation, curriculum vitae, academic records from all schools. Additional exam requirements/recommendations for international students: Required—TOEFL (minimum score 600 paper-based; 100 iBT); Recommended—IELTS (minimum score 7.5), TWE. Electronic applications accepted. *Faculty research:* Cancer and congenital malformations, nutritional epidemiology, AIDS, tuberculosis, cardiovascular disease, risk assessment.

Marquette University, Graduate School, Program in Transfusion Medicine, Milwaukee, WI 53201-1881. Offers MSTM. Program is held in collaboration with BloodCenter of Wisconsin. *Program availability:* Part-time. *Students:* 5 part-time (4 women), 1 international. Average age 35. 2 applicants, 100% accepted, 1 enrolled. In 2015, 1 master's awarded. *Entrance requirements:* For master's, official transcripts from all current and previous colleges, three letters of recommendation. Additional exam requirements/recommendations for international students: Required—TOEFL. *Application deadline:* For fall admission, 4/1 for domestic and international students. Application fee: $50. *Application contact:* Sue Johnson, E-mail: sue.johnson@bcw.edu.
Website: http://www.bcw.edu/bcw/education/sbbprogram/mstm/index.htm

McMaster University, Faculty of Health Sciences and School of Graduate Studies, Program in Medical Sciences, Blood and Vascular Area, Hamilton, ON L8S 4M2, Canada. Offers M Sc, PhD, MD/PhD. *Degree requirements:* For master's, thesis; for doctorate, comprehensive exam, thesis/dissertation. *Entrance requirements:* For master's, honors B Sc, B+ average in related field; for doctorate, M Sc, minimum B+ average, students with proven research experience and an A average may be admitted with a B Sc degree. Additional exam requirements/recommendations for international students: Required—TOEFL (minimum score 580 paper-based; 92 iBT).

Medical University of South Carolina, College of Graduate Studies, Program in Molecular and Cellular Biology and Pathobiology, Charleston, SC 29425. Offers cancer biology (PhD); cardiovascular biology (PhD); cardiovascular imaging (PhD); cell regulation (PhD); craniofacial biology (PhD); genetics and development (PhD); marine biomedicine (PhD); DMD/PhD; MD/PhD. *Degree requirements:* For doctorate, thesis/dissertation, oral and written exams. *Entrance requirements:* For doctorate, GRE General Test, interview, minimum GPA of 3.0. Additional exam requirements/

recommendations for international students: Required—TOEFL (minimum score 600 paper-based; 100 iBT). Electronic applications accepted.

Memorial University of Newfoundland, Faculty of Medicine and School of Graduate Studies, Graduate Programs in Medicine, Division of Biomedical Sciences, St. John's, NL A1C 5S7, Canada. Offers cancer (M Sc, PhD); cardiovascular (M Sc, PhD); immunology (M Sc, PhD); neuroscience (M Sc, PhD). *Program availability:* Part-time. *Degree requirements:* For master's, thesis; for doctorate, comprehensive exam, thesis/dissertation, oral defense of thesis. *Entrance requirements:* For master's, MD or B Sc; for doctorate, MD or M Sc. Additional exam requirements/recommendations for international students: Required—TOEFL. *Expenses:* Tuition, area resident: Full-time $2199 Canadian dollars. *International tuition:* $2859 Canadian dollars full-time. *Faculty research:* Neuroscience, immunology, cardiovascular, and cancer.

Midwestern University, Glendale Campus, College of Health Sciences, Arizona Campus, Program in Cardiovascular Science, Glendale, AZ 85308. Offers MCVS. *Expenses:* Contact institution.

Milwaukee School of Engineering, Department of Electrical Engineering and Computer Science, Program in Perfusion, Milwaukee, WI 53202-3109. Offers MS. *Program availability:* Part-time, evening/weekend. *Faculty:* 2 full-time (0 women), 5 part-time/adjunct (1 woman). *Students:* 10 full-time (8 women); includes 1 minority (Hispanic/Latino). 44 applicants, 14% accepted, 6 enrolled. In 2015, 7 master's awarded. *Degree requirements:* For master's, comprehensive exam, thesis, exam. *Entrance requirements:* For master's, GRE General Test or GMAT (percentiles must average 50% or better), BS in appropriate discipline (biomedical engineering, biology, biomedical sciences, etc.), 3 letters of recommendation, personal interview, observation of 2 perfusion clinical cases. Additional exam requirements/recommendations for international students: Required—TOEFL (minimum score 79 iBT), IELTS (minimum score 6.5). *Application deadline:* Applications are processed on a rolling basis. Application fee: $0. Electronic applications accepted. *Expenses:* Tuition, area resident: Full-time $34,200; part-time $760 per credit. *Financial support:* Career-related internships or fieldwork, institutionally sponsored loans, and scholarships/grants available. Financial award application deadline: 3/15; financial award applicants required to submit FAFSA. *Faculty research:* Heart medicine. *Unit head:* Dr. Ronald Gerrits, Director, 414-277-7561, Fax: 414-277-7494, E-mail: gerrits@msoe.edu. *Application contact:* Ian Dahlinghaus, Graduate Program Associate, 414-277-7208, E-mail: dahlinghaus@msoe.edu.
Website: http://www.msoe.edu/community/academics/engineering/page/1328/perfusion-overview

See Display on page 501 and Close-Up on page 533.

Queen's University at Kingston, School of Graduate Studies, Faculty of Health Sciences, Department of Anatomy and Cell Biology, Kingston, ON K7L 3N6, Canada. Offers biology of reproduction (M Sc, PhD); cancer (M Sc, PhD); cardiovascular pathophysiology (M Sc, PhD); cell and molecular biology (M Sc, PhD); drug metabolism (M Sc, PhD); endocrinology (M Sc, PhD); motor control (M Sc, PhD); neural regeneration (M Sc, PhD); neurophysiology (M Sc, PhD). *Program availability:* Part-time. *Degree requirements:* For master's, thesis; for doctorate, one foreign language, comprehensive exam, thesis/dissertation. *Entrance requirements:* Additional exam requirements/recommendations for international students: Required—TOEFL. Electronic applications accepted. *Faculty research:* Human kinetics, neuroscience, reproductive biology, cardiovascular.

Quinnipiac University, School of Health Sciences, Program in Cardiovascular Perfusion, Hamden, CT 06518-1940. Offers MHS. *Faculty:* 1 full-time (0 women), 4 part-time/adjunct (0 women). *Students:* 8 full-time (3 women), 9 part-time (3 women); includes 3 minority (2 Asian, non-Hispanic/Latino; 1 Hispanic/Latino). 48 applicants, 27% accepted, 8 enrolled. In 2015, 7 master's awarded. *Entrance requirements:* For master's, bachelor's degree in science or health-related discipline from an accredited American or Canadian college or university; 2 years of health care work experience; interview. *Application deadline:* For fall admission, 2/1 for domestic students. Applications are processed on a rolling basis. Application fee: $45. Electronic applications accepted. *Expenses:* $985 per credit tuition; $360 per semester student fee; $340 per semester (fall/spring) technology and lab fee; $75 per semester summer technology and lab fee. *Financial support:* Federal Work-Study, scholarships/grants, and unspecified assistantships available. Financial award application deadline: 6/1; financial award applicants required to submit FAFSA. *Faculty research:* Methods of preventing systemic inflammatory response syndrome (SIRS) during extracorporeal circulation of blood, investigations into the role of P-selectin in causing monocyte-platelet interaction, effect of simulated cardiopulmonary bypass on platelets and other formed elements in the blood. *Unit head:* Dr. Michael Smith, Director, 203-582-3427, E-mail: michael.smith@quinnipiac.edu. *Application contact:* Office of Graduate Admissions, 800-462-1944, Fax: 208-582-3443, E-mail: graduate@quinnipiac.edu.
Website: http://www.quinnipiac.edu/gradperfusion

Université Laval, Faculty of Medicine, Post-Professional Programs in Medical Studies, Québec, QC G1K 7P4, Canada. Offers anatomy–pathology (DESS); anesthesiology (DESS); cardiology (DESS); care of older people (Diploma); clinical research (DESS); community health (DESS); dermatology (DESS); diagnostic radiology (DESS); emergency medicine (Diploma); family medicine (DESS); general surgery (DESS); geriatrics (DESS); hematology (DESS); internal medicine (DESS); maternal and fetal medicine (Diploma); medical biochemistry (DESS); medical microbiology and infectious diseases (DESS); medical oncology (DESS); nephrology (DESS); neurology (DESS); neurosurgery (DESS); obstetrics and gynecology (DESS); ophthalmology (DESS); orthopedic surgery (DESS); oto-rhino-laryngology (DESS); palliative medicine (Diploma); pediatrics (DESS); plastic surgery (DESS); psychiatry (DESS); pulmonary medicine (DESS); radiology–oncology (DESS); thoracic surgery (DESS); urology (DESS). *Degree requirements:* For other advanced degree, comprehensive exam. *Entrance requirements:* For degree, knowledge of French. Electronic applications accepted.

University of Calgary, Cumming School of Medicine and Faculty of Graduate Studies, Program in Cardiovascular and Respiratory Sciences, Calgary, AB T2N 1N4, Canada. Offers M Sc, PhD. *Degree requirements:* For master's, thesis; for doctorate, thesis/dissertation, candidacy exam. *Entrance requirements:* For master's and doctorate, minimum GPA of 3.2. Additional exam requirements/recommendations for international students: Required—TOEFL (minimum score 600 paper-based). Electronic applications accepted. *Faculty research:* Cardiac mechanics, physiology and pharmacology; lung mechanics, physiology and pathophysiology; smooth muscle biochemistry; physiology and pharmacology.

University of Guelph, Ontario Veterinary College and Graduate Studies, Graduate Programs in Veterinary Sciences, Department of Clinical Studies, Guelph, ON N1G 2W1, Canada. Offers anesthesiology (M Sc, DV Sc); cardiology (DV Sc, Diploma); clinical studies (Diploma); dermatology (M Sc); diagnostic imaging (M Sc, DV Sc); emergency/critical care (M Sc, DV Sc, Diploma); medicine (M Sc, DV Sc); neurology (M Sc, DV Sc); ophthalmology (M Sc, DV Sc); surgery (M Sc, DV Sc). *Degree requirements:* For master's, thesis; for doctorate, comprehensive exam, thesis/ dissertation. *Entrance requirements:* Additional exam requirements/recommendations for international students: Required—TOEFL (minimum score 550 paper-based), IELTS (minimum score 6.5). Electronic applications accepted. *Faculty research:* Orthopedics, respirology, oncology, exercise physiology, cardiology.

University of Mary, School of Health Sciences, Program in Respiratory Therapy, Bismarck, ND 58504-9652. Offers MS. *Entrance requirements:* For master's, minimum GPA of 3.0, 3 letters of reference, interview. Additional exam requirements/ recommendations for international students: Required—TOEFL (minimum score 500 paper-based; 71 iBT). *Application deadline:* For fall admission, 2/15 for domestic students. Application fee: $40. Electronic applications accepted. *Financial support:* Career-related internships or fieldwork available. Financial award application deadline: 8/1; financial award applicants required to submit FAFSA.
Website: http://www.umary.edu/academics/programs/ms-respiratory-therapy.php

The University of South Dakota, Graduate School, Sanford School of Medicine and Graduate School, Biomedical Sciences Graduate Program, Cardiovascular Research Program, Vermillion, SD 57069-2390. Offers MS, PhD. *Students:* Average age 25. In 2015, 1 master's, 1 doctorate awarded. Terminal master's awarded for partial completion of doctoral program. *Degree requirements:* For master's, thesis; for doctorate, comprehensive exam, thesis/dissertation. *Entrance requirements:* For master's and doctorate, GRE General Test, minimum GPA of 3.0. Additional exam requirements/recommendations for international students: Required—TOEFL (minimum score 550 paper-based; 80 iBT), IELTS (minimum score 6). *Application deadline:* For fall admission, 4/15 priority date for domestic students, 3/15 for international students. Applications are processed on a rolling basis. Application fee: $35. Electronic applications accepted. *Expenses:* Contact institution. *Financial support:* In 2015–16, 4 students received support, including 4 fellowships with partial tuition reimbursements available (averaging $20,772 per year), research assistantships with partial tuition reimbursements available (averaging $10,386 per year); teaching assistantships and unspecified assistantships also available. Financial award application deadline: 4/15; financial award applicants required to submit FAFSA. *Faculty research:* Cardiovascular disease. *Total annual research expenditures:* $1.4 million. *Unit head:* 605-658-6322, Fax: 605-677-6381, E-mail: biomed@usd.edu.

University of South Florida, Innovative Education, Tampa, FL 33620-9951. Offers adult, career and higher education (Graduate Certificate), including college teaching, leadership in developing human resources, leadership in higher education; Africana studies (Graduate Certificate), including diasporas and health disparities, genocide and human rights; aging studies (Graduate Certificate), including gerontology; art research (Graduate Certificate), including museum studies; business foundations (Graduate Certificate); chemical and biomedical engineering (Graduate Certificate), including materials science and engineering, water, health and sustainability; child and family studies (Graduate Certificate), including positive behavior support; civil and industrial engineering (Graduate Certificate), including transportation systems analysis; community and family health (Graduate Certificate), including maternal and child health, social marketing and public health, violence and injury: prevention and intervention, women's health; criminology (Graduate Certificate), including criminal justice administration; educational measurement and research (Graduate Certificate), including evaluation; English (Graduate Certificate), including comparative literary studies, creative writing, professional and technical communication; entrepreneurship (Graduate

Certificate); environmental health (Graduate Certificate), including safety management; epidemiology and biostatistics (Graduate Certificate), including applied biostatistics, biostatistics, concepts and tools of epidemiology, epidemiology, epidemiology of infectious diseases; geography, environment and planning (Graduate Certificate), including community development, environmental policy and management, geographical information systems; geology (Graduate Certificate), including hydrogeology; global health (Graduate Certificate), including disaster management, global health and Latin American and Caribbean studies, global health practice, humanitarian assistance, infection control; government and international affairs (Graduate Certificate), including Cuban studies, globalization studies; health policy and management (Graduate Certificate), including health management and leadership, public health policy and programs; hearing specialist: early intervention (Graduate Certificate); industrial and management systems engineering (Graduate Certificate), including systems engineering, technology management; information studies (Graduate Certificate), including school library media specialist; information systems/decision sciences (Graduate Certificate), including analytics and business intelligence; instructional technology (Graduate Certificate), including distance education, Florida digital/virtual educator, instructional design, multimedia design, Web design; internal medicine, bioethics and medical humanities (Graduate Certificate), including biomedical ethics; Latin American and Caribbean studies (Graduate Certificate); mass communications (Graduate Certificate), including multimedia journalism; mathematics and statistics (Graduate Certificate), including mathematics; medicine (Graduate Certificate), including aging and neuroscience, bioinformatics, biotechnology, brain fitness and memory management, clinical investigation, health informatics, health sciences, integrative weight management, intellectual property, medicine and gender, metabolic and nutritional medicine, metabolic cardiology, pharmacy sciences; national and competitive intelligence (Graduate Certificate); psychological and social foundations (Graduate Certificate), including career counseling, college teaching, diversity in education, mental health counseling, school counseling; public affairs (Graduate Certificate), including nonprofit management, public management, research administration; public health (Graduate Certificate), including environmental health, health equity, public health generalist, translational research in adolescent behavioral health; public health practices (Graduate Certificate), including planning for healthy communities; rehabilitation and mental health counseling (Graduate Certificate), including integrative mental health care, marriage and family therapy, rehabilitation technology; secondary education (Graduate Certificate), including ESOL, foreign language education: culture and content, foreign language education: professional; social work (Graduate Certificate), including geriatric social work/clinical gerontology; special education (Graduate Certificate), including autism spectrum disorder, disabilities education: severe/profound; world languages (Graduate Certificate), including teaching English as a second language (TESL) or foreign language. *Unit head:* Kathy Barnes, Interdisciplinary Programs Coordinator, 813-974-8031, Fax: 813-974-7061, E-mail: barnesk@usf.edu. *Application contact:* Karen Tylinski, Metro Initiatives, 813-974-9943, Fax: 813-974-7061, E-mail: ktylinsk@usf.edu.
Website: http://www.usf.edu/innovative-education/

The University of Toledo, College of Graduate Studies, College of Medicine and Life Sciences, Department of Physiology and Pharmacology, Toledo, OH 43606-3390. Offers cardiovascular and metabolic diseases (MSBS, PhD); MD/MSBS; MD/PhD. Terminal master's awarded for partial completion of doctoral program. *Degree requirements:* For master's, thesis, qualifying exam; for doctorate, thesis/dissertation, qualifying exam. *Entrance requirements:* For master's and doctorate, GRE, minimum undergraduate GPA of 3.0, three letters of recommendation, statement of purpose, transcripts from all prior institutions attended, resume. Additional exam requirements/ recommendations for international students: Required—TOEFL (minimum score 550 paper-based; 80 iBT). Electronic applications accepted.

Molecular Physiology

Baylor College of Medicine, Graduate School of Biomedical Sciences, Department of Molecular Physiology and Biophysics, Houston, TX 77030-3498. Offers cardiovascular sciences (PhD); molecular physiology and biophysics (PhD); MD/PhD. *Degree requirements:* For doctorate, thesis/dissertation, public defense. *Entrance requirements:* For doctorate, GRE General Test, GRE Subject Test (strongly recommended), minimum GPA of 3.0. Additional exam requirements/recommendations for international students: Required—TOEFL. Electronic applications accepted. *Faculty research:* Cardiovascular disease; skeletal muscle disease (myasthenia gravis, muscular dystrophy, malignant hyperthermia, central core disease); cancer; Alzheimer's disease; developmental diseases of the nervous system, eye and heart; diabetes; motor neuron disease (amyotrophic lateral sclerosis and spinal muscular atrophy); asthma; autoimmune diseases.

Case Western Reserve University, School of Medicine and School of Graduate Studies, Graduate Programs in Medicine, Department of Physiology and Biophysics, Cleveland, OH 44106. Offers cell and molecular physiology (MS); cell physiology (PhD); molecular/cellular biophysics (PhD); physiology and biophysics (PhD); systems physiology (PhD); MD/PhD. Terminal master's awarded for partial completion of doctoral program. *Degree requirements:* For master's, thesis; for doctorate, thesis/dissertation. *Entrance requirements:* For master's, GRE General Test, minimum GPA of 3.28; for doctorate, GRE General Test, minimum GPA of 3.6. Additional exam requirements/ recommendations for international students: Required—TOEFL. Electronic applications accepted. *Expenses:* Tuition, area resident: Full-time $41,137; part-time $1714 per credit hour. *Required fees:* $32. Tuition and fees vary according to course load and program. *Faculty research:* Cardiovascular physiology, calcium metabolism, epithelial cell biology.

Loyola University Chicago, Graduate School, Integrated Program in Biomedical Sciences, Maywood, IL 60153. Offers biochemistry and molecular biology (MS, PhD); cell and molecular physiology (PhD); infectious disease and immunology (MS); integrative cell biology (PhD); medical physiology (MS); microbiology and immunology (MS, PhD); molecular pharmacology and therapeutics (MS, PhD); neuroscience (MS, PhD). *Students:* 135 full-time (65 women), 1 part-time (0 women); includes 28 minority (5 Black or African American, non-Hispanic/Latino; 15 Asian, non-Hispanic/Latino; 6 Hispanic/Latino; 2 Two or more races, non-Hispanic/Latino), 16 international. Average age 28. 442 applicants, 23% accepted, 55 enrolled. In 2015, 40 master's, 17 doctorates awarded. *Expenses: Tuition, area resident:* Full-time $18,054; part-time $9027 per credit hour. *Required fees:* $832; $284 per credit hour. Part-time tuition and fees vary according to course load, degree level and program. *Unit head:* Dr. Samuel Attoh, Dean, 773-508-3459, Fax: 773-508-2460, E-mail: sattoh@luc.edu. *Application contact:* Ron

Martin, Associate Director of Enrollment Management, 312-915-8950, Fax: 312-915-8905, E-mail: gradapp@luc.edu.
Website: http://ssom.luc.edu/graduate_school/degree-programs/ipbsphd/

Rutgers University–New Brunswick, Graduate School-New Brunswick, Program in Endocrinology and Animal Biosciences, Piscataway, NJ 08854-8097. Offers MS, PhD. Terminal master's awarded for partial completion of doctoral program. *Degree requirements:* For master's, thesis; for doctorate, comprehensive exam, thesis/ dissertation. *Entrance requirements:* For master's and doctorate, GRE General Test. Additional exam requirements/recommendations for international students: Required— TOEFL. Electronic applications accepted. *Faculty research:* Comparative and behavioral endocrinology, epigenetic regulation of the endocrine system, exercise physiology and immunology, fetal and neonatal developmental programming, mammary gland biology and breast cancer, neuroendocrinology and alcohol studies, reproductive and developmental toxicology.

Stony Brook University, State University of New York, Stony Brook Medicine, School of Medicine and Graduate School, Graduate Programs in Medicine, Department of Physiology and Biophysics, Stony Brook, NY 11794. Offers PhD. *Faculty:* 17 full-time (6 women). *Students:* 33 full-time (15 women), 1 part-time (0 women); includes 18 minority (6 Black or African American, non-Hispanic/Latino; 6 Asian, non-Hispanic/Latino; 5 Hispanic/Latino; 1 Two or more races, non-Hispanic/Latino), 6 international. Average age 25. 5 applicants. In 2015, 3 doctorates awarded. *Degree requirements:* For doctorate, comprehensive exam, thesis/dissertation. *Entrance requirements:* For doctorate, GRE General Test, GRE Subject Test, BS in related field, minimum GPA of 3.0, recommendation. Additional exam requirements/recommendations for international students: Required—TOEFL (minimum score 550 paper-based). *Application deadline:* For fall admission, 1/15 for domestic students; for spring admission, 10/1 for domestic students. Application fee: $100. *Expenses:* $12,421 full-time resident tuition and fees, $453 per credit hour; $23,761 full-time nonresident tuition and fees, $925 per credit hour. *Financial support:* In 2015–16, 2 research assistantships were awarded; fellowships, teaching assistantships, and Federal Work-Study also available. Financial award application deadline: 3/15. *Faculty research:* Biophysics, physiology, neuropharmacology, neurophysiology, neuroscience. *Total annual research expenditures:* $5.2 million. *Unit head:* Dr. Todd Miller, Chair, 631-444-3533, Fax: 631-444-3432, E-mail: todd.miller@stonybrook.edu. *Application contact:* Odalis Hernandez, Coordinator, 631-444-3057, Fax: 631-444-3432, E-mail: odalis.hernandez@stonybrook.edu.
Website: http://pnb.informatics.stonybrook.edu/

Molecular Physiology

University of California, Los Angeles, Graduate Division, College of Letters and Science, Program in Molecular, Cellular and Integrative Physiology, Los Angeles, CA 90095. Offers PhD. *Degree requirements:* For doctorate, thesis/dissertation, oral and written qualifying exams. *Entrance requirements:* For doctorate, GRE General Test; GRE Subject Test (biology or applicant's undergraduate major), bachelor's degree; minimum undergraduate GPA of 3.0 (or its equivalent if letter grade system not used); interview. Additional exam requirements/recommendations for international students: Required—TOEFL. Electronic applications accepted.

University of Illinois at Urbana–Champaign, Graduate College, College of Liberal Arts and Sciences, School of Molecular and Cellular Biology, Department of Molecular and Integrative Physiology, Champaign, IL 61820. Offers MS, PhD.

The University of North Carolina at Chapel Hill, School of Medicine and Graduate School, Graduate Programs in Medicine, Department of Cell and Molecular Physiology, Chapel Hill, NC 27599. Offers PhD. Terminal master's awarded for partial completion of doctoral program. *Degree requirements:* For doctorate, comprehensive exam, thesis/dissertation, ethics training. *Entrance requirements:* For doctorate, GRE General Test. Electronic applications accepted. *Faculty research:* Signal transduction; growth factors; cardiovascular diseases; neurobiology; hormones, receptors, ion channels.

University of Pittsburgh, School of Medicine, Graduate Programs in Medicine, Cell Biology and Molecular Physiology Graduate Program, Pittsburgh, PA 15260. Offers PhD. *Faculty:* 44 full-time (9 women). *Students:* 5 full-time (4 women). Average age 28. 386 applicants, 17% accepted, 25 enrolled. In 2015, 1 doctorate awarded. *Degree requirements:* For doctorate, comprehensive exam, thesis/dissertation. *Entrance requirements:* For doctorate, GRE General Test, GRE Subject Test, minimum QPA of 3.0. Additional exam requirements/recommendations for international students: Required—TOEFL (minimum score 600 paper-based; 100 iBT), IELTS (minimum score 7). *Application deadline:* For fall admission, 12/1 priority date for domestic and international students. Application fee: $50. Electronic applications accepted. Tuition and fees vary according to program. *Financial support:* In 2015–16, 5 students received support, including 3 fellowships with full tuition reimbursements available (averaging $27,000 per year), 2 research assistantships with full tuition reimbursements available (averaging $27,000 per year), teaching assistantships with full tuition reimbursements available (averaging $27,000 per year); scholarships/grants, traineeships, and health care benefits also available. *Faculty research:* Genetic disorders of ion channels, regulation of gene expression/development, membrane traffic of proteins and lipids, reproductive biology, signal transduction in diabetes and metabolism. *Unit head:* Dr.

Donna B. Stolz, Program Director, 412-383-7283, Fax: 412-648-2927, E-mail: dstolz@pitt.edu. *Application contact:* Carol Williams, Admissions and Recruiting Manager, 412-648-8957, Fax: 412-648-1077, E-mail: gradstudies@medschool.pitt.edu. Website: http://www.gradbiomed.pitt.edu

University of Virginia, School of Medicine, Department of Molecular Physiology and Biological Physics, Charlottesville, VA 22903. Offers biological and physical sciences (MS); physiology (PhD); MD/PhD. *Entrance requirements:* For doctorate, GRE General Test, GRE Subject Test. Additional exam requirements/recommendations for international students: Required—TOEFL. Electronic applications accepted.

Vanderbilt University, School of Medicine, Department of Molecular Physiology and Biophysics, Nashville, TN 37240-1001. Offers MS, PhD, MD/PhD. *Faculty:* 31 full-time (4 women). *Students:* 44 full-time (25 women); includes 7 minority (2 Black or African American, non-Hispanic/Latino; 1 Asian, non-Hispanic/Latino; 3 Hispanic/Latino; 1 Two or more races, non-Hispanic/Latino), 2 international. Average age 26. In 2015, 8 doctorates awarded. *Degree requirements:* For doctorate, comprehensive exam, thesis/dissertation, preliminary, qualifying, and final exams. *Entrance requirements:* For doctorate, GRE General Test, GRE Subject Test (recommended). Additional exam requirements/recommendations for international students: Required—TOEFL (minimum score 570 paper-based; 88 iBT). *Application deadline:* For fall admission, 1/15 for domestic and international students. Application fee: $0. Electronic applications accepted. *Financial support:* Fellowships with full tuition reimbursements, research assistantships with full tuition reimbursements, Federal Work-Study, institutionally sponsored loans, scholarships/grants, traineeships, health care benefits, and tuition waivers (partial) available. Financial award application deadline: 1/15; financial award applicants required to submit CSS PROFILE or FAFSA. *Faculty research:* Biophysics, cell signaling and gene regulation, human genetics, diabetes and obesity, neuroscience. *Unit head:* Dr. Alyssa Hasty, Director of Graduate Studies, 615-322-7000, Fax: 615-343-0490, E-mail: alyssa.hasty@vanderbilt.edu. *Application contact:* Walter B. Bieschke, Program Coordinator for Graduate Admissions, 615-342-0236, E-mail: walter.bieschke@vanderbilt.edu. Website: http://www.mc.vanderbilt.edu/root/vumc.php?site-MPB

Yale University, Graduate School of Arts and Sciences, Department of Cellular and Molecular Physiology, New Haven, CT 06520. Offers PhD. *Degree requirements:* For doctorate, thesis/dissertation. *Entrance requirements:* For doctorate, GRE General Test, GRE Subject Test.

Physiology

Albert Einstein College of Medicine, Graduate Division of Biomedical Sciences, Department of Physiology and Biophysics, Bronx, NY 10461. Offers PhD, MD/PhD. *Degree requirements:* For doctorate, thesis/dissertation. *Entrance requirements:* For doctorate, GRE General Test. Additional exam requirements/recommendations for international students: Required—TOEFL. *Faculty research:* Biophysical and biochemical basis of body function at the subcellular, cellular, organ, and whole-body level.

Augusta University, The Graduate School, Program in Physiology, Augusta, GA 30912. Offers PhD. *Degree requirements:* For doctorate, comprehensive exam, thesis/dissertation. *Entrance requirements:* For doctorate, GRE General Test. Additional exam requirements/recommendations for international students: Required—TOEFL (minimum score 550 paper-based; 79 iBT). *Application deadline:* For fall admission, 1/15 for domestic and international students. Application fee: $50. Electronic applications accepted. *Financial support:* Fellowships with partial tuition reimbursements, research assistantships with partial tuition reimbursements, Federal Work-Study, institutionally sponsored loans, scholarships/grants, and traineeships available. Support available to part-time students. Financial award application deadline: 5/31; financial award applicants required to submit FAFSA. *Faculty research:* Cardiovascular and renal physiology, behavioral neuroscience and genetics, neurophysiology, adrenal steroid endocrinology and genetics, inflammatory mediators and cardiovascular disease, hypertension, diabetes and stroke. *Unit head:* Dr. Clinton Webb, Chair and Professor, 706-721-7742, Fax: 706-721-7299, E-mail: cwebb@augusta.edu. *Application contact:* Dr. Adviye Ergul, Director, 706-721-9103, E-mail: aergul@augusta.edu. Website: http://www.augusta.edu/mcg/phy/phys_graduate.php

Ball State University, Graduate School, College of Sciences and Humanities, Department of Biology, Program in Physiology, Muncie, IN 47306. Offers physiology (MA, MS). *Program availability:* Part-time. *Students:* 23 full-time (8 women), 6 part-time (3 women); includes 6 minority (2 Black or African American, non-Hispanic/Latino; 2 Asian, non-Hispanic/Latino; 2 Hispanic/Latino), 4 international. Average age 24. 30 applicants, 70% accepted, 17 enrolled. In 2015, 10 master's awarded. *Entrance requirements:* For master's, minimum baccalaureate GPA of 2.75 or 3.0 in latter half of baccalaureate, three letters of recommendation, resume or curriculum vitae. Additional exam requirements/recommendations for international students: Required—TOEFL (minimum score 550 paper-based; 79 iBT), IELTS (minimum score 6.5). *Application deadline:* Applications are processed on a rolling basis. Application fee: $60. Electronic applications accepted. *Expenses:* Tuition, area resident: Full-time $6948; part-time $2316 per semester. Tuition, state resident: full-time $10,422; part-time $3474 per semester. Tuition, nonresident: full-time $19,062; part-time $6354 per semester. *Required fees:* $651 per semester. Tuition and fees vary according to campus/location, program and reciprocity agreements. *Financial support:* In 2015–16, 9 students received support, including 9 teaching assistantships with partial tuition reimbursements available (averaging $11,430 per year). Financial award application deadline: 3/1; financial award applicants required to submit FAFSA. *Unit head:* Dr. Kemuel Badger, Chairperson, 765-285-8820, Fax: 765-285-8804, E-mail: kbadger@bsu.edu. *Application contact:* Dr. Marianna Zamalauski-Tucker, Assistant Professor/Graduate Advisor, 765-285-8630, Fax: 765-285-8804, E-mail: mzamlaus@bsu.edu. Website: http://www.bsu.edu/biology

Boston University, College of Health and Rehabilitation Sciences: Sargent College, Department of Health Sciences, Programs in Human Physiology, Boston, MA 02215. Offers MS, PhD. *Faculty:* 10 full-time (9 women), 5 part-time/adjunct (2 women). *Students:* 10 full-time (4 women), 7 part-time (5 women); includes 5 minority (1 Black or African American, non-Hispanic/Latino; 1 Asian, non-Hispanic/Latino; 2 Hispanic/Latino; 1 Two or more races, non-Hispanic/Latino), 3 international. Average age 24. 40 applicants, 30% accepted, 9 enrolled. In 2015, 9 master's awarded. Terminal master's awarded for partial completion of doctoral program. *Degree requirements:* For master's, thesis or alternative; for doctorate, comprehensive exam, thesis/dissertation. *Entrance requirements:* For master's, GRE General Test, minimum GPA of 3.0; for doctorate,

GRE General Test. Additional exam requirements/recommendations for international students: Required—TOEFL (minimum score 550 paper-based; 84 iBT). *Application deadline:* For fall admission, 1/15 priority date for domestic and international students; for spring admission, 10/1 for domestic and international students. Applications are processed on a rolling basis. Application fee: $80. Electronic applications accepted. *Expenses:* $1,537 per credit. *Financial support:* In 2015–16, 9 students received support, including 2 research assistantships with full tuition reimbursements available (averaging $21,000 per year); career-related internships or fieldwork, Federal Work-Study, institutionally sponsored loans, and scholarships/grants also available. Support available to part-time students. Financial award application deadline: 2/15; financial award applicants required to submit FAFSA. *Faculty research:* Skeletal muscle, neural systems, smooth muscle, muscular dystrophy. Total annual research expenditures: $1.9 million. *Unit head:* Dr. Paula Quatromoni, Chair, 617-353-5797, Fax: 617-353-7567, E-mail: paulaq@bu.edu. *Application contact:* Sharon Sankey, Director, Student Services, 617-353-2713, Fax: 617-353-7500, E-mail: ssankey@bu.edu.

Boston University, School of Medicine, Division of Graduate Medical Sciences, Department of Physiology and Biophysics, Boston, MA 02118. Offers MA, PhD, MD/PhD. *Program availability:* Part-time. Terminal master's awarded for partial completion of doctoral program. *Degree requirements:* For master's, thesis; for doctorate, thesis/dissertation. *Application deadline:* For fall admission, 1/15 for domestic students; for spring admission, 10/15 for domestic students. *Faculty research:* X-ray scattering, NMR spectroscopy, protein crystallography, structural electron. *Unit head:* Dr. David Atkinson, Chairman, 617-638-4015, Fax: 617-638-4041, E-mail: atkinson@bu.edu. *Application contact:* GMS Admissions Office, 617-638-5255, E-mail: askgms@bu.edu. Website: http://www.bumc.bu.edu/phys-biophys/

Brigham Young University, Graduate Studies, College of Life Sciences, Department of Physiology and Developmental Biology, Provo, UT 84602. Offers neuroscience (MS, PhD); physiology and developmental biology (MS, PhD). *Program availability:* Part-time. *Faculty:* 20 full-time (1 woman), 4 part-time/adjunct (3 women). *Students:* 33 full-time (20 women); includes 6 minority (1 American Indian or Alaska Native, non-Hispanic/Latino; 3 Asian, non-Hispanic/Latino; 1 Hispanic/Latino; 1 Two or more races, non-Hispanic/Latino). Average age 29. 17 applicants, 29% accepted, 5 enrolled. In 2015, 6 master's, 3 doctorates awarded. Terminal master's awarded for partial completion of doctoral program. *Degree requirements:* For master's, thesis, oral exam; for doctorate, comprehensive exam, thesis/dissertation. *Entrance requirements:* For master's, GRE General Test, minimum GPA of 3.0 during previous 2 years; for doctorate, GRE General Test, minimum GPA of 3.0 overall. Additional exam requirements/recommendations for international students: Required—TOEFL (minimum score 580 paper-based; 85 iBT); Recommended—IELTS. *Application deadline:* For fall admission, 2/1 priority date for domestic and international students; for winter admission, 9/10 priority date for domestic and international students. Application fee: $50. Electronic applications accepted. *Financial support:* In 2015–16, 37 students received support, including 2 fellowships with partial tuition reimbursements available (averaging $7,100 per year), 17 research assistantships with full tuition reimbursements available (averaging $15,500 per year), 18 teaching assistantships with partial tuition reimbursements available (averaging $14,900 per year); career-related internships or fieldwork, institutionally sponsored loans, scholarships/grants, tuition waivers (full and partial), unspecified assistantships, and tuition awards also available. Financial award application deadline: 2/1. *Faculty research:* Sex differentiation of the brain, exercise physiology, developmental biology, membrane biophysics, neuroscience, heart differentiation/birth defects. Total annual research expenditures: $747,261. *Unit head:* Dr. Dixon J. Woodbury, Chair, 801-422-7562, Fax: 801-422-0004, E-mail: dixon_woodbury@byu.edu. *Application contact:* Connie L. Provost, Graduate Program Administrator, 801-422-3706, Fax: 801-422-0004, E-mail: connie_provost@byu.edu. Website: http://pdbio.byu.edu

Brown University, Graduate School, Division of Biology and Medicine, Department of Molecular Pharmacology, Physiology and Biotechnology, Providence, RI 02912. Offers biomedical engineering (Sc M, PhD); biotechnology (PhD); molecular pharmacology and physiology (PhD); MD/PhD. *Degree requirements:* For doctorate, thesis/dissertation, preliminary exam. *Entrance requirements:* For master's and doctorate, GRE General Test, GRE Subject Test. Additional exam requirements/recommendations for international students: Required—TOEFL. Electronic applications accepted. *Faculty research:* Structural biology, antiplatelet drugs, nicotinic receptor structure/function.

Case Western Reserve University, School of Medicine and School of Graduate Studies, Graduate Programs in Medicine, Department of Physiology and Biophysics, Cleveland, OH 44106. Offers cell and molecular physiology (MS); cell physiology (PhD); molecular/cellular biophysics (PhD); physiology and biophysics (PhD); systems physiology (PhD); MD/PhD. Terminal master's awarded for partial completion of doctoral program. *Degree requirements:* For master's, thesis; for doctorate, thesis/dissertation. *Entrance requirements:* For master's, GRE General Test, minimum GPA of 3.28; for doctorate, GRE General Test, minimum GPA of 3.6. Additional exam requirements/recommendations for international students: Required—TOEFL. Electronic applications accepted. *Expenses: Tuition, area resident:* Full-time $41,137; part-time $1714 per credit hour. *Required fees:* $32. Tuition and fees vary according to course load and program. *Faculty research:* Cardiovascular physiology, calcium metabolism, epithelial cell biology.

Columbia University, College of Physicians and Surgeons, Department of Physiology and Cellular Biophysics, New York, NY 10032. Offers M Phil, MA, PhD, MD/PhD. Only candidates for the PhD are admitted. Terminal master's awarded for partial completion of doctoral program. *Degree requirements:* For doctorate, thesis/dissertation. *Entrance requirements:* For master's and doctorate, GRE General Test. Additional exam requirements/recommendations for international students: Required—TOEFL. *Faculty research:* Membrane physiology, cellular biology, cardiovascular physiology, neurophysiology.

Cornell University, Graduate School, Graduate Fields of Agriculture and Life Sciences, Field of Horticulture, Ithaca, NY 14853-0001. Offers breeding of horticultural crops (MPS); horticultural crop management systems (MPS); human-plant interactions (MPS, PhD); physiology and ecology of horticultural crops (MPS, MS, PhD). *Degree requirements:* For master's, thesis (MS); for doctorate, comprehensive exam, thesis/dissertation. *Entrance requirements:* For master's and doctorate, GRE General Test, 3 letters of recommendation. Additional exam requirements/recommendations for international students: Required—TOEFL (minimum score 550 paper-based; 77 iBT). Electronic applications accepted. *Faculty research:* Plant selection/plant materials, greenhouse management, greenhouse crop production, urban landscape management, turfgrass management.

Cornell University, Graduate School, Graduate Fields of Comparative Biomedical Sciences, Field of Molecular and Integrative Physiology, Ithaca, NY 14853-0001. Offers behavioral physiology (MS, PhD); cardiovascular and respiratory physiology (MS, PhD); endocrinology (MS, PhD); environmental and comparative physiology (MS, PhD); gastrointestinal and metabolic physiology (MS, PhD); membrane and epithelial physiology (MS, PhD); molecular and cellular physiology (MS, PhD); neural and sensory physiology (MS, PhD); physiological genomics (MS, PhD); reproductive physiology (MS, PhD). *Degree requirements:* For master's, thesis; for doctorate, comprehensive exam, thesis/dissertation, 1 semester of teaching experience, seminar presentation. *Entrance requirements:* For master's and doctorate, GRE General Test, GRE Subject Test (biochemistry, cell and molecular biology, biology, or chemistry), 2 letters of recommendation. Additional exam requirements/recommendations for international students: Required—TOEFL (minimum score 550 paper-based; 77 iBT). Electronic applications accepted. *Faculty research:* Endocrinology and reproductive physiology, cardiovascular and respiratory physiology, gastrointestinal and metabolic physiology, molecular and cellular physiology, physiological genomics.

Dalhousie University, Faculty of Agriculture, Halifax, NS B3H 4R2, Canada. Offers agriculture (M Sc), including air quality, animal behavior, animal molecular genetics, animal nutrition, animal technology, aquaculture, botany, crop management, crop physiology, ecology, environmental microbiology, food science, horticulture, nutrient management, pest management, physiology, plant biotechnology, plant pathology, soil chemistry, soil fertility, waste management and composting, water quality. *Program availability:* Part-time. *Degree requirements:* For master's, thesis, ATC Exam Teaching Assistantship. *Entrance requirements:* For master's, honors B Sc, minimum GPA of 3.0. Additional exam requirements/recommendations for international students: Required—TOEFL (minimum score 580 paper-based; 92 iBT), IELTS, Michigan English Language Assessment Battery, CanTEST, CAEL. *Faculty research:* Bio-product development, organic agriculture, nutrient management, air and water quality, agricultural biotechnology.

Dalhousie University, Faculty of Medicine, Department of Physiology and Biophysics, Halifax, NS B3H 1X5, Canada. Offers M Sc, PhD, M Sc/PhD. *Degree requirements:* For master's, thesis; for doctorate, thesis/dissertation. *Entrance requirements:* For master's and doctorate, GRE Subject Test (for international students). Additional exam requirements/recommendations for international students: Required—1 of 5 approved tests: TOEFL, IELTS, CANTEST, CAEL, Michigan English Language Assessment Battery. Electronic applications accepted. *Faculty research:* Computer modeling, reproductive and endocrine physiology, cardiovascular physiology, neurophysiology, membrane biophysics.

East Carolina University, Brody School of Medicine, Department of Physiology, Greenville, NC 27858-4353. Offers PhD. *Students:* 17 full-time (5 women), 1 part-time (0 women); includes 2 minority (1 Hispanic/Latino; 1 Two or more races, non-Hispanic/Latino), 2 international. Average age 30. 12 applicants, 75% accepted, 8 enrolled. *Degree requirements:* For doctorate, comprehensive exam, thesis/dissertation. *Entrance requirements:* For doctorate, GRE General Test. Additional exam requirements/recommendations for international students: Required—TOEFL. *Application deadline:* For fall admission, 6/1 priority date for domestic students. Applications are processed on a rolling basis. Application fee: $50. *Financial support:* Fellowships with tuition reimbursements available. Financial award application deadline: 6/1. *Faculty research:* Cell and nerve biophysics; neurophysiology; cardiovascular, renal, endocrine, and gastrointestinal physiology; pulmonary/asthma. *Unit head:* Dr. Robert Lust, Chairman, 252-744-2762, Fax: 252-744-3460, E-mail: lustr@ecu.edu. *Application contact:* 252-744-2804.
Website: http://www.ecu.edu/physiology/

Eastern Michigan University, Graduate School, College of Health and Human Services, School of Health Promotion and Human Performance, Programs in Exercise Physiology, Ypsilanti, MI 48197. Offers exercise physiology (MS); sports medicine-biomechanics (MS); sports medicine-corporate adult fitness (MS); sports medicine-exercise physiology (MS). *Program availability:* Part-time, evening/weekend. *Students:* 10 full-time (8 women), 32 part-time (15 women); includes 6 minority (3 Black or African American, non-Hispanic/Latino; 1 Asian, non-Hispanic/Latino; 2 Two or more races, non-Hispanic/Latino), 3 international. Average age 32. 42 applicants, 67% accepted, 15 enrolled. In 2015, 27 master's awarded. *Degree requirements:* For master's, comprehensive exam, thesis or 450-hour internship. *Entrance requirements:* Additional exam requirements/recommendations for international students: Required—TOEFL.

Application deadline: For fall admission, 8/1 for domestic students, 5/1 for international students; for winter admission, 12/1 for domestic students, 10/1 for international students; for spring admission, 3/15 for domestic students, 3/1 for international students. Application fee: $45. *Application contact:* Dr. Stephen McGregor, Program Coordinator, 734-487-0090, Fax: 734-487-2024, E-mail: smcgregor@emich.edu.

East Stroudsburg University of Pennsylvania, Graduate College, College of Health Sciences, Department of Exercise Science, East Stroudsburg, PA 18301-2999. Offers clinical exercise physiology (MS); exercise science (MS). *Program availability:* Part-time, evening/weekend, online learning. *Faculty:* 2 full-time. *Degree requirements:* For master's, comprehensive exam, thesis or alternative, computer literacy. *Entrance requirements:* Additional exam requirements/recommendations for international students: Required—TOEFL (minimum score 560 paper-based; 83 iBT) or IELTS. *Application deadline:* For fall admission, 3/1 priority date for domestic and international students; for spring admission, 11/30 for domestic students, 10/31 for international students. Applications are processed on a rolling basis. Application fee: $50. Electronic applications accepted. *Expenses: Tuition, area resident:* Full-time $8460; part-time $5640 per year. Tuition, state resident: full-time $8460; part-time $5640 per year. Tuition, nonresident: full-time $12,690; part-time $8460 per year. *International tuition:* $15,368 full-time. *Required fees:* $2462; $1630 per unit. $815 per semester. Tuition and fees vary according to course load, campus/location and program. *Financial support:* Research assistantships with tuition reimbursements, Federal Work-Study, and institutionally sponsored loans available. Financial award application deadline: 3/1. *Unit head:* Dr. Shala Davis, Chair, 570-422-3302, Fax: 570-422-3616, E-mail: sdavis@esu.edu. *Application contact:* Dr. Chad Witmer, Graduate Coordinator, 570-422-3536, Fax: 570-422-2711, E-mail: cwitmer@esu.edu.

East Tennessee State University, James H. Quillen College of Medicine, Department of Biomedical Sciences, Johnson City, TN 37614. Offers anatomy (PhD); biochemistry (PhD); microbiology (PhD); pharmaceutical sciences (PhD); pharmacology (PhD); physiology (PhD); quantitative biosciences (PhD). *Faculty:* 30 full-time (6 women). *Students:* 35 full-time (17 women), 2 part-time (1 woman); includes 13 minority (9 Black or African American, non-Hispanic/Latino; 4 Asian, non-Hispanic/Latino), 13 international. Average age 29. 53 applicants, 17% accepted, 8 enrolled. In 2015, 8 doctorates awarded. *Degree requirements:* For doctorate, thesis/dissertation, comprehensive qualifying exam. *Entrance requirements:* For doctorate, GRE General Test, GRE Subject Test, 3 letters of recommendation. Additional exam requirements/recommendations for international students: Required—TOEFL (minimum score 550 paper-based; 79 iBT). *Application deadline:* For fall admission, 3/15 priority date for domestic students, 3/1 priority date for international students. Application fee: $35 ($45 for international students). Electronic applications accepted. *Expenses:* Contact institution. *Financial support:* In 2015-16, 30 students received support, including 27 research assistantships with full tuition reimbursements available (averaging $20,000 per year); career-related internships or fieldwork, institutionally sponsored loans, scholarships/grants, and unspecified assistantships also available. Financial award application deadline: 7/1; financial award applicants required to submit FAFSA. *Faculty research:* Cardiovascular, infectious disease, neurosciences, cancer, immunology. *Unit head:* Dr. Mitchell E. Robinson, Associate Dean/Program Director, 423-439-2031, Fax: 423-439-2140, E-mail: robinson@etsu.edu. *Application contact:* Shella Bennett, Graduate Specialist, 423-439-4708, Fax: 423-439-5624, E-mail: bennetsg@etsu.edu. Website: http://www.etsu.edu/com/dbms/

Georgetown University, Graduate School of Arts and Sciences, Department of Pharmacology and Physiology, Washington, DC 20057. Offers pharmacology (MS, PhD); physiology (MS); MD/PhD. *Degree requirements:* For doctorate, comprehensive exam, thesis/dissertation. *Entrance requirements:* For doctorate, GRE General Test, previous course work in biology and chemistry. Additional exam requirements/recommendations for international students: Required—TOEFL. *Faculty research:* Neuropharmacology, techniques in biochemistry and tissue culture.

Georgia Institute of Technology, Graduate Studies, College of Sciences, School of Biological Sciences, Program in Applied Physiology, Atlanta, GA 30332-0001. Offers PhD. *Degree requirements:* For doctorate, comprehensive exam, thesis/dissertation. *Entrance requirements:* For doctorate, GRE. Additional exam requirements/recommendations for international students: Required—TOEFL (minimum score 550 paper-based; 79 iBT). *Application deadline:* For fall admission, 2/1 for domestic and international students. Applications are processed on a rolling basis. Application fee: $75. Electronic applications accepted. *Financial support:* Fellowships, research assistantships, teaching assistantships, career-related internships or fieldwork, Federal Work-Study, institutionally sponsored loans, tuition waivers (partial), and unspecified assistantships available. Support available to part-time students. Financial award application deadline: 5/1.
Website: http://www.ap.gatech.edu/academic/PhD/

Georgia Institute of Technology, Graduate Studies, College of Sciences, School of Biological Sciences, Program in Prosthetics and Orthotics, Atlanta, GA 30332-0001. Offers MS. Terminal master's awarded for partial completion of doctoral program. *Degree requirements:* For master's, capstone research project plus minimum 500 contact hours of clinical practicum in medicine, prosthetics and orthotics, and pedorthics combined. *Entrance requirements:* For master's, GRE. Additional exam requirements/recommendations for international students: Required—TOEFL (minimum score 550 paper-based; 79 iBT). *Application deadline:* For fall admission, 1/15 priority date for domestic and international students. Applications are processed on a rolling basis. Application fee: $75. Electronic applications accepted. *Expenses:* Contact institution. *Financial support:* Fellowships, research assistantships, teaching assistantships, career-related internships or fieldwork, Federal Work-Study, institutionally sponsored loans, tuition waivers (partial), and unspecified assistantships available. Support available to part-time students. Financial award application deadline: 5/1.
Website: http://www.ap.gatech.edu/mspo

Georgia State University, College of Arts and Sciences, Department of Biology, Program in Cellular and Molecular Biology and Physiology, Atlanta, GA 30302-3083. Offers bioinformatics (MS); cellular and molecular biology and physiology (MS, PhD). *Program availability:* Part-time. Terminal master's awarded for partial completion of doctoral program. *Degree requirements:* For master's, comprehensive exam (for some programs), thesis optional; for doctorate, comprehensive exam, thesis/dissertation. *Entrance requirements:* For master's and doctorate, GRE. Additional exam requirements/recommendations for international students: Required—TOEFL (minimum score 550 paper-based; 82 iBT) or IELTS (minimum score 7). *Application deadline:* For fall admission, 7/1 priority date for domestic students, 6/1 priority date for international students; for spring admission, 11/15 priority date for domestic students, 10/15 priority date for international students. Applications are processed on a rolling basis. Application fee: $50. Electronic applications accepted. *Expenses:* Tuition, state resident: full-time $6876; part-time $382 per credit hour. Tuition, nonresident: full-time $22,374; part-time $1243 per credit hour. *Required fees:* $2128; $2128 per term. $1064 per term. Part-time tuition and fees vary according to course load and program. *Financial support:* In 2015-16, fellowships with full tuition reimbursements (averaging $22,000 per year), research assistantships with full tuition reimbursements (averaging $20,000 per year) were awarded. Financial award application deadline: 12/3. *Faculty research:* Membrane

Physiology

transport, viral infection, molecular immunology, protein modeling, gene regulation. *Unit head:* Dr. Charles Derby, Director of Graduate Studies, 404-413-5393, Fax: 404-413-5446, E-mail: cderby@gsu.edu. *Website:* http://biology.gsu.edu/

Gonzaga University, School of Nursing and Human Physiology, Spokane, WA 99258. Offers MSN, DNP, DNP-A. *Accreditation:* AACN. *Program availability:* Part-time, evening/weekend, online learning. *Faculty:* 16 full-time (14 women), 23 part-time/adjunct (18 women). *Students:* 36 full-time (22 women), 705 part-time (590 women); includes 123 minority (19 Black or African American, non-Hispanic/Latino; 6 American Indian or Alaska Native, non-Hispanic/Latino; 26 Asian, non-Hispanic/Latino; 34 Hispanic/Latino; 7 Native Hawaiian or other Pacific Islander, non-Hispanic/Latino; 31 Two or more races, non-Hispanic/Latino), 2 international. Average age 38. *Entrance requirements:* For master's, MAT, minimum B average in undergraduate course work; for doctorate, MAT or GRE within the last 5 years, curriculum vitae, personal statement, three letters of recommendation, official transcripts, copy of current RN license, practicum hours. Additional exam requirements/recommendations for international students: Required—TOEFL. *Application deadline:* For fall admission, 7/20 priority date for domestic students; for spring admission, 11/1 for domestic students. Applications are processed on a rolling basis. Application fee: $50. Electronic applications accepted. *Expenses:* Contact institution. *Financial support:* Application deadline: 2/1; applicants required to submit FAFSA. *Unit head:* Dr. Brenda Stevenson Marshall, Dean, 509-313-3569, E-mail: stevenson-marshall@gonzaga.edu. *Application contact:* Shannon Zaranski, Assistant to the Dean, 509-313-3569, E-mail: zaranski@gu.gonzaga.edu. *Website:* http://www.gonzaga.edu/Academics/Colleges-and-Schools/School-of-Nursing-Human-Physiology

Harvard University, Graduate School of Arts and Sciences, Department of Systems Biology, Cambridge, MA 02138. Offers PhD. *Degree requirements:* For doctorate, thesis/dissertation, lab rotation, qualifying examination. *Entrance requirements:* For doctorate, GRE. Additional exam requirements/recommendations for international students: Required—TOEFL. Electronic applications accepted.

Harvard University, Harvard T.H. Chan School of Public Health, Department of Environmental Health, Boston, MA 02115-6096. Offers environmental health (SM, PhD, SD); exposure, epidemiology, and risk (SM, SD); occupational health (SM, SD); physiology (PhD, SD). *Program availability:* Part-time. *Faculty:* 44 full-time (10 women), 20 part-time/adjunct (5 women). *Students:* 79 full-time (49 women); includes 11 minority (1 Black or African American, non-Hispanic/Latino; 6 Asian, non-Hispanic/Latino; 3 Hispanic/Latino; 1 Two or more races, non-Hispanic/Latino), 45 international. Average age 28. 126 applicants, 35% accepted, 34 enrolled. In 2015, 20 master's, 12 doctorates awarded. *Degree requirements:* For doctorate, thesis/dissertation, qualifying exam. *Entrance requirements:* For master's, GRE, MCAT; for doctorate, GRE. Additional exam requirements/recommendations for international students: Recommended—TOEFL (minimum score 600 paper-based; 100 iBT), IELTS (minimum score 7). *Application deadline:* For fall admission, 12/15 for domestic and international students. Application fee: $120. Electronic applications accepted. *Financial support:* Fellowships, research assistantships, teaching assistantships, career-related internships or fieldwork, Federal Work-Study, scholarships/grants, traineeships, and unspecified assistantships available. Support available to part-time students. Financial award application deadline: 2/15; financial award applicants required to submit FAFSA. *Faculty research:* Exposure assessment, epidemiology, risk assessment, environmental epidemiology, ergonomics and safety, environmental exposure assessment, occupational hygiene, industrial hygiene and occupational safety, population genetics, indoor and outdoor air pollution, cell and molecular biology of the lungs, infectious diseases. *Unit head:* Dr. Douglas Dockery, Chairman, 617-432-1270, Fax: 617-432-6913. *Application contact:* Vincent W. James, Director of Admissions, 617-432-1031, Fax: 617-432-7080, E-mail: admissions@hsph.harvard.edu. *Website:* http://www.hsph.harvard.edu/environmental-health/

Howard University, Graduate School, Department of Physiology and Biophysics, Washington, DC 20059-0002. Offers biophysics (PhD); physiology (PhD). *Degree requirements:* For doctorate, comprehensive exam, thesis/dissertation. *Entrance requirements:* For doctorate, GRE General Test, minimum B average in field. *Faculty research:* Cardiovascular physiology, pulmonary physiology, renal physiology, neurophysiology, endocrinology.

Illinois State University, Graduate School, College of Arts and Sciences, Department of Biological Sciences, Normal, IL 61790-2200. Offers animal behavior (MS); bacteriology (MS); biochemistry (MS); biological sciences (MS); biology (PhD); biophysics (MS); biotechnology (MS); botany (MS, PhD); cell biology (MS); conservation biology (MS); developmental biology (MS); ecology (MS, PhD); entomology (MS); evolutionary biology (MS); genetics (MS, PhD); immunology (MS); microbiology (MS, PhD); molecular biology (MS); molecular genetics (MS); neurobiology (MS); neuroscience (MS); parasitology (MS); physiology (MS, PhD); plant biology (MS); plant molecular biology (MS); plant sciences (MS); structural biology (MS); zoology (MS, PhD). *Program availability:* Part-time. *Degree requirements:* For master's, thesis or alternative; for doctorate, variable foreign language requirement, thesis/dissertation, 2 terms of residency. *Entrance requirements:* For master's, GRE General Test, minimum GPA of 2.6 in last 60 hours of course work; for doctorate, GRE General Test. *Application deadline:* Applications are processed on a rolling basis. Application fee: $40. *Financial support:* Research assistantships, teaching assistantships, Federal Work-Study, tuition waivers (full), and unspecified assistantships available. Financial award application deadline: 4/1. *Faculty research:* Redoc balance and drug development in schistosoma mansoni, control of the growth of listeria monocytogenes at low temperature, regulation of cell expansion and microtubule function by SPRI, CRUI: physiology and fitness consequences of different life history phenotypes. *Application contact:* Steven Juliano, Graduate Coordinator, E-mail: sajulian@ilstu.edu. *Website:* http://www.bio.ilstu.edu/

Indiana State University, College of Graduate and Professional Studies, College of Arts and Sciences, Department of Biology, Terre Haute, IN 47809. Offers cellular and molecular biology (PhD); ecology, systematics and evolution (PhD); life sciences (MS); physiology (PhD); science education (MS). *Degree requirements:* For master's, thesis optional; for doctorate, comprehensive exam, thesis/dissertation. *Entrance requirements:* For master's and doctorate, GRE General Test. Electronic applications accepted.

James Madison University, The Graduate School, College of Health and Behavioral Sciences, Program in Kinesiology, Harrisonburg, VA 22807. Offers clinical exercise physiology (MS); exercise physiology (MS); kinesiology (MAT, MS); nutrition and exercise (MS); physical and health education (MAT); sport and recreation leadership (MS). *Program availability:* Part-time, evening/weekend. *Faculty:* 9 full-time (3 women), 2 part-time/adjunct (1 woman). *Students:* 64 full-time (32 women), 7 part-time (3 women); includes 6 minority (2 Black or African American, non-Hispanic/Latino; 1 Asian, non-Hispanic/Latino; 3 Two or more races, non-Hispanic/Latino), 1 international. Average age 30. 140 applicants, 70% accepted, 44 enrolled. In 2015, 43 master's awarded. Application fee: $55. Electronic applications accepted. *Financial support:* In 2015–16, 44 students received support, including 14 teaching assistantships with full tuition reimbursements available (averaging $8,837 per year); Federal Work-Study,

unspecified assistantships, and athletic assistantships (averaging $8837); service assistantships (averaging $7530), assistantships (averaging $7530) also available. Financial award application deadline: 3/1; financial award applicants required to submit FAFSA. *Unit head:* Dr. Christopher J. Womack, Department Head, 540-568-6145, E-mail: womackcx@jmu.edu. *Application contact:* Lynette D. Michael, Director of Graduate Admissions, 540-568-6131 Ext. 6395, Fax: 540-568-7860, E-mail: michaeld@jmu.edu. *Website:* http://www.jmu.edu/kinesiology/

Johns Hopkins University, Bloomberg School of Public Health, Department of Environmental Health Sciences, Baltimore, MD 21218. Offers environmental health engineering (PhD); environmental health sciences (MHS, Dr PH); occupational and environmental health (PhD); physiology (PhD); toxicology (PhD). *Program availability:* Online learning. *Degree requirements:* For master's, essay, presentation; for doctorate, comprehensive exam, thesis/dissertation, 1-year full-time residency, oral and written exams. *Entrance requirements:* For master's, GRE General Test or MCAT, 3 letters of recommendation, transcripts; for doctorate, GRE General Test or MCAT, 3 letters of recommendation. Additional exam requirements/recommendations for international students: Required—TOEFL (minimum score 600 paper-based). Electronic applications accepted. *Faculty research:* Chemical carcinogenesis/toxicology, lung disease, occupational and environmental health, nuclear imaging, molecular epidemiology.

Johns Hopkins University, School of Medicine, Graduate Programs in Medicine, Department of Physiology, Baltimore, MD 21205. Offers cellular and molecular physiology (PhD); physiology (PhD). *Degree requirements:* For doctorate, thesis/dissertation, oral and qualifying exams. *Entrance requirements:* For doctorate, GRE General Test, previous course work in biology, calculus, chemistry, and physics. Additional exam requirements/recommendations for international students: Required—TOEFL. Electronic applications accepted. *Faculty research:* Membrane biochemistry and biophysics; signal transduction; developmental genetics and physiology; physiology and biochemistry; transporters, carriers, and ion channels.

Kansas State University, Graduate School, College of Veterinary Medicine, Department of Anatomy and Physiology, Manhattan, KS 66506. Offers physiology (PhD). Terminal master's awarded for partial completion of doctoral program. *Entrance requirements:* For doctorate, GRE. Additional exam requirements/recommendations for international students: Required—TOEFL. Electronic applications accepted. *Faculty research:* Cardiovascular and pulmonary, immunophysiology, neuroscience, pharmacology, epithelial.

Kent State University, College of Arts and Sciences, Department of Biological Sciences, Kent, OH 44242-0001. Offers biological sciences (MS, PhD), including ecology, physiology. *Program availability:* Part-time. *Faculty:* 37 full-time (12 women). *Students:* 52 full-time (33 women), 15 part-time (9 women); includes 7 minority (3 Black or African American, non-Hispanic/Latino; 2 Asian, non-Hispanic/Latino; 2 Two or more races, non-Hispanic/Latino), 20 international. Average age 30. 142 applicants, 27% accepted, 24 enrolled. In 2015, 15 master's, 9 doctorates awarded. *Degree requirements:* For master's, thesis (for some programs); for doctorate, thesis/dissertation. *Entrance requirements:* For master's and doctorate, GRE General Test, minimum GPA of 3.0, transcript, resume, statement of purpose, 3 letters of recommendation. Additional exam requirements/recommendations for international students: Required—TOEFL (minimum score: paper-based 525, iBT 71), Michigan English Language Assessment Battery (minimum score of 75), IELTS (minimum score of 6.0), PTE Academic (minimum score of 48), or completion of ELS level 112 Intensive Program. *Application deadline:* For fall admission, 12/15 for domestic students, 12/5 for international students; for spring admission, 11/29 for domestic and international students. Application fee: $45 ($70 for international students). Electronic applications accepted. *Expenses:* Tuition, state resident: full-time $10,864; part-time $495 per credit hour. Tuition, nonresident: full-time $18,380; part-time $837 per credit hour. *Financial support:* Research assistantships with full tuition reimbursements, teaching assistantships with full tuition reimbursements, career-related internships or fieldwork, Federal Work-Study, scholarships/grants, and unspecified assistantships available. Financial award application deadline: 2/1. *Unit head:* Dr. James L. Blank, Dean, 330-672-2650, E-mail: jblank@kent.edu. *Application contact:* Dr. Heather K. Caldwell, Associate Professor and Graduate Coordinator, 330-672-3636, E-mail: hcaldwel@kent.edu. *Website:* http://www.kent.edu/biology/

Kent State University, College of Arts and Sciences, School of Biomedical Sciences, Kent, OH 44242-0001. Offers biological anthropology (PhD); cellular and molecular biology (PhD), including cellular biology and structures, molecular biology and genetics; neurosciences (PhD); pharmacology (MS); physiology (PhD). *Students:* 76 full-time (46 women), 1 (woman) part-time; includes 6 minority (1 Black or African American, non-Hispanic/Latino; 2 Asian, non-Hispanic/Latino; 1 Hispanic/Latino; 2 Two or more races, non-Hispanic/Latino), 28 international. Average age 29. 223 applicants, 13% accepted, 22 enrolled. In 2015, 5 master's, 7 doctorates awarded. Terminal master's awarded for partial completion of doctoral program. *Degree requirements:* For master's, thesis; for doctorate, thesis/dissertation, candidacy exam. *Entrance requirements:* For master's and doctorate, GRE General Test, minimum GPA of 3.0, transcript, goal statement, resume, 3 letters of recommendation. Additional exam requirements/recommendations for international students: Required—TOEFL (minimum score: paper-based 525, iBT 71), Michigan English Language Assessment Battery (minimum score of 75), IELTS (minimum score of 6.0), PTE Academic (minimum score of 48), or completion of ELS level 112 Intensive Program. *Application deadline:* For fall admission, 1/1 for domestic students. Application fee: $45 ($70 for international students). Electronic applications accepted. *Expenses:* Tuition, state resident: full-time $10,864; part-time $495 per credit hour. Tuition, nonresident: full-time $18,380; part-time $837 per credit hour. *Financial support:* In 2015–16, 76 students received support. Research assistantships with full tuition reimbursements available, teaching assistantships, career-related internships or fieldwork, Federal Work-Study, and unspecified assistantships available. Financial award application deadline: 1/1. *Unit head:* Dr. Eric Mintz, Director, 330-672-2263, E-mail: emintz@kent.edu. *Application contact:* 330-672-2263, Fax: 330-672-9391, E-mail: jwearden@kent.edu. *Website:* http://www.kent.edu/biomedical/

Loma Linda University, School of Medicine, Programs in Physiology and Pharmacology, Loma Linda, CA 92350. Offers pharmacology (PhD); physiology (PhD). *Program availability:* Part-time. *Degree requirements:* For doctorate, 2 foreign languages, thesis/dissertation. *Entrance requirements:* For doctorate, GRE General Test. *Application deadline:* Applications are processed on a rolling basis. Application fee: $40. *Financial support:* Tuition waivers (full and partial) available. Support available to part-time students. *Faculty research:* Drug metabolism, biochemical pharmacology, structure and function of cell membranes, neuropharmacology. *Unit head:* Dr. John Buchholz, Vice Chair, 909-558-7026. *Application contact:* Admissions Office, 909-651-5029, Fax: 909-558-4879, E-mail: admissions.app@llu.edu.

Louisiana State University Health Sciences Center, School of Graduate Studies in New Orleans, Department of Physiology, New Orleans, LA 70112-2223. Offers PhD, MD/PhD. *Faculty:* 9 full-time (3 women). *Students:* 7 full-time (2 women); includes 1 minority (Asian, non-Hispanic/Latino). Average age 26. 3 applicants. In 2015, 1

doctorate awarded. *Degree requirements:* For doctorate, comprehensive exam, thesis/dissertation. *Entrance requirements:* For doctorate, GRE General Test. Additional exam requirements/recommendations for international students: Recommended—TOEFL, IELTS. *Application deadline:* For fall admission, 4/1 for domestic and international students. Applications are processed on a rolling basis. Application fee: $30. *Financial support:* Unspecified assistantships available. *Faculty research:* Host defense, lipoprotein metabolism, regulation of cardiopulmonary function, alcohol and drug abuse, cell to cell communication, cytokinesis, physiologic functions of nitric oxide. *Unit head:* Dr. Patricia Molina, Professor and Interim Head, 504-568-6171, Fax: 504-568-6158, E-mail: pmolin@lsuhsc.edu. *Application contact:* Dr. Scott Edwards, Graduate Coordinator and Professor, 504-568-2669, E-mail: sedwa5@lsuhsc.edu.
Website: http://www.medschool.lsuhsc.edu/physiology/

Louisiana State University Health Sciences Center at Shreveport, Department of Molecular and Cellular Physiology, Shreveport, LA 71130-3932. Offers physiology (MS, PhD); MD/PhD. *Faculty:* 8 full-time (4 women), 3 part-time/adjunct (1 woman). *Students:* 14 full-time (8 women); includes 8 minority (1 Black or African American, non-Hispanic/Latino; 7 Asian, non-Hispanic/Latino). Average age 29. 13 applicants, 46% accepted, 5 enrolled. In 2015, 1 master's, 1 doctorate awarded. *Degree requirements:* For master's, thesis; for doctorate, thesis/dissertation. *Entrance requirements:* For master's and doctorate, GRE General Test. Additional exam requirements/recommendations for international students: Required—TOEFL (minimum score 550 paper-based). *Application deadline:* For fall admission, 1/31 priority date for domestic and international students. Application fee: $0. *Expenses:* $6,467.25 resident tuition; $15,872 non-resident tuition; $410.50 student fees. *Financial support:* Fellowships with full tuition reimbursements, institutionally sponsored loans, and unspecified assistantships available. *Faculty research:* Cardiovascular, gastrointestinal, renal, and neutrophil function; cellular detoxification systems; hypoxia and mitochondria function. *Unit head:* Dr. D. Neil Granger, Head, 318-675-6011, Fax: 318-675-6005, E-mail: dgrang@lsuhsc.edu. *Application contact:* Deborah Fausto, Coordinator, 318-675-6011, Fax: 318-675-6005, E-mail: dfaust1@lsuhsc.edu.
Website: http://www.shreveportphysiology.com

Loyola University Chicago, Graduate School, Integrated Program in Biomedical Sciences, Maywood, IL 60153. Offers biochemistry and molecular biology (MS, PhD); cell and molecular physiology (PhD); infectious disease and immunology (MS); integrative cell biology (PhD); medical physiology (MS); microbiology and immunology (MS, PhD); molecular pharmacology and therapeutics (MS, PhD); neuroscience (MS, PhD). *Students:* 135 full-time (65 women), 1 part-time (0 women); includes 28 minority (5 Black or African American, non-Hispanic/Latino; 15 Asian, non-Hispanic/Latino; 6 Hispanic/Latino; 2 Two or more races, non-Hispanic/Latino), 16 international. Average age 28. 442 applicants, 23% accepted, 55 enrolled. In 2015, 40 master's, 17 doctorates awarded. *Expenses: Tuition, area resident:* Full-time $18,054; part-time $9027 per credit hour. *Required fees:* $832; $284 per credit hour. Part-time tuition and fees vary according to course load, degree level and program. *Unit head:* Dr. Samuel Attoh, Dean, 773-508-3459, Fax: 773-508-2460, E-mail: sattoh@luc.edu. *Application contact:* Ron Martin, Associate Director of Enrollment Management, 312-915-8950, Fax: 312-915-8905, E-mail: gradapp@luc.edu.
Website: http://ssom.luc.edu/graduate_school/degree-programs/ipbsphd/

Marquette University, Graduate School, College of Arts and Sciences, Department of Biology, Milwaukee, WI 53201-1881. Offers cell biology (MS, PhD); developmental biology (MS, PhD); ecology (MS, PhD); epithelial physiology (MS, PhD); genetics (MS, PhD); microbiology (MS, PhD); molecular biology (MS, PhD); muscle and exercise physiology (MS, PhD); neuroscience (MS, PhD). *Faculty:* 22 full-time (7 women), 3 part-time/adjunct (2 women). *Students:* 28 full-time (11 women), 12 part-time (4 women); includes 4 minority (1 Asian, non-Hispanic/Latino; 1 Hispanic/Latino; 2 Two or more races, non-Hispanic/Latino), 11 international. Average age 27. 72 applicants, 28% accepted, 5 enrolled. In 2015, 2 master's, 4 doctorates awarded. Terminal master's awarded for partial completion of doctoral program. *Degree requirements:* For master's, comprehensive exam, thesis, 1 year of teaching experience or equivalent; for doctorate, thesis/dissertation, 1 year of teaching experience or equivalent, qualifying exam. *Entrance requirements:* For master's and doctorate, GRE General Test, GRE Subject Test, official transcripts from all current and previous colleges/universities except Marquette, statement of professional goals and aspirations, three letters of recommendation. Additional exam requirements/recommendations for international students: Required—TOEFL (minimum score 530 paper-based). *Application deadline:* For fall admission, 12/15 for domestic and international students. Application fee: $50. Electronic applications accepted. *Financial support:* In 2015–16, 39 students received support, including 6 fellowships (averaging $1,208 per year), 4 research assistantships with full tuition reimbursements available (averaging $21,750 per year), 29 teaching assistantships with full tuition reimbursements available (averaging $21,750 per year); scholarships/grants, health care benefits, tuition waivers (full and partial), and unspecified assistantships also available. Support available to part-time students. Financial award application deadline: 2/15. *Faculty research:* Neurobiology, neuroendocrinology, epithelial physiology, neuropeptide interactions, synaptic transmission. *Total annual research expenditures:* $1.2 million. *Unit head:* Dr. Ed Blumenthal, Chair, 414-288-1748. *Application contact:* Dr. Michael Schlappi, Recruiting Contact, 414-288-1467.
Website: http://www.marquette.edu/biology/

McGill University, Faculty of Graduate and Postdoctoral Studies, Faculty of Medicine, Department of Physiology, Montréal, QC H3A 2T5, Canada. Offers M Sc, PhD.

McMaster University, Faculty of Health Sciences and School of Graduate Studies, Program in Medical Sciences, Physiology/Pharmacology Area, Hamilton, ON L8S 4M2, Canada. Offers M Sc, PhD, MD/PhD. *Degree requirements:* For master's, thesis; for doctorate, comprehensive exam, thesis/dissertation. *Entrance requirements:* For master's, honors B Sc, B+ average in related field; for doctorate, M Sc, minimum B+ average, students with proven research experience and an A average may be admitted with a B Sc degree. Additional exam requirements/recommendations for international students: Required—TOEFL (minimum score 580 paper-based; 92 iBT).

Medical College of Wisconsin, Graduate School of Biomedical Sciences, Department of Physiology, Milwaukee, WI 53226-0509. Offers PhD, MD/PhD. *Degree requirements:* For doctorate, comprehensive exam, thesis/dissertation. *Entrance requirements:* For doctorate, GRE, official transcripts, three letters of recommendation. Additional exam requirements/recommendations for international students: Required—TOEFL. *Faculty research:* Cardiovascular, respiratory, renal, and exercise physiology; mathematical modeling; molecular and cellular biology.

Michigan State University, College of Human Medicine and The Graduate School, Graduate Programs in Human Medicine, East Lansing, MI 48824. Offers biochemistry and molecular biology (MS, PhD); epidemiology (MS, PhD); microbiology (MS); microbiology and molecular genetics (PhD); pharmacology and toxicology (MS, PhD); physiology (MS, PhD); public health (MPH). *Entrance requirements:* Additional exam requirements/recommendations for international students: Required—TOEFL.

Michigan State University, College of Osteopathic Medicine and The Graduate School, Graduate Studies in Osteopathic Medicine, East Lansing, MI 48824. Offers

biochemistry and molecular biology (MS, PhD); microbiology (MS); microbiology and molecular genetics (PhD); pharmacology and toxicology (MS, PhD), including integrative pharmacology (MS), pharmacology and toxicology, pharmacology and toxicology-environmental toxicology (PhD); physiology (MS, PhD).

Michigan State University, College of Veterinary Medicine and The Graduate School, Graduate Programs in Veterinary Medicine, East Lansing, MI 48824. Offers comparative medicine and integrative biology (MS, PhD), including comparative medicine and integrative biology, comparative medicine and integrative biology–environmental toxicology (PhD); food safety and toxicology (MS), including food safety; integrative toxicology (PhD), including animal science–environmental toxicology, biochemistry and molecular biology–environmental toxicology, chemistry–environmental toxicology, crop and soil sciences–environmental toxicology, environmental engineering–environmental toxicology, environmental geosciences–environmental toxicology, fisheries and wildlife–environmental toxicology, food science–environmental toxicology, forestry–environmental toxicology, genetics–environmental toxicology, human nutrition–environmental toxicology, microbiology–environmental toxicology, pharmacology and toxicology–environmental toxicology, zoology–environmental toxicology; large animal clinical sciences (MS, PhD); microbiology and molecular genetics (MS, PhD), including industrial microbiology, microbiology, microbiology and molecular genetics, microbiology–environmental toxicology (PhD); pathobiology and diagnostic investigation (MS, PhD), including pathology, pathology–environmental toxicology (PhD); pharmacology and toxicology (MS, PhD); pharmacology and toxicology–environmental toxicology (PhD); physiology (MS, PhD); small animal clinical sciences (MS). Electronic applications accepted. *Faculty research:* Molecular genetics, food safety/toxicology, comparative orthopedics, airway disease, population medicine.

Michigan State University, The Graduate School, College of Natural Science and Graduate Programs in Human Medicine and Graduate Studies in Osteopathic Medicine, Department of Physiology, East Lansing, MI 48824. Offers MS, PhD. *Entrance requirements:* Additional exam requirements/recommendations for international students: Required—TOEFL (minimum score 600 paper-based). Electronic applications accepted.

Montclair State University, The Graduate School, College of Science and Mathematics, Program in Biology, Montclair, NJ 07043-1624. Offers biological science/education (MS); biology (MS); ecology and evolution (MS); physiology (MS). *Students:* 10 full-time (7 women), 35 part-time (27 women); includes 9 minority (6 Asian, non-Hispanic/Latino; 2 Hispanic/Latino; 1 Two or more races, non-Hispanic/Latino). Average age 28. 23 applicants, 57% accepted, 12 enrolled. In 2015, 18 master's awarded. *Expenses: Tuition, state resident:* part-time $553 per credit. *Tuition, nonresident:* part-time $854 per credit. *Required fees:* $91 per credit. Tuition and fees vary according to program. *Unit head:* Dr. Liza C. Hazard, Chairperson, 973-655-4397, E-mail: hazardl@mail.montclair.edu. *Application contact:* Amy Aiello, Director of Graduate Admissions and Operations, 973-655-5147, Fax: 973-655-7869, E-mail: graduate.school@montclair.edu.

New York Medical College, Graduate School of Basic Medical Sciences, Integrated PhD Program, Valhalla, NY 10595-1691. Offers biochemistry and molecular biology (PhD); cell biology and anatomy (PhD); microbiology and immunology (PhD); pathology (PhD); pharmacology (PhD); physiology (PhD). *Degree requirements:* For doctorate, comprehensive exam, thesis/dissertation. *Entrance requirements:* For doctorate, GRE General Test. Additional exam requirements/recommendations for international students: Required—TOEFL. Electronic applications accepted. *Expenses: Tuition, area resident:* Full-time $44,355; part-time $1025 per credit. *Required fees:* $500; $95 per year. One-time fee: $140 part-time. Tuition and fees vary according to course load and program. *Faculty research:* Cardiovascular sciences, infectious diseases, neuroscience, cancer and cell signaling.

New York Medical College, Graduate School of Basic Medical Sciences, Physiology - Master's Program, Valhalla, NY 10595-1691. Offers MS, MD/PhD. *Program availability:* Part-time, evening/weekend. *Degree requirements:* For master's, thesis. *Entrance requirements:* For master's, GRE General Test, DAT, or MCAT. Additional exam requirements/recommendations for international students: Required—TOEFL. Electronic applications accepted. *Expenses: Tuition, area resident:* Full-time $44,355; part-time $1025 per credit. *Required fees:* $500; $95 per year. One-time fee: $140 part-time. Tuition and fees vary according to course load and program. *Faculty research:* Cellular neurophysiology, regulation of sleep and awake states, neural and endocrine control of the heart and circulation microcirculation, the physiology of gene expression, heart failure and the physiological effects of oxygen metabolites.

New York University, School of Medicine and Graduate School of Arts and Science, Sackler Institute of Graduate Biomedical Sciences, Program in Neuroscience and Physiology, New York, NY 10012-1019. Offers PhD. *Degree requirements:* For doctorate, one foreign language, comprehensive exam, thesis/dissertation, qualifying exam. *Faculty research:* Rhythms in neural networks, genetic basis of neural circuit formation and function, behavior and memory formation in mouse models of neurodevelopmental disorders.

North Carolina State University, Graduate School, College of Agriculture and Life Sciences and College of Veterinary Medicine, Program in Physiology, Raleigh, NC 27695. Offers MP, MS, PhD. *Degree requirements:* For master's, thesis (for some programs); for doctorate, thesis/dissertation. *Entrance requirements:* For master's and doctorate, GRE General Test. Electronic applications accepted. *Faculty research:* Neurophysiology, gastrointestinal physiology, reproductive physiology, environmental/stress physiology, cardiovascular physiology.

Northwestern University, The Graduate School, Judd A. and Marjorie Weinberg College of Arts and Sciences, Department of Neurobiology, Evanston, IL 60208. Offers neurobiology and physiology (MS). Admissions and degrees offered through The Graduate School. *Program availability:* Part-time. *Degree requirements:* For master's, thesis. *Entrance requirements:* For master's, GRE General Test and MCAT (strongly recommended). Additional exam requirements/recommendations for international students: Required—TOEFL. Electronic applications accepted. *Expenses:* Contact institution. *Faculty research:* Sensory neurobiology and neuroendocrinology, reproductive biology, vision physiology and psychophysics, cell and developmental biology.

Ohio University, Graduate College, College of Arts and Sciences, Department of Biological Sciences, Athens, OH 45701-2979. Offers biological sciences (MS, PhD); cell biology and physiology (MS, PhD); ecology and evolutionary biology (MS, PhD); exercise physiology and muscle biology (MS, PhD); microbiology (MS, PhD); neuroscience (MS, PhD). Terminal master's awarded for partial completion of doctoral program. *Degree requirements:* For master's, comprehensive exam, thesis, 1 quarter of teaching experience; for doctorate, comprehensive exam, thesis/dissertation, 2 quarters of teaching experience. *Entrance requirements:* For master's, GRE General Test, names of three faculty members whose research interests most closely match the applicant's interest; for doctorate, GRE General Test, essay concerning prior training, research interest and career goals, plus names of three faculty members whose research interests most closely match the applicant's interest. Additional exam requirements/recommendations for international students: Required—TOEFL (minimum

Physiology

score 620 paper-based; 105 iBT) or IELTS (minimum score 7.5). Electronic applications accepted. *Faculty research:* Ecology and evolutionary biology, exercise physiology and muscle biology, neurobiology, cell biology, physiology.

Oregon Health & Science University, School of Medicine, Graduate Programs in Medicine, Program in Molecular and Cellular Biosciences, Department of Physiology and Pharmacology, Portland, OR 97239-3098. Offers PhD. *Faculty:* 15 full-time (5 women), 20 part-time/adjunct (7 women). *Students:* 9 full-time (6 women); includes 1 minority (Hispanic/Latino). Average age 27. *Degree requirements:* For doctorate, comprehensive exam, thesis/dissertation. *Entrance requirements:* For doctorate, GRE General Test (minimum scores: 153 Verbal/148 Quantitative/4.5 Analytical) or MCAT (for some programs). Additional exam requirements/recommendations for international students: Required—IELTS or TOEFL. *Application deadline:* For fall admission, 12/1 for domestic and international students. Application fee: $70. Electronic applications accepted. *Financial support:* Full tuition and stipends available. *Faculty research:* Ion conduction and gating in K+ channels, autonomic neuron plasticity, neurotransmitter/receptor expression, fetal/neonatal pharmacology, molecular pharmacology. *Unit head:* Dr. Robert Duvoisin, Program Director, 503-418-2665, E-mail: duvoisin@ohsu.edu. *Application contact:* Nermina Radaslic, Program Coordinator, 503-418-9462, E-mail: radaslic@ohsu.edu.

Penn State University Park, Graduate School, Intercollege Graduate Programs, Intercollege Graduate Program in Physiology, University Park, PA 16802. Offers physiology (MS, PhD). *Unit head:* Dr. Regina Vasilatos-Younken, Dean, 814-531-8567, Fax: 814-865-4627. *Application contact:* Lori Stania, Director, Graduate Student Services, 814-865-1795, Fax: 814-863-4627, E-mail: l-gsww@lists.psu.edu.

Purdue University, School of Veterinary Medicine and Graduate School, Graduate Programs in Veterinary Medicine, Department of Basic Medical Sciences, West Lafayette, IN 47907. Offers anatomy (MS, PhD); pharmacology (MS, PhD); physiology (MS, PhD). *Program availability:* Part-time. Terminal master's awarded for partial completion of doctoral program. *Degree requirements:* For master's, thesis; for doctorate, thesis/dissertation. *Entrance requirements:* For master's and doctorate, GRE General Test. Additional exam requirements/recommendations for international students: Required—TOEFL. Electronic applications accepted. *Faculty research:* Development and regeneration, tissue injury and shock, biomedical engineering, ovarian function, bone and cartilage biology, cell and molecular biology.

Queen's University at Kingston, School of Graduate Studies, Faculty of Health Sciences, Department of Physiology, Kingston, ON K7L 3N6, Canada. Offers M Sc, PhD. *Degree requirements:* For master's, thesis; for doctorate, comprehensive exam, thesis/dissertation. *Entrance requirements:* For master's, minimum upper B average. Additional exam requirements/recommendations for international students: Required—TOEFL. *Faculty research:* Cardiovascular and respiratory physiology, exercise, gastrointestinal physiology, neuroscience.

Rocky Mountain University of Health Professions, Doctor of Science Program in Clinical Electrophysiology, Provo, UT 84606. Offers D Sc. *Program availability:* Online learning. *Degree requirements:* For doctorate, thesis/dissertation. *Entrance requirements:* For doctorate, clinical entry-level master's or doctorate degree; professional licensure as a chiropractor, nurse practitioner, occupational therapist, physical therapist, physician or physician assistant; minimum of 100 hours experience in electroneuromyography.

Rosalind Franklin University of Medicine and Science, School of Graduate and Postdoctoral Studies - Interdisciplinary Graduate Program in Biomedical Sciences, Department of Physiology and Biophysics, North Chicago, IL 60064-3095. Offers MS, PhD, MD/PhD. Terminal master's awarded for partial completion of doctoral program. *Degree requirements:* For master's, comprehensive exam, thesis; for doctorate, comprehensive exam, thesis/dissertation. *Entrance requirements:* For master's and doctorate, GRE General Test. Additional exam requirements/recommendations for international students: Required—TOEFL, TWE. *Faculty research:* Membrane transport, mechanisms of cellular regulation, brain metabolism, peptide metabolism.

Rush University, Graduate College, Department of Molecular Biophysics and Physiology, Chicago, IL 60612-3832. Offers physiology (PhD); MD/PhD. *Degree requirements:* For doctorate, thesis/dissertation. *Entrance requirements:* For doctorate, GRE General Test. Additional exam requirements/recommendations for international students: Required—TOEFL. *Faculty research:* Physiological exocytosis, raft formation and growth, voltage-gated proton channels, molecular biophysics and physiology.

Rutgers University–Newark, Graduate School of Biomedical Sciences, Department of Pharmacology and Physiology, Newark, NJ 07107. Offers PhD. *Degree requirements:* For doctorate, thesis/dissertation, qualifying exam. *Entrance requirements:* For doctorate, GRE General Test. Additional exam requirements/recommendations for international students: Required—TOEFL. Electronic applications accepted.

Rutgers University–New Brunswick, Graduate School-New Brunswick, Program in Endocrinology and Animal Biosciences, Piscataway, NJ 08854-8097. Offers MS, PhD. Terminal master's awarded for partial completion of doctoral program. *Degree requirements:* For master's, thesis; for doctorate, comprehensive exam, thesis/dissertation. *Entrance requirements:* For master's and doctorate, GRE General Test. Additional exam requirements/recommendations for international students: Required—TOEFL. Electronic applications accepted. *Faculty research:* Comparative and behavioral endocrinology, epigenetic regulation of the endocrine system, exercise physiology and immunology, fetal and neonatal developmental programming, mammary gland biology and breast cancer, neuroendocrinology and alcohol studies, reproductive and developmental toxicology.

Rutgers University–New Brunswick, Graduate School of Biomedical Sciences, Program in Physiology and Integrative Biology, Piscataway, NJ 08854-5635. Offers MS, PhD, MD/PhD. *Entrance requirements:* Additional exam requirements/recommendations for international students: Required—TOEFL. Electronic applications accepted.

Saint Louis University, Graduate Education and School of Medicine, Graduate Program in Biomedical Sciences and Graduate Education, Department of Pharmacological and Physiological Science, St. Louis, MO 63103. Offers PhD. *Degree requirements:* For doctorate, comprehensive exam, thesis/dissertation, departmental qualifying exams. *Entrance requirements:* For doctorate, GRE General Test (GRE Subject Test optional), letters of recommendation, resume, interview. Additional exam requirements/recommendations for international students: Required—TOEFL (minimum score 525 paper-based). Electronic applications accepted. *Faculty research:* Molecular endocrinology, neuropharmacology, cardiovascular science, drug abuse, neurotransmitter and hormonal signaling mechanisms.

Salisbury University, Department of Health Sciences, Salisbury, MD 21801-6837. Offers applied health physiology (MS). *Program availability:* Part-time. *Faculty:* 4 full-time (0 women), 1 part-time/adjunct (0 women). *Students:* 36 full-time (17 women), 18 part-time (8 women); includes 4 minority (2 Black or African American, non-Hispanic/Latino; 1 Asian, non-Hispanic/Latino; 1 Hispanic/Latino), 1 international. Average age 25. 21 applicants, 100% accepted, 19 enrolled. In 2015, 18 master's awarded. *Entrance requirements:* For master's, undergraduate degree with minimum GPA of 3.0; 2 letters

of recommendation; personal statement. Additional exam requirements/recommendations for international students: Required—TOEFL (minimum score 550 paper-based, 79 iBT) or IELTS (6.5). *Application deadline:* For fall admission, 7/1 for domestic and international students; for spring admission, 12/1 for domestic and international students; for summer admission, 5/1 for domestic and international students. Applications are processed on a rolling basis. Application fee: $65. Electronic applications accepted. *Expenses:* $370 per credit hour resident; $659 per credit hour non-resident; $78 per credit hour fees. *Financial support:* In 2015–16, 5 research assistantships with full tuition reimbursements (averaging $8,500 per year) were awarded; career-related internships or fieldwork, institutionally sponsored loans, scholarships/grants, and unspecified assistantships also available. Support available to part-time students. Financial award application deadline: 3/1; financial award applicants required to submit FAFSA. *Faculty research:* Peripheral arterial disease; pulmonary rehabilitation; human performance curricular development. *Unit head:* Dr. Randy Insley, Graduate Program Director, Applied Health Physiology, 410-677-0145, Fax: 410-548-9185, E-mail: rcinsley@salisbury.edu. *Application contact:* Dr. Thomas Pellinger, Faculty, Applied Health Physiology, 410-677-0144, Fax: 410-548-9185, E-mail: tkpellinger@salisbury.edu. Website: http://www.salisbury.edu/gsr/gradstudies/MSAHPHpage.html

San Francisco State University, Division of Graduate Studies, College of Science and Engineering, Department of Biology, Program in Physiology and Behavioral Biology, San Francisco, CA 94132-1722. Offers MS. *Application deadline:* Applications are processed on a rolling basis. *Expenses:* Tuition, state resident: full-time $6738. Tuition, nonresident: full-time $15,666. *Required fees:* $1004. *Unit head:* Dr. Megurni Fuse, Coordinator, 415-405-0728, Fax: 415-338-2295, E-mail: fuse@sfsu.edu. *Application contact:* Dr. Diana Chu, Graduate Coordinator, 415-405-3487, Fax: 415-338-2295, E-mail: chud@sfsu.edu. Website: http://biology.sfsu.edu/graduate/physiology_and_behavior

San Jose State University, Graduate Studies and Research, College of Science, San Jose, CA 95192-0001. Offers biological sciences (MA, MS), including molecular biology and microbiology (MS), organismal biology, conservation and ecology (MS), physiology (MS); chemistry (MA, MS); computer science (MS); cybersecurity (Certificate); cybersecurity: core technologies (Certificate); geology (MS); marine science (MS); master biotechnology (MBT); mathematics (MA, MS), including mathematics education (MA), science; meteorology (MS); physics (MS), including computational physics, modern optics, science (MA, MS); science education (MA); statistics (MS); Unix system administration (Certificate). *Program availability:* Part-time, evening/weekend. *Students:* 118 full-time (68 women), 52 part-time (25 women); includes 125 minority (5 Black or African American, non-Hispanic/Latino; 97 Asian, non-Hispanic/Latino; 23 Hispanic/Latino), 121 international. Average age 27. 1,236 applicants, 21% accepted, 171 enrolled. In 2015, 168 master's awarded. *Entrance requirements:* For master's, GRE. *Application deadline:* For fall admission, 6/29 for domestic students; for spring admission, 11/30 for domestic students. Applications are processed on a rolling basis. Application fee: $55. Electronic applications accepted. *Financial support:* Teaching assistantships, career-related internships or fieldwork, Federal Work-Study, and institutionally sponsored loans available. Support available to part-time students. Financial award applicants required to submit FAFSA. *Faculty research:* Radiochemistry/environmental analysis, health physics, radiation effects. *Unit head:* J. Michael Parrish, Dean, 408-924-4800, Fax: 408-924-4815. *Application contact:* 408-924-2480, Fax: 408-924-2477. Website: http://www.science.sjsu.edu/

Southern Illinois University Carbondale, Graduate School, Graduate Programs in Medicine, Program in Molecular, Cellular and Systemic Physiology, Carbondale, IL 62901-4701. Offers MS. *Students:* 8 full-time (4 women), 13 part-time (11 women); includes 1 minority (Asian, non-Hispanic/Latino), 13 international. 11 applicants, 64% accepted, 4 enrolled. In 2015, 4 master's, 1 doctorate awarded. *Degree requirements:* For doctorate, thesis/dissertation. *Entrance requirements:* For master's and doctorate, GRE. *Application deadline:* For fall admission, 12/15 for domestic students. Application fee: $65. *Financial support:* In 2015–16, 17 students received support, including 3 fellowships with full tuition reimbursements available, 10 research assistantships with full tuition reimbursements available, 4 teaching assistantships with full tuition reimbursements available; unspecified assistantships also available. *Unit head:* Dr. Buck Hales, Chair, 618-453-1544, E-mail: dhales@siumed.edu. *Application contact:* Susan Sugawara, Chief Clerk, 618-453-1500, Fax: 618-453-1517, E-mail: ssugawara@siu.edu.

Southern Methodist University, Annette Caldwell Simmons School of Education and Human Development, Department of Allied Physiology and Wellness, Dallas, TX 75275. Offers sport management (MS). Program offered jointly with Cox School of Business. *Entrance requirements:* For master's, GMAT, resume, essays, transcripts from all colleges and universities attended, two references. Additional exam requirements/recommendations for international students: Required—TOEFL or PTE.

Stanford University, School of Medicine, Graduate Programs in Medicine, Department of Molecular and Cellular Physiology, Stanford, CA 94305-9991. Offers PhD. *Degree requirements:* For doctorate, thesis/dissertation, qualifying exams. *Entrance requirements:* For doctorate, GRE General Test, GRE Subject Test. Additional exam requirements/recommendations for international students: Required—TOEFL. Electronic applications accepted. *Expenses:* Tuition, area resident: Full-time $45,729. *Required fees:* $591. *Faculty research:* Signal transduction, ion channels, intracellular calcium, synaptic transmission.

State University of New York Upstate Medical University, College of Graduate Studies, Program in Physiology, Syracuse, NY 13210-2334. Offers MS, PhD, MD/PhD. Terminal master's awarded for partial completion of doctoral program. *Degree requirements:* For master's, thesis; for doctorate, comprehensive exam, thesis/dissertation. *Entrance requirements:* For master's, GRE General Test, interview; for doctorate, GRE General Test, telephone interview. Additional exam requirements/recommendations for international students: Required—TOEFL. Electronic applications accepted.

Stony Brook University, State University of New York, Stony Brook Medicine, School of Medicine and Graduate School, Graduate Programs in Medicine, Department of Physiology and Biophysics, Stony Brook, NY 11794. Offers PhD. *Faculty:* 17 full-time (6 women). *Students:* 33 full-time (15 women), 1 part-time (0 women); includes 18 minority (6 Black or African American, non-Hispanic/Latino; 6 Asian, non-Hispanic/Latino; 5 Hispanic/Latino; 1 Two or more races, non-Hispanic/Latino), 6 International. Average age 25. 5 applicants. In 2015, 3 doctorates awarded. *Degree requirements:* For doctorate, comprehensive exam, thesis/dissertation. *Entrance requirements:* For doctorate, GRE General Test, GRE Subject Test, BS in related field, minimum GPA of 3.0, recommendation. Additional exam requirements/recommendations for international students: Required—TOEFL (minimum score 550 paper-based). *Application deadline:* For fall admission, 1/15 for domestic students; for spring admission, 10/1 for domestic students. Application fee: $100. *Expenses:* $12,421 full-time resident tuition and fees, $453 per credit hour; $23,761 full-time nonresident tuition and fees, $925 per credit hour. *Financial support:* In 2015–16, 2 research assistantships were awarded; fellowships, teaching assistantships, and Federal Work-Study also available. Financial

award application deadline: 3/15. *Faculty research:* Biophysics, physiology, neuropharmacology, neurophysiology, neuroscience. *Total annual research expenditures:* $5.2 million. *Unit head:* Dr. Todd Miller, Chair, 631-444-3533, Fax: 631-444-3432, E-mail: todd.miller@stonybrook.edu. *Application contact:* Odalis Hernandez, Coordinator, 631-444-3057, Fax: 631-444-3432, E-mail: odalis.hernandez@stonybrook.edu.
Website: http://pnb.informatics.stonybrook.edu/

Syracuse University, School of Education, MS Program in Exercise Science, Syracuse, NY 13244. Offers exercise science (MS), including clinical exercise physiology (including cardiac rehabilitation), exercise physiology and fitness, research in exercise physiology. *Program availability:* Part-time. *Students:* Average age 24. *Degree requirements:* For master's, thesis or alternative. *Entrance requirements:* For master's, GRE, baccalaureate degree from regionally-accredited college/university; 8 hours each in general biology and human anatomy and physiology; 6 hours of exercise science (including physiology of exercise and general science); three letters of recommendation; personal statement; resume; transcripts. Additional exam requirements/recommendations for international students: Required—TOEFL (minimum score 100 iBT). *Application deadline:* For fall admission, 1/15 priority date for domestic and international students; for spring admission, 10/15 priority date for domestic and international students; for summer admission, 1/15 priority date for domestic and international students. Applications are processed on a rolling basis. Application fee: $75. Electronic applications accepted. *Expenses: Tuition, area resident:* Full-time $25,974; part-time $1443 per credit hour. *Required fees:* $802; $50 per course. Tuition and fees vary according to course load and program. *Financial support:* Fellowships, research assistantships with tuition reimbursements, teaching assistantships with tuition reimbursements, career-related internships or fieldwork, and scholarships/grants available. Financial award application deadline: 1/15. *Faculty research:* Bone density, obesity in females, cardiovascular functioning, attitudes toward physical education, sports management and psychology. *Unit head:* Dr. Tom Brutsaert, Chair, 315-443-9696, E-mail: tdbrutsa@syr.edu. *Application contact:* Speranza Migliore, Graduate Admissions Recruiter, 315-443-2505, E-mail: gradrcrt@syr.edu.

Teachers College, Columbia University, Department of Biobehavioral Sciences, New York, NY 10027-6696. Offers applied exercise physiology (Ed M, MA, Ed D); communication sciences and disorders (MS, Ed D, PhD); kinesiology (PhD); motor learning and control (Ed M, MA); motor learning/movement science (Ed D); neuroscience and education (MS); physical education (MA, Ed D). *Program availability:* Part-time, evening/weekend. *Students:* 121 full-time (103 women), 218 part-time (171 women); includes 157 minority (30 Black or African American, non-Hispanic/Latino; 58 Asian, non-Hispanic/Latino; 63 Hispanic/Latino; 6 Two or more races, non-Hispanic/Latino), 6 international. *Expenses: Tuition, area resident:* Part-time $1454 per credit. *Required fees:* $428 per semester. One-time fee: $475 full-time. Full-time tuition and fees vary according to course load. *Financial support:* Fellowships, teaching assistantships, career-related internships or fieldwork, Federal Work-Study, institutionally sponsored loans, traineeships, and tuition waivers (full and partial) available. Support available to part-time students. *Unit head:* Prof. Carol Garber, Chair, E-mail: garber@tc.columbia.edu. *Application contact:* David Estrella, Director of Admissions, E-mail: estrella@tc.columbia.edu.
Website: http://www.tc.columbia.edu/biobehavioral-sciences/

Tulane University, School of Medicine and School of Liberal Arts, Graduate Programs in Biomedical Sciences, Department of Physiology, New Orleans, LA 70118-5669. Offers MS. MS and PhD offered through the Graduate School. *Degree requirements:* For master's, one foreign language, thesis. *Entrance requirements:* For master's, GRE General Test, minimum B average in undergraduate course work. Additional exam requirements/recommendations for international students: Required—TOEFL. *Application deadline:* For fall admission, 2/1 for domestic students. Application fee: $45. Electronic applications accepted. *Expenses: Tuition, area resident:* Full-time $47,658; part-time $2648 per credit hour. *Required fees:* $1980; $44.50 per credit hour. $550 per term. Tuition and fees vary according to course load, degree level and program. *Financial support:* Fellowships and research assistantships available. Financial award application deadline: 2/1. *Faculty research:* Renal microcirculation, neurophysiology, NA+ transport, renin/angio tensin system, cell and molecular endocrinology.

Universidad Central del Caribe, School of Medicine, Program in Biomedical Sciences, Bayamón, PR 00960-6032. Offers anatomy and cell biology (MA, MS); biochemistry (MS); biomedical sciences (MA); cellular and molecular biology (PhD); microbiology and immunology (MA, MS); pharmacology (MS); physiology (MS).

Université de Montréal, Faculty of Medicine, Department of Physiology, Montréal, QC H3C 3J7, Canada. Offers neurological sciences (M Sc, PhD); physiology (M Sc, PhD). Terminal master's awarded for partial completion of doctoral program. *Degree requirements:* For master's, thesis; for doctorate, thesis/dissertation, general exam. *Entrance requirements:* For master's and doctorate, proficiency in French, knowledge of English. Electronic applications accepted. *Faculty research:* Cardiovascular, neuropeptides, membrane transport and biophysics, signaling pathways.

Université de Sherbrooke, Faculty of Medicine and Health Sciences, Graduate Programs in Medicine, Department of Physiology and Biophysics, Sherbrooke, QC J1H 5N4, Canada. Offers M Sc, PhD. Terminal master's awarded for partial completion of doctoral program. *Degree requirements:* For master's, thesis; for doctorate, thesis/dissertation. Electronic applications accepted. *Faculty research:* Ion channels, neurological basis of pain, insulin resistance, obesity.

Université Laval, Faculty of Medicine, Graduate Programs in Medicine, Programs in Physiology-Endocrinology, Québec, QC G1K 7P4, Canada. Offers M Sc, PhD. Terminal master's awarded for partial completion of doctoral program. *Degree requirements:* For master's, thesis; for doctorate, comprehensive exam, thesis/dissertation. Electronic applications accepted.

University at Buffalo, the State University of New York, Graduate School, School of Medicine and Biomedical Sciences, Graduate Programs in Medicine and Biomedical Sciences, Department of Physiology and Biophysics, Buffalo, NY 14214. Offers biophysics (MS, PhD), including medical physics; physiology (MA, PhD). *Faculty:* 28 full-time (4 women). *Students:* 64 full-time (28 women); includes 34 minority (4 Black or African American, non-Hispanic/Latino; 26 Asian, non-Hispanic/Latino; 1 Hispanic/Latino; 3 Two or more races, non-Hispanic/Latino), 20 international. Average age 28. 62 applicants, 18% accepted, 8 enrolled. In 2015, 7 master's, 4 doctorates awarded. Terminal master's awarded for partial completion of doctoral program. *Degree requirements:* For master's, comprehensive exam, thesis optional, oral exam, project; for doctorate, comprehensive exam, thesis/dissertation, oral and written qualifying exam or 2 research proposals. *Entrance requirements:* For master's, GRE General Test, unofficial transcripts, 3 letters of recommendation, personal statement, curriculum vitae; for doctorate, GRE General Test or MCAT, unofficial transcripts, 3 letters of recommendation, personal statement, curriculum vitae. Additional exam requirements/recommendations for international students: Required—TOEFL (minimum score 550 paper-based; 79 iBT). *Application deadline:* Applications are processed on a rolling basis. Application fee: $85. Electronic applications accepted. *Financial support:* In 2015–16, 5 students received support, including 1 research assistantship with full tuition

reimbursement available (averaging $25,000 per year); Federal Work-Study, institutionally sponsored loans, health care benefits, and unspecified assistantships also available. Financial award applicants required to submit FAFSA. *Faculty research:* Neurosciences, ion channels, cardiac physiology, renal/epithelial transport, cardiopulmonary exercise. *Total annual research expenditures:* $2.7 million. *Unit head:* Dr. Perry M. Hogan, Chair, 716-829-2738, Fax: 716-829-2344, E-mail: phogan@buffalo.edu. *Application contact:* Kara M. Rickicki, Graduate Programs Coordinator, 716-829-2417, Fax: 716-829-2344, E-mail: rickicki@buffalo.edu.
Website: http://www.smbs.buffalo.edu/phb/

University of Alberta, Faculty of Graduate Studies and Research, Department of Biological Sciences, Edmonton, AB T6G 2E1, Canada. Offers environmental biology and ecology (M Sc, PhD); microbiology and biotechnology (M Sc, PhD); molecular biology and genetics (M Sc, PhD); physiology and cell biology (M Sc, PhD); plant biology (M Sc, PhD); systematics and evolution (M Sc, PhD). Terminal master's awarded for partial completion of doctoral program. *Degree requirements:* For master's, thesis; for doctorate, thesis/dissertation. *Entrance requirements:* Additional exam requirements/recommendations for international students: Required—TOEFL.

University of Alberta, Faculty of Medicine and Dentistry and Faculty of Graduate Studies and Research, Graduate Programs in Medicine, Department of Physiology, Edmonton, AB T6G 2E1, Canada. Offers M Sc, PhD. Terminal master's awarded for partial completion of doctoral program. *Degree requirements:* For master's, thesis; for doctorate, thesis/dissertation. *Entrance requirements:* For master's and doctorate, minimum GPA of 3.0. Additional exam requirements/recommendations for international students: Required—TOEFL (minimum score 580 paper-based). Electronic applications accepted. *Faculty research:* Membrane transport, cell biology, perinatal endocrinology, neurophysiology, cardiovascular.

The University of Arizona, Graduate Interdisciplinary Programs, Graduate Interdisciplinary Program in Physiological Sciences, Tucson, AZ 85721. Offers MS, PhD. *Degree requirements:* For doctorate, thesis/dissertation. *Entrance requirements:* For master's, GRE General Test, 3 letters of recommendation, statement of purpose; for doctorate, GRE General Test, 3 letters of recommendation. Additional exam requirements/recommendations for international students: Required—TOEFL (minimum score 600 paper-based). *Application deadline:* For fall admission, 3/15 for domestic and international students. Applications are processed on a rolling basis. Application fee: $75. Electronic applications accepted. *Financial support:* Research assistantships, teaching assistantships, health care benefits, and unspecified assistantships available. *Faculty research:* Cellular transport and signaling, receptor and messenger modulation, neural interaction and biomechanics, fluid network regulation, environmental adaptation. *Unit head:* Dr. Heddwen Brooks, Department Chair, 520-626-2472, E-mail: brooksh@email.arizona.edu. *Application contact:* Holly Lopez, Information Contact, 520-626-2898, Fax: 520-626-2382, E-mail: hollyl@email.arizona.edu.
Website: http://physiological-sciences.arizona.edu/

University of Arkansas for Medical Sciences, Graduate School, Little Rock, AR 72205. Offers biochemistry and molecular biology (MS, PhD); bioinformatics (MS, PhD); cellular physiology and molecular biophysics (MS, PhD); clinical nutrition (MS); interdisciplinary biomedical sciences (MS, PhD, Certificate); interdisciplinary toxicology (MS); microbiology and immunology (PhD); neurobiology and developmental sciences (PhD); pharmacology (PhD); MD/PhD. Bioinformatics programs hosted jointly with the University of Arkansas at Little Rock. *Program availability:* Part-time. Terminal master's awarded for partial completion of doctoral program. *Degree requirements:* For master's, comprehensive exam (for some programs), thesis (for some programs); for doctorate, thesis/dissertation. *Entrance requirements:* For master's and doctorate, GRE. Additional exam requirements/recommendations for international students: Required—TOEFL. Electronic applications accepted. *Expenses:* Contact institution.

University of Calgary, Cumming School of Medicine and Faculty of Graduate Studies, Medical Science Graduate Program, Calgary, AB T2N 1N4, Canada. Offers cancer biology (M Sc, PhD); critical care medicine (M Sc, PhD); joint injury and arthritis (M Sc, PhD); molecular and medical genetics (M Sc, PhD); mountain medicine and high altitude physiology (M Sc, PhD); pathologists' assistant (M Sc, PhD). *Degree requirements:* For master's, thesis; for doctorate, thesis/dissertation, candidacy exam. *Entrance requirements:* For master's, minimum undergraduate GPA of 3.2; for doctorate, minimum graduate GPA of 3.2. Additional exam requirements/recommendations for international students: Required—TOEFL (minimum score 600 paper-based). Electronic applications accepted. *Faculty research:* Cancer biology, immunology, joint injury and arthritis, medical education, population genomics.

University of Calgary, Cumming School of Medicine and Faculty of Graduate Studies, Program in Gastrointestinal Sciences, Calgary, AB T2N 1N4, Canada. Offers M Sc, PhD. *Degree requirements:* For master's, thesis; for doctorate, thesis/dissertation, candidacy exam. *Entrance requirements:* For master's and doctorate, minimum GPA of 3.2 during previous 2 years. Additional exam requirements/recommendations for international students: Required—TOEFL. Electronic applications accepted. *Faculty research:* Physiology, biochemistry, molecular biology, pharmacology, immunology.

University of California, Berkeley, Graduate Division, College of Letters and Science, Group in Endocrinology, Berkeley, CA 94720-1500. Offers MA, PhD. *Degree requirements:* For doctorate, thesis/dissertation, oral qualifying exam. *Entrance requirements:* For master's, GRE General Test or the equivalent (MCAT), minimum GPA of 3.0, 3 letters of recommendation; for doctorate, GRE General Test or the equivalent (MCAT), minimum GPA of 3.4, 3 letters of recommendation. Additional exam requirements/recommendations for international students: Required—TOEFL.

University of California, Davis, Graduate Studies, Molecular, Cellular and Integrative Physiology Graduate Group, Davis, CA 95616. Offers MS, PhD. *Degree requirements:* For master's, comprehensive exam (for some programs), thesis (for some programs); for doctorate, thesis/dissertation. *Entrance requirements:* For master's and doctorate, GRE General Test. Additional exam requirements/recommendations for international students: Required—TOEFL (minimum score 550 paper-based). Electronic applications accepted. *Faculty research:* Systemic physiology, cellular physiology, neurophysiology, cardiovascular physiology, endocrinology.

University of California, Irvine, School of Medicine and Francisco J. Ayala School of Biological Sciences, Department of Physiology and Biophysics, Irvine, CA 92697. Offers biological sciences (PhD); MD/PhD. *Students:* 10 full-time (3 women); includes 5 minority (4 Asian, non-Hispanic/Latino; 1 Hispanic/Latino), 2 international. Average age 29. In 2015, 1 doctorate awarded. *Degree requirements:* For doctorate, thesis/dissertation. *Entrance requirements:* For doctorate, GRE General Test, GRE Subject Test, minimum GPA of 3.0. Additional exam requirements/recommendations for international students: Required—TOEFL (minimum score 550 paper-based). *Application deadline:* For fall admission, 1/15 priority date for domestic students, 1/15 for international students. Application fee: $80 ($100 for international students). Electronic applications accepted. *Financial support:* Fellowships, research assistantships with full tuition reimbursements, teaching assistantships, institutionally sponsored loans, traineeships, health care benefits, and unspecified assistantships available. Financial award application deadline: 3/1; financial award applicants required to submit FAFSA. *Faculty research:* Membrane physiology, exercise physiology, regulation of hormone

Physiology

biosynthesis and action, endocrinology, ion channels and signal transduction. *Unit head:* Prof. Michael Cahalan, Chair, 949-824-7776, Fax: 949-824-3143, E-mail: mcahalan@uci.edu. *Application contact:* Janita Parpana, Chief Administrative Officer, 949-824-6833, Fax: 949-824-8540, E-mail: jparpana@uci.edu. Website: http://www.physiology.uci.edu/

University of California, Los Angeles, David Geffen School of Medicine and Graduate Division, Graduate Programs in Medicine, Department of Physiology, Los Angeles, CA 90095. Offers PhD. *Degree requirements:* For doctorate, thesis/dissertation, oral and written qualifying exams. *Entrance requirements:* For doctorate, GRE General Test, GRE Subject Test. *Faculty research:* Membrane physiology, cell physiology, muscle physiology, neurophysiology, cardiopulmonary physiology.

University of California, Los Angeles, Graduate Division, College of Letters and Science, Department of Integrative Biology and Physiology, Los Angeles, CA 90095. Offers physiological science (MS). *Degree requirements:* For master's, thesis. *Entrance requirements:* For master's, GRE General Test or MCAT, bachelor's degree; minimum undergraduate GPA of 3.0 (or its equivalent if letter grade system not used). Additional exam requirements/recommendations for international students: Required—TOEFL. Electronic applications accepted.

University of California, Los Angeles, Graduate Division, College of Letters and Science and David Geffen School of Medicine, UCLA ACCESS to Programs in the Molecular, Cellular and Integrative Life Sciences, Los Angeles, CA 90095. Offers biochemistry and molecular biology (PhD); biological chemistry (PhD); cellular and molecular pathology (PhD); human genetics (PhD); microbiology, immunology, and molecular genetics (PhD); molecular biology (PhD); molecular toxicology (PhD); molecular, cellular and integrative physiology (PhD); neurobiology (PhD); oral biology (PhD); physiology (PhD). *Degree requirements:* For doctorate, thesis/dissertation, oral and written qualifying exams. *Entrance requirements:* For doctorate, GRE General Test, bachelor's degree; minimum undergraduate GPA of 3.0 (or its equivalent if letter grade system not used). Additional exam requirements/recommendations for international students: Required—TOEFL. Electronic applications accepted.

University of Central Florida, College of Education and Human Performance, Department of Educational and Human Sciences, Program in Sport and Exercise Science, Orlando, FL 32816. Offers applied exercise physiology (MS). *Program availability:* Part-time, evening/weekend. *Students:* 60 full-time (18 women), 27 part-time (17 women); includes 22 minority (7 Black or African American, non-Hispanic/Latino; 2 Asian, non-Hispanic/Latino; 12 Hispanic/Latino; 1 Two or more races, non-Hispanic/Latino), 1 international. Average age 26. 129 applicants, 57% accepted, 32 enrolled. In 2015, 30 master's awarded. *Entrance requirements:* For master's, GRE General Test. Additional exam requirements/recommendations for international students: Required—TOEFL. *Application deadline:* For fall admission, 7/15 for domestic students; for spring admission, 12/1 for domestic students. Application fee: $30. Electronic applications accepted. *Expenses:* Tuition, state resident: part-time $288.16 per credit hour. Tuition, nonresident: part-time $1071.31 per credit hour. *Financial support:* In 2015–16, 6 students received support, including 1 fellowship (averaging $10,000 per year), 6 research assistantships with partial tuition reimbursements available (averaging $5,000 per year), 5 teaching assistantships with partial tuition reimbursements available (averaging $3,500 per year); career-related internships or fieldwork, Federal Work-Study, institutionally sponsored loans, tuition waivers (partial), and unspecified assistantships also available. Financial award application deadline: 3/1; financial award applicants required to submit FAFSA. *Unit head:* Dr. Jeffrey Stout, Coordinator, 407-823-0211, E-mail: jeffrey.stout@ucf.edu. *Application contact:* Director, Admissions and Student Support, 407-823-2766, Fax: 407-823-6442, E-mail: gradadmissions@ucf.edu.

University of Cincinnati, Graduate School, College of Medicine, Graduate Programs in Biomedical Sciences, Department of Molecular and Cellular Physiology, Cincinnati, OH 45221. Offers physiology (PhD). *Degree requirements:* For doctorate, comprehensive exam, thesis/dissertation, publication. *Entrance requirements:* For doctorate, GRE General Test, GRE Subject Test. Additional exam requirements/recommendations for international students: Required—TOEFL (minimum score 560 paper-based). Electronic applications accepted. *Faculty research:* Endocrinology, cardiovascular physiology, muscle physiology, neurophysiology, transgenic mouse physiology.

University of Colorado Boulder, Graduate School, College of Arts and Sciences, Department of Integrative Physiology, Boulder, CO 80309. Offers MS, PhD. *Faculty:* 23 full-time (7 women). *Students:* 60 full-time (32 women), 4 part-time (1 woman); includes 8 minority (1 Asian, non-Hispanic/Latino; 5 Hispanic/Latino; 2 Two or more races, non-Hispanic/Latino), 1 international. Average age 27. 68 applicants, 21% accepted, 12 enrolled. In 2015, 20 master's, 5 doctorates awarded. Terminal master's awarded for partial completion of doctoral program. *Degree requirements:* For master's, comprehensive exam, thesis or alternative; for doctorate, thesis/dissertation. *Entrance requirements:* For master's, GRE General Test, minimum undergraduate GPA of 2.75. *Application deadline:* For fall admission, 1/15 for domestic students, 12/15 for international students. Applications are processed on a rolling basis. Application fee: $50 ($70 for international students). Electronic applications accepted. Application fee is waived when completed online. *Financial support:* In 2015–16, 138 students received support, including 14 fellowships (averaging $3,142 per year), 17 research assistantships with tuition reimbursements available (averaging $24,999 per year), 44 teaching assistantships with tuition reimbursements available (averaging $29,977 per year); institutionally sponsored loans, scholarships/grants, health care benefits, and unspecified assistantships also available. Financial award application deadline: 2/1; financial award applicants required to submit FAFSA. *Faculty research:* Aging/gerontology, human physiology, nervous system, neurophysiology, neuroscience. *Total annual research expenditures:* $5.1 million. *Application contact:* E-mail: iphygrad@colorado.edu. Website: http://www.colorado.edu/intphys/

University of Colorado Denver, School of Medicine, Program in Physiology, Aurora, CO 80045. Offers PhD. *Students:* 52 full-time (35 women), 2 part-time (both women); includes 13 minority (4 Black or African American, non-Hispanic/Latino; 1 American Indian or Alaska Native, non-Hispanic/Latino; 6 Hispanic/Latino; 2 Two or more races, non-Hispanic/Latino). Average age 26. 95 applicants, 27% accepted, 22 enrolled. In 2015, 2 doctorates awarded. *Degree requirements:* For doctorate, comprehensive exam, 30 semester credit hours each of coursework and thesis, 3 lab rotations within 1st year. *Entrance requirements:* For doctorate, GRE General Test, 2 transcripts, 4 letters of recommendation, minimum GPA of 3.2, completion of college-level mathematics through calculus, one year each of organic chemistry, physical chemistry, and physics, two years of biology. Additional exam requirements/recommendations for international students: Required—TOEFL (minimum score 550 paper-based; 80 iBT). *Application deadline:* For fall admission, 1/1 for domestic students, 12/1 for international students. Application fee: $50 ($75 for international students). Electronic applications accepted. *Expenses:* Contact institution. *Financial support:* In 2015–16, 52 students received support, including 1 fellowship with full tuition reimbursement available (averaging $25,000 per year); research assistantships, teaching assistantships, Federal Work-Study, institutionally sponsored loans, scholarships/grants, traineeships, health care benefits, tuition waivers (full), and unspecified assistantships also available. Financial award application deadline: 3/15; financial award applicants required to submit FAFSA.

Faculty research: Nicotinic receptors, immunity, molecular structure, function and regulation of ion channels, calcium influx in the function of cytotoxic T lymphocytes. *Unit head:* Dr. Angeles Ribera, Chair, 303-724-4517, E-mail: angie.ribera@ucdenver.edu. *Application contact:* Rebecca Propes, Department Operations Specialist, 303-724-4500, Fax: 303-724-4501, E-mail: rebecca.propes@ucdenver.edu. Website: http://www.ucdenver.edu/academics/colleges/medicalschool/departments/physiology/Pages/home.aspx

★ **University of Connecticut,** Graduate School, College of Liberal Arts and Sciences, Department of Physiology and Neurobiology, Storrs, CT 06269. Offers comparative physiology (MS, PhD). Terminal master's awarded for partial completion of doctoral program. *Degree requirements:* For master's, comprehensive exam; for doctorate, thesis/dissertation. *Entrance requirements:* For master's and doctorate, GRE General Test, GRE Subject Test. Additional exam requirements/recommendations for international students: Required—TOEFL (minimum score 550 paper-based). *Application deadline:* For fall admission, 2/1 priority date for domestic and international students; for spring admission, 11/1 for domestic students, 10/1 for international students. Applications are processed on a rolling basis. Application fee: $55. Electronic applications accepted. *Financial support:* Fellowships, research assistantships with full tuition reimbursements, teaching assistantships with full tuition reimbursements, Federal Work-Study, scholarships/grants, health care benefits, tuition waivers (full), and unspecified assistantships available. Financial award application deadline: 2/1. Website: http://www.pnb.uconn.edu/

See Display on next page and Close-Up on page 435.

University of Delaware, College of Arts and Sciences, Department of Biological Sciences, Newark, DE 19716. Offers biotechnology (MS); cancer biology (MS, PhD); cell and extracellular matrix biology (MS, PhD); cell and systems physiology (MS, PhD); developmental biology (MS, PhD); ecology and evolution (MS, PhD); microbiology (MS, PhD); molecular biology and genetics (MS, PhD). Terminal master's awarded for partial completion of doctoral program. *Degree requirements:* For master's, thesis, preliminary exam; for doctorate, comprehensive exam, thesis/dissertation, preliminary exam. *Entrance requirements:* For master's and doctorate, GRE General Test. Additional exam requirements/recommendations for international students: Required—TOEFL (minimum score 600 paper-based); Recommended—TWE. Electronic applications accepted. *Faculty research:* Microorganisms, bone, cancer metastasis, developmental biology, cell biology, DNA.

University of Delaware, College of Health Sciences, Department of Kinesiology and Applied Physiology, Newark, DE 19716. Offers MS, PhD.

University of Florida, College of Medicine and Graduate School, Interdisciplinary Program in Biomedical Sciences, Concentration in Physiology and Pharmacology, Gainesville, FL 32611. Offers PhD. *Degree requirements:* For doctorate, thesis/dissertation. *Entrance requirements:* For doctorate, GRE General Test, minimum GPA of 3.0, biochemistry before enrollment. Electronic applications accepted.

University of Florida, Graduate School, College of Health and Human Performance, Department of Applied Physiology and Kinesiology, Gainesville, FL 32611. Offers applied physiology and kinesiology (MS); athletic training/sports medicine (MS); bio behavioral science (MS); clinical exercise physiology (MS); exercise physiology (MS); health and human performance (PhD), including applied physiology and kinesiology, biobehavioral science, exercise physiology; human performance (MS). *Faculty:* 15 full-time, 2 part-time/adjunct. *Students:* 59 full-time (36 women), 6 part-time (1 woman); includes 13 minority (3 Black or African American, non-Hispanic/Latino; 1 American Indian or Alaska Native, non-Hispanic/Latino; 2 Asian, non-Hispanic/Latino; 7 Hispanic/Latino), 20 international. Average age 25. 125 applicants, 33% accepted, 27 enrolled. In 2015, 21 master's awarded. *Degree requirements:* For master's, comprehensive exam, thesis (for some programs); for doctorate, comprehensive exam, thesis/dissertation. *Entrance requirements:* For master's and doctorate, GRE General Test, minimum GPA of 3.0. Additional exam requirements/recommendations for international students: Required—TOEFL (minimum score 550 paper-based; 80 iBT), IELTS (minimum score 6). *Application deadline:* For fall admission, 6/1 priority date for domestic students, 6/1 for international students; for spring admission, 9/15 for domestic and international students. Applications are processed on a rolling basis. Application fee: $30. Electronic applications accepted. *Financial support:* In 2015–16, 16 research assistantships, 43 teaching assistantships were awarded; fellowships and unspecified assistantships also available. Financial award application deadline: 2/1; financial award applicants required to submit FAFSA. *Faculty research:* Cardiovascular disease; basic mechanisms that underlie exercise-induced changes in the body at the organ, tissue, cellular and molecular level; development of rehabilitation techniques for regaining motor control after stroke or as a consequence of Parkinson's disease; maintaining optimal health and delaying age-related declines in physiological function; psychomotor mechanisms impacting health and performance across the life span. *Total annual research expenditures:* $2.4 million. *Unit head:* Michael Delp, PhD, Professor and Chair, 352-392-0584 Ext. 1338, E-mail: mdelp@hhp.ufl.edu. *Application contact:* Evangelos A. Christou, PhD, Associate Professor and Graduate Coordinator, 352-294-1719 Ext. 1270, E-mail: eachristou@hhp.ufl.edu. Website: http://apk.hhp.ufl.edu/

University of Georgia, College of Veterinary Medicine, Department of Physiology and Pharmacology, Athens, GA 30602. Offers pharmacology (MS, PhD); physiology (MS, PhD). *Degree requirements:* For master's, thesis; for doctorate, one foreign language, thesis/dissertation. *Entrance requirements:* For master's and doctorate, GRE General Test. Electronic applications accepted.

University of Guelph, Ontario Veterinary College and Graduate Studies, Graduate Programs in Veterinary Sciences, Department of Biomedical Sciences, Guelph, ON N1G 2W1, Canada. Offers morphology (M Sc, DV Sc, PhD); neuroscience (M Sc, DV Sc, PhD); pharmacology (M Sc, DV Sc, PhD); physiology (M Sc, DV Sc, PhD); toxicology (M Sc, DV Sc, PhD). *Program availability:* Part-time. *Degree requirements:* For master's, thesis; for doctorate, comprehensive exam, thesis/dissertation. *Entrance requirements:* For master's, honors B Sc, minimum 75% average in last 20 courses; for doctorate, M Sc with thesis from accredited institution. Additional exam requirements/recommendations for international students: Required—TOEFL (minimum score 550 paper-based; 89 iBT). Electronic applications accepted. *Faculty research:* Cellular morphology; endocrine, vascular and reproductive physiology; clinical pharmacology; veterinary toxicology; developmental biology; neuroscience.

University of Hawaii at Manoa, John A. Burns School of Medicine, Program in Developmental and Reproductive Biology, Honolulu, HI 96813. Offers MS, PhD. *Program availability:* Part-time. *Faculty:* 24 full-time (7 women). *Students:* 11 full-time (5 women), 3 part-time (1 woman); includes 9 minority (7 Asian, non-Hispanic/Latino; 2 Two or more races, non-Hispanic/Latino), 2 international. 19 applicants, 32% accepted, 2 enrolled. In 2015, 1 master's, 1 doctorate awarded. *Degree requirements:* For doctorate, thesis/dissertation. *Entrance requirements:* For doctorate, GRE General Test, GRE Subject Test. Additional exam requirements/recommendations for international students: Recommended—TOEFL (minimum score 560 paper-based), IELTS (minimum score 5). *Application deadline:* For fall admission, 3/1 for domestic and international

students. Application fee: $100. *Financial support:* In 2015–16, 2 fellowships (averaging $4,577 per year), 10 research assistantships (averaging $16,328 per year) were awarded; teaching assistantships also available. *Faculty research:* Biology of gametes and fertilization, reproductive endocrinology. *Total annual research expenditures:* $5.4 million. *Unit head:* Dr. Yusuke Marikawa, Chair, 808-692-1411.
Website: http://www2.jabsom.hawaii.edu/Grad_DRB/

University of Illinois at Chicago, College of Medicine and Graduate College, Graduate Programs in Medicine, Department of Physiology and Biophysics, Chicago, IL 60607-7128. Offers MS, PhD. *Faculty:* 19 full-time (5 women), 3 part-time/adjunct (1 woman). *Students:* 8 full-time (3 women); includes 1 minority (Hispanic/Latino). Average age 28. Terminal master's awarded for partial completion of doctoral program. *Degree requirements:* For master's, thesis; for doctorate, thesis/dissertation. *Entrance requirements:* For master's and doctorate, GRE General Test. Additional exam requirements/recommendations for international students: Required—TOEFL. *Application deadline:* For fall admission, 1/15 priority date for domestic students, 2/15 for international students. Applications are processed on a rolling basis. Application fee: $60. Electronic applications accepted. *Expenses:* Tuition, state resident: full-time $11,480; part-time $3826 per credit. Tuition, nonresident: full-time $23,720; part-time $7906 per credit. *Required fees:* $1333 per semester. Part-time tuition and fees vary according to course load and program. *Financial support:* In 2015–16, 5 fellowships with full tuition reimbursements were awarded; research assistantships with full tuition reimbursements, teaching assistantships with full tuition reimbursements, Federal Work-Study, traineeships, and tuition waivers (full) also available. Financial award application deadline: 3/1; financial award applicants required to submit FAFSA. *Faculty research:* Neuroscience, endocrinology and reproduction, cell physiology, exercise physiology, NMR, cardiovascular physiology and metabolism, cytoskeleton and vascular biology, gastrointestinal and epithelial cell biology, reproductive and endocrine sciences. *Unit head:* Prof. R. John Solaro, Department Head, 312-996-7620, Fax: 312-996-1414, E-mail: solarorj@uic.edu. *Application contact:* Jackie Perry, Graduate College Receptionist, 312-413-2550, Fax: 312-413-0185, E-mail: gradcoll@uic.edu.
Website: http://www.physiology.uic.edu/

University of Illinois at Urbana–Champaign, Graduate College, College of Liberal Arts and Sciences, School of Molecular and Cellular Biology, Department of Molecular and Integrative Physiology, Champaign, IL 61820. Offers MS, PhD.

The University of Iowa, Roy J. and Lucille A. Carver College of Medicine and Graduate College, Graduate Programs in Medicine, Department of Molecular Physiology and Biophysics, Iowa City, IA 52242. Offers MS, PhD. *Degree requirements:* For master's, comprehensive exam; for doctorate, comprehensive exam, thesis/dissertation. *Entrance requirements:* For master's, GRE General Test; for doctorate, GRE. Additional exam requirements/recommendations for international students: Required—TOEFL. Electronic applications accepted. *Faculty research:* Cellular and molecular endocrinology, membrane structure and function, cardiac cell electrophysiology, regulation of gene expression, neurophysiology.

The University of Kansas, University of Kansas Medical Center, School of Medicine, Department of Molecular and Integrative Physiology, Kansas City, KS 66160. Offers molecular and integrative physiology (PhD); MD/PhD. *Faculty:* 44. *Students:* 19 full-time (14 women); includes 1 minority (Hispanic/Latino), 13 international. Average age 29. In 2015, 3 doctorates awarded. Terminal master's awarded for partial completion of doctoral program. *Degree requirements:* For doctorate, comprehensive exam, thesis/dissertation. *Entrance requirements:* For doctorate, GRE. Additional exam requirements/recommendations for international students: Required—TOEFL. *Application deadline:* For fall admission, 12/1 priority date for domestic and international students. Applications are processed on a rolling basis. Application fee: $60. Electronic

applications accepted. *Financial support:* Fellowships with tuition reimbursements, research assistantships with partial tuition reimbursements, teaching assistantships with tuition reimbursements, scholarships/grants, and unspecified assistantships available. Financial award application deadline: 3/1; financial award applicants required to submit FAFSA. *Faculty research:* Male reproductive physiology and contraception, ovarian development and regulation by pituitary and hypothalamus, neural control of movement and stroke recovery, cardio-pulmonary physiology and hypoxia, plasticity of the autonomic nervous system, renal physiology, exercise physiology, diabetes, cancer biology. *Total annual research expenditures:* $9.5 million. *Unit head:* Dr. Victor G. Blanco, Interim Chair, 913-588-7400, Fax: 913-588-7430, E-mail: gblanco@kumc.edu. *Application contact:* Dr. Michael W. Wolfe, Director of Graduate Studies, 913-588-7418, Fax: 913-588-7430, E-mail: mwolfe2@kumc.edu.
Website: http://www.kumc.edu/school-of-medicine/molecular-and-integrative-physiology.html

University of Kentucky, Graduate School, Graduate School Programs from the College of Medicine, Program in Physiology, Lexington, KY 40506-0032. Offers PhD. *Degree requirements:* For doctorate, comprehensive exam, thesis/dissertation. *Entrance requirements:* For doctorate, GRE General Test, minimum undergraduate GPA of 2.75, graduate 3.0. Additional exam requirements/recommendations for international students: Required—TOEFL (minimum score 550 paper-based). Electronic applications accepted.

University of Louisville, School of Medicine, Department of Physiology and Biophysics, Louisville, KY 40292-0001. Offers MS, PhD, MD/PhD. *Students:* 36 full-time (15 women), 11 part-time (1 woman); includes 12 minority (3 Black or African American, non-Hispanic/Latino; 4 Asian, non-Hispanic/Latino; 3 Hispanic/Latino; 2 Two or more races, non-Hispanic/Latino), 9 international. Average age 28. 47 applicants, 51% accepted, 20 enrolled. In 2015, 5 master's awarded *Median time to degree:* Of those who began their doctoral program in fall 2007, 85% received their degree in 8 years or less. *Degree requirements:* For doctorate, comprehensive exam, thesis/dissertation. *Entrance requirements:* For master's and doctorate, GRE General Test (minimum score of 1000 verbal and quantitative), minimum GPA of 3.0. Additional exam requirements/recommendations for international students: Required—TOEFL (minimum score 550 paper-based). *Application deadline:* For fall admission, 1/15 for domestic students; for winter admission, 2/15 for international students; for spring admission, 2/15 for domestic students. Applications are processed on a rolling basis. Application fee: $60. Electronic applications accepted. *Expenses:* Tuition, state resident: full-time $11,664; part-time $649 per credit hour. Tuition, nonresident: full-time $24,274; part-time $1350 per credit hour. *Required fees:* $196. Tuition and fees vary according to program and reciprocity agreements. *Financial support:* In 2015–16, 4 fellowships with full tuition reimbursements (averaging $23,500 per year) were awarded; health care benefits also available. Financial award application deadline: 4/15. *Faculty research:* Vascular remodeling; cerebral microcirculation; renal vasculature; cardiac regeneration. *Total annual research expenditures:* $300,388. *Unit head:* Dr. Irving G. Joshua, Chair, 502-852-5371, Fax: 502-852-6239, E-mail: igjosh01@louisville.edu. *Application contact:* Dr. William Wead, Director of Admissions, 502-852-7571, Fax: 502-852-6849, E-mail: wbwead01@gwise.louisville.edu.
Website: http://louisville.edu/medicine/departments/physiology

The University of Manchester, Faculty of Life Sciences, Manchester, United Kingdom. Offers adaptive organismal biology (M Phil, PhD); animal biology (M Phil, PhD); biochemistry (M Phil, PhD); bioinformatics (M Phil, PhD); biomolecular sciences (M Phil, PhD); biotechnology (M Phil, PhD); cell biology (M Phil, PhD); cell matrix research (M Phil, PhD); channels and transporters (M Phil, PhD); developmental biology (M Phil, PhD); Egyptology (M Phil, PhD); environmental biology (M Phil, PhD); evolutionary biology (M Phil, PhD); gene expression (M Phil, PhD); genetics (M Phil, PhD); history of

Physiology

science, technology and medicine (M Phil, PhD); immunology (M Phil, PhD); integrative neurobiology and behavior (M Phil, PhD); membrane trafficking (M Phil, PhD); microbiology (M Phil, PhD); molecular and cellular neuroscience (M Phil, PhD); molecular biology (M Phil, PhD); molecular cancer studies (M Phil, PhD); neuroscience (M Phil, PhD); ophthalmology (M Phil, PhD); optometry (M Phil, PhD); organelle function (M Phil, PhD); pharmacology (M Phil, PhD); physiology (M Phil, PhD); plant sciences (M Phil, PhD); stem cell research (M Phil, PhD); structural biology (M Phil, PhD); systems neuroscience (M Phil, PhD); toxicology (M Phil, PhD).

University of Manitoba, Faculty of Medicine and Faculty of Graduate Studies, Graduate Programs in Medicine, Department of Physiology, Winnipeg, MB R3T 2N2, Canada. Offers M Sc, PhD, MD/PhD. Terminal master's awarded for partial completion of doctoral program. *Degree requirements:* For master's, one foreign language, thesis; for doctorate, one foreign language, thesis/dissertation. *Entrance requirements:* For master's, minimum GPA of 3.5; for doctorate, minimum GPA of 3.5, M Sc. *Faculty research:* Cardiovascular research, gene technology, cell biology, neuroscience, respiration.

University of Massachusetts Amherst, Graduate School, Interdisciplinary Programs, Program in Plant Biology, Amherst, MA 01003. Offers biochemistry and metabolism (MS, PhD); cell biology and physiology (MS, PhD); environmental, ecological and integrative biology (MS, PhD); genetics and evolution (MS, PhD). *Degree requirements:* For master's, thesis; for doctorate, 2 foreign languages, comprehensive exam, thesis/dissertation. *Entrance requirements:* For master's and doctorate, GRE General Test. Additional exam requirements/recommendations for international students: Required—TOEFL (minimum score 550 paper-based; 80 iBT), IELTS (minimum score 6.5). Electronic applications accepted.

University of Miami, Graduate School, Miller School of Medicine, Graduate Programs in Medicine, Department of Physiology and Biophysics, Coral Gables, FL 33124. Offers PhD, MD/PhD. *Degree requirements:* For doctorate, thesis/dissertation, qualifying exam. *Entrance requirements:* For doctorate, GRE General Test, minimum GPA of 3.0 in sciences. Additional exam requirements/recommendations for international students: Required—TOEFL. *Faculty research:* Cell and membrane physiology, cell-to-cell communication; molecular neurobiology, neuroimmunology, neural development.

University of Michigan, Rackham Graduate School, Program in Biomedical Sciences (PIBS), Department of Molecular and Integrative Physiology, Ann Arbor, MI 48109. Offers MS, PhD. *Faculty:* 45 full-time (14 women), 11 part-time/adjunct (3 women). *Students:* 62 full-time (33 women); includes 15 minority (2 Black or African American, non-Hispanic/Latino; 1 American Indian or Alaska Native, non-Hispanic/Latino; 9 Asian, non-Hispanic/Latino; 3 Hispanic/Latino). Average age 25. 186 applicants, 41% accepted, 40 enrolled. In 2015, 28 master's, 4 doctorates awarded. *Degree requirements:* For master's, thesis (for some programs), capstone project (for some programs); for doctorate, thesis/dissertation, oral defense of dissertation, preliminary exam. *Entrance requirements:* For master's, GRE, MCAT, DAT or PCAT, minimum science and overall GPA of 3.0; for doctorate, GRE General Test, 3 letters of recommendation, research experience. Additional exam requirements/recommendations for international students: Required—TOEFL (minimum score 84 iBT) or Michigan English Language Assessment Battery. *Application deadline:* For fall admission, 12/1 for domestic and international students. Application fee: $75 ($90 for international students). Electronic applications accepted. *Financial support:* In 2015–16, 33 students received support, including 33 fellowships with full tuition reimbursements available (averaging $29,025 per year); scholarships/grants, health care benefits, tuition waivers (full), and unspecified assistantships also available. Financial award application deadline: 12/1. *Faculty research:* Ion transport, cardiovascular physiology, gene expression, hormone action, gastrointestinal physiology, endocrinology, muscle, signal transduction. *Unit head:* Dr. Bishr Omary, Chair, 734-764-4376, Fax: 734-936-8813, E-mail: mbishr@umich.edu. *Application contact:* Michelle DiMondo, Director of Student Life, 734-647-5773, Fax: 734-647-7022, E-mail: mdimondo@umich.edu. Website: http://medicine.umich.edu/dept/molecular-integrative-physiology

University of Minnesota, Duluth, Medical School, Graduate Program in Physiology, Duluth, MN 55812-2496. Offers MS, PhD. MS, PhD offered jointly with University of Minnesota, Twin Cities Campus. Terminal master's awarded for partial completion of doctoral program. *Degree requirements:* For master's, thesis; for doctorate, thesis/dissertation. *Entrance requirements:* For master's, GRE or MCAT; for doctorate, GRE or MCAT, 1 year of course work in each calculus, physics, and biology; 2 years of course work in chemistry; minimum GPA of 3.0 in science. Additional exam requirements/recommendations for international students: Required—TOEFL. *Faculty research:* Neural control of posture and locomotion, transport and metabolic phenomena in biological systems, control of organ blood flow, intracellular means of communication.

University of Minnesota, Twin Cities Campus, Graduate School, Department of Integrative Biology and Physiology, Minneapolis, MN 55455-0213. Offers PhD. *Program availability:* Part-time. *Degree requirements:* For doctorate, comprehensive exam, thesis/dissertation. *Entrance requirements:* For doctorate, GRE General Test. Electronic applications accepted. *Faculty research:* Cardiovascular physiology.

University of Mississippi Medical Center, School of Graduate Studies in the Health Sciences, Department of Physiology and Biophysics, Jackson, MS 39216-4505. Offers PhD, MD/PhD. *Degree requirements:* For doctorate, thesis/dissertation, first authored publication. *Entrance requirements:* For doctorate, GRE General Test, minimum GPA of 3.0. *Faculty research:* Cardiovascular, renal, endocrine, and cellular neurophysiology; molecular physiology.

University of Missouri, School of Medicine and Office of Research and Graduate Studies, Graduate Programs in Medicine, Department of Medical Pharmacology and Physiology, Columbia, MO 65211. Offers MS, PhD. *Degree requirements:* For master's, thesis; for doctorate, thesis/dissertation. *Entrance requirements:* For master's and doctorate, GRE General Test, minimum GPA of 3.0. Additional exam requirements/recommendations for international students: Required—TOEFL (minimum score 500 paper-based; 61 iBT). *Application deadline:* For fall admission, 1/10 priority date for domestic and international students; for winter admission, 10/10 priority date for domestic and international students. Applications are processed on a rolling basis. Application fee: $55 ($75 for international students). Electronic applications accepted. *Financial support:* Fellowships, research assistantships, teaching assistantships, institutionally sponsored loans, scholarships/grants, health care benefits, and unspecified assistantships available. Support available to part-time students. Website: http://mpp.missouri.edu/

University of Nebraska Medical Center, Department of Cellular and Integrative Physiology, Omaha, NE 68198. Offers MS, PhD. *Program availability:* Part-time. *Faculty:* 17 full-time (4 women). *Students:* 10 full-time (3 women); includes 2 minority (both Asian, non-Hispanic/Latino), 5 international. Average age 28. 6 applicants, 33% accepted, 2 enrolled. In 2015, 3 doctorates awarded. Terminal master's awarded for partial completion of doctoral program. *Degree requirements:* For master's, comprehensive exam, thesis optional; for doctorate, comprehensive exam, thesis/dissertation, at least one first-author research publication. *Entrance requirements:* For master's and doctorate, GRE General Test or MCAT, course work in biology, chemistry, mathematics, and physics. Additional exam requirements/recommendations for

international students: Required—TOEFL (minimum score 600 paper-based; 100 iBT), IELTS (minimum score 7). *Application deadline:* For fall admission, 4/1 for domestic and international students. Application fee: $45. Electronic applications accepted. *Expenses:* Tuition, state resident: full-time $7830; part-time $3915 per credit hour. Tuition, nonresident: full-time $22,410; part-time $11,205 per credit hour. *Required fees:* $521. *Financial support:* In 2015–16, fellowships with full tuition reimbursements (averaging $23,100 per year), 7 research assistantships with full tuition reimbursements (averaging $4,620 per year) were awarded; scholarships/grants, health care benefits, unspecified assistantships, and 3 partial assistantships with full tuition reimbursements (for students receiving extramural fellowships) also available. Support available to part-time students. Financial award application deadline: 2/15; financial award applicants required to submit FAFSA. *Faculty research:* Cardiovascular, neuroscience, renal physiology and pathophysiology, cardiopulmonary and renal consequences of heart failure, free radical biology, reproductive endocrinology. *Total annual research expenditures:* $4.2 million. *Unit head:* Dr. Pamela K. Carmines, Vice Chair for Graduate Education, Department of Cellular and Integrative Physiology, 402-559-9343, Fax: 402-559-4438, E-mail: pcarmines@unmc.edu. *Application contact:* Kim Kavan, Office Associate, 402-559-4426, E-mail: kimberly.kavan@unmc.edu. Website: http://www.unmc.edu/physiology/

University of Nevada, Reno, Graduate School, Interdisciplinary Program in Cellular and Molecular Pharmacology and Physiology, Reno, NV 89557. Offers PhD. *Degree requirements:* For doctorate, one foreign language, thesis/dissertation. *Entrance requirements:* For doctorate, GRE General Test or MCAT, minimum GPA of 3.0. Additional exam requirements/recommendations for international students: Required—TOEFL (minimum score 500 paper-based; 61 iBT), IELTS (minimum score 6). Electronic applications accepted. *Faculty research:* Neuropharmacology, toxicology, cardiovascular pharmacology, neuromuscular pharmacology.

University of New Mexico, Graduate Studies, Health Sciences Center, Program in Biomedical Sciences, Albuquerque, NM 87131-5196. Offers biochemistry and molecular biology (MS, PhD); cell biology and physiology (MS, PhD); molecular genetics and microbiology (MS, PhD); neuroscience (MS, PhD); pathology (MS, PhD); toxicology (MS, PhD). *Program availability:* Part-time. *Faculty:* 18 full-time (10 women), 1 part-time/adjunct (0 women). *Students:* 31 full-time (17 women), 45 part-time (26 women); includes 29 minority (1 American Indian or Alaska Native, non-Hispanic/Latino; 3 Asian, non-Hispanic/Latino; 22 Hispanic/Latino; 2 Native Hawaiian or other Pacific Islander, non-Hispanic/Latino; 1 Two or more races, non-Hispanic/Latino), 18 international. Average age 30. 98 applicants, 11% accepted, 11 enrolled. In 2015, 11 master's, 14 doctorates awarded. Terminal master's awarded for partial completion of doctoral program. *Degree requirements:* For master's, thesis; for doctorate, comprehensive exam, thesis/dissertation, qualifying exam at the end of year 1/core curriculum. *Entrance requirements:* For master's and doctorate, GRE General Test, minimum undergraduate GPA of 3.0. Additional exam requirements/recommendations for international students: Required—TOEFL. *Application deadline:* For fall admission, 3/1 priority date for domestic and international students. Applications are processed on a rolling basis. Application fee: $50. Electronic applications accepted. *Financial support:* Fellowships with tuition reimbursements, research assistantships with full tuition reimbursements, teaching assistantships, career-related internships or fieldwork, Federal Work-Study, institutionally sponsored loans, scholarships/grants, traineeships, health care benefits, and unspecified assistantships available. Financial award application deadline: 1/1; financial award applicants required to submit FAFSA. *Faculty research:* Infectious disease/immunity, cancer biology, cardiovascular and metabolic diseases, brain and behavioral illness, environmental health. *Unit head:* Dr. Helen J. Hathaway, Program Director, 505-272-1887, Fax: 505-272-2412, E-mail: hhathaway@salud.unm.edu. *Application contact:* Mary Fenton, Admissions Coordinator, 505-272-1887, Fax: 505-272-2412, E-mail: mfenton@salud.unm.edu.

University of North Dakota, Graduate School and Graduate School, Graduate Programs in Medicine, Department of Pharmacology, Physiology, and Therapeutics, Grand Forks, ND 58202. Offers pharmacology (MS, PhD); physiology (MS, PhD). *Degree requirements:* For master's, comprehensive exam, thesis; for doctorate, thesis/dissertation, written and oral exam. *Entrance requirements:* For master's, GRE General Test or MCAT, minimum GPA of 3.0; for doctorate, GRE General Test, minimum GPA of 3.5. Additional exam requirements/recommendations for international students: Required—TOEFL (minimum score 550 paper-based; 79 iBT), IELTS (minimum score 6.5). Electronic applications accepted.

University of North Texas Health Science Center at Fort Worth, Graduate School of Biomedical Sciences, Fort Worth, TX 76107-2699. Offers anatomy and cell biology (MS, PhD); biochemistry and molecular biology (MS, PhD); biomedical sciences (MS, PhD); biotechnology (MS); forensic genetics (MS); integrative physiology (MS, PhD); medical science (MS); microbiology and immunology (MS, PhD); pharmacology (MS, PhD); science education (MS); DO/MS; DO/PhD. Terminal master's awarded for partial completion of doctoral program. *Degree requirements:* For master's, thesis; for doctorate, thesis/dissertation. *Entrance requirements:* For master's and doctorate, GRE General Test. Additional exam requirements/recommendations for international students: Required—TOEFL. *Expenses:* Contact institution. *Faculty research:* Alzheimer's disease, aging, eye diseases, cancer, cardiovascular disease.

University of Notre Dame, Graduate School, College of Science, Department of Biological Sciences, Notre Dame, IN 46556. Offers aquatic ecology, evolution and environmental biology (MS, PhD); cellular and molecular biology (MS, PhD); genetics (MS, PhD); physiology (MS, PhD); vector biology and parasitology (MS, PhD). Terminal master's awarded for partial completion of doctoral program. *Degree requirements:* For master's, comprehensive exam, thesis; for doctorate, comprehensive exam, thesis/dissertation, candidacy exam. *Entrance requirements:* For master's and doctorate, GRE General Test. Additional exam requirements/recommendations for international students: Required—TOEFL (minimum score 600 paper-based; 80 iBT). Electronic applications accepted. *Faculty research:* Tropical disease, molecular genetics, neurobiology, evolutionary biology, aquatic biology.

University of Oklahoma Health Sciences Center, College of Medicine and Graduate College, Graduate Programs in Medicine, Department of Physiology, Oklahoma City, OK 73190. Offers MS, PhD. *Program availability:* Part-time. Terminal master's awarded for partial completion of doctoral program. *Degree requirements:* For master's, thesis (for some programs); for doctorate, thesis/dissertation. *Entrance requirements:* For master's, GRE General Test, statement of career goals, 3 letters of recommendation; for doctorate, GRE General Test, 3 letters of recommendation. Additional exam requirements/recommendations for international students: Required—TOEFL. *Faculty research:* Cardiopulmonary physiology, neurophysiology, exercise physiology, cell and molecular physiology.

University of Oregon, Graduate School, College of Arts and Sciences, Department of Human Physiology, Eugene, OR 97403. Offers MS, PhD. *Degree requirements:* For master's, thesis optional; for doctorate, one foreign language, thesis/dissertation. *Entrance requirements:* For master's, GRE General Test, minimum GPA of 2.75 in undergraduate course work; for doctorate, GRE General Test. *Faculty research:* Balance control, muscle fatigue, lower extremity function, knee control.

University of Pennsylvania, Perelman School of Medicine, Biomedical Graduate Studies, Graduate Group in Cell and Molecular Biology, Philadelphia, PA 19104. Offers cancer biology (PhD); cell biology, physiology, and metabolism (PhD); developmental stem cell regenerative biology (PhD); gene therapy and vaccines (PhD); genetics and gene regulation (PhD); microbiology, virology, and parasitology (PhD); MD/PhD; VMD/PhD. *Faculty:* 317. *Students:* 339 full-time (189 women); includes 100 minority (7 Black or African American, non-Hispanic/Latino; 2 American Indian or Alaska Native, non-Hispanic/Latino; 45 Asian, non-Hispanic/Latino; 34 Hispanic/Latino; 1 Native Hawaiian or other Pacific Islander, non-Hispanic/Latino; 11 Two or more races, non-Hispanic/Latino), 52 international. 493 applicants, 22% accepted, 37 enrolled. In 2015, 51 doctorates awarded. *Degree requirements:* For doctorate, thesis/dissertation. *Entrance requirements:* For doctorate, GRE General Test. Additional exam requirements/recommendations for international students: Required—TOEFL. *Application deadline:* For fall admission, 12/1 priority date for domestic and international students. Applications are processed on a rolling basis. Application fee: $80. Electronic applications accepted. *Expenses: Tuition,* area resident: Full-time $31,068; part-time $5762 per course. *Required fees:* $3200; $336 per course. Full-time tuition and fees vary according to degree level, program and student level. Part-time tuition and fees vary according to course load, degree level and program. *Financial support:* In 2015–16, 339 students received support. Fellowships, research assistantships, scholarships/grants, traineeships, and unspecified assistantships available. *Unit head:* Dr. Daniel Kessler, Graduate Group Chair, 215-898-1478. *Application contact:* Meagan Schofer, Coordinator, 215-898-4360.
Website: http://www.med.upenn.edu/camb/

University of Prince Edward Island, Atlantic Veterinary College, Graduate Program in Veterinary Medicine, Charlottetown, PE C1A 4P3, Canada. Offers anatomy (M Sc, PhD); bacteriology (M Sc, PhD); clinical pharmacology (M Sc, PhD); clinical sciences (M Sc, PhD); epidemiology (M Sc, PhD), including reproduction; fish health (M Sc, PhD); food animal nutrition (M Sc, PhD); immunology (M Sc, PhD); microanatomy (M Sc, PhD); parasitology (M Sc, PhD); pathology (M Sc, PhD); pharmacology (M Sc, PhD); physiology (M Sc, PhD); toxicology (M Sc, PhD); veterinary science (M Vet Sci); virology (M Sc, PhD). *Program availability:* Part-time. *Degree requirements:* For master's, thesis; for doctorate, thesis/dissertation. *Entrance requirements:* For master's, DVM, B Sc honors degree, or equivalent; for doctorate, M Sc. Additional exam requirements/recommendations for international students: Required—TOEFL (minimum score 550 paper-based; 80 iBT). *Expenses:* Contact institution. *Faculty research:* Animal health management, infectious diseases, fin fish and shellfish health, basic biomedical sciences, ecosystem health.

University of Puerto Rico, Medical Sciences Campus, School of Medicine, Biomedical Sciences Graduate Program, Department of Physiology, San Juan, PR 00936-5067. Offers MS, PhD. Terminal master's awarded for partial completion of doctoral program. *Degree requirements:* For master's, one foreign language, thesis; for doctorate, one foreign language, comprehensive exam, thesis/dissertation. *Entrance requirements:* For master's and doctorate, GRE General Test, GRE Subject Test, interview; course work in biology, chemistry and physics; minimum GPA of 3.0; 3 letters of recommendation. Electronic applications accepted. *Faculty research:* Respiration, neuroendocrinology, cellular and molecular physiology, cardiovascular, exercise physiology and neurobiology.

University of Rochester, School of Medicine and Dentistry, Graduate Programs in Medicine and Dentistry, Department of Pharmacology and Physiology, Programs in Physiology, Rochester, NY 14627. Offers MS, PhD. Terminal master's awarded for partial completion of doctoral program. *Degree requirements:* For master's, thesis; for doctorate, thesis/dissertation, qualifying exam. *Entrance requirements:* For master's and doctorate, GRE General Test. *Expenses: Tuition,* area resident: Full-time $47,450; part-time $1482 per credit hour. *Required fees:* $528. Tuition and fees vary according to program.

University of Saskatchewan, College of Medicine, Department of Physiology, Saskatoon, SK S7N 5A2, Canada. Offers M Sc, PhD. *Degree requirements:* For master's, thesis; for doctorate, thesis/dissertation. *Entrance requirements:* Additional exam requirements/recommendations for international students: Required—TOEFL.

University of Saskatchewan, Western College of Veterinary Medicine and College of Graduate Studies and Research, Graduate Programs in Veterinary Medicine, Department of Veterinary Biomedical Sciences, Saskatoon, SK S7N 5A2, Canada. Offers veterinary anatomy (M Sc); veterinary biomedical sciences (M Vet Sci); veterinary physiological sciences (M Sc, PhD). *Degree requirements:* For master's, thesis; for doctorate, comprehensive exam (for some programs), thesis/dissertation. *Entrance requirements:* Additional exam requirements/recommendations for international students: Required—TOEFL (minimum score 80 iBT); Recommended—IELTS (minimum score 6.5). Electronic applications accepted. *Faculty research:* Toxicology, animal reproduction, pharmacology, chloride channels, pulmonary pathobiology.

The University of South Dakota, Graduate School, Sanford School of Medicine and Graduate School, Biomedical Sciences Graduate Program, Physiology and Pharmacology Group, Vermillion, SD 57069-2390. Offers MS, PhD. *Students:* Average age 25. In 2015, 1 master's, 3 doctorates awarded. Terminal master's awarded for partial completion of doctoral program. *Degree requirements:* For master's, thesis; for doctorate, comprehensive exam, thesis/dissertation. *Entrance requirements:* For master's and doctorate, GRE General Test, minimum GPA of 3.0. Additional exam requirements/recommendations for international students: Required—TOEFL (minimum score 550 paper-based; 80 iBT), IELTS (minimum score 6). *Application deadline:* For fall admission, 4/15 priority date for domestic students, 3/15 for international students. Applications are processed on a rolling basis. Application fee: $35. Electronic applications accepted. *Expenses:* Contact institution. *Financial support:* In 2015–16, 12 students received support. Fellowships with partial tuition reimbursements available, research assistantships with partial tuition reimbursements available, scholarships/grants, and unspecified assistantships available. Financial award application deadline: 4/15; financial award applicants required to submit FAFSA. *Faculty research:* Pulmonary physiology and pharmacology, drug abuse, reproduction, signal transduction, cardiovascular physiology and pharmacology. *Unit head:* 605-658-632, Fax: 605-677-6381, E-mail: biomed@usd.edu.

University of Southern California, Keck School of Medicine and Graduate School, Graduate Programs in Medicine, Department of Physiology and Biophysics, Los Angeles, CA 90089. Offers MS. *Faculty:* 13 full-time (2 women). *Students:* 3 full-time (all women); includes 2 minority (1 Asian, non-Hispanic/Latino; 1 Hispanic/Latino). Average age 22. 7 applicants, 43% accepted, 3 enrolled. *Degree requirements:* For master's, thesis optional. *Entrance requirements:* For master's, GRE General Test, minimum GPA of 3.0. Additional exam requirements/recommendations for international students: Required—TOEFL (minimum score 600 paper-based; 100 iBT). *Application deadline:* For fall admission, 12/1 priority date for domestic and international students. Applications are processed on a rolling basis. Application fee: $85. Electronic applications accepted. *Expenses:* Contact institution. *Financial support:* Application deadline: 4/15. *Faculty research:* Endocrinology and metabolism, neurophysiology, mathematical modeling, cell transport, autoimmunity and cancer immunotherapy. *Unit head:* Dr. Berislav Zlokavic, Chair, 323-442-2566, Fax: 323-442-2230, E-mail:

zlokovic@usc.edu. *Application contact:* Jim Lee, Student Services Advisor, 323-442-0230, Fax: 323-442-1610, E-mail: jim.lee@med.usc.edu.

University of South Florida, College of Arts and Sciences, Department of Integrative Biology, Tampa, FL 33620-9951. Offers biology (MS), including ecology and evolution (MS, PhD), environmental and ecological microbiology (MS, PhD), physiology and morphology (MS, PhD); integrative biology (PhD), including ecology and evolution (MS, PhD), environmental and ecological microbiology (MS, PhD), physiology and morphology (MS, PhD). *Program availability:* Part-time. *Faculty:* 14 full-time (6 women). *Students:* 48 full-time (30 women), 6 part-time (3 women); includes 10 minority (1 American Indian or Alaska Native, non-Hispanic/Latino; 1 Asian, non-Hispanic/Latino; 7 Hispanic/Latino; 1 Two or more races, non-Hispanic/Latino), 3 international. Average age 30. 43 applicants, 37% accepted, 12 enrolled. In 2015, 8 master's, 3 doctorates awarded. *Degree requirements:* For master's, comprehensive exam, thesis (for some programs); for doctorate, comprehensive exam, thesis/dissertation. *Entrance requirements:* For master's and doctorate, GRE General Test, minimum GPA of 3.0 in last 60 hours of BS. Additional exam requirements/recommendations for international students: Required—TOEFL (minimum score 570 paper-based; 88 iBT). *Application deadline:* For fall admission, 2/15 priority date for domestic students, 1/2 for international students; for spring admission, 8/1 for domestic students, 6/1 for international students. Application fee: $30. Electronic applications accepted. *Financial support:* Research assistantships, teaching assistantships, and unspecified assistantships available. Financial award application deadline: 6/30; financial award applicants required to submit FAFSA. *Faculty research:* Marine ecology, ecosystem responses to urbanization, biomechanical and physiological mechanisms of animal movement, population biology and conservation, microbial ecology and public health microbiology, natural diversity of parasites and herbivores; ecosystems, vertebrates, disturbance ecology, functional and ecological morphology of feeding in fishes, rare amphibians and reptiles, genomics in ecological experiments, ecotoxicology, global carbon cycle, plant-animal interactions. *Total annual research expenditures:* $1.3 million. *Unit head:* Dr. Valerie Harwood, Professor and Chair, 813-974-1524, Fax: 813-974-3263, E-mail: vharwood@usf.edu. *Application contact:* Dr. Lynn Martin, Associate Professor and Graduate Program Director, 813-974-0157, Fax: 813-974-3263, E-mail: lbmartin@usf.edu.
Website: http://biology.usf.edu/ib/grad/

University of South Florida, Morsani College of Medicine and College of Graduate Studies, Graduate Programs in Medical Sciences, Tampa, FL 33620-9951. Offers advanced athletic training (MS); athletic training (MS); bioinformatics and computational biology (MSBCB); biotechnology (MSB); health informatics (MSHI); medical sciences (MSMS, PhD), including aging and neuroscience (MSMS), allergy, immunology and infectious disease (PhD), anatomy (MSMS), athletic training (MSMS), clinical and translational research, health informatics (MSMS), health science (MSMS), interdisciplinary medical sciences (MSMS), medical microbiology and immunology (MSMS), metabolic and nutritional medicine (MSMS), molecular medicine, molecular pharmacology and physiology (PhD), neurology (PhD), pathology and laboratory medicine (PhD), pharmacology and therapeutics (PhD), physiology and biophysics (PhD), women's health (MSMS). *Students:* 510 full-time (261 women), 318 part-time (208 women); includes 360 minority (108 Black or African American, non-Hispanic/Latino; 3 American Indian or Alaska Native, non-Hispanic/Latino; 101 Asian, non-Hispanic/Latino; 124 Hispanic/Latino; 1 Native Hawaiian or other Pacific Islander, non-Hispanic/Latino; 23 Two or more races, non-Hispanic/Latino), 52 international. Average age 26. 6,567 applicants, 13% accepted, 469 enrolled. In 2015, 216 master's awarded. Terminal master's awarded for partial completion of doctoral program. *Degree requirements:* For master's, comprehensive exam, thesis; for doctorate, comprehensive exam, thesis/dissertation. *Entrance requirements:* For master's, GRE General Test or GMAT, bachelor's degree or equivalent from regionally-accredited university with minimum GPA of 3.0 in upper-division sciences coursework; prerequisites in general biology, general chemistry, general physics, organic chemistry, quantitative analysis, and integral and differential calculus; for doctorate, GRE General Test, bachelor's degree from regionally-accredited university with minimum GPA of 3.0 in upper-division sciences coursework; 3 letters of recommendation; personal interview; 1-2 page personal statement; prerequisites in biology, chemistry, physics, organic chemistry, quantitative analysis, and integral/differential calculus. Additional exam requirements/recommendations for international students: Required—TOEFL (minimum score 550 paper-based; 79 iBT) or IELTS (minimum score 6.5). *Application deadline:* For fall admission, 2/15 for domestic students, 1/2 for international students. Application fee: $30. *Expenses:* Contact institution. *Faculty research:* Anatomy, biochemistry, cancer biology, cardiovascular disease, cell biology, immunology, microbiology, molecular biology, neuroscience, pharmacology, physiology. *Unit head:* Dr. Michael Barber, Professor/Associate Dean for Graduate and Postdoctoral Affairs, 813-974-9908, Fax: 813-974-4317, E-mail: mbarber@health.usf.edu. *Application contact:* Dr. Eric Bennett, Graduate Director, PhD Program in Medical Sciences, 813-974-1545, Fax: 813-974-4317, E-mail: esbennet@health.usf.edu.
Website: http://health.usf.edu/nocms/medicine/graduatestudies/

The University of Tennessee, Graduate School, College of Agricultural Sciences and Natural Resources, Department of Animal Science, Knoxville, TN 37996. Offers animal anatomy (PhD); breeding (MS, PhD); management (MS, PhD); nutrition (MS, PhD); physiology (MS, PhD). *Program availability:* Part-time. *Degree requirements:* For master's, thesis; for doctorate, thesis/dissertation. *Entrance requirements:* For master's and doctorate, GRE General Test, minimum GPA of 2.7. Additional exam requirements/recommendations for international students: Required—TOEFL. Electronic applications accepted.

The University of Texas Medical Branch, Graduate School of Biomedical Sciences, Program in Cellular Physiology and Molecular Biophysics, Galveston, TX 77555. Offers MS, PhD. *Degree requirements:* For master's, thesis or alternative; for doctorate, thesis/dissertation. *Entrance requirements:* For master's and doctorate, GRE General Test. Additional exam requirements/recommendations for international students: Required—TOEFL (minimum score 550 paper-based). Electronic applications accepted.

University of Toronto, Faculty of Medicine, Department of Physiology, Toronto, ON M5S 1A1, Canada. Offers M Sc, PhD, MD/PhD. *Degree requirements:* For master's, thesis; for doctorate, thesis/dissertation. *Entrance requirements:* For master's and doctorate, minimum B+ average in final year, 2 letters of reference. Additional exam requirements/recommendations for international students: Required—TOEFL (minimum score 600 paper-based), Michigan English Language Assessment Battery (minimum score 95), IELTS (minimum score 8), or COPE (minimum score 5). Electronic applications accepted.

University of Utah, Graduate School, College of Health, Division of Nutrition, Salt Lake City, UT 84112. Offers nutrition and integrative physiology (MS, PhD), including integrative physiology (MS), nutrition (MS). *Accreditation:* AND. *Program availability:* 100% online. *Faculty:* 4 full-time (2 women), 12 part-time/adjunct (10 women). *Students:* 36 full-time (29 women), 6 part-time (5 women); includes 3 minority (1 American Indian or Alaska Native, non-Hispanic/Latino; 1 Native Hawaiian or other Pacific Islander, non-Hispanic/Latino; 1 Two or more races, non-Hispanic/Latino), 1 international. Average age 27. 65 applicants, 26% accepted, 17 enrolled. In 2015, 17 master's awarded. Terminal master's awarded for partial completion of doctoral program. *Degree*

Physiology

requirements: For master's, comprehensive exam, thesis; for doctorate, thesis/dissertation. *Entrance requirements:* For master's, GRE General Test, minimum undergraduate GPA of 3.0; for doctorate, GRE General Test. Additional exam requirements/recommendations for international students: Required—TOEFL (minimum score 500 paper-based). *Application deadline:* For fall and winter admission, 2/15 for domestic and international students. Application fee: $55 ($65 for international students). Electronic applications accepted. *Expenses:* Contact institution. *Financial support:* In 2015–16, 22 students received support, including 2 research assistantships with partial tuition reimbursements available (averaging $7,250 per year), 10 teaching assistantships with partial tuition reimbursements available (averaging $7,250 per year); career-related internships or fieldwork, scholarships/grants, and unspecified assistantships also available. Financial award application deadline: 2/15; financial award applicants required to submit FAFSA. *Faculty research:* Cholesterol metabolism, sport nutrition education, metabolic and critical care, cardiovascular nutrition, wilderness nutrition, pediatric nutrition. *Total annual research expenditures:* $120,000. *Unit head:* Dr. Julie Metos, Director, 801-587-3024, Fax: 801-585-3874, E-mail: julie.metos@hsc.utah.edu. *Application contact:* Jean Zancanella, Academic Adviser, 801-581-5280, Fax: 801-585-3874, E-mail: jean.zancanella@health.utah.edu.
Website: http://www.health.utah.edu/fdnu

University of Utah, School of Medicine and Graduate School, Graduate Programs in Medicine, Department of Physiology, Salt Lake City, UT 84112-1107. Offers PhD. *Degree requirements:* For doctorate, thesis/dissertation, comprehensive qualifying exam, preliminary exam. *Entrance requirements:* For doctorate, GRE General Test, GRE Subject Test, minimum GPA of 3.0. Additional exam requirements/recommendations for international students: Required—TOEFL (minimum score 650 paper-based; 100 iBT); Recommended—TWE (minimum score 6). Electronic applications accepted. *Faculty research:* Cell neurobiology, chemosensory systems, cardiovascular and kidney physiology, endocrinology.

University of Virginia, School of Medicine, Department of Molecular Physiology and Biological Physics, Program in Physiology, Charlottesville, VA 22903. Offers PhD, MD/PhD. *Entrance requirements:* For doctorate, GRE General Test, 2 letters of recommendation. Additional exam requirements/recommendations for international students: Required—TOEFL. Electronic applications accepted.

University of Washington, Graduate School, School of Medicine, Graduate Programs in Medicine, Department of Physiology and Biophysics, Seattle, WA 98195. Offers PhD. *Degree requirements:* For doctorate, thesis/dissertation. *Entrance requirements:* For doctorate, GRE General Test. Additional exam requirements/recommendations for international students: Required—TOEFL (minimum score 580 paper-based; 70 iBT). *Faculty research:* Membrane and cell biophysics, neuroendocrinology, cardiovascular and respiratory physiology, systems neurophysiology and behavior, molecular physiology.

The University of Western Ontario, Faculty of Graduate Studies, Biosciences Division, Department of Physiology and Pharmacology, London, ON N6A 5B8, Canada. Offers M Sc, PhD. *Degree requirements:* For master's, thesis, seminar course; for doctorate, comprehensive exam, thesis/dissertation. *Entrance requirements:* For master's, minimum B average, honors degree; for doctorate, minimum B average, honors degree, M Sc. *Faculty research:* Reproductive and endocrine physiology, neurophysiology, cardiovascular and renal physiology, cell physiology, gastrointestinal and metabolic physiology.

University of Wisconsin–La Crosse, College of Science and Health, Department of Biology, La Crosse, WI 54601-3742. Offers aquatic sciences (MS); biology (MS); cellular and molecular biology (MS); clinical microbiology (MS); microbiology (MS); nurse anesthesia (MS); physiology (MS). *Program availability:* Part-time. *Students:* 19 full-time (12 women), 50 part-time (26 women); includes 4 minority (3 Asian, non-Hispanic/Latino; 1 Hispanic/Latino), 1 international. Average age 29. 44 applicants, 75% accepted, 27 enrolled. In 2015, 27 master's awarded. *Degree requirements:* For master's, comprehensive exam, thesis. *Entrance requirements:* For master's, GRE General Test, minimum GPA of 2.85. Additional exam requirements/recommendations for international students: Required—TOEFL (minimum score 550 paper-based; 79 iBT). *Application deadline:* For fall admission, 2/1 priority date for domestic and international students; for spring admission, 1/4 priority date for domestic and international students. Applications are processed on a rolling basis. Electronic applications accepted. *Financial support:* Research assistantships with partial tuition reimbursements, Federal Work-Study, scholarships/grants, health care benefits, and tuition waivers (partial) available. Support available to part-time students. Financial award application deadline: 3/15; financial award applicants required to submit FAFSA. *Unit head:* Dr. Mark Sandheinrich, Department Chair, 608-785-8261, E-mail: msandheinrich@uwlax.edu. *Application contact:* Brandon Schaller, Senior Graduate Student Status Examiner, 608-785-8941, E-mail: admissions@uwlax.edu.
Website: http://uwlax.edu/biology/

University of Wisconsin–Madison, School of Medicine and Public Health, Endocrinology-Reproductive Physiology Program, Madison, WI 53706. Offers MS, PhD. Terminal master's awarded for partial completion of doctoral program. *Expenses:* Tuition, state resident: full-time $5364. Tuition, nonresident: full-time $12,027. *Required fees:* $571. Tuition and fees vary according to campus/location, program and reciprocity agreements.
Website: http://www.erp.wisc.edu/

University of Wisconsin–Madison, School of Medicine and Public Health, Physiology Graduate Training Program, Madison, WI 53706. Offers PhD. *Expenses:* Tuition, state resident: full-time $5364. Tuition, nonresident: full-time $12,027. *Required fees:* $571. Tuition and fees vary according to campus/location, program and reciprocity agreements.
Website: http://www.pgtp.wisc.edu/

University of Wyoming, College of Arts and Sciences, Department of Zoology and Physiology, Laramie, WY 82071. Offers MS, PhD. *Program availability:* Part-time. *Degree requirements:* For master's, comprehensive exam (for some programs), thesis; for doctorate, comprehensive exam (for some programs), thesis/dissertation. *Entrance requirements:* For master's and doctorate, GRE General Test, minimum GPA of 3.0. Additional exam requirements/recommendations for international students: Required—TOEFL. Electronic applications accepted. *Faculty research:* Cell biology, ecology/wildlife, organismal physiology, zoology.

Virginia Commonwealth University, Graduate School, School of Allied Health Professions, Department of Physical Therapy, Richmond, VA 23284-9005. Offers advanced physical therapy (DPT); entry-level physical therapy (DPT); health related sciences (PhD); physiology/physical therapy (PhD). *Accreditation:* APTA (one or more programs are accredited). *Degree requirements:* For doctorate, thesis/dissertation. *Entrance requirements:* For doctorate, GRE General Test, Physical Therapist Centralized Application Service (PTCAS). Additional exam requirements/recommendations for international students: Required—TOEFL (minimum score 600 paper-based; 100 iBT). Electronic applications accepted. *Faculty research:* Eye movement, bilabyrinthectomy on ferret muscle fiber typing, neck disability index, cost-effective care, training effect on muscle.

Virginia Commonwealth University, Medical College of Virginia-Professional Programs, School of Medicine, School of Medicine Graduate Programs, Department of Physiology and Biophysics, Richmond, VA 23284-9005. Offers physical therapy (PhD); physiology (MS, PhD); MD/PhD. Terminal master's awarded for partial completion of doctoral program. *Degree requirements:* For master's, thesis; for doctorate, thesis/dissertation, comprehensive oral and written exams. *Entrance requirements:* For master's, GRE General Test, MCAT, or DAT; for doctorate, GRE, MCAT or DAT. Additional exam requirements/recommendations for international students: Required—TOEFL (minimum score 600 paper-based; 100 iBT). Electronic applications accepted.

Virginia Commonwealth University, Program in Pre-Medical Basic Health Sciences, Richmond, VA 23284-9005. Offers anatomy (CBHS); biochemistry (CBHS); human genetics (CBHS); microbiology (CBHS); pharmacology (CBHS); physiology (CBHS). *Entrance requirements:* For degree, GRE, MCAT or DAT, course work in organic chemistry, minimum undergraduate GPA of 2.8. Additional exam requirements/recommendations for international students: Required—TOEFL (minimum score 600 paper-based). Electronic applications accepted.

Wake Forest University, School of Medicine and Graduate School of Arts and Sciences, Graduate Programs in Medicine, Program in Physiology and Pharmacology, Winston-Salem, NC 27109. Offers pharmacology (PhD); physiology (PhD); MD/PhD. *Degree requirements:* For doctorate, thesis/dissertation. *Entrance requirements:* For doctorate, GRE General Test. Additional exam requirements/recommendations for international students: Required—TOEFL. Electronic applications accepted. *Faculty research:* Aging, substance abuse, cardiovascular control, endocrine systems, toxicology.

Wayne State University, School of Medicine, Office of Biomedical Graduate Programs, Department of Physiology, Detroit, MI 48202. Offers physiology (MS, PhD); reproductive sciences (PhD); MD/PhD. *Faculty:* 40. *Students:* 25 full-time (15 women), 5 part-time (1 woman); includes 5 minority (2 Black or African American, non-Hispanic/Latino; 1 Asian, non-Hispanic/Latino; 1 Hispanic/Latino; 1 Two or more races, non-Hispanic/Latino), 10 international. Average age 28. 42 applicants, 17% accepted, 3 enrolled. In 2015, 3 master's, 9 doctorates awarded. *Degree requirements:* For master's, thesis; for doctorate, thesis/dissertation. *Entrance requirements:* For master's, GRE General Test, minimum GPA of 2.75, personal statement, resume, three letters of recommendation, current curriculum vitae or resume; for doctorate, GRE General Test, minimum GPA of 3.0, personal statement, resume, three letters of recommendation, current curriculum vitae or resume. Additional exam requirements/recommendations for international students: Required—TOEFL. *Application deadline:* For fall admission, 2/1 priority date for domestic and international students. Applications are processed on a rolling basis. Application fee: $0. Electronic applications accepted. *Expenses:* $17,645 per year resident tuition, $33,311 non-resident tuition; $735.20 per credit hour resident tuition, $1,387.95 per credit hour non-resident tuition; fees include $47.45 per credit hour student services fee and $274.60 per semester registration fee. *Financial support:* In 2015–16, 26 students received support, including 7 fellowships with tuition reimbursements available (averaging $24,125 per year), 21 research assistantships with tuition reimbursements available (averaging $26,877 per year); scholarships/grants and unspecified assistantships also available. Financial award application deadline: 3/31. *Faculty research:* Cardiovascular pathophysiology and muscle contractility, neural regulation of peripheral organ systems, ischemia and reperfusion injury of heart and brain, basic cellular physiology of endocrine signallin, biochemical and biophysical studies of ion transport, and cellular stress responses. *Unit head:* Dr. Douglas Yingst, Graduate Program Director, 313-577-1548, E-mail: dyingst@med.wayne.edu.
Website: http://physiology.med.wayne.edu/phd.php

Weill Cornell Medicine, Weill Cornell Graduate School of Medical Sciences, Physiology, Biophysics and Systems Biology Program, New York, NY 10065. Offers MS, PhD. Terminal master's awarded for partial completion of doctoral program. *Degree requirements:* For master's, comprehensive exam; for doctorate, thesis/dissertation, final exam. *Entrance requirements:* For doctorate, GRE General Test, introductory courses in biology, inorganic and organic chemistry, physics, and mathematics. Additional exam requirements/recommendations for international students: Required—TOEFL. *Faculty research:* Receptor-mediated regulation of cell function, molecular properties of channels or receptors, bioinformatics, mathematical modeling.

Western Michigan University, Graduate College, College of Education and Human Development, Department of Health, Physical Education and Recreation, Kalamazoo, MI 49008. Offers athletic training (MS), including exercise physiology; sport management (MA), including pedagogy, special physical education.

West Virginia University, Davis College of Agriculture, Forestry and Consumer Sciences, Division of Animal and Nutritional Sciences, Program in Animal and Nutritional Sciences, Morgantown, WV 26506. Offers breeding (MS); food sciences (MS); nutrition (MS); physiology (MS); production management (MS); reproduction (MS). *Program availability:* Part-time. *Degree requirements:* For master's, thesis, oral and written exams. *Entrance requirements:* For master's, GRE, minimum GPA of 2.5. Additional exam requirements/recommendations for international students: Required—TOEFL. *Expenses:* Tuition, state resident: full-time $8568. Tuition, nonresident: full-time $22,140. Tuition and fees vary according to program. *Faculty research:* Animal nutrition, reproductive physiology, food science.

West Virginia University, Davis College of Agriculture, Forestry and Consumer Sciences, Interdisciplinary Program in Reproductive Physiology, Morgantown, WV 26506. Offers MS, PhD. *Program availability:* Part-time. Terminal master's awarded for partial completion of doctoral program. *Degree requirements:* For master's, thesis; for doctorate, comprehensive exam, thesis/dissertation. *Entrance requirements:* For master's, minimum GPA of 2.75; for doctorate, minimum GPA of 3.0. Additional exam requirements/recommendations for international students: Required—TOEFL. Electronic applications accepted. *Expenses:* Tuition, state resident: full-time $8568. Tuition, nonresident: full-time $22,140. Tuition and fees vary according to program. *Faculty research:* Uterine prostaglandins, luteal function, neural control of luteinizing hormone and follicle-stimulating hormone, follicular development, embryonic and fetal loss.

West Virginia University, School of Medicine, Graduate Programs at the Health Sciences Center, Interdisciplinary Graduate Programs in Biomedical Sciences, Program in Cellular and Integrative Physiology, Morgantown, WV 26506. Offers MS, PhD, MD/PhD. *Degree requirements:* For doctorate, comprehensive exam, thesis/dissertation. *Entrance requirements:* For doctorate, GRE General Test, minimum GPA of 3.0. Additional exam requirements/recommendations for international students: Required—TOEFL. Electronic applications accepted. *Expenses:* Tuition, state resident: full-time $8568. Tuition, nonresident: full-time $22,140. Tuition and fees vary according to program. *Faculty research:* Cell signaling and development of the microvasculature, neural control of reproduction, learning and memory, airway responsiveness and remodeling.

Wright State University, School of Graduate Studies, College of Science and Mathematics, Department of Neuroscience, Cell Biology, and Physiology, Dayton, OH 45435. Offers anatomy (MS); physiology and biophysics (MS). *Degree requirements:* For master's, thesis optional. *Entrance requirements:* Additional exam requirements/

recommendations for international students: Required—TOEFL. *Faculty research:* Reproductive cell biology, neurobiology of pain, neurohistochemistry.

Yale University, School of Medicine and Graduate School of Arts and Sciences, Combined Program in Biological and Biomedical Sciences (BBS), Physiology and Integrative Medical Biology Track, New Haven, CT 06520. Offers PhD, MD/PhD. *Entrance requirements:* Additional exam requirements/recommendations for international students: Required—TOEFL.

Youngstown State University, Graduate School, College of Science, Technology, Engineering and Mathematics, Department of Biological Sciences, Youngstown, OH 44555-0001. Offers environmental biology (MS); molecular biology, microbiology, and genetic (MS); physiology and anatomy (MS). *Program availability:* Part-time. *Degree requirements:* For master's, comprehensive exam, thesis, oral review. *Entrance requirements:* For master's, GRE General Test, minimum GPA of 2.7. Additional exam requirements/recommendations for international students: Required—TOEFL. *Faculty research:* Cell biology, neurophysiology, molecular biology, neurobiology, gene regulation.

UNIVERSITY OF CONNECTICUT
College of Liberal Arts and Sciences
Department of Physiology and Neurobiology

 For more information, visit http://petersons.to/uconn-physiology-neurobio

Programs of Study

The Department offers course work and research programs leading to M.S. and Ph.D. degrees in physiology and neurobiology with concentrations in the areas of neurobiology, endocrinology, and comparative physiology. In addition, the Department of Molecular and Cell Biology, the Department of Ecology and Evolutionary Biology, and the Biotechnology Center provide the opportunity for students to obtain a comprehensive background in biological sciences and offer the possibility of collaborative research. Graduate programs are designed to fit the individual student's background and scientific interests. In the first year, students take two courses on the foundations of physiology and neurobiology. Through the first two years, and occasionally into the third year of training, students select from a number of additional seminars and courses in their area of major interest and related areas. By the end of the first year, the student selects the area of dissertation research, and a committee consisting of a major adviser and 3 associate advisers is formed. Students may begin dissertation research during the first year (http://www.pnb.uconn. edu/pnb-home-page/graduate-program/).

Research Facilities

The Department of Physiology and Neurobiology (PNB) is located primarily in the new state-of-the-art Pharmacy/Biology Building. The Department houses both shared and individual laboratories for behavioral, cellular, electrophysiological, and molecular research in physiology. The Department also houses the University's electron microscopy facility, which contains equipment for scanning and transmission EM as well as electron probe analysis. Departmental faculty members also utilize the Marine Research Laboratories at Noank and Avery Point, Connecticut.

Financial Aid

Several types of financial support are available to graduate students. Most students are supported either on teaching assistantships or research assistantships from faculty grants. For the 2016–17 academic year, full-time teaching assistantships (nine months) pay $22,243 for beginning graduate students, $23,405 for those with an M.S. or the equivalent, and $26,021 for those who have passed the Ph.D. general examination. Both half and full graduate assistantships come with a tuition waiver with full-time registration (six credits or more and maintaining a 3.0 or better grade point average). Students may purchase health-care coverage, subsidized by the University of Connecticut. In addition, the Graduate School provides the Outstanding Scholar Award to as many as 10 incoming Ph.D. candidates during the first year of study. Several additional research fellowships and University fellowships are awarded on a competitive basis. Many labs also provide additional funding for summer research (up to $6,000).

Cost of Study

Tuition is waived for full-time graduate assistants; however, they pay the full-time University fees at the full-time rate (http://bursar.uconn.edu/2016-2017-graduate-tuition-and-fees/). Tuition is prorated for graduate assistants registering for fewer than 6 credits per semester.

Living and Housing Costs

The University is in the midst of an extraordinary period of growth. Priority is given to newly admitted international graduate students and graduate housing is only provided to graduate students enrolled at the Storrs campus. Graduate students can request access to the fall 2016 housing application via email to livingoncampus@uconn.edu. Access will only be granted if spaces are available. The University does not have family housing available for students. Single graduate student housing is offered in Northwood Apartments.

Graduate students who accept on-campus housing are financially responsible for room (and board if applicable) fees for the entire academic year, or the portion of the academic year that remains at the time of occupancy. More information and the housing contract can be found online at http://reslife. uconn.edu/housing-contract-forms. Information regarding off-campus housing is available from Off-Campus Student Services, www.offcampus. uconn.edu; offcampus@uconn.edu.

Student Group

Approximately 23,000 undergraduates and 8,000 graduate students are enrolled at the main campus at Storrs. Seventy-seven percent of the undergraduate students and 64 percent of the graduate students are from

Connecticut. The rest of the students come from forty states and more than 111 countries (http://uconn.edu/about-us/). The Department of Physiology and Neurobiology has about 40 graduate students (http://www.pnb.uconn. edu/pnb-home-page/graduate-program/).

Location

The University is located in a scenic countryside setting of small villages, streams, and rolling hills. There is easy access by car and bus to major urban and cultural centers, including Hartford, New Haven, Boston, and New York, and to other educational institutions, such as Yale, Harvard, and MIT. Recreational opportunities include skiing, fishing, sailing, hiking, ice-skating, and athletic events. The University of Connecticut offers a range of culturally—and gastronomically—rich attractions. Students can visit diverse and distinct museums; attend world-class performances in music, theater, and the performing arts; and frequent nearby Storrs Downtown, a vibrant town square featuring cafés, restaurants, and shopping galore. There are also several large shopping centers nearby.

The University

The University of Connecticut at Storrs is the state's flagship public research university and is in the midst of a $2.6 billion transformation, ensuring its place as one of the premier public research universities in the country. Perennially ranked the top public university in New England, the University of Connecticut now stands among the best public institutions in the nation. The University was founded in 1881 and is a state-supported institution. The 1,800-acre main campus at Storrs is the site of vigorous undergraduate and graduate programs in agriculture, liberal arts and sciences, fine arts, engineering, education, business administration, human development and family relations, physical education, pharmacy, nursing, and physical therapy. Extensive cultural and recreational programs and athletic facilities are available.

Applying

Prospective PNB graduate students are asked to fill out the PNB Department's preliminary questionnaire online at http://pnbfiles.uconn.edu/PNB_Base/ graduate/questionnaire.html. For admission to the fall semester, it is suggested that applications be submitted by December 15. To be considered for financial support, students should submit applications by January 15 for admission the following August. U.S. applicants must submit scores on the General Test of the Graduate Record Examinations (or MCATs) and must have maintained at least a 3.0 quality point ratio (GPA) for admission as graduate students with regular status. Applicants must request that GRE scores be sent directly to the Graduate School in Storrs, code 3915; the PNB Department code is 0217. Although there is no official deadline, applications and credentials from international students should be received by February 1 for admission in the fall semester or by October 1 for the spring semester and must include official TOEFL scores. The University does not discriminate in admission on the basis of race, gender, age, or national origin. Graduate students can apply online at http://grad.uconn.edu/prospective-students/admissions-requirements.

Correspondence and Information

Graduate Admissions Committee
Department of Physiology and Neurobiology
University of Connecticut
Box U-3156
Storrs, Connecticut 06269-3156
United States
E-mail: kathleen.kelleher@uconn.edu
Website: http://www.pnb.uconn.edu

THE FACULTY AND THEIR RESEARCH

Marie E. Cantino, Associate Professor; Ph.D., Washington (Seattle). Research in this laboratory is directed toward understanding the mechanisms of contraction in striated muscle. In particular, the lab is using electron microscopy and biochemical and mechanical assays to study the structure and organization of proteins in the contractile filaments and the mechanisms by which calcium regulates the interactions of these proteins.

Joanne Conover, Associate Professor; Ph.D., Bath (England). Research in the laboratory focuses on stem cell niche dynamics supporting neurogenesis and other reparative functions in the adult mouse brain. A combination of techniques, including cell culture of neural and embryonic stem cells,

RT-PCR–based gene expression analysis, and examination of mouse genetic models for neurodegenerative diseases and mild traumatic brain injury aid us in understanding the potential for stem cell–mediated contributions for repair and replacement in human disease and aging.

Joseph F. Crivello, Professor (joint appointment in Marine Sciences); Ph.D., Wisconsin. Research is centered in two areas. One area examines the impact of pollution on marine organisms at a biochemical and genetic level. The other area examines pollution as a selective pressure altering the genetic diversity of marine organisms.

Angel L. de Blas, Professor; Ph.D., Indiana. Molecular structure and function of neurotransmitter receptors and inhibitory synapses in the brain. Studies are being conducted on elucidating the molecular structure of GABA receptors with other synaptic proteins that determine the synaptic localization of the GABA receptors. Techniques include recombinant DNA; transgenic expression of proteins; mRNA; protein regulation; monoclonal antibodies; cell culture; and light, electron, and laser confocal microscopy.

Robert V. Gallo, Professor; Ph.D., Purdue. The objective of the research program is to understand the neuroendocrine mechanisms regulating luteinizing hormone release during different physiological conditions. In particular, the research examines the involvement of CNS neurotransmitters and endogenous opioid peptides in this process.

Alexander C. Jackson, Assistant Professor; Ph.D. Harvard. Research in the laboratory is focused on the cellular and synaptic neurophysiology of neural circuits in the mammalian hypothalamus that regulate fundamental behavioral states such as sleep, arousal and feeding. Techniques are centered on using patch-clamp electrophysiology and pharmacology in brain slices in order to elucidate the cellular and synaptic properties of specific hypothalamic cell-types and their local and long-range synaptic connectivity. This approach is carried out in concert with a toolbox of neuroanatomical methods and optogenetic strategies to manipulate the excitability of genetically targeted neurons.

Rahul N. Kanadia, Assistant Professor, Ph.D., Florida. Research is focused on deciphering the role of alternative splicing in neural development. The neural mouse retina is employed as a model system to investigate this question. Various techniques such as in situ hybridizations and molecular biology techniques are used to detect different forms of RNA. Since this is studied in development, live imaging is also used to document changes in splice pattern and its impact on cell fate determination and differentiation.

Joseph J. LoTurco, Professor and Department Head; Ph.D., Stanford. Pathophysiology related to disruptions in cerebral neocortical development, causes of epilepsy and brain tumors. Currently, a combination of molecular genetics, patch clamp electrophysiology, and cell culture are being used to study the mechanisms that regulate neurogenesis in the cerebral cortex.

Karen Menuz, Assistant Professor; Ph.D., California, San Francisco. Research is focused on the molecular basis of volatile chemical detection by olfactory receptors, neurons employing electrophysiology, genomic, genetic, molecular biology, and microscopy techniques.

Andrew Moiseff, Professor and Associate Dean for Life Sciences, CLAS; Ph.D., Cornell. The laboratory is interested in the extraction and processing of sensory information by the nervous system. We are currently focused on identifying generalizable principles of visual system organization by employing behavioral and electrophysiological techniques to study flash signaling in fireflies.

Daniel K. Mulkey, Associate Professor; Ph.D., Wright State. Research focuses on the cellular and molecular mechanisms by which the brain controls breathing, in particular, understanding the molecular mechanism by which respiratory chemoreceptors sense changes in pH to drive breathing and the cellular mechanisms that modulate activity of these cells. Another interest is the role of nitric oxide on state-dependent modulation of respiratory motor neurons for a better understanding of the mechanisms underlying respiratory control, leading to new therapeutic approaches for the treatment of disorders such as sudden infant death syndrome and sleep apnea. Techniques include cellular electrophysiology in brain slices, cell culture, and single-cell RT-PCR.

Akiko Nishiyama, Professor; M.D., Nippon Medical School; Ph.D., Niigata (Japan). Research focuses on the lineage and function of oligodendrocyte progenitor cells (NG2 cells) in the central nervous system in normal and pathological states. Current studies apply immunohistochemical, tissue culture, biochemical, and molecular biological analyses on various mouse genetic models to understand the mechanisms that regulate proliferation and differentiation of these glial cells and to explore their role in the neural network.

J. Larry Renfro, Professor; Ph.D., Oklahoma. Currently we are studying the mechanisms and regulation of epithelial transport of phosphate and xenobiotics by tissues isolated from a variety of vertebrates, including rats, birds, and fishes. Work has concentrated on ion transport and its regulation in primary monolayer cultures of renal epithelium and choroid plexus. The laboratory also studies transport by renal tubule brush border and basolateral membrane vesicles.

Daniel Schwartz, Assistant Professor; Ph.D., Harvard. Research is focused on computational and experimental techniques to discover, catalog, and functionally understand short linear protein motifs. Specific projects include: (1) the continued improvement of the motif-x and scan-x web-tools, (2) the development of experimental methodologies to uncover kinase motifs, and (3) the analysis of motif signatures on viral protein primary structure toward the goal of elucidating mechanisms of viral propagation and developing therapeutic agents.

Jianjun Sun, Assistant Professor; Ph.D., Florida State. Research in the laboratory focuses on reproductive physiology and ovarian cancer. Powerful genetic tools in *Drosophila* will be applied to decipher the formation and physiological function of the secretory cells in the female reproductive tract, the cells of origin of ovarian cancer. Another focus in the lab is to decipher the intrinsic mechanism controlling follicle rupture and ovulation, a process positively linked to ovarian cancer risk. The conserved molecular mechanisms will be further verified in mice with conditional knock-out models, which will ultimately aid in understanding the basic biology of the female reproductive system and their contributions to ovarian cancer.

Anastasios Tzingounis, Associate Professor; Ph.D., Oregon Health & Science. Research in the laboratory concentrates on the cellular and molecular mechanisms that control neuronal excitability in the mammalian brain. To study the molecules and signaling networks that tune the brain's innate ability to prevent epilepsy, a multidisciplinary approach is used that combines molecular and genetic techniques with optical imaging and electrophysiology.

Randall S. Walikonis, Associate Professor; Ph.D., Mayo. Research is directed at studying the postsynaptic signal transduction systems of excitatory synapses. The laboratory uses biochemical and molecular biological techniques to identify proteins associated with NMDA receptors and to determine their specific roles in the function of excitatory synapses. The lab also studies the role of growth factors in modifying excitatory synapses.

Li Wang, Professor; Ph.D., Research in this laboratory is focused on several related areas centered on nuclear receptor regulation of chronic liver diseases: 1) transcriptional and translational regulation of non-coding RNA (microRNA and lncRNA) in bile acid metabolism and cholestatic liver fibrosis; 2) nutrient mediated mTOR and metabolic signaling in the epigenetic control of liver cancer; 3) circadian clock control of ER stress signaling and homocysteine metabolism in alcoholic fatty liver. Our approach makes full use of system biology, molecular biology, biochemistry, and genome-wide high throughput transcriptomics (RNA-seq) and metabolomics (GC-MS). Both in vitro cell culture and in vivo single- and double-knockout mouse models are employed for our studies.

PNB graduate student conducting experiments in the Crivello Lab in the UConn PNB Department.

PNB graduate student conducting experiments in the Renfro Lab in the UConn PNB Department.

Section 19
Zoology

This section contains a directory of institutions offering graduate work in zoology. Additional information about programs listed in the directory may be obtained by writing directly to the dean of a graduate school or chair of a department at the address given in the directory.

For programs offering related work, see also in this book *Anatomy; Biochemistry; Biological and Biomedical Sciences; Cell, Molecular, and Structural Biology; Ecology, Environmental Biology, and Evolutionary Biology; Entomology; Genetics, Developmental Biology, and Reproductive Biology; Microbiological Sciences; Neuroscience and Neurobiology; Neurobiology; Physiology;* and *Veterinary Medicine and Sciences.* In the other guides in this series:

Graduate Programs in the Physical Sciences, Mathematics, Agricultural Sciences, the Environment & Natural Resources

See *Agricultural and Food Sciences, Environmental Sciences and Management,* and *Marine Sciences and Oceanography*

Graduate Programs in Engineering & Applied Sciences

See *Agricultural Engineering and Bioengineering* and *Ocean Engineering*

CONTENTS

Program Directories

Animal Behavior

Arizona State University at the Tempe campus, College of Liberal Arts and Sciences, School of Life Sciences, Tempe, AZ 85287-4601. Offers animal behavior (PhD); applied ethics (biomedical and health ethics) (MA); biology (MS, PhD), including biology, biology and society, complex adaptive systems science (PhD), plant biology and conservation (MS); environmental life sciences (PhD); evolutionary biology (PhD); history and philosophy of science (PhD); human and social dimensions of science and technology (PhD); microbiology (PhD); molecular and cellular biology (PhD); neuroscience (PhD). Terminal master's awarded for partial completion of doctoral program. *Degree requirements:* For master's, thesis (for some programs), interactive Program of Study (iPOS) submitted before completing 50 percent of required credit hours; for doctorate, variable foreign language requirement, comprehensive exam, thesis/dissertation, interactive Program of Study (iPOS) submitted before completing 50 percent of required credit hours. *Entrance requirements:* For master's and doctorate, GRE, minimum GPA of 3.0 or equivalent in last 2 years of work leading to bachelor's degree. Additional exam requirements/recommendations for international students: Required—TOEFL (minimum score 600 paper-based; 100 iBT). Electronic applications accepted.

Bucknell University, Graduate Studies, College of Arts and Sciences, Department of Animal Behavior, Lewisburg, PA 17837. Offers MS. *Degree requirements:* For master's, thesis. *Entrance requirements:* For master's, GRE General Test, GRE Subject Test, minimum GPA of 3.0. Additional exam requirements/recommendations for international students: Required—TOEFL (minimum score 600 paper-based).

Cornell University, Graduate School, Graduate Fields of Agriculture and Life Sciences, Field of Neurobiology and Behavior, Ithaca, NY 14853-0001. Offers behavioral biology (PhD), including behavioral ecology, chemical ecology, ethology, neuroethology, sociobiology; neurobiology (PhD), including cellular and molecular neurobiology, neuroanatomy, neurochemistry, neuropharmacology, neurophysiology, sensory physiology. *Degree requirements:* For doctorate, comprehensive exam, thesis/dissertation, 1 year of teaching experience, seminar presentation. *Entrance requirements:* For doctorate, GRE General Test, GRE Subject Test (biology), 3 letters of recommendation. Additional exam requirements/recommendations for international students: Required—TOEFL (minimum score 550 paper-based; 77 iBT). Electronic applications accepted. *Faculty research:* Cellular neurobiology and neuropharmacology, integrative neurobiology, social behavior, chemical ecology, neuroethology.

Emory University, Laney Graduate School, Department of Psychology, Atlanta, GA 30322-1100. Offers clinical psychology (PhD); cognition and development (PhD); neuroscience and animal behavior (PhD). *Accreditation:* APA. *Degree requirements:* For doctorate, comprehensive exam, thesis/dissertation. *Entrance requirements:* For doctorate, GRE General Test, minimum GPA of 3.25. Additional exam requirements/recommendations for international students: Required—TOEFL. Electronic applications accepted. *Faculty research:* Neuroscience and animal behavior; adult and child psychopathology, cognition development assessment.

Illinois State University, Graduate School, College of Arts and Sciences, Department of Biological Sciences, Normal, IL 61790-2200. Offers animal behavior (MS); bacteriology (MS); biochemistry (MS); biological sciences (MS); biology (PhD); biophysics (MS); biotechnology (MS); botany (MS, PhD); cell biology (MS); conservation biology (MS); developmental biology (MS); ecology (MS, PhD); entomology (MS); evolutionary biology (MS); genetics (MS, PhD); immunology (MS); microbiology (MS, PhD); molecular biology (MS); molecular genetics (MS); neurobiology (MS); neuroscience (MS); parasitology (MS); physiology (MS, PhD); plant biology (MS); plant molecular biology (MS); plant sciences (MS); structural biology (MS); zoology (MS, PhD). *Program availability:* Part-time. *Degree requirements:* For master's, thesis or alternative; for doctorate, variable foreign language requirement, thesis/dissertation, 2 terms of residency. *Entrance requirements:* For master's, GRE General Test, minimum GPA of 2.6 in last 60 hours of course work; for doctorate, GRE General Test. *Application deadline:* Applications are processed on a rolling basis. Application fee: $40. *Financial support:* Research assistantships, teaching assistantships, Federal Work-Study, tuition waivers (full), and unspecified assistantships available. Financial award application deadline: 4/1. *Faculty research:* Redoc balance and drug development in schistosoma mansoni, control of the growth of listeria monocytogenes at low temperature, regulation of cell expansion and microtubule function by SPRI, CRUI: physiology and fitness consequences of different life history phenotypes. *Application contact:* Steven Juliano, Graduate Coordinator, E-mail: sajulian@ilstu.edu. Website: http://www.bio.ilstu.edu/

University of California, Davis, Graduate Studies, Graduate Group in Animal Behavior, Davis, CA 95616. Offers PhD. *Degree requirements:* For doctorate, thesis/dissertation. *Entrance requirements:* For doctorate, GRE General Test. Additional exam requirements/recommendations for international students: Required—TOEFL (minimum score 550 paper-based), IELTS (minimum score 7). Electronic applications accepted. *Faculty research:* Wildlife behavior, conservation biology, companion animal behavior, behavioral endocrinology, animal communication.

University of Colorado Boulder, Graduate School, College of Arts and Sciences, Department of Ecology and Evolutionary Biology, Boulder, CO 80309. Offers animal behavior (MA); biology (MA, PhD); environmental biology (MA, PhD); evolutionary biology (MA, PhD); neurobiology (MA); population biology (MA); population genetics (PhD). *Faculty:* 31 full-time (12 women). *Students:* 67 full-time (31 women), 3 part-time (1 woman); includes 8 minority (1 Asian, non-Hispanic/Latino; 3 Hispanic/Latino; 4 Two or more races, non-Hispanic/Latino), 4 international. Average age 30. 119 applicants, 11% accepted, 13 enrolled. In 2015, 10 master's, 14 doctorates awarded. Terminal master's awarded for partial completion of doctoral program. *Degree requirements:* For master's, comprehensive exam, thesis or alternative; for doctorate, comprehensive exam, thesis/dissertation. *Entrance requirements:* For master's, GRE General Test, GRE Subject Test, minimum undergraduate GPA of 3.0; for doctorate, GRE General Test, GRE Subject Test. *Application deadline:* For fall admission, 12/31 for domestic students, 12/1 for international students. Application fee: $50 ($70 for international students). Electronic applications accepted. Application fee is waived when completed online. *Financial support:* In 2015–16, 138 students received support, including 14 fellowships (averaging $7,260 per year), 12 research assistantships with tuition reimbursements available (averaging $31,833 per year), 47 teaching assistantships with tuition reimbursements available (averaging $33,448 per year); institutionally sponsored loans, scholarships/grants, health care benefits, and unspecified assistantships also available. Financial award applicants required to submit FAFSA. *Faculty research:*

Ecology, botany, evolutionary biology, biological sciences, conservation biology. *Total annual research expenditures:* $6.3 million. *Application contact:* E-mail: ebiograd@colorado.edu. Website: http://ebio.colorado.edu

University of Colorado Denver, College of Liberal Arts and Sciences, Department of Integrative and Systems Biology, Denver, CO 80217. Offers animal behavior (MS); biology (MS); cell and developmental biology (MS); ecology (MS); evolutionary biology (MS); genetics (MS); integrative and systems biology (PhD); microbiology (MS); molecular biology (MS); neurobiology (MS); plant systematics (MS). *Program availability:* Part-time. *Faculty:* 21 full-time (8 women), 3 part-time/adjunct (1 woman). *Students:* 31 full-time (19 women), 7 part-time (3 women); includes 8 minority (1 Black or African American, non-Hispanic/Latino; 1 Asian, non-Hispanic/Latino; 3 Hispanic/Latino; 3 Two or more races, non-Hispanic/Latino), 1 international. Average age 28. 34 applicants, 29% accepted, 8 enrolled. In 2015, 6 master's awarded. *Degree requirements:* For master's, comprehensive exam, thesis, 30-32 credit hours; for doctorate, comprehensive exam, thesis/dissertation. *Entrance requirements:* For master's, GRE General Test (minimum score in 50th percentile in each section), BA/BS from accredited institution awarded within the last 10 years; minimum undergraduate GPA of 3.0; prerequisite courses: 1 year each of general biology and general chemistry; 1 semester each of general genetics, general ecology, and cell biology; and a structure/function course; for doctorate, GRE, minimum undergraduate GPA of 3.2, three letters of recommendation, official transcripts from all universities and colleges attended. Additional exam requirements/recommendations for international students: Required—TOEFL (minimum score 537 paper-based; 75 iBT); Recommended—IELTS (minimum score 6.5). *Application deadline:* For fall admission, 1/15 for domestic and international students. Application fee: $50 ($75 for international students). Electronic applications accepted. *Financial support:* In 2015–16, 32 students received support. Fellowships, research assistantships, teaching assistantships, Federal Work-Study, institutionally sponsored loans, scholarships/grants, and traineeships available. Financial award application deadline: 4/1; financial award applicants required to submit FAFSA. *Faculty research:* Molecular developmental biology; quantitative ecology, biogeography, and population dynamics; environmental signaling and endocrine disruption; speciation, the evolution of reproductive isolation, and hybrid zones; evolutionary, behavioral, and conservation ecology. *Unit head:* Dr. John Swallow, Chair, 303-556-6154, E-mail: john.swallow@ucdenver.edu. *Application contact:* Dr. Michael Wunder, Graduate Advisor, 303-556-8870, E-mail: michael.wunder@ucdenver.edu. Website: http://www.ucdenver.edu/academics/colleges/CLAS/Departments/biology/Programs/MasterofScience/Pages/BiologyMasterOfScience.aspx

University of Massachusetts Amherst, Graduate School, Interdisciplinary Programs, Program in Neuroscience and Behavior, Amherst, MA 01003. Offers animal behavior and learning (PhD); molecular and cellular neuroscience (PhD); neural and behavioral development (PhD); neuroendocrinology (PhD); neuroscience and behavior (MS); sensorimotor, cognitive, and computational neuroscience (PhD). Terminal master's awarded for partial completion of doctoral program. *Degree requirements:* For master's, thesis or alternative; for doctorate, comprehensive exam, thesis/dissertation. *Entrance requirements:* For master's, GRE General Test; for doctorate, GRE General Test; GRE Subject Test in psychology, biology, or mathematics (recommended). Additional exam requirements/recommendations for international students: Required—TOEFL (minimum score 550 paper-based; 80 iBT), IELTS (minimum score 6.5). Electronic applications accepted.

University of Minnesota, Twin Cities Campus, Graduate School, College of Biological Sciences, Department of Ecology, Evolution, and Behavior, St. Paul, MN 55418. Offers MS, PhD. Terminal master's awarded for partial completion of doctoral program. *Degree requirements:* For master's, comprehensive exam, thesis or projects; for doctorate, comprehensive exam, thesis/dissertation. *Entrance requirements:* For master's and doctorate, GRE General Test, minimum GPA of 3.0. Additional exam requirements/recommendations for international students: Required—TOEFL (minimum score 550 paper-based; 79 iBT), Michigan English Language Assessment Battery. Electronic applications accepted. *Faculty research:* Behavioral ecology, community ecology, community genetics, ecosystem and global change, evolution and systematics.

University of Montana, Graduate School, College of Humanities and Sciences, Department of Psychology, Missoula, MT 59812-0002. Offers clinical psychology (PhD); experimental psychology (PhD), including animal behavior psychology, developmental psychology; school psychology (MA, PhD, Ed S). *Accreditation:* APA (one or more programs are accredited). Terminal master's awarded for partial completion of doctoral program. *Degree requirements:* For master's, thesis; for doctorate, thesis/dissertation. *Entrance requirements:* For master's, doctorate, and Ed S, GRE General Test. Additional exam requirements/recommendations for international students: Required—TOEFL.

The University of Tennessee, Graduate School, College of Arts and Sciences, Department of Ecology and Evolutionary Biology, Knoxville, TN 37996. Offers behavior (MS, PhD); ecology (MS, PhD); evolutionary biology (MS, PhD). *Program availability:* Part-time. *Degree requirements:* For master's, thesis; for doctorate, thesis/dissertation. *Entrance requirements:* For master's and doctorate, GRE General Test, minimum GPA of 2.7. Additional exam requirements/recommendations for international students: Required—TOEFL. Electronic applications accepted.

The University of Texas at Austin, Graduate School, College of Natural Sciences, School of Biological Sciences, Program in Ecology, Evolution and Behavior, Austin, TX 78712-1111. Offers PhD. *Entrance requirements:* For doctorate, GRE General Test. Additional exam requirements/recommendations for international students: Required—TOEFL. Electronic applications accepted.

University of Washington, Graduate School, College of Arts and Sciences, Department of Psychology, Seattle, WA 98195. Offers animal behavior (PhD); child psychology (PhD); clinical psychology (PhD); cognition and perception (PhD); developmental psychology (PhD); quantitative psychology (PhD); social psychology and personality (PhD). *Accreditation:* APA. *Degree requirements:* For doctorate, thesis/dissertation. *Entrance requirements:* For doctorate, GRE General Test, minimum GPA of 3.0. Electronic applications accepted. *Faculty research:* Addictive behaviors, artificial intelligence, child psychopathology, mechanisms and development of vision, physiology of ingestive behaviors.

Zoology

Auburn University, Graduate School, College of Sciences and Mathematics, Department of Biological Sciences, Auburn University, AL 36849. Offers botany (MS); zoology (MS). *Faculty:* 39 full-time (14 women). *Students:* 57 full-time (36 women), 54 part-time (29 women); includes 14 minority (5 Black or African American, non-Hispanic/Latino; 4 Asian, non-Hispanic/Latino; 2 Hispanic/Latino; 3 Two or more races, non-Hispanic/Latino), 12 international. Average age 27. 83 applicants, 43% accepted, 28 enrolled. In 2015, 10 master's, 4 doctorates awarded. *Entrance requirements:* For master's and doctorate, GRE General Test. Additional exam requirements/recommendations for international students: Required—TOEFL. Application fee: $50 ($60 for international students). Electronic applications accepted. *Expenses:* Tuition, state resident: full-time $8802; part-time $489 per credit hour. Tuition, nonresident: full-time $26,406; part-time $1467 per credit hour. *Required fees:* $808 per semester. Tuition and fees vary according to degree level and program. *Financial support:* Research assistantships and teaching assistantships available. Financial award applicants required to submit FAFSA. *Unit head:* Dr. Jack W. Feminella, Chair, 334-844-3906, Fax: 334-844-1645. *Application contact:* Dr. George Flowers, Dean of the Graduate School, 334-844-2125.

Canisius College, Graduate Division, College of Arts and Sciences, Department of Animal Behavior, Ecology and Conservation, Buffalo, NY 14208-1098. Offers anthrozoology (MS). Applicants accepted in Fall only. *Program availability:* Part-time, evening/weekend, blended/hybrid learning. *Faculty:* 4 full-time (2 women), 3 part-time/adjunct (all women). *Students:* 15 full-time (14 women), 30 part-time (21 women); includes 3 minority (1 Asian, non-Hispanic/Latino; 2 Hispanic/Latino), 3 international. Average age 33. 84 applicants, 27% accepted, 18 enrolled. In 2015, 20 master's awarded. *Entrance requirements:* For master's, GRE (recommended), official transcript of all college work, bachelor's degree, minimum GPA of 3.0, three essays. Additional exam requirements/recommendations for international students: Required—TOEFL (minimum score 550 paper-based, 80 iBT), IELTS (minimum score 6.5), or CAEL (minimum score 70). *Application deadline:* For fall admission, 3/1 for domestic and international students. Applications are processed on a rolling basis. Application fee: $25. Electronic applications accepted. Application fee is waived when completed online. *Expenses:* $780 per credit hour; $644 per year full-time fees. *Financial support:* Career-related internships or fieldwork, Federal Work-Study, scholarships/grants, tuition waivers (partial), and unspecified assistantships available. Support available to part-time students. Financial award application deadline: 4/30; financial award applicants required to submit FAFSA. *Unit head:* Dr. Michael Noonan, Program Director, 716-888-2770, E-mail: noonan@canisius.edu. *Application contact:* Kathleen B. Davis, Vice President of Enrollment Management, 716-888-2500, Fax: 716-888-3195, E-mail: daviskb@canisius.edu.
Website: http://www.canisius.edu/abec/

Colorado State University, College of Natural Sciences, Department of Biology, Fort Collins, CO 80523-1878. Offers botany (MS, PhD); zoology (MS, PhD). *Faculty:* 29 full-time (9 women), 4 part-time/adjunct (3 women). *Students:* 18 full-time (8 women), 22 part-time (13 women); includes 5 minority (4 Asian, non-Hispanic/Latino; 1 Hispanic/Latino), 6 international. Average age 30. 18 applicants, 94% accepted, 11 enrolled. In 2015, 7 master's, 2 doctorates awarded. Terminal master's awarded for partial completion of doctoral program. *Degree requirements:* For master's, comprehensive exam, thesis; for doctorate, comprehensive exam, thesis/dissertation. *Entrance requirements:* For master's and doctorate, GRE General Test (minimum scores above 70th percentile), transcripts, 3 letters of recommendation, statement of purpose, minimum GPA of 3.0. Additional exam requirements/recommendations for international students: Required—TOEFL (minimum score 550 paper-based; 80 iBT), IELTS (minimum score 6.5). *Application deadline:* For fall admission, 1/15 priority date for domestic and international students; for spring admission, 11/1 priority date for domestic and international students. Applications are processed on a rolling basis. Application fee: $60 ($70 for international students). Electronic applications accepted. *Expenses:* Tuition, state resident: full-time $9348. Tuition, nonresident: full-time $22,916. *Required fees:* $2174; $473.72 per credit hour. $236.86 per semester. Tuition and fees vary according to course load and program. *Financial support:* In 2015–16, 21 fellowships (averaging $42,613 per year), 12 research assistantships with full tuition reimbursements (averaging $18,531 per year), 66 teaching assistantships with full tuition reimbursements (averaging $17,703 per year) were awarded; career-related internships or fieldwork, Federal Work-Study, scholarships/grants, traineeships, and unspecified assistantships also available. Financial award application deadline: 1/1; financial award applicants required to submit FAFSA. *Faculty research:* Global ecological change; organismal interactions in infectious disease; stream ecology; muscle protein structure; plant biotechnology. *Total annual research expenditures:* $7.8 million. *Unit head:* Dr. Michael F. Antolin, Department Chair, 970-491-7011, Fax: 970-491-0649, E-mail: michael.antolin@colostate.edu. *Application contact:* Dorothy Ramirez, Graduate Coordinator, 970-491-1923, Fax: 970-491-0649, E-mail: dramirez@colostate.edu.
Website: http://www.biology.colostate.edu/

Cornell University, Graduate School, Graduate Fields of Agriculture and Life Sciences, Field of Zoology and Wildlife Conservation, Ithaca, NY 14853-0001. Offers animal cytology (PhD); comparative and functional anatomy (PhD); developmental biology (PhD); ecology (PhD); histology (PhD); wildlife conservation (PhD). *Degree requirements:* For doctorate, comprehensive exam, thesis/dissertation, 2 semesters of teaching experience. *Entrance requirements:* For doctorate, GRE General Test, GRE Subject Test (biology), 2 letters of recommendation. Additional exam requirements/recommendations for international students: Required—TOEFL (minimum score 550 paper-based; 77 iBT). Electronic applications accepted. *Faculty research:* Organismal biology, functional morphology, biomechanics, comparative vertebrate anatomy, comparative invertebrate anatomy, paleontology.

Eastern New Mexico University, Graduate School, College of Liberal Arts and Sciences, Department of Biology, Portales, NM 88130. Offers applied ecology (MS); botany (MS); cell, molecular biology and biotechnology (MS); microbiology (MS); zoology (MS). *Program availability:* Part-time. *Degree requirements:* For master's, comprehensive exam, thesis optional. *Entrance requirements:* For master's, GRE, minimum GPA of 3.0, 2 letters of recommendation, statement of research interest, bachelor's degree related to field of study or proof of common knowledge. Additional exam requirements/recommendations for international students: Required—TOEFL (minimum score 550 paper-based; 79 iBT), IELTS (minimum score 6). Electronic applications accepted.

Emporia State University, Department of Biological Sciences, Emporia, KS 66801-5415. Offers botany (MS); environmental biology (MS); general biology (MS); microbial and cellular biology (MS); zoology (MS). *Program availability:* Part-time. *Faculty:* 14 full-time (3 women), 1 part-time/adjunct (0 women). *Students:* 26 full-time (13 women), 15 part-time (7 women); includes 1 minority (Two or more races, non-Hispanic/Latino), 24 international. 16 applicants, 100% accepted, 11 enrolled. In 2015, 17 master's awarded. *Degree requirements:* For master's, comprehensive exam or thesis. *Entrance requirements:* For master's, GRE, appropriate undergraduate degree, interview, letters of reference. Additional exam requirements/recommendations for international students: Required—TOEFL (minimum score 520 paper-based; 68 iBT). *Application deadline:* For fall admission, 8/15 priority date for domestic students. Applications are processed on a rolling basis. Application fee: $30 ($75 for international students). Electronic applications accepted. *Expenses:* Tuition, state resident: full-time $5640; part-time $235 per credit hour. Tuition, nonresident: full-time $17,544; part-time $731 per credit hour. *Required fees:* $1848; $77 per credit hour. *Financial support:* In 2015–16, 7 research assistantships with full tuition reimbursements (averaging $7,344 per year), 12 teaching assistantships with full tuition reimbursements (averaging $7,844 per year) were awarded; career-related internships or fieldwork, Federal Work-Study, institutionally sponsored loans, health care benefits, and unspecified assistantships also available. Financial award application deadline: 3/15; financial award applicants required to submit FAFSA. *Faculty research:* Fisheries, range, and wildlife management; aquatic, plant, grassland, vertebrate, and invertebrate ecology; mammalian and plant systematics, taxonomy, and evolution; immunology, virology, and molecular biology. *Unit head:* Dr. Yixin Eric Yang, Chair, 620-341-5311, Fax: 620-341-5608, E-mail: yyang@emporia.edu. Website: http://www.emporia.edu/info/degrees-courses/grad/biology

Illinois State University, Graduate School, College of Arts and Sciences, Department of Biological Sciences, Normal, IL 61790-2200. Offers animal behavior (MS); bacteriology (MS); biochemistry (MS); biological sciences (MS); biology (PhD); biophysics (MS); biotechnology (MS); botany (MS, PhD); cell biology (MS); conservation biology (MS); developmental biology (MS); ecology (MS, PhD); entomology (MS); evolutionary biology (MS); genetics (MS, PhD); immunology (MS); microbiology (MS, PhD); molecular biology (MS); molecular genetics (MS); neurobiology (MS); neuroscience (MS); parasitology (MS); physiology (MS, PhD); plant biology (MS); plant molecular biology (MS); plant sciences (MS); structural biology (MS); zoology (MS, PhD). *Program availability:* Part-time. *Degree requirements:* For master's, thesis or alternative; for doctorate, variable foreign language requirement, thesis/dissertation, 2 terms of residency. *Entrance requirements:* For master's, GRE General Test, minimum GPA of 2.6 in last 60 hours of course work; for doctorate, GRE General Test. *Application deadline:* Applications are processed on a rolling basis. Application fee: $40. *Financial support:* Research assistantships, teaching assistantships, Federal Work-Study, tuition waivers (full), and unspecified assistantships available. Financial award application deadline: 4/1. *Faculty research:* Redoc balance and drug development in schistosoma mansoni, control of the growth of listeria monocytogenes at low temperature, regulation of cell expansion and microtubule function by SPRI, CRUI: physiology and fitness consequences of different life history phenotypes. *Application contact:* Steven Juliano, Graduate Coordinator, E-mail: sajulian@ilstu.edu.
Website: http://www.bio.ilstu.edu/

Indiana University Bloomington, University Graduate School, College of Arts and Sciences, Department of Biology, Bloomington, IN 47405. Offers biology teaching (MAT); biotechnology (MA); evolution, ecology, and behavior (MA, PhD); genetics (PhD); microbiology (MA, PhD); molecular, cellular, and developmental biology (PhD); plant sciences (MA, PhD); zoology (MA, PhD). Terminal master's awarded for partial completion of doctoral program. *Degree requirements:* For master's, thesis, oral defense; for doctorate, thesis/dissertation, oral defense. *Entrance requirements:* For master's and doctorate, GRE General Test. Additional exam requirements/recommendations for international students: Required—TOEFL (minimum score 100 iBT). Electronic applications accepted. *Faculty research:* Evolution, ecology and behavior; microbiology; molecular biology and genetics; plant biology.

Michigan State University, The Graduate School, College of Natural Science, Department of Zoology, East Lansing, MI 48824. Offers zoo and aquarium management (MS); zoology (MS, PhD); zoology-environmental toxicology (PhD). *Entrance requirements:* Additional exam requirements/recommendations for international students: Required—TOEFL. Electronic applications accepted.

North Carolina State University, Graduate School, College of Agriculture and Life Sciences, Department of Zoology, Raleigh, NC 27695. Offers MS, MZS, PhD. Terminal master's awarded for partial completion of doctoral program. *Degree requirements:* For master's, thesis (for some programs), oral exam; for doctorate, thesis/dissertation, oral and written exams. *Entrance requirements:* For master's and doctorate, GRE General Test, minimum GPA of 3.0. Additional exam requirements/recommendations for international students: Required—TOEFL. Electronic applications accepted. *Faculty research:* Aquatic and terrestrial ecology, herpetology, behavioral biology, neurobiology, avian ecology.

North Dakota State University, College of Graduate and Interdisciplinary Studies, College of Science and Mathematics, Department of Biological Sciences, Fargo, ND 58102. Offers biology (MS); botany (MS, PhD); cellular and molecular biology (PhD); genomics (PhD); zoology (MS, PhD). *Degree requirements:* For master's, thesis; for doctorate, thesis/dissertation. *Entrance requirements:* For master's and doctorate, GRE General Test. Additional exam requirements/recommendations for international students: Required—TOEFL. *Application deadline:* For fall admission, 1/15 for domestic students. Applications are processed on a rolling basis. Application fee: $35. Electronic applications accepted. *Financial support:* Fellowships with full tuition reimbursements, research assistantships with full tuition reimbursements, teaching assistantships with full tuition reimbursements, career-related internships or fieldwork, Federal Work-Study, institutionally sponsored loans, scholarships/grants, tuition waivers (full), and unspecified assistantships available. Support available to part-time students. Financial award application deadline: 4/15; financial award applicants required to submit FAFSA. *Faculty research:* Comparative endocrinology, physiology, behavioral ecology, plant cell biology, aquatic biology. *Unit head:* Dr. Wendy Reed, Head, 701-231-5921, E-mail: wendy.reed@ndsu.edu. *Application contact:* Elizabeth Worth, Marketing, Recruitment, and Public Relations Coordinator, 701-231-8476, Fax: 701-231-6524, E-mail: elizabeth.worth@ndsu.edu.
Website: http://www.ndsu.edu/biology/

Oregon State University, College of Science, Program in Zoology, Corvallis, OR 97331. Offers behavioral ecology (MA, MS, PhD); behavioral endocrinology (MA, MS, PhD); cell biology (MA, MS, PhD); chemical ecology (MA, MS, PhD); conservation biology (MA, MS, PhD); developmental biology (MA, MS, PhD). *Faculty:* 21 full-time (9 women), 2 part-time/adjunct (1 woman). *Students:* 58 full-time (38 women), 1 part-time (0 women); includes 11 minority (1 Black or African American, non-Hispanic/Latino; 1 American Indian or Alaska Native, non-Hispanic/Latino; 7 Asian, non-Hispanic/Latino; 1 Hispanic/Latino; 1 Two or more races, non-Hispanic/Latino), 3 international. Average

Zoology

age 28. 75 applicants, 13% accepted, 9 enrolled. In 2015, 1 master's, 5 doctorates awarded. Terminal master's awarded for partial completion of doctoral program. *Degree requirements:* For doctorate, thesis/dissertation. *Entrance requirements:* For master's and doctorate, GRE. Additional exam requirements/recommendations for international students: Required—TOEFL (minimum score 80 iBT) (minimum score 6.5). *Application deadline:* For fall admission, 12/15 for domestic and international students. Application fee: $75 ($85 for international students). *Expenses:* Tuition, state resident: full-time $12,150; part-time $450 per credit. Tuition, nonresident: full-time $20,952; part-time $776 per credit. *Required fees:* $1572; $1443 per unit. One-time fee: $350. Tuition and fees vary according to course load, campus/location and program. *Financial support:* Fellowships, research assistantships, teaching assistantships, Federal Work-Study, and institutionally sponsored loans available. Support available to part-time students. *Faculty research:* Ecology and evolutionary biology, physiology and behavior, development and cell biology. *Unit head:* Dr. Virginia M. Weis, Professor and Chair of Integrative Biology, 541-737-4359. *Application contact:* Graduate Admissions Coordinator, 541-737-5335, E-mail: ib@science.oregonstate.edu.
Website: http://ib.oregonstate.edu/

Southern Illinois University Carbondale, Graduate School, College of Science, Department of Zoology, Carbondale, IL 62901-4701. Offers MS, PhD. *Faculty:* 25 full-time (1 woman). *Students:* 14 full-time (6 women), 65 part-time (27 women); includes 2 minority (1 Asian, non-Hispanic/Latino; 1 Hispanic/Latino), 28 international. Average age 25. 28 applicants, 54% accepted, 9 enrolled. In 2015, 17 master's, 1 doctorate awarded. *Degree requirements:* For master's, thesis; for doctorate, thesis/dissertation. *Entrance requirements:* For master's, GRE, minimum GPA of 2.7; for doctorate, GRE, minimum GPA of 3.25. Additional exam requirements/recommendations for international students: Required—TOEFL. *Application deadline:* Applications are processed on a rolling basis. Application fee: $65. *Financial support:* In 2015–16, 56 students received support, including 2 fellowships with full tuition reimbursements available, 31 research assistantships with full tuition reimbursements available, 23 teaching assistantships with full tuition reimbursements available; Federal Work-Study, institutionally sponsored loans, and tuition waivers (full) also available. Support available to part-time students. *Faculty research:* Ecology, fisheries and wildlife, systematics, behavior, vertebrate and invertebrate biology. *Unit head:* Dr. Carey Krajewski, Chairperson, 618-453-4128, E-mail: careyk@siu.edu. *Application contact:* Judy Rains, Office Systems Specialist, 618-453-4110, E-mail: jrains@zoology.siu.edu.

Texas Tech University, Graduate School, College of Arts and Sciences, Department of Biological Sciences, Lubbock, TX 79409-3131. Offers biology (MS, PhD); environmental sustainability and natural resources management (PSM); microbiology (MS); zoology (MS, PhD). *Program availability:* Part-time, blended/hybrid learning. *Faculty:* 41 full-time (12 women), 2 part-time/adjunct (1 woman). *Students:* 94 full-time (51 women), 5 part-time (3 women); includes 6 minority (1 American Indian or Alaska Native, non-Hispanic/Latino; 1 Asian, non-Hispanic/Latino; 3 Hispanic/Latino; 1 Two or more races, non-Hispanic/Latino), 53 international. Average age 29. 92 applicants, 39% accepted, 21 enrolled. In 2015, 7 master's, 9 doctorates awarded. *Degree requirements:* For master's, thesis or alternative; for doctorate, thesis/dissertation. *Entrance requirements:* For master's and doctorate, GRE General Test. Additional exam requirements/recommendations for international students: Required—TOEFL (minimum score 550 paper-based; 79 iBT). *Application deadline:* For fall admission, 6/1 priority date for domestic students, 1/15 priority date for international students; for spring admission, 9/1 priority date for domestic students, 6/15 priority date for international students. Applications are processed on a rolling basis. Application fee: $60. Electronic applications accepted. *Expenses:* Tuition, state resident: full-time $6477; part-time $269.89 per credit hour. Tuition, nonresident: full-time $15,837; part-time $659.89 per credit hour. *Required fees:* $2751; $36.50 per credit hour. $937.50 per semester. Tuition and fees vary according to course level. *Financial support:* In 2015–16, 98 students received support, including 79 fellowships (averaging $1,515 per year), 36 research assistantships (averaging $6,272 per year), 98 teaching assistantships (averaging $13,936 per year). Financial award application deadline: 4/15; financial award applicants required to submit FAFSA. *Faculty research:* Biodiversity, genomics and evolution, climate change in arid ecosystems, plant biology and biotechnology, animal communication and behavior, zoonotic and emerging diseases. *Total annual research expenditures:* $1.4 million. *Unit head:* Dr. Ron Chesser, Chair, 806-834-0121, Fax: 806-742-2963, E-mail: ron.chesser@ttu.edu. *Application contact:* Dr. Lou Densmore, Graduate Adviser, 806-834-6479, Fax: 806-742-2963, E-mail: lou.densmore@ttu.edu.
Website: http://www.depts.ttu.edu/biology/

Uniformed Services University of the Health Sciences, F. Edward Hebert School of Medicine, Graduate Programs in the Biomedical Sciences and Public Health, Bethesda, MD 20814. Offers emerging infectious diseases (PhD); medical and clinical psychology (PhD), including clinical psychology, medical psychology; medicine (MS, PhD), including health professions education; molecular and cell biology (MS, PhD); neuroscience (PhD); preventive medicine and biometrics (MPH, MS, MSPH, MTMH, Dr PH, PhD), including environmental health sciences (PhD), healthcare administration and policy (MS), medical zoology (PhD), public health (MPH, MSPH, Dr PH), tropical medicine and hygiene (MTMH). *Faculty:* 372 full-time (119 women), 4,044 part-time/adjunct (908 women). *Students:* 240 full-time (133 women); includes 40 minority (15 Black or African American, non-Hispanic/Latino; 13 Asian, non-Hispanic/Latino; 12 Hispanic/Latino), 30 international. Average age 25. 598 applicants, 17% accepted, 77 enrolled. In 2015, 19 master's, 50 doctorates awarded. Terminal master's awarded for partial completion of doctoral program. *Degree requirements:* For master's, comprehensive exam, thesis or alternative; for doctorate, comprehensive exam, thesis/dissertation, qualifying exam. *Entrance requirements:* For master's, GRE General Test; for doctorate, GRE General Test, minimum GPA of 3.0. *Application deadline:* For fall admission, 12/15 priority date for domestic students. Applications are processed on a rolling basis. Application fee: $0. Electronic applications accepted. *Financial support:* In 2015–16, 50 fellowships (averaging $43,000 per year) were awarded; research assistantships, career-related internships or fieldwork, scholarships/grants, health care benefits, and tuition waivers (full) also available. *Unit head:* Dr. Gregory Mueller, Associate Dean, 301-295-3507, E-mail: gregory.mueller@usuhs.edu. *Application contact:* Tina Finley, Administrative Officer, 301-295-3642, Fax: 301-295-6772, E-mail: netina.finley@usuhs.edu.
Website: http://www.usuhs.mil/graded

Uniformed Services University of the Health Sciences, F. Edward Hebert School of Medicine, Graduate Programs in the Biomedical Sciences and Public Health, Department of Preventive Medicine and Biometrics, Program in Medical Zoology, Bethesda, MD 20814-4799. Offers PhD. *Degree requirements:* For doctorate, comprehensive exam, thesis/dissertation, qualifying exam. *Entrance requirements:* For doctorate, GRE General Test, GRE Subject Test, minimum GPA of 3.0, U.S. citizenship. Additional exam requirements/recommendations for international students: Required—TOEFL. *Faculty research:* Epidemiology, biostatistics, tropical public health, parasitology, vector biology.

The University of British Columbia, Faculty of Science, Department of Zoology, Vancouver, BC V6T 1Z1, Canada. Offers M Sc, PhD. *Degree requirements:* For master's, thesis, final defense; for doctorate, comprehensive exam, thesis/dissertation, final defense. *Entrance requirements:* For master's and doctorate, faculty support.

Additional exam requirements/recommendations for international students: Required—TOEFL. Electronic applications accepted. *Faculty research:* Cell and developmental biology; community, environmental, and population biology; comparative physiology and biochemistry; fisheries; ecology and evolutionary biology.

University of California, Davis, Graduate Studies, Graduate Group in Avian Sciences, Davis, CA 95616. Offers MS. *Degree requirements:* For master's, comprehensive exam (for some programs), thesis (for some programs). *Entrance requirements:* For master's, GRE General Test, minimum GPA of 3.0. Additional exam requirements/recommendations for international students: Required—TOEFL (minimum score 550 paper-based). Electronic applications accepted. *Faculty research:* Reproduction, nutrition, toxicology, food products, ecology of avian species.

University of Chicago, Division of the Biological Sciences, Department of Organismal Biology and Anatomy, Chicago, IL 60637. Offers integrative biology (PhD). *Students:* 22 full-time (13 women); includes 3 minority (1 Asian, non-Hispanic/Latino; 2 Hispanic/Latino), 2 international. Average age 27. 17 applicants, 35% accepted, 4 enrolled. *Degree requirements:* For doctorate, thesis/dissertation, ethics class, 2 teaching assistantships. *Entrance requirements:* For doctorate, GRE General Test. Additional exam requirements/recommendations for international students: Required—TOEFL (minimum score 600 paper-based; 104 iBT), IELTS (minimum score 7). *Application deadline:* For fall admission, 12/1 for domestic and international students. Application fee: $90. Electronic applications accepted. *Financial support:* In 2015–16, 12 students received support, including fellowships with tuition reimbursements available (averaging $29,781 per year), research assistantships with tuition reimbursements available (averaging $29,781 per year); institutionally sponsored loans, scholarships/grants, traineeships, and health care benefits also available. Financial award applicants required to submit FAFSA. *Faculty research:* Ecological physiology, evolution of fossil reptiles, vertebrate paleontology. *Unit head:* Dr. Robert Ho, Chairman, 773-834-8423, Fax: 773-702-0037, E-mail: rkh@uchicago.edu.
Website: http://pondside.uchicago.edu/oba/

University of Florida, Graduate School, College of Liberal Arts and Sciences, Department of Biology, Gainesville, FL 32611. Offers botany (MS, MST, PhD), including botany, tropical conservation and development, wetland sciences; zoology (MS, MST, PhD), including animal molecular and cellular biology (PhD), tropical conservation and development, wetland sciences, zoology. *Faculty:* 9 full-time, 9 part-time/adjunct. *Students:* 96 full-time (41 women), 6 part-time (3 women); includes 9 minority (4 Asian, non-Hispanic/Latino; 5 Hispanic/Latino), 35 international. 77 applicants, 30% accepted, 16 enrolled. In 2015, 8 master's, 15 doctorates awarded. *Degree requirements:* For master's, comprehensive exam (for some programs), thesis; for doctorate, comprehensive exam, thesis/dissertation. *Entrance requirements:* For master's and doctorate, GRE General Test, minimum GPA of 3.0. Additional exam requirements/recommendations for international students: Required—TOEFL (minimum score 550 paper-based; 80 iBT), IELTS (minimum score 6). *Application deadline:* For fall admission, 12/1 for domestic and international students. Applications are processed on a rolling basis. Application fee: $30. Electronic applications accepted. *Financial support:* In 2015–16, 9 fellowships, 36 research assistantships, 62 teaching assistantships were awarded; unspecified assistantships also available. Financial award application deadline: 12/15; financial award applicants required to submit FAFSA. *Faculty research:* Ecology of natural populations, plant and animal genome evolution, biodiversity, plant biology, behavior. *Total annual research expenditures:* $3.6 million. *Unit head:* Marta Wayne, PhD, Professor and Chair, 352-392-9925, E-mail: mlwayne@ufl.edu. *Application contact:* William T. Barbazuk, PhD, Associate Professor/Graduate Coordinator, 352-273-8624, Fax: 352-392-3704, E-mail: bbarbazuk@ufl.edu.
Website: http://www.biology.ufl.edu/

University of Guelph, Graduate Studies, College of Biological Science, Department of Integrative Biology, Botany and Zoology, Guelph, ON N1G 2W1, Canada. Offers botany (M Sc, PhD); zoology (M Sc, PhD). *Program availability:* Part-time. *Degree requirements:* For master's, thesis, research proposal; for doctorate, thesis/dissertation, research proposal, qualifying exam. *Entrance requirements:* For master's, minimum B average during previous 2 years of course work. Additional exam requirements/recommendations for international students: Required—TOEFL (minimum score 550 paper-based), IELTS (minimum score 6.5). Electronic applications accepted. *Faculty research:* Aquatic science, environmental physiology, parasitology, wildlife biology, management.

University of Hawaii at Manoa, Graduate Division, College of Natural Sciences, Department of Biology, Honolulu, HI 96822. Offers zoology (MS, PhD). *Program availability:* Part-time. *Faculty:* 39 full-time (10 women), 2 part-time/adjunct (1 woman). *Students:* 61 full-time (32 women), 4 part-time (3 women); includes 18 minority (5 Asian, non-Hispanic/Latino; 5 Hispanic/Latino; 2 Native Hawaiian or other Pacific Islander, non-Hispanic/Latino; 6 Two or more races, non-Hispanic/Latino), 7 international. Average age 30. 25 applicants, 20% accepted, 3 enrolled. In 2015, 6 master's, 11 doctorates awarded. *Degree requirements:* For master's, one foreign language, thesis optional; for doctorate, one foreign language, comprehensive exam, thesis/dissertation, seminar. *Entrance requirements:* For master's and doctorate, GRE General Test, GRE Subject Test. Additional exam requirements/recommendations for international students: Required—TOEFL (minimum score 600 paper-based; 100 iBT), IELTS (minimum score 7). *Application deadline:* For fall admission, 12/31 for domestic and international students. Applications are processed on a rolling basis. Application fee: $100. *Financial support:* In 2015–16, 14 fellowships (averaging $1,126 per year), 44 research assistantships (averaging $20,768 per year), 27 teaching assistantships (averaging $15,699 per year) were awarded; tuition waivers (full) also available. Financial award application deadline: 2/1. *Faculty research:* Molecular evolution, reproductive biology, animal behavior, conservation biology, avian biology. *Total annual research expenditures:* $231,000. *Unit head:* William Ditto, Dean, 808-956-6451, E-mail: wditto@hawaii.edu. *Application contact:* Leslie E. Watling, Graduate Chairperson, 808-956-8621, Fax: 808-956-9812, E-mail: watling@hawaii.edu.
Website: http://manoa.hawaii.edu/biology/

University of Illinois at Urbana–Champaign, Graduate College, College of Liberal Arts and Sciences, School of Integrative Biology, Department of Animal Biology, Champaign, IL 61820. Offers animal biology (ecology, ethology and evolution) (MS, PhD).

University of Maine, Graduate School, College of Natural Sciences, Forestry, and Agriculture, School of Biology and Ecology, Orono, ME 04469. Offers biological sciences (PhD); botany and plant pathology (MS); ecology and environmental science (MS, PhD); entomology (MS); plant science (PhD); zoology (MS, PhD). *Program availability:* Part-time. *Faculty:* 24 full-time (12 women), 34 part-time/adjunct (13 women). *Students:* 64 full-time (36 women), 1 part-time (0 women); includes 4 minority (1 American Indian or Alaska Native, non-Hispanic/Latino; 1 Asian, non-Hispanic/Latino; 1 Hispanic/Latino; 1 Two or more races, non-Hispanic/Latino), 8 international. Average age 29. 52 applicants, 25% accepted, 11 enrolled. In 2015, 7 master's, 8 doctorates awarded. Terminal master's awarded for partial completion of doctoral program. *Degree requirements:* For master's, thesis (for some programs); for doctorate, comprehensive exam, thesis/dissertation. *Entrance requirements:* For master's and doctorate, GRE General Test. Additional exam requirements/recommendations for international

students: Required—TOEFL. *Application deadline:* For fall admission, 2/1 priority date for domestic students. Applications are processed on a rolling basis. Application fee: $65. Electronic applications accepted. *Financial support:* In 2015–16, 14 students received support, including 6 research assistantships with full tuition reimbursements available (averaging $14,600 per year), 8 teaching assistantships with full tuition reimbursements available (averaging $14,600 per year); career-related internships or fieldwork, Federal Work-Study, institutionally sponsored loans, and tuition waivers (full and partial) also available. Financial award application deadline: 3/1. *Faculty research:* Ecology and evolution (aquatic, terrestrial, paleo); development and genetics; biomedical research; ecophysiology and stress; invasion ecology and pest management. *Total annual research expenditures:* $3.2 million. *Unit head:* Dr. Andrei Aloykhin, Director, 207-581-2977, Fax: 207-581-2537. *Application contact:* Scott G. Delcourt, Assistant Vice President for Graduate Studies and Senior Associate Dean, 207-581-3291, Fax: 207-581-3232, E-mail: graduate@maine.edu.
Website: http://sbe.umaine.edu/

University of Manitoba, Faculty of Graduate Studies, Faculty of Science, Department of Biological Sciences, Winnipeg, MB R3T 2N2, Canada. Offers botany (M Sc, PhD); ecology (M Sc, PhD); zoology (M Sc, PhD).

University of Montana, Graduate School, College of Humanities and Sciences, Division of Biological Sciences, Program in Organismal Biology and Ecology, Missoula, MT 59812-0002. Offers MS, PhD. Terminal master's awarded for partial completion of doctoral program. *Degree requirements:* For master's, one foreign language, thesis; for doctorate, 2 foreign languages, thesis/dissertation. *Entrance requirements:* For master's and doctorate, GRE General Test. *Faculty research:* Conservation biology, ecology and behavior, evolutionary genetics, avian biology.

University of North Dakota, Graduate School, College of Arts and Sciences, Department of Biology, Grand Forks, ND 58202. Offers botany (MS, PhD); ecology (MS, PhD); entomology (MS, PhD); environmental biology (MS, PhD); fisheries/wildlife (MS, PhD); genetics (MS, PhD); zoology (MS, PhD). Terminal master's awarded for partial completion of doctoral program. *Degree requirements:* For master's, thesis, final exam; for doctorate, comprehensive exam, thesis/dissertation, final exam. *Entrance requirements:* For master's, GRE General Test, GRE Subject Test, minimum GPA of 3.0; for doctorate, GRE General Test, GRE Subject Test, minimum GPA of 3.5. Additional exam requirements/recommendations for international students: Required—TOEFL (minimum score 550 paper-based; 79 iBT), IELTS (minimum score 6.5). Electronic applications accepted. *Faculty research:* Population biology, wildlife ecology, RNA processing, hormonal control of behavior.

University of Wisconsin–Madison, Graduate School, College of Letters and Science, Department of Zoology, Madison, WI 53706-1380. Offers MA, MS, PhD. *Program availability:* Part-time. *Degree requirements:* For master's, thesis; for doctorate, one foreign language, thesis/dissertation. *Entrance requirements:* For master's and

doctorate, GRE General Test. Additional exam requirements/recommendations for international students: Required—TOEFL. Electronic applications accepted. *Expenses:* Tuition, state resident: full-time $5364. Tuition, nonresident: full-time $12,027. *Required fees:* $571. Tuition and fees vary according to campus/location, program and reciprocity agreements. *Faculty research:* Developmental biology, ecology, neurobiology, aquatic ecology, animal behavior.

University of Wisconsin–Oshkosh, Graduate Studies, College of Letters and Science, Department of Biology and Microbiology, Oshkosh, WI 54901. Offers biology (MS), including botany, microbiology, zoology. *Degree requirements:* For master's, comprehensive exam, thesis. *Entrance requirements:* For master's, GRE General Test, minimum GPA of 3.0, BS in biology. Additional exam requirements/recommendations for international students: Required—TOEFL (minimum score 550 paper-based; 79 iBT). Electronic applications accepted.

University of Wyoming, College of Arts and Sciences, Department of Zoology and Physiology, Laramie, WY 82071. Offers MS, PhD. *Program availability:* Part-time. *Degree requirements:* For master's, comprehensive exam (for some programs), thesis; for doctorate, comprehensive exam (for some programs), thesis/dissertation. *Entrance requirements:* For master's and doctorate, GRE General Test, minimum GPA of 3.0. Additional exam requirements/recommendations for international students: Required—TOEFL. Electronic applications accepted. *Faculty research:* Cell biology, ecology/wildlife, organismal physiology, zoology.

Western Illinois University, School of Graduate Studies, College of Arts and Sciences, Department of Biological Sciences, Macomb, IL 61455-1390. Offers biological sciences (MS); environmental geographic information systems (Certificate); zoo and aquarium studies (Certificate). *Program availability:* Part-time. *Students:* 57 full-time (40 women), 32 part-time (23 women); includes 5 minority (2 Black or African American, non-Hispanic/Latino; 1 Hispanic/Latino; 2 Two or more races, non-Hispanic/Latino), 25 international. Average age 28. 56 applicants, 84% accepted, 30 enrolled. In 2015, 15 master's, 11 other advanced degrees awarded. *Degree requirements:* For master's, thesis or alternative. *Entrance requirements:* Additional exam requirements/recommendations for international students: Required—TOEFL (minimum score 550 paper-based; 80 iBT); Recommended—IELTS. *Application deadline:* Applications are processed on a rolling basis. Application fee: $30. Electronic applications accepted. *Financial support:* In 2015–16, 15 research assistantships with full tuition reimbursements (averaging $7,544 per year), 15 teaching assistantships with full tuition reimbursements (averaging $8,688 per year) were awarded; unspecified assistantships also available. Financial award applicants required to submit FAFSA. *Unit head:* Dr. Charles Lydeard, Chairperson, 309-298-1546. *Application contact:* Dr. Nancy Parsons, Associate Provost and Director of Graduate Studies, 309-298-1806, Fax: 309-298-2345, E-mail: grad-office@wiu.edu.
Website: http://wiu.edu/biology

ACADEMIC AND PROFESSIONAL PROGRAMS IN HEALTH-RELATED PROFESSIONS

Section 20
Allied Health

This section contains a directory of institutions offering graduate work in allied health, followed by an in-depth entries submitted by institutions that chose to prepare detailed program descriptions. Additional information about programs listed in the directory but not augmented by an in-depth entry may be obtained by writing directly to the dean of a graduate school or chair of a department at the address given in the directory.

For programs offering related work, see also in this book *Anatomy, Biophysics, Dentistry and Dental Sciences, Health Services, Microbiological Sciences, Pathology and Pathobiology, Physiology,* and *Public Health.* In the other guides in this series:

Graduate Programs in the Humanities, Arts & Social Sciences

See *Art and Art History (Art Therapy), Family and Consumer Sciences (Gerontology), Performing Arts (Therapies),* and *Psychology and Counseling'*

Graduate Programs in the Physical Sciences, Mathematics, Agricultural Sciences, the Environment & Natural Resources

See *Physics (Acoustics)*

Graduate Programs in Engineering & Applied Sciences

See *Agricultural Engineering and Bioengineering (Bioengineering), Biomedical Engineering and Biotechnology,* and *Energy and Power Engineering (Nuclear Engineering)*

Graduate Programs in Business, Education, Information Studies, Law & Social Work

See *Administration, Instruction, and Theory (Educational Psychology); Special Focus (Education of the Multiply Handicapped); Social Work;* and *Subject Areas (Counselor Education)*

CONTENTS

Program Directories

Allied Health—General

Alabama State University, College of Health Sciences, Montgomery, AL 36101-0271. Offers MRC, MS, DPT. *Students:* 182 full-time (128 women), 24 part-time (16 women); includes 97 minority (80 Black or African American, non-Hispanic/Latino; 1 American Indian or Alaska Native, non-Hispanic/Latino; 11 Asian, non-Hispanic/Latino; 3 Hispanic/Latino; 2 Two or more races, non-Hispanic/Latino), 4 international. Average age 26. 222 applicants, 32% accepted, 66 enrolled. In 2015, 36 master's, 29 doctorates awarded. *Entrance requirements:* Additional exam requirements/recommendations for international students: Required—TOEFL (minimum score 500 paper-based). *Application deadline:* For fall admission, 7/15 for domestic students; for spring admission, 12/15 for domestic students. Applications are processed on a rolling basis. Application fee: $25. *Expenses: Tuition, area resident:* Full-time $3087; part-time $2744 per credit. Tuition, nonresident: full-time $6174; part-time $5488 per credit. *Required fees:* $2284; $1142 per credit. $571 per semester. Tuition and fees vary according to class time, course level, course load, degree level, program and student level. *Financial support:* In 2015–16, 3 students received support. Research assistantships and unspecified assistantships available. Financial award application deadline: 6/30. *Unit head:* Dr. Leon Wilsom, Acting Dean, 334-229-4232, E-mail: lwilson@alasu.edu. *Application contact:* Dr. William Person, Dean of Graduate Studies, 334-229-4274, Fax: 334-229-4928, E-mail: wperson@alasu.edu.
Website: http://www.alasu.edu/academics/colleges—departments/health-sciences/index.aspx

American College of Healthcare Sciences, Graduate Programs, Portland, OR 97239-3719. Offers aromatherapy (Graduate Certificate); complementary alternative medicine (MS, Graduate Certificate); herbal medicine (Graduate Certificate); nutrition (Graduate Certificate). *Program availability:* Part-time, evening/weekend, online learning. *Degree requirements:* For master's, capstone project. *Entrance requirements:* For master's, interview, letters of recommendation, essay.

Andrews University, School of Health Professions, Department of Medical Laboratory Sciences, Berrien Springs, MI 49104. Offers MSMLS. *Accreditation:* APTA. *Faculty:* 2 full-time (1 woman). *Students:* 5 full-time (4 women); includes 1 minority (Black or African American, non-Hispanic/Latino), 4 international. Average age 25. 21 applicants, 19% accepted, 3 enrolled. In 2015, 3 master's awarded. *Entrance requirements:* For master's, GRE. Additional exam requirements/recommendations for international students: Required—TOEFL (minimum score 550 paper-based). *Application deadline:* Applications are processed on a rolling basis. Application fee: $40. *Unit head:* Dr. Marcia A. Kilsby, Chair, 269-471-3336. *Application contact:* Monica Wringer, Supervisor of Graduate Admission, 800-253-2874, Fax: 269-471-6321, E-mail: graduate@andrews.edu.
Website: http://www.andrews.edu/shp/mls/

Athabasca University, Faculty of Health Disciplines, Athabasca, AB T9S 3A3, Canada. Offers advanced nursing practice (MN, Advanced Diploma); generalist (MN); health studies (MHS). *Program availability:* Part-time, online learning. *Faculty:* 11 full-time (all women), 1 (woman) part-time/adjunct. *Students:* 1,687 part-time. Average age 38. In 2015, 243 master's, 5 other advanced degrees awarded. *Degree requirements:* For master's, comprehensive exam (for some programs). *Entrance requirements:* For master's, bachelor's degree in health-related field and 2 years of professional health service experience (MHS); bachelor's degree in nursing and 2 years' nursing experience (MN); minimum GPA of 3.0 in final 30 credits; for Advanced Diploma, RN license, 2 years of health care experience. *Application deadline:* For fall admission, 3/1 for domestic and international students. Application fee: $80. Electronic applications accepted. *Expenses:* Contact institution. *Unit head:* Dr. Margaret Edwards, Dean, 800-788-9041 Ext. 6381, Fax: 780-675-6468, E-mail: marge@athabascau.ca. *Application contact:* Donna Dunn Hart, Academic Student Advisor, Graduate Programs, 800-788-9041 Ext. 6300, Fax: 780-675-6468, E-mail: donnad@athabascau.ca.
Website: http://fhd.athabascau.ca/

A.T. Still University, Arizona School of Health Sciences, Mesa, AZ 85206. Offers advanced occupational therapy (MS); advanced physician assistant studies (MS); athletic training (MS, DAT); audiology (Au D); occupational therapy (OTD); physical therapy (DPT); physician assistant studies (MS); transitional audiology (Au D); transitional physical therapy (DPT). *Accreditation:* AOTA (one or more programs are accredited); ASHA. *Program availability:* Part-time, evening/weekend, 100% online. *Faculty:* 54 full-time (31 women), 188 part-time/adjunct (132 women). *Students:* 509 full-time (339 women), 397 part-time (310 women); includes 203 minority (41 Black or African American, non-Hispanic/Latino; 5 American Indian or Alaska Native, non-Hispanic/Latino; 83 Asian, non-Hispanic/Latino; 57 Hispanic/Latino; 2 Native Hawaiian or other Pacific Islander, non-Hispanic/Latino; 15 Two or more races, non-Hispanic/Latino), 60 international. Average age 33. 3,902 applicants, 10% accepted, 245 enrolled. In 2015, 178 master's, 271 doctorates awarded. *Degree requirements:* For master's, thesis (for some programs); for doctorate, thesis/dissertation (for some programs). *Entrance requirements:* For master's, GRE General Test; for doctorate, GRE, Evaluation of Practicing Audiologists Capabilities (Au D), Physical Therapist Evaluation Tool (DPT), current state licensure, master's degree or equivalent (Au D). Additional exam requirements/recommendations for international students: Required—TOEFL (minimum score 80 iBT). *Application deadline:* Applications are processed on a rolling basis. Application fee: $70. Electronic applications accepted. *Expenses:* Contact institution. *Financial support:* In 2015–16, 158 students received support. Federal Work-Study and scholarships/grants available. Financial award application deadline: 5/1; financial award applicants required to submit FAFSA. *Faculty research:* Pediatric sport-related concussion, adolescent athlete health-related quality of life; geriatric and pediatric well-being, pain management for participation, practice-based research network, BMI and dental caries. *Total annual research expenditures:* $156,319. *Unit head:* Dr. Randy Danielsen, Dean, 480-219-6000, Fax: 480-219-6110, E-mail: rdanielsen@atsu.edu. *Application contact:* Donna Sparks, Associate Director, Admissions Processing, 660-626-2117, Fax: 660-626-2969, E-mail: admissions@atsu.edu.
Website: http://www.atsu.edu/ashs

Baylor University, Graduate School, Military Programs, Waco, TX 76798. Offers MHA, MS, D Sc, D Sc PA, DPT, DScPT, MHA/MBA. *Accreditation:* APTA (one or more programs are accredited). *Faculty:* 44 full-time (4 women), 21 part-time/adjunct (5 women). *Students:* 210 full-time (79 women); includes 39 minority (6 Black or African American, non-Hispanic/Latino; 1 American Indian or Alaska Native, non-Hispanic/Latino; 9 Asian, non-Hispanic/Latino; 15 Hispanic/Latino; 8 Two or more races, non-Hispanic/Latino). In 2015, 64 master's, 44 doctorates awarded. *Entrance requirements:* For master's and doctorate, GRE General Test. *Application deadline:* Applications are processed on a rolling basis. *Expenses:* Contact institution. *Unit head:* Scott Shaffer, Dean, 210-221-6457, Fax: 210-221-6457, E-mail: scott.w.shaffer.mil@mail.mil.

Application contact: Lori McNamara, Admissions Coordinator, 254-710-3588, Fax: 254-710-3870.

Belmont University, College of Health Sciences, Nashville, TN 37212-3757. Offers nursing (MSN, DNP); occupational therapy (MSOT, OTD); physical therapy (DPT). *Program availability:* Part-time, online learning. *Faculty:* 54 full-time (50 women), 92 part-time/adjunct (81 women). *Students:* 371 full-time (324 women), 10 part-time (all women); includes 30 minority (10 Black or African American, non-Hispanic/Latino; 9 Asian, non-Hispanic/Latino; 6 Hispanic/Latino; 5 Two or more races, non-Hispanic/Latino), 2 international. Average age 26. *Degree requirements:* For master's, comprehensive exam, thesis; for doctorate, comprehensive exam. *Entrance requirements:* For master's, GRE, BSN, minimum GPA of 3.0. Additional exam requirements/recommendations for international students: Required—TOEFL (minimum score 550 paper-based). *Application deadline:* Applications are processed on a rolling basis. Application fee: $50. Electronic applications accepted. *Expenses:* Contact institution. *Financial support:* Teaching assistantships with full tuition reimbursements, career-related internships or fieldwork, scholarships/grants, and traineeships available. Financial award application deadline: 3/1; financial award applicants required to submit FAFSA. *Unit head:* Dr. Cathy Taylor, Dean, 615-460-6916, Fax: 615-460-6750. *Application contact:* David Mee, Dean of Enrollment Services, 615-460-6785, Fax: 615-460-5434, E-mail: david.mee@belmont.edu.
Website: http://www.belmont.edu/healthsciences/

Bennington College, Graduate Programs, Post baccalaureate Premedical Program, Bennington, VT 05201. Offers allied and health sciences (Certificate). *Faculty:* 11 full-time (4 women). *Students:* 12 full-time (6 women), 1 international. Average age 24. 80 applicants, 38% accepted, 14 enrolled. In 2015, 11 Certificates awarded. *Application deadline:* For fall admission, 2/15 for domestic students; for summer admission, 4/1 for domestic students. Applications are processed on a rolling basis. Application fee: $60. Electronic applications accepted. *Expenses:* Contact institution. *Financial support:* Scholarships/grants available. Financial award application deadline: 4/1; financial award applicants required to submit FAFSA. *Faculty research:* Cellular functions of Hsp90, foundations of quantum mechanics, history and philosophy of physics, cytosolic quality control, forest ecology, plate tectonics of rift systems, amphibian evolutionary physiology, photochemistry of gold complexes. *Unit head:* Dr. Janet Foley, Chief Health Professions Advisor, 802-440-4463, Fax: 802-440-4461, E-mail: jfoley@bennington.edu. *Application contact:* Ferrilyn Sourdiffe, Postbaccalaureate and Graduate Admissions Counselor, 802-440-4885, Fax: 802-440-4320, E-mail: fsourdiffe@bennington.edu.
Website: http://www.bennington.edu/postbac

Boston University, College of Health and Rehabilitation Sciences: Sargent College, Boston, MA 02215. Offers MS, DPT, OTD, PhD. *Accreditation:* APTA (one or more programs are accredited). *Program availability:* Blended/hybrid learning. *Faculty:* 54 full-time (42 women), 44 part-time/adjunct (28 women). *Students:* 459 full-time (385 women), 36 part-time (33 women); includes 91 minority (5 Black or African American, non-Hispanic/Latino; 43 Asian, non-Hispanic/Latino; 26 Hispanic/Latino; 17 Two or more races, non-Hispanic/Latino), 21 international. Average age 25. 2,072 applicants, 16% accepted, 126 enrolled. In 2015, 106 master's, 63 doctorates awarded. Terminal master's awarded for partial completion of doctoral program. *Degree requirements:* For master's, comprehensive exam (for some programs), thesis optional; for doctorate, variable foreign language requirement, comprehensive exam (for some programs), thesis/dissertation. *Entrance requirements:* For master's and doctorate, GRE General Test. Additional exam requirements/recommendations for international students: Required—TOEFL (minimum score 550 paper-based; 84 iBT). *Application deadline:* For fall admission, 1/1 priority date for domestic and international students. Applications are processed on a rolling basis. Application fee: $80. Electronic applications accepted. *Expenses:* $1,537 per credit. *Financial support:* In 2015–16, 302 students received support, including 24 research assistantships with full tuition reimbursements available (averaging $21,000 per year), 18 teaching assistantships (averaging $2,500 per year); career-related internships or fieldwork, Federal Work-Study, institutionally sponsored loans, scholarships/grants, and health care benefits also available. Support available to part-time students. Financial award application deadline: 1/1; financial award applicants required to submit FAFSA. *Faculty research:* Outcome measurement, gerontology, neuroanatomy, aphasia, autism, Parkinson's Disease, psychiatric rehabilitation, obesity prevention, speech production and imaging. *Total annual research expenditures:* $8.3 million. *Unit head:* Dr. Christopher Moore, Dean, 617-353-2705, Fax: 617-353-7500, E-mail: mooreca@bu.edu. *Application contact:* Sharon Sankey, Assistant Dean, Student Services, 617-353-2713, Fax: 617-353-7500, E-mail: ssankey@bu.edu.
Website: http://www.bu.edu/sargent/

Brock University, Faculty of Graduate Studies, Faculty of Applied Health Sciences, St. Catharines, ON L2S 3A1, Canada. Offers M Sc, MA, PhD. *Degree requirements:* For master's, thesis. *Entrance requirements:* For master's, honors degree, BA and/or B Sc. Additional exam requirements/recommendations for international students: Required—TOEFL (minimum score 550 paper-based; 80 iBT), IELTS (minimum score 6.5), TWE (minimum score 4). Electronic applications accepted. *Faculty research:* Health and physical activity, aging and health, health advocacy, exercise psychology, community development.

Canisius College, Graduate Division, School of Education and Human Services, Office of Professional Studies, Buffalo, NY 14208-1098. Offers applied nutrition (MS, Certificate); community and school health (MS); health and human performance (MS); health information technology (MS); respiratory care (MS). *Program availability:* Part-time, evening/weekend, 100% online, blended/hybrid learning. *Faculty:* 1 full-time (0 women), 11 part-time/adjunct (7 women). *Students:* 23 full-time (14 women), 79 part-time (58 women); includes 13 minority (7 Black or African American, non-Hispanic/Latino; 1 American Indian or Alaska Native, non-Hispanic/Latino; 3 Asian, non-Hispanic/Latino; 2 Hispanic/Latino), 4 international. Average age 35. 62 applicants, 81% accepted, 32 enrolled. In 2015, 37 master's awarded. *Entrance requirements:* For master's, GRE (recommended), bachelor's degree transcript, two letters of recommendation, current licensure (for applied nutrition), minimum GPA of 2.7, current resume. Additional exam requirements/recommendations for international students: Required—TOEFL (minimum score 550 paper-based, 80 iBT), IELTS (minimum score 6.5), or CAEL (minimum score 70). *Application deadline:* Applications are processed on a rolling basis. Application fee: $25. Electronic applications accepted. Application fee is waived when completed online. *Expenses:* $780 per credit hour; $644 per year full-time fees. *Financial support:* Career-related internships or fieldwork, Federal Work-Study, scholarships/grants, tuition waivers (partial), and unspecified assistantships available. Support available to part-time students. Financial award application deadline: 4/30; financial award applicants required to submit FAFSA. *Faculty research:* Nutrition, community and school health; community and health; health and human performance

applied; nutrition and respiratory care. *Unit head:* Sandy McKenna, Director, Professional Studies, 716-888-8296, E-mail: mckekkas@canisius.edu. *Application contact:* Kathleen B. Davis, Vice President of Enrollment Management, 716-888-2500, Fax: 716-888-3195, E-mail: daviskb@canisius.edu.
Website: http://www.canisius.edu/graduate/

Cleveland State University, College of Graduate Studies, College of Sciences and Health Professions, School of Health Sciences, Program in Health Sciences, Cleveland, OH 44115. Offers health sciences (MS); physician assistant science (MS). *Program availability:* Part-time, evening/weekend, online learning. *Faculty:* 7 full-time (6 women), 6 part-time/adjunct (all women). *Students:* 109 full-time (80 women), 40 part-time (33 women); includes 38 minority (20 Black or African American, non-Hispanic/Latino; 1 American Indian or Alaska Native, non-Hispanic/Latino; 8 Asian, non-Hispanic/Latino; 6 Hispanic/Latino; 3 Two or more races, non-Hispanic/Latino), 2 international. Average age 30. 85 applicants, 73% accepted, 48 enrolled. In 2015, 44 master's awarded. *Degree requirements:* For master's, completion of two 3-month field placements. *Entrance requirements:* For master's, GRE (scores of 50th percentile or greater in all areas; minimum analytical writing score of 3.5), bachelor's degree from accredited institution, minimum prerequisite course GPA of 3.0, all courses completed with minimum grade of C. Additional exam requirements/recommendations for international students: Required—TOEFL (minimum score 550 paper-based; 78 iBT). *Application deadline:* For fall admission, 1/15 for domestic and international students. Electronic applications accepted. *Expenses:* Tuition, state resident: full-time $9565. Tuition, nonresident: full-time $17,980. Tuition and fees vary according to program. *Financial support:* In 2015–16, 8 research assistantships with partial tuition reimbursements (averaging $10,000 per year) were awarded; career-related internships or fieldwork, Federal Work-Study, institutionally sponsored loans, scholarships/grants, traineeships, tuition waivers (partial), and unspecified assistantships also available. Support available to part-time students. Financial award applicants required to submit FAFSA. *Faculty research:* Assisted technologies, biomechanics, clinical administration, cultural health, gerontology. *Unit head:* Dr. Stephen Slane, Chairperson and Professor Emeritus, 216-687-2379, E-mail: s.slane@csuohio.edu. *Application contact:* Karen Armstrong, Administrative Assistant, 216-687-3567, Fax: 216-687-9316, E-mail: healthsci@csuohio.edu.
Website: http://www.csuohio.edu/sciences/dept/healthsciences/graduate/index.html

The Commonwealth Medical College, Professional Program in Medicine, Scranton, PA 18509. Offers MD, MD/MHA, MD/MPH. *Entrance requirements:* For doctorate, MCAT, bachelor's degree. Application fee: $100. *Application contact:* Jillian Golaszewski, Enrollment Management Recruiter, 570-504-7000, Fax: 570-504-2794, E-mail: jgolaszewski@tcmc.edu.
Website: http://www.tcmc.edu/md

Creighton University, School of Pharmacy and Health Professions, Omaha, NE 68178-0001. Offers MS, DPT, OTD, Pharm D, Pharm D/MS. *Accreditation:* ACPE (one or more programs are accredited). *Program availability:* Online learning. *Entrance requirements:* For doctorate, PCAT (for Pharm D); GRE (for DPT). Electronic applications accepted. *Expenses:* Contact institution. *Faculty research:* Patient safety in health services research, health information technology and health services research, interdisciplinary educational research in the health professions, outcomes research in the health professions, cross-cultural care in the health professions.

Dominican College, Division of Allied Health, Orangeburg, NY 10962-1210. Offers MS, DPT. *Program availability:* Part-time, evening/weekend, online learning.

Drexel University, College of Nursing and Health Professions, Philadelphia, PA 19104-2875. Offers MA, MFT, MHS, MS, MSN, DPT, Dr NP, PPDPT, PhD, Certificate, PMC. *Accreditation:* ACEN. *Program availability:* Part-time, evening/weekend. Terminal master's awarded for partial completion of doctoral program. *Degree requirements:* For master's, comprehensive exam, thesis (for some programs); for doctorate, thesis/dissertation, qualifying exam. *Entrance requirements:* For doctorate, GRE General Test. Electronic applications accepted.

Duquesne University, John G. Rangos, Sr. School of Health Sciences, Pittsburgh, PA 15282-0001. Offers health management systems (MHMS); occupational therapy (MS, OTD); physical therapy (DPT); physician assistant studies (MPAS); rehabilitation science (MS, PhD); speech-language pathology (MS); MBA/MHMS. *Accreditation:* AOTA (one or more programs are accredited); APTA (one or more programs are accredited); ASHA. *Program availability:* Minimal on-campus study. *Faculty:* 45 full-time (32 women), 33 part-time/adjunct (17 women). *Students:* 230 full-time (180 women), 11 part-time (5 women); includes 15 minority (1 Black or African American, non-Hispanic/Latino; 3 Asian, non-Hispanic/Latino; 7 Hispanic/Latino; 4 Two or more races, non-Hispanic/Latino), 20 international. Average age 23. 685 applicants, 9% accepted, 24 enrolled. In 2015, 132 master's, 32 doctorates awarded. *Degree requirements:* For doctorate, comprehensive exam (for some programs), thesis/dissertation (for some programs). *Entrance requirements:* For master's, GRE General Test (speech-language pathology), 3 letters of recommendation; minimum GPA of 2.75 (health management systems), 3.0 (speech-language pathology); for doctorate, GRE General Test (for physical therapy and rehabilitation science), 3 letters of recommendation, minimum GPA of 3.0, personal interview. Additional exam requirements/recommendations for international students: Required—TOEFL (minimum score 550 paper-based; 90 iBT). *Application deadline:* For fall admission, 2/1 for domestic and international students; for spring admission, 7/1 for domestic and international students. Applications are processed on a rolling basis. Application fee: $0. Electronic applications accepted. *Expenses:* $1,254 per credit. *Financial support:* Federal Work-Study available. Financial award applicants required to submit FAFSA. *Faculty research:* Neuronal processing, electrical stimulation on peripheral neuropathy, central nervous system (CNS) stimulatory and inhibitory signals, behavioral genetic methodologies to development disorders of speech, neurogenic communication disorders. *Total annual research expenditures:* $38,730. *Unit head:* Dr. Gregory H. Frazer, Dean, 412-396-5303, Fax: 412-396-5554, E-mail: frazer@duq.edu. *Application contact:* Christopher R. Hilf, Recruiter/Academic Advisor, 412-396-5653, Fax: 412-396-5554, E-mail: hilfc@duq.edu.
Website: http://www.duq.edu/academics/schools/health-sciences

Duquesne University, Post-Baccalaureate Pre-Medical and Health Professions Program, Pittsburgh, PA 15282-0001. Offers Postbaccalaureate Certificate. *Expenses:* Tuition, area resident: Full-time $21,402; part-time $1189 per credit. Tuition and fees vary according to program.

East Carolina University, Graduate School, College of Allied Health Sciences, Greenville, NC 27858-4353. Offers MS, MSOT, DPT, PhD, Certificate, Au D/PhD. *Program availability:* Part-time, evening/weekend, online learning. *Students:* 466 full-time (379 women), 109 part-time (89 women); includes 70 minority (33 Black or African American, non-Hispanic/Latino; 1 American Indian or Alaska Native, non-Hispanic/Latino; 13 Asian, non-Hispanic/Latino; 14 Hispanic/Latino; 9 Two or more races, non-Hispanic/Latino), 2 international. Average age 28. 903 applicants, 31% accepted, 213 enrolled. In 2015, 127 master's, 38 doctorates awarded. *Degree requirements:* For master's, comprehensive exam. *Entrance requirements:* For master's, GRE General Test. Additional exam requirements/recommendations for international students:

Required—TOEFL. Application fee: $70. *Financial support:* Research assistantships with partial tuition reimbursements, teaching assistantships with partial tuition reimbursements, career-related internships or fieldwork, Federal Work-Study, and scholarships/grants available. Support available to part-time students. Financial award application deadline: 6/1; financial award applicants required to submit FAFSA. *Faculty research:* Hearing, stuttering, therapeutic activities, ACL injury. *Unit head:* Dr. Greg Hassler, Interim Dean, 252-744-6010, E-mail: hasslerg@ecu.edu. *Application contact:* Dean of Graduate School, 252-328-6012, Fax: 252-328-6071, E-mail: gradschool@ecu.edu.
Website: http://www.ecu.edu/cs-dhs/ah/

Eastern Kentucky University, The Graduate School, College of Health Sciences, Richmond, KY 40475-3102. Offers MPH, MS, MSN. *Program availability:* Part-time. *Entrance requirements:* For master's, GRE General Test, minimum GPA of 2.75.

East Tennessee State University, School of Graduate Studies, College of Clinical and Rehabilitative Health Sciences, Department of Allied Health Science, Johnson City, TN 37614. Offers allied health (MSAH); clinical nutrition (MS). *Program availability:* Part-time, online learning. *Faculty:* 13 full-time (9 women). *Students:* 23 full-time (22 women), 22 part-time (18 women); includes 1 minority (Asian, non-Hispanic/Latino). Average age 31. 52 applicants, 31% accepted, 16 enrolled. In 2015, 15 master's awarded. *Degree requirements:* For master's, comprehensive exam, thesis or advanced practice seminar (for MSAH); internship (for MS). *Entrance requirements:* For master's, GRE General Test, professional license in allied health discipline, minimum GPA of 2.75, and three professional letters of recommendation (for MSAH); bachelor's degree from an undergraduate didactic program in dietetics with minimum GPA of 3.0 in DPD coursework and three letters of recommendation (for MS). Additional exam requirements/recommendations for international students: Required—TOEFL (minimum score 550 paper-based; 79 iBT). *Application deadline:* For fall admission, 2/15 for domestic and international students; for spring admission, 11/1 for domestic students, 9/30 for international students. Application fee: $35 ($45 for international students). Electronic applications accepted. *Financial support:* In 2015–16, 18 students received support, including 14 research assistantships with partial tuition reimbursements available (averaging $3,000 per year), 4 teaching assistantships with partial tuition reimbursements available (averaging $3,000 per year); career-related internships or fieldwork, institutionally sponsored loans, scholarships/grants, and unspecified assistantships also available. Financial award application deadline: 7/1; financial award applicants required to submit FAFSA. *Faculty research:* Recruitment and retention of allied health professionals, relationship between APACHEE II scores and the need for a tracheotomy, health care workers, patient care, occupational stress, radiofrequency lesioning, absorption of lipophilic compounds, Vitamin D status in college-age students, childhood and adolescence obesity, nutrition education/interventions. *Unit head:* Dr. Ester Verhovsek, Chair, 423-547-4900, Fax: 423-439-4921, E-mail: verhovse@etsu.edu. *Application contact:* Mary Duncan, Graduate Specialist, 423-439-4302, Fax: 423-439-5624, E-mail: duncanm@etsu.edu.
Website: http://www.etsu.edu/crhs/alliedhealth/

East Tennessee State University, School of Graduate Studies, College of Public Health, Johnson City, TN 37614. Offers MPH, MSEH, DPH, PhD, Postbaccalaureate Certificate. *Program availability:* Part-time, online learning. *Faculty:* 43 full-time (14 women), 4 part-time/adjunct (3 women). *Students:* 105 full-time (74 women), 89 part-time (75 women); includes 45 minority (29 Black or African American, non-Hispanic/Latino; 10 Asian, non-Hispanic/Latino; 3 Hispanic/Latino; 3 Two or more races, non-Hispanic/Latino), 24 international. Average age 30. 147 applicants, 71% accepted, 60 enrolled. In 2015, 26 master's, 6 doctorates, 9 other advanced degrees awarded. *Degree requirements:* For master's, comprehensive exam, field experience; research project or thesis; environmental health practice; seminar; for doctorate, comprehensive exam, thesis/dissertation, practicum; seminar. *Entrance requirements:* For master's, GRE General Test, SOPHAS application, three letters of recommendation; for doctorate, GRE General Test, SOPHAS application, three letters of recommendation, curriculum vitae or resume; for Postbaccalaureate Certificate, minimum GPA of 2.5, three letters of recommendation, resume. Additional exam requirements/recommendations for international students: Required—TOEFL (minimum score 550 paper-based; 79 iBT), IELTS. Application fee: $35 ($45 for international students). Electronic applications accepted. *Financial support:* In 2015–16, 57 students received support, including 54 research assistantships with tuition reimbursements available (averaging $6,750 per year), 3 teaching assistantships with tuition reimbursements available (averaging $14,000 per year); career-related internships or fieldwork, institutionally sponsored loans, scholarships/grants, and unspecified assistantships also available. Financial award application deadline: 7/1; financial award applicants required to submit FAFSA. *Faculty research:* Cancer prevention, obesity and diabetes prevention, prescription drug abuse, tobacco policy, women's health. *Unit head:* Dr. Randy Wykoff, Dean, 423-439-4243, Fax: 423-439-5238, E-mail: wykoff@etsu.edu. *Application contact:* Mary Duncan, Graduate Specialist, 423-439-4302, Fax: 423-439-5624, E-mail: duncanm@etsu.edu.
Website: http://www.etsu.edu/cph/default.aspx

Emory University, School of Medicine, Programs in Allied Health Professions, Atlanta, GA 30322-1100. Offers anesthesiology assistant (MM Sc); genetic counseling (MM Sc), including human genetics and genetic counseling; physical therapy (DPT); physician assistant (MM Sc). *Entrance requirements:* For master's, GRE or MCAT; for doctorate, GRE. Electronic applications accepted. *Expenses:* Contact institution.

Ferris State University, College of Health Professions, Big Rapids, MI 49307. Offers MSN. *Program availability:* Part-time, evening/weekend, 100% online. *Faculty:* 5 full-time (all women), 2 part-time/adjunct (both women). *Students:* 95 part-time (84 women); includes 11 minority (4 Black or African American, non-Hispanic/Latino; 1 American Indian or Alaska Native, non-Hispanic/Latino; 3 Asian, non-Hispanic/Latino; 1 Hispanic/Latino; 1 Native Hawaiian or other Pacific Islander, non-Hispanic/Latino; 1 Two or more races, non-Hispanic/Latino). Average age 39. 23 applicants, 117% accepted, 13 enrolled. In 2015, 15 master's awarded. *Degree requirements:* For master's, comprehensive exam, practicum, practicum project. *Entrance requirements:* For master's, BS in nursing or bachelor's degree in related field with registered nurse license; minimum GPA of 3.0; writing sample; 3 professional references. Additional exam requirements/recommendations for international students: Required—TOEFL (minimum score 500 paper-based; 61 iBT). *Application deadline:* For fall admission, 4/15 priority date for domestic students; for spring admission, 10/15 for domestic students. Applications are processed on a rolling basis. Application fee: $0. Electronic applications accepted. Tuition and fees vary according to degree level and program. *Financial support:* In 2015–16, 3 students received support. Career-related internships or fieldwork, Federal Work-Study, and scholarships/grants available. Support available to part-time students. Financial award application deadline: 4/15; financial award applicants required to submit FAFSA. *Faculty research:* Nursing education, end of life, leadership/education introverts in nursing. *Unit head:* Dr. Susan Owens, Chair, School of Nursing, 231-591-2267, Fax: 231-591-3788, E-mail: owenss3@ferris.edu. *Application contact:* Debby Buck, Off-Campus Student Support, 231-591-2094, Fax: 231-591-3788, E-mail: buckd@ferris.edu.
Website: http://www.ferris.edu/htmls/colleges/alliedhe/

Allied Health—General

Florida Agricultural and Mechanical University, Division of Graduate Studies, Research, and Continuing Education, School of Allied Health Sciences, Tallahassee, FL 32307-3200. Offers health administration (MS); occupational therapy (MOT); physical therapy (DPT). *Degree requirements:* For master's, thesis (for some programs). *Entrance requirements:* For master's, GRE General Test or GMAT, minimum GPA of 3.0. Additional exam requirements/recommendations for international students: Required—TOEFL (minimum score 550 paper-based).

Florida Gulf Coast University, College of Health Professions and Social Work, Fort Myers, FL 33965-6565. Offers M Ed, MA, MS, MSN, MSW, DNP, DPT. *Accreditation:* AOTA. *Program availability:* Part-time, evening/weekend, online learning. *Faculty:* 58 full-time (42 women), 43 part-time/adjunct (28 women). *Students:* 225 full-time (143 women), 158 part-time (123 women); includes 94 minority (29 Black or African American, non-Hispanic/Latino; 14 Asian, non-Hispanic/Latino; 44 Hispanic/Latino; 7 Two or more races, non-Hispanic/Latino), 1 international. Average age 31. 476 applicants, 42% accepted, 153 enrolled. In 2015, 86 master's, 36 doctorates awarded. *Degree requirements:* For master's, thesis or alternative. *Entrance requirements:* For master's, GRE General Test or MAT, minimum GPA of 3.0. Additional exam requirements/recommendations for international students: Required—TOEFL (minimum score 550 paper-based). *Application deadline:* Applications are processed on a rolling basis. Application fee: $30. Electronic applications accepted. *Expenses:* Tuition, state resident: full-time $6974. Tuition, nonresident: full-time $28,170. *Required fees:* $1987. One-time fee: $10 full-time. Tuition and fees vary according to course load and degree level. *Financial support:* In 2015–16, 111 students received support. Career-related internships or fieldwork, Federal Work-Study, and institutionally sponsored loans available. Financial award application deadline: 6/30; financial award applicants required to submit FAFSA. *Faculty research:* Gerontology, health care policy, health administration, community-based services. *Total annual research expenditures:* $59,237. *Unit head:* Dr. Mitchell Cordova, Dean, 239-590-7451, Fax: 239-590-7474. *Application contact:* Lynn O'Hare, Administrative Assistant, 239-590-7451, Fax: 239-590-7474, E-mail: lohare@fgcu.edu.

Georgia Southern University, Jack N. Averitt College of Graduate Studies, College of Health and Human Sciences, Statesboro, GA 30460. Offers MS, MSN, DNP, Certificate. *Program availability:* Part-time, evening/weekend, blended/hybrid learning. *Faculty:* 76 full-time (51 women), 1 (woman) part-time/adjunct. *Students:* 110 full-time (74 women), 120 part-time (76 women); includes 60 minority (33 Black or African American, non-Hispanic/Latino; 1 American Indian or Alaska Native, non-Hispanic/Latino; 8 Asian, non-Hispanic/Latino; 10 Hispanic/Latino; 8 Two or more races, non-Hispanic/Latino), 2 international. Average age 29. 309 applicants, 49% accepted, 50 enrolled. In 2015, 98 master's, 10 doctorates, 2 other advanced degrees awarded. *Degree requirements:* For master's, comprehensive exam (for some programs), thesis (for some programs), exams; for doctorate, comprehensive exam, practicum. *Entrance requirements:* For master's, GRE General Test, MAT or GMAT; for doctorate, GRE or MAT. Additional exam requirements/recommendations for international students: Required—TOEFL (minimum score 550 paper-based; 80 iBT), IELTS (minimum score 6). *Application deadline:* For fall admission, 3/1 priority date for domestic students, 3/1 for international students; for spring admission, 10/1 priority date for domestic students, 10/1 for international students. Applications are processed on a rolling basis. Application fee: $50. Electronic applications accepted. *Expenses:* Tuition, state resident: full-time $7236; part-time $277 per semester hour. Tuition, nonresident: full-time $27,118; part-time $1105 per semester hour. *Required fees:* $2092. *Financial support:* In 2015–16, 118 students received support, including 24 fellowships with full tuition reimbursements available (averaging $7,750 per year), 9 research assistantships with full tuition reimbursements available (averaging $7,750 per year), 33 teaching assistantships with full tuition reimbursements available (averaging $7,750 per year); career-related internships or fieldwork, Federal Work-Study, scholarships/grants, traineeships, tuition waivers (full), and unspecified assistantships also available. Support available to part-time students. Financial award application deadline: 4/15; financial award applicants required to submit FAFSA. *Faculty research:* Kinesiology, sport performance, coaching, nursing, nutrition. *Total annual research expenditures:* $99,590. *Unit head:* Dr. Barry Joyner, Dean, 912-478-5322, Fax: 912-478-5349, E-mail: joyner@georgiasouthern.edu. Website: http://chhs.georgiasouthern.edu/

Georgia State University, Byrdine F. Lewis School of Nursing, Division of Respiratory Therapy, Atlanta, GA 30302-3083. Offers MS. *Faculty:* 3 full-time (2 women). *Students:* 25 full-time (13 women), 5 part-time (2 women); includes 9 minority (5 Black or African American, non-Hispanic/Latino; 2 Asian, non-Hispanic/Latino; 2 Two or more races, non-Hispanic/Latino), 12 international. Average age 27. 49 applicants, 67% accepted, 30 enrolled. In 2015, 9 master's awarded. *Degree requirements:* For master's, thesis. *Entrance requirements:* For master's, GRE, transcripts, resume, statement of goals, letters of recommendation. Additional exam requirements/recommendations for international students: Required—TOEFL (minimum score 550 paper-based; 80 iBT). *Application deadline:* For fall admission, 5/1 for domestic and international students; for spring admission, 9/15 for domestic and international students. Application fee: $50. Electronic applications accepted. *Expenses:* Tuition, state resident: full-time $6876; part-time $382 per credit hour. Tuition, nonresident: full-time $22,374; part-time $1243 per credit hour. *Required fees:* $2128; $2128 per term. $1064 per term. Part-time tuition and fees vary according to course load and program. *Financial support:* In 2015–16, research assistantships with full tuition reimbursements (averaging $2,000 per year), teaching assistantships with full tuition reimbursements (averaging $2,000 per year) were awarded; scholarships/grants and unspecified assistantships also available. Financial award application deadline: 6/1; financial award applicants required to submit FAFSA. *Faculty research:* Aerosol delivery methods, aerosol devices, smoking cessation, continuing and professional respiratory therapy education, chronic lung disease management. *Unit head:* Dr. Douglas Gardenhire, Department Head, 404-413-1270, Fax: 404-413-1230, E-mail: dgardenhire@gsu.edu. Website: http://respiratorytherapy.gsu.edu/

Grand Valley State University, College of Health Professions, Allendale, MI 49401-9403. Offers MPAS, MPH, MS, DPT. *Faculty:* 57 full-time (41 women), 20 part-time/adjunct (18 women). *Students:* 592 full-time (452 women), 33 part-time (27 women); includes 62 minority (14 Black or African American, non-Hispanic/Latino; 1 American Indian or Alaska Native, non-Hispanic/Latino; 12 Asian, non-Hispanic/Latino; 18 Hispanic/Latino; 17 Two or more races, non-Hispanic/Latino), 4 international. Average age 26. 1,332 applicants, 27% accepted, 246 enrolled. In 2015, 174 master's, 47 doctorates awarded. *Entrance requirements:* For master's, volunteer work, interview, minimum GPA of 3.0, writing sample; for doctorate, GRE, 50 hours of volunteer work, interview, minimum GPA of 3.0 in last 60 hours and in prerequisites, writing sample. Additional exam requirements/recommendations for international students: Required—TOEFL (minimum score 610 paper-based). *Application deadline:* For winter admission, 1/15 priority date for domestic and international students. Applications are processed on a rolling basis. Electronic applications accepted. *Financial support:* In 2015–16, 106 students received support, including 74 fellowships (averaging $8,745 per year), 41 research assistantships with partial tuition reimbursements available (averaging $4,439 per year); career-related internships or fieldwork, Federal Work-Study, institutionally sponsored loans, and scholarships/grants also available. Financial award application deadline: 2/15. *Faculty research:* Skeletal muscle structure, blood platelets,

thrombospondin activity, FES exercise for quadriplegics, balance. *Unit head:* Dr. Roy Olsson, Dean, 616-331-3356, Fax: 616-331-3350, E-mail: olssonr@gvsu.edu. *Application contact:* Darlene Zwart, Student Services Coordinator, 616-331-3958, E-mail: zwartda@gvsu.edu. Website: http://www.gvsu.edu/shp/

Hampton University, School of Science, Program in Medical Science, Hampton, VA 23668. Offers MS. *Degree requirements:* For master's, comprehensive exam. *Entrance requirements:* For master's, MCAT or DAT. Additional exam requirements/recommendations for international students: Required—TOEFL (minimum score 525 paper-based) or IELTS (6.5). Electronic applications accepted. *Expenses: Tuition, area resident:* Full-time $10,263; part-time $522 per credit hour. *Required fees:* $35. Tuition and fees vary according to course load and program. *Faculty research:* Cancer, health disparities, protein kinases, neurodegeneration, nanoparticles, cellular differentiation, experimental physical chemistry, laser spectroscopy, RNA biology, bioinformatics, genomics.

Harding University, College of Allied Health, Searcy, AR 72149-0001. Offers MS, DPT. *Faculty:* 27 full-time (16 women), 4 part-time/adjunct (2 women). *Students:* 240 full-time (163 women); includes 32 minority (9 Black or African American, non-Hispanic/Latino; 4 American Indian or Alaska Native, non-Hispanic/Latino; 8 Asian, non-Hispanic/Latino; 8 Hispanic/Latino; 3 Two or more races, non-Hispanic/Latino), 1 international. Average age 27. 825 applicants, 16% accepted, 92 enrolled. In 2015, 47 master's, 26 doctorates awarded. *Entrance requirements:* Additional exam requirements/recommendations for international students: Required—TOEFL. *Financial support:* In 2015–16, 6 students received support. *Application contact:* Dr. Julie Hixson-Wallace, Vice Provost, 501-279-5205, Fax: 501-279-5192, E-mail: jahixson@harding.edu. Website: http://www.harding.edu/academics/colleges-departments/allied-health

Idaho State University, Office of Graduate Studies, Kasiska College of Health Professions, Pocatello, ID 83209-8090. Offers M Coun, MHE, MOT, MPAS, MPH, MS, Au D, DPT, PhD, Certificate, Ed S, Post-Doctoral Certificate, Post-Master's Certificate, Postbaccalaureate Certificate. *Accreditation:* APTA (one or more programs are accredited). *Program availability:* Part-time. *Degree requirements:* For master's, comprehensive exam, thesis (for some programs), 8-week externship; for doctorate, comprehensive exam, thesis/dissertation, clinical rotation (for some programs); for other advanced degree, comprehensive exam, thesis, case study, oral exam. *Entrance requirements:* For master's, GRE General Test or MAT, minimum GPA of 3.0, 3 letters of recommendation; for doctorate, GRE General Test or MAT, minimum GPA of 3.0, counseling license, professional research, interview, work experience, 3 letters of recommendation; for other advanced degree, GRE General Test or MAT, master's degree in similar field of study, 3 letters of recommendation, 2 years of work experience. Additional exam requirements/recommendations for international students: Required—TOEFL (minimum score 600 paper-based; 80 iBT). Electronic applications accepted. *Expenses:* Contact institution. *Faculty research:* Mental health, information technology, dental health, nursing.

Ithaca College, School of Health Sciences and Human Performance, Ithaca, NY 14850. Offers MS, DPT. *Program availability:* Part-time. *Faculty:* 60 full-time (42 women). *Students:* 305 full-time (241 women), 21 part-time (17 women); includes 33 minority (7 Black or African American, non-Hispanic/Latino; 12 Asian, non-Hispanic/Latino; 8 Hispanic/Latino; 6 Two or more races, non-Hispanic/Latino), 5 international. Average age 23. In 2015, 97 master's, 82 doctorates awarded. *Degree requirements:* For master's, comprehensive exam (for some programs), thesis optional; for doctorate, thesis/dissertation optional. *Entrance requirements:* Additional exam requirements/recommendations for international students: Required—TOEFL (minimum score 550 paper-based; 80 iBT). *Application deadline:* Applications are processed on a rolling basis. Application fee: $40. Electronic applications accepted. *Expenses:* Contact institution. *Financial support:* In 2015–16, 216 students received support, including 61 teaching assistantships (averaging $11,982 per year); career-related internships or fieldwork, Federal Work-Study, scholarships/grants, and unspecified assistantships also available. Support available to part-time students. Financial award applicants required to submit CSS PROFILE or FAFSA. *Unit head:* Dr. Linda Petrosino, Dean, 607-274-3265, Fax: 607-274-1263, E-mail: lpetrosino@ithaca.edu. *Application contact:* Nicole Eversley Bradwell, Interim Director, Office of Admission, 607-274-3124, Fax: 607-274-1263, E-mail: admission@ithaca.edu. Website: http://www.ithaca.edu/hshp

Jacksonville University, School of Applied Health Sciences, Jacksonville, FL 32211. Offers health informatics (MS); kinesiological sciences (MS); mental health counseling (MS); speech language pathology (MS). *Expenses: Tuition, area resident:* Full-time $12,960; part-time $8640 per credit hour. One-time fee: $50. Tuition and fees vary according to course load, degree level, campus/location and program. *Application contact:* Marisol Preston, Chief Admissions Officer, 904-256-7000, E-mail: admissions@ju.edu. Website: http://www.ju.edu/chs/AHS/

Loma Linda University, School of Allied Health Professions, Loma Linda, CA 92350. Offers MOT, MPA, MS, DPT, OTD, PhD, SLPD. *Accreditation:* AOTA; APTA. *Entrance requirements:* For master's, minimum GPA of 2.0; for doctorate, minimum 2.0 GPA, associate degree in physical therapy. Additional exam requirements/recommendations for international students: Required—TOEFL (minimum score 550 paper-based). *Application deadline:* For fall admission, 8/1 for domestic and international students; for winter admission, 11/1 for domestic and international students; for spring admission, 2/1 for domestic and international students. Applications are processed on a rolling basis. Application fee: $60. Electronic applications accepted. *Unit head:* Dr. Craig R. Jackson, Dean, 909-824-4545, Fax: 909-824-4809. *Application contact:* Helen Greenwood, Director, Admissions and Records, 909-824-4599, Fax: 909-824-4809, E-mail: hgreenwood@sahp.llu.edu. Website: http://alliedhealth.llu.edu

Long Island University–LIU Post, School of Health Professions and Nursing, Brookville, NY 11548-1300. Offers biomedical sciences (MS), including applied laboratory medicine, cancer biology, medical and molecular immunology, microbiology/infectious diseases; cardiovascular perfusion (MS); dietetic internship (Advanced Certificate); family nurse practitioner (MS); forensic social work (Advanced Certificate); nursing education (MS); social work (MSW). *Program availability:* Part-time, evening/weekend, blended/hybrid learning. *Faculty:* 16 full-time (14 women), 46 part-time/adjunct (33 women). *Students:* 190 full-time (139 women), 181 part-time (157 women); includes 141 minority (51 Black or African American, non-Hispanic/Latino; 46 Asian, non-Hispanic/Latino; 41 Hispanic/Latino; 3 Two or more races, non-Hispanic/Latino), 47 international. Average age 36. 422 applicants, 64% accepted, 141 enrolled. In 2015, 96 master's, 28 other advanced degrees awarded. *Degree requirements:* For master's, comprehensive exam (for some programs), thesis (for some programs). *Entrance requirements:* Additional exam requirements/recommendations for international students: Required—TOEFL, IELTS. *Application deadline:* Applications are processed on a rolling basis. Application fee: $50. Electronic applications accepted. *Expenses:* $1,155 per credit, $934 per term full-time university fee, $442 per term part-time university fee. *Financial support:* In 2015–16, 6 research assistantships with partial tuition reimbursements were awarded; career-related internships or fieldwork, Federal

Work-Study, institutionally sponsored loans, tuition waivers (partial), and unspecified assistantships also available. Support available to part-time students. Financial award application deadline: 2/15; financial award applicants required to submit FAFSA. *Faculty research:* Breast cancer, childhood obesity, dietary beverage consumption, emotional distress, histone modification, interprofessional practice, interstitial cystitis, lung cancer, pancreatic cancer, pediatric pain management, post-traumatic growth, poverty, renal nutrition, social ethics, yeast and bacterial drug resistance. *Total annual research expenditures:* $15,000. *Unit head:* Dr. Stacy Gropack, Acting Dean, 516-299-2486, Fax: 516-299-2527, E-mail: post-shpn@liu.edu. *Application contact:* Carol Zerah, Director of Graduate and International Admissions, 516-299-2900 Ext. 3952, Fax: 516-299-2137, E-mail: post-enroll@liu.edu.
Website: http://liu.edu/post/health

Marymount University, School of Health Professions, Arlington, VA 22207-4299. Offers MS, MSN, DNP, DPT, Certificate. *Program availability:* Part-time, evening/weekend. *Faculty:* 16 full-time (13 women), 19 part-time/adjunct (16 women). *Students:* 135 full-time (95 women), 68 part-time (62 women); includes 56 minority (26 Black or African American, non-Hispanic/Latino; 14 Asian, non-Hispanic/Latino; 10 Hispanic/Latino; 1 Native Hawaiian or other Pacific Islander, non-Hispanic/Latino; 5 Two or more races, non-Hispanic/Latino), 5 international. Average age 30. 773 applicants, 26% accepted, 71 enrolled. In 2015, 25 master's, 34 doctorates awarded. *Degree requirements:* For master's, thesis or alternative. *Entrance requirements:* For master's, GRE, MAT, 2 letters of recommendation, interview, resume; for doctorate, GRE, 2 letters of recommendation, resume; for Certificate, interview. Additional exam requirements/recommendations for international students: Required—TOEFL (minimum score 600 paper-based; 96 iBT), IELTS (minimum score 6.5). *Application deadline:* For fall admission, 7/1 for international students; for spring admission, 10/15 for international students. Applications are processed on a rolling basis. Application fee: $40. Electronic applications accepted. *Expenses:* Contact institution. *Financial support:* In 2015–16, 34 students received support, including 3 research assistantships with tuition reimbursements available, 14 teaching assistantships with tuition reimbursements available; career-related internships or fieldwork, Federal Work-Study, scholarships/grants, and unspecified assistantships also available. Support available to part-time students. Financial award applicants required to submit FAFSA. *Unit head:* Dr. Jeanne Matthews, Dean, 703-284-1580, Fax: 703-284-3819, E-mail: jeanne.matthews@marymount.edu. *Application contact:* Francesca Reed, Director, Graduate Admissions, 703-284-5901, Fax: 703-527-3815, E-mail: grad.admissions@marymount.edu.
Website: http://www.marymount.edu/Academics/Malek-School-of-Health-Professions

Maryville of Saint Louis, Walker College of Health Professions, St. Louis, MO 63141-7299. Offers MARC, MMT, MOT, MSN, DNP, DPT. *Accreditation:* CORE. *Program availability:* Part-time, evening/weekend, 100% online. *Faculty:* 51 full-time (42 women), 168 part-time/adjunct (149 women). *Students:* 136 full-time (113 women), 2,891 part-time (2,588 women); includes 692 minority (338 Black or African American, non-Hispanic/Latino; 40 American Indian or Alaska Native, non-Hispanic/Latino; 126 Asian, non-Hispanic/Latino; 129 Hispanic/Latino; 8 Native Hawaiian or other Pacific Islander, non-Hispanic/Latino; 51 Two or more races, non-Hispanic/Latino), 59 international. Average age 36. In 2015, 460 master's, 62 doctorates awarded. *Entrance requirements:* Additional exam requirements/recommendations for international students: Required—TOEFL (minimum score 550 paper-based). *Application deadline:* Applications are processed on a rolling basis. Electronic applications accepted. Application fee is waived when completed online. *Expenses: Tuition, area resident:* Full-time $25,558; part-time $781 per credit hour. *Required fees:* $2400. Part-time tuition and fees vary according to course load and degree level. *Financial support:* Career-related internships or fieldwork, Federal Work-Study, and campus employment available. Financial award application deadline: 3/1; financial award applicants required to submit FAFSA. *Unit head:* Dr. Charles Gulas, Dean, 314-529-9625, Fax: 314-529-9495, E-mail: hlthprofessions@maryville.edu. *Application contact:* Crystal Jacobsmeyer, Assistant Director, Graduate Enrollment Advising, 314-529-9654, Fax: 314-529-9927, E-mail: cjacobsmeyer@maryville.edu.
Website: http://www.maryville.edu/hp/

Medical University of South Carolina, College of Health Professions, Charleston, SC 29425. Offers MHA, MS, MSNA, MSOT, DHA, DPT, PhD. *Accreditation:* CAHME (one or more programs are accredited). *Program availability:* Part-time. *Degree requirements:* For doctorate, comprehensive exam, thesis/dissertation. *Entrance requirements:* For master's, GRE. Additional exam requirements/recommendations for international students: Required—TOEFL (minimum score 600 paper-based). Electronic applications accepted. *Expenses:* Contact institution. *Faculty research:* Spinal cord injury, geriatrics, rehabilitation sciences, behavioral medicine.

Mercy College, School of Health and Natural Sciences, Dobbs Ferry, NY 10522-1189. Offers communication disorders (MS); nursing (MS), including nursing administration, nursing education; occupational therapy (MS); physical therapy (DPT); physician assistant studies (MS). *Program availability:* Part-time, evening/weekend, online learning. *Degree requirements:* For master's, comprehensive exam (for some programs), thesis (for some programs). *Entrance requirements:* For master's and doctorate, essay, interview, resume, letters of recommendation, undergraduate transcripts. Additional exam requirements/recommendations for international students: Required—TOEFL (minimum score 600 paper-based; 79 iBT), IELTS (minimum score 8). Electronic applications accepted. *Expenses:* Contact institution.

Midwestern University, Downers Grove Campus, College of Health Sciences, Illinois Campus, Doctor of Health Science Program, Downers Grove, IL 60515-1235. Offers DHS. *Program availability:* Part-time. *Entrance requirements:* For doctorate, master's or bachelor's degree, minimum cumulative GPA of 3.0.

Midwestern University, Glendale Campus, College of Health Sciences, Arizona Campus, Glendale, AZ 85308. Offers MA, MBS, MCVS, MMS, MOT, MS, DPM, DPT, Psy D. *Program availability:* Part-time. *Expenses:* Contact institution.

Minnesota State University Mankato, College of Graduate Studies and Research, College of Allied Health and Nursing, Mankato, MN 56001. Offers MA, MS, MSN, DNP, Postbaccalaureate Certificate. *Program availability:* Part-time. *Degree requirements:* For master's, comprehensive exam; for Postbaccalaureate Certificate, thesis. *Entrance requirements:* For master's, GRE (for some programs), minimum GPA of 3.0 during previous 2 years; for Postbaccalaureate Certificate, GRE General Test, minimum GPA of 3.0. Electronic applications accepted.

Misericordia University, College of Health Sciences, Dallas, PA 18612-1098. Offers MSN, MSOT, MSSLP, DNP, DPT, OTD. *Program availability:* Part-time, evening/weekend. *Faculty:* 33 full-time (27 women), 18 part-time/adjunct (14 women). *Students:* 228 full-time (167 women), 151 part-time (132 women); includes 21 minority (3 Black or African American, non-Hispanic/Latino; 5 Asian, non-Hispanic/Latino; 8 Hispanic/Latino; 5 Two or more races, non-Hispanic/Latino). Average age 28. In 2015, 91 master's, 70 doctorates awarded. *Entrance requirements:* For doctorate, interview, references. Additional exam requirements/recommendations for international students: Required—TOEFL. *Application deadline:* Applications are processed on a rolling basis. Application fee: $35. Electronic applications accepted. *Financial support:* In 2015–16, 252 students received support. Teaching assistantships, career-related internships or fieldwork,

Federal Work-Study, scholarships/grants, traineeships, and tuition waivers (partial) available. Support available to part-time students. Financial award application deadline: 6/30; financial award applicants required to submit FAFSA. *Unit head:* Dr. Leamor Kahanov, Dean, 570-674-8406, E-mail: lkahanov@misericordia.edu. *Application contact:* Maureen Sheridan, Assistant Director of Admissions, Part-Time Undergraduate and Graduate Programs, 570-674-6451, Fax: 570-674-6232, E-mail: msherida@misericordia.edu.
Website: http://www.misericordia.edu/page.cfm?p-880

Moravian College, Moravian College Comenius Center, Business and Management Programs, Bethlehem, PA 18018-6650. Offers accounting (MBA); business analytics (MBA); general management (MBA); health administration (MHA); healthcare management (MBA); human resource management (MBA); leadership (MSHRM); learning and performance management (MSHRM); supply chain management (MBA). *Program availability:* Part-time, evening/weekend. *Entrance requirements:* For master's, GMAT. Additional exam requirements/recommendations for international students: Required—TOEFL (minimum score 550 paper-based; 90 iBT). Application fee is waived when completed online. *Expenses:* Contact institution. *Faculty research:* Leadership, change management, human resources.

New Jersey City University, College of Professional Studies, Department of Health Sciences, Jersey City, NJ 07305-1597. Offers community health education (MS); health administration (MS); school health education (MS). *Program availability:* Part-time, evening/weekend. *Degree requirements:* For master's, thesis or alternative, internship. *Entrance requirements:* Additional exam requirements/recommendations for international students: Required—TOEFL (minimum score 79 iBT). *Application deadline:* For fall admission, 8/1 priority date for domestic students; for spring admission, 12/1 for domestic students. Applications are processed on a rolling basis. Application fee: $0. *Expenses.* Tuition, state resident: part-time $566.55 per credit. Tuition, nonresident: part-time $998.15 per credit. *Required fees:* $108 per credit. Part-time tuition and fees vary according to class time, degree level, campus/location and program. *Financial support:* Career-related internships or fieldwork and unspecified assistantships available.

Northeastern University, Bouvé College of Health Sciences, Boston, MA 02115-5096. Offers applied behavior analysis (MS, CAGS); audiology (Au D); biomedical nanotechnology (MS); college student development and counseling (MS, CAGS); counseling psychology (MS, PhD, CAGS); exercise science (MS); health informatics (MS); medicinal chemistry (MS); nurse anesthesia (DNP, CAGS); nursing (MS, PhD, CAGS), including administration (MS), adult-gerontology acute care nurse practitioner (MS, CAGS), adult-gerontology primary care nurse practitioner (MS, CAGS), anesthesia (MS), family nurse practitioner (MS, CAGS), neonatal nurse practitioner (MS, CAGS), pediatric nurse practitioner (MS, CAGS), psychiatric mental health nurse practitioner (MS, CAGS); nursing practice (DNP); personal health informatics (MS); pharmaceutical sciences (MS, PhD), including interdisciplinary concentration, pharmaceutics and drug delivery systems; pharmacology (MS); pharmacy (Pharm D); physical therapy (Postbaccalaureate Certificate); physician assistant (MS); population health (PhD); school psychology (MS, PhD, CAGS); speech-language pathology (MS); urban health (MPH); MS/MBA. *Accreditation:* ACPE (one or more programs are accredited). *Program availability:* Part-time, evening/weekend, online learning. *Faculty:* 194 full-time (120 women), 169 part-time/adjunct (136 women). *Students:* 1,416 full-time (1,049 women), 310 part-time (248 women). In 2015, 374 master's, 313 doctorates, 37 other advanced degrees awarded. *Degree requirements:* For doctorate, thesis/dissertation (for some programs); for other advanced degree, comprehensive exam. Application fee: $75. Electronic applications accepted. *Expenses:* Contact institution. *Financial support:* Applicants required to submit FAFSA. *Unit head:* John R. Reynolds, Professor and Interim Dean, 617-373-3323, Fax: 617-373-3030. *Application contact:* Molly Schnabel, Senior Director of Graduate Affairs, 617-373-2708, Fax: 617-373-4701, E-mail: bouvegrad@neu.edu.
Website: http://www.northeastern.edu/bouve/

Northern Arizona University, Graduate College, College of Health and Human Services, Flagstaff, AZ 86011. Offers MPAS, MS, MSN, DNP, DPT, Certificate. *Accreditation:* APTA (one or more programs are accredited). *Program availability:* Part-time. Application fee: $65. *Expenses: Tuition, area resident:* Full-time $8710. Tuition, nonresident: full-time $20,350. *Required fees:* $896. *Financial support:* Research assistantships and tuition waivers (full and partial) available. Financial award applicants required to submit FAFSA. *Unit head:* Leslie Schulz, Executive Dean, 928-523-4331, E-mail: leslie.schulz@nau.edu.
Website: http://nau.edu/chhs/

Northern Kentucky University, Office of Graduate Programs, School of Nursing and Health Professions, Program in Health Science, Highland Heights, KY 41099. Offers MS. *Program availability:* Online learning. *Degree requirements:* For master's, capstone, internship. *Entrance requirements:* For master's, official transcripts, minimum GPA of 3.0 on last 40 hours of undergraduate work, letter of intent, resume, undergraduate course in statistical methods with minimum C grade, interview. Additional exam requirements/recommendations for international students: Required—TOEFL (minimum score 79 iBT); Recommended—IELTS (minimum score 6.5).

Nova Southeastern University, College of Health Care Sciences, Fort Lauderdale, FL 33314-7796. Offers anesthesiologist assistant (MSA); audiology (Au D); health science (MH Sc, DHSc, PhD); occupational therapy (MOT, Dr OT, PhD); physical therapy (DPT, TDPT); physician assistant (MMS). *Program availability:* Online learning. *Faculty:* 109 full-time (64 women), 100 part-time/adjunct (65 women). *Students:* 1,590 full-time (1,179 women), 969 part-time (819 women); includes 831 minority (234 Black or African American, non-Hispanic/Latino; 8 American Indian or Alaska Native, non-Hispanic/Latino; 151 Asian, non-Hispanic/Latino; 378 Hispanic/Latino; 1 Native Hawaiian or other Pacific Islander, non-Hispanic/Latino; 59 Two or more races, non-Hispanic/Latino), 18 international. Average age 30. 8,133 applicants, 14% accepted, 728 enrolled. In 2015, 556 master's, 105 doctorates awarded. *Degree requirements:* For master's, thesis; for doctorate, comprehensive exam, thesis/dissertation. *Entrance requirements:* For master's, GRE General Test, MCAT; for doctorate, GRE General Test, personal interview, essay. Additional exam requirements/recommendations for international students: Required—TOEFL (minimum score 600 paper-based). *Application deadline:* For winter admission, 4/15 for domestic students; for summer admission, 12/15 for domestic and international students. Applications are processed on a rolling basis. Application fee: $50. Electronic applications accepted. *Expenses:* Contact institution. *Financial support:* In 2015–16, 151 students received support, including 4 research assistantships (averaging $3,500 per year); institutionally sponsored loans and unspecified assistantships also available. Financial award application deadline: 4/15; financial award applicants required to submit FAFSA. *Unit head:* Dr. Stanley Wilson, Dean, 954-262-1203, E-mail: swilson@nova.edu. *Application contact:* Joey Jankie, Admissions Counselor, 954-262-7249, E-mail: joey@nova.edu.
Website: http://www.nova.edu/chcs

Oakland University, Graduate Study and Lifelong Learning, School of Health Sciences, Rochester, MI 48309-4401. Offers MS, DPT, Dr Sc PT, TDPT, Graduate Certificate. *Accreditation:* APTA (one or more programs are accredited). *Faculty:* 21 full-time (13 women), 5 part-time/adjunct (2 women). *Students:* 195 full-time (145 women), 59 part-time (35 women); includes 22 minority (9 Black or African American, non-Hispanic/

Allied Health—General

Latino; 1 American Indian or Alaska Native, non-Hispanic/Latino; 6 Asian, non-Hispanic/Latino; 6 Two or more races, non-Hispanic/Latino; 17 international. Average age 26. 742 applicants, 13% accepted, 77 enrolled. In 2015, 33 master's, 41 doctorates, 15 other advanced degrees awarded. *Entrance requirements:* For master's, minimum GPA of 3.0; for doctorate, GRE General Test. Additional exam requirements/recommendations for international students: Required—TOEFL (minimum score 550 paper-based). *Application deadline:* For fall admission, 10/15 for domestic and international students. Applications are processed on a rolling basis. Application fee: $0. Electronic applications accepted. *Expenses:* Contact institution. *Financial support:* Fellowships, Federal Work-Study, institutionally sponsored loans, and tuition waivers (full) available. Financial award application deadline: 3/1; financial award applicants required to submit FAFSA. *Unit head:* Dr. Richard J. Rozek, Interim Dean/Associate Professor, 248-370-3562, Fax: 248-364-3562, E-mail: rozek@oakland.edu.

The Ohio State University, College of Medicine, School of Health and Rehabilitation Sciences, Program in Allied Health, Columbus, OH 43210. Offers MS. *Students:* 34 full-time (23 women), 10 part-time (9 women); includes 4 minority (1 American Indian or Alaska Native, non-Hispanic/Latino; 1 Asian, non-Hispanic/Latino; 2 Hispanic/Latino). Average age 26. In 2015, 19 master's awarded. *Entrance requirements:* For master's, GRE. Additional exam requirements/recommendations for international students: Required—TOEFL (minimum score 550 paper-based; 79 iBT), Michigan English Language Assessment Battery (minimum score 82); Recommended—IELTS (minimum score 7). *Application deadline:* For fall admission, 11/1 priority date for domestic students, 10/1 priority date for international students; for spring admission, 12/12 for domestic students, 11/10 for international students; for summer admission, 4/10 for domestic students, 3/13 for international students. Applications are processed on a rolling basis. Application fee: $60 ($70 for international students). Electronic applications accepted. *Unit head:* Dr. Kay Wolf, Graduate Studies Chair, 614-292-8131, E-mail: wolf.4@osu.edu. *Application contact:* Graduate and Professional Admissions, 614-292-9444, Fax: 614-292-3895, E-mail: gpadmissions@osu.edu.

Old Dominion University, College of Health Sciences, Norfolk, VA 23529. Offers MS, MSAT, MSN, DNP, DPT, PhD. *Program availability:* Part-time, evening/weekend, 100% online, blended/hybrid learning. *Faculty:* 64 full-time (42 women), 3 part-time/adjunct. *Students:* 295 full-time (223 women), 118 part-time (102 women); includes 80 minority (40 Black or African American, non-Hispanic/Latino; 1 American Indian or Alaska Native, non-Hispanic/Latino; 13 Asian, non-Hispanic/Latino; 10 Hispanic/Latino; 16 Two or more races, non-Hispanic/Latino), 15 international. Average age 33. 1,047 applicants, 25% accepted, 202 enrolled. In 2015, 108 master's, 78 doctorates awarded. *Degree requirements:* For master's, comprehensive exam; for doctorate, comprehensive exam, thesis/dissertation. *Entrance requirements:* For master's and doctorate, GRE or MAT. Additional exam requirements/recommendations for international students: Required—TOEFL (minimum score 550 paper-based; 79 iBT). *Application deadline:* Applications are processed on a rolling basis. Application fee: $50. Electronic applications accepted. *Expenses:* Tuition, state resident: full-time $11,136; part-time $464 per credit hour. Tuition, nonresident: full-time $27,840; part-time $1160 per credit hour. *Required fees:* $64 per semester. Tuition and fees vary according to campus/location, program and reciprocity agreements. *Financial support:* In 2015–16, 37 students received support, including 7 fellowships with full tuition reimbursements available (averaging $15,000 per year), 12 research assistantships with partial tuition reimbursements available (averaging $15,000 per year), 9 teaching assistantships with partial tuition reimbursements available (averaging $13,000 per year); career-related internships or fieldwork, institutionally sponsored loans, scholarships/grants, health care benefits, tuition waivers (full and partial), and unspecified assistantships also available. Support available to part-time students. Financial award application deadline: 2/15; financial award applicants required to submit FAFSA. *Faculty research:* Health promotion and wellness, health care ethics, health policy, health services, cultural competency, environmental health, global health, falls prevention, breast cancer detection. *Total annual research expenditures:* $2.7 million. *Unit head:* Dr. Shelley Mishoe, Dean, 757-683-4960, Fax: 757-683-5674, E-mail: smishoe@odu.edu. *Application contact:* William Heffelfinger, Director of Graduate Admissions, 757-683-5554, Fax: 757-683-3255, E-mail: gradadmit@odu.edu. Website: http://hs.odu.edu/

Oregon State University, Interdisciplinary/Institutional Programs, Program in Comparative Health Sciences, Corvallis, OR 97331. Offers biomedical sciences (MS, PhD); clinical sciences (MS, PhD). *Faculty:* 19 full-time (9 women), 3 part-time/adjunct (2 women). *Students:* 16 full-time (11 women), 2 part-time (1 woman); includes 2 minority (1 Black or African American, non-Hispanic/Latino; 1 Asian, non-Hispanic/Latino), 4 international. Average age 29. 24 applicants, 38% accepted, 8 enrolled. *Entrance requirements:* For master's and doctorate, GRE. Additional exam requirements/recommendations for international students: Required—TOEFL (minimum score 80 iBT), IELTS (minimum score 6.5). *Application deadline:* For fall admission, 12/10 for domestic students. Application fee: $75 ($85 for international students). *Expenses:* Tuition, state resident: full-time $12,150; part-time $450 per credit. Tuition, nonresident: full-time $20,952; part-time $776 per credit. *Required fees:* $1572; $1443 per unit. One-time fee: $350. Tuition and fees vary according to course load, campus/location and program. *Unit head:* Dr. Luiz E. Bermudez, Department Head/Professor. *Application contact:* Beth Chamblin, E-mail: beth.chamblin@oregonstate.edu.

Purdue University, Graduate School, College of Health and Human Sciences, School of Health Sciences, West Lafayette, IN 47907. Offers health physics (MS, PhD); medical physics (MS, PhD); occupational and environmental health science (MS, PhD), including aerosol deposition and lung disease, ergonomics, exposure and risk assessment, indoor air quality and bioaerosols (PhD), liver/lung toxicology; radiation biology (PhD); toxicology (PhD); MS/PhD. *Program availability:* Part-time. *Degree requirements:* For master's, thesis optional; for doctorate, one foreign language, thesis/dissertation. *Entrance requirements:* For master's and doctorate, GRE General Test, minimum undergraduate GPA of 3.0 or equivalent. Additional exam requirements/recommendations for international students: Required—TOEFL (minimum score 550 paper-based; 77 iBT); Recommended—TWE. Electronic applications accepted. *Faculty research:* Environmental toxicology, industrial hygiene, radiation dosimetry.

Quinnipiac University, School of Health Sciences, Hamden, CT 06518-1940. Offers MHS, MHS, MSW. *Accreditation:* AOTA. *Faculty:* 64 full-time (45 women), 95 part-time/adjunct (56 women). *Students:* 271 full-time (189 women), 91 part-time (68 women); includes 67 minority (27 Black or African American, non-Hispanic/Latino; 1 American Indian or Alaska Native, non-Hispanic/Latino; 17 Asian, non-Hispanic/Latino; 22 Hispanic/Latino), 16 international. 1,688 applicants, 15% accepted, 174 enrolled. In 2015, 131 master's awarded. *Entrance requirements:* Additional exam requirements/recommendations for international students: Required—TOEFL (minimum score 575 paper-based; 90 iBT), IELTS (minimum score 6.5). *Application deadline:* Applications are processed on a rolling basis. Application fee: $45. Electronic applications accepted. Tuition and fees vary according to course load and program. *Financial support:* Federal Work-Study, scholarships/grants, and unspecified assistantships available. Support available to part-time students. Financial award applicants required to submit FAFSA. *Application contact:* Office of Graduate Admissions, 800-462-1944, Fax: 203-582-3443, E-mail: graduate@quinnipiac.edu. Website: http://www.quinnipiac.edu/gradprograms

Regis University, Rueckert-Hartman College for Health Professions, Denver, CO 80221-1099. Offers addictions counseling (Post-Graduate Certificate); advanced practice nurse specialization (DNP); counseling (MA); counseling children and adolescents (Post-Graduate Certificate); counseling military families (Post-Graduate Certificate); depth psychotherapy (Post-Graduate Certificate); family nurse practitioner (MSN); health care business management (Certificate); health care quality and patient safety (Certificate); health industry leadership (MBA); health professions (Postbaccalaureate Certificate); health services administration (MS); marriage and family therapy (MA); neonatal nurse practitioner (MSN); nursing education or leadership (MSN); orthopedic manual physical therapy fellowship (Certificate); pharmacy (Pharm D); physical therapy (DPT). *Program availability:* Part-time, evening/weekend, 100% online, blended/hybrid learning. *Faculty:* 40 full-time (29 women), 116 part-time/adjunct (86 women). *Students:* 1,080 full-time (771 women), 274 part-time (239 women); includes 388 minority (59 Black or African American, non-Hispanic/Latino; 6 American Indian or Alaska Native, non-Hispanic/Latino; 109 Asian, non-Hispanic/Latino; 163 Hispanic/Latino; 1 Native Hawaiian or other Pacific Islander, non-Hispanic/Latino; 50 Two or more races, non-Hispanic/Latino), 7 international. Average age 34. 2,188 applicants, 31% accepted, 303 enrolled. In 2015, 329 master's, 160 doctorates awarded. *Degree requirements:* For master's, thesis (for some programs), internship. *Entrance requirements:* For master's, official transcript reflecting baccalaureate degree awarded from regionally-accredited college or university. Additional exam requirements/recommendations for international students: Required—TOEFL (minimum score 550 paper-based; 82 iBT). *Application deadline:* For fall admission, 8/15 priority date for domestic students; for spring admission, 1/10 priority date for domestic students; for summer admission, 5/1 priority date for domestic students. Applications are processed on a rolling basis. Application fee: $75. Electronic applications accepted. *Expenses:* Contact institution. *Financial support:* In 2015–16, 102 students received support. Federal Work-Study and scholarships/grants available. Financial award application deadline: 4/15; financial award applicants required to submit FAFSA. *Faculty research:* Normal and pathological balance and gait research, normal/pathological upper limb motor control/biomechanics, exercise energy/metabolism research, optical treatment protocols for therapeutic modalities. *Unit head:* Dr. Janet Houser, Academic Dean. *Application contact:* Cate Clark, Director of Admissions, 303-458-4900, Fax: 303-964-5534, E-mail: ruadmissions@regis.edu. Website: http://www.regis.edu/RHCHP.aspx

Rosalind Franklin University of Medicine and Science, College of Health Professions, North Chicago, IL 60064-3095. Offers MS, D Sc, DNAP, DPT, PhD, TDPT, Certificate. *Program availability:* Part-time, online learning. Terminal master's awarded for partial completion of doctoral program.

Rutgers University–Newark, School of Health Related Professions, Newark, NJ 07102. Offers MS, DCN, DPT, PhD, Certificate, DMD/MS, MD/MS. *Accreditation:* APTA (one or more programs are accredited); NAACLS. *Program availability:* Part-time. *Degree requirements:* For master's, thesis (for some programs). *Entrance requirements:* Additional exam requirements/recommendations for international students: Required—TOEFL. Electronic applications accepted. *Expenses:* Contact institution. *Faculty research:* Clinical outcomes.

Saint Louis University, Graduate Education, Doisy College of Health Sciences, St. Louis, MO 63103. Offers MAT, MMS, MOT, MS, MSN, DNP, DPT, PhD, Certificate. *Program availability:* Part-time. *Degree requirements:* For master's, comprehensive exam. *Entrance requirements:* Additional exam requirements/recommendations for international students: Required—TOEFL (minimum score 525 paper-based).

Sam Houston State University, College of Health Sciences, Department of Health Services and Promotion, Huntsville, TX 77341. Offers health (MA). *Accreditation:* NCATE. *Program availability:* Part-time. *Degree requirements:* For master's, comprehensive exam, thesis optional, internship. *Entrance requirements:* For master's, GRE General Test, MAT, letters of recommendation, statement of interest/intent. Additional exam requirements/recommendations for international students: Required—TOEFL (minimum score 550 paper-based; 79 iBT), IELTS (minimum score 6.5). Electronic applications accepted.

Seton Hall University, School of Health and Medical Sciences, Program in Health Sciences, South Orange, NJ 07079-2697. Offers PhD. *Program availability:* Part-time, evening/weekend. *Degree requirements:* For doctorate, comprehensive exam (for some programs), thesis/dissertation, candidacy exam, practicum, research projects. *Entrance requirements:* For doctorate, GRE (preferred), interview, minimum GPA of 3.0, letters of recommendation. Additional exam requirements/recommendations for international students: Required—TOEFL. Electronic applications accepted. *Faculty research:* Movement science, motor learning, dual tasks, clinical decision making, online education, teaching strategies.

Shenandoah University, School of Health Professions, Winchester, VA 22601-5195. Offers MS, DPT, Certificate. *Program availability:* Online learning. *Faculty:* 29 full-time (23 women), 14 part-time/adjunct (10 women). *Students:* 353 full-time (283 women), 115 part-time (92 women); includes 68 minority (11 Black or African American, non-Hispanic/Latino; 2 American Indian or Alaska Native, non-Hispanic/Latino; 33 Asian, non-Hispanic/Latino; 21 Hispanic/Latino; 1 Native Hawaiian or other Pacific Islander, non-Hispanic/Latino), 7 international. Average age 28. 1,574 applicants, 21% accepted, 122 enrolled. In 2015, 75 master's, 85 doctorates awarded. *Degree requirements:* For master's, comprehensive exam, thesis; for doctorate, comprehensive exam, evidence-based practice research project. *Entrance requirements:* For master's, GRE, college transcripts; thorough background in sciences, humanities and mathematics; for doctorate, GRE, PCAT. Additional exam requirements/recommendations for international students: Required—TOEFL (minimum score 550 paper-based; 79 iBT), IELTS (minimum score 6.5), Sakae Institute of Study Abroad (SISA) test (minimum score 15). *Application deadline:* For fall admission, 7/31 for domestic and international students; for summer admission, 5/1 for domestic and international students. Application fee: $30. Electronic applications accepted. *Expenses:* Tuition, area resident: Full-time $19,920; part-time $830 per credit. *Required fees:* $620; $460 per term. Tuition and fees vary according to course load and program. *Financial support:* In 2015–16, 48 students received support. Career-related internships or fieldwork, scholarships/grants, and unspecified assistantships available. Support available to part-time students. Financial award application deadline: 3/15; financial award applicants required to submit FAFSA. *Unit head:* Timothy E. Ford, PhD. *Application contact:* Andrew Woodall, Executive Director of Recruitment and Admissions, 540-665-4581, Fax: 540-665-4627, E-mail: admit@su.edu. Website: http://www.health.su.edu/

South Carolina State University, College of Graduate and Professional Studies, Department of Health Sciences, Orangeburg, SC 29117-0001. Offers speech pathology and audiology (MA). *Accreditation:* ASHA. *Program availability:* Part-time, evening/weekend. *Faculty:* 14 full-time (13 women), 2 part-time/adjunct (both women). *Students:* 42 full-time (40 women), 41 part-time (38 women); includes 50 minority (48 Black or African American, non-Hispanic/Latino; 2 Hispanic/Latino), 1 international. Average age 26. 70 applicants, 49% accepted, 27 enrolled. In 2015, 36 master's awarded. *Degree requirements:* For master's, thesis optional, departmental qualifying exam. *Entrance requirements:* For master's, GRE or NTE, minimum GPA of 3.0. *Application deadline:*

For fall admission, 6/15 for domestic and international students; for spring admission, 11/1 for domestic and international students. Application fee: $25. Electronic applications accepted. *Expenses:* Tuition, state resident: full-time $8906; part-time $495 per credit hour. Tuition, nonresident: full-time $18,674; part-time $1037 per credit hour. *Required fees:* $2497; $66 per credit hour. *Financial support:* Fellowships, career-related internships or fieldwork, Federal Work-Study, and scholarships/grants available. Financial award application deadline: 6/1. *Unit head:* Dr. Cecelia Jeffries, Chair, Department of Health Sciences, 803-536-8074, Fax: 803-536-8593, E-mail: cjeffrie@scsu.edu. *Application contact:* Curtis Foskey, Coordinator of Graduate Admission, 803-536-8419, Fax: 803-536-8812, E-mail: cfoskey@scsu.edu.

Southwestern Oklahoma State University, College of Professional and Graduate Studies, School of Behavioral Sciences and Education, Specialization in Health Sciences and Microbiology, Weatherford, OK 73096-3098. Offers M Ed.

Temple University, College of Public Health, Philadelphia, PA 19122. Offers MA, MOT, MPH, MS, MSAT, MSW, DAT, DNP, DOT, DPT, PhD, TDPT. *Accreditation:* APTA (one or more programs are accredited). *Program availability:* Part-time, evening/weekend, online learning. *Faculty:* 130 full-time (86 women), 48 part-time/adjunct (34 women). *Students:* 736 full-time (595 women), 485 part-time (384 women); includes 371 minority (199 Black or African American, non-Hispanic/Latino; 1 American Indian or Alaska Native, non-Hispanic/Latino; 60 Asian, non-Hispanic/Latino; 83 Hispanic/Latino; 3 Native Hawaiian or other Pacific Islander, non-Hispanic/Latino; 25 Two or more races, non-Hispanic/Latino), 21 international. 1,307 applicants, 44% accepted, 237 enrolled. In 2015, 365 master's, 109 doctorates awarded. *Degree requirements:* For doctorate, thesis/dissertation. *Entrance requirements:* Additional exam requirements/recommendations for international students: Required—TOEFL (minimum score 550 paper-based; 79 iBT). Application fee: $60. *Expenses:* Contact institution. *Financial support:* Fellowships, research assistantships, teaching assistantships with full tuition reimbursements, career-related internships or fieldwork, Federal Work-Study, institutionally sponsored loans, traineeships, and tuition waivers (partial) available. Support available to part-time students. Financial award application deadline: 1/15. *Total annual research expenditures:* $10.1 million. *Unit head:* Dr. Laura Siminoff, Dean, 215-707-4802, Fax: 215-707-7819.
Website: http://cph.temple.edu/

Tennessee State University, The School of Graduate Studies and Research, College of Health Sciences, Nashville, TN 37209-1561. Offers MA Ed, MOT, MPH, MS, MSN, DPT, Certificate. *Accreditation:* ASHA (one or more programs are accredited). *Program availability:* Part-time, evening/weekend. *Entrance requirements:* For master's, GRE General Test, MAT, minimum GPA of 3.5. *Application deadline:* For fall admission, 4/1 for domestic students. Applications are processed on a rolling basis. Application fee: $25. Electronic applications accepted. *Financial support:* Fellowships, research assistantships, teaching assistantships, and scholarships/grants available. Financial award application deadline: 3/15.
Website: http://www.tnstate.edu/health_sciences/

Texas A&M University, College of Medicine, Bryan, TX 77807. Offers education for healthcare professionals (MS); medical sciences (PhD); medicine (MD). *Accreditation:* LCME/AMA. *Faculty:* 113. *Students:* 897 full-time (426 women), 19 part-time (17 women); includes 413 minority (31 Black or African American, non-Hispanic/Latino; 4 American Indian or Alaska Native, non-Hispanic/Latino; 266 Asian, non-Hispanic/Latino; 103 Hispanic/Latino; 2 Native Hawaiian or other Pacific Islander, non-Hispanic/Latino; 7 Two or more races, non-Hispanic/Latino), 57 international. Average age 27. 258 applicants, 100% accepted, 220 enrolled. In 2015, 4 master's, 19 doctorates awarded. *Degree requirements:* For doctorate, comprehensive exam (for some programs); thesis/dissertation (for some programs), United States Medical Licensing Exam Steps 1 and 2 (for MD). *Entrance requirements:* For doctorate, GRE General Test (for PhD); MCAT (for MD), TMDSAS Application; letters of recommendation; official transcripts. *Application deadline:* For fall admission, 10/1 for domestic and international students. Application fee: $200. Electronic applications accepted. *Expenses:* Contact institution. *Financial support:* In 2015–16, 436 students received support, including 1 fellowship with tuition reimbursement available (averaging $1,000 per year), 108 research assistantships with tuition reimbursements available (averaging $8,949 per year), 1 teaching assistantship with tuition reimbursement available (averaging $8,167 per year); career-related internships or fieldwork, institutionally sponsored loans, scholarships/grants, traineeships, health care benefits, tuition waivers (full and partial), and unspecified assistantships also available. Support available to part-time students. Financial award applicants required to submit FAFSA. *Faculty research:* Cardiovascular medicine, fetal alcohol syndrome, molecular pathogenesis, near science membrane structure and biology. *Unit head:* Dr. Paul E. Ogden, MD, Interim Senior Vice President and Chief Operating Officer, 979-436-0202, Fax: 979-436-0092, E-mail: ogden@medicine.tamhsc.edu. *Application contact:* Filomeno G. Maldonado, Associate Dean of Admissions, 979-436-0231, Fax: 979-436-0097, E-mail: fgmaldonado@medicine.tamhsc.edu.
Website: http://medicine.tamhsc.edu/

Texas Christian University, Harris College of Nursing and Health Sciences, Fort Worth, TX 76129. Offers MHS, MS, MSN, MSW, DNP, DNP-A, Certificate. *Program availability:* Online learning. *Faculty:* 53 full-time (38 women), 6 part-time/adjunct (3 women). *Students:* 321 full-time (232 women), 50 part-time (47 women); includes 90 minority (13 Black or African American, non-Hispanic/Latino; 4 American Indian or Alaska Native, non-Hispanic/Latino; 28 Asian, non-Hispanic/Latino; 34 Hispanic/Latino; 1 Native Hawaiian or other Pacific Islander, non-Hispanic/Latino; 10 Two or more races, non-Hispanic/Latino), 2 international. Average age 32. 597 applicants, 31% accepted, 148 enrolled. In 2015, 81 master's, 58 doctorates awarded. Application fee: $60. Electronic applications accepted. *Expenses: Tuition, area resident:* Full-time $26,640; part-time $1480 per credit hour. *Required fees:* $48; $48 per unit. Tuition and fees vary according to program. *Financial support:* Applicants required to submit FAFSA. *Unit head:* Dr. Susan Weeks, Dean, 817-257-6749, E-mail: s.weeks@tcu.edu.
Website: http://www.harriscollege.tcu.edu/

Texas State University, The Graduate College, College of Health Professions, San Marcos, TX 78666. Offers MA, MHA, MHIHIM, MS, MSCD, DPT. *Program availability:* Part-time, evening/weekend. *Faculty:* 50 full-time (35 women), 18 part-time/adjunct (10 women). *Students:* 311 full-time (233 women), 24 part-time (19 women); includes 136 minority (35 Black or African American, non-Hispanic/Latino; 2 American Indian or Alaska Native, non-Hispanic/Latino; 17 Asian, non-Hispanic/Latino; 76 Hispanic/Latino; 6 Two or more races, non-Hispanic/Latino), 17 international. Average age 28. 663 applicants, 24% accepted, 106 enrolled. In 2015, 85 master's awarded. *Degree requirements:* For master's, comprehensive exam. *Entrance requirements:* For master's, GRE General Test (for some programs), baccalaureate degree from regionally-accredited institution; for doctorate, GRE (preferred minimum score of 295 with no less than 150 on the verbal and 145 on the quantitative), baccalaureate degree from regionally-accredited institution in physical therapy with minimum GPA of 3.0 on last 60 hours of undergraduate work. Additional exam requirements/recommendations for international students: Required—TOEFL (minimum score 550 paper-based; 78 iBT). *Application deadline:* For fall admission, 2/1 priority date for domestic and international students; for spring admission, 10/1 for domestic and international students.

Applications are processed on a rolling basis. Application fee: $40 ($90 for international students). Electronic applications accepted. *Expenses:* $3,615 in-state tuition (for 12 semester credit hours/1 full-time semester); $974 in-state fees. *Financial support:* In 2015–16, 184 students received support, including 3 research assistantships (averaging $10,928 per year), 45 teaching assistantships (averaging $8,461 per year); fellowships, career-related internships or fieldwork, Federal Work-Study, institutionally sponsored loans, scholarships/grants, unspecified assistantships, and stipends also available. Support available to part-time students. Financial award application deadline: 3/1; financial award applicants required to submit FAFSA. *Faculty research:* Microbiology and immunology, exploring balance and sleep function with mild traumatic brain injury, combined NMES and SS therapy for stroke patients, exploring affordable innovation to stimulate higher order learning in radiation, nursing and allied health. *Total annual research expenditures:* $130,364. *Unit head:* Dr. Ruth Welborn, Dean, 512-245-3300, Fax: 512-245-3791, E-mail: mw01@txstate.edu. *Application contact:* Dr. Andrea Golato, Dean of Graduate School, 512-245-2581, Fax: 512-245-8365, E-mail: gradcollege@txstate.edu.
Website: http://www.health.txstate.edu/

Texas Woman's University, Graduate School, College of Health Sciences, Denton, TX 76204-5527. Offers MA, MHA, MOT, MS, DPT, OTD, PhD. *Program availability:* Part-time, evening/weekend, online learning. *Faculty:* 96 full-time (72 women), 28 part-time/adjunct (24 women). *Students:* 1,030 full-time (912 women), 499 part-time (410 women); includes 523 minority (127 Black or African American, non-Hispanic/Latino; 4 American Indian or Alaska Native, non-Hispanic/Latino; 139 Asian, non-Hispanic/Latino; 219 Hispanic/Latino; 34 Two or more races, non-Hispanic/Latino), 53 international. Average age 34. 1,629 applicants, 28% accepted, 332 enrolled. In 2015, 407 master's, 115 doctorates awarded. Terminal master's awarded for partial completion of doctoral program. *Degree requirements:* For master's, comprehensive exam (for some programs), thesis (for some programs); for doctorate, comprehensive exam, thesis/dissertation, qualifying exam. *Entrance requirements:* For master's and doctorate, minimum GPA of 3.0. Additional exam requirements/recommendations for international students: Required—TOEFL (minimum score 550 paper-based; 79 iBT). *Application deadline:* For fall admission, 7/1 priority date for domestic students, 3/1 for international students; for spring admission, 12/1 priority date for domestic students, 7/1 for international students. Applications are processed on a rolling basis. Application fee: $50 ($75 for international students). Electronic applications accepted. *Expenses:* Tuition, state resident: full-time $4380; part-time $243 per credit hour. Tuition, nonresident: full-time $11,400; part-time $633 per credit hour. International tuition: $11,465 full-time. *Required fees:* $1778; $99 per credit hour. $283 per semester. One-time fee: $50. Tuition and fees vary according to course load and program. *Financial support:* In 2015–16, 747 students received support, including 59 research assistantships (averaging $11,499 per year), 15 teaching assistantships (averaging $11,499 per year); career-related internships or fieldwork, Federal Work-Study, institutionally sponsored loans, scholarships/grants, traineeships, health care benefits, and unspecified assistantships also available. Support available to part-time students. Financial award application deadline: 3/1; financial award applicants required to submit FAFSA. *Total annual research expenditures:* $690,244. *Unit head:* Ron Hovis, Interim Dean, 940-898-2852, Fax: 940-898-2853, E-mail: rhovis@twu.edu. *Application contact:* Dr. Samuel Wheeler, Assistant Director of Admissions, 940-898-3188, Fax: 940-898-3081, E-mail: wheelersr@twu.edu.
Website: http://www.twu.edu/college-health-sciences/

Towson University, Program in Health Science, Towson, MD 21252-0001. Offers MS. *Program availability:* Part-time, evening/weekend. *Students:* 10 full-time (8 women), 65 part-time (50 women); includes 33 minority (27 Black or African American, non-Hispanic/Latino; 3 Asian, non-Hispanic/Latino; 2 Hispanic/Latino; 1 Two or more races, non-Hispanic/Latino), 2 international. *Degree requirements:* For master's, thesis optional. *Entrance requirements:* For master's, undergraduate degree in a health science field or substantial upper-division course work in those fields, or experience in those same areas; minimum B grade in previous statistics course; minimum GPA of 3.0. *Application deadline:* Applications are processed on a rolling basis. Application fee: $45. Electronic applications accepted. *Expenses:* Tuition, state resident: full-time $7440; part-time $372 per unit. Tuition, nonresident: full-time $15,400; part-time $770 per unit. *Required fees:* $2360; $118 per year. $354 per term. *Financial support:* Application deadline: 4/1. *Unit head:* Dr. Susan Radius, Graduate Program Director, 410-704-4216, E-mail: sradius@towson.edu. *Application contact:* Alicia Arkell-Kleis, University Admissions, 410-704-2113, Fax: 410-704-3030, E-mail: grads@towson.edu.
Website: http://grad.towson.edu/program/master/hlth-ms/

University at Buffalo, the State University of New York, Graduate School, School of Public Health and Health Professions, Buffalo, NY 14260. Offers MA, MPH, MS, DPT, PhD, Advanced Certificate, Certificate. *Program availability:* Part-time. *Faculty:* 60 full-time (27 women), 12 part-time/adjunct (5 women). *Students:* 470 full-time (301 women), 50 part-time (32 women); includes 57 minority (13 Black or African American, non-Hispanic/Latino; 43 Asian, non-Hispanic/Latino; 1 Hispanic/Latino), 88 international. Average age 26. 775 applicants, 54% accepted, 253 enrolled. In 2015, 1,126 master's, 49 doctorates, 20 other advanced degrees awarded. Terminal master's awarded for partial completion of doctoral program. *Degree requirements:* For master's, comprehensive exam (for some programs), thesis (for some programs); for doctorate, comprehensive exam, thesis/dissertation. *Entrance requirements:* For master's and doctorate, GRE General Test. Additional exam requirements/recommendations for international students: Required—TOEFL (minimum score 79 iBT). *Application deadline:* For fall admission, 2/1 priority date for domestic and international students. Application fee: $50. Electronic applications accepted. *Financial support:* In 2015–16, 47 students received support, including 8 fellowships with full tuition reimbursements available (averaging $2,500 per year), 15 research assistantships with full tuition reimbursements available (averaging $15,000 per year), 16 teaching assistantships with full tuition reimbursements available (averaging $8,500 per year); career-related internships or fieldwork, Federal Work-Study, institutionally sponsored loans, scholarships/grants, tuition waivers (full and partial), and unspecified assistantships also available. Financial award application deadline: 3/15; financial award applicants required to submit FAFSA. *Faculty research:* Public health, epidemiology, rehabilitation, assistive technology, exercise and nutrition science. *Total annual research expenditures:* $6 million. *Unit head:* Dr. Lynn Kozlowski, Dean, 716-829-6951, Fax: 716-829-6040, E-mail: lk22@buffalo.edu.
Website: http://sphhp.buffalo.edu/

The University of Alabama at Birmingham, School of Health Professions, Birmingham, AL 35294. Offers MS, MSHA, MSHI, MSPAS, D Sc, DPT, PhD, Certificate. *Accreditation:* AANA/CANAEP (one or more programs are accredited); APTA (one or more programs are accredited); CAHME (one or more programs are accredited). *Program availability:* Part-time, online learning. *Degree requirements:* For doctorate, thesis/dissertation. Electronic applications accepted. *Expenses:* Contact institution.

University of Detroit Mercy, College of Health Professions, Detroit, MI 48221. Offers clinical nurse leader (MSN); family nurse practitioner (MSN); health services administration (MHSA); health systems management (MSN); nurse anesthesia (MS); nursing (DNP); nursing education (MSN, Certificate); nursing leadership and financial

management (Certificate); outcomes performance management (Certificate); physician assistant (MS). *Entrance requirements:* For master's, GRE General Test, minimum GPA of 3.0. *Application fee:* $30 ($50 for international students). *Expenses: Tuition, area resident:* Full-time $26,802; part-time $1489 per credit. Tuition and fees vary according to course load and program. *Financial support:* Institutionally sponsored loans and tuition waivers (partial) available. Support available to part-time students. Financial award applicants required to submit FAFSA. *Faculty research:* Research design, respiratory physiology, AIDS prevention, adolescent health, community, low income health education. *Unit head:* Dr. Christine M. Pacini, RN, Dean, 313-993-6055, Fax: 313-993-6175.
Website: http://healthprofessions.udmercy.edu/

University of Florida, Graduate School, College of Public Health and Health Professions, Gainesville, FL 32611. Offers MA, MHA, MHS, MHS, MOT, MPH, MS, Au D, DPT, PhD, Certificate, DPT/MPH, DVM/MPH, JD/MPH, MBA/MHA, MD/MPH, PhD/MPH, Pharm D/MPH. *Accreditation:* CAHME (one or more programs are accredited). *Program availability:* Part-time. *Faculty:* 124 full-time (48 women), 78 part-time/adjunct (46 women). *Students:* 644 full-time (493 women), 142 part-time (106 women); includes 180 minority (62 Black or African American, non-Hispanic/Latino; 3 American Indian or Alaska Native, non-Hispanic/Latino; 50 Asian, non-Hispanic/Latino; 65 Hispanic/Latino), 121 international. Average age 29. 1,615 applicants, 26% accepted, 196 enrolled. In 2015, 186 master's, 89 doctorates, 52 other advanced degrees awarded. Terminal master's awarded for partial completion of doctoral program. *Degree requirements:* For master's, thesis (for some programs); for doctorate, comprehensive exam, thesis/dissertation. *Entrance requirements:* For master's and doctorate, GRE General Test, minimum GPA of 3.0. Additional exam requirements/recommendations for international students: Required—TOEFL (minimum score 550 paper-based; 80 iBT), IELTS (minimum score 6). *Application deadline:* Applications are processed on a rolling basis. *Application fee:* $30. Electronic applications accepted. *Financial support:* Career-related internships or fieldwork, Federal Work-Study, institutionally sponsored loans, and unspecified assistantships available. Support available to part-time students. Financial award applicants required to submit FAFSA. *Unit head:* Dr. Michael G. Perri, Dean, 352-273-6214, Fax: 352-273-6199, E-mail: mperri@phhp.ufl.edu. *Application contact:* Office of Admissions, 352-392-1365, E-mail: webrequests@admissions.ufl.edu.
Website: http://www.phhp.ufl.edu/

University of Illinois at Chicago, College of Applied Health Sciences, Chicago, IL 60607-7128. Offers MS, DPT, OTD, PhD, CAS, Certificate. *Accreditation:* AOTA. *Program availability:* Part-time. *Faculty:* 95 full-time (58 women), 84 part-time/adjunct (54 women). *Students:* 488 full-time (371 women), 578 part-time (409 women); includes 343 minority (112 Black or African American, non-Hispanic/Latino; 132 Asian, non-Hispanic/Latino; 69 Hispanic/Latino; 2 Native Hawaiian or other Pacific Islander, non-Hispanic/Latino; 28 Two or more races, non-Hispanic/Latino), 57 international. Average age 34. 2,328 applicants, 39% accepted, 425 enrolled. In 2015, 198 master's, 66 doctorates, 40 other advanced degrees awarded. *Degree requirements:* For doctorate, thesis/dissertation. *Entrance requirements:* For master's, GRE General Test, minimum GPA of 2.75. Additional exam requirements/recommendations for international students: Required—TOEFL. *Application deadline:* For fall admission, 3/15 for domestic students, 2/15 for international students; for spring admission, 11/1 for domestic students. Applications are processed on a rolling basis. *Application fee:* $60. Electronic applications accepted. *Expenses:* Contact institution. *Financial support:* In 2015–16, 2 fellowships with full tuition reimbursements were awarded; research assistantships with full tuition reimbursements, teaching assistantships with full tuition reimbursements, career-related internships or fieldwork, Federal Work-Study, institutionally sponsored loans, traineeships, tuition waivers (full and partial), and unspecified assistantships also available. Financial award application deadline: 3/1; financial award applicants required to submit FAFSA. *Faculty research:* The impact of cultural competence training on service providers, interventions to improve the functional skills and independent living capacity of those with long term disabilities and conditions; fall prevention in the elderly and veterans with ambulatory prosthetics; helping people with chronic conditions manage their disease and prevent secondary conditions. *Unit head:* Prof. Bo Fernhall, Dean, 312-996-6695, Fax: 312-413-0086, E-mail: fernhall@uic.edu. *Application contact:* Receptionist, 312-413-2550, E-mail: gradcoll@uic.edu.
Website: http://www.ahs.uic.edu/

The University of Kansas, University of Kansas Medical Center, School of Health Professions, Kansas City, KS 66160. Offers MOT, MS, Au D, DNAP, DPT, OTD, PhD, SLPD, Graduate Certificate. *Faculty:* 107. *Students:* 396 full-time (281 women), 52 part-time (47 women); includes 48 minority (9 Black or African American, non-Hispanic/Latino; 3 American Indian or Alaska Native, non-Hispanic/Latino; 7 Asian, non-Hispanic/Latino; 15 Hispanic/Latino; 14 Two or more races, non-Hispanic/Latino), 26 international. Average age 27. In 2015, 58 master's, 76 doctorates, 21 other advanced degrees awarded. *Total annual research expenditures:* $3.4 million. *Unit head:* Dr. Abiodun Akinwuntan, Dean, 913-588-5235, Fax: 913-588-5254, E-mail: aakinwuntan@kumc.edu.
Website: http://www.kumc.edu/school-of-health-professions.html

University of Kentucky, Graduate School, College of Health Sciences, Lexington, KY 40506-0032. Offers MHA, MS, MSCD, MSHP, MSNS, MSPAS, MSPT, MSRMP, DS, PhD. *Program availability:* Part-time. *Degree requirements:* For master's, comprehensive exam, thesis (for some programs). *Entrance requirements:* For master's, GRE General Test, minimum undergraduate GPA of 2.75; for doctorate, GRE General Test, minimum undergraduate GPA of 3.0. Additional exam requirements/recommendations for international students: Required—TOEFL (minimum score 550 paper-based). Electronic applications accepted.

University of Massachusetts Lowell, College of Health Sciences, Lowell, MA 01854. Offers MS, DNP, DPT, PhD. *Accreditation:* APTA (one or more programs are accredited). *Program availability:* Part-time. *Degree requirements:* For master's, thesis optional; for doctorate, thesis/dissertation. *Entrance requirements:* For master's and doctorate, GRE General Test. *Application deadline:* Applications are processed on a rolling basis. *Application fee:* $20 ($35 for international students). *Expenses:* Tuition, state resident: full-time $14,304. Tuition, nonresident: full-time $25,853. *Required fees:* $375. Full-time tuition and fees vary according to campus/location and reciprocity agreements. *Financial support:* Fellowships with tuition reimbursements, research assistantships with full tuition reimbursements, teaching assistantships with full tuition reimbursements, career-related internships or fieldwork, Federal Work-Study, institutionally sponsored loans, scholarships/grants, and traineeships available. Support available to part-time students.
Website: http://www.uml.edu/Health-Sciences/

University of Mississippi Medical Center, School of Health Related Professions, Jackson, MS 39216-4505. Offers MOT, MPT. *Accreditation:* AOTA; NAACLS. *Program availability:* Part-time.

University of Nebraska Medical Center, School of Allied Health Professions, Omaha, NE 68198-4000. Offers MPAS, MPS, DPT, Certificate. *Accreditation:* APTA (one or more programs are accredited). *Entrance requirements:* For master's and doctorate, GRE. Additional exam requirements/recommendations for international students:

Required—TOEFL. *Expenses:* Tuition, state resident: full-time $7830; part-time $3915 per credit hour. Tuition, nonresident: full-time $22,410; part-time $11,205 per credit hour. *Required fees:* $521.

University of Nevada, Las Vegas, Graduate College, School of Allied Health Sciences, Las Vegas, NV 89154-3018. Offers MS, DMP, DPT, PhD, Advanced Certificate. *Program availability:* Part-time. *Faculty:* 22 full-time (7 women), 3 part-time/adjunct (all women). *Students:* 156 full-time (73 women), 19 part-time (4 women); includes 47 minority (2 Black or African American, non-Hispanic/Latino; 16 Asian, non-Hispanic/Latino; 14 Hispanic/Latino; 1 Native Hawaiian or other Pacific Islander, non-Hispanic/Latino; 14 Two or more races, non-Hispanic/Latino), 6 international. Average age 28. 52 applicants, 69% accepted, 21 enrolled. In 2015, 26 master's, 29 doctorates awarded. *Degree requirements:* For master's, thesis (for some programs); for doctorate, comprehensive exam (for some programs), thesis/dissertation. *Entrance requirements:* Additional exam requirements/recommendations for international students: Required—TOEFL (minimum score 550 paper-based; 80 iBT), IELTS (minimum score 7). *Application deadline:* For fall admission, 5/1 for international students; for spring admission, 10/1 for international students. *Application fee:* $60 ($95 for international students). Electronic applications accepted. *Expenses:* $264 per credit state resident full-time; $6,955 per semester; $264 per credit nonresident full-time; $555 per credit nonresident part-time. *Financial support:* In 2015–16, 43 students received support, including 21 research assistantships with partial tuition reimbursements available (averaging $12,190 per year), 22 teaching assistantships with partial tuition reimbursements available (averaging $10,909 per year); institutionally sponsored loans, scholarships/grants, health care benefits, and unspecified assistantships also available. Financial award application deadline: 3/1. *Total annual research expenditures:* $4.2 million. *Unit head:* Dr. Ronald T. Brown, Dean, 702-895-5307, Fax: 702-895-5050. *Application contact:* Graduate College Admissions Evaluator, 702-895-3367, Fax: 702-895-4180, E-mail: gradadmissions@unlv.edu.
Website: http://healthsciences.unlv.edu/

University of New Mexico, Graduate Studies, Health Sciences Center, Albuquerque, NM 87131-2039. Offers MOT, MPH, MPT, MS, MSN, DNP, DPT, MD, PhD, Pharm D, Certificate, MSN/MA. *Students:* 180 full-time (124 women), 88 part-time (61 women); includes 112 minority (7 Black or African American, non-Hispanic/Latino; 7 American Indian or Alaska Native, non-Hispanic/Latino; 12 Asian, non-Hispanic/Latino; 82 Hispanic/Latino; 2 Native Hawaiian or other Pacific Islander, non-Hispanic/Latino; 2 Two or more races, non-Hispanic/Latino), 21 international. Average age 30. *Unit head:* Dr. R. Philip Eaton, Interim Vice President. *Application contact:* Deborah Kieltyka, Associate Director, Admissions, 505-277-3140, Fax: 505-277-6686, E-mail: deborahk@unm.edu.

The University of North Carolina at Chapel Hill, School of Medicine and Graduate School, Graduate Programs in Medicine, Department of Allied Health Sciences, Chapel Hill, NC 27599. Offers human movement science (PhD); occupational science (MS, PhD), including occupational science; physical therapy (DPT), including physical therapy - off campus; physical therapy - on campus; rehabilitation counseling and psychology (MS); speech and hearing sciences (MS, Au D, PhD), including audiology (Au D), speech and hearing sciences (MS, PhD). *Accreditation:* APTA (one or more programs are accredited). *Program availability:* Online learning. *Entrance requirements:* For master's, GRE General Test; for doctorate, GRE General Test, minimum GPA of 3.0. Additional exam requirements/recommendations for international students: Required—TOEFL (minimum score 550 paper-based), TWE. Electronic applications accepted.

University of Northern Iowa, Graduate College, College of Education, Ed D Program in Education, Cedar Falls, IA 50614. Offers allied health, recreation, and community services (Ed D); curriculum and instruction (Ed D); educational leadership (Ed D). *Program availability:* Part-time, evening/weekend. *Students:* 21 full-time (16 women), 67 part-time (44 women); includes 6 minority (all Black or African American, non-Hispanic/Latino), 19 international. 31 applicants, 45% accepted, 12 enrolled. In 2015, 12 doctorates awarded. *Degree requirements:* For doctorate, thesis/dissertation. *Entrance requirements:* For doctorate, GRE, minimum GPA of 3.0, master's degree. Additional exam requirements/recommendations for international students: Required—TOEFL (minimum score 500 paper-based; 61 iBT). *Application deadline:* For fall admission, 8/1 priority date for domestic students. Applications are processed on a rolling basis. *Application fee:* $50 ($70 for international students). *Financial support:* Career-related internships or fieldwork, Federal Work-Study, and tuition waivers (full and partial) available. Support available to part-time students. Financial award application deadline: 2/1. *Unit head:* Dr. Linda Fitzgerald, Coordinator, 319-273-2214, Fax: 319-273-5886, E-mail: linda.fitzgerald@uni.edu. *Application contact:* Laurie S. Russell, Record Analyst, 319-273-2623, Fax: 319-273-2885, E-mail: laurie.russell@uni.edu.
Website: http://www.uni.edu/coe/graduate/EdDProgram/

University of Northern Iowa, Graduate College, College of Education, School of Kinesiology, Allied Health and Human Services, Cedar Falls, IA 50614. Offers athletic training (MS); health education (MA), including community health education, health promotion/fitness management, school health education; leisure, youth and human services (MA); physical education (MA), including kinesiology, teaching/coaching. *Program availability:* Part-time, evening/weekend. *Students:* 62 full-time (33 women), 45 part-time (27 women); includes 17 minority (12 Black or African American, non-Hispanic/Latino; 3 Hispanic/Latino; 2 Two or more races, non-Hispanic/Latino), 10 international. 83 applicants, 48% accepted, 30 enrolled. In 2015, 37 master's awarded. *Degree requirements:* For master's, comprehensive exam, thesis or alternative. *Entrance requirements:* For master's, minimum GPA of 3.0. Additional exam requirements/recommendations for international students: Required—TOEFL (minimum score 500 paper-based; 61 iBT). *Application deadline:* Applications are processed on a rolling basis. *Application fee:* $50 ($70 for international students). *Financial support:* Career-related internships or fieldwork, Federal Work-Study, institutionally sponsored loans, scholarships/grants, tuition waivers (full and partial), and unspecified assistantships available. Support available to part-time students. Financial award application deadline: 2/1. *Unit head:* Dr. Doris Corbett, Director, 319-273-2141, Fax: 319-273-5958, E-mail: doris.corbett@uni.edu. *Application contact:* Laurie S. Russell, Record Analyst, 319-273-2623, Fax: 319-273-2885, E-mail: laurie.russell@uni.edu.
Website: http://www.uni.edu/coe/departments/school-health-physical-education-leisure-services

University of North Florida, Brooks College of Health, Jacksonville, FL 32224. Offers MHA, MPH, MS, MSH, MSN, DNP, DPT, Certificate. *Program availability:* Part-time, evening/weekend. *Faculty:* 63 full-time (47 women), 15 part-time/adjunct (10 women). *Students:* 378 full-time (273 women), 195 part-time (150 women); includes 153 minority (54 Black or African American, non-Hispanic/Latino; 1 American Indian or Alaska Native, non-Hispanic/Latino; 28 Asian, non-Hispanic/Latino; 45 Hispanic/Latino; 1 Native Hawaiian or other Pacific Islander, non-Hispanic/Latino; 24 Two or more races, non-Hispanic/Latino), 13 international. Average age 32. 304 applicants, 46% accepted, 98 enrolled. In 2015, 137 master's, 36 doctorates awarded. *Entrance requirements:* For master's, GRE General Test, minimum GPA of 3.0 in last 60 hours. Additional exam requirements/recommendations for international students: Required—TOEFL (minimum score 500 paper-based; 61 iBT). *Application deadline:* For fall admission, 7/1 for domestic students, 5/1 for international students; for spring admission, 11/1 priority date for domestic students, 10/1 for international students. Applications are

processed on a rolling basis. Application fee: $30. Electronic applications accepted. *Expenses:* Contact institution. *Financial support:* In 2015–16, 112 students received support, including 24 research assistantships (averaging $1,505 per year), 2 teaching assistantships (averaging $1,939 per year); career-related internships or fieldwork, Federal Work-Study, scholarships/grants, and tuition waivers (partial) also available. Support available to part-time students. Financial award application deadline: 4/1; financial award applicants required to submit FAFSA. *Faculty research:* Adolescent substance abuse, detection of bacterial agents, spirituality and health, non-vitamin and non-mineral supplements, analyzing ticks and their ability to transfer diseases to humans. *Total annual research expenditures:* $226,339. *Unit head:* Dr. Pamela Chally, Dean, 904-620-2810, Fax: 904-620-1030, E-mail: pchally@unf.edu. *Application contact:* Dr. Heather Kenney, Director of Advising, 904-620-2810, Fax: 904-620-1030, E-mail: heather.kenney@unf.edu.
Website: http://www.unf.edu/brooks

University of Oklahoma Health Sciences Center, Graduate College, College of Allied Health, Oklahoma City, OK 73190. Offers MOT, MPT, MS, Au D, PhD, Certificate. *Accreditation:* AOTA; APTA. *Program availability:* Part-time. Terminal master's awarded for partial completion of doctoral program. *Degree requirements:* For master's, comprehensive exam, thesis optional; for doctorate, one foreign language, comprehensive exam, thesis/dissertation. *Entrance requirements:* For master's and doctorate, GRE General Test, 3 letters of recommendation. Additional exam requirements/recommendations for international students: Required—TOEFL.

University of Phoenix–Las Vegas Campus, College of Human Services, Las Vegas, NV 89135. Offers marriage, family, and child therapy (MSC); mental health counseling (MSC); school counseling (MSC). *Program availability:* Online learning. *Entrance requirements:* For master's, minimum undergraduate GPA of 2.5, 3 years of work experience. Additional exam requirements/recommendations for international students: Required—TOEFL (minimum score 550 paper-based; 79 iBT). Electronic applications accepted.

University of Puerto Rico, Medical Sciences Campus, School of Health Professions, San Juan, PR 00936-5067. Offers MS, Au D, Certificate. *Degree requirements:* For master's, one foreign language, thesis (for some programs). *Entrance requirements:* For master's, GRE or EXADEP, interview; for doctorate, EXADEP; for Certificate, Allied Health Professions Admissions Test, minimum GPA of 2.5, interview. Electronic applications accepted. *Faculty research:* Infantile autism, aphasia, language problems, toxicology, immunohematology, medical record documentation and quality.

University of South Alabama, Pat Capps Covey College of Allied Health Professions, Mobile, AL 36688. Offers MHS, MS, Au D, DPT, PhD. *Faculty:* 31 full-time (22 women), 10 part-time/adjunct (7 women). *Students:* 365 full-time (283 women), 2 part-time (both women); includes 19 minority (9 Black or African American, non-Hispanic/Latino; 2 American Indian or Alaska Native, non-Hispanic/Latino; 4 Asian, non-Hispanic/Latino; 3 Hispanic/Latino; 1 Native Hawaiian or other Pacific Islander, non-Hispanic/Latino), 1 international. Average age 25. 653 applicants, 40% accepted, 94 enrolled. In 2015, 88 master's, 43 doctorates awarded. *Degree requirements:* For master's, thesis optional, externship; for doctorate, thesis/dissertation, clinical internship. *Entrance requirements:* For master's, GRE General Test; for doctorate, GRE, minimum GPA of 3.0. Additional exam requirements/recommendations for international students: Required—TOEFL (minimum score 600 paper-based). *Application deadline:* For fall admission, 7/15 priority date for domestic students, 6/15 priority date for international students; for spring admission, 12/1 priority date for domestic students, 11/1 priority date for international students. Applications are processed on a rolling basis. Application fee: $35. Electronic applications accepted. *Expenses:* Contact institution. *Financial support:* Fellowships, research assistantships, teaching assistantships, career-related internships or fieldwork, Federal Work-Study, institutionally sponsored loans, scholarships/grants, and unspecified assistantships available. Support available to part-time students. Financial award application deadline: 5/31; financial award applicants required to submit FAFSA. *Unit head:* Dr. Gregory Frazer, Dean, College of Allied Health, 251-445-9250, Fax: 251-445-9259, E-mail: gfrazer@southalabama.edu. *Application contact:* Dr. Susan Gordon-Hickey, Associate Dean, College of Allied Health, 251-445-9250, Fax: 251-445-9259, E-mail: gordonhickey@southalabama.edu.
Website: http://www.southalabama.edu/colleges/alliedhealth/index.html

The University of South Dakota, Graduate School, School of Health Sciences, Vermillion, SD 57069-2390. Offers MA, MPH, MS, MSW, DPT, OTD, PhD, TDPT, Graduate Certificate. *Program availability:* Part-time. *Entrance requirements:* For master's, GRE General Test, GRE Subject Test. Application fee: $35. *Financial support:* Research assistantships, teaching assistantships, career-related internships or fieldwork, Federal Work-Study, scholarships/grants, traineeships, and unspecified assistantships available. *Faculty research:* Occupational therapy, physical therapy, vision, pediatrics, geriatrics. *Unit head:* Dr. Michael Lawler, Dean, 605-677-5000, E-mail: michael.lawler@usd.edu. *Application contact:* Graduate School, 605-658-6140, E-mail: cde@usd.edu.
Website: http://www.usd.edu/health-sciences

The University of Tennessee Health Science Center, College of Graduate Health Sciences, Memphis, TN 38163-0002. Offers biomedical engineering (MS, PhD); biomedical sciences (PhD); dental sciences (MDS); epidemiology (MS); health outcomes and policy research (PhD); laboratory research and management (MS); nursing science (PhD); pharmaceutical sciences (PhD); pharmacology (MS); speech and hearing science (PhD); DDS/PhD; DNP/PhD; MD/PhD; Pharm D/PhD. Terminal master's awarded for partial completion of doctoral program. *Degree requirements:* For master's, comprehensive exam, thesis; for doctorate, comprehensive exam, thesis/dissertation, oral and written preliminary and comprehensive exams. *Entrance requirements:* For master's and doctorate, GRE General Test, minimum GPA of 3.0. Additional exam requirements/recommendations for international students: Required—TOEFL (minimum score 79 iBT); Recommended—IELTS (minimum score 6.5). Electronic applications accepted.

The University of Tennessee Health Science Center, College of Health Professions, Memphis, TN 38163-0002. Offers audiology (MS, Au D); clinical laboratory science (MSCLS); cytopathology practice (MCP); health informatics and information management (MHIIM); occupational therapy (MOT); physical therapy (DPT, ScDPT); physician assistant (MMS); speech-language pathology (MS). *Accreditation:* AOTA; APTA. *Program availability:* Part-time, evening/weekend, online learning. Terminal master's awarded for partial completion of doctoral program. *Degree requirements:* For master's, comprehensive exam, thesis; for doctorate, comprehensive exam, residency. *Entrance requirements:* For master's, GRE (MOT, MSCLS), minimum GPA of 3.0, 3 letters of reference, national accreditation (MSCLS), GRE if GPA is less than 3.0 (MCP); for doctorate, GRE. Additional exam requirements/recommendations for international students: Required—TOEFL (minimum score 550 paper-based; 80 iBT). Electronic applications accepted. *Expenses:* Contact institution. *Faculty research:* Gait deviation, muscular dystrophy and strength, hemophilia and exercise, pediatric neurology, self-efficacy.

The University of Texas at El Paso, Graduate School, College of Health Sciences, Program in Interdisciplinary Health Sciences, El Paso, TX 79968-0001. Offers PhD. *Degree requirements:* For doctorate, thesis/dissertation. *Entrance requirements:* For doctorate, GRE, three letters of reference, relevant personal/professional experience, evidence of a master's degree (MS or MA) or other terminal degree, official transcripts. Additional exam requirements/recommendations for international students: Required—TOEFL (minimum score 550 paper-based); Recommended—IELTS. Electronic applications accepted.

The University of Texas Medical Branch, School of Health Professions, Galveston, TX 77555. Offers MOT, MPAS, MPT, DPT. *Degree requirements:* For master's, thesis or alternative; for doctorate, thesis/dissertation or alternative. *Entrance requirements:* For master's, GRE, experience in field, minimum GPA of 3.0; for doctorate, GRE, documentation of 40 hours experience. Additional exam requirements/recommendations for international students: Required—TOEFL (minimum score 550 paper-based). Electronic applications accepted.

University of Vermont, Graduate College, College of Nursing and Health Sciences, Burlington, VT 05405. Offers MS, DNP, DPT. *Degree requirements:* For master's, thesis. *Entrance requirements:* For master's and doctorate, GRE General Test. Additional exam requirements/recommendations for international students: Required—TOEFL (minimum score 550 paper-based; 80 iBT). *Application deadline:* For fall admission, 4/1 priority date for domestic students. Applications are processed on a rolling basis. Application fee: $65. Electronic applications accepted. *Financial support:* Fellowships, research assistantships, teaching assistantships, and Federal Work-Study available. Financial award application deadline: 3/1.

University of Wisconsin–Milwaukee, Graduate School, College of Health Sciences, Milwaukee, WI 53211. Offers MS, DPT, PhD, Certificate, Graduate Certificate. *Program availability:* Part-time. *Students:* 265 full-time (201 women), 44 part-time (26 women); includes 27 minority (2 Black or African American, non-Hispanic/Latino; 13 Asian, non-Hispanic/Latino; 1 Native Hawaiian or other Pacific Islander, non-Hispanic/Latino; 11 Two or more races, non-Hispanic/Latino), 26 international. Average age 28. 244 applicants, 40% accepted, 82 enrolled. In 2015, 85 master's, 24 doctorates, 5 other advanced degrees awarded. *Degree requirements:* For master's, thesis; for doctorate, comprehensive exam, thesis/dissertation. *Entrance requirements:* For doctorate, GRE General Test, master's degree. Additional exam requirements/recommendations for international students: Required—TOEFL (minimum score 600 paper-based), IELTS (minimum score 6.5). *Application deadline:* For fall admission, 1/1 priority date for domestic students; for spring admission, 9/1 for domestic students. Applications are processed on a rolling basis. Application fee: $56 ($96 for international students). *Expenses:* Contact institution. *Financial support:* Research assistantships, teaching assistantships, career-related internships or fieldwork, Federal Work-Study, and unspecified assistantships available. Support available to part-time students. Financial award application deadline: 3/30. *Unit head:* Paula M. Rhyner, PhD, Interim Dean, 414-229-4878, E-mail: prhyner@uwm.edu. *Application contact:* Roger O. Smith, General Information Contact, 414-229-6697, Fax: 414-229-6697, E-mail: smithro@uwm.edu.
Website: http://www4.uwm.edu/chs/

Virginia Commonwealth University, Graduate School, School of Allied Health Professions, Doctoral Program in Health Related Sciences, Richmond, VA 23284-9005. Offers clinical laboratory sciences (PhD); gerontology (PhD); health administration (PhD); nurse anesthesia (PhD); occupational therapy (PhD); physical therapy (PhD); radiation sciences (PhD); rehabilitation leadership (PhD). *Entrance requirements:* For doctorate, GRE General Test or MAT, minimum GPA of 3.3 in master's degree. Additional exam requirements/recommendations for international students: Required—TOEFL (minimum score 600 paper-based; 100 iBT); Recommended—IELTS (minimum score 6.5). Electronic applications accepted.

Western University of Health Sciences, College of Allied Health Professions, Pomona, CA 91766-1854. Offers MS, DPT. *Accreditation:* APTA (one or more programs are accredited). *Faculty:* 25 full-time (18 women), 4 part-time/adjunct (2 women). *Students:* 366 full-time (231 women), 52 part-time (35 women); includes 194 minority (17 Black or African American, non-Hispanic/Latino; 93 Asian, non-Hispanic/Latino; 61 Hispanic/Latino; 1 Native Hawaiian or other Pacific Islander, non-Hispanic/Latino; 22 Two or more races, non-Hispanic/Latino), 4 international. Average age 28. 3,580 applicants, 7% accepted, 180 enrolled. In 2015, 108 master's, 79 doctorates awarded. *Degree requirements:* For master's, thesis; for doctorate, comprehensive exam (for some programs). *Entrance requirements:* For master's, GRE, minimum GPA of 2.5, letters of recommendation; for doctorate, GRE, minimum GPA of 2.8, letters of recommendation, bachelor's degree. Additional exam requirements/recommendations for international students: Required—TOEFL. Electronic applications accepted. *Expenses:* $37,890 (DPT); $585 per unit (MSHS); $38,425 (MSPAS); $40 fees. *Financial support:* Scholarships/grants available. Financial award application deadline: 3/2; financial award applicants required to submit FAFSA. *Total annual research expenditures:* $148,180. *Unit head:* Dr. Stephanie Bowlin, Dean, 909-469-5390, Fax: 909-469-5438, E-mail: sbowlin@westernu.edu. *Application contact:* Karen Hutton-Lopez, Director of Admissions, 909-469-5335, Fax: 909-469-5570, E-mail: admissions@westernu.edu.
Website: http://www.westernu.edu/allied-health/

Wichita State University, Graduate School, College of Health Professions, Wichita, KS 67260. Offers MA, MPA, MSN, Au D, DNP, DPT, PhD. *Accreditation:* APTA (one or more programs are accredited). *Program availability:* Part-time. *Unit head:* Dr. Sandra C. Bibb, Dean, 316-978-3600, Fax: 316-978-3025, E-mail: sandra.bibb@wichita.edu. *Application contact:* Jordan Oleson, Admissions Coordinator, 316-978-3095, Fax: 316-978-3253, E-mail: jordan.oleson@wichita.edu.
Website: http://www.wichita.edu/chp

Anesthesiologist Assistant Studies

Case Western Reserve University, School of Medicine and School of Graduate Studies, Graduate Programs in Medicine, Department of Anesthesiology, Cleveland, OH 44106. Offers MS. *Accreditation:* AANA/CANAEP. *Degree requirements:* For master's, thesis. *Entrance requirements:* For master's, MCAT. Additional exam requirements/recommendations for international students: Required—TOEFL. Electronic applications accepted. *Expenses: Tuition, area resident:* Full-time $41,137; part-time $1714 per credit hour. *Required fees:* $32. Tuition and fees vary according to course load and program. *Faculty research:* Metabolism of bioamines, cerebral metabolism, cardiovascular hemodynamics, genetics.

Emory University, School of Medicine, Programs in Allied Health Professions, Anesthesiology Assistant Program, Atlanta, GA 30322. Offers MM Sc. *Entrance requirements:* For master's, GRE General Test, MCAT. Additional exam requirements/recommendations for international students: Required—TOEFL (minimum score 600 paper-based; 94 iBT). Electronic applications accepted. *Expenses:* Contact institution.

Nova Southeastern University, College of Health Care Sciences, Fort Lauderdale, FL 33314-7796. Offers anesthesiologist assistant (MSA); audiology (Au D); health science (MH Sc, DHSc, PhD); occupational therapy (MOT, Dr OT, PhD); physical therapy (DPT, TDPT); physician assistant (MMS). *Program availability:* Online learning. *Faculty:* 109 full-time (64 women), 100 part-time/adjunct (65 women). *Students:* 1,590 full-time (1,179 women), 969 part-time (819 women); includes 831 minority (234 Black or African American, non-Hispanic/Latino; 8 American Indian or Alaska Native, non-Hispanic/Latino; 151 Asian, non-Hispanic/Latino; 378 Hispanic/Latino; 1 Native Hawaiian or other Pacific Islander, non-Hispanic/Latino; 59 Two or more races, non-Hispanic/Latino), 18 international. Average age 30. 8,133 applicants, 14% accepted, 728 enrolled. In 2015, 556 master's, 105 doctorates awarded. *Degree requirements:* For master's, thesis; for doctorate, comprehensive exam, thesis/dissertation. *Entrance requirements:* For master's, GRE General Test, MCAT; for doctorate, GRE General Test, personal interview, essay. Additional exam requirements/recommendations for international students: Required—TOEFL (minimum score 600 paper-based). *Application deadline:* For winter admission, 4/15 for domestic students; for summer admission, 12/15 for domestic and international students. Applications are processed on a rolling basis. Application fee: $50. Electronic applications accepted. *Expenses:* Contact institution. *Financial support:* In 2015–16, 151 students received support, including 4 research assistantships (averaging $3,500 per year); institutionally sponsored loans and unspecified assistantships also available. Financial award application deadline: 4/15; financial award applicants required to submit FAFSA. *Unit head:* Dr. Stanley Wilson, Dean, 954-262-1203, E-mail: swilson@nova.edu. *Application contact:* Joey Jankie, Admissions Counselor, 954-262-7249, E-mail: joey@nova.edu.
Website: http://www.nova.edu/chcs/

Quinnipiac University, Frank H. Netter MD School of Medicine, Program for Anesthesiologist Assistant, Hamden, CT 06518-1940. Offers MMS. *Faculty:* 3 full-time (0 women), 2 part-time/adjunct (0 women). *Students:* 7 full-time (5 women); includes 4 minority (2 Black or African American, non-Hispanic/Latino; 2 Asian, non-Hispanic/Latino). Average age 26. 51 applicants, 8% accepted, 4 enrolled. *Degree requirements:* For master's, comprehensive exam. *Entrance requirements:* For master's, GRE or MCAT, bachelor's degree; official transcripts of all undergraduate and graduate course work; three letters of recommendation; essay; interview; criminal background check. Additional exam requirements/recommendations for international students: Required—TOEFL. *Application deadline:* For spring admission, 3/1 for domestic students; for summer admission, 1/15 for domestic students. Applications are processed on a rolling basis. Application fee: $45. Electronic applications accepted. *Expenses:* Contact institution. *Financial support:* Scholarships/grants available. Financial award application deadline: 6/1; financial award applicants required to submit FAFSA. *Unit head:* Dr. William Paulsen, Director, Anesthesiologist Assistant Program, 203-582-6502, E-mail: awpaulsen@quinnipiac.edu. *Application contact:* Victoria Pavasaris, Assistant Director of Operations, Anesthesiologist Assistant Program, 203-582-8726, E-mail: victoria.pavasaris@quinnipiac.edu.
Website: http://www.quinnipiac.edu/school-of-medicine/academics/anesthesiologist-assistant-program/

South University, Graduate Programs, College of Health Professions, Program in Anesthesiologist Assistant, Savannah, GA 31406. Offers MM Sc.

Université Laval, Faculty of Medicine, Post-Professional Programs in Medical Studies, Québec, QC G1K 7P4, Canada. Offers anatomy–pathology (DESS); anesthesiology (DESS); cardiology (DESS); care of older people (Diploma); clinical research (DESS); community health (DESS); dermatology (DESS); diagnostic radiology (DESS); emergency medicine (Diploma); family medicine (DESS); general surgery (DESS); geriatrics (DESS); hematology (DESS); internal medicine (DESS); maternal and fetal medicine (Diploma); medical biochemistry (DESS); medical microbiology and infectious diseases (DESS); medical oncology (DESS); nephrology (DESS); neurology (DESS); neurosurgery (DESS); obstetrics and gynecology (DESS); ophthalmology (DESS); orthopedic surgery (DESS); oto-rhino-laryngology (DESS); palliative medicine (Diploma); pediatrics (DESS); plastic surgery (DESS); psychiatry (DESS); pulmonary medicine (DESS); radiology–oncology (DESS); thoracic surgery (DESS); urology (DESS). *Degree requirements:* For other advanced degree, comprehensive exam. *Entrance requirements:* For degree, knowledge of French. Electronic applications accepted.

University of Colorado Denver, School of Medicine, Program in Anesthesiology, Aurora, CO 80045. Offers MS. *Students:* 26 full-time (10 women); includes 2 minority (1 Asian, non-Hispanic/Latino; 1 Two or more races, non-Hispanic/Latino). Average age 30. 83 applicants, 16% accepted, 13 enrolled. *Degree requirements:* For master's, seven-semester curriculum, including several rounds of anesthesiology clinical practice. *Entrance requirements:* For master's, GRE or MCAT, three letters of recommendation; curriculum vitae or resume; statement of purpose. Additional exam requirements/recommendations for international students: Required—TOEFL. *Financial support:* In 2015–16, 6 students received support. Career-related internships or fieldwork, Federal Work-Study, institutionally sponsored loans, scholarships/grants, and traineeships available. Financial award application deadline: 4/1; financial award applicants required to submit FAFSA. *Unit head:* Dr. Vesna Jevtovic-Todorovic, Professor and Chair, 720-848-6709, E-mail: vesna.jevtovic-todorovic@ucdenver.edu. *Application contact:* Carlos Rodriguez, Program Coordinator, 303-724-1764, E-mail: carlos.r.rodriguez@ucdenver.edu.
Website: http://www.ucdenver.edu/academics/colleges/medicalschool/departments/Anesthesiology/Pages/Anesthesiology.aspx

University of Guelph, Ontario Veterinary College and Graduate Studies, Graduate Programs in Veterinary Sciences, Department of Clinical Studies, Guelph, ON N1G 2W1, Canada. Offers anesthesia (M Sc, DV Sc); cardiology (DV Sc, Diploma); clinical studies (Diploma); dermatology (M Sc); diagnostic imaging (M Sc, DV Sc); emergency/critical care (M Sc, DV Sc, Diploma); medicine (M Sc, DV Sc); neurology (M Sc, DV Sc); ophthalmology (M Sc, DV Sc); surgery (M Sc, DV Sc). *Degree requirements:* For master's, thesis; for doctorate, comprehensive exam, thesis/dissertation. *Entrance requirements:* Additional exam requirements/recommendations for international students: Required—TOEFL (minimum score 550 paper-based), IELTS (minimum score 6.5). Electronic applications accepted. *Faculty research:* Orthopedics, respirology, oncology, exercise physiology, cardiology.

University of Missouri–Kansas City, School of Medicine, Kansas City, MO 64110-2499. Offers anesthesia (MS); bioinformatics (MS); health professions education (MS); medicine (MD); physician assistant (MMS); MD/PhD. *Accreditation:* LCME/AMA. *Faculty:* 41 full-time (15 women), 15 part-time/adjunct (7 women). *Students:* 483 full-time (255 women), 39 part-time (25 women); includes 254 minority (34 Black or African American, non-Hispanic/Latino; 3 American Indian or Alaska Native, non-Hispanic/Latino; 172 Asian, non-Hispanic/Latino; 16 Hispanic/Latino; 1 Native Hawaiian or other Pacific Islander, non-Hispanic/Latino; 28 Two or more races, non-Hispanic/Latino), 10 international. Average age 24. 1,004 applicants, 13% accepted, 104 enrolled. In 2015, 22 master's, 119 doctorates awarded. *Degree requirements:* For doctorate, one foreign language, United States Medical Licensing Exam Step 1 and 2. *Entrance requirements:* For doctorate, interview. *Application deadline:* For fall admission, 11/15 for domestic and international students. Application fee: $50. *Expenses:* Contact institution. *Financial support:* In 2015–16, 3 fellowships (averaging $38,566 per year), 4 research assistantships (averaging $13,200 per year) were awarded; career-related internships or fieldwork, Federal Work-Study, institutionally sponsored loans, scholarships/grants, and tuition waivers (partial) also available. Financial award application deadline: 3/1; financial award applicants required to submit FAFSA. *Faculty research:* Cardiovascular disease, women's and children's health, trauma and infectious diseases, neurological, metabolic disease. *Unit head:* Dr. Steven L. Kanter, MD, Dean, 816-235-1803, E-mail: kantersl@umkc.edu. *Application contact:* Janine Kluckhohn, Admissions Coordinator, 816-235-1870, Fax: 816-235-6579, E-mail: kluckhohnj@umkc.edu.
Website: http://www.med.umkc.edu/

Clinical Laboratory Sciences/Medical Technology

Albany College of Pharmacy and Health Sciences, School of Arts and Sciences, Albany, NY 12208. Offers clinical laboratory sciences (MS); cytotechnology and molecular cytology (MS); molecular biosciences (MS). *Degree requirements:* For master's, thesis. *Entrance requirements:* For master's, GRE, minimum GPA of 3.0. Additional exam requirements/recommendations for international students: Required—TOEFL (minimum score 84 iBT). Electronic applications accepted.

Austin Peay State University, College of Graduate Studies, College of Science and Mathematics, Department of Biology, Clarksville, TN 37044. Offers clinical laboratory science (MS). *Program availability:* Part-time. *Faculty:* 11 full-time (5 women). *Students:* 3 full-time (1 woman), 26 part-time (16 women); includes 4 minority (1 Black or African American, non-Hispanic/Latino; 3 Two or more races, non-Hispanic/Latino). Average age 26. 56 applicants, 27% accepted, 13 enrolled. In 2015, 9 master's awarded. *Degree requirements:* For master's, comprehensive exam, thesis optional. *Entrance requirements:* For master's, GRE General Test, 3 letters of recommendation, minimum undergraduate GPA of 2.75. Additional exam requirements/recommendations for international students: Required—TOEFL (minimum score 500 paper-based). *Application deadline:* For fall admission, 8/3 priority date for domestic students. Applications are processed on a rolling basis. Application fee: $25. Electronic applications accepted. *Expenses:* Tuition, state resident: full-time $8080; part-time $404 per credit hour. Tuition, nonresident: full-time $21,680; part-time 1084 per credit hour. *Required fees:* $1453; $72.65 per credit hour. *Financial support:* In 2015–16, research assistantships with full tuition reimbursements (averaging $5,184 per year) were awarded; career-related internships or fieldwork, Federal Work-Study, institutionally sponsored loans, scholarships/grants, and unspecified assistantships also available. Support available to part-time students. Financial award application deadline: 3/1; financial award applicants required to submit FAFSA. *Faculty research:* Molecular basis of microbial pathogenesis, avian ecology, aquatic toxicology, endocrinology, aquatic biology. *Unit head:* Dr. Don Dailey, Chair, 931-221-7781, Fax: 931-221-6323, E-mail: daileyd@apsu.edu. *Application contact:* June D. Lee, Graduate Coordinator, 800-859-4723, Fax: 931-221-7641, E-mail: gradadmissions@apsu.edu.
Website: http://www.apsu.edu/biology

Baylor College of Medicine, Graduate School of Biomedical Sciences, Program in Clinical Scientist Training, Houston, TX 77030-3498. Offers MS, PhD. Terminal master's awarded for partial completion of doctoral program. *Degree requirements:* For master's, thesis; for doctorate, thesis/dissertation, public defense. Electronic applications accepted. *Faculty research:* Cardiology, pulmonary, HIV, rheumatology, cancer.

The Catholic University of America, School of Arts and Sciences, Department of Biology, Washington, DC 20064. Offers biotechnology (MS); cell and microbial biology (MS, PhD), including cell biology; clinical laboratory science (MS, PhD); MSLS/MS. *Program availability:* Part-time. *Faculty:* 9 full-time (4 women), 7 part-time/adjunct (1 woman). *Students:* 29 full-time (18 women), 36 part-time (22 women); includes 8 minority (3 Black or African American, non-Hispanic/Latino; 2 Asian, non-Hispanic/Latino; 1 Hispanic/Latino; 2 Two or more races, non-Hispanic/Latino), 44 international. Average age 30. 68 applicants, 38% accepted, 13 enrolled. In 2015, 21 master's, 1

doctorate awarded. *Degree requirements:* For master's and doctorate, comprehensive exam. *Entrance requirements:* For master's and doctorate, GRE General Test, GRE Subject Test, statement of purpose, official copies of academic transcripts, three letters of recommendation. Additional exam requirements/recommendations for international students: Required—TOEFL (minimum score 550 paper-based; 80 iBT). *Application deadline:* For fall admission, 7/15 priority date for domestic students, 7/1 for international students; for spring admission, 11/15 priority date for domestic students, 11/1 for international students. Applications are processed on a rolling basis. Application fee: $55. Electronic applications accepted. *Expenses:* $20,700 per semester full-time tuition, $200 per semester full-time fees; $1,650 per credit hour part-time tuition, $145 per semester part-time fees. *Financial support:* Fellowships, research assistantships, teaching assistantships, Federal Work-Study, scholarships/grants, tuition waivers (full and partial), and unspecified assistantships available. Financial award application deadline: 2/1; financial award applicants required to submit FAFSA. *Faculty research:* Virus structure and assembly, hepatic and epithelial cell biology, drug resistance and genome stabilization in yeast, biophysics of ion-conductive nanostructures, eukaryotic gene regulation, cancer and vaccine research. *Total annual research expenditures:* $2.2 million. *Unit head:* Dr. Venigalla Rao, Chair, 202-319-5271, Fax: 202-319-5721, E-mail: rao@cua.edu. *Application contact:* Director of Graduate Admissions, 202-319-5057, Fax: 202-319-6533, E-mail: cua-admissions@cua.edu.
Website: http://biology.cua.edu/

The College of William and Mary, Faculty of Arts and Sciences, Department of Applied Science, Williamsburg, VA 23187-8795. Offers accelerator science (PhD); applied mathematics (PhD); applied mechanics (PhD); applied robotics (PhD); applied science (MS); atmospheric and environmental science (PhD); computational neuroscience (PhD); interface, thin film and surface science (PhD); lasers and optics (PhD); magnetic resonance (PhD); materials science and engineering (PhD); mathematical and computational biology (PhD); medical imaging (PhD); nanotechnology (PhD); neuroscience (PhD); non-destructive evaluation (PhD); polymer chemistry (PhD); remote sensing (PhD). *Program availability:* Part-time. *Faculty:* 7 full-time (1 woman), 1 part-time/adjunct (0 women). *Students:* 26 full-time (9 women), 3 part-time (1 woman); includes 5 minority (2 Black or African American, non-Hispanic/Latino; 1 Asian, non-Hispanic/Latino; 2 Hispanic/Latino), 12 international. Average age 28. 24 applicants, 46% accepted, 6 enrolled. In 2015, 2 master's, 6 doctorates awarded. Terminal master's awarded for partial completion of doctoral program. *Degree requirements:* For master's, comprehensive exam, thesis; for doctorate, comprehensive exam, thesis/dissertation, 4 core courses. *Entrance requirements:* For master's and doctorate, GRE General Test, GRE Subject Test. Additional exam requirements/recommendations for international students: Required—TOEFL, TWE. *Application deadline:* For fall admission, 2/3 priority date for domestic students, 2/3 for international students; for spring admission, 10/15 priority date for domestic students, 10/14 for international students. Applications are processed on a rolling basis. Application fee: $45. Electronic applications accepted. *Expenses:* $6,550 per semester; $13,100 per year. *Financial support:* Fellowships, research assistantships, teaching assistantships, Federal Work-Study, health care benefits, tuition waivers (full), and unspecified assistantships available. Financial award application deadline: 4/15; financial award applicants required to submit FAFSA. *Faculty research:* Computational biology, non-destructive evaluation, neurophysiology, lasers and optics. *Total annual research expenditures:* $1.7 million. *Unit head:* Dr. Christopher Del Negro, Chair, 757-221-7808, Fax: 757-221-2050, E-mail: cadeln@wm.edu. *Application contact:* Lianne Rios Ashburne, Graduate Program Coordinator, 757-221-2563, Fax: 757-221-2050, E-mail: lrashburne@wm.edu.
Website: http://www.wm.edu/as/appliedscience

Dominican University of California, School of Health and Natural Sciences, Program in Clinical Laboratory Sciences, San Rafael, CA 94901-2298. Offers MS. *Program availability:* Part-time, evening/weekend. *Faculty:* 5 full-time (2 women), 6 part-time/adjunct (4 women). *Students:* 1 full-time (0 women), 15 part-time (9 women); includes 13 minority (5 Black or African American, non-Hispanic/Latino; 6 Asian, non-Hispanic/Latino; 2 Native Hawaiian or other Pacific Islander, non-Hispanic/Latino), 1 international. Average age 41. 14 applicants, 93% accepted, 10 enrolled. In 2015, 9 master's awarded. *Degree requirements:* For master's, thesis. *Entrance requirements:* For master's, GRE, minimum GPA of 3.0. Additional exam requirements/recommendations for international students: Required—TOEFL (minimum score 550 paper-based; 80 iBT), IELTS (minimum score 6.5). *Application deadline:* For fall admission, 5/15 priority date for domestic and international students. Applications are processed on a rolling basis. Electronic applications accepted. Application fee is waived when completed online. *Expenses:* Contact institution. *Financial support:* Applicants required to submit FAFSA. *Unit head:* Dr. Mary Sevigny, Program Director, 415-482-3544, E-mail: mary.sevigny@dominican.edu. *Application contact:* Shannon Lovelace-White, Director, 415-485-3287, Fax: 415-485-3214, E-mail: shannon.lovelace-white@dominican.edu.

Duke University, School of Medicine, Clinical Leadership Program, Durham, NC 27701. Offers MHS. *Faculty:* 16 part-time/adjunct (8 women). *Students:* 3 part-time (2 women); includes 1 minority (Two or more races, non-Hispanic/Latino). 1 applicant, 100% accepted, 1 enrolled. In 2015, 3 master's awarded. *Degree requirements:* For master's, project. *Entrance requirements:* For master's, GRE. Additional exam requirements/recommendations for international students: Required—TOEFL. *Application deadline:* For fall admission, 7/20 for domestic students; for spring admission, 12/1 priority date for domestic students; for summer admission, 4/1 for domestic students. Applications are processed on a rolling basis. Application fee: $100. *Financial support:* Application deadline: 5/1; applicants required to submit FAFSA. *Unit head:* Dr. Anh N. Tran, Vice Chief of Education, 919-681-6079, Fax: 919-681-6899, E-mail: anh.tran@duke.edu. *Application contact:* Claudia Graham, Training Coordinator for Educational Programs, 919-681-5724, Fax: 919-681-6899, E-mail: claudia.graham@duke.edu.
Website: http://clinical-leadership.mc.duke.edu

Fairleigh Dickinson University, Metropolitan Campus, University College: Arts, Sciences, and Professional Studies, Henry P. Becton School of Nursing and Allied Health, Program in Medical Technology, Teaneck, NJ 07666-1914. Offers MS.

Inter American University of Puerto Rico, Metropolitan Campus, Graduate Programs, Program in Medical Technology, San Juan, PR 00919-1293. Offers administration of clinical laboratories (MS); molecular microbiology (MS). *Accreditation:* NAACLS. *Program availability:* Part-time. *Degree requirements:* For master's, comprehensive exam. *Entrance requirements:* For master's, BS in medical technology, minimum GPA of 2.5. Electronic applications accepted.

Medical College of Wisconsin, Graduate School of Biomedical Sciences, Program in Clinical and Translational Science, Milwaukee, WI 53226-0509. Offers MS. Program offered in collaboration with the Clinical and Translational Science Institute (CTSI) of Southeast Wisconsin. *Entrance requirements:* For master's, GRE, official transcripts, three letters of recommendation. Additional exam requirements/recommendations for international students: Required—TOEFL.

Medical College of Wisconsin, Graduate School of Biomedical Sciences, Program in Health Care Technologies Management, Milwaukee, WI 53226-0509. Offers MS. *Entrance requirements:* For master's, GRE, official transcripts, three letters of recommendation. Additional exam requirements/recommendations for international students: Required—TOEFL.

Medical College of Wisconsin, Graduate School of Biomedical Sciences, Program in Translational Science, Milwaukee, WI 53226-0509. Offers PhD. *Entrance requirements:* For doctorate, GRE, official transcripts, three letters of recommendation. Additional exam requirements/recommendations for international students: Required—TOEFL.

Michigan State University, The Graduate School, College of Natural Science, Biomedical Laboratory Diagnostics Program, East Lansing, MI 48824. Offers biomedical laboratory operations (MS); clinical laboratory sciences (MS). *Entrance requirements:* Additional exam requirements/recommendations for international students: Required—TOEFL. Electronic applications accepted.

Milwaukee School of Engineering, Department of Electrical Engineering and Computer Science, Program in Perfusion, Milwaukee, WI 53202-3109. Offers MS. *Program availability:* Part-time, evening/weekend. *Faculty:* 2 full-time (0 women), 5 part-time/adjunct (1 woman). *Students:* 10 full-time (8 women); includes 1 minority (Hispanic/Latino). 44 applicants, 14% accepted, 6 enrolled. In 2015, 7 master's awarded. *Degree requirements:* For master's, comprehensive exam, thesis, exam. *Entrance requirements:* For master's, GRE General Test or GMAT (percentiles must average 50% or better), BS in appropriate discipline (biomedical engineering, biology, biomedical sciences, etc.), 3 letters of recommendation, personal interview, observation of 2 perfusion clinical cases. Additional exam requirements/recommendations for international students: Required—TOEFL (minimum score 79 iBT), IELTS (minimum score 6.5). *Application deadline:* Applications are processed on a rolling basis. Application fee: $0. Electronic applications accepted. *Expenses: Tuition, area resident:* Full-time $34,200; part-time $760 per credit. *Financial support:* Career-related internships or fieldwork, institutionally sponsored loans, and scholarships/grants available. Financial award application deadline: 3/15; financial award applicants required to submit FAFSA. *Faculty research:* Heart medicine. *Unit head:* Dr. Ronald Gerrits, Director, 414-277-7561, Fax: 414-277-7494, E-mail: gerrits@msoe.edu. *Application contact:* Ian Dahlinghaus, Graduate Program Associate, 414-277-7208, E-mail: dahlinghaus@msoe.edu.
Website: http://www.msoe.edu/community/academics/engineering/page/1328/perfusion-overview

See Display on page 501 and Close-Up on page 533.

Northern Michigan University, Office of Graduate Education and Research, College of Health Sciences and Professional Studies, School of Clinical Sciences, Marquette, MI 49855-5301. Offers clinical molecular genetics (MS). *Program availability:* Part-time. *Degree requirements:* For master's, thesis or project to be presented as a seminar at the conclusion of the program. *Entrance requirements:* For master's, minimum undergraduate GPA of 3.0; bachelor's degree in clinical laboratory science or biology; laboratory experience; statement of intent that includes lab skills and experiences along with reason for pursuing this degree; 3 letters of recommendation (instructors or professional references). Additional exam requirements/recommendations for international students: Required—TOEFL (minimum score 550 paper-based; 79 iBT), IELTS (minimum score 6.5). Electronic applications accepted.

Northwestern University, School of Professional Studies, Program in Regulatory Compliance, Evanston, IL 60208. Offers clinical research (MS); healthcare compliance (MS); quality systems (MS). Offered in partnership with Northwestern University's Clinical and Translational Sciences Institute.

Pontifical Catholic University of Puerto Rico, College of Sciences, School of Medical Technology, Ponce, PR 00717-0777. Offers Certificate. *Entrance requirements:* For degree, letters of recommendation, interview, minimum GPA of 2.75.

Quinnipiac University, School of Health Sciences, Program for Pathologists' Assistant, Hamden, CT 06518-1940. Offers MHS. *Accreditation:* NAACLS. *Faculty:* 3 full-time (0 women), 3 part-time/adjunct (0 women). *Students:* 45 full-time (32 women); includes 3 minority (1 Black or African American, non-Hispanic/Latino; 2 Hispanic/Latino), 1 international. 111 applicants, 26% accepted, 24 enrolled. In 2015, 22 master's awarded. *Degree requirements:* For master's, residency. *Entrance requirements:* For master's, interview, coursework in biological and health sciences, minimum GPA of 3.0. *Application deadline:* For summer admission, 9/1 for domestic students. Applications are processed on a rolling basis. Application fee: $45. Electronic applications accepted. *Expenses:* $985 per credit; $360 per semester student fee; $340 per semester (fall/spring) technology and lab fee; $75 per semester summer technology and lab fee. *Financial support:* Scholarships/grants and unspecified assistantships available. Financial award application deadline: 5/1; financial award applicants required to submit FAFSA. *Faculty research:* ACL injury mechanism and running injuries and performance; transcriptional activators upstream stimulatory factor (USF); identification of novel antimicrobials; vaccines, formites and opportunistic pathogens; molecular biology of the Lyme Disease agent, Borrelia burgdorferi; molecular and microscopic techniques in host-pathogen interactions; non-invasive vascular biology, external pneumatic compression, sports performance. *Unit head:* Robert Cottrell, Program Director, 203-582-8672, E-mail: paadmissions@quinnipiac.edu. *Application contact:* Office of Graduate Admissions, 800-462-1944, Fax: 203-582-3443, E-mail: paadmissions@quinnipiac.edu.
Website: http://www.quinnipiac.edu/gradpathologists

Quinnipiac University, School of Health Sciences, Program in Medical Laboratory Sciences, Hamden, CT 06518-1940. Offers MHS. *Program availability:* Part-time, evening/weekend. *Faculty:* 10 full-time (2 women), 18 part-time/adjunct (7 women). *Students:* 41 full-time (26 women), 13 part-time (6 women); includes 14 minority (6 Black or African American, non-Hispanic/Latino; 1 American Indian or Alaska Native, non-Hispanic/Latino; 2 Asian, non-Hispanic/Latino; 5 Hispanic/Latino), 14 international. 107 applicants, 62% accepted, 34 enrolled. In 2015, 39 master's awarded. *Degree requirements:* For master's, comprehensive exam, thesis optional. *Entrance requirements:* For master's, minimum GPA of 2.75; bachelor's degree in biological, medical, or health sciences. Additional exam requirements/recommendations for international students: Required—TOEFL (minimum score 575 paper-based; 90 iBT), IELTS (minimum score 6.5). *Application deadline:* For fall admission, 7/30 priority date for domestic students, 4/30 priority date for international students; for spring admission, 12/15 priority date for domestic students, 9/30 priority date for international students. Applications are processed on a rolling basis. Application fee: $45. Electronic applications accepted. *Expenses:* $985 per credit tuition; $40 per credit student fee (not to exceed $360 per semester); $150 per semester (fall/spring) part-time technology and lab fee; $340 per semester (fall/spring) full-time technology and lab fee; $75 per semester summer technology and lab fee. *Financial support:* Federal Work-Study, scholarships/grants and unspecified assistantships available. Support available to part-time students. Financial award application deadline: 6/1; financial award applicants required to submit FAFSA. *Faculty research:* ACL injury mechanism and running injuries and performance; transcriptional activators upstream stimulatory factor (USF); identification of novel antimicrobials; vaccines, formites and opportunistic pathogens; molecular biology of the Lyme Disease agent, Borrelia burgdorferi; molecular and microscopic techniques in host-pathogen interactions; non-invasive vascular biology, external pneumatic compression, sports performance. *Unit head:* Dwayne Boucaud,

Clinical Laboratory Sciences/Medical Technology

Program Director, 203-582-3768, E-mail: graduate@quinnipiac.edu. *Application contact:* Office of Graduate Admissions, 800-462-1944, Fax: 203-582-3443, E-mail: graduate@quinnipiac.edu.
Website: http://www.quinnipiac.edu/gradmedlab

Rush University, College of Health Sciences, Department of Medical Laboratory Science, Chicago, IL 60612-3832. Offers clinical laboratory management (MS); medical laboratory science (MS). *Accreditation:* NAACLS. *Degree requirements:* For master's, comprehensive exam, project. *Entrance requirements:* For master's, 16 semester hours of chemistry, 12 semester hours of biology, 3 semester hours of mathematics, interview. Additional exam requirements/recommendations for international students: Required—TOEFL. *Application deadline:* For fall admission, 8/1 for domestic and international students; for winter admission, 12/1 for domestic and international students; for spring admission, 3/1 for domestic and international students. Applications are processed on a rolling basis. Application fee: $40. Electronic applications accepted. *Financial support:* Federal Work-Study, institutionally sponsored loans, and scholarships/grants available. Support available to part-time students. Financial award application deadline: 4/15; financial award applicants required to submit FAFSA. *Faculty research:* Hematopoietic disorders, molecular techniques, biochemistry, microbial susceptibility, immunology. *Unit head:* Dr. Maribeth Flaws, Acting Chair, 312-942-2115, E-mail: maribeth_l_flaws@rush.edu. *Application contact:* 312-942-7120, E-mail: chs_admissions@rush.edu.
Website: http://www.rushu.rush.edu/mls

Rutgers University–Newark, School of Health Related Professions, Department of Clinical Laboratory Sciences, Newark, NJ 07102. Offers MS. *Program availability:* Part-time, online learning. *Degree requirements:* For master's, project. *Entrance requirements:* For master's, two recommendations, personal statement, current resume or curriculum vita, minimum GPA of 2.75. Additional exam requirements/recommendations for international students: Required—TOEFL.

Rutgers University–New Brunswick, Graduate School of Biomedical Sciences, Program in Clinical and Translational Science, Piscataway, NJ 08854-8097. Offers MS. *Program availability:* Part-time. *Degree requirements:* For master's, thesis.

State University of New York Upstate Medical University, Program in Medical Technology, Syracuse, NY 13210-2334. Offers MS. *Accreditation:* NAACLS. *Degree requirements:* For master's, thesis. *Entrance requirements:* For master's, GRE General Test, GRE Subject Test, 2 years of medical technology experience.

Tarleton State University, College of Graduate Studies, College of Science and Technology, Department of Medical Laboratory Sciences and Public Health, Fort Worth, TX 76104. Offers medical laboratory sciences (MS). *Program availability:* Part-time, evening/weekend. *Faculty:* 6 full-time (4 women). *Students:* 4 full-time (3 women), 12 part-time (10 women); includes 8 minority (4 Black or African American, non-Hispanic/Latino; 3 Asian, non-Hispanic/Latino; 1 Hispanic/Latino), 3 international. 8 applicants, 50% accepted, 4 enrolled. In 2015, 8 master's awarded. *Degree requirements:* For master's, comprehensive exam, thesis optional. *Entrance requirements:* For master's, GRE, minimum GPA of 3.0. Additional exam requirements/recommendations for international students: Required—TOEFL (minimum score 550 paper-based; 80 iBT). *Application deadline:* For fall admission, 8/15 for domestic students; for spring admission, 1/7 for domestic students. Applications are processed on a rolling basis. Application fee: $45 ($145 for international students). Electronic applications accepted. *Expenses:* Tuition, state resident: part-time $204 per credit hour. Tuition, nonresident: part-time $594 per credit hour. *Required fees:* $1994 per unit. *Financial support:* Career-related internships or fieldwork, Federal Work-Study, and scholarships/grants available. Support available to part-time students. Financial award application deadline: 5/1; financial award applicants required to submit FAFSA. *Unit head:* Sally Lewis, Head, 817-926-1101, E-mail: slewis@tarleton.edu. *Application contact:* Information Contact, 254-968-9104, Fax: 254-968-9670, E-mail: gradoffice@tarleton.edu.
Website: http://www.tarleton.edu/degrees/masters/ms-medical-laboratory-science/

Thomas Jefferson University, Jefferson School of Health Professions, Department of Bioscience Technologies, Philadelphia, PA 19107. Offers MS. *Program availability:* Part-time, evening/weekend. *Students:* 41 full-time (30 women), 4 part-time (all women); includes 7 minority (all Black or African American, non-Hispanic/Latino). Average age 28. 67 applicants, 67% accepted, 34 enrolled. In 2015, 40 master's awarded. *Entrance requirements:* Additional exam requirements/recommendations for international students: Required—TOEFL. *Application deadline:* For fall admission, 7/15 for domestic students, 4/15 for international students; for winter admission, 12/1 for domestic students, 9/1 for international students; for spring admission, 4/1 for domestic students. Applications are processed on a rolling basis. Application fee: $95. Electronic applications accepted. *Expenses:* Contact institution. *Financial support:* In 2015–16, 27 students received support. Federal Work-Study, institutionally sponsored loans, scholarships/grants, and unspecified assistantships available. Support available to part-time students. Financial award application deadline: 4/1; financial award applicants required to submit FAFSA. *Unit head:* Dr. Barbara Goldsmith, Chair, 215-955-1327, E-mail: barbara.goldsmith@jefferson.edu. *Application contact:* Sarah McNabb, Senior Associate Director of Admissions, 215-503-1045, Fax: 215-503-7241, E-mail: sarah.mcnabb@jefferson.edu.
Website: http://www.jefferson.edu/health_professions/departments/bioscience_technologies

Universidad de las Américas Puebla, Division of Graduate Studies, School of Sciences, Program in Clinical Analysis (Biomedicine), Puebla, Mexico. Offers MS. *Program availability:* Part-time, evening/weekend. *Degree requirements:* For master's, one foreign language, thesis. *Faculty research:* Clinical techniques, clinical research.

Université de Sherbrooke, Faculty of Medicine and Health Sciences, Graduate Programs in Medicine, Program in Clinical Sciences, Sherbrooke, QC J1H 5N4, Canada. Offers M Sc, PhD. *Program availability:* Part-time. Terminal master's awarded for partial completion of doctoral program. *Degree requirements:* For master's, thesis; for doctorate, thesis/dissertation. Electronic applications accepted. *Faculty research:* Population health, health services, ethics, clinical research.

University at Buffalo, the State University of New York, Graduate School, School of Medicine and Biomedical Sciences, Graduate Programs in Medicine and Biomedical Sciences, Department of Biotechnical and Clinical Laboratory Sciences, Buffalo, NY 14214. Offers biotechnology (MS). *Accreditation:* NAACLS. *Program availability:* Part-time. *Faculty:* 7 full-time (3 women). *Students:* 12 full-time (11 women), 1 (woman) part-time, 9 international. 61 applicants, 20% accepted, 5 enrolled. In 2015, 3 master's awarded. *Degree requirement:* For master's, thesis. *Entrance requirements:* For master's, GRE General Test, minimum GPA of 3.0. Additional exam requirements/recommendations for international students: Required—TOEFL (minimum score 79 iBT), IELTS. *Application deadline:* For fall admission, 3/1 priority date for domestic students, 2/1 priority date for international students. Applications are processed on a rolling basis. Application fee: $75. Electronic applications accepted. *Financial support:* In 2015–16, 7 students received support, including 2 research assistantships with tuition reimbursements available (averaging $15,000 per year), 5 teaching assistantships with full tuition reimbursements available (averaging $10,000 per year). Financial award application deadline: 3/1. *Faculty research:* Immunology, cancer biology, toxicology, clinical chemistry, hematology, chemistry. *Total annual research expenditures:* $1.2

million. *Unit head:* Dr. Paul J. Kostyniak, Chair, 716-829-5188, Fax: 716-829-3601, E-mail: pjkost@buffalo.edu. *Application contact:* Dr. Stephen T. Koury, Director of Graduate Studies, 716-829-5188, Fax: 716-829-3601, E-mail: stvkoury@buffalo.edu.
Website: http://www.smbs.buffalo.edu/cls/biotech-ms.html

The University of Alabama at Birmingham, School of Health Professions, Program in Clinical Laboratory Science, Birmingham, AL 35294. Offers MS. *Accreditation:* NAACLS. *Degree requirements:* For master's, thesis optional. *Entrance requirements:* For master's, GRE General Test, interview, related undergraduate major, minimum undergraduate GPA of 3.0 computed from all undergraduate credits or from the last 60 semester hours of undergraduate course credit. Additional exam requirements/recommendations for international students: Required—TOEFL (minimum score 550 paper-based; 80 iBT), TWE. Electronic applications accepted. *Expenses:* Tuition, state resident: full-time $7340. Tuition, nonresident: full-time $16,628. Full-time tuition and fees vary according to course load and program. *Faculty research:* Computer-enhanced instruction, antiphospholipid antibodies, alternate site testing, technology assessment.

The University of Alabama at Birmingham, School of Public Health, Program in Public Health, Birmingham, AL 35294. Offers applied epidemiology and pharmacoepidemiology (MSPH); biostatistics (MPH); clinical and translational science (MSPH); environmental health (MPH); environmental health and toxicology (MSPH); epidemiology (MPH); general theory and practice (MPH); health behavior (MPH); health care organization (MPH); health policy quantitative policy analysis (MPH); industrial hygiene (MPH, MSPH); maternal and child health policy (Dr PH); maternal and child health policy and leadership (MPH); occupational health and safety (MPH); outcomes research (MSPH, Dr PH); public health (PhD); public health management (Dr PH); public health preparedness management (MPH). *Accreditation:* CEPH. *Program availability:* Part-time, online learning. *Degree requirements:* For doctorate, comprehensive exam, thesis/dissertation. *Entrance requirements:* For master's and doctorate, GRE. Additional exam requirements/recommendations for international students: Recommended—TOEFL (minimum score 550 paper-based; 79 iBT, IELTS (minimum score 6.5). Electronic applications accepted. *Expenses:* Tuition, state resident: full-time $7340. Tuition, nonresident: full-time $16,628. Full-time tuition and fees vary according to course load and program.

University of Alberta, Faculty of Medicine and Dentistry and Faculty of Graduate Studies and Research, Graduate Programs in Medicine, Department of Laboratory Medicine and Pathology, Edmonton, AB T6G 2E1, Canada. Offers medical sciences (M Sc, PhD). *Program availability:* Part-time. Terminal master's awarded for partial completion of doctoral program. *Degree requirements:* For master's, thesis; for doctorate, thesis/dissertation, candidacy exam. *Entrance requirements:* For master's and doctorate, 3 letters of recommendation, minimum GPA of 3.0. Additional exam requirements/recommendations for international students: Required—TOEFL. *Faculty research:* Transplantation, renal pathology, molecular mechanisms of diseases, cryobiology, immunodiagnostics, informatics/cyber medicine, neuroimmunology, microbiology.

University of California, San Diego, Graduate Division, Department of Electrical and Computer Engineering, La Jolla, CA 92093. Offers applied ocean science (MS, PhD); applied physics (MS, PhD); communication theory and systems (MS, PhD); computer engineering (MS, PhD); electronic circuits and systems (MS, PhD); intelligent systems, robotics and control (MS, PhD); medical devices and systems (MS, PhD); nanoscale devices and systems (MS, PhD); photonics (MS, PhD); signal and image processing (MS, PhD). *Students:* 503 full-time (99 women), 48 part-time (6 women); includes 79 minority (4 Black or African American, non-Hispanic/Latino; 67 Asian, non-Hispanic/Latino; 8 Hispanic/Latino), 381 international. 2,689 applicants, 21% accepted, 200 enrolled. In 2015, 97 master's, 42 doctorates awarded. *Degree requirements:* For master's, thesis or written exam; for doctorate, comprehensive exam, thesis/dissertation. *Entrance requirements:* For master's and doctorate, GRE General Test, minimum GPA of 3.0. Additional exam requirements/recommendations for international students: Required—TOEFL (minimum score 550 paper-based; 80 iBT), IELTS. *Application deadline:* For fall admission, 12/15 for domestic students. Application fee: $90 ($110 for international students). Electronic applications accepted. *Expenses:* Tuition, state resident: full-time $11,220. Tuition, nonresident: full-time $26,322. *Required fees:* $1800. *Financial support:* Fellowships, research assistantships, teaching assistantships, scholarships/grants, traineeships, and unspecified assistantships available. Financial award applicants required to submit FAFSA. *Faculty research:* Applied ocean science; applied physics; communication theory and systems; computer engineering; electronic circuits and systems; intelligent systems, robotics and control; medical devices and systems; nanoscale devices and systems; photonics; signal and image processing. *Unit head:* Truong Nguyen, Chair, 858-822-5554, E-mail: nguyent@ece.ucsd.edu. *Application contact:* Melanie Lynn, Graduate Admissions Coordinator, 858-822-3213, E-mail: ecegradapps@ece.ucsd.edu.
Website: http://ece.ucsd.edu/

University of California, San Diego, Graduate Division, Program in Medical Device Engineering, La Jolla, CA 92093. Offers MAS. *Program availability:* Part-time. *Students:* 30 part-time (9 women); includes 14 minority (1 American Indian or Alaska Native, non-Hispanic/Latino; 11 Asian, non-Hispanic/Latino; 2 Hispanic/Latino), 1 international. 34 applicants, 65% accepted, 18 enrolled. In 2015, 12 master's awarded. *Degree requirements:* For master's, capstone project. *Entrance requirements:* For master's, 3 letters of recommendation; statement of purpose; bachelor's degree in engineering, science, or mathematics; minimum undergraduate GPA of 3.0 in final two years of study; two years of relevant work experience; curriculum vitae/resume. Additional exam requirements/recommendations for international students: Required—TOEFL, IELTS. *Application deadline:* For fall admission, 1/31 priority date for domestic students. Applications are processed on a rolling basis. Application fee: $90 ($110 for international students). Electronic applications accepted. *Expenses:* Contact institution. *Financial support:* Applicants required to submit FAFSA. *Faculty research:* Mechanics and transport, anatomy and physiology, biomaterials, business processes, regulatory affairs, life science technologies. *Unit head:* Juan C. Lasheras, Director, 858-534-5437, E-mail: jlasheras@ucsd.edu. *Application contact:* Sally Binney, Program Coordinator, 858-246-1463, E-mail: mde-mas@ucsd.edu.
Website: http://maseng.ucsd.edu/mde/

University of Colorado Denver, School of Medicine, Clinical Science Graduate Program, Aurora, CO 80045. Offers clinical investigation (PhD); clinical sciences (MS); health information technology (PhD); health services research (PhD). *Students:* 38 full-time (28 women), 35 part-time (22 women); includes 12 minority (3 Black or African American, non-Hispanic/Latino; 1 American Indian or Alaska Native, non-Hispanic/Latino; 4 Asian, non-Hispanic/Latino; 2 Hispanic/Latino; 2 Two or more races, non-Hispanic/Latino), 1 international. Average age 37. 22 applicants, 68% accepted, 15 enrolled. In 2015, 13 master's, 2 doctorates awarded. *Degree requirements:* For master's, thesis, minimum of 30 credit hours, defense/final exam of thesis or publishable paper; for doctorate, comprehensive exam, thesis/dissertation, at least 30 credit hours of thesis work. *Entrance requirements:* For master's, GRE General Test or MCAT (waived if candidate has earned MS/MA or PhD from accredited U.S. school), minimum undergraduate GPA of 3.0, 3-4 letters of recommendation; for doctorate, GRE General Test or MCAT (waived if candidate has earned MS/MA or PhD from accredited U.S.

school), health care graduate, professional degree, or graduate degree related to health sciences; minimum GPA of 3.0; 3-4 letters of recommendation. Additional exam requirements/recommendations for international students: Required—TOEFL (minimum score 550 paper-based; 80 iBT). *Application deadline:* For fall admission, 2/1 for domestic students, 1/15 priority date for international students; for spring admission, 10/1 for domestic students. Application fee: $50 ($75 for international students). Electronic applications accepted. *Expenses:* Contact institution. *Financial support:* In 2015–16, 34 students received support. Fellowships, research assistantships, teaching assistantships, Federal Work-Study, institutionally sponsored loans, scholarships/grants, traineeships, and unspecified assistantships available. Financial award application deadline: 3/15; financial award applicants required to submit FAFSA. *Unit head:* Dr. Lisa Cicutto, Program Director, 303-398-1539, E-mail: cicuttol@njhealth.org. *Application contact:* Galit Mankin, Program Administrator, 720-848-6249, Fax: 303-848-7381, E-mail: galit.mankin@ucdenver.edu.
Website: http://www.ucdenver.edu/research/CCTSI/education-training/clsc/Pages/default.aspx

University of Florida, Graduate School, College of Engineering, Department of Materials Science and Engineering, Gainesville, FL 32611. Offers material science and engineering (MS), including clinical and translational science; materials science and engineering (ME, PhD); nuclear engineering (ME, PhD), including imaging science and technology (PhD), nuclear engineering sciences (ME, MS, PhD); nuclear engineering (MS), including nuclear engineering sciences (ME, MS, PhD); JD/MS. *Program availability:* Part-time, online learning. *Faculty:* 27 full-time, 23 part-time/adjunct. *Students:* 227 full-time (64 women), 34 part-time (12 women); includes 42 minority (7 Black or African American, non-Hispanic/Latino; 18 Asian, non-Hispanic/Latino; 17 Hispanic/Latino), 144 international. Average age 27. 470 applicants, 74% accepted, 93 enrolled. In 2015, 67 master's, 20 doctorates awarded. Terminal master's awarded for partial completion of doctoral program. *Degree requirements:* For master's, comprehensive exam, thesis; for doctorate, comprehensive exam, thesis/dissertation. *Entrance requirements:* For master's and doctorate, minimum GPA of 3.0. Additional exam requirements/recommendations for international students: Required—TOEFL (minimum score 550 paper-based; 80 iBT), IELTS (minimum score 6). *Application deadline:* For fall admission, 7/1 priority date for domestic students, 5/1 for international students; for spring admission, 11/1 for domestic students, 9/1 for international students. Applications are processed on a rolling basis. Application fee: $30. Electronic applications accepted. *Financial support:* In 2015–16, 2 fellowships, 101 research assistantships, 1 teaching assistantship were awarded. Financial award applicants required to submit FAFSA. *Faculty research:* Polymeric system, biomaterials and biomimetics; inorganic and organic electronic materials; functional ceramic materials for energy systems and microelectronic applications; advanced metallic systems for aerospace, transportation and biological applications; nuclear materials. *Total annual research expenditures:* $8.9 million. *Unit head:* Dr. Jim Baciak, Chair, 352-846-3782, Fax: 352-392-7219. *Application contact:* Dr. Jack Mecholsky, Jr., Graduate Coordinator, 352-846-3306, Fax: 352-846-1182, E-mail: jmech@mse.ufl.edu.
Website: http://www.mse.ufl.edu

University of Florida, Graduate School, College of Nursing, Gainesville, FL 32611. Offers clinical and translational science (PhD); clinical nursing (DNP); nursing (MSN); nursing sciences (PhD). *Accreditation:* AACN; ACNM/ACME (one or more programs are accredited). *Program availability:* Part-time. *Faculty:* 13 full-time (11 women), 5 part-time/adjunct (3 women). *Students:* 58 full-time (33 women), 31 part-time (27 women); includes 16 minority (6 Black or African American, non-Hispanic/Latino; 6 Asian, non-Hispanic/Latino; 4 Hispanic/Latino), 5 international. Average age 38. 44 applicants, 20% accepted, 8 enrolled. In 2015, 63 master's, 6 doctorates awarded. *Degree requirements:* For master's, thesis optional; for doctorate, thesis/dissertation. *Entrance requirements:* For master's and doctorate, GRE General Test, minimum GPA of 3.0. Additional exam requirements/recommendations for international students: Required—TOEFL (minimum score 550 paper-based; 80 iBT), IELTS (minimum score 6). *Application deadline:* For fall admission, 3/15 priority date for domestic students, 3/15 for international students. Applications are processed on a rolling basis. Application fee: $30. Electronic applications accepted. *Financial support:* In 2015–16, 6 fellowships, 2 research assistantships were awarded; career-related internships or fieldwork and Federal Work-Study also available. Support available to part-time students. Financial award applicants required to submit FAFSA. *Faculty research:* Aging and health: cancer survivorship, interventions to promote healthy aging, and symptom management; women's health, fetal and infant development; biobehavioral interventions: interrelationships among the biological, behavioral, psychological, social and spiritual factors that influence wellness and disease; health policy: influence of local and national policy on physical and psychological health. *Unit head:* Anna M. McDaniel, PhD, Dean, College of Nursing, 352-273-6324, Fax: 352-273-6505, E-mail: annammcdaniel@ufl.edu. *Application contact:* Bridgette Hart-Sams, Coordinator, Student Academic Services, 352-273-6331, Fax: 352-273-6440, E-mail: bhart@ufl.edu.
Website: http://nursing.ufl.edu/

University of Florida, Graduate School, College of Pharmacy and Graduate School, Graduate Programs in Pharmacy, Department of Pharmaceutics, Gainesville, FL 32611. Offers clinical and translational science (PhD); pharmaceutical science (MSP, PhD); pharmacy (MSP, PhD). *Faculty:* 2 full-time, 1 part-time/adjunct. *Students:* 30 full-time (14 women), 1 (woman) part-time; includes 1 minority (Asian, non-Hispanic/Latino), 24 international. Average age 29. 182 applicants, 57% accepted, 92 enrolled. In 2015, 4 doctorates awarded. *Degree requirements:* For doctorate, comprehensive exam, thesis/dissertation. *Entrance requirements:* For master's and doctorate, GRE General Test, minimum GPA of 3.0. Additional exam requirements/recommendations for international students: Required—TOEFL (minimum score 550 paper-based; 80 iBT), IELTS (minimum score 6). *Application deadline:* For fall admission, 2/1 priority date for domestic students, 2/1 for international students; for spring admission, 10/5 for domestic and international students. Applications are processed on a rolling basis. Application fee: $30. Electronic applications accepted. *Financial support:* In 2015–16, 3 research assistantships, 19 teaching assistantships were awarded; tuition waivers (full) and unspecified assistantships also available. Financial award applicants required to submit FAFSA. *Faculty research:* Basic, applied, and clinical investigations in pharmacokinetics/biopharmaceutics; pharmaceutical analysis, pharmaceutical biotechnology and drug delivery; herbal medicine. *Total annual research expenditures:* $2.2 million. *Unit head:* Hartmut Derendorf, PhD, Professor and Chair, 352-273-7856, Fax: 352-392-4447, E-mail: hartmut@ufl.edu. *Application contact:* Dr. Anthony Palmieri, III, Graduate Coordinator, 352-273-7868, E-mail: palmieri@cop.ufl.edu.
Website: http://www.cop.ufl.edu/pc/

University of Florida, Graduate School, College of Public Health and Health Professions, Department of Clinical and Health Psychology, Gainesville, FL 32611. Offers clinical and translational science (PhD); psychology (MS). *Accreditation:* APA (one or more programs are accredited). *Faculty:* 10 full-time, 4 part-time/adjunct. *Students:* 95 full-time (64 women), 14 part-time (13 women); includes 22 minority (10 Black or African American, non-Hispanic/Latino; 1 American Indian or Alaska Native, non-Hispanic/Latino; 3 Asian, non-Hispanic/Latino; 8 Hispanic/Latino), 2 international. 323 applicants, 5% accepted, 12 enrolled. In 2015, 13 master's, 13 doctorates awarded. *Degree requirements:* For doctorate, comprehensive exam, thesis/dissertation, pre-

doctoral internship. *Entrance requirements:* For master's and doctorate, GRE General Test, minimum GPA of 3.0. Additional exam requirements/recommendations for international students: Required—TOEFL (minimum score 550 paper-based; 80 iBT), IELTS (minimum score 6). *Application deadline:* For fall admission, 12/1 for domestic and international students. Application fee: $30. Electronic applications accepted. *Financial support:* In 2015–16, 8 teaching assistantships were awarded; career-related internships or fieldwork, Federal Work-Study, institutionally sponsored loans, scholarships/grants, and unspecified assistantships also available. Financial award application deadline: 12/1; financial award applicants required to submit FAFSA. *Faculty research:* Clinical child and pediatric psychology, medical psychology, neuropsychology, health promotion and aging. *Total annual research expenditures:* $2.8 million. *Unit head:* William W. Latimer, PhD, Professor and Chair, 352-273-6556, Fax: 352-273-6156, E-mail: wwlatimer@phhp.ufl.edu. *Application contact:* Office of Admissions, 352-392-1365, E-mail: webrequests@admissions.ufl.edu.
Website: http://www.phhp.ufl.edu/chp/

University of Florida, Graduate School, College of Public Health and Health Professions, Department of Epidemiology, Gainesville, FL 32611. Offers clinical and translational science (PhD); epidemiology (MS, PhD). *Faculty:* 5 full-time. *Students:* 28 full-time (17 women), 4 part-time (2 women); includes 8 minority (4 Black or African American, non-Hispanic/Latino; 3 Asian, non-Hispanic/Latino; 1 Hispanic/Latino), 13 international. Average age 29. 53 applicants, 32% accepted, 9 enrolled. In 2015, 1 master's, 5 doctorates awarded. *Degree requirements:* For master's, thesis; for doctorate, thesis/dissertation. *Entrance requirements:* For master's and doctorate, GRE (minimum score verbal/quantitative combined 300), minimum GPA of 3.0. Additional exam requirements/recommendations for international students: Required—TOEFL (minimum score 550 paper-based; 80 iBT), IELTS (minimum score 6). *Application deadline:* For fall admission, 2/1 for domestic and international students. Application fee: $30. *Financial support:* In 2015–16, 6 fellowships, 9 research assistantships, 11 teaching assistantships were awarded. Financial award applicants required to submit FAFSA. *Faculty research:* Substance abuse, psychiatric epidemiology, cancer epidemiology, infectious disease epidemiology, bioinformatics. *Total annual research expenditures:* $3.5 million. *Unit head:* Linda Cottler, PhD, Chair, 352-273-5468, E-mail: lbcottler@ufl.edu. *Application contact:* Betsy Jones, Program Assistant, 352-273-5961, E-mail: bjcop@ufl.edu.
Website: http://epidemiology.phhp.ufl.edu/

University of Maryland, Baltimore, Graduate School, Department of Medical and Research Technology, Baltimore, MD 21201. Offers MS. *Accreditation:* NAACLS. *Program availability:* Part-time. *Degree requirements:* For master's, thesis or management project. *Entrance requirements:* For master's, GRE General Test, minimum GPA of 3.0. Additional exam requirements/recommendations for international students: Required—TOEFL (minimum score 550 paper-based; 80 iBT) or IELTS (minimum score 7). Electronic applications accepted. Tuition and fees vary according to program. *Faculty research:* Clinical microbiology, immunology, immunohematology, hematology, clinical chemistry, molecular biology.

University of Massachusetts Dartmouth, Graduate School, College of Engineering, Program in Biomedical Engineering and Biotechnology, North Dartmouth, MA 02747-2300. Offers bioengineering (PhD); biology (PhD); biomedical engineering/biotechnology (MS, PhD); chemistry (PhD); civil engineering (PhD); computer and information science (PhD); electrical and computer engineering (PhD); mathematics (PhD); mechanical engineering (PhD); medical laboratory science (MS); physics (PhD). *Program availability:* Part-time. *Students:* 11 full-time (6 women), 14 part-time (7 women); includes 1 minority (Hispanic/Latino), 13 international. Average age 31. 33 applicants, 76% accepted, 6 enrolled. In 2015, 1 master's, 3 doctorates awarded. *Degree requirements:* For doctorate, comprehensive exam, thesis/dissertation. *Entrance requirements:* For master's and doctorate, GRE, statement of purpose (minimum of 300 words), resume, 3 letters of recommendation, official transcripts. Additional exam requirements/recommendations for international students: Required—TOEFL (minimum score 550 paper-based). *Application deadline:* For fall admission, 2/15 priority date for domestic students, 1/15 priority date for international students; for spring admission, 11/15 priority date for domestic students, 10/15 priority date for international students. Applications are processed on a rolling basis. Application fee: $60. Electronic applications accepted. *Expenses:* Tuition, state resident: full-time $2071; part-time $86.29 per credit. Tuition, nonresident: full-time $8099; part-time $337.46 per credit. *Required fees:* $18,074; $762.08 per credit. Tuition and fees vary according to course load and reciprocity agreements. *Financial support:* In 2015–16, 4 fellowships (averaging $20,000 per year), 4 research assistantships (averaging $16,440 per year), 6 teaching assistantships (averaging $10,833 per year) were awarded; Federal Work-Study and unspecified assistantships also available. Support available to part-time students. Financial award application deadline: 3/1; financial award applicants required to submit FAFSA. *Faculty research:* Comparative immunology, vaccine design, biosensors, biomimetic materials, polymer science, soft electronics, hydrogels, regenerative biological materials. *Total annual research expenditures:* $1.2 million. *Unit head:* Sankha Bhowmick, Graduate Program Director for Engineering Options, 508-999-8619, Fax: 508-999-8881, E-mail: sbhowmick@umassd.edu. *Application contact:* Steven Briggs, Director of Marketing and Recruitment for Graduate Studies, 508-999-8604, Fax: 508-999-8183, E-mail: graduate@umassd.edu.
Website: http://www.umassd.edu/engineering/graduate/doctoraldegreeprograms/biomedicalengineeringandbiotechnology/

University of Massachusetts Lowell, College of Health Sciences, Department of Clinical Laboratory and Nutritional Sciences, Lowell, MA 01854. Offers clinical laboratory sciences (MS). *Accreditation:* NAACLS. *Program availability:* Part-time, online learning. *Degree requirements:* For master's, thesis optional. *Entrance requirements:* For master's, GRE General Test, minimum GPA of 3.0, letters of recommendation. *Application deadline:* For fall admission, 4/1 priority date for domestic students; for spring admission, 10/1 for domestic students. Applications are processed on a rolling basis. Application fee: $20 ($35 for international students). *Expenses:* Tuition, state resident: full-time $14,304. Tuition, nonresident: full-time $25,853. *Required fees:* $375. Full-time tuition and fees vary according to campus/location and reciprocity agreements. *Financial support:* Research assistantships with full tuition reimbursements, teaching assistantships with full tuition reimbursements, Federal Work-Study, and institutionally sponsored loans available. Support available to part-time students. Financial award application deadline: 4/1. *Faculty research:* Cardiovascular disease, lipoprotein metabolism, micronutrient evaluation, alcohol metabolism, mycobacterial drug resistance.

University of Minnesota, Twin Cities Campus, College of Science and Engineering, Technological Leadership Institute, Program in Medical Device Innovation, Minneapolis, MN 55455-0213. Offers MS. *Entrance requirements:* Additional exam requirements/recommendations for international students: Required—TOEFL. Electronic applications accepted. *Faculty research:* Dynamics of medical device innovation, including technology innovation, project and business management, intellectual property, regulatory affairs, and public policy.

University of Nebraska Medical Center, School of Allied Health Professions, Program in Clinical Perfusion Education, Omaha, NE 68198-4144. Offers distance education

Clinical Laboratory Sciences/Medical Technology

perfusion education (MPS); perfusion science (MPS). *Accreditation:* NAACLS. *Program availability:* Online learning. *Degree requirements:* For master's, comprehensive exam, thesis. *Entrance requirements:* For master's, GRE. Electronic applications accepted. *Expenses:* Tuition, state resident: full-time $7830; part-time $3915 per credit hour. Tuition, nonresident: full-time $22,410; part-time $11,205 per credit hour. *Required fees:* $521. *Faculty research:* Platelet gel, hemoconcentrators.

University of Nebraska Medical Center, School of Allied Health Professions, Program in Cytotechnology, Omaha, NE 68198. Offers Certificate. *Accreditation:* NAACLS. *Program availability:* Online learning. Electronic applications accepted. *Expenses:* Tuition, state resident: full-time $7830; part-time $3915 per credit hour. Tuition, nonresident: full-time $22,410; part-time $11,205 per credit hour. *Required fees:* $521. *Faculty research:* HPV vaccine.

University of New Mexico, Graduate Studies, Health Sciences Center, Master's in Clinical Laboratory Science Program, Albuquerque, NM 87131. Offers education (MS); laboratory management (MS); research and development (MS). *Program availability:* Part-time. *Faculty:* 8 full-time (6 women), 2 part-time/adjunct (1 woman). *Students:* 3 full-time (1 woman); includes 1 minority (Hispanic/Latino), 1 international. Average age 31. 3 applicants, 33% accepted, 1 enrolled. *Degree requirements:* For master's, project thesis; presentation at national meeting. *Entrance requirements:* For master's, ASCP Board of Certification Exam. Additional exam requirements/recommendations for international students: Required—TOEFL. *Application deadline:* For fall admission, 7/15 priority date for domestic students, 6/15 priority date for international students. Application fee: $50. Electronic applications accepted. *Financial support:* Career-related internships or fieldwork available. Financial award application deadline: 7/15; financial award applicants required to submit FAFSA. *Faculty research:* Prostate cancer, educational techniques, online training, molecular diagnostics, laboratory medicine, laboratory management, laboratory test assessment. *Unit head:* Dr. Paul B. Roth, Dean, 505-272-8273, Fax: 505-272-6857. *Application contact:* Dr. Roberto Gomez, Associate Dean of Students, 505-272-3414, Fax: 505-272-6857, E-mail: rgomez@unm.edu. Website: http://pathology.unm.edu/medical-laboratory-sciences/program/graduate-m.s.-degree-program.html

University of New Mexico, Graduate Studies, Health Sciences Center, Program in Clinical and Translational Science, Albuquerque, NM 87131-2039. Offers Certificate. *Faculty:* 4 full-time (1 woman). *Students:* 9 full-time (5 women); includes 3 minority (1 Black or African American, non-Hispanic/Latino; 2 Asian, non-Hispanic/Latino), 1 international. Average age 33. In 2015, 6 Certificates awarded. *Unit head:* Dr. Helen J. Hathaway, Program Director, 505-272-1469, E-mail: hhathaway@salud.unm.edu. *Application contact:* Angel Cooke-Jackson, Coordinator, 505-272-1887, Fax: 505-272-8738, E-mail: acooke-jackson@salud.unm.edu.

University of North Dakota, Graduate School and Graduate School, Graduate Programs in Medicine, Department of Clinical Laboratory Science, Grand Forks, ND 58202. Offers MS. *Accreditation:* NAACLS. *Program availability:* Online learning. *Degree requirements:* For master's, comprehensive exam, thesis or alternative. *Entrance requirements:* For master's, minimum GPA of 3.0. Additional exam requirements/recommendations for international students: Required—TOEFL (minimum score 550 paper-based; 79 iBT), IELTS (minimum score 5.5). Electronic applications accepted.

University of Pennsylvania, Perelman School of Medicine, Institute for Translational Medicine and Therapeutics, Philadelphia, PA 19104. Offers MRA, MTR, MD/MTR. *Expenses:* Tuition, area resident: Full-time $31,068; part-time $5762 per course. *Required fees:* $3200; $336 per course. Full-time tuition and fees vary according to degree level, program and student level. Part-time tuition and fees vary according to course load, degree level and program. *Unit head:* Dr. Emma Meagher, MD, Director, Translational Research Programs, E-mail: itmated@mail.med.upenn.edu. *Application contact:* Rachel Bastian, Administrative Director, E-mail: itmated@mail.med.upenn.edu. Website: http://www.itmat.upenn.edu/

University of Pittsburgh, School of Medicine, Graduate Programs in Medicine, Clinical and Translational Science Graduate Program, Pittsburgh, PA 15260. Offers PhD. *Program availability:* Part-time, blended/hybrid learning. *Faculty:* 46 full-time (29 women). *Students:* 1 full-time (0 women), 10 part-time (4 women); includes 4 minority (2 Black or African American, non-Hispanic/Latino; 1 Asian, non-Hispanic/Latino; 1 Hispanic/Latino), 2 international. Average age 37. 7 applicants, 43% accepted, 3 enrolled. In 2015, 4 doctorates awarded. *Degree requirements:* For doctorate, comprehensive exam, thesis/dissertation, preliminary examination. *Entrance requirements:* For doctorate, MCAT or GRE, transcripts, curriculum vitae, personal statement, 2 letters of recommendation. Additional exam requirements/recommendations for international students: Required—TOEFL (minimum score 600 paper-based; 100 iBT), IELTS (minimum score 7). *Application deadline:* For spring admission, 1/31 priority date for domestic and international students. Application fee: $50. Electronic applications accepted. Tuition and fees vary according to program. *Faculty research:* Research design and methodology, health care outcomes and process assessment, organ and tissue transplantation and donation. *Unit head:* Dr. Wishwa Kapoor, Program Director, 412-692-4821, Fax: 412-586-9672, E-mail: kapoorwn@upmc.edu. *Application contact:* Juliana Tambellini, Program Coordinator, 412-692-2686, Fax: 412-586-9672, E-mail: tambellinijm2@upmc.edu. Website: http://www.icre.pitt.edu/phd/

University of Puerto Rico, Medical Sciences Campus, School of Health Professions, Program in Clinical Laboratory Science, San Juan, PR 00936-5067. Offers MS. *Accreditation:* NAACLS. *Program availability:* Part-time, evening/weekend. *Degree requirements:* For master's, one foreign language, thesis or alternative. *Entrance requirements:* For master's, EXADEP or GRE General Test, minimum GPA of 2.75, bachelor's degree in medical technology, 1 year lab experience, interview. *Faculty research:* Toxicology, virology, biochemistry, immunohematology, nervous system regeneration.

University of Puerto Rico, Medical Sciences Campus, School of Health Professions, Program in Cytotechnology, San Juan, PR 00936-5067. Offers Certificate. *Degree requirements:* For Certificate, one foreign language, research project. *Entrance requirements:* For degree, minimum GPA of 2.5, interview.

University of Puerto Rico, Medical Sciences Campus, School of Health Professions, Program in Medical Technology, San Juan, PR 00936-5067. Offers Certificate. *Program availability:* Part-time. *Degree requirements:* For Certificate, one foreign language, clinical practice. *Entrance requirements:* For degree, bachelor's degree in science, minimum GPA of 2.5.

University of Rhode Island, Graduate School, College of the Environment and Life Sciences, Department of Cell and Molecular Biology, Kingston, RI 02881. Offers biochemistry (MS, PhD); clinical laboratory sciences (MS), including biotechnology, clinical laboratory science, cytopathology; microbiology (MS, PhD); molecular genetics (MS, PhD). *Program availability:* Part-time. *Faculty:* 11 full-time (4 women), 1 (woman) part-time/adjunct. *Students:* 12 full-time (6 women), 36 part-time (27 women); includes 10 minority (4 Black or African American, non-Hispanic/Latino; 3 Asian, non-Hispanic/Latino; 2 Hispanic/Latino; 1 Two or more races, non-Hispanic/Latino), 8 international. In 2015, 19 master's, 1 doctorate awarded. *Degree requirements:* For master's,

comprehensive exam (for some programs), thesis optional; for doctorate, comprehensive exam, thesis/dissertation. *Entrance requirements:* For master's and doctorate, GRE, 2 letters of recommendation. Additional exam requirements/recommendations for international students: Required—TOEFL (minimum score 550 paper-based). *Application deadline:* For fall admission, 7/15 for domestic students, 2/1 for international students; for spring admission, 11/15 for domestic students, 7/15 for international students. Application fee: $65. Electronic applications accepted. *Expenses:* Tuition, state resident: full-time $11,796; part-time $655 per credit. Tuition, nonresident: full-time $24,206; part-time $1345 per credit. *Required fees:* $1546; $44 per credit. One-time fee: $155 full-time; $35 part-time. *Financial support:* In 2015–16, 3 research assistantships with tuition reimbursements (averaging $13,507 per year), 8 teaching assistantships with tuition reimbursements (averaging $13,305 per year) were awarded; traineeships also available. Financial award application deadline: 2/1; financial award applicants required to submit FAFSA. *Faculty research:* Genomics. *Total annual research expenditures:* $6.7 million. *Unit head:* Dr. Gongqing Sun, Chairperson, 401-874-5937, Fax: 401-874-2202, E-mail: gsun@mail.uri.edu. *Application contact:* Graduate Admissions, 401-874-2872, E-mail: gradadm@etal.uri.edu. Website: http://cels.uri.edu/cmb/

University of Southern Mississippi, Graduate School, College of Health, Department of Medical Laboratory Science, Hattiesburg, MS 39406-0001. Offers MLS. *Accreditation:* NAACLS. *Program availability:* Part-time, online learning. *Degree requirements:* For master's, comprehensive exam, thesis (for some programs). *Entrance requirements:* For master's, GRE General Test, minimum GPA of 2.75. Additional exam requirements/recommendations for international students: Required—TOEFL, IELTS. Electronic applications accepted. *Faculty research:* Clinical chemistry, clinical microbiology, hematology, clinical management and education, immunohematology.

The University of Tennessee Health Science Center, College of Graduate Health Sciences, Memphis, TN 38163-0002. Offers biomedical engineering (MS, PhD); biomedical sciences (PhD); dental sciences (MDS); epidemiology (MS); health outcomes and policy research (PhD); laboratory research and management (MS); nursing science (PhD); pharmaceutical sciences (PhD); pharmacology (MS); speech and hearing science (PhD); DDS/PhD; DNP/PhD; MD/PhD; Pharm D/PhD. Terminal master's awarded for partial completion of doctoral program. *Degree requirements:* For master's, comprehensive exam, thesis; for doctorate, comprehensive exam, thesis/dissertation, oral and written preliminary and comprehensive exams. *Entrance requirements:* For master's and doctorate, GRE General Test, minimum GPA of 3.0. Additional exam requirements/recommendations for international students: Required—TOEFL (minimum score 79 iBT); Recommended—IELTS (minimum score 6.5). Electronic applications accepted.

The University of Tennessee Health Science Center, College of Health Professions, Memphis, TN 38163-0002. Offers audiology (MS, Au D); clinical laboratory science (MSCLS); cytopathology practice (MCP); health informatics and information management (MHIIM); occupational therapy (MOT); physical therapy (DPT, ScDPT); physician assistant (MMS); speech-language pathology (MS). *Accreditation:* AOTA; APTA. *Program availability:* Part-time, evening/weekend, online learning. Terminal master's awarded for partial completion of doctoral program. *Degree requirements:* For master's, comprehensive exam, thesis; for doctorate, comprehensive exam, residency. *Entrance requirements:* For master's, GRE (MOT, MSCLS), minimum GPA of 3.0, 3 letters of reference, national accreditation (MSCLS), GRE if GPA is less than 3.0 (MCP); for doctorate, GRE. Additional exam requirements/recommendations for international students: Required—TOEFL (minimum score 550 paper-based; 80 iBT). Electronic applications accepted. *Expenses:* Contact institution. *Faculty research:* Gait deviation, muscular dystrophy and strength, hemophilia and exercise, pediatric neurology, self-efficacy.

The University of Texas at Austin, Graduate School, College of Pharmacy, Graduate Programs in Pharmacy, Austin, TX 78712-1111. Offers health outcomes and pharmacy practice (PhD); health outcomes and pharmacy practice (MS); medicinal chemistry (PhD); pharmaceutics (PhD); pharmacology and toxicology (PhD); pharmacotherapy (MS, PhD); translational science (PhD). PhD in translational science offered jointly with The University of Texas Health Science Center at San Antonio and The University of Texas at San Antonio. *Degree requirements:* For master's, thesis; for doctorate, thesis/dissertation. *Entrance requirements:* For master's and doctorate, GRE General Test. Electronic applications accepted. *Faculty research:* Synthetic medical chemistry, synthetic molecular biology, bio-organic chemistry, pharmacoeconomics, pharmacy practice.

The University of Texas Health Science Center at San Antonio, Graduate School of Biomedical Sciences, Translational Science Program, San Antonio, TX 78229-3900. Offers PhD. *Program availability:* Part-time. *Degree requirements:* For doctorate, comprehensive exam, thesis/dissertation.

The University of Texas Medical Branch, Graduate School of Biomedical Sciences, Program in Clinical Science, Galveston, TX 77555. Offers MS, PhD.

University of Utah, School of Medicine and Graduate School, Graduate Programs in Medicine, Department of Pathology, Program in Laboratory Medicine and Biomedical Science, Salt Lake City, UT 84112-1107. Offers MS. *Program availability:* Part-time. *Degree requirements:* For master's, comprehensive exam, thesis, thesis research. *Entrance requirements:* For master's, minimum GPA of 3.0 during last 2 years of undergraduate course work, BS in medical laboratory science or related field. Additional exam requirements/recommendations for international students: Required—TOEFL (minimum score 550 paper-based). *Faculty research:* Clinical chemistry, hematology, diagnostic microbiology, immunohematology, cell biology, immunology.

University of Vermont, College of Medicine and Graduate College, Graduate Programs in Medicine, Program in Clinical and Translational Science, Burlington, VT 05405. Offers MS, PhD, Certificate. *Entrance requirements:* For master's and doctorate, GRE. Additional exam requirements/recommendations for international students: Recommended—TOEFL (minimum score 550 paper-based; 80 iBT). *Application deadline:* For fall admission, 5/1 for domestic and international students. Applications are processed on a rolling basis. Application fee: $65. Electronic applications accepted. *Financial support:* Teaching assistantships available. *Unit head:* Dr. Alan Rubin, Director, 802-656-8228, E-mail: alan.rubin@uvm.edu. *Application contact:* Dr. Alan Rubin, Director, 802-656-8228, E-mail: alan.rubin@uvm.edu.

University of Washington, Graduate School, School of Medicine, Graduate Programs in Medicine, Department of Laboratory Medicine, Seattle, WA 98195. Offers MS. *Accreditation:* NAACLS. *Program availability:* Part-time. *Degree requirements:* For master's, thesis. *Entrance requirements:* For master's, GRE General Test, medical technology certification or specialist in an area of laboratory medicine.

Virginia Commonwealth University, Graduate School, School of Allied Health Professions, Department of Clinical Laboratory Sciences, Richmond, VA 23284-9005. Offers MS. *Accreditation:* NAACLS. *Degree requirements:* For master's, one foreign language, thesis. *Entrance requirements:* For master's, GRE General Test, major in clinical laboratory sciences, biology, or chemistry; minimum GPA of 2.7. Additional exam requirements/recommendations for international students: Required—TOEFL (minimum score 600 paper-based; 100 iBT); Recommended—IELTS (minimum score 6.5).

Electronic applications accepted. *Faculty research:* Educational outcomes assessment, virtual instrumentation development, cost-effective treatment of bacteremia using third generation cephalosporins.

Virginia Commonwealth University, Graduate School, School of Allied Health Professions, Doctoral Program in Health Related Sciences, Richmond, VA 23284-9005. Offers clinical laboratory sciences (PhD); gerontology (PhD); health administration (PhD); nurse anesthesia (PhD); occupational therapy (PhD); physical therapy (PhD); radiation sciences (PhD); rehabilitation leadership (PhD). *Entrance requirements:* For doctorate, GRE General Test or MAT, minimum GPA of 3.3 in master's degree. Additional exam requirements/recommendations for international students: Required—TOEFL (minimum score 600 paper-based; 100 iBT); Recommended—IELTS (minimum score 6.5). Electronic applications accepted.

Clinical Research

Albert Einstein College of Medicine, Graduate Division of Biomedical Sciences, Clinical Investigation Program, Bronx, NY 10461. Offers PhD.

American University of Health Sciences, School of Clinical Research, Signal Hill, CA 90755. Offers MSCR.

Augusta University, College of Allied Health Sciences, Program in Clinical Laboratory Sciences, Augusta, GA 30912. Offers MHS. Application fee: $50. *Unit head:* Dr. Barbara J. Kraj, Director, 706-721-3785, E-mail: bkraj@augusta.edu. *Application contact:* Jan Bane, Admissions Coordinator, 706-721-4176, E-mail: janb@augusta.edu.
Website: http://www.augusta.edu/alliedhealth/mlirs/cls/

Booton Univercity, School of Medicine, Division of Graduate Medical Sciences, Program in Clinical Investigation, Boston, MA 02215. Offers MA. *Degree requirements:* For master's, thesis. *Application deadline:* For spring admission, 10/15 for domestic students. *Unit head:* Dr. Susan S. Fish, Director, 617-638-7715, E-mail: sfish@bu.edu. *Application contact:* Stacey Hess Pino, GMS Admissions Office, 617-638-5255, E-mail: askgms@bu.edu.
Website: http://www.bumc.bu.edu/gms/maci/

Case Western Reserve University, School of Medicine, Clinical Research Scholars Program, Cleveland, OH 44106. Offers MS. *Expenses: Tuition, area resident:* Full-time $41,137; part-time $1714 per credit hour. *Required fees:* $32. Tuition and fees vary according to course load and program.

Clemson University, Graduate School, College of Behavioral, Social and Health Sciences, Department of Public Health Sciences, Clemson, SC 29634-0745. Offers applied health research and evaluation (MS, PhD); clinical and translational research (Certificate). *Program availability:* Part-time. *Faculty:* 21 full-time (9 women), 7 part-time/ adjunct (all women). *Students:* 10 full-time (6 women); includes 2 minority (both Asian, non-Hispanic/Latino). Average age 33. 7 applicants, 29% accepted, 1 enrolled. *Degree requirements:* For doctorate, comprehensive exam, thesis/dissertation. *Entrance requirements:* For master's and Certificate, GRE General Test, curriculum vitae, statement of career goals, letters of recommendation, unofficial transcripts; for doctorate, GRE General Test, MS/MA thesis or publications, curriculum vitae, statement of career goals, letters of recommendation, unofficial transcripts. Additional exam requirements/recommendations for international students: Required—TOEFL (minimum score 80 iBT), IELTS (minimum score 6.5). *Application deadline:* For fall admission, 4/15 for international students; for spring admission, 10/15 for international students. Applications are processed on a rolling basis. Application fee: $80 ($90 for international students). Electronic applications accepted. *Expenses:* $4,060 per semester full-time resident, $8,103 per semester full-time non-resident, $448 per credit hour part-time resident, $898 per credit hour part-time non-resident. *Financial support:* In 2015–16, 3 students received support, including 1 research assistantship with partial tuition reimbursement available (averaging $24,192 per year), 3 teaching assistantships with partial tuition reimbursements available (averaging $12,000 per year). *Faculty research:* Health promotion and behavior, epidemiology and outcomes research, public health informatics, health policy and health services research, global health, evaluation. *Unit head:* Dr. Joel Williams, Director of Graduate Studies/PhD Program Coordinator, 864-656-1017, E-mail: joel2@clemson.edu. *Application contact:* Rebecca Moses, Graduate Student Services Coordinator, 864-656-5502, E-mail: coffey2@clemson.edu.
Website: http://www.clemson.edu/hehd/departments/public-health/academics/graduate-programs/index.html

Duke University, School of Medicine, Clinical Research Program, Durham, NC 27710. Offers MHS. *Program availability:* Part-time. *Faculty:* 20 part-time/adjunct (5 women). *Students:* 11 full-time (5 women), 79 part-time (41 women); includes 20 minority (4 Black or African American, non-Hispanic/Latino; 16 Asian, non-Hispanic/Latino), 13 international. 53 applicants, 100% accepted, 53 enrolled. In 2015, 17 master's awarded. *Degree requirements:* For master's, research project. *Entrance requirements:* For master's, GRE. Additional exam requirements/recommendations for international students: Required—TOEFL, IELTS. *Application deadline:* For fall admission, 5/15 for domestic students. *Financial support:* Fellowships, research assistantships, teaching assistantships, and scholarships/grants available. Financial award application deadline: 5/1; financial award applicants required to submit FAFSA. *Unit head:* Dr. Steven C. Grambow, Director, 919-684-1292, Fax: 919-681-4569, E-mail: steven.grambow@duke.edu. *Application contact:* Gail Ladd, Program Coordinator, 919-681-4560, Fax: 919-681-4569, E-mail: gail.ladd@duke.edu.
Website: http://crtp.mc.duke.edu/

Eastern Michigan University, Graduate School, College of Health and Human Services, School of Health Sciences, Programs in Clinical Research Administration, Ypsilanti, MI 48197. Offers MS, Graduate Certificate. *Program availability:* Part-time, evening/weekend, online learning. *Students:* 7 full-time (6 women), 22 part-time (17 women); includes 3 minority (1 Black or African American, non-Hispanic/Latino; 2 Asian, non-Hispanic/Latino), 16 international. Average age 33. 31 applicants, 77% accepted, 13 enrolled. In 2015, 11 master's awarded. *Entrance requirements:* Additional exam requirements/recommendations for international students: Required—TOEFL. *Application deadline:* Applications are processed on a rolling basis. Application fee: $45. *Financial support:* Fellowships, research assistantships with full tuition reimbursements, teaching assistantships with full tuition reimbursements, career-related internships or fieldwork, Federal Work-Study, institutionally sponsored loans, scholarships/grants, tuition waivers (partial), and unspecified assistantships available. Support available to part-time students. Financial award applicants required to submit FAFSA. *Application contact:* Dr. Stephen Sonstein, Program Director, 734-487-1238, Fax: 734-487-4095, E-mail: stephen.sonstein@emich.edu.

Emory University, Laney Graduate School, Program in Clinical Research, Atlanta, GA 30322-1100. Offers MS. *Degree requirements:* For master's, thesis. *Entrance requirements:* Additional exam requirements/recommendations for international students: Recommended—TOEFL. Electronic applications accepted.

Fordham University, Graduate School of Arts and Sciences, Department of Psychology, New York, NY 10458. Offers applied developmental psychology (PhD); applied psychological methods (MS), including applied psychology methods; clinical psychology (PhD); clinical research methodology (MS); psychometrics (PhD). *Faculty:* 25 full-time (8 women), 3 part-time/adjunct (2 women). *Students:* 94 full-time (70 women), 21 part-time (14 women); includes 23 minority (9 Black or African American, non-Hispanic/Latino; 1 American Indian or Alaska Native, non-Hispanic/Latino; 13 Asian, non-Hispanic/Latino), 15 international. Average age 31. 981 applicants, 6% accepted, 24 enrolled. In 2015, 15 master's, 15 doctorates awarded. Terminal master's awarded for partial completion of doctoral program. *Degree requirements:* For master's, comprehensive exam; for doctorate, comprehensive exam, thesis/dissertation. *Entrance requirements:* For doctorate, GRE General Test, GRE Subject Test. Additional exam requirements/recommendations for international students: Required—TOEFL (minimum score 600 paper-based). *Application deadline:* For fall admission, 12/14 for domestic students. Application fee: $70. Electronic applications accepted. *Financial support:* In 2015–16, 73 students received support, including 16 fellowships with tuition reimbursements available (averaging $24,561 per year), 12 research assistantships with tuition reimbursements available (averaging $15,170 per year), 11 teaching assistantships with tuition reimbursements available (averaging $12,286 per year); career-related internships or fieldwork, institutionally sponsored loans, tuition waivers (full and partial), and unspecified assistantships also available. Financial award application deadline: 12/14; financial award applicants required to submit FAFSA. *Total annual research expenditures:* $2.8 million. *Unit head:* Dr. Barry Rosenfeld, Chair, 718-817-3794, Fax: 718-817-3699, E-mail: rosenfeld@fordham.edu. *Application contact:* Bernadette Valentino-Morrison, Director of Graduate Admissions, 718-817-4419, Fax: 718-817-3566, E-mail: valentinomor@fordham.edu.

Icahn School of Medicine at Mount Sinai, Graduate School of Biomedical Sciences, New York, NY 10029-6504. Offers biomedical sciences (MS, PhD); clinical research education (MS, PhD); community medicine (MPH); genetic counseling (MS); neurosciences (PhD); MD/PhD. Terminal master's awarded for partial completion of doctoral program. *Degree requirements:* For master's, thesis; for doctorate, comprehensive exam, thesis/dissertation. *Entrance requirements:* For master's, GRE General Test; for doctorate, GRE General Test, GRE Subject Test, 3 years of college pre-med course work. Additional exam requirements/recommendations for international students: Required—TOEFL. Electronic applications accepted. *Faculty research:* Cancer, genetics and genomics, immunology, neuroscience, developmental and stem cell biology, translational research.

Johns Hopkins University, Bloomberg School of Public Health, Graduate Training Program in Clinical Investigation, Baltimore, MD 21287. Offers MHS, Sc M, PhD. *Degree requirements:* For master's, comprehensive exam, thesis; for doctorate, comprehensive exam, thesis/dissertation. *Entrance requirements:* For master's, GRE or MCAT; United States Medical Licensing Exam, 2 letters of recommendation, curriculum vitae, transcripts, statement of purpose; for doctorate, GRE or MCAT; United States Medical Licensing Exam, 2 letters of recommendation, curriculum vitae. Additional exam requirements/recommendations for international students: Required—TOEFL (minimum score 600 paper-based). Electronic applications accepted. *Faculty research:* Ethical issues, biomedical writing, grant writing, epidemiology, biostatistics.

Loyola University Chicago, Graduate School, Program in Clinical Research Methods, Chicago, IL 60660. Offers MS. *Program availability:* Part-time. *Faculty:* 5 full-time (2 women). *Students:* 9 part-time (6 women); includes 2 minority (both Asian, non-Hispanic/Latino), 1 international. Average age 33. 8 applicants, 50% accepted, 3 enrolled. In 2015, 4 master's awarded. *Degree requirements:* For master's, research project. *Entrance requirements:* For master's, MCAT; GRE. *Application deadline:* For fall admission, 5/15 for domestic students, 5/1 for international students; for spring admission, 12/15 for domestic students, 12/1 for international students. Applications are processed on a rolling basis. Electronic applications accepted. *Expenses: Tuition, area resident:* Full-time $18,054; part-time $9027 per credit hour. *Required fees:* $832; $284 per credit hour. Part-time tuition and fees vary according to course load, degree level and program. *Financial support:* Applicants required to submit FAFSA. *Faculty research:* Genetics of hypertension and obesity, vitamin D metabolism, kidney diseases. *Unit head:* Dr. Samuel Attoh, Dean, 773-508-3459, Fax: 773-508-2460, E-mail: sattoh@luc.edu. *Application contact:* Ron Martin, Assistant Director of Enrollment Management, 312-915-8950, Fax: 312-915-8905, E-mail: gradapp@luc.edu.

Medical College of Wisconsin, Graduate School of Biomedical Sciences, Medical Scientist Training Program, Milwaukee, WI 53226-0509. Offers MD/PhD. *Entrance requirements:* Additional exam requirements/recommendations for international students: Required—TOEFL.

Medical University of South Carolina, College of Graduate Studies, South Carolina Clinical and Translational Research Institute, Charleston, SC 29425-5010. Offers MS. *Program availability:* Online learning. *Degree requirements:* For master's, thesis, oral dissertation of grant proposal. *Entrance requirements:* For master's, essay, letter of support. Additional exam requirements/recommendations for international students: Required—TOEFL (minimum score 600 paper-based; 100 iBT). Electronic applications accepted. *Faculty research:* Cardiovascular epidemiology/hypertension, cystic fibrosis, comparative effectivenessstudies, community-engaged research.

Memorial University of Newfoundland, Faculty of Medicine and School of Graduate Studies, Graduate Programs in Medicine, Division of Applied Health Services Research, St. John's, NL A1C 5S7, Canada. Offers M Sc. *Expenses: Tuition, area resident:* Full-time $2199 Canadian dollars. *International tuition:* $2859 Canadian dollars full-time.

Morehouse School of Medicine, Master of Science in Clinical Research Program, Atlanta, GA 30310-1495. Offers MS. *Program availability:* Part-time. *Degree requirements:* For master's, thesis. *Application deadline:* For fall admission, 4/6 for domestic and international students. Application fee: $50. Electronic applications accepted. *Financial support:* Applicants required to submit FAFSA. *Unit head:* Dr. Alexander Quarshie, Co-Director, 404-752-7681, E-mail: aquarshie@msm.edu. *Application contact:* Brandon Hunter, Director of Admissions, 404-752-1650, Fax: 404-752-1512, E-mail: bhunter@msm.edu.
Website: http://www.msm.edu/Education/GEBS/MSCR/index.php

Clinical Research

New York University, College of Dentistry, Program in Clinical Research, New York, NY 10010. Offers MS. *Program availability:* Part-time. *Entrance requirements:* For master's, GRE. Additional exam requirements/recommendations for international students: Required—TOEFL (minimum score 570 paper-based; 90 iBT). Electronic applications accepted.

Northwestern University, Feinberg School of Medicine, Program in Clinical Investigation, Evanston, IL 60208. Offers MSCI. *Program availability:* Part-time, evening/weekend. *Entrance requirements:* For master's, GRE or MCAT, doctoral degree in healthcare-related field. Additional exam requirements/recommendations for international students: Required—TOEFL. Electronic applications accepted. *Faculty research:* Clinical research.

Northwestern University, The Graduate School, Program in Clinical Investigation, Evanston, IL 60208. Offers MSCI, Certificate. *Program availability:* Part-time, evening/weekend.

Northwestern University, School of Professional Studies, Program in Regulatory Compliance, Evanston, IL 60208. Offers clinical research (MS); healthcare compliance (MS); quality systems (MS). Offered in partnership with Northwestern Univesity's Clinical and Translational Sciences Institute.

Oregon Health & Science University, School of Medicine, Graduate Programs in Medicine, Human Investigations Program, Portland, OR 97239-3098. Offers clinical research (MCR, Certificate). MCR program only open to those currently enrolled in the certificate program. *Program availability:* Part-time. *Faculty:* 7 part-time/adjunct (4 women). *Students:* 115 part-time (71 women); includes 29 minority (2 Black or African American, non-Hispanic/Latino; 23 Asian, non-Hispanic/Latino; 3 Hispanic/Latino; 1 Two or more races, non-Hispanic/Latino), 4 international. Average age 35. 81 applicants, 36% accepted, 28 enrolled. In 2015, 14 master's, 12 Certificates awarded. *Entrance requirements:* For master's and Certificate, MD, MD/PhD, DO, DDS, DMD, DC, Pharm D, OD, ND or PhD with clinical responsibilities or patient-oriented research; faculty or staff member, clinical or post-doctoral fellows and graduate students at OHSU, Kaiser Permanente, Portland VA Medical Center or other health care facilities in Oregon or the Northwest. *Application deadline:* For fall admission, 7/15 for domestic students; for winter admission, 12/15 for domestic students; for spring admission, 3/15 for domestic students. Applications are processed on a rolling basis. Electronic applications accepted. *Faculty research:* Clinical and translational research. *Unit head:* Dr. Cynthia Morris, Director, 503-494-3095, Fax: 503-494-5128, E-mail: morrisc@ohsu.edu. *Application contact:* Karen McCracken, Education Program Coordinator, 503-494-3095, Fax: 503-494-5128, E-mail: hip@ohsu.edu.
Website: http://www.ohsu.edu/hip

Palmer College of Chiropractic, Division of Graduate Studies, Davenport, IA 52803-5287. Offers clinical research (MS). *Faculty:* 8 full-time (3 women), 3 part-time/adjunct (2 women). *Students:* 7 full-time (2 women), 1 (woman) part-time; includes 1 minority (Black or African American, non-Hispanic/Latino). 3 applicants, 100% accepted, 3 enrolled. In 2015, 5 master's awarded. *Degree requirements:* For master's, 2 mentored practicum projects. *Entrance requirements:* For master's, GRE General Test, minimum GPA of 2.5, bachelor's and doctoral-level health professions degrees. Additional exam requirements/recommendations for international students: Required—TOEFL. *Application deadline:* For fall admission, 8/1 for domestic and international students; for spring admission, 5/28 for domestic students. Applications are processed on a rolling basis. Application fee: $50. Electronic applications accepted. *Expenses:* Contact institution. *Financial support:* In 2015–16, 7 students received support, including 7 research assistantships with full tuition reimbursements available (averaging $30,000 per year), teaching assistantships with tuition reimbursements available (averaging $6,269 per year); tuition waivers (full) and unspecified assistantships also available. Financial award application deadline: 8/1; financial award applicants required to submit FAFSA. *Faculty research:* Chiropractic clinical research. *Unit head:* Dr. Dan Weinert, Interim Vice President for Academic Affairs, 563-884-5761, Fax: 563-884-5624, E-mail: weinert_d@palmer.edu. *Application contact:* Lori Byrd, Program Coordinator, 563-884-5198, Fax: 563-884-5227, E-mail: lori.byrd@plamer.edu.

Stanford University, School of Medicine, Graduate Programs in Medicine, Department of Health Research and Policy, Program in Epidemiology and Clinical Research, Stanford, CA 94305-9991. Offers MS, PhD. *Degree requirements:* For master's, thesis; for doctorate, thesis/dissertation, qualifying examinations. *Entrance requirements:* For doctorate, GRE General Test or MCAT. Additional exam requirements/recommendations for international students: Required—TOEFL. Electronic applications accepted. *Expenses:* Tuition, area resident: Full-time $45,729. *Required fees:* $591.

Thomas Jefferson University, Jefferson College of Biomedical Sciences, Graduate Certificate Programs, Philadelphia, PA 19107. Offers clinical research and trials: implementation (Certificate); clinical research: operations (Certificate); human clinical investigation: theory (Certificate). *Program availability:* Part-time. *Faculty:* 44 full-time (14 women), 27 part-time/adjunct (11 women). *Students:* 7 part-time (6 women); includes 1 minority (Black or African American, non-Hispanic/Latino), 1 international. Average age 36. 4 applicants, 100% accepted, 4 enrolled. In 2015, 1 Certificate awarded. *Entrance requirements:* For degree, GRE General Test (recommended). Additional exam requirements/recommendations for international students: Required—TOEFL, IELTS (minimum score 7). *Application deadline:* For fall admission, 8/1 priority date for domestic students, 3/1 priority date for international students; for winter admission, 12/1 priority date for domestic students, 6/1 priority date for international students; for spring admission, 4/1 priority date for domestic students. Applications are processed on a rolling basis. Application fee: $50. *Financial support:* Federal Work-Study and institutionally sponsored loans available. Support available to part-time students. Financial award application deadline: 5/1; financial award applicants required to submit FAFSA. *Faculty research:* Epidemiology, clinical research, statistics, planning and management, disease control. *Unit head:* Dr. Dennis M. Gross, Associate Dean, 215-503-0156, Fax: 215-503-3433, E-mail: dennis.gross@jefferson.edu. *Application contact:* Marc E. Stearns, Director of Admissions, 215-503-0155, Fax: 215-503-3433, E-mail: jgsbs-info@jefferson.edu.
Website: http://www.jefferson.edu/university/biomedical-sciences/degrees-programs/graduate-certificate.html

Thomas Jefferson University, Jefferson College of Biomedical Sciences, MS Program in Clinical Research, Philadelphia, PA 19107. Offers MS. *Program availability:* Part-time, evening/weekend. *Degree requirements:* For master's, thesis, clerkship. *Entrance requirements:* For master's, GRE General Test or MCAT, minimum GPA of 3.0. Additional exam requirements/recommendations for international students: Required—TOEFL, IELTS (minimum score 7). *Application deadline:* For fall admission, 8/1 priority date for domestic students, 3/1 priority date for international students; for winter admission, 12/1 priority date for domestic students, 6/1 priority date for international students; for spring admission, 4/1 priority date for domestic students. Applications are processed on a rolling basis. Application fee: $50. Electronic applications accepted. *Financial support:* Federal Work-Study and institutionally sponsored loans available. Support available to part-time students. Financial award application deadline: 5/1; financial award applicants required to submit FAFSA. *Unit head:* Dr. Carol L. Beck, Associate Dean/Program Director, 215-503-6539, Fax: 215-503-3433, E-mail:

carol.beck@jefferson.edu. *Application contact:* Marc E. Stearns, Director of Admissions, 215-503-0155, Fax: 215-503-3433, E-mail: jgsbs-info@jefferson.edu.
Website: http://www.jefferson.edu/university/biomedical-sciences/degrees-programs/master-programs/clinical-research-MS.html

Trident University International, College of Health Sciences, Program in Health Sciences, Cypress, CA 90630. Offers clinical research administration (MS, Certificate); emergency and disaster management (MS, Certificate); environmental health science (Certificate); health care administration (PhD); health care management (MS), including health informatics; health education (MS, Certificate); health informatics (Certificate); health sciences (PhD); international health (MS); international health: educator or researcher option (PhD); international health: practitioner option (PhD); law and expert witness studies (MS, Certificate); public health (MS); quality assurance (Certificate). *Program availability:* Part-time, evening/weekend, online learning. *Degree requirements:* For doctorate, comprehensive exam, thesis/dissertation, defense of dissertation. *Entrance requirements:* For master's, minimum GPA of 2.5 (students with GPA 3.0 or greater may transfer up to 30% of graduate level credits); for doctorate, minimum GPA of 3.4, curriculum vitae, course work in research methods or statistics. Additional exam requirements/recommendations for international students: Required—TOEFL. Electronic applications accepted.

Tufts University, Sackler School of Graduate Biomedical Sciences, Clinical and Translational Science Program, Medford, MA 02155. Offers MS, PhD, Certificate. *Faculty:* 34 full-time (10 women). *Students:* 20 full-time (13 women), 1 part-time; includes 4 minority (1 Black or African American, non-Hispanic/Latino; 3 Asian, non-Hispanic/Latino), 4 international. Average age 37. 34 applicants, 47% accepted, 11 enrolled. In 2015, 3 master's, 3 doctorates, 4 other advanced degrees awarded. *Degree requirements:* For master's, thesis; for doctorate, comprehensive exam, thesis/dissertation. *Entrance requirements:* For master's, MD or PhD, strong clinical research background. Additional exam requirements/recommendations for international students: Required—TOEFL (minimum score 600 paper-based; 100 iBT). *Application deadline:* For fall admission, 4/15 for domestic and international students. Applications are processed on a rolling basis. Application fee: $90. Electronic applications accepted. *Expenses:* $26,964 per year tuition and fees. *Faculty research:* Clinical study design, mathematical modeling, meta analysis, epidemiologic research, coronary heart disease. *Unit head:* Dr. David Kent, Program Director, 617-636-3234, Fax: 617-636-8023, E-mail: dkent@tuftsmedicalcenter.edu. *Application contact:* Kellie Melchin, Associate Director of Admissions, 617-636-6767, Fax: 617-636-0375, E-mail: sackler-school@tufts.edu.
Website: http://sackler.tufts.edu/Academics/Degree-Programs/Clinical-and-Translational-Science

University of California, Berkeley, UC Berkeley Extension, Certificate Programs in Sciences, Biotechnology and Mathematics, Berkeley, CA 94720-1500. Offers clinical research conduct and management (Certificate). *Program availability:* Online learning.

University of California, Davis, Graduate Studies, Graduate Group in Clinical Research, Davis, CA 95616. Offers MAS. *Degree requirements:* For master's, comprehensive exam. *Entrance requirements:* Additional exam requirements/recommendations for international students: Required—TOEFL (minimum score 550 paper-based).

University of California, Los Angeles, David Geffen School of Medicine and Graduate Division, Graduate Programs in Medicine, Department of Biomathematics, Program in Clinical Research, Los Angeles, CA 90095. Offers MS. *Degree requirements:* For master's, thesis. *Entrance requirements:* For master's, GRE General Test, bachelor's degree; minimum undergraduate GPA of 3.0 (or its equivalent if letter grade system not used). Additional exam requirements/recommendations for international students: Required—TOEFL. Electronic applications accepted.

University of California, San Diego, School of Medicine, Program in Clinical Research, La Jolla, CA 92093. Offers MAS. *Program availability:* Part-time, evening/weekend. *Students:* 2 full-time (both women), 50 part-time (23 women); includes 20 minority (1 Black or African American, non-Hispanic/Latino; 9 Asian, non-Hispanic/Latino; 10 Hispanic/Latino), 14 international. 50 applicants, 60% accepted, 28 enrolled. In 2015, 40 master's awarded. *Degree requirements:* For master's, independent study project. *Entrance requirements:* For master's, minimum GPA of 3.0, advanced degree (recommended). Additional exam requirements/recommendations for international students: Required—TOEFL (minimum score 80 iBT), IELTS. *Application deadline:* For winter admission, 9/30 for domestic students; for summer admission, 3/29 for domestic students. Application fee: $90 ($110 for international students). Electronic applications accepted. *Expenses:* Contact institution. *Financial support:* Scholarships/grants available. Financial award applicants required to submit FAFSA. *Faculty research:* Epidemiology, bio-statistics, quantitative analysis, health services. *Unit head:* Ravindra Mehta, Chair, 619-543-7310, E-mail: rmehta@ucsd.edu. *Application contact:* Tam Nguyen, Graduate Coordinator, 858-534-9164, E-mail: clre@ucsd.edu.
Website: http://clre.ucsd.edu/

University of Colorado Denver, School of Medicine, Clinical Science Graduate Program, Aurora, CO 80045. Offers clinical investigation (PhD); clinical sciences (MS); health information technology (PhD); health services research (PhD). *Students:* 38 full-time (28 women), 35 part-time (22 women); includes 12 minority (3 Black or African American, non-Hispanic/Latino; 1 American Indian or Alaska Native, non-Hispanic/Latino; 4 Asian, non-Hispanic/Latino; 2 Hispanic/Latino; 2 Two or more races, non-Hispanic/Latino), 1 international. Average age 37. 22 applicants, 68% accepted, 15 enrolled. In 2015, 13 master's, 2 doctorates awarded. *Degree requirements:* For master's, thesis, minimum of 30 credit hours, defense/final exam of thesis or publishable paper; for doctorate, comprehensive exam, thesis/dissertation, at least 30 credit hours of thesis work. *Entrance requirements:* For master's, GRE General Test or MCAT (waived if candidate has earned MS/MA or PhD from accredited U.S. school), minimum undergraduate GPA of 3.0, 3-4 letters of recommendation; for doctorate, GRE General Test or MCAT (waived if candidate has earned MS/MA or PhD from accredited U.S. school), health care graduate, professional degree, or graduate degree related to health sciences; minimum GPA of 3.0; 3-4 letters of recommendation. Additional exam requirements/recommendations for international students: Required—TOEFL (minimum score 550 paper-based; 80 iBT). *Application deadline:* For fall admission, 2/1 for domestic students, 1/15 priority date for international students; for spring admission, 10/1 for domestic students. Application fee: $50 ($75 for international students). Electronic applications accepted. *Expenses:* Contact institution. *Financial support:* In 2015–16, 34 students received support. Fellowships, research assistantships, teaching assistantships, Federal Work-Study, institutionally sponsored loans, scholarships/grants, traineeships, and unspecified assistantships available. Financial award application deadline: 3/15; financial award applicants required to submit FAFSA. *Unit head:* Dr. Lisa Cicutto, Program Director, 303-398-1539, E-mail: cicuttol@njhealth.org. *Application contact:* Galit Mankin, Program Administrator, 720-848-6249, Fax: 303-848-7381, E-mail: galit.mankin@ucdenver.edu.
Website: http://www.ucdenver.edu/research/CCTSI/education-training/clsc/Pages/default.aspx

University of Connecticut Health Center, Graduate School, Program in Clinical and Translational Research, Farmington, CT 06030. Offers MS. *Program availability:* Part-time. *Entrance requirements:* For master's, GRE. Additional exam requirements/recommendations for international students: Required—TOEFL (minimum score 600 paper-based).

University of Florida, College of Medicine, Program in Clinical Investigation, Gainesville, FL 32611. Offers clinical investigation (MS); epidemiology (MS); public health (MPH). *Program availability:* Part-time. *Entrance requirements:* For master's, GRE, MD, PhD, DMD/DDS or Pharm D.

University of Florida, Graduate School, College of Engineering, J. Crayton Pruitt Family Department of Biomedical Engineering, Gainesville, FL 32611. Offers biomedical engineering (ME, MS, PhD, Certificate); clinical and translational science (PhD); medical physics (MS, PhD); MD/PhD. *Faculty:* 21 full-time, 19 part-time/adjunct. *Students:* 156 full-time (59 women), 13 part-time (3 women); includes 32 minority (5 Black or African American, non-Hispanic/Latino; 10 Asian, non-Hispanic/Latino; 17 Hispanic/Latino), 40 international. Average age 26. 304 applicants, 63% accepted, 55 enrolled. In 2015, 35 master's, 18 doctorates awarded. Terminal master's awarded for partial completion of doctoral program. *Degree requirements:* For master's, comprehensive exam (for some programs), thesis (for some programs); for doctorate, comprehensive exam (for some programs), thesis/dissertation (for some programs). *Entrance requirements:* Additional exam requirements/recommendations for international students: Required—TOEFL (minimum score 550 paper-based; 80 iBT), IELTS (minimum score 6). *Application deadline:* For fall admission, 12/15 priority date for domestic students, 12/15 for international students; for spring admission, 7/31 for domestic and international students. Applications are processed on a rolling basis. Application fee: $30. Electronic applications accepted. Fi…ncial support: In 2015–16, 7 fellowships, 75 research assistantships, 1 teaching assistantship were awarded. Financial award application deadline: 12/31; financial award applicants required to submit FAFSA. *Faculty research:* Neural engineering, imaging and medical physics, biomaterials and regenerative medicine, biomedical informatics and modeling. *Total annual research expenditures:* $6.2 million. *Unit head:* Christine E. Schmidt, PhD, Chair, 352-273-9222, Fax: 352-392-9791, E-mail: schmidt@bme.ufl.edu. *Application contact:* Hans Van Oostrom, PhD, Associate Professor/Associate Chair/Graduate Coordinator, 352-273-9315, Fax: 352-392-9221, E-mail: oostrom@ufl.edu.
Website: http://www.bme.ufl.edu/

The University of Iowa, Graduate College, College of Public Health, Department of Epidemiology, Iowa City, IA 52242-1316. Offers clinical investigation (MS); epidemiology (MPH, MS, PhD). *Accreditation:* CEPH. *Degree requirements:* For master's, thesis optional, exam; for doctorate, comprehensive exam, thesis/dissertation. *Entrance requirements:* For master's and doctorate, GRE General Test, minimum GPA of 3.0. Additional exam requirements/recommendations for international students: Required—TOEFL (minimum score 600 paper-based; 100 iBT). Electronic applications accepted.

The University of Kansas, University of Kansas Medical Center, School of Medicine, Department of Preventive Medicine and Public Health, Kansas City, KS 66160. Offers clinical research (MS); environmental health sciences (MPH); epidemiology (MPH); public health management (MPH); social and behavioral health (MPH); MD/MPH; PhD/MPH. *Program availability:* Part-time. *Faculty:* 70. *Students:* 48 full-time (35 women), 46 part-time (31 women); includes 31 minority (9 Black or African American, non-Hispanic/Latino; 4 American Indian or Alaska Native, non-Hispanic/Latino; 8 Asian, non-Hispanic/Latino; 6 Hispanic/Latino; 4 Two or more races, non-Hispanic/Latino), 8 international. Average age 31. 66 applicants, 68% accepted, 44 enrolled. In 2015, 31 master's awarded. *Degree requirements:* For master's, thesis, capstone practicum defense. *Entrance requirements:* For master's, GRE, MCAT, LSAT, GMAT or other equivalent graduate professional exam. Additional exam requirements/recommendations for international students: Required—TOEFL. *Application deadline:* For fall admission, 3/1 for domestic and international students. Applications are processed on a rolling basis. Application fee: $60. Electronic applications accepted. *Financial support:* In 2015–16, 9 research assistantships (averaging $15,000 per year) were awarded; career-related internships or fieldwork, Federal Work-Study, scholarships/grants, and unspecified assistantships also available. Support available to part-time students. Financial award application deadline: 3/1; financial award applicants required to submit FAFSA. *Faculty research:* Cancer screening and prevention, smoking cessation, obesity and physical activity, health services/outcomes research, health disparities. *Total annual research expenditures:* $6.6 million. *Unit head:* Dr. Edward F. Ellerbeck, Chairman, 913-588-2774, Fax: 913-588-2780, E-mail: eellerbe@kumc.edu. *Application contact:* Tanya Honderick, MPH Director, 913-588-2720, Fax: 913-588-8505, E-mail: thonderick@kumc.edu.
Website: http://www.kumc.edu/school-of-medicine/preventive-medicine-and-public-health.html

University of Kentucky, Graduate School, College of Public Health, Program in Clinical Research Design, Lexington, KY 40506-0032. Offers MS.

University of Louisville, Graduate School, School of Public Health and Information Sciences, Department of Public Health and Information Sciences, Louisville, KY 40202. Offers biostatistics (MS, PhD); clinical investigation (M Sc); epidemiology (MS); health management and systems sciences (MPH); public health sciences (PhD), including environmental health, epidemiology, health management, health promotion; public health sciences - health management (PhD). *Program availability:* Part-time. *Students:* 92 full-time (60 women), 33 part-time (19 women); includes 37 minority (16 Black or African American, non-Hispanic/Latino; 12 Asian, non-Hispanic/Latino; 6 Hispanic/Latino; 3 Two or more races, non-Hispanic/Latino), 19 international. Average age 32. 128 applicants, 77% accepted, 56 enrolled. In 2015, 38 master's, 6 doctorates awarded. *Degree requirements:* For master's, thesis optional; for doctorate, comprehensive exam, thesis/dissertation. *Entrance requirements:* For master's and doctorate, GRE General Test. Additional exam requirements/recommendations for international students: Required—TOEFL (minimum score 600 paper-based; 100 iBT). *Application deadline:* For fall admission, 5/1 for domestic and international students. Application fee: $60. Electronic applications accepted. *Expenses:* Tuition, state resident: full-time $11,664; part-time $649 per credit hour. Tuition, nonresident: full-time $24,274; part-time $1350 per credit hour. *Required fees:* $196. Tuition and fees vary according to program and reciprocity agreements. *Financial support:* In 2015–16, 718,988 students received support. Research assistantships with full tuition reimbursements available, scholarships/grants, health care benefits, and unspecified assistantships available. Financial award applicants required to submit FAFSA. *Faculty research:* Department of environmental and occupational health sciences department of health management and systems sciences department of health promotion and behavioral sciences. *Total annual research expenditures:* $2.1 million. *Unit head:* Dr. Craig Blakely, Dean, 502-852-3297, Fax: 502-852-3291, E-mail: chblak01@louisville.edu.
Website: http://louisville.edu/sphis/departments/health-management-systems-science

University of Maryland, Baltimore, Graduate School, Clinical Research Certificate Program, Baltimore, MD 21201. Offers Postbaccalaureate Certificate. *Entrance requirements:* Additional exam requirements/recommendations for international students: Required—TOEFL (minimum score 550 paper-based; 80 iBT); Recommended—IELTS (minimum score 7). Electronic applications accepted. Tuition and fees vary according to program.

University of Maryland, Baltimore, School of Medicine, Department of Epidemiology and Public Health, Baltimore, MD 21201. Offers biostatistics (MS); clinical research (MS); epidemiology and preventive medicine (MPH, MS, PhD); gerontology (PhD); human genetics and genomic medicine (MS, PhD); molecular epidemiology (MS, PhD); toxicology (MS, PhD); JD/MS; MD/PhD; MS/PhD. *Accreditation:* CEPH. *Program availability:* Part-time. *Students:* 73 full-time (58 women), 56 part-time (32 women); includes 45 minority (23 Black or African American, non-Hispanic/Latino; 12 Asian, non-Hispanic/Latino; 5 Hispanic/Latino; 5 Two or more races, non-Hispanic/Latino), 17 international. Average age 31. In 2015, 34 master's, 17 doctorates awarded. *Degree requirements:* For doctorate, comprehensive exam, thesis/dissertation. *Entrance requirements:* For master's and doctorate, GRE General Test. Additional exam requirements/recommendations for international students: Required—TOEFL (minimum score 550 paper-based; 80 iBT); Recommended—IELTS (minimum score 7). *Application deadline:* For fall admission, 1/15 for domestic and international students. Application fee: $75. Electronic applications accepted. *Expenses:* Contact institution. *Financial support:* In 2015–16, research assistantships with partial tuition reimbursements (averaging $26,000 per year) were awarded; fellowships, Federal Work-Study, scholarships/grants, and unspecified assistantships also available. Financial award application deadline: 3/1; financial award applicants required to submit FAFSA. *Unit head:* Dr. Laura Hungerford, Program Director, 410-706-8492, Fax: 410-706-4225. *Application contact:* Jessica Kelley, Program Coordinator, 410-706-8492, Fax: 410-706-4225, E-mail: jkelley@som.umaryland.edu.
Website: http://lifesciences.umaryland.edu/epidemiology/

University of Massachusetts Medical School, Graduate School of Biomedical Sciences, Worcester, MA 01655-0115. Offers biomedical sciences (PhD), including biochemistry and molecular pharmacology, bioinformatics and computational biology, cancer biology, cell biology, immunology and microbiology, interdisciplinary, neuroscience, translational science; biomedical sciences (millennium program) (PhD); clinical and population health research (PhD); clinical investigation (MS). *Faculty:* 1,339 full-time (521 women), 301 part-time/adjunct (189 women). *Students:* 363 full-time (184 women); includes 58 minority (13 Black or African American, non-Hispanic/Latino; 30 Asian, non-Hispanic/Latino; 15 Hispanic/Latino), 141 international. Average age 29. 661 applicants, 26% accepted, 51 enrolled. In 2015, 10 master's, 58 doctorates awarded. Terminal master's awarded for partial completion of doctoral program. *Degree requirements:* For master's, comprehensive exam, thesis; for doctorate, comprehensive exam, thesis/dissertation. *Entrance requirements:* For master's, MD, PhD, DVM, or PharmD; for doctorate, GRE General Test, bachelor's degree. Additional exam requirements/recommendations for international students: Required—TOEFL (minimum score 100 iBT) or IELTS (minimum score 7.5). *Application deadline:* For fall admission, 12/15 for domestic and international students; for spring admission, 5/15 for domestic students. Application fee: $80. Electronic applications accepted. *Expenses:* $6,966 resident per year; $14,182 non-resident per year. *Financial support:* In 2015–16, 383 students received support, including research assistantships with full tuition reimbursements available (averaging $30,600 per year); scholarships/grants, health care benefits, tuition waivers (full), and unspecified assistantships also available. Financial award application deadline: 5/16. *Faculty research:* RNA interference, cell/molecular/developmental biology, bioinformatics, clinical/translational research, infectious disease. *Total annual research expenditures:* $250.3 million. *Unit head:* Dr. Anthony Carruthers, Dean, 508-856-4135, E-mail: anthony.carruthers@umassmed.edu. *Application contact:* Dr. Kendall Knight, Assistant Vice Provost for Admissions, 508-856-5628, Fax: 508-856-3659, E-mail: kendall.knight@umassmed.edu.
Website: http://www.umassmed.edu/gsbs/

University of Michigan, School of Public Health, Program in Clinical Research Design and Statistical Analysis, Ann Arbor, MI 48109. Offers MS. Offered through the Rackham Graduate School; program admits applicants in odd-numbered calendar years only. *Program availability:* Evening/weekend. *Students:* 20 full-time (4 women); includes 2 minority (both Asian, non-Hispanic/Latino), 5 international. Average age 35. In 2015, 26 master's awarded. *Degree requirements:* For master's, comprehensive exam. *Entrance requirements:* For master's, GRE General Test or MCAT. Additional exam requirements/recommendations for international students: Recommended—TOEFL (minimum score 560 paper-based; 100 iBT). *Application deadline:* For fall admission, 1/15 priority date for domestic and international students. Applications are processed on a rolling basis. Application fee: $75. Electronic applications accepted. *Expenses:* Contact institution. *Financial support:* Application deadline: 3/15; applicants required to submit FAFSA. *Faculty research:* Survival analysis, missing data, Bayesian inference, health economics, quality of life. *Unit head:* Dr. Trivellore Raghunathan, Director, 734-615-9832, E-mail: teraghu@umich.edu. *Application contact:* Fatma Nedjari, Information Contact, 734-615-9812, Fax: 734-763-2215, E-mail: sph.bio.inquiries@umich.edu.
Website: http://www.sph.umich.edu/biostat/programs/clinical-stat/

University of Minnesota, Twin Cities Campus, School of Public Health, Major in Clinical Research, Minneapolis, MN 55455-0213. Offers MS. *Program availability:* Part-time. *Degree requirements:* For master's, thesis. *Entrance requirements:* For master's, advanced health professional degree. Additional exam requirements/recommendations for international students: Required—TOEFL. Electronic applications accepted. *Faculty research:* Osteoporosis prevention; heart disease prevention; role of inflammatory dental disease in the genesis of atherosclerosis; interventional research into AIDS and cancer.

The University of North Carolina Wilmington, School of Nursing, Wilmington, NC 28403-5995. Offers clinical research and product development (MS); family nurse practitioner (MSN, Post-Master's Certificate). *Accreditation:* AACN; ACEN. *Program availability:* Part-time, online learning. *Faculty:* 18 full-time (17 women). *Students:* 68 full-time (57 women), 84 part-time (73 women); includes 25 minority (15 Black or African American, non-Hispanic/Latino; 5 American Indian or Alaska Native, non-Hispanic/Latino; 2 Hispanic/Latino; 3 Two or more races, non-Hispanic/Latino). Average age 38. 222 applicants, 57 enrolled. In 2015, 33 master's awarded. *Degree requirements:* For master's, research project/presentation. *Entrance requirements:* For master's, GRE General Test. Additional exam requirements/recommendations for international students: Required—TOEFL (minimum score 79 iBT), IELTS (minimum score 6.5). *Application deadline:* For fall admission, 3/1 for domestic students. Applications are processed on a rolling basis. Application fee: $60. Electronic applications accepted. *Expenses:* $8,854.10 in-state full-time per year; $20,945.04 out-of-state full-time per year. *Financial support:* Scholarships/grants available. Financial award application deadline: 3/15; financial award applicants required to submit FAFSA. *Unit head:* Dr. Carol Heinrich, Director, 910-962-7410, Fax: 910-962-3723, E-mail: badzekl@uncw.edu. *Application contact:* Dr. Jim Lyon, Graduate Coordinator, 910-962-2936, E-mail: lyonj@uncw.edu.
Website: http://www.uncw.edu/son/

University of Pittsburgh, School of Medicine, Graduate Programs in Medicine, Clinical Research Graduate Programs, Pittsburgh, PA 15260. Offers MS, Certificate. *Program availability:* Part-time, blended/hybrid learning. *Faculty:* 46 full-time (29 women). *Students:* 81 part-time (42 women); includes 27 minority (4 Black or African American, non-Hispanic/Latino; 16 Asian, non-Hispanic/Latino; 5 Hispanic/Latino; 2 Two or more races, non-Hispanic/Latino), 13 international. Average age 33. 45 applicants, 84%

accepted, 38 enrolled. In 2015, 13 master's, 21 other advanced degrees awarded. *Degree requirements:* For master's, thesis. *Entrance requirements:* For master's, MCAT or GRE, transcripts, 2 letters of recommendation, personal statement, curriculum vitae; for Certificate, transcripts, 2 letters of recommendation, personal statement, curriculum vitae. Additional exam requirements/recommendations for international students: Required—TOEFL (minimum score 600 paper-based; 100 iBT), IELTS (minimum score 7). *Application deadline:* For fall admission, 10/31 priority date for domestic and international students; for spring admission, 2/28 priority date for domestic and international students. Application fee: $50. Electronic applications accepted. Tuition and fees vary according to program. *Faculty research:* Quality of life, mood disorders in children, pediatric palliative care, female pelvic medicines, health care disparities. *Unit head:* Dr. Wishwa Kapoor, Program Director, 412-692-4821, Fax: 412-586-9672, E-mail: kapoorwn@upmc.edu. *Application contact:* Juliana Tambellini, Program Coordinator, 412-692-2686, Fax: 412-586-9672, E-mail: tambellinijm2@upmc.edu. Website: http://www.icre.pitt.edu/degrees/

University of Puerto Rico, Medical Sciences Campus, School of Health Professions, Program in Clinical Research, San Juan, PR 00936-5067. Offers MS, Graduate Certificate.

University of Rochester, School of Medicine and Dentistry, Graduate Programs in Medicine and Dentistry, Department of Community and Preventive Medicine, Programs in Public Health and Clinical Investigation, Rochester, NY 14627. Offers clinical investigation (MS); public health (MPH); MBA/MPH; MD/MPH; MPH/MS; MPH/PhD. *Accreditation:* CEPH. *Entrance requirements:* For master's, GRE General Test. *Expenses:* Tuition, area resident: Full-time $47,450; part-time $1482 per credit hour. *Required fees:* $528. Tuition and fees vary according to program.

University of Rochester, School of Medicine and Dentistry, Graduate Programs in Medicine and Dentistry, Interdepartmental Program in Clinical Translational Research, Rochester, NY 14627. Offers MS. *Expenses:* Tuition, area resident: Full-time $47,450; part-time $1482 per credit hour. *Required fees:* $528. Tuition and fees vary according to program.

University of Southern California, Graduate School, School of Pharmacy, Regulatory Science Programs, Los Angeles, CA 90089. Offers clinical research design and management (Graduate Certificate); food safety (Graduate Certificate); patient and product safety (Graduate Certificate); preclinical drug development (Graduate Certificate); regulatory and clinical affairs (Graduate Certificate); regulatory science (MS, DRSc). *Program availability:* Part-time, evening/weekend, online learning. Terminal master's awarded for partial completion of doctoral program. *Degree requirements:* For master's, thesis optional; for doctorate, comprehensive exam, thesis/dissertation. *Entrance requirements:* For master's, GRE. Additional exam requirements/recommendations for international students: Required—TOEFL (minimum score 603 paper-based; 100 iBT). Electronic applications accepted.

University of South Florida, Innovative Education, Tampa, FL 33620-9951. Offers adult, career and higher education (Graduate Certificate), including college teaching, leadership in developing human resources, leadership in higher education; Africana studies (Graduate Certificate), including diasporas and health disparities, genocide and human rights; aging studies (Graduate Certificate), including gerontology; art research (Graduate Certificate), including museum studies; business foundations (Graduate Certificate); chemical and biomedical engineering (Graduate Certificate), including materials science and engineering, water, health and sustainability; child and family studies (Graduate Certificate), including positive behavior support; civil and industrial engineering (Graduate Certificate), including transportation systems analysis; community and family health (Graduate Certificate), including maternal and child health, social marketing and public health, violence and injury: prevention and intervention, women's health; criminology (Graduate Certificate), including criminal justice administration; educational measurement and research (Graduate Certificate), including evaluation; English (Graduate Certificate), including comparative literary studies, creative writing, professional and technical communication; entrepreneurship (Graduate Certificate); environmental health (Graduate Certificate), including safety management; epidemiology and biostatistics (Graduate Certificate), including applied biostatistics, biostatistics, concepts and tools of epidemiology, epidemiology, epidemiology of infectious diseases; geography, environment and planning (Graduate Certificate), including community development, environmental policy and management, geographical information systems; geology (Graduate Certificate), including hydrogeology; global health (Graduate Certificate), including disaster management, global health and Latin American and Caribbean studies, global health practice, humanitarian assistance, infection control; government and international affairs (Graduate Certificate), including Cuban studies, globalization studies; health policy and management (Graduate Certificate), including health management and leadership, public health policy and programs; hearing specialist: early intervention (Graduate Certificate); industrial and management systems engineering (Graduate Certificate), including systems engineering, technology management; information studies (Graduate Certificate), including school library media specialist; information systems/decision sciences (Graduate Certificate), including analytics and business intelligence; instructional technology (Graduate Certificate), including distance education, Florida digital/virtual educator, instructional design, multimedia design, Web design; internal medicine, bioethics and medical humanities (Graduate Certificate), including biomedical ethics; Latin American and Caribbean studies (Graduate Certificate); mass communications (Graduate Certificate), including multimedia journalism; mathematics and statistics (Graduate Certificate), including mathematics; medicine (Graduate Certificate), including aging and neuroscience, bioinformatics, biotechnology, brain fitness and memory management, clinical investigation, health informatics, health sciences, integrative weight management, intellectual property, medicine and gender, metabolic and nutritional medicine, metabolic cardiology, pharmacy sciences; national and competitive intelligence (Graduate Certificate); psychological and social foundations (Graduate Certificate), including career counseling, college teaching, diversity in education, mental health counseling, school counseling; public affairs (Graduate Certificate), including nonprofit management, public management, research administration; public health (Graduate Certificate), including environmental health, health equity, public health generalist, translational research in adolescent behavioral health; public health practices (Graduate Certificate), including planning for healthy communities; rehabilitation and mental health counseling (Graduate Certificate), including integrative mental health care, marriage and family therapy, rehabilitation technology; secondary education (Graduate Certificate), including ESOL, foreign language education: culture and content, foreign language education: professional; social work (Graduate Certificate), including geriatric social work/clinical gerontology; special education (Graduate Certificate), including autism spectrum disorder, disabilities education: severe/profound; world languages (Graduate Certificate), including teaching English as a second language (TESL) or foreign language. *Unit head:* Kathy Barnes, Interdisciplinary Programs Coordinator, 813-974-8031, Fax: 813-974-7061, E-mail: barnesk@usf.edu. *Application contact:* Karen Tylinski, Metro Initiatives, 813-974-9943, Fax: 813-974-7061, E-mail: ktylinsk@usf.edu. Website: http://www.usf.edu/innovative-education/

University of South Florida, Morsani College of Medicine and College of Graduate Studies, Graduate Programs in Medical Sciences, Tampa, FL 33620-9951. Offers advanced athletic training (MS); athletic training (MS); bioinformatics and computational biology (MSBCB); biotechnology (MSB); health informatics (MSHI); medical sciences (MSMS, PhD), including aging and neuroscience (MSMS), allergy, immunology and infectious disease (PhD), anatomy, athletic training (MSMS), clinical and translational research, health informatics (MSMS), health science (MSMS), interdisciplinary medical sciences (MSMS), medical microbiology and immunology (MSMS), metabolic and nutritional medicine (MSMS), molecular medicine, molecular pharmacology and physiology (PhD), neurology (PhD), pathology and laboratory medicine (PhD), pharmacology and therapeutics (PhD), physiology and biophysics (PhD), women's health (MSMS). *Students:* 510 full-time (261 women), 318 part-time (208 women); includes 360 minority (108 Black or African American, non-Hispanic/Latino; 3 American Indian or Alaska Native, non-Hispanic/Latino; 101 Asian, non-Hispanic/Latino; 124 Hispanic/Latino; 1 Native Hawaiian or other Pacific Islander, non-Hispanic/Latino; 23 Two or more races, non-Hispanic/Latino), 52 international. Average age 26. 6,567 applicants, 13% accepted, 469 enrolled. In 2015, 216 master's awarded. Terminal master's awarded for partial completion of doctoral program. *Degree requirements:* For master's, comprehensive exam, thesis; for doctorate, comprehensive exam, thesis/dissertation. *Entrance requirements:* For master's, GRE General Test or GMAT, bachelor's degree or equivalent from regionally-accredited university with minimum GPA of 3.0 in upper-division sciences coursework; prerequisites in general biology, general chemistry, general physics, organic chemistry, quantitative analysis, and integral and differential calculus; for doctorate, GRE General Test, bachelor's degree from regionally-accredited university with minimum GPA of 3.0 in upper-division sciences coursework; 3 letters of recommendation; personal interview; 1-2 page personal statement; prerequisites in biology, chemistry, physics, organic chemistry, quantitative analysis, and integral/differential calculus. Additional exam requirements/recommendations for international students: Required—TOEFL (minimum score 550 paper-based; 79 iBT) or IELTS (minimum score 6.5). *Application deadline:* For fall admission, 2/15 for domestic students, 1/2 for international students. Application fee: $30. *Expenses:* Contact institution. *Faculty research:* Anatomy, biochemistry, cancer biology, cardiovascular disease, cell biology, immunology, microbiology, molecular biology, neuroscience, pharmacology, physiology. *Unit head:* Dr. Michael Barber, Professor/Associate Dean for Graduate and Postdoctoral Affairs, 813-974-9908, Fax: 813-974-4317, E-mail: mbarber@health.usf.edu. *Application contact:* Dr. Eric Bennett, Graduate Director, PhD Program in Medical Sciences, 813-974-1545, Fax: 813-974-4317, E-mail: esbennet@health.usf.edu. Website: http://health.usf.edu/nocms/medicine/graduatestudies/

The University of Texas Health Science Center at San Antonio, Graduate School of Biomedical Sciences, Master of Science in Clinical Investigation Program, San Antonio, TX 78229-3900. Offers MS. *Program availability:* Part-time. *Degree requirements:* For master's, comprehensive exam.

University of Virginia, School of Medicine, Department of Public Health Sciences, Program in Clinical Research, Charlottesville, VA 22903. Offers clinical investigation and patient-oriented research (MS); informatics in medicine (MS). *Program availability:* Part-time. *Degree requirements:* For master's, thesis (for some programs). *Entrance requirements:* For master's, 2 letters of recommendation. Additional exam requirements/recommendations for international students: Required—TOEFL (minimum score 600 paper-based; 90 iBT). Electronic applications accepted.

University of Washington, Graduate School, School of Public Health, Department of Biostatistics, Seattle, WA 98195. Offers biostatistics (MPH, MS, PhD); clinical research (MS), including biostatistics; statistical genetics (PhD). *Program availability:* Part-time. Terminal master's awarded for partial completion of doctoral program. *Degree requirements:* For master's, comprehensive exam, thesis, practicum (MPH); for doctorate, comprehensive exam, thesis/dissertation. *Entrance requirements:* For master's and doctorate, GRE General Test, coursework on multivariate calculus, linear algebra and probability; minimum GPA of 3.0. Additional exam requirements/recommendations for international students: Required—TOEFL. Electronic applications accepted. *Expenses:* Contact institution. *Faculty research:* Statistical methods for survival data analysis, clinical trials, epidemiological case control and cohort studies, statistical genetics.

University of Washington, Graduate School, School of Public Health, Department of Epidemiology, Seattle, WA 98195. Offers clinical research (MS); epidemiology (MPH, MS, PhD); global health (MPH); maternal/child health (MPH); MPH/MPA. *Accreditation:* CEPH (one or more programs are accredited). *Degree requirements:* For master's, comprehensive exam (for some programs), thesis, formal thesis proposal; for doctorate, comprehensive exam, thesis/dissertation, general exam, dissertation proposals, final exam (dissertation defense). *Entrance requirements:* For master's, GRE (except for those holding PhD, MD, DDS, DVM, DO or equivalent from U.S. institutions); for doctorate, GRE. Additional exam requirements/recommendations for international students: Required—TOEFL (minimum score 580 paper-based, 92 iBT), IELTS (minimum score 7), or PTE (minimum score of 65). Electronic applications accepted. *Expenses:* Contact institution. *Faculty research:* Chronic disease, health disparities and social determinants of health, aging and neuroepidemiology, maternal and child health, molecular and genetic epidemiology.

University of Washington, Graduate School, School of Public Health, Department of Health Services, Seattle, WA 98195. Offers clinical research (MS); community-oriented public health practice (MPH); evaluative sciences and statistics (PhD); health behavior and social determinants of health (PhD); health economics (PhD); health informatics and health information management (MHIHIM); health services (MS, PhD); health services administration (EMHA, MHA); health systems and policy (MPH); health systems research (PhD); maternal and child health (MPH); social and behavioral sciences (MPH); JD/MHA; MHA/MBA; MHA/MD; MHA/MPA; MPH/JD; MPH/MD; MPH/MN; MPH/MPA; MPH/MS; MPH/MSD; MPH/MSW; MPH/PhD. *Program availability:* Online learning. Terminal master's awarded for partial completion of doctoral program. *Degree requirements:* For master's, thesis (for some programs), practicum (MPH); for doctorate, comprehensive exam, thesis/dissertation. *Entrance requirements:* For master's and doctorate, GRE General Test, minimum GPA of 3.0. Additional exam requirements/recommendations for international students: Required—TOEFL (minimum score 580 paper-based; 92 iBT), IELTS (minimum score 7). Electronic applications accepted. *Expenses:* Contact institution. *Faculty research:* Public health practice, health promotion and disease prevention, maternal and child health, organizational behavior and culture, health policy.

University of Wisconsin–Madison, School of Medicine and Public Health, Program in Clinical Investigation, Madison, WI 53706-1380. Offers MS, PhD. *Program availability:* Part-time, evening/weekend. *Application deadline:* For fall admission, 2/1 for domestic and international students. Electronic applications accepted. *Expenses:* Tuition, state resident: full-time $5364. Tuition, nonresident: full-time $12,027. *Required fees:* $571. Tuition and fees vary according to campus/location, program and reciprocity agreements. *Financial support:* Fellowships, research assistantships, teaching assistantships, scholarships/grants, traineeships, health care benefits, and unspecified assistantships available. Support available to part-time students. *Faculty research:*

Clinical and translational research; patient outcomes research; basic science; applied science. *Application contact:* Sally Wedde, Student Services, E-mail: sally.wedde@wisc.edu.
Website: https://ictr.wisc.edu/graduateprogram

Vanderbilt University, School of Medicine, Clinical Investigation Program, Nashville, TN 37240-1001. Offers MS. *Entrance requirements:* Additional exam requirements/recommendations for international students: Required—TOEFL. *Application deadline:* For fall admission, 2/28 for domestic students. *Financial support:* Fellowships with full tuition reimbursements and research assistantships with full tuition reimbursements available. *Unit head:* Dr. T. Alp Ikizler, Director, 615-343-6104, Fax: 615-322-4026. *Application contact:* Arnita L. King, Coordinator, 615-322-3480, Fax: 615-322-4026, E-mail: arnita.king@vanderbilt.edu.
Website: http://www.mc.vanderbilt.edu/msci/

Walden University, Graduate Programs, School of Health Sciences, Minneapolis, MN 55401. Offers clinical research administration (MS, Graduate Certificate); health education and promotion (MS, PhD), including behavioral health (PhD), disease surveillance (PhD), emergency preparedness (MS), general (MHA, MS), global health (PhD), health policy (PhD), health policy and advocacy (MS), population health (PhD); health informatics (MS); health services (PhD), including community health, healthcare administration, leadership, public health policy, self-designed; healthcare administration (MHA), including general (MHA, MS); leadership and organizational development (MHA); public health (MPH, Dr PH, PhD, Graduate Certificate), including community health education (PhD), epidemiology (PhD); systems policy (MHA). *Program availability:* Part-time, evening/weekend, online only, 100% online. *Faculty:* 14 full-time (8 women), 222 part-time/adjunct (121 women). *Students:* 2,487 full-time (1,804 women), 2,282 part-time (1,540 women); includes 2,763 minority (2,129 Black or African American, non-Hispanic/Latino; 30 American Indian or Alaska Native, non-Hispanic/Latino; 237 Asian, non-Hispanic/Latino; 268 Hispanic/Latino; 13 Native Hawaiian or other Pacific Islander, non-Hispanic/Latino; 86 Two or more races, non-Hispanic/Latino); 87 international. Average age 39. 1,205 applicants, 98% accepted, 820 enrolled. In 2015, 641 master's, 147 doctorates, 18 other advanced degrees awarded. *Degree requirements:* For doctorate, thesis/dissertation, residency. *Entrance requirements:* For master's, bachelor's degree or higher; minimum GPA of 2.5; official transcripts; goal statement (for some programs); access to computer and Internet; for doctorate, master's degree or higher; three years of related professional or academic experience

(preferred); minimum GPA of 3.0; goal statement and current resume (for select programs); official transcripts; access to computer and Internet; for Graduate Certificate, relevant work experience; access to computer and Internet. Additional exam requirements/recommendations for international students: Required—TOEFL (minimum score 550 paper-based, 79 iBT), IELTS (minimum score 6.5), Michigan English Language Assessment Battery (minimum score 82), or PTE (minimum score 53). *Application deadline:* Applications are processed on a rolling basis. Application fee: $0. Electronic applications accepted. *Financial support:* Fellowships, Federal Work-Study, scholarships/grants, unspecified assistantships, and family tuition reduction, active duty/veteran tuition reduction, group tuition reduction, interest-free payment plans, employee tuition reduction available. Support available to part-time students. Financial award applicants required to submit FAFSA. *Unit head:* Dr. Jorg Westermann, Dean, 866-492-5336. *Application contact:* Meghan Thomas, Vice President of Enrollment Management, 866-492-5336, E-mail: info@waldenu.edu.
Website: http://www.waldenu.edu/colleges-schools/school-of-health-sciences

Washington University in St. Louis, School of Medicine, Program in Clinical Investigation, St. Louis, MO 63130-4899. Offers clinical investigation (MS), including bioethics, entrepreneurship, genetics/genomics, translational medicine. *Program availability:* Part-time, evening/weekend. *Faculty:* 61 full-time (14 women), 2 part-time/adjunct (both women). *Students:* 15 full-time (5 women), 39 part-time (19 women); includes 15 minority (3 Black or African American, non-Hispanic/Latino; 8 Asian, non-Hispanic/Latino; 2 Hispanic/Latino; 2 Two or more races, non-Hispanic/Latino), 3 international. Average age 32. 34 applicants, 65% accepted, 22 enrolled. In 2015, 35 master's awarded. *Degree requirements:* For master's, thesis. *Entrance requirements:* For master's, doctoral-level degree or in process of obtaining doctoral-level degree. *Application deadline:* For fall admission, 5/15 for domestic students; for spring admission, 10/15 for domestic students. Application fee: $0. Electronic applications accepted. *Financial support:* In 2015–16, 4 students received support. Tuition waivers (partial) available. Financial award application deadline: 12/12. *Faculty research:* Anesthesiology, infectious diseases, neurology, obstetrics and gynecology, orthopedic surgery. *Unit head:* Dr. David Warren, Associate Professor of Medicine, 314-454-8225, Fax: 314-454-8279, E-mail: dwarren@wustl.edu. *Application contact:* Suzie Fragale, Curriculum and Evaluation Coordinator, 314-454-8936, Fax: 314-454-8279, E-mail: fragale@wustl.edu.
Website: http://crtc.wustl.edu/

Communication Disorders

Abilene Christian University, Graduate School, College of Education and Human Services, Department of Communication Sciences and Disorders, Abilene, TX 79699-9100. Offers MS. *Accreditation:* ASHA. *Faculty:* 7 full-time/adjunct (6 women). *Students:* 47 full-time (45 women); includes 11 minority (1 American Indian or Alaska Native, non-Hispanic/Latino; 8 Hispanic/Latino; 2 Two or more races, non-Hispanic/Latino). 245 applicants, 21% accepted, 22 enrolled. In 2015, 24 master's awarded. *Degree requirements:* For master's, one foreign language, comprehensive exam. *Entrance requirements:* For master's, GRE General Test. Additional exam requirements/recommendations for international students: Required—TOEFL (minimum score 550 paper-based; 90 iBT), IELTS (minimum score 6.5), PTE. *Application deadline:* For fall admission, 2/1 priority date for domestic students. Applications are processed on a rolling basis. Application fee: $50. Electronic applications accepted. *Financial support:* In 2015–16, 38 students received support. Research assistantships and scholarships/grants available. Financial award application deadline: 4/1; financial award applicants required to submit FAFSA. *Unit head:* Dr. Terry Baggs, Graduate Coordinator, 325-674-2420, Fax: 325-674-2552, E-mail: barnettd@acu.edu. *Application contact:* Corey Patterson, Director of Graduate Admission and Recruiting, 325-674-6566, Fax: 325-674-6717, E-mail: gradinfo@acu.edu.

Adelphi University, Ruth S. Ammon School of Education, Program in Communication Sciences and Disorders, Garden City, NY 11530-0701. Offers audiology (MS, DA); speech-language pathology (MS, DA). *Accreditation:* ASHA. *Program availability:* Part-time. *Degree requirements:* For master's, comprehensive exam, clinical practice; for doctorate, one foreign language, comprehensive exam, thesis/dissertation. *Entrance requirements:* For master's, GRE General Test, writing exam, 3 letters of recommendation, interview, resume, 19 credits of prerequisite course work or communications disorders training; for doctorate, GRE General Test, 3 letters of recommendation, interview. Additional exam requirements/recommendations for international students: Required—TOEFL (minimum score 550 paper-based; 80 iBT). Electronic applications accepted. *Faculty research:* Pediatric audiology, child speech perception with hearing loss, auditory deprivation, fluency, cultural diversity.

Alabama Agricultural and Mechanical University, School of Graduate Studies, College of Education, Humanities, and Behavioral Sciences, Department of Health Sciences, Human Performance, and Communicative Disorders, Huntsville, AL 35811. Offers physical education (MS); speech-language pathology (MS). *Program availability:* Part-time, evening/weekend. *Degree requirements:* For master's, comprehensive exam. *Entrance requirements:* For master's, GRE General Test. Additional exam requirements/recommendations for international students: Required—TOEFL (minimum score 500 paper-based; 61 iBT). Electronic applications accepted. *Faculty research:* Cardiorespiratory assessment.

Andrews University, School of Health Professions, Department of Speech-Language Pathology and Audiology, Berrien Springs, MI 49104. Offers speech-language pathology (MS). *Faculty:* 5 full-time (all women). *Students:* 26 full-time (25 women), 1 part-time (0 women); includes 12 minority (6 Black or African American, non-Hispanic/Latino; 2 Asian, non-Hispanic/Latino; 4 Hispanic/Latino), 4 international. Average age 27. 44 applicants, 36% accepted, 11 enrolled. *Unit head:* Heather Ferguson, Chair, 269-471-6369, E-mail: hferguson@andrews.edu. *Application contact:* Monica Wringer, Supervisor of Graduate Admission, 800-253-2874, Fax: 269-471-3228, E-mail: graduate@andrews.edu.
Website: http://www.andrews.edu/shp/speech/

Appalachian State University, Cratis D. Williams Graduate School, Department of Communication Sciences and Disorders, Boone, NC 28608. Offers speech-language pathology (MS). *Accreditation:* ASHA. *Program availability:* Part-time. *Degree requirements:* For master's, comprehensive exam, thesis optional. *Entrance requirements:* For master's, GRE General Test, 3 letters of recommendation. Additional exam requirements/recommendations for international students: Required—TOEFL (minimum score 570 paper-based), IELTS (minimum score 6.5). Electronic applications accepted. *Faculty research:* Clinical service delivery, voice disorders, language disorders, fluency disorders, neurogenic disorders.

Arizona State University at the Tempe campus, College of Health Solutions, Department of Speech and Hearing Science, Tempe, AZ 85287-0102. Offers audiology (Au D); communication disorders (MS); speech and hearing science (PhD). *Accreditation:* ASHA (one or more programs are accredited). *Degree requirements:* For master's, comprehensive exam (for some programs), thesis optional, interactive Program of Study (iPOS) submitted before completing 50 percent of required credit hours; for doctorate, comprehensive exam, thesis/dissertation (for some programs), academic/practicum components (Au D); interactive Program of Study (iPOS) submitted before completing 50 percent of required credit hours. *Entrance requirements:* For master's and doctorate, GRE, minimum GPA of 3.0 or equivalent in last 2 years of work leading to bachelor's degree. Additional exam requirements/recommendations for international students: Required—TOEFL, IELTS, or PTE. *Expenses:* Contact institution.

Arkansas State University, Graduate School, College of Nursing and Health Professions, Department of Communication Disorders, State University, AR 72467. Offers communication disorders (MCD); dyslexia therapy (Graduate Certificate). *Accreditation:* ASHA. *Program availability:* Part-time. *Faculty:* 5 full-time (3 women). *Students:* 52 full-time (50 women); includes 1 minority (Black or African American, non-Hispanic/Latino). Average age 25. 42 applicants, 62% accepted, 26 enrolled. In 2015, 26 master's awarded. *Degree requirements:* For master's, comprehensive exam, thesis or alternative. *Entrance requirements:* For master's, GRE General Test, appropriate bachelor's degree, letters of recommendation, official transcripts, immunization records. Additional exam requirements/recommendations for international students: Required—TOEFL (minimum score 550 paper-based; 79 iBT), IELTS (minimum score 6), PTE (minimum score 56). *Application deadline:* For fall admission, 2/15 for domestic and international students. Applications are processed on a rolling basis. Application fee: $30 ($40 for international students). Electronic applications accepted. *Expenses:* Contact institution. *Financial support:* In 2015–16, 9 students received support. Career-related internships or fieldwork, scholarships/grants, and unspecified assistantships available. Financial award application deadline: 7/1; financial award applicants required to submit FAFSA. *Unit head:* Dr. Richard Neeley, Chair, 870-972-3106, Fax: 870-972-3788, E-mail: rneeley@astate.edu. *Application contact:* Vickey Ring, Graduate Admissions Coordinator, 870-972-2737, Fax: 870-972-3917, E-mail: vickeyring@astate.edu.
Website: http://www.astate.edu/college/conhp/departments/communication-disorders

Armstrong State University, School of Graduate Studies, Program in Communication Sciences, Savannah, GA 31419-1997. Offers MS. *Accreditation:* ASHA. *Program availability:* Part-time, evening/weekend. *Faculty:* 3 full-time (all women), 2 part-time/adjunct (both women). *Students:* 40 full-time (all women); includes 3 minority (2 Black or African American, non-Hispanic/Latino; 1 Hispanic/Latino). Average age 25. 181 applicants, 12% accepted, 20 enrolled. In 2015, 24 master's awarded. *Degree requirements:* For master's, comprehensive exam, 400 client contact hours, PRAXIS II, minimum B average. *Entrance requirements:* For master's, GRE, criminal background check and drug screen, CPR certification, clinical observation hours, minimum GPA of 3.0, letter of intent, college transcript. Additional exam requirements/recommendations for international students: Required—TOEFL (minimum score 523 paper-based). *Application deadline:* For fall admission, 1/15 for domestic and international students. Application fee: $30. Electronic applications accepted. *Expenses:* Tuition, state resident: part-time $211 per credit hour. Tuition, nonresident: part-time $782 per credit hour. *Required fees:* $1224 per unit. $612 per semester. Tuition and fees vary according to course load, campus/location and program. *Financial support:* In 2015–16, research assistantships with full tuition reimbursements (averaging $5,000 per year) were awarded; Federal Work-Study, scholarships/grants, and unspecified assistantships also available. Support available to part-time students. Financial award application deadline: 3/15; financial award applicants required to submit FAFSA. *Faculty research:* Cognitive impairment and traumatic brain injury, cultural and linguistic differences, aphasia and quality of life. *Unit head:* Maya Clark, Program Coordinator/Professor, 912-344-2969, Fax: 912-344-3439, E-mail: maya.clark@armstrong.edu. *Application contact:* McKenzie

Communication Disorders

Peterman, Assistant Director of Graduate Admissions, 912-344-2503, Fax: 912-344-3417, E-mail: graduate@armstrong.edu.
Website: http://www.armstrong.edu/Health_Professions/rehabilitation_sciences/rehab_sci_ms_communication_sciences

A.T. Still University, Arizona School of Health Sciences, Mesa, AZ 85206. Offers advanced occupational therapy (MS); advanced physician assistant studies (MS); athletic training (MS, DAT); audiology (Au D); occupational therapy (OTD); physical therapy (DPT); physician assistant studies (MS); transitional audiology (Au D); transitional physical therapy (DPT). *Accreditation:* AOTA (one or more programs are accredited); ASHA. *Program availability:* Part-time, evening/weekend, 100% online. *Faculty:* 54 full-time (31 women), 188 part-time/adjunct (132 women). *Students:* 509 full-time (339 women), 397 part-time (310 women); includes 203 minority (41 Black or African American, non-Hispanic/Latino; 5 American Indian or Alaska Native, non-Hispanic/Latino; 83 Asian, non-Hispanic/Latino; 57 Hispanic/Latino; 2 Native Hawaiian or other Pacific Islander, non-Hispanic/Latino; 15 Two or more races, non-Hispanic/Latino), 60 international. Average age 33. 3,902 applicants, 10% accepted, 245 enrolled. In 2015, 178 master's, 271 doctorates awarded. *Degree requirements:* For master's, thesis (for some programs); for doctorate, thesis/dissertation (for some programs). *Entrance requirements:* For master's, GRE General Test; for doctorate, GRE, Evaluation of Practicing Audiologists Capabilities (Au D), Physical Therapist Evaluation Tool (DPT), current state licensure, master's degree or equivalent (Au D). Additional exam requirements/recommendations for international students: Required—TOEFL (minimum score 80 iBT). *Application deadline:* Applications are processed on a rolling basis. Application fee: $70. Electronic applications accepted. *Expenses:* Contact institution. *Financial support:* In 2015–16, 158 students received support. Federal Work-Study and scholarships/grants available. Financial award application deadline: 5/1; financial award applicants required to submit FAFSA. *Faculty research:* Pediatric sport-related concussion, adolescent athlete health-related quality of life; geriatric and pediatric well-being, pain management for participation, practice-based research network, BMI and dental caries. *Total annual research expenditures:* $156,319. *Unit head:* Dr. Randy Danielsen, Dean, 480-219-6000, Fax: 480-219-6110, E-mail: rdanielsen@atsu.edu. *Application contact:* Donna Sparks, Associate Director, Admissions Processing, 660-626-2117, Fax: 660-626-2969, E-mail: admissions@atsu.edu.
Website: http://www.atsu.edu/ashs

Auburn University, Graduate School, College of Liberal Arts, Department of Communication Disorders, Auburn University, AL 36849. Offers audiology (MCD, MS, Au D); speech pathology (MCD, MS). *Accreditation:* ASHA (one or more programs are accredited). *Program availability:* Part-time. *Faculty:* 16 full-time (14 women), 2 part-time/adjunct (1 woman). *Students:* 76 full-time (75 women), 5 part-time (all women); includes 6 minority (2 Black or African American, non-Hispanic/Latino; 1 American Indian or Alaska Native, non-Hispanic/Latino; 3 Hispanic/Latino). Average age 23. 253 applicants, 20% accepted, 33 enrolled. In 2015, 22 master's, 7 doctorates awarded. *Degree requirements:* For master's, comprehensive exam (MCD), thesis (MS). *Entrance requirements:* For master's, GRE General Test. *Application deadline:* Applications are processed on a rolling basis. Application fee: $50 ($60 for international students). Electronic applications accepted. *Expenses:* Tuition, state resident: full-time $8802; part-time $489 per credit hour. Tuition, nonresident: full-time $26,406; part-time $1467 per credit hour. *Required fees:* $808 per semester. Tuition and fees vary according to degree level and program. *Financial support:* Research assistantships, teaching assistantships, and Federal Work-Study available. Support available to part-time students. Financial award application deadline: 3/15; financial award applicants required to submit FAFSA. *Unit head:* Dr. Nancy Haak, Chair, 334-844-9600. *Application contact:* Dr. George Flowers, Dean of the Graduate School, 334-844-2125.
Website: http://www.cla.auburn.edu/communicationdisorders/

Baldwin Wallace University, Graduate Programs, Speech-Language Pathology Program, Berea, OH 44017-2088. Offers speech-language pathology (MS). *Faculty:* 6 full-time (all women), 2 part-time/adjunct (both women). *Students:* 16 full-time (all women); includes 1 minority (Hispanic/Latino). Average age 22. 93 applicants, 42% accepted, 16 enrolled. *Entrance requirements:* For master's, GRE, 3 letters of recommendation, bachelor's degree, 25 clinical observation hours in speech and/or language therapy or evaluation, CSDCAS online application. Additional exam requirements/recommendations for international students: Required—TOEFL. *Application deadline:* For fall admission, 1/15 for domestic students. Applications are processed on a rolling basis. Electronic applications accepted. *Expenses:* Contact institution. *Financial support:* Applicants required to submit FAFSA. *Faculty research:* Scholarship of teaching and learning, clinical training, traumatic brain injury and concussions, feeding and swallowing disorders across the life span, voice disorders. *Unit head:* Stephen D. Stahl, Provost, Academic Affairs, 440-826-2251, Fax: 440-826-2329, E-mail: sstahl@bw.edu. *Application contact:* Winifred W. Gerhardt, Director of Transfer, Adult and Graduate Admission, 440-826-2222, Fax: 440-826-3830, E-mail: slp@bw.edu.
Website: http://www.bw.edu/graduate/speech-language-pathology/index

Ball State University, Graduate School, College of Sciences and Humanities, Department of Speech Pathology and Audiology, Muncie, IN 47306. Offers audiology (Au D); speech-language pathology (MA). *Accreditation:* ASHA. *Faculty:* 16 full-time (13 women), 2 part-time/adjunct (both women). *Students:* 96 full-time (86 women), 26 part-time (all women); includes 7 minority (1 Black or African American, non-Hispanic/Latino; 2 Asian, non-Hispanic/Latino; 4 Hispanic/Latino). Average age 23. 104 applicants, 45% accepted, 38 enrolled. In 2015, 47 master's, 5 doctorates awarded. *Degree requirements:* For doctorate, comprehensive exam. *Entrance requirements:* For master's, GRE General Test (minimum preferred combined score of 900 on verbal and quantitative sections), minimum baccalaureate GPA of 3.0, three letters of reference, transcripts of all previous course work; for doctorate, GRE General Test, statement of purpose, on-campus interview. Additional exam requirements/recommendations for international students: Required—TOEFL (minimum score 550 paper-based; 79 iBT), IELTS (minimum score 6.5). *Application deadline:* For fall admission, 2/1 for domestic students; for spring admission, 10/31 for domestic students; for summer admission, 2/1 for domestic students. Applications are processed on a rolling basis. Application fee: $60. Electronic applications accepted. *Expenses: Tuition, area resident:* Full-time $6948; part-time $2316 per semester. Tuition, state resident: full-time $10,422; part-time $3474 per semester. Tuition, nonresident: full-time $19,062; part-time $6354 per semester. *Required fees:* $651 per semester. Tuition and fees vary according to campus/location, program and reciprocity agreements. *Financial support:* In 2015–16, 60 students received support, including 15 research assistantships with partial tuition reimbursements available (averaging $6,444 per year), 22 teaching assistantships with partial tuition reimbursements available (averaging $7,717 per year); unspecified assistantships also available. Financial award application deadline: 3/1; financial award applicants required to submit FAFSA. *Faculty research:* Adult neurological disorders, stuttering, tinnitus loudness, brain stem responses. *Unit head:* Dr. Mary Jo Germani, Chairperson, 765-285-8162, Fax: 765-285-5623, E-mail: mgermani@bsu.edu.
Website: http://www.bsu.edu/spaa

Barry University, School of Education, Program in Education for Teachers of Students with Hearing Impairments, Miami Shores, FL 33161-6695. Offers MS.

Baylor University, Graduate School, Robbins College of Health and Human Sciences, Department of Communication Sciences and Disorders, Waco, TX 76798-7332. Offers MA, MSCSD. *Accreditation:* ASHA (one or more programs are accredited). *Degree requirements:* For master's, comprehensive exam (for some programs), thesis (for some programs). *Entrance requirements:* For master's, GRE General Test. Additional exam requirements/recommendations for international students: Required—TOEFL. Electronic applications accepted. *Expenses:* Contact institution. *Faculty research:* Nasality, language impairment, stuttering, Spanish speech perception, language literacy.

Biola University, School of Arts and Sciences, La Mirada, CA 90639-0001. Offers Christian apologetics (MA, Certificate); science and religion (MA); speech language pathology (MA). *Program availability:* Part-time, evening/weekend, online learning. *Faculty:* 20. *Students:* 31 full-time (8 women), 262 part-time (45 women); includes 80 minority (21 Black or African American, non-Hispanic/Latino; 1 American Indian or Alaska Native, non-Hispanic/Latino; 31 Asian, non-Hispanic/Latino; 19 Hispanic/Latino; 8 Two or more races, non-Hispanic/Latino), 15 international. 168 applicants, 70% accepted, 77 enrolled. In 2015, 64 master's awarded. *Entrance requirements:* For master's, minimum GPA of 3.0, bachelor's degree from accredited college or university (in science-related field for science and religion program). Additional exam requirements/recommendations for international students: Required—TOEFL (minimum score 600 paper-based; 100 iBT). *Application deadline:* For fall admission, 7/1 for domestic students, 6/1 for international students; for spring admission, 12/1 for domestic students. Applications are processed on a rolling basis. Application fee: $65. Electronic applications accepted. *Financial support:* Scholarships/grants and unspecified assistantships available. Support available to part-time students. Financial award applicants required to submit FAFSA. *Faculty research:* Apologetics, science and religion, intelligent design. *Application contact:* Graduate Admissions Office, 562-903-4752, E-mail: graduate.admissions@biola.edu.
Website: http://www.biola.edu/academics/sas/

Bloomsburg University of Pennsylvania, School of Graduate Studies, College of Education, Department of Exceptionality Programs, Program in Education of the Deaf/Hard of Hearing, Bloomsburg, PA 17815-1301. Offers MS. *Degree requirements:* For master's, thesis, minimum QPA of 3.0, practicum. *Entrance requirements:* For master's, PRAXIS, GRE, minimum QPA of 3.0, letter of intent, 3 letters of recommendation, interview. Additional exam requirements/recommendations for international students: Required—TOEFL (minimum score 550 paper-based). Electronic applications accepted.

Bloomsburg University of Pennsylvania, School of Graduate Studies, College of Science and Technology, Department of Audiology and Speech Pathology, Program in Audiology, Bloomsburg, PA 17815-1301. Offers Au D. *Accreditation:* ASHA. *Degree requirements:* For doctorate, comprehensive exam, thesis/dissertation, minimum QPA of 3.0, practicum. *Entrance requirements:* For doctorate, GRE, 3 letters of recommendation, interview, personal statement, minimum QPA of 3.0. Additional exam requirements/recommendations for international students: Required—TOEFL. Electronic applications accepted.

Bloomsburg University of Pennsylvania, School of Graduate Studies, College of Science and Technology, Department of Audiology and Speech Pathology, Program in Speech Pathology, Bloomsburg, PA 17815-1301. Offers school-based speech-language pathology (M Ed); speech-language pathology (MS). *Accreditation:* ASHA. *Degree requirements:* For master's, thesis optional, minimum QPA of 3.0, clinical experience. *Entrance requirements:* For master's, GRE, minimum QPA of 3.0, 3 letters of recommendation, personal statement. Additional exam requirements/recommendations for international students: Required—TOEFL (minimum score 550 paper-based). Electronic applications accepted.

Boston University, College of Health and Rehabilitation Sciences: Sargent College, Department of Speech, Language and Hearing Sciences, Boston, MA 02215. Offers speech, language and hearing sciences (PhD); speech-language pathology (MS). *Accreditation:* ASHA. *Faculty:* 13 full-time (10 women), 12 part-time/adjunct (5 women). *Students:* 63 full-time (61 women), 3 part-time (all women); includes 3 minority (2 Asian, non-Hispanic/Latino; 1 Hispanic/Latino), 2 international. Average age 24. 504 applicants, 20% accepted, 24 enrolled. In 2015, 40 master's awarded. Terminal master's awarded for partial completion of doctoral program. *Degree requirements:* For master's, comprehensive exam, thesis optional; for doctorate, comprehensive exam, thesis/dissertation. *Entrance requirements:* For master's and doctorate, GRE General Test. Additional exam requirements/recommendations for international students: Required—TOEFL (minimum score 550 paper-based; 94 iBT). *Application deadline:* For fall admission, 1/1 priority date for domestic and international students. Applications are processed on a rolling basis. Application fee: $100. Electronic applications accepted. *Expenses:* $1,537 per credit. *Financial support:* In 2015–16, 58 students received support, including 14 research assistantships with full tuition reimbursements available (averaging $21,000 per year), 9 teaching assistantships (averaging $3,000 per year); career-related internships or fieldwork, Federal Work-Study, institutionally sponsored loans, scholarships/grants, and tuition waivers (full and partial) also available. Financial award application deadline: 1/1; financial award applicants required to submit FAFSA. *Faculty research:* Child language, fluency, autism, speech science, perception of complex sounds. *Total annual research expenditures:* $3.8 million. *Unit head:* Dr. Melanie Matthies, Chair, 617-353-3188, E-mail: slhs@bu.edu. *Application contact:* Sharon Sankey, Assistant Dean, Student Services, 617-353-2713, Fax: 617-353-7500, E-mail: ssankey@bu.edu.
Website: http://www.bu.edu/sargent/

Bowling Green State University, Graduate College, College of Education and Human Development, School of Education and Intervention Services, Intervention Services Division, Program in Special Education, Bowling Green, OH 43403. Offers assistive technology (M Ed); early childhood intervention (M Ed); gifted education (M Ed); hearing impaired intervention (M Ed); mild/moderate intervention (M Ed); moderate/intensive intervention (M Ed). *Accreditation:* NCATE. *Program availability:* Part-time. *Degree requirements:* For master's, thesis or alternative. *Entrance requirements:* For master's, GRE General Test. Additional exam requirements/recommendations for international students: Required—TOEFL. Electronic applications accepted. *Faculty research:* Reading and special populations, deafness, early childhood, gifted and talented, behavior disorders.

Bowling Green State University, Graduate College, College of Health and Human Services, Department of Communication Disorders, Bowling Green, OH 43403. Offers communication disorders (PhD); speech-language pathology (MS). *Accreditation:* ASHA (one or more programs are accredited). *Degree requirements:* For master's, thesis or alternative; for doctorate, comprehensive exam, thesis/dissertation, foreign language or research tool. *Entrance requirements:* For master's, GRE General Test, minimum GPA of 3.0; for doctorate, GRE General Test, minimum GPA of 3.2. Additional exam requirements/recommendations for international students: Required—TOEFL. Electronic applications accepted. *Faculty research:* Rehabilitation and mental disorders, forensic rehabilitation, rehabilitation and substance abuse, private rehabilitation and disability management, adjustment to disability.

Brigham Young University, Graduate Studies, David O. McKay School of Education, Department of Communication Disorders, Provo, UT 84602-1001. Offers MS. *Accreditation:* ASHA. *Faculty:* 11 full-time (5 women), 4 part-time/adjunct (all women). *Students:* 36 full-time (all women), 21 part-time (all women); includes 5 minority (2 Asian, non-Hispanic/Latino; 3 Hispanic/Latino). Average age 27. 88 applicants, 48% accepted, 16 enrolled. In 2015, 21 master's awarded. *Degree requirements:* For master's, comprehensive exam, thesis, exit interview, PRAXIS. *Entrance requirements:* For master's, GRE General Test, 3 letters of recommendation, statement of intent. Additional exam requirements/recommendations for international students: Required— TOEFL (minimum score 580 paper-based; 85 iBT). *Application deadline:* For fall admission, 2/1 for domestic and international students. Application fee: $50. Electronic applications accepted. *Financial support:* In 2015–16, 41 students received support, including 20 research assistantships (averaging $1,701 per year), 18 teaching assistantships (averaging $2,786 per year); fellowships, institutionally sponsored loans, and scholarships/grants also available. Financial award application deadline: 2/1. *Unit head:* Martin Fujiki, Chair, 801-422-6461, Fax: 801-422-0197, E-mail: martin_fujiki@ byu.edu. *Application contact:* Sandy Alger, Department Secretary, 801-422-5117, Fax: 801-422-0197, E-mail: sandy_alger@byu.edu. Website: http://education.byu.edu/comd/

Brooklyn College of the City University of New York, School of Humanities and Social Sciences, Department of Speech Communication Arts and Sciences, Brooklyn, NY 11210-2889. Offers audiology (Au D); speech (MA), including public communication; speech-language pathology (MS). Au D offered jointly with Hunter College of the City University of New York. *Accreditation:* ASHA (one or more programs are accredited). *Program availability:* Part-time. Terminal master's awarded for partial completion of doctoral program. *Degree requirements:* For master's, comprehensive exam, NTE. *Entrance requirements:* For master's, GRE, minimum GPA of 3.0, interview, essay. Additional exam requirements/recommendations for international students: Required— TOEFL (minimum score 500 paper-based; 61 iBT). Electronic applications accepted. *Faculty research:* Language and learning disorders, aphasia, auditory disorders, public and business communication, voice and fluency disorders.

Buffalo State College, State University of New York, The Graduate School, Faculty of Applied Science and Education, Department of Speech-Language Pathology, Buffalo, NY 14222-1095. Offers MS Ed. *Accreditation:* ASHA. *Program availability:* Part-time, evening/weekend. *Degree requirements:* For master's, thesis or alternative, project. *Entrance requirements:* For master's, minimum GPA of 3.0 in last 60 hours, 22 hours in communication disorders. Additional exam requirements/recommendations for international students: Required—TOEFL (minimum score 550 paper-based).

California Baptist University, Program in Speech Language Pathology, Riverside, CA 92504-3206. Offers MS. *Degree requirements:* For master's, comprehensive exam, capstone, PRAXIS, clinical practicum. *Entrance requirements:* For master's, minimum undergraduate GPA of 3.0, bachelor's transcripts, three letters of recommendation, essay, resume, interview. Additional exam requirements/recommendations for international students: Required—TOEFL (minimum score 80 iBT). *Application deadline:* For fall admission, 12/1 priority date for domestic students, 11/1 priority date for international students; for spring admission, 8/1 priority date for domestic students, 7/1 priority date for international students. Applications are processed on a rolling basis. Application fee: $45. Electronic applications accepted. *Expenses:* $740 per unit plus a $355 fee per semester. *Financial support:* Applicants required to submit CSS PROFILE or FAFSA. *Unit head:* Dr. Candace Vickers, Director, 951-552-8129, E-mail: cvickers@ calbaptist.edu. *Application contact:* Taylor Neece, Director of Graduate Admissions, 951-343-4871, Fax: 877-228-8877, E-mail: graduateadmissions@calbaptist.edu.

California State University, Chico, Office of Graduate Studies, College of Communication and Education, Department of Communication Arts and Sciences, Program in Communication Sciences and Disorders, Chico, CA 95929-0722. Offers MA. *Accreditation:* ASHA. *Degree requirements:* For master's, thesis or project. *Entrance requirements:* For master's, GRE General Test, 3 letters of recommendation, statement of purpose, resume. Additional exam requirements/recommendations for international students: Required—TOEFL (minimum score 550 paper-based; 80 iBT), IELTS (minimum score 6.5), PTE (minimum score 59). *Application deadline:* For fall admission, 3/1 for domestic and international students. Application fee: $55. Electronic applications accepted. *Expenses:* Tuition, area resident: Full-time $4146; part-time $2730. *Financial support:* Teaching assistantships, career-related internships or fieldwork, scholarships/grants, traineeships, and unspecified assistantships available. *Unit head:* Dr. Suzanne B. Miller, Director, 530-898-5871, Fax: 530-898-6612. *Application contact:* Judy L. Rice, Graduate Admissions Coordinator, 530-898-5416, Fax: 530-898-3342. Website: http://www.csuchico.edu/cmsd/

California State University, East Bay, Office of Graduate Studies, College of Letters, Arts, and Social Sciences, Department of Communicative Sciences and Disorders, Hayward, CA 94542-3000. Offers speech-language pathology (MS). *Accreditation:* ASHA. *Program availability:* Part-time. *Students:* 117 full-time (108 women), 12 part-time (11 women); includes 66 minority (2 Black or African American, non-Hispanic/Latino; 31 Asian, non-Hispanic/Latino; 24 Hispanic/Latino; 2 Native Hawaiian or other Pacific Islander, non-Hispanic/Latino; 7 Two or more races, non-Hispanic/Latino), 4 international. Average age 30. 399 applicants, 12% accepted, 40 enrolled. In 2015, 28 master's awarded. *Degree requirements:* For master's, comprehensive exam, internship or thesis. *Entrance requirements:* For master's, minimum GPA of 3.0 in last 2 years of course work; baccalaureate degree in speech pathology and audiology; minimum of 60 hours' supervised clinical practice. Additional exam requirements/recommendations for international students: Required—TOEFL (minimum score 550 paper-based). *Application deadline:* For fall admission, 6/30 for domestic and international students. Application fee: $55. Electronic applications accepted. *Financial support:* Fellowships, teaching assistantships, career-related internships or fieldwork, Federal Work-Study, institutionally sponsored loans, and scholarships/grants available. Support available to part-time students. Financial award application deadline: 3/2. *Faculty research:* Aphasia, autism, dementia, diversity, voice. *Unit head:* Dr. Shubha Kashinath, Interim Chair, 510-885-3090, E-mail: shubha.kashinath@csueastbay.edu. *Application contact:* Dr. Elena Dukhovny, Graduate Coordinator, 510-885-2631, Fax: 510-885-2186, E-mail: elena.dukhovny@csueastbay.edu. Website: http://www20.csueastbay.edu/class/departments/commsci/index.html

California State University, Fresno, Division of Graduate Studies, College of Health and Human Services, Department of Communicative Disorders, Fresno, CA 93740-8027. Offers communicative disorders (MA), including deaf education, speech/language pathology. *Accreditation:* ASHA. *Program availability:* Part-time. *Degree requirements:* For master's, thesis or alternative. *Entrance requirements:* For master's, GRE General Test, minimum GPA of 3.0. Additional exam requirements/recommendations for international students: Required—TOEFL. Electronic applications accepted. *Faculty research:* Disabilities education, technology, writing skills at multiple levels, stuttering treatment.

California State University, Fullerton, Graduate Studies, College of Communications, Department of Human Communications, Fullerton, CA 92834-9480. Offers communication studies (MA); communicative disorders (MA). *Accreditation:* ASHA. *Program availability:* Part-time. *Degree requirements:* For master's, comprehensive exam, thesis and alternative. *Entrance requirements:* For master's, minimum GPA of 3.0 in major. *Faculty research:* Speech therapy.

California State University, Fullerton, Graduate Studies, College of Humanities and Social Sciences, Program in Linguistics, Fullerton, CA 92834-9480. Offers analysis of specific language structures (MA); anthropological linguistics (MA); applied linguistics (MA); communication and semantics (MA); disorders of communication (MA); experimental phonetics (MA). *Program availability:* Part-time. *Degree requirements:* For master's, one foreign language, thesis or alternative, project. *Entrance requirements:* For master's, minimum GPA of 3.0, undergraduate major in linguistics or related field.

California State University, Long Beach, Graduate Studies, College of Health and Human Services, Department of Communicative Disorders, Long Beach, CA 90840. Offers MA. *Accreditation:* ASHA. *Program availability:* Part-time. *Degree requirements:* For master's, comprehensive exam or thesis. *Entrance requirements:* For master's, GRE, minimum GPA of 3.0 in last 60 units. Electronic applications accepted.

California State University, Los Angeles, Graduate Studies, College of Health and Human Services, Department of Communication Disorders, Los Angeles, CA 90032-8530. Offers speech and hearing (MA); speech-language pathology (MA). *Accreditation:* ASHA. *Program availability:* Part-time, evening/weekend. *Degree requirements:* For master's, comprehensive exam. *Entrance requirements:* For master's, undergraduate major in communication disorders or related area, minimum GPA of 2.75 in last 90 units. Additional exam requirements/recommendations for international students: Required— TOEFL (minimum score 500 paper-based). *Application deadline:* For fall admission, 5/1 for domestic and international students. Applications are processed on a rolling basis. Application fee: $55. *Financial support:* Career-related internships or fieldwork and Federal Work-Study available. Support available to part-time students. Financial award application deadline: 3/1. *Faculty research:* Language disabilities, minority child language learning. Website: http://www.calstatela.edu/dept/com_dis/

California State University, Northridge, Graduate Studies, College of Health and Human Development, Department of Communication Disorders and Sciences, Northridge, CA 91330. Offers audiology (MS); speech language pathology (MS). *Accreditation:* ASHA. *Faculty:* 7 full-time (5 women), 9 part-time/adjunct (all women). *Students:* 124 full-time (114 women), 23 part-time (21 women); includes 56 minority (3 Black or African American, non-Hispanic/Latino; 15 Asian, non-Hispanic/Latino; 31 Hispanic/Latino; 2 Native Hawaiian or other Pacific Islander, non-Hispanic/Latino; 5 Two or more races, non-Hispanic/Latino), 1 international. Average age 29. 470 applicants, 33% accepted, 46 enrolled. *Degree requirements:* For master's, PRAXIS. *Entrance requirements:* For master's, GRE or minimum GPA of 3.5. Additional exam requirements/recommendations for international students: Required—TOEFL. *Application deadline:* For fall admission, 11/30 for domestic students. Application fee: $55. *Financial support:* Application deadline: 3/1. *Faculty research:* Infant stimulation, early intervention program. *Unit head:* Dr. Patricia Seymour, Chair, 818-677-2852. Website: http://www.csun.edu/hhd/cd/

California State University, Sacramento, Office of Graduate Studies, College of Health and Human Services, Department of Speech Pathology and Audiology, Sacramento, CA 95819. Offers speech pathology (MS). *Accreditation:* ASHA. *Degree requirements:* For master's, thesis, project, or comprehensive exam; writing proficiency exam. *Entrance requirements:* For master's, GRE General Test, appropriate bachelor's degree, minimum GPA of 3.0 in last 2 years of course work. Additional exam requirements/recommendations for international students: Required—TOEFL. Electronic applications accepted.

California State University, San Marcos, College of Education, Health and Human Services, Department of Speech-Language Pathology, San Marcos, CA 92096-0001. Offers MA. *Expenses:* Contact institution.

California University of Pennsylvania, School of Graduate Studies and Research, College of Education and Human Services, Department of Communication Disorders, California, PA 15419-1394. Offers MS. *Accreditation:* ASHA. *Program availability:* Part-time, evening/weekend. *Degree requirements:* For master's, comprehensive exam, thesis optional. *Entrance requirements:* For master's, GRE General Test, minimum GPA of 3.0, references. Additional exam requirements/recommendations for international students: Required—TOEFL (minimum score 550 paper-based; 80 iBT). *Application deadline:* For fall admission, 2/15 priority date for domestic and international students. Applications are processed on a rolling basis. Application fee: $25. Electronic applications accepted. *Expenses:* Tuition, state resident: full-time $11,280; part-time $5640 per semester. Tuition, nonresident: full-time $16,920; part-time $8460 per semester. *Required fees:* $2876. Tuition and fees vary according to course load, degree level, campus/location and reciprocity agreements. *Financial support:* Career-related internships or fieldwork, scholarships/grants, traineeships, and unspecified assistantships available. Financial award applicants required to submit FAFSA. *Faculty research:* Normative voice database, communication disorders and health. *Unit head:* Dr. Barbara H. Bonfanti, Chairperson, 724-938-4175, Fax: 724-938-1526, E-mail: bonfanti@calu.edu. *Application contact:* Suzanne C. Powers, Director of Graduate Admissions and Recruitment, 724-938-4029, Fax: 724-938-5712, E-mail: powers_s@ cup.edu. Website: http://www.calu.edu/academics/colleges/education/communication-disorders/

Canisius College, Graduate Division, School of Education and Human Services, Department of Graduate Education and Leadership, Buffalo, NY 14208-1098. Offers business and marketing education (MS Ed); college student personnel (MS Ed); deaf education (MS Ed); deaf/adolescent education, grades 7-12 (MS Ed); deaf/childhood education, grades 1-6 (MS Ed); differentiated instruction (MS Ed); education administration (MS); educational administration (MS Ed); educational technologies (Certificate); gifted education extension (Certificate); literacy (MS Ed); reading (Certificate); school building leadership (MS Ed, Certificate); school district leadership (Certificate); teacher leader (Certificate); TESOL (MS Ed). *Accreditation:* NCATE. *Program availability:* Part-time, evening/weekend, 100% online, blended/hybrid learning. *Faculty:* 8 full-time (7 women), 30 part-time/adjunct (21 women). *Students:* 123 full-time (97 women), 243 part-time (188 women); includes 39 minority (18 Black or African American, non-Hispanic/Latino; 1 Asian, non-Hispanic/Latino; 16 Hispanic/Latino; 4 Two or more races, non-Hispanic/Latino), 1 international. Average age 30. 257 applicants, 88% accepted, 122 enrolled. In 2015, 152 master's, 61 other advanced degrees awarded. *Entrance requirements:* For master's, GRE (if cumulative GPA less than 2.7), transcripts, two letters of recommendation. Additional exam requirements/ recommendations for international students: Required—TOEFL (minimum score 550 paper-based, 80 iBT), IELTS (minimum score 6.5), or CAEL (minimum score 70). *Application deadline:* Applications are processed on a rolling basis. Application fee: $25. Electronic applications accepted. Application fee is waived when completed online. *Expenses:* $780 per credit hour. *Financial support:* Career-related internships or fieldwork, Federal Work-Study, scholarships/grants, tuition waivers (partial), and

Communication Disorders

unspecified assistantships available. Support available to part-time students. Financial award application deadline: 4/30; financial award applicants required to submit FAFSA. *Faculty research:* Asperger's disease, autism, private higher education, reading strategies. *Unit head:* Dr. Rosemary K. Murray, Chair/Associate Professor of Graduate Education and Leadership, 716-888-3723, E-mail: murray1@canisius.edu. *Application contact:* Kathleen B. Davis, Vice President of Enrollment Management, 716-888-2500, Fax: 716-888-3195, E-mail: daviskb@canisius.edu.
Website: http://www.canisius.edu/graduate/

Carlos Albizu University, Graduate Programs, San Juan, PR 00901. Offers clinical psychology (MS, PhD, Psy D); general psychology (PhD); industrial/organizational psychology (MS, PhD); speech and language pathology (MS). *Accreditation:* APA (one or more programs are accredited). *Program availability:* Part-time, evening/weekend. Terminal master's awarded for partial completion of doctoral program. *Degree requirements:* For master's, one foreign language, comprehensive exam, thesis; for doctorate, one foreign language, comprehensive exam, thesis/dissertation, written qualifying exams. *Entrance requirements:* For master's, GRE General Test or EXADEP, interview; minimum GPA of 2.8 (industrial/organizational psychology); for doctorate, GRE General Test or EXADEP, interview; minimum GPA of 3.0 (PhD in industrial/organizational psychology and clinical psychology), 3.25 (Psy D). *Faculty research:* Psychotherapeutic techniques for Hispanics, psychology of the aged, school dropouts, stress, violence.

Carlos Albizu University, Miami Campus, Graduate Programs, Miami, FL 33172-2209. Offers clinical psychology (PhD, Psy D); entrepreneurship (MBA); exceptional student education (MS); human services (PhD); industrial/organizational psychology (MS); marriage and family therapy (MS); mental health counseling (MS); nonprofit management (MBA); organizational management (MBA); psychology (MS); school counseling (MS); speech and language pathology (MS); teaching English for speakers of other languages (MS). *Accreditation:* APA. *Program availability:* Part-time, evening/weekend, 100% online. *Faculty:* 31 full-time (22 women), 37 part-time/adjunct (17 women). *Students:* 519 full-time (426 women), 171 part-time (143 women); includes 583 minority (55 Black or African American, non-Hispanic/Latino; 1 American Indian or Alaska Native, non-Hispanic/Latino; 8 Asian, non-Hispanic/Latino; 514 Hispanic/Latino; 5 Two or more races, non-Hispanic/Latino), 15 international. Average age 34. 189 applicants, 86% accepted, 142 enrolled. In 2015, 147 master's, 36 doctorates awarded. Terminal master's awarded for partial completion of doctoral program. *Degree requirements:* For master's, one foreign language, comprehensive exam, integrative project (for MBA); research project (for exceptional student education, teaching English as a second language); for doctorate, one foreign language, comprehensive exam, internship, project. *Entrance requirements:* For master's, 3 letters of recommendation, interview, minimum GPA of 3.0, resume, statement of purpose, official transcripts; for doctorate, 3 letters of recommendation, minimum GPA of 3.0, resume, interview, statement of purpose, official transcripts. Additional exam requirements/recommendations for international students: Required—Michigan Test of English Language Proficiency. *Application deadline:* For fall admission, 4/1 priority date for domestic students, 5/1 priority date for international students; for spring admission, 11/1 priority date for domestic students, 9/1 priority date for international students. Applications are processed on a rolling basis. Application fee: $50. Electronic applications accepted. *Expenses:* $570 per credit tuition (for master's degrees); $750 per credit tuition (for doctoral degrees); $302 per session fees. *Financial support:* In 2015–16, 158 students received support. Federal Work-Study, scholarships/grants, and tuition discounts available. Financial award application deadline: 6/1; financial award applicants required to submit FAFSA. *Faculty research:* Psychotherapy, forensic psychology, neuropsychology, marketing strategy, entrepreneurship, special education, speech-language pathology. *Unit head:* Dr. Etiony Aldarondo, Provost, 305-593-1223 Ext. 3138, Fax: 305-592-7930, E-mail: ealdarondo@albizu.edu. *Application contact:* Sonia Feliciano, Institutional Director of Student Recruitment, 305-593-1223 Ext. 3108, Fax: 305-477-8983, E-mail: sfeliciano@albizu.edu.

Case Western Reserve University, School of Graduate Studies, Psychological Sciences Department, Program in Communication Sciences, Cleveland, OH 44106. Offers speech-language pathology (MA, PhD). *Accreditation:* ASHA (one or more programs are accredited). *Program availability:* Part-time. *Faculty:* 7 full-time (all women), 6 part-time/adjunct (5 women). *Students:* 12 full-time (all women), 9 part-time (all women); includes 7 minority (2 Black or African American, non-Hispanic/Latino; 2 Asian, non-Hispanic/Latino; 1 Hispanic/Latino; 2 Two or more races, non-Hispanic/Latino). Average age 28. 54 applicants, 19% accepted, 10 enrolled. In 2015, 13 master's awarded. Terminal master's awarded for partial completion of doctoral program. *Degree requirements:* For master's, comprehensive exam, thesis optional; for doctorate, thesis/dissertation. *Entrance requirements:* For master's and doctorate, GRE General Test, statement of objectives; curriculum vitae; 3 letters of recommendation; interview. Additional exam requirements/recommendations for international students: Required—TOEFL (minimum score 577 paper-based; 90 iBT); Recommended—IELTS (minimum score 7). *Application deadline:* For fall admission, 1/31 for domestic students. Application fee: $50. Electronic applications accepted. *Expenses: Tuition, area resident:* Full-time $41,137; part-time $1714 per credit hour. *Required fees:* $32. Tuition and fees vary according to course load and program. *Financial support:* Research assistantships, tuition waivers (partial), and unspecified assistantships available. Financial award application deadline: 1/31; financial award applicants required to submit FAFSA. *Faculty research:* Traumatic brain injury, phonological disorders, child language disorders, communication problems in the aged and Alzheimer's patients, cleft palate, voice disorders. *Unit head:* Dr. Lee Thompson, Chair, 216-368-6477, Fax: 216-368-6078, E-mail: lee.thompson@case.edu. *Application contact:* Kori Kosek, Department Administrator, 216-368-6469, Fax: 216-368-6078, E-mail: cosigrad@case.edu.
Website: http://psychsciences.case.edu/graduate/

Central Michigan University, College of Graduate Studies, The Herbert H. and Grace A. Dow College of Health Professions, Department of Communication Disorders, Doctor of Audiology Program, Mount Pleasant, MI 48859. Offers Au D. *Accreditation:* ASHA. *Degree requirements:* For doctorate, comprehensive exam, thesis/dissertation or alternative. *Entrance requirements:* For doctorate, GRE, interview. Electronic applications accepted. *Faculty research:* Auditory electrophysiology, auditory process disorders, neuroanatomy, pediatric audiology, rehabilitative audiology.

Central Michigan University, College of Graduate Studies, The Herbert H. and Grace A. Dow College of Health Professions, Department of Communication Disorders, Program in Speech-Language Pathology, Mount Pleasant, MI 48859. Offers MA. *Accreditation:* ASHA. *Degree requirements:* For master's, thesis or alternative. Electronic applications accepted. *Expenses:* Contact institution. *Faculty research:* Traumatic brain injury, neuro-linguistics, multidisciplinary and transdisciplinary therapy, speech audiometry, phonological disorders.

Chapman University, Crean College of Health and Behavioral Sciences, Department of Communication Sciences and Disorders, Orange, CA 92866. Offers MS. *Program availability:* Evening/weekend. *Faculty:* 5 full-time (all women), 7 part-time/adjunct (5 women). *Students:* 65 full-time (59 women); includes 25 minority (10 Asian, non-Hispanic/Latino; 15 Hispanic/Latino). Average age 26. 380 applicants, 12% accepted, 33 enrolled. In 2015, 30 master's awarded. *Degree requirements:* For master's,

comprehensive exam, thesis, 400 hours of supervised practicum. *Entrance requirements:* For master's, GRE. Additional exam requirements/recommendations for international students: Required—TOEFL (minimum score 550 paper-based; 80 iBT). *Application deadline:* For fall admission, 1/15 for domestic students. Application fee: $60. Electronic applications accepted. *Expenses:* $875 per unit. *Financial support:* Fellowships, scholarships/grants, and unspecified assistantships available. Financial award applicants required to submit FAFSA. *Unit head:* Dr. Judy Montgomery, Director, 714-997-6844, E-mail: montgome@chapman.edu. *Application contact:* Sara Simon, Graduate Admission Counselor, 714-997-6770, E-mail: simon@chapman.edu.

Clarion University of Pennsylvania, Office of Transfer, Adult and Graduate Admissions, On-Campus Master's Programs, Clarion, PA 16214. Offers data analytics (MS); rehabilitative sciences (MS); special education (MS); speech language pathology (MS). *Accreditation:* ASHA. *Program availability:* Part-time, online learning. *Degree requirements:* For master's, comprehensive exam (for some programs), thesis or alternative. *Entrance requirements:* For master's, GRE, minimum QPA of 3.0. Additional exam requirements/recommendations for international students: Required—TOEFL (minimum score 600 paper-based; 89 iBT), IELTS (minimum score 7.5). Electronic applications accepted.

Cleveland State University, College of Graduate Studies, College of Sciences and Health Professions, School of Health Sciences, Program in Speech Pathology and Audiology, Cleveland, OH 44115. Offers MA. *Accreditation:* ASHA. *Faculty:* 7 full-time (6 women), 5 part-time/adjunct (all women). *Students:* 53 full-time (51 women); includes 5 minority (4 Black or African American, non-Hispanic/Latino; 1 Hispanic/Latino). Average age 25. 296 applicants, 39% accepted, 23 enrolled. In 2015, 19 master's awarded. *Degree requirements:* For master's, comprehensive exam, thesis optional. *Entrance requirements:* For master's, GRE. Additional exam requirements/recommendations for international students: Required—TOEFL (minimum score 550 paper-based; 78 iBT). *Application deadline:* For fall admission, 2/1 priority date for domestic and international students. Application fee: $30. Electronic applications accepted. *Expenses:* Tuition, state resident: full-time $9565. Tuition, nonresident: full-time $17,980. Tuition and fees vary according to program. *Financial support:* In 2015–16, 9 students received support, including 9 teaching assistantships with partial tuition reimbursements available; career-related internships or fieldwork, Federal Work-Study, and unspecified assistantships also available. Financial award application deadline: 2/1; financial award applicants required to submit FAFSA. *Faculty research:* Child language and literacy development, cultural diversity, variant dialects, voice disorders, neurogenic communication disorders. *Unit head:* Dr. Monica Gordon Pershey, Program Director, 216-687-4534, Fax: 216-687-6993, E-mail: m.pershey@csuohio.edu. *Application contact:* Donna Helwig, Administrative Coordinator to the Chairperson, 216-687-3807, Fax: 216-687-6993, E-mail: d.helwig@csuohio.edu.
Website: http://www.csuohio.edu/sciences/dept/healthsciences/graduate/SPH/index.html

The College of Saint Rose, Graduate Studies, School of Education, Program in Communication Sciences and Disorders, Albany, NY 12203-1419. Offers MS Ed. *Accreditation:* ASHA. *Students:* 113 full-time (108 women), 11 part-time (all women); includes 16 minority (3 Black or African American, non-Hispanic/Latino; 4 Asian, non-Hispanic/Latino; 5 Hispanic/Latino; 4 Two or more races, non-Hispanic/Latino), 11 international. Average age 24. In 2015, 46 master's awarded. *Degree requirements:* For master's, comprehensive exam (for some programs), thesis (for some programs), comprehensive exam or thesis. *Entrance requirements:* For master's, minimum undergraduate GPA of 3.0, on-campus interview, 32 undergraduate credits (if undergraduate degree is not in communication disorders). Additional exam requirements/recommendations for international students: Required—TOEFL (minimum score 550 paper-based, 80 iBT), IELTS (minimum score 6) or PTE (minimum score 56). *Application deadline:* For fall admission, 1/15 for domestic and international students; for spring admission, 9/15 for domestic and international students; for summer admission, 1/15 for domestic and international students. Application fee: $125. Electronic applications accepted. *Expenses: Tuition, area resident:* Full-time $13,968; part-time $776 per credit. *Required fees:* $790; $32 per credit hour. $85 per semester. Tuition and fees vary according to course load. *Financial support:* Career-related internships or fieldwork, scholarships/grants, tuition waivers, and unspecified assistantships available. Support available to part-time students. Financial award application deadline: 4/15; financial award applicants required to submit FAFSA. *Unit head:* Dr. Jim Feeney, Chair, 518-454-5255, E-mail: feenyj@strose.edu. *Application contact:* Cris Murray, Assistant Vice President for Graduate Recruitment and Enrollment, 518-485-3390, E-mail: grad@strose.edu.
Website: https://www.strose.edu/communication-sciences-disorders-ms/

Dalhousie University, Faculty of Health Professions, School of Human Communication Disorders, Halifax, NS B3H 1R2, Canada. Offers audiology (M Sc); speech-language pathology (M Sc). *Degree requirements:* For master's, thesis or alternative. *Entrance requirements:* Additional exam requirements/recommendations for international students: Required—TOEFL, IELTS, CANTEST, CAEL, or Michigan English Language Assessment Battery. Electronic applications accepted. *Expenses:* Contact institution. *Faculty research:* Audiology, hearing aids, speech and voice disorders, language development and disorders, treatment efficacy.

Duquesne University, John G. Rangos, Sr. School of Health Sciences, Pittsburgh, PA 15282-0001. Offers health management systems (MHMS); occupational therapy (MS, OTD); physical therapy (DPT); physician assistant studies (MPAS); rehabilitation science (MS, PhD); speech-language pathology (MS); MBA/MHMS. *Accreditation:* AOTA (one or more programs are accredited); APTA (one or more programs are accredited); ASHA. *Program availability:* Minimal on-campus study. *Faculty:* 45 full-time (32 women), 33 part-time/adjunct (17 women). *Students:* 230 full-time (180 women), 11 part-time (5 women); includes 15 minority (1 Black or African American, non-Hispanic/Latino; 3 Asian, non-Hispanic/Latino; 7 Hispanic/Latino; 4 Two or more races, non-Hispanic/Latino), 20 international. Average age 23. 685 applicants, 9% accepted, 24 enrolled. In 2015, 132 master's, 32 doctorates awarded. *Degree requirements:* For doctorate, comprehensive exam (for some programs), thesis/dissertation (for some programs). *Entrance requirements:* For master's, GRE General Test (speech-language pathology), 3 letters of recommendation; minimum GPA of 2.75 (health management systems), 3.0 (speech-language pathology); for doctorate, GRE General Test (for physical therapy and rehabilitation science), 3 letters of recommendation, minimum GPA of 3.0, personal interview. Additional exam requirements/recommendations for international students: Required—TOEFL (minimum score 550 paper-based; 90 iBT). *Application deadline:* For fall admission, 2/1 for domestic and international students; for spring admission, 7/1 for domestic and international students. Applications are processed on a rolling basis. Application fee: $0. Electronic applications accepted. *Expenses:* $1,254 per credit. *Financial support:* Federal Work-Study available. Financial award applicants required to submit FAFSA. *Faculty research:* Neuronal processing, electrical stimulation on peripheral neuropathy, central nervous system (CNS) stimulatory and inhibitory signals, behavioral genetic methodologies to development disorders of speech, neurogenic communication disorders. *Total annual research expenditures:* $38,730. *Unit head:* Dr. Gregory H. Frazer, Dean, 412-396-5303, Fax: 412-396-5554, E-mail: frazer@duq.edu. *Application contact:* Christopher R.

Hilf, Recruiter/Academic Advisor, 412-396-5653, Fax: 412-396-5554, E-mail: hilfc@duq.edu.
Website: http://www.duq.edu/academics/schools/health-sciences

East Carolina University, Graduate School, College of Allied Health Sciences, Department of Communication Sciences and Disorders, Greenville, NC 27858-4353. Offers MS, PhD, Au D/PhD. *Accreditation:* ASHA (one or more programs are accredited). *Program availability:* Online learning. *Students:* 112 full-time (106 women), 25 part-time (23 women); includes 13 minority (1 Black or African American, non-Hispanic/Latino; 4 Asian, non-Hispanic/Latino; 4 Hispanic/Latino; 4 Two or more races, non-Hispanic/Latino), 2 international. Average age 29. 303 applicants, 34% accepted, 58 enrolled. In 2015, 38 master's, 6 doctorates awarded. *Degree requirements:* For master's, comprehensive exam, thesis or alternative; for doctorate, comprehensive exam, thesis/dissertation. *Entrance requirements:* For master's and doctorate, GRE General Test. Additional exam requirements/recommendations for international students: Required—TOEFL. *Application deadline:* For fall admission, 4/1 for domestic students. Application fee: $50. *Financial support:* Research assistantships with partial tuition reimbursements, teaching assistantships with partial tuition reimbursements, and unspecified assistantships available. Financial award application deadline: 6/1. *Faculty research:* Hearing, language disorders, stuttering, reading disorder. *Unit head:* Dr. Kathleen Cox, Interim Chair, 252-744-6095, E-mail: coxka@ecu.edu. *Application contact:* Graduate School, 252-328-6012, Fax: 252-328-6071, E-mail: gradschool@ecu.edu.
Website: http://www.ecu.edu/cs-dhs/csd/index.cfm

Eastern Illinois University, Graduate School, College of Sciences, Department of Communication Disorders and Sciences, Charleston, IL 61920. Offers MS. *Accreditation:* ASHA. *Program availability:* Part-time, evening/weekend, online learning. *Degree requirements:* For master's, comprehensive exam (for some programs), thesis (for some programs). *Entrance requirements:* For master's, GMAT or GRE. Additional exam requirements/recommendations for international students: Required—TOEFL (minimum score 500 paper-based; 61 iBT), IELTS (minimum score 6). Electronic applications accepted.

Eastern Kentucky University, The Graduate School, College of Education, Department of Special Education, Program in Communication Disorders, Richmond, KY 40475-3102. Offers MA Ed. *Accreditation:* ASHA. *Degree requirements:* For master's, comprehensive exam, thesis optional, 375 clinical clock hours. *Entrance requirements:* For master's, GRE General Test, minimum GPA of 3.0. *Faculty research:* Distance learning, fluency, phonemic awareness, technology, autism.

Eastern Michigan University, Graduate School, College of Education, Department of Special Education, Program in Hearing Impairment, Ypsilanti, MI 48197. Offers MA. *Students:* 1 (woman) full-time, 1 (woman) part-time; both minorities (both Black or African American, non-Hispanic/Latino). Average age 29. Application fee: $45. *Application contact:* Linda Polter, Coordinator, 734-487-3300, Fax: 734-487-2473, E-mail: lpolter1@emich.edu.

Eastern Michigan University, Graduate School, College of Education, Department of Special Education, Program in Speech-Language Pathology, Ypsilanti, MI 48197. Offers MA. *Accreditation:* ASHA. *Program availability:* Part-time, evening/weekend, online learning. *Students:* 84 full-time (81 women), 25 part-time (23 women); includes 6 minority (1 Black or African American, non-Hispanic/Latino; 2 Asian, non-Hispanic/Latino; 2 Hispanic/Latino; 1 Two or more races, non-Hispanic/Latino), 2 international. Average age 26. 221 applicants, 43% accepted, 30 enrolled. In 2015, 39 master's awarded. *Entrance requirements:* For master's, GRE General Test. Additional exam requirements/recommendations for international students: Required—TOEFL. *Application deadline:* Applications are processed on a rolling basis. Application fee: $45. *Financial support:* Fellowships, research assistantships with full tuition reimbursements, teaching assistantships with full tuition reimbursements, career-related internships or fieldwork, Federal Work-Study, institutionally sponsored loans, scholarships/grants, tuition waivers (partial), and unspecified assistantships available. Support available to part-time students. Financial award applicants required to submit FAFSA. *Application contact:* Dr. Sarah Ginsberg, Program Director, 734-487-3300, Fax: 734-487-2473, E-mail: sginsberg@emich.edu.
Website: http://www.emich.edu/coe/slp/

Eastern New Mexico University, Graduate School, College of Liberal Arts and Sciences, Department of Health and Human Services, Portales, NM 88130. Offers nursing (MSN); speech pathology and audiology (MS). *Accreditation:* ASHA. *Program availability:* Part-time, online learning. *Degree requirements:* For master's, thesis optional, oral and written comprehensive exam, oral presentation of professional portfolio. *Entrance requirements:* For master's, GRE, three letters of recommendation, resume, two essays. Additional exam requirements/recommendations for international students: Required—TOEFL (minimum score 550 paper-based; 79 iBT), IELTS (minimum score 6). Electronic applications accepted.

Eastern Washington University, Graduate Studies, College of Science, Health and Engineering, Department of Communication Disorders, Cheney, WA 99004-2431. Offers MS. *Accreditation:* ASHA. *Degree requirements:* For master's, comprehensive exam, thesis or alternative. *Entrance requirements:* For master's, GRE General Test, minimum GPA of 3.0.

East Stroudsburg University of Pennsylvania, Graduate College, College of Health Sciences, Department of Communication Sciences and Disorders, East Stroudsburg, PA 18301-2999. Offers speech-language pathology (MS). *Accreditation:* ASHA. *Program availability:* Part-time, evening/weekend, online learning. *Degree requirements:* For master's, comprehensive exam, portfolio. *Entrance requirements:* For master's, GRE General Test, minimum undergraduate QPA of 3.0 overall and in major, 3 letters of recommendation. Additional exam requirements/recommendations for international students: Required—TOEFL (minimum score 560 paper-based; 83 iBT) or IELTS. *Application deadline:* For fall admission, 2/1 priority date for domestic and international students; for spring admission, 11/30 for domestic and international students. Applications are processed on a rolling basis. Application fee: $50. *Expenses: Tuition, area resident:* Full-time $8460; part-time $5640 per year. Tuition, state resident: full-time $8460; part-time $5640 per year. Tuition, nonresident: full-time $12,690; part-time $8460 per year. *International tuition:* $15,368 full-time. *Required fees:* $2462; $1630 per unit. $815 per semester. Tuition and fees vary according to course load, campus/location and program. *Financial support:* Research assistantships with tuition reimbursements, Federal Work-Study, and institutionally sponsored loans available. Financial award application deadline: 3/1; financial award applicants required to submit FAFSA. *Faculty research:* Computer-assisted classroom instruction. *Unit head:* Elaine Shuey, 570-422-3681, Fax: 570-422-3506, E-mail: eshuey@esu.edu. *Application contact:* Dr. LuAnn Batson-Magnuson, Graduate Coordinator, 570-422-3311, Fax: 570-422-2711, E-mail: lmagnuson@esu.edu.

East Tennessee State University, School of Graduate Studies, College of Clinical and Rehabilitative Health Sciences, Department of Audiology and Speech-Language Pathology, Johnson City, TN 37614-1710. Offers communicative disorders (MS), including speech pathology. *Accreditation:* ASHA (one or more programs are accredited). *Faculty:* 29 full-time (22 women). *Students:* 92 full-time (85 women), 3 part-time (all women); includes 4 minority (1 Asian, non-Hispanic/Latino; 3 Hispanic/Latino). Average age 24. 373 applicants, 26% accepted, 35 enrolled. In 2015, 32 master's, 7 doctorates awarded. *Degree requirements:* For master's, comprehensive exam, case study or thesis; for doctorate, comprehensive exam, externship. *Entrance requirements:* For master's, GRE General Test, minimum GPA of 3.0, three letters of recommendation, resume; for doctorate, GRE General Test, minimum GPA of 3.0, three letters of recommendation. Additional exam requirements/recommendations for international students: Required—TOEFL (minimum score 550 paper-based; 79 iBT). *Application deadline:* For fall admission, 2/1 for domestic and international students. Application fee: $35 ($45 for international students). Electronic applications accepted. *Financial support:* In 2015–16, 62 students received support, including 65 research assistantships with tuition reimbursements available (averaging $6,500 per year), 2 teaching assistantships with full tuition reimbursements available (averaging $6,000 per year); career-related internships or fieldwork, institutionally sponsored loans, scholarships/grants, and unspecified assistantships also available. Financial award application deadline: 7/1; financial award applicants required to submit FAFSA. *Faculty research:* Vestibular assessment and management, tinnitus management, speech perception, hearing amplification, early speech and language intervention for children with cleft palate, assessment and management of speech sound disorders, pediatric language intervention, voice disorders and vocal fatigue. *Unit head:* Dr. Brenda Louw, Chair, 423-439-4272, Fax: 423-439-4350, E-mail: louwb1@etsu.edu. *Application contact:* Shella Bennett, Graduate Specialist, 423-439-4708, Fax: 423-439-5624, E-mail: bennetsg@etsu.edu.
Website: http://www.etsu.edu/crhs/aslp/

Edinboro University of Pennsylvania, Department of Speech, Language and Hearing, Edinboro, PA 16444. Offers speech language pathology (MA). *Accreditation:* ASHA. *Program availability:* Part-time, evening/weekend. *Degree requirements:* For master's, thesis or alternative, competency exam. *Entrance requirements:* For master's, GRE or MAT, minimum QPA of 2.5. *Application deadline:* Applications are processed on a rolling basis. Application fee: $30. Electronic applications accepted. *Expenses:* Tuition, state resident: full-time $11,280; part-time $470 per credit hour. Tuition, nonresident: full-time $16,920; part-time $705 per credit hour. *International tuition:* $16,920 full-time. *Required fees:* $3247.20; $135.30 per credit hour. *Financial support:* Research assistantships with tuition reimbursements, career-related internships or fieldwork, Federal Work-Study, scholarships/grants, and unspecified assistantships available. Support available to part-time students. Financial award application deadline: 2/15; financial award applicants required to submit FAFSA. *Unit head:* Dr. Mary Mason-Baughman, Chairperson, 814-732-1287, E-mail: mmasonbaughman@edinboro.edu. *Application contact:* Dr. Mary Mason-Baughman, Chairperson, 814-732-1287, E-mail: mmasonbaughman@edinboro.edu.

Elmhurst College, Graduate Programs, Program in Communication Sciences and Disorders, Elmhurst, IL 60126-3296. Offers MS. *Faculty:* 6 full-time (5 women), 3 part-time/adjunct (all women). *Students:* 38 full-time (37 women); includes 3 minority (1 Asian, non-Hispanic/Latino; 2 Hispanic/Latino). Average age 24. 63 applicants, 90% accepted, 21 enrolled. In 2015, 15 master's awarded. *Degree requirements:* For master's, clinical practicum. *Entrance requirements:* For master's, GRE General Test, 3 recommendations, resume, statement of purpose. Additional exam requirements/recommendations for international students: Required—TOEFL (minimum score 550 paper-based; 79 iBT). *Application deadline:* Applications are processed on a rolling basis. Application fee: $0. Electronic applications accepted. *Expenses:* $29,000 per year comprehensive fee. *Financial support:* In 2015–16, 32 students received support. Scholarships/grants available. Financial award application deadline: 2/1; financial award applicants required to submit FAFSA. *Application contact:* Timothy J. Panfil, Director of Enrollment Management, School for Professional Studies, 630-617-3300 Ext. 3256, Fax: 630-617-6471, E-mail: panfilt@elmhurst.edu.
Website: http://www.elmhurst.edu/masters_communication_sciences_disorders

Elms College, Division of Communication Sciences and Disorders, Chicopee, MA 01013-2839. Offers autism spectrum disorders (MS, CAGS); communication sciences and disorders (CAGS). *Program availability:* Part-time. *Faculty:* 6 part-time/adjunct (5 women). *Students:* 2 full-time (1 woman), 43 part-time (38 women); includes 5 minority (3 Black or African American, non-Hispanic/Latino; 2 Hispanic/Latino). Average age 36. 20 applicants, 95% accepted, 14 enrolled. In 2015, 9 master's, 12 other advanced degrees awarded. *Entrance requirements:* For degree, minimum GPA of 3.0. Additional exam requirements/recommendations for international students: Required—TOEFL. *Application deadline:* For fall admission, 7/1 priority date for domestic students; for spring admission, 11/1 priority date for domestic students. Applications are processed on a rolling basis. Application fee: $30. *Financial support:* Applicants required to submit FAFSA. *Unit head:* Dr. Kathryn James, Chair, Division of Communication Sciences and Disorders, 413-265-2253, E-mail: jamesk@elms.edu. *Application contact:* Dr. Elizabeth Teahan Hukowicz, Dean, School of Graduate and Professional Studies, 413-265-2360, Fax: 413-265-2459, E-mail: hukowicze@elms.edu.

Emerson College, Graduate Studies, School of Communication, Department of Communication Sciences and Disorders, Program in Communication Disorders, Boston, MA 02116-4624. Offers MS. *Accreditation:* ASHA. *Faculty:* 8 full-time (5 women), 2 part-time/adjunct (1 woman). *Students:* 89 full-time (85 women), 1 (woman) part-time; includes 16 minority (7 Asian, non-Hispanic/Latino; 8 Hispanic/Latino; 1 Two or more races, non-Hispanic/Latino), 2 international. Average age 25. 634 applicants, 21% accepted, 50 enrolled. In 2015, 44 master's awarded. *Degree requirements:* For master's, comprehensive exam, thesis or alternative. *Entrance requirements:* For master's, GRE General Test. Additional exam requirements/recommendations for international students: Required—TOEFL (minimum score 550 paper-based; 80 iBT), IELTS (minimum score 6.5). *Application deadline:* For fall admission, 1/5 for domestic and international students. Applications are processed on a rolling basis. Application fee: $60 ($75 for international students). Electronic applications accepted. *Financial support:* In 2015–16, 11 students received support, including 11 fellowships with partial tuition reimbursements available (averaging $10,363 per year); research assistantships with partial tuition reimbursements available, Federal Work-Study, scholarships/grants, and unspecified assistantships also available. Financial award application deadline: 2/15; financial award applicants required to submit FAFSA. *Unit head:* Dr. Sandra Cohn Thau, Graduate Program Director, 617-824-8730, E-mail: sandra_cohn_thau@emerson.edu. *Application contact:* Leanda Ferland, Director of Graduate Admission, 617-824-8610, Fax: 617-824-8614, E-mail: gradapp@emerson.edu.
Website: http://www.emerson.edu/graduate_admission

Florida Atlantic University, College of Education, Department of Communication Sciences and Disorders, Boca Raton, FL 33431-0991. Offers speech-language pathology (MS). *Accreditation:* ASHA. *Faculty:* 4 full-time (2 women). *Students:* 50 full-time (45 women), 3 part-time (all women); includes 8 minority (3 Black or African American, non-Hispanic/Latino; 1 Asian, non-Hispanic/Latino; 3 Hispanic/Latino; 1 Two or more races, non-Hispanic/Latino). Average age 25. 288 applicants, 19% accepted, 26 enrolled. In 2015, 24 master's awarded. *Degree requirements:* For master's, thesis optional. *Entrance requirements:* For master's, GRE General Test, minimum undergraduate GPA of 3.0 in last 60 hours of course work or graduate 3.5. Additional

Communication Disorders

exam requirements/recommendations for international students: Required—TOEFL (minimum score 500 paper-based; 61 iBT), IELTS (minimum score 6). *Application deadline:* For fall admission, 2/1 for domestic and international students. Application fee: $30. *Expenses: Tuition, area resident:* Full-time $7392; part-time $369.82 per credit hour. Tuition, state resident: full-time $7392; part-time $369.82 per credit hour. Tuition, nonresident: full-time $19,432; part-time $1024.81 per credit hour. *Financial support:* Career-related internships or fieldwork available. *Faculty research:* Fluency disorders, auditory processing, child language, adult language and cognition, multicultural speech and language issues. *Unit head:* Dr. Deena Louise Wener, Chair, 561-297-2258, Fax: 561-297-2268, E-mail: wener@fau.edu. *Application contact:* Dr. Eliah Watlington, Associate Dean, 561-296-8520, Fax: 261-297-2991, E-mail: ewatling@fau.edu. Website: http://www.coe.fau.edu/academicdepartments/csd/

Florida International University, College of Nursing and Health Sciences, Department of Communication Sciences and Disorders, Miami, FL 33199. Offers speech-language pathology (MS). *Accreditation:* ASHA. *Program availability:* Part-time, evening/weekend. *Faculty:* 4 full-time (3 women), 8 part-time/adjunct (6 women). *Students:* 90 full-time (85 women), 5 part-time (all women); includes 78 minority (5 Black or African American, non-Hispanic/Latino; 1 Asian, non-Hispanic/Latino; 72 Hispanic/Latino), 1 international. Average age 27. 324 applicants, 16% accepted, 46 enrolled. In 2015, 32 master's awarded. *Degree requirements:* For master's, thesis optional. *Entrance requirements:* For master's, minimum undergraduate GPA of 3.0 in upper-level coursework; letter of intent; 2 letters of recommendation. Additional exam requirements/recommendations for international students: Required—TOEFL (minimum score 550 paper-based; 80 iBT). *Application deadline:* For fall admission, 2/1 for domestic and international students. Application fee: $30. Electronic applications accepted. *Expenses:* Tuition, state resident: full-time $10,708; part-time $455.64 per credit hour. Tuition, nonresident: full-time $23,816; part-time $1001.69 per credit hour. *Required fees:* $390; $195 per semester. Tuition and fees vary according to program. *Financial support:* Institutionally sponsored loans, scholarships/grants, and unspecified assistantships available. Financial award application deadline: 3/1; financial award applicants required to submit FAFSA. *Unit head:* Dr. Monica Hough, Chair, 305-348-2873, E-mail: mshough@fiu.edu. *Application contact:* Nanett Rojas, Manager, Admissions Operations, 305-348-7464, Fax: 305-348-7441, E-mail: gradadm@fiu.edu. Website: http://cnhs.fiu.edu/

Florida State University, The Graduate School, College of Communication and Information, School of Communication Science and Disorders, Tallahassee, FL 32306-1200. Offers MS, PhD. *Accreditation:* ASHA (one or more programs are accredited). *Program availability:* Part-time, blended/hybrid learning. *Faculty:* 19 full-time (15 women), 8 part-time/adjunct (6 women). *Students:* 73 full-time (all women), 63 part-time (59 women); includes 33 minority (7 Black or African American, non-Hispanic/Latino; 4 Asian, non-Hispanic/Latino; 20 Hispanic/Latino; 2 Two or more races, non-Hispanic/Latino), 2 international. 363 applicants, 17% accepted, 29 enrolled. In 2015, 57 master's, 3 doctorates awarded. *Degree requirements:* For master's, thesis optional; for doctorate, thesis/dissertation. *Entrance requirements:* For master's, GRE General Test, minimum GPA of 3.0; for doctorate, GRE General Test, minimum GPA of 3.0 (undergraduate), 3.5 (graduate). Additional exam requirements/recommendations for international students: Required—TOEFL (minimum score 550 paper-based; 80 iBT). *Application deadline:* For fall admission, 1/15 for domestic and international students. Application fee: $30. Electronic applications accepted. *Expenses: Tuition, area resident:* Full-time $7263; part-time $403.50 per credit hour. Tuition, nonresident: full-time $18,087; part-time $1004.85 per credit hour. *Required fees:* $1365; $75.81 per credit hour. $20 per semester. Tuition and fees vary according to campus/location. *Financial support:* In 2015–16, 2 fellowships with full tuition reimbursements (averaging $14,000 per year), 25 research assistantships with partial tuition reimbursements (averaging $8,000 per year), 21 teaching assistantships with partial tuition reimbursements (averaging $9,000 per year) were awarded; career-related internships or fieldwork, Federal Work-Study, institutionally sponsored loans, scholarships/grants, tuition waivers (partial); and unspecified assistantships also available. Financial award application deadline: 1/1; financial award applicants required to submit FAFSA. *Faculty research:* Autism, neurogenic disorders, early intervention, child language disorders, literacy development and disorders, augmentative communication, dialectal influences on language development, speech development. *Total annual research expenditures:* $1.8 million. *Unit head:* Dr. Hugh W. Catts, Director, 850-644-6566, Fax: 850-645-8994, E-mail: hugh.catts@cci.fsu.edu. *Application contact:* Jennifer Boss Kekelis, Academic Program Specialist, 850-644-2253, Fax: 850-644-8994, E-mail: jennifer.kekelis@cci.fsu.edu. Website: http://commdisorders.cci.fsu.edu/Academic-Programs-Admissions/Doctoral-Program-Admissions/?_ga-1.91886682.1375024079.1443718977

Fontbonne University, Graduate Programs, St. Louis, MO 63105-3098. Offers accounting (MS); art (MA); art (K-12) (MAT); business (MBA); computer science (MS); deaf education (MA); early intervention in deaf education (MA); education (MA), including autism spectrum disorders, curriculum and instruction, diverse learners, early childhood education, reading, special education; elementary education (MAT); family and consumer sciences (MA, MAT), including child and family studies (MA), multidisciplinary health communication studies (MA); fine arts (MFA); instructional design and technology (MS); learning technologies (MS); management (MM); middle school education (MAT); nonprofit management (MS); secondary education (MAT); special education (MAT); speech-language pathology (MS); supply chain management (MS); theatre (MA). *Program availability:* Part-time, evening/weekend, online learning. *Degree requirements:* For master's, comprehensive exam (for some programs), thesis (for some programs). *Entrance requirements:* Additional exam requirements/recommendations for international students: Required—TOEFL (minimum score 500 paper-based; 65 iBT). Electronic applications accepted.

Fort Hays State University, Graduate School, College of Health and Life Sciences, Department of Communication Disorders, Hays, KS 67601-4099. Offers speech-language pathology (MS). *Accreditation:* ASHA. *Program availability:* Part-time. *Degree requirements:* For master's, comprehensive exam, thesis optional. *Entrance requirements:* For master's, GRE General Test. Additional exam requirements/recommendations for international students: Required—TOEFL (minimum score 550 paper-based). Electronic applications accepted. *Faculty research:* Aural rehabilitation, phonological and articulation skills, middle ear diseases, output capability of stereo cassette units, language development.

Gallaudet University, The Graduate School, Washington, DC 20002-3625. Offers American Sign Language/English bilingual early childhood deaf education: birth to 5 (Certificate); audiology (Au D); clinical psychology (PhD); deaf and hard of hearing infants, toddlers, and their families (Certificate); deaf education (MA, Ed S); deaf history (Certificate); deaf studies (Certificate); educating deaf students with disabilities (Certificate); education: teacher preparation (MA), including deaf education, early childhood education and deaf education, elementary education and deaf education, secondary education and deaf education; educational neuroscience (PhD); hearing, speech and language sciences (MS, PhD); international development (MA); interpretation (MA, PhD), including combined interpreting practice and research (MA), interpreting research (MA); linguistics (MA, PhD); mental health counseling (MA); peer

mentoring (Certificate); public administration (MPA); school counseling (MA); school psychology (Psy S); sign language teaching (MA); social work (MSW); speech-language pathology (MS). *Program availability:* Part-time. *Students:* 295 full-time (229 women), 149 part-time (104 women); includes 127 minority (32 Black or African American, non-Hispanic/Latino; 2 American Indian or Alaska Native, non-Hispanic/Latino; 14 Asian, non-Hispanic/Latino; 35 Hispanic/Latino; 44 Two or more races, non-Hispanic/Latino), 26 international. Average age 31. 598 applicants, 47% accepted, 158 enrolled. In 2015, 140 master's, 17 doctorates, 8 other advanced degrees awarded. Terminal master's awarded for partial completion of doctoral program. *Degree requirements:* For master's, comprehensive exam (for some programs), thesis optional; for doctorate, comprehensive exam, thesis/dissertation. *Entrance requirements:* For master's and doctorate, GRE General Test or MAT, letters of recommendation, interviews, goals statement, American Sign Language proficiency interview, written English competency. Additional exam requirements/recommendations for international students: Required—TOEFL. *Application deadline:* For fall admission, 2/15 for domestic students. Applications are processed on a rolling basis. Application fee: $75. Electronic applications accepted. *Expenses: Tuition, area resident:* Full-time $16,596; part-time $922 per credit hour. International tuition: $33,192 full-time. *Required fees:* $3047; $263 per semester. *Financial support:* In 2015–16, 229 students received support. Fellowships, research assistantships, teaching assistantships, career-related internships or fieldwork, Federal Work-Study, scholarships/grants, tuition waivers (partial), and unspecified assistantships available. Support available to part-time students. Financial award application deadline: 7/1; financial award applicants required to submit FAFSA. *Faculty research:* Signing math dictionaries, telecommunications access, cancer genetics, linguistics, visual language and visual learning, integrated quantum materials, deaf legal discourse, advance recruitment and retention in geosciences. *Unit head:* Dr. Gaurav Mathur, Dean, Graduate School and Continuing Studies, 202-250-2380, Fax: 202-651-5027, E-mail: gaurav.mathur@gallaudet.edu. *Application contact:* Wednesday Luria, Coordinator of Prospective Graduate Student Services, 202-651-5400, Fax: 202-651-5295, E-mail: graduate.school@gallaudet.edu. Website: http://www.gallaudet.edu/x26696.xml

The George Washington University, Columbian College of Arts and Sciences, Department of Speech and Hearing Sciences, Washington, DC 20052. Offers speech-language pathology (MA). *Accreditation:* ASHA. *Faculty:* 12 full-time (7 women), 5 part-time/adjunct (4 women). *Students:* 49 full-time (45 women), 33 part-time (all women); includes 14 minority (4 Black or African American, non-Hispanic/Latino; 6 Asian, non-Hispanic/Latino; 2 Hispanic/Latino; 2 Two or more races, non-Hispanic/Latino), 2 international. Average age 25. 455 applicants, 17% accepted, 34 enrolled. In 2015, 31 master's awarded. *Degree requirements:* For master's, comprehensive exam, thesis or alternative. *Entrance requirements:* For master's, GRE General Test, interview, minimum GPA of 3.0. Additional exam requirements/recommendations for international students: Required—TOEFL (minimum score 550 paper-based; 80 iBT). *Application deadline:* For fall admission, 2/1 priority date for domestic students, 1/15 priority date for international students. Applications are processed on a rolling basis. Application fee: $75. Electronic applications accepted. *Financial support:* In 2015–16, 16 students received support. Fellowships with tuition reimbursements available, teaching assistantships with tuition reimbursements available, career-related internships or fieldwork, Federal Work-Study, and tuition waivers available. Financial award application deadline: 1/15. *Unit head:* James Mahshie, Chair, 202-994-2052, E-mail: jmahshie@gwu.edu. *Application contact:* Information Contact, 202-994-7362, Fax: 202-994-2589, E-mail: gwusphr@gwu.edu. Website: http://speechhearing.columbian.gwu.edu/

Georgia State University, College of Education, Department of Educational Psychology, Special Education, and Communication Disorders, Program in Communication Disorders, Atlanta, GA 30302-3083. Offers M Ed. *Accreditation:* ASHA; NCATE. *Entrance requirements:* For master's, GRE, minimum undergraduate GPA of 3.0. Additional exam requirements/recommendations for international students: Required—TOEFL (minimum score 550 paper-based; 79 iBT), IELTS (minimum score 6.5). *Application deadline:* For fall admission, 1/15 for domestic and international students. Application fee: $50. Electronic applications accepted. *Expenses:* Tuition, state resident: full-time $6876; part-time $382 per credit hour. Tuition, nonresident: full-time $22,374; part-time $1243 per credit hour. *Required fees:* $2128; $2128 per term. $1064 per term. Part-time tuition and fees vary according to course load and program. *Faculty research:* Dialect, aphasia, motor speech disorders, child language development, high risk populations. *Unit head:* Dr. Jacqueline Sue Laures-Gore, Program Coordinator, 404-413-8299, E-mail: jlaures@gsu.edu. *Application contact:* Sandy Vaughn, Senior Administrative Coordinator, 404-413-8318, Fax: 404-413-8043, E-mail: svaughn@gsu.edu. Website: http://esc.education.gsu.edu/academics-and-admissions/communication-sciences-and-disorders/

Georgia State University, College of Education, Department of Educational Psychology, Special Education, and Communication Disorders, Program in Education of Students with Exceptionalities, Atlanta, GA 30302-3083. Offers autism spectrum disorders (PhD); behavior disorders (PhD); communication disorders (PhD); early childhood special education (PhD); learning disabilities (PhD); mental retardation (PhD); orthopedic impairments (PhD); sensory impairments (PhD). *Accreditation:* NCATE. *Program availability:* Part-time, evening/weekend. *Degree requirements:* For doctorate, comprehensive exam, thesis/dissertation. *Entrance requirements:* Additional exam requirements/recommendations for international students: Required—TOEFL (minimum score 550 paper-based; 79 iBT) or IELTS (minimum score 6.5). *Application deadline:* For fall admission, 6/1 for domestic and international students; for winter admission, 11/1 for domestic and international students; for spring admission, 5/1 for domestic and international students. Application fee: $50. Electronic applications accepted. *Expenses:* Tuition, state resident: full-time $6876; part-time $382 per credit hour. Tuition, nonresident: full-time $22,374; part-time $1243 per credit hour. *Required fees:* $2128; $2128 per term. $1064 per term. Part-time tuition and fees vary according to course load and program. *Financial support:* In 2015–16, fellowships with full tuition reimbursements (averaging $28,000 per year), research assistantships with full tuition reimbursements (averaging $2,000 per year) were awarded; scholarships/grants, health care benefits, and unspecified assistantships also available. *Faculty research:* Academic and behavioral supports for students with emotional/behavior disorders; academic interventions for learning disabilities; cultural, socioeconomic, and linguistic diversity; language and literacy development, disorders, and instruction. *Unit head:* Dr. Kristine Jolivette, Associate Professor, 404-413-8040, Fax: 404-413-8043, E-mail: kjolivette@gsu.edu. *Application contact:* Sandy Vaughn, Senior Administrative Coordinator, 404-413-8318, Fax: 404-413-8043, E-mail: svaughn@gsu.edu. Website: http://esc.education.gsu.edu/academics-and-admissions/special-education/education-of-students-with-exceptionalities-ph-d/

Georgia State University, College of Education, Department of Educational Psychology, Special Education, and Communication Disorders, Program in Multiple and Severe Disabilities, Atlanta, GA 30302-3083. Offers early childhood special education (M Ed); special education adapted curriculum (intellectual disabilities) (M Ed); special education deaf education (M Ed); special education general and adapted curriculum (autism spectrum disorders) (M Ed); special education physical and health disabilities (orthopedic impairments) (M Ed). *Accreditation:* NCATE. *Program availability:* Part-time. *Degree requirements:* For master's, variable foreign language requirement, comprehensive exam, thesis (for some programs). *Entrance requirements:* For master's, GRE. Additional exam requirements/recommendations for international students: Required—TOEFL (minimum score 550 paper-based; 79 iBT) or IELTS (minimum score 6.5). *Application deadline:* For fall admission, 6/1 for domestic and international students; for winter admission, 11/1 for domestic and international students; for spring admission, 5/1 for domestic and international students. Application fee: $50. Electronic applications accepted. *Expenses:* Tuition, state resident: full-time $6876; part-time $382 per credit hour. Tuition, nonresident: full-time $22,374; part-time $1243 per credit hour. *Required fees:* $2128; $2128 per term. $1064 per term. Part-time tuition and fees vary according to course load and program. *Financial support:* In 2015–16, fellowships with full tuition reimbursements (averaging $25,000 per year), research assistantships with full tuition reimbursements (averaging $2,000 per year) were awarded; teaching assistantships with full tuition reimbursements, scholarships/grants, health care benefits, and unspecified assistantships also available. *Faculty research:* Literacy, language, behavioral supports. *Unit head:* Dr. Kathryn Wolff Heller, Professor, 404-413-8040, E-mail: kheller@gsu.edu. *Application contact:* Sandy Vaughn, Senior Administrative Coordinator, 404-413-8318, Fax: 404-413-8043, E-mail: svaughn@gsu.edu.

Governors State University, College of Health Professions, Program in Communication Disorders, University Park, IL 60484. Offers MHS. *Accreditation:* ASHA. *Program availability:* Part-time, evening/weekend. *Degree requirements:* For master's, comprehensive exam, thesis or alternative, practicum. *Entrance requirements:* For master's, minimum GPA of 3.3. *Faculty research:* Speech perception of hearing-impaired, effects of binaural listening, communication assessment of infants, voice characteristics of head-neck cancer patients.

The Graduate Center, City University of New York, Graduate Studies, Program in Audiology, New York, NY 10016-4039. Offers Au D. *Entrance requirements:* For doctorate, GRE General Test. Additional exam requirements/recommendations for international students: Required—TOEFL. Electronic applications accepted.

The Graduate Center, City University of New York, Graduate Studies, Program in Speech and Hearing Sciences, New York, NY 10016-4039. Offers PhD. *Accreditation:* ASHA. *Degree requirements:* For doctorate, one foreign language, thesis/dissertation. *Entrance requirements:* For doctorate, GRE General Test. Additional exam requirements/recommendations for international students: Required—TOEFL. Electronic applications accepted.

Grand Valley State University, College of Health Professions, Speech-Language Pathology Program, Allendale, MI 49401-9403. Offers MS. *Faculty:* 9 full-time (7 women), 3 part-time/adjunct (all women). *Students:* 94 full-time (80 women), 6 part-time (5 women); includes 13 minority (4 Black or African American, non-Hispanic/Latino; 1 American Indian or Alaska Native, non-Hispanic/Latino; 2 Asian, non-Hispanic/Latino; 3 Hispanic/Latino; 3 Two or more races, non-Hispanic/Latino), 1 international. Average age 25. 342 applicants, 14% accepted, 45 enrolled. In 2015, 55 master's awarded. *Financial support:* In 2015–16, 10 students received support, including 6 fellowships (averaging $1,230 per year), 5 research assistantships (averaging $5,526 per year). *Unit head:* Dr. Dan Halling, Department Chair, 616-331-5604, Fax: 616-331-5556, E-mail: halling@gvsu.edu. *Application contact:* Dr. Beth Macauley, Graduate Program Director, 616-331-5617, E-mail: macauleb@gvsu.edu.

Hampton University, School of Science, Department of Communicative Sciences and Disorders, Hampton, VA 23668. Offers speech-language pathology (MA). *Accreditation:* ASHA. *Program availability:* Part-time, online learning. *Degree requirements:* For master's, comprehensive exam. *Entrance requirements:* For master's, GRE General Test. Additional exam requirements/recommendations for international students: Required—TOEFL (minimum score 525 paper-based) or IELTS (6.5). Electronic applications accepted. *Expenses: Tuition, area resident:* Full-time $10,263; part-time $522 per credit hour. *Required fees:* $35. Tuition and fees vary according to course load and program. *Faculty research:* Language development, the scholarship of teaching and learning, post-stroke care, multicultural issues, family intervention.

Harding University, College of Allied Health, Program in Communication Sciences and Disorders, Searcy, AR 72149-0001. Offers MS. *Accreditation:* ASHA. *Faculty:* 11 full-time (9 women), 2 part-time/adjunct (1 woman). *Students:* 38 full-time (35 women); includes 4 minority (1 Black or African American, non-Hispanic/Latino; 2 Hispanic/Latino; 1 Two or more races, non-Hispanic/Latino). Average age 25. 96 applicants, 23% accepted, 19 enrolled. In 2015, 13 master's awarded. *Application deadline:* For fall admission, 3/1 for domestic and international students. Application fee: $40. *Financial support:* In 2015–16, 6 students received support. Application deadline: 3/1; applicants required to submit FAFSA. *Unit head:* Dr. Dan Tullos, Professor and Chair, 501-279-4633, Fax: 501-279-4325, E-mail: tullos@harding.edu. *Application contact:* Dr. Cheri Yecke, Dean of Graduate Programs, 501-279-4335, Fax: 501-279-5192, E-mail: cyecke@harding.edu.
Website: http://www.harding.edu/academics/colleges-departments/allied-health/communication-sciences-disorders/graduate-program

Hofstra University, School of Health Sciences and Human Services, Programs in Speech Language Pathology and Audiology, Hempstead, NY 11549. Offers audiology (Au D); speech-language pathology (MA). *Accreditation:* ASHA (one or more programs are accredited). *Students:* 97 full-time (95 women), 2 part-time (both women); includes 10 minority (5 Asian, non-Hispanic/Latino; 5 Hispanic/Latino). Average age 24. 406 applicants, 32% accepted, 40 enrolled. In 2015, 40 master's, 8 doctorates awarded. *Degree requirements:* For master's, comprehensive exam, thesis optional; for doctorate, comprehensive exam, thesis/dissertation. *Entrance requirements:* For master's, GRE, 3 letters of recommendation, essay; for doctorate, GRE or master's degree, 3 letters of recommendation, essay. Additional exam requirements/recommendations for international students: Required—TOEFL (minimum score 550 paper-based; 80 iBT). *Application deadline:* For fall admission, 1/15 for domestic and international students. Application fee: $70 ($75 for international students). Electronic applications accepted. *Financial support:* In 2015–16, 39 students received support, including 25 fellowships with tuition reimbursements available (averaging $6,199 per year); research assistantships with tuition reimbursements available, Federal Work-Study, institutionally sponsored loans, scholarships/grants, tuition waivers (full and partial), and unspecified assistantships also available. Support available to part-time students. Financial award applicants required to submit FAFSA. *Faculty research:* Efficacy of story-telling strategies in aphasia, language and literacy development in internationally adopted children, aerodynamic aspects of speech in people who stutter, second language acquisition and first language attrition, acoustic aspects of normal and disordered speech production. *Unit head:* Dr. Hope Baylow, Program Director, 516-463-5507, Fax: 516-463-5260, E-mail: hope.e.baylow@hofstra.edu. *Application contact:* Sunil Samuel, Assistant Vice President of Admissions, 516-463-4723, Fax: 516-463-4664, E-mail: graduateadmission@hofstra.edu.
Website: http://www.hofstra.edu/academics/colleges/healthscienceshumanservices/

Howard University, School of Communications, Department of Communication Sciences and Disorders, Washington, DC 20059-0002. Offers communication sciences (PhD); speech pathology (MS). Offered through the Graduate School of Arts and Sciences. *Accreditation:* ASHA (one or more programs are accredited). *Program availability:* Part-time. *Degree requirements:* For master's, comprehensive exam, thesis or alternative; for doctorate, one foreign language, comprehensive exam, thesis/dissertation. *Entrance requirements:* For master's, GRE General Test, minimum GPA of 3.2; for doctorate, GRE General Test, minimum GPA of 3.5. Additional exam requirements/recommendations for international students: Required—TOEFL. Electronic applications accepted. *Faculty research:* Multiculturalism, augmentative communication, adult neurological disorders, child language disorders.

Hunter College of the City University of New York, Graduate School, Schools of the Health Professions, School of Health Sciences, Department of Speech-Language Pathology and Audiology, New York, NY 10065-5085. Offers speech-language pathology (MS). *Accreditation:* ASHA. *Program availability:* Part-time. *Students:* 41 full-time (38 women); includes 4 minority (1 Black or African American, non-Hispanic/Latino; 3 Asian, non-Hispanic/Latino). Average age 25. In 2015, 8 master's awarded. *Degree requirements:* For master's, comprehensive exam (for some programs), NTE, research project. *Entrance requirements:* For master's, GRE, letters of reference. Additional exam requirements/recommendations for international students: Required—TOEFL. *Application deadline:* For fall admission, 4/1 for domestic students, 2/1 for international students; for spring admission, 11/1 for domestic students, 9/1 for international students. *Financial support:* In 2015–16, 11 students received support, including 3 fellowships with partial tuition reimbursements available (averaging $1,000 per year), 6 research assistantships; career-related internships or fieldwork, Federal Work-Study, institutionally sponsored loans, scholarships/grants, and tuition waivers (full and partial) also available. Support available to part-time students. Financial award application deadline: 3/1. *Faculty research:* Aging and communication disorders, fluency, speech science, diagnostic audiology, amplification. *Total annual research expenditures:* $600,000. *Unit head:* Dr. Paul Cascella, Department Chair, 212-481-3273, Fax: 212-481-4458, E-mail: paul.cascella@hunter.cuny.edu. *Application contact:* Milena Solo, Director for Graduate Admissions, 212-772-4288, E-mail: admissions@hunter.cuny.edu. Website: http://www.hunter.cuny.edu/schoolhp/comsc/index.htm

Idaho State University, Office of Graduate Studies, Kasiska College of Health Professions, Department of Communication Sciences and Disorders and Education of the Deaf, Pocatello, ID 83209-8116. Offers audiology (MS, Au D); communication sciences and disorders (Postbaccalaureate Certificate); communication sciences and disorders and education of the deaf (Certificate); deaf education (MS); speech language pathology (MS). *Accreditation:* ASHA (one or more programs are accredited). *Program availability:* Part-time. *Degree requirements:* For master's, thesis optional, written and oral comprehensive exams; for doctorate, comprehensive exam, thesis/dissertation optional, externship, 1 year full time clinical practicum, 3rd year spent in Boise. *Entrance requirements:* For master's, GRE General Test, minimum GPA of 3.0, 3 letters of recommendation; for doctorate, GRE General Test (at least 2 scores minimum 40th percentile), minimum GPA of 3.0, 3 letters of recommendation, bachelor's degree. Additional exam requirements/recommendations for international students: Required—TOEFL (minimum score 600 paper-based; 80 iBT). Electronic applications accepted. *Faculty research:* Neurogenic disorders, central auditory processing disorders, vestibular disorders, cochlear implants, language disorders, professional burnout, swallowing disorders.

Illinois State University, Graduate School, College of Arts and Sciences, Department of Communication Sciences and Disorders, Normal, IL 61790-2200. Offers MA, MS. *Accreditation:* ASHA. *Degree requirements:* For master's, thesis or alternative, 1 term of residency, 2 practica. *Entrance requirements:* For master's, GRE General Test, minimum GPA of 3.0 in last 60 hours.

Indiana State University, College of Graduate and Professional Studies, Bayh College of Education, Department of Communication Disorders and Counseling, School, and Educational Psychology, Terre Haute, IN 47809. Offers clinical mental health counseling (MS); communication disorders (MS); school counseling (M Ed); school psychology (PhD, Ed S); MA/MS. *Accreditation:* ACA; NCATE. *Program availability:* Part-time, evening/weekend. *Degree requirements:* For master's, thesis optional; for doctorate, thesis/dissertation, research tools proficiency tests. *Entrance requirements:* For master's, GRE General Test or MAT, minimum undergraduate GPA of 2.75; for doctorate, GRE General Test, master's degree, minimum undergraduate GPA of 3.5. Electronic applications accepted. *Faculty research:* Vocational development supervision.

Indiana University Bloomington, University Graduate School, College of Arts and Sciences, Department of Speech and Hearing Sciences, Clinical Program in Audiology, Bloomington, IN 47405-7000. Offers Au D. *Accreditation:* ASHA.

Indiana University Bloomington, University Graduate School, College of Arts and Sciences, Department of Speech and Hearing Sciences, Program in Speech and Hearing Sciences, Bloomington, IN 47405-7000. Offers auditory sciences (Au D, PhD); language sciences (PhD); speech and voice sciences (PhD); speech-language pathology (MA). *Accreditation:* ASHA.

Indiana University of Pennsylvania, School of Graduate Studies and Research, College of Education and Educational Technology, Department of Communication Disorders, Special Education, and Disability Services, Program in Speech-Language Pathology, Indiana, PA 15705-1087. Offers MS. *Accreditation:* ASHA. *Program availability:* Part-time. *Faculty:* 11 full-time (8 women), 2 part-time/adjunct (both women). *Students:* 43 full-time (all women), 2 part-time (both women). Average age 24. 194 applicants, 12% accepted, 22 enrolled. In 2015, 18 master's awarded. *Degree requirements:* For master's, comprehensive exam, thesis optional. *Entrance requirements:* For master's, GRE, 2 letters of recommendation, minimum undergraduate GPA of 3.0. Additional exam requirements/recommendations for international students: Required—TOEFL. *Application deadline:* For fall admission, 2/15 priority date for domestic students. Application fee: $50. Electronic applications accepted. *Financial support:* In 2015–16, 17 research assistantships with tuition reimbursements (averaging $2,720 per year) were awarded; fellowships with partial tuition reimbursements, career-related internships or fieldwork, Federal Work-Study, scholarships/grants, and unspecified assistantships also available. Support available to part-time students. Financial award application deadline: 4/15; financial award applicants required to submit FAFSA. *Unit head:* Dr. David Stein, Graduate Coordinator, 724-357-7841, E-mail: david.stein@iup.edu.
Website: http://www.iup.edu/grad/speechlanguage/default.aspx

Iona College, School of Arts and Science, Department of Speech Communication Studies, New Rochelle, NY 10801-1890. Offers communication sciences and disorders (MA). *Accreditation:* ASHA. *Degree requirements:* For master's, comprehensive exam. *Entrance requirements:* For master's, GRE, 3 letters of recommendation, personal statement, interview. Additional exam requirements/recommendations for international students: Required—TOEFL (minimum score 550 paper-based; 80 iBT). *Expenses:* Contact institution. *Faculty research:* Child language development, adult language disorders, social language disorders, neuropathology's.

Ithaca College, School of Health Sciences and Human Performance, Program in Speech-Language Pathology and Audiology, Ithaca, NY 14850. Offers speech-language pathology (MS); speech-language pathology with teacher certification (MS).

Communication Disorders

Accreditation: ASHA. Program availability: Part-time. Faculty: 10 full-time (9 women). Students: 48 full-time (46 women), 2 part-time (1 woman); includes 3 minority (2 Hispanic/Latino; 1 Two or more races, non-Hispanic/Latino), 2 international. Average age 24. 274 applicants, 32% accepted, 20 enrolled. In 2015, 25 master's awarded. Degree requirements: For master's, comprehensive exam, thesis optional, clinical experience. Entrance requirements: For master's, GRE General Test, minimum GPA of 3.0. Additional exam requirements/recommendations for international students: Required—TOEFL (minimum score 550 paper-based; 80 iBT). Application deadline: For fall admission, 2/1 priority date for domestic and international students. Applications are processed on a rolling basis. Application fee: $40. Electronic applications accepted. Expenses: Contact institution. Financial support: In 2015–16, 23 students received support, including 23 teaching assistantships (averaging $10,928 per year); career-related internships or fieldwork, Federal Work-Study, scholarships/grants, and unspecified assistantships also available. Support available to part-time students. Financial award application deadline: 2/1; financial award applicants required to submit CSS PROFILE or FAFSA. Faculty research: Learning enhancement in higher education, augmentative/alternative communication, cultural and linguistic variables in communication, language and literacy acquisition. Unit head: Dr. Luanne Andersson, Chair, 607-274-1890, E-mail: landersson@ithaca.edu. Application contact: Nicole Eversley Bradwell, Interim Director, Office of Admission, 607-274-3124, Fax: 607-274-1263, E-mail: admission@ithaca.edu.
Website: http://www.ithaca.edu/gradprograms/slpa

Jackson State University, Graduate School, College of Public Service, Department of Communicative Disorders, Jackson, MS 39217. Offers MS. Accreditation: ASHA. Degree requirements: For master's, comprehensive exam. Entrance requirements: For master's, GRE General Test. Additional exam requirements/recommendations for international students: Required—TOEFL (minimum score 520 paper-based; 67 iBT).

Jacksonville University, School of Applied Health Sciences, Jacksonville, FL 32211. Offers health informatics (MS); kinesiological sciences (MS); mental health counseling (MS); speech language pathology (MS). Expenses: Tuition, area resident: Full-time $12,960; part-time $8640 per credit hour. One-time fee: $50. Tuition and fees vary according to course load, degree level, campus/location and program. Application contact: Marisol Preston, Chief Admissions Officer, 904-256-7000, E-mail: admissions@ju.edu.
Website: http://www.ju.edu/chs/AHS/

James Madison University, The Graduate School, College of Health and Behavioral Sciences, Program in Audiology, Harrisonburg, VA 22807. Offers Au D. Accreditation: ASHA. Program availability: Part-time. Students: 24 full-time (22 women); includes 3 minority (1 Black or African American, non-Hispanic/Latino; 1 Hispanic/Latino; 1 Two or more races, non-Hispanic/Latino). Average age 30. 106 applicants, 6% accepted, 6 enrolled. In 2015, 6 doctorates awarded. Application fee: $55. Electronic applications accepted. Financial support: In 2015–16, 18 students received support, including 1 fellowship, 1 teaching assistantship (averaging $7,000 per year); Federal Work-Study, unspecified assistantships, and assistantships (averaging $5375), doctoral assistantships (average $5000) also available. Financial award application deadline: 3/1; financial award applicants required to submit FAFSA. Unit head: Dr. Cynthia R. O'Donoghue, Department Head, 540-568-6440, E-mail: odonogcr@jmu.edu. Application contact: Lynette D. Michael, Director of Graduate Admissions, 540-568-6131 Ext. 6395, Fax: 540-568-7860, E-mail: michaeld@jmu.edu.
Website: http://www.csd.jmu.edu/aud/

James Madison University, The Graduate School, College of Health and Behavioral Sciences, Program in Communication Sciences and Disorders, Harrisonburg, VA 22807. Offers PhD. Accreditation: ASHA. Program availability: Part-time.

James Madison University, The Graduate School, College of Health and Behavioral Sciences, Program in Speech-Language Pathology, Harrisonburg, VA 22807. Offers speech-language pathology (MS). Accreditation: ASHA. Program availability: Part-time. Students: 61 full-time (60 women), 52 part-time (49 women); includes 16 minority (3 Black or African American, non-Hispanic/Latino; 1 American Indian or Alaska Native, non-Hispanic/Latino; 5 Asian, non-Hispanic/Latino; 5 Hispanic/Latino; 2 Two or more races, non-Hispanic/Latino), 1 international. Average age 30. 358 applicants, 19% accepted, 32 enrolled. In 2015, 22 master's awarded. Application fee: $55. Electronic applications accepted. Financial support: In 2015–16, 28 students received support, including 2 fellowships; Federal Work-Study, unspecified assistantships, and assistantships (averaging $7300), doctoral assistantships (averaging 15,312) also available. Financial award application deadline: 3/1; financial award applicants required to submit FAFSA. Unit head: Dr. Cynthia R. O'Donoghue, Department Head, 540-568-6440, E-mail: odonogcr@jmu.edu. Application contact: Lynette D. Michael, Director of Graduate Admissions, 540-568-6131 Ext. 6395, Fax: 540-568-7860, E-mail: michaeld@jmu.edu.
Website: http://www.csd.jmu.edu/MS-SLP/

Kansas State University, Graduate School, College of Human Ecology, School of Family Studies and Human Services, Manhattan, KS 66506. Offers communication sciences and disorders (MS); conflict resolution (Graduate Certificate); early childhood education (MS); family and community service (MS); family studies (MS); life span human development (MS); marriage and family therapy (MS); personal financial planning (MS, Graduate Certificate); youth development (MS, Graduate Certificate). Accreditation: AAMFT/COAMFTE; ASHA. Program availability: Part-time, online learning. Degree requirements: For master's, comprehensive exam (for some programs), thesis optional. Entrance requirements: For master's, GRE, minimum GPA of 3.0 in last 2 years of undergraduate study. Additional exam requirements/recommendations for international students: Required—TOEFL (minimum score 600 paper-based). Electronic applications accepted. Faculty research: Health and security of military families, personal and family risk assessment and evaluation, disorders of communication and swallowing, families and health, financial decision-making.

Kean University, Nathan Weiss Graduate College, Program in Speech Language Pathology, Union, NJ 07083. Offers MA. Accreditation: ASHA. Program availability: Part-time. Faculty: 10 full-time (8 women). Students: 118 full-time (113 women), 47 part-time (42 women); includes 41 minority (9 Black or African American, non-Hispanic/Latino; 10 Asian, non-Hispanic/Latino; 18 Hispanic/Latino; 1 Native Hawaiian or other Pacific Islander, non-Hispanic/Latino; 3 Two or more races, non-Hispanic/Latino), 2 international. Average age 26. 443 applicants, 17% accepted, 74 enrolled. In 2015, 40 master's awarded. Degree requirements: For master's, comprehensive exam, thesis, six credits of research, minimum of 400 supervised clinical hours, PRAXIS. Entrance requirements: For master's, GRE General Test, minimum cumulative GPA of 3.2, official transcripts from all institutions attended, personal statement, three letters of recommendation, professional resume/curriculum vitae. Additional exam requirements/recommendations for international students: Required—TOEFL (minimum score 550 paper-based; 79 iBT), IELTS. Application deadline: For fall admission, 2/1 for domestic and international students; for summer admission, 12/1 for domestic and international students. Application fee: $75. Electronic applications accepted. Expenses: Tuition, state resident: full-time $12,835; part-time $625 per credit. Tuition, nonresident: full-time $17,396; part-time $766 per credit. Required fees: $3235; $147 per credit. Tuition and fees vary according to course level, course load, degree level and program. Financial

support: In 2015–16, 16 research assistantships with full tuition reimbursements (averaging $3,771 per year) were awarded; scholarships/grants and unspecified assistantships also available. Financial award applicants required to submit FAFSA. Unit head: Dr. Barbara D. Glazewski, Program Coordinator, 908-737-5807, E-mail: bglazews@kean.edu. Application contact: Amy Hadjusek, Program Assistant, 908-737-7100, E-mail: grad-adm@kean.edu.
Website: http://grad.kean.edu/slp

Kent State University, College of Education, Health and Human Services, School of Health Sciences, Program in Audiology, Kent, OH 44242-0001. Offers Au D, PhD. Entrance requirements: For doctorate, GRE, 3 letters of reference, goals statement. Additional exam requirements/recommendations for international students: Required—TOEFL (minimum score 550 paper-based; 80 iBT). Expenses: Tuition, state resident: full-time $10,864; part-time $495 per credit hour. Tuition, nonresident: full-time $18,380; part-time $837 per credit hour.

Kent State University, College of Education, Health and Human Services, School of Health Sciences, Program in Speech Language Pathology, Kent, OH 44242-0001. Offers MA, PhD. Accreditation: ASHA. Degree requirements: For doctorate, comprehensive exam, thesis/dissertation. Entrance requirements: For master's and doctorate, GRE, 3 letters of reference, goals statement. Additional exam requirements/recommendations for international students: Required—TOEFL (minimum score 550 paper-based; 80 iBT). Expenses: Tuition, state resident: full-time $10,864; part-time $495 per credit hour. Tuition, nonresident: full-time $18,380; part-time $837 per credit hour.

Kent State University, College of Education, Health and Human Services, School of Lifespan Development and Educational Sciences, Program in Special Education, Kent, OH 44242-0001. Offers deaf education (M Ed); early childhood education (M Ed); educational interpreter K-12 (M Ed); general special education (M Ed); mild/moderate intervention (M Ed); special education (PhD, Ed S); transition to work (M Ed). Accreditation: NCATE. Degree requirements: For doctorate, comprehensive exam, thesis/dissertation. Entrance requirements: For master's, minimum undergraduate GPA of 2.75, moral character form, 2 letters of reference, goals statement; for doctorate and Ed S, GRE General Test, goals statement, 2 letters of reference, interview, resume. Additional exam requirements/recommendations for international students: Required—TOEFL (minimum score 550 paper-based; 80 iBT). Electronic applications accepted. Expenses: Tuition, state resident: full-time $10,864; part-time $495 per credit hour. Tuition, nonresident: full-time $18,380; part-time $837 per credit hour. Faculty research: Social/emotional needs of gifted, inclusion transition services, early intervention/ecobehavioral assessments, applied behavioral analysis.

Lamar University, College of Graduate Studies, College of Fine Arts and Communication, Department of Speech and Hearing Science, Beaumont, TX 77710. Offers audiology (Au D); speech language pathology (MS). Faculty: 11 full-time (7 women), 3 part-time/adjunct (2 women). Students: 83 full-time (75 women), 15 part-time (13 women); includes 37 minority (8 Black or African American, non-Hispanic/Latino; 1 American Indian or Alaska Native, non-Hispanic/Latino; 5 Asian, non-Hispanic/Latino; 21 Hispanic/Latino; 2 Two or more races, non-Hispanic/Latino). Average age 27. 62 applicants, 81% accepted, 36 enrolled. In 2015, 36 master's, 8 doctorates awarded. Degree requirements: For master's, thesis optional; for doctorate, thesis/dissertation. Entrance requirements: For master's, GRE General Test, performance IQ score of 115 (for deaf students), minimum GPA of 2.5; for doctorate, GRE General Test, performance IQ score of 115 (for deaf students). Additional exam requirements/recommendations for international students: Required—TOEFL (minimum score 550 paper-based; 79 iBT), IELTS (minimum score 6.5). Application deadline: For fall admission, 8/10 for domestic students, 7/1 for international students; for spring admission, 1/5 for domestic students, 12/1 for international students. Applications are processed on a rolling basis. Application fee: $25 ($50 for international students). Electronic applications accepted. Expenses: Tuition, area resident: Full-time $6720; part-time $4032. Tuition, nonresident: full-time $14,880; part-time $8928. Required fees: $1900; $950 $784. Financial support: Fellowships with tuition reimbursements, teaching assistantships, and institutionally sponsored loans available. Support available to part-time students. Financial award application deadline: 4/1; financial award applicants required to submit FAFSA. Unit head: Dr. Monica Harn, Chair, 409-880-8338. Application contact: Melissa Gallien, Director, Admissions and Academic Services, 409-880-8888, Fax: 409-880-7419, E-mail: gradmissions@lamar.edu.
Website: http://fineartscomm.lamar.edu/speech-and-hearing-sciences

La Salle University, School of Nursing and Health Sciences, Program in Speech-Language Pathology, Philadelphia, PA 19141-1199. Offers MS. Accreditation: ASHA. Faculty: 5 full-time (3 women), 6 part-time/adjunct (5 women). Students: 57 full-time (54 women); includes 6 minority (2 Black or African American, non-Hispanic/Latino; 3 Asian, non-Hispanic/Latino; 1 Two or more races, non-Hispanic/Latino), 1 international. Average age 24. 327 applicants, 24% accepted, 22 enrolled. In 2015, 37 master's awarded. Degree requirements: For master's, comprehensive exam, capstone project, which includes a written manuscript suitable for publication in a scholarly journal. Entrance requirements: For master's, GRE, personal essay; 3 letters of recommendation; CSDCAS centralized application. Additional exam requirements/recommendations for international students: Required—TOEFL. Application deadline: For fall admission, 2/1 for domestic and international students. Application fee: $100. Expenses: $870 per credit hour; $150 technology fee full-time, $75 technology fee part-time; $135 general university fee. Financial support: In 2015–16, 19 students received support. Federal Work-Study and scholarships/grants available. Financial award application deadline: 8/31; financial award applicants required to submit FAFSA. Unit head: Dr. Barbara Amster, Director, 215-951-1986, Fax: 215-951-5171, E-mail: slh@lasalle.edu. Application contact: Alison McAnespey Target, Director, Graduate and Adult Enrollment, 215-951-1100, Fax: 215-951-1462, E-mail: target@lasalle.edu.
Website: http://www.lasalle.edu/master-speech-language-pathology/

Lehman College of the City University of New York, Division of Arts and Humanities, Department of Speech–Language–Hearing Sciences, Bronx, NY 10468-1589. Offers speech-language pathology and audiology (MA). Accreditation: ASHA. Program availability: Part-time, evening/weekend. Degree requirements: For master's, thesis or alternative.

Lewis & Clark College, Graduate School of Education and Counseling, Department of Teacher Education, Program in Special Education, Portland, OR 97219-7899. Offers M Ed. Accreditation: NCATE. Program availability: Part-time, evening/weekend. Entrance requirements: For master's, minimum GPA of 2.75. Additional exam requirements/recommendations for international students: Required—TOEFL (minimum score 575 paper-based). Electronic applications accepted.

Lindenwood University, Graduate Programs, School of Education, St. Charles, MO 63301-1695. Offers education (MA), including autism spectrum disorders, character education, early intervention in autism and sensory impairment, gifted, technology; educational administration (MA, Ed D, Ed S); English to speakers of other languages (MA); instructional leadership (Ed D, Ed S); library media (MA); professional counseling (MA); school administration (MA, Ed S); school counseling (MA); teaching (MA). Program availability: Part-time, evening/weekend, 100% online. Faculty: 43 full-time (27 women), 234 part-time/adjunct (154 women). *Students:* 359 full-time (267 women), 1,544 part-time (1,149 women); includes 479 minority (408 Black or African American, non-Hispanic/Latino; 7 American Indian or Alaska Native, non-Hispanic/Latino; 5 Asian, non-Hispanic/Latino; 27 Hispanic/Latino; 2 Native Hawaiian or other Pacific Islander, non-Hispanic/Latino; 30 Two or more races, non-Hispanic/Latino), 22 international. Average age 36. 609 applicants, 74% accepted, 402 enrolled. In 2015, 519 master's, 59 doctorates, 74 other advanced degrees awarded. *Degree requirements:* For master's, thesis (for some programs), minimum GPA of 3.0; for doctorate, thesis/dissertation, minimum GPA of 3.0; for Ed S, comprehensive exam, project, minimum GPA of 3.0. *Entrance requirements:* For master's, interview, minimum undergraduate cumulative GPA of 3.0, writing sample, letter of recommendation; for doctorate, GRE, minimum graduate GPA of 3.4, resume, interview, writing sample, 4 letters of recommendation; for Ed S, master's degree in education, relevant work experience. Additional exam requirements/recommendations for international students: Required—TOEFL (minimum score 550 paper-based; 80 iBT); Recommended—IELTS (minimum score 6.5). *Application deadline:* For fall admission, 8/22 priority date for domestic and international students; for spring admission, 1/9 priority date for domestic and international students; for summer admission, 5/16 priority date for domestic and international students. Applications are processed on a rolling basis. Application fee: $30 ($100 for international students). Electronic applications accepted. *Expenses: Tuition, area resident:* Full-time $15,672; part-time $453 per credit hour. *Required fees:* $205 per semester. Tuition and fees vary according to course level, course load and degree level. *Financial support:* In 2015–16, 442 students received support. Career-related internships or fieldwork, Federal Work-Study, institutionally sponsored loans, scholarships/grants, tuition waivers (partial), and unspecified assistantships available. Financial award application deadline: 6/30; financial award applicants required to submit FAFSA. *Unit head:* Dr. Cynthia Bice, Dean, School of Education, 636-949-4618, Fax: 636-949-4197, E-mail: cbice@lindenwood.edu. *Application contact:* Tyler Kostich, Director, Evening and Graduate Admissions, 636-949-4138, Fax: 636-949-4109, E-mail: adultadmissions@lindenwood.edu.

Loma Linda University, School of Allied Health Professions, Department of Communication Sciences and Disorders, Loma Linda, CA 92350. Offers speech-language pathology (MS, SLPD). *Accreditation:* ASHA (one or more programs are accredited). *Program availability:* Part-time. *Degree requirements:* For master's, thesis or alternative. *Entrance requirements:* For master's, GRE General Test. Additional exam requirements/recommendations for international students: Required—TOEFL (minimum score 550 paper-based). *Application deadline:* For fall admission, 7/31 for domestic and international students. Applications are processed on a rolling basis. Application fee: $60. Electronic applications accepted. *Financial support:* Federal Work-Study and tuition waivers (partial) available. Support available to part-time students. *Unit head:* Dr. Terry D. Douglas, Chair, 902-558-4998. *Application contact:* Helen Greenwood, Director, Admissions and Records, 909-824-4599, Fax: 909-824-4809, E-mail: hgreenwood@sahp.llu.edu.

Long Island University–LIU Brooklyn, Richard L. Conolly College of Liberal Arts and Sciences, Brooklyn, NY 11201-8423. Offers biology (MA); chemistry (MS); clinical psychology (PhD); communication sciences and disorders (MS); creative writing (MFA); English (MA); media arts (MA, MFA); political science (MA); psychology (MS); social science (MS); speech-language pathology (MS); United Nations (Advanced Certificate); urban studies (MA); writing and production for television (MFA). *Program availability:* Part-time, evening/weekend, blended/hybrid learning. *Faculty:* 90 full-time (35 women), 125 part-time/adjunct (67 women). *Students:* 382 full-time (288 women), 223 part-time (154 women); includes 257 minority (129 Black or African American, non-Hispanic/Latino; 33 Asian, non-Hispanic/Latino; 80 Hispanic/Latino; 1 Native Hawaiian or other Pacific Islander, non-Hispanic/Latino; 14 Two or more races, non-Hispanic/Latino), 93 international. Average age 33. 801 applicants, 44% accepted, 169 enrolled. In 2015, 163 master's, 16 doctorates, 9 other advanced degrees awarded. *Degree requirements:* For doctorate, thesis/dissertation. *Entrance requirements:* Additional exam requirements/recommendations for international students: Required—TOEFL (minimum score 550 paper-based; 79 iBT). *Application deadline:* Applications are processed on a rolling basis. Application fee: $50. Electronic applications accepted. *Expenses:* $1,155 per credit tuition, $934 per term full-time fees, $442 per term part-time fees. *Financial support:* In 2015–16, 221 students received support, including 135 fellowships with full tuition reimbursements available (averaging $23,986 per year), 29 research assistantships with partial tuition reimbursements available (averaging $13,860 per year), 185 teaching assistantships with full tuition reimbursements available (averaging $20,790 per year). Financial award application deadline: 2/15; financial award applicants required to submit FAFSA. *Faculty research:* Nanocrystal polymerization of cellulose using electron microscopy. *Unit head:* Dr. David Cohen, Dean, 718-488-1003, E-mail: david.cohen@liu.edu. *Application contact:* Richard Sunday, Dean of Admissions, 718-488-1011, Fax: 718-780-6110, E-mail: bkln-admissions@liu.edu.

Long Island University–LIU Post, College of Education, Information and Technology, Brookville, NY 11548-1300. Offers adolescence education (MS); archives and records management (AC); art education (MS); childhood education (MS); childhood/special education (MS); clinical mental health counseling (AC); early childhood education (MS); early childhood education/childhood education (MS); educational leadership (AC); educational technology (MS); information studies (PhD); information technology education (MS); interdisciplinary educational studies (Ed D); literacy B-6 (MS); special education (MS Ed); students with disabilities, 7-12 generalist (AC); teaching students with speech language disabilities (MA); TESOL (MA). *Accreditation:* Teacher Education Accreditation Council. *Program availability:* Part-time, evening/weekend. *Faculty:* 54 full-time (31 women), 131 part-time/adjunct (49 women). *Students:* 440 full-time (373 women), 690 part-time (545 women); includes 250 minority (96 Black or African American, non-Hispanic/Latino; 39 Asian, non-Hispanic/Latino; 105 Hispanic/Latino; 1 Native Hawaiian or other Pacific Islander, non-Hispanic/Latino; 9 Two or more races, non-Hispanic/Latino), 36 international. Average age 32. 875 applicants, 76% accepted, 344 enrolled. In 2015, 326 master's, 15 doctorates, 62 other advanced degrees awarded. Terminal master's awarded for partial completion of doctoral program. *Degree requirements:* For master's, comprehensive exam (for some programs), thesis (for some programs), minimum GPA of 3.0; for doctorate, comprehensive exam, thesis/dissertation, minimum GPA of 3.0. *Entrance requirements:* For master's, GRE, minimum GPA of 3.0. Additional exam requirements/recommendations for international students: Required—TOEFL (minimum score 550 paper-based; 79 iBT), IELTS (minimum score 6.5). *Application deadline:* Applications are processed on a rolling basis. Application fee: $50. Electronic applications accepted. *Expenses:* $1,155 per credit; $934 full-time fee per term, $442 part-time fee per term. *Financial support:* Career-related internships or fieldwork and Federal Work-Study available. Support available to part-time students. Financial award application deadline: 2/15; financial award applicants required to submit FAFSA. *Faculty research:* Career opportunities for individuals with autism spectrum disorders; Educating data management. *Total annual research expenditures:* $97,964. *Unit head:* Dr. Barbara Garii, Dean, 516-299-2210, Fax: 516-299-4167, E-mail: barbara.garii@liu.edu. *Application contact:* Carol Zerah, Director of Graduate and International Admissions, 516-299-2900 Ext. 3952, Fax: 516-299-3952, E-mail: enroll@cwpost.liu.edu.

Website: http://liu.edu/CWPost/Academics/College-of-Education-Information-and-Technology

Longwood University, College of Graduate and Professional Studies, College of Education and Human Services, Department of Social Work and Communication Sciences and Disorders, Farmville, VA 23909. Offers communication sciences and disorders (MS). *Accreditation:* ASHA. *Faculty:* 7 full-time (all women), 2 part-time/adjunct (0 women). *Students:* 43 full-time (all women), 1 (woman) part-time; includes 3 minority (1 Black or African American, non-Hispanic/Latino; 1 Asian, non-Hispanic/Latino; 1 Hispanic/Latino). 227 applicants, 36% accepted, 20 enrolled. In 2015, 25 master's awarded. *Degree requirements:* For master's, comprehensive exam, thesis optional. *Entrance requirements:* For master's, GRE, bachelor's degree from regionally-accredited institution, minimum GPA of 3.0, CSDCAS application. Additional exam requirements/recommendations for international students: Required—TOEFL (minimum score 570 paper-based), IELTS (minimum score 6.5). *Application deadline:* For fall admission, 2/1 for domestic students. Application fee: $50. Electronic applications accepted. *Expenses:* $442 per credit hour. *Financial support:* Fellowships, research assistantships, teaching assistantships, career-related internships or fieldwork, Federal Work-Study, and unspecified assistantships available. Financial award applicants required to submit FAFSA. *Unit head:* Dr. Lissa A. Power-deFur, Graduate Program Coordinator, 434-395-2369, E-mail: powerdefurea@longwood.edu. *Application contact:* College of Graduate and Professional Studies, 434-395-2380, Fax: 434-395-2750, E-mail: graduate@longwood.edu.
Website: http://www.longwood.edu/socialworkcsds/

Louisiana State University and Agricultural & Mechanical College, Graduate School, College of Humanities and Social Sciences, Department of Communication Sciences and Disorders, Baton Rouge, LA 70803. Offers MA, PhD. *Accreditation:* ASHA (one or more programs are accredited).

Louisiana State University Health Sciences Center, School of Allied Health Professions, Department of Communication Disorders, New Orleans, LA 70112-2223. Offers audiology (Au D); speech pathology (MCD). *Accreditation:* ASHA (one or more programs are accredited). *Degree requirements:* For master's, comprehensive exam or thesis. *Entrance requirements:* For master's, GRE General Test (minimum 296 combined score), minimum undergraduate GPA of 3.0, 3 letters of recommendation; for doctorate, GRE General Test (minimum 294 combined score), 3 letters of recommendation, minimum undergraduate GPA of 3.0. *Faculty research:* Hearing aids, clinical audiology, swallowing respiration, language acquisition, speech science.

Louisiana Tech University, Graduate School, College of Liberal Arts, Department of Communication Disorders, Ruston, LA 71272. Offers audiology (Au D); speech-language pathology (MA). *Accreditation:* ASHA (one or more programs are accredited). *Degree requirements:* For master's, thesis or alternative. *Entrance requirements:* For master's, GRE General Test. *Application deadline:* For fall admission, 1/15 for domestic students; for spring admission, 2/3 for domestic students. Application fee: $40. *Financial support:* Fellowships, career-related internships or fieldwork, Federal Work-Study, institutionally sponsored loans, and unspecified assistantships available. Financial award application deadline: 2/1. *Unit head:* Dr. Brenda L. Heiman, Interim Head, 318-257-4764, Fax: 318-257-4492. *Application contact:* Marilyn J. Robinson, Assistant to the Dean of the Graduate School, 318-257-2924, Fax: 318-257-4487.
Website: https://liberalarts.latech.edu/communication/language/

Loyola University Maryland, Graduate Programs, Loyola College of Arts and Sciences, Department of Speech-Language-Hearing Sciences, Baltimore, MD 21210-2699. Offers speech-language pathology (MS). *Accreditation:* ASHA. *Degree requirements:* For master's, comprehensive exam, thesis. *Entrance requirements:* Additional exam requirements/recommendations for international students: Required—TOEFL (minimum score 550 paper-based). *Application deadline:* For fall admission, 2/1 for domestic and international students. Applications are processed on a rolling basis. Application fee: $50. Electronic applications accepted. *Financial support:* Research assistantships and unspecified assistantships available. Financial award application deadline: 4/15; financial award applicants required to submit FAFSA. *Unit head:* Dr. Lisa Schoenbrodt, Chair, 410-617-2578, E-mail: lschoenbrodt@loyola.edu. *Application contact:* Maureen Faux, Executive Director, Graduate Admissions, 410-617-5020, Fax: 410-617-2002, E-mail: graduate@loyola.edu.
Website: http://www.loyola.edu/speech/

Marquette University, Graduate School, College of Health Sciences, Department of Speech Pathology and Audiology, Milwaukee, WI 53201-1881. Offers bilingual English/Spanish (Certificate); speech-language pathology (MS). *Accreditation:* ASHA (one or more programs are accredited). *Program availability:* Part-time. *Faculty:* 13 full-time (10 women), 5 part-time/adjunct (3 women). *Students:* 54 full-time (51 women), 14 part-time (all women); includes 13 minority (1 Black or African American, non-Hispanic/Latino; 3 Asian, non-Hispanic/Latino; 7 Hispanic/Latino; 2 Two or more races, non-Hispanic/Latino). Average age 24. 300 applicants, 30% accepted, 25 enrolled. In 2015, 28 master's awarded. *Degree requirements:* For master's, comprehensive exam, thesis (for some programs). *Entrance requirements:* For master's, GRE General Test, official transcripts from all current and previous colleges/universities except Marquette, three letters of recommendation, personal statement. Additional exam requirements/recommendations for international students: Required—TOEFL (minimum score 530 paper-based). *Application deadline:* For fall admission, 1/15 for domestic students. Application fee: $50. Electronic applications accepted. *Financial support:* In 2015–16, 30 students received support, including 1 fellowship with full tuition reimbursement available (averaging $20,000 per year), 4 research assistantships with full tuition reimbursements available (averaging $13,285 per year); career-related internships or fieldwork, scholarships/grants, health care benefits, tuition waivers (partial), and unspecified assistantships also available. Support available to part-time students. Financial award application deadline: 2/15. *Faculty research:* Language processing in the brain, vocal aging, early language development, birth-to-three intervention, computer applications. *Total annual research expenditures:* $6,955. *Unit head:* Dr. Linda Crowe, Chair, 414-288-5665, Fax: 414-288-3980, E-mail: edward.korabic@marquette.edu. *Application contact:* Dr. Linda Crowe, Chair, 414-288-3215.
Website: http://www.marquette.edu/chs/speech/graduate.shtml

Marshall University, Academic Affairs Division, College of Health Professions, Department of Communication Disorders, Huntington, WV 25755. Offers MS. *Accreditation:* ASHA. *Students:* 57 full-time (55 women), 1 (woman) part-time; includes 1 minority (Black or African American, non-Hispanic/Latino). Average age 24. In 2015, 20 master's awarded. *Degree requirements:* For master's, thesis optional. *Entrance requirements:* For master's, GRE General Test. Application fee: $40. *Financial support:* Fellowships available. *Unit head:* Karen McNealy, Chairperson, 304-696-3634, E-mail: mcnealy@marshall.edu. *Application contact:* Information Contact, 304-746-1900, Fax: 304-746-1902, E-mail: services@marshall.edu.

Marywood University, Academic Affairs, Reap College of Education and Human Development, Department of Communication Sciences and Disorders, Scranton, PA 18509-1598. Offers speech-language pathology (MS). *Accreditation:* ASHA. *Program availability:* Part-time. Electronic applications accepted.

Communication Disorders

Massachusetts Institute of Technology, School of Engineering, Harvard-MIT Health Sciences and Technology Program, Cambridge, MA 02139. Offers health sciences and technology (SM, PhD, Sc D), including bioastronautics (PhD, Sc D), bioinformatics and integrative genomics (PhD, Sc D), medical engineering and medical physics (PhD, Sc D), speech and hearing bioscience and technology (PhD, Sc D). *Faculty:* 125 full-time (20 women). *Students:* 271 full-time (111 women), 15 part-time (4 women); includes 79 minority (2 Black or African American, non-Hispanic/Latino; 1 American Indian or Alaska Native, non-Hispanic/Latino; 61 Asian, non-Hispanic/Latino; 12 Hispanic/Latino; 3 Two or more races, non-Hispanic/Latino), 51 international. Average age 26. 265 applicants, 11% accepted, 21 enrolled. In 2015, 3 master's, 25 doctorates awarded. Terminal master's awarded for partial completion of doctoral program. *Degree requirements:* For master's, thesis; for doctorate, comprehensive exam, thesis/dissertation. *Entrance requirements:* For doctorate, GRE General Test (for medical engineering and medical physics). Additional exam requirements/recommendations for international students: Required—TOEFL (minimum score 600 paper-based; 100 iBT), IELTS (minimum score 7). *Application deadline:* For fall admission, 12/15 for domestic and international students. Application fee: $75. Electronic applications accepted. *Expenses: Tuition:* Full-time $46,400; part-time $725 per credit. One-time fee: $304 full-time. Full-time tuition and fees vary according to course load and program. *Financial support:* In 2015–16, 128 students received support, including 57 fellowships (averaging $38,200 per year), 52 research assistantships (averaging $34,200 per year), 1 teaching assistantship (averaging $19,500 per year); Federal Work-Study, institutionally sponsored loans, scholarships/grants, traineeships, health care benefits, and unspecified assistantships also available. Support available to part-time students. Financial award application deadline: 4/15; financial award applicants required to submit FAFSA. *Faculty research:* Signal processing, biomedical imaging, drug delivery, medical devices, medical diagnostics, regenerative biomedical technologies. *Unit head:* Emery N. Brown, Director, 617-452-4091. *Application contact:* 617-253-3609, Fax: 617-253-6692, E-mail: hst-phd-admissions@mit.edu.
Website: http://hst.mit.edu/

McGill University, Faculty of Graduate and Postdoctoral Studies, Faculty of Medicine, School of Communication Sciences and Disorders, Montréal, QC H3A 2T5, Canada. Offers communication science and disorders (M Sc); communication sciences and disorders (PhD); speech-language pathology (M Sc A). *Accreditation:* ASHA.

Mercy College, School of Health and Natural Sciences, Program in Communication Disorders, Dobbs Ferry, NY 10522-1189. Offers MS. *Accreditation:* ASHA. *Program availability:* Part-time, evening/weekend. *Entrance requirements:* For master's, essay, interview, resume, 2 letters of recommendation, undergraduate transcripts. Additional exam requirements/recommendations for international students: Required—TOEFL (minimum score 600 paper-based; 100 iBT), IELTS (minimum score 8). Electronic applications accepted. *Expenses:* Contact institution. *Faculty research:* Phonology, articulation, hearing deficits, fluency, attention.

MGH Institute of Health Professions, School of Health and Rehabilitation Sciences, Department of Communication Sciences and Disorders, Boston, MA 02129. Offers reading (Certificate); speech-language pathology (MS). *Accreditation:* ASHA (one or more programs are accredited). *Program availability:* Part-time. *Degree requirements:* For master's, thesis or alternative, research proposal. *Entrance requirements:* For master's, GRE General Test, bachelor's degree from regionally-accredited college or university. Additional exam requirements/recommendations for international students: Required—TOEFL (minimum score 550 paper-based; 80 iBT). Electronic applications accepted. *Faculty research:* Children's language disorders, reading, speech disorders, voice disorders, augmentative communication, autism.

Miami University, College of Arts and Science, Department of Speech Pathology and Audiology, Oxford, OH 45056. Offers MA, MS. *Accreditation:* ASHA. *Program availability:* Part-time. *Students:* 54 full-time (53 women); includes 3 minority (1 Asian, non-Hispanic/Latino; 1 Hispanic/Latino; 1 Two or more races, non-Hispanic/Latino). Average age 23. In 2015, 35 master's awarded. *Entrance requirements:* For master's, GRE, Communication Sciences and Disorders Centralized (CSDCAS) Application; personal statement; three letters of recommendation; resume. Additional exam requirements/recommendations for international students: Recommended—TOEFL (minimum score 80 iBT), IELTS (minimum score 6.5), TSE (minimum score 54). *Application deadline:* For fall admission, 12/15 for domestic and international students. Application fee: $50. Electronic applications accepted. *Expenses:* Tuition, state resident: full-time $12,888; part-time $537 per credit hour. Tuition, nonresident: full-time $29,022; part-time $1209 per credit hour. *Required fees:* $530; $24 per credit hour. $30 per semester. Part-time tuition and fees vary according to course load and program. *Financial support:* Application deadline: 2/15; applicants required to submit FAFSA. *Unit head:* Dr. Susan Baker Brehm, Chair, 513-529-2500, E-mail: bakerse1@miamioh.edu. *Application contact:* Dr. Donna Scarborough, Director of Graduate Studies, 513-529-2506, E-mail: scarbod@miamioh.edu.
Website: http://www.MiamiOH.edu/spa/

Michigan State University, The Graduate School, College of Communication Arts and Sciences, Department of Communicative Sciences and Disorders, East Lansing, MI 48824. Offers MA, PhD. *Accreditation:* ASHA (one or more programs are accredited). *Entrance requirements:* Additional exam requirements/recommendations for international students: Required—TOEFL. Electronic applications accepted.

Minnesota State University Mankato, College of Graduate Studies and Research, College of Allied Health and Nursing, Program in Communication Disorders, Mankato, MN 56001. Offers MS. *Accreditation:* ASHA. *Program availability:* Part-time. *Degree requirements:* For master's, comprehensive exam, thesis or alternative. *Entrance requirements:* For master's, GRE General Test, minimum GPA of 3.0 during previous 2 years, references, writing sample. Additional exam requirements/recommendations for international students: Required—TOEFL. *Faculty research:* Internet/technology issues related to speech-language pathology.

Minnesota State University Moorhead, Graduate Studies, College of Education and Human Services, Moorhead, MN 56563. Offers counseling and student affairs (MS); curriculum and instruction (MS); educational leadership (MS, Ed S); special education (MS); speech-language pathology (MS). *Accreditation:* NCATE. *Program availability:* Part-time, evening/weekend, 100% online, blended/hybrid learning. *Application deadline:* For fall admission, 4/15 priority date for domestic students; for spring admission, 11/1 priority date for domestic students. Applications are processed on a rolling basis. Application fee: $20. Electronic applications accepted. *Expenses:* Tuition, state resident: full-time $9000; part-time $4500 per credit. Tuition, nonresident: full-time $18,000; part-time $9000 per credit. *Required fees:* $942; $39.25 per credit. One-time fee: $90 full-time. Full-time tuition and fees vary according to course load, degree level, program and reciprocity agreements. *Financial support:* Career-related internships or fieldwork, Federal Work-Study, and unspecified assistantships available. Financial award application deadline: 7/15; financial award applicants required to submit FAFSA. *Unit head:* Dr. Boyd Bradbury, Interim Dean, 218-477-2471. *Application contact:* Karla Wenger, Graduate Studies Office, 218-477-2344, Fax: 218-477-2482, E-mail: wengerk@mnstate.edu.
Website: http://www.mnstate.edu/cehs/

Minot State University, Graduate School, Department of Communication Disorders, Minot, ND 58707-0002. Offers speech-language pathology (MS). *Accreditation:* ASHA. *Degree requirements:* For master's, comprehensive exam (for some programs), thesis (for some programs). *Entrance requirements:* For master's, GRE General Test, minimum GPA of 3.25. Additional exam requirements/recommendations for international students: Required—TOEFL (minimum score 79 iBT), IELTS (minimum score 6). *Expenses:* Tuition, state resident: full-time $6018. Tuition, nonresident: full-time $6018. *Required fees:* $1325. *Faculty research:* Auditory evoked potentials, pathologies of auditory system, newborn hearing screening, cleft palate research, intervention, the diagnostic process, early language, the pedagogy of clinical teaching, phonology, geriatric communication problems, dysphagia, brain functioning after injury.

Minot State University, Graduate School, Program in Special Education, Minot, ND 58707-0002. Offers deaf/hard of hearing education (MS); specific learning disabilities (MS). *Accreditation:* NCATE. *Degree requirements:* For master's, comprehensive exam (for some programs), thesis (for some programs). *Entrance requirements:* For master's, minimum GPA of 2.75, bachelor's degree in education or related field, teacher licensure (for some concentrations). Additional exam requirements/recommendations for international students: Required—TOEFL (minimum score 79 iBT), IELTS (minimum score 6). *Expenses:* Tuition, state resident: full-time $6018. Tuition, nonresident: full-time $6018. *Required fees:* $1325.

Misericordia University, College of Health Sciences, Department of Speech-Language Pathology, Dallas, PA 18612-1098. Offers MSSLP. *Accreditation:* ASHA. *Faculty:* 7 full-time (5 women), 4 part-time/adjunct (3 women). *Students:* 40 full-time (37 women), 1 (woman) part-time; includes 2 minority (1 Hispanic/Latino; 1 Two or more races, non-Hispanic/Latino). Average age 23. In 2015, 32 master's awarded. *Entrance requirements:* For master's, GRE, minimum undergraduate GPA of 3.5. Additional exam requirements/recommendations for international students: Required—TOEFL. *Application deadline:* For fall admission, 2/1 priority date for domestic students. Application fee: $35. *Financial support:* Scholarships/grants available. Support available to part-time students. Financial award application deadline: 6/30; financial award applicants required to submit FAFSA. *Unit head:* Dr. Glen Tellis, Chair, 570-674-6471, E-mail: gtellis@misericordia.edu. *Application contact:* Maureen Sheridan, Assistant Director of Admissions, 570-674-6255, Fax: 570-674-6232, E-mail: msherida@misericordia.edu.
Website: http://www.misericordia.edu/page.cfm?p-659

Mississippi University for Women, Graduate School, College of Nursing and Speech Language Pathology, Columbus, MS 39701-9998. Offers nursing (MSN, PMC); speech-language pathology (MS). *Accreditation:* AACN. *Program availability:* Part-time. *Degree requirements:* For master's, comprehensive exam, thesis. *Entrance requirements:* For master's, GRE General Test, bachelor's degree in nursing, previous course work in statistics, proficiency in English.

Molloy College, Program in Speech Language Pathology, Rockville Centre, NY 11571-5002. Offers speech-language pathology (MS). *Accreditation:* ASHA. *Program availability:* Part-time, evening/weekend. *Faculty:* 7 full-time (all women), 3 part-time/adjunct (all women). *Students:* 52 full-time (51 women), 1 (woman) part-time; includes 8 minority (4 Asian, non-Hispanic/Latino; 3 Hispanic/Latino; 1 Two or more races, non-Hispanic/Latino), 1 international. Average age 24. 324 applicants, 24% accepted, 32 enrolled. In 2015, 17 master's awarded. *Entrance requirements:* Additional exam requirements/recommendations for international students: Required—TOEFL (minimum score 550 paper-based; 79 iBT). *Application deadline:* Applications are processed on a rolling basis. Application fee: $60. Electronic applications accepted. *Expenses: Tuition,* area resident: Full-time $18,450; part-time $1025 per credit. *Required fees:* $900; $740 per unit. Tuition and fees vary according to course load. *Financial support:* Applicants required to submit FAFSA. *Faculty research:* Voice in Parkinson's Disease, neurophysiology of language, cultural competency, motor speech intervention. *Unit head:* Dr. Barbara Schmidt, Associate Dean of Speech-Language Pathology, 516-323-3519, E-mail: bschmidt@molloy.edu. *Application contact:* Jaclyn Machowicz, Assistant Director for Admissions, 516-323-4010, E-mail: jmachowicz@molloy.edu.

Monmouth University, Graduate Studies, School of Education, West Long Branch, NJ 07764-1898. Offers applied behavioral analysis (Certificate); autism (Certificate); director of school counseling services (Post-Master's Certificate); initial certification (MAT), including elementary level, K-12, secondary level; learning disabilities teacher-consultant (Post-Master's Certificate); principal/school administrator (MS Ed); principal/supervisor (MS Ed); school counseling (MS Ed); special education (MS Ed), including autism, learning disabilities teacher-consultant, teaching in inclusive settings; speech-language pathology (MS Ed); student affairs and college counseling (MS Ed); supervisor (Post-Master's Certificate); teaching English to speakers of other languages (TESOL) (Certificate). *Accreditation:* NCATE. *Program availability:* Part-time, evening/weekend, 100% online, blended/hybrid learning. *Faculty:* 25 full-time (20 women), 28 part-time/adjunct (22 women). *Students:* 195 full-time (173 women), 153 part-time (126 women); includes 42 minority (12 Black or African American, non-Hispanic/Latino; 6 Asian, non-Hispanic/Latino; 21 Hispanic/Latino; 1 Native Hawaiian or other Pacific Islander, non-Hispanic/Latino; 2 Two or more races, non-Hispanic/Latino). Average age 27. 471 applicants, 54% accepted, 147 enrolled. In 2015, 124 master's, 3 other advanced degrees awarded. *Entrance requirements:* For master's, GRE taken within last 5 years (for MS Ed in speech-language pathology); SAT (minimum combined score of 1660 in 3 sections), ACT (23), GRE (minimum score of 4.0 on analytical writing section and minimum combined score of 310 on quantitative and verbal sections), or passing scores on 3 parts of Core Academic Skills Educators, minimum GPA of 3.0 in major; 2 letters of recommendation (for some programs); resume, personal statement or essay (depending on program). Additional exam requirements/recommendations for international students: Required—TOEFL (minimum score 550 paper-based; 79 iBT), IELTS (minimum score 6), Michigan English Language Assessment Battery (minimum score 77) or Certificate of Advanced English (minimum score B2). *Application deadline:* For fall admission, 7/15 priority date for domestic students, 7/1 for international students; for spring admission, 12/15 priority date for domestic students, 11/1 for international students. Applications are processed on a rolling basis. Application fee: $50. Electronic applications accepted. *Expenses:* Tuition, area resident: Part-time $1098 per credit hour. *Required fees:* $175 per semester. Tuition and fees vary according to program. *Financial support:* In 2015–16, 303 students received support, including 274 fellowships (averaging $3,853 per year), 29 research assistantships (averaging $11,874 per year); institutionally sponsored loans, scholarships/grants, and unspecified assistantships also available. Support available to part-time students. Financial award applicants required to submit FAFSA. *Faculty research:* Multicultural literacy, science and mathematics teaching strategies, teacher as reflective practitioner, children with disabilities. *Unit head:* Dr. John E. Henning, Dean of The School of Education, 732-263-5513, Fax: 732-263-5277. *Application contact:* Laurie Kuhn, Associate Director of Graduate Admission, 732-571-3452, Fax: 732-263-5123, E-mail: gradadm@monmouth.edu.
Website: http://www.monmouth.edu/academics/schools/education/default.asp

Montclair State University, The Graduate School, College of Humanities and Social Sciences, Doctoral Program in Audiology, Montclair, NJ 07043-1624. Offers Sc D. *Program availability:* Part-time, evening/weekend. *Students:* 43 full-time (38 women), 5 part-time (all women); includes 9 minority (1 Black or African American, non-Hispanic/

Latino; 1 Asian, non-Hispanic/Latino; 5 Hispanic/Latino; 2 Two or more races, non-Hispanic/Latino). Average age 25. 114 applicants, 11% accepted, 12 enrolled. In 2015, 15 doctorates awarded. *Degree requirements:* For doctorate, comprehensive exam (for some programs), thesis/dissertation (for some programs). *Entrance requirements:* For doctorate, GRE General Test, essay, 2 letters of recommendation. Additional exam requirements/recommendations for international students: Required—TOEFL (minimum score 83 iBT), IELTS (minimum score 6.5). *Application deadline:* For fall admission, 2/1 for domestic students. Applications are processed on a rolling basis. Application fee: $60. Electronic applications accepted. *Expenses:* Tuition, state resident: part-time $553 per credit. Tuition, nonresident: part-time $854 per credit. *Required fees:* $91 per credit. Tuition and fees vary according to program. *Financial support:* In 2015–16, 12 research assistantships with partial tuition reimbursements (averaging $7,500 per year) were awarded; Federal Work-Study, scholarships/grants, and unspecified assistantships also available. Support available to part-time students. Financial award application deadline: 3/1; financial award applicants required to submit FAFSA. *Faculty research:* Child language development and disorders, word finding in discourse of aphasic and non-aphasics, phonological assessment and remediation, behavioral and electrophysiological measures of aging and spatial hearing, behavioral and electrophysiological measures of bilingual speech perception. *Unit head:* Dr. Janet Koehnke, Chairperson, 973-655-3305. *Application contact:* Amy Aiello, Director of Graduate Admissions and Operations, 973-655-5147, Fax: 973-655-7869, E-mail: graduate.school@montclair.edu.

Montclair State University, The Graduate School, College of Humanities and Social Sciences, Program in Communication Sciences and Disorders, Montclair, NJ 07043-1624. Offers MA. *Program availability:* Part-time, evening/weekend. *Students:* 84 full-time (79 women), 16 part-time (15 women); includes 16 minority (2 Black or African American, non-Hispanic/Latino, 4 Asian, non-Hispanic/Latino; 7 Hispanic/Latino; 3 Two or more races, non-Hispanic/Latino). Average age 26. 518 applicants, 7% accepted, 31 enrolled. In 2015, 30 master's awarded. *Degree requirements:* For master's, comprehensive exam, thesis (for some programs). *Entrance requirements:* For master's, GRE General Test, 2 letters of recommendation, essay. Additional exam requirements/recommendations for international students: Required—TOEFL (minimum score 83 iBT), IELTS (minimum score 6.5). *Application deadline:* For fall admission, 3/1 for domestic students. Applications are processed on a rolling basis. Application fee: $60. Electronic applications accepted. *Expenses:* Tuition, state resident: part-time $553 per credit. Tuition, nonresident: part-time $854 per credit. *Required fees:* $91 per credit. Tuition and fees vary according to program. *Financial support:* In 2015–16, 7 research assistantships with full tuition reimbursements (averaging $7,000 per year) were awarded; Federal Work-Study, scholarships/grants, and unspecified assistantships also available. Support available to part-time students. Financial award application deadline: 3/1; financial award applicants required to submit FAFSA. *Faculty research:* Child language development and disorders, word finding in discourse of aphasic and non-aphasics, phonological assessment and remediation, behavioral and electrophysiological measures of aging and spatial hearing, behavioral and electrophysiological measures of bilingual speech perception. *Unit head:* Dr. Janet Koehnke, Chairperson, 973-655-3305. *Application contact:* Amy Aiello, Director of Graduate Admissions and Operations, 973-655-5147, Fax: 973-655-7869, E-mail: graduate.school@montclair.edu.
Website: http://www.montclair.edu/chss/communication-sciences-disorders/

Murray State University, College of Health Sciences and Human Services, Department of Wellness and Therapeutic Sciences, Program in Speech-Language Pathology, Murray, KY 42071. Offers MS. *Accreditation:* ASHA. *Program availability:* Part-time. *Degree requirements:* For master's, comprehensive exam, thesis optional. *Entrance requirements:* For master's, GRE General Test or MAT, minimum GPA of 3.0. Additional exam requirements/recommendations for international students: Required—TOEFL.

National University, Academic Affairs, School of Education, La Jolla, CA 92037-1011. Offers applied behavior analysis (Certificate); applied school leadership (MS); autism (Certificate); best practices (Certificate); e-teaching and learning (Certificate); early childhood education (Certificate); education (MA), including best practices (M Ed, MA), e-teaching and learning (M Ed, MA), education technology, teacher leadership (M Ed, MA), teaching and learning in a global society (M Ed, MA), teaching mathematics (M Ed, MA); education with preliminary multiple or single subject (M Ed), including best practices (M Ed, MA), e-teaching and learning (M Ed, MA), educational technology (M Ed, MA), teacher leadership (M Ed, MA), teaching and learning in a global society (M Ed, MA), teaching mathematics (M Ed, MA); educational administration (MS); educational and instructional technology (MS); educational counseling (MS); educational technology (Certificate); higher education administration (MS); innovative school leadership (MS); instructional leadership (MS); juvenile justice special education (MS); reading (Certificate); school psychology (MS); special education (MS), including deaf and hard-of-hearing, mild/moderate disabilities, moderate/severe disabilities; teacher leadership (Certificate); teaching (MA), including applied behavioral analysis, autism, best practices (M Ed, MA), e-teaching and learning (M Ed, MA), early childhood education, educational technology (M Ed, MA), reading, special education, teacher leadership (M Ed, MA), teaching and learning in a global society (M Ed, MA), teaching mathematics (M Ed, MA); teaching mathematics (Certificate). *Program availability:* Part-time, evening/weekend, 100% online, blended/hybrid learning. *Faculty:* 81 full-time (51 women), 371 part-time/adjunct (227 women). *Students:* 3,029 full-time (2,147 women), 2,210 part-time (1,524 women); includes 2,391 minority (367 Black or African American, non-Hispanic/Latino; 21 American Indian or Alaska Native, non-Hispanic/Latino; 301 Asian, non-Hispanic/Latino; 1,489 Hispanic/Latino; 31 Native Hawaiian or other Pacific Islander, non-Hispanic/Latino; 182 Two or more races, non-Hispanic/Latino). Average age 33. In 2015, 3,396 master's awarded. *Degree requirements:* For master's, thesis (for some programs). *Entrance requirements:* For master's, interview, minimum GPA of 2.5. Additional exam requirements/recommendations for international students: Required—TOEFL (minimum score 550 paper-based; 79 iBT), IELTS (minimum score 6). *Application deadline:* Applications are processed on a rolling basis. Application fee: $60 ($65 for international students). Electronic applications accepted. *Financial support:* Career-related internships or fieldwork, institutionally sponsored loans, scholarships/grants, and tuition waivers (partial) available. Support available to part-time students. Financial award application deadline: 6/30. *Faculty research:* Teacher education, special education, educational effectiveness, teaching abroad, school counseling. *Unit head:* School of Education, 800-628-8648, E-mail: soe@nu.edu. *Application contact:* Brandon Jouganatos, Vice President for Enrollment Services, 800-628-8648, E-mail: advisor@nu.edu.
Website: http://www.nu.edu/OurPrograms/SchoolOfEducation.html

Nazareth College of Rochester, Graduate Studies, Department of Speech-Language Pathology, Communication Sciences and Disorders Program, Rochester, NY 14618-3790. Offers MS. *Accreditation:* ASHA. *Program availability:* Part-time, online learning. *Degree requirements:* For master's, comprehensive exam. *Entrance requirements:* For master's, GRE General Test, minimum GPA of 3.0. *Application deadline:* For fall admission, 2/1 for domestic students; for spring admission, 10/1 for domestic students. Application fee: $40. *Financial support:* Research assistantships with partial tuition reimbursements available. Financial award application deadline: 3/1. *Unit head:* Lisa Durant-Jones, Director, 585-389-2775, E-mail: ldurant4@naz.edu. *Application contact:*

Judith G. Baker, Director, Graduate Admissions, 585-389-2050, Fax: 585-389-2817, E-mail: gradstudies@naz.edu.

New Mexico State University, College of Education, Department of Special Education and Communication Disorders, Las Cruces, NM 88003-8001. Offers autism spectrum disorders (MA); bilingual/multicultural special education (PhD); communication disorders (MA); deaf and hard of hearing (MA, Ed S); special education (MA, Ed D, PhD, Ed S), including general special education (MA); speech-language pathology (MA). *Accreditation:* ASHA (one or more programs are accredited); NCATE. *Program availability:* Part-time, evening/weekend, online learning. *Faculty:* 16 full-time (13 women), 1 (woman) part-time/adjunct. *Students:* 68 full-time (56 women), 72 part-time (61 women); includes 70 minority (4 Black or African American, non-Hispanic/Latino; 2 Asian, non-Hispanic/Latino; 61 Hispanic/Latino; 3 Two or more races, non-Hispanic/Latino), 4 international. Average age 32. 184 applicants, 33% accepted, 54 enrolled. In 2015, 46 master's, 6 doctorates awarded. *Degree requirements:* For master's, comprehensive exam, thesis optional; for doctorate, comprehensive exam, thesis/dissertation. *Entrance requirements:* For master's, GRE General Test or MAT. Additional exam requirements/recommendations for international students: Required—TOEFL (minimum score 550 paper-based; 79 iBT), IELTS (minimum score 6.5). *Application deadline:* For fall admission, 2/1 priority date for domestic students. Applications are processed on a rolling basis. Application fee: $40 ($50 for international students). Electronic applications accepted. *Expenses:* $274.50 per credit hour for in-state students, and all students enrolled in six or fewer credits; $839.30 per credit hour for out-of-state and international students enrolled in at least seven hours. *Financial support:* In 2015–16, 43 students received support, including 17 teaching assistantships (averaging $9,753 per year); career-related internships or fieldwork, Federal Work-Study, scholarships/grants, traineeships, health care benefits, and unspecified assistantships also available. Support available to part-time students. Financial award application deadline: 3/1; financial award applicants required to submit FAFSA. *Faculty research:* Multicultural special education, multicultural communication disorders, mild disability, multicultural assessment, deaf education, early childhood, bilingual special education. *Total annual research expenditures:* $413,805. *Unit head:* Dr. Marlene Salas-Provance, Assistant Dean/Department Head, 575-646-2402, Fax: 575-646-7712, E-mail: lolasas@nmsu.edu. *Application contact:* Dr. Karen Potter, Director, Special Education Program, 575-646-2402, Fax: 575-646-7712, E-mail: potterk@nmsu.edu.
Website: http://spedcd.education.nmsu.edu

New York Medical College, School of Health Sciences and Practice, Department of Speech-Language Pathology, Valhalla, NY 10595-1691. Offers MS. *Accreditation:* ASHA. *Degree requirements:* For master's, comprehensive exam, thesis or alternative. *Entrance requirements:* For master's, GRE, minimum GPA of 3.5. Additional exam requirements/recommendations for international students: Required—TOEFL (minimum score 637 paper-based; 117 iBT), IELTS (minimum score 7). Electronic applications accepted. Application fee is waived when completed online. *Expenses:* Tuition, area resident: Full-time $44,355; part-time $1025 per credit. *Required fees:* $500; $95 per year. One-time fee: $140 part-time. Tuition and fees vary according to course load and program.

New York University, Steinhardt School of Culture, Education, and Human Development, Department of Communication Sciences and Disorders, New York, NY 10003-6860. Offers MS, PhD. *Accreditation:* ASHA. *Program availability:* Part-time. *Degree requirements:* For master's, thesis (for some programs); for doctorate, thesis/dissertation. *Entrance requirements:* For master's, GRE General Test; for doctorate, GRE General Test, interview. Additional exam requirements/recommendations for international students: Required—TOEFL (minimum score 100 iBT). Electronic applications accepted. *Faculty research:* Evidence-based practice, phonological acquisition, dysphagia, child language acquisition and disorders, neuromotor disorders.

North Carolina Central University, School of Education, Department of Communication Disorders, Durham, NC 27707-3129. Offers M Ed. *Accreditation:* ASHA. *Program availability:* Part-time, evening/weekend. *Degree requirements:* For master's, comprehensive exam, thesis or alternative. *Entrance requirements:* For master's, GRE, minimum GPA of 3.0 in major, 2.5 overall. Additional exam requirements/recommendations for international students: Required—TOEFL. *Faculty research:* Vocational programs for special needs learners.

Northeastern State University, College of Science and Health Professions, Department of Health Professions, Program in Speech-Language Pathology, Tahlequah, OK 74464-2399. Offers MS. *Accreditation:* ASHA. *Program availability:* Part-time, evening/weekend. *Faculty:* 12 full-time (10 women), 1 (woman) part-time/adjunct. *Students:* 73 full-time (68 women), 1 (woman) part-time; includes 24 minority (1 Black or African American, non-Hispanic/Latino; 11 American Indian or Alaska Native, non-Hispanic/Latino; 1 Asian, non-Hispanic/Latino; 3 Hispanic/Latino; 8 Two or more races, non-Hispanic/Latino), 3 international. Average age 25. In 2015, 38 master's awarded. *Degree requirements:* For master's, thesis, capstone experience. *Entrance requirements:* For master's, GRE, minimum GPA of 2.75. Additional exam requirements/recommendations for international students: Required—TOEFL. *Application deadline:* For fall admission, 6/1 priority date for domestic students. Applications are processed on a rolling basis. Application fee: $25. Electronic applications accepted. *Expenses:* Tuition, state resident: part-time $189.60 per credit hour. Tuition, nonresident: part-time $462.60 per credit hour. *Required fees:* $37.40 per credit hour. *Financial support:* Teaching assistantships, career-related internships or fieldwork, and Federal Work-Study available. Financial award application deadline: 3/1. *Unit head:* Dr. Karen Patterson, Chair, 918-456-5111 Ext. 3778, Fax: 918-458-2351. *Application contact:* Carla Barnett, Secretary, 918-444-3775, E-mail: barnett@nsuok.edu.
Website: https://academics.nsuok.edu/healthprofessions/DegreePrograms/Speech-LangPath.aspx

Northeastern University, Bouvé College of Health Sciences, Boston, MA 02115-5096. Offers applied behavior analysis (MS, CAGS); audiology (Au D); biomedical nanotechnology (MS); college student development and counseling (MS, CAGS); counseling psychology (MS, PhD, CAGS); exercise science (MS); health informatics (MS); medicinal chemistry (MS); nurse anesthesia (DNP, CAGS); nursing (MS, PhD, CAGS), including administration (MS), adult-gerontology acute care nurse practitioner (MS, CAGS), adult-gerontology primary care nurse practitioner (MS, CAGS), anesthesia (MS), family nurse practitioner (MS, CAGS), neonatal nurse practitioner (MS, CAGS), pediatric nurse practitioner (MS, CAGS), psychiatric mental health nurse practitioner (MS, CAGS); nursing practice (DNP); personal health informatics (MS); pharmaceutical sciences (MS, PhD), including interdisciplinary concentration, pharmaceutics and drug delivery systems; pharmacology (MS); pharmacy (Pharm D); physical therapy (Postbaccalaureate Certificate); physician assistant (MS); population health (PhD); school psychology (MS, PhD, CAGS); speech-language pathology (MS); urban health (MPH); MS/MBA. *Accreditation:* ACPE (one or more programs are accredited). *Program availability:* Part-time, evening/weekend, online learning. *Faculty:* 194 full-time (120 women), 169 part-time/adjunct (136 women). *Students:* 1,416 full-time (1,049 women), 310 part-time (248 women). In 2015, 374 master's, 313 doctorates, 37 other advanced degrees awarded. *Degree requirements:* For doctorate, thesis/dissertation (for some programs); for other advanced degree, comprehensive exam. Application fee: $75. Electronic applications accepted. *Expenses:* Contact institution. *Financial support:*

Communication Disorders

Applicants required to submit FAFSA. *Unit head:* John R. Reynolds, Professor and Interim Dean, 617-373-3323, Fax: 617-373-3030. *Application contact:* Molly Schnabel, Senior Director of Graduate Affairs, 617-373-2708, Fax: 617-373-4701, E-mail: bouvegrad@neu.edu.
Website: http://www.northeastern.edu/bouve/

Northern Arizona University, Graduate College, College of Health and Human Services, Department of Communication Sciences and Disorders, Flagstaff, AZ 86011. Offers clinical speech-language pathology (MS). *Accreditation:* ASHA. *Program availability:* Part-time. *Entrance requirements:* For master's, GRE General Test, minimum GPA of 3.0. Additional exam requirements/recommendations for international students: Required—TOEFL (minimum score 550 paper-based; 80 iBT), IELTS (minimum score 7). *Application deadline:* For fall admission, 1/31 priority date for domestic students, 1/31 for international students. Application fee: $65. Electronic applications accepted. *Expenses:* Tuition, *area resident:* Full-time $8710. Tuition, nonresident: full-time $20,350. *Required fees:* $896. *Financial support:* Research assistantships, career-related internships or fieldwork, Federal Work-Study, scholarships/grants, health care benefits, tuition waivers (full and partial), and unspecified assistantships available. Financial award applicants required to submit FAFSA. *Faculty research:* Meta-analysis of language, laryngeal speech, aphasia. *Unit head:* Dr. Elise Lindstedt, Chair, 928-523-2969, E-mail: elise.lindstedt@nau.edu. *Application contact:* Joan Brakefield, Senior Program Coordinator, 928-523-7444, Fax: 928-523-0034, E-mail: speech@nau.edu.
Website: http://nau.edu/chhs/csd/

Northern Illinois University, Graduate School, College of Health and Human Sciences, School of Allied Health and Communicative Disorders, Program in Communicative Disorders, De Kalb, IL 60115-2854. Offers MA, Au D. *Accreditation:* ASHA (one or more programs are accredited); CORE. *Faculty:* 9 full-time (6 women), 2 part-time/adjunct (1 woman). *Students:* 86 full-time (77 women), 3 part-time (all women); includes 18 minority (5 Black or African American, non-Hispanic/Latino; 2 Asian, non-Hispanic/Latino; 5 Hispanic/Latino; 6 Two or more races, non-Hispanic/Latino), 1 international. Average age 26. 83 applicants, 45% accepted, 16 enrolled. In 2015, 28 master's, 7 doctorates awarded. *Degree requirements:* For master's, comprehensive exam, thesis optional, practicum; for doctorate, practicum, research project. *Entrance requirements:* For master's, GRE General Test, minimum undergraduate GPA of 3.0; for doctorate, GRE General Test, minimum undergraduate GPA of 3.2. Additional exam requirements/recommendations for international students: Required—TOEFL (minimum score 550 paper-based). *Application deadline:* For fall admission, 2/1 priority date for domestic students, 5/1 for international students; for spring admission, 9/1 priority date for domestic students, 10/1 for international students. Applications are processed on a rolling basis. Application fee: $40. Electronic applications accepted. *Financial support:* Fellowships with full tuition reimbursements, research assistantships with full tuition reimbursements, teaching assistantships with full tuition reimbursements, career-related internships or fieldwork, Federal Work-Study, scholarships/grants, tuition waivers (full), and unspecified assistantships available. Support available to part-time students. Financial award applicants required to submit FAFSA. *Faculty research:* Impact of disability employment, deaf education, American Sign Language, autism, bilingualism. *Unit head:* Dr. Sherrill Morris, Chair, 815-753-1484, Fax: 815-753-9123, E-mail: ahcd@niu.edu. *Application contact:* Graduate School Office, 815-753-0395, E-mail: gradsch@niu.edu.
Website: http://www.chhs.niu.edu/slp/graduate/index.shtml

Northwestern University, The Graduate School, School of Communication, The Roxelyn and Richard Pepper Department of Communication Sciences and Disorders, Evanston, IL 60208. Offers audiology (Au D); communication sciences and disorders (PhD); speech, language, and learning (MS). Admissions and degrees offered through The Graduate School. *Accreditation:* ASHA (one or more programs are accredited). Terminal master's awarded for partial completion of doctoral program. *Degree requirements:* For master's, seminar paper; for doctorate, thesis/dissertation, pre-dissertation research project, qualifying exam. *Entrance requirements:* For master's and doctorate, GRE General Test, letters of recommendation. Additional exam requirements/recommendations for international students: Required—TOEFL. *Faculty research:* Swallow behavior, verb structure in aphasia, language decline in dementia, cognitive processing in children, word-finding defects in children.

Nova Southeastern University, College of Health Care Sciences, Fort Lauderdale, FL 33314-7796. Offers anesthesiologist assistant (MSA); audiology (Au D); health science (MH Sc, DHSc, PhD); occupational therapy (MOT, Dr OT, PhD); physical therapy (DPT, TDPT); physician assistant (MMS). *Program availability:* Online learning. *Faculty:* 109 full-time (64 women), 100 part-time/adjunct (65 women). *Students:* 1,590 full-time (1,179 women), 969 part-time (819 women); includes 831 minority (234 Black or African American, non-Hispanic/Latino; 8 American Indian or Alaska Native, non-Hispanic/Latino; 151 Asian, non-Hispanic/Latino; 378 Hispanic/Latino; 1 Native Hawaiian or other Pacific Islander, non-Hispanic/Latino; 59 Two or more races, non-Hispanic/Latino), 18 international. Average age 30. 8,133 applicants, 14% accepted, 728 enrolled. In 2015, 556 master's, 105 doctorates awarded. *Degree requirements:* For master's, thesis; for doctorate, comprehensive exam, thesis/dissertation. *Entrance requirements:* For master's, GRE General Test, MCAT; for doctorate, GRE General Test, personal interview, essay. Additional exam requirements/recommendations for international students: Required—TOEFL (minimum score 600 paper-based). *Application deadline:* For winter admission, 4/15 for domestic students; for summer admission, 12/15 for domestic and international students. Applications are processed on a rolling basis. Application fee: $50. Electronic applications accepted. *Expenses:* Contact institution. *Financial support:* In 2015–16, 151 students received support, including 4 research assistantships (averaging $3,500 per year); institutionally sponsored loans and unspecified assistantships also available. Financial award application deadline: 4/15; financial award applicants required to submit FAFSA. *Unit head:* Dr. Stanley Wilson, Dean, 954-262-1203, E-mail: swilson@nova.edu. *Application contact:* Joey Jankie, Admissions Counselor, 954-262-7249, E-mail: joey@nova.edu.
Website: http://www.nova.edu/chcs/

The Ohio State University, Graduate School, College of Arts and Sciences, Division of Social and Behavioral Sciences, Department of Speech and Hearing Science, Columbus, OH 43210. Offers audiology (Au D, PhD); hearing science (PhD); speech hearing science (MA); speech-language pathology (MA, PhD); speech-language science (PhD). *Accreditation:* ASHA (one or more programs are accredited). *Students:* 99 full-time (89 women), 5 part-time (all women); includes 3 minority (2 Asian, non-Hispanic/Latino; 1 Two or more races, non-Hispanic/Latino), 1 international. Average age 25. In 2015, 29 master's, 14 doctorates awarded. *Degree requirements:* For master's, thesis optional; for doctorate, thesis/dissertation. *Entrance requirements:* For master's and doctorate, GRE General Test. Additional exam requirements/recommendations for international students: Required—TOEFL (minimum score 600 paper-based; 100 iBT); Recommended—IELTS (minimum score 9). *Application deadline:* For fall admission, 12/1 for domestic students, 11/30 for international students. Applications are processed on a rolling basis. Electronic applications accepted. *Financial support:* Fellowships with tuition reimbursements, research assistantships with tuition reimbursements, teaching assistantships with tuition reimbursements,

Federal Work-Study, and institutionally sponsored loans available. Support available to part-time students. *Unit head:* Dr. Robert A. Fox, Chair, 614-292-1628, E-mail: fox.2@osu.edu. *Application contact:* Graduate and Professional Admissions, 614-292-9444, E-mail: gpadmissions@osu.edu.
Website: http://sphs.osu.edu/

Ohio University, Graduate College, College of Health Sciences and Professions, School of Rehabilitation and Communication Sciences, Division of Communication Sciences and Disorders, Athens, OH 45701-2979. Offers clinical audiology (Au D); hearing science (PhD); speech language pathology (MA); speech language science (PhD). *Accreditation:* ASHA.

Oklahoma State University, College of Arts and Sciences, Department of Communication Sciences and Disorders, Stillwater, OK 74078. Offers MS. *Accreditation:* ASHA. *Faculty:* 10 full-time (7 women), 12 part-time/adjunct (all women). *Students:* 46 full-time (45 women), 2 part-time (both women); includes 13 minority (1 Black or African American, non-Hispanic/Latino; 1 American Indian or Alaska Native, non-Hispanic/Latino; 3 Hispanic/Latino; 8 Two or more races, non-Hispanic/Latino). Average age 24. 118 applicants, 24% accepted, 17 enrolled. In 2015, 29 master's awarded. *Degree requirements:* For master's, thesis or creative research project, clinical practicum experience. *Entrance requirements:* For master's, GRE, minimum GPA of 3.0 in undergraduate major. Additional exam requirements/recommendations for international students: Required—TOEFL (minimum score 550 paper-based; 79 iBT). *Application deadline:* For fall admission, 3/1 priority date for international students; for spring admission, 8/1 priority date for international students. Applications are processed on a rolling basis. Application fee: $40 ($75 for international students). Electronic applications accepted. *Expenses:* Tuition, state resident: full-time $3528; part-time $196 per credit hour. Tuition, nonresident: full-time $14,144; part-time $785.75 per credit hour. *Required fees:* $1895; $105.25 per credit hour. Tuition and fees vary according to campus/location. *Financial support:* In 2015–16, 1 research assistantship (averaging $6,180 per year), 15 teaching assistantships (averaging $6,180 per year) were awarded; career-related internships or fieldwork, Federal Work-Study, scholarships/grants, health care benefits, tuition waivers (partial), and unspecified assistantships also available. Support available to part-time students. Financial award application deadline: 3/1; financial award applicants required to submit FAFSA. *Faculty research:* Speech communications. *Unit head:* Dr. Maureen Sullivan, Interim Department Head, 405-744-8938, E-mail: maureen.sullivan@okstate.edu. *Application contact:* Abby Grantham, Graduate Advisor, 405-744-8922, E-mail: abby.l.grantham@okstate.edu.
Website: http://cdis.okstate.edu/

Old Dominion University, Darden College of Education, Program in Speech-Language Pathology, Norfolk, VA 23529. Offers MS Ed. *Accreditation:* ASHA. *Faculty:* 10 full-time (all women), 5 part-time/adjunct (all women). *Students:* 54 full-time (all women), 5 part-time (all women); includes 12 minority (6 Black or African American, non-Hispanic/Latino; 4 Hispanic/Latino; 2 Two or more races, non-Hispanic/Latino). Average age 24. 238 applicants, 28% accepted, 26 enrolled. In 2015, 24 master's awarded. *Degree requirements:* For master's, comprehensive exam, written exams, case studies paper, practica. *Entrance requirements:* For master's, GRE General Test, minimum GPA of 3.0 in major, 2.8 overall. Additional exam requirements/recommendations for international students: Required—TOEFL, IELTS. *Application deadline:* For fall admission, 2/1 for domestic and international students. Application fee: $50. Electronic applications accepted. *Expenses:* $464 in-state, $1,160 out-of-state per credit. *Financial support:* In 2015–16, 14 students received support, including 6 fellowships (averaging $6,000 per year), 4 research assistantships (averaging $9,000 per year); scholarships/grants and unspecified assistantships also available. Financial award application deadline: 2/1; financial award applicants required to submit CSS PROFILE or FAFSA. *Faculty research:* Childhood language disorders, phonological disorders, stuttering, aphasia, hearing aid outcomes, apraxia of speech, augmentative communication, auditory attention. *Total annual research expenditures:* $370,000. *Unit head:* Dr. Anastasia M. Raymer, Graduate Program Director, 757-683-4117, Fax: 757-683-5593, E-mail: sraymer@odu.edu. *Application contact:* William Heffelfinger, Director of Graduate Admissions, 757-683-5554, Fax: 757-683-3255, E-mail: gradadmit@odu.edu.
Website: http://www.odu.edu/cdse

Our Lady of the Lake University of San Antonio, School of Professional Studies, Program in Communication and Learning Disorders, San Antonio, TX 78207-4689. Offers MA. *Accreditation:* ASHA. *Program availability:* Part-time. *Faculty:* 8 full-time (7 women), 1 (woman) part-time/adjunct. *Students:* 51 full-time (50 women); includes 29 minority (2 Asian, non-Hispanic/Latino; 27 Hispanic/Latino), 1 international. Average age 27. 227 applicants, 12% accepted, 23 enrolled. In 2015, 25 master's awarded. *Degree requirements:* For master's, comprehensive exam, comprehensive clinical practicum. *Entrance requirements:* For master's, GRE General Test, official transcripts. Additional exam requirements/recommendations for international students: Required—TOEFL. *Application deadline:* For fall admission, 2/1 for domestic and international students. Application fee: $40 ($50 for international students). Electronic applications accepted. *Expenses:* Tuition, area resident: Full-time $14,796; part-time $822 per credit hour. *Required fees:* $232 per semester. Tuition and fees vary according to course load, degree level, campus/location and program. *Financial support:* In 2015–16, 6 students received support, including 4 research assistantships, 4 teaching assistantships; Federal Work-Study, scholarships/grants, unspecified assistantships, and tuition discounts also available. Support available to part-time students. Financial award application deadline: 5/1; financial award applicants required to submit FAFSA. *Unit head:* Cynthia Davila, Administrative Assistant, 210-431-3938, E-mail: cadavila@ollusa.edu. *Application contact:* Office of Graduate Admissions, 210-431-3995, Fax: 210-431-3945, E-mail: gradadm@lake.ollusa.edu.
Website: http://www.ollusa.edu/s/1190/hybrid/default-hybrid-ollu.aspx?sid=1190&gid=1&pgid=7874

Pacific University, College of Education, Forest Grove, OR 97116-1797. Offers early childhood education (MAT); education (MAE); elementary education (MAT); ESOL (MAT); high school education (MAT); middle school education (MAT); special education (MAT); speech-language pathology (MS); STEM education (MAT); talented and gifted (M Ed); visual function in learning (M Ed). *Accreditation:* NCATE. *Program availability:* Part-time, evening/weekend. *Degree requirements:* For master's, research project. *Entrance requirements:* For master's, California Basic Educational Skills Test, PRAXIS II, minimum undergraduate GPA of 2.75, 3.0 graduate. Additional exam requirements/recommendations for international students: Required—TOEFL. Electronic applications accepted. *Expenses:* Contact institution. *Faculty research:* Defining a culturally competent classroom, technology in the k-12 classroom, Socratic seminars, social studies education.

Pacific University, School of Audiology, Forest Grove, OR 97116-1797. Offers Au D.

Penn State University Park, Graduate School, College of Health and Human Development, Department of Communication Sciences and Disorders, University Park, PA 16802. Offers communication sciences and disorders (MS, PhD, Certificate). *Accreditation:* ASHA (one or more programs are accredited). *Unit head:* Dr. Ann C. Crouter, Dean, 814-865-1420, Fax: 814-865-3282. *Application contact:* Lori Stania, Director, Graduate Student Services, 814-865-1795, Fax: 814-863-4627, E-mail: l-gswww@lists.psu.edu.
Website: http://csd.hhd.psu.edu/

Portland State University, Graduate Studies, College of Liberal Arts and Sciences, Department of Speech and Hearing Sciences, Portland, OR 97207-0751. Offers speech-language pathology (MA, MS). *Accreditation:* ASHA (one or more programs are accredited). *Faculty:* 12 full-time (9 women), 9 part-time/adjunct (6 women). *Students:* 80 full-time (67 women), 7 part-time (all women); includes 17 minority (5 Asian, non-Hispanic/Latino; 10 Hispanic/Latino; 2 Two or more races, non-Hispanic/Latino), 2 international. Average age 30. 143 applicants, 29% accepted, 42 enrolled. In 2015, 48 master's awarded. *Degree requirements:* For master's, variable foreign language requirement, thesis or alternative, oral exam. *Entrance requirements:* For master's, GRE General Test, minimum GPA of 3.0 in upper-division course work or 2.75 overall, BA/BS in speech and hearing sciences. Additional exam requirements/recommendations for international students: Required—TOEFL (minimum score 550 paper-based; 80 iBT), IELTS (minimum score 6.5). *Application deadline:* For fall admission, 2/1 for domestic and international students. Application fee: $50. *Expenses:* $11,490 per year. *Financial support:* In 2015–16, 2 teaching assistantships with full tuition reimbursements (averaging $5,220 per year) were awarded; research assistantships, career-related internships or fieldwork, Federal Work-Study, and institutionally sponsored loans also available. Support available to part-time students. Financial award application deadline: 3/1; financial award applicants required to submit FAFSA. *Faculty research:* Adolescents with clefts, spectral analysis of stuttering, communication in late talkers, speech intelligibility, brainstem response in fitting hearing aids. *Total annual research expenditures:* $88,543. *Unit head:* Christina Gildersleeve Neumann, PhD, Chair, 503-725-3230, Fax: 503-725-5385, E-mail: cegn@pdx.edu. *Application contact:* Dr. Jennifer Larsen, Graduate Program Director, 503-725-3533, E-mail: larsenj@pdx.edu. Website: http://www.pdx.edu/sphr/

Purdue University, Graduate School, College of Health and Human Sciences, Department of Speech, Language, and Hearing Sciences, West Lafayette, IN 47907. Offers audiology clinic (MS, Au D, PhD); linguistics (MS, PhD); speech and hearing science (MS, PhD); speech-language pathology (MS, PhD). *Accreditation:* ASHA. *Degree requirements:* For master's, comprehensive exam (for some programs), thesis optional; for doctorate, comprehensive exam, thesis/dissertation. *Entrance requirements:* For master's and doctorate, GRE General Test, minimum undergraduate GPA of 3.0 or equivalent. Additional exam requirements/recommendations for international students: Required—TOEFL (minimum score 77 iBT). Electronic applications accepted. *Faculty research:* Psychoacoustics, speech perception, speech physiology, stuttering, child language.

Queens College of the City University of New York, Arts and Humanities Division, Department of Linguistics and Communication Disorders, Flushing, NY 11367-1597. Offers applied linguistics (MA); speech-language pathology (MA); teaching English to speakers of other languages (MS Ed). *Program availability:* Part-time. *Faculty:* 22 full-time (16 women), 19 part-time/adjunct (13 women). *Students:* 43 full-time (41 women), 152 part-time (133 women); includes 52 minority (6 Black or African American, non-Hispanic/Latino; 19 Asian, non-Hispanic/Latino; 27 Hispanic/Latino), 3 international. Average age 35. 445 applicants, 27% accepted, 85 enrolled. In 2015, 43 master's awarded. *Degree requirements:* For master's, thesis optional. *Entrance requirements:* For master's, minimum GPA of 3.0. Additional exam requirements/recommendations for international students: Required—TOEFL, IELTS. *Application deadline:* For fall admission, 4/1 for domestic students. Applications are processed on a rolling basis. Application fee: $125. Electronic applications accepted. *Expenses:* Tuition, state resident: full-time $5065; part-time $425 per credit. Tuition, nonresident: part-time $780 per credit. *Required fees:* $522. Part-time tuition and fees vary according to course load and program. *Financial support:* Career-related internships or fieldwork available. Financial award application deadline: 4/1; financial award applicants required to submit FAFSA. *Unit head:* Dr. Robert Vago, Chairperson, 718-997-2875, E-mail: robert.vago@qc.cuny.edu.

Radford University, College of Graduate and Professional Studies, Waldron College of Health and Human Services, Program in Communication Sciences and Disorders, Radford, VA 24142. Offers speech-language pathology (MA, MS). *Accreditation:* ASHA (one or more programs are accredited). *Program availability:* Part-time. *Faculty:* 9 full-time (8 women), 5 part-time/adjunct (all women). *Students:* 59 full-time (all women); includes 7 minority (1 Black or African American, non-Hispanic/Latino; 5 Hispanic/Latino; 1 Two or more races, non-Hispanic/Latino), 1 international. Average age 23. 276 applicants, 36% accepted, 32 enrolled. In 2015, 31 master's awarded. *Degree requirements:* For master's, comprehensive exam, thesis (for some programs). *Entrance requirements:* For master's, GRE, minimum GPA of 3.0; completed CSDCAS application with 3 letters of reference; personal essay; resume. Additional exam requirements/recommendations for international students: Required—TOEFL (minimum score 550 paper-based; 79 iBT), IELTS (minimum score 6.5). *Application deadline:* For fall admission, 2/1 priority date for domestic students, 12/1 for international students; for spring admission, 7/1 for international students. Applications are processed on a rolling basis. Application fee: $50. Electronic applications accepted. *Expenses:* Tuition, state resident: full-time $7640; part-time $318 per credit hour. Tuition, nonresident: full-time $16,394; part-time $683 per credit hour. *Required fees:* $3021; $127 per credit hour. Tuition and fees vary according to course load and program. *Financial support:* In 2015–16, 35 students received support, including 32 research assistantships with partial tuition reimbursements available (averaging $4,008 per year), 2 teaching assistantships with partial tuition reimbursements available (averaging $10,000 per year); career-related internships or fieldwork, Federal Work-Study, institutionally sponsored loans, scholarships/grants, and unspecified assistantships also available. Financial award application deadline: 3/1; financial award applicants required to submit FAFSA. *Unit head:* Dr. Diane C. Millar, Chair, 540-831-7735, Fax: 540-831-7699, E-mail: dcmillar@radford.edu. *Application contact:* Rebecca Conner, Director, Graduate Enrollment, 540-831-6296, Fax: 540-831-6061, E-mail: gradcollege@radford.edu. Website: http://www.radford.edu/content/wchs/home/cosd.html

Rockhurst University, College of Health and Human Services, Program in Communication Sciences and Disorders, Kansas City, MO 64110-2561. Offers communication sciences and disorders (MS). *Accreditation:* ASHA. *Program availability:* Part-time. *Faculty:* 6 full-time (all women), 2 part-time/adjunct (1 woman). *Students:* 58 full-time (56 women), 10 part-time (all women); includes 2 minority (1 Black or African American, non-Hispanic/Latino; 1 Asian, non-Hispanic/Latino). Average age 24. 156 applicants, 80% accepted, 35 enrolled. In 2015, 33 master's awarded. *Entrance requirements:* For master's, GRE General Test, interview, minimum GPA of 3.0, letters of recommendation. Additional exam requirements/recommendations for international students: Required—TOEFL (minimum score 550 paper-based; 79 iBT). *Application deadline:* Applications are processed on a rolling basis. Application fee: $25. Electronic applications accepted. Application fee is waived when completed online. *Financial support:* Applicants required to submit FAFSA. *Faculty research:* Bioacoustics, physiology, applied speech science, pediatric nutrition/dysphagia, communication/cognition. *Unit head:* Kathy Ermgodts, Chair, 816-501-4505, Fax: 816-501-4169, E-mail: kathy.ermgodts@rockhurst.edu. *Application contact:* Cheryl Hooper, Director of Graduate Admission, 816-501-4097, Fax: 816-501-4241, E-mail: cheryl.hooper@rockhurst.edu. Website: http://www.rockhurst.edu/academic/csd/index.asp

Rocky Mountain University of Health Professions, Program in Speech-Language Pathology, Provo, UT 84606. Offers Clin Sc D.

Rush University, College of Health Sciences, Department of Communication Disorders and Sciences, Chicago, IL 60612-3832. Offers audiology (Au D); speech-language pathology (MS). *Accreditation:* ASHA (one or more programs are accredited). *Degree requirements:* For master's, comprehensive exam, thesis optional; for doctorate, comprehensive exam, investigative project. *Entrance requirements:* For master's and doctorate, GRE General Test, minimum GPA of 3.0. Additional exam requirements/recommendations for international students: Required—TOEFL. *Application deadline:* For fall admission, 1/1 for domestic students. Applications are processed on a rolling basis. Application fee: $40. Electronic applications accepted. *Expenses:* Contact institution. *Financial support:* Research assistantships with partial tuition reimbursements, career-related internships or fieldwork, Federal Work-Study, institutionally sponsored loans, scholarships/grants, traineeships, tuition waivers (partial), and stipends available. Support available to part-time students. Financial award application deadline: 4/1; financial award applicants required to submit FAFSA. *Faculty research:* Electrostimulation of subthalamic nucleus, sensory feedback in speech modulation, sentence complexity in children's writing, velopharyngeal function, adult neurology. *Unit head:* Dr. Gail Kempster, Chairperson, E-mail: gail_b_kempster@rush.edu. *Application contact:* 312-942-7120, E-mail: chs_admissions@rush.edu.

Sacred Heart University, Graduate Programs, College of Health Professions, Program in Speech-Language Pathology, Fairfield, CT 06825. Offers MS. *Program availability:* Part-time, evening/weekend. *Faculty:* 7 full-time (all women). *Students:* 55 full-time (53 women); includes 8 minority (3 Black or African American, non-Hispanic/Latino; 2 Asian, non-Hispanic/Latino; 2 Hispanic/Latino; 1 Two or more races, non-Hispanic/Latino). Average age 25. 306 applicants, 25% accepted, 35 enrolled. *Entrance requirements:* For master's, bachelor's degree with minimum GPA of 3.0. Additional exam requirements/recommendations for international students: Recommended—TOEFL (minimum score 570 paper-based; 80 iBT), IELTS (minimum score 6.5). *Application deadline:* For fall admission, 1/15 for domestic students. Applications are processed on a rolling basis. Application fee: $75. Electronic applications accepted. *Expenses: Tuition, area resident:* Part-time $654 per credit hour. *Financial support:* Unspecified assistantships available. Financial award applicants required to submit FAFSA. *Unit head:* Rhea Paul, Chair/Professor of Speech Language Pathology, 203-416-3947, E-mail: paulr4@sacredheart.edu. *Application contact:* William Sweeney, Director of Graduate Admissions, 203-365-4827, E-mail: sweeneyw@sacredheart.edu. Website: http://www.sacredheart.edu/academics/collegeofhealthprofessions/academicprograms/speech-languagepathology/

St. Ambrose University, College of Education and Health Sciences, Program in Speech-Language Pathology, Davenport, IA 52803-2898. Offers MSLP. *Program availability:* Part-time, evening/weekend. *Entrance requirements:* Additional exam requirements/recommendations for international students: Required—TOEFL. Electronic applications accepted.

St. Cloud State University, School of Graduate Studies, School of Health and Human Services, Department of Communication Sciences and Disorders, St. Cloud, MN 56301-4498. Offers MS. *Accreditation:* ASHA. *Degree requirements:* For master's, comprehensive exam (for some programs), thesis or alternative. *Entrance requirements:* For master's, GRE General Test, minimum GPA of 2.75. Additional exam requirements/recommendations for international students: Required—Michigan English Language Assessment Battery; Recommended—TOEFL (minimum score 550 paper-based), IELTS (minimum score 6.5). Electronic applications accepted.

St. John's University, St. John's College of Liberal Arts and Sciences, Department of Communication Sciences and Disorders, Queens, NY 11439. Offers MA, Au D. *Accreditation:* ASHA. *Program availability:* Evening/weekend. *Degree requirements:* For master's, comprehensive exam, thesis, practicum, residency; for doctorate, practicum. *Entrance requirements:* For master's, GRE, minimum GPA of 3.0, 3 letters of recommendation, statement of goals, bachelor's degree; for doctorate, GRE, official transcript from all schools attended, minimum GPA of 3.0, 3 letters of recommendation, essay, interview. Additional exam requirements/recommendations for international students: Required—TOEFL (minimum score 600 paper-based; 100 iBT), IELTS (minimum score 7). Electronic applications accepted. *Expenses:* Contact institution. *Faculty research:* Bilingualism and adult and child language disorders, neural processing of speech, dysphagia, speech motor control, electrophysiological measurement of hearing, central auditory processing disorders, scholarship of teaching and learning, evidence-based education, developmental dyslexia.

Saint Louis University, Graduate Education, College of Arts and Sciences and Graduate Education, Department of Communication Sciences and Disorders, St. Louis, MO 63103. Offers MA, MA-R. *Accreditation:* ASHA (one or more programs are accredited). *Degree requirements:* For master's, thesis optional, comprehensive oral and written exams. *Entrance requirements:* For master's, GRE General Test, letters of recommendation, resume. Additional exam requirements/recommendations for international students: Required—TOEFL (minimum score 525 paper-based). Electronic applications accepted. *Faculty research:* Communication disorders in culturally and linguistically diverse populations, disability study-specific to World Health Organization classifications, early intervention in communication disorders and literacy skills, communication difficulties in internationally adopted children, voice and swallowing disorders secondary to cancer treatments.

Saint Mary's College, Graduate Programs, Program in Speech Language Pathology, Notre Dame, IN 46556. Offers MS. *Faculty:* 6 full-time (all women). *Students:* 24 full-time (all women). Average age 23. 152 applicants, 31% accepted, 24 enrolled. *Degree requirements:* For master's, comprehensive exam (for some programs), thesis optional, 400 hours of a supervised clinical practicum. *Entrance requirements:* For master's, GRE, bachelor's degree in communication sciences and disorders or related field, official transcripts, current resume or curriculum vitae, 3 letters of recommendation, personal statement. Additional exam requirements/recommendations for international students: Recommended—TOEFL, IELTS. *Application deadline:* For fall admission, 2/1 for domestic and international students. Application fee: $0. Electronic applications accepted. *Expenses:* $10,077 per term. *Financial support:* In 2015–16, 5 students received support. Fellowships available. Financial award application deadline: 3/1; financial award applicants required to submit FAFSA. *Faculty research:* Autism, children's develop of speech perception, auditory middle latency response in individuals with tinnitus, speech analysis app development to identify neurodegenerative disease processes. *Unit head:* Susan Latham, Program Director, Master of Science in Speech Language Pathology, 574-284-4686, E-mail: slatham@saintmarys.edu. *Application contact:* Melissa Fruscione, Graduate Admission, 574-284-5098, E-mail: graduateadmission@saintmarys.edu. Website: http://grad.saintmarys.edu/academic-programs/ms-speech-pathology

Saint Xavier University, Graduate Studies, College of Arts and Sciences, Department of Communication Sciences and Disorders, Chicago, IL 60655-3105. Offers speech-language pathology (MS). *Accreditation:* ASHA. *Entrance requirements:* For master's, GRE General Test, minimum GPA of 3.0, undergraduate course work in speech. *Expenses:* Contact institution.

SECTION 20: ALLIED HEALTH

Communication Disorders

Salus University, George S. Osborne College of Audiology, Elkins Park, PA 19027-1598. Offers Au D. *Accreditation:* ASHA. *Entrance requirements:* Additional exam requirements/recommendations for international students: Required—TOEFL. Electronic applications accepted.

Samford University, School of Health Professions, Birmingham, AL 35229. Offers athletic training (MAT); physical therapy (DPT); speech language pathology (MS). *Program availability:* Evening/weekend, online learning. *Faculty:* 11 full-time (8 women). *Students:* 53 full-time (38 women); includes 1 minority (Two or more races, non-Hispanic/Latino). Average age 24. 117 applicants, 73% accepted, 55 enrolled. *Degree requirements:* For master's, thesis or alternative; for doctorate, thesis/dissertation or alternative. *Entrance requirements:* For master's and doctorate, GRE, 3 recommendations, resume, on-campus interview, personal statement, CPR certification. Additional exam requirements/recommendations for international students: Required—TOEFL (minimum score 550 paper-based). *Application deadline:* For fall admission, 6/1 for domestic students; for spring admission, 10/1 for domestic students. Application fee: $120. Electronic applications accepted. *Expenses: Tuition, area resident:* Full-time $18,673; part-time $766 per credit hour. Tuition and fees vary according to course load, degree level and student level. *Financial support:* In 2015–16, 7 students received support. Application deadline: 3/1; applicants required to submit FAFSA. *Unit head:* Dr. Alan P. Jung, Dean, School of Health Professions, 205-726-2716, Fax: 205-726-2666, E-mail: apjung@samford.edu. *Application contact:* Dr. Marian Carter, Assistant Dean of Enrollment Management and Student Services, 205-726-2611, Fax: 205-726-2666, E-mail: mwcarter@samford.edu.
Website: http://www.samford.edu/healthprofessions/

San Diego State University, Graduate and Research Affairs, College of Health and Human Services, School of Speech, Language, and Hearing Sciences, San Diego, CA 92182. Offers audiology (Au D); communicative disorders (MA); language and communicative disorders (PhD). PhD offered jointly with University of California, San Diego. *Accreditation:* ASHA (one or more programs are accredited). *Program availability:* Part-time. *Degree requirements:* For master's, comprehensive exam (for some programs), thesis (for some programs); for doctorate, thesis/dissertation. *Entrance requirements:* For master's and doctorate, GRE General Test. Additional exam requirements/recommendations for international students: Required—TOEFL. Electronic applications accepted. *Faculty research:* Brain/behavior relationships in language development, grammatical processing and language disorders, interdisciplinary training of bilingual speech pathologists.

San Francisco State University, Division of Graduate Studies, College of Education, Department of Special Education and Communicative Disorders, Program in Communicative Disorders, San Francisco, CA 94132-1722. Offers MS. *Accreditation:* ASHA. *Expenses:* Tuition, state resident: full-time $6738. Tuition, nonresident: full-time $15,666. *Required fees:* $1004. *Unit head:* Dr. Yvonne Bui, Chair, 415-338-2503, E-mail: ybui@sfsu.edu. *Application contact:* Dr. Laura Epstein, Program Coordinator, 415-338-1058, E-mail: lepstein@sfsu.edu.
Website: http://www.sfsu.edu/~comdis/

San Jose State University, Graduate Studies and Research, Connie L. Lurie College of Education, San Jose, CA 95192-0001. Offers child and adolescent development (MA); common core mathematics (K-8) (Certificate, Credential); education (MA, Credential), including counseling and student personnel (MA), speech pathology (MA); education specialist preliminary teaching: early childhood special (Credential); educational leadership (MA, Ed D, Credential), including administration and supervision (MA), higher education (MA), preliminary administrative services (Credential); professional administrative services (Credential); elementary education (MA), including curriculum and instruction; K-12 school counseling (Credential); K-12 school counseling internship (Credential); school child welfare attendance (Credential); single subject (Credential); theory (Certificate), including knowledge and practice about autism spectrum disorders. *Accreditation:* NCATE. *Program availability:* Evening/weekend. *Students:* 146 full-time (117 women), 28 part-time (25 women); includes 253 minority (18 Black or African American, non-Hispanic/Latino; 80 Asian, non-Hispanic/Latino; 155 Hispanic/Latino), 22 international. Average age 29. 579 applicants, 39% accepted, 175 enrolled. In 2015, 218 master's awarded. *Application deadline:* For fall admission, 6/29 for domestic students; for spring admission, 11/30 for domestic students. Applications are processed on a rolling basis. Application fee: $55. Electronic applications accepted. *Financial support:* Career-related internships or fieldwork available. Financial award applicants required to submit FAFSA. *Unit head:* Elaine Chin, Dean, 408-924-3600, Fax: 408-924-3713. *Application contact:* 408-924-2480, Fax: 408-924-2477.
Website: http://www1.coe.sjsu.edu/

Seton Hall University, School of Health and Medical Sciences, Program in Speech-Language Pathology, South Orange, NJ 07079-2697. Offers MS. *Accreditation:* ASHA. *Entrance requirements:* For master's, GRE, bachelor's degree, clinical experience; minimum GPA of 3.0, undergraduate preprofessional coursework in communication sciences and disorders. Additional exam requirements/recommendations for international students: Recommended—TOEFL. Electronic applications accepted. *Faculty research:* Child language disorders, motor speech control, voice disorders, dysphagia, early intervention/teaming.

South Carolina State University, College of Graduate and Professional Studies, Department of Health Sciences, Orangeburg, SC 29117-0001. Offers speech pathology and audiology (MA). *Accreditation:* ASHA. *Program availability:* Part-time, evening/weekend. *Faculty:* 14 full-time (13 women), 2 part-time/adjunct (both women). *Students:* 42 full-time (40 women), 41 part-time (38 women); includes 50 minority (48 Black or African American, non-Hispanic/Latino; 2 Hispanic/Latino), 1 international. Average age 26. 70 applicants, 49% accepted, 27 enrolled. In 2015, 36 master's awarded. *Degree requirements:* For master's, thesis optional, departmental qualifying exam. *Entrance requirements:* For master's, GRE or NTE, minimum GPA of 3.0. *Application deadline:* For fall admission, 6/15 for domestic and international students; for spring admission, 11/1 for domestic and international students. Application fee: $25. Electronic applications accepted. *Expenses:* Tuition, state resident: full-time $8906; part-time $495 per credit hour. Tuition, nonresident: full-time $18,674; part-time $1037 per credit hour. *Required fees:* $2497; $66 per credit hour. *Financial support:* Fellowships, career-related internships or fieldwork, Federal Work-Study, and scholarships/grants available. Financial award application deadline: 6/1. *Unit head:* Dr. Cecelia Jeffries, Chair, Department of Health Sciences, 803-536-8074, Fax: 803-536-8593, E-mail: cjeffrie@scsu.edu. *Application contact:* Curtis Foskey, Coordinator of Graduate Admission, 803-536-8419, Fax: 803-536-8812, E-mail: cfoskey@scsu.edu.

Southeastern Louisiana University, College of Nursing and Health Sciences, Department of Health and Human Sciences, Hammond, LA 70402. Offers communication sciences and disorders (MS); counselor education (M Ed). *Accreditation:* ASHA; NCATE. *Faculty:* 15 full-time (all women), 1 (woman) part-time/adjunct. *Students:* 102 full-time (90 women), 41 part-time (38 women); includes 36 minority (20 Black or African American, non-Hispanic/Latino; 1 American Indian or Alaska Native, non-Hispanic/Latino; 1 Native Hawaiian or other Pacific Islander, non-Hispanic/Latino; 6 Two or more races, non-Hispanic/Latino), 1 international. Average age 26. 77 applicants, 74% accepted, 35 enrolled. In 2015, 17 master's awarded. *Degree requirements:* For master's, comprehensive exam, thesis optional, 25 clock hours of clinical observation. *Entrance requirements:* For master's, GRE (verbal and quantitative), minimum GPA of 2.75; undergraduate degree; three letters of reference; favorable criminal background check. Additional exam requirements/recommendations for international students: Required—TOEFL (minimum score 500 paper-based; 61 iBT). *Application deadline:* For fall admission, 3/1 priority date for domestic students, 6/1 for international students; for spring admission, 10/1 priority date for domestic and international students. Applications are processed on a rolling basis. Application fee: $20 ($30 for international students). Electronic applications accepted. *Expenses: Tuition, area resident:* Full-time $5551; part-time $436 per credit hour. Tuition, nonresident: full-time $18,115; part-time $1129 per credit hour. *Required fees:* $1559. *Financial support:* In 2015–16, 5 research assistantships (averaging $9,440 per year), 4 teaching assistantships (averaging $8,425 per year) were awarded; career-related internships or fieldwork, Federal Work-Study, institutionally sponsored loans, scholarships/grants, and unspecified assistantships also available. Support available to part-time students. Financial award application deadline: 5/1; financial award applicants required to submit FAFSA. *Faculty research:* Aphasia, autism spectrum disorders, child language and literacy, language and dementia, clinical supervision. *Total annual research expenditures:* $4,881. *Unit head:* Dr. Jacqueline Guendouzi, Department Head, 985-549-2309, Fax: 985-549-5030, E-mail: jguendouzi@selu.edu. *Application contact:* Amanda Harper, Graduate Admissions Analyst, 985-549-5620, Fax: 985-549-5632, E-mail: admissions@selu.edu.
Website: http://www.southeastern.edu/acad_research/depts/hhs/

Southeast Missouri State University, School of Graduate Studies, Department of Communication Disorders, Cape Girardeau, MO 63701-4799. Offers MA. *Accreditation:* ASHA. *Faculty:* 6 full-time (5 women), 2 part-time/adjunct (both women). *Students:* 29 full-time (28 women), 1 (woman) part-time; includes 1 minority (Hispanic/Latino). Average age 25. 136 applicants, 29% accepted, 15 enrolled. In 2015, 14 master's awarded. *Degree requirements:* For master's, comprehensive exam, research project or thesis. *Entrance requirements:* For master's, GRE General Test. Additional exam requirements/recommendations for international students: Required—TOEFL (minimum score 550 paper-based; 79 iBT), IELTS (minimum score 6), PTE (minimum score 53). *Application deadline:* For fall admission, 2/1 for domestic and international students. Applications are processed on a rolling basis. Application fee: $30 ($40 for international students). Electronic applications accepted. *Expenses:* Tuition, state resident: part-time $260.80 per credit hour. Tuition, nonresident: part-time $486.80 per credit hour. *Required fees:* $33.70 per credit hour. *Financial support:* In 2015–16, 11 students received support, including teaching assistantships with full tuition reimbursements available (averaging $8,467 per year); career-related internships or fieldwork, Federal Work-Study, scholarships/grants, traineeships, tuition waivers (full), and unspecified assistantships also available. Financial award application deadline: 6/30; financial award applicants required to submit FAFSA. *Faculty research:* Dysphagia, fluency disorders, voice disorders, language disorders, speech disorders, autism spectrum disorders. *Unit head:* Dr. Marcia Brown Haims, Department of Communication Disorders Chair, 573-651-2488, Fax: 573-651-2827, E-mail: mjbrown@semo.edu.
Website: http://www.semo.edu/commdisorders/

Southern Connecticut State University, School of Graduate Studies, School of Health and Human Services, Department of Communication Disorders, New Haven, CT 06515-1355. Offers speech pathology (MS). *Accreditation:* ASHA. *Program availability:* Part-time. *Faculty:* 9 full-time (7 women), 5 part-time/adjunct (4 women). *Students:* 101 full-time (96 women), 3 part-time (all women); includes 7 minority (2 Asian, non-Hispanic/Latino; 4 Hispanic/Latino; 1 Two or more races, non-Hispanic/Latino), 1 international. Average age 25. 348 applicants, 12% accepted, 42 enrolled. In 2015, 40 master's awarded. *Degree requirements:* For master's, thesis or alternative, clinical experience. *Entrance requirements:* For master's, GRE, interview, minimum QPA of 3.0. *Application deadline:* For fall admission, 3/1 for domestic students. Application fee: $50. Electronic applications accepted. *Expenses:* Tuition, state resident: full-time $4968; part-time $494 per credit hour. Tuition, nonresident: full-time $16,078; part-time $509 per credit hour. *Required fees:* $4632; $55 per semester. Tuition and fees vary according to program. *Financial support:* Career-related internships or fieldwork, scholarships/grants, and unspecified assistantships available. Financial award application deadline: 4/15; financial award applicants required to submit FAFSA. *Unit head:* Dr. Deborah Weiss, Chairperson, 203-392-6615, Fax: 203-392-5968, E-mail: weissd1@southernct.edu. *Application contact:* Lisa Galvin, Director of Graduate Admissions, 203-392-5240, Fax: 203-392-5235, E-mail: galvinl1@southernct.edu.

Southern Illinois University Carbondale, Graduate School, College of Education and Human Services, Department of Communication Disorders and Sciences, Carbondale, IL 62901-4701. Offers MS. *Accreditation:* ASHA. *Faculty:* 4 full-time (2 women). *Students:* 52 full-time (51 women), 1 (woman) part-time; includes 6 minority (2 Black or African American, non-Hispanic/Latino; 4 Asian, non-Hispanic/Latino), 12 international. Average age 29. 175 applicants, 15% accepted, 26 enrolled. In 2015, 27 master's awarded. *Degree requirements:* For master's, thesis. *Entrance requirements:* For master's, GRE, minimum GPA of 3.0. Additional exam requirements/recommendations for international students: Required—TOEFL (minimum score 550 paper-based; 80 iBT). *Application deadline:* For fall admission, 2/15 for domestic students. Application fee: $65. Electronic applications accepted. *Financial support:* In 2015–16, 16 students received support, including 2 fellowships with full tuition reimbursements available, 8 research assistantships with full tuition reimbursements available; teaching assistantships with full tuition reimbursements available, career-related internships or fieldwork, Federal Work-Study, institutionally sponsored loans, tuition waivers (full), and unspecified assistantships also available. *Faculty research:* Neurolinguistics, language processing, child language, fluency, phonology. *Unit head:* Dr. Carl Flowers, Director, 618-453-8280, E-mail: cflowers@siu.edu. *Application contact:* Sheila Dingrando, Office Support Specialist, 618-453-8262, E-mail: sding@siu.edu.

Southern Illinois University Edwardsville, Graduate School, School of Education, Health, and Human Behavior, Department of Special Education and Communication Disorders, Program in Speech-Language Pathology, Edwardsville, IL 62026. Offers MS. *Accreditation:* ASHA. *Program availability:* Part-time, evening/weekend. *Students:* 50 full-time (45 women), 1 (woman) part-time; includes 3 minority (1 Black or African American, non-Hispanic/Latino; 2 Hispanic/Latino), 1 international. 313 applicants, 32% accepted. In 2015, 29 master's awarded. *Degree requirements:* For master's, thesis (for some programs), final exam. *Entrance requirements:* For master's, GRE, minimum GPA of 3.0. Additional exam requirements/recommendations for international students: Required—TOEFL (minimum score 550 paper-based; 79 iBT), IELTS (minimum score 6.5). *Application deadline:* For fall admission, 1/15 for domestic and international students. Application fee: $30. Electronic applications accepted. *Expenses:* Tuition, state resident: full-time $5026; part-time $837 per course. Tuition, nonresident: full-time $12,566; part-time $2094 per course. *Required fees:* $1682; $474 per course. Tuition and fees vary according to course load, campus/location and program. *Financial support:* In 2015–16, 3 fellowships with full tuition reimbursements, 6 teaching assistantships with full tuition reimbursements were awarded; research assistantships with full tuition reimbursements, institutionally sponsored loans, scholarships/grants, and unspecified assistantships also available. Financial award application deadline: 3/1; financial award applicants required to submit FAFSA. *Unit head:* Dr. Steffany Chleboun, Chair, 618-650-3677, E-mail: schlebo@siue.edu. *Application contact:* Bob Skorczewski,

Coordinator of International and Graduate Recruitment, 618-650-3705, Fax: 618-650-3618, E-mail: gradadmissions@siue.edu.
Website: http://www.siue.edu/education/secd/

State University of New York at Fredonia, College of Liberal Arts and Sciences, Fredonia, NY 14063. Offers biology (MS); interdisciplinary studies (MS); speech pathology (MS); MA/MS. *Program availability:* Part-time, evening/weekend. *Degree requirements:* For master's, comprehensive exam (for some programs), thesis (for some programs). *Entrance requirements:* For master's, GRE. Additional exam requirements/recommendations for international students: Required—TOEFL (minimum score 79 iBT), IELTS (minimum score 6.5), Cambridge English Advanced (minimum score: 52) recommended. Electronic applications accepted. *Expenses:* Tuition, state resident: full-time $10,870; part-time $453 per credit. Tuition, nonresident: full-time $22,210; part-time $925 per credit. *Required fees:* $1604; $66.70 per credit. *Faculty research:* Immunology/microbiology, applied human physiology, ecology and evolution, invertebrate biology, molecular biology, biochemistry, physiology, animal behavior, science education, vertebrate physiology, cell biology, plant biology, developmental biology, aquatic ecology, bilingual language acquisition, bilingual language acquisition and disorders, augmentative and alternate communication with ALS, World War I, Zweig, environmental literature, editing, adolescent literature, pedagogy.

State University of New York at New Paltz, Graduate School, School of Liberal Arts and Sciences, Department of Communication Disorders, New Paltz, NY 12561. Offers communication disorders (MS), including speech-language disabilities, speech-language pathology. *Accreditation:* ASHA. *Program availability:* Part-time, evening/weekend. *Faculty:* 8 full-time (all women), 5 part-time/adjunct (all women). *Students:* 46 full-time (41 women), 2 part-time (both women); includes 10 minority (1 Black or African American, non-Hispanic/Latino; 4 Asian, non-Hispanic/Latino; 3 Hispanic/Latino; 2 Two or more races, non-Hispanic/Latino). Average age 26. 212 applicants, 16% accepted, 20 enrolled. In 2015, 29 master's awarded. *Degree requirements:* For master's, comprehensive exam, thesis. *Entrance requirements:* For master's, GRE General Test or MAT, minimum GPA of 3.0. Additional exam requirements/recommendations for international students: Required—TOEFL (minimum score 550 paper-based; 80 iBT), IELTS (minimum score 6.5). *Application deadline:* For fall admission, 3/1 for domestic and international students. Application fee: $50. Electronic applications accepted. *Financial support:* In 2015–16, 4 teaching assistantships with partial tuition reimbursements (averaging $5,000 per year) were awarded. Financial award application deadline: 8/1. *Unit head:* Dr. Stella Turk, Department Chair, 845-257-3620, E-mail: commdis@newpaltz.edu. *Application contact:* Dr. Anne Balant, Graduate Coordinator, 845-257-3453, E-mail: balanta@newpaltz.edu.
Website: http://www.newpaltz.edu/commdis/

State University of New York at Plattsburgh, Division of Education, Health, and Human Services, Department of Communication Disorders, Plattsburgh, NY 12901-2681. Offers speech-language pathology (MA). *Accreditation:* ASHA. *Program availability:* Part-time. *Entrance requirements:* For master's, GRE General Test, minimum GPA of 3.0. Additional exam requirements/recommendations for international students: Required—TOEFL. *Faculty research:* Autotoxins and noise effects on hearing, language impairment in Alzheimer's disease, attitudes on stuttering, diagnostic audiology.

Stephen F. Austin State University, Graduate School, College of Education, Department of Human Services, Nacogdoches, TX 75962. Offers counseling (MA); school psychology (MA); special education (M Ed); speech pathology (MS). *Accreditation:* ACA (one or more programs are accredited); ASHA (one or more programs are accredited); CORE; NCATE. *Degree requirements:* For master's, comprehensive exam, thesis (for some programs). *Entrance requirements:* For master's, GRE General Test, minimum GPA of 2.8. Additional exam requirements/recommendations for international students: Required—TOEFL.

Stockton University, Office of Graduate Studies, Program in Communication Disorders, Galloway, NJ 08205-9441. Offers MS. *Accreditation:* ASHA. *Faculty:* 5 full-time (4 women), 2 part-time/adjunct (both women). *Students:* 63 full-time (60 women), 28 part-time (26 women); includes 15 minority (2 Black or African American, non-Hispanic/Latino; 2 Asian, non-Hispanic/Latino; 5 Hispanic/Latino; 6 Two or more races, non-Hispanic/Latino). Average age 26. 261 applicants, 17% accepted, 30 enrolled. In 2015, 28 master's awarded. *Degree requirements:* For master's, comprehensive exam (for some programs), thesis optional. *Entrance requirements:* For master's, GRE, 3 letters of recommendation, official transcripts from all colleges/universities attended, minimum undergraduate cumulative GPA of 3.2. *Application deadline:* For fall admission, 2/1 for domestic students. Electronic applications accepted. *Expenses:* Tuition, state resident: full-time $13,968; part-time $582 per credit. Tuition, nonresident: full-time $21,502; part-time $895 per credit. *Required fees:* $4200; $175 per credit. Fee: $90. Tuition and fees vary according to degree level. *Financial support:* Fellowships, research assistantships with partial tuition reimbursements, career-related internships or fieldwork, Federal Work-Study, scholarships/grants, and unspecified assistantships available. Support available to part-time students. Financial award application deadline: 3/1. *Unit head:* Dr. Amy Hadley, Program Director, 609-626-3640, E-mail: graduatestudies@stockton.edu. *Application contact:* Tara Williams, Assistant Director of Enrollment Management, 609-626-3640, Fax: 609-626-6050, E-mail: gradschool@stockton.edu.

Syracuse University, College of Arts and Sciences, MS Program in Speech-Language Pathology, Syracuse, NY 13244. Offers MS. *Accreditation:* ASHA. *Program availability:* Part-time. *Students:* Average age 24. In 2015, 39 degrees awarded. *Degree requirements:* For master's, thesis or alternative. *Entrance requirements:* For master's, GRE, three letters of recommendation, personal statement, resume, transcripts. Additional exam requirements/recommendations for international students: Required—TOEFL (minimum score 100 iBT). *Application deadline:* For fall admission, 1/1 priority date for domestic and international students. Application fee: $75. Electronic applications accepted. *Expenses: Tuition, area resident:* Full-time $25,974; part-time $1443 per credit hour. *Required fees:* $802; $50 per course. Tuition and fees vary according to course load and program. *Financial support:* Fellowships with full tuition reimbursements, research assistantships with tuition reimbursements, teaching assistantships with tuition reimbursements, and scholarships/grants available. Financial award application deadline: 1/1. *Faculty research:* Auditory electrophysiology, hearing science, pediatric auditory, speech production, aphasia and psycholinguistics. *Unit head:* Dr. Karen Doherty, Professor and Chair, Communications Sciences and Disorders, 315-443-5662, E-mail: kadohert@syr.edu. *Application contact:* Jennifer Steigerwald, Information Contact, 315-443-9615, E-mail: jssteige@syr.edu.
Website: http://csd.syr.edu/

Syracuse University, College of Arts and Sciences, Programs in Audiology, Syracuse, NY 13244. Offers audiology (Au D, PhD). *Accreditation:* ASHA. *Program availability:* Part-time. *Students:* Average age 25. In 2015, 4 doctorates awarded. *Degree requirements:* For doctorate, thesis/dissertation, internship. *Entrance requirements:* For doctorate, GRE General Test, undergraduate and graduate transcripts, three letters of recommendation, resume, personal statement. Additional exam requirements/recommendations for international students: Required—TOEFL (minimum score 100 iBT). *Application deadline:* For fall admission, 1/1 priority date for domestic and

international students. Application fee: $75. Electronic applications accepted. *Expenses: Tuition, area resident:* Full-time $25,974; part-time $1443 per credit hour. *Required fees:* $802; $50 per course. Tuition and fees vary according to course load and program. *Financial support:* Fellowships with full tuition reimbursements, research assistantships with tuition reimbursements, teaching assistantships with tuition reimbursements, and scholarships/grants available. Financial award application deadline: 1/1. *Faculty research:* Auditory electrophysiology, hearing science, pediatric auditory, speech production, aphasia and psycholinguistics. *Unit head:* Dr. Karen Doherty, Department Chair, 315-443-9637, E-mail: csd@syr.edu. *Application contact:* Jennifer Steigerwald, Information Contact, 315-443-9615, E-mail: csdcasinfo@csdcas.org.
Website: http://csd.syr.edu/

Teachers College, Columbia University, Department of Biobehavioral Sciences, New York, NY 10027-6696. Offers applied exercise physiology (Ed M, MA, Ed D); communication sciences and disorders (MS, Ed D, PhD); kinesiology (PhD); motor learning and control (Ed M, MA); motor learning/movement science (Ed D); neuroscience and education (MS); physical education (MA, Ed D). *Program availability:* Part-time, evening/weekend. *Students:* 121 full-time (103 women), 218 part-time (171 women); includes 157 minority (30 Black or African American, non-Hispanic/Latino; 58 Asian, non-Hispanic/Latino; 63 Hispanic/Latino; 6 Two or more races, non-Hispanic/Latino), 6 international. *Expenses: Tuition, area resident:* Part-time $1454 per credit. *Required fees:* $428 per semester. One-time fee: $475 full-time. Full-time tuition and fees vary according to course load. *Financial support:* Fellowships, teaching assistantships, career-related internships or fieldwork, Federal Work-Study, institutionally sponsored loans, traineeships, and tuition waivers (full and partial) available. Support available to part-time students. *Unit head:* Prof. Carol Garber, Chair, E-mail: garber@tc.columbia.edu. *Application contact:* David Estrella, Director of Admissions, E-mail: estrella@tc.columbia.edu.
Website: http://www.tc.columbia.edu/biobehavioral-sciences/

Teachers College, Columbia University, Department of Health and Behavior Studies, New York, NY 10027-6696. Offers applied behavior analysis (MA, PhD); applied educational psychology: school psychology (Ed M, PhD); behavioral nutrition (PhD); including nutrition (Ed D, PhD); community health education (MS); community nutrition education (Ed M), including community nutrition education; education of deaf and hard of hearing (MA, PhD); health education (MA, Ed D); hearing impairment (Ed D); intellectual disability/autism (MA, Ed D, PhD); nursing education (Advanced Certificate); nutrition and education (MS); nutrition and exercise physiology (MS); nutrition and public health (MS); nutrition education (Ed D), including nutrition (Ed D, PhD); physical disabilities (Ed D); reading specialist (MA); severe or multiple disabilities (MA); special education (Ed M, MA, Ed D); teaching of sign language (MA). *Program availability:* Part-time, evening/weekend. *Students:* 186 full-time (168 women), 362 part-time (319 women); includes 199 minority (50 Black or African American, non-Hispanic/Latino; 1 American Indian or Alaska Native, non-Hispanic/Latino; 73 Asian, non-Hispanic/Latino; 59 Hispanic/Latino; 1 Native Hawaiian or other Pacific Islander, non-Hispanic/Latino; 15 Two or more races, non-Hispanic/Latino), 13 international. Terminal master's awarded for partial completion of doctoral program. *Expenses: Tuition, area resident:* Part-time $1454 per credit. *Required fees:* $428 per semester. One-time fee: $475 full-time. Full-time tuition and fees vary according to course load. *Unit head:* Prof. Stephen T. Peverly, Chair, 212-678-3964, Fax: 212-678-8259, E-mail: stp4@columbia.edu. *Application contact:* David Estrella, Director of Admission, 212-678-3305, E-mail: estrella@tc.columbia.edu.
Website: http://www.tc.columbia.edu/health-and-behavior-studies/

Temple University, College of Public Health, Department of Communication Sciences and Disorders, Philadelphia, PA 19122. Offers communication sciences and disorders (PhD); speech-language-hearing (MA). *Accreditation:* ASHA. *Faculty:* 13 full-time (10 women), 6 part-time/adjunct (all women). *Students:* 71 full-time (63 women), 1 (woman) part-time; includes 10 minority (2 Black or African American, non-Hispanic/Latino; 1 Asian, non-Hispanic/Latino; 7 Hispanic/Latino), 1 international. 473 applicants, 15% accepted, 26 enrolled. In 2015, 24 master's awarded. *Degree requirements:* For master's, comprehensive exam; for doctorate, comprehensive exam, thesis/dissertation. *Entrance requirements:* For master's, GRE General Test, minimum GPA of 3.0, 2 letters of reference, statement of goals; for doctorate, GRE General Test, minimum GPA of 3.0, 3 letters of reference, statement of goals, writing sample, resume. Additional exam requirements/recommendations for international students: Required—TOEFL (minimum score 550 paper-based; 79 iBT). *Application deadline:* For fall admission, 1/1 for domestic and international students; for spring admission, 11/1 for domestic students, 10/1 for international students. Application fee: $60. Electronic applications accepted. *Expenses:* Contact institution. *Financial support:* Federal Work-Study, institutionally sponsored loans, and unspecified assistantships available. Financial award application deadline: 1/15. *Faculty research:* Bilingualism; biliteracy; adult neurogenic language disorders, including aphasia; dementia; school readiness. *Unit head:* Doris Fallon Snyder, Program Director, 215-204-7543, E-mail: dfallon@temple.edu. *Application contact:* Dawn Dandridge, Academic Coordinator, 215-204-9005, E-mail: ddandrid@temple.edu.
Website: http://chpsw.temple.edu/commsci/home

Tennessee State University, The School of Graduate Studies and Research, College of Health Sciences, Speech and Hearing Science Department, Nashville, TN 37209-1561. Offers MS. *Accreditation:* ASHA. *Program availability:* Part-time, online learning. *Degree requirements:* For master's, comprehensive exam, thesis optional. *Entrance requirements:* For master's, GRE General Test or MAT, minimum GPA of 3.5. Additional exam requirements/recommendations for international students: Required—TOEFL. *Application deadline:* For fall admission, 7/1 for domestic and international students. Application fee: $25. *Financial support:* Fellowships with tuition reimbursements, research assistantships with tuition reimbursements, teaching assistantships with tuition reimbursements, scholarships/grants, traineeships, and unspecified assistantships available. Support available to part-time students. Financial award application deadline: 3/15; financial award applicants required to submit FAFSA. *Faculty research:* Assessment and management of dysphagia, early intervention language disorders, multicultural diversity. *Unit head:* Dr. Tina Smith, Head, 615-963-7057, E-mail: tsmith31@tnstate.edu. *Application contact:* Dr. Tina Smith, Head, 615-963-7057, E-mail: tsmith31@tnstate.edu.
Website: http://www.tnstate.edu/speechpath

Texas A&M University–Kingsville, College of Graduate Studies, College of Arts and Sciences, Program in Communication Sciences and Disorders, Kingsville, TX 78363. Offers MS. *Accreditation:* ASHA. *Faculty:* 6 full-time (3 women), 3 part-time/adjunct (2 women). *Students:* 42 full-time (all women), 4 part-time (all women); includes 34 minority (2 Black or African American, non-Hispanic/Latino; 31 Hispanic/Latino; 1 Native Hawaiian or other Pacific Islander, non-Hispanic/Latino). Average age 25. 95 applicants, 19% accepted, 15 enrolled. In 2015, 24 master's awarded. *Entrance requirements:* Additional exam requirements/recommendations for international students: Required—TOEFL (minimum score 550 paper-based; 79 iBT); Recommended—IELTS. *Application deadline:* Applications are processed on a rolling basis. Application fee: $35 ($50 for international students). Electronic applications accepted. *Financial support:* Research assistantships, teaching assistantships, career-related internships or fieldwork, Federal

Communication Disorders

Work-Study, institutionally sponsored loans, scholarships/grants, tuition waivers (full and partial), and unspecified assistantships available. Support available to part-time students. *Unit head:* Dr. Darin Hoskisson, Interim Department Chair, Clinical Health Sciences, 361-593-3493, E-mail: darin.hoskisson@tamuk.edu. *Application contact:* Dr. Eric Swartz, Graduate Coordinator, Communication Sciences and Disorders, 361-593-4937, E-mail: eric.swartz@tamuk.edu.

Texas Christian University, Harris College of Nursing and Health Sciences, Davies School of Communication Sciences and Disorders, Fort Worth, TX 76129. Offers speech-language pathology (MS). *Accreditation:* ASHA. *Faculty:* 7 full-time (6 women). *Students:* 39 full-time (36 women); includes 12 minority (1 Black or African American, non-Hispanic/Latino; 10 Hispanic/Latino; 1 Two or more races, non-Hispanic/Latino). Average age 23. 285 applicants, 7% accepted, 20 enrolled. In 2015, 20 master's awarded. *Degree requirements:* For master's, comprehensive exam, thesis optional. *Entrance requirements:* For master's, GRE General Test. *Application deadline:* For fall admission, 1/15 for domestic and international students. Application fee: $60. Electronic applications accepted. *Expenses: Tuition, area resident:* Full-time $26,640; part-time $1480 per credit hour. *Required fees:* $48; $48 per unit. Tuition and fees vary according to program. *Financial support:* In 2015–16, 40 students received support, including 40 research assistantships (averaging $35,000 per year); tuition waivers (partial) and unspecified assistantships also available. Financial award application deadline: 1/15; financial award applicants required to submit FAFSA. *Faculty research:* Voice disorders, hearing loss, cochlear implants, aphasia, child language. *Total annual research expenditures:* $75,000. *Unit head:* Dr. Christopher Watts, Director, 817-257-7620, E-mail: c.watts@tcu.edu. *Application contact:* Janet Smith, Administrative Assistant, 817-257-7620, E-mail: janet.smith@tcu.edu.
Website: http://csd.tcu.edu/graduate/

Texas State University, The Graduate College, College of Health Professions, Program in Communication Disorders, San Marcos, TX 78666. Offers MA, MSCD. *Accreditation:* ASHA (one or more programs are accredited). *Faculty:* 11 full-time (9 women). *Students:* 61 full-time (57 women); includes 26 minority (4 Black or African American, non-Hispanic/Latino; 22 Hispanic/Latino). Average age 24. 418 applicants, 11% accepted, 31 enrolled. In 2015, 31 master's awarded. *Degree requirements:* For master's, comprehensive exam, thesis (for some programs), practicum. *Entrance requirements:* For master's, baccalaureate degree in communication disorders from regionally-accredited institution with minimum GPA of 3.0 in communication disorders courses and in last 60 hours of course work; 2 letters of recommendation from professors in previous major; resume on form provided by department; statement of purpose. Additional exam requirements/recommendations for international students: Required—TOEFL (minimum score 550 paper-based; 78 iBT). *Application deadline:* For fall admission, 2/1 for domestic and international students. Applications are processed on a rolling basis. Application fee: $40 ($90 for international students). Electronic applications accepted. *Expenses:* $3,615 in-state tuition (for 12 semester credit hours/1 full-time semester), $974 in-state fees. *Financial support:* In 2015–16, 43 students received support, including 1 research assistantship (averaging $5,927 per year), 10 teaching assistantships (averaging $6,016 per year); fellowships, career-related internships or fieldwork, Federal Work-Study, institutionally sponsored loans, scholarships/grants, and unspecified assistantships also available. Support available to part-time students. Financial award application deadline: 3/1; financial award applicants required to submit FAFSA. *Faculty research:* Microbiology and immunology in-service, Sarcoidosis Research Initiative. *Total annual research expenditures:* $4,403. *Unit head:* Dr. Valarie Fleming, Graduate Advisor, 512-245-2330, Fax: 512-245-2029, E-mail: vf13@txstate.edu. *Application contact:* Dr. Andrea Golato, Dean of Graduate School, 512-245-2581, Fax: 512-245-8365, E-mail: gradcollege@txstate.edu.
Website: http://www.health.txstate.edu/CDIS/

Texas Tech University Health Sciences Center, School of Health Professions, Program in Speech, Language and Hearing Sciences, Lubbock, TX 79430. Offers MS, Au D, PhD. *Accreditation:* ASHA (one or more programs are accredited). *Faculty:* 19 full-time (13 women), 1 (woman) part-time/adjunct. *Students:* 121 full-time (114 women), 10 part-time (8 women); includes 29 minority (3 Black or African American, non-Hispanic/Latino; 5 Asian, non-Hispanic/Latino; 20 Hispanic/Latino; 1 Two or more races, non-Hispanic/Latino). Average age 25. 366 applicants, 14% accepted, 52 enrolled. In 2015, 38 master's, 12 doctorates awarded. *Degree requirements:* For master's, comprehensive exam, thesis optional; for doctorate, comprehensive exam, thesis/dissertation. *Entrance requirements:* For master's and doctorate, GRE. Additional exam requirements/recommendations for international students: Required—TOEFL (minimum score 550 paper-based; 79 iBT), IELTS. *Application deadline:* For fall admission, 11/1 for domestic students; for winter admission, 1/15 for domestic students; for spring admission, 2/1 for domestic students. Applications are processed on a rolling basis. Application fee: $40. Electronic applications accepted. *Financial support:* In 2015–16, 8 research assistantships (averaging $3,000 per year), 28 teaching assistantships (averaging $3,000 per year) were awarded; career-related internships or fieldwork, institutionally sponsored loans, scholarships/grants, and unspecified assistantships also available. Financial award application deadline: 9/1; financial award applicants required to submit FAFSA. *Unit head:* Dr. Rajinder Koul, Department Chair, 806-743-5678, Fax: 806-743-5670, E-mail: rajinder.koul@ttuhsc.edu. *Application contact:* Lindsay Johnson, Associate Dean for Admissions and Student Affairs, 806-743-3220, Fax: 806-742-2994, E-mail: lindsay.johnson@ttuhsc.edu.
Website: https://www.ttuhsc.edu/shp/csd/

Texas Woman's University, Graduate School, College of Health Sciences, Department of Communication Sciences and Disorders, Denton, TX 76201. Offers deaf education (MS); speech-language pathology (MS). *Accreditation:* ASHA. *Program availability:* Part-time, online learning. *Degree requirements:* For master's, comprehensive exam, thesis (for some programs). *Entrance requirements:* For master's, GRE General Test (preferred minimum score 156 [550 old version] Verbal, 140 [400 old version] Quantitative), 2 letters of reference (3 for speech/language pathology), personal essay. Additional exam requirements/recommendations for international students: Required—TOEFL (minimum score 550 paper-based; 79 iBT). *Application deadline:* For fall admission, 2/1 priority date for domestic students, 2/1 for international students. Applications are processed on a rolling basis. Application fee: $50 ($75 for international students). Electronic applications accepted. *Expenses:* Tuition, state resident: full-time $4380; part-time $243 per credit hour. Tuition, nonresident: full-time $11,400; part-time $633 per credit hour. *International tuition:* $11,465 full-time. *Required fees:* $1778; $99 per credit hour. $283 per semester. One-time fee: $50. Tuition and fees vary according to course load and program. *Financial support:* Research assistantships, career-related internships or fieldwork, Federal Work-Study, institutionally sponsored loans, scholarships/grants, traineeships, health care benefits, and unspecified assistantships available. Support available to part-time students. Financial award application deadline: 3/1; financial award applicants required to submit FAFSA. *Faculty research:* Stroke, language assessment auditory processing and relationship between speech and language, effectiveness of distance education learning, neuromodulation of recovery of aphasia. *Unit head:* Dr. Erika Armstrong, Chair, 940-898-2474, Fax: 940-898-2070, E-mail: coms@twu.edu. *Application contact:* Dr. Samuel Wheeler, Assistant Director of Admissions, 940-898-3188, Fax: 940-898-3081, E-mail: wheelersr@twu.edu.
Website: http://www.twu.edu/communication-sciences/

Touro College, School of Health Sciences, Bay Shore, NY 11706. Offers industrial-organizational psychology (MS); mental health counseling (MS); occupational therapy (MS); physical therapy (DPT); physician assistant (MS); school psychology (MS); speech-language pathology (MS). *Faculty:* 20 full-time, 94 part-time/adjunct. *Students:* 1,057 full-time (772 women), 121 part-time (88 women); includes 243 minority (59 Black or African American, non-Hispanic/Latino; 1 American Indian or Alaska Native, non-Hispanic/Latino; 102 Asian, non-Hispanic/Latino; 58 Hispanic/Latino; 1 Native Hawaiian or other Pacific Islander, non-Hispanic/Latino; 22 Two or more races, non-Hispanic/Latino), 102 international. *Expenses:* Contact institution. *Financial support:* Fellowships available. *Unit head:* Dr. Louis Primavera, Dean, School of Health Sciences, 516-673-3200, E-mail: louis.primavera@touro.edu. *Application contact:* Brian J. Diele, Director of Student Administrative Services, 631-665-1600 Ext. 6311, E-mail: brian.diele@touro.edu.

Towson University, Program in Audiology, Towson, MD 21252-0001. Offers Au D. *Accreditation:* ASHA. *Students:* 50 full-time (45 women); includes 7 minority (3 Black or African American, non-Hispanic/Latino; 1 Asian, non-Hispanic/Latino; 2 Hispanic/Latino; 1 Two or more races, non-Hispanic/Latino), 1 international. *Entrance requirements:* For doctorate, GRE, 3 letters of recommendation, minimum GPA of 3.0, interview, essay. Additional exam requirements/recommendations for international students: Required—TOEFL (minimum score 600 paper-based). *Application deadline:* For fall admission, 2/1 for domestic students. Application fee: $45. Electronic applications accepted. *Expenses:* Tuition, state resident: full-time $7440; part-time $372 per unit. Tuition, nonresident: full-time $15,400; part-time $770 per unit. *Required fees:* $2360; $118 per year. $354 per term. *Financial support:* Application deadline: 4/1. *Unit head:* Dr. Jennifer Smart, Graduate Program Director, 410-704-3105, E-mail: audiology@towson.edu. *Application contact:* Alicia Arkell-Kleis, University Admissions, 410-704-2113, Fax: 410-704-3030, E-mail: grads@towson.edu.
Website: http://grad.towson.edu/program/doctoral/acsd-aud/

Towson University, Program in Speech-Language Pathology, Towson, MD 21252-0001. Offers MS. *Accreditation:* ASHA. *Students:* 91 full-time (all women), 1 (woman) part-time; includes 4 minority (2 Black or African American, non-Hispanic/Latino; 2 Two or more races, non-Hispanic/Latino). *Degree requirements:* For master's, thesis (for some programs). *Entrance requirements:* For master's, GRE, bachelor's degree in speech-language pathology and audiology; CLEP or advanced placement (AP) examination credits in biological sciences, physical sciences, social/behavioral sciences and statistics; minimum GPA of 3.0 in major; 3 letters of recommendation; essay. Additional exam requirements/recommendations for international students: Required—TOEFL (minimum score 600 paper-based). *Application deadline:* For fall admission, 1/15 for domestic students. Applications are processed on a rolling basis. Application fee: $45. Electronic applications accepted. *Expenses:* Tuition, state resident: full-time $7440; part-time $372 per unit. Tuition, nonresident: full-time $15,400; part-time $770 per unit. *Required fees:* $2360; $118 per year. $354 per term. *Financial support:* Application deadline: 4/1. *Unit head:* Dr. Karen Fallon, Graduate Program Director, 410-704-2437, E-mail: slpgrad@towson.edu. *Application contact:* Alicia Arkell-Kleis, University Admissions, 410-704-2113, Fax: 410-704-3030, E-mail: grads@towson.edu.
Website: http://grad.towson.edu/program/master/sppa-ms/

Truman State University, Graduate School, School of Health Sciences and Education, Program in Communication Disorders, Kirksville, MO 63501-4221. Offers MA. *Accreditation:* ASHA. *Degree requirements:* For master's, comprehensive exam, thesis optional. *Entrance requirements:* For master's, GRE General Test, minimum GPA of 3.0. Additional exam requirements/recommendations for international students: Required—TOEFL (minimum score 550 paper-based). *Application deadline:* For fall admission, 6/1 for domestic and international students; for spring admission, 11/1 for domestic and international students; for summer admission, 4/1 for domestic and international students. Applications are processed on a rolling basis. Application fee: $40. Electronic applications accepted. *Expenses:* Tuition, state resident: full-time $6870; part-time $343.50 per credit hour. Tuition, nonresident: full-time $11,790; part-time $589.50 per credit hour. Tuition and fees vary according to course load and program. *Financial support:* Fellowships, career-related internships or fieldwork, and Federal Work-Study available. Financial award application deadline: 5/1; financial award applicants required to submit FAFSA. *Unit head:* Dr. Paula Cochran, Department Chair, 660-785-4677. *Application contact:* Stephanie Rudolph, Graduate Secretary, 660-785-4109, Fax: 660-785-7460, E-mail: sdunn@truman.edu.

Universidad del Turabo, Graduate Programs, School of Health Sciences, Program in Speech and Language Pathology, Gurabo, PR 00778-3030. Offers MS.

Université de Montréal, Faculty of Medicine, School of Speech Therapy and Audiology, Montréal, QC H3C 3J7, Canada. Offers audiology (PMS); speech therapy (PMS, DESS). *Degree requirements:* For master's, thesis. *Entrance requirements:* For master's, B Sc in speech-language pathology and audiology, proficiency in French. Electronic applications accepted. *Faculty research:* Aphasia in adults, dysarthria, speech and hearing-impaired children, noise-induced hearing impairment, computerized audiometry.

Université Laval, Faculty of Medicine, Graduate Programs in Medicine, Program in Speech Therapy, Québec, QC G1K 7P4, Canada. Offers M Sc. *Entrance requirements:* For master's, knowledge of French, interview. Electronic applications accepted.

University at Buffalo, the State University of New York, Graduate School, College of Arts and Sciences, Department of Communicative Disorders and Sciences, Buffalo, NY 14214. Offers audiology (Au D); communicative disorders and sciences (MA, PhD). *Accreditation:* ASHA (one or more programs are accredited). *Faculty:* 15 full-time (9 women), 1 (woman) part-time/adjunct. *Students:* 107 full-time (98 women); includes 19 minority (3 Black or African American, non-Hispanic/Latino; 1 American Indian or Alaska Native, non-Hispanic/Latino; 11 Asian, non-Hispanic/Latino; 2 Hispanic/Latino; 2 Native Hawaiian or other Pacific Islander, non-Hispanic/Latino). Average age 23. 225 applicants, 43% accepted, 41 enrolled. In 2015, 30 master's, 8 doctorates awarded. *Degree requirements:* For master's, thesis or alternative, exam; for doctorate, thesis/dissertation, exams. *Entrance requirements:* For master's and doctorate, GRE General Test, minimum GPA of 3.0. Additional exam requirements/recommendations for international students: Required—TOEFL (minimum score 550 paper-based; 79 iBT). *Application deadline:* For fall admission, 1/1 priority date for domestic and international students. Application fee: $75. Electronic applications accepted. *Expenses:* Contact institution. *Financial support:* In 2015–16, 20 students received support, including 1 research assistantship with partial tuition reimbursement available (averaging $15,000 per year), 20 teaching assistantships with tuition reimbursements available (averaging $7,000 per year); fellowships, career-related internships or fieldwork, Federal Work-Study, institutionally sponsored loans, scholarships/grants, health care benefits, tuition waivers (full and partial), and unspecified assistantships also available. Financial award applicants required to submit FAFSA. *Faculty research:* Hearing and speech science, child and adult language disorders, augmentative communication, cochlear implants, tinnitus. *Total annual research expenditures:* $2 million. *Unit head:* Dr. D. Jeffery Higginbotham, Chairperson, 716-829-5542, Fax: 716-829-3979, E-mail: cdsjeff@buffalo.edu. *Application contact:* Virginia L. Majewski, Graduate Coordinator, 716-829-5570, Fax: 716-829-3979, E-mail: vmajewsk@buffalo.edu.
Website: http://cdswebserver.med.buffalo.edu/drupal/

The University of Akron, Graduate School, College of Health Professions, School of Speech-Language Pathology and Audiology, Program in Audiology, Akron, OH 44325. Offers Au D. *Accreditation:* ASHA. *Students:* 42 full-time (38 women); includes 5 minority (1 Black or African American, non-Hispanic/Latino; 1 Asian, non-Hispanic/Latino; 2 Hispanic/Latino; 1 Two or more races, non-Hispanic/Latino), 1 international. Average age 24. 91 applicants, 21% accepted, 12 enrolled. In 2015, 9 doctorates awarded. *Degree requirements:* For doctorate, 2000 clock hours of clinical experience, academic and clinical competency-based exams. *Entrance requirements:* For doctorate, GRE, minimum GPA of 3.0, letters of recommendation, statement of purpose. Additional exam requirements/recommendations for international students: Required—TOEFL (minimum score 550 paper-based; 79 iBT), IELTS (minimum score 6.5). *Application deadline:* For fall admission, 1/15 for domestic and international students. Application fee: $45 ($70 for international students). Electronic applications accepted. *Expenses:* Tuition, state resident: full-time $7958; part-time $442 per credit hour. Tuition, nonresident: full-time $13,464; part-time $748 per credit hour. *Required fees:* $1404. *Total annual research expenditures:* $500,935. *Unit head:* Dr. Kristina English, Interim School Director, 330-972-6116, E-mail: ke3@uakron.edu. *Application contact:* Dr. James Steiger, Program Coordinator, 330-972-8190, E-mail: steiger@uakron.edu.

The University of Akron, Graduate School, College of Health Professions, School of Speech-Language Pathology and Audiology, Program in Speech-Language Pathology, Akron, OH 44325. Offers MA. *Accreditation:* ASHA. *Students:* 89 full-time (80 women), 21 part-time (19 women); includes 5 minority (2 Black or African American, non-Hispanic/Latino; 3 Two or more races, non-Hispanic/Latino). Average age 25. 291 applicants, 14% accepted, 38 enrolled. In 2015, 47 master's awarded. *Degree requirements:* For master's, thesis optional. *Entrance requirements:* For master's, GRE, baccalaureate degree in speech-language pathology, minimum GPA of 2.75, three letters of recommendation, statement of purpose, resume. Additional exam requirements/recommendations for international students: Required—TOEFL (minimum score 550 paper-based; 79 iBT). *Application deadline:* For fall admission, 1/1 for domestic and international students. Application fee: $45 ($70 for international students). Electronic applications accepted. *Expenses:* Tuition, state resident: full-time $7958; part-time $442 per credit hour. Tuition, nonresident: full-time $13,464; part-time $748 per credit hour. *Required fees:* $1404. *Unit head:* Dr. Roberta DePompei, Director, 330-972-6114, E-mail: rdepom1@uakron.edu. *Application contact:* Dr. Mark Tausig, Associate Dean, 330-972-6266, Fax: 330-972-6475, E-mail: mtausig@uakron.edu.

The University of Alabama, Graduate School, College of Arts and Sciences, Department of Communicative Disorders, Tuscaloosa, AL 35487-0242. Offers speech language pathology (MS). *Accreditation:* ASHA. *Faculty:* 8 full-time (7 women), 1 (woman) part-time/adjunct. *Students:* 68 full-time (67 women); includes 8 minority (2 Black or African American, non-Hispanic/Latino; 5 Hispanic/Latino; 1 Two or more races, non-Hispanic/Latino). Average age 24. 229 applicants, 25% accepted, 24 enrolled. In 2015, 27 master's awarded. *Degree requirements:* For master's, comprehensive exam, thesis optional. *Entrance requirements:* For master's, GRE or MAT, minimum GPA of 3.0. Additional exam requirements/recommendations for international students: Required—TOEFL. *Application deadline:* For fall and spring admission, 1/15 for domestic and international students. Application fee: $50 ($60 for international students). Electronic applications accepted. *Expenses:* Tuition, state resident: full-time $10,170. Tuition, nonresident: full-time $25,950. *Financial support:* In 2015–16, 12 students received support, including 3 fellowships with tuition reimbursements available (averaging $6,000 per year), 20 teaching assistantships with partial tuition reimbursements available (averaging $6,660 per year); career-related internships or fieldwork, Federal Work-Study, scholarships/grants, traineeships, health care benefits, and unspecified assistantships also available. Financial award application deadline: 1/15. *Faculty research:* Aphasia, cochlear implants, autism, voice, balance, multicultural, fluency, dysphagia, rural health. *Total annual research expenditures:* $350,000. *Unit head:* Dr. Marcia Jean Hay-McCutcheon, Associate Professor and Chair, 205-348-7131, Fax: 205-348-1845, E-mail: marcia.hay-mccutcheon@ua.edu. *Application contact:* Patrick D. Fuller, Senior Graduate Admissions Counselor, 205-348-5923, Fax: 205-348-0400, E-mail: patrick.d.fuller@ua.edu.
Website: http://cd.ua.edu/

University of Alberta, Faculty of Graduate Studies and Research, Department of Speech Pathology and Audiology, Edmonton, AB T6G 2E1, Canada. Offers speech pathology and audiology (PhD); speech-language pathology (M Sc). *Degree requirements:* For master's, thesis (for some programs), clinical practicum (MSLP). *Entrance requirements:* For master's, GRE, minimum GPA of 6.5 on a 9.0 scale. Additional exam requirements/recommendations for international students: Required—TOEFL. *Faculty research:* Clinical education, hearing conservation, motor speech disorders, child language, voice resonance.

The University of Arizona, College of Science, Department of Speech, Language, and Hearing Sciences, Tucson, AZ 85721. Offers MS, PhD, Certificate. *Accreditation:* ASHA (one or more programs are accredited). *Students:* Average age 28. *Degree requirements:* For master's, thesis optional; for doctorate, thesis/dissertation. *Entrance requirements:* For master's, GRE General Test, 3 letters of recommendation; for doctorate, GRE General Test, 3 letters of recommendation, personal statement, writing sample. Additional exam requirements/recommendations for international students: Required—TOEFL (minimum score 550 paper-based; 79 iBT). *Application deadline:* Applications are processed on a rolling basis. Application fee: $75. Electronic applications accepted. *Financial support:* Research assistantships, teaching assistantships, career-related internships or fieldwork, Federal Work-Study, institutionally sponsored loans, scholarships/grants, health care benefits, tuition waivers (full and partial), and unspecified assistantships available. Financial award application deadline: 2/1. *Faculty research:* Alzheimer's disease, speech motor control, auditory-evoked potentials, analyzing pathological speech. *Unit head:* Dr. Pelagie Beeson, Head, 520-621-9879, Fax: 520-621-9901, E-mail: pelagie@email.arizona.edu. *Application contact:* Dr. Pelagie Beeson, Head, 520-621-9879, Fax: 520-621-9901, E-mail: pelagie@email.arizona.edu.
Website: http://slhs.arizona.edu/

University of Arkansas, Graduate School, College of Education and Health Professions, Department of Rehabilitation, Human Resources and Communication Disorders, Program in Communication Disorders, Fayetteville, AR 72701-1201. Offers MS. *Accreditation:* ASHA. *Program availability:* Part-time. *Students:* 28 full-time (23 women), 29 part-time (28 women); includes 4 minority (1 Asian, non-Hispanic/Latino; 2 Hispanic/Latino; 1 Two or more races, non-Hispanic/Latino), 2 international. In 2015, 25 master's awarded. *Degree requirements:* For master's, thesis optional, 8-week externship. *Entrance requirements:* For master's, GRE General Test. *Application deadline:* For fall admission, 4/1 for international students; for spring admission, 10/1 for international students. Applications are processed on a rolling basis. Application fee: $40 ($50 for international students). Electronic applications accepted. *Financial support:* In 2015–16, 5 research assistantships were awarded; fellowships, teaching assistantships, career-related internships or fieldwork, and Federal Work-Study also available. Support available to part-time students. Financial award application deadline: 4/1; financial award applicants required to submit FAFSA. *Unit head:* Dr. Kate Mamiseishvili, Head, 479-575-4758, E-mail: kmamisei@uark.edu. *Application contact:*

Dr. Kimberly Baker Frazier, Graduate Coordinator, 479-575-4916, E-mail: kimfraz@uark.edu.
Website: http://cdis.uark.edu

University of Arkansas for Medical Sciences, College of Health Professions, Little Rock, AR 72205-7199. Offers audiology (Au D); communication sciences and disorders (MS, PhD); genetic counseling (MS); nuclear medicine advanced associate (MIS); physician assistant studies (MPAS); radiologist assistant (MIS). PhD offered through consortium with University of Arkansas at Little Rock and University of Central Arkansas. *Program availability:* Part-time, online learning. *Degree requirements:* For master's, thesis (for some programs); for doctorate, comprehensive exam (for some programs), thesis/dissertation (for some programs). *Entrance requirements:* For master's, GRE. Additional exam requirements/recommendations for international students: Required—TOEFL (minimum score 550 paper-based; 79 iBT). Electronic applications accepted. *Expenses:* Contact institution. *Faculty research:* Auditory-based intervention, soy diet, nutrition and cancer.

The University of British Columbia, Faculty of Medicine, School of Audiology and Speech Sciences, Vancouver, BC V6T 1Z3, Canada. Offers M Sc, PhD. *Accreditation:* ASHA. *Degree requirements:* For master's, thesis or alternative, externship; for doctorate, comprehensive exam, thesis/dissertation. *Entrance requirements:* For master's, 4-year undergraduate degree; for doctorate, master's degree, research proposal. Additional exam requirements/recommendations for international students: Required—TOEFL (minimum score 600 paper-based; 100 iBT), IELTS (minimum score 7). Electronic applications accepted. *Faculty research:* Language development, experimental phonetics, linguistic aphasiology, amplification, auditory physiology.

University of California, San Diego, Graduate Division, Interdisciplinary Program in Language and Communicative Disorders, La Jolla, CA 92093. Offers PhD. Program offered jointly with San Diego State University. *Accreditation:* ASHA. *Students:* 13 part-time (10 women); includes 3 minority (1 Asian, non-Hispanic/Latino; 2 Hispanic/Latino). In 2015, 3 doctorates awarded. *Degree requirements:* For doctorate, one foreign language, comprehensive exam, thesis/dissertation, teaching assistantship. *Entrance requirements:* For doctorate, GRE General Test, minimum GPA of 3.25. Additional exam requirements/recommendations for international students: Required—TOEFL, IELTS. *Application deadline:* For fall admission, 12/15 for domestic students. Electronic applications accepted. *Expenses:* Tuition, state resident: full-time $11,220. Tuition, nonresident: full-time $26,322. *Required fees:* $1800. *Financial support:* Teaching assistantships available. Financial award applicants required to submit FAFSA. *Faculty research:* Language acquisition and development, sign languages, bilingualism, neural bases of language use and loss, language development in disorders. *Unit head:* Seana Coulson, Program Director, 858-534-7486, E-mail: scoulson@ucsd.edu. *Application contact:* Janet Shin, Graduate Coordinator, 858-822-2698, E-mail: jshin@ucsd.edu.
Website: http://slhs.sdsu.edu/programs/phd/

University of California, San Diego, School of Medicine, Program in Audiology, La Jolla, CA 92093. Offers Au D. Program offered jointly with San Diego State University. *Students:* 9 full-time (5 women), 4 part-time (2 women); includes 7 minority (3 Asian, non-Hispanic/Latino; 4 Hispanic/Latino). In 2015, 6 doctorates awarded. *Degree requirements:* For doctorate, comprehensive exam, thesis/dissertation, 2,950 clinic hours; externship. *Entrance requirements:* For doctorate, GRE General Test, minimum GPA of 3.0; at least one course in each of the following areas: statistics, biological science, physical science, and American Sign Language; additional courses in behavioral/social sciences and biological or physical sciences. Additional exam requirements/recommendations for international students: Required—TOEFL, IELTS. *Application deadline:* For fall admission, 12/15 for domestic students. Electronic applications accepted. *Expenses:* Contact institution. *Financial support:* Fellowships, research assistantships, scholarships/grants, and unspecified assistantships available. Financial award applicants required to submit FAFSA. *Faculty research:* Peripheral auditory physiology, auditory evoked potentials, psychoacoustics, epidemiology of age-related hearing loss, aural rehabilitation. *Unit head:* Erika Zettner, Chair, 858-657-8057, E-mail: ezettner@ucsd.edu.
Website: http://slhs.sdsu.edu/programs/aud/

University of Central Arkansas, Graduate School, College of Health and Behavioral Sciences, Department of Communication Sciences and Disorders, Conway, AR 72035-0001. Offers communication sciences and disorders (PhD); speech-language pathology (MS). *Accreditation:* ASHA (one or more programs are accredited). *Degree requirements:* For master's, comprehensive exam, thesis optional, portfolio, internship. *Entrance requirements:* For master's, GRE General Test, NTE, minimum GPA of 2.7. Additional exam requirements/recommendations for international students: Required—TOEFL (minimum score 550 paper-based). Electronic applications accepted. *Expenses:* Contact institution.

University of Central Florida, College of Education and Human Performance, Education Doctoral Programs, Orlando, FL 32816. Offers communication sciences and disorders (PhD); early childhood education (PhD); education (Ed D); elementary education (PhD); exceptional education (PhD); exercise physiology (PhD); higher education (PhD); instructional technology (PhD); mathematics education (PhD); methodology, measurement and analysis (PhD); reading education (PhD); science education (PhD); social science education (PhD); TESOL (PhD). *Students:* 135 full-time (101 women), 63 part-time (47 women); includes 41 minority (19 Black or African American, non-Hispanic/Latino; 5 Asian, non-Hispanic/Latino; 13 Hispanic/Latino; 4 Two or more races, non-Hispanic/Latino), 27 international. Average age 37. 157 applicants, 35% accepted, 44 enrolled. In 2015, 51 doctorates awarded. Application fee: $30. Electronic applications accepted. *Expenses:* Tuition, state resident: part-time $288.16 per credit hour. Tuition, nonresident: part-time $1071.31 per credit hour. *Financial support:* In 2015–16, 86 students received support, including 45 fellowships with partial tuition reimbursements available (averaging $6,200 per year), 45 research assistantships with partial tuition reimbursements available (averaging $5,700 per year), 58 teaching assistantships with partial tuition reimbursements available (averaging $6,400 per year). *Unit head:* Dr. Edward Robinson, Director of Doctoral Programs, 407-823-6106, E-mail: edward.robinson@ucf.edu. *Application contact:* Associate Director, Admissions and Student Services, 407-823-2766, Fax: 407-823-6442, E-mail: gradadmissions@ucf.edu.
Website: http://education.ucf.edu/departments.cfm

University of Central Florida, College of Health and Public Affairs, Department of Communication Sciences and Disorders, Orlando, FL 32816. Offers communication sciences and disorders (MA); medical speech-language pathology (Certificate). *Accreditation:* ASHA (one or more programs are accredited). *Program availability:* Part-time, evening/weekend. *Faculty:* 24 full-time (16 women), 23 part-time/adjunct (18 women). *Students:* 171 full-time (163 women), 16 part-time (15 women); includes 30 minority (2 Black or African American, non-Hispanic/Latino; 1 American Indian or Alaska Native, non-Hispanic/Latino; 7 Asian, non-Hispanic/Latino; 16 Hispanic/Latino; 4 Two or more races, non-Hispanic/Latino). Average age 25. 379 applicants, 28% accepted, 26 enrolled. In 2015, 93 master's, 1 other advanced degree awarded. *Degree requirements:* For master's, comprehensive exam, thesis or alternative. *Entrance requirements:* For master's, GRE General Test, minimum GPA of 3.0 in last 60 hours. Additional exam requirements/recommendations for international students: Required—

Communication Disorders

TOEFL. *Application deadline:* For fall admission, 4/1 for domestic students; for spring admission, 11/1 for domestic students. Electronic applications accepted. *Expenses:* Tuition, state resident: part-time $288.16 per credit hour. Tuition, nonresident: part-time $1071.31 per credit hour. *Financial support:* In 2015–16, 15 students received support, including 3 fellowships with partial tuition reimbursements available (averaging $5,000 per year), 2 research assistantships with partial tuition reimbursements available (averaging $4,100 per year), 11 teaching assistantships with partial tuition reimbursements available (averaging $4,700 per year); career-related internships or fieldwork, Federal Work-Study, institutionally sponsored loans, and unspecified assistantships also available. Financial award application deadline: 3/1; financial award applicants required to submit FAFSA. *Unit head:* Dr. Richard Zraick, Chair, 407-823-4795, E-mail: richard.zraick@ucf.edu. *Application contact:* Director, Admissions and Student Services, 407-823-2766, Fax: 407-823-6442, E-mail: gradadmissions@ucf.edu. Website: http://www.cohpa.ucf.edu/comdis.

University of Central Missouri, The Graduate School, Warrensburg, MO 64093. Offers accountancy (MA); accounting (MBA); applied mathematics (MS); aviation safety (MA); biology (MS); business administration (MBA); career and technical education leadership (MS); college student personnel administration (MS); communication (MA); computer science (MS); counseling (MS); criminal justice (MS); educational leadership (Ed D); educational technology (MS); elementary and early childhood education (MSE); English (MA); environmental studies (MA); finance (MBA); history (MA); human services/educational technology (Ed S); human services/learning resources (Ed S); human services/professional counseling (Ed S); industrial hygiene (MS); industrial management (MS); information systems (MBA); information technology (MS); kinesiology (MS); library science and information services (MS); literacy education (MSE); marketing (MBA); mathematics (MS); music (MA); occupational safety management (MS); psychology (MS); rural family nursing (MS); school administration (MSE); social gerontology (MS); sociology (MA); special education (MSE); speech language pathology (MS); superintendency (Ed S); teaching (MAT); teaching English as a second language (MA); technology (MS); technology management (PhD); theatre (MA). *Program availability:* Part-time, 100% online, blended/hybrid learning. *Faculty:* 336 full-time (145 women), 39 part-time/adjunct (25 women). *Students:* 2,161 full-time (723 women), 2,077 part-time (1,061 women); includes 188 minority (93 Black or African American, non-Hispanic/Latino; 4 American Indian or Alaska Native, non-Hispanic/Latino; 15 Asian, non-Hispanic/Latino; 32 Hispanic/Latino; 1 Native Hawaiian or other Pacific Islander, non-Hispanic/Latino; 43 Two or more races, non-Hispanic/Latino), 2,514 international. Average age 28. 3,454 applicants, 68% accepted, 1632 enrolled. In 2015, 1,530 master's, 53 other advanced degrees awarded. *Degree requirements:* For master's and Ed S, comprehensive exam (for some programs), thesis (for some programs). *Entrance requirements:* Additional exam requirements/recommendations for international students: Required—TOEFL (minimum score 550 paper-based; 79 iBT). *Application deadline:* For fall admission, 6/1 priority date for domestic and international students; for spring admission, 10/1 priority date for domestic and international students; for summer admission, 4/1 priority date for domestic and international students. Applications are processed on a rolling basis. Application fee: $30 ($75 for international students). Electronic applications accepted. *Expenses:* Tuition, state resident: full-time $6683; part-time $278.45 per credit hour. Tuition, nonresident: full-time $13,366; part-time $556.90 per credit hour. *Required fees:* $701; $29.20 per credit hour. Tuition and fees vary according to degree level and campus/location. *Financial support:* In 2015–16, 97 students received support, including 146 research assistantships with partial tuition reimbursements available (averaging $7,500 per year), 73 teaching assistantships with partial tuition reimbursements available (averaging $7,500 per year); career-related internships or fieldwork, Federal Work-Study, scholarships/grants, and administrative and laboratory assistantships also available. Support available to part-time students. Financial award application deadline: 3/1; financial award applicants required to submit FAFSA. *Unit head:* Tina Church-Hockett, Director of Graduate School and International Admissions, 660-543-4621, Fax: 660-543-4778, E-mail: church@ucmo.edu. *Application contact:* Brittany Lawrence, Graduate Student Services Coordinator, 660-543-4621, Fax: 660-543-4778, E-mail: gradinfo@ucmo.edu. Website: http://www.ucmo.edu/graduate/

University of Central Oklahoma, The Jackson College of Graduate Studies, College of Education and Professional Studies, Department of Advanced Professional and Special Services, Edmond, OK 73034-5209. Offers educational leadership (M Ed); library media education (M Ed); reading (M Ed); school counseling (M Ed); special education (M Ed), including mild/moderate disabilities, severe-profound/multiple disabilities, special education; speech-language pathology (MS). *Program availability:* Part-time. *Degree requirements:* For master's, comprehensive exam (for some programs), thesis (for some programs). *Entrance requirements:* For master's, GRE. Additional exam requirements/recommendations for international students: Required—TOEFL (minimum score 550 paper-based; 79 iBT), IELTS (minimum score 6.5). Electronic applications accepted. *Faculty research:* Intellectual freedom, fair use copyright, technology integration, young adult literature, distance learning.

University of Cincinnati, Graduate School, College of Allied Health Sciences, Department of Communication Sciences and Disorders, Cincinnati, OH 45221. Offers MA, Au D, PhD. *Accreditation:* ASHA (one or more programs are accredited). *Degree requirements:* For master's, thesis optional; for doctorate, comprehensive exam, thesis/dissertation. *Entrance requirements:* For master's and doctorate, GRE General Test, minimum GPA of 3.0. Additional exam requirements/recommendations for international students: Required—TOEFL (minimum score 600 paper-based). Electronic applications accepted. *Faculty research:* Neurogenic speech and language disorders, speech science, linguistics, swallowing disorders, speech-language pathology.

University of Cincinnati, Graduate School, College of Education, Criminal Justice, and Human Services, Division of Teacher Education, Cincinnati, OH 45221. Offers curriculum and instruction (M Ed, Ed D); deaf studies (Certificate); early childhood education (M Ed); middle childhood education (M Ed); postsecondary literacy instruction (Certificate); reading/literacy (M Ed, Ed D); secondary education (M Ed); special education (M Ed, Ed D); teaching English as a second language (Ed D, Certificate); teaching science (MS). *Program availability:* Part-time. *Degree requirements:* For doctorate, thesis/dissertation. *Entrance requirements:* For master's, GRE General Test. Additional exam requirements/recommendations for international students: Required—TOEFL (minimum score 550 paper-based). Electronic applications accepted.

University of Colorado Boulder, Graduate School, College of Arts and Sciences, Department of Speech, Language and Hearing Sciences, Boulder, CO 80309. Offers audiology (Au D, PhD); clinical research and practice in audiology (PhD); speech, language and hearing sciences (MA, PhD); speech-language pathology (MA, PhD). *Accreditation:* ASHA (one or more programs are accredited). *Faculty:* 7 full-time (all women). *Students:* 105 full-time (98 women), 1 (woman) part-time; includes 14 minority (2 Black or African American, non-Hispanic/Latino; 2 Asian, non-Hispanic/Latino; 6 Hispanic/Latino; 4 Two or more races, non-Hispanic/Latino), 3 international. Average age 27. 577 applicants, 19% accepted, 36 enrolled. In 2015, 35 master's, 11 doctorates awarded. Terminal master's awarded for partial completion of doctoral program. *Degree requirements:* For master's, comprehensive exam, thesis or alternative; for doctorate, one foreign language, thesis/dissertation. *Entrance requirements:* For master's, GRE

General Test, minimum undergraduate GPA of 3.25; for doctorate, GRE General Test. *Application deadline:* For fall admission, 1/15 for domestic students, 12/1 for international students; for spring admission, 10/1 for domestic and international students. Applications are processed on a rolling basis. Application fee: $50 ($70 for international students). Electronic applications accepted. Application fee is waived when completed online. *Financial support:* In 2015–16, 80 students received support, including 50 fellowships (averaging $3,342 per year), 1 research assistantship with tuition reimbursement available (averaging $20,322 per year), 10 teaching assistantships with tuition reimbursements available (averaging $27,311 per year); institutionally sponsored loans, scholarships/grants, health care benefits, and unspecified assistantships also available. Financial award application deadline: 2/1; financial award applicants required to submit FAFSA. *Faculty research:* Cognitive development/processes, speech communicative disorders, speech pathology, aging/gerontology, audiology. *Total annual research expenditures:* $1.2 million. *Application contact:* E-mail: slhsgrad@colorado.edu. Website: http://slhs.colorado.edu

University of Connecticut, Graduate School, College of Liberal Arts and Sciences, Department of Communication Sciences, Program in Speech-Language Pathology, Storrs, CT 06269. Offers MA, Au D, PhD. *Accreditation:* ASHA. Terminal master's awarded for partial completion of doctoral program. *Degree requirements:* For master's, comprehensive exam, thesis optional; for doctorate, thesis/dissertation. *Entrance requirements:* For master's and doctorate, GRE General Test. Additional exam requirements/recommendations for international students: Required—TOEFL (minimum score 550 paper-based). *Application deadline:* For fall admission, 2/1 priority date for domestic and international students; for spring admission, 11/1 for domestic students, 10/1 for international students. Applications are processed on a rolling basis. Application fee: $55. Electronic applications accepted. *Financial support:* Fellowships, research assistantships with full tuition reimbursements, teaching assistantships with full tuition reimbursements, Federal Work-Study, scholarships/grants, health care benefits, and unspecified assistantships available. Financial award application deadline: 2/1; financial award applicants required to submit FAFSA.

University of Florida, Graduate School, College of Public Health and Health Professions, Department of Speech, Language and Hearing Sciences, Gainesville, FL 32611. Offers audiology (Au D); communication sciences and disorders (MA, PhD). *Accreditation:* ASHA (one or more programs are accredited). *Faculty:* 7 part-time/adjunct. *Students:* 137 full-time (116 women), 30 part-time (23 women); includes 29 minority (6 Black or African American, non-Hispanic/Latino; 1 American Indian or Alaska Native, non-Hispanic/Latino; 4 Asian, non-Hispanic/Latino; 18 Hispanic/Latino; 32 international. 409 applicants, 25% accepted, 46 enrolled. In 2015, 33 master's, 4 doctorates awarded. *Degree requirements:* For master's, thesis optional; for doctorate, comprehensive exam, thesis/dissertation. *Entrance requirements:* For master's and doctorate, GRE General Test, minimum GPA of 3.0. Additional exam requirements/recommendations for international students: Required—TOEFL (minimum score 550 paper-based; 80 iBT), IELTS (minimum score 6). *Application deadline:* For fall admission, 1/15 priority date for domestic students, 1/15 for international students. Applications are processed on a rolling basis. Application fee: $30. Electronic applications accepted. *Financial support:* In 2015–16, 2 fellowships, 33 teaching assistantships were awarded; research assistantships, career-related internships or fieldwork, and unspecified assistantships also available. Financial award application deadline: 1/15; financial award applicants required to submit FAFSA. *Faculty research:* Phonetic science, cochlear implant, dyslexia, auditory development, voice. *Total annual research expenditures:* $538,106. *Unit head:* Scott Griffiths, PhD, Associate Professor and Chair, 352-273-3725, E-mail: sgriff@ufl.edu. *Application contact:* Office of Admissions, 352-392-1365, E-mail: webrequests@admissions.ufl.edu. Website: http://slhs.phhp.ufl.edu/

University of Georgia, College of Education, Department of Communication Sciences and Special Education, Athens, GA 30602. Offers communication science and disorders (M Ed, MA, PhD, Ed S); special education (M Ed, Ed D, PhD, Ed S). *Accreditation:* ASHA (one or more programs are accredited). Terminal master's awarded for partial completion of doctoral program. *Degree requirements:* For master's, comprehensive exam (for some programs), thesis (for some programs); for doctorate, thesis/dissertation. *Entrance requirements:* For master's, doctorate, and Ed S, GRE General Test. Additional exam requirements/recommendations for international students: Required—TOEFL. Electronic applications accepted.

University of Hawaii at Manoa, John A. Burns School of Medicine, Department of Communication Sciences and Disorders, Honolulu, HI 96822. Offers MS. *Accreditation:* ASHA. *Program availability:* Part-time. *Faculty:* 2 full-time (0 women). *Students:* 54 full-time (27 women), 6 part-time; includes 11 minority (5 Asian, non-Hispanic/Latino; 1 Hispanic/Latino; 1 Native Hawaiian or other Pacific Islander, non-Hispanic/Latino; 4 Two or more races, non-Hispanic/Latino). Average age 31. 156 applicants, 17% accepted, 13 enrolled. In 2015, 3 master's awarded. *Degree requirements:* For master's, thesis optional. *Entrance requirements:* For master's, GRE General Test, minimum GPA of 3.0. Additional exam requirements/recommendations for international students: Required—TOEFL (minimum score 580 paper-based; 92 iBT), IELTS (minimum score 5). *Application deadline:* For fall admission, 3/1 for domestic and international students; for spring admission, 9/1 for domestic and international students. Application fee: $100. *Financial support:* In 2015–16, 12 students received support, including 12 fellowships (averaging $2,447 per year); research assistantships, career-related internships or fieldwork, Federal Work-Study, institutionally sponsored loans, and tuition waivers (full and partial) also available. Support available to part-time students. *Faculty research:* Emerging language (child phonology and special populations), central auditory function, developmental phonology, processing in the aging. *Total annual research expenditures:* $750,000. *Unit head:* Dr. Jerris R. Hedges, Dean, 808-692-0881. *Application contact:* Henry Lew, Graduate Chair, 808-956-5438, Fax: 808-956-5482, E-mail: jyates@hawaii.edu. Website: http://www.hawaii.edu/graduatestudies/fields/html/departments/stuz/spa/spa.htm

University of Houston, College of Liberal Arts and Social Sciences, Department of Communication Sciences and Disorders, Houston, TX 77204. Offers MA. *Accreditation:* ASHA. *Program availability:* Part-time. *Degree requirements:* For master's, comprehensive exam, thesis optional. *Entrance requirements:* For master's, GRE General Test, minimum GPA of 3.0 in last 60 hours. Additional exam requirements/recommendations for international students: Required—TOEFL (minimum score 550 paper-based; 79 iBT). *Faculty research:* Stuttering, voice disorders, language disorders, phonological processing, cognition.

University of Illinois at Urbana–Champaign, Graduate College, College of Applied Health Sciences, Department of Speech and Hearing Science, Champaign, IL 61820. Offers audiology (Au D); speech and hearing science (MA, PhD). *Accreditation:* ASHA (one or more programs are accredited).

The University of Iowa, Graduate College, College of Liberal Arts and Sciences, Department of Communication Sciences and Disorders, Iowa City, IA 52242-1316. Offers MA, Au D, PhD, Au D/PhD. *Accreditation:* ASHA. *Degree requirements:* For master's, thesis optional, exam; for doctorate, comprehensive exam (for some programs), thesis/dissertation (for some programs). *Entrance requirements:* For master's and doctorate, GRE General Test, minimum GPA of 3.0. Additional exam requirements/recommendations for international students: Required—TOEFL (minimum score 550 paper-based; 81 iBT). Electronic applications accepted.

The University of Kansas, Graduate Studies, College of Liberal Arts and Sciences, Intercampus Program in Communicative Disorders: Speech-Language Pathology, Lawrence, KS 66045. Offers speech-language pathology (MA, PhD). *Accreditation:* ASHA. *Program availability:* Part-time. *Students:* 85 full-time (80 women), 3 part-time (2 women); includes 13 minority (2 American Indian or Alaska Native, non-Hispanic/Latino; 1 Asian, non-Hispanic/Latino; 6 Hispanic/Latino; 4 Two or more races, non-Hispanic/Latino), 8 international. Average age 27. 172 applicants, 42% accepted, 36 enrolled. In 2015, 24 master's, 2 doctorates awarded. Terminal master's awarded for partial completion of doctoral program. *Entrance requirements:* For master's and doctorate, GRE General Test, minimum GPA of 3.0, bachelor's degree. Additional exam requirements/recommendations for international students: Required—TOEFL. *Application deadline:* For fall admission, 1/15 priority date for domestic and international students; for spring admission, 10/1 for domestic and international students. Application fee: $65 ($85 for international students). Electronic applications accepted. *Financial support:* Research assistantships, teaching assistantships, career-related internships or fieldwork, Federal Work-Study, institutionally sponsored loans, scholarships/grants, traineeships, and unspecified assistantships available. Support available to part-time students. Financial award application deadline: 3/1; financial award applicants required to submit FAFSA. *Faculty research:* Reading disorders, language acquisition, auditory electrophysiology, genetics of language, phonological development. *Unit head:* Holly L. Storkel, Chair, 785-864-0497, E-mail: hstorkel@ku.edu. *Application contact:* Angela Carrasco, Graduate Admissions Coordinator, 913-588-5935, Fax: 913-588-5923, E-mail: hearingspeech@kumc.edu.
Website: http://splh.ku.edu/ipcd/

The University of Kansas, University of Kansas Medical Center, School of Health Professions, Intercampus Program in Communicative Disorders: Audiology, Lawrence, KS 66045. Offers audiology (Au D, PhD). *Faculty:* 27. *Students:* 27 full-time (24 women), 13 part-time (12 women); includes 7 minority (2 Black or African American, non-Hispanic/Latino; 1 American Indian or Alaska Native, non-Hispanic/Latino; 1 Asian, non-Hispanic/Latino; 2 Hispanic/Latino; 1 Two or more races, non-Hispanic/Latino), 1 international. Average age 25. 55 applicants, 51% accepted, 12 enrolled. In 2015, 5 doctorates awarded. *Degree requirements:* For doctorate, thesis/dissertation, oral comprehensive exam (for Au D). *Entrance requirements:* For doctorate, GRE (for Au D), bachelor's degree and minimum GPA of 3.25 in communication sciences and disorders courses (for Au D). Additional exam requirements/recommendations for international students: Required—TOEFL or IELTS. *Application deadline:* For fall admission, 1/15 for domestic and international students. Application fee: $60. Electronic applications accepted. *Expenses:* Contact institution. *Financial support:* Research assistantships with partial tuition reimbursements, teaching assistantships with partial tuition reimbursements, institutionally sponsored loans, scholarships/grants, traineeships, and unspecified assistantships available. Financial award application deadline: 3/1; financial award applicants required to submit FAFSA. *Faculty research:* Child language development, diagnosis and treatment of language disorders; newborn/pediatric hearing testing and treatment of hearing loss in children; voice disorders; auditory physiology and applied electrophysiology; diagnosis and treatment for adult speech and language disorders. *Total annual research expenditures:* $408,130. *Unit head:* Dr. John A. Ferraro, Chair, Department of Hearing and Speech/Co-Director, 913-588-5937, Fax: 913-588-5923, E-mail: jferraro@kumc.edu. *Application contact:* Angela Carrasco, Admissions Coordinator, 913-588-5935, Fax: 913-588-5923, E-mail: hearingspeech@kumc.edu.
Website: http://ipcd.ku.edu

University of Kentucky, Graduate School, College of Health Sciences, Program in Communication Disorders, Lexington, KY 40506-0032. Offers MS. *Accreditation:* ASHA. *Degree requirements:* For master's, comprehensive exam. *Entrance requirements:* For master's, GRE General Test, minimum undergraduate GPA of 2.75. Additional exam requirements/recommendations for international students: Required—TOEFL (minimum score 550 paper-based). Electronic applications accepted. *Faculty research:* Swallowing disorders, infant speech development, child language intervention, augmentative communication.

University of Louisiana at Lafayette, College of Liberal Arts, Department of Communicative Disorders, Lafayette, LA 70504. Offers MS, PhD. *Accreditation:* ASHA (one or more programs are accredited). *Degree requirements:* For master's, thesis or alternative. *Entrance requirements:* For master's, GRE General Test, minimum GPA of 2.75. Additional exam requirements/recommendations for international students: Required—TOEFL (minimum score 550 paper-based).

University of Louisiana at Monroe, Graduate School, College of Health and Pharmaceutical Sciences, Department of Speech-Language Pathology, Monroe, LA 71209-0001. Offers MS. *Accreditation:* ASHA. *Degree requirements:* For master's, thesis. *Entrance requirements:* For master's, GRE, minimum GPA of 2.5. Additional exam requirements/recommendations for international students: Required—TOEFL (minimum score 500 paper-based; 61 iBT). Electronic applications accepted. *Faculty research:* Child language, stuttering, multicultural issues, ethics.

University of Louisville, School of Medicine, Department of Surgery, Louisville, KY 40292-0001. Offers audiology (Au D); communicative disorders (MS). *Students:* 92 full-time (86 women); includes 3 minority (2 Hispanic/Latino; 1 Two or more races, non-Hispanic/Latino), 1 international. Average age 26. 228 applicants, 43% accepted, 37 enrolled. In 2015, 20 master's, 8 doctorates awarded. Application fee: $60. *Expenses:* Tuition, state resident: full-time $11,664; part-time $649 per credit hour. Tuition, nonresident: full-time $24,274; part-time $1350 per credit hour. *Required fees:* $196. Tuition and fees vary according to program and reciprocity agreements. *Financial support:* In 2015–16, 179,325 students received support. *Total annual research expenditures:* $12.5 million. *Unit head:* Dr. Edward C. Halperin, Dean, 502-852-1499, Fax: 502-852-1484, E-mail: edward.halperin@louisville.edu. *Application contact:* Director of Admissions, 502-852-5793, Fax: 502-852-6849.
Website: http://louisvillesurgery.com/

University of Maine, Graduate School, College of Natural Sciences, Forestry, and Agriculture, Department of Communication Sciences and Disorders, Orono, ME 04469. Offers MA. *Accreditation:* ASHA. *Faculty:* 6 full-time (5 women), 6 part-time/adjunct (4 women). *Students:* 33 full-time (32 women); includes 1 minority (Two or more races, non-Hispanic/Latino), 7 international. Average age 25. 236 applicants, 16% accepted, 16 enrolled. In 2015, 14 master's awarded. *Degree requirements:* For master's, comprehensive exam. *Entrance requirements:* For master's, GRE General Test. Additional exam requirements/recommendations for international students: Required—TOEFL. *Application deadline:* For fall admission, 1/15 priority date for domestic students. Applications are processed on a rolling basis. Application fee: $65. Electronic applications accepted. *Financial support:* In 2015–16, 7 students received support, including 4 research assistantships (averaging $7,300 per year), 1 teaching assistantship with partial tuition reimbursement available (averaging $5,000 per year); career-related internships or fieldwork, Federal Work-Study, institutionally sponsored

loans, and tuition waivers (full and partial) also available. Support available to part-time students. Financial award application deadline: 3/1. *Faculty research:* Telepractice, stuttering, language disorders, dyslexia, aphasia. *Unit head:* Dr. Allan Smith, Chair, 207-581-2006, Fax: 207-581-1953. *Application contact:* Scott G. Delcourt, Assistant Vice President for Graduate Studies and Senior Associate Dean, 207-581-3291, Fax: 207-581-3232, E-mail: graduate@maine.edu.
Website: http://umaine.edu/comscidis/

The University of Manchester, School of Psychological Sciences, Manchester, United Kingdom. Offers audiology (M Phil, PhD); clinical psychology (M Phil, PhD, Psy D); psychology (M Phil, PhD).

University of Maryland, College Park, Academic Affairs, College of Behavioral and Social Sciences, Department of Hearing and Speech Sciences, College Park, MD 20742. Offers audiology (MA, PhD); hearing and speech sciences (Au D); language pathology (MA, PhD); neuroscience (PhD); speech (MA, PhD). *Accreditation:* ASHA (one or more programs are accredited). *Degree requirements:* For master's, thesis optional; for doctorate, thesis/dissertation, written and oral exams. *Entrance requirements:* For master's, GRE General Test, minimum GPA of 3.5, 3 letters of recommendation; for doctorate, GRE General Test, minimum GPA of 3.5. Additional exam requirements/recommendations for international students: Required—TOEFL. Electronic applications accepted. *Faculty research:* Speech perception, language acquisition, bilingualism, hearing loss.

University of Massachusetts Amherst, Graduate School, School of Public Health and Health Sciences, Department of Communication Disorders, Amherst, MA 01003. Offers audiology (Au D, PhD); clinical audiology (PhD); speech-language pathology (MA, PhD). *Accreditation:* ASHA (one or more programs are accredited). *Program availability:* Part-time. Terminal master's awarded for partial completion of doctoral program. *Degree requirements:* For master's, thesis optional; for doctorate, comprehensive exam, thesis/ dissertation. *Entrance requirements:* For master's and doctorate, GRE General Test. Additional exam requirements/recommendations for international students: Required—TOEFL (minimum score 550 paper-based; 80 iBT), IELTS (minimum score 6.5). Electronic applications accepted.

University of Memphis, Graduate School, School of Communication Sciences and Disorders, Memphis, TN 38152. Offers MA, Au D, PhD. *Accreditation:* ASHA. *Program availability:* Part-time. *Faculty:* 11 full-time (4 women), 2 part-time/adjunct (1 woman). *Students:* 86 full-time (83 women), 11 part-time (6 women); includes 8 minority (2 Black or African American, non-Hispanic/Latino; 3 Asian, non-Hispanic/Latino; 3 Two or more races, non-Hispanic/Latino), 9 international. Average age 26. 433 applicants, 23% accepted, 35 enrolled. In 2015, 37 master's, 20 doctorates awarded. Terminal master's awarded for partial completion of doctoral program. *Degree requirements:* For master's, comprehensive exam, thesis or alternative; for doctorate, thesis/dissertation, qualifying exam. *Entrance requirements:* For master's, GRE General Test or MAT, minimum GPA of 3.0, ASHA certification; for doctorate, GRE General Test, minimum GPA of 3.5, letters of recommendation. *Application deadline:* For fall admission, 2/1 for domestic students. Application fee: $35 ($60 for international students). *Financial support:* Research assistantships with full tuition reimbursements, Federal Work-Study, scholarships/ grants, and unspecified assistantships available. Financial award application deadline: 2/15; financial award applicants required to submit FAFSA. *Faculty research:* Hearing aid characteristic selection, language acquisition, speech disorders, characteristics of the aging voice, hearing science. *Total annual research expenditures:* $1.5 million. *Unit head:* Dr. Maurice Mendel, Dean, 901-678-5800, Fax: 901-525-1282, E-mail: dlluna@memphis.edu. *Application contact:* Dr. David J. Wark, Coordinator of Graduate Studies, 901-678-5891, E-mail: dwark@memphis.edu.
Website: http://www.memphis.edu/ausp

University of Minnesota, Duluth, Graduate School, College of Education and Human Service Professions, Department of Communication Sciences and Disorders, Duluth, MN 55812-2496. Offers MA. *Accreditation:* ASHA. *Program availability:* Part-time. *Degree requirements:* For master's, research project, oral exam. *Entrance requirements:* For master's, minimum GPA of 3.0, undergraduate degree in communication sciences and disorders. Additional exam requirements/ recommendations for international students: Required—TOEFL (minimum score 550 paper-based). *Faculty research:* Clinical supervision, augmentative communication, speech understanding, fluency, developmental apraxia of speech.

University of Minnesota, Twin Cities Campus, Graduate School, College of Liberal Arts, Department of Speech-Language-Hearing Sciences, Minneapolis, MN 55455. Offers audiology (Au D); speech-language pathology (MA); speech-language-hearing sciences (PhD). *Accreditation:* ASHA (one or more programs are accredited). Terminal master's awarded for partial completion of doctoral program. *Degree requirements:* For master's, thesis, 375 client contact hours; for doctorate, comprehensive exam, thesis/ dissertation. *Entrance requirements:* For master's and doctorate, GRE General Test, minimum GPA of 3.0. Additional exam requirements/recommendations for international students: Required—TOEFL. Electronic applications accepted. *Faculty research:* Normal and disordered child phonology, specific language impairment, bilingual and multicultural aspects of language, TBI, AAC.

University of Mississippi, Graduate School, School of Applied Sciences, University, MS 38677. Offers communicative disorders (MS); criminal justice (MCJ); exercise science (MS); food and nutrition services (MS); health and kinesiology (PhD); health promotion (MS); park and recreation management (MA); social work (MSW). *Faculty:* 65 full-time (36 women), 32 part-time/adjunct (23 women). *Students:* 192 full-time (148 women), 43 part-time (23 women); includes 47 minority (37 Black or African American, non-Hispanic/Latino; 2 Asian, non-Hispanic/Latino; 7 Hispanic/Latino; 1 Two or more races, non-Hispanic/Latino), 12 international. In 2015, 99 master's, 3 doctorates awarded. *Entrance requirements:* For master's, GRE General Test, minimum GPA of 3.0. Additional exam requirements/recommendations for international students: Required—TOEFL. *Application deadline:* For fall admission, 4/1 for domestic students; for spring admission, 10/1 for domestic students. Applications are processed on a rolling basis. Application fee: $40. Electronic applications accepted. *Financial support:* Scholarships/grants available. Financial award application deadline: 3/1; financial award applicants required to submit FAFSA. *Unit head:* Dr. Velmer Stanley Burton, Dean, 662-915-1081, Fax: 662-915-5717, E-mail: applsci@olemiss.edu. *Application contact:* Dr. Christy M. Wyandt, Associate Dean of Graduate School, 662-915-7474, Fax: 662-915-7577, E-mail: cwyandt@olemiss.edu.

University of Missouri, School of Health Professions, Program in Communication Science and Disorders, Columbia, MO 65211. Offers MHS, PhD. *Accreditation:* ASHA (one or more programs are accredited). *Entrance requirements:* For master's, GRE General Test, minimum GPA of 3.0. Additional exam requirements/recommendations for international students: Required—TOEFL (minimum score 600 paper-based; 100 iBT). *Application deadline:* For fall admission, 1/15 priority date for domestic and international students; for winter admission, 10/15 priority date for domestic students, 10/15 for international students. Applications are processed on a rolling basis. Application fee: $55 ($75 for international students). Electronic applications accepted. *Financial support:* Research assistantships, teaching assistantships, and institutionally sponsored loans available.
Website: http://shp.missouri.edu/csd/

University of Montevallo, College of Arts and Sciences, Department of Communication Science and Disorders, Montevallo, AL 35115. Offers speech-language pathology (MS). *Accreditation:* ASHA. *Students:* 52 full-time (51 women); includes 2 minority (both Hispanic/Latino). In 2015, 23 master's awarded. *Degree requirements:* For master's, comprehensive exam. *Entrance requirements:* For master's, GRE General Test, MAT. Additional exam requirements/recommendations for international students: Required—TOEFL (minimum score 550 paper-based). *Application deadline:* For fall admission, 7/15 for domestic students; for spring admission, 11/15 for domestic students. Application fee: $25. *Expenses:* Tuition, state resident: full-time $9384. Tuition, nonresident: full-time $19,272. *Required fees:* $670. *Financial support:* Federal Work-Study, scholarships/grants, and unspecified assistantships available. *Unit head:* Dr. Claire Edwards, Chair, 205-665-6724, E-mail: edwardsc@montevallo.edu. *Application contact:* Kevin Thornthwaite, Acting Director, Graduate Admissions and Records, 205-665-6350, E-mail: graduate@montevallo.edu.
Website: http://www.montevallo.edu/csd/

University of Nebraska at Kearney, Graduate Studies and Research, College of Education, Department of Communication Disorders, Kearney, NE 68849-0001. Offers speech/language pathology (MS Ed). *Accreditation:* ASHA. *Program availability:* Part-time. *Faculty:* 4 full-time (all women). *Students:* 25 full-time (all women), 9 part-time (8 women); includes 2 minority (both Asian, non-Hispanic/Latino). Average age 24. 74 applicants, 35% accepted, 13 enrolled. In 2015, 27 master's awarded. *Degree requirements:* For master's, comprehensive exam, thesis optional. *Entrance requirements:* For master's, GRE General Test, personal statement, letters of recommendation, phase 2 video response. Additional exam requirements/recommendations for international students: Recommended—TOEFL (minimum score 550 paper-based; 79 iBT), IELTS (minimum score 6.5). *Application deadline:* For fall admission, 1/15 for domestic and international students. Application fee: $45. Electronic applications accepted. *Expenses: Tuition, area resident:* Full-time $3965; part-time $220.25 per credit hour. Tuition, nonresident: full-time $8699; part-time $483.25 per credit hour. *Required fees:* $677; $21 per credit hour. $174. Part-time tuition and fees vary according to course load and program. *Financial support:* In 2015–16, 6 students received support, including 3 research assistantships with full tuition reimbursements available (averaging $11,500 per year), 3 teaching assistantships with full tuition reimbursements available (averaging $11,500 per year); career-related internships or fieldwork and unspecified assistantships also available. Support available to part-time students. Financial award application deadline: 2/28; financial award applicants required to submit FAFSA. *Faculty research:* Neurogenic, communication disorders in adults, phonological development and disorders, orofacial anomalies, audiologic rehabilitation of the elderly. *Unit head:* Dr. Diane Loeb, Department Chair, 308-856-8305, Fax: 308-865-8397, E-mail: loebdm@unk.edu. *Application contact:* Linda Johnson, Director, Graduate Admissions and Programs, 800-717-7881, Fax: 308-865-8837, E-mail: gradstudies@unk.edu.
Website: http://www.unk.edu/academics/cdis/index.php

University of Nebraska at Omaha, Graduate Studies, College of Education, Department of Special Education and Communication Disorders, Omaha, NE 68182. Offers special education (MA, MS); speech-language pathology (MA, MS). *Accreditation:* ASHA (one or more programs are accredited); NCATE. *Program availability:* Part-time, evening/weekend. *Faculty:* 8 full-time (7 women). *Students:* 22 full-time (all women), 80 part-time (68 women); includes 9 minority (2 Asian, non-Hispanic/Latino; 4 Hispanic/Latino; 3 Two or more races, non-Hispanic/Latino). Average age 30. 201 applicants, 11% accepted, 17 enrolled. In 2015, 35 master's awarded. *Degree requirements:* For master's, comprehensive exam, thesis (for some programs). *Entrance requirements:* For master's, minimum GPA of 3.0, statement of purpose, 2 letters of recommendation, copy of teaching certificate. Additional exam requirements/recommendations for international students: Required—TOEFL, IELTS, PTE. *Application deadline:* For fall admission, 2/1 for domestic and international students; for spring admission, 11/1 for domestic and international students; for summer admission, 4/1 for domestic and international students. Applications are processed on a rolling basis. Application fee: $45. Electronic applications accepted. *Financial support:* In 2015–16, 8 students received support, including 6 research assistantships with tuition reimbursements available, 2 teaching assistantships with tuition reimbursements available; fellowships, career-related internships or fieldwork, Federal Work-Study, institutionally sponsored loans, scholarships/grants, health care benefits, tuition waivers (partial), and unspecified assistantships also available. Support available to part-time students. Financial award application deadline: 3/1; financial award applicants required to submit FAFSA. *Unit head:* Dr. Kristine Swain, Chairperson, 402-554-2341, E-mail: graduate@unomaha.edu. *Application contact:* Dr. Philip Nordness, Graduate Program Chair, 402-554-2341, E-mail: graduate@unomaha.edu.

University of Nebraska–Lincoln, Graduate College, College of Education and Human Sciences, Department of Special Education and Communication Disorders, Program in Speech-Language Pathology and Audiology, Lincoln, NE 68588. Offers audiology and hearing science (Au D); speech-language pathology and audiology (MS). *Accreditation:* ASHA. *Degree requirements:* For master's, thesis optional. *Entrance requirements:* For master's, GRE. Additional exam requirements/recommendations for international students: Required—TOEFL (minimum score 500 paper-based). Electronic applications accepted.

University of Nevada, Reno, Graduate School, Division of Health Sciences, Department of Speech Pathology and Audiology, Reno, NV 89557. Offers speech pathology (PhD); speech pathology and audiology (MS). *Accreditation:* ASHA (one or more programs are accredited). Terminal master's awarded for partial completion of doctoral program. *Degree requirements:* For master's, thesis optional; for doctorate, thesis/dissertation. *Entrance requirements:* For master's, GRE General Test, minimum GPA of 2.75; for doctorate, GRE General Test, minimum GPA of 3.0. Additional exam requirements/recommendations for international students: Required—TOEFL (minimum score 500 paper-based; 61 iBT), IELTS (minimum score 6). Electronic applications accepted. *Faculty research:* Language impairment in children, voice disorders, stuttering.

University of New Hampshire, Graduate School, College of Health and Human Services, Department of Communication Sciences and Disorders, Durham, NH 03824. Offers adult neurogenic communication disorders (MS); communication sciences and disorders (MS); early childhood communication disorders (MS); language/literacy disorders (MS). Program offered in fall only. *Accreditation:* ASHA. *Program availability:* Part-time. *Degree requirements:* For master's, thesis or alternative. *Entrance requirements:* For master's, GRE General Test or MAT. Additional exam requirements/recommendations for international students: Required—TOEFL (minimum score 550 paper-based; 80 iBT). *Application deadline:* For fall admission, 1/15 priority date for domestic students, 4/1 for international students. Applications are processed on a rolling basis. Application fee: $65. Electronic applications accepted. *Expenses:* Tuition, state resident: full-time $13,840; part-time $770 per credit hour. Tuition, nonresident: full-time $27,130; part-time $1175 per credit hour. *Required fees:* $2080; $1040. Tuition and fees vary according to degree level and program. *Financial support:* Fellowships, research assistantships, teaching assistantships, career-related internships or fieldwork, Federal Work-Study, scholarships/grants, and tuition waivers (full and partial) available. Support

available to part-time students. Financial award application deadline: 2/15. *Faculty research:* Speech pathology. *Unit head:* Don Robin, Chair, 603-862-2125. *Application contact:* Maria Russell, Administrative Assistant III, 603-862-0144, E-mail: communication.disorders@unh.edu.
Website: http://chhs.unh.edu/csd

University of New Mexico, Graduate Studies, College of Arts and Sciences, Program in Speech and Hearing Sciences, Albuquerque, NM 87131. Offers speech-language pathology (MS). *Accreditation:* ASHA. *Faculty:* 10 full-time (9 women), 1 (woman) part-time/adjunct. *Students:* 43 full-time (34 women), 14 part-time (all women); includes 27 minority (1 American Indian or Alaska Native, non-Hispanic/Latino; 5 Asian, non-Hispanic/Latino; 20 Hispanic/Latino; 1 Two or more races, non-Hispanic/Latino). Average age 28. 104 applicants, 19% accepted, 18 enrolled. In 2015, 17 master's awarded. *Degree requirements:* For master's, comprehensive exam, thesis optional. *Entrance requirements:* For master's, GRE General Test, minimum GPA of 3.4 in speech and hearing sciences coursework. Additional exam requirements/recommendations for international students: Required—TOEFL (minimum score 550 paper-based; 80 iBT). *Application deadline:* For fall admission, 2/1 for domestic students, 1/1 for international students. Application fee: $50. Electronic applications accepted. *Financial support:* Research assistantships with partial tuition reimbursements, career-related internships or fieldwork, Federal Work-Study, scholarships/grants, health care benefits, and unspecified assistantships available. Financial award application deadline: 2/1; financial award applicants required to submit FAFSA. *Faculty research:* Augmentative and alternative communication (AAC), behavioral genetic studies of language, child language assessment, bilingual language acquisition, bilingual phonology, speech perception, swallowing disorders, transition from oral language to literacy. *Total annual research expenditures:* $172,031. *Unit head:* Dr. Barbara Rodriguez, Chair, 505-277-9728, Fax: 505-277-0968, E-mail: brodrig@unm.edu. *Application contact:* Tracy Wenzl, Department Administrator, 505-277-4453, Fax: 505-277-0968, E-mail: twenzl@unm.edu.
Website: http://shs.unm.edu

The University of North Carolina at Chapel Hill, School of Medicine and Graduate School, Graduate Programs in Medicine, Chapel Hill, NC 27599. Offers allied health sciences (MPT, MS, Au D, DPT, PhD), including human movement science (MS, PhD), occupational science (MS, PhD), physical therapy (MPT, MS, DPT), rehabilitation counseling and psychology (MS); speech and hearing sciences (MS, Au D, PhD); biochemistry and biophysics (MS, PhD); bioinformatics and computational biology (PhD); biomedical engineering (MS, PhD); cell and developmental biology (PhD); cell and molecular physiology (PhD); genetics and molecular biology (PhD); microbiology and immunology (MS, PhD), including immunology, microbiology; neurobiology (PhD); pathology and laboratory medicine (PhD), including experimental pathology; pharmacology (PhD); MD/PhD. *Program availability:* Online learning. Terminal master's awarded for partial completion of doctoral program. *Degree requirements:* For master's, comprehensive exam; for doctorate, thesis/dissertation. Electronic applications accepted. *Expenses:* Contact institution.

The University of North Carolina at Chapel Hill, School of Medicine and Graduate School, Graduate Programs in Medicine, Department of Allied Health Sciences, Division of Speech and Hearing Sciences, Chapel Hill, NC 27599. Offers audiology (Au D); speech and hearing sciences (MS, PhD). *Accreditation:* ASHA (one or more programs are accredited). *Program availability:* Online learning. *Degree requirements:* For master's, comprehensive exam, thesis optional; for doctorate, comprehensive exam, thesis/dissertation. *Entrance requirements:* For master's, GRE General Test, minimum GPA of 3.0; for doctorate, GRE, minimum GPA of 3.0. Additional exam requirements/recommendations for international students: Required—TOEFL (minimum score 550 paper-based). Electronic applications accepted. *Faculty research:* Child language and literacy, family participation in early intervention, child and adult hearing loss and treatment, vocal characteristics of African-American speakers and aging populations, adult apraxia of speech.

The University of North Carolina at Greensboro, Graduate School, School of Health and Human Sciences, Department of Communication Sciences and Disorders, Greensboro, NC 27412-5001. Offers speech language pathology (PhD); speech pathology and audiology (MA). *Accreditation:* ASHA. *Degree requirements:* For master's, thesis or alternative. *Entrance requirements:* For master's, GRE General Test. Additional exam requirements/recommendations for international students: Required—TOEFL. Electronic applications accepted.

University of North Dakota, Graduate School, College of Arts and Sciences, Department of Communication Sciences and Disorders, Grand Forks, ND 58202. Offers communication sciences and disorders (PhD); speech-language pathology (MS). *Accreditation:* ASHA (one or more programs are accredited). *Program availability:* Part-time. *Degree requirements:* For master's, comprehensive exam, thesis or alternative; for doctorate, comprehensive exam, thesis/dissertation, final exam. *Entrance requirements:* For master's and doctorate, GRE General Test, minimum GPA of 3.0. Additional exam requirements/recommendations for international students: Required—TOEFL (minimum score 550 paper-based; 79 iBT), IELTS (minimum score 6.5). Electronic applications accepted. *Faculty research:* Mass communications, journalism, community law, international communications, cultural studies.

University of Northern Colorado, Graduate School, College of Natural and Health Sciences, School of Human Sciences, Program in Audiology and Speech Language Sciences, Greeley, CO 80639. Offers audiology (Au D); speech language pathology (MA). *Accreditation:* ASHA (one or more programs are accredited). *Program availability:* Part-time, evening/weekend, online learning. *Degree requirements:* For master's, comprehensive exam, thesis or alternative; for doctorate, comprehensive exam, thesis/dissertation. *Entrance requirements:* For master's and doctorate, GRE General Test. Electronic applications accepted.

University of Northern Iowa, Graduate College, College of Humanities, Arts and Sciences, Department of Communicative Sciences and Disorders, Cedar Falls, IA 50614. Offers speech-language pathology (MA). *Accreditation:* ASHA. *Program availability:* Part-time, evening/weekend. *Students:* 100 full-time (97 women); includes 1 minority (Asian, non-Hispanic/Latino). 173 applicants, 19% accepted, 31 enrolled. In 2015, 42 master's awarded. *Degree requirements:* For master's, comprehensive exam, thesis or alternative. *Entrance requirements:* For master's, GRE, minimum GPA of 3.0. Additional exam requirements/recommendations for international students: Required—TOEFL (minimum score 500 paper-based; 61 iBT). *Application deadline:* For fall admission, 8/1 priority date for domestic students. Applications are processed on a rolling basis. Application fee: $50 ($70 for international students). *Financial support:* Career-related internships or fieldwork, Federal Work-Study, scholarships/grants, and tuition waivers (full and partial) available. Financial award application deadline: 2/1. *Unit head:* Dr. Lauren Nelson, Department Head/Associate Professor, 319-273-6806, Fax: 319-273-6384, E-mail: lauren.nelson@uni.edu. *Application contact:* Laurie S. Russell, Record Analyst, 319-273-2623, Fax: 319-273-2885, E-mail: laurie.russell@uni.edu.
Website: http://www.uni.edu/comdis

University of North Florida, College of Education and Human Services, Department of Exceptional, Deaf, and Interpreter Education, Jacksonville, FL 32224. Offers American

Sign Language/English interpreting (M Ed); applied behavior analysis (M Ed); autism (M Ed); deaf education (M Ed); disability services (M Ed); exceptional student education (M Ed). *Accreditation:* NCATE. *Program availability:* Part-time, evening/weekend. *Faculty:* 13 full-time (12 women), 3 part-time/adjunct (all women). *Students:* 35 full-time (34 women), 68 part-time (54 women); includes 26 minority (9 Black or African American, non-Hispanic/Latino; 3 Asian, non-Hispanic/Latino; 11 Hispanic/Latino; 3 Two or more races, non-Hispanic/Latino), 4 international. Average age 33. 30 applicants, 50% accepted, 13 enrolled. In 2015, 42 master's awarded. *Entrance requirements:* For master's, GRE General Test, minimum GPA of 3.0 in last 60 hours, interview, 3 letters of recommendation. Additional exam requirements/recommendations for international students: Required—TOEFL (minimum score 500 paper-based). *Application deadline:* For fall admission, 7/1 priority date for domestic students, 5/1 for international students; for spring admission, 11/1 priority date for domestic students, 10/1 for international students. Application fee: $30. Electronic applications accepted. *Expenses:* Tuition, state resident: part-time $408.10 per credit hour. Tuition, nonresident: part-time $932.61 per credit hour. *Required fees:* $111.81 per credit hour. Tuition and fees vary according to course load, campus/location and program. *Financial support:* In 2015–16, 18 students received support, including 4 research assistantships (averaging $1,709 per year); teaching assistantships, career-related internships or fieldwork, Federal Work-Study, scholarships/grants, tuition waivers (partial), and unspecified assistantships also available. Support available to part-time students. Financial award application deadline: 4/1; financial award applicants required to submit FAFSA. *Faculty research:* Transition, integrating technology into teacher education, written language development, professional school development, learning strategies. *Total annual research expenditures:* $816,202. *Unit head:* Dr. Karen Patterson, Chair, 904-620-2930, Fax: 904-620-3895, E-mail: karen.patterson@unf.edu. *Application contact:* Dr. Amanda Pascale, Director, Tho Graduate School, 904-620-1360, Fax: 904-620-1362, E-mail: graduateschool@unf.edu.
Website: http://www.unf.edu/coehs/edie/

University of North Texas, Robert B. Toulouse School of Graduate Studies, Denton, TX 76203-5459. Offers accounting (MS); applied anthropology (MA, MS); applied behavior analysis (Certificate); applied geography (MA); applied technology and performance improvement (M Ed, MS); art education (MA); art history (MA); art museum education (Certificate); arts leadership (Certificate); audiology (Au D); behavior analysis (MS); behavioral science (PhD); biochemistry and molecular biology (MA); biology (MA, MS); biomedical engineering (MS); business analysis (MS); chemistry (MS); clinical health psychology (PhD); communication studies (MA, MS); computer engineering (MS); computer science (MS); counseling (M Ed, MS), including clinical mental health counseling, college and university counseling, elementary school counseling, secondary school counseling; creative writing (MA); criminal justice (MS); curriculum and instruction (M Ed); decision sciences (MBA); design (MA, MFA), including fashion design (MFA), innovation studies, interior design (MFA); early childhood studies (MS); economics (MS); educational leadership (M Ed, Ed D); educational psychology (MS, PhD), including family studies (MS), gifted and talented (MS), human development (MS), learning and cognition (MS), research, measurement and evaluation (MS); electrical engineering (MS); emergency management (MPA); engineering technology (MS); English (MA); English as a second language (MA); environmental science (MS); finance (MBA, MS); financial management (MPA); French (MA); health services management (MBA); higher education (M Ed, Ed D); history (MA, MS); hospitality management (MS); human resources management (MPA); information science (MS); information systems (PhD); information technologies (MBA); interdisciplinary studies (MA, MS); international studies (MA); international sustainable tourism (MS); jazz studies (MM); journalism (MA, MJ, Graduate Certificate), including interactive and virtual digital communication (Graduate Certificate), narrative journalism (Graduate Certificate), public relations (Graduate Certificate); kinesiology (MS); linguistics (MA); local government management (MPA); logistics (PhD); logistics and supply chain management (MBA); long-term care, senior housing, and aging services (MA); management (PhD); marketing (MBA); mathematics (MA, MS); mechanical and energy engineering (MS, PhD); music (MA), including ethnomusicology, music theory, musicology, performance; music composition (PhD); music education (MM Ed, PhD); nonprofit management (MPA); operations and supply chain management (MBA); performance (MM, DMA); philosophy (MA); political science (MA); professional and technical communication (MA); radio, television and film (MA, MFA); rehabilitation counseling (Certificate); sociology (MA); Spanish (MA); special education (M Ed); speech-language pathology (MA); strategic management (MBA); studio art (MFA); teaching (M Ed); MBA/MS. *Program availability:* Part-time, evening/weekend, online learning. Terminal master's awarded for partial completion of doctoral program. *Degree requirements:* For master's, variable foreign language requirement, comprehensive exam (for some programs), thesis (for some programs); for doctorate, variable foreign language requirement, comprehensive exam (for some programs), thesis/dissertation; for other advanced degree, variable foreign language requirement, comprehensive exam (for some programs). *Entrance requirements:* For master's and doctorate, GRE, GMAT. Additional exam requirements/recommendations for international students: Required—TOEFL (minimum score 550 paper-based; 79 iBT). Electronic applications accepted.

University of Oklahoma Health Sciences Center, Graduate College, College of Allied Health, Department of Communication Sciences and Disorders, Oklahoma City, OK 73190. Offers audiology (MS, Au D); communication sciences and disorders (Certificate), including reading, speech-language pathology; education of the deaf (MS); speech-language pathology (MS, PhD). *Accreditation:* ASHA (one or more programs are accredited). *Program availability:* Part-time. Terminal master's awarded for partial completion of doctoral program. *Degree requirements:* For master's, comprehensive exam, thesis optional; for doctorate, one foreign language, comprehensive exam, thesis/dissertation. *Entrance requirements:* For master's and doctorate, GRE General Test, 3 letters of recommendation. Additional exam requirements/recommendations for international students: Required—TOEFL (minimum score 550 paper-based). *Faculty research:* Event-related potentials, cleft palate, fluency disorders, language disorders, hearing and speech science.

University of Ottawa, Faculty of Graduate and Postdoctoral Studies, Faculty of Health Sciences, School of Rehabilitation Sciences, Ottawa, ON K1N 6N5, Canada. Offers audiology (M Sc); orthophony (M Sc). *Program availability:* Part-time, evening/weekend. *Entrance requirements:* For master's, honors degree or equivalent, minimum B average. Electronic applications accepted.

University of Pittsburgh, School of Health and Rehabilitation Sciences, Department of Communication Science and Disorders, Pittsburgh, PA 15260. Offers MA, MS, Au D, CScD, PhD. *Accreditation:* ASHA (one or more programs are accredited). *Faculty:* 19 full-time (14 women), 8 part-time/adjunct (6 women). *Students:* 138 full-time (125 women), 17 part-time (15 women); includes 11 minority (1 Black or African American, non-Hispanic/Latino; 4 Asian, non-Hispanic/Latino; 5 Hispanic/Latino; 1 Two or more races, non-Hispanic/Latino), 9 international. Average age 27. 504 applicants, 47% accepted, 74 enrolled. In 2015, 43 master's, 21 doctorates awarded. *Degree requirements:* For master's, comprehensive exam, thesis (for some programs); for doctorate, comprehensive exam, thesis/dissertation. *Entrance requirements:* For master's and doctorate, GRE General Test. Additional exam requirements/recommendations for international students: Required—TOEFL (minimum score 550

paper-based; 80 iBT), IELTS (minimum score 6.5). *Application deadline:* For fall admission, 12/15 for domestic and international students. Applications are processed on a rolling basis. Application fee: $100. Electronic applications accepted. Tuition and fees vary according to program. *Financial support:* In 2015–16, 14 students received support, including 5 fellowships with full tuition reimbursements available (averaging $20,970 per year), 8 research assistantships with full tuition reimbursements available (averaging $20,970 per year), 1 teaching assistantship with full tuition reimbursement available (averaging $22,000 per year); Federal Work-Study and traineeships also available. *Faculty research:* Pediatric and geriatric neurogenic speech and language, pediatric hearing disorders, hearing aids, language development, speech motor control. *Total annual research expenditures:* $2.5 million. *Unit head:* Dr. Malcolm McNeil, Department Chair/Professor, 412-383-6541, Fax: 412-383-6555, E-mail: mcneil@pitt.edu. *Application contact:* Pamela Morocco, Administrator, 412-383-6540, Fax: 412-383-6555, E-mail: pjm79@pitt.edu.
Website: http://www.shrs.pitt.edu/CSDPrograms/

University of Puerto Rico, Medical Sciences Campus, School of Health Professions, Program in Audiology, San Juan, PR 00936-5067. Offers Au D. *Faculty research:* Hearing, auditory brainstem responses, otoacoustic emissions.

University of Puerto Rico, Medical Sciences Campus, School of Health Professions, Program in Speech-Language Pathology, San Juan, PR 00936-5067. Offers MS. *Accreditation:* ASHA. *Degree requirements:* For master's, one foreign language, comprehensive exam, thesis or alternative. *Entrance requirements:* For master's, EXADEP, interview; previous course work in linguistics, statistics, human development, and basic concepts in speech-language pathology; minimum GPA of 2.5. *Faculty research:* Aphasia, autism, language, aphasia, assistive technology.

University of Redlands, College of Arts and Sciences, Department of Communicative Disorders, Redlands, CA 92373-0999. Offers MS. *Accreditation:* ASHA. *Degree requirements:* For master's, final exam. *Entrance requirements:* For master's, GMAT or GRE, minimum GPA of 3.0, 3 letters of recommendation. Additional exam requirements/recommendations for international students: Required—TOEFL (minimum score 550 paper-based). Electronic applications accepted. *Expenses:* Contact institution. *Faculty research:* Neuropathy.

University of Rhode Island, Graduate School, College of Human Science and Services, Department of Communicative Disorders, Kingston, RI 02881. Offers speech-language pathology (MS). *Accreditation:* ASHA. *Program availability:* Part-time. *Faculty:* 7 full-time (5 women), 1 part-time/adjunct (0 women). *Students:* 37 full-time (all women), 8 part-time (all women); includes 3 minority (1 American Indian or Alaska Native, non-Hispanic/Latino; 1 Asian, non-Hispanic/Latino; 1 Hispanic/Latino). In 2015, 21 master's awarded. *Degree requirements:* For master's, comprehensive exam (for some programs), thesis optional. *Entrance requirements:* For master's, GRE or MAT, 2 letters of recommendation (3 recommended). Additional exam requirements/recommendations for international students: Required—TOEFL (minimum score 550 paper-based). *Application deadline:* For fall admission, 3/1 for domestic students, 2/1 for international students; for spring admission, 10/15 for domestic students, 7/15 for international students. Application fee: $65. Electronic applications accepted. *Expenses:* Tuition, state resident: full-time $11,796; part-time $655 per credit. Tuition, nonresident: full-time $24,206; part-time $1345 per credit. *Required fees:* $1546; $44 per credit. One-time fee: $155 full-time; $35 part-time. *Financial support:* In 2015–16, 4 teaching assistantships with tuition reimbursements (averaging $7,922 per year) were awarded. Financial award application deadline: 2/1; financial award applicants required to submit FAFSA. *Faculty research:* Efficacy of treatment for acquired alexia in individuals with aphasia, application of principles of neuroplasticity to individuals with motor speech disorders secondary to neurological deficits, study of the conversation factors that promote fluency or exacerbate stuttering in young children. *Unit head:* Dr. Dana Kovarsky, Chair, 401-874-2735, Fax: 401-874-4404, E-mail: dana@uri.edu. *Application contact:* Dr. Ann Weiss, Graduate Program Coordinator, 401-874-9071, Fax: 401-874-5787, E-mail: alw@uri.edu.
Website: http://www.uri.edu/hss/cmd/

University of San Diego, School of Leadership and Education Sciences, Department of Learning and Teaching, San Diego, CA 92110-2492. Offers special education with deaf and hard of hearing (M Ed); teaching (MAT); TESOL, literacy and culture (M Ed). *Program availability:* Part-time, evening/weekend. *Faculty:* 9 full-time (7 women), 25 part-time/adjunct (20 women). *Students:* 103 full-time (83 women), 162 part-time (140 women); includes 78 minority (7 Black or African American, non-Hispanic/Latino; 10 Asian, non-Hispanic/Latino; 55 Hispanic/Latino; 6 Two or more races, non-Hispanic/Latino), 8 international. Average age 32. 262 applicants, 76% accepted, 144 enrolled. In 2015, 98 master's awarded. *Degree requirements:* For master's, thesis (for some programs), international experience. *Entrance requirements:* For master's, California Basic Educational Skills Test, California Subject Examination for Teachers, minimum GPA of 2.75. Additional exam requirements/recommendations for international students: Required—TOEFL (minimum score 580 paper-based; 83 iBT), TWE. *Application deadline:* Applications are processed on a rolling basis. Application fee: $45. Electronic applications accepted. *Financial support:* In 2015–16, 42 students received support. Career-related internships or fieldwork, Federal Work-Study, institutionally sponsored loans, and stipends available. Financial award application deadline: 4/1; financial award applicants required to submit FAFSA. *Faculty research:* Action research methodology, cultural studies, instructional theories and practices, second language acquisition, school reform. *Unit head:* Dr. Lea Hubbard, Chair, 619-260-7618, E-mail: lhubbard@sandiego.edu. *Application contact:* Monica Mahon, Associate Director of Graduate Admissions, 619-260-4524, Fax: 619-260-4158, E-mail: grads@sandiego.edu.
Website: http://www.sandiego.edu/soles/departments/learning-and-teaching/

University of South Alabama, Pat Capps Covey College of Allied Health Professions, Department of Speech Pathology and Audiology, Mobile, AL 36688. Offers audiology (Au D); communication sciences and disorders (PhD); speech-language pathology (MS). *Accreditation:* ASHA. *Faculty:* 13 full-time (10 women), 1 (woman) part-time/adjunct. *Students:* 85 full-time (81 women), 1 (woman) part-time; includes 6 minority (4 Black or African American, non-Hispanic/Latino; 1 Asian, non-Hispanic/Latino; 1 Hispanic/Latino), 1 international. Average age 24. 332 applicants, 33% accepted, 31 enrolled. In 2015, 23 master's, 10 doctorates awarded. *Degree requirements:* For master's, thesis optional, externship; for doctorate, thesis/dissertation, clinical externship; minimum of 11 full-time semesters of academic study. *Entrance requirements:* For master's, GRE, bachelor's degree in communication sciences and disorders, three faculty references from undergraduate program; for doctorate, GRE, minimum GPA of 3.0. Additional exam requirements/recommendations for international students: Required—TOEFL (minimum score 525 paper-based; 71 iBT). *Application deadline:* For fall admission, 2/1 for domestic students. Application fee: $35. Electronic applications accepted. *Expenses:* Contact institution. *Financial support:* Fellowships, research assistantships, teaching assistantships, career-related internships or fieldwork, Federal Work-Study, institutionally sponsored loans, scholarships/grants, and unspecified assistantships available. Support available to part-time students. Financial award application deadline: 5/31; financial award applicants required to submit FAFSA. *Faculty research:* Adult speech and language, background noise, child language, developmental stuttering, evoked potentials and multicultural issues, vestibular

Communication Disorders

research. *Unit head:* Dr. Robert Moore, Department Chair, 251-445-9596, Fax: 251-445-9376, E-mail: rmoore@usouthal.edu. *Application contact:* Dr. Susan Gordon-Hickey, Associate Dean, Allied Health, 251-445-9250, Fax: 251-445-9259, E-mail: gordonhickey@southalabama.edu.
Website: http://www.southalabama.edu/alliedhealth/speechandhearing

University of South Carolina, The Graduate School, Arnold School of Public Health, Department of Communication Sciences and Disorders, Columbia, SC 29208. Offers MCD, MSP, PhD. *Accreditation:* ASHA (one or more programs are accredited). *Program availability:* Online learning. *Degree requirements:* For master's, thesis optional; for doctorate, comprehensive exam, thesis/dissertation. *Entrance requirements:* For master's, GRE General Test, minimum GPA of 3.0; for doctorate, GRE General Test. Electronic applications accepted. *Faculty research:* Noise-induced hearing loss, recurrent laryngeal nerve regeneration, cleft palate, child language-phonology, epidemiology of craniofacial anomalies.

The University of South Dakota, Graduate School, College of Arts and Sciences, Department of Communication Disorders, Vermillion, SD 57069-2390. Offers audiology (Au D); speech-language pathology (MA). *Accreditation:* ASHA (one or more programs are accredited). *Program availability:* Part-time. *Degree requirements:* For master's, comprehensive exam; for doctorate, comprehensive exam, thesis/dissertation. *Entrance requirements:* For master's, GRE General Test, minimum GPA of 3.0. Additional exam requirements/recommendations for international students: Required—TOEFL (minimum score 550 paper-based; 79 iBT). *Application deadline:* For fall admission, 2/1 for domestic students; for spring admission, 10/15 for domestic students. Application fee: $35. Electronic applications accepted. *Financial support:* Research assistantships with partial tuition reimbursements, teaching assistantships with partial tuition reimbursements, career-related internships or fieldwork, Federal Work-Study, scholarships/grants, and unspecified assistantships available. Support available to part-time students. Financial award application deadline: 5/1; financial award applicants required to submit FAFSA. *Faculty research:* Craniofacial anomalies, central auditory processing, phonological disorders. *Unit head:* Dr. Teri James Bellis, Chair, 605-677-6201, E-mail: teri.bellis@usd.edu. *Application contact:* Director of Disability Services, 605-677-6389, Fax: 605-677-3172, E-mail: disabilityservices@usd.edu.
Website: http://www.usd.edu/arts-and-sciences/communication-sciences-and-disorders

University of Southern Mississippi, Graduate School, College of Health, Department of Speech and Hearing Sciences, Hattiesburg, MS 39406-0001. Offers audiology (Au D); speech language pathology (MA, MS), including deaf education (MS). *Accreditation:* ASHA (one or more programs are accredited). *Degree requirements:* For master's, comprehensive exam, thesis or alternative; for doctorate, comprehensive exam, thesis/dissertation. *Entrance requirements:* For master's, GRE General Test, minimum GPA of 3.0 in field of study, 2.75 in last 60 hours; for doctorate, GRE General Test, minimum GPA of 3.5. Additional exam requirements/recommendations for international students: Required—TOEFL, IELTS. Electronic applications accepted. *Faculty research:* Voice disorders, auditory-evoked responses, acoustic analysis of speech, child language, parent-child interaction.

University of South Florida, College of Behavioral and Community Sciences, Department of Communication Sciences and Disorders, Tampa, FL 33620. Offers audiology (Au D); communication sciences and disorders (PhD), including communication sciences and disorders, hearing sciences and audiology, language and speech science, neurocommunicative science; speech-language pathology (post-bacc) (MS). *Accreditation:* ASHA (one or more programs are accredited). *Program availability:* Part-time, evening/weekend, online learning. *Faculty:* 29 full-time (23 women). *Students:* 169 full-time (156 women), 57 part-time (51 women); includes 46 minority (5 Black or African American, non-Hispanic/Latino; 6 Asian, non-Hispanic/Latino; 30 Hispanic/Latino; 5 Two or more races, non-Hispanic/Latino), 7 international. Average age 27. 694 applicants, 15% accepted, 94 enrolled. In 2015, 66 master's, 14 doctorates awarded. *Degree requirements:* For master's, comprehensive exam; for doctorate, comprehensive exam, thesis/dissertation. *Entrance requirements:* For master's, GRE General Test (for MS in speech language pathology and audiology), demonstrated competency in communication skills, 3 letters of recommendation, and letter of intent; minimum GPA of 3.2 in upper-division undergraduate course work and resume (for speech language pathology); minimum GPA of 3.0 for last 60 hours of bachelor's degree (for audiology); for doctorate, GRE General Test, minimum GPA of 3.5 during bachelor's, master's, and/or graduate study (for PhD), 3.0 during last 60 hours of bachelor's degree (for AuD); three letters of recommendation; letter of intent. Additional exam requirements/recommendations for international students: Required—TOEFL (minimum score 550 paper-based; 79 iBT) or IELTS (minimum score 6.5). *Application deadline:* For fall admission, 12/1 for domestic and international students; for spring admission, 10/15 for domestic students, 9/15 for international students. Application fee: $30. Electronic applications accepted. *Financial support:* In 2015–16, 25 students received support, including 1 research assistantship with tuition reimbursement available (averaging $10,920 per year), 15 teaching assistantships with tuition reimbursements available (averaging $10,881 per year); career-related internships or fieldwork, traineeships, health care benefits, and unspecified assistantships also available. Financial award application deadline: 2/1; financial award applicants required to submit FAFSA. *Faculty research:* Auditory perception and intervention; language and literacy; neurophysiology of hearing, speech, and language; adult neurogenics; bilingualism and language variation; language processing and intervention; speech and voice production; speech perception; translational science. *Total annual research expenditures:* $1.3 million. *Unit head:* Dr. Jennifer Lister, Interim Chair/Professor, 813-974-9712, Fax: 813-974-0822, E-mail: jlister@usf.edu. *Application contact:* Dr. Joseph Walton, PhD Program Director/Associate Professor, 813-974-4080, Fax: 813-974-0822, E-mail: jwalton1@usf.edu.
Website: http://csd.cbcs.usf.edu/

University of South Florida, Innovative Education, Tampa, FL 33620-9951. Offers adult, career and higher education (Graduate Certificate), including college teaching, leadership in developing human resources, leadership in higher education; Africana studies (Graduate Certificate), including diasporas and health disparities, genocide and human rights; aging studies (Graduate Certificate), including gerontology; art research (Graduate Certificate), including museum studies; business foundations (Graduate Certificate); chemical and biomedical engineering (Graduate Certificate), including materials science and engineering, water, health and sustainability; child and family studies (Graduate Certificate), including positive behavior support; civil and industrial engineering (Graduate Certificate), including transportation systems analysis; community and family health (Graduate Certificate), including maternal and child health, social marketing and public health, violence and injury: prevention and intervention, women's health; criminology (Graduate Certificate), including criminal justice administration; educational measurement and research (Graduate Certificate), including evaluation; English (Graduate Certificate), including comparative literary studies, creative writing, professional and technical communication; entrepreneurship (Graduate Certificate); environmental health (Graduate Certificate), including safety management; epidemiology and biostatistics (Graduate Certificate), including applied biostatistics, biostatistics, concepts and tools of epidemiology, epidemiology, epidemiology of infectious diseases; geography, environment and planning (Graduate Certificate), including community development, environmental policy and management, geographical information systems; geology (Graduate Certificate), including hydrogeology; global health (Graduate Certificate), including disaster management, global health and Latin American and Caribbean studies, global health practice, humanitarian assistance, infection control; government and international affairs (Graduate Certificate), including Cuban studies, globalization studies; health policy and management (Graduate Certificate), including health management and leadership, public health policy and programs; hearing specialist: early intervention (Graduate Certificate); industrial and management systems engineering (Graduate Certificate), including systems engineering, technology management; information studies (Graduate Certificate), including school library media specialist; information systems/decision sciences (Graduate Certificate), including analytics and business intelligence; instructional technology (Graduate Certificate), including distance education, Florida digital/virtual educator, instructional design, multimedia design, Web design; internal medicine, bioethics and medical humanities (Graduate Certificate), including biomedical ethics; Latin American and Caribbean studies (Graduate Certificate); mass communications (Graduate Certificate), including multimedia journalism; mathematics and statistics (Graduate Certificate), including mathematics; medicine (Graduate Certificate), including aging and neuroscience, bioinformatics, biotechnology, brain fitness and memory management, clinical investigation, health informatics, health sciences, integrative weight management, intellectual property, medicine and gender, metabolic and nutritional medicine, metabolic cardiology, pharmacy sciences; national and competitive intelligence (Graduate Certificate); psychological and social foundations (Graduate Certificate), including career counseling, college teaching, diversity in education, mental health counseling, school counseling; public affairs (Graduate Certificate), including nonprofit management, public management, research administration; public health (Graduate Certificate), including environmental health, health equity, public health generalist, translational research in adolescent behavioral health; public health practices (Graduate Certificate), including planning for healthy communities; rehabilitation and mental health counseling (Graduate Certificate), including integrative mental health care, marriage and family therapy, rehabilitation technology; secondary education (Graduate Certificate), including ESOL, foreign language education: culture and content, foreign language education: professional; social work (Graduate Certificate), including geriatric social work/clinical gerontology; special education (Graduate Certificate), including autism spectrum disorder, disabilities education: severe/profound; world languages (Graduate Certificate), including teaching English as a second language (TESL) or foreign language. *Unit head:* Kathy Barnes, Interdisciplinary Programs Coordinator, 813-974-8031, Fax: 813-974-7061, E-mail: barnesk@usf.edu. *Application contact:* Karen Tylinski, Metro Initiatives, 813-974-9943, Fax: 813-974-7061, E-mail: ktylinsk@usf.edu.
Website: http://www.usf.edu/innovative-education/

The University of Tennessee, Graduate School, College of Arts and Sciences, Department of Audiology and Speech Pathology, Program in Audiology, Knoxville, TN 37996. Offers MA. *Accreditation:* ASHA. *Degree requirements:* For master's, thesis or alternative. *Entrance requirements:* For master's, GRE General Test, minimum GPA of 2.7. Additional exam requirements/recommendations for international students: Required—TOEFL. Electronic applications accepted.

The University of Tennessee, Graduate School, College of Arts and Sciences, Department of Audiology and Speech Pathology, Program in Speech and Hearing Science, Knoxville, TN 37996. Offers audiology (PhD); hearing science (PhD); speech and language pathology (PhD); speech and language science (PhD). *Accreditation:* ASHA. *Degree requirements:* For doctorate, thesis/dissertation. *Entrance requirements:* For doctorate, GRE General Test, minimum GPA of 2.7. Additional exam requirements/recommendations for international students: Required—TOEFL. Electronic applications accepted.

The University of Tennessee, Graduate School, College of Arts and Sciences, Department of Audiology and Speech Pathology, Program in Speech Pathology, Knoxville, TN 37996. Offers MA. *Accreditation:* ASHA. *Degree requirements:* For master's, thesis or alternative. *Entrance requirements:* For master's, GRE General Test, minimum GPA of 2.7. Additional exam requirements/recommendations for international students: Required—TOEFL. Electronic applications accepted.

The University of Tennessee, Graduate School, College of Education, Health and Human Sciences, Program in Education, Knoxville, TN 37996. Offers art education (MS); counseling education (PhD); cultural studies in education (PhD); curriculum (MS, Ed S); curriculum, educational research and evaluation (Ed D, PhD); early childhood education (PhD); early childhood special education (MS); education of deaf and hard of hearing (MS); educational administration and policy studies (Ed D, PhD); educational administration and supervision (Ed S); educational psychology (Ed D, PhD); elementary education (MS, Ed S); elementary teaching (MS); English education (MS, Ed S); exercise science (PhD); foreign language/ESL education (MS, Ed S); instructional technology (MS, Ed D, PhD, Ed S); literacy, language and ESL education (PhD); literacy, language education, and ESL education (Ed D); mathematics education (MS, Ed S); modified and comprehensive special education (MS); reading education (MS, Ed S); school counseling (Ed S); school psychology (PhD, Ed S); science education (MS, Ed S); secondary teaching (MS); social foundations (MS); social science education (MS, Ed S); socio-cultural foundations of sports and education (PhD); special education (Ed S); teacher education (Ed D, PhD). *Accreditation:* NCATE. *Program availability:* Part-time, evening/weekend. *Degree requirements:* For master's and Ed S, thesis optional; for doctorate, variable foreign language requirement, thesis/dissertation. *Entrance requirements:* For master's, minimum GPA of 2.7; for doctorate and Ed S, GRE General Test, minimum GPA of 2.7. Additional exam requirements/recommendations for international students: Required—TOEFL. Electronic applications accepted.

The University of Tennessee Health Science Center, College of Graduate Health Sciences, Memphis, TN 38163-0002. Offers biomedical engineering (MS, PhD); biomedical sciences (PhD); dental sciences (MDS); epidemiology (MS); health outcomes and policy research (PhD); laboratory research and management (MS); nursing science (PhD); pharmaceutical sciences (PhD); pharmacology (MS); speech and hearing science (PhD); DDS/PhD; DNP/PhD; MD/PhD; Pharm D/PhD. Terminal master's awarded for partial completion of doctoral program. *Degree requirements:* For master's, comprehensive exam, thesis; for doctorate, comprehensive exam, thesis/dissertation, oral and written preliminary and comprehensive exams. *Entrance requirements:* For master's and doctorate, GRE General Test, minimum GPA of 3.0. Additional exam requirements/recommendations for international students: Required—TOEFL (minimum score 79 iBT); Recommended—IELTS (minimum score 6.5). Electronic applications accepted.

The University of Tennessee Health Science Center, College of Health Professions, Memphis, TN 38163-0002. Offers audiology (MS, Au D); clinical laboratory science (MSCLS); cytopathology practice (MCP); health informatics and information management (MHIIM); occupational therapy (MOT); physical therapy (DPT, ScDPT); physician assistant (MMS); speech-language pathology (MS). *Accreditation:* AOTA; APTA. *Program availability:* Part-time, evening/weekend, online learning. Terminal master's awarded for partial completion of doctoral program. *Degree requirements:* For master's, comprehensive exam, thesis; for doctorate, comprehensive exam, residency. *Entrance requirements:* For master's, GRE (MOT, MSCLS), minimum GPA of 3.0, 3 letters of reference, national accreditation (MSCLS), GRE if GPA is less than 3.0 (MCP); for doctorate, GRE. Additional exam requirements/recommendations for international students: Required—TOEFL (minimum score 550 paper-based; 80 iBT). Electronic applications accepted. *Expenses:* Contact institution. *Faculty research:* Gait deviation, muscular dystrophy and strength, hemophilia and exercise, pediatric neurology, self-efficacy.

The University of Texas at Austin, Graduate School, College of Communication, Department of Communication Sciences and Disorders, Austin, TX 78712-1111. Offers audiology (Au D); communication sciences and disorders (PhD); speech language pathology (MA). *Accreditation:* ASHA (one or more programs are accredited). *Entrance requirements:* For master's and doctorate, GRE General Test.

The University of Texas at Dallas, School of Behavioral and Brain Sciences, Program in Audiology, Dallas, TX 75235. Offers Au D. *Accreditation:* ASHA. *Faculty:* 8 full-time (3 women), 3 part-time/adjunct (1 woman). *Students:* 33 full-time (25 women), 9 part-time (all women); includes 9 minority (2 Black or African American, non-Hispanic/Latino; 2 Asian, non-Hispanic/Latino; 5 Hispanic/Latino). Average age 26. 130 applicants, 9% accepted, 12 enrolled. In 2015, 10 doctorates awarded. *Degree requirements:* For doctorate, research project. *Entrance requirements:* For doctorate, GRE. Additional exam requirements/recommendations for international students: Required—TOEFL (minimum score 550 paper-based). *Application deadline:* For fall admission, 7/15 for domestic students, 5/1 priority date for international students; for spring admission, 11/15 for domestic students, 9/1 priority date for international students. Applications are processed on a rolling basis. Application fee: $50 ($100 for international students). Electronic applications accepted. *Expenses:* Tuition, state resident: full-time $11,940; part-time $663 per semester hour. Tuition, nonresident: full time $22,786; part-time $1266 per semester hour. Tuition and fees vary according to course load. *Financial support:* In 2015–16, 42 students received support. Research assistantships with partial tuition reimbursements available, teaching assistantships with partial tuition reimbursements available, career-related internships or fieldwork, Federal Work-Study, institutionally sponsored loans, scholarships/grants, and unspecified assistantships available. Support available to part-time students. Financial award application deadline: 4/30; financial award applicants required to submit FAFSA. *Faculty research:* Hearing disorders, amplification of hearing aids, cochlear implants and aural habilitation. *Unit head:* Dr. Colleen Le Prell, Program Head, 214-905-3018, Fax: 972-883-2491, E-mail: colleen.leprell@utdallas.edu. *Application contact:* Cathy Bittner, Program Assistant, 214-905-3116, Fax: 972-883-2491, E-mail: cbittner@utdallas.edu. Website: http://bbs.utdallas.edu/aud

The University of Texas at Dallas, School of Behavioral and Brain Sciences, Program in Communication Sciences and Disorders, Richardson, TX 75080. Offers communication disorders (MS); communication science and disorders (PhD). *Program availability:* Part-time, evening/weekend. *Faculty:* 16 full-time (10 women), 13 part-time/adjunct (12 women). *Students:* 240 full-time (232 women), 13 part-time (all women); includes 61 minority (3 Black or African American, non-Hispanic/Latino; 19 Asian, non-Hispanic/Latino; 28 Hispanic/Latino; 11 Two or more races, non-Hispanic/Latino), 9 international. Average age 25. 565 applicants, 14% accepted, 61 enrolled. In 2015, 129 master's awarded. *Degree requirements:* For doctorate, thesis/dissertation. *Entrance requirements:* For master's and doctorate, GRE General Test, minimum GPA of 3.0 in upper-level course work in field. Additional exam requirements/recommendations for international students: Required—TOEFL (minimum score 550 paper-based). *Application deadline:* For fall admission, 7/15 for domestic students, 5/1 priority date for international students; for spring admission, 11/15 for domestic students, 9/1 priority date for international students. Applications are processed on a rolling basis. Application fee: $50 ($100 for international students). Electronic applications accepted. *Expenses:* Tuition, state resident: full-time $11,940; part-time $663 per semester hour. Tuition, nonresident: full-time $22,786; part-time $1266 per semester hour. Tuition and fees vary according to course load. *Financial support:* In 2015–16, 188 students received support, including 7 research assistantships with partial tuition reimbursements available (averaging $23,427 per year), 21 teaching assistantships with partial tuition reimbursements available (averaging $16,857 per year); fellowships, Federal Work-Study, institutionally sponsored loans, scholarships/grants, and unspecified assistantships also available. Support available to part-time students. Financial award application deadline: 4/30; financial award applicants required to submit FAFSA. *Faculty research:* Developmental neurolinguistics, brain plasticity and biofeedback treatment, autism spectrum disorders, speech production, neurogenic speech and language disorders. *Unit head:* Dr. Robert D. Stillman, Program Head, 214-905-3106, Fax: 972-883-3022, E-mail: stillman@utdallas.edu. *Application contact:* 972-883-3106, Fax: 972-883-3022, E-mail: commsciphd@utdallas.edu. Website: http://bbs.utdallas.edu/csd/

The University of Texas at El Paso, Graduate School, College of Health Sciences, Department of Speech-Language Pathology, El Paso, TX 79968-0001. Offers MS. *Accreditation:* ASHA. *Degree requirements:* For master's, comprehensive exam, thesis optional. *Entrance requirements:* For master's, GRE, minimum GPA of 3.0, resume, letters of recommendation, writing sample, interview. Additional exam requirements/recommendations for international students: Required—TOEFL; Recommended—IELTS. Electronic applications accepted. *Faculty research:* Bilingual language disorders, clinical supervision, hearing loss, traumatic brain injury, aphasia, policy, augmentative communication.

The University of Texas Health Science Center at San Antonio, School of Medicine, San Antonio, TX 78229-3900. Offers deaf education and hearing (MS); medicine (MD); MPH/MD. *Accreditation:* LCME/AMA. *Degree requirements:* For master's, comprehensive exam, practicum assignments. *Entrance requirements:* For master's, minimum GPA of 3.0, interview, 3 professional letters of recommendation; for doctorate, MCAT. Electronic applications accepted. *Expenses:* Contact institution. *Faculty research:* Geriatrics, diabetes, cancer, AIDS, obesity.

The University of Texas Rio Grande Valley, College of Health Affairs, Department of Communication Sciences and Disorders, Edinburg, TX 78539. Offers MS. *Accreditation:* ASHA. *Degree requirements:* For master's, comprehensive exam, thesis optional, NESPA exam. *Entrance requirements:* For master's, GRE General Test, minimum GPA of 3.0 in major, 3 letters of recommendation, resume. Additional exam requirements/recommendations for international students: Required—TOEFL (minimum score 550 paper-based). Electronic applications accepted. Tuition and fees vary according to course load and program. *Faculty research:* Bilingual/bicultural language development/disorders, elementary-age language disorders, voice disorders.

University of the District of Columbia, College of Arts and Sciences, Program in Speech-Language Pathology, Washington, DC 20008-1175. Offers MS. *Accreditation:* ASHA. *Program availability:* Part-time. *Degree requirements:* For master's, comprehensive exam, thesis optional. *Entrance requirements:* For master's, GRE General Test, writing proficiency exam. *Application deadline:* For fall admission, 6/15 priority date for domestic students; for spring admission, 11/1 for domestic students. Applications are processed on a rolling basis. Application fee: $50. *Financial support:* Fellowships and research assistantships available. Financial award application

deadline: 6/10. *Faculty research:* Child language, dialect variation, English as a second language.

University of the Pacific, Thomas J. Long School of Pharmacy and Health Sciences, Department of Speech-Language Pathology, Stockton, CA 95211-0197. Offers MS. *Accreditation:* ASHA. *Entrance requirements:* For master's, GRE General Test. Additional exam requirements/recommendations for international students: Required—TOEFL (minimum score 475 paper-based).

The University of Toledo, College of Graduate Studies, College of Health Sciences, Department of Rehabilitation Sciences, Toledo, OH 43606-3390. Offers occupational therapy (OTD); physical therapy (DPT); speech-language pathology (MA). *Degree requirements:* For master's, comprehensive exam, thesis; for doctorate, thesis/dissertation or alternative. *Entrance requirements:* For master's, GRE, minimum cumulative GPA of 2.7 for all previous academic work, letters of recommendation; for doctorate, GRE, minimum cumulative GPA of 3.0 for all previous academic work, letters of recommendation; OTCAS or PTCAS application and UT supplemental application (for OTD and DPT). Additional exam requirements/recommendations for international students: Required—TOEFL (minimum score 550 paper-based; 80 iBT). Electronic applications accepted.

University of Toronto, Faculty of Medicine, Department of Speech-Language Pathology, Toronto, ON M5S 1A1, Canada. Offers M Sc, MH Sc, PhD. *Program availability:* Part-time. *Degree requirements:* For master's, thesis (for some programs), clinical internship (MH Sc), oral thesis defense (M Sc); for doctorate, comprehensive exam, thesis/dissertation, oral thesis defense. *Entrance requirements:* For master's, minimum B+ average in last 2 years (MH Sc), B average in final year (M Sc); volunteer/work experience in a clinical setting (MH Sc); for doctorate, previous research experience or thesis, resume, 3 writing samples, 3 letters of recommendation. Electronic applications accepted.

The University of Tulsa, Graduate School, Kendall College of Arts and Sciences, Program in Speech-Language Pathology, Tulsa, OK 74104-3189. Offers MS. *Accreditation:* ASHA. *Program availability:* Part-time. *Faculty:* 5 full-time (all women), 3 part-time/adjunct (all women). *Students:* 39 full-time (all women); includes 8 minority (7 American Indian or Alaska Native, non-Hispanic/Latino; 1 Hispanic/Latino), 2 international. Average age 23. 114 applicants, 37% accepted, 20 enrolled. In 2015, 19 master's awarded. *Degree requirements:* For master's, thesis optional. *Entrance requirements:* For master's, GRE General Test. Additional exam requirements/recommendations for international students: Required—TOEFL (minimum score 577 paper-based; 90 iBT), IELTS (minimum score 6.5). *Application deadline:* For fall admission, 2/1 priority date for domestic students. Application fee: $55. Electronic applications accepted. *Expenses: Tuition, area resident:* Full-time $22,230; part-time $1176 per credit hour. *Required fees:* $590 per semester. Tuition and fees vary according to course load. *Financial support:* In 2015–16, 21 students received support, including 3 fellowships with full tuition reimbursements available (averaging $17,222 per year), 17 teaching assistantships with full tuition reimbursements available (averaging $8,348 per year); career-related internships or fieldwork, Federal Work-Study, scholarships/grants, traineeships, health care benefits, tuition waivers (full and partial), and unspecified assistantships also available. Support available to part-time students. Financial award application deadline: 2/1; financial award applicants required to submit FAFSA. *Faculty research:* Disorders of fluency, delayed language and literacy, aphasia, voice, speech articulation, swallowing, cognition. *Total annual research expenditures:* $183,727. *Application contact:* Dr. Paula Cadogan, Adviser, 918-631-2897, Fax: 918-631-3668, E-mail: paula-cadogan@utulsa.edu.

University of Utah, Graduate School, College of Education, Department of Special Education, Salt Lake City, UT 84112. Offers deaf and hard of hearing (M Ed); deaf/blind (M Ed, MS); early childhood deaf and hard of hearing (MS); early childhood special education (M Ed, MS, PhD); early childhood vision impairments (M Ed); mild/moderate disabilities (M Ed, MS, PhD); severe disabilities (M Ed, MS, PhD); visual impairment (M Ed, MS). *Program availability:* Part-time, evening/weekend, 100% online, blended/hybrid learning. *Faculty:* 14 full-time (11 women), 26 part-time/adjunct (19 women). *Students:* 24 full-time (19 women), 15 part-time (13 women); includes 3 minority (1 Asian, non-Hispanic/Latino; 2 Hispanic/Latino). Average age 36. 30 applicants, 97% accepted, 28 enrolled. In 2015, 22 master's awarded. Terminal master's awarded for partial completion of doctoral program. *Degree requirements:* For master's, comprehensive exam, thesis (for some programs), qualifying exam; for doctorate, thesis/dissertation, qualifying exam. *Entrance requirements:* For master's, GRE, minimum GPA of 3.0; for doctorate, GRE General Test, minimum GPA of 3.5. Additional exam requirements/recommendations for international students: Required—TOEFL (minimum score 600 paper-based; 100 iBT); Recommended—IELTS (minimum score 7). *Application deadline:* For fall admission, 3/1 for domestic and international students; for spring admission, 11/1 for domestic and international students; for summer admission, 5/16 for domestic and international students. Application fee: $55 ($65 for international students). Electronic applications accepted. *Expenses:* $1,256.83 per credit hour resident; $3,897.93 per credit hour non-resident. *Financial support:* In 2015–16, 22 students received support, including 33 fellowships with partial tuition reimbursements available (averaging $4,350 per year), 4 teaching assistantships with tuition reimbursements available (averaging $10,000 per year); career-related internships or fieldwork and health care benefits also available. Support available to part-time students. Financial award application deadline: 3/1; financial award applicants required to submit FAFSA. *Faculty research:* Inclusive education, positive behavior support, reading, instruction and intervention strategies. *Total annual research expenditures:* $139,750. *Unit head:* Dr. Robert E. O'Neill, Chair, 801-581-8121, Fax: 801-585-6476, E-mail: rob.oneill@utah.edu. *Application contact:* Patty Davis, Academic Advisor, 801-581-4764, Fax: 801-585-6476, E-mail: patty.davis@utah.edu. Website: http://special-ed.utah.edu/

University of Utah, Graduate School, College of Health, Department of Communication Sciences and Disorders, Salt Lake City, UT 84112. Offers audiology (Au D, PhD); speech-language pathology (MA, MS, PhD). *Accreditation:* ASHA (one or more programs are accredited). *Faculty:* 16 full-time (10 women), 8 part-time/adjunct (6 women). *Students:* 148 full-time (111 women), 3 part-time (2 women); includes 18 minority (1 Black or African American, non-Hispanic/Latino; 4 Asian, non-Hispanic/Latino; 11 Hispanic/Latino; 2 Two or more races, non-Hispanic/Latino), 3 international. Average age 27. 243 applicants, 49% accepted, 46 enrolled. In 2015, 38 master's, 6 doctorates awarded. Terminal master's awarded for partial completion of doctoral program. *Degree requirements:* For master's, thesis optional, written exam; for doctorate, thesis/dissertation, written and oral exams. *Entrance requirements:* For master's and doctorate, GRE General Test, minimum GPA of 3.0. Additional exam requirements/recommendations for international students: Required—TOEFL (minimum score 600 paper-based; 100 iBT). *Application deadline:* For fall admission, 1/15 for domestic and international students. Application fee: $55 ($65 for international students). Electronic applications accepted. *Expenses:* Contact institution. *Financial support:* In 2015–16, 32 students received support, including 9 research assistantships with partial tuition reimbursements available (averaging $9,333 per year); teaching assistantships, career-related internships or fieldwork, Federal Work-Study, scholarships/grants, tuition waivers (full and partial), and unspecified assistantships also

available. Financial award application deadline: 1/15; financial award applicants required to submit FAFSA. *Faculty research:* Motor speech disorders, fluency disorders, language disorders, voice disorders, speech perception, audiology disorders. *Total annual research expenditures:* $441,812. *Unit head:* Dr. Michael Blomgren, Department Chair, 801-581-6725, Fax: 801-581-7955, E-mail: michael.blomgren@hsc.utah.edu. *Application contact:* Dr. Kathy Chapman, Director of Graduate Studies, 801-581-6725, Fax: 801-581-7955, E-mail: kathy.chapman@hsc.utah.edu.
Website: http://www.health.utah.edu/csd

University of Vermont, Graduate College, College of Nursing and Health Sciences, Department of Communication Sciences and Disorders, Burlington, VT 05405. Offers MS. *Accreditation:* ASHA. *Entrance requirements:* For master's, GRE General Test. Additional exam requirements/recommendations for international students: Required—TOEFL (minimum score 550 paper-based; 80 iBT). *Application deadline:* For fall admission, 1/1 for domestic and international students. Application fee: $65. Electronic applications accepted. *Financial support:* Fellowships available. Financial award application deadline: 3/1. *Unit head:* Dr. Barry Guitar, 802-656-3858. *Application contact:* Dr. Barry Guitar, 802-656-3858.

University of Virginia, Curry School of Education, Department of Human Services, Program in Communication Disorders, Charlottesville, VA 22903. Offers M Ed. *Accreditation:* ASHA. *Entrance requirements:* For master's, GRE General Test, 2 letters of recommendation. Additional exam requirements/recommendations for international students: Required—TOEFL (minimum score 600 paper-based; 90 iBT), IELTS (minimum score 7). Electronic applications accepted.

University of Washington, Graduate School, College of Arts and Sciences, Department of Speech and Hearing Sciences, Seattle, WA 98195. Offers audiology (Au D); speech and hearing sciences (PhD); speech-language pathology (MS). *Accreditation:* ASHA (one or more programs are accredited). *Degree requirements:* For master's, comprehensive exam, thesis or alternative; for doctorate, thesis/dissertation. *Entrance requirements:* For master's and doctorate, GRE, minimum GPA of 3.0. Additional exam requirements/recommendations for international students: Required—TOEFL. Electronic applications accepted. *Faculty research:* Treatment of communication disorders across the life span, speech physiology, auditory perception, behavioral and physiologic audiology.

The University of Western Ontario, Faculty of Graduate Studies, Health Sciences Division, School of Communication Sciences and Disorders, London, ON N6A 5B8, Canada. Offers audiology (M Cl Sc, M Sc); speech-language pathology (M Cl Sc, M Sc). *Degree requirements:* For master's, thesis (for some programs), supervised clinical practicum. *Entrance requirements:* For master's, 14 hours volunteer experience in field of study, minimum B average during last 2 years, previous course work in developmental psychology and statistics, 4 year honors degree. Additional exam requirements/recommendations for international students: Required—TOEFL (minimum score 620 paper-based). *Faculty research:* Child language, voice, neurogenics; auditory function, stuttering.

University of West Georgia, College of Education, Carrollton, GA 30118. Offers business education (M Ed); early childhood education (M Ed, Ed S); educational leadership (M Ed, Ed S); media (M Ed, Ed S); professional counseling (M Ed, Ed S); professional counseling and supervision (Ed D); reading instruction (M Ed); school improvement (Ed D); secondary education (M Ed); special education (M Ed, Ed S), including teaching (M Ed); speech language pathology (M Ed); teaching (MAT). *Accreditation:* NCATE. *Program availability:* Part-time, evening/weekend, 100% online. *Faculty:* 41 full-time (27 women). *Students:* 352 full-time (280 women), 910 part-time (734 women); includes 444 minority (395 Black or African American, non-Hispanic/Latino; 1 American Indian or Alaska Native, non-Hispanic/Latino; 10 Asian, non-Hispanic/Latino; 29 Hispanic/Latino; 9 Two or more races, non-Hispanic/Latino), 11 international. Average age 34. 586 applicants, 81% accepted, 377 enrolled. In 2015, 271 master's, 31 doctorates, 161 other advanced degrees awarded. *Entrance requirements:* Additional exam requirements/recommendations for international students: Required—TOEFL (minimum score 523 paper-based; 69 iBT); Recommended—IELTS (minimum score 6.5). *Application deadline:* For fall admission, 7/21 for domestic students, 6/1 for international students; for spring admission, 11/30 for domestic students, 10/15 for international students; for summer admission, 4/15 for domestic students, 3/30 for international students. Applications are processed on a rolling basis. Application fee: $40. Electronic applications accepted. *Expenses:* $7,278 resident full-time; $222 per credit hour resident tuition and fees; $22,620 nonresident full-time; $861 per credit hour nonresident tuition and fees. *Financial support:* Fellowships, research assistantships, teaching assistantships, career-related internships or fieldwork, Federal Work-Study, institutionally sponsored loans, scholarships/grants, and unspecified assistantships available. Support available to part-time students. Financial award application deadline: 4/1; financial award applicants required to submit FAFSA. *Unit head:* Dr. Diane Hoff, Dean, 678-839-6570, Fax: 678-839-6098, E-mail: dhoff@westga.edu. *Application contact:* Dr. Toby Ziglar, Director of Graduate Studies and International Admissions, 678-839-1394, Fax: 678-839-1395, E-mail: graduate@westga.edu.
Website: http://www.westga.edu/education/

University of Wisconsin–Eau Claire, College of Education and Human Sciences, Program in Communication Sciences and Disorders, Eau Claire, WI 54702-4004. Offers MS. *Accreditation:* ASHA. *Program availability:* Part-time. *Degree requirements:* For master's, comprehensive exam, thesis optional, written or oral exam with thesis, externship. *Entrance requirements:* For master's, GRE, Wisconsin residency; minimum GPA of 3.0 in communication disorders, 2.75 overall. Additional exam requirements/recommendations for international students: Required—TOEFL (minimum score 79 iBT).

University of Wisconsin–Madison, Graduate School, College of Letters and Science, Department of Communicative Disorders, Madison, WI 53706-1380. Offers normal aspects of speech, language and hearing (MS, PhD); speech-language pathology (MS, PhD); MS/PhD. *Accreditation:* ASHA (one or more programs are accredited). *Degree requirements:* For doctorate, thesis/dissertation. *Entrance requirements:* For master's and doctorate, GRE. Electronic applications accepted. *Expenses:* Tuition, state resident: full-time $5364. Tuition, nonresident: full-time $12,027. *Required fees:* $571. Tuition and fees vary according to campus/location, program and reciprocity agreements. *Faculty research:* Language disorders in children and adults, disorders of speech production, intelligibility, fluency, hearing impairment, deafness.

University of Wisconsin–Milwaukee, Graduate School, College of Health Sciences, Department of Communication Sciences and Disorders, Milwaukee, WI 53211. Offers assistive technology and accessible design (Graduate Certificate); communication sciences and disorders (MS). *Accreditation:* ASHA (one or more programs are accredited). *Program availability:* Part-time. *Faculty:* 6 full-time (5 women), 1 (woman) part-time/adjunct. *Students:* 51 full-time (50 women), 1 (woman) part-time; includes 2 minority (both Asian, non-Hispanic/Latino). Average age 26. 65 applicants, 43% accepted, 27 enrolled. In 2015, 30 master's awarded. *Degree requirements:* For master's, comprehensive exam, thesis optional. *Entrance requirements:* For master's, GRE General Test, minimum GPA of 3.0. Additional exam requirements/recommendations for international students: Required—TOEFL (minimum score 550

paper-based; 79 iBT), IELTS (minimum score 6.5). *Application deadline:* For fall admission, 1/1 priority date for domestic students; for spring admission, 9/1 for domestic students. Applications are processed on a rolling basis. Application fee: $56 ($96 for international students). *Financial support:* In 2015–16, 1 teaching assistantship was awarded; fellowships, research assistantships, career-related internships or fieldwork, unspecified assistantships, and project assistantships also available. Support available to part-time students. Financial award application deadline: 4/15. *Unit head:* Marylou Gelfer, Department Chair, 414-229-6465, E-mail: gelfer@uwm.edu. *Application contact:* General Information Contact, 414-229-4982, Fax: 414-229-6967, E-mail: gradschool@uwm.edu.
Website: http://www4.uwm.edu/chs/academics/comm_sci_disorders/

University of Wisconsin–River Falls, Outreach and Graduate Studies, College of Education and Professional Studies, Department of Communicative Disorders, River Falls, WI 54022. Offers communicative disorders (MS); secondary education-communicative disorders (MSE). *Accreditation:* ASHA (one or more programs are accredited). *Program availability:* Part-time. *Degree requirements:* For master's, comprehensive exam. *Entrance requirements:* For master's, minimum GPA of 2.75, 3 letters of reference. Additional exam requirements/recommendations for international students: Required—TOEFL (minimum score 500 paper-based; 65 iBT), IELTS (minimum score 5.5). *Faculty research:* Voice, language, audiology.

University of Wisconsin–Stevens Point, College of Professional Studies, School of Communicative Disorders, Stevens Point, WI 54481-3897. Offers audiology (Au D); speech-language pathology (MS). *Accreditation:* ASHA (one or more programs are accredited). *Degree requirements:* For master's, thesis optional, clinical semester and capstone project; for doctorate, capstone project, full-time clinical externship. *Entrance requirements:* For master's, completion of specific course contents and practicum experiences at the undergraduate level.

University of Wisconsin–Whitewater, School of Graduate Studies, College of Education and Professional Studies, Program in Communication Sciences and Disorders, Whitewater, WI 53190-1790. Offers MS. *Accreditation:* ASHA. *Program availability:* Part-time, evening/weekend, online learning. *Degree requirements:* For master's, comprehensive exam. *Entrance requirements:* For master's, 2 letters of recommendation. Additional exam requirements/recommendations for international students: Required—TOEFL (minimum score 550 paper-based; 80 iBT), IELTS (minimum score 6). *Application deadline:* For fall admission, 2/1 for domestic and international students. Applications are processed on a rolling basis. Application fee: $56. Electronic applications accepted. *Expenses:* Tuition, state resident: full-time $9008. Tuition, nonresident: full-time $18,600. *Financial support:* Research assistantships with tuition reimbursements, Federal Work-Study, unspecified assistantships, and out-of-state fee waivers available. Support available to part-time students. Financial award application deadline: 3/15; financial award applicants required to submit FAFSA. *Faculty research:* Occupational hearing conservation.

University of Wyoming, College of Health Sciences, Division of Communication Disorders, Laramie, WY 82071. Offers speech-language pathology (MS). *Accreditation:* ASHA. *Program availability:* Part-time, online learning. *Entrance requirements:* For master's, GRE General Test, minimum GPA of 3.0. Additional exam requirements/recommendations for international students: Required—TOEFL. Electronic applications accepted. *Faculty research:* Child language, visual reinforcement audiometry, voice, auditory brain response, TBI.

Utah State University, School of Graduate Studies, Emma Eccles Jones College of Education and Human Services, Department of Communicative Disorders and Deaf Education, Logan, UT 84322. Offers audiology (Au D, Ed S); communication disorders and deaf education (M Ed); communicative disorders and deaf education (MA, MS). *Accreditation:* ASHA (one or more programs are accredited). *Program availability:* Evening/weekend, online learning. *Degree requirements:* For master's, thesis optional; for Ed S, thesis or alternative. *Entrance requirements:* For master's, GRE General Test, minimum GPA of 3.0, 3 recommendations; for doctorate, GRE General Test, interview, minimum GPA of 3.25. Additional exam requirements/recommendations for international students: Required—TOEFL. *Expenses:* Contact institution. *Faculty research:* Parent-infant intervention with hearing-impaired infants, voice disorders, language development and disorders, oto-accoustic emissions, deaf or hard-of-hearing infants.

Vanderbilt University, School of Medicine, Department of Hearing and Speech Sciences, Nashville, TN 37240-1001. Offers audiology (Au D, PhD); deaf education (MED); speech-language pathology (MS). *Students:* 28 full-time (18 women), 3 part-time (all women); includes 1 minority (Asian, non-Hispanic/Latino), 5 international. Average age 29. 27 applicants, 56% accepted, 11 enrolled. In 2015, 1 master's, 4 doctorates awarded. *Degree requirements:* For master's, thesis optional; for doctorate, thesis/dissertation, final and qualifying exams. *Entrance requirements:* For master's and doctorate, GRE General Test. Additional exam requirements/recommendations for international students: Required—TOEFL. *Application deadline:* For fall admission, 1/15 for domestic and international students. Application fee: $0. Electronic applications accepted. *Financial support:* Fellowships with full tuition reimbursements, research assistantships with full tuition reimbursements, career-related internships or fieldwork, institutionally sponsored loans, traineeships, and tuition waivers (full and partial) available. Financial award application deadline: 1/15; financial award applicants required to submit FAFSA. *Faculty research:* Child language. *Total annual research expenditures:* $3.6 million. *Unit head:* Dr. Todd Ricketts, Director of Graduate Studies, 615-936-5103, Fax: 615-936-5014, E-mail: todd.a.ricketts@vanderbilt.edu. *Application contact:* Penny Welch, Coordinator, 615-936-5103, Fax: 615-936-6914, E-mail: penny.welch@vanderbilt.edu.
Website: http://www.vanderbiltbillwilkersoncenter.com

Washington State University, College of Medicine, Program in Speech and Hearing Sciences, Spokane, WA 99210. Offers MS. Program offered at the Spokane campus. *Degree requirements:* For master's, comprehensive exam, thesis (for some programs). *Entrance requirements:* For master's, GRE, minimum GPA of 3.0, 3 letters of recommendation. Additional exam requirements/recommendations for international students: Required—TOEFL (minimum score 550 paper-based). Electronic applications accepted. *Faculty research:* Autism spectrum disorder, childhood apraxia of speech, cleft palate and craniofacial disorders, motor speech disorders in patients with neurodegenerative disease and galactosemia, early language and literacy in multicultural populations.

Washington University in St. Louis, School of Medicine, Program in Audiology and Communication Sciences, St. Louis, MO 63110. Offers audiology (Au D); deaf education (MS); speech and hearing sciences (PhD). *Accreditation:* ASHA (one or more programs are accredited). *Faculty:* 22 full-time (12 women), 18 part-time/adjunct (12 women). *Students:* 73 full-time (71 women). Average age 24. 136 applicants, 25% accepted, 24 enrolled. In 2015, 10 master's, 11 doctorates awarded. *Degree requirements:* For master's, comprehensive exam, thesis, independent study project, oral exam; for doctorate, comprehensive exam, thesis/dissertation, capstone project. *Entrance requirements:* For master's and doctorate, GRE General Test, minimum B average in previous college/university coursework (recommended). Additional exam requirements/recommendations for international students: Required—TOEFL (minimum score 100

iBT). *Application deadline:* For fall admission, 2/15 for domestic and international students. Application fee: $60 ($80 for international students). Electronic applications accepted. *Expenses:* Contact institution. *Financial support:* In 2015–16, 72 students received support, including 73 fellowships with tuition reimbursements available (averaging $15,000 per year), 6 teaching assistantships with partial tuition reimbursements available (averaging $1,000 per year); career-related internships or fieldwork, Federal Work-Study, institutionally sponsored loans, scholarships/grants, traineeships, health care benefits, tuition waivers (partial), and unspecified assistantships also available. Financial award application deadline: 2/15; financial award applicants required to submit FAFSA. *Faculty research:* Audiology, deaf education, speech and hearing sciences, sensory neuroscience. *Unit head:* Dr. William W. Clark, Program Director, 314-747-0104, Fax: 314-747-0105. *Application contact:* Beth Elliott, Director, Finance and Student Academic Affairs, 314-747-0104, Fax: 314-747-0105, E-mail: elliottb@wustl.edu.
Website: http://pacs.wustl.edu/

Wayne State University, College of Liberal Arts and Sciences, Department of Communication Sciences and Disorders, Detroit, MI 48202. Offers audiology (Au D); communication disorders and science (PhD); speech-language pathology (MA). *Accreditation:* ASHA (one or more programs are accredited). *Faculty:* 11 full-time (8 women), 13 part-time/adjunct (6 women). *Students:* 121 full-time (113 women), 4 part-time (all women); includes 7 minority (3 Black or African American, non-Hispanic/Latino; 1 Asian, non-Hispanic/Latino; 2 Hispanic/Latino; 1 Two or more races, non-Hispanic/Latino), 16 international. Average age 26. 306 applicants, 18% accepted, 53 enrolled. In 2015, 31 master's, 10 doctorates awarded. *Degree requirements:* For master's, comprehensive exam (for some programs), thesis (for some programs); for doctorate, thesis/dissertation (for some programs), written and oral comprehensive examinations. *Entrance requirements:* For master's, GRE, letters of recommendation, minimum GPA of 3.0, three letters of recommendation, written statement of intent, official transcripts, CSDCAS Centralized Application Service; for doctorate, GRE, minimum GPA of 3.0, three letters of recommendation, written statement of intent, official transcripts, CSDCAS Centralized Application Service (for audiology applicants). Additional exam requirements/recommendations for international students: Required—TOEFL (minimum score 550 paper-based; 79 iBT), TWE (minimum score 5.5), Michigan English Language Assessment Battery (minimum score 85); Recommended—IELTS (minimum score 6.5). *Application deadline:* For fall admission, 1/15 for domestic and international students. Application fee: $0. Electronic applications accepted. *Expenses:* Tuition, state resident: full-time $14,165; part-time $590.20 per credit hour. Tuition, nonresident: full-time $30,682; part-time $1278.40 per credit hour. *Required fees:* $1688; $47.45 per credit hour. $274.60 per semester. Tuition and fees vary according to course load and program. *Financial support:* In 2015–16, 41 students received support, including 2 fellowships with tuition reimbursements available (averaging $13,932 per year); research assistantships with tuition reimbursements available, scholarships/grants, and unspecified assistantships also available. Financial award application deadline: 3/31; financial award applicants required to submit FAFSA. *Faculty research:* Aphasia, stuttering/fluency, speech and auditory genetics, neuroscience, tinnitus. *Unit head:* Dr. Margaret Greenwald, Chair, 313-577-0608, E-mail: mgreenwald@wayne.edu. *Application contact:* Dr. Derek Daniels, Associate Professor/Director of Graduate Studies, 313-577-3339, E-mail: dedaniels@wayne.edu.
Website: http://clas.wayne.edu/csd/

Webster University, School of Education, Department of Communication Arts, Reading and Early Childhood, St. Louis, MO 63119-3194. Offers communication arts (MAT); reading (MA). *Entrance requirements:* For master's, minimum GPA of 2.5. Additional exam requirements/recommendations for international students: Required—TOEFL. *Expenses: Tuition, area resident:* Full-time $20,550; part-time $685 per credit hour. Tuition and fees vary according to campus/location and program.

West Chester University of Pennsylvania, College of Health Sciences, Department of Communication Sciences and Disorders, West Chester, PA 19383. Offers communicative disorders (MA). *Accreditation:* ASHA. *Program availability:* Part-time. *Faculty:* 7 full-time (all women), 2 part-time/adjunct (both women). *Students:* 48 full-time (47 women), 12 part-time (11 women); includes 1 minority (Two or more races, non-Hispanic/Latino). Average age 27. 315 applicants, 23% accepted, 28 enrolled. In 2015, 27 master's awarded. *Degree requirements:* For master's, comprehensive exam, thesis optional, 62 semester credit hours. *Entrance requirements:* For master's, GRE, two letters of recommendation, personal statement of academic and professional goals, logs of clinical observation, practicum hours. Additional exam requirements/recommendations for international students: Required—TOEFL or IELTS. *Application deadline:* For fall admission, 5/15 for international students; for spring admission, 10/15 for international students. Applications are processed on a rolling basis. Application fee: $50. Electronic applications accepted. *Expenses:* Tuition, state resident: full-time $8460; part-time $470 per credit. Tuition, nonresident: full-time $12,690; part-time $705 per credit. *Required fees:* $2312; $126.75 per credit. Tuition and fees vary according to campus/location and program. *Financial support:* Scholarships/grants and unspecified assistantships available. Financial award application deadline: 2/15; financial award applicants required to submit FAFSA. *Faculty research:* Identification/interaction with students with communicative disorders, voice therapy, autism, bilingual assessment and intervention, critical thinking, literacy development, fluency, interprofessional collaboration, scholarship of teaching. *Unit head:* Dr. Cheryl Gunter, Chair, 610-436-3401, Fax: 610-436-3388, E-mail: cgunter@wcupa.edu. *Application contact:* Dr. Mareile Koenig, Graduate Coordinator, 610-436-3218, Fax: 610-436-3388, E-mail: mkoenig@wcupa.edu.
Website: http://www.wcupa.edu/_ACADEMICS/HealthSciences/commdisorder/

Western Carolina University, Graduate School, College of Health and Human Sciences, Department of Communication Sciences and Disorders, Cullowhee, NC 28723. Offers MS. *Accreditation:* ASHA. *Program availability:* Part-time. *Degree requirements:* For master's, comprehensive exam, thesis or alternative. *Entrance requirements:* For master's, GRE, appropriate undergraduate degree with minimum GPA of 3.0, 3 letters of recommendation. Additional exam requirements/recommendations for international students: Required—TOEFL (minimum score 550 paper-based; 79 iBT). *Application deadline:* For fall admission, 2/15 for domestic students. Application fee: $50. *Financial support:* Fellowships, research assistantships, teaching assistantships, institutionally sponsored loans, traineeships, and unspecified assistantships available. Financial award application deadline: 3/31; financial award applicants required to submit FAFSA. *Faculty research:* Early assessment and intervention in language, stuttering, school-family partnerships, voice and organic disorders, accent reduction.
Website: http://www.wcu.edu/8389.asp

Western Illinois University, School of Graduate Studies, College of Fine Arts and Communication, Department of Communication Sciences and Disorders, Macomb, IL 61455-1390. Offers MS. *Accreditation:* ASHA. *Program availability:* Part-time. *Students:* 38 full-time (36 women), 2 part-time (both women); includes 1 minority (Hispanic/Latino), 1 international. Average age 24. 164 applicants, 37% accepted, 20 enrolled. In 2015, 14 master's awarded. *Degree requirements:* For master's, comprehensive exam, thesis or alternative. *Entrance requirements:* For master's, GRE, minimum GPA of 3.0. Additional

exam requirements/recommendations for international students: Required—TOEFL (minimum score 550 paper-based; 80 iBT). *Application deadline:* For fall admission, 2/1 priority date for domestic students. Applications are processed on a rolling basis. Application fee: $30. Electronic applications accepted. *Financial support:* In 2015–16, 15 students received support. Unspecified assistantships available. Financial award applicants required to submit FAFSA. *Unit head:* Dr. Stacy Betz, Chairperson, 309-298-1955. *Application contact:* Dr. Nancy Parsons, Associate Provost and Director of Graduate Studies, 309-298-1806, Fax: 309-298-2345, E-mail: grad-office@wiu.edu.
Website: http://wiu.edu/csd

Western Kentucky University, Graduate Studies, College of Health and Human Services, Department of Communication Disorders, Bowling Green, KY 42101. Offers MS. *Accreditation:* ASHA. *Program availability:* Part-time, evening/weekend, online learning. *Degree requirements:* For master's, comprehensive exam, written exam. *Entrance requirements:* For master's, GRE General Test, 3 letters of recommendation. Additional exam requirements/recommendations for international students: Required—TOEFL (minimum score 555 paper-based; 79 iBT).

Western Michigan University, Graduate College, College of Health and Human Services, Department of Speech Pathology and Audiology, Kalamazoo, MI 49008. Offers audiology (Au D); speech pathology and audiology (MA). *Accreditation:* ASHA. *Degree requirements:* For master's, thesis optional.

Western Washington University, Graduate School, College of Humanities and Social Sciences, Department of Communication Sciences and Disorders, Bellingham, WA 98225-5996. Offers MA. *Accreditation:* ASHA. *Program availability:* Part-time. *Degree requirements:* For master's, comprehensive exam, thesis optional. *Entrance requirements:* For master's, GRE General Test, minimum GPA of 3.0 in last 60 semester hours or last 90 quarter hours. Additional exam requirements/recommendations for international students: Required—TOEFL (minimum score 567 paper-based). Electronic applications accepted. *Faculty research:* Autism, stroke and stroke perception, aural rehabilitation and cochlear implants, auditory processing, speech in individuals with Parkinson's disease.

West Texas A&M University, College of Nursing and Health Sciences, Department of Communication Disorders, Canyon, TX 79016-0001. Offers MS. *Accreditation:* ASHA. *Program availability:* Part-time. *Degree requirements:* For master's, comprehensive exam, thesis optional. *Entrance requirements:* For master's, GRE General Test, minimum B average in all clinical courses, liability insurance, first aid card, immunizations. Additional exam requirements/recommendations for international students: Required—TOEFL (minimum score 550 paper-based).

West Virginia University, College of Education and Human Services, Department of Speech Pathology and Audiology, Morgantown, WV 26506. Offers audiology (Au D); speech-language pathology (MS). *Accreditation:* ASHA. *Degree requirements:* For master's, thesis optional, PRAXIS; for doctorate, thesis/dissertation or alternative, PRAXIS. *Entrance requirements:* For master's, GRE General Test, minimum GPA of 3.0, letter of recommendation; for doctorate, GRE General Test, letters of recommendation, minimum GPA of 3.0. Additional exam requirements/recommendations for international students: Required—TOEFL. Electronic applications accepted. *Expenses:* Tuition, state resident: full-time $8568. Tuition, nonresident: full-time $22,140. Tuition and fees vary according to program. *Faculty research:* Speech perception, language disorders in children, auditory skills, fluency disorders, phonological disorders in children.

Wichita State University, Graduate School, College of Health Professions, Department of Communication Sciences and Disorders, Wichita, KS 67260. Offers MA, Au D, PhD. *Accreditation:* ASHA (one or more programs are accredited). *Financial support:* Teaching assistantships available. *Unit head:* Dr. Julie Scherz, Chairperson, 316-978-3240, Fax: 316-978-3302, E-mail: julie.scherz@wichita.edu. *Application contact:* Jordan Oleson, Admissions Coordinator, 316-978-3095, Fax: 316-978-3253, E-mail: jordan.oleson@wichita.edu.
Website: http://www.wichita.edu/csd

William Paterson University of New Jersey, College of Science and Health, Wayne, NJ 07470-8420. Offers biology (MS); biotechnology (MS); communication disorders (MS); exercise and sports studies (MS); nursing (MSN); nursing practice (DNP). *Program availability:* Part-time, evening/weekend. *Faculty:* 25 full-time (11 women), 13 part-time/adjunct (4 women). *Students:* 73 full-time (58 women), 208 part-time (183 women); includes 111 minority (18 Black or African American, non-Hispanic/Latino; 40 Asian, non-Hispanic/Latino; 50 Hispanic/Latino; 3 Two or more races, non-Hispanic/Latino), 5 international. Average age 34. 495 applicants, 27% accepted, 74 enrolled. In 2015, 63 master's, 10 doctorates awarded. *Degree requirements:* For master's, comprehensive exam (for some programs), thesis (for some programs), non-thesis internship/practicum (for some programs). *Entrance requirements:* For master's, GRE/MAT, minimum GPA of 3.0; 2 or 3 letters of recommendation; personal statement; work experience (for some programs); for doctorate, GRE/MAT, minimum GPA of 3.3; work experience; 3 letters of recommendation; interview; master's degree in nursing. Additional exam requirements/recommendations for international students: Required—TOEFL (minimum score 550 paper-based; 79 iBT), IELTS (minimum score 6). *Application deadline:* For fall admission, 6/1 for domestic students, 3/1 for international students; for spring admission, 11/1 for domestic students, 10/1 for international students. Applications are processed on a rolling basis. Application fee: $50. Electronic applications accepted. *Expenses:* Tuition, state resident: full-time $11,544; part-time $577.21 per credit. Tuition, nonresident: full-time $19,024; part-time $951.21 per credit. *Required fees:* $1916; $95.79 per credit. $62.50 per semester. Tuition and fees vary according to course load and degree level. *Financial support:* Research assistantships with full tuition reimbursements, career-related internships or fieldwork, Federal Work-Study, scholarships/grants, and unspecified assistantships available. Support available to part-time students. Financial award application deadline: 4/1; financial award applicants required to submit FAFSA. *Faculty research:* Human biomechanics, autism, nanomaterials, health and environment, neurophysiology and neurobiology. *Unit head:* Dr. Kenneth Wolf, Dean, 973-720-2194, Fax: 973-720-3414, E-mail: wolfk@wpunj.edu. *Application contact:* Christina Aiello, Assistant Director, Graduate Admissions, 973-720-2506, Fax: 973-720-2035, E-mail: aielloc@wpunj.edu.
Website: http://www.wpunj.edu/cosh

Worcester State University, Graduate Studies, Program in Speech-Language Pathology, Worcester, MA 01602-2597. Offers MS. *Accreditation:* ASHA. *Program availability:* Part-time, evening/weekend. *Faculty:* 7 full-time (5 women), 4 part-time/adjunct (all women). *Students:* 51 full-time (50 women), 35 part-time (33 women); includes 8 minority (2 Black or African American, non-Hispanic/Latino; 2 Asian, non-Hispanic/Latino; 1 Hispanic/Latino; 3 Two or more races, non-Hispanic/Latino). Average age 27. 227 applicants, 35% accepted, 33 enrolled. In 2015, 27 master's awarded. *Degree requirements:* For master's, comprehensive exam, thesis, practicum; national licensing exam; clinical observation and participation in diagnostic/therapeutic work. *Entrance requirements:* For master's, GRE General Test or MAT. Additional exam requirements/recommendations for international students: Required—TOEFL (minimum score 550 paper-based; 79 iBT). *Application deadline:* For fall admission, 2/1 priority date for domestic and international students. Applications are processed on a rolling basis. Application fee: $50. Electronic applications accepted. *Expenses:* Contact institution. *Financial support:* Career-related internships or fieldwork, scholarships/grants, and unspecified assistantships available. Financial award application deadline: 3/1; financial award applicants required to submit FAFSA. *Unit head:* Dr. Sharon Antonucci, Coordinator, 508-929-8567, Fax: 508-929-8475, E-mail: sharon.antonucci@worcester.edu. *Application contact:* Sara Grady, Associate Dean of Graduate and

Continuing Education, 508-929-8787, Fax: 508-929-8100, E-mail: sara.grady@worcester.edu.

Yeshiva University, Graduate Programs in Arts and Sciences, New York, NY 10033-3201. Offers mathematical sciences (PhD); mathematics (MA); quantitative economics (MS); speech-language pathology (MS).

Dental Hygiene

Boston University, Henry M. Goldman School of Dental Medicine, Boston, MA 02118. Offers dental public health (MS, MSD, D Sc D); dentistry (DMD); endodontics (MSD, D Sc D, CAGS); operative dentistry (MSD, D Sc D, CAGS); oral and maxillofacial surgery (MSD, D Sc D, CAGS); oral biology (MSD, D Sc D); orthodontics (MSD, D Sc D); pediatric dentistry (MSD, D Sc D, CAGS); periodontology (MSD, D Sc D, CAGS); prosthodontics (D Sc D). *Accreditation:* ADA (one or more programs are accredited). *Faculty:* 136 full-time (60 women), 90 part-time/adjunct (31 women). *Students:* 812 full-time (428 women), 2 part-time (1 woman); includes 195 minority (12 Black or African American, non-Hispanic/Latino; 127 Asian, non-Hispanic/Latino; 42 Hispanic/Latino; 14 Two or more races, non-Hispanic/Latino), 316 international. Average age 28. 6,681 applicants, 8% accepted, 263 enrolled. In 2015, 23 master's, 204 doctorates, 59 other advanced degrees awarded. *Degree requirements:* For master's and CAGS, thesis; for doctorate, thesis/dissertation (for some programs). *Entrance requirements:* For doctorate, DAT (for DMD), minimum recommended GPA of 3.0 (for DMD); for CAGS, National Board Dental Exam Part 1, dental degree. Additional exam requirements/recommendations for international students: Required—TOEFL. *Application deadline:* For fall admission, 12/1 for domestic and international students. Applications are processed on a rolling basis. Application fee: $75 ($105 for international students). Electronic applications accepted. *Expenses:* Contact institution. *Financial support:* In 2015–16, 125 students received support. Career-related internships or fieldwork, institutionally sponsored loans, scholarships/grants, and stipends available. Financial award application deadline: 4/18; financial award applicants required to submit FAFSA. *Faculty research:* Defense mechanisms, bone-cell regulation, protein biochemistry, molecular biology, biomaterials. *Unit head:* Dr. Jeffrey W. Hutter, Dean, 617-638-4780. *Application contact:* Admissions Representative, 617-638-4787, Fax: 617-638-4798, E-mail: sdmadmis@bu.edu.
Website: http://www.bu.edu/dental

Eastern Washington University, Graduate Studies, College of Science, Health and Engineering, Department of Dental Hygiene, Cheney, WA 99004-2431. Offers MS.

Idaho State University, Office of Graduate Studies, Kasiska College of Health Professions, Department of Dental Hygiene, Pocatello, ID 83209-8048. Offers MS. *Program availability:* Part-time. *Degree requirements:* For master's, comprehensive exam, thesis, thesis defense, practicum experience, oral exam. *Entrance requirements:* For master's, GRE, MAT, baccalaureate degree in dental hygiene, minimum GPA of 3.0 in upper-division and dental hygiene coursework, current dental hygiene licensure in good standing. Additional exam requirements/recommendations for international students: Required—TOEFL (minimum score 600 paper-based; 80 iBT). Electronic applications accepted.

Missouri Southern State University, Program in Dental Hygiene, Joplin, MO 64801-1595. Offers MS. Program offered jointly with University of Missouri–Kansas City. *Program availability:* Part-time. *Degree requirements:* For master's, project. *Entrance requirements:* For master's, copy of current dental hygiene license. Electronic applications accepted.

The Ohio State University, College of Dentistry, Columbus, OH 43210. Offers dental anesthesiology (MS); dental hygiene (MDH); dentistry (DDS); endodontics (MS); oral and maxillofacial pathology (MS); oral and maxillofacial surgery (MS); oral biology (PhD); orthodontics (MS); pediatric dentistry (MS); periodontology (MS); prosthodontics (MS); DDS/PhD. *Accreditation:* ADA (one or more programs are accredited). *Faculty:* 77. *Students:* 520 full-time (219 women), 5 part-time (4 women); includes 95 minority (12 Black or African American, non-Hispanic/Latino; 2 American Indian or Alaska Native, non-Hispanic/Latino; 49 Asian, non-Hispanic/Latino; 18 Hispanic/Latino; 14 Two or more races, non-Hispanic/Latino), 28 international. Average age 26. In 2015, 31 master's, 112 doctorates awarded. Terminal master's awarded for partial completion of doctoral program. *Degree requirements:* For master's, thesis; for doctorate, thesis/dissertation (for some programs). *Entrance requirements:* For master's, GRE General Test (for all applicants with cumulative GPA below 3.0); for doctorate, DAT (for DDS); GRE General Test, GRE Subject Test in biology recommended (for PhD). Additional exam requirements/recommendations for international students: Required—TOEFL (minimum score 550 paper-based; 79 iBT), IELTS (minimum score 7), Michigan English Language Assessment Battery (minimum score 82). *Application deadline:* For fall admission, 10/1 for domestic and international students; for summer admission, 4/11 for domestic students, 3/10 for international students. Applications are processed on a rolling basis. Electronic applications accepted. *Expenses:* Contact institution. *Financial support:* Fellowships with tuition reimbursements, research assistantships with tuition reimbursements, teaching assistantships with tuition reimbursements, Federal Work-Study, institutionally sponsored loans, and health care benefits available. Financial award application deadline: 2/15. *Faculty research:* Neurobiology, inflammation and immunity, materials science, bone biology. *Unit head:* Dr. Patrick M. Lloyd, Dean, 614-292-9755, E-mail: lloyd.256@osu.edu.
Website: http://www.dentistry.osu.edu/

Old Dominion University, College of Health Sciences, School of Dental Hygiene, Norfolk, VA 23529. Offers MS. *Program availability:* Part-time, evening/weekend, blended/hybrid learning. *Faculty:* 10 full-time (9 women). *Students:* 9 full-time (all women), 16 part-time (all women); includes 5 minority (4 Black or African American, non-Hispanic/Latino; 1 Hispanic/Latino), 2 international. Average age 34. 12 applicants, 25% accepted, 2 enrolled. In 2015, 3 master's awarded. *Degree requirements:* For master's, comprehensive exam, thesis optional, writing proficiency exam, responsible conduct of research training. *Entrance requirements:* For master's, Dental Hygiene National Board Examination or copy of license to practice dental hygiene, BS or certificate in dental hygiene or related area, minimum GPA of 2.8 (3.0 in major), 4 letters of recommendation. Additional exam requirements/recommendations for international students: Required—TOEFL (minimum score 550 paper-based, 79 iBT) or IELTS (minimum score 6.5). *Application deadline:* For fall admission, 7/1 for domestic students, 4/15 for international students; for spring admission, 12/1 for domestic students, 10/1 for international students; for summer admission, 3/1 for domestic students, 2/1 for international students. Applications are processed on a rolling basis. Application fee: $50. Electronic applications accepted. *Expenses:* $501 per credit. *Financial support:* In

2015–16, 4 students received support, including 4 teaching assistantships with partial tuition reimbursements available (averaging $10,000 per year); scholarships/grants and health care benefits also available. Support available to part-time students. Financial award application deadline: 2/15; financial award applicants required to submit CSS PROFILE or FAFSA. *Faculty research:* Clinical dental hygiene, dental hygiene client health behaviors, dental hygiene education interventions, oral product testing, cold plasma. *Total annual research expenditures:* $43,581. *Unit head:* Deborah B. Bauman, Assistant Dean/Graduate Program Director, 757-683-6079, Fax: 757-683-4753, E-mail: dbauman@odu.edu. *Application contact:* William Heffelfinger, Director of Graduate Admissions, 757-683-5554, Fax: 757-683-3255, E-mail: gradadmit@odu.edu.
Website: http://www.odu.edu/academics/programs/masters/dental-hygiene

Université de Montréal, Faculty of Dental Medicine, Program in Stomatology Residency, Montréal, QC H3C 3J7, Canada. Offers Certificate.

University of Alberta, Faculty of Medicine and Dentistry, Department of Dentistry, Program in Dental Hygiene, Edmonton, AB T6G 2E1, Canada. Offers Diploma. Electronic applications accepted.

University of Bridgeport, Fones School of Dental Hygiene, Bridgeport, CT 06604. Offers MS. *Program availability:* Part-time, evening/weekend, online learning. *Degree requirements:* For master's, thesis. *Entrance requirements:* For master's, Dental Hygiene National Board Examination. Additional exam requirements/recommendations for international students: Recommended—TOEFL (minimum score 550 paper-based; 80 iBT), IELTS (minimum score 6.5). *Application deadline:* For fall admission, 8/1 priority date for domestic and international students; for spring admission, 12/1 priority date for domestic and international students. Application fee: $50. *Expenses:* Contact institution. *Financial support:* Applicants required to submit FAFSA.

University of Michigan, School of Dentistry and Rackham Graduate School, Graduate Programs in Dentistry, Dental Hygiene Program, Ann Arbor, MI 48109-1078. Offers MS. *Program availability:* Part-time. *Students:* 8 full-time (all women); includes 1 minority (Black or African American, non-Hispanic/Latino). 4 applicants, 100% accepted, 2 enrolled. In 2015, 5 master's awarded. *Degree requirements:* For master's, thesis. *Entrance requirements:* For master's, bachelor's degree in dental hygiene. Additional exam requirements/recommendations for international students: Required—TOEFL (minimum score 84 iBT). *Application deadline:* Applications are processed on a rolling basis. Application fee: $75 ($90 for international students). Electronic applications accepted. *Expenses:* $31,200 resident tuition part-time per degree, $53,196 nonresident tuition part-time per degree. *Unit head:* Anne Gwozdek, Director, 734-763-3392, E-mail: agwozdek@umich.edu. *Application contact:* Patricia Katcher, Associate Admissions Director, 734-763-3316, Fax: 734-764-1922, E-mail: graddentinquiry@umich.edu.
Website: http://www.dent.umich.edu/dentalhygiene/education/MShome

University of Missouri–Kansas City, School of Dentistry, Kansas City, MO 64110-2499. Offers advanced education in dentistry (Graduate Dental Certificate); dental hygiene education (MS); dentistry (DDS); endodontics (Graduate Dental Certificate); oral and maxillofacial surgery (Graduate Dental Certificate); oral biology (MS, PhD); orthodontics and dentofacial orthopedics (Graduate Dental Certificate); periodontics (Graduate Dental Certificate). PhD (interdisciplinary) offered through the School of Graduate Studies. *Accreditation:* ADA (one or more programs are accredited). *Faculty:* 84 full-time (38 women), 56 part-time/adjunct (16 women). *Students:* 432 full-time (184 women), 54 part-time (26 women); includes 99 minority (12 Black or African American, non-Hispanic/Latino; 3 American Indian or Alaska Native, non-Hispanic/Latino; 46 Asian, non-Hispanic/Latino; 28 Hispanic/Latino; 10 Two or more races, non-Hispanic/Latino), 3 international. Average age 27. 793 applicants, 17% accepted, 129 enrolled. In 2015, 7 master's, 107 doctorates, 17 other advanced degrees awarded. *Degree requirements:* For master's, thesis; for doctorate, thesis/dissertation (for some programs). *Entrance requirements:* For master's, DAT, letters of evaluation, personal interview; for doctorate, DAT (for DDS); for Graduate Dental Certificate, DDS. Additional exam requirements/recommendations for international students: Required—TOEFL (minimum score 550 paper-based; 80 iBT). *Application deadline:* For fall admission, 2/1 for domestic and international students. Application fee: $45 ($50 for international students). *Expenses:* Contact institution. *Financial support:* In 2015–16, 1 research assistantship (averaging $22,000 per year) was awarded; career-related internships or fieldwork, Federal Work-Study, institutionally sponsored loans, and tuition waivers (full and partial) also available. Support available to part-time students. Financial award application deadline: 3/1; financial award applicants required to submit FAFSA. *Faculty research:* Biomaterials, dental use of lasers, effectiveness of periodontal treatments, temporomandibular joint dysfunction. *Unit head:* Dr. Marsha Pyle, Dean, 816-235-2010, E-mail: pylem@umkc.edu. *Application contact:* Richard Bigham, Assistant Dean for Student Programs, 816-235-2082, E-mail: bighamr@umkc.edu.
Website: http://dentistry.umkc.edu/

University of New Mexico, Graduate Studies, Health Sciences Center, Program in Dental Hygiene, Albuquerque, NM 87131-2039. Offers MS. *Program availability:* Part-time, evening/weekend, online learning. *Faculty:* 1 (woman) full-time. *Students:* 6 full-time (5 women), 13 part-time (all women); includes 14 minority (1 Black or African American, non-Hispanic/Latino; 1 American Indian or Alaska Native, non-Hispanic/Latino; 1 Asian, non-Hispanic/Latino; 11 Hispanic/Latino). Average age 32. 14 applicants, 79% accepted, 7 enrolled. In 2015, 3 master's awarded. *Application deadline:* For fall admission, 4/15 for domestic and international students; for winter admission, 1/31 priority date for domestic and international students. Application fee: $50. *Total annual research expenditures:* $1.3 million. *Unit head:* Prof. Christine N. Nathe, Director, 505-272-8147, Fax: 505-272-5584, E-mail: cnathe@unm.edu. *Application contact:* Prof. Demetra D. Logothetis, Graduate Program Director, 505-272-6687, Fax: 505-272-5584, E-mail: dlogothetis@salud.unm.edu.

The University of North Carolina at Chapel Hill, School of Dentistry and Graduate School, Graduate Programs in Dentistry, Chapel Hill, NC 27599. Offers dental hygiene (MS); endodontics (MS); epidemiology (PhD); operative dentistry (MS); oral and maxillofacial pathology (MS); oral and maxillofacial radiology (MS); oral biology (PhD); orthodontics (MS); pediatric dentistry (MS); periodontology (MS); prosthodontics (MS).

Degree requirements: For master's, thesis; for doctorate, thesis/dissertation. *Entrance requirements:* For master's, GRE General Test (for orthodontics and oral biology only); National Dental Board Part I (Part II if available), dental degree (for all except dental hygiene); for doctorate, GRE General Test. Additional exam requirements/ recommendations for international students: Required—TOEFL (minimum score 550 paper-based; 79 iBT). Electronic applications accepted. *Expenses:* Contact institution. *Faculty research:* Clinical research, inflammation, immunology, neuroscience, molecular biology.

Emergency Medical Services

Baylor University, Graduate School, Military Programs, Program in Emergency Medicine, Waco, TX 76798. Offers D Sc PA. *Faculty:* 49 full-time (7 women), 19 part-time/adjunct (3 women). *Students:* 20 full-time (5 women); includes 4 minority (2 Hispanic/Latino; 2 Two or more races, non-Hispanic/Latino). In 2015, 7 doctorates awarded. *Degree requirements:* For doctorate, comprehensive exam. *Entrance requirements:* For doctorate, GRE. Additional exam requirements/recommendations for international students: Required—TOEFL, IELTS. *Unit head:* Sharon Rosser, Graduate Program Director, 210-221-6729, E-mail: sharon.l.rosser.mil@mail.mil. *Application contact:* Dr. Sue Love, 210-916-4542, Fax: 254-710-3870, E-mail: sue.love@ us.army.mil.

Creighton University, Graduate School, Program in Emergency Medical Services, Omaha, NE 68178-0001. Offers MS. Program offered jointly with School of Pharmacy and Health Professions. *Program availability:* Part-time, online only, 100% online, blended/hybrid learning. *Faculty:* 3 full-time (0 women), 2 part-time/adjunct (1 woman). *Students:* 1 full-time (0 women), 12 part-time (7 women); includes 3 minority (1 Black or African American, non-Hispanic/Latino; 1 Asian, non-Hispanic/Latino; 1 Native Hawaiian or other Pacific Islander, non-Hispanic/Latino). Average age 42. 6 applicants, 83% accepted, 3 enrolled. In 2015, 1 master's awarded. *Entrance requirements:* Additional exam requirements/recommendations for international students: Required—TOEFL (minimum score 90 iBT). *Application deadline:* For fall admission, 8/1 for domestic students, 6/1 for international students; for spring admission, 11/15 for domestic students, 10/1 for international students; for summer admission, 3/1 for domestic students, 2/1 for international students. Applications are processed on a rolling basis. Application fee: $50. Electronic applications accepted. *Expenses: Tuition, area resident:* Full-time $14,400; part-time $800 per credit hour. *Required fees:* $158 per semester. Tuition and fees vary according to course load, campus/location, program, reciprocity agreements and student's religious affiliation. *Financial support:* Scholarships/grants available. *Unit head:* Dr. Michael Miller, Director, 402-280-1189, E-mail: mikemiller@ creighton.edu. *Application contact:* Lindsay Johnson, Director of Graduate and Adult Recruitment, 402-280-2703, Fax: 402-280-2423, E-mail: gradschool@creighton.edu. Website: http://ems.creighton.edu/

Drexel University, College of Nursing and Health Professions, Emergency and Public Safety Services Program, Philadelphia, PA 19104-2875. Offers MS. *Program availability:* Part-time, evening/weekend. *Degree requirements:* For master's, comprehensive exam. *Entrance requirements:* For master's, GRE General Test, minimum GPA of 2.75.

San Diego State University, Graduate and Research Affairs, College of Health and Human Services, Graduate School of Public Health, San Diego, CA 92182. Offers environmental health (MPH); epidemiology (MPH, PhD), including biostatistics (MPH); global emergency preparedness and response (MS); global health (PhD); health behavior (PhD); health promotion (MPH); health services administration (MPH); toxicology (MS); MPH/MA; MSW/MPH. *Accreditation:* CAHME (one or more programs are accredited); CEPH (one or more programs are accredited). *Program availability:* Part-time. *Degree requirements:* For master's, comprehensive exam (for some programs), thesis (for some programs); for doctorate, thesis/dissertation. *Entrance requirements:* For master's, GMAT (MPH in health services administration), GRE General Test; for doctorate, GRE General Test. Additional exam requirements/ recommendations for international students: Required—TOEFL. *Faculty research:* Evaluation of tobacco, AIDS prevalence and prevention, mammography, infant death project, Alzheimer's in elderly Chinese.

Université Laval, Faculty of Medicine, Post-Professional Programs in Medical Studies, Québec, QC G1K 7P4, Canada. Offers anatomy–pathology (DESS); anesthesiology (DESS); cardiology (DESS); care of older people (Diploma); clinical research (DESS); community health (DESS); dermatology (DESS); diagnostic radiology (DESS); emergency medicine (Diploma); family medicine (DESS); general surgery (DESS); geriatrics (DESS); hematology (DESS); internal medicine (DESS); maternal and fetal medicine (Diploma); medical biochemistry (DESS); medical microbiology and infectious diseases (DESS); medical oncology (DESS); nephrology (DESS); neurology (DESS); neurosurgery (DESS); obstetrics and gynecology (DESS); ophthalmology (DESS); orthopedic surgery (DESS); oto-rhino-laryngology (DESS); palliative medicine (Diploma); pediatrics (DESS); plastic surgery (DESS); psychiatry (DESS); pulmonary medicine (DESS); radiology–oncology (DESS); thoracic surgery (DESS); urology (DESS). *Degree requirements:* For other advanced degree, comprehensive exam. *Entrance requirements:* For degree, knowledge of French. Electronic applications accepted.

University of Guelph, Ontario Veterinary College and Graduate Studies, Graduate Programs in Veterinary Sciences, Department of Clinical Studies, Guelph, ON N1G 2W1, Canada. Offers anesthesiology (M Sc, DV Sc); cardiology (DV Sc, Diploma); clinical studies (Diploma); dermatology (M Sc); diagnostic imaging (M Sc, DV Sc); emergency/critical care (M Sc, DV Sc, Diploma); medicine (M Sc, DV Sc); neurology (M Sc, DV Sc); ophthalmology (M Sc, DV Sc); surgery (M Sc, DV Sc). *Degree requirements:* For master's, thesis; for doctorate, comprehensive exam, thesis/ dissertation. *Entrance requirements:* Additional exam requirements/recommendations for international students: Required—TOEFL (minimum score 550 paper-based), IELTS (minimum score 6.5). Electronic applications accepted. *Faculty research:* Orthopedics, respirology, oncology, exercise physiology, cardiology.

Occupational Therapy

Abilene Christian University, Graduate School, College of Education and Human Services, Department of Occupational Therapy, Abilene, TX 79699-9100. Offers MS. *Faculty:* 3 full-time (all women), 5 part-time/adjunct (3 women). *Students:* 47 full-time (46 women); includes 14 minority (3 Black or African American, non-Hispanic/Latino; 1 American Indian or Alaska Native, non-Hispanic/Latino; 10 Hispanic/Latino). 120 applicants, 32% accepted, 25 enrolled. *Entrance requirements:* Additional exam requirements/recommendations for international students: Required—TOEFL (minimum score 550 paper-based; 90 iBT), IELTS (minimum score 6.5), PTE. Application fee: $50. *Expenses:* $810 per credit hour. *Financial support:* In 2015–16, 10 students received support. Institutionally sponsored loans, scholarships/grants, and unspecified assistantships available. Support available to part-time students. Financial award application deadline: 4/1; financial award applicants required to submit FAFSA. *Unit head:* Dr. Hope Martin, Program Director, 325-674-2474, Fax: 325-674-3707, E-mail: msot@acu.edu. *Application contact:* Corey Patterson, Director of Graduate Admission and Recruiting, 325-674-6566, Fax: 325-674-6717, E-mail: gradinfo@acu.edu.

Alabama State University, College of Health Sciences, Department of Occupational Therapy, Montgomery, AL 36101-0271. Offers MS. *Accreditation:* AOTA. *Faculty:* 5 full-time (all women). *Students:* 66 full-time (57 women), 1 (woman) part-time; includes 16 minority (12 Black or African American, non-Hispanic/Latino; 2 Asian, non-Hispanic/ Latino; 2 Hispanic/Latino). Average age 25. 41 applicants, 83% accepted, 24 enrolled. In 2015, 20 master's awarded. *Entrance requirements:* For master's, interview. Application fee: $25. Electronic applications accepted. *Expenses: Tuition, area resident:* Full-time $3087; part-time $2744 per credit. Tuition, nonresident: full-time $6174; part-time $5488 per credit. *Required fees:* $2284; $1142 per credit. $571 per semester. Tuition and fees vary according to class time, course level, course load, degree level, program and student level. *Unit head:* Dr. Susan Denham, Chair, 334-229-5611, E-mail: sdenham@ alasu.edu. *Application contact:* Dr. William Person, Dean of Graduate Studies, 334-229-4274, Fax: 334-229-4928, E-mail: wperson@alasu.edu. Website: http://www.alasu.edu/academics/colleges—departments/health-sciences/ occupational-therapy/index.aspx

Allen College, Graduate Programs, Waterloo, IA 50703. Offers acute care nurse practitioner (Post-Master's Certificate); adult nurse practitioner (Post-Master's Certificate); adult psychiatric-mental health nurse practitioner (Post-Master's Certificate); adult-gerontology acute care nurse practitioner (MSN); community public health (Post-Master's Certificate); community/public health nursing (MSN); family nurse practitioner (MSN, Post-Master's Certificate); gerontological nurse practitioner (Post-Master's Certificate); health sciences (Ed D); leadership in health care delivery (MSN, Post-Master's Certificate); nursing (DNP); occupational therapy (MS). *Accreditation:* AACN; ACEN. *Program availability:* Part-time, blended/hybrid learning. *Faculty:* 3 full-time (all women), 21 part-time/adjunct (20 women). *Students:* 61 full-time (54 women), 163 part-time (144 women); includes 9 minority (5 Black or African American, non-Hispanic/ Latino; 2 Hispanic/Latino; 2 Two or more races, non-Hispanic/Latino), 2 international. Average age 34. 212 applicants, 60% accepted, 94 enrolled. In 2015, 51 master's, 1 doctorate awarded. *Degree requirements:* For master's, thesis optional. *Entrance requirements:* For master's, minimum GPA of 3.0 in the last 60 hours of undergraduate coursework; for doctorate, minimum GPA of 3.25 in graduate coursework. Additional exam requirements/recommendations for international students: Recommended— TOEFL (minimum score 580 paper-based; 92 iBT), IELTS (minimum score 6). *Application deadline:* For fall admission, 2/1 priority date for domestic students; for spring admission, 9/1 priority date for domestic students. Applications are processed on a rolling basis. Application fee: $50. Electronic applications accepted. *Expenses:* $15,940 tuition, $1,240 fees. *Financial support:* Institutionally sponsored loans, scholarships/grants, and traineeships available. Support available to part-time students. Financial award application deadline: 8/15; financial award applicants required to submit FAFSA. *Unit head:* Nancy Kramer, Vice Chancellor for Academic Affairs, 319-226-2040, Fax: 319-226-2070, E-mail: nancy.kramer@allencollege.edu. *Application contact:* Molly Quinn, Administrative Assistant for Student Services, 319-226-2014, Fax: 319-226-2010, E-mail: admissions@allencollege.edu. Website: http://www.allencollege.edu/

Alvernia University, Graduate Studies, Program in Occupational Therapy, Reading, PA 19607-1799. Offers MSOT. *Accreditation:* AOTA. *Program availability:* Part-time, evening/weekend. *Degree requirements:* For master's, thesis optional. Electronic applications accepted.

American International College, School of Health Sciences, Occupational Therapy Program, Springfield, MA 01109-3189. Offers MSOT. *Accreditation:* AOTA. *Faculty:* 6 full-time (all women), 2 part-time/adjunct (both women). *Students:* 74 full-time (59 women), 1 part-time (0 women); includes 29 minority (12 Black or African American, non-Hispanic/Latino; 1 American Indian or Alaska Native, non-Hispanic/Latino; 6 Asian, non-Hispanic/Latino; 5 Hispanic/Latino; 2 Native Hawaiian or other Pacific Islander, non-Hispanic/Latino; 3 Two or more races, non-Hispanic/Latino), 1 international. Average age 25. 195 applicants, 29% accepted, 23 enrolled. In 2015, 21 master's awarded. *Degree requirements:* For master's, comprehensive exam, thesis (for some programs), clinical observation. *Entrance requirements:* For master's, bachelor's degree with minimum GPA of 3.0 or GRE. Additional exam requirements/recommendations for international students: Required—TOEFL (minimum score 577 paper-based; 91 iBT). *Application deadline:* For fall admission, 12/1 priority date for domestic and international students; for spring admission, 12/1 for domestic and international students. Application fee: $50. Electronic applications accepted. *Expenses:* Contact institution. *Financial support:* Career-related internships or fieldwork available. Financial award application deadline: 4/1; financial award applicants required to submit FAFSA. *Faculty research:* Occupational therapy education, use of social media in occupational therapy education, interprofessional collaboration in the health sciences. *Unit head:* Dr. Cathy Dow-Royer,

Occupational Therapy

Acting Director, 413-205-3056, Fax: 413-654-1430, E-mail: cesarina.thompson@aic.edu. *Application contact:* Kerry Barnes, Director of Graduate Admissions, 413-205-3703, Fax: 413-205-3051, E-mail: kerry.barnes@aic.edu. Website: http://www.aic.edu/academics/hs

Arkansas State University, Graduate School, College of Nursing and Health Professions, Program in Occupational Therapy, State University, AR 72467. Offers occupational therapy (DOT). *Faculty:* 4 full-time (3 women). *Students:* 28 full-time (20 women); includes 2 minority (1 Black or African American, non-Hispanic/Latino; 1 Asian, non-Hispanic/Latino). Average age 24. 29 applicants, 93% accepted, 27 enrolled. *Degree requirements:* For doctorate, comprehensive exam, thesis/dissertation. *Entrance requirements:* For doctorate, GRE or MAT, bachelor's degree; transcripts; minimum GPA of 3.0 on prerequisites, 2.5 overall; 3 letters of recommendation; CPR Certification; TB Test; immunizations; health insurance; professional liability insurance; resume; personal statement. Additional exam requirements/recommendations for international students: Required—TOEFL (minimum score 550 paper-based; 79 iBT), IELTS (minimum score 6), PTE (minimum score 56). *Application deadline:* For fall admission, 2/15 for domestic and international students. Application fee: $50. Electronic applications accepted. *Expenses:* Contact institution. *Financial support:* In 2015–16, 1 student received support. Federal Work-Study and scholarships/grants available. Financial award application deadline: 7/1; financial award applicants required to submit FAFSA. *Unit head:* Dr. Tracy Morrison, Chair/Program Director, 870-972-2610, Fax: 870-972-2040, E-mail: mmorrison@astate.edu. *Application contact:* Vickey Ring, Graduate Admissions Coordinator, 870-972-2737, Fax: 870-972-3917, E-mail: vickeyring@astate.edu. Website: http://www.astate.edu/college/conhp/departments/occupational-therapy

A.T. Still University, Arizona School of Health Sciences, Mesa, AZ 85206. Offers advanced occupational therapy (MS); advanced physician assistant studies (MS); athletic training (MS, DAT); audiology (Au D); occupational therapy (OTD); physical therapy (DPT); physician assistant studies (MS); transitional audiology (Au D); transitional physical therapy (DPT). *Accreditation:* AOTA (one or more programs are accredited); ASHA. *Program availability:* Part-time, evening/weekend, 100% online. *Faculty:* 54 full-time (31 women), 188 part-time/adjunct (132 women). *Students:* 509 full-time (339 women), 397 part-time (310 women); includes 203 minority (41 Black or African American, non-Hispanic/Latino; 5 American Indian or Alaska Native, non-Hispanic/Latino; 83 Asian, non-Hispanic/Latino; 57 Hispanic/Latino; 2 Native Hawaiian or other Pacific Islander, non-Hispanic/Latino; 15 Two or more races, non-Hispanic/Latino), 60 international. Average age 33. 3,902 applicants, 10% accepted, 245 enrolled. In 2015, 178 master's, 271 doctorates awarded. *Degree requirements:* For master's, thesis (for some programs); for doctorate, thesis/dissertation (for some programs). *Entrance requirements:* For master's, GRE General Test; for doctorate, GRE, Evaluation of Practicing Audiologists Capabilities (Au D), Physical Therapist Evaluation Tool (DPT), current state licensure, master's degree or equivalent (Au D). Additional exam requirements/recommendations for international students: Required—TOEFL (minimum score 80 iBT). *Application deadline:* Applications are processed on a rolling basis. Application fee: $70. Electronic applications accepted. *Expenses:* Contact institution. *Financial support:* In 2015–16, 158 students received support. Federal Work-Study and scholarships/grants available. Financial award application deadline: 5/1; financial award applicants required to submit FAFSA. *Faculty research:* Pediatric sport-related concussion, adolescent athlete health-related quality of life; geriatric and pediatric well-being, pain management for participation, practice-based research network, BMI and dental caries. *Total annual research expenditures:* $156,319. *Unit head:* Dr. Randy Danielsen, Dean, 480-219-6000, Fax: 480-219-6110, E-mail: rdanielsen@atsu.edu. *Application contact:* Donna Sparks, Associate Director, Admissions Processing, 660-626-2117, Fax: 660-626-2969, E-mail: admissions@atsu.edu. Website: http://www.atsu.edu/ashs

Augusta University, College of Allied Health Sciences, Department of Occupational Therapy, Augusta, GA 30912. Offers MHS. *Accreditation:* AOTA. *Program availability:* Part-time. *Degree requirements:* For master's, thesis. *Entrance requirements:* For master's, GRE General Test. Additional exam requirements/recommendations for international students: Required—TOEFL (minimum score 550 paper-based; 79 iBT). *Application deadline:* For fall admission, 2/15 for domestic students. Applications are processed on a rolling basis. Application fee: $30. Electronic applications accepted. *Financial support:* Federal Work-Study and institutionally sponsored loans available. Support available to part-time students. Financial award application deadline: 5/31; financial award applicants required to submit FAFSA. *Unit head:* Dr. Michael K. Iwama, Chair, 706-721-3641, Fax: 706-721-9718. *Application contact:* Phoebe Prestridge, Office Coordinator, 706-721-3641, Fax: 706-721-7279, E-mail: studyot@augusta.edu. Website: http://www.augusta.edu/alliedhealth/ot/

Barry University, College of Health Sciences, Program in Occupational Therapy, Miami Shores, FL 33161-6695. Offers MS. *Accreditation:* AOTA. Electronic applications accepted.

Bay Path University, Program in Occupational Therapy, Longmeadow, MA 01106-2292. Offers MOT. *Accreditation:* AOTA. *Program availability:* Part-time. *Students:* 241 full-time (219 women), 13 part-time (all women); includes 39 minority (6 Black or African American, non-Hispanic/Latino; 8 Asian, non-Hispanic/Latino; 16 Hispanic/Latino; 9 Two or more races, non-Hispanic/Latino), 1 international. Average age 26. 357 applicants, 66% accepted, 130 enrolled. In 2015, 119 master's awarded. *Degree requirements:* For master's, 78 credits and 24 weeks of full-time level II fieldwork following completion of all academic courses. *Entrance requirements:* For master's, bachelor's degree with minimum GPA of 3.0; two courses in anatomy and physiology, and one course each in developmental psychology, statistics, and sociology or culture (for occupational therapy). *Application deadline:* For fall admission, 3/1 priority date for domestic students. Applications are processed on a rolling basis. Application fee: $45. Electronic applications accepted. Application fee is waived when completed online. *Expenses:* Contact institution. *Financial support:* In 2015–16, 83 students received support. Scholarships/grants available. Financial award applicants required to submit FAFSA. *Unit head:* Dr. Lori Vaughn, Assistant Dean/Program Director, 413-565-1012, E-mail: lvaughn@baypath.edu. *Application contact:* Diane Ranaldi, Dean of Graduate Admissions, 413-565-1332, Fax: 413-565-1250, E-mail: dranaldi@baypath.edu. Website: http://graduate.baypath.edu/Graduate-Programs/Programs-On-Campus/MS-Programs/Master-of-Occupational-Therapy

Belmont University, College of Health Sciences, Nashville, TN 37212-3757. Offers nursing (MSN, DNP); occupational therapy (MSOT, OTD); physical therapy (DPT). *Program availability:* Part-time, online learning. *Faculty:* 54 full-time (50 women), 92 part-time/adjunct (81 women). *Students:* 371 full-time (324 women), 10 part-time (all women); includes 30 minority (10 Black or African American, non-Hispanic/Latino; 9 Asian, non-Hispanic/Latino; 6 Hispanic/Latino; 5 Two or more races, non-Hispanic/Latino), 2 international. Average age 26. *Degree requirements:* For master's, comprehensive exam, thesis; for doctorate, comprehensive exam. *Entrance requirements:* For master's, GRE, BSN, minimum GPA of 3.0. Additional exam requirements/recommendations for international students: Required—TOEFL (minimum score 550 paper-based). *Application deadline:* Applications are processed on a rolling

basis. Application fee: $50. Electronic applications accepted. *Expenses:* Contact institution. *Financial support:* Teaching assistantships with full tuition reimbursements, career-related internships or fieldwork, scholarships/grants, and traineeships available. Financial award application deadline: 3/1; financial award applicants required to submit FAFSA. *Unit head:* Dr. Cathy Taylor, Dean, 615-460-6916, Fax: 615-460-6750. *Application contact:* David Mee, Dean of Enrollment Services, 615-460-6785, Fax: 615-460-5434, E-mail: david.mee@belmont.edu. Website: http://www.belmont.edu/healthsciences

Boston University, College of Health and Rehabilitation Sciences: Sargent College, Department of Occupational Therapy, Boston, MA 02215. Offers occupational therapy (OTD); rehabilitation sciences (PhD). *Accreditation:* AOTA (one or more programs are accredited). *Program availability:* Blended/hybrid learning. *Faculty:* 13 full-time (all women), 2 part-time/adjunct (both women). *Students:* 151 full-time (141 women), 25 part-time (24 women); includes 36 minority (19 Asian, non-Hispanic/Latino; 10 Hispanic/Latino; 7 Two or more races, non-Hispanic/Latino), 5 international. Average age 26. 487 applicants, 20% accepted, 29 enrolled. In 2015, 5 doctorates awarded. *Degree requirements:* For doctorate, comprehensive exam, thesis/dissertation. *Entrance requirements:* For doctorate, GRE General Test. Additional exam requirements/recommendations for international students: Required—TOEFL (minimum score 550 paper-based; 84 iBT), TWE (minimum score 5). *Application deadline:* For fall admission, 1/15 priority date for domestic and international students. Applications are processed on a rolling basis. Application fee: $125. Electronic applications accepted. *Expenses:* $1,537 per credit. *Financial support:* In 2015–16, 68 students received support, including 7 research assistantships with full tuition reimbursements available (averaging $21,000 per year), 9 teaching assistantships (averaging $2,500 per year); career-related internships or fieldwork, Federal Work-Study, institutionally sponsored loans, and scholarships/grants also available. Financial award application deadline: 2/15; financial award applicants required to submit FAFSA. *Faculty research:* Sensory integration, outcomes measurement, impact of Parkinson's disease, families of people with autism. *Total annual research expenditures:* $700,000. *Unit head:* Dr. Ellen Cohn, Program Director, 617-358-1063, Fax: 617-353-2926, E-mail: ecohn@bu.edu. *Application contact:* Sharon Sankey, Assistant Dean, Student Services, 617-353-2713, Fax: 617-353-7500, E-mail: ssankey@bu.edu. Website: http://www.bu.edu/sargent/

Brenau University, Sydney O. Smith Graduate School, College of Health and Science, Gainesville, GA 30501. Offers family nurse practitioner (MSN); nurse educator (MSN); nursing management (MSN); occupational therapy (MS); psychology (MS). *Accreditation:* AOTA. *Program availability:* Part-time, evening/weekend. *Degree requirements:* For master's, comprehensive exam (for some programs), thesis (for some programs), clinical practicum hours. *Entrance requirements:* For master's, GRE General Test or MAT (for some programs), interview, writing sample, references (for some programs). Additional exam requirements/recommendations for international students: Required—TOEFL (minimum score 500 paper-based; 61 iBT); Recommended—IELTS (minimum score 5). Electronic applications accepted. *Expenses:* Contact institution.

Cabarrus College of Health Sciences, Program in Occupational Therapy, Concord, NC 28025. Offers MOT.

California State University, Dominguez Hills, College of Health, Human Services and Nursing, Program in Occupational Therapy, Carson, CA 90747-0001. Offers MS. *Accreditation:* AOTA. *Degree requirements:* For master's, comprehensive exam. *Entrance requirements:* For master's, GRE. Additional exam requirements/recommendations for international students: Required—TOEFL, TWE. *Application deadline:* For fall admission, 9/15 priority date for domestic students. Electronic applications accepted. *Faculty research:* Child school functioning, assessment, lifespan occupational development, low vision occupational therapy intervention. *Unit head:* Dr. Terry Peralta-Catipon, Department Chair, 310-243-2812, E-mail: tperalta@csudh.edu. *Application contact:* Brandy McLelland, Director of Student Information Services/Registrar, 310-243-3645, E-mail: bmclelland@csudh.edu. Website: http://www4.csudh.edu/ot/program/

Chatham University, Program in Occupational Therapy, Pittsburgh, PA 15232-2826. Offers MOT, OTD. *Accreditation:* AOTA. *Faculty:* 7 full-time (all women), 10 part-time/adjunct (all women). *Students:* 114 full-time (105 women), 29 part-time (24 women); includes 22 minority (8 Black or African American, non-Hispanic/Latino; 6 Asian, non-Hispanic/Latino; 7 Hispanic/Latino; 1 Two or more races, non-Hispanic/Latino). Average age 31. 509 applicants, 20% accepted, 66 enrolled. In 2015, 38 master's, 40 doctorates awarded. *Entrance requirements:* For master's, recommendation letter, community service, volunteer service. Additional exam requirements/recommendations for international students: Required—TOEFL (minimum score 600 paper-based; 100 iBT), IELTS (minimum score 7), TWE. *Application deadline:* For fall admission, 12/5 priority date for domestic and international students. Applications are processed on a rolling basis. Application fee: $45. Electronic applications accepted. Application fee is waived when completed online. *Expenses:* $9,952 per semester tuition; $230 per semester campus fee; $190 per semester lab and insurance fee. *Financial support:* Applicants required to submit FAFSA. *Unit head:* Dr. Joyce Salls, Director, 412-365-1177, E-mail: salls@chatham.edu. *Application contact:* Ashlee Bartko, Senior Assistant Director of Graduate Admission, 412-365-1115, Fax: 412-365-1609, E-mail: gradadmissions@chatham.edu. Website: http://www.chatham.edu/ot

Chicago State University, School of Graduate and Professional Studies, College of Health Sciences, Department of Occupational Therapy, Chicago, IL 60628. Offers MOT. *Accreditation:* AOTA. *Program availability:* Part-time. *Entrance requirements:* For master's, bachelor's degree from accredited college or university with minimum GPA of 3.0 in final 60 semester credit hours; two recommendations; human service experience; essay; interview.

Clarkson University, Graduate School, School of Arts and Sciences, Department of Occupational Therapy, Potsdam, NY 13699. Offers MS. *Faculty:* 3 full-time (2 women), 3 part-time/adjunct (all women). *Students:* 20 full-time (18 women); includes 8 minority (3 Black or African American, non-Hispanic/Latino; 4 Asian, non-Hispanic/Latino; 1 Hispanic/Latino). Average age 25. 85 applicants, 24% accepted, 20 enrolled. *Entrance requirements:* For master's, GRE, Occupational Therapy Centralized Application Service (OTCAS) application, including transcripts of all college coursework, observation/volunteer or work experience in the field of study, personal statement, and three letters of recommendation; on-campus interview (may be satisfied via tele-meeting technology). Additional exam requirements/recommendations for international students: Required—TOEFL or IELTS. *Application deadline:* Applications are processed on a rolling basis. Application fee: $190. Electronic applications accepted. *Financial support:* In 2015–16, 1 student received support. Scholarships/grants available. *Unit head:* Dr. Rondalyn Whitney, Chair, 315-268-4412, E-mail: rwhitney@clarkson.edu. *Application contact:* Melissa Roberts, Health Professions Graduate Admissions Coordinator, 315-268-7942, E-mail: mroberts@clarkson.edu. Website: http://www.clarkson.edu/ot/

Cleveland State University, College of Graduate Studies, College of Sciences and Health Professions, School of Health Sciences, Program in Occupational Therapy,

Cleveland, OH 44115. Offers MOT. *Accreditation:* AOTA. *Faculty:* 7 full-time (5 women), 2 part-time/adjunct (both women). *Students:* 88 full-time (84 women), 45 part-time (36 women); includes 10 minority (3 Black or African American, non-Hispanic/Latino; 2 Asian, non-Hispanic/Latino; 5 Hispanic/Latino), 1 international. Average age 26. 163 applicants, 30% accepted, 45 enrolled. In 2015, 29 master's awarded. *Degree requirements:* For master's, fieldwork, capstone research project. *Entrance requirements:* For master's, GRE (if overall GPA less than 3.0). Additional exam requirements/recommendations for international students: Recommended—TOEFL (minimum score 550 paper-based; 78 iBT), IELTS (minimum score 6). *Application deadline:* For fall admission, 1/15 priority date for domestic and international students. Application fee: $55. Electronic applications accepted. *Expenses:* Tuition, state resident: full-time $9565. Tuition, nonresident: full-time $17,980. Tuition and fees vary according to program. *Financial support:* In 2015–16, 9 students received support, including 9 teaching assistantships (averaging $11,000 per year); unspecified assistantships also available. Financial award application deadline: 3/15; financial award applicants required to submit FAFSA. *Faculty research:* Pediatrics, psychology, daily living, exercise physiology, neuromuscular disorders. *Total annual research expenditures:* $620,000. *Unit head:* Dr. Glenn D. Goodman, Director, 216-687-2493, Fax: 216-687-9316, E-mail: g.goodman@csuohio.edu. *Application contact:* Karen Armstrong, Administrative Assistant, 216-687-3567, Fax: 216-687-9316, E-mail: k.bradley@csuohio.edu.
Website: http://www.csuohio.edu/sciences/dept/healthsciences/graduate/MOT/index.html

College of Saint Mary, Program in Occupational Therapy, Omaha, NE 68106. Offers MOT. *Accreditation:* AOTA.

The College of St. Scholastica, Graduate Studies, Department of Occupational Therapy, Duluth, MN 55811-4199. Offers MA. *Accreditation:* AOTA. *Program availability:* Part-time. *Degree requirements:* For master's, thesis. *Entrance requirements:* Additional exam requirements/recommendations for international students: Required—TOEFL (minimum score 550 paper-based; 79 iBT). Electronic applications accepted. *Faculty research:* Gerontology, occupational therapy administration, neurorehabilitation, occupational therapy in nontraditional settings, clinical fieldwork issues.

Colorado State University, College of Health and Human Sciences, Department of Occupational Therapy, Fort Collins, CO 80523-1573. Offers MOT, MS, PhD. *Accreditation:* AOTA. *Faculty:* 10 full-time (7 women), 1 (woman) part-time/adjunct. *Students:* 117 full-time (105 women), 9 part-time (8 women); includes 17 minority (2 Asian, non-Hispanic/Latino; 12 Hispanic/Latino; 3 Two or more races, non-Hispanic/Latino), 3 international. Average age 28. 477 applicants, 12% accepted, 52 enrolled. In 2015, 48 master's awarded. *Degree requirements:* For master's, thesis (for some programs); for doctorate, comprehensive exam, thesis/dissertation. *Entrance requirements:* For master's and doctorate, GRE General Test, minimum cumulative undergraduate or master's GPA of 3.0. Additional exam requirements/recommendations for international students: Required—TOEFL (minimum score 587 paper-based). *Application deadline:* For fall admission, 1/15 for domestic and international students. Application fee: $60 ($70 for international students). Electronic applications accepted. *Expenses:* Contact institution. *Financial support:* In 2015–16, 90 students received support, including 10 research assistantships with partial tuition reimbursements available (averaging $20,636 per year), 2 teaching assistantships with partial tuition reimbursements available (averaging $7,099 per year); fellowships with partial tuition reimbursements available, scholarships/grants, and unspecified assistantships also available. Financial award application deadline: 1/15. *Faculty research:* Cognitive, motor, sensory and neurophysiological performance; everyday occupation, disability, rehabilitation and health; education from an occupation and rehabilitation science perspective. *Total annual research expenditures:* $713,229. *Unit head:* Dr. Anita Bundy, Department Head, 970-491-3105, Fax: 970-491-6290, E-mail: anita.bundy@colostate.edu. *Application contact:* Linda McDowell, MOT and MS Programs Coordinator, 970-491-6243, Fax: 970-491-6290, E-mail: linda.mcdowell@colostate.edu. Website: http://www.ot.chhs.colostate.edu/

Columbia University, College of Physicians and Surgeons, Programs in Occupational Therapy, New York, NY 10032. Offers movement science (Ed D), including occupational therapy; occupational therapy (professional) (MS); occupational therapy administration or education (post-professional) (MS); MPH/MS. *Accreditation:* AOTA. *Degree requirements:* For master's, project, 6 months of fieldwork, thesis (for post-professional students); for doctorate, comprehensive exam, thesis/dissertation. *Entrance requirements:* For master's, undergraduate course work in anatomy, physiology, statistics, psychology, social sciences, humanities, English composition; NBCOT eligibility; for doctorate, NBCOT certification, MS. Additional exam requirements/recommendations for international students: Required—TOEFL (minimum score 100 iBT), TWE (minimum score 4). Electronic applications accepted. *Expenses:* Contact institution. *Faculty research:* Community mental health, developmental tasks of late life, infant play, cognition, obesity, motor learning.

Concordia University Wisconsin, Graduate Programs, School of Human Services, Program in Occupational Therapy, Mequon, WI 53097-2402. Offers MOT. *Accreditation:* AOTA. *Degree requirements:* For master's, comprehensive exam, thesis or alternative. *Entrance requirements:* Additional exam requirements/recommendations for international students: Required—TOEFL.

Creighton University, School of Pharmacy and Health Professions, Program in Occupational Therapy, Omaha, NE 68178-0001. Offers OTD. *Accreditation:* AOTA. *Program availability:* Online learning. *Entrance requirements:* Additional exam requirements/recommendations for international students: Required—TOEFL. Electronic applications accepted. *Expenses: Tuition, area resident:* Full-time $14,400; part-time $800 per credit hour. *Required fees:* $158 per semester. Tuition and fees vary according to course load, campus/location, program, reciprocity agreements and student's religious affiliation. *Faculty research:* Patient safety in health services research, health information technology and health services research, health care services in minority and underserved populations, occupational therapy in school-based programs, educational technology use in the classroom.

Dalhousie University, Faculty of Health Professions, School of Occupational Therapy, Halifax, NS B3H3J5, Canada. Offers occupational therapy (entry to profession) (M Sc); occupational therapy (post-professional) (M Sc). *Program availability:* Part-time, evening/weekend, online learning. *Degree requirements:* For master's, thesis. *Entrance requirements:* Additional exam requirements/recommendations for international students: Required—TOEFL, IELTS, CANTEST, CAEL, or Michigan English Language Assessment Battery. Electronic applications accepted. *Faculty research:* Gender, health systems, design, geriatrics power and empowerment.

Dominican College, Division of Allied Health, Department of Occupational Therapy, Orangeburg, NY 10962-1210. Offers MS. Students enter program as undergraduates. *Accreditation:* AOTA. *Program availability:* Part-time, evening/weekend. *Degree requirements:* For master's, 2 clinical affiliations. *Entrance requirements:* For master's, minimum GPA of 3.0, writing sample, 3 letters of recommendation. Additional exam requirements/recommendations for international students: Required—TOEFL (minimum score 550 paper-based).

Dominican University of California, School of Health and Natural Sciences, Program in Occupational Therapy, San Rafael, CA 94901-2298. Offers MS. *Accreditation:* AOTA. *Faculty:* 7 full-time (6 women), 6 part-time/adjunct (all women). *Students:* 77 full-time (64 women), 20 part-time (19 women); includes 43 minority (30 Asian, non-Hispanic/Latino; 10 Hispanic/Latino; 3 Two or more races, non-Hispanic/Latino). Average age 27. 143 applicants, 31% accepted, 28 enrolled. In 2015, 49 master's awarded. *Degree requirements:* For master's, thesis. *Entrance requirements:* For master's, GRE, minimum GPA of 3.0, minimum of 60 hours of volunteer experience. Additional exam requirements/recommendations for international students: Required—TOEFL (minimum score 550 paper-based; 80 iBT), IELTS (minimum score 6.5). *Application deadline:* For fall admission, 2/1 priority date for domestic students. Electronic applications accepted. *Expenses:* Contact institution. *Financial support:* Application deadline: 3/2; applicants required to submit FAFSA. *Unit head:* Dr. Ruth Ramsey, Department Chair and Program Director, 415-257-1393, E-mail: rramsey@dominican.edu. *Application contact:* Ryan Purtill, Admissions Counselor, 415-458-3748, Fax: 415-485-3214, E-mail: ryan.purtill@dominican.edu.
Website: http://www.dominican.edu/academics/hns/ot/grad

Duquesne University, John G. Rangos, Sr. School of Health Sciences, Pittsburgh, PA 15282-0001. Offers health management systems (MHMS); occupational therapy (MS, OTD); physical therapy (DPT); physician assistant studies (MPAS); rehabilitation science (MS, PhD); speech-language pathology (MS); MBA/MHMS. *Accreditation:* AOTA (one or more programs are accredited); APTA (one or more programs are accredited); ASHA. *Program availability:* Minimal on-campus study. *Faculty:* 45 full-time (32 women), 33 part-time/adjunct (17 women). *Students:* 230 full-time (180 women), 11 part-time (5 women); includes 15 minority (1 Black or African American, non-Hispanic/Latino; 3 Asian, non-Hispanic/Latino; 7 Hispanic/Latino; 4 Two or more races, non-Hispanic/Latino), 20 international. Average age 23. 685 applicants, 9% accepted, 24 enrolled. In 2015, 132 master's, 32 doctorates awarded. *Degree requirements:* For doctorate, comprehensive exam (for some programs), thesis/dissertation (for some programs). *Entrance requirements:* For master's, GRE General Test (speech-language pathology), 3 letters of recommendation; minimum GPA of 2.75 (health management systems), 3.0 (speech-language pathology); for doctorate, GRE General Test (for physical therapy and rehabilitation science), 3 letters of recommendation, minimum GPA of 3.0, personal interview. Additional exam requirements/recommendations for international students: Required—TOEFL (minimum score 550 paper-based; 90 iBT). *Application deadline:* For fall admission, 2/1 for domestic and international students; for spring admission, 7/1 for domestic and international students. Applications are processed on a rolling basis. Application fee: $0. Electronic applications accepted. *Expenses:* $1,254 per credit. *Financial support:* Federal Work-Study available. Financial award applicants required to submit FAFSA. *Faculty research:* Neuronal processing, electrical stimulation on peripheral neuropathy, central nervous system (CNS) stimulatory and inhibitory signals, behavioral genetic methodologies to development disorders of speech, neurogenic communication disorders. *Total annual research expenditures:* $38,730. *Unit head:* Dr. Gregory H. Frazer, Dean, 412-396-5303, Fax: 412-396-5554, E-mail: frazer@duq.edu. *Application contact:* Christopher R. Hilf, Recruiter/Academic Advisor, 412-396-5653, Fax: 412-396-5554, E-mail: hilfc@duq.edu.
Website: http://www.duq.edu/academics/schools/health-sciences

D'Youville College, Occupational Therapy Department, Buffalo, NY 14201-1084. Offers MS. *Accreditation:* AOTA. *Students:* 262 full-time (242 women), 29 part-time (26 women); includes 33 minority (11 Black or African American, non-Hispanic/Latino; 1 American Indian or Alaska Native, non-Hispanic/Latino; 9 Asian, non-Hispanic/Latino; 7 Hispanic/Latino; 5 Two or more races, non-Hispanic/Latino), 9 international. Average age 23. 361 applicants, 44% accepted, 81 enrolled. In 2015, 70 master's awarded. *Degree requirements:* For master's, research project or thesis. *Entrance requirements:* For master's, minimum undergraduate GPA of 3.0. Additional exam requirements/recommendations for international students: Required—TOEFL (minimum score 500 paper-based). *Application deadline:* For fall admission, 5/1 priority date for international students; for spring admission, 9/1 priority date for international students. Applications are processed on a rolling basis. Electronic applications accepted. *Expenses: Tuition, area resident:* Full-time $21,120; part-time $880 per credit hour. *Required fees:* $235; $96. One-time fee: $100. *Financial support:* Scholarships/grants, tuition waivers (partial), and unspecified assistantships available. *Faculty research:* Learning styles, range of motion in the elderly, hospice care, culture, health, differences in education and performance of Afro-American children, autistic spectrum disorder and social stories, autistic disorders and listening programs. *Unit head:* Dr. Theresa Vallone, Chair, 716-829-7831, Fax: 716-829-8137. *Application contact:* Mark Pavone, Graduate Admissions Director, 716-829-8400, Fax: 716-829-7900, E-mail: graduateadmissions@dyc.edu.

East Carolina University, Graduate School, College of Allied Health Sciences, Department of Addictions and Rehabilitation Studies, Greenville, NC 27858-4353. Offers military and trauma counseling (Certificate); rehabilitation and career counseling (MS); rehabilitation counseling (Certificate); rehabilitation counseling and administration (PhD); substance abuse and clinical counseling (MS); substance abuse counseling (Certificate); vocational evaluation (Certificate). *Accreditation:* CORE. *Program availability:* Part-time, evening/weekend. *Students:* 77 full-time (57 women), 15 part-time (14 women); includes 23 minority (14 Black or African American, non-Hispanic/Latino; 8 Hispanic/Latino; 1 Two or more races, non-Hispanic/Latino). Average age 30. 45 applicants, 73% accepted, 25 enrolled. In 2015, 24 master's, 3 doctorates awarded. *Degree requirements:* For master's, comprehensive exam, thesis or alternative, internship. *Entrance requirements:* For master's, GRE General Test or MAT. Additional exam requirements/recommendations for international students: Required—TOEFL. *Application deadline:* For fall admission, 3/1 priority date for domestic students; for spring admission, 10/1 priority date for domestic students. Applications are processed on a rolling basis. Application fee: $50. *Financial support:* Research assistantships with partial tuition reimbursements, teaching assistantships with partial tuition reimbursements, Federal Work-Study, and scholarships/grants available. Support available to part-time students. Financial award application deadline: 3/1. *Unit head:* Dr. Paul Toriello, Chair, 252-744-6292, E-mail: toriellop@ecu.edu.
Website: http://www.ecu.edu/rehb/

East Carolina University, Graduate School, College of Allied Health Sciences, Department of Occupational Therapy, Greenville, NC 27858-4353. Offers MSOT. *Accreditation:* AOTA. *Program availability:* Part-time, online learning. *Students:* 62 full-time (57 women), 11 part-time (9 women); includes 3 minority (1 Black or African American, non-Hispanic/Latino; 1 Asian, non-Hispanic/Latino; 1 Two or more races, non-Hispanic/Latino). Average age 26. 280 applicants, 13% accepted, 24 enrolled. In 2015, 25 master's awarded. *Degree requirements:* For master's, comprehensive exam, thesis or research project. *Entrance requirements:* For master's, GRE General Test. Additional exam requirements/recommendations for international students: Required—TOEFL. *Application deadline:* For fall admission, 6/1 for domestic students. Applications are processed on a rolling basis. Application fee: $50. Electronic applications accepted. *Financial support:* Research assistantships, career-related internships or fieldwork, and Federal Work-Study available. Financial award application deadline: 6/1; financial award applicants required to submit FAFSA. *Faculty research:* Quality of life, assistive technology, environmental contributions, modifications of occupation to health,

Occupational Therapy

therapeutic activities. *Unit head:* Dr. Leonard Trujillo, Chair, 252-744-6195, E-mail: trujillol@ecu.edu. *Application contact:* Dean of Graduate School, 252-328-6012, Fax: 252-328-6071, E-mail: gradschool@ecu.edu. *Website:* http://www.ecu.edu/ot/

Eastern Kentucky University, The Graduate School, College of Health Sciences, Department of Occupational Therapy, Richmond, KY 40475-3102. Offers MS. *Accreditation:* AOTA. *Program availability:* Part-time. *Degree requirements:* For master's, thesis optional. *Entrance requirements:* For master's, GRE General Test, minimum GPA of 3.0. *Faculty research:* Rehabilitation, pediatrics, leadership issues.

Eastern Michigan University, Graduate School, College of Health and Human Services, School of Health Sciences, Programs in Occupational Therapy, Ypsilanti, MI 48197. Offers MOT, MS. *Accreditation:* AOTA. *Program availability:* Part-time, evening/ weekend, online learning. *Students:* 59 full-time (51 women), 1 (woman) part-time; includes 3 minority (1 Black or African American, non-Hispanic/Latino; 1 Asian, non-Hispanic/Latino; 1 Hispanic/Latino). Average age 28. 4 applicants. In 2015, 36 master's awarded. *Entrance requirements:* Additional exam requirements/recommendations for international students: Required—TOEFL. *Application deadline:* Applications are processed on a rolling basis. Application fee: $45. *Financial support:* Fellowships, research assistantships with full tuition reimbursements, teaching assistantships with full tuition reimbursements, career-related internships or fieldwork, Federal Work-Study, institutionally sponsored loans, scholarships/grants, tuition waivers (partial), and unspecified assistantships available. Support available to part-time students. Financial award applicants required to submit FAFSA. *Application contact:* Sharon Holt, Advisor, 734-487-4096, Fax: 734-487-4095, E-mail: ot_intent_advising@emich.edu.

Eastern Washington University, Graduate Studies, College of Science, Health and Engineering, Department of Occupational Therapy, Cheney, WA 99004-2431. Offers MOT. *Accreditation:* AOTA. *Degree requirements:* For master's, comprehensive exam.

Elizabethtown College, Department of Occupational Therapy, Elizabethtown, PA 17022-2298. Offers MS. *Accreditation:* AOTA.

Florida Agricultural and Mechanical University, Division of Graduate Studies, Research, and Continuing Education, School of Allied Health Sciences, Division of Occupational Therapy, Tallahassee, FL 32307-3200. Offers MOT. *Accreditation:* AOTA.

Florida Gulf Coast University, College of Health Professions and Social Work, Department of Occupational Therapy, Fort Myers, FL 33965-6565. Offers MS. *Accreditation:* AOTA. *Faculty:* 57 full-time (40 women), 39 part-time/adjunct (23 women). *Students:* 63 full-time (55 women); includes 10 minority (1 Asian, non-Hispanic/Latino; 6 Hispanic/Latino; 3 Two or more races, non-Hispanic/Latino). Average age 27. 223 applicants, 15% accepted, 32 enrolled. In 2015, 30 master's awarded. *Entrance requirements:* For master's, GRE General Test, MAT, minimum GPA of 3.0. Additional exam requirements/recommendations for international students: Required—TOEFL (minimum score 550 paper-based). *Application deadline:* For fall admission, 2/1 for domestic students. Applications are processed on a rolling basis. Application fee: $30. Electronic applications accepted. *Expenses:* Tuition, state resident: full-time $6974. Tuition, nonresident: full-time $28,170. *Required fees:* $1987. One-time fee: $10 full-time. Tuition and fees vary according to course load and degree level. *Financial support:* In 2015–16, 31 students received support. Application deadline: 6/30; applicants required to submit FAFSA. *Unit head:* Dr. Eric Shamus, Head, 239-590-1418, Fax: 239-590-7474, E-mail: leshamus@fgcu.edu. *Application contact:* Wanda Smith, Office Manager, 239-590-7550, Fax: 239-590-7474, E-mail: wsmith@fgcu.edu.

Florida International University, College of Nursing and Health Sciences, Department of Occupational Therapy, Miami, FL 33199. Offers MSOT. *Accreditation:* AOTA. *Program availability:* Part-time. *Faculty:* 6 full-time (5 women), 9 part-time/adjunct (6 women). *Students:* 138 full-time (118 women), 14 part-time (13 women); includes 111 minority (13 Black or African American, non-Hispanic/Latino; 4 Asian, non-Hispanic/Latino; 88 Hispanic/Latino; 6 Two or more races, non-Hispanic/Latino, 1 international. Average age 25. 287 applicants, 20% accepted, 54 enrolled. In 2015, 56 master's awarded. *Entrance requirements:* For master's, thesis or alternative. *Entrance requirements:* For master's, minimum undergraduate GPA of 3.0 in upper-level course work, letter of intent, 3 letters of recommendation, resume. Additional exam requirements/recommendations for international students: Required—TOEFL (minimum score 550 paper-based; 80 iBT). *Application deadline:* For fall admission, 2/15 for domestic and international students. Applications are processed on a rolling basis. Application fee: $30. Electronic applications accepted. *Expenses:* Contact institution. *Financial support:* Career-related internships or fieldwork, Federal Work-Study, institutionally sponsored loans, scholarships/grants, and unspecified assistantships available. Financial award application deadline: 3/1; financial award applicants required to submit FAFSA. *Faculty research:* Senior transportation and driving, foster care, adolescent transitions, independent living skills development, family and patient-centered care, aging, quality of life, social justice, cognition. *Unit head:* Dr. Lynn Richard, Interim Chair, 305-348-2921, E-mail: lyrichar@fiu.edu. *Application contact:* Nanett Rojas, Manager, Admissions Operations, 305-348-7464, Fax: 305-348-7441, E-mail: gradadm@fiu.edu. *Website:* http://cnhs.fiu.edu/index.html

Gannon University, School of Graduate Studies, Morosky College of Health Professions and Sciences, School of Health Professions, Program in Occupational Therapy, Erie, PA 16541-0001. Offers MS, OTD. *Accreditation:* AOTA. *Students:* 76 full-time (71 women); includes 4 minority (2 Black or African American, non-Hispanic/Latino; 1 Asian, non-Hispanic/Latino; 1 Two or more races, non-Hispanic/Latino). Average age 23. 7 applicants. In 2015, 40 master's awarded. *Degree requirements:* For master's, thesis, field work; for doctorate, thesis/dissertation. *Entrance requirements:* For master's, bachelor's degree, Student Self-Report Transcript Evaluation, minimum GPA of 3.0, 40 hours of volunteer experience; for doctorate, bachelor's degree from accredited college or university with minimum GPA of 3.0, transcript, minimum of 40 hours of volunteer experience in an OT setting, Student Self-Report Transcript Evaluation. Additional exam requirements/recommendations for international students: Required—TOEFL (minimum score 79 iBT). *Application deadline:* For fall admission, 1/15 for domestic students. Application fee: $25. Electronic applications accepted. Application fee is waived when completed online. *Expenses:* Contact institution. *Financial support:* Federal Work-Study and unspecified assistantships available. Financial award application deadline: 7/1; financial award applicants required to submit FAFSA. *Faculty research:* Assistive technology, autism, sexuality in occupational therapy intervention, health and wellness in Parkinson's disease, occupational science. *Unit head:* Dr. David LeVan, Chairperson, 814-871-7730, E-mail: levan005@gannon.edu. *Application contact:* Kara Morgan, Director of Graduate Admissions, 814-871-5831, Fax: 814-871-5827, E-mail: graduate@gannon.edu.

Governors State University, College of Health Professions, Program in Occupational Therapy, University Park, IL 60484. Offers MOT. *Accreditation:* AOTA. *Degree requirements:* For master's, thesis or alternative. *Entrance requirements:* For master's, minimum GPA of 3.0 in field, 2.75 overall.

Grand Valley State University, College of Health Professions, Occupational Therapy Program, Allendale, MI 49401-9403. Offers MS. *Accreditation:* AOTA. *Faculty:* 9 full-time (7 women), 4 part-time/adjunct (all women). *Students:* 131 full-time (108 women), 21 part-time (17 women); includes 15 minority (3 Black or African American, non-

Hispanic/Latino; 5 Asian, non-Hispanic/Latino; 5 Hispanic/Latino; 2 Two or more races, non-Hispanic/Latino). Average age 27. 149 applicants, 44% accepted, 57 enrolled. In 2015, 49 master's awarded. *Degree requirements:* For master's, thesis or alternative, fieldwork, project. *Entrance requirements:* For master's, interview, volunteer work, writing sample. Additional exam requirements/recommendations for international students: Required—TOEFL (minimum score 610 paper-based). *Application deadline:* For winter admission, 1/15 priority date for domestic students. Applications are processed on a rolling basis. Application fee: $30. Electronic applications accepted. *Financial support:* In 2015–16, 21 students received support, including 16 fellowships (averaging $927 per year), 5 research assistantships with tuition reimbursements available (averaging $7,469 per year); unspecified assistantships also available. Financial award application deadline: 2/15. *Faculty research:* Teaching/learning methods, continuing professional education, clinical reasoning, geriatrics, performing artists. *Unit head:* Dr. Cynthia Grapczynski, Director, 616-331-2734, Fax: 616-331-3350, E-mail: grapczyc@gvsu.edu. *Application contact:* Darlene Zwart, Student Services Coordinator, 616-331-3958, E-mail: zwartda@gvsu.edu. *Website:* http://www.gvsu.edu/ot/

Husson University, Master of Science in Occupational Therapy Program, Bangor, ME 04401-2999. Offers MSOT. *Accreditation:* AOTA. *Faculty:* 6 full-time (5 women), 1 part-time/adjunct (0 women). *Students:* 57 full-time (53 women); includes 5 minority (2 Hispanic/Latino; 1 Native Hawaiian or other Pacific Islander, non-Hispanic/Latino; 2 Two or more races, non-Hispanic/Latino). Average age 25. 64 applicants, 23% accepted, 9 enrolled. In 2015, 35 master's awarded. *Degree requirements:* For master's, research project, paper and presentation. *Entrance requirements:* For master's, GRE, BS with minimum GPA of 3.0, letters of recommendation, statement of purpose essay. Additional exam requirements/recommendations for international students: Required—TOEFL (minimum score 550 paper-based; 80 iBT). *Application deadline:* For fall admission, 5/1 for domestic students. Application fee: $50 ($0 for international students). Electronic applications accepted. *Expenses:* $18,489 per year. *Financial support:* Federal Work-Study, scholarships/grants, and unspecified assistantships available. Financial award application deadline: 4/15; financial award applicants required to submit FAFSA. *Faculty research:* College student sleep patterns and the impact on performance of student occupations, grip strength and perceived ADL performance in older adults, use of literary narratives in the training of health care students, use of art for coping and stress reduction. *Unit head:* Dr. Laurie Mouradian, Program Director, 207-404-5630, E-mail: mouradianl@husson.edu. *Application contact:* Kristen Card, Director of Graduate Admissions, 207-404-5660, E-mail: cardk@husson.edu. *Website:* http://www.husson.edu/occupational-therapy

Idaho State University, Office of Graduate Studies, Kasiska College of Health Professions, Department of Physical and Occupational Therapy, Program in Occupational Therapy, Pocatello, ID 83209-8045. Offers MOT. *Accreditation:* AOTA. *Degree requirements:* For master's, comprehensive exam, thesis, oral and written exam. *Entrance requirements:* For master's, GRE General Test, minimum GPA of 3.0, 80 hours in 2 practice settings of occupational therapy. Additional exam requirements/recommendations for international students: Required—TOEFL (minimum score 600 paper-based). Electronic applications accepted. *Expenses:* Contact institution. *Faculty research:* Human movement, health care.

Indiana State University, College of Graduate and Professional Studies, College of Nursing, Health, and Human Services, Department of Applied Medicine and Rehabilitation, Terre Haute, IN 47809. Offers athletic training (MS, DAT); occupational therapy (MS); physical therapy (DPT); physician assistant (MS). *Degree requirements:* For master's, thesis or alternative. *Entrance requirements:* For master's, GRE General Test. Electronic applications accepted.

Indiana University–Purdue University Indianapolis, School of Health and Rehabilitation Sciences, Indianapolis, IN 46202-5119. Offers health and rehabilitation sciences (PhD); health sciences (MS); nutrition and dietetics (MS); occupational therapy (MS); physical therapy (DPT); physician assistant (MPAS). *Program availability:* Part-time, evening/weekend. *Degree requirements:* For master's, thesis (for some programs). *Entrance requirements:* For master's, GRE General Test, minimum GPA of 3.0 (for MS in health sciences, nutrition and dietetics), 3.2 (for MS in occupational therapy), 3.0 cumulative and prerequisite math/science (for MPAS); for doctorate, GRE, minimum cumulative and prerequisite math/science GPA of 3.2. Additional exam requirements/recommendations for international students: Required—TOEFL (minimum score 550 paper-based; 79 iBT), IELTS (minimum score 6.5), PTE (minimum score 54). Electronic applications accepted. *Expenses:* Contact institution. *Faculty research:* Function and mobility across the lifespan, pediatric nutrition, driving and mobility rehabilitation, neurorehabilitation and biomechanics, rehabilitation and integrative therapy.

Ithaca College, School of Health Sciences and Human Performance, Program in Occupational Therapy, Ithaca, NY 14850. Offers occupational therapy (MS). *Accreditation:* AOTA. *Faculty:* 12 full-time (all women). *Students:* 61 full-time (56 women), 2 part-time (both women); includes 9 minority (2 Black or African American, non-Hispanic/Latino; 3 Asian, non-Hispanic/Latino; 3 Hispanic/Latino; 1 Two or more races, non-Hispanic/Latino). Average age 23. In 2015, 43 master's awarded. *Degree requirements:* For master's, thesis optional, clinical fieldwork. *Entrance requirements:* Additional exam requirements/recommendations for international students: Required—TOEFL (minimum score 550 paper-based; 80 iBT). *Expenses:* Contact institution. *Financial support:* In 2015–16, 45 students received support, including 11 teaching assistantships (averaging $13,853 per year); career-related internships or fieldwork, Federal Work-Study, and scholarships/grants also available. Support available to part-time students. Financial award application deadline: 3/1; financial award applicants required to submit CSS PROFILE or FAFSA. *Faculty research:* Sensory integration intervention, therapeutic listening, motor control intervention for pediatrics and adults, adult neuromuscular facilitation for individuals with neurological impairments, school-aged handwriting assessment, psychosocial community, intervention and assessment, virtual reality and robotic training for children with neurological and or sensory disorders, clinical reasoning, aging and human occupations. *Unit head:* Dr. Melinda Cozzolino, Chair, 607-274-3618, Fax: 607-274-1263, E-mail: mcozzoli@ithaca.edu. *Application contact:* Nicole Eversley Bradwell, Interim Director, Office of Admission, 607-274-3124, Fax: 607-274-1263, E-mail: admission@ithaca.edu. *Website:* http://www.ithaca.edu/gradprograms/ot

James Madison University, The Graduate School, College of Health and Behavioral Sciences, Program in Occupational Therapy, Harrisonburg, VA 22807. Offers MOT. *Accreditation:* AOTA. *Program availability:* Part-time. *Students:* 60 full-time (54 women), 1 part-time (0 women); includes 8 minority (3 Asian, non-Hispanic/Latino; 2 Hispanic/Latino; 3 Two or more races, non-Hispanic/Latino). Average age 30. 105 applicants, 23% accepted, 22 enrolled. In 2015, 25 master's awarded. Application fee: $55. Electronic applications accepted. *Financial support:* In 2015–16, 10 fellowships were awarded. Financial award application deadline: 3/1; financial award applicants required to submit FAFSA. *Unit head:* Dr. Allen Lewis, Interim Department Head, 540-568-6510, E-mail: amatohk@jmu.edu. *Application contact:* Lynette D. Michael, Director of Graduate Admissions, 540-568-6131 Ext. 6395, Fax: 540-568-7860, E-mail: michaeld@jmu.edu. *Website:* http://www.healthsci.jmu.edu/occupationaltherapy

Jefferson College of Health Sciences, Program in Occupational Therapy, Roanoke, VA 24013. Offers MS. *Accreditation:* AOTA. *Program availability:* Part-time. *Entrance requirements:* For master's, GRE. Additional exam requirements/recommendations for international students: Required—TOEFL (minimum score 550 paper-based; 80 iBT). Electronic applications accepted.

Kean University, Nathan Weiss Graduate College, Program in Occupational Therapy, Union, NJ 07083. Offers MS. *Accreditation:* AOTA. *Program availability:* Part-time. *Faculty:* 5 full-time (all women). *Students:* 71 full-time (62 women), 30 part-time (29 women); includes 27 minority (2 Black or African American, non-Hispanic/Latino; 7 Asian, non-Hispanic/Latino; 16 Hispanic/Latino; 1 Native Hawaiian or other Pacific Islander, non-Hispanic/Latino; 1 Two or more races, non-Hispanic/Latino). Average age 25. 302 applicants, 13% accepted, 37 enrolled. In 2015, 31 master's awarded. *Degree requirements:* For master's, 6 months of field work, final project. *Entrance requirements:* For master's, minimum GPA of 3.0, minimum grade of B in each prerequisite course, official transcripts from all institutions attended, three letters of recommendation (one letter must be from an occupational therapist), documented observation of occupational therapy services in two or more practice settings for a minimum of 40 hours, resume, personal statement. Additional exam requirements/recommendations for international students: Required—TOEFL (minimum score 550 paper-based; 79 iBT), IELTS. *Application deadline:* For fall admission, 2/2 for domestic and international students. Applications are processed on a rolling basis. Application fee: $75. Electronic applications accepted. *Expenses:* Tuition, state resident: full-time $12,835; part-time $625 per credit. Tuition, nonresident: full-time $17,396; part-time $766 per credit. *Required fees:* $3235; $147 per credit. Tuition and fees vary according to course level, course load, degree level and program. *Financial support:* In 2015–16, 7 research assistantships with full tuition reimbursements (averaging $3,771 per year) were awarded; scholarships/grants and unspecified assistantships also available. Financial award applicants required to submit FAFSA. *Unit head:* Dr. Laurie Knis-Matthews, Program Coordinator, 908-737-5850, Fax: 908-737-5855, E-mail: ot@kean.edu. *Application contact:* Brittany Gerstenhaber, Admissions Counselor, 908-737-7100, E-mail: grad-adm@kean.edu.
Website: http://grad.kean.edu/ot

Keuka College, Program in Occupational Therapy, Keuka Park, NY 14478-0098. Offers MS. *Accreditation:* AOTA. *Faculty:* 6 full-time (all women), 2 part-time/adjunct (0 women). *Students:* 38 full-time (32 women); includes 4 minority (2 Black or African American, non-Hispanic/Latino; 2 Asian, non-Hispanic/Latino). Average age 24. 38 applicants, 97% accepted, 37 enrolled. In 2015, 37 master's awarded. *Degree requirements:* For master's, thesis, clinical internships. *Entrance requirements:* For master's, minimum GPA of 3.0, bachelor's degree in occupational therapy from Keuka College. Additional exam requirements/recommendations for international students: Required—TOEFL (minimum score 550 paper-based). *Application deadline:* For fall admission, 8/15 priority date for domestic students; for winter admission, 12/15 priority date for domestic students; for spring admission, 4/15 priority date for domestic students. Applications are processed on a rolling basis. Application fee: $50. Electronic applications accepted. *Expenses:* Contact institution. *Financial support:* In 2015–16, 3 students received support. Scholarships/grants and tuition waivers available. Financial award applicants required to submit FAFSA. *Faculty research:* Joint mobility applications; driving competence and aging; inter-professional education; history of OT; interdisciplinary service learning. *Unit head:* Dr. Dianne Trickey-Rokenbrok, Associate Professor/Chair/Program Director, 315-279-5608, Fax: 315-279-5439, E-mail: dtrickey@keuka.edu. *Application contact:* Jennifer Nielsen, Transfer Counselor, Admissions, 315-279-5203, Fax: 315-279-5386, E-mail: jnielsen@keuka.edu.

Le Moyne College, Department of Occupational Therapy, Syracuse, NY 13214. Offers MS.

Lenoir-Rhyne University, Graduate Programs, School of Occupational Therapy, Hickory, NC 28601. Offers MS. *Accreditation:* AOTA. *Faculty:* 4 full-time (all women). *Students:* 61 full-time (59 women), 1 (woman) part-time; includes 4 minority (2 Hispanic/Latino; 2 Two or more races, non-Hispanic/Latino). Average age 25. In 2015, 19 master's awarded. *Entrance requirements:* For master's, GRE, official transcripts, three letters of recommendation, essay, criminal background check. *Application deadline:* For summer admission, 1/31 for domestic students. Application fee: $35. *Expenses:* $750 per credit hour tuition. *Financial support:* Research assistantships available. Financial award applicants required to submit FAFSA. *Unit head:* Dr. Toni Oakes, Coordinator, 828-328-7366, E-mail: oakes@lrc.edu. *Application contact:* Mary Ann Gosnell, Director of Graduate Recruiting, 828-328-3711, E-mail: maryann.gosnell@lr.edu.

Loma Linda University, School of Allied Health Professions, Department of Occupational Therapy, Loma Linda, CA 92350. Offers MOT, OTD. *Accreditation:* AOTA. Application fee: $60. *Unit head:* Dr. Liane Hewitt, Chair, 909-558-1000. *Application contact:* Helen Greenwood, Director, Admissions and Records, 909-824-4599, Fax: 909-824-4809, E-mail: hgreenwood@sahp.llu.edu.

Long Island University–LIU Brooklyn, School of Health Professions, Brooklyn, NY 11201-8423. Offers athletic training and sport sciences (MS); exercise science (MS); occupational therapy (MS); physical therapy (DPT); physician assistant (MS); public health (MPH); social work (MSW). *Faculty:* 36 full-time (26 women), 47 part-time/adjunct (19 women). *Students:* 503 full-time (326 women), 112 part-time (82 women); includes 212 minority (117 Black or African American, non-Hispanic/Latino; 35 Asian, non-Hispanic/Latino; 48 Hispanic/Latino; 12 Two or more races, non-Hispanic/Latino), 59 international. Average age 31. 1,154 applicants, 38% accepted, 227 enrolled. In 2015, 228 master's, 41 doctorates awarded. *Degree requirements:* For master's, comprehensive exam (for some programs), thesis (for some programs), research capstone; for doctorate, comprehensive exam, research capstone. *Entrance requirements:* For master's and doctorate, GRE, two letters of recommendation. Additional exam requirements/recommendations for international students: Required—TOEFL (minimum score 550 paper-based; 79 iBT). *Application deadline:* Applications are processed on a rolling basis. Application fee: $50. Electronic applications accepted. *Expenses:* $1,155 per credit tuition, $934 per term full-time fees, $442 per term part-time fees. *Financial support:* In 2015–16, 10 research assistantships with partial tuition reimbursements (averaging $12,660 per year), 40 teaching assistantships with partial tuition reimbursements (averaging $12,660 per year) were awarded. Financial award application deadline: 2/15; financial award applicants required to submit FAFSA. *Faculty research:* Manual physical therapy, Parkinson's disease response to physical activity, violence in young minority men, LGBT safety. *Unit head:* Dr. Barry S. Eckert, Dean, 718-780-6578, Fax: 718-780-4561, E-mail: barry.eckert@liu.edu. *Application contact:* Richard Sunday, Dean of Admissions, 718-488-1011, Fax: 718-780-6110, E-mail: bkln-admissions@liu.edu.
Website: http://liu.edu/brooklyn/academics/school-of-health-professions

Louisiana State University Health Sciences Center, School of Allied Health Professions, Department of Occupational Therapy, New Orleans, LA 70112-2223. Offers MOT. *Accreditation:* AOTA. *Entrance requirements:* For master's, GRE (minimum scores: 150 verbal, 141 quantitative, and 3.5 analytical), bachelor's degree; 40 hours of observation in occupational therapy; minimum cumulative GPA of 2.5, cumulative prerequisite GPA of 2.8. Electronic applications accepted.

Maryville University of Saint Louis, Walker College of Health Professions, Occupational Therapy Program, St. Louis, MO 63141-7299. Offers MOT. *Accreditation:* AOTA. *Faculty:* 8 full-time (7 women), 4 part-time/adjunct (all women). *Students:* 30 part-time (29 women); includes 1 minority (Two or more races, non-Hispanic/Latino). Average age 22. In 2015, 35 master's awarded. *Entrance requirements:* For master's, GRE or MAT, minimum cumulative GPA of 3.0, resume, interview, writing sample. Additional exam requirements/recommendations for international students: Required—TOEFL (minimum score 563 paper-based). *Application deadline:* Applications are processed on a rolling basis. Electronic applications accepted. Application fee is waived when completed online. *Expenses:* Contact institution. *Financial support:* Career-related internships or fieldwork, Federal Work-Study, and campus employment available. Financial award application deadline: 3/1; financial award applicants required to submit FAFSA. *Unit head:* Robert Cunningham, Director, 314-529-9682, Fax: 314-529-9191, E-mail: rcunningham@maryville.edu. *Application contact:* Crystal Jacobsmeyer, Assistant Director, Graduate Enrollment Advising, 314-529-9654, Fax: 314-529-9927, E-mail: cjacobsmeyer@maryville.edu.
Website: http://www.maryville.edu/hp/occupational-therapy/

McMaster University, Faculty of Health Sciences, Professional Program in Occupational Therapy, Hamilton, ON L8S 4M2, Canada. Offers M Sc. *Degree requirements:* For master's, fieldwork and independent research project. *Entrance requirements:* For master's, minimum B average over last 60 undergraduate units. Additional exam requirements/recommendations for international students: Required—TOEFL (minimum score 600 paper-based).

Medical University of South Carolina, College of Health Professions, Program in Occupational Therapy, Charleston, SC 29425. Offers MSOT. *Accreditation:* AOTA. *Degree requirements:* For master's, thesis or alternative, research project. *Entrance requirements:* For master's, GRE General Test, interview, minimum GPA of 3.0, references. Additional exam requirements/recommendations for international students: Required—TOEFL (minimum score 600 paper-based). Electronic applications accepted. *Faculty research:* Therapeutic interventions for children with cerebral palsy; function, well being, quality of life for adults with chronic conditions and health disparities; driving interventions for adults with head and neck cancer; oral health for adults with tetraplegia; interprofessional education.

Mercy College, School of Health and Natural Sciences, Program in Occupational Therapy, Dobbs Ferry, NY 10522-1189. Offers MS. *Accreditation:* AOTA. *Program availability:* Evening/weekend. *Degree requirements:* For master's, comprehensive exam (for some programs), thesis, fieldwork. *Entrance requirements:* For master's, essay, 3 letters of recommendation, interview, resume, undergraduate transcripts with minimum GPA of 3.0. Additional exam requirements/recommendations for international students: Required—TOEFL (minimum score 600 paper-based; 100 iBT), IELTS (minimum score 8). Electronic applications accepted. *Expenses:* Contact institution.

MGH Institute of Health Professions, School of Health and Rehabilitation Sciences, Department of Occupational Therapy, Boston, MA 02129. Offers OTD. *Entrance requirements:* For doctorate, GRE, bachelor's degree from regionally-accredited U.S. college or university with minimum undergraduate GPA of 3.0; official transcripts; personal statement; recommendation letters. Additional exam requirements/recommendations for international students: Required—TOEFL (minimum score 80 iBT). Electronic applications accepted.

Midwestern University, Downers Grove Campus, College of Health Sciences, Illinois Campus, Program in Occupational Therapy, Downers Grove, IL 60515-1235. Offers MOT. *Accreditation:* AOTA. *Entrance requirements:* For master's, GRE General Test. *Expenses:* Contact institution.

Midwestern University, Glendale Campus, College of Health Sciences, Arizona Campus, Program in Occupational Therapy, Glendale, AZ 85308. Offers MOT. *Accreditation:* AOTA. *Entrance requirements:* For master's, GRE. *Expenses:* Contact institution.

Milligan College, Program in Occupational Therapy, Milligan College, TN 37682. Offers MSOT. *Accreditation:* AOTA. *Faculty:* 6 full-time (4 women), 5 part-time/adjunct (4 women). *Students:* 92 full-time (82 women). Average age 30. 400 applicants, 10% accepted, 32 enrolled. In 2015, 31 master's awarded. *Degree requirements:* For master's, thesis or alternative. *Entrance requirements:* For master's, GRE. Additional exam requirements/recommendations for international students: Required—TOEFL (minimum score 550 paper-based; 80 iBT). *Application deadline:* For spring admission, 11/15 for domestic and international students. Application fee: $120. Electronic applications accepted. *Expenses:* Contact institution. *Financial support:* In 2015–16, 55 students received support. Career-related internships or fieldwork and institutionally sponsored loans available. Financial award application deadline: 4/15; financial award applicants required to submit FAFSA. *Faculty research:* Handwriting, creativity, leadership in health care and rehabilitation, prevention and rehabilitation of work-related musculoskeletal disorders, parent-child interaction therapy, community-based occupational therapy programs. *Unit head:* Dr. Jeff Snodgrass, Department Chair/Professor, 423-975-8010, Fax: 423-975-8019, E-mail: jsnodgrass@milligan.edu. *Application contact:* Kristia Brown, Office Manager and Admissions Representative, 423-975-8010, Fax: 423-975-8019, E-mail: kngarland@milligan.edu.
Website: http://www.milligan.edu/msot/

Misericordia University, College of Health Sciences, Program in Occupational Therapy, Dallas, PA 18612-1098. Offers MSOT, OTD. *Accreditation:* AOTA. *Faculty:* 8 full-time (7 women), 8 part-time/adjunct (7 women). *Students:* 32 full-time (30 women), 79 part-time (68 women); includes 7 minority (3 Asian, non-Hispanic/Latino; 2 Hispanic/Latino; 2 Two or more races, non-Hispanic/Latino). Average age 29. In 2015, 49 master's, 13 doctorates awarded. *Entrance requirements:* For master's, minimum undergraduate GPA of 2.8, 2 letters of reference; for doctorate, minimum graduate GPA of 3.0, interview, 3 letters of reference. Additional exam requirements/recommendations for international students: Required—TOEFL. *Application deadline:* Applications are processed on a rolling basis. Application fee: $35. Electronic applications accepted. *Financial support:* Career-related internships or fieldwork and scholarships/grants available. Support available to part-time students. Financial award application deadline: 6/30; financial award applicants required to submit FAFSA. *Unit head:* Dr. Grace Fisher, Chair, 570-674-8015, E-mail: gfisher@misericordia.edu. *Application contact:* Maureen Sheridan, Assistant Director of Admissions, Part-Time Undergraduate and Graduate Programs, 570-674-6451, E-mail: msherida@misericordia.edu.
Website: http://www.misericordia.edu/page.cfm?p-634

Missouri State University, Graduate College, College of Health and Human Services, Department of Sports Medicine and Athletic Training, Springfield, MO 65897. Offers athletic training (MS); occupational therapy (MOT). *Program availability:* Part-time. *Faculty:* 7 full-time (4 women), 5 part-time/adjunct (3 women). *Students:* 45 full-time (30 women), 1 part-time (0 women); includes 3 minority (2 Asian, non-Hispanic/Latino; 1 Two or more races, non-Hispanic/Latino), 2 international. Average age 24. 46 applicants, 78% accepted, 36 enrolled. In 2015, 11 master's awarded. *Degree requirements:* For master's, comprehensive exam, thesis or alternative. *Entrance requirements:* For master's, GRE, current Professional Rescuer and AED certification, BOC certification, licensure as an athletic trainer, minimum undergraduate GPA of 3.0

Occupational Therapy

(for MS); OTCAS application (for MOT). Additional exam requirements/recommendations for international students: Required—TOEFL (minimum score 550 paper-based; 79 iBT), IELTS (minimum score 6). *Application deadline:* For fall admission, 1/15 for domestic and international students. Application fee: $35 ($50 for international students). Electronic applications accepted. *Expenses:* Tuition, state resident: full-time $5500. Tuition, nonresident: full-time $10,108. *Required fees:* $1000. *Financial support:* In 2015–16, 5 teaching assistantships with partial tuition reimbursements (averaging $8,600 per year) were awarded; Federal Work-Study, institutionally sponsored loans, and unspecified assistantships also available. *Unit head:* Dr. Tona Hetzler, Head, 417-836-8924, Fax: 417-836-8554, E-mail: tonahetzler@missouristate.edu. *Application contact:* Michael Edwards, Coordinator of Graduate Admissions, 417-836-5330, Fax: 417-836-6200, E-mail: michaeledwards@missouristate.edu.
Website: http://sportsmed.missouristate.edu/

Mount Mary University, Graduate Division, Program in Occupational Therapy, Milwaukee, WI 53222-4597. Offers MS, OTD. *Accreditation:* AOTA. *Program availability:* Part-time, evening/weekend, 100% online, blended/hybrid learning. *Faculty:* 7 full-time (all women), 2 part-time/adjunct (both women). *Students:* 117 full-time (106 women), 11 part-time (10 women); includes 16 minority (2 Black or African American, non-Hispanic/Latino; 1 American Indian or Alaska Native, non-Hispanic/Latino; 6 Asian, non-Hispanic/Latino; 6 Hispanic/Latino; 1 Two or more races, non-Hispanic/Latino). Average age 33. In 2015, 62 master's awarded. *Degree requirements:* For master's, comprehensive exam, thesis or alternative, professional development portfolio. *Entrance requirements:* For master's, minimum GPA of 3.0, occupational therapy license, 1 year of work experience. Additional exam requirements/recommendations for international students: Required—TOEFL (minimum score 550 paper-based; 80 iBT); Recommended—IELTS (minimum score 6.5). *Application deadline:* For fall admission, 1/15 priority date for domestic and international students. Application fee: $45. Electronic applications accepted. *Expenses:* $700 per credit; $750 per credit (for post-professional master's program); $770 (for doctorate program). *Financial support:* Career-related internships or fieldwork and Federal Work-Study available. Support available to part-time students. Financial award application deadline: 5/1; financial award applicants required to submit FAFSA. *Faculty research:* Clinical reasoning, occupational science, sensory integration. *Unit head:* Dr. Jane Olson, Director, 414-930-3376, E-mail: olsonj@mtmary.edu. *Application contact:* Kirk Heller de Messer, Director, Graduate Admissions, 414-930-3221, E-mail: hellerk@mtmary.edu.
Website: http://www.mtmary.edu/majors-programs/graduate/occupational-therapy/index.html

New England Institute of Technology, Program in Occupational Therapy, East Greenwich, RI 02818. Offers MS. *Accreditation:* AOTA. *Program availability:* Part-time-only, evening/weekend, blended/hybrid learning. *Students:* 55 full-time (47 women), 9 part-time (6 women); includes 4 minority (1 Black or African American, non-Hispanic/Latino; 2 Asian, non-Hispanic/Latino; 1 Two or more races, non-Hispanic/Latino), 6 international. Average age 33. *Degree requirements:* For master's, fieldwork. *Entrance requirements:* Additional exam requirements/recommendations for international students: Required—TOEFL. *Application deadline:* Applications are processed on a rolling basis. Application fee: $25. Electronic applications accepted. *Expenses:* Contact institution. *Financial support:* Applicants required to submit FAFSA. *Unit head:* Michael Caruso, Director of Admissions, 401-467-7744 Ext. 3411, Fax: 401-886-0868, E-mail: mcaruso@neit.edu. *Application contact:* Michael Caruso, Director of Admissions, 401-467-7744 Ext. 3411, Fax: 401-886-0868, E-mail: mcaruso@neit.edu.
Website: http://www.neit.edu/Programs/Masters-Degree-Programs/Occupational-Therapy

New York Institute of Technology, School of Health Professions, Department of Occupational Therapy, Old Westbury, NY 11568-8000. Offers MS. *Accreditation:* AOTA. *Faculty:* 5 full-time (all women), 7 part-time/adjunct (5 women). *Students:* 67 full-time (57 women), 41 part-time (29 women); includes 37 minority (7 Black or African American, non-Hispanic/Latino; 18 Asian, non-Hispanic/Latino; 11 Hispanic/Latino; 1 Native Hawaiian or other Pacific Islander, non-Hispanic/Latino). Average age 25. 318 applicants, 13% accepted, 32 enrolled. In 2015, 41 master's awarded. *Degree requirements:* For master's, thesis. *Entrance requirements:* For master's, minimum undergraduate cumulative GPA of 3.0; 100 hours of volunteer work under the supervision of a licensed occupational therapist; 3 professional letters of recommendation; essay. Additional exam requirements/recommendations for international students: Required—TOEFL (minimum score 550 paper-based; 79 iBT), IELTS (minimum score 6). *Application deadline:* For fall admission, 10/31 for domestic and international students. Applications are processed on a rolling basis. Application fee: $50. Electronic applications accepted. *Expenses:* Tuition, area resident: Full-time $20,790; part-time $1155 per credit. *Required fees:* $95; $75 per credit. Full-time tuition and fees vary according to degree level, campus/location and program. Part-time tuition and fees vary according to course load and campus/location. *Financial support:* Research assistantships with partial tuition reimbursements, scholarships/grants, health care benefits, tuition waivers, and unspecified assistantships available. Support available to part-time students. Financial award application deadline: 3/1; financial award applicants required to submit FAFSA. *Faculty research:* Health and wellness in aging population, technology in education, caregiver burden in ALS, strategies to increase student learning. *Unit head:* Dr. Gioia Ciani, Department Chairperson, 516-686-3863, E-mail: rhamed@nyit.edu. *Application contact:* Alice Dolitsky, Director, Graduate Admissions, 516-686-7520, Fax: 516-686-1116, E-mail: nyitgrad@nyit.edu.
Website: http://www.nyit.edu/degrees/occupational_therapy

New York University, Steinhardt School of Culture, Education, and Human Development, Department of Occupational Therapy, New York, NY 10012. Offers advanced occupational therapy (MA); occupational therapy (MS, DPS); research in occupational therapy (PhD). *Accreditation:* AOTA (one or more programs are accredited). *Program availability:* Part-time. *Degree requirements:* For master's, thesis (for some programs), terminal project; fieldwork; for doctorate, thesis/dissertation, terminal project. *Entrance requirements:* For doctorate, GRE General Test, interview. Additional exam requirements/recommendations for international students: Required—TOEFL (minimum score 100 iBT). Electronic applications accepted. *Faculty research:* Pediatrics, assistive rehabilitation technology, adaptive computer technology for children with disabilities, cognitive bases of adult disablement, upper limb rehabilitation.

Northeastern State University, College of Science and Health Professions, Department of Health Professions, Program in Occupational Therapy, Tahlequah, OK 74464-2399. Offers MS. *Faculty:* 10 full-time (7 women), 2 part-time/adjunct (both women). *Students:* 27 full-time (20 women); includes 9 minority (3 American Indian or Alaska Native, non-Hispanic/Latino; 6 Two or more races, non-Hispanic/Latino). Average age 27. *Application deadline:* For fall admission, 7/1 priority date for domestic and international students. Applications are processed on a rolling basis. Electronic applications accepted. *Expenses:* Tuition, state resident: part-time $189.60 per credit hour. Tuition, nonresident: part-time $462.60 per credit hour. *Required fees:* $37.40 per credit hour. *Unit head:* Dr. Judith A. Melvin, Director, 918-444-5232, E-mail: melvin02@nsuok.edu. *Application contact:* Jenney Fleming, Administrative Assistant, 918-444-5216, E-mail: flemi001@nsuok.edu.
Website: http://academics.nsuok.edu/healthprofessions/DegreePrograms/Graduate/OccupatTherapy.aspx

Nova Southeastern University, College of Health Care Sciences, Fort Lauderdale, FL 33314-7796. Offers anesthesiologist assistant (MSA); audiology (Au D); health science (MH Sc, DHSc, PhD); occupational therapy (MOT, Dr OT, PhD); physical therapy (DPT, TDPT); physician assistant (MMS). *Program availability:* Online learning. *Faculty:* 109 full-time (64 women), 100 part-time/adjunct (65 women). *Students:* 1,590 full-time (1,179 women), 969 part-time (819 women); includes 831 minority (234 Black or African American, non-Hispanic/Latino; 8 American Indian or Alaska Native, non-Hispanic/Latino; 151 Asian, non-Hispanic/Latino; 378 Hispanic/Latino; 1 Native Hawaiian or other Pacific Islander, non-Hispanic/Latino; 59 Two or more races, non-Hispanic/Latino), 18 international. Average age 30. 8,133 applicants, 14% accepted, 728 enrolled. In 2015, 556 master's, 105 doctorates awarded. *Degree requirements:* For master's, thesis; for doctorate, comprehensive exam, thesis/dissertation. *Entrance requirements:* For master's, GRE General Test, MCAT; for doctorate, GRE General Test, personal interview, essay. Additional exam requirements/recommendations for international students: Required—TOEFL (minimum score 600 paper-based). *Application deadline:* For winter admission, 4/15 for domestic students; for summer admission, 12/15 for domestic and international students. Applications are processed on a rolling basis. Application fee: $50. Electronic applications accepted. *Expenses:* Contact institution. *Financial support:* In 2015–16, 151 students received support, including 4 research assistantships (averaging $3,500 per year); institutionally sponsored loans and unspecified assistantships also available. Financial award application deadline: 4/15; financial award applicants required to submit FAFSA. *Unit head:* Dr. Stanley Wilson, Dean, 954-262-1203, E-mail: swilson@nova.edu. *Application contact:* Joey Jankie, Admissions Counselor, 954-262-7249, E-mail: joey@nova.edu.
Website: http://www.nova.edu/chcs/

The Ohio State University, College of Medicine, School of Health and Rehabilitation Sciences, Program in Occupational Therapy, Columbus, OH 43210. Offers MOT, MOT/PhD. *Accreditation:* AOTA. *Faculty:* 8. *Students:* 123 full-time (114 women); includes 5 minority (3 Asian, non-Hispanic/Latino; 2 Two or more races, non-Hispanic/Latino). Average age 24. In 2015, 41 master's awarded. *Degree requirements:* For master's, fieldwork. *Entrance requirements:* For master's, GRE General Test. Additional exam requirements/recommendations for international students: Required—TOEFL (minimum score 550 paper-based; 79 iBT), Michigan English Language Assessment Battery (minimum score 82); Recommended—IELTS (minimum score 7). *Application deadline:* For summer admission, 11/1 for domestic and international students. Applications are processed on a rolling basis. Application fee: $60 ($70 for international students). Electronic applications accepted. *Unit head:* Dr. Amy Darragh, Program Director, 614-292-0370, Fax: 614-292-0210, E-mail: darragh.6@osu.edu. *Application contact:* Graduate and Professional Admissions, 614-292-9444, Fax: 614-292-3895, E-mail: gpadmissions@osu.edu.
Website: http://medicine.osu.edu/hrs/ot

Pacific University, School of Occupational Therapy, Forest Grove, OR 97116-1797. Offers OTD. *Accreditation:* AOTA. Electronic applications accepted. *Expenses:* Contact institution. *Faculty research:* Cultural competency development, disability policy, scholarship of teaching and learning, driver rehabilitation and older adult visual perception, neurorehabilitation and motor learning.

Philadelphia University, College of Science, Health and the Liberal Arts, Occupational Therapy Clinical Doctorate Program, Philadelphia, PA 19144. Offers OTD. *Accreditation:* AOTA. *Entrance requirements:* For doctorate, proof of occupational therapy certification or eligibility for certification in the U.S.; official transcripts from all colleges and universities attended with minimum GPA of 3.0; statistics; research methods; resume or curriculum vitae; two letters of recommendation; personal statement. Additional exam requirements/recommendations for international students: Required—TOEFL (minimum iBT score 79) or IELTS (minimum score 6.5). Electronic applications accepted.

Philadelphia University, College of Science, Health and the Liberal Arts, Program in Occupational Therapy, Philadelphia, PA 19144. *Accreditation:* AOTA. *Program availability:* Evening/weekend. *Degree requirements:* For master's, portfolio. *Entrance requirements:* For master's, GRE or MAT. Additional exam requirements/recommendations for international students: Required—TOEFL (minimum score 550 paper-based; 79 iBT). Electronic applications accepted.

Queen's University at Kingston, School of Graduate Studies, Faculty of Health Sciences, School of Rehabilitation Therapy, Kingston, ON K7L 3N6, Canada. Offers occupational therapy (M Sc OT); physical therapy (M Sc PT); rehabilitation science (M Sc, PhD). *Program availability:* Part-time. *Degree requirements:* For master's, thesis; for doctorate, comprehensive exam, thesis/dissertation. *Entrance requirements:* Additional exam requirements/recommendations for international students: Required—TOEFL. *Faculty research:* Disability, community, motor performance, rehabilitation, treatment efficiency.

Radford University, College of Graduate and Professional Studies, Waldron College of Health and Human Services, Program in Occupational Therapy, Radford, VA 24142. Offers MOT. *Accreditation:* AOTA. *Program availability:* Part-time, evening/weekend. *Faculty:* 6 full-time (5 women), 1 (woman) part-time/adjunct. *Students:* 63 full-time (56 women); includes 9 minority (2 Black or African American, non-Hispanic/Latino; 2 Asian, non-Hispanic/Latino; 3 Hispanic/Latino; 2 Two or more races, non-Hispanic/Latino). Average age 25. 72 applicants, 32% accepted, 23 enrolled. In 2015, 23 master's awarded. *Degree requirements:* For master's, comprehensive exam. *Entrance requirements:* For master's, GRE, minimum GPA of 3.25, minimum B grade in prerequisite courses, 2 letters of recommendation, professional resume, 40 hours of observation, official transcripts, completion of a college or community course to learn a new occupation. Additional exam requirements/recommendations for international students: Required—TOEFL (minimum score 550 paper-based; 79 iBT), IELTS (minimum score 6.5). *Application deadline:* For fall admission, 2/15 priority date for domestic students, 12/1 for international students; for spring admission, 7/1 for international students. Applications are processed on a rolling basis. Application fee: $50. Electronic applications accepted. *Expenses:* $451 per credit hour in-state tuition and fees; $1,011 per credit hour out-of-state tuition and fees. *Financial support:* In 2015–16, 25 students received support, including 23 research assistantships (averaging $4,500 per year); career-related internships or fieldwork, Federal Work-Study, institutionally sponsored loans, scholarships/grants, and unspecified assistantships also available. Financial award application deadline: 3/1; financial award applicants required to submit FAFSA. *Unit head:* Dr. Douglas Mitchell, Chair, 540-831-2693, Fax: 540-831-6802, E-mail: ot@radford.edu. *Application contact:* Rebecca Conner, Director, Graduate Enrollment, 540-831-6290, Fax: 540-831-6001, E-mail: gradcollege@radford.edu.
Website: http://www.radford.edu/content/wchs/home/occupational-therapy.html

Regis College, School of Nursing and Health Sciences, Weston, MA 02493. Offers applied behavior analysis (MS); biomedical sciences (MS); counseling psychology (MA); health administration (MS); molecular imaging and therapeutics (MS); nurse practitioner (Certificate); nursing (MS, DNP); nursing education (Certificate); occupational therapy (MS). *Accreditation:* ACEN. *Program availability:* Part-time, evening/weekend. *Degree requirements:* For master's, thesis. *Entrance requirements:* For master's, GRE General Test or MAT, minimum GPA of 3.0; for doctorate, MAT or GRE if GPA from master's lower than 3.5. Additional exam requirements/recommendations for international students: Required—TOEFL (minimum score 550 paper-based). *Application deadline:* Applications are processed on a rolling basis. Application fee: $50. Electronic applications accepted. *Financial support:* Research assistantships, Federal Work-Study, scholarships/grants, traineeships, and unspecified assistantships available. Support available to part-time students. Financial award applicants required to submit FAFSA. *Faculty research:* Health policy, education, aging, job satisfaction, psychiatric nursing, critical thinking. *Application contact:* Shelagh Tomaino, Associate Director, Graduate Admission, 781-768-7188, Fax: 781-768-7071, E-mail: shelagh.tomaino@ regiscollege.edu.

Rochester Institute of Technology, Graduate Enrollment Services, National Technical Institute for the Deaf, Research and Teacher Education Department, Rochester, NY 14623. Offers secondary education for the deaf and hard of hearing (MS). *Accreditation:* Teacher Education Accreditation Council. *Students:* 34 full-time (29 women), 2 part-time (1 woman); includes 4 minority (1 American Indian or Alaska Native, non-Hispanic/ Latino; 2 Hispanic/Latino; 1 Two or more races, non-Hispanic/Latino), 3 international. Average age 30. 33 applicants, 52% accepted, 15 enrolled. In 2015, 18 master's awarded. *Degree requirements:* For master's, thesis or alternative. *Entrance requirements:* For master's, minimum GPA of 3.0. Additional exam requirements/ recommendations for international students: Required—PTE (minimum score 58), TOEFL (minimum score 550 paper-based, 79 iBT) or IELTS (minimum score 6.5). *Application deadline:* For fall admission, 2/15 priority date for domestic and international students. Applications are processed on a rolling basis. Application fee: $60. Electronic applications accepted. *Expenses:* $695 per credit hour. *Financial support:* In 2015–16, 31 students received support. Fellowships with full tuition reimbursements available, research assistantships with partial tuition reimbursements available, teaching assistantships with partial tuition reimbursements available, career-related internships or fieldwork, scholarships/grants, and unspecified assistantships available. Support available to part-time students. Financial award applicants required to submit FAFSA. *Faculty research:* Applied research on the effective use of access and support services and new technologies to enhance learning for deaf and hard-of-hearing students in the mainstream classroom, STEM research and instruction. *Unit head:* Dr. Gerald C. Bateman, Director, 585-475-6480, Fax: 585-475-2525, E-mail: gcbnmp@rit.edu. *Application contact:* Diane Ellison, Assistant Vice President, Graduate Enrollment Services, 585-475-2229, Fax: 585-475-7164, E-mail: gradinfo@rit.edu. Website: http://www.ntid.rit.edu/msse/

Rockhurst University, College of Health and Human Services, Program in Occupational Therapy, Kansas City, MO 64110-2561. Offers MOT. *Accreditation:* AOTA. *Program availability:* Part-time. *Faculty:* 7 full-time (all women), 5 part-time/ adjunct (all women). *Students:* 70 full-time (65 women), 1 (woman) part-time; includes 4 minority (2 Asian, non-Hispanic/Latino; 2 Two or more races, non-Hispanic/Latino). Average age 25. 257 applicants, 55% accepted, 40 enrolled. In 2015, 35 master's awarded. *Entrance requirements:* For master's, minimum GPA of 3.0. Additional exam requirements/recommendations for international students: Required—TOEFL (minimum score 550 paper-based; 79 iBT). *Application deadline:* Applications are processed on a rolling basis. Application fee: $25. Electronic applications accepted. Application fee is waived when completed online. *Financial support:* Applicants required to submit FAFSA. *Faculty research:* Problem-based learning, cognitive rehabilitation behavioral state in infants and children, adult neurological defects and prosthetics. *Unit head:* Dr. Mylene Schriner, Interim Chair, 816-501-4635, Fax: 816-501-4643, E-mail: mylene.schriner@rockhurst.edu. *Application contact:* Cheryl Hooper, Director of Graduate Recruitment and Admission, 816-501-4097, Fax: 816-501-4241, E-mail: cheryl.hooper@rockhurst.edu.
Website: http://www.rockhurst.edu/academic/ot/index.asp

Rocky Mountain University of Health Professions, Program in Occupational Therapy, Provo, UT 84606. Offers OTD. *Program availability:* Online learning. *Entrance requirements:* For doctorate, bachelor's or master's degree from accredited institution with minimum cumulative GPA of 3.0; current U.S. occupational therapy license; resume/curriculum vitae; two letters of recommendation; official transcripts. Electronic applications accepted.

Rush University, College of Health Sciences, Department of Occupational Therapy, Chicago, IL 60612-3832. Offers MS. *Accreditation:* AOTA. *Program availability:* Part-time. *Degree requirements:* For master's, thesis optional. *Entrance requirements:* For master's, GRE General Test. *Application deadline:* For fall admission, 12/1 for domestic students. Applications are processed on a rolling basis. Application fee: $40. Electronic applications accepted. *Financial support:* Career-related internships or fieldwork, Federal Work-Study, institutionally sponsored loans, and scholarships/grants available. Support available to part-time students. Financial award application deadline: 3/15; financial award applicants required to submit FAFSA. *Faculty research:* Intervention and practice strategies in the stroke population and the impact of evidenced based interventions. *Unit head:* Dr. Linda M. Olson, Chairperson, 312-942-8721, E-mail: linda_m_olson@rush.edu. *Application contact:* 312-942-7120, E-mail: chs_admissions@rush.edu.
Website: http://www.rushu.rush.edu/occuth/

Sacred Heart University, Graduate Programs, College of Health Professions, Program in Occupational Therapy, Fairfield, CT 06825. Offers MSOT. *Accreditation:* AOTA. *Faculty:* 7 full-time (all women), 6 part-time/adjunct (all women). *Students:* 93 full-time (87 women), 2 part-time (both women); includes 8 minority (1 Black or African American, non-Hispanic/Latino; 3 Asian, non-Hispanic/Latino; 3 Hispanic/Latino; 1 Two or more races, non-Hispanic/Latino). Average age 25. 425 applicants, 19% accepted, 49 enrolled. In 2015, 46 master's awarded. *Entrance requirements:* For master's, GRE (recommended), minimum overall and prerequisites GPA of 3.2 (science 3.0) with no prerequisite course below a C; statistics and human anatomy and physiology completed in the past 10 years. Additional exam requirements/recommendations for international students: Required—TOEFL (minimum score 570 paper-based; 80 iBT), IELTS (minimum score 6.5), PTE. *Application deadline:* For fall admission, 1/15 for domestic students. Applications are processed on a rolling basis. Application fee: $75. Electronic applications accepted. *Expenses:* Contact institution. *Financial support:* Career-related internships or fieldwork, institutionally sponsored loans, and unspecified assistantships available. Financial award applicants required to submit FAFSA. *Unit head:* Dr. Jody Bortone, Associate Dean of College of Health Professions/Chair, Occupational Therapy and Health Professions/Clinical Associate Professor, 203-396-8023, Fax: 203-365-7508, E-mail: bortonej@sacredheart.edu. *Application contact:* William Sweeney, Director of Graduate Admissions, 203-365-4827, E-mail: sweeneyw@sacredheart.edu. Website: http://www.sacredheart.edu/academics/collegeofhealthprofessions/academicprograms/occupationaltherapy/

Sage Graduate School, School of Health Sciences, Program in Occupational Therapy, Troy, NY 12180-4115. Offers MS. *Accreditation:* AOTA. *Faculty:* 8 full-time (7 women), 9 part-time/adjunct (8 women). *Students:* 65 full-time (61 women), 35 part-time (34 women); includes 5 minority (1 Black or African American, non-Hispanic/Latino; 1 Asian, non-Hispanic/Latino; 1 Hispanic/Latino; 2 Two or more races, non-Hispanic/Latino). Average age 25. 202 applicants, 15% accepted, 22 enrolled. In 2015, 35 master's awarded. *Entrance requirements:* For master's, baccalaureate degree, minimum undergraduate GPA of 3.0, completion of 20 hours of clinical observation. Additional

exam requirements/recommendations for international students: Required—TOEFL (minimum score 550 paper-based). *Application deadline:* For fall admission, 2/1 for domestic students. Applications are processed on a rolling basis. Application fee: $40. Electronic applications accepted. *Expenses:* Contact institution. *Financial support:* Fellowships, research assistantships, Federal Work-Study, scholarships/grants, and unspecified assistantships available. Support available to part-time students. Financial award applicants required to submit FAFSA. *Unit head:* Dr. Theresa Hand, Dean, School of Health Sciences, 518-244-2264, Fax: 518-244-4571, E-mail: handt@ sage.edu. *Application contact:* Theresa Hand, Dean of Health Sciences/Program Director, 518-244-2264, Fax: 518-244-4524, E-mail: handt@sage.edu.

Saginaw Valley State University, College of Health and Human Services, Program in Occupational Therapy, University Center, MI 48710. Offers MSOT. *Accreditation:* AOTA. *Program availability:* Part-time, evening/weekend. *Students:* 121 full-time (105 women), 61 part-time (45 women); includes 8 minority (4 Hispanic/Latino; 4 Two or more races, non-Hispanic/Latino), 2 international. Average age 24. 2 applicants, 50% accepted. In 2015, 47 master's awarded. *Entrance requirements:* For master's, minimum GPA of 3.0. Additional exam requirements/recommendations for international students: Required— TOEFL (minimum score 525 paper-based; 71 iBT). *Application deadline:* For spring admission, 1/23 for domestic and international students. Applications are processed on a rolling basis. Application fee: $30 ($90 for international students). Electronic applications accepted. *Expenses:* Tuition, state resident: full-time $9515; part-time $514 per credit hour. Tuition, nonresident: full-time $17,899; part-time $980 per credit hour. *Required fees:* $263; $14.60 per credit hour. Tuition and fees vary according to degree level. *Financial support:* Federal Work-Study and scholarships/grants available. Support available to part-time students. *Unit head:* Dr. Ellen Herlache-Pretzer, Graduate Program Coordinator, 989-964-2187, E-mail: echerlac@svsu.edu. *Application contact:* Jenna Briggs, Director, Graduate and International Admissions, 989-964-6096, Fax: 989-964-2788, E-mail: gradadm@svsu.edu.

St. Ambrose University, College of Education and Health Sciences, Program in Occupational Therapy, Davenport, IA 52803-2898. Offers MOT. *Accreditation:* AOTA. *Degree requirements:* For master's, board exams. *Entrance requirements:* For master's, 50 hours of volunteer experience in 2 occupational therapy settings, minimum GPA of 2.7, essay or interview on campus, 3 letters of reference. Additional exam requirements/ recommendations for international students: Required—TOEFL. Electronic applications accepted.

St. Catherine University, Graduate Programs, Program in Occupational Therapy, St. Paul, MN 55105. Offers MA, OTD. *Accreditation:* AOTA. *Program availability:* Part-time, evening/weekend. *Degree requirements:* For master's, thesis. *Entrance requirements:* For master's, GRE, minimum GPA of 3.0. Additional exam requirements/ recommendations for international students: Required—Michigan English Language Assessment Battery or TOEFL. *Expenses:* Contact institution.

Saint Francis University, Department of Occupational Therapy, Loretto, PA 15940-0600. Offers MOT. *Accreditation:* AOTA. *Degree requirements:* For master's, one foreign language, thesis. *Faculty research:* Retention, technology, work injury, distance learning. *Application contact:* Dr. Peter Raymond Skoner, Associate Vice President for Academic Affairs, 814-472-3085, Fax: 814-472-3365, E-mail: pskoner@francis.edu. Website: http://www.francis.edu/ot

Saint Louis University, Graduate Education, Doisy College of Health Sciences, Department of Occupational Science and Occupational Therapy, St. Louis, MO 63103. Offers MOT. *Accreditation:* AOTA. *Degree requirements:* For master's, project. *Entrance requirements:* For master's, minimum GPA of 2.8. Additional exam requirements/ recommendations for international students: Required—TOEFL (minimum score 525 paper-based; 55 iBT). Electronic applications accepted. *Faculty research:* Autism spectrum and Asperger's disease, early intervention with children of homeless families, disability awareness program development of developing countries, environmental adaptations and universal design for persons who are disabled and/or aging, physical activity models for persons with dementia.

Salem State University, School of Graduate Studies, Program in Occupational Therapy, Salem, MA 01970-5353. Offers MS. *Accreditation:* AOTA. *Program availability:* Part-time, evening/weekend. *Entrance requirements:* For master's, GRE or MAT. Additional exam requirements/recommendations for international students: Required— TOEFL (minimum score 550 paper-based; 80 iBT), IELTS (minimum score 5.5).

Samuel Merritt University, Department of Occupational Therapy, Oakland, CA 94609-3108. Offers MOT. *Accreditation:* AOTA. *Faculty:* 9 full-time (7 women), 11 part-time/ adjunct (9 women). *Students:* 116 full-time (98 women); includes 50 minority (4 Black or African American, non-Hispanic/Latino; 22 Asian, non-Hispanic/Latino; 16 Hispanic/ Latino; 8 Two or more races, non-Hispanic/Latino). Average age 29. 249 applicants, 21% accepted, 38 enrolled. In 2015, 37 master's awarded. *Degree requirements:* For master's, project. *Entrance requirements:* For master's, GRE General Test, minimum GPA of 3.0 in science and overall; 40-70 hours of volunteer or professional occupational therapy experience; interview. Additional exam requirements/recommendations for international students: Required—TOEFL (minimum score 100 iBT). *Application deadline:* For fall admission, 10/1 priority date for domestic students. Application fee: $50. Electronic applications accepted. *Expenses:* $44,669 per year; $1,215 per unit; $50 per year student fee; $235 one-time lab fee; $160 graduation fee. *Financial support:* In 2015–16, 15 students received support. Career-related internships or fieldwork, Federal Work-Study, and scholarships/grants available. Support available to part-time students. Financial award application deadline: 3/2; financial award applicants required to submit FAFSA. *Faculty research:* Neurological rehabilitation, attention, social responsiveness, computer assisted remediation. *Unit head:* Kate Hayner, Chair, 510-869-4780, E-mail: khayner@samuelmerritt.edu. *Application contact:* Timothy Cranford, Dean of Admission, 510-869-1550, Fax: 510-869-6525, E-mail: admission@samuelmerritt.edu. Website: http://www.samuelmerritt.edu/occupational_therapy

San Jose State University, Graduate Studies and Research, College of Applied Sciences and Arts, San Jose, CA 95192-0001. Offers big data (Certificate); California library media teacher services (Credential); collaborative response to family violence (Certificate); justice studies (MS); kinesiology (MA), including applied sciences and arts (MA, MS), athletic training, exercise physiology, sport management, sport studies; library and information science (MLIS, Certificate); mass communication (MA); master of social work (MSW); nutritional science (MS); occupational therapy (MS); public health (MPH); pupil personnel services (Credential); recreation (MS), including applied sciences and arts (MA, MS), international tourism; Spanish language counseling (Certificate); strategic management of digital assets and services (Certificate). *Program availability:* Part-time, evening/weekend. *Students:* 219 full-time (155 women), 140 part-time (103 women); includes 472 minority (38 Black or African American, non-Hispanic/ Latino; 2 American Indian or Alaska Native, non-Hispanic/Latino; 190 Asian, non-Hispanic/Latino; 238 Hispanic/Latino; 4 Native Hawaiian or other Pacific Islander, non-Hispanic/Latino), 28 international. Average age 31. 1,404 applicants, 37% accepted, 360 enrolled. In 2015, 850 master's awarded. *Application deadline:* For fall admission, 6/ 29 for domestic students; for spring admission, 11/30 for domestic students. Applications are processed on a rolling basis. Application fee: $55. Electronic applications accepted. *Financial support:* Career-related internships or fieldwork,

Occupational Therapy

Federal Work-Study, institutionally sponsored loans, and scholarships/grants available. Support available to part-time students. Financial award application deadline: 6/15; financial award applicants required to submit FAFSA. *Unit head:* Dr. Mary Schutten, Dean, 408-924-2900, Fax: 408-924-2901, E-mail: mary.schutten@sjsu.edu. *Application contact:* 408-924-2480, Fax: 408-924-2477.
Website: http://www.sjsu.edu/casa/

Seton Hall University, School of Health and Medical Sciences, Program in Occupational Therapy, South Orange, NJ 07079-2697. Offers MS. *Accreditation:* AOTA. *Entrance requirements:* For master's, health care experience, minimum GPA of 3.0, 50 hours of occupational therapy volunteer work, pre-requisite courses. Additional exam requirements/recommendations for international students: Required—TOEFL. Electronic applications accepted. *Faculty research:* Occupational genesis, occupational technology, pediatric OT, community practice, families of children with special needs; family routines; complementary medicine and wellness.

Shawnee State University, Program in Occupational Therapy, Portsmouth, OH 45662-4344. Offers MOT. *Accreditation:* AOTA.

Shenandoah University, School of Health Professions, Division of Occupational Therapy, Winchester, VA 22601. Offers MS. *Accreditation:* AOTA. *Faculty:* 6 full-time (all women), 6 part-time/adjunct (all women). *Students:* 91 full-time (83 women), 27 part-time (24 women); includes 17 minority (6 Black or African American, non-Hispanic/Latino; 4 Asian, non-Hispanic/Latino; 6 Hispanic/Latino; 1 Two or more races, non-Hispanic/Latino). Average age 27. 169 applicants, 59% accepted, 48 enrolled. In 2015, 27 master's awarded. *Degree requirements:* For master's, thesis, capstone project. *Entrance requirements:* For master's, GRE, minimum GPA of 3.0, bachelor's degree, completion of prerequisite courses with minimum grade of C, writing sample, two references (from two of these three people: licensed occupational therapist, professor or employer). Additional exam requirements/recommendations for international students: Required—TOEFL (minimum score 558 paper-based; 83 iBT). *Application deadline:* For fall admission, 10/15 for domestic and international students. Application fee: $140. Electronic applications accepted. *Expenses:* $62,250 tuition; $4,165 fees (including technology fee, student services fee, and clinical fee). *Financial support:* In 2015–16, 11 students received support. Scholarships/grants and unspecified assistantships available. Financial award application deadline: 3/15; financial award applicants required to submit FAFSA. *Faculty research:* Dynamometer testing, hippotherapy with veterans, first response training, socialization for the geriatric population, caregivers of special needs. *Unit head:* Cathy F. Shanholtz, PhD, Interim Division Director, 540-678-4313, Fax: 540-665-5564, E-mail: cshanhol2@su.edu. *Application contact:* Linda Burrows, OT Admissions Coordinator, 540-665-5559, Fax: 540-665-5530, E-mail: lburrows@su.edu.
Website: http://www.su.edu/occupational-therapy/

Sonoma State University, School of Science and Technology, Department of Kinesiology, Rohnert Park, CA 94928. Offers adapted physical education (MA); interdisciplinary (MA); interdisciplinary pre-occupational therapy (MA); lifetime physical activity (MA), including coach education, fitness and wellness; physical education (MA); pre-physical therapy (MA). *Program availability:* Part-time. *Degree requirements:* For master's, thesis, oral exam. *Entrance requirements:* For master's, minimum GPA of 2.8. Additional exam requirements/recommendations for international students: Required—TOEFL (minimum score 500 paper-based).

South University, Program in Occupational Therapy, Royal Palm Beach, FL 33411. Offers OTD.

Spalding University, Graduate Studies, Kosair College of Health and Natural Sciences, Auerbach School of Occupational Therapy, Louisville, KY 40203-2188. Offers MS. *Accreditation:* AOTA. *Faculty:* 9 full-time (7 women), 2 part-time/adjunct (1 woman). *Students:* 133 full-time (113 women), 37 part-time (35 women); includes 18 minority (10 Black or African American, non-Hispanic/Latino; 1 American Indian or Alaska Native, non-Hispanic/Latino; 4 Hispanic/Latino; 3 Two or more races, non-Hispanic/Latino). Average age 28. 54 applicants, 50% accepted, 22 enrolled. In 2015, 72 master's awarded. *Entrance requirements:* For master's, interview, letters of recommendation, transcripts, writing sample, 20 observation hours in human service delivery setting, on-site writing. Additional exam requirements/recommendations for international students: Required—TOEFL (minimum score 535 paper-based). *Application deadline:* For spring admission, 6/24 priority date for domestic students. Application fee: $30. *Financial support:* In 2015–16, 9 research assistantships (averaging $5,200 per year) were awarded; scholarships/grants and unspecified assistantships also available. Financial award applicants required to submit FAFSA. *Faculty research:* High-risk youth, community-dwelling older adults, assistive technology, mother-infant relationships, community accessibility. *Unit head:* Dr. Laura Schluter Strickland, Chair, 502-873-4219, E-mail: lstrickland@spalding.edu. *Application contact:* Joe McCombs, Office Manager, 502-588-7196, E-mail: jmccombs@spalding.edu.
Website: http://spalding.edu/academics/occupational-therapy/

Springfield College, Graduate Programs, Program in Occupational Therapy, Springfield, MA 01109-3797. Offers MS. *Accreditation:* AOTA. *Program availability:* Part-time. *Degree requirements:* For master's, comprehensive exam, research project; 6 months of full-time fieldwork. *Entrance requirements:* For master's, prerequisite courses in anatomy and physiology, other physical science, intro to psychology, intro to sociology, abnormal psychology, developmental psychology, English composition, additional English course, statistics; minimum undergraduate GPA of 3.0; prior experience in/exposure to occupational therapy services. Additional exam requirements/recommendations for international students: Required—TOEFL (minimum score 550 paper-based); Recommended—IELTS (minimum score 6). Electronic applications accepted. *Expenses:* Contact institution. *Faculty research:* Gerontology and dementia, service learning in higher education, students with learning disabilities, domestic violence, pediatric assessment.

Stockton University, Office of Graduate Studies, Program in Occupational Therapy, Galloway, NJ 08205-9441. Offers MSOT. *Accreditation:* AOTA. *Faculty:* 5 full-time (all women), 1 (woman) part-time/adjunct. *Students:* 59 full-time (54 women), 26 part-time (22 women); includes 8 minority (1 Black or African American, non-Hispanic/Latino; 6 Hispanic/Latino; 1 Two or more races, non-Hispanic/Latino), 1 international. Average age 25. 277 applicants, 18% accepted, 30 enrolled. In 2015, 20 master's awarded. *Degree requirements:* For master's, fieldwork, research project. *Entrance requirements:* For master's, minimum GPA of 3.0; 60 hours of work, volunteer or community service. Additional exam requirements/recommendations for international students: Required—TOEFL. *Application deadline:* For fall admission, 11/17 for domestic and international students. Application fee: $50. Electronic applications accepted. *Expenses:* Tuition, state resident: full-time $13,968; part-time $582 per credit. Tuition, nonresident: full-time $21,502; part-time $895 per credit. *Required fees:* $4200; $175 per credit. $90. Tuition and fees vary according to degree level. *Financial support:* Fellowships, research assistantships, career-related internships or fieldwork, institutionally sponsored loans, scholarships/grants, and unspecified assistantships available. Support available to part-time students. Financial award application deadline: 3/1; financial award applicants required to submit FAFSA. *Faculty research:* Home health-based occupational therapy for women with HIV/AIDS. *Unit head:* Dr. Kim Furphy, Program Director, 609-626-3640, E-mail: msot@stockton.edu. *Application contact:* Tara Williams, Assistant Director of Graduate Enrollment Management, 609-626-3640, Fax: 609-626-6050, E-mail: gradschool@stockton.edu.

Stony Brook University, State University of New York, Stony Brook Medicine, School of Health Technology and Management, Stony Brook, NY 11794. Offers health care management (Advanced Certificate); health care policy and management (MS); occupational therapy (MS); physical therapy (DPT); physician assistant (MS). *Accreditation:* APTA. *Faculty:* 67 full-time (41 women), 64 part-time/adjunct (45 women). *Students:* 488 full-time (301 women), 99 part-time (82 women); includes 167 minority (34 Black or African American, non-Hispanic/Latino; 3 American Indian or Alaska Native, non-Hispanic/Latino; 84 Asian, non-Hispanic/Latino; 41 Hispanic/Latino; 5 Two or more races, non-Hispanic/Latino), 12 international. Average age 28. 2,646 applicants, 14% accepted, 260 enrolled. In 2015, 104 master's, 71 doctorates, 34 other advanced degrees awarded. *Degree requirements:* For master's, thesis. *Entrance requirements:* For master's, GRE General Test, minimum GPA of 3.0, work experience in field, references; for doctorate, GRE, references. Additional exam requirements/recommendations for international students: Required—TOEFL (minimum score 550 paper-based). *Application deadline:* For fall admission, 1/15 for domestic students; for spring admission, 10/1 for domestic students. Application fee: $100. *Expenses:* Contact institution. *Financial support:* Fellowships, research assistantships, teaching assistantships, career-related internships or fieldwork, Federal Work-Study, and institutionally sponsored loans available. Financial award application deadline: 3/15. *Faculty research:* Health promotion and disease prevention. *Total annual research expenditures:* $1.3 million. *Unit head:* Dr. Craig A. Lehmann, Dean, 631-444-2252, Fax: 631-444-7621, E-mail: craig.lehmann@stonybrook.edu. *Application contact:* Dr. Richard W. Johnson, Associate Dean for Graduate Studies, 631-444-3251, Fax: 631-444-7621, E-mail: richard.johnson@stonybrook.edu.
Website: http://healthtechnology.stonybrookmedicine.edu/

Temple University, College of Public Health, Department of Rehabilitation Sciences, Philadelphia, PA 19122. Offers occupational therapy (MOT, DOT); therapeutic recreation (MS), including recreation therapy. *Program availability:* Part-time. *Faculty:* 14 full-time (13 women), 6 part-time/adjunct (4 women). *Students:* 79 full-time (71 women), 17 part-time (all women); includes 13 minority (3 Black or African American, non-Hispanic/Latino; 6 Asian, non-Hispanic/Latino; 2 Hispanic/Latino; 2 Two or more races, non-Hispanic/Latino). 29 applicants, 79% accepted, 17 enrolled. In 2015, 52 master's, 4 doctorates awarded. *Degree requirements:* For doctorate, comprehensive exam (for some programs), thesis/dissertation (for some programs). *Entrance requirements:* For master's and doctorate, GRE General Test, minimum GPA of 3.0. Additional exam requirements/recommendations for international students: Required—TOEFL (minimum score 550 paper-based; 79 iBT). *Application deadline:* For fall admission, 2/1 for domestic students, 1/1 for international students; for spring admission, 11/1 for domestic students, 10/1 for international students. Applications are processed on a rolling basis. Application fee: $60. Electronic applications accepted. *Expenses:* Contact institution. *Financial support:* Career-related internships or fieldwork and Federal Work-Study available. *Faculty research:* Participation, community inclusion, disability issues, leisure/recreation, occupation, quality of life, adaptive equipment and technology. *Unit head:* Dr. Mark Salzer, Chair, 215-204-7879, E-mail: mark.salzer@temple.edu.
Website: http://cph.temple.edu/rs/home

Tennessee State University, The School of Graduate Studies and Research, College of Health Sciences, Department of Occupational Therapy, Nashville, TN 37209-1561. Offers MOT. *Accreditation:* AOTA. *Entrance requirements:* For master's, GRE taken within the last 5 years, undergraduate degree with minimum GPA of 3.0; 30 hours of observation, volunteer, or work with an occupational therapist; 3 professional and/or academic references. *Unit head:* Dr. Larry Snyder, Head, 615-963-5891, Fax: 615-963-5956, E-mail: lsnyder@tnstate.edu. *Application contact:* Deborah Chisom, Director of Graduate Admissions, 615-963-5962, Fax: 615-963-5963, E-mail: dchiscom@tnstate.edu.
Website: http://www.tnstate.edu/ot/

Texas Tech University Health Sciences Center, School of Health Professions, Program in Occupational Therapy, Lubbock, TX 79430. Offers MOT. *Accreditation:* AOTA. *Faculty:* 6 full-time (5 women). *Students:* 138 full-time (120 women); includes 42 minority (5 Black or African American, non-Hispanic/Latino; 6 Asian, non-Hispanic/Latino; 29 Hispanic/Latino; 2 Two or more races, non-Hispanic/Latino). Average age 25. 385 applicants, 13% accepted, 50 enrolled. In 2015, 36 master's awarded. *Entrance requirements:* Additional exam requirements/recommendations for international students: Required—TOEFL (minimum score 550 paper-based; 79 iBT), IELTS. *Application deadline:* For fall admission, 11/15 priority date for domestic students. Applications are processed on a rolling basis. Application fee: $40. Electronic applications accepted. *Expenses:* $66,836.50 non-resident; $29,396.50 resident. *Financial support:* Career-related internships or fieldwork, institutionally sponsored loans, and scholarships/grants available. Financial award application deadline: 9/1; financial award applicants required to submit FAFSA. *Unit head:* Dr. Sandra Whisner, Program Director, 806-743-3240, Fax: 806-743-2189, E-mail: sandra.whisner@ttuhsc.edu. *Application contact:* Lindsay Johnson, Associate Dean for Admissions and Student Affairs, 806-743-3220, Fax: 806-743-2994, E-mail: lindsay.johnson@ttuhsc.edu.
Website: http://www.ttuhsc.edu/shp/mot/

Texas Woman's University, Graduate School, College of Health Sciences, School of Occupational Therapy, Denton, TX 76201. Offers MOT, OTD, PhD. *Accreditation:* AOTA (one or more programs are accredited). *Program availability:* Part-time, evening/weekend, online learning. *Degree requirements:* For master's, thesis or alternative; for doctorate, comprehensive exam, thesis/dissertation. *Entrance requirements:* For master's, minimum GPA of 3.0 on prerequisites, interview, recommendation based on 20 hours of observation with one supervising OTR; for doctorate, GRE General Test, essay, interview, 3 letters of reference, certification and master's degree in occupational therapy or related field. Additional exam requirements/recommendations for international students: Required—TOEFL (minimum score 550 paper-based; 79 iBT). *Application deadline:* For fall admission, 9/15 priority date for domestic students, 9/15 for international students. Applications are processed on a rolling basis. Application fee: $50 ($75 for international students). Electronic applications accepted. *Expenses:* Tuition, state resident: full-time $4380; part-time $243 per credit hour. Tuition, nonresident: full-time $11,400; part-time $633 per credit hour. *International tuition:* $11,465 full-time. *Required fees:* $1778; $99 per credit hour. $283 per semester. One-time fee: $50. Tuition and fees vary according to course load and program. *Financial support:* Research assistantships, career-related internships or fieldwork, Federal Work-Study, institutionally sponsored loans, scholarships/grants, traineeships, health care benefits, and unspecified assistantships available. Support available to part-time students. Financial award application deadline: 3/1; financial award applicants required to submit FAFSA. *Faculty research:* Quality of life/wellness, Alzheimer's disease, hand rehabilitation, psychosocial dysfunction, adaptation/chronic disability, long-term care. *Unit head:* Dr. Cynthia Evetts, Director, 940-898-2815, Fax: 940-898-2806, E-mail: ot@twu.edu. *Application contact:* Dr. Samuel Wheeler, Assistant Director of Admissions, 940-898-3188, Fax: 940-898-3081, E-mail: wheelersr@twu.edu.
Website: http://www.twu.edu/occupational-therapy/

Thomas Jefferson University, Jefferson School of Health Professions, Program in Occupational Therapy, Philadelphia, PA 19107. Offers MS, OTD. *Accreditation:* AOTA. *Program availability:* Part-time. *Students:* 130 full-time (122 women), 48 part-time (45 women); includes 9 minority (5 Black or African American, non-Hispanic/Latino; 2 Asian, non-Hispanic/Latino; 2 Hispanic/Latino). Average age 29. 925 applicants, 12% accepted, 72 enrolled. In 2015, 72 master's, 7 doctorates awarded. *Degree requirements:* For master's, thesis (for some programs). *Entrance requirements:* For master's, GRE General Test or MAT. Additional exam requirements/recommendations for international students: Required—TOEFL. *Application deadline:* For fall admission, 3/1 for domestic and international students. Applications are processed on a rolling basis. Application fee: $125. Electronic applications accepted. *Expenses:* Contact institution. *Financial support:* Federal Work-Study, institutionally sponsored loans, scholarships/grants, and unspecified assistantships available. Support available to part-time students. Financial award application deadline: 4/1; financial award applicants required to submit FAFSA. *Unit head:* Dr. Roseann Schaaf, Chair, Occupational Therapy Department, 215-503-9609, Fax: 215-503-0376, E-mail: roseann.schaaf@jefferson.edu. *Application contact:* Leslie Hindman, Senior Associate Director of Admissions, Fax: 215-503-7241, E-mail: jshpadmissions@jefferson.edu.
Website: http://www.jefferson.edu/health_professions/departments/occupational_therapy

Touro College, School of Health Sciences, Bay Shore, NY 11706. Offers industrial-organizational psychology (MS); mental health counseling (MS); occupational therapy (MS); physical therapy (DPT); physician assistant (MS); school psychology (MS); speech-language pathology (MS). *Faculty:* 20 full-time, 94 part-time/adjunct. *Students:* 1,057 full-time (772 women), 121 part-time (88 women); includes 243 minority (59 Black or African American, non-Hispanic/Latino; 1 American Indian or Alaska Native, non-Hispanic/Latino; 102 Asian, non-Hispanic/Latino; 58 Hispanic/Latino; 1 Native Hawaiian or other Pacific Islander, non-Hispanic/Latino; 22 Two or more races, non-Hispanic/Latino), 102 international. *Expenses:* Contact institution. *Financial support:* Fellowships available. *Unit head:* Dr. Louis Primavera, Dean, School of Health Sciences, 516-673-3200, E-mail: louis.primavera@touro.edu. *Application contact:* Brian J. Diele, Director of Student Administrative Services, 631-665-1600 Ext. 6311, E-mail: brian.diele@touro.edu.

Towson University, Program in Occupational Therapy, Towson, MD 21252-0001. Offers MS. *Accreditation:* AOTA. *Students:* 152 full-time (145 women), 1 (woman) part-time; includes 17 minority (5 Black or African American, non-Hispanic/Latino; 5 Asian, non-Hispanic/Latino; 5 Hispanic/Latino; 2 Two or more races, non-Hispanic/Latino). *Degree requirements:* For master's, thesis optional. *Entrance requirements:* For master's, bachelor's degree with minimum GPA of 3.25, master's degree, or doctorate; 3 letters of recommendation; human service/OT observation hours; personal statement. *Application deadline:* For spring admission, 8/1 for domestic students. Applications are processed on a rolling basis. Application fee: $45. Electronic applications accepted. *Expenses:* Tuition, state resident: full-time $7440; part-time $372 per unit. Tuition, nonresident: full-time $15,400; part-time $770 per unit. *Required fees:* $2360; $118 per year. $354 per term. *Financial support:* Application deadline: 4/1. *Unit head:* Dr. Sonia Lawson, Graduate Program Director, 410-704-2313, E-mail: slawson@towson.edu. *Application contact:* Lynne Murphy, University Admissions, 410-704-2113, Fax: 410-704-3030, E-mail: grads@towson.edu.
Website: http://grad.towson.edu/program/master/octh-ms/

Tufts University, Graduate School of Arts and Sciences, Department of Occupational Therapy, Medford, MA 02155. Offers MS, OTD. *Accreditation:* AOTA. *Degree requirements:* For master's, thesis (for some programs); for doctorate, leadership project. *Entrance requirements:* For master's and doctorate, GRE General Test. Additional exam requirements/recommendations for international students: Required—TOEFL (minimum score 550 paper-based; 80 iBT), IELTS (minimum score 6.5). Electronic applications accepted. *Expenses:* Contact institution.

Tufts University, Graduate School of Arts and Sciences, Graduate Certificate Programs, Advanced Professional Study in Occupational Therapy Program, Medford, MA 02155. Offers Certificate. *Program availability:* Part-time, evening/weekend. Electronic applications accepted. *Expenses:* Contact institution.

Tuskegee University, Graduate Programs, College of Veterinary Medicine, Nursing and Allied Health, School of Nursing and Allied Health, Tuskegee, AL 36088. Offers occupational therapy (MS).

Université de Montréal, Faculty of Medicine, Programs in Ergonomics, Montréal, QC H3C 3J7, Canada. Offers occupational therapy (DESS). Program offered jointly with École Polytechnique de Montréal.

University at Buffalo, the State University of New York, Graduate School, School of Public Health and Health Professions, Department of Rehabilitation Science, Program in Occupational Therapy, Buffalo, NY 14260. Offers MS. *Accreditation:* AOTA. *Faculty:* 8 full-time (7 women). *Students:* 122 full-time (104 women), 1 part-time (0 women); includes 15 minority (4 Black or African American, non-Hispanic/Latino; 11 Asian, non-Hispanic/Latino), 1 international. Average age 23. 72 applicants, 99% accepted, 71 enrolled. In 2015, 47 master's awarded. *Degree requirements:* For master's, project. *Entrance requirements:* Additional exam requirements/recommendations for international students: Required—TOEFL (minimum score 79 iBT). *Application deadline:* For fall admission, 2/1 priority date for domestic students, 4/1 for international students; for spring admission, 11/1 priority date for domestic students, 9/1 for international students. Application fee: $50. Electronic applications accepted. *Financial support:* In 2015–16, 5 teaching assistantships with tuition reimbursements (averaging $2,750 per year) were awarded; unspecified assistantships also available. Financial award application deadline: 2/1; financial award applicants required to submit FAFSA. *Faculty research:* Sensory integration, assistive technology, aging and technology, transition for students with emotional/behavioral problems. *Total annual research expenditures:* $391,708. *Unit head:* Dr. Susan Nochajski, Graduate Program Director, 716-829-6942, Fax: 716-829-3217, E-mail: phhpadv@buffalo.edu. *Application contact:* MaryAnn Venezia, Program Coordinator, 716-829-6942, Fax: 716-829-3217, E-mail: venezia3@buffalo.edu.
Website: http://sphhp.buffalo.edu/rehabilitation-science/education/occupational-therapy-bsms.html

The University of Alabama at Birmingham, School of Health Professions, Program in Occupational Therapy, Birmingham, AL 35294. Offers low vision rehabilitation (Certificate); occupational therapy (MS). *Accreditation:* AOTA. *Program availability:* Part-time, online learning. *Entrance requirements:* Additional exam requirements/recommendations for international students: Recommended—TOEFL, IELTS. *Expenses:* Tuition, state resident: full-time $7340. Tuition, nonresident: full-time $16,628. Full-time tuition and fees vary according to course load and program.

University of Alberta, Faculty of Graduate Studies and Research, Department of Occupational Therapy, Edmonton, AB T6G 2E1, Canada. Offers M Sc, PhD. *Program availability:* Part-time. *Degree requirements:* For master's, thesis. *Entrance requirements:* For master's, bachelor's degree in occupational therapy, minimum GPA of 6.9 on a 9.0 scale. Additional exam requirements/recommendations for international

students: Required—TOEFL. Electronic applications accepted. *Faculty research:* Work evaluation, pediatrics, geriatrics, program evaluation, community-based rehabilitation.

The University of British Columbia, Faculty of Medicine, Department of Occupational Science and Occupational Therapy, Vancouver, BC V6T 1Z1, Canada. Offers MOT. *Entrance requirements:* Additional exam requirements/recommendations for international students: Required—TOEFL (minimum score 600 paper-based; 100 iBT), IELTS (minimum score 6.5). Electronic applications accepted.

University of Central Arkansas, Graduate School, College of Health and Behavioral Sciences, Department of Occupational Therapy, Conway, AR 72035-0001. Offers MS. *Accreditation:* AOTA. *Degree requirements:* For master's, thesis optional, internship. *Entrance requirements:* For master's, GRE General Test, minimum GPA of 2.7. Additional exam requirements/recommendations for international students: Required—TOEFL (minimum score 550 paper-based; 80 iBT). Electronic applications accepted. *Expenses:* Contact institution.

The University of Findlay, Office of Graduate Admissions, Findlay, OH 45840-3653. Offers athletic training (MAT); business (MBA), including health care management, hospitality management, organizational leadership, public management; education (MA Ed), including administration, children's literature, early childhood, human resource development, reading, science, special education, technology; environmental, safety and health management (MSEM); health informatics (MS); occupational therapy (MOT); pharmacy (Pharm D); physical therapy (DPT); physician assistant (MPA); rhetoric and writing (MA); teaching English to speakers of other languages (TESOL) and bilingual education (MA). *Program availability:* Part-time, evening/weekend, online learning. *Degree requirements:* For master's, thesis, cumulative project, capstone project. *Entrance requirements:* For master's, GRE/GMAT, bachelor's degree from accredited institution, minimum undergraduate GPA of 2.5 in last 64 hours of course work; for doctorate, GRE, minimum cumulative GPA of 3.0. Additional exam requirements/recommendations for international students: Required—TOEFL (minimum score 80 iBT). Electronic applications accepted.

University of Florida, Graduate School, College of Public Health and Health Professions, Department of Occupational Therapy, Gainesville, FL 32611. Offers MHS, MOT. *Accreditation:* AOTA. *Faculty:* 2 full-time, 1 part-time/adjunct. *Students:* 82 full-time (72 women), 24 part-time (22 women); includes 31 minority (5 Black or African American, non-Hispanic/Latino; 10 Asian, non-Hispanic/Latino; 16 Hispanic/Latino). Average age 26. 277 applicants, 9% accepted, 12 enrolled. In 2015, 43 master's awarded. *Degree requirements:* For master's, clinical rotations. *Entrance requirements:* For master's, GRE General Test, minimum GPA of 3.0. Additional exam requirements/recommendations for international students: Required—TOEFL (minimum score 550 paper-based; 80 iBT), IELTS (minimum score 6). *Application deadline:* For fall admission, 2/15 for domestic and international students; for spring admission, 1/15 for domestic and international students. Application fee: $30. Electronic applications accepted. *Financial support:* Career-related internships or fieldwork, institutionally sponsored loans, scholarships/grants, and unspecified assistantships available. Support available to part-time students. Financial award applicants required to submit FAFSA. *Faculty research:* Rehabilitation intervention outcomes assessment, safe driving and community participation, assessment of driving skills and impact on participation, stroke and upper extremity rehabilitation, effective rehabilitation outcomes, community participation in families and children with muscular dystrophy, assessment of the impact of MD on community participation, assistive technology, AT effectiveness and availability. *Total annual research expenditures:* $728,473. *Unit head:* William C. Mann, PhD, Professor and Chair, 352-273-6817, Fax: 352-273-6042, E-mail: wmann@phhp.ufl.edu. *Application contact:* Office of Admissions, 352-392-1365, E-mail: webrequests@admissions.ufl.edu.
Website: http://www.phhp.ufl.edu/ot/

University of Illinois at Chicago, College of Applied Health Sciences, Department of Occupational Therapy, Chicago, IL 60607-7128. Offers MS, OTD. *Accreditation:* AOTA. *Program availability:* Part-time. *Faculty:* 10 full-time (9 women), 10 part-time/adjunct (8 women). *Students:* 85 full-time (74 women), 14 part-time (13 women); includes 36 minority (6 Black or African American, non-Hispanic/Latino; 14 Asian, non-Hispanic/Latino; 14 Hispanic/Latino; 2 Two or more races, non-Hispanic/Latino), 2 international. Average age 28. *Degree requirements:* For master's, thesis. *Entrance requirements:* For master's, GRE General Test, minimum GPA of 2.75, previous course work in statistics. Additional exam requirements/recommendations for international students: Required—TOEFL. *Application deadline:* For fall admission, 12/1 priority date for domestic and international students. Application fee: $60 ($50 for international students). Electronic applications accepted. *Expenses:* Contact institution. *Financial support:* Fellowships with full tuition reimbursements, research assistantships with full tuition reimbursements, teaching assistantships with full tuition reimbursements, career-related internships or fieldwork, Federal Work-Study, traineeships, tuition waivers (full), and unspecified assistantships available. Financial award application deadline: 3/1; financial award applicants required to submit FAFSA. *Faculty research:* Sensory integration, perception, play, treatment efficacy, instrument development. *Unit head:* Dr. Yolanda Suarez-Balcazar, Head, 312-996-3051, Fax: 312-413-0256, E-mail: ysuarez@uic.edu. *Application contact:* Receptionist, 312-413-2550, E-mail: gradcoll@uic.edu.
Website: http://www.ahs.uic.edu/ot/

University of Indianapolis, Graduate Programs, College of Health Sciences, School of Occupational Therapy, Indianapolis, IN 46227-3697. Offers MOT, DHS, OTD. *Accreditation:* AOTA. *Program availability:* Part-time, evening/weekend. *Degree requirements:* For master's, thesis. *Entrance requirements:* For master's, minimum GPA of 3.0, interview; for doctorate, minimum GPA of 3.3, BA/BS or MA/MS from occupational therapy program, current state license, currently in practice as occupational therapist or have 1000 hours of practice in last 5 years. Additional exam requirements/recommendations for international students: Required—TOEFL (minimum score 550 paper-based; 92 iBT), TWE (minimum score 5). *Expenses:* Contact institution.

The University of Kansas, University of Kansas Medical Center, School of Health Professions, Department of Occupational Therapy Education, Kansas City, KS 66160. Offers occupational therapy (MOT, OTD); therapeutic science (PhD). *Accreditation:* AOTA. *Program availability:* Part-time. *Faculty:* 15 full-time (12 women), 1 part-time/adjunct. *Students:* 109 full-time (103 women), 34 part-time (29 women); includes 18 minority (4 Black or African American, non-Hispanic/Latino; 3 Asian, non-Hispanic/Latino; 8 Hispanic/Latino; 3 Two or more races, non-Hispanic/Latino), 5 international. Average age 25. 185 applicants, 23% accepted, 42 enrolled. In 2015, 38 master's, 4 doctorates awarded. *Degree requirements:* For doctorate, comprehensive exam, thesis/dissertation, oral defense. *Entrance requirements:* For master's, 40 hours of paid work or volunteer experience working directly with people with special needs, 3 letters of recommendation, personal statement, program statement of interest, bachelor's degree with 40 hours of prerequisite work, minimum GPA of 3.0; for doctorate, 24 hours of master's-level research. Additional exam requirements/recommendations for international students: Required—TOEFL. *Application deadline:* For fall admission, 12/1 for domestic students, 4/1 for international students; for summer admission, 12/1 for domestic students. Applications are processed on a rolling basis. Application fee: $60. Electronic applications accepted. *Financial support:* Research assistantships with partial tuition reimbursements, teaching assistantships with tuition reimbursements,

Occupational Therapy

traineeships, and unspecified assistantships available. Financial award application deadline: 3/1; financial award applicants required to submit FAFSA. *Faculty research:* Impact of sensory processing in everyday life; improving balance, motor skills, and independence with community nonprofit organizations serving people with special needs; improving self-confidence and self-sufficiency with poverty-based services in community; working with autism population in a community-wide aquatics program; improving quality of life of people living with cancer and chronic illness. *Unit head:* Dr. Winifred W. Dunn, Professor/Chair, 913-588-7195, Fax: 913-588-4568, E-mail: wdunn@kumc.edu. *Application contact:* Wendy Hildenbrand, Admissions Representative, 913-588-7174, Fax: 913-588-4568, E-mail: whildenb@kumc.edu.
Website: http://www.kumc.edu/school-of-health-professions/occupational-therapy-education.html

University of Louisiana at Monroe, Graduate School, College of Health and Pharmaceutical Sciences, Department of Occupational Therapy, Monroe, LA 71209-0001. Offers MOT. *Accreditation:* AOTA.

University of Manitoba, Faculty of Graduate Studies, School of Medical Rehabilitation, Winnipeg, MB R3T 2N2, Canada. Offers applied health sciences (PhD); occupational therapy (MOT); physical therapy (MPT); rehabilitation (M Sc).

University of Mary, School of Health Sciences, Program in Occupational Therapy, Bismarck, ND 58504-9652. Offers MSOT. *Accreditation:* AOTA. *Program availability:* Part-time, online learning. *Degree requirements:* For master's, thesis or alternative, seminar. *Entrance requirements:* For master's, minimum cumulative GPA of 3.0, 48 hours of volunteer experience, 3 letters of reference. Additional exam requirements/recommendations for international students: Required—TOEFL (minimum score 550 paper-based). *Application deadline:* For spring admission, 3/15 priority date for domestic and international students. Applications are processed on a rolling basis. Application fee: $40. Electronic applications accepted. *Expenses:* Contact institution. *Financial support:* Teaching assistantships with full tuition reimbursements and scholarships/grants available. Financial award application deadline: 8/1; financial award applicants required to submit FAFSA. *Faculty research:* Safe homes for well elderly, occupation and spirituality, professional development in the spiritual domain, case method instruction, ergonomics, assistive technology.
Website: http://www.umary.edu/academics/programs/ms-occupational-therapy.php

University of Mississippi Medical Center, School of Health Related Professions, Department of Occupational Therapy, Jackson, MS 39216-4505. Offers MOT. *Accreditation:* AOTA.

University of Missouri, School of Health Professions, Program in Occupational Therapy, Columbia, MO 65211. Offers MOT. *Accreditation:* AOTA. *Entrance requirements:* Additional exam requirements/recommendations for international students: Required—TOEFL (minimum score 500 paper-based; 61 iBT). *Application deadline:* For fall admission, 12/31 priority date for domestic and international students; for spring admission, 12/31 for domestic students. Applications are processed on a rolling basis. Application fee: $55 ($75 for international students). Electronic applications accepted.
Website: http://shp.missouri.edu/ot/degrees.php

University of New England, Westbrook College of Health Professions, Program in Occupational Therapy, Biddeford, ME 04005-9526. Offers MS. *Accreditation:* AOTA. *Faculty:* 10 full-time (8 women), 6 part-time/adjunct (5 women). *Students:* 100 full-time (87 women); includes 7 minority (1 Black or African American, non-Hispanic/Latino; 3 Asian, non-Hispanic/Latino; 3 Hispanic/Latino). Average age 25. 412 applicants, 20% accepted, 51 enrolled. In 2015, 40 master's awarded. *Degree requirements:* For master's, research project, clinical fieldwork. *Entrance requirements:* For master's, minimum undergraduate GPA of 3.0, prerequisite coursework in anatomy and physiology. *Application deadline:* For fall admission, 1/15 for domestic students. Applications are processed on a rolling basis. Electronic applications accepted. Tuition and fees vary according to degree level and program. *Financial support:* Application deadline: 5/1; applicants required to submit FAFSA. *Unit head:* Dr. Kathryn Loukas, Interim Director/Clinical Professor, 207-221-4103, E-mail: kloukas@une.edu. *Application contact:* Scott Steinberg, Dean of University Admission, 207-221-4225, Fax: 207-523-1925, E-mail: ssteinberg@une.edu.
Website: http://www.une.edu/wchp/ot

University of New Hampshire, Graduate School, College of Health and Human Services, Department of Occupational Therapy, Durham, NH 03824. Offers assistive technology (Postbaccalaureate Certificate); occupational therapy (MS). *Accreditation:* AOTA. *Program availability:* Part-time. *Degree requirements:* For master's, thesis or alternative. *Entrance requirements:* For master's, GRE General Test, current certification as an OTR from the American Occupational Therapy Board or World Federation of Occupational Therapy. Additional exam requirements/recommendations for international students: Required—TOEFL (minimum score 550 paper-based; 80 iBT). *Application deadline:* For fall admission, 4/1 for domestic and international students. Applications are processed on a rolling basis. Application fee: $65. Electronic applications accepted. *Expenses:* Tuition, state resident: full-time $13,840; part-time $770 per credit hour. Tuition, nonresident: full-time $27,130; part-time $1175 per credit hour. *Required fees:* $2080; $1040. Tuition and fees vary according to degree level and program. *Financial support:* Fellowships, research assistantships, teaching assistantships, career-related internships or fieldwork, Federal Work-Study, and scholarships/grants available. Support available to part-time students. Financial award application deadline: 2/15. *Unit head:* Kerryellen Vroman, Chair, 603-862-4932. *Application contact:* Kerryellen Vroman, Chair, 603-862-4932.
Website: http://www.chhs.unh.edu/ot

University of New Mexico, Graduate Studies, Health Sciences Center, Program in Occupational Therapy, Albuquerque, NM 87131-5196. Offers MOT. *Accreditation:* AOTA. *Program availability:* Part-time. *Faculty:* 8 full-time (all women), 1 (woman) part-time/adjunct. *Students:* 81 full-time (64 women), 1 (woman) part-time; includes 33 minority (1 Black or African American, non-Hispanic/Latino; 3 American Indian or Alaska Native, non-Hispanic/Latino; 2 Asian, non-Hispanic/Latino; 26 Hispanic/Latino; 1 Two or more races, non-Hispanic/Latino). Average age 31. 79 applicants, 32% accepted, 24 enrolled. In 2015, 23 master's awarded. *Degree requirements:* For master's, thesis, clinical fieldwork. *Entrance requirements:* For master's, interview, writing sample, volunteer experience. *Application deadline:* For fall admission, 12/1 priority date for domestic students. Applications are processed on a rolling basis. Application fee: $50. Electronic applications accepted. *Financial support:* Research assistantships, Federal Work-Study, institutionally sponsored loans, scholarships/grants, traineeships, and unspecified assistantships available. Financial award application deadline: 3/1; financial award applicants required to submit FAFSA. *Faculty research:* Sensory processing, scleroderma treatment, use of therapy dogs, educational scholarship. *Total annual research expenditures:* $290,062. *Unit head:* Dr. Betsy VanLeit, Director, 505-272-1753, Fax: 505-272-3583, E-mail: bvanleit@salud.unm.edu. *Application contact:* Janet Werner, Coordinator, 505-272-1753, Fax: 505-272-3583, E-mail: werner@salud.unm.edu.
Website: http://hsc.unm.edu/som/ot/

The University of North Carolina at Chapel Hill, School of Medicine and Graduate School, Graduate Programs in Medicine, Chapel Hill, NC 27599. Offers allied health sciences (MPT, MS, Au D, DPT, PhD), including human movement science (MS, PhD), occupational science (MS, PhD), physical therapy (MPT, MS, DPT), rehabilitation counseling and psychology (MS), speech and hearing sciences (MS, Au D, PhD); biochemistry and biophysics (MS, PhD); bioinformatics and computational biology (PhD); biomedical engineering (MS, PhD); cell and developmental biology (PhD); cell and molecular physiology (PhD); genetics and molecular biology (PhD); microbiology and immunology (MS, PhD), including immunology, microbiology; neurobiology (PhD); pathology and laboratory medicine (PhD), including experimental pathology; pharmacology (PhD); MD/PhD. *Program availability:* Online learning. Terminal master's awarded for partial completion of doctoral program. *Degree requirements:* For master's, comprehensive exam; for doctorate, thesis/dissertation. Electronic applications accepted. *Expenses:* Contact institution.

The University of North Carolina at Chapel Hill, School of Medicine and Graduate School, Graduate Programs in Medicine, Department of Allied Health Sciences, Division of Occupational Science and Occupational Therapy, Chapel Hill, NC 27599. Offers occupational science (PhD); occupational therapy (MS). *Accreditation:* AOTA. *Degree requirements:* For master's, comprehensive exam, thesis optional, collaborative research project; for doctorate, thesis/dissertation. *Entrance requirements:* For master's, GRE General Test; for doctorate, GRE, master's degree in occupational therapy, relevant social behavioral sciences or health field. Additional exam requirements/recommendations for international students: Required—TOEFL (minimum score 550 paper-based). Electronic applications accepted. *Faculty research:* Parents and infants in co-occupations, psychosocial dysfunction, predictors of autism, factors influencing the occupation of primates, factors influencing occupations of people with dementia, occupational development of young children.

University of North Dakota, Graduate School and Graduate School, Graduate Programs in Medicine, Department of Occupational Therapy, Grand Forks, ND 58202. Offers MOT. *Accreditation:* AOTA. *Program availability:* Part-time. *Entrance requirements:* For master's, letter of reference; volunteer or work experience, preferably from health-related field; interview; minimum GPA of 2.7. Additional exam requirements/recommendations for international students: Required—TOEFL (minimum score 550 paper-based; 79 iBT), IELTS (minimum score 6.5). Electronic applications accepted.

University of Oklahoma Health Sciences Center, Graduate College, College of Allied Health, Department of Occupational Therapy, Oklahoma City, OK 73190. Offers MOT. *Accreditation:* AOTA.

University of Pittsburgh, School of Health and Rehabilitation Sciences, Master of Occupational Therapy Program, Pittsburgh, PA 15260. Offers MOT. *Accreditation:* AOTA. *Faculty:* 8 full-time (7 women), 1 (woman) part-time/adjunct. *Students:* 102 full-time (96 women), 2 part-time (both women); includes 8 minority (2 Black or African American, non-Hispanic/Latino; 2 Asian, non-Hispanic/Latino; 3 Hispanic/Latino; 1 Two or more races, non-Hispanic/Latino), 1 international. Average age 26. 817 applicants, 12% accepted, 51 enrolled. In 2015, 50 master's awarded. *Entrance requirements:* For master's, GRE General Test, volunteer experience in occupational therapy. Additional exam requirements/recommendations for international students: Required—TOEFL (minimum score 550 paper-based; 80 iBT), IELTS (minimum score 6.5). *Application deadline:* For summer admission, 3/1 for domestic students, 2/1 for international students. Applications are processed on a rolling basis. Application fee: $125. Electronic applications accepted. Tuition and fees vary according to program. *Financial support:* In 2015–16, 2 students received support, including 2 fellowships with full tuition reimbursements available (averaging $18,134 per year); Federal Work-Study and scholarships/grants also available. *Faculty research:* Expertise in evidence-based practice, measuring occupational performance, ergonomics, geriatrics, mental health, neurorehabilitation, research. *Total annual research expenditures:* $707,351. *Unit head:* Dr. Elizabeth Skidmore, Department Chair and Associate Professor, 412-383-6617, Fax: 412-383-6613, E-mail: skidmore@pitt.edu. *Application contact:* Joyce Broadwick, Administrator, 412-383-6620, Fax: 412-383-6613, E-mail: otpitt@shrs.pitt.edu.
Website: http://www.shrs.pitt.edu/MOT/

University of Pittsburgh, School of Health and Rehabilitation Sciences, Master's Programs in Health and Rehabilitation Sciences, Pittsburgh, PA 15260. Offers health and rehabilitation sciences (MS), including health information systems, healthcare supervision and management, occupational therapy, physical therapy, rehabilitation counseling, rehabilitation science and technology, sports medicine, wellness and human performance. *Accreditation:* APTA. *Program availability:* Part-time, evening/weekend. *Faculty:* 32 full-time (21 women). *Students:* 111 full-time (73 women), 42 part-time (31 women); includes 23 minority (5 Black or African American, non-Hispanic/Latino; 8 Asian, non-Hispanic/Latino; 7 Hispanic/Latino; 3 Two or more races, non-Hispanic/Latino), 65 international. Average age 29. 330 applicants, 66% accepted, 107 enrolled. In 2015, 89 master's awarded. *Degree requirements:* For master's, comprehensive exam (for some programs), thesis optional. *Entrance requirements:* For master's, minimum GPA of 3.0. Additional exam requirements/recommendations for international students: Required—TOEFL (minimum score 550 paper-based; 80 iBT), IELTS (minimum score 6.5). *Application deadline:* For fall admission, 3/1 for international students; for spring admission, 9/1 for international students. Applications are processed on a rolling basis. Application fee: $50. Electronic applications accepted. Tuition and fees vary according to program. *Financial support:* In 2015–16, 7 students received support, including 7 fellowships with full tuition reimbursements available (averaging $17,048 per year); traineeships also available. *Faculty research:* Assistive technology, seating and wheelchair mobility, cellular neurophysiology, low back syndrome, augmentative communication. *Total annual research expenditures:* $7.7 million. *Unit head:* Dr. Anthony Delitto, Dean, 412-383-6560, Fax: 412-383-6535, E-mail: delitto@pitt.edu. *Application contact:* Jessica Maguire, Director of Admissions, 412-383-6557, Fax: 412-383-6535, E-mail: maguire@pitt.edu.

University of Puerto Rico, Medical Sciences Campus, School of Health Professions, Program in Occupational Therapy, San Juan, PR 00936-5067. Offers MS. *Accreditation:* AOTA.

University of Puget Sound, School of Occupational Therapy, Tacoma, WA 98416. Offers MSOT, Dr OT. *Accreditation:* AOTA. *Degree requirements:* For master's, thesis, publishable paper or program development project. *Entrance requirements:* For master's, GRE General Test, minimum baccalaureate GPA of 3.0, three letters of recommendation. Additional exam requirements/recommendations for international students: Required—TOEFL (minimum score 550 paper-based; 90 iBT). Electronic applications accepted. *Expenses:* Contact institution. *Faculty research:* Scope of practice for school-based occupational therapy, family occupational adaptation to autism, clinical decision-making, low vision adaptation, assistive technology.

University of St. Augustine for Health Sciences, Graduate Programs, Master of Occupational Therapy Program, St. Augustine, FL 32086. Offers MOT. *Accreditation:* AOTA. *Entrance requirements:* For master's, GRE General Test. Application fee is waived when completed online.

University of St. Augustine for Health Sciences, Graduate Programs, Post Professional Programs, St. Augustine, FL 32086. Offers health science (DH Sc); health sciences education (Ed D); occupational therapy (TOTD); physical therapy (TDPT). *Program availability:* Part-time, online learning. *Entrance requirements:* For doctorate, GRE General Test, master's degree in related field. Additional exam requirements/recommendations for international students: Required—TOEFL.

The University of Scranton, Panuska College of Professional Studies, Program in Occupational Therapy, Scranton, PA 18510. Offers MS. *Accreditation:* AOTA. *Students:* 53 full-time (48 women), 10 part-time (9 women); includes 2 minority (both Asian, non-Hispanic/Latino). Average age 22. *Degree requirements:* For master's, comprehensive exam (for some programs), thesis (for some programs), capstone experience. *Entrance requirements:* For master's, minimum GPA of 3.0, three letters of reference. Additional exam requirements/recommendations for international students: Required—TOEFL (minimum score 500 paper-based; 80 iBT), IELTS (minimum score 6.5). *Application deadline:* For fall admission, 6/1 for international students; for spring admission, 11/1 for international students; for summer admission, 3/1 for international students. Applications are processed on a rolling basis. Application fee: $0. Electronic applications accepted. *Financial support:* Applicants required to submit FAFSA. *Faculty research:* Low vision; developmental visual perception; home safety for elderly; history of occupational therapy; telehealth. *Unit head:* Dr. Carol Reinson, Chair and Program Director, 570-941-4125, Fax: 570-941-4380, E-mail: carol.reinson@scranton.edu. *Application contact:* Joseph M. Roback, Director of Admissions, 570-941-4385, Fax: 570-941-5928, E-mail: robackj2@scranton.edu.

University of South Alabama, Pat Capps Covey College of Allied Health Professions, Department of Occupational Therapy, Mobile, AL 36688. Offers MS. *Accreditation:* AOTA. *Faculty:* 2 full-time (both women), 7 part-time/adjunct (6 women). *Students:* 85 full-time (76 women); includes 5 minority (3 Black or African American, non-Hispanic/Latino; 1 American Indian or Alaska Native, non-Hispanic/Latino; 1 Asian, non-Hispanic/Latino). Average age 24. 137 applicants, 39% accepted, 26 enrolled. In 2015, 25 master's awarded. *Degree requirements:* For master's, clinical externship. *Entrance requirements:* For master's, GRE, minimum GPA of 3.0; bachelor's degree or 96 semester hours of prerequisites and electives. Additional exam requirements/recommendations for international students: Required—TOEFL (minimum score 600 paper-based), TWE (minimum score 5.5). *Application deadline:* For fall admission, 1/15 for domestic and international students. Application fee: $75. Electronic applications accepted. *Expenses:* Contact institution. *Financial support:* Fellowships, research assistantships, teaching assistantships, career-related internships or fieldwork, Federal Work-Study, institutionally sponsored loans, scholarships/grants, and unspecified assistantships available. Support available to part-time students. Financial award application deadline: 5/31; financial award applicants required to submit FAFSA. *Unit head:* Dr. Donna W. Wooster, Chair, 251-445-9222, Fax: 251-445-9211, E-mail: otdept@southalabama.edu. *Application contact:* Dr. Susan Gordon-Hickey, Associate Dean, Allied Health, 251-445-9250, Fax: 251-460-9259, E-mail: gordonhickey@southalabama.edu.
Website: http://www.southalabama.edu/alliedhealth/ot/

The University of South Dakota, Graduate School, School of Health Sciences, Department of Occupational Therapy, Vermillion, SD 57069-2390. Offers occupational therapy (MS, OTD); post-professional occupational therapy (OTD). *Accreditation:* AOTA. *Program availability:* Part-time. *Degree requirements:* For master's, thesis optional, 6 months of supervised fieldwork. *Entrance requirements:* For master's, courses in human anatomy, human physiology, general psychology, abnormal psychology, lifespan development, statistics. Additional exam requirements/recommendations for international students: Required—TOEFL (minimum score 550 paper-based). *Application deadline:* For fall admission, 11/1 priority date for domestic and international students. Applications are processed on a rolling basis. Application fee: $35. *Expenses:* Contact institution. *Financial support:* Research assistantships with partial tuition reimbursements, teaching assistantships with partial tuition reimbursements, scholarships/grants, and traineeships available. Financial award application deadline: 3/1. *Faculty research:* Low vision in youth and adults, agricultural/rural health, childhood obesity, adolescent mental health, elder health and well being. *Unit head:* Dr. Barbara L. Brockevelt, Chair, 605-677-5000, E-mail: barb.brockevelt@usd.edu. *Application contact:* Graduate School, 605-658-6140, Fax: 605-677-6118, E-mail: cde@usd.edu.
Website: http://www.usd.edu/health-sciences/occupational-therapy/graduate

University of Southern California, Graduate School, Herman Ostrow School of Dentistry, Division of Occupational Science and Occupational Therapy, Graduate Program in Occupational Science, Los Angeles, CA 90089. Offers PhD. *Accreditation:* AOTA. *Degree requirements:* For doctorate, thesis/dissertation, qualifying exam. *Entrance requirements:* For doctorate, GRE (minimum combined score of 1100), minimum GPA of 3.0. Additional exam requirements/recommendations for international students: Required—TOEFL (minimum score 600 paper-based; 100 iBT). Electronic applications accepted. *Faculty research:* Health and well-being; health disparities and cultural influences on health and recovery; family life; community re-integration and social participation; engagement, activity and neuroscience; rehabilitation science and ethics; society and social justice; autism and sensory integration; interventions; health disparities in autism diagnosis.

University of Southern California, Graduate School, Herman Ostrow School of Dentistry, Division of Occupational Science and Occupational Therapy, Graduate Programs in Occupational Therapy, Los Angeles, CA 90089. Offers MA, OTD. *Accreditation:* AOTA. *Program availability:* Part-time. *Degree requirements:* For master's, comprehensive exam (for some programs), thesis or alternative; for doctorate, residency, portfolio. *Entrance requirements:* For master's and doctorate, GRE (minimum score 1000), minimum cumulative GPA of 3.0. Additional exam requirements/recommendations for international students: Required—TOEFL (minimum score 600 paper-based; 100 iBT). Electronic applications accepted. *Faculty research:* Health and well-being; health disparities and cultural influences on health and recovery; family life; community re-integration and social participation; engagement, activity and neuroscience; rehabilitation science and ethics; society and social justice; autism and sensory integration; interventions; health disparities in autism diagnosis.

University of Southern Indiana, Graduate Studies, College of Nursing and Health Professions, Program in Occupational Therapy, Evansville, IN 47712-3590. Offers MSOT. *Accreditation:* AOTA. *Program availability:* Part-time. *Faculty:* 2 full-time (1 woman). *Students:* 54 full-time (46 women), 1 (woman) part-time; includes 2 minority (both Asian, non-Hispanic/Latino). Average age 23. In 2015, 28 master's awarded. *Entrance requirements:* For master's, minimum GPA of 3.0, two letters of recommendations (one professional letter from previous employer or practicing OT; one academic letter from a professor or advisor from undergraduate degree). Additional exam requirements/recommendations for international students: Required—TOEFL (minimum score 550 paper-based; 79 iBT), IELTS (minimum score 6). *Application deadline:* For fall admission, 2/15 for domestic and international students. Applications are processed on a rolling basis. Application fee: $40. Electronic applications accepted. *Expenses:* Contact institution. *Financial support:* Federal Work-Study, scholarships/grants, tuition waivers (full and partial), and unspecified assistantships available. Financial award application deadline: 3/1; financial award applicants required to submit FAFSA. *Unit head:* Dr. Janet Kilbane, Interim Program Chair, 812-465-1179, E-mail:

bjwilliams4@usi.edu. *Application contact:* Dr. Mayola Rowser, Director, Graduate Studies, 812-465-7016, Fax: 812-464-1956, E-mail: mrowser@usi.edu.
Website: http://www.usi.edu/health/occupational-therapy

University of Southern Maine, Lewiston-Auburn College, Program in Occupational Therapy, Lewiston, ME 04240. Offers MOT. *Accreditation:* AOTA. *Degree requirements:* For master's, fieldwork, original research. *Entrance requirements:* For master's, minimum GPA of 3.0, writing sample, interview, reference letters, job shadow observation. Electronic applications accepted. *Expenses: Tuition, area resident:* Full-time $6840; part-time $380 per credit hour. Tuition, state resident: full-time $10,260; part-time $570 per credit hour. Tuition, nonresident: full-time $18,468; part-time $1026 per credit hour. *Required fees:* $830; $83 per credit hour. Tuition and fees vary according to course load and program. *Faculty research:* Multicultural curricula, cultural competence, parents responses to fussy infants, chronic pain, early childhood eating disorders.

The University of Tennessee Health Science Center, College of Health Professions, Memphis, TN 38163-0002. Offers audiology (MS, Au D); clinical laboratory science (MSCLS); cytopathology practice (MCP); health informatics and information management (MHIIM); occupational therapy (MOT); physical therapy (DPT, ScDPT); physician assistant (MMS); speech-language pathology (MS). *Accreditation:* AOTA; APTA. *Program availability:* Part-time, evening/weekend, online learning. Terminal master's awarded for partial completion of doctoral program. *Degree requirements:* For master's, comprehensive exam, thesis; for doctorate, comprehensive exam, residency. *Entrance requirements:* For master's, GRE (MOT, MSCLS), minimum GPA of 3.0, 3 letters of reference, national accreditation (MSCLS), GRE if GPA is less than 3.0 (MCP); for doctorate, GRE. Additional exam requirements/recommendations for international students: Required—TOEFL (minimum score 550 paper-based; 80 iBT). Electronic applications accepted. *Expenses.* Contact institution. *Faculty research:* Gait deviation, muscular dystrophy and strength, hemophilia and exercise, pediatric neurology, self-efficacy.

The University of Texas at El Paso, Graduate School, College of Health Sciences, Master of Occupational Therapy (MOT) Program, El Paso, TX 79968-0001. Offers MOT. *Accreditation:* AOTA. *Degree requirements:* For master's, thesis optional. *Entrance requirements:* For master's, GRE, minimum cumulative and prerequisite GPA of 3.0, bachelor's degree, 40 clock hours of supervised observations with an OT. Additional exam requirements/recommendations for international students: Required—TOEFL; Recommended—IELTS. *Faculty research:* Falls prevention, coping of mothers with children with disabilities.

The University of Texas Health Science Center at San Antonio, School of Health Professions, San Antonio, TX 78229-3900. Offers occupational therapy (MOT); physical therapy (DPT); physician assistant studies (MS). *Accreditation:* AOTA; APTA; ARC-PA. *Degree requirements:* For master's, comprehensive exam, thesis (for some programs); for doctorate, comprehensive exam.

The University of Texas Medical Branch, School of Health Professions, Department of Occupational Therapy, Galveston, TX 77555. Offers MOT. *Accreditation:* AOTA. *Entrance requirements:* For master's, MAT, 20 volunteer hours, telephone interview, 2 references.

The University of Texas Rio Grande Valley, College of Health Affairs, Department of Occupational Therapy, Edinburg, TX 78539. Offers MS. *Accreditation:* AOTA. *Program availability:* Evening/weekend. *Entrance requirements:* For master's, Health Occupations Aptitude Examination. Tuition and fees vary according to course load and program. *Faculty research:* Parenting of children with disabilities, effects of healing touch on student stress.

University of the Sciences, Program in Occupational Therapy, Philadelphia, PA 19104-4495. Offers MOT, Dr OT. *Program availability:* Online learning. *Degree requirements:* For doctorate, capstone project. *Entrance requirements:* For doctorate, master's degree, two years of occupational therapy practice experience, 500-word essay. Electronic applications accepted.

The University of Toledo, College of Graduate Studies, College of Health Sciences, Department of Rehabilitation Sciences, Toledo, OH 43606-3390. Offers occupational therapy (OTD); physical therapy (DPT); speech-language pathology (MA). *Degree requirements:* For master's, comprehensive exam, thesis; for doctorate, thesis/dissertation or alternative. *Entrance requirements:* For master's, GRE, minimum cumulative GPA of 2.7 for all previous academic work, letters of recommendation; for doctorate, GRE, minimum cumulative GPA of 3.0 for all previous academic work, letters of recommendation; OTCAS or PTCAS application and UT supplemental application (for OTD and DPT). Additional exam requirements/recommendations for international students: Required—TOEFL (minimum score 550 paper-based; 80 iBT). Electronic applications accepted.

University of Toronto, Faculty of Medicine, Department of Occupational Science and Occupational Therapy, Toronto, ON M5S 1A1, Canada. Offers occupational therapy (M Sc OT). *Entrance requirements:* For master's, bachelor's degree with high academic standing from recognized university with minimum B average in final year, personal statement. Additional exam requirements/recommendations for international students: Required—TOEFL (minimum score 600 paper-based; 100 iBT), TWE (minimum score 5). Electronic applications accepted.

University of Utah, Graduate School, College of Health, Division of Occupational Therapy, Salt Lake City, UT 84108. Offers MOT, OTD. *Accreditation:* AOTA. *Program availability:* Part-time, evening/weekend, 100% online. *Faculty:* 10 full-time (all women), 10 part-time/adjunct (8 women). *Students:* 100 full-time (74 women), 27 part-time (23 women); includes 13 minority (2 Black or African American, non-Hispanic/Latino; 1 American Indian or Alaska Native, non-Hispanic/Latino; 6 Asian, non-Hispanic/Latino; 3 Hispanic/Latino). Average age 28. 200 applicants, 23% accepted, 34 enrolled. In 2015, 34 master's, 6 doctorates awarded. *Degree requirements:* For master's, thesis or alternative, project; for doctorate, thesis/dissertation or alternative, capstone. *Entrance requirements:* For master's, GRE General Test. Additional exam requirements/recommendations for international students: Required—TOEFL (minimum score 575 paper-based). *Application deadline:* For fall admission, 11/20 for domestic and international students. Application fee: $125. Electronic applications accepted. *Expenses:* Contact institution. *Financial support:* In 2015–16, 10 students received support. Career-related internships or fieldwork, Federal Work-Study, institutionally sponsored loans, scholarships/grants, and unspecified assistantships available. Financial award application deadline: 2/15; financial award applicants required to submit FAFSA. *Faculty research:* Community-based practice, occupational science, refugees, resilience, executive function, traumatic brain injury, pediatrics. *Total annual research expenditures:* $13,409. *Unit head:* Dr. Lorie Richards, Chairperson, 801-585-1069, Fax: 801-585-1001, E-mail: lorie.richards@hsc.utah.edu. *Application contact:* Kelly C. Brown, Academic Advisor, 801-585-0555, Fax: 801-585-1001, E-mail: kelly.brown@hsc.utah.edu.
Website: http://www.health.utah.edu/ot/

University of Washington, Graduate School, School of Medicine, Graduate Programs in Medicine, Department of Rehabilitation Medicine, Seattle, WA 98195-6490. Offers

Occupational Therapy

occupational therapy (MOT); physical therapy (DPT); prosthetics and orthotics (MPO); rehabilitation science (PhD). *Degree requirements:* For doctorate, comprehensive exam (for some programs), thesis/dissertation (for some programs). *Entrance requirements:* For master's and doctorate, GRE. Additional exam requirements/recommendations for international students: Required—TOEFL. *Faculty research:* Biomechanics, balance, brain injury, spinal cord injury, pain, degenerative diseases.

The University of Western Ontario, Faculty of Graduate Studies, Health Sciences Division, School of Occupational Therapy, London, ON N6A 5B8, Canada. Offers M Sc. *Program availability:* Part-time. *Degree requirements:* For master's, thesis. *Entrance requirements:* For master's, Canadian BA in occupational therapy or equivalent, minimum B+ average in last 2 years of 4 year degree. Additional exam requirements/recommendations for international students: Required—TOEFL (minimum score 570 paper-based). *Faculty research:* Human occupation, clumsy children, biomechanics, learning disabilities, ergonomics.

University of Wisconsin–La Crosse, College of Science and Health, Department of Health Professions, Program in Occupational Therapy, La Crosse, WI 54601-3742. Offers MS. *Accreditation:* AOTA. *Students:* 50 full-time (44 women), 27 part-time (25 women); includes 3 minority (1 Black or African American, non-Hispanic/Latino; 1 Hispanic/Latino; 1 Two or more races, non-Hispanic/Latino). Average age 25. 171 applicants, 25% accepted, 26 enrolled. In 2015, 22 master's awarded. *Degree requirements:* For master's, 6-month clinical internship. *Entrance requirements:* For master's, minimum GPA of 3.0, 20 job shadowing hours. Additional exam requirements/recommendations for international students: Required—TOEFL (minimum score 550 paper-based; 79 iBT). *Application deadline:* For fall admission, 1/4 for domestic students. Application fee: $50. Electronic applications accepted. *Expenses:* Contact institution. *Financial support:* Federal Work-Study, scholarships/grants, and health care benefits available. Support available to part-time students. Financial award application deadline: 3/15; financial award applicants required to submit FAFSA. *Unit head:* Dr. Peggy Denton, Director, 608-785-8470, E-mail: pdenton@uwlax.edu. *Application contact:* Brandon Schaller, Senior Graduate Student Status Examiner, 608-785-8941, E-mail: admissions@uwlax.edu.
Website: http://www.uwlax.edu/ot/

University of Wisconsin–Madison, Graduate School, School of Education, Department of Kinesiology, Occupational Therapy Program, Madison, WI 53706-1380. Offers MS, PhD. *Accreditation:* AOTA. *Degree requirements:* For doctorate, thesis/dissertation. *Expenses:* Tuition, state resident: full-time $5364. Tuition, nonresident: full-time $12,027. *Required fees:* $571. Tuition and fees vary according to campus/location, program and reciprocity agreements.

University of Wisconsin–Milwaukee, Graduate School, College of Health Sciences, Department of Occupational Science and Technology, Milwaukee, WI 53201-0413. Offers assistive technology and accessible design (Graduate Certificate); health sciences (PhD); occupational therapy (MS), including assistive technology and accessible design, ergonomics; therapeutic recreation (Graduate Certificate). *Accreditation:* AOTA. *Faculty:* 11 full-time (6 women), 1 (woman) part-time/adjunct. *Students:* 103 full-time (84 women), 15 part-time (12 women); includes 10 minority (1 Black or African American, non-Hispanic/Latino; 6 Asian, non-Hispanic/Latino; 3 Two or more races, non-Hispanic/Latino), 13 international. Average age 29. 122 applicants, 37% accepted, 38 enrolled. In 2015, 35 master's, 3 doctorates, 5 other advanced degrees awarded. *Degree requirements:* For master's, thesis or alternative. *Entrance requirements:* Additional exam requirements/recommendations for international students: Required—TOEFL (minimum score 550 paper-based; 79 iBT), IELTS (minimum score 6.5). *Application deadline:* For fall admission, 1/1 priority date for domestic students; for spring admission, 9/1 for domestic students. Applications are processed on a rolling basis. Application fee: $45 ($75 for international students). *Financial support:* Fellowships, research assistantships, teaching assistantships, and unspecified assistantships available. Support available to part-time students. Financial award application deadline: 4/15. *Unit head:* Jay Kapellusch, Department Chair, 414-229-5292, E-mail: kap@uwm.edu. *Application contact:* Roger O. Smith, General Information Contact, 414-229-6697, Fax: 414-229-6697, E-mail: smithro@uwm.edu.
Website: http://uwm.edu/healthsciences/academics/occupational-science-technology/

Utica College, Program in Occupational Therapy, Utica, NY 13502-4892. Offers MS. *Accreditation:* AOTA. *Program availability:* Part-time, evening/weekend. *Faculty:* 7 full-time (all women). *Students:* 94 full-time (78 women); includes 6 minority (1 Black or African American, non-Hispanic/Latino; 2 Asian, non-Hispanic/Latino; 2 Hispanic/Latino; 1 Two or more races, non-Hispanic/Latino), 1 international. Average age 26. 69 applicants, 100% accepted, 63 enrolled. In 2015, 62 master's awarded. *Degree requirements:* For master's, thesis. *Entrance requirements:* For master's, physical health exam, CPR certification, 60 hours of volunteer experience, minimum GPA of 3.0. Additional exam requirements/recommendations for international students: Required—TOEFL (minimum score 525 paper-based). *Application deadline:* Applications are processed on a rolling basis. Application fee: $50. Electronic applications accepted. *Expenses:* Contact institution. *Financial support:* Career-related internships or fieldwork, scholarships/grants, tuition waivers (partial), and unspecified assistantships available. Support available to part-time students. Financial award application deadline: 3/15; financial award applicants required to submit FAFSA. *Unit head:* Cora Bruns, Director, 315-792-3125, E-mail: cbruns@utica.edu. *Application contact:* John D. Rowe, Director of Graduate Admissions, 315-792-3824, Fax: 315-792-3003, E-mail: jrowe@utica.edu.

Virginia Commonwealth University, Graduate School, School of Allied Health Professions, Department of Occupational Therapy, Richmond, VA 23284-9005. Offers MS, MSOT, OTD. *Accreditation:* AOTA (one or more programs are accredited). *Degree requirements:* For master's, fieldwork. *Entrance requirements:* For master's, GRE General Test. Additional exam requirements/recommendations for international students: Required—TOEFL (minimum score 600 paper-based; 100 iBT); Recommended—IELTS (minimum score 6.5). Electronic applications accepted. *Faculty research:* Children with complex care needs, instrument development, carpal tunnel syndrome, development of oral-motor feeding programs, school system practice.

Virginia Commonwealth University, Graduate School, School of Allied Health Professions, Doctoral Program in Health Related Sciences, Richmond, VA 23284-9005. Offers clinical laboratory sciences (PhD); gerontology (PhD); health administration (PhD); nurse anesthesia (PhD); occupational therapy (PhD); physical therapy (PhD); radiation sciences (PhD); rehabilitation leadership (PhD). *Entrance requirements:* For doctorate, GRE General Test or MAT, minimum GPA of 3.3 in master's degree.

Additional exam requirements/recommendations for international students: Required—TOEFL (minimum score 600 paper-based; 100 iBT); Recommended—IELTS (minimum score 6.5). Electronic applications accepted.

Washington University in St. Louis, School of Medicine, Program in Occupational Therapy, Saint Louis, MO 63108. Offers MSOT, OTD. *Accreditation:* AOTA. Terminal master's awarded for partial completion of doctoral program. *Degree requirements:* For master's, fieldwork experiences; for doctorate, fieldwork and apprenticeship experiences. *Entrance requirements:* For master's and doctorate, GRE General Test, bachelor's degree in another field or enrollment in an affiliated institution. Additional exam requirements/recommendations for international students: Required—TOEFL, TWE (minimum score 5). Electronic applications accepted. *Faculty research:* Brain injury, ergonomics, work performance, care giving, quality of life, rehabilitation.

Wayne State University, Eugene Applebaum College of Pharmacy and Health Sciences, Department of Health Care Sciences, Program in Occupational Therapy, Detroit, MI 48202. Offers MOT. Students begin the program as undergraduates. *Accreditation:* AOTA. *Faculty:* 11. *Students:* 29 full-time (25 women); includes 22 minority (20 Asian, non-Hispanic/Latino; 2 Two or more races, non-Hispanic/Latino). Average age 26. In 2015, 34 master's awarded. *Entrance requirements:* For master's, minimum cumulative GPA of 3.0 and in science prerequisite coursework; personal resume; 20 contact hours under supervision of an OTR; interview; background check; OTCAS application. Additional exam requirements/recommendations for international students: Required—TOEFL (minimum score 550 paper-based; 79 iBT), Michigan English Language Assessment Battery (minimum score 85); Recommended—IELTS (minimum score 6.5), TWE (minimum score 5.5). *Application deadline:* For fall admission, 2/28 for domestic and international students. Electronic applications accepted. *Expenses:* $16,104 per year resident tuition, $32,401 non-resident tuition; $671 per credit hour resident tuition, $1,350.05 per credit hour non-resident tuition; fees include $47.45 per credit hour student services fee and $274.60 per semester registration fee. *Financial support:* Teaching assistantships and scholarships/grants available. Financial award application deadline: 3/31; financial award applicants required to submit FAFSA. *Faculty research:* Technology for neurorehabilitation, body shape and movement analysis, grasp and manipulation, methods of measurement of quality-of-life outcomes of the entire family of a person with chronic illnesses or disabilities, evaluating the efficacy of different types of family support interventions for persons of low socioeconomic status, program evaluation for persons with disabilities across the lifespan. *Unit head:* Dr. Doreen Head, Program Director, 313-577-5884, E-mail: doreen.head@wayne.edu. *Application contact:* 617-612-2860, Fax: 313-577-5822, E-mail: otcasinfo@otcas.org.
Website: http://cphs.wayne.edu/occupational-therapy/

West Coast University, Graduate Programs, North Hollywood, CA 91606. Offers advanced generalist (MSN); family nurse practitioner (MSN); health administration (MHA); occupational therapy (MS); pharmacy (Pharm D); physical therapy (DPT).

Western Michigan University, Graduate College, College of Health and Human Services, Department of Occupational Therapy, Kalamazoo, MI 49008. Offers MS. *Accreditation:* AOTA.

Western New Mexico University, Graduate Division, Program in Occupational Therapy, Silver City, NM 88062-0680. Offers MOT. *Accreditation:* AOTA. *Program availability:* Part-time.

West Virginia University, School of Medicine, Graduate Programs in Human Performance, Division of Occupational Therapy, Morgantown, WV 26506. Offers MOT. Students enter program as undergraduates. *Accreditation:* AOTA. *Program availability:* Online learning. *Degree requirements:* For master's, clinical rotation. *Entrance requirements:* For master's, interview, 2 reference forms, minimum GPA of 3.0, 60 hours of volunteer experience with people with disabilities. *Expenses:* Contact institution.

Winston-Salem State University, Department of Occupational Therapy, Winston-Salem, NC 27110-0003. Offers MS. *Accreditation:* AOTA. *Entrance requirements:* For master's, GRE, 3 letters of recommendation (one from a licensed occupational therapist where volunteer or work experiences were performed; the other two from former professors or persons acquainted with academic potential); writing sample. Additional exam requirements/recommendations for international students: Required—TOEFL. Electronic applications accepted. *Faculty research:* Assistive technology, environmental adaptations, comprehensive performance evaluations.

Worcester State University, Graduate Studies, Program in Occupational Therapy, Worcester, MA 01602-2597. Offers MOT. *Accreditation:* AOTA. *Faculty:* 4 full-time (all women), 2 part-time/adjunct (both women). *Students:* 52 full-time (42 women), 16 part-time (all women); includes 1 minority (American Indian or Alaska Native, non-Hispanic/Latino). Average age 26. 93 applicants, 34% accepted, 31 enrolled. In 2015, 22 master's awarded. *Degree requirements:* For master's, comprehensive exam (for some programs), thesis, fieldwork. *Entrance requirements:* For master's, GRE General Test or MAT, minimum undergraduate GPA of 3.0. Additional exam requirements/recommendations for international students: Required—TOEFL (minimum score 550 paper-based; 79 iBT). *Application deadline:* For fall admission, 3/1 priority date for domestic and international students. Applications are processed on a rolling basis. Application fee: $50. Electronic applications accepted. *Expenses:* Contact institution. *Financial support:* Career-related internships or fieldwork, scholarships/grants, and unspecified assistantships available. Financial award application deadline: 3/1; financial award applicants required to submit FAFSA. *Unit head:* Dr. Joanne Gallagher, Coordinator, 508-929-8783, Fax: 508-929-8178, E-mail: jgallagher@worcester.edu. *Application contact:* Sara Grady, Associate Dean of Graduate and Continuing Education, 508-929-8787, Fax: 508-929-8100, E-mail: sara.grady@worcester.edu.

Xavier University, College of Social Sciences, Health and Education, Department of Occupational Therapy, Cincinnati, OH 45207. Offers MOT. *Accreditation:* AOTA. *Degree requirements:* For master's, one foreign language, group research project. *Entrance requirements:* For master's, GRE (minimum of 33% average across all GRE sections - verbal, quantitative, analytical writing), minimum GPA of 3.0, completion of 40 volunteer hours, completion of all prerequisite courses with no more than 2 grades of C or lower; official transcript; personal statement; interview. Additional exam requirements/recommendations for international students: Required—TOEFL (minimum score 550 paper-based; 70 iBT) or IELTS. Electronic applications accepted. Application fee is waived when completed online. *Expenses:* Contact institution. *Faculty research:* Occupation, ethics, pediatric, occupational therapy interventions, pediatric occupational therapy assessment.

Perfusion

Milwaukee School of Engineering, Department of Electrical Engineering and Computer Science, Program in Perfusion, Milwaukee, WI 53202-3109. Offers MS. *Program availability:* Part-time, evening/weekend. *Faculty:* 2 full-time (0 women), 5 part-time/adjunct (1 woman). *Students:* 10 full-time (8 women); includes 1 minority (Hispanic/Latino). 44 applicants, 14% accepted, 6 enrolled. In 2015, 7 master's awarded. *Degree requirements:* For master's, comprehensive exam, thesis, exam. *Entrance requirements:* For master's, GRE General Test or GMAT (percentiles must average 50% or better), BS in appropriate discipline (biomedical engineering, biology, biomedical sciences, etc.), 3 letters of recommendation, personal interview, observation of 2 perfusion clinical cases. Additional exam requirements/recommendations for international students: Required—TOEFL (minimum score 79 iBT), IELTS (minimum score 6.5). *Application deadline:* Applications are processed on a rolling basis. Application fee: $0. Electronic applications accepted. *Expenses: Tuition, area resident:* Full-time $34,200; part-time $760 per credit. *Financial support:* Career-related internships or fieldwork, institutionally sponsored loans, and scholarships/grants available. Financial award application deadline: 3/15; financial award applicants required to submit FAFSA. *Faculty research:* Heart medicine. *Unit head:* Dr. Ronald Gerrits, Director, 414-277-7561, Fax: 414-277-7494, E-mail: gerrits@msoe.edu. *Application contact:* Ian Dahlinghaus, Graduate Program Associate, 414-277-7208, E-mail: dahlinghaus@msoe.edu.
Website: http://www.msoe.edu/community/academics/engineering/page/1328/perfusion-overview

See Display on this page and Close-Up on page 533.

Quinnipiac University, School of Health Sciences, Program in Cardiovascular Perfusion, Hamden, CT 06518-1940. Offers MHS. *Faculty:* 1 full-time (0 women), 4 part-time/adjunct (0 women). *Students:* 8 full-time (3 women), 9 part-time (3 women); includes 3 minority (2 Asian, non-Hispanic/Latino; 1 Hispanic/Latino). 48 applicants, 27% accepted, 8 enrolled. In 2015, 7 master's awarded. *Entrance requirements:* For master's, bachelor's degree in science or health-related discipline from an accredited American or Canadian college or university; 2 years of health care work experience; interview. *Application deadline:* For fall admission, 2/1 for domestic students. Applications are processed on a rolling basis. Application fee: $45. Electronic applications accepted. *Expenses:* $985 per credit tuition; $360 per semester student fee; $340 per semester (fall/spring) technology and lab fee; $75 per semester summer technology and lab fee. *Financial support:* Federal Work-Study, scholarships/grants, and unspecified assistantships available. Financial award application deadline: 6/1; financial award applicants required to submit FAFSA. *Faculty research:* Methods of preventing systemic inflammatory response syndrome (SIRS) during extracorporeal circulation of blood, investigations into the role of P-selectin in causing monocyte-platelet interaction, effect of simulated cardiopulmonary bypass on platelets and other formed elements in the blood. *Unit head:* Dr. Michael Smith, Director, 203-582-3427, E-mail: michael.smith@quinnipiac.edu. *Application contact:* Office of Graduate Admissions, 800-462-1944, Fax: 208-582-3443, E-mail: graduate@quinnipiac.edu. Website: http://www.quinnipiac.edu/gradperfusion

Rush University, College of Health Sciences, Program in Perfusion Technology, Chicago, IL 60612-3832. Offers MS. *Unit head:* Mindy Blackwell, Director, 312-942-7120, E-mail: charlotte_m_blackwell@rush.edu. *Application contact:* E-mail: chs_admissions@rush.edu.

The University of Arizona, College of Pharmacy, Department of Pharmacology and Toxicology, Graduate Program in Medical Pharmacology, Tucson, AZ 85721. Offers medical pharmacology (PhD); perfusion science (MS). *Degree requirements:* For master's, thesis; for doctorate, comprehensive exam, thesis/dissertation. *Entrance requirements:* For master's, GRE General Test, 3 letters of recommendation; for doctorate, GRE General Test, personal statement, 3 letters of recommendation. Additional exam requirements/recommendations for international students: Required—TOEFL (minimum score 550 paper-based; 79 iBT). *Application deadline:* For fall admission, 1/1 for domestic and international students. Applications are processed on a rolling basis. Application fee: $75. Electronic applications accepted. *Financial support:* Research assistantships, institutionally sponsored loans, and tuition waivers (partial) available. Financial award applicants required to submit FAFSA. *Faculty research:* Immunopharmacology, pharmacogenetics, pharmacogenomics, clinical pharmacology, ocularpharmacology and neuropharmacology. *Unit head:* Todd W. Vanderah, Director, 520-626-7801, Fax: 520-626-2204. *Application contact:* Anabel T. Moreno, Coordinator, 520-626-7218, Fax: 520-626-2204.
Website: http://www.pharmacology.arizona.edu/

University of Nebraska Medical Center, School of Allied Health Professions, Program in Clinical Perfusion Education, Omaha, NE 68198-4144. Offers distance education perfusion education (MPS); perfusion science (MPS). *Accreditation:* NAACLS. *Program availability:* Online learning. *Degree requirements:* For master's, comprehensive exam, thesis. *Entrance requirements:* For master's, GRE. Electronic applications accepted. *Expenses:* Tuition, state resident: full-time $7830; part-time $3915 per credit hour. Tuition, nonresident: full-time $22,410; part-time $11,205 per credit hour. *Required fees:* $521. *Faculty research:* Platelet gel, hemoconcentrators.

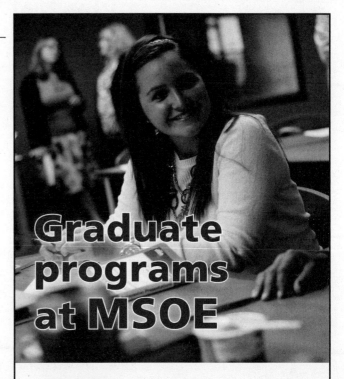

BUSINESS

- MBA
- MBA Education Leadership
- MBA STEM Leadership
- Engineering Management
- Marketing and Export Management
- New Product Management

ENGINEERING

- Architectural Engineering
- Civil Engineering
- Engineering

HEALTH PROFESSIONS

- Nursing–Health Care Systems Management
- Perfusion

Program formats vary but include blended, online and face-to-face.

Visit **msoe.edu/gpe**
Call **(800) 321-6763**
Email **gpe@msoe.edu**

Physical Therapy

Alabama State University, College of Health Sciences, Department of Physical Therapy, Montgomery, AL 36101-0271. Offers DPT. *Accreditation:* APTA. *Faculty:* 7 full-time (6 women). *Students:* 70 full-time (39 women), 18 part-time (12 women); includes 45 minority (35 Black or African American, non-Hispanic/Latino; 1 American Indian or Alaska Native, non-Hispanic/Latino; 8 Asian, non-Hispanic/Latino; 1 Two or more races, non-Hispanic/Latino), 1 international. Average age 28. 147 applicants, 16% accepted, 23 enrolled. In 2015, 29 doctorates awarded. Terminal master's awarded for partial completion of doctoral program. *Entrance requirements:* Additional exam requirements/recommendations for international students: Required—TOEFL (minimum score 500 paper-based). *Application deadline:* For fall admission, 7/15 for domestic students; for spring admission, 12/15 for domestic students. Applications are processed on a rolling basis. Application fee: $25. *Expenses: Tuition, area resident:* Full-time $3087; part-time $2744 per credit. Tuition, nonresident: full-time $6174; part-time $5488 per credit. *Required fees:* $2284; $1142 per credit. $571 per semester. Tuition and fees vary according to class time, course level, course load, degree level, program and student level. *Unit head:* Dr. Bernadette Williams-York, Chair, 334-229-4707, Fax: 334-229-4964, E-mail: asupt@alasu.edu. *Application contact:* Dr. William Person, Dean of Graduate Studies, 334-229-4274, Fax: 334-229-4928, E-mail: wperson@alasu.edu. Website: http://www.alasu.edu/academics/colleges—departments/health-sciences/physical-therapy/index.aspx

American International College, School of Health Sciences, Physical Therapy Program, Springfield, MA 01109-3189. Offers DPT. *Accreditation:* APTA. *Faculty:* 7 full-time (6 women), 3 part-time/adjunct (all women). *Students:* 90 full-time (56 women); includes 10 minority (3 Black or African American, non-Hispanic/Latino; 5 Asian, non-Hispanic/Latino; 2 Two or more races, non-Hispanic/Latino), 2 international. Average age 25. 100 applicants, 54% accepted, 30 enrolled. In 2015, 33 doctorates awarded. *Degree requirements:* For doctorate, comprehensive exam, thesis/dissertation. *Entrance requirements:* For doctorate, minimum GPA of 3.2 (recommended). *Application deadline:* For fall admission, 12/1 priority date for domestic and international students; for spring admission, 12/1 for domestic and international students. Application fee: $50. Electronic applications accepted. *Expenses:* Contact institution. *Financial support:* Career-related internships or fieldwork available. Financial award application deadline: 4/1; financial award applicants required to submit FAFSA. *Faculty research:* Ergonomics, orthopedics, teaching simulations. *Unit head:* Dr. Cindy Buchanan, Director, 413-205-3918, Fax: 413-654-1430, E-mail: cindy.buchanan@aic.edu. *Application contact:* Kerry Barnes, Director of Graduate Admissions, 413-205-3703, Fax: 413-205-3051, E-mail: kerry.barnes@aic.edu. Website: http://www.aic.edu/academics/hs/physical_therapy/dpt

Andrews University, School of Health Professions, Department of Physical Therapy, Postprofessional Physical Therapy Program, Berrien Springs, MI 49104. Offers Dr Sc PT, TDPT. *Accreditation:* APTA. *Students:* 17 full-time (10 women), 30 part-time (10 women); includes 6 minority (5 Asian, non-Hispanic/Latino; 1 Hispanic/Latino), 18 international. Average age 37. 61 applicants, 48% accepted, 22 enrolled. In 2015, 9 doctorates awarded. *Application deadline:* For fall admission, 12/1 priority date for domestic students. Applications are processed on a rolling basis. Application fee: $40. *Expenses:* Contact institution. *Financial support:* Federal Work-Study, institutionally sponsored loans, and scholarships/grants available. Financial award application deadline: 9/1; financial award applicants required to submit FAFSA. *Faculty research:* Home health patient profile, clinical education, breeding success of marine birds, trends in home health care for physical therapy, patient motivation in acute rehabilitation. *Unit head:* Kathy Berglund, Director of Professional Programs, 269-471-6076, Fax: 269-471-2866, E-mail: berglund@andrews.edu. *Application contact:* Jillian Panigot, Director of Admissions, 800-827-2878, Fax: 269-471-2867, E-mail: pt-info@andrews.edu. Website: http://www.andrews.edu/PHTH/

Angelo State University, College of Graduate Studies, Archer College of Health and Human Services, Department of Physical Therapy, San Angelo, TX 76909. Offers DPT. *Accreditation:* APTA. *Degree requirements:* For doctorate, 3 clinical placements. *Entrance requirements:* For doctorate, GRE General Test, interview, minimum undergraduate GPA of 3.0 in all prerequisite courses, essay, letters of recommendation, self-report transcript, volunteer hours. Additional exam requirements/recommendations for international students: Required—TOEFL or IELTS. *Application deadline:* For fall admission, 2/1 for domestic students, 3/10 for international students. Application fee: $40 ($50 for international students). Electronic applications accepted. *Expenses: Tuition, area resident:* Full-time $3726; part-time $2484 per year. Tuition, state resident: full-time $3726; part-time $2484 per year. Tuition, nonresident: full-time $10,746; part-time $7164 per year. International tuition: $10,746 full-time. *Required fees:* $2538; $1702 per unit. *Financial support:* Scholarships/grants available. Financial award application deadline: 3/1; financial award applicants required to submit FAFSA. *Faculty research:* Women and lipoproteins, international distance education, quadriceps femoris and the vastus medialis obliquus (VMO), ergonomics, children and obesity. *Unit head:* Dr. Shelly D. Weise, Chair, 325-486-6474, Fax: 325-942-2548, E-mail: shelly.weise@angelo.edu. *Application contact:* Amber M. Ward, Office Coordinator II, 325-486-6878, Fax: 325-942-2548, E-mail: amber.ward@angelo.edu. Website: http://www.angelo.edu/dept/physical_therapy/

Arcadia University, Graduate Studies, Department of Physical Therapy, Glenside, PA 19038-3295. Offers DPT. *Accreditation:* APTA. *Faculty:* 6 full-time (4 women), 20 part-time/adjunct (15 women). *Students:* 116 full-time (70 women), 176 part-time (125 women); includes 41 minority (4 Black or African American, non-Hispanic/Latino; 1 American Indian or Alaska Native, non-Hispanic/Latino; 28 Asian, non-Hispanic/Latino; 6 Hispanic/Latino; 1 Native Hawaiian or other Pacific Islander, non-Hispanic/Latino; 1 Two or more races, non-Hispanic/Latino), 4 international. Average age 34. 665 applicants, 32% accepted, 79 enrolled. In 2015, 133 doctorates awarded. *Application deadline:* For fall admission, 1/31 for domestic students. Application fee: $50. *Expenses:* Contact institution. *Financial support:* Career-related internships or fieldwork, tuition waivers (partial), and unspecified assistantships available. *Unit head:* Dr. Phil McClure, Chair, 215-572-2863, *Application contact:* 215-572-2910, Fax: 215-572-4049, E-mail: admiss@arcadia.edu.

Arkansas State University, Graduate School, College of Nursing and Health Professions, Department of Physical Therapy, State University, AR 72467. Offers DPT. *Accreditation:* APTA. *Program availability:* Part-time. *Faculty:* 8 full-time (4 women). *Students:* 87 full-time (44 women), 4 part-time (2 women); includes 18 minority (7 Black or African American, non-Hispanic/Latino; 4 Asian, non-Hispanic/Latino; 4 Hispanic/Latino; 1 Native Hawaiian or other Pacific Islander, non-Hispanic/Latino; 2 Two or more races, non-Hispanic/Latino), 3 international. Average age 25. 458 applicants, 7% accepted, 28 enrolled. In 2015, 31 doctorates awarded. *Degree requirements:* For doctorate, comprehensive exam, thesis/dissertation. *Entrance requirements:* For doctorate, GRE, Allied Health Professions Admissions Test, appropriate bachelor's or

master's degree, letters of reference, resume, official transcript, volunteer experience, criminal background check, immunization records, writing sample, PTCAS Application. Additional exam requirements/recommendations for international students: Required—TOEFL (minimum score 550 paper-based; 79 iBT), IELTS (minimum score 6), PTE (minimum score 56). *Application deadline:* For fall admission, 2/1 for domestic and international students. Applications are processed on a rolling basis. Application fee: $50. Electronic applications accepted. *Expenses:* Contact institution. *Financial support:* In 2015–16, 13 students received support. Fellowships, career-related internships or fieldwork, scholarships/grants, and unspecified assistantships available. Financial award application deadline: 7/1; financial award applicants required to submit FAFSA. *Unit head:* Dr. Shawn Drake, Chair, 870-972-3591, Fax: 870-972-3652, E-mail: sdrake@astate.edu. *Application contact:* Vickey Ring, Graduate Admissions Coordinator, 870-972-2737, Fax: 870-972-3917, E-mail: vickeyring@astate.edu. Website: http://www.astate.edu/college/conhp/departments/physical-therapy/

Armstrong State University, School of Graduate Studies, Program in Physical Therapy, Savannah, GA 31419-1997. Offers DPT. *Accreditation:* APTA. *Faculty:* 7 full-time (4 women). *Students:* 95 full-time (63 women); includes 6 minority (2 Black or African American, non-Hispanic/Latino; 3 Hispanic/Latino; 1 Two or more races, non-Hispanic/Latino), 1 international. Average age 26. In 2015, 20 doctorates awarded. *Degree requirements:* For doctorate, thesis/dissertation, licensure exam. *Entrance requirements:* For doctorate, GRE General Test, course work in general biology, chemistry, physical anatomy, physiology, and statistics; letters of recommendation; bachelor's degree; minimum GPA of 3.0; observation hours. Additional exam requirements/recommendations for international students: Required—TOEFL (minimum score 600 paper-based). *Application deadline:* For fall admission, 10/15 priority date for domestic students; for summer admission, 8/15 priority date for domestic students. Applications are processed on a rolling basis. Application fee: $30. Electronic applications accepted. *Expenses:* Contact institution. *Financial support:* In 2015–16, research assistantships with full tuition reimbursements (averaging $5,000 per year) were awarded; career-related internships or fieldwork, scholarships/grants, and unspecified assistantships also available. Financial award application deadline: 3/5; financial award applicants required to submit FAFSA. *Faculty research:* Therapeutic exercise, effectiveness of therapeutic interventions, injury prevention and prediction, effective teaching and learning in health professions. *Unit head:* Dr. Sara Plaspohl, Program Coordinator/Professor, 912-344-2780, Fax: 912-344-3490, E-mail: sara.plaspohl@armstrong.edu. *Application contact:* McKenzie Peterman, Assistant Director of Graduate Admissions, 912-344-2503, Fax: 912-344-3417, E-mail: graduate@armstrong.edu. Website: http://www.armstrong.edu/Health_Professions/rehabilitation_sciences/rehab_sci_doctor_physical_therapy

A.T. Still University, Arizona School of Health Sciences, Mesa, AZ 85206. Offers advanced occupational therapy (MS); advanced physician assistant studies (MS); athletic training (MS, DAT); audiology (Au D); occupational therapy (OTD); physical therapy (DPT); physician assistant studies (MS); transitional audiology (Au D); transitional physical therapy (DPT). *Accreditation:* AOTA (one or more programs are accredited); ASHA. *Program availability:* Part-time, evening/weekend, 100% online. *Faculty:* 54 full-time (31 women), 188 part-time/adjunct (132 women). *Students:* 509 full-time (339 women), 397 part-time (310 women); includes 203 minority (41 Black or African American, non-Hispanic/Latino; 5 American Indian or Alaska Native, non-Hispanic/Latino; 83 Asian, non-Hispanic/Latino; 57 Hispanic/Latino; 2 Native Hawaiian or other Pacific Islander, non-Hispanic/Latino; 15 Two or more races, non-Hispanic/Latino), 60 international. Average age 33. 3,902 applicants, 10% accepted, 245 enrolled. In 2015, 178 master's, 271 doctorates awarded. *Degree requirements:* For master's, thesis (for some programs); for doctorate, thesis/dissertation (for some programs). *Entrance requirements:* For master's, GRE General Test; for doctorate, GRE, Evaluation of Practicing Audiologists Capabilities (Au D), Physical Therapist Evaluation Tool (DPT), current state licensure, master's degree or equivalent (Au D). Additional exam requirements/recommendations for international students: Required—TOEFL (minimum score 80 iBT). *Application deadline:* Applications are processed on a rolling basis. Application fee: $70. Electronic applications accepted. *Expenses:* Contact institution. *Financial support:* In 2015–16, 158 students received support. Federal Work-Study and scholarships/grants available. Financial award application deadline: 5/1; financial award applicants required to submit FAFSA. *Faculty research:* Pediatric sport-related concussion, adolescent athlete health-related quality of life; geriatric and pediatric well-being, pain management for participation, practice-based research network, BMI and dental caries. *Total annual research expenditures:* $156,319. *Unit head:* Dr. Randy Danielsen, Dean, 480-219-6000, Fax: 480-219-6110, E-mail: rdanielsen@atsu.edu. *Application contact:* Donna Sparks, Associate Director, Admissions Processing, 660-626-2117, Fax: 660-626-2969, E-mail: admissions@atsu.edu. Website: http://www.atsu.edu/ashs

Augusta University, College of Allied Health Sciences, Department of Physical Therapy, Augusta, GA 30912. Offers DPT. *Accreditation:* APTA. *Program availability:* Part-time, online learning. *Degree requirements:* For doctorate, acute experience and rehabilitation experience. *Entrance requirements:* For doctorate, GRE, at least 100 hours of observational, volunteer or other work experiences in physical therapy settings. Additional exam requirements/recommendations for international students: Required—TOEFL (minimum score 500 paper-based; 79 iBT). *Application deadline:* For fall admission, 10/1 priority date for domestic students. Applications are processed on a rolling basis. Application fee: $25. Electronic applications accepted. *Financial support:* Federal Work-Study and institutionally sponsored loans available. Support available to part-time students. Financial award application deadline: 5/31; financial award applicants required to submit FAFSA. *Unit head:* Dr. Scott Hasson, Chairman, 706-721-2141, Fax: 706-721-3209, E-mail: shasson@augusta.edu. *Application contact:* Meisha Hudson, Office Manager, 706-721-2725, Fax: 706-721-7279, E-mail: meihudson@augusta.edu. Website: http://www.augusta.edu/alliedhealth/pt/

Azusa Pacific University, School of Behavioral and Applied Sciences, Department of Physical Therapy, Azusa, CA 91702-7000. Offers DPT. *Accreditation:* APTA. *Degree requirements:* For doctorate, thesis/dissertation. *Entrance requirements:* For doctorate, GRE General Test. Additional exam requirements/recommendations for international students: Required—TOEFL (minimum score 600 paper-based). Electronic applications accepted. *Expenses:* Contact institution. *Faculty research:* Antioxidants and endothelial function, EEG and pain, imaging ultrasound for MSK, metabolic function in obesity.

Baylor University, Graduate School, Military Programs, Program in Orthopedics, Waco, TX 76798. Offers D Sc. *Students:* 13 full-time (2 women), 4 part-time (1 woman); includes 1 minority (Hispanic/Latino). In 2015, 4 doctorates awarded. *Degree*

requirements: For doctorate, comprehensive exam. *Unit head:* Sharon Rosser, Graduate Program Director, 210-916-7142, E-mail: sharon.l.rosser.mil@mail.mil. *Application contact:* Lori McNamara, Admissions Coordinator, 254-710-3588, Fax: 254-710-3870.

Baylor University, Graduate School, Military Programs, Program in Physical Therapy, Waco, TX 76798. Offers DPT, DScPT. Program offered jointly with the U.S. Army. *Accreditation:* APTA. *Students:* 51 full-time (26 women); includes 6 minority (1 Black or African American, non-Hispanic/Latino; 2 Asian, non-Hispanic/Latino; 3 Hispanic/Latino). In 2015, 24 doctorates awarded. *Degree requirements:* For doctorate, comprehensive exam. *Application deadline:* For fall admission, 2/1 for domestic students. Applications are processed on a rolling basis. Application fee: $0. *Faculty research:* Effect of electrical stimulation on normal and immobilized muscle, effects of inversion traction. *Unit head:* Skip Gill, Graduate Program Director, 210-221-8410, Fax: 210-221-7585, E-mail: norman.w.gill2.mil@mail.mil. *Application contact:* Ted Croy, 210-221-6897, E-mail: theodore.w.croy2.mil@mail.mil.
Website: http://www.cs.amedd.army.mil/baylorpt/

Bellarmine University, Donna and Allan Lansing School of Nursing and Health Sciences, Louisville, KY 40205. Offers family nurse practitioner (MSN); health science (MHS); nursing administration (MSN); nursing education (MSN); nursing practice (DNP); physical therapy (DPT). *Accreditation:* AACN; APTA. *Program availability:* Part-time, evening/weekend. *Faculty:* 27 full-time (24 women), 8 part-time/adjunct (7 women). *Students:* 210 full-time (144 women), 91 part-time (83 women); includes 22 minority (6 Black or African American, non-Hispanic/Latino; 1 American Indian or Alaska Native, non-Hispanic/Latino; 7 Asian, non-Hispanic/Latino; 4 Hispanic/Latino; 4 Two or more races, non-Hispanic/Latino), 2 international. Average age 28. In 2015, 33 master's, 64 doctorates awarded. *Degree requirements:* For doctorate, comprehensive exam, thesis/dissertation. *Entrance requirements:* For master's, GRE General Test, RN license; for doctorate, GRE General Test, Physical Therapist Centralized Application Service (for DPT). Additional exam requirements/recommendations for international students: Required—TOEFL (minimum score 550 paper-based; 80 iBT). Application fee: $40. Electronic applications accepted. *Expenses:* Contact institution. *Financial support:* Career-related internships or fieldwork and scholarships/grants available. *Faculty research:* Nursing: pain, empathy, leadership styles, control; physical therapy: service-learning; exercise in chronic and pre-operative conditions, athletes; women's health; aging. *Unit head:* Dr. Mark Wiegand, Dean, 800-274-4723 Ext. 8368, E-mail: mwiegand@bellarmine.edu. *Application contact:* Julie Armstrong-Binnix, Health Science Recruiter, 800-274-4723 Ext. 8364, E-mail: julieab@bellarmine.edu.
Website: http://www.bellarmine.edu/lansing

Belmont University, College of Health Sciences, Nashville, TN 37212-3757. Offers nursing (MSN, DNP); occupational therapy (MSOT, OTD); physical therapy (DPT). *Program availability:* Part-time, online learning. *Faculty:* 54 full-time (50 women), 92 part-time/adjunct (81 women). *Students:* 371 full-time (324 women), 10 part-time (all women); includes 30 minority (10 Black or African American, non-Hispanic/Latino; 9 Asian, non-Hispanic/Latino; 6 Hispanic/Latino; 5 Two or more races, non-Hispanic/Latino), 2 international. Average age 26. *Degree requirements:* For master's, comprehensive exam, thesis; for doctorate, comprehensive exam. *Entrance requirements:* For master's, GRE, BSN, minimum GPA of 3.0. Additional exam requirements/recommendations for international students: Required—TOEFL (minimum score 550 paper-based). *Application deadline:* Applications are processed on a rolling basis. Application fee: $50. Electronic applications accepted. *Expenses:* Contact institution. *Financial support:* Teaching assistantships with full tuition reimbursements, career-related internships or fieldwork, scholarships/grants, and traineeships available. Financial award application deadline: 3/1; financial award applicants required to submit FAFSA. *Unit head:* Dr. Cathy Taylor, Dean, 615-460-6916, Fax: 615-460-6750. *Application contact:* David Mee, Dean of Enrollment Services, 615-460-6785, Fax: 615-460-5434, E-mail: david.mee@belmont.edu.
Website: http://www.belmont.edu/healthsciences/

Boston University, College of Health and Rehabilitation Sciences: Sargent College, Department of Physical Therapy and Athletic Training, Boston, MA 02215. Offers physical therapy (DPT); rehabilitation sciences (PhD). *Accreditation:* APTA (one or more programs are accredited). *Faculty:* 13 full-time (10 women), 26 part-time/adjunct (12 women). *Students:* 165 full-time (116 women); includes 36 minority (3 Black or African American, non-Hispanic/Latino; 14 Asian, non-Hispanic/Latino; 11 Hispanic/Latino; 8 Two or more races, non-Hispanic/Latino), 4 international. Average age 24. 867 applicants, 7% accepted, 33 enrolled. In 2015, 52 doctorates awarded. *Degree requirements:* For doctorate, comprehensive exam and thesis (for PhD). *Entrance requirements:* For doctorate, GRE General Test, master's degree (for PhD); bachelor's degree (for DPT). Additional exam requirements/recommendations for international students: Required—TOEFL (minimum score 550 paper-based; 84 iBT). *Application deadline:* For fall admission, 12/15 priority date for domestic and international students. Applications are processed on a rolling basis. Application fee: $120. Electronic applications accepted. *Expenses:* $1,537 per credit. *Financial support:* In 2015–16, 120 students received support, including 7 research assistantships with full tuition reimbursements available (averaging $21,000 per year), 6 teaching assistantships (averaging $2,500 per year); career-related internships or fieldwork, Federal Work-Study, institutionally sponsored loans, scholarships/grants, and tuition waivers (full and partial) also available. Financial award application deadline: 4/15; financial award applicants required to submit FAFSA. *Faculty research:* Gait, balance, motor control, dynamic systems analysis, spinal cord injury. *Total annual research expenditures:* $1.9 million. *Unit head:* Dr. Melanie Matthies, Department Chair, 617-353-2724, E-mail: pt@bu.edu. *Application contact:* Sharon Sankey, Assistant Dean, Student Services, 617-353-2713, Fax: 617-353-7500, E-mail: ssankey@bu.edu.
Website: http://www.bu.edu/sargent/

Bradley University, Graduate School, College of Education and Health Sciences, Department of Physical Therapy and Health Science, Peoria, IL 61625-0002. Offers physical therapy (DPT). *Accreditation:* APTA. *Entrance requirements:* For doctorate, GRE, 2 letters of recommendation. Additional exam requirements/recommendations for international students: Required—TOEFL (minimum score 600 paper-based; 100 iBT), IELTS (minimum score 6.5). Electronic applications accepted. *Expenses:* Contact institution.

California State University, Fresno, Division of Graduate Studies, College of Health and Human Services, Department of Physical Therapy, Fresno, CA 93740-8027. Offers MPT, DPT. *Accreditation:* APTA. *Degree requirements:* For master's, comprehensive exam. *Entrance requirements:* For master's, GRE General Test, minimum GPA of 3.0. Additional exam requirements/recommendations for international students: Required—TOEFL. Electronic applications accepted. *Faculty research:* Dance, occupational health, ethics.

California State University, Long Beach, Graduate Studies, College of Health and Human Services, Department of Physical Therapy, Long Beach, CA 90840. Offers DPT. *Accreditation:* APTA. *Entrance requirements:* Additional exam requirements/recommendations for international students: Required—TOEFL. Electronic applications accepted.

California State University, Northridge, Graduate Studies, College of Health and Human Development, Department of Physical Therapy, Northridge, CA 91330. Offers MPT. *Accreditation:* APTA. *Faculty:* 7 full-time (6 women), 8 part-time/adjunct (5 women). *Students:* 90 full-time (58 women); includes 47 minority (28 Asian, non-Hispanic/Latino; 10 Hispanic/Latino; 9 Two or more races, non-Hispanic/Latino). Average age 26. *Entrance requirements:* For master's, GRE General Test or minimum GPA of 3.0. Additional exam requirements/recommendations for international students: Required—TOEFL. *Application deadline:* For fall admission, 11/30 for domestic students. Application fee: $55. *Financial support:* Application deadline: 3/1. *Unit head:* Dr. Sheryl Low, Chair, 818-677-2203. *Application contact:* E-mail: pt@csun.edu.
Website: http://www.csun.edu/hhd/pt/

Campbell University, Graduate and Professional Programs, College of Pharmacy and Health Sciences, Buies Creek, NC 27506. Offers clinical research (MS); pharmaceutical sciences (MS); pharmacy (Pharm D); physician assistant (MPAP); public health (MS). *Accreditation:* ACPE. *Program availability:* Part-time, evening/weekend. *Entrance requirements:* For master's, MCAT, PCAT, GRE, bachelor's degree in health sciences or related field; for doctorate, PCAT. Additional exam requirements/recommendations for international students: Required—TOEFL (minimum score 550 paper-based; 79 iBT). Electronic applications accepted. *Expenses:* Contact institution. *Faculty research:* Immunology, medicinal chemistry, pharmaceutics, applied pharmacology.

Carroll University, Program in Physical Therapy, Waukesha, WI 53186-5593. Offers MPT, DPT. *Accreditation:* APTA. *Faculty:* 6 full-time (3 women), 5 part-time/adjunct (4 women). *Students:* 78 full-time (59 women); includes 4 minority (2 Asian, non-Hispanic/Latino; 2 Hispanic/Latino). Average age 24. 150 applicants, 69% accepted, 57 enrolled. In 2015, 33 doctorates awarded. *Degree requirements:* For master's, thesis (for some programs). *Entrance requirements:* For master's, GRE General Test, recommendations, clinical observation. Additional exam requirements/recommendations for international students: Required—TOEFL. *Application deadline:* For fall admission, 7/14 for domestic students. Applications are processed on a rolling basis. Application fee: $25. *Expenses:* Contact institution. *Financial support:* Available to part-time students. Application deadline: 3/15; applicants required to submit FAFSA. *Faculty research:* Physical therapy education, geriatrics, neural control of movement, wellness and prevention in apparently healthy individuals with disease and disability. *Unit head:* Dr. Jane F. Hopp, Dean, Natural and Health Sciences, 262-524-7294, E-mail: jhopp@carrollu.edu. *Application contact:* Tami Bartunek, Graduate Admission Counselor, 262-524-7643, E-mail: tbartune@carrollu.edu.
Website: http://www.carrollu.edu/gradprograms/physicaltherapy/default.asp

Central Michigan University, College of Graduate Studies, The Herbert H. and Grace A. Dow College of Health Professions, School of Rehabilitation and Medical Sciences, Mount Pleasant, MI 48859. Offers physical therapy (DPT); physician assistant (MS). *Accreditation:* APTA; ARC-PA. *Degree requirements:* For master's, thesis or alternative; for doctorate, thesis/dissertation or alternative. *Entrance requirements:* For master's and doctorate, GRE. Electronic applications accepted.

Chapman University, Crean College of Health and Behavioral Sciences, Department of Physical Therapy, Orange, CA 92866. Offers DPT, TDPT. *Accreditation:* APTA. *Faculty:* 16 full-time (10 women), 10 part-time/adjunct (5 women). *Students:* 137 full-time (75 women), 73 part-time (47 women); includes 90 minority (3 Black or African American, non-Hispanic/Latino; 58 Asian, non-Hispanic/Latino; 17 Hispanic/Latino; 12 Two or more races, non-Hispanic/Latino), 3 international. Average age 28. 1,500 applicants, 9% accepted, 67 enrolled. In 2015, 50 doctorates awarded. *Degree requirements:* For doctorate, 1440 hours of clinical experience. *Entrance requirements:* For doctorate, GRE, 40 hours of physical therapy observation (or paid work). Additional exam requirements/recommendations for international students: Required—TOEFL (minimum score 550 paper-based; 80 iBT), IELTS (minimum score 6.5). *Application deadline:* For fall admission, 11/16 for domestic students; for summer admission, 11/16 for domestic students. Electronic applications accepted. *Expenses:* $39,366 per year. *Financial support:* Fellowships, Federal Work-Study, and scholarships/grants available. Financial award applicants required to submit FAFSA. *Unit head:* Dr. Emmanuel John, Chair, 714-744-7906, E-mail: john@chapman.edu. *Application contact:* Adrian Rodriguez, 714-744-7620, E-mail: cudptadmissions@chapman.edu.

Chatham University, Program in Physical Therapy, Pittsburgh, PA 15232-2826. Offers DPT, TDPT. *Accreditation:* APTA. *Faculty:* 8 full-time (5 women), 1 (woman) part-time/adjunct. *Students:* 117 full-time (87 women), 1 (woman) part-time; includes 11 minority (2 Black or African American, non-Hispanic/Latino; 5 Asian, non-Hispanic/Latino; 4 Hispanic/Latino). Average age 25. 409 applicants, 18% accepted, 39 enrolled. In 2015, 37 doctorates awarded. *Entrance requirements:* For doctorate, GRE, community service, interview, minimum GPA of 3.0, writing sample, volunteer/work experience, 3 references. Additional exam requirements/recommendations for international students: Required—TOEFL (minimum score 600 paper-based; 100 iBT), IELTS (minimum score 7), TWE. *Application deadline:* For fall admission, 12/1 priority date for domestic and international students. Application fee: $45. Electronic applications accepted. Application fee is waived when completed online. *Expenses:* $10,944 per semester tuition; $230 per semester campus fee; $190 per semester lab and insurance fee. *Financial support:* Career-related internships or fieldwork available. Financial award applicants required to submit FAFSA. *Faculty research:* Stroke rehabilitation, osteoporosis and fall prevention, physical therapy for children with disabilities, evidence-based practice and decision-making, low back pain in children and adolescents. *Unit head:* Dr. Patricia Downey, Director, 412-365-1199, Fax: 412-365-1505, E-mail: downey@chatham.edu. *Application contact:* Ashlee Bartko, Senior Assistant Director of Graduate Admission, 412-365-2988, Fax: 412-365-1609, E-mail: gradadmissions@chatham.edu.
Website: http://www.chatham.edu/departments/healthmgmt/graduate/pt

Clarke University, Physical Therapy Program, Dubuque, IA 52001-3198. Offers DPT. *Accreditation:* APTA. *Faculty:* 6 full-time (4 women), 6 part-time/adjunct (3 women). *Students:* 63 full-time (42 women), 1 (woman) part-time. Average age 24. 167 applicants, 28% accepted, 33 enrolled. In 2015, 30 doctorates awarded. *Entrance requirements:* For doctorate, GRE, minimum GPA of 3.0; total of 30 hours observing in three of the following areas: pediatrics, geriatrics, inpatient, acute/subacute care, neurological rehabilitation, orthopedics, or sports medicine; three recommendations. Additional exam requirements/recommendations for international students: Required—TOEFL (minimum score 550 paper-based; 80 iBT). *Application deadline:* For fall admission, 11/2 for domestic students. Application fee: $0. Electronic applications accepted. *Expenses:* Contact institution. *Financial support:* In 2015–16, 6 students received support. Scholarships/grants and tuition waivers available. Financial award applicants required to submit FAFSA. *Faculty research:* Qualitative research, occupational health, discontinuous anaerobic studies, low back dysfunction. *Unit head:* Dr. Bill O'Dell, Chair, 319-588-6382, Fax: 319-588-8684. *Application contact:* Kara Shroeder, Academic Program Coordinator, 563-588-6354, Fax: 563-588-6789, E-mail: graduate@clarke.edu.
Website: http://www.clarke.edu/

Clarkson University, Graduate School, School of Arts and Sciences, Department of Physical Therapy, Potsdam, NY 13699. Offers DPT. *Accreditation:* APTA. *Faculty:* 9 full-time (4 women), 12 part-time/adjunct (9 women). *Students:* 73 full-time (51 women);

Physical Therapy

includes 10 minority (1 American Indian or Alaska Native, non-Hispanic/Latino; 2 Asian, non-Hispanic/Latino; 6 Hispanic/Latino; 1 Two or more races, non-Hispanic/Latino), 1 international. Average age 24. 359 applicants, 9% accepted, 25 enrolled. In 2015, 19 doctorates awarded. *Entrance requirements:* For doctorate, GRE, Physical Therapy Centralized Application Service (PTCAS) application, including transcripts of all college coursework, observation/volunteer or work experience in the field of study, two personal essays, and three letters of recommendation. Additional exam requirements/recommendations for international students: Required—TOEFL or IELTS. *Application deadline:* Applications are processed on a rolling basis. Application fee: $140. Electronic applications accepted. *Financial support:* In 2015–16, 72 students received support. Scholarships/grants and tuition waivers (partial) available. *Faculty research:* Longitudinal assessment of the risk of falling. *Total annual research expenditures:* $28,711. *Unit head:* Dr. George Fulk, Chair, 315-268-3786, Fax: 315-268-1539, E-mail: gfulk@clarkson.edu. *Application contact:* Jennifer Reed, Graduate School Coordinator, Provost's Office, 315-268-3802, Fax: 315-268-3989, E-mail: sciencegrad@clarkson.edu.
Website: http://www.clarkson.edu/pt/

Cleveland State University, College of Graduate Studies, College of Sciences and Health Professions, School of Health Sciences, Program in Physical Therapy, Cleveland, OH 44115. Offers DPT. *Accreditation:* APTA. *Faculty:* 7 full-time (6 women), 7 part-time/adjunct (5 women). *Students:* 10 full-time (9 women), 10 part-time (5 women); includes 6 minority (1 Asian, non-Hispanic/Latino; 3 Hispanic/Latino; 2 Two or more races, non-Hispanic/Latino), 1 international. Average age 25. 23 applicants, 13% accepted. In 2015, 35 doctorates awarded. *Degree requirements:* For doctorate, comprehensive exam. *Entrance requirements:* For doctorate, GRE (minimum scores: 450 verbal; 550 quantitative; 4.0 analytical writing), minimum overall GPA of 3.0. Additional exam requirements/recommendations for international students: Required—TOEFL (minimum score 550 paper-based; 78 iBT). *Application deadline:* For spring admission, 2/15 priority date for domestic and international students. Electronic applications accepted. Application fee is waived when completed online. *Expenses:* Contact institution. *Financial support:* In 2015–16, 9 research assistantships with tuition reimbursements were awarded; career-related internships or fieldwork and unspecified assistantships also available. Financial award application deadline: 1/1; financial award applicants required to submit FAFSA. *Faculty research:* Electronic gaming to increase balance, clinical education in physical therapy, use of ankle foot orthotics, function of patients on dialysis, student impressions on working with the elderly. *Unit head:* Dr. Karen Ann O'Loughlin, Director, 216-687-3581, Fax: 216-687-9316, E-mail: k.oloughlin@csuohio.edu. *Application contact:* Lisa Pistone, Associate Professor of Physical Therapy/Program Director, 216-687-3581, Fax: 216-687-9316, E-mail: s.m.giuffre@csuohio.edu.

The College of St. Scholastica, Graduate Studies, Department of Physical Therapy, Duluth, MN 55811-4199. Offers DPT. *Accreditation:* APTA. *Entrance requirements:* For doctorate, GRE. Additional exam requirements/recommendations for international students: Required—TOEFL (minimum score 550 paper-based; 79 iBT). Electronic applications accepted. *Faculty research:* Postural control, reliability and validity of spinal assessment tools, biomechanics of golf swing and low back pain, gait assessment and treatment, ethical issues.

College of Staten Island of the City University of New York, Graduate Programs, School of Health Sciences, Program in Physical Therapy, Staten Island, NY 10314-6600. Offers DPT. *Accreditation:* APTA. *Faculty:* 6 full-time, 9 part-time/adjunct. *Students:* 37 full-time. Average age 26. 203 applicants, 10% accepted, 19 enrolled. *Degree requirements:* For doctorate, 105 credits, four clinical affiliations. *Entrance requirements:* For doctorate, GRE, baccalaureate degree from regionally-accredited four-year institution by the end of the semester prior to entry. Additional exam requirements/recommendations for international students: Required—TOEFL (minimum score 550 paper-based; 79 iBT), IELTS (minimum score 6.5). *Application deadline:* For fall admission, 11/1 for domestic and international students. Application fee: $125. Electronic applications accepted. *Expenses:* Contact institution. *Financial support:* Applicants required to submit FAFSA. *Faculty research:* Spinal cord injury treatment, treatment of spasticity as a result of neurological disorders, transcranial stimulation, osteoarthritis, carpal tunnel treatment, balance & coordination evaluation and treatment. *Unit head:* Dr. Jeffrey Rothman, Chairperson, 718-982-3153, Fax: 718-982-2934, E-mail: jeffrey.rothman@csi.cuny.edu. *Application contact:* Sasha Spence, Associate Director for Graduate Admissions, 718-982-2019, Fax: 718-982-2500, E-mail: sasha.spence@csi.cuny.edu.

Columbia University, College of Physicians and Surgeons, Program in Physical Therapy, New York, NY 10032. Offers DPT. *Accreditation:* APTA. *Degree requirements:* For doctorate, fieldwork, capstone project. *Entrance requirements:* For doctorate, GRE General Test, undergraduate course work in biology, chemistry, physics, psychology, statistics and humanities. Additional exam requirements/recommendations for international students: Required—TOEFL. Electronic applications accepted. *Expenses:* Contact institution. *Faculty research:* Motor control, motion analysis, back assessment, recovery of function following neurological injury, women's health, disability awareness, pediatrics, orthopedics.

Concordia University, St. Paul, College of Education and Science, St. Paul, MN 55104-5494. Offers classroom instruction (MA Ed), including K-12 reading; criminal justice (MA); differentiated instruction (MA Ed); early childhood education (MA Ed); educational leadership (MA Ed, Ed D); educational technology (MA Ed); exercise science (MS); family science (MA); forensic mental health (MA); K-12 principal licensure (Ed S); K-12 reading (Certificate); orthotics and prosthetics (MS); physical therapy (DPT); special education (MA Ed, Certificate), including autism spectrum disorder (MA Ed), emotional and behavioral disorders (MA Ed), learning disabilities (MA Ed); sports management (MA); superintendent (Ed S); teaching (MAT). *Accreditation:* NCATE. *Program availability:* Part-time, evening/weekend, 100% online, blended/hybrid learning. *Faculty:* 15 full-time (6 women), 119 part-time/adjunct (67 women). *Students:* 1,327 full-time (944 women), 66 part-time (38 women); includes 168 minority (77 Black or African American, non-Hispanic/Latino; 12 American Indian or Alaska Native, non-Hispanic/Latino; 27 Asian, non-Hispanic/Latino; 25 Hispanic/Latino; 2 Native Hawaiian or other Pacific Islander, non-Hispanic/Latino; 25 Two or more races, non-Hispanic/Latino), 32 international. Average age 33. 924 applicants, 62% accepted, 473 enrolled. In 2015, 583 master's, 116 other advanced degrees awarded. *Degree requirements:* For master's, thesis (for some programs); for doctorate, thesis/dissertation (for some programs), clinical internships (for DPT); capstone projects (for Ed D); for other advanced degree, e-folio review of competencies. *Entrance requirements:* For master's, official transcripts from regionally-accredited institution stating the conferral of a bachelor's degree with minimum cumulative GPA of 3.0; personal statement; professional resume; practitioner in field through work or volunteerism; resume; for doctorate, GRE taken within last five years (for DPT), bachelor's degree with minimum cumulative GPA of 3.0, 100 physical therapy observation hours, and 2 letters of recommendation (for DPT); transcript, writing sample, three letters of recommendation, current resume, and on-campus interview (for Ed D); for other advanced degree, at least three years of teaching experience; master's degree; valid MN teaching license; writing sample; two letters of recommendation; resume. Additional exam requirements/

recommendations for international students: Recommended—TOEFL (minimum score 547 paper-based; 78 iBT), IELTS (minimum score 6). *Application deadline:* For fall admission, 8/1 for domestic and international students; for spring admission, 12/1 for domestic and international students; for summer admission, 5/1 for domestic and international students. Applications are processed on a rolling basis. Application fee: $50. Electronic applications accepted. *Expenses:* $36,450 (for DPT); $11,070 (for Ed D); $7,290 (for Ed S). *Financial support:* Applicants required to submit FAFSA. *Faculty research:* Teacher efficacy and its impact on reading instruction; autism in the criminal justice system; parental incarceration and its impact on children; use of video games to increase sport knowledge and game-play performance; challenges for women as leaders in college athletics. *Unit head:* Lonn Maly, Dean, 651-641-8203, E-mail: maly@csp.edu. *Application contact:* Kimberly Craig, Associate Vice President, Cohort Enrollment Management, 651-603-6223, Fax: 651-603-6320, E-mail: craig@csp.edu.

Concordia University Wisconsin, Graduate Programs, School of Human Services, Program in Physical Therapy, Mequon, WI 53097-2402. Offers MSPT, DPT. *Accreditation:* APTA. *Degree requirements:* For master's, comprehensive exam, thesis or alternative. *Entrance requirements:* Additional exam requirements/recommendations for international students: Required—TOEFL. *Expenses:* Contact institution.

Creighton University, School of Pharmacy and Health Professions, Program in Physical Therapy, Omaha, NE 68178-0001. Offers DPT. *Accreditation:* APTA. *Entrance requirements:* For doctorate, GRE. Additional exam requirements/recommendations for international students: Required—TOEFL. Electronic applications accepted. *Expenses: Tuition, area resident:* Full-time $14,400; part-time $800 per credit hour. *Required fees:* $158 per semester. Tuition and fees vary according to course load, campus/location, program, reciprocity agreements and student's religious affiliation. *Faculty research:* Patient safety in health services research, health information technology and health services research, Parkinson's rigidity and rehabilitation sciences, prion disease transmission, outcomes research in the rehabilitation sciences.

Daemen College, Department of Physical Therapy, Amherst, NY 14226-3592. Offers orthopedic manual physical therapy (Advanced Certificate); physical therapy-direct entry (DPT); transitional (DPT). *Accreditation:* APTA. *Program availability:* Part-time. *Degree requirements:* For doctorate, minimum C grade in all coursework; for Advanced Certificate, minimum GPA of 3.0; degree completion in maximum of 3 years. *Entrance requirements:* For doctorate, baccalaureate degree with minimum GPA of 2.8 in science coursework; letter of intent; resume; 2 letters of reference; 120 hours of PT exposure; transcripts; for Advanced Certificate, BS/BA; license to practice physical therapy; current registration; 2 recommendations; letter of intent; 2 years of physical therapy experience. Additional exam requirements/recommendations for international students: Required—TOEFL (minimum score 500 paper-based; 63 iBT), IELTS (minimum score 5.5). Electronic applications accepted. *Faculty research:* Athletic injuries, myofacial pain syndrome, electrical stimulation and tissue healing, lumbar spine dysfunction, temporomandibular joint syndrome.

Dalhousie University, Faculty of Health Professions, School of Physiotherapy, Halifax, NS B3H 3J5, Canada. Offers physiotherapy (entry to profession) (M Sc); physiotherapy (rehabilitation research) (M Sc). *Entrance requirements:* Additional exam requirements/recommendations for international students: Required—TOEFL, IELTS, CANTEST, CAEL, or Michigan English Language Assessment Battery. Electronic applications accepted.

Des Moines University, College of Health Sciences, Program in Physical Therapy, Des Moines, IA 50312-4104. Offers DPT. *Accreditation:* APTA. *Entrance requirements:* For doctorate, GRE. Additional exam requirements/recommendations for international students: Required—TOEFL. Electronic applications accepted. *Expenses:* Contact institution.

Dominican College, Division of Allied Health, Department of Physical Therapy, Orangeburg, NY 10962-1210. Offers MS, DPT. *Accreditation:* APTA. *Program availability:* Part-time, evening/weekend. *Degree requirements:* For master's, 3 clinical affiliations. *Entrance requirements:* For master's, minimum GPA of 3.0. Additional exam requirements/recommendations for international students: Required—TOEFL (minimum score 550 paper-based).

Drexel University, College of Nursing and Health Professions, Department of Physical Therapy and Rehabilitation Sciences, Philadelphia, PA 19102. Offers clinical biomechanics and orthopedics (PhD); hand and upper quarter rehabilitation (Certificate); hand therapy (MHS, PPDPT); orthopedics (MHS, PPDPT); pediatric rehabilitation (Certificate); pediatrics (MHS, PPDPT, PhD); physical therapy (DPT). *Accreditation:* APTA. *Program availability:* Part-time. Terminal master's awarded for partial completion of doctoral program. *Degree requirements:* For master's, comprehensive exam; for doctorate, thesis/dissertation, qualifying exam. *Entrance requirements:* For master's and doctorate, GRE General Test. Additional exam requirements/recommendations for international students: Required—TOEFL. Electronic applications accepted. *Faculty research:* Cerebral palsy, chronic low back pain, shoulder dysfunction, early intervention/community programs.

Duke University, School of Medicine, Physical Therapy Division, Durham, NC 27708. Offers DPT. *Accreditation:* APTA. *Faculty:* 17 full-time (9 women), 6 part-time/adjunct (5 women). *Students:* 212 full-time (148 women); includes 24 minority (6 Black or African American, non-Hispanic/Latino; 1 American Indian or Alaska Native, non-Hispanic/Latino; 8 Asian, non-Hispanic/Latino; 9 Hispanic/Latino), 2 international. 964 applicants, 13% accepted, 74 enrolled. In 2015, 61 doctorates awarded. *Degree requirements:* For doctorate, comprehensive exam, scholarly project. *Entrance requirements:* For doctorate, GRE, previous course work in anatomy, physiology, biological sciences, chemistry, physics, psychology, and statistics. Additional exam requirements/recommendations for international students: Recommended—TOEFL, IELTS. *Application deadline:* For fall admission, 11/1 priority date for domestic and international students. Applications are processed on a rolling basis. Application fee: $50. Electronic applications accepted. *Financial support:* In 2015–16, 11 students received support. Application deadline: 5/1; applicants required to submit FAFSA. *Faculty research:* Geriatrics, visual plasticity, educational outcomes, orthopedics, neurology. *Unit head:* Dr. Chad Cook, Program Director, 919-684-8905, Fax: 919-684-1846, E-mail: chad.cook@duke.edu. *Application contact:* Mya Shackleford, Admissions Coordinator, 919-668-5206, Fax: 919-684-1846, E-mail: mya.shackleford@duke.edu.
Website: http://dpt.duhs.duke.edu

Duquesne University, John G. Rangos, Sr. School of Health Sciences, Pittsburgh, PA 15282-0001. Offers health management systems (MHMS); occupational therapy (MS, OTD); physical therapy (DPT); physician assistant studies (MPAS); rehabilitation science (MS, PhD); speech-language pathology (MS); MBA/MHMS. *Accreditation:* AOTA (one or more programs are accredited); APTA (one or more programs are accredited); ASHA. *Program availability:* Minimal on-campus study. *Faculty:* 45 full-time (32 women), 33 part-time/adjunct (17 women). *Students:* 230 full-time (180 women), 11 part-time (5 women); includes 15 minority (1 Black or African American, non-Hispanic/Latino; 3 Asian, non-Hispanic/Latino; 7 Hispanic/Latino; 4 Two or more races, non-Hispanic/Latino), 20 international. Average age 23. 685 applicants, 9% accepted, 24 enrolled. In 2015, 132 master's, 32 doctorates awarded. *Degree requirements:* For doctorate, comprehensive exam (for some programs), thesis/dissertation (for some programs). *Entrance*

requirements: For master's, GRE General Test (speech-language pathology), 3 letters of recommendation; minimum GPA of 2.75 (health management systems), 3.0 (speech-language pathology); for doctorate, GRE General Test (for physical therapy and rehabilitation science), 3 letters of recommendation, minimum GPA of 3.0, personal interview. Additional exam requirements/recommendations for international students: Required—TOEFL (minimum score 550 paper-based; 90 iBT). *Application deadline:* For fall admission, 2/1 for domestic and international students; for spring admission, 7/1 for domestic and international students. Applications are processed on a rolling basis. Application fee: $0. Electronic applications accepted. *Expenses:* $1,254 per credit. *Financial support:* Federal Work-Study available. Financial award applicants required to submit FAFSA. *Faculty research:* Neuronal processing, electrical stimulation on peripheral neuropathy, central nervous system (CNS) stimulatory and inhibitory signals, behavioral genetic methodologies to development disorders of speech, neurogenic communication disorders. *Total annual research expenditures:* $38,730. *Unit head:* Dr. Gregory H. Frazer, Dean, 412-396-5303, Fax: 412-396-5554, E-mail: frazer@duq.edu. *Application contact:* Christopher R. Hilf, Recruiter/Academic Advisor, 412-396-5653, Fax: 412-396-5554, E-mail: hilfc@duq.edu.
Website: http://www.duq.edu/academics/schools/health-sciences

D'Youville College, Department of Physical Therapy, Buffalo, NY 14201-1084. Offers advanced orthopedic physical therapy (Certificate); manual physical therapy (Certificate); physical therapy (DPT). *Accreditation:* APTA. *Program availability:* Part-time, online learning. *Students:* 160 full-time (91 women), 4 part-time (2 women); includes 20 minority (6 Black or African American, non-Hispanic/Latino; 1 American Indian or Alaska Native, non-Hispanic/Latino; 9 Asian, non-Hispanic/Latino; 3 Hispanic/Latino; 1 Two or more races, non-Hispanic/Latino), 27 international. Average age 25. 368 applicants, 26% accepted, 57 enrolled. In 2015, 49 doctorates awarded. *Degree requirements:* For doctorate, comprehensive exam, project or thesis. *Entrance requirements:* For doctorate, bachelor's degree, minimum GPA of 3.0. Additional exam requirements/recommendations for international students: Required—TOEFL (minimum score 500 paper-based). *Application deadline:* For fall admission, 5/1 priority date for international students; for spring admission, 9/1 priority date for international students. Applications are processed on a rolling basis. Electronic applications accepted. *Expenses:* Tuition, area resident: Full-time $21,120; part-time $880 per credit hour. *Required fees:* $235; $96. One-time fee: $100. *Financial support:* Federal Work-Study and scholarships/grants available. Financial award application deadline: 3/1; financial award applicants required to submit FAFSA. *Faculty research:* Therapeutic effects of Tai Chi, orthopedics, health promotion in type 2 diabetes, athletic performance in youth and college sports, behavioral determinants in childhood obesity. *Total annual research expenditures:* $4,000. *Unit head:* Dr. Lynn Rivers, Chair, 716-829-7708, Fax: 716-829-8137, E-mail: riversl@dyc.edu. *Application contact:* Mark Pavone, Graduate Admissions Director, 716-829-8400, Fax: 716-829-7900, E-mail: graduateadmissions@dyc.edu.

East Carolina University, Graduate School, College of Allied Health Sciences, Department of Physical Therapy, Greenville, NC 27858-4353. Offers DPT. *Accreditation:* APTA. *Students:* 86 full-time (62 women); includes 7 minority (2 Black or African American, non-Hispanic/Latino; 3 Asian, non-Hispanic/Latino; 1 Hispanic/Latino; 1 Two or more races, non-Hispanic/Latino). Average age 24. 191 applicants, 18% accepted, 28 enrolled. In 2015, 29 doctorates awarded. *Entrance requirements:* Additional exam requirements/recommendations for international students: Required—TOEFL. *Application deadline:* For fall admission, 1/15 for domestic students. Application fee: $50. *Financial support:* Application deadline: 6/1. *Faculty research:* Diabetes and obesity, diabetic foot, ACL injury. *Unit head:* Dr. Walter L. Jenkins, Chair, 252-744-6234, E-mail: jenkinsw@ecu.edu. *Application contact:* Dean of Graduate School, 252-328-6012, Fax: 252-328-6071, E-mail: gradschool@ecu.edu.

Eastern Washington University, Graduate Studies, College of Science, Health and Engineering, Department of Physical Therapy, Cheney, WA 99004-2431. Offers DPT. *Accreditation:* APTA. *Degree requirements:* For doctorate, comprehensive exam, thesis/dissertation or final project. *Entrance requirements:* For doctorate, GRE General Test, minimum GPA of 3.0, 75 hours of experience, 3 letters of recommendation.

East Tennessee State University, School of Graduate Studies, College of Clinical and Rehabilitative Health Sciences, Department of Physical Therapy, Johnson City, TN 37614. Offers DPT. *Accreditation:* APTA. *Faculty:* 15 full-time (10 women), 3 part-time/adjunct (all women). *Students:* 106 full-time (57 women); includes 6 minority (1 Black or African American, non-Hispanic/Latino; 2 Asian, non-Hispanic/Latino; 2 Hispanic/Latino; 1 Two or more races, non-Hispanic/Latino). Average age 25. In 2015, 36 doctorates awarded. *Degree requirements:* For doctorate, comprehensive exam, internship. *Entrance requirements:* For doctorate, GRE General Test, minimum prerequisite GPA of 3.0, three letters of recommendation with at least one from a licensed PT, interview. Additional exam requirements/recommendations for international students: Required—TOEFL (minimum score 550 paper-based; 79 iBT). *Application deadline:* For spring admission, 3/1 priority date for domestic and international students. Application fee: $35 ($45 for international students). Electronic applications accepted. *Financial support:* In 2015–16, 17 students received support, including 18 research assistantships with tuition reimbursements available (averaging $4,200 per year); career-related internships or fieldwork, institutionally sponsored loans, scholarships/grants, and unspecified assistantships also available. Financial award application deadline: 7/1; financial award applicants required to submit FAFSA. *Faculty research:* Health and wellness across the lifespan; relationships between scapular kinematics, pain, and function; cognitive training and dual-task ability in older adult; vestibular rehabilitation and dizziness in geriatric patients; assessment tools for patients with TMJ dysfunction; proprioceptive training and gait variability in older adults. *Unit head:* Dr. Patricia King, Interim Chair, 423-439-8793, Fax: 423-439-8077, E-mail: kingpm@etsu.edu. *Application contact:* Mary Duncan, Graduate Specialist, 423-439-4302, Fax: 423-439-5624, E-mail: duncanm@etsu.edu.
Website: http://www.etsu.edu/crhs/physther/default.php

Elon University, Program in Physical Therapy, Elon, NC 27244-2010. Offers DPT. *Accreditation:* APTA. *Faculty:* 14 full-time (8 women), 10 part-time/adjunct (7 women). *Students:* 148 full-time (102 women); includes 9 minority (1 Black or African American, non-Hispanic/Latino; 2 Hispanic/Latino; 6 Two or more races, non-Hispanic/Latino). Average age 26. 992 applicants, 8% accepted, 46 enrolled. In 2015, 58 doctorates awarded. *Entrance requirements:* For doctorate, GRE General Test. Additional exam requirements/recommendations for international students: Required—TOEFL (minimum score 550 paper-based; 79 iBT). *Application deadline:* For fall admission, 11/2 for domestic students; for winter admission, 12/1 priority date for domestic students. Applications are processed on a rolling basis. Application fee: $50. Electronic applications accepted. *Financial support:* Federal Work-Study and scholarships/grants available. Financial award application deadline: 10/1; financial award applicants required to submit FAFSA. *Faculty research:* Exercise readiness in female survivors of domestic violence, animal-assisted therapy, locomotor training for multiple sclerosis patients, effect of infant positioning on the attainment of gross motor skills, physical activity levels for methadone maintenance treatment patients. *Unit head:* Dr. Stephen Folger, Chair, 336-278-6347, Fax: 336-278-6414, E-mail: folgers@elon.edu. *Application contact:* Art Fadde, Director of Graduate Admissions, 800-334-8448 Ext. 3, Fax: 336-278-7699, E-mail: afadde@elon.edu.
Website: http://www.elon.edu/dpt/

Emory University, School of Medicine, Programs in Allied Health Professions, Doctor of Physical Therapy Program, Atlanta, GA 30322. Offers DPT. *Accreditation:* APTA. *Entrance requirements:* For doctorate, GRE General Test. Additional exam requirements/recommendations for international students: Recommended—TOEFL. Electronic applications accepted. *Expenses:* Contact institution. *Faculty research:* Sensorimotor plasticity, biomechanics of walking, qualitative distinctions of moral practice, constraint induced therapy following stroke.

Florida Agricultural and Mechanical University, Division of Graduate Studies, Research, and Continuing Education, School of Allied Health Sciences, Division of Physical Therapy, Tallahassee, FL 32307-3200. Offers DPT. *Accreditation:* APTA. *Entrance requirements:* Additional exam requirements/recommendations for international students: Required—TOEFL.

Florida Gulf Coast University, College of Health Professions and Social Work, Department of Physical Therapy, Fort Myers, FL 33965-6565. Offers DPT. *Accreditation:* APTA. *Program availability:* Part-time, online learning. *Faculty:* 57 full-time (40 women), 39 part-time/adjunct (23 women). *Students:* 82 full-time (34 women), 3 part-time (1 woman); includes 13 minority (1 Black or African American, non-Hispanic/Latino; 4 Asian, non-Hispanic/Latino; 8 Hispanic/Latino). Average age 27. 42 applicants, 90% accepted, 31 enrolled. In 2015, 21 doctorates awarded. *Entrance requirements:* Additional exam requirements/recommendations for international students: Required—TOEFL (minimum score 550 paper-based). *Application deadline:* For fall admission, 1/15 priority date for domestic students. Applications are processed on a rolling basis. Application fee: $30. Electronic applications accepted. *Expenses:* Tuition, state resident: full-time $6974. Tuition, nonresident: full-time $28,170. *Required fees:* $1987. One-time fee: $10 full-time. Tuition and fees vary according to course load and degree level. *Financial support:* In 2015–16, 35 students received support. Career-related internships or fieldwork, Federal Work-Study, and institutionally sponsored loans available. Financial award application deadline: 6/30; financial award applicants required to submit FAFSA. *Faculty research:* Physical therapy practice and education. *Unit head:* Dr. Arie Van Juijn, Program Director, 239-590-7537, Fax: 239-590-7474, E-mail: avanduij@fgcu.edu. *Application contact:* MeLinda Coffey, Administrative Assistant, 239-590-7530, Fax: 239-590-7474, E-mail: mcoffey@fgcu.edu.

Florida International University, College of Nursing and Health Sciences, Department of Physical Therapy, Miami, FL 33199. Offers DPT. *Accreditation:* APTA. *Program availability:* Part-time. *Faculty:* 7 full-time (5 women), 11 part-time/adjunct (4 women). *Students:* 156 full-time (92 women), 4 part-time (all women); includes 96 minority (10 Black or African American, non-Hispanic/Latino; 18 Asian, non-Hispanic/Latino; 65 Hispanic/Latino; 1 Native Hawaiian or other Pacific Islander, non-Hispanic/Latino; 2 Two or more races, non-Hispanic/Latino), 1 international. Average age 25. 803 applicants, 9% accepted, 53 enrolled. In 2015, 54 doctorates awarded. *Degree requirements:* For doctorate, comprehensive exam. *Entrance requirements:* For doctorate, minimum undergraduate GPA of 3.0 in upper-level coursework; letter of intent; resume; at least 40 hours of observation within physical therapy clinic or facility. Additional exam requirements/recommendations for international students: Required—TOEFL (minimum score 550 paper-based; 80 iBT). *Application deadline:* For fall admission, 1/15 for domestic and international students. Application fee: $30. Electronic applications accepted. *Expenses:* Tuition, state resident: full-time $10,708; part-time $455.64 per credit hour. Tuition, nonresident: full-time $23,816; part-time $1001.69 per credit hour. *Required fees:* $390; $195 per semester. Tuition and fees vary according to program. *Financial support:* Institutionally sponsored loans, scholarships/grants, and unspecified assistantships available. Financial award application deadline: 3/1; financial award applicants required to submit FAFSA. *Faculty research:* Isokinetic test results and gait abnormalities after knee arthroscopy. *Unit head:* Dr. Mark Rossi, Interim Chair, 305-348-3478, E-mail: mark.rossi@fiu.edu. *Application contact:* Nanett Rojas, Manager, Admissions Operations, 305-348-7464, Fax: 305-348-7441, E-mail: gradadm@fiu.edu.
Website: http://cnhs.fiu.edu/index.html

Franklin Pierce University, Graduate and Professional Studies, Rindge, NH 03461-0060. Offers curriculum and instruction (M Ed); elementary education (MS Ed); emerging network technologies (Graduate Certificate); energy and sustainability studies (MBA, Graduate Certificate); health administration (MBA, Graduate Certificate); human resource management (MBA, Graduate Certificate); information technology (MBA); leadership (MBA); nursing education (MS); nursing leadership (MS); physical therapy (DPT); physician assistant studies (MPAS); special education (M Ed); sports management (MBA). *Accreditation:* APTA. *Program availability:* Part-time, online learning. *Degree requirements:* For master's, concentrated original research projects; student teaching; fieldwork and/or internship; leadership project; PRAXIS I and II (for M Ed); for doctorate, concentrated original research projects, clinical fieldwork and/or internship, leadership project. *Entrance requirements:* For master's, minimum GPA of 2.5, 3 letters of recommendation; competencies in accounting, economics, statistics, and computer skills through life experience or undergraduate coursework (for MBA); certification/e-portfolio, minimum C grade in all education courses (for M Ed); license to practice as RN (for MS in nursing); for doctorate, GRE, BA/BS, 3 letters of recommendation, personal mission statement, interview, writing sample, minimum cumulative GPA of 2.8, master's degree (for DA); 80 hours of observation/work in PT settings, completion of anatomy, chemistry, physics, and statistics, minimum GPA of 3.0 (for DPT). Additional exam requirements/recommendations for international students: Required—TOEFL (minimum score 550 paper-based; 61 iBT). *Application deadline:* Applications are processed on a rolling basis. Application fee: $0. Electronic applications accepted. *Expenses:* Tuition, area resident: Part-time $660 per credit hour. Tuition and fees vary according to program. *Financial support:* Teaching assistantships with tuition reimbursements, career-related internships or fieldwork, and unspecified assistantships available. Support available to part-time students. Financial award applicants required to submit FAFSA. *Faculty research:* Evidence-based practice in sports physical therapy, human resource management in economic crisis, leadership in nursing, innovation in sports facility management, differentiated learning and understanding by design. *Unit head:* Dr. Maria Altobello, Dean, 603-647-3509, Fax: 603-229-4580, E-mail: altobellom@franklinpierce.edu. *Application contact:* Graduate Studies, 800-325-1090, Fax: 603-626-4815, E-mail: cgps@franklinpierce.edu.
Website: http://www.franklinpierce.edu/academics/gradstudies/index.htm

Gannon University, School of Graduate Studies, Morosky College of Health Professions and Sciences, School of Health Professions, Program in Physical Therapy, Erie, PA 16541-0001. Offers DPT. *Accreditation:* APTA. *Students:* 148 full-time (81 women), 1 part-time (0 women); includes 9 minority (2 Black or African American, non-Hispanic/Latino; 2 Asian, non-Hispanic/Latino; 3 Hispanic/Latino; 2 Two or more races, non-Hispanic/Latino), 3 international. Average age 24. 224 applicants, 48% accepted, 52 enrolled. In 2015, 41 doctorates awarded. *Degree requirements:* For doctorate, thesis/dissertation or alternative, research project, practicum. *Entrance requirements:* For doctorate, baccalaureate degree from accredited college or university with minimum GPA of 3.0, interview. Additional exam requirements/recommendations for international students: Required—TOEFL (minimum score 79 iBT). *Application deadline:* For fall admission, 1/15 for domestic students. Application fee: $50. Electronic applications accepted. *Expenses:* Contact institution. *Financial support:* Scholarships/grants and unspecified assistantships available. Financial award application deadline: 7/1; financial

Physical Therapy

award applicants required to submit FAFSA. *Faculty research:* Ergonomics and cervical dysfunction, thoracic spine mobilization, anterior cruciate ligament injury in adolescent female athletes, ethics in physical therapy, admission requirements of entry-level physical therapy students. *Unit head:* Dr. Richard Johnson, Director, 814-871-4904, E-mail: johnson171@gannon.edu. *Application contact:* Bridget Philip, Director of Graduate Admissions, 814-871-7412, E-mail: graduate@gannon.edu.

George Fox University, Program in Physical Therapy, Newberg, OR 97132-2697. Offers DPT. *Accreditation:* APTA. *Entrance requirements:* For doctorate, bachelor's degree from regionally-accredited university or college, minimum GPA of 3.0. Additional exam requirements/recommendations for international students: Required—TOEFL, IELTS. *Application deadline:* For fall admission, 12/1 for domestic and international students. Application fee: $40. Electronic applications accepted. *Financial support:* Applicants required to submit FAFSA. *Unit head:* Dr. Tyler Cuddeford, Director, 503-554-2452, E-mail: tcuddeford@georgefox.edu. *Application contact:* Cristina Schmitt, Director of Graduate Admissions, 503-554-6097, Fax: 503-554-3110, E-mail: dpt@georgefox.edu.
Website: http://www.georgefox.edu/physical-therapy/index.html

The George Washington University, School of Medicine and Health Sciences, Health Sciences Programs, Program in Physical Therapy, Washington, DC 20052. Offers DPT. *Accreditation:* APTA. *Faculty:* 22 full-time (17 women), 14 part-time/adjunct (11 women). *Students:* 124 full-time (91 women), 2 part-time (1 woman); includes 32 minority (5 Black or African American, non-Hispanic/Latino; 1 American Indian or Alaska Native, non-Hispanic/Latino; 15 Asian, non-Hispanic/Latino; 7 Hispanic/Latino; 4 Two or more races, non-Hispanic/Latino), 1 international. Average age 26. 732 applicants, 18% accepted, 44 enrolled. In 2015, 33 doctorates awarded. *Entrance requirements:* Additional exam requirements/recommendations for international students: Required—TOEFL (minimum score 550 paper-based). *Application deadline:* For spring admission, 7/31 priority date for domestic students. Applications are processed on a rolling basis. Application fee: $75. *Unit head:* Dr. Joyce Maring, Director, 202-994-0053, E-mail: maringj@gwu.edu. *Application contact:* Marsha White, Program Administrator, 202-994-5105, E-mail: hsp@gwu.edu.

Georgia State University, Byrdine F. Lewis School of Nursing, Division of Physical Therapy, Atlanta, GA 30302-3083. Offers DPT. *Accreditation:* APTA. *Faculty:* 4 full-time (1 woman). *Students:* 107 full-time (61 women), 1 part-time (0 women); includes 29 minority (12 Black or African American, non-Hispanic/Latino; 15 Asian, non-Hispanic/Latino; 1 Native Hawaiian or other Pacific Islander, non-Hispanic/Latino; 1 Two or more races, non-Hispanic/Latino), 2 international. Average age 26. 343 applicants, 15% accepted, 36 enrolled. In 2015, 33 doctorates awarded. *Degree requirements:* For doctorate, comprehensive exam, thesis/dissertation or alternative, clinical education. *Entrance requirements:* For doctorate, GRE, transcripts, documentation of Physical Therapy Experience Form, statement of goals. Additional exam requirements/recommendations for international students: Required—TOEFL (minimum score 550 paper-based; 80 iBT). *Application deadline:* For fall admission, 11/15 for domestic and international students. Application fee: $50. Electronic applications accepted. *Expenses:* Contact institution. *Financial support:* In 2015–16, research assistantships with full tuition reimbursements (averaging $2,000 per year), teaching assistantships with full tuition reimbursements (averaging $2,000 per year) were awarded; scholarships/grants, tuition waivers (partial), and unspecified assistantships also available. Financial award application deadline: 4/1; financial award applicants required to submit FAFSA. *Faculty research:* Tissue regeneration, wheelchair propulsion, neurophysiology, function in cerebral palsy, musculoskeletal anatomy and function. *Unit head:* Dr. Andrew Butler, Department Head, 404-413-1415, Fax: 404-413-1230, E-mail: andrewbutler@gsu.edu. Website: http://physicaltherapy.gsu.edu/

Governors State University, College of Health Professions, Program in Physical Therapy, University Park, IL 60484. Offers MPT, DPT. *Accreditation:* APTA. *Degree requirements:* For master's, thesis or alternative. *Entrance requirements:* For master's, minimum GPA of 3.0 in field, 2.75 overall.

The Graduate Center, City University of New York, Graduate Studies, Program in Physical Therapy, New York, NY 10016-4039. Offers DPT. Program offered jointly with College of Staten Island of the City University of New York and Hunter College of the City University of New York. *Accreditation:* APTA. *Degree requirements:* For doctorate, exams, publishable research project. *Entrance requirements:* For doctorate, GRE, CPR certification, 100 hours of clinical experience, minimum undergraduate GPA of 3.0. Additional exam requirements/recommendations for international students: Required—TOEFL.

Grand Valley State University, College of Health Professions, Physical Therapy Program, Allendale, MI 49401-9403. Offers DPT. *Accreditation:* APTA. *Faculty:* 15 full-time (10 women), 6 part-time/adjunct (5 women). *Students:* 183 full-time (127 women), 6 part-time (5 women); includes 9 minority (2 Black or African American, non-Hispanic/Latino; 3 Asian, non-Hispanic/Latino; 2 Hispanic/Latino; 2 Two or more races, non-Hispanic/Latino). Average age 24. 463 applicants, 23% accepted, 77 enrolled. In 2015, 47 doctorates awarded. *Entrance requirements:* For doctorate, GRE, minimum GPA of 3.0 in most recent 60 hours and in prerequisites, 50 hours of volunteer work, interview, writing sample. Additional exam requirements/recommendations for international students: Required—TOEFL (minimum score 610 paper-based). *Application deadline:* For winter admission, 1/15 priority date for domestic and international students. Applications are processed on a rolling basis. Application fee: $30. Electronic applications accepted. *Financial support:* In 2015–16, 39 students received support, including 19 fellowships (averaging $2,031 per year), 28 research assistantships with tuition reimbursements available (averaging $3,584 per year); career-related internships or fieldwork, Federal Work-Study, institutionally sponsored loans, and unspecified assistantships also available. Financial award application deadline: 2/15. *Faculty research:* Balance deficits, motion analysis, nutritional knowledge of female athletes, trust in athletic performance, spinal functions dysfunction. *Unit head:* Dr. Daniel Vaughn, Director, 616-331-2678, Fax: 616-331-3350, E-mail: vaughnd@gvsu.edu. *Application contact:* Darlene Zwart, Student Services Coordinator, 616-331-3958, E-mail: zwartda@gvsu.edu.
Website: http://www.gvsu.edu/pt/

Hampton University, School of Science, Department of Physical Therapy, Hampton, VA 23668. Offers DPT. *Accreditation:* APTA. *Degree requirements:* For doctorate, thesis/dissertation. *Entrance requirements:* For doctorate, GRE General Test, bachelor's degree, minimum cumulative and prerequisite GPA of 3.0. Electronic applications accepted. *Expenses:* Contact institution. *Faculty research:* Physical therapy, cardiovascular disease, neuromuscular diseases and conditions, health disparities, cancer.

Harding University, College of Allied Health, Program in Physical Therapy, Searcy, AR 72149-0001. Offers DPT. *Accreditation:* APTA. *Faculty:* 9 full-time (3 women). *Students:* 95 full-time (48 women); includes 10 minority (5 Black or African American, non-Hispanic/Latino; 1 American Indian or Alaska Native, non-Hispanic/Latino; 1 Asian, non-Hispanic/Latino; 2 Hispanic/Latino; 1 Two or more races, non-Hispanic/Latino), 1 international. Average age 25. 75 applicants, 73% accepted, 37 enrolled. In 2015, 26 doctorates awarded. *Entrance requirements:* For doctorate, GRE. Additional exam requirements/recommendations for international students: Required—TOEFL (minimum score 550 paper-based). Application fee: $50. *Expenses:* Contact institution. *Unit head:* Dr. Michael McGalliard, Chair and Associate Professor, 501-279-5990, E-mail: mmcgalliard@harding.edu. *Application contact:* Dr. Cheri Yecke, Dean of Graduate Programs, 501-279-4335, Fax: 501-279-5192, E-mail: cyecke@harding.edu.
Website: http://www.harding.edu/pt/

Hardin-Simmons University, Graduate School, Holland School of Sciences and Mathematics, Department of Physical Therapy, Abilene, TX 79698. Offers DPT. *Accreditation:* APTA. *Faculty:* 8 full-time (4 women), 1 part-time/adjunct (0 women). *Students:* 82 full-time (57 women); includes 14 minority (1 Black or African American, non-Hispanic/Latino; 2 Asian, non-Hispanic/Latino; 10 Hispanic/Latino; 1 Native Hawaiian or other Pacific Islander, non-Hispanic/Latino). Average age 24. 204 applicants, 20% accepted, 28 enrolled. In 2015, 28 doctorates awarded. *Degree requirements:* For doctorate, comprehensive exam, thesis/dissertation or alternative. *Entrance requirements:* For doctorate, GRE, letters of recommendation, interview, transcripts from all colleges attended. Additional exam requirements/recommendations for international students: Required—TOEFL (minimum score 550 paper-based; 75 iBT). *Application deadline:* For fall admission, 11/1 priority date for domestic and international students. Applications are processed on a rolling basis. Application fee: $100 for international students. Electronic applications accepted. *Expenses:* Contact institution. *Financial support:* In 2015–16, 52 students received support. Scholarships/grants available. Financial award application deadline: 6/1; financial award applicants required to submit FAFSA. *Faculty research:* Upper limb tension (treatment effects); health promotion for seniors/disabled populations, sports injuries and recovery, sensory integration, postural stability, breathing techniques in tennis players. *Unit head:* Dr. Janelle K. O'Connell, Department Head/Professor, 325-670-5860, Fax: 325-670-5868, E-mail: ptoffice@hsutx.edu.
Website: http://www.hsutx.edu/academics/holland/graduate/physicaltherapy

Humboldt State University, Academic Programs, College of Professional Studies, Department of Kinesiology and Recreation Administration, Arcata, CA 95521-8299. Offers athletic training education (MS); exercise science/wellness management (MS); pre-physical therapy (MS); teaching/coaching (MS). *Degree requirements:* For master's, thesis or alternative. *Entrance requirements:* For master's, GMAT, minimum GPA of 2.5. Additional exam requirements/recommendations for international students: Required—TOEFL. *Application deadline:* For fall admission, 6/1 for domestic students; for spring admission, 12/2 for domestic students. Applications are processed on a rolling basis. Application fee: $55. *Financial support:* Teaching assistantships, career-related internships or fieldwork, Federal Work-Study, and institutionally sponsored loans available. Financial award application deadline: 3/1; financial award applicants required to submit FAFSA. *Faculty research:* Human performance, adapted physical education, physical therapy.
Website: http://www.humboldt.edu/kra/

Husson University, Doctorate in Physical Therapy Program, Bangor, ME 04401-2999. Offers DPT. *Accreditation:* APTA. *Faculty:* 10 full-time (6 women), 9 part-time/adjunct (6 women). *Students:* 74 full-time (42 women); includes 1 minority (Black or African American, non-Hispanic/Latino), 1 international. Average age 24. 428 applicants, 4% accepted, 10 enrolled. In 2015, 33 doctorates awarded. *Degree requirements:* For doctorate, group research project. *Entrance requirements:* For doctorate, GRE (minimum score of 1500), essay, minimum GPA of 3.5. Additional exam requirements/recommendations for international students: Required—TOEFL (minimum score 550 paper-based; 75 iBT). *Application deadline:* For fall admission, 4/15 for domestic and international students. Application fee: $50. Electronic applications accepted. *Expenses:* $23,514 per year. *Financial support:* Federal Work-Study and unspecified assistantships available. Financial award application deadline: 4/15; financial award applicants required to submit FAFSA. *Faculty research:* Educational and leadership processes within physical therapy programs; use of motor control and learning principles in treating clinical populations; approaches from dynamic systems to understand how social, cognitive, and physical development impact motor behavior and physical activity in children with and without disabilities; nervous system plasticity and spinal cord physiology. *Unit head:* Dr. Suzanne Gordon, Director, 207-941-7797, E-mail: gordons@husson.edu. *Application contact:* Cecile Ferguson, Administrative Assistant, 207-941-7101, E-mail: pt@fc.husson.edu.
Website: http://www.husson.edu/graduate-pt-admission

Idaho State University, Office of Graduate Studies, Kasiska College of Health Professions, Department of Physical and Occupational Therapy, Program in Physical Therapy, Pocatello, ID 83209-8045. Offers DPT. *Accreditation:* APTA. *Degree requirements:* For doctorate, comprehensive exam, thesis/dissertation, oral and written exam. *Entrance requirements:* For doctorate, GRE General Test, minimum GPA of 3.0, 80 hours in 2 practice settings of physical therapy. Additional exam requirements/recommendations for international students: Required—TOEFL (minimum score 600 paper-based). Electronic applications accepted. *Expenses:* Contact institution. *Faculty research:* Cardiovascular/pulmonary balance, neural plasticity, orthopedics, geriatrics, hypertension.

Indiana State University, College of Graduate and Professional Studies, College of Nursing, Health, and Human Services, Department of Applied Medicine and Rehabilitation, Terre Haute, IN 47809. Offers athletic training (MS, DAT); occupational therapy (MS); physical therapy (DPT); physician assistant (MS). *Degree requirements:* For master's, thesis or alternative. *Entrance requirements:* For master's, GRE General Test. Electronic applications accepted.

Indiana University–Purdue University Indianapolis, School of Health and Rehabilitation Sciences, Indianapolis, IN 46202-5119. Offers health and rehabilitation sciences (PhD); health sciences (MS); nutrition and dietetics (MS); occupational therapy (MS); physical therapy (DPT); physician assistant (MPAS). *Program availability:* Part-time, evening/weekend. *Degree requirements:* For master's, thesis (for some programs). *Entrance requirements:* For master's, GRE General Test, minimum GPA of 3.0 (for MS in health sciences, nutrition and dietetics), 3.2 (for MS in occupational therapy), 3.0 cumulative and prerequisite math/science (for MPAS); for doctorate, GRE, minimum cumulative and prerequisite math/science GPA of 3.2. Additional exam requirements/recommendations for international students: Required—TOEFL (minimum score 550 paper-based; 79 iBT), IELTS (minimum score 6.5), PTE (minimum score 54). Electronic applications accepted. *Expenses:* Contact institution. *Faculty research:* Function and mobility across the lifespan, pediatric nutrition, driving and mobility rehabilitation, neurorehabilitation and biomechanics, rehabilitation and integrative therapy.

Ithaca College, School of Health Sciences and Human Performance, Program in Physical Therapy, Ithaca, NY 14850. Offers physical therapy (DPT). *Accreditation:* APTA. *Faculty:* 17 full-time (9 women). *Students:* 167 full-time (119 women), 1 (woman) part-time; includes 18 minority (3 Black or African American, non-Hispanic/Latino; 9 Asian, non-Hispanic/Latino; 3 Hispanic/Latino; 3 Two or more races, non-Hispanic/Latino). Average age 23. In 2015, 82 doctorates awarded. *Degree requirements:* For doctorate, thesis/dissertation optional, clinical internship. *Entrance requirements:* Additional exam requirements/recommendations for international students: Required—TOEFL (minimum score 550 paper-based; 80 iBT). Tuition and fees vary according to program. *Financial support:* In 2015–16, 118 students received support. Career-related

internships or fieldwork, Federal Work-Study, and scholarships/grants available. Support available to part-time students. Financial award applicants required to submit CSS PROFILE or FAFSA. *Faculty research:* Mindful practice and failure in clinical education; relationships between patient characteristics, health behaviors and patient reported outcomes; prevention and treatment of knee injuries; use of technology in teaching and clinic; mindfulness and its role in failure within the clinical setting; evaluation and treatment of foot and ankle pathologies; shoulder impingement in individuals with spinal cord injury; cognitive-behavioral pain self-management; performing arts medicine; movement analysis. *Unit head:* Dr. Stephen Lahr, Chair, 607-274-3743, E-mail: lahr@ithaca.edu. *Application contact:* Nicole Eversley Bradwell, Interim Director, Office of Admission, 607-274-3124, Fax: 607-274-1263, E-mail: admission@ithaca.edu.
Website: http://www.ithaca.edu/gradprograms/pt/

Langston University, School of Physical Therapy, Langston, OK 73050. Offers DPT. *Accreditation:* APTA.

Lebanon Valley College, Program in Physical Therapy, Annville, PA 17003-1400. Offers DPT. *Accreditation:* APTA. *Faculty:* 9 full-time (4 women), 3 part-time/adjunct (0 women). *Students:* 76 full-time (54 women), 1 (woman) part-time; includes 9 minority (1 Black or African American, non-Hispanic/Latino; 1 American Indian or Alaska Native, non-Hispanic/Latino; 2 Hispanic/Latino; 5 Two or more races, non-Hispanic/Latino). Average age 23. 188 applicants, 27% accepted, 46 enrolled. In 2015, 30 doctorates awarded. *Degree requirements:* For doctorate, minimum GPA of 3.0. *Entrance requirements:* For doctorate, GRE, documented clinical hours. Additional exam requirements/recommendations for international students: Required—TOEFL (minimum score 80 iBT). *Application deadline:* For winter admission, 2/1 for domestic students. Electronic applications accepted. *Expenses:* $43,320 per professional year. *Financial support:* In 2015–16, 100 students received support. Scholarships/grants available. Financial award application deadline: 3/1; financial award applicants required to submit FAFSA. *Faculty research:* Concussions in athletes, exercise in autism spectrum disorders, predictors of injury in athletes, prevention and factors influencing healthcare beliefs and behaviors. *Unit head:* Dr. Stan M. Dacko, Chair of Physical Therapy, 717-867-6843, Fax: 717-867-6849, E-mail: dacko@lvc.edu. *Application contact:* EJ Smith, Assistant Director of Admission, 866-582-4236, Fax: 717-867-6026, E-mail: ejsmith@lvc.edu.
Website: http://www.lvc.edu/physical-therapy

Loma Linda University, School of Allied Health Professions, Department of Physical Therapy, Loma Linda, CA 92350. Offers physical therapy (DPT, PhD); rehabilitation (MS). *Accreditation:* APTA. *Entrance requirements:* Additional exam requirements/recommendations for international students: Required—TOEFL (minimum score 550 paper-based). *Application deadline:* For fall admission, 5/1 for domestic and international students; for winter admission, 12/1 for domestic and international students. Application fee: $60. Electronic applications accepted. *Unit head:* Chair, 909-558-1000. *Application contact:* Helen Greenwood, Director, Admissions and Records, 909-824-4599, Fax: 909-824-4809, E-mail: hgreenwood@sahp.llu.edu.

Long Island University–LIU Brooklyn, School of Health Professions, Brooklyn, NY 11201-8423. Offers athletic training and sport sciences (MS); exercise science (MS); occupational therapy (MS); physical therapy (DPT); physician assistant (MS); public health (MPH); social work (MSW). *Faculty:* 36 full-time (26 women), 47 part-time/adjunct (19 women). *Students:* 503 full-time (326 women), 112 part-time (82 women); includes 212 minority (117 Black or African American, non-Hispanic/Latino; 35 Asian, non-Hispanic/Latino; 48 Hispanic/Latino; 12 Two or more races, non-Hispanic/Latino), 59 international. Average age 31. 1,154 applicants, 38% accepted, 227 enrolled. In 2015, 228 master's, 41 doctorates awarded. *Degree requirements:* For master's, comprehensive exam (for some programs), thesis (for some programs), research capstone; for doctorate, comprehensive exam, research capstone. *Entrance requirements:* For master's and doctorate, GRE, two letters of recommendation. Additional exam requirements/recommendations for international students: Required—TOEFL (minimum score 550 paper-based; 79 iBT). *Application deadline:* Applications are processed on a rolling basis. Application fee: $50. Electronic applications accepted. *Expenses:* $1,155 per credit tuition, $934 per term full-time fees, $442 per term part-time fees. *Financial support:* In 2015–16, 10 research assistantships with partial tuition reimbursements (averaging $12,660 per year), 40 teaching assistantships with partial tuition reimbursements (averaging $12,660 per year) were awarded. Financial award application deadline: 2/15; financial award applicants required to submit FAFSA. *Faculty research:* Manual physical therapy, Parkinson's disease response to physical activity, violence in young minority men, LGBT safety. *Unit head:* Dr. Barry S. Eckert, Dean, 718-780-6578, Fax: 718-780-4561, E-mail: barry.eckert@liu.edu. *Application contact:* Richard Sunday, Dean of Admissions, 718-488-1011, Fax: 718-780-6110, E-mail: bkln-admissions@liu.edu.
Website: http://liu.edu/brooklyn/academics/school-of-health-professions

Louisiana State University Health Sciences Center, School of Allied Health Professions, Department of Physical Therapy, New Orleans, LA 70112-2223. Offers DPT. *Accreditation:* APTA. *Degree requirements:* For doctorate, thesis/dissertation optional. *Entrance requirements:* For doctorate, GRE General Test (minimum combined score: 296), 60 hours of experience in physical therapy, minimum GPA of 3.0 in math and science, bachelor's degree. Electronic applications accepted. *Faculty research:* Wound healing, spinal cord injury, pain management, geriatrics, muscle physiology, muscle damage, motor control, balance.

Lynchburg College, Graduate Studies, Doctor of Physical Therapy Program, Lynchburg, VA 24501-3199. Offers DPT. *Faculty:* 10 full-time (5 women), 1 part-time/adjunct (0 women). *Students:* 135 full-time (82 women), 1 (woman) part-time; includes 4 minority (1 American Indian or Alaska Native, non-Hispanic/Latino; 2 Asian, non-Hispanic/Latino; 1 Hispanic/Latino). Average age 25. In 2015, 45 doctorates awarded. *Degree requirements:* For doctorate, comprehensive exam. *Entrance requirements:* For doctorate, GRE, references, 4-year bachelor's degree. Additional exam requirements/recommendations for international students: Required—TOEFL. *Application deadline:* For spring admission, 2/1 priority date for domestic and international students. Applications are processed on a rolling basis. Application fee: $135. Electronic applications accepted. *Expenses:* $34,340 per year tuition and fees. *Financial support:* Scholarships/grants, tuition waivers (partial), and unspecified assistantships available. Financial award application deadline: 7/31; financial award applicants required to submit FAFSA. *Unit head:* Dr. A. Russell Smith, Jr., Associate Professor/Director of DPT Program, 434-544-8880, E-mail: smith.ar@lynchburg.edu. *Application contact:* Savannah G. Cook, Admissions Coordinator, 434-544-8885, Fax: 434-544-8887, E-mail: cook.s@lynchburg.edu.
Website: http://www.lynchburg.edu/graduate/doctor-of-physical-therapy/

Marquette University, Graduate School, College of Health Sciences, Department of Physical Therapy, Milwaukee, WI 53200. Offers DPT. *Accreditation:* APTA. *Faculty:* 18 full-time (8 women), 33 part-time/adjunct (20 women). *Students:* 94 full-time (69 women), 2 part-time (1 woman); includes 20 minority (1 Black or African American, non-Hispanic/Latino; 8 Asian, non-Hispanic/Latino; 7 Hispanic/Latino; 4 Two or more races, non-Hispanic/Latino). Average age 23. 1,311 applicants, 13% accepted, 12 enrolled. *Degree requirements:* For doctorate, clinical rotations. *Entrance requirements:*

For doctorate, GRE General Test. Additional exam requirements/recommendations for international students: Required—TOEFL. Application fee: $50. Electronic applications accepted. *Expenses:* Contact institution. *Financial support:* In 2015–16, 2 students received support, including 2 research assistantships with full tuition reimbursements available (averaging $21,750 per year); health care benefits and unspecified assistantships also available. Financial award application deadline: 2/15. *Faculty research:* Urban health issues, mechanisms and management of pain, kinesiologic principles, brain and spinal cord control of human locomotion, mechanisms of motor impairment. *Total annual research expenditures:* $905,127. *Unit head:* Dr. Lawrence Pan, Chair, 414-288-7161, Fax: 414-288-5987, E-mail: lawrence.pan@marquette.edu.
Website: http://www.marquette.edu/physical-therapy/

Marshall University, Academic Affairs Division, College of Health Professions, School of Physical Therapy, Huntington, WV 25755. Offers DPT. *Students:* 111 full-time (50 women); includes 2 minority (both Asian, non-Hispanic/Latino). Average age 25. In 2015, 25 doctorates awarded. *Application deadline:* Applications are processed on a rolling basis. *Unit head:* Dr. Penny G. Kroll, Program Director, 800-642-3463, E-mail: kroll@marshall.edu. *Application contact:* Information Contact, 304-746-1900, Fax: 304-746-1902, E-mail: services@marshall.edu.

Marymount University, School of Health Professions, Program in Physical Therapy, Arlington, VA 22207-4299. Offers DPT. *Accreditation:* APTA. *Faculty:* 8 full-time (6 women), 15 part-time/adjunct (13 women). *Students:* 118 full-time (79 women); includes 27 minority (4 Black or African American, non-Hispanic/Latino; 10 Asian, non-Hispanic/Latino; 9 Hispanic/Latino; 4 Two or more races, non-Hispanic/Latino), 4 international. Average age 27. 715 applicants, 23% accepted, 44 enrolled. In 2015, 33 doctorates awarded. *Degree requirements:* For doctorate, comprehensive exam, thesis/dissertation. *Entrance requirements:* For doctorate, GRE, 2 letters of recommendation, interview, resume, 40 hours of clinical work experience, essay, minimum GPA of 3.0 from previous university coursework. Additional exam requirements/recommendations for international students: Required—TOEFL (minimum score 600 paper-based; 96 iBT), IELTS (minimum score 6.5). *Application deadline:* For fall admission, 12/2 priority date for domestic students, 12/13 for international students. Application fee: $180. Electronic applications accepted. *Expenses:* $37,400 per year. *Financial support:* In 2015–16, 15 students received support, including 10 teaching assistantships with partial tuition reimbursements available; research assistantships with partial tuition reimbursements available, career-related internships or fieldwork, Federal Work-Study, scholarships/grants, and unspecified assistantships also available. Financial award applicants required to submit FAFSA. *Unit head:* Dr. Cathy S. Elrod, Chair, 703-284-5988, Fax: 703-284-5981, E-mail: cathy.elrod@marymount.edu. *Application contact:* Francesca Reed, Director, Graduate Admissions, 703-284-5901, Fax: 703-527-3815, E-mail: grad.admissions@marymount.edu.
Website: http://www.marymount.edu/Academics/Malek-School-of-Health-Professions/Graduate-Programs/Physical-Therapy-(D-P-T-)

Maryville University of Saint Louis, Walker College of Health Professions, Physical Therapy Program, St. Louis, MO 63141-7299. Offers DPT. *Accreditation:* APTA. *Faculty:* 16 full-time (12 women), 3 part-time/adjunct (all women). *Students:* 75 full-time (57 women), 39 part-time (29 women); includes 3 minority (2 Hispanic/Latino; 1 Two or more races, non-Hispanic/Latino). Average age 24. In 2015, 29 doctorates awarded. *Degree requirements:* For doctorate, clinical rotations. *Entrance requirements:* For doctorate, minimum cumulative GPA of 3.0 or ACT composite of 24, 2 letters of recommendation, interview, documentation of observation hours. Additional exam requirements/recommendations for international students: Required—TOEFL (minimum score 573 paper-based). *Application deadline:* Applications are processed on a rolling basis. Electronic applications accepted. Application fee is waived when completed online. *Expenses:* Tuition, area resident: Full-time $25,558; part-time $781 per credit hour. *Required fees:* $2400. Part-time tuition and fees vary according to course load and degree level. *Financial support:* Career-related internships or fieldwork, Federal Work-Study, and campus employment available. Financial award application deadline: 3/1; financial award applicants required to submit FAFSA. *Faculty research:* Memory and exercise. *Unit head:* Dr. Michelle Unterberg, Director, 314-529-9590, Fax: 314-529-9946, E-mail: munterberg@maryville.edu. *Application contact:* Crystal Jacobsmeyer, Assistant Director, Graduate Enrollment Advising, 314-529-9654, Fax: 314-529-9927, E-mail: cjacobsmeyer@maryville.edu.
Website: http://www.maryville.edu/hp/physical-therapy/

Mayo School of Health Sciences, Program in Physical Therapy, Rochester, MN 55905. Offers DPT. *Accreditation:* APTA. *Faculty:* 5 full-time (0 women), 3 part-time/adjunct (all women). *Students:* 84 full-time (57 women); includes 6 minority (3 Black or African American, non-Hispanic/Latino; 1 American Indian or Alaska Native, non-Hispanic/Latino; 1 Asian, non-Hispanic/Latino; 1 Hispanic/Latino). Average age 25. 629 applicants, 9% accepted, 28 enrolled. In 2015, 28 doctorates awarded. *Degree requirements:* For doctorate, comprehensive exam. *Entrance requirements:* For doctorate, GRE. Additional exam requirements/recommendations for international students: Required—TOEFL. *Application deadline:* For fall admission, 10/15 for domestic and international students. Applications are processed on a rolling basis. Electronic applications accepted. Full-time tuition and fees vary according to course load and program. *Financial support:* In 2015–16, 75 students received support. Scholarships/grants available. Financial award applicants required to submit FAFSA. *Faculty research:* Biomechanics, gait analysis, growth factor-mediated plasticity in muscle, musculoskeletal clinical tests and measures, Parkinson's disease, coordination testing. *Unit head:* Dr. John Hollman, Director, 507-284-9547, Fax: 507-284-0656, E-mail: hollman.john@mayo.edu. *Application contact:* Carol Cooper, Administrative Assistant, 507-284-2054, Fax: 507-284-0656, E-mail: cooper.carol@mayo.edu.
Website: http://www.mayo.edu/mshs/careers/physical-therapy/physical-therapy-doctoral-program-minnesota

McMaster University, Faculty of Health Sciences, Professional Program in Physiotherapy, Hamilton, ON L8S 4M2, Canada. Offers M Sc. *Degree requirements:* For master's, clinical placements, independent research project. *Entrance requirements:* For master's, minimum B average over last 60 undergraduate units. Additional exam requirements/recommendations for international students: Required—TOEFL (minimum score 600 paper-based).

Medical University of South Carolina, College of Health Professions, Program in Physical Therapy, Charleston, SC 29425. Offers DPT. *Accreditation:* APTA. *Program availability:* Online learning. *Entrance requirements:* For doctorate, GRE, references, minimum GPA of 3.0, volunteer hours. Additional exam requirements/recommendations for international students: Required—TOEFL (minimum score 600 paper-based). Electronic applications accepted. *Faculty research:* Low back pain, spinal cord injury.

Mercer University, Graduate Studies, Cecil B. Day Campus, College of Health Professions, Atlanta, GA 30341. Offers physical therapy (DPT); physician assistant (MM Sc); public health (MPH). *Faculty:* 27 full-time (19 women), 11 part-time/adjunct (7 women). *Students:* 286 full-time (230 women), 4 part-time (all women); includes 94 minority (69 Black or African American, non-Hispanic/Latino; 14 Asian, non-Hispanic/Latino; 7 Hispanic/Latino; 4 Two or more races, non-Hispanic/Latino), 3 international. Average age 26. In 2015, 80 master's, 32 doctorates awarded. *Expenses:* Contact institution. *Financial support:* Federal Work-Study, traineeships, and unspecified

Physical Therapy

assistantships available. *Faculty research:* Scholarship of teaching and learning, health disparities, clinical outcomes, health promotion. *Unit head:* Dr. Lisa Lundquist, Dean/Clinical Professor, 678-547-6308, E-mail: lundquist_lm@mercer.edu. *Application contact:* Laura Ellison, Director of Admissions and Student Affairs, 678-547-6391, E-mail: ellison_la@mercer.edu.
Website: http://chp.mercer.edu/

Mercy College, School of Health and Natural Sciences, Program in Physical Therapy, Dobbs Ferry, NY 10522-1189. Offers DPT. *Accreditation:* APTA. *Program availability:* Evening/weekend. *Entrance requirements:* For doctorate, interview, two letters of recommendations, official college transcripts with minimum GPA of 3.0, two-page typewritten essay on reasons for pursuing career in physical therapy, volunteer/work experience forms demonstrating at least eighty hours of volunteer work or work-related experience. Additional exam requirements/recommendations for international students: Required—TOEFL (minimum score 600 paper-based; 100 iBT), IELTS (minimum score 8). Electronic applications accepted. *Expenses:* Contact institution.

MGH Institute of Health Professions, School of Health and Rehabilitation Sciences, Doctor of Physical Therapy Program, Boston, MA 02129. Offers DPT. *Accreditation:* APTA. *Degree requirements:* For doctorate, thesis/dissertation or alternative, research project. *Entrance requirements:* For doctorate, GRE General Test, interview, minimum of 10 physical therapy observation hours, bachelor's degree from regionally-accredited college or university. Additional exam requirements/recommendations for international students: Required—TOEFL (minimum score 550 paper-based; 80 iBT). Electronic applications accepted. *Faculty research:* Disability in the elderly; gait, balance, and posture; cardiac rehabilitation: relationship of impairment to disability.

MGH Institute of Health Professions, School of Health and Rehabilitation Sciences, MS Program in Physical Therapy, Boston, MA 02129. Offers MS, Certificate. *Program availability:* Part-time, evening/weekend. *Degree requirements:* For master's, thesis, clinical preceptorship. *Entrance requirements:* For master's, GRE General Test, graduation from an approved program in physical therapy. Additional exam requirements/recommendations for international students: Required—TOEFL (minimum score 550 paper-based; 80 iBT). Electronic applications accepted. *Faculty research:* Disability in the elderly; gait, balance and posture; cardiac rehabilitation; relationship of impairment to disability; effect of muscle strengthening in the elderly.

Midwestern University, Downers Grove Campus, College of Health Sciences, Illinois Campus, Program in Physical Therapy, Downers Grove, IL 60515-1235. Offers DPT. *Accreditation:* APTA. *Entrance requirements:* For doctorate, GRE General Test. *Expenses:* Contact institution.

Midwestern University, Glendale Campus, College of Health Sciences, Arizona Campus, Program in Physical Therapy, Glendale, AZ 85308. Offers DPT. *Accreditation:* APTA. *Entrance requirements:* For doctorate, GRE General Test, bachelor's degree, minimum cumulative GPA of 2.75.

Misericordia University, College of Health Sciences, Program in Physical Therapy, Dallas, PA 18612-1098. Offers DPT. *Accreditation:* APTA. *Faculty:* 12 full-time (9 women), 5 part-time/adjunct (3 women). *Students:* 156 full-time (100 women), 7 part-time (3 women); includes 11 minority (3 Black or African American, non-Hispanic/Latino; 2 Asian, non-Hispanic/Latino; 4 Hispanic/Latino; 2 Two or more races, non-Hispanic/Latino). Average age 24. In 2015, 75 doctorates awarded. *Entrance requirements:* For doctorate, GRE General Test, minimum undergraduate GPA of 3.0, volunteer experience. Additional exam requirements/recommendations for international students: Required—TOEFL. *Application deadline:* For fall admission, 12/15 priority date for domestic students. Applications are processed on a rolling basis. Application fee: $35. Electronic applications accepted. *Financial support:* In 2015–16, 155 students received support. Career-related internships or fieldwork and scholarships/grants available. Support available to part-time students. Financial award application deadline: 6/30; financial award applicants required to submit FAFSA. *Faculty research:* Wound care, computer-assisted instruction, instruction in applied physiology, isokinetics, prosthetics. *Unit head:* Dr. Susan Barker, Chair, 570-674-6422, E-mail: sbarker@misericordia.edu. *Application contact:* Kristen Andrews, Assistant Director of Admissions, 570-674-6255, Fax: 570-674-6232, E-mail: kandrews@misericordia.edu.
Website: http://www.misericordia.edu/page.cfm?p-654

Missouri State University, Graduate College, College of Health and Human Services, Department of Physical Therapy, Springfield, MO 65897. Offers DPT. *Accreditation:* APTA. *Faculty:* 7 full-time (4 women), 13 part-time/adjunct (4 women). *Students:* 121 full-time (70 women); includes 6 minority (1 Black or African American, non-Hispanic/Latino; 1 Hispanic/Latino; 4 Two or more races, non-Hispanic/Latino). Average age 24. 69 applicants, 64% accepted, 38 enrolled. In 2015, 33 doctorates awarded. *Degree requirements:* For doctorate, comprehensive exam, thesis/dissertation or alternative. *Entrance requirements:* For doctorate, GRE, minimum GPA of 3.0, PTCAS. Additional exam requirements/recommendations for international students: Required—TOEFL (minimum score 550 paper-based; 79 iBT), IELTS (minimum score 6). *Application deadline:* For fall admission, 12/15 for domestic and international students. Application fee: $35 ($50 for international students). Electronic applications accepted. *Expenses:* Tuition, state resident: full-time $5500. Tuition, nonresident: full-time $10,108. *Required fees:* $1000. *Financial support:* Federal Work-Study, institutionally sponsored loans, and unspecified assistantships available. Financial award application deadline: 3/31; financial award applicants required to submit FAFSA. *Faculty research:* Complex regional pain syndrome (CRPS), posture and the temporomandibular joint, clinical orthopedics, aging of the motor system. *Unit head:* Dr. Jeanne Cook, Head, 417-836-6179, Fax: 417-836-6229, E-mail: physicaltherapy@missouristate.edu. *Application contact:* Misty Stewart, Coordinator of Graduate Admissions, 417-836-5330, Fax: 417-836-6200, E-mail: michaeledwards@missouristate.edu.
Website: http://www.missouristate.edu/physicaltherapy/

Mount St. Joseph University, Physical Therapy Program, Cincinnati, OH 45233-1670. Offers DPT. *Accreditation:* APTA. *Faculty:* 7 full-time (6 women), 1 part-time/adjunct (0 women). *Students:* 66 full-time (45 women), 43 part-time (13 women); includes 2 minority (1 Black or African American, non-Hispanic/Latino; 1 Two or more races, non-Hispanic/Latino). Average age 24. 148 applicants, 43% accepted, 43 enrolled. In 2015, 40 doctorates awarded. *Degree requirements:* For doctorate, clinical internship; integrative project. *Entrance requirements:* For doctorate, GRE, minimum GPA of 3.0; prerequisite coursework in sciences, humanities, social sciences, and statistics; 80 observation hours; at least 80 hours of clinical observation in 2 different physical therapy settings; PTCAS application. Additional exam requirements/recommendations for international students: Required—TOEFL (minimum score 560 paper-based; 83 iBT). *Application deadline:* For fall admission, 11/1 for domestic students. Application fee: $50. Electronic applications accepted. *Expenses:* Contact institution. *Financial support:* In 2015–16, 1 student received support. Application deadline: 6/1; applicants required to submit FAFSA. *Faculty research:* Utilizing technology in learning, neurobiology, assessment of student learning, critical thinking, effectiveness of distance education methods. *Unit head:* Dr. Rosanne Thomas, Chair, 513-244-4519, Fax: 513-451-2547, E-mail: rosanne.thomas@msj.edu. *Application contact:* Mary Brigham, Assistant Director of Graduate Recruitment, 513-244-4233, Fax: 513-244-4629, E-mail: mary.brigham@msj.edu.

Website: http://www.msj.edu/academics/graduate-programs/doctor-of-physical-therapy1/

Mount Saint Mary's University, Graduate Division, Los Angeles, CA 90049. Offers business administration (MBA); counseling psychology (MS); creative writing (MFA); education (MS, Certificate); film and television (MFA); health policy and management (MS); humanities (MA); nursing (MSN, Certificate); physical therapy (DPT); religious studies (MA). *Program availability:* Part-time, evening/weekend. *Faculty:* 115 full-time, 304 part-time. *Students:* 495 full-time (369 women), 149 part-time (121 women); includes 414 minority (73 Black or African American, non-Hispanic/Latino; 4 American Indian or Alaska Native, non-Hispanic/Latino; 60 Asian, non-Hispanic/Latino; 259 Hispanic/Latino; 7 Native Hawaiian or other Pacific Islander, non-Hispanic/Latino; 11 Two or more races, non-Hispanic/Latino), 4 international. Average age 33. 1,398 applicants, 21% accepted, 242 enrolled. In 2015, 172 master's, 26 doctorates, 23 other advanced degrees awarded. *Entrance requirements:* Additional exam requirements/recommendations for international students: Required—TOEFL. *Application deadline:* For fall admission, 6/30 priority date for domestic and international students; for spring admission, 10/30 priority date for domestic and international students; for summer admission, 3/30 priority date for domestic and international students. Applications are processed on a rolling basis. Application fee: $50. Electronic applications accepted. One-time fee: $135. Tuition and fees vary according to degree level. *Financial support:* Career-related internships or fieldwork, Federal Work-Study, institutionally sponsored loans, and tuition waivers (full and partial) available. Support available to part-time students. Financial award application deadline: 3/15; financial award applicants required to submit FAFSA. *Unit head:* Dr. Linda Moody, Graduate Dean, 213-477-2800, E-mail: gradprograms@msmu.edu. *Application contact:* Tara Wessel, Assistant Director, Graduate Admission, 213-477-2799, E-mail: gradprograms@msmu.edu.
Website: http://www.msmu.edu/graduate-programs/

Nazareth College of Rochester, Graduate Studies, Department of Physical Therapy, Doctoral Program in Physical Therapy, Rochester, NY 14618-3790. Offers DPT. *Accreditation:* APTA. *Entrance requirements:* For doctorate, minimum GPA of 3.0. *Application deadline:* For fall admission, 2/1 for domestic students. Application fee: $40. *Financial support:* Research assistantships with partial tuition reimbursements and career-related internships or fieldwork available. Support available to part-time students. Financial award application deadline: 3/1; financial award applicants required to submit FAFSA. *Unit head:* J.J. Mowder-Tinney, Associate Professor and Program Chair, 585-389-2901, E-mail: jmowder3@naz.edu. *Application contact:* Judith G. Baker, Director, Graduate Admissions, 585-389-2050, Fax: 585-389-2817, E-mail: gradstudies@naz.edu.

Neumann University, Program in Physical Therapy, Aston, PA 19014-1298. Offers DPT. *Accreditation:* APTA. *Program availability:* Evening/weekend. *Entrance requirements:* For doctorate, GRE, official transcripts, resume, three letters of recommendation, minimum of 200 hours of documented experience with a physical therapist. Additional exam requirements/recommendations for international students: Required—TOEFL. *Application deadline:* For fall admission, 11/1 for domestic students. Applications are processed on a rolling basis. Application fee: $50. Electronic applications accepted. *Expenses:* Contact institution. *Financial support:* Available to part-time students. Application deadline: 3/15; applicants required to submit FAFSA. *Unit head:* Dr. Robert Post, Director, 610-558-5233, Fax: 610-459-1370, E-mail: postr@neumann.edu. *Application contact:* Kittie D. Pain, Associate Director, Graduate and Adult Admissions, 610-558-5613, Fax: 610-558-5652, E-mail: paink@neumann.edu.

New York Institute of Technology, School of Health Professions, Department of Physical Therapy, Old Westbury, NY 11568-8000. Offers DPT. *Accreditation:* APTA. *Faculty:* 9 full-time (5 women), 13 part-time/adjunct (6 women). *Students:* 113 full-time (69 women); includes 39 minority (5 Black or African American, non-Hispanic; 21 Asian, non-Hispanic/Latino; 12 Hispanic/Latino; 1 Two or more races, non-Hispanic/Latino), 2 international. Average age 25. 1,016 applicants, 7% accepted, 43 enrolled. In 2015, 31 doctorates awarded. *Entrance requirements:* For doctorate, minimum undergraduate GPA of 3.0, interview, essay, 100 hours of volunteer or paid work under direct supervision of a physical therapist, 2 letters of recommendation. Additional exam requirements/recommendations for international students: Required—TOEFL (minimum score 550 paper-based; 79 iBT), IELTS (minimum score 6). *Application deadline:* For fall admission, 10/1 for domestic and international students. Application fee: $50. *Expenses: Tuition, area resident:* Full-time $20,790; part-time $1155 per credit. *Required fees:* $95; $75 per credit. Full-time tuition and fees vary according to degree level, campus/location and program. Part-time tuition and fees vary according to course load and campus/location. *Financial support:* Research assistantships with partial tuition reimbursements, scholarships/grants, health care benefits, tuition waivers, and unspecified assistantships available. Support available to part-time students. Financial award application deadline: 3/1; financial award applicants required to submit FAFSA. *Faculty research:* Parkinson's disease, spinal cord injury, manual therapy, educational technology, response to exercise, geriatrics, balance, virtual reality. *Unit head:* Dr. Karen Friel, Department Chair, 516-686-7651, Fax: 516-686-7699, E-mail: kfriel@nyit.edu. *Application contact:* Alice Dolitsky, Director, Graduate Admissions, 516-686-7520, Fax: 516-686-1116, E-mail: nyitgrad@nyit.edu.
Website: http://www.nyit.edu/degrees/physical_therapy

New York Medical College, School of Health Sciences and Practice, Department of Physical Therapy, Valhalla, NY 10595-1691. Offers DPT. *Accreditation:* APTA. *Degree requirements:* For doctorate, comprehensive exam, thesis/dissertation, project. *Entrance requirements:* For doctorate, GRE, minimum GPA of 3.2. Additional exam requirements/recommendations for international students: Required—TOEFL (minimum score 637 paper-based; 117 iBT), IELTS (minimum score 7). Electronic applications accepted. Application fee is waived when completed online. *Expenses:* Contact institution.

New York University, Steinhardt School of Culture, Education, and Human Development, Department of Physical Therapy, New York, NY 10010-5615. Offers orthopedic physical therapy (Advanced Certificate); physical therapy (MA, DPT, PhD), including pathokinesiology (MA). *Accreditation:* APTA (one or more programs are accredited). *Program availability:* Part-time. *Degree requirements:* For master's, thesis (for some programs); for doctorate, thesis/dissertation. *Entrance requirements:* For master's, physical therapy certificate; for doctorate, GRE General Test, interview, physical therapy certificate. Additional exam requirements/recommendations for international students: Required—TOEFL (minimum score 100 iBT). Electronic applications accepted. *Faculty research:* Motor learning and control, neuromuscular disorders, biomechanics and ergonomics, movement analysis, pathomechanics.

Northeastern University, Bouvé College of Health Sciences, Boston, MA 02115-5096. Offers applied behavior analysis (MS, CAGS); audiology (Au D); biomedical nanotechnology (MS); college student development and counseling (MS, CAGS); counseling psychology (MS, PhD, CAGS); exercise science (MS); health informatics (MS); medicinal chemistry (MS); nurse anesthesia (DNP, CAGS); nursing (MS, PhD, CAGS), including administration (MS), adult-gerontology acute care nurse practitioner (MS, CAGS), adult-gerontology primary care nurse practitioner (MS, CAGS), anesthesia (MS), family nurse practitioner (MS, CAGS), neonatal nurse practitioner (MS, CAGS), pediatric nurse practitioner (MS, CAGS), psychiatric mental health nurse practitioner

(MS, CAGS); nursing practice (DNP); personal health informatics (PhD); pharmaceutical sciences (MS, PhD), including interdisciplinary concentration, pharmaceutics and drug delivery systems; pharmacology (MS); pharmacy (Pharm D); physical therapy (Postbaccalaureate Certificate); physician assistant (MS); population health (PhD); school psychology (MS, PhD, CAGS); speech-language pathology (MS); urban health (MPH); MS/MBA. *Accreditation:* ACPE (one or more programs are accredited). *Program availability:* Part-time, evening/weekend, online learning. *Faculty:* 194 full-time (120 women), 169 part-time/adjunct (136 women). *Students:* 1,416 full-time (1,049 women), 310 part-time (248 women). In 2015, 374 master's, 313 doctorates, 37 other advanced degrees awarded. *Degree requirements:* For doctorate, thesis/dissertation (for some programs); for other advanced degree, comprehensive exam. Application fee: $75. Electronic applications accepted. *Expenses:* Contact institution. *Financial support:* Applicants required to submit FAFSA. *Unit head:* John R. Reynolds, Professor and Interim Dean, 617-373-3323, Fax: 617-373-3030. *Application contact:* Molly Schnabel, Senior Director of Graduate Affairs, 617-373-2708, Fax: 617-373-4701, E-mail: bouvegrad@neu.edu.
Website: http://www.northeastern.edu/bouve/

Northern Arizona University, Graduate College, College of Health and Human Services, Department of Physical Therapy, Flagstaff, AZ 86011. Offers DPT. *Accreditation:* APTA. *Entrance requirements:* For doctorate, GRE General Test, minimum GPA of 3.0. Additional exam requirements/recommendations for international students: Required—TOEFL (minimum score 550 paper-based; 80 iBT), IELTS (minimum score 7). *Application deadline:* For fall admission, 11/1 priority date for domestic and international students. Applications are processed on a rolling basis. Application fee: $65. Electronic applications accepted. *Expenses:* Contact institution. *Financial support:* Career-related internships or fieldwork, Federal Work-Study, scholarships/grants, health care benefits, tuition waivers (full and partial), and unspecified assistantships available. Financial award applicants required to submit FAFSA. *Unit head:* Dr. Patricia S. Pohl, Chair, 602-877-2368, E-mail: patricia.pohl@nau.edu. *Application contact:* John Hammond, Program Coordinator, 928-523-4270, Fax: 928-523-9289, E-mail: physical.therapy@nau.edu.
Website: http://nau.edu/chhs/physical-therapy/

Northern Illinois University, Graduate School, College of Health and Human Sciences, School of Allied Health and Communicative Disorders, Program in Physical Therapy, De Kalb, IL 60115-2854. Offers MPT, DPT, TDPT. *Accreditation:* APTA; CEPH. *Program availability:* Part-time. *Students:* 100 full-time (55 women), 2 part-time (both women); includes 15 minority (3 Black or African American, non-Hispanic/Latino; 2 Asian, non-Hispanic/Latino; 5 Hispanic/Latino; 5 Two or more races, non-Hispanic/Latino). Average age 26. 171 applicants, 17% accepted, 23 enrolled. In 2015, 37 doctorates awarded. *Degree requirements:* For master's, comprehensive exam, thesis optional, internship, research paper in public health. *Entrance requirements:* For master's, GRE General Test, minimum GPA of 2.75. Additional exam requirements/recommendations for international students: Required—TOEFL (minimum score 550 paper-based). *Application deadline:* For fall admission, 6/1 for domestic students, 5/1 for international students; for spring admission, 11/1 for domestic students, 10/1 for international students. Applications are processed on a rolling basis. Application fee: $40. Electronic applications accepted. *Financial support:* Fellowships with full tuition reimbursements, research assistantships with full tuition reimbursements, teaching assistantships with full tuition reimbursements, career-related internships or fieldwork, Federal Work-Study, scholarships/grants, tuition waivers (full), and unspecified assistantships available. Support available to part-time students. Financial award applicants required to submit FAFSA. *Faculty research:* Stroke rehabilitation, radon exposure prevention, environmental causes of cancer, body image in young girls. *Unit head:* Sherrill Morris, Chair, 815-753-1486, Fax: 815-753-6169, E-mail: ahcd@niu.edu. *Application contact:* Graduate School Office, 815-753-0395, E-mail: gradsch@niu.edu.
Website: http://www.chhs.niu.edu/physical_therapy/

Northwestern University, Feinberg School of Medicine, Department of Physical Therapy and Human Movement Sciences, Chicago, IL 60611-2814. Offers neuroscience (PhD), including movement and rehabilitation science; physical therapy (DPT); DPT/PhD. *Accreditation:* APTA. *Faculty:* 30 full-time, 26 part-time/adjunct. *Students:* 281 full-time (208 women); includes 56 minority (8 Black or African American, non-Hispanic/Latino; 1 American Indian or Alaska Native, non-Hispanic/Latino; 32 Asian, non-Hispanic/Latino; 12 Hispanic/Latino; 1 Native Hawaiian or other Pacific Islander, non-Hispanic/Latino; 2 Two or more races, non-Hispanic/Latino). Average age 25. 556 applicants, 34% accepted, 93 enrolled. *Degree requirements:* For doctorate, synthesis research project. *Entrance requirements:* For doctorate, GRE General Test (for DPT), baccalaureate degree with minimum GPA of 3.0 in required course work (DPT). Additional exam requirements/recommendations for international students: Required—TOEFL (minimum score 600 paper-based; 100 iBT). *Application deadline:* For fall admission, 10/3 for domestic and international students. Applications are processed on a rolling basis. Application fee: $50. Electronic applications accepted. *Expenses:* Contact institution. *Financial support:* Institutionally sponsored loans and scholarships/grants available. Financial award application deadline: 3/1; financial award applicants required to submit FAFSA. *Faculty research:* Motor control, robotics, neuromuscular imaging, student performance (academic/professional), clinical outcomes. *Unit head:* Dr. Julius P. A. Dewald, Professor and Chair, 312-908-8160, Fax: 312-908-0741. *Application contact:* Dr. Jane Sullivan, Associate Professor/Assistant Chair for Recruitment and Admissions, 312-908-8160, Fax: 312-908-0741, E-mail: dpt-admissions@northwestern.edu.
Website: http://www.feinberg.northwestern.edu/sites/pthms/

Nova Southeastern University, College of Health Care Sciences, Fort Lauderdale, FL 33314-7796. Offers anesthesiologist assistant (MSA); audiology (Au D); health science (MH Sc, DHSc, PhD); occupational therapy (MOT, Dr OT, PhD); physical therapy (DPT, TDPT); physician assistant (MMS). *Program availability:* Online learning. *Faculty:* 109 full-time (64 women), 100 part-time/adjunct (65 women). *Students:* 1,590 full-time (1,179 women), 969 part-time (819 women); includes 831 minority (234 Black or African American, non-Hispanic/Latino; 8 American Indian or Alaska Native, non-Hispanic/Latino; 151 Asian, non-Hispanic/Latino; 378 Hispanic/Latino; 1 Native Hawaiian or other Pacific Islander, non-Hispanic/Latino; 59 Two or more races, non-Hispanic/Latino), 18 international. Average age 30. 8,133 applicants, 14% accepted, 728 enrolled. In 2015, 556 master's, 105 doctorates awarded. *Degree requirements:* For master's, thesis; for doctorate, comprehensive exam, thesis/dissertation. *Entrance requirements:* For master's, GRE General Test, MCAT; for doctorate, GRE General Test, personal interview, essay. Additional exam requirements/recommendations for international students: Required—TOEFL (minimum score 600 paper-based). *Application deadline:* For winter admission, 4/15 for domestic students; for summer admission, 12/15 for domestic and international students. Applications are processed on a rolling basis. Application fee: $50. Electronic applications accepted. *Expenses:* Contact institution. *Financial support:* In 2015–16, 151 students received support, including 4 research assistantships (averaging $3,500 per year); institutionally sponsored loans and unspecified assistantships also available. Financial award application deadline: 4/15; financial award applicants required to submit FAFSA. *Unit head:* Dr. Stanley Wilson, Dean, 954-262-1203, E-mail: swilson@nova.edu. *Application contact:* Joey Jankie,

Admissions Counselor, 954-262-7249, E-mail: joey@nova.edu.
Website: http://www.nova.edu/chcs.

Oakland University, Graduate Study and Lifelong Learning, School of Health Sciences, Program in Physical Therapy, Rochester, MI 48309-4401. Offers clinical exercise science (Dr Sc PT); complementary medicine and wellness (Dr Sc PT); corporate worksite wellness (Dr Sc PT); exercise science (Dr Sc PT); neurological rehabilitation (Dr Sc PT, TDPT); orthopedic manual physical therapy (Dr Sc PT, TDPT, Graduate Certificate); orthopedic physical therapy (Graduate Certificate); orthopedics (Dr Sc PT, TDPT); pediatric rehabilitation (Dr Sc PT, TDPT); physical therapy (DPT); teaching and learning for rehabilitation professionals (Dr Sc PT, TDPT). *Accreditation:* APTA. *Faculty:* 12 full-time (9 women), 1 part-time/adjunct (0 women). *Students:* 138 full-time (100 women), 19 part-time (13 women); includes 8 minority (4 Asian, non-Hispanic/Latino; 4 Two or more races, non-Hispanic/Latino), 3 international. Average age 25. 604 applicants, 7% accepted, 42 enrolled. In 2015, 41 doctorates, 15 other advanced degrees awarded. *Entrance requirements:* For doctorate, GRE General Test. Additional exam requirements/recommendations for international students: Required—TOEFL (minimum score 550 paper-based). *Application deadline:* For fall admission, 10/15 for domestic and international students. Application fee: $0. *Expenses:* Contact institution. *Financial support:* Federal Work-Study, institutionally sponsored loans, and tuition waivers (full) available. Financial award application deadline: 3/1; financial award applicants required to submit FAFSA. *Unit head:* Dr. Kristine A. Thompson, Physical Therapy Program Director/Special Instructor, 248-364-8662, E-mail: kathomps@oakland.edu.
Website: http://www.oakland.edu/shs/pt/

The Ohio State University, College of Medicine, School of Health and Rehabilitation Sciences, Program in Physical Therapy, Columbus, OH 43210. Offers DPT. *Accreditation:* APTA. *Faculty:* 19. *Students:* 138 full-time (96 women), 1 part-time (0 women); includes 9 minority (1 Black or African American, non-Hispanic/Latino; 3 Asian, non-Hispanic/Latino; 3 Hispanic/Latino; 2 Two or more races, non-Hispanic/Latino), 1 international. Average age 24. In 2015, 56 doctorates awarded. *Degree requirements:* For doctorate, thesis/dissertation. *Entrance requirements:* For doctorate, GRE General Test. Additional exam requirements/recommendations for international students: Required—TOEFL (minimum score 550 paper-based; 79 iBT), Michigan English Language Assessment Battery (minimum score 82); Recommended—IELTS (minimum score 7). *Application deadline:* For summer admission, 10/3 for domestic and international students. Applications are processed on a rolling basis. Application fee: $60 ($70 for international students). Electronic applications accepted. *Financial support:* Fellowships with tuition reimbursements available. *Unit head:* Dr. John Buford, Program Director, 614-292-1520, Fax: 614-292-0210, E-mail: buford.5@osu.edu. *Application contact:* Graduate and Professional Admissions, 614-292-9444, Fax: 614-292-3895, E-mail: gpadmissions@osu.edu.
Website: http://medicine.osu.edu/hrs/pt

Ohio University, Graduate College, College of Health Sciences and Professions, School of Rehabilitation and Communication Sciences, Division of Physical Therapy, Athens, OH 45701-2979. Offers DPT. Applications accepted for summer term only. *Accreditation:* APTA. *Entrance requirements:* For doctorate, GRE. Additional exam requirements/recommendations for international students: Required—TOEFL (minimum score 550 paper-based; 80 iBT) or IELTS (minimum score 6.5). Electronic applications accepted. *Faculty research:* Motor control, muscle architecture, postural control, morphonetrics, sensory integration.

Old Dominion University, College of Health Sciences, School of Physical Therapy and Athletic Training, Norfolk, VA 23529. Offers athletic training (MSAT); physical therapy (DPT). *Accreditation:* APTA. *Faculty:* 13 full-time (8 women), 5 part-time/adjunct (3 women). *Students:* 130 full-time (81 women); includes 22 minority (7 Black or African American, non-Hispanic/Latino; 5 Asian, non-Hispanic/Latino; 4 Hispanic/Latino; 6 Two or more races, non-Hispanic/Latino), 1 international. Average age 25. 584 applicants, 14% accepted, 44 enrolled. In 2015, 47 doctorates awarded. *Degree requirements:* For doctorate, comprehensive exam, 5 clinical internships. *Entrance requirements:* For doctorate, GRE (minimum Verbal and Quantitative scores of 148, Analytical 3.5), 3 letters of recommendation (1 of which is from a physical therapist); 80 hours of volunteer experience in two separate physical therapy settings (i.e. hospital, private practice, rehab center, home health agency, etc.). Additional exam requirements/recommendations for international students: Required—TOEFL (minimum score 550 paper-based). *Application deadline:* For fall admission, 11/1 for domestic and international students. Application fee: $50. Electronic applications accepted. *Expenses:* $478 per credit resident; $1,195 per credit non-resident. *Financial support:* In 2015–16, 6 students received support, including 1 fellowship (averaging $15,000 per year), 4 teaching assistantships with partial tuition reimbursements available (averaging $7,500 per year); career-related internships or fieldwork, scholarships/grants, and unspecified assistantships also available. Financial award applicants required to submit FAFSA. *Faculty research:* Virtual reality and rehabilitation, rehabilitation for amputees, electromyography, biomechanics, gait and balance. *Total annual research expenditures:* $103,022. *Unit head:* Dr. George Maihafer, Graduate Program Director, 757-683-4519, Fax: 757-683-4410, E-mail: ptgpd@odu.edu. *Application contact:* William Heffelfinger, Director of Graduate Admissions, 757-683-5554, Fax: 757-683-3255, E-mail: gradadmit@odu.edu.
Website: http://www.odu.edu/ptat

Pacific University, School of Physical Therapy, Forest Grove, OR 97116-1797. Offers athletic training (MSAT); physical therapy (DPT). *Accreditation:* APTA. *Degree requirements:* For doctorate, evidence-based capstone project thesis. *Entrance requirements:* For doctorate, 100 hours of volunteer/observational hours, minimum cumulative GPA of 3.0, prerequisite courses with a C grade or better, minimum GPA of 2.5 in science/statistics. Additional exam requirements/recommendations for international students: Required—TOEFL (minimum score 600 paper-based). Electronic applications accepted. *Expenses:* Contact institution. *Faculty research:* Balance disorders, geriatrics, orthopedic treatment outcomes, obesity, women's health.

Queen's University at Kingston, School of Graduate Studies, Faculty of Health Sciences, School of Rehabilitation Therapy, Kingston, ON K7L 3N6, Canada. Offers occupational therapy (M Sc OT); physical therapy (M Sc PT); rehabilitation science (M Sc, PhD). *Program availability:* Part-time. *Degree requirements:* For master's, thesis; for doctorate, comprehensive exam, thesis/dissertation. *Entrance requirements:* Additional exam requirements/recommendations for international students: Required—TOEFL. *Faculty research:* Disability, community, motor performance, rehabilitation, treatment efficiency.

Radford University, College of Graduate and Professional Studies, Waldron College of Health and Human Services, Program in Physical Therapy, Roanoke, VA 24013. Offers DPT. *Faculty:* 7 full-time (3 women), 4 part-time/adjunct (3 women). *Students:* 73 full-time (49 women); includes 7 minority (2 Black or African American, non-Hispanic/Latino; 2 Asian, non-Hispanic/Latino; 1 Hispanic/Latino; 2 Two or more races, non-Hispanic/Latino). Average age 24. 384 applicants, 20% accepted, 27 enrolled. In 2015, 20 doctorates awarded. *Degree requirements:* For doctorate, comprehensive exam, capstone research project suitable for publication. *Entrance requirements:* For doctorate, GRE, PTCAS application with 3 letters of reference, personal essay, resume,

Physical Therapy

40 hours of clinical experience, minimum overall GPA of 3.25, 3.0 in math and science prerequisites. Additional exam requirements/recommendations for international students: Required—TOEFL (minimum score 575 paper-based; 88 iBT). *Application deadline:* For fall admission, 11/1 priority date for domestic students. Applications are processed on a rolling basis. Application fee: $50. Electronic applications accepted. *Expenses:* $540 per credit hour in-state tuition and fees; $1,004 per credit hour out-of-state tuition and fees. *Financial support:* In 2015–16, 14 students received support, including 2 research assistantships (averaging $3,697 per year). Financial award application deadline: 3/1; financial award applicants required to submit FAFSA. *Unit head:* Dr. Kristen Jagger, Chair, 540-224-6675, Fax: 540-224-6660, E-mail: dpt@radford.edu. *Application contact:* Rebecca Conner, Director, Graduate Enrollment, 540-831-6296, Fax: 540-831-6061, E-mail: gradcollege@radford.edu. *Website:* http://www.radford.edu/content/wchs/home/pt.html

Regis University, Rueckert-Hartman College for Health Professions, Denver, CO 80221-1099. Offers addictions counseling (Post-Graduate Certificate); advanced practice nurse specialization (DNP); counseling (MA); counseling children and adolescents (Post-Graduate Certificate); counseling military families (Post-Graduate Certificate); depth psychotherapy (Post-Graduate Certificate); family nurse practitioner (MSN); health care business management (Certificate); health care quality and patient safety (Certificate); health industry leadership (MBA); health professions (Postbaccalaureate Certificate); health services administration (MS); marriage and family therapy (MA); neonatal nurse practitioner (MSN); nursing education or leadership (MSN); orthopedic manual physical therapy fellowship (Certificate); pharmacy (Pharm D); physical therapy (DPT). *Program availability:* Part-time, evening/weekend, 100% online, blended/hybrid learning. *Faculty:* 40 full-time (29 women), 116 part-time/adjunct (86 women). *Students:* 1,080 full-time (771 women), 274 part-time (239 women); includes 388 minority (59 Black or African American, non-Hispanic/Latino; 6 American Indian or Alaska Native, non-Hispanic/Latino; 109 Asian, non-Hispanic/Latino; 163 Hispanic/Latino; 1 Native Hawaiian or other Pacific Islander, non-Hispanic/Latino; 50 Two or more races, non-Hispanic/Latino), 7 international. Average age 34. 2,188 applicants, 31% accepted, 303 enrolled. In 2015, 329 master's, 160 doctorates awarded. *Degree requirements:* For master's, thesis (for some programs), internship. *Entrance requirements:* For master's, official transcript reflecting baccalaureate degree awarded from regionally-accredited college or university. Additional exam requirements/recommendations for international students: Required—TOEFL (minimum score 550 paper-based; 82 iBT). *Application deadline:* For fall admission, 8/15 priority date for domestic students; for spring admission, 1/10 priority date for domestic students; for summer admission, 5/1 priority date for domestic students. Applications are processed on a rolling basis. Application fee: $75. Electronic applications accepted. *Expenses:* Contact institution. *Financial support:* In 2015–16, 102 students received support. Federal Work-Study and scholarships/grants available. Financial award application deadline: 4/15; financial award applicants required to submit FAFSA. *Faculty research:* Normal and pathological balance and gait research, normal/pathological upper limb motor control/biomechanics, exercise energy/metabolism research, optical treatment protocols for therapeutic modalities. *Unit head:* Dr. Janet Houser, Academic Dean. *Application contact:* Cate Clark, Director of Admissions, 303-458-4900, Fax: 303-964-5534, E-mail: ruadmissions@regis.edu. *Website:* http://www.regis.edu/RHCHP.aspx

Rockhurst University, College of Health and Human Services, Program in Physical Therapy, Kansas City, MO 64110-2561. Offers DPT. *Accreditation:* APTA. *Faculty:* 12 full-time (11 women), 5 part-time/adjunct (4 women). *Students:* 139 full-time (97 women), 1 (woman) part-time; includes 5 minority (1 American Indian or Alaska Native, non-Hispanic/Latino; 2 Hispanic/Latino; 2 Two or more races, non-Hispanic/Latino). Average age 25. 386 applicants, 42% accepted, 47 enrolled. In 2015, 48 doctorates awarded. *Entrance requirements:* For doctorate, 3 letters of recommendation, interview, minimum GPA of 3.0, physical therapy experience. Additional exam requirements/recommendations for international students: Required—TOEFL (minimum score 550 paper-based; 79 iBT). *Application deadline:* Applications are processed on a rolling basis. Application fee: $25. Electronic applications accepted. Application fee is waived when completed online. *Financial support:* Application deadline: 4/1; applicants required to submit FAFSA. *Faculty research:* Clinical decision-making, geriatrics, balance in persons with neurological disorders, physical rehabilitation following total joint replacement, clinical education. *Unit head:* Dr. Jean Hiebert, Chair, 816-501-4059, Fax: 816-501-4169, E-mail: jean.hiebert@rockhurst.edu. *Application contact:* Cheryl Hooper, Director of Graduate Admission, 816-501-4097, Fax: 816-501-4241, E-mail: cheryl.hooper@rockhurst.edu. *Website:* http://www.rockhurst.edu/academic/pt/index.asp

Rocky Mountain University of Health Professions, Programs in Physical Therapy, Provo, UT 84606. Offers DPT, TDPT. *Entrance requirements:* For doctorate, GRE, bachelor's degree; two courses each of general chemistry and general physics with lab (for science majors); one course each in biology, human anatomy (with lab), and physiology (with lab); three semester hours of statistics; six semester hours in the behavioral sciences (life span development preferred); minimum cumulative GPA of 3.0.

Rosalind Franklin University of Medicine and Science, College of Health Professions, Department of Physical Therapy, North Chicago, IL 60064-3095. Offers MS, DPT, TDPT. *Accreditation:* APTA. *Program availability:* Online learning. *Degree requirements:* For master's, thesis. *Entrance requirements:* For master's, physical therapy license. Additional exam requirements/recommendations for international students: Required—TOEFL. *Faculty research:* Clinical research, development/analysis of tests, measures, education.

Rush University, College of Health Sciences, Department of Respiratory Care, Chicago, IL 60612-3832. Offers MS. *Unit head:* David L. Vines, Chairperson, 312-563-2353. *Application contact:* 312-942-7120, E-mail: chs_admissions@rush.edu.

Rutgers University–Camden, Graduate School of Arts and Sciences, Program in Physical Therapy, Stratford, NJ 08084. Offers DPT. Program offered jointly with University of Medicine and Dentistry of New Jersey. *Accreditation:* APTA. *Entrance requirements:* For doctorate, GRE, physical therapy experience, 3 letters of recommendation, statement of personal, professional and academic goals, resume. Additional exam requirements/recommendations for international students: Required—TOEFL, IELTS. Electronic applications accepted. *Faculty research:* Clinical education, migrant workers, biomechanical constraints on motor control, high intensity strength training and the elderly, posture and ergonomics.

Rutgers University–Newark, School of Health Related Professions, Department of Rehabilitation and Movement Sciences, Program in Physical Therapy–Newark, Newark, NJ 07102. Offers DPT. *Accreditation:* APTA. *Entrance requirements:* For doctorate, GRE, chemistry, physics, calculus, psychology, statistics, interview, 3 reference letters. Additional exam requirements/recommendations for international students: Required—TOEFL (minimum score 500 paper-based; 79 iBT). Electronic applications accepted.

Rutgers University–Newark, School of Health Related Professions, Department of Rehabilitation and Movement Sciences, Program in Physical Therapy–Stratford, Newark, NJ 07102. Offers DPT. *Accreditation:* APTA. *Entrance requirements:* For doctorate, GRE, BS, 3 reference letters, interview. Additional exam requirements/

recommendations for international students: Required—TOEFL (minimum score 500 paper-based; 79 iBT). Electronic applications accepted.

Sacred Heart University, Graduate Programs, College of Health Professions, Department of Physical Therapy, Fairfield, CT 06825. Offers DPT, Graduate Certificate. *Accreditation:* APTA. *Faculty:* 10 full-time (5 women), 35 part-time/adjunct (27 women). *Students:* 188 full-time (152 women), 4 part-time (2 women); includes 16 minority (2 Black or African American, non-Hispanic/Latino; 1 American Indian or Alaska Native, non-Hispanic/Latino; 4 Asian, non-Hispanic/Latino; 8 Hispanic/Latino; 1 Two or more races, non-Hispanic/Latino), 2 international. Average age 24. 654 applicants, 20% accepted, 63 enrolled. In 2015, 67 doctorates awarded. *Entrance requirements:* For doctorate, GRE (recommended), minimum overall and prerequisites GPA of 3.2. Additional exam requirements/recommendations for international students: Required—PTE; Recommended—TOEFL (minimum score 570 paper-based; 80 iBT), IELTS (minimum score 6.5). *Application deadline:* For fall admission, 12/15 for domestic and international students. Applications are processed on a rolling basis. Application fee: $75. *Expenses:* Contact institution. *Financial support:* Unspecified assistantships available. Financial award applicants required to submit FAFSA. *Unit head:* Dr. Kevin Chui, Associate Professor/Chair, Physical Therapy and Human Movement, 203-371-7976, E-mail: chuik@sacredheart.edu. *Application contact:* William Sweeney, Director of Graduate Admissions, 203-396-4827, E-mail: sweeneyw@sacredheart.edu. *Website:* http://www.sacredheart.edu/academics/collegeofhealthprofessions/academicprograms/physicaltherapy/

Sage Graduate School, School of Health Sciences, Program in Physical Therapy, Troy, NY 12180-4115. Offers DPT. *Accreditation:* APTA. *Faculty:* 8 full-time (6 women), 13 part-time/adjunct (11 women). *Students:* 103 full-time (75 women); includes 16 minority (6 Black or African American, non-Hispanic/Latino; 4 Asian, non-Hispanic/Latino; 4 Hispanic/Latino; 2 Two or more races, non-Hispanic/Latino). Average age 25. 237 applicants, 20% accepted, 25 enrolled. In 2015, 38 doctorates awarded. *Entrance requirements:* For doctorate, baccalaureate degree; current resume; 2 letters of recommendation; minimum GPA of 3.0 overall and in science prerequisites; completion of 40 hours of physical therapy observation. Additional exam requirements/recommendations for international students: Required—TOEFL (minimum score 550 paper-based). *Application deadline:* Applications are processed on a rolling basis. Application fee: $40. Electronic applications accepted. *Expenses:* Contact institution. *Financial support:* Federal Work-Study, scholarships/grants, and unspecified assistantships available. Support available to part-time students. Financial award application deadline: 3/1; financial award applicants required to submit FAFSA. *Unit head:* Dr. Theresa Hand, Dean, School of Health Sciences, 518-244-2265, Fax: 518-244-4571, E-mail: handt@sage.edu. *Application contact:* Dr. James Brennan, Chair and Assistant Professor, 518-244-2058, Fax: 518-244-4524, E-mail: brennj@sage.edu.

St. Ambrose University, College of Education and Health Sciences, Department of Physical Therapy, Davenport, IA 52803-2898. Offers DPT. *Accreditation:* APTA. *Degree requirements:* For doctorate, board exams. *Entrance requirements:* For doctorate, GRE, interview. Additional exam requirements/recommendations for international students: Required—TOEFL. *Faculty research:* Human motor control, orthopedic physical therapy, cardiopulmonary physical therapy, kinesiology/biomechanics.

St. Catherine University, Graduate Programs in Physical Therapy, St. Paul, MN 55105. Offers DPT. Offered on the Minneapolis campus only. *Accreditation:* APTA. *Degree requirements:* For doctorate, research project. *Entrance requirements:* For doctorate, GRE, minimum GPA of 3.0, coursework in biology/zoology, anatomy, physiology, chemistry, physics, psychology, statistics, mathematics and medical terminology. Additional exam requirements/recommendations for international students: Required—Michigan English Language Assessment Battery or TOEFL (minimum score 600 paper-based; 100 iBT). *Expenses:* Contact institution.

Saint Francis University, Department of Physical Therapy, Loretto, PA 15940-0600. Offers DPT. *Accreditation:* APTA. *Entrance requirements:* Additional exam requirements/recommendations for international students: Required—TOEFL. *Application deadline:* For winter admission, 1/15 for domestic and international students. Application fee: $30. Electronic applications accepted. *Financial support:* Teaching assistantships with partial tuition reimbursements and unspecified assistantships available. *Faculty research:* Childhood asthma, athletic performance, energy expenditure, sports injuries, balance and falls, concussion management, physical therapy administration, orthopedic assignment. *Unit head:* Dr. Ivan J. Mulligan, Chair/Associate Professor, 814-472-3123, Fax: 814-472-3140, E-mail: imulligan@francis.edu. *Application contact:* Dr. Peter Raymond Skoner, Associate Provost, 814-472-3085, Fax: 814-472-3365, E-mail: pskoner@francis.edu.

Saint Louis University, Graduate Education, Doisy College of Health Sciences, Department of Physical Therapy, St. Louis, MO 63103. Offers athletic training (MAT); physical therapy (DPT). *Accreditation:* APTA. *Program availability:* Part-time. *Entrance requirements:* Additional exam requirements/recommendations for international students: Required—TOEFL (minimum score 525 paper-based; 55 iBT). Electronic applications accepted. *Faculty research:* Patellofemoral pain and associated risk factors; prevalence of disordered eating in physical therapy students; effects of selected interventions for children with cerebral palsy on gait and posture; hippotherapy, ankle strengthening, supported treadmill training, spirituality in physical therapy/patient care, risk factors for exercise-related leg pain in running athletes.

Samford University, School of Health Professions, Birmingham, AL 35229. Offers athletic training (MAT); physical therapy (DPT); speech language pathology (MS). *Program availability:* Evening/weekend, online learning. *Faculty:* 11 full-time (8 women). *Students:* 53 full-time (38 women); includes 1 minority (Two or more races, non-Hispanic/Latino). Average age 24. 117 applicants, 73% accepted, 55 enrolled. *Degree requirements:* For master's, thesis or alternative; for doctorate, thesis/dissertation or alternative. *Entrance requirements:* For master's and doctorate, GRE, 3 recommendations, resume, on-campus interview, personal statement, CPR certification. Additional exam requirements/recommendations for international students: Required—TOEFL (minimum score 550 paper-based). *Application deadline:* For fall admission, 6/1 for domestic students; for spring admission, 10/1 for domestic students. Application fee: $120. Electronic applications accepted. *Expenses: Tuition,* area resident: Full-time $18,673; part-time $766 per credit hour. *Required fees:* $550. Tuition and fees vary according to course load, degree level and student level. *Financial support:* In 2015–16, 7 students received support. *Application deadline:* 3/1; applicants required to submit FAFSA. *Unit head:* Dr. Alan P. Jung, Dean, School of Health Professions, 205-726-2716, Fax: 205-726-2666, E-mail: apjung@samford.edu. *Application contact:* Dr. Marian Carter, Assistant Dean of Enrollment Management and Student Services, 205-726-2611, Fax: 205-726-2666, E-mail: mwcarter@samford.edu. *Website:* http://www.samford.edu/healthprofessions/

Samuel Merritt University, Department of Physical Therapy, Oakland, CA 94609-3108. Offers DPT. *Accreditation:* APTA. *Faculty:* 11 full-time (9 women), 22 part-time/adjunct (14 women). *Students:* 104 full-time (60 women), 4 part-time (3 women); includes 54 minority (1 Black or African American, non-Hispanic/Latino; 28 Asian, non-Hispanic/Latino; 20 Hispanic/Latino; 1 Native Hawaiian or other Pacific Islander, non-Hispanic/Latino; 4 Two or more races, non-Hispanic/Latino). Average age 28. 585 applicants,

16% accepted, 34 enrolled. *Entrance requirements:* For doctorate, GRE General Test, minimum GPA of 3.0 in science and overall; related work experience; interview. Additional exam requirements/recommendations for international students: Required—TOEFL (minimum score 100 iBT). *Application deadline:* For fall admission, 10/1 priority date for domestic students. Application fee: $50. Electronic applications accepted. *Expenses:* $15,244 per semester; $50 annual student body fee; $480 lab fee; $300 graduation fee. *Financial support:* In 2015–16, 17 students received support. Career-related internships or fieldwork, Federal Work-Study, and scholarships/grants available. Financial award application deadline: 3/2; financial award applicants required to submit FAFSA. *Faculty research:* Human movement, motor control, falls prevention in the elderly. *Total annual research expenditures:* $25,000. *Unit head:* Dr. Nicole Christensen, Co-Chair, 510-869-6567, Fax: 510-869-6282, E-mail: nchristensen@samuelmerritt.edu. *Application contact:* Timothy Cranford, Dean of Admissions, 510-869-1550, Fax: 510-869-6525, E-mail: admission@samuelmerritt.edu.
Website: http://www.samuelmerritt.edu/physical_therapy

San Diego State University, Graduate and Research Affairs, College of Health and Human Services, School of Exercise and Nutritional Sciences, Program in Physical Therapy, San Diego, CA 92182. Offers DPT.

San Francisco State University, Division of Graduate Studies, College of Health and Social Sciences, Program in Physical Therapy, San Francisco, CA 94132-1722. Offers DPT, Dr Sc PT. Programs offered jointly with University of California, San Francisco. *Accreditation:* APTA. *Expenses:* Tuition, state resident: full-time $6738. Tuition, nonresident: full-time $15,666. *Required fees:* $1004. *Financial support:* Career-related internships or fieldwork and institutionally sponsored loans available. *Unit head:* Dr. Linda Wanek, Director, 415-338-2001, Fax: 415-338-0907, E-mail: lwanek@sfsu.edu. *Application contact:* Jill Lionau, Academic Office Coordinator, 415-338-2001, Fax: 415-338-0907, E-mail: jlienau@sfsu.edu.
Website: http://www.pt.sfsu.edu/

Seton Hall University, School of Health and Medical Sciences, Program in Physical Therapy, South Orange, NJ 07079-2697. Offers professional physical therapy (DPT). *Accreditation:* APTA. *Degree requirements:* For doctorate, research project. *Entrance requirements:* Additional exam requirements/recommendations for international students: Required—TOEFL. Electronic applications accepted. *Faculty research:* Electrical stimulation, motor learning, backpacks, gait and balance, orthopedic injury, women's health, pediatric obesity.

Shenandoah University, School of Health Professions, Division of Physical Therapy, Winchester, VA 22601. Offers physical therapy (DPT). *Accreditation:* APTA. *Program availability:* Minimal on-campus study. *Faculty:* 12 full-time (8 women), 2 part-time/adjunct (1 woman). *Students:* 143 full-time (105 women), 87 part-time (55 women); includes 46 minority (4 Black or African American, non-Hispanic/Latino; 1 American Indian or Alaska Native, non-Hispanic/Latino; 28 Asian, non-Hispanic/Latino; 9 Hispanic/Latino; 4 Two or more races, non-Hispanic/Latino), 11 international. Average age 30. 525 applicants, 26% accepted, 95 enrolled. In 2015, 90 doctorates awarded. *Degree requirements:* For doctorate, comprehensive exam, evidence-based practice research project. *Entrance requirements:* For doctorate, GRE General Test, minimum GPA of 2.8 in completed coursework; minimum grade of C in all prerequisites coursework; 2 letters of recommendation, one from a licensed practicing PT and one from a college professor; 40 documented hours of exposure to PT practice. Additional exam requirements/recommendations for international students: Required—TOEFL (minimum score 558 paper-based; 83 iBT). *Application deadline:* For fall admission, 10/1 for domestic and international students; for summer admission, 4/1 for domestic and international students. Application fee: $30. Electronic applications accepted. *Expenses:* $83,000 tuition, $4,760 fees (including technology fee, student services fee, and clinical fee). *Financial support:* In 2015–16, 13 students received support. Career-related internships or fieldwork, scholarships/grants, and unspecified assistantships available. Financial award application deadline: 3/15; financial award applicants required to submit FAFSA. *Faculty research:* Footwear, thoracic spine manipulation, concussions in dancers, urinary incontinence. *Unit head:* Dr. Karen Abraham, Director, 540-665-5520, Fax: 540-545-7387, E-mail: kabraham@su.edu. *Application contact:* Andrew Woodall, Executive Director of Recruitment and Admissions, 540-665-4581, Fax: 540-665-4627, E-mail: admit@su.edu.
Website: http://www.su.edu/physical-therapy/

Simmons College, School of Nursing and Health Sciences, Boston, MA 02115. Offers didactic dietetics (Certificate); dietetic internship (Certificate); health education profession (PhD); health professions education (CAGS); nursing (MS), including family nurse practitioner; nursing practice (DNP); nutrition and health promotion (MS); physical therapy (DPT); sports nutrition (Certificate). *Program availability:* Part-time, blended/hybrid learning. *Faculty:* 21 full-time (17 women), 171 part-time/adjunct (157 women). *Students:* 333 full-time (305 women), 889 part-time (813 women); includes 250 minority (88 Black or African American, non-Hispanic/Latino; 3 American Indian or Alaska Native, non-Hispanic/Latino; 65 Asian, non-Hispanic/Latino; 67 Hispanic/Latino; 2 Native Hawaiian or other Pacific Islander, non-Hispanic/Latino; 25 Two or more races, non-Hispanic/Latino), 9 international. Average age 33. 846 applicants, 66% accepted, 441 enrolled. In 2015, 70 master's, 45 doctorates awarded. *Entrance requirements:* For doctorate, GRE. Additional exam requirements/recommendations for international students: Required—TOEFL (minimum score 570 paper-based; 88 iBT). *Application deadline:* For fall admission, 6/1 for international students. Application fee: $50. Electronic applications accepted. *Expenses:* Contact institution. *Financial support:* In 2015–16, 12 research assistantships (averaging $6,000 per year) were awarded; scholarships/grants and unspecified assistantships also available. *Unit head:* Dr. Judy Beal, Dean, 617-521-2139. *Application contact:* Brett DiMarzo, Director of Graduate Admission, 617-521-2651, Fax: 617-521-3137, E-mail: brett.dimarzo@simmons.edu.
Website: http://www.simmons.edu/snhs/

Slippery Rock University of Pennsylvania, Graduate Studies (Recruitment), College of Health, Environment, and Science, School of Physical Therapy, Slippery Rock, PA 16057-1383. Offers DPT. *Accreditation:* APTA. *Faculty:* 9 full-time (6 women), 1 (woman) part-time/adjunct. *Students:* 143 full-time (100 women); includes 8 minority (2 Black or African American, non-Hispanic/Latino; 2 Asian, non-Hispanic/Latino; 3 Hispanic/Latino; 1 Native Hawaiian or other Pacific Islander, non-Hispanic/Latino). Average age 24. 297 applicants, 28% accepted, 41 enrolled. In 2015, 48 doctorates awarded. *Degree requirements:* For doctorate, clinical residency. *Entrance requirements:* For doctorate, GRE General Test, minimum GPA of 3.0, three letters of recommendation, essay, 100 hours of PT experience with licensed physical therapist, CPR certification. Additional exam requirements/recommendations for international students: Required—TOEFL (minimum score 550 paper-based; 80 iBT). *Application deadline:* For fall admission, 11/1 priority date for domestic and international students. Application fee: $35. Electronic applications accepted. *Expenses:* $629.87 per credit in-state; $912.12 per credit out-of-state. *Financial support:* In 2015–16, 60 students received support. Career-related internships or fieldwork, Federal Work-Study, institutionally sponsored loans, scholarships/grants, tuition waivers (partial), and unspecified assistantships available. Financial award application deadline: 5/1; financial award applicants required to submit FAFSA. *Unit head:* Dr. Carol Martin-Elkins, Graduate Coordinator, 724-738-2080, Fax: 724-738-2113, E-mail: carol.martin-elkins@

sru.edu. *Application contact:* Brandi Weber-Mortimer, Director of Graduate Admissions, 724-738-2051, Fax: 724-738-2146, E-mail: graduate.admissions@sru.edu.
Website: http://www.sru.edu/academics/graduate-programs/physical-therapy-doctor-of-physical-therapy

Sonoma State University, School of Science and Technology, Department of Kinesiology, Rohnert Park, CA 94928. Offers adapted physical education (MA); interdisciplinary (MA); interdisciplinary pre-occupational therapy (MA); lifetime physical activity (MA), including coach education, fitness and wellness; physical education (MA); pre-physical therapy (MA). *Program availability:* Part-time. *Degree requirements:* For master's, thesis, oral exam. *Entrance requirements:* For master's, minimum GPA of 2.8. Additional exam requirements/recommendations for international students: Required—TOEFL (minimum score 500 paper-based).

Southwest Baptist University, Program in Physical Therapy, Bolivar, MO 65613-2597. Offers DPT. *Accreditation:* APTA. *Degree requirements:* For doctorate, comprehensive exam, 3-4 clinical education experiences. *Entrance requirements:* Additional exam requirements/recommendations for international students: Required—TOEFL (minimum score 550 paper-based). *Expenses:* Contact institution. *Faculty research:* Balance and falls prevention, distance and web based learning, foot and ankle intervention, pediatrics, musculoskeletal management.

Springfield College, Graduate Programs, Program in Physical Therapy, Springfield, MA 01109-3797. Offers DPT. *Accreditation:* APTA. *Program availability:* Part-time. *Degree requirements:* For doctorate, comprehensive exam, thesis/dissertation, research project. *Entrance requirements:* For doctorate, GRE General Test. Additional exam requirements/recommendations for international students: Required—TOEFL (minimum score 550 paper-based); Recommended—IELTS (minimum score 6). Electronic applications accepted.

State University of New York Upstate Medical University, Department of Physical Therapy, Syracuse, NY 13210-2334. Offers DPT. *Accreditation:* APTA. *Program availability:* Part-time, evening/weekend, online learning. Electronic applications accepted.

Stockton University, Office of Graduate Studies, Program in Physical Therapy, Galloway, NJ 08205-9441. Offers DPT. *Accreditation:* APTA. *Faculty:* 7 full-time (5 women). *Students:* 67 full-time (40 women), 25 part-time (21 women); includes 12 minority (10 Asian, non-Hispanic/Latino; 1 Hispanic/Latino; 1 Two or more races, non-Hispanic/Latino), 1 international. Average age 29. 286 applicants, 20% accepted, 29 enrolled. In 2015, 32 doctorates awarded. *Entrance requirements:* For doctorate, GRE. Additional exam requirements/recommendations for international students: Required—TOEFL. *Application deadline:* For fall admission, 10/15 priority date for domestic students, 10/15 for international students. Application fee: $50. Electronic applications accepted. *Expenses:* Tuition, state resident: full-time $13,968; part-time $582 per credit. Tuition, nonresident: full-time $21,502; part-time $895 per credit. *Required fees:* $4200; $175 per credit. $90. Tuition and fees vary according to degree level. *Financial support:* Fellowships, research assistantships, career-related internships or fieldwork, Federal Work-Study, scholarships/grants, and unspecified assistantships available. Support available to part-time students. Financial award application deadline: 3/1; financial award applicants required to submit FAFSA. *Faculty research:* Spinal flexibility in the well elderly, use of traditional Chinese medicine concepts in physical therapy, computerized vs. traditional study in human gross anatomy. *Unit head:* Dr. Bess Kathrins, Program Director, 609-626-3640, E-mail: gradschool@stockton.edu. *Application contact:* Tara Williams, Assistant Director of Graduate Enrollment Management, 609-626-3640, Fax: 609-626-6050, E-mail: gradschool@stockton.edu.

Stony Brook University, State University of New York, Stony Brook Medicine, School of Health Technology and Management, Stony Brook, NY 11794. Offers health care management (Advanced Certificate); health care policy and management (MS); occupational therapy (MS); physical therapy (DPT); physician assistant (MS). *Accreditation:* APTA. *Faculty:* 67 full-time (41 women), 64 part-time/adjunct (45 women). *Students:* 488 full-time (301 women), 99 part-time (82 women); includes 167 minority (34 Black or African American, non-Hispanic/Latino; 3 American Indian or Alaska Native, non-Hispanic/Latino; 84 Asian, non-Hispanic/Latino; 41 Hispanic/Latino; 5 Two or more races, non-Hispanic/Latino), 12 international. Average age 28. 2,646 applicants, 14% accepted, 260 enrolled. In 2015, 104 master's, 71 doctorates, 34 other advanced degrees awarded. *Degree requirements:* For master's, thesis. *Entrance requirements:* For master's, GRE General Test, minimum GPA of 3.0, work experience in field, references; for doctorate, GRE, references. Additional exam requirements/recommendations for international students: Required—TOEFL (minimum score 550 paper-based). *Application deadline:* For fall admission, 1/15 for domestic students; for spring admission, 10/1 for domestic students. Application fee: $100. *Expenses:* Contact institution. *Financial support:* Fellowships, research assistantships, teaching assistantships, career-related internships or fieldwork, Federal Work-Study, and institutionally sponsored loans available. Financial award application deadline: 3/15. *Faculty research:* Health promotion and disease prevention. *Total annual research expenditures:* $1.3 million. *Unit head:* Dr. Craig A. Lehmann, Dean, 631-444-2252, Fax: 631-444-7621, E-mail: craig.lehmann@stonybrook.edu. *Application contact:* Dr. Richard W. Johnson, Associate Dean for Graduate Studies, 631-444-3251, Fax: 631-444-7621, E-mail: richard.johnson@stonybrook.edu.
Website: http://healthtechnology.stonybrookmedicine.edu/

Temple University, College of Public Health, Department of Physical Therapy, Philadelphia, PA 19122. Offers DPT, TDPT. *Accreditation:* APTA (one or more programs are accredited). *Program availability:* Part-time, online learning. *Faculty:* 13 full-time (7 women), 1 part-time/adjunct (0 women). *Students:* 147 full-time (113 women), 58 part-time (39 women); includes 35 minority (7 Black or African American, non-Hispanic/Latino; 16 Asian, non-Hispanic/Latino; 7 Hispanic/Latino; 1 Native Hawaiian or other Pacific Islander, non-Hispanic/Latino; 4 Two or more races, non-Hispanic/Latino), 2 international. 26 applicants, 88% accepted, 18 enrolled. In 2015, 89 doctorates awarded. *Degree requirements:* For doctorate, comprehensive exam, thesis/dissertation. *Entrance requirements:* For doctorate, GRE General Test, essay, interview, clinical experience. Additional exam requirements/recommendations for international students: Required—TOEFL (minimum score 550 paper-based; 79 iBT). *Application deadline:* For fall admission, 3/1 for domestic students, 2/1 for international students; for spring admission, 11/1 for domestic students, 10/1 for international students; for summer admission, 3/1 for domestic students, 2/1 for international students. Applications are processed on a rolling basis. Application fee: $60. Electronic applications accepted. *Expenses:* Contact institution. *Financial support:* Teaching assistantships with tuition reimbursements, career-related internships or fieldwork, Federal Work-Study, scholarships/grants, and unspecified assistantships available. Financial award application deadline: 1/1; financial award applicants required to submit FAFSA. *Faculty research:* Balance dysfunction, biomechanics, development, qualitative research, developmental neuroscience, health services. *Unit head:* Dr. Emily A. Keshner, Chair, 215-707-4815, Fax: 215-707-7500, E-mail: deptpt@temple.edu. *Application contact:* Scott Burns, Director of Program Administration/Director of Admissions/Director of the Transition DPT, 215-707-4815, E-mail: dptadmissions@temple.edu.
Website: http://chpsw.temple.edu/pt/home

Physical Therapy

Tennessee State University, The School of Graduate Studies and Research, College of Health Sciences, Department of Physical Therapy, Nashville, TN 37209-1561. Offers DPT. *Accreditation:* APTA. *Program availability:* Part-time, online learning. *Entrance requirements:* For doctorate, GRE, baccalaureate degree, 2 letters of recommendation, interview, essay. *Application deadline:* For fall admission, 1/15 for domestic and international students. Applications are processed on a rolling basis. Application fee: $25. Electronic applications accepted. *Financial support:* Fellowships with tuition reimbursements, research assistantships with tuition reimbursements, teaching assistantships with tuition reimbursements, scholarships/grants, traineeships, and unspecified assistantships available. Support available to part-time students. Financial award applicants required to submit FAFSA. *Faculty research:* Evidence-based research clinical research case studies/reports qualitative research education assessment total knee anthroplasty; ergonomics; childhood obesity. *Unit head:* Dr. Ronald Barredo, Head, 615-963-5932, Fax: 615-963-5935, E-mail: rbarredo@tnstate.edu. *Application contact:* Deborah Chisom, Director of Graduate Admissions, 615-963-5962, Fax: 615-963-5963, E-mail: dchiscom@tnstate.edu. Website: http://www.tnstate.edu/pt/

Texas State University, The Graduate College, College of Health Professions, Doctor of Physical Therapy Program, San Marcos, TX 78666. Offers DPT. *Accreditation:* APTA. *Faculty:* 14 full-time (13 women), 4 part-time/adjunct (0 women). *Students:* 118 full-time (66 women), 1 (woman) part-time; includes 38 minority (3 Black or African American, non-Hispanic/Latino; 5 Asian, non-Hispanic/Latino; 26 Hispanic/Latino; 4 Two or more races, non-Hispanic/Latino), 1 international. Average age 27. 578 applicants, 11% accepted, 41 enrolled. *Degree requirements:* For doctorate, comprehensive exam. *Entrance requirements:* For doctorate, GRE General Test (preferred minimum score of 295 with no less than 150 verbal and 145 quantitative), baccalaureate degree in physical therapy from regionally-accredited institution with minimum GPA of 3.0 on last 60 hours of undergraduate work and specific courses in the sciences (i.e., psychology, physiology, chemistry, statistics). Additional exam requirements/recommendations for international students: Required—TOEFL (minimum score 550 paper-based; 78 iBT). *Application deadline:* For summer admission, 10/15 for domestic and international students. Applications are processed on a rolling basis. Application fee: $65 ($115 for international students). Electronic applications accepted. *Expenses:* $3,615 in-state tuition (for 12 semester credit hours/1 full-time semester), $974 in-state fees. *Financial support:* In 2015–16, 92 students received support, including 18 teaching assistantships (averaging $7,156 per year); research assistantships, career-related internships or fieldwork, Federal Work-Study, institutionally sponsored loans, scholarships/grants, and unspecified assistantships also available. Support available to part-time students. Financial award application deadline: 3/1; financial award applicants required to submit FAFSA. *Faculty research:* Exploring balance and sleep function with mild traumatic brain injury, combined NMES and SS therapy for stroke patients. *Unit head:* Dr. Barbara Sanders, Graduate Advisor, 512-245-8351, Fax: 512-245-8736, E-mail: bs04@txstate.edu. *Application contact:* Dr. Andrea Golato, Dean of Graduate School, 512-245-2581, Fax: 512-245-8365, E-mail: gradcollege@txstate.edu. Website: http://www.health.txstate.edu/pt/

Texas Tech University Health Sciences Center, School of Health Professions, Program in Physical Therapy, Lubbock, TX 79430. Offers DPT, Sc D, TDPT. *Accreditation:* APTA. *Program availability:* Online learning. *Faculty:* 19 full-time (6 women), 3 part-time/adjunct (2 women). *Students:* 196 full-time (126 women), 143 part-time (71 women); includes 97 minority (5 Black or African American, non-Hispanic/Latino; 3 American Indian or Alaska Native, non-Hispanic/Latino; 27 Asian, non-Hispanic/Latino; 51 Hispanic/Latino; 1 Native Hawaiian or other Pacific Islander, non-Hispanic/Latino; 10 Two or more races, non-Hispanic/Latino), 1 international. Average age 31. 499 applicants, 23% accepted, 113 enrolled. In 2015, 89 doctorates awarded. *Entrance requirements:* For doctorate, GRE. Additional exam requirements/recommendations for international students: Required—TOEFL (minimum score 550 paper-based; 79 iBT), IELTS. *Application deadline:* For fall admission, 10/1 priority date for domestic students. Applications are processed on a rolling basis. Application fee: $40. Electronic applications accepted. *Financial support:* Career-related internships or fieldwork, institutionally sponsored loans, and scholarships/grants available. Financial award application deadline: 9/1; financial award applicants required to submit FAFSA. *Unit head:* Dr. Steven Sawyer, Department Chair, 806-743-4525, Fax: 806-743-6005, E-mail: steven.sawyer@ttuhsc.edu. *Application contact:* Lindsay Johnson, Associate Dean for Admissions and Student Affairs, 806-743-3220, Fax: 806-743-2994, E-mail: lindsay.johnson@ttuhsc.edu. Website: https://www.ttuhsc.edu/shp

Texas Woman's University, Graduate School, College of Health Sciences, School of Physical Therapy, Denton, TX 76201. Offers DPT, PhD. *Accreditation:* APTA (one or more programs are accredited). *Program availability:* Part-time. *Degree requirements:* For doctorate, comprehensive exam, thesis/dissertation. *Entrance requirements:* For doctorate, interview, resume, essay; eligibility for licensure and 2 letters of recommendation (PhD); 3 letters of recommendation on department form (DPT). Additional exam requirements/recommendations for international students: Required—TOEFL (minimum score 550 paper-based; 79 iBT). *Application deadline:* For fall admission, 10/17 priority date for domestic students, 10/17 for international students. Applications are processed on a rolling basis. Application fee: $50 ($75 for international students). Electronic applications accepted. *Expenses:* Tuition, state resident: full-time $4380; part-time $243 per credit hour. Tuition, nonresident: full-time $11,400; part-time $633 per credit hour. *International tuition:* $11,465 full-time. *Required fees:* $1778; $99 per credit hour. $283 per semester. One-time fee: $50. Tuition and fees vary according to course load and program. *Financial support:* Research assistantships, career-related internships or fieldwork, Federal Work-Study, institutionally sponsored loans, scholarships/grants, traineeships, health care benefits, and unspecified assistantships available. Support available to part-time students. Financial award application deadline: 3/1; financial award applicants required to submit FAFSA. *Faculty research:* Gait training in stroke survivors, physical activity to promote health in youth and adults, exercise training for individuals with amputation, treatment of balance and gait deficits in persons with multiple sclerosis. *Unit head:* Dr. Ann Medley, Director, 713-794-2070, Fax: 713-794-2071, E-mail: pt@twu.edu. *Application contact:* Dr. Samuel Wheeler, Assistant Director of Admissions, 940-898-3188, Fax: 940-898-3081, E-mail: wheelersr@twu.edu. Website: http://www.twu.edu/physical-therapy/

Thomas Jefferson University, Jefferson School of Health Professions, Program in Physical Therapy, Philadelphia, PA 19107. Offers DPT. *Accreditation:* APTA. *Students:* 178 full-time (129 women); includes 8 minority (7 Black or African American, non-Hispanic/Latino; 1 Asian, non-Hispanic/Latino). Average age 25. 1,419 applicants, 8% accepted, 59 enrolled. In 2015, 50 doctorates awarded. *Entrance requirements:* Additional exam requirements/recommendations for international students: Required—TOEFL. *Application deadline:* For fall admission, 3/1 priority date for domestic and international students. Applications are processed on a rolling basis. Application fee: $140. Electronic applications accepted. *Expenses:* $33,767 per year. *Financial support:* In 2015–16, 130 students received support. Federal Work-Study, institutionally sponsored loans, scholarships/grants, and unspecified assistantships available. Support available to part-time students. Financial award application deadline: 4/1; financial award applicants required to submit FAFSA. *Unit head:* Dr. Susan Wainwright, Chair,

Department of Physical Therapy, 215-503-8961, Fax: 215-503-3499, E-mail: susan.wainwright@jefferson.edu. *Application contact:* Evelyn Janick, Admissions Counselor, 215-503-1431, Fax: 215-503-7241, E-mail: jshpadmissions@jefferson.edu. Website: http://www.jefferson.edu/health_professions/departments/physical_therapy

Touro College, School of Health Sciences, Bay Shore, NY 11706. Offers industrial-organizational psychology (MS); mental health counseling (MS); occupational therapy (MS); physical therapy (DPT); physician assistant (MS); school psychology (MS); speech-language pathology (MS). *Faculty:* 20 full-time, 94 part-time/adjunct. *Students:* 1,057 full-time (772 women), 121 part-time (88 women); includes 243 minority (59 Black or African American, non-Hispanic/Latino; 1 American Indian or Alaska Native, non-Hispanic/Latino; 102 Asian, non-Hispanic/Latino; 58 Hispanic/Latino; 1 Native Hawaiian or other Pacific Islander, non-Hispanic/Latino; 22 Two or more races, non-Hispanic/Latino), 102 international. *Expenses:* Contact institution. *Financial support:* Fellowships available. *Unit head:* Dr. Louis Primavera, Dean, School of Health Sciences, 516-673-3200, E-mail: louis.primavera@touro.edu. *Application contact:* Brian J. Diele, Director of Student Administrative Services, 631-665-1600 Ext. 6311, E-mail: brian.diele@touro.edu.

University at Buffalo, the State University of New York, Graduate School, School of Public Health and Health Professions, Department of Rehabilitation Science, Program in Physical Therapy, Buffalo, NY 14260. Offers DPT. *Accreditation:* APTA. *Faculty:* 8 full-time (5 women), 1 part-time/adjunct (0 women). *Students:* 127 full-time (51 women); includes 16 minority (3 Black or African American, non-Hispanic/Latino; 12 Asian, non-Hispanic/Latino; 1 Hispanic/Latino), 2 international. Average age 24. 86 applicants, 53% accepted, 43 enrolled. In 2015, 45 doctorates awarded. *Entrance requirements:* For doctorate, GRE. Additional exam requirements/recommendations for international students: Required—TOEFL (minimum score 79 iBT). *Application deadline:* For fall admission, 11/1 for domestic and international students. Application fee: $50. Electronic applications accepted. *Financial support:* Application deadline: 2/1; applicants required to submit FAFSA. *Faculty research:* Functional limitations and rehabilitation for individuals with osteoporosis, multiple sclerosis, juvenile arthritis and aging; neuroscience concepts as they relate to rehabilitation in stroke and cerebral palsy; neural mechanisms associated with development, aging and neuromuscular disorders; sleep apnea and episodic hypoxia as it relates to muscles in the upper airway and cardiovascular system, neurobiological changes in ventilator control. *Total annual research expenditures:* $391,708. *Unit head:* Dr. Kirkwood Personious, Program Director, 716-829-6742, Fax: 716-829-3217, E-mail: phhpadv@buffalo.edu. *Application contact:* MaryAnn Venezia, Program Coordinator, 716-829-6742, Fax: 716-829-3217, E-mail: venezia3@buffalo.edu. Website: http://sphhp.buffalo.edu/rehabilitation-science/education/doctor-of-physical-therapy-dpt.html

The University of Alabama at Birmingham, School of Health Professions, Program in Physical Therapy, Birmingham, AL 35294. Offers DPT. *Accreditation:* APTA. *Entrance requirements:* For doctorate, GRE, interview; letters of recommendation; minimum GPA of 3.0 overall, in prerequisite courses, and last 60 hours; 40 hours of PT observation. Electronic applications accepted. *Expenses:* Tuition, state resident: full-time $7340. Tuition, nonresident: full-time $16,628. Full-time tuition and fees vary according to course load and program. *Faculty research:* Geriatrics, exercise physiology, aquatic therapy, industrial rehabilitation, outcome measurement.

University of Alberta, Faculty of Graduate Studies and Research, Department of Physical Therapy, Edmonton, AB T6G 2E1, Canada. Offers M Sc, PhD. *Program availability:* Part-time. *Degree requirements:* For master's, thesis. *Entrance requirements:* For master's, bachelor's degree in physical therapy, minimum GPA of 6.5 on a 9.0 scale. Additional exam requirements/recommendations for international students: Required—TOEFL. Electronic applications accepted. *Faculty research:* Spinal disorders, musculoskeletal disorders, ergonomics, sports therapy, motor development, cardiac rehabilitation/therapeutic exercise.

University of California, San Francisco, Graduate Division, Program in Physical Therapy, San Francisco, CA 94143. Offers DPT, DPTSc. Programs offered jointly with San Francisco State University. *Accreditation:* APTA. *Entrance requirements:* For doctorate, GRE General Test, letters of recommendation.

University of Central Arkansas, Graduate School, College of Health and Behavioral Sciences, Department of Physical Therapy, Conway, AR 72035-0001. Offers DPT, PhD. *Accreditation:* APTA. *Degree requirements:* For doctorate, comprehensive exam, thesis/dissertation. *Entrance requirements:* Additional exam requirements/recommendations for international students: Required—TOEFL (minimum score 550 paper-based; 80 iBT). Electronic applications accepted. *Expenses:* Contact institution.

University of Central Florida, College of Health and Public Affairs, Program in Physical Therapy, Orlando, FL 32816. Offers DPT. *Accreditation:* APTA. *Faculty:* 16 full-time (9 women), 19 part-time/adjunct (13 women). *Students:* 101 full-time (66 women); includes 27 minority (4 Black or African American, non-Hispanic/Latino; 4 Asian, non-Hispanic/Latino; 16 Hispanic/Latino; 3 Two or more races, non-Hispanic/Latino). Average age 26. In 2015, 32 doctorates awarded. Application fee: $30. Electronic applications accepted. *Expenses:* Contact institution. *Financial support:* In 2015–16, 2 students received support, including 2 fellowships with partial tuition reimbursements available (averaging $2,000 per year); teaching assistantships, career-related internships or fieldwork, institutionally sponsored loans, scholarships/grants, tuition waivers (partial), and unspecified assistantships also available. *Unit head:* Dr. Kristen Schellhase, Interim Chair, 407-823-3463, E-mail: kristen.schellhase@ucf.edu. *Application contact:* Director, Admissions and Student Services, 407-823-2766, Fax: 407-823-6442, E-mail: gradadmissions@ucf.edu. Website: https://www.cohpa.ucf.edu/hp/

University of Colorado Denver, School of Medicine, Program in Physical Therapy, Aurora, CO 80045. Offers DPT. *Accreditation:* APTA. *Program availability:* Part-time. *Students:* 196 full-time (153 women), 2 part-time (1 woman); includes 13 minority (1 American Indian or Alaska Native, non-Hispanic/Latino; 3 Asian, non-Hispanic/Latino; 9 Hispanic/Latino). Average age 26. 644 applicants, 11% accepted, 70 enrolled. In 2015, 58 doctorates awarded. *Degree requirements:* For doctorate, thesis/dissertation or alternative, 116 credit hours, 44 weeks of clinical experiences, capstone project at end of year 3. *Entrance requirements:* For doctorate, GRE, minimum GPA of 3.0; prerequisite coursework in anatomy, physiology, chemistry, physics, psychology, English composition or writing, college-level math, statistics, and upper-level science; 45 hours of observation. Additional exam requirements/recommendations for international students: Required—TOEFL (minimum score 550 paper-based). *Application deadline:* For fall admission, 10/1 for domestic students, 8/8 priority date for international students. Application fee: $120. Electronic applications accepted. *Financial support:* In 2015–16, 198 students received support. Fellowships, research assistantships, teaching assistantships, Federal Work-Study, institutionally sponsored loans, scholarships/grants, traineeships, and unspecified assistantships available. Financial award application deadline: 3/15; financial award applicants required to submit FAFSA. *Faculty research:* Interventions for early and mid-stages of Parkinson's disease, physical therapy for individuals with recurrent lower back pain. *Unit head:* Margaret Schenkman, Program Director, 303-724-9375, E-mail: margaret.schenkman@

ucdenver.edu. *Application contact:* Lauren Wahlquist, Admissions Advisor, 303-724-9144, E-mail: lauren.wahlquist@ucdenver.edu. Website: http://www.ucdenver.edu/academics/colleges/medicalschool/education/degree_programs/pt/Pages/PT.aspx

University of Connecticut, Graduate School, College of Agriculture, Health and Natural Resources, Department of Kinesiology, Program in Physical Therapy, Storrs, CT 06269. Offers DPT. *Accreditation:* APTA. *Entrance requirements:* Additional exam requirements/recommendations for international students: Required—TOEFL (minimum score 550 paper-based). *Application deadline:* For fall admission, 2/1 priority date for domestic and international students; for spring admission, 11/1 for domestic students, 10/1 for international students. Applications are processed on a rolling basis. Application fee: $55. Electronic applications accepted. *Financial support:* Research assistantships and Federal Work-Study available. Financial award application deadline: 2/1; financial award applicants required to submit FAFSA. Website: http://pt.kins.uconn.edu/

University of Dayton, Department of Physical Therapy, Dayton, OH 45469. Offers DPT. *Faculty:* 9 full-time (4 women), 23 part-time/adjunct (18 women). *Students:* 111 full-time (65 women); includes 8 minority (2 Black or African American, non-Hispanic/Latino; 1 Asian, non-Hispanic/Latino; 2 Hispanic/Latino; 3 Two or more races, non-Hispanic/Latino). Average age 24. 209 applicants, 28% accepted, 36 enrolled. In 2015, 38 doctorates awarded. *Degree requirements:* For doctorate, comprehensive exam. *Entrance requirements:* For doctorate, GRE, bachelor's degree from accredited college or university; minimum cumulative GPA of 3.0 across all schools attended; minimum of 64 semester credits and four or more prerequisite science courses with labs; minimum grade of C in all prerequisite courses. Additional exam requirements/recommendations for international students: Required—TOEFL (minimum score 89 iRT) *Application deadline:* For fall admission, 10/1 priority date for domestic students, 9/1 priority date for international students. Electronic applications accepted. *Expenses:* $10,605 per year. *Financial support:* In 2015–16, 7 research assistantships with partial tuition reimbursements (averaging $10,900 per year) were awarded; institutionally sponsored loans and health care benefits also available. Financial award application deadline: 3/1; financial award applicants required to submit FAFSA. *Faculty research:* Women's health and cancer survivors, sports medicine and orthopedics, pediatric and adult neurological rehabilitation, biomechanics, geriatric rehabilitation. *Unit head:* Dr. Philip A. Anloague, Chair/Associate Professor, 937-229-5600, Fax: 937-229-5601, E-mail: panalogue1@udayton.edu. *Application contact:* Trista Cathcart, Admissions Coordinator, 937-229-5611, Fax: 937-229-5601, E-mail: tcathcart1@udayton.edu. Website: https://www.udayton.edu/education/departments_and_programs/dpt/index.php

University of Delaware, College of Health Sciences, Department of Physical Therapy, Newark, DE 19716. Offers DPT. *Accreditation:* APTA. *Entrance requirements:* For doctorate, GRE, 100 hours clinical experience, 3 letters of recommendation. Additional exam requirements/recommendations for international students: Required—TOEFL (minimum score 550 paper-based). Electronic applications accepted. *Faculty research:* Movement sciences, applied physiology, physical rehabilitation.

University of Evansville, College of Education and Health Sciences, Department of Physical Therapy, Evansville, IN 47722. Offers DPT. *Accreditation:* APTA. *Entrance requirements:* Additional exam requirements/recommendations for international students: Required—TOEFL (minimum score 88 iBT), IELTS (minimum score 6.5).

The University of Findlay, Office of Graduate Admissions, Findlay, OH 45840-3653. Offers athletic training (MAT); business (MBA), including health care management, hospitality management, organizational leadership, public management; education (MA Ed), including administration, children's literature, early childhood, human resource development, reading, science, special education, technology; environmental, safety and health management (MSEM); health informatics (MS); occupational therapy (MOT); pharmacy (Pharm D); physical therapy (DPT); physician assistant (MPA); rhetoric and writing (MA); teaching English to speakers of other languages (TESOL) and bilingual education (MA). *Program availability:* Part-time, evening/weekend, online learning. *Degree requirements:* For master's, thesis, cumulative project, capstone project. *Entrance requirements:* For master's, GRE/GMAT, bachelor's degree from accredited institution, minimum undergraduate GPA of 2.5 in last 64 hours of course work; for doctorate, GRE, minimum cumulative GPA of 3.0. Additional exam requirements/recommendations for international students: Required—TOEFL (minimum score 80 iBT). Electronic applications accepted.

University of Florida, Graduate School, College of Public Health and Health Professions, Department of Physical Therapy, Gainesville, FL 32611. Offers DPT, DPT/MPH. *Accreditation:* APTA (one or more programs are accredited). *Entrance requirements:* For doctorate, GRE General Test, minimum GPA of 3.0. Additional exam requirements/recommendations for international students: Required—TOEFL (minimum score 515 paper-based; 80 iBT), IELTS (minimum score 6). *Application deadline:* For fall admission, 11/1 for domestic students; for spring admission, 11/1 for domestic students. Applications are processed on a rolling basis. Application fee: $30. Electronic applications accepted. *Financial support:* Career-related internships or fieldwork available. Financial award applicants required to submit FAFSA. *Faculty research:* Exercise physiology, motor control, rehabilitation, geriatrics. *Total annual research expenditures:* $4.4 million. *Unit head:* Krista Vandenborne, PhD, Department Chair/Associate Dean for Research and Planning, 352-273-6085, Fax: 352-273-6109, E-mail: kvandenb@phhp.ufl.edu. *Application contact:* Steven Z. George, PhD, Associate Professor/Assistant Department Chair, 352-273-6432, Fax: 352-273-6109, E-mail: szgeorge@phhp.ufl.edu. Website: http://pt.phhp.ufl.edu/

University of Hartford, College of Education, Nursing, and Health Professions, Program in Physical Therapy, West Hartford, CT 06117-1599. Offers MSPT, DPT. *Accreditation:* APTA. *Entrance requirements:* For master's, GRE, 3 letters of recommendation. Additional exam requirements/recommendations for international students: Required—TOEFL (minimum score 550 paper-based).

University of Illinois at Chicago, College of Applied Health Sciences, Department of Physical Therapy, Chicago, IL 60607-7128. Offers MS, DPT. *Accreditation:* APTA. *Faculty:* 20 full-time (13 women), 6 part-time/adjunct (2 women). *Students:* 184 full-time (120 women), 11 part-time (3 women); includes 29 minority (5 Black or African American, non-Hispanic/Latino; 15 Asian, non-Hispanic/Latino; 5 Hispanic/Latino; 4 Two or more races, non-Hispanic/Latino), 17 international. Average age 25. *Degree requirements:* For master's, thesis. *Entrance requirements:* For master's, GRE General Test, minimum GPA of 2.75. Additional exam requirements/recommendations for international students: Required—TOEFL. *Application deadline:* For fall admission, 2/15 for domestic and international students. Electronic applications accepted. *Expenses:* Tuition, state resident: full-time $11,480; part-time $3826 per credit. Tuition, nonresident: full-time $23,720; part-time $7906 per credit. *Required fees:* $1333 per semester. Part-time tuition and fees vary according to course load and program. *Financial support:* Fellowships with full tuition reimbursements, research assistantships with full tuition reimbursements, teaching assistantships with full tuition reimbursements, Federal Work-Study, tuition waivers (full), and tuition service fee waivers available.

Financial award applicants required to submit FAFSA. *Faculty research:* Diagnosing delayed development in high-risk infants, falling mechanics and prevention, posture and movement control in the elderly, healthy lifestyle behaviors of people with disabilities, motor dysfunction following spinal cord injury and stroke. *Unit head:* Prof. Ross Anthony Arena, Department Head, 312-996-3338, Fax: 312-996-4583, E-mail: raarena@uic.edu. *Application contact:* Alexander Aruin, Receptionist, 312-355-0904, E-mail: aaruin@uic.edu. Website: http://www.ahs.uic.edu/pt/

University of Indianapolis, Graduate Programs, College of Health Sciences, Krannert School of Physical Therapy, Indianapolis, IN 46227-3697. Offers MHS, DHS, DPT. *Accreditation:* APTA (one or more programs are accredited). *Program availability:* Part-time, evening/weekend. *Entrance requirements:* For doctorate, GRE General Test (for DPT), minimum GPA of 3.0 (for DPT), 3 letters of recommendation. Additional exam requirements/recommendations for international students: Required—TOEFL (minimum score 100 iBT), TWE (minimum score 5). Electronic applications accepted. *Expenses:* Contact institution. *Faculty research:* Patella positioning, reaction time, allocation of physical therapy resources.

The University of Iowa, Roy J. and Lucille A. Carver College of Medicine and Graduate College, Graduate Programs in Medicine, Department of Physical Therapy and Rehabilitation Science, Iowa City, IA 52242. Offers physical rehabilitation science (MA, PhD); physical therapy (DPT). *Accreditation:* APTA (one or more programs are accredited). Terminal master's awarded for partial completion of doctoral program. *Degree requirements:* For master's, thesis (for some programs); for doctorate, comprehensive exam (for some programs), thesis/dissertation (for some programs). *Entrance requirements:* For master's and doctorate, GRE. Additional exam requirements/recommendations for international students: Required—TOEFL. Electronic applications accepted. *Expenses:* Contact institution. *Faculty research:* Neuroplasticity and motor control, pain mechanisms, biomechanics and sports medicine, neuromuscular physiology, cardiovascular physiology.

University of Jamestown, Program in Physical Therapy, Jamestown, ND 58405. Offers DPT. *Entrance requirements:* For doctorate, bachelor's degree.

The University of Kansas, University of Kansas Medical Center, School of Health Professions, Department of Physical Therapy and Rehabilitation Science, Kansas City, KS 66160. Offers physical therapy (DPT); rehabilitation science (PhD). *Accreditation:* APTA. *Faculty:* 21. *Students:* 178 full-time (102 women), 2 part-time (1 woman); includes 17 minority (3 Asian, non-Hispanic/Latino; 8 Hispanic/Latino; 6 Two or more races, non-Hispanic/Latino), 16 international. Average age 25. 306 applicants, 26% accepted, 60 enrolled. In 2015, 44 doctorates awarded. *Degree requirements:* For doctorate, comprehensive exam, research project with paper. *Entrance requirements:* For doctorate, GRE General Test, minimum GPA of 3.0. Additional exam requirements/recommendations for international students: Required—TOEFL. *Application deadline:* For fall admission, 11/1 for domestic students. Application fee: $60. Electronic applications accepted. *Expenses:* Contact institution. *Financial support:* Research assistantships with tuition reimbursements, teaching assistantships with tuition reimbursements, career-related internships or fieldwork, Federal Work-Study, institutionally sponsored loans, scholarships/grants, traineeships, and unspecified assistantships available. Financial award application deadline: 3/1; financial award applicants required to submit FAFSA. *Faculty research:* Stroke rehabilitation and the effects on balance and coordination; deep brain stimulation and Parkinson's Disease; peripheral neuropathies, pain and the effects of exercise; islet transplants for Type 1 diabetes; cardiac disease associated with diabetes. *Total annual research expenditures:* $434,052. *Unit head:* Dr. Patricia Kluding, Interim Chair, 913-588-6733, Fax: 913-588-6910, E-mail: pkluding@kumc.edu. *Application contact:* Robert Bagley, Senior Coordinator, 913-588-6799, Fax: 913-588-6910, E-mail: rbagley@kumc.edu. Website: http://www.kumc.edu/school-of-health-professions/physical-therapy-and-rehabilitation-science.html

University of Kentucky, Graduate School, College of Health Sciences, Program in Physical Therapy, Lexington, KY 40506-0032. Offers DPT. *Accreditation:* APTA. *Degree requirements:* For doctorate, comprehensive exam, thesis/dissertation optional. *Entrance requirements:* For doctorate, GRE General Test, minimum undergraduate GPA of 2.75, U.S. physical therapist license. Additional exam requirements/recommendations for international students: Required—TOEFL (minimum score 550 paper-based). Electronic applications accepted. *Faculty research:* Orthopedics, biomechanics, electrophysiological stimulation, neural plasticity, brain damage and mechanism.

University of Manitoba, Faculty of Graduate Studies, School of Medical Rehabilitation, Winnipeg, MB R3T 2N2, Canada. Offers applied health sciences (PhD); occupational therapy (MOT); physical therapy (MPT); rehabilitation (M Sc).

University of Mary, School of Health Sciences, Program in Physical Therapy, Bismarck, ND 58504-9652. Offers DPT. *Accreditation:* APTA. *Degree requirements:* For doctorate, comprehensive exam, professional paper. *Entrance requirements:* For doctorate, GRE, minimum GPA of 2.75, 3.0 in core requirements; 40 hours of paid/volunteer experience; 2 letters of recommendation. Additional exam requirements/recommendations for international students: Required—TOEFL (minimum score 500 paper-based; 71 iBT). *Application deadline:* Applications are processed on a rolling basis. Application fee: $40. Electronic applications accepted. *Expenses:* Contact institution. *Financial support:* Teaching assistantships with partial tuition reimbursements and career-related internships or fieldwork available. Financial award application deadline: 8/1; financial award applicants required to submit FAFSA. Website: http://www.umary.edu/academics/programs/doctorate-physical-therapy.php

University of Mary Hardin-Baylor, Graduate Studies in Physical Therapy, Belton, TX 76513. Offers physical therapy (DPT). *Faculty:* 10 full-time (7 women), 6 part-time/adjunct (3 women). *Students:* 40 full-time (26 women); includes 8 minority (2 Black or African American, non-Hispanic/Latino; 2 Asian, non-Hispanic/Latino; 4 Hispanic/Latino). Average age 25. 100 applicants, 51% accepted, 40 enrolled. *Entrance requirements:* For doctorate, minimum GPA of 3.2 in last 60 hours of bachelor's or relevant master's degree, 3.0 in prerequisites; therapy and other healthcare-related experience; resume; letters of recommendation. Additional exam requirements/recommendations for international students: Required—TOEFL (minimum score 100 iBT), IELTS (minimum score 7). *Application deadline:* For fall admission, 6/1 for domestic students, 4/30 priority date for international students; for spring admission, 11/1 for domestic students, 9/30 priority date for international students. Applications are processed on a rolling basis. Application fee: $35 ($135 for international students). Electronic applications accepted. *Expenses: Tuition, area resident:* Part-time $815 per credit hour. Tuition and fees vary according to course load and degree level. *Financial support:* Federal Work-Study, unspecified assistantships, and scholarships for some active duty military personnel available. Financial award applicants required to submit FAFSA. *Unit head:* Dr. Barbara Gresham, Director, 254-295-4921, E-mail: bgresham@umhb.edu. *Application contact:* Melissa Williams, Director, Graduate Student Services and Engagement, 254-295-4020, Fax: 254-295-5038, E-mail: mwilliams@umhb.edu. Website: http://graduate.umhb.edu/dpt/

Physical Therapy

University of Maryland, Baltimore, School of Medicine, Department of Physical Therapy and Rehabilitation Science, Baltimore, MD 21201. Offers physical rehabilitation science (PhD); physical therapy and rehabilitation science (DPT). *Accreditation:* APTA. *Students:* 173 full-time (111 women), 2 part-time (1 woman); includes 32 minority (7 Black or African American, non-Hispanic/Latino; 10 Asian, non-Hispanic/Latino; 13 Hispanic/Latino; 2 Two or more races, non-Hispanic/Latino), 2 international. Average age 25. 154 applicants, 82% accepted, 65 enrolled. In 2015, 59 doctorates awarded. *Entrance requirements:* For doctorate, GRE General Test, BS, science coursework. Additional exam requirements/recommendations for international students: Required—TOEFL (minimum score 80 iBT). Electronic applications accepted. *Expenses:* Contact institution. *Financial support:* Career-related internships or fieldwork, Federal Work-Study, scholarships/grants, traineeships, health care benefits, and unspecified assistantships available. Financial award application deadline: 3/1; financial award applicants required to submit FAFSA. *Unit head:* Dr. Mark W. Rogers, Interim Chair, 410-706-5216, Fax: 410-706-4903, E-mail: mrodgers@som.umaryland.edu. *Application contact:* Aynsley Hamel, Program Coordinator, 410-706-0566, Fax: 410-706-6387, E-mail: ptadmissions@som.umaryland.edu.
Website: http://pt.umaryland.edu/pros.asp

University of Maryland Eastern Shore, Graduate Programs, Department of Physical Therapy, Princess Anne, MD 21853-1299. Offers DPT. *Accreditation:* APTA. *Degree requirements:* For doctorate, thesis/dissertation, clinical practicum, research project. *Entrance requirements:* For doctorate, minimum GPA of 3.0, course work in science and mathematics, interview, knowledge of the physical therapy field. Additional exam requirements/recommendations for international students: Required—TOEFL (minimum score 80 iBT). Electronic applications accepted. *Faculty research:* Allied health projects.

University of Massachusetts Lowell, College of Health Sciences, Department of Physical Therapy, Lowell, MA 01854. Offers DPT. *Accreditation:* APTA. *Entrance requirements:* For doctorate, GRE General Test, minimum GPA of 3.0, 3 letters of recommendation. Additional exam requirements/recommendations for international students: Required—TOEFL (minimum score 560 paper-based). *Application deadline:* For fall admission, 1/15 for domestic students. Application fee: $20 ($35 for international students). *Expenses:* Tuition, state resident: full-time $14,304. Tuition, nonresident: full-time $25,853. *Required fees:* $375. Full-time tuition and fees vary according to campus/location and reciprocity agreements. *Financial support:* Fellowships with full tuition reimbursements, research assistantships with full tuition reimbursements, teaching assistantships with full tuition reimbursements, career-related internships or fieldwork, Federal Work-Study, institutionally sponsored loans, scholarships/grants, and traineeships available. Support available to part-time students. Financial award application deadline: 2/15. *Faculty research:* Orthopedics, pediatrics, electrophysiology, cardiopulmonary, neurology.

University of Miami, Graduate School, Miller School of Medicine, Graduate Programs in Medicine, Department of Physical Therapy, Coral Gables, FL 33124. Offers DPT, PhD. *Accreditation:* APTA (one or more programs are accredited). *Degree requirements:* For doctorate, comprehensive exam, thesis/dissertation. *Entrance requirements:* For doctorate, GRE General Test. Additional exam requirements/recommendations for international students: Required—TOEFL. Electronic applications accepted. *Expenses:* Contact institution. *Faculty research:* Central pattern generators in SCI balance and vestibular function in children, amputee rehabilitation.

University of Michigan–Flint, School of Health Professions and Studies, Program in Physical Therapy, Flint, MI 48502-1950. Offers geriatrics (DPT, PhD, Certificate); neurology (DPT, PhD, Certificate); orthopedics (DPT, PhD, Certificate); pediatrics (DPT, PhD, Certificate); physical therapy (DPT). *Accreditation:* APTA. *Program availability:* Part-time. *Faculty:* 15 full-time (11 women), 6 part-time/adjunct (3 women). *Students:* 190 full-time (109 women), 41 part-time (28 women); includes 25 minority (1 Black or African American, non-Hispanic/Latino; 1 American Indian or Alaska Native, non-Hispanic/Latino; 13 Asian, non-Hispanic/Latino; 7 Hispanic/Latino; 3 Two or more races, non-Hispanic/Latino), 20 international. Average age 27. 531 applicants, 30% accepted, 70 enrolled. In 2015, 79 doctorates, 1 other advanced degree awarded. *Degree requirements:* For doctorate, comprehensive exam, thesis/dissertation or alternative. *Entrance requirements:* For doctorate, GRE (minimum Verbal score between 340-480; Quantitative 370-710); for Certificate, physical therapy degree from accredited institution; current physical therapy license in the United States or Canada; minimum overall GPA of 3.0 in the physical therapy degree; current CPR certification. Additional exam requirements/recommendations for international students: Required—TOEFL (minimum score 560 paper-based; 84 iBT), IELTS (minimum score 6.5). *Application deadline:* For fall admission, 5/1 for domestic students, 2/1 for international students; for winter admission, 7/31 for domestic students, 4/1 for international students; for spring admission, 3/1 for domestic students, 12/1 for international students. Application fee: $55. Electronic applications accepted. *Expenses:* Contact institution. *Financial support:* Federal Work-Study, scholarships/grants, and unspecified assistantships available. Support available to part-time students. Financial award application deadline: 3/1; financial award applicants required to submit FAFSA. *Faculty research:* Cumulative trauma disorders, oncology rehabilitation, neurological rehabilitation, musculoskeletal rehabilitation, cardiopulmonary rehabilitation. *Unit head:* Dr. Amy Yorke, Admissions Chair, 810-762-3373, E-mail: amyorke@umflint.edu. *Application contact:* Crystal Quaderer, Administrative Assistant, 810-762-3373, Fax: 810-766-6668, E-mail: quaderer@umflint.edu.
Website: https://www.umflint.edu/pt/pt_career

University of Minnesota, Twin Cities Campus, Medical School, Minneapolis, MN 55455-0213. Offers MA, MS, DPT, MD, PhD, JD/MD, MD/MBA, MD/MHI, MD/MPH, MD/MS, MD/PhD. *Accreditation:* LCME/AMA. *Program availability:* Part-time, evening/weekend. *Expenses:* Contact institution.

University of Mississippi Medical Center, School of Health Related Professions, Department of Physical Therapy, Jackson, MS 39216-4505. Offers MPT. *Accreditation:* APTA. *Faculty research:* Pain, acupressure, seating, patient satisfaction, physical therapy educational issues.

University of Missouri, School of Health Professions, Program in Physical Therapy, Columbia, MO 65211. Offers DPT. *Accreditation:* APTA. *Entrance requirements:* Additional exam requirements/recommendations for international students: Required—TOEFL (minimum score 600 paper-based; 100 iBT). *Application deadline:* For spring admission, 1/10 priority date for domestic and international students. Applications are processed on a rolling basis. Application fee: $55 ($75 for international students). Electronic applications accepted. *Financial support:* Research assistantships, teaching assistantships, and institutionally sponsored loans available.
Website: http://shp.missouri.edu/pt/index.php

University of Montana, Graduate School, College of Health Professions and Biomedical Sciences, School of Physical Therapy and Rehabilitation Science, Missoula, MT 59812-0002. Offers physical therapy (DPT). *Accreditation:* APTA. *Degree requirements:* For doctorate, professional paper. *Entrance requirements:* For doctorate, GRE General Test. Additional exam requirements/recommendations for international students: Required—TOEFL. Electronic applications accepted. *Expenses:* Contact

institution. *Faculty research:* Muscle stiffness, fitness with a disability, psychosocial aspects of disability, clinical learning, motion analysis.

University of Nebraska Medical Center, School of Allied Health Professions, Division of Physical Therapy Education, Omaha, NE 68198. Offers DPT. *Accreditation:* APTA. *Expenses:* Tuition, state resident: full-time $7830; part-time $3915 per credit hour. Tuition, nonresident: full-time $22,410; part-time $11,205 per credit hour. *Required fees:* $521.

University of Nevada, Las Vegas, Graduate College, School of Allied Health Sciences, Department of Physical Therapy, Las Vegas, NV 89154-3029. Offers DPT. *Accreditation:* APTA. *Faculty:* 6 full-time (2 women), 3 part-time/adjunct (all women). *Students:* 102 full-time (45 women); includes 30 minority (12 Asian, non-Hispanic/Latino; 8 Hispanic/Latino; 1 Native Hawaiian or other Pacific Islander, non-Hispanic/Latino; 9 Two or more races, non-Hispanic/Latino), 1 international. Average age 27. In 2015, 28 doctorates awarded. *Degree requirements:* For doctorate, comprehensive exam (for some programs), thesis/dissertation. *Entrance requirements:* For doctorate, PTCAS application, observation hours. Additional exam requirements/recommendations for international students: Required—TOEFL (minimum score 550 paper-based; 80 iBT), IELTS (minimum score 7). *Application deadline:* For fall admission, 5/1 for international students; for spring admission, 10/1 for international students; for summer admission, 11/2 priority date for domestic students. Application fee: $60 ($95 for international students). Electronic applications accepted. *Expenses:* $264 per credit state resident full-time and part-time; $6,955 per semester, $264 per credit nonresident full-time; $555 per credit nonresident part-time. *Financial support:* In 2015–16, 10 students received support, including 9 research assistantships with partial tuition reimbursements available (averaging $13,000 per year), 1 teaching assistantship with partial tuition reimbursement available (averaging $13,000 per year); institutionally sponsored loans, scholarships/grants, health care benefits, and unspecified assistantships also available. Financial award application deadline: 3/1. *Faculty research:* Pathobiomechanics of prosthetics, knee osteoarthritis, patellofemoral pain, spinal manipulation, balance assessment and impairment, falls and fall avoidance behavior, wound care and acute care delivery services, pain reduction and pain science education. *Total annual research expenditures:* $100,590. *Unit head:* Dr. Merrill Landers, Chair/Associate Professor, 702-895-1377, Fax: 702-895-4883, E-mail: merrill.landers@unlv.edu. *Application contact:* Graduate College Admissions Evaluator, 702-895-3367, Fax: 702-895-4180, E-mail: gradadmissions@unlv.edu.
Website: http://pt.unlv.edu/

University of New England, Westbrook College of Health Professions, Program in Physical Therapy, Biddeford, ME 04005-9526. Offers DPT. *Accreditation:* APTA. *Program availability:* Online learning. *Faculty:* 11 full-time (7 women), 9 part-time/adjunct (7 women). *Students:* 201 full-time (142 women); includes 24 minority (3 Black or African American, non-Hispanic/Latino; 12 Asian, non-Hispanic/Latino; 5 Hispanic/Latino; 1 Native Hawaiian or other Pacific Islander, non-Hispanic/Latino; 3 Two or more races, non-Hispanic/Latino). Average age 27. 1,215 applicants, 14% accepted, 64 enrolled. In 2015, 68 doctorates awarded. *Degree requirements:* For doctorate, clinical rotations. *Entrance requirements:* For doctorate, GRE. *Application deadline:* For fall admission, 1/15 for domestic students. Applications are processed on a rolling basis. Electronic applications accepted. Tuition and fees vary according to degree level and program. *Financial support:* Scholarships/grants available. Financial award application deadline: 5/1; financial award applicants required to submit FAFSA. *Unit head:* Dr. Michael Sheldon, Program Director/Associate Professor, 207-221-4591, Fax: 207-523-1910, E-mail: msheldon@une.edu. *Application contact:* Scott Steinberg, Dean of University Admissions, 207-221-4225, Fax: 207-523-1925, E-mail: ssteinberg@une.edu.
Website: http://www.une.edu/wchp/pt

University of New Mexico, Graduate Studies, Health Sciences Center, Division of Physical Therapy, Albuquerque, NM 87131. Offers DPT. *Accreditation:* APTA. *Faculty:* 6 full-time (4 women), 1 (woman) part-time/adjunct. *Students:* 81 full-time (64 women), 1 (woman) part-time; includes 33 minority (1 Black or African American, non-Hispanic/Latino; 3 American Indian or Alaska Native, non-Hispanic/Latino; 2 Asian, non-Hispanic/Latino; 26 Hispanic/Latino; 1 Two or more races, non-Hispanic/Latino). Average age 31. 30 applicants, 100% accepted, 30 enrolled. In 2015, 26 doctorates awarded. *Degree requirements:* For doctorate, comprehensive exam, thesis/dissertation or alternative. *Entrance requirements:* For doctorate, GRE General Test, GRE Writing Assessment Test, interview, minimum GPA of 3.0. *Application deadline:* For fall admission, 12/15 priority date for domestic students. Applications are processed on a rolling basis. Application fee: $50. *Financial support:* Fellowships, Federal Work-Study, institutionally sponsored loans, and scholarships/grants available. Financial award application deadline: 3/1; financial award applicants required to submit FAFSA. *Faculty research:* Gait analysis, motion analysis, balance, articular cartilage, quality of life. *Total annual research expenditures:* $7,428. *Unit head:* Dr. Susan A. Queen, Director, 505-272-5756, Fax: 505-272-8079, E-mail: squeen@salud.unm.edu. *Application contact:* Rosalia Loya Vejar, Administrative Assistant, 505-272-6956, Fax: 505-272-8079, E-mail: rloyavejar@salud.unm.edu.

The University of North Carolina at Chapel Hill, School of Medicine and Graduate School, Graduate Programs in Medicine, Chapel Hill, NC 27599. Offers allied health sciences (MPT, MS, Au D, DPT, PhD), including human movement science (MS, PhD), occupational science (MS, PhD), physical therapy (MPT, MS, DPT), rehabilitation counseling and psychology (MS); speech and hearing sciences (MS, Au D, PhD); biochemistry and biophysics (MS, PhD); bioinformatics and computational biology (PhD); biomedical engineering (MS, PhD); cell and developmental biology (PhD); cell and molecular physiology (PhD); genetics and molecular biology (PhD); microbiology and immunology (MS, PhD), including immunology, microbiology; neurobiology (PhD); pathology and laboratory medicine (PhD), including experimental pathology; pharmacology (PhD); MD/PhD. *Program availability:* Online learning. Terminal master's awarded for partial completion of doctoral program. *Degree requirements:* For master's, comprehensive exam; for doctorate, thesis/dissertation. Electronic applications accepted. *Expenses:* Contact institution.

The University of North Carolina at Chapel Hill, School of Medicine and Graduate School, Graduate Programs in Medicine, Department of Allied Health Sciences, Program in Physical Therapy, Chapel Hill, NC 27599. Offers physical therapy - off campus (DPT); physical therapy - on campus (DPT). *Accreditation:* APTA. *Program availability:* Part-time, evening/weekend, online learning. *Degree requirements:* For doctorate, thesis/dissertation or alternative. *Entrance requirements:* For doctorate, physical therapy license. Additional exam requirements/recommendations for international students: Required—TOEFL (minimum score 550 paper-based). Electronic applications accepted. *Faculty research:* Traumatic brain injury, quality of life after heart and/or lung transplant, cultural diversity, life care planning, rehabilitation education and supervision.

University of North Dakota, Graduate School and Graduate School, Graduate Programs in Medicine, Department of Physical Therapy, Grand Forks, ND 58202. Offers MPT, DPT. *Accreditation:* APTA. *Degree requirements:* For master's, comprehensive exam, thesis or alternative. *Entrance requirements:* For master's and doctorate, minimum GPA of 3.0, pre-physical therapy program. Additional exam requirements/recommendations for international students: Required—TOEFL (minimum score 550 paper-based; 79 iBT), IELTS (minimum score 6.5). *Faculty research:* Practice-based program.

University of North Florida, Brooks College of Health, Department of Clinical and Applied Movement Sciences, Jacksonville, FL 32224. Offers exercise science and chronic disease (MSH); physical therapy (DPT). *Accreditation:* APTA. *Program availability:* Part-time, evening/weekend. *Faculty:* 12 full-time (8 women), 7 part-time/adjunct (4 women). *Students:* 87 full-time (48 women), 2 part-time (1 woman); includes 28 minority (2 Black or African American, non-Hispanic/Latino; 4 Asian, non-Hispanic/Latino; 14 Hispanic/Latino; 8 Two or more races, non-Hispanic/Latino). Average age 25. 414 applicants, 18% accepted, 34 enrolled. In 2015, 30 doctorates awarded. *Degree requirements:* For master's, internship. *Entrance requirements:* For master's, GRE General Test, minimum GPA of 3.0 in last 60 hours, volunteer/observation experience. Additional exam requirements/recommendations for international students: Required—TOEFL (minimum score 500 paper-based). *Application deadline:* For fall admission, 2/15 for domestic students, 1/15 for international students. Application fee: $30. Electronic applications accepted. *Expenses:* Tuition, state resident: part-time $408.10 per credit hour. Tuition, nonresident: part-time $932.61 per credit hour. *Required fees:* $111.81 per credit hour. Tuition and fees vary according to course load, campus/location and program. *Financial support:* In 2015–16, 27 students received support, including 6 teaching assistantships (averaging $1,500 per year); career-related internships or fieldwork, Federal Work-Study, scholarships/grants, and tuition waivers (partial) also available. Support available to part-time students. Financial award application deadline: 4/1; financial award applicants required to submit FAFSA. *Faculty research:* Clinical outcomes related to orthopedic physical therapy interventions, instructional multimedia in physical therapy education, effect of functional electrical stimulation orthostatic hypotension in acute complete spinal cord injury individuals. *Total annual research expenditures:* $87,684. *Unit head:* Dr. Joel Beam, Chair, 904-620-1424, E-mail: jbeam@unf.edu. *Application contact:* Beth Dibble, Program Director, 904-620-2418, E-mail: ptadmissions@unf.edu.
Website: http://www.unf.edu/brooks/movement_science/

University of North Georgia, Department of Physical Therapy, Dahlonega, GA 30597. Offers DPT. *Accreditation:* APTA. *Entrance requirements:* For doctorate, GRE, interview, recommendations, physical therapy observations hours, minimum GPA of 2.8. Additional exam requirements/recommendations for international students: Required—TOEFL (minimum score 550 paper-based; 79 iBT), IELTS (minimum score 6.5). *Application deadline:* Applications are processed on a rolling basis. Application fee: $50. Electronic applications accepted. *Expenses:* Contact institution. *Financial support:* Unspecified assistantships available. Financial award application deadline: 5/1; financial award applicants required to submit CSS PROFILE or FAFSA. *Faculty research:* Ergonomics, spinal mobility measurements, electrophysiology, orthopedic physical therapy.
Website: http://ung.edu/physical-therapy/

University of Oklahoma Health Sciences Center, Graduate College, College of Allied Health, Department of Physical Therapy, Oklahoma City, OK 73190. Offers MPT. *Accreditation:* APTA.

University of Pittsburgh, School of Health and Rehabilitation Sciences, Doctor of Physical Therapy Program, Pittsburgh, PA 15260. Offers DPT. *Accreditation:* APTA. *Faculty:* 12 full-time (6 women), 3 part-time/adjunct (1 woman). *Students:* 171 full-time (114 women); includes 4 minority (2 Black or African American, non-Hispanic/Latino; 2 Two or more races, non-Hispanic/Latino), 2 international. Average age 26. 1,026 applicants, 15% accepted, 56 enrolled. In 2015, 63 doctorates awarded. *Degree requirements:* For doctorate, clinical practice. *Entrance requirements:* For doctorate, GRE General Test, volunteer work in physical therapy. Additional exam requirements/recommendations for international students: Required—TOEFL (minimum score 550 paper-based; 80 iBT), IELTS (minimum score 6.5). *Application deadline:* For summer admission, 12/15 for domestic and international students. Applications are processed on a rolling basis. Application fee: $140. Electronic applications accepted. Tuition and fees vary according to program. *Financial support:* Career-related internships or fieldwork and traineeships available. *Faculty research:* Biomechanics, neuromuscular system, sports medicine, movement analysis, validity/outcomes of clinical procedures. *Total annual research expenditures:* $3.1 million. *Unit head:* Dr. Debora L. Miller, Department Chair/Associate Professor, 412-383-6641, E-mail: dlm27@pitt.edu. *Application contact:* Corinne Grubb, Administrator, Physical Therapy Student Services, 412-383-8169, Fax: 412-648-5970, E-mail: cgrubb@pitt.edu.
Website: http://www.shrs.pitt.edu/DPT/

University of Pittsburgh, School of Health and Rehabilitation Sciences, Master's Programs in Health and Rehabilitation Sciences, Pittsburgh, PA 15260. Offers health and rehabilitation sciences (MS), including health information systems, healthcare supervision and management, occupational therapy, physical therapy, rehabilitation counseling, rehabilitation science and technology, sports medicine, wellness and human performance. *Accreditation:* APTA. *Program availability:* Part-time, evening/weekend. *Faculty:* 32 full-time (21 women). *Students:* 111 full-time (73 women), 42 part-time (31 women); includes 23 minority (5 Black or African American, non-Hispanic/Latino; 8 Asian, non-Hispanic/Latino; 7 Hispanic/Latino; 3 Two or more races, non-Hispanic/Latino), 65 international. Average age 29. 330 applicants, 66% accepted, 107 enrolled. In 2015, 89 master's awarded. *Degree requirements:* For master's, comprehensive exam (for some programs), thesis optional. *Entrance requirements:* For master's, minimum GPA of 3.0. Additional exam requirements/recommendations for international students: Required—TOEFL (minimum score 550 paper-based; 80 iBT), IELTS (minimum score 6.5). *Application deadline:* For fall admission, 3/1 for international students; for spring admission, 9/1 for international students. Applications are processed on a rolling basis. Application fee: $50. Electronic applications accepted. Tuition and fees vary according to program. *Financial support:* In 2015–16, 7 students received support, including 7 fellowships with full tuition reimbursements available (averaging $17,048 per year); traineeships also available. *Faculty research:* Assistive technology, seating and wheelchair mobility, cellular neurophysiology, low back syndrome, augmentative communication. *Total annual research expenditures:* $7.7 million. *Unit head:* Dr. Anthony Delitto, Dean, 412-383-6560, Fax: 412-383-6535, E-mail: delitto@pitt.edu. *Application contact:* Jessica Maguire, Director of Admissions, 412-383-6557, Fax: 412-383-6535, E-mail: maguire@pitt.edu.

University of Puerto Rico, Medical Sciences Campus, School of Health Professions, Program in Physical Therapy, San Juan, PR 00936-5067. Offers MS. *Accreditation:* APTA. *Program availability:* Part-time, evening/weekend. *Degree requirements:* For master's, one foreign language, thesis. *Entrance requirements:* For master's, EXADEP, minimum GPA of 2.8, interview, first aid training and CPR certification.

University of Puget Sound, School of Physical Therapy, Tacoma, WA 98416. Offers DPT. *Accreditation:* APTA. *Degree requirements:* For doctorate, comprehensive exam, thesis/dissertation or alternative, successful completion of 36 weeks of full-time internships, research project. *Entrance requirements:* For doctorate, GRE General Test, minimum baccalaureate GPA of 3.0, observation hours (at least 100 recommended), three letters of recommendation. Additional exam requirements/recommendations for international students: Required—TOEFL (minimum score 550 paper-based; 90 iBT). Electronic applications accepted. *Expenses:* Contact institution. *Faculty research:*

Manual therapy, assessment of chronic pain, movement assessment of children, pediatric gait, seating interventions, electro-physical agents, injury prevention.

University of Rhode Island, Graduate School, College of Human Science and Services, Physical Therapy Department, Kingston, RI 02881. Offers DPT. *Accreditation:* APTA. *Program availability:* Part-time. *Faculty:* 5 full-time (2 women). *Students:* 64 full-time (43 women), 28 part-time (23 women); includes 7 minority (6 Asian, non-Hispanic/Latino; 1 Hispanic/Latino), 1 international. In 2015, 35 doctorates awarded. *Degree requirements:* For doctorate, comprehensive exam. *Entrance requirements:* For doctorate, GRE, 2 letters of recommendation (one must be from a physical therapist). Additional exam requirements/recommendations for international students: Required—TOEFL (minimum score 550 paper-based). *Application deadline:* For fall admission, 12/15 for domestic and international students; for summer admission, 11/1 for domestic and international students. Application fee: $65. Electronic applications accepted. *Expenses:* Tuition, state resident: full-time $11,796; part-time $655 per credit. Tuition, nonresident: full-time $24,206; part-time $1345 per credit. *Required fees:* $1546; $44 per credit. One-time fee: $155 full-time; $35 part-time. *Financial support:* In 2015–16, 2 research assistantships (averaging $5,924 per year), 1 teaching assistantship with tuition reimbursement (averaging $5,258 per year) were awarded. Financial award application deadline: 11/1; financial award applicants required to submit FAFSA. *Total annual research expenditures:* $180,819. *Unit head:* Dr. Jeff Konin, Chair, 401-574-5627, E-mail: jkonin@mail.uri.edu. *Application contact:* Graduate Admissions, 401-874-2872, E-mail: gradadm@etal.uri.edu.
Website: http://www.uri.edu/hss/pt/

University of St. Augustine for Health Sciences, Graduate Programs, Doctor of Physical Therapy Program, St. Augustine, FL 32086. Offers DPT. *Accreditation:* APTA. *Entrance requirements:* Additional exam requirements/recommendations for international students: Required—TOEFL. Application fee is waived when completed online.

University of St. Augustine for Health Sciences, Graduate Programs, Post Professional Programs, St. Augustine, FL 32086. Offers health science (DH Sc); health sciences education (Ed D); occupational therapy (TOTD); physical therapy (TDPT). *Program availability:* Part-time, online learning. *Entrance requirements:* For doctorate, GRE General Test, master's degree in related field. Additional exam requirements/recommendations for international students: Required—TOEFL.

University of Saint Mary, Graduate Programs, Program in Physical Therapy, Leavenworth, KS 66048-5082. Offers DPT. *Accreditation:* APTA. *Students:* 119 full-time (63 women); includes 11 minority (1 Black or African American, non-Hispanic/Latino; 4 Asian, non-Hispanic/Latino; 4 Hispanic/Latino; 2 Two or more races, non-Hispanic/Latino). Average age 25. In 2015, 37 doctorates awarded. Application fee: $35. *Expenses:* $725 per hour. *Unit head:* Candace Bahner, DPT Chair, 913-758-6190, E-mail: dpt@stmary.edu. *Application contact:* Christi Sumpter, Department Secretary, 913-758-4398, Fax: 913-345-2802, E-mail: dpt@stmary.edu.
Website: http://www.stmary.edu/DPT

The University of Scranton, Panuska College of Professional Studies, Department of Physical Therapy, Scranton, PA 18510. Offers DPT. *Accreditation:* APTA. *Program availability:* Part-time. *Students:* 122 full-time (71 women), 1 (woman) part-time; includes 6 minority (3 Asian, non-Hispanic/Latino; 2 Hispanic/Latino; 1 Two or more races, non-Hispanic/Latino). Average age 23. *Degree requirements:* For doctorate, capstone experience. *Entrance requirements:* For doctorate, minimum undergraduate GPA of 3.0, minimum 60 hours of observation. Additional exam requirements/recommendations for international students: Required—TOEFL (minimum score 500 paper-based; 80 iBT), IELTS (minimum score 6.5). *Application deadline:* For fall admission, 6/1 for international students; for spring admission, 11/1 for international students; for summer admission, 3/1 for international students. Applications are processed on a rolling basis. Application fee: $0. Electronic applications accepted. *Financial support:* Applicants required to submit FAFSA. *Unit head:* Dr. Peter Leininger, Chair, 570-941-6662, Fax: 570-941-7940, E-mail: peter.leininger@scranton.edu. *Application contact:* Joseph M. Roback, Director of Admissions, 570-941-4385, Fax: 570-941-5928, E-mail: robackj2@scranton.edu.

University of South Alabama, Pat Capps Covey College of Allied Health Professions, Department of Physical Therapy, Mobile, AL 36688. Offers DPT. *Accreditation:* APTA. *Faculty:* 9 full-time (5 women), 1 part-time/adjunct (0 women). *Students:* 116 full-time (73 women), 1 (woman) part-time; includes 3 minority (2 Black or African American, non-Hispanic/Latino; 1 Hispanic/Latino). Average age 24. 184 applicants, 54% accepted, 37 enrolled. In 2015, 33 doctorates awarded. *Entrance requirements:* For doctorate, GRE, minimum GPA of 3.0. Additional exam requirements/recommendations for international students: Required—TOEFL (minimum score 600 paper-based), TWE (minimum score 4.5). *Application deadline:* For fall admission, 12/15 for domestic students, 10/15 for international students. Application fee: $75. Electronic applications accepted. *Expenses:* Contact institution. *Financial support:* Fellowships, research assistantships, teaching assistantships, career-related internships or fieldwork, Federal Work-Study, institutionally sponsored loans, scholarships/grants, and unspecified assistantships available. Support available to part-time students. Financial award application deadline: 5/31; financial award applicants required to submit FAFSA. *Unit head:* Dr. Dennis Fell, Chair, 251-445-9330, Fax: 251-445-9238, E-mail: ptdept@southalabama.edu. *Application contact:* Dr. Susan Gordon-Hickey, Associate Dean, Allied Health, 251-445-9250, Fax: 251-445-9259, E-mail: gordonhickey@southalabama.edu.
Website: http://www.southalabama.edu/alliedhealth/pt/

The University of South Dakota, Graduate School, School of Health Sciences, Department of Physical Therapy, Vermillion, SD 57069-2390. Offers DPT, TDPT. *Accreditation:* APTA. *Entrance requirements:* For doctorate, GRE General Test. Additional exam requirements/recommendations for international students: Required—TOEFL. *Application deadline:* For spring admission, 5/31 for domestic students. Applications are processed on a rolling basis. Application fee: $35. *Expenses:* Contact institution. *Financial support:* Scholarships/grants available. *Faculty research:* Physical therapy, knee rehabilitation, pediatric intervention, wound care, motion analysis. *Unit head:* Dr. Lana Svien, Director, 605-658-6359, E-mail: l.svien@usd.edu.
Website: http://www.usd.edu/health-sciences/physical-therapy/graduate

University of Southern California, Graduate School, Herman Ostrow School of Dentistry, Division of Biokinesiology and Physical Therapy, Los Angeles, CA 90089. Offers biokinesiology (MS, PhD); physical therapy (DPT). *Accreditation:* APTA (one or more programs are accredited). *Degree requirements:* For master's, comprehensive exam; for doctorate, thesis/dissertation. *Entrance requirements:* For master's and doctorate, GRE (minimum combined score 1200, verbal 600, quantitative 600). Additional exam requirements/recommendations for international students: Required—TOEFL. Electronic applications accepted. *Expenses:* Contact institution. *Faculty research:* Exercise and aging biomechanics, musculoskeletal biomechanics, exercise and hormones related to muscle wasting, computational neurorehabilitation, motor behavior and neurorehabilitation, motor development, infant motor performance.

University of South Florida, Morsani College of Medicine, School of Physical Therapy, Tampa, FL 33620-9951. Offers physical therapy (DPT); rehabilitation sciences (PhD), including chronic disease, neuromusculoskeletal disability, physical therapy, veteran's

Physical Therapy

health/reintegration. *Accreditation:* APTA. *Students:* 134 full-time (91 women), 1 part-time (0 women); includes 29 minority (6 Black or African American, non-Hispanic/Latino; 1 American Indian or Alaska Native, non-Hispanic/Latino; 9 Asian, non-Hispanic/Latino; 13 Hispanic/Latino). Average age 25. 1,300 applicants, 8% accepted, 48 enrolled. In 2015, 95 doctorates awarded. *Entrance requirements:* For doctorate, GRE General Test, bachelor's degree from regionally-accredited university with minimum GPA of 3.0 in all upper-division coursework; interview; at least 20 hours of documented volunteer or work experience in hospital outpatient/inpatient physical therapy settings; written personal statement of values and purpose for attending. Additional exam requirements/recommendations for international students: Required—TOEFL (minimum score 600 paper-based; 79 iBT). *Application deadline:* For fall admission, 9/1 for domestic students, 2/1 for international students. Application fee: $30. *Faculty research:* Veteran's reintegration and resilience, prosthetics and orthotics (microprocessor prosthetic knee), neuromusculoskeletal disorders (occupational ergonomics, fall risk and prevention, exercise adherence and compliance, and orthotic and prosthetic wear and use), human movement and function. *Total annual research expenditures:* $1 million. *Unit head:* Dr. William S. Quillen, Director, 813-974-9863, Fax: 813-974-8915, E-mail: wquillen@health.usf.edu. *Application contact:* Dr. Gina Maria Musolino, Associate Professor and Coordinator for Clinical Education, 813-974-2254, Fax: 813-974-8915, E-mail: gmusolin@health.usf.edu.
Website: http://health.usf.edu/medicine/dpt/index.htm

The University of Tennessee at Chattanooga, Program in Physical Therapy, Chattanooga, TN 37403. Offers DPT. *Accreditation:* APTA. *Faculty:* 8 full-time (5 women), 5 part-time/adjunct (3 women). *Students:* 100 full-time (64 women); includes 16 minority (3 Hispanic/Latino; 13 Two or more races, non-Hispanic/Latino). Average age 24. In 2015, 36 doctorates awarded. *Degree requirements:* For doctorate, qualifying exams, internship. *Entrance requirements:* For doctorate, interview, minimum GPA of 3.0 in science and overall. Additional exam requirements/recommendations for international students: Required—TOEFL (minimum score 79 iBT); Recommended—IELTS (minimum score 6). *Application deadline:* For fall admission, 6/13 priority date for domestic students, 6/1 for international students; for spring admission, 10/15 priority date for domestic students, 10/1 for international students. Applications are processed on a rolling basis. Application fee: $30 ($35 for international students). Electronic applications accepted. *Expenses:* Tuition, state resident: full-time $7938; part-time $441 per credit hour. Tuition, nonresident: full-time $24,056; part-time $1336 per credit hour. *Required fees:* $1732; $253 per credit hour. *Financial support:* Research assistantships, teaching assistantships, career-related internships or fieldwork, scholarships/grants, and unspecified assistantships available. Support available to part-time students. *Faculty research:* Diabetes and wound management, disabilities, animal physical therapy and rehabilitation, orthopedics. *Total annual research expenditures:* $6,850. *Unit head:* Dr. Debbie Ingram, Interim Department Head, 423-425-4767, Fax: 423-425-2215, E-mail: debbie-ingram@utc.edu. *Application contact:* Dr. J. Randy Walker, Dean of Graduate Studies, 423-425-4478, Fax: 423-425-5223, E-mail: randy-walker@utc.edu.
Website: http://www.utc.edu/Academic/PhysicalTherapy/

The University of Tennessee Health Science Center, College of Health Professions, Memphis, TN 38163-0002. Offers audiology (MS, Au D); clinical laboratory science (MSCLS); cytopathology practice (MCP); health informatics and information management (MHIIM); occupational therapy (MOT); physical therapy (DPT, ScDPT); physician assistant (MMS); speech-language pathology (MS). *Accreditation:* AOTA; APTA. *Program availability:* Part-time, evening/weekend, online learning. Terminal master's awarded for partial completion of doctoral program. *Degree requirements:* For master's, comprehensive exam, thesis; for doctorate, comprehensive exam, residency. *Entrance requirements:* For master's, GRE (MOT, MSCLS), minimum GPA of 3.0, 3 letters of reference, national accreditation (MSCLS), GRE if GPA is less than 3.0 (MCP); for doctorate, GRE. Additional exam requirements/recommendations for international students: Required—TOEFL (minimum score 550 paper-based; 80 iBT). Electronic applications accepted. *Expenses:* Contact institution. *Faculty research:* Gait deviation, muscular dystrophy and strength, hemophilia and exercise, pediatric neurology, self-efficacy.

The University of Texas at El Paso, Graduate School, College of Health Sciences, Program in Physical Therapy, El Paso, TX 79968-0001. Offers DPT. *Accreditation:* APTA. *Entrance requirements:* For doctorate, GRE General Test. Additional exam requirements/recommendations for international students: Required—TOEFL. Electronic applications accepted.

The University of Texas Health Science Center at San Antonio, School of Health Professions, San Antonio, TX 78229-3900. Offers occupational therapy (MOT); physical therapy (DPT); physician assistant studies (MS). *Accreditation:* AOTA; APTA; ARC-PA. *Degree requirements:* For master's, comprehensive exam, thesis (for some programs); for doctorate, comprehensive exam.

The University of Texas Medical Branch, School of Health Professions, Department of Physical Therapy, Galveston, TX 77555. Offers MPT, DPT. *Accreditation:* APTA. *Degree requirements:* For master's, thesis or alternative. *Entrance requirements:* For master's and doctorate, GRE, documentation of 40 hours' experience. Electronic applications accepted.

The University of Texas Southwestern Medical Center, Southwestern School of Health Professions, Physical Therapy Program, Dallas, TX 75390. Offers DPT. *Accreditation:* APTA. *Entrance requirements:* For doctorate, GRE, minimum GPA of 3.0. Additional exam requirements/recommendations for international students: Required—TOEFL (minimum score 600 paper-based). Electronic applications accepted.

University of the Pacific, Thomas J. Long School of Pharmacy and Health Sciences, Department of Physical Therapy, Stockton, CA 95211-0197. Offers MS, DPT. *Accreditation:* APTA. *Entrance requirements:* For master's, GRE General Test, minimum GPA of 3.0. Additional exam requirements/recommendations for international students: Required—TOEFL (minimum score 475 paper-based).

University of the Sciences, Doctor of Physical Therapy Program, Philadelphia, PA 19104-4495. Offers DPT. *Accreditation:* APTA. *Program availability:* Part-time, evening/weekend, online learning. *Entrance requirements:* For doctorate, interview. *Application deadline:* For spring admission, 11/1 for domestic students. Application fee: $0. *Expenses:* Contact institution. *Unit head:* Dr. Susan Wainwright, Director, 215-596-8849, Fax: 215-596-3121, E-mail: s.wainwr@usp.edu. *Application contact:* Lorraine Cella, Assistant to Dean of Graduate Studies, 215-596-8926, E-mail: l.cella@usp.edu.

The University of Toledo, College of Graduate Studies, College of Health Sciences, Department of Rehabilitation Sciences, Toledo, OH 43606-3390. Offers occupational therapy (OTD); physical therapy (DPT); speech-language pathology (MA). *Degree requirements:* For master's, comprehensive exam, thesis; for doctorate, thesis/dissertation or alternative. *Entrance requirements:* For master's, GRE, minimum cumulative GPA of 2.7 for all previous academic work, letters of recommendation; for doctorate, GRE, minimum cumulative GPA of 3.0 for all previous academic work, letters of recommendation; OTCAS or PTCAS application and UT supplemental application (for OTD and DPT). Additional exam requirements/recommendations for international

students: Required—TOEFL (minimum score 550 paper-based; 80 iBT). Electronic applications accepted.

The University of Toledo, College of Graduate Studies, College of Medicine and Life Sciences, Department of Orthopedic Surgery, Toledo, OH 43606-3390. Offers MSBS. *Degree requirements:* For master's, thesis or alternative. *Entrance requirements:* For master's, GRE, minimum undergraduate GPA of 3.0, three letters of recommendation, statement of purpose, transcripts from all prior institutions attended, resume. Additional exam requirements/recommendations for international students: Required—TOEFL (minimum score 550 paper-based; 80 iBT). Electronic applications accepted.

University of Toronto, Faculty of Medicine, Department of Physical Therapy, Toronto, ON M5S 1A1, Canada. Offers M Sc PT. *Accreditation:* APTA. *Entrance requirements:* For master's, minimum B average in final year, 2 references. Additional exam requirements/recommendations for international students: Required—TOEFL (minimum score 600 paper-based; 100 iBT), TWE (minimum score 5). Electronic applications accepted.

University of Utah, Graduate School, College of Health, Department of Physical Therapy, Salt Lake City, UT 84108. Offers physical therapy (DPT); rehabilitation science (PhD). *Accreditation:* APTA. *Faculty:* 13 full-time (5 women), 14 part-time/adjunct (7 women). *Students:* 155 full-time (82 women), 3 part-time (all women); includes 20 minority (1 Black or African American, non-Hispanic/Latino; 1 American Indian or Alaska Native, non-Hispanic/Latino; 5 Asian, non-Hispanic/Latino; 6 Hispanic/Latino; 2 Native Hawaiian or other Pacific Islander, non-Hispanic/Latino; 5 Two or more races, non-Hispanic/Latino), 5 international. Average age 28. 437 applicants, 11% accepted, 48 enrolled. In 2015, 46 doctorates awarded. *Degree requirements:* For doctorate, thesis/dissertation. *Entrance requirements:* For doctorate, GRE, minimum GPA of 3.0, volunteer work, bachelor's degree. Additional exam requirements/recommendations for international students: Required—TOEFL (minimum score 90 iBT); Recommended—IELTS (minimum score 7). *Application deadline:* For fall admission, 10/3 priority date for domestic students, 10/3 for international students. Application fee: $55 ($65 for international students). Electronic applications accepted. *Expenses:* Contact institution. *Financial support:* In 2015–16, 29 students received support. Research assistantships with full tuition reimbursements available, teaching assistantships with full tuition reimbursements available, Federal Work-Study, scholarships/grants, tuition waivers (full), and unspecified assistantships available. Financial award application deadline: 10/1; financial award applicants required to submit FAFSA. *Faculty research:* Rehabilitation and Parkinson's disease, motor control and musculoskeletal dysfunction, burns/wound care, rehabilitation and multiple sclerosis, cancer. *Total annual research expenditures:* $600,129. *Unit head:* Dr. R. Scott Ward, Chair, 801-581-4895, E-mail: scott.ward@hsc.utah.edu. *Application contact:* Dee-Dee Darby-Duffin, Academic Advisor, 801-585-9510, E-mail: d.darby-duffin@hsc.utah.edu.
Website: http://www.health.utah.edu/pt

University of Vermont, Graduate College, College of Nursing and Health Sciences, Program in Physical Therapy, Burlington, VT 05405. Offers DPT. *Accreditation:* APTA. *Entrance requirements:* For doctorate, GRE General Test. Additional exam requirements/recommendations for international students: Required—TOEFL (minimum score 550 paper-based; 80 iBT). *Application deadline:* For fall admission, 12/15 for domestic and international students. Applications are processed on a rolling basis. Application fee: $65. Electronic applications accepted. *Financial support:* Fellowships, research assistantships, teaching assistantships, and Federal Work-Study available. Financial award application deadline: 3/1. *Unit head:* Dr. Barbara Tschoepe, 802-656-3858. *Application contact:* Dr. Barbara Tschoepe, 802-656-3858.

University of Washington, Graduate School, School of Medicine, Graduate Programs in Medicine, Department of Rehabilitation Medicine, Seattle, WA 98195-6490. Offers occupational therapy (MOT); physical therapy (DPT); prosthetics and orthotics (MPO); rehabilitation science (PhD). *Degree requirements:* For doctorate, comprehensive exam (for some programs), thesis/dissertation (for some programs). *Entrance requirements:* For master's and doctorate, GRE. Additional exam requirements/recommendations for international students: Required—TOEFL. *Faculty research:* Biomechanics, balance, brain injury, spinal cord injury, pain, degenerative diseases.

The University of Western Ontario, Faculty of Graduate Studies, Biosciences Division, School of Physical Therapy, London, ON N6A 5B8, Canada. Offers manipulative therapy (CAS); physical therapy (MPT); wound healing (CAS). *Accreditation:* APTA. *Program availability:* Part-time. *Degree requirements:* For master's, thesis. *Entrance requirements:* For master's, B Sc in physical therapy. Additional exam requirements/recommendations for international students: Required—TOEFL. *Faculty research:* Muscle strength, wound healing, motor control, respiratory physiology, exercise physiology.

University of Wisconsin–La Crosse, College of Science and Health, Department of Health Professions, Program in Physical Therapy, La Crosse, WI 54601-3742. Offers DPT. *Accreditation:* APTA. *Students:* 87 full-time (63 women), 44 part-time (23 women); includes 2 minority (1 Asian, non-Hispanic/Latino; 1 Two or more races, non-Hispanic/Latino). Average age 24. 596 applicants, 10% accepted, 45 enrolled. In 2015, 44 doctorates awarded. *Entrance requirements:* Additional exam requirements/recommendations for international students: Required—TOEFL (minimum score 550 paper-based; 79 iBT). Application fee: $50. Electronic applications accepted. *Expenses:* Contact institution. *Financial support:* Federal Work-Study, scholarships/grants, and health care benefits available. Support available to part-time students. Financial award application deadline: 11/1; financial award applicants required to submit FAFSA. *Unit head:* Dr. Michele Thorman, Director, 608-785-8466, E-mail: thorman.mich@uwlax.edu. *Application contact:* Brandon Schaller, Senior Graduate Student Status Examiner, 608-785-8941, E-mail: admissions@uwlax.edu.
Website: http://www.uwlax.edu/pt/

University of Wisconsin–Madison, School of Medicine and Public Health, Doctor of Physical Therapy Program, Madison, WI 53706-1532. Offers DPT. *Faculty:* 11 full-time (8 women), 4 part-time/adjunct (3 women). *Students:* 119 full-time (72 women); includes 8 minority (1 Black or African American, non-Hispanic/Latino; 1 American Indian or Alaska Native, non-Hispanic/Latino; 1 Asian, non-Hispanic/Latino; 3 Hispanic/Latino; 2 Two or more races, non-Hispanic/Latino). Average age 25. In 2015, 40 doctorates awarded. *Entrance requirements:* For doctorate, GRE. Additional exam requirements/recommendations for international students: Required—TOEFL. Electronic applications accepted. *Expenses:* Tuition, state resident: full-time $5364. Tuition, nonresident: full-time $12,027. *Required fees:* $571. Tuition and fees vary according to campus/location, program and reciprocity agreements. *Faculty research:* Running injuries, interprofessional education, female athlete, human factors in engineering, children muscular disorders. *Application contact:* Reenie Euhardy, Admission Advisor, 608-265-4815, Fax: 608-262-7809, E-mail: euhardy@pt.wisc.edu.
Website: http://ortho.wisc.edu/Home/DoctorOfPhysicalTherapy.aspx

University of Wisconsin–Milwaukee, Graduate School, College of Health Sciences, Doctor of Physical Therapy Program, Milwaukee, WI 53201-0413. Offers DPT. *Accreditation:* APTA. *Students:* 73 full-time (42 women), 1 (woman) part-time; includes 8 minority (1 Black or African American, non-Hispanic/Latino; 2 Asian, non-Hispanic/Latino; 1 Native Hawaiian or other Pacific Islander, non-Hispanic/Latino; 4 Two or more races, non-Hispanic/Latino), 1 international. Average age 26. 4 applicants, 25% accepted, 1 enrolled. In 2015, 21 doctorates awarded. *Degree requirements:* For doctorate, thesis/dissertation optional. *Entrance requirements:* For doctorate, GRE General Test, minimum GPA of 3.0. Additional exam requirements/recommendations for international students: Required—TOEFL (minimum score 550 paper-based; 79 iBT), IELTS (minimum score 6.5). *Financial support:* In 2015–16, 1 teaching assistantship was awarded; fellowships, research assistantships, and project assistantships also available. *Unit head:* Kyle T. Ebersole, Department Chair, 414-229-6717, E-mail: ebersole@uwm.edu. *Application contact:* General Information Contact, 414-229-4982, Fax: 414-229-6967, E-mail: gradschool@uwm.edu.

Utica College, Department of Physical Therapy, Utica, NY 13502-4892. Offers DPT, TDPT. *Accreditation:* APTA. *Program availability:* Part-time, evening/weekend, online learning. *Faculty:* 10 full-time (4 women). *Students:* 81 full-time (52 women), 389 part-time (251 women); includes 293 minority (23 Black or African American, non-Hispanic/Latino; 1 American Indian or Alaska Native, non-Hispanic/Latino; 253 Asian, non-Hispanic/Latino; 13 Hispanic/Latino; 2 Native Hawaiian or other Pacific Islander, non-Hispanic/Latino; 1 Two or more races, non-Hispanic/Latino). Average age 37. 256 applicants, 97% accepted, 216 enrolled. In 2015, 263 doctorates awarded. *Degree requirements:* For doctorate, comprehensive exam, thesis/dissertation (for some programs). *Entrance requirements:* For doctorate, GRE, MCAT, DAT or OPT, BS, minimum GPA of 3.0. Additional exam requirements/recommendations for international students: Required—TOEFL (minimum score 525 paper-based). *Application deadline:* Applications are processed on a rolling basis. Application fee: $50. Electronic applications accepted. *Expenses:* $1,166 per credit hour. *Financial support:* Career-related internships or fieldwork, scholarships/grants, tuition waivers (partial), and unspecified assistantships available. Support available to part-time students. Financial award application deadline: 3/15; financial award applicants required to submit FAFSA. *Faculty research:* Forensic paleopathology, biomechanical analysis of movement, neuronal plasticity, somatosensory mechanotransduction. *Unit head:* Dr. Shauna Malta, Director, 315-792-3313, E-mail: smalta@utica.edu. *Application contact:* John D. Rowe, Director of Graduate Admissions, 315-792-3824, Fax: 315-792-3003, E-mail: jrowe@utica.edu.

Virginia Commonwealth University, Graduate School, School of Allied Health Professions, Department of Physical Therapy, Richmond, VA 23284-9005. Offers advanced physical therapy (DPT); entry-level physical therapy (DPT); health related sciences (PhD); physiology/physical therapy (PhD). *Accreditation:* APTA (one or more programs are accredited). *Degree requirements:* For doctorate, thesis/dissertation. *Entrance requirements:* For doctorate, GRE General Test, Physical Therapist Centralized Application Service (PTCAS). Additional exam requirements/recommendations for international students: Required—TOEFL (minimum score 600 paper-based; 100 iBT). Electronic applications accepted. *Faculty research:* Eye movement, bilabyrinthectomy on ferret muscle fiber typing, neck disability index, cost-effective care, training effect on muscle.

Virginia Commonwealth University, Medical College of Virginia-Professional Programs, School of Medicine, School of Medicine Graduate Programs, Department of Physiology and Biophysics, Richmond, VA 23284-9005. Offers physical therapy (PhD); physiology (MS, PhD); MD/PhD. Terminal master's awarded for partial completion of doctoral program. *Degree requirements:* For master's, thesis; for doctorate, thesis/dissertation, comprehensive oral and written exams. *Entrance requirements:* For master's, GRE General Test, MCAT, or DAT; for doctorate, GRE, MCAT or DAT. Additional exam requirements/recommendations for international students: Required—TOEFL (minimum score 600 paper-based; 100 iBT). Electronic applications accepted.

Walsh University, Graduate Studies, Program in Physical Therapy, North Canton, OH 44720-3396. Offers DPT. *Accreditation:* APTA. *Faculty:* 8 full-time (6 women), 5 part-time/adjunct (3 women). *Students:* 85 full-time (58 women); includes 5 minority (1 Black or African American, non-Hispanic/Latino; 2 Asian, non-Hispanic/Latino; 2 Hispanic/Latino). Average age 25. 245 applicants, 23% accepted, 32 enrolled. In 2015, 31 doctorates awarded. *Degree requirements:* For doctorate, comprehensive exam, research project, 3 clinical placements. *Entrance requirements:* For doctorate, GRE General Test (minimum scores: verbal 150, quantitative 150, or combined score of 291), previous coursework in anatomy, human physiology, exercise physiology, chemistry, statistics, psychology, biology, and physics; minimum GPA of 3.0. Additional exam requirements/recommendations for international students: Required—TOEFL (minimum score 500 paper-based; 61 iBT). *Application deadline:* For fall admission, 10/1 priority date for domestic students. Application fee: $25. Electronic applications accepted. Application fee is waived when completed online. *Expenses:* Contact institution. *Financial support:* In 2015–16, 5 students received support, including 5 research assistantships (averaging $6,579 per year). Financial award application deadline: 12/31; financial award applicants required to submit FAFSA. *Faculty research:* Concussion, teaching methodology, clinical decision making, diagnostic accuracy, professional education. *Total annual research expenditures:* $6,084. *Unit head:* Dr. Jaime Paz, Chair, 330-490-4760, Fax: 330-490-7371, E-mail: jpaz@walsh.edu. *Application contact:* Audra Dice, Graduate Admissions Counselor, 330-490-7181, Fax: 330-244-4680, E-mail: adice@walsh.edu.

Washington University in St. Louis, School of Medicine, Program in Physical Therapy, Saint Louis, MO 63108. Offers DPT. *Accreditation:* APTA. *Degree requirements:* For doctorate, thesis/dissertation (for some programs). *Entrance requirements:* For doctorate, GRE. Additional exam requirements/recommendations for international students: Required—TOEFL (minimum score 600 paper-based; 100 iBT), TWE (minimum score 5). Electronic applications accepted. *Expenses:* Contact institution. *Faculty research:* Movement and movement dysfunction.

Wayne State University, Eugene Applebaum College of Pharmacy and Health Sciences, Department of Health Care Sciences, Program in Physical Therapy, Detroit, MI 48202. Offers DPT. *Accreditation:* APTA. *Program availability:* Part-time. *Faculty:* 12. *Students:* 134 full-time (89 women), 10 part-time (7 women); includes 19 minority (4 Black or African American, non-Hispanic/Latino; 7 Asian, non-Hispanic/Latino; 2 Hispanic/Latino; 6 Two or more races, non-Hispanic/Latino), 56 international. Average age 26. 282 applicants, 15% accepted, 37 enrolled. In 2015, 32 doctorates awarded. *Entrance requirements:* For doctorate, GRE, interview; 90 undergraduate credit hours;

minimum GPA of 3.0 overall and in all prerequisite courses with no less than a C grade in prerequisite courses; PTCAS application; essay. Additional exam requirements/recommendations for international students: Required—TOEFL (minimum score 550 paper-based; 79 iBT), Michigan English Language Assessment Battery (minimum score 85); Recommended—IELTS (minimum score 6.5), TWE (minimum score 5.5). *Application deadline:* For fall admission, 10/15 for domestic and international students. Electronic applications accepted. *Expenses:* $16,104 per year resident tuition, $32,401 non-resident tuition; $671 per credit hour resident tuition, $1,350.05 per credit hour non-resident tuition; fees include $47.45 per credit hour student services fee and $274.60 per semester registration fee. *Financial support:* In 2015–16, 53 students received support. Scholarships/grants available. Financial award application deadline: 3/31; financial award applicants required to submit FAFSA. *Faculty research:* Muscle dysfunction, response to immobility and exercise. *Unit head:* Dr. Sara Maher, Associate Professor/Clinical and Program Director, 313-577-5630, E-mail: sara.maher@wayne.edu. *Application contact:* E-mail: cphsinfo@wayne.edu.
Website: http://cphs.wayne.edu/physical-therapy/

West Coast University, Graduate Programs, North Hollywood, CA 91606. Offers advanced generalist (MSN); family nurse practitioner (MSN); health administration (MHA); occupational therapy (MS); pharmacy (Pharm D); physical therapy (DPT).

Western Carolina University, Graduate School, College of Health and Human Sciences, Department of Physical Therapy, Cullowhee, NC 28723. Offers DPT. *Accreditation:* APTA. *Entrance requirements:* Additional exam requirements/recommendations for international students: Required—TOEFL (minimum score 550 paper-based; 79 iBT). *Application deadline:* For fall admission, 2/1 for domestic students. Applications are processed on a rolling basis. Application fee: $50. *Financial support:* Fellowships, research assistantships with full tuition reimbursements, teaching assistantships with full tuition reimbursements, Federal Work-Study, institutionally sponsored loans, scholarships/grants, and unspecified assistantships available. Financial award application deadline: 3/31; financial award applicants required to submit FAFSA. *Faculty research:* Bone density, disability in older adults, neuroanatomy, intervention of musculoskeletal conditions.
Website: http://www.wcu.edu/aps/pt/

Western Kentucky University, Graduate Studies, College of Health and Human Services, Department of Allied Health, Bowling Green, KY 42101. Offers physical therapy (DPT).

Western University of Health Sciences, College of Allied Health Professions, Program in Physical Therapy, Pomona, CA 91766-1854. Offers DPT. *Accreditation:* APTA. *Faculty:* 12 full-time (9 women), 3 part-time/adjunct (2 women). *Students:* 159 full-time (93 women), 31 part-time (16 women); includes 95 minority (6 Black or African American, non-Hispanic/Latino; 50 Asian, non-Hispanic/Latino; 27 Hispanic/Latino; 12 Two or more races, non-Hispanic/Latino), 1 international. Average age 29. 1,183 applicants, 12% accepted, 71 enrolled. In 2015, 79 doctorates awarded. *Degree requirements:* For doctorate, comprehensive exam (for some programs). *Entrance requirements:* For doctorate, GRE, bachelor's degree, letters of recommendation, volunteer or paid work experience, access to a computer meeting minimum technical standards, health screening and immunization, background check. *Application deadline:* For fall admission, 11/2 for domestic and international students. Application fee: $60. Electronic applications accepted. *Expenses:* $37,980 tuition; $40 fees. *Financial support:* Scholarships/grants available. Financial award application deadline: 3/2; financial award applicants required to submit FAFSA. *Unit head:* Dr. Dee Schilling, Chair, 909-469-3526, Fax: 909-469-5692, E-mail: dschilling@westernu.edu. *Application contact:* Karen Hutton-Lopez, Director of Admissions, 909-469-5335, Fax: 909-469-5570, E-mail: admissions@westernu.edu.
Website: http://www.westernu.edu/allied-health/allied-health-dpt/

West Virginia University, School of Medicine, Graduate Programs in Human Performance, Division of Physical Therapy, Morgantown, WV 26506. Offers DPT. *Accreditation:* APTA. *Program availability:* Evening/weekend, online learning. *Entrance requirements:* For doctorate, GRE, minimum cumulative GPA and prerequisite science GPA of 3.0; volunteer/work experience in physical therapy; letters of recommendation. *Expenses:* Contact institution.

Wheeling Jesuit University, Department of Physical Therapy, Wheeling, WV 26003-6295. Offers DPT. *Accreditation:* APTA. *Degree requirements:* For doctorate, comprehensive exam, thesis/dissertation. *Entrance requirements:* For doctorate, GRE, minimum GPA of 3.0. Additional exam requirements/recommendations for international students: Required—TOEFL (minimum score 650 paper-based). Electronic applications accepted. Application fee is waived when completed online. *Expenses:* Contact institution. *Faculty research:* Service-learning, clinical prediction rules, ergonomics, public health, pediatrics.

Wichita State University, Graduate School, College of Health Professions, Department of Physical Therapy, Wichita, KS 67260. Offers DPT. *Accreditation:* APTA. *Unit head:* Dr. Robert C. Manske, Chair, 316-978-3604, Fax: 316-978-3025, E-mail: robert.manske@wichita.edu. *Application contact:* Jordan Oleson, Admissions Coordinator, 316-978-3095, Fax: 316-978-3253, E-mail: jordan.oleson@wichita.edu.
Website: http://www.wichita.edu/pt

Widener University, School of Human Service Professions, Institute for Physical Therapy Education, Chester, PA 19013-5792. Offers MS, DPT. *Accreditation:* APTA. *Degree requirements:* For master's, thesis. *Entrance requirements:* For master's, GRE. *Expenses:* Contact institution. *Faculty research:* Social support, aquatics, children and adults with movement dysfunction, physical therapy modalities.

Winston-Salem State University, Department of Physical Therapy, Winston-Salem, NC 27110-0003. Offers DPT. *Accreditation:* APTA. Electronic applications accepted. *Faculty research:* Tissue healing; neuroimaging with functional recovery; visual, proprioceptive and vestibular sensor inputs roles.

Youngstown State University, Graduate School, Bitonte College of Health and Human Services, Department of Physical Therapy, Youngstown, OH 44555-0001. Offers DPT. *Accreditation:* APTA. *Entrance requirements:* Additional exam requirements/recommendations for international students: Required—TOEFL.

Physician Assistant Studies

Albany Medical College, Center for Physician Assistant Studies, Albany, NY 12208-3479. Offers MS. *Accreditation:* ARC-PA. *Degree requirements:* For master's, comprehensive exam, clinical portfolio. *Entrance requirements:* For master's, GRE.

Additional exam requirements/recommendations for international students: Required—TOEFL. Electronic applications accepted. *Expenses:* Contact institution. *Faculty research:* Genetics, education, informatics.

Physician Assistant Studies

Alderson Broaddus University, Program in Physician Assistant Studies, Philippi, WV 26416. Offers MPAS. *Degree requirements:* For master's, comprehensive exam, thesis. *Entrance requirements:* For master's, minimum 60 semester hours plus specific science. Electronic applications accepted.

Arcadia University, Graduate Studies, Department of Medical Science and Community Health, Glenside, PA 19038-3295. Offers health education (MA, MSHE); physician assistant (MM Sc); MM Sc/MAHE; MM Sc/MSPH. *Students:* 206 full-time (174 women); includes 36 minority (4 Black or African American, non-Hispanic/Latino; 26 Asian, non-Hispanic/Latino; 4 Hispanic/Latino; 2 Two or more races, non-Hispanic/Latino). Average age 25. 2,449 applicants, 9% accepted, 104 enrolled. In 2015, 93 master's awarded. *Entrance requirements:* For master's, GRE General Test or MCAT. Additional exam requirements/recommendations for international students: Required—TOEFL. *Application deadline:* For fall admission, 1/5 priority date for domestic students. Application fee: $50. *Expenses:* Contact institution. *Financial support:* Tuition waivers (partial) available. *Unit head:* Diana Noller, Chair, 215-517-2376. *Application contact:* 215-572-2910, Fax: 215-572-4041, E-mail: admiss@arcadia.edu.

A.T. Still University, Arizona School of Health Sciences, Mesa, AZ 85206. Offers advanced occupational therapy (MS); advanced physician assistant studies (MS); athletic training (MS, DAT); audiology (Au D); occupational therapy (OTD); physical therapy (DPT); physician assistant studies (MS); transitional audiology (Au D); transitional physical therapy (DPT). *Accreditation:* AOTA (one or more programs are accredited); ASHA. *Program availability:* Part-time, evening/weekend, 100% online. *Faculty:* 54 full-time (31 women), 188 part-time/adjunct (132 women). *Students:* 509 full-time (339 women), 397 part-time (310 women); includes 203 minority (41 Black or African American, non-Hispanic/Latino; 5 American Indian or Alaska Native, non-Hispanic/Latino; 83 Asian, non-Hispanic/Latino; 57 Hispanic/Latino; 2 Native Hawaiian or other Pacific Islander, non-Hispanic/Latino; 15 Two or more races, non-Hispanic/Latino), 60 international. Average age 33. 3,902 applicants, 10% accepted, 245 enrolled. In 2015, 178 master's, 271 doctorates awarded. *Degree requirements:* For master's, thesis (for some programs); for doctorate, thesis/dissertation (for some programs). *Entrance requirements:* For master's, GRE General Test; for doctorate, GRE, Evaluation of Practicing Audiologists Capabilities (Au D), Physical Therapist Evaluation Tool (DPT), current state licensure, master's degree or equivalent (Au D). Additional exam requirements/recommendations for international students: Required—TOEFL (minimum score 80 iBT). *Application deadline:* Applications are processed on a rolling basis. Application fee: $70. Electronic applications accepted. *Expenses:* Contact institution. *Financial support:* In 2015–16, 158 students received support. Federal Work-Study and scholarships/grants available. Financial award application deadline: 5/1; financial award applicants required to submit FAFSA. *Faculty research:* Pediatric sport-related concussion, adolescent athlete health-related quality of life; geriatric and pediatric well-being, pain management for participation, practice-based research network, BMI and dental caries. *Total annual research expenditures:* $156,319. *Unit head:* Dr. Randy Danielsen, Dean, 480-219-6000, Fax: 480-219-6110, E-mail: rdanielsen@atsu.edu. *Application contact:* Donna Sparks, Associate Director, Admissions Processing, 660-626-2117, Fax: 660-626-2969, E-mail: admissions@atsu.edu.
Website: http://www.atsu.edu/ashs

Augsburg College, Program in Physician Assistant Studies, Minneapolis, MN 55454-1351. Offers MS. *Accreditation:* ARC-PA.

Augusta University, College of Allied Health Sciences, Physician Assistant Program, Augusta, GA 30912. Offers MPA. *Accreditation:* ARC-PA. *Program availability:* Part-time. *Students:* 1 part-time. *Degree requirements:* For master's, thesis or alternative. *Entrance requirements:* For master's, GRE General Test, minimum of 100 hours of hands-on health care experience. Additional exam requirements/recommendations for international students: Required—TOEFL (minimum score 600 paper-based; 100 iBT), TWE. *Application deadline:* For fall admission, 10/15 for domestic students. Applications are processed on a rolling basis. Application fee: $30. Electronic applications accepted. *Financial support:* Research assistantships with partial tuition reimbursements, Federal Work-Study, and institutionally sponsored loans available. Support available to part-time students. Financial award application deadline: 5/31; financial award applicants required to submit FAFSA. *Unit head:* Dr. Bonnie Dadig, Chair/Program Director, 706-721-3246, Fax: 706-721-3990, E-mail: bdadig@mail.mcg.edu. *Application contact:* Lisa Daitch, Director of Admissions, 706-721-2725, Fax: 706-721-7279, E-mail: admissions@georgiahealth.edu.
Website: http://www.augusta.edu/alliedhealth/pa/

Baldwin Wallace University, Graduate Programs, Physician Assistant Program, Berea, OH 44017-2088. Offers MMS. *Faculty:* 5 full-time (2 women), 3 part-time/adjunct (1 woman). *Students:* 55 full-time (44 women); includes 4 minority (2 Hispanic/Latino; 2 Two or more races, non-Hispanic/Latino). Average age 24. 476 applicants, 8% accepted, 31 enrolled. In 2015, 17 master's awarded. *Degree requirements:* For master's, comprehensive exam, thesis or alternative, capstone project. *Entrance requirements:* For master's, GRE, 3 letters of recommendation, personal statement, 40 hours of shadowing. Additional exam requirements/recommendations for international students: Required—TOEFL. *Application deadline:* For fall admission, 11/1 for domestic and international students. Applications are processed on a rolling basis. Electronic applications accepted. *Expenses:* Contact institution. *Financial support:* Applicants required to submit FAFSA. *Unit head:* Jared R. Pennington, Director/Chair, 440-826-2221, E-mail: jpenning@bw.edu. *Application contact:* Michele Siverd, Program Support Specialist, 440-826-8585, E-mail: msiverd@bw.edu.
Website: http://www.bw.edu/graduate/physician-assistant/index

Barry University, Physician Assistant Program, Miami Shores, FL 33161-6695. Offers MCMS. *Accreditation:* ARC-PA. *Entrance requirements:* For master's, GRE General Test. Electronic applications accepted.

Baylor College of Medicine, School of Allied Health Sciences, Physician Assistant Program, Houston, TX 77030-3498. Offers MS. *Accreditation:* ARC-PA. *Degree requirements:* For master's, comprehensive exam, thesis. *Entrance requirements:* For master's, GRE General Test, bachelor's degree; minimum GPA of 3.0; prerequisite courses in general chemistry, organic chemistry, microbiology, general psychology, human anatomy, human physiology, statistics, and expository writing. Additional exam requirements/recommendations for international students: Required—TOEFL. Electronic applications accepted. *Expenses:* Contact institution. *Faculty research:* Cultural competency attainment, health behavioral counseling skills mastery, readiness for inter-professional learning, probability error in differential diagnosis, shared decision-making.

Bay Path University, Program in Physician Assistant Studies, Longmeadow, MA 01106-2292. Offers MS. *Students:* 59 full-time (29 women); includes 6 minority (1 Asian, non-Hispanic/Latino; 1 Hispanic/Latino; 4 Two or more races, non-Hispanic/Latino). Average age 28. 872 applicants, 4% accepted, 30 enrolled. In 2015, 23 master's awarded. *Degree requirements:* For master's, 116 credits with minimum cumulative GPA of 3.0 and no grade below a B. *Entrance requirements:* For master's, minimum of 500 hours of patient contact hours; minimum of 24 hours of documented PA shadowing; all prerequisite courses completed with minimum C grade and cumulative GPA of 3.0.

Additional exam requirements/recommendations for international students: Required—TOEFL (minimum score 550 paper-based; 90 iBT). *Application deadline:* For fall admission, 10/1 for domestic students. Application fee: $60. *Financial support:* Unspecified assistantships available. Financial award applicants required to submit FAFSA. *Unit head:* Theresa Riethle, Director, 413-565-1206, E-mail: triethle@baypath.edu. *Application contact:* Diane Ranaldi, Dean of Graduate Admissions, 413-565-1332, Fax: 413-565-1250, E-mail: dranaldi@baypath.edu.
Website: http://graduate.baypath.edu/Graduate-Programs/Programs-On-Campus/MS-Programs/Physician-Assistant-Studies

Bethel University, Graduate Programs, McKenzie, TN 38201. Offers administration and supervision (MA Ed); business administration (MBA); conflict resolution (MA); physician assistant studies (MS). *Program availability:* Part-time, evening/weekend. *Degree requirements:* For master's, thesis (for some programs). *Entrance requirements:* For master's, GRE General Test or MAT, minimum undergraduate GPA of 2.5.

Bethel University, Graduate School, St. Paul, MN 55112-6999. Offers business administration (MBA); child and adolescent mental health (Certificate); classroom management (Certificate); communication (MA); counseling psychology (MA); educational leadership (Ed D); gerontology (MA, Certificate); international baccalaureate teaching and learning (Certificate); K-12 education (MA); leadership foundations (Certificate); literacy education (MA); nurse educator (Certificate); nurse-midwifery (MS); nursing (MS); physician assistant (MS); special education (MA); STEM education (Certificate); strategic leadership (MA); teaching (MA). *Program availability:* Part-time, evening/weekend, 100% online, blended/hybrid learning. *Faculty:* 21 full-time (15 women), 74 part-time/adjunct (38 women). *Students:* 772 full-time (537 women), 372 part-time (232 women); includes 188 minority (94 Black or African American, non-Hispanic/Latino; 3 American Indian or Alaska Native, non-Hispanic/Latino; 43 Asian, non-Hispanic/Latino; 31 Hispanic/Latino; 1 Native Hawaiian or other Pacific Islander, non-Hispanic/Latino; 16 Two or more races, non-Hispanic/Latino), 33 international. Average age 37. 663 applicants, 49% accepted, 232 enrolled. In 2015, 272 master's, 16 doctorates, 65 other advanced degrees awarded. *Degree requirements:* For master's, comprehensive exam (for some programs), thesis (for some programs); for doctorate, comprehensive exam, thesis/dissertation. *Entrance requirements:* Additional exam requirements/recommendations for international students: Required—TOEFL (minimum score 550 paper-based, 80 iBT) or IELTS. *Application deadline:* Applications are processed on a rolling basis. Application fee: $0. Electronic applications accepted. *Expenses:* Contact institution. *Financial support:* In 2015–16, 132 students received support. Teaching assistantships, career-related internships or fieldwork, and scholarships/grants available. Support available to part-time students. Financial award applicants required to submit FAFSA. *Unit head:* Dick Crombie, Vice-President/Dean, 651-635-8000, Fax: 651-635-8004, E-mail: gs@bethel.edu. *Application contact:* Director of Admissions, 651-635-8000, Fax: 651-635-8004, E-mail: gs@bethel.edu.
Website: https://www.bethel.edu/graduate/

Boston University, School of Medicine, Division of Graduate Medical Sciences, Physician Assistant Program, Boston, MA 02215. Offers MS. *Students:* 24. *Entrance requirements:* For master's, GRE, three letters of recommendation. Additional exam requirements/recommendations for international students: Required—TOEFL (minimum score 550 paper-based; 80 iBT). *Application deadline:* For spring admission, 10/1 for domestic students. Electronic applications accepted. *Unit head:* Mary Warner, Director, 617-638-5744, E-mail: paoffice@bu.edu. *Application contact:* GMS Admissions Office, 617-638-5255, E-mail: askgms@bu.edu.
Website: http://www.bu.edu/paprogram/

Butler University, College of Pharmacy and Health Sciences, Indianapolis, IN 46208-3485. Offers pharmaceutical science (MS); pharmacy (Pharm D); physician assistant studies (MS). *Accreditation:* ACPE (one or more programs are accredited). *Faculty:* 63 full-time (44 women). *Students:* 310 full-time (219 women), 5 part-time (3 women); includes 25 minority (1 Black or African American, non-Hispanic/Latino; 1 American Indian or Alaska Native, non-Hispanic/Latino; 14 Asian, non-Hispanic/Latino; 6 Hispanic/Latino; 3 Two or more races, non-Hispanic/Latino), 8 international. Average age 24. 42 applicants, 2% accepted. In 2015, 59 master's, 132 doctorates awarded. *Degree requirements:* For master's, thesis (for some programs), research paper or thesis; for doctorate, research paper or thesis. *Entrance requirements:* For master's, GRE General Test, CASPA application, official transcripts, baccalaureate degree from accredited institution (for physician assistant studies). Additional exam requirements/recommendations for international students: Required—TOEFL (minimum score 550 paper-based; 79 iBT). *Application deadline:* For fall admission, 5/1 for domestic and international students. Electronic applications accepted. Application fee is waived when completed online. *Expenses:* Contact institution. *Financial support:* Applicants required to submit FAFSA. *Faculty research:* Cancer research; molecular pharmacology; pharmaceutics; drug delivery and targeting; neuropharmacology. *Total annual research expenditures:* $50,000. *Unit head:* Dr. Mary Graham, Dean, 317-940-8056, E-mail: mandritz@butler.edu. *Application contact:* Diane Dubord, Graduate Student Services Specialist, 317-940-8107, E-mail: ddubord@butler.edu.
Website: http://www.butler.edu/academics/graduate-cophs

California Baptist University, Program in Physician Assistant Studies, Riverside, CA 92504-3206. Offers MS. *Entrance requirements:* For master's, minimum undergraduate GPA of 3.0, bachelor's transcripts, three letters of recommendation, essay, interview. Additional exam requirements/recommendations for international students: Required—TOEFL (minimum score 80 iBT). *Application deadline:* For fall admission, 12/1 priority date for domestic students, 11/1 priority date for international students; for spring admission, 8/1 priority date for domestic students, 7/1 priority date for international students. Applications are processed on a rolling basis. Application fee: $45. Electronic applications accepted. *Expenses:* $723 per unit plus a $355 fee per semester. *Financial support:* Applicants required to submit CSS PROFILE or FAFSA. *Unit head:* Dr. Allan M. Bedashi, Director, 951-552-8838, E-mail: abedashi@calbaptist.edu. *Application contact:* Taylor Neece, Director of Graduate Admissions, 951-343-4871, Fax: 877-228-8877, E-mail: graduateadmissions@calbaptist.edu.

Campbell University, Graduate and Professional Programs, College of Pharmacy and Health Sciences, Buies Creek, NC 27506. Offers clinical research (MS); pharmaceutical sciences (MS); pharmacy (Pharm D); physician assistant (MPAP); public health (MS). *Accreditation:* ACPE. *Program availability:* Part-time, evening/weekend. *Entrance requirements:* For master's, MCAT, PCAT, GRE, bachelor's degree in health sciences or related field; for doctorate, PCAT. Additional exam requirements/recommendations for international students: Required—TOEFL (minimum score 550 paper-based; 79 iBT). Electronic applications accepted. *Expenses:* Contact institution. *Faculty research:* Immunology, medicinal chemistry, pharmaceutics, applied pharmacology.

Carroll University, Program in Physician Assistant Studies, Waukesha, WI 53186-5593. Offers MS. *Students:* 167 applicants, 16% accepted, 22 enrolled. *Entrance requirements:* For master's, GRE, three letters of reference, personal essay, documentation of college or community service activities, transcripts. Additional exam requirements/recommendations for international students: Required—TOEFL. Application fee: $0. *Expenses:* Tuition, area resident: Full-time $10,548; part-time $586 per credit. *Required fees:* $520 per semester. Tuition and fees vary according to course load, degree level and program. *Financial support:* Applicants required to submit

FAFSA. *Unit head:* Dr. Russell W. Harland, Director, 262-524-7399, E-mail: rharland@carrollu.edu. *Application contact:* Tami Bartunek, Graduate Admission Counselor, 262-524-7643, E-mail: tbartune@carrollu.edu.
Website: http://www.carrollu.edu/gradprograms/physasst/default.asp

Case Western Reserve University, School of Graduate Studies, Physician Assistant Program, Cleveland, OH 44106. Offers MA. *Degree requirements:* For master's, thesis. *Entrance requirements:* For master's, GRE, statement of objectives, letters of recommendation (minimum of 3). Additional exam requirements/recommendations for international students: Required—TOEFL (minimum score 577 paper-based; 90 iBT); Recommended—IELTS (minimum score 7). Electronic applications accepted. *Expenses:* Tuition, area resident: Full-time $41,137; part-time $1714 per credit hour. *Required fees:* $32. Tuition and fees vary according to course load and program. *Faculty research:* Culture, history, critical theory, religion and healing, social justice and urban religion, religion and cognitive science, comparative religious ethics, Judaic Studies, religion and science, and the philosophy of religion.

Central Michigan University, College of Graduate Studies, The Herbert H. and Grace A. Dow College of Health Professions, School of Rehabilitation and Medical Sciences, Mount Pleasant, MI 48859. Offers physical therapy (DPT); physician assistant (MS). *Accreditation:* APTA; ARC-PA. *Degree requirements:* For master's, thesis or alternative; for doctorate, thesis/dissertation or alternative. *Entrance requirements:* For master's and doctorate, GRE. Electronic applications accepted.

Chatham University, Program in Physician Assistant Studies, Pittsburgh, PA 15232-2826. Offers MPAS. *Accreditation:* ARC-PA. *Faculty:* 10 full-time (8 women), 12 part-time/adjunct (all women). *Students:* 147 full-time (118 women), 1 part-time (0 women); includes 16 minority (4 Black or African American, non-Hispanic/Latino; 1 American Indian or Alaska Native, non-Hispanic/Latino; 5 Asian, non-Hispanic/Latino; 5 Hispanic/Latino; 1 Two or more races, non-Hispanic/Latino). Average age 26. 592 applicants, 25% accepted, 77 enrolled. In 2015, 72 master's awarded. *Degree requirements:* For master's, thesis, clinical experience, research project. *Entrance requirements:* For master's, community service, minimum GPA of 3.0, health science work or shadowing, volunteer work experience, PA shadowing form, 3 references. Additional exam requirements/recommendations for international students: Required—TOEFL (minimum score 600 paper-based; 100 iBT), IELTS (minimum score 7), TWE. *Application deadline:* For fall admission, 10/1 priority date for domestic and international students. Application fee: $0. Electronic applications accepted. *Expenses:* $13,945 per semester tuition; $230 per semester campus fee; $190 per semester lab and insurance fee. *Financial support:* Career-related internships or fieldwork available. Financial award applicants required to submit FAFSA. *Faculty research:* Complementary and alternative medicine, education methods, physician assistant practice. *Unit head:* Carl Garrubba, Director, 412-365-1425, Fax: 412-365-1213, E-mail: cgarrubba@chatham.edu. *Application contact:* Maureen Stokan, Assistant Director of Graduate Admission, 412-365-2988, Fax: 412-365-1609, E-mail: gradadmissions@chatham.edu.
Website: http://www.chatham.edu/departments/healthmgmt/graduate/pa

Christian Brothers University, School of Sciences, Memphis, TN 38104-5581. Offers physician assistant studies (MS).

Clarkson University, Graduate School, School of Arts and Sciences, Department of Physician Assistant Studies, Potsdam, NY 13699. Offers MS. *Faculty:* 8 full-time (4 women), 21 part-time/adjunct (9 women). *Students:* 39 full-time (22 women); includes 3 minority (1 American Indian or Alaska Native, non-Hispanic/Latino; 2 Asian, non-Hispanic/Latino, 4 international. Average age 29. 701 applicants, 3% accepted, 20 enrolled. In 2015, 20 master's awarded. *Entrance requirements:* Additional exam requirements/recommendations for international students: Required—TOEFL or IELTS. *Application deadline:* Applications are processed on a rolling basis. Application fee: $225. Electronic applications accepted. *Financial support:* Scholarships/grants and tuition waivers (partial) available. *Unit head:* Dr. Keith Young, Chair, 315-268-7942, Fax: 315-268-7944, E-mail: kyoung@clarkson.edu. *Application contact:* Melissa Roberts, Health Professions Graduate Admissions Coordinator, 315-268-7942, E-mail: mroberts@clarkson.edu.
Website: http://www.clarkson.edu/pa/

Cleveland State University, College of Graduate Studies, College of Sciences and Health Professions, School of Health Sciences, Program in Health Sciences, Cleveland, OH 44115. Offers health sciences (MS); physician assistant studies (MS). *Program availability:* Part-time, evening/weekend, online learning. *Faculty:* 7 full-time (6 women), 6 part-time/adjunct (all women). *Students:* 109 full-time (80 women), 40 part-time (33 women); includes 38 minority (20 Black or African American, non-Hispanic/Latino; 1 American Indian or Alaska Native, non-Hispanic/Latino; 8 Asian, non-Hispanic/Latino; 6 Hispanic/Latino; 3 Two or more races, non-Hispanic/Latino), 2 international. Average age 30. 85 applicants, 73% accepted, 48 enrolled. In 2015, 44 master's awarded. *Degree requirements:* For master's, completion of two 3-month field placements. *Entrance requirements:* For master's, GRE (scores of 50th percentile or greater in all areas; minimum analytical writing score of 3.5), bachelor's degree from accredited institution, minimum prerequisite course GPA of 3.0, all courses completed with minimum grade of C. Additional exam requirements/recommendations for international students: Required—TOEFL (minimum score 550 paper-based; 78 iBT). *Application deadline:* For fall admission, 1/15 for domestic and international students. Electronic applications accepted. *Expenses:* Tuition, state resident: full-time $9565. Tuition, nonresident: full-time $17,980. Tuition and fees vary according to program. *Financial support:* In 2015–16, 8 research assistantships with partial tuition reimbursements (averaging $10,000 per year) were awarded; career-related internships or fieldwork, Federal Work-Study, institutionally sponsored loans, scholarships/grants, traineeships, tuition waivers (partial), and unspecified assistantships also available. Support available to part-time students. Financial award applicants required to submit FAFSA. *Faculty research:* Assisted technologies, biomechanics, clinical administration, cultural health, gerontology. *Unit head:* Dr. Stephen Slane, Chairperson and Professor Emeritus, 216-687-2379, E-mail: s.slane@csuohio.edu. *Application contact:* Karen Armstrong, Administrative Assistant, 216-687-3567, Fax: 216-687-9316, E-mail: healthsci@csuohio.edu.
Website: http://www.csuohio.edu/sciences/dept/healthsciences/graduate/index.html

Daemen College, Physician Assistant Department, Amherst, NY 14226-3592. Offers MS. *Accreditation:* ARC-PA. *Degree requirements:* For master's, 30 credits (40 weeks) in clinical clerk-ships; 2 research courses; 3 final year seminars. *Entrance requirements:* For master's, minimum GPA of 3.0 overall and in math and science prerequisites; 120 hours of direct patient contact; admission to professional phase. Additional exam requirements/recommendations for international students: Required—TOEFL (minimum score 500 paper-based; 63 iBT), IELTS (minimum score 5.5). Electronic applications accepted.

Des Moines University, College of Health Sciences, Physician Assistant Program, Des Moines, IA 50312-4104. Offers MS. *Accreditation:* ARC-PA. *Degree requirements:* For master's, research project. *Entrance requirements:* For master's, GRE, interview, minimum GPA of 2.8, related work experience. Additional exam requirements/recommendations for international students: Recommended—TOEFL. Electronic applications accepted. *Expenses:* Contact institution.

Drexel University, College of Nursing and Health Professions, Physician Assistant Department, Philadelphia, PA 19104-2875. Offers MHS. *Accreditation:* ARC-PA. Electronic applications accepted.

Duke University, School of Medicine, Physician Assistant Program, Durham, NC 27701. Offers MHS. *Accreditation:* ARC-PA. *Faculty:* 16 full-time (14 women), 2 part-time/adjunct (0 women). *Students:* 178 full-time (131 women); includes 53 minority (19 Black or African American, non-Hispanic/Latino; 2 American Indian or Alaska Native, non-Hispanic/Latino; 17 Asian, non-Hispanic/Latino; 15 Hispanic/Latino). Average age 28. 1,342 applicants, 8% accepted, 90 enrolled. In 2015, 87 master's awarded. *Entrance requirements:* For master's, GRE, bachelor's degree from regionally-accredited college; 8 core courses: anatomy, physiology, microbiology, biology (choice of 2), chemistry including labs (choice of 2), and statistics. Additional exam requirements/recommendations for international students: Recommended—TOEFL. *Application deadline:* For fall admission, 10/1 for domestic students. Application fee: $50. Electronic applications accepted. *Financial support:* In 2015–16, 49 students received support. Fellowships, research assistantships, teaching assistantships, institutionally sponsored loans, and scholarships/grants available. Financial award application deadline: 5/1; financial award applicants required to submit FAFSA. *Unit head:* Karen J. Hills, Program Director/Associate Professor, 919-681-3161, Fax: 919-681-9666, E-mail: karen.hills@duke.edu. *Application contact:* Wendy Z. Elwell, Admissions Coordinator, 919-668-4710, Fax: 919-681-9666, E-mail: wendy.elwell@duke.edu.
Website: http://pa.mc.duke.edu/

Duquesne University, John G. Rangos, Sr. School of Health Sciences, Pittsburgh, PA 15282-0001. Offers health management systems (MHMS); occupational therapy (MS, OTD); physical therapy (DPT); physician assistant studies (MPAS); rehabilitation science (MS, PhD); speech-language pathology (MS); MBA/MHMS. *Accreditation:* AOTA (one or more programs are accredited); APTA (one or more programs are accredited); ASHA. *Program availability:* Minimal on-campus study. *Faculty:* 45 full-time (32 women), 33 part-time/adjunct (17 women). *Students:* 230 full-time (180 women), 11 part-time (5 women); includes 15 minority (1 Black or African American, non-Hispanic/Latino; 3 Asian, non-Hispanic/Latino; 7 Hispanic/Latino; 4 Two or more races, non-Hispanic/Latino), 20 international. Average age 23. 685 applicants, 9% accepted, 24 enrolled. In 2015, 132 master's, 32 doctorates awarded. *Degree requirements:* For doctorate, comprehensive exam (for some programs), thesis/dissertation (for some programs). *Entrance requirements:* For master's, GRE General Test (speech-language pathology), 3 letters of recommendation; minimum GPA of 2.75 (health management systems), 3.0 (speech-language pathology); for doctorate, GRE General Test (for physical therapy and rehabilitation science), 3 letters of recommendation, minimum GPA of 3.0, personal interview. Additional exam requirements/recommendations for international students: Required—TOEFL (minimum score 550 paper-based; 90 iBT). *Application deadline:* For fall admission, 2/1 for domestic and international students; for spring admission, 7/1 for domestic and international students. Applications are processed on a rolling basis. Application fee: $0. Electronic applications accepted. *Expenses:* $1,254 per credit. *Financial support:* Federal Work-Study available. Financial award applicants required to submit FAFSA. *Faculty research:* Neuronal processing, electrical stimulation on peripheral neuropathy, central nervous system (CNS) stimulatory and inhibitory signals, behavioral genetic methodologies to development disorders of speech, neurogenic communication disorders. Total annual research expenditures: $38,730. *Unit head:* Dr. Gregory H. Frazer, Dean, 412-396-5303, Fax: 412-396-5554, E-mail: frazer@duq.edu. *Application contact:* Christopher R. Hilf, Recruiter/Academic Advisor, 412-396-5653, Fax: 412-396-5554, E-mail: hilfc@duq.edu.
Website: http://www.duq.edu/academics/schools/health-sciences

D'Youville College, Physician Assistant Department, Buffalo, NY 14201-1084. Offers MS. *Accreditation:* ARC-PA. *Students:* 154 full-time (95 women), 15 part-time (10 women); includes 20 minority (5 Black or African American, non-Hispanic/Latino; 2 American Indian or Alaska Native, non-Hispanic/Latino; 3 Asian, non-Hispanic/Latino; 7 Hispanic/Latino; 3 Two or more races, non-Hispanic/Latino), 4 international. Average age 26. 230 applicants, 29% accepted, 55 enrolled. In 2015, 35 master's awarded. *Entrance requirements:* For master's, BS, patient contact, 3 letters of recommendation. Additional exam requirements/recommendations for international students: Required—TOEFL (minimum score 500 paper-based). *Application deadline:* For fall admission, 5/1 priority date for international students; for spring admission, 9/1 priority date for international students. Applications are processed on a rolling basis. Electronic applications accepted. *Expenses:* Tuition, area resident: Full-time $21,120; part-time $880 per credit hour. *Required fees:* $235; $96. One-time fee: $100. *Unit head:* Dr. Maureen F. Finney, Chair, 716-829-7730, E-mail: finneym@dyc.edu. *Application contact:* Dr. Stephen Smith, Admissions Director, 716-829-7600, Fax: 716-829-7900, E-mail: admissions@dyc.edu.

East Carolina University, Graduate School, College of Allied Health Sciences, Department of Physician Assistant Studies, Greenville, NC 27858-4353. Offers MS. *Accreditation:* ARC-PA. *Students:* 100 full-time (75 women); includes 6 minority (1 Black or African American, non-Hispanic/Latino; 3 Asian, non-Hispanic/Latino; 2 Two or more races, non-Hispanic/Latino). Average age 26. 37 applicants, 100% accepted, 36 enrolled. In 2015, 33 master's awarded. Application fee: $50. *Unit head:* Dr. Alan Gindoff, Chair, 252-744-6271, E-mail: gindoffa@ecu.edu. *Application contact:* Dean of Graduate School, 252-328-6012, Fax: 252-328-6071, E-mail: gradschool@ecu.edu.
Website: http://www.ecu.edu/cs-dhs/pa/index.cfm

Eastern Michigan University, Graduate School, College of Health and Human Services, School of Health Promotion and Human Performance, Program in Physician Assistant Studies, Ypsilanti, MI 48197. Offers MS. *Program availability:* Part-time, evening/weekend. *Students:* 47 full-time (38 women), 1 (woman) part-time; includes 1 minority (Black or African American, non-Hispanic/Latino). Average age 28. *Entrance requirements:* Additional exam requirements/recommendations for international students: Required—TOEFL. Application fee: $45. *Financial support:* Research assistantships with full tuition reimbursements, teaching assistantships with full tuition reimbursements, career-related internships or fieldwork, Federal Work-Study, institutionally sponsored loans, scholarships/grants, tuition waivers (full and partial), and unspecified assistantships available. Support available to part-time students. *Application contact:* Linda Jerome, HPHP Academic Advisor, 734-487-0092, Fax: 734-483-1834, E-mail: ljerome@emich.edu.

Eastern Virginia Medical School, Master of Physician Assistant Program, Norfolk, VA 23501-1980. Offers MPA. *Accreditation:* ARC-PA. *Entrance requirements:* Additional exam requirements/recommendations for international students: Required—TOEFL. Electronic applications accepted. *Expenses:* Contact institution.

Elon University, Program in Physician Assistant Studies, Elon, NC 27244-2010. Offers MS. *Faculty:* 8 full-time (7 women), 6 part-time/adjunct (3 women). *Students:* 75 full-time (59 women); includes 4 minority (3 Asian, non-Hispanic/Latino; 1 Two or more races, non-Hispanic/Latino). Average age 27. 1,825 applicants, 3% accepted, 40 enrolled. In 2015, 37 master's awarded. *Entrance requirements:* Additional exam requirements/recommendations for international students: Required—TOEFL. *Application deadline:* For fall admission, 10/1 for domestic students. Applications are processed on a rolling basis. Application fee: $50. Electronic applications accepted. *Financial support:* Federal

Physician Assistant Studies

Work-Study and scholarships/grants available. Financial award application deadline: 10/1; financial award applicants required to submit FAFSA. *Unit head:* Dr. Patti Ragan, Deptartment Chair/Program Director of the School of Physician Assistant Studies, 336-278-6850, E-mail: pragan@elon.edu. *Application contact:* Art Fadde, Director of Graduate Admissions, 800-334-8448 Ext. 3, Fax: 336-278-7699, E-mail: afadde@elon.edu.
Website: http://www.elon.edu/e-web/academics/pa/

Emory University, School of Medicine, Programs in Allied Health Professions, Physician Assistant Program, Atlanta, GA 30322. Offers MM Sc. *Accreditation:* ARC-PA. *Entrance requirements:* For master's, GRE General Test. Additional exam requirements/recommendations for international students: Required—TOEFL (minimum score 69 iBT). Electronic applications accepted. *Expenses:* Contact institution. *Faculty research:* Cultural competency in medical education, farm worker health, technology in medicine, physician assistants in primary care, interprofessional education.

Florida International University, Herbert Wertheim College of Medicine, Program in Physician Assistant Studies, Miami, FL 33199. Offers MPA. *Students:* 45 full-time (37 women); includes 26 minority (1 Black or African American, non-Hispanic/Latino; 7 Asian, non-Hispanic/Latino; 18 Hispanic/Latino), 2 international. Average age 26. 378 applicants, 12% accepted, 45 enrolled. *Entrance requirements:* For master's, GRE, minimum GPA of 3.0; resume. Additional exam requirements/recommendations for international students: Required—TOEFL (minimum score 550 paper-based; 80 iBT) or IELTS (minimum score 6.5). *Application deadline:* For fall admission, 4/1 for domestic and international students; for spring admission, 10/1 for domestic students, 9/1 for international students. Application fee: $30. Electronic applications accepted. *Expenses:* Tuition, state resident: full-time $10,708; part-time $455.64 per credit hour. Tuition, nonresident: full-time $23,816; part-time $1001.69 per credit hour. *Required fees:* $390; $195 per semester. Tuition and fees vary according to program. *Financial support:* Institutionally sponsored loans and scholarships/grants available. Financial award application deadline: 3/1; financial award applicants required to submit FAFSA. *Unit head:* Dr. John Rock, Dean, 305-348-0570, E-mail: john.rock@fiu.edu. *Application contact:* Nanett Rojas, Manager, Admissions Operations, 305-348-7464, Fax: 305-348-7441, E-mail: nanett.rojas@fiu.edu.

Francis Marion University, Graduate Programs, Physician Assistant Program, Florence, SC 29502-0547. Offers MPAS. *Entrance requirements:* For master's, GRE, bachelor's degree with minimum GPA of 3.0, official transcripts, 3 letters of recommendation, 250 hours of clinical work, criminal background check, personal statement, proof of immunizations. Electronic applications accepted. *Expenses: Tuition, area resident:* Full-time $9780; part-time $489 per credit hour. Tuition, nonresident: full-time $19,560; part-time $978 per credit hour. *Required fees:* $14.40 per credit hour. $141 per semester. Tuition and fees vary according to course load and program.

Franklin Pierce University, Graduate and Professional Studies, Rindge, NH 03461-0060. Offers curriculum and instruction (M Ed); elementary education (MS Ed); emerging network technologies (Graduate Certificate); energy and sustainability studies (MBA, Graduate Certificate); health administration (MBA, Graduate Certificate); human resource management (MBA, Graduate Certificate); information technology (MBA); leadership (MBA); nursing education (MS); nursing leadership (MS); physical therapy (DPT); physician assistant studies (MPAS); special education (M Ed); sports management (MBA). *Accreditation:* APTA. *Program availability:* Part-time, online learning. *Degree requirements:* For master's, concentrated original research projects; student teaching; fieldwork and/or internship; leadership project; PRAXIS I and II (for M Ed); for doctorate, concentrated original research projects, clinical fieldwork and/or internship, leadership project. *Entrance requirements:* For master's, minimum GPA of 2.5, 3 letters of recommendation; competencies in accounting, economics, statistics, and computer skills through life experience or undergraduate coursework (for MBA); certification/e-portfolio, minimum C grade in all education courses (for M Ed); license to practice as RN (for MS in nursing); for doctorate, GRE, BA/BS, 3 letters of recommendation, personal mission statement, interview, writing sample, minimum cumulative GPA of 2.8, master's degree (for DA); 80 hours of observation/work in PT settings, completion of anatomy, chemistry, physics, and statistics, minimum GPA of 3.0 (for DPT). Additional exam requirements/recommendations for international students: Required—TOEFL (minimum score 550 paper-based; 61 iBT). *Application deadline:* Applications are processed on a rolling basis. Application fee: $0. Electronic applications accepted. *Expenses: Tuition, area resident:* Part-time $660 per credit hour. Tuition and fees vary according to program. *Financial support:* Teaching assistantships with tuition reimbursements, career-related internships or fieldwork, and unspecified assistantships available. Support available to part-time students. Financial award applicants required to submit FAFSA. *Faculty research:* Evidence-based practice in sports physical therapy, human resource management in economic crisis, leadership in nursing, innovation in sports facility management, differentiated learning and understanding by design. *Unit head:* Dr. Maria Altobello, Dean, 603-647-3509, Fax: 603-229-4580, E-mail: altobellom@franklinpierce.edu. *Application contact:* Graduate Studies, 800-325-1090, Fax: 603-626-4815, E-mail: cgps@franklinpierce.edu.
Website: http://www.franklinpierce.edu/academics/gradstudies/index.htm

Gannon University, School of Graduate Studies, Morosky College of Health Professions and Sciences, School of Health Professions, Program in Physician Assistant Science, Erie, PA 16541-0001. Offers MPAS. *Accreditation:* ARC-PA. *Students:* 72 full-time (59 women); includes 1 minority (Asian, non-Hispanic/Latino). Average age 22. 70 applicants, 21% accepted, 14 enrolled. In 2015, 46 master's awarded. *Degree requirements:* For master's, thesis or alternative, research project, practicum. *Entrance requirements:* For master's, baccalaureate degree with minimum GPA of 3.0, 3 letters of recommendation, interview, transcript, 30 hours of documented volunteer/paid medical experience or shadowing a physician assistant. Additional exam requirements/recommendations for international students: Required—TOEFL (minimum score 79 iBT). *Application deadline:* For fall admission, 1/15 for domestic students. Application fee: $25. Electronic applications accepted. Application fee is waived when completed online. *Expenses:* Contact institution. *Financial support:* Application deadline: 7/1; applicants required to submit FAFSA. *Faculty research:* Cardiology, assessment and evaluation, cervical cancer screening and prevention, simulation. *Unit head:* Michele Roth-Kauffman, Chair, 814-871-5643, E-mail: rothkauf001@gannon.edu. *Application contact:* Kara Morgan, Director of Graduate Admissions, 814-871-7412, E-mail: graduate@gannon.edu.

Gardner-Webb University, Graduate School, Program in Physician Assistant Studies, Boiling Springs, NC 28017. Offers MPAS. *Faculty:* 3 full-time (all women). *Students:* 51 full-time (33 women); includes 6 minority (4 Asian, non-Hispanic/Latino; 2 Hispanic/Latino). Average age 26. 1 applicant. *Unit head:* Dr. Franki Burch, Dean, 704-406-4723, E-mail: gradschool@gardner-webb.edu. *Application contact:* Melissa Hamrick, Secretary, 704-406-2369, Fax: 704-406-2370, E-mail: mhamrick8@gardner-webb.edu.
Website: http://www.gardner-webb.edu/academic-programs-and-resources/colleges-and-schools/health-sciences/schools-and-departments/physician-assistant-studies/%

The George Washington University, School of Medicine and Health Sciences, Health Sciences Programs, Physician Assistant Program, Washington, DC 20052. Offers MSHS. *Accreditation:* ARC-PA. *Faculty:* 22 full-time (17 women), 6 part-time/adjunct (3 women). *Students:* 142 full-time (100 women), 1 part-time (0 women); includes 38 minority (4 Black or African American, non-Hispanic/Latino; 15 Asian, non-Hispanic/Latino; 15 Hispanic/Latino; 3 Native Hawaiian or other Pacific Islander, non-Hispanic/Latino; 1 Two or more races, non-Hispanic/Latino), 1 international. Average age 29. 1,021 applicants, 11% accepted, 60 enrolled. In 2015, 67 master's awarded. *Entrance requirements:* For master's, GRE General Test, BA/BS with clinical experience. *Application deadline:* For fall admission, 10/15 for domestic students. Applications are processed on a rolling basis. Application fee: $75. Electronic applications accepted. *Unit head:* Dr. Karen Wright, Program Director, 202-994-9279, E-mail: kawright@gwu.edu. *Application contact:* Erin C. McKan Thomas, Assistant Director of Admissions and Enrollment Services, 202-994-6395, E-mail: emckan@gwu.edu.

Grand Valley State University, College of Health Professions, Physician Assistant Studies Program, Allendale, MI 49401-9403. Offers MPAS. *Accreditation:* ARC-PA. *Faculty:* 11 full-time (8 women), 3 part-time/adjunct (2 women). *Students:* 151 full-time (102 women), 6 part-time (5 women); includes 9 minority (1 Black or African American, non-Hispanic/Latino; 4 Asian, non-Hispanic/Latino; 2 Hispanic/Latino; 2 Two or more races, non-Hispanic/Latino). Average age 26. 284 applicants, 18% accepted, 51 enrolled. In 2015, 46 master's awarded. *Degree requirements:* For master's, thesis, clinical rotations, project. *Entrance requirements:* For master's, interview, 250 hours of health care experience. Additional exam requirements/recommendations for international students: Required—TOEFL (minimum score 610 paper-based). *Application deadline:* For fall admission, 11/1 for domestic and international students. Application fee: $30. Electronic applications accepted. *Financial support:* In 2015–16, 33 students received support, including 32 fellowships (averaging $18,667 per year), 1 research assistantship; institutionally sponsored loans also available. Financial award application deadline: 2/15. *Faculty research:* Women's health, pain management, PA practice issues, hematology/hemostasis, patient education. *Unit head:* Andrew Booth, Director, 616-331-5991, Fax: 616-331-5654, E-mail: bootha@gvsu.edu. *Application contact:* Darlene Zwart, Student Services Coordinator, 616-331-3958, E-mail: zwartda@gvsu.edu.
Website: http://www.gvsu.edu/pas/

Harding University, College of Allied Health, Program in Physician Assistant, Searcy, AR 72149-0001. Offers MS. *Faculty:* 7 full-time (4 women), 2 part-time/adjunct (1 woman). *Students:* 107 full-time (80 women); includes 18 minority (3 Black or African American, non-Hispanic/Latino; 3 American Indian or Alaska Native, non-Hispanic/Latino; 7 Asian, non-Hispanic/Latino; 4 Hispanic/Latino; 1 Two or more races, non-Hispanic/Latino). Average age 27. 654 applicants, 8% accepted, 36 enrolled. In 2015, 34 master's awarded. *Entrance requirements:* For master's, GRE. Additional exam requirements/recommendations for international students: Required—TOEFL. *Application deadline:* For fall admission, 11/1 for domestic and international students. Application fee: $25. *Expenses:* Contact institution. *Unit head:* Dr. Mike Murphy, Professor/Program Director, 501-279-5642, E-mail: mmurphy1@harding.edu. *Application contact:* Dr. Cheri Yecke, Dean of Graduate Programs, 501-279-4335, Fax: 501-279-5192, E-mail: cyecke@harding.edu.
Website: http://www.harding.edu/paprogram/

Hofstra University, School of Health Sciences and Human Services, Program in Physician Assistant, Hempstead, NY 11549. Offers MS. *Students:* 124 full-time (96 women); includes 17 minority (1 Black or African American, non-Hispanic/Latino; 13 Asian, non-Hispanic/Latino; 2 Hispanic/Latino; 1 Native Hawaiian or other Pacific Islander, non-Hispanic/Latino), 2 international. Average age 25. 1,340 applicants, 6% accepted, 39 enrolled. In 2015, 37 master's awarded. *Degree requirements:* For master's, comprehensive exam, minimum GPA of 3.0. *Entrance requirements:* For master's, bachelor's degree in biology or equivalent, 2 letters of recommendation, essay, minimum GPA of 3.0. Additional exam requirements/recommendations for international students: Required—TOEFL (minimum score 550 paper-based; 80 iBT). *Application deadline:* For fall admission, 11/1 for domestic students. Application fee: $70 ($75 for international students). Electronic applications accepted. *Financial support:* In 2015–16, 6 students received support, including 6 fellowships with tuition reimbursements available (averaging $8,083 per year); research assistantships with tuition reimbursements available, career-related internships or fieldwork, Federal Work-Study, institutionally sponsored loans, scholarships/grants, and tuition waivers (full and partial) also available. Support available to part-time students. Financial award applicants required to submit FAFSA. *Faculty research:* Population health, disability health, smoke cessation, remediation methods, evaluation and assessment. *Unit head:* Carlina Loscalzo, Chairperson, 516-463-4412, Fax: 516-463-5177, E-mail: bioczl@hofstra.edu. *Application contact:* Sunil Samuel, Assistant Vice President of Admissions, 516-463-4723, Fax: 516-463-4664, E-mail: graduateadmission@hofstra.edu.
Website: http://www.hofstra.edu/academics/colleges/healthscienceshumanservices/

Idaho State University, Office of Graduate Studies, Kasiska College of Health Professions, Program in Physician Assistant Studies, Pocatello, ID 83209-8253. Offers MPAS. *Accreditation:* ARC-PA. *Degree requirements:* For master's, comprehensive exam, thesis (for some programs), portfolio, clinical year, oral case presentation. *Entrance requirements:* For master's, GRE General Test, minimum GPA of 3.0, letters of reference. Additional exam requirements/recommendations for international students: Required—TOEFL (minimum score 500 paper-based). Electronic applications accepted. *Expenses:* Contact institution.

Indiana State University, College of Graduate and Professional Studies, College of Nursing, Health, and Human Services, Department of Applied Medicine and Rehabilitation, Terre Haute, IN 47809. Offers athletic training (MS, DAT); occupational therapy (MS); physical therapy (DPT); physician assistant (MS). *Degree requirements:* For master's, thesis or alternative. *Entrance requirements:* For master's, GRE General Test. Electronic applications accepted.

James Madison University, The Graduate School, College of Health and Behavioral Sciences, Program in Physician Assistant Studies, Harrisonburg, VA 22807. Offers MPAS. *Accreditation:* ARC-PA. *Program availability:* Part-time. *Students:* 83 full-time (67 women), 1 (woman) part-time; includes 7 minority (3 Black or African American, non-Hispanic/Latino; 3 Asian, non-Hispanic/Latino; 1 Hispanic/Latino). Average age 30. 377 applicants, 14% accepted, 31 enrolled. In 2015, 22 master's awarded. Application fee: $55. Electronic applications accepted. *Financial support:* In 2015–16, 5 fellowships were awarded. Financial award application deadline: 3/1; financial award applicants required to submit FAFSA. *Unit head:* Dr. Allen Lewis, Department Head, 540-568-6510, E-mail: lewis6an@jmu.edu. *Application contact:* Lynette D. Michael, Director of Graduate Admissions, 540-568-6131 Ext. 6395, Fax: 540-568-7860, E-mail: michaeld@jmu.edu.
Website: http://www.healthsci.jmu.edu/PA/index.html

Jefferson College of Health Sciences, Program in Physician Assistant, Roanoke, VA 24013. Offers MS. *Accreditation:* ARC-PA. *Degree requirements:* For master's, rotations. *Entrance requirements:* For master's, GRE. Additional exam requirements/recommendations for international students: Required—TOEFL (minimum score 550 paper-based; 80 iBT). Electronic applications accepted. *Faculty research:* Community health, chronic disease management, geriatrics, rheumatology, medically underserved populations.

Johnson & Wales University, Graduate Studies, Master of Science Program in Physician Assistant Studies, Providence, RI 02903-3703. Offers MS. *Expenses: Tuition, area resident:* Full-time $11,826; part-time $5913 per credit hour. *Application contact:* Katie Spolidoro, Admissions Counselor, 401-598-2381, E-mail: pastudies@admissions.jwu.edu.
Website: http://www.jwu.edu/PA/

Keiser University, MS in Physician Assistant Program, Ft. Lauderdale, FL 33309. Offers MS.

Kettering College, Program in Physician Assistant Studies, Kettering, OH 45429-1299. Offers MPAS.

King's College, Program in Physician Assistant Studies, Wilkes-Barre, PA 18711-0801. Offers MSPAS. *Accreditation:* ARC-PA. *Degree requirements:* For master's, thesis. *Entrance requirements:* For master's, bachelor's degree; minimum cumulative GPA of 3.2 overall and in science; 500 clinical hours of health care experience; 2 letters of reference; personal statement. Additional exam requirements/recommendations for international students: Required—TOEFL (minimum score 610 paper-based; 108 iBT). Electronic applications accepted. *Expenses:* Contact institution.

Le Moyne College, Department of Physician Assistant Studies, Syracuse, NY 13214. Offers MS. *Accreditation:* ARC-PA. *Degree requirements:* For master's, project. *Entrance requirements:* For master's, minimum GPA of 3.0, patient contact, interview, 3 letters of recommendation. Additional exam requirements/recommendations for international students: Required—TOEFL (minimum score 550 paper-based; 79 iBT); Recommended—IELTS (minimum score 6.5). Electronic applications accepted. *Expenses:* Contact institution. *Faculty research:* Cultural competence, educational outcomes, preventive medicine, health literacy.

Lenoir-Rhyne University, Graduate Programs, School of Physician Assistant Studies, Hickory, NC 28601. Offers MS. *Faculty:* 4 full-time (1 woman). *Expenses:* Contact institution. *Unit head:* Richard Ball, Chair, School of Physician Assistant Studies, 828-328-7764, E-mail: richard.ball@lr.edu. *Application contact:* Mary Ann Gosnell, Director of Graduate Recruiting, 828-328-7111, E-mail: admission@lr.edu.
Website: http://www.lr.edu/academics/programs/physician-assistant-studies

Lock Haven University of Pennsylvania, College of Natural, Behavioral and Health Sciences, Lock Haven, PA 17745-2390. Offers actuarial science (PSM); athletic training (MS); health promotion/education (MHS); healthcare management (MHS); physician assistant (MHS). Program also offered at the Clearfield, Coudersport, and Harrisburg campuses. *Accreditation:* ARC-PA. *Entrance requirements:* For master's, minimum undergraduate GPA of 3.0. Additional exam requirements/recommendations for international students: Required—TOEFL. *Application deadline:* Applications are processed on a rolling basis. Application fee: $25. Electronic applications accepted. *Expenses:* Tuition, state resident: part-time $470 per credit hour. Tuition, nonresident: part-time $705 per credit hour. *Required fees:* $203 per credit hour. $40 per semester. Tuition and fees vary according to program. *Financial support:* Unspecified assistantships available. Financial award application deadline: 8/1. *Unit head:* Dr. Scott Carnicom, Dean, 570-484-2204, E-mail: carnicom@lhup.edu. *Application contact:* Cherie Dolan, Secretary to the Dean, 570-484-2204, Fax: 570-484-2734, E-mail: cdolan1@lhup.edu.
Website: http://www.lhup.edu/colleges/natural_behavioral_health/

Loma Linda University, School of Allied Health Professions, Department of Physician Assistant Sciences, Loma Linda, CA 92350. Offers MPA. *Accreditation:* ARC-PA. *Entrance requirements:* For master's, minimum GPA of 3.0. Additional exam requirements/recommendations for international students: Required—TOEFL (minimum score 550 paper-based). *Application deadline:* For fall admission, 1/15 for domestic and international students. Application fee: $50. *Unit head:* Dr. Gerald Glavaz, Chair, 909-558-7295. *Application contact:* Helen Greenwood, Director, Admissions and Records, 909-824-4599, Fax: 909-824-4809, E-mail: hgreenwood@sahp.llu.edu.

Long Island University–LIU Brooklyn, School of Health Professions, Brooklyn, NY 11201-8423. Offers athletic training and sport sciences (MS); exercise science (MS); occupational therapy (MS); physical therapy (DPT); physician assistant (MS); public health (MPH); social work (MSW). *Faculty:* 36 full-time (26 women), 47 part-time/adjunct (19 women). *Students:* 503 full-time (326 women), 112 part-time (82 women); includes 212 minority (117 Black or African American, non-Hispanic/Latino; 35 Asian, non-Hispanic/Latino; 48 Hispanic/Latino; 12 Two or more races, non-Hispanic/Latino), 59 international. Average age 31. 1,154 applicants, 38% accepted, 227 enrolled. In 2015, 228 master's, 41 doctorates awarded. *Degree requirements:* For master's, comprehensive exam (for some programs), thesis (for some programs), research capstone; for doctorate, comprehensive exam, research capstone. *Entrance requirements:* For master's and doctorate, GRE, two letters of recommendation. Additional exam requirements/recommendations for international students: Required—TOEFL (minimum score 550 paper-based; 79 iBT). *Application deadline:* Applications are processed on a rolling basis. Application fee: $50. Electronic applications accepted. *Expenses:* $1,155 per credit tuition, $934 per term full-time fees, $442 per term part-time fees. *Financial support:* In 2015–16, 10 research assistantships with partial tuition reimbursements (averaging $12,660 per year), 40 teaching assistantships with partial tuition reimbursements (averaging $12,660 per year) were awarded. Financial award application deadline: 2/15; financial award applicants required to submit FAFSA. *Faculty research:* Manual physical therapy, Parkinson's disease response to physical activity, violence in young minority men, LGBT safety. *Unit head:* Dr. Barry S. Eckert, Dean, 718-780-6578, Fax: 718-780-4561, E-mail: barry.eckert@liu.edu. *Application contact:* Richard Sunday, Dean of Admissions, 718-488-1011, Fax: 718-780-6110, E-mail: bkln-admissions@liu.edu.
Website: http://liu.edu/brooklyn/academics/school-of-health-professions

Louisiana State University Health Sciences Center, School of Allied Health Professions, Program in Physician Assistant Studies, New Orleans, LA 70112. Offers MPAS. *Entrance requirements:* For master's, GRE (minimum score 153 verbal, 144 quantitative, and 3.5 analytical), minimum cumulative and overall science GPA of 3.0, 80 hours of documented healthcare experience. Electronic applications accepted.

Marietta College, Program in Physician Assistant Studies, Marietta, OH 45750-4000. Offers MS. *Accreditation:* ARC-PA. *Faculty:* 5 full-time (2 women), 2 part-time/adjunct (0 women). *Students:* 72 full-time (53 women); includes 12 minority (1 Black or African American, non-Hispanic/Latino; 1 American Indian or Alaska Native, non-Hispanic/Latino; 7 Asian, non-Hispanic/Latino; 2 Hispanic/Latino; 1 Two or more races, non-Hispanic/Latino). Average age 24. 877 applicants, 4% accepted, 36 enrolled. In 2015, 36 master's awarded. *Degree requirements:* For master's, capstone project. *Entrance requirements:* For master's, MCAT and/or GRE, official transcripts. Additional exam requirements/recommendations for international students: Recommended—TOEFL (minimum score 100 iBT). *Application deadline:* For fall admission, 11/1 for domestic students. Application fee: $175. Electronic applications accepted. *Expenses:* Contact institution. *Financial support:* Scholarships/grants available. *Faculty research:* Meniscal tears, radiology, oncology, clinical medicine, hospitalist care. *Unit head:* Miranda Collins, Director, 740-376-4953, E-mail: miranda.collins@marietta.edu.
Website: http://w3.marietta.edu/departments/Physician_Assistant/index.html

Marquette University, Graduate School, College of Health Sciences, Department of Physician Assistant Studies, Milwaukee, WI 53201-1881. Offers MPAS. Students enter the program as undergraduates. *Accreditation:* ARC-PA. *Faculty:* 10 full-time (6 women), 2 part-time/adjunct (both women). *Students:* 122 full-time (98 women); includes 9 minority (2 Black or African American, non-Hispanic/Latino; 5 Asian, non-Hispanic/Latino; 2 Hispanic/Latino). Average age 25. 683 applicants, 11% accepted, 56 enrolled. In 2015, 49 master's awarded. *Degree requirements:* For master's, clinical clerkship experience, capstone project. *Entrance requirements:* For master's, GRE General Test, three letters of recommendation, minimum GPA of 3.0, official transcripts from all current and previous institutions except Marquette. Additional exam requirements/recommendations for international students: Required—TOEFL (minimum score 530 paper-based). *Application deadline:* For fall admission, 10/1 for domestic students. Application fee: $50. Electronic applications accepted. *Expenses:* Contact institution. *Financial support:* Application deadline: 2/15. *Total annual research expenditures:* $37,542. *Unit head:* MaryJo Wiemiller, 414-288-7180, Fax: 414-288-7951, E-mail: maryjo.wiemiller@marquette.edu.
Website: http://www.marquette.edu/chs/pa/index.shtml

Marywood University, Academic Affairs, College of Health and Human Services, Department of Physician Assistant Studies, Scranton, PA 18509-1598. Offers MS. *Accreditation:* ARC-PA. Electronic applications accepted. *Expenses:* Contact institution.

MCPHS University, Graduate Studies, Programs in Physician Assistant Studies, Accelerated Program in Physician Assistant Studies (Manchester/Worcester), Boston, MA 02115-5896. Offers MPAS. *Accreditation:* ARC-PA. *Entrance requirements:* Additional exam requirements/recommendations for international students: Required—TOEFL (minimum score 550 paper-based; 79 iBT). Electronic applications accepted.

MCPHS University, Graduate Studies, Programs in Physician Assistant Studies, Program in Physician Assistant Studies (Boston), Boston, MA 02115 5896. Offers MPAS. *Entrance requirements:* Additional exam requirements/recommendations for international students: Required—TOEFL (minimum score 550 paper-based; 79 iBT).

Medical University of South Carolina, College of Health Professions, Physician Assistant Studies Program, Charleston, SC 29425. Offers MS. *Accreditation:* ARC-PA. *Degree requirements:* For master's, clinical clerkship, research project. *Entrance requirements:* For master's, GRE General Test, interview, minimum GPA of 3.0, 3 references. Additional exam requirements/recommendations for international students: Required—TOEFL (minimum score 600 paper-based). Electronic applications accepted. *Faculty research:* Oral health, pediatric emergency medicine, simulation technology in education, health manpower needs, cultural competency.

Mercer University, Graduate Studies, Cecil B. Day Campus, College of Health Professions, Atlanta, GA 30341. Offers physical therapy (DPT); physician assistant (MM Sc); public health (MPH). *Faculty:* 27 full-time (19 women), 14 part-time/adjunct (7 women). *Students:* 286 full-time (230 women), 4 part-time (all women); includes 94 minority (69 Black or African American, non-Hispanic/Latino; 14 Asian, non-Hispanic/Latino; 7 Hispanic/Latino; 4 Two or more races, non-Hispanic/Latino), 3 international. Average age 26. In 2015, 80 master's, 32 doctorates awarded. *Expenses:* Contact institution. *Financial support:* Federal Work-Study, traineeships, and unspecified assistantships available. *Faculty research:* Scholarship of teaching and learning, health disparities, clinical outcomes, health promotion. *Unit head:* Dr. Lisa Lundquist, Dean/Clinical Professor, 678-547-6308, E-mail: lundquist_lm@mercer.edu. *Application contact:* Laura Ellison, Director of Admissions and Student Affairs, 678-547-6391, E-mail: ellison_la@mercer.edu.
Website: http://chp.mercer.edu/

Mercy College, School of Health and Natural Sciences, Program in Physician Assistant Studies, Dobbs Ferry, NY 10522-1189. Offers MS. *Accreditation:* ARC-PA. *Program availability:* Evening/weekend. *Entrance requirements:* For master's, essay, interview, two letters of reference, undergraduate transcripts with minimum GPA of 3.0. Additional exam requirements/recommendations for international students: Required—TOEFL (minimum score 600 paper-based; 100 iBT), IELTS (minimum score 8). Electronic applications accepted. *Expenses:* Contact institution.

Mercyhurst University, Graduate Studies, Program in Physician Assistant Studies, Erie, PA 16546. Offers MS.

Methodist University, School of Graduate Studies, Program in Physician Assistant Studies, Fayetteville, NC 28311-1498. Offers MMS. *Accreditation:* ARC-PA. *Degree requirements:* For master's, comprehensive exam. *Entrance requirements:* For master's, GRE, bachelor's degree from four-year, regionally-accredited college or university; minimum of 500 hours' clinical experience with direct patient contact; minimum GPA of 3.0 on all college level work attempted, 3.2 on medical core prerequisites (recommended). Additional exam requirements/recommendations for international students: Required—TOEFL (minimum score 500 paper-based; 60 iBT).

MGH Institute of Health Professions, School of Health and Rehabilitation Sciences, Program in Physician Assistant Studies, Boston, MA 02129. Offers MPAS.

Midwestern University, Downers Grove Campus, College of Health Sciences, Illinois Campus, Program in Physician Assistant Studies, Downers Grove, IL 60515-1235. Offers MMS. *Accreditation:* ARC-PA. *Entrance requirements:* For master's, GRE General Test. *Expenses:* Contact institution.

Midwestern University, Glendale Campus, College of Health Sciences, Arizona Campus, Program in Physician Assistant Studies, Glendale, AZ 85308. Offers MMS. *Accreditation:* ARC-PA. *Entrance requirements:* For master's, GRE. *Expenses:* Contact institution.

Missouri State University, Graduate College, College of Health and Human Services, Department of Physician Assistant Studies, Springfield, MO 65897. Offers physician assistant studies (MS). *Accreditation:* ARC-PA. *Faculty:* 6 full-time (4 women), 50 part-time/adjunct (11 women). *Students:* 62 full-time (44 women); includes 9 minority (2 Black or African American, non-Hispanic/Latino; 2 Asian, non-Hispanic/Latino; 2 Hispanic/Latino; 3 Two or more races, non-Hispanic/Latino). Average age 28. 1 applicant. In 2015, 32 master's awarded. *Degree requirements:* For master's, comprehensive exam, thesis or alternative. *Entrance requirements:* For master's, GRE General Test, minimum GPA of 3.0; CASPA. Additional exam requirements/recommendations for international students: Required—TOEFL (minimum score 550 paper-based; 79 iBT), IELTS (minimum score 6). *Application deadline:* For spring admission, 8/1 for domestic and international students. Application fee: $35 ($50 for international students). Electronic applications accepted. *Expenses:* Tuition, state resident: full-time $5500. Tuition, nonresident: full-time $10,108. *Required fees:* $1000. *Financial support:* Application deadline: 3/31; applicants required to submit FAFSA. *Unit head:* Dr. Steven Dodge, Head, 417-836-6151, Fax: 417-836-6406, E-mail: physicianassststudies@missouristate.edu. *Application contact:* Misty Stewart, Coordinator of Graduate Admissions, 417-836-5033, Fax: 417-836-6200, E-mail: michaeledwards@missouristate.edu.
Website: http://www.missouristate.edu/pas/

Monmouth University, Graduate Studies, The Marjorie K. Unterberg School of Nursing and Health Studies, West Long Branch, NJ 07764-1898. Offers adult and gerontological primary care nurse practitioner (MSN); adult-gerontological primary care nurse

Physician Assistant Studies

practitioner (Post-Master's Certificate); family nurse practitioner (MSN, Post-Master's Certificate); family psychiatric and mental health advanced practice nursing (MSN); family psychiatric and mental health nurse practitioner (Post-Master's Certificate); forensic nursing (MSN, Certificate); nursing (MSN); nursing administration (MSN, Post-Master's Certificate); nursing education (MSN, Post-Master's Certificate); nursing practice (DNP); physician assistant (MS); school nursing (MSN, Certificate). *Accreditation:* AACN. *Program availability:* Part-time, evening/weekend, 100% online, blended/hybrid learning. *Faculty:* 14 full-time (13 women), 10 part-time/adjunct (5 women). *Students:* 58 full-time (46 women), 271 part-time (252 women); includes 93 minority (31 Black or African American, non-Hispanic/Latino; 40 Asian, non-Hispanic/Latino; 18 Hispanic/Latino; 1 Native Hawaiian or other Pacific Islander, non-Hispanic/Latino; 3 Two or more races, non-Hispanic/Latino), 1 international. Average age 37. 450 applicants, 32% accepted, 103 enrolled. In 2015, 68 master's, 8 doctorates, 11 other advanced degrees awarded. *Degree requirements:* For master's, practicum (for some tracks); for doctorate, practicum, capstone course. *Entrance requirements:* For master's, GRE General Test (waived for MSN applicants with minimum B grade in each of the first four courses and for MS applicants with master's degree), BSN with minimum GPA of 2.75, current RN license, proof of liability and malpractice policy, personal statement, two letters of recommendation, college course work in health assessment, resume; CASPA application (for MS); for doctorate, accredited master's nursing program degree with minimum GPA of 3.2, graduate research course in statistics, active RN license, national certification as Nurse Practitioner or Nurse Administrator, working knowledge of statistics, statement of goals and vision for change, 2 letters of recommendation (professional or academic), resume, interview. Additional exam requirements/recommendations for international students: Required—TOEFL (minimum score 550 paper-based; 79 iBT), IELTS (minimum score 6) or Michigan English Language Assessment Battery (minimum score 77). *Application deadline:* For fall admission, 7/15 priority date for domestic students, 6/1 for international students; for spring admission, 12/15 priority date for domestic students, 11/1 for international students; for summer admission, 5/1 for domestic students. Applications are processed on a rolling basis. Application fee: $50. Electronic applications accepted. *Expenses:* Contact institution. *Financial support:* In 2015–16, 241 students received support, including 220 fellowships (averaging $3,403 per year), 5 research assistantships (averaging $5,146 per year); career-related internships or fieldwork, scholarships/grants, and unspecified assistantships also available. Support available to part-time students. Financial award applicants required to submit FAFSA. *Faculty research:* School nursing, health policy, and smoking cessation in teens, Multiple Sclerosis; adherence and self-efficacy, aging issues and geriatric care. *Unit head:* Dr. Janet Mahoney, Dean, 732-571-3443, Fax: 732-263-5131, E-mail: jmahoney@monmouth.edu. *Application contact:* Lucia Fedele, Graduate Admission Counselor, 732-571-3452, Fax: 732-263-5123, E-mail: gradadm@monmouth.edu.
Website: http://www.monmouth.edu/school-of-nursing-health/graduate-nursing-programs.aspx

New York Institute of Technology, School of Health Professions, Department of Physician Assistant Studies, Old Westbury, NY 11568-8000. Offers MS. *Accreditation:* ARC-PA. *Faculty:* 6 full-time (4 women), 8 part-time/adjunct (4 women). *Students:* 148 full-time (115 women), 2 part-time (0 women); includes 40 minority (5 Black or African American, non-Hispanic/Latino; 24 Asian, non-Hispanic/Latino; 8 Hispanic/Latino; 3 Two or more races, non-Hispanic/Latino), 1 international. Average age 25. 1,623 applicants, 7% accepted, 54 enrolled. In 2015, 56 master's awarded. *Degree requirements:* For master's, thesis. *Entrance requirements:* For master's, minimum overall undergraduate GPA of 3.0, interview, minimum of 100 hours of verifiable patient care experience in the U.S. healthcare system, 3 letters of recommendation (including one from a physician assistant, osteopathic doctor, or medical doctor). Additional exam requirements/recommendations for international students: Required—TOEFL (minimum score 550 paper-based; 79 iBT), IELTS (minimum score 6). *Application deadline:* For fall admission, 10/1 for domestic and international students. Applications are processed on a rolling basis. Application fee: $50. Electronic applications accepted. *Expenses: Tuition, area resident:* Full-time $20,790; part-time $1155 per credit. *Required fees:* $95; $75 per credit. Full-time tuition and fees vary according to degree level, campus/location and program. Part-time tuition and fees vary according to course load and campus/location. *Financial support:* Research assistantships with partial tuition reimbursements, scholarships/grants, health care benefits, tuition waivers, and unspecified assistantships available. Support available to part-time students. Financial award application deadline: 3/1; financial award applicants required to submit FAFSA. *Faculty research:* Healthcare workforce issues, point-of-care ultrasound, cultural competency, palliative care, diet and disease prevention. *Unit head:* Dr. Zehra Ahmed, Interim Department Chair, 516-686-3871, E-mail: zahmed01@nyit.edu. *Application contact:* Alice Dolitsky, Director, Graduate Admissions, 516-686-7520, Fax: 516-686-1116, E-mail: nyitgrad@nyit.edu.
Website: http://www.nyit.edu/degrees/physician_assistant_studies

Northeastern University, Bouvé College of Health Sciences, Boston, MA 02115-5096. Offers applied behavior analysis (MS, CAGS); audiology (Au D); biomedical nanotechnology (MS); college student development and counseling (MS, CAGS); counseling psychology (MS, PhD, CAGS); exercise science (MS); health informatics (MS); medicinal chemistry (MS); nurse anesthesia (DNP, CAGS); nursing (MS, PhD, CAGS), including administration (MS), adult-gerontology acute care nurse practitioner (MS, CAGS), adult-gerontology primary care nurse practitioner (MS, CAGS), anesthesia (MS), family nurse practitioner (MS, CAGS), neonatal nurse practitioner (MS, CAGS), pediatric nurse practitioner (MS, CAGS), psychiatric mental health nurse practitioner (MS, CAGS); nursing practice (DNP); personal health informatics (PhD); pharmaceutical sciences (MS, PhD), including interdisciplinary concentration, pharmaceutics and drug delivery systems; pharmacology (MS); pharmacy (Pharm D); physical therapy (Postbaccalaureate Certificate); physician assistant (MS); population health (PhD); school psychology (MS, PhD, CAGS); speech-language pathology (MS); urban health (MPH); MS/MBA. *Accreditation:* ACPE (one or more programs are accredited). *Program availability:* Part-time, evening/weekend, online learning. *Faculty:* 194 full-time (120 women), 169 part-time/adjunct (136 women). *Students:* 1,416 full-time (1,049 women), 310 part-time (248 women). In 2015, 374 master's, 313 doctorates, 37 other advanced degrees awarded. *Degree requirements:* For doctorate, thesis/dissertation (for some programs); for other advanced degree, comprehensive exam. Application fee: $75. Electronic applications accepted. *Expenses:* Contact institution. *Financial support:* Applicants required to submit FAFSA. *Unit head:* John R. Reynolds, Professor and Interim Dean, 617-373-3323, Fax: 617-373-3030. *Application contact:* Molly Schnabel, Senior Director of Graduate Affairs, 617-373-2708, Fax: 617-373-4701, E-mail: bouvegrad@neu.edu.
Website: http://www.northeastern.edu/bouve/

Northern Arizona University, Graduate College, College of Health and Human Services, Physician Assistant Program, Flagstaff, AZ 86011. Offers MPAS. *Expenses: Tuition, area resident:* Full-time $8710; nonresident: full-time $20,350. *Required fees:* $896. *Unit head:* Richard Dehn, Chair, 602-827-2421, E-mail: paprog@nau.edu.
Website: http://nau.edu/CHHS/PA/

Nova Southeastern University, College of Health Care Sciences, Fort Lauderdale, FL 33314-7796. Offers anesthesiologist assistant (MSA); audiology (Au D); health science (MH Sc, DHSc, PhD); occupational therapy (MOT, Dr OT, PhD); physical therapy (DPT,

TDPT); physician assistant (MMS). *Program availability:* Online learning. *Faculty:* 109 full-time (64 women), 100 part-time/adjunct (65 women). *Students:* 1,590 full-time (1,179 women), 969 part-time (819 women); includes 831 minority (234 Black or African American, non-Hispanic/Latino; 8 American Indian or Alaska Native, non-Hispanic/Latino; 151 Asian, non-Hispanic/Latino; 378 Hispanic/Latino; 1 Native Hawaiian or other Pacific Islander, non-Hispanic/Latino; 59 Two or more races, non-Hispanic/Latino), 18 international. Average age 30. 8,133 applicants, 14% accepted, 728 enrolled. In 2015, 556 master's, 105 doctorates awarded. *Degree requirements:* For master's, thesis; for doctorate, comprehensive exam, thesis/dissertation. *Entrance requirements:* For master's, GRE General Test, MCAT; for doctorate, GRE General Test, personal interview, essay. Additional exam requirements/recommendations for international students: Required—TOEFL (minimum score 600 paper-based). *Application deadline:* For winter admission, 4/15 for domestic students; for summer admission, 12/15 for domestic and international students. Applications are processed on a rolling basis. Application fee: $50. Electronic applications accepted. *Expenses:* Contact institution. *Financial support:* In 2015–16, 151 students received support, including 4 research assistantships (averaging $3,500 per year); institutionally sponsored loans and unspecified assistantships also available. Financial award application deadline: 4/15; financial award applicants required to submit FAFSA. *Unit head:* Dr. Stanley Wilson, Dean, 954-262-1203, E-mail: swilson@nova.edu. *Application contact:* Joey Jankie, Admissions Counselor, 954-262-7249, E-mail: joey@nova.edu.
Website: http://www.nova.edu/chcs/

Ohio Dominican University, Graduate Programs, Division of Math, Computer and Natural Science, Columbus, OH 43219-2099. Offers physician assistant studies (MS). *Students:* 151 full-time (106 women); includes 7 minority (2 Black or African American, non-Hispanic/Latino; 3 Asian, non-Hispanic/Latino; 1 Hispanic/Latino; 1 Two or more races, non-Hispanic/Latino). Average age 25. 602 applicants, 13% accepted, 49 enrolled. *Entrance requirements:* For master's, GRE and/or MCAT, bachelor's degree from accredited college or university with minimum GPA of 3.0 overall and in science; minimum of 250 hours of documented patient-care experience. Additional exam requirements/recommendations for international students: Required—TOEFL (minimum score 550 paper-based), IELTS (minimum score 6.5). *Application deadline:* For fall admission, 11/1 for domestic and international students. Applications are processed on a rolling basis. Electronic applications accepted. *Expenses:* $807 per credit hour. *Financial support:* Applicants required to submit FAFSA. *Unit head:* Prof. Shonna Riedlinger, Program Director, 614-251-8988, E-mail: riedlins@ohiodominican.edu. *Application contact:* John W. Naughton, Director for Graduate Admissions, 614-251-4721, Fax: 614-251-6654, E-mail: grad@ohiodominican.edu.
Website: http://www.ohiodominican.edu/academics/graduate/mspas

Oregon Health & Science University, School of Medicine, Graduate Programs in Medicine, Division of Physician Assistant Education, Portland, OR 97239-3098. Offers physician assistant studies (MPAS). *Accreditation:* ARC-PA. *Faculty:* 7 full-time (4 women), 9 part-time/adjunct (5 women). *Students:* 87 full-time (59 women); includes 22 minority (2 Black or African American, non-Hispanic/Latino; 1 American Indian or Alaska Native, non-Hispanic/Latino; 8 Asian, non-Hispanic/Latino; 9 Hispanic/Latino; 2 Two or more races, non-Hispanic/Latino). Average age 30. 1,470 applicants, 3% accepted, 42 enrolled. In 2015, 40 master's awarded. *Application deadline:* For fall admission, 10/1 for domestic students. Electronic applications accepted. *Unit head:* Ted Ruback, Program Director/Division Head, 503-494-1408, E-mail: ruback@ohsu.edu. *Application contact:* Colleen Schierholtz, Director of Admissions, 503-494-1408, E-mail: schierhc@ohsu.edu.
Website: http://www.ohsu.edu/xd/education/schools/school-of-medicine/academic-programs/physician-assistant/index.cfm

Our Lady of the Lake College, School of Arts, Sciences and Health Professions, Baton Rouge, LA 70808. Offers health administration (MHA); physician assistant studies (MMS).

Pace University, College of Health Professions, Department of Physician Assistant Studies, New York, NY 10038. Offers physician assistant studies (MS). *Accreditation:* ARC-PA. *Faculty:* 10 full-time (all women). *Students:* 150 full-time (116 women), 45 part-time (32 women); includes 60 minority (7 Black or African American, non-Hispanic/Latino; 8 American Indian or Alaska Native, non-Hispanic/Latino; 27 Asian, non-Hispanic/Latino; 9 Hispanic/Latino; 9 Two or more races, non-Hispanic/Latino). Average age 29. 986 applicants, 16% accepted, 73 enrolled. In 2015, 119 master's awarded. *Degree requirements:* For master's, thesis. *Entrance requirements:* For master's, baccalaureate degree from accredited institution, minimum science and cumulative GPA of 3.0, minimum 200 hours of direct patient care, 3 references from professionals (1 must be a health care professional), completion of all prerequisite courses at time of CASPA e-submission, no more than 1 grade that is less than a B- in a prerequisite course. Additional exam requirements/recommendations for international students: Required—TOEFL (minimum score 100 iBT), IELTS (minimum score 7.5) or PTE (minimum score 61). *Application deadline:* For spring admission, 9/1 for domestic and international students. Application fee: $70. Electronic applications accepted. *Expenses: Tuition, area resident:* Part-time $1195 per credit. *Required fees:* $260 per semester. Tuition and fees vary according to degree level, campus/location and program. *Financial support:* Institutionally sponsored loans and scholarships/grants available. Financial award application deadline: 2/15; financial award applicants required to submit FAFSA. *Unit head:* Susan Cappelmann, Program Director, 212-618-6052, E-mail: paprogram_admissions@pace.edu. *Application contact:* Susan Ford-Goldschein, Director of Graduate Admissions, 212-346-1531, Fax: 212-346-1585, E-mail: graduateadmission@pace.edu.
Website: http://www.pace.edu/physician-assistant/

Pacific University, School of Physician Assistant Studies, Forest Grove, OR 97116-1797. Offers MS. *Accreditation:* ARC-PA. *Degree requirements:* For master's, comprehensive exam, thesis, clinical project. *Entrance requirements:* For master's, minimum of 1000 hours of direct clinical patient care, prerequisite coursework in science with minimum C average. Additional exam requirements/recommendations for international students: Required—TOEFL (minimum score 600 paper-based). *Expenses:* Contact institution. *Faculty research:* Public health, evidenced based medicine.

★ **Philadelphia College of Osteopathic Medicine,** Graduate and Professional Programs, Physician Assistant Studies Program, Philadelphia, PA 19131-1694. Offers health sciences (MS). *Accreditation:* ARC-PA. *Degree requirements:* For master's, thesis. *Entrance requirements:* For master's, minimum GPA of 3.0; 200 hours of patient contact. Additional exam requirements/recommendations for international students: Required—TOEFL (minimum score 79 iBT). Electronic applications accepted.

See Display on next page and Close-Up on page 535.

Philadelphia University, College of Science, Health and the Liberal Arts, Program in Physician Assistant Studies, Philadelphia, PA 19144. Offers MS. *Accreditation:* ARC-PA. *Entrance requirements:* For master's, MCAT, GRE, or MAT. Additional exam requirements/recommendations for international students: Required—TOEFL (minimum score 550 paper-based; 79 iBT), IELTS (minimum score 6.5).

Quinnipiac University, School of Health Sciences, Program for Pathologists' Assistant, Hamden, CT 06518-1940. Offers MHS. *Accreditation:* NAACLS. *Faculty:* 3 full-time (0 women), 3 part-time/adjunct (0 women). *Students:* 45 full-time (32 women); includes 3 minority (1 Black or African American, non-Hispanic/Latino; 2 Hispanic/Latino), 1 international. 111 applicants, 26% accepted, 24 enrolled. In 2015, 22 master's awarded. *Degree requirements:* For master's, residency. *Entrance requirements:* For master's, interview, coursework in biological and health sciences, minimum GPA of 3.0. *Application deadline:* For summer admission, 9/1 for domestic students. Applications are processed on a rolling basis. Application fee: $45. Electronic applications accepted. *Expenses:* $985 per credit; $360 per semester student fee; $340 per semester (fall/spring) technology and lab fee; $75 per semester summer technology and lab fee. *Financial support:* Scholarships/grants and unspecified assistantships available. Financial award application deadline: 5/1; financial award applicants required to submit FAFSA. *Faculty research:* ACL injury mechanism and running injuries and performance; transcriptional activators upstream stimulatory factor (USF); identification of novel antimicrobials; vaccines, formites and opportunistic pathogens; molecular biology of the Lyme Disease agent, Borrelia burgdorferi; molecular and microscopic techniques in host-pathogen interactions; non-invasive vascular biology, external pneumatic compression, sports performance. *Unit head:* Robert Cottrell, Program Director, 203-582-8672, E-mail: paadmissions@quinnipiac.edu. *Application contact:* Office of Graduate Admissions, 800-462-1944, Fax: 203-582-3443, E-mail: paadmissions@quinnipiac.edu.
Website: http://www.quinnipiac.edu/gradpathologists

Quinnipiac University, School of Health Sciences, Program for Physician Assistant, Hamden, CT 06518-1940. Offers MHS. *Accreditation:* ARC-PA. *Faculty:* 8 full-time (6 women), 24 part-time/adjunct (9 women). *Students:* 108 full-time (71 women), 4 part-time (3 women); includes 17 minority (2 Black or African American, non-Hispanic/Latino; 7 Asian, non-Hispanic/Latino; 8 Hispanic/Latino). 1,331 applicants, 5% accepted, 54 enrolled. In 2015, 58 master's awarded. *Degree requirements:* For master's, comprehensive exam. *Entrance requirements:* For master's, minimum GPA of 3.2; course work in biological, physical, and behavioral sciences; interviews; 2500 hours of direct patient care experience. *Application deadline:* For summer admission, 9/1 for domestic students. Electronic applications accepted. *Expenses:* $985 per credit tuition; $340 per semester (fall/spring) technology and lab fees; $75 per semester summer technology and lab fees. *Financial support:* Scholarships/grants and unspecified assistantships available. Financial award application deadline: 5/1; financial award applicants required to submit FAFSA. *Application contact:* Office of Graduate Admissions, 800-462-1944, Fax: 203-582-3443, E-mail: paadmissions@quinnipiac.edu.
Website: http://www.quinnipiac.edu/gradphysicianasst

Rocky Mountain College, Program in Physician Assistant Studies, Billings, MT 59102-1796. Offers MPAS. *Accreditation:* ARC-PA. *Faculty:* 4 full-time (2 women), 3 part-time/adjunct (1 woman). *Students:* 73 full-time (47 women); includes 12 minority (1 Black or African American, non-Hispanic/Latino; 6 Hispanic/Latino; 5 Two or more races, non-Hispanic/Latino). Average age 29. In 2015, 31 master's awarded. *Entrance requirements:* For master's, GRE (minimum combined verbal and quantitative score of 291). Additional exam requirements/recommendations for international students: Required—TOEFL (minimum score 570 paper-based; 88 iBT), IELTS (minimum score 6.5). *Application deadline:* Applications are processed on a rolling basis. Application fee: $35. Electronic applications accepted. *Expenses:* Contact institution. *Financial support:* Applicants required to submit FAFSA. *Unit head:* Heather Heggem, Program Director, 406-657-1190, E-mail: heather.heggem@rocky.edu. *Application contact:* Calley Thompson, PA Admissions Counselor, 406-657-1198, E-mail: calley.thompson@rocky.edu.
Website: http://rocky.edu/academics/academic-programs/graduate-programs/mpas/index.php

Rocky Mountain University of Health Professions, Program in Physician Assistant Studies, Provo, UT 84606. Offers MPAS.

Rosalind Franklin University of Medicine and Science, College of Health Professions, Physician Assistant Department, North Chicago, IL 60064-3095. Offers MS. *Accreditation:* ARC-PA. *Degree requirements:* For master's, thesis. *Entrance requirements:* For master's, GRE, writing sample. Additional exam requirements/recommendations for international students: Required—TOEFL. Electronic applications accepted. *Faculty research:* Ortho-spine, diabetes education, cultural competency, interprofessional medical education.

Rush University, College of Health Sciences, Physician Assistant Studies Program, Chicago, IL 60612-3832. Offers MS. *Entrance requirements:* For master's, GRE General Test. Additional exam requirements/recommendations for international students: Required—TOEFL (minimum score 570 paper-based; 88 iBT). *Application deadline:* For summer admission, 12/1 for domestic students. Electronic applications accepted. *Unit head:* Regina Chen, Director, 312-563-3234, E-mail: pa_admissions@rush.edu. *Application contact:* 312-942-7120, E-mail: chs_admissions@rush.edu.

Rutgers University–Newark, School of Health Related Professions, Department of Primary Care, Physician Assistant Program, Newark, NJ 07102. Offers MS. *Accreditation:* ARC-PA. *Degree requirements:* For master's, internship. *Entrance requirements:* For master's, GRE, interview, minimum GPA of 3.0, BS, 3 reference letters. Additional exam requirements/recommendations for international students: Required—TOEFL. Electronic applications accepted.

St. Catherine University, Graduate Programs, Program in Physician Assistant Studies, St. Paul, MN 55105. Offers MPAS. *Entrance requirements:* For master's, GRE, personal essay. *Expenses:* Contact institution.

Saint Francis University, Department of Physician Assistant Sciences, Loretto, PA 15940-0600. Offers physician assistant sciences (MPAS). *Accreditation:* ARC-PA. *Degree requirements:* For master's, capstone, summative evaluation. *Entrance requirements:* For master's, interview. Additional exam requirements/recommendations for international students: Required—TOEFL (minimum score 550 paper-based; 70 iBT). *Application deadline:* For fall admission, 10/1 for domestic and international students. Applications are processed on a rolling basis. Application fee: $175. Electronic applications accepted. *Financial support:* Applicants required to submit FAFSA.
Website: http://francis.edu/physician-assistant-science/

Saint Louis University, Graduate Education, Doisy College of Health Sciences, Department of Physician Assistant Education, St. Louis, MO 63103. Offers MMS. *Accreditation:* ARC-PA. *Entrance requirements:* Additional exam requirements/recommendations for international students: Required—TOEFL (minimum score 86 iBT). Electronic applications accepted.

Salus University, College of Health Sciences, Elkins Park, PA 19027-1598. Offers physician assistant (MMS); public health (MPH). *Accreditation:* ARC-PA. *Entrance requirements:* For master's, GRE (recommended). Additional exam requirements/recommendations for international students: Required—TOEFL. Electronic applications accepted.

Samuel Merritt University, Department of Physician Assistant Studies, Oakland, CA 94609-3108. Offers MPA. *Accreditation:* ARC-PA. *Faculty:* 8 full-time (5 women), 9 part-

Physician Assistant Studies

time/adjunct (4 women). *Students:* 128 full-time (93 women), 2 part-time (both women); includes 65 minority (4 Black or African American, non-Hispanic/Latino; 24 Asian, non-Hispanic/Latino; 27 Hispanic/Latino; 2 Native Hawaiian or other Pacific Islander, non-Hispanic/Latino; 8 Two or more races, non-Hispanic/Latino). Average age 32. 2,065 applicants, 3% accepted, 44 enrolled. In 2015, 39 master's awarded. *Entrance requirements:* For master's, health care experience, minimum GPA of 3.0, previous course work in statistics. Additional exam requirements/recommendations for international students: Required—TOEFL (minimum score 100 iBT). *Application deadline:* For fall admission, 10/1 priority date for domestic students. Application fee: $50. Electronic applications accepted. *Expenses:* $45,732 per year tuition; $480 lab fees; $160 graduation fee. *Financial support:* Federal Work-Study, institutionally sponsored loans, and scholarships/grants available. Financial award application deadline: 3/2; financial award applicants required to submit FAFSA. *Application contact:* Timothy Cranford, Dean of Admission, 510-869-1550, Fax: 510-869-6525, E-mail: admission@samuelmerritt.edu.
Website: http://www.samuelmerritt.edu/

Seton Hall University, School of Health and Medical Sciences, Physician Assistant Program, South Orange, NJ 07079-2697. Offers MS. *Accreditation:* ARC-PA. *Entrance requirements:* For master's, GRE, health care experience, interview, minimum GPA of 3.0. Additional exam requirements/recommendations for international students: Required—TOEFL. Electronic applications accepted.

Seton Hill University, Program in Physician Assistant, Greensburg, PA 15601. Offers MS. *Accreditation:* ARC-PA. *Entrance requirements:* For master's, minimum GPA of 3.2, transcripts, 3 letters of recommendation, personal statement. Additional exam requirements/recommendations for international students: Required—TOEFL (minimum score 650 paper-based; 114 iBT), IELTS (minimum score 7). *Application deadline:* For spring admission, 1/15 priority date for domestic students. Electronic applications accepted. *Expenses:* Tuition, area resident: Part-time $704 per credit. Part-time tuition and fees vary according to program. *Financial support:* Application deadline: 8/15; applicants required to submit FAFSA. *Unit head:* Dr. James France. *Application contact:* Lisa Glessner.
Website: http://www.setonhill.edu/academics/graduate_programs/physician_assistant

Shenandoah University, School of Health Professions, Division of Physician Assistant Studies, Winchester, VA 22602. Offers physician assistant (MS). *Accreditation:* ARC-PA. *Faculty:* 7 full-time (6 women), 7 part-time/adjunct (4 women). *Students:* 116 full-time (96 women), 2 part-time (1 woman); includes 16 minority (2 Black or African American, non-Hispanic/Latino; 8 Asian, non-Hispanic/Latino; 5 Hispanic/Latino; 1 Two or more races, non-Hispanic/Latino), 1 international. Average age 27. 827 applicants, 7% accepted, 42 enrolled. In 2015, 40 master's awarded. *Degree requirements:* For master's, comprehensive exam, capstone project. *Entrance requirements:* For master's, GRE General Test, bachelor's degree; minimum GPA of 3.0 cumulative and in BCP (biology, chemistry, physics); academic transcripts; three references. Additional exam requirements/recommendations for international students: Required—TOEFL (minimum score 558 paper-based; 83 iBT). *Application deadline:* For summer admission, 1/15 for domestic and international students. Application fee: $175. Electronic applications accepted. *Expenses:* $71,380 tuition. *Financial support:* In 2015–16, 8 students received support. Scholarships/grants and unspecified assistantships available. Financial award application deadline: 3/15; financial award applicants required to submit FAFSA. *Faculty research:* Adult learning, oral health, quality improvement, educational theory. *Unit head:* Dr. Rachel A. Carlson, Director and Associate Professor, 540-542-6208, Fax: 540-542.6210, E-mail: rcarlso2@su.edu. *Application contact:* Cathy Carr, Admissions Coordinator, 540-545-7381, Fax: 540-542-6210, E-mail: pa@su.edu.
Website: http://www.su.edu/physician-assistant/

South College, Program in Physician Assistant Studies, Knoxville, TN 37917. Offers MHS. *Accreditation:* ARC-PA.

Southern Illinois University Carbondale, Graduate School, Graduate Programs in Medicine, Program in Physician Assistant Studies, Carbondale, IL 62901-4701. Offers MSPA. *Accreditation:* ARC-PA. *Faculty:* 12 full-time (8 women). *Students:* 71 full-time (52 women), 30 international. 14 applicants. In 2015, 30 master's awarded. *Entrance requirements:* For master's, GRE, MAT, or MCAT. Additional exam requirements/recommendations for international students: Required—TOEFL. *Application deadline:* For summer admission, 11/1 for domestic students. Application fee: $65. *Unit head:* Donald Diemer, Program Director, 618-453-8850, E-mail: ddiemer@siumed.edu.

South University, Graduate Programs, College of Health Professions, Program in Physician Assistant Studies, Savannah, GA 31406. Offers MS. *Accreditation:* ARC-PA.

South University, Program in Physician Assistant Studies, Tampa, FL 33614. Offers MS.

Springfield College, Graduate Programs, Program in Physician Assistant, Springfield, MA 01109-3797. Offers MS. *Accreditation:* ARC-PA. *Program availability:* Part-time. *Degree requirements:* For master's, comprehensive exam. *Entrance requirements:* Additional exam requirements/recommendations for international students: Required—TOEFL (minimum score 550 paper-based); Recommended—IELTS (minimum score 6). Electronic applications accepted.

Stony Brook University, State University of New York, Stony Brook Medicine, School of Health Technology and Management, Stony Brook, NY 11794. Offers health care management (Advanced Certificate); health care policy and management (MS); occupational therapy (MS); physical therapy (DPT); physician assistant (MS). *Accreditation:* APTA. *Faculty:* 67 full-time (41 women), 64 part-time/adjunct (45 women). *Students:* 488 full-time (301 women), 99 part-time (82 women); includes 167 minority (34 Black or African American, non-Hispanic/Latino; 3 American Indian or Alaska Native, non-Hispanic/Latino; 84 Asian, non-Hispanic/Latino; 41 Hispanic/Latino; 5 Two or more races, non-Hispanic/Latino), 12 international. Average age 28. 2,646 applicants, 14% accepted, 260 enrolled. In 2015, 104 master's, 71 doctorates, 34 other advanced degrees awarded. *Degree requirements:* For master's, thesis. *Entrance requirements:* For master's, GRE General Test, minimum GPA of 3.0, work experience in field, references; for doctorate, GRE, references. Additional exam requirements/recommendations for international students: Required—TOEFL (minimum score 550 paper-based). *Application deadline:* For fall admission, 1/15 for domestic students; for spring admission, 10/1 for domestic students. Application fee: $100. *Expenses:* Contact institution. *Financial support:* Fellowships, research assistantships, teaching assistantships, career-related internships or fieldwork, Federal Work-Study, and institutionally sponsored loans available. Financial award application deadline: 3/15. *Faculty research:* Health promotion and disease prevention. *Total annual research expenditures:* $1.3 million. *Unit head:* Dr. Craig A. Lehmann, Dean, 631-444-2252, Fax: 631-444-7621, E-mail: craig.lehmann@stonybrook.edu. *Application contact:* Dr. Richard W. Johnson, Associate Dean for Graduate Studies, 631-444-3251, Fax: 631-444-7621, E-mail: richard.johnson@stonybrook.edu.
Website: http://healthtechnology.stonybrookmedicine.edu/

Texas Tech University Health Sciences Center, School of Health Professions, Program in Physician Assistant Studies, Midland, TX 79705. Offers MPAS. *Accreditation:* ARC-PA. *Faculty:* 4 full-time (1 woman). *Students:* 109 full-time (82 women), 2 part-time (1 woman); includes 52 minority (5 Black or African American, non-Hispanic/Latino; 27 Asian, non-Hispanic/Latino; 18 Hispanic/Latino; 1 Native Hawaiian or other Pacific Islander, non-Hispanic/Latino; 1 Two or more races, non-Hispanic/Latino). Average age 27. 576 applicants, 10% accepted, 60 enrolled. In 2015, 55 master's awarded. *Entrance requirements:* For master's, GRE. Additional exam requirements/recommendations for international students: Required—TOEFL (minimum score 550 paper-based; 79 iBT), IELTS. *Application deadline:* For fall admission, 12/1 for domestic students. Applications are processed on a rolling basis. Application fee: $40. Electronic applications accepted. *Expenses:* $56,637.80 non-resident; $25,047.80 resident. *Financial support:* Career-related internships or fieldwork, institutionally sponsored loans, and scholarships/grants available. Financial award application deadline: 9/1; financial award applicants required to submit FAFSA. *Unit head:* Christina Robohm, Program Director, 432-620-1120, Fax: 432-620-8605, E-mail: christina.robohm@ttuhsc.edu. *Application contact:* Lindsay Johnson, Associate Dean for Admissions and Student Affairs, 806-743-3220, Fax: 806-743-2994, E-mail: lindsay.johnson@ttuhsc.edu.
Website: http://www.ttuhsc.edu/shp/mpa/

Thomas Jefferson University, Jefferson School of Health Professions, Program in Physician Assistant Studies, Philadelphia, PA 19107. Offers MS. *Students:* 70 full-time (53 women), includes 2 minority (both Black or African American, non-Hispanic/Latino). Average age 27. 1,274 applicants, 5% accepted, 40 enrolled. *Entrance requirements:* Additional exam requirements/recommendations for international students: Required—TOEFL. *Application deadline:* For summer admission, 10/1 for domestic and international students. *Expenses:* Contact institution. *Financial support:* In 2015–16, 65 students received support. Application deadline: 4/1. *Unit head:* Michele Zawora, Interim Chair, 215-503-5724, Fax: 215-503-0315, E-mail: michele.zawora@jefferson.edu. *Application contact:* Amina Floyd-Murphy, Admissions Counselor, 215-503-1040, E-mail: amina.floyd-murphy@jefferson.edu.
Website: http://www.jefferson.edu/university/health_professions/departments/physician_assistant.html

Touro College, School of Health Sciences, Bay Shore, NY 11706. Offers industrial-organizational psychology (MS); mental health counseling (MS); occupational therapy (MS); physical therapy (DPT); physician assistant (MS); school psychology (MS); speech-language pathology (MS). *Faculty:* 20 full-time, 94 part-time/adjunct. *Students:* 1,057 full-time (772 women), 121 part-time (88 women); includes 243 minority (59 Black or African American, non-Hispanic/Latino; 1 American Indian or Alaska Native, non-Hispanic/Latino; 102 Asian, non-Hispanic/Latino; 58 Hispanic/Latino; 1 Native Hawaiian or other Pacific Islander, non-Hispanic/Latino; 22 Two or more races, non-Hispanic/Latino), 102 international. *Expenses:* Contact institution. *Financial support:* Fellowships available. *Unit head:* Dr. Louis Primavera, Dean, School of Health Sciences, 516-673-3200, E-mail: louis.primavera@touro.edu. *Application contact:* Brian J. Diele, Director of Student Administrative Services, 631-665-1600 Ext. 6311, E-mail: brian.diele@touro.edu.

Towson University, Program in Physician Assistant Studies, Towson, MD 21252-0001. Offers MS. *Accreditation:* ARC-PA. *Students:* 63 full-time (53 women); includes 10 minority (4 Black or African American, non-Hispanic/Latino; 3 Asian, non-Hispanic/Latino; 2 Hispanic/Latino; 1 Two or more races, non-Hispanic/Latino), 1 international. *Entrance requirements:* For master's, bachelor's degree with minimum GPA of 3.0, completion of prerequisite math and science courses, minimum of 800 hours of patient contact experience or medical/health-related experience. Additional exam requirements/recommendations for international students: Required—TOEFL (minimum score 550 paper-based; 80 iBT). *Application deadline:* Applications are processed on a rolling basis. Application fee: $45. Electronic applications accepted. *Expenses:* Contact institution. *Financial support:* Application deadline: 4/1. *Unit head:* Prof. Jack Goble, Graduate Program Director, 443-840-1159, E-mail: jgoblejr@ccbmd.edu. *Application contact:* Alicia Arkell-Kleis, University Admissions, 410-704-2113, Fax: 410-704-3030, E-mail: grads@towson.edu.
Website: http://grad.towson.edu/program/master/past-ms/

Trevecca Nazarene University, Graduate Physician Assistant Program, Nashville, TN 37210-2877. Offers MS. *Accreditation:* ARC-PA. *Faculty:* 4 full-time (all women), 1 (woman) part-time/adjunct. *Students:* 97 full-time (75 women). Average age 25. In 2015, 44 master's awarded. *Degree requirements:* For master's, comprehensive exam, successful completion of 9 clinical skills rotations, professional assessment, OSCE exam. *Entrance requirements:* For master's, GRE (minimum score: 300 combined verbal and quatitative), minimum GPA of 3.25, 3 letters of recommendation (physician or physician assistant familiar with applicant abilities/potential, college professor, employer), clinical preference (highly recommended), prerequisites in human anatomy and physiology with lab, general chemistry I and II with lab, microbiology with lab, general psychology. Additional exam requirements/recommendations for international students: Required—TOEFL (minimum score 550 paper-based; 80 iBT). *Application deadline:* For fall admission, 11/1 for domestic students. *Expenses:* Contact institution. *Financial support:* Applicants required to submit FAFSA. *Unit head:* Dr. Bret Reeves, Director, 615-248-1225, E-mail: admissions_pa@trevecca.edu. *Application contact:* 615-248-1225, E-mail: admissions_pa@trevecca.edu.
Website: http://www.trevecca.edu/pa

Tufts University, School of Medicine, Public Health and Professional Degree Programs, Boston, MA 02111. Offers biomedical sciences (MS); health communication (MS, Certificate); pain research, education and policy (MS, Certificate); physician assistant (MS); public health (MPH, Dr PH, including behavioral science (MPH), biostatistics (MPH), epidemiology (MPH), health communication (MPH), health services (MPH), management and policy (MPH), nutrition (MPH); DMD/MPH; DVM/MPH; JD/MPH; MD/MPH; MMS/MPH; MS/MBA; MS/MPH. MS programs offered jointly with Emerson College. *Accreditation:* CEPH (one or more programs are accredited). *Program availability:* Part-time, evening/weekend. *Faculty:* 78 full-time (29 women), 42 part-time/adjunct (20 women). *Students:* 457 full-time (266 women), 61 part-time (46 women); includes 187 minority (21 Black or African American, non-Hispanic/Latino; 107 Asian, non-Hispanic/Latino; 37 Hispanic/Latino; 22 Two or more races, non-Hispanic/Latino), 24 international. Average age 27. 1,599 applicants, 48% accepted, 222 enrolled. In 2015, 219 master's awarded. *Degree requirements:* For master's, thesis (for some programs); for doctorate, thesis/dissertation. *Entrance requirements:* For master's, GRE General Test, MCAT, or GMAT; for doctorate, GRE General Test or MCAT. Additional exam requirements/recommendations for international students: Required—TOEFL (minimum score 100 iBT). *Application deadline:* For fall admission, 1/15 priority date for domestic students; 12/15 priority date for international students; for spring admission, 10/25 priority date for domestic and international students. Applications are processed on a rolling basis. Application fee: $70. Electronic applications accepted. *Expenses:* Contact institution. *Financial support:* In 2015–16, 12 students received support, including 1 fellowship (averaging $3,000 per year), 50 research assistantships (averaging $1,000 per year), 65 teaching assistantships (averaging $2,000 per year); Federal Work-Study and scholarships/grants also available. Support available to part-time students. Financial award application deadline: 2/19; financial award applicants required to submit FAFSA. *Faculty research:* Environmental and occupational health, nutrition, epidemiology, health communication, biostatics, obesity/chronic disease, health policy and health care delivery, global health, health inequality and social determinants of health. *Unit head:* Dr. Aviva Must, Dean, 617-636-0935, Fax: 617-636-0898, E-mail: aviva.must@tufts.edu. *Application contact:* Emily Keily, Director of Admissions, 617-636-0935, Fax: 617-636-0898, E-mail: med-phpd@tufts.edu. Website: http://publichealth.tufts.edu

Union College, Physician Assistant Program, Lincoln, NE 68506-4300. Offers MPAS. *Accreditation:* ARC-PA. *Entrance requirements:* Additional exam requirements/recommendations for international students: Required—TOEFL (minimum score 600 paper-based; 100 iBT). Electronic applications accepted. *Faculty research:* Servant leadership, cultural competency.

The University of Alabama at Birmingham, School of Health Professions, Program in Physician Assistant Studies, Birmingham, AL 35294. Offers physician assistant studies (MSPAS). *Accreditation:* ARC-PA. *Faculty:* 10 full-time (2 women), 13 part-time/adjunct (6 women). *Students:* 183 full-time (143 women); includes 17 minority (8 Black or African American, non-Hispanic/Latino; 5 Asian, non-Hispanic/Latino; 4 Hispanic/Latino). Average age 26. 1,000 applicants, 8% accepted, 80 enrolled. In 2015, 57 master's awarded. *Entrance requirements:* For master's, GRE or MCAT, minimum GPA of 3.0. Additional exam requirements/recommendations for international students: Required—TOEFL. *Application deadline:* For fall admission, 8/1 for domestic students. Application fee: $75. Electronic applications accepted. *Expenses:* Tuition, state resident: full-time $7340. Tuition, nonresident: full-time $16,628. Full-time tuition and fees vary according to course load and program. *Financial support:* Scholarships/grants available. *Faculty research:* Primary care and public health, infectious disease/HIV, oral health. *Total annual research expenditures:* $1 million. *Unit head:* Dr. James R. Kilgore, Program Director, 205-934-9142, E-mail: jrkilgo@uab.edu. Website: http://www.uab.edu/shp/cds/physician-assistant

University of Arkansas for Medical Sciences, College of Health Professions, Little Rock, AR 72205-7199. Offers audiology (Au D); communication sciences and disorders (MS, PhD); genetic counseling (MS); nuclear medicine advanced associate (MIS); physician assistant studies (MPAS); radiologist assistant (MIS). PhD offered through consortium with University of Arkansas at Little Rock and University of Central Arkansas. *Program availability:* Part-time, online learning. *Degree requirements:* For master's, thesis (for some programs); for doctorate, comprehensive exam (for some programs), thesis/dissertation (for some programs). *Entrance requirements:* For master's, GRE. Additional exam requirements/recommendations for international students: Required—TOEFL (minimum score 550 paper-based; 79 iBT). Electronic applications accepted. *Expenses:* Contact institution. *Faculty research:* Auditory-based intervention, soy diet, nutrition and cancer.

University of Bridgeport, Physician Assistant Institute, Bridgeport, CT 06604. Offers MS. *Degree requirements:* For master's, thesis. *Entrance requirements:* Additional exam requirements/recommendations for international students: Recommended—TOEFL (minimum score 550 paper-based; 80 iBT), IELTS (minimum score 6.5). *Application deadline:* For fall admission, 8/1 for domestic and international students; for spring admission, 12/1 priority date for domestic and international students. Applications are processed on a rolling basis. Application fee: $50.

University of Charleston, Physician Assistant Program, Charleston, WV 25304-1099. Offers MPAS. *Students:* 47 full-time (36 women); includes 3 minority (all Asian, non-Hispanic/Latino), 1 international. Average age 27. *Application deadline:* Applications are processed on a rolling basis. Electronic applications accepted. *Expenses:* Tuition, area resident: Full-time $20,602; part-time $425 per credit. *Required fees:* $200. *Financial support:* Career-related internships or fieldwork available. *Unit head:* Jennifer Pack, Program Director, 304-357-4790, E-mail: jenniferpack@ucwv.edu. *Application contact:* Pam Carden, Admissions Coordinator, 304-357-4968, E-mail: pamcarden@ucwv.edu. Website: http://www.ucwv.edu/PA/

University of Colorado Denver, School of Medicine, Physician Assistant Program, Aurora, CO 80045. Offers child health associate (MPAS), including global health, leadership, education, advocacy, development, and scholarship, pediatric critical and acute care, rural health, urban/underserved populations. *Accreditation:* ARC-PA. *Students:* 131 full-time (107 women); includes 18 minority (2 Black or African American, non-Hispanic/Latino; 6 Asian, non-Hispanic/Latino; 9 Hispanic/Latino; 1 Two or more races, non-Hispanic/Latino). Average age 28. In 2015, 45 master's awarded. *Degree requirements:* For master's, comprehensive exam. *Entrance requirements:* For master's, GRE General Test, minimum GPA of 2.8; 3 letters of recommendation; prerequisite courses in chemistry, biology, general genetics, psychology and statistics; interview. Additional exam requirements/recommendations for international students: Required—TOEFL (minimum score 550 paper-based; 80 iBT). *Application deadline:* For fall admission, 9/1 for domestic students, 8/15 for international students. Application fee: $170. Electronic applications accepted. *Financial support:* In 2015–16, 130 students received support. Fellowships, research assistantships, teaching assistantships, career-related internships or fieldwork, Federal Work-Study, institutionally sponsored loans, scholarships/grants, traineeships, and unspecified assistantships available. Financial award application deadline: 3/15; financial award applicants required to submit FAFSA. *Faculty research:* Clinical genetics and genetic counseling, evidence-based medicine, pediatric allergy and asthma, childhood diabetes, standardized patient assessment. *Unit head:* Jonathan Bowser, Program Director, 303-724-1349, E-mail: jonathan.bowser@ucdenver.edu. *Application contact:* Kay Denler, Academic Services Program Manager, 303-724-7963, E-mail: kay.denler@ucdenver.edu. Website: http://www.ucdenver.edu/academics/colleges/medicalschool/education/degree_programs/PAProgram/Pages/Home.aspx

University of Dayton, Department of Physician Assistant Education, Dayton, OH 45469. Offers physician assistant education (MPAP). *Faculty:* 6 full-time (all women), 1 (woman) part-time/adjunct. *Students:* 65 full-time (47 women); includes 9 minority (1 Black or African American, non-Hispanic/Latino; 3 Asian, non-Hispanic/Latino; 4 Hispanic/Latino; 1 Two or more races, non-Hispanic/Latino). Average age 27. 611 applicants, 17% accepted, 30 enrolled. *Degree requirements:* For master's, comprehensive exam, capstone project. *Entrance requirements:* For master's, interview; health care experience; community service; PA shadowing. Additional exam requirements/recommendations for international students: Required—TOEFL (minimum score 85 iBT). *Application deadline:* For fall admission, 12/1 priority date for domestic and international students. Application fee: $175. Electronic applications accepted. *Expenses:* $11,110 per semester, $319 fees. *Financial support:* Career-related internships or fieldwork and institutionally sponsored loans available. Financial award application deadline: 3/1; financial award applicants required to submit FAFSA. *Unit head:* Susan Wulff, Founding Chair/Director, 937-229-3377, E-mail: swulff1@udayton.edu. *Application contact:* Amy Kidwell, 937-229-2900, E-mail: akidwell1@udayton.edu. Website: https://www.udayton.edu/education/departments_and_programs/pa/index.php

University of Detroit Mercy, College of Health Professions, Detroit, MI 48221. Offers clinical nurse leader (MSN); family nurse practitioner (MSN); health services administration (MHSA); health systems management (MSN); nurse anesthesia (MS); nursing (DNP); nursing education (MSN, Certificate); nursing leadership and financial management (Certificate); outcomes performance management (Certificate); physician assistant (MS). *Entrance requirements:* For master's, GRE General Test, minimum GPA of 3.0. Application fee: $30 ($50 for international students). *Expenses:* Tuition, area resident: Full-time $26,802; part-time $1489 per credit. Tuition and fees vary according to course load and program. *Financial support:* Institutionally sponsored loans and tuition waivers (partial) available. Support available to part-time students. Financial award applicants required to submit FAFSA. *Faculty research:* Research design, respiratory physiology, AIDS prevention, adolescent health, community, low income health education. *Unit head:* Dr. Christine M. Pacini, RN, Dean, 313-993-6055, Fax: 313-993-6175. Website: http://healthprofessions.udmercy.edu/

The University of Findlay, Office of Graduate Admissions, Findlay, OH 45840-3653. Offers athletic training (MAT); business (MBA), including health care management, hospitality management, organizational leadership, public management; education (MA Ed), including administration, children's literature, early childhood, human resource development, reading, science, special education, technology; environmental, safety and health management (MSEM); health informatics (MS); occupational therapy (MOT); pharmacy (Pharm D); physical therapy (DPT); physician assistant (MPA); rhetoric and writing (MA); teaching English to speakers of other languages (TESOL) and bilingual education (MA). *Program availability:* Part-time, evening/weekend, online learning. *Degree requirements:* For master's, thesis, cumulative project, capstone project. *Entrance requirements:* For master's, GRE/GMAT, bachelor's degree from accredited institution, minimum undergraduate GPA of 2.5 in last 64 hours of course work; for doctorate, GRE, minimum cumulative GPA of 3.0. Additional exam requirements/recommendations for international students: Required—TOEFL (minimum score 80 iBT). Electronic applications accepted.

University of Florida, College of Medicine, Program in Physician Assistant, Gainesville, FL 32611. Offers MPAS. *Accreditation:* ARC-PA. *Entrance requirements:* For master's, GRE General Test, interview. Electronic applications accepted.

The University of Iowa, Roy J. and Lucille A. Carver College of Medicine and Graduate College, Graduate Programs in Medicine, Department of Physician Assistant Studies and Services, Iowa City, IA 52242-1110. Offers MPAS. *Accreditation:* ARC-PA. *Degree requirements:* For master's, comprehensive exam, comprehensive clinical exam, clinical presentation. *Entrance requirements:* For master's, GRE General Test or MCAT, minimum of 1,000 hours of health care and/or research experience. Additional exam requirements/recommendations for international students: Required—TOEFL (minimum score 93 iBT). Electronic applications accepted. *Expenses:* Contact institution.

University of Kentucky, Graduate School, College of Health Sciences, Program in Physician Assistant Studies, Lexington, KY 40506-0032. Offers MSPAS. *Accreditation:* ARC-PA. *Degree requirements:* For master's, comprehensive exam. *Entrance requirements:* For master's, GRE General Test, minimum undergraduate GPA of 2.75. Additional exam requirements/recommendations for international students: Required—TOEFL (minimum score 550 paper-based). Electronic applications accepted.

University of Missouri–Kansas City, School of Medicine, Kansas City, MO 64110-2499. Offers anesthesia (MS); bioinformatics (MS); health professions education (MS); medicine (MD); physician assistant (MMS); MD/PhD. *Accreditation:* LCME/AMA. *Faculty:* 41 full-time (15 women), 15 part-time/adjunct (7 women). *Students:* 483 full-time (255 women), 39 part-time (25 women); includes 254 minority (34 Black or African American, non-Hispanic/Latino; 3 American Indian or Alaska Native, non-Hispanic/Latino; 172 Asian, non-Hispanic/Latino; 16 Hispanic/Latino; 1 Native Hawaiian or other Pacific Islander, non-Hispanic/Latino; 28 Two or more races, non-Hispanic/Latino), 10 international. Average age 24. 1,004 applicants, 13% accepted, 104 enrolled. In 2015, 22 master's, 119 doctorates awarded. *Degree requirements:* For doctorate, one foreign language, United States Medical Licensing Exam Step 1 and 2. *Entrance requirements:* For doctorate, interview. *Application deadline:* For fall admission, 11/15 for domestic and international students. Application fee: $50. *Expenses:* Contact institution. *Financial support:* In 2015–16, 3 fellowships (averaging $38,566 per year), 4 research assistantships (averaging $13,200 per year) were awarded; career-related internships or fieldwork, Federal Work-Study, institutionally sponsored loans, scholarships/grants, and tuition waivers (partial) also available. Financial award application deadline: 3/1; financial award applicants required to submit FAFSA. *Faculty research:* Cardiovascular disease, women's and children's health, trauma and infectious diseases, neurological, metabolic disease. *Unit head:* Dr. Steven L. Kanter, MD, Dean, 816-235-1803, E-mail: kantersl@umkc.edu. *Application contact:* Janine Kluckhohn, Admissions Coordinator, 816-235-1870, Fax: 816-235-6579, E-mail: kluckhohnj@umkc.edu. Website: http://www.med.umkc.edu/

University of Mount Union, Program in Physician Assistant Studies, Alliance, OH 44601-3993. Offers MS. *Faculty:* 4 full-time (3 women), 2 part-time/adjunct (1 woman). *Students:* 63 full-time (48 women); includes 2 minority (both Two or more races, non-Hispanic/Latino). Average age 25. 250 applicants, 20% accepted, 34 enrolled. In 2015, 31 master's awarded. *Entrance requirements:* For master's, interview. *Application deadline:* Applications are processed on a rolling basis. Electronic applications accepted. *Expenses:* Contact institution. *Financial support:* Applicants required to submit FAFSA. *Unit head:* Betsey Ekey, Director, 800-992-6682. *Application contact:* Jessie Canavan, Director of Admissions, 330-823-2579, E-mail: canavajl@mountunion.edu. Website: http://www.mountunion.edu/physician-assistant-program

University of Nebraska Medical Center, School of Allied Health Professions, Division of Physician Assistant Education, Omaha, NE 68198-4300. Offers MPAS. *Accreditation:* ARC-PA. *Degree requirements:* For master's, comprehensive exam, research paper. *Entrance requirements:* For master's, GRE General Test, 16 undergraduate hours of course work in both biology and chemistry, 3 in math, 6 in English, 9 in psychology; minimum GPA of 3.0. Additional exam requirements/recommendations for international students: Required—TOEFL (minimum score 600 paper-based; 100 iBT). Electronic applications accepted. *Expenses:* Tuition, state resident: full-time $7830; part-time $3915 per credit hour. Tuition, nonresident: full-time $22,410; part-time $11,205 per credit hour. *Required fees:* $521. *Faculty research:* Substance abuse, mental health, women's health, geriatrics.

University of New England, Westbrook College of Health Professions, Program in Physician Assistant, Biddeford, ME 04005-9526. Offers MS. *Accreditation:* ARC-PA. *Degree requirements:* For master's, clinical rotations. *Entrance requirements:* For master's, minimum undergraduate GPA of 3.0, prerequisite courses in anatomy and physiology. Electronic applications accepted. Tuition and fees vary according to degree level and program.

University of New Mexico, Graduate Studies, Health Sciences Center, Program in Physician Assistant Studies, Albuquerque, NM 87131. Offers MS. *Accreditation:* ARC-PA. *Faculty:* 3 full-time (2 women). *Students:* 34 full-time (20 women); includes 15 minority (1 Black or African American, non-Hispanic/Latino; 1 American Indian or Alaska Native, non-Hispanic/Latino; 1 Asian, non-Hispanic/Latino; 12 Hispanic/Latino). Average age 31. 2 applicants. In 2015, 15 master's awarded. *Degree requirements:* For master's, comprehensive exam. *Entrance requirements:* For master's, GRE. Additional exam requirements/recommendations for international students: Recommended—TOEFL. *Application deadline:* For fall admission, 8/1 for domestic and international students; for

Physician Assistant Studies

winter admission, 8/1 for domestic and international students; for spring admission, 8/8 for domestic students, 8/1 for international students. Applications are processed on a rolling basis. Application fee: $50. Electronic applications accepted. *Financial support:* Application deadline: 6/30; applicants required to submit FAFSA. *Unit head:* Dr. Nikki Katalanos, Program Director, 505-272-9864, E-mail: paprogram@salud.unm.edu. *Application contact:* Marlys Harrison, Program Manager, 505-272-9864, E-mail: mharrison@salud.unm.edu.
Website: http://fcm.unm.edu/education/physician-assistant-program/index.html

University of North Dakota, Graduate School and Graduate School, Graduate Programs in Medicine, Physician Assistant Program, Grand Forks, ND 58202. Offers MPAS. *Accreditation:* ARC-PA. *Entrance requirements:* For master's, current RN licensure, minimum of 4 years of clinical experience, current ACLS certification, interview, letters of recommendation. Additional exam requirements/recommendations for international students: Required—TOEFL (minimum score 550 paper-based; 79 iBT), IELTS (minimum score 6.5).

University of North Texas Health Science Center at Fort Worth, Texas College of Osteopathic Medicine, School of Health Professions, Fort Worth, TX 76107-2699. Offers MPAS. *Accreditation:* ARC-PA. *Degree requirements:* For master's, thesis or alternative, research paper. *Entrance requirements:* For master's, minimum GPA of 2.85. *Faculty research:* Impact of mid-level providers on medical treatment, curriculum development, pain in geriatric patients, biopsychosocial risk factors.

University of Oklahoma Health Sciences Center, College of Medicine, Program in Physician Associate, Oklahoma City, OK 73190. Offers MHS.

University of Pittsburgh, School of Health and Rehabilitation Sciences, Physician Assistant Studies Program, Pittsburgh, PA 15260. Offers MS. *Faculty:* 5 full-time (3 women), 2 part-time/adjunct (0 women). *Students:* 75 full-time (55 women), 1 (woman) part-time; includes 8 minority (1 Black or African American, non-Hispanic/Latino; 2 Asian, non-Hispanic/Latino; 5 Hispanic/Latino). Average age 28. 685 applicants, 7% accepted, 37 enrolled. In 2015, 39 master's awarded. *Entrance requirements:* For master's, GRE General Test, hands-on patient care experience, CPR certification. Additional exam requirements/recommendations for international students: Required—TOEFL (minimum score 550 paper-based; 80 iBT), IELTS (minimum score 6.5). *Application deadline:* For spring admission, 11/1 for domestic students, 9/1 for international students. Application fee: $175. Electronic applications accepted. Tuition and fees vary according to program. *Unit head:* Dr. Deborah A. Opacic, Program Director/Assistant Professor, 412-647-4646, E-mail: dopacic@pitt.edu. *Application contact:* Marsha LaCovey, Program Administrator, 412-624-6719, Fax: 412-624-7934, E-mail: mlacovey@pitt.edu.
Website: http://www.shrs.pitt.edu/PAProgram/

University of St. Francis, College of Arts and Sciences, Joliet, IL 60435-6169. Offers forensic social work (Post-Master's Certificate); physician assistant practice (MS); social work (MSW). *Faculty:* 9 full-time (8 women). *Students:* 106 full-time (83 women), 24 part-time (21 women); includes 51 minority (16 Black or African American, non-Hispanic/Latino; 1 American Indian or Alaska Native, non-Hispanic/Latino; 11 Asian, non-Hispanic/Latino; 16 Hispanic/Latino; 7 Two or more races, non-Hispanic/Latino), 2 international. Average age 30. 111 applicants, 48% accepted, 28 enrolled. In 2015, 47 master's awarded. *Entrance requirements:* For master's, GRE (for MS). Additional exam requirements/recommendations for international students: Required—TOEFL (minimum score 550 paper-based; 79 iBT), IELTS (minimum score 6). *Application deadline:* Applications are processed on a rolling basis. Application fee: $30. Electronic applications accepted. Application fee is waived when completed online. *Expenses: Tuition, area resident:* Part-time $730 per credit hour. *Required fees:* $125 per semester. Part-time tuition and fees vary according to program. *Financial support:* In 2015–16, 19 students received support. Career-related internships or fieldwork, scholarships/grants, tuition waivers (partial), and unspecified assistantships available. Support available to part-time students. Financial award applicants required to submit FAFSA. *Unit head:* Dr. Robert Kase, Dean, 815-740-3367, Fax: 815-740-6366. *Application contact:* Sandra Sloka, Director of Admissions for Graduate and Degree Completion Programs, 800-735-7500, Fax: 815-740-3431, E-mail: ssloka@stfrancis.edu.
Website: http://www.stfrancis.edu/academics/cas

University of Saint Francis, Graduate School, Department of Physician Assistant Studies, Fort Wayne, IN 46808-3994. Offers MS. *Accreditation:* ARC-PA. *Degree requirements:* For master's, comprehensive exam. *Entrance requirements:* For master's, GRE, previous coursework in biology, chemistry, and psychology; direct patient care experience. Additional exam requirements/recommendations for international students: Required—TOEFL or IELTS. *Expenses:* Contact institution.

University of South Alabama, Pat Capps Covey College of Allied Health Professions, Department of Physician Assistant Studies, Mobile, AL 36688. Offers MHS. *Accreditation:* ARC-PA. *Faculty:* 6 full-time (5 women), 1 part-time/adjunct (0 women). *Students:* 79 full-time (53 women); includes 5 minority (1 American Indian or Alaska Native, non-Hispanic/Latino; 2 Asian, non-Hispanic/Latino; 1 Hispanic/Latino; 1 Native Hawaiian or other Pacific Islander, non-Hispanic/Latino). Average age 26. In 2015, 40 master's awarded. *Degree requirements:* For master's, comprehensive exam, thesis optional, externship; 121 hours consisting of 73 credit hours of didactic course work and 48 hours of clinical work. *Entrance requirements:* For master's, GRE General Test, minimum GPA of 3.0; 500 hours in Direct Patient Contact Experience. *Application deadline:* For fall admission, 10/1 for domestic students. Application fee: $110. Electronic applications accepted. *Expenses:* Contact institution. *Financial support:* Fellowships, research assistantships, teaching assistantships, career-related internships or fieldwork, Federal Work-Study, institutionally sponsored loans, scholarships/grants, and unspecified assistantships available. Support available to part-time students. Financial award application deadline: 5/31; financial award applicants required to submit FAFSA. *Unit head:* Dr. Diane Abercrombie, Department Chair, 251-445-9334, Fax: 251-445-9336, E-mail: pastudies@southalabama.edu. *Application contact:* Dr. Nancy Dunn, Admissions Coordinator, 251-445-9334, Fax: 251-445-9336, E-mail: ndunn@southalabama.edu.
Website: http://www.southalabama.edu/alliedhealth/pa/

The University of South Dakota, Graduate School, School of Health Sciences, Department of Physician Assistant Studies, Vermillion, SD 57069-2390. Offers MS. *Accreditation:* ARC-PA. *Entrance requirements:* Additional exam requirements/recommendations for international students: Required—TOEFL (minimum score 550 paper-based). *Application deadline:* For spring admission, 10/1 for domestic and international students. Application fee: $150. Electronic applications accepted. *Expenses:* Contact institution. *Financial support:* Scholarships/grants available. Financial award application deadline: 3/15; financial award applicants required to submit FAFSA. *Faculty research:* Neuroscience, teaching techniques in physician assistant education. *Unit head:* Wade A. Nilson, Director, 605-677-6573, Fax: 605-677-6569, E-mail: wade.nilson@usd.edu. *Application contact:* Graduate School, 605-658-6140, Fax: 605-677-6118, E-mail: cde@usd.edu.
Website: http://www.usd.edu/pa

University of Southern California, Keck School of Medicine and Graduate School, Graduate Programs in Medicine, Primary Care Physician Assistant Program, Alhambra, CA 91803. Offers MPAP. *Accreditation:* ARC-PA. *Faculty:* 12 full-time (8 women), 7 part-time/adjunct (4 women). *Students:* 174 full-time (142 women); includes 91 minority (9 Black or African American, non-Hispanic/Latino; 43 Asian, non-Hispanic/Latino; 38 Hispanic/Latino; 1 Two or more races, non-Hispanic/Latino). Average age 26. 833 applicants, 9% accepted, 60 enrolled. In 2015, 55 master's awarded. *Degree requirements:* For master's, comprehensive exam, clinical training. *Entrance requirements:* For master's, GRE or MCAT, bachelor's degree; minimum cumulative GPA of 3.0, cumulative science 2.75. Additional exam requirements/recommendations for international students: Required—TOEFL (minimum score 600 paper-based; 100 iBT). *Application deadline:* For fall admission, 11/1 for domestic and international students. Applications are processed on a rolling basis. Application fee: $50. Electronic applications accepted. *Expenses:* Contact institution. *Financial support:* Institutionally sponsored loans and scholarships/grants available. Financial award application deadline: 5/4; financial award applicants required to submit FAFSA. *Faculty research:* Interprofessional education; clinical case topics and medical review; clinical education and best practices; faculty development. *Total annual research expenditures:* $450,000. *Unit head:* Dr. Kevin C. Lohenry, Program Director, 626-457-4242, Fax: 626-457-4245, E-mail: lohenry@med.usc.edu. *Application contact:* Dr. Alberto Vallejo, Chair, Physician Assistant Admissions Committee, 626-457-4240, Fax: 626-457-4245, E-mail: uscpa@usc.edu.
Website: http://www.usc.edu/schools/medicine/pa/

The University of Tennessee Health Science Center, College of Health Professions, Memphis, TN 38163-0002. Offers audiology (MS, Au D); clinical laboratory science (MSCLS); cytopathology practice (MCP); health informatics and information management (MHIIM); occupational therapy (MOT); physical therapy (DPT, ScDPT); physician assistant (MMS); speech-language pathology (MS). *Accreditation:* AOTA; APTA. *Program availability:* Part-time, evening/weekend, online learning. Terminal master's awarded for partial completion of doctoral program. *Degree requirements:* For master's, comprehensive exam, thesis; for doctorate, comprehensive exam, residency. *Entrance requirements:* For master's, GRE (MOT, MSCLS), minimum GPA of 3.0, 3 letters of reference, national accreditation (MSCLS), GRE if GPA is less than 3.0 (MCP); for doctorate, GRE. Additional exam requirements/recommendations for international students: Required—TOEFL (minimum score 550 paper-based; 80 iBT). Electronic applications accepted. *Expenses:* Contact institution. *Faculty research:* Gait deviation, muscular dystrophy and strength, hemophilia and exercise, pediatric neurology, self-efficacy.

The University of Texas Health Science Center at San Antonio, School of Health Professions, San Antonio, TX 78229-3900. Offers occupational therapy (MOT); physical therapy (DPT); physician assistant studies (MS). *Accreditation:* AOTA; APTA; ARC-PA. *Degree requirements:* For master's, comprehensive exam, thesis (for some programs); for doctorate, comprehensive exam.

The University of Texas Medical Branch, School of Health Professions, Department of Physician Assistant Studies, Galveston, TX 77555. Offers MPAS. *Accreditation:* ARC-PA. *Entrance requirements:* For master's, GRE, interview. Electronic applications accepted.

The University of Texas Southwestern Medical Center, Southwestern School of Health Professions, Physician Assistant Studies Program, Dallas, TX 75390. Offers MPAS. *Accreditation:* ARC-PA. *Entrance requirements:* For master's, GRE, minimum GPA of 3.0. Electronic applications accepted.

University of the Cumberlands, Program in Physician Assistant Studies, Williamsburg, KY 40769-1372. Offers MPAS. *Accreditation:* ARC-PA. *Entrance requirements:* Additional exam requirements/recommendations for international students: Required—TOEFL. Electronic applications accepted.

University of the Sciences, Program in Physician Assistant Studies, Philadelphia, PA 19104-4495. Offers MSPAS.

The University of Toledo, College of Graduate Studies, College of Medicine and Life Sciences, Department of Physician Assistant Studies, Toledo, OH 43606-3390. Offers MSBS. *Accreditation:* ARC-PA. *Degree requirements:* For master's, thesis or alternative, scholarly project. *Entrance requirements:* For master's, GRE, interview, minimum undergraduate GPA of 3.0, writing sample, transcripts. Additional exam requirements/recommendations for international students: Required—TOEFL (minimum score 550 paper-based; 80 iBT). Electronic applications accepted. *Expenses:* Contact institution.

University of Utah, School of Medicine and Graduate School, Graduate Programs in Medicine, Department of Family and Preventive Medicine, Utah Physician Assistant Program, Salt Lake City, UT 84112-1107. Offers MPAS. *Accreditation:* ARC-PA. *Degree requirements:* For master's, comprehensive exam, thesis or alternative. *Entrance requirements:* Additional exam requirements/recommendations for international students: Required—TOEFL (minimum score 550 paper-based). Electronic applications accepted. *Expenses:* Contact institution. *Faculty research:* Physical assistant education, evidence–based medicine, technology and education, international medicine education.

University of Wisconsin–La Crosse, College of Science and Health, Department of Health Professions, Program in Physician Assistant Studies, La Crosse, WI 54601-3742. Offers MS. *Accreditation:* ARC-PA. *Students:* 38 full-time (31 women). Average age 25. 319 applicants, 10% accepted, 19 enrolled. In 2015, 19 master's awarded. *Degree requirements:* For master's, comprehensive exam. *Entrance requirements:* For master's, GRE. Additional exam requirements/recommendations for international students: Required—TOEFL (minimum score 104 iBT). *Application deadline:* For fall admission, 8/1 for domestic and international students. Application fee: $50. Electronic applications accepted. *Expenses:* Contact institution. *Financial support:* Federal Work-Study and scholarships/grants available. Support available to part-time students. *Unit head:* Sandra Sieck, MD, Director, 608-785-6621, E-mail: ssieck@uwlax.edu. *Application contact:* Brandon Schaller, Senior Graduate Student Status Examiner, 608-785-8941, E-mail: admissions@uwlax.edu.
Website: http://www.uwlax.edu/pastudies/

University of Wisconsin–Madison, School of Medicine and Public Health, Physician Assistant Program, Madison, WI 53705. Offers MPA. *Expenses:* Tuition, state resident: full-time $5364. Tuition, nonresident: full-time $12,027. *Required fees:* $571. Tuition and fees vary according to campus/location, program and reciprocity agreements.
Website: http://www.fammed.wisc.edu/pa-program/

Wayne State University, Eugene Applebaum College of Pharmacy and Health Sciences, Department of Health Care Sciences, Program in Physician Assistant Studies, Detroit, MI 48202. Offers MS. *Accreditation:* ARC-PA. *Faculty:* 11. *Students:* 96 full-time (70 women); includes 6 minority (1 Black or African American, non-Hispanic/Latino; 2 Asian, non-Hispanic/Latino; 2 Hispanic/Latino; 1 Two or more races, non-Hispanic/Latino). Average age 27. 380 applicants, 15% accepted, 49 enrolled. In 2015, 43 master's awarded. *Entrance requirements:* For master's, GRE General Test, course work in science, 500 hours of work experience in patient care in a health-service environment, three letters of recommendation, personal statement, interview, bachelor's degree from accredited institution with minimum GPA of 3.0 overall and in prerequisites,

CASPA application. Additional exam requirements/recommendations for international students: Required—TOEFL (minimum score 550 paper-based; 79 iBT), TWE (minimum score 5.5), Michigan English Language Assessment Battery (minimum score 85); Recommended—IELTS (minimum score 6.5). *Application deadline:* For spring admission, 9/1 for domestic and international students. Application fee: $0. Electronic applications accepted. *Expenses:* $16,104 annual resident tuition, $32,401 non-resident tuition; $671 per credit hour resident tuition, $1,350.05 per credit hour non-resident tuition; fees include $47.45 per credit hour student services fee and $274.60 per semester registration fee. *Financial support:* In 2015–16, 53 students received support. Scholarships/grants available. Financial award application deadline: 3/31; financial award applicants required to submit FAFSA. *Faculty research:* Professionalism in physician assistant programs, interprofessional education, including advancements in neurological surgery, vestibular dysfunction, special needs populations. *Unit head:* John G. McGinnity, Program Director/Professor, 313-577-3707, E-mail: jmcginnity@wayne.edu. *Application contact:* E-mail: paadmit@wayne.edu.
Website: http://cphs.wayne.edu/physician-assistant/

Weill Cornell Medicine, Weill Cornell Graduate School of Medical Sciences, Physician Assistant Program, New York, NY 10022. Offers health sciences (MS), including surgery. *Accreditation:* ARC-PA. *Degree requirements:* For master's, thesis. *Entrance requirements:* For master's, GRE. Additional exam requirements/recommendations for international students: Required—TOEFL. Electronic applications accepted.

Western Michigan University, Graduate College, College of Health and Human Services, Department of Physician Assistant, Kalamazoo, MI 49008. Offers MSM. *Accreditation:* ARC-PA. *Program availability:* Part-time.

Western University of Health Sciences, College of Allied Health Professions, Program in Physician Assistant Studies, Pomona, CA 91766-1854. Offers MS. *Accreditation:* ARC-PA. *Faculty:* 11 full-time (8 women), 1 part-time/adjunct (0 women). *Students:* 194 full-time (128 women); includes 76 minority (4 Black or African American, non-Hispanic/Latino; 39 Asian, non-Hispanic/Latino; 25 Hispanic/Latino; 1 Native Hawaiian or other Pacific Islander, non-Hispanic/Latino; 7 Two or more races, non-Hispanic/Latino). Average age 28. 2,374 applicants, 5% accepted, 98 enrolled. In 2015, 98 master's awarded. *Entrance requirements:* For master's, bachelor's degree, minimum GPA of 2.7, letters of recommendation, interview, demonstrated history of ongoing community service and involvement, health screenings and immunizations, background check. *Application deadline:* For fall admission, 12/1 for domestic and international students. Application fee: $50. Electronic applications accepted. *Expenses:* $38,425 tuition, $40 fees. *Financial support:* Scholarships/grants available. Financial award application deadline: 3/2; financial award applicants required to submit FAFSA. *Unit head:* Roy Guizado, Chair, 909-469-5445, Fax: 909-469-5407, E-mail: roygpac@westernu.edu. *Application contact:* Karen Hutton-Lopez, Director of Admissions, 909-469-5335, Fax: 909-469-5570, E-mail: admissions@westernu.edu.
Website: http://www.westernu.edu/allied-health/allied-health-mspas/

Wichita State University, Graduate School, College of Health Professions, Department of Physician Assistant, Wichita, KS 67260. Offers MPA. *Accreditation:* ARC-PA. *Unit head:* Dr. Sue Nyberg, Chair, 316-978-3011, Fax: 316-978-3669, E-mail: sue.nyberg@wichita.edu. *Application contact:* Jordan Oleson, Admissions Coordinator, 316-978-3095, Fax: 316-978-3253, E-mail: jordan.oleson@wichita.edu.
Website: http://www.wichita.edu/pa

Yale University, School of Medicine, Physician Associate Program, New Haven, CT 06510. Offers MM Sc, MM Sc/MPH. *Accreditation:* ARC-PA. *Program availability:* Online learning. *Degree requirements:* For master's, thesis. *Entrance requirements:* For master's, GRE General Test, course work in science. Additional exam requirements/recommendations for international students: Required—TOEFL. Electronic applications accepted. *Expenses:* Contact institution. *Faculty research:* Correlation of GRE scores and program performance, relationship of PA programs and pharmaceutical companies, career patterns in physician assistants, PA utilization and satisfaction with care, factors influencing PAs in their decision to pursue postgraduate residencies.

Rehabilitation Sciences

Alabama State University, College of Health Sciences, Department of Prosthetics and Orthotics, Montgomery, AL 36101-0271. Offers MS. *Program availability:* Evening/weekend. *Faculty:* 3 full-time (1 woman), 1 (woman) part-time/adjunct. *Students:* 18 full-time (7 women), 1 part-time (0 women); includes 6 minority (3 Black or African American, non-Hispanic/Latino; 1 Asian, non-Hispanic/Latino; 1 Hispanic/Latino; 1 Two or more races, non-Hispanic/Latino). Average age 26. 14 applicants, 57% accepted, 8 enrolled. In 2015, 8 master's awarded. *Degree requirements:* For master's, thesis. Application fee: $25. *Expenses: Tuition, area resident:* Full-time $3087; part-time $2744 per credit. Tuition, nonresident: full-time $6174; part-time $5488 per credit. *Required fees:* $2284; $1142 per credit. $571 per semester. Tuition and fees vary according to class time, course level, course load, degree level, program and student level. *Financial support:* Applicants required to submit FAFSA. *Unit head:* Dr. John Chad Duncan, Chair, 334-229-5888, E-mail: jduncan@alasu.edu. *Application contact:* Dr. William Person, Dean of Graduate Studies, 334-229-4274, Fax: 334-229-4928, E-mail: wperson@alasu.edu.
Website: http://www.alasu.edu/academics/colleges—departments/health-sciences/prosthetics-orthotics/index.aspx

Appalachian State University, Cratis D. Williams Graduate School, Department of Health, Leisure, and Exercise Science, Boone, NC 28608. Offers exercise science (MS), including clinical exercise physiology, research, strength and conditioning. *Degree requirements:* For master's, comprehensive exam, thesis optional. *Entrance requirements:* For master's, GRE General Test, 3 letters of recommendation. Additional exam requirements/recommendations for international students: Required—TOEFL (minimum score 570 paper-based; 79 iBT), IELTS (minimum score 6.5). Electronic applications accepted. *Faculty research:* Exercise immunology, biomechanics, exercise and chronic disease, muscle damage, strength and conditioning.

Boston University, College of Health and Rehabilitation Sciences: Sargent College, Department of Occupational Therapy, Boston, MA 02215. Offers occupational therapy (OTD); rehabilitation sciences (PhD). *Accreditation:* AOTA (one or more programs are accredited). *Program availability:* Blended/hybrid learning. *Faculty:* 13 full-time (all women), 2 part-time/adjunct (both women). *Students:* 151 full-time (141 women), 25 part-time (24 women); includes 36 minority (19 Asian, non-Hispanic/Latino; 10 Hispanic/Latino; 7 Two or more races, non-Hispanic/Latino), 5 international. Average age 26. 487 applicants, 20% accepted, 29 enrolled. In 2015, 5 doctorates awarded. *Degree requirements:* For doctorate, comprehensive exam, thesis/dissertation. *Entrance requirements:* For doctorate, GRE General Test. Additional exam requirements/recommendations for international students: Required—TOEFL (minimum score 550 paper-based; 84 iBT), TWE (minimum score 5). *Application deadline:* For fall admission, 1/15 priority date for domestic and international students. Applications are processed on a rolling basis. Application fee: $125. Electronic applications accepted. *Expenses:* $1,537 per credit. *Financial support:* In 2015–16, 68 students received support, including 7 research assistantships with full tuition reimbursements available (averaging $21,000 per year), 9 teaching assistantships (averaging $2,500 per year); career-related internships or fieldwork, Federal Work-Study, institutionally sponsored loans, and scholarships/grants also available. Financial award application deadline: 2/15; financial award applicants required to submit FAFSA. *Faculty research:* Sensory integration, outcomes measurement, impact of Parkinson's disease, families of people with autism. *Total annual research expenditures:* $700,000. *Unit head:* Dr. Ellen Cohn, Program Director, 617-358-1063, Fax: 617-353-2926, E-mail: ecohn@bu.edu. *Application contact:* Sharon Sankey, Assistant Dean, Student Services, 617-353-2713, Fax: 617-353-7500, E-mail: ssankey@bu.edu.
Website: http://www.bu.edu/sargent/

Boston University, College of Health and Rehabilitation Sciences: Sargent College, Department of Physical Therapy and Athletic Training, Boston, MA 02215. Offers physical therapy (DPT); rehabilitation sciences (PhD). *Accreditation:* APTA (one or more programs are accredited). *Faculty:* 13 full-time (10 women), 26 part-time/adjunct (12 women). *Students:* 165 full-time (116 women); includes 36 minority (3 Black or African American, non-Hispanic/Latino; 14 Asian, non-Hispanic/Latino; 11 Hispanic/Latino; 8 Two or more races, non-Hispanic/Latino), 4 international. Average age 24. 867 applicants, 7% accepted, 33 enrolled. In 2015, 52 doctorates awarded. *Degree requirements:* For doctorate, comprehensive exam and thesis (for PhD). *Entrance requirements:* For doctorate, GRE General Test, master's degree (for PhD), bachelor's degree (for DPT). Additional exam requirements/recommendations for international students: Required—TOEFL (minimum score 550 paper-based; 84 iBT). *Application deadline:* For fall admission, 12/15 priority date for domestic and international students. Applications are processed on a rolling basis. Application fee: $120. Electronic applications accepted. *Expenses:* $1,537 per credit. *Financial support:* In 2015–16, 120 students received support, including 7 research assistantships with full tuition reimbursements available (averaging $21,000 per year), 6 teaching assistantships (averaging $2,500 per year); career-related internships or fieldwork, Federal Work-Study, institutionally sponsored loans, scholarships/grants, and tuition waivers (full and partial) also available. Financial award application deadline: 4/15; financial award applicants required to submit FAFSA. *Faculty research:* Gait, balance, motor control, dynamic systems analysis, spinal cord injury. *Total annual research expenditures:* $1.9 million. *Unit head:* Dr. Melanie Matthies, Department Chair, 617-353-2724, E-mail: pt@bu.edu. *Application contact:* Sharon Sankey, Assistant Dean, Student Services, 617-353-2713, Fax: 617-353-7500, E-mail: ssankey@bu.edu.
Website: http://www.bu.edu/sargent/

California University of Pennsylvania, School of Graduate Studies and Research, College of Education and Human Services, Program in Exercise Science and Health Promotion, California, PA 15419-1394. Offers performance enhancement and injury prevention (MS); rehabilitation science (MS); sport psychology (MS); wellness and fitness (MS). *Program availability:* Part-time, evening/weekend, online learning. *Degree requirements:* For master's, comprehensive exam, thesis optional. *Entrance requirements:* For master's, minimum GPA of 3.0. Additional exam requirements/recommendations for international students: Required—TOEFL (minimum score 550 paper-based; 80 iBT). *Application deadline:* For winter admission, 12/1 priority date for domestic and international students. Applications are processed on a rolling basis. Application fee: $25. Electronic applications accepted. *Expenses:* Contact institution. *Financial support:* Career-related internships or fieldwork, scholarships/grants, and unspecified assistantships available. Financial award applicants required to submit FAFSA. *Faculty research:* Reducing obesity in children, sport performance, creating unique biomechanical assessment techniques, web-based training for fitness professionals, webcams. *Unit head:* Dr. Barry E. McGlumphy, Chair, 724-938-4356, Fax: 724-938-4342, E-mail: mcglumphy@calu.edu. *Application contact:* Suzanne C. Powers, Director of Graduate Admissions and Recruitment, 724-938-4029, Fax: 724-938-5712, E-mail: powers_s@cup.edu.
Website: http://www.cup.edu/education/hsss/msExerciseScience/index.jsp

Central Michigan University, College of Graduate Studies, The Herbert H. and Grace A. Dow College of Health Professions, School of Rehabilitation and Medical Sciences, Mount Pleasant, MI 48859. Offers physical therapy (DPT); physician assistant (MS). *Accreditation:* APTA; ARC-PA. *Degree requirements:* For master's, thesis or alternative; for doctorate, thesis/dissertation or alternative. *Entrance requirements:* For master's and doctorate, GRE. Electronic applications accepted.

Clarion University of Pennsylvania, Office of Transfer, Adult and Graduate Admissions, On-Campus Master's Programs, Clarion, PA 16214. Offers data analytics (MS); rehabilitative sciences (MS); special education (MS); speech language pathology (MS). *Accreditation:* ASHA. *Program availability:* Part-time, online learning. *Degree requirements:* For master's, comprehensive exam (for some programs), thesis or alternative. *Entrance requirements:* For master's, GRE, minimum QPA of 3.0. Additional exam requirements/recommendations for international students: Required—TOEFL (minimum score 600 paper-based; 89 iBT), IELTS (minimum score 7.5). Electronic applications accepted.

Concordia University Wisconsin, Graduate Programs, School of Human Services, Program in Rehabilitation Science, Mequon, WI 53097-2402. Offers MSRS.

Duquesne University, John G. Rangos, Sr. School of Health Sciences, Pittsburgh, PA 15282-0001. Offers health management systems (MHMS); occupational therapy (MS, OTD); physical therapy (DPT); physician assistant studies (MPAS); rehabilitation science (MS, PhD); speech-language pathology (MS); MBA/MHMS. *Accreditation:* AOTA (one or more programs are accredited); APTA (one or more programs are accredited); ASHA. *Program availability:* Minimal on-campus study. *Faculty:* 45 full-time (32 women), 33 part-time/adjunct (17 women). *Students:* 230 full-time (180 women), 11 part-time (5 women); includes 15 minority (1 Black or African American, non-Hispanic/Latino; 3 Asian, non-Hispanic/Latino; 7 Hispanic/Latino; 4 Two or more races, non-Hispanic/Latino), 20 international. Average age 23. 685 applicants, 9% accepted, 24 enrolled. In 2015, 132 master's, 32 doctorates awarded. *Degree requirements:* For doctorate, comprehensive exam (for some programs), thesis/dissertation (for some

programs). *Entrance requirements:* For master's, GRE General Test (speech-language pathology), 3 letters of recommendation; minimum GPA of 2.75 (health management systems), 3.0 (speech-language pathology); for doctorate, GRE General Test (for physical therapy and rehabilitation science), 3 letters of recommendation, minimum GPA of 3.0, personal interview. Additional exam requirements/recommendations for international students: Required—TOEFL (minimum score 550 paper-based; 90 iBT). *Application deadline:* For fall admission, 2/1 for domestic and international students; for spring admission, 7/1 for domestic and international students. Applications are processed on a rolling basis. Application fee: $0. Electronic applications accepted. *Expenses:* $1,254 per credit. *Financial support:* Federal Work-Study available. Financial award applicants required to submit FAFSA. *Faculty research:* Neuronal processing, electrical stimulation on peripheral neuropathy, central nervous system (CNS) stimulatory and inhibitory signals, behavioral genetic methodologies to development disorders of speech, neurogenic communication disorders. *Total annual research expenditures:* $38,730. *Unit head:* Dr. Gregory H. Frazer, Dean, 412-396-5303, Fax: 412-396-5554, E-mail: frazer@duq.edu. *Application contact:* Christopher R. Hilf, Recruiter/Academic Advisor, 412-396-5653, Fax: 412-396-5554, E-mail: hilfc@duq.edu.
Website: http://www.duq.edu/academics/schools/health-sciences

East Carolina University, Graduate School, College of Allied Health Sciences, Department of Addictions and Rehabilitation Studies, Greenville, NC 27858-4353. Offers military and trauma counseling (Certificate); rehabilitation and career counseling (MS); rehabilitation counseling (Certificate); rehabilitation counseling and administration (PhD); substance abuse and clinical counseling (MS); substance abuse counseling (Certificate); vocational evaluation (Certificate). *Accreditation:* CORE. *Program availability:* Part-time, evening/weekend. *Students:* 77 full-time (57 women), 15 part-time (14 women); includes 23 minority (14 Black or African American, non-Hispanic/Latino; 8 Hispanic/Latino; 1 Two or more races, non-Hispanic/Latino). Average age 30. 45 applicants, 73% accepted, 25 enrolled. In 2015, 24 master's, 3 doctorates awarded. *Degree requirements:* For master's, comprehensive exam, thesis or alternative, internship. *Entrance requirements:* For master's, GRE General Test or MAT. Additional exam requirements/recommendations for international students: Required—TOEFL. *Application deadline:* For fall admission, 3/1 priority date for domestic students; for spring admission, 10/1 priority date for domestic students. Applications are processed on a rolling basis. Application fee: $50. *Financial support:* Research assistantships with partial tuition reimbursements, teaching assistantships with partial tuition reimbursements, Federal Work-Study, and scholarships/grants available. Support available to part-time students. Financial award application deadline: 3/1. *Unit head:* Dr. Paul Toriello, Chair, 252-744-6292, E-mail: toriellop@ecu.edu.
Website: http://www.ecu.edu/rehb/

East Stroudsburg University of Pennsylvania, Graduate College, College of Education, Department of Special Education and Rehabilitation, East Stroudsburg, PA 18301-2999. Offers special education (M Ed); special education: applied behavior analysis (M Ed). *Program availability:* Part-time, evening/weekend, online learning. *Degree requirements:* For master's, comprehensive exam. *Entrance requirements:* For master's, PRAXIS/teacher certification, letter of recommendation, Pennsylvania Department of Education requirements. Additional exam requirements/recommendations for international students: Required—TOEFL (minimum score 560 paper-based; 83 iBT) or IELTS. *Application deadline:* For fall admission, 7/31 priority date for domestic students, 6/30 priority date for international students; for spring admission, 11/30 for domestic students, 10/31 for international students. Applications are processed on a rolling basis. Application fee: $50. Electronic applications accepted. *Expenses:* Tuition, area resident: Full-time $8460; part-time $5640 per year. Tuition, state resident: Full-time $8460; part-time $5640 per year. Tuition, nonresident: full-time $12,690; part-time $8460 per year. *International tuition:* $15,368 full-time. *Required fees:* $2462; $1630 per unit. $815 per semester. Tuition and fees vary according to course load, campus/location and program. *Financial support:* Research assistantships with tuition reimbursements, career-related internships or fieldwork, Federal Work-Study, and institutionally sponsored loans available. Financial award application deadline: 3/1; financial award applicants required to submit FAFSA. *Unit head:* Dr. Gina Scala, Chair, 570-422-3781, Fax: 570-422-3506, E-mail: gscala@esu.edu. *Application contact:* Kevin Quintero, Graduate Admissions Coordinator, 570-422-3536, Fax: 570-422-2711, E-mail: kquintero@esu.edu.

George Mason University, College of Health and Human Services, Department of Rehabilitation Science, Fairfax, VA 22030. Offers PhD, Certificate. *Faculty:* 7 full-time (2 women), 2 part-time/adjunct (0 women). *Students:* 14 full-time (7 women), 8 part-time (6 women); includes 4 minority (1 Black or African American, non-Hispanic/Latino; 2 Asian, non-Hispanic/Latino; 1 Hispanic/Latino; 6 international. Average age 32. 20 applicants, 60% accepted, 8 enrolled. In 2015, 1 doctorate awarded. *Degree requirements:* For doctorate, comprehensive exam, thesis/dissertation. *Entrance requirements:* For doctorate, GRE, 2 official college transcripts, expanded goals statement, 3 letters of recommendation, resume. Additional exam requirements/recommendations for international students: Required—TOEFL (minimum score 570 paper-based; 88 iBT), IELTS (minimum score 6.5), PTE (minimum score 59). *Application deadline:* For fall admission, 2/1 for domestic students. Application fee: $75 ($80 for international students). Electronic applications accepted. *Expenses:* Contact institution. *Financial support:* In 2015–16, 12 students received support, including 1 fellowship (averaging $10,000 per year), 4 research assistantships (averaging $13,250 per year); career-related internships or fieldwork, Federal Work-Study, scholarships/grants, unspecified assistantships, and health care benefits (for full-time research or teaching assistantship recipients) also available. Support available to part-time students. Financial award applicants required to submit FAFSA. *Faculty research:* Physiological determinants of functional loss; biobehavioral factors that contribute to functional disablement; cardiorespiratory function and performance; human motion, function, and performance. *Total annual research expenditures:* $161,516. *Unit head:* Andrew Guccione, Professor/Founding Chair, 703-993-4650, Fax: 703-993-2695, E-mail: aguccion@gmu.edu. *Application contact:* Bowen Joshua, Program Coordinator, 703-993-1950, Fax: 703-993-6073, E-mail: jbowen6@gmu.edu.
Website: http://chhs.gmu.edu/rehabscience/

Indiana University–Purdue University Indianapolis, School of Health and Rehabilitation Sciences, Indianapolis, IN 46202-5119. Offers health and rehabilitation sciences (PhD); health sciences (MS); nutrition and dietetics (MS); occupational therapy (MS); physical therapy (DPT); physician assistant (MPAS). *Program availability:* Part-time, evening/weekend. *Degree requirements:* For master's, thesis (for some programs). *Entrance requirements:* For master's, GRE General Test, minimum GPA of 3.0 (for MS in health sciences, nutrition and dietetics), 3.2 (for MS in occupational therapy), 3.0 cumulative and prerequisite math/science (for MPAS); for doctorate, GRE, minimum cumulative and prerequisite math/science GPA of 3.2. Additional exam requirements/recommendations for international students: Required—TOEFL (minimum score 550 paper-based; 79 iBT), IELTS (minimum score 6.5), PTE (minimum score 54). Electronic applications accepted. *Expenses:* Contact institution. *Faculty research:* Function and mobility across the lifespan, pediatric nutrition, driving and mobility rehabilitation, neurorehabilitation and biomechanics, rehabilitation and integrative therapy.

Lasell College, Graduate and Professional Studies in Rehabilitation Science, Newton, MA 02466-2709. Offers rehabilitation science (MS). *Program availability:* Part-time, evening/weekend, online learning. *Entrance requirements:* For master's, one-page personal statement, 2 letters of recommendation, resume, bachelor's degree transcript. Additional exam requirements/recommendations for international students: Required—TOEFL (minimum score 550 paper-based, 79 iBT) or IELTS (minimum score 6). *Application deadline:* For fall admission, 8/31 priority date for domestic students, 6/30 priority date for international students; for spring admission, 12/31 priority date for domestic students, 10/31 priority date for international students. Applications are processed on a rolling basis. Electronic applications accepted. Application fee is waived when completed online. *Expenses:* Tuition, area resident: Full-time $10,710; part-time $595 per credit hour. *Required fees:* $160; $160 per unit. One-time fee: $40. *Financial support:* Federal Work-Study and scholarships/grants available. Support available to part-time students. Financial award application deadline: 8/31; financial award applicants required to submit FAFSA. *Unit head:* Dr. Joan Dolamore, Dean of Graduate and Professional Studies, 617-243-2485, Fax: 617-243-2450, E-mail: gradinfo@lasell.edu. *Application contact:* Adrienne Franciosi, Director of Graduate Enrollment, 617-243-2450, Fax: 617-243-2450, E-mail: gradinfo@lasell.edu.
Website: http://www.lasell.edu/academics/graduate-and-professional-studies/programs-of-study/master-of-science-in-rehabilitation-science.html

Logan University, College of Health Sciences, Chesterfield, MO 63017. Offers health informatics (MS); health professions education (DHPE); nutrition and human performance (MS); sports science and rehabilitation (MS). *Program availability:* Part-time, 100% online, blended/hybrid learning. *Faculty:* 3 full-time (2 women), 14 part-time/adjunct (5 women). *Students:* 19 full-time (15 women), 96 part-time (60 women); includes 12 minority (6 Black or African American, non-Hispanic/Latino; 1 Asian, non-Hispanic/Latino; 4 Hispanic/Latino; 1 Two or more races, non-Hispanic/Latino). Average age 31. 74 applicants, 85% accepted, 63 enrolled. In 2015, 95 master's awarded. *Entrance requirements:* For master's, minimum GPA of 2.5. Additional exam requirements/recommendations for international students: Required—TOEFL (minimum score 500 paper-based; 79 iBT); Recommended—IELTS (minimum score 6.5). *Application deadline:* Applications are processed on a rolling basis. Application fee: $50. Electronic applications accepted. *Expenses:* Contact institution. *Financial support:* In 2015–16, 4 students received support. Federal Work-Study and scholarships/grants available. Support available to part-time students. Financial award applicants required to submit FAFSA. *Faculty research:* Ankle injury prevention in high school athletes, low back pain in college football players, short arc banding and low back pain, the effects of enzymes on inflammatory blood markers, gait analysis in high school and college athletes. *Unit head:* Dr. Sherri Cole, Dean, College of Health Sciences, 636-227-2100 Ext. 2702, Fax: 636-207-2418, E-mail: sherri.cole@logan.edu. *Application contact:* Jordan LaMarca, Assistant Director of Admissions, 636-227-2100 Ext. 1973, Fax: 636-207-2425, E-mail: admissions@logan.edu.
Website: http://www.logan.edu

Loma Linda University, School of Allied Health Professions, Department of Physical Therapy, Loma Linda, CA 92350. Offers physical therapy (DPT, PhD); rehabilitation (MS). *Accreditation:* APTA. *Entrance requirements:* Additional exam requirements/recommendations for international students: Required—TOEFL (minimum score 550 paper-based). *Application deadline:* For fall admission, 5/1 for domestic and international students; for winter admission, 12/1 for domestic and international students. Application fee: $60. Electronic applications accepted. *Unit head:* Chair, 909-558-1000. *Application contact:* Helen Greenwood, Director, Admissions and Records, 909-824-4599, Fax: 909-824-4809, E-mail: hgreenwood@sahp.llu.edu.

Marquette University, Graduate School, College of Health Sciences, Clinical and Translational Rehabilitation Science Program, Milwaukee, WI 53201-1881. Offers MS, PhD. *Students:* 12 full-time (5 women), 12 part-time (3 women); includes 2 minority (both Hispanic/Latino), 3 international. Average age 29. 15 applicants, 67% accepted, 4 enrolled. In 2015, 1 master's, 1 doctorate awarded. *Entrance requirements:* For master's and doctorate, GRE, official transcripts, curriculum vitae, personal statement, three letters of recommendation, interview. Additional exam requirements/recommendations for international students: Required—TOEFL (minimum score 90 iBT). *Application deadline:* For fall admission, 8/1 for domestic students, 6/1 for international students; for spring admission, 12/15 for domestic students, 10/15 for international students. Applications are processed on a rolling basis. Application fee: $50. *Financial support:* Research assistantships available. Financial award application deadline: 2/15. *Unit head:* Dr. Lawrence Pan, Chair, 414-288-7161. *Application contact:* Dr. Paula Papanek, Associate Professor/Director of Exercise Science, 414-288-5069.

McGill University, Faculty of Graduate and Postdoctoral Studies, Faculty of Medicine, School of Physical and Occupational Therapy, Montréal, QC H3A 2T5, Canada. Offers assessing driving capability (PGC); rehabilitation science (M Sc, PhD).

McMaster University, Faculty of Health Sciences and School of Graduate Studies, Program in Rehabilitation Science (course-based), Hamilton, ON L8S 4M2, Canada. Offers M Sc. *Program availability:* Part-time. *Degree requirements:* For master's, online courses and scholarly paper. *Entrance requirements:* For master's, minimum B+ average in final year of a 4-year undergraduate health professional program or other relevant program. Additional exam requirements/recommendations for international students: Required—TOEFL (minimum score 600 paper-based).

McMaster University, Faculty of Health Sciences and School of Graduate Studies, Program in Rehabilitation Science (Thesis Option), Hamilton, ON L8S 4M2, Canada. Offers M Sc, PhD. *Program availability:* Part-time. *Degree requirements:* For master's, thesis. *Entrance requirements:* For master's, minimum B+ average in final year of a 4-year undergraduate health professional program or other relevant program. Additional exam requirements/recommendations for international students: Required—TOEFL (minimum score 600 paper-based).

Medical University of South Carolina, College of Health Professions, PhD Program in Health and Rehabilitation Science, Charleston, SC 29425. Offers PhD. *Degree requirements:* For doctorate, comprehensive exam, thesis/dissertation. *Entrance requirements:* Additional exam requirements/recommendations for international students: Required—TOEFL (minimum score 600 paper-based). Electronic applications accepted. *Faculty research:* Spinal cord injury, geriatrics, health economics, health psychology, behavioral medicine.

New York University, Steinhardt School of Culture, Education, and Human Development, Department of Nutrition, Food Studies, and Public Health, Programs in Nutrition and Dietetics, New York, NY 10003. Offers clinical nutrition (MS); nutrition and dietetics (MS, PhD); including food and nutrition (MS); rehabilitation sciences (PhD). *Program availability:* Part-time. *Degree requirements:* For master's, thesis (for some programs); for doctorate, thesis/dissertation. *Entrance requirements:* For doctorate, GRE General Test, interview. Additional exam requirements/recommendations for international students: Required—TOEFL (minimum score 100 iBT). Electronic applications accepted. *Faculty research:* Nutrition and race, childhood obesity and other eating disorders, nutritional epidemiology, nutrition policy, nutrition and health promotion.

Northwestern University, Feinberg School of Medicine, Department of Physical Therapy and Human Movement Sciences, Chicago, IL 60611-2814. Offers neuroscience (PhD), including movement and rehabilitation science; physical therapy (DPT); DPT/PhD. *Accreditation:* APTA. *Faculty:* 30 full-time, 26 part-time/adjunct. *Students:* 281 full-time (208 women); includes 56 minority (8 Black or African American, non-Hispanic/Latino; 1 American Indian or Alaska Native, non-Hispanic/Latino; 32 Asian, non-Hispanic/Latino; 12 Hispanic/Latino; 1 Native Hawaiian or other Pacific Islander, non-Hispanic/Latino; 2 Two or more races, non-Hispanic/Latino). Average age 25. 556 applicants, 34% accepted, 93 enrolled. *Degree requirements:* For doctorate, synthesis research project. *Entrance requirements:* For doctorate, GRE General Test (for DPT), baccalaureate degree with minimum GPA of 3.0 in required course work (DPT). Additional exam requirements/recommendations for international students: Required—TOEFL (minimum score 600 paper-based; 100 iBT). *Application deadline:* For fall admission, 10/3 for domestic and international students. Applications are processed on a rolling basis. Application fee: $50. Electronic applications accepted. *Expenses:* Contact institution. *Financial support:* Institutionally sponsored loans and scholarships/grants available. Financial award application deadline: 3/1; financial award applicants required to submit FAFSA. *Faculty research:* Motor control, robotics, neuromuscular imaging, student performance (academic/professional), clinical outcomes. *Unit head:* Dr. Julius P. A. Dewald, Professor and Chair, 312-908-8160, Fax: 312-908-0741. *Application contact:* Dr. Jane Sullivan, Associate Professor/Assistant Chair for Recruitment and Admissions, 312-908-8160, Fax: 312-908-0741, E-mail: dpt-admissions@northwestern.edu.
Website: http://www.feinberg.northwestern.edu/sites/pthms

The Ohio State University, College of Medicine, School of Health and Rehabilitation Sciences, Program in Health and Rehabilitation Sciences, Columbus, OH 43210. Offers PhD. *Faculty:* 28. *Students:* 14 full-time (9 women), 1 part-time (0 women). Average age 30. In 2015, 3 doctorates awarded. *Degree requirements:* For doctorate, thesis/dissertation. *Entrance requirements:* For doctorate, GRE. Additional exam requirements/recommendations for international students: Required—TOEFL (minimum score 550 paper-based; 79 iBT), Michigan English Language Assessment Battery (minimum score 82); Recommended—IELTS (minimum score 7). *Application deadline:* For fall admission, 11/1 priority date for domestic students, 10/1 priority date for international students; for spring admission, 12/12 for domestic students, 11/10 for international students; for summer admission, 4/10 for domestic students, 3/13 for international students. Applications are processed on a rolling basis. Application fee: $60 ($70 for international students). Electronic applications accepted. *Financial support:* Fellowships with tuition reimbursements, research assistantships with tuition reimbursements, and teaching assistantships with tuition reimbursements available. *Unit head:* Dr. Deborah S. Larsen, Professor and Director, 614-292-5645, Fax: 614-292-0210, E-mail: larsen.64@osu.edu. *Application contact:* Graduate and Professional Admissions, 614-292-9444, Fax: 614-292-3895, E-mail: gpadmissions@osu.edu.
Website: http://medicine.osu.edu/hrs/phd

Queen's University at Kingston, School of Graduate Studies, Faculty of Health Sciences, School of Rehabilitation Therapy, Kingston, ON K7L 3N6, Canada. Offers occupational therapy (M Sc OT); physical therapy (M Sc PT); rehabilitation science (M Sc, PhD). *Program availability:* Part-time. *Degree requirements:* For master's, thesis; for doctorate, comprehensive exam, thesis/dissertation. *Entrance requirements:* Additional exam requirements/recommendations for international students: Required—TOEFL. *Faculty research:* Disability, community, motor performance, rehabilitation, treatment efficiency.

Salus University, College of Education and Rehabilitation, Elkins Park, PA 19027-1598. Offers education of children and youth with visual and multiple impairments (M Ed, Certificate); low vision rehabilitation (MS, Certificate); orientation and mobility therapy (MS, Certificate); vision rehabilitation therapy (MS, Certificate); OD/MS. *Program availability:* Part-time, online learning. *Entrance requirements:* For master's, GRE or MAT, letters of reference (3), interviews (2). Additional exam requirements/recommendations for international students: Required—TOEFL, TWE. *Expenses:* Contact institution. *Faculty research:* Knowledge utilization, technology transfer.

Temple University, College of Public Health, Department of Rehabilitation Sciences, Philadelphia, PA 19122. Offers occupational therapy (MOT, DOT); therapeutic recreation (MS), including recreation therapy. *Program availability:* Part-time. *Faculty:* 14 full-time (13 women), 6 part-time/adjunct (4 women). *Students:* 79 full-time (71 women), 17 part-time (all women); includes 13 minority (3 Black or African American, non-Hispanic/Latino; 6 Asian, non-Hispanic/Latino; 2 Hispanic/Latino; 2 Two or more races, non-Hispanic/Latino). 29 applicants, 79% accepted, 17 enrolled. In 2015, 52 master's, 4 doctorates awarded. *Degree requirements:* For doctorate, comprehensive exam (for some programs), thesis/dissertation (for some programs). *Entrance requirements:* For master's and doctorate, GRE General Test, minimum GPA of 3.0. Additional exam requirements/recommendations for international students: Required—TOEFL (minimum score 550 paper-based; 79 iBT). *Application deadline:* For fall admission, 2/1 for domestic students, 1/1 for international students; for spring admission, 11/1 for domestic students, 10/1 for international students. Applications are processed on a rolling basis. Application fee: $60. Electronic applications accepted. *Expenses:* Contact institution. *Financial support:* Career-related internships or fieldwork and Federal Work-Study available. *Faculty research:* Participation, community inclusion, disability issues, leisure/recreation, occupation, quality of life, adaptive equipment and technology. *Unit head:* Dr. Mark Salzer, Chair, 215-204-7879, E-mail: mark.salzer@temple.edu.
Website: http://cph.temple.edu/rs/home

Texas Tech University Health Sciences Center, School of Health Professions, Program in Rehabilitation Sciences, Lubbock, TX 79430. Offers PhD. *Program availability:* Part-time. *Faculty:* 12 full-time (3 women). *Students:* 6 full-time (1 woman), 5 part-time (2 women); includes 4 minority (1 Black or African American, non-Hispanic/Latino; 3 Asian, non-Hispanic/Latino). Average age 33. 10 applicants, 40% accepted, 4 enrolled. In 2015, 1 doctorate awarded. *Entrance requirements:* For doctorate, GRE. Additional exam requirements/recommendations for international students: Required—TOEFL (minimum score 550 paper-based; 79 iBT), IELTS. *Application deadline:* For fall admission, 3/15 for domestic students; for spring admission, 10/15 for domestic students; for summer admission, 2/1 for domestic students. Applications are processed on a rolling basis. Application fee: $40. Electronic applications accepted. *Financial support:* Institutionally sponsored loans and scholarships/grants available. Financial award application deadline: 9/1; financial award applicants required to submit FAFSA. *Unit head:* Dr. Roger James, Program Director, 806-743-3226, Fax: 806-743-2189, E-mail: roger.james@ttuhsc.edu. *Application contact:* Lindsay Johnson, Associate Dean for Admissions and Student Affairs, 806-743-3220, Fax: 806-743-2994, E-mail: lindsay.johnson@ttuhsc.edu.
Website: http://www.ttuhsc.edu/shp/phdrs

Université de Montréal, Faculty of Medicine, Program in Mobility and Posture, Montréal, QC H3C 3J7, Canada. Offers DESS.

University at Buffalo, the State University of New York, Graduate School, School of Public Health and Health Professions, Department of Rehabilitation Science, Buffalo, NY 14214. Offers assistive and rehabilitation technology (Certificate); occupational therapy (MS); physical therapy (DPT); rehabilitation science (PhD). *Faculty:* 21 full-time (14 women), 6 part-time/adjunct (4 women). *Students:* 252 full-time (157 women), 2 part-time (0 women); includes 31 minority (7 Black or African American, non-Hispanic/Latino; 23 Asian, non-Hispanic/Latino; 1 Hispanic/Latino), 4 international. Average age 24. 187 applicants, 66% accepted, 116 enrolled. In 2015, 47 master's, 45 doctorates, 1 other advanced degree awarded. *Degree requirements:* For doctorate, comprehensive exam, thesis/dissertation. *Entrance requirements:* For doctorate, GRE General Test. Additional exam requirements/recommendations for international students: Required—TOEFL (minimum score 550 paper-based; 79 iBT). *Application deadline:* For fall admission, 11/1 for domestic students. Application fee: $50. *Financial support:* In 2015–16, 1 fellowship (averaging $4,000 per year), 1 teaching assistantship with tuition reimbursement (averaging $11,000 per year) were awarded; scholarships/grants and unspecified assistantships also available. *Faculty research:* Occupational therapy, physical therapy, exercise physiology. *Total annual research expenditures:* $392,087. *Unit head:* Dr. Robert Burkard, Chair, 716-829-6720, Fax: 716-829-2317, E-mail: phhpadv@buffalo.edu. *Application contact:* Debbie McDuffie, Assistant to the Chair, 716-829-6729, Fax: 716-829-3217, E-mail: dlm1@buffalo.edu.
Website: http://sphhp.buffalo.edu/rehabilitation-science.html

The University of Alabama at Birmingham, School of Health Professions, Program in Rehabilitation Science, Birmingham, AL 35294. Offers PhD. Program offered jointly by Departments of Occupational Therapy and Physical Therapy. *Faculty:* 15 full-time (5 women). *Students:* 12 full-time (10 women); includes 2 minority (both Asian, non-Hispanic/Latino), 3 international. Average age 29. 25 applicants, 20% accepted, 4 enrolled. In 2015, 1 doctorate awarded. *Degree requirements:* For doctorate, comprehensive exam, thesis/dissertation. *Entrance requirements:* For doctorate, GRE, references, minimum GPA of 3.0, interview. Additional exam requirements/recommendations for international students: Required—TOEFL (minimum score 500 paper based; 80 iBT); Recommended—IELTS (minimum score 5). *Application deadline:* For fall admission, 1/31 for domestic and international students. Applications are processed on a rolling basis. Application fee: $0 ($60 for international students). Electronic applications accepted. *Expenses:* Tuition, state resident: full-time $7340. Tuition, nonresident: full-time $16,628. Full-time tuition and fees vary according to course load and program. *Financial support:* In 2015–16, 4 students received support. Traineeships and health care benefits available. *Faculty research:* Motor control physiology occupation science adaptive physical activity exercise physiology neurological rehabilitation. *Unit head:* Dr. David A. Brown, Graduate Program Director/Professor, 205-975-2788, E-mail: dbrownpt@uab.edu. *Application contact:* Holly G. Hebard, Director of Graduate School Operations, 205-934-8227, Fax: 205-934-8413, E-mail: gradschool@uab.edu.
Website: http://www.uab.edu/shp/pt/rsphd

University of Alberta, Faculty of Graduate Studies and Research, Faculty of Rehabilitation Medicine, Edmonton, AB T6G 2E1, Canada. Offers PhD. *Degree requirements:* For doctorate, thesis/dissertation. *Entrance requirements:* For doctorate, GRE, minimum GPA of 7.0 on a 9.0 scale. Additional exam requirements/recommendations for international students: Required—TOEFL. Electronic applications accepted. *Faculty research:* Musculoskeletal disorders, neuromotor control, exercise physiology, motor speech disorders, assistive technologies, cardiac rehabilitation/therapeutic exercise.

The University of British Columbia, Faculty of Medicine, School of Rehabilitation Sciences, Vancouver, BC V6T 1Z1, Canada. Offers M Sc, MOT, MPT, MRSc, PhD. *Degree requirements:* For master's, thesis; for doctorate, comprehensive exam, thesis/dissertation. *Entrance requirements:* For master's, minimum B+ average; for doctorate, minimum B+ average, master's degree. Additional exam requirements/recommendations for international students: Required—TOEFL (minimum score 600 paper-based). Electronic applications accepted. *Faculty research:* Disability, rehabilitation and society, exercise science and rehabilitation, neurorehabilitation and motor control.

University of Cincinnati, Graduate School, College of Allied Health Sciences, Department of Rehabilitation Sciences, Cincinnati, OH 45221. Offers DPT. *Accreditation:* APTA. *Entrance requirements:* For doctorate, GRE General Test, bachelor's degree with minimum GPA of 3.0, 50 hours volunteer/work in physical therapy setting. Additional exam requirements/recommendations for international students: Required—TOEFL. Electronic applications accepted. *Faculty research:* Biomechanics, sports-related injuries, motor learning, stroke rehabilitation.

University of Colorado Denver, School of Medicine, Program in Rehabilitation Science, Aurora, CO 80045. Offers PhD. *Students:* 7 full-time (2 women). Average age 29. 11 applicants, 9% accepted, 1 enrolled. In 2015, 1 doctorate awarded. *Degree requirements:* For doctorate, comprehensive exam, 60 credit hours (30 of core coursework and 30 of thesis). *Entrance requirements:* For doctorate, GRE, bachelor's degree with minimum GPA of 3.0, research experience (preferred), three letters of recommendation, interview. Additional exam requirements/recommendations for international students: Required—TOEFL (minimum score 570 paper-based; 89 iBT). *Application deadline:* For fall admission, 1/1 for domestic students, 12/1 for international students. Application fee: $50 ($75 for international students). Electronic applications accepted. *Financial support:* In 2015–16, 7 students received support. Fellowships, research assistantships, teaching assistantships, Federal Work-Study, institutionally sponsored loans, scholarships/grants, traineeships and unspecified assistantships available. Financial award application deadline: 4/1; financial award applicants required to submit FAFSA. *Unit head:* Margaret Schenkman, Director of Physical Therapy Program, 303-724-9375, E-mail: margaret.schenkman@ucdenver.edu. *Application contact:* Vonelle Kelly, Program Administrator, 303-724-3102, E-mail: vonelle.kelly@ucdenver.edu.
Website: http://www.ucdenver.edu/academics/colleges/medicalschool/education/degree_programs/pt/EducationPrograms/PhD/Pages/Overview.aspx

University of Florida, Graduate School, College of Public Health and Health Professions, Program in Rehabilitation Science, Gainesville, FL 32611. Offers PhD, PhD/MPH. *Faculty:* 6 full-time. *Students:* 31 full-time (20 women), 1 part-time (0 women); includes 4 minority (2 Black or African American, non-Hispanic/Latino; 1 Asian, non-Hispanic/Latino; 1 Hispanic/Latino), 16 international. Average age 32. 31 applicants, 26% accepted, 7 enrolled. In 2015, 7 doctorates awarded. *Degree requirements:* For doctorate, comprehensive exam, thesis/dissertation. *Entrance requirements:* For doctorate, GRE (minimum scores: 150 Verbal, 145 Quantitative), minimum GPA of 3.0. Additional exam requirements/recommendations for international students: Required—TOEFL (minimum score 550 paper-based; 80 iBT), IELTS (minimum score 6). *Application deadline:* For fall admission, 3/15 for domestic and international students; for spring admission, 7/15 for domestic and international students. Applications are processed on a rolling basis. Application fee: $30. Electronic applications accepted. *Financial support:* In 2015–16, 2 fellowships, 18 research assistantships, 5 teaching assistantships were awarded. Financial award application deadline: 4/1; financial award applicants required to submit FAFSA. *Faculty research:* Neuroplasticity and neurorehabilitation, musculoskeletal pain, cardiopulmonary and respiratory, rehabilitation, muscle degeneration, regeneration and pathology, clinical and patient outcome measures. *Total annual research expenditures:* $19.5 million. *Unit head:* David Fuller, PhD, Professor and Program Director, 352-273-6634, Fax: 352-273-

6109, E-mail: ddf@phhp.ufl.edu. *Application contact:* Amy Ladendorf, Rehabilitation Science Program Admissions, 352-273-6507, E-mail: gradinfo@ufl.edu. Website: http://rehabsci.phhp.ufl.edu/

University of Illinois at Urbana–Champaign, Graduate College, College of Applied Health Sciences, Department of Kinesiology and Community Health, Champaign, IL 61820. Offers community health (MS, MSPH, PhD); kinesiology (MS, PhD); public health (MPH); rehabilitation (MS); PhD/MPH.

The University of Iowa, Roy J. and Lucille A. Carver College of Medicine and Graduate College, Graduate Programs in Medicine, Department of Physical Therapy and Rehabilitation Science, Iowa City, IA 52242. Offers physical rehabilitation science (MA, PhD); physical therapy (DPT). *Accreditation:* APTA (one or more programs are accredited). Terminal master's awarded for partial completion of doctoral program. *Degree requirements:* For master's, thesis (for some programs); for doctorate, comprehensive exam (for some programs), thesis/dissertation (for some programs). *Entrance requirements:* For master's and doctorate, GRE. Additional exam requirements/recommendations for international students: Required—TOEFL. Electronic applications accepted. *Expenses:* Contact institution. *Faculty research:* Neuroplasticity and motor control, pain mechanisms, biomechanics and sports medicine, neuromuscular physiology, cardiovascular physiology.

The University of Kansas, University of Kansas Medical Center, School of Health Professions, Department of Occupational Therapy Education, Kansas City, KS 66160. Offers occupational therapy (MOT, OTD); therapeutic science (PhD). *Accreditation:* AOTA. *Program availability:* Part-time. *Faculty:* 15 full-time (12 women), 1 part-time/ adjunct. *Students:* 109 full-time (103 women), 34 part-time (29 women); includes 18 minority (4 Black or African American, non-Hispanic/Latino; 3 Asian, non-Hispanic/ Latino; 8 Hispanic/Latino; 3 Two or more races, non-Hispanic/Latino), 5 international. Average age 25. 185 applicants, 23% accepted, 42 enrolled. In 2015, 38 master's, 4 doctorates awarded. *Degree requirements:* For doctorate, comprehensive exam, thesis/ dissertation, oral defense. *Entrance requirements:* For master's, 40 hours of paid work or volunteer experience working directly with people with special needs, 3 letters of recommendation, personal statement, program statement of interest, bachelor's degree with 40 hours of prerequisite work, minimum GPA of 3.0; for doctorate, 24 hours of master's-level research. Additional exam requirements/recommendations for international students: Required—TOEFL. *Application deadline:* For fall admission, 12/1 for domestic students, 4/1 for international students; for summer admission, 12/1 for domestic students. Applications are processed on a rolling basis. Application fee: $60. Electronic applications accepted. *Financial support:* Research assistantships with partial tuition reimbursements, teaching assistantships with tuition reimbursements, traineeships, and unspecified assistantships available. Financial award application deadline: 3/1; financial award applicants required to submit FAFSA. *Faculty research:* Impact of sensory processing in everyday life; improving balance, motor skills, and independence with community nonprofit organizations serving people with special needs; improving self-confidence and self-sufficiency with poverty-based services in community; working with autism population in a community-wide aquatics program; improving quality of life of people living with cancer and chronic illness. *Unit head:* Dr. Winifred W. Dunn, Professor/Chair, 913-588-7195, Fax: 913-588-4568, E-mail: wdunn@ kumc.edu. *Application contact:* Wendy Hildenbrand, Admissions Representative, 913-588-7174, Fax: 913-588-4568, E-mail: whildenb@kumc.edu.
Website: http://www.kumc.edu/school-of-health-professions/occupational-therapy-education.html

The University of Kansas, University of Kansas Medical Center, School of Health Professions, Department of Physical Therapy and Rehabilitation Science, Kansas City, KS 66160. Offers physical therapy (DPT); rehabilitation science (PhD). *Accreditation:* APTA. *Faculty:* 21. *Students:* 178 full-time (102 women), 2 part-time (1 woman); includes 17 minority (3 Asian, non-Hispanic/Latino; 8 Hispanic/Latino; 6 Two or more races, non-Hispanic/Latino), 16 international. Average age 25. 306 applicants, 26% accepted, 60 enrolled. In 2015, 44 doctorates awarded. *Degree requirements:* For doctorate, comprehensive exam, research project with paper. *Entrance requirements:* For doctorate, GRE General Test, minimum GPA of 3.0. Additional exam requirements/ recommendations for international students: Required—TOEFL. *Application deadline:* For fall admission, 11/1 for domestic students. Application fee: $60. Electronic applications accepted. *Expenses:* Contact institution. *Financial support:* Research assistantships with tuition reimbursements, teaching assistantships with tuition reimbursements, career-related internships or fieldwork, Federal Work-Study, institutionally sponsored loans, scholarships/grants, traineeships, and unspecified assistantships available. Financial award application deadline: 3/1; financial award applicants required to submit FAFSA. *Faculty research:* Stroke rehabilitation and the effects on balance and coordination; deep brain stimulation and Parkinson's Disease; peripheral neuropathies, pain and the effects of exercise; islet transplants for Type 1 diabetes; cardiac disease associated with diabetes. *Total annual research expenditures:* $434,052. *Unit head:* Dr. Patricia Kluding, Interim Chair, 913-588-6733, Fax: 913-588-6910, E-mail: pkluding@kumc.edu. *Application contact:* Robert Bagley, Senior Coordinator, 913-588-6799, Fax: 913-588-6910, E-mail: rbagley@kumc.edu. Website: http://www.kumc.edu/school-of-health-professions/physical-therapy-and-rehabilitation-science.html

University of Kentucky, Graduate School, College of Health Sciences, Program in Rehabilitation Sciences, Lexington, KY 40506-0032. Offers PhD. *Degree requirements:* For doctorate, comprehensive exam, thesis/dissertation. *Entrance requirements:* For doctorate, GRE General Test, minimum undergraduate GPA of 2.75. Additional exam requirements/recommendations for international students: Required—TOEFL (minimum score 550 paper-based). Electronic applications accepted.

University of Manitoba, Faculty of Graduate Studies, School of Medical Rehabilitation, Winnipeg, MB R3T 2N2, Canada. Offers applied health sciences (PhD); occupational therapy (MOT); physical therapy (MPT); rehabilitation (M Sc).

University of Manitoba, Faculty of Medicine and Faculty of Graduate Studies, Graduate Programs in Medicine, Department of Medical Rehabilitation, Winnipeg, MB R3T 2N2, Canada. Offers rehabilitation (M Sc). *Program availability:* Part-time. *Faculty research:* Understanding of human dynamics, motor control and neurological dysfunction, exercise physiology, functional motion of the upper extremity and effects of musculoskeletal disorders.

University of Maryland, Baltimore, Graduate School, Graduate Program in Life Sciences, Program in Physical Rehabilitation Science, Baltimore, MD 21201. Offers PhD. *Degree requirements:* For doctorate, comprehensive exam, thesis/dissertation. *Entrance requirements:* For doctorate, GRE. Additional exam requirements/ recommendations for international students: Required—TOEFL (minimum score 550 paper-based; 80 iBT); Recommended—IELTS (minimum score 7). Electronic applications accepted. Tuition and fees vary according to program. *Faculty research:* Applied physiology, biomechanics, epidemiology of disability, neuromotor control.

University of Maryland, Baltimore, School of Medicine, Department of Physical Therapy and Rehabilitation Science, Baltimore, MD 21201. Offers physical rehabilitation science (PhD); physical therapy and rehabilitation science (DPT). *Accreditation:* APTA. *Students:* 173 full-time (111 women), 2 part-time (1 woman); includes 32 minority (7

Black or African American, non-Hispanic/Latino; 10 Asian, non-Hispanic/Latino; 13 Hispanic/Latino; 2 Two or more races, non-Hispanic/Latino), 2 international. Average age 25. 154 applicants, 82% accepted, 65 enrolled. In 2015, 59 doctorates awarded. *Entrance requirements:* For doctorate, GRE General Test, BS, science coursework. Additional exam requirements/recommendations for international students: Required— TOEFL (minimum score 80 iBT). Electronic applications accepted. *Expenses:* Contact institution. *Financial support:* Career-related internships or fieldwork, Federal Work-Study, scholarships/grants, traineeships, health care benefits, and unspecified assistantships available. Financial award application deadline: 3/1; financial award applicants required to submit FAFSA. *Unit head:* Dr. Mark W. Rogers, Interim Chair, 410-706-5216, Fax: 410-706-4903, E-mail: mrodgers@som.umaryland.edu. *Application contact:* Aynsley Hamel, Program Coordinator, 410-706-0566, Fax: 410-706-6387, E-mail: ptadmissions@som.umaryland.edu.
Website: http://pt.umaryland.edu/pros.asp

University of Maryland Eastern Shore, Graduate Programs, Department of Rehabilitation Services, Princess Anne, MD 21853-1299. Offers rehabilitation counseling (MS). *Accreditation:* CORE. *Program availability:* Part-time, evening/ weekend. *Degree requirements:* For master's, internship. *Entrance requirements:* For master's, interview. Additional exam requirements/recommendations for international students: Required—TOEFL (minimum score 80 iBT). Electronic applications accepted. *Faculty research:* Long-term rehabilitation training.

University of Oklahoma Health Sciences Center, Graduate College, College of Allied Health, Department of Rehabilitation Sciences, Oklahoma City, OK 73190. Offers MS. *Degree requirements:* For master's, comprehensive exam, thesis optional. *Entrance requirements:* For master's, GRE General Test, 2 years of clinical experience, 3 letters of reference. Additional exam requirements/recommendations for international students: Required—TOEFL (minimum score 550 paper-based).

University of Ottawa, Faculty of Graduate and Postdoctoral Studies, Faculty of Health Sciences, School of Rehabilitation Sciences, Ottawa, ON K1N 6N5, Canada. Offers audiology (M Sc); orthophony (M Sc). *Program availability:* Part-time, evening/weekend. *Entrance requirements:* For master's, honors degree or equivalent, minimum B average. Electronic applications accepted.

University of Pittsburgh, School of Health and Rehabilitation Sciences, Master's Programs in Health and Rehabilitation Sciences, Pittsburgh, PA 15260. Offers health and rehabilitation sciences (MS), including health information systems, healthcare supervision and management, occupational therapy, physical therapy, rehabilitation counseling, rehabilitation science and technology, sports medicine, wellness and human performance. *Accreditation:* APTA. *Program availability:* Part-time, evening/weekend. *Faculty:* 32 full-time (21 women). *Students:* 111 full-time (73 women), 42 part-time (31 women); includes 23 minority (5 Black or African American, non-Hispanic/Latino; 8 Asian, non-Hispanic/Latino; 7 Hispanic/Latino; 3 Two or more races, non-Hispanic/ Latino), 65 international. Average age 29. 330 applicants, 66% accepted, 107 enrolled. In 2015, 89 master's awarded. *Degree requirements:* For master's, comprehensive exam (for some programs), thesis optional. *Entrance requirements:* For master's, minimum GPA of 3.0. Additional exam requirements/recommendations for international students: Required—TOEFL (minimum score 550 paper-based; 80 iBT), IELTS (minimum score 6.5). *Application deadline:* For fall admission, 3/1 for international students; for spring admission, 9/1 for international students. Applications are processed on a rolling basis. Application fee: $50. Electronic applications accepted. Tuition and fees vary according to program. *Financial support:* In 2015–16, 7 students received support, including 7 fellowships with full tuition reimbursements available (averaging $17,048 per year); traineeships also available. *Faculty research:* Assistive technology, seating and wheelchair mobility, cellular neurophysiology, low back syndrome, augmentative communication. *Total annual research expenditures:* $7.7 million. *Unit head:* Dr. Anthony Delitto, Dean, 412-383-6560, Fax: 412-383-6535, E-mail: delitto@ pitt.edu. *Application contact:* Jessica Maguire, Director of Admissions, 412-383-6557, Fax: 412-383-6535, E-mail: maguire@pitt.edu.

University of Pittsburgh, School of Health and Rehabilitation Sciences, PhD Program in Rehabilitation Science, Pittsburgh, PA 15260. Offers PhD. *Program availability:* Part-time. *Faculty:* 45 full-time (19 women). *Students:* 62 full-time (29 women), 5 part-time (3 women); includes 9 minority (4 Black or African American, non-Hispanic/Latino; 1 Asian, non-Hispanic/Latino; 2 Hispanic/Latino; 2 Two or more races, non-Hispanic/Latino), 30 international. Average age 33. 23 applicants, 35% accepted, 6 enrolled. In 2015, 11 doctorates awarded. *Degree requirements:* For doctorate, comprehensive exam, thesis/ dissertation. *Entrance requirements:* For doctorate, GRE General Test. Additional exam requirements/recommendations for international students: Required—TOEFL (minimum score 550 paper-based; 80 iBT), IELTS (minimum score 6.5). *Application deadline:* For fall admission, 3/1 for international students; for spring admission, 9/1 for international students; for summer admission, 2/1 for international students. Applications are processed on a rolling basis. Application fee: $50. Electronic applications accepted. Tuition and fees vary according to program. *Financial support:* In 2015–16, 35 students received support, including 2 fellowships with full tuition reimbursements available (averaging $21,232 per year), 31 research assistantships with full tuition reimbursements available (averaging $23,300 per year), 2 teaching assistantships with full tuition reimbursements available (averaging $26,159 per year); scholarships/grants, traineeships, and unspecified assistantships also available. *Faculty research:* Measurement and study of motion, balance disorders, human performance, neuropsychological parameters, telerehabilitation, wheelchair performance and design, injury prevention and treatment, nutrition, data mining. *Total annual research expenditures:* $11.1 million. *Unit head:* Dr. Kelley Fitzgerald, Associate Dean of Graduate Studies/Professor, 412-383-6643, Fax: 412-383-6613, E-mail: kfitzger@ pitt.edu. *Application contact:* Jessica Maguire, Director of Admissions, 412-383-6557, Fax: 412-383-6556, E-mail: maguire@pitt.edu.
Website: http://www.shrs.pitt.edu/PhDRS/

University of Pittsburgh, School of Health and Rehabilitation Sciences, Prosthetics and Orthotics Program, Pittsburgh, PA 15260. Offers MS. *Program availability:* Part-time. *Faculty:* 5 full-time (2 women), 6 part-time/adjunct (2 women). *Students:* 35 full-time (19 women), 1 (woman) part-time; includes 1 minority (Asian, non-Hispanic/Latino), 1 international. Average age 26. 126 applicants, 47% accepted, 20 enrolled. In 2015, 18 master's awarded. *Entrance requirements:* For master's, GRE General Test, volunteer experience in prosthetics and orthotics. Additional exam requirements/ recommendations for international students: Required—TOEFL (minimum score 550 paper-based; 80 iBT), IELTS (minimum score 6.5). *Application deadline:* For fall admission, 1/1 for domestic and international students. Applications are processed on a rolling basis. Application fee: $135. Electronic applications accepted. Tuition and fees vary according to program. *Unit head:* Dr. Rory Cooper, Department Chair/Professor, 412-383-6596, E-mail: rcooper@pitt.edu. *Application contact:* Meghan Wander, Academic Programs Coordinator, 412-624-6214, Fax: 412-624-6501, E-mail: mew135@ pitt.edu.
Website: http://www.shrs.pitt.edu/MSPO/

University of South Carolina, School of Medicine and The Graduate School, Graduate Programs in Medicine, Program in Rehabilitation Counseling, Columbia, SC 29208. Offers psychiatric rehabilitation (Certificate); rehabilitation counseling (MRC).

Accreditation: CORE. *Program availability:* Part-time, evening/weekend. *Degree requirements:* For master's, comprehensive exam, internship, practicum. *Entrance requirements:* For master's and Certificate, GRE General Test or GMAT. Electronic applications accepted. *Expenses:* Contact institution. *Faculty research:* Quality of life, alcohol dependency, technology for disabled, psychiatric rehabilitation, women with disabilities.

University of South Florida, Morsani College of Medicine, School of Physical Therapy, Tampa, FL 33620-9951. Offers physical therapy (DPT); rehabilitation sciences (PhD), including chronic disease, neuromusculoskeletal disability, physical therapy, veteran's health/reintegration. *Accreditation:* APTA. *Students:* 134 full-time (91 women), 1 part-time (0 women); includes 29 minority (6 Black or African American, non-Hispanic/Latino; 1 American Indian or Alaska Native, non-Hispanic/Latino; 9 Asian, non-Hispanic/Latino; 13 Hispanic/Latino). Average age 25. 1,300 applicants, 8% accepted, 48 enrolled. In 2015, 95 doctorates awarded. *Entrance requirements:* For doctorate, GRE General Test, bachelor's degree from regionally-accredited university with minimum GPA of 3.0 in all upper-division coursework; interview; at least 20 hours of documented volunteer or work experience in hospital outpatient/inpatient physical therapy settings; written personal statement of values and purpose for attending. Additional exam requirements/recommendations for international students: Required—TOEFL (minimum score 600 paper-based; 79 iBT). *Application deadline:* For fall admission, 9/1 for domestic students, 2/1 for international students. Application fee: $30. *Faculty research:* Veteran's reintegration and resilience, prosthetics and orthotics (microprocessor prosthetic knee), neuromusculoskeletal disorders (occupational ergonomics, fall risk and prevention, exercise adherence and compliance, and orthotic and prosthetic wear and use), human movement and function. *Total annual research expenditures:* $1 million. *Unit head:* Dr. William S. Quillen, Director, 813-974-9863, Fax: 813-974-8915, E-mail: wquillen@health.usf.edu. *Application contact:* Dr. Gina Maria Musolino, Associate Professor and Coordinator for Clinical Education, 813-974-2254, Fax: 813-974-8915, E-mail: gmusolin@health.usf.edu.
Website: http://health.usf.edu/medicine/dpt/index.htm

The University of Texas Medical Branch, Graduate School of Biomedical Sciences, Department of Preventive Medicine and Community Health, Galveston, TX 77555. Offers population health sciences (MS, PhD); public health (MPH); rehabilitation sciences (PhD). *Accreditation:* CEPH. *Degree requirements:* For master's, thesis; for doctorate, thesis/dissertation. *Entrance requirements:* For master's, GRE General Test or MAT; for doctorate, GRE General Test. Additional exam requirements/recommendations for international students: Required—TOEFL (minimum score 550 paper-based). Electronic applications accepted.

University of Toronto, Faculty of Medicine, Department of Rehabilitation Science, Toronto, ON M5S 1A1, Canada. Offers M Sc, PhD. *Degree requirements:* For master's, thesis. *Entrance requirements:* For master's, B Sc or equivalent; specialization in occupational therapy, physical therapy, or a related field; minimum B+ average in final 2 years. Additional exam requirements/recommendations for international students: Required—TOEFL (minimum score 580 paper-based; 93 iBT), TWE (minimum score 5). Electronic applications accepted.

University of Utah, Graduate School, College of Health, Department of Physical Therapy, Salt Lake City, UT 84108. Offers physical therapy (DPT); rehabilitation science (PhD). *Accreditation:* APTA. *Faculty:* 13 full-time (5 women), 14 part-time/adjunct (7 women). *Students:* 155 full-time (82 women), 3 part-time (all women); includes 20 minority (1 Black or African American, non-Hispanic/Latino; 1 American Indian or Alaska Native, non-Hispanic/Latino; 5 Asian, non-Hispanic/Latino; 6 Hispanic/Latino; 2 Native Hawaiian or other Pacific Islander, non-Hispanic/Latino; 5 Two or more races, non-Hispanic/Latino), 5 international. Average age 28. 437 applicants, 11% accepted, 48 enrolled. In 2015, 46 doctorates awarded. *Degree requirements:* For doctorate, thesis/dissertation. *Entrance requirements:* For doctorate, GRE, minimum GPA of 3.0, volunteer work, bachelor's degree. Additional exam requirements/recommendations for international students: Required—TOEFL (minimum score 90 iBT); Recommended—IELTS (minimum score 7). *Application deadline:* For fall admission, 10/3 priority date for domestic students, 10/3 for international students. Application fee: $55 ($65 for international students). Electronic applications accepted. *Expenses:* Contact institution. *Financial support:* In 2015–16, 29 students received support. Research assistantships with full tuition reimbursements available, teaching assistantships with full tuition reimbursements available, Federal Work-Study, scholarships/grants, tuition waivers (full), and unspecified assistantships available. Financial award application deadline: 10/1; financial award applicants required to submit FAFSA. *Faculty research:* Rehabilitation and Parkinson's disease, motor control and musculoskeletal dysfunction, burns/wound care, rehabilitation and multiple sclerosis, cancer. *Total annual research expenditures:* $600,129. *Unit head:* Dr. R. Scott Ward, Chair, 801-581-4895, E-mail: scott.ward@hsc.utah.edu. *Application contact:* Dee-Dee Darby-Duffin, Academic Advisor, 801-585-9510, E-mail: d.darby-duffin@hsc.utah.edu.
Website: http://www.health.utah.edu/pt

University of Washington, Graduate School, School of Medicine, Graduate Programs in Medicine, Department of Rehabilitation Medicine, Seattle, WA 98195-6490. Offers occupational therapy (MOT); physical therapy (DPT); prosthetics and orthotics (MPO); rehabilitation science (PhD). *Degree requirements:* For doctorate, comprehensive exam (for some programs), thesis/dissertation (for some programs). *Entrance requirements:* For master's and doctorate, GRE. Additional exam requirements/recommendations for international students: Required—TOEFL. *Faculty research:* Biomechanics, balance, brain injury, spinal cord injury, pain, degenerative diseases.

University of Wisconsin–La Crosse, College of Science and Health, Department of Exercise and Sport Science, Program in Clinical Exercise Physiology, La Crosse, WI 54601-3742. Offers MS. *Students:* 15 full-time (13 women), 1 (woman) part-time. Average age 23. 27 applicants, 56% accepted, 15 enrolled. In 2015, 15 master's awarded. *Degree requirements:* For master's, thesis optional. *Entrance requirements:* Additional exam requirements/recommendations for international students: Required—TOEFL (minimum score 550 paper-based; 79 iBT). *Application deadline:* For fall admission, 2/1 priority date for domestic and international students. Electronic applications accepted. *Financial support:* Federal Work-Study, scholarships/grants, health care benefits, and tuition waivers (partial) available. Support available to part-time students. Financial award application deadline: 3/15; financial award applicants required to submit FAFSA. *Unit head:* Dr. John Porcari, Director, 608-785-8684, Fax: 608-785-8686, E-mail: porcari.john@uwlax.edu. *Application contact:* Brandon Schaller, Senior Graduate Student Status Examiner, 608-785-8941, E-mail: admissions@uwlax.edu.
Website: http://www.uwlax.edu/sah/ess/cep/

Virginia Commonwealth University, Graduate School, School of Education, Department of Health and Human Performance, Program in Rehabilitation and Movement Science, Richmond, VA 23284-9005. Offers PhD. *Entrance requirements:* Additional exam requirements/recommendations for international students: Required—TOEFL (minimum score 600 paper-based; 100 iBT). Electronic applications accepted.

Washington University in St. Louis, School of Medicine, Program in Rehabilitation and Participation Science, St. Louis, MO 63130-4899. Offers PhD.

Western Michigan University, Graduate College, College of Health and Human Services, Department of Blindness and Low Vision Studies, Kalamazoo, MI 49008. Offers orientation and mobility (MA); orientation and mobility of children (MA); vision rehabilitation therapy (MA). *Accreditation:* CORE.

MILWAUKEE SCHOOL OF ENGINEERING
Master's Programs in Health Care Systems Management and Perfusion

Program of Study

The Milwaukee School of Engineering (MSOE) offers eleven master's degree programs.

A Master of Science in Nursing (M.S.N.) in Health Care Systems Management from MSOE, with its unique blend of nursing, business, and engineering concepts, equips graduates with the knowledge and skills necessary to function effectively in the health care environment. MSOE's M.S.N. program is based on the fact that nurses at mid-management and executive levels and nurse entrepreneurs must have the capacity to manage financial resources, analyze large data sets, manage human capital, understand complex organizational systems, and ensure quality and safety—all through the lens of nursing practice. The curriculum in the M.S.N. program meets this need by blending the expertise of the faculties of the School of Nursing and the Rader School of Business with the students' knowledge and experience. The M.S.N. in Health Care Systems Management is best described as a graduate degree in nursing, blended with business concepts.

The Master of Science in Perfusion (M.S.P.) prepares graduates to utilize their competencies in a hospital operating room. This profession requires the application of invasive surgical techniques, particularly in open-heart surgery. The M.S.P. is for full-time students only. Students start in September of each year and attend for six consecutive quarters. Upon completion of the M.S.P. program, students are eligible to sit for the Certified Clinical Perfusionist examination. The application deadline is December 15 each year for the classes that being the following September. Applications are considered until the class is full, after which applicants have the option of being considered for the waiting list as well as carrying over their application for the following year.

Research Facilities

MSOE's newest lab facility—the Ruehlow Nursing Complex—is a $3-million, 25,000-square-foot building that provides a home for the School of Nursing classrooms, labs, and faculty offices. The new space is nearly quadruple the size of the previous nursing labs, and allows faculty to enhance the already innovative education experience that is the hallmark of an MSOE education. The new nursing experiential learning and simulation center includes:

Simulation Labs: The Ruehlow Nursing Complex features four simulated hospital rooms that are connected by a central nurses station, similar to a hospital intensive care unit. The rooms feature call lights for the patients, who are high-fidelity manikins. The life-like manikins are driven by computer software that enables them to breathe, cough, talk, or change conditions based on what nursing professors have programmed. Simulations provide students with opportunities to communicate with patients, respond to patient needs, and witness the outcomes of their decision-making and clinical reasoning in a hospital-like setting.

A unique feature of the Ruehlow Nursing Complex is the direct linking of two classrooms to two simulation rooms. Students learn theoretical concepts in class and can immediately turn to the back of the classroom where an opened wall allows them to apply what they have just learned to the care of a patient in the simulated hospital.

The four simulation rooms and their patients are:

- CC-131 Sim Junior Manikin—Students learn to provide nursing care for a pediatric patient in an acute care environment. This patient might have acute or chronic health conditions.
- CC-132 Laboring Mom Manikin—Students learn to provide nursing care for a woman with maternal health needs. This mother may be in labor or delivering her baby.
- CC-133 Simman Classic Manikin—Students learn to provide nursing care for adults with acute and chronic conditions.
- CC-134 Simman Essential—This patient has an acute illness, and also can be transported into the classroom for the purposes of teaching and learning.

In two other laboratories, students experience situations regarding invasive procedures and advanced patient care.

Health Assessment Labs: In two state-of-the-art laboratories, students learn health assessment skills and about active integration of pharmacology with medication administration. These skills prepare sophomores for their first clinical experience with real patients.

Home Care Lab: The home care lab is set up like a handicap accessible studio apartment. It includes a kitchen area, table and chairs, living room furniture, a large screen TV, washer, dryer, and spacious bathroom with shower. Students take turns playing the role of the patient and teaching one another how to maneuver within the home with an illness. Students also learn how to use adaptive devices such as wheelchairs, walkers, and assistive devices within the home and simulate their patients' experience.

The center is not limited only to nursing students. Biomedical engineering, mechanical engineering, and industrial engineering students access the home care lab to test medical equipment and evaluate its technological fit and function in a patient's home. Graduate students in MSOE's perfusion program also access the simulation suite replicated as a hospital operating room.

Other Laboratories: There are more laboratories on the MSOE campus than classrooms. Information about the many other specialty labs can be found at http://www.msoe.edu/community/academics/labs/page/1464/academic-labs#sthash.ctBKYemR.dpuf

Applied Technology Center™ (ATC): This is the research arm of the university. It serves as a technology transfer catalyst among academia, business and industry, and governmental agencies. The close association between MSOE and the business and industrial community has long been one of the university's strengths; applied research serves as a renewable resource in this linkage. The ATC undertakes more than 250 company-sponsored projects per year that involve faculty, staff members, and students. Interdisciplinary capabilities provide a major advantage and can span fields such as engineering, science, health care, business, computers, and technical communication.

Financial Aid

Most graduate students receive some type of tuition reimbursement from their employers. For those students who do not have this benefit, several loan options may be available. Nonimmigrant alien graduate students are not eligible for federal or state financial assistance or MSOE loan money. MSOE offers a limited number of graduate research assistantships.

Milwaukee School of Engineering

Cost of Study

The 2016–17 tuition for all graduate programs is $760 per credit hour.

Living and Housing Costs

MSOE operates three on-campus residence halls. Although undergraduate students compose the largest segment of the resident population, the on-campus residence halls are an option for graduate students. The Housing Department can provide more information on what is available and how personal needs might be accommodated. Off-campus housing is available from the many independently owned rental units near the University.

Student Group

In fall 2015, MSOE had 2,939 full- and part-time students. Of these, 227 were graduate students. The majority of graduate students at MSOE have prior professional experience in their field.

Student areas on the campus offer the opportunity to engage in collaborative learning as well as an environment in which to socialize and relax. In addition to comfortable furniture, there is a Mondopad, which is a touch screen TV that allows for student computer use as a display screen for group work. The student area also has a refrigerator, microwave, and cabinets for storage of materials by the nursing student organizations.

Location

MSOE is located just a few blocks from Lake Michigan on the east side of downtown Milwaukee, which is approximately 90 miles north of Chicago. MSOE is in a vibrant downtown neighborhood in Milwaukee called East Town. There are countless activities within walking distance from campus including shopping, theaters, restaurants, professional sporting venues, and more.

The University

Milwaukee School of Engineering is an independent, nonprofit university with about 2,800 students that was founded in 1903. MSOE offers bachelor's and master's degrees in engineering, business, mathematics, and nursing. The university has a national academic reputation, longstanding ties to business and industry, dedicated professors with real-world experience, a 96 percent undergraduate placement rate, and the highest ROI and average starting and midcareer salaries of any Wisconsin university according to PayScale Inc. MSOE graduates are well-rounded, technologically experienced, and highly productive professionals and leaders.

The Faculty

MSOE's faculty focus is on teaching, both in the classroom and in its world-class research facilities. Unlike many educational institutions, MSOE does not utilize teaching assistants. MSOE has more than 200 full- and part-time faculty members. Small classes, a low 12:1 student-faculty ratio for undergraduate courses, and a 7:1 student-faculty ratio for graduate courses ensures that students receive personal attention.

Applying

Applicants can submit an application online for no cost at http://msoe.edu/apply.

General application requirements include an official transcript of all undergraduate and graduate course work, two or three letters of recommendation (depending on the program), and GMAT/GRE test scores, depending upon the program and/or undergraduate cumulative grade point average.

International students are required to submit additional documentation. Some programs may have additional requirements; program-specific details are available on MSOE's website.

Correspondence and Information

Graduate and Professional Education
Milwaukee School of Engineering
1025 North Broadway
Milwaukee, Wisconsin 53202-3109
United States
Phone: 800-321-6763 (toll-free)
E-mail: gpe@msoe.edu
Website: http://www.msoe.edu/graduate
Facebook: http://facebook.com/msoegpe
Twitter: http://twitter.com/msoegpe

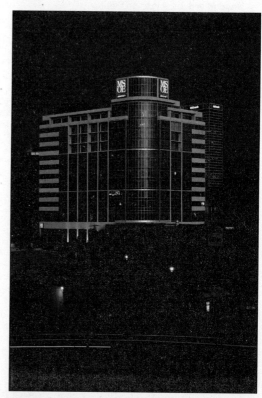

MSOE's new Grohmann Tower apartments, which opened in the fall of 2014.

PHILADELPHIA COLLEGE OF OSTEOPATHIC MEDICINE
Physician Assistant Program

 For more information, visit http://petersons.to/pcomphysicianassistant

Program of Study

The Physician Assistant (PA) Studies program is a twenty-six-month program that leads to a Master of Science degree in health sciences. Students are prepared for clinical practice, using a variety of learning strategies: formal lectures, practical laboratory classes, and clinical education. Students develop patient communication skills and advanced clinical problem-solving skills in addition to acquiring technical proficiency in areas related to professional practice. The program is highly intensive. Most of the program is provided by experienced physician assistants with clinical backgrounds in multiple specialties.

The Physician Assistant Studies program at PCOM provides students with the ability to positively affect the lives of their patients, their families, their employers, and their communities. Students become lifelong learners, developing a baseline of analytic and critical thinking skills that prepare them for the challenges of caring for the entire patient, young or old, from the emergency room to the operating room.

Accreditation

The Accreditation Review Commission on Education for the Physician Assistant (ARC-PA) has granted Accreditation-Continued status to the Philadelphia College of Osteopathic Medicine Physician Assistant Program in Philadelphia, Pennsylvania and approved a distant campus in Suwanee, Georgia. Both the main campus and distant campus programs are sponsored by Philadelphia College of Osteopathic Medicine. Accreditation-Continued is an accreditation status granted when a currently accredited program is in compliance with the ARC-PA Standards.

Accreditation remains in effect until the program closes or withdraws from the accreditation process or until accreditation is withdrawn for failure to comply with the Standards. The approximate date for the next validation review of the program by the ARC-PA is March 2018. The review date is contingent upon continued compliance with the Accreditation Standards and ARC-PA policy.

Research Facilities

PCOM's libraries feature both a well-developed collection of medical journals and texts and new capabilities for access to online medical references and Internet searching in a facility that provides individual student stations, Internet terminals, advanced audiovisual resources, and a large student computer lab.

Financial Aid

The Financial Aid Office at PCOM offers financial assistance to students through the Federal Direct Loan program, institutional grants, and various alternative private loan programs.

Cost of Study

In 2016–17, the tuition for the entire PCOM Physician Assistant Studies program is $88,633.

Living and Housing Costs

Students live off campus within the Philadelphia, Pennsylvania and Suwanee, Georgia metropolitan and suburban areas, as there is no on-campus housing. Room and board costs vary by each student's individual preferences.

Student Group

Admission to the PA Studies program is competitive and selective. The Faculty Committee on Admissions looks for academically and socially well-rounded individuals who are committed to caring for patients. The class of 2018 for the Philadelphia campus totals 55 students, 46 women and 9 men, ranging in age from 21 to 32. Twenty-one percent of the class reports their ethnicity to be Hispanic, Asian Indian, Black/African American, South or Central American, Korean, Peruvian, and Cuban. Thirty were residents of Pennsylvania. Twelve were residents of Georgia. The average GPA of the entering class was 3.73. The class of 2018 for the Georgia campus totals 20 students, 17 women and 3 men, ranging in age from 21 to 35. Thirty-five percent of the class reports their ethnicity to be Hispanic/Latino, South or Central American, Chinese, Black/African American, Korean, Hmong, Thai, and Vietnamese.

Location

Philadelphia College of Osteopathic Medicine is one of the largest of thirty-three osteopathic colleges in the United States, with campuses in both Philadelphia, Pennsylvania and Suwanee, Georgia. The Physician Assistant Studies program is offered on both the Philadelphia, Pennsylvania and Suwanee, Georgia campuses. PCOM's facilities include large lecture halls, small classrooms, labs for teaching, clinical skills, robotic and human actor simulation, and research, a state-of-the-art library, and scenic landscaping, all in a suburban setting.

The College

PCOM, chartered in 1899, enrolls approximately 2,800 students in its various programs across both campuses, and is committed to educating community-responsive, primary-care–oriented physicians and physician assistants to practice medicine in the twenty-first century. Supported by the latest in medical and educational technology, PCOM emphasizes treating the whole person, not merely the symptoms. Students have a committed, professional, humanistic faculty who are leaders in the osteopathic and physician assistant national health-care community. The PA Studies program provides a thorough foundation in health-care delivery that focuses on comprehensive, humanistic health care.

Applying

Selection for the Physician Assistant Studies program is very competitive. Applicants must complete a baccalaureate degree at a regionally accredited college or university in the United States, Canada, or the United Kingdom with a minimum science and cumulative GPA of 3.0 (on a 4.0 scale as calculated by CASPA), document in their CASPA application 200 hours of experience in volunteer or employment in or related to the health-care industry, and fulfill the following course requirements: five semesters of biology, three semesters of chemistry, one semester of physics or another health related science, two semesters of mathematics, and three semesters of social science courses. All requirements must have been completed within the last ten years, unless the applicant has completed an advanced degree or has extensive experience in the field of patient care. Applications are not accepted from graduates of medical schools. Selected applicants are invited to interview on campus. Application and deadline information is available online at http://www.caspaonline.org and http://admissions.pcom.edu/app-process/physician-assistant-studies-ms/.

In addition to admission through the standard application process, there is also one 5-year cooperative program between Philadelphia College of Osteopathic Medicine (PCOM) and University of the Sciences in Philadelphia. The programs consist of two distinct phases: the preprofessional phase and the professional phase. After successful completion of the fourth year, students earn a B.S. in health science from

University of the Sciences and an M.S. from PCOM after completion of the fifth year. The B.S. degree does not qualify the student as a PA. Students must complete the entire professional phase of the program (years four and five) and obtain an M.S. from PCOM to become eligible to be certified as a PA. PCOM has the ultimate responsibility for granting the M.S. degree. Applicants from institutions without cooperative agreements are certainly admitted into each entering class as affiliation agreement students are not provided preferential admission.

Correspondence and Information

Philadelphia College of Osteopathic Medicine
Office of Admissions
4170 City Avenue
Philadelphia, Pennsylvania 19131
Phone: 800-999-6998 (toll-free)
      215-871-6700 (local)
Fax: 215-871-6719
E-mail: admissions@pcom.edu

Georgia Campus—Philadelphia College of Osteopathic Medicine
Office of Admissions
625 Old Peachtree Road
Suwanee, Georgia 30024
Phone: 866-282-4544 (toll-free)
      678-225-7500 (local)
Fax: 678-225-7509
E-mail: GAAdmissions@pcom.edu

THE FACULTY AND THEIR RESEARCH

Full-Time Faculty

Gregory McDonald, D.O., Philadelphia College of Osteopathic Medicine. Medical Director, Department of Physician Assistant Studies. Pathology.

John Cavenagh, Ph.D., Union (Ohio); PA-C. Professor, Department of Physician Assistant Studies. Emergency medicine.

Jill Cunningham, M.H.S., Drexel; PA-C. Assistant Professor, Department of Physician Assistant Studies. Internal medicine.

Sean Guinane, D.H.Sc., A. T. Still; PA-C. Assistant Professor, Director of Outcomes, Assessment, and Technology, Department of Physician Assistant Studies. Family medicine.

Paul Krajewski, M.S., Philadelphia College of Osteopathic Medicine; PA-C. Associate Professor, Director of Clinical Studies, Department of Physician Assistant Studies. Orthopedic surgery, emergency medicine.

Kate Laramie, M.H.S., Drexel; PA-C, Assistant Professor, Department of Physician Assistant Studies. Emergency medicine.

Laura Levy, D.H.Sc., A. T. Still; PA-C. Professor, Chair, Department of Physician Assistant Studies. Family medicine, women's health.

Nancy E. McLaughlin, M.H.A., D.H.Sc., Nova Southeastern; PA-C. Associate Professor, Assistant Program Director, and Georgia Campus Site Director, Department of Physician Assistant Studies. Surgical medicine, orthopedics, ophthalmology.

Emily McSparin, M.P.A., Eastern Virginia Medical School, PA-C. Assistant Professor, Department of Physician assistant Studies. OB/GYN, internal medicine.

Christine Mount, M.S., University of Medicine and Dentistry of New Jersey; PA-C. Assistant Professor, Department of Physician Assistant Studies. Neurology, emergency medicine, trauma.

Carrie Smith-Nold, M.P.A., Medical College of Georgia; PA-C. Assistant Professor, Department of Physician Assistant Studies. Neurology.

Rebekah Thomas, Pharm.D., M.P.A., Drake; PA-C, BCPS, BC-ADM. Assistant Professor, Department of Physician Assistant Studies. Pharmacology, endocrinology, internal medicine.

Adjunct Faculty

Patrick Auth, Ph.D., Drexel; PA-C. Emergency medicine, orthopedics.

Thomas Abelew, Ph.D., UCLA. Anatomy.

Christopher Brandon, Ph.D., Georgia. Physiology.

Robert Cuzzolino, Ed.D., Temple. Academic policy.

Jeff Gutting, M.S., Philadelphia College of Osteopathic Medicine; PA-C. Cardiology.

Fred Katz, D.O., Des Moines University. Radiology.

Michael Kirifides, Ph.D., Maryland. Human physiology.

Brian Levine, M.D., Vermont. Emergency medicine.

Amanda Murphy, M.S., Philadelphia College of Osteopathic Medicine; PA-C. Dermatology.

Joseph Norris, M.S., D.C., Philadelphia College of Osteopathic Medicine; PA-C. Family medicine.

Richard Pascucci, D.O., Philadelphia College of Osteopathic Medicine; FACOI. Rheumatology.

Margaret Reinhart, M.M.A.; M.T., Penn State; ASCP. Laboratory diagnostics.

Gretchen Reynolds, M.S., Philadelphia College of Osteopathic Medicine; PA-C. Occupational health.

Lauren Tavani, M.S., Philadelphia College of Osteopathic Medicine; PA-C. Critical care.

Rosemary Vickers, D.O., Philadelphia College of Osteopathic Medicine. Pediatrics.

Tracy Offerdahl, Pharm.D., Temple. Pharmacology.

PCOM provides a collaborative learning environment for students.

Section 21
Health Sciences

This section contains a directory of institutions offering graduate work in health sciences. Additional information about programs listed in the directory may be obtained by writing directly to the dean of a graduate school or chair of a department at the address given in the directory.

For programs offering related work, see also in this book *Biological and Biomedical Sciences, Biophysics (Radiation Biology), Dentistry and Dental Sciences, Health Services, Medicine, Nursing,* and *Public Health.* In the other guides in this series:

Graduate Programs in the Physical Sciences, Mathematics, Agricultural Sciences, the Environment & Natural Resources
See *Physics*

Graduate Programs in Engineering & Applied Sciences
See *Agricultural Engineering and Bioengineering (Bioengineering), Biomedical Engineering and Biotechnology,* and *Energy and Power Engineering (Nuclear Engineering)*

CONTENTS

Program Directories

Health Physics/Radiological Health

East Carolina University, Graduate School, Thomas Harriot College of Arts and Sciences, Department of Physics, Greenville, NC 27858-4353. Offers applied physics (MS); biomedical physics (PhD); health physics (MS); medical physics (MS). *Program availability:* Part-time. *Students:* 28 full-time (5 women), 8 part-time (3 women); includes 10 minority (4 Black or African American, non-Hispanic/Latino; 3 Asian, non-Hispanic/Latino; 1 Hispanic/Latino; 2 Two or more races, non-Hispanic/Latino), 5 international. Average age 29. 48 applicants, 60% accepted, 8 enrolled. In 2015, 6 master's, 1 doctorate awarded. *Degree requirements:* For master's, one foreign language, comprehensive exam. *Entrance requirements:* For master's, GRE General Test. Additional exam requirements/recommendations for international students: Required—TOEFL. *Application deadline:* Applications are processed on a rolling basis. Application fee: $50. *Financial support:* Research assistantships with partial tuition reimbursements, teaching assistantships with partial tuition reimbursements, and Federal Work-Study available. Support available to part-time students. Financial award application deadline: 6/1. *Unit head:* Dr. John Sutherland, Chair, 252-328-6739, E-mail: sutherlandj@ecu.edu. *Application contact:* Dean of Graduate School, 252-328-6012, Fax: 252-328-6071, E-mail: gradschool@ecu.edu.
Website: http://www.ecu.edu/cs-cas/physics/Graduate-Program.cfm#

Georgetown University, Graduate School of Arts and Sciences, Department of Health Physics and Radiation Protection, Washington, DC 20057. Offers health physics (MS); nuclear nonproliferation (MS). *Degree requirements:* For master's, thesis. *Entrance requirements:* Additional exam requirements/recommendations for international students: Required—TOEFL.

Georgia Institute of Technology, Graduate Studies, College of Engineering, George W. Woodruff School of Mechanical Engineering, Nuclear and Radiological Engineering and Medical Physics Programs, Atlanta, GA 30332-0001. Offers medical physics (MS, MSMP); nuclear and radiological engineering (PhD); nuclear engineering (MSNE). *Program availability:* Part-time, online learning. Terminal master's awarded for partial completion of doctoral program. *Degree requirements:* For master's, thesis optional; for doctorate, comprehensive exam, thesis/dissertation. *Entrance requirements:* For master's and doctorate, GRE General Test, minimum GPA of 3.0. Additional exam requirements/recommendations for international students: Required—TOEFL (minimum score 580 paper-based; 94 iBT). *Application deadline:* For fall admission, 2/1 priority date for domestic and international students; for spring admission, 10/1 priority date for domestic and international students; for summer admission, 2/1 for domestic and international students. Applications are processed on a rolling basis. Application fee: $75. Electronic applications accepted. *Financial support:* Fellowships, research assistantships with tuition reimbursements, teaching assistantships with tuition reimbursements, career-related internships or fieldwork, Federal Work-Study, institutionally sponsored loans, traineeships, tuition waivers (partial), and unspecified assistantships available. Support available to part-time students. Financial award application deadline: 5/1. *Faculty research:* Reactor physics, nuclear materials, plasma physics, radiation detection, radiological assessment.
Website: http://www.nre.gatech.edu

Idaho State University, Office of Graduate Studies, College of Science and Engineering, Department of Physics, Pocatello, ID 83209-8106. Offers applied physics (PhD); health physics (MS); physics (MNS). *Program availability:* Part-time. *Degree requirements:* For master's, comprehensive exam, thesis (for some programs), oral exam (for some programs); for doctorate, comprehensive exam, thesis/dissertation (for some programs), oral exam, written qualifying exam in physics or health physics after 1st year. *Entrance requirements:* For master's, GRE General Test, 3 letters of recommendation, BS or BA in physics, teaching certificate (MNS); for doctorate, GRE General Test (minimum 50th percentile), 3 letters of recommendation, statement of career goals. Additional exam requirements/recommendations for international students: Required—TOEFL (minimum score 550 paper-based; 80 iBT). Electronic applications accepted. *Faculty research:* Ion beam applications, low-energy nuclear physics, relativity and cosmology, observational astronomy.

Illinois Institute of Technology, Graduate College, College of Science, Department of Physics, Chicago, IL 60616. Offers applied physics (MS); health physics (MAS); physics (MS, PhD). *Program availability:* Part-time, evening/weekend, online learning. Terminal master's awarded for partial completion of doctoral program. *Degree requirements:* For master's, comprehensive exam (for some programs), thesis (for some programs); for doctorate, comprehensive exam, thesis/dissertation. *Entrance requirements:* For master's, GRE General Test (minimum score 295 Quantitative and Verbal, 2.5 Analytical Writing), minimum undergraduate GPA of 3.0; for doctorate, GRE General Test (minimum score 310 Quantitative and Verbal, 3.0 Analytical Writing); GRE Subject Test in physics (strongly recommended), minimum undergraduate GPA of 3.0. Additional exam requirements/recommendations for international students: Required—TOEFL (minimum score 550 paper-based; 80 iBT). Electronic applications accepted. *Faculty research:* Elementary particle physics, condensed matter, superconductivity, experimental and computational biophysics.

McMaster University, School of Graduate Studies, Faculty of Science, Department of Medical Physics and Applied Radiation Sciences, Hamilton, ON L8S 4M2, Canada. Offers health and radiation physics (M Sc); medical physics (M Sc, PhD). *Program availability:* Part-time. *Degree requirements:* For master's, thesis or alternative. *Entrance requirements:* For master's, minimum B+ average. Additional exam requirements/recommendations for international students: Required—TOEFL (minimum score 550 paper-based). *Faculty research:* Imaging, toxicology, dosimetry, body composition, medical lasers.

Midwestern State University, Billie Doris McAda Graduate School, Robert D. and Carol Gunn College of Health Sciences and Human Services, Program in Radiologic Sciences, Wichita Falls, TX 76308. Offers MS. *Program availability:* Part-time, evening/weekend, online learning. *Degree requirements:* For master's, comprehensive exam, thesis optional. *Entrance requirements:* For master's, GRE General Test, MAT or GMAT, credentials in one of the medical imaging modalities or radiation therapy; 1 year of experience; 3 letters of recommendation from past and/or present educators and employers. Additional exam requirements/recommendations for international students: Required—TOEFL (minimum score 550 paper-based). Electronic applications accepted. *Faculty research:* Bone densitometry, radiologic dose trends, teaching of radiologic science, radiographic positioning landmarks.

Northwestern State University of Louisiana, Graduate Studies and Research, College of Nursing and School of Allied Health, Department of Radiologic Sciences, Natchitoches, LA 71497. Offers MS. *Degree requirements:* For master's, comprehensive exam, thesis (for some programs). *Entrance requirements:* Additional exam requirements/recommendations for international students: Required—TOEFL. Electronic applications accepted.

Oregon State University, College of Engineering, Program in Radiation Health Physics, Corvallis, OR 97331. Offers MHP, MS, PhD. *Program availability:* Part-time, blended/hybrid learning. *Faculty:* 12 full-time (4 women), 1 part-time/adjunct (0 women). *Students:* 16 full-time (4 women), 46 part-time (19 women); includes 6 minority (1 Black or African American, non-Hispanic/Latino; 1 Asian, non-Hispanic/Latino; 2 Hispanic/Latino; 2 Two or more races, non-Hispanic/Latino), 87 international. Average age 34. 67 applicants, 54% accepted, 25 enrolled. In 2015, 15 master's, 1 doctorate awarded. *Degree requirements:* For master's, thesis. *Entrance requirements:* For master's and doctorate, GRE. Additional exam requirements/recommendations for international students: Required—TOEFL (minimum score 80 iBT), IELTS (minimum score 6.5). *Application deadline:* For fall admission, 2/1 priority date for domestic and international students. Application fee: $75 ($85 for international students). *Expenses:* $14,130 full-time resident tuition, $22,932 full-time non-resident tuition, $1,572 fees. *Financial support:* Fellowships, research assistantships, teaching assistantships, and institutionally sponsored loans available. Support available to part-time students. Financial award application deadline: 2/1. *Faculty research:* Radioactive material transport, research reactor health physics, radiation instrumentation, radiation shielding, environmental monitoring. *Unit head:* Dr. Kathryn Higley, Department Head/Professor. *Application contact:* Radiation Health Physics Advisor, 541-737-2343, E-mail: nuc_engr@ne.oregonstate.edu.
Website: http://ne.oregonstate.edu/health-physics-program

Purdue University, Graduate School, College of Health and Human Sciences, School of Health Sciences, West Lafayette, IN 47907. Offers health physics (MS, PhD); medical physics (MS, PhD); occupational and environmental health science (MS, PhD), including aerosol deposition and lung disease, ergonomics, exposure and risk assessment, indoor air quality and bioaerosols (PhD), liver/lung toxicology; radiation biology (PhD); toxicology (PhD); MS/PhD. *Program availability:* Part-time. *Degree requirements:* For master's, thesis optional; for doctorate, one foreign language, thesis/dissertation. *Entrance requirements:* For master's and doctorate, GRE General Test, minimum undergraduate GPA of 3.0 or equivalent. Additional exam requirements/recommendations for international students: Required—TOEFL (minimum score 550 paper-based; 77 iBT); Recommended—TWE. Electronic applications accepted. *Faculty research:* Environmental toxicology, industrial hygiene, radiation dosimetry.

Quinnipiac University, School of Health Sciences, Program for Radiologist Assistant, Hamden, CT 06518-1940. Offers MHS. *Faculty:* 1 full-time (0 women), 3 part-time/adjunct (2 women). *Students:* 4 full-time (3 women), 1 (woman) part-time; includes 2 minority (1 Black or African American, non-Hispanic/Latino; 1 Asian, non-Hispanic/Latino). 6 applicants, 83% accepted, 4 enrolled. In 2015, 5 master's awarded. *Entrance requirements:* For master's, proof of certification from American Registry of Radiologic Technologists; 2000 hours of direct patient care; CPR certification. Additional exam requirements/recommendations for international students: Required—TOEFL (minimum score 575 paper-based; 90 iBT), IELTS (minimum score 6.5). *Application deadline:* For summer admission, 4/30 priority date for domestic students, 4/30 for international students. Applications are processed on a rolling basis. Application fee: $45. Electronic applications accepted. *Expenses:* $985 per credit tuition; $360 per semester student fee; $340 per semester (fall/spring) technology and lab fee; $75 per semester summer technology and lab fee. *Financial support:* Scholarships/grants and unspecified assistantships available. Financial award application deadline: 5/1; financial award applicants required to submit FAFSA. *Faculty research:* Curriculum development, assessment of student learning, radiation safety. *Unit head:* John Candler, Director, 203-582-6205, E-mail: john.candler@quinnipiac.edu. *Application contact:* Office of Graduate Admissions, 800-462-1944, Fax: 203-582-3443, E-mail: graduate@quinnipiac.edu.
Website: http://www.quinnipiac.edu/gradradiologistasst

Rutgers University–Newark, School of Health Related Professions, Department of Medical Imaging Sciences, Newark, NJ 07102. Offers radiologist assistant (MS). *Program availability:* Part-time, evening/weekend. *Entrance requirements:* For master's, BS with minimum GPA of 3.0, RT license, coursework in intro to pathopsychology, interview, all transcripts, personal statement, BCLS certification. Additional exam requirements/recommendations for international students: Required—TOEFL (minimum score 500 paper-based; 79 iBT). Electronic applications accepted.

San Diego State University, Graduate and Research Affairs, College of Sciences, Department of Physics, Program in Radiological Physics, San Diego, CA 92182. Offers MS. *Program availability:* Part-time. *Degree requirements:* For master's, thesis optional, oral or written exam. *Entrance requirements:* For master's, GRE General Test, GRE Subject Test (physics), 2 letters of recommendation. Additional exam requirements/recommendations for international students: Required—TOEFL. Electronic applications accepted. *Faculty research:* Computational radiological physics, medical physics.

Texas A&M University, College of Engineering, Department of Nuclear Engineering, College Station, TX 77843. Offers health physics (MS); nuclear engineering (M Eng, MS, PhD). *Faculty:* 16. *Students:* 115 full-time (19 women), 33 part-time (5 women); includes 35 minority (5 Black or African American, non-Hispanic/Latino; 1 American Indian or Alaska Native, non-Hispanic/Latino; 6 Asian, non-Hispanic/Latino; 21 Hispanic/Latino; 2 Two or more races, non-Hispanic/Latino), 28 international. Average age 27. 127 applicants, 45% accepted, 23 enrolled. In 2015, 24 master's, 13 doctorates awarded. *Degree requirements:* For master's, thesis or alternative; for doctorate, thesis/dissertation, departmental qualifying exams. *Entrance requirements:* For master's and doctorate, GRE General Test, 3 letters of recommendation. Additional exam requirements/recommendations for international students: Required—TOEFL (minimum score 550 paper-based; 80 iBT), IELTS (minimum score 6), PTE (minimum score 53). *Application deadline:* For fall admission, 3/1 for domestic and international students; for spring admission, 8/1 for domestic and international students. Applications are processed on a rolling basis. Application fee: $50 ($90 for international students). Electronic applications accepted. *Expenses:* Contact institution. *Financial support:* In 2015–16, 125 students received support, including 15 fellowships with tuition reimbursements available (averaging $26,334 per year), 72 research assistantships with tuition reimbursements available (averaging $8,592 per year), 16 teaching assistantships with tuition reimbursements available (averaging $9,163 per year); career-related internships or fieldwork, institutionally sponsored loans, scholarships/grants, traineeships, health care benefits, tuition waivers (full and partial), and unspecified assistantships also available. Support available to part-time students. Financial award application deadline: 3/15; financial award applicants required to submit FAFSA. *Unit head:* Dr. Yassin A. Hassan, Head, 979-845-7090, E-mail: y-hassan@tamu.edu. *Application contact:* Robb Jenson, Graduate Program Coordinator, 979-458-2072, E-mail: robb.jenson@tamu.edu.
Website: https://engineering.tamu.edu/nuclear

Thomas Jefferson University, Jefferson School of Health Professions, Department of Radiologic Sciences, Philadelphia, PA 19107. Offers radiologic and imaging sciences (MS). *Students:* 13 full-time (7 women), 3 part-time (2 women); includes 5 minority (3 Black or African American, non-Hispanic/Latino; 1 Asian, non-Hispanic/Latino; 1 Hispanic/Latino). Average age 32. 22 applicants, 64% accepted, 9 enrolled. In 2015, 23 master's awarded. *Entrance requirements:* Additional exam requirements/recommendations for international students: Required—TOEFL. *Application deadline:* For fall admission, 7/15 for domestic students. Applications are processed on a rolling basis. Application fee: $95. Electronic applications accepted. *Expenses:* $35,220 per year. *Financial support:* Scholarships/grants available. Financial award application deadline: 4/1; financial award applicants required to submit FAFSA. *Unit head:* Frances H. Gilman, Chair, 215-503-1865, E-mail: frances.gilman@jefferson.edu. *Application contact:* Dave Wood, Associate Director of Admission, 215-503-9847, Fax: 215-503-7241, E-mail: jshpadmissions@jefferson.edu.
Website: http://www.jefferson.edu/health_professions/departments/radiologic_sciences/

Université Laval, Faculty of Medicine, Post-Professional Programs in Medical Studies, Québec, QC G1K 7P4, Canada. Offers anatomy–pathology (DESS); anesthesiology (DESS); cardiology (DESS); care of older people (Diploma); clinical research (DESS); community health (DESS); dermatology (DESS); diagnostic radiology (DESS); emergency medicine (Diploma); family medicine (DESS); general surgery (DESS); geriatrics (DESS); hematology (DESS); internal medicine (DESS); maternal and fetal medicine (Diploma); medical biochemistry (DESS); medical microbiology and infectious diseases (DESS); medical oncology (DESS); nephrology (DESS); neurology (DESS); neurosurgery (DESS); obstetrics and gynecology (DESS); ophthalmology (DESS); orthopedic surgery (DESS); oto-rhino-laryngology (DESS); palliative medicine (Diploma); pediatrics (DESS); plastic surgery (DESS); psychiatry (DESS); pulmonary medicine (DESS); radiology–oncology (DESS); thoracic surgery (DESS); urology (DESS). *Degree requirements:* For other advanced degree, comprehensive exam. *Entrance requirements:* For degree, knowledge of French. Electronic applications accepted.

University of Alberta, Faculty of Medicine and Dentistry and Faculty of Graduate Studies and Research, Graduate Programs in Medicine, Department of Radiology and Diagnostic Imaging, Edmonton, AB T6G 2E1, Canada. Offers medical sciences (PhD); radiology and diagnostic imaging (M Sc). Terminal master's awarded for partial completion of doctoral program. *Degree requirements:* For master's, thesis; for doctorate, thesis/dissertation. *Entrance requirements:* For master's, minimum GPA of 6.5 on a 9.0 scale; for doctorate, M Sc. *Faculty research:* Spectroscopic attenuation correction, nuclear medicine technology, monoclonal antibody labeling, bone mineral analysis using ultrasound.

University of Arkansas for Medical Sciences, College of Health Professions, Little Rock, AR 72205-7199. Offers audiology (Au D); communication sciences and disorders (MS, PhD); genetic counseling (MS); nuclear medicine advanced associate (MIS); physician assistant studies (MPAS); radiologist assistant (MIS). PhD offered through consortium with University of Arkansas at Little Rock and University of Central Arkansas. *Program availability:* Part-time, online learning. *Degree requirements:* For master's, thesis (for some programs); for doctorate, comprehensive exam (for some programs), thesis/dissertation (for some programs). *Entrance requirements:* For master's, GRE. Additional exam requirements/recommendations for international students: Required—TOEFL (minimum score 550 paper-based; 79 iBT). Electronic applications accepted. *Expenses:* Contact institution. *Faculty research:* Auditory-based intervention, soy diet, nutrition and cancer.

University of Cincinnati, Graduate School, College of Medicine, Graduate Programs in Biomedical Sciences, Department of Radiology, Cincinnati, OH 45267. Offers medical physics (MS). *Program availability:* Part-time. *Degree requirements:* For master's, comprehensive exam, project. *Entrance requirements:* For master's, GRE General Test. Additional exam requirements/recommendations for international students: Required—TOEFL (minimum score 575 paper-based). Electronic applications accepted. *Faculty research:* Radiation oncology, radiologic imaging, dosimetry, radiation biology, radiation therapy.

University of Kentucky, Graduate School, Graduate School Programs from the College of Medicine, Program in Radiation Sciences, Lexington, KY 40506-0032. Offers MSRMP. *Program availability:* Part-time. *Degree requirements:* For master's, comprehensive exam, thesis. *Entrance requirements:* For master's, GRE General Test, minimum undergraduate GPA of 2.75. Additional exam requirements/recommendations for international students: Required—TOEFL (minimum score 550 paper-based). Electronic applications accepted. *Faculty research:* Dosimetry, manpower studies, diagnostic imaging physics, shielding.

University of Massachusetts Lowell, College of Sciences, Department of Physics, Program in Radiological Sciences and Protection, Lowell, MA 01854. Offers MS, PSM. *Degree requirements:* For master's, one foreign language, thesis. *Entrance requirements:* For master's, GRE General Test, 3 letters of reference. Additional exam requirements/recommendations for international students: Required—TOEFL. *Application deadline:* For fall admission, 4/1 for domestic students; for spring admission, 10/1 for domestic students. Applications are processed on a rolling basis. Application fee: $20 ($35 for international students). Electronic applications accepted. *Expenses:* Tuition, state resident: full-time $14,304. Tuition, nonresident: full-time $25,853. *Required fees:* $375. Full-time tuition and fees vary according to campus/location and reciprocity agreements. *Financial support:* Fellowships with tuition reimbursements, research assistantships with tuition reimbursements, teaching assistantships with tuition reimbursements, career-related internships or fieldwork, Federal Work-Study, institutionally sponsored loans, scholarships/grants, and traineeships available. Support available to part-time students. Financial award application deadline: 4/1.

University of Michigan, College of Engineering, Department of Nuclear Engineering and Radiological Sciences, Ann Arbor, MI 48109. Offers nuclear engineering (Nuc E); nuclear engineering and radiological sciences (MSE, PhD); nuclear science (MS, PhD). *Students:* 123 full-time (23 women). 134 applicants, 43% accepted, 32 enrolled. In 2015, 27 master's, 19 doctorates awarded. Terminal master's awarded for partial completion of doctoral program. *Degree requirements:* For master's, thesis optional; for doctorate, thesis/dissertation, oral defense of dissertation, preliminary exams. *Entrance requirements:* For master's and doctorate, GRE General Test. Additional exam requirements/recommendations for international students: Required—TOEFL (minimum score 560 paper-based). *Application deadline:* Applications are processed on a rolling basis. Electronic applications accepted. *Financial support:* Fellowships, research assistantships, teaching assistantships, career-related internships or fieldwork, institutionally sponsored loans, scholarships/grants, traineeships, health care benefits, and unspecified assistantships available. *Faculty research:* Radiation safety, environmental sciences, medical physics, fission systems and radiation transport, materials, plasmas and fusion, radiation measurements and imaging. *Total annual research expenditures:* $16.5 million. *Unit head:* Dr. Ronald Gilgenbach, Chair, 734-763-1261, Fax: 734-763-4540, E-mail: rongilg@umich.edu. *Application contact:* Peggy Jo Gramer, Graduate Program Coordinator, 734-615-8810, Fax: 734-763-4540, E-mail: ners-grad-admissions@umich.edu.
Website: http://www.engin.umich.edu/ners

University of Missouri, School of Health Professions, Department of Clinical and Diagnostic Sciences, Columbia, MO 65211. Offers diagnostic medical ultrasound (MHS). *Entrance requirements:* Additional exam requirements/recommendations for international students: Required—TOEFL (minimum score 500 paper-based; 61 iBT). *Application deadline:* For fall admission, 12/1 priority date for domestic and international students; for winter admission, 10/15 for domestic students. Applications are processed on a rolling basis. Application fee: $55 ($75 for international students). Electronic applications accepted.
Website: http://shp.missouri.edu/cds/index.php

University of Nevada, Las Vegas, Graduate College, School of Allied Health Sciences, Department of Health Physics and Diagnostic Sciences, Las Vegas, NV 89154-3037. Offers MS, DMP, PhD, Advanced Certificate. *Accreditation:* ABET. *Program availability:* Part-time. *Students:* 12 full-time (4 women), 5 part-time (1 woman); includes 7 minority (1 Black or African American, non-Hispanic/Latino; 1 Asian, non-Hispanic/Latino; 3 Hispanic/Latino; 2 Two or more races, non-Hispanic/Latino), 2 international. Average age 29. 15 applicants, 73% accepted, 6 enrolled. In 2015, 3 master's awarded. *Degree requirements:* For master's, thesis, professional paper, oral exam; for doctorate, comprehensive exam (for some programs), thesis/dissertation. *Entrance requirements:* For master's and doctorate, GRE General Test. Additional exam requirements/recommendations for international students: Required—TOEFL (minimum score 550 paper-based; 80 iBT), IELTS (minimum score 7). *Application deadline:* For fall admission, 6/15 for domestic students, 5/1 for international students; for spring admission, 11/15 for domestic students, 10/1 for international students. Application fee: $60 ($95 for international students). Electronic applications accepted. *Expenses:* $264 per credit state resident full-time and part-time; $6,955 per semester, $264 per credit nonresident full-time; $555 per credit nonresident part-time. *Financial support:* In 2015–16, 7 students received support, including 1 research assistantship with partial tuition reimbursement available (averaging $10,000 per year), 6 teaching assistantships with partial tuition reimbursements available (averaging $10,500 per year); institutionally sponsored loans, scholarships/grants, health care benefits, and unspecified assistantships also available. Financial award application deadline: 3/1. *Faculty research:* Fate and transport of radionuclides in the environment, radioanalytical methods and applications, biomedical optics and laser biophysics, microdosimetry and cancer initiation processes, medical imaging. *Total annual research expenditures:* $167,991. *Unit head:* Dr. Steen Madsen, Chair/Associate Professor, 702-895-1805, Fax: 702-895-4819, E-mail: steen.madsen@unlv.edu. *Application contact:* Graduate College Admissions Evaluator, 702-895-3367, Fax: 702-895-4180, E-mail: gradadmissions@unlv.edu.
Website: http://healthphysics.unlv.edu/

University of Oklahoma Health Sciences Center, College of Medicine and Graduate College, Graduate Programs in Medicine, Department of Radiological Sciences, Oklahoma City, OK 73190. Offers medical radiation physics (MS, PhD), including diagnostic radiology, nuclear medicine, radiation therapy, ultrasound. *Program availability:* Part-time. Terminal master's awarded for partial completion of doctoral program. *Degree requirements:* For master's, thesis; for doctorate, thesis/dissertation. *Entrance requirements:* For master's, GRE General Test; for doctorate, GRE General Test, 3 letters of recommendation. Additional exam requirements/recommendations for international students: Required—TOEFL. *Faculty research:* Monte Carlo applications in radiation therapy, observer-performed studies in diagnostic radiology, error analysis in gated cardiac nuclear medicine studies, nuclear medicine absorbed fraction determinations.

University of Toronto, Faculty of Medicine, Institute of Medical Science, Toronto, ON M5S 1A1, Canada. Offers bioethics (MH Sc); biomedical communications (M Sc BMC); medical radiation science (MH Sc); medical science (PhD). *Degree requirements:* For master's, thesis; for doctorate, thesis/dissertation, thesis defense. *Entrance requirements:* For master's, minimum GPA of 3.7 in 3 of 4 years (M Sc), interview; for doctorate, M Sc or equivalent, defended thesis, minimum A- average, interview. Additional exam requirements/recommendations for international students: Required—TOEFL (minimum score 600 paper-based; 93 iBT), TWE (minimum score 5). Electronic applications accepted.

Vanderbilt University, Department of Physics and Astronomy, Nashville, TN 37240-1001. Offers astronomy (MS); health physics (MA); physics (MAT, MS, PhD). *Faculty:* 26 full-time (3 women). *Students:* 55 full-time (9 women); includes 10 minority (2 Black or African American, non-Hispanic/Latino; 1 Asian, non-Hispanic/Latino; 6 Hispanic/Latino; 1 Two or more races, non-Hispanic/Latino), 18 international. Average age 27. 169 applicants, 19% accepted, 7 enrolled. In 2015, 4 master's, 12 doctorates awarded. *Degree requirements:* For master's, thesis; for doctorate, comprehensive exam, thesis/dissertation, final and qualifying exams. *Entrance requirements:* For master's, GRE General Test; for doctorate, GRE General Test, GRE Subject Test. Additional exam requirements/recommendations for international students: Required—TOEFL (minimum score 570 paper-based; 88 iBT). *Application deadline:* For fall admission, 1/15 for domestic and international students. Electronic applications accepted. *Financial support:* Fellowships with tuition reimbursements, research assistantships with full tuition reimbursements, teaching assistantships with full tuition reimbursements, career-related internships or fieldwork, Federal Work-Study, and institutionally sponsored loans available. Financial award application deadline: 1/15; financial award applicants required to submit CSS PROFILE or FAFSA. *Faculty research:* Experimental and theoretical physics, free electron laser, living-state physics, heavy-ion physics, nuclear structure. *Unit head:* Dr. Julia Velkovska, Director of Graduate Studies, 615-322-2828, Fax: 615-343-7263, E-mail: julia.velkovska@vanderbilt.edu. *Application contact:* Donald Pickert, Administrative Assistant, 615-343-1026, Fax: 615-343-7263, E-mail: donald.pickert@vanderbilt.edu.
Website: http://www.vanderbilt.edu/physics

Virginia Commonwealth University, Graduate School, School of Allied Health Professions, Doctoral Program in Health Related Sciences, Richmond, VA 23284-9005. Offers clinical laboratory sciences (PhD); gerontology (PhD); health administration (PhD); nurse anesthesia (PhD); occupational therapy (PhD); physical therapy (PhD); radiation sciences (PhD); rehabilitation leadership (PhD). *Entrance requirements:* For doctorate, GRE General Test or MAT, minimum GPA of 3.3 in master's degree. Additional exam requirements/recommendations for international students: Required—TOEFL (minimum score 600 paper-based; 100 iBT); Recommended—IELTS (minimum score 6.5). Electronic applications accepted.

Weber State University, College of Health Professions, Department of Radiologic Sciences, Ogden, UT 84408-1001. Offers MSRS. *Faculty:* 5 full-time (2 women). *Students:* 31 full-time (16 women); includes 2 minority (1 Black or African American, non-Hispanic/Latino; 1 Hispanic/Latino). Average age 37. *Entrance requirements:* Additional exam requirements/recommendations for international students: Required—TOEFL (minimum score 550 paper-based). *Application deadline:* For fall admission, 5/1 priority date for domestic and international students. Application fee: $60 ($90 for international students). Electronic applications accepted. *Expenses:* Tuition, state resident: full-time $6520; part-time $1252 per credit hour. Tuition, nonresident: full-time $15,003; part-time $2998 per credit hour. *Required fees:* $380; $180 per credit hour. $8.50 per term. Tuition and fees vary according to course level and program. *Financial*

Health Physics/Radiological Health

support: In 2015–16, 16 students received support. Scholarships/grants available. Financial award application deadline: 4/1; financial award applicants required to submit FAFSA. *Unit head:* Dr. Robert Walker, Program Director, 801-626-7156, Fax: 801-626-7683, E-mail: rwalker2@weber.edu. *Application contact:* Lonnie Lujan, Graduate Enrollment Director, 801-626-6088, Fax: 801-626-7966, E-mail: lonnielujan@weber.edu.
Website: http://www.weber.edu/msrs

Medical Imaging

Boston University, School of Medicine, Division of Graduate Medical Sciences, Program in Bio imaging, Boston, MA 02215. Offers MA. *Degree requirements:* For master's, thesis. *Financial support:* Applicants required to submit FAFSA. *Unit head:* Dr. Mark Moss, Chair, 617-638-4200, E-mail: markmoss@bu.edu. *Application contact:* GMS Admissions Office, 617-638-5255, E-mail: askgms@bu.edu.
Website: http://www.bumc.bu.edu/mbi/

Cleveland State University, College of Graduate Studies, College of Sciences and Health Professions, Department of Physics, Cleveland, OH 44115. Offers applied optics (MS); condensed matter physics (MS); medical physics (MS); optics and materials (MS); optics and medical imaging (MS). *Program availability:* Part-time, evening/weekend. *Faculty:* 4 full-time (0 women), 1 part-time/adjunct (0 women). *Students:* 10 full-time (5 women), 9 part-time (1 woman); includes 5 minority (2 Black or African American, non-Hispanic/Latino; 1 Asian, non-Hispanic/Latino; 2 Hispanic/Latino), 2 international. Average age 28. 23 applicants, 78% accepted, 6 enrolled. In 2015, 10 master's awarded. *Entrance requirements:* For master's, undergraduate degree in engineering, physics, chemistry or mathematics. Additional exam requirements/recommendations for international students: Required—TOEFL (minimum score 550 paper-based; 78 iBT). *Application deadline:* For fall admission, 7/1 priority date for domestic students, 4/1 priority date for international students. Applications are processed on a rolling basis. Application fee: $30. Electronic applications accepted. *Expenses:* Tuition, state resident: full-time $9565. Tuition, nonresident: full-time $17,980. Tuition and fees vary according to program. *Financial support:* In 2015–16, 1 research assistantship with tuition reimbursement (averaging $5,666 per year) was awarded; fellowships with tuition reimbursements, teaching assistantships, and tuition waivers (full) also available. Financial award applicants required to submit FAFSA. *Faculty research:* Statistical physics, experimental solid-state physics, theoretical optics, experimental biological physics (macromolecular crystallography), experimental optics. *Total annual research expenditures:* $350,000. *Unit head:* Dr. Miron Kaufman, Chairperson, 216-687-2436, Fax: 216-523-7268, E-mail: m.kaufman@csuohio.edu. *Application contact:* Dr. James A. Lock, Director, 216-687-2420, Fax: 216-523-7268, E-mail: j.lock@csuohio.edu.
Website: http://www.csuohio.edu/sciences/physics/physics

Illinois Institute of Technology, Graduate College, Armour College of Engineering, Department of Electrical and Computer Engineering, Chicago, IL 60616. Offers biomedical imaging and signals (MAS); computer engineering (MS, PhD); electrical engineering (MS, PhD); electricity markets (MAS); network engineering (MAS); power engineering (MAS); telecommunications and software engineering (MAS); VLSI and microelectronics (MAS); MS/MS. *Program availability:* Part-time, evening/weekend, online learning. Terminal master's awarded for partial completion of doctoral program. *Degree requirements:* For master's, comprehensive exam (for some programs), thesis (for some programs); for doctorate, comprehensive exam, thesis/dissertation. *Entrance requirements:* For master's and doctorate, GRE General Test (minimum score 1100 Quantitative and Verbal, 3.5 Analytical Writing), minimum undergraduate GPA of 3.0. Additional exam requirements/recommendations for international students: Required—TOEFL (minimum score 550 paper-based; 80 iBT); Recommended—IELTS (minimum score 5.5). Electronic applications accepted. *Faculty research:* Communication systems, wireless networks, computer systems, computer networks, wireless security, cloud computing and micro-electronics; electromagnetics and electronics; power and control systems; signal and image processing.

Medical College of Wisconsin, Graduate School of Biomedical Sciences, Program in Functional Imaging, Milwaukee, WI 53226-0509. Offers PhD.

Medical University of South Carolina, College of Graduate Studies, Program in Molecular and Cellular Biology and Pathobiology, Charleston, SC 29425. Offers cancer biology (PhD); cardiovascular biology (PhD); cardiovascular imaging (PhD); cell regulation (PhD); craniofacial biology (PhD); genetics and development (PhD); marine biomedicine (PhD); DMD/PhD; MD/PhD. *Degree requirements:* For doctorate, thesis/dissertation, oral and written exams. *Entrance requirements:* For doctorate, GRE General Test, interview, minimum GPA of 3.0. Additional exam requirements/recommendations for international students: Required—TOEFL (minimum score 600 paper-based; 100 iBT). Electronic applications accepted.

New York University, School of Medicine and Graduate School of Arts and Science, Sackler Institute of Graduate Biomedical Sciences, Program in Biomedical Imaging, New York, NY 10012-1019. Offers PhD. *Degree requirements:* For doctorate, comprehensive exam, thesis/dissertation, qualifying exam. *Faculty research:* In vivo microimaging of transgenic mice, radio frequency (RF) coil design, magnetic resonance spectroscopic imaging.

Rutgers University–Newark, School of Health Related Professions, Department of Medical Imaging Sciences, Newark, NJ 07102. Offers radiologist assistant (MS). *Program availability:* Part-time, evening/weekend. *Entrance requirements:* For master's, BS with minimum GPA of 3.0, RT license, coursework in intro to pathopsychology, interview, all transcripts, personal statement, BCLS certification. Additional exam requirements/recommendations for international students: Required—TOEFL (minimum score 500 paper-based; 79 iBT). Electronic applications accepted.

University of California, San Francisco, Graduate Division, Biomedical Imaging Graduate Program, San Francisco, CA 94143. Offers MS. *Program availability:* Part-time. *Faculty:* 14 full-time (7 women). *Students:* 21 full-time (6 women). In 2015, 19 master's awarded. *Degree requirements:* For master's, The MSBI program can be completed by taking a comprehensive exam or submitting a thesis. *Entrance requirements:* For master's, The program require applicants to provide MCAT or GRE scores. Additional exam requirements/recommendations for international students: Required—TOEFL (minimum score 550 paper-based, 80 iBT) or IELTS (minimum score 7.0). *Application deadline:* For fall admission, 2/28 for domestic and international students. Application fee: $90 ($110 for international students). Electronic applications accepted. *Financial support:* Applicants required to submit FAFSA. *Unit head:* Rukayah Abdolcader, Program Administrator, 415-514-8246, E-mail: msbi@ucsf.edu. *Application contact:* Richard Wyllie, Academic Program Coordinator, 415-476-2111, Fax: 415-514-0844, E-mail: rick.wyllie@ucsf.edu.
Website: http://radiology.ucsf.edu/education/graduate-programs/msbi-program

University of Cincinnati, Graduate School, College of Engineering and Applied Science, Department of Biomedical, Chemical and Environmental Engineering, Cincinnati, OH 45221. Offers biomechanics (PhD); chemical engineering (MS, PhD); environmental engineering (MS, PhD); environmental sciences (MS, PhD); medical imaging (PhD); tissue engineering (PhD). *Program availability:* Part-time. *Degree requirements:* For master's, thesis or alternative; for doctorate, one foreign language, thesis/dissertation. *Entrance requirements:* For master's and doctorate, GRE General Test. Additional exam requirements/recommendations for international students: Required—TOEFL (minimum score 600 paper-based).

University of Guelph, Ontario Veterinary College and Graduate Studies, Graduate Programs in Veterinary Sciences, Department of Clinical Studies, Guelph, ON N1G 2W1, Canada. Offers anesthesiology (M Sc, DV Sc); cardiology (DV Sc, Diploma); clinical studies (Diploma); dermatology (M Sc); diagnostic imaging (M Sc, DV Sc); emergency/critical care (M Sc, DV Sc, Diploma); medicine (M Sc, DV Sc); neurology (M Sc, DV Sc); ophthalmology (M Sc, DV Sc); surgery (M Sc, DV Sc). *Degree requirements:* For master's, thesis; for doctorate, comprehensive exam, thesis/dissertation. *Entrance requirements:* Additional exam requirements/recommendations for international students: Required—TOEFL (minimum score 550 paper-based), IELTS (minimum score 6.5). Electronic applications accepted. *Faculty research:* Orthopedics, respirology, oncology, exercise physiology, cardiology.

University of Southern California, Graduate School, Viterbi School of Engineering, Department of Biomedical Engineering, Los Angeles, CA 90089. Offers biomedical engineering (PhD); medical device and diagnostic engineering (MS); medical imaging and imaging informatics (MS). *Program availability:* Online learning. Terminal master's awarded for partial completion of doctoral program. *Degree requirements:* For master's, thesis optional; for doctorate, thesis/dissertation. *Entrance requirements:* For master's and doctorate, GRE General Test. Additional exam requirements/recommendations for international students: Recommended—TOEFL. Electronic applications accepted. *Faculty research:* Medical ultrasound, BioMEMS, neural prosthetics, computational bioengineering, bioengineering of vision, medical devices.

Wayne State University, College of Engineering, Department of Biomedical Engineering, Detroit, MI 48202. Offers biomedical engineering (MS, PhD), including biomedical imaging (PhD); injury biomechanics (Graduate Certificate). *Faculty:* 18. *Students:* 79 full-time (37 women), 18 part-time (7 women); includes 12 minority (4 Black or African American, non-Hispanic/Latino; 5 Asian, non-Hispanic/Latino; 3 Two or more races, non-Hispanic/Latino), 46 international. Average age 28. 197 applicants, 45% accepted, 28 enrolled. In 2015, 45 master's, 6 doctorates awarded. Terminal master's awarded for partial completion of doctoral program. *Degree requirements:* For master's, thesis optional; for doctorate, thesis/dissertation. *Entrance requirements:* For master's, GRE (recommended), bachelor's degree, minimum undergraduate GPA of 3.0, one-page statement of purpose, completion of prerequisite coursework in calculus and engineering physics; for doctorate, GRE, bachelor's degree with minimum undergraduate GPA of 3.5, undergraduate major or substantial specialized work in proposed doctoral major field, personal statement, three letters of recommendation; for Graduate Certificate, minimum undergraduate GPA of 3.0, bachelor's degree in engineering. Additional exam requirements/recommendations for international students: Required—TOEFL (minimum score 550 paper-based; 79 iBT), TWE (minimum score 5.5), Michigan English Language Assessment Battery (minimum score 85); Recommended—IELTS (minimum score 6.5). *Application deadline:* For fall admission, 6/1 priority date for domestic students, 5/1 priority date for international students; for winter admission, 10/1 priority date for domestic students, 9/1 priority date for international students; for spring admission, 2/1 priority date for domestic students, 1/1 priority date for international students. Applications are processed on a rolling basis. Application fee: $0. Electronic applications accepted. *Expenses:* $16,444 annual resident tuition, $32,915 non-resident tuition; $685 per credit hour resident tuition, $1,371.45 per credit hour non-resident tuition; fees include $47.45 per credit hour student services fee and $274.60 per semester registration fee. *Financial support:* In 2015–16, 41 students received support, including 4 fellowships with tuition reimbursements available (averaging $16,000 per year), 8 research assistantships with tuition reimbursements available (averaging $18,173 per year), 7 teaching assistantships with tuition reimbursements available (averaging $19,084 per year); Federal Work-Study, scholarships/grants, health care benefits, and unspecified assistantships also available. Support available to part-time students. Financial award application deadline: 3/31; financial award applicants required to submit FAFSA. *Faculty research:* Injury and orthopedic biomechanics, neurophysiology of pain, smart sensors, biomaterials and imaging. *Total annual research expenditures:* $3.4 million. *Unit head:* Dr. Johhn Cavanaugh, Interim Department Chair, 313-577-3916, E-mail: jmc@wayne.edu. *Application contact:* Ellen Cope, Graduate Program Coordinator, 313-577-0409, Fax: 313-577-8333, E-mail: bmeinfo@eng.wayne.edu.
Website: http://engineering.wayne.edu/bme/

Medical Physics

Cleveland State University, College of Graduate Studies, College of Sciences and Health Professions, Department of Physics, Cleveland, OH 44115. Offers applied optics (MS); condensed matter physics (MS); medical physics (MS); optics and materials (MS); optics and medical imaging (MS). *Program availability:* Part-time, evening/weekend. *Faculty:* 4 full-time (0 women), 1 part-time/adjunct (0 women). *Students:* 10 full-time (5 women), 9 part-time (1 woman); includes 5 minority (2 Black or African American, non-Hispanic/Latino; 1 Asian, non-Hispanic/Latino; 2 Hispanic/Latino), 2 international. Average age 28. 23 applicants, 78% accepted, 6 enrolled. In 2015, 10 master's awarded. *Entrance requirements:* For master's, undergraduate degree in engineering, physics, chemistry or mathematics. Additional exam requirements/recommendations for international students: Required—TOEFL (minimum score 550 paper-based; 78 iBT). *Application deadline:* For fall admission, 7/1 priority date for domestic students, 4/1 priority date for international students. Applications are processed on a rolling basis. Application fee: $30. Electronic applications accepted. *Expenses:* Tuition, state resident: full-time $9565. Tuition, nonresident: full-time $17,980. Tuition and fees vary according to program. *Financial support:* In 2015–16, 1 research assistantship with tuition reimbursement (averaging $5,666 per year) was awarded; fellowships with tuition reimbursements, teaching assistantships, and tuition waivers (full) also available. Financial award applicants required to submit FAFSA. *Faculty research:* Statistical physics, experimental solid-state physics, theoretical optics, experimental biological physics (macromolecular crystallography), experimental optics. *Total annual research expenditures:* $350,000. *Unit head:* Dr. Miron Kaufman, Chairperson, 216-687-2436, Fax: 216-523-7268, E-mail: m.kaufman@csuohio.edu. *Application contact:* Dr. James A. Lock, Director, 216-687-2420, Fax: 216-523-7268, E-mail: j.lock@csuohio.edu. Website: http://www.csuohio.edu/sciences/physics/physics

The College of William and Mary, Faculty of Arts and Sciences, Department of Applied Science, Williamsburg, VA 23187-8795. Offers accelerator science (PhD); applied mathematics (PhD); applied mechanics (PhD); applied robotics (PhD); applied science (MS); atmospheric and environmental science (PhD); computational neuroscience (PhD); interface, thin film and surface science (PhD); lasers and optics (PhD); magnetic resonance (PhD); materials science and engineering (PhD); mathematical and computational biology (PhD); medical imaging (PhD); nanotechnology (PhD); neuroscience (PhD); non-destructive evaluation (PhD); polymer chemistry (PhD); remote sensing (PhD). *Program availability:* Part-time. *Faculty:* 7 full-time (1 woman), 1 part-time/adjunct (0 women). *Students:* 26 full-time (9 women), 3 part-time (1 woman); includes 5 minority (2 Black or African American, non-Hispanic/Latino; 1 Asian, non-Hispanic/Latino; 2 Hispanic/Latino), 12 international. Average age 28. 24 applicants, 46% accepted, 6 enrolled. In 2015, 2 master's, 6 doctorates awarded. Terminal master's awarded for partial completion of doctoral program. *Degree requirements:* For master's, comprehensive exam, thesis; for doctorate, comprehensive exam, thesis/dissertation, 4 core courses. *Entrance requirements:* For master's and doctorate, GRE General Test, GRE Subject Test. Additional exam requirements/recommendations for international students: Required—TOEFL, TWE. *Application deadline:* For fall admission, 2/3 priority date for domestic students, 2/3 for international students; for spring admission, 10/15 priority date for domestic students, 10/14 for international students. Applications are processed on a rolling basis. Application fee: $45. Electronic applications accepted. *Expenses:* $6,550 per semester; $13,100 per year. *Financial support:* Fellowships, research assistantships, teaching assistantships, Federal Work-Study, health care benefits, tuition waivers (full), and unspecified assistantships available. Financial award application deadline: 4/15; financial award applicants required to submit FAFSA. *Faculty research:* Computational biology, non-destructive evaluation, neurophysiology, lasers and optics. *Total annual research expenditures:* $1.7 million. *Unit head:* Dr. Christopher Del Negro, Chair, 757-221-7808, Fax: 757-221-2050, E-mail: cadeln@wm.edu. *Application contact:* Lianne Rios Ashburne, Graduate Program Coordinator, 757-221-2563, Fax: 757-221-2050, E-mail: lrashburne@wm.edu. Website: http://www.wm.edu/as/appliedscience

Columbia University, Fu Foundation School of Engineering and Applied Science, Department of Applied Physics and Applied Mathematics, New York, NY 10027. Offers applied mathematics (MS, Eng Sc D, PhD); applied physics (MS, Eng Sc D, PhD); materials science and engineering (MS, Eng Sc D, PhD); medical physics (MS). *Program availability:* Part-time, online learning. Terminal master's awarded for partial completion of doctoral program. *Degree requirements:* For master's, comprehensive exam; for doctorate, thesis/dissertation, qualifying exam. *Entrance requirements:* For master's, GRE General Test, GRE Subject Test (strongly recommended); for doctorate, GRE General Test, GRE Subject Test (applied physics). Additional exam requirements/recommendations for international students: Required—TOEFL, IELTS, PTE. Electronic applications accepted. *Faculty research:* Plasma physics and fusion energy; optical and laser physics; atmospheric, oceanic and earth physics; applied mathematics; solid state science and processing of materials, their properties, and their structure; medical physics.

Duke University, Graduate School, Medical Physics Graduate Program, Durham, NC 27705. Offers MS, PhD. *Entrance requirements:* For master's and doctorate, GRE General Test. Additional exam requirements/recommendations for international students: Required—TOEFL (minimum score 577 paper-based; 90 iBT) or IELTS (minimum score 7). Electronic applications accepted.

East Carolina University, Graduate School, Thomas Harriot College of Arts and Sciences, Department of Physics, Greenville, NC 27858-4353. Offers applied physics (MS); biomedical physics (PhD); health physics (MS); medical physics (MS). *Program availability:* Part-time. *Students:* 28 full-time (5 women), 8 part-time (3 women); includes 10 minority (4 Black or African American, non-Hispanic/Latino; 3 Asian, non-Hispanic/Latino; 1 Hispanic/Latino; 2 Two or more races, non-Hispanic/Latino), 5 international. Average age 29. 48 applicants, 60% accepted, 8 enrolled. In 2015, 6 master's, 1 doctorate awarded. *Degree requirements:* For master's, one foreign language, comprehensive exam. *Entrance requirements:* For master's, GRE General Test. Additional exam requirements/recommendations for international students: Required—TOEFL. *Application deadline:* Applications are processed on a rolling basis. Application fee: $50. *Financial support:* Research assistantships with partial tuition reimbursements, teaching assistantships with partial tuition reimbursements, and Federal Work-Study available. Support available to part-time students. Financial award application deadline: 6/1. *Unit head:* Dr. John Sutherland, Chair, 252-328-6739, E-mail: sutherlandj@ecu.edu. *Application contact:* Dean of Graduate School, 252-328-6012, Fax: 252-328-6071, E-mail: gradschool@ecu.edu. Website: http://www.ecu.edu/cs-cas/physics/Graduate-Program.cfm#

Hampton University, School of Science, Department of Physics, Hampton, VA 23668. Offers medical physics (MS, PhD); nuclear physics (MS, PhD); optical physics (MS, PhD). *Degree requirements:* For master's, thesis optional; for doctorate, thesis/dissertation, oral defense, qualifying exam. *Entrance requirements:* For master's, GRE

General Test; for doctorate, GRE General Test, minimum GPA of 3.0 or master's degree in physics or related field. Additional exam requirements/recommendations for international students: Required—TOEFL (minimum score 525 paper-based) or IELTS (6.5). Electronic applications accepted. *Expenses: Tuition, area resident:* Full-time $10,263; part-time $522 per credit hour. *Required fees:* $35. Tuition and fees vary according to course load and program. *Faculty research:* Laser optics, remote sensing.

Harvard University, Graduate School of Arts and Sciences, Department of Physics, Cambridge, MA 02138. Offers experimental physics (PhD); medical engineering/medical physics (PhD), including applied physics, engineering sciences, physics; theoretical physics (PhD). *Degree requirements:* For doctorate, thesis/dissertation, final exams, laboratory experience. *Entrance requirements:* For doctorate, GRE General Test, GRE Subject Test. Additional exam requirements/recommendations for international students: Required—TOEFL. *Faculty research:* Particle physics, condensed matter physics, atomic physics.

Hofstra University, College of Liberal Arts and Sciences, Program in Medical Physics, Hempstead, NY 11549. Offers MS. *Program availability:* Part-time, evening/weekend. *Students:* 9 full-time (3 women); includes 2 minority (both Asian, non-Hispanic/Latino). Average age 26. 10 applicants, 80% accepted, 2 enrolled. In 2015, 4 master's awarded. *Degree requirements:* For master's, comprehensive exam, minimum GPA of 3.0. *Entrance requirements:* For master's, bachelor's degree in science, minimum GPA of 3.0, 2 letters of recommendation. Additional exam requirements/recommendations for international students: Required—TOEFL (minimum score 550 paper-based; 80 iBT). *Application deadline:* Applications are processed on a rolling basis. Application fee: $70 ($75 for international students). Electronic applications accepted. *Financial support:* In 2015–16, 7 students received support, including 2 fellowships with tuition reimbursements available (averaging $3,435 per year); research assistantships with tuition reimbursements available, Federal Work-Study, institutionally sponsored loans, scholarships/grants, and tuition waivers (full and partial) also available. Support available to part-time students. Financial award applicants required to submit FAFSA. *Faculty research:* Medical physics general; radiation therapy physics, diagnostic radiological physics; nuclear medicine; radiation protection and safety. *Unit head:* Dr. Ajay Kapur, Program Director, 516-463-5013, Fax: 516-463-3059, E-mail: ajay.kapur@hofstra.edu. *Application contact:* Sunil Samuel, Assistant Vice President of Admissions, 516-463-4723, Fax: 516-463-4664, E-mail: graduateadmission@hofstra.edu. Website: http://www.hofstra.edu/hclas

Indiana University Bloomington, University Graduate School, College of Arts and Sciences, Department of Physics, Bloomington, IN 47405. Offers medical physics (MS); physics (MAT, MS, PhD). *Program availability:* Part-time, online learning. Terminal master's awarded for partial completion of doctoral program. *Degree requirements:* For master's, comprehensive exam (for some programs), thesis (for some programs), qualifying exam; for doctorate, comprehensive exam, thesis/dissertation, qualifying exam. *Entrance requirements:* For master's and doctorate, GRE General Test, GRE Subject Test (physics), minimum GPA of 3.0. Additional exam requirements/recommendations for international students: Required—TOEFL (minimum score 550 paper-based; 80 iBT) or IELTS (minimum score 6.5). Electronic applications accepted. *Faculty research:* Accelerator physics, astrophysics and cosmology, biophysics (biocomplexity, neural networks, visual systems, chemical signaling), condensed matter physics (neutron scattering, complex fluids, quantum computing), particle physics (collider physics, hybrid mesons, lattice gauge, symmetries, collider phenomenology), neutrino physics, nuclear physics (proton and neutron physics, neutrinos, symmetries, nuclear astrophysics, hadron structure).

Louisiana State University and Agricultural & Mechanical College, Graduate School, College of Science, Department of Physics and Astronomy, Baton Rouge, LA 70803. Offers astronomy (PhD); astrophysics (PhD); medical physics (PhD); physics (MS, PhD).

Massachusetts Institute of Technology, School of Engineering, Harvard-MIT Health Sciences and Technology Program, Cambridge, MA 02139. Offers health sciences and technology (SM, PhD, Sc D), including bioastronautics (PhD, Sc D), bioinformatics and integrative genomics (PhD, Sc D), medical engineering and medical physics (PhD, Sc D), speech and hearing bioscience and technology (PhD, Sc D). *Faculty:* 125 full-time (20 women). *Students:* 271 full-time (111 women), 15 part-time (4 women); includes 79 minority (2 Black or African American, non-Hispanic/Latino; 1 American Indian or Alaska Native, non-Hispanic/Latino; 61 Asian, non-Hispanic/Latino; 12 Hispanic/Latino; 3 Two or more races, non-Hispanic/Latino), 51 international. Average age 26. 265 applicants, 11% accepted, 21 enrolled. In 2015, 3 master's, 25 doctorates awarded. Terminal master's awarded for partial completion of doctoral program. *Degree requirements:* For master's, thesis; for doctorate, comprehensive exam, thesis/dissertation. *Entrance requirements:* For doctorate, GRE General Test (for medical engineering and medical physics). Additional exam requirements/recommendations for international students: Required—TOEFL (minimum score 600 paper-based; 100 iBT), IELTS (minimum score 7). *Application deadline:* For fall admission, 12/15 for domestic and international students. Application fee: $75. Electronic applications accepted. *Expenses: Tuition:* Full-time $46,400; part-time $725 per credit. One-time fee: $304 full-time. Full-time tuition and fees vary according to course load and program. *Financial support:* In 2015–16, 128 students received support, including 57 fellowships (averaging $38,200 per year), 52 research assistantships (averaging $34,200 per year), 1 teaching assistantship (averaging $19,500 per year); Federal Work-Study, institutionally sponsored loans, scholarships/grants, traineeships, health care benefits, and unspecified assistantships also available. Support available to part-time students. Financial award application deadline: 4/15; financial award applicants required to submit FAFSA. *Faculty research:* Signal processing, biomedical imaging, drug delivery, medical devices, medical diagnostics, regenerative biomedical technologies. *Unit head:* Emery N. Brown, Director, 617-452-4091. *Application contact:* 617-253-3609, Fax: 617-253-6692, E-mail: hst-phd-admissions@mit.edu. Website: http://hst.mit.edu/

McGill University, Faculty of Graduate and Postdoctoral Studies, Faculty of Medicine, Medical Physics Unit, Montréal, QC H3A 2T5, Canada. Offers M Sc, PhD. *Entrance requirements:* Additional exam requirements/recommendations for international students: Required—TOEFL.

McMaster University, School of Graduate Studies, Faculty of Science, Department of Medical Physics and Applied Radiation Sciences, Hamilton, ON L8S 4M2, Canada. Offers health and radiation physics (M Sc); medical physics (M Sc, PhD). *Program availability:* Part-time. *Degree requirements:* For master's, thesis or alternative. *Entrance requirements:* For master's, minimum B+ average. Additional exam requirements/recommendations for international students: Required—TOEFL (minimum score 550

Medical Physics

paper-based). *Faculty research:* Imaging, toxicology, dosimetry, body composition, medical lasers.

Oakland University, Graduate Study and Lifelong Learning, College of Arts and Sciences, Department of Physics, Rochester, MI 48309-4401. Offers medical physics (PhD); physics (MS). *Faculty:* 6 full-time (0 women). *Students:* 10 full-time (5 women), 5 part-time (2 women); includes 3 minority (1 Black or African American, non-Hispanic/Latino; 2 Asian, non-Hispanic/Latino), 6 international. Average age 33. 28 applicants, 7% accepted. In 2015, 1 doctorate awarded. *Degree requirements:* For doctorate, thesis/dissertation. *Entrance requirements:* For master's, minimum GPA of 3.0; for doctorate, GRE Subject Test, GRE General Test, minimum GPA of 3.0. Additional exam requirements/recommendations for international students: Required—TOEFL (minimum score 550 paper-based). *Application deadline:* For fall admission, 7/15 priority date for domestic students, 5/1 priority date for international students; for winter admission, 12/1 priority date for domestic students, 9/1 priority date for international students; for spring admission, 3/15 priority date for domestic students. Applications are processed on a rolling basis. Application fee: $0. Electronic applications accepted. *Expenses:* Contact institution. *Financial support:* Fellowships, career-related internships or fieldwork, Federal Work-Study, institutionally sponsored loans, and tuition waivers (full) available. Financial award application deadline: 3/1; financial award applicants required to submit FAFSA. *Unit head:* Dr. Andrei Slavin, Chair, 248-370-3401, Fax: 248-370-3401, E-mail: slavin@oakland.edu.

Oregon State University, College of Engineering, Program in Medical Physics, Corvallis, OR 97331. Offers medical health physics (MMP, MS, PhD); therapeutic radiologic physics (MMP, MS, PhD). *Faculty:* 12 full-time (4 women), 1 part-time/adjunct (0 women). *Students:* 5 full-time (2 women), 3 part-time (1 woman); includes 1 minority (Asian, non-Hispanic/Latino). Average age 29. 53 applicants, 32% accepted. In 2015, 2 master's awarded. *Entrance requirements:* For master's and doctorate, GRE. Additional exam requirements/recommendations for international students: Required—TOEFL (minimum score 80 iBT), IELTS (minimum score 6.5). *Application deadline:* For fall admission, 7/1 for domestic students. Application fee: $75 ($85 for international students). *Expenses:* $21,600 full-time resident tuition, $33,336 full-time non-resident tuition; $1,572 fees. *Financial support:* Application deadline: 2/1. *Unit head:* Dr. Krystina M. Tack, Director. *Application contact:* Medical Physics Advisor, 541-737-2343, E-mail: nuc_engr@ne.oregonstate.edu.
Website: http://ne.oregonstate.edu/content/medical-physics-program

Purdue University, Graduate School, College of Health and Human Sciences, School of Health Sciences, West Lafayette, IN 47907. Offers health physics (MS, PhD); medical physics (MS, PhD); occupational and environmental health science (MS, PhD), including aerosol deposition and lung disease, ergonomics, exposure and risk assessment, indoor air quality and bioaerosols (PhD), liver/lung toxicology; radiation biology (PhD); toxicology (PhD); MS/PhD. *Program availability:* Part-time. *Degree requirements:* For master's, thesis optional; for doctorate, one foreign language, thesis/dissertation. *Entrance requirements:* For master's and doctorate, GRE General Test, minimum undergraduate GPA of 3.0 or equivalent. Additional exam requirements/recommendations for international students: Required—TOEFL (minimum score 550 paper-based; 77 iBT); Recommended—TWE. Electronic applications accepted. *Faculty research:* Environmental toxicology, industrial hygiene, radiation dosimetry.

Rush University, Graduate College, Division of Medical Physics, Chicago, IL 60612-3832. Offers MS, PhD. Terminal master's awarded for partial completion of doctoral program. *Degree requirements:* For master's, thesis, qualifying exam; for doctorate, thesis/dissertation, preliminary and qualifying exams. *Entrance requirements:* For master's, GRE General Test, BS in physics or physical science; for doctorate, GRE General Test, GRE Subject Test. Additional exam requirements/recommendations for international students: Required—TOEFL. Electronic applications accepted. *Faculty research:* Radiation therapy treatment planning, dosimetry, diagnostic radiology and nuclear imaging.

Southern Illinois University Carbondale, Graduate School, College of Applied Science, Program in Medical Dosimetry, Carbondale, IL 62901-4701. Offers MS. *Faculty:* 32 full-time (22 women). *Students:* 22 full-time (12 women), 7 part-time (2 women); includes 2 minority (1 Black or African American, non-Hispanic/Latino; 1 Asian, non-Hispanic/Latino), 14 international. Average age 25. 87 applicants, 26% accepted, 23 enrolled. In 2015, 26 master's awarded. *Entrance requirements:* Additional requirements/recommendations for international students: Required—TOEFL. *Application deadline:* For fall admission, 2/1 for domestic and international students. Application fee: $65. Electronic applications accepted. *Unit head:* Dr. K. Scott Collins, Program Director, 618-453-8800, E-mail: kscollin@siu.edu. *Application contact:* Brandie Coleman, Office Support Associate, 618-453-8869, E-mail: kcham3@siu.edu.

Stony Brook University, State University of New York, Graduate School, College of Engineering and Applied Sciences, Department of Biomedical Engineering, Program in Medical Physics, Stony Brook, NY 11794. Offers MS, PhD. *Entrance requirements:* For doctorate, GRE. Additional exam requirements/recommendations for international students: Required—TOEFL. Application fee: $100. *Expenses:* Tuition, state resident: full-time $10,870; part-time $453 per credit hour. Tuition, nonresident: full-time $22,210; part-time $925 per credit hour. *Financial support:* Fellowships available. *Unit head:* Dr. Terry Button, Director, 631-444-3841, Fax: 631-632-8577, E-mail: terry.button@sunysb.edu. *Application contact:* Jessica Anne Kuhn, Assistant to Chair/Graduate Program Coordinator, 631-632-8371, Fax: 631-632-8577, E-mail: jessica.kuhn@stonybrook.edu.
Website: http://bme.sunysb.edu/grad/medicalphysics.html

University at Buffalo, the State University of New York, Graduate School, School of Medicine and Biomedical Sciences, Graduate Programs in Medicine and Biomedical Sciences, Department of Physiology and Biophysics, Buffalo, NY 14214. Offers biophysics (MS, PhD), including medical physics; physiology (MA, PhD). *Faculty:* 28 full-time (4 women). *Students:* 64 full-time (26 women); includes 34 minority (4 Black or African American, non-Hispanic/Latino; 26 Asian, non-Hispanic/Latino; 1 Hispanic/Latino; 3 Two or more races, non-Hispanic/Latino), 20 international. Average age 28. 62 applicants, 18% accepted, 8 enrolled. In 2015, 7 master's, 4 doctorates awarded. Terminal master's awarded for partial completion of doctoral program. *Degree requirements:* For master's, comprehensive exam, thesis optional, oral exam, project; for doctorate, comprehensive exam, thesis/dissertation, oral and written qualifying exam or 2 research proposals. *Entrance requirements:* For master's, GRE General Test, unofficial transcripts, 3 letters of recommendation, personal statement, curriculum vitae; for doctorate, GRE General Test or MCAT, unofficial transcripts, 3 letters of recommendation, personal statement, curriculum vitae. Additional exam requirements/recommendations for international students: Required—TOEFL (minimum score 550 paper-based; 79 iBT). *Application deadline:* Applications are processed on a rolling basis. Application fee: $85. Electronic applications accepted. *Financial support:* In 2015–16, 5 students received support, including 1 research assistantship with full tuition reimbursement available (averaging $25,000 per year); Federal Work-Study, institutionally sponsored loans, health care benefits, and unspecified assistantships also available. Financial award applicants required to submit FAFSA. *Faculty research:* Neurosciences, ion channels, cardiac physiology, renal/epithelial transport, cardiopulmonary exercise. *Total annual research expenditures:* $2.7 million. *Unit head:*

Dr. Perry M. Hogan, Chair, 716-829-2738, Fax: 716-829-2344, E-mail: phogan@buffalo.edu. *Application contact:* Kara M. Rickicki, Graduate Programs Coordinator, 716-829-2417, Fax: 716-829-2344, E-mail: rickicki@buffalo.edu.
Website: http://www.smbs.buffalo.edu/phb/

University of Alberta, Faculty of Graduate Studies and Research, Department of Physics, Edmonton, AB T6G 2E1, Canada. Offers astrophysics (M Sc, PhD); condensed matter (M Sc, PhD); geophysics (M Sc, PhD); medical physics (M Sc, PhD); subatomic physics (M Sc, PhD). *Degree requirements:* For master's, thesis; for doctorate, thesis/dissertation. *Entrance requirements:* For master's and doctorate, minimum GPA of 7.0 on a 9.0 scale. Additional exam requirements/recommendations for international students: Required—TOEFL. *Faculty research:* Cosmology, astroparticle physics, high-intermediate energy, magnetism, superconductivity.

The University of Arizona, College of Science, Department of Physics, Medical Physics Program, Tucson, AZ 85721. Offers PSM. *Program availability:* Part-time. *Degree requirements:* For master's, thesis or alternative, internship, colloquium, business courses. *Entrance requirements:* Additional exam requirements/recommendations for international students: Required—TOEFL (minimum score 550 paper-based; 79 iBT). Application fee: $75. Electronic applications accepted. *Financial support:* Career-related internships or fieldwork, Federal Work-Study, and scholarships/grants available. *Faculty research:* Nanotechnology, optics, medical imaging, high energy physics, biophysics. *Unit head:* Christopher J. Watchman, Department Head, 520-694-5481. *Application contact:* Hildegard K. Lueders, Graduate Coordinator, 520-621-2290, Fax: 520-621-4721.
Website: http://www.physics.arizona.edu/

University of California, Los Angeles, David Geffen School of Medicine and Graduate Division, Graduate Programs in Medicine, Program in Biomedical Physics, Los Angeles, CA 90095. Offers MS, PhD. Terminal master's awarded for partial completion of doctoral program. *Degree requirements:* For master's, comprehensive exam or thesis; for doctorate, thesis/dissertation, oral and written qualifying exams. *Entrance requirements:* For master's and doctorate, GRE General Test. Additional exam requirements/recommendations for international students: Required—TOEFL. Electronic applications accepted.

University of Chicago, Division of the Biological Sciences, Committee on Medical Physics, Chicago, IL 60637-1513. Offers PhD. *Students:* 18 full-time (3 women), 4 international. Average age 28. 54 applicants, 17% accepted, 3 enrolled. In 2015, 6 doctorates awarded. *Degree requirements:* For doctorate, thesis/dissertation, ethics class, 2 teaching assistantships. *Entrance requirements:* For doctorate, GRE General Test. Additional exam requirements/recommendations for international students: Required—TOEFL (minimum score 600 paper-based; 104 iBT), IELTS (minimum score 7). *Application deadline:* For fall admission, 12/1 for domestic and international students. Application fee: $90. Electronic applications accepted. *Financial support:* In 2015–16, 20 students received support, including fellowships with full tuition reimbursements available (averaging $29,781 per year), research assistantships with full tuition reimbursements available (averaging $29,781 per year); institutionally sponsored loans, scholarships/grants, traineeships, and health care benefits also available. Financial award applicants required to submit FAFSA. *Unit head:* Dr. Samuel Armato, III, Chair. *Application contact:* Ruth Magana, Program Administrator, E-mail: rmagana@radiology.bsd.uchicago.edu.
Website: http://medicalphysics.uchicago.edu/

University of Cincinnati, Graduate School, College of Medicine, Graduate Programs in Biomedical Sciences, Department of Radiology, Cincinnati, OH 45267. Offers medical physics (MS). *Program availability:* Part-time. *Degree requirements:* For master's, comprehensive exam, project. *Entrance requirements:* For master's, GRE General Test. Additional exam requirements/recommendations for international students: Required—TOEFL (minimum score 575 paper-based). Electronic applications accepted. *Faculty research:* Radiation oncology, radiologic imaging, dosimetry, radiation biology, radiation therapy.

University of Colorado Boulder, Graduate School, College of Arts and Sciences, Department of Physics, Boulder, CO 80309. Offers chemical physics (PhD); geophysics (PhD); liquid crystal science and technology (PhD); mathematical physics (PhD); medical physics (PhD); optical sciences and engineering (PhD); physics (MS, PhD). *Faculty:* 48 full-time (8 women). *Students:* 131 full-time (22 women), 97 part-time (22 women); includes 14 minority (5 Asian, non-Hispanic/Latino; 4 Hispanic/Latino; 5 Two or more races, non-Hispanic/Latino), 61 international. Average age 26. 624 applicants, 24% accepted, 36 enrolled. In 2015, 24 master's, 29 doctorates awarded. Terminal master's awarded for partial completion of doctoral program. *Degree requirements:* For master's, comprehensive exam, thesis or alternative; for doctorate, comprehensive exam, thesis/dissertation. *Entrance requirements:* For master's and doctorate, GRE General Test, GRE Subject Test, minimum undergraduate GPA of 3.0. Additional exam requirements/recommendations for international students: Required—TOEFL. *Application deadline:* For fall admission, 12/15 for domestic students, 12/1 for international students. Applications are processed on a rolling basis. Application fee: $50 ($70 for international students). Electronic applications accepted. Application fee is waived when completed online. *Financial support:* In 2015–16, 521 students received support, including 7 fellowships (averaging $5,311 per year), 162 research assistantships with tuition reimbursements available (averaging $34,608 per year), 51 teaching assistantships with tuition reimbursements available (averaging $29,058 per year); institutionally sponsored loans, scholarships/grants, health care benefits, and unspecified assistantships also available. Financial award application deadline: 1/15; financial award applicants required to submit FAFSA. *Faculty research:* Physics, theoretical physics, high energy physics, experimental physics, solid state physics. *Total annual research expenditures:* $24.8 million. *Application contact:* E-mail: jeanne.nijhowne@colorado.edu.
Website: http://phys.colorado.edu/graduate-students

University of Florida, Graduate School, College of Engineering, J. Crayton Pruitt Family Department of Biomedical Engineering, Gainesville, FL 32611. Offers biomedical engineering (ME, MS, PhD, Certificate); clinical and translational science (PhD); medical physics (MS, PhD); MD/PhD. *Faculty:* 21 full-time, 19 part-time/adjunct. *Students:* 156 full-time (59 women), 13 part-time (3 women); includes 32 minority (5 Black or African American, non-Hispanic/Latino; 10 Asian, non-Hispanic/Latino; 17 Hispanic/Latino), 40 international. Average age 26. 304 applicants, 63% accepted, 55 enrolled. In 2015, 35 master's, 18 doctorates awarded. Terminal master's awarded for partial completion of doctoral program. *Degree requirements:* For master's, comprehensive exam (for some programs), thesis (for some programs); for doctorate, comprehensive exam (for some programs), thesis/dissertation (for some programs). *Entrance requirements:* Additional exam requirements/recommendations for international students: Required—TOEFL (minimum score 550 paper-based; 80 iBT), IELTS (minimum score 6). *Application deadline:* For fall admission, 12/15 priority date for domestic students, 12/15 for international students; for spring admission, 7/31 for domestic and international students. Applications are processed on a rolling basis. Application fee: $30. Electronic applications accepted. *Financial support:* In 2015–16, 7 fellowships, 75 research assistantships, 1 teaching assistantship were awarded. Financial award application deadline: 12/31; financial award applicants required to submit FAFSA. *Faculty research:*

Neural engineering, imaging and medical physics, biomaterials and regenerative medicine, biomedical informatics and modeling. *Total annual research expenditures:* $6.2 million. *Unit head:* Christine E. Schmidt, PhD, Chair, 352-273-9222, Fax: 352-392-9791, E-mail: schmidt@bme.ufl.edu. *Application contact:* Hans Van Oostrom, PhD, Associate Professor/Associate Chair/Graduate Coordinator, 352-273-9315, Fax: 352-392-9221, E-mail: oostrom@ufl.edu.
Website: http://www.bme.ufl.edu/

University of Kentucky, Graduate School, Graduate School Programs from the College of Medicine, Program in Radiation Sciences, Lexington, KY 40506-0032. Offers MSRMP. *Program availability:* Part-time. *Degree requirements:* For master's, comprehensive exam, thesis. *Entrance requirements:* For master's, GRE General Test, minimum undergraduate GPA of 2.75. Additional exam requirements/recommendations for international students: Required—TOEFL (minimum score 550 paper-based). Electronic applications accepted. *Faculty research:* Dosimetry, manpower studies, diagnostic imaging physics, shielding.

University of Minnesota, Twin Cities Campus, Graduate School, Program in Biophysical Sciences and Medical Physics, Minneapolis, MN 55455-0213. Offers MS, PhD. *Program availability:* Part-time. *Degree requirements:* For master's, thesis optional, research paper, oral exam; for doctorate, thesis/dissertation, oral/written preliminary exam, oral final exam. *Faculty research:* Theoretical biophysics, radiological physics, cellular and molecular biophysics.

University of Oklahoma Health Sciences Center, College of Medicine and Graduate College, Graduate Programs in Medicine, Department of Radiological Sciences, Oklahoma City, OK 73190. Offers medical radiation physics (MS, PhD), including diagnostic radiology, nuclear medicine, radiation therapy, ultrasound. *Program availability:* Part-time. Terminal master's awarded for partial completion of doctoral program. *Degree requirements:* For master's, thesis; for doctorate, thesis/dissertation. *Entrance requirements:* For master's, GRE General Test; for doctorate, GRE General Test, 3 letters of recommendation. Additional exam requirements/recommendations for international students: Required—TOEFL. *Faculty research:* Monte Carlo applications in radiation therapy, observer-performed studies in diagnostic radiology, error analysis in gated cardiac nuclear medicine studies, nuclear medicine absorbed fraction determinations.

University of Pennsylvania, School of Arts and Sciences, College of Liberal and Professional Studies, Philadelphia, PA 19104. Offers applied geosciences (MSAG); applied positive psychology (MAP); chemical sciences (MCS); environmental studies (MES); individualized study (MLA); liberal arts (M Phil); medical physics (MMP); organization dynamics (M Phil). *Students:* 135 full-time (69 women), 329 part-time (203 women); includes 85 minority (27 Black or African American, non-Hispanic/Latino; 23 Asian, non-Hispanic/Latino; 17 Hispanic/Latino; 18 Two or more races, non-Hispanic/Latino), 61 international. Average age 35. 542 applicants, 52% accepted, 173 enrolled. In 2015, 161 master's awarded. *Expenses: Tuition, area resident:* Full-time $31,068; part-time $5762 per course. *Required fees:* $3200; $336 per course. Full-time tuition and fees vary according to degree level, program and student level. Part-time tuition and fees vary according to course load, degree level and program. *Unit head:* Nora Lewis, E-mail: nlewis@sas.upenn.edu.
Website: http://www.sas.upenn.edu/lps/graduate

University of Pennsylvania, School of Arts and Sciences, Graduate Group in Physics and Astronomy, Philadelphia, PA 19104. Offers medical physics (MS); physics (PhD). *Program availability:* Part-time. *Faculty:* 43 full-time (7 women), 11 part-time/adjunct (0 women). *Students:* 100 full-time (28 women), 1 part-time (0 women); includes 18 minority (1 Black or African American, non-Hispanic/Latino; 9 Asian, non-Hispanic/Latino; 6 Hispanic/Latino; 2 Two or more races, non-Hispanic/Latino), 20 international. Average age 26. 371 applicants, 20% accepted, 28 enrolled. In 2015, 35 master's, 24 doctorates awarded. *Expenses: Tuition, area resident:* Full-time $31,068; part-time $5762 per course. *Required fees:* $3200; $336 per course. Full-time tuition and fees vary according to degree level, program and student level. Part-time tuition and fees vary according to course load, degree level and program. *Financial support:* Application deadline: 12/1.
Website: http://www.physics.upenn.edu/graduate/

University of South Florida, College of Arts and Sciences, Department of Physics, Tampa, FL 33620-9951. Offers applied physics (PhD); physics (MS), including applied physics, atmospheric physics, atomic and molecular physics, laser physics, materials physics, medical physics, optical physics, semiconductor physics, solid state physics. *Program availability:* Part-time. *Faculty:* 25 full-time (2 women). *Students:* 71 full-time (16 women), 6 part-time (1 woman); includes 14 minority (2 Black or African American, non-Hispanic/Latino; 12 Hispanic/Latino), 36 international. Average age 31. 97 applicants, 21% accepted, 12 enrolled. In 2015, 14 master's, 8 doctorates awarded. *Degree requirements:* For master's, comprehensive exam, thesis optional; for doctorate, comprehensive exam, thesis/dissertation. *Entrance requirements:* For master's and doctorate, GRE General Test; GRE Subject Test in physics (recommended), minimum GPA of 3.0, three letters of recommendation, statement of purpose. Additional exam requirements/recommendations for international students: Required—TOEFL (minimum score 550 paper-based; 79 iBT) or IELTS (minimum score 6.5). *Application deadline:* For fall admission, 2/15 priority date for domestic students, 1/2 for international students; for spring admission, 9/1 for domestic students, 7/1 for international students. Applications are processed on a rolling basis. Application fee: $30. Electronic applications accepted. *Financial support:* In 2015–16, 70 students received support, including 27 research assistantships with tuition reimbursements available (averaging $15,272 per year), 43 teaching assistantships with tuition reimbursements available (averaging $16,267 per year); unspecified assistantships also available. *Faculty research:* The molecular organization of collagen, lipid rafts in biological membranes, the formation of Alzheimer plaques, the role of cellular ion pumps in wound healing, carbon nanotubes as biological detectors, optical imaging of neuronal activity, three-dimensional imaging of intact tissues, motility of cancer cells, the optical detection of pathogens in water. *Total annual research expenditures:* $2.4 million. *Unit head:* Dr. Pritish Mukherjee, Professor and Chairperson, 813-974-3293, Fax: 813-974-5813, E-mail: pritish@usf.edu. *Application contact:* Dr. Lilia Woods, Professor and Graduate Program Director, 813-974-2862, Fax: 813-974-5813, E-mail: lmwoods@usf.edu.
Website: http://physics.usf.edu/

The University of Texas Health Science Center at Houston, Graduate School of Biomedical Sciences, Program in Medical Physics, Houston, TX 77225-0036. Offers MS, PhD, MD/PhD. *Degree requirements:* For master's, thesis; for doctorate, thesis/dissertation. *Entrance requirements:* For master's and doctorate, GRE General Test. Additional exam requirements/recommendations for international students: Required—TOEFL. Electronic applications accepted. *Faculty research:* Medical physics, radiation oncology physics, diagnostic imaging physics, medical nuclear physics, image-guided therapy.

The University of Texas Health Science Center at San Antonio, Graduate School of Biomedical Sciences, Radiological Sciences Graduate Program, San Antonio, TX 78229-3900. Offers PhD. *Degree requirements:* For doctorate, comprehensive exam, thesis/dissertation.

The University of Toledo, College of Graduate Studies, College of Medicine and Life Sciences, Program in Medical Physics, Toledo, OH 43606-3390. Offers MSBS. *Degree requirements:* For master's, thesis. *Entrance requirements:* For master's, GRE, minimum undergraduate GPA of 3.0, three letters of recommendation, statement of purpose, transcripts from all prior institutions attended, resume. Additional exam requirements/recommendations for international students: Required—TOEFL (minimum score 550 paper-based; 80 iBT). Electronic applications accepted.

The University of Toledo, College of Graduate Studies, College of Natural Sciences and Mathematics, Department of Physics and Astronomy, Toledo, OH 43606-3390. Offers photovoltaics (PSM); physics (MS, PhD), including astrophysics (PhD), materials science, medical physics (PhD); MS/PhD. *Degree requirements:* For master's, thesis; for doctorate, thesis/dissertation, departmental qualifying exam. *Entrance requirements:* For master's and doctorate, GRE General Test, GRE Subject Test, minimum cumulative point-hour ratio of 2.7 for all previous academic work, three letters of recommendation, statement of purpose, transcripts from all prior institutions attended. Additional exam requirements/recommendations for international students: Required—TOEFL (minimum score 550 paper-based; 80 iBT). Electronic applications accepted. *Faculty research:* Atomic physics, solid-state physics, materials science, astrophysics.

University of Utah, Graduate School, College of Science, Department of Physics and Astronomy, Salt Lake City, UT 84112. Offers chemical physics (PhD); medical physics (MS, PhD); physics (MA, MS, PhD); physics teaching (PhD). *Program availability:* Part-time. *Faculty:* 34 full-time (4 women), 16 part-time/adjunct (1 woman). *Students:* 79 full-time (26 women), 19 part-time (7 women); includes 7 minority (3 Asian, non-Hispanic/Latino; 4 Hispanic/Latino), 51 international. Average age 28. 141 applicants, 30% accepted, 19 enrolled. In 2015, 13 master's, 10 doctorates awarded. Terminal master's awarded for partial completion of doctoral program. *Degree requirements:* For master's, comprehensive exam (for some programs), thesis or alternative, teaching experience, departmental exam; for doctorate, comprehensive exam, thesis/dissertation, departmental qualifying exam. *Entrance requirements:* For master's and doctorate, GRE Subject Test, minimum GPA of 3.0. Additional exam requirements/recommendations for international students: Required—TOEFL (minimum score 550 paper-based; 85 iBT). *Application deadline:* For fall admission, 4/1 priority date for domestic and international students. Applications are processed on a rolling basis. Application fee: $55 ($65 for international students). Electronic applications accepted. *Financial support:* In 2015–16, 23 research assistantships with full tuition reimbursements (averaging $23,500 per year), 52 teaching assistantships with full tuition reimbursements (averaging $20,641 per year) were awarded; institutionally sponsored loans, scholarships/grants, and unspecified assistantships also available. Financial award application deadline: 2/15; financial award applicants required to submit FAFSA. *Faculty research:* High-energy, cosmic-ray, astrophysics, medical physics, condensed matter, relativity applied physics, biophysics, astronomy. *Total annual research expenditures:* $5.2 million. *Unit head:* Dr. Carleton DeTar, Chair, 801-581-3538, Fax: 801-581-4801, E-mail: detar@physics.utah.edu. *Application contact:* Jackie Hadley, Graduate Secretary, 801-581-6861, Fax: 801-581-4801, E-mail: jackie@physics.utah.edu.
Website: http://www.physics.utah.edu/

University of Victoria, Faculty of Graduate Studies, Faculty of Science, Department of Physics and Astronomy, Victoria, BC V8W 2Y2, Canada. Offers astronomy and astrophysics (M Sc, PhD); condensed matter physics (M Sc, PhD); experimental particle physics (M Sc, PhD); medical physics (M Sc, PhD); ocean physics (M Sc, PhD); theoretical physics (M Sc, PhD). *Degree requirements:* For master's, thesis; for doctorate, comprehensive exam, thesis/dissertation, candidacy exam. *Entrance requirements:* For master's and doctorate, GRE. Additional exam requirements/recommendations for international students: Required—TOEFL (minimum score 575 paper-based), IELTS (minimum score 7). Electronic applications accepted. *Faculty research:* Old stellar populations; observational cosmology and large scale structure; cp violation; atlas.

University of Wisconsin–Madison, School of Medicine and Public Health, Medical Physics Graduate Program, Madison, WI 53705-2275. Offers health physics (MS); medical physics (MS, PhD). *Program availability:* Part-time. *Faculty:* 44 full-time (4 women), 8 part-time/adjunct (0 women). *Students:* 87 full-time (24 women); includes 21 minority (2 Black or African American, non-Hispanic/Latino; 6 Asian, non-Hispanic/Latino; 11 Hispanic/Latino; 2 Two or more races, non-Hispanic/Latino), 17 international. Average age 26. 81 applicants, 30% accepted, 12 enrolled. In 2015, 17 master's, 23 doctorates awarded. Terminal master's awarded for partial completion of doctoral program. *Degree requirements:* For master's, comprehensive exam; for doctorate, comprehensive exam, thesis/dissertation. *Entrance requirements:* For master's and doctorate, GRE General Test, minimum GPA of 3.0. Additional exam requirements/recommendations for international students: Required—TOEFL or IELTS. *Application deadline:* For fall admission, 12/1 priority date for domestic students, 11/15 for international students. Application fee: $56 ($64 for international students). Electronic applications accepted. *Expenses:* Tuition, state resident: full-time $5364. Tuition, nonresident: full-time $12,027. *Required fees:* $571. Tuition and fees vary according to campus/location, program and reciprocity agreements. *Financial support:* In 2015–16, 78 students received support, including 11 fellowships with full tuition reimbursements available (averaging $23,515 per year), 74 research assistantships with full tuition reimbursements available (averaging $23,515 per year), 7 teaching assistantships with full tuition reimbursements available (averaging $15,342 per year); scholarships/grants, traineeships, health care benefits, and unspecified assistantships also available. Financial award application deadline: 11/15. *Faculty research:* Biomagnetism, anatomic and functional imaging, medical image processing, radiation therapy physics, radiation metrology, molecular imaging, novel radionuclide production. *Total annual research expenditures:* $4.5 million. *Unit head:* Dr. Edward F. Jackson, Chair, 608-262-2171, Fax: 608-262-2413, E-mail: efjackson@wisc.edu. *Application contact:* Debra A. Torgerson, Graduate Coordinator, 608-265-6504, Fax: 608-262-2413, E-mail: datorger@wisc.edu.
Website: http://www.medphysics.wisc.edu/

Virginia Commonwealth University, Graduate School, College of Humanities and Sciences, Department of Physics, Programs in Medical Physics, Richmond, VA 23284-9005. Offers MS, PhD. *Entrance requirements:* For master's and doctorate, GRE General Test. Additional exam requirements/recommendations for international students: Required—TOEFL (minimum score 600 paper-based; 100 iBT); Recommended—IELTS (minimum score 6.5). Electronic applications accepted. *Faculty research:* Functional imaging using PET and NMR, computed tomography (CT) image artifact removal and deformation, intensity-modulated radiation therapy, radiation therapy dose calculations, 4D radiation therapy, brachytherapy dose calculations.

Wayne State University, School of Medicine, Office of Biomedical Graduate Programs, Program in Medical Physics, Detroit, MI 48202. Offers MS, PhD. *Program availability:* Part-time, evening/weekend. *Faculty:* 10. *Students:* 15 full-time (1 woman), 8 part-time (3 women); includes 1 minority (Asian, non-Hispanic/Latino), 7 international. Average age 29. 60 applicants, 22% accepted, 4 enrolled. In 2015, 9 master's, 4 doctorates awarded. Terminal master's awarded for partial completion of doctoral program. *Degree requirements:* For master's, thesis, essay, exit exam, clinical internship; for doctorate, thesis/dissertation, qualifying exam, clinical internship. *Entrance requirements:* For master's and doctorate, GRE General Test, BS in physics or related area. Additional

exam requirements/recommendations for international students: Required—TOEFL; Recommended—TWE. Application fee: $0. Electronic applications accepted. *Expenses:* $17,645 per year resident tuition, $33,311 non-resident tuition; $735.20 per credit hour resident tuition, $1,387.95 per credit hour non-resident tuition; fees include $47.45 per credit hour student services fee and $274.60 per semester registration fee. *Financial support:* In 2015–16, 11 students received support, including 6 fellowships with tuition reimbursements available (averaging $17,811 per year); research assistantships with tuition reimbursements available, teaching assistantships, scholarships/grants, health care benefits, and unspecified assistantships also available. Financial award application deadline: 3/31; financial award applicants required to submit FAFSA. *Unit head:* Dr. Jay Burmeister, Program Director, 313-579-9617, Fax: 313-576-9624, E-mail: burmeist@med.wayne.edu.
Website: http://www.medicalphysics.med.wayne.edu/programinfo.php

Wright State University, School of Graduate Studies, College of Science and Mathematics, Department of Physics, Program in Physics, Dayton, OH 45435. Offers geophysics (MS); medical physics (MS). *Program availability:* Part-time, evening/weekend. *Degree requirements:* For master's, thesis. *Entrance requirements:* Additional exam requirements/recommendations for international students: Required—TOEFL. *Faculty research:* Solid-state physics, optics, geophysics.

Section 22
Health Services

This section contains a directory of institutions offering graduate work in health services. Additional information about programs listed in the directory may be obtained by writing directly to the dean of a graduate school or chair of a department at the address given in the directory.

For programs offering related work, see also in this book *Allied Health, Nursing,* and *Public Health.* In another book in this series:

Graduate Programs in Business, Education, Information Studies, Law & Social Work

See *Business Administration and Management*

CONTENTS

Program Directories

Displays and Close-Ups

See also:

Health Services Management and Hospital Administration

Adelphi University, Robert B. Willumstad School of Business, MBA Program, Garden City, NY 11530-0701. Offers accounting (MBA); finance (MBA); health services administration (MBA); human resource management (MBA); management (MBA); management information systems (MBA); marketing (MBA); sport management (MBA). *Accreditation:* AACSB. *Program availability:* Part-time, evening/weekend. *Degree requirements:* For master's, capstone course. *Entrance requirements:* For master's, GMAT, 2 letters of recommendation. Additional exam requirements/recommendations for international students: Required—TOEFL (minimum score 550 paper-based; 80 iBT). Electronic applications accepted. *Faculty research:* Supply chain management, distribution channels, productivity benchmark analysis, data envelopment analysis, financial portfolio analysis.

Alaska Pacific University, Graduate Programs, Business Administration Department, Program in Business Administration, Anchorage, AK 99508-4672. Offers business administration (MBA); health services administration (MBA). *Program availability:* Part-time, evening/weekend. *Degree requirements:* For master's, capstone course. *Entrance requirements:* For master's, GMAT or GRE General Test, minimum GPA of 3.0.

Albany State University, College of Arts and Humanities, Albany, GA 31705-2717. Offers English education (M Ed); public administration (MPA), including community and economic development administration, criminal justice administration, general administration, health administration and policy, human resources management, public policy, water resources management; social work (MSW). *Program availability:* Part-time. *Degree requirements:* For master's, comprehensive exam, professional portfolio (for MPA), internship, capstone report. *Entrance requirements:* For master's, GRE, MAT, minimum GPA of 3.0, official transcript, pre-medical record/certificate of immunization, letters of reference. Electronic applications accepted. *Faculty research:* HIV prevention for minority students.

Albany State University, College of Business, Albany, GA 31705-2717. Offers accounting (MBA); general (MBA); healthcare (MBA). *Accreditation:* ACBSP. *Program availability:* Part-time, evening/weekend. *Degree requirements:* For master's, comprehensive exam, internship, 3 hours of physical education. *Entrance requirements:* For master's, GMAT (minimum score of 450)/GRE (minimum score of 800) for those without earned master's degree or higher, minimum undergraduate GPA of 2.5, 2 letters of reference, official transcript, pre-entrance medical record and certificate of immunization. Electronic applications accepted. *Faculty research:* Diversity issues, ancestry, understanding finance through use of technology.

American InterContinental University Online, Program in Business Administration, Schaumburg, IL 60173. Offers accounting and finance (MBA); finance (MBA); healthcare management (MBA); human resource management (MBA); international business (MBA); management (MBA); marketing (MBA); operations management (MBA); organizational psychology and development (MBA); project management (MBA). *Accreditation:* ACBSP. *Program availability:* Evening/weekend, online learning. *Entrance requirements:* Additional exam requirements/recommendations for international students: Required—TOEFL (minimum score 550 paper-based). Electronic applications accepted.

American Public University System, AMU/APU Graduate Programs, Charles Town, WV 25414. Offers accounting (MBA, MS); analytics (MBA); criminal justice (MA), including business administration, emergency and disaster management, general (MA, MS); educational leadership (M Ed); emergency and disaster management (MS); entrepreneurship (MBA); environmental policy and management (MS), including environmental planning, environmental sustainability, fish and wildlife management, general (MA, MS), global environmental management; finance (MBA); general (MBA); global business management (MBA); government contracting and acquisition (MBA); health care administration (MBA); history (MA), including American history, ancient and classical history, European history, global history, public history; homeland security (MA), including business administration, counterterrorism studies, criminal justice, cyber, emergency management and public health, intelligence studies, transportation security; homeland security resource allocation (MBA); humanities (MA); information technology (MS), including digital forensics, enterprise software development, information assurance and security, IT project management; information technology management (MBA); intelligence studies (MA), including criminal intelligence, cyber, general (MA, MS), homeland security, intelligence analysis, intelligence collection, intelligence management, intelligence operations, terrorism studies; international relations and conflict resolution (MA), including comparative and security issues, conflict resolution, international and transnational security issues, peacekeeping; legal studies (MA); management (MA), including strategic consulting; marketing (MBA); military history (MA), including American military history, American Revolution, civil war, war since 1945, World War II; military studies (MA), including joint warfare, strategic leadership; national security studies (MA), including cyber, general (MA, MS), homeland security, regional security studies, security and intelligence analysis, terrorism studies; nonprofit management (MBA); political science (MA), including American politics and government, comparative government and development, general (MA, MS), international relations, public policy; psychology (MA); public administration (MPA), including disaster management, environmental policy, health policy, human resources, national security, organizational management, security management; public health (MPH); reverse logistics management (MA); school counseling (M Ed); security management (MA); space studies (MS), including aerospace science, general (MA, MS), planetary science; sports and health sciences (MS); sports management (MBA); teaching (M Ed), including autism spectrum disorder, curriculum and instruction for elementary teachers, elementary reading, English language learners, instructional leadership, online learning, special education, STEAM (STEM plus the arts); transportation and logistics management (MA). *Program availability:* Part-time, evening/weekend, online only. *Faculty:* 431 full-time (241 women), 1,839 part-time/adjunct (865 women). *Students:* 531 full-time (233 women), 9,094 part-time (3,735 women); includes 3,140 minority (1,679 Black or African American, non-Hispanic/Latino; 55 American Indian or Alaska Native, non-Hispanic/Latino; 252 Asian, non-Hispanic/Latino; 773 Hispanic/Latino; 75 Native Hawaiian or other Pacific Islander, non-Hispanic/Latino; 306 Two or more races, non-Hispanic/Latino; 111 international. Average age 37. In 2015, 3,391 master's awarded. *Degree requirements:* For master's, comprehensive exam or practicum. *Entrance requirements:* For master's, official transcript showing earned bachelor's degree from institution accredited by recognized accrediting body. Additional exam requirements/recommendations for international students: Required—TOEFL (minimum score 550 paper-based), IELTS (minimum score 6.5). *Application deadline:*

Applications are processed on a rolling basis. Application fee: $0. Electronic applications accepted. *Expenses: Tuition, area resident:* Part-time $350 per credit hour. *Financial support:* Applicants required to submit FAFSA. *Unit head:* Dr. Karan Powell, Executive Vice President and Provost, 877-468-6268, Fax: 304-724-3780. *Application contact:* Terry Grant, Vice President of Enrollment Management, 877-468-6268, Fax: 304-724-3780, E-mail: info@apus.edu.
Website: http://www.apus.edu

American Sentinel University, Graduate Programs, Aurora, CO 80014. Offers business administration (MBA); business intelligence (MS); computer science (MSCS); health information management (MS); healthcare (MBA); information systems (MSIS); nursing (MSN). *Program availability:* Part-time, evening/weekend, online learning. *Entrance requirements:* Additional exam requirements/recommendations for international students: Required—TOEFL (minimum score 600 paper-based). Electronic applications accepted.

American University of Beirut, Graduate Programs, Faculty of Health Sciences, Beirut, Lebanon. Offers environmental sciences (MS), including environmental health; epidemiology (MS); epidemiology and biostatistics (MPH); health management and policy (MPH); health promotion and community health (MPH). *Program availability:* Part-time. *Faculty:* 30 full-time (21 women), 3 part-time/adjunct (1 woman). *Students:* 49 full-time (38 women), 99 part-time (81 women). Average age 27. 115 applicants, 71% accepted, 40 enrolled. In 2015, 51 master's awarded. *Degree requirements:* For master's, one foreign language, comprehensive exam (for some programs), thesis (for some programs). *Entrance requirements:* For master's, 2 letters of recommendation, personal statement, transcripts. Additional exam requirements/recommendations for international students: Required—TOEFL (minimum score 583 paper-based; 97 iBT), IELTS (minimum score 7). *Application deadline:* For fall admission, 1/4 priority date for domestic and international students; for spring admission, 11/1 for domestic and international students. Application fee: $50. Electronic applications accepted. *Expenses: Tuition, area resident:* Full-time $16,254; part-time $903 per credit. *Required fees:* $699. Tuition and fees vary according to course load and program. *Financial support:* In 2015–16, 70 students received support. Scholarships/grants, health care benefits, and unspecified assistantships available. Financial award application deadline: 4/1. *Faculty research:* Tobacco control; health of the elderly; youth health; mental health; women's health; reproductive and sexual health, including HIV/AIDS; water quality; health systems; quality in health care delivery; health human resources; health policy; occupational and environmental health; social inequality; social determinants of health; non-communicable diseases; nutrition; refugees health; conflict and health. *Total annual research expenditures:* $2 million. *Unit head:* Iman Adel Nuwayhid, Dean, 961-1759683, Fax: 961-1744470, E-mail: nuwayhid@aub.edu.lb. *Application contact:* Mitra Tauk, Administrative Coordinator, 961-1350000 Ext. 4687, Fax: 961-1744470, E-mail: mt12@aub.edu.lb.

Aquinas College, School of Management, Grand Rapids, MI 49506-1799. Offers health care administration (MM); marketing management (MM); organizational leadership (MM); sustainable business (MM, MSB). *Program availability:* Part-time, evening/weekend. *Entrance requirements:* For master's, GMAT, minimum undergraduate GPA of 2.75, 2 years of work experience. Additional exam requirements/recommendations for international students: Required—TOEFL (minimum score 550 paper-based). *Expenses:* Contact institution.

Aquinas Institute of Theology, Graduate and Professional Programs, St. Louis, MO 63108. Offers biblical studies (Certificate); church music (MM); health care mission (MAHCM); ministry (M Div); pastoral care (Certificate); pastoral ministry (MAPM); pastoral studies (MAPS); preaching (D Min); spiritual direction (Certificate); theology (M Div, MA); Thomistic studies (Certificate); M Div/MA; MA/PhD; MAPS/MSW. *Accreditation:* ATS (one or more programs are accredited). *Program availability:* Part-time, evening/weekend, online learning. *Degree requirements:* For master's, variable foreign language requirement, comprehensive exam (for some programs), thesis (for some programs); for doctorate, thesis/dissertation. *Entrance requirements:* For master's and Certificate, MAT; for doctorate, 3 years of ministerial experience, 6 hours of graduate course work in homiletics, M Div or the equivalent, minimum GPA of 3.0. Additional exam requirements/recommendations for international students: Required—TOEFL. *Expenses:* Contact institution. *Faculty research:* Theology of preaching, hermeneutics, lay ecclesial ministry, pastoral and practical theology.

Argosy University, Atlanta, College of Business, Atlanta, GA 30328. Offers accounting (DBA); corporate compliance (MBA); customized professional concentration (MBA, DBA); finance (MBA); healthcare administration (MBA); information systems (DBA); information systems management (MBA); international business (MBA, DBA); management (MBA, MSM, DBA); marketing (MBA, DBA).

Argosy University, Chicago, College of Business, Chicago, IL 60601. Offers accounting (DBA); customized professional concentration (MBA, DBA); finance (MBA); fraud examination (MBA); global business sustainability (DBA); healthcare administration (MBA); information systems (DBA); information systems management (MBA); international business (MBA, DBA); management (MBA, MSM, DBA); marketing (MBA, DBA); organizational leadership (Ed D); public administration (MBA); sustainable management (MBA). *Program availability:* Online learning.

Argosy University, Dallas, College of Business, Farmers Branch, TX 75244. Offers accounting (DBA, AGC); corporate compliance (MBA, Graduate Certificate); customized professional concentration (MBA); finance (MBA, Graduate Certificate); fraud examination (MBA, Graduate Certificate); global business sustainability (DBA, AGC); healthcare administration (Graduate Certificate); healthcare management (MBA); information systems (MBA, DBA, AGC); information systems management (Graduate Certificate); international business (MBA, DBA, AGC, Graduate Certificate); management (MBA, DBA, AGC, Graduate Certificate); marketing (MBA, DBA, AGC, Graduate Certificate); public administration (MBA, Graduate Certificate); sustainable management (MBA, Graduate Certificate).

Argosy University, Denver, College of Business, Denver, CO 80231. Offers accounting (DBA); corporate compliance (MBA); customized professional concentration (MBA, DBA); finance (MBA); fraud examination (MBA); global business sustainability (DBA); healthcare administration (MBA); information systems (DBA); information systems management (MBA); international business (MBA, DBA); management (MBA, MSM, DBA); marketing (MBA, DBA); organizational leadership (Ed D); public administration (MBA); sustainable management (MBA).

Health Services Management and Hospital Administration

Argosy University, Hawai`i, College of Business, Honolulu, HI 96813. Offers accounting (DBA); corporate compliance (MBA); customized professional concentration (MBA, DBA); finance (MBA, Certificate); fraud examination (MBA); global business sustainability (DBA); healthcare administration (MBA, Certificate); information systems (DBA); information systems management (MBA, Certificate); international business (MBA, DBA, Certificate); management (MBA, MSM, DBA); marketing (MBA, DBA, Certificate); organizational leadership (Ed D); public administration (MBA); sustainable management (MBA).

Argosy University, Inland Empire, College of Business, Ontario, CA 91761. Offers accounting (DBA); corporate compliance (MBA); customized professional concentration (MBA, DBA); finance (MBA); fraud examination (MBA); global business sustainability (DBA); healthcare administration (MBA); information systems (DBA); information systems management (MBA); international business (MBA, DBA); management (MBA, MSM, DBA); marketing (MBA, DBA); organizational leadership (Ed D); public administration (MBA); sustainable management (MBA).

Argosy University, Los Angeles, College of Business, Santa Monica, CA 90045. Offers accounting (DBA); corporate compliance (MBA); customized professional concentration (MBA, DBA); finance (MBA); fraud examination (MBA); global business sustainability (DBA); healthcare administration (MBA); information systems (DBA); information systems management (MBA); international business (MBA, DBA); management (MBA, MSM, DBA); marketing (MBA, DBA); organizational leadership (Ed D); public administration (MBA); sustainable management (MBA).

Argosy University, Nashville, College of Business, Nashville, TN 37214. Offers accounting (DBA); customized professional concentration (MBA, DBA); finance (MBA); healthcare administration (MBA); information systems (MBA, DBA); international business (MBA, DBA); management (MBA, MSM, DBA); marketing (MBA, DBA).

Argosy University, Orange County, College of Business, Orange, CA 92868. Offers accounting (DBA, Adv C); corporate compliance (MBA); customized professional concentration (MBA, DBA); finance (MBA, Certificate); fraud examination (MBA); global business sustainability (DBA); healthcare administration (MBA, Certificate); information systems (DBA, Adv C, Certificate); information systems management (MBA); international business (MBA, DBA, Adv C, Certificate); management (MBA, MSM, DBA, Adv C); marketing (MBA, DBA, Adv C, Certificate); organizational leadership (Ed D); public administration (MBA, Certificate); sustainable management (MBA).

Argosy University, Phoenix, College of Business, Phoenix, AZ 85021. Offers accounting (DBA); corporate compliance (MBA); customized professional concentration (MBA, DBA); finance (MBA); fraud examination (MBA); global business sustainability (DBA); healthcare administration (MBA); information systems (DBA); information systems management (MBA); international business (MBA, DBA); management (MBA, DBA); marketing (MBA, DBA); public administration (MBA); sustainable management (MBA).

Argosy University, Salt Lake City, College of Business, Draper, UT 84020. Offers accounting (DBA); corporate compliance (MBA); customized professional concentration (MBA, DBA); finance (MBA); fraud examination (MBA); global business sustainability (DBA); healthcare administration (MBA); information systems (DBA); information systems management (MBA); international business (MBA, DBA); management (MBA, DBA); marketing (MBA, DBA); public administration (MBA); sustainable management (MBA).

Argosy University, San Francisco Bay Area, College of Business, Alameda, CA 94501. Offers accounting (DBA); corporate compliance (MBA); customized professional concentration (MBA, DBA); finance (MBA); fraud examination (MBA); global business sustainability (DBA); healthcare administration (MBA); information systems (DBA); information systems management (MBA); international business (MBA, DBA); management (MBA, MSM, DBA); marketing (MBA, DBA); organizational leadership (Ed D); public administration (MBA); sustainable management (MBA).

Argosy University, Sarasota, College of Business, Sarasota, FL 34235. Offers accounting (DBA, Adv C); corporate compliance (MBA, DBA, Certificate); customized professional concentration (MBA, DBA); finance (MBA, Certificate); fraud examination (MBA, Certificate); global business sustainability (DBA, Adv C); healthcare administration (MBA, Certificate); information systems (DBA, Adv C, Certificate); information systems management (MBA); international business (MBA, DBA, Adv C, Certificate); management (MBA, MSM, DBA, Adv C, Certificate); marketing (MBA, DBA, Adv C, Certificate); organizational leadership (Ed D); public administration (MBA, Certificate); sustainable management (MBA, Certificate).

Argosy University, Schaumburg, Graduate School of Business and Management, Schaumburg, IL 60173-5403. Offers accounting (DBA, Adv C); customized professional concentration (MBA, DBA); finance (MBA, Certificate); fraud examination (MBA); healthcare administration (MBA, Certificate); human resource management (MS); information systems (Adv C, Certificate); information systems management (MBA); international business (MBA, DBA, Adv C, Certificate); management (MBA, MSM, DBA, Adv C, Certificate); marketing (MBA, DBA, Adv C, Certificate); organizational leadership (MS, Ed D); public administration (MBA); sustainable management (MBA).

Argosy University, Seattle, College of Business, Seattle, WA 98121. Offers accounting (DBA); corporate compliance (MBA); customized professional concentration (MBA, DBA); finance (MBA); fraud examination (MBA); global business sustainability (DBA); healthcare administration (MBA); information systems (DBA); information systems management (MBA); international business (MBA, DBA); management (MBA, MSM, DBA); marketing (MBA, DBA); organizational leadership (Ed D); public administration (MBA); sustainable management (MBA).

Argosy University, Tampa, College of Business, Tampa, FL 33607. Offers accounting (DBA); corporate compliance (MBA); customized professional concentration (MBA, DBA); finance (MBA); fraud examination (MBA); global business sustainability (DBA); healthcare administration (MBA); information systems (DBA); information systems management (MBA); international business (MBA, DBA); management (MBA, MSM, DBA); marketing (MBA, DBA); organizational leadership (Ed D); public administration (MBA); sustainable management (MBA).

Argosy University, Twin Cities, College of Business, Eagan, MN 55121. Offers accounting (DBA); customized professional concentration (MBA, DBA); finance (MBA); fraud examination (MBA); global business sustainability (DBA); healthcare administration (MBA); information systems (DBA); information systems management (MBA); international business (MBA, DBA); management (MBA, MSM, DBA); marketing (MBA, DBA); organizational leadership (Ed D); public administration (MBA); sustainable management (MBA).

Argosy University, Twin Cities, College of Health Sciences, Eagan, MN 55121. Offers health services management (MS); public health (MPH).

Argosy University, Washington DC, College of Business, Arlington, VA 22209. Offers accounting (DBA); customized professional concentration (MBA, DBA); finance (MBA); fraud examination (MBA); global business sustainability (DBA); healthcare administration (MBA); information systems (DBA); information systems management (MBA); international business (MBA, DBA, Certificate); management (MBA, MSM,

DBA); marketing (MBA, DBA, Certificate); organizational leadership (Ed D); public administration (MBA); sustainable management (MBA).

Arizona State University at the Tempe campus, W. P. Carey School of Business, Program in Business Administration, Tempe, AZ 85287-4906. Offers entrepreneurship (MBA); finance (MBA); health sector management (MBA); international business (MBA); leadership (MBA); marketing (MBA); organizational behavior (PhD); strategic management (PhD); supply chain management (MBA, PhD); JD/MBA; MBA/M Acc; MBA/M Arch. *Accreditation:* AACSB. *Program availability:* Part-time, evening/weekend, online learning. Terminal master's awarded for partial completion of doctoral program. *Degree requirements:* For master's, thesis or alternative, internship, interactive Program of Study (iPOS) submitted before completing 50 percent of required credit hours; for doctorate, comprehensive exam, thesis/dissertation, interactive Program of Study (iPOS) submitted before completing 50 percent of required credit hours. *Entrance requirements:* For master's, GMAT, minimum GPA of 3.0 in last 2 years of work leading to bachelor's degree, 2 letters of recommendation, professional resume, official transcripts, 3 essays; for doctorate, GMAT or GRE, minimum GPA of 3.0 in last 2 years of work leading to bachelor's degree, 3 letters of recommendation, resume, personal statement/essay. Additional exam requirements/recommendations for international students: Required—TOEFL (minimum score 550 paper-based; 80 iBT), IELTS (minimum score 6.5). Electronic applications accepted. *Expenses:* Contact institution.

Arkansas State University, Graduate School, College of Nursing and Health Professions, School of Nursing, State University, AR 72467. Offers aging studies (Graduate Certificate); health care management (Graduate Certificate); health sciences (MS); health sciences education (Graduate Certificate); nurse anesthesia (MSN); nursing (MSN); nursing practice (DNP). *Accreditation:* AANA/CANAEP (one or more programs are accredited). *Program availability:* Part-time. *Faculty:* 16 full-time (14 women). *Students:* 80 full-time (30 women), 139 part-time (121 women); includes 38 minority (26 Black or African American, non-Hispanic/Latino; 3 American Indian or Alaska Native, non-Hispanic/Latino; 3 Asian, non-Hispanic/Latino; 4 Hispanic/Latino; 1 Native Hawaiian or other Pacific Islander, non-Hispanic/Latino; 1 Two or more races, non-Hispanic/Latino), 2 international. Average age 34. 147 applicants, 33% accepted, 43 enrolled. In 2015, 84 master's awarded. *Degree requirements:* For master's and Graduate Certificate, comprehensive exam, thesis or alternative; for doctorate, comprehensive exam, thesis/dissertation. *Entrance requirements:* For master's, GRE General Test or MAT, appropriate bachelor's degree, current Arkansas nursing license, CPR certification, physical examination, professional liability insurance, critical care experience, ACLS Certification, PALS Certification, interview, immunization records, personal goal statement, health assessment; for doctorate, GRE or MAT, NCLEX-RN Exam, appropriate master's degree, current Arkansas nursing license, CPR certification, physical examination, professional liability insurance, critical care experience, ACLS Certification, PALS Certification, interview, immunization records, personal goal statement, health assessment, TB skin test, background check; for Graduate Certificate, GRE or MAT, appropriate bachelor's degree, official transcripts, immunization records, proof of employment in healthcare, TB Skin Test, TB Mask Fit Test, CPR Certification. Additional exam requirements/recommendations for international students: Required—TOEFL (minimum score 550 paper-based; 79 iBT), IELTS (minimum score 6), PTE (minimum score 56). *Application deadline:* Applications are processed on a rolling basis. Electronic applications accepted. *Expenses:* Contact institution. *Financial support:* In 2015–16, 1 student received support. Fellowships, career-related internships or fieldwork, scholarships/grants, and unspecified assistantships available. Financial award application deadline: 7/1; financial award applicants required to submit FAFSA. *Unit head:* Dr. Jill Oswaks, Chair of Graduate Programs, 870-972-3074, Fax: 870-972-2954, E-mail: jdettyoswaks@astate.edu. *Application contact:* Vickey Ring, Graduate Admissions Coordinator, 870-972-2737, Fax: 870-972-3917, E-mail: vickeyring@astate.edu.
Website: http://www.astate.edu/college/conhp/departments/nursing/

Armstrong State University, School of Graduate Studies, Program in Health Services Administration, Savannah, GA 31419-1997. Offers health services administration (MHSA). *Accreditation:* CAHME; CEPH. *Program availability:* Part-time, evening/weekend. *Faculty:* 4 full-time (2 women), 1 part-time/adjunct (0 women). *Students:* 23 full-time (13 women), 12 part-time (9 women); includes 15 minority (7 Black or African American, non-Hispanic/Latino; 4 Asian, non-Hispanic/Latino; 4 Hispanic/Latino). Average age 29. 20 applicants, 80% accepted, 10 enrolled. In 2015, 8 master's awarded. *Degree requirements:* For master's, comprehensive exam, thesis optional, capstone project and internship, administration practicum, or research practicum. *Entrance requirements:* For master's, GMAT or GRE General Test, MAT, minimum GPA of 2.8, letter of intent, letters of recommendation. Additional exam requirements/recommendations for international students: Required—TOEFL (minimum score 523 paper-based). *Application deadline:* For fall admission, 6/1 priority date for domestic students, 5/1 priority date for international students; for spring admission, 11/15 priority date for domestic students, 9/15 priority date for international students; for summer admission, 4/15 for domestic students, 9/15 for international students. Applications are processed on a rolling basis. Application fee: $30. Electronic applications accepted. *Expenses:* Contact institution. *Financial support:* In 2015–16, research assistantships with full tuition reimbursements (averaging $5,000 per year) were awarded; career-related internships or fieldwork, Federal Work-Study, scholarships/grants, tuition waivers (full), and unspecified assistantships also available. Support available to part-time students. Financial award applicants required to submit FAFSA. *Faculty research:* Health administration, community health, health education. *Unit head:* Dr. Robert LeFavi, Interim Department Head, 912-344-3208, Fax: 912-344-3490, E-mail: robert.lefavi@armstrong.edu. *Application contact:* McKenzie Peterman, Assistant Director of Graduate Admissions, 912-344-2503, Fax: 912-344-3417, E-mail: graduate@armstrong.edu.
Website: http://www.armstrong.edu/Health_Professions/Health_Sciences/healthsciences_master_of_health_services_administration

Ashworth College, Graduate Programs, Norcross, GA 30092. Offers business administration (MBA); criminal justice (MS); health care administration (MBA, MS); human resource management (MBA, MS); international business (MBA); management (MS); marketing (MBA, MS).

Assumption College, Health Advocacy Program, Worcester, MA 01609-1296. Offers MA, Professional Certificate. *Program availability:* Part-time, evening/weekend, 100% online. *Faculty:* 1 (woman) full-time, 4 part-time/adjunct (0 women). *Students:* 7 part-time (all women). Average age 51. 9 applicants, 67% accepted, 4 enrolled. In 2015, 3 other advanced degrees awarded. *Degree requirements:* For master's, research course, practicum, capstone. *Entrance requirements:* For master's and Professional Certificate, three letters of recommendation, resume, official transcripts, interview, essay. Additional exam requirements/recommendations for international students: Required—TOEFL (minimum score 540 paper-based; 76 iBT), IELTS (minimum score 6). *Application deadline:* For fall admission, 5/1 for domestic and international students; for spring admission, 10/15 for domestic and international students. Applications are processed on a rolling basis. Application fee: $30. Electronic applications accepted. *Expenses:* $625 per credit. *Financial support:* In 2015–16, 1 student received support. Tuition waivers (full and partial) and institutional discounts available. Financial award applicants

Health Services Management and Hospital Administration

required to submit FAFSA. *Unit head:* Lea Christo, Director, 508-767-7503, E-mail: l.christo@assumption.edu. *Application contact:* Karen Stoyanoff, Director of Recruitment for Graduate Enrollment, 508-767-7442, Fax: 508-799-4412, E-mail: graduate@assumption.edu.
Website: http://graduate.assumption.edu/health-advocacy/graduate-programs-health-advocacy

A.T. Still University, College of Graduate Health Studies, Kirksville, MO 63501. Offers dental public health (MPH); health administration (MHA, DHA); health education (DH Ed); health sciences (DH Sc); kinesiology (MS); public health (MPH); school health education (MS). *Program availability:* Part-time, evening/weekend, 100% online, blended/hybrid learning. *Faculty:* 29 full-time (18 women), 89 part-time/adjunct (46 women). *Students:* 456 full-time (271 women), 391 part-time (232 women); includes 291 minority (126 Black or African American, non-Hispanic/Latino; 7 American Indian or Alaska Native, non-Hispanic/Latino; 71 Asian, non-Hispanic/Latino; 80 Hispanic/Latino; 4 Native Hawaiian or other Pacific Islander, non-Hispanic/Latino; 3 Two or more races, non-Hispanic/Latino), 21 international. Average age 37. 286 applicants, 99% accepted, 221 enrolled. In 2015, 130 master's, 74 doctorates awarded. *Degree requirements:* For master's, thesis, integrated terminal project, practicum; for doctorate, thesis/dissertation. *Entrance requirements:* For master's, minimum GPA of 3.0, bachelor's degree or equivalent, background check, essay, three references; for doctorate, minimum GPA of 3.0, master's or terminal degree, background check, essay, three references. Additional exam requirements/recommendations for international students: Required—TOEFL (minimum score 550 paper-based; 80 iBT). *Application deadline:* For fall admission, 5/16 for domestic and international students; for winter admission, 8/1 for domestic and international students; for spring admission, 11/7 for domestic and international students; for summer admission, 1/23 for domestic and international students. Applications are processed on a rolling basis. Application fee: $70. Electronic applications accepted. Application fee is waived when completed online. *Expenses:* Contact institution. *Financial support:* In 2015–16, 30 students received support. Scholarships/grants available. Financial award application deadline: 5/1; financial award applicants required to submit FAFSA. *Faculty research:* Public health: influence of availability of comprehensive wellness resources online, student wellness, oral health care needs assessment of community, oral health knowledge and behaviors of Medicaid-eligible pregnant women and mothers of young children in relations to early childhood caries and tooth decay, alcohol use and alcohol related problems among college students. *Unit head:* Dr. Donald Altman, Interim Dean, 660-626-2820, Fax: 660-626-2826, E-mail: daltman@atsu.edu. *Application contact:* Amie Waldemer, Associate Director, Online Admissions, 480-219-6146, E-mail: awaldemer@atsu.edu.
Website: http://www.atsu.edu/college-of-graduate-health-studies

Auburn University at Montgomery, College of Public Policy and Justice, Department of Political Science and Public Administration, Montgomery, AL 36124-4023. Offers international relations (MIR); nonprofit management and leadership (Certificate); political science (MPS); public administration (MPA); public administration and public policy (PhD); public health care administration and policy (Certificate). PhD offered jointly with Auburn University. *Accreditation:* NASPAA (one or more programs are accredited). *Program availability:* Part-time, evening/weekend. *Faculty:* 5 full-time (1 woman), 1 part-time/adjunct (0 women). *Students:* 5 full-time (3 women), 44 part-time (30 women); includes 13 minority (10 Black or African American, non-Hispanic/Latino; 2 American Indian or Alaska Native, non-Hispanic/Latino; 1 Hispanic/Latino), 1 international. Average age 29. 32 applicants, 88% accepted, 19 enrolled. In 2015, 15 master's awarded. *Degree requirements:* For master's, comprehensive exam; for doctorate, thesis/dissertation. *Entrance requirements:* For master's, GRE General Test or MAT; for doctorate, GRE General Test. *Application deadline:* Applications are processed on a rolling basis. *Expenses:* Tuition, state resident: full-time $6462; part-time $359 per credit hour. Tuition, nonresident: full-time $14,526; part-time $807 per credit hour. *Required fees:* $554. *Financial support:* In 2015–16, 1 teaching assistantship was awarded; research assistantships, career-related internships or fieldwork, and scholarships/grants also available. Support available to part-time students. Financial award application deadline: 3/1; financial award applicants required to submit FAFSA. *Unit head:* Dr. Andrew Cortell, Department Head, 334-244-3622, E-mail: acortell@aum.edu.
Website: http://www.cla.auburn.edu/polisci/graduate-programs/phd-in-public-administration-and-public-policy/

Avila University, School of Business, Kansas City, MO 64145-1698. Offers accounting (MBA); finance (MBA); health care administration (MBA); international business (MBA); management (MBA); management information systems (MBA); marketing (MBA). *Program availability:* Part-time, evening/weekend. *Faculty:* 9 full-time (4 women), 14 part-time/adjunct (4 women). *Students:* 70 full-time (29 women), 31 part-time (21 women); includes 25 minority (19 Black or African American, non-Hispanic/Latino; 2 Asian, non-Hispanic/Latino; 2 Hispanic/Latino; 2 Two or more races, non-Hispanic/Latino), 33 international. Average age 30. 35 applicants, 86% accepted, 28 enrolled. In 2015, 44 master's awarded. *Degree requirements:* For master's, comprehensive exam, capstone course. *Entrance requirements:* For master's, GMAT (minimum score 420), minimum GPA of 3.0, interview. Additional exam requirements/recommendations for international students: Required—TOEFL (minimum score 550 paper-based). *Application deadline:* For fall admission, 7/30 priority date for domestic and international students; for winter admission, 11/30 priority date for domestic and international students; for spring admission, 2/28 priority date for domestic and international students; for summer admission, 6/1 priority date for domestic and international students. Applications are processed on a rolling basis. Application fee: $0. Electronic applications accepted. *Expenses:* Contact institution. *Financial support:* In 2015–16, 12 students received support. Career-related internships or fieldwork and scholarships/grants available. Support available to part-time students. Financial award applicants required to submit FAFSA. *Faculty research:* Leadership characteristics, financial hedging, group dynamics. *Unit head:* Dr. Richard Woodall, Dean, 816-501-3720, Fax: 816-501-2463, E-mail: richard.woodall@avila.edu. *Application contact:* Sarah Belanus, MBA Admissions Director, 816-501-3601, Fax: 816-501-2463, E-mail: sarah.belanus@avila.edu.
Website: http://www.avila.edu/mba

Baker College Center for Graduate Studies–Online, Graduate Programs, Flint, MI 48507-9843. Offers accounting (MBA); business administration (DBA); finance (MBA); general business (MBA); health care management (MBA); human resources management (MBA); information management (MBA); leadership studies (MBA); management information systems (MSIS); marketing (MBA). *Program availability:* Part-time, evening/weekend, online learning. *Degree requirements:* For master's, portfolio. *Entrance requirements:* For master's, 3 years of work experience, minimum undergraduate GPA of 2.5, writing sample, 3 letters of recommendation; for doctorate, MBA or acceptable master's degree from accredited association, 5 years work experience, minimum graduate GPA of 3.25, writing sample, 3 professional references. Additional exam requirements/recommendations for international students: Required—TOEFL (minimum score 550 paper-based). Electronic applications accepted.

Baldwin Wallace University, Graduate Programs, School of Business, Program in Health Care, Berea, OH 44017-2088. Offers MBA. *Program availability:* Part-time,

evening/weekend. *Students:* 44 full-time (24 women), 10 part-time (5 women); includes 12 minority (3 Black or African American, non-Hispanic/Latino; 5 Asian, non-Hispanic/Latino; 3 Hispanic/Latino; 1 Two or more races, non-Hispanic/Latino). Average age 41. 16 applicants, 81% accepted, 11 enrolled. In 2015, 19 master's awarded. *Degree requirements:* For master's, minimum overall GPA of 3.0. *Entrance requirements:* For master's, GMAT, interview, work experience, bachelor's degree in any field. Additional exam requirements/recommendations for international students: Required—TOEFL (minimum score 550 paper-based; 79 iBT). *Application deadline:* For fall admission, 7/25 priority date for domestic students, 4/30 priority date for international students; for spring admission, 12/10 priority date for domestic students, 9/30 priority date for international students. Applications are processed on a rolling basis. Application fee: $25. Electronic applications accepted. Application fee is waived when completed online. *Expenses:* $895 per credit hour. *Financial support:* Applicants required to submit FAFSA. *Unit head:* Tom Campanella, Director, 440-826-3818, Fax: 440-826-3868, E-mail: tcampane@bw.edu. *Application contact:* Laura Spencer, Graduate Application Specialist, 440-826-2191, Fax: 440-826-3868, E-mail: lspencer@bw.edu.
Website: http://www.bw.edu/graduate/business/health-care-mba/index

Barry University, Andreas School of Business, Graduate Certificate Programs, Miami Shores, FL 33161-6695. Offers finance (Certificate); health services administration (Certificate); international business (Certificate); management (Certificate); management information systems (Certificate); marketing (Certificate).

Barry University, College of Health Sciences, Graduate Certificate Programs, Miami Shores, FL 33161-6695. Offers health care leadership (Certificate); health care planning and informatics (Certificate); histotechnology (Certificate); long term care management (Certificate); medical group practice management (Certificate); quality improvement and outcomes management (Certificate).

Barry University, College of Health Sciences, Program in Health Services Administration, Miami Shores, FL 33161-6695. Offers MS. *Program availability:* Part-time, evening/weekend. *Degree requirements:* For master's, comprehensive exam. *Entrance requirements:* For master's, GMAT or GRE General Test, 2 years of experience in the health field, minimum GPA of 3.0, 1 semester of course work in computer applications or the equivalent (business). Electronic applications accepted.

Baruch College of the City University of New York, School of Public Affairs, Program in Public Administration, New York, NY 10010-5585. Offers general public administration (MPA); health care policy (MPA); nonprofit administration (MPA); policy analysis and evaluation (MPA); public management (MPA); MS/MPA. *Accreditation:* NASPAA. *Program availability:* Part-time, evening/weekend. *Degree requirements:* For master's, thesis, capstone. *Entrance requirements:* For master's, GRE General Test. Additional exam requirements/recommendations for international students: Required—TOEFL. Electronic applications accepted. *Expenses:* Contact institution. *Faculty research:* Urbanization, population and poverty in the developing world, housing and community development, labor unions and housing, government-nongovernment relations, immigration policy, social network analysis, cross-sectoral governance, comparative healthcare systems, program evaluation, social welfare policy, health outcomes, educational policy and leadership, transnationalism, infant health, welfare reform, racial/ethnic disparities in health, urban politics, homelessness, race and ethnic relations.

Baruch College of the City University of New York, Zicklin School of Business, Zicklin Executive Programs, Baruch/Mt. Sinai Program in Health Care Administration, New York, NY 10010-5585. Offers MBA. *Accreditation:* CAHME. *Program availability:* Part-time, evening/weekend. *Entrance requirements:* For master's, GMAT, personal interview, work experience in health care. Additional exam requirements/recommendations for international students: Required—TOEFL. Electronic applications accepted. *Expenses:* Contact institution. *Faculty research:* Economics of reproductive health, multivariate point estimation.

Baylor University, Graduate School, Military Programs, Program in Health Care Administration, Waco, TX 76798. Offers MHA, MHA/MBA. Program offered jointly with the U.S. Army. *Accreditation:* CAHME. *Faculty:* 19 full-time (5 women), 18 part-time/adjunct (2 women). *Students:* 101 full-time (40 women); includes 23 minority (4 Black or African American, non-Hispanic/Latino; 1 American Indian or Alaska Native, non-Hispanic/Latino; 7 Asian, non-Hispanic/Latino; 7 Hispanic/Latino; 4 Two or more races, non-Hispanic/Latino). In 2015, 53 master's awarded. *Degree requirements:* For master's, comprehensive exam. *Entrance requirements:* For master's, GRE General Test. Additional exam requirements/recommendations for international students: Required—TOEFL, IELTS. *Application deadline:* For fall admission, 6/15 for domestic students. Applications are processed on a rolling basis. *Faculty research:* Data quality, public health policy, organizational behavior, AIDS. *Unit head:* Forest Kim, Graduate Program Director, 210-221-8857, E-mail: forest_kim@baylor.edu. *Application contact:* Rene Pryor, Program Administrator, 210-221-6443, Fax: 210-221-6010, E-mail: rene.l.pryor.civ@mail.mil.
Website: http://www.cs.amedd.army.mil/baylorhca/

Belhaven University, School of Business, Jackson, MS 39202-1789. Offers business administration (MBA); health administration (MBA, MHA); human resources (MBA, MSL); leadership (MBA); public administration (MPA); sports administration (MBA, MSA). MBA program also offered in Houston, TX, Memphis, TN and Orlando, FL. *Program availability:* Part-time, evening/weekend, online learning. *Faculty:* 26 full-time (8 women), 61 part-time/adjunct (29 women). *Students:* 22 full-time (19 women), 1,120 part-time (793 women); includes 946 minority (899 Black or African American, non-Hispanic/Latino; 6 American Indian or Alaska Native, non-Hispanic/Latino; 3 Asian, non-Hispanic/Latino; 17 Hispanic/Latino; 3 Native Hawaiian or other Pacific Islander, non-Hispanic/Latino; 18 Two or more races, non-Hispanic/Latino). Average age 36. In 2015, 274 master's awarded. *Degree requirements:* For master's, comprehensive exam (for some programs), thesis (for some programs). *Entrance requirements:* For master's, GMAT, GRE General Test or MAT, minimum GPA of 2.8. *Application deadline:* Applications are processed on a rolling basis. Application fee: $25. Electronic applications accepted. *Expenses:* Tuition, area resident: Full-time $9990; part-time $6600 per credit hour. *Financial support:* Applicants required to submit FAFSA. *Unit head:* Dr. Ralph Mason, Dean, 601-968-8949, Fax: 601-968-8951, E-mail: cmason@belhaven.edu. *Application contact:* Dr. Audrey Kelleher, Vice President of Adult and Graduate Marketing and Development, 407-804-1424, Fax: 407-620-5210, E-mail: akelleher@belhaven.edu.
Website: http://www.belhaven.edu/campuses/index.htm

Bellevue University, Graduate School, College of Arts and Sciences, Bellevue, NE 68005-3098. Offers clinical counseling (MS); healthcare administration (MHA); human services (MA); international security and intelligence studies (MS); managerial communication (MA). *Program availability:* Online learning.

Belmont University, Jack C. Massey Graduate School of Business, Nashville, TN 37212-3757. Offers accounting (M Acc); business (AMBA, PMBA); healthcare (MBA). *Accreditation:* AACSB. *Program availability:* Part-time, evening/weekend. *Faculty:* 46 full-time (16 women), 27 part-time/adjunct (11 women). *Students:* 161 full-time (71 women), 66 part-time (28 women); includes 37 minority (12 Black or African American, non-Hispanic/Latino; 12 Asian, non-Hispanic/Latino; 7 Hispanic/Latino; 6 Two or more

Health Services Management and Hospital Administration

races, non-Hispanic/Latino), 15 international. Average age 28. 148 applicants, 64% accepted, 77 enrolled. In 2015, 136 master's awarded. *Entrance requirements:* For master's, GMAT, 2 years of work experience (MBA). Additional exam requirements/recommendations for international students: Required—TOEFL (minimum score 550 paper-based). *Application deadline:* For fall admission, 7/1 for domestic and international students; for spring admission, 11/1 for domestic and international students. Applications are processed on a rolling basis. Application fee: $50. Electronic applications accepted. *Expenses:* Contact institution. *Financial support:* Scholarships/grants, tuition waivers (partial), and unspecified assistantships available. Financial award application deadline: 7/1; financial award applicants required to submit FAFSA. *Faculty research:* Music business, strategy, ethics, finance, accounting systems. *Unit head:* Dr. Patrick Raines, Dean, 615-460-6480, Fax: 615-460-6455, E-mail: pat.raines@belmont.edu. *Application contact:* Tonya Hollin, Admissions Assistant, 615-460-6480, Fax: 615-460-6353, E-mail: masseyadmissions@belmont.edu.
Website: http://www.belmont.edu/business/masseyschool/

Benedictine University, Graduate Programs, Program in Business Administration, Lisle, IL 60532. Offers accounting (MBA); entrepreneurship and managing innovation (MBA); financial management (MBA); health administration (MBA); human resource management (MBA); information systems security (MBA); international business (MBA); management consulting (MBA); management information systems (MBA); marketing management (MBA); operations management and logistics (MBA); organizational leadership (MBA). *Program availability:* Part-time, evening/weekend, online learning. *Entrance requirements:* For master's, GMAT. Additional exam requirements/recommendations for international students: Required—TOEFL (minimum score 550 paper-based). Electronic applications accepted. *Faculty research:* Strategic leadership in professional organizations, sociology of professions, organizational change, social identity theory, applications to change management.

Benedictine University, Graduate Programs, Program in Public Health, Lisle, IL 60532. Offers administration of health care institutions (MPH); dietetics (MPH); disaster management (MPH); health education (MPH); health information systems (MPH); MBA/MPH; MPH/MS. *Accreditation:* CEPH. *Program availability:* Part-time, evening/weekend, online learning. *Entrance requirements:* For master's, MAT, GRE, or GMAT. Additional exam requirements/recommendations for international students: Required—TOEFL (minimum score 550 paper-based).

Binghamton University, State University of New York, Graduate School, School of Management, Program in Business Administration, Binghamton, NY 13902-6000. Offers business administration (MBA); corporate executive (MBA); executive business administration (MBA); health care professional executive (MBA); management (PhD); professional business administration (MBA). Executive and Professional MBA programs offered in Manhattan. *Accreditation:* AACSB. *Program availability:* Part-time. *Students:* 121 full-time (50 women), 13 part-time (6 women); includes 26 minority (9 Black or African American, non-Hispanic/Latino; 14 Asian, non-Hispanic/Latino; 3 Hispanic/Latino), 46 international. Average age 26. 310 applicants, 55% accepted, 84 enrolled. In 2015, 92 master's, 7 doctorates awarded. *Degree requirements:* For doctorate, thesis/dissertation. *Entrance requirements:* For master's and doctorate, GMAT. Additional exam requirements/recommendations for international students: Required—TOEFL (minimum score 96 iBT). *Application deadline:* Applications are processed on a rolling basis. Application fee: $75. Electronic applications accepted. *Expenses:* Contact institution. *Financial support:* In 2015–16, 29 students received support, including 10 teaching assistantships with full tuition reimbursements available (averaging $17,000 per year); career-related internships or fieldwork, Federal Work-Study, institutionally sponsored loans, scholarships/grants, health care benefits, tuition waivers (full and partial), and unspecified assistantships also available. Financial award applicants required to submit FAFSA. *Unit head:* Dr. Upinder Dhillon, Dean, 607-777-4381, E-mail: dhillon@binghamton.edu. *Application contact:* Kishan Zuber, Recruiting and Admissions Coordinator, 607-777-2151, Fax: 607-777-2501, E-mail: kzuber@binghamton.edu.

Binghamton University, State University of New York, Graduate School, Thomas J. Watson School of Engineering and Applied Science, Department of Systems Science and Industrial Engineering, Binghamton, NY 13902-6000. Offers executive health systems (MS); industrial and systems engineering (M Eng); systems science and industrial engineering (MS, PhD). MS in executive health systems also offered in Manhattan. *Program availability:* Part-time, evening/weekend, online learning. *Faculty:* 20 full-time (4 women), 5 part-time/adjunct (1 woman). *Students:* 222 full-time (71 women), 114 part-time (28 women); includes 50 minority (22 Black or African American, non-Hispanic/Latino; 16 Asian, non-Hispanic/Latino; 12 Hispanic/Latino), 226 international. Average age 28. 391 applicants, 92% accepted, 124 enrolled. In 2015, 46 master's, 7 doctorates awarded. *Degree requirements:* For master's, thesis; for doctorate, thesis/dissertation. *Entrance requirements:* For master's and doctorate, GRE General Test. Additional exam requirements/recommendations for international students: Required—TOEFL (minimum score 550 paper-based; 80 iBT). *Application deadline:* For fall admission, 4/1 priority date for domestic and international students; for spring admission, 11/15 priority date for domestic and international students. Applications are processed on a rolling basis. Application fee: $75. Electronic applications accepted. *Expenses:* Contact institution. *Financial support:* In 2015–16, 89 students received support, including 1 fellowship with full tuition reimbursement available (averaging $10,000 per year), 45 research assistantships with full tuition reimbursements available (averaging $16,500 per year), 13 teaching assistantships with full tuition reimbursements available (averaging $16,500 per year); career-related internships or fieldwork, Federal Work-Study, institutionally sponsored loans, scholarships/grants, health care benefits, tuition waivers (full and partial), and unspecified assistantships also available. Financial award application deadline: 2/1; financial award applicants required to submit FAFSA. *Faculty research:* Problem restructuring, protein modeling. *Unit head:* Ellen Tilden, Coordinator of Graduate Studies, 607-777-2873, E-mail: etilden@binghamton.edu. *Application contact:* Kishan Zuber, Recruiting and Admissions Coordinator, 607-777-2151, Fax: 607-777-2501, E-mail: kzuber@binghamton.edu.
Website: http://www.ssie.binghamton.edu

Bluffton University, Programs in Business, Bluffton, OH 45817. Offers accounting and financial management (MBA); business administration (MBA); health care management (MBA); leadership (MBA); organizational management (MA); production and operations management (MBA); sport management (MBA). *Program availability:* Evening/weekend, online learning. *Entrance requirements:* For master's, current resume, official transcript, two recommendation forms, bachelor's degree, minimum GPA of 3.0, four years of professional experience, interview. Additional exam requirements/recommendations for international students: Recommended—TOEFL. *Application deadline:* For fall admission, 7/31 priority date for domestic and international students. Applications are processed on a rolling basis. Application fee: $25. Electronic applications accepted. Application fee is waived when completed online. *Expenses:* Tuition, area resident: Full-time $6420. Tuition and fees vary according to program. *Financial support:* Scholarships/grants, tuition waivers, and unspecified assistantships available. Financial award application deadline: 5/1. *Unit head:* Dr. George Lehman, Administrative Assistant for Graduate Programs in Business, 419-358-3065.
Website: http://www.bluffton.edu/grad/

Boston University, School of Medicine, Division of Graduate Medical Sciences, Program in Healthcare Emergency Management, Boston, MA 02215. Offers MS. *Financial support:* Applicants required to submit FAFSA. *Unit head:* Dr. Kevin Thomas, Director, 617-414-2316, Fax: 617-414-2332, E-mail: kipthoma@bu.edu. *Application contact:* GMS Admissions Office, 617-638-5255, E-mail: askgms@bu.edu.
Website: http://www.bumc.bu.edu/bmcm/

Boston University, School of Medicine, Division of Graduate Medical Sciences, Program in Medical Sciences, Boston, MA 02215. Offers MA, MA/MA, MBA/MA, MPH/MA. *Program availability:* Part-time. *Degree requirements:* For master's, thesis. *Entrance requirements:* For master's, MCAT or GRE. *Application deadline:* Applications are processed on a rolling basis. Application fee: $75. Electronic applications accepted. *Financial support:* Federal Work-Study available. Financial award applicants required to submit FAFSA. *Unit head:* Dr. Gwynneth D. Offner, Director, 617-638-8221, E-mail: goffner@bu.edu. *Application contact:* GMS Admissions Office, 617-638-5255, E-mail: askgms@bu.edu.
Website: http://www.bumc.bu.edu/gms/academics/masters-in-medical-sciences/

Boston University, School of Public Health, Health Law, Policy and Management Department, Boston, MA 02215. Offers health services research (MS). *Accreditation:* CAHME. *Program availability:* Part-time, evening/weekend. *Faculty:* 37 full-time, 31 part-time/adjunct. *Students:* 137 full-time (98 women), 96 part-time (76 women); includes 64 minority (16 Black or African American, non-Hispanic/Latino; 2 American Indian or Alaska Native, non-Hispanic/Latino; 27 Asian, non-Hispanic/Latino; 12 Hispanic/Latino; 7 Two or more races, non-Hispanic/Latino), 33 international. Average age 28. 507 applicants, 44% accepted, 77 enrolled. In 2015, 266 master's, 5 doctorates awarded. *Degree requirements:* For master's, comprehensive exam (for some programs), thesis (for some programs); for doctorate, comprehensive exam, thesis/dissertation. *Entrance requirements:* For master's, GRE, MCAT, GMAT; for doctorate, GRE. Additional exam requirements/recommendations for international students: Required—TOEFL (minimum score 600 paper-based; 100 iBT), IELTS (minimum score 7). *Application deadline:* For fall admission, 12/1 priority date for domestic and international students; for spring admission, 10/15 priority date for domestic students. Applications are processed on a rolling basis. Application fee: $115. Electronic applications accepted. *Financial support:* Career-related internships or fieldwork, Federal Work-Study, institutionally sponsored loans, scholarships/grants, and tuition waivers (partial) available. Support available to part-time students. Financial award application deadline: 3/1; financial award applicants required to submit FAFSA. *Faculty research:* Health policy, health law and ethics, human rights, healthcare management. *Unit head:* Dr. David Rosenbloom, Interim Chair, 617-638-5042. *Application contact:* LePhan Quan, Associate Director of Admissions, 617-638-4640, Fax: 617-638-5299, E-mail: asksph@bu.edu.
Website: http://www.bu.edu/sph/about/departments/health-law-policy-and-management/

Brandeis University, The Heller School for Social Policy and Management, Program in Nonprofit Management, Waltham, MA 02454-9110. Offers child, youth, and family management (MBA); health care management (MBA); social impact management (MBA); social policy and management (MBA); sustainable development (MBA); MBA/MA; MBA/MD. MBA/MD program offered in conjunction with Tufts University School of Medicine. *Accreditation:* AACSB. *Program availability:* Part-time. *Degree requirements:* For master's, team consulting project. *Entrance requirements:* For master's, GMAT (preferred) or GRE, 2 letters of recommendation, problem statement analysis, 3-5 years of professional experience. Additional exam requirements/recommendations for international students: Required—TOEFL (minimum score 600 paper-based; 100 iBT). Electronic applications accepted. *Expenses:* Contact institution. *Faculty research:* Health care; children and families; elder and disabled services; social impact management; organizations in the non-profit, for-profit, or public sector.

Brandman University, School of Nursing and Health Professions, Irvine, CA 92618. Offers health administration (MHA); health risk and crisis communication (MS).

Brenau University, Sydney O. Smith Graduate School, School of Business and Mass Communication, Gainesville, GA 30501. Offers accounting (MBA); business administration (MBA); healthcare management (MBA); organizational leadership (MS); project management (MBA). *Accreditation:* ACBSP. *Program availability:* Part-time, evening/weekend, online learning. *Degree requirements:* For master's, comprehensive exam (for some programs). *Entrance requirements:* For master's, resume, minimum undergraduate GPA of 2.5. Additional exam requirements/recommendations for international students: Required—TOEFL (minimum score 500 paper-based; 61 iBT); Recommended—IELTS (minimum score 5). Electronic applications accepted. *Expenses:* Contact institution.

Broadview University–West Jordan, Graduate Programs, West Jordan, UT 84088. Offers business administration (MBA); health care management (MSM); information technology (MSM); managerial leadership (MSM).

Brooklyn College of the City University of New York, School of Natural and Behavioral Sciences, Department of Health and Nutrition Sciences, Program in Public Health, Brooklyn, NY 11210-2889. Offers general public health (MPH); health care policy and administration (MPH). *Accreditation:* CEPH. *Degree requirements:* For master's, thesis or alternative, 46 credits. *Entrance requirements:* For master's, GRE, 2 letters of recommendation, essay, interview. Electronic applications accepted.

California Baptist University, Program in Business Administration, Riverside, CA 92504-3206. Offers accounting (MBA); construction management (MBA); healthcare management (MBA); management (MBA). *Accreditation:* ACBSP. *Program availability:* Part-time, evening/weekend, 100% online, blended/hybrid learning. *Faculty:* 18 full-time (5 women), 9 part-time/adjunct (1 woman). *Students:* 56 full-time (26 women), 115 part-time (55 women); includes 80 minority (20 Black or African American, non-Hispanic/Latino; 2 Asian, non-Hispanic/Latino; 55 Hispanic/Latino; 3 Two or more races, non-Hispanic/Latino), 26 international. Average age 30. 232 applicants, 71% accepted, 63 enrolled. In 2015, 48 master's awarded. *Degree requirements:* For master's, interdisciplinary capstone project. *Entrance requirements:* For master's, GMAT, minimum GPA of 2.5; two recommendations; comprehensive essay; resume; interview. Additional exam requirements/recommendations for international students: Required—TOEFL (minimum score 80 iBT). *Application deadline:* For fall admission, 8/1 priority date for domestic students, 7/1 for international students; for spring admission, 12/1 priority date for domestic students, 11/1 for international students. Applications are processed on a rolling basis. Application fee: $45. Electronic applications accepted. *Expenses:* $621 per unit, $355 fees per semester. *Financial support:* Federal Work-Study and scholarships/grants available. Financial award applicants required to submit CSS PROFILE or FAFSA. *Faculty research:* Behavioral economics, economic indicators, marketing ethics, international business, microfinance. *Unit head:* Dr. Steve Strombeck, Interim Dean, School of Business, 951-343-4701, Fax: 951-343-4361, E-mail: sstrombeck@calbaptist.edu. *Application contact:* Stephanie Fluitt, Graduate Admissions Counselor, 951-343-4696, E-mail: sfluitt@calbaptist.edu.
Website: http://www.calbaptist.edu/mba/about/

California Baptist University, Program in Nursing, Riverside, CA 92504-3206. Offers clinical nurse specialist (MSN); family nurse practitioner (MSN); healthcare systems management (MSN); teaching-learning (MSN). *Program availability:* Part-time. *Faculty:*

Health Services Management and Hospital Administration

18 full-time (17 women), 14 part-time/adjunct (11 women). *Students:* 77 full-time (63 women), 143 part-time (117 women); includes 111 minority (26 Black or African American, non-Hispanic/Latino; 3 American Indian or Alaska Native, non-Hispanic/Latino; 38 Asian, non-Hispanic/Latino; 39 Hispanic/Latino; 1 Native Hawaiian or other Pacific Islander, non-Hispanic/Latino; 4 Two or more races, non-Hispanic/Latino), 5 international. Average age 33. 44 applicants, 64% accepted, 23 enrolled. In 2015, 19 master's awarded. *Degree requirements:* For master's, comprehensive exam or directed project thesis; capstone practicum. *Entrance requirements:* For master's, GRE or California Critical Thinking Skills Test; Test of Essential Academic Skills (TEAS), minimum undergraduate GPA of 3.0; completion of prerequisite courses with minimum grade of C; CPR certification; background check clearance; health clearance; drug testing; proof of health insurance; proof of motor vehicle insurance; three letters of recommendation; 1000-word essay; interview. Additional exam requirements/recommendations for international students: Required—TOEFL (minimum score 80 iBT). *Application deadline:* For fall admission, 8/1 priority date for domestic students, 7/1 for international students; for spring admission, 12/1 priority date for domestic students, 11/1 for international students. Applications are processed on a rolling basis. Application fee: $45. Electronic applications accepted. *Expenses:* $742 per unit, $355 per semester fees. *Financial support:* Federal Work-Study and scholarships/grants available. Financial award applicants required to submit CSS PROFILE or FAFSA. *Faculty research:* Qualitative research using Parse methodology, gerontology, disaster preparedness, medical-surgical nursing, maternal-child nursing. *Unit head:* Dr. Geneva Oaks, Dean, School of Nursing, 951-343-4702, E-mail: goaks@calbaptist.edu. *Application contact:* Dr. Rebecca Meyer, Director, Graduate Program in Nursing, 951-343-4952, Fax: 951-343-5095, E-mail: rmeyer@calbaptist.edu.
Website: http://www.calbaptist.edu/explore-cbu/schools-colleges/school-nursing/master-science-nursing/

California Baptist University, Program in Public Health, Riverside, CA 92504-3206. Offers health education and promotion (MPH); health policy and administration (MPH). *Program availability:* Part-time, evening/weekend. *Faculty:* 7 full-time (4 women), 3 part-time/adjunct (2 women). *Students:* 41 full-time (36 women), 9 part-time (8 women); includes 33 minority (4 Black or African American, non-Hispanic/Latino; 1 Asian, non-Hispanic/Latino; 26 Hispanic/Latino; 2 Two or more races, non-Hispanic/Latino), 2 international. Average age 25. 41 applicants, 71% accepted, 26 enrolled. *Degree requirements:* For master's, capstone project; practicum. *Entrance requirements:* For master's, minimum undergraduate GPA of 2.75, two recommendations, 500-word essay, resume. Additional exam requirements/recommendations for international students: Required—TOEFL (minimum score 80 iBT). *Application deadline:* For fall admission, 8/1 priority date for domestic students, 7/1 for international students; for spring admission, 12/1 priority date for domestic students, 11/1 for international students. Applications are processed on a rolling basis. Application fee: $45. Electronic applications accepted. *Expenses:* $800 per unit, $355 per semester fees. *Financial support:* Federal Work-Study and scholarships/grants available. Financial award applicants required to submit CSS PROFILE or FAFSA. *Faculty research:* Epidemiology, statistical education, exercise and immunity, obesity and chronic disease. *Unit head:* Dr. David Pearson, Dean, College of Health Science, 951-343-4298, E-mail: dpearson@calbaptist.edu. *Application contact:* Dr. Robert LaChausse, Chair, Department of Public Health Sciences, 951-552-8484, E-mail: rlachausse@calbaptist.edu.
Website: http://www.calbaptist.edu/explore-cbu/schools-colleges/college-allied-health/health-sciences/master-public-health/

California Coast University, School of Administration and Management, Santa Ana, CA 92701. Offers business marketing (MBA); health care management (MBA); human resource management (MBA); management (MBA, MS). *Program availability:* Online learning. Electronic applications accepted.

California Intercontinental University, School of Healthcare, Irvine, CA 92614. Offers healthcare management and leadership (MBA, DBA).

California State University, Bakersfield, Division of Graduate Studies, School of Business and Public Administration, Program in Health Care Administration, Bakersfield, CA 93311. Offers MS. *Entrance requirements:* For master's, official transcripts, two letters of recommendation, personal statement. Additional exam requirements/recommendations for international students: Required—TOEFL (minimum score 550 paper-based; 79 iBT), IELTS (minimum score 7). *Application deadline:* Applications are processed on a rolling basis. Application fee: $55. Electronic applications accepted. *Expenses:* Tuition, area resident: Full-time $2246; part-time $1302 per semester. Tuition, state resident: full-time $2246; part-time $1302 per semester. *Unit head:* Dr. B.J. Moore, Coordinator, 661-654-3026, E-mail: bjmoore@csub.edu. *Application contact:* Debbie Blowers, Assistant Director of Admissions, 661-664-3381, E-mail: dblowers@csub.edu.

California State University, Chico, Office of Graduate Studies, College of Behavioral and Social Sciences, Political Science and Criminal Justice Department, Program in Public Administration, Chico, CA 95929-0722. Offers health administration (MPA); local government management (MPA). *Accreditation:* NASPAA. *Program availability:* Part-time. *Degree requirements:* For master's, thesis or culminating practicum. *Entrance requirements:* For master's, 2 letters of recommendation. Additional exam requirements/recommendations for international students: Required—TOEFL (minimum score 550 paper-based; 80 iBT), IELTS (minimum score 6.5). *Application deadline:* For fall admission, 3/1 priority date for domestic students, 3/1 for international students; for spring admission, 9/15 priority date for domestic students, 9/15 for international students. Applications are processed on a rolling basis. Application fee: $55. Electronic applications accepted. *Expenses:* Tuition, area resident: Full-time $4146; part-time $2730. *Financial support:* Fellowships and career-related internships or fieldwork available. *Unit head:* Mahalley Allen, Chair, 530-898-6506, Fax: 530-898-5301, E-mail: mdallen@csuchico.edu. *Application contact:* Judy L. Rice, School of Graduate, International, and Interdisciplinary Studies, 530-898-6880, Fax: 530-898-6889, E-mail: jlrice@csuchico.edu.
Website: http://catalog.csuchico.edu/viewer/12/POLS/PADMNONEMP.html

California State University, East Bay, Office of Graduate Studies, College of Letters, Arts, and Social Sciences, Department of Public Affairs and Administration, Program in Health Care Administration, Hayward, CA 94542-3000. Offers management and change in health care (MS). *Program availability:* Part-time, evening/weekend, online learning. *Students:* 4 full-time (all women), 156 part-time (126 women); includes 112 minority (29 Black or African American, non-Hispanic/Latino; 55 Asian, non-Hispanic/Latino; 21 Hispanic/Latino; 7 Two or more races, non-Hispanic/Latino), 20 international. Average age 30. 274 applicants, 36% accepted, 49 enrolled. In 2015, 88 master's awarded. *Degree requirements:* For master's, thesis or alternative, final project. *Entrance requirements:* For master's, minimum undergraduate cumulative GPA of 2.5, statement of purpose, two letters of academic or professional recommendation, professional resume/curriculum vitae, all undergraduate/graduate transcripts. Additional exam requirements/recommendations for international students: Required—TOEFL (minimum score 550 paper-based). *Application deadline:* For fall admission, 6/18 for domestic and international students. Application fee: $55. Electronic applications accepted. *Financial support:* Career-related internships or fieldwork, Federal Work-Study, institutionally

sponsored loans, and scholarships/grants available. Support available to part-time students. Financial award application deadline: 3/2; financial award applicants required to submit FAFSA. *Unit head:* Dr. Toni Fogarty, Chair/Graduate Advisor, 510-885-2268, E-mail: toni.fogarty@csueastbay.edu. *Application contact:* Prof. Michael Moon, Public Administration Graduate Advisor, 510-885-2545, Fax: 510-885-3726, E-mail: michael.moon@csueastbay.edu.

California State University, East Bay, Office of Graduate Studies, College of Letters, Arts, and Social Sciences, Department of Public Affairs and Administration, Program in Public Administration, Hayward, CA 94542-3000. Offers health care administration (MPA); public management and policy analysis (MPA). *Program availability:* Part-time, evening/weekend. *Students:* 6 full-time (all women), 176 part-time (122 women); includes 128 minority (47 Black or African American, non-Hispanic/Latino; 1 American Indian or Alaska Native, non-Hispanic/Latino; 24 Asian, non-Hispanic/Latino; 45 Hispanic/Latino; 3 Native Hawaiian or other Pacific Islander, non-Hispanic/Latino; 8 Two or more races, non-Hispanic/Latino), 15 international. Average age 32. 153 applicants, 67% accepted, 39 enrolled. In 2015, 75 master's awarded. *Degree requirements:* For master's, comprehensive exam (for some programs), comprehensive exam or thesis. *Entrance requirements:* For master's, minimum GPA of 2.5; statement of purpose; 2 letters of recommendation; professional resume/curriculum vitae. Additional exam requirements/recommendations for international students: Required—TOEFL (minimum score 550 paper-based; 79 iBT). *Application deadline:* For fall admission, 6/18 for domestic and international students. Application fee: $55. Electronic applications accepted. *Financial support:* Fellowships, teaching assistantships, career-related internships or fieldwork, Federal Work-Study, institutionally sponsored loans, and scholarships/grants available. Support available to part-time students. Financial award application deadline: 3/2; financial award applicants required to submit FAFSA. *Unit head:* Dr. Toni Fogarty, Chair, 510-885-2268, E-mail: toni.fogarty@csueastbay.edu. *Application contact:* Prof. Michael Moon, Public Administration Graduate Advisor, 510-885-2545, Fax: 510-885-3726, E-mail: michael.moon@csueastbay.edu.

California State University, Fresno, Division of Graduate Studies, College of Health and Human Services, Department of Public Health, Fresno, CA 93740-8027. Offers health policy and management (MPH); health promotion (MPH). *Accreditation:* CEPH. *Program availability:* Part-time, evening/weekend. *Degree requirements:* For master's, thesis or alternative. *Entrance requirements:* For master's, GRE General Test, minimum GPA of 2.5. Additional exam requirements/recommendations for international students: Required—TOEFL. Electronic applications accepted. *Faculty research:* Foster parent training, geriatrics, tobacco control.

California State University, Long Beach, Graduate Studies, College of Health and Human Services, Program in Health Care Administration, Long Beach, CA 90840. Offers MS. *Accreditation:* CAHME. *Program availability:* Part-time. *Degree requirements:* For master's, comprehensive exam or thesis. *Entrance requirements:* For master's, minimum GPA of 3.0. Electronic applications accepted. *Faculty research:* Long-term care, Immigration Reform Act and health care, physician reimbursement.

California State University, Los Angeles, Graduate Studies, College of Business and Economics, Department of Management, Los Angeles, CA 90032-8530. Offers health care management (MS); management (MBA). *Accreditation:* AACSB. *Program availability:* Part-time, evening/weekend. *Entrance requirements:* For master's, GMAT, minimum GPA of 2.5 during previous 2 years of course work. Additional exam requirements/recommendations for international students: Required—TOEFL (minimum score 550 paper-based). *Application deadline:* For fall admission, 5/1 for domestic and international students. Applications are processed on a rolling basis. Application fee: $55. Electronic applications accepted. *Financial support:* Application deadline: 3/1.
Website: http://cbe.calstatela.edu/mgmt/

California State University, Northridge, Graduate Studies, College of Health and Human Development, Department of Health Sciences, Northridge, CA 91330. Offers health administration (MS); public health (MPH). *Accreditation:* CEPH. *Faculty:* 14 full-time (8 women), 47 part-time/adjunct (26 women). *Students:* 107 full-time (83 women), 74 part-time (59 women); includes 63 minority (11 Black or African American, non-Hispanic/Latino; 18 Asian, non-Hispanic/Latino; 30 Hispanic/Latino; 4 Two or more races, non-Hispanic/Latino), 21 international. Average age 30. 258 applicants, 40% accepted, 52 enrolled. *Entrance requirements:* For master's, GRE General Test or minimum GPA of 3.0. Additional exam requirements/recommendations for international students: Required—TOEFL. *Application deadline:* For fall admission, 11/30 for domestic students. Application fee: $55. *Financial support:* Teaching assistantships available. Financial award application deadline: 3/1. *Faculty research:* Labor market needs assessment, health education products, dental hygiene, independent practice prototype. *Unit head:* Anita Slechta, Chair, 818-677-3101.
Website: http://www.csun.edu/hhd/hsci/

California State University, Northridge, Graduate Studies, The Tseng College of Extended Learning, Program in Health Administration, Northridge, CA 91330. Offers MPA. Offered in collaboration with the College of Health and Human Development. *Program availability:* Online learning. *Degree requirements:* For master's, comprehensive exam. *Entrance requirements:* For master's, bachelor's degree from accredited college or university, minimum cumulative GPA of 2.5, at least two years of work experience. Additional exam requirements/recommendations for international students: Required—TOEFL (minimum score of 85 iBT or 563 paper-based) or IELTS (minimum score of 7). Electronic applications accepted.

California State University, San Bernardino, Graduate Studies, College of Natural Sciences, Program in Health Services Administration, San Bernardino, CA 92407. Offers MS. *Students:* 1 full-time (0 women), 5 part-time (3 women); includes 4 minority (1 Black or African American, non-Hispanic/Latino; 3 Hispanic/Latino), 2 international. 30 applicants, 33% accepted, 5 enrolled. In 2015, 5 master's awarded. *Degree requirements:* For master's, thesis or alternative. *Entrance requirements:* Additional exam requirements/recommendations for international students: Required—TOEFL. *Application deadline:* For fall admission, 5/5 for domestic students. Application fee: $55. *Expenses:* Tuition, state resident: full-time $7843; part-time $5011.20 per year. Tuition and fees vary according to course load, degree level, program and reciprocity agreements. *Unit head:* Dr. Marsha Greer, Assistant Dean, 909-537-5339, Fax: 909-537-7037, E-mail: mgreer@csusb.edu. *Application contact:* Dr. Jeffrey Thompson, Dean of Graduate Studies, 909-537-5058, E-mail: jthompso@csusb.edu.

Cambridge College, School of Management, Cambridge, MA 02138-5304. Offers business negotiation and conflict resolution (M Mgt); general business (M Mgt); health care informatics (M Mgt); health care management (M Mgt); leadership in human and organizational dynamics (M Mgt); non-profit and public organization management (M Mgt); small business development (M Mgt); technology management (M Mgt). *Program availability:* Part-time, evening/weekend. *Degree requirements:* For master's, thesis, seminars. *Entrance requirements:* For master's, resume, 2 professional references. Additional exam requirements/recommendations for international students: Required—TOEFL (minimum score 550 paper-based; 79 iBT), Michigan English Language Assessment Battery (minimum score 85); Recommended—IELTS (minimum score 6). Electronic applications accepted. *Expenses:* Contact institution. *Faculty research:* Negotiation, mediation and conflict resolution; leadership; management of

Health Services Management and Hospital Administration

diverse organizations; case studies and simulation methodologies for management education, digital as a second language: social networking for digital immigrants, non-profit and public management.

Capella University, School of Business and Technology, Master's Programs in Business, Minneapolis, MN 55402. Offers accounting (MBA); business analysis (MS); business intelligence (MBA); entrepreneurship (MBA); finance (MBA); general business administration (MBA); general human resource management (MS); general leadership (MS); health care management (MBA); human resource management (MBA); marketing (MBA); project management (MBA, MS). *Accreditation:* ACBSP.

Capella University, School of Public Service Leadership, Doctoral Programs in Healthcare, Minneapolis, MN 55402. Offers criminal justice (PhD); emergency management (PhD); epidemiology (Dr PH); general health administration (DHA); general public administration (DPA); health advocacy and leadership (Dr PH); health care administration (PhD); health care leadership (DHA); health policy advocacy (DHA); multidisciplinary human services (PhD); nonprofit management and leadership (PhD); public safety leadership (PhD); social and community services (PhD).

Capella University, School of Public Service Leadership, Master's Programs in Healthcare, Minneapolis, MN 55402. Offers criminal justice (MS); emergency management (MS); general public health (MPH); gerontology (MS); health administration (MHA); health care operations (MHA); health management policy (MPH); health policy (MHA); homeland security (MS); multidisciplinary human services (MS); public administration (MPA); public safety leadership (MS); social and community services (MS); social behavioral sciences (MPH). MS/MPA.

Carlow University, College of Leadership and Social Change, MBA Program, Pittsburgh, PA 15213-3165. Offers fraud and forensics (MBA); healthcare management (MBA); human resource management (MBA); leadership and management (MDA); project management (MBA). *Program availability:* Part-time, evening/weekend, 100% online, blended/hybrid learning. *Students:* 85 full-time (66 women), 24 part-time (15 women); includes 25 minority (20 Black or African American, non-Hispanic/Latino; 2 Asian, non-Hispanic/Latino; 2 Hispanic/Latino; 1 Two or more races, non-Hispanic/Latino), 1 international. Average age 32. 56 applicants, 95% accepted, 39 enrolled. In 2015, 27 master's awarded. *Entrance requirements:* For master's, undergraduate GPA of 3.0 preferred; personal essay; resume; official transcripts; two professional recommendations; interview may be required. Additional exam requirements/recommendations for international students: Required—TOEFL (minimum score 550 paper-based). *Application deadline:* Applications are processed on a rolling basis. Electronic applications accepted. Application fee is waived when completed online. *Expenses: Tuition, area resident:* Full-time $11,147; part-time $801 per credit. Tuition and fees vary according to course load, degree level and program. *Unit head:* Dr. Howard Stern, Chair, MBA Program, 412-578-8828, E-mail: hastern@carlow.edu. *Application contact:* 412-578-6059, Fax: 412-578-6321, E-mail: gradstudies@carlow.edu.
Website: http://www.carlow.edu/Business_Administration.aspx

Carnegie Mellon University, H. John Heinz III College, School of Public Policy and Management, Master of Science Program in Health Care Policy and Management, Pittsburgh, PA 15213-3891. Offers MSHCPM. *Program availability:* Part-time, evening/weekend. *Degree requirements:* For master's, internship. *Entrance requirements:* For master's, GRE or GMAT, college-level course in advanced algebra/pre-calculus; college-level courses in economics and statistics (recommended). Additional exam requirements/recommendations for international students: Required—TOEFL or IELTS. Electronic applications accepted.

Carnegie Mellon University, H. John Heinz III College, School of Public Policy and Management, Programs in Medical Management, Pittsburgh, PA 15213-3891. Offers MMM.

Case Western Reserve University, Weatherhead School of Management, Program in Healthcare, Cleveland, OH 44106. Offers MSM. *Program availability:* Evening/weekend. *Entrance requirements:* For master's, GMAT/GRE, master's degree or higher in a medical to management-related field, or bachelor's degree plus 5 years of experience working in the healthcare industry, essay, current resume, letters of recommendation. Electronic applications accepted. *Expenses: Tuition, area resident:* Full-time $41,137; part-time $1714 per credit hour. *Required fees:* $32. Tuition and fees vary according to course load and program.

Central Michigan University, Central Michigan University Global Campus, Program in Administration, Mount Pleasant, MI 48859. Offers acquisitions administration (MSA, Certificate); engineering management administration (MSA, Certificate); general administration (MSA, Certificate); health services administration (MSA, Certificate); human resources administration (MSA, Certificate); information resource management (MSA); information resource management administration (Certificate); international administration (MSA, Certificate); leadership (MSA, Certificate); philanthropy and fundraising administration (MSA, Certificate); public administration (MSA, Certificate); recreation and park administration (MSA); research administration (MSA, Certificate). *Program availability:* Part-time, evening/weekend, online learning. *Entrance requirements:* For master's, minimum GPA of 2.7 in major. Electronic applications accepted.

Central Michigan University, Central Michigan University Global Campus, Program in Health Administration, Mount Pleasant, MI 48859. Offers health administration (DHA); international health (Certificate); nutrition and dietetics (MS). *Program availability:* Part-time, evening/weekend, online learning. Electronic applications accepted.

Central Michigan University, College of Graduate Studies, The Herbert H. and Grace A. Dow College of Health Professions, School of Health Sciences, Mount Pleasant, MI 48859. Offers exercise science (MA); health administration (DHA). *Program availability:* Part-time, evening/weekend, online learning. *Degree requirements:* For doctorate, comprehensive exam, thesis/dissertation. *Entrance requirements:* For doctorate, accredited master's or doctoral degree, 5 years of related work experience. Electronic applications accepted. *Faculty research:* Exercise science.

Central Michigan University, College of Graduate Studies, Interdisciplinary Administration Programs, Mount Pleasant, MI 48859. Offers acquisitions administration (MSA, Graduate Certificate); general administration (MSA, Graduate Certificate); health services administration (MSA, Graduate Certificate); human resource administration (Graduate Certificate); human resources administration (MSA); information resource management (MSA, Graduate Certificate); international administration (MSA, Graduate Certificate); leadership (MSA, Graduate Certificate); public administration (MSA, Graduate Certificate); research administration (Graduate Certificate); sport administration (MSA). *Accreditation:* AACSB. *Program availability:* Part-time, evening/weekend, online learning. *Degree requirements:* For master's, thesis or alternative. *Entrance requirements:* For master's, bachelor's degree with minimum GPA of 2.7. Electronic applications accepted. *Faculty research:* Interdisciplinary studies in acquisitions administration, health services administration, sport administration, recreation and park administration, and international administration.

Champlain College, Graduate Studies, Burlington, VT 05402-0670. Offers business (MBA); digital forensic science (MS); early childhood education (M Ed); emergent media

(MFA, MS); executive leadership (MS); health care administration (MS); information security operations (MS); law (MS); mediation and applied conflict studies (MS). MS in emergent media program held in Shanghai. *Program availability:* Part-time, online learning. *Degree requirements:* For master's, capstone project. *Entrance requirements:* Additional exam requirements/recommendations for international students: Required—TOEFL (minimum score 550 paper-based; 80 iBT). Electronic applications accepted.

Clarkson University, Graduate School, School of Business, Potsdam, NY 13699. Offers business administration (MBA); general management (Certificate); health data analytics (MS); health systems administration (MBA, Certificate); human resources (Certificate). *Program availability:* Part-time, evening/weekend, blended/hybrid learning. *Faculty:* 48 full-time (11 women), 19 part-time/adjunct (2 women). *Students:* 121 full-time (58 women), 155 part-time (65 women); includes 35 minority (7 Black or African American, non-Hispanic/Latino; 23 Asian, non-Hispanic/Latino; 3 Hispanic/Latino; 2 Two or more races, non-Hispanic/Latino), 30 international. Average age 30. 355 applicants, 29% accepted, 42 enrolled. In 2015, 121 master's, 4 other advanced degrees awarded. *Entrance requirements:* For master's, GMAT or GRE, transcripts of all college coursework, resume, personal statement, three letters of recommendation. Additional exam requirements/recommendations for international students: Required—TOEFL (minimum score 550 paper-based, 80 iBT) or IELTS (minimum score 6.5). *Application deadline:* For fall admission, 1/30 priority date for domestic and international students; for spring admission, 9/1 priority date for domestic and international students. Applications are processed on a rolling basis. Electronic applications accepted. *Financial support:* In 2015–16, 81 students received support. Scholarships/grants available. *Faculty research:* New York state farmlands, green data, environmental socioeconomic factors, Adirondack park. *Total annual research expenditures:* $104,440. *Unit head:* Dr. Dayle M. Smith, Dean, 315-268-2300, Fax: 315-268-3810, E-mail: dsmith@clarkson.edu. *Application contact:* Erin Dumers, Program Coordinator, 315-268-6613, Fax: 315-268-3810, E-mail: busgrad@clarkson.edu.
Website: http://www.clarkson.edu/business/

Cleary University, Online Program in Business Administration, Howell, MI 48843. Offers accounting (MBA); financial planning (MBA); financial planning (Graduate Certificate); green business strategy (MBA, Graduate Certificate); health care leadership (MBA); management (MBA); nonprofit management (MBA, Graduate Certificate); organizational leadership (MBA). *Program availability:* Part-time, evening/weekend, online learning. *Degree requirements:* For master's, thesis. *Entrance requirements:* For master's, bachelor's degree; minimum GPA of 2.5; professional resume indicating minimum of 2 years of management or related experience; undergraduate degree from accredited college or university with at least 18 quarter hours (or 12 semester hours) of accounting study (for MBA in accounting). Additional exam requirements/recommendations for international students: Required—TOEFL (minimum score 550 paper-based; 79 iBT), Michigan English Language Assessment Battery (minimum score 75). Electronic applications accepted.

Cleveland State University, College of Graduate Studies, Maxine Goodman Levin College of Urban Affairs, Program in Public Administration, Cleveland, OH 44115. Offers city management (MPA); economic development (MPA); healthcare administration (MPA); local and urban management (Certificate); non-profit management (MPA, Certificate); public financial management (MPA); public management (MPA); urban economic development (Certificate); JD/MPA. *Accreditation:* NASPAA. *Program availability:* Part-time, evening/weekend. *Faculty:* 16 full-time (8 women), 13 part-time/adjunct (5 women). *Students:* 16 full-time (10 women), 56 part-time (36 women); includes 28 minority (25 Black or African American, non-Hispanic/Latino; 2 Hispanic/Latino; 1 Two or more races, non-Hispanic/Latino), 3 international. Average age 32. 96 applicants, 92% accepted, 13 enrolled. In 2015, 20 master's awarded. *Degree requirements:* For master's, thesis or alternative, exit project. *Entrance requirements:* For master's, GRE General Test (minimum scores in 40th percentile verbal and quantitative, 4.0 writing), minimum GPA of 3.0. Additional exam requirements/recommendations for international students: Required—TOEFL (minimum score 550 paper-based; 78 iBT), IELTS (6.0), or International Test of English Proficiency (iTEP). *Application deadline:* For fall admission, 7/1 priority date for domestic students, 5/15 for international students; for spring admission, 11/15 for domestic students, 11/1 for international students; for summer admission, 4/1 for domestic students, 3/15 for international students. Applications are processed on a rolling basis. Application fee: $30. Electronic applications accepted. *Expenses:* Contact institution. *Financial support:* In 2015–16, 16 students received support, including 5 research assistantships with full tuition reimbursements available (averaging $7,200 per year), 1 teaching assistantship with partial tuition reimbursement available (averaging $2,400 per year); scholarships/grants, tuition waivers (full and partial), and unspecified assistantships also available. Support available to part-time students. Financial award application deadline: 3/1; financial award applicants required to submit FAFSA. *Faculty research:* City management, nonprofit management, health care administration, public management, economic development. *Unit head:* Dr. Nicholas Zingale, Director, 216-802-3389, Fax: 216-687-9342, E-mail: n.zingale@csuohio.edu. *Application contact:* David Arrighi, Graduate Academic Advisor, 216-523-7522, Fax: 216-687-5398, E-mail: d.arrighi@csuohio.edu.
Website: http://urban.csuohio.edu/academics/graduate/mpa/

Cleveland State University, College of Graduate Studies, Monte Ahuja College of Business, Department of Management, Cleveland, OH 44115. Offers health care administration (MBA); labor relations and human resources (MLRHR). *Program availability:* Part-time, evening/weekend. *Faculty:* 6 full-time (3 women), 8 part-time/adjunct (1 woman). *Students:* 10 full-time (all women), 17 part-time (14 women); includes 9 minority (8 Black or African American, non-Hispanic/Latino; 1 Asian, non-Hispanic/Latino), 1 international. Average age 32. In 2015, 30 master's awarded. *Entrance requirements:* For master's, GMAT or GRE, minimum GPA of 3.0. Additional exam requirements/recommendations for international students: Required—TOEFL (minimum score 550 paper-based; 78 iBT). *Application deadline:* For fall admission, 7/15 for domestic students; for spring admission, 12/15 for domestic students. Applications are processed on a rolling basis. Application fee: $30. Electronic applications accepted. *Expenses:* Tuition, state resident: full-time $9565. Tuition, nonresident: full-time $17,980. Tuition and fees vary according to program. *Financial support:* In 2015–16, 3 students received support. Career-related internships or fieldwork, scholarships/grants, and unspecified assistantships available. Financial award application deadline: 5/1; financial award applicants required to submit FAFSA. *Faculty research:* Employee selection, individual differences, leadership, emotions, interviews. *Unit head:* Dr. Timothy G. DeGroot, Chairperson, 216-687-4747, Fax: 216-687-4708, E-mail: t.degroot@csuohio.edu. *Application contact:* Ronald Mickler, Assistant Director, Graduate Programs, 216-687-9358, Fax: 216-687-6888, E-mail: r.mickler@csuohio.edu.
Website: https://www.csuohio.edu/business/management/management

Cleveland State University, College of Graduate Studies, Monte Ahuja College of Business, MBA Programs, Cleveland, OH 44115. Offers business administration (AMBA, MBA); executive business administration (EMBA); health care administration (MBA); JD/MBA; MSN/MBA. Programs also offered at Progressive Insurance Corporation, The Cleveland Clinic, and Metro Health Medical Center. *Accreditation:* AACSB. *Program availability:* Part-time, evening/weekend, online learning. *Faculty:* 33

Health Services Management and Hospital Administration

full-time (9 women), 16 part-time/adjunct (2 women). *Students:* 163 full-time (65 women), 369 part-time (155 women); includes 102 minority (52 Black or African American, non-Hispanic/Latino; 20 Asian, non-Hispanic/Latino; 20 Hispanic/Latino; 10 Two or more races, non-Hispanic/Latino), 91 international. Average age 30. 674 applicants, 48% accepted, 160 enrolled. In 2015, 290 master's awarded. *Degree requirements:* For master's, variable foreign language requirement, comprehensive exam (for some programs), thesis (for some programs). *Entrance requirements:* For master's, GMAT or GRE, minimum cumulative GPA of 2.75 from bachelor's degree; resume, statement of purpose and two letters of reference (for health care administration MBA). Additional exam requirements/recommendations for international students: Required—TOEFL (minimum score 550 paper-based; 78 iBT). *Application deadline:* For fall admission, 6/1 priority date for domestic students, 6/1 for international students; for spring admission, 11/1 priority date for domestic students, 11/1 for international students. Applications are processed on a rolling basis. Application fee: $30. Electronic applications accepted. *Expenses:* Tuition, state resident: full-time $9565. Tuition, nonresident: full-time $17,980. Tuition and fees vary according to program. *Financial support:* In 2015–16, 594 students received support, including 45 research assistantships with tuition reimbursements available (averaging $6,960 per year), 1 teaching assistantship with tuition reimbursement available (averaging $7,800 per year); tuition waivers (full) and unspecified assistantships also available. Financial award application deadline: 5/15; financial award applicants required to submit FAFSA. *Faculty research:* Accounting and finance, management and organizational behavior, marketing, computer information systems, international business. *Total annual research expenditures:* $70,000. *Unit head:* Ronald John Mickler, Jr., Acting Assistant Director, Graduate Programs, 216-687-3730, Fax: 216-687-5311, E-mail: cbacsu@csuohio.edu. *Application contact:* Kenneth Dippong, Director, Student Services, 216-523-7545, Fax: 216-687-9354, E-mail: k.dippong@csuohio.edu.
Website: http://www.csuohio.edu/cba/

The College at Brockport, State University of New York, School of Education and Human Services, Department of Public Administration, Brockport, NY 14420-2997. Offers arts administration (AGC); nonprofit management (AGC); public administration (MPA), including health care management, nonprofit management, public management. *Accreditation:* NASPAA. *Program availability:* Part-time, evening/weekend. *Faculty:* 5 full-time (2 women), 3 part-time/adjunct (2 women). *Students:* 65 full-time (38 women), 76 part-time (53 women); includes 30 minority (14 Black or African American, non-Hispanic/Latino; 4 Asian, non-Hispanic/Latino; 6 Hispanic/Latino; 6 Two or more races, non-Hispanic/Latino). 94 applicants, 86% accepted, 64 enrolled. In 2015, 34 master's, 4 other advanced degrees awarded. *Degree requirements:* For master's, thesis or alternative. *Entrance requirements:* For master's, GRE or minimum GPA of 3.0, letters of recommendation, statement of objectives, current resume. Additional exam requirements/recommendations for international students: Required—TOEFL (minimum score 550 paper-based; 79 iBT), IELTS (minimum score 6.5). *Application deadline:* For fall admission, 8/15 priority date for domestic and international students; for spring admission, 1/15 priority date for domestic and international students; for summer admission, 4/15 priority date for domestic and international students. Application fee: $50. Electronic applications accepted. *Expenses:* $11,840 per academic year. *Financial support:* In 2015–16, 1 fellowship with full tuition reimbursement (averaging $7,500 per year), 1 teaching assistantship with full tuition reimbursement (averaging $6,000 per year) were awarded; Federal Work-Study, scholarships/grants, and unspecified assistantships also available. Support available to part-time students. Financial award application deadline: 3/15; financial award applicants required to submit FAFSA. *Faculty research:* E-government, performance management, nonprofits and policy implementation, Medicaid and disabilities. *Unit head:* Dr. Celia Watt, Graduate Director, 585-395-5538, Fax: 585-395-2172, E-mail: cwatt@brockport.edu. *Application contact:* Danielle A. Welch, Graduate Admissions Counselor, 585-395-2525, Fax: 585-395-2515.
Website: http://www.brockport.edu/pubadmin

College of Saint Elizabeth, Health Administration Program, Morristown, NJ 07960. Offers MS. *Program availability:* Part-time. *Faculty:* 3 full-time (2 women), 4 part-time/adjunct (0 women). *Students:* 5 full-time (4 women), 45 part-time (35 women); includes 15 minority (8 Black or African American, non-Hispanic/Latino; 4 Asian, non-Hispanic/Latino; 3 Hispanic/Latino), 1 international. Average age 41. 31 applicants, 68% accepted, 14 enrolled. In 2015, 47 degrees awarded. *Degree requirements:* For master's, thesis (for some programs), culminating experience. *Entrance requirements:* For master's, GRE, minimum cumulative undergraduate GPA of 3.0, personal statement, resume, two letters of professional recommendation. Additional exam requirements/recommendations for international students: Required—TOEFL (minimum score 550 paper-based; 79 iBT), IELTS (minimum score 6.5). *Application deadline:* For fall admission, 5/1 for international students. Applications are processed on a rolling basis. Application fee: $35. Electronic applications accepted. Application fee is waived when completed online. *Expenses:* $1,001 per credit; graduation fee: $175. *Financial support:* Career-related internships or fieldwork, scholarships/grants, tuition waivers (partial), and unspecified assistantships available. Financial award applicants required to submit FAFSA. *Unit head:* Dr. David B. Tataw, Program Chair and Director, Health Care Administration, 973-290-4271, Fax: 973-290-4167, E-mail: dtataw@cse.edu. *Application contact:* Marie Scolavino, Admissions Director of Graduate and Continuing Studies, 973-290-4413, Fax: 973-290-4710, E-mail: apply@cse.edu.
Website: http://www.cse.edu/academics/prof-studies/health-administration/

Colorado Heights University, Program in International Business, Denver, CO 80236-2711. Offers accounting (MBA); corporate finance (MBA); environmental management (MBA); healthcare management (MBA). *Entrance requirements:* For master's, official transcripts, resume or curriculum vitae, two reference letters, interview.

Colorado State University–Global Campus, Graduate Programs, Greenwood Village, CO 80111. Offers criminal justice and law enforcement administration (MS); education leadership (MS); finance (MS); healthcare administration and management (MS); human resource management (MHRM); information technology management (MITM); international management (MS); management (MS); organizational leadership (MS); professional accounting (MPA); project management (MS); teaching and learning (MS). *Program availability:* Online learning.

Columbia Southern University, MBA Program, Orange Beach, AL 36561. Offers finance (MBA); health care management (MBA); human resource management (MBA); marketing (MBA); project management (MBA); public administration (MBA). *Program availability:* Part-time, evening/weekend, online learning. *Entrance requirements:* For master's, bachelor's degree from accredited/approved institution. Additional exam requirements/recommendations for international students: Required—TOEFL. Electronic applications accepted.

Columbia University, Columbia University Mailman School of Public Health, Department of Health Policy and Management, New York, NY 10032. Offers Exec MHA, Exec MPH, MHA, MPH. *Accreditation:* CAHME. *Program availability:* Part-time, evening/weekend. *Students:* 209 full-time (154 women), 162 part-time (101 women); includes 141 minority (18 Black or African American, non-Hispanic/Latino; 1 American Indian or Alaska Native, non-Hispanic/Latino; 85 Asian, non-Hispanic/Latino; 33 Hispanic/Latino; 1 Native Hawaiian or other Pacific Islander, non-Hispanic/Latino; 5 Two or more races, non-Hispanic/Latino), 44 international. Average age 30. 688 applicants, 61% accepted,

167 enrolled. In 2015, 162 master's awarded. *Degree requirements:* For master's, thesis optional. *Entrance requirements:* For master's, GRE General Test. Additional exam requirements/recommendations for international students: Required—TOEFL (minimum score 600 paper-based; 100 iBT). *Application deadline:* For fall admission, 12/1 priority date for domestic and international students. Application fee: $120. Electronic applications accepted. *Financial support:* Research assistantships, teaching assistantships, career-related internships or fieldwork, and Federal Work-Study available. Support available to part-time students. Financial award application deadline: 2/1; financial award applicants required to submit FAFSA. *Faculty research:* Health care reform, health care disparities, state and national and cross-national health policy, health care quality, organization structure and performance. *Unit head:* Dr. Michael Sparer, Chairperson, 212-305-3924. *Application contact:* Dr. Joseph Korevec, Senior Director of Admissions and Financial Aid, 212-305-8698, Fax: 212-342-1861, E-mail: ph-admit@columbia.edu.
Website: https://www.mailman.columbia.edu/become-student/departments/health-policy-and-management

Columbus State University, Graduate Studies, College of Letters and Sciences, Department of Political Science, Columbus, GA 31907-5645. Offers public administration (MPA), including criminal justice, environmental policy, government administration, health services administration, political campaigning, urban policy. *Program availability:* Part-time, evening/weekend, 100% online, blended/hybrid learning. *Faculty:* 8 full-time (2 women), 2 part-time/adjunct (0 women). *Students:* 34 full-time (15 women), 96 part-time (45 women); includes 63 minority (46 Black or African American, non-Hispanic/Latino; 2 American Indian or Alaska Native, non-Hispanic/Latino; 2 Asian, non-Hispanic/Latino; 9 Hispanic/Latino; 4 Two or more races, non-Hispanic/Latino). Average age 33. 75 applicants, 36% accepted, 23 enrolled. In 2015, 47 master's awarded. *Degree requirements:* For master's, comprehensive exam. *Entrance requirements:* For master's, GRE General Test, minimum GPA of 2.75, three letters of recommendation. Additional exam requirements/recommendations for international students: Required—TOEFL (minimum score 550 paper-based; 79 iBT). *Application deadline:* For fall admission, 6/30 for domestic students, 5/1 for international students; for spring admission, 11/1 for domestic and international students; for summer admission, 3/1 for domestic and international students. Applications are processed on a rolling basis. Application fee: $50. Electronic applications accepted. *Expenses:* Tuition, state resident: full-time $4804; part-time $2412 per semester hour. Tuition, nonresident: full-time $19,218; part-time $9612 per semester hour. *Required fees:* $1830; $1830 per unit. Tuition and fees vary according to program. *Financial support:* In 2015–16, 59 students received support, including 8 research assistantships with partial tuition reimbursements available (averaging $3,000 per year); career-related internships or fieldwork, Federal Work-Study, institutionally sponsored loans, scholarships/grants, tuition waivers (partial), and unspecified assistantships also available. Support available to part-time students. Financial award application deadline: 5/1; financial award applicants required to submit FAFSA. *Unit head:* Dr. Frederick Gordon, Director, 706-565-7875, E-mail: gordon_frederick@colstate.edu. *Application contact:* Kristin Williams, Director of International and Graduate Recruitment, 706-507-8848, Fax: 706-568-5091, E-mail: williams_kristin@columbusstate.edu.
Website: http://politicalscience.columbusstate.edu/

Concordia University, St. Paul, College of Business and Technology, St. Paul, MN 55104-5494. Offers business administration (MBA), including cyber-security leadership; business and organizational leadership (MBA); health care management (MBA); human resource management (MA); leadership and management (MA); strategic communication management (MA). *Program availability:* Evening/weekend, 100% online, blended/hybrid learning. *Faculty:* 11 full-time (3 women), 29 part-time/adjunct (13 women). *Students:* 392 full-time (252 women), 28 part-time (20 women); includes 104 minority (51 Black or African American, non-Hispanic/Latino; 1 American Indian or Alaska Native, non-Hispanic/Latino; 27 Asian, non-Hispanic/Latino; 11 Hispanic/Latino; 1 Native Hawaiian or other Pacific Islander, non-Hispanic/Latino; 13 Two or more races, non-Hispanic/Latino), 7 international. Average age 34. 417 applicants, 45% accepted, 152 enrolled. In 2015, 225 master's awarded. *Degree requirements:* For master's, thesis (for some programs). *Entrance requirements:* For master's, official transcripts from regionally-accredited institution stating the conferral of a bachelor's degree with minimum cumulative GPA of 3.0; personal statement; professional resume. Additional exam requirements/recommendations for international students: Recommended—TOEFL (minimum score 547 paper-based; 78 iBT), IELTS (minimum score 6). *Application deadline:* For fall admission, 8/1 for domestic and international students; for spring admission, 12/1 for domestic and international students; for summer admission, 5/1 for domestic and international students. Applications are processed on a rolling basis. Application fee: $50. Electronic applications accepted. *Expenses:* $26,250 per degree (for MBA); $17,100 per degree (for MA). *Financial support:* Applicants required to submit FAFSA. *Faculty research:* How innovation leads to success at Spain's oldest universities; contemporary practices in leadership development. *Unit head:* Dr. Kevin Hall, Dean, 651-603-6165, Fax: 651-641-8807, E-mail: khall@csp.edu. *Application contact:* Kimberly Craig, Associate Vice President, Cohort Enrollment Management, 651-603-6223, Fax: 651-603-6320, E-mail: craig@csp.edu.

Concordia University Wisconsin, Graduate Programs, School of Business and Legal Studies, MBA Program, Mequon, WI 53097-2402. Offers finance (MBA); health care administration (MBA); human resource management (MBA); international business (MBA); international business-bilingual English/Chinese (MBA); management (MBA); management information systems (MBA); managerial communications (MBA); marketing (MBA); public administration (MBA); risk management (MBA). *Program availability:* Online learning. *Degree requirements:* For master's, comprehensive exam, thesis or alternative. *Entrance requirements:* Additional exam requirements/recommendations for international students: Required—TOEFL. *Expenses:* Contact institution.

Copenhagen Business School, Graduate Programs, Copenhagen, Denmark. Offers business administration (Exec MBA, MBA, PhD); business administration and information systems (M Sc); business, language and culture (M Sc); economics and business administration (M Sc); health management (MHM); international business and politics (M Sc); public administration (MPA); shipping and logistics (Exec MBA); technology, market and organization (MBA).

Cornell University, Graduate School, Graduate Fields of Human Ecology, Field of Policy Analysis and Management, Ithaca, NY 14853-0001. Offers consumer policy (PhD); family and social welfare policy (PhD); health administration (MHA); health management and policy (PhD); public policy (PhD). *Degree requirements:* For master's, thesis; for doctorate, thesis/dissertation. *Entrance requirements:* For master's, GRE General Test or GMAT, 2 letters of recommendation; for doctorate, GRE General Test, 2 letters of recommendation. Additional exam requirements/recommendations for international students: Required—TOEFL (minimum score 550 paper-based; 77 iBT). Electronic applications accepted. *Faculty research:* Health policy, family policy, social welfare policy, program evaluation, consumer policy.

Daemen College, Program in Executive Leadership and Change, Amherst, NY 14226-3592. Offers business (MS); health professions (MS); not-for-profit organizations (MS). *Program availability:* Part-time, evening/weekend. *Degree requirements:* For master's,

Health Services Management and Hospital Administration

thesis, cohort learning sequence (2 years for weekend cohort; 3 years for weeknight cohort). *Entrance requirements:* For master's, 2 letters of recommendation, interview, goal statement, official transcripts, resume. Additional exam requirements/recommendations for international students: Required—TOEFL (minimum score 500 paper-based; 63 iBT), IELTS (minimum score 5.5). Electronic applications accepted.

Dalhousie University, Faculty of Health Professions, School of Health Administration, Halifax, NS B3H 1R2, Canada. Offers MAHSR, MHA, MPH, PhD, LL B/MHA, MBA/MHA, MHA/MN. *Accreditation:* CAHME. *Program availability:* Part-time, online learning. *Entrance requirements:* For master's, GMAT. Additional exam requirements/recommendations for international students: Required—TOEFL, IELTS, CANTEST, CAEL, or Michigan English Language Assessment Battery. Electronic applications accepted. *Expenses:* Contact institution. *Faculty research:* Hospital, nursing, long-term, public, and community health administration; government administration in health areas.

Dallas Baptist University, College of Business, Business Administration Program, Dallas, TX 75211-9299. Offers accounting (MBA); business communication (MBA); conflict resolution management (MBA); entrepreneurship (MBA); finance (MBA); health care management (MBA); international business (MBA); leading the non-profit organization (MBA); management (MBA); management information systems (MBA); marketing (MBA); project management (MBA); technology and engineering (MBA). *Accreditation:* ACBSP. *Program availability:* Part-time, evening/weekend. *Entrance requirements:* For master's, GMAT, minimum GPA of 3.0. Additional exam requirements/recommendations for international students: Required—TOEFL, IELTS. *Application deadline:* Applications are processed on a rolling basis. Application fee: $25. Electronic applications accepted. *Expenses: Tuition, area resident:* Full-time $14,814; part-time $823 per credit hour. *Required fees:* $250 per semester. Tuition and fees vary according to course load and degree level. *Financial support:* Federal Work-Study, institutionally sponsored loans, scholarships/grants, and tuition waivers (full and partial) available. Support available to part-time students. Financial award applicants required to submit FAFSA. *Faculty research:* Sports management, services marketing, retailing, strategic management, financial planning/investments. *Unit head:* Dr. Sandra S. Reid, Chair, 214-333-5280, Fax: 214-333-5293, E-mail: graduate@dbu.edu. *Application contact:* Kit P. Montgomery, Director of Graduate Programs, 214-333-5242, Fax: 214-333-5579, E-mail: graduate@dbu.edu.
Website: http://www3.dbu.edu/graduate/mba.asp

Dallas Baptist University, College of Business, Management Program, Dallas, TX 75211-9299. Offers conflict resolution management (MA); general management (MA); health care management (MA); human resource management (MA); management (MS); organizational communication (MA); performance management (MA); professional sales and management optimization (MA). *Program availability:* Part-time, evening/weekend. *Entrance requirements:* For master's, GRE General Test, minimum GPA of 3.0. Additional exam requirements/recommendations for international students: Required—TOEFL, IELTS. *Application deadline:* Applications are processed on a rolling basis. Application fee: $25. Electronic applications accepted. *Expenses: Tuition, area resident:* Full-time $14,814; part-time $823 per credit hour. *Required fees:* $250 per semester. Tuition and fees vary according to course load and degree level. *Financial support:* Federal Work-Study, institutionally sponsored loans, scholarships/grants, and tuition waivers (full and partial) available. Support available to part-time students. Financial award applicants required to submit FAFSA. *Faculty research:* Organizational behavior, conflict personalities. *Unit head:* Joanne Hix, Director, 214-333-5280, Fax: 214-333-5293, E-mail: graduate@dbu.edu. *Application contact:* Kit P. Montgomery, Director of Graduate Programs, 214-333-5242, Fax: 214-333-5579, E-mail: graduate@dbu.edu.

Dartmouth College, The Dartmouth Institute, Program in Health Policy and Clinical Practice, Hanover, NH 03755. Offers evaluative clinical sciences (MS, PhD). *Program availability:* Part-time. *Students:* 34 full-time (22 women), 21 part-time (10 women); includes 13 minority (2 Black or African American, non-Hispanic/Latino; 5 Asian, non-Hispanic/Latino; 3 Hispanic/Latino; 3 Two or more races, non-Hispanic/Latino), 8 international. Average age 31. 25 applicants, 8% accepted, 1 enrolled. In 2015, 40 master's awarded. *Degree requirements:* For master's, research project or practicum; for doctorate, thesis/dissertation. *Entrance requirements:* For master's and doctorate, GRE or MCAT, 3 letters of recommendation. Additional exam requirements/recommendations for international students: Required—TOEFL. *Application deadline:* For fall admission, 1/15 for domestic students. Applications are processed on a rolling basis. Application fee: $75. *Expenses: Tuition, area resident:* Full-time $48,120. *Required fees:* $296. One-time fee: $50 full-time. *Financial support:* Fellowships with tuition reimbursements, research assistantships, teaching assistantships with tuition reimbursements, institutionally sponsored loans, and scholarships/grants available. Financial award application deadline: 6/1; financial award applicants required to submit FAFSA. *Faculty research:* Prevention and treatment of cardiovascular diseases, health care cost containment, variation of delivery of care, health care improvement, decision evaluation. *Unit head:* Dr. Elliot S. Fisher, Director, 603-653-0802. *Application contact:* Courtney Theroux, Director of Recruitment and Admissions, 603-653-3234.
Website: http://tdi.dartmouth.edu/

Davenport University, Sneden Graduate School, Grand Rapids, MI 49512. Offers accounting (MBA); business administration (EMBA); finance (MBA); health care management (MBA); human resources (MBA); information assurance (MS); public health (MPH); strategic management (MBA). *Program availability:* Evening/weekend. *Entrance requirements:* For master's, GMAT, minimum undergraduate GPA of 2.75. Additional exam requirements/recommendations for international students: Required—TOEFL. Electronic applications accepted. *Faculty research:* Leadership, management, marketing, organizational culture.

Defiance College, Program in Business Administration, Defiance, OH 43512-1610. Offers criminal justice (MBA); health care (MBA); leadership (MBA); sport management (MBA). *Program availability:* Part-time, evening/weekend. *Degree requirements:* For master's, thesis. *Entrance requirements:* For master's, minimum GPA of 2.5. Additional exam requirements/recommendations for international students: Recommended—TOEFL.

Delta State University, Graduate Programs, School of Nursing, Cleveland, MS 38733. Offers family nurse practitioner (MSN); nurse administrator (MSN); nurse educator (MSN). *Accreditation:* AACN. *Program availability:* Part-time. *Degree requirements:* For master's, thesis optional. *Entrance requirements:* For master's, GRE General Test. Electronic applications accepted.

DePaul University, Charles H. Kellstadt Graduate School of Business, Chicago, IL 60604. Offers accountancy (M Acc, MS, MSA); applied economics (MBA); banking (MBA); behavioral finance (MBA); brand and product management (MBA); business development (MBA); business information technology (MS); business strategy and decision-making (MBA); computational finance (MS); consumer insights (MBA); corporate finance (MBA); economic policy analysis (MS); entrepreneurship (MBA, MS); finance (MBA, MS); financial analysis (MBA); general business (MBA); health sector management (MBA); hospitality leadership (MBA); hospitality leadership and operational performance (MS); human resource management (MBA); human resources (MS); investment management (MBA); leadership and change management (MBA); management accounting (MBA); marketing (MBA, MS); marketing analysis (MS);

marketing strategy and planning (MBA); operations management (MBA); organizational diversity (MBA); real estate (MS); real estate finance and investment (MBA); revenue management (MBA); sports management (MBA); strategic global marketing (MBA); strategy, execution and valuation (MBA); sustainable management (MBA, MS); taxation (MS); wealth management (MS); JD/MBA. *Accreditation:* AACSB. *Program availability:* Part-time, evening/weekend, online learning. *Entrance requirements:* For master's, GMAT, 2 letters of recommendation, resume, essay, official transcripts. Additional exam requirements/recommendations for international students: Required—TOEFL (minimum score 550 paper-based; 80 iBT). Electronic applications accepted. *Expenses:* Contact institution.

DeSales University, Division of Business, Center Valley, PA 18034-9568. Offers accounting (MBA); computer information systems (MBA); finance (MBA); health care systems management (MBA); human resources management (MBA); management (MBA); marketing (MBA); project management (MBA); self-design (MBA); supply chain management (MBA); DNP/MBA; MSN/MBA. *Accreditation:* ACBSP. *Program availability:* Part-time, evening/weekend, 100% online, blended/hybrid learning. *Faculty:* 13 full-time (5 women), 31 part-time/adjunct (7 women). *Students:* 61 full-time (29 women), 346 part-time (181 women); includes 65 minority (17 Black or African American, non-Hispanic/Latino; 22 Asian, non-Hispanic/Latino; 20 Hispanic/Latino; 6 Two or more races, non-Hispanic/Latino). Average age 38. In 2015, 120 master's awarded. *Entrance requirements:* For master's, GMAT (waived if undergraduate GPA is 3.0 or better), minimum GPA of 3.0 in undergraduate work, literacy in basic software, background or interest in the field of study, personal statement, 2 years of work experience. Additional exam requirements/recommendations for international students: Required—TOEFL. *Application deadline:* Applications are processed on a rolling basis. Application fee: $50. Electronic applications accepted. *Expenses:* $815 per credit hour. *Financial support:* Applicants required to submit FAFSA. *Faculty research:* Quality improvement, executive development, productivity, cross-cultural managerial differences, leadership. *Unit head:* Dr. David M. Gilfoil, Director, MBA Program, 610-282-1100 Ext. 1828, Fax: 610-282-2869, E-mail: david.gilfoil@desales.edu. *Application contact:* Abigail Wernicki, Director of Graduate Admissions, 610-282-1100 Ext. 1768, E-mail: gradadmissions@desales.edu.

Des Moines University, College of Health Sciences, Program in Healthcare Administration, Des Moines, IA 50312-4104. Offers MHA. *Program availability:* Part-time, evening/weekend. *Entrance requirements:* For master's, minimum GPA of 3.0. Additional exam requirements/recommendations for international students: Required—TOEFL (minimum score 600 paper-based). Electronic applications accepted. *Expenses:* Contact institution. *Faculty research:* Quality improvement, rural sociology, women's health, health promotion, patient education.

Dominican College, MBA Program, Orangeburg, NY 10962-1210. Offers accounting (MBA); healthcare management (MBA); management (MBA). *Program availability:* Evening/weekend. *Entrance requirements:* For master's, GMAT, 2 letters of recommendation. Additional exam requirements/recommendations for international students: Required—TOEFL. Electronic applications accepted. *Expenses:* Contact institution.

Drew University, Caspersen School of Graduate Studies, Madison, NJ 07940-1493. Offers conflict resolution and leadership (Certificate), including community leadership, moderation, peace building; history and culture (MA, PhD), including American history, book history, British history, European history, Holocaust and genocide (M Litt, MA, D Litt, PhD), intellectual history, Irish history, print culture, public history; K-12 education (MAT), including art, biology, chemistry, elementary education, English, French, Italian, math, secondary education, special education, teacher of students with disabilities; liberal studies (M Litt, D Litt), including history, Holocaust and genocide (M Litt, MA, D Litt, PhD), Irish/Irish-American studies, literature (M Litt, MMH, D Litt, DMH, CMH), religion, spirituality, teaching in the two-year college, writing; medical humanities (MMH, DMH, CMH), including arts, health, healthcare, literature (M Litt, MMH, D Litt, DMH, CMH), scientific research; poetry and poetry in translation (MFA). *Program availability:* Part-time, evening/weekend. *Faculty:* 1 full-time, 26 part-time/adjunct. *Students:* 125 full-time (82 women), 261 part-time (164 women); includes 34 minority (17 Black or African American, non-Hispanic/Latino; 6 Asian, non-Hispanic/Latino; 11 Hispanic/Latino), 6 international. Average age 42. 120 applicants, 90% accepted, 76 enrolled. In 2015, 54 master's, 36 doctorates, 9 other advanced degrees awarded. Terminal master's awarded for partial completion of doctoral program. *Degree requirements:* For master's and other advanced degree, thesis (for some programs); for doctorate, one foreign language, comprehensive exam (for some programs), thesis/dissertation. *Entrance requirements:* For master's, GRE (MA in history and culture), PRAXIS Core and Subject Area tests (MAT), resume, transcripts, writing sample, personal statement, letters of recommendation; for doctorate, GRE (PhD in history and culture), resume, transcripts, writing sample, personal statement, letters of recommendation. Additional exam requirements/recommendations for international students: Required—TOEFL (minimum score 587 paper-based; 94 iBT), IELTS (minimum score 7), TWE (minimum score 4). *Application deadline:* Applications are processed on a rolling basis. Application fee: $35. Tuition and fees vary according to program. *Financial support:* In 2015–16, 214 students received support. Fellowships, research assistantships, teaching assistantships, career-related internships or fieldwork, Federal Work-Study, scholarships/grants, and unspecified assistantships available. Support available to part-time students. Financial award applicants required to submit FAFSA. *Unit head:* Dr. Robert Ready, Dean, 973-408-3285, Fax: 973-408-3040, E-mail: gsdean@drew.edu. *Application contact:* Leanne Horinko, Interim Director of Admissions, 973-408-3110, Fax: 973-408-3110, E-mail: gradm@drew.edu.
Website: http://www.drew.edu/graduate

Duke University, The Fuqua School of Business, The Duke MBA-Cross Continent Program, Durham, NC 27708-0586. Offers business administration (MBA); energy and environment (MBA); entrepreneurship and innovation (MBA); finance (MBA); health sector management (Certificate); marketing (MBA); strategy (MBA). *Faculty:* 87 full-time (17 women), 47 part-time/adjunct (7 women). *Students:* 218 full-time (81 women); includes 60 minority (12 Black or African American, non-Hispanic/Latino; 38 Asian, non-Hispanic/Latino; 10 Hispanic/Latino), 47 international. Average age 31. In 2015, 115 master's awarded. *Entrance requirements:* For master's, GMAT or GRE, transcripts, essays, resume, recommendation letters, letter of company support, interview. *Application deadline:* For fall admission, 10/21 priority date for domestic and international students; for winter admission, 2/10 priority date for domestic and international students; for spring admission, 5/4 priority date for domestic and international students; for summer admission, 6/1 for domestic and international students. Applications are processed on a rolling basis. Application fee: $225. Electronic applications accepted. *Expenses:* Contact institution. *Financial support:* In 2015–16, 54 students received support. Institutionally sponsored loans and scholarships/grants available. Financial award applicants required to submit FAFSA. *Unit head:* John Gallagher, Associate Dean for Executive MBA Programs, 919-660-7641, Fax: 919-684-8742, E-mail: johng@duke.edu. *Application contact:* Liz Riley Hargrove, Associate Dean for Admissions, 919-660-7705, Fax: 919-681-8026, E-mail: admissions-info@fuqua.duke.edu.
Website: http://www.fuqua.duke.edu/programs/duke_mba/cross_continent/

Health Services Management and Hospital Administration

Duke University, The Fuqua School of Business, The Duke MBA-Daytime Program, Durham, NC 27708-0586. Offers academic excellence in finance (Certificate); business administration (MBA); decision sciences (MBA); energy and environment (MBA); energy finance (MBA); entrepreneurship and innovation (MBA); finance (MBA); financial analysis (MBA); health sector management (Certificate); leadership and ethics (MBA); management (MBA); marketing (MBA); operations management (MBA); social entrepreneurship (MBA); strategy (MBA). *Faculty:* 87 full-time (17 women), 47 part-time/adjunct (7 women). *Students:* 894 full-time (316 women); includes 170 minority (34 Black or African American, non-Hispanic/Latino; 5 American Indian or Alaska Native, non-Hispanic/Latino; 84 Asian, non-Hispanic/Latino; 45 Hispanic/Latino; 1 Native Hawaiian or other Pacific Islander, non-Hispanic/Latino; 1 Two or more races, non-Hispanic/Latino), 336 international. Average age 29. In 2015, 434 master's awarded. *Entrance requirements:* For master's, GMAT or GRE, transcripts, essays, resume, recommendation letters, interview. *Application deadline:* For fall admission, 9/15 for domestic and international students; for winter admission, 10/14 for domestic and international students; for spring admission, 1/5 for domestic and international students; for summer admission, 3/22 for domestic and international students. Application fee: $225. Electronic applications accepted. *Expenses:* $63,956 (first-year tuition and fees). *Financial support:* In 2015–16, 433 students received support. Institutionally sponsored loans and scholarships/grants available. Financial award applicants required to submit FAFSA. *Unit head:* Russ Morgan, Associate Dean for the Daytime MBA Program, 919-660-2931, Fax: 919-684-8742, E-mail: ruskin.morgan@duke.edu. *Application contact:* Liz Riley Hargrove, Associate Dean for Admissions, 919-660-7705, Fax: 919-681-8026, E-mail: admissions-info@fuqua.duke.edu.
Website: http://www.fuqua.duke.edu/daytime-mba/

Duke University, The Fuqua School of Business, The Duke MBA-Global Executive Program, Durham, NC 27708-0586. Offers business administration (MBA); energy and environment (MBA); entrepreneurship and innovation (MBA); finance (MBA); health sector management (Certificate); marketing (MBA); strategy (MBA). *Faculty:* 87 full-time (17 women), 47 part-time/adjunct (7 women). *Students:* 26 full-time (6 women); includes 6 minority (1 Black or African American, non-Hispanic/Latino; 3 Asian, non-Hispanic/Latino; 2 Hispanic/Latino), 9 international. Average age 40. In 2015, 35 master's awarded. *Entrance requirements:* For master's, transcripts, essays, resume, recommendation letters, letter of company support, interview. *Application deadline:* For fall admission, 9/2 priority date for domestic and international students; for winter admission, 12/2 priority date for domestic and international students; for spring admission, 3/30 priority date for domestic and international students; for summer admission, 6/1 for domestic and international students. Applications are processed on a rolling basis. Application fee: $225. Electronic applications accepted. *Expenses:* Contact institution. *Financial support:* In 2015–16, 1 student received support. Institutionally sponsored loans and scholarships/grants available. Financial award applicants required to submit FAFSA. *Unit head:* John Gallagher, Associate Dean for Executive MBA Programs, 919-660-7641, Fax: 919-684-8742, E-mail: johng@duke.edu. *Application contact:* Liz Riley Hargrove, Associate Dean for Admissions, 919-660-7705, Fax: 919-681-8026, E-mail: admissions-info@fuqua.duke.edu.
Website: http://www.fuqua.duke.edu/programs/duke_mba/global-executive/

Duke University, The Fuqua School of Business, The Duke MBA-Weekend Executive Program, Durham, NC 27708-0586. Offers business administration (MBA); energy and environment (MBA); entrepreneurship and innovation (MBA); finance (MBA); health sector management (Certificate); marketing (MBA); strategy (MBA). *Faculty:* 87 full-time (17 women), 47 part-time/adjunct (7 women). *Students:* 183 full-time (31 women); includes 77 minority (10 Black or African American, non-Hispanic/Latino; 1 American Indian or Alaska Native, non-Hispanic/Latino; 56 Asian, non-Hispanic/Latino; 10 Hispanic/Latino), 30 international. Average age 36. In 2015, 93 master's awarded. *Entrance requirements:* For master's, GMAT or GRE, transcripts, essays, resume, recommendation letters, letter of company support, interview. *Application deadline:* For fall admission, 9/2 priority date for domestic and international students; for winter admission, 10/21 priority date for domestic and international students; for spring admission, 2/10 priority date for domestic and international students; for summer admission, 3/30 for domestic and international students. Applications are processed on a rolling basis. Application fee: $225. Electronic applications accepted. *Expenses:* Contact institution. *Financial support:* In 2015–16, 24 students received support. Institutionally sponsored loans and scholarships/grants available. Financial award applicants required to submit FAFSA. *Unit head:* John Gallagher, Associate Dean for Executive MBA Programs, 919-660-7641, Fax: 919-684-8742, E-mail: johng@duke.edu. *Application contact:* Liz Riley Hargrove, Associate Dean for Admissions, 919-660-7705, Fax: 919-681-8026, E-mail: admissions-info@fuqua.duke.edu.
Website: http://www.fuqua.duke.edu/programs/duke_mba/weekend_executive/

Duquesne University, John G. Rangos, Sr. School of Health Sciences, Pittsburgh, PA 15282-0001. Offers health management systems (MHMS); occupational therapy (MS, OTD); physical therapy (DPT); physician assistant studies (MPAS); rehabilitation science (MS, PhD); speech-language pathology (MS); MBA/MHMS. *Accreditation:* AOTA (one or more programs are accredited); APTA (one or more programs are accredited); ASHA. *Program availability:* Minimal on-campus study. *Faculty:* 45 full-time (32 women), 33 part-time/adjunct (17 women). *Students:* 230 full-time (180 women), 11 part-time (5 women); includes 15 minority (1 Black or African American, non-Hispanic/Latino; 3 Asian, non-Hispanic/Latino; 7 Hispanic/Latino; 4 Two or more races, non-Hispanic/Latino), 20 international. Average age 23. 685 applicants, 9% accepted, 24 enrolled. In 2015, 132 master's, 32 doctorates awarded. *Degree requirements:* For doctorate, comprehensive exam (for some programs), thesis/dissertation (for some programs). *Entrance requirements:* For master's, GRE General Test (speech-language pathology), 3 letters of recommendation; minimum GPA of 2.75 (health management systems), 3.0 (speech-language pathology); for doctorate, GRE General Test (for physical therapy and rehabilitation science), 3 letters of recommendation, minimum GPA of 3.0, personal interview. Additional exam requirements/recommendations for international students: Required—TOEFL (minimum score 550 paper-based; 90 iBT). *Application deadline:* For fall admission, 2/1 for domestic and international students; for spring admission, 7/1 for domestic and international students. Applications are processed on a rolling basis. Application fee: $0. Electronic applications accepted. *Expenses:* $1,254 per credit. *Financial support:* Federal Work-Study available. Financial award applicants required to submit FAFSA. *Faculty research:* Neuronal processing, electrical stimulation on peripheral neuropathy, central nervous system (CNS) stimulatory and inhibitory signals, behavioral genetic methodologies to development disorders of speech, neurogenic communication disorders. *Total annual research expenditures:* $38,730. *Unit head:* Dr. Gregory H. Frazer, Dean, 412-396-5303, Fax: 412-396-5554, E-mail: frazer@duq.edu. *Application contact:* Christopher R. Hilf, Recruiter/Academic Advisor, 412-396-5653, Fax: 412-396-5554, E-mail: hilfc@duq.edu.
Website: http://www.duq.edu/academics/schools/health-sciences

D'Youville College, Department of Health Services Administration, Buffalo, NY 14201-1084. Offers clinical research associate (Certificate); health administration (Ed D); health services administration (MS, Certificate); long term care administration (Certificate). *Program availability:* Part-time, evening/weekend. *Students:* 17 full-time (9 women), 68 part-time (50 women); includes 25 minority (20 Black or African American, non-Hispanic/Latino; 2 American Indian or Alaska Native, non-Hispanic/Latino; 1 Asian, non-Hispanic/Latino; 2 Hispanic/Latino), 13 international. Average age 37. 51 applicants, 84% accepted, 25 enrolled. In 2015, 10 master's, 2 doctorates awarded. *Degree requirements:* For master's, project or thesis. *Entrance requirements:* For master's, minimum GPA of 3.0 in major. Additional exam requirements/recommendations for international students: Required—TOEFL (minimum score 500 paper-based). *Application deadline:* For fall admission, 5/1 priority date for international students; for spring admission, 9/1 priority date for international students. Applications are processed on a rolling basis. Electronic applications accepted. *Expenses: Tuition, area resident:* Full-time $21,120; part-time $880 per credit hour. *Required fees:* $235; $96. One-time fee: $100. *Financial support:* Career-related internships or fieldwork, Federal Work-Study, and scholarships/grants available. Support available to part-time students. Financial award application deadline: 3/1; financial award applicants required to submit FAFSA. *Faculty research:* Outcomes research in rehabilitation medicine, cost/benefit analysis of prospective payment systems. *Unit head:* Dr. Lisa Rafalson, Chair, 716-829-8489, Fax: 716-829-8184. *Application contact:* Mark Pavone, Graduate Admissions Director, 716-829-8400, Fax: 716-829-7900, E-mail: graduateadmissions@dyc.edu.

Eastern Kentucky University, The Graduate School, College of Arts and Sciences, Department of Government, Program in General Public Administration, Richmond, KY 40475-3102. Offers community development (MPA); community health administration (MPA); general public administration (MPA). *Accreditation:* NASPAA. *Program availability:* Part-time, evening/weekend. *Entrance requirements:* For master's, GRE General Test, minimum GPA of 2.5.

Eastern Mennonite University, Program in Business Administration, Harrisonburg, VA 22802-2462. Offers general management (MBA); health services administration (MBA); non-profit leadership (MBA). *Program availability:* Part-time, evening/weekend. *Faculty:* 1 part-time/adjunct. *Students:* 10 part-time. *Degree requirements:* For master's, final capstone course. *Entrance requirements:* For master's, GMAT, minimum GPA of 2.5, 2 years of work experience, 2 letters of reference. Additional exam requirements/recommendations for international students: Required—TOEFL (minimum score 500 paper-based). *Application deadline:* For fall admission, 3/1 priority date for domestic and international students. Applications are processed on a rolling basis. Application fee: $25. Electronic applications accepted. *Expenses:* Contact institution. *Financial support:* Application deadline: 6/30; applicants required to submit FAFSA. *Faculty research:* Information security, Anabaptist/Mennonite experiences and perspectives, limits of multi-cultural education, international development performance criteria. *Unit head:* Dr. James M. Leaman, Department Chair, 540-432-4152, Fax: 540-432-4071, E-mail: james.leaman@emu.edu. *Application contact:* Patricia S. Eckard, Administrative Coordinator, 540-432-4150, Fax: 540-432-4071, E-mail: eckardp@emu.edu.
Website: http://www.emu.edu/mba

Eastern Michigan University, Graduate School, College of Arts and Sciences, Department of Political Science, Programs in Public Administration, Ypsilanti, MI 48197. Offers general public management (Graduate Certificate); local government management (Graduate Certificate); management of public healthcare services (Graduate Certificate); nonprofit management (Graduate Certificate); public administration (MPA, Graduate Certificate); public budget management (Graduate Certificate); public land planning and development management (Graduate Certificate); public personnel management (Graduate Certificate); public policy analysis (Graduate Certificate). *Accreditation:* NASPAA. *Students:* 10 full-time (5 women), 42 part-time (19 women); includes 18 minority (14 Black or African American, non-Hispanic/Latino; 4 Hispanic/Latino). Average age 34. 43 applicants, 58% accepted, 17 enrolled. In 2015, 19 master's, 1 other advanced degree awarded. Application fee: $45. *Application contact:* Dr. Jeffrey L. Bernstein, Program Advisor, 734-487-6970, Fax: 734-487-3340, E-mail: jeffrey.bernstein@emich.edu.
Website: http://www.emich.edu/polisci

Eastern Michigan University, Graduate School, College of Health and Human Services, Interdisciplinary Program in Health and Human Services, Ypsilanti, MI 48197. Offers community building (Graduate Certificate). *Program availability:* Part-time, evening/weekend. In 2015, 1 Graduate Certificate awarded. *Entrance requirements:* Additional exam requirements/recommendations for international students: Required—TOEFL. Application fee: $45. *Unit head:* Dr. Marcia Bombyk, Program Coordinator, 734-487-0393, Fax: 734-487-8536, E-mail: marcia.bombyk@emich.edu. *Application contact:* Graduate Admissions, 734-487-2400, Fax: 734-487-6559, E-mail: graduate.admissions@emich.edu.

Eastern Michigan University, Graduate School, College of Health and Human Services, School of Health Sciences, Programs in Health Administration, Ypsilanti, MI 48197. Offers MHA, MS, Graduate Certificate. *Students:* 8 full-time (5 women), 54 part-time (38 women); includes 18 minority (13 Black or African American, non-Hispanic/Latino; 1 American Indian or Alaska Native, non-Hispanic/Latino; 3 Asian, non-Hispanic/Latino; 1 Hispanic/Latino). Average age 32. 41 applicants, 29% accepted, 5 enrolled. In 2015, 31 master's, 1 other advanced degree awarded. Application fee: $45. *Application contact:* Dr. Pamela Walsh, Program Director, 734-487-2383, Fax: 734-487-4095, E-mail: pwalsh@emich.edu.

Eastern University, School of Management Studies, St. Davids, PA 19087-3696. Offers health administration (MBA); health services management (MS); management (MBA). Programs also offered at Harrisburg location. *Program availability:* Part-time, evening/weekend, online learning. *Faculty:* 7 full-time (5 women), 40 part-time/adjunct (13 women). *Students:* 38 full-time (29 women), 176 part-time (114 women); includes 101 minority (86 Black or African American, non-Hispanic/Latino; 7 Asian, non-Hispanic/Latino; 7 Hispanic/Latino; 1 Two or more races, non-Hispanic/Latino), 23 international. Average age 35. 84 applicants, 96% accepted, 64 enrolled. In 2015, 143 master's awarded. *Entrance requirements:* Additional exam requirements/recommendations for international students: Required—TOEFL (minimum score 550 paper-based; 79 iBT). *Application deadline:* For fall admission, 8/16 for domestic students; for spring admission, 3/14 for domestic students. Applications are processed on a rolling basis. Application fee: $35. Application fee is waived when completed online. *Financial support:* In 2015–16, 34 students received support. Scholarships/grants available. Financial award applicants required to submit FAFSA. *Unit head:* Michael Dziedziak, Executive Director of Enrollment, 800-732-7669, Fax: 610-225-5601, E-mail: gpsadm@eastern.edu.
Website: http://www.eastern.edu/academics/programs/school-management-studies-sms

East Tennessee State University, School of Graduate Studies, College of Business and Technology, Department of Management and Marketing, Johnson City, TN 37614. Offers business administration (MBA, Postbaccalaureate Certificate); digital marketing (MS); entrepreneurial leadership (Postbaccalaureate Certificate); health care management (Postbaccalaureate Certificate). *Program availability:* Part-time, evening/weekend. *Faculty:* 16 full-time (3 women). *Students:* 82 full-time (44 women), 35 part-time (11 women); includes 12 minority (6 Black or African American, non-Hispanic/Latino; 2 Asian, non-Hispanic/Latino; 2 Hispanic/Latino; 2 Two or more races, non-Hispanic/Latino), 14 international. Average age 29. 187 applicants, 39% accepted, 51 enrolled. In 2015, 52 master's, 4 other advanced degrees awarded. *Degree*

Health Services Management and Hospital Administration

requirements: For master's, comprehensive exam, capstone. *Entrance requirements:* For master's, GMAT, minimum GPA of 2.5 (for MBA), 3.0 (for MS); for Postbaccalaureate Certificate, minimum GPA of 2.5. Additional exam requirements/recommendations for international students: Required—TOEFL (minimum score 550 paper-based; 79 iBT). *Application deadline:* For fall admission, 6/1 for domestic students, 4/30 for international students; for spring admission, 11/1 for domestic students, 9/30 for international students. Application fee: $35 ($45 for international students). Electronic applications accepted. *Financial support:* In 2015–16, 40 students received support, including 35 research assistantships with full tuition reimbursements available (averaging $6,000 per year), 2 teaching assistantships with full tuition reimbursements available (averaging $6,000 per year); career-related internships or fieldwork, institutionally sponsored loans, scholarships/grants, and unspecified assistantships also available. Financial award application deadline: 7/1; financial award applicants required to submit FAFSA. *Faculty research:* Sustainability, healthcare effectiveness, consumer behavior, merchandizing trends, organizational management issues. *Unit head:* Dr. Phillip E. Miller, Chair, 423-439-4422, Fax: 423-439-5661, E-mail: millerpe@etsu.edu. *Application contact:* Cindy Hill, Graduate Specialist, 423-439-6590, Fax: 423-439-5624, E-mail: hillcc@etsu.edu.
Website: http://www.etsu.edu/cbat/mgmtmkt/

Ellis University, MBA Program, Oakbrook Terrace, IL 60181. Offers e-commerce (MBA); finance (MBA); general business (MBA); global management (MBA); health care administration (MBA); leadership (MBA); management of information systems (MBA); marketing (MBA); professional accounting (MBA); project management (MBA); public accounting (MBA); risk management (MBA).

Elms College, Division of Business, Chicopee, MA 01013-2839. Offers accounting (MBA); healthcare leadership (MBA); management (MBA). *Program availability:* Part-time, evening/weekend. *Faculty:* 2 full-time (both women), 6 part-time/adjunct (4 women). *Students:* 42 part-time (27 women); includes 5 minority (4 Black or African American, non-Hispanic/Latino; 1 Hispanic/Latino), 1 international. Average age 34. 7 applicants, 100% accepted, 5 enrolled. In 2015, 30 master's awarded. *Entrance requirements:* For master's, minimum GPA of 3.0. *Application deadline:* Applications are processed on a rolling basis. Application fee: $30. *Unit head:* Dr. David Kimball, Chair, Division of Business, 413-265-2300, E-mail: kimballd@elms.edu. *Application contact:* Dr. Elizabeth Teahan Hukowicz, Dean, School of Graduate and Professional Studies, 413-265-2360 Ext. 238, Fax: 413-265-2459, E-mail: hukowicze@elms.edu.

Emory University, Rollins School of Public Health, Department of Health Policy and Management, Atlanta, GA 30322-1100. Offers health policy (MPH); health policy research (MSPH); health services management (MPH); health services research and health policy (PhD). *Program availability:* Part-time. *Degree requirements:* For master's, thesis (for some programs), practicum, capstone course. *Entrance requirements:* For master's, GRE General Test. Additional exam requirements/recommendations for international students: Required—TOEFL (minimum score 550 paper-based; 80 iBT). Electronic applications accepted. *Faculty research:* U.S. health policy and financing, healthcare organization and financing.

Excelsior College, School of Business and Technology, Albany, NY 12203-5159. Offers business administration (MBA); cybersecurity (MS); cybersecurity management (MBA, Graduate Certificate); health care management (MBA); human performance technology (MBA); human resources management (MBA); leadership (MBA); mediation and arbitration (MBA); social media management (MBA); technology management (MBA). *Program availability:* Part-time, evening/weekend, online learning. *Faculty:* 27 part-time/adjunct (10 women). *Students:* 1,698 part-time (490 women); includes 720 minority (388 Black or African American, non-Hispanic/Latino; 5 American Indian or Alaska Native, non-Hispanic/Latino; 53 Asian, non-Hispanic/Latino; 200 Hispanic/Latino; 9 Native Hawaiian or other Pacific Islander, non-Hispanic/Latino; 65 Two or more races, non-Hispanic/Latino), 11 international. Average age 39. In 2015, 153 master's awarded. *Application deadline:* Applications are processed on a rolling basis. Application fee: $110. Electronic applications accepted. *Expenses: Tuition, area resident:* Part-time $645 per credit. *Required fees:* $265 per unit. *Financial support:* Scholarships/grants available. *Unit head:* Dr. Karl Lawrence, Dean, 888-647-2388. *Application contact:* Admissions, 888-647-2388 Ext. 133, Fax: 518-464-8777, E-mail: admissions@excelsior.edu.

Fairleigh Dickinson University, College at Florham, Silberman College of Business, Executive MBA Programs, Executive MBA Program for Health Care and Life Sciences Professionals, Madison, NJ 07940-1099. Offers EMBA.

Fairleigh Dickinson University, Metropolitan Campus, Silberman College of Business, Program in Healthcare and Life Sciences, Teaneck, NJ 07666-1914. Offers EMBA.

Felician University, Program in Health Care Administration, Lodi, NJ 07644-2117. Offers MSHA. *Program availability:* Part-time, evening/weekend. *Faculty:* 5 full-time (3 women). *Students:* 3 full-time (all women), 20 part-time (8 women); includes 8 minority (5 Black or African American, non-Hispanic/Latino; 2 Hispanic/Latino; 1 Two or more races, non-Hispanic/Latino). Average age 29. 20 applicants, 95% accepted, 10 enrolled. In 2015, 7 master's awarded. Terminal master's awarded for partial completion of doctoral program. *Degree requirements:* For master's, thesis. *Entrance requirements:* For master's, MBA or GRE, resume/personal statement. Additional exam requirements/recommendations for international students: Required—TOEFL (minimum score 79 iBT), IELTS (minimum score 6.5). *Application deadline:* Applications are processed on a rolling basis. Application fee: $40. Electronic applications accepted. Application fee is waived when completed online. *Expenses: Tuition, area resident:* Part-time $965 per credit. Tuition and fees vary according to course load and program. *Financial support:* Applicants required to submit FAFSA. *Faculty research:* Healthcare communications. *Unit head:* Dr. David M. Turi, Associate Dean/Associate Professor, School of Business, 201-559-3327, E-mail: turid@felician.edu. *Application contact:* Dr. Margaret Smolin, Director, Graduate Admissions, 201-559-1451, E-mail: graduate@felician.edu.

Florida Institute of Technology, Nathan M. Bisk College of Business, Program in Healthcare Management, Melbourne, FL 32901-6975. Offers MBA. *Program availability:* Part-time, evening/weekend. *Students:* 2 full-time (both women), 1 part-time (0 women); includes 1 minority (Asian, non-Hispanic/Latino), 1 international. Average age 28. 36 applicants, 53% accepted, 2 enrolled. In 2015, 1 master's awarded. *Degree requirements:* For master's, 36 credit hours. *Entrance requirements:* For master's, GMAT, GRE (recommended). Additional exam requirements/recommendations for international students: Required—TOEFL (minimum score 550 paper-based; 79 iBT). *Application deadline:* For fall admission, 4/1 for international students; for spring admission, 9/30 for international students. Applications are processed on a rolling basis. Electronic applications accepted. *Expenses: Tuition, area resident:* Full-time $21,690; part-time $1205 per credit hour. *Required fees:* $500. Tuition and fees vary according to degree level, campus/location and program. *Financial support:* Career-related internships or fieldwork and tuition remissions available. Support available to part-time students. Financial award application deadline: 3/1; financial award applicants required to submit FAFSA. *Unit head:* Dr. S. Ann Becker, Dean, 321-674-7327, E-mail: abecker@fit.edu. *Application contact:* Cheryl A. Brown, Associate Director of Graduate Admissions, 321-674-7581, Fax: 321-723-9468, E-mail: cbrown@fit.edu.

Website: http://www.fit.edu/programs/8334/mba-healthcare-management#.VUI2Jk10ypo

Florida International University, Robert Stempel College of Public Health and Social Work, Programs in Public Health, Miami, FL 33199. Offers biostatistics (MPH); environmental and occupational health (MPH, PhD); epidemiology (MPH, PhD); health policy and management (MPH); health promotion and disease prevention (PhD); health promotion and diseases prevention (MPH). Ph D program has fall admissions only; MPH offered jointly with University of Miami. *Accreditation:* CEPH. *Program availability:* Part-time, evening/weekend, online learning. *Faculty:* 27 full-time (12 women), 2 part-time/adjunct (1 woman). *Students:* 126 full-time (80 women), 62 part-time (46 women); includes 129 minority (47 Black or African American, non-Hispanic/Latino; 10 Asian, non-Hispanic/Latino; 69 Hispanic/Latino; 3 Two or more races, non-Hispanic/Latino), 32 international. Average age 30. 298 applicants, 35% accepted, 68 enrolled. In 2015, 67 master's, 10 doctorates awarded. *Degree requirements:* For master's, thesis optional; for doctorate, comprehensive exam, thesis/dissertation. *Entrance requirements:* For master's, minimum GPA of 3.0, letters of recommendation; for doctorate, GRE, resume, minimum GPA of 3.0, letters of recommendation, letter of intent. Additional exam requirements/recommendations for international students: Required—TOEFL (minimum score 550 paper-based; 80 iBT). *Application deadline:* For fall admission, 6/1 for domestic students, 4/1 for international students; for spring admission, 10/1 for domestic students, 9/1 for international students. Applications are processed on a rolling basis. Application fee: $30. Electronic applications accepted. *Expenses:* Contact institution. *Financial support:* Institutionally sponsored loans, scholarships/grants, and tuition waivers (full) available. Financial award application deadline: 3/1; financial award applicants required to submit FAFSA. *Faculty research:* Drugs/AIDS intervention among migrant workers, provision of services for active/recovering drug users with HIV. *Unit head:* Dr. Benjamin C. Amick, III, Chair, 305-348-4903, E-mail: benjamin.amickiii@fiu.edu. *Application contact:* Dr. Vukosava Pekovic, Director, 305-348-1823, Fax: 305-348-4901, E-mail: pekovic@fiu.edu.

Florida National University, Program in Business Administration, Hialeah, FL 33012. Offers finance (MBA); general management (MBA); health services administration (MBA); marketing (MBA); public management and leadership (MBA). *Program availability:* Part-time, blended/hybrid learning. *Faculty:* 6 full-time (2 women), 2 part-time/adjunct (0 women). *Students:* 21 full-time (12 women), 2 part-time (1 woman); includes 17 minority (2 Black or African American, non-Hispanic/Latino; 15 Hispanic/Latino), 2 international. Average age 32. 8 applicants, 100% accepted, 8 enrolled. In 2015, 15 master's awarded. *Degree requirements:* For master's, capstone. *Entrance requirements:* For master's, writing assessment, bachelor's degree from accredited institution; official undergraduate transcripts; minimum undergraduate GPA of 2.5, GMAT (minimum score of 400), or GRE (minimum score of 900). Additional exam requirements/recommendations for international students: Required—TOEFL, IELTS. *Application deadline:* Applications are processed on a rolling basis. Electronic applications accepted. *Expenses:* Contact institution. *Financial support:* Federal Work-Study, institutionally sponsored loans, scholarships/grants, and tuition waivers available. Financial award applicants required to submit FAFSA. *Unit head:* Dr. Ernesto Gonzalez, Business Department Head, 305-821-3333 Ext. 1070, Fax: 305-362-0595, E-mail: egonzalez@fnu.edu. *Application contact:* Olga Rodriguez, Assistant Campus Dean, 305-821-3333 Ext. 1044, Fax: 305-362-0595, E-mail: orodriguez@fnu.edu.
Website: http://www.fnu.edu/graduate-programs/

Florida National University, Program in Health Services Administration, Hialeah, FL 33012. Offers MHSA. *Program availability:* Part-time, evening/weekend, 100% online, blended/hybrid learning. *Faculty:* 2 full-time (both women), 1 part-time/adjunct (0 women). *Students:* 18 full-time (14 women); all minorities (1 Black or African American, non-Hispanic/Latino; 17 Hispanic/Latino). Average age 32. 6 applicants, 100% accepted, 6 enrolled. *Degree requirements:* For master's, capstone project. *Entrance requirements:* For master's, writing assessment, bachelor's degree from an accredited institution; official undergraduate transcripts; minimum undergraduate GPA of 2.5, GMAT (minimum score of 400), or GRE (minimum score of 900). Additional exam requirements/recommendations for international students: Required—TOEFL, IELTS. *Application deadline:* Applications are processed on a rolling basis. Electronic applications accepted. *Expenses: Tuition, area resident:* Full-time $15,600. *Required fees:* $650. *Financial support:* Scholarships/grants available. Financial award applicants required to submit FAFSA. *Unit head:* Dr. Loreto Almonte, Allied Health Division Head, 305-821-3333 Ext. 1074, Fax: 305-362-0595, E-mail: lalmonte@fnu.edu. *Application contact:* Virginia Rabelo, Admissions supervisor, 305-821-3333 Ext. 1016, Fax: 305-362-0595, E-mail: vrabelo@fnu.edu.
Website: http://www.fnu.edu/health-services-administration-hsa-master/

Framingham State University, Continuing Education, Program in Health Care Administration, Framingham, MA 01701-9101. Offers MA. *Program availability:* Part-time, evening/weekend.

Francis Marion University, Graduate Programs, School of Business, Florence, SC 29502-0547. Offers business (MBA); health executive management (MBA). *Accreditation:* AACSB. *Program availability:* Part-time, evening/weekend. *Faculty:* 4 full-time (2 women). *Students:* 4 full-time (2 women), 34 part-time (13 women); includes 10 minority (7 Black or African American, non-Hispanic/Latino; 2 Asian, non-Hispanic/Latino; 1 Hispanic/Latino), 2 international. Average age 34. 18 applicants, 67% accepted, 12 enrolled. In 2015, 15 master's awarded. *Degree requirements:* For master's, comprehensive exam. *Entrance requirements:* For master's, GMAT or GRE, official transcripts, two letters of recommendation. Additional exam requirements/recommendations for international students: Required—TOEFL (minimum score 550 paper-based; 79 iBT). *Application deadline:* For fall admission, 3/15 for domestic and international students; for spring admission, 10/15 for domestic and international students. Applications are processed on a rolling basis. Application fee: $37. *Expenses: Tuition, area resident:* Full-time $9780; part-time $489 per credit hour. Tuition, nonresident: full-time $19,560; part-time $978 per credit hour. *Required fees:* $14.40 per credit hour. $141 per semester. Tuition and fees vary according to course load and program. *Financial support:* Research assistantships available. Support available to part-time students. Financial award application deadline: 3/1; financial award applicants required to submit FAFSA. *Faculty research:* Ethics, directions of MBA, international business, regional economics, environmental issues. *Unit head:* Dr. M. Barry O'Brien, Dean, 843-661-1419, Fax: 843-661-1432, E-mail: mobrien@fmarion.edu. *Application contact:* Jennifer Taylor, Administrative Manager, 843-661-1286, Fax: 843-661-4688, E-mail: jtaylor@fmarion.edu.
Website: http://www.fmarion.edu/academics/schoolofbusiness

Franklin Pierce University, Graduate and Professional Studies, Rindge, NH 03461-0060. Offers curriculum and instruction (M Ed); elementary education (MS Ed); emerging network technologies (Graduate Certificate); energy and sustainability studies (MBA, Graduate Certificate); health administration (MBA, Graduate Certificate); human resource management (MBA, Graduate Certificate); information technology (MBA); leadership (MBA); nursing education (MS); nursing leadership (MS); physical therapy (DPT); physician assistant studies (MPAS); special education (M Ed); sports management (MBA). *Accreditation:* APTA. *Program availability:* Part-time, online learning. *Degree requirements:* For master's, concentrated original research projects;

Health Services Management and Hospital Administration

student teaching; fieldwork and/or internship; leadership project; PRAXIS I and II (for M Ed); for doctorate, concentrated original research projects, clinical fieldwork and/or internship, leadership project. *Entrance requirements:* For master's, minimum GPA of 2.5, 3 letters of recommendation; competencies in accounting, economics, statistics, and computer skills through life experience or undergraduate coursework (for MBA); certification/e-portfolio, minimum C grade in all education courses (for M Ed); license to practice as RN (for MS in nursing); for doctorate, GRE, BA/BS, 3 letters of recommendation, personal mission statement, interview, writing sample, minimum cumulative GPA of 2.8, master's degree (for DA); 80 hours of observation/work in PT settings, completion of anatomy, chemistry, physics, and statistics, minimum GPA of 3.0 (for DPT). Additional exam requirements/recommendations for international students: Required—TOEFL (minimum score 550 paper-based; 61 iBT). *Application deadline:* Applications are processed on a rolling basis. Application fee: $0. Electronic applications accepted. *Expenses: Tuition, area resident:* Part-time $660 per credit hour. Tuition and fees vary according to program. *Financial support:* Teaching assistantships with tuition reimbursements, career-related internships or fieldwork, and unspecified assistantships available. Support available to part-time students. Financial award applicants required to submit FAFSA. *Faculty research:* Evidence-based practice in sports physical therapy, human resource management in economic crisis, leadership in nursing, innovation in sports facility management, differentiated learning and understanding by design. *Unit head:* Dr. Maria Altobello, Dean, 603-647-3509, Fax: 603-229-4580, E-mail: altobellom@franklinpierce.edu. *Application contact:* Graduate Studies, 800-325-1090, Fax: 603-626-4815, E-mail: cgps@franklinpierce.edu.
Website: http://www.franklinpierce.edu/academics/gradstudies/index.htm

Friends University, Graduate School, Wichita, KS 67213. Offers family therapy (MSFT); global business administration (MBA), including accounting, business law, change management, health care leadership, management information systems, supply chain management and logistics; health care leadership (MHCL); management information systems (MMIS); professional business administration (MBA), including accounting, business law, change management, health care leadership, management information systems, supply chain management and logistics. *Program availability:* Part-time, evening/weekend, online learning. *Degree requirements:* For master's, research project. *Entrance requirements:* For master's, bachelor's degree from accredited institution, official transcripts, interview with program director, letter(s) of recommendation. Additional exam requirements/recommendations for international students: Required—TOEFL (minimum score 560 paper-based). Electronic applications accepted.

George Mason University, College of Health and Human Services, Department of Health Administration and Policy, Fairfax, VA 22030. Offers health and medical policy (MS); health systems management (MHA). *Accreditation:* CAHME. *Faculty:* 17 full-time (6 women), 22 part-time/adjunct (11 women). *Students:* 60 full-time (38 women), 108 part-time (74 women); includes 77 minority (29 Black or African American, non-Hispanic/Latino; 35 Asian, non-Hispanic/Latino; 11 Hispanic/Latino; 1 Native Hawaiian or other Pacific Islander, non-Hispanic/Latino; 1 Two or more races, non-Hispanic/Latino), 25 international. Average age 32. 121 applicants, 67% accepted, 50 enrolled. In 2015, 62 master's awarded. *Degree requirements:* For master's, comprehensive exam, internship. *Entrance requirements:* For master's, GRE recommended if undergraduate GPA is below 3.0 (for senior housing administration MS only), 2 official transcripts; expanded goals statement; 3 letters of recommendation; resume; 1 year of work experience (for MHA in health systems management). Additional exam requirements/recommendations for international students: Required—TOEFL (minimum score 575 paper-based; 88 iBT), IELTS (minimum score 6.5), PTE (minimum score 59). *Application deadline:* For fall admission, 4/1 for domestic and international students; for spring admission, 11/1 for domestic and international students. Application fee: $75 ($80 for international students). Electronic applications accepted. *Expenses:* Contact institution. *Financial support:* In 2015–16, 6 students received support, including 12 research assistantships with tuition reimbursements available (averaging $15,900 per year), 6 teaching assistantships (averaging $3,647 per year); career-related internships or fieldwork, Federal Work-Study, scholarships/grants, unspecified assistantships, and health care benefits (for full-time research or teaching assistantship recipients) also available. Support available to part-time students. Financial award application deadline: 3/1; financial award applicants required to submit FAFSA. *Faculty research:* Universal health care, publications, relationships between malpractice pressure and rates of Cesarean section and VBAC, seniors and Wii gaming, relationships between changes in physician's incomes and practice settings and their care to Medicaid and charity patients. *Total annual research expenditures:* $687,560. *Unit head:* Dr. P. J. Maddox, Chair, 703-993-1982, Fax: 703-993-1953, E-mail: pmaddox@gmu.edu. *Application contact:* Tracy Shevlin, Department Manager, 703-993-1929, Fax: 703-993-1953, E-mail: tshevlin@gmu.edu.
Website: http://chhs.gmu.edu/hap/index

The George Washington University, College of Professional Studies, Program in Healthcare Corporate Compliance, Washington, DC 20052. Offers Graduate Certificate. Program offered jointly with Milken Institute School of Public Health and the law firm of Feldesman Tucker Leifer Fidel LLP. *Program availability:* Online learning. *Students:* 20 part-time (14 women); includes 4 minority (1 American Indian or Alaska Native, non-Hispanic/Latino; 2 Asian, non-Hispanic/Latino; 1 Hispanic/Latino). Average age 44. 41 applicants, 78% accepted, 20 enrolled. In 2015, 31 Graduate Certificates awarded. *Application deadline:* For fall admission, 8/31 for domestic students. *Unit head:* Phyllis C. Borzi, Director, 202-530-2312, E-mail: borziph@gwu.edu. *Application contact:* Kristin Williams, Assistant Vice President for Graduate and Special Enrollment Management, 202-994-0467, Fax: 202-994-0371, E-mail: ksw@gwu.edu.
Website: http://cps.gwu.edu/hcc.html

The George Washington University, Milken Institute School of Public Health, Department of Health Policy, Washington, DC 20052. Offers EMHA, MHA, MPH, MS, Graduate Certificate. *Faculty:* 33 full-time (21 women), 1 (woman) part-time/adjunct. *Students:* 46 full-time (31 women), 72 part-time (54 women); includes 42 minority (17 Black or African American, non-Hispanic/Latino; 1 American Indian or Alaska Native, non-Hispanic/Latino; 15 Asian, non-Hispanic/Latino; 7 Hispanic/Latino; 2 Two or more races, non-Hispanic/Latino), 7 international. Average age 29. 217 applicants, 78% accepted, 35 enrolled. In 2015, 50 master's, 2 other advanced degrees awarded. *Degree requirements:* For master's, case study or special project. *Entrance requirements:* For master's, GMAT, GRE General Test, or MCAT. Additional exam requirements/recommendations for international students: Required—TOEFL. *Application deadline:* For fall admission, 4/15 priority date for domestic students, 4/15 for international students; for spring admission, 11/1 for domestic and international students. Applications are processed on a rolling basis. Application fee: $75. *Financial support:* In 2015–16, 10 students received support. Tuition waivers available. Financial award application deadline: 2/15. *Unit head:* Prof. Thomas LaVeist, Chair, E-mail: toml@gwu.edu. *Application contact:* Jane Smith, Director of Admissions, 202-994-0248, Fax: 202-994-1860, E-mail: sphhsinfo@gwumc.edu.

The George Washington University, School of Medicine and Health Sciences, Health Sciences Programs, Washington, DC 20052. Offers clinical practice management (MSHS); clinical research administration (MSHS); emergency services management

(MSHS); end-of-life care (MSHS); immunohematology (MSHS); immunohematology and biotechnology (MSHS); physical therapy (DPT); physician assistant (MSHS). *Program availability:* Online learning. *Faculty:* 22 full-time (17 women), 13 part-time/adjunct (10 women). *Students:* 277 full-time (198 women), 249 part-time (182 women); includes 159 minority (54 Black or African American, non-Hispanic/Latino; 2 American Indian or Alaska Native, non-Hispanic/Latino; 53 Asian, non-Hispanic/Latino; 40 Hispanic/Latino; 3 Native Hawaiian or other Pacific Islander, non-Hispanic/Latino; 7 Two or more races, non-Hispanic/Latino), 13 international. Average age 33. 1,905 applicants, 19% accepted, 197 enrolled. In 2015, 146 master's, 35 doctorates, 5 other advanced degrees awarded. *Entrance requirements:* Additional exam requirements/recommendations for international students: Required—TOEFL (minimum score 550 paper-based). *Application deadline:* Applications are processed on a rolling basis. Application fee: $75. *Expenses:* Contact institution. *Unit head:* Jean E. Johnson, Senior Associate Dean, 202-994-3725, E-mail: jejohns@gwu.edu. *Application contact:* Joke Ogundiran, Director of Admission, 202-994-1668, Fax: 202-994-0870, E-mail: jokeogun@gwu.edu.

Georgia Institute of Technology, Graduate Studies, College of Engineering, H. Milton Stewart School of Industrial and Systems Engineering, Program in Health Systems, Atlanta, GA 30332-0001. Offers MS. *Program availability:* Part-time. *Entrance requirements:* For master's, GRE General Test. Additional exam requirements/recommendations for international students: Required—TOEFL (minimum score 550 paper-based; 79 iBT). *Application deadline:* For fall admission, 7/1 for domestic students; for spring admission, 2/1 for domestic and international students. Applications are processed on a rolling basis. Application fee: $75. Electronic applications accepted. *Financial support:* Fellowships, research assistantships, teaching assistantships, career-related internships or fieldwork, Federal Work-Study, institutionally sponsored loans, tuition waivers (partial), and unspecified assistantships available. Support available to part-time students. Financial award application deadline: 5/1. *Faculty research:* Emergency medical services, health development planning, health services evaluations. *Unit head:* Alan Erera, Director, 404-385-0358, E-mail: alan.erera@isye.gatech.edu. *Application contact:* Pam Morrison, Graduate Coordinator, 404-894-4289, E-mail: pam.morrison@isye.gatech.edu.
Website: http://www.isye.gatech.edu

Georgia Southern University, Jack N. Averitt College of Graduate Studies, Jiann-Ping Hsu College of Public Health, Program in Healthcare Administration, Statesboro, GA 30460. Offers healthcare administration (MHA). *Program availability:* Part-time, evening/weekend. *Students:* 29 full-time (19 women), 2 part-time (0 women); includes 16 minority (13 Black or African American, non-Hispanic/Latino; 2 Hispanic/Latino; 1 Two or more races, non-Hispanic/Latino). Average age 25. 38 applicants, 42% accepted, 14 enrolled. In 2015, 15 master's awarded. *Degree requirements:* For master's, practicum. *Entrance requirements:* For master's, GRE, GMAT, personal statement, minimum cumulative undergraduate GPA of 2.75, resume, 3 letters of recommendation. Additional exam requirements/recommendations for international students: Required—TOEFL (minimum score 550 paper-based; 80 iBT), IELTS (minimum score 6). *Application deadline:* For fall admission, 6/1 priority date for domestic and international students; for spring admission, 10/1 priority date for domestic students, 10/1 for international students. Electronic applications accepted. *Expenses:* $335 per credit hour. *Financial support:* In 2015–16, 20 students received support, including 23 fellowships with full tuition reimbursements available (averaging $7,750 per year), 1 research assistantship with full tuition reimbursement available (averaging $7,750 per year), 1 teaching assistantship with full tuition reimbursement available (averaging $7,750 per year); Federal Work-Study, scholarships/grants, tuition waivers (full), and unspecified assistantships also available. Financial award application deadline: 4/15; financial award applicants required to submit FAFSA. *Faculty research:* Health disparity elimination, cost effectiveness analysis, epidemiology of rural public health, health care system assessment, rural health care, health policy and healthcare financing. *Total annual research expenditures:* $57,935. *Unit head:* Dr. James Stephens, Program Director, 912-478-5958, Fax: 912-478-0171, E-mail: jstephens@georgiasouthern.edu.

Georgia Southern University, Jack N. Averitt College of Graduate Studies, Jiann-Ping Hsu College of Public Health, Program in Public Health, Statesboro, GA 30460. Offers biostatistics (MPH, Dr PH); community health behavior and education (Dr PH); community health education (MPH); environmental health sciences (MPH); epidemiology (MPH); health policy and management (MPH, Dr PH). *Accreditation:* CEPH. *Program availability:* Part-time. *Students:* 129 full-time (86 women), 41 part-time (32 women); includes 87 minority (67 Black or African American, non-Hispanic/Latino; 6 Asian, non-Hispanic/Latino; 8 Hispanic/Latino; 6 Two or more races, non-Hispanic/Latino), 30 international. Average age 30. 218 applicants, 63% accepted, 41 enrolled. In 2015, 37 master's, 8 doctorates awarded. *Degree requirements:* For master's, thesis optional, practicum; for doctorate, comprehensive exam, thesis/dissertation, practicum. *Entrance requirements:* For master's, GRE General Test, minimum GPA of 2.75, resume, 3 letters of reference; for doctorate, GRE, GMAT, MCAT, LSAT, 3 letters of reference, statement of purpose, resume or curriculum vitae. Additional exam requirements/recommendations for international students: Required—TOEFL (minimum score 550 paper-based; 80 iBT), IELTS (minimum score 6). *Application deadline:* For fall admission, 6/1 priority date for domestic and international students; for spring admission, 10/1 priority date for domestic students, 10/1 for international students. Applications are processed on a rolling basis. Application fee: $50. Electronic applications accepted. *Expenses:* $335 per credit hour. *Financial support:* In 2015–16, 93 students received support, including 23 fellowships with full tuition reimbursements available (averaging $7,750 per year), 1 research assistantship with full tuition reimbursement available (averaging $7,750 per year), 1 teaching assistantship with full tuition reimbursement available (averaging $7,750 per year); career-related internships or fieldwork, Federal Work-Study, scholarships/grants, tuition waivers (full), and unspecified assistantships also available. Support available to part-time students. Financial award application deadline: 4/15; financial award applicants required to submit FAFSA. *Faculty research:* Rural public health best practices, health disparity elimination, community initiatives to enhance public health, cost effectiveness analysis, epidemiology of rural public health, environmental health issues, health care system assessment, rural health care, health policy and healthcare financing, survival analysis, nonparametric statistics and resampling methods, micro-arrays and genomics, data imputation techniques and clinical trial methodology. *Total annual research expenditures:* $281,707. *Unit head:* Dr. Shamia Garrett, Program Coordinator, 912-478-2393, E-mail: sgarrett@georgiasouthern.edu.
Website: http://chhs.georgiasouthern.edu/health/

Georgia State University, Andrew Young School of Policy Studies, Department of Public Management and Policy, Atlanta, GA 30303. Offers criminal justice (MPA); disaster management (Certificate); disaster policy (MPA); environmental policy (PhD); health policy (PhD); management and finance (MPA); nonprofit management (MPA, Certificate); nonprofit policy (MPA); planning and economic development (MPP, Certificate); policy analysis and evaluation (MPA), including planning and economic development; public and nonprofit management (PhD); public finance and budgeting (PhD), including science and technology policy, urban and regional economic development; public finance policy (MPA), including social policy; public health (MPA). *Accreditation:* NASPAA (one or more programs are accredited). *Program availability:* Part-time. *Faculty:* 15 full-time (8 women). *Students:* 128 full-time (80 women), 78 part-

Health Services Management and Hospital Administration

time (48 women); includes 78 minority (61 Black or African American, non-Hispanic/Latino; 4 Asian, non-Hispanic/Latino; 11 Hispanic/Latino; 2 Two or more races, non-Hispanic/Latino), 31 international. Average age 30. 262 applicants, 63% accepted, 74 enrolled. In 2015, 92 master's, 2 doctorates, 6 other advanced degrees awarded. Terminal master's awarded for partial completion of doctoral program. *Degree requirements:* For master's, thesis optional; for doctorate, comprehensive exam, thesis/dissertation. *Entrance requirements:* For master's and doctorate, GRE. Additional exam requirements/recommendations for international students: Required—TOEFL (minimum score 603 paper-based; 100 iBT) or IELTS (minimum score 7). *Application deadline:* For fall admission, 1/15 for domestic and international students. Application fee: $50. Electronic applications accepted. *Expenses:* Tuition, state resident: full-time $6876; part-time $382 per credit hour. Tuition, nonresident: full-time $22,374; part-time $1243 per credit hour. *Required fees:* $2128; $2128 per term. $1064 per term. Part-time tuition and fees vary according to course load and program. *Financial support:* In 2015–16, fellowships (averaging $8,194 per year), research assistantships (averaging $8,068 per year), teaching assistantships (averaging $3,660 per year) were awarded; institutionally sponsored loans, scholarships/grants, health care benefits, and unspecified assistantships also available. Financial award application deadline: 2/1. *Faculty research:* Public budgeting and finance, public management, nonprofit management, performance measurement and management, urban development. *Unit head:* Dr. Carolyn Bourdeaux, Chair and Professor, 404-413-0013, Fax: 404-413-0104, E-mail: cbourdeaux@gsu.edu. Website: http://aysps.gsu.edu/pmap/

Georgia State University, J. Mack Robinson College of Business, Institute of Health Administration, Atlanta, GA 30302-3083. Offers health administration (MBA, MSHA); health informatics (MBA, MSCIS); MBA/MHA; PMBA/MHA. *Accreditation:* CAHME. *Program availability:* Part-time, evening/weekend. *Entrance requirements:* For master's, GRE or GMAT, transcripts from all institutions attended, resume, essays. Additional exam requirements/recommendations for international students: Required—TOEFL (minimum score 610 paper-based; 101 iBT), IELTS (minimum score 7). Electronic applications accepted. *Expenses:* Tuition, state resident: full-time $6876; part-time $382 per credit hour. Tuition, nonresident: full-time $22,374; part-time $1243 per credit hour. *Required fees:* $2128; $2128 per term. $1064 per term. Part-time tuition and fees vary according to course load and program. *Faculty research:* Health information technology, health insurance exchanges, health policy and economic impact, healthcare quality, healthcare transformation.

Globe University–Woodbury, Minnesota School of Business, Woodbury, MN 55125. Offers business administration (MBA); health care management (MSM); information technology (MSM); managerial leadership (MSM).

Goldey-Beacom College, Graduate Program, Wilmington, DE 19808-1999. Offers business administration (MBA); finance (MS); financial management (MBA); health care management (MBA); human resource management (MBA); information technology (MBA); international business management (MBA); major finance (MBA); major taxation (MBA); management (MM); marketing management (MBA); taxation (MBA, MS). *Accreditation:* ACBSP. *Program availability:* Part-time, evening/weekend. *Entrance requirements:* For master's, GMAT, MAT, GRE, minimum GPA of 3.0. Additional exam requirements/recommendations for international students: Required—TOEFL (minimum score 65 iBT); Recommended—IELTS (minimum score 6). Electronic applications accepted.

Goldfarb School of Nursing at Barnes-Jewish College, Graduate Programs, St. Louis, MO 63110. Offers adult-gerontology acute care nurse practitioner (MSN); adult-gerontology nurse practitioner (MSN); nurse anesthesia (MSN); nurse educator (MSN); nurse executive (MSN). *Accreditation:* AACN; AANA/CANAEP. *Program availability:* Part-time, online learning. *Faculty:* 51 full-time (47 women), 6 part-time/adjunct (all women). *Students:* 58 full-time (57 women), 29 part-time (24 women); includes 17 minority (11 Black or African American, non-Hispanic/Latino; 2 Asian, non-Hispanic/Latino; 3 Hispanic/Latino; 2 Two or more races, non-Hispanic/Latino). Average age 26. 41 applicants, 22% accepted, 8 enrolled. In 2015, 56 master's awarded. *Degree requirements:* For master's, thesis or alternative. *Entrance requirements:* For master's, 2 references, personal statement, curriculum vitae or resume. Additional exam requirements/recommendations for international students: Required—TOEFL (minimum score 575 paper-based; 85 iBT). *Application deadline:* For fall admission, 2/1 priority date for international students; for spring admission, 10/1 priority date for international students. Applications are processed on a rolling basis. Application fee: $50. *Expenses:* Contact institution. *Financial support:* Fellowships, research assistantships, Federal Work-Study, institutionally sponsored loans, and scholarships/grants available. Support available to part-time students. Financial award applicants required to submit FAFSA. *Faculty research:* HIV stigma, HIV symptom management, palliative care with children and their families, heart disease prevention in Hispanic women, depression in the well elderly, alternative therapies in pre-term infants. *Unit head:* Dr. Gretchen Drinkard, Dean, 314-454-7540, Fax: 314-362-9222, E-mail: gld9643@bjc.org. *Application contact:* Karen Sartorius, Admissions Specialist, 314-454-7057, Fax: 314-362-9250, E-mail: ksartorius@bjc.org. Website: http://www.barnesjewishcollege.edu/

Governors State University, College of Health Professions, Program in Health Administration, University Park, IL 60484. Offers MHA. *Accreditation:* CAHME. *Degree requirements:* For master's, comprehensive exam, field experience or internship. *Entrance requirements:* For master's, minimum GPA of 3.0 in last 60 hours of undergraduate course work or 9 hours of graduate course work.

Grambling State University, School of Graduate Studies and Research, College of Arts and Sciences, Department of Political Science and Public Administration, Grambling, LA 71270. Offers health services administration (MPA); human resource management (MPA); public management (MPA); state and local government (MPA). *Accreditation:* NASPAA. *Program availability:* Part-time. *Degree requirements:* For master's, comprehensive exam (for some programs), thesis optional. *Entrance requirements:* For master's, GRE, minimum GPA of 2.75 on last degree. Additional exam requirements/recommendations for international students: Required—TOEFL (minimum score 500 paper-based; 62 iBT). Electronic applications accepted.

Grand Canyon University, College of Business, Phoenix, AZ 85017-1097. Offers accounting (MBA); corporate business administration (MBA); disaster preparedness and crisis management (MBA); executive fire service leadership (MS); finance (MBA); general management (MBA); government and policy (MPA); health care management (MPA); health systems management (MBA); human resource management (MBA); innovation (MBA); leadership (MBA, MS); management of information system (MBA); marketing (MBA); project-based (MBA); six sigma (MBA); strategic human resource management (MBA). *Accreditation:* ACBSP. *Program availability:* Part-time, evening/weekend, online learning. *Entrance requirements:* For master's, equivalent of two years full-time professional work experience. Additional exam requirements/recommendations for international students: Required—TOEFL (minimum score 575 paper-based; 90 iBT), IELTS (minimum score 7). Electronic applications accepted.

Grand Canyon University, College of Nursing, Phoenix, AZ 85017-1097. Offers acute care nurse practitioner (MS, PMC); clinical nurse specialist (PMC), including clinical

nurse specialist, education; family nurse practitioner (MS); leadership in health care systems (MS); nurse education (MS). *Accreditation:* AACN. *Program availability:* Part-time, evening/weekend, online learning. *Degree requirements:* For master's and PMC, comprehensive exam (for some programs). *Entrance requirements:* For master's, minimum cumulative and science course undergraduate GPA of 3.0. Additional exam requirements/recommendations for international students: Required—TOEFL (minimum score 575 paper-based; 90 iBT), IELTS (minimum score 7).

Grand Canyon University, College of Nursing and Health Sciences, Phoenix, AZ 85017-1097. Offers addiction counseling (MS); health care administration (MS); health care informatics (MS); marriage and family therapy (MS); professional counseling (MS); public health (MS). *Program availability:* Part-time, evening/weekend, online learning. *Entrance requirements:* For master's, undergraduate degree with minimum GPA of 2.8. Additional exam requirements/recommendations for international students: Required—TOEFL (minimum score 575 paper-based; 90 iBT), IELTS (minimum score 7).

Grand Valley State University, College of Community and Public Service, School of Public and Nonprofit Administration, Program in Health Administration, Allendale, MI 49401-9403. Offers MHA. *Program availability:* Part-time, evening/weekend. *Students:* 43 full-time (27 women), 48 part-time (28 women); includes 11 minority (3 Black or African American, non-Hispanic/Latino; 1 American Indian or Alaska Native, non-Hispanic/Latino; 3 Asian, non-Hispanic/Latino; 3 Hispanic/Latino; 1 Two or more races, non-Hispanic/Latino), 8 international. Average age 29. 41 applicants, 78% accepted, 30 enrolled. In 2015, 20 master's awarded. *Entrance requirements:* Additional exam requirements/recommendations for international students: Required—TOEFL. *Application deadline:* For fall admission, 5/1 priority date for domestic students; for winter admission, 11/1 priority date for domestic students. Applications are processed on a rolling basis. Application fee: $30. Electronic applications accepted. *Financial support:* In 2015–16, 8 students received support, including 3 fellowships (averaging $2,978 per year), 5 research assistantships with tuition reimbursements available (averaging $9,803 per year). Financial award application deadline: 5/1. *Faculty research:* Long-term care and aging, Medicare and Medicaid finance and administration, health economics. *Unit head:* Dr. Richard Jelier, Director, 616-331-6575, Fax: 616-331-7120, E-mail: jelierr@gvsu.edu. *Application contact:* Dr. Greg Cline, Graduate Program Director, 616-331-6437, E-mail: clinegr@gvsu.edu. Website: http://www.gvsu.edu/spna

Grand Valley State University, Kirkhof College of Nursing, Allendale, MI 49401-9403. Offers advanced practice (MSN); case management (MSN); nursing administration (MSN); nursing education (MSN); nursing practice (DNP); MSN/MBA. *Accreditation:* AACN. *Program availability:* Part-time. *Faculty:* 17 full-time (16 women), 6 part-time/adjunct (5 women). *Students:* 71 full-time (59 women), 53 part-time (45 women); includes 16 minority (10 Black or African American, non-Hispanic/Latino; 2 Asian, non-Hispanic/Latino; 3 Hispanic/Latino; 1 Two or more races, non-Hispanic/Latino), 3 international. Average age 33. 64 applicants, 94% accepted, 31 enrolled. In 2015, 1 master's, 11 doctorates awarded. *Degree requirements:* For master's, thesis optional. *Entrance requirements:* For master's, GRE, minimum upper-division GPA of 3.0, course work in statistics, Michigan RN license. Additional exam requirements/recommendations for international students: Required—TOEFL. *Application deadline:* For fall admission, 3/15 priority date for domestic students. Applications are processed on a rolling basis. Application fee: $30. Electronic applications accepted. *Financial support:* In 2015–16, 58 students received support, including 39 fellowships (averaging $11,141 per year), 33 research assistantships with tuition reimbursements available (averaging $7,339 per year); career-related internships or fieldwork, Federal Work-Study, institutionally sponsored loans, and traineeships also available. Financial award application deadline: 2/15. *Faculty research:* Multigenerational health promotion, chronic disease prevention, end-of-life issues, nursing workload, family caregiver health. *Total annual research expenditures:* $36,000. *Unit head:* Dr. Cynthia McCurren, Dean, 616-331-7161, Fax: 616-331-7362. *Application contact:* Dr. Cynthia Coviak, Associate Dean of Nursing Research and Faculty Development, 616-331-7170, Fax: 616-331-7362, E-mail: coviakc@gvsu.edu. Website: http://www.gvsu.edu/kcon/

Grantham University, College of Nursing and Allied Health, Lenexa, KS 66219. Offers case management (MSN); health systems management (MHSM, MSN); healthcare administration (MHA); nursing education (MSN); nursing informatics (MSN); nursing management and organizational leadership (MSN). *Program availability:* Part-time, evening/weekend, online only, 100% online. *Faculty:* 1 (woman) full-time, 15 part-time/adjunct (11 women). *Students:* 59 full-time (42 women), 368 part-time (277 women); includes 181 minority (119 Black or African American, non-Hispanic/Latino; 2 American Indian or Alaska Native, non-Hispanic/Latino; 23 Asian, non-Hispanic/Latino; 21 Hispanic/Latino; 4 Native Hawaiian or other Pacific Islander, non-Hispanic/Latino; 12 Two or more races, non-Hispanic/Latino). Average age 41. 498 applicants, 94% accepted, 427 enrolled. In 2015, 119 master's awarded. *Degree requirements:* For master's, capstone. *Entrance requirements:* For master's, bachelor's degree from accredited degree-granting institution with minimum GPA of 2.5, BSN from accredited nursing program, valid RN license. Additional exam requirements/recommendations for international students: Required—TOEFL (minimum score 71 iBT); Recommended—IELTS (minimum score 6.5), TSE (minimum score 50). *Application deadline:* Applications are processed on a rolling basis. Electronic applications accepted. *Expenses: Tuition, area resident:* Full-time $3900; part-time $325 per credit hour. *Required fees:* $45 per term. One-time fee: $100. *Financial support:* Scholarships/grants available. *Faculty research:* Experimental exploration of the use of human patient simulation in the theory course, simulation education's impact on nursing confidence in the care of patients with Ebola virus, women's health-smoking cessation program for pregnant women, nursing and healthcare administration, business administration in healthcare. *Unit head:* Dana Basara, Dean, College of Nursing and Allied Health, 913-309-4783, Fax: 844-897-6490, E-mail: dbasara@grantham.edu. *Application contact:* Jared Parlette, Vice President of Student Enrollment, 888-947-2684, Fax: 866-908-2360, E-mail: admissions@grantham.edu. Website: http://www.grantham.edu/colleges-and-schools/college-of-nursing-and-allied-health/

Gwynedd Mercy University, School of Graduate and Professional Studies, Gwynedd Valley, PA 19437-0901. Offers health care administration (MBA); management (MSM); strategic management and leadership (MBA). *Program availability:* Part-time, evening/weekend. *Faculty:* 7 part-time/adjunct (1 woman). *Students:* 97 full-time (73 women); includes 51 minority (44 Black or African American, non-Hispanic/Latino; 2 Asian, non-Hispanic/Latino; 5 Hispanic/Latino). Average age 36. In 2015, 80 master's awarded. *Degree requirements:* For master's, thesis. *Entrance requirements:* For master's, minimum GPA of 3.0. *Application deadline:* Applications are processed on a rolling basis. *Expenses: Tuition, area resident:* Part-time $500 per credit. One-time fee: $165. Tuition and fees vary according to degree level and program. *Financial support:* Career-related internships or fieldwork, Federal Work-Study, tuition waivers (full and partial), and unspecified assistantships available. Financial award applicants required to submit FAFSA. *Unit head:* Dr. Mary Sortino, Dean, 215-646-7300, E-mail: sortino.m@gmercyu.edu. *Application contact:* Information Contact, 800-342-5462, Fax: 215-641-5556.

Health Services Management and Hospital Administration

Harding University, Paul R. Carter College of Business Administration, Searcy, AR 72149-0001. Offers health care management (MBA); information technology management (MBA); international business (MBA); leadership and organizational management (MBA). *Accreditation:* ACBSP. *Program availability:* Part-time, evening/weekend, online learning. *Faculty:* 26 part-time/adjunct (6 women). *Students:* 37 full-time (19 women), 116 part-time (48 women); includes 23 minority (16 Black or African American, non-Hispanic/Latino; 1 American Indian or Alaska Native, non-Hispanic/Latino; 4 Asian, non-Hispanic/Latino; 2 Hispanic/Latino), 13 international. Average age 37. 45 applicants, 98% accepted, 44 enrolled. In 2015, 78 master's awarded. *Degree requirements:* For master's, portfolio. *Entrance requirements:* For master's, GMAT (minimum score of 500) or GRE (minimum score of 300), minimum GPA of 3.0, 2 letters of recommendation, resume, 3 essays, all official transcripts. Additional exam requirements/recommendations for international students: Required—TOEFL (minimum score 550 paper-based; 79 iBT). *Application deadline:* For fall admission, 8/1 priority date for domestic and international students; for spring admission, 12/1 priority date for domestic and international students. Applications are processed on a rolling basis. Application fee: $40. *Financial support:* Unspecified assistantships available. Financial award application deadline: 7/30; financial award applicants required to submit FAFSA. *Unit head:* Glen Metheny, Director of Graduate Studies, 501-279-5851, Fax: 501-279-4805, E-mail: gmetheny@harding.edu. *Application contact:* Melanie Kiihnl, Recruiting Manager/Director of Marketing, 501-279-4523, Fax: 501-279-4805, E-mail: mba@harding.edu.
Website: http://www.harding.edu/mba

Harrisburg University of Science and Technology, Program in Information Systems Engineering and Management, Harrisburg, PA 17101. Offers digital government (MS); digital health (MS); entrepreneurship (MS). *Program availability:* Part-time. *Degree requirements:* For master's, comprehensive exam, thesis optional. *Entrance requirements:* For master's, baccalaureate degree. Additional exam requirements/recommendations for international students: Required—TOEFL (minimum score 520 paper-based; 80 iBT). Electronic applications accepted.

Harvard University, Graduate School of Arts and Sciences, Committee on Higher Degrees in Health Policy, Cambridge, MA 02138. Offers PhD. *Degree requirements:* For doctorate, thesis/dissertation. *Entrance requirements:* For doctorate, GMAT, GRE General Test, or MCAT. Additional exam requirements/recommendations for international students: Required—TOEFL.

Harvard University, Harvard Business School, Doctoral Programs in Management, Boston, MA 02163. Offers accounting and management (DBA); business economics (PhD); health policy management (PhD); management (DBA); marketing (DBA); organizational behavior (PhD); science, technology and management (PhD); strategy (DBA); technology and operations management (DBA). *Degree requirements:* For doctorate, comprehensive exam (for some programs), thesis/dissertation. *Entrance requirements:* For doctorate, GRE General Test or GMAT. Additional exam requirements/recommendations for international students: Required—TOEFL.

Harvard University, Harvard T.H. Chan School of Public Health, Department of Health Policy and Management, Boston, MA 02115-6096. Offers health policy and management (SM). *Program availability:* Part-time. *Faculty:* 46 full-time (12 women), 23 part-time/adjunct (9 women). *Students:* 21 full-time (13 women), 49 part-time (16 women); includes 23 minority (1 Black or African American, non-Hispanic/Latino; 17 Asian, non-Hispanic/Latino; 4 Hispanic/Latino; 1 Two or more races, non-Hispanic/Latino), 9 international. Average age 37. 38 applicants, 63% accepted, 21 enrolled. In 2015, 39 master's awarded. *Entrance requirements:* For master's, GRE, GMAT, MCAT. Additional exam requirements/recommendations for international students: Recommended—TOEFL (minimum score 600 paper-based; 100 iBT), IELTS (minimum score 7). *Application deadline:* For fall admission, 12/15 for domestic and international students. Application fee: $120. Electronic applications accepted. *Financial support:* Fellowships, research assistantships, teaching assistantships, Federal Work-Study, scholarships/grants, traineeships, and unspecified assistantships available. Support available to part-time students. Financial award application deadline: 2/15; financial award applicants required to submit FAFSA. *Faculty research:* Environmental science and risk management. *Unit head:* Dr. Arnold Epstein, Chair, 617-432-3895, Fax: 617-432-4494, E-mail: aepstein@hsph.harvard.edu. *Application contact:* Vincent W. James, Director of Admissions, 617-432-1031, Fax: 617-432-7080, E-mail: admissions@hsph.harvard.edu.
Website: http://www.hsph.harvard.edu/departments/health-policy-and-management/

Herzing University Online, Program in Business Administration, Menomonee Falls, WI 53051. Offers accounting (MBA); business administration (MBA); business management (MBA); healthcare management (MBA); human resources (MBA); marketing (MBA); project management (MBA); technology management (MBA). *Program availability:* Online learning.

Hilbert College, Program in Public Administration, Hamburg, NY 14075-1597. Offers health administration (MPA); public administration (MPA). *Program availability:* Evening/weekend. *Faculty:* 1 full-time (0 women), 4 part-time/adjunct (2 women). *Students:* 24 full-time (17 women), 11 part-time (10 women); includes 11 minority (5 Black or African American, non-Hispanic/Latino; 2 American Indian or Alaska Native, non-Hispanic/Latino; 1 Hispanic/Latino; 3 Two or more races, non-Hispanic/Latino), 1 international. Average age 34. 24 applicants, 33% accepted, 8 enrolled. In 2015, 16 master's awarded. *Degree requirements:* For master's, final capstone project. *Entrance requirements:* For master's, admissions statement/essay, official transcripts from all prior colleges, two letters of recommendation, current resume, relevant work experience, baccalaureate degree from accredited college or university with minimum cumulative GPA of 3.0, personal interview. Additional exam requirements/recommendations for international students: Recommended—TOEFL. *Application deadline:* Applications are processed on a rolling basis. Application fee: $25. Electronic applications accepted. Application fee is waived when completed online. *Expenses: Tuition, area resident:* Full-time $17,400; part-time $725 per credit. *Required fees:* $160; $20 per course. One-time fee: $50. *Financial support:* In 2015–16, 25 students received support. Scholarships/grants and tuition waivers (partial) available. Financial award application deadline: 7/1; financial award applicants required to submit FAFSA. *Unit head:* Dr. Walter Iwanenko, Dean of Graduate Studies/Professor of Public Administration, 716-649-7900 Ext. 331, E-mail: wiwanenko@hilbert.edu. *Application contact:* Kim Chiarmonte, Director, Center for Adult and Graduate Studies, 716-926-8948, Fax: 716-649-0702, E-mail: kchiarmonte@hilbert.edu.
Website: http://www.hilbert.edu/grad/mpa

Hodges University, Graduate Programs, Naples, FL 34119. Offers accounting (M Acc); business administration (MBA); clinical mental health counseling (MS); health services administration (MS); information systems management (MIS); legal studies (MS); management (MSM). *Program availability:* Part-time, evening/weekend, 100% online, blended/hybrid learning. *Faculty:* 13 full-time (8 women), 7 part-time/adjunct (0 women). *Students:* 47 full-time (30 women), 190 part-time (122 women); includes 99 minority (27 Black or African American, non-Hispanic/Latino; 6 Asian, non-Hispanic/Latino; 63 Hispanic/Latino; 3 Two or more races, non-Hispanic/Latino). Average age 38. 79 applicants, 100% accepted, 79 enrolled. In 2015, 77 master's awarded. *Degree requirements:* For master's, comprehensive exam (for some programs), thesis (for some

programs). *Entrance requirements:* For master's, essay. Additional exam requirements/recommendations for international students: Recommended—TOEFL. *Application deadline:* Applications are processed on a rolling basis. Application fee: $50. Electronic applications accepted. *Expenses: Tuition, area resident:* Part-time $660 per credit hour. *Financial support:* Federal Work-Study and scholarships/grants available. Financial award application deadline: 7/9; financial award applicants required to submit FAFSA. *Unit head:* Dr. David Borofsky, President, 239-513-1122, Fax: 239-598-6253, E-mail: dwortham@hodges.edu. *Application contact:* Brent Passey, Chief Admissions Officer, 239-513-1122, Fax: 239-598-6253, E-mail: bpassey@hodges.edu.

Hofstra University, Frank G. Zarb School of Business, Programs in Management and General Business, Hempstead, NY 11549. Offers business administration (MBA), including health services management, management, sports and entertainment management, strategic business management, strategic healthcare management; general management (Advanced Certificate); human resource management (MS, Advanced Certificate). *Program availability:* Part-time, evening/weekend, online learning. *Students:* 128 full-time (61 women), 145 part-time (59 women); includes 60 minority (24 Black or African American, non-Hispanic/Latino; 23 Asian, non-Hispanic/Latino; 12 Hispanic/Latino; 1 Native Hawaiian or other Pacific Islander, non-Hispanic/Latino), 54 international. Average age 32. 275 applicants, 75% accepted, 103 enrolled. In 2015, 102 master's awarded. *Degree requirements:* For master's, capstone course (for MBA), thesis (for MS), minimum GPA of 3.0. *Entrance requirements:* For master's, GMAT/GRE, 2 letters of recommendation, resume, essay. Additional exam requirements/recommendations for international students: Required—TOEFL (minimum score 550 paper-based; 80 iBT); Recommended—IELTS (minimum score 6). *Application deadline:* Applications are processed on a rolling basis. Application fee: $70 ($75 for international students). Electronic applications accepted. *Expenses:* Contact institution. *Financial support:* In 2015–16, 26 students received support, including 19 fellowships with tuition reimbursements available (averaging $5,035 per year); research assistantships with tuition reimbursements available, career-related internships or fieldwork, Federal Work-Study, institutionally sponsored loans, scholarships/grants, tuition waivers (full and partial), and unspecified assistantships also available. Support available to part-time students. Financial award applicants required to submit FAFSA. *Faculty research:* Organizational behavior/studies, human resources management, business ethics, nonprofit organizations; sustainability, innovation, decision-making; operations and supply chain management; learning and pedagogical issues; family business, small business, entrepreneurship. *Unit head:* Dr. Kaushik Sengupta, Chairperson, 516-463-7825, Fax: 516-463-4834, E-mail: mgbkzs@hofstra.edu. *Application contact:* Sunil Samuel, Assistant Vice President of Admissions, 516-463-4723, Fax: 516-463-4664, E-mail: graduateadmission@hofstra.edu.
Website: http://www.hofstra.edu/business/

Hofstra University, School of Health Sciences and Human Services, Programs in Health, Hempstead, NY 11549. Offers community health (MS), including adventure education, strength and conditioning; health administration (MHA); public health (MPH). *Program availability:* Part-time, evening/weekend. *Students:* 145 full-time (98 women), 96 part-time (60 women); includes 104 minority (45 Black or African American, non-Hispanic/Latino; 39 Asian, non-Hispanic/Latino; 16 Hispanic/Latino; 2 Native Hawaiian or other Pacific Islander, non-Hispanic/Latino; 2 Two or more races, non-Hispanic/Latino), 21 international. Average age 28. 174 applicants, 85% accepted, 87 enrolled. In 2015, 59 master's awarded. *Degree requirements:* For master's, internship, minimum GPA of 3.0. *Entrance requirements:* For master's, interview, 2 letters of recommendation, essay, resume. Additional exam requirements/recommendations for international students: Required—TOEFL (minimum score 550 paper-based; 80 iBT). *Application deadline:* Applications are processed on a rolling basis. Application fee: $70 ($75 for international students). Electronic applications accepted. *Financial support:* In 2015–16, 71 students received support, including 40 fellowships with tuition reimbursements available (averaging $4,332 per year), 4 research assistantships with tuition reimbursements available (averaging $8,834 per year); Federal Work-Study, institutionally sponsored loans, scholarships/grants, and tuition waivers (full and partial) also available. Support available to part-time students. Financial award applicants required to submit FAFSA. *Faculty research:* Integrated long term care and policy reform; health care policy; cost benefit analysis; chronic illness management; development and implementation of leadership in sports, physical activity and recreation. *Unit head:* Dr. Jayne Ellinger, Chairperson, 516-463-6952, Fax: 516-463-6275, E-mail: hprjmk@hofstra.edu. *Application contact:* Sunil Samuel, Assistant Vice President of Admissions, 516-463-4723, Fax: 516-463-4664, E-mail: graduateadmission@hofstra.edu.
Website: http://www.hofstra.edu/academics/colleges/healthscienceshumanservices/

Holy Family University, Division of Extended Learning, Bensalem, PA 19020. Offers business administration (MBA); finance (MBA); health care administration (MBA); human resources management (MBA). *Accreditation:* ACBSP. *Program availability:* Part-time, evening/weekend. *Faculty:* 13 part-time/adjunct (3 women). *Students:* 116 part-time (59 women); includes 4 minority (2 Black or African American, non-Hispanic/Latino; 1 Asian, non-Hispanic/Latino; 1 Hispanic/Latino). Average age 34. 25 applicants, 96% accepted, 6 enrolled. In 2015, 52 master's awarded. *Entrance requirements:* For master's, minimum GPA of 3.0, interview, essay/professional statement, 2 recommendations, current resume, official transcripts of college or university work. Additional exam requirements/recommendations for international students: Required—TOEFL (minimum score 550 paper-based; 79 iBT). *Application deadline:* For fall admission, 7/1 priority date for domestic and international students; for spring admission, 11/1 priority date for domestic and international students; for summer admission, 4/1 priority date for domestic and international students. Applications are processed on a rolling basis. Application fee: $50. Electronic applications accepted. *Financial support:* In 2015–16, 3 students received support. Available to part-time students. Applicants required to submit FAFSA. *Unit head:* Chris Quinn, Director of Academic Services, 267-341-5006, Fax: 215-633-0558, E-mail: cquinn1@holyfamily.edu. *Application contact:* Don Reinmold, Director of Admissions, 267-341-5001 Ext. 3230, Fax: 215-633-0558, E-mail: dreinmold@holyfamily.edu.

Holy Family University, Graduate and Professional Programs, School of Business Administration, Philadelphia, PA 19114. Offers accountancy (MS); finance (MBA); health care administration (MBA); human resource management (MBA); information systems management (MBA). *Accreditation:* ACBSP. *Program availability:* Part-time, evening/weekend. *Degree requirements:* For master's, comprehensive exam, thesis optional. *Entrance requirements:* For master's, minimum GPA of 3.0, interview, essay/personal statement, current resume, official transcript of all college or university work. Additional exam requirements/recommendations for international students: Required—TOEFL (minimum score 550 paper-based; 79 iBT), IELTS (minimum score 6), PTE (minimum score 54). *Application deadline:* For fall admission, 7/1 priority date for domestic and international students; for winter admission, 1/1 for domestic students; for spring admission, 11/1 priority date for domestic and international students; for summer admission, 4/1 priority date for domestic and international students. Applications are processed on a rolling basis. Application fee: $25. Electronic applications accepted. *Financial support:* Available to part-time students. Financial award application deadline: 5/1; applicants required to submit FAFSA. *Unit head:* Dr. Barry Dickinson, Dean, 267-341-3440, Fax: 215-637-5937, E-mail: jdickinson@holyfamily.edu. *Application contact:* Gidget Marie

Montelibano, Associate Director of Graduate Admissions, 267-341-3558, Fax: 215-637-1478, E-mail: gmontelibano@holyfamily.edu.
Website: http://www.holyfamily.edu/choosing-holy-family-u/academics/schools-of-study/school-of-business-administration

Hunter College of the City University of New York, Graduate School, Schools of the Health Professions, School of Health Sciences, Programs in Urban Public Health, Program in Health Policy Management, New York, NY 10065-5085. Offers MPH. *Program availability:* Part-time, evening/weekend. *Students:* 308 applicants, 39% accepted, 91 enrolled. *Degree requirements:* For master's, comprehensive exam, thesis optional, internship. *Entrance requirements:* For master's, GRE General Test, previous course work in calculus and statistics. Additional exam requirements/recommendations for international students: Required—TOEFL. *Application deadline:* For fall admission, 4/1 for domestic students; for spring admission, 11/1 for domestic students. *Financial support:* In 2015–16, 6 fellowships were awarded; career-related internships or fieldwork, Federal Work-Study, institutionally sponsored loans, and tuition waivers (partial) also available. Support available to part-time students. *Unit head:* Prof. Barbara Berney, Program Director, 212-396-7756, Fax: 212-481-5260, E-mail: bberney@hunter.cuny.edu. *Application contact:* Milena Solo, Director for Graduate Admissions, 212-772-4280, E-mail: milena.solo@hunter.cuny.edu.
Website: http://www.cuny.edu/site/sph/hunter-college/a-programs/graduate/hpm-mph.html

Husson University, Master of Business Administration Program, Bangor, ME 04401-2999. Offers biotechnology and innovation (MBA); general business administration (MBA); healthcare management (MBA); hospitality and tourism management (MBA); organizational management (MBA); risk management (MBA). *Program availability:* Part-time, evening/weekend. *Faculty:* 9 full-time (5 women), 11 part-time/adjunct (2 women). *Students:* 125 full-time (54 women), 97 part-time (56 women); includes 18 minority (4 Black or African American, non-Hispanic/Latino; 2 American Indian or Alaska Native, non-Hispanic/Latino; 7 Asian, non-Hispanic/Latino; 2 Hispanic/Latino; 3 Two or more races, non-Hispanic/Latino), 6 international. Average age 34. 143 applicants, 76% accepted, 53 enrolled. In 2015, 108 master's awarded. *Degree requirements:* For master's, comprehensive exam (for some programs), thesis optional. *Entrance requirements:* For master's, GMAT or GRE, minimum GPA of 3.0. Additional exam requirements/recommendations for international students: Required—TOEFL (minimum score 550 paper-based; 80 iBT). *Application deadline:* Applications are processed on a rolling basis. Application fee: $50. Electronic applications accepted. *Expenses:* $435 per credit. *Financial support:* Career-related internships or fieldwork, Federal Work-Study, scholarships/grants, and unspecified assistantships available. Financial award application deadline: 4/15; financial award applicants required to submit FAFSA. *Unit head:* Prof. Stephanie Shayne, Director, Graduate and Online Programs, 207-404-5632, Fax: 207-992-4987, E-mail: shaynes@husson.edu. *Application contact:* Kristen Card, Director of Graduate Admissions, 207-404-5660, Fax: 207-941-7935, E-mail: cardk@husson.edu.
Website: http://www.husson.edu/mba

Independence University, Program in Business Administration in Health Care, Salt Lake City, UT 84107. Offers health care administration (MBA). *Program availability:* Part-time, evening/weekend, online learning. *Degree requirements:* For master's, fieldwork/internship.

Independence University, Program in Health Care Administration, Salt Lake City, UT 84107. Offers MSHCA. *Program availability:* Part-time, evening/weekend, online learning. *Degree requirements:* For master's, fieldwork, internship. *Entrance requirements:* For master's, previous course work in psychology.

Independence University, Program in Health Services, Salt Lake City, UT 84107. Offers community health (MSHS); wellness promotion (MSHS). *Program availability:* Part-time, evening/weekend, online learning. *Degree requirements:* For master's, fieldwork, internship, final project (wellness promotion). *Entrance requirements:* For master's, previous course work in psychology.

Indiana Tech, Program in Business Administration, Fort Wayne, IN 46803-1297. Offers accounting (MBA); health care management (MBA); human resources (MBA); management (MBA); marketing (MBA). *Program availability:* Part-time, evening/weekend, online learning. *Students:* 160 full-time (94 women), 97 part-time (53 women); includes 69 minority (58 Black or African American, non-Hispanic/Latino; 1 Asian, non-Hispanic/Latino; 8 Hispanic/Latino; 2 Two or more races, non-Hispanic/Latino), 11 international. Average age 36. *Entrance requirements:* For master's, GMAT, bachelor's degree from regionally-accredited university; minimum undergraduate GPA of 2.5; 2 years of significant work experience; 3 letters of recommendation. *Application deadline:* Applications are processed on a rolling basis. Application fee: $25. Electronic applications accepted. *Expenses: Tuition, area resident:* Part-time $495 per credit. Part-time tuition and fees vary according to degree level and program. *Financial support:* Applicants required to submit FAFSA. *Unit head:* Dr. Andrew I. Nwanne, Associate Dean of Business/Academic Coordinator, 260-422-5561 Ext. 2214, E-mail: ainwanne@indianatech.edu. *Application contact:* Dr. Andrew I. Nwanne, Associate Dean of Business/Academic Coordinator, 260-422-5561 Ext. 2214, E-mail: ainwanne@indianatech.edu.
Website: https://www.indianatech.edu/

Indiana University Bloomington, School of Public Health, Department of Applied Health Science, Bloomington, IN 47405. Offers behavioral, social, and community health (MPH); family health (MPH); health behavior (PhD); nutrition science (MS); professional health education (MPH); public health administration (MPH); safety management (MS); school and college health education (MS). *Accreditation:* CEPH (one or more programs are accredited). *Degree requirements:* For master's, thesis optional; for doctorate, comprehensive exam, thesis/dissertation. *Entrance requirements:* For master's, GRE (for MS in nutrition science), 3 recommendations; for doctorate, GRE, 3 recommendations. Additional exam requirements/recommendations for international students: Required—TOEFL (minimum score 550 paper-based; 80 iBT). Electronic applications accepted. *Faculty research:* Cancer education, HIV/AIDS and drug education, public health, parent-child interactions, safety education, obesity, public health policy, public health administration, school health, health education, human development, nutrition, human sexuality, chronic disease, early childhood health.

Indiana University Kokomo, Department of Public Administration and Health Management, Kokomo, IN 46904-9003. Offers MPM, Graduate Certificate.

Indiana University Northwest, School of Public and Environmental Affairs, Gary, IN 46408-1197. Offers criminal justice (MPA); environmental affairs (Graduate Certificate); health services (MPA); nonprofit management (Certificate); public management (MPA). *Accreditation:* NASPAA (one or more programs are accredited). *Program availability:* Part-time. *Entrance requirements:* For master's, GRE General Test or GMAT, letters of recommendation. *Faculty research:* Employment in income security policies, evidence in criminal justice, equal employment law, social welfare policy and welfare reform, public finance in developing countries.

Indiana University of Pennsylvania, School of Graduate Studies and Research, College of Health and Human Services, Department of Employment and Labor Relations, Program in Health Services Administration, Indiana, PA 15705-1087. Offers

MS. Program offered at Northpointe Campus near Pittsburgh, PA. *Program availability:* Part-time, evening/weekend, online learning. *Faculty:* 4 full-time (1 woman). *Students:* 13 full-time (10 women), 15 part-time (14 women); includes 7 minority (1 Black or African American, non-Hispanic/Latino; 1 American Indian or Alaska Native, non-Hispanic/Latino; 2 Asian, non-Hispanic/Latino; 2 Hispanic/Latino; 1 Two or more races, non-Hispanic/Latino). Average age 33. 33 applicants, 64% accepted, 14 enrolled. In 2015, 3 master's awarded. *Degree requirements:* For master's, thesis optional. *Application deadline:* Applications are processed on a rolling basis. Application fee: $50. Electronic applications accepted. *Financial support:* In 2015–16, 2 research assistantships with tuition reimbursements (averaging $1,975 per year) were awarded; career-related internships or fieldwork, Federal Work-Study, scholarships/grants, and unspecified assistantships also available. Financial award application deadline: 4/15; financial award applicants required to submit FAFSA. *Unit head:* Dr. Scott Decker, Graduate Coordinator, 724-357-4470, E-mail: s.e.decker@iup.edu.
Website: http://www.iup.edu/elr/grad/health-services-administration-ms/default.aspx

Indiana University of Pennsylvania, School of Graduate Studies and Research, College of Health and Human Services, Department of Nursing and Allied Health, Indiana, PA 15705. Offers health service administration (MS); nursing (MS, PhD); nursing administration (MS); nursing education (MS). *Program availability:* Part-time, evening/weekend. *Faculty:* 12 full-time (11 women). *Students:* 26 full-time (22 women), 73 part-time (68 women); includes 3 minority (1 Asian, non-Hispanic/Latino; 1 Hispanic/Latino; 1 Two or more races, non-Hispanic/Latino), 27 international. Average age 37. 85 applicants, 72% accepted, 28 enrolled. In 2015, 12 master's, 4 doctorates awarded. *Degree requirements:* For master's, thesis optional; for doctorate, comprehensive exam, thesis/dissertation. *Entrance requirements:* For master's, 2 letters of recommendation; for doctorate, GRE, 2 letters of recommendation, current nursing license, current curriculum vitae. Additional exam requirements/recommendations for international students: Required—TOEFL (minimum score 540 paper-based). *Application deadline:* Applications are processed on a rolling basis. Application fee: $50. Electronic applications accepted. *Financial support:* In 2015–16, 5 research assistantships with tuition reimbursements (averaging $3,383 per year), 2 teaching assistantships with partial tuition reimbursements (averaging $23,305 per year) were awarded; fellowships with partial tuition reimbursements, career-related internships or fieldwork, Federal Work-Study, scholarships/grants, and unspecified assistantships also available. Support available to part-time students. Financial award application deadline: 4/15; financial award applicants required to submit FAFSA. *Unit head:* Dr. Theresa Gropelli, Chairperson, 724-357-2279, E-mail: theresa.gropelli@iup.edu. *Application contact:* Paula Stossel, Assistant Dean of Administration, 724-357-4511, E-mail: pstoss@iup.edu.
Website: http://www.iup.edu/rn-alliedhealth

Indiana University–Purdue University Indianapolis, School of Public Health, Indianapolis, IN 46202. Offers biostatistics (MPH); environmental health science (MPH); epidemiology (MPH, PhD); health administration (MHA); health policy and management (MPH, PhD); social and behavioral sciences (MPH). *Accreditation:* CEPH. *Expenses:* Contact institution.

Indiana Wesleyan University, College of Adult and Professional Studies, Graduate Studies in Business, Marion, IN 46953. Offers accounting (MBA, Graduate Certificate); applied management (MBA); business administration (MBA); health care (MBA, Graduate Certificate); human resources (MBA, Graduate Certificate); management (MS); organizational leadership (MA). *Program availability:* Part-time, evening/weekend, online learning. *Faculty:* 94 full-time (28 women), 6 part-time/adjunct (1 woman). *Students:* 1,564 full-time (980 women), 158 part-time (96 women); includes 715 minority (590 Black or African American, non-Hispanic/Latino; 6 American Indian or Alaska Native, non-Hispanic/Latino; 30 Asian, non-Hispanic/Latino; 57 Hispanic/Latino; 32 Two or more races, non-Hispanic/Latino), 4 international. Average age 36. *Degree requirements:* For master's, applied business or management project. *Entrance requirements:* For master's, minimum GPA of 2.5, 2 years of related work experience. Additional exam requirements/recommendations for international students: Required—TOEFL (minimum score 550 paper-based). *Application deadline:* Applications are processed on a rolling basis. Application fee: $25. Electronic applications accepted. *Financial support:* Available to part-time students. Applicants required to submit FAFSA. *Unit head:* Dr. Paul Richardson, Associate Director, 765-677-2283, Fax: 765-677-1464, E-mail: paul.richardson@indwes.edu. *Application contact:* Graduate School, 866-IWU-4-YOU, Fax: 765-677-2541, E-mail: graduate@indwes.edu.
Website: http://caps.indwes.edu/

Institute of Public Administration, Programs in Public Administration, Dublin, Ireland. Offers healthcare management (MA); local government management (MA); public management (MA, Diploma).

Iona College, Hagan School of Business, Department of Management, Business Administration and Health Care Management, New Rochelle, NY 10801-1890. Offers business administration (MBA); health care management (MBA, AC); human resource management (PMC); long term care services management (AC); management (MBA, PMC). *Program availability:* Part-time, evening/weekend. *Entrance requirements:* For master's, GMAT, 2 letters of recommendation, minimum GPA of 3.0; for other advanced degree, GMAT, minimum GPA of 3.0. Additional exam requirements/recommendations for international students: Required—TOEFL (minimum score 550 paper-based; 80 iBT), IELTS (minimum score 6.5). Electronic applications accepted. *Expenses:* Contact institution. *Faculty research:* Information systems, strategic management, corporate values and ethics.

Johns Hopkins University, Bloomberg School of Public Health, Department of Health Policy and Management, Baltimore, MD 21205-1996. Offers bioethics and policy (PhD); health and public policy (PhD); health care management and leadership (Dr PH); health economics (MHS); health economics and policy (PhD); health finance and management (MHA); health policy (MSPH); health services research and policy (PhD); public policy (MPP). *Accreditation:* CAHME (one or more programs are accredited). *Program availability:* Part-time. *Degree requirements:* For master's, thesis (for some programs), internship (for some programs); for doctorate, comprehensive exam, thesis/dissertation, 1-year full-time residency (for some programs), oral and written exams. *Entrance requirements:* For master's, GRE General Test or GMAT, 3 letters of recommendation, curriculum vitae/resume; for doctorate, GRE General Test or GMAT, 3 letters of recommendation, curriculum vitae, transcripts. Additional exam requirements/recommendations for international students: Recommended—TOEFL (minimum score 600 paper-based; 100 iBT), IELTS. Electronic applications accepted. *Faculty research:* Quality of care and health outcomes, health care finance and technology, health disparities and vulnerable populations, injury prevention, health policy and health care policy.

Johns Hopkins University, Bloomberg School of Public Health, Department of International Health, Baltimore, MD 21205. Offers global disease epidemiology and control (MHS, PhD); health systems (MHS, PhD); human nutrition (MHS, PhD); international health (MSPH, Dr PH); registered dietician (MSPH); social and behavioral interventions (MHS, PhD). *Degree requirements:* For master's, comprehensive exam, thesis (for some programs), 1-year full-time residency, 4-9 month internship; for doctorate, comprehensive exam, thesis/dissertation or alternative, 1.5 years' full-time

Health Services Management and Hospital Administration

residency, oral and written exams. *Entrance requirements:* For master's, GRE General Test or MCAT, 3 letters of recommendation, resume; for doctorate, GRE General Test or MCAT, 3 letters of recommendation, resume, transcripts. Additional exam requirements/recommendations for international students: Required—TOEFL (minimum score 600 paper-based; 100 iBT). Recommended—IELTS (minimum score 7). Electronic applications accepted. *Faculty research:* Nutrition, infectious diseases, health systems, health economics, humanitarian emergencies.

Johns Hopkins University, Carey Business School, Health Care Management Programs, Baltimore, MD 21218. Offers business of health care (Certificate); health care management (MS). *Program availability:* Part-time, evening/weekend. *Entrance requirements:* For master's, GMAT or GRE, minimum GPA of 3.0, resume, work experience, two letters of recommendation; for Certificate, minimum GPA of 3.0, resume, work experience, two letters of recommendation. Additional exam requirements/recommendations for international students: Required—TOEFL (minimum score 600 paper-based; 100 iBT). Electronic applications accepted.

Kaplan University, Davenport Campus, School of Business, Davenport, IA 52807-2095. Offers business administration (MBA); change leadership (MS); entrepreneurship (MBA); finance (MBA); health care management (MBA, MS); human resource (MBA); international business (MBA); management (MS); marketing (MBA); project management (MBA, MS); supply chain management and logistics (MBA, MS). *Accreditation:* ACBSP. *Program availability:* Part-time, evening/weekend, online learning. *Entrance requirements:* Additional exam requirements/recommendations for international students: Required—TOEFL (minimum score 550 paper-based; 80 iBT). Electronic applications accepted.

Kaplan University, Davenport Campus, School of Legal Studies, Davenport, IA 52807-2095. Offers health care delivery (MS); pathway to paralegal (Postbaccalaureate Certificate); state and local government (MS). *Program availability:* Part-time, evening/weekend, online learning. *Entrance requirements:* Additional exam requirements/recommendations for international students: Required—TOEFL (minimum score 550 paper-based; 80 iBT).

Kean University, College of Business and Public Management, Program in Public Administration, Union, NJ 07083. Offers health services administration (MPA); non-profit management (MPA); public administration (MPA). *Accreditation:* NASPAA. *Program availability:* Part-time. *Faculty:* 15 full-time (5 women). *Students:* 82 full-time (55 women), 66 part-time (44 women); includes 102 minority (74 Black or African American, non-Hispanic/Latino; 5 Asian, non-Hispanic/Latino; 21 Hispanic/Latino; 2 Two or more races, non-Hispanic/Latino), 4 international. Average age 32. 48 applicants, 71% accepted, 30 enrolled. In 2015, 46 master's awarded. *Degree requirements:* For master's, thesis, internship, research seminar. *Entrance requirements:* For master's, minimum cumulative GPA of 3.0, official transcripts from all institutions attended, two letters of recommendation, personal statement, writing sample, professional resume/curriculum vitae. Additional exam requirements/recommendations for international students: Required—TOEFL (minimum score 550 paper-based; 79 iBT). *Application deadline:* For fall admission, 6/1 for domestic and international students; for spring admission, 12/1 for domestic and international students. Applications are processed on a rolling basis. Application fee: $75 ($150 for international students). Electronic applications accepted. *Expenses:* Tuition, state resident: full-time $12,835; part-time $625 per credit. Tuition, nonresident: full-time $17,396; part-time $766 per credit. *Required fees:* $3235; $147 per credit. Tuition and fees vary according to course level, course load, degree level and program. *Financial support:* In 2015–16, 13 research assistantships with full tuition reimbursements (averaging $3,771 per year) were awarded; scholarships/grants and unspecified assistantships also available. Financial award applicants required to submit FAFSA. *Unit head:* Dr. Patricia Moore, Program Coordinator, 908-737-4314, E-mail: pmoore@kean.edu. *Application contact:* Pedro Lopes, Admissions Counselor, 908-737-7100, E-mail: grad-adm@kean.edu. Website: http://grad.kean.edu/masters-programs/public-administration

Keiser University, Master of Business Administration Program, Ft. Lauderdale, FL 33309. Offers accounting (MBA); health services management (MBA); information security management (MBA); international business (MBA); leadership for managers (MBA); marketing (MBA). All concentrations except information security management also offered in Mandarin; leadership for managers and international business also offered in Spanish. *Program availability:* Part-time, online learning.

Kennesaw State University, WellStar College of Health and Human Services, Program in Advanced Care Management and Leadership, Kennesaw, GA 30144. Offers MSN. *Program availability:* Part-time, evening/weekend, online learning. *Entrance requirements:* For master's, GRE General Test, minimum GPA of 3.0, RN license. Additional exam requirements/recommendations for international students: Required—TOEFL (minimum score 550 paper-based; 80 iBT), IELTS (minimum score 6.5). Electronic applications accepted.

King's College, William G. McGowan School of Business, Wilkes-Barre, PA 18711-0801. Offers MS. *Accreditation:* AACSB. *Program availability:* Part-time. *Entrance requirements:* Additional exam requirements/recommendations for international students: Required—TOEFL (minimum score 600 paper-based).

King University, School of Business and Economics, Bristol, TN 37620-2699. Offers accounting (MBA); finance (MBA); healthcare management (MBA); human resources management (MBA); leadership (MBA); management (MBA); marketing (MBA); project management (MBA). *Program availability:* Part-time, evening/weekend, online learning. *Degree requirements:* For master's, comprehensive exam, thesis optional. *Entrance requirements:* For master's, GMAT, 2 years of work experience. Additional exam requirements/recommendations for international students: Required—TOEFL (minimum score 550 paper-based). Electronic applications accepted. *Faculty research:* International monetary policy.

Lake Erie College, School of Business, Painesville, OH 44077-3389. Offers general management (MBA); health care administration (MBA); information technology management (MBA). *Program availability:* Part-time, evening/weekend. *Faculty:* 2 full-time (1 woman), 8 part-time/adjunct (1 woman). *Students:* 34 full-time (17 women), 144 part-time (66 women); includes 19 minority (12 Black or African American, non-Hispanic/Latino; 3 Asian, non-Hispanic/Latino; 2 Hispanic/Latino; 2 Two or more races, non-Hispanic/Latino), 6 international. Average age 33. 57 applicants, 82% accepted, 37 enrolled. In 2015, 53 master's awarded. *Entrance requirements:* For master's, GMAT or minimum GPA of 3.0, resume, personal statement. Additional exam requirements/recommendations for international students: Required—TOEFL (minimum score 550 paper-based; 79 iBT), IELTS (minimum score 6), STEP Eiken 1st and pre-1st grade level (for Japanese students). *Application deadline:* For fall admission, 8/1 priority date for domestic students, 6/1 for international students; for spring admission, 12/15 for domestic students, 10/1 for international students. Applications are processed on a rolling basis. Application fee: $30. Electronic applications accepted. Application fee is waived when completed online. *Expenses:* $550 per credit hour. *Financial support:* Career-related internships or fieldwork, tuition waivers (full and partial), and unspecified assistantships available. Financial award applicants required to submit FAFSA. *Unit head:* Dr. Robert Trebar, Dean, 440-375-7115, Fax: 440-375-7005, E-mail: rtrebar@lec.edu. *Application contact:* Marco Gaudio, Senior Assistant Director of International Recruitment, 800-533-4996, Fax: 440-375-7060, E-mail: mgaudio@lec.edu. Website: http://www.lec.edu/parkermba

Lake Forest Graduate School of Management, The Leadership MBA Program, Lake Forest, IL 60045. Offers finance (MBA); global business (MBA); healthcare management (MBA); management (MBA); marketing (MBA); organizational behavior (MBA). *Program availability:* Part-time, evening/weekend. *Entrance requirements:* For master's, 4 years of work experience in field, interview, 2 letters of recommendation. Electronic applications accepted.

Lakeland University, Graduate Studies Division, Program in Business Administration, Plymouth, WI 53073. Offers accounting (MBA); finance (MBA); healthcare management (MBA); project management (MBA). *Entrance requirements:* For master's, GMAT. *Expenses:* Contact institution.

Lamar University, College of Graduate Studies, College of Business, Beaumont, TX 77710. Offers accounting (MBA); experiential business and entrepreneurship (MBA); healthcare administration (MBA); MSA/MBA. *Accreditation:* AACSB. *Program availability:* Part-time, evening/weekend. *Faculty:* 24 full-time (7 women), 2 part-time/adjunct (0 women). *Students:* 35 full-time (20 women), 167 part-time (95 women); includes 70 minority (43 Black or African American, non-Hispanic/Latino; 11 Asian, non-Hispanic/Latino; 16 Hispanic/Latino), 51 international. Average age 31. 156 applicants, 91% accepted, 52 enrolled. In 2015, 93 master's awarded. *Degree requirements:* For master's, comprehensive exam (for some programs), thesis optional. *Entrance requirements:* For master's, GMAT. Additional exam requirements/recommendations for international students: Required—TOEFL (minimum score 550 paper-based; 79 iBT), IELTS (minimum score 6.5). *Application deadline:* For fall admission, 8/10 for domestic students, 7/1 for international students; for spring admission, 1/5 for domestic students, 12/1 for international students. Applications are processed on a rolling basis. Application fee: $25 ($50 for international students). Electronic applications accepted. *Expenses:* Tuition, area resident: Full-time $6720; part-time $4032. Tuition, nonresident: full-time $14,880; part-time $8928. *Required fees:* $1900; $950 $784. *Financial support:* Fellowships with tuition reimbursements, research assistantships with partial tuition reimbursements, career-related internships or fieldwork, Federal Work-Study, institutionally sponsored loans, scholarships/grants, and tuition waivers (partial) available. Support available to part-time students. Financial award application deadline: 4/1; financial award applicants required to submit FAFSA. *Faculty research:* Marketing, finance, quantitative methods, management information systems, legal, environmental. *Unit head:* Dr. Enrique R. Venta, Dean, 409-880-8604, Fax: 409-880-8088, E-mail: henry.venta@lamar.edu. *Application contact:* Melissa Gallien, Director, Admissions and Academic Services, 409-880-8888, Fax: 409-880-7419, E-mail: gradmissions@lamar.edu.
Website: http://business.lamar.edu

Lasell College, Graduate and Professional Studies in Management, Newton, MA 02466-2709. Offers business administration (PMBA); elder care management (MSM, Graduate Certificate); hospitality and event management (MSM, Graduate Certificate); human resources management (MSM, Graduate Certificate); management (MSM, Graduate Certificate); marketing (MSM, Graduate Certificate); non-profit management (MSM, Graduate Certificate); project management (MSM, Graduate Certificate). *Accreditation:* ACBSP. *Program availability:* Part-time, evening/weekend, 100% online, blended/hybrid learning. *Faculty:* 3 full-time (1 woman), 16 part-time/adjunct (9 women). *Students:* 69 full-time (48 women), 84 part-time (68 women); includes 37 minority (26 Black or African American, non-Hispanic/Latino; 6 Asian, non-Hispanic/Latino; 2 Hispanic/Latino; 3 Two or more races, non-Hispanic/Latino), 23 international. Average age 32. 81 applicants, 60% accepted, 34 enrolled. In 2015, 68 master's, 4 other advanced degrees awarded. *Degree requirements:* For master's, internship or research paper. *Entrance requirements:* For master's, one-page personal statement, 2 letters of recommendation, resume, and bachelor's degree transcript; proof of microeconomics and statistics (for PMBA); for Graduate Certificate, bachelor's degree transcript, 2 letters of recommendation, 1-page personal statement, resume. Additional exam requirements/recommendations for international students: Required—TOEFL (minimum score 550 paper-based, 79 iBT) or IELTS (minimum score 6). *Application deadline:* For fall admission, 8/31 priority date for domestic students, 6/30 priority date for international students; for spring admission, 12/31 priority date for domestic students, 10/31 priority date for international students. Applications are processed on a rolling basis. Electronic applications accepted. Application fee is waived when completed online. *Expenses:* $595 per credit. *Financial support:* Federal Work-Study and scholarships/grants available. Support available to part-time students. Financial award application deadline: 8/31; financial award applicants required to submit FAFSA. *Unit head:* Dr. Joan Dolamore, Dean of Graduate and Professional Studies, 617-243-2485, Fax: 617-243-2450, E-mail: gradinfo@lasell.edu. *Application contact:* Adrienne Franciosi, Director of Graduate Admission, 617-243-2214, Fax: 617-243-2450, E-mail: gradinfo@lasell.edu. Website: http://www.lasell.edu/academics/graduate-and-professional-studies/programs-of-study/master-of-science-in-management.html

Lebanon Valley College, Program in Business Administration, Annville, PA 17003-1400. Offers business administration (MBA); healthcare management (MBA). *Program availability:* Part-time, evening/weekend. *Faculty:* 7 full-time (1 woman), 10 part-time/adjunct (1 woman). *Students:* 17 full-time (13 women), 85 part-time (46 women); includes 11 minority (4 Black or African American, non-Hispanic/Latino; 2 Asian, non-Hispanic/Latino; 4 Hispanic/Latino; 1 Two or more races, non-Hispanic/Latino), 2 international. Average age 33. 17 applicants, 94% accepted, 14 enrolled. In 2015, 51 master's awarded. *Degree requirements:* For master's, capstone course. *Entrance requirements:* For master's, GMAT, 3 years of work experience, resume, professional statement. Additional exam requirements/recommendations for international students: Required—TOEFL (minimum score 80 iBT), IELTS (minimum score 6.5) or STEP Eiken (grade 1). *Application deadline:* Applications are processed on a rolling basis. Application fee: $0. Electronic applications accepted. *Expenses:* $635 per credit. *Financial support:* Scholarships/grants available. Financial award application deadline: 3/1; financial award applicants required to submit FAFSA. *Faculty research:* Research into organizational factors that contribute to organizational benefits from implementation of business analytics and the impact of experiential learning on students taking management information systems courses; research into the concept of Corporate Personhood; global learning and campus internationalization; problem-based learning pedagogy; leadership and organizational commitment. *Unit head:* Dr. David Setley, Chair of the Department of Business and Economics/MBA Director, 717-867-6104, Fax: 717-867-6018, E-mail: setley@lvc.edu. *Application contact:* Christine M. Martin, Enrollment and Operations Specialist, 717-867-6486, Fax: 717-867-6013, E-mail: cmartin@lvc.edu.
Website: http://www.lvc.edu/mba

Lehigh University, P.C. Rossin College of Engineering and Applied Science, Department of Industrial and Systems Engineering, Program in Healthcare Systems Engineering, Bethlehem, PA 18015. Offers M Eng. *Program availability:* Part-time, 100% online, blended/hybrid learning. *Faculty:* 1 (woman) full-time, 2 part-time/adjunct (0 women). *Students:* 22 full-time (11 women), 20 part-time (8 women); includes 9 minority (3 Black or African American, non-Hispanic/Latino; 3 Asian, non-Hispanic/Latino; 3 Hispanic/Latino), 9 international. Average age 29. 38 applicants, 74% accepted, 11

enrolled. In 2015, 20 degrees awarded. *Degree requirements:* For master's, 30 credits. *Entrance requirements:* For master's, GRE (minimum scores in the 75th percentile). Additional exam requirements/recommendations for international students: Required—TOEFL (minimum score 79 iBT). *Application deadline:* Applications are processed on a rolling basis. Application fee: $75. Electronic applications accepted. *Expenses:* $1,380 per credit. *Financial support:* Application deadline: 1/15. *Faculty research:* Project management; engineering economics; statistics and stochastic processes; operations research; simulation, optimization, and IT. *Unit head:* Prof. Ana Iulia Alexandrescu, Professor of Practice, 610-758-3865, Fax: 610-758-6766, E-mail: aia210@lehigh.edu. *Application contact:* Linda Wismer, Coordinator, 610-758-5867, Fax: 610-758-6766, E-mail: liw511@lehigh.edu.
Website: http://hse.lehigh.edu/

Lenoir-Rhyne University, Graduate Programs, Charles M. Snipes School of Business, Hickory, NC 28601. Offers accounting (MBA); business analytics and information technology (MBA); entrepreneurship (MBA); global business (MBA); healthcare administration (MBA); innovation and change management (MBA); leadership development (MBA). *Accreditation:* ACBSP. *Program availability:* Part-time, evening/weekend, online learning. *Faculty:* 7 full-time (2 women). *Students:* 38 full-time (13 women), 47 part-time (19 women); includes 15 minority (6 Black or African American, non-Hispanic/Latino; 1 Asian, non-Hispanic/Latino; 8 Hispanic/Latino), 7 international. Average age 30. In 2015, 18 master's awarded. *Degree requirements:* For master's, capstone course. *Entrance requirements:* For master's, GMAT, GRE, MAT, minimum undergraduate GPA of 2.7, graduate 3.0. Additional exam requirements/recommendations for international students: Required—TOEFL (minimum score 600 paper-based). *Application deadline:* Applications are processed on a rolling basis. Application fee: $35. Electronic applications accepted. *Expenses:* $550 per credit hour. *Financial support:* Scholarships/grants available. Financial award application deadline: 3/1; financial award applicants required to submit FAFSA. *Unit head:* Dr. Mary Lesser, Dean, 828-328-7078, Fax: 828-328-7368, E-mail: mary.lesser@lr.edu. *Application contact:* Mary Ann Gosnell, Director of Graduate Recruitment, 828-328-7111, Fax: 828-328-7378, E-mail: admission@lr.edu.
Website: http://bus.lr.edu/

LeTourneau University, Graduate Programs, Longview, TX 75607-7001. Offers business administration (MBA); counseling (MA); curriculum and instruction (M Ed); education administration (M Ed); engineering (ME, MS); engineering management (MEM); health care administration (MS); marriage and family therapy (MA); psychology (MA); strategic leadership (MSL); teacher leadership (M Ed); teaching and learning (M Ed). *Program availability:* Part-time, 100% online, blended/hybrid learning. *Faculty:* 24 full-time (7 women), 40 part-time/adjunct (15 women). *Students:* 82 full-time (48 women), 428 part-time (331 women); includes 234 minority (138 Black or African American, non-Hispanic/Latino; 5 American Indian or Alaska Native, non-Hispanic/Latino; 5 Asian, non-Hispanic/Latino; 50 Hispanic/Latino; 36 Two or more races, non-Hispanic/Latino), 15 international. Average age 37. 257 applicants, 60% accepted, 141 enrolled. In 2015, 136 master's awarded. *Degree requirements:* For master's, thesis for some programs). *Entrance requirements:* Additional exam requirements/recommendations for international students: Required—TOEFL. *Application deadline:* For fall admission, 8/22 for domestic students, 8/29 for international students; for winter admission, 10/10 for domestic students; for spring admission, 1/2 for domestic students, 1/10 for international students; for summer admission, 5/1 for domestic and international students. Applications are processed on a rolling basis. Electronic applications accepted. Application fee is waived when completed online. *Financial support:* Research assistantships, institutionally sponsored loans, and unspecified assistantships available. Financial award applicants required to submit FAFSA. *Application contact:* Chris Fontaine, Assistant Vice President for Global Campus Admissions, 903-233-4312, E-mail: chrisfontaine@letu.edu.
Website: http://www.letu.edu

Lewis University, College of Business, Graduate School of Management, Program in Business Administration, Romeoville, IL 60446. Offers accounting (MBA); custom elective option (MBA); e-business (MBA); finance (MBA); healthcare management (MBA); human resources management (MBA); international business (MBA); management information systems (MBA); marketing (MBA); project management (MBA); technology and operations management (MBA). *Program availability:* Part-time, evening/weekend. *Entrance requirements:* For master's, interview, bachelor's degree, resume, 2 recommendations. Additional exam requirements/recommendations for international students: Required—TOEFL (minimum score 550 paper-based). Electronic applications accepted.

Liberty University, School of Business, Lynchburg, VA 24515. Offers accounting (MBA, MS, DBA); business administration (MBA); criminal justice (MBA); cyber security (MS); executive leadership (MA); healthcare (MBA); human resources (DBA); information systems (MS), including information assurance, technology management; international business (MBA, DBA); leadership (MBA, DBA); marketing (MBA, MS, DBA), including digital marketing and advertising (MS), project management (MS), public relations (MS), sports marketing and media (MS); project management (MBA, DBA); public administration (MBA); public relations (MBA). *Program availability:* Part-time, online learning. *Students:* 1,488 full-time (825 women), 4,187 part-time (1,957 women); includes 1,252 minority (987 Black or African American, non-Hispanic/Latino; 24 American Indian or Alaska Native, non-Hispanic/Latino; 72 Asian, non-Hispanic/Latino; 53 Hispanic/Latino; 5 Native Hawaiian or other Pacific Islander, non-Hispanic/Latino; 111 Two or more races, non-Hispanic/Latino), 136 international. Average age 35. 5,375 applicants, 44% accepted, 1245 enrolled. In 2015, 1,474 master's, 63 other advanced degrees awarded. *Entrance requirements:* For master's, minimum undergraduate GPA of 3.0, 15 hours of upper-level business courses. Additional exam requirements/recommendations for international students: Required—TOEFL (minimum score 600 paper-based; 100 iBT). *Application deadline:* Applications are processed on a rolling basis. Application fee: $50. Electronic applications accepted. *Expenses:* Contact institution. *Unit head:* Dr. Scott Hicks, Dean, 434-592-4808, Fax: 434-582-2366, E-mail: smhicks@liberty.edu. *Application contact:* Jay Bridge, Director of Graduate Admissions, 800-424-9595, Fax: 800-628-7977, E-mail: gradadmissions@liberty.edu.
Website: http://www.liberty.edu/academics/business/index.cfm?PID-149

Liberty University, School of Health Sciences, Lynchburg, VA 24515. Offers biomedical sciences (MS); global health (MPH); health promotion (MPH); healthcare management (Certificate); nutrition (MPH). *Program availability:* Part-time, online learning. *Students:* 435 full-time (342 women), 609 part-time (489 women); includes 301 minority (238 Black or African American, non-Hispanic/Latino; 6 American Indian or Alaska Native, non-Hispanic/Latino; 25 Asian, non-Hispanic/Latino; 12 Hispanic/Latino; 1 Native Hawaiian or other Pacific Islander, non-Hispanic/Latino; 19 Two or more races, non-Hispanic/Latino), 71 international. Average age 33. 1,433 applicants, 43% accepted, 295 enrolled. In 2015, 50 master's, 8 other advanced degrees awarded. *Degree requirements:* For master's, thesis (for some programs). *Entrance requirements:* Additional exam requirements/recommendations for international students: Required—TOEFL (minimum score 600 paper-based; 100 iBT). Application fee: $50. *Unit head:* Dr. Ralph Linstra, Dean. *Application contact:* Jay Bridge, Director of Admissions, 800-424-9595, Fax: 800-628-7977, E-mail: gradadmissions@liberty.edu.

Lindenwood University, Graduate Programs, School of Accelerated Degree Programs, St. Charles, MO 63301-1695. Offers administration (MSA), including management, marketing, project management; business administration (MBA); communications (MA), including digital and multimedia, media management, promotions, training and development; criminal justice and administration (MS); gerontology (MA); healthcare administration (MS); human resource management (MS); information technology (Certificate); managing information security (MS); managing information technology (MS); managing virtualization and cloud computing (MS); writing (MFA). *Program availability:* Part-time, evening/weekend, 100% online. *Faculty:* 18 full-time (7 women), 72 part-time/adjunct (28 women). *Students:* 707 full-time (442 women), 143 part-time (92 women); includes 286 minority (232 Black or African American, non-Hispanic/Latino; 5 American Indian or Alaska Native, non-Hispanic/Latino; 6 Asian, non-Hispanic/Latino; 27 Hispanic/Latino; 1 Native Hawaiian or other Pacific Islander, non-Hispanic/Latino; 15 Two or more races, non-Hispanic/Latino), 21 international. Average age 35. 337 applicants, 68% accepted, 190 enrolled. In 2015, 473 master's awarded. *Degree requirements:* For master's, thesis (for some programs), minimum cumulative GPA of 3.0; for Certificate, minimum cumulative GPA of 3.0. *Entrance requirements:* For master's, resume, personal statement, official undergraduate transcript, minimum undergraduate cumulative GPA of 3.0. Additional exam requirements/recommendations for international students: Required—TOEFL (minimum score 550 paper-based; 80 iBT); Recommended—IELTS (minimum score 6.5). *Application deadline:* For fall admission, 9/28 priority date for domestic and international students; for winter admission, 1/4 priority date for domestic and international students; for spring admission, 4/4 priority date for domestic and international students; for summer admission, 7/5 priority date for domestic and international students. Applications are processed on a rolling basis. Application fee: $30 ($100 for international students). Electronic applications accepted. *Expenses:* Contact institution. *Financial support:* In 2015–16, 852 students received support. Career-related internships or fieldwork, institutionally sponsored loans, scholarships/grants, tuition waivers (partial), and unspecified assistantships available. Financial award application deadline: 6/30; financial award applicants required to submit FAFSA. *Unit head:* Dr. Gina Ganahl, Dean, Accelerated Degree Programs, 636-949-4501, Fax: 636-949-4505, E-mail: gganahl@lindenwood.edu. *Application contact:* Tyler Kostich, Director, Evening and Graduate Admissions, 636-949-4138, Fax: 636-949-4109, E-mail: adultadmissions@lindenwood.edu.
Website: http://www.lindenwood.edu/lead/index.html

Lindenwood University–Belleville, Graduate Programs, Belleville, IL 62226. Offers business administration (MBA); communications (MA), including digital and multimedia, media management, promotions, training and development; counseling (MA); criminal justice administration (MS); education (MA); healthcare administration (MS); human resource management (MS); school administration (MA); teaching (MAT).

Lipscomb University, College of Business, Nashville, TN 37204-3951. Offers accountancy (M Acc); accounting (MBA); conflict management (MBA); financial services (MBA); health care informatics (MBA); healthcare management (MBA); human resources (MHR); information security (MBA); leadership (MBA); nonprofit management (MBA); professional accountancy (Certificate); sports management (MBA); strategic human resources (MBA); sustainability (MBA); MBA/MS. *Accreditation:* ACBSP. *Program availability:* Part-time, evening/weekend. *Faculty:* 15 full-time (1 woman), 10 part-time/adjunct (2 women). *Students:* 128 full-time (67 women), 114 part-time (53 women); includes 43 minority (27 Black or African American, non-Hispanic/Latino; 4 Asian, non-Hispanic/Latino; 7 Hispanic/Latino; 5 Two or more races, non-Hispanic/Latino), 2 international. Average age 32. 225 applicants, 62% accepted, 92 enrolled. In 2015, 125 master's awarded. *Entrance requirements:* For master's, GMAT, transcripts, interview, 2 references, resume. Additional exam requirements/recommendations for international students: Required—TOEFL (minimum score 570 paper-based). *Application deadline:* For fall admission, 6/15 for domestic students, 2/1 for international students; for winter admission, 6/1 for international students; for spring admission, 11/15 for domestic students. Applications are processed on a rolling basis. Application fee: $50 ($75 for international students). Electronic applications accepted. *Expenses:* $1,290 per credit hour (for MBA); $1,190 per credit hour (for M Acc); $1,150 per credit hour (for MHR and MMGT). *Financial support:* Career-related internships or fieldwork, scholarships/grants, tuition waivers (partial), and unspecified assistantships available. Support available to part-time students. Financial award application deadline: 7/1; financial award applicants required to submit FAFSA. *Faculty research:* Impact of spirituality on organization commitment, women in corporate leadership, psychological empowerment, training. *Unit head:* Allison Duke, Associate Dean of Graduate Business Programs, 615-966-5732, Fax: 615-966-1818, E-mail: allison.duke@lipscomb.edu. *Application contact:* Lisa Shacklett, Assistant Dean of Enrollment and Marketing, 615-966-5968, E-mail: lisa.shacklett@lipscomb.edu.
Website: http://www.lipscomb.edu/business/Graduate-Programs

Lock Haven University of Pennsylvania, College of Natural, Behavioral and Health Sciences, Lock Haven, PA 17745-2390. Offers actuarial science (PSM); athletic training (MS); health promotion/education (MHS); healthcare management (MHS); physician assistant (MHS). Program also offered at the Clearfield, Coudersport, and Harrisburg campuses. *Accreditation:* ARC-PA. *Entrance requirements:* For master's, minimum undergraduate GPA of 3.0. Additional exam requirements/recommendations for international students: Required—TOEFL. *Application deadline:* Applications are processed on a rolling basis. Application fee: $25. Electronic applications accepted. *Expenses:* Tuition, state resident: part-time $470 per credit hour. Tuition, nonresident: part-time $705 per credit hour. *Required fees:* $203 per credit hour. $40 per semester. Tuition and fees vary according to program. *Financial support:* Unspecified assistantships available. Financial award application deadline: 8/1. *Unit head:* Dr. Scott Carnicom, Dean, 570-484-2204, E-mail: carnicom@lhup.edu. *Application contact:* Cherie Dolan, Secretary to the Dean, 570-484-2204, Fax: 570-484-2734, E-mail: cdolan1@lhup.edu.
Website: http://www.lhup.edu/colleges/natural_behavioral_health/

Loma Linda University, School of Public Health, Program in Healthcare Administration, Loma Linda, CA 92350. Offers MBA. *Entrance requirements:* Additional exam requirements/recommendations for international students: Required—Michigan Test of English Language Proficiency or TOEFL. *Application deadline:* Applications are processed on a rolling basis. Application fee: $100. *Financial support:* Career-related internships or fieldwork available. Financial award application deadline: 5/15. *Unit head:* Elisa Blethen, Director, 909-824-4573, Fax: 909-824-4087, E-mail: eblethen@llu.edu. *Application contact:* Wendy Genovez, Assistant Dean of Admissions and Records, 909-824-4694, Fax: 909-824-8087, E-mail: wgenovez@llu.edu.

London Metropolitan University, Graduate Programs, London, United Kingdom. Offers applied psychology (M Sc); architecture (MA); biomedical science (M Sc); blood science (M Sc); cancer pharmacology (M Sc); computer networking and cyber security (M Sc); computing and information systems (M Sc); conference interpreting (MA); counter-terrorism studies (M Sc); creative, digital and professional writing (MA); crime, violence and prevention (M Sc); criminology (M Sc); curating contemporary art (MA); data analytics (M Sc); digital media (MA); early childhood studies (MA); education (MA, Ed D); financial services law, regulation and compliance (LL M); food science (M Sc); forensic psychology (M Sc); health and social care management and policy (M Sc);

Health Services Management and Hospital Administration

human nutrition (M Sc); human resource management (MA); human rights and international conflict (MA); information technology (M Sc); intelligence and security studies (M Sc); international oil, gas and energy law (LL M); international relations (MA); interpreting (MA); learning and teaching in higher education (MA); legal practice (LL M); media and entertainment law (LL M); organizational and consumer psychology (M Sc); psychological therapy (M Sc); psychology of mental health (M Sc); public health (M Sc); public policy and management (MPA); security studies (M Sc); social work (M Sc); spatial planning and urban design (MA); sports therapy (M Sc); supporting older children and young people with dyslexia (MA); teaching languages (MA), including Arabic, English; translation (MA); woman and child abuse (MA).

Long Island University–Hudson at Westchester, Graduate School, Purchase, NY 10577. Offers adolescence education (MS Ed); autism (Advanced Certificate); childhood education (MS Ed); finance (MBA); healthcare sector management (MBA); literacy B-12 (MS Ed); management (MBA); mental health counseling (MS), including credentialed alcoholism and substance abuse counselor; school counselor (Advanced Certificate); school psychology (MS Ed); special education (MS Ed); TESOL (all grades) (MS Ed, Advanced Certificate). *Program availability:* Part-time, evening/weekend, online learning. *Faculty:* 6 full-time (5 women). *Students:* 50 full-time (35 women), 128 part-time (101 women); includes 40 minority (8 Black or African American, non-Hispanic/Latino; 1 Asian, non-Hispanic/Latino; 31 Hispanic/Latino). Average age 35. In 2015, 58 master's, 15 other advanced degrees awarded. *Entrance requirements:* Additional exam requirements/recommendations for international students: Required—TOEFL (minimum score 550 paper-based; 79 iBT). *Application deadline:* Applications are processed on a rolling basis. Application fee: $50. Electronic applications accepted. *Expenses:* $1,155 per credit; $884 per term full-time fees, $442 per term part-time fees. *Unit head:* Dr. Sylvia Blake, Dean and Chief Operating Officer, 914-831-2704, Fax: 914-251-5959, E-mail: sylvia.blake@liu.edu. *Application contact:* Cindy Pagnotta, Director of Marketing and Enrollment, 914-831-2701, Fax: 914-251-5959, E-mail: cindy.pagnotta@liu.edu.

Long Island University–LIU Brooklyn, School of Business, Public Administration and Information Sciences, Brooklyn, NY 11201-8423. Offers accounting (MBA); accounting (MS); business administration (MBA); computer science (MS); gerontology (Advanced Certificate); health administration (MPA); human resource management (Advanced Certificate); human resources management (MS); not-for-profit management (Advanced Certificate); public administration (MPA); taxation (MS); United Nations (Advanced Certificate). *Program availability:* Part-time, evening/weekend. *Faculty:* 22 full-time (12 women), 46 part-time/adjunct (10 women). *Students:* 298 full-time (178 women), 240 part-time (158 women); includes 319 minority (218 Black or African American, non-Hispanic/Latino; 2 American Indian or Alaska Native, non-Hispanic/Latino; 47 Asian, non-Hispanic/Latino; 46 Hispanic/Latino; 1 Native Hawaiian or other Pacific Islander, non-Hispanic/Latino; 5 Two or more races, non-Hispanic/Latino), 122 international. Average age 33. 756 applicants, 77% accepted, 195 enrolled. In 2015, 174 master's, 10 other advanced degrees awarded. *Degree requirements:* For master's, thesis optional. *Entrance requirements:* For master's, GMAT or GRE General Test (excluding MPA and computer science; exceptions for all other degrees if holder of advanced degree or CPA license). Additional exam requirements/recommendations for international students: Required—TOEFL (minimum score 550 paper-based; 79 iBT). *Application deadline:* Applications are processed on a rolling basis. Application fee: $50. Electronic applications accepted. *Expenses:* $1,155 per credit tuition; $934 full-time fees per term; $442 part-time fees per term. *Financial support:* In 2015–16, 94 students received support. Federal Work-Study, scholarships/grants, and unspecified assistantships available. Support available to part-time students. Financial award application deadline: 2/15; financial award applicants required to submit FAFSA. *Unit head:* Dr. Edward Rogoff, Dean, 718-488-1159, E-mail: edward.rogoff@liu.edu. *Application contact:* Richard Sunday, Dean of Admissions, 718-488-1011, Fax: 718-780-6110, E-mail: bkln-admissions@liu.edu.
Website: http://liu.edu/Brooklyn/Academics/School-of-Business-Public-Administration-and-Information-Sciences

Louisiana State University Health Sciences Center, School of Public Health, New Orleans, LA 70112. Offers behavioral and community health sciences (MPH); biostatistics (MPH, MS, PhD); community health sciences (PhD); environmental and occupational health sciences (MPH); epidemiology (MPH, PhD); health policy and systems management (MPH). *Accreditation:* CEPH. *Program availability:* Part-time. *Entrance requirements:* For master's, GRE General Test.

Louisiana State University in Shreveport, College of Business, Education, and Human Development, Program in Health Administration, Shreveport, LA 71115-2399. Offers MHA. *Program availability:* Part-time, evening/weekend, online learning. *Students:* 101 full-time (72 women), 238 part-time (171 women); includes 122 minority (79 Black or African American, non-Hispanic/Latino; 2 American Indian or Alaska Native, non-Hispanic/Latino; 12 Asian, non-Hispanic/Latino; 17 Hispanic/Latino; 12 Two or more races, non-Hispanic/Latino), 9 international. Average age 30. 296 applicants, 95% accepted, 99 enrolled. In 2015, 13 master's awarded. *Entrance requirements:* For master's, GRE or GMAT, minimum GPA of 3.0, recommendations. Additional exam requirements/recommendations for international students: Required—TOEFL (minimum score 550 paper-based; 61 iBT). *Application deadline:* For fall admission, 6/30 for domestic and international students; for spring admission, 11/30 for domestic and international students; for summer admission, 4/30 for domestic and international students. Applications are processed on a rolling basis. Application fee: $20 ($30 for international students). Electronic applications accepted. *Expenses:* Tuition, state resident: part-time $325 per credit hour. Tuition, nonresident: part-time $1019 per credit hour. *Required fees:* $52 per credit hour. Tuition and fees vary according to program. *Financial support:* In 2015–16, 3 students received support. *Faculty research:* Healthcare marketing, law and ethics, leadership. *Unit head:* Dr. John Fortenberry, Program Director, 318-212-0240, E-mail: john.fortenberry@lsus.edu. *Application contact:* Kimberly Thornton, Director of Admissions, 318-795-2403, Fax: 318-797-5286, E-mail: david.stanford@lsus.edu.

Loyola University Chicago, Institute of Pastoral Studies, Chicago, IL 60660. Offers counseling for ministry (MA); healthcare mission leadership (MA); pastoral counseling (MA); pastoral studies (M Div, MA); social justice (MA, Certificate); spirituality (MA); M Div/MA; M Div/MSN; M Div/MSW; MSW/MA. *Accreditation:* ACIPE. *Program availability:* Part-time, evening/weekend. *Faculty:* 6 full-time (1 woman), 33 part-time/adjunct (16 women). *Students:* 65 full-time (50 women), 137 part-time (99 women); includes 40 minority (17 Black or African American, non-Hispanic/Latino; 5 Asian, non-Hispanic/Latino; 15 Hispanic/Latino; 3 Two or more races, non-Hispanic/Latino), 19 international. Average age 45. 88 applicants, 99% accepted, 63 enrolled. In 2015, 58 master's, 4 other advanced degrees awarded. *Degree requirements:* For master's, thesis optional, project. *Entrance requirements:* For master's, interview. Additional exam requirements/recommendations for international students: Required—TOEFL. *Application deadline:* Applications are processed on a rolling basis. Application fee: $50. Electronic applications accepted. Application fee is waived when completed online. *Expenses:* Contact institution. *Financial support:* In 2015–16, 84 students received support. Career-related internships or fieldwork, Federal Work-Study, institutionally sponsored loans, scholarships/grants, and tuition waivers (partial) available. Support

available to part-time students. Financial award application deadline: 3/1; financial award applicants required to submit FAFSA. *Faculty research:* Catholic theology, skills of religious ministry, family ministries, spirituality and divorced men. *Unit head:* Dr. Brian J. Schmisek, Director, 312-915-7400, Fax: 312-915-7410, E-mail: bschmisek@luc.edu. *Application contact:* Dr. M. Therese Lysaught, Associate Director, 312-915-7485, Fax: 312-915-7410, E-mail: mlysaught@luc.edu.
Website: http://www.luc.edu/ips/

Loyola University Chicago, Quinlan School of Business, MBA Programs, Chicago, IL 60611. Offers accounting (MBA); business ethics (MBA); derivative markets (MBA); economics (MBA); entrepreneurship (MBA); executive business administration (MBA); finance (MBA); healthcare management (MBA); human resources management (MBA); information systems management (MBA); intercontinental (MBA); international business (MBA); marketing (MBA); operations management (MBA); risk management (MBA); JD/MBA; MBA/MSA; MBA/MSF; MBA/MSHR; MBA/MSN; MBA/MSP; MBA/MSSCM; MSIMC/MBA. *Program availability:* Part-time, evening/weekend. *Faculty:* 79 full-time (22 women), 10 part-time/adjunct (6 women). *Students:* 322 full-time (145 women), 78 part-time (38 women); includes 87 minority (23 Black or African American, non-Hispanic/Latino; 36 Asian, non-Hispanic/Latino; 23 Hispanic/Latino; 5 Two or more races, non-Hispanic/Latino), 53 international. Average age 31. 536 applicants, 49% accepted, 141 enrolled. In 2015, 238 master's awarded. *Entrance requirements:* For master's, GMAT or GRE, official transcripts, two letters of recommendation, statement of purpose, resume. Additional exam requirements/recommendations for international students: Required—TOEFL (minimum score 90 iBT) or IELTS (minimum score 6.5). *Application deadline:* For fall admission, 7/15 for domestic and international students; for winter admission, 10/1 for domestic and international students; for spring admission, 1/15 for domestic and international students; for summer admission, 4/1 for domestic and international students. Applications are processed on a rolling basis. Application fee: $50. Electronic applications accepted. Application fee is waived when completed online. *Expenses:* Contact institution. *Financial support:* Federal Work-Study, scholarships/grants, health care benefits, and unspecified assistantships available. Support available to part-time students. *Faculty research:* Social enterprise and responsibility, emerging markets, supply chain management, risk management. *Unit head:* Katherine Acles, Assistant Dean for Graduate Programs, 312-915-6124, Fax: 312-915-7207, E-mail: kacles@luc.edu. *Application contact:* Lauren Griffin, Enrollment Advisor, Quinlan School of Business Graduate Programs, 312-915-6124, Fax: 312-915-7207, E-mail: lgriffin3@luc.edu.

Loyola University New Orleans, College of Social Sciences, School of Nursing, New Orleans, LA 70118. Offers health care systems management (MSN); nursing (MSN, DNP). *Accreditation:* Teacher Education Accreditation Council. *Program availability:* Part-time, evening/weekend, online learning. *Faculty:* 14 full-time (13 women), 16 part-time/adjunct (12 women). *Students:* 350 full-time (321 women), 95 part-time (85 women); includes 139 minority (97 Black or African American, non-Hispanic/Latino; 2 American Indian or Alaska Native, non-Hispanic/Latino; 22 Asian, non-Hispanic/Latino; 15 Hispanic/Latino; 1 Native Hawaiian or other Pacific Islander, non-Hispanic/Latino; 2 Two or more races, non-Hispanic/Latino). Average age 41. 229 applicants, 76% accepted, 100 enrolled. In 2015, 139 master's, 28 doctorates awarded. *Degree requirements:* For master's, practicum; for doctorate, capstone project. *Entrance requirements:* For master's, BSN, unencumbered RN license, 1 year of work experience in clinical nursing, interview, resume, 3 recommendations, statement of purpose. Additional exam requirements/recommendations for international students: Recommended—TOEFL (minimum score 550 paper-based), IELTS. *Application deadline:* For fall admission, 8/1 priority date for domestic and international students; for winter admission, 12/15 priority date for domestic and international students; for spring admission, 5/15 priority date for domestic and international students. Applications are processed on a rolling basis. Application fee: $40. Electronic applications accepted. *Financial support:* Traineeships and Incumbent Workers Training Program grants available. Financial award application deadline: 5/1; financial award applicants required to submit FAFSA. *Faculty research:* Increasing compliance with treatment, patient satisfaction with care provided by nurse practitioners. *Unit head:* Dr. Patricia Pearce, Interim Director, 800-488-6257, Fax: 504-865-3254, E-mail: nursing@loyno.edu. *Application contact:* Deborah Smith, Executive Assistant to the Director, 504-865-2823, Fax: 504-865-3254, E-mail: dhsmith@loyno.edu.
Website: http://css.loyno.edu/nursing

Madonna University, Program in Health Services, Livonia, MI 48150-1173. Offers MSHS. *Program availability:* Part-time. *Degree requirements:* For master's, thesis or alternative. *Entrance requirements:* For master's, GRE General Test or minimum GPA of 3.25. Additional exam requirements/recommendations for international students: Required—TOEFL, TWE. Electronic applications accepted.

Marshall University, Academic Affairs Division, College of Arts and Media, Program in Journalism, Huntington, WV 25755. Offers journalism (MAJ), including health care public relations. *Faculty:* 6 full-time (2 women). *Students:* 9 full-time (7 women), 4 part-time (3 women); includes 1 minority (Two or more races, non-Hispanic/Latino), 2 international. Average age 28. In 2015, 3 master's awarded. *Degree requirements:* For master's, thesis optional. *Entrance requirements:* For master's, GRE General Test. Application fee: $40. *Unit head:* Dr. Janet Dooley, Chair, 304-696-2734, E-mail: dooley@marshall.edu. *Application contact:* Dr. Robert Rabe, Graduate Coordinator, 304-696-4636, E-mail: rabe@marshall.edu.

Marshall University, Academic Affairs Division, College of Business, Program in Health Care Administration, Huntington, WV 25755. Offers MS. *Program availability:* Part-time, evening/weekend. *Students:* 57 full-time (31 women), 20 part-time (16 women); includes 8 minority (6 Black or African American, non-Hispanic/Latino; 1 Hispanic/Latino; 1 Two or more races, non-Hispanic/Latino), 15 international. Average age 30. In 2015, 24 master's awarded. *Degree requirements:* For master's, comprehensive assessment. *Entrance requirements:* For master's, GMAT or GRE General Test. *Application deadline:* Applications are processed on a rolling basis. Application fee: $40. *Financial support:* Career-related internships or fieldwork and tuition waivers (full) available. Support available to part-time students. Financial award applicants required to submit FAFSA. *Unit head:* Dr. Margie McInerney, Associate Dean, 304-696-2575, E-mail: mcinerney@marshall.edu. *Application contact:* Wesley Spradlin, Academic Advisor, 304-746-8964, Fax: 304-746-1902, E-mail: spradlin2@marshall.edu.

Marylhurst University, Department of Business Administration, Marylhurst, OR 97036-0261. Offers health care management (MBA); real estate (MBA); sustainable business (MBA). *Program availability:* Part-time, evening/weekend, 100% online, blended/hybrid learning. *Students:* 287 (155 women); includes 57 minority (31 Black or African American, non-Hispanic/Latino; 11 Asian, non-Hispanic/Latino; 9 Hispanic/Latino; 2 Native Hawaiian or other Pacific Islander, non-Hispanic/Latino; 4 Two or more races, non-Hispanic/Latino), 5 international. Average age 38. *Degree requirements:* For master's, comprehensive exam, capstone course. *Entrance requirements:* For master's, transcripts from all institutions attended, 2 letters of recommendation, resume, 5 years of work experience, essay, interview. Additional exam requirements/recommendations for international students: Required—TOEFL (minimum score 79 iBT), IELTS (minimum score 6.5). *Application deadline:* Applications are processed on a rolling basis. Application fee: $50. Electronic applications accepted. *Expenses: Tuition, area resident:*

Part-time $463 per credit hour. *Financial support:* Scholarships/grants available. Support available to part-time students. Financial award applicants required to submit FAFSA. *Unit head:* Stuart Noble-Goodman, School of Business Director, 503-699-6315, E-mail: snoblegoodman@marylhurst.edu. *Application contact:* Maruska Lynch, Graduate Admissions Counselor, 800-634-9982 Ext. 6322, E-mail: admissions@marylhurst.edu.
Website: http://www.marylhurst.edu/

Marymount University, School of Business Administration, Program in Health Care Management, Arlington, VA 22207-4299. Offers MS, MS/MBA, MS/MS. *Accreditation:* CAHME. *Program availability:* Part-time, evening/weekend. *Faculty:* 5 full-time (3 women). *Students:* 9 full-time (7 women), 26 part-time (17 women); includes 17 minority (10 Black or African American, non-Hispanic/Latino; 4 Asian, non-Hispanic/Latino; 2 Hispanic/Latino; 1 Native Hawaiian or other Pacific Islander, non-Hispanic/Latino), 2 international. Average age 32. 21 applicants, 81% accepted, 7 enrolled. In 2015, 13 master's awarded. *Degree requirements:* For master's, thesis or alternative. *Entrance requirements:* For master's, GMAT or GRE General Test, resume. Additional exam requirements/recommendations for international students: Required—TOEFL (minimum score 600 paper-based; 96 iBT), IELTS (minimum score 6.5). *Application deadline:* For fall admission, 7/15 priority date for domestic students, 7/1 for international students; for spring admission, 11/15 priority date for domestic students, 11/15 for international students. Applications are processed on a rolling basis. Application fee: $40. Electronic applications accepted. *Expenses:* $930 per credit hour. *Financial support:* In 2015–16, 3 students received support, including 1 research assistantship with tuition reimbursement available; career-related internships or fieldwork, Federal Work-Study, scholarships/grants, and unspecified assistantships also available. Support available to part-time students. Financial award applicants required to submit FAFSA. *Unit head:* Dr. Alyson Eisenhardt, Interim Director, 703-284-4984, Fax: 703-527-3830, E-mail: alyson.eisenhardt@marymount.edu. *Application contact:* Francesca Reed, Director, Graduate Admissions, 703-284-5901, Fax: 703-527-3815, E-mail: grad.admissions@marymount.edu.
Website: http://www.marymount.edu/Academics/School-of-Business-Administration/Graduate-Programs/Health-Care-Management-(M-S-)

Maryville University of Saint Louis, The John E. Simon School of Business, St. Louis, MO 63141-7299. Offers accounting (MBA, Certificate); business studies (Certificate); cyber security (MBA); cybersecurity (Certificate); financial services (MBA, Certificate); healthcare practice management (MBA, Certificate); human resource management (MBA); information technology (MBA, Certificate); management (MBA, Certificate); management and leadership (MA); marketing (MBA, Certificate); project management (MBA); sport business management (MBA); supply chain management/logistics (MBA). *Accreditation:* ACBSP. *Program availability:* Part-time, evening/weekend, 100% online, blended/hybrid learning. *Faculty:* 3 full-time (1 woman), 42 part-time/adjunct (11 women). *Students:* 61 full-time (35 women), 131 part-time (76 women); includes 40 minority (24 Black or African American, non-Hispanic/Latino; 5 Asian, non-Hispanic/Latino; 5 Hispanic/Latino; 1 Native Hawaiian or other Pacific Islander, non-Hispanic/Latino; 5 Two or more races, non-Hispanic/Latino), 9 international. Average age 32. In 2015, 43 master's awarded. *Entrance requirements:* Additional exam requirements/recommendations for international students: Required—TOEFL (minimum score 563 paper-based; 85 iBT). *Application deadline:* Applications are processed on a rolling basis. Electronic applications accepted. Application fee is waived when completed online. *Expenses: Tuition, area resident:* Full-time $25,558; part-time $781 per credit hour. *Required fees:* $2400. Part-time tuition and fees vary according to course load and degree level. *Financial support:* Career-related internships or fieldwork, Federal Work-Study, tuition waivers (partial), and campus employment available. Financial award application deadline: 3/1; financial award applicants required to submit FAFSA. *Faculty research:* Global business, e-marketing, strategic planning, interpersonal management skills, financial analysis. *Unit head:* Interim Dean, 314-529-9680, Fax: 314-529-9975. *Application contact:* Dustin Loeffler, Director for Graduate Studies in Business, 314-529-9571, Fax: 314-529-9975, E-mail: dloeffler@maryville.edu.
Website: http://www.maryville.edu/bu/business-administration-masters/

Marywood University, Academic Affairs, College of Health and Human Services, School of Social Work and Administrative Studies, Program in Health Services Administration, Scranton, PA 18509-1598. Offers MHSA. *Program availability:* Part-time. Electronic applications accepted.

McGill University, Faculty of Graduate and Postdoctoral Studies, Faculty of Medicine, Department of Epidemiology and Biostatistics, Montréal, QC H3A 2T5, Canada. Offers community health (M Sc); environmental health (M Sc); epidemiology and biostatistics (M Sc, PhD, Diploma); health care evaluation (M Sc); medical statistics (M Sc). *Accreditation:* CEPH (one or more programs are accredited).

MCPHS University, Graduate Studies, Program in Drug Regulatory Affairs and Health Policy, Boston, MA 02115-5896. Offers MS. *Program availability:* Part-time, evening/weekend. *Degree requirements:* For master's, thesis, oral defense of thesis. *Entrance requirements:* For master's, GRE General Test, minimum GPA of 3.0. Additional exam requirements/recommendations for international students: Required—TOEFL (minimum score 550 paper-based; 79 iBT). Electronic applications accepted. *Faculty research:* Epidemiology, drug policy, drug regulation, ethics.

Medical University of South Carolina, College of Health Professions, Doctoral Program in Health Administration, Charleston, SC 29425. Offers DHA. *Degree requirements:* For doctorate, comprehensive exam, thesis/dissertation. *Entrance requirements:* For doctorate, experience in health care, interview, master's degree in relevant field, resume, 3 references. Additional exam requirements/recommendations for international students: Required—TOEFL (minimum score 600 paper-based). *Faculty research:* HIV outcomes, health outcomes and statistics, inter-professional education.

Medical University of South Carolina, College of Health Professions, Program in Health Administration-Executive, Charleston, SC 29425. Offers MHA. *Program availability:* Part-time, online learning. *Degree requirements:* For master's, 20 hours of community service. *Entrance requirements:* For master's, GRE General Test or GMAT, minimum GPA of 3.0. Additional exam requirements/recommendations for international students: Required—TOEFL (minimum score 600 paper-based). Electronic applications accepted. *Faculty research:* Electronic health records; telemedicine; fraud prediction and prevention; decision modeling; continuous quality improvement; empathy, caring, patient-centered health care and health outcomes; heath policy.

Medical University of South Carolina, College of Health Professions, Program in Health Administration-Global, Charleston, SC 29425. Offers MHA. *Entrance requirements:* Additional exam requirements/recommendations for international students: Required—TOEFL.

Medical University of South Carolina, College of Health Professions, Program in Health Administration-Residential, Charleston, SC 29425. Offers MHA. *Accreditation:* CAHME. *Program availability:* Part-time, online learning. *Degree requirements:* For master's, 20 hours of community service, internship or field project. *Entrance requirements:* For master's, GRE General Test, GMAT, minimum GPA of 3.0, 3 references, interview. Additional exam requirements/recommendations for international

students: Required—TOEFL (minimum score 550 paper-based). *Faculty research:* Electronic health records; telemedicine; fraud prediction and prevention; decision modeling; continuous quality improvement; empathy, caring, patient-centered health care; health policy; health outcomes.

Meharry Medical College, School of Graduate Studies, Division of Community Health Sciences, Nashville, TN 37208-9989. Offers occupational medicine (MSPH); public health administration (MSPH). *Accreditation:* CEPH. *Program availability:* Part-time, evening/weekend. *Degree requirements:* For master's, thesis, externship. *Entrance requirements:* For master's, GRE General Test, GMAT. *Application deadline:* For fall admission, 6/1 for domestic students. Applications are processed on a rolling basis. Application fee: $65. *Expenses:* Contact institution. *Financial support:* Career-related internships or fieldwork, Federal Work-Study, institutionally sponsored loans, and scholarships/grants available. Support available to part-time students. Financial award application deadline: 7/15; financial award applicants required to submit FAFSA.

Mercy College, School of Social and Behavioral Sciences, Program in Health Services Management, Dobbs Ferry, NY 10522-1189. Offers MPA, MS. *Program availability:* Part-time, evening/weekend, online learning. *Entrance requirements:* For master's, interview, resume, undergraduate transcript. Additional exam requirements/recommendations for international students: Required—TOEFL (minimum score 600 paper-based; 100 iBT), IELTS (minimum score 8). Electronic applications accepted. *Expenses: Tuition, area resident:* Full-time $14,904; part-time $828 per credit hour. *Required fees:* $610; $153 per term. $153 per term. Tuition and fees vary according to course load and program.

Metropolitan College of New York, Program in Business Administration, New York, NY 10013. Offers financial services (MBA); general management (MBA); health services and risk management (MBA); media management (MBA). *Accreditation:* ACBSP. *Program availability:* Evening/weekend. *Students:* 163 full-time (108 women), 33 part-time (16 women); includes 141 minority (106 Black or African American, non-Hispanic/Latino; 7 Asian, non-Hispanic/Latino; 26 Hispanic/Latino; 2 Two or more races, non-Hispanic/Latino), 27 international. Average age 35. 273 applicants, 65% accepted, 75 enrolled. In 2015, 88 master's awarded. *Degree requirements:* For master's, thesis, 10-day study abroad. *Entrance requirements:* For master's, GMAT. Additional exam requirements/recommendations for international students: Required—TOEFL (minimum score 600 paper-based). *Application deadline:* For fall admission, 7/15 priority date for domestic students; for winter admission, 11/15 priority date for domestic students; for spring admission, 3/30 priority date for domestic students. Applications are processed on a rolling basis. Application fee: $45. Electronic applications accepted. *Expenses:* Contact institution. *Financial support:* Scholarships/grants available. Financial award application deadline: 8/15; financial award applicants required to submit FAFSA. *Unit head:* Dr. Tilokie Depoo, Dean and Professor, School for Business, 212-343-1234 Ext. 2204. *Application contact:* Steebo Varghese, Assistant Director of Admissions, 212-343-1234 Ext. 2708, Fax: 212-343-8470.

Midwestern State University, Billie Doris McAda Graduate School, Robert D. and Carol Gunn College of Health Sciences and Human Services, Department of Criminal Justice and Health Services Administration, Wichita Falls, TX 76308. Offers criminal justice (MA); health information management (MHA); health services administration (Graduate Certificate); medical practice management (MHA); public and community sector health care management (MHA); rural and urban hospital management (MHA). *Program availability:* Part-time, evening/weekend. *Degree requirements:* For master's, comprehensive exam, thesis. *Entrance requirements:* For master's, GRE. Additional exam requirements/recommendations for international students: Required—TOEFL (minimum score 550 paper-based). Electronic applications accepted. *Faculty research:* Universal service policy, telehealth, bullying, healthcare financial management, public health ethics.

Milwaukee School of Engineering, Program in Health Care Systems Management, Milwaukee, WI 53202-3109. Offers MSN. *Faculty:* 1 (woman) full-time, 1 (woman) part-time/adjunct. *Students:* 4 full-time (all women), 6 part-time (all women); includes 2 minority (both Hispanic/Latino). 8 applicants, 75% accepted, 4 enrolled. *Entrance requirements:* For master's, GRE General Test or GMAT if undergraduate GPA less than 3.0, 2 letters of recommendation; BSN. Additional exam requirements/recommendations for international students: Required—TOEFL (minimum score 90 iBT), IELTS (minimum score 6.5). *Application deadline:* Applications are processed on a rolling basis. Electronic applications accepted. Application fee is waived when completed online. *Expenses: Tuition, area resident:* Full-time $34,200; part-time $760 per credit. *Financial support:* In 2015–16, 2 students received support. Scholarships/grants available. Financial award application deadline: 3/15; financial award applicants required to submit FAFSA. *Unit head:* Dr. Debra Jenks, Department Chair, 414-277-4516, E-mail: jenks@msoe.edu. *Application contact:* Ian Dahlinghaus, Graduate Admissions Counselor, 414-277-7208, E-mail: dahlinghaus@msoe.edu.
Website: http://www.msoe.edu/community/academics/nursing/page/2419/ms-in-nursing-healthcare-systems-management

See Display on page 501 and Close-Up on page 533.

Minnesota State University Moorhead, Graduate Studies, College of Science, Health and the Environment, Moorhead, MN 56563. Offers healthcare administration (MHA); nursing (MS); school psychology (MS, Psy S). *Program availability:* Part-time, evening/weekend, 100% online, blended/hybrid learning. *Application deadline:* Applications are processed on a rolling basis. Application fee: $20. Electronic applications accepted. *Expenses:* Tuition, state resident: full-time $9000; part-time $4500 per credit. Tuition, nonresident: full-time $18,000; part-time $9000 per credit. *Required fees:* $942; $39.25 per credit. One-time fee: $90 full-time. Full-time tuition and fees vary according to course load, degree level, program and reciprocity agreements. *Financial support:* Research assistantships, career-related internships or fieldwork, Federal Work-Study, and unspecified assistantships available. Financial award application deadline: 7/15; financial award applicants required to submit FAFSA. *Unit head:* Jeffrey Bodwin, Acting Dean, 218-477-5892, E-mail: bodwin@mnstate.edu. *Application contact:* Karla Wenger, Graduate Studies Office, 218-477-2344, Fax: 218-477-2482, E-mail: wengerk@mnstate.edu.
Website: http://www.mnstate.edu/cshe/

Misericordia University, College of Professional Studies and Social Sciences, Master of Business Administration Program, Dallas, PA 18612-1098. Offers accounting (MBA); healthcare management (MBA); human resources (MBA); management (MBA); sport management (MBA). *Program availability:* Part-time, evening/weekend, online learning. *Faculty:* 6 full-time (1 woman), 5 part-time/adjunct (2 women). *Students:* 86 part-time (43 women); includes 2 minority (1 Black or African American, non-Hispanic/Latino; 1 Hispanic/Latino). Average age 34. In 2015, 26 master's awarded. *Entrance requirements:* For master's, GMAT, MAT, GRE (50th percentile or higher), or minimum undergraduate GPA of 3.0, interview. Additional exam requirements/recommendations for international students: Required—TOEFL. *Application deadline:* Applications are processed on a rolling basis. Application fee: $35. Electronic applications accepted. Application fee is waived when completed online. *Financial support:* In 2015–16, 70 students received support. Scholarships/grants and unspecified assistantships available. Support available to part-time students. Financial award applicants required to

Health Services Management and Hospital Administration

submit FAFSA. *Unit head:* Dr. Corina Slaff, Chair of Business Department, 570-674-8022, E-mail: cslaff@misericordia.edu. *Application contact:* David Pasquini, Assistant Director of Admissions, 570-674-8183, Fax: 570-674-6232, E-mail: dpasquin@misericordia.edu.
Website: http://www.misericordia.edu/page.cfm?p-1360

Misericordia University, College of Professional Studies and Social Sciences, Program in Organizational Management, Dallas, PA 18612-1098. Offers healthcare management (MS); human resource management (MS); information technology management (MS); management (MS); not-for-profit management (MS). *Program availability:* Part-time, evening/weekend, online learning. *Faculty:* 3 full-time (1 woman), 8 part-time/adjunct (3 women). *Students:* 77 part-time (46 women); includes 2 minority (1 Hispanic/Latino; 1 Native Hawaiian or other Pacific Islander, non-Hispanic/Latino). Average age 34. In 2015, 35 master's awarded. *Entrance requirements:* For master's, GRE General Test, MAT (35th percentile or higher), or minimum undergraduate GPA of 3.0. Additional exam requirements/recommendations for international students: Required—TOEFL. *Application deadline:* Applications are processed on a rolling basis. Application fee: $35. Electronic applications accepted. Application fee is waived when completed online. *Expenses:* Contact institution. *Financial support:* In 2015–16, 52 students received support. Scholarships/grants available. Support available to part-time students. Financial award application deadline: 6/30; financial award applicants required to submit FAFSA. *Unit head:* Dr. Corina Slaff, Chair of Business Department, 570-674-8022, E-mail: cslaff@misericordia.edu. *Application contact:* David Pasquini, Assistant Director of Admissions, 570-674-8183, Fax: 570-674-6232, E-mail: dpasquin@misericordia.edu.
Website: http://www.misericordia.edu/page.cfm?p-652

Mississippi College, Graduate School, Program in Health Services Administration, Clinton, MS 39058. Offers MHSA. *Program availability:* Part-time. *Degree requirements:* For master's, comprehensive exam. *Entrance requirements:* For master's, GRE General Test, minimum GPA of 2.5. Additional exam requirements/recommendations for international students: Recommended—TOEFL, IELTS. Electronic applications accepted.

Missouri State University, Graduate College, College of Business Administration, Department of Management, Springfield, MO 65897. Offers health administration (MHA). *Program availability:* Part-time, evening/weekend. *Faculty:* 12 full-time (4 women). *Students:* 40 full-time (18 women), 20 part-time (8 women); includes 3 minority (2 Hispanic/Latino; 1 Two or more races, non-Hispanic/Latino), 11 international. Average age 31. 55 applicants, 35% accepted, 6 enrolled. In 2015, 62 master's awarded. *Degree requirements:* For master's, thesis optional. *Entrance requirements:* For master's, GMAT or GRE, minimum GPA of 2.75. Additional exam requirements/recommendations for international students: Required—TOEFL (minimum score 550 paper-based; 79 iBT), IELTS (minimum score 6). *Application deadline:* For fall admission, 7/20 priority date for domestic students, 5/1 for international students; for spring admission, 12/20 priority date for domestic students, 9/1 for international students; for summer admission, 5/20 priority date for domestic students. Applications are processed on a rolling basis. Application fee: $35 ($50 for international students). Electronic applications accepted. *Expenses:* Tuition, state resident: full-time $5500. Tuition, nonresident: full-time $10,108. *Required fees:* $1000. *Financial support:* Career-related internships or fieldwork, institutionally sponsored loans, scholarships/grants, tuition waivers, and unspecified assistantships available. Support available to part-time students. Financial award application deadline: 3/31; financial award applicants required to submit FAFSA. *Faculty research:* Medical tourism, performance management, entrepreneurship. *Unit head:* Dr. Barry Cobb, Interim Department Head, 417-836-4698, E-mail: management@missouristate.edu. *Application contact:* Michael Edwards, Coordinator of Graduate Admissions, 417-836-5330, E-mail: michaeledwards@missouristate.edu.
Website: http://mgt.missouristate.edu/

Molloy College, Graduate Business Program, Rockville Centre, NY 11571-5002. Offers accounting (MBA); finance (MBA); healthcare (MBA); management (MBA); marketing (MBA). *Program availability:* Part-time, evening/weekend. *Faculty:* 5 full-time (2 women), 14 part-time/adjunct (7 women). *Students:* 46 full-time (25 women), 103 part-time (51 women); includes 48 minority (27 Black or African American, non-Hispanic/Latino; 8 Asian, non-Hispanic/Latino; 12 Hispanic/Latino; 1 Native Hawaiian or other Pacific Islander, non-Hispanic/Latino), 3 international. Average age 29. 64 applicants, 84% accepted, 46 enrolled. In 2015, 55 master's awarded. *Entrance requirements:* Additional exam requirements/recommendations for international students: Required—TOEFL (minimum score 550 paper-based; 79 iBT). *Application deadline:* Applications are processed on a rolling basis. Application fee: $60. Electronic applications accepted. *Expenses:* Tuition, area resident: Full-time $18,450; part-time $1025 per credit. *Required fees:* $900; $740 per unit. Tuition and fees vary according to course load. *Financial support:* Applicants required to submit FAFSA. *Faculty research:* Building curriculum that prepares students to face ethical dilemmas in the business world; cultural influences on IFRS judgments and impact of say on pay regulations under the Dodd Frank act; relationship between marketing orientation and social responsibilities toward increased performance; leadership profiles of New Mexico Doughboys for World War I centenary; organizational behavior case book based on chapters from political novels to cover leadership, motivation, commune. *Unit head:* Dr. Maureen Mackenzie, Associate Dean/Director of Graduate Program, 516-323-3080, E-mail: mmackenzie@molloy.edu. *Application contact:* Jaclyn Machowicz, Assistant Director for Admissions, 516-323-4010, E-mail: jmachowicz@molloy.edu.
Website: http://www.molloy.edu/academics/graduate-programs/graduate-business

Montana State University Billings, College of Allied Health Professions, Department of Health Administration, Billings, MT 59101. Offers MHA. *Program availability:* Online learning. *Degree requirements:* For master's, thesis or professional paper and/or field experience. *Entrance requirements:* For master's, GRE General Test or GMAT, minimum undergraduate GPA of 3.0, graduate 3.25; 3 years' clinical or administrative experience in health care delivery or 5 years' experience in business or industry management.

Moravian College, Moravian College Comenius Center, Business and Management Programs, Bethlehem, PA 18018-6650. Offers accounting (MBA); business analytics (MBA); general management (MBA); health administration (MHA); healthcare management (MBA); human resource management (MBA); leadership (MSHRM); learning and performance management (MSHRM); supply chain management (MBA). *Program availability:* Part-time, evening/weekend. *Entrance requirements:* For master's, GMAT. Additional exam requirements/recommendations for international students: Required—TOEFL (minimum score 550 paper-based; 90 iBT). Application fee is waived when completed online. *Expenses:* Contact institution. *Faculty research:* Leadership, change management, human resources.

Mount Aloysius College, Program in Business Administration, Cresson, PA 16630. Offers accounting (MBA); health and human services administration (MBA); non-profit management (MBA); project management (MBA). *Program availability:* Part-time, evening/weekend. *Entrance requirements:* Additional exam requirements/recommendations for international students: Required—IELTS (minimum score 5.5); Recommended—TOEFL. *Application deadline:* For fall admission, 8/1 for domestic

students; for spring admission, 12/1 for domestic students. Applications are processed on a rolling basis. Application fee: $30. Electronic applications accepted. *Expenses:* Tuition, area resident: Full-time $6390; part-time $710 per credit. *Financial support:* Unspecified assistantships available. Financial award applicants required to submit FAFSA. *Application contact:* Matthew P. Bodenschatz, Director of Graduate and Continuing Education Admissions, 814-886-6406, Fax: 814-886-6441, E-mail: mbodenschatz@mtaloy.edu.
Website: http://www.mtaloy.edu

Mount Ida College, Program in Management, Newton, MA 02459. Offers healthcare management (MSM); human resource management (MSM); interior architecture (MSM); leadership in sport (MSM); management (MSM). *Program availability:* Part-time, evening/weekend, online learning. *Faculty:* 4 full-time (2 women), 2 part-time/adjunct (0 women). *Students:* 9 full-time (5 women), 23 part-time (13 women). Average age 26. 46 applicants, 46% accepted, 18 enrolled. *Entrance requirements:* For master's, resume, undergraduate transcripts, letters of reference, personal essay. Additional exam requirements/recommendations for international students: Required—TOEFL (minimum score 550 paper-based; 79 iBT); Recommended—IELTS (minimum score 5.5). *Application deadline:* For fall admission, 8/15 for domestic and international students; for spring admission, 1/10 for domestic and international students. Applications are processed on a rolling basis. Application fee: $0. Electronic applications accepted. *Expenses:* $595 per credit. *Financial support:* Federal Work-Study and unspecified assistantships available. Support available to part-time students. Financial award application deadline: 8/15; financial award applicants required to submit FAFSA. *Unit head:* Sharon McKechnie, Dean, School of Business, 617-928-7354, E-mail: smckechnie@mountida.edu. *Application contact:* Trae Alston-Swan, Associate Director of Graduate Admissions, 617-928-4508, Fax: 617-928-4507, E-mail: taswan@mountida.edu.
Website: http://msm.mountida.edu

Mount St. Joseph University, Doctor of Nursing Practice Program, Cincinnati, OH 45233-1670. Offers health systems leadership (DNP). *Program availability:* Part-time. *Faculty:* 12 full-time (11 women), 5 part-time/adjunct (all women). *Students:* Average age 51. *Entrance requirements:* For doctorate, essay; MSN from regionally-accredited university; minimum graduate GPA of 3.5; professional resume; three professional references; interview; 2 years of clinical nursing experience; active RN license; criminal background check; minimum C grade in an undergraduate statistics course; official documentation of practicum. Additional exam requirements/recommendations for international students: Required—TOEFL (minimum score 560 paper-based; 83 iBT). Application fee: $50. Electronic applications accepted. *Expenses:* Contact institution. *Financial support:* Applicants required to submit FAFSA. *Unit head:* Dr. Nancy Hinzman, Director, 513-244-4325, E-mail: nancy.hinzman@msj.edu. *Application contact:* Mary Brigham, Assistant Director for Graduate Recruitment, 513-244-4233, Fax: 513-244-4629, E-mail: mary.brigham@msj.edu.
Website: http://www.msj.edu/academics/graduate-programs/doctor-of-nursing-practice/

Mount Saint Mary's University, Graduate Division, Los Angeles, CA 90049. Offers business administration (MBA); counseling psychology (MS); creative writing (MFA); education (MS, Certificate); film and television (MFA); health policy and management (MS); humanities (MA); nursing (MSN, Certificate); physical therapy (DPT); religious studies (MA). *Program availability:* Part-time, evening/weekend. *Faculty:* 115 full-time, 304 part-time/adjunct. *Students:* 495 full-time (369 women), 149 part-time (121 women); includes 414 minority (73 Black or African American, non-Hispanic/Latino; 4 American Indian or Alaska Native, non-Hispanic/Latino; 60 Asian, non-Hispanic/Latino; 259 Hispanic/Latino; 7 Native Hawaiian or other Pacific Islander, non-Hispanic/Latino; 11 Two or more races, non-Hispanic/Latino), 4 international. Average age 33. 1,398 applicants, 21% accepted, 242 enrolled. In 2015, 172 master's, 26 doctorates, 23 other advanced degrees awarded. *Entrance requirements:* Additional exam requirements/recommendations for international students: Required—TOEFL. *Application deadline:* For fall admission, 6/30 priority date for domestic and international students; for spring admission, 10/30 priority date for domestic and international students; for summer admission, 3/30 priority date for domestic and international students. Applications are processed on a rolling basis. Application fee: $50. Electronic applications accepted. One-time fee: $135. Tuition and fees vary according to degree level. *Financial support:* Career-related internships or fieldwork, Federal Work-Study, institutionally sponsored loans, and tuition waivers (full and partial) available. Support available to part-time students. Financial award application deadline: 3/15; financial award applicants required to submit FAFSA. *Unit head:* Dr. Linda Moody, Graduate Dean, 213-477-2800, E-mail: gradprograms@msmu.edu. *Application contact:* Tara Wessel, Assistant Director, Graduate Admission, 213-477-2799, E-mail: gradprograms@msmu.edu.
Website: http://www.msmu.edu/graduate-programs/

Mount St. Mary's University, Program in Health Administration, Emmitsburg, MD 21727-7799. Offers MHA. *Program availability:* Part-time, evening/weekend. *Faculty:* 6 part-time/adjunct (1 woman). *Students:* 1 full-time (0 women), 49 part-time (31 women); includes 19 minority (7 Black or African American, non-Hispanic/Latino; 1 American Indian or Alaska Native, non-Hispanic/Latino; 5 Asian, non-Hispanic/Latino; 6 Hispanic/Latino). Average age 31. 30 applicants, 73% accepted, 16 enrolled. In 2015, 33 master's awarded. *Degree requirements:* For master's, health care field practicum. *Entrance requirements:* For master's, undergraduate degree, minimum cumulative undergraduate GPA of 2.75. Additional exam requirements/recommendations for international students: Required—TOEFL (minimum score 550 paper-based; 83 iBT). *Application deadline:* Applications are processed on a rolling basis. Application fee: $35. *Expenses:* $590 per credit hour. *Financial support:* Applicants required to submit FAFSA. *Faculty research:* Determinants of healthcare utilization, healthcare marketing. *Unit head:* Cyd Maubert, Director, 301-447-5773.
Website: http://www.msmary.edu/School_of_business/Graduate_Programs/mha/

National University, Academic Affairs, School of Health and Human Services, La Jolla, CA 92037-1011. Offers clinical affairs (MS); clinical informatics (Certificate); clinical regulatory affairs (MS); health and life science analytics (MS); health coaching (Certificate); health informatics (MS); healthcare administration (MHA); nurse anesthesia (MS); nursing (MS), including forensic nursing, nursing administration, nursing informatics; nursing administration (Certificate); nursing informatics (Certificate); nursing practice (DNP); public health (MPH), including health promotion, healthcare administration, mental health. *Program availability:* Part-time, evening/weekend, 100% online, blended/hybrid learning. *Faculty:* 31 full-time (18 women), 33 part-time/adjunct (20 women). *Students:* 353 full-time (263 women), 136 part-time (87 women); includes 322 minority (111 Black or African American, non-Hispanic/Latino; 1 American Indian or Alaska Native, non-Hispanic/Latino; 105 Asian, non-Hispanic/Latino; 72 Hispanic/Latino; 7 Native Hawaiian or other Pacific Islander, non-Hispanic/Latino; 26 Two or more races, non-Hispanic/Latino), 31 international. Average age 32. In 2015, 103 master's awarded. *Degree requirements:* For master's, thesis (for some programs). *Entrance requirements:* For master's, interview, minimum GPA of 2.5. Additional exam requirements/recommendations for international students: Required—TOEFL (minimum score 550 paper-based; 79 iBT), IELTS (minimum score 6). *Application deadline:* Applications are processed on a rolling basis. Application fee: $60 ($65 for international students). Electronic applications accepted. *Financial support:* Career-related internships or fieldwork, institutionally sponsored loans, scholarships/grants, and tuition waivers (partial) available. Support available to part-time students. Financial award application deadline: 6/30; financial award applicants required to submit FAFSA. *Faculty research:* Nursing education, obesity prevention, workforce diversity. *Unit head:* School of Health and Human Services, 800-628-8648, E-mail: shhs@nu.edu. *Application contact:* Frank Rojas, Vice President for Enrollment Services, 800-628-8648, E-mail: advisor@nu.edu. Website: http://www.nu.edu/OurPrograms/SchoolOfHealthAndHumanServices.html

Nebraska Methodist College, Program in Healthcare Operations Management, Omaha, NE 68114. Offers MS. *Program availability:* Part-time, evening/weekend, online learning. *Degree requirements:* For master's, thesis or alternative, capstone. *Entrance requirements:* Additional exam requirements/recommendations for international students: Required—TOEFL (minimum score 550 paper-based; 80 iBT).

New Charter University, College of Business, San Francisco, CA 94105. Offers finance (MBA); health care management (MBA); management (MBA). *Program availability:* Part-time, evening/weekend, online learning. *Entrance requirements:* For master's, course work in calculus, statistics, macroeconomics. Additional exam requirements/recommendations for international students: Required—TOEFL (minimum score 550 paper-based). Electronic applications accepted.

New England College, Program in Management, Henniker, NH 03242-3293. Offers accounting (MSA); healthcare administration (MS); international relations (MA); marketing management (MS); nonprofit leadership (MS); project management (MS); strategic leadership (MS). *Program availability:* Part-time, evening/weekend. *Degree requirements:* For master's, independent research project. Electronic applications accepted.

New Jersey City University, College of Professional Studies, Department of Health Sciences, Jersey City, NJ 07305-1597. Offers community health education (MS); health administration (MS); school health education (MS). *Program availability:* Part-time, evening/weekend. *Degree requirements:* For master's, thesis or alternative, internship. *Entrance requirements:* Additional exam requirements/recommendations for international students: Required—TOEFL (minimum score 79 iBT). *Application deadline:* For fall admission, 8/1 priority date for domestic students; for spring admission, 12/1 for domestic students. Applications are processed on a rolling basis. Application fee: $0. *Expenses:* Tuition, state resident: part-time $566.55 per credit. Tuition, nonresident: part-time $998.15 per credit. *Required fees:* $108 per credit. Part-time tuition and fees vary according to class time, degree level, campus/location and program. *Financial support:* Career-related internships or fieldwork and unspecified assistantships available.

New Jersey Institute of Technology, Newark College of Engineering, Newark, NJ 07102. Offers biomedical engineering (MS, PhD); chemical engineering (MS, PhD); computer engineering (MS, PhD); electrical engineering (MS, PhD); engineering management (MS); environmental engineering (PhD); healthcare systems management (MS); industrial engineering (MS, PhD); Internet engineering (MS); manufacturing engineering (MS); mechanical engineering (MS, PhD); occupational safety and health engineering (MS); pharmaceutical bioprocessing (MS); pharmaceutical engineering (MS); pharmaceutical systems management (MS); power and energy systems (MS); telecommunications (MS); transportation (MS, PhD). *Program availability:* Part-time, evening/weekend. *Faculty:* 139 full-time (22 women), 152 part-time/adjunct (18 women). *Students:* 946 full-time (226 women), 580 part-time (122 women); includes 397 minority (93 Black or African American, non-Hispanic/Latino; 136 Asian, non-Hispanic/Latino; 145 Hispanic/Latino; 23 Two or more races, non-Hispanic/Latino), 808 international. Average age 28. 3,111 applicants, 62% accepted, 591 enrolled. In 2015, 570 master's, 31 doctorates awarded. Terminal master's awarded for partial completion of doctoral program. *Degree requirements:* For master's, thesis optional; for doctorate, thesis/dissertation. *Entrance requirements:* For master's, GRE General Test; for doctorate, GRE General Test, minimum graduate GPA of 3.5. Additional exam requirements/recommendations for international students: Required—TOEFL (minimum score 550 paper-based; 79 iBT). *Application deadline:* For fall admission, 6/1 priority date for domestic students, 5/1 priority date for international students; for spring admission, 11/15 priority date for domestic and international students. Applications are processed on a rolling basis. Application fee: $75. Electronic applications accepted. *Expenses:* $28,800 per year non-resident full-time. *Financial support:* In 2015–16, fellowships with partial tuition reimbursements (averaging $3,900 per year), 68 research assistantships with partial tuition reimbursements (averaging $18,120 per year), 68 teaching assistantships with partial tuition reimbursements (averaging $13,325 per year) were awarded. Financial award application deadline: 1/15. *Total annual research expenditures:* $41.3 million. *Unit head:* Dr. Moshe Kam, Dean, 973-596-5534, E-mail: moshe.kam@njit.edu. *Application contact:* Stephen Eck, Director of Admissions, 973-596-3300, Fax: 973-596-3461, E-mail: admissions@njit.edu. Website: http://engineering.njit.edu/

New York Medical College, School of Health Sciences and Practice, Department of Health Policy and Management, Valhalla, NY 10595-1691. Offers MPH, Dr PH, Graduate Certificate. *Program availability:* Part-time, evening/weekend. *Degree requirements:* For master's, comprehensive exam, thesis, capstone; for doctorate, comprehensive exam, thesis/dissertation. *Entrance requirements:* For master's, minimum GPA of 3.0, some work experience; for doctorate, GRE, minimum graduate GPA of 3.5. Additional exam requirements/recommendations for international students: Required—TOEFL (minimum score 600 paper-based; 96 iBT), IELTS (minimum score 7); Recommended—TSE. Electronic applications accepted. *Expenses:* Tuition, area resident: Full-time $44,355; part-time $1025 per credit. *Required fees:* $500; $95 per year. One-time fee: $140 part-time. Tuition and fees vary according to course load and program.

New York University, College of Global Public Health, New York, NY 10003. Offers biological basis of public health (PhD); community and international health (MPH); global health leadership (MPH); health systems and health services research (PhD); population and community health (PhD); public health nutrition (MPH); social and behavioral sciences (MPH); socio-behavioral health (PhD). *Program availability:* Part-time, online learning. *Degree requirements:* For master's, thesis (for some programs); for doctorate, thesis/dissertation. *Entrance requirements:* For master's and doctorate, GRE. Additional exam requirements/recommendations for international students: Required—TOEFL. Electronic applications accepted.

New York University, Robert F. Wagner Graduate School of Public Service, Program in Health Policy and Management, New York, NY 10010. Offers health finance (MPA); health policy analysis (MPA); health services management (MPA); international health (MPA); MBA/MPA; MD/MPA; MPA/MPH. *Accreditation:* CAHME (one or more programs are accredited). *Program availability:* Part-time. *Degree requirements:* For master's, thesis or alternative, capstone end event. *Entrance requirements:* Additional exam requirements/recommendations for international students: Required—TOEFL (minimum score 100 iBT), IELTS (minimum score 7.5), TWE. Electronic applications accepted. *Expenses:* Contact institution.

Niagara University, Graduate Division of Business Administration, Niagara University, NY 14109. Offers accounting (MBA); business administration (MBA); finance (MBA, MS); financial planning (MBA); healthcare administration (MBA, MHA); human resources (MBA); international management (MBA); professional accountancy (MBA); strategic management (MBA); strategic marketing management (MBA); strategic wealth management (MBA). *Accreditation:* AACSB. *Program availability:* Part-time, evening/weekend. *Faculty:* 25 full-time (7 women). *Students:* 183 full-time (79 women), 63 part-time (37 women); includes 22 minority (6 Black or African American, non-Hispanic/Latino; 1 American Indian or Alaska Native, non-Hispanic/Latino; 8 Asian, non-Hispanic/Latino; 4 Hispanic/Latino; 3 Two or more races, non-Hispanic/Latino), 83 international. Average age 27. In 2015, 106 master's awarded. *Entrance requirements:* For master's, GMAT. Additional exam requirements/recommendations for international students: Required—TOEFL (minimum score 550 paper-based; 79 iBT), IELTS (minimum score 6). *Application deadline:* For fall admission, 8/1 for domestic students; for spring admission, 11/1 for domestic students. Applications are processed on a rolling basis. Application fee: $30. Electronic applications accepted. *Expenses:* $835 per credit hour. *Financial support:* Fellowships, research assistantships, career-related internships or fieldwork, and Federal Work-Study available. Support available to part-time students. Financial award application deadline: 4/15; financial award applicants required to submit FAFSA. *Faculty research:* Capital flows, Federal Reserve policy, human resource management, public policy, issues in marketing, auctions, economics of information, risk and capital markets, management strategy, consumer behavior, Internet and social media marketing. *Unit head:* Dr. Paul Richardson, MBA Director/Chair of the Marketing Department, 716-286-8169, Fax: 716-286-8206, E-mail: psr@niagara.edu. *Application contact:* Evan Pierce, Associate Director for Graduate Recruitment, 716-286-8769, Fax: 716-286-8170, E-mail: epierce@niagara.edu. Website: http://mba.niagara.edu

Northeast Ohio Medical University, College of Graduate Studies, Rootstown, OH 44272-0095. Offers bioethics (Certificate); health-system pharmacy administration (MS); integrated pharmaceutical medicine (MS, PhD); public health (MS). *Program availability:* Part-time. *Faculty:* 15 part-time/adjunct (6 women). *Students:* 15 full-time (7 women), 26 part-time (11 women); includes 7 minority (5 Asian, non-Hispanic/Latino; 2 Hispanic/Latino). Average age 27. In 2015, 9 master's, 1 doctorate awarded. *Entrance requirements:* For master's, GRE. *Application deadline:* For fall admission, 9/1 priority date for domestic students; for winter admission, 1/5 priority date for domestic students. Applications are processed on a rolling basis. Electronic applications accepted. *Expenses:* Contact institution. *Financial support:* In 2015–16, 18 students received support. *Unit head:* Dr. Walter E. Horton, Jr., Dean. *Application contact:* Heidi Terry, Executive Director, Enrollment Services, 330-325-6479, E-mail: hterry@neoucom.edu. Website: http://www.neomed.edu/academics/graduatestudies

Northwestern University, Feinberg School of Medicine and Interdepartmental Programs, Integrated Graduate Programs in the Life Sciences, Chicago, IL 60611. Offers biostatistics (PhD); epidemiology (PhD); health and biomedical informatics (PhD); health services and outcomes research (PhD); healthcare quality and patient safety (PhD); translational outcomes in science (PhD). *Degree requirements:* For doctorate, comprehensive exam, thesis/dissertation, written and oral qualifying exams. *Entrance requirements:* For doctorate, GRE General Test. Additional exam requirements/recommendations for international students: Required—TOEFL (minimum score 600 paper-based). Electronic applications accepted.

Northwestern University, The Graduate School, Kellogg School of Management, Management Programs, Evanston, IL 60208. Offers accounting information and management (MBA, PhD); analytical finance (MBA); business administration (MBA); decision sciences (MBA); entrepreneurship and innovation (MBA); finance (MBA, PhD); health enterprise management (MBA); human resources management (MBA); international business (MBA); management and organizations (MBA, PhD); management and organizations and sociology (PhD); management and strategy (MBA); management studies (MS); managerial analytics (MBA); managerial economics (MBA); managerial economics and strategy (PhD); marketing (MBA, PhD); marketing management (MBA); media management (MBA); operations management (MBA, PhD); real estate (MBA); social enterprise at Kellogg (MBA); JD/MBA. *Program availability:* Part-time, evening/weekend. Terminal master's awarded for partial completion of doctoral program. *Degree requirements:* For doctorate, thesis/dissertation, 2 years of coursework, qualifying (field) exam and candidacy, summer research papers and presentations to faculty, proposal defense, final exam/defense. *Entrance requirements:* For master's, GMAT, GRE, interview, 2 letters of recommendation, college transcripts, resume, essays, Kellogg honor code; for doctorate, GMAT, GRE, statement of purpose, transcripts, 2 letters of recommendation, resume, interview. Additional exam requirements/recommendations for international students: Required—TOEFL, IELTS. Electronic applications accepted. *Expenses:* Contact institution. *Faculty research:* Business cycles and international finance, health policy, networks, non-market strategy, consumer psychology.

Northwestern University, School of Professional Studies, Program in Public Policy and Administration, Evanston, IL 60208. Offers global policy (MA); health services policy (MA); public administration (MA); public policy (MA). *Program availability:* Online learning.

Northwest Nazarene University, Graduate Studies, Program in Business Administration, Nampa, ID 83686-5897. Offers business administration (MBA); healthcare (MBA). *Accreditation:* ACBSP. *Program availability:* Part-time, evening/weekend, online learning. *Degree requirements:* For master's, comprehensive exam, thesis or alternative. *Entrance requirements:* For master's, minimum GPA of 3.0. Electronic applications accepted. *Expenses:* Contact institution.

Ohio Dominican University, Graduate Programs, Division of Business, Program in Healthcare Administration, Columbus, OH 43219-2099. Offers MS. *Program availability:* Part-time, evening/weekend. *Students:* 11 full-time (7 women), 3 part-time (2 women); includes 10 minority (8 Black or African American, non-Hispanic/Latino; 1 Asian, non-Hispanic/Latino; 1 Two or more races, non-Hispanic/Latino). Average age 37. *Entrance requirements:* For master's, minimum GPA of 3.0 in undergraduate degree from regionally-accredited institution, or 2.7 in the last 60 semester hours of bachelor's degree and at least two years of professional experience. Additional exam requirements/recommendations for international students: Required—TOEFL (minimum score 550 paper-based), IELTS (minimum score 6.5). *Application deadline:* For fall admission, 8/15 for domestic students, 6/10 for international students; for spring admission, 1/4 for domestic students, 11/2 for international students; for summer admission, 5/30 for domestic students. Applications are processed on a rolling basis. Application fee: $25. Electronic applications accepted. *Expenses:* $580 per credit hour. *Financial support:* Applicants required to submit FAFSA. *Unit head:* Dr. Anna Parkman, Director of Graduate Business Programs, 614-251-4569, E-mail: parkmana@ohiodominican.edu. *Application contact:* John W Naughton, Director for Graduate Admissions, 614-251-4721, Fax: 614-251-6654, E-mail: grad@ohiodominican.edu. Website: http://www.ohiodominican.edu/academics/graduate/msha

The Ohio State University, College of Public Health, Columbus, OH 43210. Offers MHA, MPH, MS, PhD, DVM/MPH, JD/MHA, MHA/MBA, MHA/MD, MHA/MPA, MHA/MS, MPH/MBA, MPH/MD, MPH/MSW. *Accreditation:* CAHME; CEPH. *Program availability:* Part-time. *Faculty:* 44. *Students:* 268 full-time (189 women), 67 part-time (49 women); includes 73 minority (22 Black or African American, non-Hispanic/Latino; 1 American Indian or Alaska Native, non-Hispanic/Latino; 29 Asian, non-Hispanic/Latino; 12

Health Services Management and Hospital Administration

Hispanic/Latino; 9 Two or more races, non-Hispanic/Latino), 11 international. Average age 28. In 2015, 114 master's, 7 doctorates awarded. Terminal master's awarded for partial completion of doctoral program. *Degree requirements:* For master's, thesis optional, practicum; for doctorate, thesis/dissertation. *Entrance requirements:* For master's and doctorate, GRE. Additional exam requirements/recommendations for international students: Required—TOEFL (minimum score 550 paper-based; 79 iBT); Recommended—IELTS (minimum score 7). *Application deadline:* For fall admission, 12/1 priority date for domestic students, 11/1 priority date for international students. Applications are processed on a rolling basis. Application fee: $60 ($70 for international students). Electronic applications accepted. *Financial support:* Fellowships with tuition reimbursements and research assistantships with tuition reimbursements available. *Unit head:* Dr. William J. Martin, II, Dean and Professor, 614-292-8350, E-mail: martin.3047@osu.edu. *Application contact:* Dr. William J. Martin, II, Dean and Professor, 614-292-8350, E-mail: martin.3047@osu.edu.
Website: http://cph.osu.edu/

Ohio University, Graduate College, College of Business, Program in Business Administration, Athens, OH 45701-2979. Offers executive management (MBA); finance (MBA); healthcare (MBA). *Accreditation:* AACSB. *Program availability:* Part-time, evening/weekend, online learning. *Entrance requirements:* For master's, minimum GPA of 3.0. Additional exam requirements/recommendations for international students: Required—TOEFL (minimum score 600 paper-based). Electronic applications accepted. *Expenses:* Contact institution.

Ohio University, Graduate College, College of Health Sciences and Professions, Department of Social and Public Health, Athens, OH 45701-2979. Offers early child development and family life (MS); family studies (MS); health administration (MHA); public health (MPH); social work (MSW). *Accreditation:* CEPH. *Program availability:* Part-time, evening/weekend, online learning. *Degree requirements:* For master's, capstone (MPH). *Entrance requirements:* For master's, GMAT, GRE General Test, previous course work in accounting, management, and statistics, previous public health background (MHA, MPH). Additional exam requirements/recommendations for international students: Required—TOEFL (minimum score 550 paper-based; 80 iBT) or IELTS (minimum score 6.5). Electronic applications accepted. *Expenses:* Contact institution. *Faculty research:* Health care management, health policy, managed care, health behavior, disease prevention.

Oklahoma Christian University, Graduate School of Business, Oklahoma City, OK 73136-1100. Offers accounting (M Acc, MBA); financial services (MBA); general business (MBA); health services management (MBA); human resources (MBA); international business (MBA); leadership and organizational development (MBA); marketing (MBA); project management (MBA). *Program availability:* Part-time, 100% online. *Faculty:* 24 full-time (17 women), 4 part-time/adjunct (1 woman). *Students:* 150 full-time (100 women), 137 part-time (95 women). 374 applicants, 213 enrolled. In 2015, 188 master's awarded. *Entrance requirements:* For master's, bachelor's degree. Additional exam requirements/recommendations for international students: Required—TOEFL (minimum score 550 paper-based). Application fee: $25. Electronic applications accepted. *Expenses:* $500 per semester hour; $540 per semester hour for international students. *Unit head:* Dr. Ken Johnson, Chair, 405-425-5567, E-mail: ken.johnson@oc.edu. *Application contact:* Angie Ricketts, Graduate School Admissions Counselor, 405-425-5587, E-mail: angie.ricketts@oc.edu.
Website: http://www.oc.edu/academics/graduate/business/

Oklahoma State University Center for Health Sciences, Program in Health Care Administration, Tulsa, OK 74107-1898. Offers MS. *Program availability:* Part-time, evening/weekend, 100% online. *Faculty:* 1 full-time (0 women), 5 part-time/adjunct (2 women). *Students:* 108 full-time (74 women), 194 part-time (124 women); includes 76 minority (22 Black or African American, non-Hispanic/Latino; 26 American Indian or Alaska Native, non-Hispanic/Latino; 8 Asian, non-Hispanic/Latino; 8 Hispanic/Latino; 1 Native Hawaiian or other Pacific Islander, non-Hispanic/Latino; 11 Two or more races, non-Hispanic/Latino), 10 international. Average age 32. 64 applicants, 97% accepted, 57 enrolled. In 2015, 38 master's awarded. *Degree requirements:* For master's, thesis or alternative. *Entrance requirements:* For master's, official transcripts with minimum GPA of 3.0. Additional exam requirements/recommendations for international students: Required—TOEFL. *Application deadline:* For fall admission, 7/1 for domestic students; for spring admission, 12/1 for domestic students. Application fee: $50 ($75 for international students). *Financial support:* In 2015–16, 1 teaching assistantship with full tuition reimbursement (averaging $18,000 per year) was awarded. Financial award applicants required to submit FAFSA. *Faculty research:* Healthcare economics, emotional intelligence, leadership, organizational development. *Total annual research expenditures:* $100,000. *Unit head:* Dr. James D. Hess, Director, 918-561-1105, Fax: 918-561-1416, E-mail: jim.hess@okstate.edu. *Application contact:* Patrick Anderson, Coordinator of Graduate Admissions, 918-561-1228, Fax: 918-561-8243, E-mail: patrick.anderson@okstate.edu.
Website: http://www.healthsciences.okstate.edu/hca/index.cfm

Oregon Health & Science University, School of Medicine, Graduate Programs in Medicine, Division of Management, Portland, OR 97239-3098. Offers healthcare management (MBA, MS, Certificate). *Program availability:* Part-time. *Faculty:* 4 full-time (1 woman), 21 part-time/adjunct (5 women). *Students:* 184 part-time (107 women); includes 38 minority (3 Black or African American, non-Hispanic/Latino; 2 American Indian or Alaska Native, non-Hispanic/Latino; 21 Asian, non-Hispanic/Latino; 5 Hispanic/Latino; 7 Two or more races, non-Hispanic/Latino), 7 international. Average age 37. 119 applicants, 71% accepted, 77 enrolled. *Degree requirements:* For master's, thesis optional. *Entrance requirements:* For master's, GRE General Test (minimum scores: 153 Verbal/148 Quantitative/4.5 Analytical) or GMAT. Additional exam requirements/recommendations for international students: Required—IELTS or TOEFL (minimum score 625 paper-based). *Application deadline:* For fall admission, 7/15 for domestic and international students; for winter admission, 10/15 for domestic and international students; for spring admission, 1/15 for domestic and international students. Applications are processed on a rolling basis. Application fee: $70. Electronic applications accepted. *Financial support:* Health care benefits available. *Faculty research:* Enhancing quality and reducing cost for healthcare by improving patient activation, identifying factors in hospital readmissions using system dynamics modeling, human and organizational dimensions of creating healthy communities. *Unit head:* Jim Huntzicker, Division Head, 503-346-0368, E-mail: hcmanagement@ohsu.edu. *Application contact:* Jessica Walter, Program Coordinator, 503-346-0369, E-mail: hcmanagement@ohsu.edu.

Oregon Health & Science University, School of Nursing, Program in Health Systems and Organizational Leadership, Portland, OR 97239-3098. Offers MN, PMC.

Oregon State University, College of Public Health and Human Sciences, Program in Public Health, Corvallis, OR 97331. Offers biostatistics (MPH); environmental and occupational health and safety (MPH, PhD); epidemiology (MPH, PhD); health management and policy (MPH); health policy (PhD); health promotion and health behavior (MPH, PhD); international health (MPH). *Accreditation:* CEPH. *Program availability:* Part-time. *Faculty:* 32 full-time (18 women), 3 part-time/adjunct (0 women). *Students:* 123 full-time (91 women), 20 part-time (14 women); includes 43 minority (2 Black or African American, non-Hispanic/Latino; 2 American Indian or Alaska Native,

non-Hispanic/Latino; 9 Asian, non-Hispanic/Latino; 18 Hispanic/Latino; 1 Native Hawaiian or other Pacific Islander, non-Hispanic/Latino; 11 Two or more races, non-Hispanic/Latino), 18 international. Average age 31. 276 applicants, 65% accepted, 45 enrolled. In 2015, 59 master's, 6 doctorates awarded. Terminal master's awarded for partial completion of doctoral program. *Degree requirements:* For doctorate, one foreign language, thesis/dissertation. *Entrance requirements:* For master's and doctorate, GRE, minimum GPA of 3.0 in last 90 hours. Additional exam requirements/recommendations for international students: Required—TOEFL (minimum score 80 iBT), IELTS (minimum score 6.5). *Application deadline:* For fall admission, 12/1 priority date for domestic students. Applications are processed on a rolling basis. *Expenses:* $13,851 full-time resident tuition, $23,679 full-time non-resident tuition, $1,572 fees. *Financial support:* Fellowships, research assistantships, teaching assistantships, career-related internships or fieldwork, Federal Work-Study, and institutionally sponsored loans available. Support available to part-time students. Financial award application deadline: 12/1. *Faculty research:* Traffic safety, health safety, injury control, health promotion. *Unit head:* Dr. Sheryl Thorburn, Professor/Co-Director. *Application contact:* Amanda Armington, Public Health Program Manager, 541-737-3825, E-mail: amanda.armington@oregonstate.edu.

Our Lady of the Lake College, School of Arts, Sciences and Health Professions, Baton Rouge, LA 70808. Offers health administration (MHA); physician assistant studies (MMS).

Our Lady of the Lake University of San Antonio, School of Business and Leadership, Program in Healthcare Management, San Antonio, TX 78207-4689. Offers healthcare management (MBA). *Program availability:* Part-time, evening/weekend, 100% online, blended/hybrid learning. *Faculty:* 1 full-time (0 women), 1 part-time/adjunct (0 women). *Students:* 68 full-time (50 women), 9 part-time (8 women); includes 51 minority (11 Black or African American, non-Hispanic/Latino; 2 Asian, non-Hispanic/Latino; 36 Hispanic/Latino; 2 Two or more races, non-Hispanic/Latino). Average age 35. 37 applicants, 76% accepted, 21 enrolled. In 2015, 34 master's awarded. *Entrance requirements:* For master's, official transcripts showing six hours of coursework in economics and 3 hours of coursework in each of the following areas: statistics, management, business law, and finance; rsum including detailed work history describing managerial or professional work experience. Additional exam requirements/recommendations for international students: Required—TOEFL. *Application deadline:* For fall admission, 7/15 for domestic and international students; for spring admission, 11/15 for domestic and international students; for summer admission, 4/15 for domestic and international students. Application fee: $40 ($50 for international students). Electronic applications accepted. *Expenses: Tuition, area resident:* Full-time $14,796; part-time $822 per credit hour. *Required fees:* $232 per semester. Tuition and fees vary according to course load, degree level, campus/location and program. *Financial support:* In 2015–16, 12 students received support. Federal Work-Study, scholarships/grants, unspecified assistantships, and tuition discounts available. Support available to part-time students. Financial award application deadline: 5/1; financial award applicants required to submit FAFSA. *Application contact:* Office of Graduate Admissions, 210-431-3995, Fax: 210-431-3945, E-mail: gradadm@ollusa.edu.
Website: http://www.ollusa.edu/s/1190/hybrid/default-hybrid-ollu.aspx?sid=1190&gid=1&pgid=7873

Pace University, Dyson College of Arts and Sciences, Department of Public Administration, New York, NY 10038. Offers government management (MPA); health care administration (MPA); management for public safety and homeland security (MA); not-for-profit management (MPA). JD/MPA. Offered at White Plains, NY location only. *Program availability:* Part-time, evening/weekend, 100% online, blended/hybrid learning. *Faculty:* 6 full-time (4 women), 4 part-time/adjunct (1 woman). *Students:* 65 full-time (43 women), 78 part-time (42 women); includes 65 minority (39 Black or African American, non-Hispanic/Latino; 4 Asian, non-Hispanic/Latino; 21 Hispanic/Latino; 1 Two or more races, non-Hispanic/Latino), 31 international. Average age 30. 100 applicants, 87% accepted, 51 enrolled. In 2015, 53 master's awarded. *Degree requirements:* For master's, comprehensive exam (for some programs), thesis (for some programs). *Entrance requirements:* For master's, GRE General Test, 2 letters of recommendation, resume, personal statement, official transcripts. Additional exam requirements/recommendations for international students: Required—TOEFL (minimum score 88 iBT), IELTS (minimum score 7) or PTE (minimum score 60). *Application deadline:* For fall admission, 8/1 priority date for domestic students, 6/1 for international students; for spring admission, 12/1 priority date for domestic students, 10/1 for international students. Applications are processed on a rolling basis. Application fee: $70. Electronic applications accepted. *Expenses: Tuition, area resident:* Part-time $1195 per credit. *Required fees:* $260 per semester. Tuition and fees vary according to degree level, campus/location and program. *Financial support:* Research assistantships, career-related internships or fieldwork, Federal Work-Study, and tuition waivers (partial) available. Support available to part-time students. Financial award application deadline: 2/15; financial award applicants required to submit FAFSA. *Unit head:* Dr. Joseph Ryan, Chairperson, 914-773-3814, E-mail: jryan@pace.edu. *Application contact:* Susan Ford-Goldschein, Director of Admissions, 914-422-4283, Fax: 212-346-1585, E-mail: graduateadmission@pace.edu.
Website: http://www.pace.edu/dyson/academic-departments-and-programs/public-admin

Pacific University, Healthcare Administration Program, Forest Grove, OR 97116-1797. Offers MHA.

Park University, School of Graduate and Professional Studies, Kansas City, MO 54105. Offers adult education (M Ed); business and government leadership (Graduate Certificate); business, government, and global society (MPA); communication and leadership (MA); creative and life writing (Graduate Certificate); disaster and emergency management (MPA, Graduate Certificate); educational leadership (M Ed); finance (MBA, Graduate Certificate); general business (MBA); global business (Graduate Certificate); healthcare administration (MHA); healthcare services management and leadership (Graduate Certificate); international business (MBA); language and literacy (M Ed), including English for speakers of other languages, special reading teacher/literacy coach; leadership of international healthcare organizations (Graduate Certificate); management information systems (MBA, Graduate Certificate); music performance (ADP, Graduate Certificate), including cello (MM, ADP), piano (MM, ADP), viola (MM, ADP), violin (MM, ADP); nonprofit and community services management (MPA); nonprofit leadership (Graduate Certificate); performance (MM), including cello (MM, ADP), piano (MM, ADP), viola (MM, ADP), violin (MM, ADP); public management (MPA); social work (MSW); teacher leadership (M Ed), including curriculum and assessment, instructional leader. *Program availability:* Part-time, evening/weekend, online learning. *Degree requirements:* For master's, comprehensive exam (for some programs), thesis (for some programs), exam (for some programs). *Entrance requirements:* For master's, GRE or GMAT (for some programs), teacher certification (for some M Ed programs), letters of recommendation, essay, resume (for some programs). Additional exam requirements/recommendations for international students: Required—TOEFL (minimum score 550 paper-based; 79 iBT), IELTS (minimum score 6). Electronic applications accepted.

Penn State Great Valley, Graduate Studies, Management Division, Malvern, PA 19355-1488. Offers business administration (MBA); cyber security (Certificate); data analytics (Certificate); finance (M Fin, Certificate); health sector management (Certificate); human resource management (Certificate); information science (MSIS); leadership development (MLD); sustainable management practices (Certificate). *Accreditation:* AACSB. *Unit head:* Dr. Craig S. Edelbrock, Chancellor, 610-648-3202, Fax: 610-889-1334. *Application contact:* JoAnn Kelly, Director of Admissions, 610-648-3315, Fax: 610-725-5296, E-mail: jek2@psu.edu.
Website: http://www.sgps.psu.edu/Academics/Degrees/31885.htm

Penn State Harrisburg, Graduate School, School of Public Affairs, Middletown, PA 17057-4898. Offers criminal justice (MA); health administration (MHA); homeland security (MPS, Certificate); long term care (Certificate); non-profit administration (Certificate); public administration (MPA, PhD); public budgeting and financial management (Certificate); public sector human resource management (Certificate). *Accreditation:* NASPAA. *Unit head:* Dr. Mukund S. Kulkarni, Chancellor, 717-948-6105, Fax: 717-948-6452. *Application contact:* Robert W. Coffman, Jr., Director of Enrollment Management, Admissions, 717-948-6250, Fax: 717-948-6325, E-mail: hbgadmit@psu.edu.
Website: https://harrisburg.psu.edu/public-affairs

Penn State University Park, Graduate School, College of Health and Human Development, Department of Health Policy and Administration, University Park, PA 16802. Offers health policy and administration (MHA, MS, PhD). *Accreditation:* CAHME. *Unit head:* Dr. Ann C. Crouter, Dean, 814-865-1420, Fax: 814-865-3282. *Application contact:* Lori Stania, Director, Graduate Student Services, 814-865-1795, Fax: 814-863-4627, E-mail: l-gswww@lists.psu.edu.
Website: http://www.hhdcv.pcu.edu/hpa

Pennsylvania College of Health Sciences, Graduate Programs, Lancaster, PA 17602. Offers administration (MSN); education (MSHS, MSN); healthcare administration (MHA). *Degree requirements:* For master's, internship (for MHA, MSN in administration); practicum (for MSHS, MSN in education).

Pfeiffer University, Program in Health Administration, Misenheimer, NC 28109-0960. Offers MHA, MBA/MHA.

Point Loma Nazarene University, Fermanian School of Business, San Diego, CA 92106-2899. Offers general business (MBA); healthcare management (MBA); innovation and entrepreneurship (MBA); organizational leadership (MBA); project management (MBA). *Accreditation:* ACBSP. *Program availability:* Part-time, evening/weekend. *Faculty:* 6 full-time, 5 part-time/adjunct (1 woman). *Students:* 28 full-time (11 women), 44 part-time (21 women); includes 28 minority (4 Black or African American, non-Hispanic/Latino; 3 Asian, non-Hispanic/Latino; 17 Hispanic/Latino; 4 Two or more races, non-Hispanic/Latino), 3 international. Average age 30. 41 applicants, 95% accepted, 27 enrolled. In 2015, 67 master's awarded. *Entrance requirements:* For master's, GMAT, letters of recommendation, essay, interview. Additional exam requirements/recommendations for international students: Required—TOEFL. *Application deadline:* For fall admission, 7/26 priority date for domestic students; for spring admission, 11/29 priority date for domestic students; for summer admission, 4/2 priority date for domestic students. Applications are processed on a rolling basis. Application fee: $50. Electronic applications accepted. *Financial support:* Applicants required to submit FAFSA. *Unit head:* Dan Bothe, Dean of Graduate Business Education, 619-849-2394, E-mail: danbothe@pointloma.edu. *Application contact:* Claire Buckley, Director of Graduate Admission, 619-563-2846, E-mail: clairebuckley@pointloma.edu.
Website: http://www.pointloma.edu/discover/graduate-school-san-diego/san-diego-graduate-programs-masters-degree-san-diego/mba

Portland State University, Graduate Studies, College of Urban and Public Affairs, School of Community Health, Program in Health Studies, Portland, OR 97207-0751. Offers health administration (MPA, MPH). *Program availability:* Part-time, evening/weekend. *Faculty:* 19 full-time (14 women), 31 part-time/adjunct (15 women). *Students:* 39 full-time (33 women), 26 part-time (all women); includes 15 minority (2 Black or African American, non-Hispanic/Latino; 2 American Indian or Alaska Native, non-Hispanic/Latino; 3 Asian, non-Hispanic/Latino; 3 Hispanic/Latino; 5 Two or more races, non-Hispanic/Latino), 3 international. Average age 30. 57 applicants, 70% accepted, 25 enrolled. In 2015, 47 master's, 2 doctorates awarded. *Degree requirements:* For master's, comprehensive exam (for some programs), thesis (for some programs), internship (MPA), practicum (MPH); for doctorate, comprehensive exam, thesis/dissertation. *Entrance requirements:* For master's, GRE (for MPH program), minimum GPA of 3.0 in upper-division course work or 2.75 overall, resume, 3 recommendation letters; for doctorate, GRE, transcripts, personal statement, resume, writing sample, 3 recommendation letters. Additional exam requirements/recommendations for international students: Required—TOEFL (minimum score 550 paper-based; 80 iBT). *Application deadline:* For fall admission, 2/1 for domestic and international students. Applications are processed on a rolling basis. Application fee: $50. *Expenses:* Tuition, state resident: full-time $10,040. Tuition, nonresident: full-time $14,063. *Financial support:* In 2015–16, 4 research assistantships with tuition reimbursements (averaging $2,109 per year), 2 teaching assistantships with full tuition reimbursements (averaging $8,937 per year) were awarded; career-related internships or fieldwork, Federal Work-Study, institutionally sponsored loans, scholarships/grants, and unspecified assistantships also available. Support available to part-time students. Financial award application deadline: 3/1; financial award applicants required to submit FAFSA. *Total annual research expenditures:* $1 million. *Unit head:* Dr. Carlos J. Crespo, Director, 503-725-5120, Fax: 503-725-5100, E-mail: ccrespo@pdx.edu. *Application contact:* Elizabeth Bull, Assistant to the Director, 503-725-4592, Fax: 503-725-5100, E-mail: bulle@pdx.edu.

Post University, Program in Business Administration, Waterbury, CT 06723-2540. Offers accounting (MSA); business administration (MBA); corporate innovation (MBA); entrepreneurship (MBA); finance (MBA); healthcare (MBA); leadership (MBA); marketing (MBA); project management (MBA). *Accreditation:* ACBSP. *Program availability:* Online learning.

Queen's University at Kingston, School of Graduate Studies, Faculty of Health Sciences, Department of Community Health and Epidemiology, Kingston, ON K7L 3N6, Canada. Offers epidemiology (PhD); epidemiology and population health (M Sc); health services (M Sc); policy research and clinical epidemiology (M Sc); public health (MPH). *Program availability:* Part-time. *Degree requirements:* For master's, thesis. *Entrance requirements:* For master's, GRE General Test (strongly recommended). Additional exam requirements/recommendations for international students: Required—TOEFL (minimum score 600 paper-based). *Faculty research:* Cancer epidemiology, clinical trials, biostatistics health services research, health policy.

Quinnipiac University, School of Business and Engineering, Program in Business Administration, Hamden, CT 06518-1940. Offers chartered financial analyst (MBA); health care management (MBA); supply chain management (MBA); JD/MBA. *Accreditation:* AACSB. *Program availability:* Part-time, evening/weekend, 100% online, blended/hybrid learning. *Faculty:* 32 full-time (9 women), 11 part-time/adjunct (4 women). *Students:* 139 full-time (60 women), 299 part-time (142 women); includes 64 minority (15 Black or African American, non-Hispanic/Latino; 1 American Indian or Alaska Native, non-Hispanic/Latino; 17 Asian, non-Hispanic/Latino; 26 Hispanic/Latino; 5 Two or more races, non-Hispanic/Latino), 20 international. 270 applicants, 81% accepted, 174 enrolled. In 2015, 159 master's awarded. *Entrance requirements:* For master's, GMAT or GRE, minimum GPA of 3.0. Additional exam requirements/recommendations for international students: Required—TOEFL (minimum score 575 paper-based; 90 iBT), IELTS (minimum score 6.5). *Application deadline:* For fall admission, 7/30 priority date for domestic students, 4/30 priority date for international students; for spring admission, 12/15 priority date for domestic students, 9/15 priority date for international students. Applications are processed on a rolling basis. Application fee: $45. Electronic applications accepted. *Expenses:* $985 per credit tuition; $925 per credit tuition (for online courses); $40 per credit student fee (not to exceed $360 per semester); $150 per semester technology fee part-time (fall/spring); $340 per semester technology fee full-time (fall/spring); $75 per semester technology fee (summer). *Financial support:* Career-related internships or fieldwork, Federal Work-Study, scholarships/grants, and unspecified assistantships available. Support available to part-time students. Financial award application deadline: 6/1; financial award applicants required to submit FAFSA. *Faculty research:* Financial markets and investments, international business, supply chain management, health care management, corporate governance. *Application contact:* Office of Graduate Admissions, 800-462-1944, Fax: 203-582-3443, E-mail: graduate@quinnipiac.edu.
Website: http://www.quinnipiac.edu/mba

Regent University, Graduate School, School of Business and Leadership, Virginia Beach, VA 23464-9800. Offers business administration (MBA), including accounting, business and leadership (MA, MBA), entrepreneurship, finance and investing, franchising, general management, healthcare management (MA, MBA), human resource management, innovation management; leadership (Certificate); organizational leadership (MA, PhD), including business and leadership (MA, MBA), ecclesia leadership (PhD), entrepreneurial leadership (PhD), future studies (MA), healthcare management (MA, MBA), human resource development (PhD), interdisciplinary studies (MA), international organizations (MA), leadership coaching and mentoring (MA), not-for-profit management (MA), organizational communication (MA), organizational development consulting (MA); strategic leadership (DSL), including global consulting, leadership coaching, strategic foresight. *Program availability:* Part-time, evening/weekend, 100% online, blended/hybrid learning. *Faculty:* 8 full-time (2 women), 16 part-time/adjunct (4 women). *Students:* 79 full-time (46 women), 786 part-time (385 women); includes 389 minority (322 Black or African American, non-Hispanic/Latino; 4 American Indian or Alaska Native, non-Hispanic/Latino; 21 Asian, non-Hispanic/Latino; 33 Hispanic/Latino; 1 Native Hawaiian or other Pacific Islander, non-Hispanic/Latino; 8 Two or more races, non-Hispanic/Latino), 70 international. Average age 41. 767 applicants, 53% accepted, 268 enrolled. In 2015, 107 master's, 65 doctorates awarded. *Degree requirements:* For master's, thesis or alternative, 3 credit hour culminating experience; for doctorate, thesis/dissertation. *Entrance requirements:* For master's, college transcripts, resume, essay; for doctorate, college transcripts, resume, essay, writing sample; for Certificate, writing sample, resume, transcripts. Additional exam requirements/recommendations for international students: Required—TOEFL (minimum score 577 paper-based). *Application deadline:* For fall admission, 5/1 priority date for domestic students; for spring admission, 10/1 priority date for domestic students. Applications are processed on a rolling basis. Application fee: $50. Electronic applications accepted. *Expenses:* Contact institution. *Financial support:* Career-related internships or fieldwork, scholarships/grants, health care benefits, tuition waivers (full and partial), and unspecified assistantships available. Support available to part-time students. Financial award application deadline: 9/1; financial award applicants required to submit FAFSA. *Faculty research:* Servant leadership, global business, team effectiveness, technology utilization, leadership development. *Unit head:* Dr. Doris Gomez, Dean, 757-352-4686, Fax: 757-352-4634, E-mail: dorigom@regent.edu. *Application contact:* Heidi Cece, Executive Director of University Admissions, 800-373-5504, Fax: 757-352-4381, E-mail: admissions@regent.edu.
Website: http://www.regent.edu/acad/global/

Regis College, School of Nursing and Health Sciences, Weston, MA 02493. Offers applied behavior analysis (MS); biomedical sciences (MS); counseling psychology (MA); health administration (MS); molecular imaging and therapeutics (MS); nurse practitioner (Certificate); nursing (MS, DNP); nursing education (Certificate); occupational therapy (MS). *Accreditation:* ACEN. *Program availability:* Part-time, evening/weekend. *Degree requirements:* For master's, thesis. *Entrance requirements:* For master's, GRE General Test or MAT, minimum GPA of 3.0; for doctorate, MAT or GRE if GPA from master's lower than 3.5. Additional exam requirements/recommendations for international students: Required—TOEFL (minimum score 550 paper-based). *Application deadline:* Applications are processed on a rolling basis. Application fee: $50. Electronic applications accepted. *Financial support:* Research assistantships, Federal Work-Study, scholarships/grants, traineeships, and unspecified assistantships available. Support available to part-time students. Financial award applicants required to submit FAFSA. *Faculty research:* Health policy, education, aging, job satisfaction, psychiatric nursing, critical thinking. *Application contact:* Shelagh Tomaino, Associate Director, Graduate Admission, 781-768-7188, Fax: 781-768-7071, E-mail: shelagh.tomaino@regiscollege.edu.

Regis University, Rueckert-Hartman College for Health Professions, Denver, CO 80221-1099. Offers addictions counseling (Post-Graduate Certificate); advanced practice nurse specialization (DNP); counseling (MA); counseling children and adolescents (Post-Graduate Certificate); counseling military families (Post-Graduate Certificate); depth psychotherapy (Post-Graduate Certificate); family nurse practitioner (MSN); health care business management (Certificate); health care quality and patient safety (Certificate); health industry leadership (MBA); health professions (Postbaccalaureate Certificate); health services administration (MS); marriage and family therapy (MA); neonatal nurse practitioner (MSN); nursing education or leadership (MSN); orthopedic manual physical therapy fellowship (Certificate); pharmacy (Pharm D); physical therapy (DPT). *Program availability:* Part-time, evening/weekend, 100% online, blended/hybrid learning. *Faculty:* 40 full-time (29 women), 116 part-time/adjunct (86 women). *Students:* 1,080 full-time (771 women), 274 part-time (239 women); includes 388 minority (59 Black or African American, non-Hispanic/Latino; 6 American Indian or Alaska Native, non-Hispanic/Latino; 109 Asian, non-Hispanic/Latino; 163 Hispanic/Latino; 1 Native Hawaiian or other Pacific Islander, non-Hispanic/Latino; 50 Two or more races, non-Hispanic/Latino), 7 international. Average age 34. 2,188 applicants, 31% accepted, 303 enrolled. In 2015, 329 master's, 160 doctorates awarded. *Degree requirements:* For master's, thesis (for some programs), internship. *Entrance requirements:* For master's, official transcript reflecting baccalaureate degree awarded from regionally-accredited college or university. Additional exam requirements/recommendations for international students: Required—TOEFL (minimum score 550 paper-based; 82 iBT). *Application deadline:* For fall admission, 8/15 priority date for domestic students; for spring admission, 1/10 priority date for domestic students; for summer admission, 5/1 priority date for domestic students. Applications are processed on a rolling basis. Application fee: $75. Electronic applications accepted. *Expenses:* Contact institution. *Financial support:* In 2015–16, 102 students received support. Federal Work-Study and scholarships/grants available. Financial award application

deadline: 4/15; financial award applicants required to submit FAFSA. *Faculty research:* Normal and pathological balance and gait research, normal/pathological upper limb motor control/biomechanics, exercise energy/metabolism research, optical treatment protocols for therapeutic modalities. *Unit head:* Dr. Janet Houser, Academic Dean. *Application contact:* Cate Clark, Director of Admissions, 303-458-4900, Fax: 303-964-5534, E-mail: ruadmissions@regis.edu.
Website: http://www.regis.edu/RHCHP.aspx

Rice University, Graduate Programs, Wiess School–Professional Science Master's Programs, Professional Master's Program in Bioscience Research and Health Policy, Houston, TX 77251-1892. Offers MS.

Robert Morris University Illinois, Morris Graduate School of Management, Chicago, IL 60605. Offers accounting (MBA); accounting/finance (MBA); business analytics (MIS); design and media (MM); educational technology (MM); health care administration (MM); higher education administration (MM); human resource management (MBA); information security (MIS); information systems (MBA, MIS); law enforcement administration (MM); management (MBA); management/finance (MBA); management/human resource management (MBA); mobile computing (MIS); sports administration (MM). *Program availability:* Part-time, evening/weekend. *Faculty:* 9 full-time (4 women), 28 part-time/adjunct (10 women). *Students:* 208 full-time (113 women), 141 part-time (76 women); includes 206 minority (113 Black or African American, non-Hispanic/Latino; 1 American Indian or Alaska Native, non-Hispanic/Latino; 15 Asian, non-Hispanic/Latino; 70 Hispanic/Latino; 1 Native Hawaiian or other Pacific Islander, non-Hispanic/Latino; 6 Two or more races, non-Hispanic/Latino), 22 international. Average age 33. 206 applicants, 58% accepted, 99 enrolled. In 2015, 249 master's awarded. *Entrance requirements:* For master's, official transcripts and letters of recommendation (for some programs); written personal statement. Additional exam requirements/recommendations for international students: Required—TOEFL (minimum score 550 paper-based). *Application deadline:* Applications are processed on a rolling basis. Application fee: $20 ($100 for international students). Electronic applications accepted. *Financial support:* In 2015–16, 434 students received support. Federal Work-Study, scholarships/grants, and unspecified assistantships available. Support available to part-time students. Financial award applicants required to submit FAFSA. *Unit head:* Kayed Akkawi, Dean, 312-935-6050, Fax: 312-935-6020, E-mail: kakkawi@robertmorris.edu. *Application contact:* Danielle Naffziger, Vice President of Marketing and Graduate Enrollment, 312-935-4532, Fax: 312-935-6020, E-mail: dnaffziger@robertmorris.edu.

Roberts Wesleyan College, Health Administration Programs, Rochester, NY 14624-1997. Offers health administration (MS); healthcare informatics administration (MS). *Program availability:* Evening/weekend, online learning. *Faculty:* 2 full-time (0 women), 4 part-time/adjunct (all women). *Students:* 73 full-time (60 women). Average age 34. In 2015, 23 master's awarded. *Degree requirements:* For master's, thesis or alternative. *Entrance requirements:* For master's, minimum GPA of 3.0, verifiable work experience or recommendation. *Application deadline:* Applications are processed on a rolling basis. Application fee: $35. *Financial support:* Applicants required to submit FAFSA. *Unit head:* Joe McCarthy, Chair, 585-594-6990, Fax: 585-594-6940, E-mail: mccarthyj@roberts.edu. *Application contact:* Cheryl Johnson, Program Coordinator, 585-594-6452, Fax: 585-594-6940, E-mail: johnson_cheryl@roberts.edu.
Website: http://www.roberts.edu/health-administration-programs.aspx

Rochester Institute of Technology, Graduate Enrollment Services, College of Health Sciences and Technology, Health Sciences Department, Advanced Certificate Program in Health Care Finance, Rochester, NY 14623. Offers Advanced Certificate. *Program availability:* Part-time, evening/weekend, online only, 100% online. *Entrance requirements:* For degree, minimum GPA of 3.0 (recommended). Additional exam requirements/recommendations for international students: Required—PTE (minimum score 58), TOEFL (minimum score 550 paper-based, 79 iBT) or IELTS (minimum score 6.5). *Application deadline:* Applications are processed on a rolling basis. Application fee: $60. Electronic applications accepted. *Expenses:* $993 per credit hour. *Financial support:* Available to part-time students. Applicants required to submit FAFSA. *Faculty research:* Policy and law formation; healthcare economics, innovation, and leadership. *Unit head:* Dr. William Walence, Vice President and Dean, Institute and College of Health Sciences and Technology, 585-475-4761, E-mail: william.walence@rit.edu. *Application contact:* Diane Ellison, Associate Vice President, Graduate Enrollment Services, 585-475-2229, Fax: 585-475-7164, E-mail: gradinfo@rit.edu.
Website: https://www.rit.edu/emcs/ptgrad/program_detail.php?id-1223

Rochester Institute of Technology, Graduate Enrollment Services, College of Health Sciences and Technology, Health Sciences Department, Advanced Certificate Program in Health Systems Administration, Rochester, NY 14623-5603. Offers Advanced Certificate. *Program availability:* Part-time, evening/weekend, 100% online. *Entrance requirements:* Additional exam requirements/recommendations for international students: Required—PTE (minimum score 58), TOEFL (minimum score 550 paper-based, 79 iBT) or IELTS (minimum score 6.5). *Application deadline:* Applications are processed on a rolling basis. Application fee: $60. Electronic applications accepted. *Expenses:* $993 per credit hour. *Financial support:* Available to part-time students. Applicants required to submit FAFSA. *Unit head:* Dr. William Walence, Director, 585-475-4761, E-mail: william.walence@rit.edu. *Application contact:* Diane Ellison, Associate Vice President, Graduate Enrollment Services, 585-475-2229, Fax: 585-475-7164, E-mail: gradinfo@rit.edu.

Rochester Institute of Technology, Graduate Enrollment Services, College of Health Sciences and Technology, Health Sciences Department, MS Program in Health Systems Administration, Rochester, NY 14623. Offers MS. *Program availability:* Part-time, evening/weekend, online only, 100% online. *Students:* 5 full-time (4 women), 15 part-time (9 women); includes 3 minority (2 Black or African American, non-Hispanic/Latino; 1 Asian, non-Hispanic/Latino), 1 international. Average age 34. 22 applicants, 23% accepted, 2 enrolled. In 2015, 9 master's awarded. *Degree requirements:* For master's, thesis or alternative, capstone. *Entrance requirements:* For master's, minimum GPA of 3.0 (recommended); related professional work experience. Additional exam requirements/recommendations for international students: Required—PTE (minimum score 58), TOEFL (minimum score 550 paper-based, 79 iBT) or IELTS (minimum score 6.5). *Application deadline:* Applications are processed on a rolling basis. Application fee: $60. Electronic applications accepted. *Expenses:* $993 per credit hour. *Financial support:* In 2015–16, 4 students received support. Available to part-time students. Applicants required to submit FAFSA. *Faculty research:* Policy and law formation, healthcare economics, innovation, leadership, health systems management. *Unit head:* Dr. William Walence, Program Director, 585-475-4761, E-mail: william.walence@rit.edu. *Application contact:* Diane Ellison, Associate Vice President, Graduate Enrollment Services, 585-475-2229, Fax: 585-475-7164, E-mail: gradinfo@rit.edu.
Website: http://www.rit.edu/healthsciences/graduate-programs/health-systems-administration

Rockhurst University, Helzberg School of Management, Kansas City, MO 64110-2561. Offers accounting (MBA); business intelligence (MBA, Certificate); data science (MBA, Certificate); entrepreneurship (MBA); finance (MBA); fundraising leadership (MBA, Certificate); healthcare management (MBA, Certificate); human capital (Certificate); international business (Certificate); management (MBA, Certificate); nonprofit administration (Certificate); organizational development (Certificate); science

leadership (Certificate). *Accreditation:* AACSB. *Program availability:* Part-time, evening/weekend. *Faculty:* 19 full-time (4 women), 18 part-time/adjunct (11 women). *Students:* 122 full-time (45 women), 268 part-time (91 women); includes 61 minority (23 Black or African American, non-Hispanic/Latino; 1 American Indian or Alaska Native, non-Hispanic/Latino; 27 Asian, non-Hispanic/Latino; 9 Hispanic/Latino; 1 Two or more races, non-Hispanic/Latino), 7 international. 288 applicants, 74% accepted, 119 enrolled. In 2015, 115 master's, 16 other advanced degrees awarded. *Entrance requirements:* For master's, GMAT or GRE. Additional exam requirements/recommendations for international students: Required—TOEFL (minimum score 550 paper-based; 79 iBT). *Application deadline:* For fall admission, 7/25 priority date for domestic students; for spring admission, 12/15 priority date for domestic students. Applications are processed on a rolling basis. Application fee: $25. Electronic applications accepted. Application fee is waived when completed online. *Financial support:* Career-related internships or fieldwork available. Support available to part-time students. Financial award application deadline: 4/1; financial award applicants required to submit FAFSA. *Faculty research:* Offshoring/outsourcing, systems analysis/synthesis, work teams, multilateral trade, path dependencies/creation. *Unit head:* Cheryl McConnell, Dean, 816-501-4201, Fax: 816-501-4650, E-mail: cheryl.mcconnell@rockhurst.edu. *Application contact:* Matthew Honeycutt, Director of MBA Advising, 816-501-4823, E-mail: matthew.honeycutt@rockhurst.edu.
Website: http://www.rockhurst.edu/helzberg-school-of-management

Roger Williams University, School of Justice Studies, Bristol, RI 02809. Offers criminal justice (MS); cybersecurity (MS); leadership (MS), including health care administration (MPA, MS), public management (MPA, MS); public administration (MPA), including health care administration (MPA, MS), public management (MPA, MS); MS/JD. *Program availability:* Part-time, evening/weekend, online learning. *Faculty:* 7 full-time (3 women), 5 part-time/adjunct (0 women). *Students:* 54 full-time (30 women), 49 part-time (18 women); includes 18 minority (9 Black or African American, non-Hispanic/Latino; 3 Asian, non-Hispanic/Latino; 5 Hispanic/Latino; 1 Native Hawaiian or other Pacific Islander, non-Hispanic/Latino), 3 international. Average age 37. 58 applicants, 95% accepted, 30 enrolled. In 2015, 29 master's awarded. *Degree requirements:* For master's, comprehensive exam, thesis optional. *Entrance requirements:* For master's, 2 letters of recommendation, college transcript, resume (for MS in leadership and MPA programs). Additional exam requirements/recommendations for international students: Recommended—TOEFL (minimum score 85 iBT), IELTS. *Application deadline:* Applications are processed on a rolling basis. Application fee: $50. Electronic applications accepted. *Expenses:* Contact institution. *Financial support:* Application deadline: 6/15; applicants required to submit FAFSA. *Unit head:* Dr. Stephanie Manzi, Dean, 401-254-3021, Fax: 401-254-3431, E-mail: smanzi@rwu.edu. *Application contact:* Lori Vales, Graduate Admissions Coordinator, 401-254-6200, Fax: 401-254-3557, E-mail: gradadmit@rwu.edu.
Website: http://www.rwu.edu/academics/departments/criminaljustice.htm#graduate

Rollins College, Hamilton Holt School, Master of Health Services Administration Program, Winter Park, FL 32789-4499. Offers MHSA. *Program availability:* Part-time, evening/weekend. *Faculty:* 2 full-time (both women), 1 (woman) part-time/adjunct. *Students:* 11 full-time (8 women); includes 3 minority (1 Black or African American, non-Hispanic/Latino; 1 Asian, non-Hispanic/Latino; 1 Hispanic/Latino). Average age 41. 12 applicants, 100% accepted, 12 enrolled. *Degree requirements:* For master's, internship/field experience. *Entrance requirements:* For master's, GRE, official transcripts, two letters of recommendation, essay, current resume. Additional exam requirements/recommendations for international students: Required—TOEFL (minimum score 550 paper-based; 213 iBT). *Application deadline:* For fall admission, 7/15 for domestic students. Applications are processed on a rolling basis. Application fee: $50. *Expenses:* Contact institution. *Financial support:* Federal Work-Study, scholarships/grants, and unspecified assistantships available. Support available to part-time students. Financial award applicants required to submit FAFSA. *Unit head:* Dr. Renee Brent Hotchkiss, Director, 407-646-2480, E-mail: rhotchkiss@rollins.edu. *Application contact:* Graduate Program Admission, 407-646-2232, Fax: 407-646-1551.

Rosalind Franklin University of Medicine and Science, College of Health Professions, Department of Interprofessional Healthcare Studies, Healthcare Administration and Management Program, North Chicago, IL 60064-3095. Offers MS, Certificate. *Program availability:* Part-time, evening/weekend, online learning. *Degree requirements:* For master's, capstone portfolio. *Entrance requirements:* For master's, minimum GPA of 2.75, BS/BA from accredited college or university. Additional exam requirements/recommendations for international students: Required—TOEFL.

Royal Roads University, Graduate Studies, Applied Leadership and Management Program, Victoria, BC V9B 5Y2, Canada. Offers executive coaching (Graduate Certificate); health systems leadership (Graduate Certificate); project management (Graduate Certificate); public relations management (Graduate Certificate); strategic human resources management (Graduate Certificate).

Rush University, College of Health Sciences, Department of Health Systems Management, Chicago, IL 60612-3832. Offers MS, PhD. *Accreditation:* CAHME. *Program availability:* Part-time, evening/weekend. *Degree requirements:* For master's, thesis; for doctorate, thesis/dissertation. *Entrance requirements:* For master's, GMAT or GRE General Test, previous undergraduate course work in accounting and statistics; for doctorate, GRE General Test, master's degree preferably in a health discipline. Additional exam requirements/recommendations for international students: Required—TOEFL. *Application deadline:* For fall admission, 2/15 for domestic students, 7/1 for international students. Applications are processed on a rolling basis. Application fee: $50 ($100 for international students). Electronic applications accepted. *Financial support:* Career-related internships or fieldwork, Federal Work-Study, institutionally sponsored loans, scholarships/grants, and traineeships available. Support available to part-time students. Financial award applicants required to submit FAFSA. *Faculty research:* Organizational performance, occupational health, quality of care indicators, leadership development, entrepreneurship, health insurance and disability, managed care. *Unit head:* Peter W. Butler, Chair, 312-942-2169, Fax: 312-942-2055. *Application contact:* Dr. Andrew N. Garman, Director, 312-942-5402, Fax: 312-942-4957, E-mail: andy_n_garman@rush.edu.
Website: http://www.rushu.rush.edu/hsm

Rutgers University–Camden, School of Public Health, Stratford, NJ 08084. Offers general public health (Certificate); health systems and policy (MPH); DO/MPH. *Accreditation:* CEPH. *Program availability:* Part-time, evening/weekend. *Degree requirements:* For master's, thesis, internship. *Entrance requirements:* For master's, GRE General Test. Additional exam requirements/recommendations for international students: Required—TOEFL. Electronic applications accepted.

Rutgers University–Newark, Graduate School, Program in Public Administration, Newark, NJ 07102. Offers health care administration (MPA); human resources administration (MPA); public administration (PhD); public management (MPA); public policy analysis (MPA); urban systems and issues (MPA). *Accreditation:* NASPAA (one or more programs are accredited). *Program availability:* Part-time, evening/weekend. *Degree requirements:* For master's, comprehensive exam, thesis or alternative; for doctorate, thesis/dissertation. *Entrance requirements:* For master's, GRE, minimum undergraduate B average; for doctorate, GRE, MPA, minimum B average. Electronic

Health Services Management and Hospital Administration

applications accepted. *Faculty research:* Government finance, municipal and state government, public productivity.

Rutgers University–Newark, Rutgers Business School–Newark and New Brunswick, Program in Healthcare Services Management, Newark, NJ 07102. Offers MHSM.

Rutgers University–Newark, School of Health Related Professions, Department of Interdisciplinary Studies, Program in Health Care Management, Newark, NJ 07102. Offers MS. *Program availability:* Part-time, evening/weekend, online learning. *Entrance requirements:* For master's, minimum GPA of 3.0, bachelor's degree, statement of career goals, curriculum vitae, transcript of highest degree. Additional exam requirements/recommendations for international students: Required—TOEFL (minimum score 500 paper-based; 79 iBT). Electronic applications accepted.

Rutgers University–Newark, School of Public Health, Newark, NJ 07107-1709. Offers clinical epidemiology (Certificate); dental public health (MPH); general public health (Certificate); public policy and oral health services administration (Certificate); quantitative methods (MPH); urban health (MPH); DMD/MPH; MD/MPH; MS/MPH. *Accreditation:* CEPH. *Program availability:* Part-time, evening/weekend. *Degree requirements:* For master's, thesis, internship. *Entrance requirements:* For master's, GRE General Test. Additional exam requirements/recommendations for international students: Required—TOEFL. Electronic applications accepted.

Rutgers University–New Brunswick, School of Public Health, Piscataway, NJ 08854. Offers biostatistics (MPH, MS, Dr PH, PhD); clinical epidemiology (Certificate); environmental and occupational health (MPH, Dr PH, PhD, Certificate); epidemiology (MPH, Dr PH, PhD); general public health (Certificate); health education and behavioral science (MPH, Dr PH, PhD); health systems and policy (MPH, PhD); public health (MPH, Dr PH, PhD); public health preparedness (Certificate); DO/MPH; JD/MPH; MBA/MPH; MD/MPH; MPH/MBA; MPH/MSPA; MS/MPH; Psy D/MPH. *Accreditation:* CEPH. *Program availability:* Part-time, evening/weekend. *Degree requirements:* For master's, thesis, internship; for doctorate, comprehensive exam, thesis/dissertation. *Entrance requirements:* For master's, GRE General Test; for doctorate, GRE General Test, MPH (Dr PH); MA, MPH, or MS (PhD). Additional exam requirements/recommendations for international students: Required—TOEFL. Electronic applications accepted.

Sage Graduate School, School of Health Sciences, Department of Nursing, Troy, NY 12180-4115. Offers adult gerontology nurse practitioner (MS, Certificate); education and leadership (DNS); family nurse practitioner (MS, Post Master's Certificate), including adult gerontology acute care (Post Master's Certificate), family nurse practitioner (MS), family psychiatric mental health (Post Master's Certificate); gerontological nurse practitioner (Post Master's Certificate); nurse administrator/executive (Post Master's Certificate); psychiatric mental health nurse clinical nurse specialist (MS); psychiatric mental health nurse practitioner (MS, Post Master's Certificate), including psychiatric mental health. *Accreditation:* AACN. *Program availability:* Part-time, evening/weekend. *Faculty:* 9 full-time (all women), 27 part-time/adjunct (24 women). *Students:* 45 full-time (43 women), 198 part-time (180 women); includes 36 minority (15 Black or African American, non-Hispanic/Latino; 2 American Indian or Alaska Native, non-Hispanic/Latino; 12 Asian, non-Hispanic/Latino; 4 Hispanic/Latino; 3 Two or more races, non-Hispanic/Latino), 3 international. Average age 38. 212 applicants, 36% accepted, 45 enrolled. In 2015, 18 master's, 8 doctorates, 9 other advanced degrees awarded. *Degree requirements:* For master's, thesis or alternative. *Entrance requirements:* For master's, currently licensed as registered professional nurse in state of practice; baccalaureate degree in nursing from nationally-accredited program or its international equivalent. Additional exam requirements/recommendations for international students: Required—TOEFL (minimum score 550 paper-based). *Application deadline:* Applications are processed on a rolling basis. Application fee: $40. Electronic applications accepted. *Expenses: Tuition, area resident:* Full-time $12,240; part-time $680 per credit hour. Tuition and fees vary according to degree level and program. *Financial support:* Fellowships, research assistantships, Federal Work-Study, scholarships/grants, and unspecified assistantships available. Support available to part-time students. Financial award application deadline: 3/1; financial award applicants required to submit FAFSA. *Unit head:* Dr. Theresa Hand, Dean, School of Health Sciences, 518-244-2064, Fax: 518-244-4571, E-mail: handt@sage.edu. *Application contact:* Dr. Carol Braungart, Co-Director, Graduate Nursing Program, 518-244-2459, Fax: 518-244-2009, E-mail: braunc@sage.edu.

Sage Graduate School, School of Management, Program in Health Services Administration, Troy, NY 12180-4115. Offers gerontology (MS). *Program availability:* Part-time, evening/weekend, 100% online. *Faculty:* 3 full-time (2 women), 11 part-time/adjunct (4 women). *Students:* 5 full-time (4 women), 33 part-time (23 women); includes 8 minority (5 Black or African American, non-Hispanic/Latino; 1 Asian, non-Hispanic/Latino; 2 Hispanic/Latino). Average age 34. 47 applicants, 45% accepted, 10 enrolled. In 2015, 9 master's awarded. *Entrance requirements:* For master's, minimum GPA of 2.75, resume, 2 letters of recommendation. Additional exam requirements/recommendations for international students: Required—TOEFL (minimum score 550 paper-based). *Application deadline:* Applications are processed on a rolling basis. Application fee: $40. Electronic applications accepted. *Expenses: Tuition, area resident:* Full-time $12,240; part-time $680 per credit hour. Tuition and fees vary according to degree level and program. *Financial support:* Fellowships, research assistantships, Federal Work-Study, scholarships/grants, and unspecified assistantships available. Support available to part-time students. Financial award application deadline: 3/1; financial award applicants required to submit FAFSA. *Unit head:* Dr. Kimberly Fredericks, Dean, School of Management, 518-292-1782, Fax: 518-292-1964, E-mail: fredek1@sage.edu. *Application contact:* Wendy D. Diefendorf, Director of Graduate and Adult Admission, 518-244-2443, Fax: 518-244-6880, E-mail: diefew@sage.edu.

Saginaw Valley State University, College of Health and Human Services, Program in Health Leadership, University Center, MI 48710. Offers MS. *Program availability:* Part-time, evening/weekend. *Students:* 25 full-time (21 women), 48 part-time (29 women); includes 13 minority (9 Black or African American, non-Hispanic/Latino; 1 Asian, non-Hispanic/Latino; 1 Hispanic/Latino; 2 Two or more races, non-Hispanic/Latino), 14 international. Average age 32. 94 applicants, 52% accepted, 33 enrolled. In 2015, 22 master's awarded. *Entrance requirements:* For master's, minimum GPA of 3.0. Additional exam requirements/recommendations for international students: Required—TOEFL (minimum score 580 paper-based; 92 iBT). *Application deadline:* For fall admission, 7/15 for international students; for winter admission, 11/15 for international students; for spring admission, 4/15 for international students. Applications are processed on a rolling basis. Application fee: $30 ($90 for international students). Electronic applications accepted. *Expenses:* Tuition, state resident: full-time $9515; part-time $514 per credit hour. Tuition, nonresident: full-time $17,899; part-time $980 per credit hour. *Required fees:* $263; $14.60 per credit hour. Tuition and fees vary according to degree level. *Financial support:* Federal Work-Study and scholarships/grants available. Support available to part-time students. *Unit head:* Dr. Marilyn Skrocki, Program Coordinator, 989-964-7394, E-mail: mskrocki@svsu.edu. *Application contact:* Jenna Briggs, Director, Graduate and International Admissions, 989-964-6096, Fax: 989-964-2788, E-mail: gradadm@svsu.edu.

St. Ambrose University, College of Business, Program in Business Administration, Davenport, IA 52803-2898. Offers business administration (DBA); health care (MBA);

human resources (MBA). *Accreditation:* ACBSP. *Program availability:* Part-time, evening/weekend. *Degree requirements:* For master's, comprehensive exam (for some programs), thesis or alternative, capstone seminar; for doctorate, comprehensive exam, thesis/dissertation, oral and written exams. *Entrance requirements:* For master's, GMAT; for doctorate, GMAT, master's degree. Additional exam requirements/recommendations for international students: Required—TOEFL. Electronic applications accepted. *Expenses:* Contact institution.

St. Catherine University, Graduate Programs, Program in Business Administration, St. Paul, MN 55105. Offers healthcare (MBA); integrated marketing communications (MBA); management (MBA). *Program availability:* Part-time, evening/weekend. *Students:* 11 full-time (9 women), 64 part-time (59 women); includes 8 minority (3 Black or African American, non-Hispanic/Latino; 3 Asian, non-Hispanic/Latino; 1 Hispanic/Latino; 1 Two or more races, non-Hispanic/Latino). Average age 35. 30 applicants, 83% accepted, 22 enrolled. *Entrance requirements:* For master's, GMAT (if undergraduate GPA is less than 3.0), 2+ years' work or volunteer experience in professional setting(s). Additional exam requirements/recommendations for international students: Required—TOEFL. *Application deadline:* For fall admission, 8/1 priority date for domestic students; for spring admission, 12/15 priority date for domestic students. Application fee: $35. *Expenses:* Contact institution. *Financial support:* In 2015–16, 33 students received support. *Unit head:* Michelle Wieser, Director, 651-690-6355, E-mail: mawieser@stkate.edu. *Application contact:* 651-690-6933, Fax: 651-690-6064.

St. Joseph's College, Long Island Campus, Programs in Health Care Administration, Field in Health Care Management, Patchogue, NY 11772-2399. Offers MBA. *Program availability:* Evening/weekend. *Expenses: Tuition, area resident:* Full-time $14,850; part-time $825 per credit. *Required fees:* $440. *Unit head:* John Sardelis, Professor/Associate Chairperson, 631-687-1493, E-mail: jsardelis@sjcny.edu. *Application contact:* Jodi A. Duffy, Senior Associate Director of Graduate Admissions, 631-687-4525, E-mail: jduffy@sjcny.edu.

St. Joseph's College, Long Island Campus, Programs in Management, Field in Health Care Management, Patchogue, NY 11772-2399. Offers MS. *Program availability:* Evening/weekend. *Faculty:* 11 part-time/adjunct (3 women). *Students:* 5 full-time (4 women), 46 part-time (34 women); includes 14 minority (8 Black or African American, non-Hispanic/Latino; 1 Asian, non-Hispanic/Latino; 5 Hispanic/Latino). Average age 39. 29 applicants, 86% accepted, 21 enrolled. In 2015, 10 master's awarded. *Expenses: Tuition, area resident:* Full-time $14,850; part-time $825 per credit. *Required fees:* $440. *Unit head:* Charles Pendola, Director and Assistant Professor, 631-687-1297, E-mail: cpendola@sjcny.edu. *Application contact:* Jodi A. Duffy, Senior Associate Director of Graduate Admissions, E-mail: tsaladino@stony.edu.

St. Joseph's College, New York, Programs in Health Care Administration, Field in Health Care Management, Brooklyn, NY 11205-3688. Offers MBA. *Program availability:* Evening/weekend. *Faculty:* 2 full-time (both women), 6 part-time/adjunct (3 women). *Students:* 2 part-time (both women); includes 1 minority (Black or African American, non-Hispanic/Latino). Average age 39. 1 applicant. In 2015, 3 master's awarded. *Expenses: Tuition, area resident:* Full-time $14,850; part-time $825 per credit. *Required fees:* $440. *Unit head:* Lauren Pete, Chair, 718-940-5890, E-mail: lpete@sjcny.edu. *Application contact:* John Fitzgerald, Associate Director, Admissions, 718-940-5810, Fax: 718-636-8303, E-mail: jfitzgerald3@sjcny.edu.

St. Joseph's College, New York, Programs in Health Care Administration, Field in Health Care Management - Health Information Systems, Brooklyn, NY 11205-3688. Offers MBA. *Faculty:* 2 full-time (both women), 6 part-time/adjunct (3 women). *Students:* 4 full-time (2 women), 13 part-time (8 women); includes 15 minority (12 Black or African American, non-Hispanic/Latino; 2 Asian, non-Hispanic/Latino; 1 Hispanic/Latino). Average age 35. In 2015, 4 master's awarded. *Expenses: Tuition, area resident:* Full-time $14,850; part-time $825 per credit. *Required fees:* $440. *Unit head:* Lauren Pete, Chair, 718-940-5890, E-mail: lpete@sjcny.edu. *Application contact:* John Fitzgerald, Associate Director, Admissions, 718-940-5810, Fax: 718-636-8303, E-mail: jfitzgerald3@sjcny.edu.

St. Joseph's College, New York, Programs in Management, Field in Health Care Management, Brooklyn, NY 11205-3688. Offers MBA, MS. *Faculty:* 2 full-time (both women), 6 part-time/adjunct (3 women). *Students:* 1 (woman) full-time, 17 part-time (13 women); includes 13 minority (7 Black or African American, non-Hispanic/Latino; 1 Asian, non-Hispanic/Latino; 5 Hispanic/Latino). Average age 38. 21 applicants, 48% accepted, 8 enrolled. In 2015, 14 master's awarded. *Expenses: Tuition, area resident:* Full-time $14,850; part-time $825 per credit. *Required fees:* $440. *Unit head:* Lauren Pete, Associate Professor/Chair, 718-940-5890, E-mail: lpete@sjcny.edu. *Website:* http://www.sjcny.edu

Saint Joseph's College of Maine, Master of Health Administration Program, Standish, ME 04084. Offers MHA. Degree program is external; available only by correspondence and online. *Program availability:* Part-time, online learning. *Entrance requirements:* For master's, two years of experience in health care. Electronic applications accepted. *Faculty research:* Health care organization, policy, and management; long-term care.

Saint Joseph's University, College of Arts and Sciences, Department of Health Services, Philadelphia, PA 19131-1395. Offers health administration (MS); health education (MS); healthcare ethics (MS); long-term care administration (MS); nurse anesthesia (MS); school nurse certification (MS). *Program availability:* Part-time, evening/weekend. *Entrance requirements:* For master's, GRE (if GPA less than 3.0), 2 letters of recommendation, resume, personal statement, official transcripts. Additional exam requirements/recommendations for international students: Required—TOEFL (minimum score 550 paper-based; 80 iBT), IELTS (minimum score 6.5). Electronic applications accepted.

Saint Joseph's University, Erivan K. Haub School of Business, Professional MBA Program, Philadelphia, PA 19131-1395. Offers accounting (MBA, Postbaccalaureate Certificate); business intelligence (MBA); finance (MBA); general business (MBA); health and medical services administration (MBA); international business (MBA); international marketing (MBA); managing human capital (MBA); marketing (MBA); DO/MBA. DO/MBA offered jointly with Philadelphia College of Osteopathic Medicine. *Program availability:* Part-time, evening/weekend. *Degree requirements:* For master's and Postbaccalaureate Certificate, minimum GPA of 3.0. *Entrance requirements:* For master's, GMAT or GRE, 2 letters of recommendation, resume, personal statement, official undergraduate and graduate transcripts; for Postbaccalaureate Certificate, official master's-level transcripts. Additional exam requirements/recommendations for international students: Required—TOEFL (minimum score 550 paper-based, 80 iBT), IELTS (minimum score 6.5), or PTE (minimum score 60). Electronic applications accepted.

Saint Leo University, Graduate Business Studies, Saint Leo, FL 33574-6665. Offers accounting (M Acc, MBA); cybersecurity (MS); health care management (MBA); human resource management (MBA); information security management (MBA); marketing (MBA); marketing research and social media analytics (MBA); project management (MBA); sport business (MBA). *Accreditation:* ACBSP. *Program availability:* Part-time, evening/weekend, online learning. *Faculty:* 49 full-time (12 women), 63 part-time/adjunct (24 women). *Students:* 1,887 full-time (1,024 women), 7 part-time (3 women); includes 821 minority (603 Black or African American, non-Hispanic/Latino; 5 American Indian or

Health Services Management and Hospital Administration

Alaska Native, non-Hispanic/Latino; 35 Asian, non-Hispanic/Latino; 156 Hispanic/Latino; 2 Native Hawaiian or other Pacific Islander, non-Hispanic/Latino; 20 Two or more races, non-Hispanic/Latino; 35 international. Average age 38. In 2015, 782 master's awarded. *Entrance requirements:* For master's, GMAT (minimum score 500 if applicant has less than 3.0 in the last two years of undergraduate study), bachelor's degree with minimum GPA of 3.0 in the last 60 hours of coursework from regionally-accredited college or university; 2 years of professional work experience; resume; 2 letters of recommendation. Additional exam requirements/recommendations for international students: Required—TOEFL (minimum score 550 paper-based; 80 iBT). *Application deadline:* For fall admission, 7/1 priority date for domestic and international students; for spring admission, 11/12 priority date for domestic students, 11/1 for international students. Applications are processed on a rolling basis. Application fee: $80. Electronic applications accepted. *Expenses:* Contact institution. *Financial support:* In 2015–16, 116 students received support. Career-related internships or fieldwork, scholarships/grants, and health care benefits available. Financial award application deadline: 3/1; financial award applicants required to submit FAFSA. *Unit head:* Dr. Lorrie McGovern, Assistant Dean, Graduate Studies in Business, 352-588-7390, Fax: 352-588-8912, E-mail: mbaslu@saintleo.edu. *Application contact:* Jennifer Shelley, Senior Associate Director of Graduate Admissions, 800-707-8846, Fax: 352-588-7873, E-mail: grad.admissions@saintleo.edu.
Website: http://www.saintleo.edu/academics/graduate.aspx

Saint Louis University, Graduate Education, School of Public Health and Graduate Education, Department of Health Management and Policy, St. Louis, MO 63103. Offers health administration (MHA); health policy (MPH); public health studies (PhD). *Accreditation:* CAHME. *Program availability:* Part-time. *Degree requirements:* For master's, comprehensive exam, internship. *Entrance requirements:* For master's, GMAT or GRE General Test, LSAT, MCAT, letters of recommendation, resume. Additional exam requirements/recommendations for international students: Required—TOEFL (minimum score 525 paper-based). *Faculty research:* Management of HIV/AIDS, rural health services, prevention of asthma, genetics and health services use, health insurance and access to care.

Saint Mary's University of Minnesota, Schools of Graduate and Professional Programs, Graduate School of Health and Human Services, Health and Human Services Administration Program, Winona, MN 55987-1399. Offers MA. Tuition and fees vary according to degree level and program. *Unit head:* Susan Doherty, Director, 612-238-4549, E-mail: sdoherty@smumn.edu. *Application contact:* James Callinan, Director of Admissions for Graduate and Professional Programs, 612-728-5185, Fax: 612-728-5121, E-mail: jcallina@smumn.edu.
Website: http://www.smumn.edu/graduate-home/areas-of-study/graduate-school-of-health-human-services/ma-in-health-human-services-administration

St. Norbert College, Program in Business Administration, De Pere, WI 54115-2099. Offers business (MBA); health care (MBA); supply chain and manufacturing (MBA). *Program availability:* Part-time. *Faculty:* 4 full-time (0 women), 2 part-time/adjunct (0 women). *Students:* 31 part-time (10 women); includes 2 minority (1 American Indian or Alaska Native, non-Hispanic/Latino; 1 Two or more races, non-Hispanic/Latino). Average age 33. 35 applicants, 94% accepted, 31 enrolled. *Entrance requirements:* For master's, official transcripts, letters of recommendation, professional resume, essay. *Application deadline:* For fall admission, 8/5 for domestic students; for spring admission, 3/7 for domestic students. Applications are processed on a rolling basis. Application fee: $50. Electronic applications accepted. *Expenses:* $675 per credit; $37.50 per course technology fee. *Financial support:* Federal Work-Study available. Financial award application deadline: 3/1; financial award applicants required to submit FAFSA. *Unit head:* Lisa Gray, Executive Assistant, 920-403-3449, E-mail: lisa.gray@snc.edu. *Application contact:* Brenda Busch, Associate Director of Graduate Recruitment, 920-403-3942, Fax: 920-403-4072, E-mail: brenda.busch@snc.edu.
Website: http://www.snc.edu/mba/

Saint Peter's University, Graduate Business Programs, MBA Program, Jersey City, NJ 07306-5997. Offers finance (MBA); health care administration (MBA); human resource management (MBA); international business (MBA); management (MBA); management information systems (MBA); marketing (MBA); risk management (MBA); MBA/MS. *Program availability:* Part-time, evening/weekend. *Entrance requirements:* Additional exam requirements/recommendations for international students: Required—TOEFL. Electronic applications accepted. *Faculty research:* Finance, health care management, human resource management, international business, management, management information systems, marketing, risk management.

St. Thomas University, School of Business, Department of Management, Miami Gardens, FL 33054-6459. Offers accounting (MBA); general management (MSM, Certificate); health management (MBA, MSM, Certificate); human resource management (MBA, MSM, Certificate); international business (MBA, MIB, MSM, Certificate); justice administration (MSM, Certificate); management accounting (MSM, Certificate); public management (MSM, Certificate); sports administration (MS). *Program availability:* Part-time, evening/weekend. *Degree requirements:* For master's, comprehensive exam. *Entrance requirements:* For master's, interview, minimum GPA of 3.0 or GMAT. Additional exam requirements/recommendations for international students: Required—TOEFL (minimum score 550 paper-based; 79 iBT). Electronic applications accepted.

Saint Xavier University, Graduate Studies, Graham School of Management, Chicago, IL 60655-3105. Offers employee health benefits (Certificate); finance (MBA); financial fraud examination and management (MBA, Certificate); financial planning (MBA, Certificate); generalist/individualized (MBA); health administration (MBA); managed care (Certificate); management (MBA); marketing (MBA); project management (MBA, MBA/MS. *Accreditation:* AACSB; ACBSP. *Program availability:* Part-time, evening/weekend. *Entrance requirements:* For master's, GMAT, minimum GPA of 3.0, 2 years of work experience. Electronic applications accepted. *Expenses:* Contact institution.

Salve Regina University, Program in Business Administration, Newport, RI 02840-4192. Offers cybersecurity issues in business (MBA); entrepreneurial enterprise (MBA); health care administration and management (MBA); social ventures (MBA). *Program availability:* Part-time, evening/weekend, online learning. *Entrance requirements:* For master's, GMAT, GRE General Test, or MAT, 6 undergraduate credits each in accounting, economics, quantitative analysis and calculus or statistics. Additional exam requirements/recommendations for international students: Required—TOEFL (minimum score 000 paper-based, 100 iBT) or IELTS. Electronic applications accepted.

Salve Regina University, Program in Healthcare Administration and Management, Newport, RI 02840-4192. Offers MS, CGS. *Program availability:* Part-time, evening/weekend, online learning. *Degree requirements:* For master's, internship. *Entrance requirements:* For master's, GMAT, GRE General Test, or MAT, health care work experience or 250 internship hours. Additional exam requirements/recommendations for international students: Required—TOEFL (minimum score 600 paper-based; 100 iBT) or IELTS. Electronic applications accepted.

Samford University, Ida V. Moffett School of Nursing, Birmingham, AL 35229. Offers administration (DNP); advanced practice (DNP); family nurse practitioner (MSN); health

systems management and leadership (MSN); nurse anesthesia (MSN); nurse educator (MSN). *Accreditation:* AACN; AANA/CANAEP (one or more programs are accredited). *Program availability:* Part-time, blended/hybrid learning. *Faculty:* 19 full-time (all women), 5 part-time/adjunct (1 woman). *Students:* 300 full-time (228 women), 40 part-time (36 women); includes 65 minority (28 Black or African American, non-Hispanic/Latino; 4 American Indian or Alaska Native, non-Hispanic/Latino; 8 Asian, non-Hispanic/Latino; 13 Hispanic/Latino; 12 Two or more races, non-Hispanic/Latino). Average age 35. 69 applicants, 77% accepted, 52 enrolled. In 2015, 98 master's, 16 doctorates awarded. *Degree requirements:* For doctorate, capstone project with oral presentation. *Entrance requirements:* For master's, MAT; GRE (for nurse anesthesia), unencumbered licensure as registered nurse; BSN from CCNE, CNEA, or ACEN (formerly NLNAC) accredited program; minimum cumulative GPA of 3.0 in nursing courses; video submission; one undergraduate course in nursing research with minimum grade of C; for doctorate, unencumbered licensure as registered nurse; master's degree from CCNE, CNEA or ACEN (formerly NLNAC) accredited program in the area of advanced practice or administration; minimum master's degree cumulative GPA of 3.5; video interview submission. Additional exam requirements/recommendations for international students: Required—TOEFL (minimum score 550 paper-based; 80 iBT). *Application deadline:* For fall admission, 6/1 for domestic and international students; for spring admission, 9/1 for domestic and international students. Application fee: $65. Electronic applications accepted. *Expenses: Tuition, area resident:* Full-time $18,673; part-time $766 per credit hour. *Required fees:* $550. Tuition and fees vary according to course load, degree level and student level. *Financial support:* In 2015–16, 56 students received support. Institutionally sponsored loans, scholarships/grants, and traineeships available. Financial award application deadline: 3/1; financial award applicants required to submit FAFSA. *Faculty research:* Issues in rural health care, vulnerable populations, genetics and disabilities in pediatrics, geriatrics, parish nursing research, interprofessional education, global health disparities. *Unit head:* Dr. Nena F. Sanders, Vice Provost, College of Health Sciences/Dean/Professor, 205-726-2612, Fax: 205-726-4179, E-mail: nfsander@samford.edu. *Application contact:* Allyson Maddox, Director of Graduate Student Services, Ida V. Moffett School of Nursing, 205-726-2047, Fax: 205-726-4179, E-mail: amaddox@samford.edu.
Website: http://samford.edu/nursing

San Diego State University, Graduate and Research Affairs, College of Health and Human Services, Graduate School of Public Health, San Diego, CA 92182. Offers environmental health (MPH); epidemiology (MPH, PhD), including biostatistics (MPH); global emergency preparedness and response (MS); global health (PhD); health behavior (PhD); health promotion (MPH); health services administration (MPH); toxicology (MS); MPH/MA; MSW/MPH. *Accreditation:* CAHME (one or more programs are accredited); CEPH (one or more programs are accredited). *Program availability:* Part-time. *Degree requirements:* For master's, comprehensive exam (for some programs), thesis (for some programs); for doctorate, thesis/dissertation. *Entrance requirements:* For master's, GMAT (in health services administration), GRE General Test; for doctorate, GRE General Test. Additional exam requirements/recommendations for international students: Required—TOEFL. *Faculty research:* Evaluation of tobacco, AIDS prevalence and prevention, mammography, infant death project, Alzheimer's in elderly Chinese.

San Francisco State University, Division of Graduate Studies, College of Business, Program in Business Administration, San Francisco, CA 94132-1722. Offers decision sciences/operations research (MBA); ethics and compliance (MBA); finance (MBA); global business and innovation (MBA); healthcare administration (MBA); hospitality and tourism management (MBA); information systems (MBA); leadership (MBA); marketing (MBA); nonprofit and social enterprise leadership (MBA); sustainable business (MBA). *Accreditation:* AACSB. *Program availability:* Part-time, evening/weekend. *Faculty:* 100. *Degree requirements:* For master's, thesis, essay test. *Entrance requirements:* For master's, GMAT, minimum GPA of 2.7 in last 60 units. Additional exam requirements/recommendations for international students: Required—TOEFL (minimum score 550 paper-based). *Application deadline:* For fall admission, 5/1 priority date for domestic students, 4/1 for international students; for spring admission, 11/1 for domestic students, 10/15 for international students. Applications are processed on a rolling basis. Application fee: $55. *Expenses:* Tuition, state resident: full-time $6738. Tuition, nonresident: full-time $15,666. *Required fees:* $1004. *Financial support:* Application deadline: 3/1. *Unit head:* Dr. Bruce Patton, Faculty Director, 415-817-4363, Fax: 415-817-4340, E-mail: bpaton@sfsu.edu. *Application contact:* Manuel Maranan, Director of Admissions, Recruitment and External Relations, 415-817-4323, Fax: 415-817-4340, E-mail: mmaranan@sfsu.edu.
Website: http://cob.sfsu.edu/cob/graduate-programs/mba

Seton Hall University, College of Arts and Sciences, Department of Public and Healthcare Administration, South Orange, NJ 07079-2697. Offers nonprofit organization management (Graduate Certificate); public administration (MPA), including health policy and management, nonprofit organization management, public service: leadership, governance, and policy. *Accreditation:* CAHME; NASPAA. *Program availability:* Part-time, evening/weekend. *Degree requirements:* For master's, thesis or alternative, internship or practicum. *Entrance requirements:* Additional exam requirements/recommendations for international students: Required—TOEFL. Electronic applications accepted.

Seton Hall University, College of Nursing, South Orange, NJ 07079-2697. Offers advanced practice in primary health care (MSN, DNP), including adult/gerontological nurse practitioner, pediatric nurse practitioner; entry into practice (MSN); health systems administration (MSN, DNP); nursing (PhD); nursing case management (MSN); nursing education (MA); school nurse (MSN); MSN/MA. *Accreditation:* AACN. *Program availability:* Part-time, online learning. *Degree requirements:* For master's, research project; for doctorate, dissertation or scholarly project. *Entrance requirements:* For doctorate, GRE (waived for students with GPA of 3.5 or higher). Additional exam requirements/recommendations for international students: Required—TOEFL. Electronic applications accepted. *Faculty research:* Parent/child, adult, and gerontological nursing; breast cancer; families of children with HIV; parish nursing.

Shenandoah University, Harry F. Byrd, Jr. School of Business, Winchester, VA 22601-5195. Offers business (MBA); healthcare management (Certificate). *Accreditation:* AACSB. *Program availability:* Part-time, evening/weekend. *Faculty:* 18 full-time (6 women), 2 part-time/adjunct (0 women). *Students:* 33 full-time (12 women), 42 part-time (25 women); includes 21 minority (10 Black or African American, non-Hispanic/Latino; 2 American Indian or Alaska Native, non-Hispanic/Latino; 5 Asian, non-Hispanic/Latino; 3 Hispanic/Latino; 1 Native Hawaiian or other Pacific Islander, non-Hispanic/Latino), 16 international. Average age 31. 113 applicants, 46% accepted, 24 enrolled. In 2015, 41 master's, 2 other advanced degrees awarded. *Entrance requirements:* For master's, transcripts from all institutions of higher learning; minimum GPA of 3.0 in appropriate undergraduate course work; 2 letters of recommendation; resume; interview; brief narrative essay (2-3 pages) of career, professional development and goals, as they relate to the completion of an MBA; for Certificate, 2 letters of recommendation, resume, interview, brief narrative, transcripts from all institutions of higher learning attended. Additional exam requirements/recommendations for international students: Required—TOEFL (minimum score 550 paper-based; 79 iBT). *Application deadline:* For fall

Health Services Management and Hospital Administration

admission, 5/1 for domestic and international students; for spring admission, 11/1 for domestic and international students; for summer admission, 3/1 for domestic and international students. Application fee: $30. Electronic applications accepted. *Expenses:* $29,880 tuition, $1,240 fees (including technology fee and student services fee). *Financial support:* In 2015–16, 24 students received support. Scholarships/grants and unspecified assistantships available. Financial award application deadline: 3/15; financial award applicants required to submit FAFSA. *Faculty research:* Sustainability, green initiatives, lean manufacturing, healthcare economics. *Unit head:* Miles K. Davis, PhD, Dean, 540-665-4572, Fax: 540-665-5437, E-mail: mdavi3@su.edu. *Application contact:* Andrew Woodall, Executive Director of Recruitment and Admissions, 540-665-4581, Fax: 540-665-4627, E-mail: admit@su.edu.
Website: http://www.su.edu/business/

Siena Heights University, Graduate College, Adrian, MI 49221-1796. Offers clinical mental health counseling (MA); educational leadership (Specialist); leadership (MA), including health care leadership, organizational leadership; teacher education (MA), including early childhood education, early childhood education: Montessori, education leadership: principal, elementary education: reading K-12, leadership: higher education, secondary education: reading K-12, special education: cognitive impairment, special education: learning disabilities. *Program availability:* Part-time, evening/weekend. *Degree requirements:* For master's, thesis, presentation. *Entrance requirements:* For master's, minimum GPA of 3.0, current resume, essay, all post-secondary transcripts, 3 letters of reference, conviction disclosure form; copy of teaching certificate (for some education programs); for Specialist, master's degree, minimum GPA of 3.0, current resume, essay, all post-secondary transcripts, 3 letters of reference, conviction disclosure form; copy of teaching certificate (for some education programs). Electronic applications accepted.

Simmons College, School of Management, Boston, MA 02115. Offers business administration (MBA); health care (MBA); management (MS), including communications management, non-profit management; MBA/MSW; MS/MA. *Accreditation:* AACSB. *Program availability:* Part-time, evening/weekend. *Faculty:* 17 full-time (12 women), 9 part-time/adjunct (8 women). *Students:* 66 full-time (59 women), 144 part-time (133 women); includes 55 minority (26 Black or African American, non-Hispanic/Latino; 11 Asian, non-Hispanic/Latino; 16 Hispanic/Latino; 2 Two or more races, non-Hispanic/Latino), 18 international. Average age 32. 105 applicants, 88% accepted, 49 enrolled. In 2015, 86 master's awarded. *Entrance requirements:* For master's, GMAT or GRE. Additional exam requirements/recommendations for international students: Required—TOEFL. *Application deadline:* Applications are processed on a rolling basis. Application fee: $75. Electronic applications accepted. *Expenses:* Contact institution. *Financial support:* Scholarships/grants and unspecified assistantships available. Financial award applicants required to submit FAFSA. *Faculty research:* Gender and organizations, leadership, health care management. *Unit head:* Cathy Minehan, Dean, 617-521-2846. *Application contact:* Melissa Terrio, Director of Graduate Admissions, 617-521-3840, Fax: 617-521-3880, E-mail: somadm@simmons.edu.
Website: http://www.simmons.edu/som

Southeast Missouri State University, School of Graduate Studies, Harrison College of Business, Cape Girardeau, MO 63701-4799. Offers accounting (MBA); entrepreneurship (MBA); environmental management (MBA); financial management (MBA); general management (MBA); health administration (MBA); industrial management (MBA); international business (MBA); organizational management (MS); sport management (MBA). *Accreditation:* AACSB. *Program availability:* Part-time, evening/weekend, online learning. *Faculty:* 27 full-time (7 women), 1 (woman) part-time/adjunct. *Students:* 68 full-time (40 women), 132 part-time (46 women); includes 21 minority (9 Black or African American, non-Hispanic/Latino; 9 Asian, non-Hispanic/Latino; 2 Hispanic/Latino; 1 Two or more races, non-Hispanic/Latino), 60 international. Average age 30. In 2015, 57 master's awarded. *Degree requirements:* For master's, variable foreign language requirement, comprehensive exam (for some programs), thesis or alternative, applied research project, 33 credit hours. *Entrance requirements:* For master's, GMAT or GRE, minimum undergraduate GPA of 2.5, minimum grade of C in prerequisite courses. Additional exam requirements/recommendations for international students: Required—TOEFL (minimum score 550 paper-based; 79 iBT), IELTS (minimum score 6), PTE (minimum score 53). *Application deadline:* For fall admission, 8/1 for domestic students, 6/1 for international students; for spring admission, 11/21 for domestic students, 10/1 for international students; for summer admission, 5/15 for domestic students. Applications are processed on a rolling basis. Application fee: $30 ($40 for international students). Electronic applications accepted. *Expenses:* Tuition, state resident: part-time $260.80 per credit hour. Tuition, nonresident: part-time $486.80 per credit hour. *Required fees:* $33.70 per credit hour. *Financial support:* In 2015–16, 60 students received support. Career-related internships or fieldwork, Federal Work-Study, scholarships/grants, traineeships, tuition waivers (full), and unspecified assistantships available. Financial award application deadline: 6/30; financial award applicants required to submit FAFSA. *Faculty research:* Organizational justice, ethics, leadership, corporate finance, generational differences. *Unit head:* Dr. Kenneth A. Heischmidt, Director, Graduate Business Studies, 573-651-2912, Fax: 573-651-5032, E-mail: kheischmidt@semo.edu. *Application contact:* Gail Amick, Admissions Specialist, 573-651-2590, Fax: 573-651-5936, E-mail: gamick@semo.edu.
Website: http://www.semo.edu/mba

Southern Adventist University, School of Business and Management, Collegedale, TN 37315-0370. Offers accounting (MBA); church administration (MSA); church and nonprofit leadership (MBA); financial management (MFM); healthcare administration (MBA); management (MBA); marketing management (MBA); outdoor education (MSA). *Program availability:* Part-time, evening/weekend, online learning. *Entrance requirements:* For master's, GMAT. Additional exam requirements/recommendations for international students: Required—TOEFL (minimum score 600 paper-based; 100 iBT). Electronic applications accepted.

Southern Illinois University Carbondale, School of Law, Program in Legal Studies, Carbondale, IL 62901-4701. Offers general law (MLS); health law and policy (MLS). *Students:* 8 full-time (6 women), 2 part-time (1 woman); includes 3 minority (all Black or African American, non-Hispanic/Latino). 14 applicants, 57% accepted, 5 enrolled. In 2015, 7 master's awarded. Application fee: $65. *Unit head:* Lisa David, Admissions Coordinator, 618-453-8767, E-mail: ldavid@law.siu.edu.

Southern Nazarene University, College of Professional and Graduate Studies, School of Business, Bethany, OK 73008. Offers business administration (MBA); health care management (MBA); management (MS Mgt). *Accreditation:* ACBSP. *Program availability:* Part-time, evening/weekend, online learning. *Degree requirements:* For master's, thesis optional. *Entrance requirements:* For master's, resume. Additional exam requirements/recommendations for international students: Required—TOEFL (minimum score 550 paper-based; 80 iBT), IELTS (minimum score 7). Electronic applications accepted.

Southern New Hampshire University, School of Business, Manchester, NH 03106-1045. Offers accounting (MBA, MS, Graduate Certificate); accounting finance (MS); accounting/auditing (MS); accounting/forensic accounting (MS); accounting/taxation (MS); athletic administration (MBA, Graduate Certificate); business administration

(IMBA, MBA, Certificate, Graduate Certificate), including accounting (Certificate), business administration (MBA), business information systems (Graduate Certificate), human resource management (Certificate); corporate social responsibility (MBA); entrepreneurship (MBA); finance (MBA, MS, Graduate Certificate); finance/corporate finance (MS); finance/investments and securities (MS); forensic accounting (MBA); healthcare informatics (MBA); healthcare management (MBA); human resource management (Graduate Certificate); information technology (MS, Graduate Certificate); information technology management (MBA); international business (Graduate Certificate); international business and information technology (Graduate Certificate); international finance (Graduate Certificate); international sport management (Graduate Certificate); justice studies (MBA); leadership of nonprofit organizations (Graduate Certificate); marketing (MBA, MS, Graduate Certificate); operations and project management (MS); operations and supply chain management (MBA, Graduate Certificate); organizational leadership (MS); project management (MBA, Graduate Certificate); Six Sigma (MBA); Six Sigma quality (Graduate Certificate); social media marketing (MBA); sport management (MBA, MS, Graduate Certificate); sustainability and environmental compliance (MBA); workplace conflict management (MBA); MBA/Certificate. *Accreditation:* ACBSP. *Program availability:* Part-time, evening/weekend, online learning. Terminal master's awarded for partial completion of doctoral program. *Degree requirements:* For master's, one foreign language, comprehensive exam (for some programs), thesis or alternative. *Entrance requirements:* For master's, minimum GPA of 2.5. Additional exam requirements/recommendations for international students: Required—TOEFL (minimum score 500 paper-based). Electronic applications accepted.

South University, Graduate Programs, College of Business, Program in Healthcare Administration, Savannah, GA 31406. Offers MBA.

South University, Program in Business Administration, Royal Palm Beach, FL 33411. Offers business administration (MDA); healthcare administration (MBA)

South University, Program in Healthcare Administration, Columbia, SC 29203. Offers MBA.

South University, Program in Healthcare Administration, Montgomery, AL 36116-1120. Offers MBA.

South University, Program in Healthcare Administration, Tampa, FL 33614. Offers MBA.

Southwest Baptist University, Program in Business, Bolivar, MO 65613-2597. Offers business administration (MBA); health administration (MBA). *Accreditation:* ACBSP. *Program availability:* Part-time, online learning. *Degree requirements:* For master's, comprehensive exam. *Entrance requirements:* For master's, interviews, minimum GPA of 2.75. Additional exam requirements/recommendations for international students: Required—TOEFL (minimum score 550 paper-based).

Stevenson University, Program in Healthcare Management, Owings Mills, MD 21117. Offers project management (MS); quality management and patient safety (MS). *Program availability:* Part-time, online only, 100% online. *Faculty:* 2 full-time (both women), 7 part-time/adjunct (5 women). *Students:* 6 full-time (5 women), 25 part-time (21 women); includes 15 minority (9 Black or African American, non-Hispanic/Latino; 5 Asian, non-Hispanic/Latino; 1 Hispanic/Latino). Average age 32. 28 applicants, 32% accepted, 5 enrolled. In 2015, 2 master's awarded. *Degree requirements:* For master's, capstone course. *Entrance requirements:* For master's, official college transcripts from all previous academic work, minimum cumulative GPA of 3.0 in past academic work, minimum grade of B in statistics or an upper-level math and English composition, two professional letters of recommendation with at least one from a current or past supervisor, 250-word personal statement. Additional exam requirements/recommendations for international students: Required—TOEFL (minimum score 550 paper-based), IELTS (minimum score 6.5). *Application deadline:* Applications are processed on a rolling basis. Electronic applications accepted. *Expenses:* $670 per credit, $125 fee per semester. *Financial support:* Applicants required to submit FAFSA. *Unit head:* Sharon Buchbinder, PhD, Coordinator, 443-394-9290, Fax: 443-394-0538, E-mail: sbuchbinder@stevenson.edu. *Application contact:* Amanda Courter, Enrollment Counselor, 443-352-4243, Fax: 443-394-0538, E-mail: acourter@stevenson.edu.
Website: http://www.stevenson.edu

Stony Brook University, State University of New York, Graduate School, College of Business, Program in Business Administration, Stony Brook, NY 11794. Offers accounting (MBA); business administration (MBA); finance (MBA, Certificate); health care management (MBA); innovation, human resources, management, or operations management (MBA); marketing (MBA). *Faculty:* 37 full-time (11 women), 18 part-time/adjunct (5 women). *Students:* 190 full-time (101 women), 124 part-time (50 women); includes 73 minority (10 Black or African American, non-Hispanic/Latino; 1 American Indian or Alaska Native, non-Hispanic/Latino; 41 Asian, non-Hispanic/Latino; 16 Hispanic/Latino; 1 Native Hawaiian or other Pacific Islander, non-Hispanic/Latino; 4 Two or more races, non-Hispanic/Latino), 75 international. Average age 29. 262 applicants, 68% accepted, 81 enrolled. In 2015, 114 master's awarded. *Entrance requirements:* For master's, GMAT, 3 letters of recommendation from current or former employers or professors, transcripts, personal statement, resume. Additional exam requirements/recommendations for international students: Required—TOEFL (minimum score 550 paper-based; 90 iBT), IELTS (minimum score 6.5). *Application deadline:* For fall admission, 6/1 for domestic students, 3/15 for international students; for spring admission, 12/1 for domestic students, 11/1 for international students. Application fee: $100. *Expenses:* $15,961 per year full-time resident tuition and fees, $600 per credit hour; $25,941 per year full-time non-resident tuition and fees, $1,016 per credit hour. *Financial support:* In 2015–16, 1 teaching assistantship was awarded. *Total annual research expenditures:* $2,800. *Unit head:* Dr. Manuel London, Dean and Director, Center for Human Resource Management, 631-632-7159, Fax: 631-632-8181, E-mail: manuel.london@stonybrook.edu. *Application contact:* Dr. Jadranka Skorin-Kapov, Graduate Program Director, 631-632-7171, Fax: 631-632-8181, E-mail: jadranka.skorin-kapov@stonybrook.edu.

Stony Brook University, State University of New York, Stony Brook Medicine, School of Health Technology and Management, Stony Brook, NY 11794. Offers health care management (Advanced Certificate); health care policy and management (MS); occupational therapy (MS); physical therapy (DPT); physician assistant (MS). *Accreditation:* APTA. *Faculty:* 67 full-time (41 women), 64 part-time/adjunct (45 women). *Students:* 488 full-time (301 women), 99 part-time (82 women); includes 167 minority (34 Black or African American, non-Hispanic/Latino; 3 American Indian or Alaska Native, non-Hispanic/Latino; 84 Asian, non-Hispanic/Latino; 41 Hispanic/Latino; 5 Two or more races, non-Hispanic/Latino), 12 international. Average age 28. 2,646 applicants, 14% accepted, 260 enrolled. In 2015, 104 master's, 71 doctorates, 34 other advanced degrees awarded. *Degree requirements:* For master's, thesis. *Entrance requirements:* For master's, GRE General Test, minimum GPA of 3.0, work experience in field, references; for doctorate, GRE, references. Additional exam requirements/recommendations for international students: Required—TOEFL (minimum score 550 paper-based). *Application deadline:* For fall admission, 1/15 for domestic students; for spring admission, 10/1 for domestic students. Application fee: $100. *Expenses:* Contact institution. *Financial support:* Fellowships, research assistantships, teaching assistantships, career-related internships or fieldwork, Federal Work-Study, and

Health Services Management and Hospital Administration

institutionally sponsored loans available. Financial award application deadline: 3/15. *Faculty research:* Health promotion and disease prevention. *Total annual research expenditures:* $1.3 million. *Unit head:* Dr. Craig A. Lehmann, Dean, 631-444-2252, Fax: 631-444-7621, E-mail: craig.lehmann@stonybrook.edu. *Application contact:* Dr. Richard W. Johnson, Associate Dean for Graduate Studies, 631-444-3251, Fax: 631-444-7621, E-mail: richard.johnson@stonybrook.edu.
Website: http://healthtechnology.stonybrookmedicine.edu/

Stony Brook University, State University of New York, Stony Brook Medicine, School of Nursing, Program in Nursing Practice, Stony Brook, NY 11794. Offers DNP. *Program availability:* Part-time, blended/hybrid learning. *Students:* 35 full-time (33 women), 29 part-time (28 women); includes 30 minority (14 Black or African American, non-Hispanic/Latino; 1 American Indian or Alaska Native, non-Hispanic/Latino; 10 Asian, non-Hispanic/Latino; 5 Hispanic/Latino). Average age 41. 38 applicants, 79% accepted, 25 enrolled. In 2015, 20 doctorates awarded. *Degree requirements:* For doctorate, project. *Entrance requirements:* For doctorate, minimum GPA of 3.0. Additional exam requirements/recommendations for international students: Required—TOEFL (minimum score 90 iBT). *Application deadline:* For fall admission, 12/1 for domestic and international students. Application fee: $100. *Expenses:* $24,781 full-time resident tuition and fees, $968 per credit hour; $44,431 full-time nonresident tuition and fees, $1,787 per credit hour. *Unit head:* Corrine Jurgens, Program Director, 631-444-3236, Fax: 631-444-3136, E-mail: corrine.jurgens@stonybroko.edu. *Application contact:* Dr. Dolores Bilges, Senior Staff Assistant, 631-444-2644, Fax: 631-444-3136, E-mail: dnp.nursing@stonybrook.edu.
Website: http://www.nursing.stonybrookmedicine.edu/

Stratford University, School of Graduate Studies, Falls Church, VA 22043. Offers business administration (IMBA, MBA); cyber security (MS); cyber security leadership and policy (MS); digital forensics (MS); entrepreneurship (IMBA); finance (IMBA); global leadership (IMBA); healthcare administration (MS); information systems (MS); information technology (DIT); information technology and e-commerce (IMBA); international hospitality management (MS); marketing (IMBA); networking and telecommunications (MS); software engineering (MS). *Program availability:* Part-time, evening/weekend, 100% online, blended/hybrid learning. *Students:* 703 full-time (226 women), 189 part-time (101 women); includes 681 minority (172 Black or African American, non-Hispanic/Latino; 38 American Indian or Alaska Native, non-Hispanic/Latino; 445 Asian, non-Hispanic/Latino; 16 Hispanic/Latino; 8 Native Hawaiian or other Pacific Islander, non-Hispanic/Latino; 2 Two or more races, non-Hispanic/Latino). Average age 30. *Degree requirements:* For master's, comprehensive exam, capstone project. *Entrance requirements:* For master's, GRE or GMAT, baccalaureate degree. Additional exam requirements/recommendations for international students: Required—TOEFL (minimum score 79 iBT) or IELTS (6.5). *Application deadline:* Applications are processed on a rolling basis. Application fee: $50. Electronic applications accepted. *Expenses:* $495 per credit; $2,227.50 per course; $100 one-time student activity fee; $235 graduation fee. *Financial support:* Federal Work-Study and scholarships/grants available. Financial award applicants required to submit FAFSA. *Unit head:* Dr. Richard R. Shurtz, President, 703-539-6890, Fax: 703-539-6960. *Application contact:* Admissions, 800-444-0804, E-mail: fcadmissions@stratford.edu.

Strayer University, Graduate Studies, Washington, DC 20005-2603. Offers accounting (MS); acquisition (MBA); business administration (MBA); communications technology (MS); educational management (M Ed); finance (MBA); health services administration (MHSA); hospitality and tourism management (MBA); human resource management (MBA); information systems (MS), including computer security management, decision support system management, enterprise resource management, network management, software engineering management, systems development management; management (MBA); management information systems (MS); marketing (MBA); professional accounting (MS), including accounting information systems, controllership, taxation; public administration (MPA); supply chain management (MBA); technology in education (M Ed). Programs also offered at campus locations in Birmingham, AL; Chamblee, GA; Cobb County, GA; Morrow, GA; White Marsh, MD; Charleston, SC; Columbia, SC; Greensboro, NC; Greenville, SC; Lexington, KY; Louisville, KY; Nashville, TN; North Raleigh, NC; Washington, DC. *Program availability:* Part-time, evening/weekend, online learning. *Degree requirements:* For master's, thesis. *Entrance requirements:* For master's, GMAT, GRE General Test, bachelor's degree from an accredited college or university, minimum undergraduate GPA of 2.75. Electronic applications accepted.

Suffolk University, Sawyer Business School, Master of Business Administration Program, Boston, MA 02108-2770. Offers accounting (MBA); business administration (APC); entrepreneurship (MBA); executive business administration (EMBA); finance (MBA); global business administration (GMBA); health administration (MBA); international business (MBA); marketing (MBA); nonprofit management (MBA); organizational behavior (MBA); strategic management (MBA); supply chain management (MBA); taxation (MBA); JD/MBA; MBA/MHA; MBA/MSA; MBA/MSF; MBA/MST. *Accreditation:* AACSB. *Program availability:* Part-time, evening/weekend, online learning. *Faculty:* 25 full-time (9 women), 9 part-time/adjunct (2 women). *Students:* 117 full-time (57 women), 294 part-time (152 women); includes 86 minority (32 Black or African American, non-Hispanic/Latino; 17 Asian, non-Hispanic/Latino; 32 Hispanic/Latino; 5 Two or more races, non-Hispanic/Latino), 43 international. Average age 31. 415 applicants, 64% accepted, 114 enrolled. In 2015, 189 master's awarded. *Entrance requirements:* For master's, GMAT, minimum undergraduate GPA of 2.75 (MBA), 5 years of managerial experience (EMBA). Additional exam requirements/recommendations for international students: Required—TOEFL (minimum score 550 paper-based; 80 iBT). *Application deadline:* For fall admission, 6/15 priority date for domestic students, 6/15 for international students; for spring admission, 11/1 priority date for domestic students, 11/1 for international students. Applications are processed on a rolling basis. Application fee: $50. Electronic applications accepted. *Expenses: Tuition, area resident:* Full-time $41,440; part-time $1383 per credit hour. *Required fees:* $52; $52 per unit. Part-time tuition and fees vary according to course load and program. *Financial support:* In 2015–16, 170 students received support, including 149 fellowships with tuition reimbursements available (averaging $9,713 per year); career-related internships or fieldwork, Federal Work-Study, and institutionally sponsored loans also available. Support available to part-time students. Financial award application deadline: 4/1; financial award applicants required to submit FAFSA. *Faculty research:* Foreign investments; career strategies and boundaryless careers; corporate ethics codes; interest rates, inflation, and growth options; innovation and product development performance. *Unit head:* Jodi Detjen, Director of MBA Programs, 617-573-8306, E-mail: jdetjon@suffolk.edu. *Application contact:* Mara Marzocchi, Associate Director of Graduate Admissions, 617-573-8302, Fax: 617-305-1733, E-mail: grad.admission@suffolk.edu.
Website: http://www.suffolk.edu/mba

Suffolk University, Sawyer Business School, Program in Health Administration, Boston, MA 02108-2770. Offers MBAH, MHA. *Program availability:* Part-time, evening/weekend. *Faculty:* 5 full-time (1 woman), 6 part-time/adjunct (4 women). *Students:* 33 full-time (22 women), 63 part-time (46 women); includes 21 minority (14 Black or African American, non-Hispanic/Latino; 4 Asian, non-Hispanic/Latino; 3 Hispanic/Latino), 16 international. Average age 29. 59 applicants, 71% accepted, 24 enrolled. In 2015, 21

master's awarded. *Entrance requirements:* Additional exam requirements/recommendations for international students: Required—TOEFL (minimum score 550 paper-based; 80 iBT). *Application deadline:* For fall admission, 6/15 priority date for domestic students, 6/15 for international students; for spring admission, 11/1 priority date for domestic students, 11/1 for international students. Applications are processed on a rolling basis. Application fee: $50. Electronic applications accepted. *Expenses:* Contact institution. *Financial support:* In 2015–16, 52 students received support, including 52 fellowships (averaging $8,898 per year); career-related internships or fieldwork, Federal Work-Study, and institutionally sponsored loans also available. Support available to part-time students. Financial award application deadline: 4/1; financial award applicants required to submit FAFSA. *Faculty research:* Mental health, federal policy, health care. *Unit head:* Richard Gregg, Director of Programs in Healthcare Administration/Chair of Healthcare Department, 617-994-4246, E-mail: rgregg@suffolk.edu. *Application contact:* Mara Marzocchi, Associate Director of Graduate Admissions, 617-573-8302, Fax: 617-305-1733, E-mail: grad.admission@suffolk.edu.
Website: http://www.suffolk.edu/business/graduate/11532.php

Syracuse University, Maxwell School of Citizenship and Public Affairs, CAS Program in Health Services Management and Policy, Syracuse, NY 13244. Offers health services management and policy (CAS). *Program availability:* Part-time. In 2015, 23 CASs awarded. *Entrance requirements:* For degree, 7 years of mid-level professional experience, resume, personal statement, three letters of recommendation, official transcriptions. Additional exam requirements/recommendations for international students: Required—TOEFL (minimum score 100 iBT). *Application deadline:* For fall admission, 2/1 for domestic students, 2/1 priority date for international students; for spring admission, 8/15 priority date for domestic and international students. Applications are processed on a rolling basis. Application fee: $75. Electronic applications accepted. *Expenses:* Tuition, area resident: Full-time $25,974; part-time $1443 per credit hour. *Required fees:* $802; $50 per course. Tuition and fees vary according to course load and program. *Financial support:* Application deadline: 1/1. *Unit head:* Dr. Thomas H. Dennison, Head, 315-443-9060, Fax: 315-443-9721, E-mail: thdennis@syr.edu. *Application contact:* Margaret Lane, Assistant Director, Executive Education Programs, 315-443-1090, E-mail: melane02@maxwell.syr.edu.
Website: http://www.maxwell.syr.edu/

Temple University, Fox School of Business, MBA Programs, Philadelphia, PA 19122-6096. Offers accounting (MBA); business management (MBA); financial management (MBA); healthcare and life sciences innovation (MBA); human resource management (MBA); international business (IMBA); IT management (MBA); marketing management (MBA); pharmaceutical management (MBA); strategic management (EMBA, MBA). EMBA offered in Philadelphia, PA and Tokyo, Japan. *Accreditation:* AACSB. *Program availability:* Part-time, evening/weekend, online learning. *Entrance requirements:* For master's, GMAT, minimum undergraduate GPA of 3.0. Additional exam requirements/recommendations for international students: Required—TOEFL (minimum score 600 paper-based; 100 iBT), IELTS (minimum score 7.5).

Texas A&M University, School of Public Health, College Station, TX 77843. Offers health administration (MHA); health policy and management (MPH); health promotion and community health sciences (MPH); health services research (PhD). *Accreditation:* CEPH. *Program availability:* Part-time, blended/hybrid learning. *Faculty:* 68. *Students:* 313 full-time (189 women), 71 part-time (41 women); includes 169 minority (40 Black or African American, non-Hispanic/Latino; 38 Asian, non-Hispanic/Latino; 88 Hispanic/Latino; 3 Two or more races, non-Hispanic/Latino), 88 international. Average age 30. 138 applicants, 100% accepted, 126 enrolled. In 2015, 139 master's, 5 doctorates awarded. *Degree requirements:* For master's, thesis optional. *Entrance requirements:* For master's, GRE General Test, 3 letters of recommendation; statement of purpose; current curriculum vitae or resume; official transcripts; for doctorate, GRE General Test, 3 letters of recommendation; statement of purpose; current curriculum vitae or resume; official transcripts; interview (in some cases). Additional exam requirements/recommendations for international students: Required—TOEFL (minimum score 597 paper-based, 95 iBT) or GRE (minimum verbal score 153). *Application deadline:* For fall admission, 8/27 for domestic students; for spring admission, 1/14 for domestic students. Application fee: $120. Electronic applications accepted. *Expenses:* Contact institution. *Financial support:* In 2015–16, 186 students received support, including 2 fellowships with tuition reimbursements available (averaging $17,190 per year), 55 research assistantships with tuition reimbursements available (averaging $5,728 per year), 14 teaching assistantships with tuition reimbursements available (averaging $5,836 per year); career-related internships or fieldwork, institutionally sponsored loans, scholarships/grants, traineeships, health care benefits, tuition waivers (full and partial), and unspecified assistantships also available. Support available to part-time students. Financial award applicants required to submit FAFSA. *Unit head:* Dr. Jay Maddock, Dean, 979-436-9322, Fax: 979-458-1878, E-mail: maddock@tamhsc.edu. *Application contact:* Erin E. Schneider, Associate Director of Admissions and Recruitment, 979-436-9380, E-mail: eschneider@sph.tamhsc.edu.
Website: http://sph.tamhsc.edu

Texas A&M University–Corpus Christi, College of Graduate Studies, College of Business, Corpus Christi, TX 78412-5503. Offers accounting (M Acc); health care administration (MBA); international business (MBA). *Accreditation:* AACSB. *Program availability:* Part-time, evening/weekend, online learning. *Students:* 141 full-time (80 women), 378 part-time (173 women); includes 191 minority (27 Black or African American, non-Hispanic/Latino; 1 American Indian or Alaska Native, non-Hispanic/Latino; 28 Asian, non-Hispanic/Latino; 131 Hispanic/Latino; 4 Two or more races, non-Hispanic/Latino), 119 international. Average age 32. 414 applicants, 53% accepted, 168 enrolled. In 2015, 136 master's awarded. *Degree requirements:* For master's, comprehensive exam, thesis (for some programs). *Entrance requirements:* For master's, GMAT, GRE. Additional exam requirements/recommendations for international students: Required—TOEFL (minimum score 550 paper-based), IELTS (minimum score 6.5). *Application deadline:* For fall admission, 7/15 priority date for domestic students, 5/1 priority date for international students; for spring admission, 11/15 priority date for domestic students, 9/1 priority date for international students; for summer admission, 4/15 priority date for domestic students, 2/1 priority date for international students. Applications are processed on a rolling basis. Application fee: $50 ($70 for international students). Electronic applications accepted. *Financial support:* Research assistantships, teaching assistantships, career-related internships or fieldwork, Federal Work-Study, institutionally sponsored loans, scholarships/grants, health care benefits, and unspecified assistantships available. Support available to part-time students. Financial award application deadline: 3/15; financial award applicants required to submit FAFSA. *Unit head:* Dr. John Gamble, Dean, 361-825-6045, Fax: 361-825-2725, E-mail: john.gamble@tamucc.edu. *Application contact:* Sharon Polansky, Director, Master's Program, 361-825-3448, Fax: 361-825-2755, E-mail: gradweb@tamucc.edu.
Website: http://cob.tamucc.edu

Texas A&M University–Corpus Christi, College of Graduate Studies, College of Nursing and Health Sciences, Corpus Christi, TX 78412-5503. Offers family nurse practitioner (MSN); leadership in nursing systems (MSN); nurse educator (MSN). *Accreditation:* AACN. *Program availability:* Part-time, evening/weekend, online only,

100% online. *Students:* 12 full-time (11 women), 375 part-time (322 women); includes 200 minority (20 Black or African American, non-Hispanic/Latino; 1 American Indian or Alaska Native, non-Hispanic/Latino; 27 Asian, non-Hispanic/Latino; 142 Hispanic/Latino; 3 Native Hawaiian or other Pacific Islander, non-Hispanic/Latino; 7 Two or more races, non-Hispanic/Latino), 1 international. Average age 38. 337 applicants, 42% accepted, 128 enrolled. In 2015, 102 master's awarded. *Degree requirements:* For master's, comprehensive exam, thesis (for some programs), capstone - clinical. *Entrance requirements:* For master's, essay, resume, 3 letters of recommendation, minimum GPA of 3.0. Additional exam requirements/recommendations for international students: Required—TOEFL (minimum score 550 paper-based; 79 iBT), IELTS (minimum score 6.5). *Application deadline:* For fall admission, 4/15 priority date for domestic and international students; for spring admission, 1/7 for domestic and international students; for summer admission, 5/27 for domestic and international students. Applications are processed on a rolling basis. Application fee: $50 ($70 for international students). Electronic applications accepted. *Financial support:* Research assistantships, teaching assistantships, career-related internships or fieldwork, Federal Work-Study, institutionally sponsored loans, scholarships/grants, health care benefits, and unspecified assistantships available. Support available to part-time students. Financial award application deadline: 3/15; financial award applicants required to submit FAFSA. *Unit head:* Dr. Mary Jane Hamilton, Dean, 361-825-2469, E-mail: mary.hamilton@tamucc.edu. *Application contact:* Graduate Admissions Coordinator, 361-825-2177, Fax: 361-825-2755, E-mail: gradweb@tamucc.edu.
Website: http://conhs.tamucc.edu/

Texas A&M University–San Antonio, School of Business, San Antonio, TX 78224. Offers business administration (MBA); enterprise resource planning systems (MBA); finance (MBA); healthcare management (MBA); human resources management (MBA); information assurance and security (MBA); international business (MBA); professional accounting (MPA); project management (MBA); supply chain management (MBA). *Program availability:* Part-time, evening/weekend. *Entrance requirements:* For master's, GMAT. Additional exam requirements/recommendations for international students: Required—TOEFL (minimum score 550 paper-based; 80 iBT), IELTS (minimum score 6). Electronic applications accepted.

Texas Health and Science University, Graduate Programs, Austin, TX 78704. Offers acupuncture and Oriental medicine (MS, DAOM); business administration (MBA); healthcare management (MBA). *Accreditation:* ACAOM. *Faculty:* 8 full-time (3 women), 7 part-time/adjunct (5 women). *Students:* 102 full-time (64 women), 9 part-time (8 women); includes 43 minority (1 Black or African American, non-Hispanic/Latino; 1 American Indian or Alaska Native, non-Hispanic/Latino; 35 Asian, non-Hispanic/Latino; 6 Hispanic/Latino). Average age 34. *Entrance requirements:* For master's, 60 hours applicable to bachelor's degree. Additional exam requirements/recommendations for international students: Required—TOEFL (minimum score 500 paper-based), TWE. *Application deadline:* For fall admission, 8/25 priority date for domestic and international students; for spring admission, 12/22 priority date for domestic and international students. Applications are processed on a rolling basis. Application fee: $75 ($300 for international students). Electronic applications accepted. *Expenses: Tuition, area resident:* Full-time $10,260; part-time $7560 per trimester. *Required fees:* $1600; $1200 per trimester. $600 per trimester. One-time fee: $388. Tuition and fees vary according to course load, degree level and program. *Financial support:* Teaching assistantships with partial tuition reimbursements, career-related internships or fieldwork, Federal Work-Study, institutionally sponsored loans, scholarships/grants, and tuition waivers (partial) available. Financial award applicants required to submit FAFSA. *Unit head:* Dr. David G. Vequist, IV, Vice President of Academic Affairs, 512-444-8082. *Application contact:* Caleb Li, Admissions Coordinator, 512-444-8082, Fax: 512-444-6345, E-mail: admissions@thsu.edu.

Texas Southern University, College of Pharmacy and Health Sciences, Department of Health Sciences, Houston, TX 77004-4584. Offers health care administration (MS). *Program availability:* Online learning. *Entrance requirements:* For master's, PCAT. Electronic applications accepted.

Texas State University, The Graduate College, College of Health Professions, Program in Healthcare Administration, San Marcos, TX 78666. Offers MHA. *Program availability:* Part-time, evening/weekend. *Faculty:* 12 full-time (3 women), 1 part-time/adjunct (0 women). *Students:* 53 full-time (39 women), 17 part-time (12 women); includes 34 minority (13 Black or African American, non-Hispanic/Latino; 5 Asian, non-Hispanic/Latino; 14 Hispanic/Latino; 2 Two or more races, non-Hispanic/Latino), 15 international. Average age 27. 85 applicants, 47% accepted, 23 enrolled. In 2015, 25 master's awarded. *Degree requirements:* For master's, comprehensive exam, thesis optional, committee review. *Entrance requirements:* For master's, GRE General Test, baccalaureate degree from regionally-accredited institution, 3 letters of reference, written statement of purpose, resume. Additional exam requirements/recommendations for international students: Required—TOEFL (minimum score 550 paper-based; 78 iBT). *Application deadline:* For fall admission, 6/1 for domestic and international students; for spring admission, 10/1 for domestic and international students. Applications are processed on a rolling basis. Application fee: $40 ($90 for international students). Electronic applications accepted. *Expenses:* $3,615 in-state tuition (for 12 semester credit hours/1 full-time semester), $974 in-state fees. *Financial support:* In 2015–16, 32 students received support, including 2 research assistantships (averaging $13,428 per year), 17 teaching assistantships (averaging $11,279 per year); career-related internships or fieldwork, Federal Work-Study, institutionally sponsored loans, scholarships/grants, and unspecified assistantships also available. Support available to part-time students. Financial award application deadline: 3/1; financial award applicants required to submit FAFSA. *Unit head:* Dr. Kimberly Ann Lee, Graduate Advisor, 512-245-3492, Fax: 512-245-8712, E-mail: kl12@txstate.edu. *Application contact:* Dr. Andrea Golato, Dean of Graduate School, 512-245-2581, Fax: 512-245-8365, E-mail: gradcollege@txstate.edu.
Website: http://www.health.txstate.edu/ha/degs-progs/mha.html

Texas Tech University, Rawls College of Business Administration, Lubbock, TX 79409-2101. Offers accounting (MSA, PhD), including audit/financial reporting (MSA), taxation (MSA); business statistics (MS, PhD); data science (MS); finance (MS, PhD); general business (MBA); healthcare management (MS); information systems and operations management (PhD); management (PhD); marketing (PhD); STEM (MBA); JD/MBA; JD/MSA; MBA/M Arch; MBA/MD; MBA/MS; MBA/Pharm D. *Accreditation:* AACSB; CAHME (one or more programs are accredited). *Program availability:* Evening/weekend. *Faculty:* 67 full-time (8 women). *Students:* 931 full-time (350 women); includes 226 minority (36 Black or African American, non-Hispanic/Latino; 3 American Indian or Alaska Native, non-Hispanic/Latino; 35 Asian, non-Hispanic/Latino; 132 Hispanic/Latino; 1 Native Hawaiian or other Pacific Islander, non-Hispanic/Latino; 19 Two or more races, non-Hispanic/Latino), 172 international. Average age 29. 1,041 applicants, 38% accepted, 283 enrolled. In 2015, 363 master's, 13 doctorates awarded. *Degree requirements:* For master's, capstone course; for doctorate, comprehensive exam, thesis/dissertation, qualifying exams. *Entrance requirements:* For master's, GMAT, GRE, MCAT, PCAT, LSAT, or DAT, holistic review of academic credentials, resume, essay, letters of recommendation; for doctorate, GMAT, GRE, holistic review of academic credentials, resume, statement of purpose, letters of recommendation.

Additional exam requirements/recommendations for international students: Required—TOEFL (minimum score 550 paper-based; 79 iBT), IELTS (minimum score 6.5). *Application deadline:* For fall admission, 7/1 priority date for domestic students, 1/15 for international students; for spring admission, 12/1 priority date for domestic students, 6/15 for international students; for summer admission, 5/1 for domestic students. Applications are processed on a rolling basis. Application fee: $60. Electronic applications accepted. *Expenses:* Tuition, state resident: full-time $6477; part-time $269.89 per credit hour. Tuition, nonresident: full-time $15,837; part-time $659.89 per credit hour. *Required fees:* $2751; $36.50 per credit hour. $937.50 per semester. Tuition and fees vary according to course level. *Financial support:* In 2015–16, 157 students received support, including 25 research assistantships (averaging $22,725 per year), 27 teaching assistantships (averaging $22,725 per year); fellowships, career-related internships or fieldwork, Federal Work-Study, scholarships/grants, health care benefits, and unspecified assistantships also available. Financial award applicants required to submit FAFSA. *Faculty research:* Governmental and nonprofit accounting, securities and options futures, statistical analysis and design, leadership, consumer behavior. *Unit head:* Dr. Paul Goebel, Dean, 806-742-3188, Fax: 806-742-1092, E-mail: paul.goebel@ttu.edu. *Application contact:* Chathry Keaton, Applications Manager, Graduate and Professional Programs, 806-742-3184, Fax: 806-742-3958, E-mail: rawlsgrad@ttu.edu.
Website: http://grad.ba.ttu.edu

Texas Tech University Health Sciences Center, School of Health Professions, Program in Clinical Practice Management, Lubbock, TX 79430. Offers MS. *Accreditation:* CORE. *Program availability:* Part-time, online only, 100% online. *Faculty:* 4 full-time (2 women). *Students:* 9 full-time (6 women), 119 part-time (66 women); includes 75 minority (14 Black or African American, non-Hispanic/Latino; 17 Asian, non-Hispanic/Latino; 41 Hispanic/Latino; 3 Two or more races, non-Hispanic/Latino). Average age 37. 140 applicants, 64% accepted, 90 enrolled. In 2015, 69 master's awarded. *Entrance requirements:* Additional exam requirements/recommendations for international students: Required—TOEFL (minimum score 550 paper-based; 79 iBT), IELTS. *Application deadline:* For fall admission, 8/1 for domestic students; for spring admission, 12/1 for domestic students; for summer admission, 5/1 for domestic students. Applications are processed on a rolling basis. Application fee: $40. Electronic applications accepted. *Expenses:* $14,220 non-residents; $8,532 residents. *Financial support:* Institutionally sponsored loans available. Financial award application deadline: 9/1; financial award applicants required to submit FAFSA. *Unit head:* Sharon Hunt, Program Director, 806-743-2262, Fax: 806-743-3244, E-mail: sharon.hunt@ttuhsc.edu. *Application contact:* Lindsay Johnson, Associate Dean for Admissions and Student Affairs, 806-743-3220, Fax: 806-743-2994, E-mail: lindsay.johnson@ttuhsc.edu.
Website: http://www.ttuhsc.edu/shp/mscpm

Texas Woman's University, Graduate School, College of Health Sciences, Program in Health Care Administration, Houston, TX 77030. Offers MHA. Program offered at Texas Medical Center in Houston. *Accreditation:* CAHME. *Program availability:* Part-time, evening/weekend. *Degree requirements:* For master's, comprehensive exam, thesis or alternative. *Entrance requirements:* For master's, GMAT (preferred minimum score 450) or GRE General Test (preferred minimum scores 150 [450 old version] Verbal, 141 [450 old version] Quantitative), interview, resume, 3 letters of reference, essay. Additional exam requirements/recommendations for international students: Required—TOEFL (minimum score 550 paper-based; 79 iBT). *Application deadline:* For fall admission, 5/30 priority date for domestic students, 3/1 for international students; for spring admission, 9/30 priority date for domestic students, 7/1 for international students. Applications are processed on a rolling basis. Application fee: $50 ($75 for international students). Electronic applications accepted. *Expenses:* Tuition, state resident: full-time $4380; part-time $243 per credit hour. Tuition, nonresident: full-time $11,400; part-time $633 per credit hour. *International tuition:* $11,465 full-time. *Required fees:* $1778; $99 per credit hour. $283 per semester. One-time fee: $50. Tuition and fees vary according to course load and program. *Financial support:* Research assistantships, career-related internships or fieldwork, Federal Work-Study, institutionally sponsored loans, scholarships/grants, traineeships, health care benefits, and unspecified assistantships available. Support available to part-time students. Financial award application deadline: 3/1; financial award applicants required to submit FAFSA. *Faculty research:* Organizational culture, medical errors, ethical analysis in health care, leadership and professional development, strategic management, recruitment and retention issues, elderly health care. *Unit head:* Dr. Gerald Goodman, Director, 713-794-2361, Fax: 713-794-2350, E-mail: healthcareadmission@twu.edu. *Application contact:* Dr. Samuel Wheeler, Assistant Director of Admissions, 940-898-3188, Fax: 940-898-3081, E-mail: wheelersr@twu.edu.
Website: http://www.twu.edu/health-care-administration/

Texas Woman's University, Graduate School, College of Nursing, Denton, TX 76204-5498. Offers acute care nurse practitioner (MS); adult health clinical nurse specialist (MS); adult health nurse practitioner (MS); child health clinical nurse specialist (MS); clinical nurse leader (MS); family nurse practitioner (MS); health systems management (MS); nursing education (MS); nursing practice (DNP); nursing science (PhD); pediatric nurse practitioner (MS); women's health clinical nurse specialist (MS); women's health nurse practitioner (MS). *Accreditation:* AACN. *Program availability:* Part-time, online learning. *Faculty:* 55 full-time (51 women), 42 part-time/adjunct (35 women). *Students:* 39 full-time (37 women), 958 part-time (888 women); includes 566 minority (226 Black or African American, non-Hispanic/Latino; 8 American Indian or Alaska Native, non-Hispanic/Latino; 221 Asian, non-Hispanic/Latino; 88 Hispanic/Latino; 3 Native Hawaiian or other Pacific Islander, non-Hispanic/Latino; 20 Two or more races, non-Hispanic/Latino), 37 international. Average age 36. 430 applicants, 65% accepted, 193 enrolled. In 2015, 248 master's, 10 doctorates awarded. *Degree requirements:* For master's, comprehensive exam, thesis or alternative; for doctorate, comprehensive exam, thesis/dissertation. *Entrance requirements:* For master's, GRE or MAT, minimum GPA of 3.0 on last 60 hours in undergraduate nursing degree and overall, RN license, BS in nursing, basic statistics course; for doctorate, GRE (preferred minimum score 153 [500 old version] Verbal, 144 [500 old version] Quantitative, 4 Analytical), MS in nursing, minimum preferred GPA of 3.5, RN license, statistics, 2 letters of reference, curriculum vitae, graduate nursing-theory course, graduate research course, statement of professional goals and research interests. Additional exam requirements/recommendations for international students: Required—TOEFL (minimum score 550 paper-based; 79 iBT). *Application deadline:* For fall admission, 5/1 priority date for domestic students, 3/1 for international students; for spring admission, 9/15 priority date for domestic students, 7/1 for international students. Applications are processed on a rolling basis. Application fee: $50 ($75 for international students). Electronic applications accepted. *Expenses:* Tuition, state resident: full-time $4380; part-time $243 per credit hour. Tuition, nonresident: full-time $11,400; part-time $633 per credit hour. *International tuition:* $11,465 full-time. *Required fees:* $1778; $99 per credit hour. $283 per semester. One-time fee: $50. Tuition and fees vary according to course load and program. *Financial support:* In 2015–16, 149 students received support, including 10 research assistantships (averaging $5,600 per year), 1 teaching assistantship (averaging $5,600 per year); career-related internships or fieldwork, Federal Work-Study, institutionally sponsored loans, scholarships/grants, traineeships, health care benefits, and unspecified assistantships also available. Support available to part-time students. Financial award application deadline: 3/1; financial award applicants required

Health Services Management and Hospital Administration

to submit FAFSA. *Faculty research:* Screening, prevention, and treatment for intimate partner violence; needs of adolescents during childbirth intervention; a network analysis decision tool for nurse managers (social network analysis); support for adolescents with implantable cardioverter defibrillators; informatics: nurse staffing, safety, quality, and financial data as they relate to patient care outcomes; prevention and treatment of obesity; improving infant outcomes related to premature birth. *Total annual research expenditures:* $1.7 million. *Unit head:* Dr. Anita G. Hufft, Dean, 940-898-2401, Fax: 940-898-2437, E-mail: nursing@twu.edu. *Application contact:* Dr. Samuel Wheeler, Assistant Director of Admissions, 940-898-3188, Fax: 940-898-3081, E-mail: wheelersr@twu.edu.
Website: http://www.twu.edu/nursing/

Texas Woman's University, Graduate School, School of Management, Denton, TX 76201. Offers accounting (MBA); business administration (MBA); health systems management (MHSM). *Accreditation:* ACBSP. *Program availability:* Part-time. *Degree requirements:* For master's, thesis optional. *Entrance requirements:* For master's, 2 letters of reference, resume, 5 years of relevant experience (EMBA only). Additional exam requirements/recommendations for international students: Required—TOEFL (minimum score 550 paper-based; 79 iBT). *Application deadline:* For fall admission, 8/1 priority date for domestic students, 3/1 for international students; for spring admission, 12/1 priority date for domestic students, 7/1 for international students. Applications are processed on a rolling basis. Application fee: $50 ($75 for international students). Electronic applications accepted. *Expenses:* Tuition, state resident: full-time $4380; part-time $243 per credit hour. Tuition, nonresident: full-time $11,400; part-time $633 per credit hour. *International tuition:* $11,465 full-time. *Required fees:* $1778; $99 per credit hour. $283 per semester. One-time fee: $50. Tuition and fees vary according to course load and program. *Financial support:* Research assistantships, career-related internships or fieldwork, Federal Work-Study, institutionally sponsored loans, scholarships/grants, traineeships, health care benefits, and unspecified assistantships available. Support available to part-time students. Financial award application deadline: 3/1; financial award applicants required to submit FAFSA. *Faculty research:* Tax research, privacy issues in Web-based marketing, multitasking, leadership, women in management, global comparative studies, corporate sustainability and responsibility. *Unit head:* Dr. Margaret A. Young, Director, 940-898-2105, Fax: 940-898-2120, E-mail: myoung13@twu.edu. *Application contact:* Dr. Samuel Wheeler, Assistant Director of Admissions, 940-898-3188, Fax: 940-898-3081, E-mail: wheelersr@twu.edu.
Website: http://www.twu.edu/som/

Thomas Jefferson University, Jefferson School of Population Health, Program in Healthcare Quality and Safety, Philadelphia, PA 19107. Offers MS, PhD, Certificate. *Program availability:* Part-time, evening/weekend, online learning. *Entrance requirements:* For master's, GRE or other graduate examination, 2 letters of recommendation, interview, curriculum vitae; for doctorate, GRE (within the last 5 years), 3 letters of recommendation, interview, curriculum vitae. Additional exam requirements/recommendations for international students: Required—TOEFL.

Thomas Jefferson University, Jefferson School of Population Health, Program in Health Policy, Philadelphia, PA 19107. Offers MS, PhD, Certificate. *Program availability:* Part-time, evening/weekend, online learning. *Entrance requirements:* For master's, GRE or other graduate exam, two letters of recommendation, curriculum vitae/resume, interview; for doctorate, GRE (taken within the last 5 years), three letters of recommendation, curriculum vitae/resume, interview. Additional exam requirements/recommendations for international students: Required—TOEFL. Electronic applications accepted.

Tiffin University, Program in Business Administration, Tiffin, OH 44883-2161. Offers finance (MBA); general management (MBA); healthcare administration (MBA); human resource management (MBA); international business (MBA); leadership (MBA); marketing (MBA); non-profit management (MBA); sports management (MBA). *Accreditation:* ACBSP. *Program availability:* Part-time, evening/weekend, online learning. *Students:* 10 full-time (4 women), 497 part-time (240 women); includes 91 minority (67 Black or African American, non-Hispanic/Latino; 1 American Indian or Alaska Native, non-Hispanic/Latino; 5 Asian, non-Hispanic/Latino; 15 Hispanic/Latino; 3 Two or more races, non-Hispanic/Latino), 102 international. Average age 31. 214 applicants, 86% accepted, 146 enrolled. *Entrance requirements:* For master's, minimum undergraduate GPA of 2.5, work experience. Additional exam requirements/recommendations for international students: Required—TOEFL (minimum score 550 paper-based; 79 iBT), IELTS. *Application deadline:* For fall admission, 8/15 for domestic students, 8/1 for international students; for spring admission, 1/9 for domestic students, 12/1 for international students. Applications are processed on a rolling basis. Application fee: $50. Electronic applications accepted. Application fee is waived when completed online. *Expenses:* Tuition, area resident: Full-time $21,000. Tuition and fees vary according to program. *Financial support:* Unspecified assistantships available. Support available to part-time students. Financial award application deadline: 7/31; financial award applicants required to submit FAFSA. *Faculty research:* Small business, executive development operations, research and statistical analysis, market research, management information systems. *Unit head:* Dr. Bonnie Tiell, Dean of Graduate Studies, 419-448-3261, Fax: 419-443-5002, E-mail: btiell@tiffin.edu. *Application contact:* Nikki Hintze, Director of Graduate and Distance Education Academic Advising, 800-968-6446 Ext. 3596, Fax: 419-443-5002, E-mail: hintzenm@tiffin.edu.
Website: http://www.tiffin.edu/graduateprograms/

Towson University, Program in Clinician-Administrator Transition, Towson, MD 21252-0001. Offers MS, Postbaccalaureate Certificate. *Students:* 17 full-time (all women), 20 part-time (19 women); includes 7 minority (6 Black or African American, non-Hispanic/Latino; 1 Asian, non-Hispanic/Latino), 1 international. *Entrance requirements:* For degree, minimum GPA of 3.0; bachelor's or master's degree in a clinical field; licensure, licensure eligibility, or certificate in a clinical field. *Application deadline:* Applications are processed on a rolling basis. Application fee: $45. Electronic applications accepted. *Expenses:* Tuition, state resident: full-time $7440; part-time $372 per unit. Tuition, nonresident: full-time $15,400; part-time $770 per unit. *Required fees:* $2360; $118 per year. $354 per term. *Financial support:* Application deadline: 4/1. *Unit head:* Dr. Kathleen Ogle, Graduate Program Director, 410-704-4049, E-mail: mweinstein@towson.edu. *Application contact:* Alicia Arkell-Kleis, University Admissions, 410-704-2113, Fax: 410-704-3030, E-mail: grads@towson.edu.
Website: http://grad.towson.edu/program/master/nurs-cat-ms/index.asp

Trident University International, College of Health Sciences, Cypress, CA 90630. Offers MS, PhD, Certificate. *Program availability:* Part-time, evening/weekend, online learning. *Degree requirements:* For doctorate, comprehensive exam, thesis/dissertation. *Entrance requirements:* For master's, minimum GPA of 2.5 (students with GPA 3.0 or greater may transfer up to 30% of graduate level credits); for doctorate, minimum GPA of 3.4. Additional exam requirements/recommendations for international students: Required—TOEFL. Electronic applications accepted.

Trinity University, Department of Health Care Administration, San Antonio, TX 78212-7200. Offers health care administration (MS). *Accreditation:* CAHME. *Program availability:* Part-time, online learning. *Faculty:* 6 full-time (1 woman), 6 part-time/adjunct (0 women). *Students:* 51 full-time (26 women), 40 part-time (21 women); includes 31 minority (4 Black or African American, non-Hispanic/Latino; 1 American Indian or Alaska

Native, non-Hispanic/Latino; 7 Asian, non-Hispanic/Latino; 18 Hispanic/Latino; 1 Two or more races, non-Hispanic/Latino). Average age 28. In 2015, 29 master's awarded. *Entrance requirements:* For master's, GRE or GMAT, resume or autobiographical sketch; statement of purpose; letters of recommendation; three-credit-hour undergraduate course each in accounting, economics, and statistics with minimum B grade. *Application deadline:* Applications are processed on a rolling basis. Application fee: $50. Electronic applications accepted. *Financial support:* Fellowships, institutionally sponsored loans, scholarships/grants, and unspecified assistantships available. Support available to part-time students. Financial award application deadline: 5/1; financial award applicants required to submit FAFSA. *Unit head:* Dr. Ed Schumacher, Professor and Department Chair, 210-999-8107, E-mail: hca@trinity.edu.
Website: http://new.trinity.edu/academics/departments/health-care-administration

Trinity Western University, School of Graduate Studies, Program in Leadership, Langley, BC V2Y 1Y1, Canada. Offers business (MA, Certificate); Christian ministry (MA); education (MA, Certificate); healthcare (MA, Certificate); non-profit (MA, Certificate). *Program availability:* Online learning. *Degree requirements:* For master's, major project. *Entrance requirements:* For master's, minimum GPA of 2.7. Additional exam requirements/recommendations for international students: Required—TOEFL (minimum score 620 paper-based; 105 iBT). Electronic applications accepted. *Expenses:* Contact institution. *Faculty research:* Servant leadership.

Troy University, Graduate School, College of Arts and Sciences, Program in Public Administration, Troy, AL 36082. Offers government contracting (MPA); health care administration (MPA); justice administration (MPA); national security affairs (MPA); nonprofit management (MPA); public human resources management (MPA); public management (MPA). *Accreditation:* NASPAA. *Program availability:* Part-time, evening/weekend, online learning. *Faculty:* 15 full-time (11 women), 5 part-time/adjunct (2 women). *Students:* 38 full-time (21 women), 196 part-time (122 women); includes 143 minority (121 Black or African American, non-Hispanic/Latino; 17 American Indian or Alaska Native, non-Hispanic/Latino; 3 Asian, non-Hispanic/Latino; 2 Two or more races, non-Hispanic/Latino). Average age 33. 183 applicants, 54% accepted, 38 enrolled. In 2015, 108 master's awarded. *Degree requirements:* For master's, capstone course with minimum B grade, minimum GPA of 3.0, admission to candidacy. *Entrance requirements:* For master's, GRE (minimum score of 920 on old exam or 294 on new exam), MAT (minimum score of 400) or GMAT (minimum score of 490), bachelor's degree; minimum undergraduate GPA of 2.5 or 3.0 on last 30 semester hours, letter of recommendation; essay, resume. Additional exam requirements/recommendations for international students: Required—TOEFL (minimum score 523 paper-based; 70 iBT), IELTS (minimum score 6). *Application deadline:* Applications are processed on a rolling basis. Application fee: $50. Electronic applications accepted. *Expenses:* Tuition, state resident: full-time $7146; part-time $397 per credit hour. Tuition, nonresident: full-time $14,292; part-time $794 per credit hour. *Required fees:* $802. Tuition and fees vary according to campus/location and program. *Financial support:* Fellowships, career-related internships or fieldwork, and scholarships/grants available. Support available to part-time students. Financial award applicants required to submit FAFSA. *Unit head:* Dr. Pamela Trump Dunning, Director, 334-808-6507, Fax: 334-670-5647, E-mail: pdunningl@troy.edu. *Application contact:* Jessica A. Kimbro, Director of Graduate Admissions, 334-670-3178, E-mail: jacord@troy.edu.

Troy University, Graduate School, College of Business, Program in Business Administration, Troy, AL 36082. Offers accounting (EMBA, MBA); criminal justice (EMBA); finance (MBA); general management (EMBA, MBA); healthcare management (EMBA); information systems (EMBA, MBA); international economic development (MBA). *Accreditation:* ACBSP. *Program availability:* Part-time, evening/weekend. *Faculty:* 15 full-time (4 women), 2 part-time/adjunct (0 women). *Students:* 54 full-time (23 women), 164 part-time (80 women); includes 100 minority (74 Black or African American, non-Hispanic/Latino; 1 American Indian or Alaska Native, non-Hispanic/Latino; 14 Asian, non-Hispanic/Latino; 7 Hispanic/Latino; 4 Two or more races, non-Hispanic/Latino). Average age 30. 184 applicants, 68% accepted, 22 enrolled. In 2015, 193 master's awarded. *Degree requirements:* For master's, minimum GPA of 3.0, capstone course, research course. *Entrance requirements:* For master's, GMAT (minimum score 500) or GRE (minimum score 900 on old exam or 294 on new exam), bachelor's degree; minimum undergraduate GPA of 2.5 or 3.0 on last 30 semester hours, letter of recommendation. Additional exam requirements/recommendations for international students: Required—TOEFL (minimum score 523 paper-based; 70 iBT), IELTS (minimum score 6). *Application deadline:* Applications are processed on a rolling basis. Application fee: $50. Electronic applications accepted. *Expenses:* Tuition, state resident: full-time $7146; part-time $397 per credit hour. Tuition, nonresident: full-time $14,292; part-time $794 per credit hour. *Required fees:* $802. Tuition and fees vary according to campus/location and program. *Financial support:* Fellowships, career-related internships or fieldwork, and scholarships/grants available. Support available to part-time students. Financial award applicants required to submit FAFSA. *Unit head:* Dr. Bob Wheatley, Director, Graduate Business Programs, 334-670-3194, Fax: 334-670-3599, E-mail: rwheat@troy.edu. *Application contact:* Jessica A. Kimbro, Director of Graduate Admissions, 334-670-3178, E-mail: jacord@troy.edu.

Troy University, Graduate School, College of Business, Program in Management, Troy, AL 36082. Offers applied management (MSM); healthcare management (MSM); human resources management (MSM); information systems (MSM); international hospitality management (MSM); international management (MSM); leadership and organizational effectiveness (MSM); public management (MS, MSM). *Accreditation:* ACBSP. *Program availability:* Part-time, evening/weekend. *Faculty:* 12 full-time (5 women), 2 part-time/adjunct (1 woman). *Students:* 37 full-time (17 women), 161 part-time (90 women); includes 97 minority (84 Black or African American, non-Hispanic/Latino; 1 American Indian or Alaska Native, non-Hispanic/Latino; 5 Hispanic/Latino; 7 Two or more races, non-Hispanic/Latino). Average age 36. 124 applicants, 97% accepted, 84 enrolled. In 2015, 53 master's awarded. *Degree requirements:* For master's, Graduate Educational Testing Service Major Field Test, capstone exam, minimum GPA of 3.0. *Entrance requirements:* For master's, GRE (minimum score of 900 on old exam or 294 on new exam) or GMAT (minimum score of 500), bachelor's degree; minimum undergraduate GPA of 2.5 or 3.0 on last 30 semester hours, letter of recommendation. Additional exam requirements/recommendations for international students: Required—TOEFL (minimum score 523 paper-based; 70 iBT), IELTS (minimum score 6). *Application deadline:* Applications are processed on a rolling basis. Application fee: $50. Electronic applications accepted. *Expenses:* Contact institution. *Financial support:* Fellowships, career-related internships or fieldwork, and scholarships/grants available. Support available to part-time students. *Unit head:* Dr. Bob Wheatley, Director, Graduate Business Programs, 334-670-3143, Fax: 334-670-3599, E-mail: rwheat@troy.edu. *Application contact:* Jessica A. Kimbro, Director of Graduate Admissions, 334-670-3178, E-mail: kimbro@troy.edu.

Tufts University, School of Medicine, Public Health and Professional Degree Programs, Boston, MA 02111. Offers biomedical sciences (MS); health communication (MS, Certificate); pain research, education and policy (MS, Certificate); physician assistant (MS); public health (MPH, Dr PH), including behavioral science (MPH), biostatistics (MPH), epidemiology (MPH), health communication (MPH), health services (MPH), management and policy (MPH), nutrition (MPH); DMD/MPH; DVM/MPH; JD/

Health Services Management and Hospital Administration

MPH; MD/MPH; MMS/MPH; MS/MBA; MS/MPH. MS programs offered jointly with Emerson College. *Accreditation:* CEPH (one or more programs are accredited). *Program availability:* Part-time, evening/weekend. *Faculty:* 78 full-time (29 women), 42 part-time/adjunct (20 women). *Students:* 457 full-time (266 women), 61 part-time (46 women); includes 187 minority (21 Black or African American, non-Hispanic/Latino; 107 Asian, non-Hispanic/Latino; 37 Hispanic/Latino; 22 Two or more races, non-Hispanic/Latino), 24 international. Average age 27. 1,599 applicants, 48% accepted, 222 enrolled. In 2015, 219 master's awarded. *Degree requirements:* For master's, thesis (for some programs); for doctorate, thesis/dissertation. *Entrance requirements:* For master's, GRE General Test, MCAT, or GMAT; for doctorate, GRE General Test or MCAT. Additional exam requirements/recommendations for international students: Required—TOEFL (minimum score 100 iBT). *Application deadline:* For fall admission, 1/15 priority date for domestic students, 12/15 priority date for international students; for spring admission, 10/25 priority date for domestic and international students. Applications are processed on a rolling basis. Application fee: $70. Electronic applications accepted. *Expenses:* Contact institution. *Financial support:* In 2015–16, 12 students received support, including 1 fellowship (averaging $3,000 per year), 50 research assistantships (averaging $1,000 per year), 65 teaching assistantships (averaging $2,000 per year); Federal Work-Study and scholarships/grants also available. Support available to part-time students. Financial award application deadline: 2/19; financial award applicants required to submit FAFSA. *Faculty research:* Environmental and occupational health, nutrition, epidemiology, health communication, biostatics, obesity/chronic disease, health policy and health care delivery, global health, health inequality and social determinants of health. *Unit head:* Dr. Aviva Must, Dean, 617-636-0935, Fax: 617-636-0898, E-mail: aviva.must@tufts.edu. *Application contact:* Emily Keily, Director of Admissions, 617-636-0935, Fax: 617-636-0898, E-mail: med-phpd@tufts.edu. Website: http://publichealth.tufts.edu

Tulane University, School of Public Health and Tropical Medicine, Department of Global Health Management and Policy, New Orleans, LA 70118-5669. Offers MHA, MPH, PhD, Sc D, JD/MHA, MBA/MHA, MD/MPH, MSW/MPH. *Accreditation:* CAHME (one or more programs are accredited). *Degree requirements:* For doctorate, comprehensive exam, thesis/dissertation. *Entrance requirements:* For master's, GMAT, GRE General Test; for doctorate, GRE General Test. Additional exam requirements/recommendations for international students: Required—TOEFL. *Application deadline:* For fall admission, 4/15 priority date for domestic and international students; for spring admission, 10/15 priority date for domestic and international students. Applications are processed on a rolling basis. Application fee: $40. Electronic applications accepted. *Expenses: Tuition, area resident:* Full-time $47,658; part-time $2648 per credit hour. *Required fees:* $1980; $44.50 per credit hour. $550 per term. Tuition and fees vary according to course load, degree level and program. *Financial support:* Fellowships with tuition reimbursements, Federal Work-Study, scholarships/grants, traineeships, and tuition waivers (partial) available. Support available to part-time students. Financial award application deadline: 4/15. *Faculty research:* Health policy, organizational governance, international health administration.

Uniformed Services University of the Health Sciences, F. Edward Hebert School of Medicine, Graduate Programs in the Biomedical Sciences and Public Health, Bethesda, MD 20814. Offers emerging infectious diseases (PhD); medical and clinical psychology (PhD), including clinical psychology, medical psychology; medicine (MS, PhD), including health professions education; molecular and cell biology (MS, PhD); neuroscience (PhD); preventive medicine and biometrics (MPH, MS, MSPH, MTMH, Dr PH, PhD), including environmental health sciences (PhD), healthcare administration and policy (MS), medical zoology (PhD), public health (MPH, MSPH, Dr PH), tropical medicine and hygiene (MTMH). *Faculty:* 372 full-time (119 women), 4,044 part-time/adjunct (908 women). *Students:* 240 full-time (133 women); includes 40 minority (15 Black or African American, non-Hispanic/Latino; 13 Asian, non-Hispanic/Latino; 12 Hispanic/Latino), 30 international. Average age 25. 598 applicants, 17% accepted, 77 enrolled. In 2015, 19 master's, 50 doctorates awarded. Terminal master's awarded for partial completion of doctoral program. *Degree requirements:* For master's, comprehensive exam, thesis or alternative; for doctorate, comprehensive exam, thesis/dissertation, qualifying exam. *Entrance requirements:* For master's, GRE General Test; for doctorate, GRE General Test, minimum GPA of 3.0. *Application deadline:* For fall admission, 12/15 priority date for domestic students. Applications are processed on a rolling basis. Application fee: $0. Electronic applications accepted. *Financial support:* In 2015–16, 50 fellowships (averaging $43,000 per year) were awarded; research assistantships, career-related internships or fieldwork, scholarships/grants, health care benefits, and tuition waivers (full) also available. *Unit head:* Dr. Gregory Mueller, Associate Dean, 301-295-3507, E-mail: gregory.mueller@usuhs.edu. *Application contact:* Tina Finley, Administrative Officer, 301-295-3642, Fax: 301-295-6772, E-mail: netina.finley@usuhs.edu. Website: http://www.usuhs.mil/graded

Uniformed Services University of the Health Sciences, F. Edward Hebert School of Medicine, Graduate Programs in the Biomedical Sciences and Public Health, Department of Preventive Medicine and Biometrics, Program in Healthcare Administration and Policy, Bethesda, MD 20814-4799. Offers MS.

Universidad de Ciencias Medicas, Graduate Programs, San Jose, Costa Rica. Offers dermatology (SP); family health (MS); health service center administration (MHA); human anatomy (MS); medical and surgery (MD); occupational medicine (MS); pharmacy (Pharm D). *Program availability:* Part-time. *Degree requirements:* For master's, thesis; for doctorate and SP, comprehensive exam. *Entrance requirements:* For master's, MD or bachelor's degree; for doctorate, admissions test; for SP, admissions test, MD.

Universidad de Iberoamerica, Graduate School, San Jose, Costa Rica. Offers clinical neuropsychology (PhD); clinical psychology (M Psych); educational psychology (M Psych); forensic psychology (M Psych); hospital management (MHA); intensive care nursing (MN); medicine (MD).

Université de Montréal, Faculty of Medicine, Department of Health Administration, Montréal, QC H3C 3J7, Canada. Offers M Sc, DESS. *Accreditation:* CAHME. *Degree requirements:* For master's, thesis. *Entrance requirements:* For master's, proficiency in French. Electronic applications accepted.

University at Albany, State University of New York, Nelson A. Rockefeller College of Public Affairs and Policy, Department of Public Administration and Policy, Albany, NY 12222-0001. Offers financial management and public economics (MPA); financial market regulation (MPA); health policy (MPA); healthcare management (MPA); homeland security (MPA); human resources management (MPA); information strategy and management (MPA); local government management (MPA); nonprofit management (MPA); nonprofit management and leadership (Certificate); organizational behavior and theory (MPA, PhD); planning and policy analysis (CAS); policy analytic methods (MPA); politics and administration (PhD); public finance (PhD); public management (PhD); public policy (PhD); public sector management (Certificate); women and public policy (Certificate); JD/MPA. JD/MPA offered jointly with Albany Law School. *Accreditation:* NASPAA (one or more programs are accredited). *Degree requirements:* For doctorate, one foreign language, thesis/dissertation. *Entrance requirements:* For doctorate, GRE General Test. Additional exam requirements/recommendations for international

students: Required—TOEFL (minimum score 550 paper-based). Electronic applications accepted.

University at Albany, State University of New York, School of Public Health, Department of Health Policy, Management, and Behavior, Albany, NY 12222-0001. Offers MPH, MS, Dr PH, PhD. *Degree requirements:* For master's, thesis. *Entrance requirements:* For master's, GRE General Test. Additional exam requirements/recommendations for international students: Required—TOEFL (minimum score 550 paper-based). Electronic applications accepted.

University at Buffalo, the State University of New York, Graduate School, School of Nursing, Buffalo, NY 14214. Offers adult gerontology nurse practitioner (DNP); family nurse practitioner (DNP); health care systems and leadership (MS); nurse anesthetist (DNP); nursing (PhD); nursing education (Certificate); psychiatric/mental health nurse practitioner (DNP). *Accreditation:* AACN; AANA/CANAEP (one or more programs are accredited). *Program availability:* Part-time, 100% online. *Students:* 61 full-time (37 women), 137 part-time (114 women); includes 35 minority (17 Black or African American, non-Hispanic/Latino; 1 American Indian or Alaska Native, non-Hispanic/Latino; 17 Asian, non-Hispanic/Latino), 7 international. Average age 32. 193 applicants, 49% accepted, 75 enrolled. In 2015, 6 master's, 37 doctorates awarded. *Degree requirements:* For master's, thesis optional; for doctorate, comprehensive exam (for some programs), capstone (for DNP), dissertation (for PhD). *Entrance requirements:* For master's, GRE or MAT; for doctorate, GRE or MAT, minimum GPA of 3.0 (for DNP), 3.25 (for PhD); RN license; BS or MS in nursing; 3 references; writing sample; resume; personal statement; for Certificate, interview, minimum GPA of 3.0 or GRE General Test, RN license, MS in nursing, professional certification. Additional exam requirements/recommendations for international students: Required—TOEFL (minimum score 550 paper-based; 79 iBT), IELTS (minimum score 6.5). *Application deadline:* For fall admission, 7/1 for domestic students, 2/1 for international students; for spring admission, 12/1 for domestic students, 10/1 for international students; for summer admission, 2/1 for domestic students. Applications are processed on a rolling basis. Application fee: $75. Electronic applications accepted. *Financial support:* In 2015–16, 80 students received support, including 2 fellowships with tuition reimbursements available (averaging $17,000 per year), 4 research assistantships with tuition reimbursements available (averaging $10,600 per year), 7 teaching assistantships with tuition reimbursements available (averaging $10,600 per year); scholarships/grants, traineeships, health care benefits, and unspecified assistantships also available. Financial award application deadline: 2/1; financial award applicants required to submit FAFSA. *Faculty research:* Oncology, palliative care, gerontology, addictions, mental health, community wellness, sleep, workforce, care of underserved populations, quality and safety, person-centered care, adolescent health. *Total annual research expenditures:* $1.4 million. *Unit head:* Dr. Marsha L. Lewis, Dean and Professor, 716-829-2533, Fax: 716-829-2566, E-mail: ubnursingdean@buffalo.edu. *Application contact:* Jennifer H. VanLaeken, Director of Graduate Student Services, 716-829-3311, Fax: 716-829-2067, E-mail: jhv2@buffalo.edu. Website: http://nursing.buffalo.edu/

The University of Akron, Graduate School, College of Business Administration, Department of Management, Program in Healthcare Management, Akron, OH 44325. Offers MBA. *Students:* 14 full-time (8 women), 11 part-time (5 women); includes 4 minority (2 Black or African American, non-Hispanic/Latino; 2 Asian, non-Hispanic/Latino), 3 international. Average age 36. 17 applicants, 65% accepted, 10 enrolled. In 2015, 5 master's awarded. *Entrance requirements:* For master's, GMAT, minimum GPA of 3.0 (preferred), two letters of recommendation, resume, statement of purpose. Additional exam requirements/recommendations for international students: Required—TOEFL (minimum score 550 paper-based; 79 iBT), IELTS (minimum score 6.5). *Application deadline:* For fall admission, 7/15 for domestic and international students; for spring admission, 11/15 for domestic and international students; for summer admission, 4/15 for domestic and international students. Application fee: $45 ($75 for international students). Electronic applications accepted. *Expenses:* Tuition, state resident: full-time $7958; part-time $442 per credit hour. Tuition, nonresident: full-time $13,464; part-time $748 per credit hour. *Required fees:* $1404. *Unit head:* Dr. Steve Ash, Chair, 330-972-6429, E-mail: ash@uakron.edu. *Application contact:* Dr. William Hauser, Director of Graduate Business Programs, 330-972-7043, Fax: 330-972-6588, E-mail: whauser@uakron.edu.

The University of Alabama at Birmingham, Collat School of Business, Program in Business Administration, Birmingham, AL 35294. Offers business administration (MBA), including finance, health care management, information technology management, marketing. *Program availability:* Part-time, evening/weekend. *Entrance requirements:* For master's, GMAT. Additional exam requirements/recommendations for international students: Required—TOEFL. *Expenses:* Tuition, state resident: full-time $7340. Tuition, nonresident: full-time $16,628. Full-time tuition and fees vary according to course load and program.

The University of Alabama at Birmingham, School of Education, Community Health and Human Services Program, Birmingham, AL 35294. Offers MA Ed. *Accreditation:* NCATE. *Faculty:* 4 full-time (2 women). *Students:* 12 full-time (11 women), 12 part-time (9 women); includes 14 minority (13 Black or African American, non-Hispanic/Latino; 1 Hispanic/Latino), 1 international. Average age 33. In 2015, 14 master's awarded. *Degree requirements:* For master's, comprehensive exam (for some programs), thesis optional. *Entrance requirements:* For master's, GRE General Test or MAT, minimum GPA of 3.0, references. *Application deadline:* Applications are processed on a rolling basis. Application fee: $35 ($60 for international students). Electronic applications accepted. *Expenses:* Tuition, state resident: full-time $7340. Tuition, nonresident: full-time $16,628. Full-time tuition and fees vary according to course load and program. *Faculty research:* College student health, minority health disparities/disease, health eating. *Total annual research expenditures:* $10,000. *Unit head:* Dr. Kristi Menear, Chair, 205-975-7409, Fax: 205-975-8040, E-mail: kmenear@uab.edu. *Application contact:* Dr. Retta R. Evans, Program Coordinator, 205-996-2701, Fax: 205-975-8040, E-mail: rrevans@uab.edu.

The University of Alabama at Birmingham, School of Health Professions, Program in Administration/Health Services, Birmingham, AL 35294. Offers D Sc, PhD. *Degree requirements:* For doctorate, thesis/dissertation. *Entrance requirements:* For doctorate, GRE General Test. Additional exam requirements/recommendations for international students: Required—TOEFL. *Expenses:* Tuition, state resident: full-time $7340. Tuition, nonresident: full-time $16,628. Full-time tuition and fees vary according to course load and program. *Faculty research:* Healthcare strategic management, marketing, organization studies.

The University of Alabama at Birmingham, School of Health Professions, Program in Health Administration, Birmingham, AL 35294. Offers MSHA. *Accreditation:* CAHME. *Degree requirements:* For master's, administrative residency. *Entrance requirements:* For master's, GMAT or GRE General Test, minimum GPA of 3.0 in final 60 hours of undergraduate course work; 5 years of experience in health care organizations, either as manager or as clinical professional (for executive program). Additional exam requirements/recommendations for international students: Required—TOEFL (minimum score 550 paper-based), TWE. Electronic applications accepted. *Expenses:* Tuition,

Health Services Management and Hospital Administration

state resident: full-time $7340. Tuition, nonresident: full-time $16,628. Full-time tuition and fees vary according to course load and program.

The University of Alabama at Birmingham, School of Public Health, Program in Public Health, Birmingham, AL 35294. Offers applied epidemiology and pharmacoepidemiology (MSPH); biostatistics (MPH); clinical and translational science (MSPH); environmental health (MPH); environmental health and toxicology (MSPH); epidemiology (MPH); general theory and practice (MPH); health behavior (MPH); health care organization (MPH); health policy quantitative policy analysis (MPH); industrial hygiene (MPH, MSPH); maternal and child health policy (Dr PH); maternal and child health policy and leadership (MPH); occupational health and safety (MPH); outcomes research (MSPH, Dr PH); public health (PhD); public health management (Dr PH); public health preparedness management (MPH). *Accreditation:* CEPH. *Program availability:* Part-time, online learning. *Degree requirements:* For doctorate, comprehensive exam, thesis/dissertation. *Entrance requirements:* For master's and doctorate, GRE. Additional exam requirements/recommendations for international students: Recommended—TOEFL (minimum score 550 paper-based; 79 iBT), IELTS (minimum score 6.5). Electronic applications accepted. *Expenses:* Tuition, state resident: full-time $7340. Tuition, nonresident: full-time $16,628. Full-time tuition and fees vary according to course load and program.

The University of Alabama in Huntsville, School of Graduate Studies, College of Nursing, Huntsville, AL 35899. Offers family nurse practitioner (Certificate); nursing (MSN, DNP), including adult-gerontology acute care nurse practitioner (MSN), adult-gerontology clinical nurse specialist (MSN), family nurse practitioner (MSN), leadership in health care systems (MSN); nursing education (Certificate). DNP offered jointly with The University of Alabama at Birmingham. *Accreditation:* AACN. *Program availability:* Part-time, evening/weekend, online learning. *Degree requirements:* For master's, comprehensive exam, thesis or alternative, oral and written exams. *Entrance requirements:* For master's, MAT or GRE, Alabama RN license, BSN, minimum GPA of 3.0; for doctorate, master's degree in nursing in an advanced practice area; for Certificate, MAT or GRE, minimum GPA of 3.0. Additional exam requirements/recommendations for international students: Required—TOEFL (minimum score 500 paper-based; 80 iBT), IELTS (minimum score 6.5). *Application deadline:* For fall admission, 7/15 for domestic students, 4/1 for international students; for spring admission, 11/30 for domestic students, 9/1 for international students. Applications are processed on a rolling basis. Application fee: $50. Electronic applications accepted. *Expenses: Tuition, area resident:* Full-time $9548; part-time $547 per credit hour. Tuition, state resident: full-time $9548; part-time $547 per credit hour. Tuition, nonresident: full-time $21,402; part-time $1224 per credit hour. *International tuition:* $21,402 full-time. *Financial support:* Teaching assistantships with full tuition reimbursements, career-related internships or fieldwork, Federal Work-Study, institutionally sponsored loans, scholarships/grants, traineeships, health care benefits, and unspecified assistantships available. Support available to part-time students. Financial award application deadline: 4/1; financial award applicants required to submit FAFSA. *Faculty research:* Health care informatics, chronic illness management, maternal and child health, genetics/genomics, technology and health care. *Unit head:* Dr. Marsha Adams, Dean, 256-824-6345, Fax: 256-824-6026, E-mail: marsha.adams@uah.edu. *Application contact:* Charles Davis, Director of Graduate Admission and Advisement, 256-824-6669, Fax: 256-824-6026, E-mail: charles.davis@uah.edu. Website: http://www.uah.edu/nursing

University of Alberta, School of Public Health, Department of Public Health Sciences, Edmonton, AB T6G 2E1, Canada. Offers clinical epidemiology (M Sc, MPH); environmental and occupational health (MPH); environmental health sciences (M Sc); epidemiology (M Sc); global health (M Sc, MPH); health policy and management (MPH); health policy research (M Sc); health technology assessment (MPH); occupational health (M Sc); population health (M Sc); public health leadership (MPH); public health sciences (PhD); quantitative methods (MPH). *Accreditation:* CEPH (one or more programs are accredited). Terminal master's awarded for partial completion of doctoral program. *Degree requirements:* For master's, thesis (for some programs); for doctorate, thesis/dissertation. *Entrance requirements:* For master's, GMAT or GRE General Test. Additional exam requirements/recommendations for international students: Required—TOEFL (minimum score 550 paper-based) or IELTS (minimum score 6). Electronic applications accepted. *Faculty research:* Biostatistics, health promotion and socio-behavioral health science.

University of Arkansas for Medical Sciences, College of Public Health, Little Rock, AR 72205-7199. Offers biostatistics (MPH); environmental and occupational health (MPH, Certificate); epidemiology (MPH, PhD); health behavior and health education (MPH); health policy and management (MPH); health promotion and prevention research (PhD); health services administration (MHSA); health systems research (PhD); public health (Certificate); public health leadership (Dr PH). *Program availability:* Part-time. *Degree requirements:* For master's, preceptorship, culminating experience, internship; for doctorate, comprehensive exam, capstone. *Entrance requirements:* For master's, GRE, GMAT, LSAT, PCAT, MCAT, DAT; for doctorate, GRE. Additional exam requirements/recommendations for international students: Required—TOEFL (minimum score 80 iBT), IELTS. Electronic applications accepted. *Expenses:* Contact institution. *Faculty research:* Health systems, tobacco prevention control, obesity prevention, environmental and occupational exposure, cancer prevention.

University of Baltimore, Graduate School, College of Public Affairs, Program in Health Systems Management, Baltimore, MD 21201-5779. Offers MS. *Program availability:* Part-time, evening/weekend. *Entrance requirements:* For master's, minimum undergraduate GPA of 3.0. Additional exam requirements/recommendations for international students: Required—TOEFL (minimum score 550 paper-based).

The University of British Columbia, Faculty of Medicine, School of Population and Public Health, Vancouver, BC V6T 1Z3, Canada. Offers health administration (MHA); health care and epidemiology (MH Sc, PhD); public health (MPH). *Accreditation:* CEPH (one or more programs are accredited). *Program availability:* Online learning. *Degree requirements:* For master's, thesis (for some programs), major paper (MH Sc), research project (MHA); for doctorate, thesis/dissertation. *Entrance requirements:* For master's, GRE General Test or GMAT, PCAT, MCAT (MHA), MD or equivalent (for MH Sc); 4-year undergraduate degree from accredited university with minimum B+ overall academic average and in math or statistics course at undergraduate level (for MPH); 4-year undergraduate degree from accredited university with minimum B+ overall academic average plus work experience (for MHA); for doctorate, master's degree from accredited university with minimum B+ overall academic average and in math or statistics course at undergraduate level. Additional exam requirements/recommendations for international students: Required—TOEFL. Electronic applications accepted. *Faculty research:* Population and public health, clinical epidemiology, epidemiology and biostatistics, global health and vulnerable populations, health care services and systems, occupational and environmental health, public health emerging threats and rapid response, social and life course determinants of health, health administration.

University of California, Berkeley, Graduate Division, School of Public Health, Group in Health Policy, Berkeley, CA 94720-1500. Offers PhD. *Degree requirements:* For

doctorate, thesis/dissertation, qualifying exam. *Entrance requirements:* For doctorate, GRE General Test, minimum GPA of 3.0, 3 letters of recommendation.

University of California, Irvine, The Paul Merage School of Business, Health Care Executive MBA Program, Irvine, CA 92697. Offers MBA. *Students:* 34 full-time (16 women), 30 part-time (11 women); includes 30 minority (2 Black or African American, non-Hispanic/Latino; 7 American Indian or Alaska Native, non-Hispanic/Latino; 20 Asian, non-Hispanic/Latino; 1 Hispanic/Latino), 11 international. Average age 40. 46 applicants, 89% accepted, 25 enrolled. In 2015, 53 master's awarded. Application fee: $90 ($110 for international students). *Unit head:* Anthony Hansford, Senior Assistant Dean, 949-824-3801, E-mail: hansfora@uci.edu. *Application contact:* Jon Masciana, Senior Director, 949-824-0595, E-mail: jmascian@uci.edu. Website: http://merage.uci.edu/HealthCareExecutiveMBA/Default.aspx

University of California, Los Angeles, Graduate Division, School of Public Health, Department of Health Services, Los Angeles, CA 90095. Offers MPH, MS, Dr PH, PhD, JD/MPH, MBA/MPH, MD/MPH. *Degree requirements:* For master's, comprehensive exam or thesis; for doctorate, thesis/dissertation, oral and written qualifying exams. *Entrance requirements:* For master's, GRE General Test, minimum GPA of 3.0; for doctorate, GRE General Test, minimum undergraduate GPA of 3.0. Electronic applications accepted.

University of California, San Diego, Graduate Division, Program in Health Policy and Law, La Jolla, CA 92093. Offers MAS. Program offered jointly with School of Medicine and California Western School of Law. *Program availability:* Part-time. *Students:* 14 full-time (8 women), 10 part-time (9 women); includes 11 minority (4 Black or African American, non-Hispanic/Latino; 3 Asian, non-Hispanic/Latino; 4 Hispanic/Latino), 2 international. 30 applicants, 80% accepted, 14 enrolled. In 2015, 35 master's awarded. *Degree requirements:* For master's, capstone project. *Entrance requirements:* For master's, appropriate medical, healthcare, legal or related degree; minimum GPA of 3.0 in final two years of study; minimum 3 years of relevant work experience or equivalent. Additional exam requirements/recommendations for international students: Required—TOEFL (minimum score 550 paper-based; 80 iBT), IELTS (minimum score 7). *Application deadline:* For fall admission, 5/10 for domestic students. Applications are processed on a rolling basis. Application fee: $90 ($110 for international students). Electronic applications accepted. *Expenses:* Contact institution. *Financial support:* Scholarships/grants available. *Unit head:* Gerard Manecke, Program Co-Director, 619-543-3164, E-mail: gmanecke@ucsd.edu. *Application contact:* Jessica Nguyen, Program Coordinator, 858-534-9162, E-mail: healthpolicyandlaw@ucsd.edu. Website: http://hlaw.ucsd.edu/

University of California, San Diego, School of Medicine, Program in the Leadership of Healthcare Organizations, La Jolla, CA 92093. Offers MAS. *Program availability:* Part-time, evening/weekend. *Students:* 2 full-time (1 woman), 26 part-time (19 women); includes 8 minority (3 Black or African American, non-Hispanic/Latino; 3 Asian, non-Hispanic/Latino; 2 Hispanic/Latino), 3 international. 18 applicants, 89% accepted, 10 enrolled. In 2015, 17 master's awarded. *Degree requirements:* For master's, independent study project. *Entrance requirements:* For master's, minimum GPA of 3.0; minimum 5 years of professional work/internship in health care or a related field. Additional exam requirements/recommendations for international students: Required—TOEFL, IELTS. *Application deadline:* For fall admission, 5/24 for domestic students; for winter admission, 10/14 for domestic students; for spring admission, 1/12 for domestic students. Applications are processed on a rolling basis. Application fee: $90 ($110 for international students). Electronic applications accepted. *Expenses:* Contact institution. *Financial support:* Scholarships/grants available. Financial award applicants required to submit FAFSA. *Unit head:* Todd Gilmer, Chair, 858-534-7596, E-mail: tgilmer@ucsd.edu. *Application contact:* Jessica Nguyen, Graduate Coordinator, 858-534-9162, E-mail: lhco@ucsd.edu. Website: http://lhco.ucsd.edu/

University of Central Florida, College of Health and Public Affairs, Department of Health Management and Informatics, Orlando, FL 32816. Offers health care informatics (MS); health information administration (Certificate); health services administration (MS). *Accreditation:* CAHME. *Program availability:* Part-time, evening/weekend. *Faculty:* 19 full-time (10 women), 22 part-time/adjunct (14 women). *Students:* 142 full-time (105 women), 177 part-time (128 women); includes 168 minority (84 Black or African American, non-Hispanic/Latino; 39 Asian, non-Hispanic/Latino; 37 Hispanic/Latino; 8 Two or more races, non-Hispanic/Latino), 6 international. Average age 28. 266 applicants, 67% accepted, 116 enrolled. In 2015, 135 master's awarded. *Degree requirements:* For master's, comprehensive exam, thesis or alternative, research report. *Entrance requirements:* For master's, GRE General Test. Additional exam requirements/recommendations for international students: Required—TOEFL. *Application deadline:* For fall admission, 7/15 for domestic students; for spring admission, 10/1 for domestic students. Application fee: $30. Electronic applications accepted. *Expenses:* Tuition, state resident: part-time $288.16 per credit hour. Tuition, nonresident: part-time $1071.31 per credit hour. *Financial support:* In 2015–16, 2 students received support, including 2 research assistantships with partial tuition reimbursements available (averaging $8,200 per year); career-related internships or fieldwork, Federal Work-Study, institutionally sponsored loans, and unspecified assistantships also available. Financial award application deadline: 3/1; financial award applicants required to submit FAFSA. *Unit head:* Dr. Reid Oetjen, Interim Chair, 407-823-5668, E-mail: reid.oetjen@ucf.edu. *Application contact:* Director, Admissions and Student Services, 407-823-2766, Fax: 407-823-6442, E-mail: gradadmissions@ucf.edu. Website: http://www.cohpa.ucf.edu/hmi/

University of Chicago, Booth School of Business, Full-Time MBA Program, Chicago, IL 60637. Offers accounting (MBA); analytic finance (MBA); analytic management (MBA); econometrics and statistics (MBA); economics (MBA); entrepreneurship (MBA); finance (MBA); general management (MBA); health administration and policy (Certificate); international business (MBA); managerial and organizational behavior (MBA); marketing management (MBA); operations management (MBA); strategic management (MBA); MBA/AM; MBA/JD; MBA/MA; MBA/MD; MBA/MPP. *Accreditation:* AACSB. *Students:* 1,151 full-time (443 women), 17 part-time (9 women). Terminal master's awarded for partial completion of doctoral program. *Entrance requirements:* For master's, GMAT or GRE, transcripts, resume, 2 letters of recommendation, essay, interview. Additional exam requirements/recommendations for international students: Required—TOEFL (minimum score 600 paper-based; 104 iBT), IELTS (minimum score 7), PTE (minimum score 70). *Application deadline:* For spring admission, 4/1 for domestic and international students. Electronic applications accepted. *Expenses:* Contact institution. *Unit head:* Stacey Kole, Deputy Dean, 773-702-7121. *Application contact:* Full-time MBA Program Admissions, 773-702-7369, Fax: 773-702-9085, E-mail: admissions@chicagobooth.edu. Website: https://www.chicagobooth.edu/programs/full-time

University of Colorado Denver, Business School, Master of Business Administration Program, Denver, CO 80217. Offers bioinnovation and entrepreneurship (MBA); business intelligence (MBA); business strategy (MBA); business to business marketing (MBA); business to consumer marketing (MBA); change management (MBA); corporate financial management (MBA); enterprise technology management (MBA); entrepreneurship (MBA); health administration (MBA), including financial management,

health administration, health information technologies, international health management and policy; human resources management (MBA); international business (MBA); investment management (MBA); managing for sustainability (MBA); sports and entertainment management (MBA). *Accreditation:* AACSB. *Program availability:* Part-time, evening/weekend, 100% online, blended/hybrid learning. *Students:* 541 full-time (211 women), 135 part-time (41 women); includes 82 minority (16 Black or African American, non-Hispanic/Latino; 2 American Indian or Alaska Native, non-Hispanic/Latino; 29 Asian, non-Hispanic/Latino; 30 Hispanic/Latino; 5 Two or more races, non-Hispanic/Latino), 24 international. Average age 33. 330 applicants, 75% accepted, 175 enrolled. In 2015, 290 master's awarded. *Degree requirements:* For master's, 48 semester hours, including 30 of core courses, 3 in international business, and 15 in electives from over 50 other graduate business courses. *Entrance requirements:* For master's, GMAT, resume, official transcripts, essay, two letters of recommendation, financial statements (for international applicants). Additional exam requirements/recommendations for international students: Required—TOEFL (minimum score 560 paper-based; 83 iBT); Recommended—IELTS (minimum score 6.5). *Application deadline:* For fall admission, 4/15 priority date for domestic students, 3/15 priority date for international students; for spring admission, 10/15 priority date for domestic students, 9/15 priority date for international students; for summer admission, 2/15 priority date for domestic students, 1/15 priority date for international students. Applications are processed on a rolling basis. Application fee: $50 ($75 for international students). Electronic applications accepted. *Expenses:* Contact institution. *Financial support:* In 2015–16, 202 students received support. Fellowships, research assistantships, teaching assistantships, Federal Work-Study, institutionally sponsored loans, scholarships/grants, traineeships, and unspecified assistantships available. Financial award application deadline: 4/1; financial award applicants required to submit FAFSA. *Faculty research:* Marketing, management, entrepreneurship, finance, health administration *Unit head:* Woodrow Eckard, MBA Director, 303-315-8470, E-mail: woody.eckard@ucdenver.edu. *Application contact:* Shelly Townley, Admissions Director, Graduate Programs, 303-315-8202, E-mail: shelly.townley@ucdenver.edu.
Website: http://www.ucdenver.edu/academics/colleges/business/degrees/mba/Pages/MBA.aspx

University of Colorado Denver, Business School, Program in Health Administration, Denver, CO 80217. Offers MS. *Accreditation:* CAHME. *Program availability:* Part-time, evening/weekend. *Students:* 6 full-time (4 women), 1 (woman) part-time; includes 1 minority (Asian, non-Hispanic/Latino). Average age 33. 8 applicants, 25% accepted, 1 enrolled. In 2015, 1 master's awarded. *Degree requirements:* For master's, 30 credit hours. *Entrance requirements:* For master's, GMAT, resume, essay, two letters of reference, financial statements (for international applicants). Additional exam requirements/recommendations for international students: Required—TOEFL (minimum score 525 paper-based; 71 iBT); Recommended—IELTS (minimum score 6.5). *Application deadline:* For fall admission, 4/15 priority date for domestic students, 3/15 priority date for international students; for spring admission, 10/15 priority date for domestic students, 9/15 priority date for international students; for summer admission, 2/15 priority date for domestic students, 1/15 priority date for international students. Applications are processed on a rolling basis. Application fee: $50 ($75 for international students). Electronic applications accepted. *Expenses:* Contact institution. *Financial support:* In 2015–16, 2 students received support. Fellowships, research assistantships, teaching assistantships, Federal Work-Study, institutionally sponsored loans, scholarships/grants, and traineeships available. Financial award application deadline: 4/1; financial award applicants required to submit FAFSA. *Faculty research:* Cost containment, financial management, governance, rural health-care delivery systems. *Unit head:* Dr. Errol Biggs, Director, 303-315-8851, E-mail: errol.biggs@ucdenver.edu. *Application contact:* 303-315-8202, E-mail: bschool.admissions@ucdenver.edu.
Website: http://www.ucdenver.edu/academics/colleges/business/degrees/ms/health-admin/Pages/Health-Administration.aspx

University of Colorado Denver, Business School, Program in Information Systems, Denver, CO 80217. Offers accounting and information systems audit and control (MS); business intelligence systems (MS); digital health entrepreneurship (MS); enterprise risk management (MS); enterprise technology management (MS); geographic information systems (MS); health information technology (MS); technology innovation and entrepreneurship (MS); Web and mobile computing (MS). *Program availability:* Part-time, evening/weekend, online learning. *Students:* 104 full-time (34 women), 27 part-time (8 women); includes 22 minority (2 Black or African American, non-Hispanic/Latino; 14 Asian, non-Hispanic/Latino; 5 Hispanic/Latino; 1 Two or more races, non-Hispanic/Latino), 58 international. Average age 31. 102 applicants, 75% accepted, 36 enrolled. In 2015, 28 master's awarded. *Degree requirements:* For master's, 30 credit hours. *Entrance requirements:* For master's, GMAT, resume, essay, two letters of recommendation, financial statements (for international applicants). Additional exam requirements/recommendations for international students: Required—TOEFL (minimum score 525 paper-based; 71 iBT); Recommended—IELTS (minimum score 6.5). *Application deadline:* For fall admission, 4/15 priority date for domestic students, 3/15 priority date for international students; for spring admission, 10/15 priority date for domestic students, 9/15 priority date for international students; for summer admission, 2/15 priority date for domestic students, 1/15 priority date for international students. Applications are processed on a rolling basis. Application fee: $50 ($75 for international students). Electronic applications accepted. *Expenses:* Contact institution. *Financial support:* In 2015–16, 22 students received support. Fellowships, research assistantships, teaching assistantships, Federal Work-Study, institutionally sponsored loans, scholarships/grants, and traineeships available. Financial award application deadline: 4/1; financial award applicants required to submit FAFSA. *Faculty research:* Human-computer interaction, expert systems, database management, electronic commerce, object-oriented software development. *Unit head:* Dr. Jahangir Karimi, Director of Information Systems Programs, 303-315-8430, E-mail: jahangir.karimi@ucdenver.edu. *Application contact:* 303-315-8200, E-mail: bschool.admissions@ucdenver.edu.
Website: http://www.ucdenver.edu/academics/colleges/business/degrees/ms/IS/Pages/Information-Systems.aspx

University of Colorado Denver, Colorado School of Public Health, Program in Public Health, Aurora, CO 80045. Offers community and behavioral health (MPH, Dr PH); environmental and occupational health (MPH); epidemiology (MPH); health systems, management and policy (MPH). *Accreditation:* CEPH. *Program availability:* Part-time, evening/weekend. *Faculty:* 16 full-time (14 women), 1 (woman) part-time/adjunct. *Students:* 379 full-time (293 women), 77 part-time (69 women); includes 111 minority (10 Black or African American, non-Hispanic/Latino; 3 American Indian or Alaska Native, non-Hispanic/Latino; 36 Asian, non-Hispanic/Latino; 47 Hispanic/Latino; 1 Native Hawaiian or other Pacific Islander, non-Hispanic/Latino; 14 Two or more races, non-Hispanic/Latino), 12 international. Average age 31. 785 applicants, 25% accepted, 166 enrolled. In 2015, 144 master's awarded. *Degree requirements:* For master's, thesis or alternative, 42 credit hours; for doctorate, comprehensive exam, thesis/dissertation, 67 credit hours. *Entrance requirements:* For master's, GRE, MCAT, DAT, LSAT, PCAT, GMAT or master's degree from accredited institution, baccalaureate degree or equivalent; minimum GPA of 3.0; transcripts; references; resume; essay; for doctorate, GRE, MCAT, DAT, LSAT, PCAT or GMAT, MPH or master's or higher degree in related

field or equivalent; 2 years of previous work experience in public health; essay; resume. Additional exam requirements/recommendations for international students: Required—TOEFL (minimum score 550 paper-based; 80 iBT). *Application deadline:* For fall admission, 12/15 priority date for domestic students, 12/1 priority date for international students. Application fee: $65. Electronic applications accepted. *Expenses:* Contact institution. *Financial support:* In 2015–16, 265 students received support. Fellowships, research assistantships, teaching assistantships, Federal Work-Study, institutionally sponsored loans, scholarships/grants, traineeships, and unspecified assistantships available. Financial award application deadline: 3/15; financial award applicants required to submit FAFSA. *Faculty research:* Cancer prevention by nutrition, cancer survivorship outcomes, social and cultural factors related to health. *Total annual research expenditures:* $302,793. *Unit head:* Dr. Lori Crane, Chair, 303-724-4385, E-mail: lori.crane@ucdenver.edu. *Application contact:* 303-724-4613, E-mail: csph.studentaffairs@ucdenver.edu.
Website: http://www.ucdenver.edu/academics/colleges/PublicHealth/Academics/degreesandprograms/Pages/index.aspx

University of Connecticut, Graduate School, School of Business, Storrs, CT 06269. Offers accounting (MS, PhD); business administration (MBA, PhD); finance (PhD); health care management and insurance studies (MBA); management (PhD); management consulting (MBA); marketing (PhD); marketing intelligence (MBA). *Accreditation:* AACSB. *Degree requirements:* For master's, comprehensive exam; for doctorate, thesis/dissertation. *Entrance requirements:* For master's and doctorate, GMAT. Additional exam requirements/recommendations for international students: Required—TOEFL (minimum score 550 paper-based). *Application deadline:* For fall admission, 2/1 priority date for domestic and international students; for spring admission, 11/1 for domestic students, 10/1 for international students. Applications are processed on a rolling basis. Electronic applications accepted. *Financial support:* Fellowships, research assistantships with full tuition reimbursements, teaching assistantships with full tuition reimbursements, career-related internships or fieldwork, Federal Work-Study, scholarships/grants, health care benefits, and unspecified assistantships available. Financial award application deadline: 2/1; financial award applicants required to submit FAFSA.
Website: http://www.business.uconn.edu

University of Dallas, Satish and Yasmin Gupta College of Business, Irving, TX 75062-4736. Offers accounting (MBA, MS); business administration (DBA); business analytics (MS); business management (MBA); corporate finance (MBA); cybersecurity (MS); finance (MS); financial services (MBA); global business (MBA, MS); health services management (MBA); human resource management (MBA); information and technology managemeny (MS); information assurance (MBA); information technology (MBA); information technology service management (MBA); marketing management (MBA); organization development (MBA); project management (MBA); sports and entertainment management (MBA); strategic leadership (MBA); supply chain management (MBA). *Program availability:* Part-time, evening/weekend, online learning. *Entrance requirements:* Additional exam requirements/recommendations for international students: Required—TOEFL. Electronic applications accepted. *Expenses:* Contact institution.

University of Detroit Mercy, College of Health Professions, Detroit, MI 48221. Offers clinical nurse leader (MSN); family nurse practitioner (MSN); health services administration (MHSA); health systems management (MSN); nurse anesthesia (MS); nursing (DNP); nursing education (MSN, Certificate); nursing leadership and financial management (Certificate); outcomes performance management (Certificate); physician assistant (MS). *Entrance requirements:* For master's, GRE General Test, minimum GPA of 3.0. Application fee: $30 ($50 for international students). *Expenses:* Tuition, area resident: Full-time $26,802; part-time $1489 per credit. Tuition and fees vary according to course load and program. *Financial support:* Institutionally sponsored loans and tuition waivers (partial) available. Support available to part-time students. Financial award applicants required to submit FAFSA. *Faculty research:* Research design, respiratory physiology, AIDS prevention, adolescent health, community, low income health education. *Unit head:* Dr. Christine M. Pacini, RN, Dean, 313-993-6055, Fax: 313-993-6175.
Website: http://healthprofessions.udmercy.edu/

University of Evansville, College of Education and Health Sciences, School of Public Health, Evansville, IN 47722. Offers health services administration (MS). *Program availability:* Part-time, evening/weekend. *Entrance requirements:* Additional exam requirements/recommendations for international students: Required—TOEFL, IELTS (minimum score 6.5). *Expenses:* Contact institution.

The University of Findlay, Office of Graduate Admissions, Findlay, OH 45840-3653. Offers athletic training (MAT); business (MBA), including health care management, hospitality management, organizational leadership, public management; education (MA Ed), including administration, children's literature, early childhood, human resource development, reading, science, special education, technology; environmental, safety and health management (MSEM); health informatics (MS); occupational therapy (MOT); pharmacy (Pharm D); physical therapy (DPT); physician assistant (MPA); rhetoric and writing (MA); teaching English to speakers of other languages (TESOL) and bilingual education (MA). *Program availability:* Part-time, evening/weekend, online learning. *Degree requirements:* For master's, thesis, cumulative project, capstone project. *Entrance requirements:* For master's, GRE/GMAT, bachelor's degree from accredited institution, minimum undergraduate GPA of 2.5 in last 64 hours of course work; for doctorate, GRE, minimum cumulative GPA of 3.0. Additional exam requirements/recommendations for international students: Required—TOEFL (minimum score 80 iBT). Electronic applications accepted.

University of Florida, Graduate School, College of Pharmacy and Graduate School, Graduate Programs in Pharmacy, Department of Pharmaceutical Outcomes and Policy, Gainesville, FL 32611. Offers MSP, PhD. *Program availability:* Part-time, online learning. *Faculty:* 4 full-time, 3 part-time/adjunct. *Students:* 30 full-time (19 women), 135 part-time (85 women); includes 64 minority (37 Black or African American, non-Hispanic/Latino; 2 American Indian or Alaska Native, non-Hispanic/Latino; 15 Asian, non-Hispanic/Latino; 10 Hispanic/Latino), 25 international. Average age 38. 95 applicants, 41% accepted, 34 enrolled. In 2015, 71 master's, 4 doctorates awarded. *Degree requirements:* For doctorate, thesis/dissertation. *Entrance requirements:* For master's and doctorate, GRE General Test, minimum GPA of 3.0. Additional exam requirements/recommendations for international students: Required—TOEFL (minimum score 550 paper-based; 80 iBT), IELTS (minimum score 6). *Application deadline:* For fall admission, 1/1 priority date for domestic students, 1/1 for international students; for spring admission, 11/15 for domestic and international students. Applications are processed on a rolling basis. Application fee: $30. Electronic applications accepted. *Financial support:* In 2015–16, 2 fellowships, 2 research assistantships, 14 teaching assistantships were awarded; tuition waivers (full) also available. Financial award applicants required to submit FAFSA. *Faculty research:* Pharmacoepidemiology, patient safety and program evaluation, sociology-behavioral issues in medication use, medication safety, pharmacoeconomics, medication therapy management. *Total annual research expenditures:* $1.2 million. *Unit head:* Richard Segal, PhD, Chair, 352-273-6265, Fax: 352-273-6270, E-mail: segal@cop.health.ufl.edu. *Application contact:* Almut

Health Services Management and Hospital Administration

Winterstein, PhD, Professor and Graduate Program Director, 352-273-6258, Fax: 352-273-6270, E-mail: almut@cop.ufl.edu. Website: http://pop.pharmacy.ufl.edu/

University of Florida, Graduate School, College of Public Health and Health Professions, Department of Health Services Research, Management and Policy, Gainesville, FL 32611. Offers health administration (MHA); health services research (PhD). *Accreditation:* CAHME. *Program availability:* Part-time. *Faculty:* 2 full-time. *Students:* 7 full-time (6 women), 1 part-time (0 women); includes 16 minority (6 Black or African American, non-Hispanic/Latino; 3 Asian, non-Hispanic/Latino; 7 Hispanic/Latino), 3 international. Average age 38. 17 applicants. In 2015, 5 doctorates awarded. *Degree requirements:* For master's, internship. *Entrance requirements:* For master's, GRE General Test (minimum score 300) or GMAT (minimum score 500), minimum GPA of 3.0; for doctorate, GRE General Test, minimum GPA of 3.0. Additional exam requirements/recommendations for international students: Required—TOEFL (minimum score 550 paper-based; 80 iBT), IELTS (minimum score 6). *Application deadline:* For fall admission, 2/1 for domestic and international students. Applications are processed on a rolling basis. Application fee: $30. Electronic applications accepted. *Financial support:* In 2015–16, 1 fellowship, 4 research assistantships, 8 teaching assistantships were awarded; career-related internships or fieldwork and unspecified assistantships also available. Financial award applicants required to submit FAFSA. *Faculty research:* State health policy evaluation, health informatics for pain, family medicine, secondary data analysis, disability, mental health. *Unit head:* Dr. Arch G. Mainous, III, Department Chair/Professor, 352-273-6073, Fax: 352-273-6075, E-mail: arch.mainous@phhp.ufl.edu. *Application contact:* Barbara Ross, Student Services Coordinator, 352-273-6074, Fax: 352-273-6075, E-mail: bross@phhp.ufl.edu. Website: http://www.phhp.ufl.edu/hsrmp/

University of Florida, Graduate School, Warrington College of Business Administration, Hough Graduate School of Business, Department of Management, Gainesville, FL 32611. Offers health care risk management (MS); international business (MA); management (MS, PhD). *Accreditation:* AACSB. *Program availability:* Online learning. *Faculty:* 5 full-time, 1 part-time/adjunct. *Students:* 97 full-time (48 women), 37 part-time (27 women); includes 47 minority (1 American Indian or Alaska Native, non-Hispanic/Latino; 19 Asian, non-Hispanic/Latino; 27 Hispanic/Latino), 83 international. Average age 25. 183 applicants, 42% accepted, 50 enrolled. In 2015, 110 master's awarded. *Degree requirements:* For master's, comprehensive exam, thesis. *Entrance requirements:* For master's, GMAT (minimum score of 465) or GRE General Test, minimum GPA of 3.0. Additional exam requirements/recommendations for international students: Required—TOEFL (minimum score 550 paper-based; 80 iBT), IELTS (minimum score 6). *Application deadline:* For fall admission, 1/1 for domestic and international students. Applications are processed on a rolling basis. Application fee: $30. Electronic applications accepted. *Financial support:* In 2015–16, 4 research assistantships, 13 teaching assistantships were awarded; fellowships and unspecified assistantships also available. Financial award applicants required to submit FAFSA. *Faculty research:* Job attitudes, personality and individual differences, organizational entry and exit, knowledge management, competitive dynamics. *Total annual research expenditures:* $1,055. *Unit head:* Robert E. Thomas, PhD, Chair, 352-392-0136, Fax: 352-392-6020, E-mail: rethomas@ufl.edu. *Application contact:* Office of Admissions, 352-392-1365, E-mail: webrequests@admissions.ufl.edu. Website: http://warrington.ufl.edu/departments/mgt/

University of Georgia, College of Public Health, Department of Health Policy and Management, Athens, GA 30602. Offers MPH.

University of Houston–Clear Lake, School of Business, Program in Healthcare Administration, Houston, TX 77058-1002. Offers MHA, MHA/MBA. *Degree requirements:* For master's, thesis optional. *Entrance requirements:* For master's, GMAT. Additional exam requirements/recommendations for international students: Required—TOEFL (minimum score 550 paper-based).

University of Illinois at Chicago, School of Public Health, Division of Health Policy and Administration, Chicago, IL 60607-7128. Offers clinical and translational science (MS); health policy (PhD); health services research (PhD); healthcare administration (MHA); public health policy management (MPH). *Program availability:* Part-time. *Faculty:* 16 full-time (9 women), 18 part-time/adjunct (7 women). *Students:* 129 full-time (88 women), 149 part-time (102 women); includes 140 minority (39 Black or African American, non-Hispanic/Latino; 59 Asian, non-Hispanic/Latino; 34 Hispanic/Latino; 1 Native Hawaiian or other Pacific Islander, non-Hispanic/Latino; 7 Two or more races, non-Hispanic/Latino), 18 international. Average age 32. Terminal master's awarded for partial completion of doctoral program. *Degree requirements:* For master's, thesis, field practicum; for doctorate, thesis/dissertation, independent research, internship. *Entrance requirements:* For master's and doctorate, GRE General Test, minimum GPA of 2.75. Additional exam requirements/recommendations for international students: Required—TOEFL. *Application deadline:* For fall admission, 2/1 for domestic students, 1/1 priority date for international students. Application fee: $60. Electronic applications accepted. *Expenses:* Contact institution. *Financial support:* In 2015–16, 4 fellowships with full tuition reimbursements were awarded; research assistantships with full tuition reimbursements, teaching assistantships with full tuition reimbursements, career-related internships or fieldwork, Federal Work-Study, institutionally sponsored loans, scholarships/grants, traineeships, and unspecified assistantships also available. Support available to part-time students. Financial award application deadline: 3/1; financial award applicants required to submit FAFSA. *Faculty research:* Cancer screening in underserved populations, practices and devices used to reduce firefighter injury, the relationship between communal housing and substance abuse recovery. *Unit head:* Prof. Jack Zwanziger, Director, 312-996-1062, Fax: 312-996-5356, E-mail: jzwanzig@uic.edu. *Application contact:* Aimee Wiebel, Academic Coordinator, 312-996-7816, Fax: 312-996-5356, E-mail: aimee@uic.edu. Website: http://publichealth.uic.edu/departments/healthpolicyandadministration/

University of Illinois at Urbana–Champaign, Graduate College, School of Social Work, Champaign, IL 61820. Offers advocacy, leadership, and social change (MSW); children, youth and family services (MSW); health care (MSW); mental health (MSW); school social work (MSW); social work (PhD). *Accreditation:* CSWE (one or more programs are accredited). *Entrance requirements:* For master's and doctorate, minimum GPA of 3.0.

The University of Iowa, Graduate College, College of Public Health, Department of Health Management and Policy, Iowa City, IA 52242-1316. Offers MHA, PhD, JD/MHA, MBA/MIIA, MHA/MA, MHA/MS. *Accreditation:* CAHME (one or more programs are accredited). *Degree requirements:* For doctorate, comprehensive exam, thesis/dissertation. *Entrance requirements:* For master's, GRE General Test or equivalent, minimum GPA of 3.0; for doctorate, GRE General Test, minimum GPA of 3.0. Additional exam requirements/recommendations for international students: Required—TOEFL (minimum score 550 paper-based; 81 iBT). Electronic applications accepted. *Expenses:* Contact institution.

The University of Kansas, University of Kansas Medical Center, School of Medicine, Department of Health Policy and Management, Kansas City, KS 66160. Offers health policy and management (PhD); health services administration (MHSA); JD/MHSA; MD/MHSA;

MHSA/MS. *Accreditation:* CAHME. *Program availability:* Part-time. *Faculty:* 16. *Students:* 35 full-time (23 women), 39 part-time (23 women); includes 14 minority (1 Black or African American, non-Hispanic/Latino; 8 Asian, non-Hispanic/Latino; 3 Hispanic/Latino; 2 Two or more races, non-Hispanic/Latino), 3 international. Average age 31. 61 applicants, 62% accepted, 23 enrolled. In 2015, 16 master's awarded. *Degree requirements:* For master's, internship or research practicum; for doctorate, comprehensive exam, thesis/dissertation. *Entrance requirements:* For master's, GRE, college-level statistics; for doctorate, GRE, graduate statistics course. Additional exam requirements/recommendations for international students: Required—TOEFL. *Application deadline:* For fall admission, 3/1 for domestic and international students. Applications are processed on a rolling basis. Application fee: $60. Electronic applications accepted. *Financial support:* Fellowships with full tuition reimbursements, research assistantships with partial tuition reimbursements, teaching assistantships with full tuition reimbursements, career-related internships or fieldwork, and scholarships/grants available. Financial award application deadline: 3/1; financial award applicants required to submit FAFSA. *Faculty research:* Impacts of the Affordable Care Act and Medicaid reforms; cancer health services research; health care workforce and occupational health; implementation science and performance improvement; disparities in health outcomes. *Total annual research expenditures:* $332,070. *Unit head:* Dr. Robert H. Lee, Chair, 913-588-2689, Fax: 913-588-8236, E-mail: rlee2@kumc.edu. *Application contact:* Deborah S. Lewis, Student Support Manager, 913-588-3763, Fax: 913-588-8236, E-mail: dlewis4@kumc.edu. Website: http://www.kumc.edu/school-of-medicine/hpm.html

University of Kentucky, Graduate School, College of Health Sciences, Program in Health Administration, Lexington, KY 40506-0032. Offers MHA. *Accreditation:* CAHME. *Degree requirements:* For master's, comprehensive exam. *Entrance requirements:* For master's, GRE General Test, minimum undergraduate GPA of 2.75. Additional exam requirements/recommendations for international students: Required—TOEFL (minimum score 550 paper-based). Electronic applications accepted. *Faculty research:* Health economy, health finance, health policy.

University of La Verne, College of Business and Public Management, Graduate Programs in Business Administration, La Verne, CA 91750-4443. Offers accounting (MBA); executive management (MBA-EP); finance (MBA, MBA-EP); health services management (MBA); information technology (MBA, MBA-EP); international business (MBA, MBA-EP); leadership (MBA-EP); managed care (MBA); management (MBA, MBA-EP); marketing (MBA, MBA-EP). *Program availability:* Part-time, evening/weekend. *Faculty:* 16 full-time (9 women), 23 part-time/adjunct (7 women). *Students:* 421 full-time (212 women), 89 part-time (47 women); includes 90 minority (8 Black or African American, non-Hispanic/Latino; 15 Asian, non-Hispanic/Latino; 64 Hispanic/Latino; 1 Native Hawaiian or other Pacific Islander, non-Hispanic/Latino; 2 Two or more races, non-Hispanic/Latino), 360 international. Average age 28. In 2015, 625 master's awarded. *Entrance requirements:* For master's, GMAT, MAT, or GRE, minimum undergraduate GPA of 3.0, 2 letters of recommendation, resume, statement of purpose. Additional exam requirements/recommendations for international students: Required—TOEFL (minimum score 550 paper-based; 85 iBT). *Application deadline:* Applications are processed on a rolling basis. Application fee: $50. *Expenses:* $757 per semester hour. *Financial support:* Career-related internships or fieldwork, institutionally sponsored loans, and scholarships/grants available. Financial award application deadline: 3/2; financial award applicants required to submit FAFSA. *Unit head:* Dr. Abe Helou, Chairperson, 909-448-4455 Ext. 4455, Fax: 909-392-2704, E-mail: ihelou@laverne.edu. *Application contact:* Rina Lazarian-Chehab, Senior Associate Director of Graduate Admissions, 909-448-4317, Fax: 909-971-2295, E-mail: rlazarian@laverne.edu. Website: http://laverne.edu/business-and-public-administration/

University of La Verne, College of Business and Public Management, Program in Gerontology, La Verne, CA 91750-4443. Offers geriatric care management (MS); gerontology (Certificate); gerontology administration (MS); health services management (MS). *Program availability:* Part-time. *Faculty:* 5 full-time (4 women), 3 part-time/adjunct (1 woman). *Students:* 8 full-time (6 women), 11 part-time (8 women); includes 13 minority (3 Black or African American, non-Hispanic/Latino; 10 Hispanic/Latino), 3 international. Average age 43. In 2015, 12 master's awarded. *Entrance requirements:* For master's, bachelor's degree, minimum preferred GPA of 2.75, 2 recommendations, personal statement. Additional exam requirements/recommendations for international students: Required—TOEFL (minimum score 550 paper-based). *Application deadline:* Applications are processed on a rolling basis. Application fee: $50. *Expenses:* $757 per semester hour. *Financial support:* Federal Work-Study available. Financial award application deadline: 3/2; financial award applicants required to submit FAFSA. *Unit head:* Kelly Niles-Yokum, Program Director, 909-448-1584, E-mail: kniles-yokum@laverne.edu. *Application contact:* Barbara Cox, Program and Admissions Specialist, 909-593-3511 Ext. 4004, Fax: 909-971-2295, E-mail: bcox@laverne.edu. Website: http://laverne.edu/business-and-public-administration/m-s-in-gerontology/

University of La Verne, College of Business and Public Management, Program in Health Administration, La Verne, CA 91750-4443. Offers financial management (MHA); management and leadership (MHA); marketing and business development (MHA). *Program availability:* Part-time. *Faculty:* 5 full-time (4 women), 3 part-time/adjunct (1 woman). *Students:* 48 full-time (29 women), 34 part-time (25 women); includes 36 minority (9 Black or African American, non-Hispanic/Latino; 1 American Indian or Alaska Native, non-Hispanic/Latino; 5 Asian, non-Hispanic/Latino; 21 Hispanic/Latino), 10 international. Average age 31. In 2015, 34 master's awarded. *Entrance requirements:* For master's, bachelor's degree, experience in health services industry (preferred). Additional exam requirements/recommendations for international students: Required—TOEFL (minimum score 550 paper-based). *Application deadline:* Applications are processed on a rolling basis. Application fee: $50. *Expenses:* $757 per semester hour. *Financial support:* Federal Work-Study available. Financial award application deadline: 3/2; financial award applicants required to submit FAFSA. *Unit head:* Dr. Kathy Duncan, Program Chairperson, 909-448-4415, E-mail: kduncan2@laverne.edu. *Application contact:* Barbara Cox, Program and Admissions Specialist, 909-448-4004, Fax: 909-971-2295, E-mail: bcox@laverne.edu. Website: http://laverne.edu/business-and-public-administration/mha-2/

University of La Verne, Regional and Online Campuses, Graduate Programs, Central Coast/Vandenberg Air Force Base Campuses, La Verne, CA 91750-4443. Offers business administration for experienced professionals (MBA), including health services management, information technology; education (special emphasis) (M Ed); educational counseling (MS); educational leadership (M Ed); multiple subject (elementary) (Credential); preliminary administrative services (Credential); pupil personnel services (Credential); single subject (secondary) (Credential). *Program availability:* Part-time. *Faculty:* 3 part-time/adjunct (1 woman). *Students:* 6 full-time (1 woman), 37 part-time (20 women); includes 9 minority (1 Asian, non-Hispanic/Latino; 8 Hispanic/Latino). Average age 40. In 2015, 20 master's awarded. *Application deadline:* Applications are processed on a rolling basis. Application fee: $50. *Expenses:* Contact institution. *Financial support:* Application deadline: 3/2; applicants required to submit FAFSA. *Unit head:* Kitt Vincent, Director, Central Coast Campus, 805-788-6202, Fax: 805-788-6201, E-mail: kvincent@laverne.edu. *Application contact:* Admissions, 805-788-6200, E-mail: lavernecentralcoast@laverne.edu. Website: http://www.laverne.edu/locations

University of La Verne, Regional and Online Campuses, Graduate Programs, Inland Empire Campus, Ontario, CA 91730. Offers business administration (MBA, MBA-EP), including accounting (MBA), finance (MBA), health services management (MBA-EP), information technology (MBA-EP), international business (MBA), managed care (MBA), management and leadership (MBA-EP), marketing (MBA-EP), supply chain management (MBA); leadership and management (MS), including human resource management, nonprofit management, organizational development. *Program availability:* Part-time, evening/weekend. *Faculty:* 5 part-time/adjunct (1 woman). *Students:* 24 full-time (13 women), 72 part-time (44 women); includes 64 minority (12 Black or African American, non-Hispanic/Latino; 13 Asian, non-Hispanic/Latino; 36 Hispanic/Latino; 3 Two or more races, non-Hispanic/Latino). Average age 38. In 2015, 42 master's awarded. *Application deadline:* Applications are processed on a rolling basis. Application fee: $50. *Expenses:* Contact institution. *Financial support:* Application deadline: 3/2; applicants required to submit FAFSA. *Unit head:* Allen Stout, Campus Director, Inland Empire Regional Campus in Ontario, 909-937-6987, E-mail: astout@laverne.edu. *Application contact:* Karen Schumann, Senior Associate Director of Admissions, Inland Empire Regional Campus in Ontario, 909-937-6991, E-mail: kschumann@laverne.edu.
Website: http://laverne.edu/locations/inland-empire/

University of La Verne, Regional and Online Campuses, Graduate Programs, Kern County Campus, Bakersfield, CA 93301. Offers business administration for experienced professionals (MBA-EP); education (special emphasis) (M Ed); educational counseling (MS); educational leadership (M Ed); health administration (MHA); leadership and management (MS); mild/moderate education specialist (Credential); multiple subject (elementary) (Credential); organizational leadership (Ed D); preliminary administrative services (Credential); single subject (secondary) (Credential); special education studies (MS). *Program availability:* Part-time, evening/weekend. *Faculty:* 2 part-time/adjunct (1 woman). *Students:* 5 full-time (2 women), 10 part-time (5 women); includes 6 minority (5 Hispanic/Latino; 1 Two or more races, non-Hispanic/Latino). Average age 36. In 2015, 3 master's awarded. *Application deadline:* Applications are processed on a rolling basis. Application fee: $50. *Expenses:* Contact institution. *Financial support:* Institutionally sponsored loans available. Financial award application deadline: 3/2; financial award applicants required to submit FAFSA. *Unit head:* Nora Dominguez, Regional Campus Director, 661-861-6802, E-mail: ndominguez@laverne.edu. *Application contact:* Rebecca Murillo, Associate Director of Admissions, 661-861-6807, E-mail: rmurillo@laverne.edu.
Website: http://laverne.edu/locations/bakersfield/

University of La Verne, Regional and Online Campuses, Graduate Programs, Orange County Campus, Irvine, CA 92840. Offers business administration for experienced professionals (MBA); educational counseling (MS); educational leadership (M Ed); health administration (MHA); leadership and management (MS); preliminary administrative services (Credential); pupil personnel services (Credential). *Program availability:* Part-time. *Faculty:* 9 part-time/adjunct (2 women). *Students:* 19 full-time (11 women), 51 part-time (30 women); includes 53 minority (12 Black or African American, non-Hispanic/Latino; 2 American Indian or Alaska Native, non-Hispanic/Latino; 12 Asian, non-Hispanic/Latino; 27 Hispanic/Latino). Average age 39. In 2015, 43 master's awarded. *Application deadline:* Applications are processed on a rolling basis. Application fee: $50. *Expenses:* Contact institution. *Financial support:* Application deadline: 3/2; applicants required to submit FAFSA. *Unit head:* Alison Rodriguez-Balles, Interim Campus Director, 714-505-6943, E-mail: arodriguez2@laverne.edu. *Application contact:* Oscar Cancio, Associate Director of Admissions, 714-505-6939, E-mail: ocancio@laverne.edu.
Website: http://laverne.edu/locations/irvine/

University of Louisville, Graduate School, College of Business, MBA Programs, Louisville, KY 40292-0001. Offers entrepreneurship (MBA); global business (MBA); health sector management (MBA). *Accreditation:* AACSB. *Program availability:* Part-time, evening/weekend. *Students:* 215 full-time (64 women), 30 part-time (8 women); includes 26 minority (8 Black or African American, non-Hispanic/Latino; 1 American Indian or Alaska Native, non-Hispanic/Latino; 9 Asian, non-Hispanic/Latino; 8 Hispanic/Latino); 13 international. Average age 31. 284 applicants, 65% accepted, 156 enrolled. In 2015, 69 master's awarded. *Degree requirements:* For master's, international learning experience. *Entrance requirements:* For master's, GMAT, 2 letters of reference, personal interview, resume, personal statement, college transcript(s). Additional exam requirements/recommendations for international students: Required—TOEFL (minimum score 83 iBT). *Application deadline:* For fall admission, 7/1 for domestic students; for spring admission, 12/1 for domestic students. Applications are processed on a rolling basis. Application fee: $60. *Expenses:* Tuition, state resident: full-time $11,664; part-time $649 per credit hour. Tuition, nonresident: full-time $24,274; part-time $1350 per credit hour. *Required fees:* $196. Tuition and fees vary according to program and reciprocity agreements. *Financial support:* In 2015–16, 919,859 students received support. Fellowships with full tuition reimbursements available, research assistantships with full tuition reimbursements available, health care benefits, and unspecified assistantships available. Financial award application deadline: 3/31; financial award applicants required to submit FAFSA. *Faculty research:* Entrepreneurship, venture capital, retailing/franchising, corporate governance and leadership, supply chain management. *Total annual research expenditures:* $1.2 million. *Unit head:* Dr. Carolyn M. Callahan, Dean, 502-852-6440, Fax: 502-852-7557, E-mail: cmcall04@louisville.edu. *Application contact:* Susan E. Hildebrand, Program Director, 502-852-7257, Fax: 502-852-4901, E-mail: s.hildebrand@louisville.edu.
Website: http://business.louisville.edu/mba

University of Management and Technology, Program in Health Administration, Arlington, VA 22209. Offers MHA. *Application contact:* Kenny Hickey, Admissions, 703-516-0035, Fax: 703-516-0985, E-mail: admissions@umtweb.edu.

University of Mary, Gary Tharaldson School of Business, Bismarck, ND 58504-9652. Offers business administration (MBA); energy management (MBA, MS); executive (MBA, MS); health care (MBA, MS); human resource management (MBA); project management (MBA, MPM, MS); virtuous leadership (MBA, MPM, MS). *Program availability:* Part-time, evening/weekend. *Entrance requirements:* For master's, minimum GPA of 2.5. Additional exam requirements/recommendations for international students: Required—TOEFL (minimum score 550 paper-based; 80 iBT). *Application deadline:* Applications are processed on a rolling basis. Application fee: $45. Electronic applications accepted. *Financial support:* Application deadline: 8/1; applicants required to submit FAFSA.
Website: http://www.umary.edu/academics/schools/business.php

University of Maryland, Baltimore County, The Graduate School, College of Arts, Humanities and Social Sciences, Department of Emergency Health Services, Baltimore, MD 21250. Offers administration, planning, and policy (MS); education (MS); emergency health services (MS); emergency management (Postbaccalaureate Certificate); preventive medicine and epidemiology (MS). *Program availability:* Part-time, evening/weekend, 100% online, blended/hybrid learning. *Faculty:* 3 full-time (1 woman), 8 part-time/adjunct (2 women). *Students:* 24 full-time (14 women), 11 part-time (5 women); includes 8 minority (2 Black or African American, non-Hispanic/Latino; 3 Asian, non-Hispanic/Latino; 3 Hispanic/Latino), 14 international. Average age 26. 18 applicants,

56% accepted, 7 enrolled. In 2015, 13 master's awarded. *Degree requirements:* For master's, comprehensive exam, thesis (for some programs), capstone project. *Entrance requirements:* For master's, GRE General Test, minimum GPA of 3.2. Additional exam requirements/recommendations for international students: Required—TOEFL (minimum score 85 iBT) or IELTS. *Application deadline:* For fall admission, 6/15 for domestic students, 3/1 for international students; for spring admission, 11/1 for domestic students, 10/1 for international students. Applications are processed on a rolling basis. Application fee: $50. Electronic applications accepted. *Expenses:* Tuition, state resident: full-time $12,816. Tuition, nonresident: full-time $19,710. *Financial support:* In 2015–16, 2 students received support, including 1 fellowship with tuition reimbursement available (averaging $70,000 per year), 1 research assistantship with tuition reimbursement available (averaging $26,800 per year); career-related internships or fieldwork, Federal Work-Study, scholarships/grants, health care benefits, and unspecified assistantships also available. Financial award application deadline: 5/30; financial award applicants required to submit FAFSA. *Faculty research:* EMS management, disaster health services, emergency management, epidemiology, risk profiles. *Total annual research expenditures:* $50,000. *Unit head:* Dr. Bruce J. Walz, Chairman, 410-455-3216, Fax: 410-455-3045, E-mail: walz@umbc.edu. *Application contact:* Dr. Rick Bissell, Program Director, 410-455-3776, Fax: 410-455-3045, E-mail: bissell@umbc.edu.
Website: http://ehs.umbc.edu/

University of Maryland, Baltimore County, The Graduate School, College of Arts, Humanities and Social Sciences, School of Public Policy, Baltimore, MD 21250. Offers public policy (MPP, PhD), including economics (PhD), educational policy, evaluation and analytical methods, health policy, policy history (PhD), public management, urban policy. *Accreditation:* NASPAA (one or more programs are accredited). *Program availability:* Part-time, evening/weekend. *Faculty:* 8 full-time (2 women), 1 part-time/adjunct (0 women). *Students:* 49 full-time (25 women), 66 part-time (33 women); includes 22 minority (8 Black or African American, non-Hispanic/Latino; 10 Asian, non-Hispanic/Latino; 3 Hispanic/Latino; 1 Two or more races, non-Hispanic/Latino), 5 international. Average age 36. 75 applicants, 69% accepted, 29 enrolled. In 2015, 14 master's, 9 doctorates awarded. Terminal master's awarded for partial completion of doctoral program. *Degree requirements:* For master's, thesis optional, policy analysis paper, internship for pre-service; for doctorate, comprehensive exam, thesis/ dissertation, comprehensive and field qualifying exams. *Entrance requirements:* For master's and doctorate, GRE General Test, 3 academic letters of reference, resume, research paper, official transcripts. Additional exam requirements/recommendations for international students: Required—TOEFL (minimum score 550 paper-based; 80 iBT). *Application deadline:* For fall admission, 1/15 priority date for domestic students, 1/1 priority date for international students; for spring admission, 11/1 priority date for domestic students, 5/1 priority date for international students. Applications are processed on a rolling basis. Application fee: $50. Electronic applications accepted. *Expenses:* $708 per credit hour in-state; $1,091 per credit hour out-of-state. *Financial support:* In 2015–16, 23 students received support, including 1 fellowship with full tuition reimbursement available (averaging $14,000 per year), 22 research assistantships with full tuition reimbursements available (averaging $20,000 per year); career-related internships or fieldwork, Federal Work-Study, scholarships/grants, health care benefits, tuition waivers, and unspecified assistantships also available. Support available to part-time students. Financial award application deadline: 1/15; financial award applicants required to submit FAFSA. *Faculty research:* Education policy, health policy, urban policy, public management, evaluation and analytical method. *Unit head:* Dr. Donald F. Norris, Director, 410-455-3201, Fax: 410-455-1172, E-mail: norris@umbc.edu. *Application contact:* Sally F. Helms, Administrator of Academic Affairs, 410-455-3202, Fax: 410-455-1172, E-mail: gradpubpol@umbc.edu.
Website: http://publicpolicy.umbc.edu/

University of Maryland, Baltimore County, The Graduate School, Erickson School of Aging Studies, Baltimore, MD 21228. Offers management of aging services (MA). *Faculty:* 4 full-time (1 woman), 7 part-time/adjunct (1 woman). *Students:* 18 full-time (11 women); includes 9 minority (8 Black or African American, non-Hispanic/Latino; 1 Hispanic/Latino). Average age 30. 23 applicants, 91% accepted, 18 enrolled. In 2015, 13 master's awarded. *Degree requirements:* For master's, thesis or alternative. *Entrance requirements:* For master's, essays. *Application deadline:* Applications are processed on a rolling basis. Application fee: $50. Electronic applications accepted. *Expenses:* Contact institution. *Financial support:* In 2015–16, 15 students received support, including 1 teaching assistantship with full tuition reimbursement available (averaging $21,600 per year). Financial award applicants required to submit FAFSA. *Faculty research:* Policy implications of entitlement programs, demographic impact of aging population, person-centered care for dementia, changing culture in long-term care. *Unit head:* Bill Holman, Graduate Program Director, 443-543-5603, E-mail: bholman@sagepointcare.org. *Application contact:* Michelle Howell, Administrative Assistant, 443-543-5607, E-mail: mhowell@umbc.edu.
Website: http://www.umbc.edu/erickson/

University of Maryland, College Park, Academic Affairs, School of Public Health, Department of Health Services Administration, College Park, MD 20742. Offers MHA, PhD.

University of Maryland University College, The Graduate School, Program in Health Care Administration, Adelphi, MD 20783. Offers MS, Certificate. *Program availability:* Part-time, evening/weekend, online learning. *Students:* 10 full-time (all women), 664 part-time (527 women); includes 420 minority (313 Black or African American, non-Hispanic/Latino; 1 American Indian or Alaska Native, non-Hispanic/Latino; 52 Asian, non-Hispanic/Latino; 35 Hispanic/Latino; 3 Native Hawaiian or other Pacific Islander, non-Hispanic/Latino; 16 Two or more races, non-Hispanic/Latino), 15 international. Average age 33. 211 applicants, 100% accepted, 157 enrolled. In 2015, 131 master's awarded. *Degree requirements:* For master's, thesis or alternative. *Application deadline:* Applications are processed on a rolling basis. Application fee: $50. Electronic applications accepted. *Financial support:* Federal Work-Study and scholarships/grants available. Support available to part-time students. Financial award application deadline: 6/1; financial award applicants required to submit FAFSA. *Unit head:* Monica Bruenn, Program Director, 240-684-2400, Fax: 240-684-2401, E-mail: monica.sava@umuc.edu. *Application contact:* Coordinator, Graduate Admissions, 800-888-8682, Fax: 240-684-2151, E-mail: newgrad@umuc.edu.
Website: http://www.umuc.edu/academic-programs/masters-degrees/health-care-administration.cfm

University of Massachusetts Amherst, Graduate School, Isenberg School of Management, Program in Management, Amherst, MA 01003. Offers accounting (PhD); business administration (MBA); entrepreneurship (MBA); finance (MBA, PhD); healthcare administration (MBA); hospitality and tourism management (PhD); management science (PhD); marketing (MBA, PhD); organization studies (PhD); sport management (PhD); strategic management (PhD); MBA/MS. *Accreditation:* AACSB. *Program availability:* Part-time, evening/weekend, online learning. Terminal master's awarded for partial completion of doctoral program. *Degree requirements:* For doctorate, comprehensive exam, thesis/dissertation. *Entrance requirements:* For master's and doctorate, GMAT or GRE General Test. Additional exam requirements/

Health Services Management and Hospital Administration

recommendations for international students: Required—TOEFL (minimum score 550 paper-based; 80 iBT), IELTS (minimum score 6.5). Electronic applications accepted.

University of Massachusetts Amherst, Graduate School, School of Public Health and Health Sciences, Department of Public Health, Amherst, MA 01003. Offers biostatistics (MPH, MS, PhD); community health education (MPH, MS, PhD); environmental health sciences (MPH, MS, PhD); epidemiology (MPH, MS, PhD); health policy and management (MPH, MS, PhD); nutrition (MPH, PhD); public health practice (MPH); MPH/MPPA. *Accreditation:* CEPH (one or more programs are accredited). *Program availability:* Part-time, evening/weekend, online learning. Terminal master's awarded for partial completion of doctoral program. *Degree requirements:* For master's, thesis (for some programs); for doctorate, comprehensive exam, thesis/dissertation. *Entrance requirements:* For master's and doctorate, GRE General Test. Additional exam requirements/recommendations for international students: Required—TOEFL (minimum score 550 paper-based; 80 iBT), IELTS (minimum score 6.5). Electronic applications accepted.

University of Massachusetts Dartmouth, Graduate School, Charlton College of Business, Department of Decision and Information Sciences, North Dartmouth, MA 02747-2300. Offers healthcare management (MS); technology management (MS). *Program availability:* Part-time, 100% online. *Faculty:* 12 full-time (5 women), 3 part-time/adjunct (1 woman). *Students:* 3 full-time (all women), 7 part-time (5 women); includes 3 minority (1 Black or African American, non-Hispanic/Latino; 1 Asian, non-Hispanic/Latino; 1 Two or more races, non-Hispanic/Latino), 2 international. Average age 34. 14 applicants, 93% accepted, 9 enrolled. *Degree requirements:* For master's, thesis or project as alternative to course electives. *Entrance requirements:* For master's, GMAT, statement of purpose (minimum 300 words), resume, official transcripts, 2 letters of recommendation. Additional exam requirements/recommendations for international students: Required—TOEFL (minimum score 533 paper-based; 72 iBT). *Application deadline:* For fall admission, 8/1 priority date for domestic students, 6/1 priority date for international students; for spring admission, 11/15 priority date for domestic students, 10/15 priority date for international students. Applications are processed on a rolling basis. Application fee: $60. *Expenses:* Tuition, state resident: full-time $2071; part-time $86.29 per credit. Tuition, nonresident: full-time $8099; part-time $337.46 per credit. *Required fees:* $18,074; $762.08 per credit. Tuition and fees vary according to course load and reciprocity agreements. *Financial support:* Career-related internships or fieldwork, scholarships/grants, and unspecified assistantships available. Financial award application deadline: 3/1; financial award applicants required to submit FAFSA. *Faculty research:* Healthcare management and policy, process management, supply chain management, project management, particularly project team work processes, technology-mediated learning, the use of IT in organizations, leadership in health systems, decision models for adaptation of the advanced manufacturing technologies. *Unit head:* Dr. Laura Forker, Program Coordinator, 508-999-9259, E-mail: lforker@umassd.edu. *Application contact:* Steven Briggs, Director of Marketing and Recruitment for Graduate Studies, 508-999-8604, Fax: 508-999-8183, E-mail: graduate@umassd.edu.
Website: http://www.umassd.edu/charlton/programs/graduate/

University of Memphis, Graduate School, School of Public Health, Memphis, TN 38152. Offers biostatistics (MPH); environmental health (MPH); epidemiology (MPH); health systems management (MPH); public health (MHA); social and behavioral sciences (MPH). *Program availability:* Part-time, evening/weekend, online learning. *Faculty:* 117 full-time (5 women), 5 part-time/adjunct (1 woman). *Students:* 100 full-time (68 women), 48 part-time (35 women); includes 63 minority (33 Black or African American, non-Hispanic/Latino; 20 Asian, non-Hispanic/Latino; 7 Hispanic/Latino; 3 Two or more races, non-Hispanic/Latino), 17 international. Average age 30. 114 applicants, 83% accepted, 37 enrolled. In 2015, 55 master's awarded. *Degree requirements:* For master's, comprehensive exam, thesis. *Entrance requirements:* For master's, GRE, letters of recommendation. Additional exam requirements/recommendations for international students: Required—TOEFL. *Application deadline:* For fall admission, 4/1 for domestic students; for spring admission, 11/1 for domestic students. Application fee: $35 ($60 for international students). Electronic applications accepted. *Financial support:* In 2015–16, 46 students received support. Research assistantships with full tuition reimbursements available, Federal Work-Study, scholarships/grants, and unspecified assistantships available. Financial award application deadline: 2/15; financial award applicants required to submit FAFSA. *Faculty research:* Health and medical savings accounts, adoption rates, health informatics, Telehealth technologies, biostatistics, environmental health, epidemiology, health systems management, social and behavioral sciences. *Unit head:* Dr. Lisa M. Klesges, Director, 901-678-4637, E-mail: lmklsges@memphis.edu. *Application contact:* Dr. Karen Weddle-West, Information Contact, 901-678-2531, Fax: 901-678-5023, E-mail: gradsch@memphis.edu.
Website: http://www.memphis.edu/sph/

University of Michigan, School of Public Health, Department of Health Management and Policy, Ann Arbor, MI 48109. Offers health management and policy (MHSA, MPH); health services organization and policy (PhD); JD/MHSA; MD/MPH; MHSA/MBA; MHSA/MPP; MHSA/MSIOE; MPH/JD; MPH/MBA; MPH/MPP. PhD and MS offered through the Rackham Graduate School. *Accreditation:* CAHME (one or more programs are accredited). *Program availability:* Evening/weekend. *Faculty:* 21 full-time (9 women), 40 part-time/adjunct (12 women). *Students:* 165 full-time (99 women), 6 part-time (4 women); includes 46 minority (9 Black or African American, non-Hispanic/Latino; 30 Asian, non-Hispanic/Latino; 5 Hispanic/Latino; 2 Two or more races, non-Hispanic/Latino), 20 international. Average age 28. 646 applicants, 27% accepted, 90 enrolled. In 2015, 83 master's, 8 doctorates awarded. *Degree requirements:* For doctorate, thesis/dissertation, oral defense of dissertation, preliminary exam. *Entrance requirements:* For master's, GMAT, GRE General Test; for doctorate, GRE General Test. Additional exam requirements/recommendations for international students: Required—TOEFL (minimum score 600 paper-based; 100 iBT). *Application deadline:* For fall admission, 12/15 priority date for domestic students, 1/15 for international students. Applications are processed on a rolling basis. Application fee: $75. Electronic applications accepted. *Financial support:* Fellowships, research assistantships, teaching assistantships, career-related internships or fieldwork, Federal Work-Study, institutionally sponsored loans, scholarships/grants, traineeships, health care benefits, and unspecified assistantships available. *Faculty research:* Health insurance, long-term care and aging, tobacco policy, health information technology, understanding organization. *Unit head:* Prof. Kyle Grazier, Chair, 734-936-1222, Fax: 734-764-4338, E-mail: kgrazier@umich.edu. *Application contact:* Charlita Daniels, Program Coordinator, 734-936-5944, Fax: 734-764-4338, E-mail: dancharl@umich.edu.
Website: http://www.sph.umich.edu/hmp/

University of Michigan–Flint, Graduate Programs, Program in Public Administration, Flint, MI 48502-1950. Offers administration of non-profit agencies (MPA); criminal justice administration (MPA); educational administration (MPA); general public administration (MPA); healthcare administration (MPA). *Program availability:* Part-time. *Faculty:* 1 full-time (0 women), 5 part-time/adjunct (3 women). *Students:* 7 full-time (6 women), 110 part-time (75 women); includes 36 minority (27 Black or African American, non-Hispanic/Latino; 1 Asian, non-Hispanic/Latino; 5 Hispanic/Latino; 1 Native Hawaiian or other Pacific Islander, non-Hispanic/Latino; 2 Two or more races, non-Hispanic/Latino), 3

international. Average age 34. 68 applicants, 65% accepted, 29 enrolled. In 2015, 44 master's awarded. *Degree requirements:* For master's, thesis or alternative, internship. *Entrance requirements:* For master's, bachelor's degree from accredited institution, minimum overall undergraduate GPA of 3.0. Additional exam requirements/recommendations for international students: Required—TOEFL (minimum score 560 paper-based; 84 iBT), IELTS (minimum score 6.5). *Application deadline:* For fall admission, 8/1 for domestic students, 5/1 for international students; for winter admission, 11/15 for domestic students, 9/1 for international students; for spring admission, 3/15 for domestic students, 1/1 for international students; for summer admission, 5/15 for domestic students. Applications are processed on a rolling basis. Application fee: $55. Electronic applications accepted. *Expenses:* Contact institution. *Financial support:* Career-related internships or fieldwork, Federal Work-Study, and scholarships/grants available. Support available to part-time students. Financial award application deadline: 3/1; financial award applicants required to submit FAFSA. *Unit head:* Dr. Kathryn Schellenberg, Director, 810-762-3340, E-mail: kathsch@umflint.edu. *Application contact:* Bradley T. Maki, Director of Graduate Admissions, 810-762-3171, Fax: 810-766-6789, E-mail: bmaki@umflint.edu.
Website: http://www.umflint.edu/graduateprograms/public-administration-mpa

University of Michigan–Flint, School of Health Professions and Studies, Program in Public Health, Flint, MI 48502-1950. Offers health administration (MPH); health education (MPH). *Program availability:* Part-time. *Faculty:* 6 full-time (2 women), 5 part-time/adjunct (2 women). *Students:* 23 full-time (15 women), 43 part-time (34 women); includes 20 minority (13 Black or African American, non-Hispanic/Latino; 2 American Indian or Alaska Native, non-Hispanic/Latino; 4 Asian, non-Hispanic/Latino; 1 Hispanic/Latino), 11 international. Average age 31. 87 applicants, 64% accepted, 25 enrolled. In 2015, 2 master's awarded. *Entrance requirements:* For master's, bachelor's degree from accredited institution with sufficient preparation in algebra to succeed in epidemiology and biostatistics; minimum overall undergraduate GPA of 3.0. Additional exam requirements/recommendations for international students: Required—TOEFL (minimum score 560 paper-based; 84 iBT), IELTS (minimum score 6.5). *Application deadline:* For fall admission, 8/1 for domestic students, 5/1 for international students; for winter admission, 11/15 for domestic students, 8/15 for international students; for spring admission, 3/15 for domestic students, 1/15 for international students. Applications are processed on a rolling basis. Application fee: $55. Electronic applications accepted. *Financial support:* Federal Work-Study, scholarships/grants, and unspecified assistantships available. Support available to part-time students. Financial award application deadline: 3/1; financial award applicants required to submit FAFSA. *Unit head:* Dr. Suzanne Selig, Director, 810-762-3172, E-mail: sselig@umflint.edu. *Application contact:* Bradley T. Maki, Director of Graduate Admissions, 810-762-3171, Fax: 810-766-6789, E-mail: bmaki@umflint.edu.
Website: http://www.umflint.edu/graduateprograms/public-health-mph

University of Michigan–Flint, School of Management, Program in Business Administration, Flint, MI 48502-1950. Offers accounting (MBA); computer information systems (MBA); finance (MBA); general business administration (MBA); health care management (MBA); international business (MBA); lean manufacturing (MBA); marketing (MBA); organizational leadership (MBA). *Program availability:* Part-time, evening/weekend, online learning. *Faculty:* 2 full-time (0 women), 3 part-time/adjunct (1 woman). *Students:* 15 full-time (4 women), 146 part-time (57 women); includes 34 minority (12 Black or African American, non-Hispanic/Latino; 3 American Indian or Alaska Native, non-Hispanic/Latino; 14 Asian, non-Hispanic/Latino; 1 Hispanic/Latino; 1 Native Hawaiian or other Pacific Islander, non-Hispanic/Latino; 3 Two or more races, non-Hispanic/Latino), 24 international. Average age 33. 117 applicants, 56% accepted, 36 enrolled. In 2015, 70 degrees awarded. *Degree requirements:* For master's, thesis or alternative. *Entrance requirements:* For master's, GMAT or GRE, bachelor's degree in arts, sciences, engineering, or business administration from accredited college or university with minimum GPA of 3.0. Additional exam requirements/recommendations for international students: Required—TOEFL (minimum score 560 paper-based; 84 iBT), IELTS (minimum score 6.5). *Application deadline:* For fall admission, 8/1 for domestic students, 5/1 for international students; for winter admission, 11/1 for domestic students, 9/1 for international students. Applications are processed on a rolling basis. Application fee: $55. Electronic applications accepted. *Financial support:* Federal Work-Study, scholarships/grants, and unspecified assistantships available. Support available to part-time students. Financial award application deadline: 3/1; financial award applicants required to submit FAFSA. *Unit head:* Dr. Scott Johnson, Dean, School of Management, 810-762-3164, Fax: 810-237-6685, E-mail: scotjohn@umflint.edu. *Application contact:* Bradley T. Maki, Director of Graduate Admissions, 810-762-3171, E-mail: bmaki@umflint.edu.
Website: http://www.umflint.edu/graduateprograms/business-administration-mba

University of Minnesota, Twin Cities Campus, Carlson School of Management, Carlson Full-Time MBA Program, Minneapolis, MN 55455. Offers applied economics (MBA); business analytics (MBA); finance (MBA); human resources and industrial relations (MBA); information technology (MBA); management (MBA); marketing (MBA); medical industry orientation (MBA); supply chain and operations (MBA); JD/MBA; MBA/MPP; MD/MBA; MHA/MBA; Pharm D/MBA. *Accreditation:* AACSB. *Faculty:* 143 full-time (42 women), 24 part-time/adjunct (6 women). *Students:* 195 full-time (53 women); includes 28 minority (3 Black or African American, non-Hispanic/Latino; 1 American Indian or Alaska Native, non-Hispanic/Latino; 10 Asian, non-Hispanic/Latino; 7 Hispanic/Latino; 1 Native Hawaiian or other Pacific Islander, non-Hispanic/Latino; 6 Two or more races, non-Hispanic/Latino), 44 international. Average age 28. 594 applicants, 39% accepted, 86 enrolled. In 2015, 107 master's awarded. *Entrance requirements:* For master's, GMAT or GRE. Additional exam requirements/recommendations for international students: Required—TOEFL (minimum score 580 paper-based; 84 iBT), IELTS (minimum score 7), PTE. *Application deadline:* For fall admission, 4/1 for domestic students, 2/1 for international students. Application fee: $60 ($90 for international students). Electronic applications accepted. *Expenses:* $36,140 per year tuition resident; $46,500 per year tuition nonresident; $2,270 per year fees; additional $318 per year international fees; $1,998 per year hospitalization insurance fees. *Financial support:* In 2015–16, 126 students received support, including 126 fellowships with tuition reimbursements available (averaging $23,898 per year); research assistantships with partial tuition reimbursements available, teaching assistantships with partial tuition reimbursements available, career-related internships or fieldwork, Federal Work-Study, institutionally sponsored loans, scholarships/grants, health care benefits, and unspecified assistantships also available. Financial award application deadline: 4/1; financial award applicants required to submit FAFSA. *Faculty research:* Market regulation and asset pricing, social networks and data analytics, consumer behavior, innovation and entrepreneurship, workplace wellbeing and labor relationships. *Total annual research expenditures:* $577,440. *Unit head:* Philip J. Miller, Assistant Dean, MBA Programs and Graduate Business Career Center, 612-625-5555, Fax: 612-625-1012, E-mail: mba@umn.edu. *Application contact:* Linh Gilles, Director of Admissions and Recruiting, 612-625-5555, Fax: 612-625-1012, E-mail: ftmba@umn.edu.
Website: http://www.csom.umn.edu/MBA/full-time/

University of Minnesota, Twin Cities Campus, Carlson School of Management, Carlson Part-Time MBA Program, Minneapolis, MN 55455. Offers finance (MBA); information technology (MBA); management (MBA); marketing (MBA); medical industry

orientation (MBA); supply chain and operations (MBA). *Program availability:* Part-time, evening/weekend. *Faculty:* 143 full-time (42 women), 26 part-time/adjunct (6 women). *Students:* 1,047 part-time (338 women); includes 99 minority (16 Black or African American, non-Hispanic/Latino; 3 American Indian or Alaska Native, non-Hispanic/Latino; 50 Asian, non-Hispanic/Latino; 15 Hispanic/Latino; 15 Two or more races, non-Hispanic/Latino; 55 international. Average age 28. 225 applicants, 82% accepted, 155 enrolled. In 2015, 297 master's awarded. *Entrance requirements:* For master's, GMAT or GRE. Additional exam requirements/recommendations for international students: Required—TOEFL (minimum score 580 paper-based; 84 iBT), IELTS (minimum score 7), PTE. *Application deadline:* For fall admission, 5/15 priority date for domestic and international students; for spring admission, 10/15 priority date for domestic and international students. Applications are processed on a rolling basis. Application fee: $60 ($90 for international students). Electronic applications accepted. *Expenses:* $1,302 tuition per credit; $326 fees per semester. *Financial support:* Applicants required to submit FAFSA. *Faculty research:* Market regulation and asset pricing, social networks and data analytics, consumer behavior, innovation and entrepreneurship, workplace wellbeing and labor relationships. *Total annual research expenditures:* $577,440. *Unit head:* Philip J. Miller, Assistant Dean, MBA Programs and Graduate Business Career Center, 612-624-2039, Fax: 612-625-1012, E-mail: mba@umn.edu. *Application contact:* Linh Gilles, Director of Admissions and Recruiting, 612-625-5555, Fax: 612-625-1012, E-mail: ptmba@umn.edu.
Website: http://www.carlsonschool.umn.edu/ptmba

University of Minnesota, Twin Cities Campus, Graduate School, Program in Health Informatics, Minneapolis, MN 55455-0213. Offers MHI, MS, PhD, MD/MHI. *Program availability:* Part-time. *Degree requirements:* For master's, thesis or alternative; for doctorate, thesis/dissertation. *Entrance requirements:* For master's and doctorate, GRE General Test, previous course work in life sciences, programming, calculus. Additional exam requirements/recommendations for international students: Required—TOEFL (minimum score 550 paper-based). Electronic applications accepted. *Faculty research:* Medical decision making, physiological control systems, population studies, clinical information systems, telemedicine.

University of Minnesota, Twin Cities Campus, School of Public Health, Major in Health Services Research, Policy, and Administration, Minneapolis, MN 55455-0213. Offers MS, PhD, JD/MS, JD/PhD, MD/PhD, MPP/MS. *Program availability:* Part-time. Terminal master's awarded for partial completion of doctoral program. *Degree requirements:* For master's, thesis, internship, final oral exam; for doctorate, thesis/dissertation, teaching experience, written preliminary exam, final oral exam, dissertation. *Entrance requirements:* For master's, GRE General Test, course work in mathematics; for doctorate, GRE General Test, prerequisite courses in calculus and statistics. Additional exam requirements/recommendations for international students: Required—TOEFL (minimum score 600 paper-based; 100 iBT). *Faculty research:* Outcomes, economics and statistics, sociology, health care management.

University of Minnesota, Twin Cities Campus, School of Public Health, Major in Public Health Administration and Policy, Minneapolis, MN 55455-0213. Offers MPH, MPH/JD, MPH/MSN. *Program availability:* Part-time. *Degree requirements:* For master's, thesis, field experience. *Entrance requirements:* For master's, GRE General Test. Additional exam requirements/recommendations for international students: Required—TOEFL. Electronic applications accepted. *Faculty research:* Community health service organizations, nursing services, dental services, the elderly, insurance coverage.

University of Minnesota, Twin Cities Campus, School of Public Health, Program in Healthcare Administration, Minneapolis, MN 55455-0213. Offers MHA. *Accreditation:* AACSB; CAHME. *Program availability:* Part-time, evening/weekend, online learning. *Degree requirements:* For master's, thesis, project. *Entrance requirements:* For master's, GMAT or GRE General Test, minimum GPA of 3.0. Additional exam requirements/recommendations for international students: Required—TOEFL (minimum score 600 paper-based; 100 iBT). Electronic applications accepted. *Expenses:* Contact institution. *Faculty research:* Managed care, physician payment, structure and performance of healthcare systems, long-term care.

University of Missouri, Office of Research and Graduate Studies, Department of Health Management and Informatics, Columbia, MO 65211. Offers health administration (MHA); health informatics (MS, Certificate). *Accreditation:* CAHME. *Program availability:* Part-time. *Entrance requirements:* For master's, GRE General Test or GMAT, minimum GPA of 3.0. Additional exam requirements/recommendations for international students: Required—TOEFL (minimum score 500 paper-based; 61 iBT). *Application deadline:* Applications are processed on a rolling basis. Application fee: $55 ($75 for international students). Electronic applications accepted. *Financial support:* Fellowships, research assistantships, teaching assistantships, institutionally sponsored loans, scholarships/grants, traineeships, health care benefits, and unspecified assistantships available. Support available to part-time students.
Website: http://www.hmi.missouri.edu/

University of Missouri, Office of Research and Graduate Studies, Master of Public Health Program, Columbia, MO 65211. Offers global public health (Graduate Certificate); health promotion and policy (MPH); public health (Graduate Certificate); veterinary public health (MPH); DVM/MPH; MPH/MA; MPH/MPA. *Accreditation:* CEPH. *Entrance requirements:* Additional exam requirements/recommendations for international students: Required—TOEFL (minimum score 550 paper-based; 80 iBT). *Application deadline:* For fall admission, 6/30 priority date for domestic and international students. Applications are processed on a rolling basis. Application fee: $55 ($75 for international students). Electronic applications accepted. *Financial support:* Fellowships with tuition reimbursements, research assistantships with tuition reimbursements, teaching assistantships with tuition reimbursements, scholarships/grants, traineeships, health care benefits, and unspecified assistantships available. Support available to part-time students.
Website: http://publichealth.missouri.edu/

University of Missouri, School of Medicine and Office of Research and Graduate Studies, Graduate Programs in Medicine, Columbia, MO 65211. Offers family and community medicine (MS); health administration (MS); medical pharmacology and physiology (MS, PhD); molecular microbiology and immunology (MS, PhD); pathology and anatomical sciences (MS). *Program availability:* Part-time. *Degree requirements:* For doctorate, thesis/dissertation. *Entrance requirements:* For master's and doctorate, GRE General Test, minimum GPA of 3.0. Additional exam requirements/recommendations for international students: Required—TOEFL. *Application deadline:* Applications are processed on a rolling basis. Application fee: $55 ($75 for international students). *Expenses:* Contact institution. *Financial support:* Fellowships, research assistantships, teaching assistantships, career-related internships or fieldwork, and institutionally sponsored loans available.
Website: http://som.missouri.edu/departments.shtml

University of Nevada, Las Vegas, Graduate College, School of Community Health Sciences, Department of Health Care Administration and Policy, Las Vegas, NV 89154-3023. Offers MHA. *Faculty:* 4 full-time, 2 part-time/adjunct (both women). *Students:* 15 full-time (9 women), 20 part-time (12 women); includes 12 minority (2 Black or African

American, non-Hispanic/Latino; 4 Asian, non-Hispanic/Latino; 2 Hispanic/Latino; 1 Native Hawaiian or other Pacific Islander, non-Hispanic/Latino; 3 Two or more races, non-Hispanic/Latino), 4 international. Average age 32. 17 applicants, 71% accepted, 6 enrolled. In 2015, 21 master's awarded. *Degree requirements:* For master's, thesis (for some programs). *Entrance requirements:* Additional exam requirements/recommendations for international students: Required—TOEFL (minimum score 550 paper-based; 80 iBT), IELTS (minimum score 7). *Application deadline:* For fall admission, 4/1 for domestic students, 5/1 for international students; for spring admission, 11/1 for domestic students, 10/1 for international students. Application fee: $60 ($95 for international students). Electronic applications accepted. *Expenses:* $264 per credit resident full-time and part-time; $6,955 per semester nonresident full-time, $264 per credit; $555 per credit nonresident part-time. *Financial support:* In 2015–16, 2 students received support, including 2 research assistantships with partial tuition reimbursements available (averaging $10,000 per year); institutionally sponsored loans, scholarships/grants, health care benefits, and unspecified assistantships also available. Financial award application deadline: 3/1. *Faculty research:* Effects of the EHR on healthcare outcome, quality and financial performance; patient satisfactions on hospital services; mediation errors, medical home performance, ER use among patients with mental illness. *Total annual research expenditures:* $11,335. *Unit head:* Dr. Chris Cochran, Chair/Associate Professor, 702-895-1400, Fax: 702-895-3979, E-mail: chris.cochran@unlv.edu. *Application contact:* Graduate College Admissions Evaluator, 702-895-3367, Fax: 702-895-4180, E-mail: gradadmissions@unlv.edu.
Website: http://hca.unlv.edu

University of New Haven, Graduate School, College of Business, Program in Health Care Administration, West Haven, CT 06516-1916. Offers health care administration (MS); health care management (Graduate Certificate); health care marketing (MS); health policy and finance (MS); human resource management in health care (MS); long-term care (MS); long-term health care (Graduate Certificate); managed care (MS); medical group management (MS). *Program availability:* Part-time, evening/weekend. *Students:* 67 full-time (44 women), 71 part-time (56 women); includes 43 minority (27 Black or African American, non-Hispanic/Latino; 7 Asian, non-Hispanic/Latino; 5 Hispanic/Latino; 4 Two or more races, non-Hispanic/Latino), 35 international. Average age 33. 147 applicants, 78% accepted, 56 enrolled. In 2015, 38 master's, 2 other advanced degrees awarded. *Entrance requirements:* Additional exam requirements/recommendations for international students: Required—TOEFL (minimum score 80 iBT), IELTS, PTE. *Application deadline:* For fall admission, 5/31 for international students; for winter admission, 10/15 for international students; for spring admission, 1/15 for international students. Applications are processed on a rolling basis. Application fee: $75. Electronic applications accepted. Application fee is waived when completed online. *Expenses:* Tuition, area resident: Full-time $15,282; part-time $849 per credit hour. *Required fees:* $150; $60 per term. Tuition and fees vary according to program. *Financial support:* Research assistantships with partial tuition reimbursements, teaching assistantships with partial tuition reimbursements, career-related internships or fieldwork, Federal Work-Study, scholarships/grants, and unspecified assistantships available. Support available to part-time students. Financial award applicants required to submit FAFSA. *Unit head:* Dr. Summer McGee, Associate Professor, 203-479-4104, E-mail: smcgee@newhaven.edu. *Application contact:* Michelle Mason, Director of Graduate Enrollment, 203-932-7067, E-mail: mmason@newhaven.edu.
Website: http://www.newhaven.edu/6848/

University of New Haven, Graduate School, Henry C. Lee College of Criminal Justice and Forensic Sciences, Program in Public Administration, West Haven, CT 06516-1916. Offers city management (MPA); community-clinical services (MPA); health care management (MPA); long-term health care (MPA); personnel and labor relations (MPA); public administration (MPA, Graduate Certificate); MBA/MPA. *Program availability:* Part-time, evening/weekend. *Students:* 22 full-time (10 women), 19 part-time (14 women); includes 11 minority (7 Black or African American, non-Hispanic/Latino; 1 Asian, non-Hispanic/Latino; 3 Hispanic/Latino), 8 international. Average age 32. 36 applicants, 86% accepted, 10 enrolled. In 2015, 24 master's, 10 other advanced degrees awarded. *Degree requirements:* For master's, thesis or alternative. *Entrance requirements:* Additional exam requirements/recommendations for international students: Required—TOEFL (minimum score 80 iBT), IELTS, PTE. *Application deadline:* For fall admission, 5/31 for international students; for winter admission, 10/15 for international students; for spring admission, 1/15 for international students. Applications are processed on a rolling basis. Application fee: $75. Electronic applications accepted. Application fee is waived when completed online. *Expenses:* Contact institution. *Financial support:* Research assistantships with partial tuition reimbursements, teaching assistantships with partial tuition reimbursements, career-related internships or fieldwork, Federal Work-Study, scholarships/grants, and unspecified assistantships available. Support available to part-time students. Financial award application deadline: 5/1; financial award applicants required to submit FAFSA. *Unit head:* Dr. Cynthia Conrad, Associate Professor, 203-932-7486, E-mail: cconrad@newhaven.edu. *Application contact:* Michelle Mason, Director of Graduate Enrollment, 203-932-7067, E-mail: mmason@newhaven.edu.
Website: http://www.newhaven.edu/6854/

University of New Mexico, Graduate Studies, Health Sciences Center, Program in Public Health, Albuquerque, NM 87131-5196. Offers community health (MPH); epidemiology (MPH); health systems, services and policy (MPH). *Accreditation:* CEPH. *Program availability:* Part-time, online learning. *Faculty:* 9 full-time (7 women), 3 part-time/adjunct (2 women). *Students:* 25 full-time (17 women), 20 part-time (16 women); includes 17 minority (3 Black or African American, non-Hispanic/Latino; 1 American Indian or Alaska Native, non-Hispanic/Latino; 2 Asian, non-Hispanic/Latino; 10 Hispanic/Latino), 1 international. Average age 31. 32 applicants, 63% accepted, 16 enrolled. In 2015, 13 master's awarded. *Degree requirements:* For master's, thesis. *Entrance requirements:* For master's, GRE, MCAT, 2 years of experience in health field. Additional exam requirements/recommendations for international students: Required—TOEFL. *Application deadline:* For fall admission, 2/1 for domestic students. Application fee: $50. *Financial support:* Fellowships, research assistantships with tuition reimbursements, and Federal Work-Study available. Financial award application deadline: 12/15; financial award applicants required to submit FAFSA. *Faculty research:* Epidemiology, rural health, environmental health, Native American health issues. *Unit head:* Dr. Kristine Tollestrup, Director, 505-272-4173, Fax: 505-272-4494, E-mail: ktollestrup@salud.unm.edu. *Application contact:* Gayle Garcia, Education Coordinator, 505-272-3982, Fax: 505-272-4494, E-mail: garciag@salud.unm.edu.
Website: http://fcm.unm.edu/

University of New Mexico, Graduate Studies, School of Public Administration, Program in Health Administration, Albuquerque, NM 87131-2039. Offers MHA. *Faculty:* 3 full-time (0 women), 1 (woman) part-time/adjunct. *Students:* 24 full-time (17 women), 25 part-time (16 women); includes 24 minority (4 Black or African American, non-Hispanic/Latino; 4 American Indian or Alaska Native, non-Hispanic/Latino; 1 Asian, non-Hispanic/Latino; 14 Hispanic/Latino; 1 Two or more races, non-Hispanic/Latino), 2 international. Average age 37. 18 applicants, 100% accepted, 17 enrolled. In 2015, 1 master's awarded. *Entrance requirements:* For master's, baccalaureate degree from accredited college or university with minimum undergraduate GPA of 3.0 for last 60 hours or overall major; letter of intent; three letters of recommendation; resume; official transcripts. *Application deadline:* For fall admission, 4/1 for domestic students, 3/1 for international students. Application fee: $50. Electronic applications accepted. *Unit head:* Dr. Uday Desai, Director, 505-277-1092, Fax: 505-277-2529, E-mail: ucdesai@unm.edu. *Application contact:* Gene V. Henley, Associate Director and Graduate Academic Advisor, 505-277-9196, Fax: 505-277-2529, E-mail: spadvise@unm.edu. Website: http://spa.unm.edu/mha-graduate-program/

University of New Orleans, Graduate School, College of Business Administration, Program in Health Care Management, New Orleans, LA 70148. Offers MS. *Degree requirements:* For master's, thesis optional. *Entrance requirements:* For master's, GRE or GMAT. Additional exam requirements/recommendations for international students: Required—TOEFL (minimum score 550 paper-based; 79 iBT). Electronic applications accepted.

University of North Alabama, College of Business, Florence, AL 35632-0001. Offers business administration (MBA), including accounting, enterprise resource planning systems, executive, finance, health care management, information systems, international business, project management. *Accreditation:* ACBSP. *Program availability:* Part-time, 100% online, blended/hybrid learning. *Faculty:* 15 full-time (1 woman), 5 part-time/adjunct (1 woman). *Students:* 127 full-time (56 women), 272 part-time (132 women); includes 133 minority (55 Black or African American, non-Hispanic/Latino; 4 American Indian or Alaska Native, non-Hispanic/Latino; 66 Asian, non-Hispanic/Latino; 2 Hispanic/Latino; 4 Native Hawaiian or other Pacific Islander, non-Hispanic/Latino; 2 Two or more races, non-Hispanic/Latino), 33 international. Average age 35. 268 applicants, 76% accepted, 140 enrolled. In 2015, 133 master's awarded. *Entrance requirements:* For master's, GMAT, GRE, minimum GPA of 2.75 in last 60 hours, 2.5 overall (on a 3.0 scale); 27 hours of course work in business and economics. Additional exam requirements/recommendations for international students: Required—TOEFL (minimum score 79 iBT), IELTS (minimum score 6), PTE (minimum score 54). *Application deadline:* Applications are processed on a rolling basis. Application fee: $50 ($100 for international students). Electronic applications accepted. *Expenses:* Tuition, state resident: full-time $2286; part-time $1524 per semester. Tuition, nonresident: full-time $4572; part-time $3048 per semester. *Required fees:* $801; $579 per semester. Tuition and fees vary according to course load. *Financial support:* In 2015–16, 1 student received support. Scholarships/grants available. Financial award application deadline: 2/1; financial award applicants required to submit FAFSA. *Unit head:* Dr. Gregory A. Carnes, Dean, 256-765-4261, Fax: 256-765-4170, E-mail: gacarnes@una.edu. *Application contact:* Hillary N. Coats, Graduate Admissions Coordinator, 256-765-4447, E-mail: graduate@una.edu. Website: http://www.una.edu/business/

The University of North Carolina at Chapel Hill, Graduate School, Gillings School of Global Public Health, Department of Health Policy and Management, Chapel Hill, NC 27599. Offers MHA, MPH, MSPH, Dr PH, PhD, JD/MPH, MBA/MSPH, MHA/MBA, MHA/MCRP, MHA/MSIS, MHA/MSLS, MSPH/MCRP, MSPH/MSIS, MSPH/MSLS. *Accreditation:* CAHME (one or more programs are accredited). *Program availability:* Part-time, online learning. *Students:* 331 full-time (218 women); includes 100 minority (35 Black or African American, non-Hispanic/Latino; 1 American Indian or Alaska Native, non-Hispanic/Latino; 25 Asian, non-Hispanic/Latino; 11 Hispanic/Latino; 1 Native Hawaiian or other Pacific Islander, non-Hispanic/Latino; 27 Two or more races, non-Hispanic/Latino), 33 international. Average age 33. 456 applicants, 43% accepted, 118 enrolled. *Degree requirements:* For master's, comprehensive exam, capstone course or paper; for doctorate, comprehensive exam, thesis/dissertation. *Entrance requirements:* For master's and doctorate, GRE General Test, minimum GPA of 3.0 (recommended). Additional exam requirements/recommendations for international students: Required—TOEFL, IELTS. *Application deadline:* For fall admission, 12/10 priority date for domestic and international students. Applications are processed on a rolling basis. Application fee: $85. Electronic applications accepted. *Financial support:* Fellowships with tuition reimbursements, research assistantships with tuition reimbursements, teaching assistantships with tuition reimbursements, career-related internships or fieldwork, Federal Work-Study, institutionally sponsored loans, scholarships/grants, traineeships, health care benefits, and unspecified assistantships available. Financial award application deadline: 12/10; financial award applicants required to submit FAFSA. *Faculty research:* Organizational behavior; human resource management in healthcare; health services finance; mental health economics, service, and research; strategic planning and marketing. *Unit head:* Dr. Daniel Lee, Chair, 919-966-6328, Fax: 919-843-6308, E-mail: sylee@unc.edu. *Application contact:* Lynnette Jones, Student Services Manager, 919-966-7391, Fax: 919-843-4980, E-mail: ljones3@email.unc.edu. Website: http://sph.unc.edu/hpm/health-policy-and-management-home/

The University of North Carolina at Charlotte, College of Health and Human Services, Department of Public Health Sciences, Charlotte, NC 28223-0001. Offers community health (Certificate); health administration (MHA); public health (MSPH); public health core concepts (Graduate Certificate); public health sciences (PhD). *Accreditation:* CAHME. *Program availability:* Part-time. *Faculty:* 18 full-time (9 women), 6 part-time/adjunct (4 women). *Students:* 96 full-time (78 women), 22 part-time (18 women); includes 46 minority (26 Black or African American, non-Hispanic/Latino; 1 American Indian or Alaska Native, non-Hispanic/Latino; 11 Asian, non-Hispanic/Latino; 7 Hispanic/Latino; 1 Two or more races, non-Hispanic/Latino), 15 international. Average age 26. 154 applicants, 66% accepted, 55 enrolled. In 2015, 47 master's, 4 other advanced degrees awarded. *Degree requirements:* For master's, thesis (for some programs), thesis or project; internship; for doctorate, thesis/dissertation. *Entrance requirements:* For master's, GRE or MCAT (for MSPH); GRE or GMAT (for MHA); for doctorate, GRE, master's degree in public health or a related field with minimum GPA of 3.5 in all graduate work; statement of purpose detailing why applicant wants to pursue a PhD in public health sciences in the specified concentration at UNC Charlotte; three letters of recommendation (including at least two letters from former professors); for other advanced degree, bachelor's degree from regionally-accredited university; minimum GPA of 2.75 on all post-secondary work attempted; transcripts; personal statement outlining why the applicant seeks admission to the program. Additional exam requirements/recommendations for international students: Required—TOEFL (minimum score 557 paper-based, 83 iBT) or IELTS (minimum score 6.5). *Application deadline:* For fall admission, 1/10 for domestic and international students; for spring admission, 9/15 for domestic and international students; for summer admission, 2/15 for domestic and international students. Applications are processed on a rolling basis. Application fee: $75. Electronic applications accepted. *Expenses:* Contact institution. *Financial support:* In 2015–16, 18 students received support, including 1 fellowship (averaging $42,000 per year), 15 research assistantships (averaging $6,031 per year); career-related internships or fieldwork, Federal Work-Study, institutionally sponsored loans, scholarships/grants, unspecified assistantships, and administrative assistantships also available. Support available to part-time students. Financial award application deadline: 3/1; financial award applicants required to submit FAFSA. *Faculty research:* Pediatric asthma self-management, reproductive epidemiology, social aspects of injury prevention, chronic illness self-care, competency-based professional education, cognitive health, aging and dementia, infant health outcomes, policing and suicide, data mining for health executive decision support, segmentation analyses in identifying patient satisfaction problems in the primary care setting, enhancing community capacity through data sharing. *Total annual research expenditures:* $573,805. *Unit head:* Dr. Susan M. Sell, Interim Chair, 704-687-7191, Fax: 704-687-1644, E-mail: ssell@

uncc.edu. *Application contact:* Kathy B. Giddings, Director of Graduate Admissions, 704-687-5503, Fax: 704-687-1668, E-mail: gradadm@uncc.edu. Website: http://publichealth.uncc.edu/

University of North Florida, Brooks College of Health, Department of Public Health, Jacksonville, FL 32224. Offers aging services (Certificate); community health (MPH); geriatric management (MSH); health administration (MHA); rehabilitation counseling (MS). *Accreditation:* CEPH. *Program availability:* Part-time, evening/weekend. *Faculty:* 19 full-time (14 women), 3 part-time/adjunct (all women). *Students:* 149 full-time (109 women), 59 part-time (40 women); includes 58 minority (28 Black or African American, non-Hispanic/Latino; 10 Asian, non-Hispanic/Latino; 11 Hispanic/Latino; 9 Two or more races, non-Hispanic/Latino), 9 international. Average age 29. 244 applicants, 43% accepted, 75 enrolled. In 2015, 74 master's awarded. *Degree requirements:* For master's, thesis optional. *Entrance requirements:* For master's, GRE General Test (MSH, MS, MPH); GMAT or GRE General Test (MHA), minimum GPA of 3.0 in last 60 hours. Additional exam requirements/recommendations for international students: Required—TOEFL (minimum score 500 paper-based). *Application deadline:* For fall admission, 7/1 for domestic students, 5/1 for international students; for spring admission, 11/1 for domestic students, 10/1 for international students. Application fee: $30. Electronic applications accepted. *Expenses:* Tuition, state resident: part-time $408.10 per credit hour. Tuition, nonresident: part-time $932.61 per credit hour. *Required fees:* $111.81 per credit hour. Tuition and fees vary according to course load, campus/location and program. *Financial support:* In 2015–16, 33 students received support, including 10 teaching assistantships (averaging $1,500 per year); research assistantships, career-related internships or fieldwork, Federal Work-Study, scholarships/grants, and tuition waivers (partial) also available. Support available to part-time students. Financial award application deadline: 4/1; financial award applicants required to submit FAFSA. *Faculty research:* Dietary supplements; alcohol, tobacco, and other drug use prevention; turnover among health professionals; aging; psychosocial aspects of disabilities. *Total annual research expenditures:* $57,986. *Unit head:* Dr. Jeffrey Harrison, Chair, 904-620-1440, Fax: 904-620-2848, E-mail: jeffrey.harrison@unf.edu. *Application contact:* Dr. Heather Kenney, Director of Advising, 904-620-2810, Fax: 904-620-1030, E-mail: heather.kenney@unf.edu. Website: http://www.unf.edu/brooks/public_health/

University of North Texas, Robert B. Toulouse School of Graduate Studies, Denton, TX 76203-5459. Offers accounting (MS); applied anthropology (MA, MS); applied behavior analysis (Certificate); applied geography (MA); applied technology and performance improvement (M Ed, MS); art education (MA); art history (MA); art museum education (Certificate); arts leadership (Certificate); audiology (Au D); behavior analysis (MS); behavioral science (PhD); biochemistry and molecular biology (MS); biology (MA, MS); biomedical engineering (MS); business analysis (MS); chemistry (MS); clinical health psychology (PhD); communication studies (MA, MS); computer engineering (MS); computer science (MS); counseling (M Ed, MS), including clinical mental health counseling (MS), college and university counseling, elementary school counseling, secondary school counseling; creative writing (MA); criminal justice (MS); curriculum and instruction (M Ed); decision sciences (MBA); design (MA, MFA), including fashion design (MFA), innovation studies, interior design (MFA); early childhood studies (MS); economics (MS); educational leadership (M Ed, Ed D); educational psychology (MS, PhD), including family studies (MS), gifted and talented (MS), human development (MS), learning and cognition (MS), research, measurement and evaluation (MS); electrical engineering (MS); emergency management (MPA); engineering technology (MS); English (MA); English as a second language (MA); environmental science (MS); finance (MBA, MS); financial management (MPA); French (MA); health services management (MBA); higher education (M Ed, Ed D); history (MA, MS); hospitality management (MS); human resources management (MPA); information science (MS); information systems (PhD); information technologies (MBA); interdisciplinary studies (MA, MS); international studies (MA); international sustainable tourism (MS); jazz studies (MM); journalism (MA, MJ, Graduate Certificate), including interactive and virtual digital communication (Graduate Certificate), narrative journalism (Graduate Certificate), public relations (Graduate Certificate); kinesiology (MS); linguistics (MS); local government management (MPA); logistics (PhD); logistics and supply chain management (MBA); long-term care, senior housing, and aging services (MA); management (PhD); marketing (MBA); mathematics (MA, MS); mechanical and energy engineering (MS, PhD); music (MA), including ethnomusicology, music theory, musicology, performance; music composition (PhD); music education (MM Ed, PhD); nonprofit management (MPA); operations and supply chain management (MBA); performance (MM, DMA); philosophy (MA); political science (MA); professional and technical communication (MA); radio, television and film (MA, MFA); rehabilitation counseling (Certificate); sociology (MA); Spanish (MA); special education (M Ed); speech-language pathology (MA); strategic management (MBA); studio art (MFA); teaching (M Ed); MBA/MS. *Program availability:* Part-time, evening/weekend, online learning. Terminal master's awarded for partial completion of doctoral program. *Degree requirements:* For master's, variable foreign language requirement, comprehensive exam (for some programs), thesis (for some programs); for doctorate, variable foreign language requirement, comprehensive exam (for some programs), thesis/dissertation; for other advanced degree, variable foreign language requirement, comprehensive exam (for some programs). *Entrance requirements:* For master's and doctorate, GRE, GMAT. Additional exam requirements/recommendations for international students: Required—TOEFL (minimum score 550 paper-based; 79 iBT). Electronic applications accepted.

University of North Texas Health Science Center at Fort Worth, School of Public Health, Fort Worth, TX 76107-2699. Offers biostatistics (MPH); community health (MPH); disease control and prevention (Dr PH); environmental and occupational health sciences (MPH); epidemiology (MPH); health administration (MHA); health policy and management (MPH, Dr PH); DO/MPH; MS/MPH; MSN/MPH. MPH offered jointly with University of North Texas; DO/MPH with Texas College of Osteopathic Medicine. *Accreditation:* CEPH. *Program availability:* Part-time, evening/weekend. *Degree requirements:* For master's, thesis or alternative, supervised internship; for doctorate, thesis/dissertation, supervised internship. *Entrance requirements:* For master's, GRE General Test. Additional exam requirements/recommendations for international students: Required—TOEFL. Electronic applications accepted.

University of Oklahoma, College of Liberal Studies, Norman, OK 73019. Offers administrative leadership (MA, Graduate Certificate); corrections management (Graduate Certificate); criminal justice (MS); liberal studies (MA), including human and health services administration, integrated studies, museum studies; prevention science (MPS); restorative justice administration (Graduate Certificate). *Program availability:* Part-time, online only, 100% online, blended/hybrid learning. *Faculty:* 15 full-time (10 women), 2 part-time/adjunct (0 women). *Students:* 65 full-time (38 women), 602 part-time (299 women); includes 184 minority (57 Black or African American, non-Hispanic/Latino; 49 American Indian or Alaska Native, non-Hispanic/Latino; 6 Asian, non-Hispanic/Latino; 39 Hispanic/Latino; 1 Native Hawaiian or other Pacific Islander, non-Hispanic/Latino; 32 Two or more races, non-Hispanic/Latino), 1 international. Average age 35. 205 applicants, 97% accepted, 137 enrolled. In 2015, 166 master's, 5 other advanced degrees awarded. *Degree requirements:* For master's, comprehensive exam, thesis optional, 33 credit hours; project/internship (for museum studies program only); for Graduate Certificate, 12 credit hours. *Entrance requirements:* For master's and

Graduate Certificate, minimum GPA of 3.0 in last 60 undergraduate hours; statement of goals; resume. Additional exam requirements/recommendations for international students: Required—TOEFL (minimum score 79 iBT) or IELTS (minimum score 6.5). *Application deadline:* For fall admission, 7/1 for domestic and international students; for winter admission, 12/1 for domestic and international students; for spring admission, 5/1 for domestic and international students. Applications are processed on a rolling basis. Application fee: $50 ($100 for international students). Electronic applications accepted. *Expenses:* Tuition, state resident: full-time $4577; part-time $190.70 per credit hour. Tuition, nonresident: full-time $17,758; part-time $739.90 per credit hour. *Required fees:* $3060; $115.70 per credit hour. $141.50 per semester. *Financial support:* In 2015–16, 120 students received support. Career-related internships or fieldwork, institutionally sponsored loans, scholarships/grants, health care benefits, and tuition waivers (partial) available. Support available to part-time students. Financial award application deadline: 6/1; financial award applicants required to submit FAFSA. *Faculty research:* Ethics and leadership; leadership and management in policing; neuro-psychology of addiction; disproportionate minority contact; ethnic identity and nationalism. *Unit head:* Dr. James Pappas, Vice President, University Outreach/Dean, College of Liberal Studies, 405-325-6361, E-mail: jpappas@ou.edu. *Application contact:* Michelle Shults, Academic Advisement Services Coordinator, 405-325-2928, Fax: 405-325-7132, E-mail: mshults@ou.edu.
Website: http://www.ou.edu/cls/

University of Oklahoma Health Sciences Center, Graduate College, College of Public Health, Department of Health Administration and Policy, Oklahoma City, OK 73190. Offers MHA, MPH, MS, Dr PH, PhD, JD/MPH, MBA/MPH. MBA/MPH offered jointly with Oklahoma State University; JD/MPH with University of Oklahoma. *Accreditation:* CAHME. *Program availability:* Part-time. *Degree requirements:* For master's, comprehensive exam, thesis (for some programs); for doctorate, 2 foreign languages, comprehensive exam, thesis/dissertation. *Entrance requirements:* For master's, 3 letters of recommendation, resume; for doctorate, GRE General Test, letters of recommendation. Additional exam requirements/recommendations for international students: Required—TOEFL (minimum score 570 paper-based). *Faculty research:* Public health administration, health institutions management, public policy and the aged, injury control.

University of Ottawa, Faculty of Graduate and Postdoctoral Studies, Telfer School of Management, Health Administration Program, Ottawa, ON K1N 6N5, Canada. Offers MHA. *Program availability:* Part-time. *Degree requirements:* For master's, thesis optional, residency. *Entrance requirements:* For master's, GMAT, bachelor's degree or equivalent, minimum B average. Additional exam requirements/recommendations for international students: Recommended—TOEFL. Electronic applications accepted.

University of Pennsylvania, Wharton School, Health Care Management Department, Philadelphia, PA 19104. Offers MBA, PhD. *Degree requirements:* For doctorate, comprehensive exam, thesis/dissertation. *Entrance requirements:* For master's, GMAT; for doctorate, GMAT or GRE. Electronic applications accepted. *Expenses: Tuition, area resident:* Full-time $31,068; part-time $5762 per course. *Required fees:* $3200; $336 per course. Full-time tuition and fees vary according to degree level, program and student level. Part-time tuition and fees vary according to course load, degree level and program. *Faculty research:* Health economics, health policy, health care management, health insurance and financing.

University of Phoenix–Atlanta Campus, College of Nursing, Sandy Springs, GA 30350-4147. Offers health administration (MHA); nursing (MSN); nursing/health care education (MSN); MSN/MBA; MSN/MHA. *Program availability:* Evening/weekend, online learning. *Degree requirements:* For master's, thesis (for some programs). *Entrance requirements:* For master's, minimum undergraduate GPA of 2.5, 3 years of work experience. Additional exam requirements/recommendations for international students: Required—TOEFL (minimum score 550 paper-based; 79 iBT). Electronic applications accepted.

University of Phoenix–Augusta Campus, College of Nursing, Augusta, GA 30909-4583. Offers health administration (MHA); nursing (MSN); nursing/health care education (MSN); MSN/MBA; MSN/MHA. *Program availability:* Online learning.

University of Phoenix–Bay Area Campus, School of Business, San Jose, CA 95134-1805. Offers accountancy (MS); accounting (MBA); business administration (MBA, DBA); energy management (MBA); global management (MBA); health care management (MBA); human resource management (MBA); human resources management (MM); management (MM); marketing (MBA); organizational leadership (DM); project management (MBA); public administration (MPA); technology management (MBA). *Program availability:* Evening/weekend, online learning. *Degree requirements:* For master's, thesis (for some programs). *Entrance requirements:* For master's, minimum undergraduate GPA of 3.0, 3 years of work experience. Additional exam requirements/recommendations for international students: Required—TOEFL (minimum score 550 paper-based; 79 iBT). Electronic applications accepted.

University of Phoenix–Central Valley Campus, College of Nursing, Fresno, CA 93720-1552. Offers education (MHA); gerontology (MHA); health administration (MHA); nursing (MSN); MSN/MBA.

University of Phoenix–Charlotte Campus, College of Nursing, Charlotte, NC 28273-3409. Offers education (MHA); gerontology (MHA); health administration (MHA); informatics (MHA, MSN); nursing (MSN); nursing/health care education (MSN). *Program availability:* Evening/weekend. *Degree requirements:* For master's, thesis (for some programs). *Entrance requirements:* For master's, minimum undergraduate GPA of 2.5, 3 years work experience. Additional exam requirements/recommendations for international students: Required—TOEFL (minimum score 550 paper-based; 79 iBT). Electronic applications accepted.

University of Phoenix–Colorado Campus, College of Nursing, Lone Tree, CO 80124-5453. Offers health administration (MHA); nursing (MSN); MSN/MBA; MSN/MHA. *Program availability:* Evening/weekend, online learning. *Degree requirements:* For master's, thesis (for some programs). *Entrance requirements:* For master's, minimum undergraduate GPA of 2.5, 3 years work experience, RN license. Additional exam requirements/recommendations for international students: Required—TOEFL (minimum score 550 paper-based; 79 iBT). Electronic applications accepted.

University of Phoenix–Colorado Springs Downtown Campus, College of Nursing, Colorado Springs, CO 80903. Offers education (MHA); gerontology (MHA); health administration (MHA); nursing (MSN); MSN/MBA. *Program availability:* Evening/weekend. *Degree requirements:* For master's, thesis (for some programs). *Entrance requirements:* For master's, minimum undergraduate GPA of 2.5, 3 years of work experience, RN license. Additional exam requirements/recommendations for international students: Required—TOEFL (minimum score 550 paper-based; 79 iBT). Electronic applications accepted.

University of Phoenix–Hawaii Campus, College of Nursing, Honolulu, HI 96813-3800. Offers education (MHA); family nurse practitioner (MSN); gerontology (MHA); health administration (MHA); nursing (MSN); nursing/health care education (MSN); MSN/MBA. *Program availability:* Evening/weekend. *Degree requirements:* For master's, thesis (for some programs). *Entrance requirements:* For master's, minimum undergraduate GPA of

2.5, 3 years of work experience, RN license. Additional exam requirements/recommendations for international students: Required—TOEFL (minimum score 550 paper-based; 79 iBT). Electronic applications accepted.

University of Phoenix–Houston Campus, College of Nursing, Houston, TX 77079-2004. Offers health administration (MHA). *Program availability:* Online learning. *Degree requirements:* For master's, thesis (for some programs). *Entrance requirements:* For master's, minimum undergraduate GPA of 2.5, 3 years of work experience. Additional exam requirements/recommendations for international students: Required—TOEFL (minimum score 550 paper-based; 79 iBT). Electronic applications accepted.

University of Phoenix–New Mexico Campus, College of Nursing, Albuquerque, NM 87113-1570. Offers health administration (MHA); health care education (MSN); nursing (MSN); MSN/MBA. *Program availability:* Evening/weekend. *Degree requirements:* For master's, thesis (for some programs). *Entrance requirements:* For master's, minimum undergraduate GPA of 2.5, 3 years of work experience, RN license. Additional exam requirements/recommendations for international students: Required—TOEFL (minimum score 550 paper-based; 79 iBT). Electronic applications accepted.

University of Phoenix–North Florida Campus, College of Nursing, Jacksonville, FL 32216-0959. Offers health administration (MHA); health care education (MSN); nursing (MSN); MSN/MBA; MSN/MHA. *Program availability:* Evening/weekend. *Degree requirements:* For master's, thesis (for some programs). *Entrance requirements:* For master's, minimum undergraduate GPA of 2.5, 3 years work experience, RN license. Additional exam requirements/recommendations for international students: Required—TOEFL (minimum score 550 paper-based; 79 iBT). Electronic applications accepted.

University of Phoenix–Online Campus, School of Advanced Studies, Phoenix, AZ 85034-7209. Offers business administration (DBA); education (Ed S); educational leadership (Ed D), including curriculum and instruction, education technology, educational leadership; health administration (DHA); higher education administration (PhD); industrial/organizational psychology (PhD); nursing (PhD); organizational leadership (DM), including information systems and technology, organizational leadership. *Program availability:* Evening/weekend, online learning. *Degree requirements:* For doctorate, thesis/dissertation. *Entrance requirements:* Additional exam requirements/recommendations for international students: Required—TOEFL, TOEIC (Test of English as an International Communication), Berlitz Online English Proficiency Exam, PTE, or IELTS. Electronic applications accepted. *Expenses:* Contact institution.

University of Phoenix–Online Campus, School of Business, Phoenix, AZ 85034-7209. Offers accountancy (MS); accounting (MBA, Certificate); business administration (MBA); energy management (MBA); global management (MBA); health care management (MBA); human resource management (MBA, Certificate); human resources management (MM); management (MM); marketing (MBA, Certificate); project management (MBA, Certificate); public administration (MBA, MM); technology management (MBA). *Program availability:* Evening/weekend, online learning. *Entrance requirements:* Additional exam requirements/recommendations for international students: Required—TOEFL, TOEIC (Test of English as an International Communication), Berlitz Online English Proficiency Exam, PTE, or IELTS. Electronic applications accepted. *Expenses:* Contact institution.

University of Phoenix–Phoenix Campus, School of Business, Tempe, AZ 85282-2371. Offers accounting (MBA, MS, Certificate); business administration (MBA); energy management (MBA); global management (MBA); health care management (MBA); human resource management (MBA, Certificate); management (MM); marketing (MBA); project management (MBA); technology management (MBA). *Program availability:* Evening/weekend, online learning. *Entrance requirements:* Additional exam requirements/recommendations for international students: Required—TOEFL, TOEIC (Test of English as an International Communication), Berlitz Online English Proficiency Exam, PTE, or IELTS. Electronic applications accepted. *Expenses:* Contact institution.

University of Phoenix–Sacramento Valley Campus, College of Nursing, Sacramento, CA 95833-4334. Offers family nurse practitioner (MSN); health administration (MHA); health care education (MSN); nursing (MSN); MSN/MBA. *Program availability:* Evening/weekend. *Degree requirements:* For master's, thesis (for some programs). *Entrance requirements:* For master's, RN license, minimum undergraduate GPA of 2.5, 3 years work experience. Additional exam requirements/recommendations for international students: Required—TOEFL (minimum score 550 paper-based; 79 iBT). Electronic applications accepted.

University of Phoenix–San Antonio Campus, College of Nursing, San Antonio, TX 78230. Offers health administration (MHA).

University of Phoenix–Southern California Campus, School of Business, Costa Mesa, CA 92626. Offers accounting (MBA); business administration (MBA); energy management (MBA); global management (MBA); health care management (MBA); human resource management (MBA); management (MM); marketing (MBA); project management (MBA); technology management (MBA). *Program availability:* Evening/weekend, online learning. *Entrance requirements:* Additional exam requirements/recommendations for international students: Required—TOEFL, TOEIC (Test of English as an International Communication), Berlitz Online English Proficiency Exam, PTE, or IELTS. Electronic applications accepted. *Expenses:* Contact institution.

University of Phoenix–South Florida Campus, College of Nursing, Miramar, FL 33027-4145. Offers health administration (MHA); health care education (MSN); nursing (MSN); MSN/MBA; MSN/MHA. *Program availability:* Evening/weekend. *Degree requirements:* For master's, thesis (for some programs). *Entrance requirements:* For master's, minimum undergraduate GPA of 2.5, 3 years work experience, RN license. Additional exam requirements/recommendations for international students: Required—TOEFL (minimum score 550 paper-based; 79 iBT). Electronic applications accepted.

University of Phoenix–Washington D.C. Campus, College of Nursing, Washington, DC 20001. Offers education (MHA); gerontology (MHA); health administration (MHA, DHA); informatics (MHA, MSN); nursing (MSN, PhD); nursing/health care education (MSN); MSN/MBA; MSN/MHA.

University of Pittsburgh, Graduate School of Public Health, Department of Behavioral and Community Health Sciences, Pittsburgh, PA 15261. Offers applied research and leadership (Dr PH); applied social and behavioral concepts in public health (MPH); community-based participatory research (Certificate); health equity (Certificate); LGBT health and wellness (Certificate); maternal and child health (MPH); program evaluation (Certificate); MID/MPH; MPH/MPA; MPH/MSW; MPH/PhD. *Accreditation:* CAHME (one or more programs are accredited). *Program availability:* Part-time. *Faculty:* 15 full-time (9 women), 15 part-time/adjunct (4 women). *Students:* 48 full-time (38 women), 69 part-time (56 women); includes 29 minority (9 Black or African American, non-Hispanic/Latino; 8 Asian, non-Hispanic/Latino; 7 Hispanic/Latino; 5 Two or more races, non-Hispanic/Latino), 6 international. Average age 28. 311 applicants, 56% accepted, 23 enrolled. In 2015, 26 master's, 4 doctorates awarded. *Degree requirements:* For master's, thesis, 200 contact hour practicum; for doctorate, comprehensive exam, thesis/dissertation, preliminary exam. *Entrance requirements:* For master's, GRE, bachelor's degree; for doctorate, GRE, master's degree in public health or related field; for Certificate, GRE. Additional exam requirements/recommendations for international

Health Services Management and Hospital Administration

students: Required—TOEFL (minimum score 550 paper-based; 80 iBT), IELTS (minimum score 6.5). *Application deadline:* For fall admission, 1/15 for domestic and international students; for spring admission, 10/15 for domestic students, 8/1 for international students. Applications are processed on a rolling basis. Application fee: $120. Electronic applications accepted. *Expenses:* $12,834 per term in-state; $20,872 per term out-of-state. *Financial support:* In 2015–16, 14 students received support, including 6 fellowships with partial tuition reimbursements available (averaging $3,775 per year), 8 research assistantships with tuition reimbursements available (averaging $21,922 per year); teaching assistantships with tuition reimbursements available, scholarships/grants, traineeships, and health care benefits also available. Financial award applicants required to submit FAFSA. *Faculty research:* Community-based participatory research, health equity, evaluation science, LGBT health, aging, violence prevention. *Total annual research expenditures:* $3.3 million. *Unit head:* Dr. Steven M. Albert, Chair, 412-624-3102, Fax: 412-648-5975, E-mail: smalbert@pitt.edu. *Application contact:* Miriam P. Fagan, Academic Administrator, 412-624-3107, Fax: 412-624-5510, E-mail: mpfagan@pitt.edu.
Website: http://www.bchs.pitt.edu/

University of Pittsburgh, Graduate School of Public Health, Department of Health Policy and Management, Pittsburgh, PA 15261. Offers decision sciences (MS); health policy and economics (MS); health policy and management (MHA, MPH, PhD); JD/MPH. *Accreditation:* CAHME. *Program availability:* Part-time. *Faculty:* 16 full-time (7 women), 29 part-time/adjunct (8 women). *Students:* 62 full-time (42 women), 20 part-time (13 women); includes 17 minority (5 Black or African American, non-Hispanic/Latino; 7 Asian, non-Hispanic/Latino; 3 Hispanic/Latino; 2 Two or more races, non-Hispanic/Latino), 10 international. Average age 28. 202 applicants, 49% accepted, 34 enrolled. In 2015, 35 master's, 2 doctorates awarded. Terminal master's awarded for partial completion of doctoral program. *Degree requirements:* For master's, comprehensive exam (for some programs), essay, practicum; for doctorate, comprehensive exam, thesis/dissertation, preliminary exam, dissertation overview. *Entrance requirements:* For master's, GRE, one college-level mathematics or statistics course; at least two courses in the social sciences, preferably one in microeconomics and biology; bachelor's degree; recommendations; professional statement; transcripts; minimum QPA of 3.0; for doctorate, GRE (60th percentile or higher), bachelor's degree, recommendations, professional statement, transcripts, college-level calculus course with minimum B grade; minimum QPA of 3.3. Additional exam requirements/recommendations for international students: Required—TOEFL (minimum score 550 paper-based; 80 iBT) or IELTS (minimum score 6.5). *Application deadline:* For fall admission, 1/15 for domestic and international students. Applications are processed on a rolling basis. Application fee: $120. Electronic applications accepted. *Expenses:* $12,464 per term full-time in-state, $20,502 per term full-time out-of-state, $1,016 per credit part-time in-state, $1,680 per credit part-time out-of-state; $400 full-time fees, $205 part-time fees. *Financial support:* In 2015–16, 16 students received support, including 2 fellowships (averaging $3,775 per year), 11 research assistantships (averaging $23,911 per year), 4 teaching assistantships (averaging $14,978 per year); scholarships/grants, health care benefits, and unspecified assistantships also available. Financial award application deadline: 1/15; financial award applicants required to submit FAFSA. *Faculty research:* Decision analysis and cost-effectiveness, long-term care, health policy, organ donation, Medicare and Medicaid. *Total annual research expenditures:* $2.9 million. *Unit head:* Dr. Mark S. Roberts, Chair, 412-383-7049, Fax: 412-624-3146, E-mail: mroberts@pitt.edu. *Application contact:* Jessica Dornin, Recruitment and Academic Affairs Administrator, 412-624-3625, Fax: 412-624-3146, E-mail: jld115@pitt.edu.
Website: http://www.hpm.pitt.edu/

University of Pittsburgh, School of Health and Rehabilitation Sciences, Master's Programs in Health and Rehabilitation Sciences, Pittsburgh, PA 15260. Offers health and rehabilitation sciences (MS), including health information systems, healthcare supervision and management, occupational therapy, physical therapy, rehabilitation counseling, rehabilitation science and technology, sports medicine, wellness and human performance. *Accreditation:* APTA. *Program availability:* Part-time, evening/weekend. *Faculty:* 32 full-time (21 women). *Students:* 111 full-time (73 women), 42 part-time (31 women); includes 23 minority (5 Black or African American, non-Hispanic/Latino; 8 Asian, non-Hispanic/Latino; 7 Hispanic/Latino; 3 Two or more races, non-Hispanic/Latino), 65 international. Average age 29. 330 applicants, 66% accepted, 107 enrolled. In 2015, 89 master's awarded. *Degree requirements:* For master's, comprehensive exam (for some programs), thesis optional. *Entrance requirements:* For master's, minimum GPA of 3.0. Additional exam requirements/recommendations for international students: Required—TOEFL (minimum score 550 paper-based; 80 iBT), IELTS (minimum score 6.5). *Application deadline:* For fall admission, 3/1 for international students; for spring admission, 9/1 for international students. Applications are processed on a rolling basis. Application fee: $50. Electronic applications accepted. Tuition and fees vary according to program. *Financial support:* In 2015–16, 7 students received support, including 7 fellowships with full tuition reimbursements available (averaging $17,048 per year); traineeships also available. *Faculty research:* Assistive technology, seating and wheelchair mobility, cellular neurophysiology, low back syndrome, augmentative communication. *Total annual research expenditures:* $7.7 million. *Unit head:* Dr. Anthony Delitto, Dean, 412-383-6560, Fax: 412-383-6535, E-mail: delitto@pitt.edu. *Application contact:* Jessica Maguire, Director of Admissions, 412-383-6557, Fax: 412-383-6535, E-mail: maguire@pitt.edu.

University of Portland, Dr. Robert B. Pamplin, Jr. School of Business, Portland, OR 97203-5798. Offers entrepreneurship (MBA); finance (MBA, MS); health care management (MBA); marketing (MBA); nonprofit management (EMBA); operations and technology management (MBA, MS); sustainability (MBA). *Accreditation:* AACSB. *Program availability:* Part-time, evening/weekend. *Entrance requirements:* For master's, GMAT, minimum GPA of 3.0, resume, 2 letters of recommendation. Additional exam requirements/recommendations for international students: Required—TOEFL (minimum score 570 paper-based; 89 iBT), IELTS (minimum score 7). *Expenses:* Contact institution.

University of Puerto Rico, Medical Sciences Campus, Graduate School of Public Health, Department of Health Services Administration, Program in Health Services Administration, San Juan, PR 00936-5067. Offers MHSA. *Accreditation:* CAHME. *Program availability:* Part-time. *Degree requirements:* For master's, thesis. *Entrance requirements:* For master's, GRE, previous course work in accounting, statistics, economics, algebra, and managerial finance.

University of Regina, Faculty of Graduate Studies and Research, Johnson-Shoyama Graduate School of Public Policy, Regina, SK S4S 0A2, Canada. Offers economic analysis for public policy (Master's Certificate); health administration (MHA); health systems management (Master's Certificate); public management (MPA, Master's Certificate); public policy (MPA, MPP, PhD); public policy analysis (Master's Certificate). *Program availability:* Part-time. *Degree requirements:* For master's, thesis (for some programs); for doctorate, thesis/dissertation. *Entrance requirements:* For doctorate, master's degree, intended research program in an area of public policy. Additional exam requirements/recommendations for international students: Required—TOEFL (minimum score 580 paper-based; 80 iBT), IELTS (minimum score 6.5), PTE (minimum score 59).

Electronic applications accepted. *Expenses:* Contact institution. *Faculty research:* Governance and administration, public finance, public policy analysis, non-governmental organizations and alternative service delivery, micro-economics for policy analysis.

University of Rhode Island, Graduate School, College of Business Administration, Kingston, RI 02881. Offers accounting (MS); business administration (PhD), including finance and insurance, marketing, supply chain management; finance (MBA, MS); general business (MBA); health care management (MBA); management (MBA); marketing (MBA); oceanography (MBA); strategic innovation (MBA); supply chain management (MBA); Pharm D/MBA. *Accreditation:* AACSB. *Program availability:* Part-time, evening/weekend. *Faculty:* 55 full-time (22 women), 7 part-time/adjunct (3 women). *Students:* 87 full-time (35 women), 182 part-time (89 women); includes 43 minority (9 Black or African American, non-Hispanic/Latino; 2 American Indian or Alaska Native, non-Hispanic/Latino; 19 Asian, non-Hispanic/Latino; 7 Hispanic/Latino; 6 Two or more races, non-Hispanic/Latino), 23 international. In 2015, 117 master's, 2 doctorates awarded. *Degree requirements:* For master's, comprehensive exam (for some programs), thesis optional; for doctorate, comprehensive exam, thesis/dissertation. *Entrance requirements:* For master's, GMAT or GRE, 2 letters of recommendation, resume; for doctorate, GMAT or GRE, 3 letters of recommendation, resume. Additional exam requirements/recommendations for international students: Required—TOEFL (minimum score 575 paper-based; 91 iBT). *Application deadline:* For fall admission, 4/15 for domestic students, 2/15 for international students. Application fee: $65. Electronic applications accepted. *Expenses:* Tuition, state resident: full-time $11,796; part-time $655 per credit. Tuition, nonresident: full-time $24,206; part-time $1345 per credit. *Required fees:* $1546; $44 per credit. One-time fee: $155 full-time; $35 part-time. *Financial support:* In 2015–16, 3 research assistantships (averaging $15,996 per year), 11 teaching assistantships with tuition reimbursements (averaging $15,414 per year) were awarded. Financial award application deadline: 4/15; financial award applicants required to submit FAFSA. *Total annual research expenditures:* $66,948. *Unit head:* Dr. Maling Ebrahimpour, Dean, 401-874-4348, Fax: 401-874-4312, E-mail: mebrahimpour@uri.edu. *Application contact:* Lisa Lancellotta, Coordinator, MBA Programs, 401-874-4241, Fax: 401-874-4312, E-mail: mba@uri.edu.
Website: http://www.cba.uri.edu/

University of Rochester, School of Nursing, Rochester, NY 14642. Offers adult gerontological acute care nurse practitioner (MS); clinical nurse leader (MS); family nurse practitioner (MS); family psychiatric mental health nurse practitioner (MS); health care organization management and leadership (MS); health practice research (PhD); nursing (DNP); nursing education (MS); pediatric nurse practitioner (MS); pediatric nurse practitioner/neonatal nurse practitioner (MS). *Accreditation:* AACN. *Program availability:* Part-time, online learning. *Faculty:* 56 full-time (45 women), 63 part-time/adjunct (55 women). *Students:* 21 full-time (20 women), 212 part-time (175 women); includes 35 minority (12 Black or African American, non-Hispanic/Latino; 1 American Indian or Alaska Native, non-Hispanic/Latino; 10 Asian, non-Hispanic/Latino; 7 Hispanic/Latino; 5 Two or more races, non-Hispanic/Latino), 2 international. Average age 35. 111 applicants, 68% accepted, 71 enrolled. In 2015, 52 master's, 9 doctorates awarded. Terminal master's awarded for partial completion of doctoral program. *Degree requirements:* For master's, comprehensive exam (for some programs); for doctorate, thesis/dissertation. *Entrance requirements:* For master's, BS in nursing, minimum GPA of 3.0, course work in statistics; for doctorate, GRE General Test (for PhD), MS in nursing, minimum GPA of 3.5. Additional exam requirements/recommendations for international students: Required—TOEFL (minimum score 560 paper-based; 88 iBT) or IELTS (minimum score 6.5) recommended. *Application deadline:* For fall admission, 4/1 for domestic and international students; for spring admission, 9/1 for domestic and international students; for summer admission, 1/2 for domestic and international students. Application fee: $50. Electronic applications accepted. *Expenses:* Tuition, area resident: Full-time $47,450; part-time $1482 per credit hour. *Required fees:* $528. Tuition and fees vary according to program. *Financial support:* In 2015–16, 52 students received support, including 2 fellowships with tuition reimbursements available (averaging $30,000 per year); scholarships/grants, traineeships, health care benefits, tuition waivers (full and partial), and unspecified assistantships also available. Support available to part-time students. Financial award application deadline: 6/30. *Faculty research:* Symptom assessment and self-management of chronic illness, health promotion and illness prevention, nursing intervention research with vulnerable populations, palliative care, aging. *Total annual research expenditures:* $2.1 million. *Unit head:* Dr. Kathy H. Rideout, Dean, 585-273-8902, Fax: 585-273-1268, E-mail: kathy_rideout@urmc.rochester.edu. *Application contact:* Elaine Andolina, Director of Admissions, 585-275-2375, Fax: 585-756-8299, E-mail: elaine_andolina@urmc.rochester.edu.
Website: http://www.son.rochester.edu

University of Rochester, Simon Business School, Full-Time Master's Program in Business Administration, Rochester, NY 14627. Offers accounting and information systems (MBA); business environment and public policy (MBA); business systems consulting (MBA); competitive and organizational strategy - pricing (MBA); computers and information systems (MBA); corporate accounting (MBA); electronic commerce (MBA); entrepreneurship (MBA); finance (MBA); health sciences management (MBA); international management (MBA); marketing - brand management and pricing (MBA); operations management - manufacturing (MBA); operations management - services (MBA); public accounting (MBA). *Accreditation:* AACSB. *Program availability:* Part-time, evening/weekend. *Entrance requirements:* For master's, GMAT/GRE, previous course work in calculus. Additional exam requirements/recommendations for international students: Required—TOEFL. Electronic applications accepted. *Expenses:* Tuition, area resident: Full-time $47,450; part-time $1482 per credit hour. *Required fees:* $528. Tuition and fees vary according to program.

University of Rochester, Simon Business School, Part-Time MBA Program, Rochester, NY 14627. Offers accounting and information systems (MBA); business environment and public policy (MBA); business systems consulting (MBA); competitive and organizational strategy (MBA); computers and information systems (MBA); corporate accounting (MBA); electronic commerce (MBA); entrepreneurship (MBA); finance (MBA); health sciences management (MBA); international management (MBA); manufacturing management (MBA); marketing (MBA); operations management - services (MBA); public accounting (MBA). *Program availability:* Part-time, evening/weekend. *Entrance requirements:* For master's, GRE or GMAT, resume, recommendation letters, essays, transcripts. Electronic applications accepted. *Expenses:* Tuition, area resident: Full-time $47,450; part-time $1482 per credit hour. *Required fees:* $528. Tuition and fees vary according to program.

University of St. Francis, College of Business and Health Administration, School of Health Administration, Joliet, IL 60435-6169. Offers health administration (MS). *Program availability:* Part-time, evening/weekend, 100% online. *Faculty:* 6 full-time (3 women), 8 part-time/adjunct (4 women). *Students:* 97 full-time (82 women), 118 part-time (90 women); includes 62 minority (31 Black or African American, non-Hispanic/Latino; 4 Asian, non-Hispanic/Latino; 22 Hispanic/Latino; 5 Two or more races, non-Hispanic/Latino), 9 international. Average age 41. 104 applicants, 70% accepted, 51 enrolled. In 2015, 114 master's awarded. *Degree requirements:* For master's, comprehensive exam.

Entrance requirements: Additional exam requirements/recommendations for international students: Required—TOEFL (minimum score 550 paper-based; 79 iBT), IELTS (minimum score 6). *Application deadline:* Applications are processed on a rolling basis. Application fee: $30. Electronic applications accepted. Application fee is waived when completed online. *Expenses: Tuition, area resident:* Part-time $730 per credit hour. *Required fees:* $125 per semester. Part-time tuition and fees vary according to program. *Financial support:* In 2015–16, 83 students received support. Tuition waivers (partial) and unspecified assistantships available. Support available to part-time students. Financial award applicants required to submit FAFSA. *Unit head:* Dr. Orlando Griego, Dean, 815-740-3395, Fax: 815-740-3537, E-mail: ogriego@stfrancis.edu. *Application contact:* Sandra Sloka, Director of Admissions for Graduate and Degree Completion Programs, 800-735-7500, Fax: 815-740-3431, E-mail: ssloka@stfrancis.edu.
Website: http://www.stfrancis.edu/academics/college-of-business-health-administration/

University of Saint Francis, Graduate School, Keith Busse School of Business and Entrepreneurial Leadership, Fort Wayne, IN 46808-3994. Offers business administration (MBA); environmental health (MEH); healthcare administration (MHA); sustainability (MBA). *Accreditation:* ACBSP. *Program availability:* Part-time, evening/weekend, online learning. *Entrance requirements:* For master's, minimum cumulative GPA of 2.75. Additional exam requirements/recommendations for international students: Required—TOEFL or IELTS. Electronic applications accepted. *Expenses:* Contact institution.

University of Saint Mary, Graduate Programs, Program in Business Administration, Leavenworth, KS 66048-5082. Offers enterprise risk management (MBA); general management (MBA); health care management (MBA); human resource management (MBA); marketing and advertising management (MBA). *Program availability:* Part-time, evening/weekend, 100% online, blended/hybrid learning. *Students:* 186 full-time (108 women), 65 part-time (40 women); Includes 79 minority (34 Black or African American, non-Hispanic/Latino; 3 American Indian or Alaska Native, non-Hispanic/Latino; 12 Asian, non-Hispanic/Latino; 24 Hispanic/Latino; 1 Native Hawaiian or other Pacific Islander, non-Hispanic/Latino; 5 Two or more races, non-Hispanic/Latino), 5 international. Average age 34. In 2015, 58 master's awarded. *Degree requirements:* For master's, thesis. *Entrance requirements:* For master's, minimum undergraduate GPA of 2.75, official transcripts, two letters of recommendation. *Application deadline:* Applications are processed on a rolling basis. Application fee: $25. *Expenses:* $595 per credit hour. *Unit head:* Rick Gunter, Director, 913-319-3007. *Application contact:* Mark Harvey, Program Manager, 913-319-3007, E-mail: mark.harvey@stmary.edu.
Website: http://www.stmary.edu/success/Grad-Program/Master-of-Business-Administration-MBA.aspx

University of St. Thomas, Graduate Studies, Opus College of Business, Health Care UST MBA Program, Minneapolis, MN 55403. Offers MBA. *Accreditation:* CAHME. *Program availability:* Online learning. *Entrance requirements:* For master's, minimum 5 years of work experience in related field, letters of recommendation, essays, interview. Additional exam requirements/recommendations for international students: Required—TOEFL (minimum score 80 iBT), IELTS, or Michigan English Language Assessment Battery. Electronic applications accepted. *Expenses:* Contact institution.

University of San Francisco, School of Management, Master of Public Administration Program, San Francisco, CA 94105. Offers health services administration (MPA); public administration (MPA). *Program availability:* Part-time, evening/weekend, online learning. *Faculty:* 12 full-time (2 women), 7 part-time/adjunct (2 women). *Students:* 205 full-time (128 women), 13 part-time (8 women); includes 128 minority (28 Black or African American, non-Hispanic/Latino; 39 Asian, non-Hispanic/Latino; 49 Hispanic/Latino; 4 Native Hawaiian or other Pacific Islander, non-Hispanic/Latino; 8 Two or more races, non-Hispanic/Latino). Average age 33. 153 applicants, 84% accepted, 79 enrolled. In 2015, 64 master's awarded. *Entrance requirements:* For master's, resume demonstrating minimum of two years of professional work experience, transcripts from each college or university attended, two letters of recommendation, personal statement. Additional exam requirements/recommendations for international students: Required—TOEFL (minimum score 600 paper-based, 100 iBT), IELTS (minimum score 7) or PTE (minimum score 68). *Application deadline:* For fall admission, 6/15 for domestic students, 5/15 for international students. Application fee: $55. Electronic applications accepted. *Expenses: Tuition, area resident:* Full-time $22,410; part-time $1245 per credit. Tuition and fees vary according to course load, degree level and campus/location. *Financial support:* In 2015–16, 13 students received support. Scholarships/grants available. Financial award application deadline: 3/2; financial award applicants required to submit FAFSA. *Unit head:* Dr. Catherine Horiuchi, Director, 415-422-2221, E-mail: management@usfca.edu. *Application contact:* Office of Graduate Recruiting and Admissions, 415-422-2221, Fax: 415-422-6315, E-mail: management@usfca.edu.
Website: http://www.usfca.edu/mpa

University of Saskatchewan, College of Graduate Studies and Research, Edwards School of Business, Program in Business Administration, Saskatoon, SK S7N 5A2, Canada. Offers agribusiness management (MBA); biotechnology management (MBA); health services management (MBA); indigenous management (MBA); international business management (MBA).

The University of Scranton, Kania School of Management, Program in Business Administration, Scranton, PA 18510. Offers accounting (MBA); finance (MBA); general business administration (MBA); health care management (MBA); international business (MBA); management information systems (MBA); marketing (MBA); operations management (MBA). *Accreditation:* AACSB. *Program availability:* Part-time, evening/weekend, 100% online. *Students:* 107 full-time (27 women), 398 part-time (172 women); includes 89 minority (41 Black or African American, non-Hispanic/Latino; 1 American Indian or Alaska Native, non-Hispanic/Latino; 24 Asian, non-Hispanic/Latino; 17 Hispanic/Latino; 6 Two or more races, non-Hispanic/Latino), 64 international. Average age 34. *Entrance requirements:* For master's, GMAT (for MBA). *Financial support:* Applicants required to submit FAFSA. *Faculty research:* Financial markets, strategic impact of total quality management, internal accounting controls, consumer preference, information systems and the Internet. *Unit head:* Dr. Robyn Lawrence, Director, 570-941-7786, Fax: 570-941-4342, E-mail: robyn.lawrence@scranton.edu. *Application contact:* Joseph M. Roback, Director of Admissions, 570-941-4385, Fax: 570-941-5928, E-mail: robackj2@scranton.edu.
Website: https://www.scranton.edu/academics/cgce/grad-programs/busad.shtml

The University of Scranton, Panuska College of Professional Studies, Department of Health Administration and Human Resources, Program in Health Administration, Scranton, PA 18510. Offers MHA. *Accreditation:* CAHME. *Program availability:* Part-time, evening/weekend, online only, 100% online. *Students:* 53 full-time (32 women), 74 part-time (39 women); includes 28 minority (8 Black or African American, non-Hispanic/Latino; 11 Asian, non-Hispanic/Latino; 8 Hispanic/Latino; 1 Two or more races, non-Hispanic/Latino), 12 international. Average age 28. *Financial support:* Applicants required to submit FAFSA. *Unit head:* Steven J. Szydlowski, Director, 570-941-4367, Fax: 570-941-4201, E-mail: sjs14@scranton.edu. *Application contact:* Joseph M. Roback, Director of Admissions, 570-941-4385, Fax: 570-941-5928, E-mail: robackj2@scranton.edu.

University of Sioux Falls, Vucurevich School of Business, Sioux Falls, SD 57105-1699. Offers entrepreneurial leadership (MBA); general management (MBA); health care management (MBA); marketing (MBA). *Program availability:* Part-time, evening/weekend. *Degree requirements:* For master's, project. *Entrance requirements:* For master's, minimum GPA of 3.0. Additional exam requirements/recommendations for international students: Required—TOEFL. *Expenses:* Contact institution.

University of South Africa, College of Human Sciences, Pretoria, South Africa. Offers adult education (M Ed); African languages (MA, PhD); African politics (MA, PhD); Afrikaans (MA, PhD); ancient history (MA, PhD); ancient Near Eastern studies (MA, PhD); anthropology (MA, PhD); applied linguistics (MA); Arabic (MA, PhD); archaeology (MA); art history (MA); Biblical archaeology (MA); Biblical studies (M Th, D Th, PhD); Christian spirituality (M Th, D Th); church history (M Th, D Th); classical studies (MA, PhD); clinical psychology (MA); communication (MA, PhD); comparative education (M Ed, Ed D); consulting psychology (D Admin, D Com, PhD); curriculum studies (M Ed, Ed D); development studies (M Admin, MA, D Admin, PhD); didactics (M Ed, Ed D); education (M Tech); education management (M Ed, Ed D); educational psychology (M Ed); English (MA); environmental education (M Ed); French (MA, PhD); German (MA, PhD); Greek (MA); guidance and counseling (M Ed); health studies (MA, PhD), including health sciences education (MA), health services management (MA), medical and surgical nursing science (critical care general) (MA), midwifery and neonatal nursing science (MA), trauma and emergency care (MA); history (MA, PhD); history of education (Ed D); inclusive education (M Ed, Ed D); information and communications technology policy and regulation (MA); information science (MA, MIS, PhD); international politics (MA, PhD); Islamic studies (MA, PhD); Italian (MA, PhD); Judaica (MA, PhD); linguistics (MA, PhD); mathematical education (M Ed); mathematics education (MA); missiology (M Th, D Th); modern Hebrew (MA, PhD); musicology (MA, MMus, D Mus, PhD); natural science education (M Ed); New Testament (M Th, D Th); Old Testament (D Th); pastoral therapy (M Th, D Th); philosophy (MA); philosophy of education (M Ed, Ed D); politics (MA, PhD); Portuguese (MA, PhD); practical theology (M Th, D Th); psychology (MA, MS, PhD); psychology of education (M Ed, Ed D); public health (MA); religious studies (MA, D Th, PhD); Romance languages (MA); Russian (MA, PhD); Semitic languages (MA, PhD); social behavior studies in HIV/AIDS (MA); social science (mental health) (MA); social science in development studies (MA); social science in psychology (MA); social science in social work (MA); social science in sociology (MA); social work (MSW, DSW, PhD); socio-education (M Ed, Ed D); sociolinguistics (MA); sociology (MA, PhD); Spanish (MA, PhD); systematic theology (M Th, D Th); TESOL (teaching English to speakers of other languages) (MA); theological ethics (M Th, D Th); theory of literature (MA, PhD); urban ministries (D Th); urban ministry (M Th).

University of South Carolina, The Graduate School, Arnold School of Public Health, Department of Health Services Policy and Management, Columbia, SC 29208. Offers MHA, MPH, Dr PH, PhD, JD/MHA, MPH/MSN, MSW/MPH. *Accreditation:* CAHME (one or more programs are accredited). *Program availability:* Part-time, evening/weekend. *Degree requirements:* For master's, comprehensive exam, thesis or alternative, internship (MHA); for doctorate, comprehensive exam, thesis/dissertation. *Entrance requirements:* For master's, GMAT (MHA), GRE General Test (MPH); for doctorate, GRE General Test. Additional exam requirements/recommendations for international students: Required—TOEFL (minimum score 570 paper-based). Electronic applications accepted. *Faculty research:* Health systems management, evaluation, and planning; forecast applications in health care; Medicaid process to health care services.

The University of South Dakota, Graduate School, Beacom School of Business, Department of Business Administration, Vermillion, SD 57069-2390. Offers business administration (MBA); business analytics (MBA); health services administration (MBA); JD/MBA. *Accreditation:* AACSB. *Program availability:* Part-time, evening/weekend, online learning. *Degree requirements:* For master's, thesis or alternative. *Entrance requirements:* For master's, GMAT, minimum GPA of 2.7, resume. Additional exam requirements/recommendations for international students: Required—TOEFL (minimum score 550 paper-based; 79 iBT). *Application deadline:* For fall admission, 6/1 priority date for domestic students, 5/1 priority date for international students; for spring admission, 10/1 priority date for domestic students, 9/1 priority date for international students. Applications are processed on a rolling basis. Application fee: $35. Electronic applications accepted. *Expenses:* Contact institution. *Financial support:* Research assistantships with partial tuition reimbursements, teaching assistantships with partial tuition reimbursements, career-related internships or fieldwork, Federal Work-Study, and unspecified assistantships available. Financial award applicants required to submit FAFSA. *Unit head:* Dr. Venky Venkatachalam, Dean, 605-677-5455, Fax: 605-677-5058, E-mail: venky.venkatachalam@usd.edu. *Application contact:* Dr. Venky Venkatachalam, Dean, 605-677-5455, Fax: 605-677-5058, E-mail: venky.venkatachalam@usd.edu.
Website: http://www.usd.edu/business/business-administration/graduate

The University of South Dakota, Graduate School, College of Arts and Sciences, Program in Administrative Studies, Vermillion, SD 57069-2390. Offers alcohol and drug studies (MSA); criminal justice (MSA); health services administration (MSA); human resource management (MSA); interdisciplinary (MSA); long term care administration (MSA); organizational leadership (MSA). *Program availability:* Part-time, evening/weekend, online learning. *Degree requirements:* For master's, thesis or alternative. *Entrance requirements:* For master's, 3 years of work or experience, minimum GPA of 2.7, resume. Additional exam requirements/recommendations for international students: Required—TOEFL (minimum score 550 paper-based; 79 iBT). *Application deadline:* Applications are processed on a rolling basis. Application fee: $35. Electronic applications accepted. *Financial support:* Teaching assistantships with partial tuition reimbursements available. *Application contact:* Graduate School, 605-658-6140, Fax: 605-677-6118, E-mail: cde@usd.edu.
Website: http://www.usd.edu/usd-online/online-programs/master-of-science-in-administration

University of Southern California, Graduate School, School of Policy, Planning, and Development, Executive Master of Health Administration Program, Los Angeles, CA 90089. Offers EMHA. *Program availability:* Part-time, evening/weekend, online learning. *Entrance requirements:* Additional exam requirements/recommendations for international students: Required—TOEFL (minimum score 600 paper-based; 100 iBT). Electronic applications accepted. *Expenses:* Contact institution. *Faculty research:* Health management and policy, health care systems, health care economics and financing, health care access, community health, healthy communities.

University of Southern California, Graduate School, School of Policy, Planning, and Development, Master of Health Administration Program, Los Angeles, CA 90089. Offers ambulatory care (Graduate Certificate); health administration (MHA); long-term care (Graduate Certificate); MHA/MS. *Accreditation:* CAHME. *Program availability:* Part-time. *Degree requirements:* For master's, residency placement. *Entrance requirements:* For master's, GRE, GMAT. Additional exam requirements/recommendations for international students: Required—TOEFL (minimum score 600 paper-based; 100 iBT). Electronic applications accepted. *Faculty research:* Health administration, health management and policy, health care economics and financing, health care access, community health, healthy communities.

Health Services Management and Hospital Administration

University of Southern Indiana, Graduate Studies, College of Nursing and Health Professions, Program in Health Administration, Evansville, IN 47712-3590. Offers MHA. *Program availability:* Part-time, online learning. *Faculty:* 2 full-time (1 woman), 1 part-time/adjunct (0 women). *Students:* 3 full-time (2 women), 33 part-time (28 women); includes 3 minority (1 Black or African American, non-Hispanic/Latino; 2 Hispanic/Latino). Average age 32. In 2015, 18 master's awarded. *Entrance requirements:* For master's, GRE, minimum GPA of 3.0, curriculum vitae, letter of intent, three professional references, focused essay(s). Additional exam requirements/recommendations for international students: Required—TOEFL (minimum score 550 paper-based; 79 iBT), IELTS (minimum score 6). *Application deadline:* For fall admission, 6/1 for domestic students, 1/1 priority date for international students. Applications are processed on a rolling basis. Application fee: $40. Electronic applications accepted. *Expenses:* Tuition, state resident: full-time $8110. Tuition, nonresident: full-time $15,989. *Required fees:* $340; $115 per semester. Tuition and fees vary according to program. *Financial support:* Federal Work-Study, scholarships/grants, tuition waivers (full and partial), and unspecified assistantships available. Financial award application deadline: 3/1; financial award applicants required to submit FAFSA. *Unit head:* Dr. Kevin Valadares, Program Chair, 812-461-5277, E-mail: kvaladar@usi.edu. *Application contact:* Dr. Mayola Rowser, Director, Graduate Studies, 812-465-7016, Fax: 812-464-1956, E-mail: mrowser@usi.edu.
Website: http://www.usi.edu/health/master-of-health-administration

University of Southern Maine, College of Management and Human Service, School of Business, Portland, ME 04104-9300. Offers accounting (MBA); business administration (MBA); finance (MBA); health management and policy (MBA); sustainability (MBA); JD/MBA; MBA/MSA; MBA/MSN; MS/MBA. *Accreditation:* AACSB. *Program availability:* Part-time, evening/weekend. *Entrance requirements:* For master's, GMAT or GRE, minimum AACSB index of 1100. Additional exam requirements/recommendations for international students: Required—TOEFL (minimum score 550 paper-based; 79 iBT). Electronic applications accepted. *Expenses: Tuition, area resident:* Full-time $6840; part-time $380 per credit hour. Tuition, state resident: full-time $10,260; part-time $570 per credit hour. Tuition, nonresident: full-time $18,468; part-time $1026 per credit hour. *Required fees:* $830; $83 per credit hour. Tuition and fees vary according to course load and program. *Faculty research:* Economic development, management information systems, real options, system dynamics, simulation.

University of Southern Mississippi, Graduate School, College of Health, Department of Public Health, Hattiesburg, MS 39406-0001. Offers epidemiology and biostatistics (MPH); health education (MPH); health policy and administration (MPH). *Accreditation:* CEPH. *Program availability:* Part-time, evening/weekend. *Degree requirements:* For master's, comprehensive exam, thesis (for some programs). *Entrance requirements:* For master's, GRE General Test, minimum GPA of 2.75 in last 60 hours. Additional exam requirements/recommendations for international students: Required—TOEFL, IELTS. Electronic applications accepted. *Faculty research:* Rural health care delivery, school health, nutrition of pregnant teens, risk factor reduction, sexually transmitted diseases.

University of South Florida, College of Public Health, Department of Health Policy and Management, Tampa, FL 33620-9951. Offers MHA, MPH, MSPH, PhD. *Accreditation:* CAHME. *Program availability:* Part-time, evening/weekend. *Degree requirements:* For master's, comprehensive exam, thesis (for some programs); for doctorate, comprehensive exam, thesis/dissertation. *Entrance requirements:* For master's, GRE General Test or GMAT, minimum GPA of 3.0 in upper-level course work, 3 professional letters of recommendation, resume/curriculum vitae; for doctorate, GRE General Test, minimum GPA of 3.0 in upper-level course work, goal statement letter, three professional letters of recommendation, resume/curriculum vitae, writing sample. Additional exam requirements/recommendations for international students: Required—TOEFL (minimum score 550 paper-based; 79 iBT). Electronic applications accepted. *Faculty research:* Tracking community health, inpatient care, discharge policies, stroke education, leadership practices.

University of South Florida, Innovative Education, Tampa, FL 33620-9951. Offers adult, career and higher education (Graduate Certificate), including college teaching, leadership in developing human resources, leadership in higher education; Africana studies (Graduate Certificate), including diasporas and health disparities, genocide and human rights; aging studies (Graduate Certificate), including gerontology; art research (Graduate Certificate), including museum studies; business foundations (Graduate Certificate); chemical and biomedical engineering (Graduate Certificate), including materials science and engineering, water, health and sustainability; child and family studies (Graduate Certificate), including positive behavior support; civil and industrial engineering (Graduate Certificate), including transportation systems analysis; community and family health (Graduate Certificate), including maternal and child health, social marketing and public health, violence and injury: prevention and intervention, women's health; criminology (Graduate Certificate), including criminal justice administration; educational measurement and research (Graduate Certificate), including evaluation; English (Graduate Certificate), including comparative literary studies, creative writing, professional and technical communication; entrepreneurship (Graduate Certificate); environmental health (Graduate Certificate), including safety management; epidemiology and biostatistics (Graduate Certificate), including applied biostatistics, biostatistics, concepts and tools of epidemiology, epidemiology, epidemiology of infectious diseases; geography, environment and planning (Graduate Certificate), including community development, environmental policy and management, geographical information systems; geology (Graduate Certificate), including hydrogeology; global health (Graduate Certificate), including disaster management, global health and Latin American and Caribbean studies, global health practice, humanitarian assistance, infection control; government and international affairs (Graduate Certificate), including Cuban studies, globalization studies; health policy and management (Graduate Certificate), including health management and leadership, public health policy and programs; hearing specialist: early intervention (Graduate Certificate); industrial and management systems engineering (Graduate Certificate), including systems engineering, technology management; information studies (Graduate Certificate), including school library media specialist; information systems/decision sciences (Graduate Certificate), including analytics and business intelligence; instructional technology (Graduate Certificate), including distance education, Florida digital/virtual educator, instructional design, multimedia design, Web design; internal medicine, bioethics and medical humanities (Graduate Certificate), including biomedical ethics; Latin American and Caribbean studies (Graduate Certificate); mass communications (Graduate Certificate), including multimedia journalism; mathematics and statistics (Graduate Certificate), including mathematics; medicine (Graduate Certificate), including aging and neuroscience, bioinformatics, biotechnology, brain fitness and memory management, clinical investigation, health informatics, health sciences, integrative weight management, intellectual property, medicine and gender, metabolic and nutritional medicine, metabolic cardiology, pharmacy sciences; national and competitive intelligence (Graduate Certificate); psychological and social foundations (Graduate Certificate), including career counseling, college teaching, diversity in education, mental health counseling, school counseling; public affairs (Graduate Certificate), including nonprofit management, public management, research administration; public health (Graduate Certificate), including environmental health, health equity, public health generalist, translational research in adolescent behavioral

health; public health practices (Graduate Certificate), including planning for healthy communities; rehabilitation and mental health counseling (Graduate Certificate), including integrative mental health care, marriage and family therapy, rehabilitation technology; secondary education (Graduate Certificate), including ESOL, foreign language education: culture and content, foreign language education: professional; social work (Graduate Certificate), including geriatric social work/clinical gerontology; special education (Graduate Certificate), including autism spectrum disorder, disabilities education: severe/profound; world languages (Graduate Certificate), including teaching English as a second language (TESL) or foreign language. *Unit head:* Kathy Barnes, Interdisciplinary Programs Coordinator, 813-974-8031, Fax: 813-974-7061, E-mail: barnesk@usf.edu. *Application contact:* Karen Tylinski, Metro Initiatives, 813-974-9943, Fax: 813-974-7061, E-mail: ktylinsk@usf.edu.
Website: http://www.usf.edu/innovative-education/

The University of Tennessee, Graduate School, College of Education, Health and Human Sciences, Program in Public Health, Knoxville, TN 37996. Offers community health education (MPH); gerontology (MPH); health planning/administration (MPH); MS/MPH. *Accreditation:* CEPH. *Degree requirements:* For master's, thesis optional. *Entrance requirements:* For master's, minimum GPA of 2.7. Additional exam requirements/recommendations for international students: Required—TOEFL. Electronic applications accepted.

The University of Texas at Arlington, Graduate School, College of Business, Program in Health Care Administration, Arlington, TX 76019. Offers MS. *Program availability:* Part-time, evening/weekend. *Degree requirements:* For master's, one foreign language, thesis optional. *Entrance requirements:* For master's, GRE General Test or GMAT, minimum GPA of 3.0, official undergraduate and graduate transcripts, current professional resume, personal statement, three letters of recommendation. Additional exam requirements/recommendations for international students: Required—TOEFL (minimum score 550 paper-based; 79 iBT).

The University of Texas at Dallas, Naveen Jindal School of Management, Program in Business Administration, Richardson, TX 75080. Offers business administration (MBA); executive business administration (EMBA); global leadership (EMBA); healthcare management for physicians (EMBA); project management (EMBA); MS/MBA. *Accreditation:* AACSB. *Program availability:* Part-time, evening/weekend, online learning. *Faculty:* 63 full-time (15 women), 74 part-time/adjunct (23 women). *Students:* 366 full-time (140 women), 600 part-time (207 women); includes 318 minority (57 Black or African American, non-Hispanic/Latino; 3 American Indian or Alaska Native, non-Hispanic/Latino; 159 Asian, non-Hispanic/Latino; 74 Hispanic/Latino; 25 Two or more races, non-Hispanic/Latino), 200 international. Average age 33. 812 applicants, 44% accepted, 304 enrolled. In 2015, 384 master's awarded. *Degree requirements:* For master's, thesis optional. *Entrance requirements:* For master's, GMAT, 10 years of business experience (EMBA), minimum GPA of 3.0. Additional exam requirements/recommendations for international students: Required—TOEFL (minimum score 550 paper-based). *Application deadline:* For fall admission, 7/15 for domestic students, 5/1 priority date for international students; for spring admission, 11/15 for domestic students, 9/1 priority date for international students. Applications are processed on a rolling basis. Application fee: $50 ($100 for international students). Electronic applications accepted. *Expenses:* Contact institution. *Financial support:* In 2015–16, 393 students received support, including 8 teaching assistantships with partial tuition reimbursements available (averaging $11,625 per year); research assistantships with partial tuition reimbursements available, career-related internships or fieldwork, Federal Work-Study, institutionally sponsored loans, scholarships/grants, and unspecified assistantships also available. Support available to part-time students. Financial award application deadline: 4/30; financial award applicants required to submit FAFSA. *Faculty research:* Production scheduling, trade and finance, organizational decision-making, life/work planning. *Unit head:* Lisa Shatz, Assistant Dean, MBA Programs, 972-883-6191, E-mail: lisa.shatz@utdallas.edu. *Application contact:* Brooke Scarborough, Academic Support Coordinator, 972-883-5899, E-mail: bes016100@utdallas.edu.
Website: http://jindal.utdallas.edu/mba-programs/

The University of Texas at Dallas, Naveen Jindal School of Management, Program in Organizations, Strategy and International Management, Richardson, TX 75080. Offers healthcare management (MS); innovation and entrepreneurship (MS); international management studies (MS, PhD); management and administrative sciences (MS); project management (MS); systems engineering and management (MS). *Program availability:* Part-time, evening/weekend. *Faculty:* 14 full-time (4 women), 13 part-time/adjunct (4 women). *Students:* 107 full-time (62 women), 156 part-time (84 women); includes 93 minority (23 Black or African American, non-Hispanic/Latino; 43 Asian, non-Hispanic/Latino; 16 Hispanic/Latino; 1 Native Hawaiian or other Pacific Islander, non-Hispanic/Latino; 10 Two or more races, non-Hispanic/Latino), 67 international. Average age 35. 309 applicants, 48% accepted, 84 enrolled. In 2015, 148 master's, 2 doctorates awarded. *Degree requirements:* For doctorate, thesis/dissertation. *Entrance requirements:* For master's and doctorate, GMAT. Additional exam requirements/recommendations for international students: Required—TOEFL (minimum score 550 paper-based). *Application deadline:* For fall admission, 7/15 for domestic students, 5/1 priority date for international students; for spring admission, 11/15 for domestic students, 9/1 priority date for international students. Applications are processed on a rolling basis. Application fee: $50 ($100 for international students). Electronic applications accepted. *Expenses:* Tuition, state resident: full-time $11,940; part-time $663 per semester hour. Tuition, nonresident: full-time $22,786; part-time $1266 per semester hour. Tuition and fees vary according to course load. *Financial support:* In 2015–16, 79 students received support, including 5 research assistantships with partial tuition reimbursements available (averaging $24,000 per year), 16 teaching assistantships with partial tuition reimbursements available (averaging $18,469 per year); Federal Work-Study, institutionally sponsored loans, scholarships/grants, and unspecified assistantships also available. Support available to part-time students. Financial award application deadline: 4/30; financial award applicants required to submit FAFSA. *Faculty research:* International accounting, international trade and finance, economic development, international economics. *Unit head:* Dr. Mike Peng, Area Coordinator, 972-883-2714, Fax: 972-883-5977, E-mail: mikepeng@utdallas.edu. *Application contact:* Maria Hasenhuttl, Assistant Area Coordinator, 972-883-5898, Fax: 972-883-5977, E-mail: maria.hasenhuttl@utdallas.edu.
Website: http://jindal.utdallas.edu/osim/

The University of Texas at El Paso, Graduate School, School of Nursing, El Paso, TX 79968-0001. Offers family nurse practitioner (MSN); health care leadership and management (Certificate); interdisciplinary health sciences (PhD); nursing (DNP); nursing education (MSN, Certificate); nursing systems management (MSN). *Accreditation:* AACN. *Program availability:* Online learning. *Degree requirements:* For master's, thesis optional; for doctorate, thesis/dissertation. *Entrance requirements:* For master's, minimum GPA of 3.0, resume; for doctorate, GRE, letters of reference, relevant personal/professional experience; master's degree in nursing (for DNP); for Certificate, bachelor's degree in nursing. Additional exam requirements/recommendations for international students: Required—TOEFL; Recommended—IELTS. Electronic applications accepted.

The University of Texas at Tyler, College of Business and Technology, School of Business Administration, Tyler, TX 75799-0001. Offers business administration (MBA); general management (MBA); health care (MBA). *Program availability:* Part-time, online learning. *Entrance requirements:* Additional exam requirements/recommendations for international students: Required—TOEFL (minimum score 550 paper-based). *Faculty research:* General business, inventory control, institutional markets, service marketing, product distribution, accounting fraud, financial reporting and recognition.

University of the Incarnate Word, School of Graduate Studies and Research, H-E-B School of Business and Administration, Program in Health Administration, San Antonio, TX 78209-6397. Offers MHA. *Accreditation:* CAHME. *Program availability:* Part-time, evening/weekend. *Faculty:* 13 full-time (5 women), 14 part-time/adjunct (5 women). *Students:* 35 full-time (20 women); includes 24 minority (3 Black or African American, non-Hispanic/Latino; 3 Asian, non-Hispanic/Latino; 17 Hispanic/Latino; 1 Two or more races, non-Hispanic/Latino), 1 international. Average age 30. 42 applicants, 69% accepted, 17 enrolled. In 2015, 22 master's awarded. *Entrance requirements:* For master's, GRE or GMAT if applicant has GPA of at least 2.5 but less than 3.0, baccalaureate degree with minimum GPA of 3.5, official transcripts of all undergraduate work, letter of intent, interview and evaluation by MHA admissions committee. Additional exam requirements/recommendations for international students: Required—TOEFL (minimum score 560 paper-based; 83 iBT). *Expenses: Tuition, area resident:* Part-time $885 per credit hour. *Required fees:* $40 per credit hour. Tuition and fees vary according to course load, degree level, campus/location, program and student level. *Financial support:* Scholarships/grants, tuition waivers, and unspecified assistantships available. *Unit head:* Dr. Daniel G. Dominguez, Director, 210-829-3180, E-mail: domingue@uiwtx.edu. *Application contact:* Johnny Garcia, Assistant Director of Graduate Admissions, 210-805-3554, Fax: 210-829-3921, E-mail: jsgarcia@uiwtx.edu. Website: http://www.uiw.edu/mha/

University of the Sciences, Program in Health Policy, Philadelphia, PA 19104-4495. Offers MS, PhD. *Program availability:* Part-time, evening/weekend, online learning. *Degree requirements:* For doctorate, comprehensive exam, thesis/dissertation. *Entrance requirements:* For master's and doctorate, GRE General Test. Additional exam requirements/recommendations for international students: Required—TOEFL, TWE. *Application deadline:* For fall admission, 6/1 for domestic students, 5/1 for international students; for winter admission, 12/1 for domestic students, 10/1 for international students; for spring admission, 3/1 for international students. Applications are processed on a rolling basis. Application fee: $50. *Expenses:* Contact institution. *Financial support:* Tuition waivers (partial) and unspecified assistantships available. Support available to part-time students. Financial award application deadline: 5/1. *Unit head:* Dr. Stephen Metraux, Interim Director, 215-596-7614, E-mail: s.metrau@usciences.edu. *Application contact:* Dr. Stephen Metraux, Interim Director, 215-596-7614, E-mail: s.metrau@usciences.edu.

The University of Toledo, College of Graduate Studies, College of Languages, Literature and Social Sciences, Department of Political Science and Public Administration, Toledo, OH 43606-3390. Offers health care policy and administration (Certificate); management of non-profit organizations (Certificate); municipal administration (Certificate); political science (MA); public administration (MPA); JD/MPA. *Accreditation:* NASPAA. *Program availability:* Part-time. *Degree requirements:* For master's, comprehensive exam (for some programs), thesis. *Entrance requirements:* For master's, GRE General Test, minimum cumulative point-hour ratio of 2.7 (3.0 for MPA) for all previous academic work, three letters of recommendation, statement of purpose, transcripts from all prior institutions attended; for Certificate, minimum cumulative point-hour ratio of 2.7 for all previous academic work, three letters of recommendation, statement of purpose, transcripts from all prior institutions attended. Additional exam requirements/recommendations for international students: Required—TOEFL (minimum score 550 paper-based; 80 iBT). Electronic applications accepted. *Faculty research:* Economic development, health care, Third World, criminal justice, Eastern Europe.

The University of Toledo, College of Graduate Studies, College of Medicine and Life Sciences, Department of Public Health and Preventative Medicine, Toledo, OH 43606-3390. Offers biostatistics and epidemiology (Certificate); contemporary gerontological practice (Certificate); environmental and occupational health and safety (MPH); epidemiology (Certificate); global public health (Certificate); health promotion and education (MPH); industrial hygiene (MSOH); medical and health science teaching and learning (Certificate); occupational health (Certificate); public health administration (MPH); public health and emergency response (Certificate); public health epidemiology (MPH); public health nutrition (MPH); MD/MPH. *Program availability:* Part-time, evening/weekend. *Degree requirements:* For master's, thesis or alternative. *Entrance requirements:* For master's, GRE, minimum undergraduate GPA of 3.0, three letters of recommendation, statement of purpose, transcripts from all prior institutions attended, resume; for Certificate, minimum undergraduate GPA of 3.0, three letters of recommendation, statement of purpose, transcripts from all prior institutions attended, resume. Additional exam requirements/recommendations for international students: Required—TOEFL (minimum score 550 paper-based; 80 iBT), IELTS (minimum score 6.5). Electronic applications accepted.

University of Toronto, Faculty of Medicine, Institute of Health Policy, Management and Evaluation, Program in Health Administration, Toronto, ON M5S 1A1, Canada. Offers MH Sc. *Entrance requirements:* For master's, minimum B+ average on each of the last two years of a four-year undergraduate program, minimum of three years relevant clinical or management experience. Additional exam requirements/recommendations for international students: Required—TOEFL (minimum score 580 paper-based; 93 iBT), TWE (minimum score 5). Electronic applications accepted.

University of Utah, Graduate School, College of Pharmacy, Department of Pharmacotherapy, Salt Lake City, UT 84112. Offers health system pharmacy administration (MS); outcomes research and health policy (PhD). *Faculty:* 6 full-time (4 women), 26 part-time/adjunct (18 women). *Students:* 8 full-time (5 women), 5 part-time (3 women), 5 international. Average age 28. 26 applicants, 19% accepted, 4 enrolled. In 2015, 3 master's awarded. Terminal master's awarded for partial completion of doctoral program. *Degree requirements:* For master's, comprehensive exam, thesis or alternative, project; for doctorate, comprehensive exam, thesis/dissertation. *Entrance requirements:* For doctorate, GRE. Additional exam requirements/recommendations for international students: Required—TOEFL (minimum score 550 paper-based; 80 iBT). *Application deadline:* For fall admission, 1/10 for domestic students, 12/15 for international students. Application fee: $55 ($65 for international students). *Financial support:* In 2015–16, 7 students received support, including 9 research assistantships with full tuition reimbursements available (averaging $21,400 per year); health care benefits also available. Financial award application deadline: 12/15. *Faculty research:* Outcomes in pharmacy, pharmacotherapy. *Total annual research expenditures:* $131,217. *Unit head:* Dr. Diana I. Brixner, Department Chair and Professor, 801-581-6731. *Application contact:* Sara Ray, Academic Program Manager, 801-581-5984, Fax: 801-585-6160, E-mail: sara.ray@pharm.utah.edu. Website: http://www.pharmacy.utah.edu/pharmacotherapy/

University of Utah, Graduate School, David Eccles School of Business, Master in Healthcare Administration Program, Salt Lake City, UT 84112. Offers MHA, MBA/MHA, MHA/MPA, MPH/MHA, PMBA/MHA. *Accreditation:* CAHME. *Program availability:* Part-

time. *Faculty:* 1 (woman) full-time, 2 part-time/adjunct (0 women). *Students:* 12 full-time (5 women). Average age 27. 51 applicants, 55% accepted, 28 enrolled. In 2015, 20 master's awarded. *Degree requirements:* For master's, administrative internship. *Entrance requirements:* For master's, GMAT, GRE, statistics course with minimum B grade; minimum undergraduate GPA of 3.0. Additional exam requirements/recommendations for international students: Required—TOEFL (minimum score 600 paper-based), IELTS (minimum score 7). *Application deadline:* For fall admission, 2/15 priority date for domestic and international students. Applications are processed on a rolling basis. Application fee: $55 ($65 for international students). Electronic applications accepted. *Expenses:* Contact institution. *Financial support:* In 2015–16, 15 students received support, including 15 fellowships with partial tuition reimbursements available (averaging $13,000 per year); scholarships/grants and unspecified assistantships also available. Financial award application deadline: 2/15; financial award applicants required to submit FAFSA. *Faculty research:* Healthcare leadership, problem-solving, primary care delivery redesign, patient engagement, patient-reported outcomes. *Unit head:* Dr. Debra Scammon, Professor, 801-581-4754, Fax: 801-581-3666, E-mail: debra.scammon@business.utah.edu. *Application contact:* Aislynn Schultz, Graduate Admissions Specialist, 801-581-7785, Fax: 801-581-7785, E-mail: mastersinfo@business.utah.edu.

University of Virginia, School of Medicine, Department of Public Health Sciences, Charlottesville, VA 22903. Offers clinical research (MS), including clinical investigation and patient-oriented research, informatics in medicine; public health (MPH); MPP/MPH. *Program availability:* Part-time. *Entrance requirements:* For master's, GRE General Test or MCAT. Additional exam requirements/recommendations for international students: Required—TOEFL. Electronic applications accepted.

University of Washington, Graduate School, School of Public Health, Department of Health Services, Programs in Health Services Administration, Seattle, WA 98195. Offers EMHA, MHA, JD/MHA, MHA/MBA, MHA/MD, MHA/MPA. *Accreditation:* CAHME. *Program availability:* Part-time. *Degree requirements:* For master's, capstone project. *Entrance requirements:* For master's, GRE General Test or GMAT (for MHA), minimum GPA of 3.0. Additional exam requirements/recommendations for international students: Required—TOEFL (minimum score 580 paper-based; 92 iBT), IELTS (minimum score 7). Electronic applications accepted. *Expenses:* Contact institution. *Faculty research:* Health economics, health information management, research design in health services, health policy, clinical effectiveness.

The University of Western Ontario, Richard Ivey School of Business, London, ON N6A 3K7, Canada. Offers business (EMBA, PhD); corporate strategy and leadership elective (MBA); entrepreneurship elective (MBA); finance elective (MBA); health sector stream (MBA); international management elective (MBA); marketing elective (MBA); JD/MBA. *Degree requirements:* For master's, thesis (for some programs); for doctorate, thesis/dissertation. *Entrance requirements:* For master's, GMAT, 2 years of full-time work experience, interview. Additional exam requirements/recommendations for international students: Required—TOEFL (minimum score 100 iBT) or IELTS (minimum score 6). Electronic applications accepted. *Faculty research:* Strategy, organizational behavior, international business, finance, operations management.

University of West Georgia, Tanner Health System School of Nursing, Carrollton, GA 30118. Offers health systems leadership (Post-Master's Certificate); nursing (MSN); nursing education (Ed D, Post-Master's Certificate). *Accreditation:* AACN. *Program availability:* Part-time, evening/weekend, 100% online. *Faculty:* 13 full-time (all women). *Students:* 58 full-time (51 women), 69 part-time (61 women); includes 33 minority (29 Black or African American, non-Hispanic/Latino; 1 Asian, non-Hispanic/Latino; 3 Hispanic/Latino). Average age 42. 78 applicants, 90% accepted, 58 enrolled. In 2015, 32 master's, 1 other advanced degree awarded. *Entrance requirements:* Additional exam requirements/recommendations for international students: Required—TOEFL (minimum score 523 paper-based; 69 iBT); Recommended—IELTS (minimum score 6.5). *Application deadline:* For fall admission, 2/1 priority date for domestic and international students. Applications are processed on a rolling basis. Application fee: $40. Electronic applications accepted. *Expenses:* Contact institution. *Financial support:* Fellowships, research assistantships, teaching assistantships, career-related internships or fieldwork, Federal Work-Study, institutionally sponsored loans, scholarships/grants, and unspecified assistantships available. Support available to part-time students. Financial award application deadline: 4/1; financial award applicants required to submit FAFSA. *Unit head:* Dr. Jennifer Schuessler, Dean, 678-839-5640, Fax: 678-839-6553, E-mail: jschuess@westga.edu. *Application contact:* Dr. Toby Ziglar, Director of Graduate and International Admissions, 678-839-1390, Fax: 678-839-1395, E-mail: graduate@westga.edu. Website: http://nursing.westga.edu

University of Wisconsin–Oshkosh, Graduate Studies, College of Letters and Science, Department of Public Administration, Oshkosh, WI 54901. Offers general agency (MPA); health care (MPA). *Program availability:* Part-time, evening/weekend. *Degree requirements:* For master's, thesis or alternative. *Entrance requirements:* For master's, public service-related experience, resume, sample of written work. Additional exam requirements/recommendations for international students: Required—TOEFL (minimum score 550 paper-based; 79 iBT). Electronic applications accepted. *Faculty research:* Drug policy, local government state revenues and expenditures, health care regulation.

University of Wyoming, College of Health Sciences, School of Pharmacy, Laramie, WY 82071. Offers health services administration (MS); pharmacy (Pharm D). *Accreditation:* ACPE (one or more programs are accredited). *Program availability:* Online learning. *Entrance requirements:* For doctorate, PCAT. Additional exam requirements/recommendations for international students: Required—TOEFL.

Utica College, Program in Health Care Administration, Utica, NY 13502-4892. Offers MS. *Program availability:* Part-time, evening/weekend, online learning. *Students:* 4 full-time (all women), 158 part-time (130 women); includes 35 minority (20 Black or African American, non-Hispanic/Latino; 7 Asian, non-Hispanic/Latino; 6 Hispanic/Latino; 2 Two or more races, non-Hispanic/Latino). Average age 34. 82 applicants, 95% accepted, 67 enrolled. In 2015, 70 master's awarded. *Degree requirements:* For master's, capstone (internship or research/program development project). *Entrance requirements:* For master's, BS, minimum GPA of 3.0, 2 recommendation letters, personal essay. Additional exam requirements/recommendations for international students: Required—TOEFL (minimum score 525 paper-based). *Application deadline:* Applications are processed on a rolling basis. Application fee: $50. Electronic applications accepted. *Expenses:* $675 per credit hour. *Financial support:* Application deadline: 3/15; applicants required to submit FAFSA. *Unit head:* Dr. Dana Hart, Head, 315-792-3375, E-mail: dhart@utica.edu. *Application contact:* John D. Rowe, Director of Graduate Admissions, 315-792-3824, Fax: 315-792-3003, E-mail: jrowe@utica.edu.

Valdosta State University, Masters of Business Administration Program, Valdosta, GA 31698. Offers business administration (MBA); healthcare administration (MBA). Program is a member of the Georgia WebMBA. *Accreditation:* AACSB. *Program availability:* Part-time, evening/weekend, 100% online, blended/hybrid learning. *Faculty:* 7 full-time (0 women). *Students:* 18 full-time (12 women), 53 part-time (29 women); includes 21 minority (18 Black or African American, non-Hispanic/Latino; 3 Two or more races, non-Hispanic/Latino), 8 international. Average age 24. 38 applicants, 79%

Health Services Management and Hospital Administration

accepted, 25 enrolled. In 2015, 32 master's awarded. *Degree requirements:* For master's, comprehensive written and/or oral exams. *Entrance requirements:* For master's, GMAT or GRE, minimum GPA of 2.75. Additional exam requirements/recommendations for international students: Required—TOEFL (minimum score 523 paper-based); Recommended—IELTS. *Application deadline:* For fall admission, 7/1 for domestic and international students; for spring admission, 11/1 for domestic and international students. Applications are processed on a rolling basis. Application fee: $35. Electronic applications accepted. *Expenses:* $243 per credit hour in-state; $875 per credit hour out-of-state; $970 per semester fees; $739 per credit hour (for WebMBA). *Financial support:* In 2015–16, 5 students received support, including 4 research assistantships with full tuition reimbursements available (averaging $3,652 per year); institutionally sponsored loans and scholarships/grants also available. Support available to part-time students. Financial award application deadline: 7/1; financial award applicants required to submit FAFSA. *Unit head:* Dr. Mel Schnake, Director, 229-245-2233, Fax: 229-245-2795, E-mail: mschnake@valdosta.edu. *Application contact:* Jessica Powers, Admissions Specialist, 229-333-5694, Fax: 229-245-3853, E-mail: jldevane@valdosta.edu.
Website: http://www.valdosta.edu/academics/graduate-school/our-programs/business-administration.php

Valparaiso University, Graduate School, Program in Health Administration, Valparaiso, IN 46383. Offers MHA, MS. *Program availability:* Part-time, evening/weekend. *Students:* 15 full-time (6 women), 68 part-time (44 women); includes 17 minority (13 Black or African American, non-Hispanic/Latino; 2 Asian, non-Hispanic/Latino; 2 Hispanic/Latino), 20 international. Average age 34. In 2015, 5 master's awarded. *Degree requirements:* For master's, practicum, internship. *Entrance requirements:* For master's, minimum overall GPA of 3.0 or 5 years of work experience in the field; basic course in statistics; official transcripts; two letters of recommendation; essay. Additional exam requirements/recommendations for international students: Required—TOEFL (minimum score 550 paper-based; 80 iBT), IELTS (minimum score 6). *Application deadline:* Applications are processed on a rolling basis. Application fee: $30 ($50 for international students). Electronic applications accepted. *Financial support:* Available to part-time students. Applicants required to submit FAFSA. *Unit head:* Dr. Jennifer A. Ziegler, Dean, Graduate School and Continuing Education, 219-464-5313, Fax: 219-464-5381, E-mail: jennifer.ziegler@valpo.edu. *Application contact:* Jessica Choquette, Graduate Admissions Specialist, 219-464-6510, Fax: 219-464-5381, E-mail: jessica.choquette@valpo.edu.
Website: http://www.valpo.edu/grad/healthadmin/index.php

Vanderbilt University, Vanderbilt University Owen Graduate School of Management, Master of Management in Health Care Program, Nashville, TN 37203. Offers healthcare (MM). *Faculty:* 10 full-time (1 woman), 3 part-time/adjunct (0 women). *Students:* 38 full-time (23 women); includes 7 minority (2 Black or African American, non-Hispanic/Latino; 4 Asian, non-Hispanic/Latino; 1 Hispanic/Latino), 1 international. Average age 40. 45 applicants, 87% accepted, 38 enrolled. In 2015, 29 master's awarded. *Entrance requirements:* For master's, GMAT or GRE (recommended), undergraduate transcript, five years of relevant work experience, interview. *Application deadline:* For fall admission, 6/1 priority date for domestic students. Applications are processed on a rolling basis. Application fee: $140. Electronic applications accepted. *Expenses:* Contact institution. *Unit head:* Lawrence Van Horn, Executive Director, 615-322-6046, E-mail: larry.vanhorn@owen.vanderbilt.edu. *Application contact:* Burch S. Wood, Director of Healthcare Programs, 615-875-8312, E-mail: burch.wood@owen.vanderbilt.edu.
Website: http://www.owen.vanderbilt.edu/programs/mm-health-care

Vanderbilt University, Vanderbilt University Owen Graduate School of Management, Vanderbilt MBA Program, Nashville, TN 37203. Offers accounting (MBA); finance (MBA); general management (MBA); health care (MBA); human and organizational performance (MBA); marketing (MBA); operations (MBA); strategy (MBA); MBA/JD; MBA/M Div; MBA/MD; MBA/MSN; MBA/MTS; MBA/PhD. *Accreditation:* AACSB. *Faculty:* 48 full-time (9 women), 26 part-time/adjunct (0 women). *Students:* 343 full-time (95 women); includes 37 minority (11 Black or African American, non-Hispanic/Latino; 9 Asian, non-Hispanic/Latino; 7 Hispanic/Latino; 10 Two or more races, non-Hispanic/Latino), 68 international. Average age 28. 888 applicants, 42% accepted, 174 enrolled. In 2015, 172 master's awarded. *Degree requirements:* For master's, 62 credit hours of coursework; completion of ethics course; minimum GPA of 3.0. *Entrance requirements:* For master's, GMAT (preferred) or GRE, 2 years of work experience (recommended). Additional exam requirements/recommendations for international students: Required—TOEFL (minimum score 100 iBT). *Application deadline:* For fall admission, 10/27 priority date for domestic and international students; for winter admission, 1/12 priority date for domestic and international students; for spring admission, 3/1 priority date for domestic and international students; for summer admission, 5/3 for domestic and international students. Applications are processed on a rolling basis. Application fee: $175. Electronic applications accepted. *Expenses:* $50,380 per year tuition and fees. *Financial support:* In 2015–16, 240 students received support. Scholarships/grants available. Financial award application deadline: 5/12; financial award applicants required to submit FAFSA. *Faculty research:* Accounting and finance, business strategy and economics, marketing, operations management, organization studies. *Unit head:* Nancy Lea Hyer, Associate Dean, 615-322-2530, Fax: 615-343-7110, E-mail: nancy.lea.hyer@owen.vanderbilt.edu. *Application contact:* Dinah Webster, Administrative Assistant, 615-322-6469, Fax: 615-343-1175, E-mail: mba@owen.vanderbilt.edu.
Website: http://www.owen.vanderbilt.edu/programs/mba

Villanova University, Villanova School of Business, MBA - The Fast Track Program, Villanova, PA 19085. Offers finance (MBA); health care management (MBA); international business (MBA); management information systems (MBA); marketing (MBA); real estate (MBA); strategic management (MBA). *Accreditation:* AACSB. *Program availability:* Part-time, evening/weekend. *Faculty:* 108 full-time (37 women), 32 part-time/adjunct (8 women). *Students:* 144 part-time (50 women); includes 20 minority (3 Black or African American, non-Hispanic/Latino; 13 Asian, non-Hispanic/Latino; 4 Hispanic/Latino), 3 international. Average age 29. 105 applicants, 78% accepted, 65 enrolled. In 2015, 69 master's awarded. *Degree requirements:* For master's, minimum GPA of 3.0. *Entrance requirements:* For master's, GMAT or GRE, work experience. Additional exam requirements/recommendations for international students: Required—TOEFL (minimum score 550 paper-based; 90 iBT). *Application deadline:* For fall admission, 6/30 for domestic and international students. Application fee: $50. Electronic applications accepted. *Expenses:* $1,095 per credit (includes cost of international trip), plus $50 general fee each semester. *Financial support:* Scholarships/grants available. Financial award application deadline: 6/30; financial award applicants required to submit FAFSA. *Faculty research:* Business analytics; creativity; innovation and entrepreneurship; global leadership; real estate; church management; business ethics; marketing and consumer insights. *Unit head:* Michael L. Capella, Associate Dean of Graduate and Executive Business Programs, 610-519-4336, Fax: 610-519-6273, E-mail: michael.l.capella@villanova.edu. *Application contact:* Meredith L. Lockyer, Manager of Recruiting, 610-519-7016, Fax: 610-519-6273, E-mail: meredith.lockyer@villanova.edu.
Website: http://www1.villanova.edu/villanova/business/graduate/mba.html

Villanova University, Villanova School of Business, MBA - The Flex Track Program, Villanova, PA 19085. Offers finance (MBA); health care management (MBA); international business (MBA); management information systems (MBA); marketing (MBA); real estate (MBA); strategic management (MBA); JD/MBA. *Accreditation:* AACSB. *Program availability:* Part-time, evening/weekend, online learning. *Faculty:* 108 full-time (37 women), 32 part-time/adjunct (8 women). *Students:* 16 full-time (5 women), 410 part-time (129 women); includes 68 minority (16 Black or African American, non-Hispanic/Latino; 1 American Indian or Alaska Native, non-Hispanic/Latino; 32 Asian, non-Hispanic/Latino; 13 Hispanic/Latino; 1 Native Hawaiian or other Pacific Islander, non-Hispanic/Latino; 5 Two or more races, non-Hispanic/Latino), 12 international. Average age 31. 78 applicants, 87% accepted, 61 enrolled. In 2015, 133 master's awarded. *Degree requirements:* For master's, minimum GPA of 3.0. *Entrance requirements:* For master's, GMAT or GRE, work experience. Additional exam requirements/recommendations for international students: Required—TOEFL (minimum score 550 paper-based; 90 iBT). *Application deadline:* For fall admission, 6/30 for domestic and international students; for winter admission, 11/15 for domestic and international students; for spring admission, 11/15 for domestic and international students; for summer admission, 3/31 for domestic and international students. Applications are processed on a rolling basis. Application fee: $50. Electronic applications accepted. *Expenses:* $970 per credit, plus a $50 general fee each semester. *Financial support:* In 2015–16, 13 research assistantships with full tuition reimbursements (averaging $13,100 per year) were awarded; scholarships/grants and unspecified assistantships also available. Financial award application deadline: 6/30; financial award applicants required to submit FAFSA. *Faculty research:* Business analytics; creativity, innovation and entrepreneurship; global leadership; real estate; church management; business ethics. *Unit head:* Michael L. Capella, Associate Dean of Graduate and Executive Business Programs, 610-610-4336, Fax: 610-519-6273, E-mail: michael.l.capella@villanova.edu. *Application contact:* Claire Bruno, Director of Recruitment and Enrollment Management, 610-519-4336, Fax: 610-519-6273, E-mail: claire.bruno@villanova.edu.
Website: http://www1.villanova.edu/villanova/business/graduate/mba.html

Virginia College in Birmingham, Program in Business Administration, Birmingham, AL 35209. Offers healthcare (MBA); management (MBA). *Program availability:* Part-time, evening/weekend, online learning. *Entrance requirements:* For master's, bachelor's degree in related academic area.

Virginia Commonwealth University, Graduate School, School of Allied Health Professions, Department of Health Administration, Doctoral Program in Health Services Organization and Research, Richmond, VA 23284-9005. Offers PhD. *Degree requirements:* For doctorate, thesis/dissertation, residency. *Entrance requirements:* For doctorate, GMAT or GRE General Test, minimum graduate GPA of 3.0. Additional exam requirements/recommendations for international students: Required—TOEFL (minimum score 600 paper-based; 100 iBT). Electronic applications accepted. *Faculty research:* Organizational studies, theory, associated analytical techniques.

Virginia Commonwealth University, Graduate School, School of Allied Health Professions, Department of Health Administration, Master's Program in Health Administration, Richmond, VA 23284-9005. Offers MHA, JD/MHA, MD/MHA. *Accreditation:* CAHME. *Degree requirements:* For master's, residency. *Entrance requirements:* For master's, GMAT or GRE General Test (preferred minimum score of 5.0 on analytical writing), course work in accounting, economics, and statistics; minimum GPA of 3.0. Additional exam requirements/recommendations for international students: Required—TOEFL (minimum score 600 paper-based; 100 iBT). Electronic applications accepted.

Virginia Commonwealth University, Graduate School, School of Allied Health Professions, Department of Health Administration, Professional Online Master of Science in Health Administration Program, Richmond, VA 23284-9005. Offers MSHA. *Accreditation:* CAHME. *Program availability:* Online learning. *Degree requirements:* For master's, residency. *Entrance requirements:* For master's, GMAT or GRE General Test. Additional exam requirements/recommendations for international students: Required—TOEFL (minimum score 600 paper-based; 100 iBT). Electronic applications accepted.

Virginia Commonwealth University, Graduate School, School of Allied Health Professions, Doctoral Program in Health Related Sciences, Richmond, VA 23284-9005. Offers clinical laboratory sciences (PhD); gerontology (PhD); health administration (PhD); nurse anesthesia (PhD); occupational therapy (PhD); physical therapy (PhD); radiation sciences (PhD); rehabilitation leadership (PhD). *Entrance requirements:* For doctorate, GRE General Test or MAT, minimum GPA of 3.3 in master's degree. Additional exam requirements/recommendations for international students: Required—TOEFL (minimum score 600 paper-based; 100 iBT); Recommended—IELTS (minimum score 6.5). Electronic applications accepted.

Virginia Commonwealth University, Medical College of Virginia-Professional Programs, School of Medicine, School of Medicine Graduate Programs, Department of Healthcare Policy and Research, Richmond, VA 23284-9005. Offers PhD. *Entrance requirements:* For doctorate, GRE General Test. Additional exam requirements/recommendations for international students: Required—TOEFL (minimum score 600 paper-based; 100 iBT). Electronic applications accepted. *Faculty research:* Evaluation of healthcare services and systems to enhance quality of care and patient safety outcomes; examination of chronic disease (e.g. cancer, HIV/AIDS) policies and practices to improve health outcomes and economic efficiency; impact of uninsurance, public insurance (such as Medicaid) and the safety net on access to care and the health of low-income, underserved, and foreign-born populations; the study of labor supply and healthcare coverage in response to health behaviors and shocks.

Virginia International University, School of Business, Fairfax, VA 22030. Offers accounting (MBA, MS); entrepreneurship (MBA); executive management (Graduate Certificate); global logistics (MBA); health care management (MBA); hospitality and tourism management (MBA); human resources management (MBA); international business management (MBA); international finance (MBA); marketing management (MBA); mass media and public relations (MBA); project management (MBA, MS). *Program availability:* Part-time, online learning. *Entrance requirements:* For master's and Graduate Certificate, bachelor's degree. Additional exam requirements/recommendations for international students: Required—TOEFL (minimum score 550 paper-based; 80 iBT), IELTS (minimum score 6). Electronic applications accepted.

Viterbo University, Master of Business Administration Program, La Crosse, WI 54601-4797. Offers general business administration (MBA); health care management (MBA); international business (MBA); leadership (MBA); project management (MBA). *Accreditation:* ACBSP. *Program availability:* Part-time, evening/weekend. *Faculty:* 6 full-time (2 women), 2 part-time/adjunct (1 woman). *Students:* 101 full-time (58 women), 14 part-time (11 women); includes 6 minority (1 Black or African American, non-Hispanic/Latino; 1 Asian, non-Hispanic/Latino; 3 Hispanic/Latino; 1 Two or more races, non-Hispanic/Latino), 9 international. Average age 33. In 2015, 47 master's awarded. *Degree requirements:* For master's, 34 semester credits. *Entrance requirements:* For master's, bachelor's degree, transcripts, minimum undergraduate cumulative GPA of 3.0, 2 letters of reference, 3-5 page essay. Additional exam requirements/recommendations for international students: Recommended—TOEFL (minimum score

Health Services Management and Hospital Administration

550 paper-based). *Application deadline:* Applications are processed on a rolling basis. Electronic applications accepted. *Expenses:* $570 per credit. *Financial support:* Applicants required to submit FAFSA. *Unit head:* Sara Cook, MBA Director, 608-796-3374, E-mail: slcook@viterbo.edu. *Application contact:* Tiffany Morey, MBA Coordinator, 608-796-3379, E-mail: tlmorey@viterbo.edu.

Wagner College, Division of Graduate Studies, Department of Business Administration, Staten Island, NY 10301-4495. Offers accounting (MS); business administration (MBA); finance (MBA); health care administration (MBA); international business (MBA); management (Exec MBA); marketing (MBA). *Accreditation:* ACBSP. *Program availability:* Part-time, evening/weekend. *Degree requirements:* For master's, thesis optional. *Entrance requirements:* For master's, minimum GPA of 2.75, proficiency in computers and math. Additional exam requirements/recommendations for international students: Required—TOEFL (minimum score 550 paper-based; 79 iBT).

Walden University, Graduate Programs, School of Health Sciences, Minneapolis, MN 55401. Offers clinical research administration (MS, Graduate Certificate); health education and promotion (MS, PhD), including behavioral health (PhD); disease surveillance (PhD); emergency preparedness (MS); general (MHA, MS); global health (PhD); health policy (PhD); health policy and advocacy (MS); population health (PhD); health informatics (MS); health services (PhD), including community health, healthcare administration, leadership, public health policy, self-designed; healthcare administration (MHA), including general (MHA, MS); leadership and organizational development (MHA); public health (MPH, Dr PH, PhD, Graduate Certificate), including community health education (PhD), epidemiology (PhD); systems policy (MHA). *Program availability:* Part-time, evening/weekend, online only, 100% online. *Faculty:* 14 full-time (8 women), 222 part-time/adjunct (121 women). *Students:* 2,487 full-time (1,804 women), 2,282 part-time (1,540 women); includes 2,763 minority (2,129 Black or African American, non-Hispanic/Latino; 30 American Indian or Alaska Native, non-Hispanic/Latino; 237 Asian, non-Hispanic/Latino; 268 Hispanic/Latino; 13 Native Hawaiian or other Pacific Islander, non-Hispanic/Latino; 86 Two or more races, non-Hispanic/Latino; 87 international. Average age 39. 1,205 applicants, 98% accepted, 820 enrolled. In 2015, 641 master's, 147 doctorates, 18 other advanced degrees awarded. *Degree requirements:* For doctorate, thesis/dissertation, residency. *Entrance requirements:* For master's, bachelor's degree or higher; minimum GPA of 2.5; official transcripts; goal statement (for some programs); access to computer and Internet; for doctorate, master's degree or higher; three years of related professional or academic experience (preferred); minimum GPA of 3.0; goal statement and current resume (for select programs); official transcripts; access to computer and Internet; for Graduate Certificate, relevant work experience; access to computer and Internet. Additional exam requirements/recommendations for international students: Required—TOEFL (minimum score 550 paper-based, 79 iBT), IELTS (minimum score 6.5), Michigan English Language Assessment Battery (minimum score 82), or PTE (minimum score 53). *Application deadline:* Applications are processed on a rolling basis. Application fee: $0. Electronic applications accepted. *Financial support:* Fellowships, Federal Work-Study, scholarships/grants, unspecified assistantships, and family tuition reduction, active duty/veteran tuition reduction, group tuition reduction, interest-free payment plans, employee tuition reduction available. Support available to part-time students. Financial award applicants required to submit FAFSA. *Unit head:* Dr. Jorg Westermann, Dean, 866-492-5336. *Application contact:* Meghan Thomas, Vice President of Enrollment Management, 866-492-5336, E-mail: info@waldenu.edu.
Website: http://www.waldenu.edu/colleges-schools/school-of-health-sciences

Walden University, Graduate Programs, School of Management, Minneapolis, MN 55401. Offers accounting (MBA, MS, DBA), including accounting for the professional (MS), accounting with CPA emphasis (MS), self-designed (MS); advanced project management (Graduate Certificate); applied project management (Graduate Certificate); auditing (Graduate Certificate); bridge to business administration (Post-Doctoral Certificate); bridge to management (Post-Doctoral Certificate); business management (Graduate Certificate); communication (MBA); corporate finance (MBA); digital marketing (Graduate Certificate); entrepreneurship (DBA); entrepreneurship and small business (MBA); finance (MS, DBA), including finance for the professional (MS), finance with CFA/investment (MS), finance with CPA emphasis (MS); global supply chain management (DBA); healthcare management (MBA, DBA); human resource management (MBA, MS, Graduate Certificate), including functional human resource management (MS), general program (MS), integrating functional and strategic human resource management (MS), organizational strategy (MS); human resources management (DBA); information systems management (DBA); international business (MBA, DBA); leadership (MBA, MS, DBA, Graduate Certificate), including general program (MS), human resource leadership (MS), leader development (MS), self-designed (MS); management (MS, PhD), including communications (MS), finance (PhD), general program (MS), healthcare management (MS), human resource management (MS), human resources management (PhD), information systems management (PhD), international business (MS), leadership (MS), leadership and organizational change (PhD), marketing (MS), project management (MS), strategy and operations (MS); managerial accounting (Graduate Certificate); marketing (MBA, MS, DBA); project management (MBA, MS, DBA); self-designed (MBA, DBA); social impact management (DBA); technology entrepreneurship (DBA). *Program availability:* Part-time, evening/weekend, online only, 100% online. *Faculty:* 22 full-time (8 women), 292 part-time/adjunct (115 women). *Students:* 4,351 full-time (2,480 women), 2,750 part-time (1,591 women); includes 4,010 minority (3,368 Black or African American, non-Hispanic/Latino; 31 American Indian or Alaska Native, non-Hispanic/Latino; 159 Asian, non-Hispanic/Latino; 265 Hispanic/Latino; 14 Native Hawaiian or other Pacific Islander, non-Hispanic/Latino; 173 Two or more races, non-Hispanic/Latino; 69 international. Average age 41. 2,163 applicants, 100% accepted, 1643 enrolled. In 2015, 862 master's, 149 doctorates, 138 other advanced degrees awarded. *Degree requirements:* For master's, thesis (for some programs), residency (for EMBA); for doctorate, thesis/dissertation (for some programs), residency. *Entrance requirements:* For master's, bachelor's degree or higher; minimum GPA of 2.5; official transcripts; goal statement (for some programs); access to computer and Internet; for doctorate, master's degree or higher; three years of related professional or academic experience (preferred); minimum GPA of 3.0; goal statement and current resume (for select programs); official transcripts; access to computer and Internet; for other advanced degree, relevant work experience; access to computer and Internet. Additional exam requirements/recommendations for international students: Required—TOEFL (minimum score 550 paper-based, 79 iBT), IELTS (minimum score 6.5), Michigan English Language Assessment Battery (minimum score 82), or PTE (minimum score 53). *Application deadline:* Applications are processed on a rolling basis. Application fee: $0. Electronic applications accepted. *Financial support:* Fellowships, Federal Work-Study, scholarships/grants, unspecified assistantships, and family tuition reduction, active duty/veteran tuition reduction, group tuition reduction, interest-free payment plans, employee tuition reduction available. Support available to part-time students. Financial award applicants required to submit FAFSA. *Unit head:* Dr. Freda Turner, Dean, 866-492-5336. *Application contact:* Meghan Thomas, Vice President of Enrollment Management, 866-492-5336, E-mail: info@waldenu.edu.
Website: http://www.waldenu.edu/programs/colleges-schools/management

Walden University, Graduate Programs, School of Nursing, Minneapolis, MN 55401. Offers adult-gerontology acute care nurse practitioner (MSN); adult-gerontology nurse practitioner (MSN); education (MSN); family nurse practitioner (MSN); informatics (MSN); leadership and management (MSN); nursing (PhD, Post-Master's Certificate), including education (PhD), healthcare administration (PhD), interdisciplinary health (PhD), leadership (PhD), nursing education (Post-Master's Certificate), nursing informatics (Post-Master's Certificate), nursing leadership and management (Post-Master's Certificate), public health policy (PhD); nursing practice (DNP); psychiatric-mental health (MSN). *Accreditation:* AACN. *Program availability:* Part-time, evening/weekend, online only, 100% online. *Faculty:* 22 full-time (18 women), 540 part-time/adjunct (487 women). *Students:* 4,320 full-time (3,773 women), 5,250 part-time (4,740 women); includes 3,550 minority (2,360 Black or African American, non-Hispanic/Latino; 29 American Indian or Alaska Native, non-Hispanic/Latino; 523 Asian, non-Hispanic/Latino; 421 Hispanic/Latino; 25 Native Hawaiian or other Pacific Islander, non-Hispanic/Latino; 192 Two or more races, non-Hispanic/Latino; 221 international. Average age 40. 2,057 applicants, 100% accepted, 1507 enrolled. In 2015, 3,022 master's, 86 doctorates, 34 other advanced degrees awarded. *Degree requirements:* For doctorate, thesis/dissertation (for some programs), residency (for some programs), field experience (for some programs). *Entrance requirements:* For master's, bachelor's degree or equivalent in related field or RN; minimum GPA of 2.5; official transcripts; goal statement (for some programs); access to computer and Internet; for doctorate, master's degree or higher; RN; three years of related professional or academic experience; goal statement; access to computer and Internet; for Post-Master's Certificate, relevant work experience; access to computer and Internet. Additional exam requirements/recommendations for international students: Required—TOEFL (minimum score 550 paper-based, 79 iBT), IELTS (minimum score 6.5), Michigan English Language Assessment Battery (minimum score 82), or PTE (minimum score 53). *Application deadline:* Applications are processed on a rolling basis. Application fee: $0. Electronic applications accepted. *Financial support:* Fellowships, Federal Work-Study, scholarships/grants, unspecified assistantships, and family tuition reduction, active duty/veteran tuition reduction, group tuition reduction, interest-free payment plans, employee tuition reduction available. Support available to part-time students. Financial award applicants required to submit FAFSA. *Unit head:* Dr. Andrea Lindell, Dean, 866-492-5336. *Application contact:* Meghan Thomas, Vice President of Enrollment Management, 866-492-5336, E-mail: info@waldenu.edu.
Website: http://www.waldenu.edu/programs/colleges-schools/nursing

Walden University, Graduate Programs, School of Public Policy and Administration, Minneapolis, MN 55401. Offers criminal justice (MPA, MPP, MS, Graduate Certificate), including emergency management (MS, PhD), general program (MS), global leadership (MS, PhD), homeland security and policy coordination (MS, PhD), law and public policy (MS, PhD), policy analysis (MS, PhD), public management and leadership (MS, PhD), self-designed (MS), terrorism, mediation, and peace (MS, PhD); criminal justice and executive management (MS), including global leadership (MS, PhD); criminal justice leadership and executive management (MS), including emergency management (MS, PhD), general program, homeland security and policy coordination (MS, PhD), law and public policy (MS, PhD), policy analysis (MS, PhD), public management and leadership (MS, PhD), self-designed, terrorism, mediation, and peace (MS, PhD); emergency management (MPA, MPP, MS), including criminal justice (MS, PhD), general program (MS), homeland security (MS), public management and leadership (MS, PhD), terrorism and emergency management (MS); general program (MPA, MPP); global leadership (MPA, MPP); government management (Graduate Certificate); health policy (MPA, MPP); homeland security (Graduate Certificate); homeland security and policy coordination (MPA, MPP); international nongovernmental organizations (MPA, MPP); law and public policy (MPA, MPP); local government management for sustainable communities (MPA, MPP); nonprofit management (Graduate Certificate); nonprofit management and leadership (MPA, MPP, MS), including global leadership (MS, PhD), international nongovernmental organization (MS), local government for sustainable communities (MS), self designed (MS); online teaching in higher education (Post-Master's Certificate); policy analysis (MPA); public management and leadership (MPA, MPP, Graduate Certificate); public policy (Graduate Certificate); public policy and administration (PhD), including criminal justice (MS, PhD), emergency management (MS, PhD), global leadership (MS, PhD), health policy, homeland security and policy coordination (MS, PhD), international nongovernmental organizations, law and public policy (MS, PhD), local government management for sustainable communities, nonprofit management and leadership, policy analysis (MS, PhD), public management and leadership (MS, PhD), terrorism, mediation, and peace (MS, PhD); strategic planning and public policy (Graduate Certificate); terrorism, mediation, and peace (MPA, MPP). *Program availability:* Part-time, evening/weekend, online only, 100% online. *Faculty:* 7 full-time (2 women), 107 part-time/adjunct (46 women). *Students:* 1,025 full-time (619 women), 1,788 part-time (983 women); includes 1,640 minority (1,375 Black or African American, non-Hispanic/Latino; 18 American Indian or Alaska Native, non-Hispanic/Latino; 42 Asian, non-Hispanic/Latino; 130 Hispanic/Latino; 10 Native Hawaiian or other Pacific Islander, non-Hispanic/Latino; 65 Two or more races, non-Hispanic/Latino; 23 international. Average age 43. 637 applicants, 100% accepted, 478 enrolled. In 2015, 298 master's, 79 doctorates, 32 other advanced degrees awarded. *Degree requirements:* For doctorate, thesis/dissertation, residency. *Entrance requirements:* For master's, bachelor's degree or higher; minimum GPA of 2.5; official transcripts; goal statement (for some programs); access to computer and Internet; for doctorate, master's degree or higher; three years of related professional or academic experience (preferred); minimum GPA of 3.0; goal statement and current resume (for select programs); official transcripts; access to computer and Internet; for other advanced degree, relevant work experience; access to computer and Internet. Additional exam requirements/recommendations for international students: Required—TOEFL (minimum score 550 paper-based, 79 iBT), IELTS (minimum score 6.5), Michigan English Language Assessment Battery (minimum score 82), or PTE (minimum score 53). *Application deadline:* Applications are processed on a rolling basis. Application fee: $0. Electronic applications accepted. *Financial support:* Fellowships, Federal Work-Study, scholarships/grants, unspecified assistantships, and family tuition reduction, active duty/veteran tuition reduction, group tuition reduction, interest-free payment plans, employee tuition reduction available. Support available to part-time students. Financial award applicants required to submit FAFSA. *Unit head:* Dr. Shana Garrett, Dean, 866-492-5336. *Application contact:* Meghan Thomas, Vice President of Enrollment Management, 866-492-5336, E-mail: info@waldenu.edu.
Website: http://www.waldenu.edu/programs/colleges-schools/public-policy-and-administration

Walsh University, Graduate Studies, MBA Program, North Canton, OH 44720-3396. Offers healthcare management (MBA); management (MBA); marketing (MBA). *Program availability:* Part-time, evening/weekend, online learning. *Faculty:* 10 full-time (4 women), 17 part-time/adjunct (3 women). *Students:* 24 full-time (12 women), 107 part-time (72 women); includes 10 minority (7 Black or African American, non-Hispanic/Latino; 1 Asian, non-Hispanic/Latino; 2 Hispanic/Latino), 3 international. Average age 35. 61 applicants, 87% accepted, 46 enrolled. In 2015, 58 master's awarded. *Degree requirements:* For master's, capstone course in strategic management. *Entrance requirements:* For master's, GMAT (minimum score of 490), minimum GPA of 3.0.

Health Services Management and Hospital Administration

Additional exam requirements/recommendations for international students: Required—TOEFL (minimum score 500 paper-based; 61 iBT). *Application deadline:* For fall admission, 7/15 priority date for domestic students. Applications are processed on a rolling basis. Application fee: $25. Electronic applications accepted. Application fee is waived when completed online. *Expenses: Tuition,* area resident: Full-time $11,610; part-time $7740 per credit hour. Full-time tuition and fees vary according to program. *Financial support:* In 2015–16, 6 students received support, including 6 research assistantships with partial tuition reimbursements available (averaging $7,395 per year); tuition discounts also available. Financial award application deadline: 12/31; financial award applicants required to submit FAFSA. *Faculty research:* Leadership, entrepreneurship, medical tourist, healthcare management, pedagogy. *Total annual research expenditures:* $3,000. *Unit head:* Dr. Michael Petrochuk, Director of the MBA Program/Assistant Professor, 330-244-4764, Fax: 330-490-7359, E-mail: mpetrochuk@walsh.edu. *Application contact:* Audra Dice, Graduate and Transfer Admissions Counselor, 330-490-7181, Fax: 330-244-4925, E-mail: adice@walsh.edu.
Website: http://www.walsh.edu/mba-program

Walsh University, Graduate Studies, Program in Healthcare Management, North Canton, OH 44720-3396. Offers Graduate Certificate. *Students:* 2 part-time (1 woman); includes 1 minority (Black or African American, non-Hispanic/Latino). Average age 38. *Entrance requirements:* For degree, minimum GPA of 3.0, official transcripts, current resume. Application fee: $25. *Expenses: Tuition,* area resident: Full-time $11,610; part-time $7740 per credit hour. Full-time tuition and fees vary according to program. *Unit head:* Dr. Michael Petrochuk, Director of the MBA Program, 330-244-4764, Fax: 330-490-7371, E-mail: mpetrochuk@walsh.edu. *Application contact:* Audra Dice, Assistant Director for Graduate and Transfer Admissions, 330-490-7181, Fax: 330-244-4925, E-mail: adice@walsh.edu.
Website: http://www.walsh.edu/certificate-in-healthcare-management

Washington Adventist University, Program in Health Care Administration, Takoma Park, MD 20912. Offers MA. *Program availability:* Part-time. *Entrance requirements:* Additional exam requirements/recommendations for international students: Required—TOEFL (minimum score 550 paper-based), IELTS (minimum score 5).

Washington State University, College of Pharmacy, Department of Health Policy and Administration, Spokane, WA 99210. Offers MHPA. Programs offered at the Spokane campus. *Accreditation:* CAHME. *Program availability:* Part-time, evening/weekend. *Degree requirements:* For master's, comprehensive exam (for some programs), thesis (for some programs), oral exam. *Entrance requirements:* For master's, GRE General Test or GMAT, minimum GPA of 3.0, 3 letters of recommendation. Additional exam requirements/recommendations for international students: Required—TOEFL (minimum score 550 paper-based) or IELTS (minimum score 7).

Wayland Baptist University, Graduate Programs, Programs in Business Administration/Management, Plainview, TX 79072-6998. Offers accounting (MBA); general business (MBA); health care administration (MAM, MBA); human resource management (MAM, MBA); international management (MBA); management (MBA, D Mgt); management information systems (MBA); organization management (MAM); project management (MBA). *Program availability:* Part-time, evening/weekend, online learning. *Faculty:* 30 full-time (5 women), 38 part-time/adjunct (9 women). *Students:* 39 full-time (19 women), 614 part-time (298 women); includes 325 minority (140 Black or African American, non-Hispanic/Latino; 6 American Indian or Alaska Native, non-Hispanic/Latino; 26 Asian, non-Hispanic/Latino; 121 Hispanic/Latino; 9 Native Hawaiian or other Pacific Islander, non-Hispanic/Latino; 23 Two or more races, non-Hispanic/Latino), 4 international. Average age 40. 106 applicants, 94% accepted, 42 enrolled. In 2015, 263 master's awarded. *Degree requirements:* For master's, capstone course. *Entrance requirements:* For master's, GMAT, GRE or MAT. Additional exam requirements/recommendations for international students: Required—TOEFL (minimum score 500 paper-based; 61 iBT). *Application deadline:* Applications are processed on a rolling basis. Application fee: $50. Electronic applications accepted. *Financial support:* Federal Work-Study, institutionally sponsored loans, and scholarships/grants available. Support available to part-time students. Financial award application deadline: 5/1; financial award applicants required to submit FAFSA. *Unit head:* Dr. Barry Evans, Chairman, 806-291-1020, Fax: 806-291-1957, E-mail: evansb@wbu.edu. *Application contact:* Amanda Stanton, Graduate Studies, 806-291-3423, Fax: 806-291-1950, E-mail: stanton@wbu.edu.

Waynesburg University, Graduate and Professional Studies, Canonsburg, PA 15370. Offers business (MBA), including energy management, finance, health systems, human resources, leadership, market development; counseling (MA), including addictions counseling, clinical mental health; counselor education and supervision (PhD); criminal investigation (MA); education (M Ed), including autism, curriculum and instruction, educational leadership, online teaching; nursing (MSN), including administration, education, informatics; nursing practice (DNP); special education (M Ed); technology (M Ed); MSN/MBA. *Accreditation:* AACN. *Program availability:* Part-time, evening/weekend. *Degree requirements:* For doctorate, thesis/dissertation. *Entrance requirements:* Additional exam requirements/recommendations for international students: Required—TOEFL. Electronic applications accepted.

Wayne State University, College of Liberal Arts and Sciences, Department of Political Science, Detroit, MI 48202. Offers political science (MA, PhD); public administration (MPA), including economic development policy and management, health and human services policy and management, human and fiscal resource management, nonprofit policy and management, organizational behavior and management, urban and metropolitan policy and management; JD/MA. *Accreditation:* NASPAA. *Faculty:* 23. *Students:* 57 full-time (20 women), 79 part-time (54 women); includes 41 minority (24 Black or African American, non-Hispanic/Latino; 3 Asian, non-Hispanic/Latino; 5 Hispanic/Latino; 9 Two or more races, non-Hispanic/Latino), 10 international. Average age 33. 148 applicants, 30% accepted, 22 enrolled. In 2015, 12 master's, 7 doctorates awarded. *Degree requirements:* For master's, comprehensive exam; for doctorate, thesis/dissertation. *Entrance requirements:* For master's, GRE General Test, substantial undergraduate preparation in the social sciences, minimum upper-division undergraduate GPA of 3.0, two letters of recommendation, personal statement; for doctorate, GRE General Test, 3 letters of recommendation; personal statement; interview. Additional exam requirements/recommendations for international students: Required—TOEFL (minimum score 550 paper-based; 79 iBT), TWE (minimum score 5.5), Michigan English Language Assessment Battery (minimum score 85); Recommended—IELTS (minimum score 6.5). *Application deadline:* For fall admission, 5/1 priority date for domestic and international students; for winter admission, 10/1 priority date for domestic students, 9/1 priority date for international students; for spring admission, 2/1 priority date for domestic students, 1/1 priority date for international students. Applications are processed on a rolling basis. Application fee: $0. Electronic applications accepted. *Expenses:* Tuition, state resident: full-time $14,165; part-time $590.20 per credit hour. Tuition, nonresident: full-time $30,682; part-time $1278.40 per credit hour. *Required fees:* $1688; $47.45 per credit hour. $274.60 per semester. Tuition and fees vary according to course load and program. *Financial support:* In 2015–16, 46 students received support, including 4 fellowships with tuition reimbursements available (averaging $14,524 per year), 13 teaching assistantships with tuition reimbursements available (averaging $17,427 per year); research assistantships with tuition

reimbursements available, scholarships/grants, health care benefits, and unspecified assistantships also available. Financial award application deadline: 3/31; financial award applicants required to submit FAFSA. *Faculty research:* American government and politics, comparative politics, political methodology, political theory, public administration, public law, public policy, world politics/international relations, formal theory/modeling, gender and politics, international law, peace research, political economy, political psychology, politics of developing countries, race, religion, and ethnicity, urban politics. *Unit head:* Dr. Daniel Geller, Professor and Chair, 313-577-6328, E-mail: dgeller@wayne.edu. *Application contact:* Dr. Sharon Lean, Graduate Director, E-mail: gradpolisci@wayne.edu.
Website: http://clas.wayne.edu/politicalscience/

Weber State University, College of Health Professions, Program of Health Administration, Ogden, UT 84408-1001. Offers MHA. *Accreditation:* CAHME. *Program availability:* Part-time, evening/weekend. *Faculty:* 3 full-time (2 women), 1 part-time/adjunct (0 women). *Students:* 58 full-time (19 women), 15 part-time (3 women); includes 4 minority (all Hispanic/Latino), 1 international. Average age 33. In 2015, 24 master's awarded. *Entrance requirements:* For master's, GMAT or GRE. Additional exam requirements/recommendations for international students: Required—TOEFL (minimum score 550 paper-based). *Application deadline:* For fall admission, 3/15 for domestic students, 2/20 for international students. Applications are processed on a rolling basis. Application fee: $60 ($95 for international students). Electronic applications accepted. *Expenses:* Tuition, state resident: full-time $6520; part-time $1252 per credit hour. Tuition, nonresident: full-time $15,003; part-time $2998 per credit hour. *Required fees:* $380; $180 per credit hour. $8.50 per term. Tuition and fees vary according to course level and program. *Financial support:* In 2015–16, 7 students received support. Scholarships/grants available. Financial award application deadline: 4/1; financial award applicants required to submit FAFSA. *Unit head:* Pat Shaw, Associate Professor/Chair, Health Administrative Services, 801-626-7989, Fax: 801-626-6475, E-mail: pshaw@weber.edu. *Application contact:* Cory Moss, Assistant Professor, 801-626-7237, Fax: 801-626-6475, E-mail: cmoss@weber.edu.
Website: http://www.weber.edu/MHA/

Webster University, George Herbert Walker School of Business and Technology, Department of Management, St. Louis, MO 63119-3194. Offers business and organizational security management (MA); health administration (MHA); health care management (MA); health services management (MA); human resources development (MA); human resources management (MA); information technology management (MS); management and leadership (MA); marketing (MA); nonprofit leadership (MA); procurement and acquisitions management (MA); public administration (MPA); space systems operations management (MS). *Program availability:* Part-time, evening/weekend, online learning. *Degree requirements:* For master's, thesis (for some programs). *Entrance requirements:* Additional exam requirements/recommendations for international students: Required—TOEFL. *Expenses: Tuition,* area resident: Full-time $20,550; part-time $685 per credit hour. Tuition and fees vary according to campus/location and program.

West Chester University of Pennsylvania, College of Health Sciences, Department of Health, West Chester, PA 19383. Offers community health (MPH); emergency preparedness (Certificate); environmental health (MPH); gerontology (Certificate); health care management (MPH, Certificate); integrative health (Certificate); school health (M Ed). *Accreditation:* CEPH. *Program availability:* Part-time, evening/weekend. *Faculty:* 12 full-time (7 women), 4 part-time/adjunct (3 women). *Students:* 98 full-time (74 women), 85 part-time (59 women); includes 73 minority (60 Black or African American, non-Hispanic/Latino; 8 Asian, non-Hispanic/Latino; 4 Hispanic/Latino; 1 Two or more races, non-Hispanic/Latino), 26 international. Average age 30. 118 applicants, 86% accepted, 60 enrolled. In 2015, 72 master's, 17 other advanced degrees awarded. *Degree requirements:* For master's, thesis or alternative, minimum GPA of 3.0; research report (for M Ed); major project and practicum (for MPH); for Certificate, minimum GPA of 3.0. *Entrance requirements:* For master's, goal statement, two letters of recommendation, undergraduate introduction to statistics course; for Certificate, minimum undergraduate GPA of 2.8 (for gerontology). Additional exam requirements/recommendations for international students: Required—TOEFL or IELTS. *Application deadline:* For fall admission, 5/15 for international students; for spring admission, 10/15 for international students. Applications are processed on a rolling basis. Application fee: $50. Electronic applications accepted. *Expenses:* Tuition, state resident: full-time $8460; part-time $470 per credit. Tuition, nonresident: full-time $12,690; part-time $705 per credit. *Required fees:* $2312; $126.75 per credit. Tuition and fees vary according to campus/location and program. *Financial support:* Scholarships/grants and unspecified assistantships available. Financial award application deadline: 2/15; financial award applicants required to submit FAFSA. *Faculty research:* Healthy school communities, community health issues and evidence-based programs, environment and health, nutrition and health, integrative health. *Unit head:* Dr. Bethann Cinelli, Chair, 610-436-2267, E-mail: bcinelli@wcupa.edu. *Application contact:* Dr. Lynn Carson, Graduate Coordinator, 610-436-2138, E-mail: lcarson@wcupa.edu.
Website: http://www.wcupa.edu/_ACADEMICS/HealthSciences/health/

West Coast University, Graduate Programs, North Hollywood, CA 91606. Offers advanced generalist (MSN); family nurse practitioner (MSN); health administration (MHA); occupational therapy (MS); pharmacy (Pharm D); physical therapy (DPT).

Western Carolina University, Graduate School, College of Health and Human Sciences, School of Health Sciences, Cullowhee, NC 28723. Offers MHS. *Program availability:* Part-time, evening/weekend. *Degree requirements:* For master's, thesis or alternative. *Entrance requirements:* For master's, GRE General Test, appropriate undergraduate degree with minimum GPA of 3.0, 3 letters of recommendation. Additional exam requirements/recommendations for international students: Required—TOEFL (minimum score 550 paper-based; 79 iBT). *Application deadline:* For fall admission, 5/1 priority date for domestic students; for spring admission, 9/1 priority date for domestic students. Applications are processed on a rolling basis. Application fee: $50. *Financial support:* Fellowships, research assistantships with tuition reimbursements, teaching assistantships with tuition reimbursements, institutionally sponsored loans, scholarships/grants, and unspecified assistantships available. Financial award application deadline: 3/31; financial award applicants required to submit FAFSA. *Faculty research:* Epidemiology, dietetics, public health, environmental technology, water quality, occupational health.
Website: http://www.wcu.edu/4626.asp

Western Connecticut State University, Division of Graduate Studies, Ancell School of Business, Program in Health Administration, Danbury, CT 06810-6885. Offers MHA. *Program availability:* Part-time. *Degree requirements:* For master's, comprehensive exam, completion of program within 6 years. *Entrance requirements:* For master's, GMAT, GRE, or MAT, minimum GPA of 2.5. Additional exam requirements/recommendations for international students: Recommended—TOEFL (minimum score 550 paper-based; 79 iBT), IELTS (minimum score 6). *Expenses:* Tuition, state resident: full-time $6188; part-time $343 per credit hour. Tuition, nonresident: full-time $17,240; part-time $350 per credit hour. *Required fees:* $4399; $173 per credit hour. One-time fee: $60 part-time. Tuition and fees vary according to degree level and program. *Faculty research:* Organizational behavior, human resource management, health delivery systems, health services financial management, managing health services organizations, health services quality management, health policy and strategic management for health services, long-term care administration, health services marketing, health care law.

Western Governors University, College of Health Professions, Salt Lake City, UT 84107. Offers healthcare management (MBA); leadership and management (MSN); nursing education (MSN). *Program availability:* Evening/weekend. *Degree requirements:* For master's, capstone project. *Entrance requirements:* For master's, Readiness Assessment, transcripts. Additional exam requirements/recommendations for international students: Required—TOEFL (minimum score 450 paper-based; 80 iBT). Electronic applications accepted.

Western Illinois University, School of Graduate Studies, College of Education and Human Services, Department of Health Sciences, Macomb, IL 61455-1390. Offers health sciences (MS); health services administration (Certificate). *Accreditation:* NCATE. *Program availability:* Part-time. *Students:* 26 full-time (22 women), 17 part-time (10 women); includes 11 minority (7 Black or African American, non-Hispanic/Latino; 3 Hispanic/Latino; 1 Two or more races, non-Hispanic/Latino), 12 international. Average age 32. 41 applicants, 83% accepted, 17 enrolled. In 2015, 13 master's, 7 other advanced degrees awarded. *Degree requirements:* For master's, comprehensive exam, thesis or alternative. *Entrance requirements:* Additional exam requirements/recommendations for international students: Required—TOEFL (minimum score 550 paper-based; 80 iBT). *Application deadline:* Applications are processed on a rolling basis. Application fee: $30. Electronic applications accepted. *Financial support:* In 2015–16, 6 students received support, including 1 teaching assistantship with full tuition reimbursement available (averaging $8,688 per year); unspecified assistantships also available. Financial award applicants required to submit FAFSA. *Unit head:* Dr. Lorette Oden, Interim Chairperson, 309-298-1076. *Application contact:* Dr. Nancy Parsons, Associate Provost and Director of Graduate Studies, 309-298-1806, Fax: 309-298-2345, E-mail: grad-office@wiu.edu.
Website: http://wiu.edu/health

Western Kentucky University, Graduate Studies, College of Health and Human Services, Department of Public Health, Bowling Green, KY 42101. Offers healthcare administration (MHA); public health (MPH). *Accreditation:* CEPH. *Program availability:* Part-time, evening/weekend. *Degree requirements:* For master's, comprehensive exam, thesis or alternative. *Entrance requirements:* For master's, GRE General Test, minimum GPA of 2.75. Additional exam requirements/recommendations for international students: Required—TOEFL (minimum score 555 paper-based; 79 iBT). *Faculty research:* Health education training, driver traffic safety, community readiness, occupational injuries, local health departments.

Western Michigan University, Graduate College, College of Arts and Sciences, School of Public Affairs and Administration, Kalamazoo, MI 49008. Offers health care administration (MPA, Graduate Certificate); nonprofit leadership and administration (Graduate Certificate); public administration (PhD). *Accreditation:* NASPAA (one or more programs are accredited). *Degree requirements:* For doctorate, thesis/dissertation.

Widener University, School of Business Administration, Program in Health and Medical Services Administration, Chester, PA 19013-5792. Offers MBA, MHA, MD/MBA, MD/MHA, Psy D/MBA, Psy D/MHA. *Accreditation:* CAHME (one or more programs are accredited). *Program availability:* Part-time, evening/weekend, 100% online, blended/hybrid learning. *Faculty:* 3 full-time (1 woman), 6 part-time/adjunct (1 woman). *Students:* 11 full-time (4 women), 46 part-time (23 women); includes 13 minority (6 Black or African American, non-Hispanic/Latino; 3 Asian, non-Hispanic/Latino; 4 Hispanic/Latino), 7 international. 30 applicants, 80% accepted. In 2015, 1 master's awarded. *Degree requirements:* For master's, clerkship, residency. *Entrance requirements:* For master's, GMAT, interview, minimum GPA of 2.5. *Application deadline:* For fall admission, 8/1 priority date for domestic students; for spring admission, 12/1 for domestic students. Applications are processed on a rolling basis. Application fee: $25 ($300 for international students). Electronic applications accepted. Tuition and fees vary according to degree level and program. *Financial support:* Research assistantships, career-related internships or fieldwork, and traineeships available. Support available to part-time students. Financial award application deadline: 5/1. *Faculty research:* Cost containment in health care, reimbursement of hospitals, strategic behavior. *Unit head:* Dr. Jose Proenca, Director, 610-499-4330. *Application contact:* Ann Seltzer, Graduate Enrollment Administrator, 610-499-4305, E-mail: apseltzer@widener.edu.
Website: http://www.widener.edu

Widener University, School of Human Service Professions, Institute for Graduate Clinical Psychology, Program in Clinical Psychology and Health and Medical Services Administration, Chester, PA 19013-5792. Offers Psy D/MBA, Psy D/MHA. *Accreditation:* APA (one or more programs are accredited); CAHME. Electronic applications accepted. Tuition and fees vary according to degree level and program. *Faculty research:* Psychosocial competence, family systems, medical care systems and financing.

Wilkes University, College of Graduate and Professional Studies, Jay S. Sidhu School of Business and Leadership, Wilkes-Barre, PA 18766-0002. Offers accounting (MBA); entrepreneurship (MBA); finance (MBA); health care administration (MBA); human resource management (MBA); international business (MBA); marketing (MBA); operations management (MBA); organizational leadership and development (MBA). *Accreditation:* ACBSP. *Program availability:* Part-time, evening/weekend. *Students:* 46 full-time (19 women), 122 part-time (59 women); includes 15 minority (5 Black or African American, non-Hispanic/Latino; 2 Asian, non-Hispanic/Latino; 5 Hispanic/Latino; 3 Two or more races, non-Hispanic/Latino), 18 international. Average age 30. In 2015, 59 master's awarded. *Entrance requirements:* For master's, GMAT. Additional exam requirements/recommendations for international students: Required—TOEFL (minimum score 550 paper-based; 79 iBT). *Application deadline:* Applications are processed on a rolling basis. Application fee: $45 ($65 for international students). Electronic applications accepted. *Expenses:* Contact institution. *Financial support:* Unspecified assistantships available. Financial award application deadline: 3/1; financial award applicants required to submit FAFSA. *Unit head:* Dr. Jennifer Edmonds, Interim Dean, 570-408-4725, Fax: 570-408-7846, E-mail: jennifer.edmonds@wilkes.edu. *Application contact:* Joanne Thomas, Director of Graduate Enrollment, 570-408-4234, Fax: 570-408-7846, E-mail: joanne.thomas1@wilkes.edu.
Website: http://www.wilkes.edu/academics/colleges/sidhu-school-of-business-leadership/index.aspx

William Woods University, Graduate and Adult Studies, Fulton, MO 65251-1098. Offers administration (M Ed, Ed S); athletic/activities administration (M Ed); curriculum and instruction (M Ed, Ed S); educational leadership (Ed D); equestrian education (M Ed); health management (MBA); human resources (MBA); leadership (MBA); marketing, advertising, and public relations (MBA); teaching and technology (M Ed). *Program availability:* Part-time, evening/weekend. *Degree requirements:* For master's, capstone course (MBA), action research (M Ed); for Ed S, field experience. *Entrance requirements:* Additional exam requirements/recommendations for international students: Required—TOEFL (minimum score 550 paper-based). Electronic applications accepted. *Expenses:* Contact institution.

Wilmington University, College of Business, New Castle, DE 19720-6491. Offers accounting (MBA, MS); business administration (MBA, DBA); environmental stewardship (MBA); finance (MBA); health care administration (MBA, MSM); homeland security (MBA, MSM); human resource management (MSM); management information systems (MBA, MSN); marketing (MSM); marketing management (MBA); military leadership (MSM); organizational leadership (MBA, MSM); public administration (MSM). *Program availability:* Part-time, evening/weekend. *Entrance requirements:* Additional exam requirements/recommendations for international students: Required—TOEFL (minimum score 500 paper-based). Electronic applications accepted.

Wilson College, Graduate Programs, Chambersburg, PA 17201-1285. Offers accounting (M Acc); choreography and visual art (MFA); education (M Ed); healthcare management for sustainability (MHM); humanities (MA), including art and culture, critical/cultural theory, English language and literature, women's studies; nursing (MSN), including nursing education, nursing leadership and management. *Program availability:* Evening/weekend. *Degree requirements:* For master's, project. *Entrance requirements:* For master's, PRAXIS, minimum undergraduate cumulative GPA of 3.0, 2 letters of recommendation, current certification for eligibility to teach in grades K-12, resume, personal interview. Electronic applications accepted.

Winston-Salem State University, Program in Health Administration, Winston-Salem, NC 27110-0003. Offers MHA. *Entrance requirements:* For master's, baccalaureate degree, minimum cumulative undergraduate GPA of 3.0, personal statement, three letters of recommendation, interview.

Worcester State University, Graduate Studies, Program in Health Care Administration, Worcester, MA 01602-2597. Offers MS. *Program availability:* Part-time. *Faculty:* 1 full-time (0 women), 3 part-time/adjunct (1 woman). *Students:* 5 full-time (all women), 16 part-time (9 women); includes 6 minority (3 Black or African American, non-Hispanic/Latino; 1 Asian, non-Hispanic/Latino; 1 Hispanic/Latino; 1 Two or more races, non-Hispanic/Latino), 3 international. Average age 35. 21 applicants, 62% accepted, 3 enrolled. In 2015, 7 master's awarded. *Degree requirements:* For master's, comprehensive exam (for some programs), thesis optional, capstone. *Entrance requirements:* For master's, GMAT (preferred), GRE. Additional exam requirements/recommendations for international students: Required—TOEFL (minimum score 550 paper-based; 79 iBT). *Application deadline:* For fall admission, 6/15 for domestic and international students; for spring admission, 11/1 for domestic and international students; for summer admission, 4/1 for domestic and international students. Applications are processed on a rolling basis. Application fee: $50. Electronic applications accepted. *Expenses:* Tuition, state resident: part-time $150 per credit. Tuition, nonresident: part-time $150 per credit. *Financial support:* Career-related internships or fieldwork, scholarships/grants, and unspecified assistantships available. Financial award application deadline: 3/1; financial award applicants required to submit FAFSA. *Unit head:* Dr. Elizabeth Wark, Coordinator, 508-929-8743, Fax: 508-929-8175, E-mail: ewark@worcester.edu. *Application contact:* Sara Grady, Associate Dean of Graduate and Continuing Education, 508-929-8787, Fax: 508-929-8100, E-mail: sara.grady@worcester.edu.

Wright State University, School of Graduate Studies, Raj Soin College of Business, Department of Management, Dayton, OH 45435. Offers flexible business (MBA); health care management (MBA); international business (MBA); management, innovation and change (MBA); project management (MBA); supply chain management (MBA); MBA/MS. *Entrance requirements:* For master's, GMAT, minimum AACSB index of 1000. Additional exam requirements/recommendations for international students: Required—TOEFL.

★ **Xavier University,** College of Social Sciences, Health and Education, Department of Health Services Administration, Cincinnati, OH 45207. Offers MHSA, MHSA/MBA. *Accreditation:* CAHME. *Program availability:* Part-time. *Degree requirements:* For master's, thesis, residency, project. *Entrance requirements:* For master's, GMAT or GRE, resume, two letters of recommendation, statement of intent, official transcripts, interview, minimum accounting and statistics grade of C. Additional exam requirements/recommendations for international students: Required—TOEFL (minimum score 550 paper-based; 80 iBT). Electronic applications accepted. Application fee is waived when completed online. *Expenses:* Contact institution. *Faculty research:* Success factors of ethics committees in health care, early hospital readmission and quality, health and labor economics, clinical emergency medicine and uncompensated care.

See Display on next page and Close-Up on page 597.

Xavier University, Williams College of Business, Master of Business Administration Program, Cincinnati, OH 45207. Offers business administration (Exec MBA, MBA); business intelligence (MBA); finance (MBA); health industry (MBA); international business (MBA); marketing (MBA); values-based leadership (MBA); MBA/MHSA; MSN/MBA. *Accreditation:* AACSB. *Program availability:* Part-time, evening/weekend. *Degree requirements:* For master's, capstone course. *Entrance requirements:* For master's, GMAT or GRE, official transcript; resume. Additional exam requirements/recommendations for international students: Required—TOEFL (minimum score 550 paper-based; 79 iBT). Electronic applications accepted. Application fee is waived when completed online. *Expenses:* Contact institution.

Yale University, School of Medicine, Yale School of Public Health, New Haven, CT 06520. Offers applied biostatistics and epidemiology (APMPH); biostatistics (MPH, MS, PhD), including global health (MPH); chronic disease epidemiology (MPH, PhD), including global health (MPH); environmental health sciences (MPH, PhD), including global health (MPH); epidemiology of microbial diseases (MPH, PhD), including global health (MPH); global health (APMPH); health management (MPH), including global health; health policy (MPH), including global health; health policy and administration (APMPH, PhD); occupational and environmental medicine (APMPH); preventive medicine (APMPH); social and behavioral sciences (APMPH, MPH), including global health (MPH); JD/MPH; M Div/MPH; MBA/MPH; MD/MPH; MEM/MPH; MFS/MPH; MM Sc/MPH; MPH/MA; MSN/MPH. MS and PhD offered through the Graduate School. *Accreditation:* CEPH. *Program availability:* Part-time. Terminal master's awarded for partial completion of doctoral program. *Degree requirements:* For master's, thesis, summer internship; for doctorate, comprehensive exam, thesis/dissertation, residency. *Entrance requirements:* For master's, GMAT, GRE, or MCAT, two years of undergraduate coursework in math and science; for doctorate, GRE General Test. Additional exam requirements/recommendations for international students: Required—TOEFL (minimum score 100 iBT). Electronic applications accepted. *Expenses:* Contact institution. *Faculty research:* Genetic and emerging infections epidemiology, virology, cost/quality, vector biology, quantitative methods, aging, asthma, cancer.

York College of Pennsylvania, Graham School of Business, York, PA 17405-7199. Offers continuous improvement (MBA); financial management (MBA); health care management (MBA); management (MBA); marketing (MBA); self-designed (MBA). *Accreditation:* ACBSP. *Program availability:* Part-time, evening/weekend. *Faculty:* 8 full-time (2 women), 3 part-time/adjunct (0 women). *Students:* 4 full-time (0 women), 79 part-time (31 women); includes 7 minority (2 Black or African American, non-Hispanic/Latino; 2 Asian, non-Hispanic/Latino; 3 Two or more races, non-Hispanic/Latino). Average age 32. 44 applicants, 66% accepted, 8 enrolled. In 2015, 22 master's awarded. *Entrance* *requirements:* For master's, GMAT. Additional exam requirements/recommendations for international students: Required—TOEFL (minimum score 530 paper-based; 72 iBT), IELTS (minimum score 6). *Application deadline:* For fall admission, 7/15 priority date for domestic students; for spring admission, 11/15 priority date for domestic students; for summer admission, 4/15 priority date for domestic students. Applications are processed on a rolling basis. Application fee: $0. Electronic applications accepted. *Expenses: Tuition, area resident:* Full-time $13,770. *Required fees:* $1750; $380. Tuition and fees vary according to degree level. *Financial support:* Scholarships/grants available. Financial award application deadline: 4/15; financial award applicants required to submit FAFSA. *Unit head:* Nicole Cornell Sadowski, MBA Director, 717-815-1491, Fax: 717-

600-3999, E-mail: ncornell@ycp.edu. *Application contact:* MBA Office, 717-815-1491, Fax: 717-600-3999, E-mail: mba@ycp.edu.
Website: http://www.ycp.edu/mba

Youngstown State University, Graduate School, Bitonte College of Health and Human Services, Department of Health Professions, Youngstown, OH 44555-0001. Offers health and human services (MHHS); public health (MPH). *Accreditation:* NAACLS. *Program availability:* Part-time, evening/weekend. *Degree requirements:* For master's, thesis optional. *Entrance requirements:* For master's, GRE General Test, minimum GPA of 3.0. Additional exam requirements/recommendations for international students: Required—TOEFL. *Faculty research:* Drug prevention, multiskilling in health care, organizational behavior, health care management, health behaviors, research management.

Health Services Research

Albany College of Pharmacy and Health Sciences, School of Pharmacy and Pharmaceutical Sciences, Albany, NY 12208. Offers health outcomes research (MS); pharmaceutical sciences (MS), including pharmaceutics, pharmacology; pharmacy (Pharm D). *Accreditation:* ACPE. *Degree requirements:* For master's, thesis; for doctorate, practice experience. *Entrance requirements:* For master's, GRE, minimum GPA of 3.0; for doctorate, PCAT, minimum GPA of 2.5. Additional exam requirements/recommendations for international students: Required—TOEFL (minimum score 84 iBT). Electronic applications accepted. *Faculty research:* Therapeutic use of drugs, pharmacokinetics, drug delivery and design.

Brown University, Graduate School, Division of Biology and Medicine, School of Public Health, Department of Health Services, Policy and Practice, Providence, RI 02912. Offers PhD.

Case Western Reserve University, School of Medicine and School of Graduate Studies, Graduate Programs in Medicine, Department of Epidemiology and Biostatistics, Program in Health Services Research, Cleveland, OH 44106. Offers MS, PhD. *Degree requirements:* For master's, comprehensive exam, thesis; for doctorate, comprehensive exam, thesis/dissertation. *Entrance requirements:* For master's and doctorate, GRE. Additional exam requirements/recommendations for international students: Required—TOEFL (minimum score 550 paper-based). *Expenses: Tuition, area resident:* Full-time $41,137; part-time $1714 per credit hour. *Required fees:* $32. Tuition and fees vary according to course load and program.

Clarkson University, Graduate School, School of Arts and Sciences, Program in Basic Science, Potsdam, NY 13699. Offers MS. *Program availability:* Part-time. *Students:* 2 full-time (0 women), 1 international. Average age 26. 5 applicants, 80% accepted, 1 enrolled. In 2015, 3 master's awarded. *Entrance requirements:* For master's, GRE, transcripts of all college coursework, resume, personal statement, three letters of recommendation. Additional exam requirements/recommendations for international students: Required—TOEFL or IELTS. *Application deadline:* For fall admission, 1/30 priority date for domestic and international students; for spring admission, 9/1 priority date for domestic and international students. Applications are processed on a rolling basis. Application fee: $25 ($35 for international students). Electronic applications accepted. *Financial support:* In

2015–16, 2 students received support, including research assistantships with full tuition reimbursements available (averaging $24,510 per year), teaching assistantships with full tuition reimbursements available (averaging $24,510 per year); scholarships/grants, tuition waivers (partial), and unspecified assistantships also available. *Faculty research:* Health science, environmental health. *Unit head:* Dr. Peter Turner, Dean, 315-268-6544, Fax: 315-268-3989, E-mail: pturner@clarkson.edu. *Application contact:* Jennifer Reed, Graduate School Coordinator, Provost's Office, 315-268-3802, Fax: 315-268-3989, E-mail: sciencegrad@clarkson.edu.
Website: http://www.clarkson.edu/artsandsci/grad/admissions/basic_sci.html

Dartmouth College, The Dartmouth Institute, Hanover, NH 03755. Offers MPH, MS, PhD. *Program availability:* Part-time. *Faculty:* 60 full-time (28 women), 99 part-time/adjunct (39 women). *Students:* 40 full-time (26 women), 37 part-time (17 women); includes 15 minority (2 Black or African American, non-Hispanic/Latino; 6 Asian, non-Hispanic/Latino; 4 Hispanic/Latino; 3 Two or more races, non-Hispanic/Latino), 7 international. Average age 33. In 2015, 51 master's awarded. *Degree requirements:* For master's, research project or practicum; for doctorate, thesis/dissertation. *Entrance requirements:* For master's, GRE, GMAT or MCAT, 2 letters of recommendation, current resume or curriculum vitae; for doctorate, GRE, 3 letters of recommendation, current resume or curriculum vitae. *Application deadline:* For fall admission, 1/15 for domestic students. Application fee: $75. *Expenses: Tuition, area resident:* Full-time $48,120. *Required fees:* $296. One-time fee: $50 full-time. *Financial support:* In 2015–16, fellowships with full tuition reimbursements (averaging $28,200 per year) were awarded; scholarships/grants also available. *Unit head:* Dr. Elliot S. Fisher, Director, 603-653-0802, Fax: 603-650-1900. *Application contact:* Courtney Theroux, Director of Recruitment and Admissions, 603-653-3234, Fax: 603-650-1900.
Website: http://tdi.dartmouth.edu/

Emory University, Rollins School of Public Health, Department of Health Policy and Management, Atlanta, GA 30322-1100. Offers health policy (MPH); health policy research (MSPH); health services management (MPH); health services research and health policy (PhD). *Program availability:* Part-time. *Degree requirements:* For master's, thesis (for some programs), practicum, capstone course. *Entrance requirements:* For

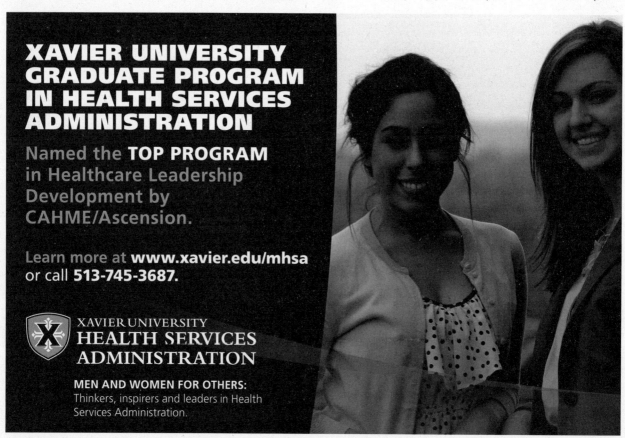

master's, GRE General Test. Additional exam requirements/recommendations for international students: Required—TOEFL (minimum score 550 paper-based; 80 iBT). Electronic applications accepted. *Faculty research:* U.S. health policy and financing, healthcare organization and financing.

Florida Agricultural and Mechanical University, Division of Graduate Studies, Research, and Continuing Education, College of Pharmacy and Pharmaceutical Sciences, Graduate Programs in Pharmaceutical Sciences, Tallahassee, FL 32307-3200. Offers environmental toxicology (PhD); health outcomes research and pharmacoeconomics (PhD); medicinal chemistry (MS, PhD); pharmaceutics (MS, PhD); pharmacology/toxicology (MS, PhD); pharmacy administration (MS). *Accreditation:* CEPH. *Degree requirements:* For master's, comprehensive exam, thesis, publishable paper; for doctorate, comprehensive exam, thesis/dissertation, publishable paper. *Entrance requirements:* For master's and doctorate, GRE General Test, minimum GPA of 3.0 in last 60 hours. Additional exam requirements/recommendations for international students: Required—TOEFL. *Faculty research:* Anticancer agents, anti-inflammatory drugs, chronopharmacology, neuroendocrinology, microbiology.

The George Washington University, School of Medicine and Health Sciences, Health Sciences Programs, Washington, DC 20052. Offers clinical practice management (MSHS); clinical research administration (MSHS); emergency services management (MSHS); end-of-life care (MSHS); immunohematology (MSHS); immunohematology and biotechnology (MSHS); physical therapy (DPT); physician assistant (MSHS). *Program availability:* Online learning. *Faculty:* 22 full-time (17 women), 13 part-time/adjunct (10 women). *Students:* 277 full-time (198 women), 249 part-time (182 women); includes 159 minority (54 Black or African American, non-Hispanic/Latino; 2 American Indian or Alaska Native, non-Hispanic/Latino; 53 Asian, non-Hispanic/Latino; 40 Hispanic/Latino; 3 Native Hawaiian or other Pacific Islander, non-Hispanic/Latino; 7 Two or more races, non-Hispanic/Latino), 13 international. Average age 33. 1,905 applicants, 19% accepted, 197 enrolled. In 2015, 146 master's, 35 doctorates, 5 other advanced degrees awarded. *Entrance requirements:* Additional exam requirements/recommendations for international students: Required—TOEFL (minimum score 550 paper-based). *Application deadline:* Applications are processed on a rolling basis. Application fee: $75. *Expenses:* Contact institution. *Unit head:* Jean E. Johnson, Senior Associate Dean, 202-994-3725, E-mail: jejohns@gwu.edu. *Application contact:* Joke Ogundiran, Director of Admission, 202-994-1668, Fax: 202-994-0870, E-mail: jokeogun@gwu.edu.

Johns Hopkins University, Bloomberg School of Public Health, Department of Health Policy and Management, Baltimore, MD 21205-1996. Offers bioethics and policy (PhD); health and public policy (PhD); health care management and leadership (Dr PH); health economics (MHS); health economics and policy (PhD); health finance and management (MHA); health policy (MSPH); health services research and policy (PhD); public policy (MPP). *Accreditation:* CAHME (one or more programs are accredited). *Program availability:* Part-time. *Degree requirements:* For master's, thesis (for some programs), internship (for some programs); for doctorate, comprehensive exam, thesis/dissertation, 1-year full-time residency (for some programs), oral and written exams. *Entrance requirements:* For master's, GRE General Test or GMAT, 3 letters of recommendation, curriculum vitae/resume; for doctorate, GRE General Test or GMAT, 3 letters of recommendation, curriculum vitae, transcripts. Additional exam requirements/recommendations for international students: Recommended—TOEFL (minimum score 600 paper-based; 100 iBT), IELTS. Electronic applications accepted. *Faculty research:* Quality of care and health outcomes, health care finance and technology, health disparities and vulnerable populations, injury prevention, health policy and health care policy.

Lakehead University, Graduate Studies, Faculty of Social Sciences and Humanities, Department of Sociology, Thunder Bay, ON P7B 5E1, Canada. Offers gerontology (MA); health services and policy research (MA); sociology (MA); women's studies (MA). *Program availability:* Part-time, evening/weekend. *Degree requirements:* For master's, research project or thesis. *Entrance requirements:* For master's, minimum B average. Additional exam requirements/recommendations for international students: Required—TOEFL. *Faculty research:* Sociology of medicine, cultural and social change, health human resources, gerontology, women's studies.

McMaster University, Faculty of Health Sciences and School of Graduate Studies, Program in Health Research Methodology (course-based), Hamilton, ON L8S 4M2, Canada. Offers M Sc. *Program availability:* Part-time. *Degree requirements:* For master's, research internship, scholarly paper courses. *Entrance requirements:* For master's, 4 year honors degree, minimum B+ average in last year of course work. Additional exam requirements/recommendations for international students: Required—TOEFL (minimum score 580 paper-based).

McMaster University, Faculty of Health Sciences and School of Graduate Studies, Program in Health Research Methodology (thesis), Hamilton, ON L8S 4M2, Canada. Offers M Sc, PhD. *Program availability:* Part-time. *Degree requirements:* For master's, thesis; for doctorate, comprehensive exam, thesis/dissertation. *Entrance requirements:* For master's, honors degree, minimum B+ average in last year of undergraduate course work; for doctorate, M Sc, minimum B+ average. Additional exam requirements/recommendations for international students: Required—TOEFL (minimum score 580 paper-based; 92 iBT).

Northwestern University, Feinberg School of Medicine and Interdepartmental Programs, Integrated Graduate Programs in the Life Sciences, Chicago, IL 60611. Offers biostatistics (PhD); epidemiology (PhD); health and biomedical informatics (PhD); health services and outcomes research (PhD); healthcare quality and patient safety (PhD); translational outcomes in science (PhD). *Degree requirements:* For doctorate, comprehensive exam, thesis/dissertation, written and oral qualifying exams. *Entrance requirements:* For doctorate, GRE General Test. Additional exam requirements/recommendations for international students: Required—TOEFL (minimum score 600 paper-based). Electronic applications accepted.

Old Dominion University, College of Health Sciences, Program in Health Services Research, Norfolk, VA 23529. Offers health services research (PhD). *Faculty:* 12 full-time (8 women), 10 part-time/adjunct (5 women). *Students:* 9 full-time (5 women), 18 part-time (17 women); includes 5 minority (2 Black or African American, non-Hispanic/Latino; 2 Asian, non-Hispanic/Latino; 1 Hispanic/Latino), 5 international. Average age 36. 16 applicants, 31% accepted, 5 enrolled. In 2015, 4 doctorates awarded. *Degree requirements:* For doctorate, comprehensive exam, thesis/dissertation, oral presentation of dissertation. *Entrance requirements:* For doctorate, GRE, minimum GPA of 3.25, master's degree, degree in health profession or health services, interview. Additional exam requirements/recommendations for international students: Required—TOEFL (minimum score 550 paper-based; 79 iBT). *Application deadline:* For fall admission, 3/1 for domestic students, 2/1 for international students. Applications are processed on a rolling basis. Application fee: $50. Electronic applications accepted. *Expenses:* $478 per credit for residents; $1,195 per credit for non-residents. *Financial support:* In 2015–16, 7 students received support, including 3 fellowships with full tuition reimbursements available (averaging $15,000 per year), 4 research assistantships with partial tuition reimbursements available (averaging $15,000 per year); unspecified assistantships also available. Financial award application deadline: 7/1; financial award applicants required to submit FAFSA. *Faculty research:* Access to health services, women's health,

domestic violence, health policy and planning, economics of obesity, substance abuse, health disparities, global health, injury prevention. *Unit head:* Dr. Bonnie Van Lunen, Graduate Program Director, 757-683-3516, Fax: 757-683-4410, E-mail: bvanlune@odu.edu. *Application contact:* William Heffelfinger, Director of Graduate Admissions, 757-683-5554, Fax: 757-683-3255, E-mail: gradadmit@odu.edu. Website: http://hs.odu.edu/commhealth/academics/phd/

Penn State Hershey Medical Center, College of Medicine, Graduate School Programs in the Biomedical Sciences, Graduate Program in Public Health Sciences, Hershey, PA 17033. Offers MS. *Program availability:* Part-time. *Students:* 10 full-time (7 women); includes 1 minority (Asian, non-Hispanic/Latino), 3 international. 26 applicants, 12% accepted, 9 enrolled. In 2015, 9 master's awarded. *Degree requirements:* For master's, thesis or alternative. *Entrance requirements:* Additional exam requirements/recommendations for international students: Required—TOEFL (minimum score 550 paper-based). *Application deadline:* For fall admission, 1/31 priority date for domestic students, 2/1 priority date for international students. Applications are processed on a rolling basis. Application fee: $65. Electronic applications accepted. *Financial support:* Fellowships available. Financial award applicants required to submit FAFSA. *Faculty research:* Clinical trials, statistical methods in genetic epidemiology, genetic factors in nicotine dependence and dementia syndromes, health economics, cancer. *Unit head:* Dr. Douglas Leslie, Director, 717-531-7178, Fax: 717-531-5779, E-mail: hes-grad-hmc@psu.edu. *Application contact:* Mardi Sawyer, Program Administrator, 717-531-7178, Fax: 717-531-5779, E-mail: hes-grad-hmc@psu.edu. Website: http://www2.med.psu.edu/phs/graduate-programs/master-of-science-in-public-health-sciences-program-ms-phs/

Stanford University, School of Medicine, Graduate Programs in Medicine, Department of Health Research and Policy, Stanford, CA 94305-9991. Offers biostatistics (PhD); epidemiology and clinical research (MS, PhD); health policy (MS, PhD). *Degree requirements:* For master's, thesis. Electronic applications accepted. *Expenses:* Tuition, area resident: Full-time $45,729. *Required fees:* $591. *Faculty research:* Cost and quality of life in cardiovascular disease, technology assessment, physician decision-making.

Texas A&M University, School of Public Health, College Station, TX 77843. Offers health administration (MHA); health policy and management (MPH); health promotion and community health sciences (MPH); health services research (PhD). *Accreditation:* CEPH. *Program availability:* Part-time, blended/hybrid learning. *Faculty:* 68. *Students:* 313 full-time (189 women), 71 part-time (41 women); includes 169 minority (40 Black or African American, non-Hispanic/Latino; 38 Asian, non-Hispanic/Latino; 88 Hispanic/Latino; 3 Two or more races, non-Hispanic/Latino), 88 international. Average age 30. 138 applicants, 100% accepted, 126 enrolled. In 2015, 139 master's, 5 doctorates awarded. *Degree requirements:* For master's, thesis optional. *Entrance requirements:* For master's, GRE General Test, 3 letters of recommendation; statement of purpose; current curriculum vitae or resume; official transcripts; for doctorate, GRE General Test, 3 letters of recommendation; statement of purpose; current curriculum vitae or resume; official transcripts; interview (in some cases). Additional exam requirements/recommendations for international students: Required—TOEFL (minimum score 597 paper-based, 95 iBT) or GRE (minimum verbal score 153). *Application deadline:* For fall admission, 8/27 for domestic students; for spring admission, 1/14 for domestic students. Application fee: $120. Electronic applications accepted. *Expenses:* Contact institution. *Financial support:* In 2015–16, 186 students received support, including 2 fellowships with tuition reimbursements available (averaging $17,190 per year), 55 research assistantships with tuition reimbursements available (averaging $5,728 per year), 14 teaching assistantships with tuition reimbursements available (averaging $5,836 per year); career-related internships or fieldwork, institutionally sponsored loans, scholarships/grants, traineeships, health care benefits, tuition waivers (full and partial), and unspecified assistantships also available. Support available to part-time students. Financial award applicants required to submit FAFSA. *Unit head:* Dr. Jay Maddock, Dean, 979-436-9322, Fax: 979-458-1878, E-mail: maddock@tamhsc.edu. *Application contact:* Erin E. Schneider, Associate Director of Admissions and Recruitment, 979-436-9380, E-mail: eschneider@sph.tamhsc.edu. Website: http://sph.tamhsc.edu/

Thomas Jefferson University, Jefferson College of Biomedical Sciences, Certificate Program in Patient-Centered Research, Philadelphia, PA 19107. Offers Certificate. *Program availability:* Part-time. *Students:* 1 (woman) part-time. 1 applicant, 100% accepted, 1 enrolled. *Entrance requirements:* For degree, GRE General Test (recommended). Additional exam requirements/recommendations for international students: Required—TOEFL, IELTS (minimum score 7). *Application deadline:* For fall admission, 8/1 priority date for domestic students, 3/1 priority date for international students; for winter admission, 12/1 priority date for domestic students, 6/1 priority date for international students; for spring admission, 4/1 priority date for domestic students. Applications are processed on a rolling basis. Application fee: $50. *Financial support:* Federal Work-Study and institutionally sponsored loans available. Support available to part-time students. Financial award application deadline: 5/1; financial award applicants required to submit FAFSA. *Unit head:* Dr. Carol L. Beck, Associate Dean/Program Director, 215-503-6539, Fax: 215-503-3433, E-mail: carol.beck@jefferson.edu. *Application contact:* Marc E. Stearns, Director of Admissions, 215-503-0155, Fax: 215-503-3433, E-mail: jgsbs-info@jefferson.edu. Website: http://www.jefferson.edu/university/biomedical-sciences/degrees-programs/graduate-certificate.html

Thomas Jefferson University, Jefferson College of Biomedical Sciences, Graduate Certificate Programs, Philadelphia, PA 19107. Offers clinical research and trials: implementation (Certificate); clinical research: operations (Certificate); human clinical investigation: theory (Certificate). *Program availability:* Part-time. *Faculty:* 44 full-time (14 women), 27 part-time/adjunct (11 women). *Students:* 7 part-time (6 women); includes 1 minority (Black or African American, non-Hispanic/Latino), 1 international. Average age 36. 4 applicants, 100% accepted, 4 enrolled. In 2015, 1 Certificate awarded. *Entrance requirements:* For degree, GRE General Test (recommended). Additional exam requirements/recommendations for international students: Required—TOEFL, IELTS (minimum score 7). *Application deadline:* For fall admission, 8/1 priority date for domestic students, 3/1 priority date for international students; for winter admission, 12/1 priority date for domestic students, 6/1 priority date for international students; for spring admission, 4/1 priority date for domestic students. Applications are processed on a rolling basis. Application fee: $50. *Financial support:* Federal Work-Study and institutionally sponsored loans available. Support available to part-time students. Financial award application deadline: 5/1; financial award applicants required to submit FAFSA. *Faculty research:* Epidemiology, clinical research, statistics, planning and management, disease control. *Unit head:* Dr. Dennis M. Gross, Associate Dean, 215-503-0156, Fax: 215-503-3433, E-mail: dennis.gross@jefferson.edu. *Application contact:* Marc E. Stearns, Director of Admissions, 215-503-0155, Fax: 215-503-3433, E-mail: jgsbs-info@jefferson.edu. Website: http://www.jefferson.edu/university/biomedical-sciences/degrees-programs/graduate-certificate.html

Thomas Jefferson University, Jefferson School of Population Health, Philadelphia, PA 19107. Offers applied health economics and outcomes research (MS, PhD, Certificate);

Health Services Research

behavioral health science (PhD); health policy (MS, Certificate); healthcare quality and safety (MS, PhD); population health (Certificate); public health (MPH, Certificate). *Program availability:* Part-time, evening/weekend, online learning. Terminal master's awarded for partial completion of doctoral program. *Degree requirements:* For master's, thesis; for doctorate, comprehensive exam, thesis/dissertation. *Entrance requirements:* For master's, GRE or other graduate entrance exam (MCAT, LSAT, DAT, etc.), two letters of recommendation, curriculum vitae, transcripts from all undergraduate and graduate institutions; for doctorate, GRE (taken within the last 5 years), three letters of recommendation, curriculum vitae, transcripts from all undergraduate and graduate institutions. Additional exam requirements/recommendations for international students: Required—TOEFL. Electronic applications accepted. *Faculty research:* Applied health economics and outcomes research, behavioral and health sciences, chronic disease management, health policy, healthcare quality and patient safety, wellness and prevention.

The University of Alabama at Birmingham, School of Public Health, Program in Public Health, Birmingham, AL 35294. Offers applied epidemiology and pharmacoepidemiology (MSPH); biostatistics (MPH); clinical and translational science (MSPH); environmental health (MPH); environmental health and toxicology (MSPH); epidemiology (MPH); general theory and practice (MPH); health behavior (MPH); health care organization (MPH); health policy quantitative policy analysis (MPH); industrial hygiene (MPH, MSPH); maternal and child health policy (Dr PH); maternal and child health policy and leadership (MPH); occupational health and safety (MPH); outcomes research (MSPH, Dr PH); public health (PhD); public health management (Dr PH); public health preparedness management (MPH). *Accreditation:* CEPH. *Program availability:* Part-time, online learning. *Degree requirements:* For doctorate, comprehensive exam, thesis/dissertation. *Entrance requirements:* For master's and doctorate, GRE. Additional exam requirements/recommendations for international students: Recommended—TOEFL (minimum score 550 paper-based; 79 iBT), IELTS (minimum score 6.5). Electronic applications accepted. *Expenses:* Tuition, state resident: full-time $7340. Tuition, nonresident: full-time $16,628. Full-time tuition and fees vary according to course load and program.

University of Alberta, School of Public Health, Department of Public Health Sciences, Edmonton, AB T6G 2E1, Canada. Offers clinical epidemiology (M Sc, MPH); environmental and occupational health (MPH); environmental health sciences (M Sc); epidemiology (M Sc); global health (M Sc, MPH); health policy and management (MPH); health policy research (M Sc); health technology assessment (MPH); occupational health (M Sc); population health (M Sc); public health leadership (MPH); public health sciences (PhD); quantitative methods (MPH). *Accreditation:* CEPH (one or more programs are accredited). Terminal master's awarded for partial completion of doctoral program. *Degree requirements:* For master's, thesis (for some programs); for doctorate, thesis/dissertation. *Entrance requirements:* For master's, GMAT or GRE General Test. Additional exam requirements/recommendations for international students: Required—TOEFL (minimum score 550 paper-based) or IELTS (minimum score 6). Electronic applications accepted. *Faculty research:* Biostatistics, health promotion and socio-behavioral health science.

University of Arkansas for Medical Sciences, College of Public Health, Little Rock, AR 72205-7199. Offers biostatistics (MPH); environmental and occupational health (MPH, Certificate); epidemiology (MPH, PhD); health behavior and health education (MPH); health policy and management (MPH); health promotion and prevention research (PhD); health services administration (MHSA); health systems research (PhD); public health (Certificate); public health leadership (Dr PH). *Program availability:* Part-time. *Degree requirements:* For master's, preceptorship, culminating experience, internship; for doctorate, comprehensive exam, capstone. *Entrance requirements:* For master's, GRE, GMAT, LSAT, PCAT, MCAT, DAT; for doctorate, GRE. Additional exam requirements/recommendations for international students: Required—TOEFL (minimum score 80 iBT), IELTS. Electronic applications accepted. *Expenses:* Contact institution. *Faculty research:* Health systems, tobacco prevention control, obesity prevention, environmental and occupational exposure, cancer prevention.

University of Cincinnati, Graduate School, College of Medicine, Graduate Programs in Biomedical Sciences, Program in Biomedical Research, Cincinnati, OH 45221. Offers MS.

University of Colorado Denver, Colorado School of Public Health, Health Services Research Program, Aurora, CO 80045. Offers PhD. *Program availability:* Part-time. *Faculty:* 8 full-time (3 women), 7 part-time/adjunct (6 women). *Students:* 21 full-time (17 women), 5 part-time (4 women); includes 8 minority (2 Black or African American, non-Hispanic/Latino; 3 Asian, non-Hispanic/Latino; 3 Hispanic/Latino), 3 international. Average age 33. 23 applicants, 17% accepted, 3 enrolled. In 2015, 1 doctorate awarded. *Degree requirements:* For doctorate, comprehensive exam, thesis/dissertation, minimum of 65 credit hours including 30 credit hours for thesis research. *Entrance requirements:* For doctorate, GRE, MCAT, or MA, MS or PhD from an accredited school, minimum undergraduate GPA of 3.0. Additional exam requirements/recommendations for international students: Required—TOEFL (minimum score 550 paper-based; 80 iBT). *Application deadline:* For fall admission, 2/1 for domestic students, 1/15 for international students. Application fee: $65. Electronic applications accepted. *Expenses:* Contact institution. *Financial support:* In 2015–16, 14 students received support. Fellowships, research assistantships, teaching assistantships, Federal Work-Study, institutionally sponsored loans, scholarships/grants, traineeships, and unspecified assistantships available. Financial award application deadline: 3/1; financial award applicants required to submit FAFSA. *Faculty research:* Drug safety and risk management, health care financing and cost, health interaction with environmental factors, quality improvement and strategic research, cardiovascular health promotion. *Unit head:* Dr. Adam Atherly, Chair, 303-724-4471, E-mail: adam.atherly@ucdenver.edu. *Application contact:* Mary Baitinger, 303-724-6698.
Website: http://www.ucdenver.edu/academics/colleges/PublicHealth/departments/HealthSystems/Pages/welcome.aspx

University of Colorado Denver, School of Medicine, Clinical Science Graduate Program, Aurora, CO 80045. Offers clinical investigation (PhD); clinical sciences (MS); health information technology (PhD); health services research (PhD). *Students:* 38 full-time (28 women), 35 part-time (22 women); includes 12 minority (3 Black or African American, non-Hispanic/Latino; 1 American Indian or Alaska Native, non-Hispanic/Latino; 4 Asian, non-Hispanic/Latino; 2 Hispanic/Latino; 2 Two or more races, non-Hispanic/Latino), 1 international. Average age 37. 22 applicants, 68% accepted, 15 enrolled. In 2015, 13 master's, 2 doctorates awarded. *Degree requirements:* For master's, thesis, minimum of 30 credit hours, defense/final exam of thesis or publishable paper; for doctorate, comprehensive exam, thesis/dissertation, at least 30 credit hours of thesis work. *Entrance requirements:* For master's, GRE General Test or MCAT (waived if candidate has earned MS/MA or PhD from accredited U.S. school), minimum undergraduate GPA of 3.0, 3-4 letters of recommendation; for doctorate, GRE General Test or MCAT (waived if candidate has earned MS/MA or PhD from accredited U.S. school), health care graduate, professional degree, or graduate degree related to health sciences; minimum GPA of 3.0; 3-4 letters of recommendation. Additional exam requirements/recommendations for international students: Required—TOEFL (minimum score 550 paper-based; 80 iBT). *Application deadline:* For fall admission, 2/1 for

domestic students, 1/15 priority date for international students; for spring admission, 10/1 for domestic students. Application fee: $50 ($75 for international students). Electronic applications accepted. *Expenses:* Contact institution. *Financial support:* In 2015–16, 34 students received support. Fellowships, research assistantships, teaching assistantships, Federal Work-Study, institutionally sponsored loans, scholarships/grants, traineeships, and unspecified assistantships available. Financial award application deadline: 3/15; financial award applicants required to submit FAFSA. *Unit head:* Dr. Lisa Cicutto, Program Director, 303-398-1539, E-mail: cicuttol@njhealth.org. *Application contact:* Galit Mankin, Program Administrator, 720-848-6249, Fax: 303-848-7381, E-mail: galit.mankin@ucdenver.edu.
Website: http://www.ucdenver.edu/research/CCTSI/education-training/clsc/Pages/default.aspx

University of Florida, Graduate School, College of Public Health and Health Professions, Department of Health Services Research, Management and Policy, Gainesville, FL 32611. Offers health administration (MHA); health services research (PhD). *Accreditation:* CAHME. *Program availability:* Part-time. *Faculty:* 2 full-time. *Students:* 7 full-time (6 women), 1 part-time (0 women); includes 16 minority (6 Black or African American, non-Hispanic/Latino; 3 Asian, non-Hispanic/Latino; 7 Hispanic/Latino), 3 international. Average age 38. 17 applicants. In 2015, 5 doctorates awarded. *Degree requirements:* For master's, internship. *Entrance requirements:* For master's, GRE General Test (minimum score 300) or GMAT (minimum score 500), minimum GPA of 3.0; for doctorate, GRE General Test, minimum GPA of 3.0. Additional exam requirements/recommendations for international students: Required—TOEFL (minimum score 550 paper-based; 80 iBT), IELTS (minimum score 6). *Application deadline:* For fall admission, 2/1 for domestic and international students. Applications are processed on a rolling basis. Application fee: $30. Electronic applications accepted. *Financial support:* In 2015–16, 1 fellowship, 4 research assistantships, 8 teaching assistantships were awarded; career-related internships or fieldwork and unspecified assistantships also available. Financial award applicants required to submit FAFSA. *Faculty research:* State health policy evaluation, health informatics for pain, family medicine, secondary data analysis, disability, mental health. *Unit head:* Dr. Arch G. Mainous, III, Department Chair/Professor, 352-273-6073, Fax: 352-273-6075, E-mail: arch.mainous@phhp.ufl.edu. *Application contact:* Barbara Ross, Student Services Coordinator, 352-273-6074, Fax: 352-273-6075, E-mail: bross@phhp.ufl.edu.
Website: http://www.phhp.ufl.edu/hsrmp/

University of Illinois at Chicago, School of Public Health, Division of Health Policy and Administration, Chicago, IL 60607-7128. Offers clinical and translational science (MS); health policy (PhD); health services research (PhD); healthcare administration (MHA); public health policy management (MPH). *Program availability:* Part-time. *Faculty:* 16 full-time (9 women), 18 part-time/adjunct (7 women). *Students:* 129 full-time (88 women), 149 part-time (102 women); includes 140 minority (39 Black or African American, non-Hispanic/Latino; 59 Asian, non-Hispanic/Latino; 34 Hispanic/Latino; 1 Native Hawaiian or other Pacific Islander, non-Hispanic/Latino; 7 Two or more races, non-Hispanic/Latino), 18 international. Average age 32. Terminal master's awarded for partial completion of doctoral program. *Degree requirements:* For master's, thesis, field practicum; for doctorate, thesis/dissertation, independent research, internship. *Entrance requirements:* For master's and doctorate, GRE General Test, minimum GPA of 2.75. Additional exam requirements/recommendations for international students: Required—TOEFL. *Application deadline:* For fall admission, 2/1 for domestic students, 1/1 priority date for international students. Application fee: $60. Electronic applications accepted. *Expenses:* Contact institution. *Financial support:* In 2015–16, 4 fellowships with full tuition reimbursements were awarded; research assistantships with full tuition reimbursements, teaching assistantships with full tuition reimbursements, career-related internships or fieldwork, Federal Work-Study, institutionally sponsored loans, scholarships/grants, traineeships, and unspecified assistantships also available. Support available to part-time students. Financial award application deadline: 3/1; financial award applicants required to submit FAFSA. *Faculty research:* Cancer screening in underserved populations, practices and devices used to reduce firefighter injury, the relationship between communal housing and substance abuse recovery. *Unit head:* Prof. Jack Zwanziger, Director, 312-996-1062, Fax: 312-996-5356, E-mail: jzwanzig@uic.edu. *Application contact:* Aimee Wiebel, Academic Coordinator, 312-996-7816, Fax: 312-996-5356, E-mail: aimee@uic.edu.
Website: http://publichealth.uic.edu/departments/healthpolicyandadministration/

University of La Verne, College of Business and Public Management, Program in Health Administration, La Verne, CA 91750-4443. Offers financial management (MHA); management and leadership (MHA); marketing and business development (MHA). *Program availability:* Part-time. *Faculty:* 5 full-time (4 women), 3 part-time/adjunct (1 woman). *Students:* 48 full-time (29 women), 34 part-time (25 women); includes 36 minority (9 Black or African American, non-Hispanic/Latino; 1 American Indian or Alaska Native, non-Hispanic/Latino; 5 Asian, non-Hispanic/Latino; 21 Hispanic/Latino), 10 international. Average age 31. In 2015, 34 master's awarded. *Entrance requirements:* For master's, bachelor's degree, experience in health services industry (preferred). Additional exam requirements/recommendations for international students: Required—TOEFL (minimum score 550 paper-based). *Application deadline:* Applications are processed on a rolling basis. Application fee: $50. *Expenses:* $757 per semester hour. *Financial support:* Federal Work-Study available. Financial award application deadline: 3/2; financial award applicants required to submit FAFSA. *Unit head:* Dr. Kathy Duncan, Program Chairperson, 909-448-4415, E-mail: kduncan2@laverne.edu. *Application contact:* Barbara Cox, Program and Admissions Specialist, 909-448-4004, Fax: 909-971-2295, E-mail: bcox@laverne.edu.
Website: http://laverne.edu/business-and-public-administration/mha-2/

University of Maryland, Baltimore, Graduate School, Graduate Programs in Pharmacy, Department of Pharmaceutical Health Service Research, Baltimore, MD 21201. Offers epidemiology (MS); pharmacy administration (PhD); Pharm D/PhD. *Degree requirements:* For doctorate, comprehensive exam, thesis/dissertation. *Entrance requirements:* For doctorate, GRE General Test. Additional exam requirements/recommendations for international students: Required—TOEFL, IELTS. Electronic applications accepted. Tuition and fees vary according to program. *Faculty research:* Pharmacoeconomics, outcomes research, public health policy, drug therapy and aging.

University of Massachusetts Medical School, Graduate School of Biomedical Sciences, Worcester, MA 01655-0115. Offers biomedical sciences (PhD), including biochemistry and molecular pharmacology, bioinformatics and computational biology, cancer biology, cell biology, immunology and microbiology, interdisciplinary, neuroscience, translational science; biomedical sciences (millennium program) (PhD); clinical and population health research (PhD); clinical investigation (MS). *Faculty:* 1,339 full-time (521 women), 301 part-time/adjunct (189 women). *Students:* 363 full-time (184 women); includes 58 minority (13 Black or African American, non-Hispanic/Latino; 30 Asian, non-Hispanic/Latino; 15 Hispanic/Latino), 141 international. Average age 29. 661 applicants, 26% accepted, 51 enrolled. In 2015, 10 master's, 58 doctorates awarded. Terminal master's awarded for partial completion of doctoral program. *Degree requirements:* For master's, comprehensive exam, thesis; for doctorate, comprehensive exam, thesis/dissertation. *Entrance requirements:* For master's, MD, PhD, DVM, or

PharmD; for doctorate, GRE General Test, bachelor's degree. Additional exam requirements/recommendations for international students: Required—TOEFL (minimum score 100 iBT) or IELTS (minimum score 7.5). *Application deadline:* For fall admission, 12/15 for domestic and international students; for spring admission, 5/15 for domestic students. Application fee: $80. Electronic applications accepted. *Expenses:* $6,966 resident per year; $14,182 non-resident per year. *Financial support:* In 2015–16, 383 students received support, including research assistantships with full tuition reimbursements available (averaging $30,600 per year); scholarships/grants, health care benefits, tuition waivers (full), and unspecified assistantships also available. Financial award application deadline: 5/16. *Faculty research:* RNA interference, cell/molecular/developmental biology, bioinformatics, clinical/translational research, infectious disease. *Total annual research expenditures:* $250.3 million. *Unit head:* Dr. Anthony Carruthers, Dean, 508-856-4135, E-mail: anthony.carruthers@umassmed.edu. *Application contact:* Dr. Kendall Knight, Assistant Vice Provost for Admissions, 508-856-5628, Fax: 508-856-3659, E-mail: kendall.knight@umassmed.edu.
Website: http://www.umassmed.edu/gsbs/

University of Minnesota, Twin Cities Campus, School of Public Health, Major in Health Services Research, Policy, and Administration, Minneapolis, MN 55455-0213. Offers MS, PhD, JD/MS, JD/PhD, MD/PhD, MPP/MS. *Program availability:* Part-time. Terminal master's awarded for partial completion of doctoral program. *Degree requirements:* For master's, thesis, internship, final oral exam; for doctorate, thesis/dissertation, teaching experience, written preliminary exam, final oral exam, dissertation. *Entrance requirements:* For master's, GRE General Test, course work in mathematics; for doctorate, GRE General Test, prerequisite courses in calculus and statistics. Additional exam requirements/recommendations for international students: Required—TOEFL (minimum score 600 paper-based; 100 iBT). *Faculty research:* Outcomes, economics and statistics, sociology, health care management.

University of Nebraska Medical Center, Department of Health Services Research and Administration, Omaha, NE 68198. Offers health services research, administration, and policy (PhD). *Faculty:* 9 full-time (4 women), 1 part-time/adjunct. *Students:* 13 full-time (10 women), 3 part-time (2 women); includes 1 minority (Two or more races, non-Hispanic/Latino), 10 international. Average age 31. 11 applicants, 36% accepted, 4 enrolled. In 2015, 5 doctorates awarded. *Degree requirements:* For doctorate, comprehensive exam, thesis/dissertation. *Entrance requirements:* For doctorate, GRE, official transcripts, resume or curriculum vitae, three letters of recommendation, statement of intent. Additional exam requirements/recommendations for international students: Required—TOEFL (minimum score 550 paper-based; 80 iBT). *Application deadline:* For fall admission, 6/1 for domestic students, 4/1 for international students. Application fee: $45. Electronic applications accepted. *Expenses:* Tuition, state resident: full-time $7830; part-time $3915 per credit hour. Tuition, nonresident: full-time $22,410; part-time $11,205 per credit hour. *Required fees:* $521. *Financial support:* In 2015–16, 5 students received support, including 1 research assistantship with full tuition reimbursement available (averaging $23,100 per year); scholarships/grants and unspecified assistantships also available. Financial award application deadline: 2/15; financial award applicants required to submit FAFSA. *Unit head:* Dr. Fernando Wilson, Associate Professor, 402-552-6948, E-mail: fernando.wilson@unmc.edu. *Application contact:* Denise Howard, Coordinator, 402-559-5260, E-mail: denise.howard@unmc.edu.
Website: http://www.unmc.edu/publichealth/departments/healthservices/

University of New Brunswick Fredericton, School of Graduate Studies, Applied Health Services Research Program, Fredericton, NB E3B 5A3, Canada. Offers MAHSR. *Program availability:* Part-time, online learning. *Faculty:* 3 full-time (1 woman). *Students:* 9 full-time (7 women), 5 part-time (all women). In 2015, 1 master's awarded. *Degree requirements:* For master's, thesis. *Entrance requirements:* For master's, honors BA, minimum GPA of 3.0. Additional exam requirements/recommendations for international students: Required—TWE (minimum score 4), TOEFL (minimum score 600 paper-based; 100 iBT) or IELTS (minimum score 7). *Application deadline:* For winter admission, 3/31 for domestic and international students. Applications are processed on a rolling basis. Application fee: $50 Canadian dollars. Electronic applications accepted. *Faculty research:* Applied health services research. *Unit head:* Dr. Linda Eyre, Assistant Dean of Graduate Studies, 506-447-3044, Fax: 506-453-4817, E-mail: gradidst@unb.ca. *Application contact:* Janet Amirault, Graduate Secretary, 506-458-7558, Fax: 506-453-4817, E-mail: jamiraul@unb.ca.
Website: http://www.artc-hsr.ca

The University of North Carolina at Charlotte, College of Health and Human Services, Program in Health Services Research, Charlotte, NC 28223-0001. Offers PhD. *Program availability:* Part-time. *Students:* 22 full-time (11 women), 8 part-time (2 women); includes 6 minority (4 Black or African American, non-Hispanic/Latino; 1 Asian, non-Hispanic/Latino; 1 Two or more races, non-Hispanic/Latino), 8 international. Average age 40. 16 applicants, 56% accepted, 8 enrolled. In 2015, 1 doctorate awarded. *Degree requirements:* For doctorate, thesis/dissertation. *Entrance requirements:* For doctorate, GRE (minimum score of 153 verbal, 144 quantitative, 4.0 analytical), master's or doctoral degree from regionally-accredited university in a health-related field, including, but not limited to, public health, nursing, medicine, social work, kinesiology, health psychology, public administration, business administration, and nutrition; minimum graduate GPA of 3.5. Additional exam requirements/recommendations for international students: Required—TOEFL (minimum score 557 paper-based, 83 iBT) or IELTS (minimum score 6.5). *Application deadline:* For fall admission, 2/1 for domestic and international students. Applications are processed on a rolling basis. Application fee: $75. Electronic applications accepted. *Expenses:* Tuition, state resident: full-time $4128. Tuition, nonresident: full-time $16,799. *Required fees:* $2904. Tuition and fees vary according to course load and program. *Financial support:* Career-related internships or fieldwork, institutionally sponsored loans, scholarships/grants, and unspecified assistantships available. Support available to part-time students. Financial award application deadline: 3/1; financial award applicants required to submit FAFSA. *Faculty research:* Epidemiology of asthma, mental health services research, healthcare disparities, building research capacity within organizations, health policy and administration, reproductive epidemiology, data warehousing/mining of large scale databases for decision support, program evaluation, health care ethics, informatics and technology, health economics. *Unit head:* Dr. Nancy Fey-Yensan, Dean, 704-687-7917, E-mail: fey-yensan@uncc.edu. *Application contact:* Kathy B. Giddings, Director of Graduate Admissions, 704-687-5503, Fax: 704-687-1668, E-mail: gradadm@uncc.edu.
Website: http://health.uncc.edu/degrees-and-programs/hsr-phd

University of Ottawa, Faculty of Graduate and Postdoctoral Studies, Interdisciplinary Programs, Ottawa, ON K1N 6N5, Canada. Offers e-business (Certificate); e-commerce (Certificate); finance (Certificate); health services and policies research (Diploma); population health (PhD); population health risk assessment and management (Certificate); public management and governance (Certificate); systems science (Certificate).

University of Pennsylvania, Perelman School of Medicine, Program in Health Policy Research, Philadelphia, PA 19104. Offers MS, MD/MS, MD/MSHP. *Program availability:* Part-time, online learning. *Faculty:* 22 full-time (10 women). *Students:* 37 full-time (22 women); includes 17 minority (3 Black or African American, non-Hispanic/Latino; 10

Asian, non-Hispanic/Latino; 2 Hispanic/Latino; 2 Two or more races, non-Hispanic/Latino). Average age 33. 23 applicants, 83% accepted, 18 enrolled. In 2015, 27 master's awarded. *Degree requirements:* For master's, thesis. *Entrance requirements:* For master's, MCAT/GRE (depending on applicant's terminal degree). Additional exam requirements/recommendations for international students: Required—TOEFL. *Application deadline:* For fall admission, 11/30 for domestic and international students. Electronic applications accepted. *Expenses: Tuition, area resident:* Full-time $31,068; part-time $5762 per course. *Required fees:* $3200; $336 per course. Full-time tuition and fees vary according to degree level, program and student level. Part-time tuition and fees vary according to course load, degree level and program. *Financial support:* In 2015–16, 17 fellowships with partial tuition reimbursements were awarded; scholarships/grants also available. *Faculty research:* Disparities in health care; cost effectiveness analysis; outcomes research; biological, clinical, behavioral and environmental factors in health care; diffusion of health care innovation; medical ethics; innovation; lay support with peer mentors and community health workers; evaluating medical homes; quality improvement research, health literacy, health numeracy, medical decision-making. *Unit head:* Dr. Judy Shea, Co-Director, 215-573-5111, E-mail: sheaja@mail.med.upenn.edu. *Application contact:* Suzanne Mosko, E-mail: suzannej@mail.med.upenn.edu.
Website: http://www.med.upenn.edu/mshp/

University of Puerto Rico, Medical Sciences Campus, Graduate School of Public Health, Department of Health Services Administration, Program in Evaluative Research of Health Systems, San Juan, PR 00936-5067. Offers MS. *Program availability:* Part-time. *Degree requirements:* For master's, thesis. *Entrance requirements:* For master's, GRE, previous course work in algebra and statistics. *Expenses:* Contact institution.

University of Rochester, School of Medicine and Dentistry, Graduate Programs in Medicine and Dentistry, Department of Community and Preventive Medicine, Program in Health Services Research and Policy, Rochester, NY 14627. Offers PhD, MPH/PhD. *Degree requirements:* For doctorate, thesis/dissertation, qualifying exam. *Entrance requirements:* For doctorate, GRE General Test. *Expenses: Tuition, area resident:* Full-time $47,450; part-time $1482 per credit hour. *Required fees:* $528. Tuition and fees vary according to program.

University of Rochester, School of Nursing, Rochester, NY 14642. Offers adult gerontological acute care nurse practitioner (MS); clinical nurse leader (MS); family nurse practitioner (MS); family psychiatric mental health nurse practitioner (MS); health care organization management and leadership (MS); health practice research (PhD); nursing (DNP); nursing education (MS); pediatric nurse practitioner (MS); pediatric nurse practitioner/neonatal nurse practitioner (MS). *Accreditation:* AACN. *Program availability:* Part-time, online learning. *Faculty:* 56 full-time (45 women), 63 part-time/adjunct (55 women). *Students:* 21 full-time (20 women), 212 part-time (175 women); includes 35 minority (12 Black or African American, non-Hispanic/Latino; 1 American Indian or Alaska Native, non-Hispanic/Latino; 10 Asian, non-Hispanic/Latino; 7 Hispanic/Latino; 5 Two or more races, non-Hispanic/Latino), 2 international. Average age 35. 111 applicants, 68% accepted, 71 enrolled. In 2015, 52 master's, 9 doctorates awarded. Terminal master's awarded for partial completion of doctoral program. *Degree requirements:* For master's, comprehensive exam (for some programs); for doctorate, thesis/dissertation. *Entrance requirements:* For master's, BS in nursing, minimum GPA of 3.0, course work in statistics; for doctorate, GRE General Test (for PhD), MS in nursing, minimum GPA of 3.5. Additional exam requirements/recommendations for international students: Required—TOEFL (minimum score 560 paper-based; 88 iBT) or IELTS (minimum score 6.5) recommended. *Application deadline:* For fall admission, 4/1 for domestic and international students; for spring admission, 9/1 for domestic and international students; for summer admission, 1/2 for domestic and international students. Application fee: $50. Electronic applications accepted. *Expenses: Tuition, area resident:* Full-time $47,450; part-time $1482 per credit hour. *Required fees:* $528. Tuition and fees vary according to program. *Financial support:* In 2015–16, 52 students received support, including 2 fellowships with tuition reimbursements available (averaging $30,000 per year); scholarships/grants, traineeships, health care benefits, tuition waivers (full and partial), and unspecified assistantships also available. Support available to part-time students. Financial award application deadline: 6/30. *Faculty research:* Symptom assessment and self-management of chronic illness, health promotion and illness prevention, nursing intervention research with vulnerable populations, palliative care, aging. *Total annual research expenditures:* $2.1 million. *Unit head:* Dr. Kathy H. Rideout, Dean, 585-273-8902, Fax: 585-273-1268, E-mail: kathy_rideout@urmc.rochester.edu. *Application contact:* Elaine Andolina, Director of Admissions, 585-275-2375, Fax: 585-756-8299, E-mail: elaine_andolina@urmc.rochester.edu.
Website: http://www.son.rochester.edu

University of Southern California, Keck School of Medicine and Graduate School, Graduate Programs in Medicine, Department of Preventive Medicine, Program in Health Behavior Research, Los Angeles, CA 90032. Offers PhD. *Faculty:* 21 full-time (13 women), 1 (woman) part-time/adjunct. *Students:* 33 full-time (20 women), 1 part-time (0 women); includes 16 minority (2 Black or African American, non-Hispanic/Latino; 9 Asian, non-Hispanic/Latino; 4 Hispanic/Latino; 1 Two or more races, non-Hispanic/Latino), 2 international. Average age 31. 42 applicants, 17% accepted, 4 enrolled. In 2015, 1 doctorate awarded. *Degree requirements:* For doctorate, comprehensive exam, thesis/dissertation. *Entrance requirements:* For doctorate, GRE General Test (minimum preferred score for combined Verbal and Quantitative of 311), minimum GPA of 3.0 (3.5 preferred). Additional exam requirements/recommendations for international students: Required—TOEFL (minimum score 600 paper-based; 100 iBT). *Application deadline:* For fall admission, 12/1 priority date for domestic and international students. Application fee: $85. Electronic applications accepted. *Financial support:* In 2015–16, 30 students received support, including 11 fellowships with full tuition reimbursements available (averaging $32,000 per year), 7 research assistantships with tuition reimbursements available (averaging $32,000 per year), 7 teaching assistantships with tuition reimbursements available (averaging $32,000 per year); institutionally sponsored loans, scholarships/grants, traineeships, health care benefits, and unspecified assistantships also available. Financial award application deadline: 5/12; financial award applicants required to submit CSS PROFILE or FAFSA. *Faculty research:* Obesity prevention; etiology and prevention of substance abuse, other addictive behaviors, and chronic diseases; health disparities; translational research. *Unit head:* Dr. Jennifer Unger, Director, 323-442-8234, E-mail: unger@usc.edu. *Application contact:* Marny Barovich, Program Manager, 323-442-8299, E-mail: barovich@hsc.usc.edu.
Website: http://phdhbr.usc.edu

The University of Tennessee Health Science Center, College of Graduate Health Sciences, Memphis, TN 38163-0002. Offers biomedical engineering (MS, PhD); biomedical sciences (PhD); dental sciences (MDS); epidemiology (MS); health outcomes and policy research (PhD); laboratory research and management (MS); nursing science (PhD); pharmaceutical sciences (PhD); pharmacology (MS); speech and hearing science (PhD); DDS/PhD; DNP/PhD; MD/PhD; Pharm D/PhD. Terminal master's awarded for partial completion of doctoral program. *Degree requirements:* For master's, comprehensive exam, thesis; for doctorate, comprehensive exam, thesis/dissertation, oral and written preliminary and comprehensive exams. *Entrance*

Health Services Research

requirements: For master's and doctorate, GRE General Test, minimum GPA of 3.0. Additional exam requirements/recommendations for international students: Required—TOEFL (minimum score 79 iBT); Recommended—IELTS (minimum score 6.5). Electronic applications accepted.

University of Utah, Graduate School, College of Pharmacy, Department of Pharmacotherapy, Salt Lake City, UT 84112. Offers health system pharmacy administration (MS); outcomes research and health policy (PhD). *Faculty:* 6 full-time (4 women), 26 part-time/adjunct (18 women). *Students:* 8 full-time (5 women), 5 part-time (3 women), 5 international. Average age 28. 26 applicants, 19% accepted, 4 enrolled. In 2015, 3 master's awarded. Terminal master's awarded for partial completion of doctoral program. *Degree requirements:* For master's, comprehensive exam, thesis or alternative, project; for doctorate, comprehensive exam, thesis/dissertation. *Entrance requirements:* For doctorate, GRE. Additional exam requirements/recommendations for international students: Required—TOEFL (minimum score 550 paper-based; 80 iBT). *Application deadline:* For fall admission, 1/10 for domestic students, 12/15 for international students. Application fee: $55 ($65 for international students). *Financial support:* In 2015–16, 7 students received support, including 9 research assistantships with full tuition reimbursements available (averaging $21,400 per year); health care benefits also available. Financial award application deadline: 12/15. *Faculty research:* Outcomes in pharmacy, pharmacotherapy. *Total annual research expenditures:* $131,217. *Unit head:* Dr. Diana I. Brixner, Department Chair and Professor, 801-581-6731. *Application contact:* Sara Ray, Academic Program Manager, 801-581-5984, Fax: 801-585-6160, E-mail: sara.ray@pharm.utah.edu.
Website: http://www.pharmacy.utah.edu/pharmacotherapy/

University of Virginia, School of Medicine, Department of Public Health Sciences, Charlottesville, VA 22903. Offers clinical research (MS), including clinical investigation and patient-oriented research, informatics in medicine; public health (MPH); MPP/MPH. *Program availability:* Part-time. *Entrance requirements:* For master's, GRE General Test or MCAT. Additional exam requirements/recommendations for international students: Required—TOEFL. Electronic applications accepted.

University of Washington, Graduate School, School of Public Health, Department of Health Services, Seattle, WA 98195. Offers clinical research (MS); community-oriented public health practice (MPH); evaluative sciences and statistics (PhD); health behavior and social determinants of health (PhD); health economics (PhD); health informatics and health information management (MHIHIM); health services (MS, PhD); health services administration (EMHA, MHA); health systems and policy (MPH); health systems research (PhD); maternal and child health (MPH); social and behavioral sciences (MPH); JD/MHA; MHA/MBA; MHA/MD; MHA/MPA; MPH/JD; MPH/MD; MPH/MN; MPH/MPA; MPH/MS; MPH/MSD; MPH/MSW; MPH/PhD. *Program availability:* Online learning. Terminal master's awarded for partial completion of doctoral program. *Degree requirements:* For master's, thesis (for some programs), practicum (MPH); for doctorate, comprehensive exam, thesis/dissertation. *Entrance requirements:* For master's and doctorate, GRE General Test, minimum GPA of 3.0. Additional exam requirements/recommendations for international students: Required—TOEFL (minimum score 580 paper-based; 92 iBT), IELTS (minimum score 7). Electronic applications accepted.

Expenses: Contact institution. *Faculty research:* Public health practice, health promotion and disease prevention, maternal and child health, organizational behavior and culture, health policy.

Virginia Commonwealth University, Graduate School, School of Allied Health Professions, Department of Health Administration, Doctoral Program in Health Services Organization and Research, Richmond, VA 23284-9005. Offers PhD. *Degree requirements:* For doctorate, thesis/dissertation, residency. *Entrance requirements:* For doctorate, GMAT or GRE General Test, minimum graduate GPA of 3.0. Additional exam requirements/recommendations for international students: Required—TOEFL (minimum score 600 paper-based; 100 iBT). Electronic applications accepted. *Faculty research:* Organizational studies, theory, associated analytical techniques.

Virginia Commonwealth University, Medical College of Virginia-Professional Programs, School of Medicine, School of Medicine Graduate Programs, Department of Healthcare Policy and Research, Richmond, VA 23284-9005. Offers PhD. *Entrance requirements:* For doctorate, GRE General Test. Additional exam requirements/recommendations for international students: Required—TOEFL (minimum score 600 paper-based; 100 iBT). Electronic applications accepted. *Faculty research:* Evaluation of healthcare services and systems to enhance quality of care and patient safety outcomes; examination of chronic disease (e.g. cancer, HIV/AIDS) policies and practices to improve health outcomes and economic efficiency; impact of uninsurance, public insurance (such as Medicaid) and the safety net on access to care and the health of low-income, underserved, and foreign-born populations; the study of labor supply and healthcare coverage in response to health behaviors and shocks.

Wake Forest University, School of Medicine and Graduate School of Arts and Sciences, Graduate Programs in Medicine, Program in Health Sciences Research, Winston-Salem, NC 27109. Offers MS. *Degree requirements:* For master's, thesis. *Entrance requirements:* For master's, GRE General Test. Additional exam requirements/recommendations for international students: Required—TOEFL. Electronic applications accepted. *Faculty research:* Research methodologies, statistical methods, measurement of health outcomes, health economics.

Washington University in St. Louis, School of Medicine, Program in Applied Health Behavior Research, Saint Louis, MO 63110. Offers health behavior planning and evaluation (Graduate Certificate); health behavior research (MS); health education, program planning and evaluation (MS). *Program availability:* Part-time, evening/weekend. *Entrance requirements:* For master's and Graduate Certificate, baccalaureate degree in psychology, biology, social work, public health, anthropology or other related field; experience working in the health care field, including health promotion research, social research, or community programs. Additional exam requirements/recommendations for international students: Required—TOEFL. *Faculty research:* Health behavior, health disparities, health education, program management, program evaluation.

Weill Cornell Medicine, Weill Cornell Graduate School of Medical Sciences, Program in Clinical Epidemiology and Health Services Research, New York, NY 10021. Offers MS. *Degree requirements:* For master's, thesis. *Entrance requirements:* For master's, 3 years of work experience, MD or RN certificate. *Faculty research:* Research methodology, biostatistical techniques, data management, decision analysis, health economics.

XAVIER UNIVERSITY
Graduate Program in Health Services Administration

 For more information, visit http://petersons.to/xavier-healthservices

Health Services Administration

Programs of Study

The Xavier University graduate program in Health Services Administration, named the Top Program for Excellence in Healthcare Administration by CAHME/Ascension Health, offers a rigorous curriculum that integrates both theory and practical experience. This combination fully equips its students to hold management, executive, and other leadership positions in a wide range of fields in the health services industry, including hospitals, health systems, group practice, insurance, consulting, government, and the military. Xavier's Master of Health Services Administration (M.H.S.A.) program is accredited by the Commission on the Accreditation of Healthcare Management Education (CAHME) and is one of only a handful of M.H.S.A. programs still requiring the eight to twelve month residency. As the nation's tenth-oldest accredited health administration program, the M.H.S.A. degree from Xavier has a tradition of excellence recognized throughout the healthcare industry since 1958.

The M.H.S.A. program offers both full-time and part-time degree options, both of which can be completed in three years. The program also offers a concurrent degree with M.B.A.

The M.H.S.A. full-time day program prepares students for administrative and executive positions in healthcare organizations. This option consists of four semesters of on-campus coursework over a two year period. After completing this coursework, students begin the required eight to twelve month paid residency (the average stipend in 2016 is $42,000) at a healthcare organization. With more than 150 approved residency sites across the country, the residency provides students with the opportunity to apply the knowledge and skills from their coursework to a real-world setting under the guidance of a senior manager.

The M.H.S.A. part-time evening program enables individuals who are already working in health care to learn the administrative skills needed to progress in their careers and increase their value to their employers. This track consists of nine consecutive semesters of part-time, on-campus coursework. During this time, students will also complete a practicum, which is a guided field experience conducted within the student's place of employment in a healthcare setting.

The concurrent degree option provides an opportunity for students to pursue a business (M.B.A.) degree in addition to an M.H.S.A. degree. Students in this track must apply and be accepted into both programs. An M.B.A. may be earned over a two-year period by pursuing additional hours of M.B.A. graduate-level course work in the Williams College of Business at Xavier. The concurrent degree is designed to be completed within three years.

Research Facilities

The McDonald Library at Xavier University contains most of the library's collections, including archives and special collections. Connected to this building is the Conaton Learning Commons (CLC), which hosts the "Connection Center," an integrated service point, blending library and help desk services. The library and CLC both provide study, lounge, conference, and instruction space along with access to photocopiers, computer workstations, and printers. The library emphasizes individual study while the CLC focuses on collaboration, housing thirteen group study rooms; nine of these rooms have plasma screen projection with Internet access. A food kiosk, vending machines, and kitchenette are available for students. The Connection Center in the CLC brings together at one desk circulation, traditional reserves, research, computer technology, and classroom support services. Other student support services in the CLC include the Learning Assistance Center, Writing Center, Language Resource Center, Academic Advising, and Digital Media Lab.

Financial Aid

Internal scholarships are available from M.H.S.A. endowed funds. These awards are granted to students based on academic merit or a scholarship application. When available, graduate assistantships are awarded which may include tuition remission and an hourly rate for work as determined by the University. Students who file a FAFSA and enroll at least half time may qualify for a Direct Loan, which is a long-term, low-interest loan. These students may also apply for a Graduate PLUS loan, which is credit-based. Various alternative loans are available for students who need additional assistance. Further information is available from the Financial Aid Office (phone: 513-745-3142) or by e-mailing hellkampal@xavier.edu.

Cost of Study

Tuition for 2016–17 is $620 per credit hour. There is a $175 admissions fee for all M.H.S.A. students upon acceptance. Textbooks are an additional cost.

Living and Housing Costs

Xavier University does not provide graduate-specific housing on campus, as most graduate students live in neighboring areas of Cincinnati at affordable prices. Information regarding apartments located on campus is available at http://liveatustation.com.

Student Group

There are between 24 and 30 students in each of the three full-time cohorts, while the part-time program consists of 6 to 10 students per cohort. The average age is 24 for full-time students and 32 for part-time students.

Location

Xavier is located just north of downtown Cincinnati, Ohio which was named one of America's most livable cities (according to *Places Rated Almanac*). Cincinnati is known for great restaurants, shops, a major amusement park, and culture with Broadway theater, museums, a zoo, and aquarium. The city is home to major sports teams, the Cincinnati Reds and the Cincinnati Bengals, plus a new professional soccer team, FC Cincinnati.

The University

Founded in 1831, Xavier is a private, coed university. As one of 28 Jesuit colleges/universities in the U.S., Xavier provides

Xavier University

an education in the Jesuit Catholic tradition of preparing the whole person, developing knowledge, values, spiritual growth, and responsibility for others. The University's focus on ethics and values helps students ready themselves for moral decisions they must make in their lives and careers. Xavier has 4,485 undergraduate students and 2,165 graduate students.

The Faculty

M.H.S.A. Full-Time Faculty

- Nancy Linenkugel, Department Chair and Program Director; D.M., OSF, Weatherhead School of Management, 1999.
- Rick Browne, Assistant Professor; Ph.D., Indiana University, 2002.
- Lin Guo, Associate Professor; Ph.D., University of Cincinnati, 1995.
- Edmond Hooker, Associate Professor; M.D., Eastern Virginia Medical School, 1985.
- Karen Kent, Visiting Assistant Professor; M.S., Rush University, 1990.
- Thomas Ruthemeyer, Clinical Professor; M.B.A., Xavier University, 1984.

M.H.S.A. Adjunct Faculty

- Chris Boue, Adjunct Faculty; M.B.A., Florida Metropolitan University, 1993.
- Donald Brennan, Adjunct Faculty; Ph.D., Walden University, 2013.
- William Freedman, Adjunct Faculty; J.D., Harvard Law School, 1973.
- Gayle Heintzelman, Adjunct Faculty; M.Ed., Xavier University.
- Jim O'Reilly, Adjunct Faculty; J.D., University of Virginia, 1974.
- Richard Schuster, Adjunct Faculty; Ph.D., Ohio State University; J.D., University of Virginia.
- Karen Tepe, Adjunct Faculty; M.H.S.A., Xavier University, 1999; M.B.A., Xavier University, 2004.
- Amy Thompson, Adjunct Faculty; M.H.S.A., Xavier University, 2005.
- ReNae Wright, Adjunct Faculty; M.H.S.A., Xavier University, 2011.

Applying

M.H.S.A. students matriculate in the fall each year. Deadlines to apply are January 1 for international students and June 1 for domestic students of the year in which they plan to enroll. Application requirements include a completed online application form, two recommendation letters, a statement of intent, resume, official transcripts from all previous college work, and GRE or GMAT scores. Prerequisites include accounting and statistics. An on-campus interview is required for admission. Additional documents are required for international students.

Correspondence and Information

Amy Hellkamp
Recruitment and Marketing Coordinator
Xavier University
Department of Health Services Administration
3800 Victory Parkway
Cincinnati, Ohio 45207-5141
Phone: 513-745-3687
E-mail: hellkampal@xavier.edu
Website: http://www.xavier.edu/mhsa/

Hinkle Hall, Xavier University.

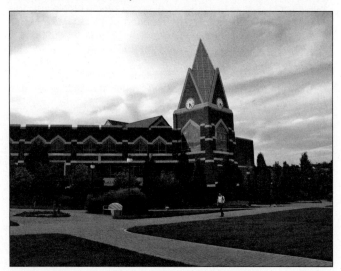

Gallagher Student Center, Xavier University Green Space.

Section 23
Nursing

This section contains a directory of institutions offering graduate work in nursing. Additional information about programs listed in the directory may be obtained by writing directly to the dean of a graduate school or chair of a department at the address given in the directory.

For programs offering related work, see also in this book *Health Services* and *Public Health.* In another guide in this series:

Graduate Programs in the Humanities, Arts & Social Sciences
See *Family and Consumer Sciences (Gerontology)*

CONTENTS

Program Directories

Display and Close-Ups

See:

Nursing—General

Adelphi University, College of Nursing and Public Health, PhD in Nursing Program, Garden City, NY 11530-0701. Offers PhD.

Albany State University, College of Sciences and Health Professions, Albany, GA 31705-2717. Offers criminal justice (MS), including corrections, forensic science, law enforcement, public administration; mathematics education (M Ed); nursing (MSN), including RN to MSN family nurse practitioner, RN to MSN nurse educator; science education (M Ed). *Accreditation:* ACEN. *Program availability:* Part-time, evening/weekend, online learning. *Degree requirements:* For master's, comprehensive exam, thesis. *Entrance requirements:* For master's, GRE or MAT, official transcript, letters of recommendations, pre-medical/certificate of immunizations. Electronic applications accepted.

Alcorn State University, School of Graduate Studies, School of Nursing, Natchez, MS 39122-8399. Offers rural nursing (MSN). *Accreditation:* AACN; ACEN.

Allen College, Graduate Programs, Waterloo, IA 50703. Offers acute care nurse practitioner (Post-Master's Certificate); adult nurse practitioner (Post-Master's Certificate); adult psychiatric-mental health nurse practitioner (Post-Master's Certificate); adult-gerontology acute care nurse practitioner (MSN); community public health (Post-Master's Certificate); community/public health nursing (MSN); family nurse practitioner (MSN, Post-Master's Certificate); gerontological nurse practitioner (Post-Master's Certificate); health sciences (Ed D); leadership in health care delivery (MSN, Post-Master's Certificate); nursing (DNP); occupational therapy (MS). *Accreditation:* AACN; ACEN. *Program availability:* Part-time, blended/hybrid learning. *Faculty:* 3 full-time (all women), 21 part-time/adjunct (20 women). *Students:* 61 full-time (54 women), 163 part-time (144 women); includes 9 minority (5 Black or African American, non-Hispanic/Latino; 2 Hispanic/Latino; 2 Two or more races, non-Hispanic/Latino), 2 international. Average age 34. 212 applicants, 60% accepted, 94 enrolled. In 2015, 51 master's, 1 doctorate awarded. *Degree requirements:* For master's, thesis optional. *Entrance requirements:* For master's, minimum GPA of 3.0 in the last 60 hours of undergraduate coursework; for doctorate, minimum GPA of 3.25 in graduate coursework. Additional exam requirements/recommendations for international students: Recommended—TOEFL (minimum score 580 paper-based; 92 iBT), IELTS (minimum score 6). *Application deadline:* For fall admission, 2/1 priority date for domestic students; for spring admission, 9/1 priority date for domestic students. Applications are processed on a rolling basis. Application fee: $50. Electronic applications accepted. *Expenses:* $15,940 tuition, $1,240 fees. *Financial support:* Institutionally sponsored loans, scholarships/grants, and traineeships available. Support available to part-time students. Financial award application deadline: 8/15; financial award applicants required to submit FAFSA. *Unit head:* Nancy Kramer, Vice Chancellor for Academic Affairs, 319-226-2040, Fax: 319-226-2070, E-mail: nancy.kramer@allencollege.edu. *Application contact:* Molly Quinn, Administrative Assistant for Student Services, 319-226-2014, Fax: 319-226-2010, E-mail: admissions@allencollege.edu.
Website: http://www.allencollege.edu/

Alverno College, JoAnn McGrath School of Nursing, Milwaukee, WI 53234-3922. Offers clinical nurse specialist (MSN); family nurse practitioner (MSN); mental health nurse practitioner (MSN). *Accreditation:* AACN. *Program availability:* Part-time, evening/weekend. *Faculty:* 8 full-time (all women), 8 part-time/adjunct (4 women). *Students:* 97 full-time (90 women), 87 part-time (82 women); includes 43 minority (18 Black or African American, non-Hispanic/Latino; 11 Asian, non-Hispanic/Latino; 9 Hispanic/Latino; 5 Two or more races, non-Hispanic/Latino), 1 international. Average age 36. 73 applicants, 95% accepted, 45 enrolled. In 2015, 33 master's awarded. *Degree requirements:* For master's, 500 clinical hours, capstone. *Entrance requirements:* For master's, BSN, current license. Additional exam requirements/recommendations for international students: Required—TOEFL. *Application deadline:* For fall admission, 7/15 priority date for domestic and international students; for spring admission, 12/15 priority date for domestic and international students. Applications are processed on a rolling basis. Application fee: $0. Electronic applications accepted. *Expenses:* Contact institution. *Financial support:* In 2015–16, 1 student received support. Federal Work-Study and scholarships/grants available. Support available to part-time students. Financial award applicants required to submit FAFSA. *Faculty research:* Impact of stroke on sexuality, children's asthma management, factors affecting baccalaureate student success. *Unit head:* Margaret Rauschenberger, Interim Dean, 414-382-6276, Fax: 414-382-6354, E-mail: margaret.rauschenberger@alverno.edu. *Application contact:* Dr. Carol Sabel, RN, Graduate Program Director, 414-382-6309, Fax: 414-382-6354, E-mail: carol.sabel@alverno.edu.
Website: http://www.alverno.edu/academics/academicdepartments/joannmcgrathschoolofnursing/

American International College, School of Health Sciences, Master of Science in Nursing Program, Springfield, MA 01109-3189. Offers family nurse practitioner (MSN); nursing administration (MSN); nursing education (MSN). *Accreditation:* AACN. *Program availability:* Part-time, evening/weekend, online only, blended/hybrid learning. *Faculty:* 1 (woman) full-time, 1 (woman) part-time/adjunct. *Students:* 52 full-time (49 women), 4 part-time (all women); includes 18 minority (12 Black or African American, non-Hispanic/Latino; 1 Asian, non-Hispanic/Latino; 4 Hispanic/Latino; 1 Two or more races, non-Hispanic/Latino). Average age 36. 66 applicants, 53% accepted, 27 enrolled. In 2015, 8 master's awarded. *Entrance requirements:* For master's, BSN, minimum GPA of 3.0. Additional exam requirements/recommendations for international students: Required—TOEFL, IELTS. *Application deadline:* For fall admission, 8/20 for domestic students, 7/1 priority date for international students; for spring admission, 1/4 for domestic students, 12/1 priority date for international students. Applications are processed on a rolling basis. Application fee: $50. Electronic applications accepted. *Expenses:* Contact institution. *Financial support:* Applicants required to submit FAFSA. *Unit head:* Dr. Ellen Furman, Associate Director of Graduate Nursing, 413-205-3918, Fax: 413-654-1430, E-mail: ellen.furman@aic.edu. *Application contact:* Kerry Barnes, Director of Graduate Admissions, 413-205-3703, Fax: 413-205-3051, E-mail: kerry.barnes@aic.edu.
Website: http://www.aic.edu/academics/hs/nursing

American Sentinel University, Graduate Programs, Aurora, CO 80014. Offers business administration (MBA); business intelligence (MS); computer science (MSCS); health information management (MS); healthcare (MBA); information systems (MSIS); nursing (MSN). *Program availability:* Part-time, evening/weekend, online learning. *Entrance requirements:* Additional exam requirements/recommendations for international students: Required—TOEFL (minimum score 600 paper-based). Electronic applications accepted.

American University of Beirut, Graduate Programs, Rafic Hariri School of Nursing, Beirut, Lebanon. Offers psychiatric mental health nursing (MSN). *Accreditation:* AACN. *Program availability:* Part-time. *Faculty:* 9 full-time (8 women), 13 part-time/adjunct (11 women). *Students:* 2 full-time (both women), 56 part-time (49 women). Average age 29.

22 applicants, 100% accepted, 10 enrolled. In 2015, 11 master's awarded. *Degree requirements:* For master's, one foreign language, comprehensive exam, thesis optional. *Entrance requirements:* For master's, letter of recommendation. Additional exam requirements/recommendations for international students: Required—TOEFL (minimum score 583 paper-based; 97 iBT); Recommended—IELTS. *Application deadline:* For fall admission, 4/1 for domestic and international students; for spring admission, 11/1 for domestic and international students. Applications are processed on a rolling basis. Application fee: $50. Electronic applications accepted. *Expenses:* Contact institution. *Financial support:* In 2015–16, 17 teaching assistantships with partial tuition reimbursements were awarded; unspecified assistantships also available. Financial award application deadline: 12/20. *Faculty research:* Pain management and palliative care, stress and post-traumatic stress disorder, health benefits and chronic illness, health promotion and community interventions. *Unit head:* Dr. Huda Huijer Abu-Saad, Director, 961-1374374 Ext. 5952, Fax: 961-1744476, E-mail: hh35@aub.edu.lb. *Application contact:* Dr. Salim Kanaan, Director, Admissions Office, 961-1350000 Ext. 2594, Fax: 961-1750775, E-mail: sk00@aub.edu.lb.
Website: http://staff.aub.edu.lb/~webson

Andrews University, School of Health Professions, Department of Nursing, Berrien Springs, MI 49104. Offers MS, DNP. *Accreditation:* ACEN. *Program availability:* Part-time, evening/weekend. *Faculty:* 3 full-time (all women), 1 (woman) part-time/adjunct. *Students:* 8 full-time (7 women), 6 part-time (all women); includes 12 minority (11 Black or African American, non-Hispanic/Latino; 1 Asian, non-Hispanic/Latino), 1 international. Average age 44. 24 applicants, 67% accepted, 11 enrolled. *Degree requirements:* For master's, thesis. *Entrance requirements:* For master's, GRE, minimum GPA of 2.5, 1 year of nursing experience, RN license. Additional exam requirements/recommendations for international students: Required—TOEFL (minimum score 550 paper-based). *Application deadline:* Applications are processed on a rolling basis. Application fee: $40. *Financial support:* Institutionally sponsored loans available. *Faculty research:* Theory for nursing, salary equitability. *Unit head:* Dr. Karen A. Allen, Chairperson, 269-471-3364. *Application contact:* Monica Wringer, Supervisor of Graduate Admission, 800-253-2874, Fax: 269-471-6321, E-mail: graduate@andrews.edu.
Website: http://www.andrews.edu/shp/nursing/

Angelo State University, College of Graduate Studies, Archer College of Health and Human Services, Department of Nursing, San Angelo, TX 76909. Offers family nurse practitioner (MSN); nurse educator (MSN). *Accreditation:* ACEN. *Program availability:* Part-time, evening/weekend, online learning. *Degree requirements:* For master's, comprehensive exam. *Entrance requirements:* For master's, essay, three letters of recommendation. Additional exam requirements/recommendations for international students: Required—TOEFL or IELTS. *Application deadline:* For fall admission, 4/1 priority date for domestic students, 6/10 for international students; for spring admission, 9/1 priority date for domestic students, 11/1 for international students. Applications are processed on a rolling basis. Application fee: $40 ($50 for international students). Electronic applications accepted. *Expenses: Tuition, area resident:* Full-time $3726; part-time $2484 per year. Tuition, state resident: full-time $3726; part-time $2484 per year. Tuition, nonresident: full-time $10,746; part-time $7164 per year. *International tuition:* $10,746 full-time. *Required fees:* $2538; $1702 per unit. *Financial support:* Research assistantships, career-related internships or fieldwork, Federal Work-Study, and scholarships/grants available. Support available to part-time students. Financial award application deadline: 3/1. *Unit head:* Dr. Wrennah L. Gabbert, Chair, 325-942-2224, Fax: 325-942-2236, E-mail: wrennah.gabbert@angelo.edu. *Application contact:* Dr. Molly J. Walker, Graduate Advisor, 325-486-6872, Fax: 325-942-2236, E-mail: molly.walker@angelo.edu.
Website: http://www.angelo.edu/dept/nursing/

Aquinas College, School of Nursing, Nashville, TN 37205-2005. Offers nursing education (MSN).

Arizona State University at the Tempe campus, College of Nursing and Health Innovation, Phoenix, AZ 85004. Offers advanced nursing practice (DNP); clinical research management (MS); community and public health practice (Graduate Certificate); family mental health nurse practitioner (Graduate Certificate); family nurse practitioner (Graduate Certificate); geriatric nursing (Graduate Certificate); healthcare innovation (MHI); nurse education in academic and practice settings (Graduate Certificate); nurse educator (MS); nursing and healthcare innovation (PhD). *Accreditation:* AACN. *Program availability:* Online learning. *Degree requirements:* For master's, comprehensive exam (for some programs), thesis (for some programs), interactive Program of Study (iPOS) submitted before completing 50 percent of required credit hours; for doctorate, comprehensive exam, thesis/dissertation, interactive Program of Study (iPOS) submitted before completing 50 percent of required credit hours. *Entrance requirements:* For master's and doctorate, GRE, minimum GPA of 3.0 or equivalent in last 2 years of work leading to bachelor's degree. Additional exam requirements/recommendations for international students: Required—TOEFL, IELTS, or PTE. Electronic applications accepted. *Expenses:* Contact institution.

Arkansas State University, Graduate School, College of Nursing and Health Professions, School of Nursing, State University, AR 72467. Offers aging studies (Graduate Certificate); health care management (Graduate Certificate); health sciences (MS); health sciences education (Graduate Certificate); nurse anesthesia (MSN); nursing (MSN); nursing practice (DNP). *Accreditation:* AANA/CANAEP (one or more programs are accredited); ACEN. *Program availability:* Part-time. *Faculty:* 16 full-time (14 women). *Students:* 80 full-time (30 women), 139 part-time (121 women); includes 38 minority (26 Black or African American, non-Hispanic/Latino; 3 American Indian or Alaska Native, non-Hispanic/Latino; 3 Asian, non-Hispanic/Latino; 4 Hispanic/Latino; 1 Native Hawaiian or other Pacific Islander, non-Hispanic/Latino; 1 Two or more races, non-Hispanic/Latino), 2 international. Average age 34. 147 applicants, 33% accepted, 43 enrolled. In 2015, 84 master's awarded. *Degree requirements:* For master's and Graduate Certificate, comprehensive exam, thesis or alternative; for doctorate, comprehensive exam, thesis/dissertation. *Entrance requirements:* For master's, GRE General Test or MAT, appropriate bachelor's degree, current Arkansas nursing license, CPR certification, physical examination, professional liability insurance, critical care experience, ACLS Certification, PALS Certification, interview, immunization records, personal goal statement, health assessment; for doctorate, GRE or MAT, NCLEX-RN Exam, appropriate master's degree, current Arkansas nursing license, CPR certification, physical examination, professional liability insurance, critical care experience, ACLS Certification, PALS Certification, interview, immunization records, personal goal statement, health assessment, TB skin test, background check; for Graduate Certificate, GRE or MAT, appropriate bachelor's degree, official transcripts, immunization records, proof of employment in healthcare, TB Skin Test, TB Mask Fit Test, CPR Certification. Additional exam requirements/recommendations for international students: Required—TOEFL (minimum score 550

paper-based; 79 iBT), IELTS (minimum score 6), PTE (minimum score 56). *Application deadline:* Applications are processed on a rolling basis. Electronic applications accepted. *Expenses:* Contact institution. *Financial support:* In 2015–16, 1 student received support. Fellowships, career-related internships or fieldwork, scholarships/grants, and unspecified assistantships available. Financial award application deadline: 7/1; financial award applicants required to submit FAFSA. *Unit head:* Dr. Jill Oswaks, Chair of Graduate Programs, 870-972-3074, Fax: 870-972-2954, E-mail: jdettyoswaks@astate.edu. *Application contact:* Vickey Ring, Graduate Admissions Coordinator, 870-972-2737, Fax: 870-972-3917, E-mail: vickeyring@astate.edu.
Website: http://www.astate.edu/college/conhp/departments/nursing/

Arkansas Tech University, College of Natural and Health Sciences, Russellville, AR 72801. Offers fisheries and wildlife biology (MS); health informatics (MS); nursing (MSN). *Program availability:* Part-time. *Students:* 7 full-time (4 women), 49 part-time (29 women); includes 9 minority (6 Black or African American, non-Hispanic/Latino; 1 Asian, non-Hispanic/Latino; 2 Two or more races, non-Hispanic/Latino), 1 international. Average age 36. In 2015, 15 master's awarded. *Degree requirements:* For master's, thesis (for some programs), project. *Entrance requirements:* For master's, GRE General Test. Additional exam requirements/recommendations for international students: Required—TOEFL (minimum score 550 paper-based; 79 iBT), IELTS (minimum score 6). *Application deadline:* For fall admission, 3/1 priority date for domestic students, 5/1 priority date for international students; for spring admission, 10/1 priority date for domestic and international students. Applications are processed on a rolling basis. Application fee: $25 ($75 for international students). Electronic applications accepted. *Financial support:* In 2015–16, research assistantships with full tuition reimbursements (averaging $4,800 per year), teaching assistantships with full tuition reimbursements (averaging $4,800 per year) were awarded; career-related internships or fieldwork, Federal Work-Study, scholarships/grants, health care benefits, and unspecified assistantships also available. Support available to part-time students. Financial award application deadline: 4/15; financial award applicants required to submit FAFSA. *Unit head:* Dr. Jeff Robertson, Dean, 479-968-0498, E-mail: jrobertson@atu.edu. *Application contact:* Dr. Mary B. Gunter, Dean of Graduate College, 479-968-0398, Fax: 479-964-0542, E-mail: gradcollege@atu.edu.
Website: http://www.atu.edu/nhs/

Armstrong State University, School of Graduate Studies, Program in Nursing, Savannah, GA 31419-1997. Offers adult-gerontological acute care nurse practitioner (Certificate); adult-gerontological clinical nurse specialist (Certificate); adult-gerontological primary care nurse practitioner (Certificate); family nurse practitioner (MSN). *Accreditation:* AACN. *Program availability:* Part-time, evening/weekend. *Faculty:* 5 full-time (all women), 1 (woman) part-time/adjunct. *Students:* 35 full-time (32 women), 19 part-time (16 women); includes 13 minority (10 Black or African American, non-Hispanic/Latino; 2 Hispanic/Latino; 1 Two or more races, non-Hispanic/Latino), 1 international. Average age 35. 23 applicants, 83% accepted, 16 enrolled. In 2015, 19 master's awarded. *Degree requirements:* For master's, comprehensive exam, project or thesis. *Entrance requirements:* For master's, GRE General Test or MAT, minimum GPA of 3.0, letter of recommendation, letter of intent. Additional exam requirements/recommendations for international students: Required—TOEFL (minimum score 523 paper-based; 70 iBT). *Application deadline:* For fall admission, 2/28 for domestic and international students; for spring admission, 11/15 for domestic students, 9/15 for international students. Applications are processed on a rolling basis. Application fee: $30. Electronic applications accepted. *Expenses:* Tuition, state resident: part-time $211 per credit hour. Tuition, nonresident: part-time $782 per credit hour. *Required fees:* $1224 per unit. $612 per semester. Tuition and fees vary according to course load, campus/location and program. *Financial support:* In 2015–16, research assistantships with full tuition reimbursements (averaging $5,000 per year) were awarded; Federal Work-Study, scholarships/grants, and unspecified assistantships also available. Support available to part-time students. Financial award application deadline: 3/1; financial award applicants required to submit FAFSA. *Faculty research:* Midwifery, mental health, nursing simulation, smoking cessation during pregnancy, asthma education, vulnerable populations, geriatrics, disaster nursing, complementary and alternative modalities, nephrology. *Unit head:* Dr. Catherine Gilbert, Department Head, 912-344-3145, E-mail: catherine.gilbert@armstrong.edu. *Application contact:* McKenzie Peterman, Assistant Director of Graduate Admissions, 912-344-2503, Fax: 912-344-3417, E-mail: graduate@armstrong.edu.
Website: http://www.armstrong.edu/Health_professions/nursing/nursing_graduate_programs

Athabasca University, Faculty of Health Disciplines, Athabasca, AB T9S 3A3, Canada. Offers advanced nursing practice (MN, Advanced Diploma); generalist (MN); health studies (MHS). *Program availability:* Part-time, online learning. *Faculty:* 11 full-time (all women), 1 (woman) part-time/adjunct. *Students:* 1,687 part-time. Average age 38. In 2015, 243 master's, 5 other advanced degrees awarded. *Degree requirements:* For master's, comprehensive exam (for some programs). *Entrance requirements:* For master's, bachelor's degree in health-related field and 2 years of professional health service experience (MHS); bachelor's degree in nursing and 2 years' nursing experience (MN); minimum GPA of 3.0 in final 30 credits; for Advanced Diploma, RN license, 2 years of health care experience. *Application deadline:* For fall admission, 3/1 for domestic and international students. Application fee: $80. Electronic applications accepted. *Expenses:* Contact institution. *Unit head:* Dr. Margaret Edwards, Dean, 800-788-9041 Ext. 6381, Fax: 780-675-6468, E-mail: marge@athabascau.ca. *Application contact:* Donna Dunn Hart, Academic Student Advisor, Graduate Programs, 800-788-9041 Ext. 6300, Fax: 780-675-6468, E-mail: donnad@athabascau.ca.
Website: http://fhd.athabascau.ca/

Auburn University, Graduate School, School of Nursing, Auburn University, AL 36849. Offers nursing educator (MSN); primary care practitioner (MSN). *Accreditation:* AACN. *Faculty:* 21 full-time (18 women). *Students:* 13 full-time (all women), 107 part-time (101 women); includes 21 minority (14 Black or African American, non-Hispanic/Latino; 1 American Indian or Alaska Native, non-Hispanic/Latino; 2 Asian, non-Hispanic/Latino; 1 Hispanic/Latino; 3 Two or more races, non-Hispanic/Latino), 1 international. Average age 34. 78 applicants, 53% accepted, 35 enrolled. In 2015, 32 master's awarded. *Expenses:* Tuition, state resident: full-time $8802; part-time $489 per credit hour. Tuition, nonresident: full-time $26,406; part-time $1467 per credit hour. *Required fees:* $808 per semester. Tuition and fees vary according to degree level and program. *Unit head:* Dr. Gregg Newschwander, Dean, 334-844-3658, E-mail: gen0002@auburn.edu. *Application contact:* Dr. George Flowers, Dean of the Graduate School, 334-844-4700, E-mail: gradadm@auburn.edu.
Website: http://www.auburn.edu/academic/nursing/

Auburn University at Montgomery, College of Nursing and Health Sciences, Montgomery, AL 36124-4023. Offers nurse educator (MSN); nurse practitioner (MSN). *Expenses:* Tuition, state resident: full-time $6462; part-time $359 per credit hour. Tuition, nonresident: full-time $14,526; part-time $807 per credit hour. *Required fees:* $554. *Unit head:* Dr. Jean Leuner, Dean, 334-244-3658, E-mail: jleuner@aum.edu. *Application contact:* Dr. Barbara Wilder, Graduate Program Director, 334-844-6766, E-mail: wildebf@auburn.edu.
Website: http://www.nursing.aum.edu/

Augsburg College, Programs in Nursing, Minneapolis, MN 55454-1351. Offers MA, DNP. *Accreditation:* AACN. *Degree requirements:* For master's, thesis or alternative.

Augusta University, The Graduate School, Doctor of Nursing Practice Program, Augusta, GA 30912. Offers adult gerontology acute care nurse practitioner (DNP); family nurse practitioner (DNP); nursing (DNP); nursing anesthesia (DNP); pediatric nurse practitioner (DNP); psychiatric mental health nurse practitioner (DNP). *Students:* 40 part-time. *Degree requirements:* For doctorate, thesis/dissertation or alternative. *Entrance requirements:* For doctorate, GRE General Test or MAT, master's degree in nursing or related field, current professional nurse licensure. Additional exam requirements/recommendations for international students: Required—TOEFL (minimum score 600 paper-based; 100 iBT). *Application deadline:* For fall admission, 3/1 for domestic and international students; for spring admission, 7/1 for domestic and international students. Applications are processed on a rolling basis. Application fee: $50. Electronic applications accepted. *Unit head:* Dr. Marguerite Murphy, RN, Director, 706-721-3676, Fax: 706-721-8169. *Application contact:* Karen Sturgill, Program Manager, 706-721-3676, Fax: 706-721-8169, E-mail: dnp@augusta.edu.
Website: http://www.augusta.edu/nursing/dnp_programs.php

Augusta University, The Graduate School, Nursing PhD Program, Augusta, GA 30912. Offers PhD. *Degree requirements:* For doctorate, thesis/dissertation. *Entrance requirements:* For doctorate, GRE General Test, current GA nurse licensure. Additional exam requirements/recommendations for international students: Required—TOEFL (minimum score 550 paper-based; 79 iBT). *Application deadline:* For fall admission, 5/1 for domestic and international students; for spring admission, 10/1 for domestic and international students. Application fee: $50. Electronic applications accepted. *Financial support:* Research assistantships with partial tuition reimbursements available. Financial award applicants required to submit FAFSA. *Unit head:* Dr. Julie Zadinsky, Director, 706 721 0740, Fax: 706 721 8160. *Application contact:* Bridgett Hill, Program Manager, 706-721-9749, Fax: 706-721-7390.
Website: http://www.augusta.edu/nursing/phdnursing.php

Aurora University, School of Nursing and Allied Health, Aurora, IL 60506-4892. Offers applied behavior analysis (MS); nursing (MSN). *Program availability:* Part-time, evening/weekend. *Faculty:* 4 full-time (3 women), 6 part-time/adjunct (5 women). *Students:* 16 full-time (all women), 86 part-time (83 women); includes 20 minority (5 Black or African American, non-Hispanic/Latino; 3 Asian, non-Hispanic/Latino; 11 Hispanic/Latino; 1 Two or more races, non-Hispanic/Latino). Average age 37. 64 applicants, 89% accepted, 38 enrolled. In 2015, 15 master's awarded. *Entrance requirements:* Additional exam requirements/recommendations for international students: Required—TOEFL (minimum score 550 paper-based; 79 iBT). *Application deadline:* For fall admission, 6/1 for international students; for spring admission, 10/1 for international students. Applications are processed on a rolling basis. Application fee: $0. Electronic applications accepted. *Expenses:* Tuition, area resident: Full-time $10,800; part-time $600 per credit hour. Tuition and fees vary according to degree level, campus/location and program. *Financial support:* In 2015–16, 28 students received support. Federal Work-Study, scholarships/grants, and unspecified assistantships available. Support available to part-time students. Financial award applicants required to submit FAFSA. *Unit head:* Dr. Brenda Shostrom, Executive Director, 630-844-5135, E-mail: bshostrom@aurora.edu. *Application contact:* Jason Harmon, Director of Orchard Center and Graduate Enrollment, 630-947-8905, E-mail: jharmon@aurora.edu.
Website: http://www.aurora.edu/academics/colleges-schools/nursing/

Austin Peay State University, College of Graduate Studies, College of Behavioral and Health Sciences, School of Nursing, Clarksville, TN 37044. Offers family nurse practitioner (MSN); nursing administration (MSN); nursing education (MSN); nursing informatics (MSN). *Program availability:* Part-time, online learning. *Faculty:* 11 full-time (all women), 6 part-time/adjunct (all women). *Students:* 23 full-time (20 women), 142 part-time (125 women); includes 27 minority (19 Black or African American, non-Hispanic/Latino; 4 Hispanic/Latino; 4 Two or more races, non-Hispanic/Latino). Average age 35. 25 applicants, 76% accepted, 14 enrolled. In 2015, 67 master's awarded. *Degree requirements:* For master's, comprehensive exam. *Entrance requirements:* For master's, minimum GPA of 3.0, RN license eligibility, 3 letters of recommendation. Additional exam requirements/recommendations for international students: Required—TOEFL (minimum score 500 paper-based). *Application deadline:* For fall admission, 8/3 priority date for domestic students. Applications are processed on a rolling basis. Application fee: $25. Electronic applications accepted. *Expenses:* Tuition, state resident: full-time $8080; part-time $404 per credit hour. Tuition, nonresident: full-time $21,680; part-time $1084 per credit hour. *Required fees:* $1453; $72.65 per credit hour. *Financial support:* In 2015–16, research assistantships with full tuition reimbursements (averaging $5,184 per year) were awarded; career-related internships or fieldwork, Federal Work-Study, institutionally sponsored loans, scholarships/grants, and unspecified assistantships also available. Support available to part-time students. Financial award application deadline: 3/1; financial award applicants required to submit FAFSA. *Unit head:* Dr. Grace Moodt, Interim Director, 931-221-6290, Fax: 931-221-7595, E-mail: moodtg@apsu.edu. *Application contact:* June D. Lee, Graduate Coordinator, 800-859-4723, Fax: 931-221-7641, E-mail: gradadmissions@apsu.edu.
Website: http://www.apsu.edu/nursing

Azusa Pacific University, School of Nursing, Azusa, CA 91702-7000. Offers nursing (MSN); nursing education (PhD). *Accreditation:* AACN. *Program availability:* Part-time, evening/weekend. *Degree requirements:* For master's, thesis optional. *Entrance requirements:* For master's, BSN.

Ball State University, Graduate School, College of Applied Sciences and Technology, School of Nursing, Muncie, IN 47306. Offers adult/gerontology nurse practitioner (Post Master's Certificate); evidence-based clinical practice (Postbaccalaureate Certificate); family nurse practitioner (Post Master's Certificate); family nurse practitioner for the adult nurse practitioner or adult/gerontology nurse practitioner (Post Master's Certificate); nurse educator (Post Master's Certificate); nursing (MS), including family nurse practitioner, nurse administrator, nurse educator; nursing education (Postbaccalaureate Certificate); nursing practice (DNP). *Accreditation:* AACN. *Program availability:* Part-time-only, online only, 100% online. *Faculty:* 12 full-time (all women), 7 part-time/adjunct (6 women). *Students:* 9 full-time (8 women), 334 part-time (311 women); includes 23 minority (11 Black or African American, non-Hispanic/Latino; 5 Asian, non-Hispanic/Latino; 6 Hispanic/Latino; 1 Two or more races, non-Hispanic/Latino). Average age 33. 88 applicants, 85% accepted, 63 enrolled. In 2015, 115 master's, 8 doctorates awarded. *Entrance requirements:* For master's, bachelor's degree in nursing, minimum GPA of 3.0, minimum C grade in at least 2 quarter or semester hours in an undergraduate research course, unencumbered license as a registered nurse in state of practice; for doctorate, advanced practice nurse (nurse practitioner, clinical nurse specialist, nurse midwife); master's degree in nursing from accredited prorgam with minimum GPA of 3.2; graduate-level statistics, nursing research, and health assessment courses; unencumbered license as registered nurse in state of practice. Additional exam requirements/recommendations for international students: Required—TOEFL (minimum score 550 paper-based; 79 iBT), IELTS (minimum score 6.5). *Application deadline:* For fall admission, 2/9 for domestic students; for spring admission, 8/9 for domestic students. Applications are processed on a rolling basis. Application fee: $60. Electronic applications accepted. *Expenses:* Contact institution. *Financial support:* Application

Nursing—General

deadline: 3/1; applicants required to submit FAFSA. *Unit head:* Dr. Linda Siktberg, Director, 765-285-8718, Fax: 765-285-2169, E-mail: lsiktberg@bsu.edu. *Application contact:* Shantelle Estes, Graduate Advisor, 765-285-9130, Fax: 765-285-2169, E-mail: smestes@bsu.edu.
Website: http://www.bsu.edu/nursing

Barry University, School of Adult and Continuing Education, Division of Nursing, Miami Shores, FL 33161-6695. Offers MSN, PhD, Certificate, MSN/MBA. *Program availability:* Part-time, evening/weekend. *Degree requirements:* For master's, research project or thesis; for doctorate, thesis/dissertation. *Entrance requirements:* For master's, GRE General Test or MAT, BSN, minimum GPA of 3.0, course work in statistics and research, Florida RN license; for doctorate, GRE General Test or MAT, minimum GPA of 3.3, MSN. Electronic applications accepted. *Faculty research:* Adult education, nurse practitioner, stress reduction in pregnancy, prevention of cardiac problems, in children, level of school age children.

Baylor University, Graduate School, Louise Herrington School of Nursing, Dallas, TX 75246. Offers family nurse practitioner (MSN); neonatal nurse practitioner (MSN); nurse-midwifery (DNP). *Accreditation:* AACN. *Program availability:* Part-time, online learning. *Degree requirements:* For doctorate, comprehensive exam (for some programs), capstone project. *Entrance requirements:* For master's, GRE General Test or MAT; for doctorate, GRE General Test. Additional exam requirements/recommendations for international students: Required—TOEFL. Electronic applications accepted. *Faculty research:* Women and strokes, obesity and pregnancy, educational environmental factors, international undeserved populations, midwifery.

Bellarmine University, Donna and Allan Lansing School of Nursing and Health Sciences, Louisville, KY 40205. Offers family nurse practitioner (MSN); health science (MHS); nursing administration (MSN); nursing education (MSN); nursing practice (DNP); physical therapy (DPT). *Accreditation:* AACN; APTA. *Program availability:* Part-time, evening/weekend. *Faculty:* 27 full-time (24 women), 8 part-time/adjunct (7 women). *Students:* 210 full-time (144 women), 91 part-time (83 women); includes 22 minority (6 Black or African American, non-Hispanic/Latino; 1 American Indian or Alaska Native, non-Hispanic/Latino; 7 Asian, non-Hispanic/Latino; 4 Hispanic/Latino; 4 Two or more races, non-Hispanic/Latino), 2 international. Average age 28. In 2015, 33 master's, 64 doctorates awarded. *Degree requirements:* For doctorate, comprehensive exam, thesis/dissertation. *Entrance requirements:* For master's, GRE General Test, RN license; for doctorate, GRE General Test, Physical Therapist Centralized Application Service (for DPT). Additional exam requirements/recommendations for international students: Required—TOEFL (minimum score 550 paper-based; 80 iBT). Application fee: $40. Electronic applications accepted. *Expenses:* Contact institution. *Financial support:* Career-related internships or fieldwork and scholarships/grants available. *Faculty research:* Nursing: pain, empathy, leadership styles, control; physical therapy: service-learning; exercise in chronic and pre-operative conditions, athletes; women's health; aging. *Unit head:* Dr. Mark Wiegand, Dean, 800-274-4723 Ext. 8368, E-mail: mwiegand@bellarmine.edu. *Application contact:* Julie Armstrong-Binnix, Health Science Recruiter, 800-274-4723 Ext. 8364, E-mail: julieab@bellarmine.edu.
Website: http://www.bellarmine.edu/lansing

Bellin College, School of Nursing, Green Bay, WI 54305. Offers family nurse practitioner (MSN); nurse educator (MSN). *Accreditation:* AACN.

Belmont University, College of Health Sciences, Nashville, TN 37212-3757. Offers nursing (MSN, DNP); occupational therapy (MSOT, OTD); physical therapy (DPT). *Program availability:* Part-time, online learning. *Faculty:* 54 full-time (50 women), 92 part-time/adjunct (81 women). *Students:* 371 full-time (324 women), 10 part-time (all women); includes 30 minority (10 Black or African American, non-Hispanic/Latino; 9 Asian, non-Hispanic/Latino; 6 Hispanic/Latino; 5 Two or more races, non-Hispanic/Latino), 2 international. Average age 26. *Degree requirements:* For master's, comprehensive exam, thesis; for doctorate, comprehensive exam. *Entrance requirements:* For master's, GRE, BSN, minimum GPA of 3.0. Additional exam requirements/recommendations for international students: Required—TOEFL (minimum score 550 paper-based). *Application deadline:* Applications are processed on a rolling basis. Application fee: $50. Electronic applications accepted. *Expenses:* Contact institution. *Financial support:* Teaching assistantships with full tuition reimbursements, career-related internships or fieldwork, scholarships/grants, and traineeships available. Financial award application deadline: 3/1; financial award applicants required to submit FAFSA. *Unit head:* Dr. Cathy Taylor, Dean, 615-460-6916, Fax: 615-460-6750. *Application contact:* David Mee, Dean of Enrollment Services, 615-460-6785, Fax: 615-460-5434, E-mail: david.mee@belmont.edu.
Website: http://www.belmont.edu/healthsciences/

Benedictine University, Graduate Programs, Program in Nursing, Lisle, IL 60532. Offers MSN. *Accreditation:* AACN.

Bethel College, Adult and Graduate Programs, Program in Nursing, Mishawaka, IN 46545-5591. Offers MSN. *Accreditation:* ACEN. *Program availability:* Part-time, evening/weekend. *Faculty:* 4 part-time/adjunct (3 women). *Students:* 22 part-time (21 women); includes 4 minority (2 Black or African American, non-Hispanic/Latino; 1 American Indian or Alaska Native, non-Hispanic/Latino; 1 Two or more races, non-Hispanic/Latino), 2 international. 11 applicants, 100% accepted, 10 enrolled. In 2015, 5 master's awarded. *Degree requirements:* For master's, thesis. *Entrance requirements:* Additional exam requirements/recommendations for international students: Required—TOEFL (minimum score 540 paper-based). *Application deadline:* For fall admission, 8/15 for domestic students, 5/1 for international students; for spring admission, 10/1 for international students. Electronic applications accepted. *Expenses: Tuition, area resident:* Full-time $6480; part-time $3240 per credit hour. *Required fees:* $75 per semester. Tuition and fees vary according to course load and program. *Financial support:* Career-related internships or fieldwork available. Financial award applicants required to submit FAFSA. *Unit head:* Dr. Deborah Gillum, Dean of Nursing, 574-807-7015, E-mail: gillumd@bethelcollege.edu. *Application contact:* Dr. Rebecca Zellers, Director, 574-807-7809, E-mail: zellerr@bethelcollege.edu.

Bethel University, Graduate School, St. Paul, MN 55112-6999. Offers business administration (MBA); child and adolescent mental health (Certificate); classroom management (Certificate); communication (MA); counseling psychology (MA); educational leadership (Ed D); gerontology (MA, Certificate); international baccalaureate teaching and learning (Certificate); K-12 education (MA); leadership foundations (Certificate); literacy education (MA); nurse educator (Certificate); nurse-midwifery (MS); nursing (MS); physician assistant (MS); special education (MA); STEM education (Certificate); strategic leadership (MA); teaching (MA). *Program availability:* Part-time, evening/weekend, 100% online, blended/hybrid learning. *Faculty:* 21 full-time (15 women), 74 part-time/adjunct (38 women). *Students:* 772 full-time (537 women), 379 part-time (232 women); includes 188 minority (94 Black or African American, non-Hispanic/Latino; 3 American Indian or Alaska Native, non-Hispanic/Latino; 43 Asian, non-Hispanic/Latino; 31 Hispanic/Latino; 1 Native Hawaiian or other Pacific Islander, non-Hispanic/Latino; 16 Two or more races, non-Hispanic/Latino), 33 international. Average age 37. 663 applicants, 49% accepted, 232 enrolled. In 2015, 272 master's, 16 doctorates, 65 other advanced degrees awarded. *Degree requirements:* For master's, comprehensive exam (for some programs), thesis (for some programs); for doctorate,

comprehensive exam, thesis/dissertation. *Entrance requirements:* Additional exam requirements/recommendations for international students: Required—TOEFL (minimum score 550 paper-based, 80 iBT) or IELTS. *Application deadline:* Applications are processed on a rolling basis. Application fee: $0. Electronic applications accepted. *Expenses:* Contact institution. *Financial support:* In 2015–16, 132 students received support. Teaching assistantships, career-related internships or fieldwork, and scholarships/grants available. Support available to part-time students. Financial award applicants required to submit FAFSA. *Unit head:* Dick Crombie, Vice-President/Dean, 651-635-8000, Fax: 651-635-8004, E-mail: gs@bethel.edu. *Application contact:* Director of Admissions, 651-635-8000, Fax: 651-635-8004, E-mail: gs@bethel.edu.
Website: https://www.bethel.edu/graduate/

Binghamton University, State University of New York, Graduate School, Decker School of Nursing, Binghamton, NY 13902-6000. Offers MS, DNP, PhD, Certificate. *Accreditation:* AACN. *Program availability:* Part-time, evening/weekend. *Faculty:* 43 full-time (40 women), 21 part-time/adjunct (14 women). *Students:* 75 full-time (64 women), 111 part-time (93 women); includes 28 minority (13 Black or African American, non-Hispanic/Latino; 1 American Indian or Alaska Native, non-Hispanic/Latino; 7 Asian, non-Hispanic/Latino; 7 Hispanic/Latino), 10 international. Average age 37. 96 applicants, 79% accepted, 45 enrolled. In 2015, 61 master's, 13 doctorates, 9 other advanced degrees awarded. Terminal master's awarded for partial completion of doctoral program. *Degree requirements:* For master's, comprehensive exam, thesis; for doctorate, comprehensive exam (for some programs), thesis/dissertation. *Entrance requirements:* For master's and doctorate, GRE General Test, nursing licensure. Additional exam requirements/recommendations for international students: Required—TOEFL (minimum score 90 iBT). Application fee: $75. Electronic applications accepted. *Expenses:* Contact institution. *Financial support:* In 2015–16, 35 students received support, including 1 fellowship with partial tuition reimbursement available (averaging $16,500 per year), research assistantships with full tuition reimbursements available (averaging $12,500 per year), 1 teaching assistantship with full tuition reimbursement available (averaging $16,500 per year); career-related internships or fieldwork, Federal Work-Study, institutionally sponsored loans, traineeships, health care benefits, tuition waivers (full and partial), and unspecified assistantships also available. Financial award applicants required to submit FAFSA. *Unit head:* Dr. Pamela Stewart-Fahs, Dean, 607-777-2311, Fax: 607-777-4440, E-mail: psfahs@binghamton.edu. *Application contact:* Kishan Zuber, Director of Graduate Studies, 607-777-2151, Fax: 607-777-2501, E-mail: kzuber@binghamton.edu.
Website: http://www.binghamton.edu/dson/

Blessing-Rieman College of Nursing, Program in Nursing, Quincy, IL 62305-7005. Offers MSN. *Accreditation:* AACN. *Program availability:* Part-time. *Degree requirements:* For master's, thesis. *Entrance requirements:* For master's, proof of RN license; BSN from CCNE- or NLNAC-accredited program; minimum GPA of 3.0 for last 60 semester hours of undergraduate course work; completion of statistics, nursing research, physical assessment or equivalent with minimum grade of C. Additional exam requirements/recommendations for international students: Required—TOEFL. Electronic applications accepted.

Blessing–Rieman College of Nursing and Health Sciences, Master of Science in Nursing Program, Quincy, IL 62305-7005. Offers nursing administration (MSN); nursing education (MSN). *Program availability:* Part-time-only, online only, 100% online. In 2015, 8 master's awarded. *Degree requirements:* For master's, thesis or project. *Entrance requirements:* Additional exam requirements/recommendations for international students: Required—TOEFL (minimum score 500 paper-based; 80 iBT). *Application deadline:* Applications are processed on a rolling basis. Electronic applications accepted. *Expenses:* Contact institution. *Financial support:* In 2015–16, 20,350 students received support. Scholarships/grants available. Financial award application deadline: 4/30; financial award applicants required to submit FAFSA. *Unit head:* Dr. Karen Mayville, Administrative Coordinator, Accreditation, 217-228-5520 Ext. 6968, Fax: 217-223-4661, E-mail: kmayville@brcn.edu. *Application contact:* Heather Mutter, Admissions Counselor, 217-228-5520 Ext. 6964, Fax: 217-223-1781, E-mail: hmutter@brcn.edu.
Website: http://brcn.edu

Bloomsburg University of Pennsylvania, School of Graduate Studies, College of Science and Technology, Department of Nursing, Bloomsburg, PA 17815. Offers adult and family nurse practitioner (MSN); community health (MSN); nurse anesthesia (MSN); nursing (MSN); nursing administration (MSN). *Accreditation:* AACN; AANA/CANAEP. *Degree requirements:* For master's, thesis (for some programs), clinical experience. *Entrance requirements:* For master's, minimum QPA of 3.0, personal statement, 2 letters of recommendation, nursing license. Additional exam requirements/recommendations for international students: Required—TOEFL. Electronic applications accepted.

Boise State University, College of Health Sciences, School of Nursing, Boise, ID 83725-1840. Offers acute care adult gerontology (Graduate Certificate); adult gerontology acute care (MSN); adult gerontology primary care (MSN); healthcare simulation (Graduate Certificate); nursing practice (DNP); primary care adult gerontology (Graduate Certificate). *Students:* 1 (woman) full-time, 91 part-time (73 women); includes 11 minority (5 Black or African American, non-Hispanic/Latino; 2 Asian, non-Hispanic/Latino; 3 Hispanic/Latino; 1 Native Hawaiian or other Pacific Islander, non-Hispanic/Latino). Average age 43. 32 applicants, 44% accepted, 12 enrolled. In 2015, 3 master's awarded. *Entrance requirements:* For master's, minimum GPA of 3.0. Additional exam requirements/recommendations for international students: Required—TOEFL (minimum score 550 paper-based; 80 iBT), IELTS (minimum score 6). *Application deadline:* For spring admission, 10/15 priority date for domestic and international students. Applications are processed on a rolling basis. Application fee: $65 ($95 for international students). Electronic applications accepted. *Expenses:* Tuition, state resident: full-time $6058; part-time $358 per credit hour. Tuition, nonresident: full-time $20,108; part-time $608 per credit hour. *Required fees:* $2108. Tuition and fees vary according to program. *Financial support:* In 2015–16, 1 student received support. Scholarships/grants and unspecified assistantships available. Financial award application deadline: 10/15; financial award applicants required to submit FAFSA. *Unit head:* Dr. Ann Hubbert, Director, 208-426-3404, E-mail: annhubbert@boisestate.edu. *Application contact:* Dr. Dawn Weiler, Program Coordinator, 208-426-1239, E-mail: dweiler@boisestate.edu.
Website: http://hs.boisestate.edu/nursing/

Boston College, William F. Connell School of Nursing, Chestnut Hill, MA 02467. Offers adult-gerontology nursing (MS); family health nursing (MS); forensic nursing (MS); nurse anesthesia (MS); nursing (PhD); pediatric nursing (MS), including pediatric and women's health; psychiatric-mental health nursing (MS); women's health nursing (MS); MBA/MS; MS/MA; MS/PhD. *Accreditation:* AACN; AANA/CANAEP (one or more programs are accredited). *Program availability:* Part-time. *Faculty:* 53 full-time (48 women), 61 part-time/adjunct (44 women). *Students:* 185 full-time (167 women), 66 part-time (56 women); includes 31 minority (10 Black or African American, non-Hispanic/Latino; 12 Asian, non-Hispanic/Latino; 7 Hispanic/Latino; 2 Two or more races, non-Hispanic/Latino), 7 international. Average age 32. 313 applicants, 66% accepted, 91 enrolled. In 2015, 98 master's, 5 doctorates awarded. *Degree requirements:* For master's,

comprehensive exam; for doctorate, comprehensive exam, thesis/dissertation, computer literacy exam or foreign language. *Entrance requirements:* For master's, bachelor's degree in nursing; for doctorate, GRE General Test, MS in nursing. Additional exam requirements/recommendations for international students: Required—TOEFL (minimum score 600 paper-based; 100 iBT), IELTS (minimum score 7.5). *Application deadline:* For fall admission, 9/30 for domestic and international students; for winter admission, 1/15 for domestic and international students; for spring admission, 3/15 for domestic and international students. Applications are processed on a rolling basis. Application fee: $40. Electronic applications accepted. *Expenses:* Contact institution. *Financial support:* In 2015–16, 1 fellowship with full tuition reimbursement (averaging $23,700 per year), 25 teaching assistantships (averaging $4,370 per year) were awarded; research assistantships, scholarships/grants, health care benefits, tuition waivers (partial), and unspecified assistantships also available. Support available to part-time students. Financial award application deadline: 3/1; financial award applicants required to submit FAFSA. *Faculty research:* Sexual and reproductive health, health promotion/illness prevention, aging, eating disorders, symptom management. *Total annual research expenditures:* $1 million. *Unit head:* Dr. Susan Gennaro, Dean, 617-552-4251, Fax: 617-552-0931, E-mail: susan.gennaro@bc.edu. *Application contact:* MaryBeth Crowley, Graduate Programs Assistant, 617-552-4928, Fax: 617-552-2121, E-mail: csongrad@bc.edu.
Website: http://www.bc.edu/schools/son/

Bowie State University, Graduate Programs, Department of Nursing, Bowie, MD 20715-9465. Offers administration of nursing services (MS); family nurse practitioner (MS); nursing education (MS). *Accreditation:* ACEN. *Program availability:* Part-time. *Degree requirements:* For master's, comprehensive exam, thesis, research paper. *Entrance requirements:* For master's, minimum GPA of 2.5. Electronic applications accepted. *Expenses:* Tuition, state resident: full-time $9384, part-time $2046 per year. Tuition, nonresident: full-time $16,344; part-time $4086 per year. *Required fees:* $2552; $325 per semester. *Faculty research:* Minority health, women's health, gerontology, leadership management.

Bradley University, Graduate School, College of Education and Health Sciences, Department of Nursing, Peoria, IL 61625-0002. Offers nursing (DNP, Certificate); nursing administration (MSN); nursing education (MSN). *Accreditation:* ACEN. *Program availability:* Part-time, evening/weekend. *Degree requirements:* For master's, comprehensive exam, thesis optional. *Entrance requirements:* For master's, GRE General Test or MAT, interview, Illinois RN license, advanced cardiac life support certification, pediatric advanced life support certification, 3 letters of recommendation. Additional exam requirements/recommendations for international students: Required—TOEFL (minimum score 550 paper-based; 79 iBT), IELTS (minimum score 6.5). Electronic applications accepted.

Briar Cliff University, Program in Nursing, Sioux City, IA 51104-0100. Offers MSN. *Accreditation:* AACN. *Program availability:* Part-time, evening/weekend. *Degree requirements:* For master's, thesis optional. *Entrance requirements:* For master's, minimum undergraduate GPA of 3.0 for last 60 undergraduate credits; current RN license. *Expenses:* Contact institution. *Faculty research:* The process/experience of trying something new (or change), the experience of taking a risk.

Brigham Young University, Graduate Studies, College of Nursing, Provo, UT 84602. Offers family nurse practitioner (MS). *Accreditation:* AACN. *Faculty:* 10 full-time (7 women), 1 part-time/adjunct (0 women). *Students:* 29 full-time (19 women); includes 1 minority (Hispanic/Latino). Average age 35. 48 applicants, 31% accepted, 15 enrolled. In 2015, 12 master's awarded. *Degree requirements:* For master's, thesis. *Entrance requirements:* For master's, GRE, minimum GPA of 3.0 in last 60 hours, interview, BS in nursing, pathophysiology class within undergraduate program, course work in basic statistics. Additional exam requirements/recommendations for international students: Required—TOEFL; Recommended—IELTS. *Application deadline:* For spring admission, 12/1 for domestic students. Applications are processed on a rolling basis. Application fee: $50. Electronic applications accepted. *Financial support:* In 2015–16, 29 students received support, including 2 research assistantships with tuition reimbursements available (averaging $10,000 per year), 3 teaching assistantships with tuition reimbursements available (averaging $10,000 per year); institutionally sponsored loans, scholarships/grants, tuition waivers (full), and unspecified assistantships also available. Support available to part-time students. Financial award application deadline: 2/1; financial award applicants required to submit FAFSA. *Faculty research:* Critical care issues, end of life, childhood immunizations, children with diabetes, global health. *Total annual research expenditures:* $3,592. *Unit head:* Dr. Patricia Ravert, Dean, 801-422-1167, Fax: 801-422-0536, E-mail: patricia_ravert@byu.edu. *Application contact:* Lynette Jakins, Graduate Secretary, 801-422-4142, Fax: 801-422-0538, E-mail: lynette-jakins@byu.edu.
Website: http://nursing.byu.edu/

California Baptist University, Doctor of Nursing Practice Program, Riverside, CA 92504-3206. Offers DNP. *Program availability:* Part-time. *Faculty:* 5 full-time (4 women). *Students:* 2 part-time (both women). Average age 49. 9 applicants, 33% accepted, 2 enrolled. *Degree requirements:* For doctorate, thesis/dissertation or alternative, translational capstone project. *Entrance requirements:* For doctorate, MA in nursing, minimum cumulative GPA of 3.3, current California RN license, interview, official transcripts, three references, written statement about potential project, professional resume or curriculum vitae, writing sample. Additional exam requirements/recommendations for international students: Required—TOEFL (minimum score 80 iBT). *Application deadline:* For fall admission, 8/1 priority date for domestic students, 7/1 priority date for international students; for spring admission, 12/1 priority date for domestic students, 11/1 priority date for international students. Applications are processed on a rolling basis. Application fee: $45. Electronic applications accepted. *Expenses:* $1,200 per unit. *Financial support:* Federal Work-Study and scholarships/grants available. Financial award applicants required to submit CSS PROFILE or FAFSA. *Faculty research:* Community health, gerontology, male health, interprofessional education, global healthcare technology. *Unit head:* Dr. Geneva Oaks, Dean, School of Nursing, 951-343-4702, E-mail: goaks@calbaptist.edu. *Application contact:* Dr. Lisa Bursch, DNP Program Director, 951-343-4940, E-mail: lbursch@calbaptist.edu.
Website: http://www.calbaptist.edu/academics/schools-colleges/school-nursing/doctor-nursing-practice/

California Baptist University, Program in Nursing, Riverside, CA 92504-3206. Offers clinical nurse specialist (MSN); family nurse practitioner (MSN); healthcare systems management (MSN); teaching-learning (MSN). *Program availability:* Part-time. *Faculty:* 18 full-time (17 women), 14 part-time/adjunct (11 women). *Students:* 77 full-time (63 women), 143 part-time (117 women); includes 111 minority (26 Black or African American, non-Hispanic/Latino; 3 American Indian or Alaska Native, non-Hispanic/Latino; 38 Asian, non-Hispanic/Latino; 39 Hispanic/Latino; 1 Native Hawaiian or other Pacific Islander, non-Hispanic/Latino; 4 Two or more races, non-Hispanic/Latino), 5 international. Average age 33. 44 applicants, 64% accepted, 23 enrolled. In 2015, 19 master's awarded. *Degree requirements:* For master's, comprehensive exam or directed project thesis; capstone practicum. *Entrance requirements:* For master's, GRE or California Critical Thinking Skills Test; Test of Essential Academic Skills (TEAS);

minimum undergraduate GPA of 3.0; completion of prerequisite courses with minimum grade of C; CPR certification; background check clearance; health clearance; drug testing; proof of health insurance; proof of motor vehicle insurance; three letters of recommendation; 1000-word essay; interview. Additional exam requirements/recommendations for international students: Required—TOEFL (minimum score 80 iBT). *Application deadline:* For fall admission, 8/1 priority date for domestic students, 7/1 for international students; for spring admission, 12/1 priority date for domestic students, 11/1 for international students. Applications are processed on a rolling basis. Application fee: $45. Electronic applications accepted. *Expenses:* $742 per unit, $355 per semester fees. *Financial support:* Federal Work-Study and scholarships/grants available. Financial award applicants required to submit CSS PROFILE or FAFSA. *Faculty research:* Qualitative research using Parse methodology, gerontology, disaster preparedness, medical-surgical nursing, maternal-child nursing. *Unit head:* Dr. Geneva Oaks, Dean, School of Nursing, 951-343-4702, E-mail: goaks@calbaptist.edu. *Application contact:* Dr. Rebecca Meyer, Director, Graduate Program in Nursing, 951-343-4952, Fax: 951-343-5095, E-mail: rmeyer@calbaptist.edu.
Website: http://www.calbaptist.edu/explore-cbu/schools-colleges/school-nursing/master-science-nursing/

California State University, Chico, Office of Graduate Studies, College of Natural Sciences, School of Nursing, Chico, CA 95929. Offers MSN. *Accreditation:* AACN. *Program availability:* Part-time, online learning. *Students:* 20 part-time. *Degree requirements:* For master's, project or thesis and oral exam. *Entrance requirements:* For master's, GRE, statement of purpose, course work in statistics in the last seven years, BSN, California nursing license. Additional exam requirements/recommendations for international students: Required—TOEFL (minimum score 550 paper-based; 80 iBT), IELTS (minimum score 6.5), PTE (minimum score 59). *Application deadline:* For fall admission, 3/1 for domestic and international students. Application fee: $55. Electronic applications accepted. *Expenses:* Tuition, area resident: Full-time $4146; part-time $2730. *Financial support:* Career-related internships or fieldwork and scholarships/grants available. Financial award application deadline: 3/1; financial award applicants required to submit FAFSA. *Unit head:* Peggy Rowberg, Director, 530-898-5891. *Application contact:* Judy L. Rice, Graduate Admissions Coordinator, 530-898-5416, Fax: 530-898-3342, E-mail: jlrice@csuchico.edu.
Website: http://www.csuchico.edu/nurs/

California State University, Dominguez Hills, College of Health, Human Services and Nursing, Program in Nursing, Carson, CA 90747-0001. Offers MSN. *Accreditation:* AACN. *Program availability:* Part-time, online learning. *Degree requirements:* For master's, comprehensive exam. *Entrance requirements:* For master's, minimum GPA of 2.5, 3.0 in prior coursework in statistics, research, pathophysiology and assessment. Additional exam requirements/recommendations for international students: Required—TOEFL. *Application deadline:* For fall admission, 6/1 for domestic students; for spring admission, 11/1 for domestic students. Applications are processed on a rolling basis. Application fee: $55. Electronic applications accepted. *Faculty research:* AIDS/HIV, health promotion, elderly. *Unit head:* Dr. Kathleen Chai, Interim Director, School of Nursing, 310-243-1050, E-mail: kchai@csudh.edu.
Website: http://www4.csudh.edu/son/programs/msn/index

California State University, Fresno, Division of Graduate Studies, College of Health and Human Services, Department of Nursing, Fresno, CA 93740-8027. Offers nursing (MS), including clinical nurse, primary care nurse practitioner, specialist/nurse educator. *Accreditation:* AACN. *Program availability:* Part-time, evening/weekend. *Degree requirements:* For master's, thesis or alternative. *Entrance requirements:* For master's, GRE General Test, 1 year of clinical practice, previous course work in statistics, BSN, minimum GPA of 3.0 in nursing. Additional exam requirements/recommendations for international students: Required—TOEFL. Electronic applications accepted. *Faculty research:* Training grant, HIV assessment.

California State University, Fullerton, Graduate Studies, College of Health and Human Development, Department of Nursing, Fullerton, CA 92834-9480. Offers leadership (MSN); nurse anesthesia (MSN); nurse educator (MSN); nursing (DNP); women's health care (MSN). *Accreditation:* AACN; AANA/CANAEP. *Program availability:* Part-time.

California State University, Long Beach, Graduate Studies, College of Health and Human Services, School of Nursing, Long Beach, CA 90840. Offers MSN, DNP, MSN/MPH. DNP offered jointly with California State University, Fullerton and California State University, Los Angeles. *Accreditation:* AACN. *Program availability:* Part-time. *Degree requirements:* For master's, thesis optional. *Entrance requirements:* For master's, minimum GPA of 3.0. Electronic applications accepted. *Faculty research:* Newborns of drug-dependent mothers, abuse of residents in nursing homes, interventions in care of Alzheimer's patients.

California State University, Los Angeles, Graduate Studies, College of Health and Human Services, School of Nursing, Los Angeles, CA 90032-8530. Offers nursing (MS). *Accreditation:* AACN. *Program availability:* Part-time, evening/weekend. *Degree requirements:* For master's, comprehensive exam, project or thesis. *Entrance requirements:* For master's, minimum GPA of 3.0 in nursing, course work in nursing and statistics. Additional exam requirements/recommendations for international students: Required—TOEFL (minimum score 500 paper-based). *Application deadline:* For fall admission, 5/1 for domestic and international students. Applications are processed on a rolling basis. Application fee: $55. *Financial support:* Federal Work-Study available. Support available to part-time students. Financial award application deadline: 3/1. *Faculty research:* Family stress, geripsychiatric nursing, self-care counseling, holistic nursing, adult health.
Website: http://web.calstatela.edu/academic/hhs/nursing/

California State University, Sacramento, Office of Graduate Studies, College of Health and Human Services, Division of Nursing, Sacramento, CA 95819. Offers MS. *Accreditation:* AACN. *Program availability:* Part-time. *Degree requirements:* For master's, thesis or project; writing proficiency exam. *Entrance requirements:* For master's, GRE, bachelor's degree in nursing, minimum GPA of 3.0. Additional exam requirements/recommendations for international students: Required—TOEFL. Electronic applications accepted.

California State University, San Bernardino, Graduate Studies, College of Natural Sciences, Program in Nursing, San Bernardino, CA 92407. Offers MSN. *Accreditation:* AACN. *Students:* 6 full-time (4 women), 21 part-time (17 women); includes 15 minority (4 Black or African American, non-Hispanic/Latino; 4 Asian, non-Hispanic/Latino; 7 Hispanic/Latino), 1 international. 28 applicants, 32% accepted, 6 enrolled. In 2015, 15 master's awarded. *Degree requirements:* For master's, thesis optional. *Entrance requirements:* Additional exam requirements/recommendations for international students: Required—TOEFL. *Application deadline:* For fall admission, 7/16 for domestic students; for winter admission, 10/16 for domestic students; for spring admission, 1/22 for domestic students. Application fee: $55. *Expenses:* Tuition, state resident: full-time $7843; part-time $5011.20 per year. Tuition and fees vary according to course load, degree level, program and reciprocity agreements. *Unit head:* Mary Anne Schultz, Chair, 909-537-5385, Fax: 909-537-7089, E-mail: mschultz@csusb.edu. *Application contact:*

Nursing—General

Dr. Jeffrey Thompson, Dean of Graduate Studies, 909-537-5058, E-mail: jthompso@csusb.edu.

California State University, Stanislaus, College of Human and Health Sciences, Program in Nursing (MS), Turlock, CA 95382. Offers gerontological nursing (MS); nursing education (MS). *Accreditation:* AACN. *Program availability:* Part-time. *Degree requirements:* For master's, comprehensive exam, thesis or alternative. *Entrance requirements:* For master's, GRE or MAT, minimum GPA of 3.0, 3 letters of reference, RN. Additional exam requirements/recommendations for international students: Required—TOEFL (minimum score 550 paper-based). Electronic applications accepted.

Capella University, School of Public Service Leadership, Doctoral Programs in Nursing, Minneapolis, MN 55402. Offers nursing education (PhD); nursing practice (DNP).

Capella University, School of Public Service Leadership, Master's Programs in Nursing, Minneapolis, MN 55402. Offers diabetes nursing (MSN); general nursing (MSN); gerontology nursing (MSN); health information management (MS); nurse educator (MSN); nursing leadership and administration (MSN).

Capital University, School of Nursing, Columbus, OH 43209-2394. Offers administration (MSN); legal studies (MSN); theological studies (MSN); JD/MSN; MBA/MSN; MSN/MTS. *Accreditation:* AACN. *Program availability:* Part-time, evening/weekend. *Degree requirements:* For master's, thesis or alternative. *Entrance requirements:* For master's, BSN, current RN license, minimum GPA of 3.0, undergraduate courses in statistics and research. Additional exam requirements/recommendations for international students: Required—TOEFL (minimum score 550 paper-based). *Expenses:* Contact institution. *Faculty research:* Bereavement, wellness/health promotion, emergency cardiac care, critical thinking, complementary and alternative healthcare.

Cardinal Stritch University, Ruth S. Coleman College of Nursing and Health Sciences, Milwaukee, WI 53217-3985. Offers MSN. *Accreditation:* ACEN. *Program availability:* Part-time, evening/weekend. *Degree requirements:* For master's, thesis. *Entrance requirements:* For master's, interview; minimum GPA of 3.0; RN license; 3 letters of recommendation; undergraduate coursework in statistics and nursing research; computer literacy; curriculum vitae. *Application deadline:* For fall admission, 6/15 priority date for domestic students; for spring admission, 11/15 priority date for domestic students. Applications are processed on a rolling basis. Application fee: $25. Electronic applications accepted. *Expenses:* Contact institution. *Financial support:* Federal Work-Study and scholarships/grants available. Financial award applicants required to submit FAFSA. *Unit head:* Kelly J. Dries, Dean, 414-410-4397. *Application contact:* 800-347-8822 Ext. 4042, E-mail: gradadm@stritch.edu.

Carlow University, College of Health and Wellness, Doctor of Nursing Practice Program, Pittsburgh, PA 15213. Offers DNP. *Program availability:* Part-time, evening/weekend, low-residency. *Students:* 20 full-time (17 women), 19 part-time (17 women); includes 7 minority (3 Black or African American, non-Hispanic/Latino; 1 Asian, non-Hispanic/Latino; 2 Hispanic/Latino; 1 Two or more races, non-Hispanic/Latino). Average age 47. 19 applicants, 89% accepted, 12 enrolled. In 2015, 16 doctorates awarded. *Degree requirements:* For doctorate, 3-semester scholarly inquiry. *Entrance requirements:* For doctorate, master's degree with minimum GPA of 3.0; BSN; current RN license; official transcripts from all undergraduate and graduate institutions; copy of RN license; current curriculum vitae; two letters of academic and/or professional recommendation; reflective essay describing career goals and expectations for education. Additional exam requirements/recommendations for international students: Required—TOEFL (minimum score 550 paper-based). *Application deadline:* For fall admission, 4/1 priority date for domestic students. Applications are processed on a rolling basis. Electronic applications accepted. Application fee is waived when completed online. *Expenses:* Contact institution. *Unit head:* Dr. Renee Ingel, PhD, RN, Director, DNP Program, 412-578-6103, Fax: 412-578-6114, E-mail: rmingel@carlow.edu.
Website: http://www.carlow.edu/Nursing_Doctoral_Offering.aspx

Carlow University, College of Health and Wellness, MSN-MBA Dual Degree Program, Pittsburgh, PA 15213-3165. Offers MSN/MBA. *Program availability:* Part-time, 100% online. *Students:* 23 full-time (16 women), 4 part-time (all women); includes 2 minority (1 Asian, non-Hispanic/Latino; 1 Hispanic/Latino). Average age 35. 15 applicants, 100% accepted, 9 enrolled. *Entrance requirements:* Additional exam requirements/recommendations for international students: Required—TOEFL. *Application deadline:* Applications are processed on a rolling basis. Electronic applications accepted. Application fee is waived when completed online. *Expenses:* Contact institution. *Financial support:* Applicants required to submit FAFSA. *Unit head:* Dr. Renee Ingel, PhD, RN, Program Director, 412-578-6103, E-mail: rmingel@carlow.edu. *Application contact:* E-mail: gradstudies@carlow.edu.
Website: http://www.carlow.edu/MSN-MBA_Dual_Degree.aspx

Carson-Newman University, Department of Nursing, Jefferson City, TN 37760. Offers family nurse practitioner (MSN); nurse educator (MSN). *Accreditation:* AACN. *Program availability:* Part-time. *Faculty:* 4 full-time (3 women), 1 (woman) part-time/adjunct. *Students:* 9 full-time (8 women), 34 part-time (31 women); includes 1 minority (Black or African American, non-Hispanic/Latino). Average age 33. 14 applicants, 100% accepted, 9 enrolled. In 2015, 19 master's awarded. *Degree requirements:* For master's, comprehensive exam, thesis optional. *Entrance requirements:* For master's, GRE (minimum score of 290 within ten years of application), minimum GPA of 3.0 for all undergraduate work. Additional exam requirements/recommendations for international students: Recommended—TOEFL (minimum score 79 iBT), IELTS (minimum score 6.5), TSE (minimum score 53). *Application deadline:* For fall admission, 3/15 for domestic students; for spring admission, 10/15 for domestic students. Applications are processed on a rolling basis. Application fee: $50. *Expenses: Tuition, area resident:* Full-time $10,142; part-time $461 per credit hour. *Required fees:* $300; $461 per credit hour. $150 per semester. One-time fee: $150. *Financial support:* Federal Work-Study and tuition waivers (full and partial) available. Financial award applicants required to submit FAFSA. *Unit head:* Dr. Kimberly Bolton, Director, 865-471-4056, E-mail: kbolton@cn.edu. *Application contact:* Nilma Stewart, Graduate Admissions and Services Adviser, 865-471-3230, Fax: 865-471-3875, E-mail: adults@cn.edu.
Website: http://www.cn.edu/adult-graduate-studies/programs/new/nursing

Case Western Reserve University, Frances Payne Bolton School of Nursing, Doctor of Nursing Practice Program, Cleveland, OH 44106. Offers DNP. *Accreditation:* AACN. *Students:* 64 full-time (63 women), 79 part-time (76 women); includes 27 minority (13 Black or African American, non-Hispanic/Latino; 8 Asian, non-Hispanic/Latino; 6 Hispanic/Latino). Average age 50. 31 applicants, 84% accepted, 22 enrolled. In 2015, 48 doctorates awarded. Terminal master's awarded for partial completion of doctoral program. *Degree requirements:* For doctorate, thesis/dissertation. *Entrance requirements:* Additional exam requirements/recommendations for international students: Required—TOEFL (minimum score 577 paper-based; 90 iBT), IELTS (minimum score 7). *Application deadline:* For fall admission, 6/1 priority date for domestic students, 6/1 for international students; for spring admission, 10/1 for domestic and international students; for summer admission, 3/1 for domestic and international students. Applications are processed on a rolling basis. Application fee: $75. Electronic

applications accepted. *Expenses: Tuition, area resident:* Full-time $41,137; part-time $1714 per credit hour. *Required fees:* $32. Tuition and fees vary according to course load and program. *Financial support:* In 2015–16, 45 students received support, including 2 teaching assistantships with partial tuition reimbursements available (averaging $8,510 per year); traineeships and Nurse Faculty Loan Program also available. Support available to part-time students. Financial award application deadline: 5/15; financial award applicants required to submit FAFSA. *Faculty research:* Symptom science, family/community care, aging across the lifespan, self-management of health and illness, neuroscience. *Unit head:* Dr. Donna Dowling, Director, 216-368-1869, Fax: 216-368-3542, E-mail: dad10@case.edu. *Application contact:* Donna Hassik, Admissions Coordinator, 216-368-5253, Fax: 216-368-0124, E-mail: dmh7@case.edu.
Website: http://fpb.case.edu/DNP/

Case Western Reserve University, Frances Payne Bolton School of Nursing, Master's Programs in Nursing, Cleveland, OH 44106. Offers nurse anesthesia (MSN); nurse educator (MSN); nurse midwifery (MSN); nurse practitioner (MSN), including acute care cardiovascular nursing, acute care nurse practitioner, acute care pediatric nurse practitioner, acute care/flight nurse, adult gerontology acute care nurse practitioner, adult gerontology nurse practitioner, adult gerontology oncology and palliative care, family nurse practitioner, family systems psychiatric mental health nursing, neonatal nurse practitioner, pediatric nurse practitioner, women's health nurse practitioner; nursing (MN). *Accreditation:* ACEN. *Program availability:* Part-time, blended/hybrid learning. *Students:* 147 full-time (120 women), 140 part-time (108 women); includes 54 minority (20 Black or African American, non-Hispanic/Latino; 20 Asian, non-Hispanic/Latino; 9 Hispanic/Latino; 5 Two or more races, non-Hispanic/Latino). Average age 35. 174 applicants, 66% accepted, 66 enrolled. In 2015, 125 master's awarded. Terminal master's awarded for partial completion of doctoral program. *Entrance requirements:* For master's, GRE General Test or MAT, CCRN certification (for nurse anesthesia). Additional exam requirements/recommendations for international students: Required—TOEFL (minimum score 577 paper-based; 90 iBT), IELTS (minimum score 7). *Application deadline:* For fall admission, 6/1 for domestic and international students; for spring admission, 10/1 for domestic and international students. Applications are processed on a rolling basis. Application fee: $75. *Expenses:* $1,891 per credit hour. *Financial support:* In 2015–16, 44 students received support, including 17 teaching assistantships with tuition reimbursements available (averaging $17,019 per year); scholarships/grants and traineeships also available. Financial award application deadline: 6/30; financial award applicants required to submit FAFSA. *Faculty research:* Symptom science, family/community care, aging across the lifespan, self-management of health and illness, neuroscience. *Unit head:* Dr. Carol Savrin, Director, 216-368-5304, Fax: 215-368-3542, E-mail: cls18@case.edu. *Application contact:* Donna Hassik, Admissions Coordinator, 216-368-5253, Fax: 216-368-0124, E-mail: dmh7@case.edu.
Website: http://fpb.case.edu/MSN/

Case Western Reserve University, Frances Payne Bolton School of Nursing, PhD in Nursing Program, Cleveland, OH 44106. Offers PhD. *Program availability:* Part-time. *Students:* 43 full-time (31 women), 6 part-time (5 women); includes 4 minority (1 Black or African American, non-Hispanic/Latino; 1 American Indian or Alaska Native, non-Hispanic/Latino; 1 Asian, non-Hispanic/Latino; 1 Two or more races, non-Hispanic/Latino), 18 international. Average age 40. 22 applicants, 32% accepted, 6 enrolled. In 2015, 45 doctorates awarded. *Degree requirements:* For doctorate, comprehensive exam, thesis/dissertation, 240-hour research practicum. *Entrance requirements:* Additional exam requirements/recommendations for international students: Required—TOEFL (minimum score 577 paper-based, 90 iBT) or IELTS (minimum score 7.0). *Application deadline:* For fall admission, 4/1 priority date for domestic students, 4/1 for international students; for spring admission, 10/1 for domestic and international students. Applications are processed on a rolling basis. Application fee: $50. Electronic applications accepted. *Expenses:* $1,714 per credit hour. *Financial support:* In 2015–16, 17 students received support, including 16 fellowships with full tuition reimbursements available (averaging $30,852 per year), 9 research assistantships with partial tuition reimbursements available (averaging $15,388 per year); traineeships also available. Financial award application deadline: 5/15; financial award applicants required to submit FAFSA. *Faculty research:* Neuroscience, self-management, symptom science, aging across the lifespan, and family/community care. *Unit head:* Dr. Jaclene A. Zauszniewski, Director, 216-368-3612, Fax: 215-368-3542, E-mail: jaz@case.edu. *Application contact:* Donna Hassik, Admissions Coordinator, Graduate Programs, 216-368-5253, Fax: 216-368-0124, E-mail: donna.hassik@case.edu.
Website: http://fpb.cwru.edu/PhD/

The Catholic University of America, School of Nursing, Washington, DC 20064. Offers MSN, DNP, PhD, Certificate. *Accreditation:* AACN. *Program availability:* Part-time. *Faculty:* 19 full-time (all women), 48 part-time/adjunct (43 women). *Students:* 35 full-time (33 women), 212 part-time (197 women); includes 82 minority (59 Black or African American, non-Hispanic/Latino; 10 Asian, non-Hispanic/Latino; 7 Hispanic/Latino; 6 Two or more races, non-Hispanic/Latino), 10 international. Average age 40. 144 applicants, 67% accepted, 60 enrolled. In 2015, 14 master's, 4 doctorates, 3 other advanced degrees awarded. *Degree requirements:* For master's, comprehensive exam, thesis optional; for doctorate, comprehensive exam, thesis/dissertation, minimum GPA of 3.0, oral proposal defense. *Entrance requirements:* For master's, GRE General Test, 3 letters of recommendation, BA in nursing, RN registration, official copies of academic transcripts, some post-baccalaureate nursing experience; for doctorate, GRE General Test, BA in nursing, professional portfolio (including statements, resume, copy of RN license, 3 letters of recommendation, narrative description of clinical practice, proposal), copy of research/scholarly paper related to clinical nursing; for Certificate, GRE General Test. Additional exam requirements/recommendations for international students: Required—TOEFL (minimum score 550 paper-based; 80 iBT). *Application deadline:* For fall admission, 7/15 priority date for domestic students, 7/1 for international students; for spring admission, 11/15 priority date for domestic students, 11/1 for international students. Applications are processed on a rolling basis. Application fee: $55. Electronic applications accepted. *Expenses:* $20,700 per semester full-time tuition, $200 per semester full-time fees; $1,650 per credit hour part-time tuition, $145 per semester part-time fees; $875 per credit hour part-time online tuition. *Financial support:* Fellowships, research assistantships, teaching assistantships, Federal Work-Study, scholarships/grants, tuition waivers (full and partial), and unspecified assistantships available. Financial award application deadline: 2/1; financial award applicants required to submit FAFSA. *Faculty research:* Community involvement in health care services, primary health care services, pediatrics, chronic illness, cardiovascular disease. *Total annual research expenditures:* $235,247. *Unit head:* Dr. Patricia McMullen, Dean, 202-319-5403, Fax: 202-319-6485, E-mail: mcmullep@cua.edu. *Application contact:* Director of Graduate Admissions, 202-319-5057, Fax: 202-319-6533, E-mail: cua-admissions@cua.edu.
Website: http://nursing.cua.edu/

Cedar Crest College, Program in Nursing, Allentown, PA 18104-6196. Offers nursing administration (MS); nursing education (MS). *Program availability:* Part-time. *Faculty:* 4 full-time (all women), 1 part-time/adjunct (0 women). *Students:* 12 part-time (all women); includes 1 minority (Hispanic/Latino). Average age 35. In 2015, 15 master's awarded. *Application deadline:* Applications are processed on a rolling basis. Electronic applications accepted. *Expenses:* Contact institution. *Unit head:* Dr. Wendy Robb,

Director, 610-606-4666, E-mail: wjrobb@cedarcrest.edu. *Application contact:* Mary Ellen Hickes, Director of School of Adult and Graduate Education, 610-606-4666, E-mail: sage@cedarcrest.edu.
Website: http://sage.cedarcrest.edu/degrees/graduate/nursing-science/

Central Methodist University, College of Graduate and Extended Studies, Fayette, MO 65248-1198. Offers clinical counseling (MS); clinical nurse leader (MSN); education (M Ed); music education (MME); nurse educator (MSN). *Program availability:* Part-time, evening/weekend, online learning. *Degree requirements:* For master's, thesis. *Entrance requirements:* For master's, GRE General Test, minimum GPA of 2.75. Electronic applications accepted.

Chatham University, Nursing Programs, Pittsburgh, PA 15232-2826. Offers education/ leadership (MSN); nursing (DNP). *Accreditation:* AACN. *Program availability:* Online learning. *Faculty:* 11 full-time (10 women), 23 part-time/adjunct (18 women). *Students:* 64 full-time (58 women), 80 part-time (73 women); includes 50 minority (31 Black or African American, non-Hispanic/Latino; 9 Asian, non-Hispanic/Latino; 5 Hispanic/Latino; 1 Native Hawaiian or other Pacific Islander, non-Hispanic/Latino; 4 Two or more races, non-Hispanic/Latino), 10 international. Average age 44. 181 applicants, 50% accepted, 61 enrolled. In 2015, 9 master's, 76 doctorates awarded. *Entrance requirements:* For master's, RN license, BSN, minimum GPA of 3.0; for doctorate, RN license, MSN. Additional exam requirements/recommendations for international students: Required— TOEFL (minimum score 600 paper-based; 100 iBT), IELTS (minimum score 6.5), TWE. *Application deadline:* For fall admission, 5/1 priority date for domestic and international students. Applications are processed on a rolling basis. Application fee: $0. Electronic applications accepted. *Expenses: Tuition, area resident:* Full-time $15,786; part-time $877 per credit hour. *Required fees:* $468; $26 per credit hour. *Financial support:* Applicants required to submit FAFSA. *Unit head:* Dr. Diane Hunker, Director, 412-365- 1738, E-mail: dhunker@chatham.edu. *Application contact:* Patricia Golla, Assistant Director of Graduate Admissions, 412-365-1386, Fax: 412-365-1720, E-mail: pgolla@ chatham.edu.
Website: http://www.chatham.edu/nursing

Chicago State University, School of Graduate and Professional Studies, College of Health Sciences, Department of Nursing, Chicago, IL 60628. Offers MSN.

Clarion University of Pennsylvania, Office of Transfer, Adult and Graduate Admissions, Master of Science in Nursing Program, Clarion, PA 16214. Offers family nurse practitioner (MSN); nurse educator (MSN). Program offered jointly with Slippery Rock University of Pennsylvania. *Accreditation:* ACEN. *Program availability:* Part-time, online learning. *Degree requirements:* For master's, comprehensive exam, thesis. *Entrance requirements:* For master's, minimum QPA of 2.75. Additional exam requirements/recommendations for international students: Required—TOEFL (minimum score 550 paper-based; 80 iBT). Electronic applications accepted.

Clarke University, Department of Nursing and Health, Dubuque, IA 52001-3198. Offers family nurse practitioner (DNP). *Accreditation:* AACN. *Program availability:* Part-time. *Faculty:* 6 full-time (all women), 1 (woman) part-time/adjunct. *Students:* 54 full-time (53 women), 9 part-time (8 women); includes 1 minority (Asian, non-Hispanic/Latino). Average age 36. 45 applicants, 58% accepted, 20 enrolled. In 2015, 8 doctorates awarded. *Degree requirements:* For doctorate, comprehensive exam, thesis/ dissertation. *Entrance requirements:* For doctorate, GRE (if GPA under 3.0), three recommendation forms, sample of scholarly writing, statement of goals, transcripts, copy of nursing license. Additional exam requirements/recommendations for international students: Required—TOEFL. *Application deadline:* For fall admission, 2/1 priority date for domestic students. Application fee: $35. Electronic applications accepted. *Expenses:* Contact institution. *Financial support:* In 2015–16, 7 students received support. Scholarships/grants and tuition waivers available. Financial award applicants required to submit FAFSA. *Faculty research:* Narrative pedagogy, ethics, end-of-life care, pedagogy, family systems, simulation. *Unit head:* Dr. Jan Lee, Chair, 563-588-6339, Fax: 563-584-8684. *Application contact:* Kara Shroeder, Graduate Studies Coordinator, 563-588-6635, Fax: 563-588-6789, E-mail: graduate@clarke.edu.
Website: http://www.clarke.edu/

Clarkson College, Master of Science in Nursing Program, Omaha, NE 68131. Offers adult nurse practitioner (MSN, Post-Master's Certificate); family nurse practitioner (MSN, Post-Master's Certificate); nursing education (MSN, Post-Master's Certificate); nursing health care leadership (MSN, Post-Master's Certificate). *Accreditation:* AANA/CANAEP; ACEN. *Program availability:* Part-time, evening/weekend, online learning. *Degree requirements:* For master's, on-campus skills assessment (family nurse practitioner, adult nurse practitioner), comprehensive exam or thesis. *Entrance requirements:* For master's, minimum GPA of 3.0, 2 references, resume. Additional exam requirements/ recommendations for international students: Required—TOEFL (minimum score 600 paper-based; 100 iBT). Electronic applications accepted.

Clayton State University, School of Graduate Studies, College of Health, Program in Nursing, Morrow, GA 30260-0285. Offers family nurse practitioner (MSN). *Accreditation:* AACN. *Faculty:* 7 full-time (all women). *Students:* 5 full-time (4 women), 15 part-time (12 women); includes 12 minority (11 Black or African American, non-Hispanic/Latino; 1 Asian, non-Hispanic/Latino). Average age 41. 7 applicants, 100% accepted, 6 enrolled. *Degree requirements:* For master's, thesis. *Entrance requirements:* For master's, GRE, official transcript, 3 letters of recommendation, statement of purpose, on-campus interview, 1-2 years of clinical nursing experience (preferred). Additional exam requirements/recommendations for international students: Required—TOEFL (minimum score 550 paper-based; 80 iBT). *Application deadline:* For fall admission, 6/15 priority date for domestic students, 5/1 for international students; for spring admission, 11/15 priority date for domestic students, 9/1 for international students. Applications are processed on a rolling basis. Application fee: $75. Electronic applications accepted. *Expenses:* Contact institution. *Financial support:* Application deadline: 7/1; applicants required to submit FAFSA. *Unit head:* Dr. Betty Glenn Lane, Program Director, Master of Science in Nursing, 678-466-4953, Fax: 678-466-4999, E-mail: katherinewillock@ clayton.edu. *Application contact:* Christy Hicks, Coordinator, 678-466-4901, Fax: 678- 466-4999, E-mail: christyhicks@clayton.edu.
Website: http://nursing.clayton.edu/MSN/

Clemson University, Graduate School, College of Behavioral, Social and Health Sciences, School of Nursing, Clemson, SC 29634-0743. Offers healthcare genetics (PhD); nursing (MS). *Accreditation:* AACN. *Program availability:* Part-time. *Faculty:* 30 full-time (28 women), 2 part-time/adjunct (both women). *Students:* 33 full-time (29 women), 76 part-time (65 women); includes 10 minority (3 Black or African American, non-Hispanic/Latino; 1 American Indian or Alaska Native, non-Hispanic/Latino; 2 Hispanic/Latino; 4 Two or more races, non-Hispanic/Latino), 6 international. Average age 39. 20 applicants, 85% accepted, 13 enrolled. In 2015, 40 master's, 1 doctorate awarded. *Degree requirements:* For master's, comprehensive exam, thesis or alternative; for doctorate, comprehensive exam, thesis/dissertation. *Entrance requirements:* For master's, GRE General Test, South Carolina RN license, unofficial transcripts, resume, letters of recommendation; for doctorate, GRE General Test, unofficial transcripts, MS/MA thesis or publications, curriculum vitae, statement of career goals, letters of recommendation. Additional exam requirements/recommendations for international students: Required—TOEFL (minimum score 80 iBT), IELTS (minimum

score 6.5). *Application deadline:* For fall admission, 3/1 priority date for domestic and international students; for spring admission, 10/1 priority date for domestic and international students. Application fee: $80 ($90 for international students). Electronic applications accepted. *Expenses:* $5,349 per semester full-time resident, $10,683 per semester full-time non-resident, $663 per credit hour part-time resident, $1,327 per credit hour part-time non-resident. *Financial support:* In 2015–16, 37 students received support, including 4 fellowships with partial tuition reimbursements available (averaging $6,848 per year), 2 research assistantships with partial tuition reimbursements available (averaging $8,874 per year), 26 teaching assistantships with partial tuition reimbursements available (averaging $6,877 per year); career-related internships or fieldwork, health care benefits, and unspecified assistantships also available. Financial award application deadline: 3/1. *Faculty research:* Breast cancer, healthcare, genetics, international healthcare, educational innovation and technology. *Total annual research expenditures:* $503,531. *Unit head:* Dr. Rosanne Pruitt, Director and Associate College Dean, 864-656-7622, Fax: 864-656-5488, E-mail: prosan@clemson.edu. *Application contact:* Dr. Stephanie Davis, Graduate Studies Coordinator, 864-656-2588, Fax: 864- 656-5488, E-mail: stephad@clemson.edu.
Website: http://www.clemson.edu/nursing/

Cleveland State University, College of Graduate Studies, School of Nursing, Cleveland, OH 44115. Offers clinical nurse leader (MSN); forensic nursing (MSN); nursing education (MSN); specialized population (MSN); urban education (PhD), including nursing education; MSN/MBA. *Accreditation:* AACN. *Program availability:* Part- time, 100% online. *Faculty:* 7 full-time (all women). *Students:* 7 full-time (all women), 43 part-time (42 women); includes 14 minority (12 Black or African American, non-Hispanic/ Latino; 1 Asian, non-Hispanic/Latino; 1 Hispanic/Latino). Average age 37. 60 applicants, 62% accepted, 26 enrolled. In 2015, 11 master's awarded. *Degree requirements:* For master's, thesis optional, portfolio, capstone practicum project; for doctorate, comprehensive exam, thesis/dissertation. *Entrance requirements:* For master's, RN license in the U.S., BSN with minimum cumulative GPA of 3.0, recent (within last 5 years) course work in statistics; for doctorate, GRE, MSN with minimum cumulative GPA of 3.25. Additional exam requirements/recommendations for international students: Required—TOEFL (minimum score 550 paper-based; 78 iBT), IELTS (minimum score 6). *Application deadline:* For fall admission, 3/1 priority date for domestic and international students. Application fee: $55. Electronic applications accepted. *Expenses:* Tuition, state resident: full-time $9565. Tuition, nonresident: full-time $17,980. Tuition and fees vary according to program. *Financial support:* Tuition waivers (full) and unspecified assistantships available. Financial award application deadline: 5/1; financial award applicants required to submit FAFSA. *Faculty research:* Diabetes management, African-American elders medication compliance, risk in home visiting, suffering, COPD and stress, nursing education, disaster health preparedness. *Total annual research expenditures:* $330,000. *Unit head:* Dr. Vida Lock, Dean, 216-523-7237, Fax: 216-687- 3556, E-mail: v.lock@csuohio.edu. *Application contact:* Maureen Mitchell, Assistant Professor and Graduate Program Director, 216-523-7128, Fax: 216-687-3556, E-mail: m.m.mitchell1@csuohio.edu.
Website: http://www.csuohio.edu/nursing/

College of Mount Saint Vincent, School of Professional and Continuing Studies, Department of Nursing, Riverdale, NY 10471-1093. Offers adult nurse practitioner (MSN, PMC); family nurse practitioner (MSN, PMC); nurse educator (PMC); nursing administration (MSN); nursing for the adult and aged (MSN). *Accreditation:* AACN. *Program availability:* Part-time. *Entrance requirements:* For master's, BSN, interview, RN license, minimum GPA of 3.0, letters of reference. Additional exam requirements/ recommendations for international students: Required—TOEFL. *Expenses:* Contact institution.

The College of New Jersey, Graduate Studies, School of Nursing, Health and Exercise Science, Program in Nursing, Ewing, NJ 08628. Offers MSN, Certificate. *Accreditation:* AACN. *Program availability:* Part-time. *Students:* 5 full-time (2 women), 41 part-time (37 women); includes 15 minority (7 Black or African American, non-Hispanic/Latino; 6 Asian, non-Hispanic/Latino; 1 Hispanic/Latino; 1 Two or more races, non-Hispanic/ Latino). 37 applicants, 76% accepted, 23 enrolled. In 2015, 9 master's awarded. *Degree requirements:* For master's, comprehensive exam. *Entrance requirements:* For master's, GRE, minimum GPA of 3.0 in field or 2.75 overall. Additional exam requirements/recommendations for international students: Required—TOEFL. *Application deadline:* For fall admission, 2/1 priority date for domestic students; for spring admission, 10/1 priority date for domestic students. Application fee: $75. Electronic applications accepted. *Financial support:* Tuition waivers (partial) and unspecified assistantships available. Financial award application deadline: 5/1; financial award applicants required to submit FAFSA. *Unit head:* Dr. Constance Kartoz, Graduate Coordinator, 609-771-2591, Fax: 609-637-5159, E-mail: kartoz@tcnj.edu. *Application contact:* Susan L. Hydro, Director of Graduate and Intersession Programs, 609-771- 2300, Fax: 609-637-5105, E-mail: graduate@tcnj.edu.

The College of New Rochelle, Graduate School, Program in Nursing, New Rochelle, NY 10805-2308. Offers acute care nurse practitioner (MS, Certificate); clinical specialist in holistic nursing (MS, Certificate); family nurse practitioner (MS, Certificate); nursing and health care management (MS); nursing education (Certificate). *Accreditation:* AACN. *Program availability:* Part-time. *Faculty:* 3 full-time (2 women), 6 part-time/ adjunct (4 women). *Students:* 116 part-time (104 women); includes 79 minority (58 Black or African American, non-Hispanic/Latino; 11 Asian, non-Hispanic/Latino; 10 Hispanic/ Latino). Average age 38. In 2015, 25 master's awarded. *Entrance requirements:* For master's, GRE General Test or MAT, BSN, malpractice insurance, minimum GPA of 3.0, RN license. *Application deadline:* For fall admission, 8/15 priority date for domestic students; for spring admission, 12/1 priority date for domestic students. Applications are processed on a rolling basis. Application fee: $35. Electronic applications accepted. *Expenses: Tuition, area resident:* Part-time $894 per credit. *Required fees:* $350 per semester. *Financial support:* Traineeships available. Support available to part-time students. Financial award application deadline: 8/15; financial award applicants required to submit FAFSA. *Unit head:* Dr. H. Michael Dreher, Dean, School of Nursing, 914-654- 5441, Fax: 914-654-5256, E-mail: hdreher@cnr.edu. *Application contact:* Michael Petri, Interim Director of Graduate Admissions, 914-654-5256, E-mail: mpetri@cnr.edu.

College of Saint Elizabeth, Department of Nursing, Morristown, NJ 07960-6989. Offers MSN. *Accreditation:* ACEN. *Program availability:* Part-time. *Faculty:* 5 part-time/adjunct (all women). *Students:* 2 full-time (1 woman), 40 part-time (34 women); includes 21 minority (6 Black or African American, non-Hispanic/Latino; 8 Asian, non-Hispanic/ Latino; 7 Hispanic/Latino). Average age 44. 18 applicants, 89% accepted, 14 enrolled. In 2015, 16 master's awarded. *Entrance requirements:* For master's, GRE, GMAT, TOEFL, minimum cumulative undergraduate GPA of 3.0. Additional exam requirements/ recommendations for international students: Required—TOEFL (minimum score 550 paper-based; 210 iBT), IELTS (minimum score 6.5). Application fee: $35. Electronic applications accepted. Application fee is waived when completed online. *Expenses:* $1,001 per credit; $175 graduation fee. *Financial support:* Career-related internships or fieldwork, scholarships/grants, tuition waivers (partial), and unspecified assistantships available. Financial award applicants required to submit FAFSA. *Unit head:* Dr. Sarah Arnold, Interim Nursing Administrator, 973-290-4037, E-mail: sarnold@cse.edu. *Application contact:* Deborah S. Cobo, Associate Director for Graduate Admissions,

Nursing—General

973-290-4194, Fax: 973-290-4710, E-mail: dscobo@cse.edu.
Website: http://cse.smartcatalogiq.com/en/2015-2016/academic-catalog/academic-programs/nursing/ms-in-nursing

College of Saint Mary, Program in Nursing, Omaha, NE 68106. Offers MSN. *Accreditation:* ACEN. *Program availability:* Part-time. *Entrance requirements:* For master's, bachelor's degree in nursing, Nebraska RN license, essay or scholarly writing, minimum cumulative GPA of 3.0, 2 references. Additional exam requirements/recommendations for international students: Required—TOEFL.

The College of St. Scholastica, Graduate Studies, Department of Nursing, Duluth, MN 55811-4199. Offers MA, PMC. *Accreditation:* AACN. *Program availability:* Part-time, online learning. *Degree requirements:* For master's, thesis. *Entrance requirements:* For master's, GRE General Test. Additional exam requirements/recommendations for international students: Required—TOEFL (minimum score 550 paper-based; 79 iBT). Electronic applications accepted. *Faculty research:* Critical thinking and professional development, social organization of responsibility, rural health HIV/AIDS prevention, Web-based instruction in nursing.

College of Staten Island of the City University of New York, Graduate Programs, School of Health Sciences, Staten Island, NY 10314-6600. Offers adult-gerontological nursing (MS, Advanced Certificate), including clinical nurse practitioner, clinical nurse specialist; cultural competence (Advanced Certificate); nursing practice (DNP); physical therapy (DPT). *Accreditation:* ACEN. *Faculty:* 11 full-time, 16 part-time/adjunct. *Students:* 37 full-time, 77 part-time. Average age 34. In 2015, 18 master's, 4 other advanced degrees awarded. *Entrance requirements:* Additional exam requirements/recommendations for international students: Required—TOEFL (minimum score 550 paper-based; 79 iBT), IELTS (minimum score 6.5). *Expenses:* Tuition, state resident: full-time $10,130; part-time $425 per credit. Tuition, nonresident: full-time $18,720; part-time $780 per credit. *Required fees:* $181.10 per semester. Tuition and fees vary according to program. *Unit head:* Dr. Maureen Becker, Interim Founding Dean, 718-982-3690, Fax: 718-982-3813, E-mail: schoolhealthscience@csi.cuny.edu. *Application contact:* Sasha Spence, Associate Director for Graduate Recruitment and Admissions, 718-982-2019, Fax: 718-982-2500, E-mail: sasha.spence@csi.cuny.edu. Website: http://www.csi.cuny.edu/schoolofhealthsciences/

Colorado Mesa University, Department of Health Sciences, Grand Junction, CO 81501-3122. Offers advanced nursing practice (MSN); family nurse practitioner (DNP); health information technology systems (Graduate Certificate); nursing education (MSN). *Program availability:* Part-time, evening/weekend, online learning. *Degree requirements:* For master's and doctorate, Capstone. *Entrance requirements:* For master's and doctorate, Minimum GPA of 3.0 in BSN Program. Additional exam requirements/recommendations for international students: Required—TOEFL (minimum score 550 paper-based). Electronic applications accepted.

Colorado State University–Pueblo, College of Education, Engineering and Professional Studies, Nursing Department, Pueblo, CO 81001-4901. Offers MS. *Accreditation:* ACEN. *Degree requirements:* For master's, comprehensive exam or thesis. *Entrance requirements:* Additional exam requirements/recommendations for international students: Required—TOEFL.

Columbia University, School of Nursing, New York, NY 10032. Offers MS, DNP, PhD, Adv C, MBA/MS, MPH/MS. *Accreditation:* AACN. *Program availability:* Part-time. *Degree requirements:* For doctorate, thesis/dissertation. *Entrance requirements:* For master's, GRE General Test, bachelor's degree, 1 year of clinical experience (preferred for most, required for some); for doctorate, GRE General Test. Additional exam requirements/recommendations for international students: Required—TOEFL. Electronic applications accepted. *Expenses:* Contact institution. *Faculty research:* HIV/AIDS, health promotion/disease prevention, health policies, advanced practice, urban health.

Columbus State University, Graduate Studies, College of Education and Health Professions, School of Nursing, Columbus, GA 31907-5645. Offers family nurse practitioner (MSN); nursing (MSN), including nurse educator, nurse informatics, nurse leader. Program offered in collaboration with Georgia Southwestern University. *Program availability:* Part-time, online only, 100% online. *Faculty:* 7 full-time (all women), 1 part-time/adjunct (0 women). *Students:* 29 full-time (24 women), 44 part-time (43 women); includes 35 minority (25 Black or African American, non-Hispanic/Latino; 1 Asian, non-Hispanic/Latino; 3 Hispanic/Latino; 6 Two or more races, non-Hispanic/Latino). Average age 38. 66 applicants, 59% accepted, 32 enrolled. In 2015, 6 master's awarded. *Entrance requirements:* For master's, GRE, BSN, minimum undergraduate GPA of 3.0. Additional exam requirements/recommendations for international students: Required—TOEFL (minimum score 550 paper-based; 79 iBT). *Application deadline:* For fall admission, 5/1 for domestic and international students; for spring admission, 11/1 for domestic and international students; for summer admission, 3/1 for domestic and international students. Applications are processed on a rolling basis. Application fee: $50. Electronic applications accepted. *Expenses:* Contact institution. *Financial support:* In 2015–16, 51 students received support. Institutionally sponsored loans available. Financial award application deadline: 5/1; financial award applicants required to submit FAFSA. *Unit head:* Latonya Sanot, Interim Director, 706-507-8576, E-mail: santo_latonya@columbusstate.edu. *Application contact:* Kristin Williams, Director of International and Graduate Recruitment, 706-507-8848, Fax: 706-568-5091, E-mail: williams_kristin@columbusstate.edu.
Website: http://nursing.columbusstate.edu/

Concordia University Wisconsin, Graduate Programs, School of Human Services, Program in Nursing, Mequon, WI 53097-2402. Offers family nurse practitioner (MSN); geriatric nurse practitioner (MSN); nurse educator (MSN). *Accreditation:* AACN. *Program availability:* Online learning. *Degree requirements:* For master's, comprehensive exam, thesis or alternative. *Entrance requirements:* Additional exam requirements/recommendations for international students: Required—TOEFL. *Expenses:* Contact institution.

Coppin State University, Division of Graduate Studies, Helene Fuld School of Nursing, Baltimore, MD 21216-3698. Offers family nurse practitioner (PMC); nursing (MSN). *Accreditation:* AACN; ACEN. *Program availability:* Part-time, evening/weekend. *Degree requirements:* For master's, comprehensive exam, thesis, clinical internship. *Entrance requirements:* For master's, GRE, bachelor's degree in nursing, interview, minimum GPA of 3.0, RN license. Additional exam requirements/recommendations for international students: Required—TOEFL (minimum score 550 paper-based).

Cox College, Programs in Nursing, Springfield, MO 65802. Offers clinical nurse leader (MSN); family nurse practitioner (MSN); nurse educator (MSN). *Accreditation:* AACN. *Entrance requirements:* For master's, RN license, essay, 2 letters of recommendation, official transcripts. Electronic applications accepted.

Creighton University, College of Nursing, Omaha, NE 68178-0001. Offers adult acute care nurse practitioner (Post-Master's Certificate); adult gerontology acute care nurse practitioner (DNP); adult gerontology nurse practitioner (DNP); clinical nurse leader (MSN, Post-Graduate Certificate); clinical systems administration (MSN, DNP); family nurse practitioner (DNP, Post-Master's Certificate); neonatal nurse practitioner (DNP, Post-Master's Certificate); pediatric acute care nurse practitioner (DNP, Post-Master's

Certificate); psychiatric mental health nurse practitioner (DNP). *Accreditation:* AACN. *Program availability:* Part-time, blended/hybrid learning. *Faculty:* 10 full-time (all women), 48 part-time/adjunct (45 women). *Students:* 132 full-time (120 women), 228 part-time (212 women); includes 38 minority (10 Black or African American, non-Hispanic/Latino; 3 American Indian or Alaska Native, non-Hispanic/Latino; 11 Asian, non-Hispanic/Latino; 1 Hispanic/Latino; 2 Native Hawaiian or other Pacific Islander, non-Hispanic/Latino; 11 Two or more races, non-Hispanic/Latino). Average age 31. 66 applicants, 91% accepted, 43 enrolled. In 2015, 54 master's, 17 doctorates, 1 other advanced degree awarded. *Degree requirements:* For master's, capstone project; for doctorate, scholarly project. *Entrance requirements:* For master's and doctorate, BSN from an ACEN- or CCNE-accredited nursing school, minimum cumulative GPA of 3.0, personal statement, current unencumbered RN license with NE eligibility, undergraduate statistics course, physical assessment course or equivalent; for other advanced degree, MSN or MS in nursing, minimum cumulative GPA of 3.0, current unencumbered RN license with NE eligibility. Additional exam requirements/recommendations for international students: Required—TOEFL (minimum score 600 paper-based; 100 iBT). *Application deadline:* For fall admission, 6/15 priority date for domestic and international students; for spring admission, 11/15 priority date for domestic and international students; for summer admission, 4/15 for domestic and international students. Applications are processed on a rolling basis. Application fee: $50. Electronic applications accepted. *Expenses:* $800 per credit hour tuition; $904 per semester full-time fees; $207 per semester part-time fees; $50 one-time drug screen fee. *Financial support:* In 2015–16, 7 students received support. Scholarships/grants available. Financial award applicants required to submit FAFSA. *Faculty research:* Obesity prevention in children, evaluation of simulated clinical experiences, vitamin D3 and calcium for cancer risk education in post menopausal women, online support and education to reduce stress for prenatal patients on bed rest, health literacy, immunization research. *Total annual research expenditures:* $162,085. *Unit head:* Dr. Catherine Todero, Dean, 402-280-2004, Fax: 402-280-2045. *Application contact:* Shannon Cox, Enrollment Specialist, 402-280-2067, Fax: 402-280-2045, E-mail: shannoncox@creighton.edu.
Website: http://nursing.creighton.edu/

Curry College, Graduate Studies, Program in Nursing, Milton, MA 02186-9984. Offers MSN. *Accreditation:* AACN.

Daemen College, Department of Nursing, Amherst, NY 14226-3592. Offers adult nurse practitioner (MS, Post Master's Certificate); nurse executive leadership (Post Master's Certificate); nursing education (MS, Post Master's Certificate); nursing executive leadership (MS); nursing practice (DNP); palliative care nursing (Post Master's Certificate). *Accreditation:* ACEN. *Program availability:* Part-time. *Degree requirements:* For master's, thesis or alternative, degree completed in 4 years; minimum GPA of 3.0; for doctorate, degree completed in 5 years; 500 post-master's clinical hours. *Entrance requirements:* For master's, BN, 1 year medical/surgical experience, RN license and state registration, statistics course with minimum C grade, 3 letters of recommendation, minimum GPA of 3.25, interview; for doctorate, MS in advance nursing practice; New York state RN license; goal statement; resume; interview; statistics course with minimum grade of 'C'; for Post Master's Certificate, master's degree in clinical area; RN license and current registration; one year of clinical experience; statistics course with minimum grade of 'C'; 3 letters of recommendation; interview; letter of intent. Additional exam requirements/recommendations for international students: Required—TOEFL (minimum score 500 paper-based; 63 iBT), IELTS (minimum score 5.5). Electronic applications accepted. *Faculty research:* Professional stress, client behavior, drug therapy, treatment modalities and pulmonary cancers, chemical dependency.

Dalhousie University, Faculty of Health Professions, School of Nursing, Halifax, NS B3H 3J5, Canada. Offers MN, PhD, MN/MHSA. *Program availability:* Part-time, online learning. *Degree requirements:* For master's, thesis optional. *Entrance requirements:* For master's, minimum GPA of 3.0; for doctorate, written support of faculty member who has agreed to be thesis supervisor. Additional exam requirements/recommendations for international students: Required—TOEFL, IELTS, CANTEST, CAEL, or Michigan English Language Assessment Battery. Electronic applications accepted. *Faculty research:* Coping, social support, health promotion, aging, feminist studies.

Delaware State University, Graduate Programs, College of Education, Health and Public Policy, Department of Nursing, Dover, DE 19901-2277. Offers MS. *Entrance requirements:* Additional exam requirements/recommendations for international students: Required—TOEFL (minimum score 550 paper-based). Electronic applications accepted.

Delta State University, Graduate Programs, School of Nursing, Cleveland, MS 38733. Offers family nurse practitioner (MSN); nurse administrator (MSN); nurse educator (MSN). *Accreditation:* AACN. *Program availability:* Part-time. *Degree requirements:* For master's, thesis optional. *Entrance requirements:* For master's, GRE General Test. Electronic applications accepted.

DePaul University, College of Science and Health, Chicago, IL 60614. Offers applied mathematics (MS); applied statistics (MS); biological sciences (MA, MS); chemistry (MS); mathematics education (MA); mathematics for teaching (MS); nursing (MS); nursing practice (DNP); physics (MS); psychology (MS); pure mathematics (MS); science education (MS); MA/PhD. Electronic applications accepted.

DeSales University, Division of Healthcare, Center Valley, PA 18034-9568. Offers adult-gerontology acute care (Post Master's Certificate); adult-gerontology acute care nurse practitioner (MSN); adult-gerontology acute certified nurse practitioner (Post Master's Certificate); adult-gerontology clinical nurse specialist (MSN, Post Master's Certificate); clinical leadership (DNP); family nurse practitioner (MSN, Post Master's Certificate); general nursing practice (DNP); health care information management (MSIS); network security (MSIS); nurse anesthetists (MSN); nurse educator (Post Master's Certificate, Postbaccalaureate Certificate); nurse midwives (MSN); nurse practitioner (MSN); project management (MSIS); psychiatric-mental health nurse practitioner (MSN, Post Master's Certificate); DNP/MBA. *Accreditation:* ACEN. *Program availability:* Part-time. *Faculty:* 22 full-time (14 women), 37 part-time/adjunct (29 women). *Students:* 244 full-time (178 women), 55 part-time (50 women); includes 24 minority (7 Black or African American, non-Hispanic/Latino; 9 Asian, non-Hispanic/Latino; 6 Hispanic/Latino; 2 Two or more races, non-Hispanic/Latino). Average age 31. 68 applicants, 85% accepted, 52 enrolled. In 2015, 73 master's awarded. *Degree requirements:* For master's, minimum GPA of 3.0, portfolio; for doctorate, minimum GPA of 3.0, scholarly capstone project. *Entrance requirements:* For master's, GRE or MAT (waived if applicant has an undergraduate GPA of 3.0 or higher), BSN from ACEN- or CCNE-accredited program, minimum undergraduate GPA of 3.0, active RN license or eligibility, two letters of recommendation, essay, health care experience, personal interview; for doctorate, BSN or MSN from ACEN- or CCNE-accredited institution, minimum GPA of 3.3 in graduate program, current licensure as an RN. Additional exam requirements/recommendations for international students: Required—TOEFL (minimum score 104 iBT). *Application deadline:* Applications are processed on a rolling basis. Application fee: $50. Electronic applications accepted. *Expenses:* Contact institution. *Financial support:* Applicants required to submit FAFSA. *Unit head:* Fr. Dr. Peter Leonard, OSFS, Dean of Graduate Education, 610-282-1100 Ext. 1289, E-mail: peter.leonard@desales.edu. *Application contact:* Abigail Wernicki, Director of Graduate

Admissions, 610-282-1100 Ext. 1768, Fax: 610-282-2869, E-mail: gradadmissions@desales.edu.

Drexel University, College of Nursing and Health Professions, Division of Graduate Nursing, Philadelphia, PA 19104-2875. Offers adult acute care (MSN); adult psychiatric/mental health (MSN); advanced practice nursing (MSN); clinical trials research (MSN); family nurse practitioner (MSN); leadership in health systems management (MSN); nursing education (MSN); pediatric primary care (MSN); women's health (MSN). *Accreditation:* AACN. Electronic applications accepted.

Drexel University, College of Nursing and Health Professions, Doctor of Nursing Practice Program, Philadelphia, PA 19104-2875. Offers Dr NP.

Duke University, School of Nursing, PhD Program in Nursing, Durham, NC 27708-0586. Offers PhD. *Faculty:* 30 full-time (24 women). *Students:* 33 full-time (29 women); includes 11 minority (7 Black or African American, non-Hispanic/Latino; 4 Asian, non-Hispanic/Latino), 2 international. Average age 31. 37 applicants, 27% accepted, 9 enrolled. In 2015, 2 doctorates awarded. *Degree requirements:* For doctorate, comprehensive exam, thesis/dissertation. *Entrance requirements:* For doctorate, GRE General Test, resume, personal statement, minimum cumulative undergraduate GPA of 3.0, recommendations, previous work in nursing, research course, graduate-level statistics course. Additional exam requirements/recommendations for international students: Required—TOEFL (minimum score 577 paper-based; 90 iBT), IELTS (minimum score 7). *Application deadline:* For fall admission, 12/1 priority date for domestic and international students; for spring admission, 5/1 for domestic and international students. Application fee: $80. Electronic applications accepted. *Financial support:* Institutionally sponsored loans, scholarships/grants, and health care benefits available. *Faculty research:* Nursing management practices, adolescents and families undergoing intense treatments, psychosocial and chronic disease. *Unit head:* Dr. Debra H. Brandon, Director, PhD in Nursing Program, 919-684-3813, Fax: 919-681-8899, E-mail: debra.brandon@duke.edu. *Application contact:* Revonda P. Huppert, Senior Program Coordinator, 919-668-4797, Fax: 919-681-8899, E-mail: revonda.huppert@duke.edu.
Website: http://nursing.duke.edu/academics/programs/phd/phd-program

Duquesne University, School of Nursing, Doctor of Nursing Practice Program, Pittsburgh, PA 15282-0001. Offers DNP. *Program availability:* Part-time, evening/weekend, minimal on-campus study. *Faculty:* 12 full-time (all women). *Students:* 17 full-time (16 women); includes 3 minority (2 Black or African American, non-Hispanic/Latino; 1 Hispanic/Latino). Average age 47. 27 applicants, 30% accepted, 7 enrolled. In 2015, 30 doctorates awarded. *Entrance requirements:* For doctorate, current RN license; BSN; master's degree with minimum GPA of 3.5; current certifications; phone interview. Additional exam requirements/recommendations for international students: Required—TOEFL (minimum score 600 paper-based; 100 iBT). *Application deadline:* For fall admission, 2/1 for domestic and international students. Application fee: $0. Electronic applications accepted. *Expenses:* $1,218 per credit. *Financial support:* In 2015–16, 18 students received support. Research assistantships with partial tuition reimbursements available, teaching assistantships with partial tuition reimbursements available, institutionally sponsored loans, scholarships/grants, traineeships, and unspecified assistantships available. Support available to part-time students. Financial award application deadline: 7/1; financial award applicants required to submit FAFSA. *Faculty research:* Vulnerable populations, social justice, cultural competence, health disparities, wellness within chronic illness, forensics. *Unit head:* Dr. Alison Colbert, Associate Professor/Associate Dean of Academic Affairs, 412-396-1511, Fax: 412-396-1821, E-mail: colberta@duq.edu. *Application contact:* Susan Hardner, Nurse Recruiter, 412-396-4945, Fax: 412-396-6346, E-mail: nursing@duq.edu.
Website: http://www.duq.edu/academics/schools/nursing/graduate-programs/doctor-of-nursing-practice

Duquesne University, School of Nursing, Doctor of Philosophy in Nursing Program, Pittsburgh, PA 15282-0001. Offers PhD. *Program availability:* Part-time, evening/weekend, minimal on-campus study. *Faculty:* 8 full-time (7 women), 1 part-time/adjunct (0 women). *Students:* 38 full-time (33 women), 17 part-time (16 women); includes 11 minority (7 Black or African American, non-Hispanic/Latino; 1 Asian, non-Hispanic/Latino; 2 Hispanic/Latino; 1 Two or more races, non-Hispanic/Latino), 3 international. Average age 48. 48 applicants, 31% accepted, 12 enrolled. In 2015, 7 doctorates awarded. *Degree requirements:* For doctorate, thesis/dissertation, preliminary exam. *Entrance requirements:* For doctorate, current RN license; BSN; master's degree with minimum GPA of 3.5; phone interview. Additional exam requirements/recommendations for international students: Required—TOEFL (minimum score 600 paper-based; 100 iBT). *Application deadline:* For fall admission, 1/15 for domestic and international students. Application fee: $0. Electronic applications accepted. *Expenses:* $1,218 per credit. *Financial support:* In 2015–16, 31 students received support, including 3 research assistantships with partial tuition reimbursements available (averaging $4,450 per year), 1 teaching assistantship with partial tuition reimbursement available (averaging $1,100 per year); institutionally sponsored loans, scholarships/grants, traineeships, and unspecified assistantships also available. Support available to part-time students. Financial award application deadline: 7/1; financial award applicants required to submit FAFSA. *Faculty research:* Vulnerable populations, social justice, cultural competence, health disparities, wellness within chronic illness, forensics. *Total annual research expenditures:* $246,973. *Unit head:* Dr. Alison Colbert, Associate Professor/Associate Dean of Academic Affairs, 412-396-1511, Fax: 412-396-1821, E-mail: colberta@duq.edu. *Application contact:* Susan Hardner, Nurse Recruiter, 412-396-4945, Fax: 412-396-6346, E-mail: nursing@duq.edu.
Website: http://www.duq.edu/academics/schools/nursing/graduate-programs/phd-in-nursing

Duquesne University, School of Nursing, Master of Science in Nursing Program, Pittsburgh, PA 15282-0001. Offers family (individual across the life span) nurse practitioner (MSN); forensic nursing (MSN); nursing education (MSN). *Accreditation:* AACN. *Program availability:* Part-time, evening/weekend, minimal on-campus study. *Faculty:* 13 full-time (11 women), 9 part-time/adjunct (all women). *Students:* 91 full-time (84 women), 87 part-time (76 women); includes 31 minority (16 Black or African American, non-Hispanic/Latino; 4 Asian, non-Hispanic/Latino; 7 Hispanic/Latino; 4 Two or more races, non-Hispanic/Latino), 1 international. Average age 34. 280 applicants, 34% accepted, 79 enrolled. In 2015, 39 master's awarded. *Entrance requirements:* For master's, current RN license; BSN with minimum GPA of 3.0; minimum of 1 year of full-time work experience as RN prior to registration in clinical or specialty course. Additional exam requirements/recommendations for international students: Required—TOEFL (minimum score 600 paper-based; 100 iBT). *Application deadline:* For fall admission, 3/1 for domestic and international students. Application fee: $0. Electronic applications accepted. *Expenses:* $1,218 per credit. *Financial support:* In 2015–16, 11 students received support, including 2 research assistantships with partial tuition reimbursements available (averaging $2,200 per year), 7 teaching assistantships with partial tuition reimbursements available (averaging $1,100 per year); scholarships/grants, traineeships, and tuition waivers (partial) also available. Support available to part-time students. Financial award application deadline: 7/1; financial award applicants required to submit FAFSA. *Faculty research:* Vulnerable populations, social justice, cultural competence, health disparities, wellness within chronic illness, forensics. *Total annual*

research expenditures: $246,973. *Unit head:* Dr. Alison Colbert, Associate Professor/Associate Dean of Academic Affairs, 412-396-1511, Fax: 412-396-1821, E-mail: colberta@duq.edu. *Application contact:* Susan Hardner, Nurse Recruiter, 412-396-4945, Fax: 412-396-6346, E-mail: nursing@duq.edu.
Website: http://www.duq.edu/academics/schools/nursing/graduate-programs/master-science-nursing

Duquesne University, School of Nursing, Post Master's Certificate Program, Pittsburgh, PA 15282-0001. Offers family (individual across the life span) nurse practitioner (Post-Master's Certificate); forensic nursing (Post-Master's Certificate); nursing education and faculty role (Post-Master's Certificate). *Program availability:* Part-time, evening/weekend, minimal on-campus study. *Faculty:* 3 full-time (all women), 7 part-time/adjunct (all women). *Students:* 2 full-time (both women), 10 part-time (9 women); includes 4 minority (3 Black or African American, non-Hispanic/Latino; 1 Hispanic/Latino). Average age 42. 28 applicants, 36% accepted, 5 enrolled. In 2015, 4 Post-Master's Certificates awarded. *Entrance requirements:* For degree, current RN license, BSN, MSN. Additional exam requirements/recommendations for international students: Required—TOEFL (minimum score 600 paper-based; 100 iBT). *Application deadline:* For fall admission, 3/1 for domestic and international students. Application fee: $0. Electronic applications accepted. *Expenses:* $1,218 per credit. *Financial support:* Teaching assistantships with partial tuition reimbursements, scholarships/grants, traineeships, and tuition waivers (partial) available. Support available to part-time students. Financial award application deadline: 7/1; financial award applicants required to submit FAFSA. *Faculty research:* Vulnerable populations, social justice, cultural competence, health disparities, wellness within chronic illness, forensics. *Total annual research expenditures:* $296,973. *Unit head:* Dr. Alison Colbert, Associate Professor/Associate Dean of Academic Affairs, 412-396-1511, Fax: 412-396-1821, E-mail: colberta@duq.edu. *Application contact:* Susan Hardner, Nurse Recruiter, 412-396-4945, Fax: 412-396-6346, E-mail: nursing@duq.edu.
Website: http://www.duq.edu/academics/schools/nursing/graduate-programs/post-masters-certificates

D'Youville College, School of Nursing, Buffalo, NY 14201-1084. Offers advanced practice nursing (DNP); family nurse practitioner (MSN, Certificate); nursing and health-related professions education (Certificate). *Accreditation:* AACN. *Program availability:* Part-time. *Faculty:* 36 full-time (35 women), 15 part-time/adjunct (13 women). *Students:* 75 full-time (70 women), 136 part-time (119 women); includes 21 minority (12 Black or African American, non-Hispanic/Latino; 1 American Indian or Alaska Native, non-Hispanic/Latino; 6 Asian, non-Hispanic/Latino; 2 Hispanic/Latino), 64 international. Average age 35. 197 applicants, 88% accepted, 119 enrolled. In 2015, 48 master's, 1 doctorate, 2 other advanced degrees awarded. *Degree requirements:* For master's, thesis or alternative. *Entrance requirements:* For master's, BS in nursing, minimum GPA of 3.0, course work in statistics and computers; for doctorate, BS in nursing, MS in advanced practice nursing specialty, minimum GPA of 3.25. Additional exam requirements/recommendations for international students: Required—TOEFL (minimum score 500 paper-based). *Application deadline:* For fall admission, 5/1 priority date for international students; for spring admission, 9/1 priority date for international students. Applications are processed on a rolling basis. Electronic applications accepted. *Expenses:* Tuition, area resident: Full-time $21,120; part-time $880 per credit hour. *Required fees:* $235; $96. One-time fee: $100. *Financial support:* Federal Work-Study, scholarships/grants, traineeships, and unspecified assistantships available. Support available to part-time students. Financial award application deadline: 3/1; financial award applicants required to submit FAFSA. *Faculty research:* Nursing curriculum, nursing theory-testing, wellness research, communication and socialization patterns. *Unit head:* Dr. Ann Caughill, Chair, 716-829-7892, Fax: 716-829-8159. *Application contact:* Mark Pavone, Graduate Admissions Director, 716-829-8400, Fax: 716-829-7900, E-mail: graduateadmissions@dyc.edu.
Website: http://www.dyc.edu/academics/nursing/

East Carolina University, Graduate School, College of Nursing, Greenville, NC 27858-4353. Offers MSN, DNP, PhD, PMC. *Accreditation:* AACN; AANA/CANAEP (one or more programs are accredited); ACNM/ACME (one or more programs are accredited). *Program availability:* Part-time. *Students:* 138 full-time (120 women), 379 part-time (351 women); includes 111 minority (72 Black or African American, non-Hispanic/Latino; 5 American Indian or Alaska Native, non-Hispanic/Latino; 12 Asian, non-Hispanic/Latino; 13 Hispanic/Latino; 9 Two or more races, non-Hispanic/Latino). Average age 38. 221 applicants, 89% accepted, 172 enrolled. In 2015, 108 master's, 11 doctorates, 7 other advanced degrees awarded. *Degree requirements:* For master's, comprehensive exam, thesis optional. *Entrance requirements:* For master's, GRE General Test or MAT, bachelor's degree in nursing, professional license, minimum B average in nursing. *Application deadline:* For fall admission, 6/1 priority date for domestic students. Applications are processed on a rolling basis. Application fee: $70. *Financial support:* Research assistantships with partial tuition reimbursements, teaching assistantships with partial tuition reimbursements, and Federal Work-Study available. Support available to part-time students. Financial award application deadline: 6/1. *Unit head:* Dr. Sylvia Brown, Dean, 252-744-6372, E-mail: brownsy@ecu.edu. *Application contact:* Dean of Graduate School, 252-328-6012, Fax: 252-328-6071, E-mail: gradschool@ecu.edu.
Website: http://www.ecu.edu/nursing/

Eastern Kentucky University, The Graduate School, College of Health Sciences, Department of Nursing, Richmond, KY 40475-3102. Offers rural community health care (MSN); rural health family nurse practitioner (MSN). *Accreditation:* AACN. *Entrance requirements:* For master's, GRE General Test, minimum GPA of 2.75.

Eastern Mennonite University, Program in Nursing, Harrisonburg, VA 22802-2462. Offers leadership and management (MSN); leadership and school nursing (MSN). *Accreditation:* AACN. *Program availability:* Part-time, online learning. *Degree requirements:* For master's, leadership project. *Entrance requirements:* For master's, RN license, one year of full-time work experience as RN, minimum GPA of 3.0. Additional exam requirements/recommendations for international students: Required—TOEFL. *Application deadline:* For fall admission, 6/1 for domestic students. Applications are processed on a rolling basis. Application fee: $25. *Expenses: Tuition, area resident:* Part-time $600 per credit hour. *Required fees:* $25 per unit. Part-time tuition and fees vary according to course load and program. *Financial support:* Federal Work-Study and scholarships/grants available. Financial award applicants required to submit FAFSA. *Faculty research:* Community health, international health, effectiveness of the nursing school environment, development of caring ability in nursing students, international nursing students. *Unit head:* Ann Hershberger, Coordinator, 540-432-4192, E-mail: hershbea@emu.edu. *Application contact:* Don A. Yoder, Director of Seminary and Graduate Admissions, 540-432-4257, Fax: 540-432-4598, E-mail: yoderda@emu.edu.

Eastern New Mexico University, Graduate School, College of Liberal Arts and Sciences, Department of Health and Human Services, Portales, NM 88130. Offers nursing (MSN); speech pathology and audiology (MS). *Accreditation:* ASHA. *Program availability:* Part-time, online learning. *Degree requirements:* For master's, thesis optional, oral and written comprehensive exam, oral presentation of professional portfolio. *Entrance requirements:* For master's, GRE, three letters of recommendation, resume, two essays. Additional exam requirements/recommendations for international

Nursing—General

students: Required—TOEFL (minimum score 550 paper-based; 79 iBT), IELTS (minimum score 6). Electronic applications accepted.

East Tennessee State University, School of Graduate Studies, College of Nursing, Johnson City, TN 37614. Offers family nurse practitioner (DNP); nursing (MSN, PhD, Post-Master's Certificate). *Accreditation:* AACN. *Program availability:* Part-time, evening/weekend, online learning. *Faculty:* 27 full-time (26 women), 7 part-time/adjunct (all women). *Students:* 107 full-time (91 women), 331 part-time (294 women); includes 37 minority (18 Black or African American, non-Hispanic/Latino; 1 American Indian or Alaska Native, non-Hispanic/Latino; 6 Asian, non-Hispanic/Latino; 4 Hispanic/Latino; 2 Native Hawaiian or other Pacific Islander, non-Hispanic/Latino; 6 Two or more races, non-Hispanic/Latino). Average age 36. 280 applicants, 42% accepted, 83 enrolled. In 2015, 80 master's, 13 doctorates, 10 other advanced degrees awarded. *Degree requirements:* For master's and Post-Master's Certificate, comprehensive exam, practicum; for doctorate, comprehensive exam, thesis/dissertation (for some programs), practicum, internship. *Entrance requirements:* For master's, bachelor's degree, minimum GPA of 3.0, current RN license and eligibility to practice, resume, three letters of recommendation; for doctorate, GRE General Test, MSN (for PhD), BSN or MSN (for DNP), current RN license and eligibility to practice, 2 years of full-time registered nurse work experience or equivalent, three letters of recommendation, resume or curriculum vitae, interview, writing sample; for Post-Master's Certificate, MSN, minimum GPA of 3.0, current RN license and eligibility to practice, three letters of recommendation, resume or curriculum vitae. Additional exam requirements/recommendations for international students: Required—TOEFL (minimum score 550 paper-based; 79 iBT). *Application deadline:* For fall admission, 2/1 for domestic and international students; for spring admission, 7/1 for domestic and international students. Application fee: $35 ($45 for international students). Electronic applications accepted. *Financial support:* In 2015–16, 3 students received support, including 9 research assistantships with tuition reimbursements available (averaging $4,500 per year), 1 teaching assistantship (averaging $6,000 per year); career-related internships or fieldwork, institutionally sponsored loans, scholarships/grants, and unspecified assistantships also available. Financial award application deadline: 7/1; financial award applicants required to submit FAFSA. *Faculty research:* Improving health of rural and underserved populations (low income elders living in public housing, rural caregivers, Hispanic populations), health services and systems research (quality outcomes of nurse-managed primary care, in-home, and rural health care), nursing education (experiences of second-degree BSN students, well-being of BSN students). *Unit head:* Dr. Wendy Nehring, Dean, 423-439-7051, Fax: 423-439-4522, E-mail: nursing@etsu.edu. *Application contact:* Linda Raines, School of Graduate Studies, 423-439-6158, Fax: 423-439-5624, E-mail: raineslt@etsu.edu.
Website: http://www.etsu.edu/nursing/

Edgewood College, Henry Predolin School of Nursing, Madison, WI 53711. Offers administration (MSN); education (MSN); nursing (DNP). *Accreditation:* AACN. *Students:* 11 full-time (10 women), 60 part-time (55 women); includes 4 minority (1 Asian, non-Hispanic/Latino; 3 Hispanic/Latino). Average age 39. In 2015, 25 master's, 5 doctorates awarded. *Degree requirements:* For master's, practicum, research project; for doctorate, practicum, capstone project. *Entrance requirements:* For master's, minimum GPA of 3.0, 2 letters of reference, current RN license. Additional exam requirements/recommendations for international students: Required—TOEFL. *Application deadline:* For fall admission, 8/15 priority date for domestic students, 5/1 for international students; for spring admission, 1/8 priority date for domestic students, 11/1 for international students. Applications are processed on a rolling basis. Application fee: $30. Electronic applications accepted. *Unit head:* Dr. Margaret Noreuil, Dean, 608-663-2820, Fax: 608-663-3291, E-mail: mnoreuil@edgewood.edu. *Application contact:* Tracy Kantor, Enrollment and Applications Manager, 608-663-3297, Fax: 608-663-3496, E-mail: gps@edgewood.edu.
Website: http://www.edgewood.edu/Academics/School-of-Nursing

Edinboro University of Pennsylvania, Department of Nursing, Edinboro, PA 16444. Offers advanced practice nursing (DNP); family nurse practitioner (MSN); nurse educator (MSN). *Program availability:* Part-time, evening/weekend. *Degree requirements:* For master's, thesis, competency exam. *Entrance requirements:* For master's, GRE or MAT, minimum QPA of 2.5. *Application deadline:* Applications are processed on a rolling basis. Application fee: $30. Electronic applications accepted. *Expenses:* Tuition, state resident: full-time $11,280; part-time $470 per credit hour. Tuition, nonresident: full-time $16,920; part-time $705 per credit hour. *International tuition:* $16,920 full-time. *Required fees:* $3247.20; $135.30 per credit hour. *Financial support:* Research assistantships with tuition reimbursements, career-related internships or fieldwork, Federal Work-Study, scholarships/grants, and unspecified assistantships available. Support available to part-time students. Financial award application deadline: 2/15; financial award applicants required to submit FAFSA. *Unit head:* Dr. Amy McClune, Chair, 814-732-2619, E-mail: amcclune@edinboro.edu. *Application contact:* Dr. Amy McClune, Chair, 814-732-2619, E-mail: amcclune@edinboro.edu.
Website: http://www.edinboro.edu/departments/nursing/nursing.dot

EDP University of Puerto Rico–San Sebastian, Graduate School, San Sebastian, PR 00685. Offers nursing science (MS).

Elmhurst College, Graduate Programs, Nursing Master's Entry Program, Elmhurst, IL 60126-3296. Offers MS. *Faculty:* 8 full-time (7 women), 1 (woman) part-time/adjunct. *Students:* 27 full-time (24 women); includes 9 minority (2 Black or African American, non-Hispanic/Latino; 1 Asian, non-Hispanic/Latino; 5 Hispanic/Latino; 1 Two or more races, non-Hispanic/Latino). Average age 30. 47 applicants, 49% accepted, 16 enrolled. *Entrance requirements:* For master's, baccalaureate degree with minimum GPA of 3.0. Additional exam requirements/recommendations for international students: Required—TOEFL (minimum score 550 paper-based; 79 iBT). *Application deadline:* Applications are processed on a rolling basis. Application fee: $0. Electronic applications accepted. *Expenses:* $28,500 per year comprehensive fee. *Financial support:* In 2015–16, 17 students received support. Scholarships/grants available. Financial award application deadline: 6/1; financial award applicants required to submit FAFSA. *Unit head:* Timothy J. Panfil, Director of Enrollment Management, School for Professional Studies, 630-617-3300 Ext. 3256, Fax: 630-617-6471, E-mail: panfilt@elmhurst.edu.
Website: http://www.elmhurst.edu/nursing_masters_entry

Elmhurst College, Graduate Programs, Program in Nursing, Elmhurst, IL 60126-3296. Offers MSN. *Accreditation:* AACN. *Program availability:* Part-time, evening/weekend. *Faculty:* 4 full-time (all women), 1 (woman) part-time/adjunct. *Students:* 41 part-time (36 women); includes 10 minority (1 Black or African American, non-Hispanic/Latino; 2 Asian, non-Hispanic/Latino; 6 Hispanic/Latino; 1 Two or more races, non-Hispanic/Latino). Average age 34. 24 applicants, 67% accepted, 12 enrolled. In 2015, 18 master's awarded. *Entrance requirements:* For master's, 3 recommendations, resume, statement of purpose, current RN licensure in Illinois, interview. Additional exam requirements/recommendations for international students: Required—TOEFL (minimum score 550 paper-based; 79 iBT). *Application deadline:* Applications are processed on a rolling basis. Application fee: $0. Electronic applications accepted. *Expenses:* $725 per semester hour. *Financial support:* In 2015–16, 2 students received support.

Scholarships/grants available. Support available to part-time students. Financial award application deadline: 6/1; financial award applicants required to submit FAFSA. *Application contact:* Timothy J. Panfil, Director of Enrollment Management, School for Professional Studies, 630-617-3300 Ext. 3256, Fax: 630-617-6471, E-mail: panfilt@elmhurst.edu.
Website: http://www.elmhurst.edu/nrs

Elms College, School of Nursing, Chicopee, MA 01013-2839. Offers nursing and health services management (MSN); nursing education (MSN). *Accreditation:* AACN. *Program availability:* Part-time, evening/weekend. *Faculty:* 4 full-time (all women), 5 part-time/adjunct (4 women). *Students:* 99 part-time (91 women); includes 6 minority (2 Black or African American, non-Hispanic/Latino; 1 American Indian or Alaska Native, non-Hispanic/Latino; 3 Hispanic/Latino). Average age 40. 43 applicants, 81% accepted, 27 enrolled. In 2015, 16 master's awarded. *Entrance requirements:* Additional exam requirements/recommendations for international students: Required—TOEFL. *Application deadline:* For fall admission, 7/1 priority date for domestic students; for spring admission, 11/1 priority date for domestic students. Applications are processed on a rolling basis. Application fee: $30. *Financial support:* Applicants required to submit FAFSA. *Unit head:* Dr. Kathleen Scoble, Dean, School of Nursing, 413-265-2204, E-mail: scoblek@elms.edu. *Application contact:* Dr. Cynthia L. Dakin, Director of Graduate Nursing Studies, 413-265-2455, Fax: 413-265-2335, E-mail: dakinc@elms.edu.

Emmanuel College, Graduate and Professional Programs, Graduate Program in Nursing, Boston, MA 02115. Offers education (MSN, Graduate Certificate); management (MSN, Graduate Certificate). *Program availability:* Part-time, evening/weekend. *Faculty:* 4 full-time (all women), 7 part-time/adjunct (all women). *Students:* 43 part-time (42 women); includes 3 minority (1 Black or African American, non-Hispanic/Latino; 1 Hispanic/Latino; 1 Two or more races, non-Hispanic/Latino). Average age 44. In 2015, 9 master's awarded. *Degree requirements:* For master's, 36 credits, including 6-credit practicum. *Entrance requirements:* For master's and Graduate Certificate, transcripts from all regionally-accredited institutions attended (showing proof of bachelor's degree completion), proof of RN license, 2 letters of recommendation, essay, resume. *Application deadline:* For fall admission, 7/30 for domestic students. Applications are processed on a rolling basis. Electronic applications accepted. Application fee is waived when completed online. *Expenses:* $2,581 per course. *Financial support:* Applicants required to submit FAFSA. *Unit head:* Diane Shea, Associate Dean for Nursing/Professor of Nursing Practice, 617-732-1604, E-mail: shead@emmanuel.edu. *Application contact:* Helen Muterperl, Assistant Director of Graduate Admissions, 617-735-9700, Fax: 617-507-0434, E-mail: gpp@emmanuel.edu.
Website: http://www.emmanuel.edu/graduate-professional-programs/academics/nursing.html

Emory University, Laney Graduate School, Program in Nursing, Atlanta, GA 30322-1100. Offers PhD. *Accreditation:* AACN. *Degree requirements:* For doctorate, comprehensive exam, thesis/dissertation. *Entrance requirements:* For doctorate, GRE General Test. Additional exam requirements/recommendations for international students: Required—TOEFL. Electronic applications accepted. *Faculty research:* Symptoms, self management, care-giving, biobehavioral approaches, women's health.

Emory University, Nell Hodgson Woodruff School of Nursing, Atlanta, GA 30322-1100. Offers adult nurse practitioner (MSN); emergency nurse practitioner (MSN); family nurse practitioner (MSN); family nurse-midwife (MSN); health systems leadership (MSN); nurse-midwifery (MSN); pediatric nurse practitioner acute and primary care (MSN); women's health care (Title X) (MSN); women's health nurse practitioner (MSN); MSN/MPH. *Accreditation:* AACN; ACNM/ACME (one or more programs are accredited). *Program availability:* Part-time. *Entrance requirements:* For master's, GRE General Test or MAT, minimum GPA of 3.0, BS in nursing from an accredited institution, RN license and additional course work, 3 letters of recommendation. Additional exam requirements/recommendations for international students: Required—TOEFL (minimum score 600 paper-based; 100 iBT). Electronic applications accepted. *Expenses:* Contact institution. *Faculty research:* Older adult falls and injuries, minority health issues, cardiac symptoms and quality of life, bio-ethics and decision-making, menopausal issues.

Endicott College, Van Loan School of Graduate and Professional Studies, Program in Nursing, Beverly, MA 01915-2096. Offers MSN, PhD. *Program availability:* Part-time. *Faculty:* 5 full-time (4 women), 9 part-time/adjunct (all women). *Students:* 27 full-time (25 women), 61 part-time (56 women); includes 7 minority (5 Black or African American, non-Hispanic/Latino; 1 Asian, non-Hispanic/Latino; 1 Hispanic/Latino). Average age 39. 39 applicants, 100% accepted, 31 enrolled. In 2015, 22 master's awarded. *Degree requirements:* For master's, thesis, practicum; for doctorate, thesis/dissertation. *Entrance requirements:* For master's, MAT or GRE, statement of professional goals, official transcripts of all undergraduate and graduate course work, two letters of recommendation, photocopy of current and unrestricted RN license, basic statistics course, interview. Additional exam requirements/recommendations for international students: Required—TOEFL. *Application deadline:* Applications are processed on a rolling basis. Application fee: $50. Electronic applications accepted. *Expenses:* Contact institution. *Financial support:* Applicants required to submit FAFSA. *Unit head:* Dr. Kelly Fisher, Dean, 978-232-2328, Fax: 978-232-3000, E-mail: kfisher@endicott.edu. *Application contact:* Ian Menchini, Director, Graduate Enrollment and Advising, 978-232-5292, Fax: 978-232-3000, E-mail: imenchin@endicott.edu.
Website: http://www.endicott.edu/nursing.aspx

Excelsior College, School of Nursing, Albany, NY 12203-5159. Offers nursing (MS); nursing education (MS); nursing informatics (MS); nursing leadership and administration of health care systems (MS). *Accreditation:* ACEN. *Program availability:* Part-time, evening/weekend, online learning. *Faculty:* 18 part-time/adjunct (14 women). *Students:* 938 part-time (770 women); includes 295 minority (166 Black or African American, non-Hispanic/Latino; 8 American Indian or Alaska Native, non-Hispanic/Latino; 36 Asian, non-Hispanic/Latino; 60 Hispanic/Latino; 8 Native Hawaiian or other Pacific Islander, non-Hispanic/Latino; 17 Two or more races, non-Hispanic/Latino; 2 international). Average age 45. In 2015, 200 master's awarded. *Entrance requirements:* For master's, RN license. *Application deadline:* Applications are processed on a rolling basis. Application fee: $110. Electronic applications accepted. *Expenses:* Tuition, area resident: Part-time $645 per credit. *Required fees:* $265 per unit. *Financial support:* Scholarships/grants available. *Unit head:* Dr. Barbara Pieper, Associate Dean, Graduate Program in Nursing, 518-464-8500, Fax: 518-464-8777, E-mail: msn@excelsior.edu. *Application contact:* Admissions Counselor, 518-464-8500, Fax: 518-464-0777, E-mail: admissions@excelsior.edu.

Fairfield University, Marion Peckham Egan School of Nursing and Health Studies, Fairfield, CT 06824. Offers advanced practice (DNP); family nurse practitioner (MSN, DNP); nurse anesthesia (DNP); nursing leadership (MSN); psychiatric nurse practitioner (MSN, DNP). *Accreditation:* AACN; AANA/CANAEP. *Program availability:* Part-time, evening/weekend. *Faculty:* 8 full-time (all women), 9 part-time/adjunct (7 women). *Students:* 43 full-time (35 women), 181 part-time (163 women); includes 52 minority (20 Black or African American, non-Hispanic/Latino; 1 American Indian or Alaska Native, non-Hispanic/Latino; 11 Asian, non-Hispanic/Latino; 16 Hispanic/Latino; 4 Two or more races, non-Hispanic/Latino, 1 international. Average age 36. 103 applicants, 67% accepted, 43 enrolled. In 2015, 12 master's, 21 doctorates awarded. *Degree

requirements: For master's, capstone project. *Entrance requirements:* For master's, minimum QPA of 3.0, RN license, resume, 2 recommendations; for doctorate, MSN (minimum QPA of 3.2) or BSN (minimum QPA of 3.0); critical care nursing experience (for nurse anesthesia DNP candidates). Additional exam requirements/ recommendations for international students: Required—TOEFL (minimum score 550 paper-based; 80 iBT) or IELTS (minimum score 6.5). *Application deadline:* For fall admission, 5/15 for international students; for spring admission, 10/15 for international students. Applications are processed on a rolling basis. Application fee: $60. Electronic applications accepted. *Expenses:* $850 per credit hour (for MSN); $900-$1,000 per credit hour (for DNP). *Financial support:* In 2015–16, 51 students received support. Unspecified assistantships available. Financial award applicants required to submit FAFSA. *Faculty research:* Aging, spiritual care, palliative and end of life care, psychiatric mental health, pediatric trauma. *Unit head:* Dr. Meredith Wallace Kazer, Dean, 203-254-4000 Ext. 2701, Fax: 203-254-4126, E-mail: mkazer@fairfield.edu. *Application contact:* Marianne Gumpper, Director of Graduate and Continuing Studies Admission, 203-254-4184, Fax: 203-254-4073, E-mail: gradadmis@fairfield.edu.
Website: http://fairfield.edu/son

Fairleigh Dickinson University, Metropolitan Campus, University College: Arts, Sciences, and Professional Studies, Henry P. Becton School of Nursing and Allied Health, Program in Nursing, Teaneck, NJ 07666-1914. Offers MSN, Certificate. *Accreditation:* AACN.

Fairleigh Dickinson University, Metropolitan Campus, University College: Arts, Sciences, and Professional Studies, Henry P. Becton School of Nursing and Allied Health, Program in Nursing Practice, Teaneck, NJ 07666-1914. Offers DNP.

Felician University, Doctor of Nursing Practice Program, Lodi, NJ 07644-2117. Offers advanced practice (DNP); executive leadership (DNP). *Program availability:* Evening/ weekend, online learning. *Faculty:* 1 (woman) full-time, 1 (woman) part-time/adjunct. *Students:* 16 part-time (14 women); includes 9 minority (5 Black or African American, non-Hispanic/Latino; 2 Asian, non-Hispanic/Latino; 1 Hispanic/Latino; 1 Native Hawaiian or other Pacific Islander, non-Hispanic/Latino). Average age 53. 16 applicants, 75% accepted, 8 enrolled. In 2015, 6 doctorates awarded. *Degree requirements:* For doctorate, scholarly project. *Entrance requirements:* Additional exam requirements/ recommendations for international students: Recommended—TOEFL (minimum score 79 iBT). *Application deadline:* Applications are processed on a rolling basis. Application fee: $40. Electronic applications accepted. Application fee is waived when completed online. *Expenses: Tuition, area resident:* Part-time $965 per credit. Tuition and fees vary according to course load and program. *Financial support:* Applicants required to submit FAFSA. *Unit head:* Dr. Ann Tritak, Associate Dean, Department of Graduate Nursing, 201-559-6151, E-mail: tritaka@felician.edu. *Application contact:* Dr. Margaret Smolin, Director, Graduate Admissions, 201-559-1451, E-mail: graduate@felician.edu.

Felician University, Master of Science in Nursing Program, Lodi, NJ 07644-2117. Offers adult-gerontology nurse practitioner (MSN, PMC); executive leadership (MSN, PMC); family nurse practitioner (MSN, PMC); nursing education (MSN, PMC). *Accreditation:* AACN. *Program availability:* Part-time, evening/weekend, online learning. *Faculty:* 11 full-time (9 women), 2 part-time/adjunct (both women). *Students:* 1 (woman) full-time, 121 part-time (112 women); includes 60 minority (23 Black or African American, non-Hispanic/Latino; 1 American Indian or Alaska Native, non-Hispanic/ Latino; 19 Asian, non-Hispanic/Latino; 17 Hispanic/Latino). Average age 40. 111 applicants, 83% accepted, 52 enrolled. In 2015, 18 master's awarded. *Entrance requirements:* For master's, BS in nursing or equivalent, minimum GPA of 3.0, 2 letters of recommendation, RN license; for PMC, RN license, minimum GPA of 3.0. Additional exam requirements/recommendations for international students: Recommended— TOEFL (minimum score 79 iBT). *Application deadline:* Applications are processed on a rolling basis. Application fee: $40. Electronic applications accepted. Application fee is waived when completed online. *Expenses: Tuition, area resident:* Part-time $965 per credit. Tuition and fees vary according to course load and program. *Financial support:* In 2015–16, 10 students received support. Traineeships available. Financial award applicants required to submit FAFSA. *Faculty research:* Anxiety and fear, curriculum innovation, health promotion. *Unit head:* Dr. Ann Tritak, Associate Dean, Department of Graduate Nursing, 201-201-559-6151, E-mail: tritaka@felician.edu. *Application contact:* Dr. Margaret Smolin, Director, Graduate Admissions, 201-559-1451, E-mail: graduate@felician.edu.

Ferris State University, College of Health Professions, School of Nursing, Big Rapids, MI 49307. Offers nursing (MSN); nursing administration (MSN); nursing education (MSN); nursing informatics (MSN). *Accreditation:* ACEN. *Program availability:* Part-time, evening/weekend, 100% online. *Faculty:* 5 full-time (all women), 2 part-time/adjunct (both women). *Students:* 95 part-time (84 women); includes 11 minority (4 Black or African American, non-Hispanic/Latino; 1 American Indian or Alaska Native, non-Hispanic/Latino; 3 Asian, non-Hispanic/Latino; 1 Hispanic/Latino; 1 Native Hawaiian or other Pacific Islander, non-Hispanic/Latino; 1 Two or more races, non-Hispanic/Latino). Average age 39. 23 applicants, 74% accepted, 13 enrolled. In 2015, 15 master's awarded. *Degree requirements:* For master's, comprehensive exam, practicum, practicum project. *Entrance requirements:* For master's, BS in nursing (for nursing education track); BS in nursing or related field (for nursing administration and nursing informatics tracks); registered nurse license, writing sample, letters of reference, 2 years' clinical experience (recommended). Additional exam requirements/ recommendations for international students: Required—TOEFL (minimum score 550 paper-based; 61 iBT). *Application deadline:* For fall admission, 4/15 priority date for domestic students; for spring admission, 10/15 for domestic students. Application fee: $0. Electronic applications accepted. Tuition and fees vary according to degree level and program. *Financial support:* In 2015–16, 3 students received support. Fellowships, research assistantships, teaching assistantships, career-related internships or fieldwork, and scholarships/grants available. Financial award application deadline: 4/15; financial award applicants required to submit FAFSA. *Faculty research:* Nursing education, end of life, leadership/education introverts in nursing. *Unit head:* Dr. Susan Owens, Chair, School of Nursing, 231-591-2267, Fax: 231-591-2325, E-mail: owenss3@ferris.edu. *Application contact:* Debby Buck, Off-Campus Program Secretary, 231-591-2270, Fax: 231-591-3788, E-mail: buckd@ferris.edu.
Website: http://www.ferris.edu/htmls/colleges/alliedhe/Nursing/homepage.htm

Florida Agricultural and Mechanical University, Division of Graduate Studies, Research, and Continuing Education, School of Nursing, Tallahassee, FL 32307-3200. Offers MSN, PhD. *Accreditation:* ACEN. *Entrance requirements:* Additional exam requirements/recommendations for international students: Required—TOEFL.

Florida Atlantic University, Christine E. Lynn College of Nursing, Boca Raton, FL 33431. Offers administrative and financial leadership in nursing and health care (Post Master's Certificate); nursing (PhD); nursing practice (DNP). *Accreditation:* AACN. *Program availability:* Part-time. *Degree requirements:* For master's, thesis or alternative; for doctorate, comprehensive exam, thesis/dissertation. *Entrance requirements:* For master's, GRE General Test or MAT, bachelor's degree in nursing, Florida RN license, minimum GPA of 3.0, resume/curriculum vitae, letter of recommendation; for doctorate, GRE General Test or MAT, curriculum vitae, Florida RN license, minimum GPA of 3.5, master's degree in nursing, three letters of recommendation. *Application deadline:* For fall admission, 6/1 for domestic students, 2/15 for international students; for spring

admission, 10/1 for domestic students, 7/15 for international students. Applications are processed on a rolling basis. Application fee: $30. *Expenses: Tuition, area resident:* Full-time $7392; part-time $369.82 per credit hour. Tuition, state resident: full-time $7392; part-time $369.82 per credit hour. Tuition, nonresident: full-time $19,432; part-time $1024.81 per credit hour. *Financial support:* Research assistantships with partial tuition reimbursements, teaching assistantships with partial tuition reimbursements, career-related internships or fieldwork, Federal Work-Study, institutionally sponsored loans, scholarships/grants, and traineeships available. Support available to part-time students. *Faculty research:* Econometrics of nurse-patient relationship, Alzheimer's disease, community-based programs, falls, self-healing.
Website: http://nursing.fau.edu/

Florida International University, College of Nursing and Health Sciences, Nursing Program, Miami, FL 33199. Offers MSN, DNP, PhD. *Accreditation:* AACN; AANA/ CANAEP. *Program availability:* Part-time, evening/weekend. *Students:* 267 full-time (188 women), 97 part-time (82 women); includes 285 minority (69 Black or African American, non-Hispanic/Latino; 28 Asian, non-Hispanic/Latino; 183 Hispanic/Latino; 1 Native Hawaiian or other Pacific Islander, non-Hispanic/Latino; 4 Two or more races, non-Hispanic/ Latino); 4 international. Average age 38. 342 applicants, 42% accepted, 129 enrolled. In 2015, 175 master's, 8 doctorates awarded. *Degree requirements:* For master's, thesis or alternative; for doctorate, comprehensive exam, thesis/dissertation. *Entrance requirements:* For master's, bachelor's degree in nursing, minimum undergraduate GPA of 3.0 in upper-level coursework, letters of recommendation; for doctorate, GRE, letters of recommendation, minimum undergraduate GPA of 3.0 in upper-level coursework, interview. Additional exam requirements/recommendations for international students: Required—TOEFL (minimum score 550 paper-based; 80 iBT). *Application deadline:* For fall admission, 6/1 for domestic students, 4/1 for international students; for spring admission, 10/1 for domestic students, 9/1 for international students. Applications are processed on a rolling basis. Application fee: $30. Electronic applications accepted. *Expenses:* Tuition, state resident: full-time $10,708; part-time $455.64 per credit hour. Tuition, nonresident: full-time $23,816; part-time $1001.69 per credit hour. *Required fees:* $390; $195 per semester. Tuition and fees vary according to program. *Financial support:* Institutionally sponsored loans and scholarships/grants available. Financial award application deadline: 3/1; financial award applicants required to submit FAFSA. *Faculty research:* Adult health nursing. *Unit head:* Dr. Yhovana Gordon, Director, 305-348-7733, E-mail: gordony@fiu.edu. *Application contact:* Nanett Rojas, Manager, Admissions Operations, 305-348-7464, Fax: 305-348-7441, E-mail: gradadm@fiu.edu. Website: http://cnhs.fiu.edu/

Florida National University, Program in Nursing, Hialeah, FL 33012. Offers family nurse practitioner (MSN); nurse educator (MSN); nurse leadership and management (MSN). *Degree requirements:* For master's, practicum. *Entrance requirements:* For master's, active registered nurse license, BSN from accredited institution. *Expenses: Tuition, area resident:* Full-time $15,600. *Required fees:* $650.

Florida Southern College, Program in Nursing, Lakeland, FL 33801-5698. Offers adult gerontology clinical nurse specialist (MSN); adult gerontology primary care nurse practitioner (MSN); nurse educator (MSN); nursing administration (MSN). *Accreditation:* AACN. *Program availability:* Part-time, evening/weekend. *Entrance requirements:* For master's, Florida RN license, 3 letters of recommendation, personal statement, minimum GPA of 3.0, resume. Additional exam requirements/recommendations for international students: Required—TOEFL (minimum score 550 paper-based). *Expenses:* Contact institution. *Faculty research:* End of life care, dementia, health promotion.

Florida State University, The Graduate School, College of Nursing, Tallahassee, FL 32306-4310. Offers family nurse practitioner (DNP); nurse educator (MSN, Certificate); nurse leader (MSN); nursing leadership (Certificate). *Accreditation:* AACN. *Program availability:* Part-time, online learning. *Faculty:* 13 full-time (12 women). *Students:* 56 full-time (49 women), 25 part-time (23 women); includes 25 minority (13 Black or African American, non-Hispanic/Latino; 4 Asian, non-Hispanic/Latino; 7 Hispanic/Latino; 1 Two or more races, non-Hispanic/Latino). Average age 38. 90 applicants, 50% accepted, 44 enrolled. In 2015, 2 master's, 20 doctorates awarded. *Degree requirements:* For master's, thesis optional; for doctorate, thesis/dissertation, evidence-based project. *Entrance requirements:* For master's, GRE General Test, MAT, minimum GPA of 3.0, BSN, United States RN license; for doctorate, GRE General Test, MAT, minimum GPA of 3.0, BSN or MSN, Florida RN license. Additional exam requirements/ recommendations for international students: Required—TOEFL (minimum score 550 paper-based). *Application deadline:* For fall admission, 4/15 for domestic and international students. Application fee: $30. Electronic applications accepted. *Expenses: Tuition, area resident:* Full-time $7263; part-time $403.50 per credit hour. Tuition, nonresident: full-time $18,087; part-time $1004.85 per credit hour. *Required fees:* $1365; $75.81 per credit hour. $20 per semester. Tuition and fees vary according to campus/location. *Financial support:* In 2015–16, 75 students received support, including fellowships with partial tuition reimbursements available (averaging $6,300 per year), research assistantships with partial tuition reimbursements available (averaging $3,000 per year), 3 teaching assistantships with partial tuition reimbursements available (averaging $3,000 per year); career-related internships or fieldwork, Federal Work-Study, institutionally sponsored loans, scholarships/grants, traineeships, and tuition waivers (partial) also available. Financial award application deadline: 4/15; financial award applicants required to submit FAFSA. *Faculty research:* Cardiac, women's health, health promotion and prevention, educational strategies, infectious diseases. *Unit head:* Dr. Judith McFetridge-Durdle, Dean, 850-644-6846, Fax: 850-644-7660, E-mail: jdurdle@nursing.fsu.edu. *Application contact:* Carlos Urrutia, Assistant Director for Student Services, 850-644-5638, Fax: 850-645-7249, E-mail: currutia@fsu.edu.
Website: http://nursing.fsu.edu/

Fort Hays State University, Graduate School, College of Health and Life Sciences, Department of Nursing, Hays, KS 67601-4099. Offers MSN. *Accreditation:* AACN. *Degree requirements:* For master's, comprehensive exam, thesis optional. *Entrance requirements:* For master's, GRE General Test or MAT. Additional exam requirements/ recommendations for international students: Required—TOEFL (minimum score 550 paper-based). Electronic applications accepted.

Framingham State University, Continuing Education, Program in Nursing, Framingham, MA 01701-9101. Offers nursing education (MSN); nursing leadership (MSN). *Accreditation:* AACN. *Entrance requirements:* For master's, BSN; minimum cumulative undergraduate GPA of 3.0, 3.25 in nursing courses; coursework in statistics; 2 letters of recommendation; interview. Electronic applications accepted.

Franciscan University of Steubenville, Graduate Programs, Department of Nursing, Steubenville, OH 43952-1763. Offers MSN. *Accreditation:* ACEN. *Program availability:* Part-time, evening/weekend. *Entrance requirements:* For master's, thesis. *Entrance requirements:* For master's, GRE General Test, MAT. Additional exam requirements/ recommendations for international students: Required—TOEFL. Electronic applications accepted. Application fee is waived when completed online. *Expenses: Tuition, area resident:* Full-time $12,330; part-time $685 per credit hour. *Required fees:* $288; $16 per credit hour. Tuition and fees vary according to course level and program.

Nursing—General

Francis Marion University, Graduate Programs, Department of Nursing, Florence, SC 29502-0547. Offers family nurse practitioner (MSN); family nurse practitioner with nurse educator certificate (MSN); nurse educator (MSN). *Program availability:* Part-time. *Faculty:* 7 full-time (all women). *Students:* 52 full-time (40 women), 28 part-time (23 women); includes 19 minority (16 Black or African American, non-Hispanic/Latino; 1 American Indian or Alaska Native, non-Hispanic/Latino; 1 Asian, non-Hispanic/Latino; 1 Two or more races, non-Hispanic/Latino). Average age 34. 37 applicants, 84% accepted, 27 enrolled. In 2015, 27 master's awarded. *Entrance requirements:* For master's, GRE, official transcripts, two letters of recommendation from professional associates or former professors, written statement of applicant's career goals, current nursing license. Additional exam requirements/recommendations for international students: Required—TOEFL (minimum score 550 paper-based; 79 iBT). *Application deadline:* For fall admission, 3/1 for domestic and international students; for spring admission, 10/1 for domestic and international students. Applications are processed on a rolling basis. Application fee: $37. Electronic applications accepted. *Expenses:* Contact institution. *Financial support:* Available to part-time students. Application deadline: 3/1; applicants required to submit FAFSA. *Unit head:* Dr. Ruth Wittmann-Price, Chair, 843-661-4625, E-mail: rwittmannprice@fmarion.edu. *Application contact:* Jennifer Taylor, Administrative Manager, Provost's Office, 843-661-1286, Fax: 843-661-4688, E-mail: jtaylor@fmarion.edu.

Fresno Pacific University, Graduate Programs, Program in Nursing, Fresno, CA 93702-4709. Offers family nurse practitioner (MSN). *Entrance requirements:* For master's, official transcripts verifying BSN from accredited nursing program; minimum cumulative GPA of 3.0; three reference forms; statement of intent; resume or curriculum vitae; personal interview; active California RN license; completion of statistics, chemistry and upper-division writing. *Expenses:* Contact institution.

Frontier Nursing University, Graduate Programs, Hyden, KY 41749. Offers family nurse practitioner (MSN, DNP, Post Master's Certificate); nurse-midwifery (MSN, DNP, Post Master's Certificate); women's health care nurse practitioner (MSN, DNP, Post Master's Certificate). *Accreditation:* ACEN; ACNM. *Degree requirements:* For doctorate, capstone project, practicum.

Frostburg State University, Graduate School, College of Liberal Arts and Sciences, Department of Nursing, Frostburg, MD 21532-1099. Offers nursing administration (MSN); nursing education (MSN). *Program availability:* Part-time, online learning.

Gannon University, School of Graduate Studies, Morosky College of Health Professions and Sciences, School of Health Professions, Erie, PA 16541-0001. Offers athletic training (MAT); nursing administration (MSN), including nursing administration; nursing practice (DNP), including nursing; occupational therapy (MS, OTD); physical therapy (DPT); physician assistant science (MPAS); sport and exercise science (MS), including human performance. *Accreditation:* APTA (one or more programs are accredited). *Program availability:* Part-time, evening/weekend, 100% online. *Faculty:* 36 full-time (31 women), 11 part-time/adjunct (8 women). *Students:* 227 full-time (162 women), 4 part-time (all women); includes 8 minority (2 Black or African American, non-Hispanic/Latino; 5 Asian, non-Hispanic/Latino; 1 Hispanic/Latino), 3 international. Average age 24. 239 applicants, 52% accepted, 57 enrolled. In 2015, 83 master's, 42 doctorates awarded. *Degree requirements:* For master's, thesis (for some programs); for doctorate, thesis/dissertation (for some programs), research project. *Entrance requirements:* For master's, GRE, bachelor's degree from accredited institution, letters of recommendation, transcripts, teaching certificate (for some programs); for doctorate, letters of recommendation. Additional exam requirements/recommendations for international students: Required—TOEFL (minimum score 79 iBT). *Application deadline:* Applications are processed on a rolling basis. Application fee: $25. Electronic applications accepted. *Financial support:* Teaching assistantships, Federal Work-Study, scholarships/grants, and unspecified assistantships available. Financial award application deadline: 7/1; financial award applicants required to submit FAFSA. *Faculty research:* Assistive technology, cervical cancer screening and prevention, ergonomics and cervical dysfunction, thoracic spine mobilization. *Unit head:* Dr. Carolyn Masters, Dean, 814-871-7568, E-mail: masters004@gannon.edu. *Application contact:* Bridget Philip, Director of Graduate Admissions, 814-871-7412, E-mail: graduate@gannon.edu.

Gannon University, School of Graduate Studies, Morosky College of Health Professions and Sciences, Villa Maria School of Nursing, Program in Nursing Practice, Erie, PA 16541-0001. Offers DNP. *Program availability:* Part-time, evening/weekend, online only, 100% online. *Students:* 5 part-time (2 women); includes 2 minority (1 Hispanic/Latino; 1 Two or more races, non-Hispanic/Latino). Average age 47. 4 applicants, 75% accepted, 2 enrolled. In 2015, 4 doctorates awarded. *Entrance requirements:* For doctorate, MSN; Nurse Practitioner, Nurse Midwife, or Nurse Anesthetist certification; transcripts; 3 letters of recommendation; portfolio (resume, copy of current license and advanced practice license, evidence of active certification and current CEU's, evidence of a thesis or evidence-based practice project, and an essay); minimum GPA of 3.5. Additional exam requirements/recommendations for international students: Required—TOEFL (minimum score 79 iBT). *Application deadline:* For fall admission, 1/15 for domestic students. Application fee: $50. Electronic applications accepted. *Expenses:* Contact institution. *Financial support:* Federal Work-Study available. Financial award applicants required to submit FAFSA. *Unit head:* Dr. Kathleen Patterson, Director, 814-871-5547, E-mail: patterso018@gannon.edu. *Application contact:* Bridget Philip, Director of Graduate Admissions, 814-871-7412, E-mail: graduate@gannon.edu.

Gardner-Webb University, Graduate School, School of Nursing, Boiling Springs, NC 28017. Offers MSN, DNP. *Accreditation:* ACEN. *Program availability:* Part-time, online learning. *Faculty:* 10 full-time (9 women), 11 part-time/adjunct (9 women). *Students:* 1 (woman) full-time, 241 part-time (224 women); includes 38 minority (28 Black or African American, non-Hispanic/Latino; 3 American Indian or Alaska Native, non-Hispanic/Latino; 5 Asian, non-Hispanic/Latino; 2 Hispanic/Latino). Average age 40. 263 applicants, 39% accepted, 89 enrolled. In 2015, 51 master's, 11 doctorates awarded. *Entrance requirements:* For master's, GRE or MAT, minimum undergraduate GPA of 2.7; unrestricted licensure to practice as an RN. *Unit head:* Dr. Sharon Starr, Dean, 704-406-4358, Fax: 704-406-4329, E-mail: gradschool@gardner-webb.edu. *Application contact:* Office of Graduate Admissions, 877-498-4723, Fax: 704-406-3895, E-mail: gradinfo@gardner-webb.edu.

George Mason University, College of Health and Human Services, School of Nursing, Fairfax, VA 22030. Offers nursing (PhD). *Faculty:* 31 full-time (30 women), 41 part-time/adjunct (40 women). *Students:* 54 full-time (45 women), 192 part-time (172 women); includes 98 minority (43 Black or African American, non-Hispanic/Latino; 1 American Indian or Alaska Native, non-Hispanic/Latino; 31 Asian, non-Hispanic/Latino; 18 Hispanic/Latino; 1 Native Hawaiian or other Pacific Islander, non-Hispanic/Latino; 4 Two or more races, non-Hispanic/Latino), 10 international. Average age 39. 214 applicants, 53% accepted, 83 enrolled. In 2015, 48 master's, 27 doctorates, 1 other advanced degree awarded. *Degree requirements:* For master's, comprehensive exam (for some programs), thesis in clinical classes; for doctorate, comprehensive exam (for some programs), thesis/dissertation (for some programs). *Entrance requirements:* For master's, 2 official transcripts; expanded goals statement; resume; BSN from accredited institution; minimum GPA of 3.0 in last 60 credits of undergraduate work; 2 letters of recommendation; completion of undergraduate statistics and graduate-level bivariate

statistics; certification in professional CPR; for doctorate, GRE, 2 official transcripts; expanded goals statement; resume; 3 recommendation letters; nursing license; at least 1 year of work experience as an RN; interview; writing sample; evidence of graduate-level course in applied statistics; master's in nursing with minimum GPA of 3.5; for Certificate, 2 official transcripts; expanded goals statement; resume; master's degree from accredited institution or currently enrolled with minimum GPA of 3.0. Additional exam requirements/recommendations for international students: Required—TOEFL (minimum score 570 paper-based; 88 iBT), IELTS (minimum score 6.5), PTE (minimum score 59). *Application deadline:* For fall admission, 2/1 for domestic and international students. Application fee: $75 ($80 for international students). Electronic applications accepted. *Expenses:* Contact institution. *Financial support:* In 2015–16, 19 students received support, including 1 fellowship (averaging $20,000 per year), 7 research assistantships with tuition reimbursements available (averaging $13,143 per year); career-related internships or fieldwork, Federal Work-Study, scholarships/grants, unspecified assistantships, and health care benefits (for full-time research or teaching assistantship recipients) also available. Financial award application deadline: 3/1; financial award applicants required to submit FAFSA. *Faculty research:* Research in health care, nursing science. *Total annual research expenditures:* $313,216. *Unit head:* Carol Urban, Director, 703-993-2991, Fax: 703-993-1949, E-mail: curban@gmu.edu. *Application contact:* Janice Lee-Beverly, Program Support, 703-993-1947, Fax: 703-993-1943, E-mail: jleebev1@gmu.edu. Website: http://chhs.gmu.edu/nursing

Georgetown University, Graduate School of Arts and Sciences, School of Nursing and Health Studies, Washington, DC 20057. Offers acute care nurse practitioner (MS); clinical nurse specialist (MS); family nurse practitioner (MS); nurse anesthesia (MS); nurse-midwifery (MS); nursing (DNP); nursing education (MS). *Accreditation:* AACN; AANA/CANAEP (one or more programs are accredited); ACNM/ACME (one or more programs are accredited). *Degree requirements:* For master's, thesis optional. *Entrance requirements:* For master's, GRE General Test or MAT, bachelor's degree in nursing from NLN-accredited school, minimum undergraduate GPA of 3.0. Additional exam requirements/recommendations for international students: Required—TOEFL.

The George Washington University, School of Nursing, Washington, DC 20052. Offers adult nurse practitioner (MSN, DNP, Post-Master's Certificate); clinical research administration (MSN); family nurse practitioner (MSN, Post-Master's Certificate); health care quality (MSN, Post-Master's Certificate); nursing leadership and management (MSN); nursing practice (DNP), including nursing education; palliative care nurse practitioner (Post-Master's Certificate). *Accreditation:* AACN. *Faculty:* 42 full-time (all women), 71 part-time/adjunct (66 women). *Students:* 52 full-time (48 women), 519 part-time (463 women); includes 162 minority (72 Black or African American, non-Hispanic/Latino; 4 American Indian or Alaska Native, non-Hispanic/Latino; 52 Asian, non-Hispanic/Latino; 31 Hispanic/Latino; 3 Two or more races, non-Hispanic/Latino), 2 international. Average age 37. 465 applicants, 69% accepted, 187 enrolled. In 2015, 121 master's, 35 doctorates, 1 other advanced degree awarded. *Unit head:* Pamela R. Jeffries, Dean, 202-994-3725, E-mail: pjeffries@gwu.edu. *Application contact:* Kristin Williams, Associate Provost for Graduate Enrollment Management, 202-994-0467, Fax: 202-994-0371, E-mail: ksw@gwu.edu. Website: http://nursing.gwumc.edu/

Georgia College & State University, Graduate School, College of Health Sciences, Georgia Nursing Program, Milledgeville, GA 31061. Offers nursing (MSN); nursing practice (DNP). *Accreditation:* ACEN. *Program availability:* Part-time, evening/weekend, 100% online. *Students:* 111 part-time (101 women); includes 29 minority (19 Black or African American, non-Hispanic/Latino; 4 Asian, non-Hispanic/Latino; 4 Hispanic/Latino; 2 Two or more races, non-Hispanic/Latino), 1 international. Average age 36. 7 applicants, 100% accepted, 3 enrolled. In 2015, 21 master's, 9 doctorates awarded. *Degree requirements:* For master's, comprehensive exam, minimum GPA of 3.0, electronic portfolio, completion of requirements within a period of 7 years; for doctorate, capstone project, complete all required courses within a period of 7 years. *Entrance requirements:* For master's, GRE (taken within last 5 years), bachelor's degree in nursing, RN license, 1 year of clinical experience, minimum GPA of 2.75, statistics course, interview, 2 letters of reference, transcript, resume; for doctorate, master's degree in nursing or anesthesia, minimum graduate GPA of 3.2 in MN program, unencumbered RN licensure, 500 faculty-supervised clinical hours in master's program, interview, computer access. Additional exam requirements/recommendations for international students: Recommended—TOEFL (minimum score 550 paper-based; 79 iBT). *Application deadline:* For fall admission, 7/1 priority date for domestic students; for spring admission, 11/1 priority date for domestic students; for summer admission, 4/1 priority date for domestic students. Applications are processed on a rolling basis. Application fee: $40. Electronic applications accepted. *Expenses:* $8,300 per year full-time tuition and fees. *Financial support:* Unspecified assistantships available. Financial award applicants required to submit FAFSA. *Unit head:* Dr. Deborah MacMillan, School of Nursing Programs Director, 478-445-5122, E-mail: debby.macmillan@gcsu.edu. Website: http://catalog.gcsu.edu/en/2015-2016/Graduate-Catalog/College-of-Health-Sciences

Georgia Southern University, Jack N. Averitt College of Graduate Studies, College of Health and Human Sciences, School of Nursing, Program in Nursing Science, Statesboro, GA 30460. Offers DNP. *Program availability:* Part-time, online learning. *Students:* 1 (woman) full-time, 17 part-time (16 women); includes 3 minority (all Black or African American, non-Hispanic/Latino). Average age 33. 1 applicant. In 2015, 10 doctorates awarded. *Degree requirements:* For doctorate, comprehensive exam (for some programs), thesis/dissertation (for some programs). *Entrance requirements:* Additional exam requirements/recommendations for international students: Required—TOEFL (minimum score 550 paper-based; 80 iBT), IELTS (minimum score 6). *Application deadline:* For fall admission, 6/1 priority date for domestic and international students; for spring admission, 10/1 priority date for domestic students, 10/1 for international students. Applications are processed on a rolling basis. Application fee: $50. Electronic applications accepted. *Expenses:* Tuition, state resident: full-time $7236; part-time $277 per semester hour. Tuition, nonresident: full-time $27,118; part-time $1105 per semester hour. *Required fees:* $2092. *Financial support:* In 2015–16, 18 students received support. Career-related internships or fieldwork, Federal Work-Study, scholarships/grants, traineeships, and tuition waivers available. Support available to part-time students. Financial award application deadline: 4/15; financial award applicants required to submit FAFSA. *Faculty research:* Vulnerable populations, breast cancer, diabetes, mellitus, advanced practice nursing issues. *Unit head:* Dr. Deborah Allen, Chair, 912-478-5770, Fax: 912-478-0536, E-mail: debbieallen@georgiasouthern.edu.

Georgia State University, Byrdine F. Lewis School of Nursing, Atlanta, GA 30303. Offers adult health clinical nurse specialist/nurse practitioner (MS, Certificate); child health clinical nurse specialist/pediatric nurse practitioner (MS, Certificate); family nurse practitioner (MS, Certificate); family psychiatric mental health nurse practitioner (MS, Certificate); nursing (PhD); nursing leadership in healthcare innovations (MS), including nursing administration, nursing informatics; nutrition (MS); perinatal nurse specialist/women's health nurse practitioner (MS, Certificate); physical therapy (DPT); respiratory therapy (MS). *Accreditation:* AACN. *Program availability:* Part-time, blended/

hybrid learning. *Faculty:* 18 full-time (11 women). *Students:* 275 full-time (195 women), 230 part-time (204 women); includes 192 minority (123 Black or African American, non-Hispanic/Latino; 49 Asian, non-Hispanic/Latino; 12 Hispanic/Latino; 2 Native Hawaiian or other Pacific Islander, non-Hispanic/Latino; 6 Two or more races, non-Hispanic/Latino), 35 international. Average age 33. 240 applicants, 61% accepted, 95 enrolled. In 2015, 115 master's, 40 doctorates, 19 other advanced degrees awarded. *Degree requirements:* For doctorate, comprehensive exam, thesis/dissertation. *Entrance requirements:* For doctorate, GRE. Additional exam requirements/recommendations for international students: Required—TOEFL. *Application deadline:* For fall admission, 2/1 priority date for domestic and international students; for spring admission, 9/15 for domestic and international students. Applications are processed on a rolling basis. Application fee: $50. Electronic applications accepted. *Expenses:* Contact institution. *Financial support:* In 2015–16, research assistantships with tuition reimbursements (averaging $1,666 per year), teaching assistantships with tuition reimbursements (averaging $1,920 per year) were awarded; scholarships/grants, tuition waivers (full and partial), and unspecified assistantships also available. Support available to part-time students. Financial award application deadline: 8/1; financial award applicants required to submit FAFSA. *Faculty research:* Stroke intervention for caregivers, stroke prevention in African-Americans; relationships between psychological distress and health outcomes in parents with a medically ill infant; medically fragile children; nursing expertise and patient outcomes. *Unit head:* Nancy Kropf, Dean of Nursing, 404-413-1101, Fax: 404-413-1090, E-mail: nkropf@gsu.edu.
Website: http://nursing.gsu.edu/

Goldfarb School of Nursing at Barnes-Jewish College, Graduate Programs, St. Louis, MO 63110. Offers adult-gerontology acute care nurse practitioner (MSN); adult-gerontology nurse practitioner (MSN); nurse anesthesia (MSN); nurse educator (MSN); nurse executive (MSN). *Accreditation:* AACN; AANA/CANAEP. *Program availability:* Part-time, online learning. *Faculty:* 51 full-time (47 women), 6 part-time/adjunct (all women). *Students:* 58 full-time (57 women), 29 part-time (24 women); includes 17 minority (11 Black or African American, non-Hispanic/Latino; 2 Asian, non-Hispanic/Latino; 2 Hispanic/Latino; 2 Two or more races, non-Hispanic/Latino). Average age 26. 41 applicants, 22% accepted, 8 enrolled. In 2015, 56 master's awarded. *Degree requirements:* For master's, thesis or alternative. *Entrance requirements:* For master's, 2 references, personal statement, curriculum vitae or resume. Additional exam requirements/recommendations for international students: Required—TOEFL (minimum score 575 paper-based; 85 iBT). *Application deadline:* For fall admission, 2/1 priority date for international students; for spring admission, 10/1 priority date for international students. Applications are processed on a rolling basis. Application fee: $50. *Expenses:* Contact institution. *Financial support:* Fellowships, research assistantships, Federal Work-Study, institutionally sponsored loans, and scholarships/grants available. Support available to part-time students. Financial award applicants required to submit FAFSA. *Faculty research:* HIV stigma, HIV symptom management, palliative care with children and their families, heart disease prevention in Hispanic women, depression in the well elderly, alternative therapies in pre-term infants. *Unit head:* Dr. Gretchen Drinkard, Dean, 314-454-7540, Fax: 314-362-9222, E-mail: gld9643@bjc.org. *Application contact:* Karen Sartorius, Admissions Specialist, 314-454-7057, Fax: 314-362-9250, E-mail: ksartorius@bjc.org.
Website: http://www.barnesjewishcollege.edu/

Gonzaga University, School of Nursing and Human Physiology, Spokane, WA 99258. Offers MSN, DNP, DNP-A. *Accreditation:* AACN. *Program availability:* Part-time, evening/weekend, online learning. *Faculty:* 16 full-time (14 women), 23 part-time/adjunct (18 women). *Students:* 36 full-time (22 women), 705 part-time (590 women); includes 123 minority (19 Black or African American, non-Hispanic/Latino; 6 American Indian or Alaska Native, non-Hispanic/Latino; 26 Asian, non-Hispanic/Latino; 34 Hispanic/Latino; 7 Native Hawaiian or other Pacific Islander, non-Hispanic/Latino; 31 Two or more races, non-Hispanic/Latino), 2 international. Average age 38. *Entrance requirements:* For master's, MAT, minimum B average in undergraduate course work; for doctorate, MAT or GRE within the last 5 years, curriculum vitae, personal statement, three letters of recommendation, official transcripts, copy of current RN license, practicum hours. Additional exam requirements/recommendations for international students: Required—TOEFL. *Application deadline:* For fall admission, 7/20 priority date for domestic students; for spring admission, 11/1 for domestic students. Applications are processed on a rolling basis. Application fee: $50. Electronic applications accepted. *Expenses:* Contact institution. *Financial support:* Application deadline: 2/1; applicants required to submit FAFSA. *Unit head:* Dr. Brenda Stevenson Marshall, Dean, 509-313-3569, E-mail: stevenson-marshall@gonzaga.edu. *Application contact:* Shannon Zaranski, Assistant to the Dean, 509-313-3569, E-mail: zaranski@gu.gonzaga.edu.
Website: http://www.gonzaga.edu/Academics/Colleges-and-Schools/School-of-Nursing-Human-Physiology

Goshen College, Program in Nursing, Goshen, IN 46526-4794. Offers family nurse practitioner (MSN). *Accreditation:* AACN. *Program availability:* Part-time, evening/weekend. *Degree requirements:* For master's, comprehensive exam (for some programs). *Entrance requirements:* For master's, minimum GPA of 3.0, curriculum vitae, bachelor's degree in nursing, active RN license in Indiana or Michigan, three professional references, essay, one year of clinical experience, statistics course, interview with program director. Additional exam requirements/recommendations for international students: Required—TOEFL (minimum score 600 paper-based; 100 iBT), IELTS (minimum score 6.5). *Application deadline:* For fall admission, 3/15 priority date for domestic students. Electronic applications accepted. *Expenses:* Contact institution. *Financial support:* Scholarships/grants available. *Unit head:* Ruth Stoltzfus, Director, 574-535-7973, E-mail: ruthas@goshen.edu. *Application contact:* Ruth Stoltzfus, Director, 574-535-7973, E-mail: ruthas@goshen.edu.
Website: http://www.goshen.edu/graduate/nursing/

Governors State University, College of Health Professions, Program in Nursing, University Park, IL 60484. Offers MSN. *Accreditation:* ACEN. *Degree requirements:* For master's, comprehensive exam, thesis or alternative, practicum. *Entrance requirements:* For master's, GRE General Test, minimum GPA of 3.0 in upper-division nursing course work, 2.5 overall; BSN verification of AAS or employment as registered nurse; Illinois licensure; BSN from NLN-accredited institution.

Graceland University, School of Nursing, Independence, MO 64050-3434. Offers family nurse practitioner (MSN, PMC); nurse educator (MSN, PMC); organizational leadership (DNP). *Program availability:* Part-time, online learning. *Faculty:* 14 full-time (12 women), 21 part-time/adjunct (20 women). *Students:* 489 full-time (441 women); includes 75 minority (41 Black or African American, non-Hispanic/Latino; 5 American Indian or Alaska Native, non-Hispanic/Latino; 15 Asian, non-Hispanic/Latino; 2 Native Hawaiian or other Pacific Islander, non-Hispanic/Latino; 12 Two or more races, non-Hispanic/Latino), 1 international. Average age 39. 140 applicants, 69% accepted, 69 enrolled. In 2015, 137 master's, 11 doctorates awarded. *Degree requirements:* For master's, comprehensive exam (for some programs), thesis optional, scholarly project; for doctorate, capstone project. *Entrance requirements:* For master's, BSN from nationally-accredited program, RN license, minimum GPA of 3.0, satisfactory criminal background check; for doctorate, MSN from nationally-accredited program, RN license, minimum GPA of 3.2, criminal background check. Additional exam requirements/

recommendations for international students: Recommended—TOEFL. *Application deadline:* For fall admission, 6/1 priority date for domestic students; for winter admission, 10/1 priority date for domestic students; for spring admission, 10/1 priority date for domestic students; for summer admission, 2/1 for domestic students. Application fee: $50. Electronic applications accepted. *Expenses:* Contact institution. *Financial support:* Institutionally sponsored loans available. Support available to part-time students. Financial award applicants required to submit FAFSA. *Faculty research:* International nursing, family care-giving, health promotion. *Unit head:* Dr. Claudia D. Horton, Dean, 816-423-4670, Fax: 816-423-4753, E-mail: horton@graceland.edu. *Application contact:* Nick Walker, Admissions Representative, 816-423-4717, Fax: 816-833-2990, E-mail: nowalker@graceland.edu.
Website: http://www.graceland.edu/nursing

The Graduate Center, City University of New York, Graduate Studies, Program in Nursing Science, New York, NY 10016-4039. Offers DNS. *Degree requirements:* For doctorate, thesis/dissertation, exams. *Entrance requirements:* For doctorate, GRE, 2 letters of recommendation. Additional exam requirements/recommendations for international students: Required—TOEFL. Electronic applications accepted.

Grambling State University, School of Graduate Studies and Research, College of Professional Studies, School of Nursing, Grambling, LA 71245. Offers family nurse practitioner (PMC); nursing (MSN). *Accreditation:* ACEN. *Program availability:* Part-time. *Degree requirements:* For master's, comprehensive exam (for some programs), thesis (for some programs). *Entrance requirements:* For master's, GRE, minimum GPA of 3.0 on last degree, interview, 2 years of experience as RN. Additional exam requirements/recommendations for international students: Required—TOEFL (minimum score 500 paper-based; 62 iBT). Electronic applications accepted.

Grand Canyon University, College of Nursing, Phoenix, AZ 85017-1097. Offers acute care nurse practitioner (MS, PMC); clinical nurse specialist (PMC), including clinical nurse specialist, education; family nurse practitioner (MS); leadership in health care systems (MS); nurse education (MS). *Accreditation:* AACN. *Program availability:* Part-time, evening/weekend, online learning. *Degree requirements:* For master's and PMC, comprehensive exam (for some programs). *Entrance requirements:* For master's, minimum cumulative and science course undergraduate GPA of 3.0. Additional exam requirements/recommendations for international students: Required—TOEFL (minimum score 575 paper-based; 90 iBT), IELTS (minimum score 7).

Grand Valley State University, Kirkhof College of Nursing, Allendale, MI 49401-9403. Offers advanced practice (MSN); case management (MSN); nursing administration (MSN); nursing education (MSN); nursing practice (DNP); MSN/MBA. *Accreditation:* AACN. *Program availability:* Part-time. *Faculty:* 17 full-time (16 women), 6 part-time/adjunct (5 women). *Students:* 71 full-time (59 women), 53 part-time (45 women); includes 16 minority (10 Black or African American, non-Hispanic/Latino; 2 Asian, non-Hispanic/Latino; 3 Hispanic/Latino; 1 Two or more races, non-Hispanic/Latino), 3 international. Average age 33. 64 applicants, 94% accepted, 31 enrolled. In 2015, 1 master's, 11 doctorates awarded. *Degree requirements:* For master's, thesis optional. *Entrance requirements:* For master's, GRE, minimum upper-division GPA of 3.0, course work in statistics, Michigan RN license. Additional exam requirements/recommendations for international students: Required—TOEFL. *Application deadline:* For fall admission, 3/15 priority date for domestic students. Applications are processed on a rolling basis. Application fee: $30. Electronic applications accepted. *Financial support:* In 2015–16, 58 students received support, including 39 fellowships (averaging $11,141 per year), 33 research assistantships with tuition reimbursements available (averaging $7,339 per year); career-related internships or fieldwork, Federal Work-Study, institutionally sponsored loans, and traineeships also available. Financial award application deadline: 2/15. *Faculty research:* Multigenerational health promotion, chronic disease prevention, end-of-life issues, nursing workload, family caregiver health. *Total annual research expenditures:* $36,000. *Unit head:* Dr. Cynthia McCurren, Dean, 616-331-7161, Fax: 616-331-7362. *Application contact:* Dr. Cynthia Coviak, Associate Dean of Nursing Research and Faculty Development, 616-331-7170, Fax: 616-331-7362, E-mail: coviakc@gvsu.edu.
Website: http://www.gvsu.edu/kcon/

Grand View University, Master of Science in Innovative Leadership Program, Des Moines, IA 50316-1599. Offers business (MS); education (MS); nursing (MS). *Program availability:* Part-time, evening/weekend. *Degree requirements:* For master's, completion of all required coursework in common core and selected track with minimum cumulative GPA of 3.0 and no more than two grades of C. *Entrance requirements:* For master's, GRE, GMAT, or essay, minimum undergraduate GPA of 3.0, professional resume, 3 letters of recommendation, interview. Additional exam requirements/recommendations for international students: Required—TOEFL (minimum score 550 paper-based). Electronic applications accepted.

Gwynedd Mercy University, Frances M. Maguire School of Nursing and Health Professions, Gwynedd Valley, PA 19437-0901. Offers clinical nurse specialist (MSN), including gerontology, oncology, pediatrics; nurse educator (MSN); nurse practitioner (MSN), including adult health, pediatric health; nursing (DNP). *Accreditation:* ACEN. *Program availability:* Part-time, online learning. *Faculty:* 3 full-time (all women), 2 part-time/adjunct (both women). *Students:* 28 full-time (23 women), 68 part-time (62 women); includes 27 minority (18 Black or African American, non-Hispanic/Latino; 7 Asian, non-Hispanic/Latino; 2 Hispanic/Latino). Average age 37. 72 applicants, 25% accepted, 16 enrolled. In 2015, 7 master's awarded. *Degree requirements:* For master's, thesis optional; for doctorate, evidence-based scholarly project. *Entrance requirements:* For master's, GRE General Test or MAT, current nursing experience, physical assessment, course work in statistics, BSN from NLNAC-accredited program, 2 letters of recommendation, personal interview. Additional exam requirements/recommendations for international students: Required—TOEFL (minimum score 575 paper-based). *Application deadline:* For fall admission, 8/1 priority date for domestic students; for winter admission, 12/1 priority date for domestic students. Applications are processed on a rolling basis. Electronic applications accepted. *Expenses:* Contact institution. *Financial support:* In 2015–16, 21 students received support. Scholarships/grants, traineeships, and unspecified assistantships available. Financial award application deadline: 8/30. *Faculty research:* Critical thinking, primary care, domestic violence, multiculturalism, nursing centers. *Unit head:* Dr. Andrea D. Hollingsworth, Dean, 215-646-7300 Ext. 539, Fax: 215-641-5517, E-mail: hollingsworth.a@gmc.edu. *Application contact:* Dr. Barbara A. Jones, Director, 215-646-7300 Ext. 407, Fax: 215-641-5564, E-mail: jones.b@gmc.edu.
Website: http://www.gmercyu.edu/academics/graduate-programs/nursing

Hampton University, School of Nursing, Hampton, VA 23668. Offers advanced adult nursing (MS); community health nursing (MS); community mental health/psychiatric nursing (MS); family nursing (MS); gerontological nursing for the nurse practitioner (MS); nursing (PhD); women's health nursing (MS). *Accreditation:* AACN. *Program availability:* Part-time, online learning. *Degree requirements:* For master's, comprehensive exam, thesis optional; for doctorate, comprehensive exam, thesis/dissertation. *Entrance requirements:* For master's, GRE General Test. Additional exam requirements/recommendations for international students: Required—TOEFL (minimum score 525 paper-based) or IELTS (6.5). Electronic applications accepted. *Expenses: Tuition, area resident:* Full-time $10,263; part-time $522 per credit hour. *Required fees:* $35. Tuition

Nursing—General

and fees vary according to course load and program. *Faculty research:* African-American stress, HIV education, pediatric obesity, hypertension, breast cancer.

Hardin-Simmons University, Graduate School, Patty Hanks Shelton School of Nursing, Abilene, TX 79698-0001. Offers advanced healthcare delivery (MSN); family nurse practitioner (MSN). Programs offered jointly with Abilene Christian University and McMurry University. *Accreditation:* AACN. *Program availability:* Part-time. *Faculty:* 5 full-time (all women), 1 (woman) part-time/adjunct. *Students:* 18 part-time (15 women); includes 5 minority (2 Black or African American, non-Hispanic/Latino; 1 American Indian or Alaska Native, non-Hispanic/Latino; 2 Hispanic/Latino). Average age 33. In 2015, 4 master's awarded. *Degree requirements:* For master's, comprehensive exam, thesis or alternative. *Entrance requirements:* For master's, GRE, minimum undergraduate GPA of 3.0 in major, 2.8 overall; interview; upper-level course work in statistics; CPR certification; letters of recommendation. Additional exam requirements/recommendations for international students: Required—TOEFL (minimum score 550 paper-based; 75 iBT). *Application deadline:* For fall admission, 8/15 priority date for domestic students, 4/1 for international students; for spring admission, 1/5 priority date for domestic students, 9/1 for international students. Applications are processed on a rolling basis. Application fee: $50. Electronic applications accepted. *Expenses:* Contact institution. *Financial support:* In 2015–16, 17 students received support. Career-related internships or fieldwork and scholarships/grants available. Support available to part-time students. Financial award application deadline: 6/30; financial award applicants required to submit FAFSA. *Faculty research:* Child abuse, alternative medicine, pediatric chronic disease, health promotion. *Unit head:* Dr. Nina Ouimette, Dean, 325-671-2357, Fax: 325-671-2386, E-mail: nouimette@phssn.edu. *Application contact:* Dr. Nancy Kucinski, Dean of Graduate Studies, 325-670-1298, Fax: 325-670-1564, E-mail: gradoff@hsutx.edu.
Website: http://www.phssn.edu/

Hawai'i Pacific University, College of Health and Society, Program in Nursing, Honolulu, HI 96813. Offers MSN. *Program availability:* Part-time, evening/weekend. *Faculty:* 5 full-time (all women), 3 part-time/adjunct (2 women). *Students:* 35 full-time (28 women), 20 part-time (18 women); includes 28 minority (3 Black or African American, non-Hispanic/Latino; 12 Asian, non-Hispanic/Latino; 7 Hispanic/Latino; 2 Native Hawaiian or other Pacific Islander, non-Hispanic/Latino; 4 Two or more races, non-Hispanic/Latino), 7 international. Average age 35. 38 applicants, 89% accepted, 22 enrolled. In 2015, 20 master's awarded. *Entrance requirements:* For master's, BN with minimum GPA of 3.0, proof of valid Hawai'i RN license. Additional exam requirements/recommendations for international students: Recommended—TOEFL (minimum score 550 paper-based; 80 iBT), IELTS (minimum score 6), TWE (minimum score 5). *Application deadline:* For fall admission, 2/15 priority date for domestic students; for spring admission, 10/15 priority date for domestic students. Applications are processed on a rolling basis. Application fee: $50. Electronic applications accepted. *Expenses:* $1,275 per credit. *Financial support:* In 2015–16, 23 students received support. Research assistantships, career-related internships or fieldwork, Federal Work-Study, scholarships/grants, tuition waivers, and unspecified assistantships available. Financial award application deadline: 3/1; financial award applicants required to submit FAFSA. *Unit head:* Dr. Diane Knight, Department Chair, 808-236-5847, Fax: 808-236-3524, E-mail: dknight@hpu.edu. *Application contact:* Danny Lam, Assistant Director of Graduate Admissions, 808-544-1135, Fax: 808-544-0280, E-mail: graduate@hpu.edu.
Website: http://www.hpu.edu/CNHS/MSN/index.html

Herzing University Online, Program in Nursing, Menomonee Falls, WI 53051. Offers nursing (MSN); nursing education (MSN); nursing management (MSN). *Accreditation:* AACN. *Program availability:* Online learning.

Holy Family University, Graduate and Professional Programs, School of Nursing and Allied Health Professions, Philadelphia, PA 19114. Offers nursing administration (MSN); nursing education (MSN). *Accreditation:* AACN. *Program availability:* Part-time, evening/weekend. *Faculty:* 7 full-time (all women). *Students:* 42 part-time (39 women); includes 9 minority (4 Black or African American, non-Hispanic/Latino; 4 Asian, non-Hispanic/Latino; 1 Hispanic/Latino). Average age 36. 17 applicants, 82% accepted, 6 enrolled. In 2015, 12 master's awarded. *Degree requirements:* For master's, thesis or alternative, comprehensive portfolio, clinical practicum. *Entrance requirements:* For master's, BSN or RN from appropriately-accredited program, minimum GPA of 3.0, professional references, official transcripts of all college or university work, essay/personal statement, current resume, completion of one undergraduate statistics course with minimum grade of C. Additional exam requirements/recommendations for international students: Required—TOEFL (minimum score 550 paper-based; 79 iBT), IELTS (minimum score 6), or PTE (minimum score 54). *Application deadline:* For fall admission, 7/1 priority date for domestic and international students; for winter admission, 1/1 for domestic students; for spring admission, 11/1 priority date for domestic and international students; for summer admission, 4/1 priority date for domestic and international students. Applications are processed on a rolling basis. Application fee: $25. Electronic applications accepted. *Financial support:* In 2015–16, 1 student received support. Available to part-time students. Application deadline: 2/15; applicants required to submit FAFSA. *Unit head:* Dr. Ana Maria Catanzaro, Dean, 267-341-3292, Fax: 215-637-6598, E-mail: acatanzaro@holyfamily.edu. *Application contact:* Gidget Matie Montelibano, Associate Director of Graduate Admissions, 267-341-3558, Fax: 215-637-1478, E-mail: gmontelibano@holyfamily.edu.
Website: http://www.holyfamily.edu/choosing-holy-family-u/academics/schools-of-study/school-of-nursing

Holy Names University, Graduate Division, Department of Nursing, Oakland, CA 94619-1699. Offers administration/management (MSN, PMC); clinical faculty (MSN, PMC); community health nursing/case manager (MSN); family nurse practitioner (MSN, PMC); MSN/MA; MSN/MBA. *Accreditation:* AACN. *Program availability:* Part-time, evening/weekend. *Entrance requirements:* For master's, bachelor's degree in nursing or related field; California RN license or eligibility; minimum cumulative GPA of 2.8, 3.0 in nursing courses from baccalaureate program; courses in pathophysiology, statistics, and research at the undergraduate level. Additional exam requirements/recommendations for international students: Required—TOEFL (minimum score 500 paper-based; 79 iBT). Electronic applications accepted. Application fee is waived when completed online. *Expenses:* Tuition, area resident: Full-time $25,272; part-time $936 per credit hour. *Required fees:* $500; $250 per credit hour. *Faculty research:* Women's reproductive health, gerontology, attitudes about aging, schizophrenic families, international health issues.

Howard University, College of Nursing and Allied Health Sciences, Division of Nursing, Washington, DC 20059-0002. Offers nurse practitioner (Certificate); primary family health nursing (MSN). *Accreditation:* AACN. *Program availability:* Part-time. *Degree requirements:* For master's, comprehensive exam, thesis optional. *Entrance requirements:* For master's, RN license, minimum GPA of 3.0, BS in nursing. *Faculty research:* Urinary incontinence, breast cancer prevention, depression in the elderly, adolescent pregnancy.

Hunter College of the City University of New York, Graduate School, Schools of the Health Professions, Hunter-Bellevue School of Nursing, New York, NY 10010. Offers MS, AC, MS/MPH. *Accreditation:* AACN. *Program availability:* Part-time. *Students:* 4 full-time (all women), 335 part-time (291 women); includes 135 minority (72 Black or African American, non-Hispanic/Latino; 37 Asian, non-Hispanic/Latino; 26 Hispanic/Latino), 16 international. *Degree requirements:* For master's, practicum, portfolio. *Entrance requirements:* For master's, BSN, minimum GPA of 3.0, New York RN license, course work in basic statistics, resume; for AC, MSN, minimum GPA of 3.0. Additional exam requirements/recommendations for international students: Required—TOEFL. *Application deadline:* For fall admission, 4/1 for domestic students; for spring admission, 11/1 for domestic students. Applications are processed on a rolling basis. *Financial support:* In 2015–16, 9 students received support. Federal Work-Study, scholarships/grants, traineeships, and tuition waivers (partial) available. Support available to part-time students. Financial award application deadline: 5/1; financial award applicants required to submit FAFSA. *Faculty research:* Aging, high-risk mothers and babies, adolescent health, care of HIV/AIDS clients, critical care nursing. *Unit head:* Dr. Gail McCain, Dean, 212-481-7596, Fax: 212-481-5078, E-mail: gmccain@hunter.cuny.edu. *Application contact:* Milena Solo, Director for Graduate Admissions, 212-772-4288, E-mail: milena.solo@hunter.cuny.edu.
Website: http://www.hunter.cuny.edu/nursing/

Husson University, Graduate Nursing Program, Bangor, ME 04401-2999. Offers advanced practice psychiatric nursing (MSN, PMC); family and community nurse practitioner (MSN, PMC); nursing education (MSN, PMC). *Accreditation:* AACN. *Program availability:* Part-time. *Faculty:* 6 full-time (all women), 2 part-time/adjunct (1 woman). *Students:* 27 full-time (26 women), 10 part-time (9 women); includes 4 minority (2 Asian, non-Hispanic/Latino; 2 Two or more races, non-Hispanic/Latino). Average age 39. 70 applicants, 27% accepted, 13 enrolled. In 2015, 9 master's awarded. *Degree requirements:* For master's, comprehensive exam (for some programs), research project. *Entrance requirements:* For master's, MAT or GRE, BSN. Additional exam requirements/recommendations for international students: Required—TOEFL (minimum score 550 paper-based; 80 iBT). *Application deadline:* For fall admission, 3/31 for domestic students; for spring admission, 10/30 for domestic students. Application fee: $40. Electronic applications accepted. *Expenses:* Contact institution. *Financial support:* Research assistantships, Federal Work-Study, institutionally sponsored loans, traineeships, and unspecified assistantships available. Financial award application deadline: 3/31; financial award applicants required to submit FAFSA. *Faculty research:* Health disparities and methods to better identify and provide healthcare services to those most in need. *Unit head:* Prof. Mary Jude, Director, Graduate Nursing, 207-941-7769, Fax: 207-941-7198, E-mail: judem@husson.edu. *Application contact:* Kristen Card, Director of Graduate Admissions, 207-404-5660, Fax: 207-941-7935, E-mail: cardk@husson.edu.
Website: http://www.husson.edu/nursing-msn

Idaho State University, Office of Graduate Studies, Kasiska College of Health Professions, Department of Nursing, Pocatello, ID 83209-8101. Offers nursing (MS, Post-Master's Certificate). *Accreditation:* AACN. *Program availability:* Part-time. *Degree requirements:* For master's, comprehensive exam, thesis optional, practicum and/or clinical hours; for Post-Master's Certificate, comprehensive exam, thesis optional, practicum. *Entrance requirements:* For master's, GRE General Test, interview, 3 letters of reference, active RN license; for Post-Master's Certificate, GRE General Test, 3 letters of reference, practicum or nursing license, graduate degree. Additional exam requirements/recommendations for international students: Required—TOEFL (minimum score 600 paper-based). Electronic applications accepted. *Faculty research:* Health promotions, health of homeless, exercise and elderly, student stress, midwifery.

Illinois State University, Graduate School, Mennonite College of Nursing, Normal, IL 61790. Offers family nurse practitioner (PMC); nursing (MSN, PhD). *Accreditation:* AACN. Application fee: $40. *Faculty research:* Expanding the teaching-nursing home culture in the state of Illinois, advanced education nursing traineeship program, collaborative doctoral program-caring for older adults. *Application contact:* Caroline Mallory, 309-438-2659, E-mail: cmmallo@ilstu.edu.
Website: http://www.mcn.ilstu.edu/

Immaculata University, College of Graduate Studies, Division of Nursing, Immaculata, PA 19345. Offers nursing administration (MSN); nursing education (MSN). *Accreditation:* AACN. *Program availability:* Part-time, evening/weekend. *Entrance requirements:* For master's, MAT or GRE, BSN, minimum undergraduate GPA of 3.0. Additional exam requirements/recommendations for international students: Required—TOEFL.

Independence University, Program in Nursing, Salt Lake City, UT 84107. Offers community health (MSN); gerontology (MSN); nursing administration (MSN); wellness promotion (MSN).

Indiana State University, College of Graduate and Professional Studies, College of Nursing, Health, and Human Services, Department of Advanced Practice Nursing, Terre Haute, IN 47809. Offers advanced practice nursing (DNP); family nurse practitioner (MS); nursing administration (MS); nursing education (MS). *Accreditation:* ACEN. *Program availability:* Part-time. *Degree requirements:* For master's, thesis or alternative. *Entrance requirements:* For master's, BSN, RN license, minimum undergraduate GPA of 3.0. Electronic applications accepted. *Faculty research:* Nursing faculty-student interactions, clinical evaluation, program evaluation, sexual dysfunction, faculty attitudes.

Indiana University East, School of Nursing, Richmond, IN 47374-1289. Offers MSN.

Indiana University Kokomo, School of Nursing, Kokomo, IN 46904-9003. Offers nurse administrator (MSN); nurse educator (MSN).

Indiana University of Pennsylvania, School of Graduate Studies and Research, College of Health and Human Services, Department of Nursing and Allied Health, Nursing DNP to PhD Pathway Program, Indiana, PA 15705-1087. Offers PhD. *Accreditation:* AACN. *Program availability:* Part-time, evening/weekend. *Faculty:* 12 full-time (11 women). *Students:* 3 part-time (all women). Average age 43. 5 applicants, 20% accepted. *Degree requirements:* For doctorate, comprehensive exam, thesis/dissertation. *Entrance requirements:* For doctorate, nursing license. *Application deadline:* Applications are processed on a rolling basis. Application fee: $50. Electronic applications accepted. *Financial support:* Fellowships with full tuition reimbursements, career-related internships or fieldwork, Federal Work-Study, scholarships/grants, and unspecified assistantships available. Financial award application deadline: 4/15; financial award applicants required to submit FAFSA. *Unit head:* Dr. Susan Poorman, Doctoral Coordinator, 724-357-3258, E-mail: susan.poorman@iup.edu.
Website: http://www.iup.edu/rn-alliedhealth/programs/nursingphd/default.aspx

Indiana University of Pennsylvania, School of Graduate Studies and Research, College of Health and Human Services, Department of Nursing and Allied Health, PhD in Nursing Program, Indiana, PA 15705-1087. Offers PhD. *Program availability:* Part-time. *Faculty:* 12 full-time (11 women). *Students:* 36 part-time (all women); includes 3 minority (1 Asian, non-Hispanic/Latino; 1 Hispanic/Latino; 1 Two or more races, non-Hispanic/Latino). Average age 45. 26 applicants, 77% accepted, 7 enrolled. In 2015, 4 doctorates awarded. *Degree requirements:* For doctorate, comprehensive exam, thesis/dissertation. *Entrance requirements:* For doctorate, GRE. Additional exam requirements/recommendations for international students: Required—TOEFL (minimum score 540 paper-based). *Application deadline:* Applications are processed on a rolling basis. Application fee: $50. Electronic applications accepted. *Financial support:* In

2015–16, 1 research assistantship (averaging $3,315 per year), 2 teaching assistantships with partial tuition reimbursements (averaging $23,305 per year) were awarded; fellowships with full tuition reimbursements, career-related internships or fieldwork, Federal Work-Study, scholarships/grants, and unspecified assistantships also available. Financial award application deadline: 4/15; financial award applicants required to submit FAFSA. *Unit head:* Dr. Susan Poorman, Doctoral Coordinator, 724-357-3258, E-mail: susan.poorman@iup.edu. Website: http://www.iup.edu/grad/nursingphd/default.aspx

Indiana University–Purdue University Fort Wayne, College of Health and Human Services, Department of Nursing, Fort Wayne, IN 46805-1499. Offers adult-gerontology primary care nurse practitioner (MS); family nurse practitioner (MS); nurse executive (MS); nursing administration (Certificate); nursing education (MS). *Accreditation:* ACEN. *Program availability:* Part-time. *Faculty:* 8 full-time (all women). *Students:* 6 full-time (all women), 79 part-time (70 women); includes 8 minority (2 Black or African American, non-Hispanic/Latino; 3 Asian, non-Hispanic/Latino; 3 Hispanic/Latino). Average age 36. 14 applicants, 100% accepted, 10 enrolled. In 2015, 17 master's awarded. *Entrance requirements:* For master's, GRE Writing Test (if GPA below 3.0), BS in nursing, eligibility for Indiana RN license, minimum GPA of 3.0, essay, copy of resume, three references, undergraduate course work in research and statistics within last 5 years. Additional exam requirements/recommendations for international students: Required—TOEFL (minimum score 550 paper-based; 79 iBT); Recommended—TWE. *Application deadline:* For fall admission, 5/1 priority date for domestic and international students; for spring admission, 11/15 priority date for domestic students. Applications are processed on a rolling basis. Application fee: $55 ($60 for international students). Electronic applications accepted. *Financial support:* In 2015–16, 12 teaching assistantships with partial tuition reimbursements (averaging $13,522 per year) were awarded; scholarships/grants also available. Support available to part-time students. Financial award application deadline: 3/1; financial award applicants required to submit FAFSA. *Faculty research:* Community engagement, cervical screening, evidence-based practice. *Total annual research expenditures:* $22,966. *Unit head:* Dr. Lee-Ellen Kirkhorn, Chair/Professor, 260-481-6789, Fax: 260-481-5767, E-mail: kirkhorl@ipfw.edu. *Application contact:* Dr. Deb Poling, Director of Graduate Program, 260-481-6276, Fax: 260-481-5767, E-mail: polingd@ipfw.edu. Website: http://www.ipfw.edu/nursing/

Indiana University–Purdue University Indianapolis, School of Nursing, Doctor of Nursing Practice Program, Indianapolis, IN 46202. Offers DNP. *Degree requirements:* For doctorate, comprehensive exam, inquiry project: evidence-based practice implementation or intervention. *Entrance requirements:* For doctorate, background check. Additional exam requirements/recommendations for international students: Required—TOEFL, IELTS. Electronic applications accepted.

Indiana University–Purdue University Indianapolis, School of Nursing, MSN Program in Nursing, Indianapolis, IN 46202. Offers nursing education (MSN); nursing leadership in health systems (MSN). *Program availability:* Part-time, online learning. *Degree requirements:* For master's, thesis. *Entrance requirements:* For master's, minimum GPA of 3.0, RN license, background check, statistics. Additional exam requirements/recommendations for international students: Required—TOEFL (minimum score 550 paper-based; 79 iBT). *Expenses:* Contact institution. *Faculty research:* Clinical science, health systems.

Indiana University–Purdue University Indianapolis, School of Nursing, PhD Program in Nursing Science, Indianapolis, IN 46202. Offers PhD. *Program availability:* Part-time, online learning. *Degree requirements:* For doctorate, comprehensive exam, thesis/dissertation. *Entrance requirements:* For doctorate, GRE. Additional exam requirements/recommendations for international students: Required—TOEFL, IELTS. Electronic applications accepted.

Indiana University South Bend, Vera Z. Dwyer College of Health Sciences, School of Nursing, South Bend, IN 46634-7111. Offers family nurse practitioner (MSN). *Program availability:* Part-time, evening/weekend. *Entrance requirements:* For master's, GRE General Test, minimum GPA of 3.0.

Indiana Wesleyan University, Graduate School, School of Nursing, Marion, IN 46953-4974. Offers nursing administration (MS); nursing education (MS); primary care nursing (MS); MSN/MBA. *Accreditation:* AACN. *Program availability:* Part-time, online learning. *Students:* 884 full-time (818 women), 27 part-time (all women); includes 148 minority (92 Black or African American, non-Hispanic/Latino; 5 American Indian or Alaska Native, non-Hispanic/Latino; 18 Asian, non-Hispanic/Latino; 16 Hispanic/Latino; 17 Two or more races, non-Hispanic/Latino), 2 international. Average age 38. *Degree requirements:* For master's, capstone project or thesis. *Entrance requirements:* For master's, writing sample, RN license, 1 year of related experience, graduate statistics course. Additional exam requirements/recommendations for international students: Required—TOEFL. *Application deadline:* Applications are processed on a rolling basis. *Expenses:* Contact institution. *Financial support:* Fellowships, career-related internships or fieldwork, scholarships/grants, and traineeships available. Support available to part-time students. Financial award application deadline: 3/15; financial award applicants required to submit FAFSA. *Faculty research:* Primary health care with international emphasis, international nursing. *Unit head:* Dr. Barbara Ihrke, Dean, 765-677-2813, Fax: 765-677-1768, E-mail: barbara.ihrke@indwes.edu. *Application contact:* Graduate School, 866-IWU-4-YOU, Fax: 765-677-2541, E-mail: graduate@indwes.edu. Website: http://graduatenursing.indwes.edu

Inter American University of Puerto Rico, Arecibo Campus, Program in Nursing, Arecibo, PR 00614-4050. Offers critical care nursing (MSN); surgical nursing (MSN). *Entrance requirements:* For master's, EXADEP or GRE General Test or MAT, 2 letters of recommendation, bachelor's degree in nursing, minimum GPA of 2.5 in last 60 credits, minimum 1 year nursing experience, nursing license.

Jacksonville State University, College of Graduate Studies and Continuing Education, College of Nursing, Jacksonville, AL 36265-1602. Offers MSN. *Accreditation:* AACN. *Program availability:* Part-time, evening/weekend. *Faculty:* 3 full-time (all women), 1 part-time/adjunct (0 women). *Students:* 10 full-time (all women), 43 part-time (41 women); includes 6 minority (all Black or African American, non-Hispanic/Latino). Average age 41. 19 applicants, 63% accepted, 10 enrolled. In 2015, 14 master's awarded. *Degree requirements:* For master's, comprehensive exam, thesis (for some programs). *Entrance requirements:* For master's, GRE General Test or MAT. Additional exam requirements/recommendations for international students: Required—TOEFL (minimum score 500 paper-based; 61 iBT). *Application deadline:* Applications are processed on a rolling basis. Application fee: $35. Electronic applications accepted. *Financial support:* Available to part-time students. Application deadline: 4/1; applicants required to submit FAFSA. *Unit head:* Dr. Sarah Latham, Dean, 256-782-5431, E-mail: slatham@jsu.edu. *Application contact:* Dr. Jean Pugliese, Associate Dean, 256-782-8278, Fax: 256-782-5321, E-mail: pugliese@jsu.edu. Website: http://www.jsu.edu/nursing/

Jacksonville University, School of Nursing, Jacksonville, FL 32211. Offers MSN, DNP. *Accreditation:* AACN. *Program availability:* Part-time. *Degree requirements:* For master's, thesis. *Entrance requirements:* For master's, GRE General Test, BS in nursing from an accredited program, course work in statistics within last 5 years, Florida nursing

license. Additional exam requirements/recommendations for international students: Required—TOEFL (minimum score 550 paper-based). Application fee: $50. *Expenses:* Contact institution. *Financial support:* Federal Work-Study, institutionally sponsored loans, and scholarships/grants available. Support available to part-time students. Financial award application deadline: 3/15. *Unit head:* Dr. Leigh B. Hart, Assistant Dean, 904-256-7600, E-mail: lhart@ju.edu. *Application contact:* Marisol Preston, Chief Admissions Officer, 904-256-7000, E-mail: admissions@ju.edu. Website: http://www.ju.edu/chs/Nursing/Pages/default.aspx

James Madison University, The Graduate School, College of Health and Behavioral Sciences, Program in Nursing, Harrisonburg, VA 22807. Offers adult/gerontology primary care nurse practitioner (MSN); clinical nurse leader (MSN); family nurse practitioner (MSN); nurse administrator (MSN); nurse midwifery (MSN); nursing (MSN, DNP). *Accreditation:* AACN. *Program availability:* Part-time, 100% online, blended/hybrid learning. *Faculty:* 15 full-time (all women), 1 (woman) part-time/adjunct. *Students:* 14 full-time (all women), 54 part-time (43 women); includes 6 minority (2 Black or African American, non-Hispanic/Latino; 1 Asian, non-Hispanic/Latino; 1 Hispanic/Latino; 2 Two or more races, non-Hispanic/Latino), 1 international. Average age 30. 49 applicants, 67% accepted, 31 enrolled. In 2015, 14 master's awarded. Application fee: $55. Electronic applications accepted. *Financial support:* In 2015–16, 2 students received support. Federal Work-Study, unspecified assistantships, and 2 assistantships (averaging $7530) available. Financial award application deadline: 3/1; financial award applicants required to submit FAFSA. *Unit head:* Dr. Julie T. Sanford, Department Head, 540-568-6314, E-mail: sanforjt@jmu.edu. *Application contact:* Lynette D. Michael, Director of Graduate Admissions and Student Records, 540-568-6131 Ext. 6395, Fax: 540-568-7860, E-mail: michaeld@jmu.edu. Website: http://www.nursing.jmu.edu

Jefferson College of Health Sciences, Program in Nursing, Roanoke, VA 24013. Offers nursing education (MSN); nursing management (MSN). *Accreditation:* AACN. *Program availability:* Part-time. *Degree requirements:* For master's, project. *Entrance requirements:* For master's, MAT. Additional exam requirements/recommendations for international students: Required—TOEFL (minimum score 550 paper-based; 80 iBT). Electronic applications accepted. *Faculty research:* Nursing, teaching and learning techniques, cultural competence, spirituality and nursing.

Johns Hopkins University, School of Nursing, Certificate Programs in Nursing, Baltimore, MD 21218. Offers Certificate.

Johns Hopkins University, School of Nursing, Doctoral Programs in Nursing, Baltimore, MD 21218. Offers DNP, PhD.

Johns Hopkins University, School of Nursing, Master's Programs in Nursing, Baltimore, MD 21218. Offers MSN, MSN/MBA, MSN/MPH.

Kaplan University, Davenport Campus, School of Nursing, Davenport, IA 52807-2095. Offers nurse administrator (MS); nurse educator (MS). *Program availability:* Part-time, evening/weekend, online learning. *Entrance requirements:* For master's, RN. Additional exam requirements/recommendations for international students: Required—TOEFL (minimum score 550 paper-based).

Kean University, College of Natural, Applied and Health Sciences, Program in Nursing, Union, NJ 07083. Offers clinical management (MSN); community health nursing (MSN); school nursing (MSN). *Accreditation:* ACEN. *Program availability:* Part-time. *Faculty:* 9 full-time (all women). *Students:* 10 full-time (all women), 120 part-time (114 women); includes 63 minority (47 Black or African American, non-Hispanic/Latino; 11 Asian, non-Hispanic/Latino; 3 Hispanic/Latino; 2 Two or more races, non-Hispanic/Latino), 1 international. Average age 44. 64 applicants, 63% accepted, 22 enrolled. In 2015, 46 master's awarded. *Degree requirements:* For master's, thesis or alternative, clinical field experience. *Entrance requirements:* For master's, minimum GPA of 3.0; BS in nursing; RN license; 2 letters of recommendation; interview; official transcripts from all institutions attended. Additional exam requirements/recommendations for international students: Required—TOEFL (minimum score 550 paper-based; 79 iBT), IELTS. *Application deadline:* For fall admission, 6/1 for domestic and international students; for spring admission, 12/1 for domestic and international students. Applications are processed on a rolling basis. Application fee: $75 ($150 for international students). Electronic applications accepted. *Expenses:* Tuition, state resident: full-time $12,835; part-time $625 per credit. Tuition, nonresident: full-time $17,396; part-time $766 per credit. *Required fees:* $235; $147 per credit. Tuition and fees vary according to course level, course load, degree level and program. *Financial support:* In 2015–16, research assistantships with full tuition reimbursements (averaging $3,771 per year) were awarded; scholarships/grants and unspecified assistantships also available. Financial award applicants required to submit FAFSA. *Unit head:* Dr. Portia Johnson, Program Coordinator, 908-737-3386, E-mail: johnsonpo@kean.edu. *Application contact:* Pedro Lopes, Admissions Counselor, 908-737-7100, E-mail: grad-adm@kean.edu. Website: http://grad.kean.edu/masters-programs/nursing-clinical-management

Keiser University, Master of Science in Nursing Program, Ft. Lauderdale, FL 33309. Offers MSN.

Kennesaw State University, WellStar College of Health and Human Services, Doctor of Nursing Science Program, Kennesaw, GA 30144. Offers DNS. *Program availability:* Part-time. *Degree requirements:* For doctorate, comprehensive exam, thesis/dissertation. *Entrance requirements:* For doctorate, GRE, master's degree in nursing, RN licensure. Additional exam requirements/recommendations for international students: Required—TOEFL (minimum score 550 paper-based; 80 iBT), IELTS (minimum score 6.5). Electronic applications accepted.

Kennesaw State University, WellStar College of Health and Human Services, Program in Primary Care Nurse Practitioner, Kennesaw, GA 30144. Offers MSN. *Accreditation:* AACN. *Program availability:* Part-time, evening/weekend. *Entrance requirements:* For master's, GRE General Test, minimum GPA of 2.5, RN license, 3 years of professional experience. Additional exam requirements/recommendations for international students: Required—TOEFL (minimum score 550 paper-based), IELTS (minimum score 6.5). Electronic applications accepted.

Kent State University, College of Nursing, Kent, OH 44242. Offers advanced nursing practice (DNP), including adult gerontology acute care nurse practitioner (MSN, DNP), adult gerontology clinical nurse specialist (MSN, DNP), family nurse practitioner (MSN, DNP); nursing (MSN, PhD), including adult gerontology acute care nurse practitioner (MSN, DNP), adult gerontology clinical nurse specialist (MSN, DNP), family nurse practitioner (MSN, DNP), nurse educator (MSN), nursing healthcare management (MSN), primary care adult nurse practitioner (MSN), primary care pediatric clinical nurse specialist (MSN), primary care pediatric nurse practitioner (MSN), psychiatric mental health practitioner (MSN), women's health nurse practitioner (MSN); nursing education (Certificate); primary care pediatric nurse practitioner (Certificate); women's health nurse practitioner (Certificate). PhD program offered jointly with The University of Akron. *Accreditation:* AACN. *Program availability:* Part-time, online learning. *Faculty:* 52 full-time (48 women). *Students:* 78 full-time (56 women), 414 part-time (365 women); includes 63 minority (34 Black or African American, non-Hispanic/Latino; 1 American Indian or Alaska Native, non-Hispanic/Latino; 12 Asian, non-Hispanic/Latino; 12 Hispanic/Latino; 4 Two or more races, non-Hispanic/Latino), 16 international. Average

age 37. 653 applicants, 54% accepted, 309 enrolled. In 2015, 140 master's, 1 doctorate, 13 other advanced degrees awarded. *Degree requirements:* For master's, thesis optional, practicum; for doctorate, comprehensive exam (for some programs), thesis/dissertation (for some programs), practicum and scholarly project (for DNP programs); for Certificate, practicum. *Entrance requirements:* For master's, minimum GPA of 3.0, transcripts, active unrestricted RN license, essay/goal statement, interview, 3 letters of recommendation; for doctorate, GRE (for PhD), minimum GPA of 3.0, transcripts, 3 letters of recommendation, interview; active unrestricted RN license, clinical experience and hours record (for DNP); goal statement, sample of written work, curriculum vitae, statement of research interests, and eligibility for RN license (for PhD); for Certificate, MSN, minimum GPA of 3.0, transcripts. Additional exam requirements/recommendations for international students: Required—TOEFL (minimum score: paper-based 525, iBT 71), Michigan English Language Assessment Battery (minimum score of 75), IELTS (minimum score of 6.0), PTE Academic (minimum score of 48), or completion of ELS level 112 Intensive Program. *Application deadline:* For fall admission, 2/1 for domestic students; for spring admission, 11/1 for domestic students. Application fee: $45 ($70 for international students). Electronic applications accepted. *Expenses:* Tuition, state resident: full-time $10,864; part-time $495 per credit hour. Tuition, nonresident: full-time $18,380; part-time $837 per credit hour. *Financial support:* Research assistantships with full tuition reimbursements, teaching assistantships with full tuition reimbursements, career-related internships or fieldwork, Federal Work-Study, traineeships, and unspecified assistantships available. Financial award application deadline: 2/1. *Unit head:* Dr. Barbara Broome, Dean, 330-672-3777, E-mail: bbroome1@kent.edu. *Application contact:* Dr. Wendy A. Umberger, Associate Dean for Graduate Programs/Professor, 330-672-8813, E-mail: wlewando@kent.edu.
Website: http://www.kent.edu/nursing

Kentucky State University, College of Professional Studies, Frankfort, KY 40601. Offers nursing (DNP); public administration (MPA), including human resource management; special education (MA). *Program availability:* Part-time, evening/weekend, blended/hybrid learning. *Faculty:* 7 full-time (3 women), 2 part-time/adjunct (both women). *Students:* 34 full-time (22 women), 34 part-time (24 women); includes 47 minority (45 Black or African American, non-Hispanic/Latino; 1 Asian, non-Hispanic/Latino; 1 Two or more races, non-Hispanic/Latino), 3 international. Average age 36. 35 applicants, 83% accepted, 22 enrolled. In 2015, 23 master's awarded. *Degree requirements:* For master's, comprehensive exam, thesis optional; for doctorate, comprehensive exam, thesis/dissertation optional, 180 clinical hours. *Entrance requirements:* For master's, GMAT, GRE; for doctorate, RN license. Additional exam requirements/recommendations for international students: Required—TOEFL (minimum score 525 paper-based). *Application deadline:* Applications are processed on a rolling basis. Application fee: $30 ($100 for international students). Electronic applications accepted. *Expenses:* Tuition, state resident: full-time $7524; part-time $418 per credit hour. Tuition, nonresident: full-time $11,322; part-time $629 per credit hour. Tuition and fees vary according to course load. *Financial support:* In 2015–16, 34 students received support, including 1 research assistantship (averaging $15,599 per year); scholarships/grants, tuition waivers (partial), and unspecified assistantships also available. Financial award application deadline: 4/15; financial award applicants required to submit FAFSA. *Faculty research:* Risk assessment and failure modeling for the public sector implication of property rights on economic development, the social stability of communities, civil peace of nations. *Total annual research expenditures:* $265,485. *Unit head:* Dr. Lynda Brown-Wright, Vice President of Academic Affairs, 502-597-6442, E-mail: lynda.brownwright@kysu.edu. *Application contact:* Dr. James Obielodan, Director of Graduate Studies, 502-597-4723, E-mail: james.obielodan@kysu.edu.
Website: http://kysu.edu/academics/college-of-professional-studies/

Keuka College, Program in Nursing, Keuka Park, NY 14478-0098. Offers adult gerontology nurse practitioner (MS); nursing (MS). *Accreditation:* AACN. *Faculty:* 8 full-time (all women), 23 part-time/adjunct (22 women). *Students:* 68 full-time (62 women); includes 8 minority (6 Black or African American, non-Hispanic/Latino; 1 Asian, non-Hispanic/Latino; 1 Hispanic/Latino). Average age 36. In 2015, 20 master's awarded. *Degree requirements:* For master's, exam or thesis. *Entrance requirements:* For master's, bachelor's degree from accredited institution, minimum GPA of 3.0, unencumbered NY State license, and current registration as RN (for nusirng); currently full-time or part-time working RN and 2 clinical letters of recommendation (for adult gerontology nurse practitioner). Additional exam requirements/recommendations for international students: Required—TOEFL (minimum score 550 paper-based). *Application deadline:* Applications are processed on a rolling basis. Application fee: $50. Electronic applications accepted. *Expenses:* Contact institution. *Financial support:* Scholarships/grants and tuition waivers available. Financial award applicants required to submit FAFSA. *Unit head:* Dr. Debra Gates, Chair, 315-279-5115 Ext. 5273, E-mail: dgates@keuka.edu. *Application contact:* Graduate Admissions, 866-255-3852, Fax: 315-279-5386, E-mail: asapadvisor@keuka.edu.
Website: http://academics.keuka.edu/asap/programs/ms_nursing

Lamar University, College of Graduate Studies, College of Arts and Sciences, JoAnne Gay Dishman Department of Nursing, Beaumont, TX 77710. Offers nursing administration (MSN); nursing education (MSN); MSN/MBA. *Accreditation:* ACEN. *Program availability:* Part-time, evening/weekend, online learning. *Faculty:* 8 full-time (all women), 2 part-time/adjunct (both women). *Students:* 2 full-time (both women), 73 part-time (64 women); includes 32 minority (17 Black or African American, non-Hispanic/Latino; 7 Asian, non-Hispanic/Latino; 6 Hispanic/Latino; 2 Two or more races, non-Hispanic/Latino). Average age 38. 47 applicants, 77% accepted, 14 enrolled. In 2015, 14 master's awarded. *Degree requirements:* For master's, comprehensive exam, practicum project presentation, evidence-based project. *Entrance requirements:* For master's, GRE General Test, MAT, criminal background check, RN license, NLN-accredited BSN, college course work in statistics in past 5 years, letters of recommendation, minimum undergraduate GPA of 3.0. Additional exam requirements/recommendations for international students: Required—TOEFL (minimum score 550 paper-based; 79 iBT), IELTS (minimum score 6.5). *Application deadline:* For fall admission, 8/10 for domestic students, 7/1 for international students; for spring admission, 1/5 for domestic students, 12/1 for international students. Applications are processed on a rolling basis. Application fee: $25 ($50 for international students). Electronic applications accepted. *Expenses: Tuition, area resident:* Full-time $6720; part-time $4032. Tuition, nonresident: full-time $14,880; part-time $8928. *Required fees:* $1900; $950 $784. *Financial support:* In 2015–16, 3 students received support. Teaching assistantships, scholarships/grants, and traineeships available. Financial award application deadline: 4/1; financial award applicants required to submit FAFSA. *Faculty research:* Student retention, theory, care giving, online course and research. *Unit head:* Cynthia Stinson, Interim Chair, 409-880-8817, Fax: 409-880-8698. *Application contact:* Melissa Gallien, Director, Admissions and Academic Services, 409-880-8888, Fax: 409-880-7419, E-mail: gradmissions@lamar.edu.
Website: http://artssciences.lamar.edu/nursing

Lander University, Graduate Studies, Greenwood, SC 29649-2099. Offers clinical nurse leader (MSN); emergency management (MS); Montessori education (M Ed); teaching and learning (M Ed). *Accreditation:* NCATE. *Program availability:* Part-time, online learning. *Degree requirements:* For master's, comprehensive exam, thesis or alternative. *Entrance requirements:* For master's, GRE General Test. Additional exam requirements/recommendations for international students: Required—TOEFL (minimum score 550 paper-based). Electronic applications accepted.

La Roche College, School of Graduate Studies and Adult Education, Program in Nursing, Pittsburgh, PA 15237-5898. Offers nursing education (MSN); nursing management (MSN). *Accreditation:* AANA/CANAEP; ACEN. *Program availability:* Part-time, evening/weekend, online only, 100% online. *Faculty:* 3 full-time (all women), 1 part-time/adjunct (0 women). *Students:* 14 full-time (all women), 8 part-time (all women), 2 international. Average age 40. 20 applicants, 75% accepted, 11 enrolled. In 2015, 3 master's awarded. *Degree requirements:* For master's, thesis optional, internship, practicum. *Entrance requirements:* For master's, GRE General Test, BSN, nursing license, work experience. Additional exam requirements/recommendations for international students: Recommended—TOEFL (minimum score 550 paper-based). *Application deadline:* For fall admission, 8/15 priority date for domestic students, 8/15 for international students; for spring admission, 12/15 priority date for domestic students, 12/15 for international students. Applications are processed on a rolling basis. Application fee: $50. Electronic applications accepted. *Expenses:* Contact institution. *Financial support:* Application deadline: 3/31; applicants required to submit FAFSA. *Faculty research:* Patient education, perception. *Unit head:* Dr. Terri Liberto, Division Chair, 412-847-1813, Fax: 412-536-1175, E-mail: terri.liberto@laroche.edu. *Application contact:* Hope Schiffgens, Director of Graduate Studies and Adult Education, 412-536-1266, Fax: 412-536-1283, E-mail: schombh1@laroche.edu.

La Salle University, School of Nursing and Health Sciences, Program in Nursing, Philadelphia, PA 19141-1199. Offers adult gerontology primary care nurse practitioner (MSN, Certificate); adult health and illness clinical nurse specialist (MSN); adult-gerontology clinical nurse specialist (MSN); clinical nurse leader (MSN); family primary care nurse practitioner (MSN, Certificate); gerontology (Certificate); nurse anesthetist (MSN, Certificate); nursing (MSN, Certificate); nursing administration (MSN, Certificate); nursing education (Certificate); nursing practice (DNP); nursing service administration (MSN); public health nursing (MSN, Certificate); school nursing (Certificate); MSN/MBA; MSN/MPH. *Accreditation:* AANA/CANAEP. *Program availability:* Part-time, evening/weekend, 100% online. *Faculty:* 13 full-time (all women), 9 part-time/adjunct (8 women). *Students:* 368 part-time (56 women); includes 103 minority (62 Black or African American, non-Hispanic/Latino; 1 American Indian or Alaska Native, non-Hispanic/Latino; 26 Asian, non-Hispanic/Latino; 9 Hispanic/Latino; 5 Two or more races, non-Hispanic/Latino), 5 international. Average age 36. 98 applicants, 85% accepted, 53 enrolled. In 2015, 87 master's, 3 doctorates, 10 other advanced degrees awarded. *Degree requirements:* For doctorate, minimum of 1,000 hours of post baccalaureate clinical practice supervised by preceptors. *Entrance requirements:* For master's, GRE, MAT, or GMAT (for students with BSN GPA of less than 3.2), baccalaureate degree in nursing from an NLNAC- or CCNE-accredited program or an MSN Bridge program; Pennsylvania RN license; 2 letters of reference; resume; statement of philosophy articulating professional values and future educational goal; 1 year of work experience as a registered nurse; for doctorate, GRE (waived for applicants with MSN cumulative GPA of 3.7 or above), MSN from nationally-accredited program or master's degree, MBA or MHA from nationally-accredited program; resume or curriculum vitae; 2 letters of reference; interview; for Certificate, GRE, MAT, or GMAT (for students with BSN GPA of less than 3.2, baccalaureate degree in nursing from an NLNAC- or CCNE-accredited program or an MSN Bridge program; Pennsylvania RN license; 2 letters of reference; resume; statement of philosophy articulating professional values and future educational goal; 1 year of work experience as a registered nurse. Additional exam requirements/recommendations for international students: Required—TOEFL. *Application deadline:* For fall admission, 8/15 priority date for domestic students, 7/15 for international students; for spring admission, 12/15 priority date for domestic students, 11/15 for international students; for summer admission, 4/15 priority date for domestic students, 3/15 for international students. Applications are processed on a rolling basis. Application fee: $35. Electronic applications accepted. Application fee is waived when completed online. *Expenses:* $870 per credit hour (for MSN); $930 per credit hour (for DNP); $150 technology fee full-time, $75 part-time; $135 general university fee. *Financial support:* In 2015–16, 13 students received support. Scholarships/grants and traineeships available. Support available to part-time students. Financial award application deadline: 8/31; financial award applicants required to submit FAFSA. *Unit head:* Dr. Patricia M. Dillon, Director, 215-951-1322, Fax: 215-951-1896, E-mail: msnapn@lasalle.edu. *Application contact:* Alison McAnespey Target, Director, Graduate and Adult Enrollment, 215-951-1100, Fax: 215-951-1462, E-mail: reilly@lasalle.edu.
Website: http://www.lasalle.edu/nursing/program-options/

Laurentian University, School of Graduate Studies and Research, Programme in Nursing, Sudbury, ON P3E 2C6, Canada. Offers M Sc N.

Lehman College of the City University of New York, School of Natural and Social Sciences, Department of Nursing, Bronx, NY 10468-1589. Offers adult health nursing (MS); nursing of older adults (MS); parent-child nursing (MS); pediatric nurse practitioner (MS). *Accreditation:* AACN. *Program availability:* Part-time, evening/weekend. *Entrance requirements:* For master's, bachelor's degree in nursing, New York RN license.

Le Moyne College, Department of Nursing, Syracuse, NY 13214. Offers informatics (MS, CAS); nursing administration (MS, CAS); nursing education (MS, CAS); nursing gerontology (MS, CAS); palliative care (MS, CAS). *Accreditation:* AACN. *Program availability:* Part-time, evening/weekend. *Degree requirements:* For master's, scholarly project. *Entrance requirements:* For master's, bachelor's degree, interview, minimum GPA of 3.0, New York RN license, 2 letters of recommendation, writing sample, transcripts. *Expenses:* Contact institution. *Faculty research:* Inter-profession education, gerontology, utilization of free healthcare services by the insured, health promotion education, innovative undergraduate nursing education models, patient and family education, horizontal violence.

Lenoir-Rhyne University, Graduate Programs, School of Nursing, Program in Nursing, Hickory, NC 28601. Offers nursing administration (MSN); nursing education (MSN). *Program availability:* Online learning. *Faculty:* 7 full-time (all women). *Students:* 4 full-time (all women), 46 part-time (45 women); includes 4 minority (2 Black or African American, non-Hispanic/Latino; 2 Hispanic/Latino). Average age 39. In 2015, 11 master's awarded. *Degree requirements:* For master's, comprehensive exam, thesis optional. *Entrance requirements:* For master's, official transcripts, two recommendations, essay, resume, unrestricted RN license, criminal background check. Additional exam requirements/recommendations for international students: Required—TOEFL (minimum score 600 paper-based). Application fee: $35. Electronic applications accepted. *Expenses:* $550 per credit hour. *Unit head:* Dr. Kerry Thompson, Chair, School of Nursing, 828-328-7282, Fax: 828-328-7368, E-mail: thompsonk@lr.edu. *Application contact:* Mary Ann Gosnell, Director of Graduate Recruiting, 828-328-7300, E-mail: admission@lr.edu.
Website: http://www.lr.edu/academics/programs/nursing-0

Lewis University, College of Nursing and Health Professions, Program in Nursing, Romeoville, IL 60446. Offers adult nurse practitioner (MSN); nursing administration (MSN); nursing education (MSN). *Accreditation:* AACN. *Program availability:* Part-time, evening/weekend, online learning. *Degree requirements:* For master's, clinical practicum. *Entrance requirements:* For master's, minimum undergraduate GPA of 3.0, degree in nursing, RN license, letter of recommendation, interview, resume or curriculum vitae. Additional exam requirements/recommendations for international students: Required—TOEFL (minimum score 550 paper-based; 80 iBT). Electronic applications accepted. *Faculty research:* Cancer prevention, phenomenological methods, public policy analysis.

Lewis University, College of Nursing and Health Professions and College of Business, Program in Nursing/Business, Romeoville, IL 60446. Offers MSN/MBA. *Program availability:* Part-time, evening/weekend. *Entrance requirements:* Additional exam requirements/recommendations for international students: Required—TOEFL (minimum score 550 paper-based; 80 iBT). Electronic applications accepted. *Faculty research:* Cancer prevention, phenomenological methods, public policy analysis.

Liberty University, School of Nursing, Lynchburg, VA 24515. Offers family nurse practitioner (DNP); nurse educator (MSN); nursing administration (MSN). *Program availability:* Part-time, online learning. *Students:* 108 full-time (100 women), 508 part-time (454 women); includes 106 minority (84 Black or African American, non-Hispanic/Latino; 3 American Indian or Alaska Native, non-Hispanic/Latino; 8 Asian, non-Hispanic/Latino; 1 Hispanic/Latino; 10 Two or more races, non-Hispanic/Latino), 7 international. Average age 39. 577 applicants, 30% accepted, 119 enrolled. In 2015, 161 master's awarded. *Entrance requirements:* For master's, minimum cumulative undergraduate GPA of 3.0; for doctorate, minimum GPA of 3.25 in most current nursing program completed. Additional exam requirements/recommendations for international students: Recommended—TOEFL. *Application deadline:* Applications are processed on a rolling basis. Application fee: $50. Electronic applications accepted. *Unit head:* Dr. Deanna Britt, Dean, 434-582-2519, E-mail: dbritt@liberty.edu. *Application contact:* Jay Bridge, Director of Admissions, 800-424-9595, Fax: 800-628-7977, E-mail: gradadmissions@liberty.edu.

Lincoln Memorial University, Caylor School of Nursing, Harrogate, TN 37752-1901. Offers family nurse practitioner (MSN); nurse anesthesia (MSN); psychiatric mental health nurse practitioner (MSN). *Accreditation:* AANA/CANAEP; ACEN. *Program availability:* Part-time. *Entrance requirements:* For master's, GRE.

Lindenwood University, Graduate Programs, School of Nursing and Allied Health Sciences, St. Charles, MO 63301-1695. Offers nursing (MS). *Program availability:* Part-time, blended/hybrid learning. *Faculty:* 2 full-time (both women). *Students:* 1 (woman) full-time, 17 part-time (all women); includes 1 minority (Black or African American, non-Hispanic/Latino). Average age 45. 23 applicants, 61% accepted, 11 enrolled. *Degree requirements:* For master's, minimum cumulative GPA of 3.0. *Entrance requirements:* For master's, BSN with 1 year of clinical experience as an RN, minimum cumulative GPA of 3.0. Additional exam requirements/recommendations for international students: Required—TOEFL (minimum score 550 paper-based; 80 iBT); Recommended—IELTS (minimum score 6.5). *Application deadline:* For fall admission, 8/22 priority date for domestic and international students; for spring admission, 1/9 priority date for domestic and international students; for summer admission, 5/16 priority date for domestic and international students. Applications are processed on a rolling basis. Application fee: $30 ($100 for international students). Electronic applications accepted. *Expenses: Tuition,* area resident: Full-time $15,672; part-time $453 per credit hour. *Required fees:* $205 per semester. Tuition and fees vary according to course level, course load and degree level. *Financial support:* In 2015–16, 30 students received support. Career-related internships or fieldwork, Federal Work-Study, institutionally sponsored loans, scholarships/grants, tuition waivers (partial), and unspecified assistantships available. Financial award application deadline: 6/30; financial award applicants required to submit FAFSA. *Unit head:* Dr. Peggy Ellis, Dean, School of Nursing and Allied Science, 636-949-2907, E-mail: pellis@lindenwood.edu. *Application contact:* Tyler Kostich, Director, Evening and Graduate Admissions, 636-949-4138, Fax: 636-949-4109, E-mail: adultadmissions@lindenwood.edu.

Website: http://www.lindenwood.edu/nursing/

Loma Linda University, School of Nursing, Program in Nursing, Loma Linda, CA 92350. Offers DNP, PhD. *Accreditation:* AACN. *Program availability:* Part-time. *Entrance requirements:* Additional exam requirements/recommendations for international students: Required—TOEFL. *Application deadline:* For fall admission, 8/1 for domestic and international students; for winter admission, 11/1 for domestic and international students; for spring admission, 2/1 for domestic and international students. Application fee: $60. Electronic applications accepted. *Financial support:* Career-related internships or fieldwork, Federal Work-Study, institutionally sponsored loans, and scholarships/grants available. Support available to part-time students. Financial award application deadline: 6/1. *Faculty research:* Family coping in chronic illness; women, identity, and career/family issues. *Unit head:* Director, 909-824-4360. *Application contact:* Admissions Office, 909-651-5029, Fax: 909-558-4879, E-mail: admissions.app@llu.edu.

Long Island University–LIU Brooklyn, Harriet Rothkopf Heilbrunn School of Nursing, Brooklyn, NY 11201-8423. Offers adult nurse practitioner (MS, Advanced Certificate); family nurse practitioner (MS, Advanced Certificate); nurse educator (MS). *Accreditation:* AACN. *Program availability:* Part-time, evening/weekend, blended/hybrid learning. *Faculty:* 6 full-time (4 women), 5 part-time/adjunct (4 women). *Students:* 1 (woman) full-time, 215 part-time (192 women); includes 136 minority (89 Black or African American, non-Hispanic/Latino; 28 Asian, non-Hispanic/Latino; 13 Hispanic/Latino; 2 Native Hawaiian or other Pacific Islander, non-Hispanic/Latino; 4 Two or more races, non-Hispanic/Latino), 1 international. Average age 43. 167 applicants, 57% accepted, 63 enrolled. In 2015, 23 master's, 5 other advanced degrees awarded. *Entrance requirements:* For master's and Advanced Certificate, New York RN license, two letters of recommendation. Additional exam requirements/recommendations for international students: Required—TOEFL (minimum score 550 paper-based; 79 iBT), IELTS (minimum score 6.5). *Application deadline:* Applications are processed on a rolling basis. Application fee: $50. Electronic applications accepted. *Expenses:* $1,155 per credit tuition; $934 per term full-time fees; $442 per term part-time fees. *Financial support:* In 2015–16, 24 students received support. Scholarships/grants and unspecified assistantships available. Support available to part-time students. Financial award application deadline: 2/15; financial award applicants required to submit FAFSA. *Faculty research:* Cultural competency, high fidelity simulation to improve nursing assessment and increase patient safety, relationship of diabetes to stress, end of life care, geriatric issues, foreign nurse's adaptation to the United States. *Unit head:* Dr. Loretta Knapp, Interim Dean, 718-488-1508, Fax: 718-780-4019, E-mail: lori.knapp@liu.edu. *Application contact:* Richard Sunday, Dean of Admissions, 718-488-1011, Fax: 718-780-6110, E-mail: bkln-admissions@liu.edu.

Website: http://liu.edu/Brooklyn/Academics/Harriet-Rothkopf-Heilbrunn-School-of-Nursing

Louisiana State University Health Sciences Center, School of Nursing, New Orleans, LA 70112. Offers adult gerontology clinical nurse specialist (Post-Master's Certificate); clinical nurse leader (MSN); executive nurse leader (Post-Master's Certificate); neonatal nurse practitioner (Post-Master's Certificate); nurse anesthesia (Post-Master's Certificate); nurse educator (MSN); nursing (DNS); primary care family nurse practitioner (Post-Master's Certificate); public/community health nursing (Post-Master's Certificate). *Accreditation:* AACN; AANA/CANAEP (one or more programs are accredited). *Program availability:* Part-time. *Faculty:* 22 full-time (19 women), 21 part-time/adjunct (8 women). *Students:* 254 (185 women); includes 68 minority (44 Black or African American, non-Hispanic/Latino; 12 Asian, non-Hispanic/Latino; 12 Hispanic/Latino). Average age 33. 144 applicants, 54% accepted, 73 enrolled. In 2015, 84 master's, 6 doctorates awarded. *Degree requirements:* For master's, thesis optional; for doctorate, thesis/dissertation. *Entrance requirements:* For master's, GRE General Test, MAT, minimum GPA of 3.0; for doctorate, GRE General Test, minimum GPA of 3.5. Additional exam requirements/recommendations for international students: Required—TOEFL (minimum score 550 paper-based; 79 iBT). *Application deadline:* Applications are processed on a rolling basis. Application fee: $250. Electronic applications accepted. *Expenses:* $9,136.50 per year; $19,633.50 per year (for DNP). *Financial support:* Federal Work-Study, institutionally sponsored loans, scholarships/grants, and traineeships available. Financial award applicants required to submit FAFSA. *Faculty research:* Advanced clinical practice, nursing education, health, social support, nursing administration. *Unit head:* Dr. Demetrius James Porche, Dean, 504-568-4106, Fax: 504-599-0573, E-mail: dporch@lsuhsc.edu. *Application contact:* Tracie Gravolet, Director, Office of Student Affairs, 504-568-4114, Fax: 504-568-5711, E-mail: tgravo@lsuhsc.edu.

Website: http://nursing.lsuhsc.edu/

Loyola University Chicago, Graduate School, Marcella Niehoff School of Nursing, Maywood, IL 60153. Offers adult gerontology acute care clinical nurse specialist (MSN), including emergency care (MSN, Certificate); adult gerontology acute care nurse practitioner (MSN), including oncology (MSN, Certificate); adult gerontology clinical nurse specialist (MSN), including oncology (MSN, Certificate); adult gerontology nursing (Certificate), including oncology (MSN, Certificate); adult nurse practitioner (Certificate); dietetics (MS); family nurse practitioner (MSN, Certificate), including emergency care; informatics (MSN); leadership (DNP), including healthcare quality using education in safety and technology, infection prevention; nursing science (PhD); women's health nurse practitioner (MSN); women's health nursing (Certificate). *Accreditation:* AACN. *Program availability:* Part-time, blended/hybrid learning. *Faculty:* 27 full-time (25 women), 12 part-time/adjunct (10 women). *Students:* 174 full-time (161 women), 232 part-time (221 women); includes 95 minority (19 Black or African American, non-Hispanic/Latino; 2 American Indian or Alaska Native, non-Hispanic/Latino; 38 Asian, non-Hispanic/Latino; 28 Hispanic/Latino; 2 Native Hawaiian or other Pacific Islander, non-Hispanic/Latino; 6 Two or more races, non-Hispanic/Latino), 3 international. Average age 35. 209 applicants, 52% accepted, 83 enrolled. In 2015, 78 master's, 10 doctorates, 17 other advanced degrees awarded. *Degree requirements:* For master's, comprehensive exam; for doctorate, thesis/dissertation, qualifying examination (for PhD); capstone project (for DNP). *Entrance requirements:* For master's, BSN, minimum nursing GPA of 3.0, Illinois RN license, 3 letters of recommendation, 1000 hours of experience in area of specialty prior to starting clinical rotations, personal statement; for doctorate, GRE General Test (for PhD), BSN or MSN, minimum GPA of 3.0, professional nursing license, 3 letters of recommendation, personal statement. Additional exam requirements/recommendations for international students: Required—TOEFL (minimum score 550 paper-based; 79 iBT), IELTS (minimum score 6.5). *Application deadline:* For fall admission, 6/1 priority date for domestic and international students; for spring admission, 11/15 priority date for domestic and international students; for summer admission, 3/15 priority date for domestic and international students. Applications are processed on a rolling basis. Application fee: $50. Electronic applications accepted. Application fee is waived when completed online. *Expenses:* $1,081 per credit hour. *Financial support:* In 2015–16, 10 students received support, including 3 research assistantships with full tuition reimbursements available (averaging $18,000 per year), 1 teaching assistantship with full tuition reimbursement available (averaging $18,000 per year); scholarships/grants, unspecified assistantships, and nurse faculty loan program also available. Financial award application deadline: 5/1; financial award applicants required to submit FAFSA. *Faculty research:* Epigenetics and social determinants of health, women's health, vitamin D, interprofessional education, prevention and self-management of chronic disease. *Total annual research expenditures:* $649,606. *Unit head:* Dr. Vicky Keough, Dean, 708-216-5448, Fax: 708-216-9555, E-mail: vkeough@luc.edu. *Application contact:* Toni Topalova, Enrollment Advisor, 708-216-3751, Fax: 708-216-9555, E-mail: atopalova@luc.edu.

Website: http://www.luc.edu/nursing/

Loyola University New Orleans, College of Social Sciences, School of Nursing, New Orleans, LA 70118. Offers health care systems management (MSN); nursing (MSN, DNP). *Accreditation:* ACEN. *Program availability:* Part-time, evening/weekend, online learning. *Faculty:* 14 full-time (13 women), 16 part-time/adjunct (12 women). *Students:* 350 full-time (321 women), 95 part-time (85 women); includes 139 minority (97 Black or African American, non-Hispanic/Latino; 2 American Indian or Alaska Native, non-Hispanic/Latino; 22 Asian, non-Hispanic/Latino; 15 Hispanic/Latino; 1 Native Hawaiian or other Pacific Islander, non-Hispanic/Latino; 2 Two or more races, non-Hispanic/Latino). Average age 41. 229 applicants, 76% accepted, 100 enrolled. In 2015, 139 master's, 28 doctorates awarded. *Degree requirements:* For master's, practicum; for doctorate, capstone project. *Entrance requirements:* For master's, BSN, unencumbered RN license, 1 year of work experience in clinical nursing, interview, resume, 3 recommendations, statement of purpose. Additional exam requirements/recommendations for international students: Recommended—TOEFL (minimum score 550 paper-based), IELTS. *Application deadline:* For fall admission, 8/1 priority date for domestic and international students; for winter admission, 12/15 priority date for domestic and international students; for spring admission, 5/15 priority date for domestic and international students. Applications are processed on a rolling basis. Application fee: $40. Electronic applications accepted. *Financial support:* Traineeships and Incumbent Workers Training Program grants available. Financial award application deadline: 5/1; financial award applicants required to submit FAFSA. *Faculty research:* Increasing compliance with treatment, patient satisfaction with care provided by nurse practitioners. *Unit head:* Dr. Patricia Pearce, Interim Director, 800-488-6257, Fax: 504-865-3254, E-mail: nursing@loyno.edu. *Application contact:* Deborah Smith, Executive Assistant to the Director, 504-865-2823, Fax: 504-865-3254, E-mail: dhsmith@loyno.edu.

Website: http://css.loyno.edu/nursing

Lynchburg College, Graduate Studies, MS Program in Nursing, Lynchburg, VA 24501-3199. Offers clinical nurse leader (MS). *Accreditation:* AACN. *Program availability:* Part-time, evening/weekend, online only, 100% online. *Faculty:* 1 (woman) full-time, 2 part-time/adjunct (both women). *Students:* 2 full-time (both women), 32 part-time (30 women); includes 4 minority (3 Black or African American, non-Hispanic/Latino; 1 Hispanic/Latino). Average age 40. In 2015, 6 master's awarded. *Degree requirements:* For master's, practicum. *Entrance requirements:* For master's, GRE or 2 years of professional nursing experience, official transcripts, personal essay, 3 letters of recommendation, current unrestricted registered nurse license in Virginia. Additional exam requirements/recommendations for international students: Required—TOEFL (minimum score 550 paper-based; 79 iBT), IELTS (minimum score 6.5). *Application deadline:* For fall admission, 7/31 for domestic students, 6/1 for international students; for spring admission, 11/30 for domestic students, 10/15 for international students. Applications are processed on a rolling basis. Application fee: $30. Electronic applications accepted. Application fee is waived when completed online. *Expenses:* $8,550. *Financial support:* Federal Work-Study, scholarships/grants, health care benefits, and unspecified assistantships available. Support available to part-time

Nursing—General

students. Financial award application deadline: 7/31; financial award applicants required to submit FAFSA. *Unit head:* Dr. Jenna Lloyd, Director of MSN Program, 434-544-8461, E-mail: lloyd.j@lynchburg.edu.
Website: http://www.lynchburg.edu/graduate/online-master-of-science-in-nursing/

Madonna University, Program in Nursing, Livonia, MI 48150-1173. Offers adult health: chronic health conditions (MSN); adult nurse practitioner (MSN); nursing administration (MSN); MSN/MSBA. *Accreditation:* AACN. *Program availability:* Part-time. *Degree requirements:* For master's, thesis or alternative. *Entrance requirements:* For master's, GRE General Test, Michigan nursing license. Electronic applications accepted. *Faculty research:* Coping, caring.

Malone University, Graduate Program in Nursing, Canton, OH 44709. Offers family nurse practitioner (MSN). *Accreditation:* AACN. *Program availability:* Part-time, evening/weekend. *Degree requirements:* For master's, thesis. *Entrance requirements:* For master's, minimum GPA of 3.0 from BSN program, interview, Ohio RN license. Additional exam requirements/recommendations for international students: Required—TOEFL (minimum score 550 paper-based; 79 iBT). *Expenses:* Contact institution. *Faculty research:* Home heath care and geriatrics, community settings, culture, Hispanics, tuberculosis, geriatrics, Neuman Systems Model, nursing education.

Mansfield University of Pennsylvania, Graduate Studies, Program in Nursing, Mansfield, PA 16933. Offers MSN. *Accreditation:* ACEN. *Program availability:* Part-time, evening/weekend, online learning. *Degree requirements:* For master's, comprehensive exam, thesis optional. *Entrance requirements:* For master's, minimum GPA of 3.0. Additional exam requirements/recommendations for international students: Required—TOEFL (minimum score 550 paper-based). Electronic applications accepted. *Faculty research:* Women's health, gyniatrics, art therapy, nursing empowerment.

Marian University, School of Nursing and Health Professions, Fond du Lac, WI 54935-4699. Offers adult nurse practitioner (MSN); nurse educator (MSN). *Accreditation:* AACN. *Program availability:* Part-time, evening/weekend. *Faculty:* 6 full-time (all women), 4 part-time/adjunct (2 women). *Students:* 21 full-time (20 women), 95 part-time (85 women); includes 10 minority (6 Black or African American, non-Hispanic/Latino; 2 Asian, non-Hispanic/Latino; 2 Hispanic/Latino). Average age 40. In 2015, 26 master's awarded. *Degree requirements:* For master's, thesis, 675 clinical practicum hours. *Entrance requirements:* For master's, 3 letters of professional recommendation; undergraduate work in nursing research, statistics, health assessment. Additional exam requirements/recommendations for international students: Required—TOEFL (minimum score 525 paper-based; 70 iBT). *Application deadline:* Applications are processed on a rolling basis. Application fee: $50. Electronic applications accepted. *Expenses:* Contact institution. *Financial support:* In 2015–16, 3 students received support. Institutionally sponsored loans and scholarships/grants available. Support available to part-time students. Financial award application deadline: 3/1; financial award applicants required to submit FAFSA. *Unit head:* Dr. Linda Matheson, Dean, 920-923-7668, Fax: 920-923-8770, E-mail: lkmatheson85@marianuniversity.edu. *Application contact:* Selina Scoles, Admissions Counselor, 920-923-8938, Fax: 920-923-8770, E-mail: sascoles30@marianuniversity.edu.
Website: http://www.marianuniversity.edu/nursing/

Marquette University, Graduate School, College of Nursing, Milwaukee, WI 53201-1881. Offers acute care nurse practitioner (Certificate); adult clinical nurse specialist (Certificate); adult nurse practitioner (Certificate); advanced practice nursing (MSN, DNP), including adult-older adult acute care (DNP), adults (MSN), adults-older adults (DNP), clinical nurse leader (MSN), health care systems leadership (DNP), nurse-midwifery (MSN), older adults (MSN), pediatrics-acute care, pediatrics-primary care, primary care (DNP), systems leadership and healthcare quality (MSN); family nurse practitioner (Certificate); nurse-midwifery (Certificate); nursing (PhD); pediatric acute care (Certificate); pediatric primary care (Certificate); systems leadership and healthcare quality (Certificate). *Accreditation:* AACN. *Faculty:* 35 full-time (all women), 56 part-time/adjunct (55 women). *Students:* 123 full-time (112 women), 242 part-time (220 women); includes 34 minority (9 Black or African American, non-Hispanic/Latino; 12 Asian, non-Hispanic/Latino; 10 Hispanic/Latino; 3 Two or more races, non-Hispanic/Latino), 4 international. Average age 30. 269 applicants, 61% accepted, 98 enrolled. In 2015, 84 master's, 5 doctorates, 22 other advanced degrees awarded. Terminal master's awarded for partial completion of doctoral program. *Degree requirements:* For master's, comprehensive exam, thesis or alternative. *Entrance requirements:* For master's, GRE General Test, BSN, Wisconsin RN license, official transcripts from all current and previous colleges/universities except Marquette, three completed recommendation forms, resume, written statement of professional goals; for doctorate, GRE General Test, official transcripts from all current and previous colleges/universities except Marquette, three letters of recommendation, resume, written statement of professional goals, sample of scholarly writing. Additional exam requirements/recommendations for international students: Required—TOEFL (minimum score 530 paper-based). *Application deadline:* For fall admission, 2/15 for domestic and international students. Electronic applications accepted. *Financial support:* In 2015–16, 41 students received support, including 1 fellowship with partial tuition reimbursement available (averaging $17,500 per year), 2 research assistantships with full tuition reimbursements available (averaging $13,285 per year), 8 teaching assistantships with full tuition reimbursements available (averaging $13,912 per year); career-related internships or fieldwork, Federal Work-Study, scholarships/grants, health care benefits, tuition waivers (partial), and unspecified assistantships also available. Support available to part-time students. Financial award application deadline: 2/15. *Faculty research:* Psychosocial adjustment to chronic illness, gerontology, reminiscence, health policy: uninsured and access, hospital care delivery systems. *Total annual research expenditures:* $480,591. *Unit head:* Dr. Donna McCarthy, Interim Chair, 414-288-3800, Fax: 414-288-1578. *Application contact:* Dr. Maureen O'Brien, Associate Dean/Clinical Associate Professor, 414-288-3823.

Marshall University, Academic Affairs Division, College of Health Professions, Department of Nursing, Huntington, WV 25755. Offers MSN. *Students:* 8 full-time (7 women), 102 part-time (92 women); includes 5 minority (4 Black or African American, non-Hispanic/Latino; 1 Hispanic/Latino), 2 international. Average age 31. In 2015, 46 master's awarded. *Entrance requirements:* For master's, GRE General Test. Application fee: $40. *Unit head:* Dr. Diana Stotts, Associate Dean, 304-696-2623, E-mail: stotts@marshall.edu. *Application contact:* Information Contact, 304-746-1900, Fax: 304-746-1902, E-mail: services@marshall.edu.

Marymount University, School of Health Professions, Program in Nursing, Arlington, VA 22207-4299. Offers family nurse practitioner (MSN, Certificate); nursing (DNP). *Accreditation:* AACN. *Program availability:* Part-time, evening/weekend. *Faculty:* 7 full-time (all women), 3 part-time/adjunct (2 women). *Students:* 12 full-time (11 women), 58 part-time (53 women); includes 25 minority (18 Black or African American, non-Hispanic/Latino; 4 Asian, non-Hispanic/Latino; 1 Hispanic/Latino; 1 Native Hawaiian or other Pacific Islander, non-Hispanic/Latino; 1 Two or more races, non-Hispanic/Latino), 1 international. Average age 36. 47 applicants, 57% accepted, 20 enrolled. In 2015, 19 master's, 1 doctorate awarded. *Degree requirements:* For master's, comprehensive exam; for doctorate, thesis/dissertation or alternative. *Entrance requirements:* For master's, 2 letters of recommendation, interview, resume, RN license, personal

statement; for doctorate, 2 letters of recommendation, interview, resume, RN license, minimum MSN GPA of 3.5 or BSN 3.3; for Certificate, interview, master's degree in nursing. Additional exam requirements/recommendations for international students: Required—TOEFL (minimum score 600 paper-based; 96 iBT), IELTS (minimum score 6.5). *Application deadline:* For fall admission, 5/1 for domestic students, 7/1 for international students; for spring admission, 11/1 for domestic students, 9/16 for international students. Application fee: $40. Electronic applications accepted. *Expenses:* Tuition, area resident: Part-time $910 per credit hour. *Required fees:* $10 per credit hour. One-time fee: $230 part-time. Tuition and fees vary according to program. *Financial support:* In 2015–16, 15 students received support, including 4 teaching assistantships with partial tuition reimbursements available; career-related internships or fieldwork, Federal Work-Study, scholarships/grants, and unspecified assistantships also available. Support available to part-time students. Financial award applicants required to submit FAFSA. *Unit head:* Dr. Shelli Wolfe Mayer, Chair, 703-284-6886, Fax: 703-284-3819, E-mail: michelle.wolfe@marymount.edu. *Application contact:* Francesca Reed, Director, Graduate Admissions, 703-284-5901, Fax: 703-527-3815, E-mail: grad.admissions@marymount.edu.
Website: http://www.marymount.edu/Academics/Malek-School-of-Health-Professions/Graduate-Programs/Nursing-(M-S-N)

Maryville University of Saint Louis, Walker College of Health Professions, The Catherine McAuley School of Nursing, St. Louis, MO 63141-7299. Offers acute care nurse practice (MSN); adult gerontology nurse practitioner (MSN); advanced practice nursing (DNP); family nurse practitioner (MSN); pediatric nurse practice (MSN). *Accreditation:* AACN. *Program availability:* 100% online. *Faculty:* 18 full-time (all women), 158 part-time/adjunct (141 women). *Students:* 38 full-time (35 women), 2,802 part-time (2,511 women); includes 681 minority (332 Black or African American, non-Hispanic/Latino; 40 American Indian or Alaska Native, non-Hispanic/Latino; 126 Asian, non-Hispanic/Latino; 126 Hispanic/Latino; 8 Native Hawaiian or other Pacific Islander, non-Hispanic/Latino; 49 Two or more races, non-Hispanic/Latino), 58 international. Average age 37. In 2015, 413 master's, 33 doctorates awarded. *Degree requirements:* For master's, practicum. *Entrance requirements:* For master's, BSN, current licensure, minimum GPA of 3.0, 3 letters of recommendation, curriculum vitae. Additional exam requirements/recommendations for international students: Required—TOEFL (minimum score 550 paper-based). *Application deadline:* Applications are processed on a rolling basis. Electronic applications accepted. Application fee is waived when completed online. *Expenses:* Tuition, area resident: Full-time $25,558; part-time $781 per credit hour. *Required fees:* $2400. Part-time tuition and fees vary according to course load and degree level. *Financial support:* Federal Work-Study and campus employment available. Support available to part-time students. Financial award application deadline: 3/1; financial award applicants required to submit FAFSA. *Unit head:* Dr. Elizabeth Buck, Director, 314-529-9453, Fax: 314-529-9139, E-mail: ebuck@maryville.edu. *Application contact:* Crystal Jacobsmeyer, Assistant Director, Graduate Enrollment Advising, 314-929-9654, Fax: 314-529-9927, E-mail: cjacobsmeyer@maryville.edu.
Website: http://www.maryville.edu/hp/nursing/

McGill University, Faculty of Graduate and Postdoctoral Studies, Faculty of Medicine, School of Nursing, Montréal, QC H3A 2T5, Canada. Offers nurse practitioner (Graduate Diploma); nursing (M Sc A, PhD). PhD offered jointly with Université du Québec à Montréal.

McKendree University, Graduate Programs, Master of Science in Nursing Program, Lebanon, IL 62254-1299. Offers nursing education (MSN); nursing management/administration (MSN). *Accreditation:* AACN. *Program availability:* Part-time, evening/weekend, online learning. *Degree requirements:* For master's, research project or thesis. *Entrance requirements:* For master's, resume, references, valid Professional Registered Nurse license. Additional exam requirements/recommendations for international students: Required—TOEFL. Electronic applications accepted.

McMaster University, Faculty of Health Sciences and School of Graduate Studies, Program in Nursing (course-based), Hamilton, ON L8S 4M2, Canada. Offers M Sc. *Degree requirements:* For master's, scholarly paper. *Entrance requirements:* For master's, 4 year honors BSCN, minimum B+ average in last 60 units. Additional exam requirements/recommendations for international students: Required—TOEFL (minimum score 580 paper-based; 92 iBT).

McMaster University, Faculty of Health Sciences and School of Graduate Studies, Program in Nursing (thesis), Hamilton, ON L8S 4M2, Canada. Offers M Sc, PhD. *Degree requirements:* For master's, thesis; for doctorate, comprehensive exam, thesis/dissertation. *Entrance requirements:* For master's, honors B Sc N, B+ average in last 60 units; for doctorate, M Sc, minimum B+ average. Additional exam requirements/recommendations for international students: Required—TOEFL (minimum score 580 paper-based; 92 iBT).

McMurry University, Graduate Studies, Abilene, TX 79697. Offers education (MSN); family nurse practitioner (MSN).

McNeese State University, Doré School of Graduate Studies, College of Nursing, Lake Charles, LA 70609. Offers MSN, PMC, Postbaccalaureate Certificate. Program offered jointly with Southeastern Louisiana University and Southern University and Agricultural and Mechanical College. *Accreditation:* AACN. *Degree requirements:* For master's, comprehensive exam. *Entrance requirements:* For master's, GRE, eligibility for unencumbered licensure as RN in Louisiana.

McNeese State University, Doré School of Graduate Studies, College of Nursing, Department of Graduate Nursing, Nursing Program, Lake Charles, LA 70609. Offers family nurse practitioner (MSN); family psychiatric/mental health nurse practitioner (MSN); nurse educator (MSN); nurse executive (MSN). *Degree requirements:* For master's, comprehensive exam. *Entrance requirements:* For master's, GRE, baccalaureate degree in nursing, minimum overall GPA of 2.7 for all undergraduate coursework, eligibility for unencumbered licensure as Registered Nurse in Louisiana or Texas, course in introductory statistics with minimum C grade, physical assessment skills, two letters of professional reference, 500-word essay, current resume.

MCPHS University, Graduate Studies, Program in Nursing, Boston, MA 02115-5896. Offers MS. *Accreditation:* AACN. *Program availability:* Part-time, online learning. *Entrance requirements:* For master's, BSN. Additional exam requirements/recommendations for international students: Required—TOEFL (minimum score 550 paper-based; 79 iBT). Electronic applications accepted.

Medical University of South Carolina, College of Nursing, PhD in Nursing Program, Charleston, SC 29425. Offers PhD. *Accreditation:* AACN. *Program availability:* Part-time, online learning. *Degree requirements:* For doctorate, comprehensive exam, thesis/dissertation, mentored teaching and research seminar. *Entrance requirements:* For doctorate, BSN or MSN from accredited NLNAC or CCNE program, minimum GPA of 3.5, documentation of RN license from state of residence, curriculum vitae, personal statement, 3 references, interview, evidence of computer literacy. Additional exam requirements/recommendations for international students: Required—TOEFL (minimum score 550 paper-based; 80 iBT). Electronic applications accepted. *Faculty research:* Rare diseases, vascular ulcer prevention, health disparities, community engagement, health services.

Medical University of South Carolina, College of Nursing, Post-MSN Doctor of Nursing Practice Program, Charleston, SC 29425. Offers advanced practice nursing (DNP). *Program availability:* Part-time, online learning. *Degree requirements:* For doctorate, final project. *Entrance requirements:* For doctorate, BSN and MSN from nationally-accredited program, minimum cumulative GPA of 3.0 for undergraduate and graduate coursework, active APRN License and specialty certification, 3 confidential references, current curriculum vitae or resume, statement of goals. Additional exam requirements/recommendations for international students: Required—TOEFL (minimum score 550 paper-based; 80 iBT). Electronic applications accepted. *Faculty research:* Women's health cardiovascular, hospital roles, HPV, guidelines implementation, adolescent family obesity.

Memorial University of Newfoundland, School of Graduate Studies, School of Nursing, St. John's, NL A1C 5S7, Canada. Offers MN, PhD. *Program availability:* Part-time. *Degree requirements:* For master's, thesis optional. *Entrance requirements:* For master's, bachelor's degree in nursing, 1 year of experience in nursing practice, practicing license. *Application deadline:* For fall admission, 2/15 priority date for domestic and international students. Applications are processed on a rolling basis. Application fee: $50 Canadian dollars ($100 Canadian dollars for international students). Electronic applications accepted. *Expenses: Tuition, area resident:* Full-time $2199 Canadian dollars. *International tuition:* $2859 Canadian dollars full-time. *Financial support:* Fellowships, research assistantships, and teaching assistantships available. Financial award application deadline: 12/31. *Faculty research:* Women's health, infant feeding practices, nursing management, care of the elderly, children's health. *Unit head:* Dr. Alice Gaudine, Dean, 709-777-6912, Fax: 709-777-7037, E-mail: agaudine@mun.ca. *Application contact:* Dr. Donna Moralejo, Graduate Officer, 709-777-6527, E-mail: mnson@mun.ca.
Website: http://www.mun.ca/nursing/grad

Mercer University, Graduate Studies, Cecil B. Day Campus, Georgia Baptist College of Nursing, Atlanta, GA 30341. Offers adult gerontology acute care nurse practitioner (MSN, Certificate); family nurse practitioner (MSN); nursing (PhD); nursing practice (DNP), including adult gerontology acute care nurse practitioner. *Accreditation:* AACN. *Program availability:* Part-time, blended/hybrid learning. *Faculty:* 10 full-time (9 women), 1 (woman) part-time/adjunct. *Students:* 78 full-time (71 women), 42 part-time (39 women); includes 44 minority (21 Black or African American, non-Hispanic/Latino; 16 Asian, non-Hispanic/Latino; 6 Hispanic/Latino; 1 Native Hawaiian or other Pacific Islander, non-Hispanic/Latino), 5 international. Average age 35. 65 applicants, 66% accepted, 30 enrolled. In 2015, 36 master's, 5 doctorates awarded. *Degree requirements:* For master's, thesis or alternative; for doctorate, comprehensive exam (for some programs), thesis/dissertation (for some programs). *Entrance requirements:* For master's, MAT or GRE, bachelor's degree from accredited nursing program, registered unencumbered GA nursing license, essay, three professional references; for doctorate, GRE (for PhD), master's degree from accredited nursing program, RN licensure, graduate statistics course, three professional references. Additional exam requirements/recommendations for international students: Required—TOEFL (minimum score 100 iBT). *Application deadline:* For fall admission, 5/1 for domestic students, 3/1 for international students; for winter admission, 11/1 for domestic students, 9/1 for international students; for spring admission, 11/1 for domestic students, 10/1 for international students; for summer admission, 3/1 for domestic and international students. Applications are processed on a rolling basis. Application fee: $50. Electronic applications accepted. *Expenses:* Contact institution. *Financial support:* In 2015–16, 59 students received support. Scholarships/grants and traineeships available. Financial award application deadline: 6/30; financial award applicants required to submit FAFSA. *Faculty research:* Cognitive competence, cancer survivorship, interprofessional education, cultural competence, clopidogrel adherence, high fidelity simulation, self-awareness practices, simulation. *Unit head:* Dr. Linda Streit, Dean/Professor, 678-547-6793, Fax: 678-547-6796, E-mail: streit_la@mercer.edu. *Application contact:* Janda Anderson, Director of Admissions, 678-547-6700, Fax: 678-547-6794, E-mail: anderson_j@mercer.edu.
Website: http://www.mercer.edu/nursing

Mercy College, School of Health and Natural Sciences, Programs in Nursing, Dobbs Ferry, NY 10522-1189. Offers nursing administration (MS); nursing education (MS). *Accreditation:* AACN. *Program availability:* Part-time, evening/weekend, online learning. *Degree requirements:* For master's, comprehensive exam (for some programs), written comprehensive exam or the production of a comprehensive project. *Entrance requirements:* For master's, interview, two letters of reference, bachelor's degree, RN registration in the U.S. Additional exam requirements/recommendations for international students: Required—TOEFL (minimum score 600 paper-based; 100 iBT), IELTS (minimum score 8). Electronic applications accepted. *Expenses: Tuition, area resident:* Full-time $14,904; part-time $828 per credit hour. *Required fees:* $610; $153 per term. $153 per term. Tuition and fees vary according to course load and program.

Metropolitan State University, College of Health, Community and Professional Studies, St. Paul, MN 55106-5000. Offers advanced dental therapy (MS); leadership and management (MSN); nurse educator (MSN); nursing (DNP); psychology (MA). *Accreditation:* AACN. *Program availability:* Part-time. *Degree requirements:* For master's, thesis or alternative; for doctorate, thesis/dissertation or alternative. *Entrance requirements:* For master's, GRE General Test, minimum GPA of 3.0, RN license, BS/BA; for doctorate, minimum GPA of 3.0; RN license, MSN. Additional exam requirements/recommendations for international students: Required—TOEFL (minimum score 550 paper-based). *Faculty research:* Women's health, gerontology.

MGH Institute of Health Professions, School of Nursing, Boston, MA 02129. Offers advanced practice nursing (MSN); gerontological nursing (MSN); nursing (DNP); pediatric nursing (MSN); psychiatric nursing (MSN); teaching and learning for health care education (Certificate); women's health nursing (MSN). *Accreditation:* AACN. *Degree requirements:* For master's, thesis or alternative. *Entrance requirements:* For master's, GRE General Test, bachelor's degree from regionally-accredited college or university. Additional exam requirements/recommendations for international students: Required—TOEFL (minimum score 550 paper-based; 80 iBT). Electronic applications accepted. *Faculty research:* Biobehavioral nursing, HIV/AIDS, gerontological nursing, women's health, vulnerable populations, health systems.

Michigan State University, The Graduate School, College of Nursing, East Lansing, MI 48824. Offers MSN, PhD. *Accreditation:* AACN; AANA/CANAEP. *Program availability:* Part-time, online learning. *Entrance requirements:* Additional exam requirements/recommendations for international students: Required—TOEFL (minimum score 580 paper-based), Michigan State University ELT (minimum score 85), Michigan English Language Assessment Battery (minimum score 83). Electronic applications accepted. *Faculty research:* Hormone replacement therapy, end of life research, human-animal bond, chronic disease, family home care for cancer.

Middle Tennessee State University, College of Graduate Studies, College of Behavioral and Health Sciences, School of Nursing, Murfreesboro, TN 37132. Offers MSN, Graduate Certificate. *Program availability:* Part-time, evening/weekend, online learning. *Entrance requirements:* Additional exam requirements/recommendations for international students: Required—TOEFL (minimum score 525 paper-based; 71 iBT) or IELTS (minimum score 6). Electronic applications accepted.

Midwestern State University, Billie Doris McAda Graduate School, Robert D. and Carol Gunn College of Health Sciences and Human Services, Wilson School of Nursing, Wichita Falls, TX 76308. Offers family nurse practitioner (MSN); family psychiatric mental health nurse practitioner (MSN); nurse educator (MSN). *Accreditation:* AACN. *Program availability:* Part-time, evening/weekend. *Degree requirements:* For master's, comprehensive exam, thesis optional. *Entrance requirements:* For master's, GRE General Test or MAT. Additional exam requirements/recommendations for international students: Required—TOEFL (minimum score 550 paper-based). Electronic applications accepted. *Faculty research:* Infant feeding, musculoskeletal disorders, diabetes, community health education, water quality reporting.

Millersville University of Pennsylvania, College of Graduate Studies and Adult Learning, College of Science and Technology, Department of Nursing, Millersville, PA 17551-0302. Offers family nurse practitioner (MSN); nursing education (MSN). *Accreditation:* ACEN. *Program availability:* Part-time, evening/weekend. *Faculty:* 6 full-time (all women), 4 part-time/adjunct (all women). *Students:* 1 (woman) full-time, 78 part-time (69 women); includes 9 minority (2 Black or African American, non-Hispanic/Latino; 3 Asian, non-Hispanic/Latino; 3 Hispanic/Latino; 1 Native Hawaiian or other Pacific Islander, non-Hispanic/Latino), 2 international. 50 applicants, 54% accepted, 27 enrolled. In 2015, 26 master's awarded. *Degree requirements:* For master's, internship, scholarly project. *Entrance requirements:* For master's, resume, copy of RN license, minimum GPA of 3.0, all transfer transcripts, interview. Additional exam requirements/recommendations for international students: Required—TOEFL (minimum score 600 paper-based), IELTS (minimum score 6). *Application deadline:* Applications are processed on a rolling basis. Application fee: $40. Electronic applications accepted. *Expenses:* Tuition, state resident: full-time $8460; part-time $470 per credit. Tuition, nonresident: full-time $12,690; part-time $705 per credit. *Required fees:* $2471; $133.75 per credit. Tuition and fees vary according to course load, degree level and program. *Financial support:* Application deadline: 3/15; applicants required to submit FAFSA. *Faculty research:* Family nurse practitioner, nurse education, primary care, health promotion. *Unit head:* Dr. Kelly A. Kuhns, Chair, 717-871-5276, Fax: 717-871-4877, E-mail: kelly.kuhns@millersville.edu. *Application contact:* Dr. Victor S. DeSantis, Dean of College of Graduate Studies and Adult Learning/Associate Provost for Civic and Community Engagement, 717-871-7619, Fax: 717-871-7954, E-mail: victor.desantis@millersville.edu.
Website: http://www.millersville.edu/nursing/

Millikin University, School of Nursing, Decatur, IL 62522-2084. Offers entry into nursing practice (MSN); nurse anesthesia (DNP); nurse educator (MSN); nursing practice (DNP). *Accreditation:* AACN; AANA/CANAEP. *Program availability:* Part-time. *Faculty:* 11 full-time (all women), 4 part-time/adjunct (3 women). *Students:* 44 full-time (27 women), 14 part-time (13 women); includes 9 minority (5 Black or African American, non-Hispanic/Latino; 1 American Indian or Alaska Native, non-Hispanic/Latino; 1 Asian, non-Hispanic/Latino; 1 Hispanic/Latino; 1 Two or more races, non-Hispanic/Latino), 1 international. Average age 32. 117 applicants, 29% accepted, 26 enrolled. In 2015, 15 master's awarded. *Degree requirements:* For master's, thesis or alternative, scholarly project; for doctorate, thesis/dissertation or alternative, scholarly project. *Entrance requirements:* For master's, GRE, official academic transcript(s), essay, immunizations, statistics course, 3 letters of recommendation, CPR certification, professional liability/malpractice insurance; for doctorate, GRE (if undergraduate cumulative GPA is below 3.0), official academic transcript(s); undergraduate courses in nursing research, health assessment, inorganic and organic chemistry, intro to statistics; graduate-level statistics; 3 written recommendations; Assessment of Critical Care Skills form; written statement; resume or curriculum vitae. Additional exam requirements/recommendations for international students: Required—TOEFL (minimum score 650 paper-based; 81 iBT). *Application deadline:* For spring admission, 7/1 priority date for domestic and international students; for summer admission, 11/1 priority date for domestic and international students. Applications are processed on a rolling basis. Application fee: $0. Electronic applications accepted. *Expenses:* Contact institution. *Financial support:* Traineeships and unspecified assistantships available. Financial award applicants required to submit FAFSA. *Faculty research:* Quality of life, transcultural nursing issues, teaching/learning strategies, clinical simulation. *Unit head:* Dr. Pamela Lindsey, Director, 217-424-6348, Fax: 217-420-6731, E-mail: plindsey@millikin.edu. *Application contact:* Bonnie Niemeyer, Administrative Assistant, 800-373-7733 Ext. 5034, Fax: 217-420-6677, E-mail: bniemeyer@millikin.edu.
Website: http://www.millikin.edu/grad-nursing

Minnesota State University Mankato, College of Graduate Studies and Research, College of Allied Health and Nursing, School of Nursing, Mankato, MN 56001. Offers family nursing (MSN), including family nurse practitioner; nursing (DNP). MSN offered jointly with Metropolitan State University; DNP with Metropolitan State University, Minnesota State University Moorhead, Winona State University. *Accreditation:* AACN. *Degree requirements:* For master's, comprehensive exam, internships, research project or thesis; for doctorate, capstone project. *Entrance requirements:* For master's, GRE General Test or on-campus essay, minimum GPA of 3.0 during previous 2 years, BSN or equivalent references; for doctorate, master's degree in nursing. Additional exam requirements/recommendations for international students: Required—TOEFL. Electronic applications accepted. *Faculty research:* Psychosocial nursing, computers in nursing, family adaptation.

Minnesota State University Moorhead, Graduate Studies, College of Science, Health and the Environment, Moorhead, MN 56563. Offers healthcare administration (MHA); nursing (MS); school psychology (MS, Psy S). *Program availability:* Part-time, evening/weekend, 100% online, blended/hybrid learning. *Application deadline:* Applications are processed on a rolling basis. Application fee: $20. Electronic applications accepted. *Expenses:* Tuition, state resident: full-time $9000; part-time $4500 per credit. Tuition, nonresident: full-time $18,000; part-time $9000 per credit. *Required fees:* $942; $39.25 per credit. One-time fee: $90 full-time. Full-time tuition and fees vary according to course load, degree level, program and reciprocity agreements. *Financial support:* Research assistantships, career-related internships or fieldwork, Federal Work-Study, and unspecified assistantships available. Financial award application deadline: 7/15; financial award applicants required to submit FAFSA. *Unit head:* Jeffrey Bodwin, Acting Dean, 218-477-5892, E-mail: bodwin@mnstate.edu. *Application contact:* Karla Wenger, Graduate Studies Office, 218-477-2344, Fax: 218-477-2482, E-mail: wengerk@mnstate.edu.
Website: http://www.mnstate.edu/cshe/

Misericordia University, College of Health Sciences, Department of Nursing, Dallas, PA 18612. Offers MSN, DNP. *Accreditation:* AACN. *Program availability:* Part-time, evening/weekend, online learning. *Faculty:* 6 full-time (all women), 1 (woman) part-time/adjunct. *Students:* 64 part-time (60 women); includes 2 minority (1 Hispanic/Latino; 1 Two or more races, non-Hispanic/Latino). Average age 33. In 2015, 13 master's awarded. *Degree requirements:* For master's, thesis optional, practicum. *Entrance requirements:* For master's, interview, minimum GPA of 3.0; for doctorate, official transcripts of all previous college work, MSN from CCNE- or NLN-accredited institution, copy of unencumbered RN license, license to practice as an advanced practice nurse, minimum graduate GPA of 3.0, two letters of reference, 500-word statement/writing sample of personal and professional goals, telephone interview. Additional exam

Nursing—General

requirements/recommendations for international students: Required—TOEFL. *Application deadline:* For fall admission, 8/7 priority date for domestic students; for spring admission, 1/3 for domestic students. Applications are processed on a rolling basis. Application fee: $35. Electronic applications accepted. *Expenses:* Contact institution. *Financial support:* In 2015–16, 28 students received support. Career-related internships or fieldwork and scholarships/grants available. Support available to part-time students. Financial award application deadline: 6/30; financial award applicants required to submit FAFSA. *Faculty research:* Quality of life, maternal-child, spirituality, critical thinking, adult health. *Unit head:* Dr. Brenda Hage, Coordinator of Graduate Nursing, 570-674-6760, E-mail: bhage@misericordia.edu. *Application contact:* Maureen Sheridan, Assistant Director of Admissions, Part-Time Undergraduate and Graduate Programs, 570-674-6451, Fax: 570-674-6232, E-mail: msherida@misericordia.edu. Website: http://www.misericordia.edu/page.cfm?p-1253

Mississippi University for Women, Graduate School, College of Nursing and Speech Language Pathology, Columbus, MS 39701-9998. Offers nursing (MSN, PMC); speech-language pathology (MS). *Accreditation:* AACN. *Program availability:* Part-time. *Degree requirements:* For master's, comprehensive exam, thesis. *Entrance requirements:* For master's, GRE General Test, bachelor's degree in nursing, previous course work in statistics, proficiency in English.

Missouri Southern State University, Program in Nursing, Joplin, MO 64801-1595. Offers MSN. Program offered jointly with University of Missouri–Kansas City. *Accreditation:* AACN. *Program availability:* Part-time. *Entrance requirements:* For master's, minimum cumulative GPA of 3.2 for the last 60 hours of the BSN program, resume, RN licensure, CPR certification, course work in statistics and health assessment. Electronic applications accepted.

Missouri State University, Graduate College, College of Health and Human Services, Department of Nursing, Springfield, MO 65897. Offers nursing (MSN), including family nurse practitioner, nurse educator; nursing practice (DNP). *Accreditation:* AACN. *Program availability:* 100% online, blended/hybrid learning. *Faculty:* 9 full-time (all women), 16 part-time/adjunct (13 women). *Students:* 27 full-time (23 women), 23 part-time (all women); includes 8 minority (3 Black or African American, non-Hispanic/Latino; 1 American Indian or Alaska Native, non-Hispanic/Latino; 2 Asian, non-Hispanic/Latino; 2 Two or more races, non-Hispanic/Latino). Average age 35. 13 applicants, 46% accepted, 1 enrolled. In 2015, 1 master's, 1 doctorate awarded. *Degree requirements:* For master's, comprehensive exam, thesis or alternative. *Entrance requirements:* For master's, GRE General Test, minimum GPA of 3.0, RN license (for MSN), 1 year of work experience (for MPH). Additional exam requirements/recommendations for international students: Required—TOEFL (minimum score 550 paper-based; 79 iBT), IELTS (minimum score 6). *Application deadline:* For fall admission, 12/1 priority date for domestic students, 5/1 for international students. Applications are processed on a rolling basis. Application fee: $35 ($50 for international students). Electronic applications accepted. *Expenses:* Tuition, state resident: full-time $5500. Tuition, nonresident: full-time $10,108. *Required fees:* $1000. *Financial support:* In 2015–16, 2 teaching assistantships with partial tuition reimbursements (averaging $8,600 per year) were awarded; Federal Work-Study, institutionally sponsored loans, scholarships/grants, and unspecified assistantships also available. Financial award application deadline: 3/31; financial award applicants required to submit FAFSA. *Faculty research:* Preconceptual health, women's health, nursing satisfaction, nursing education. *Unit head:* Dr. Kathryn Hope, Head, 417-836-5310, Fax: 417-836-5484, E-mail: nursing@missouristate.edu. *Application contact:* Michael Edwards, Coordinator of Graduate Admissions, 417-836-5330, Fax: 417-836-6200, E-mail: michaeledwards@missouristate.edu. Website: http://www.missouristate.edu/nursing/

Missouri Western State University, Program in Nursing, St. Joseph, MO 64507-2294. Offers health care leadership (MSN); nurse educator (MSN, Graduate Certificate). *Program availability:* Part-time. *Students:* 31 part-time (30 women). Average age 34. 17 applicants, 100% accepted, 14 enrolled. In 2015, 2 master's awarded. *Entrance requirements:* For master's, minimum GPA of 2.75, interview. Additional exam requirements/recommendations for international students: Recommended—TOEFL (minimum score 79 iBT), IELTS (minimum score 6). *Application deadline:* For fall admission, 7/15 for domestic and international students; for spring admission, 11/1 for domestic students, 10/15 for international students; for summer admission, 4/29 for domestic students. Applications are processed on a rolling basis. Application fee: $45 ($50 for international students). Electronic applications accepted. *Expenses:* Tuition, state resident: full-time $6290; part-time $314 per credit hour. Tuition, nonresident: full-time $11,490; part-time $574 per credit hour. *Required fees:* $542; $99 per credit hour. $176 per semester. One-time fee: $45. Tuition and fees vary according to course load and program. *Financial support:* Scholarships/grants and unspecified assistantships available. Support available to part-time students. *Unit head:* Dr. Carolyn Brose, Associate Professor, 816-271-5912, E-mail: brose@missouriwestern.edu. *Application contact:* Dr. Benjamin D. Caldwell, Dean of the Graduate School, 816-271-4394, Fax: 816-271-4525, E-mail: graduate@missouriwestern.edu. Website: https://www.missouriwestern.edu/nursing/master-of-science-in-nursing/

Molloy College, Division of Nursing, Rockville Centre, NY 11571-5002. Offers adult-gerontology primary care nurse practitioner (MS); clinical nurse specialist (MS), including adult-gerontology health; clinical nurse specialist: adult-gerontology (Advanced Certificate), including adult-gerontology; family nurse practitioner (MS, Advanced Certificate), including primary care; family psychiatric mental health nurse practitioner (MS); nursing (DNP, PhD); nursing administration (MS), including informatics; nursing education (MS); pediatric nurse practitioner (MS), including primary care (MS, Advanced Certificate). *Accreditation:* AACN. *Program availability:* Part-time, evening/weekend. *Faculty:* 26 full-time (all women), 12 part-time/adjunct (9 women). *Students:* 13 full-time (all women), 550 part-time (515 women); includes 316 minority (169 Black or African American, non-Hispanic/Latino; 1 American Indian or Alaska Native, non-Hispanic/Latino; 88 Asian, non-Hispanic/Latino; 56 Hispanic/Latino; 2 Native Hawaiian or other Pacific Islander, non-Hispanic/Latino). Average age 43. 208 applicants, 69% accepted, 121 enrolled. In 2015, 116 master's, 1 doctorate, 6 other advanced degrees awarded. *Degree requirements:* For master's, thesis optional. *Entrance requirements:* For master's, 3 letters of reference, BS in nursing, minimum undergraduate GPA of 3.0; for Advanced Certificate, 3 letters of reference, master's degree in nursing. Additional exam requirements/recommendations for international students: Required—TOEFL (minimum score 550 paper-based; 79 iBT). *Application deadline:* For fall admission, 9/2 priority date for domestic students; for spring admission, 1/20 priority date for domestic students. Applications are processed on a rolling basis. Application fee: $60. Electronic applications accepted. *Expenses: Tuition, area resident:* Full-time $18,450; part-time $1025 per credit. *Required fees:* $900; $740 per unit. Tuition and fees vary according to course load. *Financial support:* Research assistantships with partial tuition reimbursements, teaching assistantships with partial tuition reimbursements, institutionally sponsored loans, scholarships/grants, and unspecified assistantships available. Support available to part-time students. Financial award application deadline: 4/1; financial award applicants required to submit FAFSA. *Unit head:* Dr. Jeannine Muldoon, Dean of Nursing, 516-323-3651, E-mail: jmuldoon@molloy.edu. *Application contact:* Jaclyn Machowicz, Assistant Director for Admissions, 516-323-4010, E-mail: jmachowicz@molloy.edu.

Monmouth University, Graduate Studies, The Marjorie K. Unterberg School of Nursing and Health Studies, West Long Branch, NJ 07764-1898. Offers adult and gerontological primary care nurse practitioner (MSN); adult-gerontological primary care nurse practitioner (Post-Master's Certificate); family nurse practitioner (MSN, Post-Master's Certificate); family psychiatric and mental health advanced practice nursing (MSN); family psychiatric and mental health nurse practitioner (Post-Master's Certificate); forensic nursing (MSN, Certificate); nursing (MSN); nursing administration (MSN, Post-Master's Certificate); nursing education (MSN, Post-Master's Certificate); nursing practice (DNP); physician assistant (MS); school nursing (MSN, Certificate). *Accreditation:* AACN. *Program availability:* Part-time, evening/weekend, 100% online, blended/hybrid learning. *Faculty:* 14 full-time (13 women), 10 part-time/adjunct (5 women). *Students:* 58 full-time (46 women), 271 part-time (252 women); includes 93 minority (31 Black or African American, non-Hispanic/Latino; 40 Asian, non-Hispanic/Latino; 18 Hispanic/Latino; 1 Native Hawaiian or other Pacific Islander, non-Hispanic/Latino; 3 Two or more races, non-Hispanic/Latino), 1 international. Average age 37. 450 applicants, 32% accepted, 103 enrolled. In 2015, 68 master's, 8 doctorates, 11 other advanced degrees awarded. *Degree requirements:* For master's, practicum (for some tracks); for doctorate, practicum, capstone course. *Entrance requirements:* For master's, GRE General Test (waived for MSN applicants with minimum B grade in each of the first four courses and for MS applicants with master's degree), BSN with minimum GPA of 2.75, current RN license, proof of liability and malpractice policy, personal statement, two letters of recommendation, college course work in health assessment, resume; CASPA application (for MS); for doctorate, accredited master's nursing program degree with minimum GPA of 3.2, graduate research course in statistics, active RN license, national certification as Nurse Practitioner or Nurse Administrator, working knowledge of statistics, statement of goals and vision for change, 2 letters of recommendation (professional or academic), resume, interview. Additional exam requirements/recommendations for international students: Required—TOEFL (minimum score 550 paper-based; 79 iBT), IELTS (minimum score 6) or Michigan English Language Assessment Battery (minimum score 77). *Application deadline:* For fall admission, 7/15 priority date for domestic students, 6/1 for international students; for spring admission, 12/15 priority date for domestic students, 11/1 for international students; for summer admission, 5/1 for domestic students. Applications are processed on a rolling basis. Application fee: $50. Electronic applications accepted. *Expenses:* Contact institution. *Financial support:* In 2015–16, 241 students received support, including 220 fellowships (averaging $3,403 per year), 5 research assistantships (averaging $5,146 per year); career-related internships or fieldwork, scholarships/grants, and unspecified assistantships also available. Support available to part-time students. Financial award applicants required to submit FAFSA. *Faculty research:* School nursing, health policy, and smoking cessation in teens, Multiple Sclerosis; adherence and self-efficacy, aging issues and geriatric care. *Unit head:* Dr. Janet Mahoney, Dean, 732-571-3443, Fax: 732-263-5131, E-mail: jmahoney@monmouth.edu. *Application contact:* Lucia Fedele, Graduate Admission Counselor, 732-571-3452, Fax: 732-263-5123, E-mail: gradadm@monmouth.edu. Website: http://www.monmouth.edu/school-of-nursing-health/graduate-nursing-programs.aspx

Moravian College, Moravian College Comenius Center, St. Luke's School of Nursing, Bethlehem, PA 18018-6650. Offers clinical nurse leader (MS); nurse administrator (MS); nurse educator (MS). *Accreditation:* AACN. *Program availability:* Part-time, evening/weekend. *Degree requirements:* For master's, comprehensive exam (for some programs), evidence-based practice project. *Entrance requirements:* For master's, GRE or MAT. Additional exam requirements/recommendations for international students: Required—TOEFL (minimum score 550 paper-based; 90 iBT).

Morgan State University, School of Graduate Studies, School of Community Health and Policy, Program in Nursing, Baltimore, MD 21251. Offers MS.

Mount Carmel College of Nursing, Nursing Program, Columbus, OH 43222. Offers adult gerontology acute care nurse practitioner (MS); adult health clinical nurse specialist (MS); family nurse practitioner (MS); nursing (DNP); nursing administration (MS); nursing education (MS). *Accreditation:* AACN. *Program availability:* Part-time. *Faculty:* 8 full-time (all women), 5 part-time/adjunct (4 women). *Students:* 72 full-time (63 women), 92 part-time (84 women); includes 15 minority (7 Black or African American, non-Hispanic/Latino; 3 Asian, non-Hispanic/Latino; 2 Hispanic/Latino; 3 Two or more races, non-Hispanic/Latino). Average age 37. 140 applicants, 45% accepted, 50 enrolled. In 2015, 50 master's awarded. *Degree requirements:* For master's, professional manuscript; for doctorate, practicum. *Entrance requirements:* For master's, letters of recommendation, statement of purpose, current resume, baccalaureate degree in nursing, current Ohio RN license, minimum cumulative GPA of 3.0; for doctorate, master's degree in nursing from program accredited by either NLNAC/ACEN or CCNE. Additional exam requirements/recommendations for international students: Required—TOEFL (minimum score 550 paper-based; 80 iBT). *Application deadline:* For fall admission, 6/1 priority date for domestic students; for winter admission, 11/1 for domestic students; for spring admission, 10/1 priority date for domestic students; for summer admission, 3/1 for domestic students. Applications are processed on a rolling basis. Application fee: $30. *Expenses: Tuition, area resident:* Full-time $9480; part-time $474 per credit. One-time fee: $120. Tuition and fees vary according to course load, degree level and program. *Financial support:* In 2015–16, 5 students received support. Institutionally sponsored loans and scholarships/grants available. Financial award applicants required to submit FAFSA. *Unit head:* Dr. Jill Kilanowski, 614-234-5237, Fax: 614-234-2875, E-mail: jkilanowski@mccn.edu. *Application contact:* Dr. Kim Campbell, Director of Recruitment and Admissions, 614-234-5144, Fax: 614-234-5427, E-mail: kcampbell@mccn.edu. Website: http://www.mccn.edu/

Mount Marty College, Graduate Studies Division, Yankton, SD 57078-3724. Offers business administration (MBA); nurse anesthesia (MS); nursing (MSN); pastoral ministries (MPM). *Accreditation:* AANA/CANAEP (one or more programs are accredited). *Degree requirements:* For master's, thesis or alternative. *Entrance requirements:* For master's, GRE General Test, minimum GPA of 3.0. Electronic applications accepted. *Faculty research:* Clinical anesthesia, professional characteristics, motivations of applicants.

Mount Mercy University, Program in Nursing, Cedar Rapids, IA 52402-4797. Offers health advocacy (MSN); nurse administration (MSN); nurse education (MSN). *Program availability:* Evening/weekend. *Degree requirements:* For master's, project/practicum.

Mount St. Joseph University, Doctor of Nursing Practice Program, Cincinnati, OH 45233-1670. Offers health systems leadership (DNP). *Program availability:* Part-time. *Faculty:* 12 full-time (11 women), 5 part-time/adjunct (all women). *Students:* Average age 51. *Entrance requirements:* For doctorate, essay; MSN from regionally-accredited university; minimum graduate GPA of 3.5; professional resume; three professional references; interview; 2 years of clinical nursing experience; active RN license; criminal background check; minimum C grade in an undergraduate statistics course; official documentation of practicum. Additional exam requirements/recommendations for international students: Required—TOEFL (minimum score 560 paper-based; 83 iBT). Application fee: $50. Electronic applications accepted. *Expenses:* Contact institution. *Financial support:* Applicants required to submit FAFSA. *Unit head:* Dr. Nancy

Hinzman, Director, 513-244-4325, E-mail: nancy.hinzman@msj.edu. *Application contact:* Mary Brigham, Assistant Director for Graduate Recruitment, 513-244-4233, Fax: 513-244-4629, E-mail: mary.brigham@msj.edu. Website: http://www.msj.edu/academics/graduate-programs/doctor-of-nursing-practice/

Mount St. Joseph University, Master of Science in Nursing Program, Cincinnati, OH 45233-1670. Offers administration (MSN); clinical nurse leader (MSN); education (MSN). *Program availability:* Part-time. *Faculty:* 12 full-time (11 women), 5 part-time/adjunct (all women). *Students:* 53 full-time (all women), 2 part-time (both women); includes 4 minority (all Black or African American, non-Hispanic/Latino). Average age 44. 148 applicants, 68% accepted, 58 enrolled. In 2015, 65 master's awarded. *Entrance requirements:* For master's, essay; BSN from regionally-accredited university; minimum undergraduate GPA of 3.25 or GRE; professional resume; three professional references; interview; 2 years of clinical nursing experience; active RN license; criminal background check. Additional exam requirements/recommendations for international students: Required—TOEFL (minimum score 560 paper-based; 83 iBT). Application fee: $50. Electronic applications accepted. *Expenses:* Tuition, area resident: Full-time $15,255; part-time $565 per credit hour. *Required fees:* $500; $100 per term. $100 per semester. Full-time tuition and fees vary according to course load, degree level and program. *Financial support:* In 2015–16, 3 students received support. Application deadline: 3/1; applicants required to submit FAFSA. *Unit head:* Dr. Nancy Hinzman, MSN/DNP Director, 513-244-4325, E-mail: nancy.hinzman@msj.edu. *Application contact:* Mary Brigham, Assistant Director for Graduate Recruitment, 513-244-4233, Fax: 513-244-4629, E-mail: mary.brigham@msj.edu. Website: http://www.msj.edu/academics/graduate-programs/master-of-science-in-nursing/

Mount St. Joseph University, Master's Graduate Entry-Level into Nursing (MAGELIN) Program, Cincinnati, OH 45233-1670. Offers MSN. *Accreditation:* AACN. *Faculty:* 11 full-time (all women), 5 part-time/adjunct (4 women). *Students:* 96 full-time (78 women), 1 (woman) part-time; includes 19 minority (13 Black or African American, non-Hispanic/Latino; 3 Asian, non-Hispanic/Latino; 3 Two or more races, non-Hispanic/Latino). Average age 23. 36 applicants, 111% accepted, 34 enrolled. In 2015, 61 master's awarded. *Degree requirements:* For master's, evidence-based project, preceptorship. *Entrance requirements:* For master's, GRE or minimum GPA of 3.0, interview; course work in chemistry, anatomy, physiology, microbiology, psychology, sociology, statistics, life span development, and nutrition; non-nursing bachelor's degree; statement of goals; transcripts; criminal background check. Additional exam requirements/recommendations for international students: Required—TOEFL (minimum score 560 paper-based; 83 iBT). *Application deadline:* Applications are processed on a rolling basis. Application fee: $50. Electronic applications accepted. *Expenses:* Contact institution. *Financial support:* In 2015–16, 6 students received support. Scholarships/grants available. Financial award application deadline: 3/1; financial award applicants required to submit FAFSA. *Faculty research:* Utilizing technology in learning, assessment of student learning, critical thinking, women's health and nursing education. *Unit head:* Mary Kishman, Program Director, 513-244-4726, Fax: 513-441-2547, E-mail: mary.kishman@msj.edu. *Application contact:* Mary Brigham, Assistant Director of Graduate Recruitment, 513-244-4233, Fax: 513-244-4629, E-mail: mary.brigham@msj.edu. Website: http://www.msj.edu/academics/graduate-programs/magelin-masters-graduate-entry-level-into-nursing/

Mount Saint Mary College, School of Nursing, Newburgh, NY 12550-3494. Offers adult nurse practitioner (MS, Advanced Certificate), including nursing education (MS), nursing management (MS); clinical nurse specialist-adult health (MS), including nursing education, nursing management; family nurse practitioner (Advanced Certificate). *Accreditation:* AACN. *Program availability:* Part-time, evening/weekend, blended/hybrid learning. *Faculty:* 6 full-time (all women), 1 (woman) part-time/adjunct. *Students:* 5 full-time (4 women), 117 part-time (105 women); includes 42 minority (18 Black or African American, non-Hispanic/Latino; 2 American Indian or Alaska Native, non-Hispanic/Latino; 8 Asian, non-Hispanic/Latino; 12 Hispanic/Latino; 2 Native Hawaiian or other Pacific Islander, non-Hispanic/Latino). Average age 38. 44 applicants, 84% accepted, 25 enrolled. In 2015, 25 master's, 4 other advanced degrees awarded. *Degree requirements:* For master's, research utilization project. *Entrance requirements:* For master's, BSN, minimum GPA of 3.0, RN license. Additional exam requirements/recommendations for international students: Required—TOEFL (minimum score 80 iBT). *Application deadline:* For fall admission, 6/3 priority date for domestic students; for spring admission, 10/31 priority date for domestic students. Applications are processed on a rolling basis. Application fee: $45. Electronic applications accepted. Application fee is waived when completed online. *Expenses:* Tuition, area resident: Part-time $750 per credit. *Required fees:* $40 per semester. *Financial support:* In 2015–16, 14 students received support. Unspecified assistantships available. Financial award application deadline: 4/15; financial award applicants required to submit FAFSA. *Unit head:* Christine Berte, Graduate Coordinator, 845-569-3141, Fax: 845-562-6762, E-mail: christine.berte@msmc.edu. *Application contact:* Lisa Gallina, Director of Admissions for Graduate Programs and Adult Degree Completion, 845-569-3166, Fax: 845-569-3450, E-mail: lisa.gallina@msmc.edu. Website: http://www.msmc.edu/Academics/Graduate_Programs/Master_of_Science_in_Nursing

Mount Saint Mary's University, Graduate Division, Los Angeles, CA 90049. Offers business administration (MBA); counseling psychology (MS); creative writing (MFA); education (MS, Certificate); film and television (MFA); health policy and management (MS); humanities (MA); nursing (MSN, Certificate); physical therapy (DPT); religious studies (MA). *Program availability:* Part-time, evening/weekend. *Faculty:* 115 full-time, 304 part-time/adjunct. *Students:* 495 full-time (369 women), 149 part-time (121 women); includes 414 minority (73 Black or African American, non-Hispanic/Latino; 4 American Indian or Alaska Native, non-Hispanic/Latino; 60 Asian, non-Hispanic/Latino; 259 Hispanic/Latino; 7 Native Hawaiian or other Pacific Islander, non-Hispanic/Latino; 11 Two or more races, non-Hispanic/Latino; 4 international. Average age 33. 1,398 applicants, 21% accepted, 242 enrolled. In 2015, 172 master's, 26 doctorates, 23 other advanced degrees awarded. *Entrance requirements:* Additional exam requirements/recommendations for international students: Required—TOEFL. *Application deadline:* For fall admission, 6/30 priority date for domestic and international students; for spring admission, 10/30 priority date for domestic and international students; for summer admission, 3/30 priority date for domestic and international students. Applications are processed on a rolling basis. Application fee: $50. Electronic applications accepted. One-time fee: $135. Tuition and fees vary according to degree level. *Financial support:* Career-related internships or fieldwork, Federal Work-Study, institutionally sponsored loans, and tuition waivers (full and partial) available. Support available to part-time students. Financial award application deadline: 3/15; financial award applicants required to submit FAFSA. *Unit head:* Dr. Linda Moody, Graduate Dean, 213-477-2800, E-mail: gradprograms@msmu.edu. *Application contact:* Tara Wessel, Assistant Director, Graduate Admission, 213-477-2799, E-mail: gradprograms@msmu.edu. Website: http://www.msmu.edu/graduate-programs/

Murray State University, College of Health Sciences and Human Services, Program in Nursing, Murray, KY 42071. Offers clinical nurse specialist (MSN); family nurse practitioner (MSN); nurse anesthesia (MSN). *Accreditation:* AACN; AANA/CANAEP. *Degree requirements:* For master's, research project. *Entrance requirements:* For master's, GRE General Test, BSN, interview, RN licensure. Additional exam requirements/recommendations for international students: Required—TOEFL (minimum score 550 paper-based). *Faculty research:* Fibromyalgis, primary care, rural health.

National University, Academic Affairs, School of Health and Human Services, La Jolla, CA 92037-1011. Offers clinical affairs (MS); clinical informatics (Certificate); clinical regulatory affairs (MS); health and life science analytics (MS); health coaching (Certificate); health informatics (MS); healthcare administration (MHA); nurse anesthesia (MS); nursing (MS), including forensic nursing, nursing administration, nursing informatics; nursing administration (Certificate); nursing informatics (Certificate); nursing practice (DNP); public health (MPH), including health promotion, healthcare administration, mental health. *Program availability:* Part-time, evening/weekend, 100% online, blended/hybrid learning. *Faculty:* 31 full-time (18 women), 33 part-time/adjunct (20 women). *Students:* 353 full-time (263 women), 136 part-time (87 women); includes 322 minority (111 Black or African American, non-Hispanic/Latino; 1 American Indian or Alaska Native, non-Hispanic/Latino; 105 Asian, non-Hispanic/Latino; 72 Hispanic/Latino; 7 Native Hawaiian or other Pacific Islander, non-Hispanic/Latino; 26 Two or more races, non-Hispanic/Latino), 31 international. Average age 32. In 2015, 103 master's awarded. *Degree requirements:* For master's, thesis (for some programs). *Entrance requirements:* For master's, interview, minimum GPA of 2.5. Additional exam requirements/recommendations for international students: Required—TOEFL (minimum score 550 paper-based; 79 iBT), IELTS (minimum score 6). *Application deadline:* Applications are processed on a rolling basis. Application fee: $60 ($65 for international students). Electronic applications accepted. *Financial support:* Career-related internships or fieldwork, institutionally sponsored loans, scholarships/grants, and tuition waivers (partial) available. Support available to part-time students. Financial award application deadline: 6/30; financial award applicants required to submit FAFSA. *Faculty research:* Nursing education, obesity prevention, workforce diversity. *Unit head:* School of Health and Human Services, 800-628-8648, E-mail: shhs@nu.edu. *Application contact:* Frank Rojas, Vice President for Enrollment Services, 800-628-8648, E-mail: advisor@nu.edu. Website: http://www.nu.edu/OurPrograms/SchoolOfHealthAndHumanServices.html

Nebraska Methodist College, Program in Nursing, Omaha, NE 68114. Offers nurse educator (MSN); nurse executive (MSN). *Accreditation:* AACN. *Program availability:* Evening/weekend, online learning. *Degree requirements:* For master's, thesis or alternative, Evidence Based Practice (EBP) project. *Entrance requirements:* For master's, interview. Additional exam requirements/recommendations for international students: Required—TOEFL (minimum score 550 paper-based; 80 iBT). *Faculty research:* Spirituality, student outcomes, service-learning, leadership and administration, women's issues.

Nebraska Wesleyan University, University College, Program in Nursing, Lincoln, NE 68504-2796. Offers MSN. *Accreditation:* ACEN. *Program availability:* Part-time.

Neumann University, Program in Nursing, Aston, PA 19014. Offers adult-gerontology nurse practitioner (MS); nurse educator (MS). *Accreditation:* ACEN. *Program availability:* Part-time. *Students:* 18 part-time. *Entrance requirements:* For master's, GRE or MAT. Additional exam requirements/recommendations for international students: Required—TOEFL. *Application deadline:* Applications are processed on a rolling basis. Application fee: $50. *Expenses:* Contact institution. *Financial support:* Available to part-time students. Application deadline: 3/15; applicants required to submit FAFSA. *Unit head:* Dr. Kathleen Hoover, Dean, Division of Nursing and Health Sciences, 610-558-5560, Fax: 610-459-1370, E-mail: hooverk@neumann.edu. *Application contact:* Kittie D. Pain, Associate Director, Graduate and Adult Admissions, 610-558-5613, Fax: 610-558-5652, E-mail: paink@neumann.edu.

New Mexico State University, College of Health and Social Services, School of Nursing, Las Cruces, NM 88003. Offers adult/geriatric nursing (DNP); family nurse practitioner (DNP); family/psychiatric mental health nursing (DNP); nursing administration (MSN); nursing science (PhD); public/community health nursing (DNP). *Accreditation:* AACN. *Program availability:* Blended/hybrid learning. *Faculty:* 16 full-time (15 women). *Students:* 24 full-time (18 women), 90 part-time (80 women); includes 49 minority (10 Black or African American, non-Hispanic/Latino; 1 American Indian or Alaska Native, non-Hispanic/Latino; 4 Asian, non-Hispanic/Latino; 32 Hispanic/Latino; 2 Two or more races, non-Hispanic/Latino), 1 international. Average age 43. 40 applicants, 58% accepted, 17 enrolled. In 2015, 6 master's, 11 doctorates awarded. *Degree requirements:* For master's, comprehensive exam, thesis optional, clinical practice; for doctorate, comprehensive exam, thesis/dissertation. *Entrance requirements:* For master's, NCLEX, BSN, minimum GPA of 3.0, course work in statistics, 3 letters of reference, writing sample, RN license, CPR certification, proof of liability, immunizations, criminal background check; for doctorate, NCLEX, MSN, minimum GPA of 3.0, 3 letters of reference, writing sample, RN license, CPR certification, proof of liability, immunizations, criminal background check, statistics course. Additional exam requirements/recommendations for international students: Required—TOEFL (minimum score 550 paper-based; 79 iBT), IELTS (minimum score 6.5). *Application deadline:* For fall admission, 1/15 for domestic students; for spring admission, 1/15 priority date for domestic students; for summer admission, 1/15 for domestic students. Application fee: $40 ($50 for international students). Electronic applications accepted. *Expenses:* $274.50 per credit hour for in-state students, and all students enrolled in six or fewer credits; $839.30 per credit hour for out-of-state and international students enrolled in at least seven hours. *Financial support:* In 2015–16, 23 students received support, including 1 teaching assistantship (averaging $9,473 per year); career-related internships or fieldwork, Federal Work-Study, scholarships/grants, traineeships, health care benefits, and unspecified assistantships also available. Support available to part-time students. Financial award application deadline: 3/1. *Faculty research:* Women's health, community health, health disparities, nursing informatics and health care technologies, health care and nursing administration. *Total annual research expenditures:* $127,778. *Unit head:* Dr. Kathleen Huttlinger, Department Head, 575-646-3812, Fax: 575-646-2167, E-mail: khuttlin@nmsu.edu. *Application contact:* Dr. Teresa Keller, Director of Graduate Studies, 575-646-4370, Fax: 575-646-2167, E-mail: tkeller@nmsu.edu. Website: http://schoolofnursing.nmsu.edu

New York University, Rory Meyers College of Nursing, Doctor of Nursing Practice Program, New York, NY 10012-1019. Offers nursing (DNP), including adult acute care, adult primary care, family, mental health nursing, nurse-midwifery, pediatrics. *Program availability:* Part-time, evening/weekend. *Faculty:* 14 full-time (13 women). *Students:* 2 full-time (both women), 32 part-time (27 women); includes 8 minority (3 Black or African American, non-Hispanic/Latino; 4 Asian, non-Hispanic/Latino; 1 Hispanic/Latino), 1 international. Average age 40. 47 applicants, 51% accepted, 16 enrolled. In 2015, 17 doctorates awarded. *Degree requirements:* For doctorate, thesis/dissertation, project. *Entrance requirements:* For doctorate, MAT or GRE (either taken within past 5 years), MS, RN license, interview, Nurse Practitioner Certification, writing sample. Additional exam requirements/recommendations for international students: Required—TOEFL (minimum score 90 iBT), IELTS (minimum score 7). *Application deadline:* For fall admission, 3/1 for domestic and international students. Applications are processed on a rolling basis. Application fee: $80. Electronic applications accepted. *Expenses:* Contact

Nursing—General

institution. *Financial support:* In 2015–16, 12 students received support. Scholarships/grants available. Support available to part-time students. Financial award application deadline: 2/1; financial award applicants required to submit FAFSA. *Faculty research:* Workforce, LGBT, breast cancer, HIV. *Unit head:* Dr. Rona Levin, Director, 212-998-5319, Fax: 212-995-3143, E-mail: rfl2039@nyu.edu. *Application contact:* Samantha Jaser, Assistant Director, Graduate Student Affairs and Admissions, 212-992-7653, Fax: 212-995-4302, E-mail: saj283@nyu.edu.

New York University, Rory Meyers College of Nursing, Doctor of Philosophy in Nursing Program, New York, NY 10012-1019. Offers research and theory development in nursing science (PhD). *Program availability:* Part-time. *Faculty:* 29 full-time (27 women). *Students:* 5 full-time (all women), 32 part-time (26 women); includes 11 minority (2 Black or African American, non-Hispanic/Latino; 5 Asian, non-Hispanic/Latino; 4 Hispanic/Latino), 5 international. Average age 40. 24 applicants, 50% accepted, 7 enrolled. In 2015, 2 doctorates awarded. *Degree requirements:* For doctorate, thesis/dissertation, candidacy exam. *Entrance requirements:* For doctorate, GRE General Test, interview. Additional exam requirements/recommendations for international students: Required—TOEFL (minimum score 90 iBT), IELTS (minimum score 7). *Application deadline:* For fall admission, 1/15 for domestic and international students. Applications are processed on a rolling basis. Application fee: $80. Electronic applications accepted. *Expenses:* Contact institution. *Financial support:* In 2015–16, 13 students received support, including 8 research assistantships with full tuition reimbursements available (averaging $26,330 per year); scholarships/grants also available. Support available to part-time students. Financial award application deadline: 2/1; financial award applicants required to submit FAFSA. *Faculty research:* Geriatrics, infectious diseases/global public health, chronic disease prevention and management, nursing workforce, technology. *Unit head:* Dr. Deborah Chyun, Executive Associate Dean, 212-998-5264, E-mail: dc116@nyu.edu. *Application contact:* Samantha Jaser, Assistant Director, Graduate Student Affairs and Admissions, 212-992-7653, Fax: 212-995-4302, E-mail: saj283@nyu.edu.

New York University, Rory Meyers College of Nursing, Programs in Advanced Practice Nursing, New York, NY 10012-1019. Offers adult-gerontology acute care nurse practitioner (MS, Advanced Certificate); adult-gerontology primary care nurse practitioner (MS, Advanced Certificate); family nurse practitioner (MS, Advanced Certificate); gerontology nurse practitioner (Advanced Certificate); nurse-midwifery (MS, Advanced Certificate); nursing administration (MS, Advanced Certificate); nursing education (MS, Advanced Certificate); nursing informatics (MS, Advanced Certificate); pediatrics nurse practitioner (MS, Advanced Certificate); psychiatric-mental health nurse practitioner (MS, Advanced Certificate); MS/MPH. *Accreditation:* AACN; ACNM/ACME. *Program availability:* Part-time. *Faculty:* 24 full-time (all women), 76 part-time/adjunct (65 women). *Students:* 46 full-time (26 women), 586 part-time (513 women); includes 242 minority (68 Black or African American, non-Hispanic/Latino; 3 American Indian or Alaska Native, non-Hispanic/Latino; 117 Asian, non-Hispanic/Latino; 38 Hispanic/Latino; 3 Native Hawaiian or other Pacific Islander, non-Hispanic/Latino; 13 Two or more races, non-Hispanic/Latino), 23 international. Average age 32. 402 applicants, 69% accepted, 138 enrolled. In 2015, 198 master's, 5 other advanced degrees awarded. *Degree requirements:* For master's, thesis (for some programs). *Entrance requirements:* For master's, BS in nursing, AS in nursing with another BS/BA, interview, RN license, 1 year of clinical experience (3 for the MS in nursing education program); for Advanced Certificate, master's degree. Additional exam requirements/recommendations for international students: Required—TOEFL (minimum score 90 iBT), IELTS (minimum score 7). *Application deadline:* For fall admission, 6/15 for domestic and international students; for spring admission, 12/1 for domestic and international students; for summer admission, 3/1 for domestic and international students. Application fee: $80. Electronic applications accepted. *Expenses:* Contact institution. *Financial support:* In 2015–16, 101 students received support. Career-related internships or fieldwork, Federal Work-Study, and scholarships/grants available. Support available to part-time students. Financial award application deadline: 3/1; financial award applicants required to submit FAFSA. *Faculty research:* Geriatrics, HIV, families and illness, oral systemic connection, symptom management. *Unit head:* Dr. James Pace, Senior Associate Dean for Academic Programs, 212-992-7343, E-mail: james.pace@nyu.edu. *Application contact:* Samantha Jaser, Assistant Director, Graduate Student Affairs and Admissions, 212-992-7653, Fax: 212-995-4302, E-mail: saj283@nyu.edu.

Nicholls State University, Graduate Studies, College of Nursing and Allied Health, Thibodaux, LA 70310. Offers family nurse practitioner (MSN); nurse executive (MSN); nursing education (MSN); psychiatric/mental health nurse practitioner (MSN). Website: http://www.nicholls.edu/cona/

North Dakota State University, College of Graduate and Interdisciplinary Studies, College of Health Professions, School of Nursing, Fargo, ND 58102. Offers MS, DNP. *Accreditation:* AACN. *Program availability:* Part-time, online learning. *Faculty:* 8 full-time, 2 part-time/adjunct. *Degree requirements:* For master's, thesis or alternative, oral defense; for doctorate, thesis/dissertation or alternative, oral defense. *Entrance requirements:* For master's, bachelor's degree with nursing major, minimum GPA of 3.0 in nursing courses, RN license; for doctorate, bachelor's or master's degree with a nursing major, minimum GPA of 3.0 in nursing courses, RN license. Additional exam requirements/recommendations for international students: Required—TOEFL, IELTS. *Application deadline:* For fall admission, 5/1 priority date for domestic students; for spring admission, 11/1 priority date for domestic students. Applications are processed on a rolling basis. Application fee: $35. Electronic applications accepted. *Expenses:* Contact institution. *Financial support:* Research assistantships with full tuition reimbursements, teaching assistantships with full tuition reimbursements, traineeships, and unspecified assistantships available. Financial award application deadline: 8/15; financial award applicants required to submit CSS PROFILE or FAFSA. *Faculty research:* Prevention of farmers' hearing loss, breast cancer in Native American women, colon cancer, quality improvement in a wellness center. *Unit head:* Dr. Carla Gross, Chair, 701-231-7772, Fax: 701-231-7606, E-mail: carla.gross@ndsu.edu. *Application contact:* Dr. Carla Gross, Chair, 701-231-7772, Fax: 701-231-7606, E-mail: carla.gross@ndsu.edu. Website: http://www.ndsu.edu/nursing/

Northeastern University, Bouvé College of Health Sciences, Boston, MA 02115-5096. Offers applied behavior analysis (MS, CAGS); audiology (Au D); biomedical nanotechnology (MS); college student development and counseling (MS, CAGS); counseling psychology (MS, PhD, CAGS); exercise science (MS); health informatics (MS); medicinal chemistry (MS); nurse anesthesia (DNP, CAGS); nursing (MS, PhD, CAGS), including administration (MS), adult-gerontology acute care nurse practitioner (MS, CAGS), adult-gerontology primary care nurse practitioner (MS, CAGS), anesthesia (MS), family nurse practitioner (MS, CAGS), neonatal nurse practitioner (MS, CAGS), pediatric nurse practitioner (MS, CAGS), psychiatric mental health nurse practitioner (MS, CAGS); nursing practice (DNP); personal health informatics (PhD); pharmaceutical sciences (MS, PhD), including interdisciplinary concentration, pharmaceutics and drug delivery systems; pharmacology (MS); pharmacy (Pharm D); physical therapy (Postbaccalaureate Certificate); physician assistant (MS); population health (PhD); school psychology (MS, PhD, CAGS); speech-language pathology (MS); urban health (MPH); MS/MBA. *Accreditation:* ACPE (one or more programs are accredited). *Program availability:* Part-time, evening/weekend, online learning. *Faculty:* 194 full-time (120

women), 169 part-time/adjunct (136 women). *Students:* 1,416 full-time (1,049 women), 310 part-time (248 women). In 2015, 374 master's, 313 doctorates, 37 other advanced degrees awarded. *Degree requirements:* For doctorate, thesis/dissertation (for some programs); for other advanced degree, comprehensive exam. Application fee: $75. Electronic applications accepted. *Expenses:* Contact institution. *Financial support:* Applicants required to submit FAFSA. *Unit head:* John R. Reynolds, Professor and Interim Dean, 617-373-3323, Fax: 617-373-3030. *Application contact:* Molly Schnabel, Senior Director of Graduate Affairs, 617-373-2708, Fax: 617-373-4701, E-mail: bouvegrad@neu.edu. Website: http://www.northeastern.edu/bouve

Northern Arizona University, Graduate College, College of Health and Human Services, School of Nursing, Flagstaff, AZ 86011. Offers family nurse practitioner (MSN, Certificate); nurse generalist (MSN); nursing practice (DNP). *Accreditation:* AACN. *Program availability:* Part-time. *Degree requirements:* For master's, thesis (for some programs), project or thesis. *Entrance requirements:* For master's, GRE General Test or minimum GPA of 3.0, undergraduate statistics or health assessment with minimum grade of B in last 5 years or 3 years of RN experience (for nursing education). Additional exam requirements/recommendations for international students: Required—TOEFL (minimum score 550 paper-based; 80 iBT), IELTS (minimum score 7). *Application deadline:* For fall admission, 1/15 priority date for domestic and international students. Applications are processed on a rolling basis. Application fee: $65. Electronic applications accepted. *Expenses: Tuition, area resident:* Full-time $8710. *Tuition, nonresident:* full-time $20,350. *Required fees:* $896. *Financial support:* Career-related internships or fieldwork, Federal Work-Study, scholarships/grants, traineeships, health care benefits, tuition waivers, and unspecified assistantships available. Financial award applicants required to submit FAFSA. *Unit head:* Dr. Debera Thomas, Dean, 928-523-2656, Fax: 928-523-7171, E-mail: debera.thomas@nau.edu. *Application contact:* Penny Walior, Student Academic Specialist, 928-523-6770, Fax: 928-523-9155, E-mail: graduatenursing@nau.edu. Website: http://nau.edu/CHHS/Nursing/

Northern Illinois University, Graduate School, College of Health and Human Sciences, School of Nursing and Health Studies, De Kalb, IL 60115-2854. Offers nursing (MS); public health (MPH). *Accreditation:* AACN. *Program availability:* Part-time. *Faculty:* 12 full-time (11 women), 1 (woman) part-time/adjunct. *Students:* 29 full-time (22 women), 200 part-time (179 women); includes 48 minority (12 Black or African American, non-Hispanic/Latino; 21 Asian, non-Hispanic/Latino; 10 Hispanic/Latino; 5 Two or more races, non-Hispanic/Latino), 5 international. Average age 35. 177 applicants, 40% accepted, 36 enrolled. In 2015, 102 master's awarded. *Degree requirements:* For master's, thesis optional, internship. *Entrance requirements:* For master's, minimum GPA of 3.0 in last 60 hours, BA in nursing, nursing license. Additional exam requirements/recommendations for international students: Required—TOEFL (minimum score 550 paper-based). *Application deadline:* For fall admission, 6/1 for domestic students, 5/1 for international students; for spring admission, 11/1 for domestic students, 10/1 for international students. Applications are processed on a rolling basis. Application fee: $40. Electronic applications accepted. *Financial support:* In 2015–16, 1 research assistantship with full tuition reimbursement, 22 teaching assistantships with full tuition reimbursements were awarded; fellowships with full tuition reimbursements, career-related internships or fieldwork, Federal Work-Study, scholarships/grants, tuition waivers (full), and unspecified assistantships also available. Support available to part-time students. Financial award applicants required to submit FAFSA. *Faculty research:* Neonatal intensive care, stress and coping, refugee and immigrant issues, older adults, autoimmune disorders. *Unit head:* Dr. Janice Strom, Chair, 815-753-6550, Fax: 815-753-0814, E-mail: jstrom@niu.edu. *Application contact:* Graduate School Office, 815-753-0395, E-mail: gradsch@niu.edu. Website: http://www.chhs.niu.edu/nursing/

Northern Kentucky University, Office of Graduate Programs, School of Nursing and Health Professions, Online Doctor of Nursing Practice Program, Highland Heights, KY 41099. Offers DNP. *Program availability:* Part-time, online learning. *Degree requirements:* For doctorate, thesis/dissertation. *Entrance requirements:* For doctorate, RN license, master's degree in nursing, minimum GPA of 3.25, course in upper-division statistics, course in informatics, 3 professional recommendations (2 from nurses), resume or curriculum vitae, all official transcripts, graduate paper of intent, interview. Additional exam requirements/recommendations for international students: Required—TOEFL (minimum score 79 iBT); Recommended—IELTS (minimum score 6.5). *Expenses:* Contact institution. *Faculty research:* Pathways to nursing degree, lead poisoning in children, predictors for NCLEX success in BSN and ABSN programs, work-life balance and deans of baccalaureate nursing programs, heart failure self management.

Northern Kentucky University, Office of Graduate Programs, School of Nursing and Health Professions, Program in Nursing, Highland Heights, KY 41099. Offers MSHS, MSN, Certificate, Post-Master's Certificate. *Accreditation:* ACEN. *Program availability:* Part-time, evening/weekend, online learning. *Degree requirements:* For master's, comprehensive exam, thesis optional. *Entrance requirements:* For master's, BS in nursing, letter from employer on letterhead indicating a minimum of 1,000 clinical hours of RN practice, updated resume, letter of purpose, official transcripts, proof of current licensure, minimum GPA of 3.0, two electronic letters of reference, successful completion of elementary statistics. Additional exam requirements/recommendations for international students: Required—TOEFL (minimum score 550 paper-based; 79 iBT); Recommended—IELTS (minimum score 6.5). Electronic applications accepted. *Faculty research:* Career planning for middle school students, technology skills for workforce, diabetes, factors affecting NCLEX scores.

Northern Michigan University, Office of Graduate Education and Research, College of Health Sciences and Professional Studies, School of Nursing, Marquette, MI 49855-5301. Offers MSN, DNP. *Accreditation:* AACN. *Program availability:* Part-time, online learning. *Entrance requirements:* For doctorate, Michigan RN license; minimum undergraduate GPA of 3.0; 3 letters of recommendation; written personal goal statement. Additional exam requirements/recommendations for international students: Required—TOEFL (minimum score 550 paper-based; 79 iBT), IELTS (minimum score 6.5). Electronic applications accepted. *Faculty research:* Grief experiences in Alzheimer's caregivers, nursing students attitudes towards the elderly, using Facebook as a means of simulation and educational means for pediatric undergraduate nursing students, use of a nurse practitioner student educational intervention to reduce sugar sweetened beverage consumption in rural adolescents.

North Park University, School of Nursing, Chicago, IL 60625-4895. Offers advanced practice nursing (MS); leadership and management (MS); MBA/MS; MM/MSN; MS/MHR; MS/MNA. *Accreditation:* AACN. *Program availability:* Part-time, evening/weekend. *Degree requirements:* For master's, thesis. *Entrance requirements:* For master's, GMAT, MAT. *Faculty research:* Aging, consultation roles, critical thinking skills, family breakdown, science of caring.

Northwestern State University of Louisiana, Graduate Studies and Research, College of Nursing and School of Allied Health, Shreveport, LA 71101-4653. Offers MS, MSN. *Accreditation:* AACN. *Program availability:* Part-time. *Degree requirements:* For master's, comprehensive exam, thesis or alternative. *Entrance requirements:* For master's, GRE General Test, 6 months of clinical nursing experience, BS in nursing, minimum GPA of 3.0. Additional exam requirements/recommendations for international students: Required—TOEFL. Electronic applications accepted.

Norwich University, College of Graduate and Continuing Studies, Master of Science in Nursing Program, Northfield, VT 05663. Offers nursing administration (MSN); nursing education (MSN). *Accreditation:* AACN. *Program availability:* Evening/weekend, mostly all online with a week-long residency requirement. *Faculty:* 10 part-time/adjunct (7 women). *Students:* 84 full-time (78 women); includes 11 minority (8 Black or African American, non-Hispanic/Latino; 2 Asian, non-Hispanic/Latino; 1 Hispanic/Latino). Average age 40. 33 applicants, 100% accepted, 29 enrolled. In 2015, 57 master's awarded. *Entrance requirements:* For master's, minimum undergraduate GPA of 3.0. Additional exam requirements/recommendations for international students: Required—TOEFL (minimum score 550 paper-based; 80 iBT), IELTS (minimum score 6.5). *Application deadline:* For fall admission, 8/15 for domestic and international students; for winter admission, 11/14 for domestic and international students; for spring admission, 2/13 for domestic and international students; for summer admission, 5/15 for domestic and international students. Applications are processed on a rolling basis. Electronic applications accepted. *Expenses:* Contact institution. *Financial support:* In 2015–16, 22 students received support. Scholarships/grants available. Financial award application deadline: 8/5; financial award applicants required to submit FAFSA. *Unit head:* Dr. Sharon Richie-Melvan, Director, 802-485-2600, E-mail: srichiem@norwich.edu. *Application contact:* Rija Ramahatra, Associate Program Director, 802-485-2892, Fax: 802-485-2533, E-mail: rramahatr@norwich.edu.
Website: http://online.norwich.edu/degree-programs/masters/master-science-nursing/overview

Nova Southeastern University, College of Nursing, Fort Lauderdale, FL 33314-7796. Offers advanced practice registered nurse (APRN) (MSN); nursing (PhD); nursing (MSN); nursing practice (DNP). *Accreditation:* AACN. *Program availability:* Part-time, evening/weekend, 100% online, blended/hybrid learning, online PhD program with annual one-week summer institute that is delivered face-to-face on the main campus. *Faculty:* 23 full-time (22 women), 40 part-time/adjunct (35 women). *Students:* 1 (woman) full-time, 506 part-time (461 women); includes 329 minority (163 Black or African American, non-Hispanic/Latino; 34 Asian, non-Hispanic/Latino; 122 Hispanic/Latino; 1 Native Hawaiian or other Pacific Islander, non-Hispanic/Latino; 9 Two or more races, non-Hispanic/Latino), 2 international. Average age 39. In 2015, 91 master's, 15 doctorates awarded. *Degree requirements:* For doctorate, comprehensive exam, thesis/dissertation. *Entrance requirements:* For master's, minimum GPA of 3.0, RN, BSN, BS or BA; for doctorate, minimum GPA of 3.5, MSN, RN. Additional exam requirements/recommendations for international students: Recommended—TOEFL. *Application deadline:* For fall admission, 3/1 priority date for domestic students, 3/1 for international students; for winter admission, 11/1 for domestic and international students. Applications are processed on a rolling basis. Application fee: $50. Electronic applications accepted. *Expenses:* Contact institution. *Financial support:* In 2015–16, 41 students received support. Traineeships available. Financial award application deadline: 4/15; financial award applicants required to submit FAFSA. *Faculty research:* Nursing education, curriculum, clinical research, interdisciplinary research. *Unit head:* Dr. Marcella Rutherford, Dean, 954-262-1963, E-mail: rmarcell@nova.edu.
Website: http://www.nova.edu/nursing/

Oakland University, Graduate Study and Lifelong Learning, School of Nursing, Rochester, MI 48309-4401. Offers MSN, DNP, PMC. *Accreditation:* AACN. *Program availability:* Part-time, evening/weekend. *Faculty:* 17 full-time (all women), 5 part-time/adjunct (2 women). *Students:* 150 full-time (123 women), 71 part-time (62 women); includes 144 minority (16 Black or African American, non-Hispanic/Latino; 2 American Indian or Alaska Native, non-Hispanic/Latino; 99 Asian, non-Hispanic/Latino; 14 Hispanic/Latino; 13 Two or more races, non-Hispanic/Latino), 19 international. Average age 34. 400 applicants, 22% accepted, 73 enrolled. In 2015, 75 master's, 9 doctorates, 2 other advanced degrees awarded. *Entrance requirements:* For master's, GRE General Test, minimum GPA of 3.0. Application fee: $0. Electronic applications accepted. *Expenses:* Tuition, area resident: Part-time $655 per credit. Tuition and fees vary according to program. *Financial support:* Federal Work-Study, institutionally sponsored loans, and tuition waivers (full) available. Financial award application deadline: 3/1; financial award applicants required to submit FAFSA. *Unit head:* Dr. Gary Moore, Interim Dean/Associate Professor, 248-364-8787, E-mail: moore@oakland.edu.

The Ohio State University, Graduate School, College of Nursing, Columbus, OH 43210. Offers MS, DNP, PhD. *Accreditation:* AACN; ACNM/ACME. *Program availability:* Part-time. *Faculty:* 43. *Students:* 496 full-time (413 women), 218 part-time (200 women); includes 108 minority (42 Black or African American, non-Hispanic/Latino; 32 Asian, non-Hispanic/Latino; 20 Hispanic/Latino; 14 Two or more races, non-Hispanic/Latino), 5 international. Average age 33. In 2015, 164 master's, 28 doctorates awarded. *Degree requirements:* For master's, thesis optional; for doctorate, thesis/dissertation. *Entrance requirements:* For doctorate, GRE (for PhD). Additional exam requirements/recommendations for international students: Required—TOEFL (minimum score 600 paper-based; 100 iBT); Recommended—IELTS (minimum score 8). *Application deadline:* For fall admission, 12/13 priority date for domestic students, 11/30 priority date for international students; for summer admission, 10/12 for domestic and international students. Applications are processed on a rolling basis. Application fee: $60 ($70 for international students). Electronic applications accepted. *Financial support:* Fellowships, research assistantships, teaching assistantships, Federal Work-Study, institutionally sponsored loans, and unspecified assistantships available. Support available to part-time students. *Unit head:* Dr. Bernadette M. Melnyk, Dean, 614-292-4844, Fax: 614-292-4535, E-mail: melnyk.15@osu.edu. *Application contact:* Graduate and Professional Admissions, 614-292-9444, Fax: 614-292-3895, E-mail: gpadmissions@osu.edu.
Website: http://nursing.osu.edu/

Ohio University, Graduate College, College of Health Sciences and Professions, School of Nursing, Athens, OH 45701-2979. Offers acute care nurse practitioner (MSN); acute care nurse practitioner and family nurse practitioner (MSN); acute care nurse practitioner and nurse administrator (MSN); acute care nurse practitioner and nurse educator (MSN); family nurse practitioner (MSN); nurse administrator (MSN); nurse administrator and family nurse practitioner (MSN); nurse educator (MSN); nurse educator and family nurse practitioner (MSN); nurse educator and nurse administrator (MSN). *Accreditation:* AACN. *Degree requirements:* For master's, capstone project. *Entrance requirements:* For master's, GRE, bachelor's degree in nursing from an accredited college or university, minimum overall undergraduate GPA of 3.0, official transcripts, statement of goals and objectives, resume, 3 letters of recommendation. Additional exam requirements/recommendations for international students: Required—TOEFL (minimum score 550 paper-based; 80 iBT) or IELTS (minimum score 6.5). Electronic applications accepted.

Oklahoma Baptist University, Program in Nursing, Shawnee, OK 74804. Offers global nursing (MSN); nursing education (MSN). *Accreditation:* AACN.

Oklahoma City University, Kramer School of Nursing, Oklahoma City, OK 73106-1402. Offers clinical nurse leader (MSN); nursing (DNP, PhD); nursing education (MSN). *Accreditation:* ACEN. *Program availability:* Part-time, evening/weekend, online learning.

Faculty: 11 full-time (all women), 6 part-time/adjunct (5 women). *Students:* 125 full-time (107 women), 30 part-time (29 women); includes 46 minority (13 Black or African American, non-Hispanic/Latino; 11 American Indian or Alaska Native, non-Hispanic/Latino; 10 Asian, non-Hispanic/Latino; 5 Hispanic/Latino; 7 Two or more races, non-Hispanic/Latino), 19 international. Average age 38. 54 applicants, 78% accepted, 31 enrolled. In 2015, 17 master's, 7 doctorates awarded. *Degree requirements:* For master's, thesis, minimum GPA of 3.0; for doctorate, comprehensive exam, thesis/dissertation, minimum GPA of 3.0. *Entrance requirements:* For master's, registered nurse licensure, minimum undergraduate GPA of 3.0, BSN from nationally-accredited nursing program, completion of courses in health assessment and statistics; for doctorate, GRE, current RN licensure; bachelor's and master's degrees from accredited programs (at least one of which must be in nursing); minimum graduate GPA of 3.5; personal essay; approved scholarly paper or published article/paper in a refereed journal. Additional exam requirements/recommendations for international students: Required—TOEFL (minimum score 550 paper-based; 80 iBT), IELTS (minimum score 6). *Application deadline:* Applications are processed on a rolling basis. Application fee: $50. Electronic applications accepted. *Expenses:* $13,320 tuition and general fee per year for full-time study. *Financial support:* In 2015–16, 89 students received support. Federal Work-Study, institutionally sponsored loans, scholarships/grants, and tuition waivers (full and partial) available. Support available to part-time students. Financial award application deadline: 3/1; financial award applicants required to submit FAFSA. *Unit head:* Dr. Lois Salmeron, Dean, Kramer School of Nursing, 405-208-5900, Fax: 405-208-5914, E-mail: lsalmeron@okcu.edu. *Application contact:* Michael Harrington, Director of Graduate Admissions, 800-633-7242, Fax: 405-208-5916, E-mail: gadmissions@okcu.edu.
Website: http://www.okcu.edu/nursing/

Old Dominion University, College of Health Sciences, School of Nursing, Norfolk, VA 23529. Offers adult gerontology clinical nurse specialist/educator role (MSN); advanced practice nursing (DNP); family nurse practitioner (MSN), including adult-gerontology clinical nurse specialist/educator, neonatal nurse practitioner, pediatric nurse practitioner; nurse anesthesia (MSN); nurse educator (MSN), including neonatal nurse practitioner, pediatric nurse practitioner; nurse executive (MSN), including neonatal nurse practitioner, pediatric nurse practitioner; nurse midwifery (MSN). *Accreditation:* AACN; AANA/CANAEP (one or more programs are accredited). *Program availability:* Part-time, 100% online, blended/hybrid learning. *Faculty:* 6 full-time (5 women), 17 part-time/adjunct (15 women). *Students:* 116 full-time (105 women), 72 part-time (61 women); includes 34 minority (18 Black or African American, non-Hispanic/Latino; 1 American Indian or Alaska Native, non-Hispanic/Latino; 5 Asian, non-Hispanic/Latino; 2 Hispanic/Latino; 8 Two or more races, non-Hispanic/Latino), 7 international. Average age 39. 199 applicants, 42% accepted, 74 enrolled. In 2015, 67 master's, 27 doctorates awarded. *Degree requirements:* For master's, comprehensive exam; for doctorate, capstone project. *Entrance requirements:* For master's, GRE or MAT, BSN, minimum GPA of 3.0 in nursing and overall. Additional exam requirements/recommendations for international students: Required—TOEFL. *Application deadline:* For fall admission, 3/1 for domestic students, 4/15 for international students; for spring admission, 9/15 for domestic students. Application fee: $50. Electronic applications accepted. *Expenses:* Tuition, state resident: full-time $11,136; part-time $464 per credit hour. Tuition, nonresident: full-time $27,840; part-time $1160 per credit hour. *Required fees:* $64 per semester. Tuition and fees vary according to campus/location, program and reciprocity agreements. *Financial support:* In 2015–16, 18 students received support, including 2 research assistantships with partial tuition reimbursements available (averaging $10,000 per year), 1 teaching assistantship (averaging $2,500 per year); career-related internships or fieldwork, scholarships/grants, traineeships, and tuition waivers (partial) also available. Support available to part-time students. Financial award application deadline: 2/15; financial award applicants required to submit FAFSA. *Faculty research:* Health and culture, cardiovascular health, transition of military families, genetics, cultural diversity. *Total annual research expenditures:* $231,117. *Unit head:* Dr. Karen Karlowicz, Chair, 757-683-5262, Fax: 757-683-5253, E-mail: nursgpd@odu.edu. *Application contact:* Sue Parker, Coordinator, Graduate Student Services, 757-683-4298, Fax: 757-683-5253, E-mail: sparker@odu.edu.
Website: http://www.odu.edu/nursing

Oregon Health & Science University, School of Nursing, Portland, OR 97239-3098. Offers MN, MPH, MS, DNP, PhD, Post Master's Certificate. *Accreditation:* AACN; ACNM/ACME (one or more programs are accredited). *Program availability:* Part-time. *Degree requirements:* For master's, thesis optional; for doctorate, thesis/dissertation. *Entrance requirements:* For master's, GRE General Test, bachelor's degree in nursing, minimum undergraduate GPA of 3.0, previous course work in statistics; for doctorate, GRE General Test, master's degree in nursing; minimum undergraduate GPA of 3.0, 3.5 graduate; for Post Master's Certificate, master's degree in nursing. Electronic applications accepted. *Expenses:* Contact institution. *Faculty research:* Nursing care of older persons; families in health, illness, and transition; family caregiving; end of life care/decision making; mother-infant interactions; pregnancy outcomes; enteral feeding; psychoactive drugs in long-term care.

Otterbein University, Department of Nursing, Westerville, OH 43081. Offers advanced practice nurse educator (Certificate); clinical nurse leader (MSN); family nurse practitioner (MSN, Certificate); nurse anesthesia (MSN, Certificate); nursing (DNP); nursing service administration (MSN). *Accreditation:* AACN; AANA/CANAEP; ACEN. *Program availability:* Part-time, evening/weekend, online learning. *Degree requirements:* For master's, comprehensive exam (for some programs), thesis (for some programs). *Entrance requirements:* For master's, 2 reference forms, resume; for Certificate, official transcripts, 2 reference forms, essay, resumé. Additional exam requirements/recommendations for international students: Required—TOEFL (minimum score 550 paper-based; 79 iBT). *Faculty research:* Patient education, women's health, trauma curriculum development, administration.

Our Lady of the Lake College, School of Nursing, Baton Rouge, LA 70808. Offers nurse anesthesia (MS); nursing (MS), including administration, education. *Accreditation:* ACEN.

Pace University, College of Health Professions, Lienhard School of Nursing, New York, NY 10038. Offers family nurse practitioner (MS); nurse education (Advanced Certificate); nursing education (MS); nursing leadership (Advanced Certificate); nursing practice (DNP). *Accreditation:* AACN. *Program availability:* Part-time, evening/weekend, blended/hybrid learning. *Faculty:* 11 full-time (10 women), 31 part-time/adjunct (27 women). *Students:* 3 full-time (all women), 415 part-time (385 women); includes 196 minority (97 Black or African American, non-Hispanic/Latino; 2 American Indian or Alaska Native, non-Hispanic/Latino; 57 Asian, non-Hispanic/Latino; 33 Hispanic/Latino; 7 Two or more races, non-Hispanic/Latino), 2 international. Average age 34. 291 applicants, 69% accepted, 129 enrolled. In 2015, 129 master's, 20 doctorates, 7 other advanced degrees awarded. *Degree requirements:* For doctorate, thesis/dissertation. *Entrance requirements:* For master's, RN license, resume, personal statement, 2 letters of recommendation, official transcripts; for doctorate, RN license, resume, personal statement, 2 letters of recommendation, official transcripts, accredited master's degree in nursing, minimum GPA of 3.3, national certification; for Advanced Certificate, RN license, completion of 2nd degree in nursing. Additional exam requirements/recommendations for international students: Required—TOEFL (minimum score 100

Nursing—General

iBT), IELTS or PTE. *Application deadline:* For fall admission, 3/1 for domestic and international students. Applications are processed on a rolling basis. Application fee: $70. Electronic applications accepted. *Expenses:* Contact institution. *Financial support:* Research assistantships, teaching assistantships, career-related internships or fieldwork, Federal Work-Study, tuition waivers (partial), and unspecified assistantships available. Support available to part-time students. Financial award application deadline: 2/15; financial award applicants required to submit FAFSA. *Unit head:* Dr. Harriet R. Feldman, Dean, College of Health Professions, 914-773-3341, E-mail: hfeldman@pace.edu. *Application contact:* Susan Ford-Goldschein, Director of Graduate Admissions, 212-346-1531, Fax: 212-346-1585, E-mail: graduateadmission@pace.edu. Website: http://www.pace.edu/lienhard

Pacific Lutheran University, School of Nursing, Tacoma, WA 98447. Offers MSN, DNP. *Accreditation:* AACN. *Faculty:* 6 full-time (5 women), 7 part-time/adjunct (all women). *Students:* 49 full-time (39 women), 15 part-time (13 women); includes 20 minority (3 Black or African American, non-Hispanic/Latino; 2 American Indian or Alaska Native, non-Hispanic/Latino; 6 Asian, non-Hispanic/Latino; 5 Hispanic/Latino; 4 Two or more races, non-Hispanic/Latino), 1 international. Average age 34. 124 applicants, 35% accepted, 31 enrolled. In 2015, 23 master's awarded. *Degree requirements:* For master's, thesis or alternative. *Entrance requirements:* For master's, GRE General Test, minimum undergraduate GPA of 3.0. Additional exam requirements/recommendations for international students: Required—TOEFL (minimum score 550 paper-based; 86 iBT). *Application deadline:* For fall admission, 11/15 priority date for domestic and international students. Applications are processed on a rolling basis. Application fee: $55. Electronic applications accepted. *Expenses:* Contact institution. *Financial support:* In 2015–16, 60 students received support, including 14 fellowships (averaging $643 per year); Federal Work-Study, scholarships/grants, and health care benefits also available. Financial award application deadline: 3/1; financial award applicants required to submit FAFSA. *Unit head:* Dr. Teri Woo, Associate Dean of Graduate Nursing Programs/Associate Professor of Nursing, 253-535-7686, Fax: 253-535-7590, E-mail: gradnurs@plu.edu. *Application contact:* Marie Boisvert, Director, Graduate Admission, 253-535-8570, Fax: 253-536-5136, E-mail: gradadmission@plu.edu.

Palm Beach Atlantic University, School of Nursing, West Palm Beach, FL 33416-4708. Offers family nurse practitioner (DNP); health systems leadership (MSN). *Program availability:* Part-time. *Faculty:* 5 part-time/adjunct (4 women). *Students:* 43 full-time (37 women), 1 (woman) part-time; includes 22 minority (11 Black or African American, non-Hispanic/Latino; 2 Asian, non-Hispanic/Latino; 8 Hispanic/Latino; 1 Two or more races, non-Hispanic/Latino). Average age 32. 34 applicants, 100% accepted, 24 enrolled. *Entrance requirements:* For master's, minimum GPA of 3.0; for doctorate, minimum GPA of 3.0; one year of experience as an RN; personal interview. Additional exam requirements/recommendations for international students: Required—TOEFL (minimum score 550 paper-based; 79 iBT). *Application deadline:* Applications are processed on a rolling basis. Application fee: $50. Electronic applications accepted. *Expenses:* Tuition, area resident: Part-time $525 per credit hour. *Financial support:* In 2015–16, 13 students received support. Scholarships/grants and employee education grants available. Financial award application deadline: 5/1; financial award applicants required to submit FAFSA. *Unit head:* Joanne Masella, Dean, 561-803-2827. *Application contact:* Graduate Admissions, 888-468-6722, E-mail: grad@pba.edu. Website: http://www.pba.edu/school-of-nursing

Penn State University Park, Graduate School, College of Nursing, University Park, PA 16802. Offers MS, MSN, DNP, PhD. *Accreditation:* AACN; ACEN. *Program availability:* Part-time, evening/weekend, online learning. *Students:* 69 full-time (57 women), 50 part-time (45 women). Average age 32. 69 applicants, 55% accepted, 34 enrolled. *Entrance requirements:* Additional exam requirements/recommendations for international students: Required—TOEFL (minimum score 550 paper-based; 80 iBT), IELTS. *Application deadline:* Applications are processed on a rolling basis. Application fee: $65. Electronic applications accepted. *Financial support:* Fellowships, research assistantships, teaching assistantships, career-related internships or fieldwork, Federal Work-Study, scholarships/grants, traineeships, health care benefits, and unspecified assistantships available. Support available to part-time students. Financial award application deadline: 3/1; financial award applicants required to submit FAFSA. *Unit head:* Dr. Paula F. Milone-Nuzzo, Dean, 814-863-0245, Fax: 814-865-3779. *Application contact:* Lori Stania, Director, Graduate Student Services, 814-865-1795, Fax: 814-863-4627, E-mail: l-gswww@lists.psu.edu. Website: http://www.nursing.psu.edu/

Pittsburg State University, Graduate School, College of Arts and Sciences, School of Nursing, Pittsburg, KS 66762. Offers MSN. *Accreditation:* AACN. *Program availability:* Part-time. *Students:* 34 (31 women); includes 15 minority (2 Black or African American, non-Hispanic/Latino; 3 American Indian or Alaska Native, non-Hispanic/Latino; 1 Hispanic/Latino; 9 Two or more races, non-Hispanic/Latino). In 2015, 25 master's awarded. *Degree requirements:* For master's, thesis optional. *Entrance requirements:* For master's, GRE General Test. Additional exam requirements/recommendations for international students: Required—TOEFL (minimum score 550 paper-based; 79 iBT), IELTS (minimum score 6.5), PTE (minimum score 53). *Application deadline:* For fall admission, 6/1 for international students; for spring admission, 10/15 for international students; for summer admission, 4/1 for international students. Applications are processed on a rolling basis. Application fee: $35 ($60 for international students). Electronic applications accepted. *Expenses:* $305 per credit for residents; $711 per credit for non-residents; $434 (for DNP students). *Financial support:* In 2015–16, 3 teaching assistantships with full tuition reimbursements (averaging $5,500 per year) were awarded. Financial award application deadline: 2/1; financial award applicants required to submit FAFSA. *Unit head:* Dr. Mary Carol Pomatto, Chairperson, 620-235-4432, E-mail: mpomatto@pittstate.edu. *Application contact:* Lisa Allen, Assistant Director, 620-235-4223, Fax: 620-235-4219, E-mail: lallen@pittstate.edu.

Point Loma Nazarene University, School of Nursing, San Diego, CA 92106-2899. Offers adult/gerontology nursing (MSN); family/individual health (MSN); general nursing (MSN); nursing (Post-MSN Certificate); pediatric nursing (MSN); psychiatric mental health (MSN). *Accreditation:* AACN. *Program availability:* Part-time. *Faculty:* 6 full-time (5 women), 2 part-time/adjunct (both women). *Students:* 1 (woman) full-time, 74 part-time (61 women); includes 35 minority (4 Black or African American, non-Hispanic/Latino; 15 Asian, non-Hispanic/Latino; 10 Hispanic/Latino; 3 Native Hawaiian or other Pacific Islander, non-Hispanic/Latino; 3 Two or more races, non-Hispanic/Latino), 2 international. Average age 38. 34 applicants, 88% accepted, 18 enrolled. In 2015, 40 master's awarded. *Entrance requirements:* For master's, NCLEX, ADN or BSN in nursing, interview, RN license, essay, letters of recommendation, interview. *Application deadline:* For fall admission, 7/5 priority date for domestic students; for spring admission, 11/1 priority date for domestic students; for summer admission, 3/22 priority date for domestic students. Applications are processed on a rolling basis. Application fee: $50. *Financial support:* Applicants required to submit FAFSA. *Unit head:* Dr. Barb Taylor, Dean of the School of Nursing, 619-849-2766, E-mail: bataylor@pointloma.edu. *Application contact:* Claire Buckley, Director of Graduate Admissions, 619-563-2846, E-mail: clairebuckley@pointloma.edu. Website: http://www.pointloma.edu/discover/graduate-school/graduate-programs/master-science-nursing-and-post-msn-certification

Pontifical Catholic University of Puerto Rico, College of Sciences, Department of Nursing, Ponce, PR 00717-0777. Offers medical-surgical nursing (MSN); mental health and psychiatric nursing (MSN). *Accreditation:* ACEN. *Program availability:* Part-time, evening/weekend. *Degree requirements:* For master's, comprehensive exam (for some programs), thesis, clinical research paper. *Entrance requirements:* For master's, GRE General Test, 2 letters of recommendation, interview, minimum GPA of 2.5. Electronic applications accepted.

Prairie View A&M University, College of Nursing, Houston, TX 77030. Offers family nurse practitioner (MSN); nursing administration (MSN); nursing education (MSN). *Accreditation:* AACN; ACEN. *Program availability:* Part-time, evening/weekend. *Faculty:* 11 full-time (all women), 7 part-time/adjunct (6 women). *Students:* 65 full-time (58 women), 78 part-time (71 women); includes 128 minority (94 Black or African American, non-Hispanic/Latino; 24 Asian, non-Hispanic/Latino; 9 Hispanic/Latino; 1 Two or more races, non-Hispanic/Latino), 5 international. Average age 35. 84 applicants, 44% accepted, 25 enrolled. In 2015, 63 master's awarded. *Degree requirements:* For master's, comprehensive exam, thesis. *Entrance requirements:* For master's, MAT or GRE, BS in nursing; minimum 1 year of experience as registered nurse; minimum GPA of 2.75, 3 letters of recommendation from professional nurses. Additional exam requirements/recommendations for international students: Required—TOEFL (minimum score 550 paper-based; 79 iBT). *Application deadline:* For fall admission, 7/1 priority date for domestic students, 6/1 priority date for international students; for spring admission, 11/1 priority date for domestic students, 10/1 priority date for international students; for summer admission, 3/1 priority date for domestic students, 2/1 priority date for international students. Applications are processed on a rolling basis. Application fee: $50. Electronic applications accepted. *Expenses:* Tuition, state resident: full-time $4243; part-time $237.29 per credit hour. Tuition, nonresident: full-time $11,798; part-time $657 per credit hour. *Required fees:* $2762; $172.10 per credit hour. *Financial support:* Career-related internships or fieldwork, Federal Work-Study, institutionally sponsored loans, scholarships/grants, and traineeships available. Support available to part-time students. Financial award application deadline: 4/1; financial award applicants required to submit FAFSA. *Faculty research:* Software development and violence prevention, health promotion and disease prevention. *Unit head:* Dr. Betty N. Adams, Dean, 713-797-7009, Fax: 713-797-7013, E-mail: bnadams@pvamu.edu. *Application contact:* Dr. Forest Smith, Director of Student Services and Admissions, 713-797-7031, Fax: 713-797-7012, E-mail: fdsmith@pvamu.edu. Website: http://www.pvamu.edu/nursing/

Purdue University Northwest, Graduate Studies Office, School of Nursing, Hammond, IN 46323-2094. Offers adult health clinical nurse specialist (MS); critical care clinical nurse specialist (MS); family nurse practitioner (MS); nurse executive (MS). *Accreditation:* AACN; ACEN. *Program availability:* Part-time, online learning. *Entrance requirements:* For master's, BSN. Additional exam requirements/recommendations for international students: Required—TOEFL. Electronic applications accepted. *Faculty research:* Adult health, cardiovascular and pulmonary nursing.

Queen's University at Kingston, School of Graduate Studies, Faculty of Health Sciences, School of Nursing, Kingston, ON K7L 3N6, Canada. Offers health and chronic illness (M Sc); nurse scientist (PhD); primary health care nurse practitioner (Certificate); women's and children's health (M Sc). *Degree requirements:* For master's, thesis. *Entrance requirements:* For master's, RN license. Additional exam requirements/recommendations for international students: Required—TOEFL. *Faculty research:* Women and children's health, health and chronic illness.

Queens University of Charlotte, Presbyterian School of Nursing, Charlotte, NC 28274-0002. Offers clinical nurse leader (MSN); nurse educator (MSN); nursing administrator (MSN). *Accreditation:* AACN. *Degree requirements:* For master's, research project. *Entrance requirements:* For master's, minimum GPA of 3.0. Additional exam requirements/recommendations for international students: Required—TOEFL. Electronic applications accepted. *Expenses:* Contact institution.

Quinnipiac University, School of Nursing, Hamden, CT 06518-1940. Offers MSN, DNP. *Program availability:* Part-time. *Faculty:* 19 full-time (18 women), 13 part-time/adjunct (9 women). *Students:* 72 full-time (64 women), 151 part-time (136 women); includes 45 minority (19 Black or African American, non-Hispanic/Latino; 15 Asian, non-Hispanic/Latino; 10 Hispanic/Latino; 1 Two or more races, non-Hispanic/Latino), 1 international. 182 applicants, 65% accepted, 86 enrolled. In 2015, 16 doctorates awarded. *Degree requirements:* For master's, thesis optional, clinical practicum. *Entrance requirements:* For master's, RN license, minimum GPA of 3.0. Additional exam requirements/recommendations for international students: Required—TOEFL (minimum score 575 paper-based; 90 iBT), IELTS (minimum score 6.5). *Application deadline:* Applications are processed on a rolling basis. Application fee: $45. Electronic applications accepted. Tuition and fees vary according to course load and program. *Financial support:* Federal Work-Study, scholarships/grants, and unspecified assistantships available. Support available to part-time students. Financial award application deadline: 6/1; financial award applicants required to submit FAFSA. *Faculty research:* Decreasing social isolation of older adults, high fidelity simulation as a teaching method, teaching end of life care to nursing students, nurses with disabilities and practice roles, improving depression care of older home care patients, determining hip labral tears with new physical examination technique. Website: http://www.quinnipiac.edu/gradnursing

Radford University, College of Graduate and Professional Studies, Waldron College of Health and Human Services, Program in Nursing Practice, Radford, VA 24142. Offers DNP. *Accreditation:* AACN. *Program availability:* Part-time, evening/weekend, online learning. *Faculty:* 9 full-time (8 women), 2 part-time/adjunct (both women). *Students:* 4 full-time (all women), 35 part-time (28 women); includes 8 minority (4 Black or African American, non-Hispanic/Latino; 1 Asian, non-Hispanic/Latino; 1 Hispanic/Latino; 2 Two or more races, non-Hispanic/Latino). Average age 40. 15 applicants, 93% accepted, 11 enrolled. In 2015, 11 doctorates awarded. *Degree requirements:* For doctorate, thesis/dissertation. *Entrance requirements:* For doctorate, GRE, current license to practice as RN; minimum undergraduate GPA of 3.0, graduate 3.5; 3-5 page essay; professional writing sample; three letters of reference; personal interview; resume or curriculum vitae; official transcripts; 2000 hours of RN clinical experience; certification in BLS or ACLS; BSN; MSN (for some areas, eliminating GRE requirement). Additional exam requirements/recommendations for international students: Required—TOEFL (minimum score 550 paper-based; 79 iBT), IELTS (minimum score 6.5). *Application deadline:* For fall admission, 2/15 priority date for domestic students, 12/1 for international students; for spring admission, 7/1 for international students. Applications are processed on a rolling basis. Application fee: $50. Electronic applications accepted. *Expenses:* $461 per credit hour in-state tuition and fees; $931 per credit hour out-of-state tuition and fees. *Financial support:* In 2015–16, 32 students received support. Career-related internships or fieldwork, Federal Work-Study, institutionally sponsored loans, scholarships/grants, and unspecified assistantships available. Financial award application deadline: 3/1; financial award applicants required to submit FAFSA. *Unit head:* Dr. Ginger Burggraf, Coordinator, 540-831-7714, Fax: 540-831-7716, E-mail: vburggraf2@radford.edu. *Application contact:* Rebecca Conner, Director, Graduate Enrollment, 540-831-6296, Fax: 540-831-6061, E-mail: gradcollege@radford.edu. Website: http://www.radford.edu/content/wchs/home/dnp.html

Ramapo College of New Jersey, Master of Science in Nursing Program, Mahwah, NJ 07430. Offers nursing education (MSN). *Accreditation:* ACEN. *Program availability:* Part-time. *Faculty:* 3 full-time (all women), 1 part-time/adjunct (0 women). *Students:* 1 full-time (0 women), 49 part-time (43 women); includes 16 minority (4 Black or African American, non-Hispanic/Latino; 8 Asian, non-Hispanic/Latino; 3 Hispanic/Latino; 1 Two or more races, non-Hispanic/Latino). Average age 35. 36 applicants, 81% accepted, 25 enrolled. In 2015, 6 master's awarded. *Entrance requirements:* For master's, official transcript; personal statement; 2 letters of recommendation; resume; current licensure as a Registered Nurse, or eligibility for licensure; evidence of one year of recent experience as RN prior to entry into clinical practicum courses; evidence of undergraduate statistics course; criminal background check. Additional exam requirements/recommendations for international students: Required—TOEFL (minimum score 550 paper-based; 90 iBT); Recommended—IELTS (minimum score 6). *Application deadline:* For fall admission, 5/1 for domestic and international students; for spring admission, 12/1 for domestic and international students. Applications are processed on a rolling basis. Application fee: $60. Electronic applications accepted. *Expenses:* $597.05 per credit tuition, $129.45 per credit fees. *Financial support:* Career-related internships or fieldwork available. Financial award application deadline: 3/1; financial award applicants required to submit FAFSA. *Faculty research:* Learning styles and critical thinking, evidence-based education, outcomes measurement. *Unit head:* Dr. Kathleen M. Burke, Assistant Dean in Charge of Nursing Programs/Professor, 201-684-7737, Fax: 201-684-7954, E-mail: kmburke@ramapo.edu. *Application contact:* Anthony Dovi, Associate Director of Admissions, Adult Learners and Graduate Programs, 201-684-7305, Fax: 201-684-7964, E-mail: adovi@ramapo.edu.
Website: http://www.ramapo.edu/msn/

Regis College, School of Nursing and Health Sciences, Weston, MA 02493. Offers applied behavior analysis (MS); biomedical sciences (MS); counseling psychology (MA); health administration (MS); molecular imaging and therapeutics (MS); nurse practitioner (Certificate); nursing (MS, DNP); nursing education (Certificate); occupational therapy (MS). *Accreditation:* ACEN. *Program availability:* Part-time, evening/weekend. *Degree requirements:* For master's, thesis. *Entrance requirements:* For master's, GRE General Test or MAT, minimum GPA of 3.0; for doctorate, MAT or GRE if GPA from master's lower than 3.5. Additional exam requirements/recommendations for international students: Required—TOEFL (minimum score 550 paper-based). *Application deadline:* Applications are processed on a rolling basis. Application fee: $50. Electronic applications accepted. *Financial support:* Research assistantships, Federal Work-Study, scholarships/grants, traineeships, and unspecified assistantships available. Support available to part-time students. Financial award applicants required to submit FAFSA. *Faculty research:* Health policy, education, aging, job satisfaction, psychiatric nursing, critical thinking. *Application contact:* Shelagh Tomaino, Associate Director, Graduate Admission, 781-768-7188, Fax: 781-768-7071, E-mail: shelagh.tomaino@regiscollege.edu.

Research College of Nursing, Nursing Program, Kansas City, MO 64132. Offers adult-gerontological nurse practitioner (MSN); executive practice and healthcare leadership (MSN); family nurse practitioner (MSN); nursing (MSN). *Accreditation:* AACN. *Program availability:* Part-time, 100% online. *Faculty:* 9 full-time (all women), 5 part-time/adjunct (2 women). *Students:* 4 full-time (2 women), 148 part-time (132 women); includes 15 minority (9 Black or African American, non-Hispanic/Latino; 1 American Indian or Alaska Native, non-Hispanic/Latino; 3 Asian, non-Hispanic/Latino; 1 Native Hawaiian or other Pacific Islander, non-Hispanic/Latino; 1 Two or more races, non-Hispanic/Latino). In 2015, 34 master's awarded. *Degree requirements:* For master's, research project. *Entrance requirements:* For master's, 3 letters of recommendation, official transcripts, resume, personal statement/writing sample. *Application deadline:* Applications are processed on a rolling basis. Application fee: $65. Electronic applications accepted. *Expenses:* $525 per credit hour; $25 per credit hour clinical fee. *Financial support:* Applicants required to submit FAFSA. *Unit head:* Dr. Nancy O. DeBasio, President and Dean, 816-995-2815, Fax: 816-995-2817, E-mail: nancy.debasio@researchcollege.edu. *Application contact:* Leslie Burry, Director of Transfer and Graduate Recruitment, 816-995-2820, Fax: 816-995-2813, E-mail: leslie.burry@researchcollege.edu.

Resurrection University, Nursing Program, Chicago, IL 60622. Offers MSN. *Accreditation:* AACN. *Entrance requirements:* For master's, letter of recommendation.

Rhode Island College, School of Graduate Studies, School of Nursing, Providence, RI 02908-1991. Offers MSN. *Accreditation:* AACN. *Program availability:* Part-time. *Faculty:* 7 full-time (all women), 13 part-time/adjunct (all women). *Students:* 11 full-time (6 women), 78 part-time (68 women); includes 11 minority (3 Black or African American, non-Hispanic/Latino; 4 Asian, non-Hispanic/Latino; 3 Hispanic/Latino; 1 Two or more races, non-Hispanic/Latino), 2 international. Average age 36. In 2015, 13 master's awarded. *Entrance requirements:* For master's, GRE, undergraduate transcripts; minimum undergraduate GPA of 3.0; 3 letters of recommendation; evidence of current unrestricted Rhode Island RN licensure; professional resume; letter of intent. Additional exam requirements/recommendations for international students: Recommended—TOEFL (minimum score 550 paper-based; 79 iBT). *Application deadline:* For fall admission, 2/15 for domestic students. Applications are processed on a rolling basis. Application fee: $50. Electronic applications accepted. *Expenses:* Tuition, state resident: full-time $8928; part-time $372 per credit. Tuition, nonresident: full-time $17,376; part-time $724 per credit. *Required fees:* $604; $22 per credit. One-time fee: $74. *Financial support:* In 2015–16, 5 teaching assistantships with full tuition reimbursements (averaging $1,800 per year) were awarded; Federal Work-Study, scholarships/grants, health care benefits, and unspecified assistantships also available. Support available to part-time students. Financial award application deadline: 5/15; financial award applicants required to submit FAFSA. *Unit head:* Dr. Jane Williams, Dean, 401-456-8013, Fax: 401-456-9608, E-mail: jwilliams@ric.edu. *Application contact:* Graduate Studies, 401-456-8700.
Website: http://www.ric.edu/nursing/

Rivier University, School of Graduate Studies, Division of Nursing, Nashua, NH 03060. Offers adult psychiatric/mental health practitioner (MS); family nurse practitioner (MS); nursing education (MS). *Accreditation:* ACEN. *Program availability:* Part-time, evening/weekend. *Entrance requirements:* For master's, GRE, MAT. Electronic applications accepted.

Robert Morris University, Graduate Studies, School of Nursing and Health Sciences, Moon Township, PA 15108. Offers MSN, DNP. *Accreditation:* AACN. *Program availability:* Part-time, evening/weekend. *Faculty:* 15 full-time (12 women), 6 part-time/adjunct (all women). *Students:* 222 part-time (186 women); includes 26 minority (18 Black or African American, non-Hispanic/Latino; 1 Asian, non-Hispanic/Latino; 1 Hispanic/Latino; 6 Two or more races, non-Hispanic/Latino), 1 international. Average age 37. 151 applicants, 59% accepted, 76 enrolled. In 2015, 10 master's, 30 doctorates awarded. *Entrance requirements:* For master's, letters of recommendation. Additional exam requirements/recommendations for international students: Required—TOEFL (minimum score 550 paper-based; 79 iBT). *Application deadline:* For fall admission, 7/1 priority date for domestic and international students; for spring admission, 11/1 priority date for domestic and international students. Applications are processed on a rolling basis. Application fee: $35. Electronic applications accepted. *Expenses:* Contact institution. *Financial support:* Federal Work-Study, institutionally sponsored loans, and unspecified assistantships available. Financial award application deadline: 5/1; financial award applicants required to submit FAFSA. *Unit head:* Dr. Valerie M. Howard, Dean, 412-397-6801, Fax: 412-397-3277, E-mail: howardv@rmu.edu.
Website: http://www.rmu.edu/web/cms/schools/snhs/

Roberts Wesleyan College, Department of Nursing, Rochester, NY 14624-1997. Offers nursing education (MSN); nursing leadership and administration (MSN). *Accreditation:* AACN. *Program availability:* Evening/weekend, online learning. *Faculty:* 6 full-time (all women), 5 part-time/adjunct (3 women). *Students:* 66 full-time (64 women); includes 9 minority (6 Black or African American, non-Hispanic/Latino; 1 American Indian or Alaska Native, non-Hispanic/Latino; 2 Hispanic/Latino), 9 international. Average age 35. 53 applicants, 83% accepted, 41 enrolled. In 2015, 2 master's awarded. *Degree requirements:* For master's, thesis. *Entrance requirements:* For master's, minimum GPA of 3.0; BS in nursing; interview; RN license; resume; course work in statistics. Additional exam requirements/recommendations for international students: Required—TOEFL (minimum score 90 iBT), IELTS (minimum score 6.5). *Application deadline:* Applications are processed on a rolling basis. Application fee: $0. Electronic applications accepted. *Financial support:* In 2015–16, 49 students received support. Scholarships/grants available. Financial award applicants required to submit FAFSA. *Unit head:* Dr. Cheryl B. Crotser, Chairperson/Director of Graduate Program, 585-594-6668, E-mail: crotser_cheryl@roberts.edu. *Application contact:* Brenda Mutton, Admissions Coordinator, 585-594-6686, E-mail: mutton_brenda@roberts.edu.
Website: http://www.roberts.edu/gradnursing

Rowan University, Graduate School, College of Science and Mathematics, Department of Nursing, Glassboro, NJ 08028-1701. Offers MS. *Accreditation:* Electronic applications accepted. *Expenses:* Tuition, area resident: Full-time $8710; part-time $871 per credit. Tuition, state resident: full-time $8710; part-time $871 per credit. Tuition, nonresident: full-time $8710; part-time $871 per credit. *International tuition:* $8710 full-time. *Required fees:* $1510; $151 per credit.

Rush University, College of Nursing, Chicago, IL 60612. Offers MSN, DNP, PhD, Post-Graduate Certificate. *Accreditation:* AACN; AANA/CANAEP (one or more programs are accredited). *Program availability:* Part-time, online learning. *Faculty:* 43 full-time (40 women), 52 part-time/adjunct (49 women). *Students:* 368 full-time (314 women), 722 part-time (664 women); includes 252 minority (83 Black or African American, non-Hispanic/Latino; 4 American Indian or Alaska Native, non-Hispanic/Latino; 77 Asian, non-Hispanic/Latino; 86 Hispanic/Latino; 2 Native Hawaiian or other Pacific Islander, non-Hispanic/Latino). Average age 31. In 2015, 249 master's, 68 doctorates awarded. *Degree requirements:* For master's, thesis, capstone project; for doctorate, leadership project (for DNP); dissertation (for PhD). *Entrance requirements:* For master's, GRE General Test (waived if cumulative GPA is 3.25 or greater, nursing GPA is 3.0 or greater, or completed graduate program GPA is 3.5 or greater), interview, 3 letters of recommendation, personal statement, current resume; for doctorate, GRE General Test (for DNP in nurse anesthesia and PhD; waived for DNP if cumulative GPA is 3.25 or greater, nursing GPA is 3.0 or greater, or a completed graduate program GPA is 3.5 or greater), interview, 3 letters of recommendation, personal statement, current resume; for Post-Graduate Certificate, MSN in a clinical discipline, 3 letters of recommendation, personal statement, current resume, interview. Additional exam requirements/recommendations for international students: Required—TOEFL (minimum score 94 iBT). *Application deadline:* For fall admission, 1/2 for domestic students; for winter admission, 10/15 for domestic students; for spring admission, 8/3 for domestic students; for summer admission, 12/1 for domestic students. Applications are processed on a rolling basis. Application fee: $100. Electronic applications accepted. *Expenses:* Contact institution. *Financial support:* Research assistantships, teaching assistantships, Federal Work-Study, scholarships/grants, traineeships, and health care benefits available. Support available to part-time students. Financial award application deadline: 3/1; financial award applicants required to submit FAFSA. *Faculty research:* Physical activity adherence in African-American women; reduction of health disparities; evidence-based interventions for caregivers; benefit of human milk feedings for low birth weight infants; patient-centered quality assessment of psychiatric inpatient environments. *Total annual research expenditures:* $3.1 million. *Unit head:* Dr. Marquis Foreman, Dean, 312-942-7117, Fax: 312-942-3043, E-mail: marquis_d_foreman@rush.edu. *Application contact:* Jennifer Thorndyke, Admissions Specialist for the College of Nursing, 312-563-7526, E-mail: jennifer_thorndyke@rush.edu.
Website: http://www.rushu.rush.edu/nursing/

Rutgers University–Newark, Rutgers School of Nursing, Newark, NJ 07107-3001. Offers adult health (MSN); adult occupational health (MSN); advanced practice nursing (MSN, Post Master's Certificate); family nurse practitioner (MSN); nurse anesthesia (MSN); nursing (MSN); nursing informatics (MSN); urban health (PhD); women's health practitioner (MSN). *Accreditation:* AANA/CANAEP. *Program availability:* Part-time. *Entrance requirements:* For master's, GRE, RN license; basic life support, statistics, and health assessment experience. Additional exam requirements/recommendations for international students: Required—TOEFL. Electronic applications accepted. *Expenses:* Contact institution. *Faculty research:* HIV/AIDS, diabetes education, learned helplessness, nursing science, psychoeducation.

Sacred Heart University, Graduate Programs, College of Nursing, Fairfield, CT 06825. Offers clinical nurse leader (MSN); clinical practice (DNP); family nurse practitioner (MSN, Graduate Certificate); leadership (DNP); nurse educator (MSN); nursing management and executive leadership (MSN); patient care services (MSN). *Accreditation:* AACN. *Program availability:* Part-time, evening/weekend, online learning. *Faculty:* 17 full-time (all women), 21 part-time/adjunct (18 women). *Students:* 19 full-time (18 women), 777 part-time (711 women); includes 144 minority (56 Black or African American, non-Hispanic/Latino; 2 American Indian or Alaska Native, non-Hispanic/Latino; 33 Asian, non-Hispanic/Latino; 41 Hispanic/Latino; 2 Native Hawaiian or other Pacific Islander, non-Hispanic/Latino; 10 Two or more races, non-Hispanic/Latino). Average age 38. 116 applicants, 53% accepted, 50 enrolled. In 2015, 192 master's, 13 doctorates awarded. *Degree requirements:* For master's, thesis, 500 clinical hours. *Entrance requirements:* For master's, minimum GPA of 3.0, BSN or RN plus BS (for MSN); for doctorate, minimum GPA of 3.0, MSN or BSN plus MS in related field (for DNP). Additional exam requirements/recommendations for international students: Required—PTE; Recommended—TOEFL (minimum score 570 paper-based; 80 iBT), IELTS (minimum score 6.5). *Application deadline:* For fall admission, 2/15 for domestic and international students. Applications are processed on a rolling basis. Application fee: $75. Electronic applications accepted. *Expenses:* Contact institution. *Financial support:* Unspecified assistantships available. Financial award applicants required to submit FAFSA. *Unit head:* Mary Alice Donius, Dean of Nursing, 203-365-4508, E-mail: doniusm@sacredheart.edu. *Application contact:* William Sweeney, Director of Graduate Admissions Operations, 203-365-4716, Fax: 203-365-4732, E-mail: gradstudies@sacredheart.edu.
Website: http://www.sacredheart.edu/academics/collegeofhealthprofessions/academicprograms/nursing/nursingprograms/graduateprograms/

Sage Graduate School, School of Health Sciences, Department of Nursing, Troy, NY 12180-4115. Offers adult gerontology nurse practitioner (MS, Certificate); education and leadership (DNS); family nurse practitioner (MS, Post Master's Certificate), including adult gerontology acute care (Post Master's Certificate), family nurse practitioner (MS),

Nursing—General

family psychiatric mental health (Post Master's Certificate); gerontological nurse practitioner (Post Master's Certificate); nurse administrator/executive (Post Master's Certificate); psychiatric mental health nurse clinical nurse specialist (MS); psychiatric mental health nurse practitioner (MS, Post Master's Certificate), including psychiatric mental health. *Accreditation:* AACN. *Program availability:* Part-time, evening/weekend. *Faculty:* 9 full-time (all women), 27 part-time/adjunct (24 women). *Students:* 45 full-time (43 women), 198 part-time (180 women); includes 36 minority (15 Black or African American, non-Hispanic/Latino; 2 American Indian or Alaska Native, non-Hispanic/Latino; 12 Asian, non-Hispanic/Latino; 4 Hispanic/Latino; 3 Two or more races, non-Hispanic/Latino), 3 international. Average age 38. 212 applicants, 36% accepted, 45 enrolled. In 2015, 18 master's, 8 doctorates, 9 other advanced degrees awarded. *Degree requirements:* For master's, thesis or alternative. *Entrance requirements:* For master's, currently licensed as registered professional nurse in state of practice; baccalaureate degree in nursing from nationally-accredited program or its international equivalent. Additional exam requirements/recommendations for international students: Required—TOEFL (minimum score 550 paper-based). *Application deadline:* Applications are processed on a rolling basis. Application fee: $40. Electronic applications accepted. *Expenses: Tuition, area resident:* Full-time $12,240; part-time $680 per credit hour. Tuition and fees vary according to degree level and program. *Financial support:* Fellowships, research assistantships, Federal Work-Study, scholarships/grants, and unspecified assistantships available. Support available to part-time students. Financial award application deadline: 3/1; financial award applicants required to submit FAFSA. *Unit head:* Dr. Theresa Hand, Dean, School of Health Sciences, 518-244-2064, Fax: 518-244-4571, E-mail: handt@sage.edu. *Application contact:* Dr. Carol Braungart, Co-Director, Graduate Nursing Program, 518-244-2459, Fax: 518-244-2009, E-mail: braunc@sage.edu.

Saginaw Valley State University, College of Health and Human Services, Program in Clinical Nurse Specialist, University Center, MI 48710. Offers MSN. *Accreditation:* AACN. *Program availability:* Part-time, evening/weekend. *Degree requirements:* For master's, thesis optional. *Entrance requirements:* Additional exam requirements/recommendations for international students: Required—TOEFL (minimum score 580 paper-based; 92 iBT). *Application deadline:* For fall admission, 7/15 for international students; for winter admission, 11/15 for international students; for spring admission, 4/15 for international students. Applications are processed on a rolling basis. Application fee: $30 ($90 for international students). Electronic applications accepted. *Expenses:* Tuition, state resident: full-time $9515; part-time $514 per credit hour. Tuition, nonresident: full-time $17,899; part-time $980 per credit hour. *Required fees:* $263; $14.60 per credit hour. Tuition and fees vary according to degree level. *Financial support:* Federal Work-Study and scholarships/grants available. Support available to part-time students. Financial award application deadline: 4/1; financial award applicants required to submit FAFSA. *Unit head:* Dr. Karen Brown-Fackler, Coordinator, 989-964-7112, Fax: 989-964-4925, E-mail: kmbrown4@svsu.edu. *Application contact:* Jenna Briggs, Director, Graduate and International Admissions, 989-964-6096, Fax: 989-964-2788, E-mail: gradadm@svsu.edu.

Saginaw Valley State University, College of Health and Human Services, Program in Nursing, University Center, MI 48710. Offers MSN. *Accreditation:* AACN. *Program availability:* Part-time, evening/weekend. *Students:* 1 (woman) full-time, 17 part-time (15 women); includes 2 minority (1 Hispanic/Latino; 1 Two or more races, non-Hispanic/Latino). Average age 35. 4 applicants, 100% accepted, 4 enrolled. In 2015, 3 master's awarded. *Entrance requirements:* For master's, GRE, minimum GPA of 3.0. Additional exam requirements/recommendations for international students: Required—TOEFL (minimum score 580 paper-based; 92 iBT). *Application deadline:* For fall admission, 7/15 for international students; for winter admission, 11/15 for international students; for spring admission, 4/15 for international students. Applications are processed on a rolling basis. Application fee: $30 ($90 for international students). Electronic applications accepted. *Expenses:* Tuition, state resident: full-time $9515; part-time $514 per credit hour. Tuition, nonresident: full-time $17,899; part-time $980 per credit hour. *Required fees:* $263; $14.60 per credit hour. Tuition and fees vary according to degree level. *Financial support:* Federal Work-Study and scholarships/grants available. Support available to part-time students. *Unit head:* Dr. Karen Brown-Fackler, Coordinator, 989-964-2185, Fax: 989-964-4925, E-mail: kmbrown4@svsu.edu. *Application contact:* Jenna Briggs, Director, Graduate and International Admissions, 989-964-6096, Fax: 989-964-2788, E-mail: gradadm@svsu.edu.

St. Ambrose University, College of Education and Health Sciences, Program in Nursing, Davenport, IA 52803-2898. Offers MSN. *Accreditation:* AACN. *Program availability:* Part-time, evening/weekend. *Entrance requirements:* Additional exam requirements/recommendations for international students: Required—TOEFL. Electronic applications accepted.

Saint Anthony College of Nursing, Graduate Program, Rockford, IL 61108-2468. Offers MSN. *Accreditation:* AACN. *Program availability:* Part-time.

St. Catherine University, Graduate Programs, Program in Nursing, St. Paul, MN 55105. Offers adult gerontological nurse practitioner (MS); neonatal nurse practitioner (MS); nurse educator (MS); nursing (DNP); nursing: entry-level (MS); pediatric nurse practitioner (MS). *Accreditation:* ACEN. *Program availability:* Part-time, evening/weekend. *Degree requirements:* For master's, thesis; for doctorate, portfolio, systems change project. *Entrance requirements:* For master's, GRE General Test, bachelor's degree in nursing, current nursing license, 2 years of recent clinical practice; for doctorate, master's degree in nursing, RN license, advanced nursing position. Additional exam requirements/recommendations for international students: Required—TOEFL (minimum score 600 paper-based; 100 iBT). *Expenses:* Contact institution.

Saint Francis Medical Center College of Nursing, Graduate Programs, Peoria, IL 61603-3783. Offers adult gerontology (MSN); clinical nurse leader (MSN); family nurse practitioner (MSN); family psychiatric mental health nurse practitioner (MSN); neonatal nurse practitioner (MSN); nurse clinician (Post-Graduate Certificate); nurse educator (MSN, Post-Graduate Certificate); nursing (DNP); nursing management leadership (MSN). *Accreditation:* ACEN. *Program availability:* Part-time, 100% online, blended/hybrid learning. *Faculty:* 14 full-time (all women), 5 part-time/adjunct (all women). *Students:* 13 full-time (12 women), 257 part-time (228 women); includes 23 minority (14 Black or African American, non-Hispanic/Latino; 3 Asian, non-Hispanic/Latino; 4 Hispanic/Latino; 2 Two or more races, non-Hispanic/Latino). Average age 37. 86 applicants, 86% accepted, 44 enrolled. In 2015, 61 master's, 6 doctorates awarded. *Degree requirements:* For master's, research experience, portfolio, practicum; for doctorate, practicum hours. *Entrance requirements:* For master's, nursing research, health assessment, graduate course work in statistics, RN license; for doctorate, master's degree in nursing, professional portfolio, graduate statistics, transcripts, RN license. Additional exam requirements/recommendations for international students: Required—TOEFL (minimum score 550 paper-based; 79 iBT). *Application deadline:* For fall admission, 6/1 priority date for domestic and international students; for spring admission, 11/15 priority date for domestic and international students. Applications are processed on a rolling basis. Application fee: $50. *Financial support:* In 2015–16, 18 students received support. Scholarships/grants and tuition waivers (partial) available. Support available to part-time students. Financial award application deadline: 6/15; financial award applicants required to submit FAFSA. *Faculty research:* Outcome and

curriculum planning, health promotion, NCLEX-RN results, decision-making program evaluation. *Unit head:* Dr. Patti A. Stockert, President of the College, 309-655-4124, Fax: 309-624-8973, E-mail: patricia.a.stockert@osfhealthcare.org. *Application contact:* Dr. Kim A. Mitchell, Dean, Graduate Program, 309-655-2201, Fax: 309-624-8973, E-mail: kim.a.mitchell@osfhealthcare.org.
Website: http://www.sfmccon.edu/graduate-programs/

St. John Fisher College, Wegmans School of Nursing, Advanced Practice Nursing Program, Rochester, NY 14618-3597. Offers advanced practice nursing (MS); clinical nurse specialist (Certificate); family nurse practitioner (Certificate). *Accreditation:* AACN. *Program availability:* Part-time, evening/weekend. *Faculty:* 11 full-time (10 women), 7 part-time/adjunct (6 women). *Students:* 7 full-time (all women), 129 part-time (122 women); includes 18 minority (10 Black or African American, non-Hispanic/Latino; 3 Asian, non-Hispanic/Latino; 5 Hispanic/Latino), 2 international. Average age 32. 76 applicants, 50% accepted, 29 enrolled. In 2015, 25 master's awarded. *Degree requirements:* For master's, clinical practice, project; for Certificate, clinical practice. *Entrance requirements:* For master's, BSN; undergraduate course work in statistics, health assessment, and nursing research; current New York State RN license; 2 letters of recommendation; current resume. Additional exam requirements/recommendations for international students: Required—TOEFL (minimum score 575 paper-based; 80 iBT). *Application deadline:* Applications are processed on a rolling basis. Application fee: $30. Electronic applications accepted. *Expenses:* $860 per credit hour. *Financial support:* Scholarships/grants and traineeships available. Financial award applicants required to submit FAFSA. *Faculty research:* Chronic illness, pediatric injury, women's health, public health policy, health care teams. *Unit head:* Dr. Colleen Donegan, Graduate Director, 585-899-3788, Fax: 585-385-8466, E-mail: cdonegan@sjfc.edu. *Application contact:* Rebecca Norman, Associate Director of Transfer and Graduate Admissions, 585-385-8064, E-mail: rnorman@sjfc.edu.

St. John Fisher College, Wegmans School of Nursing, Doctor of Nursing Practice Program, Rochester, NY 14618-3597. Offers DNP. *Program availability:* Part-time, evening/weekend. *Faculty:* 5 full-time (4 women), 3 part-time/adjunct (2 women). *Students:* 15 full-time (14 women), 12 part-time (11 women); includes 6 minority (4 Black or African American, non-Hispanic/Latino; 2 Asian, non-Hispanic/Latino). Average age 37. 9 applicants, 89% accepted, 7 enrolled. In 2015, 4 doctorates awarded. *Degree requirements:* For doctorate, 1,000 hours of clinical practice, clinical scholarship project. *Entrance requirements:* For doctorate, New York State RN License; New York State Certificate as advanced practice nurse (APN) or eligibility and National Professional Certification in APN specialty; currently practicing as APN; 2 letters of recommendation; writing sample. *Application deadline:* For fall admission, 8/1 for domestic students; for spring admission, 12/1 for domestic students. Applications are processed on a rolling basis. Application fee: $0. Electronic applications accepted. *Expenses:* $1,200 per credit hour. *Financial support:* Scholarships/grants available. Financial award applicants required to submit FAFSA. *Unit head:* Dr. John Kirchgessner, Program Director, 585-899-3739, E-mail: jKirchgessner@sjfc.edu. *Application contact:* Rebecca Norman, Associate Director of Transfer and Graduate Admissions, 585-385-8064, E-mail: rnorman@sjfc.edu.
Website: http://www.sjfc.edu/academics/nursing/departments/dnp/

St. Joseph's College, Long Island Campus, Program in Nursing, Patchogue, NY 11772-2399. Offers MS. *Faculty:* 1 (woman) part-time/adjunct. *Students:* 18 part-time (17 women); includes 6 minority (2 Black or African American, non-Hispanic/Latino; 2 Asian, non-Hispanic/Latino; 2 Hispanic/Latino). Average age 44. 10 applicants, 90% accepted, 8 enrolled. In 2015, 3 master's awarded. *Expenses: Tuition, area resident:* Full-time $14,850; part-time $825 per credit. *Required fees:* $440. *Unit head:* Florence Jerdan, Associate Chair/Director, 631-687-5180, E-mail: fjerdan@sjcny.edu.
Website: http://www.sjcny.edu

St. Joseph's College, New York, Program in Nursing, Brooklyn, NY 11205-3688. Offers MS. *Accreditation:* ACEN. *Faculty:* 1 (woman) part-time/adjunct. *Students:* 33 part-time (30 women); includes 30 minority (27 Black or African American, non-Hispanic/Latino; 1 Hispanic/Latino; 2 Two or more races, non-Hispanic/Latino). Average age 44. 13 applicants, 85% accepted, 10 enrolled. In 2015, 7 master's awarded. *Expenses: Tuition, area resident:* Full-time $14,850; part-time $825 per credit. *Required fees:* $440. *Unit head:* Florence Jerdan, Associate Professor/Director, 718-940-9892, E-mail: fjerdan@sjcny.edu.
Website: http://www.sjcny.edu

Saint Joseph's College of Maine, Master of Science in Nursing Program, Standish, ME 04084. Offers administration (MSN); education (MSN); family nurse practitioner (MSN); nursing administration and leadership (Certificate); nursing and health care education (Certificate). *Accreditation:* AACN. *Program availability:* Part-time, online learning. *Entrance requirements:* For master's, MAT. Electronic applications accepted.

Saint Louis University, Graduate Education, Doisy College of Health Sciences, School of Nursing, St. Louis, MO 63104-1099. Offers MSN, DNP, PhD, Certificate. *Accreditation:* AACN. *Program availability:* Part-time, online learning. *Degree requirements:* For master's, comprehensive exam, thesis optional; for doctorate, comprehensive exam, thesis/dissertation, preliminary exams. *Entrance requirements:* For master's, 3 letters of recommendation, resumé, transcripts; for doctorate, GRE General Test, 3 letters of recommendation, curriculum vitae; for Certificate, 3 letters of recommendation, resumé, transcripts, copy of RN license, personal statement. Additional exam requirements/recommendations for international students: Required—TOEFL (minimum score 525 paper-based). Electronic applications accepted. *Faculty research:* Sensory enhancement to the elderly, fall prevention in elderly, tube feeding placement and gastroenterology, patient outcomes, exercise behavior in the older adult.

Saint Mary's College, Graduate Programs, Doctorate of Nursing Practice Program, Notre Dame, IN 46556. Offers DNP. *Program availability:* Part-time-only, online only, blended/hybrid learning. *Faculty:* 8 full-time (all women). *Students:* 8 part-time (7 women). Average age 30. 17 applicants, 76% accepted, 8 enrolled. *Degree requirements:* For doctorate, comprehensive exam, thesis/dissertation. *Entrance requirements:* For doctorate, BSN or MSN, unencumbered RN license or eligibility for RN licensure. Additional exam requirements/recommendations for international students: Recommended—TOEFL, IELTS. *Application deadline:* For fall admission, 6/15 priority date for domestic and international students. Applications are processed on a rolling basis. Application fee: $0. Electronic applications accepted. *Expenses:* $5,012 per term. *Financial support:* Application deadline: 3/1; applicants required to submit FAFSA. *Faculty research:* Suicide prevention, infant death prevention, delirium management, teaching methodologies, and nurses' perceptions of care. *Unit head:* Linda Paskiewicz, Director of the Department of Nursing, 574-284-4679, E-mail: lpaskie@saintmarys.edu. *Application contact:* Melissa Fruscione, Graduate Admission, 574-284-5098, E-mail: graduateadmission@saintmarys.edu.
Website: https://grad.saintmarys.edu/academic-programs/doctorate-nursing-practice

Saint Peter's University, School of Nursing, Nursing Program, Jersey City, NJ 07306-5997. Offers adult nurse practitioner (MSN, Certificate); advanced practice (DNP); case management (MSN, DNP). *Accreditation:* AACN. *Program availability:* Part-time, evening/weekend. *Entrance requirements:* Additional exam requirements/recommendations for international students: Required—TOEFL. Electronic applications accepted.

Saint Xavier University, Graduate Studies, School of Nursing, Chicago, IL 60655-3105. Offers MSN, Certificate, MBA/MS. *Accreditation:* AACN. *Program availability:* Part-time, evening/weekend. *Entrance requirements:* For master's, GRE General Test or MAT, minimum GPA of 3.0, RN license.

Salem State University, School of Graduate Studies, Program in Nursing, Salem, MA 01970-5353. Offers adult-gerontology primary care nursing (MSN); nursing administration (MSN); nursing education (MSN); MBA/MSN. *Accreditation:* AACN. *Program availability:* Part-time, evening/weekend. *Entrance requirements:* For master's, GRE or MAT. Additional exam requirements/recommendations for international students: Required—TOEFL (minimum score 550 paper-based; 80 iBT) or IELTS (minimum score 5.5).

Salisbury University, DNP in Nursing Program, Salisbury, MD 21801-6837. Offers family nurse practitioner (DNP); nursing (DNP); nursing leadership (DNP). *Accreditation:* AACN. *Program availability:* Part-time. *Faculty:* 7 full-time (5 women). *Students:* 22 full-time (20 women), 1 (woman) part-time; includes 9 minority (7 Black or African American, non-Hispanic/Latino; 1 Hispanic/Latino; 1 Two or more races, non-Hispanic/Latino). Average age 35. 16 applicants, 56% accepted, 6 enrolled. In 2015, 8 doctorates awarded. Terminal master's awarded for partial completion of doctoral program. *Entrance requirements:* For doctorate, undergraduate nursing degree with minimum cumulative GPA of 3.0; current and active United States Registered Nurse license; current resume or curriculum vitae; essay; 3 letters of recommendation. Additional exam requirements/recommendations for international students: Required—TOEFL (minimum score 550 paper-based, 79 iBT) or IELTS (6.5). *Application deadline:* For fall admission, 5/15 priority date for domestic students, 3/15 priority date for international students. Applications are processed on a rolling basis. Application fee: $65. Electronic applications accepted. *Expenses:* $620 per credit hour resident; $787 per credit hour non-resident; $78 per credit hour fees. *Financial support:* In 2015–16, 18 students received support. Career-related internships or fieldwork, institutionally sponsored loans, scholarships/grants, and unspecified assistantships available. Support available to part-time students. Financial award application deadline: 3/1; financial award applicants required to submit FAFSA. *Faculty research:* Intimate partner violence; telehealth; nursing faculty shortage; oral health needs; gerontology. *Unit head:* Dr. Lisa Seldomridge, Graduate Program Director, Nursing (DNP), 410-543-6344, Fax: 410-548-3313, E-mail: laseldomridge@salisbury.edu. *Application contact:* Carmel Boger, Administrative Assistant, 410-543-6420, Fax: 410-548-3313, E-mail: ciboger@salisbury.edu.
Website: http://www.salisbury.edu/gsr/gradstudies/DNPpage.html

Salisbury University, MS in Nursing Program, Salisbury, MD 21801-6837. Offers clinical nurse educator (MS); health care leadership (MS); nursing (MS). *Program availability:* Part-time. *Faculty:* 5 full-time (3 women). *Students:* 6 part-time (5 women); includes 1 minority (Black or African American, non-Hispanic/Latino). Average age 33. 1 applicant. In 2015, 6 master's awarded. *Degree requirements:* For master's, thesis. *Entrance requirements:* For master's, BS in nursing with minimum cumulative GPA of 3.0; current and active United States Registered Nursing license; current resume or curriculum vitae; personal statement; 2 letters of reference; interview. Additional exam requirements/recommendations for international students: Required—TOEFL (minimum score 550 paper-based, 79 iBT) or IELTS (6.5). *Application deadline:* For fall admission, 5/15 priority date for domestic and international students. Applications are processed on a rolling basis. Application fee: $65. Electronic applications accepted. *Expenses:* $620 per credit hour resident; $787 per credit hour non-resident; $78 per credit hour fees. *Financial support:* In 2015–16, 18 students received support, including 1 research assistantship with full tuition reimbursement available (averaging $8,000 per year); career-related internships or fieldwork, institutionally sponsored loans, scholarships/grants, and unspecified assistantships also available. Support available to part-time students. Financial award application deadline: 3/1; financial award applicants required to submit FAFSA. *Faculty research:* Gerontology; epidemiology; palliative care; global health; depression. *Unit head:* Dr. Lisa Seldomridge, Graduate Program Director, Nursing, 410-543-6344, Fax: 410-548-3313, E-mail: laseldomridge@salisbury.edu. *Application contact:* Carmel Boger, Administrative Assistant, 410-543-6420, Fax: 410-548-3313, E-mail: ciboger@salisbury.edu.
Website: http://www.salisbury.edu/gsr/gradstudies/MSNpage.html

Salve Regina University, Program in Nursing, Newport, RI 02840-4192. Offers DNP. *Program availability:* Part-time, evening/weekend. *Entrance requirements:* For doctorate, BS in nursing with minimum cumulative GPA of 3.0, unencumbered license or eligibility for RN licensure in the state of Rhode Island, clear criminal background check, course in statistics. Electronic applications accepted.

Samford University, Ida V. Moffett School of Nursing, Birmingham, AL 35229. Offers administration (DNP); advanced practice (DNP); family nurse practitioner (MSN); health systems management and leadership (MSN); nurse anesthesia (MSN); nurse educator (MSN). *Accreditation:* AACN; AANA/CANAEP (one or more programs are accredited). *Program availability:* Part-time, blended/hybrid learning. *Faculty:* 19 full-time (all women), 5 part-time/adjunct (1 woman). *Students:* 300 full-time (228 women), 40 part-time (36 women); includes 65 minority (28 Black or African American, non-Hispanic/Latino; 4 American Indian or Alaska Native, non-Hispanic/Latino; 8 Asian, non-Hispanic/Latino; 13 Hispanic/Latino; 12 Two or more races, non-Hispanic/Latino). Average age 35. 69 applicants, 77% accepted, 52 enrolled. In 2015, 98 master's, 16 doctorates awarded. *Degree requirements:* For doctorate, capstone project with oral presentation. *Entrance requirements:* For master's, MAT; GRE (for nurse anesthesia), unencumbered licensure as registered nurse; BSN from CCNE, CNEA, or ACEN (formerly NLNAC) accredited program; minimum cumulative GPA of 3.0 in nursing courses; video submission; one undergraduate course in nursing research with minimum grade of C; for doctorate, unencumbered licensure as registered nurse; master's degree from CCNE, CNEA or ACEN (formerly NLNAC) accredited program in the area of advanced practice or administration; minimum master's degree cumulative GPA of 3.5; video interview submission. Additional exam requirements/recommendations for international students: Required—TOEFL (minimum score 550 paper-based; 80 iBT). *Application deadline:* For fall admission, 6/1 for domestic and international students; for spring admission, 9/1 for domestic and international students. Application fee: $65. Electronic applications accepted. *Expenses: Tuition,* area resident: Full-time $18,673; part-time $766 per credit hour. *Required fees:* $550. Tuition and fees vary according to course load, degree level and student level. *Financial support:* In 2015–16, 56 students received support. Institutionally sponsored loans, scholarships/grants, and traineeships available. Financial award application deadline: 3/1; financial award applicants required to submit FAFSA. *Faculty research:* Issues in rural health care, vulnerable populations, genetics and disabilities in pediatrics, geriatrics, parish nursing research, interprofessional education, global health disparities. *Unit head:* Dr. Nena F. Sanders, Vice Provost, College of Health Sciences/Dean/Professor, 205-726-2612, Fax: 205-726-4179, E-mail: nfsander@samford.edu. *Application contact:* Allyson Maddox, Director of Graduate Student Services, Ida V. Moffett School of Nursing, 205-726-2047, Fax: 205-726-4179, E-mail: amaddox@samford.edu.
Website: http://samford.edu/nursing

Samuel Merritt University, School of Nursing, Oakland, CA 94609. Offers case management (MSN); family nurse practitioner (MSN, Certificate); nurse anesthetist (MSN, Certificate); nursing (DNP). *Accreditation:* AACN; AANA/CANAEP (one or more programs are accredited). *Program availability:* Part-time, evening/weekend, 100% online, blended/hybrid learning. *Faculty:* 47 full-time (40 women), 50 part-time/adjunct (43 women). *Students:* 437 full-time (350 women), 59 part-time (45 women); includes 327 minority (29 Black or African American, non-Hispanic/Latino; 3 American Indian or Alaska Native, non-Hispanic/Latino; 163 Asian, non-Hispanic/Latino; 95 Hispanic/Latino; 9 Native Hawaiian or other Pacific Islander, non-Hispanic/Latino; 28 Two or more races, non-Hispanic/Latino). Average age 33. 392 applicants, 43% accepted, 126 enrolled. In 2015, 31 master's awarded. *Degree requirements:* For master's, thesis or alternative. *Entrance requirements:* For master's, minimum GPA of 2.5 in science, 3.0 overall; previous course work in statistics; current RN license. Additional exam requirements/recommendations for international students: Required—TOEFL (minimum score 100 iBT). *Application deadline:* For fall admission, 1/1 priority date for domestic students; for spring admission, 7/1 for domestic students; for summer admission, 1/1 for domestic students. Applications are processed on a rolling basis. Application fee: $50. Electronic applications accepted. *Expenses:* $61,299 tuition; $240 lab fees; $160 graduation fee. *Financial support:* In 2015–16, 34 students received support. Career-related internships or fieldwork, Federal Work-Study, scholarships/grants, and traineeships available. Support available to part-time students. Financial award application deadline: 3/2; financial award applicants required to submit FAFSA. *Faculty research:* Gerontology, community health, maternal-child health, sexually transmitted diseases, substance abuse, oncology. *Total annual research expenditures:* $35,000. *Unit head:* Dr. Audrey Berman, Graduate Coordinator, 510-869-6733, Fax: 510-869-6525. *Application contact:* Timothy Cranford, Dean of Admission, 510-869-6576, Fax: 510-869-6525, E-mail: admission@samuelmerritt.edu.
Website: http://www.samuelmerritt.edu/nursing

San Diego State University, Graduate and Research Affairs, College of Health and Human Services, School of Nursing, San Diego, CA 92182. Offers MS. *Accreditation:* AACN; ACNM/ACME. *Program availability:* Part-time, evening/weekend. *Entrance requirements:* For master's, GRE General Test, previous course work in statistics and physical assessment, 3 letters of recommendation, California RN license. Additional exam requirements/recommendations for international students: Required—TOEFL. Electronic applications accepted. *Faculty research:* Health promotion, nursing systems and leadership, maternal-child nursing, advanced practice nursing, child oral health.

San Francisco State University, Division of Graduate Studies, College of Health and Social Sciences, School of Nursing, San Francisco, CA 94132-1722. Offers adult acute care (MS); clinical nurse specialist (MS); community/public health nursing (MS); family nurse practitioner (MS, Certificate); nursing administration (MS); pediatrics (MS); women's health (MS). *Accreditation:* AACN. *Program availability:* Part-time. *Application deadline:* Applications are processed on a rolling basis. *Expenses:* Tuition, state resident: full-time $6738. Tuition, nonresident: full-time $15,666. *Required fees:* $1004. *Financial support:* Career-related internships or fieldwork available. *Unit head:* Dr. Mary-Ann van Dam, Director, 415-338-1802, Fax: 415-338-0555, E-mail: vandam@sfsu.edu. *Application contact:* Connie Carr, Graduate Coordinator, 415-338-6856, Fax: 415-338-0555, E-mail: ccarr@sfsu.edu.
Website: http://nursing.sfsu.edu

Seattle Pacific University, MS in Nursing Program, Seattle, WA 98119-1997. Offers administration (MSN); adult/gerontology nurse practitioner (MSN); clinical nurse specialist (MSN); family nurse practitioner (MSN, Certificate); informatics (MSN); nurse educator (MSN). *Accreditation:* AACN. *Program availability:* Part-time. *Students:* 39 full-time (36 women), 30 part-time (25 women); includes 14 minority (3 Black or African American, non-Hispanic/Latino; 7 Asian, non-Hispanic/Latino; 3 Hispanic/Latino; 1 Two or more races, non-Hispanic/Latino), 1 international. Average age 38. 60 applicants, 48% accepted, 29 enrolled. In 2015, 23 master's awarded. *Degree requirements:* For master's, thesis. *Entrance requirements:* For master's, personal statement, transcripts, undergraduate nursing degree, proof of undergraduate statistics course with minimum GPA of 2.0, 2 recommendations. *Application deadline:* For fall admission, 1/15 priority date for domestic students; for spring admission, 1/15 for domestic students. Applications are processed on a rolling basis. Application fee: $50. Electronic applications accepted. *Expenses:* Contact institution. *Financial support:* Fellowships and scholarships/grants available. Financial award applicants required to submit FAFSA. *Unit head:* Dr. Christine Hoyle, Associate Dean, 206-281-2469, E-mail: hoylec@spu.edu.
Website: http://spu.edu/depts/health-sciences/grad/index.asp

Seattle University, College of Nursing, Doctor of Nursing Practice Program, Seattle, WA 98122-1090. Offers DNP. *Program availability:* Evening/weekend. *Degree requirements:* For doctorate, capstone project. *Entrance requirements:* For doctorate, letter of intent.

Seattle University, College of Nursing, Program in Advanced Practice Nursing Immersion, Seattle, WA 98122-1090. Offers adult/gerontological nurse practitioner (MSN); advanced community public health nursing (MSN); family nurse practitioner (MSN); family psychiatric mental health nurse practitioner (MSN); nurse midwifery (MSN). *Degree requirements:* For master's, thesis or scholarly project. *Entrance requirements:* For master's, GRE, bachelor's degree, minimum GPA of 3.0, professional resume, two recommendations, letter of intent. Additional exam requirements/recommendations for international students: Required—TOEFL (minimum score 92 iBT), IELTS. Electronic applications accepted.

Seattle University, College of Nursing, Program in Nursing, Seattle, WA 98122-1090. Offers adult/gerontological nurse practitioner (MSN); advanced community public health (MSN); psychiatric mental health nurse practitioner (MSN). *Degree requirements:* For master's, thesis or scholarly project. *Entrance requirements:* For master's, GRE, bachelor's degree in nursing or associate degree in nursing with baccalaureate in different major, 5-quarter statistics course, minimum cumulative GPA of 3.0, professional resume, two recommendations, letter of intent, copy of current RN license or ability to obtain RN license in WA state. Additional exam requirements/recommendations for international students: Required—TOEFL (minimum score 92 iBT), IELTS. Electronic applications accepted.

Seton Hall University, College of Nursing, South Orange, NJ 07079-2697. Offers advanced practice in primary health care (MSN, DNP), including adult/gerontological nurse practitioner, pediatric nurse practitioner; entry into practice (MSN); health systems administration (MSN, DNP); nursing (PhD); nursing case management (MSN); nursing education (MA); school nurse (MSN); MSN/MA. *Accreditation:* AACN. *Program availability:* Part-time, online learning. *Degree requirements:* For master's, research project; for doctorate, dissertation or scholarly project. *Entrance requirements:* For doctorate, GRE (waived for students with GPA of 3.5 or higher). Additional exam requirements/recommendations for international students: Required—TOEFL. Electronic applications accepted. *Faculty research:* Parent/child, adult, and gerontological nursing; breast cancer; families of children with HIV; parish nursing.

Shenandoah University, Eleanor Wade Custer School of Nursing, Winchester, VA 22601. Offers family nurse practitioner (MSN, DNP, Post-Graduate Certificate); health informatics (Certificate); health systems leadership (DNP); nurse midwifery (MSN, Post-Graduate Certificate); nursing education (Post-Graduate Certificate); psychiatric mental

Nursing—General

health nurse practitioner (MSN, DNP, Post-Graduate Certificate). *Accreditation:* AACN; ACNM/ACME. *Faculty:* 10 full-time (all women), 7 part-time/adjunct (4 women). *Students:* 33 full-time (31 women), 62 part-time (57 women); includes 21 minority (17 Black or African American, non-Hispanic/Latino; 3 Asian, non-Hispanic/Latino; 1 Hispanic/Latino). Average age 36. 55 applicants, 87% accepted, 39 enrolled. In 2015, 32 master's, 3 doctorates, 19 other advanced degrees awarded. *Degree requirements:* For master's, research project, clinical hours; for doctorate, scholarly project, clinical hours; for other advanced degree, clinical hours. *Entrance requirements:* For master's, United States RN license; minimum GPA of 3.0; 2080 hours of clinical experience; curriculum vitae; 3 letters of recommendation from a former dean, a faculty member or advisor familiar with the applicant, and a former or current supervisor; two- to three-page essay on a specified topic; for doctorate, MSN, minimum GPA of 3.0, 3 letters of recommendation, 500-word statement, interview, BSN; for other advanced degree, MSN, minimum GPA of 3.0, 2 letters of recommendation, minimum of one year (2080 hours) of clinical nursing experience, interview. Additional exam requirements/recommendations for international students: Required—TOEFL (minimum score 558 paper-based; 83 iBT). *Application deadline:* For fall admission, 1/15 priority date for domestic and international students; for spring admission, 11/1 for domestic and international students; for summer admission, 3/15 for domestic and international students. Application fee: $30. Electronic applications accepted. *Expenses:* Contact institution. *Financial support:* In 2015–16, 13 students received support, including 3 fellowships (averaging $1,000 per year); scholarships/grants and unspecified assistantships also available. Financial award application deadline: 3/15; financial award applicants required to submit FAFSA. *Faculty research:* Primary care providers and their unique position in geriatric, pre-operative education and its effects on post-operative, variables associated with a woman's multidimensional childbirth, interdisciplinary communication, research on health policy. *Unit head:* Kathryn Ganske, PhD, RN, Dean, 540-678-4374, Fax: 540-665-5519, E-mail: kganske@su.edu. *Application contact:* Andrew Woodall, Executive Director of Recruitment and Admissions, 540-665-4581, Fax: 540-665-4627, E-mail: admit@su.edu.
Website: http://www.su.edu/nursing/

Simmons College, School of Nursing and Health Sciences, Boston, MA 02115. Offers didactic dietetics (Certificate); dietetic internship (Certificate); health education profession (PhD); health professions education (CAGS); nursing (MS), including family nurse practitioner; nursing practice (DNP); nutrition and health promotion (MS); physical therapy (DPT); sports nutrition (Certificate). *Program availability:* Part-time, blended/hybrid learning. *Faculty:* 21 full-time (17 women), 171 part-time/adjunct (157 women). *Students:* 333 full-time (305 women), 889 part-time (813 women); includes 250 minority (88 Black or African American, non-Hispanic/Latino; 3 American Indian or Alaska Native, non-Hispanic/Latino; 65 Asian, non-Hispanic/Latino; 67 Hispanic/Latino; 2 Native Hawaiian or other Pacific Islander, non-Hispanic/Latino; 25 Two or more races, non-Hispanic/Latino), 9 international. Average age 33. 846 applicants, 66% accepted, 441 enrolled. In 2015, 70 master's, 45 doctorates awarded. *Entrance requirements:* For doctorate, GRE. Additional exam requirements/recommendations for international students: Required—TOEFL (minimum score 570 paper-based; 88 iBT). *Application deadline:* For fall admission, 6/1 for international students. Application fee: $50. Electronic applications accepted. *Expenses:* Contact institution. *Financial support:* In 2015–16, 12 research assistantships (averaging $6,000 per year) were awarded; scholarships/grants and unspecified assistantships also available. *Unit head:* Dr. Judy Beal, Dean, 617-521-2139. *Application contact:* Brett DiMarzo, Director of Graduate Admission, 617-521-2651, Fax: 617-521-3137, E-mail: brett.dimarzo@simmons.edu. Website: http://www.simmons.edu/snhs/

Sonoma State University, School of Science and Technology, Family Nurse Practitioner Program, Rohnert Park, CA 94928. Offers MSN. *Accreditation:* ACEN. *Program availability:* Part-time. *Degree requirements:* For master's, comprehensive exam, thesis or alternative, oral exams. *Entrance requirements:* For master's, GRE General Test, BSN, minimum GPA of 3.0, course work in statistics, physical assessment, RN license. Additional exam requirements/recommendations for international students: Required—TOEFL (minimum score 500 paper-based). *Faculty research:* Neonatal ethics.

South Dakota State University, Graduate School, College of Nursing, Brookings, SD 57007. Offers MS, PhD. *Accreditation:* AACN. *Program availability:* Part-time, evening/weekend, online learning. *Degree requirements:* For master's, comprehensive exam, thesis (for some programs), oral exam. *Entrance requirements:* For master's, nurse registration; for doctorate, nurse registration, MS. Additional exam requirements/recommendations for international students: Required—TOEFL (minimum score 525 paper-based; 71 iBT). *Expenses:* Contact institution. *Faculty research:* Rural health, aging, health promotion, Native American health, woman's health, underserved populations, quality of life.

Southeast Missouri State University, School of Graduate Studies, Department of Nursing, Cape Girardeau, MO 63701-4799. Offers MSN. *Accreditation:* AACN. *Faculty:* 9 full-time (all women), 1 (woman) part-time/adjunct. *Students:* 12 full-time (10 women), 15 part-time (all women); includes 3 minority (2 Black or African American, non-Hispanic/Latino; 1 Hispanic/Latino). Average age 32. 21 applicants, 62% accepted, 12 enrolled. In 2015, 10 degrees awarded. *Degree requirements:* For master's, comprehensive exam, scholarly paper. *Entrance requirements:* For master's, baccalaureate degree with upper-division major in nursing from program accredited by the National League for Nursing or the Commission on Collegiate Nursing Education; minimum GPA of 3.25; current Missouri license as registered professional nurse; evidence of professional liability insurance. Additional exam requirements/recommendations for international students: Required—TOEFL (minimum score 550 paper-based; 79 iBT), IELTS (minimum score 6), PTE (minimum score 53). *Application deadline:* For fall admission, 4/1 for domestic and international students; for spring admission, 11/21 for domestic students, 10/1 for international students. Applications are processed on a rolling basis. Application fee: $30 ($40 for international students). Electronic applications accepted. *Expenses:* Tuition, state resident: part-time $260.80 per credit hour. Tuition, nonresident: part-time $486.80 per credit hour. *Required fees:* $33.70 per credit hour. *Financial support:* In 2015–16, 6 students received support, including 7 teaching assistantships with full tuition reimbursements available (averaging $8,467 per year); career-related internships or fieldwork, Federal Work-Study, scholarships/grants, traineeships, tuition waivers (full), and unspecified assistantships also available. Financial award application deadline: 6/30; financial award applicants required to submit FAFSA. *Faculty research:* Rural health, domestic abuse, substance abuse, use of simulation for nursing education, student retention and success. *Unit head:* Dr. Gloria Green, Chair, 573-651-5961, Fax: 573-651-2141, E-mail: gjgreen@semo.edu. *Application contact:* Dr. Elaine Jackson, Graduate Program Coordinator, 573-651-2871, Fax: 573-651-2141, E-mail: ejackson@semo.edu.
Website: http://www.semo.edu/nursing/

Southern Adventist University, School of Nursing, Collegedale, TN 37315-0370. Offers acute care nurse practitioner (MSN); adult nurse practitioner (MSN); family nurse practitioner (MSN); nurse educator (MSN); MSN/MSBA. *Accreditation:* ACEN. *Program availability:* Part-time. *Degree requirements:* For master's, thesis or project. *Entrance requirements:* For master's, RN license. Additional exam requirements/

recommendations for international students: Required—TOEFL (minimum score 600 paper-based). Electronic applications accepted. *Faculty research:* Pain management, ethics, corporate wellness, caring spirituality, stress.

Southern Connecticut State University, School of Graduate Studies, School of Health and Human Services, Department of Nursing, New Haven, CT 06515-1355. Offers family nurse practitioner (MSN); nursing education (MSN). *Accreditation:* AACN. *Program availability:* Part-time, evening/weekend. *Faculty:* 12 full-time (all women), 2 part-time/adjunct (both women). *Students:* 7 full-time (6 women), 80 part-time (70 women); includes 20 minority (8 Black or African American, non-Hispanic/Latino; 5 Asian, non-Hispanic/Latino; 6 Hispanic/Latino; 1 Two or more races, non-Hispanic/Latino). Average age 36. 112 applicants, 11% accepted, 11 enrolled. In 2015, 15 master's awarded. *Degree requirements:* For master's, thesis. *Entrance requirements:* For master's, GRE, MAT, interview, minimum QPA of 2.8, RN license, minimum 1 year of professional nursing experience. *Application deadline:* For fall admission, 7/15 priority date for domestic students. Applications are processed on a rolling basis. Application fee: $50. Electronic applications accepted. *Expenses:* Tuition, state resident: full-time $4968; part-time $494 per credit hour. Tuition, nonresident: full-time $16,078; part-time $509 per credit hour. *Required fees:* $4632; $55 per semester. Tuition and fees vary according to program. *Financial support:* Career-related internships or fieldwork, scholarships/grants, and unspecified assistantships available. Financial award application deadline: 4/15; financial award applicants required to submit FAFSA. *Unit head:* Dr. Lisa Rebeschi, Chairperson, 203-392-6485, E-mail: rebeschi1@southernct.edu. *Application contact:* Lisa Galvin, Director of Graduate Admissions, 203-392-5240, Fax: 203-392-5235, E-mail: galvinl1@southernct.edu.

Southern Illinois University Edwardsville, Graduate School, School of Nursing, Edwardsville, IL 62026. Offers MS, DNP, Post-Master's Certificate. *Accreditation:* AACN. *Program availability:* Part-time, evening/weekend. *Students:* 76 full-time (50 women), 180 part-time (165 women); includes 29 minority (12 Black or African American, non-Hispanic/Latino; 7 Asian, non-Hispanic/Latino; 6 Hispanic/Latino; 4 Two or more races, non-Hispanic/Latino). 87 applicants, 86% accepted. In 2015, 136 master's, 5 doctorates, 1 other advanced degree awarded. *Degree requirements:* For master's, comprehensive exam (for some programs), thesis or alternative; for doctorate, thesis/dissertation or alternative, project. *Entrance requirements:* For master's, appropriate bachelor's degree, RN license; for Post-Master's Certificate, minimum graduate nursing GPA of 3.0, completion of graduate-level statistics and epidemiology courses with minimum B grade, current unencumbered RN licensure. Additional exam requirements/recommendations for international students: Required—TOEFL (minimum score 550 paper-based; 79 iBT), IELTS (minimum score 6.5). *Application deadline:* For fall admission, 3/1 for domestic and international students; for summer admission, 6/1 for domestic and international students. Application fee: $30. Electronic applications accepted. *Expenses:* Tuition, state resident: full-time $5026; part-time $837 per course. Tuition, nonresident: full-time $12,566; part-time $2094 per course. *Required fees:* $1682; $474 per course. Tuition and fees vary according to course load, campus/location and program. *Financial support:* In 2015–16, 5 teaching assistantships with full tuition reimbursements were awarded; fellowships with full tuition reimbursements, research assistantships with full tuition reimbursements, institutionally sponsored loans, scholarships/grants, and unspecified assistantships also available. Financial award application deadline: 3/1; financial award applicants required to submit FAFSA. *Unit head:* Dr. Laura Bernaix, Interim Dean, 618-650-3956, Fax: 618-650-3854, E-mail: lbernai@siue.edu. *Application contact:* Bob Skorczewski, Coordinator of International and Graduate Recruitment, 618-650-3705, Fax: 618-650-3854, E-mail: gradadmissions@siue.edu.
Website: http://www.siue.edu/nursing/graduate

Southern Nazarene University, College of Professional and Graduate Studies, School of Nursing, Bethany, OK 73008. Offers nursing education (MS); nursing leadership (MS). *Accreditation:* AACN. *Program availability:* Part-time, evening/weekend. *Degree requirements:* For master's, thesis. *Entrance requirements:* For master's, minimum undergraduate cumulative GPA of 3.0; baccalaureate degree in nursing from nationally-accredited program; current unencumbered registered nurse licensure in Oklahoma or eligibility for same; documentation of basic computer skills; basic statistics course; statement of professional goals; three letters of recommendation. Additional exam requirements/recommendations for international students: Required—TOEFL (minimum score 550 paper-based).

Southern University and Agricultural and Mechanical College, School of Nursing, Baton Rouge, LA 70813. Offers educator/administrator (PhD); family health nursing (MSN); family nurse practitioner (Post Master's Certificate); geriatric nurse practitioner/gerontology (PhD). *Accreditation:* AACN. *Program availability:* Part-time. *Degree requirements:* For master's, comprehensive exam, thesis; for doctorate, comprehensive exam, thesis/dissertation. *Entrance requirements:* For master's, GRE General Test, BSN, minimum GPA of 2.7; for doctorate, GRE General Test; for Post Master's Certificate, MSN. Additional exam requirements/recommendations for international students: Required—TOEFL (minimum score 525 paper-based). *Faculty research:* Health promotions, vulnerable populations, (community-based) cardiovascular participating research, health disparities chronic diseases, care of the elderly.

South University, Graduate Programs, College of Nursing, Savannah, GA 31406. Offers nurse educator (MS).

South University, Program in Nursing, Tampa, FL 33614. Offers adult health nurse practitioner (MS); family nurse practitioner (MS); nurse educator (MS).

South University, Program in Nursing, Royal Palm Beach, FL 33411. Offers family nurse practitioner (MS).

South University, Program in Nursing, Montgomery, AL 36116-1120. Offers MSN.

South University, Program in Nursing, Columbia, SC 29203. Offers MSN.

South University, Program in Nursing, Novi, MI 48377. Offers MSN.

South University, Program in Nursing, Glen Allen, VA 23060. Offers MSN.

South University, Program in Nursing, Virginia Beach, VA 23452. Offers family nurse practitioner (MSN).

Spalding University, Graduate Studies, Kosair College of Health and Natural Sciences, School of Nursing, Louisville, KY 40203-2188. Offers adult nurse practitioner (MSN, PMC); family nurse practitioner (MSN, PMC); leadership in nursing and healthcare (MSN); pediatric nurse practitioner (MSN, PMC). *Accreditation:* AACN. *Program availability:* Part-time, evening/weekend. *Faculty:* 10 full-time (9 women), 8 part-time/adjunct (7 women). *Students:* 101 full-time (94 women), 9 part-time (all women); includes 20 minority (14 Black or African American, non-Hispanic/Latino; 3 Asian, non-Hispanic/Latino; 1 Native Hawaiian or other Pacific Islander, non-Hispanic/Latino; 2 Two or more races, non-Hispanic/Latino). Average age 36. 10 applicants, 30% accepted, 2 enrolled. In 2015, 43 master's awarded. *Degree requirements:* For master's, comprehensive exam (for some programs), thesis. *Entrance requirements:* For master's, GRE General Test, BSN or bachelor's degree in related field, RN licensure, autobiographical statement, transcripts, letters of recommendation. Additional exam requirements/recommendations for international students: Required—TOEFL (minimum score 535 paper-based). *Application deadline:* For fall admission, 2/1 priority date for

domestic students. Application fee: $30. *Financial support:* Career-related internships or fieldwork, scholarships/grants, and traineeships available. Support available to part-time students. Financial award application deadline: 3/30; financial award applicants required to submit FAFSA. *Faculty research:* Nurse educational administration, gerontology, bioterrorism, healthcare ethics, leadership. *Unit head:* Dr. Patricia Spurr, Chair, 502-873-4304, E-mail: pspurr@spalding.edu. *Application contact:* Dr. Pam King, Program Director, 502-873-4292, E-mail: pking@spalding.edu.
Website: http://www.spalding.edu/nursing/

Spring Arbor University, School of Human Services, Spring Arbor, MI 49283-9799. Offers counseling (MAC); family studies (MAFS); nursing (MSN). *Program availability:* Part-time, evening/weekend, online learning. *Entrance requirements:* For master's, bachelor's degree from regionally-accredited college or university, minimum GPA of 3.0 for at least the last two years of the bachelor's degree, at least two recommendations from professional/academic individuals. Additional exam requirements/recommendations for international students: Required—TOEFL (minimum score 600 paper-based). Electronic applications accepted.

Spring Hill College, Graduate Programs, Program in Nursing, Mobile, AL 36608-1791. Offers clinical nurse leader (MSN, Post-Master's Certificate). *Accreditation:* AACN. *Program availability:* Part-time, evening/weekend, online learning. *Faculty:* 2 full-time (both women), 1 (woman) part-time/adjunct. *Students:* 13 part-time (12 women); includes 6 minority (5 Black or African American, non-Hispanic/Latino; 1 Hispanic/Latino). Average age 45. In 2015, 8 master's awarded. *Degree requirements:* For master's, comprehensive exam, capstone courses, completion of program within 6 calendar years; for Post-Master's Certificate, 460 clinical integration hours. *Entrance requirements:* For master's, RN license in state where practicing nursing; 1 year of clinical nursing experience; work in clinical setting or access to health care facility for clinical integration/research; 3 written references; employer verification; resume, 500-word essay explaining how becoming a CNL will help applicant achieve personal and professional goals; for Post-Master's Certificate, RN license; master's degree in nursing. Additional exam requirements/recommendations for international students: Required—TOEFL (minimum score 550 paper-based; 80 iBT), IELTS (minimum score 6.5), CPE or CAE (minimum score C), Michigan English Language Assessment Battery (minimum score 90). *Application deadline:* For fall admission, 8/1 priority date for domestic and international students; for spring admission, 12/1 priority date for domestic and international students. Applications are processed on a rolling basis. Application fee: $25 ($35 for international students). Electronic applications accepted. *Expenses:* Contact institution. *Financial support:* Applicants required to submit FAFSA. *Unit head:* Dr. Ola H. Fox, Director, 251-380-4486, Fax: 251-460-4495, E-mail: ofox@shc.edu. *Application contact:* Robert Stewart, Vice President of Enrollment, 251-380-3030, Fax: 251-460-2186, E-mail: rstewart@shc.edu.
Website: http://ug.shc.edu/graduate-degrees/master-science-nursing/

State University of New York Downstate Medical Center, College of Nursing, Graduate Program in Nursing, Brooklyn, NY 11203-2098. Offers clinical nurse specialist (MS, Post Master's Certificate); nurse anesthesia (MS); nurse midwifery (MS, Post Master's Certificate); nurse practitioner (MS, Post Master's Certificate); nursing (MS). *Accreditation:* AACN. *Program availability:* Part-time. *Degree requirements:* For master's, thesis optional, clinical research project. *Entrance requirements:* For master's, GRE, BSN; minimum GPA of 3.0; previous undergraduate course work in statistics, health assessment, and nursing research; RN license; for Post Master's Certificate, BSN; minimum GPA of 3.0; RN license; previous undergraduate course work in statistics, health assessment, and nursing research. *Faculty research:* AIDS, continuity of care, case management, self-care.

State University of New York Upstate Medical University, College of Nursing, Syracuse, NY 13210-2334. Offers nurse practitioner (Post Master's Certificate); nursing (MS). *Accreditation:* AACN. *Program availability:* Part-time, online learning. *Degree requirements:* For master's, thesis or alternative. *Entrance requirements:* For master's, 3 years of work experience. Electronic applications accepted.

Stevenson University, Program in Nursing, Owings Mills, MD 21117. Offers nursing education (MS); nursing leadership/management (MS); population-based care coordination (MS). *Program availability:* Part-time, blended/hybrid learning. *Faculty:* 4 full-time (all women), 7 part-time/adjunct (all women). *Students:* 178 part-time (169 women); includes 67 minority (53 Black or African American, non-Hispanic/Latino; 12 Asian, non-Hispanic/Latino; 2 Hispanic/Latino). Average age 40. 83 applicants, 75% accepted, 44 enrolled. In 2015, 37 master's awarded. *Degree requirements:* For master's, capstone course. *Entrance requirements:* For master's, bachelor's degree from regionally-accredited institution, current registered nurse's license in good standing, official college transcripts from all previous academic work, minimum cumulative GPA of 3.0 in past academic work, personal statement (250-350 words), two professional letters of recommendation, resume. Additional exam requirements/recommendations for international students: Required—TOEFL (minimum score 550 paper-based), IELTS (minimum score 6.5). *Application deadline:* Applications are processed on a rolling basis. Application fee: $0. Electronic applications accepted. *Expenses:* $625 per credit, $125 per semester. *Financial support:* Applicants required to submit FAFSA. *Unit head:* Judith Feustle, PhD, Associate Dean, 443-352-4292, Fax: 443-394-0538, E-mail: jfeustle@stevenson.edu. *Application contact:* Amanda Courter, Enrollment Counselor, 443-352-4243, Fax: 443-394-0538, E-mail: acourter@stevenson.edu.
Website: http://www.stevenson.edu

Stockton University, Office of Graduate Studies, Program in Nursing, Galloway, NJ 08205-9441. Offers MSN. *Accreditation:* AACN. *Program availability:* Part-time. *Faculty:* 6 full-time (4 women). *Students:* 1 (woman) full-time, 28 part-time (23 women); includes 6 minority (1 Black or African American, non-Hispanic/Latino; 3 Asian, non-Hispanic/Latino; 2 Hispanic/Latino). Average age 36. 19 applicants, 53% accepted, 9 enrolled. In 2015, 15 master's awarded. *Degree requirements:* For master's, 300 clinical hours. *Entrance requirements:* For master's, CPR certification, minimum GPA of 3.0, RN license. Additional exam requirements/recommendations for international students: Required—TOEFL. *Application deadline:* For fall admission, 5/1 for domestic and international students; for spring admission, 12/1 for domestic and 11/1 for international students. Applications are processed on a rolling basis. Application fee: $50. Electronic applications accepted. *Expenses:* Tuition, state resident: full-time $13,968; part-time $582 per credit. Tuition, nonresident: full-time $21,502; part-time $895 per credit. *Required fees:* $4200; $175 per credit. $90. Tuition and fees vary according to degree level. *Financial support:* Fellowships, research assistantships, career-related internships or fieldwork, Federal Work-Study, scholarships/grants, and unspecified assistantships available. Support available to part-time students. Financial award application deadline: 3/1; financial award applicants required to submit FAFSA. *Faculty research:* Psychoneuroimmunology, relationship of nutrition and disease, mental health as affected by chronic disease states, home care for elderly relatives. *Unit head:* Dr. Edward Walton, Program Director, 609-626-3640, E-mail: edward.walton@stockton.edu. *Application contact:* Tara Williams, Associate Director of Admissions, 609-626-3640, Fax: 609-626-6050, E-mail: gradschool@stockton.edu.

Stony Brook University, State University of New York, Stony Brook Medicine, School of Nursing, Stony Brook, NY 11794. Offers MS, DNP, Certificate. *Accreditation:* AACN/

ACNM/ACME. *Program availability:* Blended/hybrid learning. *Faculty:* 37 full-time (34 women), 43 part-time/adjunct (37 women). *Students:* 52 full-time (49 women), 811 part-time (724 women); includes 302 minority (125 Black or African American, non-Hispanic/Latino; 2 American Indian or Alaska Native, non-Hispanic/Latino; 105 Asian, non-Hispanic/Latino; 62 Hispanic/Latino; 8 Two or more races, non-Hispanic/Latino), 6 international. Average age 37. 708 applicants, 63% accepted, 367 enrolled. In 2015, 143 master's, 20 doctorates, 15 other advanced degrees awarded. *Degree requirements:* For master's, thesis. *Entrance requirements:* For master's, BSN, minimum GPA of 3.0, course work in statistics. Additional exam requirements/recommendations for international students: Required—TOEFL (minimum score 90 iBT). *Application deadline:* For fall admission, 12/3 for domestic students. Application fee: $100. *Expenses:* $24,781 full-time resident tuition and fees, $968 per credit hour; $44,431 full-time nonresident tuition and fees, $1,787 per credit hour. *Financial support:* Fellowships, research assistantships, teaching assistantships, career-related internships or fieldwork, Federal Work-Study, institutionally sponsored loans, and traineeships available. Financial award application deadline: 3/15. Total annual research expenditures: $1.2 million. *Unit head:* Dr. Lee Anne Xippolitos, Dean, 631-444-3200, Fax: 631-444-6628, E-mail: lee.xippolitos@stonybrook.edu. *Application contact:* Karen Allard, Admissions Coordinator, 631-444-6628, Fax: 631-444-3136, E-mail: karen.allard@stonybrook.edu.
Website: http://www.nursing.stonybrookmedicine.edu/

Tarleton State University, College of Graduate Studies, College of Science and Technology, Department of Nursing, Stephenville, TX 76402. Offers nursing administration (MSN); nursing education (MSN). *Program availability:* Part-time, evening/weekend. *Faculty:* 3 full-time (all women). *Students:* 19 part-time (17 women); includes 6 minority (3 Black or African American, non-Hispanic/Latino; 3 Hispanic/Latino). 12 applicants, 83% accepted, 8 enrolled. In 2015, 8 master's awarded. *Degree requirements:* For master's, comprehensive exam. *Entrance requirements:* For master's, GRE General Test, minimum GPA of 3.0. Additional exam requirements/recommendations for international students: Required—TOEFL (minimum score 550 paper-based; 80 iBT). *Application deadline:* For fall admission, 8/15 priority date for domestic students; for spring admission, 1/7 for domestic students. Applications are processed on a rolling basis. Application fee: $45 ($145 for international students). Electronic applications accepted. *Expenses:* Tuition, state resident: part-time $204 per credit hour. Tuition, nonresident: part-time $594 per credit hour. *Required fees:* $1994 per unit. *Financial support:* Career-related internships or fieldwork, Federal Work-Study, and institutionally sponsored loans available. Support available to part-time students. Financial award applicants required to submit FAFSA. *Unit head:* Dr. Susan Rugari, Department Head, 254-968-9139, E-mail: rugari@tarleton.edu. *Application contact:* Information Contact, 254-968-9104, Fax: 254-968-9670, E-mail: gradoffice@tarleton.edu.
Website: http://www.tarleton.edu/nursing/degrees_grad.html

Temple University, College of Public Health, Department of Nursing, Philadelphia, PA 19122. Offers adult-gerontology primary care (DNP); family-individual across the lifespan (DNP); nursing (DNP). *Accreditation:* AACN. *Program availability:* Part-time. *Faculty:* 12 full-time (11 women), 1 (woman) part-time/adjunct. *Students:* 7 full-time (all women), 61 part-time (50 women); includes 37 minority (23 Black or African American, non-Hispanic/Latino; 8 Asian, non-Hispanic/Latino; 4 Hispanic/Latino; 2 Two or more races, non-Hispanic/Latino). 28 applicants, 64% accepted, 9 enrolled. In 2015, 8 doctorates awarded. *Degree requirements:* For doctorate, evidence-based practice project. *Entrance requirements:* For doctorate, GRE General Test or MAT, 2 letters of reference, RN license, interview, statement of purpose, resume. Additional exam requirements/recommendations for international students: Required—TOEFL (minimum score 600 paper-based; 100 iBT). *Application deadline:* For fall admission, 2/15 priority date for domestic students, 1/15 for international students; for spring admission, 10/15 for domestic students, 9/15 for international students. Applications are processed on a rolling basis. Application fee: $60. Electronic applications accepted. *Expenses:* Contact institution. *Financial support:* Federal Work-Study, scholarships/grants, traineeships, and tuition waivers available. Support available to part-time students. Financial award application deadline: 1/15. *Faculty research:* Health promotion, chronic illness, family support systems, primary care, health policy, community health services, evidence-based practice. *Unit head:* Dr. Nancy Rothman, RN, Interim Chair, 215-707-5436, E-mail: rothman@temple.edu. *Application contact:* Audrey Scriven, Academic Coordinator, Graduate Program, 215-204-4618, E-mail: tunurse@temple.edu.

Tennessee State University, The School of Graduate Studies and Research, College of Health Sciences, School of Nursing, Nashville, TN 37209-1561. Offers family nurse practitioner (MSN, Certificate); holistic nurse practitioner (MSN); holistic nursing (Certificate); nursing education (MSN, Certificate). *Accreditation:* ACEN. *Entrance requirements:* For master's, GRE General Test or MAT, BSN, current RN license, minimum GPA of 3.0. *Application deadline:* For fall admission, 4/1 priority date for domestic students. Applications are processed on a rolling basis. Application fee: $25. *Financial support:* Research assistantships and teaching assistantships available. *Unit head:* Dr. Maria Revell, 615-963-5252, E-mail: mrevell1@tnstate.edu. *Application contact:* Dr. Maria Revell, 615-963-5252, E-mail: mrevell1@tnstate.edu.
Website: http://www.tnstate.edu/nursing/

Tennessee Technological University, Whitson-Hester School of Nursing, Cookeville, TN 38505. Offers family nurse practitioner (MSN); informatics (MSN); nursing administration (MSN); nursing education (MSN). *Program availability:* Part-time, evening/weekend, online learning. *Students:* 21 full-time (20 women), 95 part-time (80 women); includes 5 minority (2 Black or African American, non-Hispanic/Latino; 1 Asian, non-Hispanic/Latino; 1 Hispanic/Latino; 1 Two or more races, non-Hispanic/Latino). 42 applicants, 57% accepted, 15 enrolled. In 2015, 47 master's awarded. *Degree requirements:* For master's, comprehensive exam, thesis or alternative. *Entrance requirements:* Additional exam requirements/recommendations for international students: Required—TOEFL (minimum score 600 paper-based; 100 iBT), IELTS (minimum score 5.5), PTE, or TOEIC (Test of English as an International Communication). *Application deadline:* For fall admission, 8/1 for domestic students, 5/1 for international students; for spring admission, 12/1 for domestic students, 10/1 for international students; for summer admission, 5/1 for domestic students, 2/1 for international students. Applications are processed on a rolling basis. Application fee: $35 ($40 for international students). Electronic applications accepted. *Expenses:* Tuition, state resident: full-time $8961; part-time $6132 per credit hour. Tuition, nonresident: full-time $23,121; part-time $14,608 per credit hour. *Financial support:* Application deadline: 4/1. *Unit head:* Dr. Huey-Ming Tzeng, Dean, 931-372-3547, Fax: 931-372-6244, E-mail: htzeng@tntech.edu. *Application contact:* Shelia K. Kendrick, Coordinator of Graduate Studies, 931-372-3808, Fax: 931-372-3497, E-mail: skendrick@tntech.edu.

Texas A&M International University, Office of Graduate Studies and Research, College of Nursing and Health Sciences, Laredo, TX 78041-1900. Offers family nurse practitioner (MSN). *Accreditation:* ACEN. *Entrance requirements:* Additional exam requirements/recommendations for international students: Required—TOEFL (minimum score 550 paper-based; 79 iBT).

Texas A&M University, College of Nursing, Bryan, TX 77807. Offers family nurse practitioner (MSN); nursing education (MSN). *Faculty:* 47. *Students:* 10 full-time (8 women), 27 part-time (23 women); includes 4 minority (2 Black or African American,

Nursing—General

non-Hispanic/Latino; 1 Asian, non-Hispanic/Latino; 1 Hispanic/Latino). Average age 35. 30 applicants, 100% accepted, 30 enrolled. *Expenses:* Contact institution. *Financial support:* In 2015–16, 4 students received support. Career-related internships or fieldwork, institutionally sponsored loans, scholarships/grants, traineeships, health care benefits, tuition waivers (full and partial), and unspecified assistantships available. Support available to part-time students. Financial award applicants required to submit FAFSA. *Unit head:* Dr. Sharon A. Wilkerson, Founding Dean, 979-436-0111, Fax: 979-436-0098, E-mail: wilkerson@tamhsc.edu. *Application contact:* Jennifer Frank, Program Coordinator for Recruitment and Admission, 979-436-0110, E-mail: conadmissions@tamhsc.edu.
Website: http://nursing.tamhsc.edu/

Texas A&M University–Corpus Christi, College of Graduate Studies, College of Nursing and Health Sciences, Corpus Christi, TX 78412-5503. Offers family nurse practitioner (MSN); leadership in nursing systems (MSN); nurse educator (MSN). *Accreditation:* AACN. *Program availability:* Part-time, evening/weekend, online only, 100% online. *Students:* 12 full-time (11 women), 375 part-time (322 women); includes 200 minority (20 Black or African American, non-Hispanic/Latino; 1 American Indian or Alaska Native, non-Hispanic/Latino; 27 Asian, non-Hispanic/Latino; 142 Hispanic/Latino; 3 Native Hawaiian or other Pacific Islander, non-Hispanic/Latino; 7 Two or more races, non-Hispanic/Latino), 1 international. Average age 38. 337 applicants, 42% accepted, 128 enrolled. In 2015, 102 master's awarded. *Degree requirements:* For master's, comprehensive exam, thesis (for some programs), capstone - clinical. *Entrance requirements:* For master's, essay, resume, 3 letters of recommendation, minimum GPA of 3.0. Additional exam requirements/recommendations for international students: Required—TOEFL (minimum score 550 paper-based; 79 iBT), IELTS (minimum score 6.5). *Application deadline:* For fall admission, 4/15 priority date for domestic and international students; for spring admission, 1/7 for domestic and international students; for summer admission, 5/27 for domestic and international students. Applications are processed on a rolling basis. Application fee: $50 ($70 for international students). Electronic applications accepted. *Financial support:* Research assistantships, teaching assistantships, career-related internships or fieldwork, Federal Work-Study, institutionally sponsored loans, scholarships/grants, health care benefits, and unspecified assistantships available. Support available to part-time students. Financial award application deadline: 3/15; financial award applicants required to submit FAFSA. *Unit head:* Dr. Mary Jane Hamilton, Dean, 361-825-2469, E-mail: mary.hamilton@tamucc.edu. *Application contact:* Graduate Admissions Coordinator, 361-825-2177, Fax: 361-825-2755, E-mail: gradweb@tamucc.edu.
Website: http://conhs.tamucc.edu/

Texas Christian University, Harris College of Nursing and Health Sciences, Doctor of Nursing Practice Program, Fort Worth, TX 76129. Offers advanced practice registered nurse (DNP); nursing administration (DNP). *Program availability:* Part-time. *Faculty:* 20 full-time (17 women), 2 part-time/adjunct (both women). *Students:* 19 full-time (17 women), 26 part-time (23 women); includes 9 minority (4 Black or African American, non-Hispanic/Latino; 1 American Indian or Alaska Native, non-Hispanic/Latino; 2 Asian, non-Hispanic/Latino; 2 Hispanic/Latino). Average age 46. 24 applicants, 58% accepted, 13 enrolled. In 2015, 24 doctorates awarded. *Degree requirements:* For doctorate, thesis/dissertation or alternative, practicum. *Entrance requirements:* For doctorate, three reference letters, essay, resume, two official transcripts from each institution attended, APRN recognition or MSN with experience in nursing administration. *Application deadline:* For summer admission, 11/15 for domestic and international students. Application fee: $60. Electronic applications accepted. *Expenses: Tuition, area resident:* Full-time $26,640; part-time $1480 per credit hour. *Required fees:* $48; $48 per unit. Tuition and fees vary according to program. *Financial support:* Teaching assistantships and scholarships/grants available. Financial award application deadline: 2/15; financial award applicants required to submit FAFSA. *Faculty research:* Geriatrics, cancer survivorship, health literacy, endothelial cells, clinical simulation outcomes. *Unit head:* Dr. Kenneth Lowrance, Director, Post Master's DNP Program and CNS Program, 817-257-6729, Fax: 817-257-8383, E-mail: k.w.lowrance@tcu.edu. *Application contact:* Mary Jane Allred, Administrative Program Specialist, 817-257-6726, Fax: 817-257-8383, E-mail: m.allred@tcu.edu.
Website: http://dnp.tcu.edu/

Texas Christian University, Harris College of Nursing and Health Sciences, Master's Program in Nursing, Fort Worth, TX 76129. Offers clinical nurse leader (MSN, Certificate); clinical nurse specialist (MSN), including adult/gerontology nursing, pediatrics; nursing education (MSN). *Accreditation:* AACN; AANA/CANAEP (one or more programs are accredited). *Program availability:* Part-time, online only, 100% online. *Faculty:* 20 full-time (17 women), 2 part-time/adjunct (both women). *Students:* 47 full-time (40 women), 24 part-time (all women); includes 19 minority (3 Black or African American, non-Hispanic/Latino; 1 American Indian or Alaska Native, non-Hispanic/Latino; 10 Asian, non-Hispanic/Latino; 2 Hispanic/Latino; 1 Native Hawaiian or other Pacific Islander, non-Hispanic/Latino; 2 Two or more races, non-Hispanic/Latino), 1 international. Average age 39. 34 applicants, 82% accepted, 23 enrolled. In 2015, 14 master's awarded. *Degree requirements:* For master's, thesis or alternative, practicum. *Entrance requirements:* For master's, GRE General Test, 3 letters of reference, essay, resume, two official transcripts from every institution attended. *Application deadline:* For fall admission, 4/1 for domestic and international students; for spring admission, 9/1 for domestic and international students; for summer admission, 2/1 for domestic and international students. Applications are processed on a rolling basis. Application fee: $60. Electronic applications accepted. *Expenses:* $1,415 per semester hour; $112 fee per course. *Financial support:* In 2015–16, 71 students received support. Teaching assistantships and scholarships/grants available. Financial award application deadline: 2/15; financial award applicants required to submit FAFSA. *Faculty research:* Geriatrics, cancer survivorship, health literacy, endothelial cells, clinical simulation outcomes. *Unit head:* Dr. Kathy Baker, Director, Division of Nursing Graduate Studies and Scholarship, 817-257-6726, Fax: 817-257-8383, E-mail: kathy.baker@tcu.edu. *Application contact:* Mary Jane Allred, Administrative Program Specialist, 817-257-6726, Fax: 817-257-8383, E-mail: m.allred@tcu.edu.
Website: http://www.nursing.tcu.edu/graduate.asp

Texas Tech University Health Sciences Center, School of Nursing, Lubbock, TX 79430. Offers acute care nurse practitioner (MSN, Certificate); administration (MSN); advanced practice (DNP); education (MSN); executive leadership (DNP); family nurse practitioner (MSN, Certificate); geriatric nurse practitioner (MSN, Certificate); pediatric nurse practitioner (MSN, Certificate). *Accreditation:* AACN. *Program availability:* Part-time, online learning. *Degree requirements:* For master's, thesis optional. *Entrance requirements:* For master's, minimum GPA of 3.0, 3 letters of reference, BSN, RN license; for Certificate, minimum GPA of 3.0, 3 letters of reference, RN license. Additional exam requirements/recommendations for international students: Required—TOEFL (minimum score 550 paper-based). *Faculty research:* Diabetes/obesity, nurse competency, disease management, intervention and measurements, health disparities.

Texas Woman's University, Graduate School, College of Nursing, Denton, TX 76204-5498. Offers acute care nurse practitioner (MS); adult health clinical nurse specialist (MS); adult health nurse practitioner (MS); child health clinical nurse specialist (MS); clinical nurse leader (MS); family nurse practitioner (MS); health systems management (MS); nursing education (MS); nursing practice (DNP); nursing science (PhD); pediatric nurse practitioner (MS); women's health clinical nurse specialist (MS); women's health nurse practitioner (MS). *Accreditation:* AACN. *Program availability:* Part-time, online learning. *Faculty:* 55 full-time (51 women), 42 part-time/adjunct (35 women). *Students:* 39 full-time (37 women), 958 part-time (888 women); includes 566 minority (226 Black or African American, non-Hispanic/Latino; 8 American Indian or Alaska Native, non-Hispanic/Latino; 221 Asian, non-Hispanic/Latino; 88 Hispanic/Latino; 3 Native Hawaiian or other Pacific Islander, non-Hispanic/Latino; 20 Two or more races, non-Hispanic/Latino), 37 international. Average age 36. 430 applicants, 65% accepted, 193 enrolled. In 2015, 248 master's, 10 doctorates awarded. *Degree requirements:* For master's, comprehensive exam, thesis or alternative; for doctorate, comprehensive exam, thesis/dissertation. *Entrance requirements:* For master's, GRE or MAT, minimum GPA of 3.0 on last 60 hours in undergraduate nursing degree and overall, RN license, BS in nursing, basic statistics course; for doctorate, GRE (preferred minimum score 153 [500 old version] Verbal, 144 [500 old version] Quantitative, 4 Analytical), MS in nursing, minimum preferred GPA of 3.5, RN license, statistics, 2 letters of reference, curriculum vitae, graduate nursing-theory course, graduate research course, statement of professional goals and research interests. Additional exam requirements/recommendations for international students: Required—TOEFL (minimum score 550 paper-based; 79 iBT). *Application deadline:* For fall admission, 5/1 priority date for domestic students, 3/1 for international students; for spring admission, 9/15 priority date for domestic students, 7/1 for international students. Applications are processed on a rolling basis. Application fee: $50 ($75 for international students). Electronic applications accepted. *Expenses:* Tuition, state resident: full-time $4380; part-time $243 per credit hour. Tuition, nonresident: full-time $11,400; part-time $633 per credit hour. International tuition: $11,465 full-time. *Required fees:* $1778; $99 per credit hour. $283 per semester. One-time fee: $50. Tuition and fees vary according to course load and program. *Financial support:* In 2015–16, 149 students received support, including 10 research assistantships (averaging $5,600 per year), 1 teaching assistantship (averaging $5,600 per year); career-related internships or fieldwork, Federal Work-Study, institutionally sponsored loans, scholarships/grants, traineeships, health care benefits, and unspecified assistantships also available. Support available to part-time students. Financial award application deadline: 3/1; financial award applicants required to submit FAFSA. *Faculty research:* Screening, prevention, and treatment for intimate partner violence; needs of adolescents during childbirth intervention; a network analysis decision tool for nurse managers (social network analysis); support for adolescents with implantable cardioverter defibrillators; informatics: nurse staffing, safety, quality, and financial data as they relate to patient care outcomes; prevention and treatment of obesity; improving infant outcomes related to premature birth. *Total annual research expenditures:* $1.7 million. *Unit head:* Dr. Anita G. Hufft, Dean, 940-898-2401, Fax: 940-898-2437, E-mail: nursing@twu.edu. *Application contact:* Dr. Samuel Wheeler, Assistant Director of Admissions, 940-898-3188, Fax: 940-898-3081, E-mail: wheelersr@twu.edu.
Website: http://www.twu.edu/nursing/

Thomas Edison State University, W. Cary Edwards School of Nursing, Program in Nursing, Trenton, NJ 08608-1176. Offers MSN, DNP. *Accreditation:* AACN; ACEN. *Program availability:* Part-time, online learning. *Degree requirements:* For master's, nursing education seminar, onground practicum, online practicum. *Entrance requirements:* For master's, BSN. Additional exam requirements/recommendations for international students: Required—TOEFL (minimum score 550 paper-based; 79 iBT). Electronic applications accepted.

Thomas Jefferson University, Jefferson College of Nursing, Philadelphia, PA 19107. Offers MS, DNP. *Accreditation:* AACN; AANA/CANAEP. *Program availability:* Part-time, online learning. *Faculty:* 39 full-time (38 women). *Students:* 65 full-time (49 women), 401 part-time (360 women); includes 75 minority (38 Black or African American, non-Hispanic/Latino; 27 Asian, non-Hispanic/Latino; 10 Hispanic/Latino), 2 international. Average age 33. 325 applicants, 65% accepted, 139 enrolled. In 2015, 194 master's, 10 doctorates awarded. *Entrance requirements:* For master's, GRE or MAT, BSN or equivalent, CPR certification, professional RN license, previous undergraduate course work in statistics and nursing research, minimum GPA of 3.0. Additional exam requirements/recommendations for international students: Required—TOEFL. *Application deadline:* For fall admission, 4/1 priority date for domestic and international students; for spring admission, 9/1 priority date for domestic and international students; for summer admission, 1/2 priority date for domestic and international students. Applications are processed on a rolling basis. Electronic applications accepted. *Expenses:* $1,075 per credit. *Financial support:* In 2015–16, 337 students received support. Federal Work-Study, institutionally sponsored loans, and scholarships/grants available. Support available to part-time students. Financial award application deadline: 4/1; financial award applicants required to submit FAFSA. *Faculty research:* Interdisciplinary primary care, women and HIV, health promotion and disease prevention, psychosocial impact of disability, ethical decision-making. *Unit head:* Dr. Ksenia Zukowsky, Associate Dean, Graduate Programs, 215-503-9426, E-mail: ksenia.zukowsky@jefferson.edu. *Application contact:* Tina Heuges, Associate Director of Admissions, 215-503-1754, Fax: 215-503-7241, E-mail: tina.heuges@jefferson.edu.
Website: http://www.jefferson.edu/nursing

Thomas University, Department of Nursing, Thomasville, GA 31792-7499. Offers MSN. *Accreditation:* ACEN. *Program availability:* Part-time. *Entrance requirements:* For master's, resume, 3 academic/professional references. Additional exam requirements/recommendations for international students: Required—TOEFL (minimum score 600 paper-based). Electronic applications accepted.

Towson University, Program in Nursing, Towson, MD 21252-0001. Offers nursing (MS); nursing education (Postbaccalaureate Certificate). *Accreditation:* AACN. *Program availability:* Part-time. *Students:* 12 full-time (10 women), 45 part-time (43 women); includes 19 minority (15 Black or African American, non-Hispanic/Latino; 2 Asian, non-Hispanic/Latino; 1 Hispanic/Latino; 1 Two or more races, non-Hispanic/Latino), 3 international. *Degree requirements:* For master's, thesis optional. *Entrance requirements:* For master's, minimum GPA of 3.0, copy of current nursing license, bachelor's degree in nursing, current resume or curriculum vitae, completion of an elementary statistics and/or nursing research course, completion of an approved physical assessment course; for Postbaccalaureate Certificate, minimum GPA of 3.0, copy of current nursing license, current resume or curriculum vitae, bachelor's degree, completion of an elementary statistics and/or nursing research course, completion of an approved physical assessment course, personal statement. *Application deadline:* Applications are processed on a rolling basis. Application fee: $45. Electronic applications accepted. *Expenses:* Tuition, state resident: full-time $7440; part-time $372 per unit. Tuition, nonresident: full-time $15,400; part-time $770 per unit. *Required fees:* $2360; $118 per year. $354 per term. *Financial support:* Application deadline: 4/1. *Unit head:* Dr. Nikki Austin, Graduate Program Director, 410-704-4389, E-mail: nursinggradprogram@towson.edu. *Application contact:* Alicia Arkell-Kleis, University Admissions, 410-704-2113, Fax: 410-704-3030, E-mail: grads@towson.edu.
Website: http://grad.towson.edu/program/master/nurs-ms/

Trinity Western University, School of Graduate Studies, School of Nursing, Langley, BC V2Y 1Y1, Canada. Offers MSN.

Troy University, Graduate School, College of Health and Human Services, Program in Nursing, Troy, AL 36082. Offers adult health (MSN); clinical nurse specialist adult health (DNP); clinical nurse specialist maternal infant (DNP); family nurse practitioner (MSN, DNP, PMC); informatics specialist (MSN); maternal infant (MSN). *Accreditation:* ACEN. *Program availability:* Part-time, evening/weekend. *Faculty:* 13 full-time (12 women), 11 part-time/adjunct (all women). *Students:* 75 full-time (62 women), 202 part-time (179 women); includes 91 minority (72 Black or African American, non-Hispanic/Latino; 1 Asian, non-Hispanic/Latino; 8 Hispanic/Latino; 10 Two or more races, non-Hispanic/Latino). Average age 34. 50 applicants, 96% accepted. In 2015, 43 master's, 13 doctorates, 15 other advanced degrees awarded. *Degree requirements:* For master's, comprehensive exam, minimum GPA of 3.0, candidacy; for doctorate, minimum GPA of 3.0, submission of approved comprehensive e-portfolio, completion of residency synthesis project, minimum of 1000 hours of clinical practice, qualifying exam. *Entrance requirements:* For master's, GRE (minimum score of 850 on old exam or 290 on new exam) or MAT (minimum score of 396), minimum GPA of 3.0, BSN, current RN licensure, 2 letters of reference, undergraduate health assessment course; for doctorate, GRE (minimum score of 850 on old exam or 294 on new exam), BSN or MSN, minimum GPA of 3.0, 2 letters of reference, current RN licensure, essay. Additional exam requirements/recommendations for international students: Required—TOEFL (minimum score 523 paper-based; 70 iBT), IELTS (minimum score 6). *Application deadline:* Applications are processed on a rolling basis. Application fee: $50. Electronic applications accepted. *Expenses:* Tuition, state resident: full-time $7146; part-time $397 per credit hour. Tuition, nonresident: full-time $14,292; part-time $794 per credit hour. *Required fees:* $802. Tuition and fees vary according to campus/location and program. *Financial support:* Fellowships, career-related internships or fieldwork, and scholarships/grants available. Support available to part-time students. Financial award applicants required to submit FAFSA. *Unit head:* Dr. Diane Weed, Director, School of Nursing, 334-670-5864, Fax: 334-070-0745, E-mail: lwccd@troy.odu. *Application contact:* Crystal G. Bishop, Director of Graduate Admissions, School of Nursing, 334-241-8631, E-mail: cdgodwin@troy.edu.

Uniformed Services University of the Health Sciences, Daniel K. Inouye Graduate School of Nursing, Bethesda, MD 20814. Offers adult-gerontology clinical nurse specialist (MSN, DNP); family nurse practitioner (DNP); nurse anesthesia (DNP); nursing science (PhD); psychiatric mental health nurse practitioner (DNP); women's health nurse practitioner (DNP). MSN and DNP programs available to military officers only; PhD to military and DoD students only. *Accreditation:* AACN; AANA/CANAEP. *Faculty:* 38 full-time (22 women), 2 part-time/adjunct (1 woman). *Students:* 51 full-time (29 women); includes 17 minority (8 Black or African American, non-Hispanic/Latino; 4 Asian, non-Hispanic/Latino; 4 Hispanic/Latino; 1 Two or more races, non-Hispanic/Latino). Average age 34. 75 applicants, 68% accepted, 51 enrolled. In 2015, 4 master's, 24 doctorates awarded. *Degree requirements:* For master's, thesis or alternative; for doctorate, thesis/dissertation or alternative. *Entrance requirements:* For master's, GRE, BSN, clinical experience, minimum GPA of 3.0, previous course work in science; for doctorate, GRE, BSN, clinical experience, minimum GPA of 3.0, previous course work in sciences, and writing paper (for DNP); MSN (for PhD). *Application deadline:* For fall admission, 7/1 for domestic students; for winter admission, 2/15 for domestic students. Application fee: $0. Electronic applications accepted. *Faculty research:* Prenatal care, military health care, military readiness, distance learning. *Unit head:* Dr. Diane C. Seibert, Associate Dean for Academic Affairs, 301-295-1080, Fax: 301-295-1707, E-mail: diane.seibert@usuhs.edu. *Application contact:* Terry Lynn Malavakis, Recording Secretary for Admissions Committee/Registrar/Program Analyst, 301-295-1055, Fax: 301-295-1707, E-mail: terry.malavakis@usuhs.edu.
Website: http://www.usuhs.edu/gsn/

Union University, School of Nursing, Jackson, TN 38305-3697. Offers executive leadership (DNP); nurse anesthesia (DNP); nurse practitioner (DNP); nursing education (MSN, PMC). *Accreditation:* AACN; AANA/CANAEP. *Degree requirements:* For master's, thesis or alternative. *Entrance requirements:* For master's, GRE, 3 letters of reference, bachelor's degree in nursing, minimum GPA of 3.0. Additional exam requirements/recommendations for international students: Required—TOEFL (minimum score 560 paper-based). Electronic applications accepted. *Faculty research:* Children's health, occupational rehabilitation, informatics, health promotion.

Universidad Metropolitana, School of Health Sciences, Department of Nursing, San Juan, PR 00928-1150. Offers case management (Certificate); nursing (MSN); oncology nursing (Certificate). *Accreditation:* ACEN.

Université de Montréal, Faculty of Nursing, Montréal, QC H3C 3J7, Canada. Offers M Sc, PhD, Certificate, DESS. PhD offered jointly with McGill University. *Program availability:* Part-time. *Degree requirements:* For master's, one foreign language, thesis optional; for doctorate, thesis/dissertation, general exam; for other advanced degree, one foreign language. *Entrance requirements:* For master's, doctorate, and other advanced degree, proficiency in French. Electronic applications accepted. *Faculty research:* Mental and physical care of chronic patients, care of the hospitalized aged, cancer nursing, home care of caregivers, AIDS patients.

Université du Québec à Rimouski, Graduate Programs, Program in Nursing Studies, Rimouski, QC G5L 3A1, Canada. Offers M Sc, Diploma. Programs offered jointly with Université du Québec à Chicoutimi, Université du Québec à Trois-Rivières, and Université du Québec en Outaouais.

Université du Québec à Trois-Rivières, Graduate Programs, Program in Nursing Sciences, Trois-Rivières, QC G9A 5H7, Canada. Offers M Sc, DESS. *Program availability:* Part-time.

Université du Québec en Outaouais, Graduate Programs, Program in Nursing, Gatineau, QC J8X 3X7, Canada. Offers M Sc, DESS, Diploma. *Program availability:* Part-time, evening/weekend. *Degree requirements:* For master's, thesis (for some programs). *Entrance requirements:* For master's, appropriate bachelor's degree, proficiency in French.

Université Laval, Faculty of Nursing, Programs in Nursing, Québec, QC G1K 7P4, Canada. Offers M Sc, PhD, DESS, Diploma. *Degree requirements:* For master's, thesis (for some programs). *Entrance requirements:* For master's, French exam, knowledge of English; for other advanced degree, knowledge of French. Electronic applications accepted.

University at Buffalo, the State University of New York, Graduate School, School of Nursing, Buffalo, NY 14214. Offers adult gerontology nurse practitioner (DNP); family nurse practitioner (DNP); health care systems and leadership (MS); nurse anesthetist (DNP); nursing (PhD); nursing education (Certificate); psychiatric/mental health nurse practitioner (DNP). *Accreditation:* AACN; AANA/CANAEP (one or more programs are accredited). *Program availability:* Part-time, 100% online. *Students:* 61 full-time (37 women), 137 part-time (114 women); includes 35 minority (17 Black or African American, non-Hispanic/Latino; 1 American Indian or Alaska Native, non-Hispanic/Latino; 17 Asian, non-Hispanic/Latino), 7 international. Average age 32. 193 applicants, 49% accepted, 75 enrolled. In 2015, 6 master's, 37 doctorates awarded. *Degree requirements:* For master's, thesis optional; for doctorate, comprehensive exam (for some programs), capstone (for DNP), dissertation (for PhD). *Entrance requirements:* For master's, GRE or MAT; for doctorate, GRE or MAT, minimum GPA of 3.0 (for DNP),

3.25 (for PhD); RN license; BS or MS in nursing; 3 references; writing sample; resume; personal statement; for Certificate, interview, minimum GPA of 3.0 or GRE General Test, RN license, MS in nursing, professional certification. Additional exam requirements/recommendations for international students: Required—TOEFL (minimum score 550 paper-based; 79 iBT), IELTS (minimum score 6.5). *Application deadline:* For fall admission, 7/1 for domestic students, 2/1 for international students; for spring admission, 12/1 for domestic students, 10/1 for international students; for summer admission, 2/1 for domestic students. Applications are processed on a rolling basis. Application fee: $75. Electronic applications accepted. *Financial support:* In 2015–16, 80 students received support, including 2 fellowships with tuition reimbursements available (averaging $17,000 per year), 4 research assistantships with tuition reimbursements available (averaging $10,600 per year), 7 teaching assistantships with tuition reimbursements available (averaging $10,600 per year); scholarships/grants, traineeships, health care benefits, and unspecified assistantships also available. Financial award application deadline: 2/1; financial award applicants required to submit FAFSA. *Faculty research:* Oncology, palliative care, gerontology, addictions, mental health, community wellness, sleep, workforce, care of underserved populations, quality and safety, person-centered care, adolescent health. *Total annual research expenditures:* $1.4 million. *Unit head:* Dr. Marsha L. Lewis, Dean and Professor, 716-829-2533, Fax: 716-829-2566, E-mail: ubnursingdean@buffalo.edu. *Application contact:* Jennifer H. VanLaeken, Director of Graduate Student Services, 716-829-3311, Fax: 716-829-2067, E-mail: jhv2@buffalo.edu.
Website: http://nursing.buffalo.edu/

The University of Akron, Graduate School, College of Health Professions, School of Nursing, Akron, OH 44325-3701. Offers nursing (MSN, PhD); nursing practice (DNP); public health (MPH). PhD offered jointly with Kent State University. *Accreditation:* AACN; AANA/CANAEP (one or more programs are accredited). *Program availability:* Part-time. *Faculty:* 13 full-time (12 women), 37 part-time/adjunct (35 women). *Students:* 40 full-time (27 women), 286 part-time (223 women); includes 45 minority (19 Black or African American, non-Hispanic/Latino; 10 Asian, non-Hispanic/Latino; 10 Hispanic/Latino; 6 Two or more races, non-Hispanic/Latino), 4 international. Average age 37. 140 applicants, 56% accepted, 64 enrolled. In 2015, 101 master's, 2 doctorates awarded. *Degree requirements:* For doctorate, one foreign language, thesis/dissertation, qualifying exam. *Entrance requirements:* For master's, current Ohio state license as registered nurse, three letters of reference, 300-word essay, interview with program coordinator; for doctorate, GRE, minimum GPA of 3.0, MSN, nursing license or eligibility for licensure, writing sample, letters of recommendation, interview, resume, personal statement of research interests and career goals. Additional exam requirements/recommendations for international students: Required—TOEFL (minimum score 550 paper-based; 79 iBT), IELTS (minimum score 6.5). *Application deadline:* For fall admission, 7/15 for domestic and international students. Applications are processed on a rolling basis. Application fee: $45 ($70 for international students). Electronic applications accepted. *Expenses:* Tuition, state resident: full-time $7958; part-time $442 per credit hour. Tuition, nonresident: full-time $13,464; part-time $748 per credit hour. *Required fees:* $1404. *Financial support:* In 2015–16, 11 teaching assistantships with full tuition reimbursements were awarded. *Faculty research:* Health promotion and chronic disease prevention, mental health and psychosocial resilience, gerontological health, trauma and violence, gut oxygenation during shock and trauma, simulation and the pedagogy of teaching and learning. *Total annual research expenditures:* $476,886. *Unit head:* Dr. Marlene Huff, Interim Director, 330-972-5930, E-mail: mhuff@uakron.edu.
Website: http://www.uakron.edu/nursing/

The University of Alabama, Graduate School, Capstone College of Nursing, Tuscaloosa, AL 35487. Offers MSN, DNP, Ed D, MSN/Ed D. *Accreditation:* AACN. *Program availability:* Part-time, online learning. *Faculty:* 23 full-time (20 women), 1 part-time/adjunct (0 women). *Students:* 124 full-time (100 women), 209 part-time (181 women); includes 112 minority (76 Black or African American, non-Hispanic/Latino; 1 American Indian or Alaska Native, non-Hispanic/Latino; 9 Asian, non-Hispanic/Latino; 22 Hispanic/Latino; 1 Native Hawaiian or other Pacific Islander, non-Hispanic/Latino; 3 Two or more races, non-Hispanic/Latino), 2 international. Average age 43. 303 applicants, 57% accepted, 128 enrolled. In 2015, 42 master's, 54 doctorates awarded. *Degree requirements:* For master's, thesis optional; for doctorate, comprehensive exam, thesis/dissertation, scholarly practice project. *Entrance requirements:* For master's, GRE or MAT (if GPA is below 3.0), BSN, RN licensure, minimum GPA of 3.0; for doctorate, GRE or MAT, MSN, RN licensure, minimum GPA of 3.0, references, writing sample, curriculum vitae. Additional exam requirements/recommendations for international students: Required—TOEFL. *Application deadline:* For fall admission, 6/1 priority date for domestic students; for winter admission, 11/1 for domestic students; for spring admission, 4/1 priority date for domestic students. Applications are processed on a rolling basis. Application fee: $50 ($60 for international students). Electronic applications accepted. *Expenses:* Tuition, state resident: full-time $10,170. Tuition, nonresident: full-time $25,950. *Financial support:* In 2015–16, 2 fellowships with full tuition reimbursements (averaging $15,000 per year) were awarded. Scholarships/grants also available. Financial award application deadline: 7/1; financial award applicants required to submit FAFSA. *Faculty research:* Diabetes education, childhood asthma, HIV/AIDS prevention and care, breast cancer in rural minority women, nursing labor cost, nursing case management, sleep, gerontology, health disparities of rural children. *Total annual research expenditures:* $7,500. *Unit head:* Dr. Suzanne Prevost, Dean, 205-348-1040, Fax: 205-348-5559, E-mail: sprevost@ua.edu. *Application contact:* Dr. Marsha H. Adams, Senior Associate Dean, 205-348-1044, Fax: 205-348-5559, E-mail: madams@ua.edu.
Website: http://nursing.ua.edu/

The University of Alabama at Birmingham, School of Nursing, Birmingham, AL 35294. Offers nurse anesthesia (MSN); nursing (MSN, DNP, PhD). *Accreditation:* AACN. *Program availability:* Part-time. Terminal master's awarded for partial completion of doctoral program. *Degree requirements:* For doctorate, thesis/dissertation, research mentorship experience. *Entrance requirements:* For master's, GRE, GMAT, or MAT, BS in nursing, interview; for doctorate, GRE General Test, computer literacy, course work in statistics, interview, minimum GPA of 3.0, MS in nursing, references, writing sample. Additional exam requirements/recommendations for international students: Required—TOEFL. Electronic applications accepted. *Expenses:* Contact institution.

The University of Alabama in Huntsville, School of Graduate Studies, College of Nursing, Huntsville, AL 35899. Offers family nurse practitioner (Certificate); nursing (MSN, DNP), including adult-gerontology acute care nurse practitioner (MSN), adult-gerontology clinical nurse specialist (MSN), family nurse practitioner (MSN), leadership in health care systems (MSN), nursing education (Certificate). DNP offered jointly with The University of Alabama at Birmingham. *Accreditation:* AACN. *Program availability:* Part-time, evening/weekend, online learning. *Degree requirements:* For master's, comprehensive exam, thesis or alternative, oral and written exams. *Entrance requirements:* For master's, MAT or GRE, Alabama RN license, BSN, minimum GPA of 3.0; for doctorate, master's degree in nursing in an advanced practice area; for Certificate, MAT or GRE, minimum GPA of 3.0. Additional exam requirements/recommendations for international students: Required—TOEFL (minimum score 500 paper-based; 80 iBT), IELTS (minimum score 6.5). *Application deadline:* For fall admission, 7/15 for domestic students, 4/1 for international students; for spring

Nursing—General

admission, 11/30 for domestic students, 9/1 for international students. Applications are processed on a rolling basis. Application fee: $50. Electronic applications accepted. *Expenses: Tuition, area resident:* Full-time $9548; part-time $547 per credit hour. Tuition, state resident: full-time $9548; part-time $547 per credit hour. Tuition, nonresident: full-time $21,402; part-time $1224 per credit hour. *International tuition:* $21,402 full-time. *Financial support:* Teaching assistantships with full tuition reimbursements, career-related internships or fieldwork, Federal Work-Study, institutionally sponsored loans, scholarships/grants, traineeships, health care benefits, and unspecified assistantships available. Support available to part-time students. Financial award application deadline: 4/1; financial award applicants required to submit FAFSA. *Faculty research:* Health care informatics, chronic illness management, maternal and child health, genetics/genomics, technology and health care. *Unit head:* Dr. Marsha Adams, Dean, 256-824-6345, Fax: 256-824-6026, E-mail: marsha.adams@uah.edu. *Application contact:* Charles Davis, Director of Graduate Admission and Advisement, 256-824-6669, Fax: 256-824-6026, E-mail: charles.davis@uah.edu. Website: http://www.uah.edu/nursing

University of Alaska Anchorage, College of Health, School of Nursing, Anchorage, AK 99508. Offers MS. *Accreditation:* ACEN. *Program availability:* Part-time, evening/weekend. *Degree requirements:* For master's, comprehensive exam, individual project. *Entrance requirements:* For master's, GRE or MAT, BS in nursing, interview, minimum GPA of 3.0, RN license, 1 year of part-time or 6 months of full-time clinical experience. Additional exam requirements/recommendations for international students: Required—TOEFL (minimum score 550 paper-based).

University of Alberta, Faculty of Graduate Studies and Research, Faculty of Nursing, Edmonton, AB T6G 2E1, Canada. Offers MN, PhD. *Program availability:* Part-time. *Degree requirements:* For master's, thesis optional, clinical practice; for doctorate, thesis/dissertation. *Entrance requirements:* For master's, B Sc N, 1 year of clinical nursing experience in specialty area; for doctorate, MN. Additional exam requirements/recommendations for international students: Required—TOEFL (minimum score 550 paper-based). *Faculty research:* Symptom management, healthy human development, health policy, teaching excellence and information.

The University of Arizona, College of Nursing, Tucson, AZ 85721. Offers health care informatics (Certificate); nurse practitioner (MS); nursing (DNP, PhD). *Accreditation:* AACN. *Program availability:* Part-time, online learning. Terminal master's awarded for partial completion of doctoral program. *Degree requirements:* For master's, thesis optional; for doctorate, comprehensive exam, thesis/dissertation. *Entrance requirements:* For master's, BSN, eligibility for RN license; for doctorate, BSN; for Certificate, GRE General Test, Arizona RN license, BSN, minimum GPA of 3.0. Additional exam requirements/recommendations for international students: Required—TOEFL (minimum score 550 paper-based; 79 iBT). *Application deadline:* For fall admission, 1/15 for domestic and international students. Applications are processed on a rolling basis. Application fee: $75. Electronic applications accepted. *Expenses:* Contact institution. *Financial support:* Research assistantships, teaching assistantships, career-related internships or fieldwork, institutionally sponsored loans, scholarships/grants, traineeships, health care benefits, tuition waivers (full), and unspecified assistantships available. Financial award application deadline: 6/1. *Faculty research:* Vulnerable populations, injury mechanisms and biobehavioral responses, health care systems, informatics, rural health. *Unit head:* Dr. Joan Shaver, Dean, 520-626-7124, Fax: 520-626-6424, E-mail: cmurdaugh@nursing.arizona.edu. *Application contact:* Dr. Joan Shaver, Dean, 520-626-7124, Fax: 520-626-6424, E-mail: cmurdaugh@nursing.arizona.edu. Website: http://www.nursing.arizona.edu/

University of Arkansas, Graduate School, College of Education and Health Professions, Eleanor Mann School of Nursing, Fayetteville, AR 72701-1201. Offers MSN. *Accreditation:* AACN. *Program availability:* Online learning. *Students:* 44 full-time (40 women), 37 part-time (34 women); includes 12 minority (7 Black or African American, non-Hispanic/Latino; 1 American Indian or Alaska Native, non-Hispanic/Latino; 2 Hispanic/Latino; 2 Two or more races, non-Hispanic/Latino). In 2015, 4 master's awarded. *Application deadline:* For fall admission, 4/1 for international students; for spring admission, 10/1 for international students. Applications are processed on a rolling basis. Application fee: $40 ($50 for international students). Electronic applications accepted. *Financial support:* Fellowships, research assistantships, and teaching assistantships available. *Unit head:* Dr. Pegge Bell, Director, 479-575-3904, Fax: 479-575-3218, E-mail: plbell@uark.edu. *Application contact:* Dr. Kathleen Barta, Graduate Admissions, 479-575-5871, E-mail: kbarta@uark.edu. Website: http://nurs.uark.edu/

University of Arkansas for Medical Sciences, College of Nursing, Little Rock, AR 72205-7199. Offers PhD. *Accreditation:* AACN. *Program availability:* Part-time. *Entrance requirements:* For doctorate, GRE. Additional exam requirements/recommendations for international students: Required—TOEFL. *Expenses:* Contact institution.

The University of British Columbia, Faculty of Applied Science, Program in Nursing, Vancouver, BC V6T 1Z1, Canada. Offers MSN, PhD. *Program availability:* Part-time. *Degree requirements:* For master's, essay or thesis; for doctorate, comprehensive exam, thesis/dissertation. *Entrance requirements:* For master's, GRE, bachelor's degree in nursing; for doctorate, GRE, master's degree in nursing. Additional exam requirements/recommendations for international students: Required—TOEFL. Electronic applications accepted. *Faculty research:* Women and children, aging, critical care, cross-cultural.

University of Calgary, Faculty of Graduate Studies, Faculty of Nursing, Calgary, AB T2N 1N4, Canada. Offers MN, PhD, PMD. *Program availability:* Part-time. *Degree requirements:* For master's, comprehensive exam (for some programs), thesis (for some programs); for doctorate, thesis/dissertation; for PMD, comprehensive exam. *Entrance requirements:* For master's and PMD, nursing experience, nursing registration; for doctorate, nursing registration. Additional exam requirements/recommendations for international students: Required—TOEFL (minimum score 600 paper-based), IELTS (minimum score 7), Michigan English Language Assessment Battery. Electronic applications accepted. *Expenses:* Contact institution. *Faculty research:* Health outcomes across multiple populations and multiple settings including patients and families with chronic health problems, culturally diverse, and vulnerable populations; family health; core processes; professional, educational and health services delivery.

University of California, Irvine, Programs in Health Sciences, Program in Nursing Science, Irvine, CA 92607. Offers MSN. *Accreditation:* AACN. *Students:* 21 full-time (19 women), 20 part-time (17 women); includes 23 minority (14 Asian, non-Hispanic/Latino; 5 Hispanic/Latino; 4 Two or more races, non-Hispanic/Latino). Average age 32. 69 applicants, 39% accepted, 21 enrolled. In 2015, 15 master's awarded. Application fee: $90 ($110 for international students). *Unit head:* E. Alison Holman, Interim Director, 949-824-8932, E-mail: aholman@uci.edu. *Application contact:* Julie Aird, Manager of Student Affairs, 949-824-1514, Fax: 949-824-3650, E-mail: jaird@uci.edu. Website: http://www.nursing.uci.edu/

University of California, Los Angeles, Graduate Division, School of Nursing, Los Angeles, CA 90095. Offers MSN, PhD, MBA/MSN. *Accreditation:* AACN. *Degree*

requirements: For master's, comprehensive exam; for doctorate, thesis/dissertation, oral and written qualifying exams. *Entrance requirements:* For master's, bachelor's degree in nursing; minimum undergraduate GPA of 3.0 (or its equivalent if letter grade system not used); for doctorate, bachelor's degree in nursing; minimum undergraduate GPA of 3.5 (or its equivalent if letter grade system not used); writing sample. Additional exam requirements/recommendations for international students: Required—TOEFL. Electronic applications accepted. *Expenses:* Contact institution.

University of California, San Francisco, Graduate Division, School of Nursing, Program in Nursing, San Francisco, CA 94143. Offers MS, PhD. *Accreditation:* AACN; ACNM/ACME (one or more programs are accredited). *Degree requirements:* For master's, comprehensive exam, thesis or alternative; for doctorate, thesis/dissertation. *Entrance requirements:* For master's and doctorate, GRE General Test. *Expenses:* Contact institution.

University of Central Arkansas, Graduate School, College of Health and Behavioral Sciences, Department of Nursing, Conway, AR 72035-0001. Offers adult nurse practitioner (PMC); clinical nurse leader (PMC); clinical nurse specialist (MSN); family nurse practitioner (PMC); nurse educator (PMC); nurse practitioner (MSN). *Accreditation:* AACN. *Program availability:* Part-time, evening/weekend, online learning. *Degree requirements:* For master's, comprehensive exam, thesis optional, clinicals. *Entrance requirements:* For master's, GRE General Test, minimum GPA of 2.7. Additional exam requirements/recommendations for international students: Required—TOEFL (minimum score 550 paper-based; 80 iBT). Electronic applications accepted. *Expenses:* Contact institution.

University of Central Florida, College of Nursing, Orlando, FL 32816. Offers MSN, DNP, PhD, Post-Master's Certificate. *Accreditation:* AACN. *Program availability:* Part-time, evening/weekend. *Faculty:* 47 full-time (41 women), 74 part-time/adjunct (72 women). *Students:* 55 full-time (50 women), 245 part-time (219 women); includes 82 minority (31 Black or African American, non-Hispanic/Latino; 2 American Indian or Alaska Native, non-Hispanic/Latino; 12 Asian, non-Hispanic/Latino; 35 Hispanic/Latino; 1 Native Hawaiian or other Pacific Islander, non-Hispanic/Latino; 1 Two or more races, non-Hispanic/Latino), 1 international. Average age 38. 169 applicants, 60% accepted, 76 enrolled. In 2015, 90 master's, 16 doctorates, 3 other advanced degrees awarded. *Degree requirements:* For master's, thesis or alternative. *Entrance requirements:* For master's, GRE General Test, minimum GPA of 3.0 in last 60 hours. Additional exam requirements/recommendations for international students: Required—TOEFL. *Application deadline:* For fall admission, 2/15 for domestic students; for spring admission, 9/15 for domestic students. Application fee: $30. Electronic applications accepted. *Expenses:* Tuition, state resident: part-time $288.16 per credit hour. Tuition, nonresident: part-time $1071.31 per credit hour. *Financial support:* In 2015–16, 27 students received support, including 26 fellowships with partial tuition reimbursements available (averaging $9,010 per year), 1 research assistantship with partial tuition reimbursement available (averaging $14,400 per year), 1 teaching assistantship with partial tuition reimbursement available (averaging $12,100 per year); career-related internships or fieldwork, Federal Work-Study, institutionally sponsored loans, traineeships, and unspecified assistantships also available. Financial award application deadline: 3/1; financial award applicants required to submit FAFSA. *Unit head:* Dr. Mary Lou Sole, Dean, 407-823-5496, Fax: 407-823-5675, E-mail: mary.sole@ucf.edu. *Application contact:* Director, Admissions and Student Services, 407-823-2766, Fax: 407-823-6442, E-mail: gradadmissions@ucf.edu. Website: http://nursing.ucf.edu/

University of Central Missouri, The Graduate School, Warrensburg, MO 64093. Offers accountancy (MA); accounting (MBA); applied mathematics (MS); aviation safety (MA); biology (MS); business administration (MBA); career and technical education leadership (MS); college student personnel administration (MS); communication (MA); computer science (MS); counseling (MS); criminal justice (MS); educational leadership (Ed D); educational technology (MS); elementary and early childhood education (MSE); English (MA); environmental studies (MA); finance (MBA); history (MA); human services/educational technology (Ed S); human services/learning resources (Ed S); human services/professional counseling (Ed S); industrial hygiene (MS); industrial management (MS); information systems (MBA); information technology (MS); kinesiology (MS); library science and information services (MS); literacy education (MSE); marketing (MBA); mathematics (MS); music (MA); occupational safety management (MS); psychology (MS); rural family nursing (MS); school administration (MSE); social gerontology (MS); sociology (MA); special education (MSE); speech language pathology (MS); superintendency (Ed S); teaching (MAT); teaching English as a second language (MA); technology (MS); technology management (PhD); theatre (MA). *Program availability:* Part-time, 100% online, blended/hybrid learning. *Faculty:* 336 full-time (145 women), 39 part-time/adjunct (25 women). *Students:* 2,161 full-time (723 women), 2,077 part-time (1,061 women); includes 188 minority (93 Black or African American, non-Hispanic/Latino; 4 American Indian or Alaska Native, non-Hispanic/Latino; 15 Asian, non-Hispanic/Latino; 32 Hispanic/Latino; 1 Native Hawaiian or other Pacific Islander, non-Hispanic/Latino; 43 Two or more races, non-Hispanic/Latino), 2,514 international. Average age 28. 3,454 applicants, 68% accepted, 1632 enrolled. In 2015, 1,530 master's, 53 other advanced degrees awarded. *Degree requirements:* For master's and Ed S, comprehensive exam (for some programs), thesis (for some programs). *Entrance requirements:* Additional exam requirements/recommendations for international students: Required—TOEFL (minimum score 550 paper-based; 79 iBT). *Application deadline:* For fall admission, 6/1 priority date for domestic and international students; for spring admission, 10/1 priority date for domestic and international students; for summer admission, 4/1 priority date for domestic and international students. Applications are processed on a rolling basis. Application fee: $30 ($75 for international students). Electronic applications accepted. *Expenses:* Tuition, state resident: full-time $6683; part-time $278.45 per credit hour. Tuition, nonresident: full-time $13,366; part-time $556.90 per credit hour. *Required fees:* $701; $29.20 per credit hour. Tuition and fees vary according to degree level and campus/location. *Financial support:* In 2015–16, 97 students received support, including 146 research assistantships with partial tuition reimbursements available (averaging $7,500 per year), 73 teaching assistantships with partial tuition reimbursements available (averaging $7,500 per year); career-related internships or fieldwork, Federal Work-Study, scholarships/grants, and administrative and laboratory assistantships also available. Support available to part-time students. Financial award application deadline: 3/1; financial award applicants required to submit FAFSA. *Unit head:* Tina Church-Hockett, Director of Graduate School and International Admissions, 660-543-4621, Fax: 660-543-4778, E-mail: church@ucmo.edu. *Application contact:* Brittany Lawrence, Graduate Student Services Coordinator, 660-543-4621, Fax: 660-543-4778, E-mail: gradinfo@ucmo.edu. Website: http://www.ucmo.edu/graduate/

University of Central Oklahoma, The Jackson College of Graduate Studies, College of Mathematics and Science, Department of Nursing, Edmond, OK 73034-5209. Offers MS. *Program availability:* Part-time. *Entrance requirements:* For master's, minimum undergraduate GPA of 3.0 in nursing; bachelor's degree in nursing; license as an RN. Electronic applications accepted.

University of Cincinnati, Graduate School, College of Nursing, Cincinnati, OH 45221-0038. Offers clinical nurse specialist (MSN), including adult health, community health, neonatal, nursing administration, occupational health, pediatric health, psychiatric nursing, women's health; nurse anesthesia (MSN); nurse midwifery (MSN); nurse practitioner (MSN), including acute care, ambulatory care, family, family/psychiatric, women's health; nursing (PhD); MBA/MSN. *Accreditation:* AACN; AANA/CANAEP (one or more programs are accredited). *Program availability:* Part-time, online learning. Terminal master's awarded for partial completion of doctoral program. *Degree requirements:* For master's, thesis or alternative; for doctorate, comprehensive exam, thesis/dissertation. *Entrance requirements:* For master's and doctorate, GRE General Test. Additional exam requirements/recommendations for international students: Required—TOEFL (minimum score 520 paper-based). Electronic applications accepted. *Faculty research:* Substance abuse, injury and violence, symptom management.

University of Colorado Colorado Springs, Helen and Arthur E. Johnson Beth-El College of Nursing and Health Sciences, Colorado Springs, CO 80918. Offers nursing practice (DNP); primary care nurse practitioner (MSN). *Accreditation:* AACN. *Program availability:* Part-time, 100% online, blended/hybrid learning. *Faculty:* 10 full-time (9 women), 8 part-time/adjunct (6 women). *Students:* 65 full-time (43 women), 137 part-time (129 women); includes 34 minority (5 Black or African American, non-Hispanic/Latino; 6 Asian, non-Hispanic/Latino; 19 Hispanic/Latino; 4 Two or more races, non-Hispanic/Latino), 1 international. Average age 34. 113 applicants, 55% accepted, 31 enrolled. In 2015, 39 master's, 7 doctorates awarded. *Degree requirements:* For master's, comprehensive exam, thesis optional; for doctorate, capstone project. *Entrance requirements:* For master's, GRE General Test or MAT, minimum overall GPA of 2.75 for all undergraduate course work, minimum BSN GPA of 3.3; for doctorate, interview; active RN license; MA; minimum GPA of 3.3; National Certification as nurse practitioner or clinical nurse specialist; portfolio. Additional exam requirements/recommendations for international students: Required—TOEFL (minimum score 550 paper-based; 80 iBT). *Application deadline:* For fall admission, 3/15 priority date for domestic students, 3/15 for international students; for spring admission, 8/15 for domestic and international students. Applications are processed on a rolling basis. Application fee: $60 ($100 for international students). Electronic applications accepted. *Expenses:* $11,734 per year resident, $20,068 per year non-resident. *Financial support:* In 2015–16, 58 students received support. Career-related internships or fieldwork, Federal Work-Study, and scholarships/grants available. Support available to part-time students. Financial award application deadline: 3/1; financial award applicants required to submit FAFSA. *Faculty research:* Behavioral interventions to reduce stroke risk factors in older adults, interprofessional models of health promotion for older adults, nurse practitioner education, practice and policy, cardiology, cardiac and pulmonary rehab, heart failure and stroke, community health prevention, veterans studies, anger management, sports medicine, sports nutrition. *Unit head:* Dr. Amy Silva-Smith, Graduate Department Chairperson, 719-255-4490, Fax: 719-255-4416, E-mail: asilvasm@uccs.edu. *Application contact:* Diane Busch, Program Assistant II, 719-255-4424, Fax: 719-255-4416, E-mail: dbusch@uccs.edu.
Website: http://www.uccs.edu/bethel/index.html

University of Colorado Denver, College of Nursing, Aurora, CO 80045. Offers adult clinical nurse specialist (MS); adult nurse practitioner (MS); family nurse practitioner (MS); family psychiatric mental health nurse practitioner (MS); health care informatics (MS); nurse-midwifery (MS); nursing (DNP, PhD); nursing leadership and health care systems (MS); pediatric nurse practitioner (MS); special studies (MS); women's health (MS); MS/PhD. *Accreditation:* ACNM/ACME (one or more programs are accredited). *Program availability:* Part-time, evening/weekend, online learning. *Faculty:* 109 full-time (100 women), 55 part-time/adjunct (50 women). *Students:* 367 full-time (332 women), 141 part-time (118 women); includes 79 minority (16 Black or African American, non-Hispanic/Latino; 2 American Indian or Alaska Native, non-Hispanic/Latino; 8 Asian, non-Hispanic/Latino; 37 Hispanic/Latino; 16 Two or more races, non-Hispanic/Latino), 6 international. Average age 36. 321 applicants, 53% accepted, 145 enrolled. In 2015, 151 master's, 36 doctorates awarded. Terminal master's awarded for partial completion of doctoral program. *Degree requirements:* For master's, thesis optional; for doctorate, comprehensive exam, thesis/dissertation, 42 credits of coursework. *Entrance requirements:* For master's, GRE if cumulative undergraduate GPA is less than 3.0, undergraduate nursing degree from NLNAC- or CCNE-accredited school or university; completion of research and statistics courses with minimum grade of C; copy of current and unencumbered nursing license; for doctorate, GRE, bachelor's and/or master's degrees in nursing from NLN- or CCNE-accredited institution; portfolio; minimum undergraduate GPA of 3.0, graduate 3.5; graduate-level intermediate statistics and master's-level nursing theory courses with minimum B grade; interview. Additional exam requirements/recommendations for international students: Required—TOEFL (minimum score 560 paper-based; 83 iBT). *Application deadline:* For fall admission, 2/15 for domestic students, 1/15 for international students; for spring admission, 7/1 for domestic students, 6/1 for international students. Application fee: $50 ($75 for international students). Electronic applications accepted. *Expenses:* Contact institution. *Financial support:* In 2015–16, 148 students received support. Fellowships, research assistantships, teaching assistantships, Federal Work-Study, institutionally sponsored loans, scholarships/grants, traineeships, and unspecified assistantships available. Support available to part-time students. Financial award application deadline: 4/1; financial award applicants required to submit FAFSA. *Faculty research:* Biological and behavioral phenomena in pregnancy and postpartum; patterns of glycaemia during the insulin resistance of pregnancy; obesity, gestational diabetes, and relationship to neonatal adiposity; men's awareness and knowledge of male breast cancer; cognitive-behavioral therapy for chronic insomnia after breast cancer treatment; massage therapy for the treatment of tension-type headaches. *Total annual research expenditures:* $5.9 million. *Unit head:* Dr. Sarah Thompson, Dean, 303-724-1679, E-mail: sarah.a.thompson@ucdenver.edu. *Application contact:* Judy Campbell, Graduate Programs Coordinator, 303-724-8503, E-mail: judy.campbell@ucdenver.edu.
Website: http://www.ucdenver.edu/academics/colleges/nursing/Pages/default.aspx

University of Connecticut, Graduate School, School of Nursing, Storrs, CT 06269. Offers MS, DNP, PhD, Post-Master's Certificate. *Accreditation:* AACN. *Degree requirements:* For master's, comprehensive exam; for doctorate, thesis/dissertation. *Entrance requirements:* Additional exam requirements/recommendations for international students: Required—TOEFL (minimum score 550 paper-based). *Application deadline:* For fall admission, 5/1 for domestic and international students; for spring admission, 11/1 for domestic students, 10/1 for international students. Applications are processed on a rolling basis. Application fee: $55. Electronic applications accepted. *Financial support:* Fellowships, research assistantships with full tuition reimbursements, teaching assistantships with full tuition reimbursements, Federal Work-Study, scholarships/grants, health care benefits, and unspecified assistantships available. Financial award application deadline: 2/1; financial award applicants required to submit FAFSA.
Website: http://www.nursing.uconn.edu/

University of Delaware, College of Health Sciences, School of Nursing, Newark, DE 19716. Offers adult nurse practitioner (MSN, PMC); cardiopulmonary clinical nurse specialist (MSN, PMC); cardiopulmonary clinical nurse specialist/adult nurse practitioner (MSN, PMC); family nurse practitioner (MSN, PMC); gerontology clinical nurse specialist (MSN, PMC); gerontology clinical nurse specialist geriatric nurse practitioner (PMC); gerontology clinical nurse specialist/geriatric nurse practitioner (MSN); health services

administration (MSN, PMC); nursing of children clinical nurse specialist (MSN, PMC); nursing of children clinical nurse specialist/pediatric nurse practitioner (MSN, PMC); oncology/immune deficiency clinical nurse specialist (MSN, PMC); oncology/immune deficiency clinical nurse specialist/adult nurse practitioner (MSN, PMC); perinatal/women's health clinical nurse specialist (MSN, PMC); perinatal/women's health clinical nurse specialist/women's health nurse practitioner (MSN, PMC); psychiatric nursing clinical nurse specialist (MSN, PMC). *Accreditation:* AACN. *Program availability:* Part-time, evening/weekend, online learning. *Degree requirements:* For master's, thesis optional. *Entrance requirements:* For master's, BSN, interview, RN license. Electronic applications accepted. *Faculty research:* Marriage and chronic illness, health promotion, congestive heart failure patient outcomes, school nursing, diabetes in children, culture, health disparities, cardiovascular, prison nursing, oncology, public policy, child obesity, smoking and teen pregnancy, blood pressure measurements, men's health.

University of Detroit Mercy, College of Health Professions, Detroit, MI 48221. Offers clinical nurse leader (MSN); family nurse practitioner (MSN); health services administration (MHSA); health systems management (MSN); nurse anesthesia (MS); nursing (DNP); nursing education (MSN, Certificate); nursing leadership and financial management (Certificate); outcomes performance management (Certificate); physician assistant (MS). *Entrance requirements:* For master's, GRE General Test, minimum GPA of 3.0. Application fee: $30 ($50 for international students). *Expenses: Tuition, area resident:* Full-time $26,802; part-time $1489 per credit. Tuition and fees vary according to course load and program. *Financial support:* Institutionally sponsored loans and tuition waivers (partial) available. Support available to part-time students. Financial award applicants required to submit FAFSA. *Faculty research:* Research design, respiratory physiology, AIDS prevention, adolescent health, community, low income health education. *Unit head:* Dr. Christine M. Pacini, RN, Dean, 313-993-6055, Fax: 313-993-6175.
Website: http://healthprofessions.udmercy.edu/

University of Florida, Graduate School, College of Nursing, Gainesville, FL 32611. Offers clinical and translational science (PhD); clinical nursing (DNP); nursing (MSN); nursing sciences (PhD). *Accreditation:* AACN; ACNM/ACME (one or more programs are accredited). *Program availability:* Part-time. *Faculty:* 13 full-time (11 women), 5 part-time/adjunct (3 women). *Students:* 58 full-time (33 women), 31 part-time (27 women); includes 16 minority (6 Black or African American, non-Hispanic/Latino; 6 Asian, non-Hispanic/Latino; 4 Hispanic/Latino), 5 international. Average age 38. 44 applicants, 20% accepted, 8 enrolled. In 2015, 63 master's, 6 doctorates awarded. *Degree requirements:* For master's, thesis optional; for doctorate, thesis/dissertation. *Entrance requirements:* For master's and doctorate, GRE General Test, minimum GPA of 3.0. Additional exam requirements/recommendations for international students: Required—TOEFL (minimum score 550 paper-based; 80 iBT), IELTS (minimum score 6). *Application deadline:* For fall admission, 3/15 priority date for domestic students, 3/15 for international students. Applications are processed on a rolling basis. Application fee: $30. Electronic applications accepted. *Financial support:* In 2015–16, 6 fellowships, 2 research assistantships were awarded; career-related internships or fieldwork and Federal Work-Study also available. Support available to part-time students. Financial award applicants required to submit FAFSA. *Faculty research:* Aging and health: cancer survivorship, interventions to promote healthy aging, and symptom management; women's health, fetal and infant development; biobehavioral interventions: interrelationships among the biological, behavioral, psychological, social and spiritual factors that influence wellness and disease; health policy: influence of local and national policy on physical and psychological health. *Unit head:* Anna M. McDaniel, PhD, Dean, College of Nursing, 352-273-6324, Fax: 352-273-6505, E-mail: annammcdaniel@ufl.edu. *Application contact:* Bridgette Hart-Sams, Coordinator, Student Academic Services, 352-273-6331, Fax: 352-273-6440, E-mail: bhart@ufl.edu.
Website: http://nursing.ufl.edu/

University of Hartford, College of Education, Nursing, and Health Professions, Program in Nursing, West Hartford, CT 06117-1599. Offers community/public health nursing (MSN); nursing education (MSN); nursing management (MSN). *Accreditation:* AACN. *Program availability:* Part-time, evening/weekend. *Degree requirements:* For master's, research project. *Entrance requirements:* For master's, BSN, Connecticut RN license. Additional exam requirements/recommendations for international students: Required—TOEFL (minimum score 550 paper-based). Electronic applications accepted. *Expenses:* Contact institution. *Faculty research:* Child development, women in doctoral study, applying feminist theory in teaching methods, near death experience, grandmothers as primary care providers.

University of Hawaii at Hilo, Program in Nursing Practice, Hilo, HI 96720-4091. Offers DNP. *Entrance requirements:* Additional exam requirements/recommendations for international students: Required—TOEFL, IELTS. Electronic applications accepted.

University of Hawaii at Manoa, Graduate Division, School of Nursing and Dental Hygiene, Honolulu, HI 96822. Offers clinical nurse specialist (MS), including adult health, community mental health; nurse practitioner (MS), including adult health, community mental health, family nurse practitioner; nursing (PhD, Graduate Certificate); nursing administration (MS). *Accreditation:* AACN. *Program availability:* Part-time, online learning. *Faculty:* 32 full-time (27 women), 22 part-time/adjunct (11 women). *Students:* 167 full-time (145 women), 118 part-time (104 women); includes 128 minority (3 Black or African American, non-Hispanic/Latino; 1 American Indian or Alaska Native, non-Hispanic/Latino; 57 Asian, non-Hispanic/Latino; 14 Hispanic/Latino; 4 Native Hawaiian or other Pacific Islander, non-Hispanic/Latino; 49 Two or more races, non-Hispanic/Latino), 2 international. Average age 41. 253 applicants, 42% accepted, 88 enrolled. In 2015, 20 master's, 8 doctorates awarded. *Degree requirements:* For master's, thesis optional; for doctorate, comprehensive exam, thesis/dissertation. *Entrance requirements:* For master's, Hawaii RN license. Additional exam requirements/recommendations for international students: Required—TOEFL (minimum score 580 paper-based; 92 iBT), IELTS (minimum score 5). *Application deadline:* For fall admission, 2/1 for domestic and international students. Application fee: $100. *Expenses:* Contact institution. *Financial support:* In 2015–16, 78 fellowships (averaging $1,277 per year), 3 research assistantships (averaging $16,824 per year), 2 teaching assistantships (averaging $14,382 per year) were awarded. *Total annual research expenditures:* $1.8 million. *Unit head:* Mary Boland, Dean, 808-956-8522, Fax: 808-956-3257, E-mail: mgboland@hawaii.edu. *Application contact:* Maureen Shannon, Graduate Chair, 808-956-5201, Fax: 808-956-3257, E-mail: maureens@hawaii.edu.
Website: http://www.hawaii.edu/graduatestudies/fields/html/departments/mno/nursing/nursing.htm

University of Houston, School of Nursing, Houston, TX 77204. Offers family nurse practitioner (MSN); nursing administration (MSN); nursing education (MSN). *Accreditation:* AACN. *Entrance requirements:* For master's, GRE or MAT, minimum GPA of 3.0 in last 60 hours of academic course work, valid Texas RN licensure, 2 letters of recommendation. Electronic applications accepted.

University of Illinois at Chicago, College of Nursing, Chicago, IL 60607-7128. Offers MS, DNP, PhD, Certificate, MBA/MS, MPH/MS. *Accreditation:* AACN. *Program availability:* Part-time. *Faculty:* 103 full-time (93 women), 88 part-time/adjunct (81 women). *Students:* 379 full-time (345 women), 544 part-time (487 women); includes 243 minority (70 Black or African American, non-Hispanic/Latino; 87 Asian, non-Hispanic/

Nursing—General

Latino; 71 Hispanic/Latino; 1 Native Hawaiian or other Pacific Islander, non-Hispanic/Latino; 14 Two or more races, non-Hispanic/Latino), 39 international. Average age 33. 425 applicants, 53% accepted, 151 enrolled. In 2015, 193 master's, 29 doctorates, 4 other advanced degrees awarded. *Degree requirements:* For master's, thesis or alternative; for doctorate, thesis/dissertation. *Entrance requirements:* For master's and doctorate, GRE General Test, minimum GPA of 2.75. Additional exam requirements/recommendations for international students: Required—TOEFL. *Application deadline:* For fall admission, 5/15 for domestic students, 2/1 for international students; for spring admission, 10/15 for domestic students. Applications are processed on a rolling basis. Application fee: $60 ($50 for international students). Electronic applications accepted. *Expenses:* Contact institution. *Financial support:* In 2015–16, 3 fellowships with full tuition reimbursements were awarded; research assistantships with full tuition reimbursements, teaching assistantships with full tuition reimbursements, career-related internships or fieldwork, Federal Work-Study, institutionally sponsored loans, scholarships/grants, traineeships, tuition waivers (full and partial), and unspecified assistantships also available. Support available to part-time students. Financial award application deadline: 3/1; financial award applicants required to submit FAFSA. *Faculty research:* Health promotion and disease prevention, quality of life and symptom management, end-of-life, health disparities and health equity, pregnancy outcomes. *Total annual research expenditures:* $7.8 million. *Unit head:* Dr. Terri E. Weaver, Dean, 312-996-7808, Fax: 312-996-8066, E-mail: teweaver@uic.edu. *Application contact:* Receptionist, 312-413-2550, E-mail: gradcoll@uic.edu.
Website: http://www.nursing.uic.edu

University of Indianapolis, Graduate Programs, School of Nursing, Indianapolis, IN 46227-3697. Offers advanced practice nursing (DNP); family nurse practitioner (MSN); gerontological nurse practitioner (MSN); neonatal nurse practitioner (MSN); nurse-midwifery (MSN); nursing (MSN); nursing and health systems leadership (MSN); nursing education (MSN); women's health nurse practitioner (MSN); MBA/MSN. *Accreditation:* AACN; ACNM. *Entrance requirements:* For master's, minimum GPA of 3.0, interview, letters of recommendation, resume, IN nursing license, 1 year of professional practice; for doctorate, graduate of NLNAC- or CCNE-accredited nursing program; MSN or MA with nursing major and minimum cumulative GPA of 3.25; unencumbered RN license with eligibility for licensure in Indiana; completion of graduate-level statistics course within last 5 years with minimum grade of B; resume; essay; official transcripts from all academic institutions. Additional exam requirements/recommendations for international students: Required—TOEFL (minimum score 550 paper-based). Electronic applications accepted.

The University of Iowa, Graduate College, College of Nursing, Iowa City, IA 52242-1316. Offers MSN, DNP, PhD. *Accreditation:* AACN; AANA/CANAEP (one or more programs are accredited). *Degree requirements:* For master's, thesis optional, portfolio, project; for doctorate, comprehensive exam, thesis/dissertation. *Entrance requirements:* For master's, minimum GPA of 3.0; for doctorate, GRE General Test, minimum GPA of 3.0. Additional exam requirements/recommendations for international students: Required—TOEFL (minimum score 550 paper-based; 81 iBT). Electronic applications accepted. *Expenses:* Contact institution.

The University of Kansas, University of Kansas Medical Center, School of Nursing, Kansas City, KS 66160. Offers adult/gerontological clinical nurse specialist (PMC); adult/gerontological nurse practitioner (PMC); clinical research management (PMC); health care informatics (PMC); health professions educator (PMC); nurse midwife (PMC); nursing (MS, DNP, PhD); organizational leadership (PMC); psychiatric/mental health nurse practitioner (PMC); public health nursing (PMC). *Accreditation:* AACN; ACNM/ACME. *Program availability:* Part-time, 100% online, blended/hybrid learning. *Faculty:* 59. *Students:* 44 full-time (42 women), 261 part-time (238 women); includes 54 minority (22 Black or African American, non-Hispanic/Latino; 1 American Indian or Alaska Native, non-Hispanic/Latino; 12 Asian, non-Hispanic/Latino; 10 Hispanic/Latino; 9 Two or more races, non-Hispanic/Latino), 1 international. Average age 38. 95 applicants, 97% accepted, 74 enrolled. In 2015, 71 master's, 24 doctorates, 6 other advanced degrees awarded. Terminal master's awarded for partial completion of doctoral program. *Degree requirements:* For master's, comprehensive exam, thesis (for some programs), general oral exam; for doctorate, variable foreign language requirement, thesis/dissertation or alternative, comprehensive oral exam (for DNP); comprehensive written and oral exam, or three publications (for PhD). *Entrance requirements:* For master's, bachelor's degree in nursing, minimum GPA of 3.0, 1 year of clinical experience, RN license in KS and MO; for doctorate, GRE General Test (for PhD only), bachelor's degree in nursing, minimum GPA of 3.5, RN license in KS and MO. Additional exam requirements/recommendations for international students: Required—TOEFL. *Application deadline:* For fall admission, 4/1 for domestic and international students; for spring admission, 9/1 for domestic and international students. Application fee: $60. Electronic applications accepted. *Financial support:* Research assistantships with tuition reimbursements, teaching assistantships with tuition reimbursements, scholarships/grants, and traineeships available. Financial award application deadline: 3/1; financial award applicants required to submit FAFSA. *Faculty research:* Breastfeeding practices of teen mothers, national database of nursing quality indicators, caregiving of families of patients using technology in the home, simulation in nursing education, diaphragm fatigue. *Total annual research expenditures:* $4.6 million. *Unit head:* Dr. Sally Maliski, Dean, 913-588-1601, Fax: 913-588-1660, E-mail: smaliski@kumc.edu. *Application contact:* Dr. Pamela K. Barnes, Associate Dean, Student Affairs, 913-588-1619, Fax: 913-588-1615, E-mail: pbarnes2@kumc.edu.
Website: http://nursing.kumc.edu

University of Kentucky, Graduate School, College of Nursing, Lexington, KY 40506-0032. Offers DNP, PhD. *Degree requirements:* For doctorate, comprehensive exam, thesis/dissertation. *Entrance requirements:* For doctorate, GRE General Test, minimum undergraduate GPA of 3.0. Additional exam requirements/recommendations for international students: Required—TOEFL (minimum score 550 paper-based). Electronic applications accepted.

University of Lethbridge, School of Graduate Studies, Lethbridge, AB T1K 3M4, Canada. Offers addictions counseling (M Sc); agricultural biotechnology (M Sc); agricultural studies (M Sc, MA); anthropology (MA); archaeology (M Sc, MA); art (MA, MFA); biochemistry (M Sc); biological sciences (M Sc); biomolecular science (PhD); biosystems and biodiversity (PhD); Canadian studies (MA); chemistry (M Sc); computer science (M Sc); computer science and geographical information science (M Sc); counseling (MC); counseling psychology (M Ed); dramatic arts (MA); earth, space, and physical science (PhD); economics (MA); education (MA, PhD); educational leadership (M Ed); English (MA); environmental science (M Sc); evolution and behavior (PhD); exercise science (M Sc); French (MA); French/German (MA); French/Spanish (MA); general education (M Ed); geography (M Sc, MA); German (MA); health sciences (M Sc); individualized multidisciplinary (M Sc, MA); kinesiology (M Sc, MA); management (M Sc), including accounting, finance, human resource management and labor relations, information systems, international management, marketing, policy and strategy; mathematics (M Sc); music (M Mus, MA); Native American studies (MA); neuroscience (M Sc, PhD); new media (MA, MFA); nursing (M Sc, MN); philosophy (MA); physics (M Sc); political science (MA); psychology (M Sc, MA); religious studies (MA); sociology (MA); theatre and dramatic arts (MFA); theoretical and computational

science (PhD); urban and regional studies (MA); women and gender studies (MA). *Program availability:* Part-time, evening/weekend. *Students:* 448 full-time (249 women), 110 part-time (64 women). Average age 32. 285 applicants, 36% accepted, 96 enrolled. In 2015, 154 master's, 11 doctorates awarded. *Degree requirements:* For master's, thesis (for some programs); for doctorate, comprehensive exam, thesis/dissertation. *Entrance requirements:* For master's, GMAT (for M Sc in management), bachelor's degree in related field, minimum GPA of 3.0 during previous 20 graded semester courses, 2 years' teaching or related experience (M Ed); for doctorate, master's degree, minimum graduate GPA of 3.5. Additional exam requirements/recommendations for international students: Required—TOEFL (minimum score 580 paper-based; 93 iBT). Application fee: $100 Canadian dollars ($140 Canadian dollars for international students). Electronic applications accepted. *Financial support:* Fellowships, research assistantships, teaching assistantships, scholarships/grants, health care benefits, and unspecified assistantships available. *Faculty research:* Movement and brain plasticity, gibberellin physiology, photosynthesis, carbon cycling, molecular properties of main-group ring components. *Unit head:* Kathleen Schrage, Manager, School of Graduate Studies, 403-329-2121, E-mail: schrage@uleth.ca. *Application contact:* School of Graduate Studies, 403-329-5194, E-mail: sgsinquiries@uleth.ca.
Website: http://www.uleth.ca/graduate-studies/

University of Louisiana at Lafayette, College of Nursing, Lafayette, LA 70504. Offers MSN. Program offered jointly with Southern Louisiana University, McNeese State University, Southern University and Agricultural and Mechanical College. *Accreditation:* AACN. *Degree requirements:* For master's, thesis or alternative. *Entrance requirements:* For master's, GRE General Test, minimum GPA of 2.75. Additional exam requirements/recommendations for international students: Required—TOEFL (minimum score 550 paper-based). Electronic applications accepted.

University of Louisville, Graduate School, School of Nursing, Louisville, KY 40202. Offers adult gerontology nurse practitioner (MSN, DNP); education and administration (MSN); family nurse practitioner (MSN, DNP); neonatal nurse practitioner (MSN, DNP); nursing research (PhD); psychiatric/mental health nurse practitioner (MSN, DNP); women's health nurse practitioner (MSN). *Accreditation:* AACN. *Program availability:* Part-time. *Faculty:* 53 full-time (48 women), 27 part-time/adjunct (23 women). *Students:* 110 full-time (99 women), 33 part-time (29 women); includes 17 minority (11 Black or African American, non-Hispanic/Latino; 1 Asian, non-Hispanic/Latino; 2 Hispanic/Latino; 3 Two or more races, non-Hispanic/Latino), 5 international. Average age 34. 62 applicants, 68% accepted, 40 enrolled. In 2015, 41 master's awarded. *Degree requirements:* For doctorate, comprehensive exam (for some programs), thesis/dissertation (for some programs). *Entrance requirements:* For master's, bachelor's degree in nursing, minimum GPA of 3.0, RN license; for doctorate, GRE General Test (for PhD), 3 letters of professional reference. Additional exam requirements/recommendations for international students: Required—TOEFL (minimum score 560 paper-based; 79 iBT). *Application deadline:* For fall admission, 3/1 priority date for domestic students, 3/1 for international students. Applications are processed on a rolling basis. Application fee: $60. Electronic applications accepted. *Expenses:* Tuition, state resident: full-time $11,664; part-time $649 per credit hour. Tuition, nonresident: full-time $24,274; part-time $1350 per credit hour. *Required fees:* $196. Tuition and fees vary according to program and reciprocity agreements. *Financial support:* In 2015–16, 722,568 students received support, including 10 research assistantships with full tuition reimbursements available (averaging $20,000 per year), 2 teaching assistantships with full tuition reimbursements available (averaging $15,000 per year); fellowships with full tuition reimbursements available, scholarships/grants, and unspecified assistantships also available. Financial award application deadline: 2/15; financial award applicants required to submit FAFSA. *Faculty research:* Children and adolescents with chronic illnesses, women's mental health and parenting, asthma and environmental health, type 2 diabetes self-management in adults, health disparities and community engagement. *Total annual research expenditures:* $722,568. *Unit head:* Dr. Marcia J. Hern, Dean, 502-852-8300, Fax: 502-852-8783, E-mail: m.hern@louisville.edu. *Application contact:* Trish Hart, Assistant Dean for Student Affairs, 502-852-5825, Fax: 502-852-8783, E-mail: trish.hart@louisville.edu.
Website: http://www.louisville.edu/nursing/

University of Maine, Graduate School, College of Natural Sciences, Forestry, and Agriculture, School of Nursing, Orono, ME 04469. Offers individualized (MS); nursing education (CGS); rural health family nurse practitioner (MS, CAS). *Accreditation:* AACN. *Faculty:* 6 full-time (all women), 3 part-time/adjunct (1 woman). *Students:* 12 full-time (10 women), 3 part-time (all women); includes 2 minority (1 American Indian or Alaska Native, non-Hispanic/Latino; 1 Hispanic/Latino). Average age 41. 7 applicants, 43% accepted, 2 enrolled. In 2015, 7 master's, 1 other advanced degree awarded. *Entrance requirements:* For master's, GRE General Test; for other advanced degree, master's degree. Additional exam requirements/recommendations for international students: Required—TOEFL. *Application deadline:* For fall admission, 2/1 for domestic students. Applications are processed on a rolling basis. Application fee: $65. Electronic applications accepted. *Financial support:* In 2015–16, 1 student received support. Career-related internships or fieldwork, Federal Work-Study, institutionally sponsored loans, tuition waivers (full and partial), and unspecified assistantships available. Support available to part-time students. Financial award application deadline: 3/1. *Faculty research:* Work experiences of chief nursing officers, fatigue related to radiation therapy in oncology patients, patients' perceptions of nurses' caring behaviors, health disparities of rural Maine older women. *Unit head:* Dr. Nancy Fishwick, Director, 207-581-2505, Fax: 207-581-2585. *Application contact:* Scott G. Delcourt, Assistant Vice President for Graduate Studies and Senior Associate Dean, 207-581-3291, Fax: 207-581-3232, E-mail: graduate@maine.edu.
Website: http://umaine.edu/nursing/

The University of Manchester, School of Nursing, Midwifery and Social Work, Manchester, United Kingdom. Offers nursing (M Phil, PhD); social work (M Phil, PhD).

University of Manitoba, Faculty of Graduate Studies, Faculty of Nursing, Winnipeg, MB R3T 2N2, Canada. Offers cancer nursing (MN); nursing (MN). *Degree requirements:* For master's, thesis.

University of Mary, School of Health Sciences, Division of Nursing, Bismarck, ND 58504-9652. Offers family nurse practitioner (DNP); nurse administrator (MSN); nursing educator (MSN); MSN/MBA. *Accreditation:* AACN. *Program availability:* Part-time, evening/weekend, online learning. *Degree requirements:* For master's, comprehensive exam (for some programs), thesis (for some programs), internship (family nurse practitioner), teaching practice. *Entrance requirements:* For master's, minimum GPA of 2.75 in nursing, interview, letters of recommendation, criminal background check, immunizations, statement of professional goals. Additional exam requirements/recommendations for international students: Required—TOEFL (minimum score 500 paper-based; 71 iBT). *Application deadline:* Applications are processed on a rolling basis. Application fee: $40. Electronic applications accepted. *Financial support:* Fellowships with partial tuition reimbursements and teaching assistantships with partial tuition reimbursements available. Financial award application deadline: 8/1; financial award applicants required to submit FAFSA. *Faculty research:* Gerontology issues, rural nursing, health policy, primary care, women's health.

University of Mary Hardin-Baylor, Graduate Studies in Nursing, Belton, TX 76513. Offers clinical nurse leader (MSN); family nurse practitioner (MSN, Post-Master's Certificate); nurse educator (Post-Master's Certificate); nursing education (MSN). *Accreditation:* AACN. *Program availability:* Part-time, evening/weekend. *Faculty:* 6 full-time (all women), 3 part-time/adjunct (2 women). *Students:* 54 full-time (47 women), 2 part-time (1 woman); includes 14 minority (10 Black or African American, non-Hispanic/Latino; 3 Hispanic/Latino; 1 Two or more races, non-Hispanic/Latino), 1 international. Average age 32. 46 applicants, 70% accepted, 26 enrolled. In 2015, 47 master's awarded. *Degree requirements:* For master's, practicum. *Entrance requirements:* For master's, full-time RN for 1 year, BSN, minimum GPA of 3.0 in last 60 hours of undergraduate program, two letters of recommendation. Additional exam requirements/recommendations for international students: Required—TOEFL (minimum score 100 iBT), IELTS (minimum score 7). *Application deadline:* For fall admission, 4/15 for domestic students, 4/30 priority date for international students; for spring admission, 11/1 for domestic students, 9/30 priority date for international students. Applications are processed on a rolling basis. Application fee: $35 ($135 for international students). Electronic applications accepted. *Expenses: Tuition, area resident:* Part-time $815 per credit hour. Tuition and fees vary according to course load and degree level. *Financial support:* Applicants required to submit FAFSA. *Unit head:* Dr. Carrie Johnson, Associate Professor/Director, Master of Science in Nursing Programs, 254-295-4178, E-mail: cjohnson@umhb.edu. *Application contact:* Melissa Williams, Director, Graduate Student Services and Engagement, 254-295-4020, Fax: 254-295-5038, E-mail: mwilliams@umhb.edu.
Website: http://graduate.umhb.edu/nursing/

University of Maryland, Baltimore, Graduate School, School of Nursing, Doctoral Program in Nursing, Baltimore, MD 21201. Offers PhD. *Degree requirements:* For doctorate, thesis/dissertation. *Entrance requirements:* For doctorate, GRE General Test, minimum GPA of 3.0, MS in nursing. Additional exam requirements/recommendations for international students: Required—TOEFL (minimum score 550 paper-based; 80 iBT); Recommended—IELTS (minimum score 7). Electronic applications accepted. Tuition and fees vary according to program. *Faculty research:* Aging populations, cardiovascular health, health systems outcomes, implementation science, occupational health, pain and symptom science, palliative and end-of-life care.

University of Maryland, Baltimore, Graduate School, School of Nursing, Doctor of Nursing Practice Program, Baltimore, MD 21201. Offers DNP. Tuition and fees vary according to program.

University of Maryland, Baltimore, Graduate School, School of Nursing, Master's Program in Nursing, Baltimore, MD 21201. Offers community health nursing (MS); gerontological nursing (MS); maternal-child nursing (MS); medical-surgical nursing (MS); nurse-midwifery education (MS); nursing administration (MS); nursing education (MS); nursing health policy (MS); primary care nursing (MS); psychiatric nursing (MS); MS/MBA. MS/MBA offered jointly with University of Baltimore. *Accreditation:* AACN; AANA/CANAEP. *Program availability:* Part-time. *Degree requirements:* For master's, comprehensive exam (for some programs), thesis or alternative. *Entrance requirements:* For master's, minimum GPA of 2.75, course work in statistics, BS in nursing. Additional exam requirements/recommendations for international students: Required—TOEFL (minimum score 550 paper-based; 80 iBT); Recommended—IELTS (minimum score 7). Electronic applications accepted. Tuition and fees vary according to program.

University of Maryland, Baltimore, Graduate School, School of Nursing, Post Baccalaureate Certificate Program in Nursing, Baltimore, MD 21201. Offers Postbaccalaureate Certificate. *Entrance requirements:* Additional exam requirements/recommendations for international students: Required—TOEFL (minimum score 550 paper-based; 80 iBT); Recommended—IELTS (minimum score 7). Electronic applications accepted. Tuition and fees vary according to program.

University of Massachusetts Amherst, Graduate School, College of Nursing, Amherst, MA 01003. Offers adult gerontology primary care nurse practitioner (DNP); clinical nurse leader (MS); family nurse practitioner (DNP); nursing (PhD); public health nurse leader (DNP). *Accreditation:* AACN. *Program availability:* Part-time, online learning. Terminal master's awarded for partial completion of doctoral program. *Degree requirements:* For master's, thesis optional; for doctorate, comprehensive exam, thesis/dissertation. *Entrance requirements:* Additional exam requirements/recommendations for international students: Required—TOEFL (minimum score 550 paper-based; 80 iBT), IELTS (minimum score 6.5). Electronic applications accepted. *Faculty research:* Health of older adults and their caretakers, mental health of individuals and families, health of children and adolescents, power and decision-making, transcultural health.

University of Massachusetts Boston, College of Nursing and Health Sciences, Boston, MA 02125-3393. Offers MS, DNP, PhD. *Accreditation:* AACN. *Program availability:* Part-time, evening/weekend. *Degree requirements:* For master's, comprehensive exam; for doctorate, comprehensive exam, thesis/dissertation. *Entrance requirements:* For master's, minimum GPA of 2.75; for doctorate, GRE General Test, master's degree, minimum GPA of 3.3. *Application deadline:* For fall admission, 3/1 for domestic students; for spring admission, 11/1 for domestic students. *Expenses:* Tuition, state resident: full-time $2590. Tuition, nonresident: full-time $9758. *Required fees:* $13,525. *Financial support:* Research assistantships with full tuition reimbursements, teaching assistantships with full tuition reimbursements, career-related internships or fieldwork, Federal Work-Study, and unspecified assistantships available. Support available to part-time students. Financial award application deadline: 3/1; financial award applicants required to submit FAFSA. *Faculty research:* Domestic abuse and pregnancy, health policy and home health care, caregiving burdens of families, the chronically ill, health care delivery models and their impact on outcomes, health promotion and disease prevention among the elderly. *Unit head:* Dr. Greer Glazer, Dean, 617-287-7500. *Application contact:* Peggy Roldan Patel, Graduate Admissions Coordinator, 617-287-6400, Fax: 617-287-6236, E-mail: bos.gadm@dpc.umassp.edu.

University of Massachusetts Dartmouth, Graduate School, Programs in Nursing, North Dartmouth, MA 02747-2300. Offers adult health (MS); community health (MS); nursing (PhD); nursing practice (DNP). *Program availability:* Part-time. *Faculty:* 26 full-time (all women), 39 part-time/adjunct (38 women). *Students:* 1 (woman) full-time, 115 part-time (108 women); includes 11 minority (4 Black or African American, non-Hispanic/Latino; 3 Asian, non-Hispanic/Latino; 4 Hispanic/Latino). Average age 40. 55 applicants, 91% accepted, 36 enrolled. In 2015, 18 master's, 5 doctorates awarded. *Degree requirements:* For master's, thesis, capstone project; for doctorate, comprehensive exam or thesis (for PhD only); project (for DNP only). *Entrance requirements:* For master's, GRE (if fewer than 45 credits at baccalaureate degree granting school), statement of purpose (minimum of 300 words), resume, 3 letters of recommendation, official transcripts, copy of RN license; for doctorate, GRE (for PHD, if fewer than 45 credits at baccalaureate degree granting school for DNP), statement of purpose (minimum of 300 words), resume, 3 letters of recommendation, official transcripts, copy of RN license, scholarly writing sample (minimum 10 pages for PhD). Additional exam requirements/recommendations for international students: Required—TOEFL (minimum score 533 paper-based; 72 iBT), IELTS (minimum score 6). *Application deadline:* For fall admission, 2/15 priority date for domestic and international students; for spring admission, 12/1 priority date for domestic students, 11/1 priority date for international students. Applications are processed on a rolling basis. Application fee: $60. Electronic

applications accepted. *Expenses:* Tuition, state resident: full-time $2071; part-time $86.29 per credit. Tuition, nonresident: full-time $8099; part-time $337.46 per credit. *Required fees:* $18,074; $762.08 per credit. Tuition and fees vary according to course load and reciprocity agreements. *Financial support:* In 2015–16, 1 fellowship with full tuition reimbursement (averaging $24,000 per year), 3 teaching assistantships with full tuition reimbursements (averaging $4,333 per year) were awarded; Federal Work-Study and unspecified assistantships also available. Support available to part-time students. Financial award application deadline: 3/1; financial award applicants required to submit FAFSA. *Faculty research:* Pathophysiology, aging with spinal cord injury, patient care, self care management, nursing education, reflective practice, breast cancer and quality of life of ethnically diverse populations, community based action research among vulnerable populations, care giver experiences. *Total annual research expenditures:* $61,000. *Unit head:* Kerry Fater, Graduate Program Director, 508-999-8525, Fax: 508-999-9127, E-mail: kfater@umassd.edu. *Application contact:* Steven Briggs, Director of Marketing and Recruitment for Graduate Studies, 508-999-8604, Fax: 508-999-8183, E-mail: graduate@umassd.edu.
Website: http://www.umassd.edu/nursing/graduateprograms

University of Massachusetts Lowell, College of Health Sciences, School of Nursing, Lowell, MA 01854. Offers adult/gerontological nursing (MS); family health nursing (MS); nursing (DNP, PhD). *Accreditation:* AACN. *Degree requirements:* For master's, thesis optional; for doctorate, thesis/dissertation. *Entrance requirements:* For master's and doctorate, GRE General Test. *Application deadline:* For fall admission, 4/1 priority date for domestic students; for spring admission, 10/1 for domestic students. Applications are processed on a rolling basis. Application fee: $20 ($35 for international students). *Expenses:* Tuition, state resident: full-time $14,304. Tuition, nonresident: full-time $25,853. *Required fees:* $375. Full-time tuition and fees vary according to campus/location and reciprocity agreements. *Financial support:* Fellowships with tuition reimbursements, research assistantships with full tuition reimbursements, teaching assistantships with full tuition reimbursements, career-related internships or fieldwork, Federal Work-Study, institutionally sponsored loans, scholarships/grants, and traineeships available. Support available to part-time students. Financial award application deadline: 4/1. *Faculty research:* Gerontology, women's health issues, long-term care, alcoholism, health promotion.
Website: http://www.uml.edu/Health-Sciences/Nursing/

University of Massachusetts Medical School, Graduate School of Nursing, Worcester, MA 01655-0115. Offers adult gerontological acute care nurse practitioner (DNP, Post Master's Certificate); adult gerontological primary care nurse practitioner (DNP, Post Master's Certificate); family nursing practitioner (DNP); nurse administrator (DNP); nurse educator (MS, Post Master's Certificate); nursing (PhD); nursing practitioner (DNP); population health (MS). *Accreditation:* AACN. *Faculty:* 18 full-time (15 women), 28 part-time/adjunct (22 women). *Students:* 143 full-time (119 women), 27 part-time (25 women); includes 28 minority (15 Black or African American, non-Hispanic/Latino; 10 Asian, non-Hispanic/Latino; 3 Hispanic/Latino), 1 international. Average age 34. 129 applicants, 68% accepted, 56 enrolled. In 2015, 43 master's, 10 doctorates, 2 other advanced degrees awarded. *Degree requirements:* For doctorate, thesis/dissertation (for some programs), comprehensive exam (for PhD); capstone project and manuscript (for DNP). *Entrance requirements:* For master's, GRE General Test, bachelor's degree in nursing, course work in statistics, unrestricted Massachusetts license as registered nurse; for doctorate, GRE General Test, bachelor's or master's degree; for Post Master's Certificate, GRE General Test, MS in nursing. Additional exam requirements/recommendations for international students: Required—TOEFL. *Application deadline:* For fall admission, 12/1 priority date for domestic students. Applications are processed on a rolling basis. Application fee: $60. Electronic applications accepted. *Expenses:* $10,994 resident per year; $18,210 non-resident per year. *Financial support:* In 2015–16, 31 students received support. Institutionally sponsored loans, scholarships/grants, traineeships, and tuition waivers (partial) available. Support available to part-time students. Financial award application deadline: 5/16; financial award applicants required to submit FAFSA. *Faculty research:* Health literacy, social justice, HIV prevention, cancer-related decision making, nursing education. *Total annual research expenditures:* $650,993. *Unit head:* Dr. Joan Vitello-Cicciu, Dean, 508-856-5081, Fax: 508-856-6552, E-mail: joan.vitello@umassmed.edu. *Application contact:* Diane Brescia, Admissions Coordinator, 508-856-3488, Fax: 508-856-5851, E-mail: diane.brescia@umassmed.edu.
Website: http://www.umassmed.edu/gsn/

University of Memphis, Loewenberg College of Nursing, Memphis, TN 38152. Offers executive leadership (MSN); family nurse practitioner (MSN); nursing (Graduate Certificate); nursing administration (MSN); nursing education (MSN). *Accreditation:* AACN. *Program availability:* Part-time, evening/weekend, online learning. *Faculty:* 12 full-time (all women), 3 part-time/adjunct (2 women). *Students:* 34 full-time (32 women), 220 part-time (196 women); includes 91 minority (80 Black or African American, non-Hispanic/Latino; 8 Asian, non-Hispanic/Latino; 1 Hispanic/Latino; 2 Two or more races, non-Hispanic/Latino). Average age 36. 165 applicants, 48% accepted, 27 enrolled. In 2015, 73 master's, 3 other advanced degrees awarded. *Degree requirements:* For master's, comprehensive exam, thesis optional, scholarly project; completion of clinical practicum hours. *Entrance requirements:* For master's, NCLEX Exam, interview. Additional exam requirements/recommendations for international students: Required—TOEFL (minimum score 550 paper-based; 79 iBT). *Application deadline:* For fall admission, 2/15 for domestic and international students; for spring admission, 10/1 for domestic and international students. Application fee: $35 ($60 for international students). *Financial support:* In 2015–16, 147 students received support. Federal Work-Study and scholarships/grants available. Financial award application deadline: 2/15; financial award applicants required to submit FAFSA. *Faculty research:* Technology in nursing, nurse retention, cultural competence, health policy, health access. *Total annual research expenditures:* $560,619. *Unit head:* Dr. Robert Koch, Associate Dean, 901-678-3908, Fax: 901-678-4907, E-mail: rakoch@memphis.edu. *Application contact:* Dr. Karen Weddle-West, Information Contact, 901-678-2531, Fax: 901-678-5023, E-mail: gradsch@memphis.edu.
Website: http://www.memphis.edu/nursing

University of Miami, Graduate School, School of Nursing and Health Studies, Coral Gables, FL 33124. Offers acute care (MSN), including acute care nurse practitioner, nurse anesthesia; nursing (PhD); primary care (MSN), including adult nurse practitioner, family nurse practitioner, nurse midwifery, women's health practitioner. *Accreditation:* AACN; AANA/CANAEP; ACNM/ACME (one or more programs are accredited). *Program availability:* Part-time. *Degree requirements:* For master's, thesis optional; for doctorate, thesis/dissertation. *Entrance requirements:* For master's, GRE General Test, BSN, minimum GPA of 3.0, Florida RN license; for doctorate, GRE General Test, BSN or MSN, minimum GPA of 3.0. Additional exam requirements/recommendations for international students: Required—TOEFL (minimum score 550 paper-based). Electronic applications accepted. *Faculty research:* Transcultural nursing, exercise and depression in Alzheimer's disease, infectious diseases/HIV–AIDS, postpartum depression, outcomes assessment.

University of Michigan, Rackham Graduate School, School of Nursing, Ann Arbor, MI 48109. Offers acute care pediatric nurse practitioner (MS); nursing (DNP, PhD, Post

Nursing—General

Master's Certificate). *Accreditation:* AACN; ACNM/ACME (one or more programs are accredited). *Program availability:* Part-time, online learning. Terminal master's awarded for partial completion of doctoral program. *Degree requirements:* For doctorate, thesis/dissertation. *Faculty research:* Preparation of clinical nurse researchers, biobehavior, women's health, health promotion, substance abuse, psychobiology of menopause, fertility, obesity, health care systems. *Unit head:* Dr. Kathleen Potempa, Dean, 734-764-7185, Fax: 734-764-7186. *Application contact:* E-mail: sn-osams@umich.edu. Website: http://www.nursing.umich.edu/

University of Michigan–Flint, School of Health Professions and Studies, Program in Nursing, Flint, MI 48502-1950. Offers adult-gerontology acute care (DNP); adult-gerontology primary care (DNP); family nurse practitioner (MSN, DNP); psychiatric mental health (DNP); psychiatric mental health nurse practitioner (Certificate). *Accreditation:* AACN. *Program availability:* Part-time. *Faculty:* 32 full-time (31 women), 77 part-time/adjunct (69 women). *Students:* 131 full-time (114 women), 81 part-time (71 women); includes 59 minority (35 Black or African American, non-Hispanic/Latino; 2 American Indian or Alaska Native, non-Hispanic/Latino; 7 Asian, non-Hispanic/Latino; 7 Hispanic/Latino; 8 Two or more races, non-Hispanic/Latino), 2 international. Average age 38. 108 applicants, 75% accepted, 56 enrolled. In 2015, 16 master's, 29 doctorates awarded. *Degree requirements:* For master's, thesis. *Entrance requirements:* For master's, BSN from accredited college or university with minimum overall undergraduate GPA of 3.2; for doctorate, BSN or MSN (with APRN certification) from accredited college or university; for Certificate, completion of nurse practitioner program with MS from accredited college or university and minimum overall GPA of 3.2; current unencumbered RN license in the United States; current unencumbered license as nurse practitioner. Additional exam requirements/recommendations for international students: Required—TOEFL (minimum score 560 paper-based; 84 iBT), IELTS (minimum score 6.5). *Application deadline:* For fall admission, 8/1 for domestic students, 5/1 for international students; for winter admission, 11/15 for domestic students, 9/1 for international students; for spring admission, 3/15 for domestic students, 1/1 for international students. Applications are processed on a rolling basis. Application fee: $55. Electronic applications accepted. *Financial support:* Federal Work-Study, scholarships/grants, and unspecified assistantships available. Support available to part-time students. Financial award application deadline: 3/1; financial award applicants required to submit FAFSA. *Faculty research:* Family system stress, self breast exam, family roads evaluation, causal model testing for psychosocial development, basic needs. *Unit head:* Dr. Constance J. Creech, Director, 810-762-3420, Fax: 810-766-6851, E-mail: ccreech@umflint.edu. *Application contact:* Bradley T. Maki, Director of Graduate Admissions, 810-762-3171, Fax: 810-766-6789, E-mail: bmaki@umflint.edu. Website: https://www.umflint.edu/nursing

University of Minnesota, Twin Cities Campus, Graduate School, School of Nursing, Minneapolis, MN 55455-0213. Offers MN, MS, DNP, PhD. *Accreditation:* AACN; AANA/CANAEP; ACNM/ACME (one or more programs are accredited). *Program availability:* Part-time, online learning. Terminal master's awarded for partial completion of doctoral program. *Degree requirements:* For master's, final oral exam, project or thesis; for doctorate, thesis/dissertation. *Entrance requirements:* For master's and doctorate, GRE General Test. Additional exam requirements/recommendations for international students: Required—TOEFL (minimum score 586 paper-based). *Expenses:* Contact institution. *Faculty research:* Child and family health promotion, nursing research on elders.

University of Mississippi Medical Center, School of Nursing, Jackson, MS 39216-4505. Offers MSN, DNP, PhD. *Accreditation:* AACN. *Program availability:* Part-time, evening/weekend, online learning. *Degree requirements:* For master's, thesis optional; for doctorate, comprehensive exam, thesis/dissertation, publishable paper. *Entrance requirements:* For master's, GRE, 1 year of clinical experience (acute care nurse practitioner only), RN license; for doctorate, GRE, RN license, professional nursing experience. Additional exam requirements/recommendations for international students: Required—TOEFL (minimum score 550 paper-based; 79 iBT). Electronic applications accepted. *Expenses:* Contact institution. *Faculty research:* Predictive biomarkers for head and neck cancer; cellular events in response to demyelization in diseases; health care disparities (various diseases); childhood obesity; psychosocial adaptations to pregnancy and birth.

University of Missouri, Office of Research and Graduate Studies, Sinclair School of Nursing, Columbia, MO 65211. Offers adult-gerontology clinical nurse specialist (DNP, Certificate); family nurse practitioner (DNP); family psychiatric and mental health nurse practitioner (DNP); nursing (MS, PhD); nursing leadership and innovations in health care (DNP); pediatric clinical nurse specialist (DNP, Certificate); pediatric nurse practitioner (DNP). *Accreditation:* AACN. *Program availability:* Part-time. *Degree requirements:* For master's, thesis optional, oral exam; for doctorate, thesis/dissertation. *Entrance requirements:* For master's, GRE General Test, BSN, minimum GPA of 3.0 during last 60 hours, nursing license. Additional exam requirements/recommendations for international students: Required—TOEFL (minimum score 550 paper-based; 79 iBT). *Application deadline:* For fall admission, 2/1 priority date for domestic and international students. Applications are processed on a rolling basis. Application fee: $55 ($75 for international students). Electronic applications accepted. *Financial support:* Fellowships, research assistantships, teaching assistantships, career-related internships or fieldwork, institutionally sponsored loans, scholarships/grants, traineeships, health care benefits, tuition waivers (full), and unspecified assistantships available. Support available to part-time students. Website: http://nursing.missouri.edu/

University of Missouri–Kansas City, School of Nursing and Health Studies, Kansas City, MO 64108. Offers adult clinical nurse specialist (MSN), including adult nurse practitioner, women's health nurse practitioner (MSN, DNP); adult clinical nursing practice (DNP), including adult gerontology nurse practitioner, women's health nurse practitioner (MSN, DNP); clinical nursing practice (DNP), including family nurse practitioner; family nurse practitioner (MSN); neonatal nurse practitioner (MSN); nurse educator (MSN); nurse executive (MSN); nursing (PhD); nursing practice (DNP); pediatric clinical nursing practice (DNP), including pediatric nurse practitioner; pediatric nurse practitioner (MSN). *Accreditation:* AACN. *Program availability:* Part-time, online learning. *Faculty:* 44 full-time (40 women), 47 part-time/adjunct (45 women). *Students:* 62 full-time (43 women), 259 part-time (239 women); includes 61 minority (28 Black or African American, non-Hispanic/Latino; 3 American Indian or Alaska Native, non-Hispanic/Latino; 16 Asian, non-Hispanic/Latino; 10 Hispanic/Latino; 4 Two or more races, non-Hispanic/Latino). Average age 35. 102 applicants, 35% accepted, 36 enrolled. In 2015, 116 master's, 23 doctorates awarded. *Degree requirements:* For master's, thesis or alternative. *Entrance requirements:* For master's, minimum undergraduate GPA of 3.2; for doctorate, GRE, 3 letters of reference. Additional exam requirements/recommendations for international students: Required—TOEFL (minimum score 550 paper-based; 80 iBT). *Application deadline:* For fall admission, 2/1 priority date for domestic and international students; for spring admission, 9/1 priority date for domestic and international students. Application fee: $45 ($50 for international students). *Financial support:* In 2015–16, 2 teaching assistantships with partial tuition reimbursements (averaging $6,650 per year) were awarded; fellowships, research assistantships, career-related internships or fieldwork, Federal Work-Study,

institutionally sponsored loans, and tuition waivers (full and partial) also available. Support available to part-time students. Financial award application deadline: 3/1; financial award applicants required to submit FAFSA. *Faculty research:* Geriatrics/gerontology, children's pain, neonatology, Alzheimer's care, cancer caregivers. *Unit head:* Dr. Ann Cary, Dean, 816-235-1723, Fax: 816-235-1701, E-mail: caryah@umkc.edu. *Application contact:* Judy Jellison, Coordinator for Admissions and Recruitment, 816-235-1740, Fax: 816-235-1701, E-mail: jellisonj@umkc.edu. Website: http://nursing.umkc.edu/

University of Missouri–St. Louis, College of Nursing, St. Louis, MO 63121-4400. Offers adult/geriatric nurse practitioner (Post Master's Certificate); family nurse practitioner (Post Master's Certificate); nurse educator (MSN); nurse practitioner (MSN); nursing (DNP, PhD); pediatric nurse practitioner (Post Master's Certificate); psychiatric-mental health nurse practitioner (Post Master's Certificate); women's health nurse practitioner (Post Master's Certificate). *Accreditation:* AACN. *Program availability:* Part-time. *Faculty:* 21 full-time (19 women), 6 part-time/adjunct (5 women). *Students:* 18 full-time (17 women), 227 part-time (215 women); includes 34 minority (22 Black or African American, non-Hispanic/Latino; 8 Asian, non-Hispanic/Latino; 3 Hispanic/Latino; 1 Two or more races, non-Hispanic/Latino), 1 international. Average age 35. 152 applicants, 69% accepted, 83 enrolled. *Degree requirements:* For doctorate, comprehensive exam, thesis/dissertation; for Post Master's Certificate, thesis. *Entrance requirements:* For master's, 2 recommendation letters; minimum GPA of 3.0; BSN; nursing licensure; statement of purpose; course in differential/inferential statistics; for doctorate, GRE, 2 letters of recommendation, MSN, minimum GPA 3.2, course in differential/inferential statistics; for Post Master's Certificate, 2 recommendation letters; MSN; advanced practice certificate; minimum GPA of 3.0; essay. Additional exam requirements/recommendations for international students: Recommended—TOEFL (minimum score 550 paper-based; 79 iBT), IELTS (minimum score 6.5). *Application deadline:* For fall admission, 2/15 for domestic and international students. Application fee: $50 ($40 for international students). Electronic applications accepted. *Financial support:* Research assistantships with tuition reimbursements available. Financial award application deadline: 4/1; financial award applicants required to submit FAFSA. *Faculty research:* Health promotion and restoration, family disruption, violence, abuse, battered women, health survey methods. *Unit head:* Dr. Roberta Lavin, Director, 314-516-6066. *Application contact:* 314-516-5458, Fax: 314-516-6996, E-mail: gradadm@umsl.edu. Website: http://www.umsl.edu/divisions/nursing/

University of Mobile, Graduate Programs, Program in Nursing, Mobile, AL 36613. Offers MSN. *Accreditation:* AACN. *Program availability:* Part-time, evening/weekend. *Faculty:* 2 full-time (both women), 1 (woman) part-time/adjunct. *Students:* 8 full-time (all women), 7 part-time (6 women); includes 9 minority (6 Black or African American, non-Hispanic/Latino; 3 Asian, non-Hispanic/Latino). Average age 37. 14 applicants, 79% accepted, 11 enrolled. In 2015, 4 master's awarded. *Degree requirements:* For master's, comprehensive exam, thesis or alternative. *Entrance requirements:* For master's, GRE. Additional exam requirements/recommendations for international students: Required—TOEFL (minimum score 550 paper-based; 80 iBT). *Application deadline:* For fall admission, 8/3 priority date for domestic and international students; for spring admission, 12/23 priority date for domestic and international students. Applications are processed on a rolling basis. Application fee: $40 ($50 for international students). Electronic applications accepted. *Expenses:* Tuition, area resident: Full-time $9036; part-time $6024 per credit hour. *Required fees:* $400. *Financial support:* Application deadline: 8/1; applicants required to submit FAFSA. *Faculty research:* Nursing management, transcultural nursing, spiritual aspects, educational expectations. *Unit head:* Dr. Jan Wood, Dean, School of Nursing, 251-442-2446, Fax: 251-442-2520, E-mail: jwood@umobile.edu. *Application contact:* Danielle M. Riley, Administrative Assistant for Academic Affairs/Graduate Enrollment Counselor, 251-442-2270, Fax: 251-442-2523, E-mail: driley@umobile.edu. Website: http://www.umobile.edu/

University of Nebraska Medical Center, Program in Nursing, Omaha, NE 68198. Offers PhD. *Accreditation:* AACN. *Program availability:* Part-time, online learning. *Faculty:* 52 full-time (51 women), 8 part-time/adjunct (all women). *Students:* 18 full-time (16 women), 7 part-time (all women); includes 4 minority (2 Black or African American, non-Hispanic/Latino; 1 Hispanic/Latino; 1 Two or more races, non-Hispanic/Latino), 2 international. Average age 39. 2 applicants, 100% accepted, 2 enrolled. In 2015, 7 doctorates awarded. *Degree requirements:* For doctorate, comprehensive exam, thesis/dissertation. *Entrance requirements:* For doctorate, GRE General Test, minimum GPA of 3.2. Additional exam requirements/recommendations for international students: Required—TOEFL (minimum score 550 paper-based; 80 iBT). *Application deadline:* For fall admission, 4/1 for domestic and international students; for spring admission, 8/1 for domestic and international students. Applications are processed on a rolling basis. Application fee: $45. Electronic applications accepted. *Expenses:* Contact institution. *Financial support:* In 2015–16, 1 fellowship with full tuition reimbursement (averaging $23,100 per year), 1 research assistantship with full tuition reimbursement (averaging $23,100 per year), teaching assistantships with full tuition reimbursements (averaging $9,000 per year) were awarded; scholarships/grants also available. Support available to part-time students. Financial award application deadline: 2/1; financial award applicants required to submit FAFSA. *Faculty research:* Health promotion, sleep and fatigue in cancer patients, symptoms management in cardiovascular disease, prevention of osteoporosis in breast cancer survivors, impact of quality end of life care in nursing homes. *Unit head:* Dr. Kathleen Hanna, Professor, 402-559-5468, E-mail: kathy.hanna@unmc.edu. *Application contact:* Denise Ott, Office Associate, 402-559-2150, E-mail: denise.ott@unmc.edu. Website: http://www.unmc.edu/nursing/

University of Nevada, Las Vegas, Graduate College, School of Nursing, Las Vegas, NV 89154-3018. Offers family nurse practitioner (Advanced Certificate); nursing (MS, DNP). *Accreditation:* AACN. *Program availability:* Part-time, online learning. *Faculty:* 10 full-time (all women), 10 part-time/adjunct (9 women). *Students:* 42 full-time (36 women), 87 part-time (77 women); includes 42 minority (2 Black or African American, non-Hispanic/Latino; 21 Asian, non-Hispanic/Latino; 10 Hispanic/Latino; 9 Two or more races, non-Hispanic/Latino), 11 international. Average age 38. 135 applicants, 51% accepted, 53 enrolled. In 2015, 26 master's, 14 doctorates, 1 other advanced degree awarded. *Degree requirements:* For master's, comprehensive exam, thesis; for doctorate, comprehensive exam (for some programs), thesis/dissertation. *Entrance requirements:* For doctorate, GRE General Test. Additional exam requirements/recommendations for international students: Recommended—TOEFL (minimum score 550 paper-based; 80 iBT), IELTS (minimum score 7). *Application deadline:* For fall admission, 2/1 for domestic students, 5/1 for international students. Application fee: $60 ($95 for international students). Electronic applications accepted. *Expenses:* $264 per credit state resident full-time and part-time; $6,955 per semester nonresident full-time, $264 per credit; $555 per credit nonresident part-time. *Financial support:* In 2015–16, 6 students received support, including 6 teaching assistantships with partial tuition reimbursements available (averaging $11,500 per year); institutionally sponsored loans, scholarships/grants, health care benefits, and unspecified assistantships also available. Financial award application deadline: 3/1. *Faculty research:* Chronic diseases and health promotion in diabetes, cardiovascular disease, pain, and obesity; informal caregiver stress and risk factors; technology enhanced interventions; symptom and self-

management. *Total annual research expenditures:* $581,273. *Unit head:* Dr. Carolyn Yucha, Dean, 702-895-5307, Fax: 702-895-4807, E-mail: carolyn.yucha@unlv.edu. *Application contact:* Graduate College Admissions Evaluator, 702-895-3367, Fax: 702-895-4180, E-mail: gradadmissions@unlv.edu.
Website: http://nursing.unlv.edu/

University of Nevada, Reno, Graduate School, Division of Health Sciences, Orvis School of Nursing, Reno, NV 89557. Offers MSN, DNP, MPH/MSN. *Accreditation:* AACN. *Degree requirements:* For master's, thesis optional. *Entrance requirements:* For master's, minimum GPA of 3.0 in bachelor's degree from accredited school. Additional exam requirements/recommendations for international students: Required—TOEFL (minimum score 500 paper-based; 61 iBT), IELTS (minimum score 6). Electronic applications accepted. *Faculty research:* Analysis and evaluation of nursing theory, strategies for nursing applications.

University of New Brunswick Fredericton, School of Graduate Studies, Faculty of Nursing, Fredericton, NB E3B 5A3, Canada. Offers nurse educator (MN); nurse practitioner (MN); nursing (MN). *Program availability:* Part-time, online learning. *Faculty:* 19 full-time (18 women). *Students:* 14 full-time (13 women), 30 part-time (29 women). In 2015, 18 master's awarded. *Degree requirements:* For master's, comprehensive exam (for some programs), thesis (for some programs). *Entrance requirements:* For master's, undergraduate coursework in statistics and nursing research, minimum GPA of 3.3, registration as a nurse (or eligibility) in New Brunswick. Additional exam requirements/recommendations for international students: Required—TOEFL (minimum score 600 paper-based). *Application deadline:* For winter admission, 1/2 priority date for domestic students. Application fee: $50 Canadian dollars. Electronic applications accepted. *Financial support:* In 2015–16, 7 fellowships, 2 research assistantships were awarded. *Faculty research:* Intimate partner violence; abuse; healthy child development, chronic illness and addiction; rural populations' access to health care and primary healthcare; teaching and learning in the classroom, clinical lab, and by distance; Aboriginal nursing; workplace bullying; eating disorders; women's health; lesbian health; nurse managed primary care clinics; HIV/AIDS; returning to work after depression; adolescent mental health; cancer survivorship. *Unit head:* Kathy Wilson, Assistant Dean of Graduate and Advanced RN Studies, 506-458-7640, Fax: 506-447-3057, E-mail: kewilson@unb.ca. *Application contact:* Francis Perry, Graduate Secretary, 506-451-6844, Fax: 506-447-3057, E-mail: fperry@unb.ca.
Website: http://www.unb.ca/fredericton/nursing/graduate/

University of New Hampshire, Graduate School, College of Health and Human Services, Department of Nursing, Durham, NH 03824. Offers family practitioner (Postbaccalaureate Certificate); nursing (MS, DNP). *Accreditation:* AACN. *Program availability:* Part-time. *Degree requirements:* For master's, thesis or alternative. *Entrance requirements:* For master's, GRE General Test or MAT. Additional exam requirements/recommendations for international students: Required—TOEFL (minimum score 550 paper-based; 80 iBT). *Application deadline:* For fall admission, 4/1 priority date for domestic students, 4/1 for international students; for spring admission, 11/1 for domestic students. Applications are processed on a rolling basis. Application fee: $65. Electronic applications accepted. *Expenses:* Tuition, state resident: full-time $13,840; part-time $770 per credit hour. Tuition, nonresident: full-time $27,130; part-time $1175 per credit hour. *Required fees:* $2080; $1040. Tuition and fees vary according to degree level and program. *Financial support:* Fellowships, research assistantships, teaching assistantships, Federal Work-Study, scholarships/grants, and tuition waivers (full and partial) available. Financial award application deadline: 2/15. *Faculty research:* Adult health, nursing administration, family nurse practitioner. *Unit head:* Dr. Gene Harkless, Chair, 603-862-2285. *Application contact:* Jane Dufresne, Administrative Assistant, 603-862-2299, E-mail: nursing.department@unh.edu.
Website: http://www.chhs.unh.edu/nursing

University of New Mexico, Graduate Studies, Health Sciences Center, Program in Nursing, Albuquerque, NM 87131-0001. Offers MSN, DNP, PhD. *Accreditation:* AACN; ACNM/ACME (one or more programs are accredited). *Program availability:* Part-time, online learning. *Faculty:* 22 full-time (20 women), 3 part-time/adjunct (all women). *Students:* 77 full-time (67 women), 62 part-time (54 women); includes 62 minority (3 Black or African American, non-Hispanic/Latino; 9 American Indian or Alaska Native, non-Hispanic/Latino; 7 Asian, non-Hispanic/Latino; 40 Hispanic/Latino; 1 Native Hawaiian or other Pacific Islander, non-Hispanic/Latino; 2 Two or more races, non-Hispanic/Latino). Average age 42. 112 applicants, 62% accepted, 49 enrolled. In 2015, 70 master's, 8 doctorates awarded. *Degree requirements:* For master's, comprehensive exam, thesis optional; for doctorate, comprehensive exam, thesis/dissertation. *Entrance requirements:* For master's, minimum GPA of 3.0, course work in statistics (recommended), interview (for some concentrations), BSN or RN with BA; for doctorate, interview, minimum GPA of 3.0, writing sample, MSN or BSN with MA. Additional exam requirements/recommendations for international students: Required—TOEFL. Application fee: $60. Electronic applications accepted. *Financial support:* Fellowships, research assistantships with partial tuition reimbursements, teaching assistantships with partial tuition reimbursements, institutionally sponsored loans, scholarships/grants, and unspecified assistantships available. Support available to part-time students. Financial award application deadline: 3/1; financial award applicants required to submit FAFSA. *Faculty research:* Women's and children's health, pregnancy prevention in teens, vulnerable populations, nursing education, chronic illness, symptom appraisal and management. *Unit head:* Dr. Nancy Ridenour, Dean, 505-272-6284, Fax: 505-272-4343, E-mail: nridenour@salud.unm.edu. *Application contact:* Nissane Capps, Senior Academic Advisor, 505-272-4223, Fax: 505-272-3970, E-mail: ncapps@salud.unm.edu.
Website: http://nursing.unm.edu/

University of North Alabama, College of Nursing and Allied Health, Florence, AL 35632-0001. Offers MSN. *Accreditation:* AACN. *Program availability:* 100% online, blended/hybrid learning. *Faculty:* 4 full-time (all women). *Students:* 47 full-time (44 women), 53 part-time (47 women); includes 20 minority (18 Black or African American, non-Hispanic/Latino; 1 American Indian or Alaska Native, non-Hispanic/Latino; 1 Asian, non-Hispanic/Latino). Average age 39. 38 applicants, 89% accepted, 26 enrolled. In 2015, 24 master's awarded. *Entrance requirements:* Additional exam requirements/recommendations for international students: Required—TOEFL (minimum score 79 iBT), IELTS (minimum score 6), PTE (minimum score 54). *Application deadline:* Applications are processed on a rolling basis. Application fee: $50 ($100 for international students). Electronic applications accepted. *Expenses:* Tuition, state resident: full-time $2286; part-time $1524 per semester. Tuition, nonresident: full-time $4572; part-time $3048 per semester. *Required fees:* $801; $579 per semester. Tuition and fees vary according to course load. *Financial support:* In 2015–16, 4 students received support. Scholarships/grants available. Financial award application deadline: 2/1; financial award applicants required to submit FAFSA. *Unit head:* Dr. Vicky G. Pierce, Dean, 256-765-6301, E-mail: vgpierce@una.edu. *Application contact:* Hillary N. Coats, Graduate Admissions Coordinator, 256-465-4447, E-mail: graduate@una.edu.
Website: http://www.una.edu/nursing/

The University of North Carolina at Chapel Hill, School of Nursing, Chapel Hill, NC 27599-7460. Offers advanced practice registered nurse (DNP); health care systems (DNP); nursing (MSN, PhD, PMC), including administration (MSN), adult gerontology primary care nurse practitioner (MSN), clinical nurse leader (MSN), education (MSN),

informatics (MSN, PMC), nursing leadership (PMC), outcomes management (MSN), primary care family nurse practitioner (MSN), primary care pediatric nurse practitioner (MSN), psychiatric/mental health nurse practitioner (MSN, PMC). *Accreditation:* AACN; ACEN (one or more programs are accredited). *Program availability:* Part-time. *Faculty:* 86 full-time (78 women), 44 part-time/adjunct (40 women). *Students:* 208 full-time (186 women), 128 part-time (116 women); includes 109 minority (49 Black or African American, non-Hispanic/Latino; 4 American Indian or Alaska Native, non-Hispanic/Latino; 32 Asian, non-Hispanic/Latino; 7 Hispanic/Latino; 17 Two or more races, non-Hispanic/Latino), 17 international. Average age 33. 624 applicants, 25% accepted, 150 enrolled. In 2015, 91 master's, 14 doctorates awarded. *Degree requirements:* For master's, comprehensive exam, thesis; for doctorate, thesis/dissertation, 3 exams; for PMC, thesis. *Entrance requirements:* Additional exam requirements/recommendations for international students: Required—TOEFL (minimum score 575 paper-based; 89 iBT), IELTS (minimum score 8). *Application deadline:* For fall admission, 12/15 for domestic and international students. Application fee: $85. Electronic applications accepted. *Financial support:* In 2015–16, 8 fellowships with full tuition reimbursements, 6 research assistantships with partial tuition reimbursements (averaging $8,000 per year), 10 teaching assistantships with partial tuition reimbursements (averaging $8,000 per year) were awarded; scholarships/grants, traineeships, health care benefits, and unspecified assistantships also available. Support available to part-time students. Financial award application deadline: 3/1; financial award applicants required to submit FAFSA. *Faculty research:* Preventing and managing chronic illness, reducing health disparities, Improving healthcare quality and patient outcomes, understanding biobehavioral and genetic bases of health and illness, developing innovative ways to enhance science and its clinical translation. *Unit head:* Donna S. Havens, PhD, RN, Dean/Professor, 919-966-3731, Fax: 919-966-3540, E-mail: dhavens@email.unc.edu. *Application contact:* Emily Sayed, Assistant Director, Graduate Admissions, 919-966-4260, Fax: 919-966-3540, E-mail: sayed@unc.edu.
Website: http://nursing.unc.edu

The University of North Carolina at Charlotte, College of Health and Human Services, School of Nursing, Charlotte, NC 28223-0001. Offers adult-gerontology acute care nurse practitioner (MSN, Post-Master's Certificate); advanced clinical nursing (MSN); community public health nursing (MSN); family nurse practitioner across the lifespan (MSN, Post-Master's Certificate); nurse administrator (MSN, Graduate Certificate); nurse anesthesia (MSN, Post-Master's Certificate); nurse educator (MSN, Graduate Certificate); nursing (DNP); nursing systems/population (MSN). *Accreditation:* AACN. *Program availability:* Part-time, blended/hybrid learning. *Faculty:* 26 full-time (25 women), 4 part-time/adjunct (3 women). *Students:* 109 full-time (89 women), 112 part-time (107 women); includes 46 minority (37 Black or African American, non-Hispanic/Latino; 3 Asian, non-Hispanic/Latino; 5 Hispanic/Latino; 1 Two or more races, non-Hispanic/Latino). Average age 33. 321 applicants, 34% accepted, 84 enrolled. In 2015, 76 master's, 4 doctorates, 7 other advanced degrees awarded. Terminal master's awarded for partial completion of doctoral program. *Degree requirements:* For master's, practicum, synthesis and integration or thesis, residency, internship (varies by program); for doctorate, thesis/dissertation or alternative, residency; for other advanced degree, practicum. *Entrance requirements:* For master's, GRE General Test, unencumbered license as Registered Nurse in North Carolina; BSN from nationally-accredited program; one year of professional nursing practice in acute/critical care; minimum overall GPA of 3.0 in the last degree and 60 hours of nursing coursework; completion of an undergraduate statistics course with minimum grade of C; statement of purpose; for doctorate, GRE or MAT, master's degree in nursing in an advanced nursing practice specialty from nationally-accredited program; minimum overall GPA of 3.5 in MSN program; current RN licensure in U.S. at time of application with eligibility for NC licensure; for other advanced degree, GRE. Additional exam requirements/recommendations for international students: Required—TOEFL (minimum score 557 paper-based, 83 iBT) or IELTS (minimum score 6.5). *Application deadline:* For fall admission, 2/1 for domestic and international students; for spring admission, 10/1 priority date for domestic and international students; for summer admission, 4/1 priority date for domestic and international students. Applications are processed on a rolling basis. Application fee: $75. Electronic applications accepted. *Expenses:* Contact institution. *Financial support:* In 2015–16, 9 students received support, including 5 research assistantships (averaging $4,850 per year), 3 teaching assistantships (averaging $2,911 per year); career-related internships or fieldwork, institutionally sponsored loans, scholarships/grants, traineeships, unspecified assistantships, and administrative assistantships also available. Support available to part-time students. Financial award application deadline: 3/1; financial award applicants required to submit FAFSA. *Faculty research:* Improving care outcomes for the elderly; vulnerable populations; symptom management; self management/health promotion strategies of older adults; migration and maternal child health; health disparities, health literacy, and access to healthcare in Latino adults with diabetes; psychiatric nursing. *Total annual research expenditures:* $875,169. *Unit head:* Dr. Dee Baldwin, Associate Dean, 704-687-7952, Fax: 704-687-6017, E-mail: dbaldwi5@uncc.edu. *Application contact:* Kathy B. Giddings, Director of Graduate Admissions, 704-687-5503, Fax: 704-687-1668, E-mail: gradadm@uncc.edu.
Website: http://nursing.uncc.edu/

The University of North Carolina at Greensboro, Graduate School, School of Nursing, Greensboro, NC 27412-5001. Offers adult clinical nurse specialist (MSN, PMC); adult/gerontological nurse practitioner (MSN, PMC); nurse anesthesia (MSN, PMC); nursing (PhD); nursing administration (MSN); nursing education (MSN); MSN/MBA. *Accreditation:* AACN; AANA/CANAEP; ACEN. *Degree requirements:* For master's, thesis or alternative. *Entrance requirements:* For master's, GRE General Test or MAT, BSN, clinical experience, liability insurance, RN license; for PMC, liability insurance, MSN, RN license. Additional exam requirements/recommendations for international students: Required—TOEFL. Electronic applications accepted.

The University of North Carolina at Pembroke, Graduate School, Department of Nursing, Pembroke, NC 28372-1510. Offers clinical nurse leader (MSN); nurse educator (MSN); rural case manager (MSN). *Program availability:* Part-time. Application fee: $45 ($60 for international students). *Unit head:* Dr. Jennifer W. Twaddell, Interim Chair, 910-775-4142, Fax: 910-521-6751, E-mail: jennifer.twaddell@uncp.edu. *Application contact:* Dr. Jennifer W. Twaddell, Interim Chair, 910-775-4142, Fax: 910-521-6751, E-mail: jennifer.twaddell@uncp.edu.
Website: http://www.uncp.edu/nursing/

The University of North Carolina Wilmington, School of Nursing, Wilmington, NC 28403-5995. Offers clinical research and product development (MS); family nurse practitioner (MSN, Post-Master's Certificate). *Accreditation:* AACN; ACEN. *Program availability:* Part-time, online learning. *Faculty:* 18 full-time (17 women). *Students:* 58 full-time (57 women), 84 part-time (73 women); includes 25 minority (15 Black or African American, non-Hispanic/Latino; 5 American Indian or Alaska Native, non-Hispanic/Latino; 2 Hispanic/Latino; 3 Two or more races, non-Hispanic/Latino). Average age 38. 222 applicants, 57 enrolled. In 2015, 33 master's awarded. *Degree requirements:* For master's, research project/presentation. *Entrance requirements:* For master's, GRE General Test. Additional exam requirements/recommendations for international students: Required—TOEFL (minimum score 79 iBT), IELTS (minimum score 6.5). *Application deadline:* For fall admission, 3/1 for domestic students. Applications are

processed on a rolling basis. Application fee: $60. Electronic applications accepted. *Expenses:* $8,854.10 in-state full-time per year; $20,945.04 out-of-state full-time per year. *Financial support:* Scholarships/grants available. Financial award application deadline: 3/15; financial award applicants required to submit FAFSA. *Unit head:* Dr. Carol Heinrich, Director, 910-962-7410, Fax: 910-962-3723, E-mail: badzekl@uncw.edu. *Application contact:* Dr. Jim Lyon, Graduate Coordinator, 910-962-2936, E-mail: lyonj@uncw.edu.
Website: http://www.uncw.edu/son/

University of North Dakota, Graduate School, College of Nursing, Department of Nursing, Grand Forks, ND 58202. Offers adult-gerontological nurse practitioner (MSN); advanced public health nurse (MSN); family nurse practitioner (MSN); nurse anesthesia (MSN); nurse educator (MSN); nursing (DNP, PhD); psychiatric and mental health nurse practitioner (MSN).

University of Northern Colorado, Graduate School, College of Natural and Health Sciences, School of Nursing, Greeley, CO 80639. Offers clinical nurse specialist in chronic illness (MS); family nurse practitioner (MS); nursing education (MS, PhD). *Accreditation:* AACN. *Program availability:* Online learning. *Degree requirements:* For master's, comprehensive exam, thesis or alternative; for doctorate, comprehensive exam, thesis/dissertation. *Entrance requirements:* For master's and doctorate, GRE General Test, minimum GPA of 3.0 in last 60 hours, BS in nursing, 2 letters of recommendation. Electronic applications accepted.

University of North Florida, Brooks College of Health, School of Nursing, Jacksonville, FL 32224. Offers clinical nurse leader (MSN); clinical nurse specialist (MSN); family nurse practitioner (Certificate); nurse anesthetist (MSN); nursing practice (DNP); primary care nurse practitioner (MSN). *Accreditation:* AACN; AANA/CANAEP. *Program availability:* Part-time. *Faculty:* 23 full-time (17 women), 2 part-time/adjunct (1 woman). *Students:* 108 full-time (90 women), 117 part-time (93 women); includes 54 minority (17 Black or African American, non-Hispanic/Latino; 1 American Indian or Alaska Native, non-Hispanic/Latino; 13 Asian, non-Hispanic/Latino; 17 Hispanic/Latino; 1 Native Hawaiian or other Pacific Islander, non-Hispanic/Latino; 5 Two or more races, non-Hispanic/Latino), 3 international. Average age 36. 136 applicants, 81% accepted, 74 enrolled. In 2015, 46 master's, 6 doctorates awarded. *Degree requirements:* For master's, thesis optional. *Entrance requirements:* For master's, GRE General Test, minimum GPA of 3.0 in last 60 hours of course work, BSN, clinical experience, resume; for doctorate, GRE, master's degree in nursing specialty from nationally-accredited program; national certification in one of the following APRN roles: CNE, CNM, CNS, CRNA, CNP; minimum graduate GPA of 3.3; three letters of reference which address academic ability and clinical skills; active license as registered nurse or advanced practice registered nurse. Additional exam requirements/recommendations for international students: Required—TOEFL (minimum score 500 paper-based; 61 iBT). *Application deadline:* For fall admission, 3/15 for domestic students, 4/1 for international students. Application fee: $30. Electronic applications accepted. *Expenses:* Tuition, state resident: part-time $408.10 per credit hour. Tuition, nonresident: part-time $932.61 per credit hour. *Required fees:* $111.81 per credit hour. Tuition and fees vary according to course load, campus/location and program. *Financial support:* In 2015–16, 35 students received support. Research assistantships available. Financial award application deadline: 4/1; financial award applicants required to submit FAFSA. *Faculty research:* Teen pregnancy, diabetes, ethical decision-making, family caregivers. *Total annual research expenditures:* $39,413. *Unit head:* Dr. Li Loriz, Chair, 904-620-1053, E-mail: lloriz@unf.edu. *Application contact:* Beth Dibble, Assistant Director of Admissions for Nursing and Physical Therapy, 904-620-2684, Fax: 904-620-1832, E-mail: nursingadmissions@unf.edu.
Website: http://www.unf.edu/brooks/nursing

University of Oklahoma Health Sciences Center, Graduate College, College of Nursing, Oklahoma City, OK 73190. Offers MS, MS/MBA. MS/MBA offered jointly with Oklahoma State University and University of Oklahoma. *Accreditation:* ACEN. *Program availability:* Part-time. *Degree requirements:* For master's, comprehensive exam, thesis optional. *Entrance requirements:* For master's, 3 letters of recommendation, Oklahoma RN license, statistics course, research methods, computer course or completion of a computer literacy test. *Faculty research:* Parenting and Native Americans, elderly reminiscence, diabetes in Native Americans.

University of Ottawa, Faculty of Graduate and Postdoctoral Studies, Faculty of Health Sciences, School of Nursing, Ottawa, ON K1N 6N5, Canada. Offers nurse practitioner (Certificate); nursing (M Sc, PhD); nursing/primary health care (M Sc). *Program availability:* Part-time, evening/weekend. *Degree requirements:* For master's, thesis or alternative. *Entrance requirements:* For master's, honors degree or equivalent, minimum B average. Electronic applications accepted. *Faculty research:* Decision making in nursing, evaluating complete nursing interventions.

University of Pennsylvania, School of Nursing, Philadelphia, PA 19104. Offers MSN, PhD, Certificate, MBA/MSN, MBA/PhD, MSN/PhD. *Accreditation:* AACN; AANA/CANAEP. *Program availability:* Part-time, online learning. *Faculty:* 55 full-time (48 women), 34 part-time/adjunct (32 women). *Students:* 262 full-time (225 women), 364 part-time (335 women); includes 171 minority (46 Black or African American, non-Hispanic/Latino; 1 American Indian or Alaska Native, non-Hispanic/Latino; 63 Asian, non-Hispanic/Latino; 42 Hispanic/Latino; 19 Two or more races, non-Hispanic/Latino), 15 international. Average age 31. 749 applicants, 62% accepted, 307 enrolled. In 2015, 294 master's, 13 doctorates awarded. Terminal master's awarded for partial completion of doctoral program. *Expenses: Tuition, area resident:* Full-time $31,068; part-time $5762 per course. *Required fees:* $3200; $336 per course. Full-time tuition and fees vary according to degree level, program and student level. Part-time tuition and fees vary according to course load, degree level and program. *Unit head:* Dr. Christina Costanzo Clark, Assistant Dean for Admissions and Academic Affairs, 215-898-4271, Fax: 215-573-8439, E-mail: costanzo@nursing.upenn.edu. *Application contact:* Sylvia English, Enrollment Management Coordinator, 215-898-8439, Fax: 215-573-8439, E-mail: sylviaj@nursing.upenn.edu.
Website: http://www.nursing.upenn.edu/

University of Phoenix–Atlanta Campus, College of Nursing, Sandy Springs, GA 30350-4147. Offers health administration (MHA); nursing (MSN); nursing/health care education (MSN); MSN/MBA; MSN/MHA. *Program availability:* Evening/weekend, online learning. *Degree requirements:* For master's, thesis (for some programs). *Entrance requirements:* For master's, minimum undergraduate GPA of 2.5, 3 years of work experience. Additional exam requirements/recommendations for international students: Required—TOEFL (minimum score 550 paper-based; 79 iBT). Electronic applications accepted.

University of Phoenix–Augusta Campus, College of Nursing, Augusta, GA 30909-4583. Offers health administration (MHA); nursing (MSN); nursing/health care education (MSN); MSN/MBA; MSN/MHA. *Program availability:* Online learning.

University of Phoenix–Bay Area Campus, College of Nursing, San Jose, CA 95134-1805. Offers education (MHA); gerontology (MHA); health administration (MHA, DHA); informatics (MHA, MSN); nursing (MSN, PhD); nursing/health care education (MSN); MSN/MBA. *Program availability:* Evening/weekend, online learning. *Degree requirements:* For master's, thesis (for some programs). *Entrance requirements:* For

master's, minimum undergraduate GPA of 2.5, 3 years of work experience, RN license. Additional exam requirements/recommendations for international students: Required—TOEFL (minimum score 550 paper-based; 79 iBT). Electronic applications accepted.

University of Phoenix–Central Valley Campus, College of Nursing, Fresno, CA 93720-1552. Offers education (MHA); gerontology (MHA); health administration (MHA); nursing (MSN); MSN/MBA.

University of Phoenix–Charlotte Campus, College of Nursing, Charlotte, NC 28273-3409. Offers education (MHA); gerontology (MHA); health administration (MHA); informatics (MHA, MSN); nursing (MSN); nursing/health care education (MSN). *Program availability:* Evening/weekend. *Degree requirements:* For master's, thesis (for some programs). *Entrance requirements:* For master's, minimum undergraduate GPA of 2.5, 3 years work experience. Additional exam requirements/recommendations for international students: Required—TOEFL (minimum score 550 paper-based; 79 iBT). Electronic applications accepted.

University of Phoenix–Colorado Campus, College of Nursing, Lone Tree, CO 80124-5453. Offers health administration (MHA); nursing (MSN); MSN/MBA; MSN/MHA. *Program availability:* Evening/weekend, online learning. *Degree requirements:* For master's, thesis (for some programs). *Entrance requirements:* For master's, minimum undergraduate GPA of 2.5, 3 years work experience, RN license. Additional exam requirements/recommendations for international students: Required—TOEFL (minimum score 550 paper-based; 79 iBT). Electronic applications accepted.

University of Phoenix–Colorado Springs Downtown Campus, College of Nursing, Colorado Springs, CO 80903. Offers education (MHA); gerontology (MHA); health administration (MHA); nursing (MSN); MSN/MBA. *Program availability:* Evening/weekend. *Degree requirements:* For master's, thesis (for some programs). *Entrance requirements:* For master's, minimum undergraduate GPA of 2.5, 3 years of work experience, RN license. Additional exam requirements/recommendations for international students: Required—TOEFL (minimum score 550 paper-based; 79 iBT). Electronic applications accepted.

University of Phoenix–Columbus Georgia Campus, College of Nursing, Columbus, GA 31909. Offers health administration (MHA); nursing (MSN). *Program availability:* Online learning. *Degree requirements:* For master's, thesis (for some programs). *Entrance requirements:* For master's, minimum undergraduate GPA of 2.5, 3 years of work experience. Additional exam requirements/recommendations for international students: Required—TOEFL (minimum score 550 paper-based; 79 iBT). Electronic applications accepted.

University of Phoenix–Hawaii Campus, College of Nursing, Honolulu, HI 96813-3800. Offers education (MHA); family nurse practitioner (MSN); gerontology (MHA); health administration (MHA); nursing (MSN); nursing/health care education (MSN); MSN/MBA. *Program availability:* Evening/weekend. *Degree requirements:* For master's, thesis (for some programs). *Entrance requirements:* For master's, minimum undergraduate GPA of 2.5, 3 years of work experience, RN license. Additional exam requirements/recommendations for international students: Required—TOEFL (minimum score 550 paper-based; 79 iBT). Electronic applications accepted.

University of Phoenix–Houston Campus, College of Nursing, Houston, TX 77079-2004. Offers health administration (MHA). *Program availability:* Online learning. *Degree requirements:* For master's, thesis (for some programs). *Entrance requirements:* For master's, minimum undergraduate GPA of 2.5, 3 years of work experience. Additional exam requirements/recommendations for international students: Required—TOEFL (minimum score 550 paper-based; 79 iBT). Electronic applications accepted.

University of Phoenix–New Mexico Campus, College of Nursing, Albuquerque, NM 87113-1570. Offers health administration (MHA); health care education (MSN); nursing (MSN); MSN/MBA. *Program availability:* Evening/weekend. *Degree requirements:* For master's, thesis (for some programs). *Entrance requirements:* For master's, minimum undergraduate GPA of 2.5, 3 years of work experience, RN license. Additional exam requirements/recommendations for international students: Required—TOEFL (minimum score 550 paper-based; 79 iBT). Electronic applications accepted.

University of Phoenix–North Florida Campus, College of Nursing, Jacksonville, FL 32216-0959. Offers health administration (MHA); health care education (MSN); nursing (MSN); MSN/MBA; MSN/MHA. *Program availability:* Evening/weekend. *Degree requirements:* For master's, thesis (for some programs). *Entrance requirements:* For master's, minimum undergraduate GPA of 2.5, 3 years work experience, RN license. Additional exam requirements/recommendations for international students: Required—TOEFL (minimum score 550 paper-based; 79 iBT). Electronic applications accepted.

University of Phoenix–Online Campus, College of Health Sciences and Nursing, Phoenix, AZ 85034-7209. Offers family nurse practitioner (Certificate); health care (Certificate); health care education (Certificate); health care informatics (Certificate); informatics (MSN); nursing (MSN); nursing and health care education (MSN); MSN/MBA; MSN/MHA. *Accreditation:* AACN. *Program availability:* Evening/weekend, online learning. *Entrance requirements:* Additional exam requirements/recommendations for international students: Required—TOEFL, TOEIC (Test of English as an International Communication), Berlitz Online English Proficiency Exam, PTE, or IELTS. Electronic applications accepted. *Expenses:* Contact institution.

University of Phoenix–Online Campus, School of Advanced Studies, Phoenix, AZ 85034-7209. Offers business administration (DBA); education (Ed S); educational leadership (Ed D), including curriculum and instruction, education technology, educational leadership; health administration (DHA); higher education administration (PhD); industrial/organizational psychology (PhD); nursing (PhD); organizational leadership (DM), including information systems and technology, organizational leadership. *Program availability:* Evening/weekend, online learning. *Degree requirements:* For doctorate, thesis/dissertation. *Entrance requirements:* Additional exam requirements/recommendations for international students: Required—TOEFL, TOEIC (Test of English as an International Communication), Berlitz Online English Proficiency Exam, PTE, or IELTS. Electronic applications accepted. *Expenses:* Contact institution.

University of Phoenix–Phoenix Campus, College of Health Sciences and Nursing, Tempe, AZ 85282-2371. Offers family nurse practitioner (MSN, Certificate); gerontology health care (Certificate); health care education (MSN, Certificate); health care informatics (Certificate); informatics (MSN); nursing (MSN); MSN/MHA. *Program availability:* Evening/weekend, online learning. *Entrance requirements:* Additional exam requirements/recommendations for international students: Required—TOEFL, TOEIC (Test of English as an International Communication), Berlitz Online English Proficiency Exam, PTE, or IELTS. Electronic applications accepted. *Expenses:* Contact institution.

University of Phoenix–Sacramento Valley Campus, College of Nursing, Sacramento, CA 95833-4334. Offers family nurse practitioner (MSN); health administration (MHA); health care education (MSN); nursing (MSN); MSN/MBA. *Program availability:* Evening/weekend. *Degree requirements:* For master's, thesis (for some programs). *Entrance requirements:* For master's, RN license, minimum undergraduate GPA of 2.5, 3 years work experience. Additional exam requirements/recommendations for international students: Required—TOEFL (minimum score 550 paper-based; 79 iBT). Electronic applications accepted.

University of Phoenix–San Antonio Campus, College of Nursing, San Antonio, TX 78230. Offers health administration (MHA).

University of Phoenix–San Diego Campus, College of Nursing, San Diego, CA 92123. Offers health care education (MSN); nursing (MSN); MSN/MBA. *Program availability:* Evening/weekend. *Degree requirements:* For master's, thesis (for some programs). *Entrance requirements:* For master's, minimum undergraduate GPA of 2.5, 3 years work experience, RN license. Additional exam requirements/recommendations for international students: Required—TOEFL (minimum score 550 paper-based; 79 iBT). Electronic applications accepted.

University of Phoenix–Southern California Campus, College of Health Sciences and Nursing, Costa Mesa, CA 92626. Offers family nurse practitioner (MSN, Certificate); health care (Certificate); informatics (MSN); nursing (MSN); nursing/health care education (MSN, Certificate); MSN/MBA; MSN/MHA. *Program availability:* Evening/weekend, online learning. *Entrance requirements:* Additional exam requirements/recommendations for international students: Required—TOEFL, TOEIC (Test of English as an International Communication), Berlitz Online English Proficiency Exam, PTE, or IELTS. Electronic applications accepted. *Expenses:* Contact institution.

University of Phoenix–South Florida Campus, College of Nursing, Miramar, FL 33027-4145. Offers health administration (MHA); health care education (MSN); nursing (MSN); MSN/MBA; MSN/MHA. *Program availability:* Evening/weekend. *Degree requirements:* For master's, thesis (for some programs). *Entrance requirements:* For master's, minimum undergraduate GPA of 2.5, 3 years work experience, RN license. Additional exam requirements/recommendations for international students: Required—TOEFL (minimum score 550 paper-based; 79 iBT). Electronic applications accepted.

University of Phoenix–Utah Campus, College of Nursing, Salt Lake City, UT 84123-4642. Offers health care education (MSN); nursing (MSN); MSN/MBA. *Program availability:* Evening/weekend. *Degree requirements:* For master's, thesis (for some programs). *Entrance requirements:* For master's, minimum undergraduate GPA of 2.5, 3 years work experience, RN license. Additional exam requirements/recommendations for international students: Required—TOEFL (minimum score 550 paper-based; 79 iBT). Electronic applications accepted.

University of Phoenix–Washington D.C. Campus, College of Nursing, Washington, DC 20001. Offers education (MHA); gerontology (MHA); health administration (MHA, DHA); informatics (MHA, MSN); nursing (MSN, PhD); nursing/health care education (MSN); MSN/MBA; MSN/MHA.

University of Pittsburgh, School of Nursing, Clinical Nurse Specialist Program, Pittsburgh, PA 15260. Offers adult-gerontology (DNP); psychiatric mental health (DNP). *Accreditation:* AACN. *Program availability:* Part-time. *Students:* 1 (woman) full-time, 8 part-time (6 women); includes 2 minority (both Black or African American, non-Hispanic/Latino). Average age 47. 1 applicant, 100% accepted. In 2015, 4 doctorates awarded. *Entrance requirements:* Additional exam requirements/recommendations for international students: Required—TOEFL (minimum score 600 paper-based; 100 iBT). *Application deadline:* For fall admission, 5/1 priority date for domestic students, 2/15 priority date for international students. Application fee: $50. Electronic applications accepted. *Expenses:* Contact institution. *Financial support:* In 2015–16, 2 students received support, including 2 fellowships with tuition reimbursements available (averaging $11,294 per year); research assistantships, teaching assistantships, scholarships/grants, health care benefits, and unspecified assistantships also available. Support available to part-time students. Financial award application deadline: 3/15. *Faculty research:* Behavioral management of chronic disorders, patient management in critical care, consumer informatics, genetic applications (molecular genetics and psychosocial implications), technology for nurses and patients to improve care. *Unit head:* Dr. Sandra Engberg, Associate Dean for Clinical Education, 412-624-3835, Fax: 412-624-8521, E-mail: sje1@pitt.edu. *Application contact:* Laurie Lapsley, Administrator of Graduate Student Services, 412-624-9670, Fax: 412-624-2409, E-mail: lapsleyl@pitt.edu.

University of Pittsburgh, School of Nursing, PhD Program in Nursing, Pittsburgh, PA 15261. Offers PhD. *Program availability:* Part-time. *Students:* 31 full-time (29 women), 4 part-time (3 women); includes 1 minority (Asian, non-Hispanic/Latino), 13 international. Average age 32. 21 applicants, 52% accepted, 9 enrolled. In 2015, 5 doctorates awarded. *Degree requirements:* For doctorate, comprehensive exam, thesis/dissertation. *Entrance requirements:* For doctorate, GRE General Test, BSN/MSN, 3 letters of recommendation, resume, course work in statistics. Additional exam requirements/recommendations for international students: Required—TOEFL (minimum score 600 paper-based; 100 iBT), TOEFL (minimum score 600 paper-based; 100 iBT) or IELTS (minimum score 7.0). *Application deadline:* For fall admission, 5/1 for domestic students, 2/1 priority date for international students. Application fee: $50. Electronic applications accepted. *Expenses:* Contact institution. *Financial support:* In 2015–16, 28 students received support, including 13 fellowships with tuition reimbursements available (averaging $15,620 per year), 12 research assistantships with tuition reimbursements available (averaging $13,310 per year), 3 teaching assistantships with tuition reimbursements available (averaging $15,620 per year); scholarships/grants, traineeships, health care benefits, and unspecified assistantships also available. Support available to part-time students. *Faculty research:* Behavioral management of chronic disorders, patient management in critical care, consumer informatics, genetic applications, technology. *Unit head:* Dr. Catherine Bender, Coordinator, 412-624-3594, Fax: 412-624-2401, E-mail: cbe100@pitt.edu. *Application contact:* Laurie Lapsley, Administrator of Graduate Student Services, 412-624-9670, Fax: 412-624-2409, E-mail: lapsleyl@pitt.edu.
Website: http://www.nursing.pitt.edu/

University of Portland, School of Nursing, Portland, OR 97203. Offers clinical nurse leader (MS); family nurse practitioner (DNP); nurse educator (MS). *Accreditation:* AACN. *Program availability:* Part-time, evening/weekend, online learning. *Entrance requirements:* For master's, GRE General Test or MAT, Oregon RN license, BSN, course work in statistics, resume, letters of recommendation, writing sample; for doctorate, GRE General Test or MAT, Oregon RN license, BSN or MSN, 2 letters of recommendation, resume, writing sample, official transcripts. Additional exam requirements/recommendations for international students: Required—TOEFL (minimum score 550 paper-based; 80 iBT), IELTS (minimum score 7). *Expenses:* Contact institution.

University of Puerto Rico, Medical Sciences Campus, School of Nursing, San Juan, PR 00936-5067. Offers adult and elderly nursing (MSN); child and adolescent nursing (MSN); critical care nursing (MSN); family and community nursing (MSN); family nurse practitioner (MSN); maternity nursing (MSN); mental health and psychiatric nursing (MSN). *Accreditation:* AACN. *Entrance requirements:* For master's, GRE or EXADEP, interview, Puerto Rico RN license or professional license for international students, general and specific point average, article analysis. Electronic applications accepted. *Faculty research:* HIV, health disparities, teen violence, women and violence, neurological disorders.

University of Regina, Faculty of Graduate Studies and Research, Faculty of Nursing, Regina, SK S4S 0A2, Canada. Offers MN. *Entrance requirements:* For master's, proof of licensure or registration as an RN including registration number in a Canadian province or territory, 2 years of clinical practice within last 5 years, essay, minimum overall GPA of 75% in all 3rd- and 4th-year nursing courses taken at a Canadian-accredited or provincially-approved baccalaureate nursing education program. Additional exam requirements/recommendations for international students: Required—TOEFL (minimum score 580 paper-based; 80 iBT), IELTS (minimum score 6.5), PTE (minimum score 59). Electronic applications accepted. *Expenses:* Contact institution.

University of Rhode Island, Graduate School, College of Nursing, Kingston, RI 02881. Offers acute care nurse practitioner (MS); adult-gerontological nurse practitioner/clinical nurse specialist (MS); family nurse practitioner (MS); nursing (PhD); nursing education (MS); nursing practice (DNP). *Accreditation:* AACN; ACNM/ACME (one or more programs are accredited). *Program availability:* Part-time. *Faculty:* 11 full-time (all women). *Students:* 51 full-time (41 women), 77 part-time (70 women); includes 18 minority (11 Black or African American, non-Hispanic/Latino; 2 Asian, non-Hispanic/Latino; 4 Hispanic/Latino; 1 Two or more races, non-Hispanic/Latino), 5 international. In 2015, 19 master's, 7 doctorates awarded. *Degree requirements:* For master's, comprehensive exam; for doctorate, comprehensive exam, thesis/dissertation. *Entrance requirements:* For master's, GRE or MAT, 2 letters of recommendation, scholarly papers; for doctorate, GRE, 3 letters of recommendation, scholarly papers. Additional exam requirements/recommendations for international students: Required—TOEFL (minimum score 550 paper-based). *Application deadline:* For fall admission, 2/15 for domestic students, 2/1 for international students; for spring admission, 10/15 for domestic students, 7/15 for international students. Application fee: $65. Electronic applications accepted. *Expenses:* Tuition, state resident: full-time $11,796; part-time $655 per credit. Tuition, nonresident: full-time $24,206; part-time $1345 per credit. *Required fees:* $1546; $44 per credit. One-time fee: $155 full-time; $35 part-time. *Financial support:* In 2015–16, 2 research assistantships (averaging $12,111 per year), 7 teaching assistantships with tuition reimbursements (averaging $13,112 per year) were awarded. Financial award application deadline: 2/15, financial award applicants required to submit FAFSA. *Faculty research:* Group intervention for grieving women in prison, translating best practice in non-drug interventions for postoperative pain management, further development and testing of the pain assessment inventory, preschool motor and functional performance of two cohorts, neuroactivation of brain motor areas in preterm children. *Unit head:* Dr. Mary Sullivan, Interim Dean, 401-874-5339, Fax: 401-874-2061, E-mail: mcsullivan@uri.edu. *Application contact:* Graduate Admission, 401-874-2872, E-mail: gradadm@etal.uri.edu.
Website: http://www.uri.edu/nursing

University of Rochester, School of Nursing, Rochester, NY 14642. Offers adult gerontological acute care nurse practitioner (MS); clinical nurse leader (MS); family nurse practitioner (MS); family psychiatric mental health nurse practitioner (MS); health care organization management and leadership (MS); health practice research (PhD); nursing (DNP); nursing education (MS); pediatric nurse practitioner (MS); pediatric nurse practitioner/neonatal nurse practitioner (MS). *Accreditation:* AACN. *Program availability:* Part-time, online learning. *Faculty:* 56 full-time (45 women), 63 part-time/adjunct (55 women). *Students:* 21 full-time (20 women), 212 part-time (175 women); includes 35 minority (12 Black or African American, non-Hispanic/Latino; 1 American Indian or Alaska Native, non-Hispanic/Latino; 10 Asian, non-Hispanic/Latino; 7 Hispanic/Latino; 5 Two or more races, non-Hispanic/Latino), 2 international. Average age 35. 111 applicants, 68% accepted, 71 enrolled. In 2015, 52 master's, 9 doctorates awarded. Terminal master's awarded for partial completion of doctoral program. *Degree requirements:* For master's, comprehensive exam (for some programs); for doctorate, thesis/dissertation. *Entrance requirements:* For master's, BS in nursing, minimum GPA of 3.0, course work in statistics; for doctorate, GRE General Test (for PhD), MS in nursing, minimum GPA of 3.5. Additional exam requirements/recommendations for international students: Required—TOEFL (minimum score 560 paper-based; 88 iBT) or IELTS (minimum score 6.5) recommended. *Application deadline:* For fall admission, 4/1 for domestic and international students; for spring admission, 9/1 for domestic and international students; for summer admission, 1/2 for domestic and international students. Application fee: $50. Electronic applications accepted. *Expenses:* Tuition, area resident: Full-time $47,450; part-time $1482 per credit hour. *Required fees:* $528. Tuition and fees vary according to program. *Financial support:* In 2015–16, 52 students received support, including 2 fellowships with tuition reimbursements available (averaging $30,000 per year); scholarships/grants, traineeships, health care benefits, tuition waivers (full and partial), and unspecified assistantships also available. Support available to part-time students. Financial award application deadline: 6/30. *Faculty research:* Symptom assessment and self-management of chronic illness, health promotion and illness prevention, nursing intervention research with vulnerable populations, palliative care, aging. *Total annual research expenditures:* $2.1 million. *Unit head:* Dr. Kathy H. Rideout, Dean, 585-273-8902, Fax: 585-273-1268, E-mail: kathy_rideout@urmc.rochester.edu. *Application contact:* Elaine Andolina, Director of Admissions, 585-275-2375, Fax: 585-756-8299, E-mail: elaine_andolina@urmc.rochester.edu.
Website: http://www.son.rochester.edu

University of Saint Francis, Graduate School, Department of Nursing, Fort Wayne, IN 46808-3994. Offers family nurse practitioner (MSN, Post Master's Certificate). *Accreditation:* AACN. *Program availability:* Part-time, evening/weekend, online learning. *Degree requirements:* For master's, research project. *Entrance requirements:* For master's, GRE (if undergraduate GPA is less than 3.0), minimum undergraduate GPA of 3.2; ASN or BSN from regionally-accredited U.S. institutions; current license as registered nurse; completed graduate or undergraduate statistics course within last five years; for Post Master's Certificate, GRE (if undergraduate GPA is less than 3.0), minimum undergraduate GPA of 3.2; MSN from regionally-accredited U.S. institution; current license as registered nurse; completed graduate or undergraduate statistics course within last five years. Additional exam requirements/recommendations for international students: Required—TOEFL or IELTS. Electronic applications accepted. *Expenses:* Contact institution.

University of St. Francis, Leach College of Nursing, Joliet, IL 60435-6169. Offers family nurse practitioner (MSN, Post-Master's Certificate); family psychology/mental health nurse practitioner (MSN, Post-Master's Certificate); nursing administration (MSN); nursing education (MSN); nursing practice (DNP); teaching in nursing (Certificate). *Accreditation:* AACN. *Program availability:* Part-time, evening/weekend, 100% online. *Faculty:* 7 full-time (all women), 16 part-time/adjunct (13 women). *Students:* 82 full-time (72 women), 356 part-time (325 women); includes 147 minority (62 Black or African American, non-Hispanic/Latino; 1 American Indian or Alaska Native, non-Hispanic/Latino; 27 Asian, non-Hispanic/Latino; 45 Hispanic/Latino; 3 Native Hawaiian or other Pacific Islander, non-Hispanic/Latino; 9 Two or more races, non-Hispanic/Latino). Average age 41. 338 applicants, 42% accepted, 100 enrolled. In 2015, 91 master's, 9 doctorates, 6 other advanced degrees awarded. *Entrance requirements:* Additional exam requirements/recommendations for international students: Required—TOEFL (minimum score 550 paper-based; 79 iBT), IELTS (minimum score 6). *Application deadline:* Applications are processed on a rolling basis. Application fee: $30. Electronic applications accepted. Application fee is waived when completed online. *Expenses:* Contact institution. *Financial support:* In 2015–16, 149 students received support. Career-related internships or fieldwork, scholarships/grants, and tuition waivers (partial) available. Support available to part-time students. Financial award applicants

Nursing—General

required to submit FAFSA. *Unit head:* Dr. Carol Wilson, Dean, 815-740-3840, Fax: 815-740-4243, E-mail: cwilson@stfrancis.edu. *Application contact:* Sandra Sloka, Director of Admissions for Graduate and Degree Completion Programs, 800-735-7500, Fax: 815-740-3431, E-mail: ssloka@stfrancis.edu.
Website: http://www.stfrancis.edu/academics/college-of-nursing/

University of Saint Joseph, Department of Nursing, West Hartford, CT 06117-2700. Offers family nurse practitioner (MS); family psychiatric/mental health nurse practitioner (MS); nurse educator (MS); nursing practice (DNP). *Accreditation:* AACN. *Program availability:* Part-time, evening/weekend. *Degree requirements:* For master's, thesis. *Entrance requirements:* For master's, 2 letters of recommendation. *Application deadline:* Applications are processed on a rolling basis. Application fee: $50. Electronic applications accepted. Application fee is waived when completed online. *Financial support:* Career-related internships or fieldwork and unspecified assistantships available. Support available to part-time students. Financial award applicants required to submit FAFSA.
Website: http://www.usj.edu/academics/schools/school-of-health-natural-sciences/nursing/

University of Saint Mary, Graduate Programs, Program in Nursing, Leavenworth, KS 66048-5082. Offers nurse administrator (MSN); nurse educator (MSN). *Program availability:* Part-time, online only, 100% online. *Students:* 19 full-time (all women), 12 part-time (11 women); includes 5 minority (3 Black or African American, non-Hispanic/Latino; 1 Hispanic/Latino; 1 Two or more races, non-Hispanic/Latino). Average age 41. *Degree requirements:* For master's, practicum. *Entrance requirements:* For master's, BSN from CCNE- or NLNAC-accredited baccalaureate nursing program at regionally-accredited institution. Application fee: $25. *Expenses:* $580 per credit hour. *Unit head:* Karen R. Kidder, Chair, 877-307-4915, Fax: 913-345-2802. *Application contact:* Dr. Linda King, Director, 877-307-4915, Fax: 913-345-2802.
Website: http://online.stmary.edu/msn

University of San Diego, Hahn School of Nursing and Health Science, San Diego, CA 92110-2492. Offers adult-gerontology clinical nurse specialist (MSN); adult-gerontology nurse practitioner/family nurse practitioner (MSN); executive nurse leader (MSN); family nurse practitioner (MSN); family/lifespan psychiatric/mental health nurse practitioner (MSN); healthcare informatics (MS, MSN); nursing (PhD); nursing practice (DNP). *Accreditation:* AACN. *Program availability:* Part-time, evening/weekend. *Faculty:* 27 full-time (23 women), 46 part-time/adjunct (41 women). *Students:* 178 full-time (151 women), 157 part-time (131 women); includes 143 minority (25 Black or African American, non-Hispanic/Latino; 2 American Indian or Alaska Native, non-Hispanic/Latino; 53 Asian, non-Hispanic/Latino; 49 Hispanic/Latino; 4 Native Hawaiian or other Pacific Islander, non-Hispanic/Latino; 10 Two or more races, non-Hispanic/Latino), 5 international. Average age 36. In 2015, 122 master's, 43 doctorates awarded. *Degree requirements:* For doctorate, thesis/dissertation (for some programs), residency (DNP). *Entrance requirements:* For master's, GRE General Test (for entry-level nursing), BSN, current California RN licensure (except for entry-level nursing); minimum GPA of 3.0; for doctorate, minimum GPA of 3.5, MSN, current California RN licensure. Additional exam requirements/recommendations for international students: Required—TOEFL (minimum score 580 paper-based; 83 iBT), TWE. *Application deadline:* Applications are processed on a rolling basis. Application fee: $45. Electronic applications accepted. *Financial support:* In 2015–16, 217 students received support. Scholarships/grants and traineeships available. Support available to part-time students. Financial award application deadline: 4/1; financial award applicants required to submit FAFSA. *Faculty research:* Maternal/neonatal health, palliative and end of life care, adolescent obesity, health disparities, cognitive dysfunction. *Unit head:* Dr. Sally Hardin, Dean, 619-260-4550, Fax: 619-260-6814. *Application contact:* Monica Mahon, Associate Director of Graduate Admissions, 619-260-4524, Fax: 619-260-4158, E-mail: grads@sandiego.edu.
Website: http://www.sandiego.edu/nursing/

University of San Francisco, School of Nursing and Health Professions, San Francisco, CA 94117-1080. Offers MPH, MSBH, MSN, DNP, Psy D. *Accreditation:* AACN. *Program availability:* Part-time, 100% online, blended/hybrid learning. *Faculty:* 43 full-time (33 women), 59 part-time/adjunct (50 women). *Students:* 576 full-time (471 women), 184 part-time (156 women); includes 419 minority (70 Black or African American, non-Hispanic/Latino; 1 American Indian or Alaska Native, non-Hispanic/Latino; 196 Asian, non-Hispanic/Latino; 99 Hispanic/Latino; 17 Native Hawaiian or other Pacific Islander, non-Hispanic/Latino; 36 Two or more races, non-Hispanic/Latino), 25 international. Average age 35. 663 applicants, 63% accepted, 260 enrolled. In 2015, 201 master's, 31 doctorates awarded. *Entrance requirements:* For master's, minimum GPA of 3.0. *Application deadline:* Applications are processed on a rolling basis. *Expenses: Tuition, area resident:* Full-time $22,410; part-time $1245 per credit. Tuition and fees vary according to course load, degree level and campus/location. *Financial support:* In 2015–16, 108 students received support. Institutionally sponsored loans available. Financial award application deadline: 3/2. *Faculty research:* Direct patient/client care, providers of health care. *Unit head:* Dr. Judith Karshmer, Dean, 415-422-6681, Fax: 415-422-6877, E-mail: nursing@usfca.edu. *Application contact:* Ingrid McVanner, Information Contact, 415-422-2746, Fax: 415-422-2217.
Website: http://www.usfca.edu/nursing/

University of Saskatchewan, College of Graduate Studies and Research, College of Nursing, Saskatoon, SK S7N 5E5, Canada. Offers MN. *Program availability:* Part-time. *Entrance requirements:* Additional exam requirements/recommendations for international students: Required—TOEFL.

The University of Scranton, Panuska College of Professional Studies, Department of Nursing, Scranton, PA 18510-4595. Offers family nurse practitioner (MSN, PMC); nurse anesthesia (MSN, PMC); nursing leadership (DNP). Applicants accepted in odd-numbered years only. *Accreditation:* AACN; AANA/CANAEP. *Program availability:* Part-time, evening/weekend. *Students:* 58 full-time (46 women), 22 part-time (all women); includes 16 minority (12 Black or African American, non-Hispanic/Latino; 1 Asian, non-Hispanic/Latino; 2 Hispanic/Latino; 1 Two or more races, non-Hispanic/Latino). Average age 33. 104 applicants, 51% accepted, 45 enrolled. *Degree requirements:* For master's, comprehensive exam (for some programs), thesis (for some programs), capstone experience. *Entrance requirements:* For master's, minimum GPA of 3.0, three letters of reference; for doctorate, RN licensure and evidence of certification in advanced practice nursing specialty. Additional exam requirements/recommendations for international students: Required—TOEFL (minimum score 500 paper-based; 80 iBT), IELTS (minimum score 6.5). *Application deadline:* For fall admission, 9/1 for domestic students, 6/1 for international students; for spring admission, 11/1 for international students; for summer admission, 3/1 for international students. Applications are processed on a rolling basis. Application fee: $0. Electronic applications accepted. *Financial support:* Applicants required to submit FAFSA. *Faculty research:* Home care, doctoral education, health care of women and children, pain, health promotion and adolescence. *Unit head:* Dr. Dona Carpenter, Chair, 570-941-7673, Fax: 570-941-4201, E-mail: dona.carpenter@scranton.edu. *Application contact:* Dr. Mary Jane Hanson, Director, 570-941-4060, Fax: 570-941-4201, E-mail: hansonm2@scranton.edu.
Website: http://www.scranton.edu/academics/pcps/nursing/index.shtml

University of South Alabama, College of Nursing, Mobile, AL 36688. Offers nursing (MSN, DNP); nursing administration (Certificate); nursing education (MAIA); nursing practice (Certificate). *Accreditation:* AACN. *Program availability:* Part-time, online learning. *Faculty:* 69 full-time (63 women), 97 part-time/adjunct (89 women). *Students:* 2,489 full-time (2,179 women), 341 part-time (297 women); includes 789 minority (520 Black or African American, non-Hispanic/Latino; 26 American Indian or Alaska Native, non-Hispanic/Latino; 118 Asian, non-Hispanic/Latino; 82 Hispanic/Latino; 9 Native Hawaiian or other Pacific Islander, non-Hispanic/Latino; 34 Two or more races, non-Hispanic/Latino), 7 international. Average age 35. 1,923 applicants, 51% accepted, 722 enrolled. In 2015, 572 master's, 90 doctorates, 79 other advanced degrees awarded. *Degree requirements:* For master's, thesis optional; for doctorate, final project. *Entrance requirements:* For master's, BSN, RN licensure, minimum GPA of 3.0, resume documenting clinical experience, background check, drug screening; for doctorate, MSN, RN licensure, minimum GPA of 3.0; for Certificate, MSN/DN/DNP, RN licensure, minimum GPA of 3.0, resume documenting clinical experience, background check, drug screening. *Application deadline:* For fall admission, 3/15 for domestic students; for spring admission, 7/15 priority date for domestic students; for summer admission, 1/15 priority date for domestic students. Applications are processed on a rolling basis. Application fee: $85. Electronic applications accepted. *Expenses:* Tuition, state resident: full-time $9480; part-time $395 per credit hour. Tuition, nonresident: full-time $18,960; part-time $790 per credit hour. *Financial support:* Fellowships, research assistantships, teaching assistantships, career-related internships or fieldwork, Federal Work-Study, institutionally sponsored loans, scholarships/grants, and unspecified assistantships available. Support available to part-time students. Financial award application deadline: 5/31; financial award applicants required to submit FAFSA. *Unit head:* Dr. Debra Davis, Dean, College of Nursing, 251-445-9400, Fax: 251-445-9416, E-mail: ddavis@southalabama.edu. *Application contact:* Gail Soles, Academic Records Specialist, 251-445-9400, Fax: 251-445-9416, E-mail: gsoles@southalabama.edu.
Website: http://www.southalabama.edu/colleges/con/index.html

University of South Carolina, The Graduate School, College of Nursing, Program in Advanced Practice Clinical Nursing, Columbia, SC 29208. Offers acute care nurse practitioner (Certificate); advanced practice clinical nursing (MSN). *Accreditation:* AACN. *Program availability:* Part-time, online learning. *Entrance requirements:* For master's, master's degree in nursing, RN license; for Certificate, MSN. Additional exam requirements/recommendations for international students: Required—TOEFL (minimum score 570 paper-based). Electronic applications accepted. *Faculty research:* Systems research, evidence based practice, breast cancer, violence.

University of South Carolina, The Graduate School, College of Nursing, Program in Advanced Practice Nursing in Primary Care, Columbia, SC 29208. Offers MSN, Certificate. *Accreditation:* AACN. *Entrance requirements:* For master's, master's degree in nursing, RN license; for Certificate, MSN. Additional exam requirements/recommendations for international students: Required—TOEFL (minimum score 570 paper-based). Electronic applications accepted. *Faculty research:* Systems research, evidence based practice, breast cancer, violence.

University of Southern Indiana, Graduate Studies, College of Nursing and Health Professions, Program in Nursing, Evansville, IN 47712-3590. Offers MSN, DNP. *Program availability:* Part-time, online learning. *Faculty:* 9 full-time (8 women), 2 part-time/adjunct (both women). *Students:* 399 part-time (346 women); includes 34 minority (16 Black or African American, non-Hispanic/Latino; 3 American Indian or Alaska Native, non-Hispanic/Latino; 3 Asian, non-Hispanic/Latino; 10 Hispanic/Latino; 2 Two or more races, non-Hispanic/Latino), 3 international. Average age 36. In 2015, 105 master's, 16 doctorates awarded. *Entrance requirements:* For master's, BSN from nationally-accredited school; minimum cumulative GPA of 3.0; satisfactory completion of a course in undergraduate statistics (minimum grade C); one year of full-time experience or 2000 hours of clinical practice as an RN (recommended); for doctorate, minimum GPA of 3.0, completion of graduate research course with minimum B grade, unencumbered RN license, resume/curriculum vitae, three professional references, 1-2 page narrative of practice experience and professional goals, Capstone Project Information form. Additional exam requirements/recommendations for international students: Required—TOEFL (minimum score 550 paper-based; 79 iBT), IELTS (minimum score 6). *Application deadline:* For fall admission, 2/1 for domestic students, 1/1 priority date for international students. Applications are processed on a rolling basis. Application fee: $40. Electronic applications accepted. *Expenses:* Contact institution. *Financial support:* Federal Work-Study, scholarships/grants, tuition waivers (full and partial), and unspecified assistantships available. Financial award application deadline: 3/1; financial award applicants required to submit FAFSA. *Unit head:* Dr. Mellisa Hall, Chair of the Master of Science in Nursing Program, 812-465-1168, E-mail: mrowser@usi.edu. *Application contact:* Dr. Mayola Rowser, Director, Graduate Studies, 812-465-7016, Fax: 812-464-1956, E-mail: mrowser@usi.edu.
Website: https://www.usi.edu/health/nursing/degrees-and-programs

University of Southern Maine, College of Science, Technology, and Health, School of Nursing, Portland, ME 04103. Offers adult-gerontology primary care nurse practitioner (MS, PMC); education (MS); family nurse practitioner (MS, PMC); family psychiatric/mental health nurse practitioner (MS); management (MS); nursing (CAS, CGS); psychiatric-mental health nurse practitioner (PMC). *Accreditation:* AACN. *Program availability:* Part-time. *Degree requirements:* For master's, thesis optional. *Entrance requirements:* For master's, GRE General Test or MAT, minimum GPA of 3.0; for doctorate, GRE. Additional exam requirements/recommendations for international students: Required—TOEFL (minimum score 550 paper-based). Electronic applications accepted. *Expenses: Tuition, area resident:* Full-time $6840; part-time $380 per credit hour. Tuition, state resident: full-time $10,260; part-time $570 per credit hour. Tuition, nonresident: full-time $18,468; part-time $1026 per credit hour. *Required fees:* $830; $83 per credit hour. Tuition and fees vary according to course load and program. *Faculty research:* Women's health, nursing history, weight control, community services, substance abuse.

University of Southern Mississippi, Graduate School, College of Nursing, Hattiesburg, MS 39406-0001. Offers family nurse practitioner (MSN, Graduate Certificate); family psychiatric-mental health nurse practitioner (Graduate Certificate); nursing (DNP, PhD); psychiatric-mental health nurse practitioner (Graduate Certificate). *Accreditation:* AACN. *Program availability:* Part-time, evening/weekend. *Degree requirements:* For master's, comprehensive exam, thesis optional; for doctorate, comprehensive exam, thesis/dissertation. *Entrance requirements:* For master's, GRE General Test, minimum GPA of 2.75 during last 60 hours, nursing license, BS in nursing; for doctorate, GRE General Test, master's degree in nursing, minimum GPA of 3.5. Additional exam requirements/recommendations for international students: Required—TOEFL, IELTS. Electronic applications accepted. *Faculty research:* Gerontology, caregivers, HIV, bereavement, pain, nursing leadership.

University of South Florida, College of Nursing, Tampa, FL 33612. Offers advanced pain management (Graduate Certificate); nursing (MS, DNP), including adult gerontology acute care (DNP), adult gerontology acute care nursing (MS), adult gerontology primary care (DNP), adult gerontology primary care nursing (MS), adult gerontology primary care/occupational health nursing (MS), adult gerontology primary care/oncology nursing (MS), clinical nurse leader (MS), family health nursing, nurse

anesthesia (MS), nursing education (MS), nursing practice (DNP), occupational health/adult-gerontology (DNP), oncology/adult-gerontology primary care (DNP), pediatric health (DNP), pediatric nurse practitioner (MS); nursing education (Post Master's Certificate); nursing science (PhD). *Accreditation:* AACN; AANA/CANAEP. *Program availability:* Part-time. *Faculty:* 43 full-time (38 women), 7 part-time/adjunct (4 women). *Students:* 159 full-time (135 women), 721 part-time (625 women); includes 292 minority (119 Black or African American, non-Hispanic/Latino; 2 American Indian or Alaska Native, non-Hispanic/Latino; 60 Asian, non-Hispanic/Latino; 90 Hispanic/Latino; 1 Native Hawaiian or other Pacific Islander, non-Hispanic/Latino; 20 Two or more races, non-Hispanic/Latino), 12 international. Average age 35. 636 applicants, 44% accepted, 215 enrolled. In 2015, 333 master's, 18 doctorates awarded. *Degree requirements:* For master's, comprehensive exam, thesis optional; for doctorate, comprehensive exam, thesis/dissertation. *Entrance requirements:* For master's, GRE General Test, bachelor's degree from accredited program with minimum GPA of 3.0 in all upper-division coursework; current license as Registered Nurse; 3 letters of recommendation; personal statement of goals; resume or curriculum vitae; personal interview; for doctorate, GRE General Test (recommended), bachelor's degree in nursing from a CCNA/NLNAC regionally-accredited institution with minimum GPA of 3.0 in all coursework or in all upper-division coursework; current license as Registered Nurse in Florida; undergraduate statistics course with minimum B grade; 3 letters of recommendation; statement of goals; resume; interview. Average age 35. Additional exam requirements/recommendations for international students: Required—TOEFL (minimum score 550 paper-based; 79 iBT). *Application deadline:* For fall admission, 2/15 for domestic students, 1/2 for international students; for spring admission, 10/1 for domestic students, 6/1 for international students. Application fee: $30. Electronic applications accepted. *Financial support:* In 2015–16, 36 students received support, including 7 research assistantships with tuition reimbursements available (averaging $18,035 per year), 29 teaching assistantships with tuition reimbursements available (averaging $30,814 per year); tuition waivers (partial) and unspecified assistantships also available. Financial award application deadline: 2/1; financial award applicants required to submit FAFSA. *Faculty research:* Women's health, palliative and end-of-life care, cardiac rehabilitation, complementary therapies for chronic illness and cancer. *Total annual research expenditures:* $2.6 million. *Unit head:* Dr. Dianne C. Morrison-Beedy, Dean and Professor, College of Nursing, 813-974-9091, Fax: 813-974-5418, E-mail: dmbeedy@health.usf.edu. *Application contact:* Dr. Brian Graves, Assistant Professor/Assistant Dean, 813-974-8054, Fax: 813-974-5418, E-mail: bgraves1@health.usf.edu.
Website: http://health.usf.edu/nursing/index.htm

The University of Tampa, Program in Nursing, Tampa, FL 33606-1490. Offers adult nursing practitioner (MSN); family nursing practitioner (MSN); nursing (MS). *Accreditation:* ACEN. *Program availability:* Part-time, evening/weekend. *Faculty:* 15 full-time (13 women), 4 part-time/adjunct (3 women). *Students:* 1 (woman) full-time, 152 part-time (130 women); includes 27 minority (9 Black or African American, non-Hispanic/Latino; 1 American Indian or Alaska Native, non-Hispanic/Latino; 9 Asian, non-Hispanic/Latino; 8 Two or more races, non-Hispanic/Latino). Average age 33. 112 applicants, 54% accepted, 32 enrolled. In 2015, 33 master's awarded. *Degree requirements:* For master's, comprehensive exam, oral exam, practicum. *Entrance requirements:* For master's, GMAT or GRE, current licensure as registered nurse in state of Florida; minimum GPA of 3.0 in last 60 credit hours; minimum of one year of direct patient care experience within the past five years (recommended). Additional exam requirements/recommendations for international students: Required—TOEFL (minimum score 577 paper-based; 90 iBT), IELTS (minimum score 7.5). *Application deadline:* Applications are processed on a rolling basis. Application fee: $40. Electronic applications accepted. *Expenses:* $573 per credit tuition, $80 per term fees. *Financial support:* In 2015–16, 5 students received support. Career-related internships or fieldwork, scholarships/grants, and unspecified assistantships available. Financial award applicants required to submit FAFSA. *Faculty research:* Vaccinations and public health, osteoporosis, cultural diversity, ethics, nursing practice. *Unit head:* Dr. Cathy Kessenich, Director, 813-257-3160, Fax: 813-258-7214, E-mail: ckessenich@ut.edu. *Application contact:* Chanelle Cox, Staff Assistant, Admissions for Graduate and Continuing Studies, 813-253-6249, E-mail: ccox@ut.edu.

The University of Tennessee, Graduate School, College of Nursing, Knoxville, TN 37996. Offers MSN, PhD. *Accreditation:* AACN; AANA/CANAEP. *Program availability:* Part-time. *Degree requirements:* For master's, thesis or alternative; for doctorate, thesis/dissertation. *Entrance requirements:* For master's and doctorate, GRE General Test, minimum GPA of 2.7. Additional exam requirements/recommendations for international students: Required—TOEFL. Electronic applications accepted.

The University of Tennessee at Chattanooga, School of Nursing, Chattanooga, TN 37403. Offers administration (MSN); certified nurse anesthetist (Post-Master's Certificate); education (MSN); family nurse practitioner (MSN, Post-Master's Certificate); health care informatics (Post-Master's Certificate); nurse anesthesia (MSN); nurse education (Post-Master's Certificate); nursing (DNP). *Accreditation:* AACN; AANA/CANAEP (one or more programs are accredited). *Faculty:* 9 full-time (7 women), 2 part-time/adjunct (1 woman). *Students:* 50 full-time (25 women), 43 part-time (37 women); includes 14 minority (7 Black or African American, non-Hispanic/Latino; 1 American Indian or Alaska Native, non-Hispanic/Latino; 2 Asian, non-Hispanic/Latino; 2 Two or more races, non-Hispanic/Latino). Average age 34. In 2015, 40 master's, 12 doctorates, 1 other advanced degree awarded. *Degree requirements:* For master's, thesis optional, qualifying exams, professional project; for Post-Master's Certificate, thesis or alternative, practicum, seminar. *Entrance requirements:* For master's, GRE General Test, MAT, BSN, minimum GPA of 3.0, eligibility for Tennessee RN license, 1 year of direct patient care experience; for Post-Master's Certificate, GRE General Test, MAT, MSN, minimum GPA of 3.0, eligibility for Tennessee RN license, one year of direct patient care experience. Additional exam requirements/recommendations for international students: Required—TOEFL (minimum score 79 iBT), IELTS (minimum score 6). *Application deadline:* For fall admission, 6/13 priority date for domestic students, 6/1 for international students; for spring admission, 10/15 priority date for domestic students, 10/1 for international students. Applications are processed on a rolling basis. Application fee: $30 ($35 for international students). Electronic applications accepted. *Expenses:* Tuition, state resident: full-time $7938; part-time $441 per credit hour. Tuition, nonresident: full-time $24,056; part-time $1336 per credit hour. *Required fees:* $1732; $253 per credit hour. *Financial support:* Career-related internships or fieldwork and scholarships/grants available. Support available to part-time students. *Faculty research:* Diabetes in women, health care for elderly, alternative medicine, hypertension, nurse anesthesia. *Total annual research expenditures:* $2.6 million. *Unit head:* Dr. Chris Smith, Interim Director, 423-425-1741, Fax: 423-425-4668, E-mail: chris-smith@utc.edu. *Application contact:* Dr. J. Randy Walker, Interim Dean of Graduate Studies, 423-425-4478, Fax: 423-425-5223, E-mail: randy-walker@utc.edu.
Website: http://www.utc.edu/Academic/Nursing/

The University of Tennessee Health Science Center, College of Graduate Health Sciences, Memphis, TN 38163-0002. Offers biomedical engineering (MS, PhD); biomedical sciences (PhD); dental sciences (MDS); epidemiology (MS); health outcomes and policy research (PhD); laboratory research and management (MS); nursing science (PhD); pharmaceutical sciences (PhD); pharmacology (MS); speech and hearing science (PhD); DDS/PhD; DNP/PhD; MD/PhD; Pharm D/PhD. Terminal

master's awarded for partial completion of doctoral program. *Degree requirements:* For master's, comprehensive exam, thesis; for doctorate, comprehensive exam, thesis/dissertation, oral and written preliminary and comprehensive exams. *Entrance requirements:* For master's and doctorate, GRE General Test, minimum GPA of 3.0. Additional exam requirements/recommendations for international students: Required—TOEFL (minimum score 79 iBT); Recommended—IELTS (minimum score 6.5). Electronic applications accepted.

The University of Tennessee Health Science Center, College of Nursing, Memphis, TN 38163. Offers adult-gerontology acute care nurse practitioner (Certificate); advanced practice nursing (DNP); clinical nurse leader (MSN). *Accreditation:* AACN; AANA/CANAEP. *Program availability:* Part-time, online learning. *Degree requirements:* For master's, thesis, portfolio; for doctorate, portfolio. *Entrance requirements:* For master's, minimum GPA of 3.0; for doctorate, RN license, minimum GPA of 3.0; for Certificate, MSN, APN license, minimum GPA of 3.0. Additional exam requirements/recommendations for international students: Required—TOEFL (minimum score 550 paper-based; 80 iBT). Electronic applications accepted. *Expenses:* Contact institution. *Faculty research:* Efficacy of a cognitive behavioral group intervention and its influence on symptoms of depression and anxiety as well as caregiver function; ability of newly-developed assays to aid in the diagnosis of preeclampsia; quality of life and sexual function in women who undergo vulvar surgeries; influence of prenatal and early childhood environments on health and developmental trajectories across childhood; interaction between physical activity, diet, genetics, insulin resistance, and obesity.

The University of Texas at Arlington, Graduate School, College of Nursing, Arlington, TX 76019. Offers nurse practitioner (MSN); nursing administration (MSN); nursing education (MSN); nursing practice (DNP); nursing science (PhD). *Accreditation:* AACN. *Program availability:* Part-time, evening/weekend, online learning. *Degree requirements:* For master's, practicum course; for doctorate, comprehensive exam (for some programs), thesis/dissertation (for some programs), proposal defense dissertation (for PhD); scholarship project (for DNP). *Entrance requirements:* For master's, GRE General Test if GPA less than 3.0, minimum GPA of 3.0, Texas nursing license, minimum C grade in undergraduate statistics course; for doctorate, GRE General Test (waived for MSN-to-PhD applicants), minimum undergraduate, graduate and statistics GPA of 3.0; Texas RN license; interview; written statement of goals. Additional exam requirements/recommendations for international students: Required—TOEFL (minimum score 550 paper-based), IELTS (minimum score 7). *Faculty research:* Simulation in clinical education and practice, cultural diversity, vulnerable populations, substance abuse.

The University of Texas at Austin, Graduate School, School of Nursing, Austin, TX 78712-1111. Offers adult - gerontology clinical nurse specialist (MSN); child health (MSN), including administration, public health nursing, teaching; family nurse practitioner (MSN); family psychiatric/mental health nurse practitioner (MSN); holistic adult health (MSN), including administration, teaching; maternity (MSN), including administration, public health nursing, teaching; nursing (PhD); nursing administration and healthcare systems management (MSN); nursing practice (DNP); pediatric nurse practitioner (MSN); public health nursing (MSN). *Accreditation:* AACN. *Program availability:* Part-time. *Degree requirements:* For master's, thesis optional; for doctorate, thesis/dissertation. *Entrance requirements:* For master's and doctorate, GRE General Test. Additional exam requirements/recommendations for international students: Required—TOEFL (minimum score 550 paper-based). Electronic applications accepted. *Faculty research:* Chronic illness management, memory and aging, health promotion, women's health, adolescent health.

The University of Texas at El Paso, Graduate School, School of Nursing, El Paso, TX 79968-0001. Offers family nurse practitioner (MSN); health care leadership and management (Certificate); interdisciplinary health sciences (PhD); nursing (DNP); nursing education (MSN, Certificate); nursing systems management (MSN). *Accreditation:* AACN. *Program availability:* Online learning. *Degree requirements:* For master's, thesis optional; for doctorate, thesis/dissertation. *Entrance requirements:* For master's, minimum GPA of 3.0, resume; for doctorate, GRE, letters of reference, relevant personal/professional experience; master's degree in nursing (for DNP); for Certificate, bachelor's degree in nursing. Additional exam requirements/recommendations for international students: Required—TOEFL; Recommended—IELTS. Electronic applications accepted.

The University of Texas at Tyler, College of Nursing and Health Sciences, Program in Nursing, Tyler, TX 75799-0001. Offers nurse practitioner (MSN); nursing (PhD); nursing administration (MSN); nursing education (MSN); MSN/MBA. *Accreditation:* AACN. *Program availability:* Part-time, evening/weekend, online learning. *Degree requirements:* For master's, comprehensive exam (for some programs), thesis (for some programs); for doctorate, thesis/dissertation. *Entrance requirements:* For master's, GRE General Test or MAT, GMAT, minimum undergraduate GPA of 3.0, course work in statistics, RN license, BSN. Additional exam requirements/recommendations for international students: Required—TOEFL. Electronic applications accepted. *Faculty research:* Psychosocial adjustment, aging, support/commitment of caregivers, psychological abuse and violence, hope/hopelessness, professional values, end of life care, suicidology, clinical supervision, workforce retention and issues, global health issues, health promotion.

The University of Texas Health Science Center at Houston, School of Nursing, Houston, TX 77030. Offers MSN, DNP, PhD, MSN/MPH. *Accreditation:* AACN; AANA/CANAEP. *Program availability:* Part-time. *Degree requirements:* For master's, thesis, research project, or clinical project; for doctorate, thesis/dissertation. *Entrance requirements:* For master's, GRE or MAT, BSN, Texas RN license, related work experience, interview, writing sample; for doctorate, GRE, interview, Texas RN license, portfolio, master's degree. Additional exam requirements/recommendations for international students: Required—TOEFL (minimum score 550 paper-based; 86 iBT). Electronic applications accepted. *Faculty research:* Malnutrition in institutionalized elderly, defining nursing, sensitive outcome measures, substance abuse in mothers during pregnancy, psychoeducational intervention among caregivers of stroke patients.

The University of Texas Health Science Center at San Antonio, Graduate School of Biomedical Sciences, Program in Nursing Science, San Antonio, TX 78229-3900. Offers PhD.

The University of Texas Health Science Center at San Antonio, School of Nursing, San Antonio, TX 78229-3900. Offers administrative management (MSN); adult-gerontology acute care nurse practitioner (PGC); advanced practice leadership (DNP); clinical nurse leader (MSN); executive administrative management (DNP); family nurse practitioner (MSN, PGC); nursing (MSN, PhD); nursing education (MSN, PGC); pediatric nurse practitioner primary care (PGC); psychiatric mental health nurse practitioner (PGC); public health nurse leader (DNP). *Accreditation:* AACN. *Program availability:* Part-time. Terminal master's awarded for partial completion of doctoral program. *Degree requirements:* For master's, thesis optional; for doctorate, comprehensive exam, thesis/dissertation.

The University of Texas Medical Branch, Graduate School of Biomedical Sciences, Doctoral Program in Nursing, Galveston, TX 77555. Offers PhD. *Degree requirements:* For doctorate, comprehensive exam, thesis/dissertation. *Entrance requirements:* For doctorate, GRE General Test, minimum GPA of 3.0, BSN and MSN or equivalent

Nursing—General

advanced degree, 2 writing samples, 3 letters of reference, curriculum vitae or resume. Additional exam requirements/recommendations for international students: Required—TOEFL (minimum score 550 paper-based). Electronic applications accepted.

The University of Texas Medical Branch, School of Nursing, Master's Program in Nursing, Galveston, TX 77555. Offers MSN. *Program availability:* Part-time, online learning. *Entrance requirements:* For master's, GRE General Test or MAT, minimum BSN GPA of 3.0, 3 references, interview, 1 year nursing experience. Additional exam requirements/recommendations for international students: Required—TOEFL (minimum score 550 paper-based).

The University of Texas Rio Grande Valley, College of Health Affairs, School of Nursing, Edinburg, TX 78539. Offers adult health nursing (MSN); family nurse practitioner (MSN). *Accreditation:* AACN. *Program availability:* Part-time, evening/weekend. *Degree requirements:* For master's, thesis optional. *Entrance requirements:* For master's, Texas RN licensure, undergraduate physical statistic course. Additional exam requirements/recommendations for international students: Required—TOEFL (minimum score 550 paper-based). Electronic applications accepted. *Expenses:* Contact institution. *Faculty research:* Health promotion, adolescent pregnancy, herbal and nontraditional approaches, healing touch stress.

University of the Incarnate Word, School of Graduate Studies and Research, School of Nursing and Health Professions, Program in Nursing, San Antonio, TX 78209-6397. Offers clinical nursing leader (MSN); clinical nursing specialist (MSN); nursing (DNP). *Accreditation:* AACN. *Program availability:* Part-time, evening/weekend. *Faculty:* 7 full-time (all women), 1 (woman) part-time/adjunct. *Students:* 3 full-time (all women), 66 part-time (55 women); includes 42 minority (5 Black or African American, non-Hispanic/Latino; 1 American Indian or Alaska Native, non-Hispanic/Latino; 3 Asian, non-Hispanic/Latino; 31 Hispanic/Latino; 2 Two or more races, non-Hispanic/Latino), 3 international. Average age 39. 7 applicants, 100% accepted, 6 enrolled. In 2015, 10 master's awarded. *Degree requirements:* For master's, capstone, clinical hours. *Entrance requirements:* For master's, baccalaureate degree in nursing from CCNE- or NLN-accredited program including courses in statistics and health assessment; minimum undergraduate cumulative GPA of 2.5, 3.0 in upper-division nursing courses; three professional references; license to practice nursing in Texas or recognized state. Additional exam requirements/recommendations for international students: Required—TOEFL (minimum score 560 paper-based; 83 iBT). *Application deadline:* Applications are processed on a rolling basis. Application fee: $20. Electronic applications accepted. *Expenses: Tuition, area resident:* Part-time $885 per credit hour. *Required fees:* $40 per credit hour. Tuition and fees vary according to course load, degree level, campus/location, program and student level. *Financial support:* Federal Work-Study, scholarships/grants, traineeships, and unspecified assistantships available. Support available to part-time students. Financial award applicants required to submit FAFSA. *Unit head:* Dr. Holly Cassells, Chair, Graduate Programs, 210-829-3977, Fax: 210-829-3174, E-mail: cassells@uiwtx.edu. *Application contact:* Johnny Garcia, Graduate Admissions Counselor, 210-805-3554, Fax: 210-829-3921, E-mail: admis@uiwtx.edu. Website: http://uiw.edu/nursing/msn-program/

The University of Toledo, College of Graduate Studies, College of Nursing, Toledo, OH 43614. Offers MSN, DNP, Certificate. *Accreditation:* AACN. *Program availability:* Part-time, online learning. *Degree requirements:* For master's, thesis or scholarly project; for doctorate, thesis/dissertation or alternative, evidence-based project. *Entrance requirements:* For master's, GRE, BS in nursing, minimum undergraduate GPA of 3.0, statement of purpose, two letters of recommendation, transcripts from all prior institutions attended, resume, Nursing CAS application, UT supplemental application; for doctorate, minimum undergraduate GPA of 3.0, statement of purpose, three letters of recommendation, transcripts from all prior institutions attended, resume, Nursing CAS application, UT supplemental application. Additional exam requirements/recommendations for international students: Required—TOEFL (minimum score 550 paper-based; 80 iBT). Electronic applications accepted. *Expenses:* Contact institution. *Faculty research:* Sexuality issues, prenatal testing, health care of homeless, nursing education, chronic/acute pain, eating disorders, low birth weight infants.

University of Toronto, School of Graduate Studies, Department of Nursing Science, Toronto, ON M5S 1A1, Canada. Offers MN, PhD, MHSc/MN. *Program availability:* Part-time. *Degree requirements:* For doctorate, thesis/dissertation, departmental and final oral exam/thesis defense. *Entrance requirements:* For master's, B Sc N or equivalent, minimum B average in next-to-final year, resume, 3 letters of reference; for doctorate, minimum B+ average, master's degree in nursing or a related area, resume, 2 letters of recommendation. Additional exam requirements/recommendations for international students: Required—TOEFL (minimum score 580 paper-based; 93 iBT), TWE (minimum score 5). Electronic applications accepted. *Expenses:* Contact institution.

University of Utah, Graduate School, College of Nursing, Program in Nursing, Salt Lake City, UT 84112. Offers MS, DNP, PhD. *Program availability:* Part-time, evening/weekend, online learning. *Students:* 284 full-time (219 women), 63 part-time (49 women); includes 51 minority (8 Black or African American, non-Hispanic/Latino; 1 American Indian or Alaska Native, non-Hispanic/Latino; 19 Asian, non-Hispanic/Latino; 17 Hispanic/Latino; 6 Two or more races, non-Hispanic/Latino), 9 international. Average age 36. 262 applicants, 56% accepted, 122 enrolled. In 2015, 29 master's, 17 doctorates awarded. *Degree requirements:* For master's, thesis (for some programs), thesis or synthesis; for doctorate, comprehensive exam, thesis/dissertation. *Entrance requirements:* For master's, GRE General Test (if cumulative GPA less than 3.2), RN licensure in one of the jurisdictions of the National Council of State Boards of Nursing, goal statement, professional references; for doctorate, GRE General Test, interview, curriculum vitae/resume, goal statement, professional and academic references, writing sample. Additional exam requirements/recommendations for international students: Required—TOEFL (minimum score 500 paper-based; 85 iBT). *Application deadline:* For fall admission, 1/15 for domestic and international students. Application fee: $55 ($65 for international students). Electronic applications accepted. *Expenses:* Contact institution. *Financial support:* In 2015–16, 73 students received support, including 73 fellowships with tuition reimbursements available (averaging $10,000 per year), 4 research assistantships with tuition reimbursements available (averaging $13,000 per year), 9 teaching assistantships with partial tuition reimbursements available (averaging $11,555 per year); scholarships/grants, traineeships, health care benefits, and unspecified assistantships also available. Support available to part-time students. Financial award application deadline: 1/15; financial award applicants required to submit FAFSA. *Faculty research:* Symptom management, patient-provider communication, patient safety/informatics, gerontology/geriatric nursing, end-of-life bereavement. *Total annual research expenditures:* $2.2 million. *Unit head:* Patricia Morton, RN, PhD, Dean, 801-581-8262, Fax: 801-581-4642, E-mail: patricia.morton@nurs.utah.edu. *Application contact:* Carrie Radmall, Program Administrator, 801-581-8798, Fax: 801-585-3414, E-mail: carrie.radmall@nurs.utah.edu. Website: http://www.nursing.utah.edu/

University of Vermont, Graduate College, College of Nursing and Health Sciences, Department of Nursing, Burlington, VT 05405. Offers MS, DNP. *Accreditation:* AACN. *Entrance requirements:* For master's, GRE General Test. Additional exam requirements/recommendations for international students: Required—TOEFL (minimum score 550 paper-based; 80 iBT). *Application deadline:* For fall admission, 4/3 for domestic and

international students. Applications are processed on a rolling basis. Application fee: $65. Electronic applications accepted. *Financial support:* Application deadline: 3/1. *Unit head:* Dr. Carol Buck-Rolland, 802-656-3858. *Application contact:* Dr. Carol Buck-Rolland, 802-656-3858.

University of Victoria, Faculty of Graduate Studies, Faculty of Human and Social Development, School of Nursing, Victoria, BC V8W 2Y2, Canada. Offers advanced nursing practice (advanced practice leadership option) (MN); advanced nursing practice (nurse educator option) (MN); advanced nursing practice (nurse practitioner option) (MN); nursing (PhD). *Program availability:* Part-time, online learning. *Entrance requirements:* Additional exam requirements/recommendations for international students: Required—TOEFL (minimum score 575 paper-based), IELTS (minimum score 7). Electronic applications accepted.

University of Virginia, School of Nursing, Charlottesville, VA 22903. Offers acute and specialty care (MSN); acute care nurse practitioner (MSN); clinical nurse leadership (MSN); community-public health leadership (MSN); nursing (DNP, PhD); psychiatric mental health counseling (MSN); MSN/MBA. *Accreditation:* AACN. *Program availability:* Part-time. *Degree requirements:* For doctorate, comprehensive exam (for some programs), capstone project (DNP), dissertation (PhD). *Entrance requirements:* For master's, GRE General Test, MAT; for doctorate, GRE General Test. Additional exam requirements/recommendations for international students: Required—TOEFL, IELTS. Electronic applications accepted. *Expenses:* Contact institution.

University of Washington, Graduate School, School of Nursing, Seattle, WA 98195. Offers MN, MS, DNP, PhD, Graduate Certificate, MN/MPH. *Accreditation:* AACN; ACNM/ACME (one or more programs are accredited). *Program availability:* Part-time. *Degree requirements:* For master's, thesis (for some programs); for doctorate, thesis/dissertation. *Entrance requirements:* For master's, GRE, minimum GPA of 3.0, resume; for doctorate, GRE, minimum GPA of 3.0. Additional exam requirements/recommendations for international students: Required—TOEFL. *Faculty research:* High risk youth, pain management, women's health, oncology, sleep.

University of Washington, Bothell, Program in Nursing, Bothell, WA 98011-8246. Offers MN. *Program availability:* Part-time. *Degree requirements:* For master's, scholarly project. *Entrance requirements:* For master's, BSN (or other bachelor's degree with additional prerequisite work); current license as registered nurse in Washington state; minimum GPA of 3.0 in last 90 college credits, 2.0 in college statistics course. Additional exam requirements/recommendations for international students: Required—TOEFL (minimum score 580 paper-based). Electronic applications accepted. *Expenses:* Contact institution. *Faculty research:* Health of special populations, nursing education, higher education technology, healing through patient's narratives, women's health care issues, end of life issues in nursing.

University of Washington, Tacoma, Graduate Programs, Program in Nursing, Tacoma, WA 98402-3100. Offers communities, populations and health (MN); leadership in healthcare (MN); nurse educator (MN). *Program availability:* Part-time. *Degree requirements:* For master's, thesis (for some programs), advance fieldwork. *Entrance requirements:* For master's, Washington State NCLEX exam, minimum GPA of 3.0. Additional exam requirements/recommendations for international students: Required—TOEFL (minimum score 580 paper-based; 70 iBT); Recommended—IELTS (minimum score 7). *Faculty research:* Hospice and palliative care; clinical trial decision-making; minority nurse retention; asthma and public health; injustice, suffering, difference: Linking Them to Us; adolescent health.

The University of Western Ontario, Faculty of Graduate Studies, Health Sciences Division, School of Nursing, London, ON N6A 5B8, Canada. Offers M Sc N, MN NP, PhD. *Program availability:* Part-time. *Degree requirements:* For master's, thesis; for doctorate, thesis/dissertation. *Entrance requirements:* Additional exam requirements/recommendations for international students: Required—TOEFL. *Faculty research:* Empowerment, self-efficacy, family health, community health, gerontology.

University of West Florida, College of Science and Engineering, School of Allied Health and Life Sciences, Department of Nursing, Pensacola, FL 32514-5750. Offers MSN. *Program availability:* Part-time, evening/weekend. *Entrance requirements:* For master's, GRE or MAT, letter of intent; current curriculum vitae/resume. Additional exam requirements/recommendations for international students: Required—TOEFL (minimum score 550 paper-based).

University of West Georgia, Tanner Health System School of Nursing, Carrollton, GA 30118. Offers health systems leadership (Post-Master's Certificate); nursing (MSN); nursing education (Ed D, Post-Master's Certificate). *Accreditation:* AACN. *Program availability:* Part-time, evening/weekend, 100% online. *Faculty:* 13 full-time (all women). *Students:* 58 full-time (51 women), 69 part-time (61 women); includes 33 minority (29 Black or African American, non-Hispanic/Latino; 1 Asian, non-Hispanic/Latino; 3 Hispanic/Latino). Average age 42. 78 applicants, 90% accepted, 58 enrolled. In 2015, 32 master's, 1 other advanced degree awarded. *Entrance requirements:* Additional exam requirements/recommendations for international students: Required—TOEFL (minimum score 523 paper-based; 69 iBT); Recommended—IELTS (minimum score 6.5). *Application deadline:* For fall admission, 2/1 priority date for domestic and international students. Applications are processed on a rolling basis. Application fee: $40. Electronic applications accepted. *Expenses:* Contact institution. *Financial support:* Fellowships, research assistantships, teaching assistantships, career-related internships or fieldwork, Federal Work-Study, institutionally sponsored loans, scholarships/grants, and unspecified assistantships available. Support available to part-time students. Financial award application deadline: 4/1; financial award applicants required to submit FAFSA. *Unit head:* Dr. Jennifer Schuessler, Dean, 678-839-5640, Fax: 678-839-6553, E-mail: jschuess@westga.edu. *Application contact:* Dr. Toby Ziglar, Director of Graduate and International Admissions, 678-839-1390, Fax: 678-839-1395, E-mail: graduate@westga.edu. Website: http://nursing.westga.edu

University of Windsor, Faculty of Graduate Studies, Faculty of Nursing, Windsor, ON N9B 3P4, Canada. Offers M Sc, MN. *Degree requirements:* For master's, thesis or alternative. *Entrance requirements:* For master's, minimum B average, certificate of competence (nurse registration). Additional exam requirements/recommendations for international students: Required—TOEFL (minimum score 560 paper-based). Electronic applications accepted.

University of Wisconsin–Eau Claire, College of Nursing and Health Sciences, Program in Nursing, Eau Claire, WI 54702-4004. Offers adult-gerontological administration (DNP); adult-gerontological clinical nurse specialist (DNP); adult-gerontological education (MSN); adult-gerontological primary care nurse practitioner (DNP); family health administration (DNP); family health in education (MSN); family health nurse practitioner (DNP); nursing (MSN); nursing practice (DNP). *Program availability:* Part-time. Terminal master's awarded for partial completion of doctoral program. *Degree requirements:* For master's, thesis optional, 500-600 hours clinical practicum, oral and written exams. *Entrance requirements:* For master's, Wisconsin RN license, minimum GPA of 3.0, undergraduate statistics, course work in health assessment. Additional exam requirements/recommendations for international students: Required—TOEFL (minimum score 79 iBT). *Expenses:* Contact institution.

University of Wisconsin–Madison, School of Nursing, Madison, WI 53706-1380. Offers adult/gerontology (DNP); nursing (PhD); pediatrics (DNP); psychiatric mental health (DNP); MS/MPH. *Accreditation:* AACN. *Program availability:* Part-time. *Degree requirements:* For doctorate, comprehensive exam, thesis/dissertation. *Entrance requirements:* For doctorate, GRE General Test, 2 samples of scholarly written work, BS in nursing from an accredited program, minimum undergraduate GPA of 3.0 in last 60 credits (for PhD); licensure as professional nurse (for DNP). Additional exam requirements/recommendations for international students: Required—TOEFL (minimum score 600 paper-based; 100 iBT). Electronic applications accepted. *Expenses:* Tuition, state resident: full-time $5364. Tuition, nonresident: full-time $12,027. *Required fees:* $571. Tuition and fees vary according to campus/location, program and reciprocity agreements. *Faculty research:* Nursing informatics to promote self-care and disease management skills among patients and caregivers; quality of care to frail, vulnerable, and chronically ill populations; study of health-related and health-seeking behaviors; eliminating health disparities; pain and symptom management for patients with cancer.

University of Wisconsin–Milwaukee, Graduate School, College of Nursing, Milwaukee, WI 53201-0413. Offers clinical nurse specialist (Certificate); family nurse practitioner (Certificate); nursing (MN, MS, PhD); nursing practice (DNP). *Accreditation:* AACN. *Program availability:* Part-time. *Students:* 168 full-time (144 women), 126 part-time (115 women); includes 47 minority (16 Black or African American, non-Hispanic/Latino; 16 Asian, non-Hispanic/Latino; 3 Hispanic/Latino; 12 Two or more races, non-Hispanic/Latino), 12 international. Average age 36. 146 applicants, 64% accepted, 59 enrolled. In 2015, 22 master's, 28 doctorates, 15 other advanced degrees awarded. *Degree requirements:* For master's, thesis; for doctorate, thesis/dissertation. *Entrance requirements:* For master's, GRE General Test or MAT, autobiographical sketch; for doctorate, GRE, minimum GPA of 3.2. Additional exam requirements/recommendations for international students: Required—TOEFL (minimum score 550 paper-based; 79 iBT), IELTS (minimum score 6.5). *Application deadline:* For fall admission, 1/1 priority date for domestic students; for spring admission, 9/1 for domestic students. Applications are processed on a rolling basis. Application fee: $56 ($96 for international students). Electronic applications accepted. *Financial support:* Fellowships, research assistantships, teaching assistantships, career-related internships or fieldwork, Federal Work-Study, health care benefits, unspecified assistantships, and project assistantships available. Support available to part-time students. Financial award application deadline: 4/15; financial award applicants required to submit FAFSA. *Unit head:* Dr. Sally Lundeen, Dean, 414-229-4189, E-mail: slundeen@uwm.edu. *Application contact:* Kim Litwack, Representative, 414-229-5098.
Website: http://www.uwm.edu/Dept/Nursing/

University of Wisconsin–Oshkosh, Graduate Studies, College of Nursing, Oshkosh, WI 54901. Offers adult health and illness (MSN); family nurse practitioner (MSN). *Accreditation:* AACN. *Program availability:* Part-time. *Degree requirements:* For master's, thesis or alternative, clinical paper. *Entrance requirements:* For master's, RN license, BSN, previous course work in statistics and health assessment, minimum undergraduate GPA of 3.0, letters of recommendation. Additional exam requirements/recommendations for international students: Required—TOEFL (minimum score 550 paper-based; 79 iBT). Electronic applications accepted. *Faculty research:* Adult health and illness, nurse practitioners practice, health care service, advanced practitioner roles, natural alternative complementary healthcare.

University of Wyoming, College of Health Sciences, Fay W. Whitney School of Nursing, Laramie, WY 82071. Offers MS. *Accreditation:* AACN. *Program availability:* Part-time, online learning. *Degree requirements:* For master's, thesis. *Entrance requirements:* For master's, GRE General Test, BSN from CCNE or NCN-accredited school, minimum GPA of 3.0. Additional exam requirements/recommendations for international students: Required—TOEFL. *Faculty research:* Support systems for the elderly, fetal alcohol syndrome, teen pregnancy, rehabilitation with chronic mental illness, global peace building among women.

Urbana University, College of Nursing and Allied Health, Urbana, OH 43078-2091. Offers nursing (MSN). *Accreditation:* AACN. *Entrance requirements:* For master's, baccalaureate degree in nursing with minimum cumulative undergraduate GPA of 3.0, official transcripts, Ohio RN license, background check, statement of goals and objectives, resume, 3 letters of recommendation, interview.

Ursuline College, School of Graduate Studies, Programs in Nursing, Pepper Pike, OH 44124-4398. Offers adult nurse practitioner (MSN); adult-gerontology clinical nurse specialist (MSN); family nurse practitioner (MSN); nursing (DNP); nursing education (MSN); palliative care (MSN). *Accreditation:* AACN. *Program availability:* Part-time. *Faculty:* 5 full-time (all women), 26 part-time/adjunct (21 women). *Students:* 150 full-time (141 women), 108 part-time (99 women); includes 66 minority (50 Black or African American, non-Hispanic/Latino; 6 Asian, non-Hispanic/Latino; 6 Hispanic/Latino; 4 Two or more races, non-Hispanic/Latino), 5 international. Average age 37. 115 applicants, 95% accepted, 73 enrolled. In 2015, 69 master's, 2 doctorates awarded. *Degree requirements:* For master's, comprehensive exam. *Entrance requirements:* For master's, minimum undergraduate GPA of 3.0, bachelor's degree in nursing, eligibility for or current Ohio RN license. Additional exam requirements/recommendations for international students: Required—TOEFL (minimum score 500 paper-based). *Application deadline:* For fall admission, 8/1 priority date for domestic students. Applications are processed on a rolling basis. Application fee: $25. Electronic applications accepted. *Expenses: Tuition, area resident:* Full-time $18,036; part-time $6012 per semester. *Required fees:* $290; $210 per credit. $105 per semester. Tuition and fees vary according to program. *Financial support:* In 2015–16, 12 students received support. Scholarships/grants available. Financial award application deadline: 3/1; financial award applicants required to submit FAFSA. *Unit head:* Dr. Janet Baker, Director, 440-864-8172, Fax: 440-684-6053, E-mail: jbaker@ursuline.edu. *Application contact:* Stephanie Pratt McRoberts, Graduate Admission Coordinator, 440-646-8119, Fax: 440-684-6138, E-mail: graduateadmissions@ursuline.edu.

Utah Valley University, Program in Nursing, Orem, UT 84058-5999. Offers MSN. *Accreditation:* ACEN. *Program availability:* Part-time, online learning. Terminal master's awarded for partial completion of doctoral program. *Degree requirements:* For master's, project or thesis. *Entrance requirements:* For master's, GRE, baccalaureate degree in nursing, nurse licensure, undergraduate course in statistics, minimum undergraduate GPA of 3.2 overall or in last 60 semester hours of coursework, 3 letters of recommendation. Additional exam requirements/recommendations for international students: Required—TOEFL (minimum score 83 iBT). *Application deadline:* For fall admission, 4/1 for domestic and international students. Application fee: $45 ($100 for international students). Electronic applications accepted. *Expenses:* Contact institution. *Financial support:* Application deadline: 5/1; applicants required to submit FAFSA. *Unit head:* Dale Maughan, Department Chair, 801-863-7411, E-mail: dale.maughan@uvu.edu. *Application contact:* Diane Evans, Administrative Assistant, 801-863-8199, E-mail: dianee@uvu.edu.
Website: http://www.uvu.edu/nursing/

Valparaiso University, Graduate School, College of Nursing and Health Professions, Valparaiso, IN 46383. Offers nursing (DNP); nursing education (MSN, Certificate); public health (MPH); MSN/MHA. *Accreditation:* AACN. *Program availability:* Part-time, evening/weekend, online learning. *Faculty:* 13 part-time/adjunct (all women). *Students:* 52 full-time (43 women), 33 part-time (30 women); includes 9 minority (4 Black or African American, non-Hispanic/Latino; 1 Asian, non-Hispanic/Latino; 4 Hispanic/Latino), 22 international. Average age 33. In 2015, 9 master's, 16 doctorates awarded. *Entrance requirements:* For master's, minimum GPA of 3.0, undergraduate major in nursing, Indiana registered nursing license, undergraduate courses in research and statistics. Additional exam requirements/recommendations for international students: Required—TOEFL (minimum score 550 paper-based; 80 iBT), IELTS (minimum score 6). *Application deadline:* Applications are processed on a rolling basis. Application fee: $30 ($50 for international students). Electronic applications accepted. *Expenses:* Contact institution. *Financial support:* Available to part-time students. Applicants required to submit FAFSA. *Unit head:* Dr. Janet Brown, Dean, 219-464-5289, Fax: 219-464-5425, E-mail: janet.brown@valpo.edu. *Application contact:* Jessica Choquette, Graduate Admissions Specialist, 219-464-6510, Fax: 219-464-5381, E-mail: jessica.choquette@valpo.edu.
Website: http://www.valpo.edu/nursing/

Vanderbilt University, Program in Nursing Science, Nashville, TN 37240-1001. Offers PhD. *Faculty:* 20 full-time (16 women), 1 part-time/adjunct (0 women). *Students:* 26 full-time (20 women), 5 part-time (4 women); includes 3 minority (1 Black or African American, non-Hispanic/Latino; 1 Hispanic/Latino; 1 Native Hawaiian or other Pacific Islander, non-Hispanic/Latino). Average age 39. 39 applicants, 18% accepted, 6 enrolled. In 2015, 3 doctorates awarded. *Degree requirements:* For doctorate, comprehensive exam, thesis/dissertation, final and qualifying exams. *Entrance requirements:* For doctorate, GRE General Test. Additional exam requirements/recommendations for international students: Required—TOEFL (minimum score 570 paper-based; 88 iBT). *Application deadline:* For fall admission, 1/15 for domestic and international students. Electronic applications accepted. *Financial support:* Fellowships with full tuition reimbursements, research assistantships with full tuition reimbursements, teaching assistantships with full tuition reimbursements, career-related internships or fieldwork, Federal Work-Study, institutionally sponsored loans, scholarships/grants, health care benefits, and tuition waivers (full and partial) available. Financial award application deadline: 1/15; financial award applicants required to submit CSS PROFILE or FAFSA. *Faculty research:* Adaptation to chronic illness/conditions, health problems related to stress and coping, vulnerable childbearing and child rearing families. *Unit head:* Sheila Ridner, Director of Graduate Studies, 615-322-3800, Fax: 615-343-5898, E-mail: sheila.ridner@vanderbilt.edu. *Application contact:* Irene McKirgan, Administrative Manager, 615-322-7410, E-mail: irene.mckirgan@vanderbilt.edu.
Website: http://www.nursing.vanderbilt.edu/

Vanderbilt University, Vanderbilt University School of Nursing, Nashville, TN 37240. Offers adult-gerontology acute care nurse practitioner (MSN), including hospitalist, intensivist; adult-gerontology primary care nurse practitioner (MSN); emergency nurse practitioner (MSN); family nurse practitioner (MSN); healthcare leadership (MSN); neonatal nurse practitioner (MSN); nurse midwifery (MSN); nurse midwifery/family nurse practitioner (MSN); nursing (Post-Master's Certificate); nursing informatics (MSN); nursing practice (DNP); nursing science (PhD); pediatric acute care nurse practitioner (MSN); pediatric primary care nurse practitioner (MSN); psychiatric-mental health nurse practitioner (MSN); women's health nurse practitioner (MSN); women's health nurse practitioner/adult gerontology primary care nurse practitioner (MSN); MSN/M Div; MSN/MTS. *Accreditation:* ACEN (one or more programs are accredited); ACNM/ACME. *Program availability:* Part-time, 100% online, blended/hybrid learning. *Faculty:* 258 full-time (232 women), 363 part-time/adjunct (271 women). *Students:* 478 full-time (424 women), 342 part-time (317 women); includes 140 minority (36 Black or African American, non-Hispanic/Latino; 3 American Indian or Alaska Native, non-Hispanic/Latino; 24 Asian, non-Hispanic/Latino; 43 Hispanic/Latino; 3 Native Hawaiian or other Pacific Islander, non-Hispanic/Latino; 31 Two or more races, non-Hispanic/Latino), 11 international. Average age 31. 1,268 applicants, 49% accepted, 477 enrolled. In 2015, 343 master's, 55 doctorates awarded. *Degree requirements:* For master's, comprehensive exam, thesis/dissertation. *Entrance requirements:* For master's, GRE General Test (taken within the past 5 years), minimum B average in undergraduate course work, 3 letters of recommendation; for doctorate, GRE General Test, interview, 3 letters of recommendation from doctorally-prepared faculty, MSN, essay. Additional exam requirements/recommendations for international students: Required—TOEFL (minimum score 570 paper-based), IELTS (minimum score 6.5). *Application deadline:* For fall admission, 11/1 priority date for domestic and international students. Applications are processed on a rolling basis. Application fee: $50. Electronic applications accepted. *Expenses:* Contact institution. *Financial support:* In 2015–16, 585 students received support. Scholarships/grants available. Financial award application deadline: 3/15; financial award applicants required to submit FAFSA. *Faculty research:* Lymphedema, palliative care and bereavement, health services research including workforce, safety and quality of care, gerontology, better birth outcomes including nutrition. *Total annual research expenditures:* $2 million. *Unit head:* Dr. Linda Norman, Dean, 615-343-8876, Fax: 615-343-7711, E-mail: linda.norman@vanderbilt.edu. *Application contact:* Patricia Peerman, Assistant Dean for Enrollment Management, 615-322-3800, Fax: 615-343-0333, E-mail: vusn-admissions@vanderbilt.edu.
Website: http://www.nursing.vanderbilt.edu

Vanguard University of Southern California, Graduate Program in Nursing, Costa Mesa, CA 92626-9601. Offers MS. *Program availability:* Part-time, evening/weekend. *Degree requirements:* For master's, thesis, two 55-hour practicums. *Entrance requirements:* For master's, free and clear RN license in California. *Expenses:* Contact institution.

Villanova University, College of Nursing, Villanova, PA 19085-1699. Offers adult nurse practitioner (MSN, Post Master's Certificate); family nurse practitioner (MSN, Post Master's Certificate); nurse anesthetist (MSN, Post Master's Certificate); nursing (PhD); nursing education (MSN, Post Master's Certificate); nursing practice (DNP); pediatric nurse practitioner (MSN, Post Master's Certificate). *Accreditation:* AACN; AANA/CANAEP. *Program availability:* Part-time, online learning. *Faculty:* 16 full-time (15 women), 9 part-time/adjunct (7 women). *Students:* 219 full-time (198 women), 108 part-time (96 women); includes 36 minority (25 Black or African American, non-Hispanic/Latino; 9 Asian, non-Hispanic/Latino; 2 Hispanic/Latino), 16 international. Average age 31. 147 applicants, 78% accepted, 106 enrolled. In 2015, 64 master's, 8 doctorates, 9 other advanced degrees awarded. *Degree requirements:* For master's, independent study project; for doctorate, comprehensive exam, thesis/dissertation; for Post Master's Certificate, scholarly project. *Entrance requirements:* For master's, GRE or MAT, BSN, 1 year of recent nursing experience, physical assessment, course work in statistics; for doctorate, GRE, MSN. Additional exam requirements/recommendations for international students: Required—TOEFL (minimum score 540 paper-based; 83 iBT), IELTS (minimum score 6.5). *Application deadline:* For fall admission, 7/1 priority date for domestic students, 7/1 for international students; for spring admission, 11/1 priority date for domestic students, 11/1 for international students; for summer admission, 4/1 priority date for domestic students, 3/1 for international students. Applications are processed on a rolling basis. Application fee: $50. Electronic applications accepted. *Expenses:* $837 per credit (MSN); $1,049 per credit (PhD); $1,375 per credit (DNP). *Financial support:* In 2015–16, 22 students received support, including 5 teaching assistantships with full tuition reimbursements available (averaging $15,475 per year); institutionally sponsored

Nursing—General

loans, scholarships/grants, traineeships, tuition waivers (full), and unspecified assistantships also available. Financial award application deadline: 7/1; financial award applicants required to submit FAFSA. *Faculty research:* Genetics, ethics, cognitive development of students, women with disabilities, nursing leadership. *Unit head:* Dr. Marguerite K. Schlag, Assistant Dean/Director, Graduate Programs, 610-519-4907, Fax: 610-519-7650, E-mail: marguerite.schlag@villanova.edu. *Application contact:* Rebecca Harold, Administrative Assistant, 610-519-4934, Fax: 610-519-7650, E-mail: rebecca.harold@villanova.edu.
Website: http://www.nursing.villanova.edu/

Virginia Commonwealth University, Graduate School, School of Nursing, Richmond, VA 23284-9005. Offers adult health acute nursing (MS); adult health primary nursing (MS); biobehavioral clinical research (PhD); child health nursing (MS); clinical nurse leader (MS); family health nursing (MS); nurse educator (MS); nurse practitioner (MS); nursing (Certificate); nursing administration (MS), including clinical nurse manager; psychiatric-mental health nursing (MS); quality and safety in health care (DNP); women's health nursing (MS). *Accreditation:* ACEN (one or more programs are accredited). *Program availability:* Part-time, evening/weekend, online learning. *Degree requirements:* For master's, thesis optional; for doctorate, thesis/dissertation. *Entrance requirements:* For master's, GRE General Test, GRE General Test, minimum GPA of 2.8; for doctorate, GRE General Test. Additional exam requirements/recommendations for international students: Required—TOEFL (minimum score 600 paper-based; 100 iBT). Electronic applications accepted.

Viterbo University, Graduate Program in Nursing, La Crosse, WI 54601-4797. Offers DNP. *Accreditation:* AACN. *Program availability:* Part-time. *Faculty:* 4 full-time (all women), 15 part-time/adjunct (14 women). *Students:* 26 full-time (23 women), 24 part-time (all women); includes 6 minority (3 Black or African American, non-Hispanic/Latino; 1 American Indian or Alaska Native, non-Hispanic/Latino; 1 Asian, non-Hispanic/Latino; 1 Hispanic/Latino). Average age 35. 25 applicants, 96% accepted, 19 enrolled. *Degree requirements:* For doctorate, project. *Entrance requirements:* For doctorate, GRE General Test or MAT, bachelor's degree in nursing, minimum GPA of 3.0, RN license, one year of practice as an RN prior to beginning classes. *Application deadline:* For spring admission, 1/15 priority date for domestic students. Applications are processed on a rolling basis. Application fee: $0. Electronic applications accepted. *Expenses:* Contact institution. *Financial support:* In 2015–16, 7 students received support. Institutionally sponsored loans, scholarships/grants, and tuition remission available. Financial award application deadline: 3/1; financial award applicants required to submit FAFSA. *Faculty research:* Mild cognitive impairment, education pedagogy. *Unit head:* Dr. Mary E. Stolder, Graduate Nursing Program Director, 608-796-3625, Fax: 608-796-3668, E-mail: mestolder@viterbo.edu. *Application contact:* Bobbi Hundt, Graduate Nursing Program Administrative Assistant, 608-796-3671, Fax: 608-796-3668, E-mail: bmhundt@viterbo.edu.
Website: http://www.viterbo.edu/gradnursing

Walden University, Graduate Programs, School of Nursing, Minneapolis, MN 55401. Offers adult-gerontology acute care nurse practitioner (MSN); adult-gerontology nurse practitioner (MSN); education (MSN); family nurse practitioner (MSN); informatics (MSN); leadership and management (MSN); nursing (PhD, Post-Master's Certificate), including education (PhD), healthcare administration (PhD), interdisciplinary health (PhD), leadership (PhD), nursing education (Post-Master's Certificate), nursing informatics (Post-Master's Certificate), nursing leadership and management (Post-Master's Certificate), public health policy (PhD); nursing practice (DNP); psychiatric mental health (MSN). *Accreditation:* AACN. *Program availability:* Part-time, evening/weekend, online only, 100% online. *Faculty:* 22 full-time (18 women), 540 part-time/adjunct (487 women). *Students:* 4,320 full-time (3,773 women), 5,250 part-time (4,740 women); includes 3,550 minority (2,360 Black or African American, non-Hispanic/Latino; 29 American Indian or Alaska Native, non-Hispanic/Latino; 523 Asian, non-Hispanic/Latino; 421 Hispanic/Latino; 25 Native Hawaiian or other Pacific Islander, non-Hispanic/Latino; 192 Two or more races, non-Hispanic/Latino), 221 international. Average age 40. 2,057 applicants, 100% accepted, 1507 enrolled. In 2015, 3,022 master's, 86 doctorates, 34 other advanced degrees awarded. *Degree requirements:* For doctorate, thesis/dissertation (for some programs), residency (for some programs), field experience (for some programs). *Entrance requirements:* For master's, bachelor's degree or equivalent in related field or RN; minimum GPA of 2.5; official transcripts; goal statement (for some programs); access to computer and Internet; for doctorate, master's degree or higher; RN; three years of related professional or academic experience; goal statement; access to computer and Internet; for Post-Master's Certificate, relevant work experience; access to computer and Internet. Additional exam requirements/recommendations for international students: Required—TOEFL (minimum score 550 paper-based, 79 iBT), IELTS (minimum score 6.5), Michigan English Language Assessment Battery (minimum score 82), or PTE (minimum score 53). *Application deadline:* Applications are processed on a rolling basis. Application fee: $0. Electronic applications accepted. *Financial support:* Fellowships, Federal Work-Study, scholarships/grants, unspecified assistantships and family tuition reduction, active duty/veteran tuition reduction, group tuition reduction, interest-free payment plans, employee tuition reduction available. Support available to part-time students. Financial award applicants required to submit FAFSA. *Unit head:* Dr. Andrea Lindell, Dean, 866-492-5336. *Application contact:* Meghan Thomas, Vice President of Enrollment Management, 866-492-5336, E-mail: info@waldenu.edu.
Website: http://www.waldenu.edu/programs/colleges-schools/nursing

Walsh University, Graduate Studies, Gary and Linda Byers School of Nursing, North Canton, OH 44720-3396. Offers academic nurse educator (MSN); clinical nurse leader (MSN); nursing practice (DNP). *Program availability:* Part-time, evening/weekend, online only, 100% online. *Faculty:* 6 full-time (all women), 6 part-time/adjunct (4 women). *Students:* 25 full-time (20 women), 38 part-time (34 women); includes 2 minority (1 Black or African American, non-Hispanic/Latino; 1 Hispanic/Latino). Average age 36. 45 applicants, 71% accepted, 22 enrolled. In 2015, 9 master's, 5 doctorates awarded. *Degree requirements:* For doctorate, scholarly project; residency practicum. *Entrance requirements:* For master's, undergraduate nursing degree, current unencumbered RN license, completion of an undergraduate or graduate statistics course, essay, interview, recommendations; for doctorate, BSN; master's degree; statistics and research courses; essay; interview. Additional exam requirements/recommendations for international students: Required—TOEFL. *Application deadline:* Applications are processed on a rolling basis. Application fee: $25. Electronic applications accepted. *Expenses: Tuition, area resident:* Full-time $11,610; part-time $7740 per credit hour. Full-time tuition and fees vary according to program. *Financial support:* In 2015–16, 1 student received support, including 1 research assistantship (averaging $3,870 per year). Financial award application deadline: 12/31; financial award applicants required to submit FAFSA. *Faculty research:* Faith community nursing, gerontology, women's health, global nursing education, nursing assessment, grief and reconstitution, health needs of psychiatric patients, psychometric testing, nursing education, clinical reasoning. *Unit head:* Dr. Maris Pappas-Rogich, Director of Graduate Nursing Programs, 330-490-7283, Fax: 330-490-7371, E-mail: mpappas@walsh.edu. *Application contact:* Audra Dice, Graduate and Transfer Admissions Counselor, 330-490-7181, Fax: 330-244-4680, E-mail: adice@walsh.edu.
Website: http://www.walsh.edu/master-of-science-in-nursing

Washburn University, School of Nursing, Topeka, KS 66621. Offers clinical nurse leader (MSN); nursing (DNP); psychiatric mental health nurse practitioner (Post-Graduate Certificate). *Accreditation:* AACN. *Program availability:* Part-time. *Students:* 17 full-time (15 women), 110 part-time (96 women). Average age 37. In 2015, 43 master's, 1 doctoral, 11 other advanced degrees awarded. *Entrance requirements:* Additional exam requirements/recommendations for international students: Required—TOEFL (minimum score 550 paper-based). *Application deadline:* For fall admission, 3/15 for domestic and international students. Application fee: $40. *Expenses:* Tuition, state resident: full-time $6426; part-time $357 per credit hour. Tuition, nonresident: full-time $13,086; part-time $727 per credit hour. *Required fees:* $110; $55 per semester. Tuition and fees vary according to degree level and program. *Financial support:* Application deadline: 2/15; applicants required to submit FAFSA. *Unit head:* Dr. Monica S. Scheibmeir, Dean, 785-670-1526, E-mail: monica.scheibmeir@washburn.edu. *Application contact:* Mary V. Allen, Director of Student Services, 785-670-1533, E-mail: mary.allen@washburn.edu.
Website: http://www.washburn.edu/sonu

Washington Adventist University, Program in Nursing - Business Leadership, Takoma Park, MD 20912. Offers MSN. *Program availability:* Part-time. *Entrance requirements:* Additional exam requirements/recommendations for international students: Required—TOEFL (minimum score 550 paper-based), IELTS (minimum score 5).

Washington State University, College of Nursing, Spokane, WA 99210. Offers advanced population health (MN, DNP); family nurse practitioner (MN, DNP); nursing (PhD); psychiatric/mental health nurse practitioner (DNP); psychiatric/mental health practitioner (MN). Programs offered at the Spokane, Tri-Cities, and Vancouver campuses. *Accreditation:* AACN. *Degree requirements:* For master's, comprehensive exam (for some programs), thesis (for some programs), oral exam, research project. *Entrance requirements:* For master's, minimum GPA of 3.0, Washington state RN license, physical assessment skills, course work in statistics, recommendations, written interview (for nurse practitioner). *Faculty research:* Cardiovascular and Type 2 diabetes in children, evaluation of strategies to increase physical activity in sedentary people.

Waynesburg University, Graduate and Professional Studies, Canonsburg, PA 15370. Offers business (MBA), including energy management, finance, health systems, human resources, leadership, market development; counseling (MA), including addictions counseling, clinical mental health; counselor education and supervision (PhD); criminal investigation (MA); education (M Ed), including autism, curriculum and instruction, educational leadership, online teaching; nursing (MSN), including administration, education, informatics; nursing practice (DNP); special education (M Ed); technology (M Ed); MSN/MBA. *Accreditation:* AACN. *Program availability:* Part-time, evening/weekend. *Degree requirements:* For doctorate, thesis/dissertation. *Entrance requirements:* Additional exam requirements/recommendations for international students: Required—TOEFL. Electronic applications accepted.

Wayne State University, College of Nursing, Doctor Program of Nursing Practice, Detroit, MI 48202. Offers adult gerontology nurse practitioner - acute care (DNP); adult gerontology nurse practitioner - primary care (DNP); family nurse practitioner (DNP); infant mental health (DNP); neonatal nurse practitioner (DNP); nurse midwifery (DNP); nursing practice (DNP); pediatric nurse practitioner - acute care (DNP); pediatric nurse practitioner - primary care (DNP); psychiatric mental health nurse practitioner (DNP). *Students:* 56 full-time (50 women), 37 part-time (32 women); includes 32 minority (19 Black or African American, non-Hispanic/Latino; 6 Asian, non-Hispanic/Latino; 3 Hispanic/Latino; 4 Two or more races, non-Hispanic/Latino), 6 international. Average age 35. 44 applicants, 66% accepted, 18 enrolled. In 2015, 16 doctorates awarded. *Entrance requirements:* For doctorate, official transcripts, two professional references, curriculum vitae or resume, statement of goals, BSN or MSN, current Michigan RN license, criminal background check, interview, on-site writing example. Additional exam requirements/recommendations for international students: Required—TOEFL (minimum score 600 paper-based; 101 iBT); Recommended—IELTS (minimum score 7). *Application deadline:* For fall admission, 1/31 for domestic and international students. Electronic applications accepted. *Expenses:* $19,325 per year resident tuition, $35,114 non-resident tuition; $805.20 per credit hour resident tuition, $1,463.10 per credit hour non-resident tuition; fees include $47.45 per credit hour student services fee and $274.60 per semester registration fee. *Financial support:* In 2015–16, 22 students received support. Fellowships, research assistantships, teaching assistantships, institutionally sponsored loans, and scholarships/grants available. Financial award applicants required to submit FAFSA. *Unit head:* Dr. Laurie Lauzon Clabo, Dean and Professor, 313-577-4104, E-mail: laurie.lauzon.clabo@wayne.edu. *Application contact:* Dr. Nancy George, Director of DNP Program, 313-577-8300.
Website: http://nursing.wayne.edu/dnp/index.php

Wayne State University, College of Nursing, Program in Nursing, Detroit, MI 48202. Offers PhD. *Program availability:* Part-time. *Students:* 21 full-time (all women), 4 part-time (3 women); includes 6 minority (4 Black or African American, non-Hispanic/Latino; 1 Asian, non-Hispanic/Latino; 1 Two or more races, non-Hispanic/Latino), 6 international. Average age 40. 24 applicants, 33% accepted, 5 enrolled. In 2015, 4 doctorates awarded. *Degree requirements:* For doctorate, thesis/dissertation. *Entrance requirements:* For doctorate, minimum GPA of 3.3, bachelor's or master's degree in nursing from NLN- or CCNE-accredited program, current RN license, interview, goals statement, curriculum vitae, reference letters from three doctorally-prepared individuals. Additional exam requirements/recommendations for international students: Required—TOEFL (minimum score 550 paper-based; 79 iBT); Recommended—TWE. *Application deadline:* For fall admission, 1/31 for domestic and international students. Electronic applications accepted. *Expenses:* $19,325 annual resident tuition, $35,114 non-resident tuition; $805.20 per credit hour resident tuition, $1,463.10 per credit hour non-resident tuition; fees include $47.45 per credit hour student services fee and $274.60 per semester registration fee. *Financial support:* In 2015–16, 12 students received support. Fellowships with tuition reimbursements available, research assistantships with tuition reimbursements available, teaching assistantships with tuition reimbursements available, scholarships/grants, and unspecified assistantships available. Support available to part-time students. Financial award applicants required to submit FAFSA. *Unit head:* Dr. Laurie Lauzon Clabo, Dean, 313-577-4104, Fax: 313-577-4104, E-mail: laurie.lauzon.clabo@wayne.edu. *Application contact:* Dr. April Hazard Vallerand, Interim Director, PhD Program, 313-577-0359, E-mail: april.vallerand@wayne.edu.
Website: http://nursing.wayne.edu/phd/index.php

Weber State University, College of Health Professions, School of Nursing, Ogden, UT 84408-1001. Offers MSN. *Faculty:* 4 full-time (all women), 2 part-time/adjunct (both women). *Students:* 45 full-time (37 women), 3 part-time (1 woman); includes 10 minority (all Asian, non-Hispanic/Latino). Average age 35. In 2015, 27 master's awarded. *Application deadline:* For fall admission, 4/1 priority date for domestic students. Application fee: $60 ($90 for international students). Electronic applications accepted. *Expenses:* Tuition, state resident: full-time $6520; part-time $1252 per credit hour. Tuition, nonresident: full-time $15,003; part-time $2998 per credit hour. *Required fees:* $380; $180 per credit hour. $8.50 per term. Tuition and fees vary according to course level and program. *Financial support:* Scholarships/grants available. Financial award application deadline: 4/1; financial award applicants required to submit FAFSA. *Unit* *head:* Dr. Melissa Neville, MSN Program Director, 801-626-6204, Fax: 801-626-6397, E-mail: mneville@weber.edu. *Application contact:* Robert Holt, Director of Enrollment, 801-626-7774, Fax: 801-626-6397, E-mail: rholt@weber.edu. Website: http://www.weber.edu/nursing

Webster University, College of Arts and Sciences, Department of Nursing, St. Louis, MO 63119-3194. Offers nurse educator (MSN); nurse leader (MSN). *Accreditation:* ACEN. *Degree requirements:* For master's, comprehensive exam. *Entrance requirements:* For master's, 1 year of clinical experience, BSN, interview, minimum C+ average in statistics and physical assessment, minimum GPA of 3.0, RN license. Additional exam requirements/recommendations for international students: Required—TOEFL. *Expenses: Tuition, area resident:* Full-time $20,550; part-time $685 per credit hour. Tuition and fees vary according to campus/location and program. *Faculty research:* Health teaching.

Wesley College, Nursing Program, Dover, DE 19901-3875. Offers MSN. *Accreditation:* ACEN. *Program availability:* Part-time, evening/weekend. *Degree requirements:* For master's, thesis optional, portfolio. *Entrance requirements:* For master's, GRE or MAT. Electronic applications accepted. *Faculty research:* Childhood obesity, organizational behavior, health promotion and wellness.

West Chester University of Pennsylvania, College of Health Sciences, Department of Nursing, West Chester, PA 19383. Offers adult-gerontology clinical nurse specialist (MSN); nursing (DNP); nursing education (MSN); school nurse (Certificate). *Accreditation:* AACN. *Program availability:* Part-time, evening/weekend, blended/hybrid learning. *Faculty:* 7 full-time (6 women), 1 (woman) part-time/adjunct. *Students:* 2 full-time (1 woman), 85 part-time (78 women); includes 10 minority (7 Black or African American, non-Hispanic/Latino; 3 Asian, non-Hispanic/Latino). Average age 45. 30 applicants, 90% accepted, 20 enrolled. In 2015, 10 master's, 3 other advanced degrees awarded. *Entrance requirements:* For master's, goals statement; official academic transcript(s) from all colleges and universities attended demonstrating minimum cumulative undergraduate GPA of 2.8 with successful completion of BSN and courses in statistics and physical assessment; documentation of current clinical experience; for doctorate, master's degree in nursing in an advanced nursing specialty from nationally-accredited program; minimum master's GPA of 3.0; licensed Registered Nurse. Additional exam requirements/recommendations for international students: Required—TOEFL or IELTS. *Application deadline:* For fall admission, 5/15 for international students; for spring admission, 10/15 for international students. Applications are processed on a rolling basis. Application fee: $50. Electronic applications accepted. *Expenses:* Tuition, state resident: full-time $8460; part-time $470 per credit. Tuition, nonresident: full-time $12,690; part-time $705 per credit. *Required fees:* $2312; $126.75 per credit. Tuition and fees vary according to campus/location and program. *Financial support:* Scholarships/grants and unspecified assistantships available. Financial award application deadline: 2/15; financial award applicants required to submit FAFSA. *Unit head:* Dr. Charlotte Mackey, Chair, 610-436-3474, Fax: 610-436-3083, E-mail: cmackey@wcupa.edu. *Application contact:* Dr. Cheryl Schlamb, Graduate Coordinator, 610-436-2219, E-mail: cschlamb@wcupa.edu. Website: http://www.wcupa.edu/_ACADEMICS/HealthSciences/nursing/

West Coast University, Graduate Programs, North Hollywood, CA 91606. Offers advanced generalist (MSN); family nurse practitioner (MSN); health administration (MHA); occupational therapy (MS); pharmacy (Pharm D); physical therapy (DPT).

Western Carolina University, Graduate School, College of Health and Human Sciences, School of Nursing, Cullowhee, NC 28723. Offers MS, DNP, Post-Master's Certificate, Postbaccalaureate Certificate. *Accreditation:* AACN; AANA/CANAEP. *Program availability:* Part-time, evening/weekend. *Degree requirements:* For master's, comprehensive exam, thesis or alternative. *Entrance requirements:* For master's, GRE General Test, BSN with minimum GPA of 3.0, 3 references, 1 year of clinical experience. Additional exam requirements/recommendations for international students: Required—TOEFL (minimum score 550 paper-based; 79 iBT). *Application deadline:* For fall admission, 2/15 for domestic students; for spring admission, 6/15 for domestic students. Applications are processed on a rolling basis. Application fee: $50. *Financial support:* Fellowships, research assistantships with tuition reimbursements, teaching assistantships with tuition reimbursements, career-related internships or fieldwork, institutionally sponsored loans, scholarships/grants, and unspecified assistantships available. Financial award application deadline: 3/31; financial award applicants required to submit FAFSA.

Western Connecticut State University, Division of Graduate Studies, School of Professional Studies, Nursing Department, Danbury, CT 06810-6885. Offers adult gerontology clinical nurse specialist (MSN); adult gerontology nurse practitioner (MSN); nursing education (Ed D). *Accreditation:* AACN. *Program availability:* Part-time. *Degree requirements:* For master's, clinical component, thesis or research project, completion of program in 6 years. *Entrance requirements:* For master's, MAT (if GPA less than 3.0), bachelor's degree in nursing, minimum GPA of 3.0, previous course work in statistics and nursing research, RN license. Additional exam requirements/recommendations for international students: Recommended—TOEFL (minimum score 550 paper-based; 79 iBT), IELTS (minimum score 6). *Expenses:* Contact institution. *Faculty research:* Evaluating effectiveness of Reiki and acupressure on stress reduction.

Western Kentucky University, Graduate Studies, College of Health and Human Services, School of Nursing, Bowling Green, KY 42101. Offers MSN. *Accreditation:* AACN. *Program availability:* Part-time, evening/weekend. *Degree requirements:* For master's, comprehensive exam, thesis optional. *Entrance requirements:* For master's, GRE General Test, minimum GPA of 2.75. Additional exam requirements/recommendations for international students: Required—TOEFL (minimum score 555 paper-based; 79 iBT). *Faculty research:* Folic acid, disease and injury prevention, rural mobile health, mental health issues.

Western Michigan University, Graduate College, College of Health and Human Services, Bronson School of Nursing, Kalamazoo, MI 49008. Offers MSN. *Accreditation:* AACN.

Western University of Health Sciences, College of Graduate Nursing, Doctor of Nursing Practice Program, Pomona, CA 91766-1854. Offers DNP. *Program availability:* Part-time, blended/hybrid learning. *Faculty:* 3 full-time (2 women), 6 part-time/adjunct (4 women). *Students:* 33 full-time (30 women), 12 part-time (10 women); includes 20 minority (1 Black or African American, non-Hispanic/Latino; 15 Asian, non-Hispanic/Latino; 2 Hispanic/Latino; 2 Two or more races, non-Hispanic/Latino). Average age 47. 26 applicants, 69% accepted, 14 enrolled. In 2015, 23 doctorates awarded. *Degree requirements:* For doctorate, thesis/dissertation, dissertation project. *Entrance requirements:* For doctorate, MSN from a National League of Nursing (NLN) or Commission on Collegiate Nursing Education (CCNE) accredited program. Additional exam requirements/recommendations for international students: Required—TOEFL (minimum score 80 iBT). *Application deadline:* For fall admission, 3/1 for domestic and international students. Application fee: $60. Electronic applications accepted. *Expenses:* $18,798 per unit tuition; $1,836 clinical fees; $40 student body fee. *Financial support:* Fellowships, research assistantships, and scholarships/grants available. Support available to part-time students. Financial award application deadline: 3/2; financial award applicants required to submit FAFSA. *Unit head:* Dr. Karen J. Hanford, Dean,

909-469-5523, Fax: 909-469-5521, E-mail: khanford@westernu.edu. *Application contact:* Kathryn Ford, Director of Admissions/International Student Advisor, 909-469-5335, Fax: 909-469-5570, E-mail: admissions@westernu.edu. Website: http://www.westernu.edu/nursing-dnp

Western University of Health Sciences, College of Graduate Nursing, Master of Science in Nursing Program, Pomona, CA 91766-1854. Offers administrative nurse leader (MSN); ambulatory care (MSN); clinical nurse leader (MSN); family nurse practitioner (MSN); nursing (MSN). *Program availability:* Blended/hybrid learning. *Faculty:* 15 full-time (all women), 13 part-time/adjunct (7 women). *Students:* 243 full-time (206 women), 13 part-time (10 women); includes 155 minority (6 Black or African American, non-Hispanic/Latino; 76 Asian, non-Hispanic/Latino; 54 Hispanic/Latino; 19 Two or more races, non-Hispanic/Latino, 1 international. Average age 30. 467 applicants, 36% accepted, 93 enrolled. In 2015, 97 master's awarded. *Degree requirements:* For master's, comprehensive exam (for some programs), thesis (for some programs), project. *Entrance requirements:* For master's, personal statement, BSN, minimum GPA of 3.0, 3 letters of recommendation, resume/curriculum vitae, official transcripts of all schools attended. Additional exam requirements/recommendations for international students: Required—TOEFL (minimum score 80 iBT). *Application deadline:* For fall admission, 11/1 for domestic and international students. Application fee: $60. Electronic applications accepted. *Expenses:* $1,026 per unit tuition; $1,836 clinical fees; $40 student body fee. *Financial support:* Fellowships, research assistantships, teaching assistantships, and scholarships/grants available. Support available to part-time students. Financial award application deadline: 3/2; financial award applicants required to submit FAFSA. *Unit head:* Dr. Karen J. Hanford, Dean, 909-469-5523, Fax: 909-469-5521, E-mail: khanford@westernu.edu. *Application contact:* Kathryn Ford, Director of Admissions/International Student Advisor, 909-469-5335, Fax: 909-469-5570, E-mail: admissions@westernu.edu.

Westminster College, School of Nursing and Health Sciences, Salt Lake City, UT 84105-3697. Offers family nurse practitioner (MSN); nurse anesthesia (MSNA); nurse education (MSNED); public health (MPH). *Accreditation:* AACN; AANA/CANAEP. *Faculty:* 15 full-time (9 women), 7 part-time/adjunct (2 women). *Students:* 120 full-time (79 women), 3 part-time (all women); includes 18 minority (1 Black or African American, non-Hispanic/Latino; 3 Asian, non-Hispanic/Latino; 10 Hispanic/Latino; 4 Two or more races, non-Hispanic/Latino), 3 international. Average age 32. 157 applicants, 40% accepted, 45 enrolled. In 2015, 56 master's awarded. *Degree requirements:* For master's, clinical practicum, 504 clinical practice hours. *Entrance requirements:* For master's, GRE, personal statement, resume, 3 professional recommendations, copy of unrestricted Utah license to practice professional nursing, background check, minimum cumulative GPA of 3.0, documentation of current immunizations, physical and mental health certificate signed by primary care provider. Additional exam requirements/ recommendations for international students: Required—TOEFL (minimum score 600 paper-based; 100 iBT), IELTS (minimum score 7.5). Application fee: $50. Electronic applications accepted. *Expenses:* Contact institution. *Financial support:* In 2015–16, 8 students received support. Career-related internships or fieldwork, unspecified assistantships, and tuition reimbursements, tuition remission available. Support available to part-time students. Financial award applicants required to submit FAFSA. *Faculty research:* Intellectual empathy, professional boundaries, learned optimism, collaborative testing in nursing: student outcomes and perspectives, implementing new educational paradigms into pre-licensure nursing curricula. *Unit head:* Dr. Sheryl Steadman, Dean, 801-832-2164, Fax: 801-832-3110, E-mail: ssteadman@westminstercollege.edu. *Application contact:* Dr. John Baworowsky, Vice President of Enrollment Management, 801-832-2200, Fax: 801-832-3101, E-mail: admission@westminstercollege.edu. Website: http://www.westminstercollege.edu/msn

West Texas A&M University, College of Nursing and Health Sciences, Department of Nursing, Canyon, TX 79016-0001. Offers family nurse practitioner (MSN); nursing (MSN). *Accreditation:* AACN. *Program availability:* Part-time, online learning. *Degree requirements:* For master's, comprehensive exam, thesis optional. *Entrance requirements:* For master's, GRE General Test, bachelor's degree in nursing, minimum GPA of 3.0 in last 60 hours. Additional exam requirements/recommendations for international students: Required—TOEFL (minimum score 550 paper-based). Electronic applications accepted. *Faculty research:* Family-focused nursing, nursing traineeship, professional nursing.

West Virginia University, School of Nursing, Morgantown, WV 26506-9600. Offers nurse practitioner (Certificate); nursing (MSN, DNP, PhD). *Accreditation:* AACN. *Program availability:* Part-time, online learning. *Faculty:* 20 full-time (all women), 9 part-time/adjunct (all women). *Students:* 53 full-time (48 women), 96 part-time (88 women); includes 9 minority (2 Black or African American, non-Hispanic/Latino; 1 Hispanic/Latino; 6 Two or more races, non-Hispanic/Latino). Average age 36. In 2015, 44 master's, 10 doctorates awarded. *Degree requirements:* For master's, thesis or alternative; for doctorate, comprehensive exam, thesis/dissertation. *Entrance requirements:* For master's, GRE General Test, minimum GPA of 3.0, current U.S. RN license, BSN, course work in statistics and physical assessment; for doctorate, GRE General Test (for PhD), minimum graduate GPA of 3.0, minimum grade of B in graduate statistics course work. Additional exam requirements/recommendations for international students: Required—TOEFL (minimum score 550 paper-based). *Application deadline:* For fall admission, 6/1 for domestic students. Application fee: $60. Electronic applications accepted. *Expenses:* Contact institution. *Financial support:* Teaching assistantships, Federal Work-Study, institutionally sponsored loans, health care benefits, tuition waivers (partial), and administrative assistantships available. Financial award application deadline: 2/1; financial award applicants required to submit FAFSA. *Faculty research:* Rural primary health/health promotion, parent/child/women's health, cardiovascular risk reduction, complementary health modalities, breast cancer detection-care. *Unit head:* Dr. Tara Hulsey, Dean, 304-293-6521, Fax: 304-293-6826, E-mail: tmhulsey@hsc.wvu.edu. *Application contact:* Brandy Sue Toothman, Program Assistant III, 304-293-4298, Fax: 304-293-2546, E-mail: btoothman@hsc.wvu.edu. Website: https://nursing.hsc.wvu.edu

West Virginia Wesleyan College, Department of Nursing, Buckhannon, WV 26201. Offers family nurse practitioner (Post Master's Certificate); family nurse practitoner (MS); nurse administrator (MS); nurse educator (MS); nurse-midwifery (MS); nursing administration (Post Master's Certificate); nursing education (Post Master's Certificate); psychiatric mental health nurse practitioner (MS); MSN/MBA. *Accreditation:* ACEN.

Wheeling Jesuit University, Department of Nursing, Wheeling, WV 26003-6295. Offers MSN. *Accreditation:* AACN. *Program availability:* Part-time, evening/weekend, online learning. *Degree requirements:* For master's, comprehensive exam (for some programs), thesis (for some programs). *Entrance requirements:* For master's, GRE General Test or MAT, BSN, minimum GPA of 3.0, course work in research and statistics, U.S. nursing license. Additional exam requirements/recommendations for international students: Required—TOEFL (minimum score 600 paper-based; 100 iBT). Electronic applications accepted. Application fee is waived when completed online. *Faculty research:* Obesity in women, underserved populations, spirituality.

Wichita State University, Graduate School, College of Health Professions, School of Nursing, Wichita, KS 67260. Offers nursing (MSN); nursing practice (DNP).

Accreditation: AACN. *Program availability:* Part-time, online learning. *Unit head:* Dr. Victoria Mosack, Chairperson, 316-978-3610, Fax: 316-978-3025, E-mail: victoria.mosack@wichita.edu. *Application contact:* Jordan Oleson, Admissions Coordinator, 316-978-3095, Fax: 316-978-3253, E-mail: jordan.oleson@wichita.edu. Website: http://www.wichita.edu/nursing

Widener University, School of Nursing, Chester, PA 19013. Offers MSN, DN Sc, PhD, PMC. *Accreditation:* AACN. *Program availability:* Part-time, evening/weekend. *Faculty:* 12 full-time (all women), 4 part-time/adjunct (3 women). *Students:* 43 full-time (42 women), 157 part-time (141 women); includes 65 minority (46 Black or African American, non-Hispanic/Latino; 13 Asian, non-Hispanic/Latino; 3 Hispanic/Latino; 3 Two or more races, non-Hispanic/Latino), 6 international. Average age 33. 64 applicants, 47% accepted, 25 enrolled. In 2015, 64 master's, 12 doctorates awarded. *Degree requirements:* For doctorate, thesis/dissertation. *Entrance requirements:* For master's, GRE General Test, BSN, undergraduate course in statistics; for doctorate, GRE General Test, MSN, undergraduate course in statistics. *Application deadline:* For fall admission, 7/1 for domestic students; for winter admission, 3/1 for domestic students; for spring admission, 11/1 for domestic students. Applications are processed on a rolling basis. Application fee: $25 ($300 for international students). Electronic applications accepted. *Expenses:* Contact institution. *Financial support:* Career-related internships or fieldwork, Federal Work-Study, and traineeships available. Support available to part-time students. Financial award application deadline: 4/1. *Faculty research:* Women's health leadership, nursing education, research utilization, program evaluation, health promotion. *Unit head:* Dr. Laura Dzurec, Dean, 610-499-4214, E-mail: lcdzurec@widener.edu.

Wilkes University, College of Graduate and Professional Studies, Passan School of Nursing, Wilkes-Barre, PA 18766-0002. Offers MSN, DNP. *Accreditation:* AACN. *Program availability:* Part-time, evening/weekend, 100% online. *Students:* 11 full-time (9 women), 545 part-time (494 women); includes 136 minority (81 Black or African American, non-Hispanic/Latino; 2 American Indian or Alaska Native, non-Hispanic/Latino; 13 Asian, non-Hispanic/Latino; 29 Hispanic/Latino; 5 Native Hawaiian or other Pacific Islander, non-Hispanic/Latino; 6 Two or more races, non-Hispanic/Latino). Average age 43. In 2015, 16 master's, 21 doctorates awarded. *Entrance requirements:* Additional exam requirements/recommendations for international students: Required—TOEFL (minimum score 550 paper-based; 79 iBT). *Application deadline:* Applications are processed on a rolling basis. Application fee: $45. Electronic applications accepted. *Financial support:* Unspecified assistantships available. Financial award application deadline: 3/1; financial award applicants required to submit FAFSA. *Unit head:* Dr. Deborah Zbegner, Dean, 570-408-4086, Fax: 570-408-7807, E-mail: deborah.zbegner@wilkes.edu. *Application contact:* Joanne Thomas, Director of Graduate Enrollment, 570-408-4234, Fax: 570-408-7846, E-mail: joanne.thomas1@wilkes.edu. Website: http://www.wilkes.edu/academics/colleges/school-of-nursing/index.aspx

William Carey University, School of Nursing, Hattiesburg, MS 39401-5499. Offers MSN. *Accreditation:* AACN. *Program availability:* Part-time. *Degree requirements:* For master's, thesis or alternative. *Entrance requirements:* For master's, GRE, minimum GPA of 3.0, RN license. Additional exam requirements/recommendations for international students: Required—TOEFL (minimum score 500 paper-based).

William Paterson University of New Jersey, College of Science and Health, Wayne, NJ 07470-8420. Offers biology (MS); biotechnology (MS); communication disorders (MS); exercise and sports studies (MS); nursing (MSN); nursing practice (DNP). *Program availability:* Part-time, evening/weekend. *Faculty:* 25 full-time (11 women), 13 part-time/adjunct (4 women). *Students:* 73 full-time (58 women), 208 part-time (183 women); includes 111 minority (18 Black or African American, non-Hispanic/Latino; 40 Asian, non-Hispanic/Latino; 50 Hispanic/Latino; 3 Two or more races, non-Hispanic/Latino), 5 international. Average age 34. 495 applicants, 27% accepted, 74 enrolled. In 2015, 63 master's, 10 doctorates awarded. *Degree requirements:* For master's, comprehensive exam (for some programs), thesis (for some programs), non-thesis internship/practicum (for some programs). *Entrance requirements:* For master's, GRE/MAT, minimum GPA of 3.0; 2 or 3 letters of recommendation; personal statement; work experience (for some programs); for doctorate, GRE/MAT, minimum GPA of 3.3; work experience; 3 letters of recommendation; interview; master's degree in nursing. Additional exam requirements/recommendations for international students: Required—TOEFL (minimum score 550 paper-based; 79 iBT), IELTS (minimum score 6). *Application deadline:* For fall admission, 6/1 for domestic students, 3/1 for international students; for spring admission, 11/1 for domestic students, 10/1 for international students. Applications are processed on a rolling basis. Application fee: $50. Electronic applications accepted. *Expenses:* Tuition, state resident: full-time $11,544; part-time $577.21 per credit. Tuition, nonresident: full-time $19,024; part-time $951.21 per credit. *Required fees:* $1916; $95.79 per credit. $62.50 per semester. Tuition and fees vary according to course load and degree level. *Financial support:* Research assistantships with full tuition reimbursements, career-related internships or fieldwork, Federal Work-Study, scholarships/grants, and unspecified assistantships available. Support available to part-time students. Financial award application deadline: 4/1; financial award applicants required to submit FAFSA. *Faculty research:* Human biomechanics, autism, nanomaterials, health and environment, neurophysiology and neurobiology. *Unit head:* Dr. Kenneth Wolf, Dean, 973-720-2194, Fax: 973-720-3414, E-mail: wolfk@wpunj.edu. *Application contact:* Christina Aiello, Assistant Director, Graduate Admissions, 973-720-2506, Fax: 973-720-2035, E-mail: aielloc@wpunj.edu. Website: http://www.wpunj.edu/cosh

Wilmington University, College of Health Professions, New Castle, DE 19720-6491. Offers adult nurse practitioner (MSN); family nurse practitioner (MSN); gerontology nurse practitioner (MSN); nursing (MSN); nursing leadership (MSN); nursing practice (DNP). *Accreditation:* AACN. *Program availability:* Part-time. *Degree requirements:* For master's, thesis. *Entrance requirements:* For master's, BSN, RN license, interview, 3 letters of recommendation. Additional exam requirements/recommendations for international students: Required—TOEFL (minimum score 500 paper-based). Electronic applications accepted. *Faculty research:* Outcomes assessment, student writing ability.

Wilson College, Graduate Programs, Chambersburg, PA 17201-1285. Offers accounting (M Acc); choreography and visual art (MFA); education (M Ed); healthcare management for sustainability (MHM); humanities (MA), including art and culture,

critical/cultural theory, English language and literature, women's studies; nursing (MSN), including nursing education, nursing leadership and management. *Program availability:* Evening/weekend. *Degree requirements:* For master's, project. *Entrance requirements:* For master's, PRAXIS, minimum undergraduate cumulative GPA of 3.0, 2 letters of recommendation, current certification for eligibility to teach in grades K-12, resume, personal interview. Electronic applications accepted.

Winona State University, College of Nursing and Health Sciences, Winona, MN 55987. Offers adult nurse practitioner (MS, Post Master's Certificate); clinical nurse specialist (MS, Post Master's Certificate); family nurse practitioner (MS, Post Master's Certificate); nurse administrator (MS); nurse educator (MS, Post Master's Certificate); nursing (DNP). *Accreditation:* AACN. *Program availability:* Part-time, online learning. *Degree requirements:* For master's, thesis; for doctorate, capstone. *Entrance requirements:* For master's, GRE (if GPA less than 3.0). Additional exam requirements/recommendations for international students: Required—TOEFL (minimum score 550 paper-based).

Winston-Salem State University, Program in Nursing, Winston-Salem, NC 27110-0003. Offers advanced nurse educator (MSN); family nurse practitioner (MSN); nursing (DNP). *Accreditation:* AACN. *Program availability:* Part-time, evening/weekend, online learning. *Entrance requirements:* For master's, GRE, MAT, resume, NC or state compact license, 3 letters of recommendation. Electronic applications accepted. *Faculty research:* Elimination of health care disparities.

Wright State University, School of Graduate Studies, College of Nursing and Health, Program in Nursing, Dayton, OH 45435. Offers acute care nurse practitioner (MS); administration of nursing and health care systems (MS); adult health (MS); child and adolescent health (MS); community health (MS); family nurse practitioner (MS); nurse practitioner (MS); school nurse (MS); MBA/MS. *Accreditation:* AACN. *Program availability:* Part-time, evening/weekend. *Degree requirements:* For master's, thesis or alternative. *Entrance requirements:* For master's, GRE General Test, BSN from NLN-accredited college, Ohio RN license. Additional exam requirements/recommendations for international students: Required—TOEFL. *Faculty research:* Clinical nursing and health, teaching, caring, pain administration, informatics and technology.

Xavier University, College of Social Sciences, Health and Education, School of Nursing, Cincinnati, OH 45207. Offers MSN, DNP, PMC, MSN/M Ed, MSN/MBA, MSN/MS. *Accreditation:* AACN. *Program availability:* Part-time, evening/weekend. *Degree requirements:* For master's, thesis, scholarly project; for doctorate, thesis/dissertation, scholarly project; for PMC, practicum. *Entrance requirements:* For master's, GRE, resume; statement of purpose and/or portfolio; RN licensure or bachelor's degree; official transcript; 3 references/recommendations; for doctorate, MSN from CCNE- or ACEN-accredited school or master's degree in other field (must have BSN from a CCNE-, ACEN-, or regionally-accredited institution); basic statistics course; one year of professional nursing work experience; RN licensure; official transcript; 1-3 page personal statement; published work or paper; resume; 3 professional references; for PMC, RN licensure; master's degree in nursing; licensed in state where participating in clinical experiences; official transcript. Additional exam requirements/recommendations for international students: Required—TOEFL (minimum score 550 paper-based; 79 iBT). Electronic applications accepted. Application fee is waived when completed online. *Expenses:* Contact institution. *Faculty research:* Clinical nurse leader, simulation, employment satisfaction, nontraditional students, holistic nursing.

Yale University, School of Nursing, West Haven, CT 06516. Offers MSN, DNP, PhD, Post Master's Certificate, MAR/MSN, MSN/M Div, MSN/MPH. *Accreditation:* AACN. *Program availability:* Part-time, online learning. Terminal master's awarded for partial completion of doctoral program. *Degree requirements:* For master's, thesis; for doctorate, comprehensive exam, thesis/dissertation. *Entrance requirements:* For master's, GRE General Test, bachelor's degree; for doctorate, GRE General Test, MSN; for Post Master's Certificate, MSN. Additional exam requirements/recommendations for international students: Required—TOEFL or IELTS. Electronic applications accepted. *Expenses:* Contact institution. *Faculty research:* Family-based care, chronic illness, primary care, development, policy.

York College of Pennsylvania, Department of Nursing, York, PA 17405-7199. Offers adult gerontology clinical nurse specialist (MS), including administration, education; adult gerontology nurse practitioner (MS); nurse anesthetist (MS); nurse educator (MS); nursing practice (DNP). *Accreditation:* AACN; AANA/CANAEP. *Program availability:* Part-time, evening/weekend. *Faculty:* 9 full-time (all women), 5 part-time/adjunct (2 women). *Students:* 36 full-time (26 women), 55 part-time (47 women); includes 14 minority (4 Black or African American, non-Hispanic/Latino; 2 American Indian or Alaska Native, non-Hispanic/Latino; 5 Asian, non-Hispanic/Latino; 2 Hispanic/Latino; 1 Two or more races, non-Hispanic/Latino), 1 international. Average age 33. 115 applicants, 28% accepted, 28 enrolled. In 2015, 24 master's, 4 doctorates awarded. *Entrance requirements:* For master's, GRE General Test (for nurse anesthetist program), minimum GPA of 3.0 from CCNE- or NLNAC-accredited institution; for doctorate, master's degree in nursing from a CCNE- or NLNAC-accredited institution; minimum GPA of 3.5. Additional exam requirements/recommendations for international students: Required—TOEFL (minimum score 530 paper-based; 72 iBT). *Application deadline:* Applications are processed on a rolling basis. Application fee: $0. Electronic applications accepted. *Expenses:* Tuition, area resident: Full-time $13,770. *Required fees:* $1750; $380. Tuition and fees vary according to degree level. *Financial support:* Federal Work-Study available. *Faculty research:* Student stress response to simulation versus clinical, evidence-based practice in all clinical settings. *Unit head:* Dr. Kimberly Fenstermacher, Graduate Program Director, 717-815-1383, E-mail: kfenster@ycp.edu. *Application contact:* Allison Malachosky, Administrative Assistant, 717-815-1243, E-mail: amalacho@ycp.edu. Website: http://www.ycp.edu/academics/academic-departments/nursing/

York University, Faculty of Graduate Studies, Faculty of Health, Program in Nursing, Toronto, ON M3J 1P3, Canada. Offers M Sc N.

Youngstown State University, Graduate School, Bitonte College of Health and Human Services, Department of Nursing, Youngstown, OH 44555-0001. Offers MSN. *Accreditation:* ACEN. *Program availability:* Part-time, evening/weekend. *Degree requirements:* For master's, thesis optional. *Entrance requirements:* For master's, GRE General Test, BSN, CPR certification. Additional exam requirements/recommendations for international students: Required—TOEFL.

Acute Care/Critical Care Nursing

Allen College, Graduate Programs, Waterloo, IA 50703. Offers acute care nurse practitioner (Post-Master's Certificate); adult nurse practitioner (Post-Master's Certificate); adult psychiatric-mental health nurse practitioner (Post-Master's Certificate);

adult-gerontology acute care nurse practitioner (MSN); community public health (Post-Master's Certificate); community/public health nursing (MSN); family nurse practitioner (MSN, Post-Master's Certificate); gerontological nurse practitioner (Post-Master's

Certificate); health sciences (Ed D); leadership in health care delivery (MSN, Post-Master's Certificate); nursing (DNP); occupational therapy (MS). *Accreditation:* AACN; ACEN. *Program availability:* Part-time, blended/hybrid learning. *Faculty:* 3 full-time (all women), 21 part-time/adjunct (20 women). *Students:* 61 full-time (54 women), 163 part-time (144 women); includes 9 minority (5 Black or African American, non-Hispanic/Latino; 2 Hispanic/Latino; 2 Two or more races, non-Hispanic/Latino), 2 international. Average age 34. 212 applicants, 60% accepted, 94 enrolled. In 2015, 51 master's, 1 doctorate awarded. *Degree requirements:* For master's, thesis optional. *Entrance requirements:* For master's, minimum GPA of 3.0 in the last 60 hours of undergraduate coursework; for doctorate, minimum GPA of 3.25 in graduate coursework. Additional exam requirements/recommendations for international students: Recommended—TOEFL (minimum score 580 paper-based; 92 iBT), IELTS (minimum score 6). *Application deadline:* For fall admission, 2/1 priority date for domestic students; for spring admission, 9/1 priority date for domestic students. Applications are processed on a rolling basis. Application fee: $50. Electronic applications accepted. *Expenses:* $15,940 tuition, $1,240 fees. *Financial support:* Institutionally sponsored loans, scholarships/grants, and traineeships available. Support available to part-time students. Financial award application deadline: 8/15; financial award applicants required to submit FAFSA. *Unit head:* Nancy Kramer, Vice Chancellor for Academic Affairs, 319-226-2040, Fax: 319-226-2070, E-mail: nancy.kramer@allencollege.edu. *Application contact:* Molly Quinn, Administrative Assistant for Student Services, 319-226-2014, Fax: 319-226-2010, E-mail: admissions@allencollege.edu.
Website: http://www.allencollege.edu/

Augusta University, The Graduate School, Doctor of Nursing Practice Program, Augusta, GA 30912. Offers adult gerontology acute care nurse practitioner (DNP); family nurse practitioner (DNP); nursing (DNP); nursing anesthesia (DNP); pediatric nurse practitioner (DNP); psychiatric mental health nurse practitioner (DNP). *Students:* 40 part-time. *Degree requirements:* For doctorate, thesis/dissertation or alternative. *Entrance requirements:* For doctorate, GRE General Test or MAT, master's degree in nursing or related field, current professional nurse licensure. Additional exam requirements/recommendations for international students: Required—TOEFL (minimum score 600 paper-based; 100 iBT). *Application deadline:* For fall admission, 3/1 for domestic and international students; for spring admission, 7/1 for domestic and international students. Applications are processed on a rolling basis. Application fee: $50. Electronic applications accepted. *Unit head:* Dr. Marguerite Murphy, RN, Director, 706-721-3676, Fax: 706-721-8169. *Application contact:* Karen Sturgill, Program Manager, 706-721-3676, Fax: 706-721-8169, E-mail: dnp@augusta.edu.
Website: http://www.augusta.edu/nursing/dnp_programs.php

Barry University, School of Adult and Continuing Education, Division of Nursing, Program in Nurse Practitioner, Miami Shores, FL 33161-6695. Offers acute care nurse practitioner (MSN); family nurse practitioner (MSN); nurse practitioner (Certificate). *Accreditation:* AACN. *Program availability:* Part-time, evening/weekend. *Degree requirements:* For master's, research project or thesis. *Entrance requirements:* For master's, GRE General Test or MAT, BSN, minimum GPA of 3.0, course work in statistics. Electronic applications accepted. *Faculty research:* Child abuse, health beliefs, teenage pregnancy, cultural and clinical studies across the lifespan.

Case Western Reserve University, Frances Payne Bolton School of Nursing, Master's Programs in Nursing, Nurse Practitioner Program, Cleveland, OH 44106. Offers acute care cardiovascular nursing (MSN); acute care nurse practitioner (MSN); acute care pediatric nurse practitioner (MSN); acute care/flight nurse (MSN); adult gerontology acute care nurse practitioner (MSN); adult gerontology oncology and palliative care (MSN); adult gerontology primary care nurse practitioner (MSN); family nurse practitioner (MSN); family systems psychiatric mental health nursing (MSN); neonatal nurse practitioner (MSN); pediatric nurse practitioner (MSN); women's health nurse practitioner (MSN). *Accreditation:* ACEN. *Program availability:* Part-time, online learning. *Students:* 52 full-time (45 women), 78 part-time (68 women); includes 31 minority (10 Black or African American, non-Hispanic/Latino; 14 Asian, non-Hispanic/Latino; 7 Hispanic/Latino). Average age 35. 64 applicants, 66% accepted, 29 enrolled. In 2015, 45 master's awarded. *Degree requirements:* For master's, thesis optional. *Entrance requirements:* For master's, GRE General Test or MAT. Additional exam requirements/recommendations for international students: Required—TOEFL (minimum score 577 paper-based; 90 iBT), IELTS (minimum score 7). *Application deadline:* For fall admission, 6/1 for domestic students; for spring admission, 10/1 for domestic students. Applications are processed on a rolling basis. Application fee: $75. *Expenses:* $1,891 per credit hour. *Financial support:* In 2015–16, 54 students received support, including 17 teaching assistantships with partial tuition reimbursements available (averaging $17,019 per year); scholarships/grants and traineeships also available. Financial award application deadline: 6/30; financial award applicants required to submit FAFSA. *Faculty research:* Symptom science, family/community care, aging across the lifespan, self-management of health and illness, neuroscience. *Unit head:* Dr. Carol Savrin, Director, 216-368-5304, Fax: 216-368-3542, E-mail: cls18@case.edu. *Application contact:* Donna Hassik, Admissions Coordinator, 216-368-5253, Fax: 216-368-0124, E-mail: dmh7@case.edu.
Website: http://fpb.cwru.edu/MSN/majors.shtm

The College of New Rochelle, Graduate School, Program in Nursing, New Rochelle, NY 10805-2308. Offers acute care nurse practitioner (MS, Certificate); clinical specialist in holistic nursing (MS, Certificate); family nurse practitioner (MS, Certificate); nursing and health care management (MS); nursing education (Certificate). *Accreditation:* AACN. *Program availability:* Part-time. *Faculty:* 3 full-time (2 women), 6 part-time/adjunct (4 women). *Students:* 116 part-time (104 women); includes 79 minority (58 Black or African American, non-Hispanic/Latino; 11 Asian, non-Hispanic/Latino; 10 Hispanic/Latino). Average age 38. In 2015, 25 master's awarded. *Entrance requirements:* For master's, GRE General Test or MAT, BSN, malpractice insurance, minimum GPA of 3.0, RN license. *Application deadline:* For fall admission, 8/15 priority date for domestic students; for spring admission, 12/1 priority date for domestic students. Applications are processed on a rolling basis. Application fee: $35. Electronic applications accepted. *Expenses:* Tuition, area resident: Part-time $894 per credit. *Required fees:* $350 per semester. *Financial support:* Traineeships available. Support available to part-time students. Financial award application deadline: 8/15; financial award applicants required to submit FAFSA. *Unit head:* Dr. H. Michael Dreher, Dean, School of Nursing, 914-654-5441, E-mail: hdreher@cnr.edu. *Application contact:* Michael Petri, Interim Director of Graduate Admissions, 914-654-5256, E-mail: mpetri@cnr.edu.

Columbia University, School of Nursing, Program in Adult-Gerontology Acute Care Nurse Practitioner, New York, NY 10032. Offers MS, Adv C. *Accreditation:* AACN. *Program availability:* Part-time. *Entrance requirements:* For master's, GRE General Test, NCLEX, 1 year of clinical experience, BSN; for Adv C, MSN. Additional exam requirements/recommendations for international students: Required—TOEFL (minimum score 100 iBT). Electronic applications accepted.

Drexel University, College of Nursing and Health Professions, Division of Graduate Nursing, Philadelphia, PA 19104-2875. Offers adult acute care (MSN); adult psychiatric/mental health (MSN); advanced practice nursing (MSN); clinical trials research (MSN); family nurse practitioner (MSN); leadership in health systems management (MSN);

nursing education (MSN); pediatric primary care (MSN); women's health (MSN). *Accreditation:* AACN. Electronic applications accepted.

Duke University, School of Nursing, Durham, NC 27708-0586. Offers acute care pediatric nurse practitioner (MSN, Post Master's Certificate); adult-gerontology nurse practitioner (MSN, Post Master's Certificate), including acute care, primary care; family nurse practitioner (MSN, Post Master's Certificate); neonatal nurse practitioner (MSN, Post Master's Certificate); nurse anesthesia (DNP); nurse practitioner (DNP); nursing (PhD); nursing and health care leadership (MSN); nursing education (MSN); nursing informatics (MSN, Post Master's Certificate); pediatric nurse practitioner (MSN, Post Master's Certificate), including primary care; women's health nurse practitioner (MSN, Post Master's Certificate). *Accreditation:* AACN; AANA/CANAEP. *Program availability:* Part-time, evening/weekend, online learning. *Faculty:* 74 full-time (63 women). *Students:* 179 full-time (152 women), 528 part-time (466 women); includes 145 minority (42 Black or African American, non-Hispanic/Latino; 3 American Indian or Alaska Native, non-Hispanic/Latino; 44 Asian, non-Hispanic/Latino; 35 Hispanic/Latino; 1 Native Hawaiian or other Pacific Islander, non-Hispanic/Latino; 20 Two or more races, non-Hispanic/Latino), 7 international. Average age 33. 619 applicants, 46% accepted, 201 enrolled. In 2015, 243 master's, 62 doctorates, 26 other advanced degrees awarded. Terminal master's awarded for partial completion of doctoral program. *Degree requirements:* For master's, thesis optional; for doctorate, capstone project. *Entrance requirements:* For master's, GRE General Test (waived if undergraduate GPA of 3.4 or higher), 1 year of nursing experience (recommended), BSN, minimum GPA of 3.0, previous course work in statistics; for doctorate, GRE General Test (waived if undergraduate GPA of 3.4 or higher), BSN or MSN, minimum GPA of 3.0, portfolio, resume, personal statement, undergraduate statistics course, current licensure as a registered nurse, transcripts from all post-secondary institutions; for Post Master's Certificate, MSN, licensure or eligibility as a professional nurse, transcripts from all post-secondary institutions, previous course work in statistics. Additional exam requirements/recommendations for international students: Required—TOEFL (minimum score 100 iBT), IELTS (minimum score 7). *Application deadline:* For fall admission, 12/1 for domestic and international students; for spring admission, 5/1 for domestic and international students. Application fee: $50. Electronic applications accepted. *Expenses:* Contact institution. *Financial support:* Career-related internships or fieldwork, institutionally sponsored loans, scholarships/grants, traineeships, and tuition waivers (partial) available. Support available to part-time students. Financial award applicants required to submit FAFSA. *Faculty research:* Cardiovascular disease, caregiver skill training, data mining, prostate cancer, neonatal immune system. *Unit head:* Dr. Marion E. Broome, Dean/Vice Chancellor for Nursing Affairs/Associate Vice President for Academic Affairs for Nursing, 919-684-9446, Fax: 919-684-9414, E-mail: marion.broome@duke.edu. *Application contact:* Dr. Ernie Rushing, Director of Admissions and Recruitment, 919-668-6274, Fax: 919-668-4693, E-mail: ernie.rushing@dm.duke.edu.
Website: http://www.nursing.duke.edu/

Georgetown University, Graduate School of Arts and Sciences, School of Nursing and Health Studies, Washington, DC 20057. Offers acute care nurse practitioner (MS); clinical nurse specialist (MS); family nurse practitioner (MS); nurse anesthesia (MS); nurse-midwifery (MS); nursing (DNP); nursing education (MS). *Accreditation:* AACN; AANA/CANAEP (one or more programs are accredited); ACNM/ACME (one or more programs are accredited). *Degree requirements:* For master's, thesis optional. *Entrance requirements:* For master's, GRE General Test or MAT, bachelor's degree in nursing from NLN-accredited school, minimum undergraduate GPA of 3.0. Additional exam requirements/recommendations for international students: Required—TOEFL.

Goldfarb School of Nursing at Barnes-Jewish College, Graduate Programs, St. Louis, MO 63110. Offers adult-gerontology acute care nurse practitioner (MSN); adult-gerontology nurse practitioner (MSN); nurse anesthesia (MSN); nurse educator (MSN); nurse executive (MSN). *Accreditation:* AACN; AANA/CANAEP. *Program availability:* Part-time, online learning. *Faculty:* 51 full-time (47 women), 6 part-time/adjunct (all women). *Students:* 58 full-time (57 women), 29 part-time (24 women); includes 17 minority (11 Black or African American, non-Hispanic/Latino; 2 Asian, non-Hispanic/Latino; 2 Hispanic/Latino; 2 Two or more races, non-Hispanic/Latino). Average age 26. 41 applicants, 22% accepted, 8 enrolled. In 2015, 56 master's awarded. *Degree requirements:* For master's, thesis or alternative. *Entrance requirements:* For master's, 2 references, personal statement, curriculum vitae or resume. Additional exam requirements/recommendations for international students: Required—TOEFL (minimum score 575 paper-based; 85 iBT). *Application deadline:* For fall admission, 2/1 priority date for international students; for spring admission, 10/1 priority date for international students. Applications are processed on a rolling basis. Application fee: $50. *Expenses:* Contact institution. *Financial support:* Fellowships, research assistantships, Federal Work-Study, institutionally sponsored loans, and scholarships/grants available. Support available to part-time students. Financial award applicants required to submit FAFSA. *Faculty research:* HIV stigma, HIV symptom management, palliative care with children and their families, heart disease prevention in Hispanic women, depression in the well elderly, alternative therapies in pre-term infants. *Unit head:* Dr. Gretchen Drinkard, Dean, 314-454-7540, Fax: 314-362-9222, E-mail: gld9643@bjc.org. *Application contact:* Karen Sartorius, Admissions Specialist, 314-454-7057, Fax: 314-362-9250, E-mail: ksartorius@bjc.org.
Website: http://www.barnesjewishcollege.edu/

Grand Canyon University, College of Nursing, Phoenix, AZ 85017-1097. Offers acute care nurse practitioner (MS, PMC); clinical nurse specialist (PMC), including clinical nurse specialist, education; family nurse practitioner (MS); leadership in health care systems (MS); nurse education (MS). *Accreditation:* AACN. *Program availability:* Part-time, evening/weekend, online learning. *Degree requirements:* For master's and PMC, comprehensive exam (for some programs). *Entrance requirements:* For master's, minimum cumulative and science course undergraduate GPA of 3.0. Additional exam requirements/recommendations for international students: Required—TOEFL (minimum score 575 paper-based; 90 iBT), IELTS (minimum score 7).

Inter American University of Puerto Rico, Arecibo Campus, Program in Nursing, Arecibo, PR 00614-4050. Offers critical care nursing (MSN); surgical nursing (MSN). *Entrance requirements:* For master's, EXADEP or GRE General Test or MAT, 2 letters of recommendation, bachelor's degree in nursing, minimum GPA of 2.5 in last 60 credits, minimum 1 year nursing experience, nursing license.

Marquette University, Graduate School, College of Nursing, Milwaukee, WI 53201-1881. Offers acute care nurse practitioner (Certificate); adult clinical nurse specialist (Certificate); adult nurse practitioner (Certificate); advanced practice nursing (MSN, DNP), including adult-older adult acute care (DNP), adults (MSN), adults-older adults (DNP), clinical nurse leader (MSN), health care systems leadership (DNP), nurse-midwifery (MSN), older adults (MSN), pediatrics-acute care, pediatrics-primary care, primary care (DNP), systems leadership and healthcare quality (MSN); family nurse practitioner (Certificate); nurse-midwifery (Certificate); nursing (PhD); pediatric acute care (Certificate); pediatric primary care (Certificate); systems leadership and healthcare quality (Certificate). *Accreditation:* AACN. *Faculty:* 35 full-time (all women), 56 part-time/adjunct (55 women). *Students:* 123 full-time (112 women), 242 part-time (220 women); includes 34 minority (9 Black or African American, non-Hispanic/Latino; 12 Asian, non-Hispanic/Latino; 10 Hispanic/Latino; 3 Two or more races, non-Hispanic/Latino), 4 international. Average age 30. 269 applicants, 61% accepted, 98 enrolled. In 2015, 84 master's, 5 doctorates, 22 other advanced degrees awarded. Terminal master's awarded for partial completion of doctoral program. *Degree requirements:* For master's, comprehensive exam, thesis or alternative. *Entrance requirements:* For master's, GRE General Test, BSN, Wisconsin RN license, official transcripts from all current and previous colleges/universities except Marquette, three completed recommendation forms, resume, written statement of professional goals; for doctorate, GRE General Test, official transcripts from all current and previous colleges/universities except Marquette, three letters of recommendation, resume, written statement of professional goals, sample of scholarly writing. Additional exam requirements/recommendations for international students: Required—TOEFL (minimum score 530 paper-based). *Application deadline:* For fall admission, 2/15 for domestic and international students. Electronic applications accepted. *Financial support:* In 2015–16, 41 students received support, including 1 fellowship with partial tuition reimbursement available (averaging $17,500 per year), 2 research assistantships with full tuition reimbursements available (averaging $13,285 per year), 8 teaching assistantships with full tuition reimbursements available (averaging $13,912 per year); career-related internships or fieldwork, Federal Work-Study, scholarships/grants, health care benefits, tuition waivers (partial), and unspecified assistantships also available. Support available to part-time students. Financial award application deadline: 2/15. *Faculty research:* Psychosocial adjustment to chronic illness, gerontology, reminiscence, health policy: uninsured and access, hospital care delivery systems. *Total annual research expenditures:* $480,591. *Unit head:* Dr. Donna McCarthy, Interim Chair, 414-288-3800, Fax: 414-288-1578. *Application contact:* Dr. Maureen O'Brien, Associate Dean/Clinical Associate Professor, 414-288-3823.

Maryville University of Saint Louis, Walker College of Health Professions, The Catherine McAuley School of Nursing, St. Louis, MO 63141-7299. Offers acute care nurse practice (MSN); adult gerontology nurse practitioner (MSN); advanced practice nursing (DNP); family nurse practitioner (MSN); pediatric nurse practice (MSN). *Accreditation:* AACN. *Program availability:* 100% online. *Faculty:* 18 full-time (all women), 158 part-time/adjunct (141 women). *Students:* 38 full-time (35 women), 2,802 part-time (2,511 women); includes 681 minority (332 Black or African American, non-Hispanic/Latino; 40 American Indian or Alaska Native, non-Hispanic/Latino; 126 Asian, non-Hispanic/Latino; 126 Hispanic/Latino; 8 Native Hawaiian or other Pacific Islander, non-Hispanic/Latino; 49 Two or more races, non-Hispanic/Latino), 58 international. Average age 37. In 2015, 413 master's, 33 doctorates awarded. *Degree requirements:* For master's, practicum. *Entrance requirements:* For master's, BSN, current licensure, minimum GPA of 3.0, 3 letters of recommendation, curriculum vitae. Additional exam requirements/recommendations for international students: Required—TOEFL (minimum score 550 paper-based). *Application deadline:* Applications are processed on a rolling basis. Electronic applications accepted. Application fee is waived when completed online. *Expenses: Tuition,* area resident: Full-time $25,558; part-time $781 per credit hour. *Required fees:* $2400. Part-time tuition and fees vary according to course load and degree level. *Financial support:* Federal Work-Study and campus employment available. Support available to part-time students. Financial award application deadline: 3/1; financial award applicants required to submit FAFSA. *Unit head:* Dr. Elizabeth Buck, Director, 314-529-9453, Fax: 314-529-9139, E-mail: ebuck@maryville.edu. *Application contact:* Crystal Jacobsmeyer, Assistant Director, Graduate Enrollment Advising, 314-929-9654, Fax: 314-529-9927, E-mail: cjacobsmeyer@maryville.edu.
Website: http://www.maryville.edu/hp/nursing/

Mount Carmel College of Nursing, Nursing Program, Columbus, OH 43222. Offers adult gerontology acute care nurse practitioner (MS); adult health clinical nurse specialist (MS); family nurse practitioner (MS); nursing (DNP); nursing administration (MS); nursing education (MS). *Accreditation:* AACN. *Program availability:* Part-time. *Faculty:* 8 full-time (all women), 5 part-time/adjunct (4 women). *Students:* 72 full-time (63 women), 92 part-time (84 women); includes 15 minority (7 Black or African American, non-Hispanic/Latino; 3 Asian, non-Hispanic/Latino; 2 Hispanic/Latino; 3 Two or more races, non-Hispanic/Latino). Average age 37. 140 applicants, 45% accepted, 50 enrolled. In 2015, 50 master's awarded. *Degree requirements:* For master's, professional manuscript; for doctorate, practicum. *Entrance requirements:* For master's, letters of recommendation, statement of purpose, current resume, baccalaureate degree in nursing, current Ohio RN license, minimum cumulative GPA of 3.0; for doctorate, master's degree in nursing from program accredited by either NLNAC/ACEN or CCNE. Additional exam requirements/recommendations for international students: Required—TOEFL (minimum score 550 paper-based; 80 iBT). *Application deadline:* For fall admission, 6/1 priority date for domestic students; for winter admission, 11/1 for domestic students; for spring admission, 10/1 priority date for domestic students; for summer admission, 3/1 for domestic students. Applications are processed on a rolling basis. Application fee: $30. *Expenses: Tuition,* area resident: Full-time $9480; part-time $474 per credit. One-time fee: $120. Tuition and fees vary according to course load, degree level and program. *Financial support:* In 2015–16, 5 students received support. Institutionally sponsored loans and scholarships/grants available. Financial award applicants required to submit FAFSA. *Unit head:* Dr. Jill Kilanowski, 614-234-5237, Fax: 614-234-2875, E-mail: jkilanowski@mccn.edu. *Application contact:* Dr. Kim Campbell, Director of Recruitment and Admissions, 614-234-5144, Fax: 614-234-5427, E-mail: kcampbell@mccn.edu.
Website: http://www.mccn.edu/

New York University, Rory Meyers College of Nursing, Doctor of Nursing Practice Program, New York, NY 10012-1019. Offers nursing (DNP), including adult acute care, adult primary care, family, mental health nursing, nurse-midwifery, pediatrics. *Program availability:* Part-time, evening/weekend. *Faculty:* 14 full-time (13 women). *Students:* 2 full-time (both women), 32 part-time (27 women); includes 8 minority (3 Black or African American, non-Hispanic/Latino; 4 Asian, non-Hispanic/Latino; 1 Hispanic/Latino), 1 international. Average age 40. 47 applicants, 51% accepted, 16 enrolled. In 2015, 17 doctorates awarded. *Degree requirements:* For doctorate, thesis/dissertation, project. *Entrance requirements:* For doctorate, MAT or GRE (either taken within past 5 years), MS, RN license, interview, Nurse Practitioner Certification, writing sample. Additional exam requirements/recommendations for international students: Required—TOEFL (minimum score 90 iBT), IELTS (minimum score 7). *Application deadline:* For fall admission, 3/1 for domestic and international students. Applications are processed on a rolling basis. Application fee: $80. Electronic applications accepted. *Expenses:* Contact institution. *Financial support:* In 2015–16, 12 students received support. Scholarships/grants available. Support available to part-time students. Financial award application deadline: 2/1; financial award applicants required to submit FAFSA. *Faculty research:* Workforce, LGBT, breast cancer, HIV. *Unit head:* Dr. Rona Levin, Director, 212-998-5319, Fax: 212-995-3143, E-mail: rfl2039@nyu.edu. *Application contact:* Samantha Jaser, Assistant Director, Graduate Student Affairs and Admissions, 212-992-7653, Fax: 212-995-4302, E-mail: saj283@nyu.edu.

New York University, Rory Meyers College of Nursing, Programs in Advanced Practice Nursing, New York, NY 10012-1019. Offers adult-gerontology acute care nurse practitioner (MS, Advanced Certificate); adult-gerontology primary care nurse practitioner (MS, Advanced Certificate); family nurse practitioner (MS, Advanced Certificate); gerontology nurse practitioner (Advanced Certificate); nurse-midwifery (MS, Advanced Certificate); nursing administration (MS, Advanced Certificate); nursing education (MS, Advanced Certificate); nursing informatics (MS, Advanced Certificate); pediatrics nurse practitioner (MS, Advanced Certificate); psychiatric-mental health nurse practitioner (MS, Advanced Certificate); MS/MPH. *Accreditation:* AACN; ACNM/ACME. *Program availability:* Part-time. *Faculty:* 24 full-time (all women), 76 part-time/adjunct (65 women). *Students:* 46 full-time (26 women), 586 part-time (513 women); includes 242 minority (68 Black or African American, non-Hispanic/Latino; 3 American Indian or Alaska Native, non-Hispanic/Latino; 117 Asian, non-Hispanic/Latino; 38 Hispanic/Latino; 3 Native Hawaiian or other Pacific Islander, non-Hispanic/Latino; 13 Two or more races, non-Hispanic/Latino), 23 international. Average age 32. 402 applicants, 69% accepted, 138 enrolled. In 2015, 198 master's, 5 other advanced degrees awarded. *Degree requirements:* For master's, thesis (for some programs). *Entrance requirements:* For master's, BS in nursing, AS in nursing with another BS/BA, interview, RN license, 1 year of clinical experience (3 for the MS in nursing education program); for Advanced Certificate, master's degree. Additional exam requirements/recommendations for international students: Required—TOEFL (minimum score 90 iBT), IELTS (minimum score 7). *Application deadline:* For fall admission, 6/15 for domestic and international students; for spring admission, 12/1 for domestic and international students; for summer admission, 3/1 for domestic and international students. Application fee: $80. Electronic applications accepted. *Expenses:* Contact institution. *Financial support:* In 2015–16, 101 students received support. Career-related internships or fieldwork, Federal Work-Study, and scholarships/grants available. Support available to part-time students. Financial award application deadline: 3/1; financial award applicants required to submit FAFSA. *Faculty research:* Geriatrics, HIV, families and illness, oral systemic connection, symptom management. *Unit head:* Dr. James Pace, Senior Associate Dean for Academic Programs, 212-992-7343, E-mail: james.pace@nyu.edu. *Application contact:* Samantha Jaser, Assistant Director, Graduate Student Affairs and Admissions, 212-992-7653, Fax: 212-995-4302, E-mail: saj283@nyu.edu.

Northeastern University, Bouvé College of Health Sciences, Boston, MA 02115-5096. Offers applied behavior analysis (MS, CAGS); audiology (Au D); biomedical nanotechnology (MS); college student development and counseling (MS, CAGS); counseling psychology (MS, PhD, CAGS); exercise science (MS); health informatics (MS); medicinal chemistry (MS); nurse anesthesia (DNP, CAGS); nursing (MS, PhD, CAGS), including administration (MS), adult-gerontology acute care nurse practitioner (MS, CAGS), adult-gerontology primary care nurse practitioner (MS, CAGS), anesthesia (MS), family nurse practitioner (MS, CAGS), neonatal nurse practitioner (MS, CAGS), pediatric nurse practitioner (MS, CAGS), psychiatric mental health nurse practitioner (MS, CAGS); nursing practice (DNP); personal health informatics (PhD); pharmaceutical sciences (MS, PhD), including interdisciplinary concentration, pharmaceutics and drug delivery systems; pharmacology (MS); pharmacy (Pharm D); physical therapy (Postbaccalaureate Certificate); physician assistant (MS); population health (PhD); school psychology (MS, PhD, CAGS); speech-language pathology (MS); urban health (MPH); MS/MBA. *Accreditation:* ACPE (one or more programs are accredited). *Program availability:* Part-time, evening/weekend, online learning. *Faculty:* 194 full-time (120 women), 169 part-time/adjunct (136 women). *Students:* 1,416 full-time (1,049 women), 310 part-time (248 women). In 2015, 374 master's, 313 doctorates, 37 other advanced degrees awarded. *Degree requirements:* For doctorate, thesis/dissertation (for some programs); for other advanced degree, comprehensive exam. Application fee: $75. Electronic applications accepted. *Expenses:* Contact institution. *Financial support:* Applicants required to submit FAFSA. *Unit head:* John R. Reynolds, Professor and Interim Dean, 617-373-3323, Fax: 617-373-3030. *Application contact:* Molly Schnabel, Senior Director of Graduate Affairs, 617-373-2708, Fax: 617-373-4701, E-mail: bouvegrad@neu.edu.
Website: http://www.northeastern.edu/bouve/

Ohio University, Graduate College, College of Health Sciences and Professions, School of Nursing, Athens, OH 45701-2979. Offers acute care nurse practitioner (MSN); acute care nurse practitioner and family nurse practitioner (MSN); acute care nurse practitioner and nurse administrator (MSN); acute care nurse practitioner and nurse educator (MSN); family nurse practitioner (MSN); nurse administrator (MSN); nurse administrator and family nurse practitioner (MSN); nurse educator (MSN); nurse educator and family nurse practitioner (MSN); nurse educator and nurse administrator (MSN). *Accreditation:* AACN. *Degree requirements:* For master's, capstone project. *Entrance requirements:* For master's, GRE, bachelor's degree in nursing from an accredited college or university, minimum overall undergraduate GPA of 3.0, official transcripts, statement of goals and objectives, resume, 3 letters of recommendation. Additional exam requirements/recommendations for international students: Required—TOEFL (minimum score 550 paper-based; 80 iBT) or IELTS (minimum score 6.5). Electronic applications accepted.

Purdue University Northwest, Graduate Studies Office, School of Nursing, Hammond, IN 46323-2094. Offers adult health clinical nurse specialist (MS); critical care clinical nurse specialist (MS); family nurse practitioner (MS); nurse executive (MS). *Accreditation:* AACN; ACEN. *Program availability:* Part-time, online learning. *Entrance requirements:* For master's, BSN. Additional exam requirements/recommendations for international students: Required—TOEFL. Electronic applications accepted. *Faculty research:* Adult health, cardiovascular and pulmonary nursing.

San Francisco State University, Division of Graduate Studies, College of Health and Social Sciences, School of Nursing, San Francisco, CA 94132-1722. Offers adult acute care (MS); clinical nurse specialist (MS); community/public health nursing (MS); family nurse practitioner (MS, Certificate); nursing administration (MS); pediatrics (MS); women's health (MS). *Accreditation:* AACN. *Program availability:* Part-time. *Application deadline:* Applications are processed on a rolling basis. *Expenses:* Tuition, state resident: full-time $6738. Tuition, nonresident: full-time $15,666. *Required fees:* $1004. *Financial support:* Career-related internships or fieldwork available. *Unit head:* Dr. Mary-Ann van Dam, Director, 415-338-1802, Fax: 415-338-0555, E-mail: vandam@sfsu.edu. *Application contact:* Connie Carr, Graduate Coordinator, 415-338-6856, Fax: 415-338-0555, E-mail: ccarr@sfsu.edu.
Website: http://nursing.sfsu.edu

Southern Adventist University, School of Nursing, Collegedale, TN 37315-0370. Offers acute care nurse practitioner (MSN); adult nurse practitioner (MSN); family nurse practitioner (MSN); nurse educator (MSN); MSN/MSBA. *Accreditation:* ACEN. *Program availability:* Part-time. *Degree requirements:* For master's, thesis or project. *Entrance requirements:* For master's, RN license. Additional exam requirements/recommendations for international students: Required—TOEFL (minimum score 600 paper-based). Electronic applications accepted. *Faculty research:* Pain management, ethics, corporate wellness, caring spirituality, stress.

Texas Tech University Health Sciences Center, School of Nursing, Lubbock, TX 79430. Offers acute care nurse practitioner (MSN, Certificate); administration (MSN); advanced practice (DNP); education (MSN); executive leadership (DNP); family nurse practitioner (MSN, Certificate); geriatric nurse practitioner (MSN, Certificate); pediatric nurse practitioner (MSN, Certificate). *Accreditation:* AACN. *Program availability:* Part-time, online learning. *Degree requirements:* For master's, thesis optional. *Entrance requirements:* For master's, minimum GPA of 3.0, 3 letters of reference, BSN, RN license; for Certificate, minimum GPA of 3.0, 3 letters of reference, RN license. Additional exam requirements/recommendations for international students: Required—

TOEFL (minimum score 550 paper-based). *Faculty research:* Diabetes/obesity, nurse competency, disease management, intervention and measurements, health disparities.

Texas Woman's University, Graduate School, College of Nursing, Denton, TX 76204-5498. Offers acute care nurse practitioner (MS); adult health clinical nurse specialist (MS); adult health nurse practitioner (MS); child health clinical nurse specialist (MS); clinical nurse leader (MS); family nurse practitioner (MS); health systems management (MS); nursing education (MS); nursing practice (DNP); nursing science (PhD); pediatric nurse practitioner (MS); women's health clinical nurse specialist (MS); women's health nurse practitioner (MS). *Accreditation:* AACN. *Program availability:* Part-time, online learning. *Faculty:* 55 full-time (51 women), 42 part-time/adjunct (35 women). *Students:* 39 full-time (37 women), 958 part-time (888 women); includes 566 minority (226 Black or African American, non-Hispanic/Latino; 8 American Indian or Alaska Native, non-Hispanic/Latino; 221 Asian, non-Hispanic/Latino; 88 Hispanic/Latino; 3 Native Hawaiian or other Pacific Islander, non-Hispanic/Latino; 20 Two or more races, non-Hispanic/Latino), 37 international. Average age 36. 430 applicants, 65% accepted, 193 enrolled. In 2015, 248 master's, 10 doctorates awarded. *Degree requirements:* For master's, comprehensive exam, thesis or alternative; for doctorate, comprehensive exam, thesis/dissertation. *Entrance requirements:* For master's, GRE or MAT, minimum GPA of 3.0 on last 60 hours in undergraduate nursing degree and overall, RN license, BS in nursing, basic statistics course; for doctorate, GRE (preferred minimum score 153 [500 old version] Verbal, 144 [500 old version] Quantitative, 4 Analytical), MS in nursing, minimum preferred GPA of 3.5, RN license, statistics, 2 letters of reference, curriculum vitae, graduate nursing-theory course, graduate research course, statement of professional goals and research interests. Additional exam requirements/recommendations for international students: Required—TOEFL (minimum score 550 paper-based; 79 iBT). *Application deadline:* For fall admission, 5/1 priority date for domestic students, 3/1 for international students; for spring admission, 9/15 priority date for domestic students, 7/1 for international students. Applications are processed on a rolling basis. Application fee: $50 ($75 for international students). Electronic applications accepted. *Expenses:* Tuition, state resident: full-time $4380; part-time $243 per credit hour. Tuition, nonresident: full-time $11,400; part-time $633 per credit hour. *International tuition:* $11,465 full-time. *Required fees:* $1778; $99 per credit hour. $283 per semester. One-time fee: $50. Tuition and fees vary according to course load and program. *Financial support:* In 2015–16, 149 students received support, including 10 research assistantships (averaging $5,600 per year), 1 teaching assistantship (averaging $5,600 per year); career-related internships or fieldwork, Federal Work-Study, institutionally sponsored loans, scholarships/grants, traineeships, health care benefits, and unspecified assistantships also available. Support available to part-time students. Financial award application deadline: 3/1; financial award applicants required to submit FAFSA. *Faculty research:* Screening, prevention, and treatment for intimate partner violence; needs of adolescents during childbirth intervention; a network analysis decision tool for nurse managers (social network analysis); support for adolescents with implantable cardioverter defibrillators; informatics: nurse staffing, safety, quality, and financial data as they relate to patient care outcomes; prevention and treatment of obesity; improving infant outcomes related to premature birth. *Total annual research expenditures:* $1.7 million. *Unit head:* Dr. Anita G. Hufft, Dean, 940-898-2401, Fax: 940-898-2437, E-mail: nursing@twu.edu. *Application contact:* Dr. Samuel Wheeler, Assistant Director of Admissions, 940-898-3188, Fax: 940-898-3081, E-mail: wheelersr@twu.edu.
Website: http://www.twu.edu/nursing/

Universidad de Iberoamerica, Graduate School, San Jose, Costa Rica. Offers clinical neuropsychology (PhD); clinical psychology (M Psych); educational psychology (M Psych); forensic psychology (M Psych); hospital management (MHA); intensive care nursing (MN); medicine (MD).

The University of Alabama in Huntsville, School of Graduate Studies, College of Nursing, Huntsville, AL 35899. Offers family nurse practitioner (Certificate); nursing (MSN, DNP), including adult-gerontology acute care nurse practitioner (MSN), adult-gerontology clinical nurse specialist (MSN), family nurse practitioner (MSN), leadership in health care systems (MSN); nursing education (Certificate). DNP offered jointly with The University of Alabama at Birmingham. *Accreditation:* AACN. *Program availability:* Part-time, evening/weekend, online learning. *Degree requirements:* For master's, comprehensive exam, thesis or alternative, oral and written exams. *Entrance requirements:* For master's, MAT or GRE, Alabama RN license, BSN, minimum GPA of 3.0; for doctorate, master's degree in nursing in an advanced practice area; for Certificate, MAT or GRE, minimum GPA of 3.0. Additional exam requirements/recommendations for international students: Required—TOEFL (minimum score 500 paper-based; 80 iBT), IELTS (minimum score 6.5). *Application deadline:* For fall admission, 7/15 for domestic students, 4/1 for international students; for spring admission, 11/30 for domestic students, 9/1 for international students. Applications are processed on a rolling basis. Application fee: $50. Electronic applications accepted. *Expenses:* Tuition, area resident: Full-time $9548; part-time $547 per credit hour. Tuition, state resident: full-time $9548; part-time $547 per credit hour. Tuition, nonresident: full-time $21,402; part-time $1224 per credit hour. *International tuition:* $21,402 full-time. *Financial support:* Teaching assistantships with full tuition reimbursements, career-related internships or fieldwork, Federal Work-Study, institutionally sponsored loans, scholarships/grants, traineeships, health care benefits, and unspecified assistantships available. Support available to part-time students. Financial award application deadline: 4/1; financial award applicants required to submit FAFSA. *Faculty research:* Health care informatics, chronic illness management, maternal and child health, genetics/genomics, technology and health care. *Unit head:* Dr. Marsha Adams, Dean, 256-824-6345, Fax: 256-824-6026, E-mail: marsha.adams@uah.edu. *Application contact:* Charles Davis, Director of Graduate Admission and Advisement, 256-824-6669, Fax: 256-824-6026, E-mail: charles.davis@uah.edu.
Website: http://www.uah.edu/nursing

University of Cincinnati, Graduate School, College of Nursing, Cincinnati, OH 45221-0038. Offers clinical nurse specialist (MSN), including adult health, community health, neonatal, nursing administration, occupational health, pediatric health, psychiatric nursing, women's health; nurse anesthesia (MSN); nurse midwifery (MSN); nurse practitioner (MSN), including acute care, ambulatory care, family, family/psychiatric, women's health; nursing (PhD); MBA/MSN. *Accreditation:* AACN; AANA/CANAEP (one or more programs are accredited); ACNM/ACME. *Program availability:* Part-time, online learning. Terminal master's awarded for partial completion of doctoral program. *Degree requirements:* For master's, thesis or alternative; for doctorate, comprehensive exam, thesis/dissertation. *Entrance requirements:* For master's and doctorate, GRE General Test. Additional exam requirements/recommendations for international students: Required—TOEFL (minimum score 520 paper-based). Electronic applications accepted. *Faculty research:* Substance abuse, injury and violence, symptom management.

University of Guelph, Ontario Veterinary College and Graduate School, Graduate Programs in Veterinary Sciences, Department of Clinical Studies, Guelph, ON N1G 2W1, Canada. Offers anesthesiology (M Sc, DV Sc); cardiology (DV Sc, Diploma); clinical studies (Diploma); dermatology (M Sc); diagnostic imaging (M Sc, DV Sc); emergency/critical care (M Sc, DV Sc, Diploma); medicine (M Sc, DV Sc); neurology (M Sc, DV Sc); ophthalmology (M Sc, DV Sc); surgery (M Sc, DV Sc). *Degree*

requirements: For master's, thesis; for doctorate, comprehensive exam, thesis/dissertation. *Entrance requirements:* Additional exam requirements/recommendations for international students: Required—TOEFL (minimum score 550 paper-based), IELTS (minimum score 6.5). Electronic applications accepted. *Faculty research:* Orthopedics, respirology, oncology, exercise physiology, cardiology.

University of Illinois at Chicago, College of Nursing, Program in Nursing, Chicago, IL 60607-7128. Offers acute care clinical nurse specialist (MS); administrative nursing leadership (Certificate); adult nurse practitioner (MS); adult/geriatric nurse practitioner (MS); advanced community health nurse specialist (MS); family nurse practitioner (MS); geriatric clinical nurse specialist (MS); geriatric nurse practitioner (MS); nurse midwifery (MS); occupational health/advanced community health nurse specialist (MS); occupational health/family nurse practitioner (MS); pediatric nurse practitioner (MS); perinatal clinical nurse specialist (MS); school/advanced community health nurse specialist (MS); school/family nurse practitioner (MS); women's health nurse practitioner (MS). *Accreditation:* AACN. *Program availability:* Part-time. *Faculty:* 100 full-time (93 women), 89 part-time/adjunct (82 women). *Students:* 359 full-time (326 women), 280 part-time (249 women); includes 169 minority (43 Black or African American, non-Hispanic/Latino; 62 Asian, non-Hispanic/Latino; 56 Hispanic/Latino; 1 Native Hawaiian or other Pacific Islander, non-Hispanic/Latino; 7 Two or more races, non-Hispanic/Latino), 12 international. Average age 32. In 2015, 4 other advanced degrees awarded. *Degree requirements:* For master's, thesis or alternative. *Entrance requirements:* For master's, GRE General Test, minimum GPA of 2.75. Additional exam requirements/recommendations for international students: Required—TOEFL. *Application deadline:* For fall admission, 5/15 for domestic students, 2/15 for international students; for spring admission, 11/1 for domestic students, 7/15 for international students. Applications are processed on a rolling basis. Application fee: $60. Electronic applications accepted. *Expenses:* Tuition, state resident: full-time $11,480; part-time $3826 per credit. Tuition, nonresident: full-time $23,720; part-time $7906 per credit. *Required fees:* $1333 per semester. Part-time tuition and fees vary according to course load and program. *Financial support:* Fellowships with full tuition reimbursements, research assistantships with full tuition reimbursements, teaching assistantships with full tuition reimbursements, career-related internships or fieldwork, Federal Work-Study, institutionally sponsored loans, scholarships/grants, traineeships, tuition waivers (full and partial), and unspecified assistantships available. Support available to part-time students. Financial award application deadline: 3/1; financial award applicants required to submit FAFSA. *Unit head:* Dr. Terri E. Weaver, Dean, 312-996-7808, E-mail: teweaver@uic.edu. *Application contact:* Receptionist, 312-413-2550, E-mail: gradcoll@uic.edu.
Website: http://www.nursing.uic.edu/academics-admissions/master-science#program-overview

University of Miami, Graduate School, School of Nursing and Health Studies, Coral Gables, FL 33124. Offers acute care (MSN), including acute care nurse practitioner, nurse anesthesia; nursing (PhD); primary care (MSN), including adult nurse practitioner, family nurse practitioner, nurse midwifery, women's health practitioner. *Accreditation:* AACN; AANA/CANAEP; ACNM/ACME (one or more programs are accredited). *Program availability:* Part-time. *Degree requirements:* For master's, thesis optional; for doctorate, thesis/dissertation. *Entrance requirements:* For master's, GRE General Test, BSN, minimum GPA of 3.0, Florida RN license; for doctorate, GRE General Test, BSN or MSN, minimum GPA of 3.0. Additional exam requirements/recommendations for international students: Required—TOEFL (minimum score 550 paper-based). Electronic applications accepted. *Faculty research:* Transcultural nursing, exercise and depression in Alzheimer's disease, infectious diseases/HIV–AIDS, postpartum depression, outcomes assessment.

The University of North Carolina at Charlotte, College of Health and Human Services, School of Nursing, Charlotte, NC 28223-0001. Offers adult-gerontology acute care nurse practitioner (MSN, Post-Master's Certificate); advanced clinical nursing (MSN); community public health nursing (MSN); family nurse practitioner across the lifespan (MSN, Post-Master's Certificate); nurse administrator (MSN, Graduate Certificate); nurse anesthesia (MSN, Post-Master's Certificate); nurse educator (MSN, Graduate Certificate); nursing (DNP); nursing systems/population (MSN). *Accreditation:* AACN. *Program availability:* Part-time, blended/hybrid learning. *Faculty:* 26 full-time (25 women), 4 part-time/adjunct (3 women). *Students:* 109 full-time (89 women), 112 part-time (107 women); includes 46 minority (37 Black or African American, non-Hispanic/Latino; 3 Asian, non-Hispanic/Latino; 5 Hispanic/Latino; 1 Two or more races, non-Hispanic/Latino). Average age 33. 321 applicants, 34% accepted, 84 enrolled. In 2015, 76 master's, 4 doctorates, 7 other advanced degrees awarded. Terminal master's awarded for partial completion of doctoral program. *Degree requirements:* For master's, practicum, synthesis and integration or thesis, residency, internship (varies by program); for doctorate, thesis/dissertation or alternative, residency; for other advanced degree, practicum. *Entrance requirements:* For master's, GRE General Test, unencumbered license as Registered Nurse in North Carolina; BSN from nationally-accredited program; one year of professional nursing practice in acute/critical care; minimum overall GPA of 3.0 in the last degree and 60 hours of nursing coursework; completion of an undergraduate statistics course with minimum grade of C; statement of purpose; for doctorate, GRE or MAT, master's degree in nursing in an advanced nursing practice specialty from nationally-accredited program; minimum overall GPA of 3.5 in MSN program; current RN licensure in U.S. at time of application with eligibility for NC licensure; for other advanced degree, GRE. Additional exam requirements/recommendations for international students: Required—TOEFL (minimum score 557 paper-based, 83 iBT) or IELTS (minimum score 6.5). *Application deadline:* For fall admission, 2/1 for domestic and international students; for spring admission, 10/1 priority date for domestic and international students; for summer admission, 4/1 priority date for domestic and international students. Applications are processed on a rolling basis. Application fee: $75. Electronic applications accepted. *Expenses:* Contact institution. *Financial support:* In 2015–16, 9 students received support, including 5 research assistantships (averaging $4,850 per year), 3 teaching assistantships (averaging $2,911 per year); career-related internships or fieldwork, institutionally sponsored loans, scholarships/grants, traineeships, unspecified assistantships, and administrative assistantships also available. Support available to part-time students. Financial award application deadline: 3/1; financial award applicants required to submit FAFSA. *Faculty research:* Improving care outcomes for the elderly; vulnerable populations; symptom management; self management/health promotion strategies of older adults; migration and maternal child health; health disparities, health literacy, and access to healthcare in Latino adults with diabetes; psychiatric nursing. *Total annual research expenditures:* $875,169. *Unit head:* Dr. Dee Baldwin, Associate Dean, 704-687-7952, Fax: 704-687-6017, E-mail: dbaldwi5@uncc.edu. *Application contact:* Kathy B. Giddings, Director of Graduate Admissions, 704-687-5503, Fax: 704-687-1668, E-mail: gradadm@uncc.edu.
Website: http://nursing.uncc.edu/

University of Pennsylvania, School of Nursing, Adult-Gerontology Acute Care Nurse Practitioner Program, Philadelphia, PA 19104. Offers MSN. *Accreditation:* AACN. *Program availability:* Part-time. *Students:* 43 full-time (35 women), 148 part-time (127 women); includes 42 minority (7 Black or African American, non-Hispanic/Latino; 1 American Indian or Alaska Native, non-Hispanic/Latino; 16 Asian, non-Hispanic/Latino; 10 Hispanic/Latino; 8 Two or more races, non-Hispanic/Latino), 2 international. 157

Acute Care/Critical Care Nursing

applicants, 54% accepted, 78 enrolled. In 2015, 85 master's awarded. *Entrance requirements:* For master's, GRE General Test. *Expenses: Tuition, area resident:* Full-time $31,068; part-time $5762 per course. *Required fees:* $3200; $336 per course. Full-time tuition and fees vary according to degree level, program and student level. Part-time tuition and fees vary according to course load, degree level and program. *Financial support:* Application deadline: 4/1. *Faculty research:* Post-injury disability, bereavement and attributions in fire survivors, stress in staff nurses. *Unit head:* Assistant Dean of Admissions and Financial Aid, 866-867-6877, Fax: 215-573-8439, E-mail: admissions@nursing.upenn.edu. *Application contact:* Deborah Becker, Program Director, 215-898-0432, E-mail: debecker@nursing.upenn.edu.
Website: http://www.nursing.upenn.edu/

University of Pennsylvania, School of Nursing, Pediatric Acute Care Nurse Practitioner Program, Philadelphia, PA 19104. Offers MSN. *Accreditation:* AACN. *Program availability:* Part-time, online learning. *Students:* 10 full-time (all women), 37 part-time (all women); includes 11 minority (3 Black or African American, non-Hispanic/Latino; 5 Asian, non-Hispanic/Latino; 1 Hispanic/Latino; 2 Two or more races, non-Hispanic/Latino). Average age 28. 56 applicants, 71% accepted, 24 enrolled. In 2015, 31 master's awarded. *Expenses: Tuition, area resident:* Full-time $31,068; part-time $5762 per course. *Required fees:* $3200; $336 per course. Full-time tuition and fees vary according to degree level, program and student level. Part-time tuition and fees vary according to course load, degree level and program.

University of Pittsburgh, School of Nursing, Nurse Practitioner Program, Pittsburgh, PA 15261. Offers adult-gerontology acute care (DNP); adult-gerontology primary care (DNP); family (individual across the lifespan) (DNP); neonatal (MSN, DNP); pediatric primary care (DNP); psychiatric mental health (DNP). *Accreditation:* AACN. *Program availability:* Part-time. *Students:* 74 full-time (65 women), 59 part-time (51 women); includes 14 minority (5 Black or African American, non-Hispanic/Latino; 2 American Indian or Alaska Native, non-Hispanic/Latino; 6 Asian, non-Hispanic/Latino; 1 Hispanic/Latino). Average age 30. 65 applicants, 55% accepted, 28 enrolled. In 2015, 14 master's, 19 doctorates awarded. *Degree requirements:* For master's, comprehensive exam, thesis optional. *Entrance requirements:* For master's, GRE General Test or MAT, BSN, RN license, letters of recommendation, resume, course work in statistics, 1-3 years of nursing experience; for doctorate, GRE General Test, BSN, RN license, minimum GPA of 3.5, 3 letters of recommendation. Additional exam requirements/recommendations for international students: Required—TOEFL (minimum score 600 paper-based; 100 iBT). *Application deadline:* For fall admission, 5/1 priority date for domestic students, 2/15 priority date for international students. Application fee: $50. Electronic applications accepted. *Expenses:* Contact institution. *Financial support:* In 2015–16, 16 students received support, including 7 fellowships with tuition reimbursements available (averaging $11,278 per year), 9 teaching assistantships with tuition reimbursements available (averaging $10,879 per year); scholarships/grants, traineeships, health care benefits, and unspecified assistantships also available. Support available to part-time students. Financial award application deadline: 3/15. *Faculty research:* Behavioral management of chronic disorders, patient management in critical care, consumer informatics, genetic applications (molecular genetics and psychosocial implications), technology for nurses and patients to improve care. *Unit head:* Dr. Sandra Engberg, Associate Dean for Clinical Education, 412-624-3835, Fax: 412-624-8521, E-mail: sje1@pitt.edu. *Application contact:* Laurie Lapsley, Administrator of Graduate Student Services, 412-624-9670, Fax: 412-624-2409, E-mail: lapsleyl@pitt.edu.
Website: http://www.nursing.pitt.edu

University of Puerto Rico, Medical Sciences Campus, School of Nursing, San Juan, PR 00936-5067. Offers adult and elderly nursing (MSN); child and adolescent nursing (MSN); critical care nursing (MSN); family and community nursing (MSN); family nurse practitioner (MSN); maternity nursing (MSN); mental health and psychiatric nursing (MSN). *Accreditation:* AACN. *Entrance requirements:* For master's, GRE or EXADEP, interview, Puerto Rico RN license or professional license for international students, general and specific point average, article analysis. Electronic applications accepted. *Faculty research:* HIV, health disparities, teen violence, women and violence, neurological disorders.

University of Rhode Island, Graduate School, College of Nursing, Kingston, RI 02881. Offers acute care nurse practitioner (MS); adult-gerontological nurse practitioner/clinical nurse specialist (MS); family nurse practitioner (MS); nursing (PhD); nursing education (MS); nursing practice (DNP). *Accreditation:* AACN; ACNM/ACME (one or more programs are accredited). *Program availability:* Part-time. *Faculty:* 11 full-time (all women). *Students:* 51 full-time (41 women), 77 part-time (70 women); includes 18 minority (11 Black or African American, non-Hispanic/Latino; 2 Asian, non-Hispanic/Latino; 4 Hispanic/Latino; 1 Two or more races, non-Hispanic/Latino), 5 international. In 2015, 19 master's, 7 doctorates awarded. *Degree requirements:* For master's, comprehensive exam; for doctorate, comprehensive exam, thesis/dissertation. *Entrance requirements:* For master's, GRE or MAT, 2 letters of recommendation, scholarly papers; for doctorate, GRE, 3 letters of recommendation, scholarly papers. Additional exam requirements/recommendations for international students: Required—TOEFL (minimum score 550 paper-based). *Application deadline:* For fall admission, 2/15 for domestic students, 2/1 for international students; for spring admission, 10/15 for domestic students, 7/15 for international students. Application fee: $65. Electronic applications accepted. *Expenses:* Tuition, state resident: full-time $11,796; part-time $655 per credit. Tuition, nonresident: full-time $24,206; part-time $1345 per credit. *Required fees:* $1546; $44 per credit. One-time fee: $155 full-time; $35 part-time. *Financial support:* In 2015–16, 2 research assistantships (averaging $12,111 per year), 7 teaching assistantships with tuition reimbursements (averaging $13,112 per year) were awarded. Financial award application deadline: 2/15; financial award applicants required to submit FAFSA. *Faculty research:* Group intervention for grieving women in prison, translating best practice in non-drug interventions for postoperative pain management, further development and testing of the pain assessment inventory, preschool motor and functional performance of two cohorts, neuroactivation of brain motor areas in preterm children. *Unit head:* Dr. Mary Sullivan, Interim Dean, 401-874-5339, Fax: 401-874-2061, E-mail: mcsullivan@uri.edu. *Application contact:* Graduate Admission, 401-874-2872, E-mail: gradadm@etal.uri.edu.
Website: http://www.uri.edu/nursing/

University of Rochester, School of Nursing, Rochester, NY 14642. Offers adult gerontological acute care nurse practitioner (MS); clinical nurse leader (MS); family nurse practitioner (MS); family psychiatric mental health nurse practitioner (MS); health care organization management and leadership (MS); health practice research (PhD); nursing (DNP); nursing education (MS); pediatric nurse practitioner (MS); pediatric nurse practitioner/neonatal nurse practitioner (MS). *Accreditation:* AACN. *Program availability:* Part-time, online learning. *Faculty:* 56 full-time (45 women), 63 part-time/adjunct (55 women). *Students:* 21 full-time (20 women), 212 part-time (175 women); includes 35 minority (12 Black or African American, non-Hispanic/Latino; 1 American Indian or Alaska Native, non-Hispanic/Latino; 10 Asian, non-Hispanic/Latino; 7 Hispanic/Latino; 5 Two or more races, non-Hispanic/Latino), 2 international. Average age 35. 111 applicants, 68% accepted, 71 enrolled. In 2015, 52 master's, 9 doctorates awarded. Terminal master's awarded for partial completion of doctoral program. *Degree*

requirements: For master's, comprehensive exam (for some programs); for doctorate, thesis/dissertation. *Entrance requirements:* For master's, BS in nursing, minimum GPA of 3.0, course work in statistics; for doctorate, GRE General Test (for PhD), MS in nursing, minimum GPA of 3.5. Additional exam requirements/recommendations for international students: Required—TOEFL (minimum score 560 paper-based; 88 iBT) or IELTS (minimum score 6.5) recommended. *Application deadline:* For fall admission, 4/1 for domestic and international students; for spring admission, 9/1 for domestic and international students; for summer admission, 1/2 for domestic and international students. Application fee: $50. Electronic applications accepted. *Expenses: Tuition, area resident:* Full-time $47,450; part-time $1482 per credit hour. *Required fees:* $528. Tuition and fees vary according to program. *Financial support:* In 2015–16, 52 students received support, including 2 fellowships with tuition reimbursements available (averaging $30,000 per year); scholarships/grants, traineeships, health care benefits, tuition waivers (full and partial), and unspecified assistantships also available. Support available to part-time students. Financial award application deadline: 6/30. *Faculty research:* Symptom assessment and self-management of chronic illness, health promotion and illness prevention, nursing intervention research with vulnerable populations, palliative care, aging. *Total annual research expenditures:* $2.1 million. *Unit head:* Dr. Kathy H. Rideout, Dean, 585-273-8902, Fax: 585-273-1268, E-mail: kathy_rideout@urmc.rochester.edu. *Application contact:* Elaine Andolina, Director of Admissions, 585-275-2375, Fax: 585-756-8299, E-mail: elaine_andolina@urmc.rochester.edu.
Website: http://www.son.rochester.edu

University of South Africa, College of Human Sciences, Pretoria, South Africa. Offers adult education (M Ed); African languages (MA, PhD); African politics (MA, PhD); Afrikaans (MA, PhD); ancient history (MA, PhD); ancient Near Eastern studies (MA, PhD); anthropology (MA, PhD); applied linguistics (MA); Arabic (MA, PhD); archaeology (MA); art history (MA); Biblical archaeology (MA); Biblical studies (M Th, D Th, PhD); Christian spirituality (M Th, D Th); church history (M Th, D Th); classical studies (MA, PhD); clinical psychology (MA); communication (MA, PhD); comparative education (M Ed, Ed D); consulting psychology (D Admin, D Com, PhD); curriculum studies (M Ed, Ed D); development studies (M Admin, MA, D Admin, PhD); didactics (M Ed, Ed D); education (M Tech); education management (M Ed, Ed D); educational psychology (M Ed); English (MA); environmental education (M Ed); French (MA, PhD); German (MA, PhD); Greek (MA); guidance and counseling (M Ed); health studies (MA, PhD), including health sciences education (MA), health services management (MA), medical and surgical nursing science (critical care general) (MA), midwifery and neonatal nursing science (MA), trauma and emergency care (MA); history (MA, PhD); history of education (Ed D); inclusive education (M Ed, Ed D); information and communications technology policy and regulation (MA); information science (MA, MIS, PhD); international politics (MA, PhD); Islamic studies (MA, PhD); Italian (MA, PhD); Judaica (MA, PhD); linguistics (MA, PhD); mathematical education (M Ed); mathematics education (MA); missiology (M Th, D Th); modern Hebrew (MA, PhD); musicology (MA, MMus, D Mus, PhD); natural science education (M Ed); New Testament (M Th, D Th); Old Testament (D Th); pastoral therapy (M Th, D Th); philosophy (MA); philosophy of education (M Ed, Ed D); politics (MA, PhD); Portuguese (MA, PhD); practical theology (M Th, D Th); psychology (MA, MS, PhD); psychology of education (M Ed, Ed D); public health (MA); religious studies (MA, D Th, PhD); Romance languages (MA); Russian (MA, PhD); Semitic languages (MA, PhD); social behavior studies in HIV/AIDS (MA); social science (mental health) (MA); social science in development studies (MA); social science in psychology (MA); social science in social work (MA); social science in sociology (MA); social work (MSW, DSW, PhD); socio-education (M Ed, Ed D); sociolinguistics (MA); sociology (MA, PhD); Spanish (MA, PhD); systematic theology (M Th, D Th); TESOL (teaching English to speakers of other languages) (MA); theological ethics (M Th, D Th); theory of literature (MA, PhD); urban ministries (D Th); urban ministry (M Th).

University of South Carolina, The Graduate School, College of Nursing, Program in Advanced Practice Clinical Nursing, Columbia, SC 29208. Offers acute care nurse practitioner (Certificate); advanced practice clinical nursing (MSN). *Accreditation:* AACN. *Program availability:* Part-time, online learning. *Entrance requirements:* For master's, master's degree in nursing, RN license; for Certificate, MSN. Additional exam requirements/recommendations for international students: Required—TOEFL (minimum score 570 paper-based). Electronic applications accepted. *Faculty research:* Systems research, evidence based practice, breast cancer, violence.

University of South Carolina, The Graduate School, College of Nursing, Program in Clinical Nursing, Columbia, SC 29208. Offers acute care clinical specialist (MSN); acute care nurse practitioner (MSN); women's health nurse practitioner (MSN). *Accreditation:* AACN. *Program availability:* Part-time. *Degree requirements:* For master's, thesis or alternative. *Entrance requirements:* For master's, GRE General Test or MAT, BS in nursing, RN licensure. Additional exam requirements/recommendations for international students: Required—TOEFL (minimum score 570 paper-based). Electronic applications accepted. *Faculty research:* Systems research, evidence based practice, breast cancer, violence.

University of South Florida, College of Nursing, Tampa, FL 33612. Offers advanced pain management (Graduate Certificate); nursing (MS, DNP), including adult gerontology acute care (DNP), adult gerontology acute care nursing (MS), adult gerontology primary care (DNP), adult gerontology primary care nursing (MS), adult gerontology primary care/occupational health nursing (MS), adult gerontology primary care/oncology nursing (MS), clinical nurse leader (MS), family health nursing, nurse anesthesia (MS), nursing education (MS), nursing practice (DNP), occupational health/adult-gerontology (DNP), oncology/adult-gerontology primary care (DNP), pediatric health (DNP), pediatric nurse practitioner (MS); nursing education (Post Master's Certificate); nursing science (PhD). *Accreditation:* AACN; AANA/CANAEP. *Program availability:* Part-time. *Faculty:* 43 full-time (38 women), 7 part-time/adjunct (4 women). *Students:* 159 full-time (135 women), 721 part-time (625 women); includes 292 minority (119 Black or African American, non-Hispanic/Latino; 2 American Indian or Alaska Native, non-Hispanic/Latino; 60 Asian, non-Hispanic/Latino; 90 Hispanic/Latino; 1 Native Hawaiian or other Pacific Islander, non-Hispanic/Latino; 20 Two or more races, non-Hispanic/Latino), 12 international. Average age 35. 636 applicants, 44% accepted, 215 enrolled. In 2015, 333 master's, 18 doctorates awarded. *Degree requirements:* For master's, comprehensive exam, thesis optional; for doctorate, comprehensive exam, thesis/dissertation. *Entrance requirements:* For master's, GRE General Test, bachelor's degree from accredited program with minimum GPA of 3.0 in all upper-division coursework; current license as Registered Nurse; 3 letters of recommendation; personal statement of goals; resume or curriculum vitae; personal interview; for doctorate, GRE General Test (recommended), bachelor's degree in nursing from a CCNA/NLNAC regionally-accredited institution with minimum GPA of 3.0 in all coursework or in all upper-division coursework; current license as Registered Nurse in Florida; undergraduate statistics course with minimum B grade; 3 letters of recommendation; statement of goals; resume; interview. Additional exam requirements/recommendations for international students: Required—TOEFL (minimum score 550 paper-based; 79 iBT). *Application deadline:* For fall admission, 2/15 for domestic students, 1/2 for international students; for spring admission, 10/1 for domestic students, 6/1 for international students. Application fee: $30. Electronic applications accepted. *Financial support:* In 2015–16, 36 students received support, including 7 research assistantships with tuition

reimbursements available (averaging $18,935 per year), 29 teaching assistantships with tuition reimbursements available (averaging $30,814 per year); tuition waivers (partial) and unspecified assistantships also available. Financial award application deadline: 2/1; financial award applicants required to submit FAFSA. *Faculty research:* Women's health, palliative and end-of-life care, cardiac rehabilitation, complementary therapies for chronic illness and cancer. *Total annual research expenditures:* $2.6 million. *Unit head:* Dr. Dianne C. Morrison-Beedy, Dean and Professor, College of Nursing, 813-974-9091, Fax: 813-974-5418, E-mail: dmbeedy@health.usf.edu. *Application contact:* Dr. Brian Graves, Assistant Professor/Assistant Dean, 813-974-8054, Fax: 813-974-5418, E-mail: bgraves1@health.usf.edu.
Website: http://health.usf.edu/nursing/index.htm

The University of Texas Health Science Center at San Antonio, School of Nursing, San Antonio, TX 78229-3900. Offers administrative management (MSN); adult-gerontology acute care nurse practitioner (PGC); advanced practice leadership (DNP); clinical nurse leader (MSN); executive administrative management (DNP); family nurse practitioner (MSN, PGC); nursing (MSN, PhD); nursing education (MSN, PGC); pediatric nurse practitioner primary care (PGC); psychiatric mental health nurse practitioner (PGC); public health nurse leader (DNP). *Accreditation:* AACN. *Program availability:* Part-time. Terminal master's awarded for partial completion of doctoral program. *Degree requirements:* For master's, thesis optional; for doctorate, comprehensive exam, thesis/ dissertation.

University of Virginia, School of Nursing, Charlottesville, VA 22903. Offers acute and specialty care (MSN); acute care nurse practitioner (MSN); clinical nurse leadership (MSN); community-public health leadership (MSN); nursing (DNP, PhD); psychiatric mental health counseling (MSN); MSN/MBA. *Accreditation:* AACN. *Program availability:* Part-time. *Degree requirements:* For doctorate, comprehensive exam (for some programs), capstone project (DNP), dissertation (PhD). *Entrance requirements:* For master's, GRE General Test, MAT; for doctorate, GRE General Test. Additional exam requirements/recommendations for international students: Required—TOEFL, IELTS. Electronic applications accepted. *Expenses:* Contact institution.

Vanderbilt University, Vanderbilt University School of Nursing, Nashville, TN 37240. Offers adult-gerontology acute care nurse practitioner (MSN), including hospitalist, intensivist; adult-gerontology primary care nurse practitioner (MSN); emergency nurse practitioner (MSN); family nurse practitioner (MSN); healthcare leadership (MSN); neonatal nurse practitioner (MSN); nurse midwifery (MSN); nurse midwifery/family nurse practitioner (MSN); nursing (Post-Master's Certificate); nursing informatics (MSN); nursing practice (DNP); nursing science (PhD); pediatric acute care nurse practitioner (MSN); pediatric primary care nurse practitioner (MSN); psychiatric-mental health nurse practitioner (MSN); women's health nurse practitioner (MSN); women's health nurse practitioner/adult gerontology primary care nurse practitioner (MSN); MSN/M Div; MSN/ MTS. *Accreditation:* ACEN (one or more programs are accredited); ACNM/ACME. *Program availability:* Part-time, 100% online, blended/hybrid learning. *Faculty:* 258 full-time (232 women), 363 part-time/adjunct (271 women). *Students:* 478 full-time (424 women), 342 part-time (317 women); includes 140 minority (36 Black or African American, non-Hispanic/Latino; 3 American Indian or Alaska Native, non-Hispanic/ Latino; 24 Asian, non-Hispanic/Latino; 43 Hispanic/Latino; 3 Native Hawaiian or other Pacific Islander, non-Hispanic/Latino; 31 Two or more races, non-Hispanic/Latino), 11 international. Average age 31. 1,268 applicants, 49% accepted, 477 enrolled. In 2015, 343 master's, 55 doctorates awarded. *Degree requirements:* For doctorate, comprehensive exam, thesis/dissertation. *Entrance requirements:* For master's, GRE General Test (taken within the past 5 years), minimum B average in undergraduate course work, 3 letters of recommendation; for doctorate, GRE General Test, interview, 3 letters of recommendation from doctorally-prepared faculty, MSN, essay. Additional exam requirements/recommendations for international students: Required—TOEFL (minimum score 570 paper-based), IELTS (minimum score 6.5). *Application deadline:* For fall admission, 11/1 priority date for domestic and international students. Applications are processed on a rolling basis. Application fee: $50. Electronic applications accepted. *Expenses:* Contact institution. *Financial support:* In 2015–16, 585 students received support. Scholarships/grants available. Financial award application deadline: 3/15; financial award applicants required to submit FAFSA. *Faculty research:* Lymphedema, palliative care and bereavement, health services research including workforce, safety and quality of care, gerontology, better birth outcomes including nutrition. *Total annual research expenditures:* $2 million. *Unit head:* Dr. Linda Norman, Dean, 615-343-8876, Fax: 615-343-7711, E-mail: linda.norman@vanderbilt.edu. *Application contact:* Patricia Peerman, Assistant Dean for Enrollment Management, 615-322-3800, Fax: 615-343-0333, E-mail: vusn-admissions@vanderbilt.edu.
Website: http://www.nursing.vanderbilt.edu

Wayne State University, College of Nursing, Doctor Program of Nursing Practice, Detroit, MI 48202. Offers adult gerontology nurse practitioner - acute care (DNP); adult gerontology nurse practitioner - primary care (DNP); family nurse practitioner (DNP); infant mental health (DNP); neonatal nurse practitioner (DNP); nurse midwifery (DNP); nursing practice (DNP); pediatric nurse practitioner - acute care (DNP); pediatric nurse practitioner - primary care (DNP); psychiatric mental health nurse practitioner (DNP). *Students:* 56 full-time (50 women), 37 part-time (32 women); includes 32 minority (19 Black or African American, non-Hispanic/Latino; 6 Asian, non-Hispanic/Latino; 3 Hispanic/Latino; 4 Two or more races, non-Hispanic/Latino), 6 international. Average age 35. 44 applicants, 66% accepted, 18 enrolled. In 2015, 16 doctorates awarded. *Entrance requirements:* For doctorate, official transcripts, two professional references, curriculum vitae or resume, statement of goals, BSN or MSN, current Michigan RN license, criminal background check, interview, on-site writing example. Additional exam requirements/recommendations for international students: Required—TOEFL (minimum score 600 paper-based; 101 iBT); Recommended—IELTS (minimum score 7). *Application deadline:* For fall admission, 1/31 for domestic and international students. Electronic applications accepted. *Expenses:* $19,325 per year resident tuition, $35,114 non-resident tuition; $805.20 per credit hour resident tuition, $1,463.10 per credit hour non-resident tuition; fees include $47.45 per credit hour student services fee and $274.60 per semester registration fee. *Financial support:* In 2015–16, 22 students received support. Fellowships, research assistantships, teaching assistantships, institutionally sponsored loans, and scholarships/grants available. Financial award applicants required to submit FAFSA. *Unit head:* Dr. Laurie Lauzon Clabo, Dean and Professor, 313 577-4104, E-mail: laurie.lauzon.clabo@wayne.edu. *Application contact:* Dr. Nancy George, Director of DNP Program, 313-577-8300.
Website: http://nursing.wayne.edu/dnp/index.php

Wayne State University, College of Nursing, Graduate Certificates Program in Clinical Specialties, Detroit, MI 48202. Offers acute care nurse practitioner (Graduate Certificate); nurse midwifery (Graduate Certificate); pediatric nurse practitioner - acute care (Graduate Certificate); pediatric nurse practitioner - primary care (Graduate Certificate); psychiatric mental health nurse practitioner (Graduate Certificate). *Accreditation:* AACN. *Program availability:* Part-time. *Students:* 2 full-time (both women), 7 part-time (all women). Average age 43. 67 applicants, 12% accepted, 5 enrolled. *Entrance requirements:* For degree, master's or doctoral degree in nursing from nationally-accredited institution, current RN license, three letters of reference, personal statement. Additional exam requirements/recommendations for international students: Required—TOEFL (minimum score 600 paper-based; 101 iBT), TWE, Michigan English Language Assessment Battery (minimum score 85); Recommended—IELTS (minimum score 7). *Application deadline:* For fall admission, 6/1 priority date for domestic students, 5/1 priority date for international students; for winter admission, 10/1 priority date for domestic students, 9/1 priority date for international students; for spring admission, 2/1 priority date for domestic students, 1/1 priority date for international students. Application fee: $0. Electronic applications accepted. *Expenses:* $19,325 annual resident tuition, $35,114 non-resident tuition; $805.20 per credit hour resident tuition, $1,463.10 per credit hour non-resident tuition; fees include $47.45 per credit hour student services fee and $274.60 per semester registration fee. *Financial support:* Scholarships/grants available. Financial award application deadline: 3/31; financial award applicants required to submit FAFSA. *Unit head:* Dr. Laurie Lauzon Clabo, Dean and Professor, 313-577-4104, E-mail: laurie.lauzon.clabo@wayne.edu. *Application contact:* Leanne Nantais-Smith, Director, MSN Program and Graduate Certificates, E-mail: ar2446@wayne.edu.
Website: http://nursing.wayne.edu/gradcert/specialties.php

Wright State University, School of Graduate Studies, College of Nursing and Health, Program in Nursing, Dayton, OH 45435. Offers acute care nurse practitioner (MS); administration of nursing and health care systems (MS); adult health (MS); child and adolescent health (MS); community health (MS); family nurse practitioner (MS); nurse practitioner (MS); school nurse (MS); MBA/MS. *Accreditation:* AACN. *Program availability:* Part-time, evening/weekend. *Degree requirements:* For master's, thesis or alternative. *Entrance requirements:* For master's, GRE General Test, BSN from NLN-accredited college, Ohio RN license. Additional exam requirements/recommendations for international students: Required—TOEFL. *Faculty research:* Clinical nursing and health, teaching, caring, pain administration, informatics and technology.

Adult Nursing

Adelphi University, College of Nursing and Public Health, Program in Adult Health Nurse, Garden City, NY 11530-0701. Offers MS.

Allen College, Graduate Programs, Waterloo, IA 50703. Offers acute care nurse practitioner (Post-Master's Certificate); adult nurse practitioner (Post-Master's Certificate); adult psychiatric-mental health nurse practitioner (Post-Master's Certificate); adult-gerontology acute care nurse practitioner (MSN); community public health (Post-Master's Certificate); community/public health nursing (MSN); family nurse practitioner (MSN, Post-Master's Certificate); gerontological nurse practitioner (Post-Master's Certificate); health sciences (Ed D); leadership in health care delivery (MSN, Post-Master's Certificate); nursing (DNP); occupational therapy (MS). *Accreditation:* AACN; ACEN. *Program availability:* Part-time, blended/hybrid learning. *Faculty:* 3 full-time (all women), 21 part-time/adjunct (20 women). *Students:* 61 full-time (54 women), 163 part-time (144 women); includes 9 minority (5 Black or African American, non-Hispanic/ Latino; 2 Hispanic/Latino; 2 Two or more races, non-Hispanic/Latino), 2 international. Average age 34. 212 applicants, 60% accepted, 94 enrolled. In 2015, 51 master's, 1 doctorate awarded. *Degree requirements:* For master's, thesis optional. *Entrance requirements:* For master's, minimum GPA of 3.0 in the last 60 hours of undergraduate coursework; for doctorate, minimum GPA of 3.25 in graduate coursework. Additional exam requirements/recommendations for international students: Recommended—TOEFL (minimum score 500 paper-based; 92 iBT), IELTS (minimum score 6). *Application deadline:* For fall admission, 2/1 priority date for domestic students; for spring admission, 9/1 priority date for domestic students. Applications are processed on a rolling basis. Application fee: $50. Electronic applications accepted. *Expenses:* $15,940 tuition, $1,240 fees. *Financial support:* Institutionally sponsored loans, scholarships/grants, and traineeships available. Support available to part-time students. Financial award application deadline: 8/15; financial award applicants required to submit FAFSA. *Unit head:* Nancy Kramer, Vice Chancellor for Academic Affairs, 319-226-2040, Fax: 319-226-2070, E-mail: nancy.kramer@allencollege.edu. *Application contact:* Molly Quinn, Administrative Assistant for Student Services, 319-226-2014, Fax: 319-226-2010, E-mail: admissions@allencollege.edu.
Website: http://www.allencollege.edu/

Armstrong State University, School of Graduate Studies, Program in Nursing, Savannah, GA 31419-1997. Offers adult-gerontological acute care nurse practitioner (Certificate); adult-gerontological clinical nurse specialist (Certificate); adult-gerontological primary care nurse practitioner (Certificate); family nurse practitioner (MSN). *Accreditation:* AACN. *Program availability:* Part-time, evening/weekend. *Faculty:* 5 full-time (all women), 1 (woman) part-time/adjunct. *Students:* 35 full-time (32 women), 19 part-time (16 women); includes 13 minority (10 Black or African American, non-Hispanic/Latino; 2 Hispanic/Latino; 1 Two or more races, non-Hispanic/Latino), 1 international. Average age 35. 23 applicants, 83% accepted, 16 enrolled. In 2015, 19 master's awarded. *Degree requirements:* For master's, comprehensive exam, project or thesis. *Entrance requirements:* For master's, GRE General Test or MAT, minimum GPA of 3.0, letter of recommendation, letter of intent. Additional exam requirements/ recommendations for international students: Required—TOEFL (minimum score 523 paper-based; 70 iBT). *Application deadline:* For fall admission, 2/28 for domestic and international students; for spring admission, 11/15 for domestic students, 9/15 for international students. Applications are processed on a rolling basis. Application fee: $30. Electronic applications accepted. *Expenses:* Tuition, state resident: part-time $211 per credit hour. Tuition, nonresident: part-time $782 per credit hour. *Required fees:* $1224 per unit. $612 per semester. Tuition and fees vary according to course load, campus/location and program. *Financial support:* In 2015–16, research assistantships with full tuition reimbursements (averaging $5,000 per year) were awarded; Federal Work-Study, scholarships/grants, and unspecified assistantships also available. Support available to part-time students. Financial award application deadline: 3/1; financial award applicants required to submit FAFSA. *Faculty research:* Midwifery, mental health, nursing simulation, smoking cessation during pregnancy, asthma education, vulnerable

Adult Nursing

populations, geriatrics, disaster nursing, complementary and alternative modalities, nephrology. *Unit head:* Dr. Catherine Gilbert, Department Head, 912-344-3145, E-mail: catherine.gilbert@armstrong.edu. *Application contact:* McKenzie Peterman, Assistant Director of Graduate Admissions, 912-344-2503, Fax: 912-344-3417, E-mail: graduate@armstrong.edu.
Website: http://www.armstrong.edu/Health_professions/nursing/nursing_graduate_programs

Bloomsburg University of Pennsylvania, School of Graduate Studies, College of Science and Technology, Department of Nursing, Bloomsburg, PA 17815. Offers adult and family nurse practitioner (MSN); community health (MSN); nurse anesthesia (MSN); nursing (MSN); nursing administration (MSN). *Accreditation:* AACN; AANA/CANAEP. *Degree requirements:* For master's, thesis (for some programs), clinical experience. *Entrance requirements:* For master's, minimum QPA of 3.0, personal statement, 2 letters of recommendation, nursing license. Additional exam requirements/recommendations for international students: Required—TOEFL. Electronic applications accepted.

Boston College, William F. Connell School of Nursing, Chestnut Hill, MA 02467. Offers adult-gerontology nursing (MS); family health nursing (MS); forensic nursing (MS); nurse anesthesia (MS); nursing (PhD); pediatric nursing (MS), including pediatric and women's health; psychiatric-mental health nursing (MS); women's health nursing (MS); MBA/MS; MS/MA; MS/PhD. *Accreditation:* AACN; AANA/CANAEP (one or more programs are accredited). *Program availability:* Part-time. *Faculty:* 53 full-time (48 women), 47 part-time/adjunct (44 women). *Students:* 185 full-time (167 women), 66 part-time (56 women); includes 31 minority (10 Black or African American, non-Hispanic/Latino; 12 Asian, non-Hispanic/Latino; 7 Hispanic/Latino; 2 Two or more races, non-Hispanic/Latino), 7 international. Average age 32. 313 applicants, 66% accepted, 91 enrolled. In 2015, 98 master's, 5 doctorates awarded. *Degree requirements:* For master's, comprehensive exam; for doctorate, comprehensive exam, thesis/dissertation, computer literacy exam or foreign language. *Entrance requirements:* For master's, bachelor's degree in nursing; for doctorate, GRE General Test, MS in nursing. *Application deadline:* For fall admission, 9/30 for domestic and international students; for winter admission, 1/15 for domestic and international students; for spring admission, 3/15 for domestic and international students. Applications are processed on a rolling basis. Application fee: $40. Electronic applications accepted. *Expenses:* Contact institution. *Financial support:* In 2015–16, 1 fellowship with full tuition reimbursement (averaging $23,700 per year), 25 teaching assistantships (averaging $4,370 per year) were awarded; research assistantships, scholarships/grants, health care benefits, tuition waivers (partial), and unspecified assistantships also available. Support available to part-time students. Financial award application deadline: 3/1; financial award applicants required to submit FAFSA. *Faculty research:* Sexual and reproductive health, health promotion/illness prevention, aging, eating disorders, symptom management. *Total annual research expenditures:* $1 million. *Unit head:* Dr. Susan Gennaro, Dean, 617-552-4251, Fax: 617-552-0931, E-mail: susan.gennaro@bc.edu. *Application contact:* MaryBeth Crowley, Graduate Programs Assistant, 617-552-4928, Fax: 617-552-2121, E-mail: csongrad@bc.edu.
Website: http://www.bc.edu/schools/son/

California Baptist University, Program in Nursing, Riverside, CA 92504-3206. Offers clinical nurse specialist (MSN); family nurse practitioner (MSN); healthcare systems management (MSN); teaching-learning (MSN). *Program availability:* Part-time. *Faculty:* 18 full-time (17 women), 14 part-time/adjunct (11 women). *Students:* 77 full-time (63 women), 143 part-time (117 women); includes 111 minority (26 Black or African American, non-Hispanic/Latino; 3 American Indian or Alaska Native, non-Hispanic/Latino; 38 Asian, non-Hispanic/Latino; 39 Hispanic/Latino; 1 Native Hawaiian or other Pacific Islander, non-Hispanic/Latino; 4 Two or more races, non-Hispanic/Latino), 5 international. Average age 33. 44 applicants, 64% accepted, 23 enrolled. In 2015, 19 master's awarded. *Degree requirements:* For master's, comprehensive exam or directed project thesis; capstone practicum. *Entrance requirements:* For master's, GRE or California Critical Thinking Skills Test; Test of Essential Academic Skills (TEAS), minimum undergraduate GPA of 3.0; completion of prerequisite courses with minimum grade of C; CPR certification; background check clearance; health clearance; drug testing; proof of health insurance; proof of motor vehicle insurance; three letters of recommendation; 1000-word essay; interview. Additional exam requirements/recommendations for international students: Required—TOEFL (minimum score 80 iBT). *Application deadline:* For fall admission, 8/1 priority date for domestic students, 7/1 for international students; for spring admission, 12/1 priority date for domestic students, 11/1 for international students. Applications are processed on a rolling basis. Application fee: $45. Electronic applications accepted. *Expenses:* $742 per unit, $355 per semester fees. *Financial support:* Federal Work-Study and scholarships/grants available. Financial award applicants required to submit CSS PROFILE or FAFSA. *Faculty research:* Qualitative research using Parse methodology, gerontology, disaster preparedness, medical-surgical nursing, maternal-child nursing. *Unit head:* Dr. Geneva Oaks, Dean, School of Nursing, 951-343-4702, E-mail: goaks@calbaptist.edu. *Application contact:* Dr. Rebecca Meyer, Director, Graduate Program in Nursing, 951-343-4952, Fax: 951-343-5095, E-mail: rmeyer@calbaptist.edu.
Website: http://www.calbaptist.edu/explore-cbu/schools-colleges/school-nursing/master-science-nursing/

Clarkson College, Master of Science in Nursing Program, Omaha, NE 68131. Offers adult nurse practitioner (MSN, Post-Master's Certificate); family nurse practitioner (MSN, Post-Master's Certificate); nursing education (MSN, Post-Master's Certificate); nursing health care leadership (MSN, Post-Master's Certificate). *Accreditation:* AANA/CANAEP; ACEN. *Program availability:* Part-time, evening/weekend, online learning. *Degree requirements:* For master's, on-campus skills assessment (family nurse practitioner, adult nurse practitioner), comprehensive exam or thesis. *Entrance requirements:* For master's, minimum GPA of 3.0, 2 references, resume. Additional exam requirements/recommendations for international students: Required—TOEFL (minimum score 600 paper-based; 100 iBT). Electronic applications accepted.

College of Mount Saint Vincent, School of Professional and Continuing Studies, Department of Nursing, Riverdale, NY 10471-1093. Offers adult nurse practitioner (MSN, PMC); family nurse practitioner (MSN, PMC); nurse educator (PMC); nursing administration (MSN); nursing for the adult and aged (MSN). *Accreditation:* AACN. *Program availability:* Part-time. *Entrance requirements:* For master's, BSN, interview, RN license, minimum GPA of 3.0, letters of reference. Additional exam requirements/recommendations for international students: Required—TOEFL. *Expenses:* Contact institution.

College of Staten Island of the City University of New York, Graduate Programs, School of Health Sciences, Program in Adult-Gerontological Nursing, Staten Island, NY 10314-6600. Offers clinical nurse practitioner (MS, Advanced Certificate); clinical nurse specialist (MS, Advanced Certificate). *Program availability:* Part-time, evening/weekend. *Faculty:* 5 full-time, 7 part-time/adjunct. *Students:* Average age 38. In 2015, 18 master's, 4 other advanced degrees awarded. *Degree requirements:* For master's, thesis optional. *Entrance requirements:* For master's, bachelor's degree in nursing with minimum GPA

of 3.0 in nursing major, two letters of recommendation, personal statement, current New York State RN license, minimum of one year of full-time experience as a registered nurse; for Advanced Certificate, master's degree in nursing; master's-level courses in pathophysiology, health assessment and pharmacology. Additional exam requirements/recommendations for international students: Required—TOEFL (minimum score 550 paper-based; 79 iBT), IELTS (minimum score 6.5). *Application deadline:* For spring admission, 10/15 priority date for domestic and international students. Applications are processed on a rolling basis. Application fee: $125. Electronic applications accepted. *Expenses:* Tuition, state resident: full-time $10,130; part-time $425 per credit. Tuition, nonresident: full-time $18,720; part-time $780 per credit. *Required fees:* $181.10 per semester. Tuition and fees vary according to program. *Financial support:* Applicants required to submit FAFSA. *Faculty research:* Cardiac, health literacy, role stress, cancer survivorship, older adults and end of life: decision making, dying, palliative, and hospice care. *Unit head:* Dr. June Como, Graduate and Clinical Doctorate in Nursing Practice Programs Coordinator, 718-982-3823, Fax: 718-982-3813, E-mail: june.como@csi.cuny.edu. *Application contact:* Sasha Spence, Associate Director for Graduate Admissions, 718-982-2019, Fax: 718-982-2500, E-mail: sasha.spence@csi.cuny.edu.
Website: http://www.csi.cuny.edu/nursing/graduate.html

Columbia University, School of Nursing, Program in Adult-Gerontology Primary Care Nurse Practitioner, New York, NY 10032. Offers MS, Adv C. *Accreditation:* AACN. *Program availability:* Part-time. *Entrance requirements:* For master's, GRE General Test, NCLEX, BSN, 1 year of clinical experience (preferred); for Adv C, MSN. Additional exam requirements/recommendations for international students: Required—TOEFL (minimum score 100 iBT). Electronic applications accepted.

Creighton University, College of Nursing, Omaha, NE 68178-0001. Offers adult acute care nurse practitioner (Post-Master's Certificate); adult gerontology acute care nurse practitioner (DNP); adult gerontology nurse practitioner (DNP); clinical nurse leader (MSN, Post-Graduate Certificate); clinical systems administration (MSN, DNP); family nurse practitioner (DNP, Post-Master's Certificate); neonatal nurse practitioner (DNP, Post-Master's Certificate); pediatric acute care nurse practitioner (DNP, Post-Master's Certificate); psychiatric mental health nurse practitioner (DNP). *Accreditation:* AACN. *Program availability:* Part-time, blended/hybrid learning. *Faculty:* 10 full-time (all women), 48 part-time/adjunct (45 women). *Students:* 132 full-time (120 women), 228 part-time (212 women); includes 38 minority (10 Black or African American, non-Hispanic/Latino; 3 American Indian or Alaska Native, non-Hispanic/Latino; 11 Asian, non-Hispanic/Latino; 1 Hispanic/Latino; 2 Native Hawaiian or other Pacific Islander, non-Hispanic/Latino; 11 Two or more races, non-Hispanic/Latino). Average age 31. 66 applicants, 91% accepted, 43 enrolled. In 2015, 54 master's, 17 doctorates, 1 other advanced degree awarded. *Degree requirements:* For master's, capstone project; for doctorate, scholarly project. *Entrance requirements:* For master's and doctorate, BSN from an ACEN- or CCNE-accredited nursing school, minimum cumulative GPA of 3.0, personal statement, current unencumbered RN license with NE eligibility, undergraduate statistics course, physical assessment course or equivalent; for other advanced degree, MSN or MS in nursing, minimum cumulative GPA of 3.0, current unencumbered RN license with NE eligibility. Additional exam requirements/recommendations for international students: Required—TOEFL (minimum score 600 paper-based; 100 iBT). *Application deadline:* For fall admission, 6/15 priority date for domestic and international students; for spring admission, 11/15 priority date for domestic and international students; for summer admission, 4/15 for domestic and international students. Applications are processed on a rolling basis. Application fee: $50. Electronic applications accepted. *Expenses:* $800 per credit hour tuition; $904 per semester full-time fees; $207 per semester part-time fees; $50 one-time drug screen fee. *Financial support:* In 2015–16, 7 students received support. Scholarships/grants available. Financial award applicants required to submit FAFSA. *Faculty research:* Obesity prevention in children, evaluation of simulated clinical experiences, vitamin D3 and calcium for cancer risk education in post menopausal women, online support and education to reduce stress for prenatal patients on bed rest, health literacy, immunization research. *Total annual research expenditures:* $162,085. *Unit head:* Dr. Catherine Todero, Dean, 402-280-2004, Fax: 402-280-2045. *Application contact:* Shannon Cox, Enrollment Specialist, 402-280-2067, Fax: 402-280-2045, E-mail: shannoncox@creighton.edu.
Website: http://nursing.creighton.edu/

Daemen College, Department of Nursing, Amherst, NY 14226-3592. Offers adult nurse practitioner (MS, Post Master's Certificate); nurse executive leadership (Post Master's Certificate); nursing education (MS, Post Master's Certificate); nursing executive leadership (MS); nursing practice (DNP); palliative care nursing (Post Master's Certificate). *Accreditation:* ACEN. *Program availability:* Part-time. *Degree requirements:* For master's, thesis or alternative, degree completed in 4 years; minimum GPA of 3.0; for doctorate, degree completed in 5 years; 500 post-master's clinical hours. *Entrance requirements:* For master's, BN, 1 year medical/surgical experience, RN license and state registration, statistics course with minimum C grade, 3 letters of recommendation, minimum GPA of 3.25, interview; for doctorate, MS in advance nursing practice; New York state RN license; goal statement; resume; interview; statistics course with minimum grade of 'C'; for Post Master's Certificate, master's degree in clinical area; RN license and current registration; one year of clinical experience; statistics course with minimum grade of 'C'; 3 letters of recommendation; interview; letter of intent. Additional exam requirements/recommendations for international students: Required—TOEFL (minimum score 500 paper-based; 63 iBT), IELTS (minimum score 5.5). Electronic applications accepted. *Faculty research:* Professional stress, client behavior, drug therapy, treatment modalities and pulmonary cancers, chemical dependency.

Duke University, School of Nursing, Durham, NC 27708-0586. Offers acute care pediatric nurse practitioner (MSN, Post Master's Certificate); adult-gerontology nurse practitioner (MSN, Post Master's Certificate), including acute care, primary care; family nurse practitioner (MSN, Post Master's Certificate); neonatal nurse practitioner (MSN, Post Master's Certificate); nurse anesthesia (DNP); nurse practitioner (DNP); nursing (PhD); nursing and health care leadership (MSN); nursing education (MSN); nursing informatics (MSN, Post Master's Certificate); pediatric nurse practitioner (MSN, Post Master's Certificate), including primary care; women's health nurse practitioner (MSN, Post Master's Certificate). *Accreditation:* AACN; AANA/CANAEP. *Program availability:* Part-time, evening/weekend, online learning. *Faculty:* 74 full-time (63 women). *Students:* 179 full-time (152 women), 528 part-time (466 women); includes 145 minority (42 Black or African American, non-Hispanic/Latino; 3 American Indian or Alaska Native, non-Hispanic/Latino; 44 Asian, non-Hispanic/Latino; 35 Hispanic/Latino; 1 Native Hawaiian or other Pacific Islander, non-Hispanic/Latino; 20 Two or more races, non-Hispanic/Latino), 7 international. Average age 33. 619 applicants, 46% accepted, 201 enrolled. In 2015, 243 master's, 62 doctorates, 26 other advanced degrees awarded. Terminal master's awarded for partial completion of doctoral program. *Degree requirements:* For master's, thesis optional; for doctorate, capstone project. *Entrance requirements:* For master's, GRE General Test (waived if undergraduate GPA of 3.4 or higher), 1 year of nursing experience (recommended), BSN, minimum GPA of 3.0, previous course work in statistics; for doctorate, GRE General Test (waived if undergraduate GPA of 3.4 or higher), BSN or MSN, minimum GPA of 3.0, portfolio, resume, personal statement, undergraduate statistics course, current licensure as a registered nurse, transcripts from all post-secondary institutions; for Post Master's Certificate, MSN, licensure or eligibility

as a professional nurse, transcripts from all post-secondary institutions, previous course work in statistics. Additional exam requirements/recommendations for international students: Required—TOEFL (minimum score 100 iBT), IELTS (minimum score 7). *Application deadline:* For fall admission, 12/1 for domestic and international students; for spring admission, 5/1 for domestic and international students. Application fee: $50. Electronic applications accepted. *Expenses:* Contact institution. *Financial support:* Career-related internships or fieldwork, institutionally sponsored loans, scholarships/grants, traineeships, and tuition waivers (partial) available. Support available to part-time students. Financial award applicants required to submit FAFSA. *Faculty research:* Cardiovascular disease, caregiver skill training, data mining, prostate cancer, neonatal immune system. *Unit head:* Dr. Marion E. Broome, Dean/Vice Chancellor for Nursing Affairs/Associate Vice President for Academic Affairs for Nursing, 919-684-9446, Fax: 919-684-9414, E-mail: marion.broome@duke.edu. *Application contact:* Dr. Ernie Rushing, Director of Admissions and Recruitment, 919-668-6274, Fax: 919-668-4693, E-mail: ernie.rushing@dm.duke.edu.
Website: http://www.nursing.duke.edu/

Eastern Michigan University, Graduate School, College of Health and Human Services, School of Nursing, Ypsilanti, MI 48197. Offers nursing (MSN); teaching in health care systems (MSN, Graduate Certificate). *Accreditation:* AACN. *Program availability:* Part-time, evening/weekend, online learning. *Faculty:* 29 full-time (26 women). *Students:* 6 full-time (5 women), 22 part-time (19 women); includes 8 minority (6 Black or African American, non-Hispanic/Latino; 2 Asian, non-Hispanic/Latino). Average age 41. 24 applicants, 25% accepted, 2 enrolled. In 2015, 12 master's, 9 other advanced degrees awarded. *Degree requirements:* For master's, thesis optional. *Entrance requirements:* For master's, GRE General Test, Michigan RN license. Additional exam requirements/recommendations for international students: Required—TOEFL. *Application deadline:* Applications are processed on a rolling basis. Application fee: $45. *Financial support:* Fellowships, research assistantships with full tuition reimbursements, teaching assistantships with full tuition reimbursements, career-related internships or fieldwork, Federal Work-Study, institutionally sponsored loans, scholarships/grants, tuition waivers (partial), and unspecified assistantships available. Support available to part-time students. Financial award applicants required to submit FAFSA. *Unit head:* Dr. Michael Williams, Director, 734-487-2310, Fax: 734-487-6946, E-mail: mwilliams@emich.edu. *Application contact:* Roberta (Bobbi) Towne, Coordinator, School of Nursing, 734-487-2340, Fax: 734-487-6946, E-mail: rtowne1@emich.edu.
Website: http://www.emich.edu/nursing

Emory University, Nell Hodgson Woodruff School of Nursing, Atlanta, GA 30322-1100. Offers adult nurse practitioner (MSN); emergency nurse practitioner (MSN); family nurse practitioner (MSN); family nurse-midwife (MSN); health systems leadership (MSN); nurse-midwifery (MSN); pediatric nurse practitioner acute and primary care (MSN); women's health care (Title X) (MSN); women's health nurse practitioner (MSN); MSN/MPH. *Accreditation:* AACN; ACNM/ACME (one or more programs are accredited). *Program availability:* Part-time. *Entrance requirements:* For master's, GRE General Test or MAT, minimum GPA of 3.0, BS in nursing from an accredited institution, RN license and additional course work, 3 letters of recommendation. Additional exam requirements/recommendations for international students: Required—TOEFL (minimum score 600 paper-based; 100 iBT). Electronic applications accepted. *Expenses:* Contact institution. *Faculty research:* Older adult falls and injuries, minority health issues, cardiac symptoms and quality of life, bio-ethics and decision-making, menopausal issues.

Felician University, Master of Science in Nursing Program, Lodi, NJ 07644-2117. Offers adult-gerontology nurse practitioner (MSN, PMC); executive leadership (MSN, PMC); family nurse practitioner (MSN, PMC); nursing education (MSN, PMC). *Accreditation:* AACN. *Program availability:* Part-time, evening/weekend, online learning. *Faculty:* 11 full-time (9 women), 2 part-time/adjunct (both women). *Students:* 1 (woman) full-time, 121 part-time (112 women); includes 60 minority (23 Black or African American, non-Hispanic/Latino; 1 American Indian or Alaska Native, non-Hispanic/Latino; 19 Asian, non-Hispanic/Latino; 17 Hispanic/Latino). Average age 40. 111 applicants, 83% accepted, 52 enrolled. In 2015, 18 master's awarded. *Entrance requirements:* For master's, BS in nursing or equivalent, minimum GPA of 3.0, 2 letters of recommendation, RN license; for PMC, RN license, minimum GPA of 3.0. Additional exam requirements/recommendations for international students: Recommended—TOEFL (minimum score 79 iBT). *Application deadline:* Applications are processed on a rolling basis. Application fee: $40. Electronic applications accepted. Application fee is waived when completed online. *Expenses:* Tuition, area resident: Part-time $965 per credit. Tuition and fees vary according to course load and program. *Financial support:* In 2015–16, 10 students received support. Traineeships available. Financial award applicants required to submit FAFSA. *Faculty research:* Anxiety and fear, curriculum innovation, health promotion. *Unit head:* Dr. Ann Tritak, Associate Dean, Department of Graduate Nursing, 201-201-559-6151, E-mail: tritaka@felician.edu. *Application contact:* Dr. Margaret Smolin, Director, Graduate Admissions, 201-559-1451, E-mail: graduate@felician.edu.

Florida Southern College, Program in Nursing, Lakeland, FL 33801-5698. Offers adult gerontology clinical nurse specialist (MSN); adult gerontology primary care nurse practitioner (MSN); nurse educator (MSN); nursing administration (MSN). *Accreditation:* AACN. *Program availability:* Part-time, evening/weekend. *Entrance requirements:* For master's, Florida RN license, 3 letters of recommendation, personal statement, minimum GPA of 3.0, resume. Additional exam requirements/recommendations for international students: Required—TOEFL (minimum score 550 paper-based). *Expenses:* Contact institution. *Faculty research:* End of life care, dementia, health promotion.

The George Washington University, School of Nursing, Washington, DC 20052. Offers adult nurse practitioner (MSN, DNP, Post-Master's Certificate); clinical research administration (MSN); family nurse practitioner (MSN, Post-Master's Certificate); health care quality (MSN, Post-Master's Certificate); nursing leadership and management (MSN); nursing practice (DNP), including nursing education; palliative care nurse practitioner (Post-Master's Certificate). *Accreditation:* AACN. *Faculty:* 42 full-time (all women), 71 part-time/adjunct (66 women). *Students:* 52 full-time (48 women), 519 part-time (463 women); includes 162 minority (72 Black or African American, non-Hispanic/Latino; 4 American Indian or Alaska Native, non-Hispanic/Latino; 52 Asian, non-Hispanic/Latino; 31 Hispanic/Latino; 3 Two or more races, non-Hispanic/Latino), 2 international. Average age 37. 465 applicants, 69% accepted, 187 enrolled. In 2015, 121 master's, 35 doctorates, 1 other advanced degree awarded. *Unit head:* Pamela R. Jeffries, Dean, 202-994-3725, E-mail: pjeffries@gwu.edu. *Application contact:* Kristin Williams, Associate Provost for Graduate Enrollment Management, 202-994-0467, Fax: 202-994-0371, E-mail: ksw@gwu.edu.
Website: http://nursing.gwumc.edu/

Georgia State University, Byrdine F. Lewis School of Nursing, Atlanta, GA 30303. Offers adult health clinical nurse specialist/nurse practitioner (MS, Certificate); child health clinical nurse specialist/pediatric nurse practitioner (MS, Certificate); family nurse practitioner (MS, Certificate); family psychiatric mental health nurse practitioner (MS, Certificate); nursing (PhD); nursing leadership in healthcare innovations (MS), including nursing administration, nursing informatics; nutrition (MS); perinatal clinical nurse specialist/women's health nurse practitioner (MS, Certificate); physical therapy (DPT);

respiratory therapy (MS). *Accreditation:* AACN. *Program availability:* Part-time, blended/hybrid learning. *Faculty:* 18 full-time (11 women). *Students:* 275 full-time (195 women), 230 part-time (204 women); includes 192 minority (123 Black or African American, non-Hispanic/Latino; 49 Asian, non-Hispanic/Latino; 12 Hispanic/Latino; 2 Native Hawaiian or other Pacific Islander, non-Hispanic/Latino; 6 Two or more races, non-Hispanic/Latino), 35 international. Average age 33. 240 applicants, 61% accepted, 95 enrolled. In 2015, 115 master's, 40 doctorates, 19 other advanced degrees awarded. *Degree requirements:* For doctorate, comprehensive exam, thesis/dissertation. *Entrance requirements:* For doctorate, GRE. Additional exam requirements/recommendations for international students: Required—TOEFL. *Application deadline:* For fall admission, 2/1 priority date for domestic and international students; for spring admission, 9/15 for domestic and international students. Applications are processed on a rolling basis. Application fee: $50. Electronic applications accepted. *Expenses:* Contact institution. *Financial support:* In 2015–16, research assistantships with tuition reimbursements (averaging $1,666 per year), teaching assistantships with tuition reimbursements (averaging $1,920 per year) were awarded; scholarships/grants, tuition waivers (full and partial), and unspecified assistantships also available. Support available to part-time students. Financial award application deadline: 8/1; financial award applicants required to submit FAFSA. *Faculty research:* Stroke intervention for caregivers, stroke prevention in African-Americans; relationships between psychological distress and health outcomes in parents with a medically ill infant; medically fragile children; nursing expertise and patient outcomes. *Unit head:* Nancy Kropf, Dean of Nursing, 404-413-1101, Fax: 404-413-1090, E-mail: nkropf@gsu.edu.
Website: http://nursing.gsu.edu/

Goldfarb School of Nursing at Barnes-Jewish College, Graduate Programs, St. Louis, MO 63110. Offers adult-gerontology acute care nurse practitioner (MSN); adult-gerontology nurse practitioner (MSN); nurse anesthesia (MSN); nurse educator (MSN); nurse executive (MSN). *Accreditation:* AACN; AANA/CANAEP. *Program availability:* Part-time, online learning. *Faculty:* 51 full-time (47 women), 6 part-time/adjunct (all women). *Students:* 58 full-time (57 women), 29 part-time (24 women); includes 17 minority (11 Black or African American, non-Hispanic/Latino; 2 Asian, non-Hispanic/Latino; 2 Hispanic/Latino; 2 Two or more races, non-Hispanic/Latino). Average age 26. 41 applicants, 22% accepted, 8 enrolled. In 2015, 56 master's awarded. *Degree requirements:* For master's, thesis or alternative. *Entrance requirements:* For master's, 2 references, personal statement, curriculum vitae or resume. Additional exam requirements/recommendations for international students: Required—TOEFL (minimum score 575 paper-based; 85 iBT). *Application deadline:* For fall admission, 2/1 priority date for international students; for spring admission, 10/1 priority date for international students. Applications are processed on a rolling basis. Application fee: $50. *Expenses:* Contact institution. *Financial support:* Fellowships, research assistantships, Federal Work-Study, institutionally sponsored loans, and scholarships/grants available. Support available to part-time students. Financial award applicants required to submit FAFSA. *Faculty research:* HIV stigma, HIV symptom management, palliative care with children and their families, heart disease prevention in Hispanic women, depression in the well elderly, alternative therapies in pre-term infants. *Unit head:* Dr. Gretchen Drinkard, Dean, 314-454-7540, Fax: 314-362-9222, E-mail: gld9643@bjc.org. *Application contact:* Karen Sartorius, Admissions Specialist, 314-454-7057, Fax: 314-362-9250, E-mail: ksartorius@bjc.org.
Website: http://www.barnesjewishcollege.edu/

Gwynedd Mercy University, Frances M. Maguire School of Nursing and Health Professions, Gwynedd Valley, PA 19437-0901. Offers clinical nurse specialist (MSN), including gerontology, oncology, pediatrics; nurse educator (MSN); nurse practitioner (MSN), including adult health, pediatric health; nursing (DNP). *Accreditation:* ACEN. *Program availability:* Part-time, online learning. *Faculty:* 3 full-time (all women), 2 part-time/adjunct (both women). *Students:* 28 full-time (23 women), 68 part-time (62 women); includes 27 minority (18 Black or African American, non-Hispanic/Latino; 7 Asian, non-Hispanic/Latino; 2 Hispanic/Latino). Average age 37. 72 applicants, 25% accepted, 16 enrolled. In 2015, 7 master's awarded. *Degree requirements:* For master's, thesis optional; for doctorate, evidence-based scholarly project. *Entrance requirements:* For master's, GRE General Test or MAT, current nursing experience, physical assessment, course work in statistics, BSN from NLNAC-accredited program, 2 letters of recommendation, personal interview. Additional exam requirements/recommendations for international students: Required—TOEFL (minimum score 575 paper-based). *Application deadline:* For fall admission, 8/1 priority date for domestic students; for winter admission, 12/1 priority date for domestic students. Applications are processed on a rolling basis. Electronic applications accepted. *Expenses:* Contact institution. *Financial support:* In 2015–16, 21 students received support. Scholarships/grants, traineeships, and unspecified assistantships available. Financial award application deadline: 8/30. *Faculty research:* Critical thinking, primary care, domestic violence, multiculturalism, nursing centers. *Unit head:* Dr. Andrea D. Hollingsworth, Dean, 215-646-7300 Ext. 539, Fax: 215-641-5517, E-mail: hollingsworth.a@gmc.edu. *Application contact:* Dr. Barbara A. Jones, Director, 215-646-7300 Ext. 407, Fax: 215-641-5564, E-mail: jones.b@gmc.edu.
Website: http://www.gmercyu.edu/academics/graduate-programs/nursing

Hampton University, School of Nursing, Hampton, VA 23668. Offers advanced adult nursing (MS); community health nursing (MS); community mental health/psychiatric nursing (MS); family nursing (MS); gerontological nursing for the nurse practitioner (MS); nursing (PhD); women's health nursing (MS). *Accreditation:* AACN. *Program availability:* Part-time, online learning. *Degree requirements:* For master's, comprehensive exam, thesis optional; for doctorate, comprehensive exam, thesis/dissertation. *Entrance requirements:* For master's, GRE General Test. Additional exam requirements/recommendations for international students: Required—TOEFL (minimum score 525 paper-based) or IELTS (6.5). Electronic applications accepted. *Expenses:* Tuition, area resident: Full-time $10,263; part-time $522 per credit hour. *Required fees:* $35. Tuition and fees vary according to course load and program. *Faculty research:* African-American stress, HIV education, pediatric obesity, hypertension, breast cancer.

Hunter College of the City University of New York, Graduate School, Schools of the Health Professions, Hunter-Bellevue School of Nursing, Program in Adult Nurse Practitioner, New York, NY 10065-5085. Offers MS. *Accreditation:* AACN. *Students:* 2 part-time (both women); includes 1 minority (Black or African American, non-Hispanic/Latino). Average age 34. 25 applicants, 44% accepted, 11 enrolled. In 2015, 8 master's awarded. *Degree requirements:* For master's, practicum. *Entrance requirements:* For master's, minimum GPA of 3.0, New York RN license, 2 years of professional practice experience, BSN. Additional exam requirements/recommendations for international students: Required—TOEFL. *Application deadline:* For fall admission, 4/1 for domestic students, 2/1 for international students; for spring admission, 11/1 for domestic students, 9/1 for international students. Applications are processed on a rolling basis. *Financial support:* Federal Work-Study, scholarships/grants, and traineeships available. Support available to part-time students. Financial award application deadline: 5/1. *Unit head:* Dr. Anita Nirenberg, Interim Specialization Coordinator, 212-481-4359, Fax: 212-481-5078, E-mail: anirenbe@hunter.cuny.edu. *Application contact:* Milena Solo, Director for Graduate Admissions, 212-772-4480, E-mail: admissions@hunter.cuny.edu.
Website: http://www.hunter.cuny.edu/nursing/repository/files/graduate-fact-sheets/fsGNPANP8113.pdf

Adult Nursing

Indiana University–Purdue University Fort Wayne, College of Health and Human Services, Department of Nursing, Fort Wayne, IN 46805-1499. Offers adult-gerontology primary care nurse practitioner (MS); family nurse practitioner (MS); nurse executive (MS); nursing administration (Certificate); nursing education (MS). *Accreditation:* ACEN. *Program availability:* Part-time. *Faculty:* 8 full-time (all women). *Students:* 6 full-time (all women), 79 part-time (70 women); includes 8 minority (2 Black or African American, non-Hispanic/Latino; 3 Asian, non-Hispanic/Latino; 3 Hispanic/Latino). Average age 36. 14 applicants, 100% accepted, 10 enrolled. In 2015, 17 master's awarded. *Entrance requirements:* For master's, GRE Writing Test (if GPA below 3.0), BS in nursing, eligibility for Indiana RN license, minimum GPA of 3.0, essay, copy of resume, three references, undergraduate course work in research and statistics within last 5 years. Additional exam requirements/recommendations for international students: Required—TOEFL (minimum score 550 paper-based; 79 iBT); Recommended—TWE. *Application deadline:* For fall admission, 5/1 priority date for domestic and international students; for spring admission, 11/15 priority date for domestic students. Applications are processed on a rolling basis. Application fee: $55 ($60 for international students). Electronic applications accepted. *Financial support:* In 2015–16, 12 teaching assistantships with partial tuition reimbursements (averaging $13,522 per year) were awarded; scholarships/grants also available. Support available to part-time students. Financial award application deadline: 3/1; financial award applicants required to submit FAFSA. *Faculty research:* Community engagement, cervical screening, evidence-based practice. *Total annual research expenditures:* $22,966. *Unit head:* Dr. Lee-Ellen Kirkhorn, Chair/Professor, 260-481-6789, Fax: 260-481-5767, E-mail: kirkhorl@ipfw.edu. *Application contact:* Dr. Deb Poling, Director of Graduate Program, 260-481-6276, Fax: 260-481-5767, E-mail: polingd@ipfw.edu.
Website: http://www.ipfw.edu/nursing/

Kent State University, College of Nursing, Kent, OH 44242. Offers advanced nursing practice (DNP), including adult gerontology acute care nurse practitioner (MSN, DNP), adult gerontology clinical nurse specialist (MSN, DNP), family nurse practitioner (MSN, DNP); nursing (MSN, PhD), including adult gerontology acute care nurse practitioner (MSN, DNP), adult gerontology clinical nurse specialist (MSN, DNP), family nurse practitioner (MSN, DNP), nurse educator (MSN), nursing healthcare management (MSN), primary care adult nurse practitioner (MSN), primary care pediatric clinical nurse specialist (MSN), primary care pediatric nurse practitioner (MSN), psychiatric mental health practitioner (MSN), women's health nurse practitioner (MSN); nursing education (Certificate); primary care pediatric nurse practitioner (Certificate); women's health nurse practitioner (Certificate). PhD program offered jointly with The University of Akron. *Accreditation:* AACN. *Program availability:* Part-time, online learning. *Faculty:* 52 full-time (48 women). *Students:* 78 full-time (56 women), 414 part-time (365 women); includes 63 minority (34 Black or African American, non-Hispanic/Latino; 1 American Indian or Alaska Native, non-Hispanic/Latino; 12 Asian, non-Hispanic/Latino; 12 Hispanic/Latino; 4 Two or more races, non-Hispanic/Latino, 16 international. Average age 37. 653 applicants, 54% accepted, 309 enrolled. In 2015, 140 master's, 1 doctorate, 13 other advanced degrees awarded. *Degree requirements:* For master's, thesis optional, practicum; for doctorate, comprehensive exam (for some programs), thesis/dissertation (for some programs), practicum and scholarly project (for DNP programs); for Certificate, practicum. *Entrance requirements:* For master's, minimum GPA of 3.0, transcripts, active unrestricted RN license, essay/goal statement, interview, 3 letters of recommendation; for doctorate, GRE (for PhD), minimum GPA of 3.0, transcripts, 3 letters of recommendation, interview; active unrestricted RN license, clinical experience and hours record (for DNP); goal statement, sample of written work, curriculum vitae, statement of research interests, and eligibility for RN license (for PhD); for Certificate, MSN, minimum GPA of 3.0, transcripts. Additional exam requirements/recommendations for international students: Required—TOEFL (minimum score: paper-based 525, iBT 71), Michigan English Language Assessment Battery (minimum score of 75), IELTS (minimum score of 6.0), PTE Academic (minimum score of 48), or completion of ELS level 112 Intensive Program. *Application deadline:* For fall admission, 2/1 for domestic students; for spring admission, 11/1 for domestic students. Application fee: $45 ($70 for international students). Electronic applications accepted. *Expenses:* Tuition, state resident: full-time $10,864; part-time $495 per credit hour. Tuition, nonresident: full-time $18,380; part-time $837 per credit hour. *Financial support:* Research assistantships with full tuition reimbursements, teaching assistantships with full tuition reimbursements, career-related internships or fieldwork, Federal Work-Study, traineeships, and unspecified assistantships available. Financial award application deadline: 2/1. *Unit head:* Dr. Barbara Broome, Dean, 330-672-3777, E-mail: bbroome1@kent.edu. *Application contact:* Dr. Wendy A. Umberger, Associate Dean for Graduate Programs/Professor, 330-672-8813, E-mail: wlewando@kent.edu.
Website: http://www.kent.edu/nursing/

La Salle University, School of Nursing and Health Sciences, Program in Nursing, Philadelphia, PA 19141-1199. Offers adult gerontology primary care nurse practitioner (MSN, Certificate); adult health and illness clinical nurse specialist (MSN); adult-gerontology clinical nurse specialist (MSN, Certificate); clinical nurse leader (MSN); family primary care nurse practitioner (MSN, Certificate); gerontology (Certificate); nurse anesthetist (MSN, Certificate); nursing (MSN, Certificate); nursing administration (MSN, Certificate); nursing education (Certificate); nursing practice (DNP); nursing service administration (MSN); public health nursing (MSN, Certificate); school nursing (Certificate); MSN/MBA; MSN/MPH. *Accreditation:* AANA/CANAEP. *Program availability:* Part-time, evening/weekend, 100% online. *Faculty:* 13 full-time (all women), 9 part-time/adjunct (8 women). *Students:* 368 part-time (56 women); includes 103 minority (62 Black or African American, non-Hispanic/Latino; 1 American Indian or Alaska Native, non-Hispanic/Latino; 26 Asian, non-Hispanic/Latino; 9 Hispanic/Latino; 5 Two or more races, non-Hispanic/Latino), 5 international. Average age 36. 98 applicants, 85% accepted, 53 enrolled. In 2015, 87 master's, 3 doctorates, 10 other advanced degrees awarded. *Degree requirements:* For doctorate, minimum of 1,000 hours of post baccalaureate clinical practice supervised by preceptors. *Entrance requirements:* For master's, GRE, MAT, or GMAT (for students with BSN GPA of less than 3.2), baccalaureate degree in nursing from an NLNAC- or CCNE-accredited program or an MSN Bridge program; Pennsylvania RN license; 2 letters of reference; resume; statement of philosophy articulating professional values and future educational goal; 1 year of work experience as a registered nurse; for doctorate, GRE (waived for applicants with MSN cumulative GPA of 3.7 or above), MSN from nationally-accredited program or master's degree, MBA or MHA from nationally-accredited program; resume or curriculum vitae; 2 letters of reference; interview; for Certificate, GRE, MAT, or GMAT (for students with BSN GPA of less than 3.2, baccalaureate degree in nursing from an NLNAC- or CCNE-accredited program or an MSN Bridge program; Pennsylvania RN license; 2 letters of reference; resume; statement of philosophy articulating professional values and future educational goal; 1 year of work experience as a registered nurse. Additional exam requirements/recommendations for international students: Required—TOEFL. *Application deadline:* For fall admission, 8/15 priority date for domestic students, 7/15 for international students; for spring admission, 12/15 priority date for domestic students, 11/15 for international students; for summer admission, 4/15 priority date for domestic students, 3/15 for international students. Applications are processed on a rolling basis. Application fee: $35. Electronic applications accepted. Application fee is waived when completed online. *Expenses:* $870 per credit hour (for MSN); $930 per

credit hour (for DNP); $150 technology fee full-time, $75 part-time; $135 general university fee. *Financial support:* In 2015–16, 13 students received support. Scholarships/grants and traineeships available. Support available to part-time students. Financial award application deadline: 8/31; financial award applicants required to submit FAFSA. *Unit head:* Dr. Patricia M. Dillon, Director, 215-951-1322, Fax: 215-951-1896, E-mail: msnapn@lasalle.edu. *Application contact:* Alison McAnespey Target, Director, Graduate and Adult Enrollment, 215-951-1100, Fax: 215-951-1462, E-mail: reilly@lasalle.edu.
Website: http://www.lasalle.edu/nursing/program-options/

Lehman College of the City University of New York, School of Natural and Social Sciences, Department of Nursing, Bronx, NY 10468-1589. Offers adult health nursing (MS); nursing of older adults (MS); parent-child nursing (MS); pediatric nurse practitioner (MS). *Accreditation:* AACN. *Program availability:* Part-time, evening/weekend. *Entrance requirements:* For master's, bachelor's degree in nursing, New York RN license.

Lewis University, College of Nursing and Health Professions, Program in Nursing, Romeoville, IL 60446. Offers adult nurse practitioner (MSN); nursing administration (MSN); nursing education (MSN). *Accreditation:* AACN. *Program availability:* Part-time, evening/weekend, online learning. *Degree requirements:* For master's, clinical practicum. *Entrance requirements:* For master's, minimum undergraduate GPA of 3.0, degree in nursing, RN license, letter of recommendation, interview, resume or curriculum vitae. Additional exam requirements/recommendations for international students: Required—TOEFL (minimum score 550 paper-based; 80 iBT). Electronic applications accepted. *Faculty research:* Cancer prevention, phenomenological methods, public policy analysis.

Loma Linda University, School of Nursing, Program in Nurse Educator, Loma Linda, CA 92350. Offers adult/gerontology (MS); obstetrics-pediatrics (MS). *Accreditation:* AACN. *Program availability:* Part-time. *Degree requirements:* For master's, thesis or alternative. *Entrance requirements:* For master's, GRE General Test, BSN, minimum GPA of 3.0, RN license. Additional exam requirements/recommendations for international students: Required—TOEFL. *Application deadline:* For fall admission, 8/1 for domestic and international students; for winter admission, 11/1 for domestic and international students; for spring admission, 2/1 for domestic and international students. Application fee: $60. Electronic applications accepted. *Financial support:* Career-related internships or fieldwork, Federal Work-Study, institutionally sponsored loans, and scholarships/grants available. Support available to part-time students. Financial award application deadline: 6/1. *Faculty research:* Coping, integration of research. *Unit head:* Coordinator, 909-824-4360. *Application contact:* Admissions Office, 909-651-5029, Fax: 909-558-4879, E-mail: admissions.app@llu.edu.

Long Island University–LIU Brooklyn, Harriet Rothkopf Heilbrunn School of Nursing, Brooklyn, NY 11201-8423. Offers adult nurse practitioner (MS, Advanced Certificate); family nurse practitioner (MS, Advanced Certificate); nurse educator (MS). *Accreditation:* AACN. *Program availability:* Part-time, evening/weekend, blended/hybrid learning. *Faculty:* 6 full-time (4 women), 5 part-time/adjunct (4 women). *Students:* 1 (woman) full-time, 215 part-time (192 women); includes 136 minority (89 Black or African American, non-Hispanic/Latino; 28 Asian, non-Hispanic/Latino; 13 Hispanic/Latino; 2 Native Hawaiian or other Pacific Islander, non-Hispanic/Latino; 4 Two or more races, non-Hispanic/Latino), 1 international. Average age 43. 167 applicants, 57% accepted, 63 enrolled. In 2015, 23 master's, 5 other advanced degrees awarded. *Entrance requirements:* For master's and Advanced Certificate, New York RN license, two letters of recommendation. Additional exam requirements/recommendations for international students: Required—TOEFL (minimum score 550 paper-based; 79 iBT), IELTS (minimum score 6.5). *Application deadline:* Applications are processed on a rolling basis. Application fee: $50. Electronic applications accepted. *Expenses:* $1,155 per credit tuition; $934 per term full-time fees; $442 per term part-time fees. *Financial support:* In 2015–16, 24 students received support. Scholarships/grants and unspecified assistantships available. Support available to part-time students. Financial award application deadline: 2/15; financial award applicants required to submit FAFSA. *Faculty research:* Cultural competency, high fidelity simulation to improve nursing assessment and increase patient safety, relationship of diabetes to stress, end of life care, geriatric issues, foreign nurse's adaptation to the United States. *Unit head:* Dr. Loretta Knapp, Interim Dean, 718-488-1508, Fax: 718-780-4019, E-mail: lori.knapp@liu.edu. *Application contact:* Richard Sunday, Dean of Admissions, 718-488-1011, Fax: 718-780-6110, E-mail: bkln-admissions@liu.edu.
Website: http://liu.edu/Brooklyn/Academics/Harriet-Rothkopf-Heilbrunn-School-of-Nursing

Loyola University Chicago, Graduate School, Marcella Niehoff School of Nursing, Maywood, IL 60153. Offers adult gerontology acute care clinical nurse specialist (MSN), including emergency care (MSN, Certificate); adult gerontology acute care nurse practitioner (MSN), including oncology (MSN, Certificate); adult gerontology clinical nurse specialist (MSN), including oncology (MSN, Certificate); adult gerontology nursing (Certificate), including oncology (MSN, Certificate); adult nurse practitioner (Certificate); dietetics (MS); family nurse practitioner (MSN, Certificate), including emergency care; informatics (MSN); leadership (DNP), including healthcare quality using education in safety and technology, infection prevention; nursing science (PhD); women's health nurse practitioner (MSN); women's health nursing (Certificate). *Accreditation:* AACN. *Program availability:* Part-time, blended/hybrid learning. *Faculty:* 27 full-time (25 women), 12 part-time/adjunct (10 women). *Students:* 174 full-time (161 women), 232 part-time (221 women); includes 95 minority (19 Black or African American, non-Hispanic/Latino; 2 American Indian or Alaska Native, non-Hispanic/Latino; 38 Asian, non-Hispanic/Latino; 28 Hispanic/Latino; 2 Native Hawaiian or other Pacific Islander, non-Hispanic/Latino; 6 Two or more races, non-Hispanic/Latino), 3 international. Average age 35. 209 applicants, 52% accepted, 83 enrolled. In 2015, 78 master's, 10 doctorates, 17 other advanced degrees awarded. *Degree requirements:* For master's, comprehensive exam; for doctorate, thesis/dissertation, qualifying examination (for PhD); capstone project (for DNP). *Entrance requirements:* For master's, BSN, minimum nursing GPA of 3.0, Illinois RN license, 3 letters of recommendation, 1000 hours of experience in area of specialty prior to starting clinical rotations, personal statement; for doctorate, GRE General Test (for PhD), BSN or MSN, minimum GPA of 3.0, professional nursing license, 3 letters of recommendation, personal statement. Additional exam requirements/recommendations for international students: Required—TOEFL (minimum score 550 paper-based; 79 iBT), IELTS (minimum score 6.5). *Application deadline:* For fall admission, 6/1 priority date for domestic and international students; for spring admission, 11/15 priority date for domestic and international students; for summer admission, 3/15 priority date for domestic and international students. Applications are processed on a rolling basis. Application fee: $50. Electronic applications accepted. Application fee is waived when completed online. *Expenses:* $1,081 per credit hour. *Financial support:* In 2015–16, 10 students received support, including 3 research assistantships with full tuition reimbursements available (averaging $18,000 per year), 1 teaching assistantship with full tuition reimbursement available (averaging $18,000 per year); scholarships/grants, unspecified assistantships, and nurse faculty loan program also available. Financial award application deadline: 5/1; financial award applicants required to submit FAFSA. *Faculty research:* Epigenetics and social determinants of health, women's health, vitamin D, interprofessional education, prevention and self-management of chronic disease. *Total annual research expenditures:* $649,606. *Unit head:* Dr. Vicky Keough, Dean, 708-216-5448, Fax: 708-216-9555, E-mail: vkeough@luc.edu. *Application contact:* Toni Topalova, Enrollment Advisor, 708-216-3751, Fax: 708-216-9555, E-mail: atopalova@luc.edu. *Website:* http://www.luc.edu/nursing/

Madonna University, Program in Nursing, Livonia, MI 48150-1173. Offers adult health: chronic health conditions (MSN); adult nurse practitioner (MSN); nursing administration (MSN); MSN/MSBA. *Accreditation:* AACN. *Program availability:* Part-time. *Degree requirements:* For master's, thesis or alternative. *Entrance requirements:* For master's, GRE General Test, Michigan nursing license. Electronic applications accepted. *Faculty research:* Coping, caring.

Marian University, School of Nursing and Health Professions, Fond du Lac, WI 54935-4699. Offers adult nurse practitioner (MSN); nurse educator (MSN). *Accreditation:* AACN. *Program availability:* Part-time, evening/weekend. *Faculty:* 6 full-time (all women), 4 part-time/adjunct (2 women). *Students:* 21 full-time (20 women), 95 part-time (85 women); includes 10 minority (6 Black or African American, non-Hispanic/Latino; 2 Asian, non-Hispanic/Latino; 2 Hispanic/Latino). Average age 40. In 2015, 26 master's awarded. *Degree requirements:* For master's, thesis, 675 clinical practicum hours. *Entrance requirements:* For master's, 3 letters of professional recommendation; undergraduate work in nursing research, statistics, health assessment. Additional exam requirements/recommendations for international students: Required—TOEFL (minimum score 525 paper-based; 70 iBT). *Application deadline:* Applications are processed on a rolling basis. Application fee: $50. Electronic applications accepted. *Expenses:* Contact institution. *Financial support:* In 2015–16, 3 students received support. Institutionally sponsored loans and scholarships/grants available. Support available to part-time students. Financial award application deadline: 3/1; financial award applicants required to submit FAFSA. *Unit head:* Dr. Linda Matheson, Dean, 920-923-7668, Fax: 920-923-8770, E-mail: lkmatheson85@marianuniversity.edu. *Application contact:* Selina Scoles, Admissions Counselor, 920-923-8938, Fax: 920-923-8770, E-mail: sascoles30@marianuniversity.edu.
Website: http://www.marianuniversity.edu/nursing/

Marquette University, Graduate School, College of Nursing, Milwaukee, WI 53201-1881. Offers acute care nurse practitioner (Certificate); adult clinical nurse specialist (Certificate); adult nurse practitioner (Certificate); advanced practice nursing (MSN, DNP), including adult-older adult acute care (DNP), adults (MSN), adults-older adults (DNP), clinical nurse leader (MSN), health care systems leadership (DNP), nurse-midwifery (MSN), older adults (MSN), pediatrics-acute care, pediatrics-primary care, primary care (DNP), systems leadership and healthcare quality (MSN); family nurse practitioner (Certificate); nurse-midwifery (Certificate); nursing (PhD); pediatric acute care (Certificate); pediatric primary care (Certificate); systems leadership and healthcare quality (Certificate). *Accreditation:* AACN. *Faculty:* 35 full-time (all women), 56 part-time/adjunct (55 women). *Students:* 123 full-time (112 women), 242 part-time (220 women); includes 34 minority (9 Black or African American, non-Hispanic/Latino; 12 Asian, non-Hispanic/Latino; 10 Hispanic/Latino; 3 Two or more races, non-Hispanic/Latino), 4 international. Average age 30. 269 applicants, 61% accepted, 98 enrolled. In 2015, 84 master's, 5 doctorates, 22 other advanced degrees awarded. Terminal master's awarded for partial completion of doctoral program. *Degree requirements:* For master's, comprehensive exam, thesis or alternative. *Entrance requirements:* For master's, GRE General Test, BSN, Wisconsin RN license, official transcripts from all current and previous colleges/universities except Marquette, three completed recommendation forms, resume, written statement of professional goals; for doctorate, GRE General Test, official transcripts from all current and previous colleges/universities except Marquette, three letters of recommendation, resume, written statement of professional goals, sample of scholarly writing. Additional exam requirements/recommendations for international students: Required—TOEFL (minimum score 530 paper-based). *Application deadline:* For fall admission, 2/15 for domestic and international students. Electronic applications accepted. *Financial support:* In 2015–16, 41 students received support, including 1 fellowship with partial tuition reimbursement available (averaging $17,500 per year), 2 research assistantships with full tuition reimbursements available (averaging $13,285 per year), 8 teaching assistantships with full tuition reimbursements available (averaging $13,912 per year); career-related internships or fieldwork, Federal Work-Study, scholarships/grants, health care benefits, tuition waivers (partial), and unspecified assistantships also available. Support available to part-time students. Financial award application deadline: 2/15. *Faculty research:* Psychosocial adjustment to chronic illness, gerontology, reminiscence, health policy: uninsured and access, hospital care delivery systems. *Total annual research expenditures:* $480,591. *Unit head:* Dr. Donna McCarthy, Interim Chair, 414-288-3800, Fax: 414-288-1578. *Application contact:* Dr. Maureen O'Brien, Associate Dean/Clinical Associate Professor, 414-288-3823.

Maryville University of Saint Louis, Walker College of Health Professions, The Catherine McAuley School of Nursing, St. Louis, MO 63141-7299. Offers acute care nurse practice (MSN); adult gerontology nurse practitioner (MSN); advanced practice nursing (DNP); family nurse practitioner (MSN); pediatric nurse practice (MSN). *Accreditation:* AACN. *Program availability:* 100% online. *Faculty:* 18 full-time (all women), 158 part-time/adjunct (141 women). *Students:* 38 full-time (35 women), 2,802 part-time (2,511 women); includes 681 minority (332 Black or African American, non-Hispanic/Latino; 40 American Indian or Alaska Native, non-Hispanic/Latino; 126 Asian, non-Hispanic/Latino; 126 Hispanic/Latino; 8 Native Hawaiian or other Pacific Islander, non-Hispanic/Latino; 49 Two or more races, non-Hispanic/Latino), 58 international. Average age 37. In 2015, 413 master's, 33 doctorates awarded. *Degree requirements:* For master's, practicum. *Entrance requirements:* For master's, BSN, current licensure, minimum GPA of 3.0, 3 letters of recommendation, curriculum vitae. Additional exam requirements/recommendations for international students: Required—TOEFL (minimum score 550 paper-based). *Application deadline:* Applications are processed on a rolling basis. Electronic applications accepted. Application fee is waived when completed online. *Expenses: Tuition, area resident:* Full-time $25,558; part-time $781 per credit hour. *Required fees:* $2400. Part-time tuition and fees vary according to course load and degree level. *Financial support:* Federal Work-Study and campus employment available. Support available to part-time students. Financial award application deadline: 3/1; financial award applicants required to submit FAFSA. *Unit head:* Dr. Elizabeth Buck, Director, 314-529-9453, Fax: 314-529-9139, E-mail: ebuck@maryville.edu. *Application contact:* Crystal Jacobsmeyer, Assistant Director, Graduate Enrollment Advising, 314-929-9654, Fax: 314-529-9927, E-mail: cjacobsmeyer@maryville.edu.
Website: http://www.maryville.edu/hp/nursing/

Medical University of South Carolina, College of Nursing, Adult-Gerontology Health Nurse Practitioner Program, Charleston, SC 29425. Offers MSN, DNP. *Program availability:* Part-time, online learning. *Degree requirements:* For master's, comprehensive exam (for some programs), thesis optional; for doctorate, final project. *Entrance requirements:* For master's, BSN from nationally-accredited program, minimum nursing and cumulative GPA of 3.0, undergraduate-level statistics course, active RN License, 3 confidential references, current curriculum vitae or resume, essay; for doctorate, BSN from nationally-accredited program, minimum nursing and cumulative GPA of 3.0, undergraduate-level statistics course, active RN License, 3

confidential references, current curriculum vitae or resume, personal essay (for DNP). Additional exam requirements/recommendations for international students: Required—TOEFL (minimum score 550 paper-based; 80 iBT). Electronic applications accepted. *Faculty research:* Palliative care, dementia, hospital acquired infections, diabetes, advance practice nurse utilization.

Molloy College, Division of Nursing, Rockville Centre, NY 11571-5002. Offers adult-gerontology primary care nurse practitioner (MS); clinical nurse specialist (MS), including adult-gerontology health; clinical nurse specialist: adult-gerontology (Advanced Certificate), including adult-gerontology; family nurse practitioner (MS, Advanced Certificate), including primary care; family psychiatric mental health nurse practitioner (MS); nursing (DNP, PhD); nursing administration (MS), including informatics; nursing education (MS); pediatric nurse practitioner (MS), including primary care (MS, Advanced Certificate). *Accreditation:* AACN. *Program availability:* Part-time, evening/weekend. *Faculty:* 26 full-time (all women), 12 part-time/adjunct (9 women). *Students:* 13 full-time (all women), 550 part-time (515 women); includes 316 minority (169 Black or African American, non-Hispanic/Latino; 1 American Indian or Alaska Native, non-Hispanic/Latino; 88 Asian, non-Hispanic/Latino; 56 Hispanic/Latino; 2 Native Hawaiian or other Pacific Islander, non-Hispanic/Latino). Average age 43. 208 applicants, 69% accepted, 121 enrolled. In 2015, 116 master's, 1 doctorate, 6 other advanced degrees awarded. *Degree requirements:* For master's, thesis optional. *Entrance requirements:* For master's, 3 letters of reference, BS in nursing, minimum undergraduate GPA of 3.0; for Advanced Certificate, 3 letters of reference, master's degree in nursing. Additional exam requirements/recommendations for international students: Required—TOEFL (minimum score 550 paper-based; 79 iBT). *Application deadline:* For fall admission, 9/2 priority date for domestic students; for spring admission, 1/20 priority date for domestic students. Applications are processed on a rolling basis. Application fee: $60. Electronic applications accepted. *Expenses: Tuition, area resident:* Full-time $18,450; part-time $1025 per credit. *Required fees:* $900; $740 per unit. Tuition and fees vary according to course load. *Financial support:* Research assistantships with partial tuition reimbursements, teaching assistantships with partial tuition reimbursements, institutionally sponsored loans, scholarships/grants, and unspecified assistantships available. Support available to part-time students. Financial award application deadline: 4/1; financial award applicants required to submit FAFSA. *Unit head:* Dr. Jeannine Muldoon, Dean of Nursing, 516-323-3651, E-mail: jmuldoon@molloy.edu. *Application contact:* Jaclyn Machowicz, Assistant Director for Admissions, 516-323-4010, E-mail: jmachowicz@molloy.edu.

Monmouth University, Graduate Studies, The Marjorie K. Unterberg School of Nursing and Health Studies, West Long Branch, NJ 07764-1898. Offers adult and gerontological primary care nurse practitioner (MSN); adult-gerontological primary care nurse practitioner (Post-Master's Certificate); family nurse practitioner (MSN, Post-Master's Certificate); family psychiatric and mental health advanced practice nursing (MSN); family psychiatric and mental health nurse practitioner (Post-Master's Certificate); forensic nursing (MSN, Certificate); nursing (MSN); nursing administration (MSN, Post-Master's Certificate); nursing education (MSN, Post-Master's Certificate); nursing practice (DNP); physician assistant (MS); school nursing (MSN, Certificate). *Accreditation:* AACN. *Program availability:* Part-time, evening/weekend, 100% online, blended/hybrid learning. *Faculty:* 14 full-time (13 women), 10 part-time/adjunct (5 women). *Students:* 58 full-time (46 women), 271 part-time (252 women); includes 93 minority (31 Black or African American, non-Hispanic/Latino; 40 Asian, non-Hispanic/Latino; 18 Hispanic/Latino; 1 Native Hawaiian or other Pacific Islander, non-Hispanic/Latino; 3 Two or more races, non-Hispanic/Latino), 1 international. Average age 37. 450 applicants, 32% accepted, 103 enrolled. In 2015, 68 master's, 8 doctorates, 11 other advanced degrees awarded. *Degree requirements:* For master's, practicum (for some tracks); for doctorate, practicum, capstone course. *Entrance requirements:* For master's, GRE General Test (waived for MSN applicants with minimum B grade in each of the first four courses and for MS applicants with master's degree), BSN with minimum GPA of 2.75, current RN license, proof of liability and malpractice policy, personal statement, two letters of recommendation, college course work in health assessment, resume; CASPA application (for MS); for doctorate, accredited master's nursing program degree with minimum GPA of 3.2, graduate research course in statistics, active RN license, national certification as Nurse Practitioner or Nurse Administrator, working knowledge of statistics, statement of goals and vision for change, 2 letters of recommendation (professional or academic), resume, interview. Additional exam requirements/recommendations for international students: Required—TOEFL (minimum score 550 paper-based; 79 iBT), IELTS (minimum score 6) or Michigan English Language Assessment Battery (minimum score 77). *Application deadline:* For fall admission, 7/15 priority date for domestic students, 6/1 for international students; for spring admission, 12/15 priority date for domestic students, 11/1 for international students; for summer admission, 5/1 for domestic students. Applications are processed on a rolling basis. Application fee: $50. Electronic applications accepted. *Expenses:* Contact institution. *Financial support:* In 2015–16, 241 students received support, including 220 fellowships (averaging $3,403 per year), 5 research assistantships (averaging $5,146 per year); career-related internships or fieldwork, scholarships/grants, and unspecified assistantships also available. Support available to part-time students. Financial award applicants required to submit FAFSA. *Faculty research:* School nursing, health policy, and smoking cessation in teens, Multiple Sclerosis; adherence and self-efficacy, aging issues and geriatric care. *Unit head:* Dr. Janet Mahoney, Dean, 732-571-3443, Fax: 732-263-5131, E-mail: jmahoney@monmouth.edu. *Application contact:* Lucia Fedele, Graduate Admission Counselor, 732-571-3452, Fax: 732-263-5123, E-mail: gradadm@monmouth.edu.
Website: http://www.monmouth.edu/school-of-nursing-health/graduate-nursing-programs.aspx

Mount Carmel College of Nursing, Nursing Program, Columbus, OH 43222. Offers adult gerontology acute care nurse practitioner (MS); adult health clinical nurse specialist (MS); family nurse practitioner (MS); nursing (DNP); nursing administration (MS); nursing education (MS). *Accreditation:* AACN. *Program availability:* Part-time. *Faculty:* 8 full-time (all women), 5 part-time/adjunct (4 women). *Students:* 72 full-time (63 women), 92 part-time (84 women); includes 15 minority (7 Black or African American, non-Hispanic/Latino; 3 Asian, non-Hispanic/Latino; 2 Hispanic/Latino; 3 Two or more races, non-Hispanic/Latino). Average age 37. 140 applicants, 45% accepted, 50 enrolled. In 2015, 50 master's awarded. *Degree requirements:* For master's, professional manuscript; for doctorate, practicum. *Entrance requirements:* For master's, letters of recommendation, statement of purpose, current resume, baccalaureate degree in nursing, current Ohio RN license, minimum cumulative GPA of 3.0; for doctorate, master's degree in nursing from program accredited by either NLNAC/ACEN or CCNE. Additional exam requirements/recommendations for international students: Required—TOEFL (minimum score 550 paper-based; 80 iBT). *Application deadline:* For fall admission, 6/1 priority date for domestic students; for winter admission, 11/1 for domestic students; for spring admission, 10/1 priority date for domestic students; for summer admission, 3/1 for domestic students. Applications are processed on a rolling basis. Application fee: $30. *Expenses: Tuition, area resident:* Full-time $9480; part-time $474 per credit. One-time fee: $120. Tuition and fees vary according to course load, degree level and program. *Financial support:* In 2015–16, 5 students received support. Institutionally sponsored loans and scholarships/grants available. Financial award

Adult Nursing

applicants required to submit FAFSA. *Unit head:* Dr. Jill Kilanowski, 614-234-5237, Fax: 614-234-2875, E-mail: jkilanowski@mccn.edu. *Application contact:* Dr. Kim Campbell, Director of Recruitment and Admissions, 614-234-5144, Fax: 614-234-5427, E-mail: kcampbell@mccn.edu.
Website: http://www.mccn.edu/

Mount Saint Mary College, School of Nursing, Newburgh, NY 12550-3494. Offers adult nurse practitioner (MS, Advanced Certificate), including nursing education (MS), nursing management (MS); clinical nurse specialist-adult health (MS), including nursing education, nursing management; family nurse practitioner (Advanced Certificate). *Accreditation:* AACN. *Program availability:* Part-time, evening/weekend, blended/hybrid learning. *Faculty:* 6 full-time (all women), 1 (woman) part-time/adjunct. *Students:* 5 full-time (4 women), 117 part-time (105 women); includes 42 minority (18 Black or African American, non-Hispanic/Latino; 2 American Indian or Alaska Native, non-Hispanic/Latino; 8 Asian, non-Hispanic/Latino; 12 Hispanic/Latino; 2 Native Hawaiian or other Pacific Islander, non-Hispanic/Latino). Average age 38. 44 applicants, 84% accepted, 25 enrolled. In 2015, 25 master's, 4 other advanced degrees awarded. *Degree requirements:* For master's, research utilization project. *Entrance requirements:* For master's, BSN, minimum GPA of 3.0, RN license. Additional exam requirements/recommendations for international students: Required—TOEFL (minimum score 80 iBT). *Application deadline:* For fall admission, 6/3 priority date for domestic students; for spring admission, 10/31 priority date for domestic students. Applications are processed on a rolling basis. Application fee: $45. Electronic applications accepted. Application fee is waived when completed online. *Expenses: Tuition, area resident:* Part-time $750 per credit. *Required fees:* $40 per semester. *Financial support:* In 2015–16, 14 students received support. Unspecified assistantships available. Financial award application deadline: 4/15; financial award applicants required to submit FAFSA. *Unit head:* Christine Berte, Graduate Coordinator, 845-569-3141, Fax: 845-562-6762, E-mail: christine.berte@msmc.edu. *Application contact:* Lisa Gallina, Director of Admissions for Graduate Programs and Adult Degree Completion, 845-569-3166, Fax: 845-569-3450, E-mail: lisa.gallina@msmc.edu.
Website: http://www.msmc.edu/Academics/Graduate_Programs/Master_of_Science_in_Nursing

New York University, Rory Meyers College of Nursing, Doctor of Nursing Practice Program, New York, NY 10012-1019. Offers nursing (DNP), including adult acute care, adult primary care, family, mental health nursing, nurse-midwifery, pediatrics. *Program availability:* Part-time, evening/weekend. *Faculty:* 14 full-time (13 women). *Students:* 2 full-time (both women), 32 part-time (27 women); includes 8 minority (3 Black or African American, non-Hispanic/Latino; 4 Asian, non-Hispanic/Latino; 1 Hispanic/Latino), 1 international. Average age 40. 47 applicants, 51% accepted, 16 enrolled. In 2015, 17 doctorates awarded. *Degree requirements:* For doctorate, thesis/dissertation, project. *Entrance requirements:* For doctorate, MAT or GRE (either taken within past 5 years), MS, RN license, interview, Nurse Practitioner Certification, writing sample. Additional exam requirements/recommendations for international students: Required—TOEFL (minimum score 90 iBT), IELTS (minimum score 7). *Application deadline:* For fall admission, 3/1 for domestic and international students. Applications are processed on a rolling basis. Application fee: $80. Electronic applications accepted. *Expenses:* Contact institution. *Financial support:* In 2015–16, 12 students received support. Scholarships/grants available. Support available to part-time students. Financial award application deadline: 2/1; financial award applicants required to submit FAFSA. *Faculty research:* Workforce, LGBT, breast cancer, HIV. *Unit head:* Dr. Rona Levin, Director, 212-998-5319, Fax: 212-995-3143, E-mail: rfl2039@nyu.edu. *Application contact:* Samantha Jaser, Assistant Director, Graduate Student Affairs and Admissions, 212-992-7653, Fax: 212-995-4302, E-mail: saj283@nyu.edu.

New York University, Rory Meyers College of Nursing, Programs in Advanced Practice Nursing, New York, NY 10012-1019. Offers adult-gerontology acute care nurse practitioner (MS, Advanced Certificate); adult-gerontology primary care nurse practitioner (MS, Advanced Certificate); family nurse practitioner (MS, Advanced Certificate); gerontology nurse practitioner (Advanced Certificate); nurse-midwifery (MS, Advanced Certificate); nursing administration (MS, Advanced Certificate); nursing education (MS, Advanced Certificate); nursing informatics (MS, Advanced Certificate); pediatrics nurse practitioner (MS, Advanced Certificate); psychiatric-mental health nurse practitioner (MS, Advanced Certificate); MS/MPH. *Accreditation:* AACN; ACNM/ACME. *Program availability:* Part-time. *Faculty:* 24 full-time (all women), 76 part-time/adjunct (65 women). *Students:* 46 full-time (26 women), 586 part-time (513 women); includes 242 minority (68 Black or African American, non-Hispanic/Latino; 3 American Indian or Alaska Native, non-Hispanic/Latino; 117 Asian, non-Hispanic/Latino; 38 Hispanic/Latino; 3 Native Hawaiian or other Pacific Islander, non-Hispanic/Latino; 13 Two or more races, non-Hispanic/Latino), 23 international. Average age 32. 402 applicants, 69% accepted, 138 enrolled. In 2015, 198 master's, 5 other advanced degrees awarded. *Degree requirements:* For master's, thesis (for some programs). *Entrance requirements:* For master's, BS in nursing, AS in nursing with another BS/BA, interview, RN license, 1 year of clinical experience (3 for the MS in nursing education program); for Advanced Certificate, master's degree. Additional exam requirements/recommendations for international students: Required—TOEFL (minimum score 90 iBT), IELTS (minimum score 7). *Application deadline:* For fall admission, 6/15 for domestic and international students; for spring admission, 12/1 for domestic and international students; for summer admission, 3/1 for domestic and international students. Application fee: $80. Electronic applications accepted. *Expenses:* Contact institution. *Financial support:* In 2015–16, 101 students received support. Career-related internships or fieldwork, Federal Work-Study, and scholarships/grants available. Support available to part-time students. Financial award application deadline: 3/1; financial award applicants required to submit FAFSA. *Faculty research:* Geriatrics, HIV, families and illness, oral systemic connection, symptom management. *Unit head:* Dr. James Pace, Senior Associate Dean for Academic Programs, 212-992-7343, E-mail: james.pace@nyu.edu. *Application contact:* Samantha Jaser, Assistant Director, Graduate Student Affairs and Admissions, 212-992-7653, Fax: 212-995-4302, E-mail: saj283@nyu.edu.

North Park University, School of Nursing, Chicago, IL 60625-4895. Offers advanced practice nursing (MS); leadership and management (MS); MBA/MS; MM/MSN; MS/MHR; MS/MNA. *Accreditation:* AACN. *Program availability:* Part-time, evening/weekend. *Degree requirements:* For master's, thesis. *Entrance requirements:* For master's, GMAT, MAT. *Faculty research:* Aging, consultation roles, critical thinking skills, family breakdown, science of caring.

Old Dominion University, College of Health Sciences, School of Nursing, Family Nurse Practitioner Emphasis, Norfolk, VA 23529. Offers adult-gerontology clinical nurse specialist/educator (MSN); neonatal nurse practitioner (MSN); pediatric nurse practitioner (MSN). *Program availability:* Blended/hybrid learning. *Faculty:* 3 full-time (all women), 9 part-time/adjunct (all women). *Students:* 53 full-time (52 women), 5 part-time (all women); includes 14 minority (9 Black or African American, non-Hispanic/Latino; 2 Asian, non-Hispanic/Latino; 1 Hispanic/Latino; 2 Two or more races, non-Hispanic/Latino). Average age 35. 53 applicants, 66% accepted, 23 enrolled. In 2015, 60 master's awarded. *Degree requirements:* For master's, comprehensive exam. *Entrance requirements:* For master's, GRE or MAT (waived with a GPA above 3.5), 3 letters of recommendation, essay, resume, transcripts. Additional exam requirements/

recommendations for international students: Required—TOEFL. *Application deadline:* For fall admission, 3/1 priority date for domestic students, 4/15 priority date for international students. Application fee: $50. Electronic applications accepted. *Expenses:* Tuition, state resident: full-time $11,136; part-time $464 per credit hour. Tuition, nonresident: full-time $27,840; part-time $1160 per credit hour. *Required fees:* $64 per semester. Tuition and fees vary according to campus/location, program and reciprocity agreements. *Financial support:* In 2015–16, research assistantships with partial tuition reimbursements (averaging $10,000 per year) were awarded; career-related internships or fieldwork, scholarships/grants, and traineeships also available. Support available to part-time students. *Faculty research:* Military families, nurse practitioner student reaching modalities, gerontology, pediatrics, ethics. *Unit head:* Dr. Carolyn M. Rutledge, Associate Chair for Graduate Programs, 757-683-5009, Fax: 757-683-5253, E-mail: crutledg@odu.edu. *Application contact:* Sue Parker, Graduate Program Coordinator, 757-683-4298, Fax: 757-683-5253, E-mail: sparker@odu.edu.
Website: http://catalog.odu.edu/graduate/collegeofhealthsciences/schoolofnursing/#masterofscienceinnursing013familynursepractitionerrole

Purdue University Northwest, Graduate Studies Office, School of Nursing, Hammond, IN 46323-2094. Offers adult health clinical nurse specialist (MS); critical care clinical nurse specialist (MS); family nurse practitioner (MS); nurse executive (MS). *Accreditation:* AACN; ACEN. *Program availability:* Part-time, online learning. *Entrance requirements:* For master's, BSN. Additional exam requirements/recommendations for international students: Required—TOEFL. Electronic applications accepted. *Faculty research:* Adult health, cardiovascular and pulmonary nursing.

Quinnipiac University, School of Nursing, Adult Nurse Practitioner Track, Hamden, CT 06518-1940. Offers MSN, DNP. *Accreditation:* ACEN. *Program availability:* Part-time. *Faculty:* 19 full-time (18 women), 13 part-time/adjunct (9 women). *Students:* 26 full-time (25 women), 38 part-time (33 women); includes 12 minority (6 Black or African American, non-Hispanic/Latino; 4 Asian, non-Hispanic/Latino; 2 Hispanic/Latino), 1 international. 33 applicants, 76% accepted, 18 enrolled. In 2015, 16 master's awarded. *Degree requirements:* For master's, thesis optional, clinical practicum. *Entrance requirements:* For master's, RN license, minimum GPA of 3.0. Additional exam requirements/recommendations for international students: Required—TOEFL (minimum score 575 paper-based; 90 iBT), IELTS (minimum score 6.5). *Application deadline:* For fall admission, 5/1 priority date for domestic students, 4/30 for international students. Applications are processed on a rolling basis. Application fee: $45. Electronic applications accepted. *Expenses:* $985 per credit tuition; $40 per credit student fee (not to exceed $360 per semester); $150 per semester (fall/spring) part-time technology and lab fee; $340 per semester (fall/spring) full-time technology and lab fee; $75 per semester summer technology and lab fee. *Financial support:* Federal Work-Study, scholarships/grants, and unspecified assistantships available. Support available to part-time students. Financial award application deadline: 6/1; financial award applicants required to submit FAFSA. *Unit head:* Laima Karosas, Program Director, 203-582-8672, E-mail: graduate@quinnipiac.edu. *Application contact:* Office of Graduate Admissions, 203-582-8672, Fax: 203-582-3443, E-mail: graduate@quinnipiac.edu.
Website: http://www.quinnipiac.edu/gradnursing

Research College of Nursing, Nursing Program, Kansas City, MO 64132. Offers adult-gerontological nurse practitioner (MSN); executive practice and healthcare leadership (MSN); family nurse practitioner (MSN); nursing (MSN). *Accreditation:* AACN. *Program availability:* Part-time, 100% online. *Faculty:* 9 full-time (all women), 5 part-time/adjunct (2 women). *Students:* 4 full-time (2 women), 148 part-time (132 women); includes 15 minority (9 Black or African American, non-Hispanic/Latino; 1 American Indian or Alaska Native, non-Hispanic/Latino; 3 Asian, non-Hispanic/Latino; 1 Native Hawaiian or other Pacific Islander, non-Hispanic/Latino; 1 Two or more races, non-Hispanic/Latino). In 2015, 34 master's awarded. *Degree requirements:* For master's, research project. *Entrance requirements:* For master's, 3 letters of recommendation, official transcripts, resume, personal statement/writing sample. *Application deadline:* Applications are processed on a rolling basis. Application fee: $65. Electronic applications accepted. *Expenses:* $525 per credit hour; $25 per credit hour clinical fee. *Financial support:* Applicants required to submit FAFSA. *Unit head:* Dr. Nancy O. DeBasio, President and Dean, 816-995-2815, Fax: 816-995-2817, E-mail: nancy.debasio@researchcollege.edu. *Application contact:* Leslie Burry, Director of Transfer and Graduate Recruitment, 816-995-2820, Fax: 816-995-2813, E-mail: leslie.burry@researchcollege.edu.

Rush University, College of Nursing, Department of Adult Health and Gerontological Nursing, Chicago, IL 60612. Offers adult gerontology acute care clinical nurse specialist (DNP); adult gerontology acute care nurse practitioner (DNP); adult gerontology primary care clinical nurse specialist (DNP); adult gerontology primary care nurse practitioner (DNP); nurse anesthesia (DNP). *Accreditation:* AACN; AANA/CANAEP. *Program availability:* Part-time, 100% online. *Faculty:* 43 full-time (40 women), 52 part-time/adjunct (49 women). *Students:* 50 full-time (33 women), 193 part-time (171 women); includes 52 minority (11 Black or African American, non-Hispanic/Latino; 27 Asian, non-Hispanic/Latino; 14 Hispanic/Latino). Average age 33. 167 applicants, 41% accepted, 47 enrolled. *Degree requirements:* For doctorate, capstone project (for DNP); dissertation (for PhD). *Entrance requirements:* For doctorate, GRE General Test (for DNP in nurse anesthesia; waived if cumulative GPA is 3.25 or greater, nursing GPA is 3.0 or greater, or a completed graduate program GPA is 3.5 or greater), interview, 3 letters of recommendation, personal statement, current resume. Additional exam requirements/recommendations for international students: Required—TOEFL (minimum score 94 iBT). *Application deadline:* For fall admission, 1/2 for domestic students; for spring admission, 8/3 for domestic students; for summer admission, 12/1 for domestic students. Applications are processed on a rolling basis. Application fee: $100. Electronic applications accepted. *Expenses:* Contact institution. *Financial support:* Research assistantships, teaching assistantships, Federal Work-Study, institutionally sponsored loans, scholarships/grants, traineeships, and health care benefits available. Support available to part-time students. Financial award application deadline: 3/1; financial award applicants required to submit FAFSA. *Faculty research:* Physical activity adherence in African-American women; reduction of health disparities; evidence-based interventions for caregivers; fish oil for HIV-related immunosenescence; BAILA: Being Active, Increasing Latinos Health Aging. *Unit head:* Dr. Elizabeth Carlson, Chairperson, 312-942-7117, E-mail: elizabeth_carlson@rush.edu. *Application contact:* Jennifer Thorndyke, Admissions Specialist, 312-563-7526, E-mail: jennifer_thorndyke@rush.edu.
Website: http://www.rushu.rush.edu/servlet/Satellite?c=RushUnivLevel1Page&cid=1204497838852&pagename=Rush%2FRushUnivLevel1Page%2FLevel_1_College_Home_Page

Rutgers University–Newark, Rutgers School of Nursing, Newark, NJ 07107-3001. Offers adult health (MSN); adult occupational health (MSN); advanced practice nursing (MSN, Post Master's Certificate); family nurse practitioner (MSN); nurse anesthesia (MSN); nursing (MSN); nursing informatics (MSN); urban health (PhD); women's health practitioner (MSN). *Accreditation:* AANA/CANAEP. *Program availability:* Part-time. *Entrance requirements:* For master's, GRE, RN license; basic life support, statistics, and health assessment experience. Additional exam requirements/recommendations for international students: Required—TOEFL. Electronic applications accepted. *Expenses:*

Contact institution. *Faculty research:* HIV/AIDS, diabetes education, learned helplessness, nursing science, psychoeducation.

Sage Graduate School, School of Health Sciences, Department of Nursing, Troy, NY 12180-4115. Offers adult gerontology nurse practitioner (MS, Certificate); education and leadership (DNS); family nurse practitioner (MS, Post Master's Certificate), including adult gerontology acute care (Post Master's Certificate), family nurse practitioner (MS), family psychiatric mental health (Post Master's Certificate); gerontological nurse practitioner (Post Master's Certificate); nurse administrator/executive (Post Master's Certificate); psychiatric mental health nurse clinical nurse specialist (MS); psychiatric mental health nurse practitioner (MS, Post Master's Certificate), including psychiatric mental health. *Accreditation:* AACN. *Program availability:* Part-time, evening/weekend. *Faculty:* 9 full-time (all women), 27 part-time/adjunct (24 women). *Students:* 45 full-time (43 women), 198 part-time (180 women); includes 36 minority (15 Black or African American, non-Hispanic/Latino; 2 American Indian or Alaska Native, non-Hispanic/Latino; 12 Asian, non-Hispanic/Latino; 4 Hispanic/Latino; 3 Two or more races, non-Hispanic/Latino), 3 international. Average age 38. 212 applicants, 36% accepted, 45 enrolled. In 2015, 18 master's, 8 doctorates, 9 other advanced degrees awarded. *Degree requirements:* For master's, thesis or alternative. *Entrance requirements:* For master's, currently licensed as registered professional nurse in state of practice; baccalaureate degree in nursing from nationally-accredited program or its international equivalent. Additional exam requirements/recommendations for international students: Required—TOEFL (minimum score 550 paper-based). *Application deadline:* Applications are processed on a rolling basis. Application fee: $40. Electronic applications accepted. *Expenses: Tuition, area resident:* Full-time $12,240; part-time $680 per credit hour. Tuition and fees vary according to degree level and program. *Financial support:* Fellowships, research assistantships, Federal Work-Study, scholarships/grants, and unspecified assistantships available. Support available to part-time students. Financial award application deadline: 3/1; financial award applicants required to submit FAFSA. *Unit head:* Dr. Theresa Hand, Dean, School of Health Sciences, 518-244-2064, Fax: 518-244-4571, E-mail: handt@sage.edu. *Application contact:* Dr. Carol Braungart, Co-Director, Graduate Nursing Program, 518-244-2459, Fax: 518-244-2009, E-mail: braunc@sage.edu.

St. Catherine University, Graduate Programs, Program in Nursing, St. Paul, MN 55105. Offers adult gerontological nurse practitioner (MS); neonatal nurse practitioner (MS); nurse educator (MS); nursing (DNP); nursing: entry-level (MS); pediatric nurse practitioner (MS). *Accreditation:* ACEN. *Program availability:* Part-time, evening/weekend. *Degree requirements:* For master's, thesis; for doctorate, portfolio, systems change project. *Entrance requirements:* For master's, GRE General Test, bachelor's degree in nursing, current nursing license, 2 years of recent clinical practice; for doctorate, master's degree in nursing, RN license, advanced nursing position. Additional exam requirements/recommendations for international students: Required—TOEFL (minimum score 600 paper-based; 100 iBT). *Expenses:* Contact institution.

Saint Peter's University, School of Nursing, Nursing Program, Jersey City, NJ 07306-5997. Offers adult nurse practitioner (MSN, Certificate); advanced practice (DNP); case management (MSN, DNP). *Accreditation:* AACN. *Program availability:* Part-time, evening/weekend. *Entrance requirements:* Additional exam requirements/recommendations for international students: Required—TOEFL. Electronic applications accepted.

Seattle Pacific University, MS in Nursing Program, Seattle, WA 98119-1997. Offers administration (MSN); adult/gerontology nurse practitioner (MSN); clinical nurse specialist (MSN); family nurse practitioner (MSN, Certificate); informatics (MSN); nurse educator (MSN). *Accreditation:* AACN. *Program availability:* Part-time. *Students:* 39 full-time (36 women), 30 part-time (25 women); includes 14 minority (3 Black or African American, non-Hispanic/Latino; 7 Asian, non-Hispanic/Latino; 3 Hispanic/Latino; 1 Two or more races, non-Hispanic/Latino), 1 international. Average age 38. 60 applicants, 48% accepted, 29 enrolled. In 2015, 23 master's awarded. *Degree requirements:* For master's, thesis. *Entrance requirements:* For master's, personal statement, transcripts, undergraduate nursing degree, proof of undergraduate statistics course with minimum GPA of 2.0, 2 recommendations. *Application deadline:* For fall admission, 1/15 priority date for domestic students; for spring admission, 1/15 for domestic students. Applications are processed on a rolling basis. Application fee: $50. Electronic applications accepted. *Expenses:* Contact institution. *Financial support:* Fellowships and scholarships/grants available. Financial award applicants required to submit FAFSA. *Unit head:* Dr. Christine Hoyle, Associate Dean, 206-281-2469, E-mail: hoylec@spu.edu.
Website: http://spu.edu/depts/health-sciences/grad/index.asp

Seattle University, College of Nursing, Program in Advanced Practice Nursing Immersion, Seattle, WA 98122-1090. Offers adult/gerontological nurse practitioner (MSN); advanced community public health nursing (MSN); family nurse practitioner (MSN); family psychiatric mental health nurse practitioner (MSN); nurse midwifery (MSN). *Degree requirements:* For master's, thesis or scholarly project. *Entrance requirements:* For master's, GRE, bachelor's degree, minimum GPA of 3.0, professional resume, two recommendations, letter of intent. Additional exam requirements/recommendations for international students: Required—TOEFL (minimum score 92 iBT), IELTS. Electronic applications accepted.

Seattle University, College of Nursing, Program in Nursing, Seattle, WA 98122-1090. Offers adult/gerontological nurse practitioner (MSN); advanced community public health (MSN); psychiatric mental health nurse practitioner (MSN). *Degree requirements:* For master's, thesis or scholarly project. *Entrance requirements:* For master's, GRE, bachelor's degree in nursing or associate degree in nursing with baccalaureate in different major, 5-quarter statistics course, minimum cumulative GPA of 3.0, professional resume, two recommendations, letter of intent, copy of current RN license or ability to obtain RN license in WA state. Additional exam requirements/recommendations for international students: Required—TOEFL (minimum score 92 iBT), IELTS. Electronic applications accepted.

Seton Hall University, College of Nursing, South Orange, NJ 07079-2697. Offers advanced practice in primary health care (MSN, DNP), including adult/gerontological nurse practitioner, pediatric nurse practitioner; entry into practice (MSN); health systems administration (MSN, DNP); nursing (PhD); nursing case management (MSN); nursing education (MA); school nurse (MSN); MSN/MA. *Accreditation:* AACN. *Program availability:* Part-time, online learning. *Degree requirements:* For master's, research project; for doctorate, dissertation or scholarly project. *Entrance requirements:* For doctorate, GRE (waived for students with GPA of 3.5 or higher). Additional exam requirements/recommendations for international students: Required—TOEFL. Electronic applications accepted. *Faculty research:* Parent/child, adult, and gerontological nursing; breast cancer; families of children with HIV; parish nursing.

Southern Adventist University, School of Nursing, Collegedale, TN 37315-0370. Offers acute care nurse practitioner (MSN); adult nurse practitioner (MSN); family nurse practitioner (MSN); nurse educator (MSN); MSN/MSBA. *Accreditation:* ACEN. *Program availability:* Part-time. *Degree requirements:* For master's, thesis or project. *Entrance requirements:* For master's, RN license. Additional exam requirements/recommendations for international students: Required—TOEFL (minimum score 600

paper-based). Electronic applications accepted. *Faculty research:* Pain management, ethics, corporate wellness, caring spirituality, stress.

South University, Program in Nursing, Tampa, FL 33614. Offers adult health nurse practitioner (MS); family nurse practitioner (MS); nurse educator (MS).

Spalding University, Graduate Studies, Kosair College of Health and Natural Sciences, School of Nursing, Louisville, KY 40203-2188. Offers adult nurse practitioner (MSN, PMC); family nurse practitioner (MSN, PMC); leadership in nursing and healthcare (MSN); pediatric nurse practitioner (MSN, PMC). *Accreditation:* AACN. *Program availability:* Part-time, evening/weekend. *Faculty:* 10 full-time (9 women), 8 part-time/adjunct (7 women). *Students:* 101 full-time (94 women), 9 part-time (all women); includes 20 minority (14 Black or African American, non-Hispanic/Latino; 3 Asian, non-Hispanic/Latino; 1 Native Hawaiian or other Pacific Islander, non-Hispanic/Latino; 2 Two or more races, non-Hispanic/Latino). Average age 36. 10 applicants, 30% accepted, 2 enrolled. In 2015, 43 master's awarded. *Degree requirements:* For master's, comprehensive exam (for some programs), thesis. *Entrance requirements:* For master's, GRE General Test, BSN or bachelor's degree in related field, RN licensure, autobiographical statement, transcripts, letters of recommendation. Additional exam requirements/recommendations for international students: Required—TOEFL (minimum score 535 paper-based). *Application deadline:* For fall admission, 2/1 priority date for domestic students. Application fee: $30. *Financial support:* Career-related internships or fieldwork, scholarships/grants, and traineeships available. Support available to part-time students. Financial award application deadline: 3/30; financial award applicants required to submit FAFSA. *Faculty research:* Nurse educational administration, gerontology, bioterrorism, healthcare ethics, leadership. *Unit head:* Dr. Patricia Spurr, Chair, 502-873-4304, E-mail: pspurr@spalding.edu. *Application contact:* Dr. Pam King, Program Director, 502-873-4292, E-mail: pking@spalding.edu.
Website: http://www.spalding.edu/nursing/

Stony Brook University, State University of New York, Stony Brook Medicine, School of Nursing, Program in Adult-Gerontological Health/Primary Care Nursing, Stony Brook, NY 11794. Offers adult health nurse practitioner (Certificate); adult health/primary care nursing (MS, DNP). *Accreditation:* AACN. *Program availability:* Part-time, blended/hybrid learning. *Students:* 18 full-time (16 women), 289 part-time (254 women); includes 115 minority (35 Black or African American, non-Hispanic/Latino; 55 Asian, non-Hispanic/Latino; 23 Hispanic/Latino; 2 Two or more races, non-Hispanic/Latino), 2 international. 164 applicants, 62% accepted, 88 enrolled. In 2015, 57 master's, 13 doctorates, 1 other advanced degree awarded. *Degree requirements:* For master's, thesis. *Entrance requirements:* For master's, BSN, minimum GPA of 3.0, course work in statistics. Additional exam requirements/recommendations for international students: Required—TOEFL (minimum score 90 iBT). *Application deadline:* For fall admission, 12/1 for domestic students. Application fee: $100. *Expenses:* $24,781 full-time resident tuition and fees per year, $968 per credit hour; $44,431 full-time nonresident tuition and fees per year, $1,787 per credit hour. *Financial support:* Application deadline: 3/15. *Unit head:* Justin M. Waryold, Program Director, 631-444-3074, Fax: 631-444-3136, E-mail: justin.waryold@stonybrook.edu. *Application contact:* Dr. Dolores C. Bilges, Senior Staff Assistant, 631-444-2644, Fax: 631-444-3136, E-mail: dnp.nursing@stonybrook.edu.
Website: http://www.nursing.stonybrookmedicine.edu/about

Temple University, College of Public Health, Department of Nursing, Philadelphia, PA 19122. Offers adult-gerontology primary care (DNP); family-individual across the lifespan (DNP); nursing (DNP). *Accreditation:* AACN. *Program availability:* Part-time. *Faculty:* 12 full-time (11 women), 1 (woman) part-time/adjunct. *Students:* 7 full-time (all women), 61 part-time (50 women); includes 37 minority (23 Black or African American, non-Hispanic/Latino; 8 Asian, non-Hispanic/Latino; 4 Hispanic/Latino; 2 Two or more races, non-Hispanic/Latino). 28 applicants, 64% accepted, 9 enrolled. In 2015, 8 doctorates awarded. *Degree requirements:* For doctorate, evidence-based practice project. *Entrance requirements:* For doctorate, GRE General Test or MAT, 2 letters of reference, RN license, interview, statement of purpose, resume. Additional exam requirements/recommendations for international students: Required—TOEFL (minimum score 600 paper-based; 100 iBT). *Application deadline:* For fall admission, 2/15 priority date for domestic students, 1/15 for international students; for spring admission, 10/15 for domestic students, 9/15 for international students. Applications are processed on a rolling basis. Application fee: $60. Electronic applications accepted. *Expenses:* Contact institution. *Financial support:* Federal Work-Study, scholarships/grants, traineeships, and tuition waivers available. Support available to part-time students. Financial award application deadline: 1/15. *Faculty research:* Health promotion, chronic illness, family support systems, primary care, health policy, community health services, evidence-based practice. *Unit head:* Dr. Nancy Rothman, RN, Interim Chair, 215-707-5436, E-mail: rothman@temple.edu. *Application contact:* Audrey Scriven, Academic Coordinator, Graduate Program, 215-204-4618, E-mail: tunurse@temple.edu.

Texas Christian University, Harris College of Nursing and Health Sciences, Master's Program in Nursing, Fort Worth, TX 76129. Offers clinical nurse leader (MSN, Certificate); clinical nurse specialist (MSN), including adult/gerontology nursing, pediatrics; nursing education (MSN). *Accreditation:* AACN; AANA/CANAEP (one or more programs are accredited). *Program availability:* Part-time, online only, 100% online. *Faculty:* 20 full-time (17 women), 2 part-time/adjunct (both women). *Students:* 47 full-time (40 women), 24 part-time (all women); includes 19 minority (3 Black or African American, non-Hispanic/Latino; 1 American Indian or Alaska Native, non-Hispanic/Latino; 10 Asian, non-Hispanic/Latino; 2 Hispanic/Latino; 1 Native Hawaiian or other Pacific Islander, non-Hispanic/Latino; 2 Two or more races, non-Hispanic/Latino), 1 international. Average age 39. 34 applicants, 82% accepted, 23 enrolled. In 2015, 14 master's awarded. *Degree requirements:* For master's, thesis or alternative, practicum. *Entrance requirements:* For master's, GRE General Test, 3 letters of reference, essay, resume, two official transcripts from every institution attended. *Application deadline:* For fall admission, 4/1 for domestic and international students; for spring admission, 9/1 for domestic and international students; for summer admission, 2/1 for domestic and international students. Applications are processed on a rolling basis. Application fee: $60. Electronic applications accepted. *Expenses:* $1,415 per semester hour; $112 fee per course. *Financial support:* In 2015–16, 71 students received support. Teaching assistantships and scholarships/grants available. Financial award application deadline: 2/15; financial award applicants required to submit FAFSA. *Faculty research:* Geriatrics, cancer survivorship, health literacy, endothelial cells, clinical simulation outcomes. *Unit head:* Dr. Kathy Baker, Director, Division of Nursing Graduate Studies and Scholarship, 817-257-6726, Fax: 817-257-8383, E-mail: kathy.baker@tcu.edu. *Application contact:* Mary Jane Allred, Administrative Program Specialist, 817-257-6726, Fax: 817-257-8383, E-mail: m.allred@tcu.edu.
Website: http://www.nursing.tcu.edu/graduate.asp

Texas Woman's University, Graduate School, College of Nursing, Denton, TX 76204-5498. Offers acute care nurse practitioner (MS); adult health clinical nurse specialist (MS); adult health nurse practitioner (MS); child health clinical nurse specialist (MS); clinical nurse leader (MS); family nurse practitioner (MS); health systems management (MS); nursing education (MS); nursing practice (DNP); nursing science (PhD); pediatric nurse practitioner (MS); women's health clinical nurse specialist (MS); women's health nurse practitioner (MS). *Accreditation:* AACN. *Program availability:* Part-time, online learning. *Faculty:* 55 full-time (51 women), 42 part-time/adjunct (35 women). *Students:*

Adult Nursing

39 full-time (37 women), 958 part-time (888 women); includes 566 minority (226 Black or African American, non-Hispanic/Latino; 8 American Indian or Alaska Native, non-Hispanic/Latino; 221 Asian, non-Hispanic/Latino; 88 Hispanic/Latino; 3 Native Hawaiian or other Pacific Islander, non-Hispanic/Latino; 20 Two or more races, non-Hispanic/Latino), 37 international. Average age 36. 430 applicants, 65% accepted, 193 enrolled. In 2015, 248 master's, 10 doctorates awarded. *Degree requirements:* For master's, comprehensive exam, thesis or alternative; for doctorate, comprehensive exam, thesis/dissertation. *Entrance requirements:* For master's, GRE or MAT, minimum GPA of 3.0 on last 60 hours in undergraduate nursing degree and overall, RN license, BS in nursing, basic statistics course; for doctorate, GRE (preferred minimum score 153 [500 old version] Verbal, 144 [500 old version] Quantitative, 4 Analytical), MS in nursing, minimum preferred GPA of 3.5, RN license, statistics, 2 letters of reference, curriculum vitae, graduate nursing-theory course, graduate research course, statement of professional goals and research interests. Additional exam requirements/recommendations for international students: Required—TOEFL (minimum score 550 paper-based; 79 iBT). *Application deadline:* For fall admission, 5/1 priority date for domestic students, 3/1 for international students; for spring admission, 9/15 priority date for domestic students, 7/1 for international students. Applications are processed on a rolling basis. Application fee: $50 ($75 for international students). Electronic applications accepted. *Expenses:* Tuition, state resident: full-time $4380; part-time $243 per credit hour. Tuition, nonresident: full-time $11,400; part-time $633 per credit hour. *International tuition:* $11,465 full-time. *Required fees:* $1778; $99 per credit hour. $283 per semester. One-time fee: $50. Tuition and fees vary according to course load and program. *Financial support:* In 2015–16, 149 students received support, including 10 research assistantships (averaging $5,600 per year), 1 teaching assistantship (averaging $5,600 per year); career-related internships or fieldwork, Federal Work-Study, institutionally sponsored loans, scholarships/grants, traineeships, health care benefits, and unspecified assistantships also available. Support available to part-time students. Financial award application deadline: 3/1; financial award applicants required to submit FAFSA. *Faculty research:* Screening, prevention, and treatment for intimate partner violence; needs of adolescents during childbirth intervention; a network analysis decision tool for nurse managers (social network analysis); support for adolescents with implantable cardioverter defibrillators; informatics: nurse staffing, safety, quality, and financial data as they relate to patient care outcomes; prevention and treatment of obesity; improving infant outcomes related to premature birth. *Total annual research expenditures:* $1.7 million. *Unit head:* Dr. Anita G. Hufft, Dean, 940-898-2401, Fax: 940-898-2437, E-mail: nursing@twu.edu. *Application contact:* Dr. Samuel Wheeler, Assistant Director of Admissions, 940-898-3188, Fax: 940-898-3081, E-mail: wheelersr@twu.edu.
Website: http://www.twu.edu/nursing/

Troy University, Graduate School, College of Health and Human Services, Program in Nursing, Troy, AL 36082. Offers adult health (MSN); clinical nurse specialist adult health (DNP); clinical nurse specialist maternal infant (DNP); family nurse practitioner (MSN, DNP, PMC); informatics specialist (MSN); maternal infant (MSN). *Accreditation:* ACEN. *Program availability:* Part-time, evening/weekend. *Faculty:* 13 full-time (12 women), 11 part-time/adjunct (all women). *Students:* 75 full-time (62 women), 202 part-time (179 women); includes 91 minority (72 Black or African American, non-Hispanic/Latino; 1 Asian, non-Hispanic/Latino; 8 Hispanic/Latino; 10 Two or more races, non-Hispanic/Latino). Average age 34. 50 applicants, 96% accepted. In 2015, 43 master's, 13 doctorates, 15 other advanced degrees awarded. *Degree requirements:* For master's, comprehensive exam, minimum GPA of 3.0, candidacy; for doctorate, minimum GPA of 3.0, submission of approved comprehensive e-portfolio, completion of residency synthesis project, minimum of 1000 hours of clinical practice, qualifying exam. *Entrance requirements:* For master's, GRE (minimum score of 850 on old exam or 290 on new exam) or MAT (minimum score of 396), minimum GPA of 3.0, BSN, current RN licensure, 2 letters of reference, undergraduate health assessment course; for doctorate, GRE (minimum score of 850 on old exam or 294 on new exam), BSN or MSN, minimum GPA of 3.0, 2 letters of reference, current RN licensure, essay. Additional exam requirements/recommendations for international students: Required—TOEFL (minimum score 523 paper-based; 70 iBT), IELTS (minimum score 6). *Application deadline:* Applications are processed on a rolling basis. Application fee: $50. Electronic applications accepted. *Expenses:* Tuition, state resident: full-time $7146; part-time $397 per credit hour. Tuition, nonresident: full-time $14,292; part-time $794 per credit hour. *Required fees:* $802. Tuition and fees vary according to campus/location and program. *Financial support:* Fellowships, career-related internships or fieldwork, and scholarships/grants available. Support available to part-time students. Financial award applicants required to submit FAFSA. *Unit head:* Dr. Diane Weed, Director, School of Nursing, 334-670-5864, Fax: 334-670-3745, E-mail: lweed@troy.edu. *Application contact:* Crystal G. Bishop, Director of Graduate Admissions, School of Nursing, 334-241-8631, E-mail: cdgodwin@troy.edu.

Universidad del Turabo, Graduate Programs, School of Health Sciences, Programs in Nursing, Program in Family Nurse Practitioner - Adult Nursing, Gurabo, PR 00778-3030. Offers MSN, Certificate.

University at Buffalo, the State University of New York, Graduate School, School of Nursing, Buffalo, NY 14214. Offers adult gerontology nurse practitioner (DNP); family nurse practitioner (DNP); health care systems and leadership (MS); nurse anesthetist (DNP); nursing (PhD); nursing education (Certificate); psychiatric/mental health nurse practitioner (DNP). *Accreditation:* AACN; AANA/CANAEP (one or more programs are accredited). *Program availability:* Part-time, 100% online. *Students:* 61 full-time (37 women), 137 part-time (114 women); includes 35 minority (17 Black or African American, non-Hispanic/Latino; 1 American Indian or Alaska Native, non-Hispanic/Latino; 17 Asian, non-Hispanic/Latino), 7 international. Average age 32. 193 applicants, 49% accepted, 75 enrolled. In 2015, 6 master's, 37 doctorates awarded. *Degree requirements:* For master's, thesis optional; for doctorate, comprehensive exam (for some programs), capstone (for DNP), dissertation (for PhD). *Entrance requirements:* For master's, GRE or MAT; for doctorate, GRE or MAT, minimum GPA of 3.0 (for DNP), 3.25 (for PhD); RN license; BS or MS in nursing; 3 references; writing sample; resume; personal statement; for Certificate, interview, minimum GPA of 3.0 or GRE General Test, RN license, MS in nursing, professional certification. Additional exam requirements/recommendations for international students: Required—TOEFL (minimum score 550 paper-based; 79 iBT), IELTS (minimum score 6.5). *Application deadline:* For fall admission, 7/1 for domestic students, 2/1 for international students; for spring admission, 12/1 for domestic students, 10/1 for international students; for summer admission, 2/1 for domestic students. Applications are processed on a rolling basis. Application fee: $75. Electronic applications accepted. *Financial support:* In 2015–16, 80 students received support, including 2 fellowships with tuition reimbursements available (averaging $17,000 per year), 4 research assistantships with tuition reimbursements available (averaging $10,600 per year), 7 teaching assistantships with tuition reimbursements available (averaging $10,600 per year); scholarships/grants, traineeships, health care benefits, and unspecified assistantships also available. Financial award application deadline: 2/1; financial award applicants required to submit FAFSA. *Faculty research:* Oncology, palliative care, gerontology, addictions, mental health, community wellness, sleep, workforce, care of underserved populations, quality and safety, person-centered care, adolescent health. *Total annual research*

expenditures: $1.4 million. *Unit head:* Dr. Marsha L. Lewis, Dean and Professor, 716-829-2533, Fax: 716-829-2566, E-mail: ubnursingdean@buffalo.edu. *Application contact:* Jennifer H. VanLaeken, Director of Graduate Student Services, 716-829-3311, Fax: 716-829-2067, E-mail: jhv2@buffalo.edu.
Website: http://nursing.buffalo.edu/

University of Central Arkansas, Graduate School, College of Health and Behavioral Sciences, Department of Nursing, Conway, AR 72035-0001. Offers adult nurse practitioner (PMC); clinical nurse leader (PMC); clinical nurse specialist (MSN); family nurse practitioner (PMC); nurse educator (PMC); nurse practitioner (MSN). *Accreditation:* AACN. *Program availability:* Part-time, evening/weekend, online learning. *Degree requirements:* For master's, comprehensive exam, thesis optional, clinicals. *Entrance requirements:* For master's, GRE General Test, minimum GPA of 2.7. Additional exam requirements/recommendations for international students: Required—TOEFL (minimum score 550 paper-based; 80 iBT). Electronic applications accepted. *Expenses:* Contact institution.

University of Cincinnati, Graduate School, College of Nursing, Cincinnati, OH 45221-0038. Offers clinical nurse specialist (MSN), including adult health, community health, neonatal, nursing administration, occupational health, pediatric health, psychiatric nursing, women's health; nurse anesthesia (MSN); nurse midwifery (MSN); nurse practitioner (MSN), including acute care, ambulatory care, family, family/psychiatric, women's health; nursing (PhD); MBA/MSN. *Accreditation:* AACN; AANA/CANAEP (one or more programs are accredited); ACNM/ACME. *Program availability:* Part-time, online learning. Terminal master's awarded for partial completion of doctoral program. *Degree requirements:* For master's, thesis or alternative; for doctorate, comprehensive exam, thesis/dissertation. *Entrance requirements:* For master's and doctorate, GRE General Test. Additional exam requirements/recommendations for international students: Required—TOEFL (minimum score 520 paper-based). Electronic applications accepted. *Faculty research:* Substance abuse, injury and violence, symptom management.

University of Colorado Colorado Springs, Helen and Arthur E. Johnson Beth-El College of Nursing and Health Sciences, Colorado Springs, CO 80918. Offers nursing practice (DNP); primary care nurse practitioner (MSN). *Accreditation:* AACN. *Program availability:* Part-time, 100% online, blended/hybrid learning. *Faculty:* 10 full-time (9 women), 8 part-time/adjunct (6 women). *Students:* 65 full-time (43 women), 137 part-time (129 women); includes 34 minority (5 Black or African American, non-Hispanic/Latino; 6 Asian, non-Hispanic/Latino; 19 Hispanic/Latino; 4 Two or more races, non-Hispanic/Latino), 1 international. Average age 34. 113 applicants, 55% accepted, 31 enrolled. In 2015, 39 master's, 7 doctorates awarded. *Degree requirements:* For master's, comprehensive exam, thesis optional; for doctorate, capstone project. *Entrance requirements:* For master's, GRE General Test or MAT, minimum overall GPA of 2.75 for all undergraduate course work, minimum BSN GPA of 3.3; for doctorate, interview; active RN license; MA; minimum GPA of 3.3; National Certification as nurse practitioner or clinical nurse specialist; portfolio. Additional exam requirements/recommendations for international students: Required—TOEFL (minimum score 550 paper-based; 80 iBT). *Application deadline:* For fall admission, 3/15 priority date for domestic students, 3/15 for international students; for spring admission, 8/15 for domestic and international students. Applications are processed on a rolling basis. Application fee: $60 ($100 for international students). Electronic applications accepted. *Expenses:* $11,734 per year resident, $20,068 per year non-resident. *Financial support:* In 2015–16, 58 students received support. Career-related internships or fieldwork, Federal Work-Study, and scholarships/grants available. Support available to part-time students. Financial award application deadline: 3/1; financial award applicants required to submit FAFSA. *Faculty research:* Behavioral interventions to reduce stroke risk factors in older adults, interprofessional models of health promotion for older adults, nurse practitioner education, practice and policy, cardiology, cardiac and pulmonary rehab, heart failure and stroke, community health prevention, veterans studies, anger management, sports medicine, sports nutrition. *Unit head:* Dr. Amy Silva-Smith, Graduate Department Chairperson, 719-255-4490, Fax: 719-255-4416, E-mail: asilvasm@uccs.edu. *Application contact:* Diane Busch, Program Assistant II, 719-255-4424, Fax: 719-255-4416, E-mail: dbusch@uccs.edu.
Website: http://www.uccs.edu/bethel/index.html

University of Colorado Denver, College of Nursing, Aurora, CO 80045. Offers adult clinical nurse specialist (MS); adult nurse practitioner (MS); family nurse practitioner (MS); family psychiatric mental health nurse practitioner (MS); health care informatics (MS); nurse-midwifery (MS); nursing (DNP, PhD); nursing leadership and health care systems (MS); pediatric nurse practitioner (MS); special studies (MS); women's health (MS); MS/PhD. *Accreditation:* ACNM/ACME (one or more programs are accredited). *Program availability:* Part-time, evening/weekend, online learning. *Faculty:* 109 full-time (100 women), 55 part-time/adjunct (50 women). *Students:* 367 full-time (332 women), 141 part-time (118 women); includes 79 minority (16 Black or African American, non-Hispanic/Latino; 2 American Indian or Alaska Native, non-Hispanic/Latino; 8 Asian, non-Hispanic/Latino; 37 Hispanic/Latino; 16 Two or more races, non-Hispanic/Latino), 6 international. Average age 36. 321 applicants, 53% accepted, 145 enrolled. In 2015, 151 master's, 36 doctorates awarded. Terminal master's awarded for partial completion of doctoral program. *Degree requirements:* For master's, thesis optional; for doctorate, comprehensive exam, thesis/dissertation, 42 credits of coursework. *Entrance requirements:* For master's, GRE if cumulative undergraduate GPA is less than 3.0, undergraduate nursing degree from NLNAC- or CCNE-accredited school or university; completion of research and statistics courses with minimum grade of C; copy of current and unencumbered nursing license; for doctorate, GRE, bachelor's and/or master's degrees in nursing from NLN- or CCNE-accredited institution; portfolio; minimum undergraduate GPA of 3.0, graduate 3.5; graduate-level intermediate statistics and master's-level nursing theory courses with minimum B grade; interview. Additional exam requirements/recommendations for international students: Required—TOEFL (minimum score 560 paper-based; 83 iBT). *Application deadline:* For fall admission, 2/15 for domestic students, 1/15 for international students; for spring admission, 7/1 for domestic students, 6/1 for international students. Application fee: $50 ($75 for international students). Electronic applications accepted. *Expenses:* Contact institution. *Financial support:* In 2015–16, 148 students received support. Fellowships, research assistantships, teaching assistantships, Federal Work-Study, institutionally sponsored loans, scholarships/grants, traineeships, and unspecified assistantships available. Support available to part-time students. Financial award application deadline: 4/1; financial award applicants required to submit FAFSA. *Faculty research:* Biological and behavioral phenomena in pregnancy and postpartum; patterns of glycaemia during the insulin resistance of pregnancy; obesity, gestational diabetes, and relationship to neonatal adiposity; men's awareness and knowledge of male breast cancer; cognitive-behavioral therapy for chronic insomnia after breast cancer treatment; massage therapy for the treatment of tension-type headaches. *Total annual research expenditures:* $5.9 million. *Unit head:* Dr. Sarah Thompson, Dean, 303-724-1679, E-mail: sarah.a.thompson@ucdenver.edu. *Application contact:* Judy Campbell, Graduate Programs Coordinator, 303-724-8503, E-mail: judy.campbell@ucdenver.edu.
Website: http://www.ucdenver.edu/academics/colleges/nursing/Pages/default.aspx

University of Delaware, College of Health Sciences, School of Nursing, Newark, DE 19716. Offers adult nurse practitioner (MSN, PMC); cardiopulmonary clinical nurse specialist (MSN, PMC); cardiopulmonary clinical nurse specialist/adult nurse practitioner (MSN, PMC); family nurse practitioner (MSN, PMC); gerontology clinical nurse specialist (MSN, PMC); gerontology clinical nurse specialist geriatric nurse practitioner (PMC); gerontology clinical nurse specialist/geriatric nurse practitioner (MSN); health services administration (MSN, PMC); nursing of children clinical nurse specialist (MSN, PMC); nursing of children clinical nurse specialist/pediatric nurse practitioner (MSN, PMC); oncology/immune deficiency clinical nurse specialist (MSN, PMC); oncology/immune deficiency clinical nurse specialist/adult nurse practitioner (MSN, PMC); perinatal/women's health clinical nurse specialist (MSN, PMC); perinatal/women's health clinical nurse specialist/women's health nurse practitioner (MSN, PMC); psychiatric nursing clinical nurse specialist (MSN, PMC). *Accreditation:* AACN. *Program availability:* Part-time, evening/weekend, online learning. *Degree requirements:* For master's, thesis optional. *Entrance requirements:* For master's, BSN, interview, RN license. Electronic applications accepted. *Faculty research:* Marriage and chronic illness, health promotion, congestive heart failure patient outcomes, school nursing, diabetes in children, culture, health disparities, cardiovascular, prison nursing, oncology, public policy, child obesity, smoking and teen pregnancy, blood pressure measurements, men's health.

University of Hawaii at Manoa, Graduate Division, School of Nursing and Dental Hygiene, Honolulu, HI 96822. Offers clinical nurse specialist (MS), including adult health, community mental health; nurse practitioner (MS), including adult health, community mental health, family nurse practitioner; nursing (PhD, Graduate Certificate); nursing administration (MS). *Accreditation:* AACN. *Program availability:* Part-time, online learning. *Faculty:* 32 full-time (27 women), 22 part-time/adjunct (11 women). *Students:* 167 full-time (145 women), 118 part-time (104 women); includes 128 minority (3 Black or African American, non-Hispanic/Latino; 1 American Indian or Alaska Native, non-Hispanic/Latino; 57 Asian, non-Hispanic/Latino; 14 Hispanic/Latino; 4 Native Hawaiian or other Pacific Islander, non-Hispanic/Latino; 49 Two or more races, non-Hispanic/Latino), 2 international. Average age 41. 253 applicants, 42% accepted, 88 enrolled. In 2015, 20 master's, 8 doctorates awarded. *Degree requirements:* For master's, thesis optional; for doctorate, comprehensive exam, thesis/dissertation. *Entrance requirements:* For master's, Hawaii RN license. Additional exam requirements/recommendations for international students: Required—TOEFL (minimum score 580 paper-based; 92 iBT), IELTS (minimum score 5). *Application deadline:* For fall admission, 2/1 for domestic and international students. Application fee: $100. *Expenses:* Contact institution. *Financial support:* In 2015–16, 78 fellowships (averaging $1,277 per year), 3 research assistantships (averaging $16,824 per year), 2 teaching assistantships (averaging $14,382 per year) were awarded. *Total annual research expenditures:* $1.8 million. *Unit head:* Mary Boland, Dean, 808-956-8522, Fax: 808-956-3257, E-mail: mgboland@hawaii.edu. *Application contact:* Maureen Shannon, Graduate Chair, 808-956-5201, Fax: 808-956-3257, E-mail: maureens@hawaii.edu.
Website: http://www.hawaii.edu/graduatestudies/fields/html/departments/mno/nursing/nursing.htm

University of Illinois at Chicago, College of Nursing, Program in Nursing, Chicago, IL 60607-7128. Offers acute care clinical nurse specialist (MS); administrative nursing leadership (Certificate); adult nurse practitioner (MS); adult/geriatric nurse practitioner (MS); advanced community health nurse specialist (MS); family nurse practitioner (MS); geriatric clinical nurse specialist (MS); geriatric nurse practitioner (MS); nurse midwifery (MS); occupational health/advanced community health nurse specialist (MS); occupational health/family nurse practitioner (MS); pediatric nurse practitioner (MS); perinatal clinical nurse specialist (MS); school/advanced community health nurse specialist (MS); school/family nurse practitioner (MS); women's health nurse practitioner (MS). *Accreditation:* AACN. *Program availability:* Part-time. *Faculty:* 100 full-time (93 women), 89 part-time/adjunct (82 women). *Students:* 359 full-time (326 women), 280 part-time (249 women); includes 169 minority (43 Black or African American, non-Hispanic/Latino; 62 Asian, non-Hispanic/Latino; 56 Hispanic/Latino; 1 Native Hawaiian or other Pacific Islander, non-Hispanic/Latino; 7 Two or more races, non-Hispanic/Latino), 12 international. Average age 32. In 2015, 4 other advanced degrees awarded. *Degree requirements:* For master's, thesis or alternative. *Entrance requirements:* For master's, GRE General Test, minimum GPA of 2.75. Additional exam requirements/recommendations for international students: Required—TOEFL. *Application deadline:* For fall admission, 5/15 for domestic students, 2/15 for international students; for spring admission, 11/1 for domestic students, 7/15 for international students. Applications are processed on a rolling basis. Application fee: $60. Electronic applications accepted. *Expenses:* Tuition, state resident: full-time $11,480; part-time $3826 per credit. Tuition, nonresident: full-time $23,720; part-time $7906 per credit. *Required fees:* $1333 per semester. Part-time tuition and fees vary according to course load and program. *Financial support:* Fellowships with full tuition reimbursements, research assistantships with full tuition reimbursements, teaching assistantships with full tuition reimbursements, career-related internships or fieldwork, Federal Work-Study, institutionally sponsored loans, scholarships/grants, traineeships, tuition waivers (full and partial), and unspecified assistantships available. Support available to part-time students. Financial award application deadline: 3/1; financial award applicants required to submit FAFSA. *Unit head:* Dr. Terri E. Weaver, Dean, 312-996-7808, E-mail: teweaver@uic.edu. *Application contact:* Receptionist, 312-413-2550, E-mail: gradcoll@uic.edu.
Website: http://www.nursing.uic.edu/academics-admissions/master-science#program-overview

The University of Kansas, University of Kansas Medical Center, School of Nursing, Kansas City, KS 66160. Offers adult/gerontological clinical nurse specialist (PMC); adult/gerontological nurse practitioner (PMC); clinical research management (PMC); health care informatics (PMC); health professions educator (PMC); nurse midwife (PMC); nursing (MS, DNP, PhD); organizational leadership (PMC); psychiatric/mental health nurse practitioner (PMC); public health nursing (PMC). *Accreditation:* AACN; ACNM/ACME. *Program availability:* Part-time, 100% online, blended/hybrid learning. *Faculty:* 59. *Students:* 44 full-time (42 women), 261 part-time (238 women); includes 54 minority (22 Black or African American, non-Hispanic/Latino; 1 American Indian or Alaska Native, non-Hispanic/Latino; 12 Asian, non-Hispanic/Latino; 10 Hispanic/Latino; 9 Two or more races, non-Hispanic/Latino), 1 international. Average age 38. 95 applicants, 97% accepted, 74 enrolled. In 2015, 71 master's, 24 doctorates, 6 other advanced degrees awarded. Terminal master's awarded for partial completion of doctoral program. *Degree requirements:* For master's, comprehensive exam, thesis (for some programs), general oral exam; for doctorate, variable foreign language requirement, thesis/dissertation or alternative, comprehensive oral exam (for DNP); comprehensive written and oral exam, or three publications (for PhD). *Entrance requirements:* For master's, bachelor's degree in nursing, minimum GPA of 3.0, 1 year of clinical experience, RN license in KS and MO; for doctorate, GRE General Test (for PhD only), bachelor's degree in nursing, minimum GPA of 3.5, RN license in KS and MO. Additional exam requirements/recommendations for international students: Required—TOEFL. *Application deadline:* For fall admission, 4/1 for domestic and international students; for spring admission, 9/1 for domestic and international students. Application fee: $60. Electronic applications accepted. *Financial support:* Research assistantships with tuition reimbursements, teaching assistantships with tuition reimbursements, scholarships/grants, and traineeships available. Financial award application deadline: 3/1; financial award applicants required to submit FAFSA. *Faculty research:* Breastfeeding practices of teen mothers, national database of nursing quality indicators, caregiving of families of patients using technology in the home, simulation in nursing education, diaphragm fatigue. *Total annual research expenditures:* $4.6 million. *Unit head:* Dr. Sally Maliski, Dean, 913-588-1601, Fax: 913-588-1660, E-mail: smaliski@kumc.edu. *Application contact:* Dr. Pamela K. Barnes, Associate Dean, Student Affairs, 913-588-1619, Fax: 913-588-1615, E-mail: pbarnes2@kumc.edu.
Website: http://nursing.kumc.edu

University of Massachusetts Amherst, Graduate School, College of Nursing, Amherst, MA 01003. Offers adult gerontology primary care nurse practitioner (DNP); clinical nurse leader (MS); family nurse practitioner (DNP); nursing (PhD); public health nurse leader (DNP). *Accreditation:* AACN. *Program availability:* Part-time, online learning. Terminal master's awarded for partial completion of doctoral program. *Degree requirements:* For master's, thesis optional; for doctorate, comprehensive exam, thesis/dissertation. *Entrance requirements:* Additional exam requirements/recommendations for international students: Required—TOEFL (minimum score 550 paper-based; 80 iBT), IELTS (minimum score 6.5). Electronic applications accepted. *Faculty research:* Health of older adults and their caretakers, mental health of individuals and families, health of children and adolescents, power and decision-making, transcultural health.

University of Massachusetts Dartmouth, Graduate School, Programs in Nursing, North Dartmouth, MA 02747-2300. Offers adult health (MS); community health (MS); nursing (PhD); nursing practice (DNP). *Program availability:* Part-time. *Faculty:* 26 full-time (all women), 39 part-time/adjunct (38 women). *Students:* 1 (woman) full-time, 115 part-time (108 women); includes 11 minority (4 Black or African American, non-Hispanic/Latino; 3 Asian, non-Hispanic/Latino; 4 Hispanic/Latino). Average age 40. 55 applicants, 91% accepted, 36 enrolled. In 2015, 18 master's, 5 doctorates awarded. *Degree requirements:* For master's, thesis, capstone project; for doctorate, comprehensive exam or thesis (for PhD only); project (for DNP only). *Entrance requirements:* For master's, GRE (if fewer than 45 credits at baccalaureate degree granting school), statement of purpose (minimum of 300 words), resume, 3 letters of recommendation, official transcripts, copy of RN license; for doctorate, GRE (for PHD, if fewer than 45 credits at baccalaureate degree granting school for DNP), statement of purpose (minimum of 300 words), resume, 3 letters of recommendation, official transcripts, copy of RN license, scholarly writing sample (minimum 10 pages for PhD). Additional exam requirements/recommendations for international students: Required—TOEFL (minimum score 533 paper-based; 72 iBT), IELTS (minimum score 6). *Application deadline:* For fall admission, 2/15 priority date for domestic and international students; for spring admission, 12/1 priority date for domestic students, 11/1 priority date for international students. Applications are processed on a rolling basis. Application fee: $60. Electronic applications accepted. *Expenses:* Tuition, state resident: full-time $2071; part-time $86.29 per credit. Tuition, nonresident: full-time $8099; part-time $337.46 per credit. *Required fees:* $18,074; $762.08 per credit. Tuition and fees vary according to course load and reciprocity agreements. *Financial support:* In 2015–16, 1 fellowship with full tuition reimbursement (averaging $24,000 per year), 3 teaching assistantships with full tuition reimbursements (averaging $4,333 per year) were awarded; Federal Work-Study and unspecified assistantships also available. Support available to part-time students. Financial award application deadline: 3/1; financial award applicants required to submit FAFSA. *Faculty research:* Pathophysiology, aging with spinal cord injury, patient care, self care management, nursing education, reflective practice, breast cancer and quality of life of ethnically diverse populations, community based action research among vulnerable populations, care giver experiences. *Total annual research expenditures:* $61,000. *Unit head:* Kerry Fater, Graduate Program Director, 508-999-8525, Fax: 508-999-9127, E-mail: kfater@umassd.edu. *Application contact:* Steven Briggs, Director of Marketing and Recruitment for Graduate Studies, 508-999-8604, Fax: 508-999-8183, E-mail: graduate@umassd.edu.
Website: http://www.umassd.edu/nursing/graduateprograms

University of Massachusetts Medical School, Graduate School of Nursing, Worcester, MA 01655-0115. Offers adult gerontological acute care nurse practitioner (DNP, Post Master's Certificate); adult gerontological primary care nurse practitioner (DNP, Post Master's Certificate); family nursing practitioner (DNP); nurse administrator (DNP); nurse educator (MS, Post Master's Certificate); nursing (PhD); nursing practitioner (DNP); population health (MS). *Accreditation:* AACN. *Faculty:* 18 full-time (15 women), 28 part-time/adjunct (22 women). *Students:* 143 full-time (119 women), 27 part-time (25 women); includes 28 minority (15 Black or African American, non-Hispanic/Latino; 10 Asian, non-Hispanic/Latino; 3 Hispanic/Latino), 1 international. Average age 34. 129 applicants, 68% accepted, 56 enrolled. In 2015, 43 master's, 10 doctorates, 2 other advanced degrees awarded. *Degree requirements:* For doctorate, thesis/dissertation (for some programs), comprehensive exam (for PhD); capstone project and manuscript (for DNP). *Entrance requirements:* For master's, GRE General Test, bachelor's degree in nursing, course work in statistics, unrestricted Massachusetts license as registered nurse; for doctorate, GRE General Test, bachelor's or master's degree; for Post Master's Certificate, GRE General Test, MS in nursing. Additional exam requirements/recommendations for international students: Required—TOEFL. *Application deadline:* For fall admission, 12/1 priority date for domestic students. Applications are processed on a rolling basis. Application fee: $60. Electronic applications accepted. *Expenses:* $10,994 resident per year; $18,210 non-resident per year. *Financial support:* In 2015–16, 31 students received support. Institutionally sponsored loans, scholarships/grants, traineeships, and tuition waivers (partial) available. Support available to part-time students. Financial award application deadline: 5/16; financial award applicants required to submit FAFSA. *Faculty research:* Health literacy, social justice, HIV prevention, cancer-related decision making, nursing education. *Total annual research expenditures:* $650,993. *Unit head:* Dr. Joan Vitello-Cicciu, Dean, 508-856-5081, Fax: 508-856-6552, E-mail: joan.vitello@umassmed.edu. *Application contact:* Diane Brescia, Admissions Coordinator, 508-856-3488, Fax: 508-856-5851, E-mail: diane.brescia@umassmed.edu.
Website: http://www.umassmed.edu/gsn/

University of Miami, Graduate School, School of Nursing and Health Studies, Coral Gables, FL 33124. Offers acute care (MSN), including acute care nurse practitioner, nurse anesthesia; nursing (PhD); primary care (MSN), including adult nurse practitioner, family nurse practitioner, nurse midwifery, women's health practitioner. *Accreditation:* AACN; AANA/CANAEP; ACNM/ACME (one or more programs are accredited). *Program availability:* Part-time. *Degree requirements:* For master's, thesis optional; for doctorate, thesis/dissertation. *Entrance requirements:* For master's, GRE General Test, BSN, minimum GPA of 3.0, Florida RN license; for doctorate, GRE General Test, BSN or MSN, minimum GPA of 3.0. Additional exam requirements/recommendations for international students: Required—TOEFL (minimum score 550 paper-based). Electronic applications accepted. *Faculty research:* Transcultural nursing, exercise and depression in Alzheimer's disease, infectious diseases/HIV–AIDS, postpartum depression, outcomes assessment.

University of Minnesota, Twin Cities Campus, Graduate School, School of Nursing, Program in Adult Health Clinical Nurse Specialist, Minneapolis, MN 55455-0213. Offers MS. *Accreditation:* AACN. *Degree requirements:* For master's, final oral exam, project or thesis. *Entrance requirements:* Additional exam requirements/recommendations for international students: Required—TOEFL (minimum score 586 paper-based).

Adult Nursing

University of Missouri, Office of Research and Graduate Studies, Sinclair School of Nursing, Columbia, MO 65211. Offers adult-gerontology clinical nurse specialist (DNP, Certificate); family nurse practitioner (DNP); family psychiatric and mental health nurse practitioner (DNP); nursing (MS, PhD); nursing leadership and innovations in health care (DNP); pediatric clinical nurse specialist (DNP, Certificate); pediatric nurse practitioner (DNP). *Accreditation:* AACN. *Program availability:* Part-time. *Degree requirements:* For master's, thesis optional, oral exam; for doctorate, thesis/dissertation. *Entrance requirements:* For master's, GRE General Test, BSN, minimum GPA of 3.0 during last 60 hours, nursing license. Additional exam requirements/recommendations for international students: Required—TOEFL (minimum score 550 paper-based; 79 iBT). *Application deadline:* For fall admission, 2/1 priority date for domestic and international students. Applications are processed on a rolling basis. Application fee: $55 ($75 for international students). Electronic applications accepted. *Financial support:* Fellowships, research assistantships, teaching assistantships, career-related internships or fieldwork, institutionally sponsored loans, scholarships/grants, traineeships, health care benefits, tuition waivers (full), and unspecified assistantships available. Support available to part-time students. Website: http://nursing.missouri.edu/

University of Missouri–Kansas City, School of Nursing and Health Studies, Kansas City, MO 64108. Offers adult clinical nurse specialist (MSN), including adult nurse practitioner, women's health nurse practitioner (MSN, DNP); adult clinical nursing practice (DNP), including adult gerontology nurse practitioner, women's health nurse practitioner (MSN, DNP); clinical nursing practice (DNP), including family nurse practitioner; family nurse practitioner (MSN); neonatal nurse practitioner (MSN); nurse educator (MSN); nurse executive (MSN); nursing (PhD); nursing practice (DNP); pediatric clinical nursing practice (DNP), including pediatric nurse practitioner; pediatric nurse practitioner (MSN). *Accreditation:* AACN. *Program availability:* Part-time, online learning. *Faculty:* 44 full-time (40 women), 47 part-time/adjunct (45 women). *Students:* 62 full-time (43 women), 259 part-time (239 women); includes 61 minority (28 Black or African American, non-Hispanic/Latino; 3 American Indian or Alaska Native, non-Hispanic/Latino; 16 Asian, non-Hispanic/Latino; 10 Hispanic/Latino; 4 Two or more races, non-Hispanic/Latino). Average age 35. 102 applicants, 35% accepted, 36 enrolled. In 2015, 116 master's, 23 doctorates awarded. *Degree requirements:* For master's, thesis or alternative. *Entrance requirements:* For master's, minimum undergraduate GPA of 3.2; for doctorate, GRE, 3 letters of reference. Additional exam requirements/recommendations for international students: Required—TOEFL (minimum score 550 paper-based; 80 iBT). *Application deadline:* For fall admission, 2/1 priority date for domestic and international students; for spring admission, 9/1 priority date for domestic and international students. Application fee: $45 ($50 for international students). *Financial support:* In 2015–16, 2 teaching assistantships with partial tuition reimbursements (averaging $6,650 per year) were awarded; fellowships, research assistantships, career-related internships or fieldwork, Federal Work-Study, institutionally sponsored loans, and tuition waivers (full and partial) also available. Support available to part-time students. Financial award application deadline: 3/1; financial award applicants required to submit FAFSA. *Faculty research:* Geriatrics/gerontology, children's pain, neonatology, Alzheimer's care, cancer caregivers. *Unit head:* Dr. Ann Cary, Dean, 816-235-1723, Fax: 816-235-1701, E-mail: caryah@umkc.edu. *Application contact:* Judy Jellison, Coordinator for Admissions and Recruitment, 816-235-1740, Fax: 816-235-1701, E-mail: jellisonj@umkc.edu. Website: http://nursing.umkc.edu/

University of Missouri–St. Louis, College of Nursing, St. Louis, MO 63121-4400. Offers adult/geriatric nurse practitioner (Post Master's Certificate); family nurse practitioner (Post Master's Certificate); nurse educator (MSN); nurse practitioner (MSN); nursing (DNP, PhD); pediatric nurse practitioner (Post Master's Certificate); psychiatric-mental health nurse practitioner (Post Master's Certificate); women's health nurse practitioner (Post Master's Certificate). *Accreditation:* AACN. *Program availability:* Part-time. *Faculty:* 21 full-time (19 women), 6 part-time/adjunct (5 women). *Students:* 18 full-time (17 women), 227 part-time (215 women); includes 34 minority (22 Black or African American, non-Hispanic/Latino; 8 Asian, non-Hispanic/Latino; 3 Hispanic/Latino; 1 Two or more races, non-Hispanic/Latino), 1 international. Average age 35. 152 applicants, 69% accepted, 83 enrolled. *Degree requirements:* For doctorate, comprehensive exam, thesis/dissertation; for Post Master's Certificate, thesis. *Entrance requirements:* For master's, 2 recommendation letters; minimum GPA of 3.0; BSN; nursing licensure; statement of purpose; course in differential/inferential statistics; for doctorate, GRE, 2 letters of recommendation, MSN, minimum GPA of 3.2, course in differential/inferential statistics; for Post Master's Certificate, 2 recommendation letters; MSN; advanced practice certificate; minimum GPA of 3.0; essay. Additional exam requirements/recommendations for international students: Recommended—TOEFL (minimum score 550 paper-based; 79 iBT), IELTS (minimum score 6.5). *Application deadline:* For fall admission, 2/15 for domestic and international students. Application fee: $50 ($40 for international students). Electronic applications accepted. *Financial support:* Research assistantships with tuition reimbursements available. Financial award application deadline: 4/1; financial award applicants required to submit FAFSA. *Faculty research:* Health promotion and restoration, family disruption, violence, abuse, battered women, health survey methods. *Unit head:* Dr. Roberta Lavin, Director, 314-516-6066. *Application contact:* 314-516-5458, Fax: 314-516-6996, E-mail: gradadm@umsl.edu. Website: http://www.umsl.edu/divisions/nursing

The University of North Carolina at Chapel Hill, School of Nursing, Chapel Hill, NC 27599-7460. Offers advanced practice registered nurse (DNP); health care systems (DNP); nursing (MSN, PhD, PMC), including administration (MSN), adult gerontology primary care nurse practitioner (MSN), clinical nurse leader (MSN), education (MSN), informatics (MSN, PMC), nursing leadership (PMC), outcomes management (MSN), primary care family nurse practitioner (MSN), primary care pediatric nurse practitioner (MSN), psychiatric/mental health nurse practitioner (MSN, PMC). *Accreditation:* AACN; ACEN (one or more programs are accredited). *Program availability:* Part-time. *Faculty:* 86 full-time (78 women), 44 part-time/adjunct (40 women). *Students:* 208 full-time (186 women), 128 part-time (116 women); includes 109 minority (49 Black or African American, non-Hispanic/Latino; 4 American Indian or Alaska Native, non-Hispanic/Latino; 32 Asian, non-Hispanic/Latino; 7 Hispanic/Latino; 17 Two or more races, non-Hispanic/Latino), 17 international. Average age 33. 624 applicants, 25% accepted, 150 enrolled. In 2015, 91 master's, 14 doctorates awarded. *Degree requirements:* For master's, comprehensive exam, thesis; for doctorate, thesis/dissertation, 3 exams; for PMC, thesis. *Entrance requirements:* Additional exam requirements/recommendations for international students: Required—TOEFL (minimum score 575 paper-based; 89 iBT), IELTS (minimum score 8). *Application deadline:* For fall admission, 12/15 for domestic and international students. Application fee: $85. Electronic applications accepted. *Financial support:* In 2015–16, 8 fellowships with full tuition reimbursements, 6 research assistantships with partial tuition reimbursements (averaging $8,000 per year), 10 teaching assistantships with partial tuition reimbursements (averaging $8,000 per year) were awarded; scholarships/grants, traineeships, health care benefits, and unspecified assistantships also available. Support available to part-time students. Financial award application deadline: 3/1; financial award applicants required to submit FAFSA. *Faculty research:* Preventing and managing chronic illness, reducing health disparities, Improving healthcare quality and patient outcomes, understanding biobehavioral and

genetic bases of health and illness, developing innovative ways to enhance science and its clinical translation. *Unit head:* Donna S. Havens, PhD, RN, Dean/Professor, 919-966-3731, Fax: 919-966-3540, E-mail: dhavens@email.unc.edu. *Application contact:* Emily Sayed, Assistant Director, Graduate Admissions, 919-966-4260, Fax: 919-966-3540, E-mail: sayed@unc.edu. Website: http://nursing.unc.edu

The University of North Carolina at Greensboro, Graduate School, School of Nursing, Greensboro, NC 27412-5001. Offers adult clinical nurse specialist (MSN, PMC); adult/gerontological nurse practitioner (MSN, PMC); nurse anesthesia (MSN, PMC); nursing (PhD); nursing administration (MSN); nursing education (MSN); MSN/MBA. *Accreditation:* AACN; AANA/CANAEP; ACEN. *Degree requirements:* For master's, thesis or alternative. *Entrance requirements:* For master's, GRE General Test or MAT, BSN, clinical experience, liability insurance, RN license; for PMC, liability insurance, MSN, RN license. Additional exam requirements/recommendations for international students: Required—TOEFL. Electronic applications accepted.

University of North Florida, Brooks College of Health, School of Nursing, Jacksonville, FL 32224. Offers clinical nurse leader (MSN); clinical nurse specialist (MSN); family nurse practitioner (Certificate); nurse anesthetist (MSN); nursing practice (DNP); primary care nurse practitioner (MSN). *Accreditation:* AACN; AANA/CANAEP. *Program availability:* Part-time. *Faculty:* 23 full-time (17 women), 2 part-time/adjunct (1 woman). *Students:* 108 full-time (90 women), 117 part-time (93 women); includes 54 minority (17 Black or African American, non-Hispanic/Latino; 1 American Indian or Alaska Native, non-Hispanic/Latino; 13 Asian, non-Hispanic/Latino; 17 Hispanic/Latino; 1 Native Hawaiian or other Pacific Islander, non-Hispanic/Latino; 5 Two or more races, non-Hispanic/Latino), 3 international. Average age 36. 136 applicants, 81% accepted, 74 enrolled. In 2015, 46 master's, 6 doctorates awarded. *Degree requirements:* For master's, thesis optional. *Entrance requirements:* For master's, GRE General Test, minimum GPA of 3.0 in last 60 hours of course work, BSN, clinical experience, resume; for doctorate, GRE, master's degree in nursing specialty from nationally-accredited program; national certification in one of the following APRN roles: CNE, CNM, CNS, CRNA, CNP; minimum graduate GPA of 3.3; three letters of reference which address academic ability and clinical skills; active license as registered nurse or advanced practice registered nurse. Additional exam requirements/recommendations for international students: Required—TOEFL (minimum score 500 paper-based; 61 iBT). *Application deadline:* For fall admission, 3/15 for domestic students, 4/1 for international students. Application fee: $30. Electronic applications accepted. *Expenses:* Tuition, state resident: part-time $408.10 per credit hour. Tuition, nonresident: part-time $932.61 per credit hour. *Required fees:* $111.81 per credit hour. Tuition and fees vary according to course load, campus/location and program. *Financial support:* In 2015–16, 35 students received support. Research assistantships available. Financial award application deadline: 4/1; financial award applicants required to submit FAFSA. *Faculty research:* Teen pregnancy, diabetes, ethical decision-making, family caregivers. *Total annual research expenditures:* $39,413. *Unit head:* Dr. Li Loriz, Chair, 904-620-1053, E-mail: lloriz@unf.edu. *Application contact:* Beth Dibble, Assistant Director of Admissions for Nursing and Physical Therapy, 904-620-2684, Fax: 904-620-1832, E-mail: nursingadmissions@unf.edu. Website: http://www.unf.edu/brooks/nursing

University of Pennsylvania, School of Nursing, Adult-Gerontology Acute Care Nurse Practitioner Program, Philadelphia, PA 19104. Offers MSN. *Accreditation:* AACN. *Program availability:* Part-time. *Students:* 43 full-time (35 women), 148 part-time (127 women); includes 42 minority (7 Black or African American, non-Hispanic/Latino; 1 American Indian or Alaska Native, non-Hispanic/Latino; 16 Asian, non-Hispanic/Latino; 10 Hispanic/Latino; 8 Two or more races, non-Hispanic/Latino), 2 international. 157 applicants, 54% accepted, 78 enrolled. In 2015, 85 master's awarded. *Entrance requirements:* For master's, GRE General Test. *Expenses: Tuition,* area resident: Full-time $31,068; part-time $5762 per course. *Required fees:* $3200; $336 per course. Full-time tuition and fees vary according to degree level, program and student level. Part-time tuition and fees vary according to course load, degree level and program. *Financial support:* Application deadline: 4/1. *Faculty research:* Post-injury disability, bereavement and attributions in fire survivors, stress in staff nurses. *Unit head:* Assistant Dean of Admissions and Financial Aid, 866-867-6877, Fax: 215-573-8439, E-mail: admissions@nursing.upenn.edu. *Application contact:* Deborah Becker, Program Director, 215-898-0432, E-mail: debecker@nursing.upenn.edu. Website: http://www.nursing.upenn.edu/

University of Puerto Rico, Medical Sciences Campus, School of Nursing, San Juan, PR 00936-5067. Offers adult and elderly nursing (MSN); child and adolescent nursing (MSN); critical care nursing (MSN); family and community nursing (MSN); family nurse practitioner (MSN); maternity nursing (MSN); mental health and psychiatric nursing (MSN). *Accreditation:* AACN. *Entrance requirements:* For master's, GRE or EXADEP, interview, Puerto Rico RN license or professional license for international students, general and specific point average, article analysis. Electronic applications accepted. *Faculty research:* HIV, health disparities, teen violence, women and violence, neurological disorders.

University of San Diego, Hahn School of Nursing and Health Science, San Diego, CA 92110-2492. Offers adult-gerontology clinical nurse specialist (MSN); adult-gerontology nurse practitioner/family nurse practitioner (MSN); executive nurse leader (MSN); family nurse practitioner (MSN); family/lifespan psychiatric-mental health nurse practitioner (MSN); healthcare informatics (MS, MSN); nursing (PhD); nursing practice (DNP). *Accreditation:* AACN. *Program availability:* Part-time, evening/weekend. *Faculty:* 27 full-time (23 women), 46 part-time/adjunct (41 women). *Students:* 178 full-time (151 women), 157 part-time (131 women); includes 143 minority (25 Black or African American, non-Hispanic/Latino; 2 American Indian or Alaska Native, non-Hispanic/Latino; 53 Asian, non-Hispanic/Latino; 49 Hispanic/Latino; 4 Native Hawaiian or other Pacific Islander, non-Hispanic/Latino; 10 Two or more races, non-Hispanic/Latino), 5 international. Average age 36. In 2015, 122 master's, 43 doctorates awarded. *Degree requirements:* For doctorate, thesis/dissertation (for some programs), residency (DNP). *Entrance requirements:* For master's, GRE General Test (for entry-level nursing), BSN, current California RN licensure (except for entry-level nursing); minimum GPA of 3.0; for doctorate, minimum GPA of 3.5, MSN, current California RN licensure. Additional exam requirements/recommendations for international students: Required—TOEFL (minimum score 580 paper-based; 83 iBT), TWE. *Application deadline:* Applications are processed on a rolling basis. Application fee: $45. Electronic applications accepted. *Financial support:* In 2015-16, 217 students received support. Scholarships/grants and traineeships available. Support available to part-time students. Financial award application deadline: 4/1; financial award applicants required to submit FAFSA. *Faculty research:* Maternal/neonatal health, palliative and end of life care, adolescent obesity, health disparities, cognitive dysfunction. *Unit head:* Dr. Sally Hardin, Dean, 619-260-4550, Fax: 619-260-6814. *Application contact:* Monica Mahon, Associate Director of Graduate Admissions, 619-260-4524, Fax: 619-260-4158, E-mail: grads@sandiego.edu. Website: http://www.sandiego.edu/nursing/

University of South Carolina, The Graduate School, College of Nursing, Program in Health Nursing, Columbia, SC 29208. Offers adult nurse practitioner (MSN); community/

public health clinical nurse specialist (MSN); family nurse practitioner (MSN); pediatric nurse practitioner (MSN). *Accreditation:* AACN. *Program availability:* Part-time. *Degree requirements:* For master's, thesis or alternative. *Entrance requirements:* For master's, GRE General Test or MAT, BS in nursing, nursing license. Additional exam requirements/recommendations for international students: Required—TOEFL (minimum score 570 paper-based). Electronic applications accepted. *Faculty research:* System research, evidence based practice, breast cancer, violence.

University of Southern Maine, College of Science, Technology, and Health, School of Nursing, Portland, ME 04103. Offers adult-gerontology primary care nurse practitioner (MS, PMC); education (MS); family nurse practitioner (MS, PMC); family psychiatric/ mental health nurse practitioner (MS); management (MS); nursing (CAS, CGS); psychiatric-mental health nurse practitioner (PMC). *Accreditation:* AACN. *Program availability:* Part-time. *Degree requirements:* For master's, thesis optional. *Entrance requirements:* For master's, GRE General Test or MAT, minimum GPA of 3.0; for doctorate, GRE. Additional exam requirements/recommendations for international students: Required—TOEFL (minimum score 550 paper-based). Electronic applications accepted. *Expenses: Tuition, area resident:* Full-time $6840; part-time $380 per credit hour. Tuition, state resident: full-time $10,260; part-time $570 per credit hour. Tuition, nonresident: full-time $18,468; part-time $1026 per credit hour. *Required fees:* $830; $83 per credit hour. Tuition and fees vary according to course load and program. *Faculty research:* Women's health, nursing history, weight control, community services, substance abuse.

University of South Florida, College of Nursing, Tampa, FL 33612. Offers advanced pain management (Graduate Certificate); nursing (MS, DNP), including adult gerontology acute care (DNP), adult gerontology acute care nursing (MS), adult gerontology primary care (DNP), adult gerontology primary care nursing (MS), adult gerontology primary care/occupational health nursing (MS), adult gerontology primary care/oncology nursing (MS), clinical nurse leader (MS), family health nursing, nurse anesthesia (MS), nursing education (MS), nursing practice (DNP), occupational health/ adult-gerontology (DNP), oncology/adult-gerontology primary care (DNP), pediatric health (DNP), pediatric nurse practitioner (MS); nursing education (Post Master's Certificate); nursing science (PhD). *Accreditation:* AACN; AANA/CANAEP. *Program availability:* Part-time. *Faculty:* 43 full-time (38 women), 7 part-time/adjunct (4 women). *Students:* 159 full-time (135 women), 721 part-time (625 women); includes 292 minority (119 Black or African American, non-Hispanic/Latino; 2 American Indian or Alaska Native, non-Hispanic/Latino; 60 Asian, non-Hispanic/Latino; 90 Hispanic/Latino; 1 Native Hawaiian or other Pacific Islander, non-Hispanic/Latino; 20 Two or more races, non-Hispanic/Latino), 12 international. Average age 35. 636 applicants, 44% accepted, 215 enrolled. In 2015, 333 master's, 18 doctorates awarded. *Degree requirements:* For master's, comprehensive exam, thesis optional; for doctorate, comprehensive exam, thesis/dissertation. *Entrance requirements:* For master's, GRE General Test, bachelor's degree from accredited program with minimum GPA of 3.0 in all upper-division coursework; current license as Registered Nurse; 3 letters of recommendation; personal statement of goals; resume or curriculum vitae; personal interview; for doctorate, GRE General Test (recommended), bachelor's degree in nursing from a CCNA/NLNAC regionally-accredited institution with minimum GPA of 3.0 in all coursework or in all upper-division coursework; current license as Registered Nurse in Florida; undergraduate statistics course with minimum B grade; 3 letters of recommendation; statement of goals; resume; interview. Additional exam requirements/recommendations for international students: Required—TOEFL (minimum score 550 paper-based; 79 iBT). *Application deadline:* For fall admission, 2/15 for domestic students, 1/2 for international students; for spring admission, 10/1 for domestic students, 6/1 for international students. Application fee: $30. Electronic applications accepted. *Financial support:* In 2015–16, 36 students received support, including 7 research assistantships with tuition reimbursements available (averaging $18,935 per year), 29 teaching assistantships with tuition reimbursements available (averaging $30,814 per year); tuition waivers (partial) and unspecified assistantships also available. Financial award application deadline: 2/1; financial award applicants required to submit FAFSA. *Faculty research:* Women's health, palliative and end-of-life care, cardiac rehabilitation, complementary therapies for chronic illness and cancer. *Total annual research expenditures:* $2.6 million. *Unit head:* Dr. Dianne C. Morrison-Beedy, Dean and Professor, College of Nursing, 813-974-9091, Fax: 813-974-5418, E-mail: dmbeedy@health.usf.edu. *Application contact:* Dr. Brian Graves, Assistant Professor/Assistant Dean, 813-974-8054, Fax: 813-974-5418, E-mail: bgraves1@health.usf.edu.
Website: http://health.usf.edu/nursing/index.htm

The University of Tampa, Program in Nursing, Tampa, FL 33606-1490. Offers adult nursing practitioner (MSN); family nursing practitioner (MSN); nursing (MS). *Accreditation:* ACEN. *Program availability:* Part-time, evening/weekend. *Faculty:* 15 full-time (13 women), 4 part-time/adjunct (3 women). *Students:* 1 (woman) full-time, 152 part-time (130 women); includes 27 minority (9 Black or African American, non-Hispanic/ Latino; 1 American Indian or Alaska Native, non-Hispanic/Latino; 9 Asian, non-Hispanic/ Latino; 8 Two or more races, non-Hispanic/Latino). Average age 33. 112 applicants, 54% accepted, 32 enrolled. In 2015, 33 master's awarded. *Degree requirements:* For master's, comprehensive exam, oral exam, practicum. *Entrance requirements:* For master's, GMAT or GRE, current licensure as registered nurse in state of Florida; minimum GPA of 3.0 in last 60 credit hours; minimum of one year of direct patient care experience within the past five years (recommended). Additional exam requirements/ recommendations for international students: Required—TOEFL (minimum score 577 paper-based; 90 iBT), IELTS (minimum score 7.5). *Application deadline:* Applications are processed on a rolling basis. Application fee: $40. Electronic applications accepted. *Expenses:* $573 per credit tuition, $80 per term fees. *Financial support:* In 2015–16, 5 students received support. Career-related internships or fieldwork, scholarships/grants, and unspecified assistantships available. Financial award applicants required to submit FAFSA. *Faculty research:* Vaccinations and public health, osteoporosis, cultural diversity, ethics, nursing practice. *Unit head:* Dr. Cathy Kessenich, Director, 813-257-3160, Fax: 813-258-7214, E-mail: ckessenich@ut.edu. *Application contact:* Chanelle Cox, Staff Assistant, Admissions for Graduate and Continuing Studies, 813-253-6249, E-mail: ccox@ut.edu.

The University of Texas at Austin, Graduate School, School of Nursing, Austin, TX 78712-1111. Offers adult - gerontology clinical nurse specialist (MSN); child health (MSN), including administration, public health nursing, teaching; family nurse practitioner (MSN); family psychiatric/mental health nurse practitioner (MSN); holistic adult health (MSN), including administration, teaching; maternity (MSN), including administration, public health nursing, teaching; nursing (PhD); nursing administration and healthcare systems management (MSN); nursing practice (DNP); pediatric nurse practitioner (MSN); public health nursing (MSN). *Accreditation:* AACN. *Program availability:* Part-time. *Degree requirements:* For master's, thesis optional; for doctorate, thesis/dissertation. *Entrance requirements:* For master's and doctorate, GRE General Test. Additional exam requirements/recommendations for international students: Required—TOEFL (minimum score 550 paper-based). Electronic applications accepted. *Faculty research:* Chronic illness management, memory and aging, health promotion, women's health, adolescent health.

The University of Texas Rio Grande Valley, College of Health Affairs, School of Nursing, Edinburg, TX 78539. Offers adult health nursing (MSN); family nurse practitioner (MSN). *Accreditation:* AACN. *Program availability:* Part-time, evening/ weekend. *Degree requirements:* For master's, thesis optional. *Entrance requirements:* For master's, Texas RN licensure, undergraduate physical statistic course. Additional exam requirements/recommendations for international students: Required—TOEFL (minimum score 550 paper-based). Electronic applications accepted. *Expenses:* Contact institution. *Faculty research:* Health promotion, adolescent pregnancy, herbal and nontraditional approaches, healing touch stress.

University of Wisconsin–Eau Claire, College of Nursing and Health Sciences, Program in Nursing, Eau Claire, WI 54702-4004. Offers adult-gerontological administration (DNP); adult-gerontological clinical nurse specialist (DNP); adult-gerontological education (MSN); adult-gerontological primary care nurse practitioner (DNP); family health administration (DNP); family health in education (MSN); family health nurse practitioner (DNP); nursing (MSN); nursing practice (DNP). *Program availability:* Part-time. Terminal master's awarded for partial completion of doctoral program. *Degree requirements:* For master's, thesis optional, 500-600 hours clinical practicum, oral and written exams. *Entrance requirements:* For master's, Wisconsin RN license, minimum GPA of 3.0, undergraduate statistics, course work in health assessment. Additional exam requirements/recommendations for international students: Required—TOEFL (minimum score 79 iBT). *Expenses:* Contact institution.

University of Wisconsin–Madison, School of Nursing, Madison, WI 53706-1380. Offers adult/gerontology (DNP); nursing (PhD); pediatrics (DNP); psychiatric mental health (DNP); MS/MPH. *Accreditation:* AACN. *Program availability:* Part-time. *Degree requirements:* For doctorate, comprehensive exam, thesis/dissertation. *Entrance requirements:* For doctorate, GRE General Test, 2 samples of scholarly written work, BS in nursing from an accredited program, minimum undergraduate GPA of 3.0 in last 60 credits (for PhD); licensure as professional nurse (for DNP). Additional exam requirements/recommendations for international students: Required—TOEFL (minimum score 600 paper-based; 100 iBT). Electronic applications accepted. *Expenses:* Tuition, state resident: $5364. Tuition, nonresident: full-time $12,027. *Required fees:* $571. Tuition and fees vary according to campus/location, program and reciprocity agreements. *Faculty research:* Nursing informatics to promote self-care and disease management skills among patients and caregivers; quality of care to frail, vulnerable, and chronically ill populations; study of health-related and health-seeking behaviors; eliminating health disparities; pain and symptom management for patients with cancer.

University of Wisconsin–Oshkosh, Graduate Studies, College of Nursing, Oshkosh, WI 54901. Offers adult health and illness (MSN); family nurse practitioner (MSN). *Accreditation:* AACN. *Program availability:* Part-time. *Degree requirements:* For master's, thesis or alternative, clinical paper. *Entrance requirements:* For master's, RN license, BSN, previous course work in statistics and health assessment, minimum undergraduate GPA of 3.0, letters of recommendation. Additional exam requirements/ recommendations for international students: Required—TOEFL (minimum score 550 paper-based; 79 iBT). Electronic applications accepted. *Faculty research:* Adult health and illness, nurse practitioners practice, health care service, advanced practitioner roles, natural alternative complementary healthcare.

Ursuline College, School of Graduate Studies, Programs in Nursing, Pepper Pike, OH 44124-4398. Offers adult nurse practitioner (MSN); adult-gerontology clinical nurse specialist (MSN); family nurse practitioner (MSN); nursing (DNP); nursing education (MSN); palliative care (MSN). *Accreditation:* AACN. *Program availability:* Part-time. *Faculty:* 5 full-time (all women), 26 part-time/adjunct (21 women). *Students:* 150 full-time (141 women), 108 part-time (99 women); includes 66 minority (50 Black or African American, non-Hispanic/Latino; 6 Asian, non-Hispanic/Latino; 6 Hispanic/Latino; 4 Two or more races, non-Hispanic/Latino), 5 international. Average age 37. 115 applicants, 95% accepted, 73 enrolled. In 2015, 69 master's, 2 doctorates awarded. *Degree requirements:* For master's, comprehensive exam. *Entrance requirements:* For master's, minimum undergraduate GPA of 3.0, bachelor's degree in nursing, eligibility for or current Ohio RN license. Additional exam requirements/recommendations for international students: Required—TOEFL (minimum score 500 paper-based). *Application deadline:* For fall admission, 8/1 priority date for domestic students. Applications are processed on a rolling basis. Application fee: $25. Electronic applications accepted. *Expenses: Tuition, area resident:* Full-time $18,036; part-time $6012 per semester. *Required fees:* $290; $210 per credit. $105 per semester. Tuition and fees vary according to program. *Financial support:* In 2015–16, 12 students received support. Scholarships/grants available. Financial award application deadline: 3/ 1; financial award applicants required to submit FAFSA. *Unit head:* Dr. Janet Baker, Director, 440-864-8172, Fax: 440-684-6053, E-mail: jbaker@ursuline.edu. *Application contact:* Stephanie Pratt McRoberts, Graduate Admission Coordinator, 440-646-8119, Fax: 440-684-6138, E-mail: graduateadmissions@ursuline.edu.

Vanderbilt University, Vanderbilt University School of Nursing, Nashville, TN 37240. Offers adult-gerontology acute care nurse practitioner (MSN), including hospitalist, intensivist; adult-gerontology primary care nurse practitioner (MSN); emergency nurse practitioner (MSN); family nurse practitioner (MSN); healthcare leadership (MSN); neonatal nurse practitioner (MSN); nurse midwifery (MSN); nurse midwifery/family nurse practitioner (MSN); nursing (Post-Master's Certificate); nursing informatics (MSN); nursing practice (DNP); nursing science (PhD); pediatric acute care nurse practitioner (MSN); pediatric primary care nurse practitioner (MSN); psychiatric-mental health nurse practitioner (MSN); women's health nurse practitioner (MSN); women's health nurse practitioner/adult gerontology primary care nurse practitioner (MSN); MSN/M Div; MSN/ MTS. *Accreditation:* ACEN (one or more programs are accredited); ACNM/ACME. *Program availability:* Part-time, 100% online, blended/hybrid learning. *Faculty:* 258 full-time (232 women), 363 part-time/adjunct (271 women). *Students:* 478 full-time (424 women), 342 part-time (317 women); includes 140 minority (36 Black or African American, non-Hispanic/Latino; 3 American Indian or Alaska Native, non-Hispanic/ Latino; 24 Asian, non-Hispanic/Latino; 43 Hispanic/Latino; 3 Native Hawaiian or other Pacific Islander, non-Hispanic/Latino; 31 Two or more races, non-Hispanic/Latino), 11 international. Average age 31. 1,268 applicants, 49% accepted, 477 enrolled. In 2015, 343 master's, 55 doctorates awarded. *Degree requirements:* For doctorate, comprehensive exam, thesis/dissertation. *Entrance requirements:* For master's, GRE General Test (taken within the past 5 years), minimum B average in undergraduate course work, 3 letters of recommendation; for doctorate, GRE General Test, interview, 3 letters of recommendation from doctorally-prepared faculty, MSN, essay. Additional exam requirements/recommendations for international students: Required—TOEFL (minimum score 570 paper-based), IELTS (minimum score 6.5). *Application deadline:* For fall admission, 11/1 priority date for domestic and international students. Applications are processed on a rolling basis. Application fee: $50. Electronic applications accepted. *Expenses:* Contact institution. *Financial support:* In 2015–16, 585 students received support. Scholarships/grants available. Financial award application deadline: 3/15; financial award applicants required to submit FAFSA. *Faculty research:* Lymphedema, palliative care and bereavement, health services research including workforce, safety and quality of care, gerontology, better birth outcomes including nutrition. *Total annual research expenditures:* $2 million. *Unit head:* Dr. Linda Norman, Dean, 615-343-8876, Fax: 615-343-7711, E-mail: linda.norman@

Adult Nursing

vanderbilt.edu. *Application contact:* Patricia Peerman, Assistant Dean for Enrollment Management, 615-322-3800, Fax: 615-343-0333, E-mail: vusn-admissions@vanderbilt.edu. Website: http://www.nursing.vanderbilt.edu

Villanova University, College of Nursing, Villanova, PA 19085-1699. Offers adult nurse practitioner (MSN, Post Master's Certificate); family nurse practitioner (MSN, Post Master's Certificate); nurse anesthetist (MSN, Post Master's Certificate); nursing (PhD); nursing education (MSN, Post Master's Certificate); nursing practice (DNP); pediatric nurse practitioner (MSN, Post Master's Certificate). *Accreditation:* AACN; AANA/CANAEP. *Program availability:* Part-time, online learning. *Faculty:* 16 full-time (15 women), 9 part-time/adjunct (7 women). *Students:* 219 full-time (198 women), 108 part-time (96 women); includes 36 minority (25 Black or African American, non-Hispanic/Latino; 9 Asian, non-Hispanic/Latino; 2 Hispanic/Latino), 16 international. Average age 31. 147 applicants, 78% accepted, 106 enrolled. In 2015, 64 master's, 8 doctorates, 9 other advanced degrees awarded. *Degree requirements:* For master's, independent study project; for doctorate, comprehensive exam, thesis/dissertation; for Post Master's Certificate, scholarly project. *Entrance requirements:* For master's, GRE or MAT, BSN, 1 year of recent nursing experience, physical assessment, course work in statistics; for doctorate, GRE, MSN. Additional exam requirements/recommendations for international students: Required—TOEFL (minimum score 540 paper-based; 83 iBT), IELTS (minimum score 6.5). *Application deadline:* For fall admission, 7/1 priority date for domestic students, 7/1 for international students; for spring admission, 11/1 priority date for domestic students, 11/1 for international students; for summer admission, 4/1 priority date for domestic students, 3/1 for international students. Applications are processed on a rolling basis. Application fee: $50. Electronic applications accepted. *Expenses:* $837 per credit (MSN); $1,049 per credit (PhD); $1,375 per credit (DNP). *Financial support:* In 2015–16, 22 students received support, including 5 teaching assistantships with full tuition reimbursements available (averaging $15,475 per year); institutionally sponsored loans, scholarships/grants, traineeships, tuition waivers (full), and unspecified assistantships also available. Financial award application deadline: 7/1; financial award applicants required to submit FAFSA. *Faculty research:* Genetics, ethics, cognitive development of students, women with disabilities, nursing leadership. *Unit head:* Dr. Marguerite K. Schlag, Assistant Dean/Director, Graduate Programs, 610-519-4907, Fax: 610-519-7650, E-mail: marguerite.schlag@villanova.edu. *Application contact:* Rebecca Harold, Administrative Assistant, 610-519-4934, Fax: 610-519-7650, E-mail: rebecca.harold@villanova.edu. Website: http://www.nursing.villanova.edu/

Virginia Commonwealth University, Graduate School, School of Nursing, Richmond, VA 23284-9005. Offers adult health acute nursing (MS); adult health primary nursing (MS); biobehavioral clinical research (PhD); child health nursing (MS); clinical nurse leader (MS); family health nursing (MS); nurse educator (MS); nurse practitioner (MS); nursing (Certificate); nursing administration (MS), including clinical nurse manager; psychiatric-mental health nursing (MS); quality and safety in health care (DNP); women's health nursing (MS). *Accreditation:* ACEN (one or more programs are accredited). *Program availability:* Part-time, evening/weekend, online learning. *Degree requirements:* For master's, thesis optional; for doctorate, thesis/dissertation. *Entrance requirements:* For master's, GRE General Test, BSN, minimum GPA of 2.8; for doctorate, GRE General Test. Additional exam requirements/recommendations for international students: Required—TOEFL (minimum score 600 paper-based; 100 iBT). Electronic applications accepted.

Walden University, Graduate Programs, School of Nursing, Minneapolis, MN 55401. Offers adult-gerontology acute care nurse practitioner (MSN); adult-gerontology nurse practitioner (MSN); education (MSN); family nurse practitioner (MSN); informatics (MSN); leadership and management (MSN); nursing (PhD, Post-Master's Certificate), including education (PhD), healthcare administration (PhD), interdisciplinary health (PhD), leadership (PhD), nursing education (Post-Master's Certificate), nursing informatics (Post-Master's Certificate), nursing leadership and management (Post-Master's Certificate), public health policy (PhD); nursing practice (DNP); psychiatric mental health (MSN). *Accreditation:* AACN. *Program availability:* Part-time, evening/weekend, online only, 100% online. *Faculty:* 22 full-time (18 women), 540 part-time/adjunct (487 women). *Students:* 4,320 full-time (3,773 women), 5,250 part-time (4,740 women); includes 3,550 minority (2,360 Black or African American, non-Hispanic/Latino; 29 American Indian or Alaska Native, non-Hispanic/Latino; 523 Asian, non-Hispanic/Latino; 421 Hispanic/Latino; 25 Native Hawaiian or other Pacific Islander, non-Hispanic/Latino; 192 Two or more races, non-Hispanic/Latino), 221 international. Average age 40. 2,057 applicants, 100% accepted, 1507 enrolled. In 2015, 3,022 master's, 86 doctorates, 34 other advanced degrees awarded. *Degree requirements:* For doctorate, thesis/dissertation (for some programs), residency (for some programs), field experience (for some programs). *Entrance requirements:* For master's, bachelor's degree or equivalent in related field or RN; minimum GPA of 2.5; official transcripts; goal statement (for some programs); access to computer and Internet; for doctorate, master's degree or higher; RN; three years of related professional or academic experience; goal statement; access to computer and Internet; for Post-Master's Certificate, relevant work experience; access to computer and Internet. Additional exam requirements/recommendations for international students: Required—TOEFL (minimum score 550 paper-based, 79 iBT), IELTS (minimum score 6.5), Michigan English Language Assessment Battery (minimum score 82), or PTE (minimum score 53). *Application deadline:* Applications are processed on a rolling basis. Application fee: $0. Electronic applications accepted. *Financial support:* Fellowships, Federal Work-Study, scholarships/grants, unspecified assistantships, and family tuition reduction, active duty/veteran tuition reduction, group tuition reduction, interest-free payment plans, employee tuition reduction available. Support available to part-time students. Financial award applicants required to submit FAFSA. *Unit head:* Dr. Andrea Lindell, Dean, 866-492-5336. *Application contact:* Meghan Thomas, Vice President of Enrollment Management, 866-492-5336, E-mail: info@waldenu.edu. Website: http://www.waldenu.edu/programs/colleges-schools/nursing

Wayne State University, College of Nursing, Doctor Program of Nursing Practice, Detroit, MI 48202. Offers adult gerontology nurse practitioner - acute care (DNP); adult gerontology nurse practitioner - primary care (DNP); family nurse practitioner (DNP); infant mental health (DNP); neonatal nurse practitioner (DNP); nurse midwifery (DNP); nursing practice (DNP); pediatric nurse practitioner - acute care (DNP); pediatric nurse practitioner - primary care (DNP); psychiatric mental health nurse practitioner (DNP). *Students:* 56 full-time (50 women), 37 part-time (32 women); includes 32 minority (19 Black or African American, non-Hispanic/Latino; 6 Asian, non-Hispanic/Latino; 3 Hispanic/Latino; 4 Two or more races, non-Hispanic/Latino), 6 international. Average age 35. 44 applicants, 66% accepted, 18 enrolled. In 2015, 16 doctorates awarded. *Entrance requirements:* For doctorate, official transcripts, two professional references, curriculum vitae or resume, statement of goals, BSN or MSN, current Michigan RN license, criminal background check, interview, on-site writing example. Additional exam requirements/recommendations for international students: Required—TOEFL (minimum score 600 paper-based; 101 iBT); Recommended—IELTS (minimum score 7). *Application deadline:* For fall admission, 1/31 for domestic and international students. Electronic applications accepted. *Expenses:* $19,325 per year resident tuition, $35,114 non-resident tuition; $805.20 per credit hour resident tuition, $1,463.10 per credit hour non-resident tuition; fees include $47.45 per credit hour student services fee and $274.60 per semester registration fee. *Financial support:* In 2015–16, 22 students received support. Fellowships, research assistantships, teaching assistantships, institutionally sponsored loans, and scholarships/grants available. Financial award applicants required to submit FAFSA. *Unit head:* Dr. Laurie Lauzon Clabo, Dean and Professor, 313-577-4104, E-mail: laurie.lauzon.clabo@wayne.edu. *Application contact:* Dr. Nancy George, Director of DNP Program, 313-577-8300. Website: http://nursing.wayne.edu/dnp/index.php

Western Connecticut State University, Division of Graduate Studies, School of Professional Studies, Nursing Department, Danbury, CT 06810-6885. Offers adult gerontology clinical nurse specialist (MSN); adult gerontology nurse practitioner (MSN); nursing education (Ed D). *Accreditation:* AACN. *Program availability:* Part-time. *Degree requirements:* For master's, clinical component, thesis or research project, completion of program in 6 years. *Entrance requirements:* For master's, MAT (if GPA less than 3.0), bachelor's degree in nursing, minimum GPA of 3.0, previous course work in statistics and nursing research, RN license. Additional exam requirements/recommendations for international students: Recommended—TOEFL (minimum score 550 paper-based; 79 iBT), IELTS (minimum score 6). *Expenses:* Contact institution. *Faculty research:* Evaluating effectiveness of Reiki and acupressure on stress reduction.

Wilmington University, College of Health Professions, New Castle, DE 19720-6491. Offers adult nurse practitioner (MSN); family nurse practitioner (MSN); gerontology nurse practitioner (MSN); nursing (MSN); nursing leadership (MSN); nursing practice (DNP). *Accreditation:* AACN. *Program availability:* Part-time. *Degree requirements:* For master's, thesis. *Entrance requirements:* For master's, BSN, RN license, interview, 3 letters of recommendation. Additional exam requirements/recommendations for international students: Required—TOEFL (minimum score 500 paper-based). Electronic applications accepted. *Faculty research:* Outcomes assessment, student writing ability.

Winona State University, College of Nursing and Health Sciences, Winona, MN 55987. Offers adult nurse practitioner (MS, Post Master's Certificate); clinical nurse specialist (MS, Post Master's Certificate); family nurse practitioner (MS, Post Master's Certificate); nurse administrator (MS); nurse educator (MS, Post Master's Certificate); nursing (DNP). *Accreditation:* AACN. *Program availability:* Part-time, online learning. *Degree requirements:* For master's, thesis; for doctorate, capstone. *Entrance requirements:* For master's, GRE (if GPA less than 3.0). Additional exam requirements/recommendations for international students: Required—TOEFL (minimum score 550 paper-based).

Wright State University, School of Graduate Studies, College of Nursing and Health, Program in Nursing, Dayton, OH 45435. Offers acute care nurse practitioner (MS); administration of nursing and health care systems (MS); adult health (MS); child and adolescent health (MS); community health (MS); family nurse practitioner (MS); nurse practitioner (MS); school nurse (MS); MBA/MS. *Accreditation:* AACN. *Program availability:* Part-time, evening/weekend. *Degree requirements:* For master's, thesis or alternative. *Entrance requirements:* For master's, GRE General Test, BSN from NLN-accredited college, Ohio RN license. Additional exam requirements/recommendations for international students: Required—TOEFL. *Faculty research:* Clinical nursing and health, teaching, caring, pain administration, informatics and technology.

York College of Pennsylvania, Department of Nursing, York, PA 17405-7199. Offers adult gerontology clinical nurse specialist (MS), including administration, education; adult gerontology nurse practitioner (MS); nurse anesthetist (MS); nurse educator (MS); nursing practice (DNP). *Accreditation:* AACN; AANA/CANAEP. *Program availability:* Part-time, evening/weekend. *Faculty:* 9 full-time (all women), 5 part-time/adjunct (2 women). *Students:* 36 full-time (26 women), 55 part-time (47 women); includes 14 minority (4 Black or African American, non-Hispanic/Latino; 2 American Indian or Alaska Native, non-Hispanic/Latino; 5 Asian, non-Hispanic/Latino; 2 Hispanic/Latino; 1 Two or more races, non-Hispanic/Latino), 1 international. Average age 33. 115 applicants, 28% accepted, 28 enrolled. In 2015, 24 master's, 4 doctorates awarded. *Entrance requirements:* For master's, GRE General Test (for nurse anesthetist program), minimum GPA of 3.0 from CCNE- or NLNAC-accredited institution; for doctorate, master's degree in nursing from a CCNE- or NLNAC-accredited institution; minimum GPA of 3.5. Additional exam requirements/recommendations for international students: Required—TOEFL (minimum score 530 paper-based; 72 iBT). *Application deadline:* Applications are processed on a rolling basis. Application fee: $0. Electronic applications accepted. *Expenses: Tuition,* area resident: Full-time $13,770. *Required fees:* $1750; $380. Tuition and fees vary according to degree level. *Financial support:* Federal Work-Study available. *Faculty research:* Student stress response to simulation versus clinical, evidence-based practice in all clinical settings. *Unit head:* Dr. Kimberly Fenstermacher, Graduate Program Director, 717-815-1383, E-mail: kfenster@ycp.edu. *Application contact:* Allison Malachosky, Administrative Assistant, 717-815-1243, E-mail: amalacho@ycp.edu. Website: http://www.ycp.edu/academics/academic-departments/nursing/

Community Health Nursing

Allen College, Graduate Programs, Waterloo, IA 50703. Offers acute care nurse practitioner (Post-Master's Certificate); adult nurse practitioner (Post-Master's Certificate); adult psychiatric-mental health nurse practitioner (Post-Master's Certificate); adult-gerontology acute care nurse practitioner (Post-Master's Certificate); community public health (Post-Master's Certificate); community/public health nursing (MSN); family nurse practitioner (MSN, Post-Master's Certificate); gerontological nurse practitioner (Post-Master's Certificate); health sciences (Ed D); leadership in health care delivery (MSN, Post-Master's Certificate); nursing (DNP); occupational therapy (MS). *Accreditation:* AACN; ACEN. *Program availability:* Part-time, blended/hybrid learning. *Faculty:* 3 full-time (all women), 21 part-time/adjunct (20 women). *Students:* 61 full-time (54 women), 163 part-time (144 women); includes 9 minority (5 Black or African American, non-Hispanic/Latino; 2 Hispanic/Latino; 2 Two or more races, non-Hispanic/Latino), 2 international.

Average age 34. 212 applicants, 60% accepted, 94 enrolled. In 2015, 51 master's, 1 doctorate awarded. *Degree requirements:* For master's, thesis optional. *Entrance requirements:* For master's, minimum GPA of 3.0 in the last 60 hours of undergraduate coursework; for doctorate, minimum GPA of 3.25 in graduate coursework. Additional exam requirements/recommendations for international students: Recommended— TOEFL (minimum score 580 paper-based; 92 iBT), IELTS (minimum score 6). *Application deadline:* For fall admission, 2/1 priority date for domestic students; for spring admission, 9/1 priority date for domestic students. Applications are processed on a rolling basis. Application fee: $50. Electronic applications accepted. *Expenses:* $15,940 tuition, $1,240 fees. *Financial support:* Institutionally sponsored loans, scholarships/grants, and traineeships available. Support available to part-time students. Financial award application deadline: 8/15; financial award applicants required to submit FAFSA. *Unit head:* Nancy Kramer, Vice Chancellor for Academic Affairs, 319-226-2040, Fax: 319-226-2070, E-mail: nancy.kramer@allencollege.edu. *Application contact:* Molly Quinn, Administrative Assistant for Student Services, 319-226-2014, Fax: 319-226-2010, E-mail: admissions@allencollege.edu.
Website: http://www.allencollege.edu/

Cleveland State University, College of Graduate Studies, School of Nursing, Cleveland, OH 44115. Offers clinical nurse leader (MSN); forensic nursing (MSN); nursing education (MSN); specialized population (MSN); urban education (PhD), including nursing education; MSN/MBA. *Accreditation:* AACN. *Program availability:* Part-time, 100% online. *Faculty:* 7 full-time (all women). *Students:* 7 full-time (all women), 43 part-time (42 women); includes 14 minority (12 Black or African American, non-Hispanic/Latino; 1 Asian, non-Hispanic/Latino; 1 Hispanic/Latino). Average age 37. 60 applicants, 62% accepted, 26 enrolled. In 2015, 11 master's awarded. *Degree requirements:* For master's, thesis optional, portfolio, capstone practicum project; for doctorate, comprehensive exam, thesis/dissertation. *Entrance requirements:* For master's, RN license in the U.S., BSN with minimum cumulative GPA of 3.0, recent (within last 5 years) course work in statistics; for doctorate, GRE, MSN with minimum cumulative GPA of 3.25. Additional exam requirements/recommendations for international students: Required—TOEFL (minimum score 550 paper-based; 78 iBT), IELTS (minimum score 6). *Application deadline:* For fall admission, 3/1 priority date for domestic and international students. Application fee: $55. Electronic applications accepted. *Expenses:* Tuition, state resident: full-time $9565. Tuition, nonresident: full-time $17,980. Tuition and fees vary according to program. *Financial support:* Tuition waivers (full) and unspecified assistantships available. Financial award application deadline: 5/1; financial award applicants required to submit FAFSA. *Faculty research:* Diabetes management, African-American elders medication compliance, risk in home visiting, suffering, COPD and stress, nursing education, disaster health preparedness. *Total annual research expenditures:* $330,000. *Unit head:* Dr. Vida Lock, Dean, 216-523-7237, Fax: 216-687-3556, E-mail: v.lock@csuohio.edu. *Application contact:* Maureen Mitchell, Assistant Professor and Graduate Program Director, 216-523-7128, Fax: 216-687-3556, E-mail: m.m.mitchell1@csuohio.edu.
Website: http://www.csuohio.edu/nursing/

Hampton University, School of Nursing, Hampton, VA 23668. Offers advanced adult nursing (MS); community health nursing (MS); community mental health/psychiatric nursing (MS); family nursing (MS); gerontological nursing for the nurse practitioner (MS); nursing (PhD); women's health nursing (MS). *Accreditation:* AACN. *Program availability:* Part-time, online learning. *Degree requirements:* For master's, comprehensive exam, thesis optional; for doctorate, comprehensive exam, thesis/dissertation. *Entrance requirements:* For master's, GRE General Test. Additional exam requirements/ recommendations for international students: Required—TOEFL (minimum score 525 paper-based) or IELTS (6.5). Electronic applications accepted. *Expenses: Tuition, area resident:* Full-time 10,263; part-time $522 per credit hour. *Required fees:* $35. Tuition and fees vary according to course load and program. *Faculty research:* African-American stress, HIV education, pediatric obesity, hypertension, breast cancer.

Holy Names University, Graduate Division, Department of Nursing, Oakland, CA 94619-1699. Offers administration/management (MSN, PMC); clinical faculty (MSN, PMC); community health nursing/case manager (MSN); family nurse practitioner (MSN, PMC); MSN/MA; MSN/MBA. *Accreditation:* AACN. *Program availability:* Part-time, evening/weekend. *Entrance requirements:* For master's, bachelor's degree in nursing or related field; California RN license or eligibility; minimum cumulative GPA of 2.8, 3.0 in nursing courses from baccalaureate program; courses in pathophysiology, statistics, and research at the undergraduate level. Additional exam requirements/ recommendations for international students: Required—TOEFL (minimum score 500 paper-based; 79 iBT). Electronic applications accepted. Application fee is waived when completed online. *Expenses: Tuition, area resident:* Full-time $25,272; part-time $936 per credit hour. *Required fees:* $500; $250 per credit hour. *Faculty research:* Women's reproductive health, gerontology, attitudes about aging, schizophrenic families, international health issues.

Hunter College of the City University of New York, Graduate School, Schools of the Health Professions, Hunter-Bellevue School of Nursing, Advanced Public Health Nursing/Urban Public Health Program, New York, NY 10065-5085. Offers MS/MPH. *Accreditation:* AACN. *Program availability:* Part-time. *Students:* Average age 30. 6 applicants, 83% accepted, 4 enrolled. *Entrance requirements:* Additional exam requirements/recommendations for international students: Required—TOEFL. *Application deadline:* For fall admission, 4/1 for domestic students, 2/1 for international students; for spring admission, 11/1 for domestic students, 9/1 for international students. Applications are processed on a rolling basis. *Financial support:* Federal Work-Study, scholarships/grants, traineeships, and tuition waivers (partial) available. Support available to part-time students. Financial award application deadline: 5/1; financial award applicants required to submit FAFSA. *Faculty research:* Health promotion with vulnerable populations, immigrant health. *Unit head:* Judith Aponte, Specialization Coordinator, 212-481-7568, Fax: 212-481-5078, E-mail: jap@hunter.cuny.edu. *Application contact:* Milena Solo, Director for Graduate Admissions, 212-772-4288, E-mail: admissions@hunter.cuny.edu.
Website: http://www.hunter.cuny.edu/nursing/admissions/graduate

Hunter College of the City University of New York, Graduate School, Schools of the Health Professions, Hunter-Bellevue School of Nursing, Community Health Nursing Program, New York, NY 10065-5085. Offers MS. *Accreditation:* AACN. *Program availability:* Part-time. *Students:* 38 part-time (32 women); includes 22 minority (19 Black or African American, non-Hispanic/Latino; 2 Asian, non-Hispanic/Latino; 1 Hispanic/ Latino), 3 international. Average age 34. 6 applicants, 83% accepted, 4 enrolled. In 2015, 2 master's awarded. *Degree requirements:* For master's, practicum. *Entrance requirements:* For master's, minimum GPA of 3.0, New York RN license, BSN. Additional exam requirements/recommendations for international students: Required— TOEFL. *Application deadline:* For fall admission, 4/1 for domestic students, 2/1 for international students; for spring admission, 11/1 for domestic students, 9/1 for international students. Applications are processed on a rolling basis. *Financial support:* Federal Work-Study, scholarships/grants, traineeships, and tuition waivers (partial) available. Support available to part-time students. Financial award application deadline: 5/1; financial award applicants required to submit FAFSA. *Faculty research:* HIV/AIDS, health promotion with vulnerable populations. *Unit head:* Judith Aponte, Specialization

Coordinator, 212-481-7568, E-mail: jap@hunter.cuny.edu. *Application contact:* Milena Solo, Director for Graduate Admissions, 212-772-4480, E-mail: admissions@hunter.cuny.edu.

Husson University, Graduate Nursing Program, Bangor, ME 04401-2999. Offers advanced practice psychiatric nursing (MSN, PMC); family and community nurse practitioner (MSN, PMC); nursing education (MSN, PMC). *Accreditation:* AACN. *Program availability:* Part-time. *Faculty:* 6 full-time (all women), 2 part-time/adjunct (1 woman). *Students:* 27 full-time (26 women), 10 part-time (9 women); includes 4 minority (2 Asian, non-Hispanic/Latino; 2 Two or more races, non-Hispanic/Latino). Average age 39. 70 applicants, 27% accepted, 13 enrolled. In 2015, 9 master's awarded. *Degree requirements:* For master's, comprehensive exam (for some programs), research project. *Entrance requirements:* For master's, MAT or GRE, BSN. Additional exam requirements/recommendations for international students: Required—TOEFL (minimum score 550 paper-based; 80 iBT). *Application deadline:* For fall admission, 3/31 for domestic students; for spring admission, 10/30 for domestic students. Application fee: $40. Electronic applications accepted. *Expenses:* Contact institution. *Financial support:* Research assistantships, Federal Work-Study, institutionally sponsored loans, traineeships, and unspecified assistantships available. Financial award application deadline: 3/31; financial award applicants required to submit FAFSA. *Faculty research:* Health disparities and methods to better identify and provide healthcare services to those most in need. *Unit head:* Prof. Mary Jude, Director, Graduate Nursing, 207-941-7769, Fax: 207-941-7198, E-mail: judem@husson.edu. *Application contact:* Kristen Card, Director of Graduate Admissions, 207-404-5660, Fax: 207-941-7935, E-mail: cardk@husson.edu.
Website: http://www.husson.edu/nursing-msn

Independence University, Program in Nursing, Salt Lake City, UT 84107. Offers community health (MSN); gerontology (MSN); nursing administration (MSN); wellness promotion (MSN).

Kean University, College of Natural, Applied and Health Sciences, Program in Nursing, Union, NJ 07083. Offers clinical management (MSN); community health nursing (MSN); school nursing (MSN). *Accreditation:* ACEN. *Program availability:* Part-time. *Faculty:* 9 full-time (all women). *Students:* 10 full-time (all women), 120 part-time (114 women); includes 63 minority (47 Black or African American, non-Hispanic/Latino; 11 Asian, non-Hispanic/Latino; 3 Hispanic/Latino; 2 Two or more races, non-Hispanic/Latino), 1 international. Average age 44. 64 applicants, 63% accepted, 22 enrolled. In 2015, 46 master's awarded. *Degree requirements:* For master's, thesis or alternative, clinical field experience. *Entrance requirements:* For master's, minimum GPA of 3.0; BS in nursing; RN license; 2 letters of recommendation; interview; official transcripts from all institutions attended. Additional exam requirements/recommendations for international students: Required—TOEFL (minimum score 550 paper-based; 79 iBT), IELTS. *Application deadline:* For fall admission, 6/1 for domestic and international students; for spring admission, 12/1 for domestic and international students. Applications are processed on a rolling basis. Application fee: $75 ($150 for international students). Electronic applications accepted. *Expenses:* Tuition, state resident: full-time $12,835; part-time $625 per credit. Tuition, nonresident: full-time $17,396; part-time $766 per credit. *Required fees:* $3235; $147 per credit. Tuition and fees vary according to course level, course load, degree level and program. *Financial support:* In 2015–16, research assistantships with full tuition reimbursements (averaging $3,771 per year) were awarded; scholarships/grants and unspecified assistantships also available. Financial award applicants required to submit FAFSA. *Unit head:* Dr. Portia Johnson, Program Coordinator, 908-737-3386, E-mail: johnsonpo@kean.edu. *Application contact:* Pedro Lopes, Admissions Counselor, 908-737-7100, E-mail: grad-adm@kean.edu.
Website: http://grad.kean.edu/masters-programs/nursing-clinical-management

La Salle University, School of Nursing and Health Sciences, Program in Nursing, Philadelphia, PA 19141-1199. Offers adult gerontology primary care nurse practitioner (MSN, Certificate); adult health and illness clinical nurse specialist (MSN); adult-gerontology clinical nurse specialist (MSN, Certificate); clinical nurse leader (MSN); family primary care nurse practitioner (MSN, Certificate); gerontology (Certificate); nurse anesthetist (MSN, Certificate); nursing (MSN, Certificate); nursing administration (MSN, Certificate); nursing education (Certificate); nursing practice (DNP); nursing service administration (MSN); public health nursing (MSN, Certificate); school nursing (Certificate); MSN/MBA; MSN/MPH. *Accreditation:* AANA/CANAEP. *Program availability:* Part-time, evening/weekend, 100% online. *Faculty:* 13 full-time (all women), 9 part-time/adjunct (8 women). *Students:* 368 part-time (56 women); includes 103 minority (62 Black or African American, non-Hispanic/Latino; 1 American Indian or Alaska Native, non-Hispanic/Latino; 26 Asian, non-Hispanic/Latino; 9 Hispanic/Latino; 5 Two or more races, non-Hispanic/Latino), 5 international. Average age 36. 98 applicants, 85% accepted, 53 enrolled. In 2015, 87 master's, 3 doctorates, 10 other advanced degrees awarded. *Degree requirements:* For doctorate, minimum of 1,000 hours of post baccalaureate clinical practice supervised by preceptors. *Entrance requirements:* For master's, GRE, MAT, or GMAT (for students with BSN GPA of less than 3.2), baccalaureate degree in nursing from an NLNAC- or CCNE-accredited program or an MSN Bridge program; Pennsylvania RN license; 2 letters of reference; resume; statement of philosophy articulating professional values and future educational goal; 1 year of work experience as a registered nurse; for doctorate, GRE (waived for applicants with MSN cumulative GPA of 3.7 or above), MSN from nationally-accredited program or master's degree, MBA or MHA from nationally-accredited program; resume or curriculum vitae; 2 letters of reference; interview; for Certificate, GRE, MAT, or GMAT (for students with BSN GPA of less than 3.2, baccalaureate degree in nursing from an NLNAC- or CCNE-accredited program or an MSN Bridge program; Pennsylvania RN license; 2 letters of reference; resume; statement of philosophy articulating professional values and future educational goal; 1 year of work experience as a registered nurse. Additional exam requirements/recommendations for international students: Required— TOEFL. *Application deadline:* For fall admission, 8/15 priority date for domestic students, 7/15 for international students; for spring admission, 12/15 priority date for domestic students, 11/15 for international students; for summer admission, 4/15 priority date for domestic students, 3/15 for international students. Applications are processed on a rolling basis. Application fee: $35. Electronic applications accepted. Application fee is waived when completed online. *Expenses:* $870 per credit hour (for MSN); $930 per credit hour (for DNP); $150 technology fee full-time, $75 part-time; $135 general university fee. *Financial support:* In 2015–16, 13 students received support. Scholarships/grants and traineeships available. Support available to part-time students. Financial award application deadline: 8/31; financial award applicants required to submit FAFSA. *Unit head:* Dr. Patricia M. Dillon, Director, 215-951-1322, Fax: 215-951-1896, E-mail: msnapn@lasalle.edu. *Application contact:* Alison McAnespey Target, Director, Graduate and Adult Enrollment, 215-951-1100, Fax: 215-951-1462, E-mail: reilly@lasalle.edu.
Website: http://www.lasalle.edu/nursing/program-options/

Louisiana State University Health Sciences Center, School of Nursing, New Orleans, LA 70112. Offers adult gerontology clinical nurse specialist (Post-Master's Certificate); clinical nurse leader (MSN); executive nurse leader (Post-Master's Certificate); neonatal nurse practitioner (Post-Master's Certificate); nurse anesthesia (Post-Master's Certificate); nurse educator (MSN); nursing (DNS); primary care family nurse

Community Health Nursing

practitioner (Post-Master's Certificate); public/community health nursing (Post-Master's Certificate). *Accreditation:* AACN; AANA/CANAEP (one or more programs are accredited). *Program availability:* Part-time. *Faculty:* 22 full-time (19 women), 21 part-time/adjunct (8 women). *Students:* 254 (185 women); includes 68 minority (44 Black or African American, non-Hispanic/Latino; 12 Asian, non-Hispanic/Latino; 12 Hispanic/Latino). Average age 33. 144 applicants, 54% accepted, 73 enrolled. In 2015, 84 master's, 6 doctorates awarded. *Degree requirements:* For master's, thesis optional; for doctorate, thesis/dissertation. *Entrance requirements:* For master's, GRE General Test, MAT, minimum GPA of 3.0; for doctorate, GRE General Test, minimum GPA of 3.5. Additional exam requirements/recommendations for international students: Required—TOEFL (minimum score 550 paper-based; 79 iBT). *Application deadline:* Applications are processed on a rolling basis. Application fee: $250. Electronic applications accepted. *Expenses:* $9,136.50 per year; $19,633.50 per year (for DNP). *Financial support:* Federal Work-Study, institutionally sponsored loans, scholarships/grants, and traineeships available. Financial award applicants required to submit FAFSA. *Faculty research:* Advanced clinical practice, nursing education, health, social support, nursing administration. *Unit head:* Dr. Demetrius James Porche, Dean, 504-568-4106, Fax: 504-599-0573, E-mail: dporch@lsuhsc.edu. *Application contact:* Tracie Gravolet, Director, Office of Student Affairs, 504-568-4114, Fax: 504-568-5711, E-mail: tgravo@lsuhsc.edu.
Website: http://nursing.lsuhsc.edu/

New Mexico State University, College of Health and Social Services, School of Nursing, Las Cruces, NM 88003. Offers adult/geriatric nursing (DNP); family nurse practitioner (DNP); family/psychiatric mental health nursing (DNP); nursing administration (MSN); nursing science (PhD); public/community health nursing (DNP). *Accreditation:* AACN. *Program availability:* Blended/hybrid learning. *Faculty:* 16 full-time (15 women). *Students:* 24 full-time (18 women), 90 part-time (80 women); includes 49 minority (10 Black or African American, non-Hispanic/Latino; 1 American Indian or Alaska Native, non-Hispanic/Latino; 4 Asian, non-Hispanic/Latino; 32 Hispanic/Latino; 2 Two or more races, non-Hispanic/Latino), 1 international. Average age 43. 40 applicants, 58% accepted, 17 enrolled. In 2015, 6 master's, 11 doctorates awarded. *Degree requirements:* For master's, comprehensive exam, thesis optional, clinical practice; for doctorate, comprehensive exam, thesis/dissertation. *Entrance requirements:* For master's, NCLEX, BSN, minimum GPA of 3.0, course work in statistics, 3 letters of reference, writing sample, RN license, CPR certification, proof of liability, immunizations, criminal background check; for doctorate, NCLEX, MSN, minimum GPA of 3.0, 3 letters of reference, writing sample, RN license, CPR certification, proof of liability, immunizations, criminal background check, statistics course. Additional exam requirements/recommendations for international students: Required—TOEFL (minimum score 550 paper-based; 79 iBT), IELTS (minimum score 6.5). *Application deadline:* For fall admission, 1/15 for domestic students; for spring admission, 1/15 priority date for domestic students; for summer admission, 1/15 for domestic students. Application fee: $40 ($50 for international students). Electronic applications accepted. *Expenses:* $274.50 per credit hour for in-state students, and all students enrolled in six or fewer credits; $839.30 per credit hour for out-of-state and international students enrolled in at least seven hours. *Financial support:* In 2015–16, 23 students received support, including 1 teaching assistantship (averaging $9,473 per year); career-related internships or fieldwork, Federal Work-Study, scholarships/grants, traineeships, health care benefits, and unspecified assistantships also available. Support available to part-time students. Financial award application deadline: 3/1. *Faculty research:* Women's health, community health, health disparities, nursing informatics and health care technologies, health care and nursing administration. *Total annual research expenditures:* $127,778. *Unit head:* Dr. Kathleen Huttlinger, Department Head, 575-646-3812, Fax: 575-646-2167, E-mail: khuttlin@nmsu.edu. *Application contact:* Dr. Teresa Keller, Director of Graduate Studies, 575-646-4370, Fax: 575-646-2167, E-mail: tkeller@nmsu.edu.
Website: http://schoolofnursing.nmsu.edu

Oregon Health & Science University, School of Nursing, Program in Nursing Education, Portland, OR 97239-3098. Offers MN, MS, Post Master's Certificate.

Rush University, College of Nursing, Department of Community, Systems, and Mental Health Nursing, Chicago, IL 60612. Offers advanced public health nursing (DNP); family nurse practitioner (DNP); leadership to enhance population health outcomes (DNP); nursing science (PhD); psychiatric mental health nurse practitioner (DNP); systems leadership (DNP). *Accreditation:* AACN. *Program availability:* Part-time, 100% online. *Faculty:* 43 full-time (40 women), 52 part-time/adjunct (49 women). *Students:* 18 full-time (17 women), 341 part-time (314 women); includes 85 minority (38 Black or African American, non-Hispanic/Latino; 2 American Indian or Alaska Native, non-Hispanic/Latino; 21 Asian, non-Hispanic/Latino; 22 Hispanic/Latino; 2 Native Hawaiian or other Pacific Islander, non-Hispanic/Latino). Average age 35. 177 applicants, 62% accepted, 96 enrolled. *Degree requirements:* For doctorate, capstone project (for DNP); dissertation (for PhD). *Entrance requirements:* For doctorate, GRE General Test (waived for DNP if cumulative GPA is 3.25 or greater, nursing GPA is 3.0 or greater, or a completed graduate program GPA is 3.5 or greater), interview, 3 letters of recommendation, personal statement, current resume. Additional exam requirements/recommendations for international students: Required—TOEFL (minimum score 94 iBT). *Application deadline:* For fall admission, 1/2 for domestic students; for winter admission, 10/15 for domestic students; for spring admission, 8/4 for domestic students; for summer admission, 12/1 for domestic students. Applications are processed on a rolling basis. Application fee: $100. Electronic applications accepted. *Expenses:* Contact institution. *Financial support:* Research assistantships, teaching assistantships, Federal Work-Study, scholarships/grants, traineeships, and health care benefits available. Support available to part-time students. Financial award application deadline: 3/1; financial award applicants required to submit FAFSA. *Faculty research:* Reduction of health disparities; evidence-based interventions for caregivers; patient-centered quality assessment of psychiatric inpatient environments; digital delivery of a parent-training program for urban, low-income parents; patient-centered predictors and outcomes of inter-professional care coordination. *Unit head:* Dr. Mona Shattell, Chairperson, 312-942-7117, E-mail: mona_shattell@rush.edu. *Application contact:* Jennifer Thorndyke, Admissions Specialist, 312-563-7526, E-mail: jennifer_thorndyke@rush.edu.
Website: http://www.rushu.rush.edu/servlet/ Satellite?c=content_block&cid=1320160764996&pagename=CollegeOfNursing%2Fcontent_block%2FContentBlockDetail&rendermod

San Francisco State University, Division of Graduate Studies, College of Health and Social Sciences, School of Nursing, San Francisco, CA 94132-1722. Offers adult acute care (MS); clinical nurse specialist (MS); community/public health nursing (MS); family nurse practitioner (MS, Certificate); nursing administration (MS); pediatrics (MS); women's health (MS). *Accreditation:* AACN. *Program availability:* Part-time. *Application deadline:* Applications are processed on a rolling basis. *Expenses:* Tuition, state resident: full-time $6738. Tuition, nonresident: full-time $15,666. *Required fees:* $1004. *Financial support:* Career-related internships or fieldwork available. *Unit head:* Dr. Mary-Ann van Dam, Director, 415-338-1802, Fax: 415-338-0555, E-mail: vandam@sfsu.edu. *Application contact:* Connie Carr, Graduate Coordinator, 415-338-6856, Fax: 415-338-0555, E-mail: ccarr@sfsu.edu.
Website: http://nursing.sfsu.edu

Seattle University, College of Nursing, Program in Advanced Practice Nursing Immersion, Seattle, WA 98122-1090. Offers adult/gerontological nurse practitioner (MSN); advanced community public health nursing (MSN); family nurse practitioner (MSN); family psychiatric mental health nurse practitioner (MSN); nurse midwifery (MSN). *Degree requirements:* For master's, thesis or scholarly project. *Entrance requirements:* For master's, GRE, bachelor's degree, minimum GPA of 3.0, professional resume, two recommendations, letter of intent. Additional exam requirements/recommendations for international students: Required—TOEFL (minimum score 92 iBT), IELTS. Electronic applications accepted.

Seattle University, College of Nursing, Program in Nursing, Seattle, WA 98122-1090. Offers adult/gerontological nurse practitioner (MSN); advanced community public health (MSN); psychiatric mental health nurse practitioner (MSN). *Degree requirements:* For master's, thesis or scholarly project. *Entrance requirements:* For master's, GRE, bachelor's degree in nursing or associate degree in nursing with baccalaureate in different major, 5-quarter statistics course, minimum cumulative GPA of 3.0, professional resume, two recommendations, letter of intent, copy of current RN license or ability to obtain RN license in WA state. Additional exam requirements/recommendations for international students: Required—TOEFL (minimum score 92 iBT), IELTS. Electronic applications accepted.

University of Cincinnati, Graduate School, College of Nursing, Cincinnati, OH 45221-0038. Offers clinical nurse specialist (MSN), including adult health, community health, neonatal, nursing administration, occupational health, pediatric health, psychiatric nursing, women's health; nurse anesthesia (MSN); nurse midwifery (MSN); nurse practitioner (MSN), including acute care, ambulatory care, family, family/psychiatric, women's health; nursing (PhD); MBA/MSN. *Accreditation:* AACN; AANA/CANAEP (one or more programs are accredited); ACNM/ACME. *Program availability:* Part-time, online learning. Terminal master's awarded for partial completion of doctoral program. *Degree requirements:* For master's, thesis or alternative; for doctorate, comprehensive exam, thesis/dissertation. *Entrance requirements:* For master's and doctorate, GRE General Test. Additional exam requirements/recommendations for international students: Required—TOEFL (minimum score 520 paper-based). Electronic applications accepted. *Faculty research:* Substance abuse, injury and violence, symptom management.

University of Hartford, College of Education, Nursing, and Health Professions, Program in Nursing, West Hartford, CT 06117-1599. Offers community/public health nursing (MSN); nursing education (MSN); nursing management (MSN). *Accreditation:* AACN. *Program availability:* Part-time, evening/weekend. *Degree requirements:* For master's, research project. *Entrance requirements:* For master's, BSN, Connecticut RN license. Additional exam requirements/recommendations for international students: Required—TOEFL (minimum score 550 paper-based). Electronic applications accepted. *Expenses:* Contact institution. *Faculty research:* Child development, women in doctoral study, applying feminist theory in teaching methods, near death experience, grandmothers as primary care providers.

University of Hawaii at Manoa, Graduate Division, School of Nursing and Dental Hygiene, Honolulu, HI 96822. Offers clinical nurse specialist (MS), including adult health, community mental health; nurse practitioner (MS), including adult health, community mental health, family nurse practitioner; nursing (PhD, Graduate Certificate); nursing administration (MS). *Accreditation:* AACN. *Program availability:* Part-time, online learning. *Faculty:* 32 full-time (27 women), 22 part-time/adjunct (11 women). *Students:* 167 full-time (145 women), 118 part-time (104 women); includes 128 minority (3 Black or African American, non-Hispanic/Latino; 1 American Indian or Alaska Native, non-Hispanic/Latino; 57 Asian, non-Hispanic/Latino; 14 Hispanic/Latino; 4 Native Hawaiian or other Pacific Islander, non-Hispanic/Latino; 49 Two or more races, non-Hispanic/Latino), 2 international. Average age 41. 253 applicants, 42% accepted, 88 enrolled. In 2015, 20 master's, 8 doctorates awarded. *Degree requirements:* For master's, thesis optional; for doctorate, comprehensive exam, thesis/dissertation. *Entrance requirements:* For master's, Hawaii RN license. Additional exam requirements/recommendations for international students: Required—TOEFL (minimum score 580 paper-based; 92 iBT), IELTS (minimum score 5). *Application deadline:* For fall admission, 2/1 for domestic and international students. Application fee: $100. *Expenses:* Contact institution. *Financial support:* In 2015–16, 78 fellowships (averaging $1,277 per year), 3 research assistantships (averaging $16,824 per year), 2 teaching assistantships (averaging $14,382 per year) were awarded. *Total annual research expenditures:* $1.8 million. *Unit head:* Mary Boland, Dean, 808-956-8522, Fax: 808-956-3257, E-mail: mgboland@hawaii.edu. *Application contact:* Maureen Shannon, Graduate Chair, 808-956-5201, Fax: 808-956-3257, E-mail: maureens@hawaii.edu.
Website: http://www.hawaii.edu/graduatestudies/fields/html/departments/mno/nursing/nursing.htm

University of Illinois at Chicago, College of Nursing, Program in Nursing, Chicago, IL 60607-7128. Offers acute care clinical nurse specialist (MS); administrative nursing leadership (Certificate); adult nurse practitioner (MS); adult/geriatric nurse practitioner (MS); advanced community health nurse specialist (MS); family nurse practitioner (MS); geriatric clinical nurse specialist (MS); geriatric nurse practitioner (MS); nurse midwifery (MS); occupational health/advanced community health nurse specialist (MS); occupational health/family nurse practitioner (MS); pediatric nurse practitioner (MS); perinatal clinical nurse specialist (MS); school/advanced community health nurse specialist (MS); school/family nurse practitioner (MS); women's health nurse practitioner (MS). *Accreditation:* AACN. *Program availability:* Part-time. *Faculty:* 100 full-time (93 women), 89 part-time/adjunct (82 women). *Students:* 359 full-time (326 women), 280 part-time (249 women); includes 169 minority (43 Black or African American, non-Hispanic/Latino; 62 Asian, non-Hispanic/Latino; 56 Hispanic/Latino; 1 Native Hawaiian or other Pacific Islander, non-Hispanic/Latino; 7 Two or more races, non-Hispanic/Latino), 12 international. Average age 32. In 2015, 4 other advanced degrees awarded. *Degree requirements:* For master's, thesis or alternative. *Entrance requirements:* For master's, GRE General Test, minimum GPA of 2.75. Additional exam requirements/recommendations for international students: Required—TOEFL. *Application deadline:* For fall admission, 5/15 for domestic students, 2/15 for international students; for spring admission, 11/1 for domestic students, 7/15 for international students. Applications are processed on a rolling basis. Application fee: $60. Electronic applications accepted. *Expenses:* Tuition, state resident: full-time $11,480; part-time $3826 per credit. Tuition, nonresident: full-time $23,720; part-time $7906 per credit. *Required fees:* $1333 per semester. Part-time tuition and fees vary according to course load and program. *Financial support:* Fellowships with full tuition reimbursements, research assistantships with full tuition reimbursements, teaching assistantships with full tuition reimbursements, career-related internships or fieldwork, Federal Work-Study, institutionally sponsored loans, scholarships/grants, traineeships, tuition waivers (full and partial), and unspecified assistantships available. Support available to part-time students. Financial award application deadline: 3/1; financial award applicants required to submit FAFSA. *Unit head:* Dr. Terri E. Weaver, Dean, 312-996-7808, E-mail: teweaver@uic.edu. *Application contact:* Receptionist, 312-413-2550, E-mail: gradcoll@uic.edu.
Website: http://www.nursing.uic.edu/academics-admissions/master-science#program-overview

The University of Kansas, University of Kansas Medical Center, School of Nursing, Kansas City, KS 66160. Offers adult/gerontological clinical nurse specialist (PMC);

adult/gerontological nurse practitioner (PMC); clinical research management (PMC); health care informatics (PMC); health professions educator (PMC); nurse midwife (PMC); nursing (MS, DNP, PhD); organizational leadership (PMC); psychiatric/mental health nurse practitioner (PMC); public health nursing (PMC). *Accreditation:* AACN; ACNM/ACME. *Program availability:* Part-time, 100% online, blended/hybrid learning. *Faculty:* 59. *Students:* 44 full-time (42 women), 261 part-time (238 women); includes 54 minority (22 Black or African American, non-Hispanic/Latino; 1 American Indian or Alaska Native, non-Hispanic/Latino; 12 Asian, non-Hispanic/Latino; 10 Hispanic/Latino; 9 Two or more races, non-Hispanic/Latino), 1 international. Average age 38. 95 applicants, 97% accepted, 74 enrolled. In 2015, 71 master's, 24 doctorates, 6 other advanced degrees awarded. Terminal master's awarded for partial completion of doctoral program. *Degree requirements:* For master's, comprehensive exam, thesis (for some programs), general oral exam; for doctorate, variable foreign language requirement, thesis/dissertation or alternative, comprehensive oral exam (for DNP); comprehensive written and oral exam, or three publications (for PhD). *Entrance requirements:* For master's, bachelor's degree in nursing, minimum GPA of 3.0, 1 year of clinical experience, RN license in KS and MO; for doctorate, GRE General Test (for PhD only), bachelor's degree in nursing, minimum GPA of 3.5, RN license in KS and MO. Additional exam requirements/recommendations for international students: Required—TOEFL. *Application deadline:* For fall admission, 4/1 for domestic and international students; for spring admission, 9/1 for domestic and international students. Application fee: $60. Electronic applications accepted. *Financial support:* Research assistantships with tuition reimbursements, teaching assistantships with tuition reimbursements, scholarships/grants, and traineeships available. Financial award application deadline: 3/1; financial award applicants required to submit FAFSA. *Faculty research:* Breastfeeding practices of teen mothers, national database of nursing quality indicators, caregiving of families of patients using technology in the home, simulation in nursing education, diaphragm fatigue. *Total annual research expenditures:* $4.6 million. *Unit head:* Dr. Sally Maliski, Dean, 913-588-1601, Fax: 913-588-1660, E-mail: smaliski@kumc.edu. *Application contact:* Dr. Pamela K. Barnes, Associate Dean, Student Affairs, 913-588-1619, Fax: 913-588-1615, E-mail: pbarnes2@kumc.edu. Website: http://nursing.kumc.edu

University of Maryland, Baltimore, Graduate School, School of Nursing, Master's Program in Nursing, Baltimore, MD 21201. Offers community health nursing (MS); gerontological nursing (MS); maternal-child nursing (MS); medical-surgical nursing (MS); nurse-midwifery education (MS); nursing administration (MS); nursing education (MS); nursing health policy (MS); primary care nursing (MS); psychiatric nursing (MS); MS/MBA. MS/MBA offered jointly with University of Baltimore. *Accreditation:* AACN; AANA/CANAEP. *Program availability:* Part-time. *Degree requirements:* For master's, comprehensive exam (for some programs), thesis or alternative. *Entrance requirements:* For master's, minimum GPA of 2.75, course work in statistics, BS in nursing. Additional exam requirements/recommendations for international students: Required—TOEFL (minimum score 550 paper-based; 80 iBT); Recommended—IELTS (minimum score 7). Electronic applications accepted. Tuition and fees vary according to program.

University of Massachusetts Amherst, Graduate School, College of Nursing, Amherst, MA 01003. Offers adult gerontology primary care nurse practitioner (DNP); clinical nurse leader (MS); family nurse practitioner (DNP); nursing (PhD); public health nurse leader (DNP). *Accreditation:* AACN. *Program availability:* Part-time, online learning. Terminal master's awarded for partial completion of doctoral program. *Degree requirements:* For master's, thesis optional; for doctorate, comprehensive exam, thesis/dissertation. *Entrance requirements:* Additional exam requirements/recommendations for international students: Required—TOEFL (minimum score 550 paper-based; 80 iBT), IELTS (minimum score 6.5). Electronic applications accepted. *Faculty research:* Health of older adults and their caretakers, mental health of individuals and families, health of children and adolescents, power and decision-making, transcultural health.

University of Massachusetts Dartmouth, Graduate School, Programs in Nursing, North Dartmouth, MA 02747-2300. Offers adult health (MS); community health (MS); nursing (PhD); nursing practice (DNP). *Program availability:* Part-time. *Faculty:* 26 full-time (all women), 39 part-time/adjunct (38 women). *Students:* 1 (woman) full-time, 115 part-time (108 women); includes 11 minority (4 Black or African American, non-Hispanic/Latino; 3 Asian, non-Hispanic/Latino; 4 Hispanic/Latino). Average age 40. 55 applicants, 91% accepted, 36 enrolled. In 2015, 18 master's, 5 doctorates awarded. *Degree requirements:* For master's, thesis, capstone project; for doctorate, comprehensive exam or thesis (for PhD only); project (for DNP only). *Entrance requirements:* For master's, GRE (if fewer than 45 credits at baccalaureate degree granting school), statement of purpose (minimum of 300 words), resume, 3 letters of recommendation, official transcripts, copy of RN license; for doctorate, GRE (for PHD, if fewer than 45 credits at baccalaureate degree granting school for DNP), statement of purpose (minimum of 300 words), resume, 3 letters of recommendation, official transcripts, copy of RN license, scholarly writing sample (minimum 10 pages for PhD). Additional exam requirements/recommendations for international students: Required—TOEFL (minimum score 533 paper-based; 72 iBT), IELTS (minimum score 6). *Application deadline:* For fall admission, 2/15 priority date for domestic and international students; for spring admission, 12/1 priority date for domestic students, 11/1 priority date for international students. Applications are processed on a rolling basis. Application fee: $60. Electronic applications accepted. *Expenses:* Tuition, state resident: full-time $2071; part-time $86.29 per credit. Tuition, nonresident: full-time $8099; part-time $337.46 per credit. *Required fees:* $18,074; $762.08 per credit. Tuition and fees vary according to course load and reciprocity agreements. *Financial support:* In 2015–16, 1 fellowship with full tuition reimbursement (averaging $24,000 per year), 3 teaching assistantships with full tuition reimbursements (averaging $4,333 per year) were awarded; Federal Work-Study and unspecified assistantships also available. Support available to part-time students. Financial award application deadline: 3/1; financial award applicants required to submit FAFSA. *Faculty research:* Pathophysiology, aging with spinal cord injury, patient care, self care management, nursing education, reflective practice, breast cancer and quality of life of ethnically diverse populations, community based action research among vulnerable populations, care giver experiences. *Total annual research expenditures:* $61,000. *Unit head:* Kerry Fater, Graduate Program Director, 508-999-8525, Fax: 508-999-9127, E-mail: kfater@umassd.edu. *Application contact:* Steven Briggs, Director of Marketing and Recruitment for Graduate Studies, 508-999-8604, Fax: 508-999-8183, E-mail: graduate@umassd.edu. Website: http://www.umassd.edu/nursing/graduateprograms

University of Minnesota, Twin Cities Campus, Graduate School, School of Nursing, Program in Public Health Nursing, Minneapolis, MN 55455-0213. Offers MS. *Accreditation:* AACN. *Program availability:* Part-time, online learning. *Degree requirements:* For master's, final oral exam, project or thesis. *Entrance requirements:* Additional exam requirements/recommendations for international students: Required—TOEFL (minimum score 586 paper-based).

The University of North Carolina at Charlotte, College of Health and Human Services, School of Nursing, Charlotte, NC 28223-0001. Offers adult-gerontology acute care nurse practitioner (MSN, Post-Master's Certificate); advanced clinical nursing (MSN); community public health nursing (MSN); family nurse practitioner across the lifespan (MSN, Post-Master's Certificate); nurse administrator (MSN, Graduate

Certificate); nurse anesthesia (MSN, Post-Master's Certificate); nurse educator (MSN, Graduate Certificate); nursing (DNP); nursing systems/population (MSN). *Accreditation:* AACN. *Program availability:* Part-time, blended/hybrid learning. *Faculty:* 26 full-time (25 women), 4 part-time/adjunct (3 women). *Students:* 109 full-time (89 women), 112 part-time (107 women); includes 46 minority (37 Black or African American, non-Hispanic/Latino; 3 Asian, non-Hispanic/Latino; 5 Hispanic/Latino; 1 Two or more races, non-Hispanic/Latino). Average age 33. 321 applicants, 34% accepted, 84 enrolled. In 2015, 76 master's, 4 doctorates, 7 other advanced degrees awarded. Terminal master's awarded for partial completion of doctoral program. *Degree requirements:* For master's, practicum, synthesis and integration or thesis, residency, internship (varies by program); for doctorate, thesis/dissertation or alternative, residency; for other advanced degree, practicum. *Entrance requirements:* For master's, GRE General Test, unencumbered license as Registered Nurse in North Carolina; BSN from nationally-accredited program; one year of professional nursing practice in acute/critical care; minimum overall GPA of 3.0 in the last degree and 60 hours of nursing coursework; completion of an undergraduate statistics course with minimum grade of C; statement of purpose; for doctorate, GRE or MAT, master's degree in nursing in an advanced nursing practice specialty from nationally-accredited program; minimum overall GPA of 3.5 in MSN program; current RN licensure in U.S. at time of application with eligibility for NC licensure; for other advanced degree, GRE. Additional exam requirements/recommendations for international students: Required—TOEFL (minimum score 557 paper-based, 83 iBT) or IELTS (minimum score 6.5). *Application deadline:* For fall admission, 2/1 for domestic and international students; for spring admission, 10/1 priority date for domestic and international students; for summer admission, 4/1 priority date for domestic and international students. Applications are processed on a rolling basis. Application fee: $75. Electronic applications accepted. *Expenses:* Contact institution. *Financial support:* In 2015–16, 9 students received support, including 5 research assistantships (averaging $4,850 per year), 3 teaching assistantships (averaging $2,911 per year); career-related internships or fieldwork, institutionally sponsored loans, scholarships/grants, traineeships, unspecified assistantships, and administrative assistantships also available. Support available to part-time students. Financial award application deadline: 3/1; financial award applicants required to submit FAFSA. *Faculty research:* Improving care outcomes for the elderly; vulnerable populations; symptom management; self management/health promotion strategies of older adults; migration and maternal child health; health disparities, health literacy, and access to healthcare in Latino adults with diabetes; psychiatric nursing. *Total annual research expenditures:* $875,169. *Unit head:* Dr. Dee Baldwin, Associate Dean, 704-687-7952, Fax: 704-687-6017, E-mail: dbaldwi5@uncc.edu. *Application contact:* Kathy B. Giddings, Director of Graduate Admissions, 704-687-5503, Fax: 704-687-1668, E-mail: gradadm@uncc.edu. Website: http://nursing.uncc.edu/

University of North Dakota, Graduate School, College of Nursing, Grand Forks, ND 58202. Offers advanced public health nursing (MS); family nurse practitioner (MS); gerontological nursing (MS); nurse anesthesia (MS); nursing (MS, PhD); nursing education (MS); psychiatric and mental health (MS). *Accreditation:* AACN; AANA/CANAEP (one or more programs are accredited). *Program availability:* Part-time, evening/weekend, online learning. *Degree requirements:* For master's, thesis or alternative. *Entrance requirements:* For master's, minimum GPA of 3.0; for doctorate, GRE or MAT, minimum GPA of 3.0. Additional exam requirements/recommendations for international students: Required—TOEFL (minimum score 550 paper-based; 79 iBT), IELTS (minimum score 6.5). Electronic applications accepted. *Faculty research:* Adult health, anesthesia, rural health, health administration, family nurse practitioner.

University of Puerto Rico, Medical Sciences Campus, School of Nursing, San Juan, PR 00936-5067. Offers adult and elderly nursing (MSN); child and adolescent nursing (MSN); critical care nursing (MSN); family and community nursing (MSN); family nurse practitioner (MSN); maternity nursing (MSN); mental health and psychiatric nursing (MSN). *Accreditation:* AACN. *Entrance requirements:* For master's, GRE or EXADEP, interview, Puerto Rico RN license or professional license for international students, general and specific point average, article analysis. Electronic applications accepted. *Faculty research:* HIV, health disparities, teen violence, women and violence, neurological disorders.

University of South Carolina, The Graduate School, College of Nursing, Program in Health Nursing, Columbia, SC 29208. Offers adult nurse practitioner (MSN); community/public health clinical nurse specialist (MSN); family nurse practitioner (MSN); pediatric nurse practitioner (MSN). *Accreditation:* AACN. *Program availability:* Part-time. *Degree requirements:* For master's, thesis or alternative. *Entrance requirements:* For master's, GRE General Test or MAT, BS in nursing, nursing license. Additional exam requirements/recommendations for international students: Required—TOEFL (minimum score 570 paper-based). Electronic applications accepted. *Faculty research:* System research, evidence based practice, breast cancer, violence.

University of South Carolina, The Graduate School, College of Nursing, Program in Nursing and Public Health, Columbia, SC 29208. Offers MPH/MSN. *Accreditation:* AACN; CEPH. *Program availability:* Part-time. *Entrance requirements:* Additional exam requirements/recommendations for international students: Required—TOEFL (minimum score 570 paper-based). Electronic applications accepted. *Faculty research:* System research, evidence based practice, breast cancer, violence.

The University of Texas at Austin, Graduate School, School of Nursing, Austin, TX 78712-1111. Offers adult - gerontology clinical nurse specialist (MSN); child health (MSN), including administration, public health nursing, teaching; family nurse practitioner (MSN); family psychiatric/mental health nurse practitioner (MSN); holistic adult health (MSN), including administration, teaching; maternity (MSN), including administration, public health nursing, teaching; nursing (PhD); nursing administration and healthcare systems management (MSN); nursing practice (DNP); pediatric nurse practitioner (MSN); public health nursing (MSN). *Accreditation:* AACN. *Program availability:* Part-time. *Degree requirements:* For master's, thesis optional; for doctorate, thesis/dissertation. *Entrance requirements:* For master's and doctorate, GRE General Test. Additional exam requirements/recommendations for international students: Required—TOEFL (minimum score 550 paper-based). Electronic applications accepted. *Faculty research:* Chronic illness management, memory and aging, health promotion, women's health, adolescent health.

The University of Texas Health Science Center at San Antonio, School of Nursing, San Antonio, TX 78229-3900. Offers administrative management (MSN); adult-gerontology acute care nurse practitioner (PGC); advanced practice leadership (DNP); clinical nurse leader (MSN); executive administrative management (DNP); family nurse practitioner (MSN, PGC); nursing (MSN, PhD); nursing education (MSN, PGC); pediatric nurse practitioner primary care (PGC); psychiatric mental health nurse practitioner (PGC); public health nurse leader (DNP). *Accreditation:* AACN. *Program availability:* Part-time. Terminal master's awarded for partial completion of doctoral program. *Degree requirements:* For master's, thesis optional; for doctorate, comprehensive exam, thesis/dissertation.

The University of Toledo, College of Graduate Studies, College of Nursing, Department of Population and Community Care, Toledo, OH 43606-3390. Offers clinical nurse leader (MSN); family nurse practitioner (MSN, Certificate); nurse educator (MSN,

Community Health Nursing

Certificate); pediatric nurse practitioner (MSN, Certificate). *Program availability:* Part-time. *Degree requirements:* For master's, thesis or alternative. *Entrance requirements:* For master's, GRE, BS in nursing, minimum undergraduate GPA of 3.0, statement of purpose, three letters of recommendation, transcripts from all prior institutions attended, Nursing CAS application, UT supplemental application; for Certificate, BS in nursing, minimum undergraduate GPA of 3.0, statement of purpose, three letters of recommendation, transcripts from all prior institutions attended. Additional exam requirements/recommendations for international students: Required—TOEFL (minimum score 550 paper-based; 80 iBT). Electronic applications accepted.

University of Washington, Tacoma, Graduate Programs, Program in Nursing, Tacoma, WA 98402-3100. Offers communities, populations and health (MN); leadership in healthcare (MN); nurse educator (MN). *Program availability:* Part-time. *Degree requirements:* For master's, thesis (for some programs), advance fieldwork. *Entrance requirements:* For master's, Washington State NCLEX exam, minimum GPA of 3.0. Additional exam requirements/recommendations for international students: Required—TOEFL (minimum score 580 paper-based; 70 iBT); Recommended—IELTS (minimum score 7). *Faculty research:* Hospice and palliative care; clinical trial decision-making; minority nurse retention; asthma and public health; injustice, suffering, difference: Linking Them to Us; adolescent health.

Worcester State University, Graduate Studies, Department of Nursing, Program in Community and Public Health Nursing, Worcester, MA 01602-2597. Offers MSN. *Accreditation:* AACN. *Program availability:* Part-time. *Faculty:* 4 full-time (all women), 2 part-time/adjunct (1 woman). *Students:* 4 full-time (all women), 28 part-time (all women); includes 2 minority (1 Black or African American, non-Hispanic/Latino; 1 Hispanic/Latino). Average age 43. 30 applicants, 73% accepted, 6 enrolled. In 2015, 13 master's

awarded. *Degree requirements:* For master's, final project, practicum. *Entrance requirements:* For master's, unencumbered license to practice as a Registered Nurse in Massachusetts. Additional exam requirements/recommendations for international students: Required—TOEFL (minimum score 500 paper-based; 79 iBT). *Application deadline:* For fall admission, 6/15 for domestic and international students; for spring admission, 11/1 for domestic and international students; for summer admission, 4/1 for domestic and international students. Applications are processed on a rolling basis. Application fee: $50. Electronic applications accepted. *Expenses:* Tuition, state resident: part-time $150 per credit. Tuition, nonresident: part-time $150 per credit. *Financial support:* Career-related internships or fieldwork, scholarships/grants, and unspecified assistantships available. Financial award application deadline: 3/1; financial award applicants required to submit FAFSA. *Unit head:* Dr. Stephanie Chalupka, Coordinator, 508-929-8680, E-mail: schalupka@worcester.edu. *Application contact:* Sara Grady, Associate Dean of Graduate and Continuing Education, 508-929-8787, Fax: 508-929-8100, E-mail: sara.grady@worcester.edu.

Wright State University, School of Graduate Studies, College of Nursing and Health, Program in Nursing, Dayton, OH 45435. Offers acute care nurse practitioner (MS); administration of nursing and health care systems (MS); adult health (MS); child and adolescent health (MS); community health (MS); family nurse practitioner (MS); nurse practitioner (MS); school nurse (MS); MBA/MS. *Accreditation:* AACN. *Program availability:* Part-time, evening/weekend. *Degree requirements:* For master's, thesis or alternative. *Entrance requirements:* For master's, GRE General Test, BSN from NLN-accredited college, Ohio RN license. Additional exam requirements/recommendations for international students: Required—TOEFL. *Faculty research:* Clinical nursing and health, teaching, caring, pain administration, informatics and technology.

Family Nurse Practitioner Studies

Albany State University, College of Sciences and Health Professions, Albany, GA 31705-2717. Offers criminal justice (MS), including corrections, forensic science, law enforcement, public administration; mathematics education (M Ed); nursing (MSN), including RN to MSN family nurse practitioner, RN to MSN nurse educator; science education (M Ed). *Accreditation:* ACEN. *Program availability:* Part-time, evening/weekend, online learning. *Degree requirements:* For master's, comprehensive exam, thesis. *Entrance requirements:* For master's, GRE or MAT, official transcript, letters of recommendations, pre-medical/certificate of immunizations. Electronic applications accepted.

Allen College, Graduate Programs, Waterloo, IA 50703. Offers acute care nurse practitioner (Post-Master's Certificate); adult nurse practitioner (Post-Master's Certificate); adult psychiatric-mental health nurse practitioner (Post-Master's Certificate); adult-gerontology acute care nurse practitioner (MSN); community public health (Post-Master's Certificate); community/public health nursing (MSN); family nurse practitioner (MSN, Post-Master's Certificate); gerontological nurse practitioner (Post-Master's Certificate); health sciences (Ed D); leadership in health care delivery (MSN, Post-Master's Certificate); nursing (DNP); occupational therapy (MS). *Accreditation:* AACN, ACEN. *Program availability:* Part-time, blended/hybrid learning. *Faculty:* 3 full-time (all women), 21 part-time/adjunct (20 women). *Students:* 61 full-time (54 women), 163 part-time (144 women); includes 9 minority (5 Black or African American, non-Hispanic/Latino; 2 Hispanic/Latino; 2 Two or more races, non-Hispanic/Latino), 2 international. Average age 34. 212 applicants, 60% accepted, 94 enrolled. In 2015, 51 master's, 1 doctorate awarded. *Degree requirements:* For master's, thesis optional. *Entrance requirements:* For master's, minimum GPA of 3.0 in the last 60 hours of undergraduate coursework; for doctorate, minimum GPA of 3.25 in graduate coursework. Additional exam requirements/recommendations for international students: Recommended—TOEFL (minimum score 580 paper-based; 92 iBT), IELTS (minimum score 6). *Application deadline:* For fall admission, 2/1 priority date for domestic students; for spring admission, 9/1 priority date for domestic students. Applications are processed on a rolling basis. Application fee: $50. Electronic applications accepted. *Expenses:* $15,940 tuition, $1,240 fees. *Financial support:* Institutionally sponsored loans, scholarships/grants, and traineeships available. Support available to part-time students. Financial award application deadline: 8/15; financial award applicants required to submit FAFSA. *Unit head:* Nancy Kramer, Vice Chancellor for Academic Affairs, 319-226-2040, Fax: 319-226-2070, E-mail: nancy.kramer@allencollege.edu. *Application contact:* Molly Quinn, Administrative Assistant for Student Services, 319-226-2014, Fax: 319-226-2010, E-mail: admissions@allencollege.edu.
Website: http://www.allencollege.edu/

Alverno College, JoAnn McGrath School of Nursing, Milwaukee, WI 53234-3922. Offers clinical nurse specialist (MSN); family nurse practitioner (MSN); mental health nurse practitioner (MSN). *Accreditation:* AACN. *Program availability:* Part-time, evening/weekend. *Faculty:* 8 full-time (all women), 8 part-time/adjunct (4 women). *Students:* 97 full-time (90 women), 87 part-time (82 women); includes 43 minority (18 Black or African American, non-Hispanic/Latino; 9 Hispanic/Latino; 5 Two or more races, non-Hispanic/Latino), 1 international. Average age 36. 73 applicants, 95% accepted, 45 enrolled. In 2015, 33 master's awarded. *Degree requirements:* For master's, 500 clinical hours, capstone. *Entrance requirements:* For master's, BSN, current license. Additional exam requirements/recommendations for international students: Required—TOEFL. *Application deadline:* For fall admission, 7/15 priority date for domestic and international students; for spring admission, 12/15 priority date for domestic and international students. Applications are processed on a rolling basis. Application fee: $0. Electronic applications accepted. *Expenses:* Contact institution. *Financial support:* In 2015–16, 1 student received support. Federal Work-Study and scholarships/grants available. Support available to part-time students. Financial award applicants required to submit FAFSA. *Faculty research:* Impact of stroke on sexuality, children's asthma management, factors affecting baccalaureate student success. *Unit head:* Margaret Rauschenberger, Interim Dean, 414-382-6276, Fax: 414-382-6354, E-mail: margaret.rauschenberger@alverno.edu. *Application contact:* Dr. Carol Sabel, RN, Graduate Program Director, 414-382-0309, Fax: 414-382-6354, E-mail: carol.sabel@alverno.edu.
Website: http://www.alverno.edu/academics/academicdepartments/joannmcgrathschoolofnursing/

American International College, School of Health Sciences, Master of Science in Nursing Program, Springfield, MA 01109-3189. Offers family nurse practitioner (MSN); nursing administration (MSN); nursing education (MSN). *Accreditation:* AACN. *Program availability:* Part-time, evening/weekend, online only, blended/hybrid learning. *Faculty:* 1 (woman) full-time, 1 (woman) part-time/adjunct. *Students:* 52 full-time (49 women), 4 part-time (all women); includes 18 minority (12 Black or African American, non-Hispanic/

Latino; 1 Asian, non-Hispanic/Latino; 4 Hispanic/Latino; 1 Two or more races, non-Hispanic/Latino). Average age 36. 66 applicants, 53% accepted, 27 enrolled. In 2015, 8 master's awarded. *Entrance requirements:* For master's, BSN, minimum GPA of 3.0. Additional exam requirements/recommendations for international students: Required—TOEFL, IELTS. *Application deadline:* For fall admission, 8/20 for domestic students, 7/1 priority date for international students; for spring admission, 1/4 for domestic students, 12/1 priority date for international students. Applications are processed on a rolling basis. Application fee: $50. Electronic applications accepted. *Expenses:* Contact institution. *Financial support:* Applicants required to submit FAFSA. *Unit head:* Dr. Ellen Furman, Associate Director of Graduate Nursing, 413-205-3918, Fax: 413-654-1430, E-mail: ellen.furman@aic.edu. *Application contact:* Kerry Barnes, Director of Graduate Admissions, 413-205-3703, Fax: 413-205-3051, E-mail: kerry.barnes@aic.edu.
Website: http://www.aic.edu/academics/hs/nursing

Angelo State University, College of Graduate Studies, Archer College of Health and Human Services, Department of Nursing, San Angelo, TX 76909. Offers family nurse practitioner (MSN); nurse educator (MSN). *Accreditation:* ACEN. *Program availability:* Part-time, evening/weekend, online learning. *Degree requirements:* For master's, comprehensive exam. *Entrance requirements:* For master's, essay, three letters of recommendation. Additional exam requirements/recommendations for international students: Required—TOEFL or IELTS. *Application deadline:* For fall admission, 4/1 priority date for domestic students, 6/10 for international students; for spring admission, 9/1 priority date for domestic students, 11/1 for international students. Applications are processed on a rolling basis. Application fee: $40 ($50 for international students). Electronic applications accepted. *Expenses: Tuition, area resident:* Full-time $3726; part-time $2484 per year. *Tuition, state resident:* full-time $3726; part-time $2484 per year. *Tuition, nonresident:* full-time $10,746; part-time $7164 per year. *International tuition:* $10,746 full-time. *Required fees:* $2538; $1702 per unit. *Financial support:* Research assistantships, career-related internships or fieldwork, Federal Work-Study, and scholarships/grants available. Support available to part-time students. Financial award application deadline: 3/1. *Unit head:* Dr. Wrennah L. Gabbert, Chair, 325-942-2224, Fax: 325-942-2236, E-mail: wrennah.gabbert@angelo.edu. *Application contact:* Dr. Molly J. Walker, Graduate Advisor, 325-486-6872, Fax: 325-942-2236, E-mail: molly.walker@angelo.edu.
Website: http://www.angelo.edu/dept/nursing/

Arizona State University at the Tempe campus, College of Nursing and Health Innovation, Phoenix, AZ 85004. Offers advanced nursing practice (DNP); clinical research management (MS); community and public health practice (Graduate Certificate); family mental health nurse practitioner (Graduate Certificate); family nurse practitioner (Graduate Certificate); geriatric nursing (Graduate Certificate); healthcare innovation (MHI); nurse education in academic and practice settings (Graduate Certificate); nurse educator (MS); nursing and healthcare innovation (PhD). *Accreditation:* AACN. *Program availability:* Online learning. *Degree requirements:* For master's, comprehensive exam (for some programs), thesis (for some programs), interactive Program of Study (iPOS) submitted before completing 50 percent of required credit hours; for doctorate, comprehensive exam, thesis/dissertation, interactive Program of Study (iPOS) submitted before completing 50 percent of required credit hours. *Entrance requirements:* For master's and doctorate, GRE, minimum GPA of 3.0 or equivalent in last 2 years of work leading to bachelor's degree. Additional exam requirements/recommendations for international students: Required—TOEFL, IELTS, or PTE. Electronic applications accepted. *Expenses:* Contact institution.

Armstrong State University, School of Graduate Studies, Program in Nursing, Savannah, GA 31419-1997. Offers adult-gerontological acute care nurse practitioner (Certificate); adult-gerontological clinical nurse specialist (Certificate); adult-gerontological primary care nurse practitioner (Certificate); family nurse practitioner (MSN). *Accreditation:* AACN. *Program availability:* Part-time, evening/weekend. *Faculty:* 5 full-time (all women), 1 (woman) part-time/adjunct. *Students:* 35 full-time (32 women), 19 part-time (16 women); includes 13 minority (10 Black or African American, non-Hispanic/Latino; 2 Hispanic/Latino; 1 Two or more races, non-Hispanic/Latino), 1 international. Average age 35. 23 applicants, 83% accepted, 16 enrolled. In 2015, 19 master's awarded. *Degree requirements:* For master's, comprehensive exam, project or thesis. *Entrance requirements:* For master's, GRE General Test or MAT, minimum GPA of 3.0, letter of recommendation, letter of intent. Additional exam requirements/recommendations for international students: Required—TOEFL (minimum score 523 paper-based; 70 iBT). *Application deadline:* For fall admission, 2/28 for domestic and international students; for spring admission, 11/15 for domestic students, 9/15 for international students. Applications are processed on a rolling basis. Application fee: $30. Electronic applications accepted. *Expenses:* Tuition, state resident: part-time $211 per credit hour. Tuition, nonresident: part-time $782 per credit hour. *Required fees:*

$1224 per unit. $612 per semester. Tuition and fees vary according to course load, campus/location and program. *Financial support:* In 2015–16, research assistantships with full tuition reimbursements (averaging $5,000 per year) were awarded; Federal Work-Study, scholarships/grants, and unspecified assistantships also available. Support available to part-time students. Financial award application deadline: 3/1; financial award applicants required to submit FAFSA. *Faculty research:* Midwifery, mental health, nursing simulation, smoking cessation during pregnancy, asthma education, vulnerable populations, geriatrics, disaster nursing, complementary and alternative modalities, nephrology. *Unit head:* Dr. Catherine Gilbert, Department Head, 912-344-3145, E-mail: catherine.gilbert@armstrong.edu. *Application contact:* McKenzie Peterman, Assistant Director of Graduate Admissions, 912-344-2503, Fax: 912-344-3417, E-mail: graduate@armstrong.edu.
Website: http://www.armstrong.edu/Health_professions/nursing/nursing_graduate_programs

Augsburg College, Programs in Nursing, Minneapolis, MN 55454-1351. Offers MA, DNP. *Accreditation:* AACN. *Degree requirements:* For master's, thesis or alternative.

Augusta University, The Graduate School, Doctor of Nursing Practice Program, Augusta, GA 30912. Offers adult gerontology acute care nurse practitioner (DNP); family nurse practitioner (DNP); nursing (DNP); nursing anesthesia (DNP); pediatric nurse practitioner (DNP); psychiatric mental health nurse practitioner (DNP). *Students:* 40 part-time. *Degree requirements:* For doctorate, thesis/dissertation or alternative. *Entrance requirements:* For doctorate, GRE General Test or MAT, master's degree in nursing or related field, current professional nurse licensure. Additional exam requirements/recommendations for international students: Required—TOEFL (minimum score 600 paper-based; 100 iBT). *Application deadline:* For fall admission, 3/1 for domestic and international students; for spring admission, 7/1 for domestic and international students. Applications are processed on a rolling basis. Application fee: $50. Electronic applications accepted. *Unit head:* Dr. Marguerite Murphy, RN, Director, 706-721-3676, Fax: 706-721-8169. *Application contact:* Karen Sturgill, Program Manager, 706-721-3676, Fax: 706-721-8169, E-mail: dnp@augusta.edu.
Website: http://www.augusta.edu/nursing/dnp_programs.php

Augusta University, The Graduate School, Family Nurse Practitioner Program, Augusta, GA 30912. Offers MSN, Post-Master's Certificate. *Entrance requirements:* For master's, GRE General Test or MAT, Georgia registered professional nurse license. Additional exam requirements/recommendations for international students: Required—TOEFL (minimum score 550 paper-based; 79 iBT). *Application deadline:* For fall admission, 2/1 for domestic and international students; for spring admission, 10/1 for domestic and international students. Application fee: $50. Electronic applications accepted. *Unit head:* Dr. Lucy Marion, Dean, 706-721-3771, Fax: 706-721-8169, E-mail: lumarion@georgiahealth.edu. *Application contact:* Karen Sturgill, Program Coordinator, 706-721-3676, Fax: 706-721-8169.
Website: http://www.augusta.edu/nursing/programs.php

Austin Peay State University, College of Graduate Studies, College of Behavioral and Health Sciences, School of Nursing, Clarksville, TN 37044. Offers family nurse practitioner (MSN); nursing administration (MSN); nursing education (MSN); nursing informatics (MSN). *Program availability:* Part-time, online learning. *Faculty:* 11 full-time (all women), 6 part-time/adjunct (all women). *Students:* 23 full-time (20 women), 142 part-time (125 women); includes 27 minority (19 Black or African American, non-Hispanic/Latino; 4 Hispanic/Latino; 4 Two or more races, non-Hispanic/Latino). Average age 35. 25 applicants, 76% accepted, 14 enrolled. In 2015, 67 master's awarded. *Degree requirements:* For master's, comprehensive exam. *Entrance requirements:* For master's, minimum GPA of 3.0, RN license eligibility, 3 letters of recommendation. Additional exam requirements/recommendations for international students: Required—TOEFL (minimum score 500 paper-based). *Application deadline:* For fall admission, 8/3 priority date for domestic students. Applications are processed on a rolling basis. Application fee: $25. Electronic applications accepted. *Expenses:* Tuition, state resident: full-time $8080; part-time $404 per credit hour. Tuition, nonresident: full-time $21,680; part-time $1084 per credit hour. *Required fees:* $1453; $72.65 per credit hour. *Financial support:* In 2015–16, research assistantships with full tuition reimbursements (averaging $5,184 per year) were awarded; career-related internships or fieldwork, Federal Work-Study, institutionally sponsored loans, scholarships/grants, and unspecified assistantships also available. Support available to part-time students. Financial award application deadline: 3/1; financial award applicants required to submit FAFSA. *Unit head:* Dr. Grace Moodt, Interim Director, 931-221-6290, Fax: 931-221-7595, E-mail: moodtg@apsu.edu. *Application contact:* June D. Lee, Graduate Coordinator, 800-859-4723, Fax: 931-221-7641, E-mail: gradadmissions@apsu.edu.
Website: http://www.apsu.edu/nursing

Ball State University, Graduate School, College of Applied Sciences and Technology, School of Nursing, Muncie, IN 47306. Offers adult/gerontology nurse practitioner (Post Master's Certificate); evidence-based clinical practice (Postbaccalaureate Certificate); family nurse practitioner (Post Master's Certificate); family nurse practitioner for the adult nurse practitioner or adult/gerontology nurse practitioner (Post Master's Certificate); nurse educator (Post Master's Certificate); nursing (MS), including family nurse practitioner, nurse administrator, nurse educator; nursing education (Postbaccalaureate Certificate); nursing practice (DNP). *Accreditation:* AACN. *Program availability:* Part-time-only, online only, 100% online. *Faculty:* 12 full-time (all women), 7 part-time/adjunct (6 women). *Students:* 9 full-time (8 women), 334 part-time (311 women); includes 23 minority (11 Black or African American, non-Hispanic/Latino; 5 Asian, non-Hispanic/Latino; 6 Hispanic/Latino; 1 Two or more races, non-Hispanic/Latino). Average age 33. 88 applicants, 85% accepted, 63 enrolled. In 2015, 115 master's, 8 doctorates awarded. *Entrance requirements:* For master's, bachelor's degree in nursing, minimum GPA of 3.0, minimum C grade in at least 1 quarter or semester hours in an undergraduate research course, unencumbered license as a registered nurse in state of practice; for doctorate, advanced practice nurse (nurse practitioner, clinical nurse specialist, nurse midwife); master's degree in nursing from accredited program with minimum GPA of 3.2; graduate-level statistics, nursing research, and health assessment courses; unencumbered license as registered nurse in state of practice. Additional exam requirements/recommendations for international students: Required—TOEFL (minimum score 550 paper-based; 79 iBT), IELTS (minimum score 6.5). *Application deadline:* For fall admission, 2/9 for domestic students; for spring admission, 8/9 for domestic students. Applications are processed on a rolling basis. Application fee: $60. Electronic applications accepted. *Expenses:* Contact institution. *Financial support:* Application deadline: 3/1; applicants required to submit FAFSA. *Unit head:* Dr. Linda Siktberg, Director, 765-285-8718, Fax: 765-285-2169, E-mail: lsiktberg@bsu.edu. *Application contact:* Shantele Estes, Graduate Advisor, 765-285-9130, Fax: 765-285-2169, E-mail: smestes@bsu.edu.
Website: http://www.bsu.edu/nursing/

Barry University, School of Adult and Continuing Education, Division of Nursing, Program in Nurse Practitioner, Miami Shores, FL 33161-6695. Offers acute care nurse practitioner (MSN); family nurse practitioner (MSN); nurse practitioner (Certificate). *Accreditation:* AACN. *Program availability:* Part-time, evening/weekend. *Degree requirements:* For master's, research project or thesis. *Entrance requirements:* For master's, GRE General Test or MAT, BSN, minimum GPA of 3.0, course work in

statistics. Electronic applications accepted. *Faculty research:* Child abuse, health beliefs, teenage pregnancy, cultural and clinical studies across the lifespan.

Baylor University, Graduate School, Louise Herrington School of Nursing, Dallas, TX 75246. Offers family nurse practitioner (MSN); neonatal nurse practitioner (MSN); nurse-midwifery (DNP). *Accreditation:* AACN. *Program availability:* Part-time, online learning. *Degree requirements:* For doctorate, comprehensive exam (for some programs), capstone project. *Entrance requirements:* For master's, GRE General Test or MAT; for doctorate, GRE General Test. Additional exam requirements/recommendations for international students: Required—TOEFL. Electronic applications accepted. *Faculty research:* Women and strokes, obesity and pregnancy, educational environmental factors, international undeserved populations, midwifery.

Bellarmine University, Donna and Allan Lansing School of Nursing and Health Sciences, Louisville, KY 40205. Offers family nurse practitioner (MSN); health science (MHS); nursing administration (MSN); nursing education (MSN); nursing practice (DNP); physical therapy (DPT). *Accreditation:* AACN; APTA. *Program availability:* Part-time, evening/weekend. *Faculty:* 27 full-time (24 women), 8 part-time/adjunct (7 women). *Students:* 210 full-time (144 women), 91 part-time (83 women); includes 22 minority (6 Black or African American, non-Hispanic/Latino; 1 American Indian or Alaska Native, non-Hispanic/Latino; 7 Asian, non-Hispanic/Latino; 4 Hispanic/Latino; 4 Two or more races, non-Hispanic/Latino), 2 international. Average age 28. In 2015, 33 master's, 64 doctorates awarded. *Degree requirements:* For doctorate, comprehensive exam, thesis/dissertation. *Entrance requirements:* For master's, GRE General Test, RN license; for doctorate, GRE General Test, Physical Therapist Centralized Application Service (for DPT). Additional exam requirements/recommendations for international students: Required—TOEFL (minimum score 550 paper-based; 80 iBT). Application fee: $40. Electronic applications accepted. *Expenses:* Contact institution. *Financial support:* Career-related internships or fieldwork and scholarships/grants available. *Faculty research:* Nursing: pain, empathy, leadership styles, control; physical therapy: service-learning; exercise in chronic and pre-operative conditions, athletes; women's health; aging. *Unit head:* Dr. Mark Wiegand, Dean, 800-274-4723 Ext. 8368, E-mail: mwiegand@bellarmine.edu. *Application contact:* Julie Armstrong-Binnix, Health Science Recruiter, 800-274-4723 Ext. 8364, E-mail: julieab@bellarmine.edu.
Website: http://www.bellarmine.edu/lansing

Bellin College, School of Nursing, Green Bay, WI 54305. Offers family nurse practitioner (MSN); nurse educator (MSN). *Accreditation:* AACN.

Bloomsburg University of Pennsylvania, School of Graduate Studies, College of Science and Technology, Department of Nursing, Bloomsburg, PA 17815. Offers adult and family nurse practitioner (MSN); community health (MSN); nurse anesthesia (MSN); nursing (MSN); nursing administration (MSN). *Accreditation:* AACN; AANA/CANAEP. *Degree requirements:* For master's, thesis (for some programs), clinical experience. *Entrance requirements:* For master's, minimum QPA of 3.0, personal statement, 2 letters of recommendation, nursing license. Additional exam requirements/recommendations for international students: Required—TOEFL. Electronic applications accepted.

Bowie State University, Graduate Programs, Department of Nursing, Bowie, MD 20715-9465. Offers administration of nursing services (MS); family nurse practitioner (MS); nursing education (MS). *Accreditation:* ACEN. *Program availability:* Part-time. *Degree requirements:* For master's, comprehensive exam, thesis, research paper. *Entrance requirements:* For master's, minimum GPA of 2.5. Electronic applications accepted. *Expenses:* Tuition, state resident: full-time $9384; part-time $2346 per year. Tuition, nonresident: full-time $16,344; part-time $4086 per year. *Required fees:* $2552; $325 per semester. *Faculty research:* Minority health, women's health, gerontology, leadership management.

Brenau University, Sydney O. Smith Graduate School, College of Health and Science, Gainesville, GA 30501. Offers family nurse practitioner (MSN); nurse educator (MSN); nursing management (MSN); occupational therapy (MS); psychology (MS). *Accreditation:* AOTA. *Program availability:* Part-time, evening/weekend. *Degree requirements:* For master's, comprehensive exam (for some programs), thesis (for some programs), clinical practicum hours. *Entrance requirements:* For master's, GRE General Test or MAT (for some programs), interview, writing sample, references (for some programs). Additional exam requirements/recommendations for international students: Required—TOEFL (minimum score 500 paper-based; 61 iBT); Recommended—IELTS (minimum score 5). Electronic applications accepted. *Expenses:* Contact institution.

Brigham Young University, Graduate Studies, College of Nursing, Provo, UT 84602. Offers family nurse practitioner (MS). *Accreditation:* AACN. *Faculty:* 10 full-time (7 women), 1 part-time/adjunct (0 women). *Students:* 29 full-time (19 women); includes 1 minority (Hispanic/Latino). Average age 35. 48 applicants, 31% accepted, 15 enrolled. In 2015, 12 master's awarded. *Degree requirements:* For master's, thesis. *Entrance requirements:* For master's, GRE, minimum GPA of 3.0 in last 60 hours, interview, BS in nursing, pathophysiology class within undergraduate program, course work in basic statistics. Additional exam requirements/recommendations for international students: Required—TOEFL; Recommended—IELTS. *Application deadline:* For spring admission, 12/1 for domestic students. Applications are processed on a rolling basis. Application fee: $50. Electronic applications accepted. *Financial support:* In 2015–16, 29 students received support, including 2 research assistantships with tuition reimbursements available (averaging $10,000 per year), 3 teaching assistantships with tuition reimbursements available (averaging $10,000 per year); institutionally sponsored loans, scholarships/grants, tuition waivers (full), and unspecified assistantships also available. Support available to part-time students. Financial award application deadline: 2/1; financial award applicants required to submit FAFSA. *Faculty research:* Critical care issues, end of life, childhood immunizations, children with diabetes, global health. *Total annual research expenditures:* $3,592. *Unit head:* Dr. Patricia Ravert, Dean, 801-422-1167, Fax: 801-422-0536, E-mail: patricia_ravert@byu.edu. *Application contact:* Lynette Jakins, Graduate Secretary, 801-422-4142, Fax: 801-422-0538, E-mail: lynette-jakins@byu.edu.
Website: http://nursing.byu.edu/

California Baptist University, Program in Nursing, Riverside, CA 92504-3206. Offers clinical nurse specialist (MSN); family nurse practitioner (MSN); healthcare systems management (MSN); teaching-learning (MSN). *Program availability:* Part-time. *Faculty:* 18 full-time (17 women), 14 part-time/adjunct (11 women). *Students:* 77 full-time (63 women), 143 part-time (117 women); includes 111 minority (26 Black or African American, non-Hispanic/Latino; 3 American Indian or Alaska Native, non-Hispanic/Latino; 38 Asian, non-Hispanic/Latino; 39 Hispanic/Latino; 1 Native Hawaiian or other Pacific Islander, non-Hispanic/Latino; 4 Two or more races, non-Hispanic/Latino), 5 international. Average age 33. 44 applicants, 64% accepted, 23 enrolled. In 2015, 19 master's awarded. *Degree requirements:* For master's, comprehensive exam or directed project thesis; capstone practicum. *Entrance requirements:* For master's, GRE or California Critical Thinking Skills Test; Test of Essential Academic Skills (TEAS), minimum undergraduate GPA of 3.0; completion of prerequisite courses with minimum grade of C; CPR certification; background check clearance; health clearance; drug testing; proof of health insurance; proof of motor vehicle insurance; three letters of recommendation; 1000-word essay; interview. Additional exam requirements/

Family Nurse Practitioner Studies

recommendations for international students: Required—TOEFL (minimum score 80 iBT). *Application deadline:* For fall admission, 8/1 priority date for domestic students, 7/1 for international students; for spring admission, 12/1 priority date for domestic students, 11/1 for international students. Applications are processed on a rolling basis. Application fee: $45. Electronic applications accepted. *Expenses:* $742 per unit, $355 per semester fees. *Financial support:* Federal Work-Study and scholarships/grants available. Financial award applicants required to submit CSS PROFILE or FAFSA. *Faculty research:* Qualitative research using Parse methodology, gerontology, disaster preparedness, medical-surgical nursing, maternal-child nursing. *Unit head:* Dr. Geneva Oaks, Dean, School of Nursing, 951-343-4702, E-mail: goaks@calbaptist.edu. *Application contact:* Dr. Rebecca Meyer, Director, Graduate Program in Nursing, 951-343-4952, Fax: 951-343-5095, E-mail: rmeyer@calbaptist.edu.
Website: http://www.calbaptist.edu/explore-cbu/schools-colleges/school-nursing/master-science-nursing/

California State University, Fresno, Division of Graduate Studies, College of Health and Human Services, Department of Nursing, Fresno, CA 93740-8027. Offers nursing (MS), including clinical nurse, primary care nurse practitioner, specialist/nurse educator. *Accreditation:* AACN. *Program availability:* Part-time, evening/weekend. *Degree requirements:* For master's, thesis or alternative. *Entrance requirements:* For master's, GRE General Test, 1 year of clinical practice, previous course work in statistics, BSN, minimum GPA of 3.0 in nursing. Additional exam requirements/recommendations for international students: Required—TOEFL. Electronic applications accepted. *Faculty research:* Training grant, HIV assessment.

Carlow University, College of Health and Wellness, Program in Family Nurse Practitioner, Pittsburgh, PA 15213-3165. Offers MSN, Certificate. *Program availability:* Part-time. *Students:* 204 full-time (189 women), 24 part-time (22 women); includes 12 minority (4 Black or African American, non-Hispanic/Latino; 2 American Indian or Alaska Native, non-Hispanic/Latino; 4 Asian, non-Hispanic/Latino; 2 Hispanic/Latino), 1 international. Average age 33. 82 applicants, 89% accepted, 52 enrolled. In 2015, 63 master's, 3 other advanced degrees awarded. *Entrance requirements:* For master's, minimum undergraduate GPA of 3.0 from accredited BSN program; current license as RN in Pennsylvania; at least one year of recent clinical (bedside) nursing experience; course in statistics in past 6 years; two recommendations; personal statement; personal interview. Additional exam requirements/recommendations for international students: Required—TOEFL (minimum score 550 paper-based). *Application deadline:* Applications are processed on a rolling basis. Electronic applications accepted. Application fee is waived when completed online. *Expenses:* Contact institution. *Unit head:* Dr. Deborah Mitchum, Director, Family Nurse Practitioner Program, 412-578-6586, Fax: 412-578-6114, E-mail: dlmitchum@carlow.edu. *Application contact:* E-mail: gradstudies@carlow.edu.
Website: http://www.carlow.edu/Master_of_Science_in_Nursing_Family_Nurse_Practitioner.aspx

Carson-Newman University, Department of Nursing, Jefferson City, TN 37760. Offers family nurse practitioner (MSN); nurse educator (MSN). *Accreditation:* AACN. *Program availability:* Part-time. *Faculty:* 4 full-time (3 women), 1 (woman) part-time/adjunct. *Students:* 9 full-time (8 women), 34 part-time (31 women); includes 1 minority (Black or African American, non-Hispanic/Latino). Average age 33. 14 applicants, 100% accepted, 9 enrolled. In 2015, 19 master's awarded. *Degree requirements:* For master's, comprehensive exam, thesis optional. *Entrance requirements:* For master's, GRE (minimum score of 290 within ten years of application), minimum GPA of 3.0 for all undergraduate work. Additional exam requirements/recommendations for international students: Recommended—TOEFL (minimum score 79 iBT), IELTS (minimum score 6.5), TSE (minimum score 53). *Application deadline:* For fall admission, 3/15 for domestic students; for spring admission, 10/15 for domestic students. Applications are processed on a rolling basis. Application fee: $50. *Expenses:* Tuition, area resident: Full-time $10,142; part-time $461 per credit hour. *Required fees:* $300; $461 per credit hour. $150 per semester. One-time fee: $150. *Financial support:* Federal Work-Study and tuition waivers (full and partial) available. Financial award applicants required to submit FAFSA. *Unit head:* Dr. Kimberly Bolton, Director, 865-471-4056, E-mail: kbolton@cn.edu. *Application contact:* Nilma Stewart, Graduate Admissions and Services Adviser, 865-471-3230, Fax: 865-471-3875, E-mail: adults@cn.edu.
Website: http://www.cn.edu/adult-graduate-studies/programs/new/nursing

Case Western Reserve University, Frances Payne Bolton School of Nursing, Master's Programs in Nursing, Nurse Practitioner Program, Cleveland, OH 44106. Offers acute care cardiovascular nursing (MSN); acute care nurse practitioner (MSN); acute care pediatric nurse practitioner (MSN); acute care/flight nurse (MSN); adult gerontology acute care nurse practitioner (MSN); adult gerontology oncology and palliative care (MSN); adult gerontology primary care nurse practitioner (MSN); family nurse practitioner (MSN); family systems psychiatric mental health nursing (MSN); neonatal nurse practitioner (MSN); pediatric nurse practitioner (MSN); women's health nurse practitioner (MSN). *Accreditation:* ACEN. *Program availability:* Part-time, online learning. *Students:* 52 full-time (45 women), 78 part-time (68 women); includes 31 minority (10 Black or African American, non-Hispanic/Latino; 14 Asian, non-Hispanic/Latino; 7 Hispanic/Latino). Average age 35. 64 applicants, 66% accepted, 29 enrolled. In 2015, 45 master's awarded. *Degree requirements:* For master's, thesis optional. *Entrance requirements:* For master's, GRE General Test or MAT. Additional exam requirements/recommendations for international students: Required—TOEFL (minimum score 577 paper-based; 90 iBT), IELTS (minimum score 7). *Application deadline:* For fall admission, 6/1 for domestic students; for spring admission, 10/1 for domestic students. Applications are processed on a rolling basis. Application fee: $75. *Expenses:* $1,891 per credit hour. *Financial support:* In 2015–16, 54 students received support, including 17 teaching assistantships with partial tuition reimbursements available (averaging $17,019 per year); scholarships/grants and traineeships also available. Financial award application deadline: 6/30; financial award applicants required to submit FAFSA. *Faculty research:* Symptom science, family/community care, aging across the lifespan, self-management of health and illness, neuroscience. *Unit head:* Dr. Carol Savrin, Director, 216-368-5304, Fax: 216-368-3542, E-mail: cls18@case.edu. *Application contact:* Donna Hassik, Admissions Coordinator, 216-368-5253, Fax: 216-368-0124, E-mail: dmh7@case.edu.
Website: http://fpb.cwru.edu/MSN/majors.shtm

Cedarville University, Graduate Programs, Cedarville, OH 45314-0601. Offers business administration (MBA); curriculum (M Ed); educational administration (M Ed); family nurse practitioner (MSN); global health ministries (MSN); instruction (M Ed); ministry (M Min); pharmacy (Pharm D). *Program availability:* Part-time, evening/weekend, online learning. *Faculty:* 61 full-time (26 women), 7 part-time/adjunct (2 women). *Students:* 201 full-time (116 women), 100 part-time (71 women); includes 53 minority (32 Black or African American, non-Hispanic/Latino; 3 American Indian or Alaska Native, non-Hispanic/Latino; 15 Asian, non-Hispanic/Latino; 2 Hispanic/Latino; 1 Native Hawaiian or other Pacific Islander, non-Hispanic/Latino), 5 international. Average age 30. 142 applicants, 58% accepted, 57 enrolled. In 2015, 41 degrees awarded. *Degree requirements:* For master's, thesis. *Entrance requirements:* For master's, GRE, 2 professional recommendations; for doctorate, PCAT, professional recommendation from a practicing pharmacist or current employer/supervisor, resume, essay, interview.

Additional exam requirements/recommendations for international students: Required—TOEFL (minimum score 550 paper-based; 80 iBT). *Application deadline:* For fall admission, 5/1 priority date for domestic and international students; for spring admission, 11/1 priority date for domestic and international students. Applications are processed on a rolling basis. Application fee: $0. Electronic applications accepted. *Expenses:* Contact institution. *Financial support:* In 2015–16, 129 students received support. Scholarships/grants and unspecified assistantships available. Support available to part-time students. Financial award applicants required to submit FAFSA. *Unit head:* Dr. Mark McClain, Dean of Graduate Studies, 937-766-7700, E-mail: mcclain@cedarville.edu. *Application contact:* Roscoe Smith, Associate Vice President for University Admissions, 937-766-7700, Fax: 937-766-7575, E-mail: smithr@cedarville.edu.
Website: http://www.cedarville.edu/academics/graduate/

Clarion University of Pennsylvania, Office of Transfer, Adult and Graduate Admissions, Master of Science in Nursing Program, Clarion, PA 16214. Offers family nurse practitioner (MSN); nurse educator (MSN). Program offered jointly with Slippery Rock University of Pennsylvania. *Accreditation:* ACEN. *Program availability:* Part-time, online learning. *Degree requirements:* For master's, comprehensive exam, thesis. *Entrance requirements:* For master's, minimum QPA of 2.75. Additional exam requirements/recommendations for international students: Required—TOEFL (minimum score 550 paper-based; 80 iBT). Electronic applications accepted.

Clarion University of Pennsylvania, Office of Transfer, Adult and Graduate Admissions, Online Certificate Programs, Clarion, PA 16214. Offers family nurse practitioner (Post-Master's Certificate); library science (CAS); nurse educator (Post-Master's Certificate); public relations (Certificate). *Accreditation:* ALA (one or more programs are accredited at the [master's] level). *Program availability:* Part-time, online learning. *Entrance requirements:* Additional exam requirements/recommendations for international students: Required—TOEFL (minimum score 550 paper-based; 80 iBT), IELTS (minimum score 7). Electronic applications accepted.

Clarke University, Department of Nursing and Health, Dubuque, IA 52001-3198. Offers family nurse practitioner (DNP). *Accreditation:* AACN. *Program availability:* Part-time. *Faculty:* 6 full-time (all women), 1 (woman) part-time/adjunct. *Students:* 54 full-time (53 women), 9 part-time (8 women); includes 1 minority (Asian, non-Hispanic/Latino). Average age 36. 45 applicants, 58% accepted, 20 enrolled. In 2015, 8 doctorates awarded. *Degree requirements:* For doctorate, comprehensive exam, thesis/dissertation. *Entrance requirements:* For doctorate, GRE (if GPA under 3.0), three recommendation forms, sample of scholarly writing, statement of goals, transcripts, copy of nursing license. Additional exam requirements/recommendations for international students: Required—TOEFL. *Application deadline:* For fall admission, 2/1 priority date for domestic students. Application fee: $35. Electronic applications accepted. *Expenses:* Contact institution. *Financial support:* In 2015–16, 7 students received support. Scholarships/grants and tuition waivers available. Financial award applicants required to submit FAFSA. *Faculty research:* Narrative pedagogy, ethics, end-of-life care, pedagogy, family systems, simulation. *Unit head:* Dr. Jan Lee, Chair, 563-588-6339, Fax: 319-584-8684. *Application contact:* Kara Shroeder, Graduate Studies Coordinator, 563-588-6635, Fax: 563-588-6789, E-mail: graduate@clarke.edu.
Website: http://www.clarke.edu/

Clarkson College, Master of Science in Nursing Program, Omaha, NE 68131. Offers adult nurse practitioner (MSN, Post-Master's Certificate); family nurse practitioner (MSN, Post-Master's Certificate); nursing education (MSN, Post-Master's Certificate); nursing health care leadership (MSN, Post-Master's Certificate). *Accreditation:* AANA/CANAEP; ACEN. *Program availability:* Part-time, evening/weekend, online learning. *Degree requirements:* For master's, on-campus skills assessment (family nurse practitioner, adult nurse practitioner), comprehensive exam or thesis. *Entrance requirements:* For master's, minimum GPA of 3.0, 2 references, resume. Additional exam requirements/recommendations for international students: Required—TOEFL (minimum score 600 paper-based; 100 iBT). Electronic applications accepted.

Clayton State University, School of Graduate Studies, College of Health, Program in Nursing, Morrow, GA 30260-0285. Offers family nurse practitioner (MSN). *Accreditation:* AACN. *Faculty:* 7 full-time (all women). *Students:* 5 full-time (4 women), 15 part-time (12 women); includes 12 minority (11 Black or African American, non-Hispanic/Latino; 1 Asian, non-Hispanic/Latino). Average age 41. 7 applicants, 100% accepted, 6 enrolled. *Degree requirements:* For master's, thesis. *Entrance requirements:* For master's, GRE, official transcript, 3 letters of recommendation, statement of purpose, on-campus interview, 1-2 years of clinical nursing experience (preferred). Additional exam requirements/recommendations for international students: Required—TOEFL (minimum score 550 paper-based; 80 iBT). *Application deadline:* For fall admission, 6/15 priority date for domestic students, 5/1 for international students; for spring admission, 11/15 priority date for domestic students, 9/1 for international students. Applications are processed on a rolling basis. Application fee: $75. Electronic applications accepted. *Expenses:* Contact institution. *Financial support:* Application deadline: 7/1; applicants required to submit FAFSA. *Unit head:* Dr. Betty Glenn Lane, Program Director, Master of Science in Nursing, 678-466-4953, Fax: 678-466-4999, E-mail: katherinewillock@clayton.edu. *Application contact:* Christy Hicks, Coordinator, 678-466-4901, Fax: 678-466-4999, E-mail: christyhicks@clayton.edu.
Website: http://nursing.clayton.edu/MSN/

College of Mount Saint Vincent, School of Professional and Continuing Studies, Department of Nursing, Riverdale, NY 10471-1093. Offers adult nurse practitioner (MSN, PMC); family nurse practitioner (MSN, PMC); nurse educator (PMC); nursing administration (MSN); nursing for the adult and aged (MSN). *Accreditation:* AACN. *Program availability:* Part-time. *Entrance requirements:* For master's, BSN, interview, RN license, minimum GPA of 3.0, letters of reference. Additional exam requirements/recommendations for international students: Required—TOEFL. *Expenses:* Contact institution.

The College of New Rochelle, Graduate School, Program in Nursing, New Rochelle, NY 10805-2308. Offers acute care nurse practitioner (MS, Certificate); clinical specialist in holistic nursing (MS, Certificate); family nurse practitioner (MS, Certificate); nursing and health care management (MS); nursing education (Certificate). *Accreditation:* AACN. *Program availability:* Part-time. *Faculty:* 3 full-time (2 women), 6 part-time/adjunct (4 women). *Students:* 116 part-time (104 women); includes 79 minority (58 Black or African American, non-Hispanic/Latino; 11 Asian, non-Hispanic/Latino; 10 Hispanic/Latino). Average age 38. In 2015, 25 master's awarded. *Entrance requirements:* For master's, GRE General Test or MAT, BSN, malpractice insurance, minimum GPA of 3.0, RN license. *Application deadline:* For fall admission, 8/15 priority date for domestic students; for spring admission, 12/1 priority date for domestic students. Applications are processed on a rolling basis. Application fee: $35. Electronic applications accepted. *Expenses:* Tuition, area resident: Part-time $894 per credit. *Required fees:* $350 per semester. *Financial support:* Traineeships available. Support available to part-time students. Financial award application deadline: 8/15; financial award applicants required to submit FAFSA. *Unit head:* Dr. H. Michael Dreher, Dean, School of Nursing, 914-654-5441, E-mail: hdreher@cnr.edu. *Application contact:* Michael Petri, Interim Director of Graduate Admissions, 914-654-5256, E-mail: mpetri@cnr.edu.

College of Staten Island of the City University of New York, Graduate Programs, School of Health Sciences, Program in Doctorate of Nursing Practice, Staten Island, NY 10314-6600. Offers DNP. *Program availability:* Part-time. *Entrance requirements:* Additional exam requirements/recommendations for international students: Required—TOEFL (minimum score 550 paper-based; 79 iBT), IELTS (minimum score 6.5). *Application deadline:* For fall admission, 12/1 priority date for domestic and international students. Applications are processed on a rolling basis. Application fee: $125. Electronic applications accepted. *Expenses:* Contact institution. *Financial support:* Applicants required to submit FAFSA. *Faculty research:* Cardiac, health literacy, autism caregivers, gastro-enterology, burn survivors. *Unit head:* Dr. June Como, Director, 718-982-3818, E-mail: june.como@csi.cuny.edu. *Application contact:* Sasha Spence, Associate Director for Graduate Recruitment and Admissions, 718-982-2019, Fax: 718-982-2500, E-mail: sasha.spence@csi.cuny.edu.
Website: http://www.csi.cuny.edu/catalog/graduate/clinical-doctorate-programs-in-nursing.htm

Colorado Mesa University, Department of Health Sciences, Grand Junction, CO 81501-3122. Offers advanced nursing practice (MSN); family nurse practitioner (DNP); health information technology systems (Graduate Certificate); nursing education (MSN). *Program availability:* Part-time, evening/weekend, online learning. *Degree requirements:* For master's and doctorate, Capstone. *Entrance requirements:* For master's and doctorate, Minimum GPA of 3.0 in BSN Program. Additional exam requirements/recommendations for international students: Required—TOEFL (minimum score 550 paper-based). Electronic applications accepted.

Columbia University, School of Nursing, Program in Family Nurse Practitioner, New York, NY 10032. Offers MS, Adv C. *Accreditation:* AACN. *Program availability:* Part-time. *Entrance requirements:* For master's, GRE General Test, NCLEX, BSN, 1 year of clinical experience (preferred); for Adv C, MSN. Additional exam requirements/recommendations for international students: Required—TOEFL (minimum score 100 iBT). Electronic applications accepted.

Columbus State University, Graduate Studies, College of Education and Health Professions, School of Nursing, Columbus, GA 31907-5645. Offers family nurse practitioner (MSN); nursing (MSN), including nurse educator, nurse informatics, nurse leader. Program offered in collaboration with Georgia Southwestern University. *Program availability:* Part-time, online only, 100% online. *Faculty:* 7 full-time (all women), 1 part-time/adjunct (0 women). *Students:* 29 full-time (24 women), 44 part-time (43 women); includes 35 minority (25 Black or African American, non-Hispanic/Latino; 1 Asian, non-Hispanic/Latino; 3 Hispanic/Latino; 6 Two or more races, non-Hispanic/Latino). Average age 38. 66 applicants, 59% accepted, 32 enrolled. In 2015, 6 master's awarded. *Entrance requirements:* For master's, GRE, BSN, minimum undergraduate GPA of 3.0. Additional exam requirements/recommendations for international students: Required—TOEFL (minimum score 550 paper-based; 79 iBT). *Application deadline:* For fall admission, 5/1 for domestic and international students; for spring admission, 11/1 for domestic and international students; for summer admission, 3/1 for domestic and international students. Applications are processed on a rolling basis. Application fee: $50. Electronic applications accepted. *Expenses:* Contact institution. *Financial support:* In 2015–16, 51 students received support. Institutionally sponsored loans available. Financial award application deadline: 5/1; financial award applicants required to submit FAFSA. *Unit head:* Latonya Sanot, Interim Director, 706-507-8576, E-mail: santo_latonya@columbusstate.edu. *Application contact:* Kristin Williams, Director of International and Graduate Recruitment, 706-507-8848, Fax: 706-568-5091, E-mail: williams_kristin@columbusstate.edu.
Website: http://nursing.columbusstate.edu/

Concordia University Wisconsin, Graduate Programs, School of Human Services, Program in Nursing, Mequon, WI 53097-2402. Offers family nurse practitioner (MSN); geriatric nurse practitioner (MSN); nurse educator (MSN). *Accreditation:* AACN. *Program availability:* Online learning. *Degree requirements:* For master's, comprehensive exam, thesis or alternative. *Entrance requirements:* Additional exam requirements/recommendations for international students: Required—TOEFL. *Expenses:* Contact institution.

Coppin State University, Division of Graduate Studies, Helene Fuld School of Nursing, Baltimore, MD 21216-3698. Offers family nurse practitioner (PMC); nursing (MSN). *Accreditation:* AACN; ACEN. *Program availability:* Part-time, evening/weekend. *Degree requirements:* For master's, comprehensive exam, thesis, clinical internship. *Entrance requirements:* For master's, GRE, bachelor's degree in nursing, interview, minimum GPA of 3.0, RN license. Additional exam requirements/recommendations for international students: Required—TOEFL (minimum score 550 paper-based).

Cox College, Programs in Nursing, Springfield, MO 65802. Offers clinical nurse leader (MSN); family nurse practitioner (MSN); nurse educator (MSN). *Accreditation:* AACN. *Entrance requirements:* For master's, RN license, essay, 2 letters of recommendation, official transcripts. Electronic applications accepted.

Creighton University, College of Nursing, Omaha, NE 68178-0001. Offers adult acute care nurse practitioner (Post-Master's Certificate); adult gerontology acute care nurse practitioner (DNP); adult gerontology nurse practitioner (DNP); clinical nurse leader (MSN, Post-Graduate Certificate); clinical systems administration (MSN, DNP); family nurse practitioner (DNP, Post-Master's Certificate); neonatal nurse practitioner (DNP, Post-Master's Certificate); pediatric acute care nurse practitioner (DNP, Post-Master's Certificate); psychiatric mental health nurse practitioner (DNP). *Accreditation:* AACN. *Program availability:* Part-time, blended/hybrid learning. *Faculty:* 10 full-time (all women), 48 part-time/adjunct (45 women). *Students:* 132 full-time (120 women), 228 part-time (212 women); includes 38 minority (10 Black or African American, non-Hispanic/Latino; 3 American Indian or Alaska Native, non-Hispanic/Latino; 11 Asian, non-Hispanic/Latino; 1 Hispanic/Latino; 2 Native Hawaiian or other Pacific Islander, non-Hispanic/Latino; 11 Two or more races, non-Hispanic/Latino). Average age 31. 66 applicants, 91% accepted, 43 enrolled. In 2015, 54 master's, 17 doctorates, 1 other advanced degree awarded. *Degree requirements:* For master's, capstone project; for doctorate, scholarly project. *Entrance requirements:* For master's and doctorate, BSN from an ACEN- or CCNE-accredited nursing school, minimum cumulative GPA of 3.0, personal statement, current unencumbered RN license with NE eligibility, undergraduate statistics course, physical assessment course or equivalent; for other advanced degree, MSN or MS in nursing, minimum cumulative GPA of 3.0, current unencumbered RN license with NE eligibility. Additional exam requirements/recommendations for international students: Required—TOEFL (minimum score 600 paper-based; 100 iBT). *Application deadline:* For fall admission, 6/15 priority date for domestic and international students; for spring admission, 11/15 priority date for domestic and international students; for summer admission, 4/15 for domestic and international students. Applications are processed on a rolling basis. Application fee: $50. Electronic applications accepted. *Expenses:* $800 per credit hour tuition; $904 per semester full-time fees; $207 per semester part-time fees; $50 one-time drug screen fee. *Financial support:* In 2015–16, 7 students received support. Scholarships/grants available. Financial award applicants required to submit FAFSA. *Faculty research:* Obesity prevention in children, evaluation of simulated clinical experiences, vitamin D3 and calcium for cancer risk education in post menopausal women, online support and education to reduce stress for prenatal patients on bed rest, health literacy,

immunization research. *Total annual research expenditures:* $162,085. *Unit head:* Dr. Catherine Todero, Dean, 402-280-2004, Fax: 402-280-2045. *Application contact:* Shannon Cox, Enrollment Specialist, 402-280-2067, Fax: 402-280-2045, E-mail: shannoncox@creighton.edu.
Website: http://nursing.creighton.edu/

Delta State University, Graduate Programs, School of Nursing, Cleveland, MS 38733. Offers family nurse practitioner (MSN); nurse administrator (MSN); nurse educator (MSN). *Accreditation:* AACN. *Program availability:* Part-time. *Degree requirements:* For master's, thesis optional. *Entrance requirements:* For master's, GRE General Test. Electronic applications accepted.

DePaul University, College of Science and Health, Chicago, IL 60614. Offers applied mathematics (MS); applied statistics (MS); biological sciences (MA, MS); chemistry (MS); mathematics education (MA); mathematics for teaching (MS); nursing (MS); nursing practice (DNP); physics (MS); psychology (MS); pure mathematics (MS); science education (MS); MA/PhD. Electronic applications accepted.

DeSales University, Division of Healthcare, Center Valley, PA 18034-9568. Offers adult-gerontology acute care (Post Master's Certificate); adult-gerontology acute care nurse practitioner (MSN); adult-gerontology acute certified nurse practitioner (Post Master's Certificate); adult-gerontology clinical nurse specialist (MSN, Post Master's Certificate); clinical leadership (DNP); family nurse practitioner (MSN, Post Master's Certificate); general nursing practice (DNP); health care information management (MSIS); network security (MSIS); nurse anesthetists (MSIS); nurse educator (Post Master's Certificate, Postbaccalaureate Certificate); nurse midwives (MSN); nurse practitioner (MSN); project management (MSIS); psychiatric-mental health nurse practitioner (MSN, Post Master's Certificate); DNP/MBA. *Accreditation:* ACEN. *Program availability:* Part-time. *Faculty:* 22 full-time (14 women), 37 part-time/adjunct (29 women). *Students:* 244 full-time (170 women), 55 part-time (50 women); includes 24 minority (7 Black or African American, non-Hispanic/Latino; 9 Asian, non-Hispanic/Latino; 6 Hispanic/Latino; 2 Two or more races, non-Hispanic/Latino). Average age 31. 68 applicants, 85% accepted, 52 enrolled. In 2015, 73 master's awarded. *Degree requirements:* For master's, minimum GPA of 3.0, portfolio; for doctorate, minimum GPA of 3.0, scholarly capstone project. *Entrance requirements:* For master's, GRE or MAT (waived if applicant has an undergraduate GPA of 3.0 or higher), BSN from ACEN- or CCNE-accredited program, minimum undergraduate GPA of 3.0, active RN license or eligibility, two letters of recommendation, essay, health care experience, personal interview; for doctorate, BSN or MSN from ACEN- or CCNE-accredited institution, minimum GPA of 3.3 in graduate program, current licensure as an RN. Additional exam requirements/recommendations for international students: Required—TOEFL (minimum score 104 iBT). *Application deadline:* Applications are processed on a rolling basis. Application fee: $50. Electronic applications accepted. *Expenses:* Contact institution. *Financial support:* Applicants required to submit FAFSA. *Unit head:* Fr. Dr. Peter Leonard, OSFS, Dean of Graduate Education, 610-282-1100 Ext. 1289, E-mail: peter.leonard@desales.edu. *Application contact:* Abigail Wernicki, Director of Graduate Admissions, 610-282-1100 Ext. 1768, Fax: 610-282-2869, E-mail: gradadmissions@desales.edu.

Dominican College, Division of Nursing, Orangeburg, NY 10962-1210. Offers MSN, DNP. *Program availability:* Part-time, evening/weekend. *Degree requirements:* For master's, guided research project, 750 hours of clinical practice with a final written project. *Entrance requirements:* For master's, RN license with 1 year of experience; minimum undergraduate GPA of 3.0; 3 letters of recommendation. Additional exam requirements/recommendations for international students: Required—TOEFL (minimum score 550 paper-based).

Drexel University, College of Nursing and Health Professions, Division of Graduate Nursing, Philadelphia, PA 19104-2875. Offers adult acute care (MSN); adult psychiatric/mental health (MSN); advanced practice nursing (MSN); clinical trials research (MSN); family nurse practitioner (MSN); leadership in health systems management (MSN); nursing education (MSN); pediatric primary care (MSN); women's health (MSN). *Accreditation:* AACN. Electronic applications accepted.

Duke University, School of Nursing, Durham, NC 27708-0586. Offers acute care pediatric nurse practitioner (MSN, Post Master's Certificate); adult-gerontology nurse practitioner (MSN, Post Master's Certificate), including acute care, primary care; family nurse practitioner (MSN, Post Master's Certificate); neonatal nurse practitioner (MSN, Post Master's Certificate); nurse anesthesia (DNP); nurse practitioner (DNP); nursing (PhD); nursing and health care leadership (MSN); nursing education (MSN); nursing informatics (MSN, Post Master's Certificate); pediatric nurse practitioner (MSN, Post Master's Certificate), including primary care; women's health nurse practitioner (MSN, Post Master's Certificate). *Accreditation:* AACN; AANA/CANAEP. *Program availability:* Part-time, evening/weekend, online learning. *Faculty:* 74 full-time (63 women). *Students:* 179 full-time (152 women), 528 part-time (466 women); includes 145 minority (42 Black or African American, non-Hispanic/Latino; 3 American Indian or Alaska Native, non-Hispanic/Latino; 44 Asian, non-Hispanic/Latino; 35 Hispanic/Latino; 1 Native Hawaiian or other Pacific Islander, non-Hispanic/Latino; 20 Two or more races, non-Hispanic/Latino), 7 international. Average age 33. 619 applicants, 46% accepted, 201 enrolled. In 2015, 243 master's, 62 doctorates, 26 other advanced degrees awarded. Terminal master's awarded for partial completion of doctoral program. *Degree requirements:* For master's, thesis optional; for doctorate, capstone project. *Entrance requirements:* For master's, GRE General Test (waived if undergraduate GPA of 3.4 or higher), 1 year of nursing experience (recommended), BSN, minimum GPA of 3.0, previous course work in statistics; for doctorate, GRE General Test (waived if undergraduate GPA of 3.4 or higher), BSN or MSN, minimum GPA of 3.0, portfolio, resume, personal statement, undergraduate statistics course, current licensure as a registered nurse, transcripts from all post-secondary institutions; for Post Master's Certificate, MSN, licensure or eligibility as a professional nurse, transcripts from all post-secondary institutions, previous course work in statistics. Additional exam requirements/recommendations for international students: Required—TOEFL (minimum score 100 iBT), IELTS (minimum score 7). *Application deadline:* For fall admission, 12/1 for domestic and international students; for spring admission, 5/1 for domestic and international students. Application fee: $50. Electronic applications accepted. *Expenses:* Contact institution. *Financial support:* Career-related internships or fieldwork, institutionally sponsored loans, scholarships/grants, traineeships, and tuition waivers (partial) available. Support available to part-time students. Financial award applicants required to submit FAFSA. *Faculty research:* Cardiovascular disease, caregiver skill training, data mining, prostate cancer, neonatal immune system. *Unit head:* Dr. Marion E. Broome, Dean/Vice Chancellor for Nursing Affairs/Associate Vice President for Academic Affairs for Nursing, 919-684-9446, Fax: 919-684-9414, E-mail: marion.broome@duke.edu. *Application contact:* Dr. Ernie Rushing, Director of Admissions and Recruitment, 919-668-6274, Fax: 919-668-4693, E-mail: ernie.rushing@dm.duke.edu.
Website: http://www.nursing.duke.edu/

Duquesne University, School of Nursing, Master of Science in Nursing Program, Pittsburgh, PA 15282-0001. Offers family (individual across the life span) nurse practitioner (MSN); forensic nursing (MSN); nursing education (MSN). *Accreditation:* AACN. *Program availability:* Part-time, evening/weekend, minimal on-campus study. *Faculty:* 13 full-time (11 women), 9 part-time/adjunct (all women). *Students:* 91 full-time

Family Nurse Practitioner Studies

(84 women), 87 part-time (76 women); includes 31 minority (16 Black or African American, non-Hispanic/Latino; 4 Asian, non-Hispanic/Latino; 7 Hispanic/Latino; 4 Two or more races, non-Hispanic/Latino), 1 international. Average age 34. 280 applicants, 34% accepted, 73 enrolled. In 2015, 39 master's awarded. *Entrance requirements:* For master's, current RN license; BSN with minimum GPA of 3.0; minimum of 1 year of full-time work experience as RN prior to registration in clinical or specialty course. Additional exam requirements/recommendations for international students: Required—TOEFL (minimum score 600 paper-based; 100 iBT). *Application deadline:* For fall admission, 3/1 for domestic and international students. Application fee: $0. Electronic applications accepted. *Expenses:* $1,218 per credit. *Financial support:* In 2015–16, 11 students received support, including 2 research assistantships with partial tuition reimbursements available (averaging $2,200 per year), 7 teaching assistantships with partial tuition reimbursements available (averaging $1,100 per year); scholarships/grants, traineeships, and tuition waivers (partial) also available. Support available to part-time students. Financial award application deadline: 7/1; financial award applicants required to submit FAFSA. *Faculty research:* Vulnerable populations, social justice, cultural competence, health disparities, wellness within chronic illness, forensics. *Total annual research expenditures:* $246,973. *Unit head:* Dr. Alison Colbert, Associate Professor/Associate Dean of Academic Affairs, 412-396-1511, Fax: 412-396-1821, E-mail: colberta@duq.edu. *Application contact:* Susan Hardner, Nurse Recruiter, 412-396-4945, Fax: 412-396-6346, E-mail: nursing@duq.edu.
Website: http://www.duq.edu/academics/schools/nursing/graduate-programs/master-science-nursing

Duquesne University, School of Nursing, Post Master's Certificate Program, Pittsburgh, PA 15282-0001. Offers family (individual across the life span) nurse practitioner (Post-Master's Certificate); forensic nursing (Post-Master's Certificate); nursing education and faculty role (Post-Master's Certificate). *Program availability:* Part-time, evening/weekend, minimal on-campus study. *Faculty:* 3 full-time (all women), 7 part-time/adjunct (all women). *Students:* 2 full-time (both women), 10 part-time (9 women); includes 4 minority (3 Black or African American, non-Hispanic/Latino; 1 Hispanic/Latino). Average age 42. 28 applicants, 36% accepted, 5 enrolled. In 2015, 4 Post-Master's Certificates awarded. *Entrance requirements:* For degree, current RN license, BSN, MSN. Additional exam requirements/recommendations for international students: Required—TOEFL (minimum score 600 paper-based; 100 iBT). *Application deadline:* For fall admission, 3/1 for domestic and international students. Application fee: $0. Electronic applications accepted. *Expenses:* $1,218 per credit. *Financial support:* Teaching assistantships with partial tuition reimbursements, scholarships/grants, traineeships, and tuition waivers (partial) available. Support available to part-time students. Financial award application deadline: 7/1; financial award applicants required to submit FAFSA. *Faculty research:* Vulnerable populations, social justice, cultural competence, health disparities, wellness within chronic illness, forensics. *Total annual research expenditures:* $296,973. *Unit head:* Dr. Alison Colbert, Associate Professor/Associate Dean of Academic Affairs, 412-396-1511, Fax: 412-396-1821, E-mail: colberta@duq.edu. *Application contact:* Susan Hardner, Nurse Recruiter, 412-396-4945, Fax: 412-396-6346, E-mail: nursing@duq.edu.
Website: http://www.duq.edu/academics/schools/nursing/graduate-programs/post-masters-certificates

D'Youville College, School of Nursing, Buffalo, NY 14201-1084. Offers advanced practice nursing (DNP); family nurse practitioner (MSN, Certificate); nursing and health-related professions education (Certificate). *Accreditation:* AACN. *Program availability:* Part-time. *Faculty:* 36 full-time (35 women), 15 part-time/adjunct (13 women). *Students:* 75 full-time (70 women), 136 part-time (119 women); includes 21 minority (12 Black or African American, non-Hispanic/Latino; 1 American Indian or Alaska Native, non-Hispanic/Latino; 6 Asian, non-Hispanic/Latino; 2 Hispanic/Latino), 64 international. Average age 35. 197 applicants, 88% accepted, 119 enrolled. In 2015, 48 master's, 1 doctorate, 2 other advanced degrees awarded. *Degree requirements:* For master's, thesis or alternative. *Entrance requirements:* For master's, BS in nursing, minimum GPA of 3.0, course work in statistics and computers; for doctorate, BS in nursing, MS in advanced practice nursing specialty, minimum GPA of 3.25. Additional exam requirements/recommendations for international students: Required—TOEFL (minimum score 500 paper-based). *Application deadline:* For fall admission, 5/1 priority date for international students; for spring admission, 9/1 priority date for international students. Applications are processed on a rolling basis. Electronic applications accepted. *Expenses:* Tuition, area resident: Full-time $21,120; part-time $880 per credit hour. *Required fees:* $235; $96. One-time fee: $100. *Financial support:* Federal Work-Study, scholarships/grants, traineeships, and unspecified assistantships available. Support available to part-time students. Financial award application deadline: 3/1; financial award applicants required to submit FAFSA. *Faculty research:* Nursing curriculum, nursing theory-testing, wellness research, communication and socialization patterns. *Unit head:* Dr. Ann Caughill, Chair, 716-829-7892, Fax: 716-829-8159. *Application contact:* Mark Pavone, Graduate Admissions Director, 716-829-8400, Fax: 716-829-7900, E-mail: graduateadmissions@dyc.edu.
Website: http://www.dyc.edu/academics/nursing/

Eastern Kentucky University, The Graduate School, College of Health Sciences, Department of Nursing, Richmond, KY 40475-3102. Offers rural community health care (MSN); rural health family nurse practitioner (MSN). *Accreditation:* AACN. *Entrance requirements:* For master's, GRE General Test, minimum GPA of 2.75.

East Tennessee State University, School of Graduate Studies, College of Nursing, Johnson City, TN 37614. Offers family nurse practitioner (DNP); nursing (MSN, PhD, Post-Master's Certificate). *Accreditation:* AACN. *Program availability:* Part-time, evening/weekend, online learning. *Faculty:* 27 full-time (26 women), 7 part-time/adjunct (all women). *Students:* 107 full-time (91 women), 331 part-time (294 women); includes 37 minority (18 Black or African American, non-Hispanic/Latino; 1 American Indian or Alaska Native, non-Hispanic/Latino; 6 Asian, non-Hispanic/Latino; 4 Hispanic/Latino; 2 Native Hawaiian or other Pacific Islander, non-Hispanic/Latino; 6 Two or more races, non-Hispanic/Latino). Average age 36. 280 applicants, 42% accepted, 83 enrolled. In 2015, 80 master's, 13 doctorates, 10 other advanced degrees awarded. *Degree requirements:* For master's and Post-Master's Certificate, comprehensive exam, practicum; for doctorate, comprehensive exam, thesis/dissertation (for some programs), practicum, internship. *Entrance requirements:* For master's, bachelor's degree, minimum GPA of 3.0, current RN license and eligibility to practice, resume, three letters of recommendation; for doctorate, GRE General Test, MSN (for PhD), BSN or MSN (for DNP), current RN license and eligibility to practice, 2 years of full-time registered nurse work experience or equivalent, three letters of recommendation, resume or curriculum vitae, interview, writing sample; for Post-Master's Certificate, MSN, minimum GPA of 3.0, current RN license and eligibility to practice, three letters of recommendation, resume or curriculum vitae. Additional exam requirements/recommendations for international students: Required—TOEFL (minimum score 550 paper-based; 79 iBT). *Application deadline:* For fall admission, 2/1 for domestic and international students; for spring admission, 7/1 for domestic and international students. Application fee: $35 ($45 for international students). Electronic applications accepted. *Financial support:* In 2015–16, 3 students received support, including 9 research assistantships with tuition reimbursements available (averaging $4,500 per year), 1 teaching assistantship (averaging $6,000 per year); career-related internships or fieldwork, institutionally

sponsored loans, scholarships/grants, and unspecified assistantships also available. Financial award application deadline: 7/1; financial award applicants required to submit FAFSA. *Faculty research:* Improving health of rural and underserved populations (low income elders living in public housing, rural caregivers, Hispanic populations), health services and systems research (quality outcomes of nurse-managed primary care, in-home, and rural health care), nursing education (experiences of second-degree BSN students, well-being of BSN students). *Unit head:* Dr. Wendy Nehring, Dean, 423-439-7051, Fax: 423-439-4522, E-mail: nursing@etsu.edu. *Application contact:* Linda Raines, School of Graduate Studies, 423-439-6158, Fax: 423-439-5624, E-mail: raineslt@etsu.edu.
Website: http://www.etsu.edu/nursing/

Edinboro University of Pennsylvania, Department of Nursing, Edinboro, PA 16444. Offers advanced practice nursing (DNP); family nurse practitioner (MSN); nurse educator (MSN). *Program availability:* Part-time, evening/weekend. *Degree requirements:* For master's, thesis, competency exam. *Entrance requirements:* For master's, GRE or MAT, minimum QPA of 2.5. *Application deadline:* Applications are processed on a rolling basis. Application fee: $30. Electronic applications accepted. *Expenses:* Tuition, state resident: full-time $11,280; part-time $470 per credit hour. Tuition, nonresident: full-time $16,920; part-time $705 per credit hour. International tuition: $16,920 full-time. *Required fees:* $3247.20; $135.30 per credit hour. *Financial support:* Research assistantships with tuition reimbursements, career-related internships or fieldwork, Federal Work-Study, scholarships/grants, and unspecified assistantships available. Support available to part-time students. Financial award application deadline: 2/15; financial award applicants required to submit FAFSA. *Unit head:* Dr. Amy McClune, Chair, 814-732-2619, E-mail: amcclune@edinboro.edu. *Application contact:* Dr. Amy McClune, Chair, 814-732-2619, E-mail: amcclune@edinboro.edu.
Website: http://www.edinboro.edu/departments/nursing/nursing.dot

Emory University, Nell Hodgson Woodruff School of Nursing, Atlanta, GA 30322-1100. Offers adult nurse practitioner (MSN); emergency nurse practitioner (MSN); family nurse practitioner (MSN); family nurse-midwife (MSN); health systems leadership (MSN); nurse-midwifery (MSN); pediatric nurse practitioner acute and primary care (MSN); women's health care (Title X) (MSN); women's health nurse practitioner (MSN); MSN/MPH. *Accreditation:* AACN; ACNM/ACME (one or more programs are accredited). *Program availability:* Part-time. *Entrance requirements:* For master's, GRE General Test or MAT, minimum GPA of 3.0, BS in nursing from an accredited institution, RN license and additional course work, 3 letters of recommendation. Additional exam requirements/recommendations for international students: Required—TOEFL (minimum score 600 paper-based; 100 iBT). Electronic applications accepted. *Expenses:* Contact institution. *Faculty research:* Older adult falls and injuries, minority health issues, cardiac symptoms and quality of life, bio-ethics and decision-making, menopausal issues.

Fairfield University, Marion Peckham Egan School of Nursing and Health Studies, Fairfield, CT 06824. Offers advanced practice (DNP); family nurse practitioner (MSN, DNP); nurse anesthesia (DNP); nursing leadership (MSN); psychiatric nurse practitioner (MSN, DNP). *Accreditation:* AACN; AANA/CANAEP. *Program availability:* Part-time, evening/weekend. *Faculty:* 8 full-time (all women), 9 part-time/adjunct (7 women). *Students:* 43 full-time (35 women), 181 part-time (163 women); includes 52 minority (20 Black or African American, non-Hispanic/Latino; 1 American Indian or Alaska Native, non-Hispanic/Latino; 11 Asian, non-Hispanic/Latino; 16 Hispanic/Latino; 4 Two or more races, non-Hispanic/Latino), 1 international. Average age 36. 103 applicants, 67% accepted, 43 enrolled. In 2015, 12 master's, 21 doctorates awarded. *Degree requirements:* For master's, capstone project. *Entrance requirements:* For master's, minimum QPA of 3.0, RN license, resume, 2 recommendations; for doctorate, MSN (minimum QPA of 3.2) or BSN (minimum QPA of 3.0); critical care nursing experience (for nurse anesthesia DNP candidates). Additional exam requirements/recommendations for international students: Required—TOEFL (minimum score 550 paper-based; 80 iBT) or IELTS (minimum score 6.5). *Application deadline:* For fall admission, 5/15 for international students; for spring admission, 10/15 for international students. Applications are processed on a rolling basis. Application fee: $60. Electronic applications accepted. *Expenses:* $850 per credit hour (for MSN); $900-$1,000 per credit hour (for DNP). *Financial support:* In 2015–16, 51 students received support. Unspecified assistantships available. Financial award applicants required to submit FAFSA. *Faculty research:* Aging, spiritual care, palliative and end of life care, psychiatric mental health, pediatric trauma. *Unit head:* Dr. Meredith Wallace Kazer, Dean, 203-254-4000 Ext. 2701, Fax: 203-254-4126, E-mail: mkazer@fairfield.edu. *Application contact:* Marianne Gumpper, Director of Graduate and Continuing Studies Admission, 203-254-4184, Fax: 203-254-4073, E-mail: gradadmis@fairfield.edu.
Website: http://fairfield.edu/son

Felician University, Master of Science in Nursing Program, Lodi, NJ 07644-2117. Offers adult-gerontology nurse practitioner (MSN, PMC); executive leadership (MSN, PMC); family nurse practitioner (MSN, PMC); nursing education (MSN, PMC). *Accreditation:* AACN. *Program availability:* Part-time, evening/weekend, online learning. *Faculty:* 11 full-time (9 women), 2 part-time/adjunct (both women). *Students:* 1 (woman) full-time, 121 part-time (112 women); includes 60 minority (23 Black or African American, non-Hispanic/Latino; 1 American Indian or Alaska Native, non-Hispanic/Latino; 19 Asian, non-Hispanic/Latino; 17 Hispanic/Latino). Average age 40. 111 applicants, 83% accepted, 52 enrolled. In 2015, 18 master's awarded. *Entrance requirements:* For master's, BS in nursing or equivalent, minimum QPA of 3.0, 2 letters of recommendation, RN license; for PMC, RN license, minimum GPA of 3.0. Additional exam requirements/recommendations for international students: Recommended—TOEFL (minimum score 79 iBT). *Application deadline:* Applications are processed on a rolling basis. Application fee: $40. Electronic applications accepted. Application fee is waived when completed online. *Expenses:* Tuition, area resident: Part-time $965 per credit. Tuition and fees vary according to course load and program. *Financial support:* In 2015–16, 10 students received support. Traineeships available. Financial award applicants required to submit FAFSA. *Faculty research:* Anxiety and fear, curriculum innovation, health promotion. *Unit head:* Dr. Ann Tritak, Associate Dean, Department of Graduate Nursing, 201-201-559-6151, E-mail: tritaka@felician.edu. *Application contact:* Dr. Margaret Smolin, Director, Graduate Admissions, 201-559-1451, E-mail: graduate@felician.edu.

Florida National University, Program in Nursing, Hialeah, FL 33012. Offers family nurse practitioner (MSN); nurse educator (MSN); nurse leadership and management (MSN). *Degree requirements:* For master's, practicum. *Entrance requirements:* For master's, active registered nurse license, BSN from accredited institution. *Expenses:* Tuition, area resident: Full-time $15,600. *Required fees:* $650.

Florida State University, The Graduate School, College of Nursing, Tallahassee, FL 32306-4310. Offers family nurse practitioner (DNP); nurse educator (MSN, Certificate); nurse leader (MSN); nursing leadership (Certificate). *Accreditation:* AACN. *Program availability:* Part-time, online learning. *Faculty:* 13 full-time (12 women). *Students:* 56 full-time (49 women), 25 part-time (23 women); includes 25 minority (13 Black or African American, non-Hispanic/Latino; 4 Asian, non-Hispanic/Latino; 7 Hispanic/Latino; 1 Two or more races, non-Hispanic/Latino). Average age 38. 90 applicants, 50% accepted, 44 enrolled. In 2015, 2 master's, 20 doctorates awarded. *Degree requirements:* For master's, thesis optional; for doctorate, thesis/dissertation, evidence-based project. *Entrance requirements:* For master's, GRE General Test, MAT, minimum GPA of 3.0, BSN, United States RN license; for doctorate, GRE General Test, MAT, minimum GPA of 3.0, BSN or MSN, Florida RN license. Additional exam requirements/recommendations for international students: Required—TOEFL (minimum score 550 paper-based). *Application deadline:* For fall admission, 4/15 for domestic and international students. Application fee: $30. Electronic applications accepted. *Expenses: Tuition, area resident:* Full-time $7263; part-time $403.50 per credit hour. Tuition, nonresident: full-time $18,087; part-time $1004.85 per credit hour. *Required fees:* $1365; $75.81 per credit hour. $20 per semester. Tuition and fees vary according to campus/location. *Financial support:* In 2015–16, 75 students received support, including fellowships with partial tuition reimbursements available (averaging $6,300 per year), research assistantships with partial tuition reimbursements available (averaging $3,000 per year), 3 teaching assistantships with partial tuition reimbursements available (averaging $3,000 per year); career-related internships or fieldwork, Federal Work-Study, institutionally sponsored loans, scholarships/grants, traineeships, and tuition waivers (partial) also available. Financial award application deadline: 4/15; financial award applicants required to submit FAFSA. *Faculty research:* Cardiac, women's health, health promotion and prevention, educational strategies, infectious diseases. *Unit head:* Dr. Judith McFetridge-Durdle, Dean, 850-644-6846, Fax: 850-644-7660, E-mail: jdurdle@nursing.fsu.edu. *Application contact:* Carlos Urrutia, Assistant Director for Student Services, 850-644-5638, Fax: 850-645-7249, E-mail: currutia@fsu.edu. Website: http://nursing.fsu.edu/

Francis Marion University, Graduate Programs, Department of Nursing, Florence, SC 29502-0547. Offers family nurse practitioner (MSN); family nurse practitioner with nurse educator certificate (MSN); nurse educator (MSN). *Program availability:* Part-time. *Faculty:* 7 full-time (all women). *Students:* 52 full-time (40 women), 28 part-time (23 women); includes 19 minority (16 Black or African American, non-Hispanic/Latino; 1 American Indian or Alaska Native, non-Hispanic/Latino; 1 Asian, non-Hispanic/Latino; 1 Two or more races, non-Hispanic/Latino). Average age 34. 37 applicants, 84% accepted, 27 enrolled. In 2015, 27 master's awarded. *Entrance requirements:* For master's, GRE, official transcripts, two letters of recommendation from professional associates or former professors, written statement of applicant's career goals, current nursing license. Additional exam requirements/recommendations for international students: Required—TOEFL (minimum score 550 paper-based; 79 iBT). *Application deadline:* For fall admission, 3/1 for domestic and international students; for spring admission, 10/1 for domestic and international students. Applications are processed on a rolling basis. Application fee: $37. Electronic applications accepted. *Expenses:* Contact institution. *Financial support:* Available to part-time students. Application deadline: 3/1; applicants required to submit FAFSA. *Unit head:* Dr. Ruth Wittmann-Price, Chair, 843-661-4625, E-mail: rwittmannprice@fmarion.edu. *Application contact:* Jennifer Taylor, Administrative Manager, Provost's Office, 843-661-1286, Fax: 843-661-4688, E-mail: jtaylor@fmarion.edu.

Fresno Pacific University, Graduate Programs, Program in Nursing, Fresno, CA 93702-4709. Offers family nurse practitioner (MSN). *Entrance requirements:* For master's, official transcripts verifying BSN from accredited nursing program; minimum cumulative GPA of 3.0; three reference forms; statement of intent; resume or curriculum vitae; personal interview; active California RN license; completion of statistics, chemistry and upper-division writing. *Expenses:* Contact institution.

Frontier Nursing University, Graduate Programs, Hyden, KY 41749. Offers family nurse practitioner (MSN, DNP, Post Master's Certificate); nurse-midwifery (MSN, DNP, Post Master's Certificate); women's health care nurse practitioner (MSN, DNP, Post Master's Certificate). *Accreditation:* ACEN; ACNM. *Degree requirements:* For doctorate, capstone project, practicum.

Gannon University, School of Graduate Studies, Morosky College of Health Professions and Sciences, Villa Maria School of Nursing, Program in Family Nurse Practitioner, Erie, PA 16541-0001. Offers MSN, Certificate. *Program availability:* Part-time, evening/weekend. *Students:* 1 (woman) full-time, 22 part-time (19 women); includes 1 minority (American Indian or Alaska Native, non-Hispanic/Latino), 1 international. Average age 33. 17 applicants, 71% accepted, 6 enrolled. *Degree requirements:* For master's, thesis (for some programs), practicum. *Entrance requirements:* For master's, BS in nursing, transcripts, 3 letters of recommendation, interview, evidence of fulfillment of legal requirements for practice of nursing in the United States; for Certificate, GRE, interview. Additional exam requirements/recommendations for international students: Required—TOEFL (minimum score 79 iBT). *Application deadline:* Applications are processed on a rolling basis. Application fee: $25. Electronic applications accepted. *Unit head:* Dr. Kathleen Patterson, Director, 814-871-5547, E-mail: patterso018@gannon.edu. *Application contact:* Bridget Philip, Director of Graduate Admissions, 814-871-7412, E-mail: graduate@gannon.edu.

Georgetown University, Graduate School of Arts and Sciences, School of Nursing and Health Studies, Washington, DC 20057. Offers acute care nurse practitioner (MS); clinical nurse specialist (MS); family nurse practitioner (MS); nurse anesthesia (MS); nurse-midwifery (MS); nursing (DNP); nursing education (MS). *Accreditation:* AACN; AANA/CANAEP (one or more programs are accredited); ACNM/ACME (one or more programs are accredited). *Degree requirements:* For master's, thesis optional. *Entrance requirements:* For master's, GRE General Test or MAT, bachelor's degree in nursing from NLN-accredited school, minimum undergraduate GPA of 3.0. Additional exam requirements/recommendations for international students: Required—TOEFL.

The George Washington University, School of Nursing, Washington, DC 20052. Offers adult nurse practitioner (MSN, DNP, Post-Master's Certificate); clinical research administration (MSN); family nurse practitioner (MSN, Post-Master's Certificate); health care quality (MSN, Post-Master's Certificate); nursing leadership and management (MSN); nursing practice (DNP), including nursing education; palliative care nurse practitioner (Post-Master's Certificate). *Accreditation:* AACN. *Faculty:* 42 full-time (all women), 71 part-time/adjunct (66 women). *Students:* 52 full-time (48 women), 519 part-time (463 women); includes 162 minority (72 Black or African American, non-Hispanic/Latino; 4 American Indian or Alaska Native, non-Hispanic/Latino; 52 Asian, non-Hispanic/Latino; 31 Hispanic/Latino; 3 Two or more races, non-Hispanic/Latino), 2 international. Average age 37. 465 applicants, 69% accepted, 187 enrolled. In 2015, 121 master's, 35 doctorates, 1 other advanced degree awarded. *Unit head:* Pamela R. Jeffries, Dean, 202-994-3725, E-mail: pjeffries@gwu.edu. *Application contact:* Kristin Williams, Associate Provost for Graduate Enrollment Management, 202-994-0467, Fax: 202-994-0371, E-mail: ksw@gwu.edu.
Website: http://nursing.gwumc.edu/

Georgia Southern University, Jack N. Averitt College of Graduate Studies, College of Health and Human Sciences, School of Nursing, Program in Nurse Practitioner, Statesboro, GA 30458. Offers family nurse practitioner (MSN); psychiatric mental health nurse practitioner (MSN). *Program availability:* Part-time, blended/hybrid learning. *Students:* 30 full-time (26 women), 25 part-time (21 women); includes 17 minority (10 Black or African American, non-Hispanic/Latino; 4 Asian, non-Hispanic/Latino; 2 Hispanic/Latino; 1 Two or more races, non-Hispanic/Latino). Average age 38. 58 applicants, 71% accepted, 15 enrolled. In 2015, 19 master's awarded. *Entrance requirements:* For master's, minimum GPA of 3.0, Georgia nursing license, 2 years of

clinical experience, CPR certification. Additional exam requirements/recommendations for international students: Required—TOEFL (minimum score 550 paper-based; 80 iBT), IELTS (minimum score 6). *Application deadline:* For fall admission, 7/31 priority date for domestic and international students; for spring admission, 11/30 priority date for domestic students, 11/30 for international students; for summer admission, 3/31 for domestic and international students. Applications are processed on a rolling basis. Application fee: $50. Electronic applications accepted. *Expenses:* Tuition, state resident: full-time $7236; part-time $277 per semester hour. Tuition, nonresident: full-time $27,118; part-time $1105 per semester hour. *Required fees:* $2092. *Financial support:* In 2015–16, 26 students received support, including 5 fellowships with full tuition reimbursements available (averaging $7,750 per year); career-related internships or fieldwork, Federal Work-Study, scholarships/grants, traineeships, tuition waivers (full), and unspecified assistantships also available. Support available to part-time students. Financial award application deadline: 4/15; financial award applicants required to submit FAFSA. *Faculty research:* Vulnerable populations, breast cancer, diabetes, mellitus, advanced practice nursing issues. *Unit head:* Dr. Deborah Allen, Graduate Program Director, 912-478-5056, Fax: 912-478-5036, E-mail: debbieallen@georgiasouthern.edu.

Georgia State University, Byrdine F. Lewis School of Nursing, Atlanta, GA 30303. Offers adult health clinical nurse specialist/nurse practitioner (MS, Certificate); child health clinical nurse specialist/pediatric nurse practitioner (MS, Certificate); family nurse practitioner (MS, Certificate); family psychiatric mental health nurse practitioner (MS, Certificate); nursing (PhD); nursing leadership in healthcare innovations (MS), including nursing administration, nursing informatics; nutrition (MS); perinatal clinical nurse specialist/women's health nurse practitioner (MS, Certificate); physical therapy (DPT); respiratory therapy (MS). *Accreditation:* AACN. *Program availability:* Part-time, blended/hybrid learning. *Faculty:* 18 full-time (11 women). *Students:* 275 full-time (195 women), 230 part-time (204 women); includes 192 minority (123 Black or African American, non-Hispanic/Latino; 49 Asian, non-Hispanic/Latino; 12 Hispanic/Latino; 2 Native Hawaiian or other Pacific Islander, non-Hispanic/Latino; 6 Two or more races, non-Hispanic/Latino), 35 international. Average age 33. 240 applicants, 61% accepted, 95 enrolled. In 2015, 115 master's, 40 doctorates, 19 other advanced degrees awarded. *Degree requirements:* For doctorate, comprehensive exam, thesis/dissertation. *Entrance requirements:* For doctorate, GRE. Additional exam requirements/recommendations for international students: Required—TOEFL. *Application deadline:* For fall admission, 2/1 priority date for domestic and international students; for spring admission, 9/15 for domestic and international students. Applications are processed on a rolling basis. Application fee: $50. Electronic applications accepted. *Expenses:* Contact institution. *Financial support:* In 2015–16, research assistantships with tuition reimbursements (averaging $1,666 per year), teaching assistantships with tuition reimbursements (averaging $1,920 per year) were awarded; scholarships/grants, tuition waivers (full and partial), and unspecified assistantships also available. Support available to part-time students. Financial award application deadline: 8/1; financial award applicants required to submit FAFSA. *Faculty research:* Stroke intervention for caregivers, stroke prevention in African-Americans; relationships between psychological distress and health outcomes in parents with a medically ill infant; medically fragile children; nursing expertise and patient outcomes. *Unit head:* Nancy Kropf, Dean of Nursing, 404-413-1101, Fax: 404-413-1090, E-mail: nkropf@gsu.edu.
Website: http://nursing.gsu.edu/

Goshen College, Program in Nursing, Goshen, IN 46526-4794. Offers family nurse practitioner (MSN). *Accreditation:* AACN. *Program availability:* Part-time, evening/weekend. *Degree requirements:* For master's, comprehensive exam (for some programs). *Entrance requirements:* For master's, minimum GPA of 3.0, curriculum vitae, bachelor's degree in nursing, active RN license in Indiana or Michigan, three professional references, essay, one year of clinical experience, statistics course, interview with program director. Additional exam requirements/recommendations for international students: Required—TOEFL (minimum score 600 paper-based; 100 iBT), IELTS (minimum score 6.5). *Application deadline:* For fall admission, 3/15 priority date for domestic students. Electronic applications accepted. *Expenses:* Contact institution. *Financial support:* Scholarships/grants available. *Unit head:* Ruth Stoltzfus, Director, 574-535-7973, E-mail: ruthas@goshen.edu. *Application contact:* Ruth Stoltzfus, Director, 574-535-7973, E-mail: ruthas@goshen.edu.
Website: http://www.goshen.edu/graduate/nursing/

Graceland University, School of Nursing, Independence, MO 64050-3434. Offers family nurse practitioner (MSN, PMC); nurse educator (MSN, PMC); organizational leadership (DNP). *Program availability:* Part-time, online learning. *Faculty:* 14 full-time (12 women), 21 part-time/adjunct (20 women). *Students:* 489 full-time (441 women); includes 75 minority (41 Black or African American, non-Hispanic/Latino; 5 American Indian or Alaska Native, non-Hispanic/Latino; 15 Asian, non-Hispanic/Latino; 2 Native Hawaiian or other Pacific Islander, non-Hispanic/Latino; 12 Two or more races, non-Hispanic/Latino), 1 international. Average age 39. 140 applicants, 69% accepted, 69 enrolled. In 2015, 137 master's, 11 doctorates awarded. *Degree requirements:* For master's, comprehensive exam (for some programs), thesis optional, scholarly project; for doctorate, capstone project. *Entrance requirements:* For master's, BSN from nationally-accredited program, RN license, minimum GPA of 3.0, satisfactory criminal background check; for doctorate, MSN from nationally-accredited program, RN license, minimum GPA of 3.2, criminal background check. Additional exam requirements/recommendations for international students: Recommended—TOEFL. *Application deadline:* For fall admission, 6/1 priority date for domestic students; for winter admission, 10/1 priority date for domestic students; for spring admission, 10/1 priority date for domestic students; for summer admission, 2/1 for domestic students. Application fee: $50. Electronic applications accepted. *Expenses:* Contact institution. *Financial support:* Institutionally sponsored loans available. Support available to part-time students. Financial award applicants required to submit FAFSA. *Faculty research:* International nursing, family care-giving, health promotion. *Unit head:* Dr. Claudia D. Horton, Dean, 816-423-4670, Fax: 816-423-4753, E-mail: horton@graceland.edu. *Application contact:* Nick Walker, Admissions Representative, 816-423-4717, Fax: 816-833-2990, E-mail: nowalker@graceland.edu.
Website: http://www.graceland.edu/nursing

Grambling State University, School of Graduate Studies and Research, College of Professional Studies, School of Nursing, Grambling, LA 71245. Offers family nurse practitioner (PMC); nursing (MSN). *Accreditation:* ACEN. *Program availability:* Part-time. *Degree requirements:* For master's, comprehensive exam (for some programs), thesis (for some programs). *Entrance requirements:* For master's, GRE, minimum GPA of 3.0 on last degree, interview, 2 years of experience as RN. Additional exam requirements/recommendations for international students: Required—TOEFL (minimum score 500 paper-based; 62 iBT). Electronic applications accepted.

Grand Canyon University, College of Nursing, Phoenix, AZ 85017-1097. Offers acute care nurse practitioner (MS, PMC); clinical nurse specialist (PMC), including clinical nurse specialist, education; family nurse practitioner (MS); leadership in health care systems (MS); nurse education (MS). *Accreditation:* AACN. *Program availability:* Part-time, evening/weekend, online learning. *Degree requirements:* For master's and PMC, comprehensive exam (for some programs). *Entrance requirements:* For master's,

Family Nurse Practitioner Studies

minimum cumulative and science course undergraduate GPA of 3.0. Additional exam requirements/recommendations for international students: Required—TOEFL (minimum score 575 paper-based; 90 iBT), IELTS (minimum score 7).

Gwynedd Mercy University, Frances M. Maguire School of Nursing and Health Professions, Gwynedd Valley, PA 19437-0901. Offers clinical nurse specialist (MSN), including gerontology, oncology, pediatrics; nurse educator (MSN); nurse practitioner (MSN), including adult health, pediatric health; nursing (DNP). *Accreditation:* ACEN. *Program availability:* Part-time, online learning. *Faculty:* 3 full-time (all women), 2 part-time/adjunct (both women). *Students:* 28 full-time (23 women), 68 part-time (62 women); includes 27 minority (18 Black or African American, non-Hispanic/Latino; 7 Asian, non-Hispanic/Latino; 2 Hispanic/Latino). Average age 37. 72 applicants, 25% accepted, 16 enrolled. In 2015, 7 master's awarded. *Degree requirements:* For master's, thesis optional; for doctorate, evidence-based scholarly project. *Entrance requirements:* For master's, GRE General Test or MAT, current nursing experience, physical assessment, course work in statistics, BSN from NLNAC-accredited program, 2 letters of recommendation, personal interview. Additional exam requirements/recommendations for international students: Required—TOEFL (minimum score 575 paper-based). *Application deadline:* For fall admission, 8/1 priority date for domestic students; for winter admission, 12/1 priority date for domestic students. Applications are processed on a rolling basis. Electronic applications accepted. *Expenses:* Contact institution. *Financial support:* In 2015–16, 21 students received support. Scholarships/grants, traineeships, and unspecified assistantships available. Financial award application deadline: 8/30. *Faculty research:* Critical thinking, primary care, domestic violence, multiculturalism, nursing centers. *Unit head:* Dr. Andrea D. Hollingsworth, Dean, 215-646-7300 Ext. 539, Fax: 215-641-5517, E-mail: hollingsworth.a@gmc.edu. *Application contact:* Dr. Barbara A. Jones, Director, 215-646-7300 Ext. 407, Fax: 215-641-5564, E-mail: jones.b@gmc.edu.
Website: http://www.gmercyu.edu/academics/graduate-programs/nursing

Hardin-Simmons University, Graduate School, Patty Hanks Shelton School of Nursing, Abilene, TX 79698-0001. Offers advanced healthcare delivery (MSN); family nurse practitioner (MSN). Programs offered jointly with Abilene Christian University and McMurry University. *Accreditation:* AACN. *Program availability:* Part-time. *Faculty:* 5 full-time (all women), 1 (woman) part-time/adjunct. *Students:* 18 part-time (15 women); includes 5 minority (2 Black or African American, non-Hispanic/Latino; 1 American Indian or Alaska Native, non-Hispanic/Latino; 2 Hispanic/Latino). Average age 33. In 2015, 4 master's awarded. *Degree requirements:* For master's, comprehensive exam, thesis or alternative. *Entrance requirements:* For master's, GRE, minimum undergraduate GPA of 3.0 in major, 2.8 overall; interview; upper-level course work in statistics; CPR certification; letters of recommendation. Additional exam requirements/recommendations for international students: Required—TOEFL (minimum score 550 paper-based; 75 iBT). *Application deadline:* For fall admission, 8/15 priority date for domestic students, 4/1 for international students; for spring admission, 1/5 priority date for domestic students, 9/1 for international students. Applications are processed on a rolling basis. Application fee: $50. Electronic applications accepted. *Expenses:* Contact institution. *Financial support:* In 2015–16, 17 students received support. Career-related internships or fieldwork and scholarships/grants available. Support available to part-time students. Financial award application deadline: 6/30; financial award applicants required to submit FAFSA. *Faculty research:* Child abuse, alternative medicine, pediatric chronic disease, health promotion. *Unit head:* Dr. Nina Ouimette, Dean, 325-671-2357, Fax: 325-671-2386, E-mail: nouimette@phssn.edu. *Application contact:* Dr. Nancy Kucinski, Dean of Graduate Studies, 325-670-1298, Fax: 325-670-1564, E-mail: gradoff@hsutx.edu.
Website: http://www.phssn.edu/

Holy Names University, Graduate Division, Department of Nursing, Oakland, CA 94619-1699. Offers administration/management (MSN, PMC); clinical faculty (MSN, PMC); community health nursing/case manager (MSN); family nurse practitioner (MSN, PMC; MSN/MA; MSN/MBA. *Accreditation:* AACN. *Program availability:* Part-time, evening/weekend. *Entrance requirements:* For master's, bachelor's degree in nursing or related field; California RN license or eligibility; minimum cumulative GPA of 2.8, 3.0 in nursing courses from baccalaureate program; courses in pathophysiology, statistics, and research at the undergraduate level. Additional exam requirements/recommendations for international students: Required—TOEFL (minimum score 500 paper-based; 79 iBT). Electronic applications accepted. Application fee is waived when completed online. *Expenses:* Tuition, area resident: Full-time $25,272; part-time $936 per credit hour. *Required fees:* $500; $250 per credit hour. *Faculty research:* Women's reproductive health, gerontology, attitudes about aging, schizophrenic families, international health issues.

Howard University, College of Nursing and Allied Health Sciences, Division of Nursing, Washington, DC 20059-0002. Offers nurse practitioner (Certificate); primary family health nursing (MSN). *Accreditation:* AACN. *Program availability:* Part-time. *Degree requirements:* For master's, comprehensive exam, thesis optional. *Entrance requirements:* For master's, RN license, minimum GPA of 3.0, BS in nursing. *Faculty research:* Urinary incontinence, breast cancer prevention, depression in the elderly, adolescent pregnancy.

Husson University, Graduate Nursing Program, Bangor, ME 04401-2999. Offers advanced practice psychiatric nursing (MSN, PMC); family and community nurse practitioner (MSN, PMC); nursing education (MSN, PMC). *Accreditation:* AACN. *Program availability:* Part-time. *Faculty:* 6 full-time (all women), 2 part-time/adjunct (1 woman). *Students:* 27 full-time (26 women), 10 part-time (9 women); includes 4 minority (2 Asian, non-Hispanic/Latino; 2 Two or more races, non-Hispanic/Latino). Average age 39. 70 applicants, 27% accepted, 13 enrolled. In 2015, 9 master's awarded. *Degree requirements:* For master's, comprehensive exam (for some programs), research project. *Entrance requirements:* For master's, MAT or GRE, BSN. Additional exam requirements/recommendations for international students: Required—TOEFL (minimum score 550 paper-based; 80 iBT). *Application deadline:* For fall admission, 3/31 for domestic students; for spring admission, 10/30 for domestic students. Application fee: $40. Electronic applications accepted. *Expenses:* Contact institution. *Financial support:* Research assistantships, Federal Work-Study, institutionally sponsored loans, traineeships, and unspecified assistantships available. Financial award application deadline: 3/31; financial award applicants required to submit FAFSA. *Faculty research:* Health disparities and methods to better identify and provide healthcare services to those most in need. *Unit head:* Prof. Mary Jude, Director, Graduate Nursing, 207-941-7769, Fax: 207-941-7198, E-mail: judem@husson.edu. *Application contact:* Kristen Card, Director of Graduate Admissions, 207-404-5660, Fax: 207-941-7935, E-mail: cardk@husson.edu.
Website: http://www.husson.edu/nursing-msn

Illinois State University, Graduate School, Mennonite College of Nursing, Normal, IL 61790. Offers family nurse practitioner (PMC); nursing (MSN, PhD). *Accreditation:* AACN. Application fee: $40. *Faculty research:* Expanding the teaching-nursing home culture in the state of Illinois, advanced education nursing traineeship program, collaborative doctoral program-caring for older adults. *Application contact:* Caroline Mallory, 309-438-2659, E-mail: cmmallo@ilstu.edu.
Website: http://www.mcn.ilstu.edu/

Indiana State University, College of Graduate and Professional Studies, College of Nursing, Health, and Human Services, Department of Advanced Practice Nursing, Terre Haute, IN 47809. Offers advanced practice nursing (DNP); family nurse practitioner (MS); nursing administration (MS); nursing education (MS). *Accreditation:* ACEN. *Program availability:* Part-time. *Degree requirements:* For master's, thesis or alternative. *Entrance requirements:* For master's, BSN, RN license, minimum undergraduate GPA of 3.0. Electronic applications accepted. *Faculty research:* Nursing faculty-student interactions, clinical evaluation, program evaluation, sexual dysfunction, faculty attitudes.

Indiana University–Purdue University Fort Wayne, College of Health and Human Services, Department of Nursing, Fort Wayne, IN 46805-1499. Offers adult-gerontology primary care nurse practitioner (MS); family nurse practitioner (MS); nurse executive (MS); nursing administration (Certificate); nursing education (MS). *Accreditation:* ACEN. *Program availability:* Part-time. *Faculty:* 8 full-time (all women). *Students:* 6 full-time (all women), 79 part-time (70 women); includes 8 minority (2 Black or African American, non-Hispanic/Latino; 3 Asian, non-Hispanic/Latino; 3 Hispanic/Latino). Average age 36. 14 applicants, 100% accepted, 10 enrolled. In 2015, 17 master's awarded. *Entrance requirements:* For master's, GRE Writing Test (if GPA below 3.0), BS in nursing, eligibility for Indiana RN license, minimum GPA of 3.0, essay, copy of resume, three references, undergraduate course work in research and statistics within last 5 years. Additional exam requirements/recommendations for international students: Required—TOEFL (minimum score 550 paper-based; 79 iBT); Recommended—TWE. *Application deadline:* For fall admission, 5/1 priority date for domestic and international students; for spring admission, 11/15 priority date for domestic students. Applications are processed on a rolling basis. Application fee: $55 ($60 for international students). Electronic applications accepted. *Financial support:* In 2015–16, 12 teaching assistantships with partial tuition reimbursements (averaging $13,522 per year) were awarded; scholarships/grants also available. Support available to part-time students. Financial award application deadline: 3/1; financial award applicants required to submit FAFSA. *Faculty research:* Community engagement, cervical screening, evidence-based practice. *Total annual research expenditures:* $22,966. *Unit head:* Dr. Lee-Ellen Kirkhorn, Chair/Professor, 260-481-6789, Fax: 260-481-5767, E-mail: kirkhorl@ipfw.edu. *Application contact:* Dr. Deb Poling, Director of Graduate Program, 260-481-6276, Fax: 260-481-5767, E-mail: polingd@ipfw.edu.
Website: http://www.ipfw.edu/nursing/

Indiana University South Bend, Vera Z. Dwyer College of Health Sciences, School of Nursing, South Bend, IN 46634-7111. Offers family nurse practitioner (MSN). *Program availability:* Part-time, evening/weekend. *Entrance requirements:* For master's, GRE General Test, minimum GPA of 3.0.

James Madison University, The Graduate School, College of Health and Behavioral Sciences, Program in Nursing, Harrisonburg, VA 22807. Offers adult/gerontology primary care nurse practitioner (MSN); clinical nurse leader (MSN); family nurse practitioner (MSN); nurse administrator (MSN); nurse midwifery (MSN); nursing (MSN, DNP). *Accreditation:* AACN. *Program availability:* Part-time, 100% online, blended/hybrid learning. *Faculty:* 15 full-time (all women), 1 (woman) part-time/adjunct. *Students:* 14 full-time (all women), 54 part-time (43 women); includes 6 minority (2 Black or African American, non-Hispanic/Latino; 1 Asian, non-Hispanic/Latino; 1 Hispanic/Latino; 2 Two or more races, non-Hispanic/Latino), 1 international. Average age 30. 49 applicants, 67% accepted, 31 enrolled. In 2015, 14 master's awarded. Application fee: $55. Electronic applications accepted. *Financial support:* In 2015–16, 2 students received support. Federal Work-Study, unspecified assistantships, and 2 assistantships (averaging $7530) available. Financial award application deadline: 3/1; financial award applicants required to submit FAFSA. *Unit head:* Dr. Julie T. Sanford, Department Head, 540-568-6314, E-mail: sanforjt@jmu.edu. *Application contact:* Lynette D. Michael, Director of Graduate Admissions and Student Records, 540-568-6131 Ext. 6395, Fax: 540-568-7860, E-mail: michaeld@jmu.edu.
Website: http://www.nursing.jmu.edu

Kent State University, College of Nursing, Kent, OH 44242. Offers advanced nursing practice (DNP), including adult gerontology acute care nurse practitioner (MSN, DNP), adult gerontology clinical nurse specialist (MSN, DNP), family nurse practitioner (MSN, DNP); nursing (MSN, PhD), including adult gerontology acute care nurse practitioner (MSN, DNP), adult gerontology clinical nurse specialist (MSN, DNP), family nurse practitioner (MSN, DNP), nurse educator (MSN), nursing healthcare management (MSN), primary care adult nurse practitioner (MSN), primary care pediatric clinical nurse specialist (MSN), primary care pediatric nurse practitioner (MSN), psychiatric mental health practitioner (MSN), women's health nurse practitioner (MSN); nursing education (Certificate); primary care pediatric nurse practitioner (Certificate); women's health nurse practitioner (Certificate). PhD program offered jointly with The University of Akron. *Accreditation:* AACN. *Program availability:* Part-time, online learning. *Faculty:* 52 full-time (48 women). *Students:* 78 full-time (56 women), 414 part-time (365 women); includes 63 minority (34 Black or African American, non-Hispanic/Latino; 1 American Indian or Alaska Native, non-Hispanic/Latino; 12 Asian, non-Hispanic/Latino; 12 Hispanic/Latino; 4 Two or more races, non-Hispanic/Latino), 16 international. Average age 37. 653 applicants, 54% accepted, 309 enrolled. In 2015, 140 master's, 1 doctorate, 13 other advanced degrees awarded. *Degree requirements:* For master's, thesis optional, practicum; for doctorate, comprehensive exam (for some programs), thesis/dissertation (for some programs), practicum and scholarly project (for DNP programs); for Certificate, practicum. *Entrance requirements:* For master's, minimum GPA of 3.0, transcripts, active unrestricted RN license, essay/goal statement, interview, 3 letters of recommendation; for doctorate, GRE (for PhD), minimum GPA of 3.0, transcripts, 3 letters of recommendation, interview; active unrestricted RN license, clinical experience and hours record (for DNP); goal statement, sample of written work, curriculum vitae, statement of research interests, and eligibility for RN license (for PhD); for Certificate, MSN, minimum GPA of 3.0, transcripts. Additional exam requirements/recommendations for international students: Required—TOEFL (minimum score: paper-based 525, iBT 71), Michigan English Language Assessment Battery (minimum score of 75), IELTS (minimum score of 6.0), PTE Academic (minimum score of 48), or completion of ELS level 112 Intensive Program. *Application deadline:* For fall admission, 2/1 for domestic students; for spring admission, 11/1 for domestic students. Application fee: $45 ($70 for international students). Electronic applications accepted. *Expenses:* Tuition, state resident: full-time $10,864; part-time $495 per credit hour. Tuition, nonresident: full-time $18,380; part-time $837 per credit hour. *Financial support:* Research assistantships with full tuition reimbursements, teaching assistantships with full tuition reimbursements, career-related internships or fieldwork, Federal Work-Study, traineeships, and unspecified assistantships available. Financial award application deadline: 2/1. *Unit head:* Dr. Barbara Broome, Dean, 330-672-3777, E-mail: bbroome1@kent.edu. *Application contact:* Dr. Wendy A. Umberger, Associate Dean for Graduate Programs/Professor, 330-672-8813, E-mail: wlewando@kent.edu.
Website: http://www.kent.edu/nursing/

La Salle University, School of Nursing and Health Sciences, Program in Nursing, Philadelphia, PA 19141-1199. Offers adult-gerontology primary care nurse practitioner (MSN, Certificate); adult health and illness clinical nurse specialist (MSN); adult-gerontology clinical nurse specialist (MSN, Certificate); clinical nurse leader (MSN);

family primary care nurse practitioner (MSN, Certificate); gerontology (Certificate); nurse anesthetist (MSN, Certificate); nursing (MSN, Certificate); nursing administration (MSN, Certificate); nursing education (Certificate); nursing practice (DNP); nursing service administration (MSN); public health nursing (MSN, Certificate); school nursing (Certificate); MSN/MBA; MSN/MPH. *Accreditation:* AANA/CANAEP. *Program availability:* Part-time, evening/weekend, 100% online. *Faculty:* 13 full-time (all women), 9 part-time/adjunct (8 women). *Students:* 368 part-time (56 women); includes 103 minority (62 Black or African American, non-Hispanic/Latino; 1 American Indian or Alaska Native, non-Hispanic/Latino; 26 Asian, non-Hispanic/Latino; 9 Hispanic/Latino; 5 Two or more races, non-Hispanic/Latino), 5 international. Average age 36. 98 applicants, 85% accepted, 53 enrolled. In 2015, 87 master's, 3 doctorates, 10 other advanced degrees awarded. *Degree requirements:* For doctorate, minimum of 1,000 hours of post baccalaureate clinical practice supervised by preceptors. *Entrance requirements:* For master's, GRE, MAT, or GMAT (for students with BSN GPA of less than 3.2), baccalaureate degree in nursing from an NLNAC- or CCNE-accredited program or an MSN Bridge program; Pennsylvania RN license; 2 letters of reference; resume; statement of philosophy articulating professional values and future educational goal; 1 year of work experience as a registered nurse; for doctorate, GRE (waived for applicants with MSN cumulative GPA of 3.7 or above), MSN from nationally-accredited program or master's degree, MBA or MHA from nationally-accredited program; resume or curriculum vitae; 2 letters of reference; interview; for Certificate, GRE, MAT, or GMAT (for students with BSN GPA of less than 3.2, baccalaureate degree in nursing from an NLNAC- or CCNE-accredited program or an MSN Bridge program; Pennsylvania RN license; 2 letters of reference; resume; statement of philosophy articulating professional values and future educational goal; 1 year of work experience as a registered nurse. Additional exam requirements/recommendations for international students: Required—TOEFL. *Application deadline:* For fall admission, 8/15 priority date for domestic students, 7/15 for international students; for spring admission, 12/15 priority date for domestic students, 11/15 for international students; for summer admission, 4/15 priority date for domestic students, 3/15 for international students. Applications are processed on a rolling basis. Application fee: $35. Electronic applications accepted. Application fee is waived when completed online. *Expenses:* $870 per credit hour (for MSN); $930 per credit hour (for DNP); $150 technology fee full-time, $75 part-time; $135 general university fee. *Financial support:* In 2015–16, 13 students received support. Scholarships/grants and traineeships available. Support available to part-time students. Financial award application deadline: 8/31; financial award applicants required to submit FAFSA. *Unit head:* Dr. Patricia M. Dillon, Director, 215-951-1322, Fax: 215-951-1896, E-mail: msnapn@lasalle.edu. *Application contact:* Alison McAnespey Target, Director, Graduate and Adult Enrollment, 215-951-1100, Fax: 215-951-1462, E-mail: reilly@lasalle.edu.
Website: http://www.lasalle.edu/nursing/program-options/

Liberty University, School of Nursing, Lynchburg, VA 24515. Offers family nurse practitioner (DNP); nurse educator (MSN); nursing administration (MSN). *Program availability:* Part-time, online learning. *Students:* 108 full-time (100 women), 508 part-time (454 women); includes 106 minority (84 Black or African American, non-Hispanic/Latino; 3 American Indian or Alaska Native, non-Hispanic/Latino; 8 Asian, non-Hispanic/Latino; 1 Hispanic/Latino; 10 Two or more races, non-Hispanic/Latino), 7 international. Average age 39. 577 applicants, 30% accepted, 119 enrolled. In 2015, 161 master's awarded. *Entrance requirements:* For master's, minimum cumulative undergraduate GPA of 3.0; for doctorate, minimum GPA of 3.25 in most current nursing program completed. Additional exam requirements/recommendations for international students: Recommended—TOEFL. *Application deadline:* Applications are processed on a rolling basis. Application fee: $50. Electronic applications accepted. *Unit head:* Dr. Deanna Britt, Dean, 434-582-2519, E-mail: dbritt@liberty.edu. *Application contact:* Jay Bridge, Director of Admissions, 800-424-9595, Fax: 800-628-7977, E-mail: gradadmissions@liberty.edu.

Lincoln Memorial University, Caylor School of Nursing, Harrogate, TN 37752-1901. Offers family nurse practitioner (MSN); nurse anesthesia (MSN); psychiatric mental health nurse practitioner (MSN). *Accreditation:* AANA/CANAEP; ACEN. *Program availability:* Part-time. *Entrance requirements:* For master's, GRE.

Long Island University–LIU Brooklyn, Harriet Rothkopf Heilbrunn School of Nursing, Brooklyn, NY 11201-8423. Offers adult nurse practitioner (MS, Advanced Certificate); family nurse practitioner (MS, Advanced Certificate); nurse educator (MS). *Accreditation:* AACN. *Program availability:* Part-time, evening/weekend, blended/hybrid learning. *Faculty:* 6 full-time (4 women), 5 part-time/adjunct (4 women). *Students:* 1 (woman) full-time, 215 part-time (192 women); includes 136 minority (89 Black or African American, non-Hispanic/Latino; 28 Asian, non-Hispanic/Latino; 13 Hispanic/Latino; 2 Native Hawaiian or other Pacific Islander, non-Hispanic/Latino; 4 Two or more races, non-Hispanic/Latino), 1 international. Average age 43. 167 applicants, 57% accepted, 63 enrolled. In 2015, 23 master's, 5 other advanced degrees awarded. *Entrance requirements:* For master's and Advanced Certificate, New York RN license, two letters of recommendation. Additional exam requirements/recommendations for international students: Required—TOEFL (minimum score 550 paper-based; 79 iBT), IELTS (minimum score 6.5). *Application deadline:* Applications are processed on a rolling basis. Application fee: $50. Electronic applications accepted. *Expenses:* $1,155 per credit tuition; $934 per term full-time fees; $442 per term part-time fees. *Financial support:* In 2015–16, 24 students received support. Scholarships/grants and unspecified assistantships available. Support available to part-time students. Financial award application deadline: 2/15; financial award applicants required to submit FAFSA. *Faculty research:* Cultural competency, high fidelity simulation to improve nursing assessment and increase patient safety, relationship of diabetes to stress, end of life care, geriatric issues, foreign nurse's adaptation to the United States. *Unit head:* Dr. Loretta Knapp, Interim Dean, 718-488-1508, Fax: 718-780-4019, E-mail: lori.knapp@liu.edu. *Application contact:* Richard Sunday, Dean of Admissions, 718-488-1011, Fax: 718-780-6110, E-mail: bkln-admissions@liu.edu.
Website: http://liu.edu/Brooklyn/Academics/Harriet-Rothkopf-Heilbrunn-School-of-Nursing

Long Island University–LIU Post, School of Health Professions and Nursing, Brookville, NY 11548-1300. Offers biomedical sciences (MS), including applied laboratory medicine, cancer biology, medical and molecular immunology, microbiology/infectious diseases; cardiovascular perfusion (MS); dietetic internship (Advanced Certificate); family nurse practitioner (MS); forensic social work (Advanced Certificate); nursing education (MS); social work (MSW). *Program availability:* Part-time, evening/weekend, blended/hybrid learning. *Faculty:* 16 full-time (14 women), 46 part-time/adjunct (33 women). *Students:* 190 full-time (139 women), 181 part-time (157 women); includes 141 minority (51 Black or African American, non-Hispanic/Latino; 46 Asian, non-Hispanic/Latino; 41 Hispanic/Latino; 3 Two or more races, non-Hispanic/Latino), 47 international. Average age 36. 422 applicants, 64% accepted, 141 enrolled. In 2015, 96 master's, 28 other advanced degrees awarded. *Degree requirements:* For master's, comprehensive exam (for some programs), thesis (for some programs). *Entrance requirements:* Additional exam requirements/recommendations for international students: Required—TOEFL, IELTS. *Application deadline:* Applications are processed on a rolling basis. Application fee: $50. Electronic applications accepted. *Expenses:* $1,155 per credit, $934 per term full-time university fee, $442 per term part-time

university fee. *Financial support:* In 2015–16, 6 research assistantships with partial tuition reimbursements were awarded; career-related internships or fieldwork, Federal Work-Study, institutionally sponsored loans, tuition waivers (partial), and unspecified assistantships also available. Support available to part-time students. Financial award application deadline: 2/15; financial award applicants required to submit FAFSA. *Faculty research:* Breast cancer, childhood obesity, dietary beverage consumption, emotional distress, histone modification, interprofessional practice, interstitial cystitis, lung cancer, pancreatic cancer, pediatric pain management, post-traumatic growth, poverty, renal nutrition, social ethics, yeast and bacterial drug resistance. *Total annual research expenditures:* $15,000. *Unit head:* Dr. Stacy Gropack, Acting Dean, 516-299-2486, Fax: 516-299-2527, E-mail: post-shpn@liu.edu. *Application contact:* Carol Zerah, Director of Graduate and International Admissions, 516-299-2900 Ext. 3952, Fax: 516-299-2137, E-mail: post-enroll@liu.edu.
Website: http://liu.edu/post/health

Louisiana State University Health Sciences Center, School of Nursing, New Orleans, LA 70112. Offers adult gerontology clinical nurse specialist (Post-Master's Certificate); clinical nurse leader (MSN); executive nurse leader (Post-Master's Certificate); neonatal nurse practitioner (Post-Master's Certificate); nurse anesthesia (Post-Master's Certificate); nurse educator (MSN); nursing (DNS); primary care family nurse practitioner (Post-Master's Certificate); public/community health nursing (Post-Master's Certificate). *Accreditation:* AACN; AANA/CANAEP (one or more programs are accredited). *Program availability:* Part-time. *Faculty:* 22 full-time (19 women), 21 part-time/adjunct (8 women). *Students:* 254 (185 women); includes 68 minority (44 Black or African American, non-Hispanic/Latino; 12 Asian, non-Hispanic/Latino; 12 Hispanic/Latino). Average age 33. 144 applicants, 54% accepted, 73 enrolled. In 2015, 84 master's, 6 doctorates awarded. *Degree requirements:* For master's, thesis optional; for doctorate, thesis/dissertation. *Entrance requirements:* For master's, GRE General Test, MAT, minimum GPA of 3.0; for doctorate, GRE General Test, minimum GPA of 3.5. Additional exam requirements/recommendations for international students: Required—TOEFL (minimum score 550 paper-based; 79 iBT). *Application deadline:* Applications are processed on a rolling basis. Application fee: $250. Electronic applications accepted. *Expenses:* $9,136.50 per year; $19,633.50 per year (for DNP). *Financial support:* Federal Work-Study, institutionally sponsored loans, scholarships/grants, and traineeships available. Financial award applicants required to submit FAFSA. *Faculty research:* Advanced clinical practice, nursing education, health, social support, nursing administration. *Unit head:* Dr. Demetrius James Porche, Dean, 504-568-4106, Fax: 504-599-0573, E-mail: dporch@lsuhsc.edu. *Application contact:* Tracie Gravolet, Director, Office of Student Affairs, 504-568-4114, Fax: 504-568-5711, E-mail: tgravo@lsuhsc.edu.
Website: http://nursing.lsuhsc.edu/

Loyola University Chicago, Graduate School, Marcella Niehoff School of Nursing, Maywood, IL 60153. Offers adult gerontology acute care clinical nurse specialist (MSN), including emergency care (MSN, Certificate); adult gerontology acute care nurse practitioner (MSN), including oncology (MSN, Certificate); adult gerontology clinical nurse specialist (MSN), including oncology (MSN, Certificate); adult gerontology nurse practitioner (Certificate), including oncology (MSN, Certificate); adult nurse practitioner (Certificate); dietetics (MS); family nurse practitioner (MSN, Certificate), including emergency care; informatics (MSN); leadership (DNP), including healthcare quality using education in safety and technology, infection prevention; nursing science (PhD); women's health nurse practitioner (MSN); women's health nursing (Certificate). *Accreditation:* AACN. *Program availability:* Part-time, blended/hybrid learning. *Faculty:* 27 full-time (25 women), 12 part-time/adjunct (10 women). *Students:* 174 full-time (161 women), 232 part-time (221 women); includes 95 minority (19 Black or African American, non-Hispanic/Latino; 2 American Indian or Alaska Native, non-Hispanic/Latino; 38 Asian, non-Hispanic/Latino; 28 Hispanic/Latino; 2 Native Hawaiian or other Pacific Islander, non-Hispanic/Latino; 6 Two or more races, non-Hispanic/Latino), 3 international. Average age 35. 209 applicants, 52% accepted, 83 enrolled. In 2015, 78 master's, 10 doctorates, 17 other advanced degrees awarded. *Degree requirements:* For master's, comprehensive exam; for doctorate, thesis/dissertation, qualifying examination (for PhD); capstone project (for DNP). *Entrance requirements:* For master's, BSN, minimum nursing GPA of 3.0, Illinois RN license, 3 letters of recommendation, 1000 hours of experience in area of specialty prior to starting clinical rotations, personal statement; for doctorate, GRE General Test (for PhD), BSN or MSN, minimum GPA of 3.0, professional nursing license, 3 letters of recommendation, personal statement. Additional exam requirements/recommendations for international students: Required—TOEFL (minimum score 550 paper-based; 79 iBT), IELTS (minimum score 6.5). *Application deadline:* For fall admission, 6/1 priority date for domestic and international students; for spring admission, 11/15 priority date for domestic and international students; for summer admission, 3/15 priority date for domestic and international students. Applications are processed on a rolling basis. Application fee: $50. Electronic applications accepted. Application fee is waived when completed online. *Expenses:* $1,081 per credit hour. *Financial support:* In 2015–16, 10 students received support, including 3 research assistantships with full tuition reimbursements available (averaging $18,000 per year), 1 teaching assistantship with full tuition reimbursement available (averaging $18,000 per year); scholarships/grants, unspecified assistantships, and nurse faculty loan program also available. Financial award applicants required to submit FAFSA. *Faculty research:* Epigenetics and social determinants of health, women's health, vitamin D, interprofessional education, prevention and self-management of chronic disease. *Total annual research expenditures:* $649,606. *Unit head:* Dr. Vicky Keough, Dean, 708-216-5448, Fax: 708-216-9555, E-mail: vkeough@luc.edu. *Application contact:* Toni Topalova, Enrollment Advisor, 708-216-3751, Fax: 708-216-9555, E-mail: atopalova@luc.edu.
Website: http://www.luc.edu/nursing/

Malone University, Graduate Program in Nursing, Canton, OH 44709. Offers family nurse practitioner (MSN). *Accreditation:* AACN. *Program availability:* Part-time, evening/weekend. *Degree requirements:* For master's, thesis. *Entrance requirements:* For master's, minimum GPA of 3.0 from BSN program, interview, Ohio RN license. Additional exam requirements/recommendations for international students: Required—TOEFL (minimum score 550 paper-based; 79 iBT). *Expenses:* Contact institution. *Faculty research:* Home heath care and geriatrics, community settings, culture, Hispanics, tuberculosis, geriatrics, Neuman Systems Model, nursing education.

Marquette University, Graduate School, College of Nursing, Milwaukee, WI 53201-1881. Offers acute care nurse practitioner (Certificate); adult clinical nurse specialist (Certificate); adult nurse practitioner (Certificate); advanced practice nursing (MSN, DNP), including adult-older adult acute care (DNP), adults (MSN), adults-older adults (DNP), clinical nurse leader (MSN), health care systems leadership (DNP), nurse-midwifery (MSN), older adults (MSN), pediatrics-acute care, pediatrics-primary care, primary care (DNP), systems leadership and healthcare quality (MSN); family nurse practitioner (Certificate); nurse-midwifery (Certificate); nursing (PhD); pediatric acute care (Certificate); pediatric primary care (Certificate); systems leadership and healthcare quality (Certificate). *Accreditation:* AACN. *Faculty:* 35 full-time (all women), 56 part-time/adjunct (55 women). *Students:* 123 full-time (112 women), 242 part-time (220 women); includes 34 minority (9 Black or African American, non-Hispanic/Latino; 12 Asian, non-Hispanic/Latino; 10 Hispanic/Latino; 3 Two or more races, non-Hispanic/Latino), 4

Family Nurse Practitioner Studies

international. Average age 30. 269 applicants, 61% accepted, 98 enrolled. In 2015, 84 master's, 5 doctorates, 22 other advanced degrees awarded. Terminal master's awarded for partial completion of doctoral program. *Degree requirements:* For master's, comprehensive exam, thesis or alternative. *Entrance requirements:* For master's, GRE General Test, BSN, Wisconsin RN license, official transcripts from all current and previous colleges/universities except Marquette, three completed recommendation forms, resume, written statement of professional goals; for doctorate, GRE General Test, official transcripts from all current and previous colleges/universities except Marquette, three letters of recommendation, resume, written statement of professional goals, sample of scholarly writing. Additional exam requirements/recommendations for international students: Required—TOEFL (minimum score 530 paper-based). *Application deadline:* For fall admission, 2/15 for domestic and international students. Electronic applications accepted. *Financial support:* In 2015–16, 41 students received support, including 1 fellowship with partial tuition reimbursement available (averaging $17,500 per year), 2 research assistantships with full tuition reimbursements available (averaging $13,285 per year), 8 teaching assistantships with full tuition reimbursements available (averaging $13,912 per year); career-related internships or fieldwork, Federal Work-Study, scholarships/grants, health care benefits, tuition waivers (partial), and unspecified assistantships also available. Support available to part-time students. Financial award application deadline: 2/15. *Faculty research:* Psychosocial adjustment to chronic illness, gerontology, reminiscence, health policy: uninsured and access, hospital care delivery systems. *Total annual research expenditures:* $480,591. *Unit head:* Dr. Donna McCarthy, Interim Chair, 414-288-3800, Fax: 414-288-1578. *Application contact:* Dr. Maureen O'Brien, Associate Dean/Clinical Associate Professor, 414-288-3823.

Marymount University, School of Health Professions, Program in Nursing, Arlington, VA 22207-4299. Offers family nurse practitioner (MSN, Certificate); nursing (DNP). *Accreditation:* AACN. *Program availability:* Part-time, evening/weekend. *Faculty:* 7 full-time (all women), 3 part-time/adjunct (2 women). *Students:* 12 full-time (11 women), 58 part-time (53 women); includes 25 minority (18 Black or African American, non-Hispanic/Latino; 4 Asian, non-Hispanic/Latino; 1 Hispanic/Latino; 1 Native Hawaiian or other Pacific Islander, non-Hispanic/Latino; 1 Two or more races, non-Hispanic/Latino), 1 international. Average age 36. 47 applicants, 57% accepted, 20 enrolled. In 2015, 19 master's, 1 doctorate awarded. *Degree requirements:* For master's, comprehensive exam; for doctorate, thesis/dissertation or alternative. *Entrance requirements:* For master's, 2 letters of recommendation, interview, resume, RN license, personal statement; for doctorate, 2 letters of recommendation, interview, resume, RN license, minimum MSN GPA of 3.5 or BSN 3.3; for Certificate, interview, master's degree in nursing. Additional exam requirements/recommendations for international students: Required—TOEFL (minimum score 600 paper-based; 96 iBT), IELTS (minimum score 6.5). *Application deadline:* For fall admission, 5/1 for domestic students, 7/1 for international students; for spring admission, 11/1 for domestic students, 9/16 for international students. Application fee: $40. Electronic applications accepted. *Expenses: Tuition, area resident:* Part-time $910 per credit hour. *One-time fee:* $230 part-time. Tuition and fees vary according to program. *Financial support:* In 2015–16, 15 students received support, including 4 teaching assistantships with partial tuition reimbursements available; career-related internships or fieldwork, Federal Work-Study, scholarships/grants, and unspecified assistantships also available. Support available to part-time students. Financial award applicants required to submit FAFSA. *Unit head:* Dr. Shelli Wolfe Mayer, Chair, 703-284-6886, Fax: 703-284-3819, E-mail: michelle.wolfe@marymount.edu. *Application contact:* Francesca Reed, Director, Graduate Admissions, 703-284-5901, Fax: 703-527-3815, E-mail: grad.admissions@marymount.edu.
Website: http://www.marymount.edu/Academics/Malek-School-of-Health-Professions/Graduate-Programs/Nursing-(M-S-N-)

Maryville University of Saint Louis, Walker College of Health Professions, The Catherine McAuley School of Nursing, St. Louis, MO 63141-7299. Offers acute care nurse practice (MSN); adult gerontology nurse practitioner (MSN); advanced practice nursing (DNP); family nurse practitioner (MSN); pediatric nurse practice (MSN). *Accreditation:* AACN. *Program availability:* 100% online. *Faculty:* 18 full-time (all women), 158 part-time/adjunct (141 women). *Students:* 38 full-time (35 women), 2,802 part-time (2,511 women); includes 681 minority (332 Black or African American, non-Hispanic/Latino; 40 American Indian or Alaska Native, non-Hispanic/Latino; 126 Asian, non-Hispanic/Latino; 126 Hispanic/Latino; 8 Native Hawaiian or other Pacific Islander, non-Hispanic/Latino; 49 Two or more races, non-Hispanic/Latino), 58 international. Average age 37. In 2015, 413 master's, 33 doctorates awarded. *Degree requirements:* For master's, practicum. *Entrance requirements:* For master's, BSN, current licensure, minimum GPA of 3.0, 3 letters of recommendation, curriculum vitae. Additional exam requirements/recommendations for international students: Required—TOEFL (minimum score 550 paper-based). *Application deadline:* Applications are processed on a rolling basis. Electronic applications accepted. Application fee is waived when completed online. *Expenses: Tuition, area resident:* Full-time $25,558; part-time $781 per credit hour. *Required fees:* $2400. Part-time tuition and fees vary according to course load and degree level. *Financial support:* Federal Work-Study and campus employment available. Support available to part-time students. Financial award application deadline: 3/1; financial award applicants required to submit FAFSA. *Unit head:* Dr. Elizabeth Buck, Director, 314-529-9453, Fax: 314-529-9139, E-mail: ebuck@maryville.edu. *Application contact:* Crystal Jacobsmeyer, Assistant Director, Graduate Enrollment Advising, 314-929-9654, Fax: 314-529-9927, E-mail: cjacobsmeyer@maryville.edu.
Website: http://www.maryville.edu/hp/nursing/

McGill University, Faculty of Graduate and Postdoctoral Studies, Faculty of Medicine, School of Nursing, Montréal, QC H3A 2T5, Canada. Offers nurse practitioner (Graduate Diploma); nursing (M Sc A, PhD). PhD offered jointly with Université du Québec à Montréal.

McMurry University, Graduate Studies, Abilene, TX 79697. Offers education (MSN); family nurse practitioner (MSN).

McNeese State University, Doré School of Graduate Studies, College of Nursing, Department of Graduate Nursing, Family Nurse Practitioner Program, Lake Charles, LA 70609. Offers PMC. *Degree requirements:* For PMC, thesis. *Entrance requirements:* For degree, GRE, MSN, eligible for unencumbered licensure as RN in Louisiana.

McNeese State University, Doré School of Graduate Studies, College of Nursing, Department of Graduate Nursing, Nursing Program, Lake Charles, LA 70609. Offers family nurse practitioner (MSN); family psychiatric/mental health nurse practitioner (MSN); nurse educator (MSN); nurse executive (MSN). *Degree requirements:* For master's, comprehensive exam. *Entrance requirements:* For master's, GRE, baccalaureate degree in nursing, minimum overall GPA of 2.7 for all undergraduate coursework, eligibility for unencumbered licensure as Registered Nurse in Louisiana or Texas, course in introductory statistics with minimum C grade, physical assessment skills, two letters of professional reference, 500-word essay, current resume.

Medical University of South Carolina, College of Nursing, Family Nurse Practitioner Program, Charleston, SC 29425. Offers MSN, DNP. *Program availability:* Part-time, online learning. *Degree requirement:* For master's, thesis optional; for doctorate, final project. *Entrance requirements:* For master's, BSN from nationally-accredited program,

minimum nursing and cumulative GPA of 3.0, undergraduate-level statistics course, active RN License, 3 confidential references, current curriculum vitae or resume, essay; for doctorate, BSN from nationally-accredited program, minimum nursing and cumulative GPA of 3.0, undergraduate-level statistics course, active RN License, 3 confidential references, current curriculum vitae or resume, personal essay (for DNP). Additional exam requirements/recommendations for international students: Required—TOEFL (minimum score 550 paper-based; 80 iBT). Electronic applications accepted. *Faculty research:* Primary care, smoking cessation, patient navigation, informatics, depression.

Middle Tennessee State University, College of Graduate Studies, College of Behavioral and Health Sciences, School of Nursing, Program in Family Nurse Practitioner, Murfreesboro, TN 37132. Offers MSN, Graduate Certificate. *Program availability:* Part-time, evening/weekend, online learning. *Entrance requirements:* Additional exam requirements/recommendations for international students: Required—TOEFL (minimum score 525 paper-based; 71 iBT) or IELTS (minimum score 6). Electronic applications accepted.

Midwestern State University, Billie Doris McAda Graduate School, Robert D. and Carol Gunn College of Health Sciences and Human Services, Wilson School of Nursing, Wichita Falls, TX 76308. Offers family nurse practitioner (MSN); family psychiatric mental health nurse practitioner (MSN); nurse educator (MSN). *Accreditation:* AACN. *Program availability:* Part-time, evening/weekend. *Degree requirements:* For master's, comprehensive exam, thesis optional. *Entrance requirements:* For master's, GRE General Test or MAT. Additional exam requirements/recommendations for international students: Required—TOEFL (minimum score 550 paper-based). Electronic applications accepted. *Faculty research:* Infant feeding, musculoskeletal disorders, diabetes, community health education, water quality reporting.

Millersville University of Pennsylvania, College of Graduate Studies and Adult Learning, College of Science and Technology, Department of Nursing, Program in Family Nurse Practitioner, Millersville, PA 17551-0302. Offers MSN. *Program availability:* Part-time, evening/weekend. *Faculty:* 6 full-time (all women), 4 part-time/adjunct (all women). *Students:* 70 part-time (61 women); includes 8 minority (1 Black or African American, non-Hispanic/Latino; 3 Asian, non-Hispanic/Latino; 3 Hispanic/Latino; 1 Native Hawaiian or other Pacific Islander, non-Hispanic/Latino), 2 international. 48 applicants, 54% accepted, 26 enrolled. In 2015, 22 master's awarded. *Degree requirements:* For master's, internship, scholarly project. *Entrance requirements:* For master's, resume, copy of RN license, minimum GPA of 3.0, all transfer transcripts, interview. Additional exam requirements/recommendations for international students: Required—TOEFL (minimum score 600 paper-based), IELTS (minimum score 6). *Application deadline:* For fall admission, 1/15 for domestic and international students. Applications are processed on a rolling basis. Application fee: $40. Electronic applications accepted. *Expenses:* Tuition, state resident: full-time $8460; part-time $470 per credit. Tuition, nonresident: full-time $12,690; part-time $705 per credit. *Required fees:* $2471; $133.75 per credit. Tuition and fees vary according to course load, degree level and program. *Financial support:* Application deadline: 3/15; applicants required to submit FAFSA. *Faculty research:* Family nurse practitioner, primary care, health promotion, disease prevention. *Unit head:* Dr. Jenny Monn, Coordinator, 717-871-7454, E-mail: jenny.monn@millersville.edu. *Application contact:* Dr. Victor S. DeSantis, Dean of College of Graduate Studies and Adult Learning/Associate Provost for Civic and Community Engagement, 717-871-7619, Fax: 717-871-7954, E-mail: victor.desantis@millersville.edu.
Website: http://www.millersville.edu/nursing/msn/nurse-practitioner.php

Minnesota State University Mankato, College of Graduate Studies and Research, College of Allied Health and Nursing, School of Nursing, Mankato, MN 56001. Offers family nursing (MSN), including family nurse practitioner; nursing (DNP). MSN offered jointly with Metropolitan State University; DNP with Metropolitan State University, Minnesota State University Moorhead, Winona State University. *Accreditation:* AACN. *Degree requirements:* For master's, comprehensive exam, internships, research project or thesis; for doctorate, capstone project. *Entrance requirements:* For master's, GRE General Test or on-campus essay, minimum GPA of 3.0 during previous 2 years, BSN or equivalent references; for doctorate, master's degree in nursing. Additional exam requirements/recommendations for international students: Required—TOEFL. Electronic applications accepted. *Faculty research:* Psychosocial nursing, computers in nursing, family adaptation.

Missouri State University, Graduate College, College of Health and Human Services, Department of Nursing, Springfield, MO 65897. Offers nursing (MSN), including family nurse practitioner, nurse educator; nursing (DNP). *Accreditation:* AACN. *Program availability:* 100% online, blended/hybrid learning. *Faculty:* 9 full-time (all women), 16 part-time/adjunct (13 women). *Students:* 27 full-time (23 women), 23 part-time (all women); includes 8 minority (3 Black or African American, non-Hispanic/Latino; 1 American Indian or Alaska Native, non-Hispanic/Latino; 2 Asian, non-Hispanic/Latino; 2 Two or more races, non-Hispanic/Latino). Average age 35. 13 applicants, 46% accepted, 1 enrolled. In 2015, 1 master's, 1 doctorate awarded. *Degree requirements:* For master's, comprehensive exam, thesis or alternative. *Entrance requirements:* For master's, GRE General Test, minimum GPA of 3.0, RN license (for MSN), 1 year of work experience (for MPH). Additional exam requirements/recommendations for international students: Required—TOEFL (minimum score 550 paper-based; 79 iBT), IELTS (minimum score 6). *Application deadline:* For fall admission, 12/1 priority date for domestic students, 5/1 for international students. Applications are processed on a rolling basis. Application fee: $35 ($50 for international students). Electronic applications accepted. *Expenses:* Tuition, state resident: full-time $5500. Tuition, nonresident: full-time $10,108. *Required fees:* $1000. *Financial support:* In 2015–16, 2 teaching assistantships with partial tuition reimbursements (averaging $8,600 per year) were awarded; Federal Work-Study, institutionally sponsored loans, scholarships/grants, and unspecified assistantships also available. Financial award application deadline: 3/31; financial award applicants required to submit FAFSA. *Faculty research:* Preconceptual health, women's health, nursing satisfaction, nursing education. *Unit head:* Dr. Kathryn Hope, Head, 417-836-5310, Fax: 417-836-5484, E-mail: nursing@missouristate.edu. *Application contact:* Michael Edwards, Coordinator of Graduate Admissions, 417-836-5330, Fax: 417-836-6200, E-mail: michaeledwards@missouristate.edu.
Website: http://www.missouristate.edu/nursing/

Molloy College, Division of Nursing, Rockville Centre, NY 11571-5002. Offers adult-gerontology primary care nurse practitioner (MS); clinical nurse specialist (MS), including adult-gerontology health; clinical nurse specialist: adult-gerontology (Advanced Certificate), including adult-gerontology; family nurse practitioner (MS, Advanced Certificate), including primary care; family psychiatric mental health nurse practitioner (MS); nursing (DNP, PhD); nursing administration (MS), including informatics; nursing education (MS); pediatric nurse practitioner (MS), including primary care (MS, Advanced Certificate). *Accreditation:* AACN. *Program availability:* Part-time, evening/weekend. *Faculty:* 26 full-time (all women), 12 part-time/adjunct (9 women). *Students:* 13 full-time (all women), 550 part-time (515 women); includes 316 minority (169 Black or African American, non-Hispanic/Latino; 1 American Indian or Alaska Native, non-Hispanic/Latino; 88 Asian, non-Hispanic/Latino; 56 Hispanic/Latino; 2 Native Hawaiian or other Pacific Islander, non-Hispanic/Latino). Average age 43. 208 applicants, 69% accepted,

121 enrolled. In 2015, 116 master's, 1 doctorate, 6 other advanced degrees awarded. *Degree requirements:* For master's, thesis optional. *Entrance requirements:* For master's, 3 letters of reference, BS in nursing, minimum undergraduate GPA of 3.0; for Advanced Certificate, 3 letters of reference, master's degree in nursing. Additional exam requirements/recommendations for international students: Required—TOEFL (minimum score 550 paper-based; 79 iBT). *Application deadline:* For fall admission, 9/2 priority date for domestic students; for spring admission, 1/20 priority date for domestic students. Applications are processed on a rolling basis. Application fee: $60. Electronic applications accepted. *Expenses: Tuition, area resident:* Full-time $18,450; part-time $1025 per credit. *Required fees:* $900; $740 per unit. Tuition and fees vary according to course load. *Financial support:* Research assistantships with partial tuition reimbursements, teaching assistantships with partial tuition reimbursements, institutionally sponsored loans, scholarships/grants, and unspecified assistantships available. Support available to part-time students. Financial award application deadline: 4/1; financial award applicants required to submit FAFSA. *Unit head:* Dr. Jeannine Muldoon, Dean of Nursing, 516-323-3651, E-mail: jmuldoon@molloy.edu. *Application contact:* Jaclyn Machowicz, Assistant Director for Admissions, 516-323-4010, E-mail: jmachowicz@molloy.edu.

Monmouth University, Graduate Studies, The Marjorie K. Unterberg School of Nursing and Health Studies, West Long Branch, NJ 07764-1898. Offers adult and gerontological primary care nurse practitioner (MSN); adult-gerontological primary care nurse practitioner (Post-Master's Certificate); family nurse practitioner (MSN, Post-Master's Certificate); family psychiatric and mental health advanced practice nursing (MSN); family psychiatric and mental health nurse practitioner (Post-Master's Certificate); forensic nursing (MSN, Certificate); nursing (MSN); nursing administration (MSN, Post-Master's Certificate); nursing education (MSN, Post-Master's Certificate); nursing practice (DNP); physician assistant (MS); school nursing (MSN, Certificate). *Accreditation:* AACN. *Program availability:* Part-time, evening/weekend, 100% online, blended/hybrid learning. *Faculty:* 14 full-time (13 women), 10 part-time/adjunct (5 women). *Students:* 58 full-time (46 women), 271 part-time (252 women); includes 93 minority (31 Black or African American, non-Hispanic/Latino; 40 Asian, non-Hispanic/Latino; 18 Hispanic/Latino; 1 Native Hawaiian or other Pacific Islander, non-Hispanic/Latino; 3 Two or more races, non-Hispanic/Latino), 1 international. Average age 37. 450 applicants, 32% accepted, 103 enrolled. In 2015, 68 master's, 8 doctorates, 11 other advanced degrees awarded. *Degree requirements:* For master's, practicum (for some tracks); for doctorate, practicum, capstone course. *Entrance requirements:* For master's, GRE General Test (waived for MSN applicants with minimum B grade in each of the first four courses and for MS applicants with master's degree), BSN with minimum GPA of 2.75, current RN license, proof of liability and malpractice policy, personal statement, two letters of recommendation, college course work in health assessment, resume; CASPA application (for MS); for doctorate, accredited master's nursing program degree with minimum GPA of 3.2, graduate research course in statistics, active RN license, national certification as Nurse Practitioner or Nurse Administrator, working knowledge of statistics, statement of goals and vision for change, 2 letters of recommendation (professional or academic), resume, interview. Additional exam requirements/recommendations for international students: Required—TOEFL (minimum score 550 paper-based; 79 iBT), IELTS (minimum score 6) or Michigan English Language Assessment Battery (minimum score 77). *Application deadline:* For fall admission, 7/15 priority date for domestic students, 6/1 for international students; for spring admission, 12/15 priority date for domestic students, 11/1 for international students; for summer admission, 5/1 for domestic students. Applications are processed on a rolling basis. Application fee: $50. Electronic applications accepted. *Expenses:* Contact institution. *Financial support:* In 2015–16, 241 students received support, including 220 fellowships (averaging $3,403 per year), 5 research assistantships (averaging $5,146 per year); career-related internships or fieldwork, scholarships/grants, and unspecified assistantships also available. Support available to part-time students. Financial award applicants required to submit FAFSA. *Faculty research:* School nursing, health policy, and smoking cessation in teens, Multiple Sclerosis; adherence and self-efficacy, aging issues and geriatric care. *Unit head:* Dr. Janet Mahoney, Dean, 732-571-3443, Fax: 732-263-5131, E-mail: jmahoney@monmouth.edu. *Application contact:* Lucia Fedele, Graduate Admission Counselor, 732-571-3452, Fax: 732-263-5123, E-mail: gradadm@monmouth.edu.
Website: http://www.monmouth.edu/school-of-nursing-health/graduate-nursing-programs.aspx

Montana State University, The Graduate School, College of Nursing, Bozeman, MT 59717. Offers clinical nurse leader (MN); family and individual nurse practitioner (DNP); family nurse practitioner (MN, Post-Master's Certificate); nursing education (Certificate, Post-Master's Certificate); psychiatric mental health nurse practitioner (DNP). *Accreditation:* AACN. *Program availability:* Part-time, online learning. *Degree requirements:* For master's, comprehensive exam, thesis (for some programs); for doctorate, thesis/dissertation, 1,125 hours in clinical settings. *Entrance requirements:* For master's, GRE General Test, minimum GPA of 3.0 for undergraduate and post-baccalaureate work. Additional exam requirements/recommendations for international students: Required—TOEFL (minimum score 580 paper-based). Electronic applications accepted. *Faculty research:* Rural nursing, health disparities, environmental/public health, oral health, resilience.

Mount Carmel College of Nursing, Nursing Program, Columbus, OH 43222. Offers adult gerontology acute care nurse practitioner (MS); adult health clinical nurse specialist (MS); family nurse practitioner (MS); nursing (DNP); nursing administration (MS); nursing education (MS). *Accreditation:* AACN. *Program availability:* Part-time. *Faculty:* 8 full-time (all women), 5 part-time/adjunct (4 women). *Students:* 72 full-time (63 women), 92 part-time (84 women); includes 15 minority (7 Black or African American, non-Hispanic/Latino; 3 Asian, non-Hispanic/Latino; 2 Hispanic/Latino; 3 Two or more races, non-Hispanic/Latino). Average age 37. 140 applicants, 45% accepted, 50 enrolled. In 2015, 50 master's awarded. *Degree requirements:* For master's, professional manuscript; for doctorate, practicum. *Entrance requirements:* For master's, letters of recommendation, statement of purpose, current resume, baccalaureate degree in nursing, current Ohio RN license, minimum cumulative GPA of 3.0; for doctorate, master's degree in nursing from program accredited by either NLNAC/ACEN or CCNE. Additional exam requirements/recommendations for international students: Required—TOEFL (minimum score 550 paper-based; 80 iBT). *Application deadline:* For fall admission, 6/1 priority date for domestic students; for winter admission, 11/1 for domestic students; for spring admission, 10/1 priority date for domestic students; for summer admission, 3/1 for domestic students. Applications are processed on a rolling basis. Application fee: $30. *Expenses: Tuition, area resident:* Full-time $9480; part-time $474 per credit. One-time fee: $120. Tuition and fees vary according to course load, degree level and program. *Financial support:* In 2015–16, 5 students received support. Institutionally sponsored loans and scholarships/grants available. Financial award applicants required to submit FAFSA. *Unit head:* Dr. Jill Kilanowski, 614-234-5237, Fax: 614-234-2875, E-mail: jkilanowski@mccn.edu. *Application contact:* Dr. Kim Campbell, Director of Recruitment and Admissions, 614-234-5144, Fax: 614-234-5427, E-mail: kcampbell@mccn.edu.
Website: http://www.mccn.edu/

Mount Saint Mary College, School of Nursing, Newburgh, NY 12550-3494. Offers adult nurse practitioner (MS, Advanced Certificate), including nursing education (MS), nursing management (MS); clinical nurse specialist-adult health (MS), including nursing education, nursing management; family nurse practitioner (Advanced Certificate). *Accreditation:* AACN. *Program availability:* Part-time, evening/weekend, blended/hybrid learning. *Faculty:* 6 full-time (all women), 1 (woman) part-time/adjunct. *Students:* 5 full-time (4 women), 117 part-time (105 women); includes 42 minority (18 Black or African American, non-Hispanic/Latino; 2 American Indian or Alaska Native, non-Hispanic/Latino; 8 Asian, non-Hispanic/Latino; 12 Hispanic/Latino; 2 Native Hawaiian or other Pacific Islander, non-Hispanic/Latino). Average age 38. 44 applicants, 84% accepted, 25 enrolled. In 2015, 25 master's, 4 other advanced degrees awarded. *Degree requirements:* For master's, research utilization project. *Entrance requirements:* For master's, BSN, minimum GPA of 3.0, RN license. Additional exam requirements/recommendations for international students: Required—TOEFL (minimum score 80 iBT). *Application deadline:* For fall admission, 6/3 priority date for domestic students; for spring admission, 10/31 priority date for domestic students. Applications are processed on a rolling basis. Application fee: $45. Electronic applications accepted. Application fee is waived when completed online. *Expenses: Tuition, area resident:* Part-time $750 per credit. *Required fees:* $40 per semester. *Financial support:* In 2015–16, 14 students received support. Unspecified assistantships available. Financial award application deadline: 4/15; financial award applicants required to submit FAFSA. *Unit head:* Christine Berte, Graduate Coordinator, 845-569-3141, Fax: 845-562-6762, E-mail: christine.berte@msmc.edu. *Application contact:* Lisa Gallina, Director of Admissions for Graduate Programs and Adult Degree Completion, 845-569-3166, Fax: 845-569-3450, E-mail: lisa.gallina@msmc.edu.
Website: http://www.msmc.edu/Academics/Graduate_Programs/Master_of_Science_in_Nursing

Murray State University, College of Health Sciences and Human Services, Program in Nursing, Murray, KY 42071. Offers clinical nurse specialist (MSN); family nurse practitioner (MSN); nurse anesthesia (MSN). *Accreditation:* AACN; AANA/CANAEP. *Degree requirements:* For master's, research project. *Entrance requirements:* For master's, GRE General Test, BSN, interview, RN licensure. Additional exam requirements/recommendations for international students: Required—TOEFL (minimum score 550 paper-based). *Faculty research:* Fibromyalgis, primary care, rural health.

New Mexico State University, College of Health and Social Services, School of Nursing, Las Cruces, NM 88003. Offers adult/geriatric nursing (DNP); family nurse practitioner (DNP); family/psychiatric mental health nursing (DNP); nursing administration (MSN); nursing science (PhD); public/community health nursing (DNP). *Accreditation:* AACN. *Program availability:* Blended/hybrid learning. *Faculty:* 16 full-time (15 women). *Students:* 24 full-time (18 women), 90 part-time (80 women); includes 49 minority (10 Black or African American, non-Hispanic/Latino; 1 American Indian or Alaska Native, non-Hispanic/Latino; 4 Asian, non-Hispanic/Latino; 32 Hispanic/Latino; 2 Two or more races, non-Hispanic/Latino), 1 international. Average age 43. 40 applicants, 58% accepted, 17 enrolled. In 2015, 6 master's, 11 doctorates awarded. *Degree requirements:* For master's, comprehensive exam, thesis optional, clinical practice; for doctorate, comprehensive exam, thesis/dissertation. *Entrance requirements:* For master's, NCLEX, BSN, minimum GPA of 3.0, course work in statistics, 3 letters of reference, writing sample, RN license, CPR certification, proof of liability, immunizations, criminal background check; for doctorate, NCLEX, MSN, minimum GPA of 3.0, 3 letters of reference, writing sample, RN license, CPR certification, proof of liability, immunizations, criminal background check, statistics course. Additional exam requirements/recommendations for international students: Required—TOEFL (minimum score 550 paper-based; 79 iBT), IELTS (minimum score 6.5). *Application deadline:* For fall admission, 1/15 for domestic students; for spring admission, 1/15 priority date for domestic students; for summer admission, 1/15 for domestic students. Application fee: $40 ($50 for international students). Electronic applications accepted. *Expenses:* $274.50 per credit hour for in-state students, and all students enrolled in six or fewer credits; $839.30 per credit hour for out-of-state and international students enrolled in at least seven hours. *Financial support:* In 2015–16, 23 students received support, including 1 teaching assistantship (averaging $9,473 per year); career-related internships or fieldwork, Federal Work-Study, scholarships/grants, traineeships, health care benefits, and unspecified assistantships also available. Support available to part-time students. Financial award application deadline: 3/1. *Faculty research:* Women's health, community health, health disparities, nursing informatics and health care technologies, health care and nursing administration. *Total annual research expenditures:* $127,778. *Unit head:* Dr. Kathleen Huttlinger, Department Head, 575-646-3812, Fax: 575-646-2167, E-mail: khuttlin@nmsu.edu. *Application contact:* Dr. Teresa Keller, Director of Graduate Studies, 575-646-4370, Fax: 575-646-2167, E-mail: tkeller@nmsu.edu.
Website: http://schoolofnursing.nmsu.edu

New York University, Rory Meyers College of Nursing, Doctor of Nursing Practice Program, New York, NY 10012-1019. Offers nursing (DNP), including adult acute care, adult primary care, family, mental health nursing, nurse-midwifery, pediatrics. *Program availability:* Part-time, evening/weekend. *Faculty:* 14 full-time (13 women). *Students:* 2 full-time (both women), 32 part-time (27 women); includes 8 minority (3 Black or African American, non-Hispanic/Latino; 4 Asian, non-Hispanic/Latino; 1 Hispanic/Latino), 1 international. Average age 40. 47 applicants, 51% accepted, 16 enrolled. In 2015, 17 doctorates awarded. *Degree requirements:* For doctorate, thesis/dissertation, project. *Entrance requirements:* For doctorate, MAT or GRE (either taken within past 5 years), MS, RN license, interview, Nurse Practitioner Certification, writing sample. Additional exam requirements/recommendations for international students: Required—TOEFL (minimum score 90 iBT), IELTS (minimum score 7). *Application deadline:* For fall admission, 3/1 for domestic and international students. Applications are processed on a rolling basis. Application fee: $80. Electronic applications accepted. *Expenses:* Contact institution. *Financial support:* In 2015–16, 12 students received support. Scholarships/grants available. Support available to part-time students. Financial award application deadline: 2/1; financial award applicants required to submit FAFSA. *Faculty research:* Workforce, LGBT, breast cancer, HIV. *Unit head:* Dr. Rona Levin, Director, 212-998-5319, Fax: 212-995-3143, E-mail: rfl2039@nyu.edu. *Application contact:* Samantha Jaser, Assistant Director, Graduate Student Affairs and Admissions, 212-992-7653, Fax: 212-995-4302, E-mail: saj283@nyu.edu.

New York University, Rory Meyers College of Nursing, Programs in Advanced Practice Nursing, New York, NY 10012-1019. Offers adult-gerontology acute care nurse practitioner (MS, Advanced Certificate); adult-gerontology primary care nurse practitioner (MS, Advanced Certificate); family nurse practitioner (MS, Advanced Certificate); gerontology nurse practitioner (Advanced Certificate); nurse-midwifery (MS, Advanced Certificate); nursing administration (MS, Advanced Certificate); nursing education (MS, Advanced Certificate); nursing informatics (MS, Advanced Certificate); pediatrics nurse practitioner (MS, Advanced Certificate); psychiatric-mental health nurse practitioner (MS, Advanced Certificate); MS/MPH. *Accreditation:* AACN; ACNM/ACME. *Program availability:* Part-time. *Faculty:* 24 full-time (all women), 76 part-time/adjunct (65 women). *Students:* 46 full-time (26 women), 586 part-time (513 women); includes 242 minority (68 Black or African American, non-Hispanic/Latino; 3 American Indian or Alaska Native, non-Hispanic/Latino; 117 Asian, non-Hispanic/Latino; 38 Hispanic/Latino;

Family Nurse Practitioner Studies

3 Native Hawaiian or other Pacific Islander, non-Hispanic/Latino; 13 Two or more races, non-Hispanic/Latino; 23 international. Average age 32. 402 applicants, 69% accepted, 138 enrolled. In 2015, 198 master's, 5 other advanced degrees awarded. *Degree requirements:* For master's, thesis (for some programs). *Entrance requirements:* For master's, BS in nursing, AS in nursing with another BS/BA, interview, RN license, 1 year of clinical experience (3 for the MS in nursing education program); for Advanced Certificate, master's degree. Additional exam requirements/recommendations for international students: Required—TOEFL (minimum score 90 iBT), IELTS (minimum score 7). *Application deadline:* For fall admission, 6/15 for domestic and international students; for spring admission, 12/1 for domestic and international students; for summer admission, 3/1 for domestic and international students. Application fee: $80. Electronic applications accepted. *Expenses:* Contact institution. *Financial support:* In 2015–16, 101 students received support. Career-related internships or fieldwork, Federal Work-Study, and scholarships/grants available. Support available to part-time students. Financial award application deadline: 3/1; financial award applicants required to submit FAFSA. *Faculty research:* Geriatrics, HIV, families and illness, oral systemic connection, symptom management. *Unit head:* Dr. James Pace, Senior Associate Dean for Academic Programs, 212-992-7343, E-mail: james.pace@nyu.edu. *Application contact:* Samantha Jaser, Assistant Director, Graduate Student Affairs and Admissions, 212-992-7653, Fax: 212-995-4302, E-mail: saj283@nyu.edu.

Nicholls State University, Graduate Studies, College of Nursing and Allied Health, Thibodaux, LA 70310. Offers family nurse practitioner (MSN); nurse executive (MSN); nursing education (MSN); psychiatric/mental health nurse practitioner (MSN). Website: http://www.nicholls.edu/cona/

Northeastern University, Bouvé College of Health Sciences, Boston, MA 02115-5096. Offers applied behavior analysis (MS, CAGS); audiology (Au D); biomedical nanotechnology (MS); college student development and counseling (MS, CAGS); counseling psychology (MS, PhD, CAGS); exercise science (MS); health informatics (MS); medicinal chemistry (MS); nurse anesthesia (DNP, CAGS); nursing (MS, PhD, CAGS, including administration (MS), adult-gerontology acute care nurse practitioner (MS, CAGS), adult-gerontology primary care nurse practitioner (MS, CAGS), anesthesia (MS), family nurse practitioner (MS, CAGS), neonatal nurse practitioner (MS, CAGS), pediatric nurse practitioner (MS, CAGS), psychiatric mental health nurse practitioner (MS, CAGS); nursing practice (DNP); personal health informatics (PhD); pharmaceutical sciences (MS, PhD), including interdisciplinary concentration, pharmaceutics and drug delivery systems; pharmacology (MS); pharmacy (Pharm D); physical therapy (Postbaccalaureate Certificate); physician assistant (MS); population health (PhD); school psychology (MS, PhD, CAGS); speech-language pathology (MS); urban health (MPH); MS/MBA. *Accreditation:* ACPE (one or more programs are accredited). *Program availability:* Part-time, evening/weekend, online learning. *Faculty:* 194 full-time (120 women), 169 part-time/adjunct (136 women). *Students:* 1,416 full-time (1,049 women), 310 part-time (248 women). In 2015, 374 master's, 313 doctorates, 37 other advanced degrees awarded. *Degree requirements:* For doctorate, thesis/dissertation (for some programs); for other advanced degree, comprehensive exam. Application fee: $75. Electronic applications accepted. *Expenses:* Contact institution. *Financial support:* Applicants required to submit FAFSA. *Unit head:* John R. Reynolds, Professor and Interim Dean, 617-373-3323, Fax: 617-373-3030. *Application contact:* Molly Schnabel, Senior Director of Graduate Affairs, 617-373-2708, Fax: 617-373-4701, E-mail: bouvegrad@neu.edu.
Website: http://www.northeastern.edu/bouve/

Northern Arizona University, Graduate College, College of Health and Human Services, School of Nursing, Flagstaff, AZ 86011. Offers family nurse practitioner (MSN, Certificate); nurse generalist (MSN); nursing practice (DNP). *Accreditation:* AACN. *Program availability:* Part-time. *Degree requirements:* For master's, thesis (for some programs), project or thesis. *Entrance requirements:* For master's, GRE General Test or minimum GPA of 3.0, undergraduate statistics or health assessment with minimum grade of B in last 5 years or 3 years of RN experience (for nursing education). Additional exam requirements/recommendations for international students: Required—TOEFL (minimum score 550 paper-based; 80 iBT), IELTS (minimum score 7). *Application deadline:* For fall admission, 1/15 priority date for domestic and international students. Applications are processed on a rolling basis. Application fee: $65. Electronic applications accepted. *Expenses: Tuition, area resident:* Full-time $8710. Tuition, nonresident: full-time $20,350. *Required fees:* $896. *Financial support:* Career-related internships or fieldwork, Federal Work-Study, scholarships/grants, traineeships, health care benefits, tuition waivers, and unspecified assistantships available. Financial award applicants required to submit FAFSA. *Unit head:* Dr. Debera Thomas, Dean, 928-523-2656, Fax: 928-523-7171, E-mail: debera.thomas@nau.edu. *Application contact:* Penny Walior, Student Academic Specialist, 928-523-6770, Fax: 928-523-9155, E-mail: graduatenursing@nau.edu.
Website: http://nau.edu/CHHS/Nursing/

Northern Michigan University, Office of Graduate Education and Research, College of Health Sciences and Professional Studies, School of Nursing, Marquette, MI 49855-5301. Offers MSN, DNP. *Accreditation:* AACN. *Program availability:* Part-time, online learning. *Entrance requirements:* For doctorate, Michigan RN license; minimum undergraduate GPA of 3.0; 3 letters of recommendation; written personal goal statement. Additional exam requirements/recommendations for international students: Required—TOEFL (minimum score 550 paper-based; 79 iBT), IELTS (minimum score 6.5). Electronic applications accepted. *Faculty research:* Grief experiences in Alzheimer's caregivers, nursing students attitudes towards the elderly, using Facebook as a means of simulation and educational means for pediatric undergraduate nursing students, use of a nurse practitioner student educational intervention to reduce sugar sweetened beverage consumption in rural adolescents.

Oakland University, Graduate Study and Lifelong Learning, School of Nursing, Program in Family Nurse Practitioner, Rochester, MI 48309-4401. Offers family nurse practitioner (MSN, PMC). *Accreditation:* AACN. *Students:* 54 full-time (49 women), 28 part-time (25 women); includes 8 minority (4 Black or African American, non-Hispanic/Latino; 2 Asian, non-Hispanic/Latino; 1 Hispanic/Latino; 1 Two or more races, non-Hispanic/Latino), 1 international. Average age 33. 163 applicants, 21% accepted, 30 enrolled. In 2015, 44 master's, 1 other advanced degree awarded. *Degree requirements:* For master's, thesis. *Entrance requirements:* For master's, GRE General Test, minimum GPA of 3.0. Additional exam requirements/recommendations for international students: Required—TOEFL (minimum score 550 paper-based). *Application deadline:* For fall admission, 8/1 for domestic students, 5/1 priority date for international students; for winter admission, 11/15 for domestic students, 9/1 priority date for international students. Applications are processed on a rolling basis. Application fee: $0. Electronic applications accepted. *Expenses:* Contact institution. *Financial support:* Federal Work-Study, institutionally sponsored loans, and tuition waivers (full) available. Financial award application deadline: 3/1; financial award applicants required to submit FAFSA. *Unit head:* Dr. Colleen Meade Ripper, Interim Director of the Nurse Practitioner Program, 248-364-8724, E-mail: cmripper@oakland.edu.

Ohio University, Graduate College, College of Health Sciences and Professions, School of Nursing, Athens, OH 45701-2979. Offers acute care nurse practitioner (MSN); acute care nurse practitioner and family nurse practitioner (MSN); acute care nurse

practitioner and nurse administrator (MSN); acute care nurse practitioner and nurse educator (MSN); family nurse practitioner (MSN); nurse administrator (MSN); nurse administrator and family nurse practitioner (MSN); nurse educator (MSN); nurse educator and family nurse practitioner (MSN); nurse educator and nurse administrator (MSN). *Accreditation:* AACN. *Degree requirements:* For master's, capstone project. *Entrance requirements:* For master's, GRE, bachelor's degree in nursing from an accredited college or university, minimum overall undergraduate GPA of 3.0, official transcripts, statement of goals and objectives, resume, 3 letters of recommendation. Additional exam requirements/recommendations for international students: Required—TOEFL (minimum score 550 paper-based; 80 iBT) or IELTS (minimum score 6.5). Electronic applications accepted.

Old Dominion University, College of Health Sciences, Doctor of Nursing Practice Program, Norfolk, VA 23529. Offers advance practice (DNP); nurse executive (DNP). *Program availability:* Part-time, blended/hybrid learning. *Faculty:* 4 full-time (all women), 3 part-time/adjunct (2 women). *Students:* 19 full-time (18 women), 42 part-time (38 women); includes 9 minority (5 Black or African American, non-Hispanic/Latino; 2 Asian, non-Hispanic/Latino; 2 Two or more races, non-Hispanic/Latino). Average age 46. 55 applicants, 67% accepted, 36 enrolled. In 2015, 27 doctorates awarded. Terminal master's awarded for partial completion of doctoral program. *Degree requirements:* For doctorate, thesis/dissertation, capstone project. *Entrance requirements:* For doctorate, 3 letters of recommendation, essay, resume, transcripts. Additional exam requirements/ recommendations for international students: Required—TOEFL. *Application deadline:* For spring admission, 9/15 priority date for domestic students, 4/15 priority date for international students. Applications are processed on a rolling basis. Application fee: $50. Electronic applications accepted. *Expenses:* Tuition, state resident: full-time $11,136; part-time $464 per credit hour. Tuition, nonresident: full-time $27,840; part-time $1160 per credit hour. *Required fees:* $64 per semester. Tuition and fees vary according to campus/location, program and reciprocity agreements. *Financial support:* In 2015–16, 2 fellowships with full tuition reimbursements (averaging $15,000 per year), 1 teaching assistantship with full tuition reimbursement (averaging $15,000 per year) were awarded; scholarships/grants, traineeships, and unspecified assistantships also available. *Faculty research:* Cultural competency, sleep disorders, self-care in HIV positive African-American women, ethical decision-making in pediatric cases. *Unit head:* Dr. Carolyn M. Rutledge, Associate Chair of Graduate Program, 757-683-5009, Fax: 757-683-5253, E-mail: crutledg@odu.edu. *Application contact:* Sue Parker, Graduate Program Coordinator, 757-683-4298, Fax: 757-683-5253, E-mail: sparker@odu.edu.
Website: http://www.odu.edu/academics/programs/doctoral/nursing-practice

Old Dominion University, College of Health Sciences, School of Nursing, Family Nurse Practitioner Emphasis, Norfolk, VA 23529. Offers adult-gerontology clinical nurse specialist/educator (MSN); neonatal nurse practitioner (MSN); pediatric nurse practitioner (MSN). *Program availability:* Blended/hybrid learning. *Faculty:* 3 full-time (all women), 9 part-time/adjunct (all women). *Students:* 53 full-time (52 women), 5 part-time (all women); includes 14 minority (9 Black or African American, non-Hispanic/Latino; 2 Asian, non-Hispanic/Latino; 1 Hispanic/Latino; 2 Two or more races, non-Hispanic/Latino). Average age 35. 53 applicants, 66% accepted, 23 enrolled. In 2015, 60 master's awarded. *Degree requirements:* For master's, comprehensive exam. *Entrance requirements:* For master's, GRE or MAT (waived with a GPA above 3.5), 3 letters of recommendation, essay, resume, transcripts. Additional exam requirements/ recommendations for international students: Required—TOEFL. *Application deadline:* For fall admission, 3/1 priority date for domestic students, 4/15 priority date for international students. Application fee: $50. Electronic applications accepted. *Expenses:* Tuition, state resident: full-time $11,136; part-time $464 per credit hour. Tuition, nonresident: full-time $27,840; part-time $1160 per credit hour. *Required fees:* $64 per semester. Tuition and fees vary according to campus/location, program and reciprocity agreements. *Financial support:* In 2015–16, research assistantships with partial tuition reimbursements (averaging $10,000 per year) were awarded; career-related internships or fieldwork, scholarships/grants, and traineeships also available. Support available to part-time students. *Faculty research:* Military families, nurse practitioner student reaching modalities, gerontology, pediatrics, ethics. *Unit head:* Dr. Carolyn M. Rutledge, Associate Chair for Graduate Programs, 757-683-5009, Fax: 757-683-5253, E-mail: crutledg@odu.edu. *Application contact:* Sue Parker, Graduate Program Coordinator, 757-683-4298, Fax: 757-683-5253, E-mail: sparker@odu.edu.
Website: http://catalog.odu.edu/graduate/collegeofhealthsciences/schoolofnursing/#masterofscienceinnursing013familynursepractitionerrole

Oregon Health & Science University, School of Nursing, Family Nurse Practitioner Program, Portland, OR 97239-2941. Offers MN, MS, DNP, Post Master's Certificate. *Program availability:* Online learning. *Degree requirements:* For doctorate, thesis/dissertation (for some programs). *Entrance requirements:* For master's and doctorate, GRE, BSN, statistics within the last 5 years; for Post Master's Certificate, master's degree in nursing, statistics in the last 5 years. Additional exam requirements/ recommendations for international students: Required—TOEFL (minimum score 83 iBT). Electronic applications accepted.

Otterbein University, Department of Nursing, Westerville, OH 43081. Offers advanced practice nurse educator (Certificate); clinical nurse leader (MSN); family nurse practitioner (MSN, Certificate); nurse anesthesia (MSN, Certificate); nursing (DNP); nursing service administration (MSN). *Accreditation:* AACN; AANA/CANAEP; ACEN. *Program availability:* Part-time, evening/weekend, online learning. *Degree requirements:* For master's, comprehensive exam (for some programs), thesis (for some programs). *Entrance requirements:* For master's, 2 reference forms, resume; for Certificate, official transcripts, 2 reference forms, essay, resumé. Additional exam requirements/ recommendations for international students: Required—TOEFL (minimum score 550 paper-based; 79 iBT). *Faculty research:* Patient education, women's health, trauma curriculum development, administration.

Pace University, College of Health Professions, Lienhard School of Nursing, New York, NY 10038. Offers family nurse practitioner (MS); nurse education (Advanced Certificate); nursing education (MS); nursing leadership (Advanced Certificate); nursing practice (DNP). *Accreditation:* AACN. *Program availability:* Part-time, evening/weekend, blended/hybrid learning. *Faculty:* 11 full-time (10 women), 31 part-time/adjunct (27 women). *Students:* 3 full-time (all women), 415 part-time (385 women); includes 196 minority (97 Black or African American, non-Hispanic/Latino; 2 American Indian or Alaska Native, non-Hispanic/Latino; 57 Asian, non-Hispanic/Latino; 33 Hispanic/Latino; 7 Two or more races, non-Hispanic/Latino), 2 international. Average age 34. 291 applicants, 60% accepted, 129 enrolled. In 2015, 129 master's, 20 doctorates, 7 other advanced degrees awarded. *Degree requirements:* For doctorate, thesis/dissertation. *Entrance requirements:* For master's, RN license, resume, personal statement, 2 letters of recommendation, official transcripts; for doctorate, RN license, resume, personal statement, 2 letters of recommendation, official transcripts, accredited master's degree in nursing, minimum GPA of 3.2, national certification; for Advanced Certificate, RN license, completion of 2nd degree in nursing. Additional exam requirements/ recommendations for international students: Required—TOEFL (minimum score 100 iBT), IELTS or PTE. *Application deadline:* For fall admission, 3/1 for domestic and international students. Applications are processed on a rolling basis. Application fee: $70. Electronic applications accepted. *Expenses:* Contact institution. *Financial support:*

Research assistantships, teaching assistantships, career-related internships or fieldwork, Federal Work-Study, tuition waivers (partial), and unspecified assistantships available. Support available to part-time students. Financial award application deadline: 2/15; financial award applicants required to submit FAFSA. *Unit head:* Dr. Harriet R. Feldman, Dean, College of Health Professions, 914-773-3341, E-mail: hfeldman@ pace.edu. *Application contact:* Susan Ford-Goldschein, Director of Graduate Admissions, 212-346-1531, Fax: 212-346-1585, E-mail: graduateadmission@pace.edu. Website: http://www.pace.edu/lienhard

Pacific Lutheran University, School of Nursing, DNP Program, Tacoma, WA 98447. Offers DNP. Program designed for the working nurse; classes typically held Thursday evenings and all day Friday. *Accreditation:* AACN. *Faculty:* 6 full-time (5 women), 7 part-time/adjunct (all women). *Students:* 9 full-time (8 women), 6 part-time (all women); includes 4 minority (1 Black or African American, non-Hispanic/Latino; 1 Asian, non-Hispanic/Latino; 2 Hispanic/Latino), 1 international. Average age 38. 22 applicants, 77% accepted, 11 enrolled. *Entrance requirements:* Additional exam requirements/ recommendations for international students: Required—TOEFL (minimum score 550 paper-based; 86 iBT). *Application deadline:* For fall admission, 11/15 priority date for domestic and international students. Applications are processed on a rolling basis. Application fee: $55. Electronic applications accepted. *Expenses:* Contact institution. *Financial support:* In 2015–16, 3 students received support, including 1 fellowship (averaging $2,000 per year); Federal Work-Study, scholarships/grants, and health care benefits also available. Support available to part-time students. Financial award application deadline: 3/1; financial award applicants required to submit FAFSA. *Unit head:* Dr. Sheila Smith, Associate Dean of Graduate Nursing Programs/Associate Professor of Nursing, 253-535-7674, E-mail: gradnrs@plu.edu. *Application contact:* Marie Boisvert, Director, Graduate Admission, 253-535-8570, Fax: 253-536-5136, E-mail: gradadmission@plu.edu

Palm Beach Atlantic University, School of Nursing, West Palm Beach, FL 33416-4708. Offers family nurse practitioner (DNP); health systems leadership (MSN). *Program availability:* Part-time. *Faculty:* 5 part-time/adjunct (4 women). *Students:* 43 full-time (37 women), 1 (woman) part-time; includes 22 minority (11 Black or African American, non-Hispanic/Latino; 2 Asian, non-Hispanic/Latino; 8 Hispanic/Latino; 1 Two or more races, non-Hispanic/Latino). Average age 32. 34 applicants, 100% accepted, 24 enrolled. *Entrance requirements:* For master's, minimum GPA of 3.0; for doctorate, minimum GPA of 3.0; one year of experience as an RN; personal interview. Additional exam requirements/recommendations for international students: Required—TOEFL (minimum score 550 paper-based; 79 iBT). *Application deadline:* Applications are processed on a rolling basis. Application fee: $50. Electronic applications accepted. *Expenses:* Tuition, area resident: Part-time $525 per credit hour. *Financial support:* In 2015–16, 13 students received support. Scholarships/grants and employee education grants available. Financial award application deadline: 5/1; financial award applicants required to submit FAFSA. *Unit head:* Joanne Masella, Dean, 561-803-2827. *Application contact:* Graduate Admissions, 888-468-6722, E-mail: grad@pba.edu. Website: http://www.pba.edu/school-of-nursing

Point Loma Nazarene University, School of Nursing, San Diego, CA 92106-2899. Offers adult/gerontology nursing (MSN); family/individual health (MSN); general nursing (MSN); nursing (Post-MSN Certificate); pediatric nursing (MSN); psychiatric mental health (MSN). *Accreditation:* AACN. *Program availability:* Part-time. *Faculty:* 6 full-time (5 women), 2 part-time/adjunct (both women). *Students:* 1 (woman) full-time, 74 part-time (61 women); includes 35 minority (4 Black or African American, non-Hispanic/ Latino; 15 Asian, non-Hispanic/Latino; 10 Hispanic/Latino; 3 Native Hawaiian or other Pacific Islander, non-Hispanic/Latino; 3 Two or more races, non-Hispanic/Latino), 2 international. Average age 38. 34 applicants, 88% accepted, 18 enrolled. In 2015, 40 master's awarded. *Entrance requirements:* For master's, NCLEX, ADN or BSN in nursing, interview, RN license, essay, letters of recommendation, interview. *Application deadline:* For fall admission, 7/5 priority date for domestic students; for spring admission, 11/1 priority date for domestic students; for summer admission, 3/22 priority date for domestic students. Applications are processed on a rolling basis. Application fee: $50. *Financial support:* Applicants required to submit FAFSA. *Unit head:* Dr. Barb Taylor, Dean of the School of Nursing, 619-849-2766, E-mail: bataylor@pointloma.edu. *Application contact:* Claire Buckley, Director of Graduate Admissions, 619-563-2846, E-mail: clairebuckley@pointloma.edu. Website: http://www.pointloma.edu/discover/graduate-school/graduate-programs/ master-science-nursing-and-post-msn-certification

Prairie View A&M University, College of Nursing, Houston, TX 77030. Offers family nurse practitioner (MSN); nursing administration (MSN); nursing education (MSN). *Accreditation:* AACN; ACEN. *Program availability:* Part-time, evening/weekend. *Faculty:* 11 full-time (all women), 7 part-time/adjunct (6 women). *Students:* 65 full-time (58 women), 78 part-time (71 women); includes 128 minority (94 Black or African American, non-Hispanic/Latino; 24 Asian, non-Hispanic/Latino; 9 Hispanic/Latino; 1 Two or more races, non-Hispanic/Latino), 5 international. Average age 35. 84 applicants, 44% accepted, 25 enrolled. In 2015, 63 master's awarded. *Degree requirements:* For master's, comprehensive exam, thesis. *Entrance requirements:* For master's, MAT or GRE, BS in nursing; minimum 1 year of experience as registered nurse; minimum GPA of 2.75, 3 letters of recommendation from professional nurses. Additional exam requirements/recommendations for international students: Required—TOEFL (minimum score 550 paper-based; 79 iBT). *Application deadline:* For fall admission, 7/1 priority date for domestic students, 6/1 priority date for international students; for spring admission, 11/1 priority date for domestic students, 10/1 priority date for international students; for summer admission, 3/1 priority date for domestic students, 2/1 priority date for international students. Applications are processed on a rolling basis. Application fee: $50. Electronic applications accepted. *Expenses:* Tuition, state resident: full-time $4243; part-time $237.29 per credit hour. Tuition, nonresident: full-time $11,798; part-time $657 per credit hour. *Required fees:* $2762; $172.10 per credit hour. *Financial support:* Career-related internships or fieldwork, Federal Work-Study, institutionally sponsored loans, scholarships/grants, and traineeships available. Support available to part-time students. Financial award application deadline: 4/1; financial award applicants required to submit FAFSA. *Faculty research:* Software development and violence prevention, health promotion and disease prevention. *Unit head:* Dr. Betty N. Adams, Dean, 713-797-7009, Fax: 713-797-7013, E-mail: bnadams@pvamu.edu. *Application contact:* Dr. Forest Smith, Director of Student Services and Admissions, 713-797-7031, Fax: 713-797-7012, E-mail: fdsmith@pvamu.edu. Website: http://www.pvamu.edu/nursing/

Purdue University Northwest, Graduate Studies Office, School of Nursing, Hammond, IN 46323-2094. Offers adult health clinical nurse specialist (MS); critical care clinical nurse specialist (MS); family nurse practitioner (MS); nurse executive (MS). *Accreditation:* AACN; ACEN. *Program availability:* Part-time, online learning. *Entrance requirements:* For master's, BSN. Additional exam requirements/recommendations for international students: Required—TOEFL. Electronic applications accepted. *Faculty research:* Adult health, cardiovascular and pulmonary nursing.

Queen's University at Kingston, School of Graduate Studies, Faculty of Health Sciences, School of Nursing, Kingston, ON K7L 3N6, Canada. Offers health and chronic illness (M Sc); nurse scientist (PhD); primary health care nurse practitioner (Certificate); women's and children's health (M Sc). *Degree requirements:* For master's, thesis. *Entrance requirements:* For master's, RN license. Additional exam requirements/ recommendations for international students: Required—TOEFL. *Faculty research:* Women and children's health, health and chronic illness.

Quinnipiac University, School of Nursing, Family Nurse Practitioner Track, Hamden, CT 06518-1940. Offers MSN, DNP. *Accreditation:* ACEN. *Faculty:* 19 full-time (18 women), 13 part-time/adjunct (9 women). *Students:* 28 full-time (26 women), 44 part-time (41 women); includes 16 minority (5 Black or African American, non-Hispanic/ Latino; 7 Asian, non-Hispanic/Latino; 4 Hispanic/Latino). 51 applicants, 53% accepted, 17 enrolled. *Degree requirements:* For master's, thesis optional, clinical practicum. *Entrance requirements:* For master's, RN license, minimum GPA of 3.0. Additional exam requirements/recommendations for international students: Required—TOEFL (minimum score 575 paper-based; 90 iBT), IELTS (minimum score 6.5). *Application deadline:* For fall admission, 5/1 for domestic students, 4/30 for international students. Applications are processed on a rolling basis. Application fee: $45. Electronic applications accepted. *Expenses:* $985 per credit tuition; $40 per credit student fee (not to exceed $360 per semester); $150 per semester (fall/spring) part-time technology and lab fee; $340 per semester (fall/spring) full-time technology and lab fee; $75 per semester summer technology and lab fee. *Financial support:* Federal Work-Study, scholarships/grants, and unspecified assistantships available. Support available to part-time students. Financial award application deadline: 6/1; financial award applicants required to submit FAFSA. *Unit head:* Dr. Lynn Price, Program Director, E-mail: graduate@quinnipiac.edu. *Application contact:* Office of Graduate Admissions, 800-462-1944, Fax: 203-582-3443, E-mail: graduate@quinnipiac.edu. Website: http://www.quinnipiac.edu/gradnursing

Regis College, School of Nursing and Health Sciences, Weston, MA 02493. Offers applied behavior analysis (MS); biomedical sciences (MS); counseling psychology (MA); health administration (MS); molecular imaging and therapeutics (MS); nurse practitioner (Certificate); nursing (MS, DNP); nursing education (Certificate); occupational therapy (MS). *Accreditation:* ACEN. *Program availability:* Part-time, evening/weekend. *Degree requirements:* For master's, thesis. *Entrance requirements:* For master's, GRE General Test or MAT, minimum GPA of 3.0; for doctorate, MAT or GRE if GPA from master's lower than 3.5. Additional exam requirements/recommendations for international students: Required—TOEFL (minimum score 550 paper-based). *Application deadline:* Applications are processed on a rolling basis. Application fee: $50. Electronic applications accepted. *Financial support:* Research assistantships, Federal Work-Study, scholarships/grants, traineeships, and unspecified assistantships available. Support available to part-time students. Financial award applicants required to submit FAFSA. *Faculty research:* Health policy, education, aging, job satisfaction, psychiatric nursing, critical thinking. *Application contact:* Shelagh Tomaino, Associate Director, Graduate Admission, 781-768-7188, Fax: 781-768-7071, E-mail: shelagh.tomaino@ regiscollege.edu.

Regis University, Rueckert-Hartman College for Health Professions, Denver, CO 80221-1099. Offers addictions counseling (Post-Graduate Certificate); advanced practice nurse specialization (DNP); counseling (MA); counseling children and adolescents (Post-Graduate Certificate); counseling military families (Post-Graduate Certificate); depth psychotherapy (Post-Graduate Certificate); family nurse practitioner (MSN); health care business management (Certificate); health care quality and patient safety (Certificate); health industry leadership (MBA); health professions (Postbaccalaureate Certificate); health services administration (MS); marriage and family therapy (MA); neonatal nurse practitioner (MSN); nursing education or leadership (MSN); orthopedic manual physical therapy fellowship (Certificate); pharmacy (Pharm D); physical therapy (DPT). *Program availability:* Part-time, evening/weekend, 100% online, blended/hybrid learning. *Faculty:* 40 full-time (29 women), 116 part-time/ adjunct (86 women). *Students:* 1,080 full-time (771 women), 274 part-time (239 women); includes 388 minority (59 Black or African American, non-Hispanic/Latino; 6 American Indian or Alaska Native, non-Hispanic/Latino; 109 Asian, non-Hispanic/Latino; 163 Hispanic/Latino; 1 Native Hawaiian or other Pacific Islander, non-Hispanic/Latino; 50 Two or more races, non-Hispanic/Latino), 7 international. Average age 34. 2,188 applicants, 31% accepted, 303 enrolled. In 2015, 329 master's, 160 doctorates awarded. *Degree requirements:* For master's, thesis (for some programs), internship. *Entrance requirements:* For master's, official transcript reflecting baccalaureate degree awarded from regionally-accredited college or university. Additional exam requirements/ recommendations for international students: Required—TOEFL (minimum score 550 paper-based; 82 iBT). *Application deadline:* For fall admission, 8/15 priority date for domestic students; for spring admission, 1/10 priority date for domestic students; for summer admission, 5/1 priority date for domestic students. Applications are processed on a rolling basis. Application fee: $75. Electronic applications accepted. *Expenses:* Contact institution. *Financial support:* In 2015–16, 102 students received support. Federal Work-Study and scholarships/grants available. Financial award application deadline: 4/15; financial award applicants required to submit FAFSA. *Faculty research:* Normal and pathological balance and gait research, normal/pathological upper limb motor control/biomechanics, exercise energy/metabolism research, optical treatment protocols for therapeutic modalities. *Unit head:* Dr. Janet Houser, Academic Dean. *Application contact:* Cate Clark, Director of Admissions, 303-458-4900, Fax: 303-964-5534, E-mail: ruadmissions@regis.edu. Website: http://www.regis.edu/RHCHP.aspx

Research College of Nursing, Nursing Program, Kansas City, MO 64132. Offers adult-gerontological nurse practitioner (MSN); executive practice and healthcare leadership (MSN); family nurse practitioner (MSN); nursing (MSN). *Accreditation:* AACN. *Program availability:* Part-time, 100% online. *Faculty:* 9 full-time (all women), 5 part-time/adjunct (2 women). *Students:* 4 full-time (2 women), 148 part-time (132 women); includes 15 minority (9 Black or African American, non-Hispanic/Latino; 1 American Indian or Alaska Native, non-Hispanic/Latino; 3 Asian, non-Hispanic/Latino; 1 Native Hawaiian or other Pacific Islander, non-Hispanic/Latino; 1 Two or more races, non-Hispanic/Latino). In 2015, 34 master's awarded. *Degree requirements:* For master's, research project. *Entrance requirements:* For master's, 3 letters of recommendation, official transcripts, resume, personal statement/writing sample. *Application deadline:* Applications are processed on a rolling basis. Application fee: $65. Electronic applications accepted. *Expenses:* $525 per credit hour; $25 per credit hour clinical fee. *Financial support:* Applicants required to submit FAFSA. *Unit head:* Dr. Nancy O. DeBasio, President and Dean, 816-995-2815, Fax: 816-995-2817, E-mail: nancy.debasio@researchcollege.edu. *Application contact:* Leslie Burry, Director of Transfer and Graduate Recruitment, 816-995-2820, Fax: 816-995-2813, E-mail: leslie.burry@researchcollege.edu.

Rivier University, School of Graduate Studies, Division of Nursing, Nashua, NH 03060. Offers adult psychiatric/mental health practitioner (MS); family nurse practitioner (MS); nursing education (MS). *Accreditation:* ACEN. *Program availability:* Part-time, evening/ weekend. *Entrance requirements:* For master's, GRE, MAT. Electronic applications accepted.

Rocky Mountain University of Health Professions, Doctor of Nursing Practice Program, Provo, UT 84606. Offers DNP.

Rush University, College of Nursing, Department of Community, Systems, and Mental Health Nursing, Chicago, IL 60612. Offers advanced public health nursing (DNP); family

Family Nurse Practitioner Studies

nurse practitioner (DNP); leadership to enhance population health outcomes (DNP); nursing science (PhD); psychiatric mental health nurse practitioner (DNP); systems leadership (DNP). *Accreditation:* AACN. *Program availability:* Part-time, 100% online. *Faculty:* 43 full-time (40 women), 52 part-time/adjunct (49 women). *Students:* 18 full-time (17 women), 341 part-time (314 women); includes 85 minority (38 Black or African American, non-Hispanic/Latino; 2 American Indian or Alaska Native, non-Hispanic/Latino; 21 Asian, non-Hispanic/Latino; 22 Hispanic/Latino; 2 Native Hawaiian or other Pacific Islander, non-Hispanic/Latino). Average age 35. 177 applicants, 62% accepted, 96 enrolled. *Degree requirements:* For doctorate, capstone project (for DNP); dissertation (for PhD). *Entrance requirements:* For doctorate, GRE General Test (waived for DNP if cumulative GPA is 3.25 or greater, nursing GPA is 3.0 or greater, or a completed graduate program GPA is 3.5 or greater), interview, 3 letters of recommendation, personal statement, current resume. Additional exam requirements/recommendations for international students: Required—TOEFL (minimum score 94 iBT). *Application deadline:* For fall admission, 1/2 for domestic students; for winter admission, 10/15 for domestic students; for spring admission, 8/4 for domestic students; for summer admission, 12/1 for domestic students. Applications are processed on a rolling basis. Application fee: $100. Electronic applications accepted. *Expenses:* Contact institution. *Financial support:* Research assistantships, teaching assistantships, Federal Work-Study, scholarships/grants, traineeships, and health care benefits available. Support available to part-time students. Financial award application deadline: 3/1; financial award applicants required to submit FAFSA. *Faculty research:* Reduction of health disparities; evidence-based interventions for caregivers; patient-centered quality assessment of psychiatric inpatient environments; digital delivery of a parent-training program for urban, low-income parents; patient-centered predictors and outcomes of inter-professional care coordination. *Unit head:* Dr. Mona Shattell, Chairperson, 312-942-7117, E-mail: mona_shattell@rush.edu. *Application contact:* Jennifer Thorndyke, Admissions Specialist, 312-563-7526, E-mail: jennifer_thorndyke@rush.edu. Website: http://www.rushu.rush.edu/servlet/Satellite?c=content_block&cid=1320160764996&pagename=CollegeOfNursing%2Fcontent_block%2FContentBlockDetail&rendermod

Rutgers University–Newark, Rutgers School of Nursing, Newark, NJ 07107-3001. Offers adult health (MSN); adult occupational health (MSN); advanced practice nursing (MSN, Post Master's Certificate); family nurse practitioner (MSN); nurse anesthesia (MSN); nursing (MSN); nursing informatics (MSN); urban health (PhD); women's health practitioner (MSN). *Accreditation:* AANA/CANAEP. *Program availability:* Part-time. *Entrance requirements:* For master's, GRE, RN license; basic life support, statistics, and health assessment experience. Additional exam requirements/recommendations for international students: Required—TOEFL. Electronic applications accepted. *Expenses:* Contact institution. *Faculty research:* HIV/AIDS, diabetes education, learned helplessness, nursing science, psychoeducation.

Sacred Heart University, Graduate Programs, College of Nursing, Fairfield, CT 06825. Offers clinical nurse leader (MSN); clinical practice (DNP); family nurse practitioner (MSN, Graduate Certificate); leadership (DNP); nurse educator (MSN); nursing management and executive leadership (MSN); patient care services (MSN). *Accreditation:* AACN. *Program availability:* Part-time, evening/weekend, online learning. *Faculty:* 17 full-time (all women), 21 part-time/adjunct (18 women). *Students:* 19 full-time (18 women), 777 part-time (711 women); includes 144 minority (56 Black or African American, non-Hispanic/Latino; 2 American Indian or Alaska Native, non-Hispanic/Latino; 33 Asian, non-Hispanic/Latino; 41 Hispanic/Latino; 2 Native Hawaiian or other Pacific Islander, non-Hispanic/Latino; 10 Two or more races, non-Hispanic/Latino). Average age 38. 116 applicants, 53% accepted, 50 enrolled. In 2015, 192 master's, 13 doctorates awarded. *Degree requirements:* For master's, thesis, 500 clinical hours. *Entrance requirements:* For master's, minimum GPA of 3.0, BSN or RN plus BS (for MSN); for doctorate, minimum GPA of 3.0, MSN or BSN plus MS in related field (for DNP). Additional exam requirements/recommendations for international students: Required—PTE; Recommended—TOEFL (minimum score 570 paper-based; 80 iBT), IELTS (minimum score 6.5). *Application deadline:* For fall admission, 2/15 for domestic and international students. Applications are processed on a rolling basis. Application fee: $75. Electronic applications accepted. *Expenses:* Contact institution. *Financial support:* Unspecified assistantships available. Financial award applicants required to submit FAFSA. *Unit head:* Mary Alice Donius, Dean of Nursing, 203-365-4508, E-mail: doniusm@sacredheart.edu. *Application contact:* William Sweeney, Director of Graduate Admissions Operations, 203-365-4716, Fax: 203-365-4732, E-mail: gradstudies@sacredheart.edu. Website: http://www.sacredheart.edu/academics/collegeofhealthprofessions/academicprograms/nursing/nursingprograms/graduateprograms/

Sage Graduate School, School of Health Sciences, Department of Nursing, Program in Family Nurse Practitioner, Troy, NY 12180-4115. Offers adult gerontology acute care (Post Master's Certificate); family nurse practitioner (MS); family psychiatric mental health (Post Master's Certificate). *Accreditation:* AACN. *Program availability:* Part-time, evening/weekend. *Faculty:* 9 full-time (all women), 27 part-time/adjunct (24 women). *Students:* 24 full-time (23 women), 110 part-time (99 women); includes 24 minority (11 Black or African American, non-Hispanic/Latino; 2 American Indian or Alaska Native, non-Hispanic/Latino; 8 Asian, non-Hispanic/Latino; 2 Hispanic/Latino; 1 Two or more races, non-Hispanic/Latino). Average age 34. 114 applicants, 28% accepted, 25 enrolled. In 2015, 4 master's, 6 other advanced degrees awarded. *Degree requirements:* For master's, thesis or alternative. *Entrance requirements:* For master's, currently licensed as registered professional nurse in state of practice; baccalaureate degree in nursing from nationally-accredited program or its international equivalent. Additional exam requirements/recommendations for international students: Required—TOEFL (minimum score 550 paper-based). *Application deadline:* Applications are processed on a rolling basis. Application fee: $40. Electronic applications accepted. *Expenses:* Tuition, area resident: Full-time $12,240; part-time $680 per credit hour. Tuition and fees vary according to degree level and program. *Financial support:* Fellowships, research assistantships, teaching assistantships, Federal Work-Study, scholarships/grants, and unspecified assistantships available. Support available to part-time students. Financial award application deadline: 3/1; financial award applicants required to submit FAFSA. *Unit head:* Dr. Theresa Hand, Dean, School of Health Sciences, 518-244-2264, Fax: 518-244-4571, E-mail: handt@sage.edu. *Application contact:* Dr. Carol Braungart, Co-Director, Graduate Nursing Program, 518-244-2459, Fax: 518-244-2009, E-mail: braunc@sage.edu.

Saginaw Valley State University, College of Health and Human Services, Program in Nurse Practitioner, University Center, MI 48710. Offers MSN, DNP. *Accreditation:* AACN. *Program availability:* Part-time, evening/weekend, online learning. *Students:* 8 full-time (6 women), 63 part-time (54 women); includes 4 minority (1 Black or African American, non-Hispanic/Latino; 1 American Indian or Alaska Native, non-Hispanic/Latino; 1 Asian, non-Hispanic/Latino; 1 Hispanic/Latino), 1 international. Average age 32. 41 applicants, 73% accepted, 25 enrolled. In 2015, 28 master's awarded. *Degree requirements:* For master's, thesis optional. *Entrance requirements:* For master's, GRE, minimum GPA of 3.0, license to practice nursing in MI; for doctorate, GRE, minimum GPA of 3.3, college chemistry with minimum C grade, college statistics with minimum B grade, employed as RN with current license in MI. Additional exam requirements/recommendations for international students: Required—TOEFL (minimum score 580

paper-based; 92 iBT). *Application deadline:* For fall admission, 7/15 for international students; for winter admission, 11/15 for international students; for spring admission, 4/15 for international students. Applications are processed on a rolling basis. Application fee: $30 ($90 for international students). Electronic applications accepted. *Expenses:* Tuition, state resident: full-time $9515; part-time $514 per credit hour. Tuition, nonresident: full-time $17,899; part-time $980 per credit hour. *Required fees:* $263; $14.60 per credit hour. Tuition and fees vary according to degree level. *Financial support:* Federal Work-Study and scholarships/grants available. Support available to part-time students. Financial award application deadline: 4/1; financial award applicants required to submit FAFSA. *Unit head:* Dr. Karen Brown-Fackler, Coordinator, 989-964-2185, Fax: 989-964-4925, E-mail: kmbrown4@svsu.edu. *Application contact:* Jenna Briggs, Director, Graduate and International Admissions, 989-964-6096, Fax: 989-964-2788, E-mail: gradadm@svsu.edu.

Saint Francis Medical Center College of Nursing, Graduate Programs, Peoria, IL 61603-3783. Offers adult gerontology (MSN); clinical nurse leader (MSN); family nurse practitioner (MSN); family psychiatric mental health nurse practitioner (MSN); neonatal nurse practitioner (MSN); nurse clinician (Post-Graduate Certificate); nurse educator (MSN, Post-Graduate Certificate); nursing (DNP); nursing management leadership (MSN). *Accreditation:* ACEN. *Program availability:* Part-time, 100% online, blended/hybrid learning. *Faculty:* 14 full-time (all women), 5 part-time/adjunct (all women). *Students:* 13 full-time (12 women), 257 part-time (228 women); includes 23 minority (14 Black or African American, non-Hispanic/Latino; 3 Asian, non-Hispanic/Latino; 4 Hispanic/Latino; 2 Two or more races, non-Hispanic/Latino). Average age 37. 86 applicants, 86% accepted, 44 enrolled. In 2015, 61 master's, 6 doctorates awarded. *Degree requirements:* For master's, research experience, portfolio, practicum; for doctorate, practicum hours. *Entrance requirements:* For master's, nursing research, health assessment, graduate course work in statistics, RN license; for doctorate, master's degree in nursing, professional portfolio, graduate statistics, transcripts, RN license. Additional exam requirements/recommendations for international students: Required—TOEFL (minimum score 550 paper-based; 79 iBT). *Application deadline:* For fall admission, 6/1 priority date for domestic and international students; for spring admission, 11/15 priority date for domestic and international students. Applications are processed on a rolling basis. Application fee: $50. *Financial support:* In 2015–16, 18 students received support. Scholarships/grants and tuition waivers (partial) available. Support available to part-time students. Financial award application deadline: 6/15; financial award applicants required to submit FAFSA. *Faculty research:* Outcome and curriculum planning, health promotion, NCLEX-RN results, decision-making program evaluation. *Unit head:* Dr. Patti A. Stockert, President of the College, 309-655-4124, Fax: 309-624-8973, E-mail: patricia.a.stockert@osfhealthcare.org. *Application contact:* Dr. Kim A. Mitchell, Dean, Graduate Program, 309-655-2201, Fax: 309-624-8973, E-mail: kim.a.mitchell@osfhealthcare.org. Website: http://www.sfmccon.edu/graduate-programs/

St. John Fisher College, Wegmans School of Nursing, Advanced Practice Nursing Program, Rochester, NY 14618-3597. Offers advanced practice nursing (MS); clinical nurse specialist (Certificate); family nurse practitioner (Certificate). *Accreditation:* AACN. *Program availability:* Part-time, evening/weekend. *Faculty:* 11 full-time (10 women), 7 part-time/adjunct (6 women). *Students:* 7 full-time (all women), 129 part-time (122 women); includes 18 minority (10 Black or African American, non-Hispanic/Latino; 3 Asian, non-Hispanic/Latino; 5 Hispanic/Latino), 2 international. Average age 32. 76 applicants, 50% accepted, 29 enrolled. In 2015, 25 master's awarded. *Degree requirements:* For master's, clinical practice, project; for Certificate, clinical practice. *Entrance requirements:* For master's, BSN; undergraduate course work in statistics, health assessment, and nursing research; current New York State RN license; 2 letters of recommendation; current resume. Additional exam requirements/recommendations for international students: Required—TOEFL (minimum score 575 paper-based; 80 iBT). *Application deadline:* Applications are processed on a rolling basis. Application fee: $30. Electronic applications accepted. *Expenses:* $860 per credit hour. *Financial support:* Scholarships/grants and traineeships available. Financial award applicants required to submit FAFSA. *Faculty research:* Chronic illness, pediatric injury, women's health, public health policy, health care teams. *Unit head:* Dr. Colleen Donegan, Graduate Director, 585-899-3788, Fax: 585-385-8466, E-mail: cdonegan@sjfc.edu. *Application contact:* Rebecca Norman, Associate Director of Transfer and Graduate Admissions, 585-385-8064, E-mail: rnorman@sjfc.edu.

Saint Joseph's College of Maine, Master of Science in Nursing Program, Standish, ME 04084. Offers administration (MSN); education (MSN); family nurse practitioner (MSN); nursing administration and leadership (Certificate); nursing and health care education (Certificate). *Accreditation:* AACN. *Program availability:* Part-time, online learning. *Entrance requirements:* For master's, MAT. Electronic applications accepted.

Salisbury University, DNP in Nursing Program, Salisbury, MD 21801-6837. Offers family nurse practitioner (DNP); nursing (DNP); nursing leadership (DNP). *Accreditation:* AACN. *Program availability:* Part-time. *Faculty:* 7 full-time (5 women). *Students:* 22 full-time (20 women), 1 (woman) part-time; includes 9 minority (7 Black or African American, non-Hispanic/Latino; 1 Hispanic/Latino; 1 Two or more races, non-Hispanic/Latino). Average age 35. 16 applicants, 56% accepted, 6 enrolled. In 2015, 8 doctorates awarded. Terminal master's awarded for partial completion of doctoral program. *Entrance requirements:* For doctorate, undergraduate nursing degree with minimum cumulative GPA of 3.0; current and active United States Registered Nurse license; current resume or curriculum vitae; essay; 3 letters of recommendation. Additional exam requirements/recommendations for international students: Required—TOEFL (minimum score 550 paper-based, 79 iBT) or IELTS (6.5). *Application deadline:* For fall admission, 5/15 priority date for domestic students, 3/15 priority date for international students. Applications are processed on a rolling basis. Application fee: $65. Electronic applications accepted. *Expenses:* $620 per credit hour resident; $787 per credit hour non-resident; $78 per credit hour fees. *Financial support:* In 2015–16, 18 students received support. Career-related internships or fieldwork, institutionally sponsored loans, scholarships/grants, and unspecified assistantships available. Support available to part-time students. Financial award application deadline: 3/1; financial award applicants required to submit FAFSA. *Faculty research:* Intimate partner violence; telehealth; nursing faculty shortage; oral health needs; gerontology. *Unit head:* Dr. Lisa Seldomridge, Graduate Program Director, Nursing (DNP), 410-543-6344, Fax: 410-548-3313, E-mail: laseldomridge@salisbury.edu. *Application contact:* Carmel Boger, Administrative Assistant, 410-543-6420, Fax: 410-548-3313, E-mail: ciboger@salisbury.edu. Website: http://www.salisbury.edu/gsr/gradstudies/DNPpage.html

Samford University, Ida V. Moffett School of Nursing, Birmingham, AL 35229. Offers administration (DNP); advanced practice (DNP); family nurse practitioner (MSN); health systems management and leadership (MSN); nurse anesthesia (MSN); nurse educator (MSN). *Accreditation:* AACN; AANA/CANAEP (one or more programs are accredited). *Program availability:* Part-time, blended/hybrid learning. *Faculty:* 19 full-time (all women), 5 part-time/adjunct (1 woman). *Students:* 300 full-time (228 women), 40 part-time (36 women); includes 65 minority (28 Black or African American, non-Hispanic/Latino; 4 American Indian or Alaska Native, non-Hispanic/Latino; 8 Asian, non-Hispanic/Latino; 13 Hispanic/Latino; 12 Two or more races, non-Hispanic/Latino). Average

35. 69 applicants, 77% accepted, 52 enrolled. In 2015, 98 master's, 16 doctorates awarded. *Degree requirements:* For doctorate, capstone project with oral presentation. *Entrance requirements:* For master's, MAT; GRE (for nurse anesthesia), unencumbered licensure as registered nurse; BSN from CCNE, CNEA, or ACEN (formerly NLNAC) accredited program; minimum cumulative GPA of 3.0 in nursing courses; video submission; one undergraduate course in nursing research with minimum grade of C; for doctorate, unencumbered licensure as registered nurse; master's degree from CCNE, CNEA or ACEN (formerly NLNAC) accredited program in the area of advanced practice or administration; minimum master's degree cumulative GPA of 3.5; video interview submission. Additional exam requirements/recommendations for international students: Required—TOEFL (minimum score 550 paper-based; 80 iBT). *Application deadline:* For fall admission, 6/1 for domestic and international students; for spring admission, 9/1 for domestic and international students. Application fee: $65. Electronic applications accepted. *Expenses: Tuition, area resident:* Full-time $18,673; part-time $766 per credit hour. *Required fees:* $550. Tuition and fees vary according to course load, degree level and student level. *Financial support:* In 2015–16, 56 students received support. Institutionally sponsored loans, scholarships/grants, and traineeships available. Financial award application deadline: 3/1; financial award applicants required to submit FAFSA. *Faculty research:* Issues in rural health care, vulnerable populations, genetics and disabilities in pediatrics, geriatrics, parish nursing research, interprofessional education, global health disparities. *Unit head:* Dr. Nena F. Sanders, Vice Provost, College of Health Sciences/Dean/Professor, 205-726-2612, Fax: 205-726-4179, E-mail: nfsander@samford.edu. *Application contact:* Allyson Maddox, Director of Graduate Student Services, Ida V. Moffett School of Nursing, 205-726-2047, Fax: 205-726-4179, E-mail: amaddox@samford.edu.
Website: http://samford.edu/nursing

Samuel Merritt University, School of Nursing, Oakland, CA 94609. Offers case management (MSN); family nurse practitioner (MSN, Certificate); nurse anesthetist (MSN, Certificate); nursing (DNP). *Accreditation:* AACN; AANA/CANAEP (one or more programs are accredited). *Program availability:* Part-time, evening/weekend, 100% online, blended/hybrid learning. *Faculty:* 47 full-time (40 women), 50 part-time/adjunct (43 women). *Students:* 437 full-time (350 women), 59 part-time (45 women); includes 327 minority (29 Black or African American, non-Hispanic/Latino; 3 American Indian or Alaska Native, non-Hispanic/Latino; 163 Asian, non-Hispanic/Latino; 95 Hispanic/Latino; 9 Native Hawaiian or other Pacific Islander, non-Hispanic/Latino; 28 Two or more races, non-Hispanic/Latino). Average age 33. 392 applicants, 43% accepted, 126 enrolled. In 2015, 31 master's awarded. *Degree requirements:* For master's, thesis or alternative. *Entrance requirements:* For master's, minimum GPA of 2.5 in science, 3.0 overall; previous course work in statistics; current RN license. Additional exam requirements/recommendations for international students: Required—TOEFL (minimum score 100 iBT). *Application deadline:* For fall admission, 1/1 priority date for domestic students; for spring admission, 7/1 for domestic students; for summer admission, 1/1 for domestic students. Applications are processed on a rolling basis. Application fee: $50. Electronic applications accepted. *Expenses:* $61,299 tuition; $240 lab fees; $160 graduation fee. *Financial support:* In 2015–16, 34 students received support. Career-related internships or fieldwork, Federal Work-Study, scholarships/grants, and traineeships available. Support available to part-time students. Financial award application deadline: 3/2; financial award applicants required to submit FAFSA. *Faculty research:* Gerontology, community health, maternal-child health, sexually transmitted diseases, substance abuse, oncology. *Total annual research expenditures:* $35,000. *Unit head:* Dr. Audrey Berman, Graduate Coordinator, 510-869-6733, Fax: 510-869-6525. *Application contact:* Timothy Cranford, Dean of Admission, 510-869-6576, Fax: 510-869-6525, E-mail: admission@samuelmerritt.edu.
Website: http://www.samuelmerritt.edu/nursing

San Francisco State University, Division of Graduate Studies, College of Health and Social Sciences, School of Nursing, San Francisco, CA 94132-1722. Offers adult acute care (MS); clinical nurse specialist (MS); community/public health nursing (MS); family nurse practitioner (MS, Certificate); nursing administration (MS); pediatrics (MS); women's health (MS). *Accreditation:* AACN. *Program availability:* Part-time. *Application deadline:* Applications are processed on a rolling basis. *Expenses:* Tuition, state resident: full-time $6738. Tuition, nonresident: full-time $15,666. *Required fees:* $1004. *Financial support:* Career-related internships or fieldwork available. *Unit head:* Dr. Mary-Ann van Dam, Director, 415-338-1802, Fax: 415-338-0555, E-mail: vandam@sfsu.edu. *Application contact:* Connie Carr, Graduate Coordinator, 415-338-6856, Fax: 415-338-0555, E-mail: ccarr@sfsu.edu.
Website: http://nursing.sfsu.edu

Seattle Pacific University, MS in Nursing Program, Seattle, WA 98119-1997. Offers administration (MSN); adult/gerontology nurse practitioner (MSN); clinical nurse specialist (MSN); family nurse practitioner (MSN, Certificate); informatics (MSN); nurse educator (MSN). *Accreditation:* AACN. *Program availability:* Part-time. *Students:* 39 full-time (36 women), 30 part-time (25 women); includes 14 minority (3 Black or African American, non-Hispanic/Latino; 7 Asian, non-Hispanic/Latino; 3 Hispanic/Latino; 1 Two or more races, non-Hispanic/Latino), 1 international. Average age 38. 60 applicants, 48% accepted, 29 enrolled. In 2015, 23 master's awarded. *Degree requirements:* For master's, thesis. *Entrance requirements:* For master's, personal statement, transcripts, undergraduate nursing degree, proof of undergraduate statistics course with minimum GPA of 2.0, 2 recommendations. *Application deadline:* For fall admission, 1/15 priority date for domestic students; for spring admission, 1/15 for domestic students. Applications are processed on a rolling basis. Application fee: $50. Electronic applications accepted. *Expenses:* Contact institution. *Financial support:* Fellowships and scholarships/grants available. Financial award applicants required to submit FAFSA. *Unit head:* Dr. Christine Hoyle, Associate Dean, 206-281-2469, E-mail: hoylec@spu.edu.
Website: http://spu.edu/depts/health-sciences/grad/index.asp

Seattle University, College of Nursing, Program in Advanced Practice Nursing Immersion, Seattle, WA 98122-1090. Offers adult/gerontological nurse practitioner (MSN); advanced community public health nursing (MSN); family nurse practitioner (MSN); family psychiatric mental health nurse practitioner (MSN); nurse midwifery (MSN). *Degree requirements:* For master's, thesis or scholarly project. *Entrance requirements:* For master's, GRE, bachelor's degree, minimum GPA of 3.0, professional resume, two recommendations, letter of intent. Additional exam requirements/recommendations for international students: Required—TOEFL (minimum score 92 iBT), IELTS. Electronic applications accepted.

Shenandoah University, Eleanor Wade Custer School of Nursing, Winchester, VA 22601. Offers family nurse practitioner (MSN, DNP, Post-Graduate Certificate); health informatics (Certificate); health systems leadership (DNP); nurse midwifery (MSN, Post-Graduate Certificate); nursing education (Post-Graduate Certificate); psychiatric mental health nurse practitioner (MSN, DNP, Post-Graduate Certificate). *Accreditation:* AACN; ACNM/ACME. *Faculty:* 10 full-time (all women), 7 part-time/adjunct (4 women). *Students:* 33 full-time (31 women), 62 part-time (57 women); includes 21 minority (17 Black or African American, non-Hispanic/Latino; 3 Asian, non-Hispanic/Latino; 1 Hispanic/Latino). Average age 36. 55 applicants, 87% accepted, 39 enrolled. In 2015, 32 master's, 3 doctorates, 19 other advanced degrees awarded. *Degree requirements:*

For master's, research project, clinical hours; for doctorate, scholarly project, clinical hours; for other advanced degree, clinical hours. *Entrance requirements:* For master's, United States RN license; minimum GPA of 3.0; 2080 hours of clinical experience; curriculum vitae; 3 letters of recommendation from a former dean, a faculty member or advisor familiar with the applicant, and a former or current supervisor; two- to three-page essay on a specified topic; for doctorate, MSN, minimum GPA of 3.0, 3 letters of recommendation, 500-word statement, interview, BSN; for other advanced degree, MSN, minimum GPA of 3.0, 2 letters of recommendation, minimum of one year (2080 hours) of clinical nursing experience, interview. Additional exam requirements/recommendations for international students: Required—TOEFL (minimum score 558 paper-based; 83 iBT). *Application deadline:* For fall admission, 1/15 priority date for domestic and international students; for spring admission, 11/1 for domestic and international students; for summer admission, 3/15 for domestic and international students. Application fee: $30. Electronic applications accepted. *Expenses:* Contact institution. *Financial support:* In 2015–16, 13 students received support, including 3 fellowships (averaging $1,000 per year); scholarships/grants and unspecified assistantships also available. Financial award application deadline: 3/15; financial award applicants required to submit FAFSA. *Faculty research:* Primary care providers and their unique position in geriatric, pre-operative education and its effects on post-operative, variables associated with a woman's multidimensional childbirth, interdisciplinary communication, research on health policy. *Unit head:* Kathryn Ganske, PhD, RN, Dean, 540-678-4374, Fax: 540-665-5519, E-mail: kganske@su.edu. *Application contact:* Andrew Woodall, Executive Director of Recruitment and Admissions, 540-665-4581, Fax: 540-665-4627, E-mail: admit@su.edu.
Website: http://www.su.edu/nursing/

Simmons College, School of Nursing and Health Sciences, Boston, MA 02115. Offers didactic dietetics (Certificate); dietetic internship (Certificate); health education profession (PhD); health professions education (CAGS); nursing (MS), including family nurse practitioner, nursing practice (DNP); nutrition and health promotion (MS); physical therapy (DPT); sports nutrition (Certificate). *Program availability:* Part-time, blended/hybrid learning. *Faculty:* 21 full-time (17 women), 171 part-time/adjunct (157 women). *Students:* 333 full-time (305 women), 889 part-time (813 women); includes 250 minority (88 Black or African American, non-Hispanic/Latino; 3 American Indian or Alaska Native, non-Hispanic/Latino; 65 Asian, non-Hispanic/Latino; 67 Hispanic/Latino; 2 Native Hawaiian or other Pacific Islander, non-Hispanic/Latino; 25 Two or more races, non-Hispanic/Latino), 9 international. Average age 33. 846 applicants, 66% accepted, 441 enrolled. In 2015, 70 master's, 45 doctorates awarded. *Entrance requirements:* For doctorate, GRE. Additional exam requirements/recommendations for international students: Required—TOEFL (minimum score 570 paper-based; 88 iBT). *Application deadline:* For fall admission, 6/1 for international students. Application fee: $50. Electronic applications accepted. *Expenses:* Contact institution. *Financial support:* In 2015–16, 12 research assistantships (averaging $6,000 per year) were awarded; scholarships/grants and unspecified assistantships also available. *Unit head:* Dr. Judy Beal, Dean, 617-521-2139. *Application contact:* Brett DiMarzo, Director of Graduate Admission, 617-521-2651, Fax: 617-521-3137, E-mail: brett.dimarzo@simmons.edu.
Website: http://www.simmons.edu/snhs/

Sonoma State University, School of Science and Technology, Family Nurse Practitioner Program, Rohnert Park, CA 94928. Offers MSN. *Accreditation:* ACEN. *Program availability:* Part-time. *Degree requirements:* For master's, comprehensive exam, thesis or alternative, oral exams. *Entrance requirements:* For master's, GRE General Test, BSN, minimum GPA of 3.0, course work in statistics, physical assessment, RN license. Additional exam requirements/recommendations for international students: Required—TOEFL (minimum score 500 paper-based). *Faculty research:* Neonatal ethics.

Southern Adventist University, School of Nursing, Collegedale, TN 37315-0370. Offers acute care nurse practitioner (MSN); adult nurse practitioner (MSN); family nurse practitioner (MSN); nurse educator (MSN); MSN/MSBA. *Accreditation:* ACEN. *Program availability:* Part-time. *Degree requirements:* For master's, thesis or project. *Entrance requirements:* For master's, RN license. Additional exam requirements/recommendations for international students: Required—TOEFL (minimum score 600 paper-based). Electronic applications accepted. *Faculty research:* Pain management, ethics, corporate wellness, caring spirituality, stress.

Southern Connecticut State University, School of Graduate Studies, School of Health and Human Services, Department of Nursing, New Haven, CT 06515-1355. Offers family nurse practitioner (MSN); nursing education (MSN). *Accreditation:* AACN. *Program availability:* Part-time, evening/weekend. *Faculty:* 12 full-time (all women), 2 part-time/adjunct (both women). *Students:* 7 full-time (6 women), 80 part-time (70 women); includes 20 minority (8 Black or African American, non-Hispanic/Latino; 5 Asian, non-Hispanic/Latino; 6 Hispanic/Latino; 1 Two or more races, non-Hispanic/Latino). Average age 36. 112 applicants, 11% accepted, 11 enrolled. In 2015, 15 master's awarded. *Degree requirements:* For master's, thesis. *Entrance requirements:* For master's, GRE, MAT, interview, minimum QPA of 2.8, RN license, minimum 1 year of professional nursing experience. *Application deadline:* For fall admission, 7/15 priority date for domestic students. Applications are processed on a rolling basis. Application fee: $50. Electronic applications accepted. *Expenses:* Tuition, state resident: full-time $4968; part-time $494 per credit hour. Tuition, nonresident: full-time $16,078; part-time $509 per credit hour. *Required fees:* $4632; $55 per semester. Tuition and fees vary according to program. *Financial support:* Career-related internships or fieldwork, scholarships/grants, and unspecified assistantships available. Financial award application deadline: 4/15; financial award applicants required to submit FAFSA. *Unit head:* Dr. Lisa Rebeschi, Chairperson, 203-392-6485, E-mail: rebeschil1@southernct.edu. *Application contact:* Lisa Galvin, Director of Graduate Admissions, 203-392-5240, Fax: 203-392-5235, E-mail: galvinl1@southernct.edu.

Southern Illinois University Edwardsville, Graduate School, School of Nursing, Doctor of Nursing Practice Program, Edwardsville, IL 62026. Offers family nurse practitioner (DNP); nurse anesthesia (DNP); nursing (DNP). *Program availability:* Part-time, evening/weekend. *Students:* 37 full-time (25 women), 33 part-time (31 women); includes 14 minority (6 Black or African American, non-Hispanic/Latino; 3 Asian, non-Hispanic/Latino; 4 Hispanic/Latino; 1 Two or more races, non-Hispanic/Latino). 57 applicants, 79% accepted. In 2015, 5 doctorates awarded. *Degree requirements:* For doctorate, thesis/dissertation or alternative, project. *Entrance requirements:* Additional exam requirements/recommendations for international students: Required—TOEFL (minimum score 550 paper-based; 79 iBT), IELTS (minimum score 6.5). *Application deadline:* For fall and spring admission, 3/1 for domestic and international students; for summer admission, 3/1 for domestic and international students. Application fee: $30. Electronic applications accepted. *Expenses:* Tuition, state resident: full-time $5026; part-time $837 per course. Tuition, nonresident: full-time $12,566; part-time $2094 per course. *Required fees:* $1682; $474 per course. Tuition and fees vary according to course load, campus/location and program. *Financial support:* Institutionally sponsored loans, scholarships/grants, and unspecified assistantships available. Financial award application deadline: 3/1; financial award applicants required to submit FAFSA. *Unit head:* Dr. Kathy Ketchum, Assistant Dean for Graduate Programs, 618-650-3975, Fax: 618-650-3854, E-mail: kketchu@siue.edu. *Application contact:* Bob Skorczewski,

Family Nurse Practitioner Studies

Coordinator of International and Graduate Recruitment, 618-650-3705, Fax: 618-650-3618, E-mail: gradadmissions@siue.edu. Website: http://www.siue.edu/nursing/graduate/dnp/

Southern Illinois University Edwardsville, Graduate School, School of Nursing, Program in Family Nurse Practitioner, Edwardsville, IL 62026. Offers MS, Post-Master's Certificate. *Accreditation:* AACN. *Program availability:* Part-time, evening/weekend. *Students:* 81 part-time (74 women); includes 6 minority (2 Black or African American, non-Hispanic/Latino; 3 Asian, non-Hispanic/Latino; 1 Two or more races, non-Hispanic/Latino). In 2015, 23 master's, 1 other advanced degree awarded. *Degree requirements:* For master's, comprehensive exam. *Entrance requirements:* For master's, appropriate bachelor's degree, RN license. Additional exam requirements/recommendations for international students: Required—TOEFL (minimum score 550 paper-based; 79 iBT), IELTS (minimum score 6.5). *Application deadline:* For fall admission, 3/1 for domestic and international students. Application fee: $30. Electronic applications accepted. *Expenses:* Tuition, state resident: full-time $5026; part-time $837 per course. Tuition, nonresident: full-time $12,566; part-time $2094 per course. *Required fees:* $1682; $474 per course. Tuition and fees vary according to course load, campus/location and program. *Financial support:* In 2015–16, 2 teaching assistantships with full tuition reimbursements were awarded; fellowships with full tuition reimbursements, research assistantships, institutionally sponsored loans, scholarships/grants, and unspecified assistantships also available. Financial award application deadline: 3/1; financial award applicants required to submit FAFSA. *Unit head:* Dr. Kathy Ketchum, Associate Dean for Graduate Programs, 618-650-3936, Fax: 618-650-3864, E-mail: kketchu@siue.edu. *Application contact:* Bob Skorczewski, Coordinator of International and Graduate Recruitment, 618-650-3705, Fax: 618-650-3618, E-mail: gradadmissions@siue.edu. Website: http://www.siue.edu/nursing/graduate

Southern University and Agricultural and Mechanical College, School of Nursing, Baton Rouge, LA 70813. Offers educator/administrator (PhD); family health nursing (MSN); family nurse practitioner (Post Master's Certificate); geriatric nurse practitioner/gerontology (PhD). *Accreditation:* AACN. *Program availability:* Part-time. *Degree requirements:* For master's, comprehensive exam, thesis; for doctorate, comprehensive exam, thesis/dissertation. *Entrance requirements:* For master's, GRE General Test, BSN, minimum GPA of 2.7; for doctorate, GRE General Test; for Post Master's Certificate, MSN. Additional exam requirements/recommendations for international students: Required—TOEFL (minimum score 525 paper-based). *Faculty research:* Health promotions, vulnerable populations, (community-based) cardiovascular participating research, health disparities chronic diseases, care of the elderly.

South University, Program in Nursing, Tampa, FL 33614. Offers adult health nurse practitioner (MS); family nurse practitioner (MS); nurse educator (MS).

South University, Program in Nursing, Royal Palm Beach, FL 33411. Offers family nurse practitioner (MS).

South University, Program in Nursing, Virginia Beach, VA 23452. Offers family nurse practitioner (MSN).

Spalding University, Graduate Studies, Kosair College of Health and Natural Sciences, School of Nursing, Louisville, KY 40203-2188. Offers adult nurse practitioner (MSN, PMC); family nurse practitioner (MSN, PMC); leadership in nursing and healthcare (MSN); pediatric nurse practitioner (MSN, PMC). *Accreditation:* AACN. *Program availability:* Part-time, evening/weekend. *Faculty:* 10 full-time (9 women), 8 part-time/adjunct (7 women). *Students:* 101 full-time (94 women), 9 part-time (all women); includes 20 minority (14 Black or African American, non-Hispanic/Latino; 3 Asian, non-Hispanic/Latino; 1 Native Hawaiian or other Pacific Islander, non-Hispanic/Latino; 2 Two or more races, non-Hispanic/Latino). Average age 36. 10 applicants, 30% accepted, 2 enrolled. In 2015, 43 master's awarded. *Degree requirements:* For master's, comprehensive exam (for some programs), thesis. *Entrance requirements:* For master's, GRE General Test, BSN or bachelor's degree in related field, RN licensure, autobiographical statement, transcripts, letters of recommendation. Additional exam requirements/recommendations for international students: Required—TOEFL (minimum score 535 paper-based). *Application deadline:* For fall admission, 2/1 priority date for domestic students. Application fee: $30. *Financial support:* Career-related internships or fieldwork, scholarships/grants, and traineeships available. Support available to part-time students. Financial award application deadline: 3/30; financial award applicants required to submit FAFSA. *Faculty research:* Nurse educational administration, gerontology, bioterrorism, healthcare ethics, leadership. *Unit head:* Dr. Patricia Spurr, Chair, 502-873-4304, E-mail: pspurr@spalding.edu. *Application contact:* Dr. Pam King, Program Director, 502-873-4292, E-mail: pking@spalding.edu. Website: http://www.spalding.edu/nursing/

State University of New York Downstate Medical Center, College of Nursing, Graduate Program in Nursing, Nurse Practitioner Program, Brooklyn, NY 11203-2098. Offers MS, Post Master's Certificate. *Accreditation:* AACN. *Program availability:* Part-time. *Degree requirements:* For master's, thesis optional. *Entrance requirements:* For master's, GRE, BSN; minimum GPA of 3.0; previous undergraduate course work in statistics, health assessment, and nursing research; RN license; for Post Master's Certificate, BSN; minimum GPA of 3.0; RN license; previous undergraduate course work in statistics, health assessment, and nursing research. *Faculty research:* Women's health.

State University of New York Polytechnic Institute, Program in Family Nurse Practitioner, Utica, NY 13504-3050. Offers MS, CAS. *Accreditation:* AACN. *Program availability:* Part-time, online learning. *Degree requirements:* For master's, culminating seminar. *Entrance requirements:* For master's, minimum GPA of 3.0 in last 30 undergraduate hours, bachelor's degree in nursing, 1 year of professional experience, RN license, 2 letters of reference, resume, educational objective; for CAS, master's degree in nursing. Additional exam requirements/recommendations for international students: Required—TOEFL (minimum score 550 paper-based; 79 iBT), IELTS (minimum score 6.5). Electronic applications accepted. *Faculty research:* Adult and family healthcare, critical thinking, epidemiology, refugee and women's health, child obesity.

State University of New York Upstate Medical University, College of Nursing, Syracuse, NY 13210-2334. Offers nurse practitioner (Post Master's Certificate); nursing (MS). *Accreditation:* AACN. *Program availability:* Part-time, online learning. *Degree requirements:* For master's, thesis or alternative. *Entrance requirements:* For master's, 3 years of work experience. Electronic applications accepted.

Stony Brook University, State University of New York, Stony Brook Medicine, School of Nursing, Program in Family Nurse Practitioner, Stony Brook, NY 11794. Offers MS, DNP, Certificate. *Accreditation:* AACN. *Program availability:* Part-time, blended/hybrid learning. *Students:* 6 full-time (all women), 98 part-time (85 women); includes 44 minority (20 Black or African American, non-Hispanic/Latino; 1 American Indian or Alaska Native, non-Hispanic/Latino; 14 Asian, non-Hispanic/Latino; 9 Hispanic/Latino). 226 applicants, 43% accepted, 76 enrolled. In 2015, 6 doctorates awarded. *Degree requirements:* For master's, thesis. *Entrance requirements:* For master's, BSN, minimum GPA of 3.0, course work in statistics. Additional exam requirements/recommendations for international students: Required—TOEFL (minimum score 90 iBT). *Application deadline:* For fall admission, 1/15 for domestic students. Application fee: $100. *Expenses:* $24,781 per year full-time resident tuition and fees, $968 per credit hour; $44,431 per year full-time non-resident tuition and fees, $1,787 per credit hour. *Financial support:* Application deadline: 3/15. *Unit head:* Cheryl Meddles-Torres, Program Director, 631-444-6334, Fax: 631-444-3136, E-mail: cheryl.meddles-torres@stonybrook.edu. *Application contact:* Crystal Garcia, Staff Assistant, 631-444-3392, Fax: 631-444-3136, E-mail: crystal.garcia@stonybrook.edu. Website: http://www.nursing.stonybrookmedicine.edu/about

Stony Brook University, State University of New York, Stony Brook Medicine, School of Nursing, Program in Perinatal Women's Health Nursing, Stony Brook, NY 11794. Offers MS, DNP, Certificate. *Accreditation:* AACN. *Program availability:* Blended/hybrid learning. *Students:* 1 (woman) full-time, 21 part-time (all women); includes 4 minority (1 Black or African American, non-Hispanic/Latino; 1 American Indian or Alaska Native, non-Hispanic/Latino; 1 Asian, non-Hispanic/Latino; 1 Hispanic/Latino). In 2015, 11 master's awarded. *Degree requirements:* For master's, thesis. *Entrance requirements:* For master's, BSN, minimum GPA of 3.0, course work in statistics. Additional exam requirements/recommendations for international students: Required—TOEFL (minimum score 90 iBT). *Application deadline:* For fall admission, 1/1 for domestic students. Application fee: $100. *Expenses:* $24,781 full-time resident tuition and fees, $968 per credit hour; $44,431 full-time nonresident tuition and fees, $1,787 per credit hour. *Financial support:* Application deadline: 3/15. *Unit head:* Prof. Elizabeth Collins, Director, 631-444-3296, Fax: 631-444-3136, E-mail: elizabeth.collins@stonybrook.edu. *Application contact:* Crystal Garcia, Staff Assistant, 631-632-3392, Fax: 631-632-3136, E-mail: crystal.garcia@stonybrook.edu. Website: http://www.nursing.stonybrookmedicine.edu/

Temple University, College of Public Health, Department of Nursing, Philadelphia, PA 19122. Offers adult-gerontology primary care (DNP); family-individual across the lifespan (DNP); nursing (DNP). *Accreditation:* AACN. *Program availability:* Part-time. *Faculty:* 12 full-time (11 women), 1 (woman) part-time/adjunct. *Students:* 7 full-time (all women), 61 part-time (50 women); includes 37 minority (23 Black or African American, non-Hispanic/Latino; 8 Asian, non-Hispanic/Latino; 4 Hispanic/Latino; 2 Two or more races, non-Hispanic/Latino). 28 applicants, 64% accepted, 9 enrolled. In 2015, 8 doctorates awarded. *Degree requirements:* For doctorate, evidence-based practice project. *Entrance requirements:* For doctorate, GRE General Test or MAT, 2 letters of reference, RN license, interview, statement of purpose, resume. Additional exam requirements/recommendations for international students: Required—TOEFL (minimum score 600 paper-based; 100 iBT). *Application deadline:* For fall admission, 2/15 priority date for domestic students, 1/15 for international students; for spring admission, 10/15 for domestic students, 9/15 for international students. Applications are processed on a rolling basis. Application fee: $60. Electronic applications accepted. *Expenses:* Contact institution. *Financial support:* Federal Work-Study, scholarships/grants, traineeships, and tuition waivers available. Support available to part-time students. Financial award application deadline: 1/15. *Faculty research:* Health promotion, chronic illness, family support systems, primary care, health policy, community health services, evidence-based practice. *Unit head:* Dr. Nancy Rothman, RN, Interim Chair, 215-707-5436, E-mail: rothman@temple.edu. *Application contact:* Audrey Scriven, Academic Coordinator, Graduate Program, 215-204-4618, E-mail: tunurse@temple.edu.

Tennessee State University, The School of Graduate Studies and Research, College of Health Sciences, School of Nursing, Nashville, TN 37209-1561. Offers family nurse practitioner (MSN, Certificate); holistic nursing practitioner (MSN); holistic nursing (Certificate); nursing education (MSN, Certificate). *Accreditation:* ACEN. *Entrance requirements:* For master's, GRE General Test or MAT, BSN, current RN license, minimum GPA of 3.0. *Application deadline:* For fall admission, 4/1 priority date for domestic students. Applications are processed on a rolling basis. Application fee: $25. *Financial support:* Research assistantships and teaching assistantships available. *Unit head:* Dr. Maria Revell, 615-963-5252, E-mail: mrevell1@tnstate.edu. *Application contact:* Dr. Maria Revell, 615-963-5252, E-mail: mrevell1@tnstate.edu. Website: http://www.tnstate.edu/nursing/

Tennessee Technological University, Whitson-Hester School of Nursing, Cookeville, TN 38505. Offers family nurse practitioner (MSN); informatics (MSN); nursing administration (MSN); nursing education (MSN). *Program availability:* Part-time, evening/weekend, online learning. *Students:* 21 full-time (20 women), 95 part-time (80 women); includes 5 minority (2 Black or African American, non-Hispanic/Latino; 1 Asian, non-Hispanic/Latino; 1 Hispanic/Latino; 1 Two or more races, non-Hispanic/Latino). 42 applicants, 57% accepted, 15 enrolled. In 2015, 47 master's awarded. *Degree requirements:* For master's, comprehensive exam, thesis or alternative. *Entrance requirements:* Additional exam requirements/recommendations for international students: Required—TOEFL (minimum score 600 paper-based; 100 iBT), IELTS (minimum score 5.5), PTE, or TOEIC (Test of English as an International Communication). *Application deadline:* For fall admission, 8/1 for domestic students, 5/1 for international students; for spring admission, 12/1 for domestic students, 10/1 for international students; for summer admission, 5/1 for domestic students, 2/1 for international students. Applications are processed on a rolling basis. Application fee: $35 ($40 for international students). Electronic applications accepted. *Expenses:* Tuition, state resident: full-time $8961; part-time $6132 per credit hour. Tuition, nonresident: full-time $23,121; part-time $14,608 per credit hour. *Financial support:* Application deadline: 4/1. *Unit head:* Dr. Huey-Ming Tzeng, Dean, 931-372-3547, Fax: 931-372-6244, E-mail: htzeng@tntech.edu. *Application contact:* Shelia K. Kendrick, Coordinator of Graduate Studies, 931-372-3808, Fax: 931-372-3497, E-mail: skendrick@tntech.edu.

Texas A&M International University, Office of Graduate Studies and Research, College of Nursing and Health Sciences, Laredo, TX 78041-1900. Offers family nurse practitioner (MSN). *Accreditation:* ACEN. *Entrance requirements:* Additional exam requirements/recommendations for international students: Required—TOEFL (minimum score 550 paper-based; 79 iBT).

Texas A&M University, College of Nursing, Bryan, TX 77807. Offers family nurse practitioner (MSN); nursing education (MSN). *Faculty:* 47. *Students:* 10 full-time (8 women), 27 part-time (23 women); includes 4 minority (2 Black or African American, non-Hispanic/Latino; 1 Asian, non-Hispanic/Latino; 1 Hispanic/Latino). Average age 35. 30 applicants, 100% accepted, 30 enrolled. *Expenses:* Contact institution. *Financial support:* In 2015–16, 4 students received support. Career-related internships or fieldwork, institutionally sponsored loans, scholarships/grants, traineeships, health care benefits, tuition waivers (full and partial), and unspecified assistantships available. Support available to part-time students. Financial award applicants required to submit FAFSA. *Unit head:* Dr. Sharon A. Wilkerson, Founding Dean, 979-436-0111, Fax: 979-436-0098, E-mail: wilkerson@tamhsc.edu. *Application contact:* Jennifer Frank, Program Coordinator for Recruitment and Admission, 979-436-0110, E-mail: conadmissions@tamhsc.edu. Website: http://nursing.tamhsc.edu/

Texas A&M University–Corpus Christi, College of Graduate Studies, College of Nursing and Health Sciences, Corpus Christi, TX 78412-5503. Offers family nurse practitioner (MSN); leadership in nursing systems (MSN); nurse educator (MSN). *Accreditation:* AACN. *Program availability:* Part-time, evening/weekend, online only, 100% online. *Students:* 12 full-time (11 women), 375 part-time (322 women); includes

200 minority (20 Black or African American, non-Hispanic/Latino; 1 American Indian or Alaska Native, non-Hispanic/Latino; 27 Asian, non-Hispanic/Latino; 142 Hispanic/Latino; 3 Native Hawaiian or other Pacific Islander, non-Hispanic/Latino; 7 Two or more races, non-Hispanic/Latino), 1 international. Average age 38. 337 applicants, 42% accepted, 128 enrolled. In 2015, 102 master's awarded. *Degree requirements:* For master's, comprehensive exam, thesis (for some programs), capstone - clinical. *Entrance requirements:* For master's, essay, resume, 3 letters of recommendation, minimum GPA of 3.0. Additional exam requirements/recommendations for international students: Required—TOEFL (minimum score 550 paper-based; 79 iBT), IELTS (minimum score 6.5). *Application deadline:* For fall admission, 4/15 priority date for domestic and international students; for spring admission, 1/7 for domestic and international students; for summer admission, 5/27 for domestic and international students. Applications are processed on a rolling basis. Application fee: $50 ($70 for international students). Electronic applications accepted. *Financial support:* Research assistantships, teaching assistantships, career-related internships or fieldwork, Federal Work-Study, institutionally sponsored loans, scholarships/grants, health care benefits, and unspecified assistantships available. Support available to part-time students. Financial award application deadline: 3/15; financial award applicants required to submit FAFSA. *Unit head:* Dr. Mary Jane Hamilton, Dean, 361-825-2469, E-mail: mary.hamilton@tamucc.edu. *Application contact:* Graduate Admissions Coordinator, 361-825-2177, Fax: 361-825-2755, E-mail: gradweb@tamucc.edu.
Website: http://conhs.tamucc.edu/

Texas State University, The Graduate College, College of Health Professions, Family Nurse Practitioner Program, San Marcos, TX 78666. Offers MS. *Accreditation:* CAHME. *Program availability:* Part-time, evening/weekend. *Faculty:* 9 full-time (all women), 3 part-time/adjunct (all women). *Students:* 68 full-time (60 women), 1 (woman) part-time; includes 26 minority (7 Black or African American, non-Hispanic/Latino; 2 American Indian or Alaska Native, non-Hispanic/Latino; 7 Asian, non-Hispanic/Latino; 10 Hispanic/Latino), 1 international. Average age 33. 141 applicants, 38% accepted, 36 enrolled. In 2015, 25 master's awarded. *Degree requirements:* For master's, comprehensive exam, thesis optional. *Entrance requirements:* For master's, BSN from institution accredited by nationally-recognized nursing education accrediting body (i.e., NLNAC, CCNE) with minimum GPA of 3.0 in nursing courses and last 60 hours of undergraduate course work; current valid unencumbered RN license or multi-state privilege to practice as a registered nurse. Additional exam requirements/recommendations for international students: Required—TOEFL (minimum score 550 paper-based; 78 iBT). *Application deadline:* For fall admission, 2/15 priority date for domestic and international students. Applications are processed on a rolling basis. Application fee: $40 ($90 for international students). Electronic applications accepted. *Expenses:* $3,615 in-state tuition (for 12 semester credit hours/1 full-time semester), $974 in-state fees. *Financial support:* In 2015–16, 11 students received support. Research assistantships, teaching assistantships, career-related internships or fieldwork, Federal Work-Study, institutionally sponsored loans, scholarships/grants, and unspecified assistantships available. Support available to part-time students. Financial award application deadline: 3/1; financial award applicants required to submit FAFSA. *Faculty research:* Nursing and allied health. *Total annual research expenditures:* $119,782. *Unit head:* Dr. Shirley Levenson, Program Director, 512-716-2957, Fax: 512-716-2911, E-mail: sal111@txstate.edu. *Application contact:* Dr. Andrea Golato, Dean of Graduate School, 512-245-2581, Fax: 512-245-8365, E-mail: gradcollege@txstate.edu.
Website: http://www.health.txstate.edu/hsr

Texas Tech University Health Sciences Center, School of Nursing, Lubbock, TX 79430. Offers acute care nurse practitioner (MSN, Certificate); administration (MSN); advanced practice (DNP); education (MSN); executive leadership (DNP); family nurse practitioner (MSN, Certificate); geriatric nurse practitioner (MSN, Certificate); pediatric nurse practitioner (MSN, Certificate). *Accreditation:* AACN. *Program availability:* Part-time, online learning. *Degree requirements:* For master's, thesis optional. *Entrance requirements:* For master's, minimum GPA of 3.0, 3 letters of reference, BSN, RN license; for Certificate, minimum GPA of 3.0, 3 letters of reference, RN license. Additional exam requirements/recommendations for international students: Required—TOEFL (minimum score 550 paper-based). *Faculty research:* Diabetes/obesity, nurse competency, disease management, intervention and measurements, health disparities.

Texas Woman's University, Graduate School, College of Nursing, Denton, TX 76204-5498. Offers acute care nurse practitioner (MS); adult health clinical nurse specialist (MS); adult health nurse practitioner (MS); child health clinical nurse specialist (MS); clinical nurse leader (MS); family nurse practitioner (MS); health systems management (MS); nursing education (MS); nursing practice (DNP); nursing science (PhD); pediatric nurse practitioner (MS); women's health clinical nurse specialist (MS); women's health nurse practitioner (MS). *Accreditation:* AACN. *Program availability:* Part-time, online learning. *Faculty:* 55 full-time (51 women), 42 part-time/adjunct (35 women). *Students:* 39 full-time (37 women), 958 part-time (888 women); includes 566 minority (226 Black or African American, non-Hispanic/Latino; 8 American Indian or Alaska Native, non-Hispanic/Latino; 221 Asian, non-Hispanic/Latino; 88 Hispanic/Latino; 3 Native Hawaiian or other Pacific Islander, non-Hispanic/Latino; 20 Two or more races, non-Hispanic/Latino), 37 international. Average age 36. 430 applicants, 65% accepted, 193 enrolled. In 2015, 248 master's, 10 doctorates awarded. *Degree requirements:* For master's, comprehensive exam, thesis or alternative; for doctorate, comprehensive exam, thesis/dissertation. *Entrance requirements:* For master's, GRE or MAT, minimum GPA of 3.0 on last 60 hours in undergraduate nursing degree and overall, RN license, BS in nursing, basic statistics course; for doctorate, GRE (preferred minimum score 153 [500 old version] Verbal, 144 [500 old version] Quantitative, 4 Analytical), MS in nursing, minimum preferred GPA of 3.5, RN license, statistics, 2 letters of reference, curriculum vitae, graduate nursing-theory course, graduate research course, statement of professional goals and research interests. Additional exam requirements/recommendations for international students: Required—TOEFL (minimum score 550 paper-based; 79 iBT). *Application deadline:* For fall admission, 5/1 priority date for domestic students, 3/1 for international students; for spring admission, 9/15 priority date for domestic students, 7/1 for international students. Applications are processed on a rolling basis. Application fee: $50 ($75 for international students). Electronic applications accepted. *Expenses:* Tuition, state resident: full-time $4380; part-time $243 per credit hour. Tuition, nonresident: full-time $11,400; part-time $633 per credit hour. *International tuition:* $11,465 full-time. *Required fees:* $1778; $99 per credit hour. $283 per semester. One-time fee: $50. Tuition and fees vary according to course load and program. *Financial support:* In 2015–16, 149 students received support, including 10 research assistantships (averaging $5,600 per year), 1 teaching assistantship (averaging $5,600 per year); career-related internships or fieldwork, Federal Work-Study, institutionally sponsored loans, scholarships/grants, traineeships, health care benefits, and unspecified assistantships also available. Support available to part-time students. Financial award application deadline: 3/1; financial award applicants required to submit FAFSA. *Faculty research:* Screening, prevention, and treatment for intimate partner violence; needs of adolescents during childbirth intervention; a network analysis decision tool for nurse managers (social network analysis); support for adolescents with implantable cardioverter defibrillators; informatics: nurse staffing, safety, quality, and financial data as they relate to patient care outcomes; prevention and treatment of obesity; improving infant outcomes related to premature birth. *Total annual research*

expenditures: $1.7 million. *Unit head:* Dr. Anita G. Hufft, Dean, 940-898-2401, Fax: 940-898-2437, E-mail: nursing@twu.edu. *Application contact:* Dr. Samuel Wheeler, Assistant Director of Admissions, 940-898-3188, Fax: 940-898-3081, E-mail: wheelersr@twu.edu.
Website: http://www.twu.edu/nursing/

Troy University, Graduate School, College of Health and Human Services, Program in Nursing, Troy, AL 36082. Offers adult health (MSN); clinical nurse specialist adult health (DNP); clinical nurse specialist maternal infant (DNP); family nurse practitioner (MSN, DNP, PMC); informatics specialist (MSN); maternal infant (MSN). *Accreditation:* ACEN. *Program availability:* Part-time, evening/weekend. *Faculty:* 13 full-time (12 women), 11 part-time/adjunct (all women). *Students:* 75 full-time (62 women), 202 part-time (179 women); includes 91 minority (72 Black or African American, non-Hispanic/Latino; 1 Asian, non-Hispanic/Latino; 8 Hispanic/Latino; 10 Two or more races, non-Hispanic/Latino). Average age 34. 50 applicants, 96% accepted. In 2015, 43 master's, 13 doctorates, 15 other advanced degrees awarded. *Degree requirements:* For master's, comprehensive exam, minimum GPA of 3.0, candidacy; for doctorate, minimum GPA of 3.0, submission of approved comprehensive e-portfolio, completion of residency synthesis project, minimum of 1000 hours of clinical practice, qualifying exam. *Entrance requirements:* For master's, GRE (minimum score of 850 on old exam or 290 on new exam) or MAT (minimum score of 396), minimum GPA of 3.0, BSN, current RN licensure, 2 letters of reference, undergraduate health assessment course; for doctorate, GRE (minimum score of 850 on old exam or 294 on new exam), BSN or MSN, minimum GPA of 3.0, 2 letters of reference, current RN licensure, essay. Additional exam requirements/recommendations for international students: Required—TOEFL (minimum score 523 paper-based; 70 iBT), IELTS (minimum score 6). *Application deadline:* Applications are processed on a rolling basis. Application fee: $50. Electronic applications accepted. *Expenses:* Tuition, state resident: full-time $7146; part-time $397 per credit hour. Tuition, nonresident: full-time $14,292; part-time $794 per credit hour. *Required fees:* $802. Tuition and fees vary according to campus/location and program. *Financial support:* Fellowships, career-related internships or fieldwork, and scholarships/grants available. Support available to part-time students. Financial award applicants required to submit FAFSA. *Unit head:* Dr. Diane Weed, Director, School of Nursing, 334-670-5864, Fax: 334-670-3745, E-mail: lweed@troy.edu. *Application contact:* Crystal G. Bishop, Director of Graduate Admissions, School of Nursing, 334-241-8631, E-mail: cdgodwin@troy.edu.

Uniformed Services University of the Health Sciences, Daniel K. Inouye Graduate School of Nursing, Bethesda, MD 20814. Offers adult-gerontology clinical nurse specialist (MSN, DNP); family nurse practitioner (DNP); nurse anesthesia (DNP); nursing science (PhD); psychiatric mental health nurse practitioner (DNP); women's health nurse practitioner (DNP). MSN and DNP programs available to military officers only; PhD to military and DoD students only. *Accreditation:* AACN; AANA/CANAEP. *Faculty:* 38 full-time (22 women), 2 part-time/adjunct (1 woman). *Students:* 51 full-time (29 women); includes 17 minority (8 Black or African American, non-Hispanic/Latino; 4 Asian, non-Hispanic/Latino; 4 Hispanic/Latino; 1 Two or more races, non-Hispanic/Latino). Average age 34. 75 applicants, 68% accepted, 51 enrolled. In 2015, 4 master's, 24 doctorates awarded. *Degree requirements:* For master's, thesis or alternative; for doctorate, thesis/dissertation or alternative. *Entrance requirements:* For master's, GRE, BSN, clinical experience, minimum GPA of 3.0, previous course work in science; for doctorate, GRE, BSN, clinical experience, minimum GPA of 3.0, previous course work in sciences, and writing paper (for DNP); MSN (for PhD). *Application deadline:* For fall admission, 7/1 for domestic students; for winter admission, 2/15 for domestic students. Application fee: $0. Electronic applications accepted. *Faculty research:* Prenatal care, military health care, military readiness, distance learning. *Unit head:* Dr. Diane C. Seibert, Associate Dean for Academic Affairs, 301-295-1080, Fax: 301-295-1707, E-mail: diane.seibert@usuhs.edu. *Application contact:* Terry Lynn Malavakis, Recording Secretary for Admissions Committee/Registrar/Program Analyst, 301-295-1055, Fax: 301-295-1707, E-mail: terry.malavkis@usuhs.edu.
Website: http://www.usuhs.edu/gsn/

Union University, School of Nursing, Jackson, TN 38305-3697. Offers executive leadership (DNP); nurse anesthesia (DNP); nurse practitioner (DNP); nursing education (MSN, PMC). *Accreditation:* AACN; AANA/CANAEP. *Degree requirements:* For master's, thesis or alternative. *Entrance requirements:* For master's, GRE, 3 letters of reference, bachelor's degree in nursing, minimum GPA of 3.0. Additional exam requirements/recommendations for international students: Required—TOEFL (minimum score 560 paper-based). Electronic applications accepted. *Faculty research:* Children's health, occupational rehabilitation, informatics, health promotion.

United States University, Family Nurse Practitioner Program, Chula Vista, CA 91911. Offers MSN. *Degree requirements:* For master's, project. *Entrance requirements:* For master's, RN license, minimum cumulative undergraduate GPA of 2.5, background check, official transcripts, personal goal statement. Additional exam requirements/recommendations for international students: Required—TOEFL (minimum score 550 paper-based; 80 iBT).

Universidad del Turabo, Graduate Programs, School of Health Sciences, Programs in Nursing, Program in Family Nurse Practitioner, Gurabo, PR 00778-3030. Offers MSN.

University at Buffalo, the State University of New York, Graduate School, School of Nursing, Buffalo, NY 14214. Offers adult gerontology nurse practitioner (DNP); family nurse practitioner (DNP); health care systems and leadership (MS); nurse anesthetist (DNP); nursing (PhD); nursing education (Certificate); psychiatric/mental health nurse practitioner (DNP). *Accreditation:* AACN; AANA/CANAEP (one or more programs are accredited). *Program availability:* Part-time, 100% online. *Students:* 61 full-time (37 women), 137 part-time (114 women); includes 35 minority (17 Black or African American, non-Hispanic/Latino; 1 American Indian or Alaska Native, non-Hispanic/Latino; 17 Asian, non-Hispanic/Latino), 7 international. Average age 32. 193 applicants, 49% accepted, 75 enrolled. In 2015, 6 master's, 37 doctorates awarded. *Degree requirements:* For master's, thesis optional; for doctorate, comprehensive exam (for some programs), capstone (for DNP), dissertation (for PhD). *Entrance requirements:* For master's, GRE or MAT; for doctorate, GRE or MAT, minimum GPA of 3.0 (for DNP), 3.25 (for PhD); RN license; BS or MS in nursing; 3 references; writing sample; resume; personal statement; for Certificate, interview, minimum GPA of 3.0 or GRE General Test, RN license, MS in nursing, professional certification. Additional exam requirements/recommendations for international students: Required—TOEFL (minimum score 550 paper-based; 79 iBT), IELTS (minimum score 6.5). *Application deadline:* For fall admission, 7/1 for domestic students, 2/1 for international students; for spring admission, 12/1 for domestic students, 10/1 for international students; for summer admission, 2/1 for domestic students. Applications are processed on a rolling basis. Application fee: $75. Electronic applications accepted. *Financial support:* In 2015–16, 80 students received support, including 2 fellowships with tuition reimbursements available (averaging $17,000 per year), 4 research assistantships with tuition reimbursements available (averaging $10,600 per year), 7 teaching assistantships with tuition reimbursements available (averaging $10,600 per year); scholarships/grants, traineeships, health care benefits, and unspecified assistantships also available. Financial award application deadline: 2/1; financial award applicants required to submit FAFSA. *Faculty research:* Oncology, palliative care, gerontology, addictions, mental

Family Nurse Practitioner Studies

health, community wellness, sleep, workforce, care of underserved populations, quality and safety, person-centered care, adolescent health. *Total annual research expenditures:* $1.4 million. *Unit head:* Dr. Marsha L. Lewis, Dean and Professor, 716-829-2533, Fax: 716-829-2566, E-mail: ubnursingdean@buffalo.edu. *Application contact:* Jennifer H. VanLaeken, Director of Graduate Student Services, 716-829-3311, Fax: 716-829-2067, E-mail: jhv2@buffalo.edu.
Website: http://nursing.buffalo.edu/

The University of Alabama in Huntsville, School of Graduate Studies, College of Nursing, Huntsville, AL 35899. Offers family nurse practitioner (Certificate); nursing (MSN, DNP), including adult-gerontology acute care nurse practitioner (MSN), adult-gerontology clinical nurse specialist (MSN), family nurse practitioner (MSN), leadership in health care systems (MSN); nursing education (Certificate). DNP offered jointly with The University of Alabama at Birmingham. *Accreditation:* AACN. *Program availability:* Part-time, evening/weekend, online learning. *Degree requirements:* For master's, comprehensive exam, thesis or alternative, oral and written exams. *Entrance requirements:* For master's, MAT or GRE, Alabama RN license, BSN, minimum GPA of 3.0; for doctorate, master's degree in nursing in an advanced practice area; for Certificate, MAT or GRE, minimum GPA of 3.0. Additional exam requirements/recommendations for international students: Required—TOEFL (minimum score 500 paper-based; 80 iBT), IELTS (minimum score 6.5). *Application deadline:* For fall admission, 7/15 for domestic students, 4/1 for international students; for spring admission, 11/30 for domestic students, 9/1 for international students. Applications are processed on a rolling basis. Application fee: $50. Electronic applications accepted. *Expenses: Tuition, area resident:* Full-time $9548; part-time $547 per credit hour. Tuition, state resident: full-time $9548; part-time $547 per credit hour. Tuition, nonresident: full-time $21,402; part-time $1224 per credit hour. *International tuition:* $21,402 full-time. *Financial support:* Teaching assistantships with full tuition reimbursements, career-related internships or fieldwork, Federal Work-Study, institutionally sponsored loans, scholarships/grants, traineeships, health care benefits, and unspecified assistantships available. Support available to part-time students. Financial award application deadline: 4/1; financial award applicants required to submit FAFSA. *Faculty research:* Health care informatics, chronic illness management, maternal and child health, genetics/genomics, technology and health care. *Unit head:* Dr. Marsha Adams, Dean, 256-824-6345, Fax: 256-824-6026, E-mail: marsha.adams@uah.edu. *Application contact:* Charles Davis, Director of Graduate Admission and Advisement, 256-824-6669, Fax: 256-824-6026, E-mail: charles.davis@uah.edu.
Website: http://www.uah.edu/nursing

The University of Arizona, College of Nursing, Tucson, AZ 85721. Offers health care informatics (Certificate); nurse practitioner (MS); nursing (DNP, PhD). *Accreditation:* AACN. *Program availability:* Part-time, online learning. Terminal master's awarded for partial completion of doctoral program. *Degree requirements:* For master's, thesis optional; for doctorate, comprehensive exam, thesis/dissertation. *Entrance requirements:* For master's, BSN, eligibility for RN license; for doctorate, BSN; for Certificate, GRE General Test, Arizona RN license, BSN, minimum GPA of 3.0. Additional exam requirements/recommendations for international students: Required—TOEFL (minimum score 550 paper-based; 79 iBT). *Application deadline:* For fall admission, 1/15 for domestic and international students. Applications are processed on a rolling basis. Application fee: $75. Electronic applications accepted. *Expenses:* Contact institution. *Financial support:* Research assistantships, teaching assistantships, career-related internships or fieldwork, institutionally sponsored loans, scholarships/grants, traineeships, health care benefits, tuition waivers (full), and unspecified assistantships available. Financial award application deadline: 6/1. *Faculty research:* Vulnerable populations, injury mechanisms and biobehavioral responses, health care systems, informatics, rural health. *Unit head:* Dr. Joan Shaver, Dean, 520-626-7124, Fax: 520-626-6424, E-mail: cmurdaugh@nursing.arizona.edu. *Application contact:* Dr. Joan Shaver, Dean, 520-626-7124, Fax: 520-626-6424, E-mail: cmurdaugh@nursing.arizona.edu.
Website: http://www.nursing.arizona.edu/

University of Central Arkansas, Graduate School, College of Health and Behavioral Sciences, Department of Nursing, Conway, AR 72035-0001. Offers adult nurse practitioner (PMC); clinical nurse leader (PMC); clinical nurse specialist (MSN); family nurse practitioner (PMC); nurse educator (PMC); nurse practitioner (MSN). *Accreditation:* AACN. *Program availability:* Part-time, evening/weekend, online learning. *Degree requirements:* For master's, comprehensive exam, thesis optional, clinicals. *Entrance requirements:* For master's, GRE General Test, minimum GPA of 2.7. Additional exam requirements/recommendations for international students: Required—TOEFL (minimum score 550 paper-based; 80 iBT). Electronic applications accepted. *Expenses:* Contact institution.

University of Colorado Denver, College of Nursing, Aurora, CO 80045. Offers adult clinical nurse specialist (MS); adult nurse practitioner (MS); family nurse practitioner (MS); family psychiatric mental health nurse practitioner (MS); health care informatics (MS); nurse-midwifery (MS); nursing (DNP, PhD); nursing leadership and health care systems (MS); pediatric nurse practitioner (MS); special studies (MS); women's health (MS); MS/PhD. *Accreditation:* ACNM/ACME (one or more programs are accredited). *Program availability:* Part-time, evening/weekend, online learning. *Faculty:* 109 full-time (100 women), 55 part-time/adjunct (50 women). *Students:* 367 full-time (332 women), 141 part-time (118 women); includes 79 minority (16 Black or African American, non-Hispanic/Latino; 2 American Indian or Alaska Native, non-Hispanic/Latino; 8 Asian, non-Hispanic/Latino; 37 Hispanic/Latino; 16 Two or more races, non-Hispanic/Latino), 6 international. Average age 36. 321 applicants, 53% accepted, 145 enrolled. In 2015, 151 master's, 36 doctorates awarded. Terminal master's awarded for partial completion of doctoral program. *Degree requirements:* For master's, thesis optional; for doctorate, comprehensive exam, thesis/dissertation, 42 credits of coursework. *Entrance requirements:* For master's, GRE if cumulative undergraduate GPA is less than 3.0, undergraduate nursing degree from NLNAC- or CCNE-accredited school or university; completion of research and statistics courses with minimum grade of C; copy of current and unencumbered nursing license; for doctorate, GRE, bachelor's and/or master's degrees in nursing from NLN- or CCNE-accredited institution; portfolio; minimum undergraduate GPA of 3.0, graduate 3.5; graduate-level intermediate statistics and master's-level nursing theory courses with minimum B grade; interview. Additional exam requirements/recommendations for international students: Required—TOEFL (minimum score 560 paper-based; 83 iBT). *Application deadline:* For fall admission, 2/15 for domestic students, 1/15 for international students; for spring admission, 7/1 for domestic students, 6/1 for international students. Application fee: $50 ($75 for international students). Electronic applications accepted. *Expenses:* Contact institution. *Financial support:* In 2015–16, 148 students received support. Fellowships, research assistantships, teaching assistantships, Federal Work-Study, institutionally sponsored loans, scholarships/grants, traineeships, and unspecified assistantships available. Support available to part-time students. Financial award application deadline: 4/1; financial award applicants required to submit FAFSA. *Faculty research:* Biological and behavioral phenomena in pregnancy and postpartum; patterns of glycaemia during the insulin resistance of pregnancy; obesity, gestational diabetes, and relationship to neonatal adiposity; men's awareness and knowledge of male breast cancer; cognitive-behavioral therapy for chronic insomnia after breast cancer treatment; massage therapy

for the treatment of tension-type headaches. *Total annual research expenditures:* $5.9 million. *Unit head:* Dr. Sarah Thompson, Dean, 303-724-1679, E-mail: sarah.a.thompson@ucdenver.edu. *Application contact:* Judy Campbell, Graduate Programs Coordinator, 303-724-8503, E-mail: judy.campbell@ucdenver.edu.
Website: http://www.ucdenver.edu/academics/colleges/nursing/Pages/default.aspx

University of Delaware, College of Health Sciences, School of Nursing, Newark, DE 19716. Offers adult nurse practitioner (MSN, PMC); cardiopulmonary clinical nurse specialist (MSN, PMC); cardiopulmonary clinical nurse specialist/adult nurse practitioner (MSN, PMC); family nurse practitioner (MSN, PMC); gerontology clinical nurse specialist (MSN, PMC); gerontology clinical nurse specialist geriatric nurse practitioner (PMC); gerontology clinical nurse specialist/geriatric nurse practitioner (MSN); health services administration (MSN, PMC); nursing of children clinical nurse specialist (MSN, PMC); nursing of children clinical nurse specialist/pediatric nurse practitioner (MSN, PMC); oncology/immune deficiency clinical nurse specialist (MSN, PMC); oncology/immune deficiency clinical nurse specialist/adult nurse practitioner (MSN, PMC); perinatal/women's health clinical nurse specialist (MSN, PMC); perinatal/women's health clinical nurse specialist/women's health nurse practitioner (MSN, PMC); psychiatric nursing clinical nurse specialist (MSN, PMC). *Accreditation:* AACN. *Program availability:* Part-time, evening/weekend, online learning. *Degree requirements:* For master's, thesis optional. *Entrance requirements:* For master's, BSN, interview, RN license. Electronic applications accepted. *Faculty research:* Marriage and chronic illness, health promotion, congestive heart failure patient outcomes, school nursing, diabetes in children, culture, health disparities, cardiovascular, prison nursing, oncology, public policy, child obesity, smoking and teen pregnancy, blood pressure measurements, men's health.

University of Detroit Mercy, College of Health Professions, Detroit, MI 48221. Offers clinical nurse leader (MSN); family nurse practitioner (MSN); health services administration (MHSA); health systems management (MSN); nurse anesthesia (MS); nursing (DNP); nursing education (MSN, Certificate); nursing leadership and financial management (Certificate); outcomes performance management (Certificate); physician assistant (MS). *Entrance requirements:* For master's, GRE General Test, minimum GPA of 3.0. Application fee: $30 ($50 for international students). *Expenses: Tuition, area resident:* Full-time $26,802; part-time $1489 per credit. Tuition and fees vary according to course load and program. *Financial support:* Institutionally sponsored loans and tuition waivers (partial) available. Support available to part-time students. Financial award applicants required to submit FAFSA. *Faculty research:* Research design, respiratory physiology, AIDS prevention, adolescent health, community, low income health education. *Unit head:* Dr. Christine M. Pacini, RN, Dean, 313-993-6055, Fax: 313-993-6175.
Website: http://healthprofessions.udmercy.edu/

University of Hawaii at Manoa, Graduate Division, School of Nursing and Dental Hygiene, Honolulu, HI 96822. Offers clinical nurse specialist (MS), including adult health, community mental health; nurse practitioner (MS), including adult health, community mental health, family nurse practitioner; nursing (PhD, Graduate Certificate); nursing administration (MS). *Accreditation:* AACN. *Program availability:* Part-time, online learning. *Faculty:* 32 full-time (27 women), 22 part-time/adjunct (11 women). *Students:* 167 full-time (145 women), 118 part-time (104 women); includes 128 minority (3 Black or African American, non-Hispanic/Latino; 1 American Indian or Alaska Native, non-Hispanic/Latino; 57 Asian, non-Hispanic/Latino; 14 Hispanic/Latino; 4 Native Hawaiian or other Pacific Islander, non-Hispanic/Latino; 49 Two or more races, non-Hispanic/Latino), 2 international. Average age 41. 253 applicants, 42% accepted, 88 enrolled. In 2015, 20 master's, 8 doctorates awarded. *Degree requirements:* For master's, thesis optional; for doctorate, comprehensive exam, thesis/dissertation. *Entrance requirements:* For master's, Hawaii RN license. Additional exam requirements/recommendations for international students: Required—TOEFL (minimum score 580 paper-based; 92 iBT), IELTS (minimum score 5). *Application deadline:* For fall admission, 2/1 for domestic and international students. Application fee: $100. *Expenses:* Contact institution. *Financial support:* In 2015–16, 78 fellowships (averaging $1,277 per year), 3 research assistantships (averaging $16,824 per year), 2 teaching assistantships (averaging $14,382 per year) were awarded. *Total annual research expenditures:* $1.8 million. *Unit head:* Mary Boland, Dean, 808-956-8522, Fax: 808-956-3257, E-mail: mgboland@hawaii.edu. *Application contact:* Maureen Shannon, Graduate Chair, 808-956-5201, Fax: 808-956-3257, E-mail: maureens@hawaii.edu.
Website: http://www.hawaii.edu/graduatestudies/fields/html/departments/mno/nursing/nursing.htm

University of Houston, School of Nursing, Houston, TX 77204. Offers family nurse practitioner (MSN); nursing administration (MSN); nursing education (MSN). *Accreditation:* AACN. *Entrance requirements:* For master's, GRE or MAT, minimum GPA of 3.0 in last 60 hours of academic course work, valid Texas RN licensure, 2 letters of recommendation. Electronic applications accepted.

University of Illinois at Chicago, College of Nursing, Program in Nursing, Chicago, IL 60607-7128. Offers acute care clinical nurse specialist (MS); administrative nursing leadership (Certificate); adult nurse practitioner (MS); adult/geriatric nurse practitioner (MS); advanced community health nurse specialist (MS); family nurse practitioner (MS); geriatric clinical nurse specialist (MS); geriatric nurse practitioner (MS); nurse midwifery (MS); occupational health/advanced community health nurse specialist (MS); occupational health/family nurse practitioner (MS); pediatric nurse practitioner (MS); perinatal clinical nurse specialist (MS); school/advanced community health nurse specialist (MS); school/family nurse practitioner (MS); women's health nurse practitioner (MS). *Accreditation:* AACN. *Program availability:* Part-time. *Faculty:* 100 full-time (93 women), 89 part-time/adjunct (82 women). *Students:* 359 full-time (326 women), 280 part-time (249 women); includes 169 minority (43 Black or African American, non-Hispanic/Latino; 62 Asian, non-Hispanic/Latino; 56 Hispanic/Latino; 1 Native Hawaiian or other Pacific Islander, non-Hispanic/Latino; 7 Two or more races, non-Hispanic/Latino), 12 international. Average age 32. In 2015, 4 other advanced degrees awarded. *Degree requirements:* For master's, thesis or alternative. *Entrance requirements:* For master's, GRE General Test, minimum GPA of 2.75. Additional exam requirements/recommendations for international students: Required—TOEFL. *Application deadline:* For fall admission, 5/15 for domestic students, 2/15 for international students; for spring admission, 11/1 for domestic students, 7/15 for international students. Applications are processed on a rolling basis. Application fee: $60. Electronic applications accepted. *Expenses:* Tuition, state resident: full-time $11,480; part-time $3826 per credit. Tuition, nonresident: full-time $23,720; part-time $7906 per credit. *Required fees:* $1333 per semester. Part time tuition and fees vary according to course load and program. *Financial support:* Fellowships with full tuition reimbursements, research assistantships with full tuition reimbursements, teaching assistantships with full tuition reimbursements, career-related internships or fieldwork, Federal Work-Study, institutionally sponsored loans, scholarships/grants, traineeships, tuition waivers (full and partial), and unspecified assistantships available. Support available to part-time students. Financial award application deadline: 3/1; financial award applicants required to submit FAFSA. *Unit head:* Dr. Terri E. Weaver, Dean, 312-996-7808, E-mail: teweaver@uic.edu. *Application contact:* Receptionist, 312-413-2550, E-mail: gradcoll@uic.edu.
Website: http://www.nursing.uic.edu/academics-admissions/master-science#program-overview

University of Indianapolis, Graduate Programs, School of Nursing, Indianapolis, IN 46227-3697. Offers advanced practice nursing (DNP); family nurse practitioner (MSN); gerontological nurse practitioner (MSN); neonatal nurse practitioner (MSN); nurse-midwifery (MSN); nursing (MSN); nursing and health systems leadership (MSN); nursing education (MSN); women's health nurse practitioner (MSN); MBA/MSN. *Accreditation:* AACN; ACNM. *Entrance requirements:* For master's, minimum GPA of 3.0, interview, letters of recommendation, resume, IN nursing license, 1 year of professional practice; for doctorate, graduate of NLNAC- or CCNE-accredited nursing program; MSN or MA with nursing major and minimum cumulative GPA of 3.25; unencumbered RN license with eligibility for licensure in Indiana; completion of graduate-level statistics course within last 5 years with minimum grade of B; resume; essay; official transcripts from all academic institutions. Additional exam requirements/recommendations for international students: Required—TOEFL (minimum score 550 paper-based). Electronic applications accepted.

University of Louisville, Graduate School, School of Nursing, Louisville, KY 40202. Offers adult gerontology nurse practitioner (MSN, DNP); education and administration (MSN); family nurse practitioner (MSN, DNP); neonatal nurse practitioner (MSN, DNP); nursing research (PhD); psychiatric/mental health nurse practitioner (MSN, DNP); women's health nurse practitioner (MSN). *Accreditation:* AACN. *Program availability:* Part-time. *Faculty:* 53 full-time (48 women), 27 part-time/adjunct (23 women). *Students:* 110 full-time (99 women), 33 part-time (29 women); includes 17 minority (11 Black or African American, non-Hispanic/Latino; 1 Asian, non-Hispanic/Latino; 2 Hispanic/Latino; 3 Two or more races, non-Hispanic/Latino), 5 international. Average age 34. 62 applicants, 68% accepted, 40 enrolled. In 2015, 41 master's awarded. *Degree requirements:* For doctorate, comprehensive exam (for some programs), thesis/dissertation (for some programs). *Entrance requirements:* For master's, bachelor's degree in nursing, minimum GPA of 3.0, RN license; for doctorate, GRE General Test (for PhD), 3 letters of professional reference. Additional exam requirements/recommendations for international students: Required—TOEFL (minimum score 560 paper-based; 79 iBT). *Application deadline:* For fall admission, 3/1 priority date for domestic students, 3/1 for international students. Applications are processed on a rolling basis. Application fee: $60. Electronic applications accepted. *Expenses:* Tuition, state resident: full-time $11,664; part-time $649 per credit hour. Tuition, nonresident: full-time $24,274; part-time $1350 per credit hour. *Required fees:* $196. Tuition and fees vary according to program and reciprocity agreements. *Financial support:* In 2015–16, 722,568 students received support, including 10 research assistantships with full tuition reimbursements available (averaging $20,000 per year), 2 teaching assistantships with full tuition reimbursements available (averaging $15,000 per year); fellowships with full tuition reimbursements available, scholarships/grants, and unspecified assistantships also available. Financial award application deadline: 2/15; financial award applicants required to submit FAFSA. *Faculty research:* Children and adolescents with chronic illnesses, women's mental health and parenting, asthma and environmental health, type 2 diabetes self-management in adults, health disparities and community engagement. *Total annual research expenditures:* $722,568. *Unit head:* Dr. Marcia J. Hern, Dean, 502-852-8300, Fax: 502-852-8783, E-mail: m.hern@louisville.edu. *Application contact:* Trish Hart, Assistant Dean for Student Affairs, 502-852-5825, Fax: 502-852-8783, E-mail: trish.hart@louisville.edu.
Website: http://www.louisville.edu/nursing/

University of Maine, Graduate School, College of Natural Sciences, Forestry, and Agriculture, School of Nursing, Orono, ME 04469. Offers individualized (MS); nursing education (CGS); rural health family nurse practitioner (MS, CAS). *Accreditation:* AACN. *Faculty:* 6 full-time (all women), 3 part-time/adjunct (1 woman). *Students:* 12 full-time (10 women), 3 part-time (all women); includes 2 minority (1 American Indian or Alaska Native, non-Hispanic/Latino; 1 Hispanic/Latino). Average age 41. 7 applicants, 43% accepted, 2 enrolled. In 2015, 7 master's, 1 other advanced degree awarded. *Entrance requirements:* For master's, GRE General Test; for other advanced degree, master's degree. Additional exam requirements/recommendations for international students: Required—TOEFL. *Application deadline:* For fall admission, 2/1 for domestic students. Applications are processed on a rolling basis. Application fee: $65. Electronic applications accepted. *Financial support:* In 2015–16, 1 student received support. Career-related internships or fieldwork, Federal Work-Study, institutionally sponsored loans, tuition waivers (full and partial), and unspecified assistantships available. Support available to part-time students. Financial award application deadline: 3/1. *Faculty research:* Work experiences of chief nursing officers, fatigue related to radiation therapy in oncology patients, patients' perceptions of nurses' caring behaviors, health disparities of rural Maine older women. *Unit head:* Dr. Nancy Fishwick, Director, 207-581-2505, Fax: 207-581-2585. *Application contact:* Scott G. Delcourt, Assistant Vice President for Graduate Studies and Senior Associate Dean, 207-581-3291, Fax: 207-581-3232, E-mail: graduate@maine.edu.
Website: http://umaine.edu/nursing/

University of Mary, School of Health Sciences, Division of Nursing, Bismarck, ND 58504-9652. Offers family nurse practitioner (DNP); nurse administrator (MSN); nursing educator (MSN); MSN/MBA. *Accreditation:* AACN. *Program availability:* Part-time, evening/weekend, online learning. *Degree requirements:* For master's, comprehensive exam (for some programs), thesis (for some programs), internship (family nurse practitioner), teaching practice. *Entrance requirements:* For master's, minimum GPA of 2.75 in nursing, interview, letters of recommendation, criminal background check, immunizations, statement of professional goals. Additional exam requirements/recommendations for international students: Required—TOEFL (minimum score 500 paper-based; 71 iBT). *Application deadline:* Applications are processed on a rolling basis. Application fee: $40. Electronic applications accepted. *Financial support:* Fellowships with partial tuition reimbursements and teaching assistantships with partial tuition reimbursements available. Financial award application deadline: 8/1; financial award applicants required to submit FAFSA. *Faculty research:* Gerontology issues, rural nursing, health policy, primary care, women's health.

University of Mary Hardin-Baylor, Graduate Studies in Nursing, Belton, TX 76513. Offers clinical nurse leader (MSN); family nurse practitioner (MSN, Post-Master's Certificate); nurse educator (Post-Master's Certificate); nursing education (MSN). *Accreditation:* AACN. *Program availability:* Part-time, evening/weekend. *Faculty:* 6 full-time (all women), 3 part-time/adjunct (2 women). *Students:* 54 full-time (47 women), 2 part-time (1 woman); includes 14 minority (10 Black or African American, non-Hispanic/Latino; 3 Hispanic/Latino; 1 Two or more races, non-Hispanic/Latino), 1 international. Average age 32. 46 applicants, 70% accepted, 26 enrolled. In 2015, 47 master's awarded. *Degree requirements:* For master's, practicum. *Entrance requirements:* For master's, full-time RN for 1 year, BSN, minimum GPA of 3.0 in last 60 hours of undergraduate program, two letters of recommendation. Additional exam requirements/recommendations for international students: Required—TOEFL (minimum score 100 iBT), IELTS (minimum score 7). *Application deadline:* For fall admission, 4/15 for domestic students, 4/30 priority date for international students; for spring admission, 11/1 for domestic students, 9/30 priority date for international students. Applications are processed on a rolling basis. Application fee: $35 ($135 for international students). Electronic applications accepted. *Expenses:* Tuition, area resident: Part-time $815 per credit hour. Tuition and fees vary according to course load and degree level. *Financial support:* Applicants required to submit FAFSA. *Unit head:* Dr. Carrie Johnson,

Associate Professor/Director, Master of Science in Nursing Programs, 254-295-4178, E-mail: cjohnson@umhb.edu. *Application contact:* Melissa Williams, Director, Graduate Student Services and Engagement, 254-295-4020, Fax: 254-295-5038, E-mail: mwilliams@umhb.edu.
Website: http://graduate.umhb.edu/nursing/

University of Massachusetts Amherst, Graduate School, College of Nursing, Amherst, MA 01003. Offers adult gerontology primary care nurse practitioner (DNP); clinical nurse leader (MS); family nurse practitioner (DNP); nursing (PhD); public health nurse leader (DNP). *Accreditation:* AACN. *Program availability:* Part-time, online learning. Terminal master's awarded for partial completion of doctoral program. *Degree requirements:* For master's, thesis optional; for doctorate, comprehensive exam, thesis/dissertation. *Entrance requirements:* Additional exam requirements/recommendations for international students: Required—TOEFL (minimum score 550 paper-based; 80 iBT), IELTS (minimum score 6.5). Electronic applications accepted. *Faculty research:* Health of older adults and their caretakers, mental health of individuals and families, health of children and adolescents, power and decision-making, transcultural health.

University of Massachusetts Lowell, College of Health Sciences, School of Nursing, Program in Family Health Nursing, Lowell, MA 01854. Offers MS. *Accreditation:* AACN. *Degree requirements:* For master's, thesis optional. *Entrance requirements:* For master's, GRE General Test, minimum GPA of 3.0, MA nursing license, interview, 3 letters of recommendation. *Application deadline:* For fall admission, 4/1 priority date for domestic students; for spring admission, 10/1 for domestic students. Applications are processed on a rolling basis. Application fee: $20 ($35 for international students). *Expenses:* Tuition, state resident: full-time $14,304. Tuition, nonresident: full-time $25,853. *Required fees:* $375. Full-time tuition and fees vary according to campus/location and reciprocity agreements. *Financial support:* Fellowships with tuition reimbursements, research assistantships with full tuition reimbursements, teaching assistantships with full tuition reimbursements, career-related internships or fieldwork, Federal Work-Study, institutionally sponsored loans, scholarships/grants, and traineeships available. Support available to part-time students. Financial award application deadline: 4/1.

University of Massachusetts Medical School, Graduate School of Nursing, Worcester, MA 01655-0115. Offers adult gerontological acute care nurse practitioner (DNP, Post Master's Certificate); adult gerontological primary care nurse practitioner (DNP, Post Master's Certificate); family nursing practitioner (DNP); nurse administrator (DNP); nurse educator (MS, Post Master's Certificate); nursing (PhD); nursing practitioner (DNP); population health (MS). *Accreditation:* AACN. *Faculty:* 18 full-time (15 women), 28 part-time/adjunct (22 women). *Students:* 143 full-time (119 women), 27 part-time (25 women); includes 28 minority (15 Black or African American, non-Hispanic/Latino; 10 Asian, non-Hispanic/Latino; 3 Hispanic/Latino), 1 international. Average age 34. 129 applicants, 68% accepted, 56 enrolled. In 2015, 43 master's, 10 doctorates, 2 other advanced degrees awarded. *Degree requirements:* For doctorate, thesis/dissertation (for some programs), comprehensive exam (for PhD); capstone project and manuscript (for DNP). *Entrance requirements:* For master's, GRE General Test, bachelor's degree in nursing, course work in statistics, unrestricted Massachusetts license as registered nurse; for doctorate, GRE General Test, bachelor's or master's degree; for Post Master's Certificate, GRE General Test, MS in nursing. Additional exam requirements/recommendations for international students: Required—TOEFL. *Application deadline:* For fall admission, 12/1 priority date for domestic students. Applications are processed on a rolling basis. Application fee: $60. Electronic applications accepted. *Expenses:* $10,994 resident per year; $18,210 non-resident per year. *Financial support:* In 2015–16, 31 students received support. Institutionally sponsored loans, scholarships/grants, traineeships, and tuition waivers (partial) available. Support available to part-time students. Financial award application deadline: 5/16; financial award applicants required to submit FAFSA. *Faculty research:* Health literacy, social justice, HIV prevention, cancer-related decision making, nursing education. *Total annual research expenditures:* $650,993. *Unit head:* Dr. Joan Vitello-Cicciu, Dean, 508-856-5081, Fax: 508-856-6552, E-mail: joan.vitello@umassmed.edu. *Application contact:* Diane Brescia, Admissions Coordinator, 508-856-3488, Fax: 508-856-5851, E-mail: diane.brescia@umassmed.edu.
Website: http://www.umassmed.edu/gsn/

University of Memphis, Loewenberg College of Nursing, Memphis, TN 38152. Offers executive leadership (MSN); family nurse practitioner (MSN); nursing (Graduate Certificate); nursing administration (MSN); nursing education (MSN). *Accreditation:* AACN. *Program availability:* Part-time, evening/weekend, online learning. *Faculty:* 12 full-time (all women), 3 part-time/adjunct (2 women). *Students:* 34 full-time (32 women), 220 part-time (196 women); includes 91 minority (80 Black or African American, non-Hispanic/Latino; 8 Asian, non-Hispanic/Latino; 1 Hispanic/Latino; 2 Two or more races, non-Hispanic/Latino). Average age 36. 165 applicants, 48% accepted, 27 enrolled. In 2015, 73 master's, 3 other advanced degrees awarded. *Degree requirements:* For master's, comprehensive exam, thesis optional, scholarly project; completion of clinical practicum hours. *Entrance requirements:* For master's, NCLEX Exam, interview. Additional exam requirements/recommendations for international students: Required—TOEFL (minimum score 550 paper-based; 79 iBT). *Application deadline:* For fall admission, 2/15 for domestic and international students; for spring admission, 10/1 for domestic and international students. Application fee: $35 ($60 for international students). *Financial support:* In 2015–16, 147 students received support. Federal Work-Study and scholarships/grants available. Financial award application deadline: 2/15; financial award applicants required to submit FAFSA. *Faculty research:* Technology in nursing, nurse retention, cultural competence, health policy, health access. *Total annual research expenditures:* $560,619. *Unit head:* Dr. Robert Koch, Associate Dean, 901-678-3908, Fax: 901-678-4907, E-mail: rakoch@memphis.edu. *Application contact:* Dr. Karen Weddle-West, Information Contact, 901-678-2531, Fax: 901-678-5023, E-mail: gradsch@memphis.edu.
Website: http://www.memphis.edu/nursing

University of Miami, Graduate School, School of Nursing and Health Studies, Coral Gables, FL 33124. Offers acute care (MSN), including acute care nurse practitioner, nurse anesthesia; nursing (PhD); primary care (MSN), including adult nurse practitioner, family nurse practitioner, nurse midwifery, women's health practitioner. *Accreditation:* AACN; AANA/CANAEP; ACNM/ACME (one or more programs are accredited). *Program availability:* Part-time. *Degree requirements:* For master's, thesis optional; for doctorate, thesis/dissertation. *Entrance requirements:* For master's, GRE General Test, BSN, minimum GPA of 3.0, Florida RN license; for doctorate, GRE General Test, BSN or MSN, minimum GPA of 3.0. Additional exam requirements/recommendations for international students: Required—TOEFL (minimum score 550 paper-based). Electronic applications accepted. *Faculty research:* Transcultural nursing, exercise and depression in Alzheimer's disease, infectious diseases/HIV–AIDS, postpartum depression, outcomes assessment.

University of Michigan–Flint, School of Health Professions and Studies, Program in Nursing, Flint, MI 48502-1950. Offers adult-gerontology acute care (DNP); adult-gerontology primary care (DNP); family nurse practitioner (MSN, DNP); psychiatric mental health (DNP); psychiatric mental health nurse practitioner (Certificate). *Accreditation:* AACN. *Program availability:* Part-time. *Faculty:* 32 full-time (31 women),

Family Nurse Practitioner Studies

77 part-time/adjunct (69 women). *Students:* 131 full-time (114 women), 81 part-time (71 women); includes 59 minority (35 Black or African American, non-Hispanic/Latino; 2 American Indian or Alaska Native, non-Hispanic/Latino; 7 Asian, non-Hispanic/Latino; 7 Hispanic/Latino; 8 Two or more races, non-Hispanic/Latino), 2 international. Average age 38. 108 applicants, 75% accepted, 56 enrolled. In 2015, 16 master's, 29 doctorates awarded. *Degree requirements:* For master's, thesis. *Entrance requirements:* For master's, BSN from accredited college or university with minimum overall undergraduate GPA of 3.2; for doctorate, BSN or MSN (with APRN certification) from accredited college or university; for Certificate, completion of nurse practitioner program with MS from accredited college or university and minimum overall GPA of 3.2; current unencumbered RN license in the United States; current unencumbered license as nurse practitioner. Additional exam requirements/recommendations for international students: Required—TOEFL (minimum score 560 paper-based; 84 iBT), IELTS (minimum score 6.5). *Application deadline:* For fall admission, 8/1 for domestic students, 5/1 for international students; for winter admission, 11/15 for domestic students, 9/1 for international students; for spring admission, 3/15 for domestic students, 1/1 for international students. Applications are processed on a rolling basis. Application fee: $55. Electronic applications accepted. *Financial support:* Federal Work-Study, scholarships/grants, and unspecified assistantships available. Support available to part-time students. Financial award application deadline: 3/1; financial award applicants required to submit FAFSA. *Faculty research:* Family system stress, self breast exam, family roads evaluation, causal model testing for psychosocial development, basic needs. *Unit head:* Dr. Constance J. Creech, Director, 810-762-3420, Fax: 810-766-6851, E-mail: ccreech@umflint.edu. *Application contact:* Bradley T. Maki, Director of Graduate Admissions, 810-762-3171, Fax: 810-766-6789, E-mail: bmaki@umflint.edu. Website: https://www.umflint.edu/nursing

University of Minnesota, Twin Cities Campus, Graduate School, School of Nursing, Family Nurse Practitioner Program, Minneapolis, MN 55455-0213. Offers MS. *Accreditation:* AACN. *Degree requirements:* For master's, final oral exam, project or thesis. *Entrance requirements:* Additional exam requirements/recommendations for international students: Required—TOEFL (minimum score 586 paper-based).

University of Missouri, Office of Research and Graduate Studies, Sinclair School of Nursing, Columbia, MO 65211. Offers adult-gerontology clinical nurse specialist (DNP, Certificate); family nurse practitioner (DNP); family psychiatric and mental health nurse practitioner (DNP); nursing (MS, PhD); nursing leadership and innovations in health care (DNP); pediatric clinical nurse specialist (DNP, Certificate); pediatric nurse practitioner (DNP). *Accreditation:* AACN. *Program availability:* Part-time. *Degree requirements:* For master's, thesis optional, oral exam; for doctorate, thesis/dissertation. *Entrance requirements:* For master's, GRE General Test, BSN, minimum GPA of 3.0 during last 60 hours, nursing license. Additional exam requirements/recommendations for international students: Required—TOEFL (minimum score 550 paper-based; 79 iBT). *Application deadline:* For fall admission, 2/1 priority date for domestic and international students. Applications are processed on a rolling basis. Application fee: $55 ($75 for international students). Electronic applications accepted. *Financial support:* Fellowships, research assistantships, teaching assistantships, career-related internships or fieldwork, institutionally sponsored loans, scholarships/grants, traineeships, health care benefits, tuition waivers (full), and unspecified assistantships available. Support available to part-time students. Website: http://nursing.missouri.edu/

University of Missouri–Kansas City, School of Nursing and Health Studies, Kansas City, MO 64108. Offers adult clinical nurse specialist (MSN), including adult nurse practitioner, women's health nurse practitioner (MSN, DNP); adult clinical nursing practice (DNP), including adult gerontology nurse practitioner, women's health nurse practitioner (MSN, DNP); clinical nursing practice (DNP), including family nurse practitioner; family nurse practitioner (MSN); neonatal nurse practitioner (MSN); nurse educator (MSN); nurse executive (MSN); nursing (PhD); nursing practice (DNP); pediatric clinical nursing practice (DNP), including pediatric nurse practitioner; pediatric nurse practitioner (MSN). *Accreditation:* AACN. *Program availability:* Part-time, online learning. *Faculty:* 44 full-time (40 women), 47 part-time/adjunct (45 women). *Students:* 62 full-time (43 women), 259 part-time (239 women); includes 61 minority (28 Black or African American, non-Hispanic/Latino; 3 American Indian or Alaska Native, non-Hispanic/Latino; 16 Asian, non-Hispanic/Latino; 10 Hispanic/Latino; 4 Two or more races, non-Hispanic/Latino). Average age 35. 102 applicants, 35% accepted, 36 enrolled. In 2015, 116 master's, 23 doctorates awarded. *Degree requirements:* For master's, thesis or alternative. *Entrance requirements:* For master's, minimum undergraduate GPA of 3.2; for doctorate, GRE, 3 letters of reference. Additional exam requirements/recommendations for international students: Required—TOEFL (minimum score 550 paper-based; 80 iBT). *Application deadline:* For fall admission, 2/1 priority date for domestic and international students; for spring admission, 9/1 priority date for domestic and international students. Application fee: $45 ($50 for international students). *Financial support:* In 2015–16, 2 teaching assistantships with partial tuition reimbursements (averaging $6,650 per year) were awarded; fellowships, research assistantships, career-related internships or fieldwork, Federal Work-Study, institutionally sponsored loans, and tuition waivers (full and partial) also available. Support available to part-time students. Financial award application deadline: 3/1; financial award applicants required to submit FAFSA. *Faculty research:* Geriatrics/gerontology, children's pain, neonatology, Alzheimer's care, cancer caregivers. *Unit head:* Dr. Ann Cary, Dean, 816-235-1723, Fax: 816-235-1701, E-mail: caryah@umkc.edu. *Application contact:* Judy Jellison, Coordinator for Admissions and Recruitment, 816-235-1740, Fax: 816-235-1701, E-mail: jellisonj@umkc.edu. Website: http://nursing.umkc.edu/

University of Missouri–St. Louis, College of Nursing, St. Louis, MO 63121-4400. Offers adult/geriatric nurse practitioner (Post Master's Certificate); family nurse practitioner (Post Master's Certificate); nurse educator (MSN); nurse practitioner (MSN); nursing (DNP, PhD); pediatric nurse practitioner (Post Master's Certificate); psychiatric-mental health nurse practitioner (Post Master's Certificate); women's health nurse practitioner (Post Master's Certificate). *Accreditation:* AACN. *Program availability:* Part-time. *Faculty:* 21 full-time (19 women), 6 part-time/adjunct (5 women). *Students:* 18 full-time (17 women), 227 part-time (215 women); includes 34 minority (22 Black or African American, non-Hispanic/Latino; 8 Asian, non-Hispanic/Latino; 3 Hispanic/Latino; 1 Two or more races, non-Hispanic/Latino), 1 international. Average age 35. 152 applicants, 69% accepted, 83 enrolled. *Degree requirements:* For doctorate, comprehensive exam, thesis/dissertation; for Post Master's Certificate, thesis. *Entrance requirements:* For master's, 2 recommendation letters; minimum GPA of 3.0; BSN; nursing licensure; statement of purpose; course in differential/inferential statistics; for doctorate, GRE, 2 letters of recommendation, MSN, minimum GPA of 3.2, course in differential/inferential statistics; for Post Master's Certificate, 2 recommendation letters; MSN; advanced practice certificate; minimum GPA of 3.0; essay. Additional exam requirements/recommendations for international students: Recommended—TOEFL (minimum score 550 paper-based; 79 iBT), IELTS (minimum score 6.5). *Application deadline:* For fall admission, 2/15 for domestic and international students. Application fee: $50 ($40 for international students). Electronic applications accepted. *Financial support:* Research assistantships with tuition reimbursements available. Financial award application deadline: 4/1; financial award applicants required to submit FAFSA. *Faculty research:*

Health promotion and restoration, family disruption, violence, abuse, battered women, health survey methods. *Unit head:* Dr. Roberta Lavin, Director, 314-516-6066. *Application contact:* 314-516-5458, Fax: 314-516-6996, E-mail: gradadm@umsl.edu. Website: http://www.umsl.edu/divisions/nursing/

University of Nevada, Las Vegas, Graduate College, School of Nursing, Las Vegas, NV 89154-3018. Offers family nurse practitioner (Advanced Certificate); nursing (MS, DNP). *Accreditation:* AACN. *Program availability:* Part-time, online learning. *Faculty:* 10 full-time (all women), 10 part-time/adjunct (9 women). *Students:* 42 full-time (36 women), 87 part-time (77 women); includes 42 minority (2 Black or African American, non-Hispanic/Latino; 21 Asian, non-Hispanic/Latino; 10 Hispanic/Latino; 9 Two or more races, non-Hispanic/Latino), 11 international. Average age 38. 135 applicants, 51% accepted, 53 enrolled. In 2015, 26 master's, 14 doctorates, 1 other advanced degree awarded. *Degree requirements:* For master's, comprehensive exam, thesis; for doctorate, comprehensive exam (for some programs), thesis/dissertation. *Entrance requirements:* For doctorate, GRE General Test. Additional exam requirements/recommendations for international students: Recommended—TOEFL (minimum score 550 paper-based; 80 iBT), IELTS (minimum score 7). *Application deadline:* For fall admission, 2/1 for domestic students, 5/1 for international students. Application fee: $60 ($95 for international students). Electronic applications accepted. *Expenses:* $264 per credit state resident full-time and part-time; $6,955 per semester nonresident full-time, $264 per credit; $555 per credit nonresident part-time. *Financial support:* In 2015–16, 6 students received support, including 6 teaching assistantships with partial tuition reimbursements available (averaging $11,500 per year); institutionally sponsored loans, scholarships/grants, health care benefits, and unspecified assistantships also available. Financial award application deadline: 3/1. *Faculty research:* Chronic diseases and health promotion in diabetes, cardiovascular disease, pain, and obesity; informal caregiver stress and risk factors; technology enhanced interventions; symptom and self-management. *Total annual research expenditures:* $581,273. *Unit head:* Dr. Carolyn Yucha, Dean, 702-895-5307, Fax: 702-895-4807, E-mail: carolyn.yucha@unlv.edu. *Application contact:* Graduate College Admissions Evaluator, 702-895-3367, Fax: 702-895-4180, E-mail: gradadmissions@unlv.edu. Website: http://nursing.unlv.edu/

University of New Hampshire, Graduate School, College of Health and Human Services, Department of Nursing, Durham, NH 03824. Offers family practitioner (Postbaccalaureate Certificate); nursing (MS, DNP). *Accreditation:* AACN. *Program availability:* Part-time. *Degree requirements:* For master's, thesis or alternative. *Entrance requirements:* For master's, GRE General Test or MAT. Additional exam requirements/recommendations for international students: Required—TOEFL (minimum score 550 paper-based; 80 iBT). *Application deadline:* For fall admission, 4/1 priority date for domestic students, 4/1 for international students; for spring admission, 11/1 for domestic students. Applications are processed on a rolling basis. Application fee: $65. Electronic applications accepted. *Expenses:* Tuition, state resident: full-time $13,840; part-time $770 per credit hour. Tuition, nonresident: full-time $27,130; part-time $1175 per credit hour. *Required fees:* $2080; $1040. Tuition and fees vary according to degree level and program. *Financial support:* Fellowships, research assistantships, teaching assistantships, Federal Work-Study, scholarships/grants, and tuition waivers (full and partial) available. Financial award application deadline: 2/15. *Faculty research:* Adult health, nursing administration, family nurse practitioner. *Unit head:* Dr. Gene Harkless, Chair, 603-862-2285. *Application contact:* Jane Dufresne, Administrative Assistant, 603-862-2299, E-mail: nursing.department@unh.edu. Website: http://www.chhs.unh.edu/nursing

The University of North Carolina at Chapel Hill, School of Nursing, Chapel Hill, NC 27599-7460. Offers advanced practice registered nurse (DNP); health care systems (DNP); nursing (MSN, PhD, PMC), including administration (MSN), adult gerontology primary care nurse practitioner (MSN), clinical nurse leader (MSN), education (MSN), informatics (MSN, PMC), nursing leadership (PMC), outcomes management (MSN), primary care family nurse practitioner (MSN), primary care pediatric nurse practitioner (MSN), psychiatric/mental health nurse practitioner (MSN, PMC). *Accreditation:* AACN; ACEN (one or more programs are accredited). *Program availability:* Part-time. *Faculty:* 86 full-time (78 women), 44 part-time/adjunct (40 women). *Students:* 208 full-time (186 women), 128 part-time (116 women); includes 109 minority (49 Black or African American, non-Hispanic/Latino; 4 American Indian or Alaska Native, non-Hispanic/Latino; 32 Asian, non-Hispanic/Latino; 7 Hispanic/Latino; 17 Two or more races, non-Hispanic/Latino), 17 international. Average age 33. 624 applicants, 25% accepted, 150 enrolled. In 2015, 91 master's, 14 doctorates awarded. *Degree requirements:* For master's, comprehensive exam, thesis; for doctorate, thesis/dissertation, 3 exams; for PMC, thesis. *Entrance requirements:* Additional exam requirements/recommendations for international students: Required—TOEFL (minimum score 575 paper-based; 89 iBT), IELTS (minimum score 8). *Application deadline:* For fall admission, 12/15 for domestic and international students. Application fee: $85. Electronic applications accepted. *Financial support:* In 2015–16, 8 fellowships with full tuition reimbursements, 6 research assistantships with partial tuition reimbursements (averaging $8,000 per year), 10 teaching assistantships with partial tuition reimbursements (averaging $8,000 per year) were awarded; scholarships/grants, traineeships, health care benefits, and unspecified assistantships also available. Support available to part-time students. Financial award application deadline: 3/1; financial award applicants required to submit FAFSA. *Faculty research:* Preventing and managing chronic illness, reducing health disparities, Improving healthcare quality and patient outcomes, understanding biobehavioral and genetic bases of health and illness, developing innovative ways to enhance science and its clinical translation. *Unit head:* Donna S. Havens, PhD, RN, Dean/Professor, 919-966-3731, Fax: 919-966-3540, E-mail: dhavens@email.unc.edu. *Application contact:* Emily Sayed, Assistant Director, Graduate Admissions, 919-966-4260, Fax: 919-966-3540, E-mail: sayed@unc.edu. Website: http://nursing.unc.edu

The University of North Carolina at Charlotte, College of Health and Human Services, School of Nursing, Charlotte, NC 28223-0001. Offers adult-gerontology acute care nurse practitioner (MSN, Post-Master's Certificate); advanced clinical nursing (MSN); community public health nursing (MSN); family nurse practitioner across the lifespan (MSN, Post-Master's Certificate); nurse administrator (MSN, Graduate Certificate); nurse anesthesia (MSN, Post-Master's Certificate); nurse educator (MSN, Graduate Certificate); nursing (DNP); nursing systems/population (MSN). *Accreditation:* AACN. *Program availability:* Part-time, blended/hybrid learning. *Faculty:* 26 full-time (25 women), 4 part-time/adjunct (3 women). *Students:* 109 full-time (89 women), 112 part-time (107 women); includes 46 minority (37 Black or African American, non-Hispanic/Latino; 3 Asian, non-Hispanic/Latino; 5 Hispanic/Latino; 1 Two or more races, non-Hispanic/Latino). Average age 33. 321 applicants, 34% accepted, 84 enrolled. In 2015, 76 master's, 4 doctorates, 7 other advanced degrees awarded. Terminal master's awarded for partial completion of doctoral program. *Degree requirements:* For master's, practicum, synthesis and integration or thesis, residency, internship (varies by program); for doctorate, thesis/dissertation or alternative, residency; for other advanced degree, practicum. *Entrance requirements:* For master's, GRE General Test, unencumbered license as Registered Nurse in North Carolina; BSN from nationally-accredited program; one year of professional nursing practice in acute/critical care; minimum overall GPA of 3.0 in the last degree and 60 hours of nursing coursework; completion of an

undergraduate statistics course with minimum grade of C; statement of purpose; for doctorate, GRE or MAT, master's degree in nursing in an advanced nursing practice specialty from nationally-accredited program; minimum overall GPA of 3.5 in MSN program; current RN licensure in U.S. at time of application with eligibility for NC licensure; for other advanced degree, GRE. Additional exam requirements/recommendations for international students: Required—TOEFL (minimum score 557 paper-based, 83 iBT) or IELTS (minimum score 6.5). *Application deadline:* For fall admission, 2/1 for domestic and international students; for spring admission, 10/1 priority date for domestic and international students; for summer admission, 4/1 priority date for domestic and international students. Applications are processed on a rolling basis. Application fee: $75. Electronic applications accepted. *Expenses:* Contact institution. *Financial support:* In 2015–16, 9 students received support, including 5 research assistantships (averaging $4,850 per year), 3 teaching assistantships (averaging $2,911 per year); career-related internships or fieldwork, institutionally sponsored loans, scholarships/grants, traineeships, unspecified assistantships, and administrative assistantships also available. Support available to part-time students. Financial award application deadline: 3/1; financial award applicants required to submit FAFSA. *Faculty research:* Improving care outcomes for the elderly; vulnerable populations; symptom management; self management/health promotion strategies of older adults; migration and maternal child health; health disparities, health literacy, and access to healthcare in Latino adults with diabetes; psychiatric nursing. *Total annual research expenditures:* $875,169. *Unit head:* Dr. Dee Baldwin, Associate Dean, 704-687-7952, Fax: 704-687-6017, E-mail: dbaldwi5@uncc.edu. *Application contact:* Kathy B. Giddings, Director of Graduate Admissions, 704-687-5503, Fax: 704-687-1668, E-mail: gradadm@uncc.edu.
Website: http://nursing.uncc.edu/

The University of North Carolina Wilmington, School of Nursing, Wilmington, NC 28403-5995. Offers clinical research and product development (MS); family nurse practitioner (MSN, Post-Master's Certificate). *Accreditation:* AACN; ACEN. *Program availability:* Part-time, online learning. *Faculty:* 18 full-time (17 women). *Students:* 68 full-time (57 women), 84 part-time (73 women); includes 25 minority (15 Black or African American, non-Hispanic/Latino; 5 American Indian or Alaska Native, non-Hispanic/Latino; 2 Hispanic/Latino; 3 Two or more races, non-Hispanic/Latino). Average age 38. 222 applicants, 57 enrolled. In 2015, 33 master's awarded. *Degree requirements:* For master's, research project/presentation. *Entrance requirements:* For master's, GRE General Test. Additional exam requirements/recommendations for international students: Required—TOEFL (minimum score 79 iBT), IELTS (minimum score 6.5). *Application deadline:* For fall admission, 3/1 for domestic students. Applications are processed on a rolling basis. Application fee: $60. Electronic applications accepted. *Expenses:* $8,854.10 in-state full-time per year; $20,945.04 out-of-state full-time per year. *Financial support:* Scholarships/grants available. Financial award application deadline: 3/15; financial award applicants required to submit FAFSA. *Unit head:* Dr. Carol Heinrich, Director, 910-962-7410, Fax: 910-962-3723, E-mail: badzekl@uncw.edu. *Application contact:* Dr. Jim Lyon, Graduate Coordinator, 910-962-2936, E-mail: lyonj@uncw.edu.
Website: http://www.uncw.edu/son/

University of North Dakota, Graduate School, College of Nursing, Department of Nursing, Grand Forks, ND 58202. Offers adult-gerontological nurse practitioner (MSN); advanced public health nurse (MSN); family nurse practitioner (MSN); nurse anesthesia (MSN); nurse educator (MSN); nursing (DNP, PhD); psychiatric and mental health nurse practitioner (MSN).

University of Northern Colorado, Graduate School, College of Natural and Health Sciences, School of Nursing, Greeley, CO 80639. Offers clinical nurse specialist in chronic illness (MS); family nurse practitioner (MS); nursing education (MS, PhD). *Accreditation:* AACN. *Program availability:* Online learning. *Degree requirements:* For master's, comprehensive exam, thesis or alternative; for doctorate, comprehensive exam, thesis/dissertation. *Entrance requirements:* For master's and doctorate, GRE General Test, minimum GPA of 3.0 in last 60 hours, BS in nursing, 2 letters of recommendation. Electronic applications accepted.

University of North Florida, Brooks College of Health, School of Nursing, Jacksonville, FL 32224. Offers clinical nurse leader (MSN); clinical nurse specialist (MSN); family nurse practitioner (Certificate); nurse anesthetist (MSN); nursing practice (DNP); primary care nurse practitioner (MSN). *Accreditation:* AACN; AANA/CANAEP. *Program availability:* Part-time. *Faculty:* 23 full-time (17 women), 2 part-time/adjunct (1 woman). *Students:* 108 full-time (90 women), 117 part-time (93 women); includes 54 minority (17 Black or African American, non-Hispanic/Latino; 1 American Indian or Alaska Native, non-Hispanic/Latino; 13 Asian, non-Hispanic/Latino; 17 Hispanic/Latino; 1 Native Hawaiian or other Pacific Islander, non-Hispanic/Latino; 5 Two or more races, non-Hispanic/Latino), 3 international. Average age 36. 136 applicants, 81% accepted, 74 enrolled. In 2015, 46 master's, 6 doctorates awarded. *Degree requirements:* For master's, thesis optional. *Entrance requirements:* For master's, GRE General Test, minimum GPA of 3.0 in last 60 hours of course work, BSN, clinical experience, resume; for doctorate, GRE, master's degree in nursing specialty from nationally-accredited program; national certification in one of the following APRN roles: CNE, CNM, CNS, CRNA, CNP; minimum graduate GPA of 3.3; three letters of reference which address academic ability and clinical skills; active license as registered nurse or advanced practice registered nurse. Additional exam requirements/recommendations for international students: Required—TOEFL (minimum score 500 paper-based; 61 iBT). *Application deadline:* For fall admission, 3/15 for domestic students, 4/1 for international students. Application fee: $30. Electronic applications accepted. *Expenses:* Tuition, state resident: part-time $408.10 per credit hour; nonresident: part-time $932.61 per credit hour. *Required fees:* $111.81 per credit hour. Tuition and fees vary according to course load, campus/location and program. *Financial support:* In 2015–16, 35 students received support. Research assistantships available. Financial award application deadline: 4/1; financial award applicants required to submit FAFSA. *Faculty research:* Teen pregnancy, diabetes, ethical decision-making, family caregivers. *Total annual research expenditures:* $39,413. *Unit head:* Dr. Li Loriz, Chair, 904-620-1053, E-mail: lloriz@unf.edu. *Application contact:* Beth Dibble, Assistant Director of Admissions for Nursing and Physical Therapy, 904-620-2684, Fax: 904-620-1832, E-mail: nursingadmissions@unf.edu.
Website: http://www.unf.edu/brooks/nursing

University of North Georgia, Department of Nursing, Dahlonega, GA 30597. Offers family nurse practitioner (MS, Post-Master's Certificate). *Accreditation:* ACEN. *Program availability:* Part-time. *Degree requirements:* For master's, one foreign language, comprehensive exam, thesis. *Entrance requirements:* For master's, GRE General Test or MAT, minimum GPA of 2.5, 3 letters of recommendation, essay, current Georgia RN license, 1 year of post-licensure work, BSN, ASN. Additional exam requirements/recommendations for international students: Required—TOEFL (minimum score 550 paper-based; 79 iBT), IELTS (minimum score 6.5). *Application deadline:* For fall admission, 7/1 priority date for domestic students, 6/1 for international students. Application fee: $40. Electronic applications accepted. *Expenses:* Tuition, area resident: Full-time $2025; part-time $1350 per credit hour. Tuition, state resident: full-time $2025; part-time $1350 per credit hour. Tuition, nonresident: full-time $8082; part-time $5388

per credit hour. *International tuition:* $8082 full-time. *Required fees:* $620.50; $620.50 per semester. Tuition and fees vary according to degree level and program. *Financial support:* Career-related internships or fieldwork and unspecified assistantships available. Financial award application deadline: 5/1; financial award applicants required to submit CSS PROFILE or FAFSA.
Website: http://ung.edu/nursing/

University of Pennsylvania, School of Nursing, Family Nurse Practitioner Program, Philadelphia, PA 19104. Offers MSN, Certificate. *Accreditation:* AACN. *Program availability:* Part-time. *Students:* 31 full-time (24 women), 42 part-time (39 women); includes 25 minority (7 Black or African American, non-Hispanic/Latino; 1 American Indian or Alaska Native, non-Hispanic/Latino; 6 Asian, non-Hispanic/Latino; 9 Hispanic/Latino; 2 Two or more races, non-Hispanic/Latino). Average age 29. 96 applicants, 64% accepted, 41 enrolled. In 2015, 25 master's awarded. *Expenses: Tuition, area resident:* Full-time $31,068; part-time $5762 per course. *Required fees:* $3200; $336 per course. Full-time tuition and fees vary according to degree level, program and student level. Part-time tuition and fees vary according to course load, degree level and program. *Financial support:* Application deadline: 4/1.

University of Phoenix–Hawaii Campus, College of Nursing, Honolulu, HI 96813-3800. Offers education (MHA); family nurse practitioner (MSN); gerontology (MHA); health administration (MHA); nursing (MSN); nursing/health care education (MSN); MSN/MBA. *Program availability:* Evening/weekend. *Degree requirements:* For master's, thesis (for some programs). *Entrance requirements:* For master's, minimum undergraduate GPA of 2.5, 3 years of work experience, RN license. Additional exam requirements/recommendations for international students: Required—TOEFL (minimum score 550 paper-based; 79 iBT). Electronic applications accepted.

University of Phoenix–Online Campus, College of Health Sciences and Nursing, Phoenix, AZ 85034-7209. Offers family nurse practitioner (Certificate); health care (Certificate); health care education (Certificate); health care informatics (Certificate); informatics (MSN); nursing (MSN); nursing and health care education (MSN); MSN/MBA; MSN/MHA. *Accreditation:* AACN. *Program availability:* Evening/weekend, online learning. *Entrance requirements:* Additional exam requirements/recommendations for international students: Required—TOEFL, TOEIC (Test of English as an International Communication), Berlitz Online English Proficiency Exam, PTE, or IELTS. Electronic applications accepted. *Expenses:* Contact institution.

University of Phoenix–Phoenix Campus, College of Health Sciences and Nursing, Tempe, AZ 85282-2371. Offers family nurse practitioner (MSN, Certificate); gerontology health care (Certificate); health care education (MSN, Certificate); health care informatics (Certificate); informatics (MSN); nursing (MSN); MSN/MHA. *Program availability:* Evening/weekend, online learning. *Entrance requirements:* Additional exam requirements/recommendations for international students: Required—TOEFL, TOEIC (Test of English as an International Communication), Berlitz Online English Proficiency Exam, PTE, or IELTS. Electronic applications accepted. *Expenses:* Contact institution.

University of Phoenix–Sacramento Valley Campus, College of Nursing, Sacramento, CA 95833-4334. Offers family nurse practitioner (MSN); health administration (MHA); health care education (MSN); nursing (MSN); MSN/MBA. *Program availability:* Evening/weekend. *Degree requirements:* For master's, thesis (for some programs). *Entrance requirements:* For master's, RN license, minimum undergraduate GPA of 2.5, 3 years work experience. Additional exam requirements/recommendations for international students: Required—TOEFL (minimum score 550 paper-based; 79 iBT). Electronic applications accepted.

University of Phoenix–Southern California Campus, College of Health Sciences and Nursing, Costa Mesa, CA 92626. Offers family nurse practitioner (MSN, Certificate); health care (Certificate); informatics (MSN); nursing (MSN); nursing/health care education (MSN, Certificate); MSN/MBA; MSN/MHA. *Program availability:* Evening/weekend, online learning. *Entrance requirements:* Additional exam requirements/recommendations for international students: Required—TOEFL, TOEIC (Test of English as an International Communication), Berlitz Online English Proficiency Exam, PTE, or IELTS. Electronic applications accepted. *Expenses:* Contact institution.

University of Pittsburgh, School of Nursing, Nurse Practitioner Program, Pittsburgh, PA 15261. Offers adult-gerontology acute care (DNP); adult-gerontology primary care (DNP); family (individual across the lifespan) (DNP); neonatal (MSN, DNP); pediatric primary care (DNP); psychiatric mental health (DNP). *Accreditation:* AACN. *Program availability:* Part-time. *Students:* 74 full-time (65 women), 59 part-time (51 women); includes 14 minority (5 Black or African American, non-Hispanic/Latino; 2 American Indian or Alaska Native, non-Hispanic/Latino; 6 Asian, non-Hispanic/Latino; 1 Hispanic/Latino). Average age 30. 65 applicants, 55% accepted, 28 enrolled. In 2015, 14 master's, 19 doctorates awarded. *Degree requirements:* For master's, comprehensive exam, thesis optional. *Entrance requirements:* For master's, GRE General Test or MAT, BSN, RN license, letters of recommendation, resume, course work in statistics, 1-3 years of nursing experience; for doctorate, GRE General Test, BSN, RN license, minimum GPA of 3.5, 3 letters of recommendation. Additional exam requirements/recommendations for international students: Required—TOEFL (minimum score 600 paper-based; 100 iBT). *Application deadline:* For fall admission, 5/1 priority date for domestic students, 2/15 priority date for international students. Application fee: $50. Electronic applications accepted. *Expenses:* Contact institution. *Financial support:* In 2015–16, 16 students received support, including 7 fellowships with tuition reimbursements available (averaging $11,278 per year), 9 teaching assistantships with tuition reimbursements available (averaging $10,879 per year); scholarships/grants, traineeships, health care benefits, and unspecified assistantships also available. Support available to part-time students. Financial award application deadline: 3/15. *Faculty research:* Behavioral management of chronic disorders, patient management in critical care, consumer informatics, genetic applications (molecular genetics and psychosocial implications), technology for nurses and patients to improve care. *Unit head:* Dr. Sandra Engberg, Associate Dean for Clinical Education, 412-624-3835, Fax: 412-624-8521, E-mail: sje1@pitt.edu. *Application contact:* Laurie Lapsley, Administrator of Graduate Student Services, 412-624-9670, Fax: 412-624-2409, E-mail: lapsleyl@pitt.edu.
Website: http://www.nursing.pitt.edu

University of Portland, School of Nursing, Portland, OR 97203. Offers clinical nurse leader (MS); family nurse practitioner (DNP); nurse educator (MS). *Accreditation:* AACN. *Program availability:* Part-time, evening/weekend, online learning. *Entrance requirements:* For master's, GRE General Test or MAT, Oregon RN license, BSN, course work in statistics, resume, letters of recommendation, writing sample; for doctorate, GRE General Test or MAT, Oregon RN license, BSN or MSN, 2 letters of recommendation, resume, writing sample, official transcripts. Additional exam requirements/recommendations for international students: Required—TOEFL (minimum score 550 paper-based; 80 iBT), IELTS (minimum score 7). *Expenses:* Contact institution.

University of Puerto Rico, Medical Sciences Campus, School of Nursing, San Juan, PR 00936-5067. Offers adult and elderly nursing (MSN); child and adolescent nursing (MSN); critical care nursing (MSN); family and community nursing (MSN); family nurse practitioner (MSN); maternity nursing (MSN); mental health and psychiatric nursing

Family Nurse Practitioner Studies

(MSN). *Accreditation:* AACN. *Entrance requirements:* For master's, GRE or EXADEP, interview, Puerto Rico RN license or professional license for international students, general and specific point average, article analysis. Electronic applications accepted. *Faculty research:* HIV, health disparities, teen violence, women and violence, neurological disorders.

University of Rhode Island, Graduate School, College of Nursing, Kingston, RI 02881. Offers acute care nurse practitioner (MS); adult-gerontological nurse practitioner/clinical nurse specialist (MS); family nurse practitioner (MS); nursing (PhD); nursing education (MS); nursing practice (DNP). *Accreditation:* AACN; ACNM/ACME (one or more programs are accredited). *Program availability:* Part-time. *Faculty:* 11 full-time (all women). *Students:* 51 full-time (41 women), 77 part-time (70 women); includes 18 minority (11 Black or African American, non-Hispanic/Latino; 2 Asian, non-Hispanic/Latino; 4 Hispanic/Latino; 1 Two or more races, non-Hispanic/Latino), 5 international. In 2015, 19 master's, 7 doctorates awarded. *Degree requirements:* For master's, comprehensive exam; for doctorate, comprehensive exam, thesis/dissertation. *Entrance requirements:* For master's, GRE or MAT, 2 letters of recommendation, scholarly papers; for doctorate, GRE, 3 letters of recommendation, scholarly papers. Additional exam requirements/recommendations for international students: Required—TOEFL (minimum score 550 paper-based). *Application deadline:* For fall admission, 2/15 for domestic students, 2/1 for international students; for spring admission, 10/15 for domestic students, 7/15 for international students. Application fee: $65. Electronic applications accepted. *Expenses:* Tuition, state resident: full-time $11,796; part-time $655 per credit. Tuition, nonresident: full-time $24,206; part-time $1345 per credit. *Required fees:* $1546; $44 per credit. One-time fee: $155 full-time; $35 part-time. *Financial support:* In 2015–16, 2 research assistantships (averaging $12,111 per year), 7 teaching assistantships with tuition reimbursements (averaging $13,112 per year) were awarded. Financial award application deadline: 2/15; financial award applicants required to submit FAFSA. *Faculty research:* Group intervention for grieving women in prison, translating best practice in non-drug interventions for postoperative pain management, further development and testing of the pain assessment inventory, preschool motor and functional performance of two cohorts, neuroactivation of brain motor areas in preterm children. *Unit head:* Dr. Mary Sullivan, Interim Dean, 401-874-5339, Fax: 401-874-2061, E-mail: mcsullivan@uri.edu. *Application contact:* Graduate Admission, 401-874-2872, E-mail: gradadm@etal.uri.edu.
Website: http://www.uri.edu/nursing/

University of Rochester, School of Nursing, Rochester, NY 14642. Offers adult gerontological acute care nurse practitioner (MS); clinical nurse leader (MS); family nurse practitioner (MS); family psychiatric mental health nurse practitioner (MS); health care organization management and leadership (MS); health practice research (PhD); nursing (DNP); nursing education (MS); pediatric nurse practitioner (MS); pediatric nurse practitioner/neonatal nurse practitioner (MS). *Accreditation:* AACN. *Program availability:* Part-time, online learning. *Faculty:* 56 full-time (45 women), 63 part-time/adjunct (55 women). *Students:* 21 full-time (20 women), 212 part-time (175 women); includes 35 minority (12 Black or African American, non-Hispanic/Latino; 1 American Indian or Alaska Native, non-Hispanic/Latino; 10 Asian, non-Hispanic/Latino; 7 Hispanic/Latino; 5 Two or more races, non-Hispanic/Latino), 2 international. Average age 35. 111 applicants, 68% accepted, 71 enrolled. In 2015, 52 master's, 9 doctorates awarded. Terminal master's awarded for partial completion of doctoral program. *Degree requirements:* For master's, comprehensive exam (for some programs); for doctorate, thesis/dissertation. *Entrance requirements:* For master's, BS in nursing, minimum GPA of 3.0, course work in statistics; for doctorate, GRE General Test (for PhD), MS in nursing, minimum GPA of 3.5. Additional exam requirements/recommendations for international students: Required—TOEFL (minimum score 560 paper-based; 88 iBT) or IELTS (minimum score 6.5) recommended. *Application deadline:* For fall admission, 4/1 for domestic and international students; for spring admission, 9/1 for domestic and international students; for summer admission, 1/2 for domestic and international students. Application fee: $50. Electronic applications accepted. *Expenses: Tuition, area resident:* Full-time $47,450; part-time $1482 per credit hour. *Required fees:* $528. Tuition and fees vary according to program. *Financial support:* In 2015–16, 52 students received support, including 2 fellowships with tuition reimbursements available (averaging $30,000 per year); scholarships/grants, traineeships, health care benefits, tuition waivers (full and partial), and unspecified assistantships also available. Support available to part-time students. Financial award application deadline: 6/30. *Faculty research:* Symptom assessment and self-management of chronic illness, health promotion and illness prevention, nursing intervention research with vulnerable populations, palliative care, aging. *Total annual research expenditures:* $2.1 million. *Unit head:* Dr. Kathy H. Rideout, Dean, 585-273-8902, Fax: 585-273-1268, E-mail: kathy_rideout@urmc.rochester.edu. *Application contact:* Elaine Andolina, Director of Admissions, 585-275-2375, Fax: 585-756-8299, E-mail: elaine_andolina@urmc.rochester.edu.
Website: http://www.son.rochester.edu

University of Saint Francis, Graduate School, Department of Nursing, Fort Wayne, IN 46808-3994. Offers family nurse practitioner (MSN, Post Master's Certificate). *Accreditation:* AACN. *Program availability:* Part-time, evening/weekend, online learning. *Degree requirements:* For master's, research project. *Entrance requirements:* For master's, GRE (if undergraduate GPA is less than 3.0), minimum undergraduate GPA of 3.2; ASN or BSN from regionally-accredited U.S. institutions; current license as registered nurse; completed graduate or undergraduate statistics course within last five years; for Post Master's Certificate, GRE (if undergraduate GPA is less than 3.0), minimum undergraduate GPA of 3.2; MSN from regionally-accredited U.S. institution; current license as registered nurse; completed graduate or undergraduate statistics course within last five years. Additional exam requirements/recommendations for international students: Required—TOEFL or IELTS. Electronic applications accepted. *Expenses:* Contact institution.

University of St. Francis, Leach College of Nursing, Joliet, IL 60435-6169. Offers family nurse practitioner (MSN, Post-Master's Certificate); family psychology/mental health nurse practitioner (MSN, Post-Master's Certificate); nursing administration (MSN); nursing education (MSN); nursing practice (DNP); teaching in nursing (Certificate). *Accreditation:* AACN. *Program availability:* Part-time, evening/weekend, 100% online. *Faculty:* 7 full-time (all women), 16 part-time/adjunct (13 women). *Students:* 82 full-time (72 women), 356 part-time (325 women); includes 147 minority (62 Black or African American, non-Hispanic/Latino; 1 American Indian or Alaska Native, non-Hispanic/Latino; 27 Asian, non-Hispanic/Latino; 45 Hispanic/Latino; 3 Native Hawaiian or other Pacific Islander, non-Hispanic/Latino; 9 Two or more races, non-Hispanic/Latino). Average age 41. 338 applicants, 42% accepted, 100 enrolled. In 2015, 91 master's, 9 doctorates, 6 other advanced degrees awarded. *Entrance requirements:* Additional exam requirements/recommendations for international students: Required—TOEFL (minimum score 550 paper-based; 79 iBT), IELTS (minimum score 6). *Application deadline:* Applications are processed on a rolling basis. Application fee: $30. Electronic applications accepted. Application fee is waived when completed online. *Expenses:* Contact institution. *Financial support:* In 2015–16, 149 students received support. Career-related internships or fieldwork, scholarships/grants, and tuition waivers (partial) available. Support available to part-time students. Financial award applicants required to submit FAFSA. *Unit head:* Dr. Carol Wilson, Dean, 815-740-3840, Fax: 815-

740-4243, E-mail: cwilson@stfrancis.edu. *Application contact:* Sandra Sloka, Director of Admissions for Graduate and Degree Completion Programs, 800-735-7500, Fax: 815-740-3431, E-mail: ssloka@stfrancis.edu.
Website: http://www.stfrancis.edu/academics/college-of-nursing/

University of Saint Joseph, Department of Nursing, West Hartford, CT 06117-2700. Offers family nurse practitioner (MS); family psychiatric/mental health nurse practitioner (MS); nurse educator (MS); nursing practice (DNP). *Accreditation:* AACN. *Program availability:* Part-time, evening/weekend. *Degree requirements:* For master's, thesis. *Entrance requirements:* For master's, 2 letters of recommendation. *Application deadline:* Applications are processed on a rolling basis. Application fee: $50. Electronic applications accepted. Application fee is waived when completed online. *Financial support:* Career-related internships or fieldwork and unspecified assistantships available. Support available to part-time students. Financial award applicants required to submit FAFSA.
Website: http://www.usj.edu/academics/schools/school-of-health-natural-sciences/nursing/

University of San Diego, Hahn School of Nursing and Health Science, San Diego, CA 92110-2492. Offers adult-gerontology clinical nurse specialist (MSN); adult-gerontology nurse practitioner/family nurse practitioner (MSN); executive nurse leader (MSN); family nurse practitioner (MSN); family/lifespan psychiatric-mental health nurse practitioner (MSN); healthcare informatics (MS, MSN); nursing (PhD); nursing practice (DNP). *Accreditation:* AACN. *Program availability:* Part-time, evening/weekend. *Faculty:* 27 full-time (23 women), 46 part-time/adjunct (41 women). *Students:* 178 full-time (151 women), 157 part-time (131 women); includes 143 minority (25 Black or African American, non-Hispanic/Latino; 2 American Indian or Alaska Native, non-Hispanic/Latino; 53 Asian, non-Hispanic/Latino; 49 Hispanic/Latino; 4 Native Hawaiian or other Pacific Islander, non-Hispanic/Latino; 10 Two or more races, non-Hispanic/Latino), 5 international. Average age 36. In 2015, 122 master's, 43 doctorates awarded. *Degree requirements:* For doctorate, thesis/dissertation (for some programs), residency (DNP). *Entrance requirements:* For master's, GRE General Test (for entry-level nursing), BSN, current California RN licensure (except for entry-level nursing); minimum GPA of 3.0; for doctorate, minimum GPA of 3.5, MSN, current California RN licensure. Additional exam requirements/recommendations for international students: Required—TOEFL (minimum score 580 paper-based; 83 iBT), TWE. *Application deadline:* Applications are processed on a rolling basis. Application fee: $45. Electronic applications accepted. *Financial support:* In 2015–16, 217 students received support. Scholarships/grants and traineeships available. Support available to part-time students. Financial award application deadline: 4/1; financial award applicants required to submit FAFSA. *Faculty research:* Maternal/neonatal health, palliative and end of life care, adolescent obesity, health disparities, cognitive dysfunction. *Unit head:* Dr. Sally Hardin, Dean, 619-260-4550, Fax: 619-260-6814. *Application contact:* Monica Mahon, Associate Director of Graduate Admissions, 619-260-4524, Fax: 619-260-4158, E-mail: grads@sandiego.edu.
Website: http://www.sandiego.edu/nursing/

University of San Francisco, School of Nursing and Health Professions, Doctoral Programs, San Francisco, CA 94117-1080. Offers executive leadership (DNP); family nurse practitioner (DNP); healthcare systems leadership (DNP); psychiatric mental health nurse practitioner (DNP). *Faculty:* 19 full-time (13 women), 15 part-time/adjunct (11 women). *Students:* 150 full-time (114 women), 54 part-time (46 women); includes 114 minority (25 Black or African American, non-Hispanic/Latino; 1 American Indian or Alaska Native, non-Hispanic/Latino; 56 Asian, non-Hispanic/Latino; 21 Hispanic/Latino; 3 Native Hawaiian or other Pacific Islander, non-Hispanic/Latino; 8 Two or more races, non-Hispanic/Latino), 2 international. Average age 38. 121 applicants, 81% accepted, 70 enrolled. In 2015, 31 doctorates awarded. *Entrance requirements:* For doctorate, nursing bachelor's degree, valid RN license in California. Electronic applications accepted. *Expenses: Tuition, area resident:* Full-time $22,410; part-time $1245 per credit. Tuition and fees vary according to course load, degree level and campus/location. *Financial support:* In 2015–16, 43 students received support. *Unit head:* Dr. Judith Karshmer, Dean, 415-422-6681, Fax: 415-422-6877, E-mail: nursing@usfca.edu. *Application contact:* Ingrid McVanner, Information Contact, 415-422-2746, Fax: 415-422-2217.

The University of Scranton, Panuska College of Professional Studies, Department of Nursing, Scranton, PA 18510-4595. Offers family nurse practitioner (MSN, PMC); nurse anesthesia (MSN, PMC); nursing leadership (DNP). Applicants accepted in odd-numbered years only. *Accreditation:* AACN; AANA/CANAEP. *Program availability:* Part-time, evening/weekend. *Students:* 58 full-time (46 women), 22 part-time (all women); includes 16 minority (12 Black or African American, non-Hispanic/Latino; 1 Asian, non-Hispanic/Latino; 2 Hispanic/Latino; 1 Two or more races, non-Hispanic/Latino). Average age 33. 104 applicants, 51% accepted, 45 enrolled. *Degree requirements:* For master's, comprehensive exam (for some programs), thesis (for some programs), capstone experience. *Entrance requirements:* For master's, minimum GPA of 3.0, three letters of reference; for doctorate, RN licensure and evidence of certification in advanced practice nursing specialty. Additional exam requirements/recommendations for international students: Required—TOEFL (minimum score 500 paper-based; 80 iBT), IELTS (minimum score 6.5). *Application deadline:* For fall admission, 9/1 for domestic students, 6/1 for international students; for spring admission, 11/1 for international students; for summer admission, 3/1 for international students. Applications are processed on a rolling basis. Application fee: $0. Electronic applications accepted. *Financial support:* Applicants required to submit FAFSA. *Faculty research:* Home care, doctoral education, health care of women and children, pain, health promotion and adolescence. *Unit head:* Dr. Dona Carpenter, Chair, 570-941-7673, Fax: 570-941-4201, E-mail: dona.carpenter@scranton.edu. *Application contact:* Dr. Mary Jane Hanson, Director, 570-941-4060, Fax: 570-941-4201, E-mail: hansonm2@scranton.edu.
Website: http://www.scranton.edu/academics/pcps/nursing/index.shtml

University of South Carolina, The Graduate School, College of Nursing, Program in Health Nursing, Columbia, SC 29208. Offers adult nurse practitioner (MSN); community/public health clinical nurse specialist (MSN); family nurse practitioner (MSN); pediatric nurse practitioner (MSN). *Accreditation:* AACN. *Program availability:* Part-time. *Degree requirements:* For master's, thesis or alternative. *Entrance requirements:* For master's, GRE General Test or MAT, BS in nursing, nursing license. Additional exam requirements/recommendations for international students: Required—TOEFL (minimum score 570 paper-based). Electronic applications accepted. *Faculty research:* System research, evidence based practice, breast cancer, violence.

University of Southern Maine, College of Science, Technology, and Health, School of Nursing, Portland, ME 04103. Offers adult-gerontology primary care nurse practitioner (MS, PMC); education (MS); family nurse practitioner (MS, PMC); family psychiatric/mental health nurse practitioner (MS); management (MS); nursing (CAS, CGS); psychiatric-mental health nurse practitioner (PMC). *Accreditation:* AACN. *Program availability:* Part-time. *Degree requirements:* For master's, thesis optional. *Entrance requirements:* For master's, GRE General Test or MAT, minimum GPA of 3.0; for doctorate, GRE. Additional exam requirements/recommendations for international students: Required—TOEFL (minimum score 550 paper-based). Electronic applications accepted. *Expenses: Tuition, area resident:* Full-time $6840; part-time $380 per credit hour. Tuition, state resident: full-time $10,260; part-time $570 per credit hour. Tuition, nonresident: full-time $18,468; part-time $1026 per credit hour. *Required fees:* $830; $83 per credit hour. Tuition and fees vary according to course load and program. *Faculty research:* Women's health, nursing history, weight control, community services, substance abuse.

University of Southern Mississippi, Graduate School, College of Nursing, Hattiesburg, MS 39406-0001. Offers family nurse practitioner (MSN, Graduate Certificate); family psychiatric-mental health nurse practitioner (Graduate Certificate); nursing (DNP, PhD); psychiatric-mental health nurse practitioner (Graduate Certificate). *Accreditation:* AACN. *Program availability:* Part-time, evening/weekend. *Degree requirements:* For master's, comprehensive exam, thesis optional; for doctorate, comprehensive exam, thesis/dissertation. *Entrance requirements:* For master's, GRE General Test, minimum GPA of 2.75 during last 60 hours, nursing license, BS in nursing; for doctorate, GRE General Test, master's degree in nursing, minimum GPA of 3.5. Additional exam requirements/recommendations for international students: Required—TOEFL, IELTS. Electronic applications accepted. *Faculty research:* Gerontology, caregivers, HIV, bereavement, pain, nursing leadership.

University of South Florida, College of Nursing, Tampa, FL 33612. Offers advanced pain management (Graduate Certificate); nursing (MS, DNP), including adult gerontology acute care (DNP), adult gerontology acute care nursing (MS), adult gerontology primary care (DNP), adult gerontology primary care nursing (MS), adult gerontology primary care/occupational health nursing (MS), adult gerontology primary care/oncology nursing (MS), clinical nurse leader (MS), family health nursing, nurse anesthesia (MS), nursing education (MS), nursing practice (DNP), occupational health/adult-gerontology (DNP), oncology/adult-gerontology primary care (DNP), pediatric health (DNP), pediatric nurse practitioner (MS); nursing education (Post Master's Certificate); nursing science (PhD). *Accreditation:* AACN; AANA/CANAEP. *Program availability:* Part-time. *Faculty:* 43 full-time (38 women), 7 part-time/adjunct (4 women). *Students:* 159 full-time (135 women), 721 part-time (625 women); includes 292 minority (119 Black or African American, non-Hispanic/Latino; 2 American Indian or Alaska Native, non-Hispanic/Latino; 60 Asian, non-Hispanic/Latino; 90 Hispanic/Latino; 1 Native Hawaiian or other Pacific Islander, non-Hispanic/Latino; 20 Two or more races, non-Hispanic/Latino), 12 international. Average age 35. 636 applicants, 44% accepted, 215 enrolled. In 2015, 333 master's, 18 doctorates awarded. *Degree requirements:* For master's, comprehensive exam, thesis optional; for doctorate, comprehensive exam, thesis/dissertation. *Entrance requirements:* For master's, GRE General Test, bachelor's degree from accredited program with minimum GPA of 3.0 in all upper-division coursework; current license as Registered Nurse; 3 letters of recommendation; personal statement of goals; resume or curriculum vitae; personal interview; for doctorate, GRE General Test (recommended), bachelor's degree in nursing from a CCNA/NLNAC regionally-accredited institution with minimum GPA of 3.0 in all coursework or in all upper-division coursework; current license as Registered Nurse in Florida; undergraduate statistics course with minimum B grade; 3 letters of recommendation; statement of goals; resume; interview. Additional exam requirements/recommendations for international students: Required—TOEFL (minimum score 550 paper-based; 79 iBT). *Application deadline:* For fall admission, 2/15 for domestic students, 1/2 for international students; for spring admission, 10/1 for domestic students, 6/1 for international students. Application fee: $30. Electronic applications accepted. *Financial support:* In 2015–16, 36 students received support, including 7 research assistantships with tuition reimbursements available (averaging $18,935 per year), 29 teaching assistantships with tuition reimbursements available (averaging $30,814 per year); tuition waivers (partial) and unspecified assistantships also available. Financial award application deadline: 2/1; financial award applicants required to submit FAFSA. *Faculty research:* Women's health, palliative and end-of-life care, cardiac rehabilitation, complementary therapies for chronic illness and cancer. *Total annual research expenditures:* $2.6 million. *Unit head:* Dr. Dianne C. Morrison-Beedy, Dean and Professor, College of Nursing, 813-974-9091, Fax: 813-974-5418, E-mail: dmbeedy@health.usf.edu. *Application contact:* Dr. Brian Graves, Assistant Professor/Assistant Dean, 813-974-8054, Fax: 813-974-5418, E-mail: bgraves1@health.usf.edu.
Website: http://health.usf.edu/nursing/index.htm

The University of Tampa, Program in Nursing, Tampa, FL 33606-1490. Offers adult nursing practitioner (MSN); family nursing practitioner (MSN); nursing (MS). *Accreditation:* ACEN. *Program availability:* Part-time, evening/weekend. *Faculty:* 15 full-time (13 women), 4 part-time/adjunct (3 women). *Students:* 1 (woman) full-time, 152 part-time (130 women); includes 27 minority (9 Black or African American, non-Hispanic/Latino; 1 American Indian or Alaska Native, non-Hispanic/Latino; 9 Asian, non-Hispanic/Latino; 8 Two or more races, non-Hispanic/Latino). Average age 39. 112 applicants, 54% accepted, 32 enrolled. In 2015, 33 master's awarded. *Degree requirements:* For master's, comprehensive exam, oral exam, practicum. *Entrance requirements:* For master's, GMAT or GRE, current licensure as registered nurse in state of Florida; minimum GPA of 3.0 in last 60 credit hours; minimum of one year of direct patient care experience within the past five years (recommended). Additional exam requirements/recommendations for international students: Required—TOEFL (minimum score 577 paper-based; 90 iBT), IELTS (minimum score 7.5). *Application deadline:* Applications are processed on a rolling basis. Application fee: $40. Electronic applications accepted. *Expenses:* $573 per credit tuition, $80 per term fees. *Financial support:* In 2015–16, 5 students received support. Career-related internships or fieldwork, scholarships/grants, and unspecified assistantships available. Financial award applicants required to submit FAFSA. *Faculty research:* Vaccinations and public health, osteoporosis, cultural diversity, ethics, nursing practice. *Unit head:* Dr. Cathy Kessenich, Director, 813-257-3160, Fax: 813-258-7214, E-mail: ckessenich@ut.edu. *Application contact:* Chanelle Cox, Staff Assistant, Admissions for Graduate and Continuing Studies, 813-253-6249, E-mail: ccox@ut.edu.

The University of Tennessee at Chattanooga, School of Nursing, Chattanooga, TN 37403. Offers administration (MSN); certified nurse anesthetist (Post-Master's Certificate); education (MSN); family nurse practitioner (MSN, Post-Master's Certificate); health care informatics (Post-Master's Certificate); nurse anesthesia (MSN); nurse education (Post-Master's Certificate); nursing (DNP). *Accreditation:* AACN; AANA/CANAEP (one or more programs are accredited). *Faculty:* 9 full-time (7 women), 2 part-time/adjunct (1 woman). *Students:* 50 full-time (25 women), 43 part-time (37 women); includes 14 minority (7 Black or African American, non-Hispanic/Latino; 1 American Indian or Alaska Native, non-Hispanic/Latino; 4 Asian, non-Hispanic/Latino; 2 Two or more races, non-Hispanic/Latino). Average age 34. In 2015, 40 master's, 12 doctorates, 1 other advanced degree awarded. *Degree requirements:* For master's, thesis optional, qualifying exams, professional project; for Post-Master's Certificate, thesis or alternative, practicum, seminar. *Entrance requirements:* For master's, GRE General Test, MAT, BSN, minimum GPA of 3.0, eligibility for Tennessee RN license, 1 year of direct patient care experience; for Post-Master's Certificate, GRE General Test, MAT, MSN, minimum GPA of 3.0, eligibility for Tennessee RN license, one year of direct patient care experience. Additional exam requirements/recommendations for international students: Required—TOEFL (minimum score 79 iBT), IELTS (minimum score 6). *Application deadline:* For fall admission, 6/13 priority date for domestic students, 6/1 for international students; for spring admission, 10/15 priority date for domestic students, 10/1 for international students. Applications are processed on a rolling basis. Application fee:

$30 ($35 for international students). Electronic applications accepted. *Expenses:* Tuition, state resident: full-time $7938; part-time $441 per credit hour. Tuition, nonresident: full-time $24,056; part-time $1336 per credit hour. *Required fees:* $1732; $253 per credit hour. *Financial support:* Career-related internships or fieldwork and scholarships/grants available. Support available to part-time students. *Faculty research:* Diabetes in women, health care for elderly, alternative medicine, hypertension, nurse anesthesia. *Total annual research expenditures:* $2.6 million. *Unit head:* Dr. Chris Smith, Interim Director, 423-425-1741, Fax: 423-425-4668, E-mail: chris-smith@utc.edu. *Application contact:* Dr. J. Randy Walker, Interim Dean of Graduate Studies, 423-425-4478, Fax: 423-425-5223, E-mail: randy-walker@utc.edu.
Website: http://www.utc.edu/Academic/Nursing/

The University of Texas at Arlington, Graduate School, College of Nursing, Arlington, TX 76019. Offers nurse practitioner (MSN); nursing administration (MSN); nursing education (MSN); nursing practice (DNP); nursing science (PhD). *Accreditation:* AACN. *Program availability:* Part-time, evening/weekend, online learning. *Degree requirements:* For master's, practicum course; for doctorate, comprehensive exam (for some programs), thesis/dissertation (for some programs), proposal defense dissertation (for PhD); scholarship project (for DNP). *Entrance requirements:* For master's, GRE General Test if GPA less than 3.0, minimum GPA of 3.0, Texas nursing license, minimum C grade in undergraduate statistics course; for doctorate, GRE General Test (waived for MSN-to-PhD applicants), minimum undergraduate, graduate and statistics GPA of 3.0; Texas RN license; interview; written statement of goals. Additional exam requirements/recommendations for international students: Required—TOEFL (minimum score 550 paper-based), IELTS (minimum score 7). *Faculty research:* Simulation in clinical education and practice, cultural diversity, vulnerable populations, substance abuse.

The University of Texas at Austin, Graduate School, School of Nursing, Austin, TX 78712-1111. Offers adult - gerontology clinical nurse specialist (MSN); child health (MSN), including administration, public health nursing, teaching; family nurse practitioner (MSN); family psychiatric/mental health nurse practitioner (MSN); holistic adult health (MSN), including administration, teaching; maternity (MSN), including administration, public health nursing, teaching; nursing (PhD); nursing administration and healthcare systems management (MSN); nursing practice (DNP); pediatric nurse practitioner (MSN); public health nursing (MSN). *Accreditation:* AACN. *Program availability:* Part-time. *Degree requirements:* For master's, thesis optional; for doctorate, thesis/dissertation. *Entrance requirements:* For master's and doctorate, GRE General Test. Additional exam requirements/recommendations for international students: Required—TOEFL (minimum score 550 paper-based). Electronic applications accepted. *Faculty research:* Chronic illness management, memory and aging, health promotion, women's health, adolescent health.

The University of Texas at El Paso, Graduate School, School of Nursing, El Paso, TX 79968-0001. Offers family nurse practitioner (MSN); health care leadership and management (Certificate); interdisciplinary health sciences (PhD); nursing (DNP); nursing education (MSN, Certificate); nursing systems management (MSN). *Accreditation:* AACN. *Program availability:* Online learning. *Degree requirements:* For master's, thesis optional; for doctorate, thesis/dissertation. *Entrance requirements:* For master's, minimum GPA of 3.0, resume; for doctorate, GRE, letters of reference, relevant personal/professional experience; master's degree in nursing (for DNP); for Certificate, bachelor's degree in nursing. Additional exam requirements/recommendations for international students: Required—TOEFL; Recommended—IELTS. Electronic applications accepted.

The University of Texas at Tyler, College of Nursing and Health Sciences, Program in Nursing, Tyler, TX 75799-0001. Offers nurse practitioner (MSN); nursing (PhD); nursing administration (MSN); nursing education (MSN); MSN/MBA. *Accreditation:* AACN. *Program availability:* Part-time, evening/weekend, online learning. *Degree requirements:* For master's, comprehensive exam (for some programs), thesis (for some programs); for doctorate, thesis/dissertation. *Entrance requirements:* For master's, GRE General Test or MAT, GMAT, minimum undergraduate GPA of 3.0, course work in statistics, RN license, BSN. Additional exam requirements/recommendations for international students: Required—TOEFL. Electronic applications accepted. *Faculty research:* Psychosocial adjustment, aging, support/commitment of caregivers, psychological abuse and violence, hope/hopelessness, professional values, end of life care, suicidology, clinical supervision, workforce retention and issues, global health issues, health promotion.

The University of Texas Health Science Center at San Antonio, School of Nursing, San Antonio, TX 78229-3900. Offers administrative management (MSN); adult-gerontology acute care nurse practitioner (PGC); advanced practice leadership (DNP); clinical nurse leader (MSN); executive administrative management (DNP); family nurse practitioner (MSN, PGC); nursing (MSN, PhD); nursing education (MSN, PGC); pediatric nurse practitioner primary care (PGC); psychiatric mental health nurse practitioner (PGC); public health nurse leader (DNP). *Accreditation:* AACN. *Program availability:* Part-time. Terminal master's awarded for partial completion of doctoral program. *Degree requirements:* For master's, thesis optional; for doctorate, comprehensive exam, thesis/dissertation.

The University of Texas Rio Grande Valley, College of Health Affairs, School of Nursing, Edinburg, TX 78539. Offers adult health nursing (MSN); family nurse practitioner (MSN). *Accreditation:* AACN. *Program availability:* Part-time, evening/weekend. *Degree requirements:* For master's, thesis optional. *Entrance requirements:* For master's, Texas RN licensure, undergraduate physical statistic course. Additional exam requirements/recommendations for international students: Required—TOEFL (minimum score 550 paper-based). Electronic applications accepted. *Expenses:* Contact institution. *Faculty research:* Health promotion, adolescent pregnancy, herbal and nontraditional approaches, healing touch stress.

The University of Toledo, College of Graduate Studies, College of Nursing, Department of Population and Community Care, Toledo, OH 43606-3390. Offers clinical nurse leader (MSN); family nurse practitioner (MSN, Certificate); nurse educator (MSN, Certificate); pediatric nurse practitioner (MSN, Certificate). *Program availability:* Part-time. *Degree requirements:* For master's, thesis or alternative. *Entrance requirements:* For master's, GRE, BS in nursing, minimum undergraduate GPA of 3.0, statement of purpose, three letters of recommendation, transcripts from all prior institutions attended, Nursing CAS application, UT supplemental application; for Certificate, BS in nursing, minimum undergraduate GPA of 3.0, statement of purpose, three letters of recommendation, transcripts from all prior institutions attended. Additional exam requirements/recommendations for international students: Required—TOEFL (minimum score 550 paper-based; 80 iBT). Electronic applications accepted.

University of Victoria, Faculty of Graduate Studies, Faculty of Human and Social Development, School of Nursing, Victoria, BC V8W 2Y2, Canada. Offers advanced nursing practice (advanced practice leadership option) (MN); advanced nursing practice (nurse educator option) (MN); advanced nursing practice (nurse practitioner option) (MN); nursing (PhD). *Program availability:* Part-time, online learning. *Entrance requirements:* Additional exam requirements/recommendations for international students: Required—TOEFL (minimum score 575 paper-based), IELTS (minimum score 7). Electronic applications accepted.

Family Nurse Practitioner Studies

University of Wisconsin–Eau Claire, College of Nursing and Health Sciences, Program in Nursing, Eau Claire, WI 54702-4004. Offers adult-gerontological administration (DNP); adult-gerontological clinical nurse specialist (DNP); adult-gerontological education (MSN); adult-gerontological primary care nurse practitioner (DNP); family health administration (DNP); family health in education (MSN); family health nurse practitioner (DNP); nursing (MSN); nursing practice (DNP). *Program availability:* Part-time. Terminal master's awarded for partial completion of doctoral program. *Degree requirements:* For master's, thesis optional, 500-600 hours clinical practicum, oral and written exams. *Entrance requirements:* For master's, Wisconsin RN license, minimum GPA of 3.0, undergraduate statistics, course work in health assessment. Additional exam requirements/recommendations for international students: Required—TOEFL (minimum score 79 iBT). *Expenses:* Contact institution.

University of Wisconsin–Milwaukee, Graduate School, College of Nursing, Milwaukee, WI 53201-0413. Offers clinical nurse specialist (Certificate); family nurse practitioner (Certificate); nursing (MN, MS, PhD); nursing practice (DNP). *Accreditation:* AACN. *Program availability:* Part-time. *Students:* 168 full-time (144 women), 126 part-time (115 women); includes 47 minority (16 Black or African American, non-Hispanic/Latino; 16 Asian, non-Hispanic/Latino; 3 Hispanic/Latino; 12 Two or more races, non-Hispanic/Latino), 12 international. Average age 36. 146 applicants, 64% accepted, 59 enrolled. In 2015, 22 master's, 28 doctorates, 15 other advanced degrees awarded. *Degree requirements:* For master's, thesis; for doctorate, thesis/dissertation. *Entrance requirements:* For master's, GRE General Test or MAT, autobiographical sketch; for doctorate, GRE, minimum GPA of 3.2. Additional exam requirements/recommendations for international students: Required—TOEFL (minimum score 550 paper-based; 79 iBT), IELTS (minimum score 6.5). *Application deadline:* For fall admission, 1/1 priority date for domestic students; for spring admission, 9/1 for domestic students. Applications are processed on a rolling basis. Application fee: $56 ($96 for international students). Electronic applications accepted. *Financial support:* Fellowships, research assistantships, teaching assistantships, career-related internships or fieldwork, Federal Work-Study, health care benefits, unspecified assistantships, and project assistantships available. Support available to part-time students. Financial award application deadline: 4/15; financial award applicants required to submit FAFSA. *Unit head:* Dr. Sally Lundeen, Dean, 414-229-4189, E-mail: slundeen@uwm.edu. *Application contact:* Kim Litwack, Representative, 414-229-5098.
Website: http://www.uwm.edu/Dept/Nursing/

University of Wisconsin–Oshkosh, Graduate Studies, College of Nursing, Oshkosh, WI 54901. Offers adult health and illness (MSN); family nurse practitioner (MSN). *Accreditation:* AACN. *Program availability:* Part-time. *Degree requirements:* For master's, thesis or alternative, clinical paper. *Entrance requirements:* For master's, RN license, BSN, previous course work in statistics and health assessment, minimum undergraduate GPA of 3.0, letters of recommendation. Additional exam requirements/recommendations for international students: Required—TOEFL (minimum score 550 paper-based; 79 iBT). Electronic applications accepted. *Faculty research:* Adult health and illness, nurse practitioners practice, health care service, advanced practitioner roles, natural alternative complementary healthcare.

Ursuline College, School of Graduate Studies, Programs in Nursing, Pepper Pike, OH 44124-4398. Offers adult nurse practitioner (MSN); adult-gerontology clinical nurse specialist (MSN); family nurse practitioner (MSN); nursing (DNP); nursing education (MSN); palliative care (MSN). *Accreditation:* AACN. *Program availability:* Part-time. *Faculty:* 5 full-time (all women), 26 part-time/adjunct (21 women). *Students:* 150 full-time (141 women), 108 part-time (99 women); includes 66 minority (50 Black or African American, non-Hispanic/Latino; 6 Asian, non-Hispanic/Latino; 6 Hispanic/Latino; 4 Two or more races, non-Hispanic/Latino), 5 international. Average age 37. 115 applicants, 95% accepted, 73 enrolled. In 2015, 69 master's, 2 doctorates awarded. *Degree requirements:* For master's, comprehensive exam. *Entrance requirements:* For master's, minimum undergraduate GPA of 3.0, bachelor's degree in nursing, eligibility for or current Ohio RN license. Additional exam requirements/recommendations for international students: Required—TOEFL (minimum score 500 paper-based). *Application deadline:* For fall admission, 8/1 priority date for domestic students. Applications are processed on a rolling basis. Application fee: $25. Electronic applications accepted. *Expenses:* Tuition, area resident: Full-time $18,036; part-time $6012 per semester. *Required fees:* $290; $210 per credit. $105 per semester. Tuition and fees vary according to program. *Financial support:* In 2015–16, 12 students received support. Scholarships/grants available. Financial award application deadline: 3/1; financial award applicants required to submit FAFSA. *Unit head:* Dr. Janet Baker, Director, 440-864-8172, Fax: 440-684-6053, E-mail: jbaker@ursuline.edu. *Application contact:* Stephanie Pratt McRoberts, Graduate Admission Coordinator, 440-646-8119, Fax: 440-684-6138, E-mail: graduateadmissions@ursuline.edu.

Vanderbilt University, Vanderbilt University School of Nursing, Nashville, TN 37240. Offers adult-gerontology acute care nurse practitioner (MSN), including hospitalist, intensivist; adult-gerontology primary care nurse practitioner (MSN); emergency nurse practitioner (MSN); family nurse practitioner (MSN); healthcare leadership (MSN); neonatal nurse practitioner (MSN); nurse midwifery (MSN); nurse midwifery/family nurse practitioner (MSN); nursing (Post-Master's Certificate); nursing informatics (MSN); nursing practice (DNP); nursing science (PhD); pediatric acute care nurse practitioner (MSN); pediatric primary care nurse practitioner (MSN); psychiatric-mental health nurse practitioner (MSN); women's health nurse practitioner (MSN); women's health nurse practitioner/adult gerontology primary care nurse practitioner (MSN); MSN/M Div; MSN/MTS. *Accreditation:* ACEN (one or more programs are accredited); ACNM/ACME. *Program availability:* Part-time, 100% online, blended/hybrid learning. *Faculty:* 258 full-time (232 women), 363 part-time/adjunct (271 women). *Students:* 478 full-time (424 women), 342 part-time (317 women); includes 140 minority (36 Black or African American, non-Hispanic/Latino; 3 American Indian or Alaska Native, non-Hispanic/Latino; 24 Asian, non-Hispanic/Latino; 43 Hispanic/Latino; 3 Native Hawaiian or other Pacific Islander, non-Hispanic/Latino; 31 Two or more races, non-Hispanic/Latino), 11 international. Average age 31. 1,268 applicants, 49% accepted, 477 enrolled. In 2015, 343 master's, 55 doctorates awarded. *Degree requirements:* For doctorate, comprehensive exam, thesis/dissertation. *Entrance requirements:* For master's, GRE General Test (taken within the past 5 years), minimum B average in undergraduate course work, 3 letters of recommendation; for doctorate, GRE General Test, interview, 3 letters of recommendation from doctorally-prepared faculty, MSN, essay. Additional exam requirements/recommendations for international students: Required—TOEFL (minimum score 570 paper-based), IELTS (minimum score 6.5). *Application deadline:* For fall admission, 11/1 priority date for domestic and international students. Applications are processed on a rolling basis. Application fee: $50. Electronic applications accepted. *Expenses:* Contact Institution. *Financial support:* In 2015–16, 585 students received support. Scholarships/grants available. Financial award application deadline: 3/15; financial award applicants required to submit FAFSA. *Faculty research:* Lymphedema, palliative care and bereavement, health services research including workforce, safety and quality of care, gerontology, better birth outcomes including nutrition. *Total annual research expenditures:* $2 million. *Unit head:* Dr. Linda Norman, Dean, 615-343-8876, Fax: 615-343-7711, E-mail: linda.norman@vanderbilt.edu. *Application contact:* Patricia Peerman, Assistant Dean for Enrollment Management, 615-322-3800, Fax: 615-343-0333, E-mail: vusn-admissions@vanderbilt.edu.
Website: http://www.nursing.vanderbilt.edu

Villanova University, College of Nursing, Villanova, PA 19085-1699. Offers adult nurse practitioner (MSN, Post Master's Certificate); family nurse practitioner (MSN, Post Master's Certificate); nurse anesthetist (MSN, Post Master's Certificate); nursing (PhD); nursing education (MSN, Post Master's Certificate); nursing practice (DNP); pediatric nurse practitioner (MSN, Post Master's Certificate). *Accreditation:* AACN; AANA/CANAEP. *Program availability:* Part-time, online learning. *Faculty:* 16 full-time (15 women), 9 part-time/adjunct (7 women). *Students:* 219 full-time (198 women), 108 part-time (96 women); includes 36 minority (25 Black or African American, non-Hispanic/Latino; 9 Asian, non-Hispanic/Latino; 2 Hispanic/Latino), 16 international. Average age 31. 147 applicants, 78% accepted, 106 enrolled. In 2015, 64 master's, 8 doctorates, 9 other advanced degrees awarded. *Degree requirements:* For master's, independent study project; for doctorate, comprehensive exam, thesis/dissertation; for Post Master's Certificate, scholarly project. *Entrance requirements:* For master's, GRE or MAT, BSN, 1 year of recent nursing experience, physical assessment, course work in statistics; for doctorate, GRE, MSN. Additional exam requirements/recommendations for international students: Required—TOEFL (minimum score 540 paper-based; 83 iBT), IELTS (minimum score 6.5). *Application deadline:* For fall admission, 7/1 priority date for domestic students, 7/1 for international students; for spring admission, 11/1 priority date for domestic students, 11/1 for international students; for summer admission, 4/1 priority date for domestic students, 3/1 for international students. Applications are processed on a rolling basis. Application fee: $50. Electronic applications accepted. *Expenses:* $837 per credit (MSN); $1,049 per credit (PhD); $1,375 per credit (DNP). *Financial support:* In 2015–16, 22 students received support, including 5 teaching assistantships with full tuition reimbursements available (averaging $15,475 per year); institutionally sponsored loans, scholarships/grants, traineeships, tuition waivers (full), and unspecified assistantships also available. Financial award application deadline: 7/1; financial award applicants required to submit FAFSA. *Faculty research:* Genetics, ethics, cognitive development of students, women with disabilities, nursing leadership. *Unit head:* Dr. Marguerite K. Schlag, Assistant Dean/Director, Graduate Programs, 610-519-4907, Fax: 610-519-7650, E-mail: marguerite.schlag@villanova.edu. *Application contact:* Rebecca Harold, Administrative Assistant, 610-519-4934, Fax: 610-519-7650, E-mail: rebecca.harold@villanova.edu.
Website: http://www.nursing.villanova.edu/

Virginia Commonwealth University, Graduate School, School of Nursing, Nurse Practitioner Program, Richmond, VA 23284-9005. Offers MS, Certificate. *Program availability:* Part-time. *Entrance requirements:* For master's, GRE General Test, minimum GPA of 2.8. Additional exam requirements/recommendations for international students: Required—TOEFL (minimum score 600 paper-based; 100 iBT). Electronic applications accepted.

Walden University, Graduate Programs, School of Nursing, Minneapolis, MN 55401. Offers adult-gerontology acute care nurse practitioner (MSN); adult-gerontology nurse practitioner (MSN); education (MSN); family nurse practitioner (MSN); informatics (MSN); leadership and management (MSN); nursing (PhD, Post-Master's Certificate), including education (PhD), healthcare administration (PhD), interdisciplinary health (PhD), leadership (PhD), nursing education (Post-Master's Certificate), nursing informatics (Post-Master's Certificate), nursing leadership and management (Post-Master's Certificate), public health policy (PhD); nursing practice (DNP); psychiatric mental health (MSN). *Accreditation:* AACN. *Program availability:* Part-time, evening/weekend, online only, 100% online. *Faculty:* 22 full-time (18 women), 540 part-time/adjunct (487 women). *Students:* 4,320 full-time (3,773 women), 5,250 part-time (4,740 women); includes 3,550 minority (2,360 Black or African American, non-Hispanic/Latino; 29 American Indian or Alaska Native, non-Hispanic/Latino; 523 Asian, non-Hispanic/Latino; 421 Hispanic/Latino; 25 Native Hawaiian or other Pacific Islander, non-Hispanic/Latino; 192 Two or more races, non-Hispanic/Latino), 221 international. Average age 40. 2,057 applicants, 100% accepted, 1507 enrolled. In 2015, 3,022 master's, 86 doctorates, 34 other advanced degrees awarded. *Degree requirements:* For doctorate, thesis/dissertation (for some programs), residency (for some programs), field experience (for some programs). *Entrance requirements:* For master's, bachelor's degree or equivalent in related field or RN; minimum GPA of 2.5; official transcripts; goal statement (for some programs); access to computer and Internet; for doctorate, master's degree or higher; RN; three years of related professional or academic experience; goal statement; access to computer and Internet; for Post-Master's Certificate, relevant work experience; access to computer and Internet. Additional exam requirements/recommendations for international students: Required—TOEFL (minimum score 550 paper-based, 79 iBT), IELTS (minimum score 6.5), Michigan English Language Assessment Battery (minimum score 82), or PTE (minimum score 53). *Application deadline:* Applications are processed on a rolling basis. Application fee: $0. Electronic applications accepted. *Financial support:* Fellowships, Federal Work-Study, scholarships/grants, unspecified assistantships, and family tuition reduction, active duty/veteran tuition reduction, group tuition reduction, interest-free payment plans, employee tuition reduction available. Support available to part-time students. Financial award applicants required to submit FAFSA. *Unit head:* Dr. Andrea Lindell, Dean, 866-492-5336. *Application contact:* Meghan Thomas, Vice President of Enrollment Management, 866-492-5336, E-mail: info@waldenu.edu.
Website: http://www.waldenu.edu/programs/colleges-schools/nursing

Washington State University, College of Nursing, Spokane, WA 99210. Offers advanced population health (MN, DNP); family nurse practitioner (MN, DNP); nursing (PhD); psychiatric/mental health nurse practitioner (DNP); psychiatric/mental health practitioner (MN). Programs offered at the Spokane, Tri-Cities, and Vancouver campuses. *Accreditation:* AACN. *Degree requirements:* For master's, comprehensive exam (for some programs), thesis (for some programs), oral exam, research project. *Entrance requirements:* For master's, minimum GPA of 3.0, Washington state RN license, physical assessment skills, course work in statistics, recommendations, written interview (for nurse practitioner). *Faculty research:* Cardiovascular and Type 2 diabetes in children, evaluation of strategies to increase physical activity in sedentary people.

Wayne State University, College of Nursing, Doctor Program of Nursing Practice, Detroit, MI 48202. Offers adult gerontology nurse practitioner - acute care (DNP); adult gerontology nurse practitioner - primary care (DNP); family nurse practitioner (DNP); infant mental health (DNP); neonatal nurse practitioner (DNP); nurse midwifery (DNP); nursing practice (DNP); pediatric nurse practitioner - acute care (DNP); pediatric nurse practitioner - primary care (DNP); psychiatric mental health nurse practitioner (DNP). *Students:* 56 full-time (50 women), 37 part-time (32 women); includes 32 minority (19 Black or African American, non-Hispanic/Latino; 6 Asian, non-Hispanic/Latino; 3 Hispanic/Latino; 4 Two or more races, non-Hispanic/Latino), 6 international. Average age 35. 44 applicants, 66% accepted, 18 enrolled. In 2015, 16 doctorates awarded. *Entrance requirements:* For doctorate, official transcripts, two professional references, curriculum vitae or resume, statement of goals, BSN or MSN, current Michigan RN license, criminal background check, interview, on-site writing example. Additional exam requirements/recommendations for international students: Required—TOEFL (minimum score 600 paper-based; 101 iBT); Recommended—IELTS (minimum score 7). *Application deadline:* For fall admission, 1/31 for domestic and international students. Electronic applications accepted. *Expenses:* $19,325 per year resident tuition, $35,114 non-resident tuition; $805.20 per credit hour resident tuition, $1,463.10 per credit hour non-resident tuition; fees include $47.45 per credit hour student services fee and

$274.60 per semester registration fee. *Financial support:* In 2015–16, 22 students received support. Fellowships, research assistantships, teaching assistantships, institutionally sponsored loans, and scholarships/grants available. Financial award applicants required to submit FAFSA. *Unit head:* Dr. Laurie Lauzon Clabo, Dean and Professor, 313-577-4104, E-mail: laurie.lauzon.clabo@wayne.edu. *Application contact:* Dr. Nancy George, Director of DNP Program, 313-577-8300.
Website: http://nursing.wayne.edu/dnp/index.php

West Coast University, Graduate Programs, North Hollywood, CA 91606. Offers advanced generalist (MSN); family nurse practitioner (MSN); health administration (MHA); occupational therapy (MS); pharmacy (Pharm D); physical therapy (DPT).

Western University of Health Sciences, College of Graduate Nursing, Master of Science in Nursing Program, Pomona, CA 91766-1854. Offers administrative nurse leader (MSN); ambulatory care (MSN); clinical nurse leader (MSN); family nurse practitioner (MSN); nursing (MSN). *Program availability:* Blended/hybrid learning. *Faculty:* 15 full-time (all women), 13 part-time/adjunct (7 women). *Students:* 243 full-time (206 women), 13 part-time (10 women); includes 155 minority (6 Black or African American, non-Hispanic/Latino; 76 Asian, non-Hispanic/Latino; 54 Hispanic/Latino; 19 Two or more races, non-Hispanic/Latino), 1 international. Average age 30. 467 applicants, 36% accepted, 93 enrolled. In 2015, 97 master's awarded. *Degree requirements:* For master's, comprehensive exam (for some programs), thesis (for some programs), project. *Entrance requirements:* For master's, personal statement, BSN, minimum GPA of 3.0, 3 letters of recommendation, resume/curriculum vitae, official transcripts of all schools attended. Additional exam requirements/recommendations for international students: Required—TOEFL (minimum score 80 iBT). *Application deadline:* For fall admission, 11/1 for domestic and international students. Application fee: $60. Electronic applications accepted. *Expenses:* $1,026 per unit tuition; $1,836 clinical fees; $40 student body fee. *Financial support:* Fellowships, research assistantships, teaching assistantships, and scholarships/grants available. Support available to part-time students. Financial award application deadline: 3/2; financial award applicants required to submit FAFSA. *Unit head:* Dr. Karen J. Hanford, Dean, 909-469-5523, Fax: 909-469-5521, E-mail: khanford@westernu.edu. *Application contact:* Kathryn Ford, Director of Admissions/International Student Advisor, 909-469-5335, Fax: 909-469-5570, E-mail: admissions@westernu.edu.

Westminster College, School of Nursing and Health Sciences, Salt Lake City, UT 84105-3697. Offers family nurse practitioner (MSN); nurse anesthesia (MSN); nurse education (MSNED); public health (MPH). *Accreditation:* AACN; AANA/CANAEP. *Faculty:* 15 full-time (9 women), 7 part-time/adjunct (2 women). *Students:* 120 full-time (79 women), 3 part-time (all women); includes 18 minority (1 Black or African American, non-Hispanic/Latino; 3 Asian, non-Hispanic/Latino; 10 Hispanic/Latino; 4 Two or more races, non-Hispanic/Latino), 3 international. Average age 32. 157 applicants, 40% accepted, 45 enrolled. In 2015, 56 master's awarded. *Degree requirements:* For master's, clinical practicum, 504 clinical practice hours. *Entrance requirements:* For master's, GRE, personal statement, resume, 3 professional recommendations, copy of unrestricted Utah license to practice professional nursing, background check, minimum cumulative GPA of 3.0, documentation of current immunizations, physical and mental health certificate signed by primary care provider. Additional exam requirements/recommendations for international students: Required—TOEFL (minimum score 600 paper-based; 100 iBT), IELTS (minimum score 7.5). Application fee: $50. Electronic applications accepted. *Expenses:* Contact institution. *Financial support:* In 2015–16, 8 students received support. Career-related internships or fieldwork, unspecified assistantships, and tuition reimbursements, tuition remission available. Support available to part-time students. Financial award applicants required to submit FAFSA. *Faculty research:* Intellectual empathy, professional boundaries, learned optimism, collaborative testing in nursing: student outcomes and perspectives, implementing new

educational paradigms into pre-licensure nursing curricula. *Unit head:* Dr. Sheryl Steadman, Dean, 801-832-2164, Fax: 801-832-3110, E-mail: ssteadman@westminstercollege.edu. *Application contact:* Dr. John Baworowsky, Vice President of Enrollment Management, 801-832-2200, Fax: 801-832-3101, E-mail: admission@westminstercollege.edu.
Website: http://www.westminstercollege.edu/msn

West Texas A&M University, College of Nursing and Health Sciences, Department of Nursing, Canyon, TX 79016-0001. Offers family nurse practitioner (MSN); nursing (MSN). *Accreditation:* AACN. *Program availability:* Part-time, online learning. *Degree requirements:* For master's, comprehensive exam, thesis optional. *Entrance requirements:* For master's, GRE General Test, bachelor's degree in nursing, minimum GPA of 3.0 in last 60 hours. Additional exam requirements/recommendations for international students: Required—TOEFL (minimum score 550 paper-based). Electronic applications accepted. *Faculty research:* Family-focused nursing, nursing traineeship, professional nursing.

West Virginia Wesleyan College, Department of Nursing, Buckhannon, WV 26201. Offers family nurse practitioner (Post Master's Certificate); family nurse practitioner (MS); nurse administrator (MS); nurse educator (MS); nurse-midwifery (MS); nursing administration (Post Master's Certificate); nursing education (Post Master's Certificate); psychiatric mental health nurse practitioner (MS); MSN/MBA. *Accreditation:* ACEN.

Wilmington University, College of Health Professions, New Castle, DE 19720-6491. Offers adult nurse practitioner (MSN); family nurse practitioner (MSN); gerontology nurse practitioner (MSN); nursing (MSN); nursing leadership (MSN); nursing practice (DNP). *Accreditation:* AACN. *Program availability:* Part-time. *Degree requirements:* For master's, thesis. *Entrance requirements:* For master's, BSN, RN license, interview, 3 letters of recommendation. Additional exam requirements/recommendations for international students: Required—TOEFL (minimum score 500 paper-based). Electronic applications accepted. *Faculty research:* Outcomes assessment, student writing ability.

Winona State University, College of Nursing and Health Sciences, Winona, MN 55987. Offers adult nurse practitioner (MS, Post Master's Certificate); clinical nurse specialist (MS, Post Master's Certificate); family nurse practitioner (MS, Post Master's Certificate); nurse administrator (MS, Post Master's Certificate); nurse educator (MS, Post Master's Certificate); nursing (DNP). *Accreditation:* AACN. *Program availability:* Part-time, online learning. *Degree requirements:* For master's, thesis; for doctorate, capstone. *Entrance requirements:* For master's, GRE (if GPA less than 3.0). Additional exam requirements/recommendations for international students: Required—TOEFL (minimum score 550 paper-based).

Winston-Salem State University, Program in Nursing, Winston-Salem, NC 27110-0003. Offers advanced nurse educator (MSN); family nurse practitioner (MSN); nursing (DNP). *Accreditation:* AACN. *Program availability:* Part-time, evening/weekend, online learning. *Entrance requirements:* For master's, GRE, MAT, resume, NC or state compact license, 3 letters of recommendation. Electronic applications accepted. *Faculty research:* Elimination of health care disparities.

Wright State University, School of Graduate Studies, College of Nursing and Health, Program in Nursing, Dayton, OH 45435. Offers acute care nurse practitioner (MS); administration of nursing and health care systems (MS); adult health (MS); child and adolescent health (MS); community health (MS); family nurse practitioner (MS); nurse practitioner (MS); school nurse (MS); MBA/MS. *Accreditation:* AACN. *Program availability:* Part-time, evening/weekend. *Degree requirements:* For master's, thesis or alternative. *Entrance requirements:* For master's, GRE General Test, BSN from NLN-accredited college, Ohio RN license. Additional exam requirements/recommendations for international students: Required—TOEFL. *Faculty research:* Clinical nursing and health, teaching, caring, pain administration, informatics and technology.

Forensic Nursing

Boston College, William F. Connell School of Nursing, Chestnut Hill, MA 02467. Offers adult-gerontology nursing (MS); family health nursing (MS); forensic nursing (MS); nurse anesthesia (MS); nursing (PhD); pediatric nursing (MS), including pediatric and women's health; psychiatric-mental health nursing (MS); women's health nursing (MS); MBA/MS; MS/MA; MS/PhD. *Accreditation:* AACN; AANA/CANAEP (one or more programs are accredited). *Program availability:* Part-time. *Faculty:* 53 full-time (48 women), 47 part-time/adjunct (44 women). *Students:* 185 full-time (167 women), 66 part-time (56 women); includes 31 minority (10 Black or African American, non-Hispanic/Latino; 12 Asian, non-Hispanic/Latino; 7 Hispanic/Latino; 2 Two or more races, non-Hispanic/Latino), 7 international. Average age 32. 313 applicants, 66% accepted, 91 enrolled. In 2015, 98 master's, 5 doctorates awarded. *Degree requirements:* For master's, comprehensive exam; for doctorate, comprehensive exam, thesis/dissertation, computer literacy exam or foreign language. *Entrance requirements:* For master's, bachelor's degree in nursing; for doctorate, GRE General Test, MS in nursing. Additional exam requirements/recommendations for international students: Required—TOEFL (minimum score 600 paper-based; 100 iBT), IELTS (minimum score 7.5). *Application deadline:* For fall admission, 9/30 for domestic and international students; for winter admission, 1/15 for domestic and international students; for spring admission, 3/15 for domestic and international students. Applications are processed on a rolling basis. Application fee: $40. Electronic applications accepted. *Expenses:* Contact institution. *Financial support:* In 2015–16, 1 fellowship with full tuition reimbursement (averaging $23,700 per year), 25 teaching assistantships (averaging $4,370 per year) were awarded; research assistantships, scholarships/grants, health care benefits, tuition waivers (partial), and unspecified assistantships also available. Support available to part-time students. Financial award application deadline: 3/1; financial award applicants required to submit FAFSA. *Faculty research:* Sexual and reproductive health, health promotion/illness prevention, aging, eating disorders, symptom management. *Total annual research expenditures:* $1 million. *Unit head:* Dr. Susan Gennaro, Dean, 617-552-4251, Fax: 617-552-0931, E-mail: susan.gennaro@bc.edu. *Application contact:* MaryBeth Crowley, Graduate Programs Assistant, 617-552-4928, Fax: 617-552-2121, E-mail: csongrad@bc.edu.
Website: http://www.bc.edu/schools/son/

Cleveland State University, College of Graduate Studies, School of Nursing, Cleveland, OH 44115. Offers clinical nurse leader (MSN); forensic nursing (MSN); nursing education (MSN); specialized population (MSN); urban education (PhD), including nursing education; MSN/MBA. *Accreditation:* AACN. *Program availability:* Part-time, 100% online. *Faculty:* 7 full-time (all women). *Students:* 7 full-time (all women), 43 part-time (42 women); includes 14 minority (12 Black or African American, non-Hispanic/Latino; 1 Asian, non-Hispanic/Latino; 1 Hispanic/Latino). Average age 37. 60 applicants,

62% accepted, 26 enrolled. In 2015, 11 master's awarded. *Degree requirements:* For master's, thesis optional, portfolio, capstone practicum project; for doctorate, comprehensive exam, thesis/dissertation. *Entrance requirements:* For master's, RN license in the U.S., BSN with minimum cumulative GPA of 3.0, recent (within last 5 years) course work in statistics; for doctorate, GRE, MSN with minimum cumulative GPA of 3.25. Additional exam requirements/recommendations for international students: Required—TOEFL (minimum score 550 paper-based; 78 iBT), IELTS (minimum score 6). *Application deadline:* For fall admission, 3/1 priority date for domestic and international students. Application fee: $55. Electronic applications accepted. *Expenses:* Tuition, state resident: full-time $9565. Tuition, nonresident: full-time $17,980. Tuition and fees vary according to program. *Financial support:* Tuition waivers (full) and unspecified assistantships available. Financial award application deadline: 5/1; financial award applicants required to submit FAFSA. *Faculty research:* Diabetes management, African-American elders medication compliance, risk in home visiting, suffering, COPD and stress, nursing education, disaster health preparedness. *Total annual research expenditures:* $330,000. *Unit head:* Dr. Vida Lock, Dean, 216-523-7237, Fax: 216-687-3556, E-mail: v.lock@csuohio.edu. *Application contact:* Maureen Mitchell, Assistant Professor and Graduate Program Director, 216-523-7128, Fax: 216-687-3556, E-mail: m.m.mitchell1@csuohio.edu.
Website: http://www.csuohio.edu/nursing/

Duquesne University, School of Nursing, Master of Science in Nursing Program, Pittsburgh, PA 15282-0001. Offers family (individual across the life span) nurse practitioner (MSN); forensic nursing (MSN); nursing education (MSN). *Accreditation:* AACN. *Program availability:* Part-time, evening/weekend, minimal on-campus study. *Faculty:* 13 full-time (11 women), 9 part-time/adjunct (all women). *Students:* 91 full-time (84 women), 87 part-time (76 women); includes 31 minority (16 Black or African American, non-Hispanic/Latino; 4 Asian, non-Hispanic/Latino; 7 Hispanic/Latino; 4 Two or more races, non-Hispanic/Latino), 1 international. Average age 34. 280 applicants, 34% accepted, 73 enrolled. In 2015, 39 master's awarded. *Entrance requirements:* For master's, current RN license; BSN with minimum GPA of 3.0; minimum of 1 year of full-time work experience as RN prior to registration in clinical or specialty course. Additional exam requirements/recommendations for international students: Required—TOEFL (minimum score 600 paper-based; 100 iBT). *Application deadline:* For fall admission, 3/1 for domestic and international students. Application fee: $0. Electronic applications accepted. *Expenses:* $1,218 per credit. *Financial support:* In 2015–16, 11 students received support, including 2 research assistantships with partial tuition reimbursements available (averaging $2,200 per year), 7 teaching assistantships with partial tuition reimbursements available (averaging $1,100 per year); scholarships/grants, traineeships, and tuition waivers (partial) also available. Support available to part-time

Forensic Nursing

students. Financial award application deadline: 7/1; financial award applicants required to submit FAFSA. *Faculty research:* Vulnerable populations, social justice, cultural competence, health disparities, wellness within chronic illness, forensics. *Total annual research expenditures:* $246,973. *Unit head:* Dr. Alison Colbert, Associate Professor/ Associate Dean of Academic Affairs, 412-396-1511, Fax: 412-396-1821, E-mail: colberta@duq.edu. *Application contact:* Susan Hardner, Nurse Recruiter, 412-396-4945, Fax: 412-396-6346, E-mail: nursing@duq.edu.
Website: http://www.duq.edu/academics/schools/nursing/graduate-programs/master-science-nursing

Duquesne University, School of Nursing, Post Master's Certificate Program, Pittsburgh, PA 15282-0001. Offers family (individual across the life span) nurse practitioner (Post-Master's Certificate); forensic nursing (Post-Master's Certificate); nursing education and faculty role (Post-Master's Certificate). *Program availability:* Part-time, evening/weekend, minimal on-campus study. *Faculty:* 3 full-time (all women), 7 part-time/adjunct (all women). *Students:* 2 full-time (both women), 10 part-time (9 women); includes 4 minority (3 Black or African American, non-Hispanic/Latino; 1 Hispanic/Latino). Average age 42. 28 applicants, 36% accepted, 5 enrolled. In 2015, 4 Post-Master's Certificates awarded. *Entrance requirements:* For degree, current RN license, BSN, MSN. Additional exam requirements/recommendations for international students: Required—TOEFL (minimum score 600 paper-based; 100 iBT). *Application deadline:* For fall admission, 3/1 for domestic and international students. Application fee: $0. Electronic applications accepted. *Expenses:* $1,218 per credit. *Financial support:* Teaching assistantships with partial tuition reimbursements, scholarships/grants, traineeships, and tuition waivers (partial) available. Support available to part-time students. Financial award application deadline: 7/1; financial award applicants required to submit FAFSA. *Faculty research:* Vulnerable populations, social justice, cultural competence, health disparities, wellness within chronic illness, forensics. *Total annual research expenditures:* $296,973. *Unit head:* Dr. Alison Colbert, Associate Professor/ Associate Dean of Academic Affairs, 412-396-1511, Fax: 412-396-1821, E-mail: colberta@duq.edu. *Application contact:* Susan Hardner, Nurse Recruiter, 412-396-4945, Fax: 412-396-6346, E-mail: nursing@duq.edu.
Website: http://www.duq.edu/academics/schools/nursing/graduate-programs/post-masters-certificates

Fitchburg State University, Division of Graduate and Continuing Education, Program in Forensic Nursing, Fitchburg, MA 01420-2697. Offers MS, Certificate. *Accreditation:* AACN. *Program availability:* Part-time, evening/weekend, online learning. *Students:* 33 part-time (31 women); includes 6 minority (3 Black or African American, non-Hispanic/ Latino; 1 American Indian or Alaska Native, non-Hispanic/Latino; 2 Asian, non-Hispanic/ Latino). Average age 38. 4 applicants, 100% accepted, 2 enrolled. In 2015, 6 master's awarded. *Entrance requirements:* Additional exam requirements/recommendations for international students: Required—TOEFL (minimum score 550 paper-based; 79 iBT). *Application deadline:* For fall admission, 7/15 for international students; for spring admission, 12/1 for international students. Applications are processed on a rolling basis. Application fee: $25 ($50 for international students). Electronic applications accepted. *Expenses:* Tuition, state resident: full-time $3006; part-time $1002 per year. Tuition, nonresident: full-time $3006; part-time $1002 per year. *Required fees:* $2468. *Financial support:* In 2015–16, research assistantships with partial tuition reimbursements (averaging $5,500 per year) were awarded; Federal Work-Study, scholarships/grants, and unspecified assistantships also available. Support available to part-time students. Financial award application deadline: 3/1; financial award applicants required to submit FAFSA. *Unit head:* Dr. Robert Dumas, Chair, 978-665-3026, Fax: 978-665-3658, E-mail: gce@fitchburgstate.edu. *Application contact:* Sean Ganas, Director of Admissions, 978-665-3144, Fax: 978-665-4540, E-mail: admissions@fitchburgstate.edu.
Website: http://www.fitchburgstate.edu/

Monmouth University, Graduate Studies, The Marjorie K. Unterberg School of Nursing and Health Studies, West Long Branch, NJ 07764-1898. Offers adult and gerontological primary care nurse practitioner (MSN); adult-gerontological primary care nurse practitioner (Post-Master's Certificate); family nurse practitioner (MSN, Post-Master's Certificate); family psychiatric and mental health advanced practice nursing (MSN); family psychiatric and mental health nurse practitioner (Post-Master's Certificate); forensic nursing (MSN, Certificate); nursing (MSN); nursing administration (MSN, Post-Master's Certificate); nursing education (MSN, Post-Master's Certificate); nursing practice (DNP); physician assistant (MS); school nursing (MSN, Certificate). *Accreditation:* AACN. *Program availability:* Part-time, evening/weekend, 100% online,

blended/hybrid learning. *Faculty:* 14 full-time (13 women), 10 part-time/adjunct (5 women). *Students:* 58 full-time (46 women), 271 part-time (252 women); includes 93 minority (31 Black or African American, non-Hispanic/Latino; 40 Asian, non-Hispanic/ Latino; 18 Hispanic/Latino; 1 Native Hawaiian or other Pacific Islander, non-Hispanic/ Latino; 3 Two or more races, non-Hispanic/Latino), 1 international. Average age 37. 450 applicants, 32% accepted, 103 enrolled. In 2015, 68 master's, 8 doctorates, 11 other advanced degrees awarded. *Degree requirements:* For master's, practicum (for some tracks); for doctorate, practicum, capstone course. *Entrance requirements:* For master's, GRE General Test (waived for MSN applicants with minimum B grade in each of the first four courses and for MS applicants with master's degree), BSN with minimum GPA of 2.75, current RN license, proof of liability and malpractice policy, personal statement, two letters of recommendation, college course work in health assessment, resume; CASPA application (for MS); for doctorate, accredited master's nursing program degree with minimum GPA of 3.2, graduate research course in statistics, active RN license, national certification as Nurse Practitioner or Nurse Administrator, working knowledge of statistics, statement of goals and vision for change, 2 letters of recommendation (professional or academic), resume, interview. Additional exam requirements/ recommendations for international students: Required—TOEFL (minimum score 550 paper-based; 79 iBT), IELTS (minimum score 6) or Michigan English Language Assessment Battery (minimum score 77). *Application deadline:* For fall admission, 7/15 priority date for domestic students, 6/1 for international students; for spring admission, 12/15 priority date for domestic students, 11/1 for international students; for summer admission, 5/1 for domestic students. Applications are processed on a rolling basis. Application fee: $50. Electronic applications accepted. *Expenses:* Contact institution. *Financial support:* In 2015–16, 241 students received support, including 220 fellowships (averaging $3,403 per year), 5 research assistantships (averaging $5,146 per year); career-related internships or fieldwork, scholarships/grants, and unspecified assistantships also available. Support available to part-time students. Financial award applicants required to submit FAFSA. *Faculty research:* School nursing, health policy, and smoking cessation in teens, Multiple Sclerosis; adherence and self-efficacy, aging issues and geriatric care. *Unit head:* Dr. Janet Mahoney, Dean, 732-571-3443, Fax: 732-263-5131, E-mail: jmahoney@monmouth.edu. *Application contact:* Lucia Fedele, Graduate Admission Counselor, 732-571-3452, Fax: 732-263-5123, E-mail: gradadm@ monmouth.edu.
Website: http://www.monmouth.edu/school-of-nursing-health/graduate-nursing-programs.aspx

National University, Academic Affairs, School of Health and Human Services, La Jolla, CA 92037-1011. Offers clinical affairs (MS); clinical informatics (Certificate); clinical regulatory affairs (MS); health and life science analytics (MS); health coaching (Certificate); health informatics (MS); healthcare administration (MHA); nurse anesthesia (MS); nursing (MS), including forensic nursing, nursing administration, nursing informatics; nursing administration (Certificate); nursing informatics (Certificate); nursing practice (DNP); public health (MPH), including health promotion, healthcare administration, mental health. *Program availability:* Part-time, evening/weekend, 100% online, blended/hybrid learning. *Faculty:* 31 full-time (18 women), 33 part-time/adjunct (20 women). *Students:* 353 full-time (263 women), 136 part-time (87 women); includes 322 minority (111 Black or African American, non-Hispanic/Latino; 1 American Indian or Alaska Native, non-Hispanic/Latino; 105 Asian, non-Hispanic/Latino; 72 Hispanic/Latino; 7 Native Hawaiian or other Pacific Islander, non-Hispanic/Latino; 26 Two or more races, non-Hispanic/Latino), 31 international. Average age 32. In 2015, 103 master's awarded. *Degree requirements:* For master's, thesis (for some programs). *Entrance requirements:* For master's, interview, minimum GPA of 2.5. Additional exam requirements/ recommendations for international students: Required—TOEFL (minimum score 550 paper-based; 79 iBT), IELTS (minimum score 6). *Application deadline:* Applications are processed on a rolling basis. Application fee: $60 ($65 for international students). Electronic applications accepted. *Financial support:* Career-related internships or fieldwork, institutionally sponsored loans, scholarships/grants, and tuition waivers (partial) available. Support available to part-time students. Financial award application deadline: 6/30; financial award applicants required to submit FAFSA. *Faculty research:* Nursing education, obesity prevention, workforce diversity. *Unit head:* School of Health and Human Services, 800-628-8648, E-mail: shhs@nu.edu. *Application contact:* Frank Rojas, Vice President for Enrollment Services, 800-628-8648, E-mail: advisor@nu.edu. Website: http://www.nu.edu/OurPrograms/SchoolOfHealthAndHumanServices.html

Gerontological Nursing

Allen College, Graduate Programs, Waterloo, IA 50703. Offers acute care nurse practitioner (Post-Master's Certificate); adult nurse practitioner (Post-Master's Certificate); adult psychiatric-mental health nurse practitioner (Post-Master's Certificate); adult-gerontology acute care nurse practitioner (MSN); community public health (Post-Master's Certificate); community/public health nursing (MSN); family nurse practitioner (MSN, Post-Master's Certificate); gerontological nurse practitioner (Post-Master's Certificate); health sciences (Ed D); leadership in health care delivery (MSN, Post-Master's Certificate); nursing (DNP); occupational therapy (MS). *Accreditation:* AACN; ACEN. *Program availability:* Part-time, blended/hybrid learning. *Faculty:* 3 full-time (all women), 21 part-time/adjunct (20 women). *Students:* 61 full-time (54 women), 163 part-time (144 women); includes 9 minority (5 Black or African American, non-Hispanic/ Latino; 2 Hispanic/Latino; 2 Two or more races, non-Hispanic/Latino), 2 international. Average age 34. 212 applicants, 60% accepted, 94 enrolled. In 2015, 51 master's, 1 doctorate awarded. *Degree requirements:* For master's, thesis optional. *Entrance requirements:* For master's, minimum GPA of 3.0 in the last 60 hours of undergraduate coursework; for doctorate, minimum GPA of 3.25 in graduate coursework. Additional exam requirements/recommendations for international students: Recommended— TOEFL (minimum score 580 paper-based; 92 iBT), IELTS (minimum score 6). *Application deadline:* For fall admission, 2/1 priority date for domestic students; for spring admission, 9/1 priority date for domestic students. Applications are processed on a rolling basis. Application fee: $50. Electronic applications accepted. *Expenses:* $15,940 tuition, $1,240 fees. *Financial support:* Institutionally sponsored loans, scholarships/grants, and traineeships available. Support available to part-time students. Financial award application deadline: 8/15; financial award applicants required to submit FAFSA. *Unit head:* Nancy Kramer, Vice Chancellor for Academic Affairs, 319-226-2040, Fax: 319-226-2070, E-mail: nancy.kramer@allencollege.edu. *Application contact:* Molly Quinn, Administrative Assistant for Student Services, 319-226-2014, Fax: 319-226-2010, E-mail: admissions@allencollege.edu.
Website: http://www.allencollege.edu/

Arizona State University at the Tempe campus, College of Nursing and Health Innovation, Phoenix, AZ 85004. Offers advanced nursing practice (DNP); clinical research management (MS); community and public health practice (Graduate Certificate); family mental health nurse practitioner (Graduate Certificate); family nurse practitioner (Graduate Certificate); geriatric nursing (Graduate Certificate); healthcare innovation (MHI); nurse education in academic and practice settings (Graduate Certificate); nurse educator (MS); nursing and healthcare innovation (PhD). *Accreditation:* AACN. *Program availability:* Online learning. *Degree requirements:* For master's, comprehensive exam (for some programs), thesis (for some programs), interactive Program of Study (iPOS) submitted before completing 50 percent of required credit hours; for doctorate, comprehensive exam, thesis/dissertation, interactive Program of Study (iPOS) submitted before completing 50 percent of required credit hours. *Entrance requirements:* For master's and doctorate, GRE, minimum GPA of 3.0 or equivalent in last 2 years of work leading to bachelor's degree. Additional exam requirements/recommendations for international students: Required—TOEFL, IELTS, or PTE. Electronic applications accepted. *Expenses:* Contact institution.

Armstrong State University, School of Graduate Studies, Program in Nursing, Savannah, GA 31419-1997. Offers adult-gerontological acute care nurse practitioner (Certificate); adult-gerontological clinical nurse specialist (Certificate); adult-gerontological primary care nurse practitioner (Certificate); family nurse practitioner (MSN). *Accreditation:* AACN. *Program availability:* Part-time, evening/weekend. *Faculty:* 5 full-time (all women), 1 (woman) part-time/adjunct. *Students:* 35 full-time (32 women), 19 part-time (16 women); includes 13 minority (10 Black or African American, non-Hispanic/Latino; 2 Hispanic/Latino; 1 Two or more races, non-Hispanic/Latino), 1 international. Average age 35. 23 applicants, 83% accepted, 16 enrolled. In 2015, 19 master's awarded. *Degree requirements:* For master's, comprehensive exam, project or thesis. *Entrance requirements:* For master's, GRE General Test or MAT, minimum GPA of 3.0, letter of recommendation, letter of intent. Additional exam requirements/ recommendations for international students: Required—TOEFL (minimum score 523

paper-based; 70 iBT). *Application deadline:* For fall admission, 2/28 for domestic and international students; for spring admission, 11/15 for domestic students, 9/15 for international students. Applications are processed on a rolling basis. Application fee: $30. Electronic applications accepted. *Expenses:* Tuition, state resident: part-time $211 per credit hour. Tuition, nonresident: part-time $782 per credit hour. *Required fees:* $1224 per unit. $612 per semester. Tuition and fees vary according to course load, campus/location and program. *Financial support:* In 2015–16, research assistantships with full tuition reimbursements (averaging $5,000 per year) were awarded; Federal Work-Study, scholarships/grants, and unspecified assistantships also available. Support available to part-time students. Financial award application deadline: 3/1; financial award applicants required to submit FAFSA. *Faculty research:* Midwifery, mental health, nursing simulation, smoking cessation during pregnancy, asthma education, vulnerable populations, geriatrics, disaster nursing, complementary and alternative modalities, nephrology. *Unit head:* Dr. Catherine Gilbert, Department Head, 912-344-3145, E-mail: catherine.gilbert@armstrong.edu. *Application contact:* McKenzie Peterman, Assistant Director of Graduate Admissions, 912-344-2503, Fax: 912-344-3417, E-mail: graduate@armstrong.edu.
Website: http://www.armstrong.edu/Health_professions/nursing/nursing_graduate_programs

Augusta University, The Graduate School, Doctor of Nursing Practice Program, Augusta, GA 30912. Offers adult gerontology acute care nurse practitioner (DNP); family nurse practitioner (DNP); nursing (DNP); nursing anesthesia (DNP); pediatric nurse practitioner (DNP); psychiatric mental health nurse practitioner (DNP). *Students:* 40 part-time. *Degree requirements:* For doctorate, thesis/dissertation or alternative. *Entrance requirements:* For doctorate, GRE General Test or MAT, master's degree in nursing or related field, current professional nurse licensure. Additional exam requirements/recommendations for international students: Required—TOEFL (minimum score 600 paper-based; 100 iBT). *Application deadline:* For fall admission, 3/1 for domestic and international students; for spring admission, 7/1 for domestic and international students. Applications are processed on a rolling basis. Application fee: $50. Electronic applications accepted. *Unit head:* Dr. Marguerite Murphy, RN, Director, 706-721-3676, Fax: 706-721-8169. *Application contact:* Karen Sturgill, Program Manager, 706-721-3676, Fax: 706-721-8169, E-mail: dnp@augusta.edu.
Website: http://www.augusta.edu/nursing/dnp_programs.php

Ball State University, Graduate School, College of Applied Sciences and Technology, School of Nursing, Muncie, IN 47306. Offers adult/gerontology nurse practitioner (Post Master's Certificate); evidence-based clinical practice (Postbaccalaureate Certificate); family nurse practitioner (Post Master's Certificate); family nurse practitioner for the adult nurse practitioner or adult/gerontology nurse practitioner (Post Master's Certificate); nurse educator (Post Master's Certificate); nursing (MS), including family nurse practitioner, nurse administrator, nurse educator; nursing education (Postbaccalaureate Certificate); nursing practice (DNP). *Accreditation:* AACN. *Program availability:* Part-time-only, online only, 100% online. *Faculty:* 12 full-time (all women), 7 part-time/adjunct (6 women). *Students:* 9 full-time (8 women), 334 part-time (311 women); includes 23 minority (11 Black or African American, non-Hispanic/Latino; 5 Asian, non-Hispanic/Latino; 6 Hispanic/Latino; 1 Two or more races, non-Hispanic/Latino). Average age 33. 88 applicants, 85% accepted, 63 enrolled. In 2015, 115 master's, 8 doctorates awarded. *Entrance requirements:* For master's, bachelor's degree in nursing, minimum GPA of 3.0, minimum C grade in at least 2 quarter or semester hours in an undergraduate research course, unencumbered license as a registered nurse in state of practice; for doctorate, advanced practice nurse (nurse practitioner, clinical nurse specialist, nurse midwife); master's degree in nursing from accredited prorgam with minimum GPA of 3.2; graduate-level statistics, nursing research, and health assessment courses; unencumbered license as registered nurse in state of practice. Additional exam requirements/recommendations for international students: Required—TOEFL (minimum score 550 paper-based; 79 iBT), IELTS (minimum score 6.5). *Application deadline:* For fall admission, 2/9 for domestic students; for spring admission, 8/9 for domestic students. Applications are processed on a rolling basis. Application fee: $60. Electronic applications accepted. *Expenses:* Contact institution. *Financial support:* Application deadline: 3/1; applicants required to submit FAFSA. *Unit head:* Dr. Linda Siktberg, Director, 765-285-8718, Fax: 765-285-2169, E-mail: lsiktberg@bsu.edu. *Application contact:* Shantelle Estes, Graduate Advisor, 765-285-9130, Fax: 765-285-2169, E-mail: smestes@bsu.edu.
Website: http://www.bsu.edu/nursing/

Boise State University, College of Health Sciences, School of Nursing, Boise, ID 83725-1840. Offers acute care adult gerontology (Graduate Certificate); adult gerontology acute care (MSN); adult gerontology primary care (MSN); healthcare simulation (Graduate Certificate); nursing practice (DNP); primary care adult gerontology (Graduate Certificate). *Students:* 1 (woman) full-time, 91 part-time (73 women); includes 11 minority (5 Black or African American, non-Hispanic/Latino; 2 Asian, non-Hispanic/Latino; 3 Hispanic/Latino; 1 Native Hawaiian or other Pacific Islander, non-Hispanic/Latino). Average age 43. 32 applicants, 44% accepted, 12 enrolled. In 2015, 3 master's awarded. *Entrance requirements:* For master's, minimum GPA of 3.0. Additional exam requirements/recommendations for international students: Required—TOEFL (minimum score 550 paper-based; 80 iBT), IELTS (minimum score 6). *Application deadline:* For spring admission, 10/15 priority date for domestic and international students. Applications are processed on a rolling basis. Application fee: $65 ($95 for international students). Electronic applications accepted. *Expenses:* Tuition, state resident: full-time $6058; part-time $358 per credit hour. Tuition, nonresident: full-time $20,108; part-time $608 per credit hour. *Required fees:* $2108. Tuition and fees vary according to program. *Financial support:* In 2015–16, 1 student received support. Scholarships/grants and unspecified assistantships available. Financial award application deadline: 10/15; financial award applicants required to submit FAFSA. *Unit head:* Dr. Ann Hubbert, Director, 208-426-3404, E-mail: annhubbert@boisestate.edu. *Application contact:* Dr. Dawn Weiler, Program Coordinator, 208-426-1239, E-mail: dweiler@boisestate.edu.
Website: http://hs.boisestate.edu/nursing/

Boston College, William F. Connell School of Nursing, Chestnut Hill, MA 02467. Offers adult-gerontology nursing (MS); family health nursing (MS); forensic nursing (MS); nurse anesthesia (MS); nursing (PhD); pediatric nursing (MS), including pediatric and women's health; psychiatric-mental health nursing (MS); women's health nursing (MS); MBA/MS; MS/MA; MS/PhD. *Accreditation:* AACN; AANA/CANAEP (one or more programs are accredited). *Program availability:* Part-time. *Faculty:* 53 full-time (48 women), 47 part-time/adjunct (44 women). *Students:* 185 full-time (167 women), 66 part-time (56 women); includes 31 minority (10 Black or African American, non-Hispanic/Latino; 12 Asian, non-Hispanic/Latino; 7 Hispanic/Latino; 2 Two or more races, non-Hispanic/Latino), 7 international. Average age 32. 313 applicants, 66% accepted, 91 enrolled. In 2015, 98 master's, 5 doctorates awarded. *Degree requirements:* For master's, comprehensive exam; for doctorate, comprehensive exam, thesis/dissertation, computer literacy exam or foreign language. *Entrance requirements:* For master's, bachelor's degree in nursing; for doctorate, GRE General Test, MS in nursing. Additional exam requirements/recommendations for international students: Required—TOEFL (minimum score 600 paper-based; 100 iBT), IELTS (minimum score 7.5). *Application deadline:* For fall admission, 9/30 for domestic and international students; for winter admission, 1/15

for domestic and international students; for spring admission, 3/15 for domestic and international students. Applications are processed on a rolling basis. Application fee: $40. Electronic applications accepted. *Expenses:* Contact institution. *Financial support:* In 2015–16, 1 fellowship with full tuition reimbursement (averaging $23,700 per year), 25 teaching assistantships (averaging $4,370 per year) were awarded; research assistantships, scholarships/grants, health care benefits, tuition waivers (partial), and unspecified assistantships also available. Support available to part-time students. Financial award application deadline: 3/1; financial award applicants required to submit FAFSA. *Faculty research:* Sexual and reproductive health, health promotion/illness prevention, aging, eating disorders, symptom management. *Total annual research expenditures:* $1 million. *Unit head:* Dr. Susan Gennaro, Dean, 617-552-4251, Fax: 617-552-0931, E-mail: susan.gennaro@bc.edu. *Application contact:* MaryBeth Crowley, Graduate Programs Assistant, 617-552-4928, Fax: 617-552-2121, E-mail: csongrad@bc.edu.
Website: http://www.bc.edu/schools/son/

California State University, Stanislaus, College of Human and Health Sciences, Program in Nursing (MS), Turlock, CA 95382. Offers gerontological nursing (MS); nursing education (MS). *Accreditation:* AACN. *Program availability:* Part-time. *Degree requirements:* For master's, comprehensive exam, thesis or alternative. *Entrance requirements:* For master's, GRE or MAT, minimum GPA of 3.0, 3 letters of reference, RN. Additional exam requirements/recommendations for international students: Required—TOEFL (minimum score 550 paper-based). Electronic applications accepted.

Capella University, School of Public Service Leadership, Master's Programs in Nursing, Minneapolis, MN 55402. Offers diabetes nursing (MSN); general nursing (MSN); gerontology nursing (MSN); health information management (MS); nurse educator (MSN); nursing leadership and administration (MSN).

Caribbean University, Graduate School, Bayamón, PR 00960-0493. Offers administration and supervision (MA Ed); criminal justice (MA); curriculum and instruction (MA Ed, PhD), including elementary education (MA Ed), English education (MA Ed), history education (MA Ed), mathematics education (MA Ed), primary education (MA Ed), science education (MA Ed), Spanish education (MA Ed); educational technology in instructional systems (MA Ed); gerontology (MSN); human resources (MBA); museology, archiving and art history (MA Ed); neonatal pediatrics (MSN); physical education (MA Ed); special education (MA Ed). *Entrance requirements:* For master's, interview, minimum GPA of 2.5.

Case Western Reserve University, Frances Payne Bolton School of Nursing, Master's Programs in Nursing, Nurse Practitioner Program, Cleveland, OH 44106. Offers acute care cardiovascular nursing (MSN); acute care nurse practitioner (MSN); acute care pediatric nurse practitioner (MSN); adult gerontology acute care nurse practitioner (MSN); adult gerontology oncology and palliative care (MSN); adult gerontology primary care nurse practitioner (MSN); family nurse practitioner (MSN); family systems psychiatric mental health nursing (MSN); neonatal nurse practitioner (MSN); pediatric nurse practitioner (MSN); women's health nurse practitioner (MSN). *Accreditation:* ACEN. *Program availability:* Part-time, online learning. *Students:* 52 full-time (45 women), 78 part-time (68 women); includes 31 minority (10 Black or African American, non-Hispanic/Latino; 14 Asian, non-Hispanic/Latino; 7 Hispanic/Latino). Average age 35. 64 applicants, 66% accepted, 29 enrolled. In 2015, 45 master's awarded. *Degree requirements:* For master's, thesis optional. *Entrance requirements:* For master's, GRE General Test or MAT. Additional exam requirements/recommendations for international students: Required—TOEFL (minimum score 577 paper-based; 90 iBT), IELTS (minimum score 7). *Application deadline:* For fall admission, 6/1 for domestic students; for spring admission, 10/1 for domestic students. Applications are processed on a rolling basis. Application fee: $75. *Expenses:* $1,891 per credit hour. *Financial support:* In 2015–16, 54 students received support, including 17 teaching assistantships with partial tuition reimbursements available (averaging $17,019 per year); scholarships/grants and traineeships also available. Financial award application deadline: 6/30; financial award applicants required to submit FAFSA. *Faculty research:* Symptom science, family/community care, aging across the lifespan, self-management of health and illness, neuroscience. *Unit head:* Dr. Carol Savrin, Director, 216-368-5304, Fax: 216-368-3542, E-mail: cls18@case.edu. *Application contact:* Donna Hassik, Admissions Coordinator, 216-368-5253, Fax: 216-368-0124, E-mail: dmh7@case.edu.
Website: http://fpb.cwru.edu/MSN/majors.shtm

College of Mount Saint Vincent, School of Professional and Continuing Studies, Department of Nursing, Riverdale, NY 10471-1093. Offers adult nurse practitioner (MSN, PMC); family nurse practitioner (MSN, PMC); nurse educator (PMC); nursing administration (MSN); nursing for the adult and aged (MSN). *Accreditation:* AACN. *Program availability:* Part-time. *Entrance requirements:* For master's, BSN, interview, RN license, minimum GPA of 3.0, letters of reference. Additional exam requirements/recommendations for international students: Required—TOEFL. *Expenses:* Contact institution.

College of Staten Island of the City University of New York, Graduate Programs, School of Health Sciences, Program in Adult-Gerontological Nursing, Staten Island, NY 10314-6600. Offers clinical nurse practitioner (MS, Advanced Certificate); clinical nurse specialist (MS, Advanced Certificate). *Program availability:* Part-time, evening/weekend. *Faculty:* 5 full-time, 7 part-time/adjunct. *Students:* Average age 38. In 2015, 18 master's, 4 other advanced degrees awarded. *Degree requirements:* For master's, thesis optional. *Entrance requirements:* For master's, bachelor's degree in nursing with minimum GPA of 3.0 in nursing major, two letters of recommendation, personal statement, current New York State RN license, minimum of one year of full-time experience as a registered nurse; for Advanced Certificate, master's degree in nursing; master's-level courses in pathophysiology, health assessment and pharmacology. Additional exam requirements/recommendations for international students: Required—TOEFL (minimum score 550 paper-based; 79 iBT), IELTS (minimum score 6.5). *Application deadline:* For spring admission, 10/15 priority date for domestic and international students. Applications are processed on a rolling basis. Application fee: $125. Electronic applications accepted. *Expenses:* Tuition, state resident: full-time $10,130; part-time $425 per credit. Tuition, nonresident: full-time $18,720; part-time $780 per credit. *Required fees:* $181.10 per semester. Tuition and fees vary according to program. *Financial support:* Applicants required to submit FAFSA. *Faculty research:* Cardiac, health literacy, role stress, cancer survivorship, older adults and end of life: decision making, dying, palliative, and hospice care. *Unit head:* Dr. June Como, Graduate and Clinical Doctorate in Nursing Practice Programs Coordinator, 718-982-3823, Fax: 718-982-3813, E-mail: june.como@csi.cuny.edu. *Application contact:* Sasha Spence, Associate Director for Graduate Admissions, 718-982-2019, Fax: 718-982-2500, E-mail: sasha.spence@csi.cuny.edu.
Website: http://www.csi.cuny.edu/nursing/graduate.html

Columbia University, School of Nursing, Program in Adult-Gerontology Primary Care Nurse Practitioner, New York, NY 10032. Offers MS, Adv C. *Accreditation:* AACN. *Program availability:* Part-time. *Entrance requirements:* For master's, GRE General Test, NCLEX, BSN, 1 year of clinical experience (preferred); for Adv C, MSN. Additional exam requirements/recommendations for international students: Required—TOEFL (minimum score 100 iBT). Electronic applications accepted.

Gerontological Nursing

Concordia University Wisconsin, Graduate Programs, School of Human Services, Program in Nursing, Mequon, WI 53097-2402. Offers family nurse practitioner (MSN); geriatric nurse practitioner (MSN); nurse educator (MSN). *Accreditation:* AACN. *Program availability:* Online learning. *Degree requirements:* For master's, comprehensive exam, thesis or alternative. *Entrance requirements:* Additional exam requirements/recommendations for international students: Required—TOEFL. *Expenses:* Contact institution.

Creighton University, College of Nursing, Omaha, NE 68178-0001. Offers adult acute care nurse practitioner (Post-Master's Certificate); adult gerontology acute care nurse practitioner (DNP); adult gerontology nurse practitioner (DNP); clinical nurse leader (MSN, Post-Graduate Certificate); clinical systems administration (MSN, DNP); family nurse practitioner (DNP, Post-Master's Certificate); neonatal nurse practitioner (DNP, Post-Master's Certificate); pediatric acute care nurse practitioner (DNP, Post-Master's Certificate); psychiatric mental health nurse practitioner (DNP). *Accreditation:* AACN. *Program availability:* Part-time, blended/hybrid learning. *Faculty:* 10 full-time (all women), 48 part-time/adjunct (45 women). *Students:* 132 full-time (120 women), 228 part-time (212 women); includes 38 minority (10 Black or African American, non-Hispanic/Latino; 3 American Indian or Alaska Native, non-Hispanic/Latino; 11 Asian, non-Hispanic/Latino; 1 Hispanic/Latino; 2 Native Hawaiian or other Pacific Islander, non-Hispanic/Latino; 11 Two or more races, non-Hispanic/Latino). Average age 31. 66 applicants, 91% accepted, 43 enrolled. In 2015, 54 master's, 17 doctorates, 1 other advanced degree awarded. *Degree requirements:* For master's, capstone project; for doctorate, scholarly project. *Entrance requirements:* For master's and doctorate, BSN from an ACEN- or CCNE-accredited nursing school, minimum cumulative GPA of 3.0, personal statement, current unencumbered RN license with NE eligibility, undergraduate statistics course, physical assessment course or equivalent; for other advanced degree, MSN or MS in nursing, minimum cumulative GPA of 3.0, current unencumbered RN license with NE eligibility. Additional exam requirements/recommendations for international students: Required—TOEFL (minimum score 600 paper-based; 100 iBT). *Application deadline:* For fall admission, 6/15 priority date for domestic and international students; for spring admission, 11/15 priority date for domestic and international students; for summer admission, 4/15 for domestic and international students. Applications are processed on a rolling basis. Application fee: $50. Electronic applications accepted. *Expenses:* $800 per credit hour tuition; $904 per semester full-time fees; $207 per semester part-time fees; $50 one-time drug screen fee. *Financial support:* In 2015–16, 7 students received support. Scholarships/grants available. Financial award applicants required to submit FAFSA. *Faculty research:* Obesity prevention in children, evaluation of simulated clinical experiences, vitamin D3 and calcium for cancer risk education in post menopausal women, online support and education to reduce stress for prenatal patients on bed rest, health literacy, immunization research. *Total annual research expenditures:* $162,085. *Unit head:* Dr. Catherine Todero, Dean, 402-280-2004, Fax: 402-280-2045. *Application contact:* Shannon Cox, Enrollment Specialist, 402-280-2067, Fax: 402-280-2045, E-mail: shannoncox@creighton.edu.
Website: http://nursing.creighton.edu/

Duke University, School of Nursing, Durham, NC 27708-0586. Offers acute care pediatric nurse practitioner (MSN, Post Master's Certificate); adult-gerontology nurse practitioner (MSN, Post Master's Certificate), including acute care, primary care; family nurse practitioner (MSN, Post Master's Certificate); neonatal nurse practitioner (MSN, Post Master's Certificate); nurse anesthesia (DNP); nurse practitioner (DNP); nursing (PhD); nursing and health care leadership (MSN); nursing education (MSN); nursing informatics (MSN, Post Master's Certificate); pediatric nurse practitioner (MSN, Post Master's Certificate), including primary care; women's health nurse practitioner (MSN, Post Master's Certificate). *Accreditation:* AACN; AANA/CANAEP. *Program availability:* Part-time, evening/weekend, online learning. *Faculty:* 74 full-time (63 women). *Students:* 179 full-time (152 women), 528 part-time (466 women); includes 145 minority (42 Black or African American, non-Hispanic/Latino; 3 American Indian or Alaska Native, non-Hispanic/Latino; 44 Asian, non-Hispanic/Latino; 35 Hispanic/Latino; 1 Native Hawaiian or other Pacific Islander, non-Hispanic/Latino; 20 Two or more races, non-Hispanic/Latino), 7 international. Average age 33. 619 applicants, 46% accepted, 201 enrolled. In 2015, 243 master's, 62 doctorates, 26 other advanced degrees awarded. Terminal master's awarded for partial completion of doctoral program. *Degree requirements:* For master's, thesis optional; for doctorate, capstone project. *Entrance requirements:* For master's, GRE General Test (waived if undergraduate GPA of 3.4 or higher), 1 year of nursing experience (recommended), BSN, minimum GPA of 3.0, previous course work in statistics; for doctorate, GRE General Test (waived if undergraduate GPA of 3.4 or higher), BSN or MSN, minimum GPA of 3.0, portfolio, resume, personal statement, undergraduate statistics course, current licensure as a registered nurse, transcripts from all post-secondary institutions; for Post Master's Certificate, MSN, licensure or eligibility as a professional nurse, transcripts from all post-secondary institutions, previous course work in statistics. Additional exam requirements/recommendations for international students: Required—TOEFL (minimum score 100 iBT), IELTS (minimum score 7). *Application deadline:* For fall admission, 12/1 for domestic and international students; for spring admission, 5/1 for domestic and international students. Application fee: $50. Electronic applications accepted. *Expenses:* Contact institution. *Financial support:* Career-related internships or fieldwork, institutionally sponsored loans, scholarships/grants, traineeships, and tuition waivers (partial) available. Support available to part-time students. Financial award applicants required to submit FAFSA. *Faculty research:* Cardiovascular disease, caregiver skill training, data mining, prostate cancer, neonatal immune system. *Unit head:* Dr. Marion E. Broome, Dean/Vice Chancellor for Nursing Affairs/Associate Vice President for Academic Affairs for Nursing, 919-684-9446, Fax: 919-684-9414, E-mail: marion.broome@duke.edu. *Application contact:* Dr. Ernie Rushing, Director of Admissions and Recruitment, 919-668-6274, Fax: 919-668-4693, E-mail: ernie.rushing@dm.duke.edu.
Website: http://www.nursing.duke.edu/

Felician University, Master of Science in Nursing Program, Lodi, NJ 07644-2117. Offers adult-gerontology nurse practitioner (MSN, PMC); executive leadership (MSN, PMC); family nurse practitioner (MSN, PMC); nursing education (MSN, PMC). *Accreditation:* AACN. *Program availability:* Part-time, evening/weekend, online learning. *Faculty:* 11 full-time (9 women), 2 part-time/adjunct (both women). *Students:* 1 (woman) full-time, 121 part-time (112 women); includes 60 minority (23 Black or African American, non-Hispanic/Latino; 1 American Indian or Alaska Native, non-Hispanic/Latino; 19 Asian, non-Hispanic/Latino; 17 Hispanic/Latino). Average age 40. 111 applicants, 83% accepted, 52 enrolled. In 2015, 18 master's awarded. *Entrance requirements:* For master's, BS in nursing or equivalent, minimum GPA of 3.0, 2 letters of recommendation, RN license; for PMC, RN license, minimum GPA of 3.0. Additional exam requirements/recommendations for international students: Recommended—TOEFL (minimum score 79 iBT). *Application deadline:* Applications are processed on a rolling basis. Application fee: $40. Electronic applications accepted. Application fee is waived when completed online. *Expenses:* Tuition, area resident: Part-time $965 per credit. Tuition and fees vary according to course load and program. *Financial support:* In 2015–16, 10 students received support. Traineeships available. Financial award applicants required to submit FAFSA. *Faculty research:* Anxiety and fear, curriculum innovation, health promotion. *Unit head:* Dr. Ann Tritak, Associate Dean, Department of

Graduate Nursing, 201-201-559-6151, E-mail: tritaka@felician.edu. *Application contact:* Dr. Margaret Smolin, Director, Graduate Admissions, 201-559-1451, E-mail: graduate@felician.edu.

Florida Southern College, Program in Nursing, Lakeland, FL 33801-5698. Offers adult gerontology clinical nurse specialist (MSN); adult gerontology primary care nurse practitioner (MSN); nurse educator (MSN); nursing administration (MSN). *Accreditation:* AACN. *Program availability:* Part-time, evening/weekend. *Entrance requirements:* For master's, Florida RN license, 3 letters of recommendation, personal statement, minimum GPA of 3.0, resume. Additional exam requirements/recommendations for international students: Required—TOEFL (minimum score 550 paper-based). *Expenses:* Contact institution. *Faculty research:* End of life care, dementia, health promotion.

Goldfarb School of Nursing at Barnes-Jewish College, Graduate Programs, St. Louis, MO 63110. Offers adult-gerontology acute care nurse practitioner (MSN); adult-gerontology nurse practitioner (MSN); nurse anesthesia (MSN); nurse educator (MSN); nurse executive (MSN). *Accreditation:* AACN; AANA/CANAEP. *Program availability:* Part-time, online learning. *Faculty:* 51 full-time (47 women), 6 part-time/adjunct (all women). *Students:* 58 full-time (57 women), 29 part-time (24 women); includes 17 minority (11 Black or African American, non-Hispanic/Latino; 2 Asian, non-Hispanic/Latino; 2 Hispanic/Latino; 2 Two or more races, non-Hispanic/Latino). Average age 26. 41 applicants, 22% accepted, 8 enrolled. In 2015, 56 master's awarded. *Degree requirements:* For master's, thesis or alternative. *Entrance requirements:* For master's, 2 references, personal statement, curriculum vitae or resume. Additional exam requirements/recommendations for international students: Required—TOEFL (minimum score 575 paper-based; 85 iBT). *Application deadline:* For fall admission, 2/1 priority date for international students; for spring admission, 10/1 priority date for international students. Applications are processed on a rolling basis. Application fee: $50. *Expenses:* Contact institution. *Financial support:* Fellowships, research assistantships, Federal Work-Study, institutionally sponsored loans, and scholarships/grants available. Support available to part-time students. Financial award applicants required to submit FAFSA. *Faculty research:* HIV stigma, HIV symptom management, palliative care with children and their families, heart disease prevention in Hispanic women, depression in the well elderly, alternative therapies in pre-term infants. *Unit head:* Dr. Gretchen Drinkard, Dean, 314-454-7540, Fax: 314-362-9222, E-mail: gld9643@bjc.org. *Application contact:* Karen Sartorius, Admissions Specialist, 314-454-7057, Fax: 314-362-9250, E-mail: ksartorius@bjc.org.
Website: http://www.barnesjewishcollege.edu/

Gwynedd Mercy University, Frances M. Maguire School of Nursing and Health Professions, Gwynedd Valley, PA 19437-0901. Offers clinical nurse specialist (MSN), including gerontology, oncology, pediatrics; nurse educator (MSN); nurse practitioner (MSN), including adult health, pediatric health; nursing (DNP). *Accreditation:* ACEN. *Program availability:* Part-time, online learning. *Faculty:* 3 full-time (all women), 2 part-time/adjunct (both women). *Students:* 28 full-time (23 women), 68 part-time (62 women); includes 27 minority (18 Black or African American, non-Hispanic/Latino; 7 Asian, non-Hispanic/Latino; 2 Hispanic/Latino). Average age 37. 72 applicants, 25% accepted, 16 enrolled. In 2015, 7 master's awarded. *Degree requirements:* For master's, thesis optional; for doctorate, evidence-based scholarly project. *Entrance requirements:* For master's, GRE General Test or MAT, current nursing experience, physical assessment, course work in statistics, BSN from NLNAC-accredited program, 2 letters of recommendation, personal interview. Additional exam requirements/recommendations for international students: Required—TOEFL (minimum score 575 paper-based). *Application deadline:* For fall admission, 8/1 priority date for domestic students; for winter admission, 12/1 priority date for domestic students. Applications are processed on a rolling basis. Electronic applications accepted. *Expenses:* Contact institution. *Financial support:* In 2015–16, 21 students received support. Scholarships/grants, traineeships, and unspecified assistantships available. Financial award application deadline: 8/30. *Faculty research:* Critical thinking, primary care, domestic violence, multiculturalism, nursing centers. *Unit head:* Dr. Andrea D. Hollingsworth, Dean, 215-646-7300 Ext. 539, Fax: 215-641-5517, E-mail: hollingsworth.a@gmc.edu. *Application contact:* Dr. Barbara A. Jones, Director, 215-646-7300 Ext. 407, Fax: 215-641-5564, E-mail: jones.b@gmc.edu.
Website: http://www.gmercyu.edu/academics/graduate-programs/nursing

Hampton University, School of Nursing, Hampton, VA 23668. Offers advanced adult nursing (MS); community health nursing (MS); community mental health/psychiatric nursing (MS); family nursing (MS); gerontological nursing for the nurse practitioner (MS); nursing (PhD); women's health nursing (MS). *Accreditation:* AACN. *Program availability:* Part-time, online learning. *Degree requirements:* For master's, comprehensive exam, thesis optional; for doctorate, comprehensive exam, thesis/dissertation. *Entrance requirements:* For master's, GRE General Test. Additional exam requirements/recommendations for international students: Required—TOEFL (minimum score 525 paper-based) or IELTS (6.5). Electronic applications accepted. *Expenses:* Tuition, area resident: Full-time $10,263; part-time $522 per credit hour. *Required fees:* $35. Tuition and fees vary according to course load and program. *Faculty research:* African-American stress, HIV education, pediatric obesity, hypertension, breast cancer.

Hunter College of the City University of New York, Graduate School, Schools of the Health Professions, Hunter-Bellevue School of Nursing, Gerontological Nurse Practitioner Program, New York, NY 10065-5085. Offers MS. *Accreditation:* AACN. *Program availability:* Part-time. *Students:* 2 full-time (both women), 204 part-time (186 women); includes 80 minority (26 Black or African American, non-Hispanic/Latino; 35 Asian, non-Hispanic/Latino; 19 Hispanic/Latino), 12 international. Average age 34. 176 applicants, 24% accepted, 30 enrolled. In 2015, 59 master's awarded. *Degree requirements:* For master's, practicum. *Entrance requirements:* For master's, minimum GPA of 3.0, New York RN license, 2 years of professional practice experience, BSN. Additional exam requirements/recommendations for international students: Required—TOEFL. *Application deadline:* For fall admission, 4/1 for domestic students, 2/1 for international students; for spring admission, 11/1 for domestic students, 9/1 for international students. Applications are processed on a rolling basis. *Financial support:* Federal Work-Study, scholarships/grants, traineeships, and tuition waivers (partial) available. Support available to part-time students. Financial award application deadline: 5/1; financial award applicants required to submit FAFSA. *Unit head:* Dr. Anita Nerenberg, Interim Specialization Coordinator, 212-481-4359, Fax: 212-481-5078, E-mail: anerenbe@hunter.cuny.edu. *Application contact:* Milena Solo, Director for Graduate Admissions, 212-772-4482, E-mail: admissions@hunter.cuny.edu.
Website: http://www.hunter.cuny.edu/nursing/admissions/graduate

Independence University, Program in Nursing, Salt Lake City, UT 84107. Offers community health (MSN); gerontology (MSN); nursing administration (MSN); wellness promotion (MSN).

Indiana University–Purdue University Fort Wayne, College of Health and Human Services, Department of Nursing, Fort Wayne, IN 46805-1499. Offers adult-gerontology primary care nurse practitioner (MS); family nurse practitioner (MS); nurse executive (MS); nursing administration (Certificate); nursing education (MS). *Accreditation:* ACEN. *Program availability:* Part-time. *Faculty:* 8 full-time (all women). *Students:* 6 full-time (all women), 79 part-time (70 women); includes 8 minority (2 Black or African American,

non-Hispanic/Latino; 3 Asian, non-Hispanic/Latino; 3 Hispanic/Latino). Average age 36. 14 applicants, 100% accepted, 10 enrolled. In 2015, 17 master's awarded. *Entrance requirements:* For master's, GRE Writing Test (if GPA below 3.0), BS in nursing, eligibility for Indiana RN license, minimum GPA of 3.0, essay, copy of resume, three references, undergraduate course work in research and statistics within last 5 years. Additional exam requirements/recommendations for international students: Required—TOEFL (minimum score 550 paper-based; 79 iBT); Recommended—TWE. *Application deadline:* For fall admission, 5/1 priority date for domestic and international students; for spring admission, 11/15 priority date for domestic students. Applications are processed on a rolling basis. Application fee: $55 ($60 for international students). Electronic applications accepted. *Financial support:* In 2015–16, 12 teaching assistantships with partial tuition reimbursements (averaging $13,522 per year) were awarded; scholarships/grants also available. Support available to part-time students. Financial award application deadline: 3/1; financial award applicants required to submit FAFSA. *Faculty research:* Community engagement, cervical screening, evidence-based practice. *Total annual research expenditures:* $22,966. *Unit head:* Dr. Lee-Ellen Kirkhorn, Chair/Professor, 260-481-6789, Fax: 260-481-5767, E-mail: kirkhorl@ipfw.edu. *Application contact:* Dr. Deb Poling, Director of Graduate Program, 260-481-6276, Fax: 260-481-5767, E-mail: polingd@ipfw.edu.
Website: http://www.ipfw.edu/nursing/

James Madison University, The Graduate School, College of Health and Behavioral Sciences, Program in Nursing, Harrisonburg, VA 22807. Offers adult/gerontology primary care nurse practitioner (MSN); clinical nurse leader (MSN); family nurse practitioner (MSN); nurse administrator (MSN); nurse midwifery (MSN); nursing (MSN, DNP). *Accreditation:* AACN. *Program availability:* Part-time, 100% online, blended/hybrid learning. *Faculty:* 15 full-time (all women), 1 (woman) part-time/adjunct. *Students:* 14 full-time (all women), 54 part-time (43 women); includes 6 minority (2 Black or African American, non-Hispanic/Latino; 1 Asian, non-Hispanic/Latino; 1 Hispanic/Latino; 2 Two or more races, non-Hispanic/Latino), 1 international. Average age 30. 49 applicants, 67% accepted, 31 enrolled. In 2015, 14 master's awarded. Application fee: $55. Electronic applications accepted. *Financial support:* In 2015–16, 2 students received support. Federal Work-Study, unspecified assistantships, and 2 assistantships (averaging $7530) available. Financial award application deadline: 3/1; financial award applicants required to submit FAFSA. *Unit head:* Dr. Julie T. Sanford, Department Head, 540-568-6314, E-mail: sanforjt@jmu.edu. *Application contact:* Lynette D. Michael, Director of Graduate Admissions and Student Records, 540-568-6131 Ext. 6395, Fax: 540-568-7860, E-mail: michaeld@jmu.edu.
Website: http://www.nursing.jmu.edu

Kent State University, College of Nursing, Kent, OH 44242. Offers advanced nursing practice (DNP), including adult gerontology acute care nurse practitioner (MSN, DNP), adult gerontology clinical nurse specialist (MSN, DNP), family nurse practitioner (MSN, DNP); nursing (MSN, PhD), including adult gerontology acute care nurse practitioner (MSN, DNP), adult gerontology clinical nurse specialist (MSN, DNP), family nurse practitioner (MSN, DNP), nurse educator (MSN), nursing healthcare management (MSN), primary care adult nurse practitioner (MSN), primary care pediatric clinical nurse specialist (MSN), primary care pediatric nurse practitioner (MSN), psychiatric mental health practitioner (MSN), women's health nurse practitioner (MSN); nursing education (Certificate); primary care pediatric nurse practitioner (Certificate); women's health nurse practitioner (Certificate). PhD program offered jointly with The University of Akron. *Accreditation:* AACN. *Program availability:* Part-time, online learning. *Faculty:* 52 full-time (48 women). *Students:* 78 full-time (56 women), 414 part-time (365 women); includes 63 minority (34 Black or African American, non-Hispanic/Latino; 1 American Indian or Alaska Native, non-Hispanic/Latino; 12 Asian, non-Hispanic/Latino; 12 Hispanic/Latino; 4 Two or more races, non-Hispanic/Latino), 16 international. Average age 37. 653 applicants, 54% accepted, 309 enrolled. In 2015, 140 master's, 1 doctorate, 13 other advanced degrees awarded. *Degree requirements:* For master's, thesis optional, practicum; for doctorate, comprehensive exam (for some programs), thesis/dissertation (for some programs), practicum and scholarly project (for DNP programs); for Certificate, practicum. *Entrance requirements:* For master's, minimum GPA of 3.0, transcripts, active unrestricted RN license, essay/goal statement, interview, 3 letters of recommendation; for doctorate, GRE (for PhD), minimum GPA of 3.0, transcripts, 3 letters of recommendation, interview; active unrestricted RN license, clinical experience and hours record (for DNP); goal statement, sample of written work, curriculum vitae, statement of research interests, and eligibility for RN license (for PhD); for Certificate, MSN, minimum GPA of 3.0, transcripts. Additional exam requirements/recommendations for international students: Required—TOEFL (minimum score: paper-based 525, iBT 71), Michigan English Language Assessment Battery (minimum score of 75), IELTS (minimum score of 6.0), PTE Academic (minimum score of 48), or completion of ELS level 112 Intensive Program. *Application deadline:* For fall admission, 2/1 for domestic students; for spring admission, 11/1 for domestic students. Application fee: $45 ($70 for international students). Electronic applications accepted. *Expenses:* Tuition, state resident: full-time $10,864; part-time $495 per credit hour. Tuition, nonresident: full-time $18,380; part-time $837 per credit hour. *Financial support:* Research assistantships with full tuition reimbursements, teaching assistantships with full tuition reimbursements, career-related internships or fieldwork, Federal Work-Study, traineeships, and unspecified assistantships available. Financial award application deadline: 2/1. *Unit head:* Dr. Barbara Broome, Dean, 330-672-3777, E-mail: bbroome1@kent.edu. *Application contact:* Dr. Wendy A. Umberger, Associate Dean for Graduate Programs/Professor, 330-672-8813, E-mail: wlewando@kent.edu.
Website: http://www.kent.edu/nursing/

Keuka College, Program in Nursing, Keuka Park, NY 14478-0098. Offers adult gerontology nurse practitioner (MS); nursing (MS). *Accreditation:* AACN. *Faculty:* 8 full-time (all women), 23 part-time/adjunct (22 women). *Students:* 68 full-time (62 women); includes 8 minority (6 Black or African American, non-Hispanic/Latino; 1 Asian, non-Hispanic/Latino; 1 Hispanic/Latino). Average age 36. In 2015, 20 master's awarded. *Degree requirements:* For master's, exam or thesis. *Entrance requirements:* For master's, bachelor's degree from accredited institution, minimum GPA of 3.0, unencumbered NY State license, and current registration as RN (for nusirng); currently full-time or part-time working RN and 2 clinical letters of recommendation (for adult gerontology nurse practitioner). Additional exam requirements/recommendations for international students: Required—TOEFL (minimum score 550 paper-based). *Application deadline:* Applications are processed on a rolling basis. Application fee: $50. Electronic applications accepted. *Expenses:* Contact institution. *Financial support:* Scholarships/grants and tuition waivers available. Financial award applicants required to submit FAFSA. *Unit head:* Dr. Debra Gates, Chair, 315-279-5115 Ext. 5273, E-mail: dgates@keuka.edu. *Application contact:* Graduate Admissions, 866-255-3852, Fax: 315-279-5386, E-mail: asapadvisor@keuka.edu.
Website: http://academics.keuka.edu/asap/programs/ms_nursing

La Salle University, School of Nursing and Health Sciences, Program in Nursing, Philadelphia, PA 19141-1199. Offers adult gerontology primary care nurse practitioner (MSN, Certificate); adult health and illness clinical nurse specialist (MSN); adult-gerontology clinical nurse specialist (MSN, Certificate); clinical nurse leader (MSN); family primary care nurse practitioner (MSN, Certificate); gerontology (Certificate); nurse anesthetist (MSN, Certificate); nursing (MSN, Certificate); nursing administration (MSN,

Certificate); nursing education (Certificate); nursing practice (DNP); nursing service administration (MSN); public health nursing (MSN, Certificate); school nursing (Certificate); MSN/MBA; MSN/MPH. *Accreditation:* AANA/CANAEP. *Program availability:* Part-time, evening/weekend, 100% online. *Faculty:* 13 full-time (all women), 9 part-time/adjunct (8 women). *Students:* 368 part-time (56 women); includes 103 minority (62 Black or African American, non-Hispanic/Latino; 1 American Indian or Alaska Native, non-Hispanic/Latino; 26 Asian, non-Hispanic/Latino; 9 Hispanic/Latino; 5 Two or more races, non-Hispanic/Latino), 5 international. Average age 36. 98 applicants, 85% accepted, 53 enrolled. In 2015, 87 master's, 3 doctorates, 10 other advanced degrees awarded. *Degree requirements:* For doctorate, minimum of 1,000 hours of post baccalaureate clinical practice supervised by preceptors. *Entrance requirements:* For master's, GRE, MAT, or GMAT (for students with BSN GPA of less than 3.2), baccalaureate degree in nursing from an NLNAC- or CCNE-accredited program or an MSN Bridge program; Pennsylvania RN license; 2 letters of reference; resume; statement of philosophy articulating professional values and future educational goal; 1 year of work experience as a registered nurse; for doctorate, GRE (waived for applicants with MSN cumulative GPA of 3.7 or above), MSN from nationally-accredited program or master's degree, MBA or MHA from nationally-accredited program; resume or curriculum vitae; 2 letters of reference; interview; for Certificate, GRE, MAT, or GMAT (for students with BSN GPA of less than 3.2, baccalaureate degree in nursing from an NLNAC- or CCNE-accredited program or an MSN Bridge program; Pennsylvania RN license; 2 letters of reference; resume; statement of philosophy articulating professional values and future educational goal; 1 year of work experience as a registered nurse. Additional exam requirements/recommendations for international students: Required—TOEFL. *Application deadline:* For fall admission, 8/15 priority date for domestic students, 7/15 for international students; for spring admission, 12/15 priority date for domestic students, 11/15 for international students; for summer admission, 4/15 priority date for domestic students, 3/15 for international students. Applications are processed on a rolling basis. Application fee: $35. Electronic applications accepted. Application fee is waived when completed online. *Expenses:* $870 per credit hour (for MSN); $930 per credit hour (for DNP); $150 technology fee full-time, $75 part-time; $135 general university fee. *Financial support:* In 2015–16, 13 students received support. Scholarships/grants and traineeships available. Support available to part-time students. Financial award application deadline: 8/31; financial award applicants required to submit FAFSA. *Unit head:* Dr. Patricia M. Dillon, Director, 215-951-1322, Fax: 215-951-1896, E-mail: msnapn@lasalle.edu. *Application contact:* Alison McAnespey Target, Director, Graduate and Adult Enrollment, 215-951-1100, Fax: 215-951-1462, E-mail: reilly@lasalle.edu.
Website: http://www.lasalle.edu/nursing/program-options/

Lehman College of the City University of New York, School of Natural and Social Sciences, Department of Nursing, Bronx, NY 10468-1589. Offers adult health nursing (MS); nursing of older adults (MS); parent-child nursing (MS); pediatric nurse practitioner (MS). *Accreditation:* AACN. *Program availability:* Part-time, evening/weekend. *Entrance requirements:* For master's, bachelor's degree in nursing, New York RN license.

Le Moyne College, Department of Nursing, Syracuse, NY 13214. Offers informatics (MS, CAS); nursing administration (MS, CAS); nursing education (MS, CAS); nursing gerontology (MS, CAS); palliative care (MS, CAS). *Accreditation:* AACN. *Program availability:* Part-time, evening/weekend. *Degree requirements:* For master's, scholarly project. *Entrance requirements:* For master's, bachelor's degree, interview, minimum GPA of 3.0, New York RN license, 2 letters of recommendation, writing sample, transcripts. *Expenses:* Contact institution. *Faculty research:* Inter-profession education, gerontology, utilization of free healthcare services by the insured, health promotion education, innovative undergraduate nursing education models, patient and family education, horizontal violence.

Loma Linda University, School of Nursing, Program in Nurse Educator, Loma Linda, CA 92350. Offers adult/gerontology (MS); obstetrics-pediatrics (MS). *Accreditation:* AACN. *Program availability:* Part-time. *Degree requirements:* For master's, thesis or alternative. *Entrance requirements:* For master's, GRE General Test, BSN, minimum GPA of 3.0, RN license. Additional exam requirements/recommendations for international students: Required—TOEFL. *Application deadline:* For fall admission, 8/1 for domestic and international students; for winter admission, 11/1 for domestic and international students; for spring admission, 2/1 for domestic and international students. Application fee: $60. Electronic applications accepted. *Financial support:* Career-related internships or fieldwork, Federal Work-Study, institutionally sponsored loans, and scholarships/grants available. Support available to part-time students. Financial award application deadline: 6/1. *Faculty research:* Coping, integration of research. *Unit head:* Coordinator, 909-824-4360. *Application contact:* Admissions Office, 909-651-5029, Fax: 909-558-4879, E-mail: admissions.app@llu.edu.

Louisiana State University Health Sciences Center, School of Nursing, New Orleans, LA 70112. Offers adult gerontology clinical nurse specialist (Post-Master's Certificate); clinical nurse leader (MSN); executive nurse leader (Post-Master's Certificate); neonatal nurse practitioner (Post-Master's Certificate); nurse anesthesia (Post-Master's Certificate); nurse educator (MSN); nursing (DNS); primary care family nurse practitioner (Post-Master's Certificate); public/community health nursing (Post-Master's Certificate). *Accreditation:* AACN; AANA/CANAEP (one or more programs are accredited). *Program availability:* Part-time. *Faculty:* 22 full-time (19 women), 21 part-time/adjunct (8 women). *Students:* 254 (185 women); includes 68 minority (44 Black or African American, non-Hispanic/Latino; 12 Asian, non-Hispanic/Latino; 12 Hispanic/Latino). Average age 33. 144 applicants, 54% accepted, 73 enrolled. In 2015, 84 master's, 6 doctorates awarded. *Degree requirements:* For master's, thesis optional; for doctorate, thesis/dissertation. *Entrance requirements:* For master's, GRE General Test, MAT, minimum GPA of 3.0; for doctorate, GRE General Test, minimum GPA of 3.5. Additional exam requirements/recommendations for international students: Required—TOEFL (minimum score 550 paper-based; 79 iBT). *Application deadline:* Applications are processed on a rolling basis. Application fee: $250. Electronic applications accepted. *Expenses:* $9,136.50 per year; $19,633.50 per year (for DNP). *Financial support:* Federal Work-Study, institutionally sponsored loans, scholarships/grants, and traineeships available. Financial award applicants required to submit FAFSA. *Faculty research:* Advanced clinical practice, nursing education, health, social support, nursing administration. *Unit head:* Dr. Demetrius James Porche, Dean, 504-568-4106, Fax: 504-599-0573, E-mail: dporch@lsuhsc.edu. *Application contact:* Tracie Gravolet, Director, Office of Student Affairs, 504-568-4114, Fax: 504-568-5711, E-mail: tgravo@lsuhsc.edu.
Website: http://nursing.lsuhsc.edu/

Loyola University Chicago, Graduate School, Marcella Niehoff School of Nursing, Maywood, IL 60153. Offers adult gerontology acute care clinical nurse specialist (MSN), including emergency care (MSN, Certificate); adult gerontology acute care nurse practitioner (MSN), including oncology (MSN, Certificate); adult gerontology clinical nurse specialist (MSN), including oncology (MSN, Certificate); adult gerontology nursing (Certificate), including oncology (MSN, Certificate); adult nurse practitioner (Certificate); dietetics (MS); family nurse practitioner (MSN, Certificate), including emergency care; informatics (MSN); leadership (DNP), including healthcare quality using education in safety and technology, infection prevention; nursing science (PhD); women's health

Gerontological Nursing

nurse practitioner (MSN); women's health nursing (Certificate). *Accreditation:* AACN. *Program availability:* Part-time, blended/hybrid learning. *Faculty:* 27 full-time (25 women), 12 part-time/adjunct (10 women). *Students:* 174 full-time (161 women), 232 part-time (221 women); includes 95 minority (19 Black or African American, non-Hispanic/Latino; 2 American Indian or Alaska Native, non-Hispanic/Latino; 38 Asian, non-Hispanic/Latino; 28 Hispanic/Latino; 2 Native Hawaiian or other Pacific Islander, non-Hispanic/Latino; 6 Two or more races, non-Hispanic/Latino), 3 international. Average age 35. 209 applicants, 52% accepted, 83 enrolled. In 2015, 78 master's, 10 doctorates, 17 other advanced degrees awarded. *Degree requirements:* For master's, comprehensive exam; for doctorate, thesis/dissertation, qualifying examination (for PhD); capstone project (for DNP). *Entrance requirements:* For master's, BSN, minimum nursing GPA of 3.0, Illinois RN license, 3 letters of recommendation, 1000 hours of experience in area of specialty prior to starting clinical rotations, personal statement; for doctorate, GRE General Test (for PhD), BSN or MSN, minimum GPA of 3.0, professional nursing license, 3 letters of recommendation, personal statement. Additional exam requirements/recommendations for international students: Required—TOEFL (minimum score 550 paper-based; 79 iBT), IELTS (minimum score 6.5). *Application deadline:* For fall admission, 6/1 priority date for domestic and international students; for spring admission, 11/15 priority date for domestic and international students; for summer admission, 3/15 priority date for domestic and international students. Applications are processed on a rolling basis. Application fee: $50. Electronic applications accepted. Application fee is waived when completed online. *Expenses:* $1,081 per credit hour. *Financial support:* In 2015–16, 10 students received support, including 3 research assistantships with full tuition reimbursements available (averaging $18,000 per year), 1 teaching assistantship with full tuition reimbursement available (averaging $18,000 per year); scholarships/grants, unspecified assistantships, and nurse faculty loan program also available. Financial award application deadline: 5/1; financial award applicants required to submit FAFSA. *Faculty research:* Epigenetics and social determinants of health, women's health, vitamin D, interprofessional education, prevention and self-management of chronic disease. *Total annual research expenditures:* $649,606. *Unit head:* Dr. Vicky Keough, Dean, 708-216-5448, Fax: 708-216-9555, E-mail: vkeough@luc.edu. *Application contact:* Toni Topalova, Enrollment Advisor, 708-216-3751, Fax: 708-216-9555, E-mail: atopalova@luc.edu. Website: http://www.luc.edu/nursing/

Marquette University, Graduate School, College of Nursing, Milwaukee, WI 53201-1881. Offers acute care nurse practitioner (Certificate); adult clinical nurse specialist (Certificate); adult nurse practitioner (Certificate); advanced practice nursing (MSN, DNP), including adult-older adult acute care (DNP), adults (MSN), adults-older adults (DNP), clinical nurse leader (MSN), health care systems leadership (DNP), nurse-midwifery (MSN), older adults (MSN), pediatrics-acute care, pediatrics-primary care, primary care (DNP), systems leadership and healthcare quality (MSN); family nurse practitioner (Certificate); nurse-midwifery (Certificate); nursing (PhD); pediatric acute care (Certificate); pediatric primary care (Certificate); systems leadership and healthcare quality (Certificate). *Accreditation:* AACN. *Faculty:* 35 full-time (all women), 56 part-time/adjunct (55 women). *Students:* 123 full-time (112 women), 242 part-time (220 women); includes 34 minority (9 Black or African American, non-Hispanic/Latino; 12 Asian, non-Hispanic/Latino; 10 Hispanic/Latino; 3 Two or more races, non-Hispanic/Latino), 4 international. Average age 30. 269 applicants, 61% accepted, 98 enrolled. In 2015, 84 master's, 5 doctorates, 22 other advanced degrees awarded. Terminal master's awarded for partial completion of doctoral program. *Degree requirements:* For master's, comprehensive exam, thesis or alternative. *Entrance requirements:* For master's, GRE General Test, BSN, Wisconsin RN license, official transcripts from all current and previous colleges/universities except Marquette, three completed recommendation forms, resume, written statement of professional goals; for doctorate, GRE General Test, official transcripts from all current and previous colleges/universities except Marquette, three letters of recommendation, resume, written statement of professional goals, sample of scholarly writing. Additional exam requirements/recommendations for international students: Required—TOEFL (minimum score 530 paper-based). *Application deadline:* For fall admission, 2/15 for domestic and international students. Electronic applications accepted. *Financial support:* In 2015–16, 41 students received support, including 1 fellowship with partial tuition reimbursement available (averaging $17,500 per year), 2 research assistantships with full tuition reimbursements available (averaging $13,285 per year), 8 teaching assistantships with full tuition reimbursements available (averaging $13,912 per year); career-related internships or fieldwork, Federal Work-Study, scholarships/grants, health care benefits, tuition waivers (partial), and unspecified assistantships also available. Support available to part-time students. Financial award application deadline: 2/15. *Faculty research:* Psychosocial adjustment to chronic illness, gerontology, reminiscence, health policy: uninsured and access, hospital care delivery systems. *Total annual research expenditures:* $480,591. *Unit head:* Dr. Donna McCarthy, Interim Chair, 414-288-3800, Fax: 414-288-1578. *Application contact:* Dr. Maureen O'Brien, Associate Dean/Clinical Associate Professor, 414-288-3823.

Maryville University of Saint Louis, Walker College of Health Professions, The Catherine McAuley School of Nursing, St. Louis, MO 63141-7299. Offers acute care nurse practice (MSN); adult gerontology nurse practitioner (MSN); advanced practice nursing (DNP); family nurse practitioner (MSN); pediatric nurse practice (MSN). *Accreditation:* AACN. *Program availability:* 100% online. *Faculty:* 18 full-time (all women), 158 part-time/adjunct (141 women). *Students:* 38 full-time (35 women), 2,802 part-time (2,511 women); includes 681 minority (332 Black or African American, non-Hispanic/Latino; 40 American Indian or Alaska Native, non-Hispanic/Latino; 126 Asian, non-Hispanic/Latino; 126 Hispanic/Latino; 8 Native Hawaiian or other Pacific Islander, non-Hispanic/Latino; 49 Two or more races, non-Hispanic/Latino), 58 international. Average age 37. In 2015, 413 master's, 33 doctorates awarded. *Degree requirements:* For master's, practicum. *Entrance requirements:* For master's, BSN, current licensure, minimum GPA of 3.0, 3 letters of recommendation, curriculum vitae. Additional exam requirements/recommendations for international students: Required—TOEFL (minimum score 550 paper-based). *Application deadline:* Applications are processed on a rolling basis. Electronic applications accepted. Application fee is waived when completed online. *Expenses:* Tuition, area resident: Full-time $25,558; part-time $781 per credit hour. *Required fees:* $2400. Part-time tuition and fees vary according to course load and degree level. *Financial support:* Federal Work-Study and campus employment available. Support available to part-time students. Financial award application deadline: 3/1; financial award applicants required to submit FAFSA. *Unit head:* Dr. Elizabeth Buck, Director, 314-529-9453, Fax: 314-529-9139, E-mail: ebuck@maryville.edu. *Application contact:* Crystal Jacobsmeyer, Assistant Director, Graduate Enrollment Advising, 314-929-9654, Fax: 314-529-9927, E-mail: cjacobsmeyer@maryville.edu. Website: http://www.maryville.edu/hp/nursing/

Medical University of South Carolina, College of Nursing, Adult-Gerontology Health Nurse Practitioner Program, Charleston, SC 29425. Offers MSN, DNP. *Program availability:* Part-time, online learning. *Degree requirements:* For master's, comprehensive exam (for some programs), thesis optional; for doctorate, final project. *Entrance requirements:* For master's, BSN from nationally-accredited program, minimum nursing and cumulative GPA of 3.0, undergraduate-level statistics course, active RN License, 3 confidential references, current curriculum vitae or resume, essay;

for doctorate, BSN from nationally-accredited program, minimum nursing and cumulative GPA of 3.0, undergraduate-level statistics course, active RN License, 3 confidential references, current curriculum vitae or resume, personal essay (for DNP). Additional exam requirements/recommendations for international students: Required—TOEFL (minimum score 550 paper-based; 80 iBT). Electronic applications accepted. *Faculty research:* Palliative care, dementia, hospital acquired infections, diabetes, advance practice nurse utilization.

Mercer University, Graduate Studies, Cecil B. Day Campus, Georgia Baptist College of Nursing, Atlanta, GA 30341. Offers adult gerontology acute care nurse practitioner (MSN, Certificate); family nurse practitioner (MSN); nursing (PhD); nursing practice (DNP), including adult gerontology acute care nurse practitioner. *Accreditation:* AACN. *Program availability:* Part-time, blended/hybrid learning. *Faculty:* 10 full-time (9 women), 1 (woman) part-time/adjunct. *Students:* 78 full-time (71 women), 42 part-time (39 women); includes 44 minority (21 Black or African American, non-Hispanic/Latino; 16 Asian, non-Hispanic/Latino; 6 Hispanic/Latino; 1 Native Hawaiian or other Pacific Islander, non-Hispanic/Latino), 5 international. Average age 35. 65 applicants, 66% accepted, 30 enrolled. In 2015, 36 master's, 5 doctorates awarded. *Degree requirements:* For master's, thesis or alternative; for doctorate, comprehensive exam (for some programs), thesis/dissertation (for some programs). *Entrance requirements:* For master's, MAT or GRE, bachelor's degree from accredited nursing program, registered unencumbered GA nursing license, essay, three professional references; for doctorate, GRE (for PhD), master's degree from accredited nursing program, RN licensure, graduate statistics course, three professional references. Additional exam requirements/recommendations for international students: Required—TOEFL (minimum score 100 iBT). *Application deadline:* For fall admission, 5/1 for domestic students, 3/1 for international students; for winter admission, 11/1 for domestic students, 9/1 for international students; for spring admission, 11/1 for domestic students, 10/1 for international students; for summer admission, 3/1 for domestic and international students. Applications are processed on a rolling basis. Application fee: $50. Electronic applications accepted. *Expenses:* Contact institution. *Financial support:* In 2015–16, 59 students received support. Scholarships/grants and traineeships available. Financial award application deadline: 6/30; financial award applicants required to submit FAFSA. *Faculty research:* Cognitive competence, cancer survivorship, interprofessional education, cultural competence, clopidogrel adherence, high fidelity simulation, self-awareness practices, simulation. *Unit head:* Dr. Linda Streit, Dean/Professor, 678-547-6793, Fax: 678-547-6796, E-mail: streit_la@mercer.edu. *Application contact:* Janda Anderson, Director of Admissions, 678-547-6700, Fax: 678-547-6794, E-mail: anderson_j@mercer.edu. Website: http://www.mercer.edu/nursing

MGH Institute of Health Professions, School of Nursing, Boston, MA 02129. Offers advanced practice nursing (MSN); gerontological nursing (MSN); nursing (DNP); pediatric nursing (MSN); psychiatric nursing (MSN); teaching and learning for health care education (Certificate); women's health nursing (MSN). *Accreditation:* AACN. *Degree requirements:* For master's, thesis or alternative. *Entrance requirements:* For master's, GRE General Test, bachelor's degree from regionally-accredited college or university. Additional exam requirements/recommendations for international students: Required—TOEFL (minimum score 550 paper-based; 80 iBT). Electronic applications accepted. *Faculty research:* Biobehavioral nursing, HIV/AIDS, gerontological nursing, women's health, vulnerable populations, health systems.

Middle Georgia State University, Office of Graduate Studies, Macon, GA 31206. Offers adult/gerontology acute care nurse practitioner (MSN); information technology (MS), including health informatics, information security and digital forensics, software development. *Entrance requirements:* For master's, GRE. Additional exam requirements/recommendations for international students: Required—TOEFL (minimum score 523 paper-based; 69 iBT). *Application deadline:* For fall admission, 5/27 priority date for domestic students; for spring admission, 9/16 priority date for domestic students. Application fee: $40. *Expenses:* $255 per credit hour; $250 institutional fee per term; $46 technology fee per term. *Financial support:* Application deadline: 3/15; applicants required to submit FAFSA. *Unit head:* Dr. Loretta Clayton, Interim Dean, 478-471-4762, Fax: 478-929-6714, E-mail: loretta.clayton@mga.edu. *Application contact:* Melinda Rodgers, Graduate Admissions, 478-471-2312, E-mail: graduate.admissions@mga.edu. Website: http://www.mga.edu/graduate-studies/

Molloy College, Division of Nursing, Rockville Centre, NY 11571-5002. Offers adult-gerontology primary care nurse practitioner (MS); clinical nurse specialist (MS), including adult-gerontology health; clinical nurse specialist: adult-gerontology (Advanced Certificate), including adult-gerontology; family nurse practitioner (MS, Advanced Certificate), including primary care; family psychiatric mental health nurse practitioner (MS); nursing (DNP, PhD); nursing administration (MS), including informatics; nursing education (MS); pediatric nurse practitioner (MS), including primary care (MS, Advanced Certificate). *Accreditation:* AACN. *Program availability:* Part-time, evening/weekend. *Faculty:* 26 full-time (all women), 12 part-time/adjunct (9 women). *Students:* 13 full-time (all women), 550 part-time (515 women); includes 316 minority (169 Black or African American, non-Hispanic/Latino; 1 American Indian or Alaska Native, non-Hispanic/Latino; 88 Asian, non-Hispanic/Latino; 56 Hispanic/Latino; 2 Native Hawaiian or other Pacific Islander, non-Hispanic/Latino). Average age 43. 208 applicants, 69% accepted, 121 enrolled. In 2015, 116 master's, 1 doctorate, 6 other advanced degrees awarded. *Degree requirements:* For master's, thesis optional. *Entrance requirements:* For master's, 3 letters of reference, BS in nursing, minimum undergraduate GPA of 3.0; for Advanced Certificate, 3 letters of reference, master's degree in nursing. Additional exam requirements/recommendations for international students: Required—TOEFL (minimum score 550 paper-based; 79 iBT). *Application deadline:* For fall admission, 9/2 priority date for domestic students; for spring admission, 1/20 priority date for domestic students. Applications are processed on a rolling basis. Application fee: $60. Electronic applications accepted. *Expenses:* Tuition, area resident: Full-time $18,450; part-time $1025 per credit. *Required fees:* $900; $740 per unit. Tuition and fees vary according to course load. *Financial support:* Research assistantships with partial tuition reimbursements, teaching assistantships with partial tuition reimbursements, institutionally sponsored loans, scholarships/grants, and unspecified assistantships available. Support available to part-time students. Financial award application deadline: 4/1; financial award applicants required to submit FAFSA. *Unit head:* Dr. Jeannine Muldoon, Dean of Nursing, 516-323-3651, E-mail: jmuldoon@molloy.edu. *Application contact:* Jaclyn Machowioz, Assistant Director for Admissions, 516-323-4010, E-mail: jmachowicz@molloy.edu.

Monmouth University, Graduate Studies, The Marjorie K. Unterberg School of Nursing and Health Studies, West Long Branch, NJ 07764-1898. Offers adult and gerontological primary care nurse practitioner (MSN); adult-gerontological primary care nurse practitioner (Post-Master's Certificate); family nurse practitioner (MSN, Post-Master's Certificate); family psychiatric and mental health advanced practice nursing (MSN); family psychiatric and mental health nurse practitioner (Post-Master's Certificate); forensic nursing (MSN, Certificate); nursing (MSN); nursing administration (MSN, Post-Master's Certificate); nursing education (MSN, Post-Master's Certificate); nursing practice (DNP); physician assistant (MS); school nursing (MSN, Certificate).

Accreditation: AACN. *Program availability:* Part-time, evening/weekend, 100% online, blended/hybrid learning. *Faculty:* 14 full-time (13 women), 10 part-time/adjunct (5 women). *Students:* 58 full-time (46 women), 271 part-time (252 women); includes 93 minority (31 Black or African American, non-Hispanic/Latino; 40 Asian, non-Hispanic/Latino; 18 Hispanic/Latino; 1 Native Hawaiian or other Pacific Islander, non-Hispanic/Latino; 3 Two or more races, non-Hispanic/Latino), 1 international. Average age 37. 450 applicants, 32% accepted, 103 enrolled. In 2015, 68 master's, 8 doctorates, 11 other advanced degrees awarded. *Degree requirements:* For master's, practicum (for some tracks); for doctorate, practicum, capstone course. *Entrance requirements:* For master's, GRE General Test (waived for MSN applicants with minimum B grade in each of the first four courses and for MS applicants with master's degree), BSN with minimum GPA of 2.75, current RN license, proof of liability and malpractice policy, personal statement, two letters of recommendation, graduate course work in health assessment, resume; CASPA application (for MS); for doctorate, accredited master's nursing program degree with minimum GPA of 3.2, graduate research course in statistics, active RN license, national certification as Nurse Practitioner or Nurse Administrator, working knowledge of statistics, statement of goals and vision for change, 2 letters of recommendation (professional or academic), resume, interview. Additional exam requirements/recommendations for international students: Required—TOEFL (minimum score 550 paper-based; 79 iBT), IELTS (minimum score 6) or Michigan English Language Assessment Battery (minimum score 77). *Application deadline:* For fall admission, 7/15 priority date for domestic students, 6/1 for international students; for spring admission, 12/15 priority date for domestic students, 11/1 for international students; for summer admission, 5/1 for domestic students. Applications are processed on a rolling basis. Application fee: $50. Electronic applications accepted. *Expenses:* Contact institution. *Financial support:* In 2015–16, 241 students received support, including 220 fellowships (averaging $3,403 per year), 5 research assistantships (averaging $5,146 per year); career-related internships or fieldwork, scholarships/grants, and unspecified assistantships also available. Support available to part-time students. Financial award applicants required to submit FAFSA. *Faculty research:* School nursing, health policy, and smoking cessation in teens, Multiple Sclerosis; adherence and self-efficacy, aging issues and geriatric care. *Unit head:* Dr. Janet Mahoney, Dean, 732-571-3443, Fax: 732-263-5131, E-mail: jmahoney@monmouth.edu. *Application contact:* Lucia Fedele, Graduate Admission Counselor, 732-571-3452, Fax: 732-263-5123, E-mail: gradadm@monmouth.edu.
Website: http://www.monmouth.edu/school-of-nursing-health/graduate-nursing-programs.aspx

Mount Carmel College of Nursing, Nursing Program, Columbus, OH 43222. Offers adult gerontology acute care nurse practitioner (MS); adult health clinical nurse specialist (MS); family nurse practitioner (MS); nursing (DNP); nursing administration (MS); nursing education (MS). *Accreditation:* AACN. *Program availability:* Part-time. *Faculty:* 8 full-time (all women), 5 part-time/adjunct (4 women). *Students:* 72 full-time (63 women), 92 part-time (84 women); includes 15 minority (7 Black or African American, non-Hispanic/Latino; 3 Asian, non-Hispanic/Latino; 2 Hispanic/Latino; 3 Two or more races, non-Hispanic/Latino). Average age 37. 140 applicants, 45% accepted, 50 enrolled. In 2015, 50 master's awarded. *Degree requirements:* For master's, professional manuscript; for doctorate, practicum. *Entrance requirements:* For master's, letters of recommendation, statement of purpose, current resume, baccalaureate degree in nursing, current Ohio RN license, minimum cumulative GPA of 3.0; for doctorate, master's degree in nursing from program accredited by either NLNAC/ACEN or CCNE. Additional exam requirements/recommendations for international students: Required—TOEFL (minimum score 550 paper-based; 80 iBT). *Application deadline:* For fall admission, 6/1 priority date for domestic students; for winter admission, 11/1 for domestic students; for spring admission, 10/1 priority date for domestic students; for summer admission, 3/1 for domestic students. Applications are processed on a rolling basis. Application fee: $30. *Expenses: Tuition, area resident:* Full-time $9480; part-time $474 per credit. One-time fee: $120. Tuition and fees vary according to course load, degree level and program. *Financial support:* In 2015–16, 5 students received support. Institutionally sponsored loans and scholarships/grants available. Financial award applicants required to submit FAFSA. *Unit head:* Dr. Jill Kilanowski, 614-234-5237, Fax: 614-234-2875, E-mail: jkilanowski@mccn.edu. *Application contact:* Dr. Kim Campbell, Director of Recruitment and Admissions, 614-234-5144, Fax: 614-234-5427, E-mail: kcampbell@mccn.edu.
Website: http://www.mccn.edu/

Neumann University, Program in Nursing, Aston, PA 19014. Offers adult-gerontology nurse practitioner (MS); nurse educator (MS). *Accreditation:* ACEN. *Program availability:* Part-time. *Students:* 18 part-time. *Entrance requirements:* For master's, GRE or MAT. Additional exam requirements/recommendations for international students: Required—TOEFL. *Application deadline:* Applications are processed on a rolling basis. Application fee: $50. *Expenses:* Contact institution. *Financial support:* Available to part-time students. Application deadline: 3/15; applicants required to submit FAFSA. *Unit head:* Dr. Kathleen Hoover, Dean, Division of Nursing and Health Sciences, 610-558-5560, Fax: 610-459-1370, E-mail: hooverk@neumann.edu. *Application contact:* Kittie D. Pain, Associate Director, Graduate and Adult Admissions, 610-558-5613, Fax: 610-558-5652, E-mail: paink@neumann.edu.

New Mexico State University, College of Health and Social Services, School of Nursing, Las Cruces, NM 88003. Offers adult/geriatric nursing (DNP); family nurse practitioner (DNP); family/psychiatric mental health nursing (DNP); nursing administration (MSN); nursing science (PhD); public/community health nursing (DNP). *Accreditation:* AACN. *Program availability:* Blended/hybrid learning. *Faculty:* 16 full-time (15 women). *Students:* 24 full-time (18 women), 90 part-time (80 women); includes 49 minority (10 Black or African American, non-Hispanic/Latino; 1 American Indian or Alaska Native, non-Hispanic/Latino; 4 Asian, non-Hispanic/Latino; 32 Hispanic/Latino; 2 Two or more races, non-Hispanic/Latino), 1 international. Average age 43. 40 applicants, 58% accepted, 17 enrolled. In 2015, 6 master's, 11 doctorates awarded. *Degree requirements:* For master's, comprehensive exam, thesis optional, clinical practice; for doctorate, comprehensive exam, thesis/dissertation. *Entrance requirements:* For master's, NCLEX, BSN, minimum GPA of 3.0, course work in statistics, 3 letters of reference, writing sample, RN license, CPR certification, proof of liability, immunizations, criminal background check; for doctorate, NCLEX, MSN, minimum GPA of 3.0, 3 letters of reference, writing sample, RN license, CPR certification, proof of liability, immunizations, criminal background check, statistics course. Additional exam requirements/recommendations for international students: Required—TOEFL (minimum score 550 paper-based; 79 iBT), IELTS (minimum score 6.5). *Application deadline:* For fall admission, 1/15 for domestic students; for spring admission, 1/15 priority date for domestic students; for summer admission, 1/15 for domestic students. Application fee: $40 ($50 for international students). Electronic applications accepted. *Expenses:* $274.50 per credit hour for in-state students, and all students enrolled in six or fewer credits; $839.30 per credit hour for out-of-state and international students enrolled in at least seven hours. *Financial support:* In 2015–16, 23 students received support, including 1 teaching assistantship (averaging $9,473 per year); career-related internships or fieldwork, Federal Work-Study, scholarships/grants, traineeships, health care benefits, and unspecified assistantships also available. Support available to part-time students. Financial award application deadline: 3/1.

Faculty research: Women's health, community health, health disparities, nursing informatics and health care technologies, health care and nursing administration. *Total annual research expenditures:* $127,778. *Unit head:* Dr. Kathleen Huttlinger, Department Head, 575-646-3812, Fax: 575-646-2167, E-mail: khuttlin@nmsu.edu. *Application contact:* Dr. Teresa Keller, Director of Graduate Studies, 575-646-4370, Fax: 575-646-2167, E-mail: tkeller@nmsu.edu.
Website: http://schoolofnursing.nmsu.edu

New York University, Rory Meyers College of Nursing, Programs in Advanced Practice Nursing, New York, NY 10012-1019. Offers adult-gerontology acute care nurse practitioner (MS, Advanced Certificate); adult-gerontology primary care nurse practitioner (MS, Advanced Certificate); family nurse practitioner (MS, Advanced Certificate); gerontology nurse practitioner (Advanced Certificate); nurse-midwifery (MS, Advanced Certificate); nursing administration (MS, Advanced Certificate); nursing education (MS, Advanced Certificate); nursing informatics (MS, Advanced Certificate); pediatrics nurse practitioner (MS, Advanced Certificate); psychiatric-mental health nurse practitioner (MS, Advanced Certificate); MS/MPH. *Accreditation:* AACN; ACNM/ACME. *Program availability:* Part-time. *Faculty:* 24 full-time (all women), 76 part-time/adjunct (65 women). *Students:* 46 full-time (26 women), 586 part-time (513 women); includes 242 minority (68 Black or African American, non-Hispanic/Latino; 3 American Indian or Alaska Native, non-Hispanic/Latino; 117 Asian, non-Hispanic/Latino; 38 Hispanic/Latino; 3 Native Hawaiian or other Pacific Islander, non-Hispanic/Latino; 13 Two or more races, non-Hispanic/Latino), 23 international. Average age 32. 402 applicants, 69% accepted, 138 enrolled. In 2015, 198 master's, 5 other advanced degrees awarded. *Degree requirements:* For master's, thesis (for some programs). *Entrance requirements:* For master's, BS in nursing, AS in nursing with another BS/BA, interview, RN license, 1 year of clinical experience (3 for the MS in nursing education program); for Advanced Certificate, master's degree. Additional exam requirements/recommendations for international students: Required—TOEFL (minimum score 90 iBT), IELTS (minimum score 7). *Application deadline:* For fall admission, 6/15 for domestic and international students; for spring admission, 12/1 for domestic and international students; for summer admission, 3/1 for domestic and international students. Application fee: $80. Electronic applications accepted. *Expenses:* Contact institution. *Financial support:* In 2015–16, 101 students received support. Career-related internships or fieldwork, Federal Work-Study, and scholarships/grants available. Support available to part-time students. Financial award application deadline: 3/1; applicants required to submit FAFSA. *Faculty research:* Geriatrics, HIV, families and illness, oral systemic connection, symptom management. *Unit head:* Dr. James Pace, Senior Associate Dean for Academic Programs, 212-992-7343, E-mail: james.pace@nyu.edu. *Application contact:* Samantha Jaser, Assistant Director, Graduate Student Affairs and Admissions, 212-992-7653, Fax: 212-995-4302, E-mail: saj283@nyu.edu.

Northeastern University, Bouvé College of Health Sciences, Boston, MA 02115-5096. Offers applied behavior analysis (MS, CAGS); audiology (Au D); biomedical nanotechnology (MS); college student development and counseling (MS, CAGS); counseling psychology (MS, PhD, CAGS); exercise science (MS); health informatics (MS); medicinal chemistry (MS); nurse anesthesia (DNP, CAGS); nursing (MS, PhD, CAGS), including administration (MS), adult-gerontology acute care nurse practitioner (MS, CAGS), adult-gerontology primary care nurse practitioner (MS, CAGS), anesthesia (MS), family nurse practitioner (MS, CAGS), neonatal nurse practitioner (MS, CAGS), pediatric nurse practitioner (MS, CAGS), psychiatric mental health nurse practitioner (MS, CAGS); nursing practice (DNP); personal health informatics (PhD); pharmaceutical sciences (MS, PhD), including interdisciplinary concentration, pharmaceutics and drug delivery systems; pharmacology (MS); pharmacy (Pharm D); physical therapy (Postbaccalaureate Certificate); physician assistant (MS); population health (PhD); school psychology (MS, PhD, CAGS); speech-language pathology (MS); urban health (MPH); MS/MBA. *Accreditation:* ACPE (one or more programs are accredited). *Program availability:* Part-time, evening/weekend, online learning. *Faculty:* 194 full-time (120 women), 169 part-time/adjunct (136 women). *Students:* 1,416 full-time (1,049 women), 310 part-time (248 women). In 2015, 374 master's, 313 doctorates, 37 other advanced degrees awarded. *Degree requirements:* For doctorate, thesis/dissertation (for some programs); for other advanced degree, comprehensive exam. Application fee: $75. Electronic applications accepted. *Expenses:* Contact institution. *Financial support:* Applicants required to submit FAFSA. *Unit head:* John R. Reynolds, Professor and Interim Dean, 617-373-3323, Fax: 617-373-3030. *Application contact:* Molly Schnabel, Senior Director of Graduate Affairs, 617-373-2708, Fax: 617-373-4701, E-mail: bouvegrad@neu.edu.
Website: http://www.northeastern.edu/bouve/

Oakland University, Graduate Study and Lifelong Learning, School of Nursing, Adult Gerontological Nurse Practitioner Program, Rochester, MI 48309-4401. Offers adult gerontological nurse practitioner (MSN, PMC). *Students:* 28 full-time (27 women), 11 part-time (10 women); includes 3 minority (all Black or African American, non-Hispanic/Latino), 1 international. Average age 34. 41 applicants, 12% accepted, 5 enrolled. In 2015, 7 master's, 1 other advanced degree awarded. Application fee: $0. *Expenses: Tuition, area resident:* Part-time $655 per credit. Tuition and fees vary according to program. *Unit head:* Dr. Linda Thompson. *Application contact:* Mary Bray, Graduate Program Coordinator, 248-370-4482.

Old Dominion University, College of Health Sciences, School of Nursing, Adult Gerontology Clinical Nurse Specialist/Educator Role Emphasis, Norfolk, VA 23529. Offers MSN. *Program availability:* Evening/weekend, blended/hybrid learning. *Faculty:* 2 full-time (both women), 2 part-time/adjunct (both women). *Students:* 9 full-time (all women), 10 part-time (7 women); includes 4 minority (2 Black or African American, non-Hispanic/Latino; 1 American Indian or Alaska Native, non-Hispanic/Latino; 1 Asian, non-Hispanic/Latino). Average age 38. 8 applicants, 100% accepted, 7 enrolled. In 2015, 7 master's awarded. *Degree requirements:* For master's, comprehensive exam, internship, practicum. *Entrance requirements:* For master's, GRE or MAT (waived with a GPA above 3.5), undergraduate health/physical assessment course, statistics, 3 letters of recommendation, essay, resume, transcripts. Additional exam requirements/recommendations for international students: Required—TOEFL. *Application deadline:* For fall admission, 6/1 priority date for domestic students, 4/15 priority date for international students. Applications are processed on a rolling basis. Application fee: $50. Electronic applications accepted. *Expenses: Tuition, state resident:* full-time $11,136; part-time $464 per credit hour. Tuition, nonresident: full-time $27,840; part-time $1160 per credit hour. *Required fees:* $64 per semester. Tuition and fees vary according to campus/location, program and reciprocity agreements. *Financial support:* Unspecified assistantships available. *Unit head:* Dr. Tina Haney, Program Director, 757-683-5262683-5428, Fax: 757-683-5253, E-mail: thaney@odu.edu. *Application contact:* Sue Parker, Graduate Program Coordinator, 757-683-4298, Fax: 757-683-5253, E-mail: sparker@odu.edu.

Old Dominion University, College of Health Sciences, School of Nursing, Family Nurse Practitioner Emphasis, Norfolk, VA 23529. Offers adult-gerontology clinical nurse specialist/educator (MSN); neonatal nurse practitioner (MSN); pediatric nurse practitioner (MSN). *Program availability:* Blended/hybrid learning. *Faculty:* 18 full-time (all women), 9 part-time/adjunct (all women). *Students:* 53 full-time (52 women), 5 part-time (all women); includes 14 minority (9 Black or African American, non-Hispanic/Latino; 2

Gerontological Nursing

Asian, non-Hispanic/Latino; 1 Hispanic/Latino; 2 Two or more races, non-Hispanic/Latino). Average age 35. 53 applicants, 66% accepted, 23 enrolled. In 2015, 60 master's awarded. *Degree requirements:* For master's, comprehensive exam. *Entrance requirements:* For master's, GRE or MAT (waived with a GPA above 3.5), 3 letters of recommendation, essay, resume, transcripts. Additional exam requirements/recommendations for international students: Required—TOEFL. *Application deadline:* For fall admission, 3/1 priority date for domestic students, 4/15 priority date for international students. Application fee: $50. Electronic applications accepted. *Expenses:* Tuition, state resident: full-time $11,136; part-time $464 per credit hour. Tuition, nonresident: full-time $27,840; part-time $1160 per credit hour. *Required fees:* $64 per semester. Tuition and fees vary according to campus/location, program and reciprocity agreements. *Financial support:* In 2015–16, research assistantships with partial tuition reimbursements (averaging $10,000 per year) were awarded; career-related internships or fieldwork, scholarships/grants, and traineeships also available. Support available to part-time students. *Faculty research:* Military families, nurse practitioner student reaching modalities, gerontology, pediatrics, ethics. *Unit head:* Dr. Carolyn M. Rutledge, Associate Chair for Graduate Programs, 757-683-5009, Fax: 757-683-5253, E-mail: crutledg@odu.edu. *Application contact:* Sue Parker, Graduate Program Coordinator, 757-683-4298, Fax: 757-683-5253, E-mail: sparker@odu.edu.
Website: http://catalog.odu.edu/graduate/collegeofhealthsciences/schoolofnursing/#masterofscienceinnursing013familynursepractitionerrole

Oregon Health & Science University, School of Nursing, Program in Adult-Gerontology Acute Care Nurse Practitioner, Portland, OR 97239-3098. Offers MN, DNP, PMC.

Point Loma Nazarene University, School of Nursing, San Diego, CA 92106-2899. Offers adult/gerontology nursing (MSN); family/individual health (MSN); general nursing (MSN); nursing (Post-MSN Certificate); pediatric nursing (MSN); psychiatric mental health (MSN). *Accreditation:* AACN. *Program availability:* Part-time. *Faculty:* 6 full-time (5 women), 2 part-time/adjunct (both women). *Students:* 1 (woman) full-time, 74 part-time (61 women); includes 35 minority (4 Black or African American, non-Hispanic/Latino; 15 Asian, non-Hispanic/Latino; 10 Hispanic/Latino; 3 Native Hawaiian or other Pacific Islander, non-Hispanic/Latino; 3 Two or more races, non-Hispanic/Latino), 2 international. Average age 38. 34 applicants, 88% accepted, 18 enrolled. In 2015, 40 master's awarded. *Entrance requirements:* For master's, NCLEX, ADN or BSN in nursing, interview, RN license, essay, letters of recommendation, interview. *Application deadline:* For fall admission, 7/5 priority date for domestic students; for spring admission, 11/1 priority date for domestic students; for summer admission, 3/22 priority date for domestic students. Applications are processed on a rolling basis. Application fee: $50. *Financial support:* Applicants required to submit FAFSA. *Unit head:* Dr. Barb Taylor, Dean of the School of Nursing, 619-849-2766, E-mail: bataylor@pointloma.edu. *Application contact:* Claire Buckley, Director of Graduate Admissions, 619-563-2846, E-mail: clairebuckley@pointloma.edu.
Website: http://www.pointloma.edu/discover/graduate-school/graduate-programs/master-science-nursing-and-post-msn-certification

Research College of Nursing, Nursing Program, Kansas City, MO 64132. Offers adult-gerontological nurse practitioner (MSN); executive practice and healthcare leadership (MSN); family nurse practitioner (MSN); nursing (MSN). *Accreditation:* AACN. *Program availability:* Part-time, 100% online. *Faculty:* 9 full-time (all women), 5 part-time/adjunct (2 women). *Students:* 4 full-time (2 women), 148 part-time (132 women); includes 15 minority (9 Black or African American, non-Hispanic/Latino; 1 American Indian or Alaska Native, non-Hispanic/Latino; 3 Asian, non-Hispanic/Latino; 1 Native Hawaiian or other Pacific Islander, non-Hispanic/Latino; 1 Two or more races, non-Hispanic/Latino). In 2015, 34 master's awarded. *Degree requirements:* For master's, research project. *Entrance requirements:* For master's, 3 letters of recommendation, official transcripts, resume, personal statement/writing sample. *Application deadline:* Applications are processed on a rolling basis. Application fee: $65. Electronic applications accepted. *Expenses:* $525 per credit hour; $25 per credit hour clinical fee. *Financial support:* Applicants required to submit FAFSA. *Unit head:* Dr. Nancy O. DeBasio, President and Dean, 816-995-2815, Fax: 816-995-2817, E-mail: nancy.debasio@researchcollege.edu. *Application contact:* Leslie Burry, Director of Transfer and Graduate Recruitment, 816-995-2820, Fax: 816-995-2813, E-mail: leslie.burry@researchcollege.edu.

Rush University, College of Nursing, Department of Adult Health and Gerontological Nursing, Chicago, IL 60612. Offers adult gerontology acute care clinical nurse specialist (DNP); adult gerontology acute care nurse practitioner (DNP); adult gerontology primary care clinical nurse specialist (DNP); adult gerontology primary care nurse practitioner (DNP); nurse anesthesia (DNP). *Accreditation:* AACN; AANA/CANAEP. *Program availability:* Part-time, 100% online. *Faculty:* 43 full-time (40 women), 52 part-time/adjunct (49 women). *Students:* 50 full-time (33 women), 193 part-time (171 women); includes 52 minority (11 Black or African American, non-Hispanic/Latino; 27 Asian, non-Hispanic/Latino; 14 Hispanic/Latino). Average age 33. 167 applicants, 41% accepted, 47 enrolled. *Degree requirements:* For doctorate, capstone project (for DNP); dissertation (for PhD). *Entrance requirements:* For doctorate, GRE General Test (for DNP in nurse anesthesia; waived if cumulative GPA is 3.25 or greater, nursing GPA is 3.0 or greater, or a completed graduate program GPA is 3.5 or greater), interview, 3 letters of recommendation, personal statement, current resume. Additional exam requirements/recommendations for international students: Required—TOEFL (minimum score 94 iBT). *Application deadline:* For fall admission, 1/2 for domestic students; for spring admission, 8/3 for domestic students; for summer admission, 12/1 for domestic students. Applications are processed on a rolling basis. Application fee: $100. Electronic applications accepted. *Expenses:* Contact institution. *Financial support:* Research assistantships, teaching assistantships, Federal Work-Study, institutionally sponsored loans, scholarships/grants, traineeships, and health care benefits available. Support available to part-time students. Financial award application deadline: 3/1; financial award applicants required to submit FAFSA. *Faculty research:* Physical activity adherence in African-American women; reduction of health disparities; evidence-based interventions for caregivers; fish oil for HIV-related immunosenescence; BAILA: Being Active, Increasing Latinos Health Aging. *Unit head:* Dr. Elizabeth Carlson, Chairperson, 312-942-7117, E-mail: elizabeth_carlson@rush.edu. *Application contact:* Jennifer Thorndyke, Admissions Specialist, 312-563-7526, E-mail: jennifer_thorndyke@rush.edu.
Website: http://www.rushu.rush.edu/servlet/Satellite?c=RushUnivLevel1Page&cid=1204497838852&pagename=Rush%2FRushUnivLevel1Page%2FLevel_1_College_Home_Page

Sage Graduate School, School of Health Sciences, Department of Nursing, Program in Adult Gerontology Nurse Practitioner, Troy, NY 12180-4115. Offers MS, Certificate. *Program availability:* Part-time, evening/weekend. *Faculty:* 9 full-time (all women), 27 part-time/adjunct (24 women). *Students:* 7 full-time (all women), 17 part-time (14 women); includes 5 minority (2 Black or African American, non-Hispanic/Latino; 2 Asian, non-Hispanic/Latino; 1 Two or more races, non-Hispanic/Latino). Average age 39. 13 applicants, 46% accepted, 2 enrolled. *Entrance requirements:* For master's, currently licensed as registered professional nurse in state of practice; baccalaureate degree in nursing from nationally-accredited program or its international equivalent. Additional exam requirements/recommendations for international students: Required—TOEFL

(minimum score 550 paper-based). *Application deadline:* Applications are processed on a rolling basis. Application fee: $40. Electronic applications accepted. *Expenses: Tuition, area resident:* Full-time $12,240; part-time $680 per credit hour. Tuition and fees vary according to degree level and program. *Financial support:* Fellowships, research assistantships, Federal Work-Study, scholarships/grants, and unspecified assistantships available. Support available to part-time students. Financial award application deadline: 3/1; financial award applicants required to submit FAFSA. *Unit head:* Dr. Theresa Hand, Dean, School of Health Sciences, 518-244-2264, Fax: 518-244-4571, E-mail: handt@sage.edu. *Application contact:* Dr. Carol Braungart, Co-Director, Graduate Program in Nursing, 518-244-2459, Fax: 518-244-2009, E-mail: braunc@sage.edu.

Sage Graduate School, School of Health Sciences, Department of Nursing, Program in Family Nurse Practitioner, Troy, NY 12180-4115. Offers adult gerontology acute care (Post Master's Certificate); family nurse practitioner (MS); family psychiatric mental health (Post Master's Certificate). *Accreditation:* AACN. *Program availability:* Part-time, evening/weekend. *Faculty:* 9 full-time (all women), 27 part-time/adjunct (24 women). *Students:* 24 full-time (23 women), 110 part-time (99 women); includes 24 minority (11 Black or African American, non-Hispanic/Latino; 2 American Indian or Alaska Native, non-Hispanic/Latino; 8 Asian, non-Hispanic/Latino; 2 Hispanic/Latino; 1 Two or more races, non-Hispanic/Latino). Average age 34. 114 applicants, 28% accepted, 25 enrolled. In 2015, 4 master's, 6 other advanced degrees awarded. *Degree requirements:* For master's, thesis or alternative. *Entrance requirements:* For master's, currently licensed as registered professional nurse in state of practice; baccalaureate degree in nursing from nationally-accredited program or its international equivalent. Additional exam requirements/recommendations for international students: Required—TOEFL (minimum score 550 paper-based). *Application deadline:* Applications are processed on a rolling basis. Application fee: $40. Electronic applications accepted. *Expenses: Tuition, area resident:* Full-time $12,240; part-time $680 per credit hour. Tuition and fees vary according to degree level and program. *Financial support:* Fellowships, research assistantships, teaching assistantships, Federal Work-Study, scholarships/grants, and unspecified assistantships available. Support available to part-time students. Financial award application deadline: 3/1; financial award applicants required to submit FAFSA. *Unit head:* Dr. Theresa Hand, Dean, School of Health Sciences, 518-244-2264, Fax: 518-244-4571, E-mail: handt@sage.edu. *Application contact:* Dr. Carol Braungart, Co-Director, Graduate Nursing Program, 518-244-2459, Fax: 518-244-2009, E-mail: braunc@sage.edu.

St. Catherine University, Graduate Programs, Program in Nursing, St. Paul, MN 55105. Offers adult gerontological nurse practitioner (MS); neonatal nurse practitioner (MS); nurse educator (MS); nursing (DNP); nursing: entry-level (MS); pediatric nurse practitioner (MS). *Accreditation:* ACEN. *Program availability:* Part-time, evening/weekend. *Degree requirements:* For master's, thesis; for doctorate, portfolio, systems change project. *Entrance requirements:* For master's, GRE General Test, bachelor's degree in nursing, current nursing license, 2 years of recent clinical practice; for doctorate, master's degree in nursing, RN license, advanced nursing position. Additional exam requirements/recommendations for international students: Required—TOEFL (minimum score 600 paper-based; 100 iBT). *Expenses:* Contact institution.

Saint Francis Medical Center College of Nursing, Graduate Programs, Peoria, IL 61603-3783. Offers adult gerontology (MSN); clinical nurse leader (MSN); family nurse practitioner (MSN); family psychiatric mental health nurse practitioner (MSN); neonatal nurse practitioner (MSN); nurse clinician (Post-Graduate Certificate); nurse educator (MSN, Post-Graduate Certificate); nursing (DNP); nursing management leadership (MSN). *Accreditation:* ACEN. *Program availability:* Part-time, 100% online, blended/hybrid learning. *Faculty:* 14 full-time (all women), 5 part-time/adjunct (all women). *Students:* 13 full-time (12 women), 257 part-time (228 women); includes 23 minority (14 Black or African American, non-Hispanic/Latino; 3 Asian, non-Hispanic/Latino; 4 Hispanic/Latino; 2 Two or more races, non-Hispanic/Latino). Average age 37. 86 applicants, 86% accepted, 44 enrolled. In 2015, 61 master's, 6 doctorates awarded. *Degree requirements:* For master's, research experience, portfolio, practicum; for doctorate, practicum hours. *Entrance requirements:* For master's, nursing research, health assessment, graduate course work in statistics, RN license; for doctorate, master's degree in nursing, professional portfolio, graduate statistics, transcripts, RN license. Additional exam requirements/recommendations for international students: Required—TOEFL (minimum score 550 paper-based; 79 iBT). *Application deadline:* For fall admission, 6/1 priority date for domestic and international students; for spring admission, 11/15 priority date for domestic and international students. Applications are processed on a rolling basis. Application fee: $50. *Financial support:* In 2015–16, 18 students received support. Scholarships/grants and tuition waivers (partial) available. Support available to part-time students. Financial award application deadline: 6/15; financial award applicants required to submit FAFSA. *Faculty research:* Outcome and curriculum planning, health promotion, NCLEX-RN results, decision-making program evaluation. *Unit head:* Dr. Patti A. Stockert, President of the College, 309-655-4124, Fax: 309-624-8973, E-mail: patricia.a.stockert@osfhealthcare.org. *Application contact:* Dr. Kim A. Mitchell, Dean, Graduate Program, 309-655-2201, Fax: 309-624-8973, E-mail: kim.a.mitchell@osfhealthcare.org.
Website: http://www.sfmccon.edu/graduate-programs/

Salem State University, School of Graduate Studies, Program in Nursing, Salem, MA 01970-5353. Offers adult-gerontology primary care nursing (MSN); nursing administration (MSN); nursing education (MSN); MBA/MSN. *Accreditation:* AACN. *Program availability:* Part-time, evening/weekend. *Entrance requirements:* For master's, GRE or MAT. Additional exam requirements/recommendations for international students: Required—TOEFL (minimum score 550 paper-based; 80 iBT) or IELTS (minimum score 5.5).

Seattle Pacific University, MS in Nursing Program, Seattle, WA 98119-1997. Offers administration (MSN); adult/gerontology nurse practitioner (MSN); clinical nurse specialist (MSN); family nurse practitioner (MSN, Certificate); informatics (MSN); nurse educator (MSN). *Accreditation:* AACN. *Program availability:* Part-time. *Students:* 39 full-time (36 women), 30 part-time (25 women); includes 14 minority (3 Black or African American, non-Hispanic/Latino; 7 Asian, non-Hispanic/Latino; 3 Hispanic/Latino; 1 Two or more races, non-Hispanic/Latino), 1 international. Average age 38. 60 applicants, 48% accepted, 29 enrolled. In 2015, 23 master's awarded. *Degree requirements:* For master's, thesis. *Entrance requirements:* For master's, personal statement, transcripts, undergraduate nursing degree, proof of undergraduate statistics course with minimum GPA of 2.0, 2 recommendations. *Application deadline:* For fall admission, 1/15 priority date for domestic students; for spring admission, 1/15 for domestic students. Applications are processed on a rolling basis. Application fee: $50. Electronic applications accepted. *Expenses:* Contact institution. *Financial support:* Fellowships and scholarships/grants available. Financial award applicants required to submit FAFSA. *Unit head:* Dr. Christine Hoyle, Associate Dean, 206-281-2469, E-mail: hoylec@spu.edu.
Website: http://spu.edu/depts/health-sciences/grad/index.asp

Seattle University, College of Nursing, Program in Advanced Practice Nursing Immersion, Seattle, WA 98122-1090. Offers adult/gerontological nurse practitioner (MSN); advanced community public health nursing (MSN); family nurse practitioner

(MSN); family psychiatric mental health nurse practitioner (MSN); nurse midwifery (MSN). *Degree requirements:* For master's, thesis or scholarly project. *Entrance requirements:* For master's, GRE, bachelor's degree, minimum GPA of 3.0, professional resume, two recommendations, letter of intent. Additional exam requirements/recommendations for international students: Required—TOEFL (minimum score 92 iBT), IELTS. Electronic applications accepted.

Seattle University, College of Nursing, Program in Nursing, Seattle, WA 98122-1090. Offers adult/gerontological nurse practitioner (MSN); advanced community public health (MSN); psychiatric mental health nurse practitioner (MSN). *Degree requirements:* For master's, thesis or scholarly project. *Entrance requirements:* For master's, GRE, bachelor's degree in nursing or associate degree in nursing with baccalaureate in different major, 5-quarter statistics course, minimum cumulative GPA of 3.0, professional resume, two recommendations, letter of intent, copy of current RN license or ability to obtain RN license in WA state. Additional exam requirements/recommendations for international students: Required—TOEFL (minimum score 92 iBT), IELTS. Electronic applications accepted.

Seton Hall University, College of Nursing, South Orange, NJ 07079-2697. Offers advanced practice in primary health care (MSN, DNP), including adult/gerontological nurse practitioner, pediatric nurse practitioner; entry into practice (MSN); health systems administration (MSN, DNP); nursing (PhD); nursing case management (MSN); nursing education (MA); school nurse (MSN); MSN/MA. *Accreditation:* AACN. *Program availability:* Part-time, online learning. *Degree requirements:* For master's, research project; for doctorate, dissertation or scholarly project. *Entrance requirements:* For doctorate, GRE (waived for students with GPA of 3.5 or higher). Additional exam requirements/recommendations for international students: Required—TOEFL. Electronic applications accepted. *Faculty research:* Parent/child, adult, and gerontological nursing; breast cancer; families of children with HIV; parish nursing.

Southern University and Agricultural and Mechanical College, School of Nursing, Baton Rouge, LA 70813. Offers educator/administrator (PhD); family health nursing (MSN); family nurse practitioner (Post Master's Certificate); geriatric nurse practitioner/gerontology (PhD). *Accreditation:* AACN. *Program availability:* Part-time. *Degree requirements:* For master's, comprehensive exam, thesis; for doctorate, comprehensive exam, thesis/dissertation. *Entrance requirements:* For master's, GRE General Test, BSN, minimum GPA of 2.7; for doctorate, GRE General Test; for Post Master's Certificate, MSN. Additional exam requirements/recommendations for international students: Required—TOEFL (minimum score 525 paper-based). *Faculty research:* Health promotions, vulnerable populations, (community-based) cardiovascular participating research, health disparities chronic diseases, care of the elderly.

Stony Brook University, State University of New York, Stony Brook Medicine, School of Nursing, Program in Adult-Gerontological Health/Primary Care Nursing, Stony Brook, NY 11794. Offers adult health nurse practitioner (Certificate); adult health/primary care nursing (MS, DNP). *Accreditation:* AACN. *Program availability:* Part-time, blended/hybrid learning. *Students:* 18 full-time (16 women), 289 part-time (254 women); includes 115 minority (35 Black or African American, non-Hispanic/Latino; 55 Asian, non-Hispanic/Latino; 23 Hispanic/Latino; 2 Two or more races, non-Hispanic/Latino), 2 international. 164 applicants, 62% accepted, 88 enrolled. In 2015, 57 master's, 13 doctorates, 1 other advanced degree awarded. *Degree requirements:* For master's, thesis. *Entrance requirements:* For master's, BSN, minimum GPA of 3.0, course work in statistics. Additional exam requirements/recommendations for international students: Required—TOEFL (minimum score 90 iBT). *Application deadline:* For fall admission, 12/1 for domestic students. Application fee: $100. *Expenses:* $24,781 full-time resident tuition and fees per year, $968 per credit hour; $44,431 full-time nonresident tuition and fees per year, $1,787 per credit hour. *Financial support:* Application deadline: 3/15. *Unit head:* Justin M. Waryold, Program Director, 631-444-3074, Fax: 631-444-3136, E-mail: justin.waryold@stonybrook.edu. *Application contact:* Dr. Dolores C. Bilges, Senior Staff Assistant, 631-444-2644, Fax: 631-444-3136, E-mail: dnp.nursing@stonybrook.edu. Website: http://www.nursing.stonybrookmedicine.edu/about

Texas Christian University, Harris College of Nursing and Health Sciences, Master's Program in Nursing, Fort Worth, TX 76129. Offers clinical nurse leader (MSN, Certificate); clinical nurse specialist (MSN), including adult/gerontology nursing, pediatrics; nursing education (MSN). *Accreditation:* AACN; AANA/CANAEP (one or more programs are accredited). *Program availability:* Part-time, online only, 100% online. *Faculty:* 20 full-time (17 women), 2 part-time/adjunct (both women). *Students:* 47 full-time (40 women), 24 part-time (all women); includes 19 minority (3 Black or African American, non-Hispanic/Latino; 1 American Indian or Alaska Native, non-Hispanic/Latino; 10 Asian, non-Hispanic/Latino; 2 Hispanic/Latino; 1 Native Hawaiian or other Pacific Islander, non-Hispanic/Latino; 2 Two or more races, non-Hispanic/Latino), 1 international. Average age 39. 34 applicants, 82% accepted, 23 enrolled. In 2015, 14 master's awarded. *Degree requirements:* For master's, thesis or alternative, practicum. *Entrance requirements:* For master's, GRE General Test, 3 letters of reference, essay, resume, two official transcripts from every institution attended. *Application deadline:* For fall admission, 4/1 for domestic and international students; for spring admission, 9/1 for domestic and international students; for summer admission, 2/1 for domestic and international students. Applications are processed on a rolling basis. Application fee: $60. Electronic applications accepted. *Expenses:* $1,415 per semester hour; $112 fee per course. *Financial support:* In 2015–16, 71 students received support. Teaching assistantships and scholarships/grants available. Financial award application deadline: 2/15; financial award applicants required to submit FAFSA. *Faculty research:* Geriatrics, cancer survivorship, health literacy, endothelial cells, clinical simulation outcomes. *Unit head:* Dr. Kathy Baker, Director, Division of Nursing Graduate Studies and Scholarship, 817-257-6726, Fax: 817-257-8383, E-mail: kathy.baker@tcu.edu. *Application contact:* Mary Jane Allred, Administrative Program Specialist, 817-257-6726, Fax: 817-257-8383, E-mail: m.allred@tcu.edu.
Website: http://www.nursing.tcu.edu/graduate.asp

Texas Tech University Health Sciences Center, School of Nursing, Lubbock, TX 79430. Offers acute care nurse practitioner (MSN, Certificate); administration (MSN); advanced practice (DNP); education (MSN); executive leadership (DNP); family nurse practitioner (MSN, Certificate); geriatric nurse practitioner (MSN, Certificate); pediatric nurse practitioner (MSN, Certificate). *Accreditation:* AACN. *Program availability:* Part-time, online learning. *Degree requirements:* For master's, thesis optional. *Entrance requirements:* For master's, minimum GPA of 3.0, 3 letters of reference, BSN, RN license; for Certificate, minimum GPA of 3.0, 3 letters of reference, RN license. Additional exam requirements/recommendations for international students: Required—TOEFL (minimum score 550 paper-based). *Faculty research:* Diabetes/obesity, nurse competency, disease management, intervention and measurements, health disparities.

Uniformed Services University of the Health Sciences, Daniel K. Inouye Graduate School of Nursing, Bethesda, MD 20814. Offers adult-gerontology clinical nurse specialist (MSN, DNP); family nurse practitioner (DNP); nurse anesthesia (DNP); nursing science (PhD); psychiatric mental health nurse practitioner (DNP); women's health nurse practitioner (DNP). MSN and DNP programs available to military officers only; PhD to military and DoD students only. *Accreditation:* AACN; AANA/CANAEP. *Faculty:* 38 full-time (22 women), 2 part-time/adjunct (1 woman). *Students:* 51 full-time (29 women); includes 17 minority (8 Black or African American, non-Hispanic/Latino; 4 Asian, non-Hispanic/Latino; 4 Hispanic/Latino; 1 Two or more races, non-Hispanic/Latino). Average age 34. 75 applicants, 68% accepted, 51 enrolled. In 2015, 4 master's, 24 doctorates awarded. *Degree requirements:* For master's, thesis or alternative; for doctorate, thesis/dissertation or alternative. *Entrance requirements:* For master's, GRE, BSN, clinical experience, minimum GPA of 3.0, previous course work in science; for doctorate, GRE, BSN, clinical experience, minimum GPA of 3.0, previous course work in sciences, and writing paper (for DNP); MSN (for PhD). *Application deadline:* For fall admission, 7/1 for domestic students; for winter admission, 2/15 for domestic students. Application fee: $0. Electronic applications accepted. *Faculty research:* Prenatal care, military health care, military readiness, distance learning. *Unit head:* Dr. Diane C. Seibert, Associate Dean for Academic Affairs, 301-295-1080, Fax: 301-295-1707, E-mail: diane.seibert@usuhs.edu. *Application contact:* Terry Lynn Malavakis, Recording Secretary for Admissions Committee/Registrar/Program Analyst, 301-295-1055, Fax: 301-295-1707, E-mail: terry.malavakis@usuhs.edu.
Website: http://www.usuhs.edu/gsn/

University at Buffalo, the State University of New York, Graduate School, School of Nursing, Buffalo, NY 14214. Offers adult gerontology nurse practitioner (DNP); family nurse practitioner (DNP); health care systems and leadership (MS); nurse anesthetist (DNP); nursing (PhD); nursing education (Certificate); psychiatric/mental health nurse practitioner (DNP). *Accreditation:* AACN; AANA/CANAEP (one or more programs are accredited). *Program availability:* Part-time, 100% online. *Students:* 61 full-time (37 women), 137 part-time (114 women); includes 35 minority (17 Black or African American, non-Hispanic/Latino; 1 American Indian or Alaska Native, non-Hispanic/Latino; 17 Asian, non-Hispanic/Latino), 7 international. Average age 32. 193 applicants, 49% accepted, 75 enrolled. In 2015, 6 master's, 37 doctorates awarded. *Degree requirements:* For master's, thesis optional; for doctorate, comprehensive exam (for some programs), capstone (for DNP), dissertation (for PhD) *Entrance requirements:* For master's, GRE or MAT; for doctorate, GRE or MAT, minimum GPA of 3.0 (for DNP), 3.25 (for PhD); RN license; BS or MS in nursing; 3 references; writing sample; resume; personal statement; for Certificate, interview, minimum GPA of 3.0 or GRE General Test, RN license, MS in nursing, professional certification. Additional exam requirements/recommendations for international students: Required—TOEFL (minimum score 550 paper-based; 79 iBT), IELTS (minimum score 6.5). *Application deadline:* For fall admission, 7/1 for domestic students, 2/1 for international students; for spring admission, 12/1 for domestic students, 10/1 for international students; for summer admission, 2/1 for domestic students. Applications are processed on a rolling basis. Application fee: $75. Electronic applications accepted. *Financial support:* In 2015–16, 80 students received support, including 2 fellowships with tuition reimbursements available (averaging $17,000 per year), 4 research assistantships with tuition reimbursements available (averaging $10,600 per year), 7 teaching assistantships with tuition reimbursements available (averaging $10,600 per year); scholarships/grants, traineeships, health care benefits, and unspecified assistantships also available. Financial award application deadline: 2/1; financial award applicants required to submit FAFSA. *Faculty research:* Oncology, palliative care, gerontology, addictions, mental health, community wellness, sleep, workforce, care of underserved populations, quality and safety, person-centered care, adolescent health. *Total annual research expenditures:* $1.4 million. *Unit head:* Dr. Marsha L. Lewis, Dean and Professor, 716-829-2533, Fax: 716-829-2566, E-mail: ubnursingdean@buffalo.edu. *Application contact:* Jennifer H. VanLaeken, Director of Graduate Student Services, 716-829-3311, Fax: 716-829-2067, E-mail: jhv2@buffalo.edu.
Website: http://nursing.buffalo.edu/

The University of Alabama in Huntsville, School of Graduate Studies, College of Nursing, Huntsville, AL 35899. Offers family nurse practitioner (Certificate); nursing (MSN, DNP), including adult-gerontology acute care nurse practitioner (MSN), adult-gerontology clinical nurse specialist (MSN), family nurse practitioner (MSN), leadership in health care systems (MSN); nursing education (Certificate). DNP offered jointly with The University of Alabama at Birmingham. *Accreditation:* AACN. *Program availability:* Part-time, evening/weekend, online learning. *Degree requirements:* For master's, comprehensive exam, thesis or alternative, oral and written exams. *Entrance requirements:* For master's, MAT or GRE, Alabama RN license, BSN, minimum GPA of 3.0; for doctorate, master's degree in nursing in an advanced practice area; for Certificate, MAT or GRE, minimum GPA of 3.0. Additional exam requirements/recommendations for international students: Required—TOEFL (minimum score 500 paper-based; 80 iBT), IELTS (minimum score 6.5). *Application deadline:* For fall admission, 7/15 for domestic students, 4/1 for international students; for spring admission, 11/30 for domestic students, 9/1 for international students. Applications are processed on a rolling basis. Application fee: $50. Electronic applications accepted. *Expenses: Tuition, area resident:* Full-time $9548; part-time $547 per credit hour. Tuition, state resident: full-time $9548; part-time $547 per credit hour. Tuition, nonresident: full-time $21,402; part-time $1224 per credit hour. International tuition: $21,402 full-time. *Financial support:* Teaching assistantships with full tuition reimbursements, career-related internships or fieldwork, Federal Work-Study, institutionally sponsored loans, scholarships/grants, traineeships, health care benefits, and unspecified assistantships available. Support available to part-time students. Financial award application deadline: 4/1; financial award applicants required to submit FAFSA. *Faculty research:* Health care informatics, chronic illness management, maternal and child health, genetics/genomics, technology and health care. *Unit head:* Dr. Marsha Adams, Dean, 256-824-6345, Fax: 256-824-6026, E-mail: marsha.adams@uah.edu. *Application contact:* Charles Davis, Director of Graduate Admission and Advisement, 256-824-6669, Fax: 256-824-6026, E-mail: charles.davis@uah.edu.
Website: http://www.uah.edu/nursing

University of Colorado Colorado Springs, Helen and Arthur E. Johnson Beth-El College of Nursing and Health Sciences, Colorado Springs, CO 80918. Offers nursing practice (DNP); primary care nurse practitioner (MSN). *Accreditation:* AACN. *Program availability:* Part-time, 100% online, blended/hybrid learning. *Faculty:* 10 full-time (9 women), 8 part-time/adjunct (6 women). *Students:* 65 full-time (43 women), 137 part-time (129 women); includes 34 minority (5 Black or African American, non-Hispanic/Latino; 6 Asian, non-Hispanic/Latino; 19 Hispanic/Latino; 4 Two or more races, non-Hispanic/Latino), 1 international. Average age 34. 113 applicants, 55% accepted, 31 enrolled. In 2015, 39 master's, 7 doctorates awarded. *Degree requirements:* For master's, comprehensive exam, thesis optional; for doctorate, capstone project. *Entrance requirements:* For master's, GRE General Test or MAT, minimum overall GPA of 2.75 for all undergraduate course work, minimum BSN GPA of 3.3; for doctorate, interview; active RN license; MA; minimum GPA of 3.3; National Certification as nurse practitioner or clinical nurse specialist; portfolio. Additional exam requirements/recommendations for international students: Required—TOEFL (minimum score 550 paper-based; 80 iBT). *Application deadline:* For fall admission, 3/15 priority date for domestic students, 3/15 for international students; for spring admission, 8/15 for domestic and international students. Applications are processed on a rolling basis. Application fee: $60 ($100 for international students). Electronic applications accepted. *Expenses:* $11,734 per year resident, $20,068 per year non-resident. *Financial support:* In 2015–16, 58 students received support. Career-related internships or fieldwork, Federal Work-Study, and scholarships/grants available. Support available to part-time students. Financial award application deadline: 3/1; financial award applicants required

Gerontological Nursing

to submit FAFSA. *Faculty research:* Behavioral interventions to reduce stroke risk factors in older adults, interprofessional models of health promotion for older adults, nurse practitioner education, practice and policy, cardiology, advanced cardiac and pulmonary rehab, heart failure and stroke, community health prevention, veterans studies, anger management, sports medicine, sports nutrition. *Unit head:* Dr. Amy Silva-Smith, Graduate Department Chairperson, 719-255-4490, Fax: 719-255-4416, E-mail: asilvasm@uccs.edu. *Application contact:* Diane Busch, Program Assistant II, 719-255-4424, Fax: 719-255-4416, E-mail: dbusch@uccs.edu.
Website: http://www.uccs.edu/bethel/index.html

University of Delaware, College of Health Sciences, School of Nursing, Newark, DE 19716. Offers adult nurse practitioner (MSN, PMC); cardiopulmonary clinical nurse specialist (MSN, PMC); cardiopulmonary clinical nurse specialist/adult nurse practitioner (MSN, PMC); family nurse practitioner (MSN, PMC); gerontology clinical nurse specialist (MSN, PMC); gerontology clinical nurse specialist geriatric nurse practitioner (PMC); gerontology clinical nurse specialist/geriatric nurse practitioner (MSN); health services administration (MSN, PMC); nursing of children clinical nurse specialist (MSN, PMC); nursing of children clinical nurse specialist/pediatric nurse practitioner (MSN, PMC); oncology/immune deficiency clinical nurse specialist (MSN, PMC); oncology/immune deficiency clinical nurse specialist/adult nurse practitioner (MSN, PMC); perinatal/women's health clinical nurse specialist (MSN, PMC); perinatal/women's health clinical nurse specialist/women's health nurse practitioner (MSN, PMC); psychiatric nursing clinical nurse specialist (MSN, PMC). *Accreditation:* AACN. *Program availability:* Part-time, evening/weekend, online learning. *Degree requirements:* For master's, thesis optional. *Entrance requirements:* For master's, BSN, interview, RN license. Electronic applications accepted. *Faculty research:* Marriage and chronic illness, health promotion, congestive heart failure patient outcomes, school nursing, diabetes in children, culture, health disparities, cardiovascular, prison nursing, oncology, public policy, child obesity, smoking and teen pregnancy, blood pressure measurements, men's health.

University of Illinois at Chicago, College of Nursing, Program in Nursing, Chicago, IL 60607-7128. Offers acute care clinical nurse specialist (MS); administrative nursing leadership (Certificate); adult nurse practitioner (MS); adult/geriatric nurse practitioner (MS); advanced community health nurse specialist (MS); family nurse practitioner (MS); geriatric clinical nurse specialist (MS); geriatric nurse practitioner (MS); nurse midwifery (MS); occupational health/advanced community health nurse specialist (MS); occupational health/family nurse practitioner (MS); pediatric nurse practitioner (MS); perinatal clinical nurse specialist (MS); school/advanced community health nurse specialist (MS); school/family nurse practitioner (MS); women's health nurse practitioner (MS). *Accreditation:* AACN. *Program availability:* Part-time. *Faculty:* 100 full-time (93 women), 89 part-time/adjunct (82 women). *Students:* 359 full-time (326 women), 280 part-time (249 women); includes 169 minority (43 Black or African American, non-Hispanic/Latino; 62 Asian, non-Hispanic/Latino; 56 Hispanic/Latino; 1 Native Hawaiian or other Pacific Islander, non-Hispanic/Latino; 7 Two or more races, non-Hispanic/Latino), 12 international. Average age 32. In 2015, 4 other advanced degrees awarded. *Degree requirements:* For master's, thesis or alternative. *Entrance requirements:* For master's, GRE General Test, minimum GPA of 2.75. Additional exam requirements/recommendations for international students: Required—TOEFL. *Application deadline:* For fall admission, 5/15 for domestic students, 2/15 for international students; for spring admission, 11/1 for domestic students, 7/15 for international students. Applications are processed on a rolling basis. Application fee: $60. Electronic applications accepted. *Expenses:* Tuition, state resident: full-time $11,480; part-time $3826 per credit. Tuition, nonresident: full-time $23,720; part-time $7906 per credit. *Required fees:* $1333 per semester. Part-time tuition and fees vary according to course load and program. *Financial support:* Fellowships with full tuition reimbursements, research assistantships with full tuition reimbursements, teaching assistantships with full tuition reimbursements, career-related internships or fieldwork, Federal Work-Study, institutionally sponsored loans, scholarships/grants, traineeships, tuition waivers (full and partial), and unspecified assistantships available. Support available to part-time students. Financial award application deadline: 3/1; financial award applicants required to submit FAFSA. *Unit head:* Dr. Terri E. Weaver, Dean, 312-996-7808, E-mail: teweaver@uic.edu. *Application contact:* Receptionist, 312-413-2550, E-mail: gradcoll@uic.edu.
Website: http://www.nursing.uic.edu/academics-admissions/master-science#program-overview

The University of Kansas, University of Kansas Medical Center, School of Nursing, Kansas City, KS 66160. Offers adult/gerontological clinical nurse specialist (PMC); adult/gerontological nurse practitioner (PMC); clinical research management (PMC); health care informatics (PMC); health professions educator (PMC); nurse midwife (PMC); nursing (MS, DNP, PhD); organizational leadership (PMC); psychiatric/mental health nurse practitioner (PMC); public health nursing (PMC). *Accreditation:* AACN; ACNM/ACME. *Program availability:* Part-time, 100% online, blended/hybrid learning. *Faculty:* 59. *Students:* 44 full-time (42 women), 261 part-time (238 women); includes 54 minority (22 Black or African American, non-Hispanic/Latino; 1 American Indian or Alaska Native, non-Hispanic/Latino; 12 Asian, non-Hispanic/Latino; 10 Hispanic/Latino; 9 Two or more races, non-Hispanic/Latino), 1 international. Average age 38. 95 applicants, 97% accepted, 74 enrolled. In 2015, 71 master's, 24 doctorates, 6 other advanced degrees awarded. Terminal master's awarded for partial completion of doctoral program. *Degree requirements:* For master's, comprehensive exam, thesis (for some programs), general oral exam; for doctorate, variable foreign language requirement, thesis/dissertation or alternative, comprehensive oral exam (for DNP); comprehensive written and oral exam, or three publications (for PhD). *Entrance requirements:* For master's, bachelor's degree in nursing, minimum GPA of 3.0, 1 year of clinical experience, RN license in KS and MO; for doctorate, GRE General Test (for PhD only), bachelor's degree in nursing, minimum GPA of 3.5, RN license in KS and MO. Additional exam requirements/recommendations for international students: Required—TOEFL. *Application deadline:* For fall admission, 4/1 for domestic and international students; for spring admission, 9/1 for domestic and international students. Application fee: $60. Electronic applications accepted. *Financial support:* Research assistantships with tuition reimbursements, teaching assistantships with tuition reimbursements, scholarships/grants, and traineeships available. Financial award application deadline: 3/1; financial award applicants required to submit FAFSA. *Faculty research:* Breastfeeding practices of teen mothers, national database of nursing quality indicators, caregiving of families of patients using technology in the home, simulation in nursing education, diaphragm fatigue. *Total annual research expenditures:* $4.6 million. *Unit head:* Dr. Sally Maliski, Dean, 913-588-1601, Fax: 913-588-1660, E-mail: smaliski@kumc.edu. *Application contact:* Dr. Pamela K. Barnes, Associate Dean, Student Affairs, 913-588-1619, Fax: 913-588-1615, E-mail: pbarnes2@kumc.edu.
Website: http://nursing.kumc.edu

University of Louisville, Graduate School, School of Nursing, Louisville, KY 40202. Offers adult gerontology nurse practitioner (MSN, DNP); education and administration (MSN); family nurse practitioner (MSN, DNP); neonatal nurse practitioner (MSN, DNP); nursing research (PhD); psychiatric/mental health nurse practitioner (MSN, DNP); women's health nurse practitioner (MSN). *Accreditation:* AACN. *Program availability:* Part-time. *Faculty:* 53 full-time (48 women), 27 part-time/adjunct (23 women). *Students:* 110 full-time (99 women), 33 part-time (29 women); includes 17 minority (11 Black or African American, non-Hispanic/Latino; 1 Asian, non-Hispanic/Latino; 2 Hispanic/Latino;

3 Two or more races, non-Hispanic/Latino), 5 international. Average age 34. 62 applicants, 68% accepted, 40 enrolled. In 2015, 41 master's awarded. *Degree requirements:* For doctorate, comprehensive exam (for some programs), thesis/dissertation (for some programs). *Entrance requirements:* For master's, bachelor's degree in nursing, minimum GPA 3.0, RN license; for doctorate, GRE General Test (for PhD), 3 letters of professional reference. Additional exam requirements/recommendations for international students: Required—TOEFL (minimum score 560 paper-based; 79 iBT). *Application deadline:* For fall admission, 3/1 priority date for domestic students, 3/1 for international students. Applications are processed on a rolling basis. Application fee: $60. Electronic applications accepted. *Expenses:* Tuition, state resident: full-time $11,664; part-time $649 per credit hour. Tuition, nonresident: full-time $24,274; part-time $1350 per credit hour. *Required fees:* $196. Tuition and fees vary according to program and reciprocity agreements. *Financial support:* In 2015–16, 722,568 students received support, including 10 research assistantships with full tuition reimbursements available (averaging $20,000 per year), 2 teaching assistantships with full tuition reimbursements available (averaging $15,000 per year); fellowships with full tuition reimbursements available, scholarships/grants, and unspecified assistantships also available. Financial award application deadline: 2/15; financial award applicants required to submit FAFSA. *Faculty research:* Children and adolescents with chronic illnesses, women's mental health and parenting, asthma and environmental health, type 2 diabetes self-management in adults, health disparities and community engagement. *Total annual research expenditures:* $722,568. *Unit head:* Dr. Marcia J. Hern, Dean, 502-852-8300, Fax: 502-852-8783, E-mail: m.hern@louisville.edu. *Application contact:* Trish Hart, Assistant Dean for Student Affairs, 502-852-5825, Fax: 502-852-8783, E-mail: trish.hart@louisville.edu.
Website: http://www.louisville.edu/nursing/

University of Maryland, Baltimore, Graduate School, School of Nursing, Master's Program in Nursing, Baltimore, MD 21201. Offers community health nursing (MS); gerontological nursing (MS); maternal-child nursing (MS); medical-surgical nursing (MS); nurse-midwifery education (MS); nursing administration (MS); nursing education (MS); nursing health policy (MS); primary care nursing (MS); psychiatric nursing (MS); MS/MBA. MS/MBA offered jointly with University of Baltimore. *Accreditation:* AACN; AANA/CANAEP. *Program availability:* Part-time. *Degree requirements:* For master's, comprehensive exam (for some programs), thesis or alternative. *Entrance requirements:* For master's, minimum GPA of 2.75, course work in statistics, BS in nursing. Additional exam requirements/recommendations for international students: Required—TOEFL (minimum score 550 paper-based; 80 iBT); Recommended—IELTS (minimum score 7). Electronic applications accepted. Tuition and fees vary according to program.

University of Massachusetts Amherst, Graduate School, College of Nursing, Amherst, MA 01003. Offers adult gerontology primary care nurse practitioner (DNP); clinical nurse leader (MS); family nurse practitioner (DNP); nursing (PhD); public health nurse leader (DNP). *Accreditation:* AACN. *Program availability:* Part-time, online learning. Terminal master's awarded for partial completion of doctoral program. *Degree requirements:* For master's, thesis optional; for doctorate, comprehensive exam, thesis/dissertation. *Entrance requirements:* Additional exam requirements/recommendations for international students: Required—TOEFL (minimum score 550 paper-based; 80 iBT), IELTS (minimum score 6.5). Electronic applications accepted. *Faculty research:* Health of older adults and their caretakers, mental health of individuals and families, health of children and adolescents, power and decision-making, transcultural health.

University of Massachusetts Lowell, College of Health Sciences, School of Nursing, Program in Adult/Gerontological Nursing, Lowell, MA 01854. Offers MS. *Accreditation:* AACN. *Degree requirements:* For master's, thesis optional. *Entrance requirements:* For master's, GRE General Test, minimum GPA of 3.0, MA nursing license, interview, 3 letters of recommendation. *Application deadline:* For fall admission, 4/1 priority date for domestic students; for spring admission, 10/1 for domestic students. Applications are processed on a rolling basis. Application fee: $20 ($35 for international students). *Expenses:* Tuition, state resident: full-time $14,304. Tuition, nonresident: full-time $25,853. *Required fees:* $375. Full-time tuition and fees vary according to campus/location and reciprocity agreements. *Financial support:* Fellowships, research assistantships with full tuition reimbursements, teaching assistantships with full tuition reimbursements, career-related internships or fieldwork, Federal Work-Study, institutionally sponsored loans, scholarships/grants, and traineeships available. Support available to part-time students. Financial award application deadline: 4/1.

University of Massachusetts Medical School, Graduate School of Nursing, Worcester, MA 01655-0115. Offers adult gerontological acute care nurse practitioner (DNP, Post Master's Certificate); adult gerontological primary care nurse practitioner (DNP, Post Master's Certificate); family nursing practitioner (DNP); nurse administrator (DNP); nurse educator (MS, Post Master's Certificate); nursing (PhD); nursing practitioner (DNP); population health (MS). *Accreditation:* AACN. *Faculty:* 18 full-time (15 women), 28 part-time/adjunct (22 women). *Students:* 143 full-time (119 women), 27 part-time (25 women); includes 28 minority (15 Black or African American, non-Hispanic/Latino; 10 Asian, non-Hispanic/Latino; 3 Hispanic/Latino), 1 international. Average age 34. 129 applicants, 68% accepted, 56 enrolled. In 2015, 43 master's, 10 doctorates, 2 other advanced degrees awarded. *Degree requirements:* For doctorate, thesis/dissertation (for some programs), comprehensive exam (for PhD); capstone project and manuscript (for DNP). *Entrance requirements:* For master's, GRE General Test, bachelor's degree in nursing, course work in statistics, unrestricted Massachusetts license as registered nurse; for doctorate, GRE General Test, bachelor's or master's degree; for Post Master's Certificate, GRE General Test, MS in nursing. Additional exam requirements/recommendations for international students: Required—TOEFL. *Application deadline:* For fall admission, 12/1 priority date for domestic students. Applications are processed on a rolling basis. Application fee: $60. Electronic applications accepted. *Expenses:* $10,994 resident per year; $18,210 non-resident per year. *Financial support:* In 2015–16, 31 students received support. Institutionally sponsored loans, scholarships/grants, traineeships, and tuition waivers (partial) available. Support available to part-time students. Financial award application deadline: 5/16; financial award applicants required to submit FAFSA. *Faculty research:* Health literacy, social justice, HIV prevention, cancer-related decision making, nursing education. *Total annual research expenditures:* $650,993. *Unit head:* Dr. Joan Vitello-Cicciu, Dean, 508-856-5081, Fax: 508-856-6552, E-mail: joan.vitello@umassmed.edu. *Application contact:* Diane Brescia, Admissions Coordinator, 508-856-3488, Fax: 508-856-5851, E-mail: diane.brescia@umassmed.edu.
Website: http://www.umassmed.edu/gsn/

University of Minnesota, Twin Cities Campus, Graduate School, School of Nursing, Gerontological Nurse Practitioner Program, Minneapolis, MN 55455-0213. Offers MS. *Accreditation:* AACN. *Degree requirements:* For master's, final oral exam, project or thesis. *Entrance requirements:* Additional exam requirements/recommendations for international students: Required—TOEFL (minimum score 586 paper-based).

University of Minnesota, Twin Cities Campus, Graduate School, School of Nursing, Program in Gerontological Clinical Nurse Specialist, Minneapolis, MN 55455-0213. Offers advanced clinical specialist in gerontology (MS). *Accreditation:* AACN. *Program availability:* Part-time. *Degree requirements:* For master's, final oral exam, project or thesis. *Entrance requirements:* Additional exam requirements/recommendations for international students: Required—TOEFL (minimum score 586 paper-based).

University of Missouri, Office of Research and Graduate Studies, Sinclair School of Nursing, Columbia, MO 65211. Offers adult-gerontology clinical nurse specialist (DNP, Certificate); family nurse practitioner (DNP); family psychiatric and mental health nurse practitioner (DNP); nursing (MS, PhD); nursing leadership and innovations in health care (DNP); pediatric clinical nurse specialist (DNP, Certificate); pediatric nurse practitioner (DNP). *Accreditation:* AACN. *Program availability:* Part-time. *Degree requirements:* For master's, thesis optional, oral exam; for doctorate, thesis/dissertation. *Entrance requirements:* For master's, GRE General Test, BSN, minimum GPA of 3.0 during last 60 hours, nursing license. Additional exam requirements/recommendations for international students: Required—TOEFL (minimum score 550 paper-based; 79 iBT). *Application deadline:* For fall admission, 2/1 priority date for domestic and international students. Applications are processed on a rolling basis. Application fee: $55 ($75 for international students). Electronic applications accepted. *Financial support:* Fellowships, research assistantships, teaching assistantships, career-related internships or fieldwork, institutionally sponsored loans, scholarships/grants, traineeships, health care benefits, tuition waivers (full), and unspecified assistantships available. Support available to part-time students. Website: http://nursing.missouri.edu/

University of Missouri–Kansas City, School of Nursing and Health Studies, Kansas City, MO 64108. Offers adult clinical nurse specialist (MSN), including adult nurse practitioner, women's health nurse practitioner (MSN, DNP); adult clinical nursing practice (DNP), including adult gerontology nurse practitioner, women's health nurse practitioner (MSN, DNP); clinical nursing practice (DNP), including family nurse practitioner; family nurse practitioner (MSN); neonatal nurse practitioner (MSN); nurse educator (MSN); nurse executive (MSN); nursing (PhD); nursing practice (DNP); pediatric clinical nursing practice (DNP), including pediatric nurse practitioner; pediatric nurse practitioner (MSN). *Accreditation:* AACN. *Program availability:* Part-time, online learning. *Faculty:* 44 full-time (40 women), 47 part-time/adjunct (45 women). *Students:* 62 full-time (43 women), 259 part-time (239 women); includes 61 minority (28 Black or African American, non-Hispanic/Latino; 3 American Indian or Alaska Native, non-Hispanic/Latino; 16 Asian, non-Hispanic/Latino; 10 Hispanic/Latino; 4 Two or more races, non-Hispanic/Latino). Average age 35. 102 applicants, 35% accepted, 36 enrolled. In 2015, 116 master's, 23 doctorates awarded. *Degree requirements:* For master's, thesis or alternative. *Entrance requirements:* For master's, minimum undergraduate GPA of 3.2; for doctorate, GRE, 3 letters of reference. Additional exam requirements/recommendations for international students: Required—TOEFL (minimum score 550 paper-based; 80 iBT). *Application deadline:* For fall admission, 2/1 priority date for domestic and international students; for spring admission, 9/1 priority date for domestic and international students. Application fee: $45 ($50 for international students). *Financial support:* In 2015–16, 2 teaching assistantships with partial tuition reimbursements (averaging $6,650 per year) were awarded; fellowships, research assistantships, career-related internships or fieldwork, Federal Work-Study, institutionally sponsored loans, and tuition waivers (full and partial) also available. Support available to part-time students. Financial award application deadline: 3/1; financial award applicants required to submit FAFSA. *Faculty research:* Geriatrics/gerontology, children's pain, neonatology, Alzheimer's care, cancer caregivers. *Unit head:* Dr. Ann Cary, Dean, 816-235-1723, Fax: 816-235-1701, E-mail: caryah@umkc.edu. *Application contact:* Judy Jellison, Coordinator for Admissions and Recruitment, 816-235-1740, Fax: 816-235-1701, E-mail: jellisonj@umkc.edu. Website: http://nursing.umkc.edu/

University of Missouri–St. Louis, College of Nursing, St. Louis, MO 63121-4400. Offers adult/geriatric nurse practitioner (Post Master's Certificate); family nurse practitioner (Post Master's Certificate); nurse educator (MSN); nurse practitioner (MSN); nursing (DNP, PhD); pediatric nurse practitioner (Post Master's Certificate); psychiatric-mental health nurse practitioner (Post Master's Certificate); women's health nurse practitioner (Post Master's Certificate). *Accreditation:* AACN. *Program availability:* Part-time. *Faculty:* 21 full-time (19 women), 6 part-time/adjunct (5 women). *Students:* 18 full-time (17 women), 227 part-time (215 women); includes 34 minority (22 Black or African American, non-Hispanic/Latino; 8 Asian, non-Hispanic/Latino; 3 Hispanic/Latino; 1 Two or more races, non-Hispanic/Latino), 1 international. Average age 35. 152 applicants, 69% accepted, 83 enrolled. *Degree requirements:* For doctorate, comprehensive exam, thesis/dissertation; for Post Master's Certificate, thesis. *Entrance requirements:* For master's, 2 recommendation letters; minimum GPA of 3.0; BSN; nursing licensure; statement of purpose; course in differential/inferential statistics; for doctorate, GRE, 2 letters of recommendation, MSN, minimum GPA of 3.2, course in differential/inferential statistics; for Post Master's Certificate, 2 recommendation letters; MSN; advanced practice certificate; minimum GPA of 3.0; essay. Additional exam requirements/recommendations for international students: Recommended—TOEFL (minimum score 550 paper-based; 79 iBT), IELTS (minimum score 6.5). *Application deadline:* For fall admission, 2/15 for domestic and international students. Application fee: $50 ($40 for international students). Electronic applications accepted. *Financial support:* Research assistantships with tuition reimbursements available. Financial award application deadline: 4/1; financial award applicants required to submit FAFSA. *Faculty research:* Health promotion and restoration, family disruption, violence, abuse, battered women, health survey methods. *Unit head:* Dr. Roberta Lavin, Director, 314-516-6066. *Application contact:* 314-516-5458, Fax: 314-516-6996, E-mail: gradadm@umsl.edu. Website: http://www.umsl.edu/divisions/nursing/

The University of North Carolina at Chapel Hill, School of Nursing, Chapel Hill, NC 27599-7460. Offers advanced practice registered nurse (DNP); health care systems (DNP); nursing (MSN, PhD, PMC), including administration (MSN), adult gerontology primary care nurse practitioner (MSN), clinical nurse leader (MSN), education (MSN), informatics (MSN, PMC), nursing leadership (PMC), outcomes management (MSN), primary care family nurse practitioner (MSN), primary care pediatric nurse practitioner (MSN), psychiatric/mental health nurse practitioner (MSN, PMC). *Accreditation:* AACN; ACEN (one or more programs are accredited). *Program availability:* Part-time. *Faculty:* 86 full-time (78 women), 44 part-time/adjunct (40 women). *Students:* 208 full-time (186 women), 128 part-time (116 women); includes 109 minority (49 Black or African American, non-Hispanic/Latino; 4 American Indian or Alaska Native, non-Hispanic/Latino; 32 Asian, non-Hispanic/Latino; 7 Hispanic/Latino; 17 Two or more races, non-Hispanic/Latino), 17 international. Average age 33. 624 applicants, 25% accepted, 150 enrolled. In 2015, 91 master's, 14 doctorates awarded. *Degree requirements:* For master's, comprehensive exam, thesis; for doctorate, thesis/dissertation, 3 exams; for PMC, thesis. *Entrance requirements:* Additional exam requirements/recommendations for international students: Required—TOEFL (minimum score 575 paper-based; 89 iBT), IELTS (minimum score 8). *Application deadline:* For fall admission, 12/15 for domestic and international students. Application fee: $85. Electronic applications accepted. *Financial support:* In 2015–16, 8 fellowships with full tuition reimbursements, 6 research assistantships with partial tuition reimbursements (averaging $8,000 per year), 10 teaching assistantships with partial tuition reimbursements (averaging $8,000 per year) were awarded; scholarships/grants, traineeships, health care benefits, and unspecified assistantships also available. Support available to part-time students. Financial award application deadline: 3/1; financial award applicants required to submit FAFSA. *Faculty*

research: Preventing and managing chronic illness, reducing health disparities, improving healthcare quality and patient outcomes, understanding biobehavioral and genetic bases of health and illness, developing innovative ways to enhance science and its clinical translation. *Unit head:* Donna S. Havens, PhD, RN, Dean/Professor, 919-966-3731, Fax: 919-966-3540, E-mail: dhavens@email.unc.edu. *Application contact:* Emily Sayed, Assistant Director, Graduate Admissions, 919-966-4260, Fax: 919-966-3540, E-mail: sayed@unc.edu.
Website: http://nursing.unc.edu

The University of North Carolina at Charlotte, College of Health and Human Services, School of Nursing, Charlotte, NC 28223-0001. Offers adult-gerontology acute care nurse practitioner (MSN, Post-Master's Certificate); advanced clinical nursing (MSN); community public health nursing (MSN); family nurse practitioner across the lifespan (MSN, Post-Master's Certificate); nurse administrator (MSN, Graduate Certificate); nurse anesthesia (MSN, Post-Master's Certificate); nurse educator (MSN, Graduate Certificate); nursing (DNP); nursing systems/population (MSN). *Accreditation:* AACN. *Program availability:* Part-time, blended/hybrid learning. *Faculty:* 26 full-time (25 women), 4 part-time/adjunct (3 women). *Students:* 109 full-time (89 women), 112 part-time (107 women); includes 46 minority (37 Black or African American, non-Hispanic/Latino; 3 Asian, non-Hispanic/Latino; 5 Hispanic/Latino; 1 Two or more races, non-Hispanic/Latino). Average age 33. 321 applicants, 34% accepted, 84 enrolled. In 2015, 76 master's, 4 doctorates, 7 other advanced degrees awarded. Terminal master's awarded for partial completion of doctoral program. *Degree requirements:* For master's, practicum, synthesis and integration or thesis, residency, internship (varies by program); for doctorate, thesis/dissertation or alternative, residency; for other advanced degree, practicum. *Entrance requirements:* For master's, GRE General Test, unencumbered license as Registered Nurse in North Carolina; BSN from nationally-accredited program; one year of professional nursing practice in acute/critical care; minimum overall GPA of 3.0 in the last degree and 60 hours of nursing coursework; completion of an undergraduate statistics course with minimum grade of C; statement of purpose; for doctorate, GRE or MAT, master's degree in nursing in an advanced nursing practice specialty from nationally-accredited program; minimum overall GPA of 3.5 in MSN program; current RN licensure in U.S. at time of application with eligibility for NC licensure; for other advanced degree, GRE. Additional exam requirements/recommendations for international students: Required—TOEFL (minimum score 557 paper-based, 83 iBT) or IELTS (minimum score 6.5). *Application deadline:* For fall admission, 2/1 for domestic and international students; for spring admission, 10/1 priority date for domestic and international students; for summer admission, 4/1 priority date for domestic and international students. Applications are processed on a rolling basis. Application fee: $75. Electronic applications accepted. *Expenses:* Contact institution. *Financial support:* In 2015–16, 9 students received support, including 5 research assistantships (averaging $4,850 per year), 3 teaching assistantships (averaging $2,911 per year); career-related internships or fieldwork, institutionally sponsored loans, scholarships/grants, traineeships, unspecified assistantships, and administrative assistantships also available. Support available to part-time students. Financial award application deadline: 3/1; financial award applicants required to submit FAFSA. *Faculty research:* Improving care outcomes for the elderly; vulnerable populations; symptom management; self management/health promotion strategies of older adults; migration and maternal child health; health disparities, health literacy, and access to healthcare in Latino adults with diabetes; psychiatric nursing. *Total annual research expenditures:* $875,169. *Unit head:* Dr. Dee Baldwin, Associate Dean, 704-687-7952, Fax: 704-687-6017, E-mail: dbaldwi5@uncc.edu. *Application contact:* Kathy B. Giddings, Director of Graduate Admissions, 704-687-5503, Fax: 704-687-1668, E-mail: gradadm@uncc.edu.
Website: http://nursing.uncc.edu/

The University of North Carolina at Greensboro, Graduate School, School of Nursing, Greensboro, NC 27412-5001. Offers adult clinical nurse specialist (MSN, PMC); adult/gerontological nurse practitioner (MSN, PMC); nurse anesthesia (MSN, PMC); nursing (PhD); nursing administration (MSN); nursing education (MSN); MSN/MBA. *Accreditation:* AACN; AANA/CANAEP; ACEN. *Degree requirements:* For master's, thesis or alternative. *Entrance requirements:* For master's, GRE General Test or MAT, BSN, clinical experience, liability insurance, RN license; for PMC, liability insurance, MSN, RN license. Additional exam requirements/recommendations for international students: Required—TOEFL. Electronic applications accepted.

University of North Dakota, Graduate School, College of Nursing, Department of Nursing, Grand Forks, ND 58202. Offers adult-gerontological nurse practitioner (MSN); advanced public health nurse (MSN); family nurse practitioner (MSN); nurse anesthesia (MSN); nurse educator (MSN); nursing (DNP, PhD); psychiatric and mental health nurse practitioner (MSN).

University of Pennsylvania, School of Nursing, Adult Gerontology Clinical Nurse Specialist Program, Philadelphia, PA 19104. Offers MSN. *Students:* 3 full-time (2 women), 5 part-time (all women); includes 4 minority (1 Black or African American, non-Hispanic/Latino; 1 Asian, non-Hispanic/Latino; 2 Hispanic/Latino), 1 international. Average age 34. 10 applicants, 60% accepted, 4 enrolled. In 2015, 10 master's awarded. *Expenses:* Tuition, area resident: Full-time $31,068; part-time $5762 per course. *Required fees:* $3200; $336 per course. Full-time tuition and fees vary according to degree level, program and student level. Part-time tuition and fees vary according to course load, degree level and program. Website: http://www.nursing.upenn.edu/ahcns/

University of Pennsylvania, School of Nursing, Adult-Gerontology Primary Care Nurse Practitioner Program, Philadelphia, PA 19104. Offers MSN. *Program availability:* Part-time. *Students:* 17 full-time (15 women), 9 part-time (all women); includes 8 minority (2 Black or African American, non-Hispanic/Latino; 4 Asian, non-Hispanic/Latino; 2 Two or more races, non-Hispanic/Latino), 2 international. Average age 30. 41 applicants, 78% accepted, 21 enrolled. In 2015, 28 master's awarded. *Expenses:* Tuition, area resident: Full-time $31,068; part-time $5762 per course. *Required fees:* $3200; $336 per course. Full-time tuition and fees vary according to degree level, program and student level. Part-time tuition and fees vary according to course load, degree level and program.

University of Phoenix–Bay Area Campus, College of Nursing, San Jose, CA 95134-1805. Offers education (MHA); gerontology (MHA); health administration (MHA, DHA); informatics (MHA, MSN); nursing (MSN, PhD); nursing/health care education (MSN); MSN/MBA. *Program availability:* Evening/weekend, online learning. *Degree requirements:* For master's, thesis (for some programs). *Entrance requirements:* For master's, minimum undergraduate GPA of 2.5, 3 years of work experience, RN license. Additional exam requirements/recommendations for international students: Required—TOEFL (minimum score 550 paper-based; 79 iBT). Electronic applications accepted.

University of Phoenix–Phoenix Campus, College of Health Sciences and Nursing, Tempe, AZ 85282-2371. Offers family nurse practitioner (MSN, Certificate); gerontology health care (Certificate); health care education (MSN, Certificate); health care informatics (Certificate); informatics (MSN); nursing (MSN); MSN/MHA. *Program availability:* Evening/weekend, online learning. *Entrance requirements:* Additional exam requirements/recommendations for international students: Required—TOEFL, TOEIC (Test of English as an International Communication), Berlitz Online English Proficiency Exam, PTE, or IELTS. Electronic applications accepted. *Expenses:* Contact institution.

Gerontological Nursing

University of Pittsburgh, School of Nursing, Clinical Nurse Specialist Program, Pittsburgh, PA 15260. Offers adult-gerontology (DNP); psychiatric mental health (DNP). *Accreditation:* AACN. *Program availability:* Part-time. *Students:* 1 (woman) full-time, 8 part-time (6 women); includes 2 minority (both Black or African American, non-Hispanic/ Latino). Average age 47. 1 applicant, 100% accepted. In 2015, 4 doctorates awarded. *Entrance requirements:* Additional exam requirements/recommendations for international students: Required—TOEFL (minimum score 600 paper-based; 100 iBT). *Application deadline:* For fall admission, 5/1 priority date for domestic students, 2/15 priority date for international students. Application fee: $50. Electronic applications accepted. *Expenses:* Contact institution. *Financial support:* In 2015–16, 2 students received support, including 2 fellowships with tuition reimbursements available (averaging $11,294 per year); research assistantships, teaching assistantships, scholarships/grants, health care benefits, and unspecified assistantships also available. Support available to part-time students. Financial award application deadline: 3/15. *Faculty research:* Behavioral management of chronic disorders, patient management in critical care, consumer informatics, genetic applications (molecular genetics and psychosocial implications), technology for nurses and patients to improve care. *Unit head:* Dr. Sandra Engberg, Associate Dean for Clinical Education, 412-624-3835, Fax: 412-624-8521, E-mail: sje1@pitt.edu. *Application contact:* Laurie Lapsley, Administrator of Graduate Student Services, 412-624-9670, Fax: 412-624-2409, E-mail: lapsleyl@pitt.edu.

University of Pittsburgh, School of Nursing, Nurse Practitioner Program, Pittsburgh, PA 15261. Offers adult-gerontology acute care (DNP); adult-gerontology primary care (DNP); family (individual across the lifespan) (DNP); neonatal (MSN, DNP); pediatric primary care (DNP); psychiatric mental health (DNP). *Accreditation:* AACN. *Program availability:* Part-time. *Students:* 74 full-time (65 women), 59 part-time (51 women); includes 14 minority (5 Black or African American, non-Hispanic/Latino; 2 American Indian or Alaska Native, non-Hispanic/Latino; 6 Asian, non-Hispanic/Latino; 1 Hispanic/ Latino). Average age 30. 65 applicants, 55% accepted, 28 enrolled. In 2015, 14 master's, 19 doctorates awarded. *Degree requirements:* For master's, comprehensive exam, thesis optional. *Entrance requirements:* For master's, GRE General Test or MAT, BSN, RN license, letters of recommendation, resume, course work in statistics, 1-3 years of nursing experience; for doctorate, GRE General Test, BSN, RN license, minimum GPA of 3.5, 3 letters of recommendation. Additional exam requirements/ recommendations for international students: Required—TOEFL (minimum score 600 paper-based; 100 iBT). *Application deadline:* For fall admission, 5/1 priority date for domestic students, 2/15 priority date for international students. Application fee: $50. Electronic applications accepted. *Expenses:* Contact institution. *Financial support:* In 2015–16, 16 students received support, including 7 fellowships with tuition reimbursements available (averaging $11,278 per year), 9 teaching assistantships with tuition reimbursements available (averaging $10,879 per year); scholarships/grants, traineeships, health care benefits, and unspecified assistantships also available. Support available to part-time students. Financial award application deadline: 3/15. *Faculty research:* Behavioral management of chronic disorders, patient management in critical care, consumer informatics, genetic applications (molecular genetics and psychosocial implications), technology for nurses and patients to improve care. *Unit head:* Dr. Sandra Engberg, Associate Dean for Clinical Education, 412-624-3835, Fax: 412-624-8521, E-mail: sje1@pitt.edu. *Application contact:* Laurie Lapsley, Administrator of Graduate Student Services, 412-624-9670, Fax: 412-624-2409, E-mail: lapsleyl@pitt.edu.
Website: http://www.nursing.pitt.edu

University of Puerto Rico, Medical Sciences Campus, School of Nursing, San Juan, PR 00936-5067. Offers adult and elderly nursing (MSN); child and adolescent nursing (MSN); critical care nursing (MSN); family and community nursing (MSN); family nurse practitioner (MSN); maternity nursing (MSN); mental health and psychiatric nursing (MSN). *Accreditation:* AACN. *Entrance requirements:* For master's, GRE or EXADEP, interview, Puerto Rico RN license or professional license for international students, general and specific point average, article analysis. Electronic applications accepted. *Faculty research:* HIV, health disparities, teen violence, women and violence, neurological disorders.

University of Rhode Island, Graduate School, College of Nursing, Kingston, RI 02881. Offers acute care nurse practitioner (MS); adult-gerontological nurse practitioner/clinical nurse specialist (MS); family nurse practitioner (MS); nursing (PhD); nursing education (MS); nursing practice (DNP). *Accreditation:* AACN; ACNM/ACME (one or more programs are accredited). *Program availability:* Part-time. *Faculty:* 11 full-time (all women). *Students:* 51 full-time (41 women), 77 part-time (70 women); includes 18 minority (11 Black or African American, non-Hispanic/Latino; 2 Asian, non-Hispanic/ Latino; 4 Hispanic/Latino; 1 Two or more races, non-Hispanic/Latino), 5 international. In 2015, 19 master's, 7 doctorates awarded. *Degree requirements:* For master's, comprehensive exam; for doctorate, comprehensive exam, thesis/dissertation. *Entrance requirements:* For master's, GRE or MAT, 2 letters of recommendation, scholarly papers; for doctorate, GRE, 3 letters of recommendation, scholarly papers. Additional exam requirements/recommendations for international students: Required—TOEFL (minimum score 550 paper-based). *Application deadline:* For fall admission, 2/15 for domestic students, 2/1 for international students; for spring admission, 10/15 for domestic students, 7/15 for international students. Application fee: $65. Electronic applications accepted. *Expenses:* Tuition, state resident: full-time $11,796; part-time $655 per credit. Tuition, nonresident: full-time $24,206; part-time $1345 per credit. *Required fees:* $1546; $44 per credit. One-time fee: $155 full-time; $35 part-time. *Financial support:* In 2015–16, 2 research assistantships (averaging $12,111 per year), 7 teaching assistantships with tuition reimbursements (averaging $13,112 per year) were awarded. Financial award application deadline: 2/15; financial award applicants required to submit FAFSA. *Faculty research:* Group intervention for grieving women in prison, translating best practice in non-drug interventions for postoperative pain management, further development and testing of the pain assessment inventory, preschool motor and functional performance of two cohorts, neuroactivation of brain motor areas in preterm children. *Unit head:* Dr. Mary Sullivan, Interim Dean, 401-874-5339, Fax: 401-874-2061, E-mail: mcsullivan@uri.edu. *Application contact:* Graduate Admission, 401-874-2872, E-mail: gradadm@etal.uri.edu.
Website: http://www.uri.edu/nursing/

University of Rochester, School of Nursing, Rochester, NY 14642. Offers adult gerontological acute care nurse practitioner (MS); clinical nurse leader (MS); family nurse practitioner (MS); family psychiatric mental health nurse practitioner (MS); health care organization management and leadership (MS); health promotion (PhD); nursing (DNP); nursing education (MS); pediatric nurse practitioner (MS); pediatric nurse practitioner/neonatal nurse practitioner (MS). *Accreditation:* AACN. *Program availability:* Part-time, online learning. *Faculty:* 56 full-time (45 women), 63 part-time/ adjunct (55 women). *Students:* 21 full-time (20 women), 212 part-time (175 women); includes 35 minority (12 Black or African American, non-Hispanic/Latino; 1 American Indian or Alaska Native, non-Hispanic/Latino; 10 Asian, non-Hispanic/Latino; 7 Hispanic/ Latino; 5 Two or more races, non-Hispanic/Latino), 2 international. Average age 35. 111 applicants, 68% accepted, 71 enrolled. In 2015, 52 master's, 9 doctorates awarded. Terminal master's awarded for partial completion of doctoral program. *Degree requirements:* For master's, comprehensive exam (for some programs); for doctorate,

thesis/dissertation. *Entrance requirements:* For master's, BS in nursing, minimum GPA of 3.0, course work in statistics; for doctorate, GRE General Test (for PhD), MS in nursing, minimum GPA of 3.5. Additional exam requirements/recommendations for international students: Required—TOEFL (minimum score 560 paper-based; 88 iBT) or IELTS (minimum score 6.5) recommended. *Application deadline:* For fall admission, 4/1 for domestic and international students; for spring admission, 9/1 for domestic and international students; for summer admission, 1/2 for domestic and international students. Application fee: $50. Electronic applications accepted. *Expenses: Tuition, area resident:* Full-time $47,450; part-time $1482 per credit hour. *Required fees:* $528. Tuition and fees vary according to program. *Financial support:* In 2015–16, 52 students received support, including 2 fellowships with tuition reimbursements available (averaging $30,000 per year); scholarships/grants, traineeships, health care benefits, tuition waivers (full and partial), and unspecified assistantships also available. Support available to part-time students. Financial award application deadline: 6/30. *Faculty research:* Symptom assessment and self-management of chronic illness, health promotion and illness prevention, nursing intervention research with vulnerable populations, palliative care, aging. *Total annual research expenditures:* $2.1 million. *Unit head:* Dr. Kathy H. Rideout, Dean, 585-273-8902, Fax: 585-273-1268, E-mail: kathy_rideout@urmc.rochester.edu. *Application contact:* Elaine Andolina, Director of Admissions, 585-275-2375, Fax: 585-756-8299, E-mail: elaine_andolina@urmc.rochester.edu.
Website: http://www.son.rochester.edu

University of San Diego, Hahn School of Nursing and Health Science, San Diego, CA 92110-2492. Offers adult-gerontology clinical nurse specialist (MSN); adult-gerontology nurse practitioner/family nurse practitioner (MSN); executive nurse leader (MSN); family nurse practitioner (MSN); family/lifespan psychiatric-mental health nurse practitioner (MSN); healthcare informatics (MS, MSN); nursing (PhD); nursing practice (DNP). *Accreditation:* AACN. *Program availability:* Part-time, evening/weekend. *Faculty:* 27 full-time (23 women), 46 part-time/adjunct (41 women). *Students:* 178 full-time (151 women), 157 part-time (131 women); includes 143 minority (25 Black or African American, non-Hispanic/Latino; 2 American Indian or Alaska Native, non-Hispanic/ Latino; 53 Asian, non-Hispanic/Latino; 49 Hispanic/Latino; 4 Native Hawaiian or other Pacific Islander, non-Hispanic/Latino; 10 Two or more races, non-Hispanic/Latino), 5 international. Average age 36. In 2015, 122 master's, 43 doctorates awarded. *Degree requirements:* For doctorate, thesis/dissertation (for some programs), residency (DNP). *Entrance requirements:* For master's, GRE General Test (for entry-level nursing), BSN, current California RN licensure (except for entry-level nursing); minimum GPA of 3.0; for doctorate, minimum GPA of 3.5, MSN, current California RN licensure. Additional exam requirements/recommendations for international students: Required—TOEFL (minimum score 580 paper-based; 83 iBT), TWE. *Application deadline:* Applications are processed on a rolling basis. Application fee: $45. Electronic applications accepted. *Financial support:* In 2015–16, 217 students received support. Scholarships/grants and traineeships available. Support available to part-time students. Financial award application deadline: 4/1; financial award applicants required to submit FAFSA. *Faculty research:* Maternal/neonatal health, palliative and end of life care, adolescent obesity, health disparities, cognitive dysfunction. *Unit head:* Dr. Sally Hardin, Dean, 619-260-4550, Fax: 619-260-6814. *Application contact:* Monica Mahon, Associate Director of Graduate Admissions, 619-260-4524, Fax: 619-260-4158, E-mail: grads@sandiego.edu.
Website: http://www.sandiego.edu/nursing/

University of Southern Maine, College of Science, Technology, and Health, School of Nursing, Portland, ME 04103. Offers adult-gerontology primary care nurse practitioner (MS, PMC); education (MS); family nurse practitioner (MS, PMC); family psychiatric/ mental health nurse practitioner (MS); management (MS); nursing (CAS, CGS); psychiatric-mental health nurse practitioner (PMC). *Accreditation:* AACN. *Program availability:* Part-time. *Degree requirements:* For master's, thesis optional. *Entrance requirements:* For master's, GRE General Test or MAT, minimum GPA of 3.0; for doctorate, GRE. Additional exam requirements/recommendations for international students: Required—TOEFL (minimum score 550 paper-based). Electronic applications accepted. *Expenses: Tuition, area resident:* Full-time $6840; part-time $380 per credit hour. Tuition, state resident: full-time $10,260; part-time $570 per credit hour. Tuition, nonresident: full-time $18,468; part-time $1026 per credit hour. *Required fees:* $830; $83 per credit hour. Tuition and fees vary according to course load and program. *Faculty research:* Women's health, nursing history, weight control, community services, substance abuse.

University of South Florida, College of Nursing, Tampa, FL 33612. Offers advanced pain management (Graduate Certificate); nursing (MS, DNP), including adult gerontology acute care (DNP), adult gerontology acute care nursing (MS), adult gerontology primary care (DNP), adult gerontology primary care nursing (MS), adult gerontology primary care/occupational health nursing (MS), adult gerontology primary care/oncology nursing (MS), clinical nurse leader (MS), family health nursing, nurse anesthesia (MS), nursing education (MS), nursing practice (DNP), occupational health/ adult-gerontology (DNP), oncology/adult-gerontology primary care (DNP), pediatric health (DNP), pediatric nurse practitioner (MS); nursing education (Post Master's Certificate); nursing science (PhD). *Accreditation:* AACN; AANA/CANAEP. *Program availability:* Part-time. *Faculty:* 43 full-time (38 women), 7 part-time/adjunct (4 women). *Students:* 159 full-time (135 women), 721 part-time (625 women); includes 292 minority (119 Black or African American, non-Hispanic/Latino; 2 American Indian or Alaska Native, non-Hispanic/Latino; 60 Asian, non-Hispanic/Latino; 90 Hispanic/Latino; 1 Native Hawaiian or other Pacific Islander, non-Hispanic/Latino; 20 Two or more races, non-Hispanic/Latino), 12 international. Average age 35. 636 applicants, 44% accepted, 215 enrolled. In 2015, 333 master's, 18 doctorates awarded. *Degree requirements:* For master's, comprehensive exam, thesis optional; for doctorate, comprehensive exam, thesis/dissertation. *Entrance requirements:* For master's, GRE General Test, bachelor's degree from accredited program with minimum GPA of 3.0 in all upper-division coursework; current license as Registered Nurse; 3 letters of recommendation; personal statement of goals; resume or curriculum vitae; personal interview; for doctorate, GRE General Test (recommended), bachelor's degree in nursing from a CCNA/NLNAC regionally-accredited institution with minimum GPA of 3.0 in all coursework or in all upper-division coursework; current license as Registered Nurse in Florida; undergraduate statistics course with minimum B grade; 3 letters of recommendation; statement of goals; resume; interview. Additional exam requirements/recommendations for international students: Required—TOEFL (minimum score 550 paper-based; 79 iBT). *Application deadline:* For fall admission, 2/15 for domestic students, 1/2 for international students; for spring admission, 10/1 for domestic students, 6/1 for international students. Application fee: $30. Electronic applications accepted. *Financial support:* In 2015–16, 36 students received support, including 7 research assistantships with tuition reimbursements available (averaging $18,935 per year), 29 teaching assistantships with tuition reimbursements available (averaging $30,814 per year); tuition waivers (partial) and unspecified assistantships also available. Financial award application deadline: 2/1; financial award applicants required to submit FAFSA. *Faculty research:* Women's health, palliative and end-of-life care, cardiac rehabilitation, complementary therapies for chronic illness and cancer. *Total annual research expenditures:* $2.6 million. *Unit head:* Dr. Dianne C. Morrison-Beedy, Dean and Professor, College of Nursing, 813-974-9091,

Fax: 813-974-5418, E-mail: dmbeedy@health.usf.edu. *Application contact:* Dr. Brian Graves, Assistant Professor/Assistant Dean, 813-974-8054, Fax: 813-974-5418, E-mail: bgraves1@health.usf.edu.
Website: http://health.usf.edu/nursing/index.htm

The University of Tennessee Health Science Center, College of Nursing, Memphis, TN 38163. Offers adult-gerontology acute care nurse practitioner (Certificate); advanced practice nursing (DNP); clinical nurse leader (MSN). *Accreditation:* AACN; AANA/ CANAEP. *Program availability:* Part-time, online learning. *Degree requirements:* For master's, thesis, portfolio; for doctorate, portfolio. *Entrance requirements:* For master's, minimum GPA of 3.0; for doctorate, RN license, minimum GPA of 3.0; for Certificate, MSN, APN license, minimum GPA of 3.0. Additional exam requirements/ recommendations for international students: Required—TOEFL (minimum score 550 paper-based; 80 iBT). Electronic applications accepted. *Expenses:* Contact institution. *Faculty research:* Efficacy of a cognitive behavioral group intervention and its influence on symptoms of depression and anxiety as well as caregiver function; ability of newly-developed assays to aid in the diagnosis of preeclampsia; quality of life and sexual function in women who undergo vulvar surgeries; influence of prenatal and early childhood environments on health and developmental trajectories across childhood; interaction between physical activity, diet, genetics, insulin resistance, and obesity.

The University of Texas at Austin, Graduate School, School of Nursing, Austin, TX 78712-1111. Offers adult - gerontology clinical nurse specialist (MSN); child health (MSN), including administration, public health nursing, teaching; family nurse practitioner (MSN); family psychiatric/mental health nurse practitioner (MSN); holistic adult health (MSN), including administration, teaching; maternity (MSN), including administration, public health nursing, teaching; nursing (PhD); nursing administration and healthcare systems management (MSN); nursing practice (DNP); pediatric nurse practitioner (MSN); public health nursing (MSN). *Accreditation:* AACN. *Program availability:* Part-time. *Degree requirements:* For master's, thesis optional; for doctorate, thesis/dissertation. *Entrance requirements:* For master's and doctorate, GRE General Test. Additional exam requirements/recommendations for international students: Required—TOEFL (minimum score 550 paper-based). Electronic applications accepted. *Faculty research:* Chronic illness management, memory and aging, health promotion, women's health, adolescent health.

The University of Texas Health Science Center at San Antonio, School of Nursing, San Antonio, TX 78229-3900. Offers administrative management (MSN); adult-gerontology acute care nurse practitioner (PGC); advanced practice leadership (DNP); clinical nurse leader (MSN); executive administrative management (DNP); family nurse practitioner (MSN, PGC); nursing (MSN, PhD); nursing education (MSN, PGC); pediatric nurse practitioner primary care (PGC); psychiatric mental health nurse practitioner (PGC); public health nurse leader (DNP). *Accreditation:* AACN. *Program availability:* Part-time. Terminal master's awarded for partial completion of doctoral program. *Degree requirements:* For master's, thesis optional; for doctorate, comprehensive exam, thesis/ dissertation.

University of Utah, Graduate School, College of Nursing, Gerontology Interdisciplinary Program, Salt Lake City, UT 84112. Offers MS, Certificate. *Accreditation:* AACN. *Program availability:* Part-time, evening/weekend, online learning. *Students:* 6 full-time (5 women), 6 part-time (all women); includes 2 minority (1 Black or African American, non-Hispanic/Latino; 1 Two or more races, non-Hispanic/Latino). Average age 42. 11 applicants, 91% accepted, 7 enrolled. In 2015, 9 master's awarded. *Degree requirements:* For master's, thesis or project. *Entrance requirements:* For master's, GRE General Test (if cumulative GPA is less than 3.2), minimum undergraduate GPA of 3.0. Additional exam requirements/recommendations for international students: Required— TOEFL (minimum score 500 paper-based; 85 iBT). *Application deadline:* For fall admission, 1/15 for domestic and international students. Applications are processed on a rolling basis. Application fee: $55 ($65 for international students). Electronic applications accepted. *Expenses:* Contact institution. *Financial support:* In 2015–16, 8 students received support, including 8 fellowships with partial tuition reimbursements available (averaging $5,040 per year), 1 teaching assistantship with partial tuition reimbursement available (averaging $20,250 per year); scholarships/grants and health care benefits also available. Support available to part-time students. Financial award application deadline: 1/15; financial award applicants required to submit FAFSA. *Faculty research:* Spousal bereavement, family caregiving, health promotion and self-care, geriatric care management, technology and aging. *Unit head:* Kara Dassel, Director, 801-585-7438, Fax: 801-587-7697, E-mail: kara.dassel@nurs.utah.edu. *Application contact:* Arminka Zeljkovic, Program Manager, 801-581-8198, Fax: 801-585-9705, E-mail: arminka.zeljkovic@nurs.utah.edu.
Website: http://www.nursing.utah.edu/gerontology/

University of Wisconsin–Eau Claire, College of Nursing and Health Sciences, Program in Nursing, Eau Claire, WI 54702-4004. Offers adult-gerontological administration (DNP); adult-gerontological clinical nurse specialist (DNP); adult-gerontological education (MSN); adult-gerontological primary care nurse practitioner (DNP); family health administration (DNP); family health in education (MSN); family health nurse practitioner (DNP); nursing (MSN); nursing practice (DNP). *Program availability:* Part-time. Terminal master's awarded for partial completion of doctoral program. *Degree requirements:* For master's, thesis optional, 500-600 hours clinical practicum, oral and written exams. *Entrance requirements:* For master's, Wisconsin RN license, minimum GPA of 3.0, undergraduate statistics, course work in health assessment. Additional exam requirements/recommendations for international students: Required—TOEFL (minimum score 79 iBT). *Expenses:* Contact institution.

University of Wisconsin–Madison, School of Nursing, Madison, WI 53706-1380. Offers adult/gerontology (DNP); nursing (PhD); pediatrics (DNP); psychiatric mental health (DNP); MS/MPH. *Accreditation:* AACN. *Program availability:* Part-time. *Degree requirements:* For doctorate, comprehensive exam, thesis/dissertation. *Entrance requirements:* For doctorate, GRE General Test, 2 samples of scholarly written work, BS in nursing from an accredited program, minimum undergraduate GPA of 3.0 in last 60 credits (for PhD); licensure as professional nurse (for DNP). Additional exam requirements/recommendations for international students: Required—TOEFL (minimum score 600 paper-based; 100 iBT). Electronic applications accepted. *Expenses:* Tuition, state resident: full-time $5364. Tuition, nonresident: full-time $12,027. *Required fees:* $571. Tuition and fees vary according to campus/location, program and reciprocity agreements. *Faculty research:* Nursing informatics to promote self-care and disease management skills among patients and caregivers; quality of care to frail, vulnerable, and chronically ill populations; study of health-related and health-seeking behaviors; eliminating health disparities; pain and symptom management for patients with cancer.

Ursuline College, School of Graduate Studies, Programs in Nursing, Pepper Pike, OH 44124-4398. Offers adult nurse practitioner (MSN); adult-gerontology clinical nurse specialist (MSN); family nurse practitioner (MSN); nursing (DNP); nursing education (MSN); palliative care (MSN). *Accreditation:* AACN. *Program availability:* Part-time. *Faculty:* 5 full-time (all women), 26 part-time/adjunct (21 women). *Students:* 150 full-time (141 women), 108 part-time (99 women); includes 66 minority (50 Black or African American, non-Hispanic/Latino; 6 Asian, non-Hispanic/Latino; 6 Hispanic/Latino; 4 Two or more races, non-Hispanic/Latino), 5 international. Average age 37. 115 applicants, 95% accepted, 73 enrolled. In 2015, 69 master's, 2 doctorates awarded. *Degree*

requirements: For master's, comprehensive exam. *Entrance requirements:* For master's, minimum undergraduate GPA of 3.0, bachelor's degree in nursing, eligibility for or current Ohio RN license. Additional exam requirements/recommendations for international students: Required—TOEFL (minimum score 500 paper-based). *Application deadline:* For fall admission, 8/1 priority date for domestic students. Applications are processed on a rolling basis. Application fee: $25. Electronic applications accepted. *Expenses: Tuition, area resident:* Full-time $18,036; part-time $6012 per semester. *Required fees:* $290; $210 per credit. $105 per semester. Tuition and fees vary according to program. *Financial support:* In 2015–16, 12 students received support. Scholarships/grants available. Financial award application deadline: 3/ 1; financial award applicants required to submit FAFSA. *Unit head:* Dr. Janet Baker, Director, 440-864-8172, Fax: 440-684-6053, E-mail: jbaker@ursuline.edu. *Application contact:* Stephanie Pratt McRoberts, Graduate Admission Coordinator, 440-646-8119, Fax: 440-684-6138, E-mail: graduateadmissions@ursuline.edu.

Vanderbilt University, Vanderbilt University School of Nursing, Nashville, TN 37240. Offers adult-gerontology acute care nurse practitioner (MSN), including hospitalist, intensivist; adult-gerontology primary care nurse practitioner (MSN); emergency nurse practitioner (MSN); family nurse practitioner (MSN); healthcare leadership (MSN); neonatal nurse practitioner (MSN); nurse midwifery (MSN); nurse midwifery/family nurse practitioner (MSN); nursing (Post-Master's Certificate); nursing informatics (MSN); nursing practice (DNP); nursing science (PhD); pediatric acute care nurse practitioner (MSN); pediatric primary care nurse practitioner (MSN); psychiatric-mental health nurse practitioner (MSN); women's health nurse practitioner (MSN); women's health nurse practitioner/adult gerontology primary care nurse practitioner (MSN); MSN/M Div; MSN/ MTS. *Accreditation:* ACEN (one or more programs are accredited); ACNM/ACME. *Program availability:* Part-time, 100% online, blended/hybrid learning. *Faculty:* 258 full-time (232 women), 363 part-time/adjunct (271 women). *Students:* 478 full-time (424 women), 342 part-time (317 women); includes 140 minority (36 Black or African American, non-Hispanic/Latino; 3 American Indian or Alaska Native, non-Hispanic/Latino; 24 Asian, non-Hispanic/Latino; 43 Hispanic/Latino; 3 Native Hawaiian or other Pacific Islander, non-Hispanic/Latino; 31 Two or more races, non-Hispanic/Latino), 11 international. Average age 31. 1,268 applicants, 49% accepted, 477 enrolled. In 2015, 343 master's, 55 doctorates awarded. *Degree requirements:* For doctorate, comprehensive exam, thesis/ dissertation. *Entrance requirements:* For master's, GRE General Test (taken within the past 5 years), minimum B average in undergraduate course work, 3 letters of recommendation; for doctorate, GRE General Test, interview, 3 letters of recommendation from doctorally-prepared faculty, MSN, essay. Additional exam requirements/ recommendations for international students: Required—TOEFL (minimum score 570 paper-based), IELTS (minimum score 6.5). *Application deadline:* For fall admission, 11/1 priority date for domestic and international students. Applications are processed on a rolling basis. Application fee: $50. Electronic applications accepted. *Expenses:* Contact institution. *Financial support:* In 2015–16, 585 students received support. Scholarships/ grants available. Financial award application deadline: 3/15; financial award applicants required to submit FAFSA. *Faculty research:* Lymphedema, palliative care and bereavement, health services research including workforce, safety and quality of care, gerontology, better birth outcomes including nutrition. *Total annual research expenditures:* $2 million. *Unit head:* Dr. Linda Norman, Dean, 615-343-8876, Fax: 615-343-7711, E-mail: linda.norman@vanderbilt.edu. *Application contact:* Patricia Peerman, Assistant Dean for Enrollment Management, 615-322-3800, Fax: 615-343-0333, E-mail: vusn-admissions@ vanderbilt.edu.
Website: http://www.nursing.vanderbilt.edu

Walden University, Graduate Programs, School of Nursing, Minneapolis, MN 55401. Offers adult-gerontology acute care nurse practitioner (MSN); adult-gerontology nurse practitioner (MSN); education (MSN); family nurse practitioner (MSN); informatics (MSN); leadership and management (MSN); nursing (PhD, Post-Master's Certificate), including education (PhD), healthcare administration (PhD), interdisciplinary health (PhD), leadership (PhD), nursing education (Post-Master's Certificate), nursing informatics (Post-Master's Certificate), nursing leadership and management (Post-Master's Certificate), public health policy (PhD); nursing practice (DNP); psychiatric mental health (MSN). *Accreditation:* AACN. *Program availability:* Part-time, evening/ weekend, online only, 100% online. *Faculty:* 22 full-time (18 women), 540 part-time/ adjunct (487 women). *Students:* 4,320 full-time (3,773 women), 5,250 part-time (4,740 women); includes 3,550 minority (2,360 Black or African American, non-Hispanic/Latino; 29 American Indian or Alaska Native, non-Hispanic/Latino; 523 Asian, non-Hispanic/ Latino; 421 Hispanic/Latino; 25 Native Hawaiian or other Pacific Islander, non-Hispanic/ Latino; 192 Two or more races, non-Hispanic/Latino), 221 international. Average age 40. 2,057 applicants, 100% accepted, 1507 enrolled. In 2015, 3,022 master's, 86 doctorates, 34 other advanced degrees awarded. *Degree requirements:* For doctorate, thesis/dissertation (for some programs), residency (for some programs), field experience (for some programs). *Entrance requirements:* For master's, bachelor's degree or equivalent in related field or RN; minimum GPA of 2.5; official transcripts; goal statement (for some programs); access to computer and Internet; for doctorate, master's degree or higher; RN; three years of related professional or academic experience; goal statement; access to computer and Internet; for Post-Master's Certificate, relevant work experience; access to computer and Internet. Additional exam requirements/ recommendations for international students: Required—TOEFL (minimum score 550 paper-based, 79 iBT), IELTS (minimum score 6.5), Michigan English Language Assessment Battery (minimum score 82), or PTE (minimum score 53). *Application deadline:* Applications are processed on a rolling basis. Application fee: $0. Electronic applications accepted. *Financial support:* Fellowships, Federal Work-Study, scholarships/grants, unspecified assistantships, and family tuition reduction, active duty/ veteran tuition reduction, group tuition reduction, interest-free payment plans, employee tuition reduction available. Support available to part-time students. Financial award applicants required to submit FAFSA. *Unit head:* Dr. Andrea Lindell, Dean, 866-492-5336. *Application contact:* Meghan Thomas, Vice President of Enrollment Management, 866-492-5336, E-mail: info@waldenu.edu.
Website: http://www.waldenu.edu/programs/colleges-schools/nursing

Wayne State University, College of Nursing, Doctor Program of Nursing Practice, Detroit, MI 48202. Offers adult gerontology nurse practitioner - acute care (DNP); adult gerontology nurse practitioner - primary care (DNP); family nurse practitioner (DNP); infant mental health (DNP); neonatal nurse practitioner (DNP); nurse midwifery (DNP); nursing practice (DNP); pediatric nurse practitioner - acute care (DNP); pediatric nurse practitioner - primary care (DNP); psychiatric mental health nurse practitioner (DNP). *Students:* 56 full-time (50 women), 37 part-time (32 women); includes 32 minority (19 Black or African American, non-Hispanic/Latino; 6 Asian, non-Hispanic/Latino; 3 Hispanic/Latino; 4 Two or more races, non-Hispanic/Latino), 6 international. Average age 35. 44 applicants, 66% accepted, 18 enrolled. In 2015, 16 doctorates awarded. *Entrance requirements:* For doctorate, official transcripts, two professional references, curriculum vitae or resume, statement of goals, BSN or MSN, current Michigan RN license, criminal background check, interview, on-site writing example. Additional exam requirements/recommendations for international students: Required—TOEFL (minimum score 600 paper-based; 101 iBT); Recommended—IELTS (minimum score 7). *Application deadline:* For fall admission, 1/31 for domestic and international students. Electronic applications accepted. *Expenses:* $19,325 per year resident tuition, $35,114

Gerontological Nursing

non-resident tuition; $805.20 per credit hour resident tuition, $1,463.10 per credit hour non-resident tuition; fees include $47.45 per credit hour student services fee and $274.60 per semester registration fee. *Financial support:* In 2015–16, 22 students received support. Fellowships, research assistantships, teaching assistantships, institutionally sponsored loans, and scholarships/grants available. Financial award applicants required to submit FAFSA. *Unit head:* Dr. Laurie Lauzon Clabo, Dean and Professor, 313-577-4104, E-mail: laurie.lauzon.clabo@wayne.edu. *Application contact:* Dr. Nancy George, Director of DNP Program, 313-577-8300.
Website: http://nursing.wayne.edu/dnp/index.php

West Chester University of Pennsylvania, College of Health Sciences, Department of Nursing, West Chester, PA 19383. Offers adult-gerontology clinical nurse specialist (MSN); nursing (DNP); nursing education (MSN); school nurse (Certificate). *Accreditation:* AACN. *Program availability:* Part-time, evening/weekend, blended/hybrid learning. *Faculty:* 7 full-time (6 women), 1 (woman) part-time/adjunct. *Students:* 2 full-time (1 woman), 85 part-time (78 women); includes 10 minority (7 Black or African American, non-Hispanic/Latino; 3 Asian, non-Hispanic/Latino). Average age 45. 30 applicants, 90% accepted, 20 enrolled. In 2015, 10 master's, 3 other advanced degrees awarded. *Entrance requirements:* For master's, goals statement; official academic transcript(s) from all colleges and universities attended demonstrating minimum cumulative undergraduate GPA of 2.8 with successful completion of BSN and courses in statistics and physical assessment; documentation of current clinical experience; for doctorate, master's degree in nursing in an advanced nursing specialty from nationally-accredited program; minimum master's GPA of 3.0; licensed Registered Nurse. Additional exam requirements/recommendations for international students: Required—TOEFL or IELTS. *Application deadline:* For fall admission, 5/15 for international students; for spring admission, 10/15 for international students. Applications are processed on a rolling basis. Application fee: $50. Electronic applications accepted. *Expenses:* Tuition, state resident: full-time $8460; part-time $470 per credit. Tuition, nonresident: full-time $12,690; part-time $705 per credit. *Required fees:* $2312; $126.75 per credit. Tuition and fees vary according to campus/location and program. *Financial support:* Scholarships/grants and unspecified assistantships available. Financial award application deadline: 2/15; financial award applicants required to submit FAFSA. *Unit head:* Dr. Charlotte Mackey, Chair, 610-436-3474, Fax: 610-436-3083, E-mail: cmackey@wcupa.edu. *Application contact:* Dr. Cheryl Schlamb, Graduate Coordinator, 610-436-2219, E-mail: cschlamb@wcupa.edu.
Website: http://www.wcupa.edu/_ACADEMICS/HealthSciences/nursing/

Western Connecticut State University, Division of Graduate Studies, School of Professional Studies, Nursing Department, Danbury, CT 06810-6885. Offers adult gerontology clinical nurse specialist (MSN); adult gerontology nurse practitioner (MSN);

nursing education (Ed D). *Accreditation:* AACN. *Program availability:* Part-time. *Degree requirements:* For master's, clinical component, thesis or research project, completion of program in 6 years. *Entrance requirements:* For master's, MAT (if GPA less than 3.0), bachelor's degree in nursing, minimum GPA of 3.0, previous course work in statistics and nursing research, RN license. Additional exam requirements/recommendations for international students: Recommended—TOEFL (minimum score 550 paper-based; 79 iBT), IELTS (minimum score 6). *Expenses:* Contact institution. *Faculty research:* Evaluating effectiveness of Reiki and acupressure on stress reduction.

Wilmington University, College of Health Professions, New Castle, DE 19720-6491. Offers adult nurse practitioner (MSN); family nurse practitioner (MSN); gerontology nurse practitioner (MSN); nursing (MSN); nursing leadership (MSN); nursing practice (DNP). *Accreditation:* AACN. *Program availability:* Part-time. *Degree requirements:* For master's, thesis. *Entrance requirements:* For master's, BSN, RN license, interview, 3 letters of recommendation. Additional exam requirements/recommendations for international students: Required—TOEFL (minimum score 500 paper-based). Electronic applications accepted. *Faculty research:* Outcomes assessment, student writing ability.

York College of Pennsylvania, Department of Nursing, York, PA 17405-7199. Offers adult gerontology clinical nurse specialist (MS), including administration, education; adult gerontology nurse practitioner (MS); nurse anesthetist (MS); nurse educator (MS); nursing practice (DNP). *Accreditation:* AACN; AANA/CANAEP. *Program availability:* Part-time, evening/weekend. *Faculty:* 9 full-time (all women), 5 part-time/adjunct (2 women). *Students:* 36 full-time (26 women), 55 part-time (47 women); includes 14 minority (4 Black or African American, non-Hispanic/Latino; 2 American Indian or Alaska Native, non-Hispanic/Latino; 5 Asian, non-Hispanic/Latino; 2 Hispanic/Latino; 1 Two or more races, non-Hispanic/Latino), 1 international. Average age 33. 115 applicants, 28% accepted, 28 enrolled. In 2015, 24 master's, 4 doctorates awarded. *Entrance requirements:* For master's, GRE General Test (for nurse anesthetist program), minimum GPA of 3.0 from CCNE- or NLNAC-accredited institution; for doctorate, master's degree in nursing from a CCNE- or NLNAC-accredited institution; minimum GPA of 3.5. Additional exam requirements/recommendations for international students: Required—TOEFL (minimum score 530 paper-based; 72 iBT). *Application deadline:* Applications are processed on a rolling basis. Application fee: $0. Electronic applications accepted. *Expenses: Tuition, area resident:* Full-time $13,770. *Required fees:* $1750; $380. Tuition and fees vary according to degree level. *Financial support:* Federal Work-Study available. *Faculty research:* Student stress response to simulation versus clinical, evidence-based practice in all clinical settings. *Unit head:* Dr. Kimberly Fenstermacher, Graduate Program Director, 717-815-1383, E-mail: kfenster@ycp.edu. *Application contact:* Allison Malachosky, Administrative Assistant, 717-815-1243, E-mail: amalacho@ycp.edu.
Website: http://www.ycp.edu/academics/academic-departments/nursing/

HIV/AIDS Nursing

University of Delaware, College of Health Sciences, School of Nursing, Newark, DE 19716. Offers adult nurse practitioner (MSN, PMC); cardiopulmonary clinical nurse specialist (MSN, PMC); cardiopulmonary clinical nurse specialist/adult nurse practitioner (MSN, PMC); family nurse practitioner (MSN, PMC); gerontology clinical nurse specialist (MSN, PMC); gerontology clinical nurse specialist geriatric nurse practitioner (PMC); gerontology clinical nurse specialist/geriatric nurse practitioner (MSN); health services administration (MSN, PMC); nursing of children clinical nurse specialist (MSN, PMC); nursing of children clinical nurse specialist/pediatric nurse practitioner (MSN, PMC); oncology/immune deficiency clinical nurse specialist (MSN, PMC); oncology/immune deficiency clinical nurse specialist/adult nurse practitioner (MSN, PMC); perinatal/

women's health clinical nurse specialist (MSN, PMC); perinatal/women's health clinical nurse specialist/women's health nurse practitioner (MSN, PMC); psychiatric nursing clinical nurse specialist (MSN, PMC). *Accreditation:* AACN. *Program availability:* Part-time, evening/weekend, online learning. *Degree requirements:* For master's, thesis optional. *Entrance requirements:* For master's, BSN, interview, RN license. Electronic applications accepted. *Faculty research:* Marriage and chronic illness, health promotion, congestive heart failure patient outcomes, school nursing, diabetes in children, culture, health disparities, cardiovascular, prison nursing, oncology, public policy, child obesity, smoking and teen pregnancy, blood pressure measurements, men's health.

Hospice Nursing

Madonna University, Program in Hospice, Livonia, MI 48150-1173. Offers MSH. *Program availability:* Part-time, evening/weekend. *Degree requirements:* For master's, thesis or alternative. *Entrance requirements:* For master's, GRE General Test, minimum undergraduate GPA of 3.0, 2 letters of recommendation, interview. Electronic applications accepted.

Maternal and Child/Neonatal Nursing

Baylor University, Graduate School, Louise Herrington School of Nursing, Dallas, TX 75246. Offers family nurse practitioner (MSN); neonatal nurse practitioner (MSN); nurse-midwifery (DNP). *Accreditation:* AACN. *Program availability:* Part-time, online learning. *Degree requirements:* For doctorate, comprehensive exam (for some programs), capstone project. *Entrance requirements:* For master's, GRE General Test or MAT; for doctorate, GRE General Test. Additional exam requirements/recommendations for international students: Required—TOEFL. Electronic applications accepted. *Faculty research:* Women and strokes, obesity and pregnancy, educational environmental factors, international undeserved populations, midwifery.

Boston College, William F. Connell School of Nursing, Chestnut Hill, MA 02467. Offers adult-gerontology nursing (MS); family health nursing (MS); forensic nursing (MS); nurse anesthesia (MS); nursing (PhD); pediatric nursing (MS), including pediatric and women's health; psychiatric-mental health nursing (MS); women's health nursing (MS); MBA/MS; MS/MA; MS/PhD. *Accreditation:* AACN; AANA/CANAEP (one or more programs are accredited). *Program availability:* Part-time. *Faculty:* 53 full-time (48 women), 47 part-time/adjunct (44 women). *Students:* 185 full-time (167 women), 66 part-time (56 women); includes 31 minority (10 Black or African American, non-Hispanic/Latino; 12 Asian, non-Hispanic/Latino; 7 Hispanic/Latino; 2 Two or more races, non-Hispanic/Latino), 7 international. Average age 32. 313 applicants, 66% accepted, 91 enrolled. In 2015, 98 master's, 5 doctorates awarded. *Degree requirements:* For master's, comprehensive exam; for doctorate, comprehensive exam, thesis/dissertation, computer

literacy exam or foreign language. *Entrance requirements:* For master's, bachelor's degree in nursing; for doctorate, GRE General Test, MS in nursing. Additional exam requirements/recommendations for international students: Required—TOEFL (minimum score 600 paper-based; 100 iBT), IELTS (minimum score 7.5). *Application deadline:* For fall admission, 9/30 for domestic and international students; for winter admission, 1/15 for domestic and international students; for spring admission, 3/15 for domestic and international students. Applications are processed on a rolling basis. Application fee: $40. Electronic applications accepted. *Expenses:* Contact institution. *Financial support:* In 2015–16, 1 fellowship with full tuition reimbursement (averaging $23,700 per year), 25 teaching assistantships (averaging $4,370 per year) were awarded; research assistantships, scholarships/grants, health care benefits, tuition waivers (partial), and unspecified assistantships also available. Support available to part-time students. Financial award application deadline: 3/1; financial award applicants required to submit FAFSA. *Faculty research:* Sexual and reproductive health, health promotion/illness prevention, aging, eating disorders, symptom management. *Total annual research expenditures:* $1 million. *Unit head:* Dr. Susan Gennaro, Dean, 617-552-4251, Fax: 617-552-0931, E-mail: susan.gennaro@bc.edu. *Application contact:* MaryBeth Crowley, Graduate Programs Assistant, 617-552-4928, Fax: 617-552-2121, E-mail: csongrad@bc.edu.
Website: http://www.bc.edu/schools/son/

Case Western Reserve University, Frances Payne Bolton School of Nursing, Master's Programs in Nursing, Nurse Practitioner Program, Cleveland, OH 44106. Offers acute care cardiovascular nursing (MSN); acute care nurse practitioner (MSN); acute care pediatric nurse practitioner (MSN); acute care/flight nurse (MSN); adult gerontology acute care nurse practitioner (MSN); adult gerontology oncology and palliative care (MSN); adult gerontology primary care nurse practitioner (MSN); family nurse practitioner (MSN); family systems psychiatric mental health nursing (MSN); neonatal nurse practitioner (MSN); pediatric nurse practitioner (MSN); women's health nurse practitioner (MSN). *Accreditation:* ACEN. *Program availability:* Part-time, online learning. *Students:* 52 full-time (45 women), 78 part-time (68 women); includes 31 minority (10 Black or African American, non-Hispanic/Latino; 14 Asian, non-Hispanic/Latino; 7 Hispanic/Latino). Average age 35. 64 applicants, 66% accepted, 29 enrolled. In 2015, 45 master's awarded. *Degree requirements:* For master's, thesis optional. *Entrance requirements:* For master's, GRE General Test or MAT. Additional exam requirements/recommendations for international students: Required—TOEFL (minimum score 577 paper-based; 90 iBT), IELTS (minimum score 7). *Application deadline:* For fall admission, 6/1 for domestic students; for spring admission, 10/1 for domestic students. Applications are processed on a rolling basis. Application fee: $75. *Expenses:* $1,891 per credit hour. *Financial support:* In 2015–16, 54 students received support, including 17 teaching assistantships with partial tuition reimbursements available (averaging $17,019 per year); scholarships/grants and traineeships also available. Financial award application deadline: 6/30; financial award applicants required to submit FAFSA. *Faculty research:* Symptom science, family/community care, aging across the lifespan, self-management of health and illness, neuroscience. *Unit head:* Dr. Carol Savrin, Director, 216-368-5304, Fax: 216-368-3542, E-mail: cls18@case.edu. *Application contact:* Donna Hassik, Admissions Coordinator, 216-368-5253, Fax: 216-368-0124, E-mail: dmh7@case.edu.
Website: http://fpb.cwru.edu/MSN/majors.shtm

Creighton University, College of Nursing, Omaha, NE 68178-0001. Offers adult acute care nurse practitioner (Post-Master's Certificate); adult gerontology acute care nurse practitioner (DNP); adult gerontology nurse practitioner (DNP); clinical nurse leader (MSN, Post-Graduate Certificate); clinical systems administration (MSN, DNP); family nurse practitioner (DNP, Post-Master's Certificate); neonatal nurse practitioner (DNP, Post-Master's Certificate); pediatric acute care nurse practitioner (DNP, Post-Master's Certificate); psychiatric mental health nurse practitioner (DNP). *Accreditation:* AACN. *Program availability:* Part-time, blended/hybrid learning. *Faculty:* 10 full-time (all women), 48 part-time/adjunct (45 women). *Students:* 132 full-time (120 women), 228 part-time (212 women); includes 38 minority (10 Black or African American, non-Hispanic/Latino; 3 American Indian or Alaska Native, non-Hispanic/Latino; 11 Asian, non-Hispanic/Latino; 1 Hispanic/Latino; 2 Native Hawaiian or other Pacific Islander, non-Hispanic/Latino; 11 Two or more races, non-Hispanic/Latino). Average age 31. 66 applicants, 91% accepted, 43 enrolled. In 2015, 54 master's, 17 doctorates, 1 other advanced degree awarded. *Degree requirements:* For master's, capstone project; for doctorate, scholarly project. *Entrance requirements:* For master's and doctorate, BSN from an ACEN- or CCNE-accredited nursing school, minimum cumulative GPA of 3.0, personal statement, current unencumbered RN license with NE eligibility, undergraduate statistics course, physical assessment course or equivalent; for other advanced degree, MSN or MS in nursing, minimum cumulative GPA of 3.0, current unencumbered RN license with NE eligibility. Additional exam requirements/recommendations for international students: Required—TOEFL (minimum score 600 paper-based; 100 iBT). *Application deadline:* For fall admission, 6/15 priority date for domestic and international students; for spring admission, 11/15 priority date for domestic and international students; for summer admission, 4/15 for domestic and international students. Applications are processed on a rolling basis. Application fee: $50. Electronic applications accepted. *Expenses:* $800 per credit hour tuition; $904 per semester full-time fees; $207 per semester part-time fees; $50 one-time drug screen fee. *Financial support:* In 2015–16, 7 students received support. Scholarships/grants available. Financial award applicants required to submit FAFSA. *Faculty research:* Obesity prevention in children, evaluation of simulated clinical experiences, vitamin D3 and calcium for cancer risk education in post menopausal women, online support and education to reduce stress for prenatal patients on bed rest, health literacy, immunization research. *Total annual research expenditures:* $162,085. *Unit head:* Dr. Catherine Todero, Dean, 402-280-2004, Fax: 402-280-2045. *Application contact:* Shannon Cox, Enrollment Specialist, 402-280-2067, Fax: 402-280-2045, E-mail: shannoncox@creighton.edu.
Website: http://nursing.creighton.edu/

Duke University, School of Nursing, Durham, NC 27708-0586. Offers acute care pediatric nurse practitioner (MSN, Post Master's Certificate); adult-gerontology nurse practitioner (MSN, Post Master's Certificate), including acute care, primary care; family nurse practitioner (MSN, Post Master's Certificate); neonatal nurse practitioner (MSN, Post Master's Certificate); nurse anesthesia (DNP); nurse practitioner (DNP); nursing (PhD); nursing and health care leadership (MSN); nursing education (MSN); nursing informatics (MSN, Post Master's Certificate); pediatric nurse practitioner (MSN, Post Master's Certificate), including primary care; women's health nurse practitioner (MSN, Post Master's Certificate). *Accreditation:* AACN; AANA/CANAEP. *Program availability:* Part-time, evening/weekend, online learning. *Faculty:* 74 full-time (63 women). *Students:* 179 full-time (152 women), 528 part-time (466 women); includes 145 minority (42 Black or African American, non-Hispanic/Latino; 3 American Indian or Alaska Native, non-Hispanic/Latino; 44 Asian, non-Hispanic/Latino; 35 Hispanic/Latino; 1 Native Hawaiian or other Pacific Islander, non-Hispanic/Latino; 20 Two or more races, non-Hispanic/Latino; 7 international. Average age 33. 619 applicants, 46% accepted, 201 enrolled. In 2015, 243 master's, 62 doctorates, 26 other advanced degrees awarded. Terminal master's awarded for partial completion of doctoral program. *Degree requirements:* For master's, thesis optional; for doctorate, capstone project. *Entrance requirements:* For master's, GRE General Test (waived if undergraduate GPA of 3.4 or higher), 1 year of nursing experience (recommended), BSN, minimum GPA of 3.0, previous course work in statistics; for doctorate, GRE General Test (waived if undergraduate GPA of 3.4 or higher), BSN or MSN, minimum GPA of 3.0, portfolio, resume, personal statement, undergraduate statistics course, current licensure as a registered nurse, transcripts from all post-secondary institutions; for Post Master's Certificate, MSN, licensure or eligibility as a professional nurse, transcripts from all post-secondary institutions, previous course work in statistics. Additional exam requirements/recommendations for international students: Required—TOEFL (minimum score 100 iBT), IELTS (minimum score 7). *Application deadline:* For fall admission, 12/1 for domestic and international students; for spring admission, 5/1 for domestic and international students. Application fee: $50. Electronic applications accepted. *Expenses:* Contact institution. *Financial support:* Career-related internships or fieldwork, institutionally sponsored loans, scholarships/grants, traineeships, and tuition waivers (partial) available. Support available to part-time students. Financial award applicants required to submit FAFSA. *Faculty research:* Cardiovascular disease, caregiver skill training, data mining, prostate cancer, neonatal immune system. *Unit head:* Dr. Marion E. Broome, Dean/Vice Chancellor for Nursing Affairs/Associate Vice President for Academic Affairs for Nursing, 919-684-9446, Fax: 919-684-9414, E-mail: marion.broome@duke.edu. *Application contact:* Dr. Ernie Rushing, Director of Admissions and Recruitment, 919-668-6274, Fax: 919-668-4693,

E-mail: ernie.rushing@dm.duke.edu.
Website: http://www.nursing.duke.edu/

Hardin-Simmons University, Graduate School, Patty Hanks Shelton School of Nursing, Abilene, TX 79698-0001. Offers advanced healthcare delivery (MSN); family nurse practitioner (MSN). Programs offered jointly with Abilene Christian University and McMurry University. *Accreditation:* AACN. *Program availability:* Part-time. *Faculty:* 5 full-time (all women), 1 (woman) part-time/adjunct. *Students:* 18 part-time (15 women); includes 5 minority (2 Black or African American, non-Hispanic/Latino; 1 American Indian or Alaska Native, non-Hispanic/Latino; 2 Hispanic/Latino). Average age 33. In 2015, 4 master's awarded. *Degree requirements:* For master's, comprehensive exam, thesis or alternative. *Entrance requirements:* For master's, GRE, minimum undergraduate GPA of 3.0 in major, 2.8 overall; interview; upper-level course work in statistics; CPR certification; letters of recommendation. Additional exam requirements/recommendations for international students: Required—TOEFL (minimum score 550 paper-based; 75 iBT). *Application deadline:* For fall admission, 8/15 priority date for domestic students, 4/1 for international students; for spring admission, 1/5 priority date for domestic students, 9/1 for international students. Applications are processed on a rolling basis. Application fee: $50. Electronic applications accepted. *Expenses:* Contact institution. *Financial support:* In 2015–16, 17 students received support. Career-related internships or fieldwork and scholarships/grants available. Support available to part-time students. Financial award application deadline: 6/30; financial award applicants required to submit FAFSA. *Faculty research:* Child abuse, alternative medicine, pediatric chronic disease, health promotion. *Unit head:* Dr. Nina Ouimette, Dean, 325-671-2357, Fax: 325-671-2386, E-mail: nouimette@phssn.edu. *Application contact:* Dr. Nancy Kucinski, Dean of Graduate Studies, 325-670-1298, Fax: 325-670-1564, E-mail: gradoff@hsutx.edu.
Website: http://www.phssn.edu/

Lehman College of the City University of New York, School of Natural and Social Sciences, Department of Nursing, Bronx, NY 10468-1589. Offers adult health nursing (MS); nursing of older adults (MS); parent-child nursing (MS); pediatric nurse practitioner (MS). *Accreditation:* AACN. *Program availability:* Part-time, evening/weekend. *Entrance requirements:* For master's, bachelor's degree in nursing, New York RN license.

Louisiana State University Health Sciences Center, School of Nursing, New Orleans, LA 70112. Offers adult gerontology clinical nurse specialist (Post-Master's Certificate); clinical nurse leader (MSN); executive nurse leader (Post-Master's Certificate); neonatal nurse practitioner (Post-Master's Certificate); nurse anesthesia (Post-Master's Certificate); nurse educator (MSN); nursing (DNS); primary care family nurse practitioner (Post-Master's Certificate); public/community health nursing (Post-Master's Certificate). *Accreditation:* AACN; AANAEP (one or more programs are accredited). *Program availability:* Part-time. *Faculty:* 22 full-time (19 women), 21 part-time/adjunct (8 women). *Students:* 254 (185 women); includes 68 minority (44 Black or African American, non-Hispanic/Latino; 12 Asian, non-Hispanic/Latino; 12 Hispanic/Latino). Average age 33. 144 applicants, 54% accepted, 73 enrolled. In 2015, 84 master's, 6 doctorates awarded. *Degree requirements:* For master's, thesis optional; for doctorate, thesis/dissertation. *Entrance requirements:* For master's, GRE General Test, MAT, minimum GPA of 3.0; for doctorate, GRE General Test, minimum GPA of 3.5. Additional exam requirements/recommendations for international students: Required—TOEFL (minimum score 550 paper-based; 79 iBT). *Application deadline:* Applications are processed on a rolling basis. Application fee: $250. Electronic applications accepted. *Expenses:* $9,136.50 per year; $19,633.50 per year (for DNP). *Financial support:* Federal Work-Study, institutionally sponsored loans, scholarships/grants, and traineeships available. Financial award applicants required to submit FAFSA. *Faculty research:* Advanced clinical practice, nursing education, health, social support, nursing administration. *Unit head:* Dr. Demetrius James Porche, Dean, 504-568-4106, Fax: 504-599-0573, E-mail: dporch@lsuhsc.edu. *Application contact:* Tracie Gravolet, Director, Office of Student Affairs, 504-568-4114, Fax: 504-568-5711, E-mail: tgravo@lsuhsc.edu.
Website: http://nursing.lsuhsc.edu/

Medical University of South Carolina, College of Nursing, Pediatric Nurse Practitioner Program, Charleston, SC 29425. Offers MSN, DNP. *Accreditation:* AACN. *Program availability:* Part-time, online learning. *Degree requirements:* For master's, comprehensive exam (for some programs), thesis optional; for doctorate, final project. *Entrance requirements:* For master's, BSN from nationally-accredited program, minimum nursing and cumulative GPA of 3.0, undergraduate-level statistics course, active RN License, 3 confidential references, current curriculum vitae or resume, essay; for doctorate, BSN from nationally-accredited program, minimum nursing and cumulative GPA of 3.0, undergraduate-level statistics course, active RN License, 3 confidential references, current curriculum vitae or resume, personal essay (for DNP). Additional exam requirements/recommendations for international students: Required—TOEFL (minimum score 550 paper-based; 80 iBT). Electronic applications accepted. *Faculty research:* School based clinics, epilepsy, caregiver burden, ADD/ADHD, developmental disorders.

Northeastern University, Bouvé College of Health Sciences, Boston, MA 02115-5096. Offers applied behavior analysis (MS, CAGS); audiology (Au D); biomedical nanotechnology (MS); college student development and counseling (MS, CAGS); counseling psychology (MS, PhD, CAGS); exercise science (MS); health informatics (MS); medicinal chemistry (MS); nurse anesthesia (DNP, CAGS); nursing (MS, PhD, CAGS), including administration (MS), adult-gerontology acute care nurse practitioner (MS, CAGS), adult-gerontology primary care nurse practitioner (MS, CAGS), anesthesia (MS), family nurse practitioner (MS, CAGS), neonatal nurse practitioner (MS, CAGS), pediatric nurse practitioner (MS, CAGS), psychiatric mental health nurse practitioner (MS, CAGS); nursing practice (DNP); personal health informatics (MS); pharmaceutical sciences (MS, PhD), including interdisciplinary concentration, pharmaceutics and drug delivery systems; pharmacology (MS); pharmacy (Pharm D); physical therapy (Postbaccalaureate Certificate); physician assistant (MS); population health (PhD); school psychology (MS, PhD, CAGS); speech-language pathology (MS); urban health (MPH); MS/MBA. *Accreditation:* ACPE (one or more programs are accredited). *Program availability:* Part-time, evening/weekend, online learning. *Faculty:* 194 full-time (120 women), 169 part-time/adjunct (136 women). *Students:* 1,416 full-time (1,049 women), 310 part-time (248 women). In 2015, 374 master's, 313 doctorates, 37 other advanced degrees awarded. *Degree requirements:* For doctorate, thesis/dissertation (for some programs); for other advanced degree, comprehensive exam. Application fee: $75. Electronic applications accepted. *Expenses:* Contact institution. *Financial support:* Applicants required to submit FAFSA. *Unit head:* John R. Reynolds, Professor and Interim Dean, 617-373-3323, Fax: 617-373-3030. *Application contact:* Molly Schnabel, Senior Director of Graduate Affairs, 617-373-2708, Fax: 617-373-4701, E-mail: bouvegrad@neu.edu.
Website: http://www.northeastern.edu/bouve/

Old Dominion University, College of Health Sciences, School of Nursing, Family Nurse Practitioner Emphasis, Norfolk, VA 23529. Offers adult-gerontology clinical nurse specialist/educator (MSN); neonatal nurse practitioner (MSN); pediatric nurse practitioner (MSN). *Program availability:* Blended/hybrid learning. *Faculty:* 3 full-time (all women), 9 part-time/adjunct (all women). *Students:* 53 full-time (52 women), 5 part-time

(all women); includes 14 minority (9 Black or African American, non-Hispanic/Latino; 2 Asian, non-Hispanic/Latino; 1 Hispanic/Latino; 2 Two or more races, non-Hispanic/Latino). Average age 35. 53 applicants, 66% accepted, 23 enrolled. In 2015, 60 master's awarded. *Degree requirements:* For master's, comprehensive exam. *Entrance requirements:* For master's, GRE or MAT (waived with a GPA above 3.5), 3 letters of recommendation, essay, resume, transcripts. Additional exam requirements/recommendations for international students: Required—TOEFL. *Application deadline:* For fall admission, 3/1 priority date for domestic students, 4/15 priority date for international students. Application fee: $50. Electronic applications accepted. *Expenses:* Tuition, state resident: full-time $11,136; part-time $464 per credit hour. Tuition, nonresident: full-time $27,840; part-time $1160 per credit hour. *Required fees:* $64 per semester. Tuition and fees vary according to campus/location, program and reciprocity agreements. *Financial support:* In 2015–16, research assistantships with partial tuition reimbursements (averaging $10,000 per year) were awarded; career-related internships or fieldwork, scholarships/grants, and traineeships also available. Support available to part-time students. *Faculty research:* Military families, nurse practitioner student reaching modalities, gerontology, pediatrics, ethics. *Unit head:* Dr. Carolyn M. Rutledge, Associate Chair for Graduate Programs, 757-683-5009, Fax: 757-683-5253, E-mail: crutledg@odu.edu. *Application contact:* Sue Parker, Graduate Program Coordinator, 757-683-4298, Fax: 757-683-5253, E-mail: sparker@odu.edu.
Website: http://catalog.odu.edu/graduate/collegeofhealthsciences/schoolofnursing/#masterofscienceinnursing013familynursepractitionerrole

Old Dominion University, College of Health Sciences, School of Nursing, Nurse Educator Emphasis, Norfolk, VA 23529. Offers neonatal nurse practitioner (MSN); pediatric nurse practitioner (MSN). *Program availability:* Part-time, online learning. *Faculty:* 1 (woman) full-time, 2 part-time/adjunct (both women). *Students:* 9 full-time (7 women), 17 part-time (11 women); includes 5 minority (1 Black or African American, non-Hispanic/Latino; 1 American Indian or Alaska Native, non-Hispanic/Latino; 3 Two or more races, non-Hispanic/Latino), 7 international. Average age 36. In 2015, 7 master's awarded. *Degree requirements:* For master's, comprehensive exam, thesis optional. *Entrance requirements:* For master's, GRE or MAT (waived if GPA is above 3.5), 3 letters of recommendation, essay, resume, transcripts. Additional exam requirements/recommendations for international students: Required—TOEFL. *Application deadline:* For fall admission, 4/15 priority date for international students. Application fee: $50. *Expenses:* Tuition, state resident: full-time $11,136; part-time $464 per credit hour. Tuition, nonresident: full-time $27,840; part-time $1160 per credit hour. *Required fees:* $64 per semester. Tuition and fees vary according to campus/location, program and reciprocity agreements. *Financial support:* Fellowships, research assistantships, teaching assistantships, and unspecified assistantships available. *Faculty research:* Technology in nursing education, evidence-based instructional strategies, clinical judgment and decision-making. *Total annual research expenditures:* $35,726. *Unit head:* Dr. Kimberly Adams-Tufts, Graduate Program Director, 757-683-5011, E-mail: ktufts@odu.edu. *Application contact:* Sue Parker, Graduate Program Coordinator, 757-683-4298, Fax: 757-683-5253, E-mail: sparker@odu.edu.

Point Loma Nazarene University, School of Nursing, San Diego, CA 92106-2899. Offers adult/gerontology nursing (MSN); family/individual health (MSN); general nursing (MSN); nursing (Post-MSN Certificate); pediatric nursing (MSN); psychiatric mental health (MSN). *Accreditation:* AACN. *Program availability:* Part-time. *Faculty:* 6 full-time (5 women), 2 part-time/adjunct (both women). *Students:* 1 (woman) full-time, 74 part-time (61 women); includes 35 minority (4 Black or African American, non-Hispanic/Latino; 15 Asian, non-Hispanic/Latino; 10 Hispanic/Latino; 3 Native Hawaiian or other Pacific Islander, non-Hispanic/Latino; 3 Two or more races, non-Hispanic/Latino), 2 international. Average age 38. 34 applicants, 88% accepted, 18 enrolled. In 2015, 40 master's awarded. *Entrance requirements:* For master's, NCLEX, ADN or BSN in nursing, interview, RN license, essay, letters of recommendation, interview. *Application deadline:* For fall admission, 7/5 priority date for domestic students; for spring admission, 11/1 priority date for domestic students; for summer admission, 3/22 priority date for domestic students. Applications are processed on a rolling basis. Application fee: $50. *Financial support:* Applicants required to submit FAFSA. *Unit head:* Dr. Barb Taylor, Dean of the School of Nursing, 619-849-2766, E-mail: bataylor@pointloma.edu. *Application contact:* Claire Buckley, Director of Graduate Admissions, 619-563-2846, E-mail: clairebuckley@pointloma.edu.
Website: http://www.pointloma.edu/discover/graduate-school/graduate-programs/master-science-nursing-and-post-msn-certificate

Regis University, Rueckert-Hartman College for Health Professions, Denver, CO 80221-1099. Offers addictions counseling (Post-Graduate Certificate); advanced practice nurse specialization (DNP); counseling (MA); counseling children and adolescents (Post-Graduate Certificate); counseling military families (Post-Graduate Certificate); depth psychotherapy (Post-Graduate Certificate); family nurse practitioner (MSN); health care business management (Certificate); health care quality and patient safety (Certificate); health industry leadership (MBA); health professions (Postbaccalaureate Certificate); health services administration (MS); marriage and family therapy (MA); neonatal nurse practitioner (MSN); nursing education or leadership (MSN); orthopedic manual physical therapy fellowship (Certificate); pharmacy (Pharm D); physical therapy (DPT). *Program availability:* Part-time, evening/weekend, 100% online, blended/hybrid learning. *Faculty:* 40 full-time (29 women), 116 part-time/adjunct (86 women). *Students:* 1,080 full-time (771 women), 274 part-time (239 women); includes 388 minority (59 Black or African American, non-Hispanic/Latino; 6 American Indian or Alaska Native, non-Hispanic/Latino; 109 Asian, non-Hispanic/Latino; 163 Hispanic/Latino; 1 Native Hawaiian or other Pacific Islander, non-Hispanic/Latino; 50 Two or more races, non-Hispanic/Latino), 7 international. Average age 34. 2,188 applicants, 31% accepted, 303 enrolled. In 2015, 329 master's, 160 doctorates awarded. *Degree requirements:* For master's, thesis (for some programs), internship. *Entrance requirements:* For master's, official transcript reflecting baccalaureate degree awarded from regionally-accredited college or university. Additional exam requirements/recommendations for international students: Required—TOEFL (minimum score 550 paper-based; 82 iBT). *Application deadline:* For fall admission, 8/15 priority date for domestic students; for spring admission, 1/10 priority date for domestic students; for summer admission, 5/1 priority date for domestic students. Applications are processed on a rolling basis. Application fee: $75. Electronic applications accepted. *Expenses:* Contact institution. *Financial support:* In 2015–16, 102 students received support. Federal Work-Study and scholarships/grants available. Financial award application deadline: 4/15; financial award applicants required to submit FAFSA. *Faculty research:* Normal and pathological balance and gait research, normal/pathological upper limb motor control/biomechanics, exercise energy/metabolism research, optical treatment protocols for therapeutic modalities. *Unit head:* Dr. Janet Houser, Academic Dean. *Application contact:* Cate Clark, Director of Admissions, 303-458-4900, Fax: 303-964-5534, E-mail: ruadmissions@regis.edu.
Website: http://www.regis.edu/RHCHP.aspx

Rush University, College of Nursing, Department of Women, Children, and Family Nursing, Chicago, IL 60612. Offers neonatal clinical nurse specialist (DNP); neonatal nurse practitioner (DNP, Post-Graduate Certificate); nursing science (PhD); pediatric acute care nurse practitioner (DNP, Post-Graduate Certificate); pediatric clinical nurse specialist (DNP); pediatric primary care nurse practitioner (DNP); pediatric primary nurse practitioner (Post-Graduate Certificate); systems leadership (DNP). *Accreditation:* AACN. *Program availability:* Part-time, online learning. *Faculty:* 43 full-time (40 women), 52 part-time/adjunct (49 women). *Students:* 11 full-time (all women), 143 part-time (140 women); includes 20 minority (3 Black or African American, non-Hispanic/Latino; 1 American Indian or Alaska Native, non-Hispanic/Latino; 7 Asian, non-Hispanic/Latino; 9 Hispanic/Latino). Average age 32. 58 applicants, 91% accepted, 40 enrolled. In 2015, 19 doctorates awarded. *Degree requirements:* For doctorate, leadership project (for DNP); dissertation (for PhD). *Entrance requirements:* For doctorate, GRE General Test (waived for DNP if cumulative GPA is 3.25 or greater, nursing GPA is 3.0 or greater, or a completed graduate program GPA is 3.5 or greater), interview, 3 letters of recommendation, personal statement, current resume; for Post-Graduate Certificate, MSN in a clinical discipline, 3 letters of recommendation, personal statement, current resume, interview. Additional exam requirements/recommendations for international students: Required—TOEFL (minimum score 94 iBT). *Application deadline:* For fall admission, 1/2 for domestic students; for winter admission, 10/15 for domestic students; for spring admission, 8/3 for domestic students; for summer admission, 12/1 for domestic students. Applications are processed on a rolling basis. Application fee: $100. Electronic applications accepted. *Expenses:* Contact institution. *Financial support:* Research assistantships, teaching assistantships with tuition reimbursements, Federal Work-Study, scholarships/grants, traineeships, and health care benefits available. Support available to part-time students. Financial award application deadline: 3/1; financial award applicants required to submit FAFSA. *Faculty research:* Reduction of health disparities; benefit of human milk feedings for low birth weight infants; decision-making when living with a BRCA mutation over 5-8 year time period; accelerating adoption of comparative effectiveness research in premature infants. *Unit head:* Dr. Wrenetha Julion, Chairperson, 312-942-7117, E-mail: wrenetha_a_julion@rush.edu. *Application contact:* Jennifer Thorndyke, Admissions Specialist, 312-563-7526, E-mail: jennifer_thorndyke@rush.edu.
Website: http://www.rushu.rush.edu/servlet/Satellite?c=content_block&cid=1320160764996&pagename=CollegeOfNursing%2Fcontent_block%2FContentBlockDetail&rendermod

St. Catherine University, Graduate Programs, Program in Nursing, St. Paul, MN 55105. Offers adult gerontological nurse practitioner (MS); neonatal nurse practitioner (MS); nurse educator (MS); nursing (DNP); nursing: entry-level (MS); pediatric nurse practitioner (MS). *Accreditation:* ACEN. *Program availability:* Part-time, evening/weekend. *Degree requirements:* For master's, thesis; for doctorate, portfolio, systems change project. *Entrance requirements:* For master's, GRE General Test, bachelor's degree in nursing, current nursing license, 2 years of recent clinical practice; for doctorate, master's degree in nursing, RN license, advanced nursing position. Additional exam requirements/recommendations for international students: Required—TOEFL (minimum score 600 paper-based; 100 iBT). *Expenses:* Contact institution.

Saint Francis Medical Center College of Nursing, Graduate Programs, Peoria, IL 61603-3783. Offers adult gerontology (MSN); clinical nurse leader (MSN); family nurse practitioner (MSN); family psychiatric mental health nurse practitioner (MSN); neonatal nurse practitioner (MSN); nurse clinician (Post-Graduate Certificate); nurse educator (MSN, Post-Graduate Certificate); nursing (DNP); nursing management leadership (MSN). *Accreditation:* ACEN. *Program availability:* Part-time, 100% online, blended/hybrid learning. *Faculty:* 14 full-time (all women), 5 part-time/adjunct (all women). *Students:* 13 full-time (12 women), 257 part-time (228 women); includes 23 minority (14 Black or African American, non-Hispanic/Latino; 3 Asian, non-Hispanic/Latino; 4 Hispanic/Latino; 2 Two or more races, non-Hispanic/Latino). Average age 37. 86 applicants, 86% accepted, 44 enrolled. In 2015, 61 master's, 6 doctorates awarded. *Degree requirements:* For master's, research experience, portfolio, practicum; for doctorate, practicum hours. *Entrance requirements:* For master's, nursing research, health assessment, graduate course work in statistics, RN license; for doctorate, master's degree in nursing, professional portfolio, graduate statistics, transcripts, RN license. Additional exam requirements/recommendations for international students: Required—TOEFL (minimum score 550 paper-based; 79 iBT). *Application deadline:* For fall admission, 6/1 priority date for domestic and international students; for spring admission, 11/15 priority date for domestic and international students. Applications are processed on a rolling basis. Application fee: $50. *Financial support:* In 2015–16, 18 students received support. Scholarships/grants and tuition waivers (partial) available. Support available to part-time students. Financial award application deadline: 6/15; financial award applicants required to submit FAFSA. *Faculty research:* Outcome and curriculum planning, health promotion, NCLEX-RN results, decision-making program evaluation. *Unit head:* Dr. Patti A. Stockert, President of the College, 309-655-4124, Fax: 309-624-8973, E-mail: patricia.a.stockert@osfhealthcare.org. *Application contact:* Dr. Kim A. Mitchell, Dean, Graduate Program, 309-655-2201, Fax: 309-624-8973, E-mail: kim.a.mitchell@osfhealthcare.org.
Website: http://www.sfmccon.edu/graduate-programs/

Stony Brook University, State University of New York, Stony Brook Medicine, School of Nursing, Program in Neonatal Nursing, Stony Brook, NY 11794. Offers neonatal nurse practitioner (Certificate); neonatal nursing (MS, DNP). *Accreditation:* AACN. *Program availability:* Part-time, blended/hybrid learning. *Students:* 8 full-time (all women), 45 part-time (44 women); includes 17 minority (3 Black or African American, non-Hispanic/Latino; 11 Asian, non-Hispanic/Latino; 2 Hispanic/Latino; 1 Two or more races, non-Hispanic/Latino), 2 international. 31 applicants, 77% accepted, 21 enrolled. In 2015, 17 master's, 3 other advanced degrees awarded. *Degree requirements:* For master's, thesis. *Entrance requirements:* For master's, BSN, minimum GPA of 3.0, course work in statistics. Additional exam requirements/recommendations for international students: Required—TOEFL (minimum score 90 iBT). *Application deadline:* For fall admission, 12/1 for domestic students. Application fee: $100. *Expenses:* $24,781 full-time resident tuition and fees, $968 per credit hour; $44,431 full-time nonresident tuition and fees, $1,787 per credit hour. *Financial support:* Application deadline: 3/15. *Unit head:* Dr. Paula M. Timoney, Program Director, 631-444-3298, Fax: 631-444-3136, E-mail: paula.timoney@stonybrook.edu. *Application contact:* Crystal Garcia, Staff Assistant, 631-632-3392, Fax: 631-444-3136, E-mail: crystal.garcia@stonybrook.edu.
Website: http://www.nursing.stonybrookmedicine.edu/

Stony Brook University, State University of New York, Stony Brook Medicine, School of Nursing, Program in Perinatal Women's Health Nursing, Stony Brook, NY 11794. Offers MS, DNP, Certificate. *Accreditation:* AACN. *Program availability:* Blended/hybrid learning. *Students:* 1 (woman) full-time, 21 part-time (all women); includes 4 minority (1 Black or African American, non-Hispanic/Latino; 1 American Indian or Alaska Native, non-Hispanic/Latino; 1 Asian, non-Hispanic/Latino; 1 Hispanic/Latino). In 2015, 11 master's awarded. *Degree requirements:* For master's, thesis. *Entrance requirements:* For master's, BSN, minimum GPA of 3.0, course work in statistics. Additional exam requirements/recommendations for international students: Required—TOEFL (minimum score 90 iBT). *Application deadline:* For fall admission, 12/1 for domestic students. Application fee: $100. *Expenses:* $24,781 full-time resident tuition and fees, $968 per credit hour; $44,431 full-time nonresident tuition and fees, $1,787 per credit hour. *Financial support:* Application deadline: 3/15. *Unit head:* Prof. Elizabeth Collins, Director, 631-444-3296, Fax: 631-444-3136, E-mail: elizabeth.collins@stonybrook.edu. *Application contact:* Crystal Garcia, Staff Assistant, 631-632-3392, Fax: 631-632-3136,

E-mail: crystal.garcia@stonybrook.edu.
Website: http://www.nursing.stonybrookmedicine.edu/

University of Alberta, Faculty of Medicine and Dentistry and Faculty of Graduate Studies and Research, Graduate Programs in Medicine, Department of Obstetrics and Gynecology, Edmonton, AB T6G 2E1, Canada. Offers MD. *Entrance requirements:* Additional exam requirements/recommendations for international students: Required—TOEFL. *Faculty research:* Parturition, fetal/neonatal lung development, nitric oxide, vascular reactivity, pre-eclampsia gestational diabetes.

University of Cincinnati, Graduate School, College of Nursing, Cincinnati, OH 45221-0038. Offers clinical nurse specialist (MSN), including adult health, community health, neonatal, nursing administration, occupational health, pediatric health, psychiatric nursing, women's health; nurse anesthesia (MSN); nurse midwifery (MSN); nurse practitioner (MSN), including acute care, ambulatory care, family, family/psychiatric, women's health; nursing (PhD); MBA/MSN. *Accreditation:* AACN; AANA/CANAEP (one or more programs are accredited); ACNM/ACME. *Program availability:* Part-time, online learning. Terminal master's awarded for partial completion of doctoral program. *Degree requirements:* For master's, thesis or alternative; for doctorate, comprehensive exam, thesis/dissertation. *Entrance requirements:* For master's and doctorate, GRE General Test. Additional exam requirements/recommendations for international students: Required—TOEFL (minimum score 520 paper-based). Electronic applications accepted. *Faculty research:* Substance abuse, injury and violence, symptom management.

University of Delaware, College of Health Sciences, School of Nursing, Newark, DE 19716. Offers adult nurse practitioner (MSN, PMC); cardiopulmonary clinical nurse specialist (MSN, PMC); cardiopulmonary clinical nurse specialist/adult nurse practitioner (MSN, PMC); family nurse practitioner (MSN, PMC); gerontology clinical nurse specialist (MSN, PMC); gerontology clinical nurse specialist geriatric nurse practitioner (PMC); gerontology clinical nurse specialist/geriatric nurse practitioner (MSN); health services administration (MSN, PMC); nursing of children clinical nurse specialist (MSN, PMC); nursing of children clinical nurse specialist/pediatric nurse practitioner (MSN, PMC); oncology/immune deficiency clinical nurse specialist (MSN, PMC); oncology/immune deficiency clinical nurse specialist/adult nurse practitioner (MSN, PMC); perinatal/women's health clinical nurse specialist (MSN, PMC); perinatal/women's health clinical nurse specialist/women's health nurse practitioner (MSN, PMC); psychiatric nursing clinical nurse specialist (MSN, PMC). *Accreditation:* AACN. *Program availability:* Part-time, evening/weekend, online learning. *Degree requirements:* For master's, thesis optional. *Entrance requirements:* For master's, BSN, interview, RN license. Electronic applications accepted. *Faculty research:* Marriage and chronic illness, health promotion, congestive heart failure patient outcomes, school nursing, diabetes in children, culture, health disparities, cardiovascular, prison nursing, oncology, public policy, child obesity, smoking and teen pregnancy, blood pressure measurements, men's health.

University of Illinois at Chicago, College of Nursing, Program in Nursing, Chicago, IL 60607-7128. Offers acute care clinical nurse specialist (MS); administrative nursing leadership (Certificate); adult nurse practitioner (MS); adult/geriatric nurse practitioner (MS); advanced community health nurse specialist (MS); family nurse practitioner (MS); geriatric clinical nurse specialist (MS); geriatric nurse practitioner (MS); nurse midwifery (MS); occupational health/advanced community health nurse specialist (MS); occupational health/family nurse practitioner (MS); pediatric nurse practitioner (MS); perinatal clinical nurse specialist (MS); school/advanced community health nurse specialist (MS); school/family nurse practitioner (MS); women's health nurse practitioner (MS). *Accreditation:* AACN. *Program availability:* Part-time. *Faculty:* 100 full-time (93 women), 89 part-time/adjunct (82 women). *Students:* 359 full-time (326 women), 280 part-time (249 women); includes 169 minority (43 Black or African American, non-Hispanic/Latino; 62 Asian, non-Hispanic/Latino; 56 Hispanic/Latino; 1 Native Hawaiian or other Pacific Islander, non-Hispanic/Latino; 7 Two or more races, non-Hispanic/Latino), 12 international. Average age 32. In 2015, 4 other advanced degrees awarded. *Degree requirements:* For master's, thesis or alternative. *Entrance requirements:* For master's, GRE General Test, minimum GPA of 2.75. Additional exam requirements/recommendations for international students: Required—TOEFL. *Application deadline:* For fall admission, 5/15 for domestic students, 2/15 for international students; for spring admission, 11/1 for domestic students, 7/15 for international students. Applications are processed on a rolling basis. Application fee: $60. Electronic applications accepted. *Expenses:* Tuition, state resident: full-time $11,480; part-time $3826 per credit. Tuition, nonresident: full-time $23,720; part-time $7906 per credit. *Required fees:* $1333 per semester. Part-time tuition and fees vary according to course load and program. *Financial support:* Fellowships with full tuition reimbursements, research assistantships with full tuition reimbursements, teaching assistantships with full tuition reimbursements, career-related internships or fieldwork, Federal Work-Study, institutionally sponsored loans, scholarships/grants, traineeships, tuition waivers (full and partial), and unspecified assistantships available. Support available to part-time students. Financial award application deadline: 3/1; financial award applicants required to submit FAFSA. *Unit head:* Dr. Terri E. Weaver, Dean, 312-996-7808, E-mail: teweaver@uic.edu. *Application contact:* Receptionist, 312-413-2550, E-mail: gradcoll@uic.edu. Website: http://www.nursing.uic.edu/academics-admissions/master-science#program-overview

University of Indianapolis, Graduate Programs, School of Nursing, Indianapolis, IN 46227-3697. Offers advanced practice nursing (DNP); family nurse practitioner (MSN); gerontological nurse practitioner (MSN); neonatal nurse practitioner (MSN); nurse-midwifery (MSN); nursing (MSN); nursing and health systems leadership (MSN); nursing education (MSN); women's health nurse practitioner (MSN); MBA/MSN. *Accreditation:* AACN; ACNM. *Entrance requirements:* For master's, minimum GPA of 3.0, interview, letters of recommendation, resume, IN nursing license, 1 year of professional practice; for doctorate, graduate of NLNAC- or CCNE-accredited nursing program; MSN or MA with nursing major and minimum cumulative GPA of 3.25; unencumbered RN license with eligibility for licensure in Indiana; completion of graduate-level statistics course within last 5 years with minimum grade of B; resume; essay; official transcripts from all academic institutions. Additional exam requirements/recommendations for international students: Required—TOEFL (minimum score 550 paper-based). Electronic applications accepted.

University of Louisville, Graduate School, School of Nursing, Louisville, KY 40202. Offers adult gerontology nurse practitioner (MSN, DNP); education and administration (MSN); family nurse practitioner (MSN, DNP); neonatal nurse practitioner (MSN, DNP); nursing research (PhD); psychiatric/mental health nurse practitioner (MSN, DNP); women's health nurse practitioner (MSN). *Accreditation:* AACN. *Program availability:* Part-time. *Faculty:* 53 full-time (48 women), 27 part-time/adjunct (23 women). *Students:* 110 full-time (99 women), 33 part-time (29 women); includes 17 minority (11 Black or African American, non-Hispanic/Latino; 1 Asian, non-Hispanic/Latino; 2 Hispanic/Latino; 3 Two or more races, non-Hispanic/Latino), 5 international. Average age 34. 62 applicants, 68% accepted, 40 enrolled. In 2015, 41 master's awarded. *Degree requirements:* For doctorate, comprehensive exam (for some programs), thesis/dissertation (for some programs). *Entrance requirements:* For master's, bachelor's degree in nursing, minimum GPA of 3.0, RN license; for doctorate, GRE General Test (for PhD), 3 letters of professional reference. Additional exam requirements/recommendations for international students: Required—TOEFL (minimum score 560

paper-based; 79 iBT). *Application deadline:* For fall admission, 3/1 priority date for domestic students, 3/1 for international students. Applications are processed on a rolling basis. Application fee: $60. Electronic applications accepted. *Expenses:* Tuition, state resident: full-time $11,664; part-time $649 per credit hour. Tuition, nonresident: full-time $24,274; part-time $1350 per credit hour. *Required fees:* $196. Tuition and fees vary according to program and reciprocity agreements. *Financial support:* In 2015–16, 722,568 students received support, including 10 research assistantships with full tuition reimbursements available (averaging $20,000 per year), 2 teaching assistantships with full tuition reimbursements available (averaging $15,000 per year); fellowships with full tuition reimbursements available, scholarships/grants, and unspecified assistantships also available. Financial award application deadline: 2/15; financial award applicants required to submit FAFSA. *Faculty research:* Children and adolescents with chronic illnesses, women's mental health and parenting, asthma and environmental health, type 2 diabetes self-management in adults, health disparities and community engagement. *Total annual research expenditures:* $722,568. *Unit head:* Dr. Marcia J. Hern, Dean, 502-852-8300, Fax: 502-852-8783, E-mail: m.hern@louisville.edu. *Application contact:* Trish Hart, Assistant Dean for Student Affairs, 502-852-5825, Fax: 502-852-8783, E-mail: trish.hart@louisville.edu.
Website: http://www.louisville.edu/nursing/

University of Maryland, Baltimore, Graduate School, School of Nursing, Master's Program in Nursing, Baltimore, MD 21201. Offers community health nursing (MS); gerontological nursing (MS); maternal-child nursing (MS); medical-surgical nursing (MS); nurse-midwifery education (MS); nursing administration (MS); nursing education (MS); nursing health policy (MS); primary care nursing (MS); psychiatric nursing (MS); MS/MBA. MS/MBA offered jointly with University of Baltimore. *Accreditation:* AACN; AANA/CANAEP. *Program availability:* Part-time. *Degree requirements:* For master's, comprehensive exam (for some programs), thesis or alternative. *Entrance requirements:* For master's, minimum GPA of 2.75, course work in statistics, BS in nursing. Additional exam requirements/recommendations for international students: Required—TOEFL (minimum score 550 paper-based; 80 iBT); Recommended—IELTS (minimum score 7). Electronic applications accepted. Tuition and fees vary according to program.

University of Missouri–Kansas City, School of Nursing and Health Studies, Kansas City, MO 64108. Offers adult clinical nurse specialist (MSN), including adult nurse practitioner, women's health nurse practitioner (MSN, DNP); adult clinical nursing practice (DNP), including adult gerontology nurse practitioner, women's health nurse practitioner (MSN, DNP); clinical nursing practice (DNP), including family nurse practitioner; family nurse practitioner (MSN); neonatal nurse practitioner (MSN); nurse educator (MSN); nurse executive (MSN); nursing (PhD); nursing practice (DNP); pediatric clinical nursing practice (DNP), including pediatric nurse practitioner; pediatric nurse practitioner (MSN). *Accreditation:* AACN. *Program availability:* Part-time, online learning. *Faculty:* 44 full-time (40 women), 47 part-time/adjunct (45 women). *Students:* 62 full-time (43 women), 259 part-time (239 women); includes 61 minority (28 Black or African American, non-Hispanic/Latino; 3 American Indian or Alaska Native, non-Hispanic/Latino; 16 Asian, non-Hispanic/Latino; 10 Hispanic/Latino; 4 Two or more races, non-Hispanic/Latino). Average age 35. 102 applicants, 35% accepted, 36 enrolled. In 2015, 116 master's, 23 doctorates awarded. *Degree requirements:* For master's, thesis or alternative. *Entrance requirements:* For master's, minimum undergraduate GPA of 3.2; for doctorate, GRE, 3 letters of reference. Additional exam requirements/recommendations for international students: Required—TOEFL (minimum score 550 paper-based; 80 iBT). *Application deadline:* For fall admission, 2/1 priority date for domestic and international students; for spring admission, 9/1 priority date for domestic and international students. Application fee: $45 ($50 for international students). *Financial support:* In 2015–16, 2 teaching assistantships with partial tuition reimbursements (averaging $6,650 per year) were awarded; fellowships, research assistantships, career-related internships or fieldwork, Federal Work-Study, institutionally sponsored loans, and tuition waivers (full and partial) also available. Support available to part-time students. Financial award application deadline: 3/1; financial award applicants required to submit FAFSA. *Faculty research:* Geriatrics/gerontology, children's pain, neonatology, Alzheimer's care, cancer caregivers. *Unit head:* Dr. Ann Cary, Dean, 816-235-1723, Fax: 816-235-1701, E-mail: caryah@umkc.edu. *Application contact:* Judy Jellison, Coordinator for Admissions and Recruitment, 816-235-1740, Fax: 816-235-1701, E-mail: jellisonj@umkc.edu.
Website: http://nursing.umkc.edu/

University of Pennsylvania, School of Nursing, Neonatal Clinical Nurse Specialist Program, Philadelphia, PA 19104. Offers MSN. *Program availability:* Part-time. *Students:* 2 full-time (both women). Average age 34. 3 applicants. In 2015, 3 master's awarded. *Expenses: Tuition, area resident:* Full-time $31,068; part-time $5762 per course. *Required fees:* $3200; $336 per course. Full-time tuition and fees vary according to degree level, program and student level. Part-time tuition and fees vary according to course load, degree level and program.

University of Pennsylvania, School of Nursing, Neonatal Nurse Practitioner Program, Philadelphia, PA 19104. Offers MSN. *Accreditation:* AACN. *Program availability:* Part-time. *Students:* 2 full-time (both women), 6 part-time (all women); includes 2 minority (both Asian, non-Hispanic/Latino). Average age 26. 9 applicants, 56% accepted, 5 enrolled. In 2015, 7 master's awarded. *Expenses: Tuition, area resident:* Full-time $31,068; part-time $5762 per course. *Required fees:* $3200; $336 per course. Full-time tuition and fees vary according to degree level, program and student level. Part-time tuition and fees vary according to course load, degree level and program.

University of Pittsburgh, School of Nursing, Nurse Practitioner Program, Pittsburgh, PA 15261. Offers adult-gerontology acute care (DNP); adult-gerontology primary care (DNP); family (individual across the lifespan) (DNP); neonatal (MSN, DNP); pediatric primary care (DNP); psychiatric mental health (DNP). *Accreditation:* AACN. *Program availability:* Part-time. *Students:* 74 full-time (65 women), 59 part-time (51 women); includes 14 minority (5 Black or African American, non-Hispanic/Latino; 2 American Indian or Alaska Native, non-Hispanic/Latino; 6 Asian, non-Hispanic/Latino; 1 Hispanic/Latino). Average age 30. 65 applicants, 55% accepted, 28 enrolled. In 2015, 14 master's, 19 doctorates awarded. *Degree requirements:* For master's, comprehensive exam, thesis optional. *Entrance requirements:* For master's, GRE General Test or MAT, BSN, RN license, letters of recommendation, resume, course work in statistics, 1-3 years of nursing experience; for doctorate, GRE General Test, BSN, RN license, minimum GPA of 3.5, 3 letters of recommendation. Additional exam requirements/recommendations for international students: Required—TOEFL (minimum score 600 paper-based; 100 iBT). *Application deadline:* For fall admission, 5/1 priority date for domestic students, 2/15 priority date for international students. Application fee: $50. Electronic applications accepted. *Expenses:* Contact institution. *Financial support:* In 2015–16, 16 students received support, including 7 fellowships with tuition reimbursements available (averaging $11,278 per year), 9 teaching assistantships with tuition reimbursements available (averaging $10,879 per year); scholarships/grants, traineeships, health care benefits, and unspecified assistantships also available. Support available to part-time students. Financial award application deadline: 3/15. *Faculty research:* Behavioral management of chronic disorders, patient management in critical care, consumer informatics, genetic applications (molecular genetics and psychosocial implications), technology for nurses and patients to improve care. *Unit*

Maternal and Child/Neonatal Nursing

head: Dr. Sandra Engberg, Associate Dean for Clinical Education, 412-624-3835, Fax: 412-624-8521, E-mail: sje1@pitt.edu. *Application contact:* Laurie Lapsley, Administrator of Graduate Student Services, 412-624-9670, Fax: 412-624-2409, E-mail: lapsleyl@pitt.edu.
Website: http://www.nursing.pitt.edu

University of Puerto Rico, Medical Sciences Campus, School of Nursing, San Juan, PR 00936-5067. Offers adult and elderly nursing (MSN); child and adolescent nursing (MSN); critical care nursing (MSN); family and community nursing (MSN); family nurse practitioner (MSN); maternity nursing (MSN); mental health and psychiatric nursing (MSN). *Accreditation:* AACN. *Entrance requirements:* For master's, GRE or EXADEP, interview, Puerto Rico RN license or professional license for international students, general and specific point average, article analysis. Electronic applications accepted. *Faculty research:* HIV, health disparities, teen violence, women and violence, neurological disorders.

University of Rochester, School of Nursing, Rochester, NY 14642. Offers adult gerontological acute care nurse practitioner (MS); clinical nurse leader (MS); family nurse practitioner (MS); family psychiatric mental health nurse practitioner (MS); health care organization management and leadership (MS); health practice research (PhD); nursing (DNP); nursing education (MS); pediatric nurse practitioner (MS); pediatric nurse practitioner/neonatal nurse practitioner (MS). *Accreditation:* AACN. *Program availability:* Part-time, online learning. *Faculty:* 56 full-time (45 women), 63 part-time/adjunct (55 women). *Students:* 21 full-time (20 women), 212 part-time (175 women); includes 35 minority (12 Black or African American, non-Hispanic/Latino; 1 American Indian or Alaska Native, non-Hispanic/Latino; 10 Asian, non-Hispanic/Latino; 7 Hispanic/Latino; 5 Two or more races, non-Hispanic/Latino), 2 international. Average age 35. 111 applicants, 68% accepted, 71 enrolled. In 2015, 52 master's, 9 doctorates awarded. Terminal master's awarded for partial completion of doctoral program. *Degree requirements:* For master's, comprehensive exam (for some programs); for doctorate, thesis/dissertation. *Entrance requirements:* For master's, BS in nursing, minimum GPA of 3.0, course work in statistics; for doctorate, GRE General Test (for PhD), MS in nursing, minimum GPA of 3.5. Additional exam requirements/recommendations for international students: Required—TOEFL (minimum score 560 paper-based; 88 iBT) or IELTS (minimum score 6.5) recommended. *Application deadline:* For fall admission, 4/1 for domestic and international students; for spring admission, 9/1 for domestic and international students; for summer admission, 1/2 for domestic and international students. Application fee: $50. Electronic applications accepted. *Expenses: Tuition, area resident:* Full-time $47,450; part-time $1482 per credit hour. *Required fees:* $528. Tuition and fees vary according to program. *Financial support:* In 2015–16, 52 students received support, including 2 fellowships with tuition reimbursements available (averaging $30,000 per year); scholarships/grants, traineeships, health care benefits, tuition waivers (full and partial), and unspecified assistantships also available. Support available to part-time students. Financial award application deadline: 6/30. *Faculty research:* Symptom assessment and self-management of chronic illness, health promotion and illness prevention, nursing intervention research with vulnerable populations, palliative care, aging. *Total annual research expenditures:* $2.1 million. *Unit head:* Dr. Kathy H. Rideout, Dean, 585-273-8902, Fax: 585-273-1268, E-mail: kathy_rideout@urmc.rochester.edu. *Application contact:* Elaine Andolina, Director of Admissions, 585-275-2375, Fax: 585-756-8299, E-mail: elaine_andolina@urmc.rochester.edu.
Website: http://www.son.rochester.edu

University of South Africa, College of Human Sciences, Pretoria, South Africa. Offers adult education (M Ed); African languages (MA, PhD); African politics (MA, PhD); Afrikaans (MA, PhD); ancient history (MA, PhD); ancient Near Eastern studies (MA, PhD); anthropology (MA, PhD); applied linguistics (MA); Arabic (MA, PhD); archaeology (MA); art history (MA); Biblical archaeology (MA); Biblical studies (M Th, D Th, PhD); Christian spirituality (M Th, D Th); church history (M Th, D Th); classical studies (MA, PhD); clinical psychology (MA); communication (MA, PhD); comparative education (M Ed, Ed D); consulting psychology (D Admin, D Com, PhD); curriculum studies (M Ed, Ed D); development studies (M Admin, MA, D Admin, PhD); didactics (M Ed, Ed D); education (M Tech); education management (M Ed, Ed D); educational psychology (M Ed); English (MA); environmental education (M Ed); French (MA, PhD); German (MA, PhD); Greek (MA); guidance and counseling (M Ed); health studies (MA, PhD), including health sciences education (MA), health services management (MA), medical and surgical nursing science (critical care general) (MA), midwifery and neonatal nursing science (MA), trauma and emergency care (MA); history (MA, PhD); history of education (Ed D); inclusive education (M Ed, Ed D); information and communications technology policy and regulation (MA); information science (MA, MIS, PhD); international politics (MA, PhD); Islamic studies (MA, PhD); Italian (MA, PhD); Judaica (MA, PhD); linguistics (MA, PhD); mathematical education (M Ed); mathematics education (MA); missiology (M Th, D Th); modern Hebrew (MA, PhD); musicology (MA, MMus, D Mus, PhD); natural science education (M Ed); New Testament (M Th, D Th); Old Testament (D Th); pastoral therapy (M Th, D Th); philosophy (MA); philosophy of education (M Ed, Ed D); politics (MA, PhD); Portuguese (MA, PhD); practical theology (M Th, D Th); psychology (MA, MS, PhD); psychology of education (M Ed, Ed D); public health (MA); religious studies (MA, D Th, PhD); Romance languages (MA); Russian (MA, PhD); Semitic languages (MA, PhD); social behavior studies in HIV/AIDS (MA); social science (mental health) (MA); social science in development studies (MA); social science in psychology (MA); social science in social work (MA); social science in sociology (MA); social work (MSW, DSW, PhD); socio-education (M Ed, Ed D); sociolinguistics (MA); sociology (MA, PhD); Spanish (MA, PhD); systematic theology (M Th, D Th); TESOL (teaching English to speakers of other languages) (MA); theological ethics (M Th, D Th); theory of literature (MA, PhD); urban ministries (D Th); urban ministry (M Th).

University of Southern Mississippi, Graduate School, College of Nursing, Hattiesburg, MS 39406-0001. Offers family nurse practitioner (MSN, Graduate Certificate); family psychiatric-mental health nurse practitioner (Graduate Certificate); nursing (DNP, PhD); psychiatric-mental health nurse practitioner (Graduate Certificate). *Accreditation:* AACN. *Program availability:* Part-time, evening/weekend. *Degree requirements:* For master's, comprehensive exam, thesis optional; for doctorate, comprehensive exam, thesis/dissertation. *Entrance requirements:* For master's, GRE General Test, minimum GPA of 2.75 during last 60 hours, nursing license, BS in nursing; for doctorate, GRE General Test, master's degree in nursing, minimum GPA of 3.5. Additional exam requirements/recommendations for international students. Required—TOEFL, IELTS. Electronic applications accepted. *Faculty research:* Gerontology, caregivers, HIV, bereavement, pain, nursing leadership.

The University of Texas at Austin, Graduate School, School of Nursing, Austin, TX 78712-1111. Offers adult - gerontology clinical nurse specialist (MSN); child health (MSN), including administration, public health nursing, teaching; family nurse practitioner (MSN); family psychiatric/mental health nurse practitioner (MSN); holistic adult health (MSN), including administration, teaching; maternity (MSN), including administration, public health nursing, teaching; nursing (PhD); nursing administration and healthcare systems management (MSN); nursing practice (DNP); pediatric nurse

practitioner (MSN); public health nursing (MSN). *Accreditation:* AACN. *Program availability:* Part-time. *Degree requirements:* For master's, thesis optional; for doctorate, thesis/dissertation. *Entrance requirements:* For master's and doctorate, GRE General Test. Additional exam requirements/recommendations for international students: Required—TOEFL (minimum score 550 paper-based). Electronic applications accepted. *Faculty research:* Chronic illness management, memory and aging, health promotion, women's health, adolescent health.

Vanderbilt University, Vanderbilt University School of Nursing, Nashville, TN 37240. Offers adult-gerontology acute care nurse practitioner (MSN), including hospitalist, intensivist; adult-gerontology primary care nurse practitioner (MSN); emergency nurse practitioner (MSN); family nurse practitioner (MSN); healthcare leadership (MSN); neonatal nurse practitioner (MSN); nurse midwifery (MSN); nurse midwifery/family nurse practitioner (MSN); nursing (Post-Master's Certificate); nursing informatics (MSN); nursing practice (DNP); nursing science (PhD); pediatric acute care nurse practitioner (MSN); pediatric primary care nurse practitioner (MSN); psychiatric-mental health nurse practitioner (MSN); women's health nurse practitioner (MSN); women's health nurse practitioner/adult gerontology primary care nurse practitioner (MSN); MSN/M Div; MSN/MTS. *Accreditation:* ACEN (one or more programs are accredited); ACNM/ACME. *Program availability:* Part-time, 100% online, blended/hybrid learning. *Faculty:* 258 full-time (232 women), 363 part-time/adjunct (271 women). *Students:* 478 full-time (424 women), 342 part-time (317 women); includes 140 minority (36 Black or African American, non-Hispanic/Latino; 3 American Indian or Alaska Native, non-Hispanic/Latino; 24 Asian, non-Hispanic/Latino; 43 Hispanic/Latino; 3 Native Hawaiian or other Pacific Islander, non-Hispanic/Latino; 31 Two or more races, non-Hispanic/Latino), 11 international. Average age 31. 1,268 applicants, 49% accepted, 477 enrolled. In 2015, 343 master's, 55 doctorates awarded. *Degree requirements:* For doctorate, comprehensive exam, thesis/dissertation. *Entrance requirements:* For master's, GRE General Test (taken within the past 5 years), minimum B average in undergraduate course work, 3 letters of recommendation; for doctorate, GRE General Test, interview, 3 letters of recommendation from doctorally-prepared faculty, MSN, essay. Additional exam requirements/recommendations for international students: Required—TOEFL (minimum score 570 paper-based), IELTS (minimum score 6.5). *Application deadline:* For fall admission, 11/1 priority date for domestic and international students. Applications are processed on a rolling basis. Application fee: $50. Electronic applications accepted. *Expenses:* Contact institution. *Financial support:* In 2015–16, 585 students received support. Scholarships/grants available. Financial award application deadline: 3/15; financial award applicants required to submit FAFSA. *Faculty research:* Lymphedema, palliative care and bereavement, health services research including workforce, safety and quality of care, gerontology, better birth outcomes including nutrition. *Total annual research expenditures:* $2 million. *Unit head:* Dr. Linda Norman, Dean, 615-343-8876, Fax: 615-343-7711, E-mail: linda.norman@vanderbilt.edu. *Application contact:* Patricia Peerman, Assistant Dean for Enrollment Management, 615-322-3800, Fax: 615-343-0333, E-mail: vusn-admissions@vanderbilt.edu.
Website: http://www.nursing.vanderbilt.edu

Wayne State University, College of Nursing, Doctor Program of Nursing Practice, Detroit, MI 48202. Offers adult gerontology nurse practitioner - acute care (DNP); adult gerontology nurse practitioner - primary care (DNP); family nurse practitioner (DNP); infant mental health (DNP); neonatal nurse practitioner (DNP); nurse midwifery (DNP); nursing practice (DNP); pediatric nurse practitioner - acute care (DNP); pediatric nurse practitioner - primary care (DNP); psychiatric mental health nurse practitioner (DNP). *Students:* 56 full-time (50 women), 37 part-time (32 women); includes 32 minority (19 Black or African American, non-Hispanic/Latino; 6 Asian, non-Hispanic/Latino; 3 Hispanic/Latino; 4 Two or more races, non-Hispanic/Latino), 6 international. Average age 35. 44 applicants, 66% accepted, 18 enrolled. In 2015, 16 doctorates awarded. *Entrance requirements:* For doctorate, official transcripts, two professional references, curriculum vitae or resume, statement of goals, BSN or MSN, current Michigan RN license, criminal background check, interview, on-site writing example. Additional exam requirements/recommendations for international students: Required—TOEFL (minimum score 600 paper-based; 101 iBT); Recommended—IELTS (minimum score 7). *Application deadline:* For fall admission, 1/31 for domestic and international students. Electronic applications accepted. *Expenses:* $19,325 per year resident tuition, $35,114 non-resident tuition; $805.20 per credit hour resident tuition, $1,463.10 per credit hour non-resident tuition; fees include $47.45 per credit hour student services fee and $274.60 per semester registration fee. *Financial support:* In 2015–16, 22 students received support. Fellowships, research assistantships, teaching assistantships, institutionally sponsored loans, and scholarships/grants available. Financial award applicants required to submit FAFSA. *Unit head:* Dr. Laurie Lauzon Clabo, Dean and Professor, 313-577-4104, E-mail: laurie.lauzon.clabo@wayne.edu. *Application contact:* Dr. Nancy George, Director of DNP Program, 313-577-8300.
Website: http://nursing.wayne.edu/dnp/index.php

Wayne State University, College of Nursing, Program in Advanced Practice Nursing with Women, Neonates and Children, Detroit, MI 48202. Offers MSN, DNP. *Accreditation:* AACN. *Program availability:* Part-time. *Degree requirements:* For master's, thesis or alternative. *Entrance requirements:* For master's, BSN from NLN- or CCNE-accredited program with minimum GPA of 3.0; three references; current RN license; personal statement; for doctorate, GRE General Test (for applicants without a master's degree), resume or curriculum vitae; current RN license; goals statement; bachelor's or master's degree in nursing from NLN- or CCNE-accredited program with minimum GPA of 3.0; writing sample and interview (for DNP); reference letters (3 for PhD, 2 for DNP). Additional exam requirements/recommendations for international students: Required—TOEFL (minimum score 101 iBT); Recommended—TWE (minimum score 7). *Application deadline:* For fall admission, 6/1 priority date for domestic students, 5/1 priority date for international students; for winter admission, 10/1 priority date for domestic students, 9/1 priority date for international students; for spring admission, 2/1 priority date for domestic students, 1/1 priority date for international students. Electronic applications accepted. *Expenses:* $19,325 annual resident tuition, $35,114 non-resident tuition; $805.20 per credit hour resident tuition, $1,463.10 per credit hour non-resident tuition; fees include $47.45 per credit hour student services fee and $274.60 per semester registration fee. *Financial support:* Fellowships with tuition reimbursements, research assistantships with tuition reimbursements, teaching assistantships with tuition reimbursements, scholarships/grants, and unspecified assistantships available. Financial award application deadline: 3/31; financial award applicants required to submit FAFSA. *Faculty research:* Acculturation and parenting, domestic violence, evidence-based midwifery practice, pain in children, trauma and community violence. *Unit head:* Dr. Laurie Lauzon Clabo, Dean and Professor, 313-577-4104, E-mail: laurie.lauzon.clabo@wayne.edu. *Application contact:* Dr. Janet Harden, Associate Professor/Interim Dean, Office of Student Affairs, 313-577-4082, E-mail: nursinginfo@wayne.edu.
Website: http://nursing.wayne.edu/programs/index.php

Medical/Surgical Nursing

Daemen College, Department of Nursing, Amherst, NY 14226-3592. Offers adult nurse practitioner (MS, Post Master's Certificate); nurse executive leadership (Post Master's Certificate); nursing education (MS, Post Master's Certificate); nursing executive leadership (MS); nursing practice (DNP); palliative care nursing (Post Master's Certificate). *Accreditation:* ACEN. *Program availability:* Part-time. *Degree requirements:* For master's, thesis or alternative, degree completed in 4 years; minimum GPA of 3.0; for doctorate, degree completed in 5 years; 500 post-master's clinical hours. *Entrance requirements:* For master's, BN, 1 year medical/surgical experience, RN license and state registration, statistics course with minimum C grade, 3 letters of recommendation, minimum GPA of 3.25, interview; for doctorate, MS in advance nursing practice; New York state RN license; goal statement; resume; interview; statistics course with minimum grade of 'C'; for Post Master's Certificate, master's degree in clinical area; RN license and current registration; one year of clinical experience; statistics course with minimum grade of 'C'; 3 letters of recommendation; interview; letter of intent. Additional exam requirements/recommendations for international students: Required—TOEFL (minimum score 500 paper-based; 63 iBT), IELTS (minimum score 5.5). Electronic applications accepted. *Faculty research:* Professional stress, client behavior, drug therapy, treatment modalities and pulmonary cancers, chemical dependency.

Eastern Virginia Medical School, Master of Surgical Assisting Program, Norfolk, VA 23501-1980. Offers MSA. Electronic applications accepted. *Expenses:* Contact institution.

Inter American University of Puerto Rico, Arecibo Campus, Program in Nursing, Arecibo, PR 00614-4050. Offers critical care nursing (MSN); surgical nursing (MSN). *Entrance requirements:* For master's, EXADEP or GRE General Test or MAT, 2 letters of recommendation, bachelor's degree in nursing, minimum GPA of 2.5 in last 60 credits, minimum 1 year nursing experience, nursing license.

Pontifical Catholic University of Puerto Rico, College of Sciences, Department of Nursing, Program in Medical-Surgical Nursing, Ponce, PR 00717-0777. Offers MSN. *Program availability:* Part-time, evening/weekend. *Degree requirements:* For master's, comprehensive exam (for some programs), thesis, clinical research paper. *Entrance requirements:* For master's, GRE General Test, 2 letters of recommendation, interview, minimum GPA of 2.75. Electronic applications accepted.

Saint Francis Medical Center College of Nursing, Graduate Programs, Peoria, IL 61603-3783. Offers adult gerontology (MSN); clinical nurse leader (MSN); family nurse practitioner (MSN); family psychiatric mental health nurse practitioner (MSN); neonatal nurse practitioner (MSN); nurse clinician (Post-Graduate Certificate); nurse educator (MSN, Post-Graduate Certificate); nursing (DNP); nursing management leadership (MSN). *Accreditation:* ACEN. *Program availability:* Part-time, 100% online, blended/hybrid learning. *Faculty:* 14 full-time (all women), 5 part-time/adjunct (all women). *Students:* 13 full-time (12 women), 257 part-time (228 women); includes 23 minority (14 Black or African American, non-Hispanic/Latino; 3 Asian, non-Hispanic/Latino; 4 Hispanic/Latino; 2 Two or more races, non-Hispanic/Latino). Average age 37. 86 applicants, 86% accepted, 44 enrolled. In 2015, 61 master's, 6 doctorates awarded. *Degree requirements:* For master's, research experience, portfolio, practicum; for doctorate, practicum hours. *Entrance requirements:* For master's, nursing research, health assessment, graduate course work in statistics, RN license; for doctorate, master's degree in nursing, professional portfolio, graduate statistics, transcripts, RN license. Additional exam requirements/recommendations for international students: Required—TOEFL (minimum score 550 paper-based; 79 iBT). *Application deadline:* For fall admission, 6/1 priority date for domestic and international students; for spring admission, 11/15 priority date for domestic and international students. Applications are processed on a rolling basis. Application fee: $50. *Financial support:* In 2015–16, 18 students received support. Scholarships/grants and tuition waivers (partial) available. Support available to part-time students. Financial award application deadline: 6/15; financial award applicants required to submit FAFSA. *Faculty research:* Outcome and curriculum planning, health promotion, NCLEX-RN results, decision-making program evaluation. *Unit head:* Dr. Patti A. Stockert, President of the College, 309-655-4124, Fax: 309-624-8973, E-mail: patricia.a.stockert@osfhealthcare.org. *Application contact:* Dr. Kim A. Mitchell, Dean, Graduate Program, 309-655-2201, Fax: 309-624-8973, E-mail: kim.a.mitchell@osfhealthcare.org.
Website: http://www.sfmccon.edu/graduate-programs/

State University of New York Downstate Medical Center, College of Nursing, Graduate Program in Nursing, Program in Clinical Nurse Specialist, Brooklyn, NY 11203-2098. Offers MS, Post Master's Certificate.

Universidad Adventista de las Antillas, EGECED Department, Mayagüez, PR 00681-0118. Offers curriculum and instruction (M Ed); medical surgical nursing (MN); school administration and supervision (M Ed). *Degree requirements:* For master's, comprehensive exam (for some programs), thesis (for some programs). *Entrance requirements:* For master's, EXADEP or GRE General Test, recommendations. Electronic applications accepted.

University of Maryland, Baltimore, Graduate School, School of Nursing, Master's Program in Nursing, Baltimore, MD 21201. Offers community health nursing (MS); gerontological nursing (MS); maternal-child nursing (MS); medical-surgical nursing

(MS); nurse-midwifery education (MS); nursing administration (MS); nursing education (MS); nursing health policy (MS); primary care nursing (MS); psychiatric nursing (MS); MS/MBA. MS/MBA offered jointly with University of Baltimore. *Accreditation:* AACN; AANA/CANAEP. *Program availability:* Part-time. *Degree requirements:* For master's, comprehensive exam (for some programs), thesis or alternative. *Entrance requirements:* For master's, minimum GPA of 2.75, course work in statistics, BS in nursing. Additional exam requirements/recommendations for international students: Required—TOEFL (minimum score 550 paper-based; 80 iBT); Recommended—IELTS (minimum score 7). Electronic applications accepted. Tuition and fees vary according to program.

University of South Africa, College of Human Sciences, Pretoria, South Africa. Offers adult education (M Ed); African languages (MA, PhD); African politics (MA, PhD); Afrikaans (MA, PhD); ancient history (MA, PhD); ancient Near Eastern studies (MA, PhD); anthropology (MA, PhD); applied linguistics (MA); Arabic (MA, PhD); archaeology (MA); art history (MA); Biblical archaeology (MA); Biblical studies (M Th, D Th, PhD); Christian spirituality (M Th, D Th); church history (M Th, D Th); classical studies (MA, PhD); clinical psychology (MA); communication (MA, PhD); comparative education (M Ed, Ed D); consulting psychology (D Admin, D Com, PhD); curriculum studies (M Ed, Ed D); development studies (M Admin, MA, D Admin, PhD); didactics (M Ed, Ed D); education (M Tech); education management (M Ed, Ed D); educational psychology (M Ed); English (MA); environmental education (M Ed); French (MA, PhD); German (MA, PhD); Greek (MA); guidance and counseling (M Ed); health studies (MA, PhD), including health sciences education (MA), health services management (MA), medical and surgical nursing science (critical care general) (MA), midwifery and neonatal nursing science (MA), trauma and emergency care (MA); history (MA, PhD); history of education (Ed D); inclusive education (M Ed, Ed D); information and communications technology policy and regulation (MA); information science (MA, MIS, PhD); international politics (MA, PhD); Islamic studies (MA, PhD); Italian (MA, PhD); Judaica (MA, PhD); linguistics (MA, PhD); mathematical education (M Ed); mathematics education (MA); missiology (M Th, D Th); modern Hebrew (MA, PhD); musicology (MA, MMus, D Mus, PhD); natural science education (M Ed); New Testament (M Th, D Th); Old Testament (D Th); pastoral therapy (M Th, D Th); philosophy (MA); philosophy of education (M Ed, Ed D); politics (MA, PhD); Portuguese (MA, PhD); practical theology (M Th, D Th); psychology (MA, MS, PhD); psychology of education (M Ed, Ed D); public health (MA); religious studies (MA, D Th, PhD); Romance languages (MA); Russian (MA, PhD); Semitic languages (MA, PhD); social behavior studies in HIV/AIDS (MA); social science (mental health) (MA); social science in development studies (MA); social science in psychology (MA); social science in social work (MA); social science in sociology (MA); social work (MSW, DSW, PhD); socio-education (M Ed, Ed D); sociolinguistics (MA); sociology (MA, PhD); Spanish (MA, PhD); systematic theology (M Th, D Th); TESOL (teaching English to speakers of other languages) (MA); theological ethics (M Th, D Th); theory of literature (MA, PhD); urban ministries (D Th); urban ministry (M Th).

University of South Carolina, The Graduate School, College of Nursing, Program in Clinical Nursing, Columbia, SC 29208. Offers acute care clinical specialist (MSN); acute care nurse practitioner (MSN); women's health nurse practitioner (MSN). *Accreditation:* AACN. *Program availability:* Part-time. *Degree requirements:* For master's, thesis or alternative. *Entrance requirements:* For master's, GRE General Test or MAT, BS in nursing, RN licensure. Additional exam requirements/recommendations for international students: Required—TOEFL (minimum score 570 paper-based). Electronic applications accepted. *Faculty research:* Systems research, evidence based practice, breast cancer, violence.

Ursuline College, School of Graduate Studies, Programs in Nursing, Pepper Pike, OH 44124-4398. Offers adult nurse practitioner (MSN); adult-gerontology clinical nurse specialist (MSN); family nurse practitioner (MSN); nursing (DNP); nursing education (MSN); palliative care (MSN). *Accreditation:* AACN. *Program availability:* Part-time. *Faculty:* 5 full-time (all women), 26 part-time/adjunct (21 women). *Students:* 150 full-time (141 women), 108 part-time (99 women); includes 66 minority (50 Black or African American, non-Hispanic/Latino; 6 Asian, non-Hispanic/Latino; 6 Hispanic/Latino; 4 Two or more races, non-Hispanic/Latino), 5 international. Average age 37. 115 applicants, 95% accepted, 73 enrolled. In 2015, 69 master's, 2 doctorates awarded. *Degree requirements:* For master's, comprehensive exam. *Entrance requirements:* For master's, minimum undergraduate GPA of 3.0, bachelor's degree in nursing, eligibility for or current Ohio RN license. Additional exam requirements/recommendations for international students: Required—TOEFL (minimum score 500 paper-based). *Application deadline:* For fall admission, 8/1 priority date for domestic students. Applications are processed on a rolling basis. Application fee: $25. Electronic applications accepted. *Expenses: Tuition,* area resident: Full-time $18,036; part-time $6012 per semester. *Required fees:* $290; $210 per credit. $105 per semester. Tuition and fees vary according to program. *Financial support:* In 2015–16, 12 students received support. Scholarships/grants available. Financial award application deadline: 3/1; financial award applicants required to submit FAFSA. *Unit head:* Dr. Janet Baker, Director, 440-864-8172, Fax: 440-684-6053, E-mail: jbaker@ursuline.edu. *Application contact:* Stephanie Pratt McRoberts, Graduate Admission Coordinator, 440-646-8119, Fax: 440-684-6138, E-mail: graduateadmissions@ursuline.edu.

Nurse Anesthesia

Adventist University of Health Sciences, Program in Nurse Anesthesia, Orlando, FL 32803. Offers MS. *Accreditation:* AANA/CANAEP. *Entrance requirements:* For master's, GRE or MAT, minimum undergraduate cumulative GPA of 3.0, 1 year of intensive critical care nursing experience, 3 recommendations, interview.

Albany Medical College, Center for Nurse Anesthesiology, Albany, NY 12208. Offers anesthesia (MS). *Accreditation:* AANA/CANAEP. *Degree requirements:* For master's, thesis, thesis proposal/clinical research. *Entrance requirements:* For master's, GRE General Test, BSN or appropriate bachelor's degree, current RN license, critical care experience, organic chemistry, research methods. Electronic applications accepted. *Expenses:* Contact institution.

Arkansas State University, Graduate School, College of Nursing and Health Professions, School of Nursing, State University, AR 72467. Offers aging studies

(Graduate Certificate); health care management (Graduate Certificate); health sciences (MS); health sciences education (Graduate Certificate); nurse anesthesia (MSN); nursing (MSN); nursing practice (DNP). *Accreditation:* AANA/CANAEP (one or more programs are accredited); ACEN. *Program availability:* Part-time. *Faculty:* 16 full-time (14 women). *Students:* 80 full-time (30 women), 139 part-time (121 women); includes 38 minority (26 Black or African American, non-Hispanic/Latino; 3 American Indian or Alaska Native, non-Hispanic/Latino; 3 Asian, non-Hispanic/Latino; 4 Hispanic/Latino; 1 Native Hawaiian or other Pacific Islander, non-Hispanic/Latino; 1 Two or more races, non-Hispanic/Latino), 2 international. Average age 34. 147 applicants, 33% accepted, 43 enrolled. In 2015, 84 master's awarded. *Degree requirements:* For master's and Graduate Certificate, comprehensive exam, thesis or alternative; for doctorate, comprehensive exam, thesis/dissertation. *Entrance requirements:* For master's, GRE General Test or MAT, appropriate bachelor's degree, current Arkansas nursing license,

Nurse Anesthesia

CPR certification, physical examination, professional liability insurance, critical care experience, ACLS Certification, PALS Certification, interview, immunization records, personal goal statement, health assessment; for doctorate, GRE or MAT, NCLEX-RN Exam, appropriate master's degree, current Arkansas nursing license, CPR certification, physical examination, professional liability insurance, critical care experience, ACLS Certification, PALS Certification, interview, immunization records, personal goal statement, health assessment, TB skin test, background check; for Graduate Certificate, GRE or MAT, appropriate bachelor's degree, official transcripts, immunization records, proof of employment in healthcare, TB Skin Test, TB Mask Fit Test, CPR Certification. Additional exam requirements/recommendations for international students: Required— TOEFL (minimum score 550 paper-based; 79 iBT), IELTS (minimum score 6), PTE (minimum score 56). *Application deadline:* Applications are processed on a rolling basis. Electronic applications accepted. *Expenses:* Contact institution. *Financial support:* In 2015–16, 1 student received support. Fellowships, career-related internships or fieldwork, scholarships/grants, and unspecified assistantships available. Financial award application deadline: 7/1; financial award applicants required to submit FAFSA. *Unit head:* Dr. Jill Oswaks, Chair of Graduate Programs, 870-972-3074, Fax: 870-972-2954, E-mail: jdettyoswaks@astate.edu. *Application contact:* Vickey Ring, Graduate Admissions Coordinator, 870-972-2737, Fax: 870-972-3917, E-mail: vickeyring@astate.edu.
Website: http://www.astate.edu/college/conhp/departments/nursing/

Augusta University, The Graduate School, Doctor of Nursing Practice Program, Augusta, GA 30912. Offers adult gerontology acute care nurse practitioner (DNP); family nurse practitioner (DNP); nursing (DNP); nursing anesthesia (DNP); pediatric nurse practitioner (DNP); psychiatric mental health nurse practitioner (DNP). *Students:* 40 part-time. *Degree requirements:* For doctorate, thesis/dissertation or alternative. *Entrance requirements:* For doctorate, GRE General Test or MAT, master's degree in nursing or related field, current professional nurse licensure. Additional exam requirements/recommendations for international students: Required—TOEFL (minimum score 600 paper-based; 100 iBT). *Application deadline:* For fall admission, 3/1 for domestic and international students; for spring admission, 7/1 for domestic and international students. Applications are processed on a rolling basis. Application fee: $50. Electronic applications accepted. *Unit head:* Dr. Marguerite Murphy, RN, Director, 706-721-3676, Fax: 706-721-8169. *Application contact:* Karen Sturgill, Program Manager, 706-721-3676, Fax: 706-721-8169, E-mail: dnp@augusta.edu.
Website: http://www.augusta.edu/nursing/dnp_programs.php

Barry University, College of Health Sciences, Program in Anesthesiology, Miami Shores, FL 33161-6695. Offers MS. *Accreditation:* AANA/CANAEP. *Degree requirements:* For master's, comprehensive exam. *Entrance requirements:* For master's, GRE General Test, minimum GPA of 3.0; 2 courses in chemistry (1 with lab); minimum 1 year critical care experience; BSN or RN; 4-year bachelor's degree in health sciences, nursing, biology, or chemistry. Electronic applications accepted. *Faculty research:* Use of computers in education, psychological well-bring of health care providers.

Baylor College of Medicine, School of Allied Health Sciences, Graduate Program in Nurse Anesthesia, Houston, TX 77030-3498. Offers DNP. *Accreditation:* AANA/CANAEP. *Degree requirements:* For doctorate, comprehensive exam, thesis/dissertation. *Entrance requirements:* For doctorate, GRE General Test, Texas nursing license, 1 year of work experience in critical care nursing, minimum GPA of 3.0, BSN, statistics, organic chemistry. Electronic applications accepted. *Expenses:* Contact institution. *Faculty research:* Education, simulation.

Bloomsburg University of Pennsylvania, School of Graduate Studies, College of Science and Technology, Department of Nursing, Bloomsburg, PA 17815. Offers adult and family nurse practitioner (MSN); community health (MSN); nurse anesthesia (MSN); nursing (MSN); nursing administration (MSN). *Accreditation:* AACN; AANA/CANAEP. *Degree requirements:* For master's, thesis (for some programs), clinical experience. *Entrance requirements:* For master's, minimum QPA of 3.0, personal statement, 2 letters of recommendation, nursing license. Additional exam requirements/ recommendations for international students: Required—TOEFL. Electronic applications accepted.

Boston College, William F. Connell School of Nursing, Chestnut Hill, MA 02467. Offers adult-gerontology nursing (MS); family health nursing (MS); forensic nursing (MS); nurse anesthesia (MS); nursing (PhD); pediatric nursing (MS), including pediatric and women's health; psychiatric-mental health nursing (MS); women's health nursing (MS); MBA/MS; MS/MA; MS/PhD. *Accreditation:* AACN; AANA/CANAEP (one or more programs are accredited). *Program availability:* Part-time. *Faculty:* 53 full-time (48 women), 47 part-time/adjunct (44 women). *Students:* 185 full-time (167 women), 66 part-time (56 women); includes 31 minority (10 Black or African American, non-Hispanic/Latino; 12 Asian, non-Hispanic/Latino; 7 Hispanic/Latino; 2 Two or more races, non-Hispanic/Latino), 7 international. Average age 32. 313 applicants, 66% accepted, 91 enrolled. In 2015, 98 master's, 5 doctorates awarded. *Degree requirements:* For master's, comprehensive exam; for doctorate, comprehensive exam, thesis/dissertation, computer literacy exam or foreign language. *Entrance requirements:* For master's, bachelor's degree in nursing; for doctorate, GRE General Test, MS in nursing. Additional exam requirements/recommendations for international students: Required—TOEFL (minimum score 600 paper-based; 100 iBT), IELTS (minimum score 7.5). *Application deadline:* For fall admission, 9/30 for domestic and international students; for winter admission, 1/15 for domestic and international students; for spring admission, 3/15 for domestic and international students. Applications are processed on a rolling basis. Application fee: $40. Electronic applications accepted. *Expenses:* Contact institution. *Financial support:* In 2015–16, 1 fellowship with full tuition reimbursement (averaging $23,700 per year), 25 teaching assistantships (averaging $4,370 per year) were awarded; research assistantships, scholarships/grants, health care benefits, tuition waivers (partial), and unspecified assistantships also available. Support available to part-time students. Financial award application deadline: 3/1; financial award applicants required to submit FAFSA. *Faculty research:* Sexual and reproductive health, health promotion/illness prevention, aging, eating disorders, symptom management. *Total annual research expenditures:* $1 million. *Unit head:* Dr. Susan Gennaro, Dean, 617-552-4251, Fax: 617-552-0931, E-mail: susan.gennaro@bc.edu. *Application contact:* MaryBeth Crowley, Graduate Programs Assistant, 617-552-4928, Fax: 617-552-2121, E-mail: csongrad@bc.edu.
Website: http://www.bc.edu/schools/son/

Bryan College of Health Sciences, School of Nurse Anesthesia, Lincoln, NE 68506-1398. Offers MS. *Accreditation:* AANA/CANAEP.

California State University, Fullerton, Graduate Studies, College of Health and Human Development, Department of Nursing, Fullerton, CA 92834-9480. Offers leadership (MSN); nurse anesthesia (MSN); nurse educator (MSN); nursing (DNP); women's health care (MSN). *Accreditation:* AACN; AANA/CANAEP. *Program availability:* Part-time.

Case Western Reserve University, Frances Payne Bolton School of Nursing, Master's Programs in Nursing, Program in Nurse Anesthesia, Cleveland, OH 44106. Offers MSN. *Accreditation:* AANA/CANAEP. *Program availability:* Part-time. *Students:* 23 full-time (18 women), 50 part-time (28 women); includes 8 minority (4 Black or African American, non-Hispanic/Latino; 2 Asian, non-Hispanic/Latino; 2 Hispanic/Latino). Average age 30. 69 applicants, 57% accepted, 30 enrolled. In 2015, 24 master's awarded. Terminal master's awarded for partial completion of doctoral program. *Entrance requirements:* For master's, GRE General Test or MAT, CCRN certification. Additional exam requirements/recommendations for international students: Required—TOEFL (minimum score 577 paper-based; 90 iBT), IELTS (minimum score 7). *Application deadline:* For fall admission, 1/15 for domestic students; for summer admission, 7/15 for domestic students. Application fee: $75. *Expenses:* $1,891 per credit hour. *Financial support:* Scholarships/grants and traineeships available. Financial award application deadline: 6/30. *Faculty research:* Mechanical ventilation antioxidant trial, intravenous function and mechanical ventilation, impact of taxane on peripheral nerve function. *Unit head:* Dr. Sonya Moore, Director, 216-368-6659, Fax: 216-368-3542, E-mail: sdm37@case.edu. *Application contact:* Donna Hassik, Admissions Coordinator, 216-368-5253, Fax: 216-368-0124, E-mail: dmh7@case.edu.
Website: http://fpb.cwru.edu/MSN/anesthesia.shtm

Central Connecticut State University, School of Graduate Studies, School of Engineering, Science and Technology, Department of Biology, New Britain, CT 06050-4010. Offers biological sciences (MA, MS), including anesthesia (MS), ecology and environmental sciences (MA), general biology (MA), health sciences (MS), professional education (MS); biology (Certificate). *Program availability:* Part-time, evening/weekend. *Faculty:* 7 full-time (2 women), 2 part-time/adjunct (both women). *Students:* 113 full-time (69 women), 12 part-time (9 women); includes 24 minority (10 Black or African American, non-Hispanic/Latino; 9 Asian, non-Hispanic/Latino; 2 Hispanic/Latino; 3 Two or more races, non-Hispanic/Latino), 1 international. Average age 31. 20 applicants, 60% accepted, 2 enrolled. In 2015, 43 master's, 1 other advanced degree awarded. *Degree requirements:* For master's, comprehensive exam, thesis or alternative; for Certificate, qualifying exam. *Entrance requirements:* For master's and Certificate, minimum undergraduate GPA of 2.7, essay, letters of recommendation. Additional exam requirements/recommendations for international students: Required—TOEFL (minimum score 550 paper-based; 79 iBT). *Application deadline:* For fall admission, 6/1 for domestic students, 5/1 for international students; for spring admission, 11/1 for domestic and international students. Applications are processed on a rolling basis. Application fee: $50. Electronic applications accepted. *Expenses: Tuition, area resident:* Full-time $6188. Tuition, state resident: full-time $9284; part-time $577 per credit. Tuition, nonresident: full-time $17,240; part-time $592 per credit. *Required fees:* $4266; $234 per credit. *Financial support:* In 2015–16, 6 students received support, including 1 research assistantship; career-related internships or fieldwork, Federal Work-Study, scholarships/grants, and unspecified assistantships also available. Support available to part-time students. Financial award application deadline: 3/1; financial award applicants required to submit FAFSA. *Faculty research:* Environmental science, anesthesia, health sciences, zoology, animal behavior. *Unit head:* Dr. Douglas Carter, Chair, 860-832-2645, E-mail: carterd@ccsu.edu. *Application contact:* Patricia Gardner, Associate Director of Graduate Studies, 860-832-2350, Fax: 860-832-2362, E-mail: graduateadmissions@ccsu.edu.
Website: http://web.ccsu.edu/biodept/

Columbia University, School of Nursing, Program in Nurse Anesthesia, New York, NY 10032. Offers MS, Adv C. *Accreditation:* AACN; AANA/CANAEP. *Entrance requirements:* For master's, GRE General Test, NCLEX, BSN, 1 year of intensive care unit experience; for Adv C, MSN, 1 year of intensive care unit experience. Additional exam requirements/recommendations for international students: Required—TOEFL (minimum score 100 iBT). Electronic applications accepted.

DeSales University, Division of Healthcare, Center Valley, PA 18034-9568. Offers adult-gerontology acute care (Post Master's Certificate); adult-gerontology acute care nurse practitioner (MSN); adult-gerontology acute certified nurse practitioner (Post Master's Certificate); adult-gerontology clinical nurse specialist (MSN, Post Master's Certificate); clinical leadership (DNP); family nurse practitioner (MSN, Post Master's Certificate); general nursing practice (DNP); health care information management (MSIS); network security (MSIS); nurse anesthetists (MSN); nurse educator (Post Master's Certificate, Postbaccalaureate Certificate); nurse midwives (MSN); nurse practitioner (MSN); project management (MSIS); psychiatric-mental health nurse practitioner (MSN, Post Master's Certificate); DNP/MBA. *Accreditation:* ACEN. *Program availability:* Part-time. *Faculty:* 22 full-time (14 women), 37 part-time/adjunct (29 women). *Students:* 244 full-time (178 women), 55 part-time (50 women); includes 24 minority (7 Black or African American, non-Hispanic/Latino; 9 Asian, non-Hispanic/Latino; 6 Hispanic/Latino; 2 Two or more races, non-Hispanic/Latino). Average age 31. 68 applicants, 85% accepted, 52 enrolled. In 2015, 73 master's awarded. *Degree requirements:* For master's, minimum GPA of 3.0, portfolio; for doctorate, minimum GPA of 3.0, scholarly capstone project. *Entrance requirements:* For master's, GRE or MAT (waived if applicant has an undergraduate GPA of 3.0 or higher), BSN from ACEN- or CCNE-accredited program, minimum undergraduate GPA of 3.0, active RN license or eligibility, two letters of recommendation, essay, health care experience, personal interview; for doctorate, BSN or MSN from ACEN- or CCNE-accredited institution, minimum GPA of 3.3 in graduate program, current licensure as an RN. Additional exam requirements/recommendations for international students: Required—TOEFL (minimum score 104 iBT). *Application deadline:* Applications are processed on a rolling basis. Application fee: $50. Electronic applications accepted. *Expenses:* Contact institution. *Financial support:* Applicants required to submit FAFSA. *Unit head:* Fr. Dr. Peter Leonard, OSFS, Dean of Graduate Education, 610-282-1100 Ext. 1289, E-mail: peter.leonard@desales.edu. *Application contact:* Abigail Wernicki, Director of Graduate Admissions, 610-282-1100 Ext. 1768, Fax: 610-282-2869, E-mail: gradadmissions@desales.edu.

Drexel University, College of Nursing and Health Professions, Department of Nurse Anesthesia, Philadelphia, PA 19104-2875. Offers MSN. *Accreditation:* AACN; AANA/CANAEP. Electronic applications accepted.

Duke University, School of Nursing, Durham, NC 27708-0586. Offers acute care pediatric nurse practitioner (MSN, Post Master's Certificate); adult-gerontology nurse practitioner (MSN, Post Master's Certificate), including acute care, primary care; family nurse practitioner (MSN, Post Master's Certificate); neonatal nurse practitioner (MSN, Post Master's Certificate); nurse anesthesia (DNP); nurse practitioner (DNP); nursing (PhD); nursing and health care leadership (MSN); nursing education (MSN); nursing informatics (MSN, Post Master's Certificate); pediatric nurse practitioner (MSN, Post Master's Certificate), including primary care, women's health nurse practitioner (MSN, Post Master's Certificate). *Accreditation:* AACN; AANA/CANAEP. *Program availability:* Part-time, evening/weekend, online learning. *Faculty:* 74 full-time (63 women). *Students:* 179 full-time (152 women), 528 part-time (466 women); includes 145 minority (42 Black or African American, non-Hispanic/Latino; 3 American Indian or Alaska Native, non-Hispanic/Latino; 44 Asian, non-Hispanic/Latino; 35 Hispanic/Latino; 1 Native Hawaiian or other Pacific Islander, non-Hispanic/Latino; 20 Two or more races, non-Hispanic/Latino), 7 international. Average age 33. 619 applicants, 46% accepted, 201 enrolled. In 2015, 243 master's, 26 doctorates, 26 other advanced degrees awarded. Terminal master's awarded for partial completion of doctoral program. *Degree requirements:* For master's, thesis optional; for doctorate, capstone project. *Entrance requirements:* For

master's, GRE General Test (waived if undergraduate GPA of 3.4 or higher), 1 year of nursing experience (recommended), BSN, minimum GPA of 3.0, previous course work in statistics; for doctorate, GRE General Test (waived if undergraduate GPA of 3.4 or higher), BSN or MSN, minimum GPA of 3.0, portfolio, resume, personal statement, undergraduate statistics course, current licensure as a registered nurse, transcripts from all post-secondary institutions; for Post Master's Certificate, MSN, licensure or eligibility as a professional nurse, transcripts from all post-secondary institutions, previous course work in statistics. Additional exam requirements/recommendations for international students: Required—TOEFL (minimum score 100 iBT), IELTS (minimum score 7). *Application deadline:* For fall admission, 12/1 for domestic and international students; for spring admission, 5/1 for domestic and international students. Application fee: $50. Electronic applications accepted. *Expenses:* Contact institution. *Financial support:* Career-related internships or fieldwork, institutionally sponsored loans, scholarships/ grants, traineeships, and tuition waivers (partial) available. Support available to part-time students. Financial award applicants required to submit FAFSA. *Faculty research:* Cardiovascular disease, caregiver skill training, data mining, prostate cancer, neonatal immune system. *Unit head:* Dr. Marion E. Broome, Dean/Vice Chancellor for Nursing Affairs/Associate Vice President for Academic Affairs for Nursing, 919-684-9446, Fax: 919-684-9414, E-mail: marion.broome@duke.edu. *Application contact:* Dr. Ernie Rushing, Director of Admissions and Recruitment, 919-668-6274, Fax: 919-668-4693, E-mail: ernie.rushing@dm.duke.edu.
Website: http://www.nursing.duke.edu/

Fairfield University, Marion Peckham Egan School of Nursing and Health Studies, Fairfield, CT 06824. Offers advanced practice (DNP); family nurse practitioner (MSN, DNP); nurse anesthesia (DNP); nursing leadership (MSN); psychiatric nurse practitioner (MSN, DNP). *Accreditation:* AACN; AANA/CANAEP. *Program availability:* Part-time, evening/weekend. *Faculty:* 8 full-time (all women), 9 part time/adjunct (7 women). *Students:* 43 full-time (35 women), 181 part-time (163 women); includes 52 minority (20 Black or African American, non-Hispanic/Latino; 1 American Indian or Alaska Native, non-Hispanic/Latino; 11 Asian, non-Hispanic/Latino; 16 Hispanic/Latino; 4 Two or more races, non-Hispanic/Latino), 1 international. Average age 36. 103 applicants, 67% accepted, 43 enrolled. In 2015, 12 master's, 21 doctorates awarded. *Degree requirements:* For master's, capstone project. *Entrance requirements:* For master's, minimum QPA of 3.0, RN license, resume, 2 recommendations; for doctorate, MSN (minimum QPA of 3.2) or BSN (minimum QPA of 3.0); critical care nursing experience (for nurse anesthesia DNP candidates). Additional exam requirements/ recommendations for international students: Required—TOEFL (minimum score 550 paper-based; 80 iBT) or IELTS (minimum score 6.5). *Application deadline:* For fall admission, 5/15 for international students; for spring admission, 10/15 for international students. Applications are processed on a rolling basis. Application fee: $60. Electronic applications accepted. *Expenses:* $850 per credit hour (for MSN); $900-$1,000 per credit hour (for DNP). *Financial support:* In 2015–16, 51 students received support. Unspecified assistantships available. Financial award applicants required to submit FAFSA. *Faculty research:* Aging, spiritual care, palliative and end of life care, psychiatric mental health, pediatric trauma. *Unit head:* Dr. Meredith Wallace Kazer, Dean, 203-254-4000 Ext. 2701, Fax: 203-254-4126, E-mail: mkazer@fairfield.edu. *Application contact:* Marianne Gumpper, Director of Graduate and Continuing Studies Admission, 203-254-4184, Fax: 203-254-4073, E-mail: gradadmis@fairfield.edu.
Website: http://fairfield.edu/son

Florida Gulf Coast University, College of Health Professions and Social Work, Program in Nurse Anesthesia, Fort Myers, FL 33965-6565. Offers MSN. *Accreditation:* AACN; AANA/CANAEP. *Program availability:* Part-time. *Faculty:* 57 full-time (40 women), 39 part-time/adjunct (23 women). *Students:* 29 full-time (15 women); includes 10 minority (2 Black or African American, non-Hispanic/Latino; 4 Asian, non-Hispanic/ Latino; 4 Hispanic/Latino), 1 international. Average age 32. In 2015, 10 master's awarded. *Degree requirements:* For master's, thesis or alternative. *Entrance requirements:* For master's, GRE General Test, MAT, minimum GPA of 3.0. Additional exam requirements/recommendations for international students: Required—TOEFL (minimum score 550 paper-based). *Application deadline:* For fall admission, 4/15 priority date for domestic students; for spring admission, 6/1 for domestic students. Applications are processed on a rolling basis. Application fee: $30. Electronic applications accepted. *Expenses:* Tuition, state resident: full-time $6974. Tuition, nonresident: full-time $28,170. *Required fees:* $1987. One-time fee: $10 full-time. Tuition and fees vary according to course load and degree level. *Financial support:* In 2015–16, 8 students received support. Application deadline: 6/30; applicants required to submit FAFSA. *Faculty research:* Gerontology, community health, ethical and legal aspects of health care, critical care. *Total annual research expenditures:* $181,623. *Unit head:* Dr. Rosann Spiegel, Program Director, 239-590-4298, Fax: 239-590-7474, E-mail: rspiegel@ fgcu.edu. *Application contact:* MeLinda Coffey, Administrative Assistant, 239-590-7530, Fax: 239-590-7474, E-mail: mcoffey@fgcu.edu.

Gannon University, School of Graduate Studies, Morosky College of Health Professions and Sciences, Villa Maria School of Nursing, Program in Nurse Anesthesia, Erie, PA 16541-0001. Offers MSN, Certificate. *Program availability:* Part-time, evening/ weekend. *Students:* 40 part-time (23 women); includes 3 minority (1 Asian, non-Hispanic/Latino; 1 Hispanic/Latino; 1 Two or more races, non-Hispanic/Latino), 1 international. Average age 30. In 2015, 1 other advanced degree awarded. *Degree requirements:* For master's, thesis (for some programs), practicum. *Entrance requirements:* For master's, GRE, BSN with minimum GPA of 3.0, transcripts, evidence of fulfillment of legal requirements for practice of nursing in the United States, 4 letters of recommendation, at least 2 years of clinical experience in which critical judgments are made, interview; for Certificate, completion of statistics and research courses, minimum GPA of 3.0, 4 letters of recommendation, 2 years of clinical experience, interview. Additional exam requirements/recommendations for international students: Required— TOEFL (minimum score 79 iBT). *Application deadline:* For winter admission, 5/1 for domestic students. Application fee: $25. Electronic applications accepted. *Financial support:* Federal Work-Study available. *Unit head:* Dr. Kathleen Patterson, Director, 814-871-5547, E-mail: patterso018@gannon.edu. *Application contact:* Bridget Philip, Director of Graduate Admissions, 814-871-7412, E-mail: graduate@gannon.edu.

Georgetown University, Graduate School of Arts and Sciences, School of Nursing and Health Studies, Washington, DC 20057. Offers acute care nurse practitioner (MS); clinical nurse specialist (MS); family nurse practitioner (MS); nurse anesthesia (MS); nurse-midwifery (MS); nursing (DNP); nursing education (MS). *Accreditation:* AACN; AANA/CANAEP (one or more programs are accredited); ACNM/ACME (one or more programs are accredited). *Degree requirements:* For master's, thesis optional. *Entrance requirements:* For master's, GRE General Test or MAT, bachelor's degree in nursing from NLN-accredited school, minimum undergraduate GPA of 3.0. Additional exam requirements/recommendations for international students: Required—TOEFL.

Goldfarb School of Nursing at Barnes-Jewish College, Graduate Programs, St. Louis, MO 63110. Offers adult-gerontology acute care nurse practitioner (MSN); adult-gerontology nurse practitioner (MSN); nurse anesthesia (MSN); nurse educator (MSN); nurse executive (MSN). *Accreditation:* AACN; AANA/CANAEP. *Program availability:* Part-time, online learning. *Faculty:* 51 full-time (47 women), 6 part-time/adjunct (all women). *Students:* 58 full-time (57 women), 29 part-time (24 women); includes 17

minority (11 Black or African American, non-Hispanic/Latino; 2 Asian, non-Hispanic/ Latino; 2 Hispanic/Latino; 2 Two or more races, non-Hispanic/Latino). Average age 26. 41 applicants, 22% accepted, 8 enrolled. In 2015, 56 master's awarded. *Degree requirements:* For master's, thesis or alternative. *Entrance requirements:* For master's, 2 references, personal statement, curriculum vitae or resume. Additional exam requirements/recommendations for international students: Required—TOEFL (minimum score 575 paper-based; 85 iBT). *Application deadline:* For fall admission, 2/1 priority date for international students; for spring admission, 10/1 priority date for international students. Applications are processed on a rolling basis. Application fee: $50. *Expenses:* Contact institution. *Financial support:* Fellowships, research assistantships, Federal Work-Study, institutionally sponsored loans, and scholarships/grants available. Support available to part-time students. Financial award applicants required to submit FAFSA. *Faculty research:* HIV stigma, HIV symptom management, palliative care with children and their families, heart disease prevention in Hispanic women, depression in the well elderly, alternative therapies in pre-term infants. *Unit head:* Dr. Gretchen Drinkard, Dean, 314-454-7540, Fax: 314-362-9222, E-mail: gld9643@bjc.org. *Application contact:* Karen Sartorius, Admissions Specialist, 314-454-7057, Fax: 314-362-9250, E-mail: ksartorius@bjc.org.
Website: http://www.barnesjewishcollege.edu/

Inter American University of Puerto Rico, Arecibo Campus, Program in Anesthesia, Arecibo, PR 00614-4050. Offers MS. *Accreditation:* AANA/CANAEP. *Degree requirements:* For master's, comprehensive exam, thesis optional. *Entrance requirements:* For master's, GRE, EXADEP, 2 letters of recommendation, bachelor's degree in nursing, interview, minimum GPA of 3.0 in last 60 credits, minimum 1 year experience.

La Roche College, School of Graduate Studies and Adult Education, Program in Health Sciences, Pittsburgh, PA 15237-5898. Offers nurse anesthesia (MS). *Accreditation:* AANA/CANAEP. *Faculty:* 2 full-time (0 women), 2 part-time/adjunct (1 woman). *Students:* 30 full-time (22 women). Average age 30. 17 applicants, 100% accepted, 17 enrolled. In 2015, 20 master's awarded. *Degree requirements:* For master's, thesis optional. *Entrance requirements:* For master's, GRE General Test, prior acceptance to the Allegheny Valley School of Anesthesia. *Application deadline:* For fall admission, 12/ 31 for domestic students. Application fee: $50. Electronic applications accepted. *Expenses:* Tuition, area resident: Full-time $12,240; part-time $680 per credit. *Required fees:* $25 per semester. *Financial support:* Application deadline: 3/31; applicants required to submit FAFSA. *Unit head:* Dr. Don Fujito, Coordinator, 412-536-1157, Fax: 412-536-1175, E-mail: fujitod1@laroche.edu. *Application contact:* Hope Schiffgens, Director of Graduate Studies and Adult Education, 412-536-1266, Fax: 412-536-1283, E-mail: schombh1@laroche.edu.

La Salle University, School of Nursing and Health Sciences, Program in Nursing, Philadelphia, PA 19141-1199. Offers adult gerontology primary care nurse practitioner (MSN, Certificate); adult health and illness clinical nurse specialist (MSN); adult-gerontology clinical nurse specialist (MSN, Certificate); clinical nurse leader (MSN); family primary care nurse practitioner (MSN, Certificate); gerontology (Certificate); nurse anesthetist (MSN, Certificate); nursing (MSN, Certificate); nursing administration (MSN, Certificate); nursing education (Certificate); nursing practice (DNP); nursing service administration (MSN); public health nursing (MSN, Certificate); school nursing (Certificate); MSN/MBA; MSN/MPH. *Accreditation:* AANA/CANAEP. *Program availability:* Part-time, evening/weekend, 100% online. *Faculty:* 13 full-time (all women), 9 part-time/adjunct (8 women). *Students:* 368 part-time (56 women); includes 103 minority (62 Black or African American, non-Hispanic/Latino; 1 American Indian or Alaska Native, non-Hispanic/Latino; 26 Asian, non-Hispanic/Latino; 9 Hispanic/Latino; 5 Two or more races, non-Hispanic/Latino), 5 international. Average age 36. 98 applicants, 85% accepted, 53 enrolled. In 2015, 87 master's, 3 doctorates, 10 other advanced degrees awarded. *Degree requirements:* For doctorate, minimum of 1,000 hours of post baccalaureate clinical practice supervised by preceptors. *Entrance requirements:* For master's, GRE, MAT, or GMAT (for students with BSN GPA of less than 3.2), baccalaureate degree in nursing from an NLNAC- or CCNE-accredited program or an MSN Bridge program; Pennsylvania RN license; 2 letters of reference; resume; statement of philosophy articulating professional values and future educational goal; 1 year of work experience as a registered nurse; for doctorate, GRE (waived for applicants with MSN cumulative GPA of 3.7 or above), MSN from nationally-accredited program or master's degree, MBA or MHA from nationally-accredited program; resume or curriculum vitae; 2 letters of reference; interview; for Certificate, GRE, MAT, or GMAT (for students with BSN GPA of less than 3.2, baccalaureate degree in nursing from an NLNAC- or CCNE-accredited program or an MSN Bridge program; Pennsylvania RN license; 2 letters of reference; resume; statement of philosophy articulating professional values and future educational goal; 1 year of work experience as a registered nurse. Additional exam requirements/recommendations for international students: Required— TOEFL. *Application deadline:* For fall admission, 8/15 priority date for domestic students, 7/15 for international students; for spring admission, 12/15 priority date for domestic students, 11/15 for international students; for summer admission, 4/15 priority date for domestic students, 3/15 for international students. Applications are processed on a rolling basis. Application fee: $35. Electronic applications accepted. Application fee is waived when completed online. *Expenses:* $870 per credit hour (for MSN); $930 per credit hour (for DNP); $150 technology fee full-time, $75 part-time; $135 general university fee. *Financial support:* In 2015–16, 13 students received support. Scholarships/grants and traineeships available. Support available to part-time students. Financial award application deadline: 8/31; financial award applicants required to submit FAFSA. *Unit head:* Dr. Patricia M. Dillon, Director, 215-951-1322, Fax: 215-951-1896, E-mail: msnapn@lasalle.edu. *Application contact:* Alison McAnespey Target, Director, Graduate and Adult Enrollment, 215-951-1100, Fax: 215-951-1462, E-mail: reilly@ lasalle.edu.
Website: http://www.lasalle.edu/nursing/program-options/

Lincoln Memorial University, Caylor School of Nursing, Harrogate, TN 37752-1901. Offers family nurse practitioner (MSN); nurse anesthesia (MSN); psychiatric mental health nurse practitioner (MSN). *Accreditation:* AANA/CANAEP; ACEN. *Program availability:* Part-time. *Entrance requirements:* For master's, GRE.

Louisiana State University Health Sciences Center, School of Nursing, New Orleans, LA 70112. Offers adult gerontology clinical nurse specialist (Post-Master's Certificate); clinical nurse leader (MSN); executive nurse leader (Post-Master's Certificate); neonatal nurse practitioner (Post-Master's Certificate); nurse anesthesia (Post-Master's Certificate); nurse educator (MSN); nursing (DNS); primary care family nurse practitioner (Post-Master's Certificate); public/community health nursing (Post-Master's Certificate). *Accreditation:* AACN; AANA/CANAEP (one or more programs are accredited). *Program availability:* Part-time. *Faculty:* 22 full-time (19 women), 21 part-time/adjunct (8 women). *Students:* 254 (185 women); includes 68 minority (44 Black or African American, non-Hispanic/Latino; 12 Asian, non-Hispanic/Latino; 12 Hispanic/ Latino). Average age 33. 144 applicants, 54% accepted, 73 enrolled. In 2015, 84 master's, 6 doctorates awarded. *Degree requirements:* For master's, thesis optional; for doctorate, thesis/dissertation. *Entrance requirements:* For master's, GRE General Test, MAT, minimum GPA of 3.0; for doctorate, GRE General Test, minimum GPA of 3.5. Additional exam requirements/recommendations for international students: Required—

Nurse Anesthesia

TOEFL (minimum score 550 paper-based; 79 iBT). *Application deadline:* Applications are processed on a rolling basis. Application fee: $250. Electronic applications accepted. *Expenses:* $9,136.50 per year; $19,633.50 per year (for DNP). *Financial support:* Federal Work-Study, institutionally sponsored loans, scholarships/grants, and traineeships available. Financial award applicants required to submit FAFSA. *Faculty research:* Advanced clinical practice, nursing education, health, social support, nursing administration. *Unit head:* Dr. Demetrius James Porche, Dean, 504-568-4106, Fax: 504-599-0573, E-mail: dporch@lsuhsc.edu. *Application contact:* Tracie Gravolet, Director, Office of Student Affairs, 504-568-4114, Fax: 504-568-5711, E-mail: tgravo@lsuhsc.edu.
Website: http://nursing.lsuhsc.edu/

Lourdes University, Graduate School, Sylvania, OH 43560-2898. Offers business (MBA); leadership (M Ed); nurse anesthesia (MSN); nurse educator (MSN); nurse leader (MSN); organizational leadership (MOL); reading (M Ed); teaching and curriculum (M Ed); theology (MA). *Program availability:* Evening/weekend. *Entrance requirements:* Additional exam requirements/recommendations for international students: Required—TOEFL.

Marshall University, Academic Affairs Division, College of Business, Program in Nurse Anesthesia, Huntington, WV 25755. Offers DMPNA. Program offered jointly with Charleston Area Medical Center. *Students:* 81 full-time (47 women); includes 7 minority (2 Black or African American, non-Hispanic/Latino; 2 Asian, non-Hispanic/Latino; 2 Hispanic/Latino; 1 Two or more races, non-Hispanic/Latino). Average age 31. In 2015, 26 doctorates awarded. *Unit head:* Dr. Nancy Tierney, Director, 304-388-9950, E-mail: nancy.tierney@camc.org. *Application contact:* Information Contact, Graduate Admissions, 304-746-1900, Fax: 304-746-1902, E-mail: services@marshall.edu.
Website: http://camcinstitute.org/anesthesia

Mayo School of Health Sciences, Doctor of Nurse Anesthesia Practice Program, Rochester, MN 55905. Offers DNAP. *Accreditation:* AANA/CANAEP. *Faculty:* 3 part-time/adjunct. *Degree requirements:* For doctorate, comprehensive exam, research project. *Entrance requirements:* For doctorate, GRE General Test. Additional exam requirements/recommendations for international students: Required—TOEFL. *Application deadline:* For fall admission, 9/1 for domestic students. Application fee: $50. Electronic applications accepted. *Expenses:* Contact institution. *Financial support:* Scholarships/grants, health care benefits, and stipends available. Financial award applicants required to submit FAFSA. *Unit head:* Dr. Mary E. Marienau, Director, 507-284-8331, Fax: 507-284-2818, E-mail: marienau.mary@mayo.edu. *Application contact:* Julie Predmore, Administrative Assistant, 507-286-4163, Fax: 507-284-2818, E-mail: predmore.julie@mayo.edu.
Website: http://www.mayo.edu/mshs

Medical University of South Carolina, College of Health Professions, Anesthesia for Nurses Program, Charleston, SC 29425. Offers MSNA. *Accreditation:* AANA/CANAEP. *Degree requirements:* For master's, comprehensive exam, research project, clinical practica. *Entrance requirements:* For master's, GRE General Test, interview, minimum GPA of 3.0, 2 years of RN (ICU) experience, RN license. Additional exam requirements/recommendations for international students: Required—TOEFL (minimum score 600 paper-based). Electronic applications accepted. *Faculty research:* Stress in nurse anesthesia, economic changes and continuing education.

Middle Tennessee School of Anesthesia, Graduate Programs, Madison, TN 37116. Offers anesthesia (MS, DNAP). *Accreditation:* AANA/CANAEP. *Faculty:* 6 full-time (2 women), 13 part-time/adjunct (4 women). *Students:* 144 full-time (72 women). *Degree requirements:* For master's, project; for doctorate, capstone project. *Entrance requirements:* For master's, GRE General Test, RN license, 1 year of critical-care nursing experience, BSN, general chemistry (minimum of 3 semester hours). *Application deadline:* For fall admission, 10/31 for domestic students. Applications are processed on a rolling basis. *Financial support:* Traineeships available. *Unit head:* Dr. Chris Hulin, Dean and Program Administrator, 615-732-7841, Fax: 615-732-7676, E-mail: chris.hulin@mtsa.edu. *Application contact:* Pam Nimmo, Admissions, 615-868-6503, Fax: 615-732-7662, E-mail: pam@mtsa.edu.
Website: http://www.mtsa.edu/

Midwestern University, Glendale Campus, College of Health Sciences, Arizona Campus, Program in Nurse Anesthesia, Glendale, AZ 85308. Offers MS. *Accreditation:* AANA/CANAEP. *Expenses:* Contact institution.

Millikin University, School of Nursing, Decatur, IL 62522-2084. Offers entry into nursing practice (MSN); nurse anesthesia (DNP); nurse educator (MSN); nursing practice (DNP). *Accreditation:* AACN; AANA/CANAEP. *Program availability:* Part-time. *Faculty:* 11 full-time (all women), 4 part-time/adjunct (3 women). *Students:* 44 full-time (27 women), 14 part-time (13 women); includes 9 minority (5 Black or African American, non-Hispanic/Latino; 1 American Indian or Alaska Native, non-Hispanic/Latino; 1 Asian, non-Hispanic/Latino; 1 Hispanic/Latino; 1 Two or more races, non-Hispanic/Latino), 1 international. Average age 32. 117 applicants, 29% accepted, 26 enrolled. In 2015, 15 master's awarded. *Degree requirements:* For master's, thesis or alternative, scholarly project; for doctorate, thesis/dissertation or alternative, scholarly project. *Entrance requirements:* For master's, GRE, official academic transcript(s), essay, immunizations, statistics course, 3 letters of recommendation, CPR certification, professional liability/malpractice insurance; for doctorate, GRE (if undergraduate cumulative GPA is below 3.0), official academic transcript(s); undergraduate courses in nursing research, health assessment, inorganic and organic chemistry, intro to statistics; graduate-level statistics; 3 written recommendations; Assessment of Critical Care Skills form; written statement; resume or curriculum vitae. Additional exam requirements/recommendations for international students: Required—TOEFL (minimum score 650 paper-based; 81 iBT). *Application deadline:* For spring admission, 7/1 priority date for domestic and international students; for summer admission, 11/1 priority date for domestic and international students. Applications are processed on a rolling basis. Application fee: $0. Electronic applications accepted. *Expenses:* Contact institution. *Financial support:* Traineeships and unspecified assistantships available. Financial award applicants required to submit FAFSA. *Faculty research:* Quality of life, transcultural nursing issues, teaching/learning strategies, clinical simulation. *Unit head:* Dr. Pamela Lindsey, Director, 217-424-6348, Fax: 217-420-6731, E-mail: plindsey@millikin.edu. *Application contact:* Bonnie Niemeyer, Administrative Assistant, 800-373-7733 Ext. 5034, Fax: 217-420-6677, E-mail: bniemeyer@millikin.edu.
Website: http://www.millikin.edu/grad-nursing

Missouri State University, Graduate College, College of Health and Human Services, Department of Biomedical Sciences, Program in Nurse Anesthesia, Springfield, MO 65897. Offers DNAP. *Accreditation:* AANA/CANAEP. *Students:* 48 full-time (27 women), 24 part-time (19 women); includes 8 minority (4 Black or African American, non-Hispanic/Latino; 2 American Indian or Alaska Native, non-Hispanic/Latino; 1 Asian, non-Hispanic/Latino; 1 Hispanic/Latino). Average age 34. 26 applicants. *Entrance requirements:* Additional exam requirements/recommendations for international students: Required—TOEFL (minimum score 550 paper-based; 79 iBT), IELTS (minimum score 6). *Application deadline:* For fall admission, 11/1 for domestic and international students; for spring admission, 7/1 for domestic and international students. Application fee: $35 ($50 for international students). Electronic applications accepted.

Expenses: Tuition, state resident: full-time $5500. Tuition, nonresident: full-time $10,108. *Required fees:* $1000. *Financial support:* In 2015–16, 2 teaching assistantships with full tuition reimbursements (averaging $8,600 per year) were awarded; career-related internships or fieldwork and institutionally sponsored loans also available. Support available to part-time students. Financial award application deadline: 3/31; financial award applicants required to submit FAFSA. *Unit head:* Monika Feeney, Program Director, 417-838-5603, Fax: 417-836-5588, E-mail: monikafeeney@missouristate.edu.

Mount Marty College, Graduate Studies Division, Yankton, SD 57078-3724. Offers business administration (MBA); nurse anesthesia (MS); nursing (MSN); pastoral ministries (MPM). *Accreditation:* AANA/CANAEP (one or more programs are accredited). *Degree requirements:* For master's, thesis or alternative. *Entrance requirements:* For master's, GRE General Test, minimum GPA of 3.0. Electronic applications accepted. *Faculty research:* Clinical anesthesia, professional characteristics, motivations of applicants.

Murray State University, College of Health Sciences and Human Services, Program in Nursing, Murray, KY 42071. Offers clinical nurse specialist (MSN); family nurse practitioner (MSN); nurse anesthesia (MSN). *Accreditation:* AACN; AANA/CANAEP. *Degree requirements:* For master's, research project. *Entrance requirements:* For master's, GRE General Test, BSN, interview, RN licensure. Additional exam requirements/recommendations for international students: Required—TOEFL (minimum score 550 paper-based). *Faculty research:* Fibromyalgis, primary care, rural health.

National University, Academic Affairs, School of Health and Human Services, La Jolla, CA 92037-1011. Offers clinical affairs (MS); clinical informatics (Certificate); clinical regulatory affairs (MS); health and life science analytics (MS); health coaching (Certificate); health informatics (MS); healthcare administration (MHA); nurse anesthesia (MS); nursing (MS), including forensic nursing, nursing administration, nursing informatics; nursing administration (Certificate); nursing informatics (Certificate); nursing practice (DNP); public health (MPH), including health promotion, healthcare administration, mental health. *Program availability:* Part-time, evening/weekend, 100% online, blended/hybrid learning. *Faculty:* 31 full-time (18 women), 33 part-time/adjunct (20 women). *Students:* 353 full-time (263 women), 136 part-time (87 women); includes 322 minority (111 Black or African American, non-Hispanic/Latino; 1 American Indian or Alaska Native, non-Hispanic/Latino; 105 Asian, non-Hispanic/Latino; 72 Hispanic/Latino; 7 Native Hawaiian or other Pacific Islander, non-Hispanic/Latino; 26 Two or more races, non-Hispanic/Latino), 31 international. Average age 36. In 2015, 103 master's awarded. *Degree requirements:* For master's, thesis (for some programs). *Entrance requirements:* For master's, interview, minimum GPA of 2.5. Additional exam requirements/recommendations for international students: Required—TOEFL (minimum score 550 paper-based; 79 iBT), IELTS (minimum score 6). *Application deadline:* Applications are processed on a rolling basis. Application fee: $60 ($65 for international students). Electronic applications accepted. *Financial support:* Career-related internships or fieldwork, institutionally sponsored loans, scholarships/grants, and tuition waivers (partial) available. Support available to part-time students. Financial award application deadline: 6/30; financial award applicants required to submit FAFSA. *Faculty research:* Nursing education, obesity prevention, workforce diversity. *Unit head:* School of Health and Human Services, 800-628-8648, E-mail: shhs@nu.edu. *Application contact:* Frank Rojas, Vice President for Enrollment Services, 800-628-8648, E-mail: advisor@nu.edu.
Website: http://www.nu.edu/OurPrograms/SchoolOfHealthAndHumanServices.html

Newman University, School of Nursing and Allied Health, Wichita, KS 67213-2097. Offers nurse anesthesia (MS). *Accreditation:* AANA/CANAEP. *Degree requirements:* For master's, thesis optional. *Entrance requirements:* For master's, GRE General Test, registered professional nursing license in Kansas, 3 professional recommendations, 1-page letter detailing professional and educational goals, BSN, statistics course, 1 year of employment, interview. Additional exam requirements/recommendations for international students: Required—TOEFL (minimum score 600 paper-based; 100 iBT). Electronic applications accepted. *Expenses:* Contact institution.

Northeastern University, Bouvé College of Health Sciences, Boston, MA 02115-5096. Offers applied behavior analysis (MS, CAGS); audiology (Au D); biomedical nanotechnology (MS); college student development and counseling (MS, CAGS); counseling psychology (MS, PhD, CAGS); exercise science (MS); health informatics (MS); medicinal chemistry (MS); nurse anesthesia (DNP, CAGS); nursing (MS, PhD, CAGS), including administration (MS), adult-gerontology acute care nurse practitioner (MS, CAGS), adult-gerontology primary care nurse practitioner (MS, CAGS), anesthesia (MS), family nurse practitioner (MS, CAGS), neonatal nurse practitioner (MS, CAGS), pediatric nurse practitioner (MS, CAGS), psychiatric mental health nurse practitioner (MS, CAGS); nursing practice (DNP); personal health informatics (PhD); pharmaceutical sciences (MS, PhD), including interdisciplinary concentration, pharmaceutics and drug delivery systems; pharmacology (MS); pharmacy (Pharm D); physical therapy (Postbaccalaureate Certificate); physician assistant (MS); population health (PhD); school psychology (MS, PhD, CAGS); speech-language pathology (MS); urban health (MPH); MS/MBA. *Accreditation:* ACPE (one or more programs are accredited). *Program availability:* Part-time, evening/weekend, online learning. *Faculty:* 194 full-time (120 women), 169 part-time/adjunct (136 women). *Students:* 1,416 full-time (1,049 women), 310 part-time (248 women). In 2015, 374 master's, 313 doctorates, 37 other advanced degrees awarded. *Degree requirements:* For doctorate, thesis/dissertation (for some programs); for other advanced degree, comprehensive exam. Application fee: $75. Electronic applications accepted. *Expenses:* Contact institution. *Financial support:* Applicants required to submit FAFSA. *Unit head:* John R. Reynolds, Professor and Interim Dean, 617-373-3323, Fax: 617-373-3030. *Application contact:* Molly Schnabel, Senior Director of Graduate Affairs, 617-373-2708, Fax: 617-373-4701, E-mail: bouvegrad@neu.edu.
Website: http://www.northeastern.edu/bouve/

Oakland University, Graduate Study and Lifelong Learning, School of Nursing, Program in Nurse Anesthetist, Rochester, MI 48309-4401. Offers nurse anesthesia (MSN, PMC). Programs offered jointly with Beaumont Hospital Corporation. *Accreditation:* AACN; AANA/CANAEP. *Students:* 55 full-time (34 women), 4 part-time (3 women); includes 4 minority (1 Black or African American, non-Hispanic/Latino; 3 Asian, non-Hispanic/Latino). Average age 29. 159 applicants, 18% accepted, 20 enrolled. In 2015, 17 master's awarded. *Degree requirements:* For master's, thesis (for some programs). *Entrance requirements:* For master's, GRE General Test. Additional exam requirements/recommendations for international students: Required—TOEFL (minimum score 550 paper-based). *Application deadline:* For fall admission, 10/15 for domestic and international students. Application fee: $0. Electronic applications accepted. *Expenses:* Contact institution. *Financial support:* Federal Work-Study, institutionally sponsored loans, and tuition waivers (full) available. Financial award application deadline: 3/1; financial award applicants required to submit FAFSA. *Unit head:* Dr. Anne Hranchook, Assistant Professor/Director of the Nurse Anesthesia Program, 248-364-8708, E-mail: hranchoo@oakland.edu.

Old Dominion University, College of Health Sciences, School of Nursing, Nurse Anesthesia Program, Norfolk, VA 23464. Offers MSN. *Faculty:* 2 full-time (1 woman), 2 part-time/adjunct (1 woman). *Students:* 35 full-time (29 women), 1 part-time (0 women); includes 6 minority (2 Black or African American, non-Hispanic/Latino; 1

Asian, non-Hispanic/Latino; 2 Hispanic/Latino; 1 Two or more races, non-Hispanic/Latino). Average age 32. 45 applicants, 33% accepted, 13 enrolled. In 2015, 9 master's awarded. *Degree requirements:* For master's, comprehensive exam, statistics, organic chemistry. *Entrance requirements:* For master's, GRE. *Application deadline:* For fall admission, 10/1 priority date for domestic students; for spring admission, 3/15 for domestic and international students. Applications are processed on a rolling basis. Application fee: $50. Electronic applications accepted. *Expenses:* Contact institution. *Faculty research:* Wellness, pain, anesthesia hand off. *Unit head:* Dr. Nathaniel Michael Apatov, Graduate Program Director, 757-368-4174, Fax: 757-386-4176, E-mail: napatov@odu.edu. *Application contact:* Sue Parker, Coordinator, Graduate Student Services, 757-683-4298, Fax: 757-683-5253, E-mail: sparker@odu.edu.
Website: http://catalog.odu.edu/graduate/collegeofhealthsciences/schoolofnursing/#masterofscienceinnursing013nurseanesthesiarole

Oregon Health & Science University, School of Nursing, Program in Nurse Anesthesia, Portland, OR 97239-3098. Offers MN, MS. *Accreditation:* AANA/CANAEP.

Otterbein University, Department of Nursing, Westerville, OH 43081. Offers advanced practice nurse educator (Certificate); clinical nurse leader (MSN); family nurse practitioner (MSN, Certificate); nurse anesthesia (MSN, Certificate); nursing (DNP); nursing service administration (MSN). *Accreditation:* AACN; AANA/CANAEP; ACEN. *Program availability:* Part-time, evening/weekend, online learning. *Degree requirements:* For master's, comprehensive exam (for some programs), thesis (for some programs). *Entrance requirements:* For master's, 2 reference forms, resume; for Certificate, official transcripts, 2 reference forms, essay, resumé. Additional exam requirements/recommendations for international students: Required—TOEFL (minimum score 550 paper-based; 79 iBT). *Faculty research:* Patient education, women's health, trauma curriculum development, administration.

Our Lady of the Lake College, School of Nursing, Program in Nurse Anesthesia, Baton Rouge, LA 70808. Offers MS. *Accreditation:* AANA/CANAEP. *Degree requirements:* For master's, clinical practicum. *Entrance requirements:* For master's, GRE, current RN license; baccalaureate degree in nursing; 1 year of full-time experience (2 years preferred) as RN in adult critical care setting (adult intensive care unit preferred); minimum cumulative GPA of 3.0; one undergraduate or graduate chemistry course. Additional exam requirements/recommendations for international students: Required—TOEFL.

Quinnipiac University, School of Nursing, Post-Bachelor's Nurse Anesthesia Track, Hamden, CT 06518-1940. Offers DNP. *Faculty:* 19 full-time (18 women), 13 part-time/adjunct (9 women). *Students:* 16 full-time (11 women); includes 6 minority (2 Black or African American, non-Hispanic/Latino; 3 Asian, non-Hispanic/Latino; 1 Hispanic/Latino). 41 applicants, 41% accepted, 11 enrolled. *Application deadline:* For summer admission, 10/15 for domestic students. Applications are processed on a rolling basis. Application fee: $45. Electronic applications accepted. *Expenses:* $985 per credit tuition; $40 per credit student fee (not to exceed $360 per semester); $340 per semester (fall/spring) full-time technology and lab fee; $75 per semester summer technology and lab fee. *Financial support:* Federal Work-Study, scholarships/grants, and unspecified assistantships available. Financial award applicants required to submit FAFSA. *Unit head:* Judy Thompson, Program Director, E-mail: judy.thompson@quinnipiac.edu. *Application contact:* Office of Graduate Admissions, 800-462-1944, Fax: 203-582-3443, E-mail: graduate@quinnipiac.edu.
Website: http://www.quinnipiac.edu/academics/colleges-schools-and-departments/school-of-nursing/programs-of-study/graduate-programs/doctor-of-nursing-practice/

Quinnipiac University, School of Nursing, Post-Master's Nurse Anesthesia Track, Hamden, CT 06518-1940. Offers DNP. *Program availability:* Part-time, online only. *Faculty:* 19 full-time (18 women), 13 part-time/adjunct (9 women). *Students:* 11 part-time (7 women); includes 3 minority (all Black or African American, non-Hispanic/Latino). 8 applicants, 88% accepted, 6 enrolled. *Entrance requirements:* For doctorate, bachelor's degree in nursing or another field; master's degree; CRNA, BCLS, and ACLS certifications. *Application deadline:* Applications are processed on a rolling basis. Application fee: $45. Electronic applications accepted. *Expenses:* $985 per credit tuition; $40 per credit student fee (not to exceed $360 per semester); $340 per semester (fall/spring) part-time technology and lab fee; $75 per semester summer technology and lab fee. *Financial support:* Federal Work-Study and scholarships/grants available. Support available to part-time students. Financial award application deadline: 6/1; financial award applicants required to submit FAFSA. *Unit head:* Judy Thompson, 203-582-8875, E-mail: judy.thompson@quinnipiac.edu. *Application contact:* Quinnipiac University Online Admissions Office, 203-582-3918, E-mail: quonlineadmissions@quinnipiac.edu.
Website: https://quonline.quinnipiac.edu/online-programs/online-doctorate-programs/doctor-of-nursing-practice/nurse-anesthesia-track/

Rosalind Franklin University of Medicine and Science, College of Health Professions, Nurse Anesthesia Department, North Chicago, IL 60064-3095. Offers DNAP. *Accreditation:* AANA/CANAEP. *Entrance requirements:* For doctorate, interview. Additional exam requirements/recommendations for international students: Required—TOEFL. Electronic applications accepted. *Faculty research:* Patient safety, pediatric anesthesia, instructional technology.

Rush University, College of Nursing, Department of Adult Health and Gerontological Nursing, Chicago, IL 60612. Offers adult gerontology acute care clinical nurse specialist (DNP); adult gerontology acute care nurse practitioner (DNP); adult gerontology primary care clinical nurse specialist (DNP); adult gerontology primary care nurse practitioner (DNP); nurse anesthesia (DNP). *Accreditation:* AACN; AANA/CANAEP. *Program availability:* Part-time, 100% online. *Faculty:* 43 full-time (40 women), 52 part-time/adjunct (49 women). *Students:* 50 full-time (33 women), 193 part-time (171 women); includes 52 minority (11 Black or African American, non-Hispanic/Latino; 27 Asian, non-Hispanic/Latino; 14 Hispanic/Latino). Average age 33. 167 applicants, 41% accepted, 47 enrolled. *Degree requirements:* For doctorate, capstone project (for DNP); dissertation (for PhD). *Entrance requirements:* For doctorate, GRE General Test (for DNP in nurse anesthesia; waived if cumulative GPA is 3.25 or greater, nursing GPA is 3.0 or greater, or a completed graduate program GPA is 3.5 or greater), interview, 3 letters of recommendation, personal statement, current resume. Additional exam requirements/recommendations for international students: Required—TOEFL (minimum score 94 iBT). *Application deadline:* For fall admission, 1/2 for domestic students; for spring admission, 8/3 for domestic students; for summer admission, 12/1 for domestic students. Applications are processed on a rolling basis. Application fee: $100. Electronic applications accepted. *Expenses:* Contact institution. *Financial support:* Research assistantships, teaching assistantships, Federal Work-Study, institutionally sponsored loans, scholarships/grants, traineeships, and health care benefits available. Support available to part-time students. Financial award application deadline: 3/1; financial award applicants required to submit FAFSA. *Faculty research:* Physical activity adherence in African-American women; reduction of health disparities; evidence-based interventions for caregivers; fish oil for HIV-related immunosenescence; BAILA: Being Active, Increasing Latinos Health Aging. *Unit head:* Dr. Elizabeth Carlson, Chairperson, 312-942-7117, E-mail: elizabeth_carlson@rush.edu. *Application contact:* Jennifer Thorndyke, Admissions Specialist, 312-563-7526, E-mail: jennifer_thorndyke@rush.edu.
Website: http://www.rushu.rush.edu/servlet/

Satellite?c=RushUnivLevel1Page&cid=1204497838852&pagename=Rush%2FRushUnivLevel1Page%2FLevel_1_College_Home_Page

Rutgers University–Newark, Rutgers School of Nursing, Newark, NJ 07107-3001. Offers adult health (MSN); adult occupational health (MSN); advanced practice nursing (MSN, Post Master's Certificate); family nurse practitioner (MSN); nurse anesthesia (MSN); nursing (MSN); nursing informatics (MSN); urban health (PhD); women's health practitioner (MSN). *Accreditation:* AANA/CANAEP. *Program availability:* Part-time. *Entrance requirements:* For master's, GRE, RN license; basic life support, statistics, and health assessment experience. Additional exam requirements/recommendations for international students: Required—TOEFL. Electronic applications accepted. *Expenses:* Contact institution. *Faculty research:* HIV/AIDS, diabetes education, learned helplessness, nursing science, psychoeducation.

Saint Joseph's University, College of Arts and Sciences, Department of Health Services, Philadelphia, PA 19131-1395. Offers health administration (MS); health education (MS); healthcare ethics (MS); long-term care administration (MS); nurse anesthesia (MS); school nurse certification (MS). *Program availability:* Part-time, evening/weekend. *Entrance requirements:* For master's, GRE (if GPA less than 3.0), 2 letters of recommendation, resume, personal statement, official transcripts. Additional exam requirements/recommendations for international students: Required—TOEFL (minimum score 550 paper-based; 80 iBT), IELTS (minimum score 6.5). Electronic applications accepted.

Saint Mary's University of Minnesota, Schools of Graduate and Professional Programs, Graduate School of Health and Human Services, Nurse Anesthesia Program, Winona, MN 55987-1399. Offers MS. Program offered jointly with the Minneapolis School of Anesthesia. *Accreditation:* AANA/CANAEP. Tuition and fees vary according to degree level and program. *Unit head:* Merri Moody, Director, 612-728-5133. *Application contact:* James Callinan, Director of Admissions for Graduate and Professional Programs, 612-728-5185, Fax: 612-728-5121, E-mail: jcallina@smumn.edu.
Website: http://www.smumn.edu/graduate-home/areas-of-study/graduate-school-of-health-human-services/ms-in-nurse-anesthesia

Saint Vincent College, Program in Health Science, Latrobe, PA 15650-2690. Offers nurse anesthesia (MS).

Samford University, Ida V. Moffett School of Nursing, Birmingham, AL 35229. Offers administration (DNP); advanced practice (DNP); family nurse practitioner (MSN); health systems management and leadership (MSN); nurse anesthesia (MSN); nurse educator (MSN). *Accreditation:* AACN; AANA/CANAEP (one or more programs are accredited). *Program availability:* Part-time, blended/hybrid learning. *Faculty:* 19 full-time (all women), 5 part-time/adjunct (1 woman). *Students:* 300 full-time (228 women), 40 part-time (36 women); includes 65 minority (28 Black or African American, non-Hispanic/Latino; 4 American Indian or Alaska Native, non-Hispanic/Latino; 8 Asian, non-Hispanic/Latino; 13 Hispanic/Latino; 12 Two or more races, non-Hispanic/Latino). Average age 35. 69 applicants, 77% accepted, 52 enrolled. In 2015, 98 master's, 16 doctorates awarded. *Degree requirements:* For doctorate, capstone project with oral presentation. *Entrance requirements:* For master's, MAT; GRE (for nurse anesthesia), unencumbered licensure as registered nurse; BSN from CCNE, CNEA, or ACEN (formerly NLNAC) accredited program; minimum cumulative GPA of 3.0 in nursing courses; video submission; one undergraduate course in nursing research with minimum grade of C; for doctorate, unencumbered licensure as registered nurse; master's degree from CCNE, CNEA or ACEN (formerly NLNAC) accredited program in the area of advanced practice or administration; minimum master's degree cumulative GPA of 3.5; video interview submission. Additional exam requirements/recommendations for international students: Required—TOEFL (minimum score 550 paper-based; 80 iBT). *Application deadline:* For fall admission, 6/1 for domestic and international students; for spring admission, 9/1 for domestic and international students. Application fee: $65. Electronic applications accepted. *Expenses:* Tuition, area resident: Full-time $18,673; part-time $766 per credit hour. *Required fees:* $550. Tuition and fees vary according to course load, degree level and student level. *Financial support:* In 2015–16, 56 students received support. Institutionally sponsored loans, scholarships/grants, and traineeships available. Financial award application deadline: 3/1; financial award applicants required to submit FAFSA. *Faculty research:* Issues in rural health care, vulnerable populations, genetics and disabilities in pediatrics, geriatrics, parish nursing research, interprofessional education, global health disparities. *Unit head:* Dr. Nena F. Sanders, Vice Provost, College of Health Sciences/Dean/Professor, 205-726-2612, Fax: 205-726-4179, E-mail: nfsander@samford.edu. *Application contact:* Allyson Maddox, Director of Graduate Student Services, Ida V. Moffett School of Nursing, 205-726-2047, Fax: 205-726-4179, E-mail: amaddox@samford.edu.
Website: http://samford.edu/nursing

Samuel Merritt University, School of Nursing, Oakland, CA 94609. Offers case management (MSN); family nurse practitioner (MSN, Certificate); nurse anesthetist (MSN, Certificate); nursing (DNP). *Accreditation:* AACN; AANA/CANAEP (one or more programs are accredited). *Program availability:* Part-time, evening/weekend, 100% online, blended/hybrid learning. *Faculty:* 47 full-time (40 women), 50 part-time/adjunct (43 women). *Students:* 437 full-time (350 women), 59 part-time (45 women); includes 327 minority (29 Black or African American, non-Hispanic/Latino; 3 American Indian or Alaska Native, non-Hispanic/Latino; 163 Asian, non-Hispanic/Latino; 95 Hispanic/Latino; 9 Native Hawaiian or other Pacific Islander, non-Hispanic/Latino; 28 Two or more races, non-Hispanic/Latino). Average age 33. 392 applicants, 43% accepted, 126 enrolled. In 2015, 31 master's awarded. *Degree requirements:* For master's, thesis or alternative. *Entrance requirements:* For master's, minimum GPA of 2.5 in science, 3.0 overall; previous course work in statistics; current RN license. Additional exam requirements/recommendations for international students: Required—TOEFL (minimum score 100 iBT). *Application deadline:* For fall admission, 1/1 priority date for domestic students; for spring admission, 7/1 for domestic students; for summer admission, 1/1 for domestic students. Applications are processed on a rolling basis. Application fee: $50. Electronic applications accepted. *Expenses:* $61,299 tuition; $240 lab fees; $160 graduation fee. *Financial support:* In 2015–16, 34 students received support. Career-related internships or fieldwork, Federal Work-Study, scholarships/grants, and traineeships available. Support available to part-time students. Financial award application deadline: 3/2; financial award applicants required to submit FAFSA. *Faculty research:* Gerontology, community health, maternal-child health, sexually transmitted diseases, substance abuse, oncology. *Total annual research expenditures:* $35,000. *Unit head:* Dr. Audrey Berman, Graduate Coordinator, 510-869-6733, Fax: 510-869-6525. *Application contact:* Timothy Cranford, Dean of Admission, 510-869-6576, Fax: 510-869-6525, E-mail: admission@samuelmerritt.edu.
Website: http://www.samuelmerritt.edu/nursing

Southern Illinois University Edwardsville, Graduate School, School of Nursing, Doctor of Nursing Practice Program, Edwardsville, IL 62026. Offers family nurse practitioner (DNP); nurse anesthesia (DNP); nursing (DNP). *Program availability:* Part-time, evening/weekend. *Students:* 37 full-time (25 women), 33 part-time (31 women); includes 14 minority (6 Black or African American, non-Hispanic/Latino; 3 Asian, non-Hispanic/Latino; 4 Hispanic/Latino; 1 Two or more races, non-Hispanic/Latino). 57 applicants, 79% accepted. In 2015, 5 doctorates awarded. *Degree requirements:* For doctorate, thesis/dissertation or alternative, project. *Entrance requirements:* Additional

Nurse Anesthesia

exam requirements/recommendations for international students: Required—TOEFL (minimum score 550 paper-based; 79 iBT), IELTS (minimum score 6.5). *Application deadline:* For fall and spring admission, 3/1 for domestic and international students; for summer admission, 3/1 for domestic and international students. Application fee: $30. Electronic applications accepted. *Expenses:* Tuition, state resident: full-time $5026; part-time $837 per course. Tuition, nonresident: full-time $12,566; part-time $2094 per course. *Required fees:* $1682; $474 per course. Tuition and fees vary according to course load, campus/location and program. *Financial support:* Institutionally sponsored loans, scholarships/grants, and unspecified assistantships available. Financial award application deadline: 3/1; financial award applicants required to submit FAFSA. *Unit head:* Dr. Kathy Ketchum, Assistant Dean for Graduate Programs, 618-650-3975, Fax: 618-650-3854, E-mail: kketchu@siue.edu. *Application contact:* Bob Skorczewski, Coordinator of International and Graduate Recruitment, 618-650-3705, Fax: 618-650-3618, E-mail: gradadmissions@siue.edu.
Website: http://www.siue.edu/nursing/graduate/dnp/

State University of New York Downstate Medical Center, College of Nursing, Graduate Program in Nursing, Program in Nurse Anesthesia, Brooklyn, NY 11203-2098. Offers MS. *Accreditation:* AACN; AANA/CANAEP. *Degree requirements:* For master's, thesis optional. *Entrance requirements:* For master's, GRE, BSN; minimum GPA of 3.0; previous undergraduate course work in statistics, health assessment, and nursing research; RN license.

Texas Christian University, Harris College of Nursing and Health Sciences, School of Nurse Anesthesia, Fort Worth, TX 76129. Offers DNP-A. *Faculty:* 11 full-time (5 women). *Students:* 168 full-time (104 women); includes 33 minority (2 Black or African American, non-Hispanic/Latino; 2 American Indian or Alaska Native, non-Hispanic/Latino; 13 Asian, non-Hispanic/Latino; 12 Hispanic/Latino; 4 Two or more races, non-Hispanic/Latino). Average age 30. 194 applicants, 40% accepted, 63 enrolled. In 2015, 34 doctorates awarded. *Entrance requirements:* For doctorate, GRE General Test, writing sample. Additional exam requirements/recommendations for international students: Required—TOEFL (minimum score 600 paper-based; 94 iBT). *Application deadline:* For fall and spring admission, 7/1 for domestic and international students. Applications are processed on a rolling basis. Application fee: $60. Electronic applications accepted. *Expenses:* Contact institution. *Financial support:* Applicants required to submit FAFSA. *Faculty research:* Anesthesia, genetics. *Unit head:* Dr. Kay K. Sanders, Director, 817-257-7887, Fax: 817-257-5472, E-mail: k.sanders@tcu.edu. *Application contact:* Renee Gist, Administrative Assistant, 817-257-7887, Fax: 817-257-5472, E-mail: r.gist@tcu.edu.
Website: http://www.crna.tcu.edu/

Texas Wesleyan University, Graduate Programs, Programs in Nurse Anesthesia, Fort Worth, TX 76105-1536. Offers MHS, MSNA, DNAP. *Accreditation:* AANA/CANAEP (one or more programs are accredited). *Faculty:* 9 full-time (4 women), 1 part-time/adjunct (0 women). *Students:* 392 full-time (207 women); includes 109 minority (18 Black or African American, non-Hispanic/Latino; 4 American Indian or Alaska Native, non-Hispanic/Latino; 29 Asian, non-Hispanic/Latino; 48 Hispanic/Latino; 10 Two or more races, non-Hispanic/Latino), 1 international. Average age 32. 470 applicants, 34% accepted, 142 enrolled. In 2015, 103 master's, 22 doctorates awarded. *Entrance requirements:* For master's, GRE General Test, bachelor's degree, minimum GPA of 3.0, college-level chemistry within three years of start date, current unrestricted RN license valid in one of the 50 states or U.S. territories, minimum of one year of full-time critical care, current ACLS and PALS certifications; for doctorate, master's degree, RN license, CRNA Certification/Recertification, minimum GPA of 3.0 overall or on last 60 hours, graduate-level research course with minimum grade of B, current curriculum vitae. *Application deadline:* For fall admission, 10/15 priority date for domestic students. Applications are processed on a rolling basis. Application fee: $58. Electronic applications accepted. *Expenses:* $1,083 per credit hour (master's porgram); $1,094 per credit hour (doctoral program). *Financial support:* Federal Work-Study, institutionally sponsored loans, scholarships/grants, and tuition waivers (full and partial) available. Support available to part-time students. Financial award application deadline: 3/15; financial award applicants required to submit FAFSA. *Unit head:* Debra Maloy, Director, 817-531-4406, Fax: 817-531-6508, E-mail: dmaloy@txwes.edu. *Application contact:* Tommie Kates, Coordinator, 817-531-4279, Fax: 817-531-6508, E-mail: tkates@txwes.edu.
Website: http://www.txwes.edu/academics/gpna

Uniformed Services University of the Health Sciences, Daniel K. Inouye Graduate School of Nursing, Bethesda, MD 20814. Offers adult-gerontology clinical nurse specialist (MSN, DNP); family nurse practitioner (DNP); nurse anesthesia (DNP); nursing science (PhD); psychiatric mental health nurse practitioner (DNP); women's health nurse practitioner (DNP). MSN and DNP programs available to military officers only; PhD to military and DoD students only. *Accreditation:* AACN; AANA/CANAEP. *Faculty:* 38 full-time (22 women), 2 part-time/adjunct (1 woman). *Students:* 51 full-time (29 women); includes 17 minority (8 Black or African American, non-Hispanic/Latino; 4 Asian, non-Hispanic/Latino; 4 Hispanic/Latino; 1 Two or more races, non-Hispanic/Latino). Average age 34. 75 applicants, 68% accepted, 51 enrolled. In 2015, 4 master's, 24 doctorates awarded. *Degree requirements:* For master's, thesis or alternative; for doctorate, thesis/dissertation or alternative. *Entrance requirements:* For master's, GRE, BSN, clinical experience, minimum GPA of 3.0, previous course work in science; for doctorate, GRE, BSN, clinical experience, minimum GPA of 3.0, previous course work in sciences, and writing paper (for DNP); MSN (for PhD). *Application deadline:* For fall admission, 7/1 for domestic students; for winter admission, 2/15 for domestic students. Application fee: $0. Electronic applications accepted. *Faculty research:* Prenatal care, military health care, military readiness, distance learning. *Unit head:* Dr. Diane C. Seibert, Associate Dean for Academic Affairs, 301-295-1080, Fax: 301-295-1707, E-mail: diane.seibert@usuhs.edu. *Application contact:* Terry Lynn Malavakis, Recording Secretary for Admissions Committee/Registrar/Program Analyst, 301-295-1055, Fax: 301-295-1707, E-mail: terry.malavakis@usuhs.edu.
Website: http://www.usuhs.edu/gsn/

Union University, School of Nursing, Jackson, TN 38305-3697. Offers executive leadership (DNP); nurse anesthesia (DNP); nurse practitioner (DNP); nursing education (MSN, PMC). *Accreditation:* AACN; AANA/CANAEP. *Degree requirements:* For master's, thesis or alternative. *Entrance requirements:* For master's, GRE, 3 letters of reference, bachelor's degree in nursing, minimum GPA of 3.0. Additional exam requirements/recommendations for international students: Required—TOEFL (minimum score 560 paper-based). Electronic applications accepted. *Faculty research:* Children's health, occupational rehabilitation, informatics, health promotion.

University at Buffalo, the State University of New York, Graduate School, School of Nursing, Buffalo, NY 14214. Offers adult gerontology nurse practitioner (DNP); family nurse practitioner (DNP); health care systems and leadership (MS); nurse anesthetist (DNP); nursing (PhD); nursing education (Certificate); psychiatric/mental health nurse practitioner (DNP). *Accreditation:* AACN; AANA/CANAEP (one or more programs are accredited). *Program availability:* Part-time, 100% online. *Students:* 61 full-time (37 women), 137 part-time (114 women); includes 35 minority (17 Black or African American, non-Hispanic/Latino; 1 American Indian or Alaska Native, non-Hispanic/Latino; 17 Asian, non-Hispanic/Latino), 7 international. Average age 32. 193 applicants, 49% accepted, 75 enrolled. In 2015, 6 master's, 37 doctorates awarded. *Degree*

requirements: For master's, thesis optional; for doctorate, comprehensive exam (for some programs), capstone (for DNP), dissertation (for PhD). *Entrance requirements:* For master's, GRE or MAT; for doctorate, GRE or MAT, minimum GPA of 3.0 (for DNP), 3.25 (for PhD); RN license; BS or MS in nursing; 3 references; writing sample; resume; personal statement; for Certificate, interview, minimum GPA of 3.0 or GRE General Test, RN license, MS in nursing, professional certification. Additional exam requirements/recommendations for international students: Required—TOEFL (minimum score 550 paper-based; 79 iBT), IELTS (minimum score 6.5). *Application deadline:* For fall admission, 7/1 for domestic students, 2/1 for international students; for spring admission, 12/1 for domestic students, 10/1 for international students; for summer admission, 2/1 for domestic students. Applications are processed on a rolling basis. Application fee: $75. Electronic applications accepted. *Financial support:* In 2015–16, 80 students received support, including 2 fellowships with tuition reimbursements available (averaging $17,000 per year), 4 research assistantships with tuition reimbursements available (averaging $10,600 per year), 7 teaching assistantships with tuition reimbursements available (averaging $10,600 per year); scholarships/grants, traineeships, health care benefits, and unspecified assistantships also available. Financial award application deadline: 2/1; financial award applicants required to submit FAFSA. *Faculty research:* Oncology, palliative care, gerontology, addictions, mental health, community wellness, sleep, workforce, care of underserved populations, quality and safety, person-centered care, adolescent health. *Total annual research expenditures:* $1.4 million. *Unit head:* Dr. Marsha L. Lewis, Dean and Professor, 716-829-2533, Fax: 716-829-2566, E-mail: ubnursingdean@buffalo.edu. *Application contact:* Jennifer H. VanLaeken, Director of Graduate Student Services, 716-829-3311, Fax: 716-829-2067, E-mail: jhv2@buffalo.edu.
Website: http://nursing.buffalo.edu/

The University of Alabama at Birmingham, School of Nursing, Birmingham, AL 35294. Offers nurse anesthesia (MSN); nursing (MSN, DNP, PhD). *Accreditation:* AACN. *Program availability:* Part-time. Terminal master's awarded for partial completion of doctoral program. *Degree requirements:* For doctorate, thesis/dissertation, research mentorship experience. *Entrance requirements:* For master's, GRE, GMAT, or MAT, BS in nursing; for doctorate, GRE General Test, computer literacy, course work in statistics, interview, minimum GPA of 3.0, MS in nursing, references, writing sample. Additional exam requirements/recommendations for international students: Required—TOEFL. Electronic applications accepted. *Expenses:* Contact institution.

The University of British Columbia, Faculty of Medicine, Department of Anesthesiology, Pharmacology and Therapeutics, Vancouver, BC V6T 1Z3, Canada. Offers M Sc, PhD. Terminal master's awarded for partial completion of doctoral program. *Degree requirements:* For master's, thesis; for doctorate, comprehensive exam, thesis/dissertation. *Entrance requirements:* For master's, MD or appropriate bachelor's degree; for doctorate, MD or M Sc. Additional exam requirements/recommendations for international students: Required—TOEFL (minimum score 600 paper-based; 100 iBT). Electronic applications accepted. *Faculty research:* Cellular, biochemical, autonomic, and cardiovascular pharmacology; neuropharmacology and pulmonary pharmacology.

University of Cincinnati, Graduate School, College of Nursing, Cincinnati, OH 45221-0038. Offers clinical nurse specialist (MSN), including adult health, community health, neonatal, nursing administration, occupational health, pediatric health, psychiatric nursing, women's health; nurse anesthesia (MSN); nurse midwifery (MSN); nurse practitioner (MSN), including acute care, ambulatory care, family, family/psychiatric, women's health; nursing (PhD); MBA/MSN. *Accreditation:* AACN; AANA/CANAEP (one or more programs are accredited); ACNM/ACME. *Program availability:* Part-time, online learning. Terminal master's awarded for partial completion of doctoral program. *Degree requirements:* For master's, thesis or alternative; for doctorate, comprehensive exam, thesis/dissertation. *Entrance requirements:* For master's and doctorate, GRE General Test. Additional exam requirements/recommendations for international students: Required—TOEFL (minimum score 520 paper-based). Electronic applications accepted. *Faculty research:* Substance abuse, injury and violence, symptom management.

University of Detroit Mercy, College of Health Professions, Detroit, MI 48221. Offers clinical nurse leader (MSN); family nurse practitioner (MSN); health services administration (MHSA); health systems management (MSN); nurse anesthesia (MS); nursing (DNP); nursing education (MSN, Certificate); nursing leadership and financial management (Certificate); outcomes performance management (Certificate); physician assistant (MS). *Entrance requirements:* For master's, GRE General Test, minimum GPA of 3.0. Application fee: $30 ($50 for international students). *Expenses:* Tuition, area resident: Full-time $26,802; part-time $1489 per credit. Tuition and fees vary according to course load and program. *Financial support:* Institutionally sponsored loans and tuition waivers (partial) available. Support available to part-time students. Financial award applicants required to submit FAFSA. *Faculty research:* Research design, respiratory physiology, AIDS prevention, adolescent health, community, low income health education. *Unit head:* Dr. Christine M. Pacini, RN, Dean, 313-993-6055, Fax: 313-993-6175.
Website: http://healthprofessions.udmercy.edu/

The University of Kansas, University of Kansas Medical Center, School of Health Professions, Department of Nurse Anesthesia Education, Kansas City, KS 66160. Offers DNAP. *Accreditation:* AANA/CANAEP. *Faculty:* 21. *Students:* 71 full-time (46 women); includes 14 minority (7 Black or African American, non-Hispanic/Latino; 2 American Indian or Alaska Native, non-Hispanic/Latino; 2 Asian, non-Hispanic/Latino; 1 Hispanic/Latino; 2 Two or more races, non-Hispanic/Latino). Average age 30. 94 applicants, 30% accepted, 24 enrolled. In 2015, 21 doctorates awarded. *Degree requirements:* For doctorate, comprehensive exam, thesis/dissertation or alternative. *Entrance requirements:* For doctorate, bachelor's degree in nursing or related field, RN license, 2 years of experience as an RN including 1 year of experience in ICU; five science classes (anatomy, physiology, microbiology and 2 chemistry) and statistics. Additional exam requirements/recommendations for international students: Required—TOEFL. *Application deadline:* For summer admission, 7/15 for domestic and international students. Application fee: $60. Electronic applications accepted. *Expenses:* Contact institution. *Financial support:* In 2015–16, 15 students received support. Application deadline: 3/1; applicants required to submit FAFSA. *Faculty research:* Simulation training. *Unit head:* Dr. Donna S. Nyght, Chair, 913-588-6612, Fax: 913-588-3334, E-mail: dnyght@kumc.edu. *Application contact:* Carrie Hewitt, Administrative Officer, 913-588-6612, Fax: 913-588-3334, E-mail: na@kumc.edu.
Website: http://www.kumc.edu/school-of-health-professions/nurse-anesthesia-education.html

University of Miami, Graduate School, School of Nursing and Health Studies, Coral Gables, FL 33124. Offers acute care (MSN), including acute care nurse practitioner, nurse anesthesia; nursing (PhD); primary care (MSN), including adult nurse practitioner, family nurse practitioner, nurse midwifery, women's health practitioner. *Accreditation:* AACN; AANA/CANAEP; ACNM/ACME (one or more programs are accredited). *Program availability:* Part-time. *Degree requirements:* For master's, thesis optional; for doctorate, thesis/dissertation. *Entrance requirements:* For master's, GRE General Test, BSN, minimum GPA of 3.0, Florida RN license; for doctorate, GRE General Test, BSN or MSN, minimum GPA of 3.0. Additional exam requirements/recommendations for international students: Required—TOEFL (minimum score 550 paper-based). Electronic applications accepted. *Faculty research:* Transcultural nursing, exercise and depression in Alzheimer's disease, infectious diseases/HIV–AIDS, postpartum depression, outcomes assessment.

University of Michigan–Flint, School of Health Professions and Studies, Program in Anesthesia, Flint, MI 48502-1950. Offers MS, DrAP. *Accreditation:* AACN; AANA/ CANAEP. *Program availability:* Part-time. *Faculty:* 2 full-time (1 woman), 11 part-time/ adjunct (5 women). *Students:* 39 full-time (21 women), 47 part-time (31 women); includes 14 minority (3 Black or African American, non-Hispanic/Latino; 5 Asian, non-Hispanic/Latino; 3 Hispanic/Latino; 3 Two or more races, non-Hispanic/Latino), 1 international. Average age 37. 109 applicants, 38% accepted, 31 enrolled. In 2015, 21 master's, 1 doctorate awarded. *Degree requirements:* For master's, thesis. *Entrance requirements:* For master's, GRE, current, unrestricted licensure as Registered Nurse in Michigan or one of the United States or protectorates; bachelor's degree in nursing; for doctorate, master's degree in science, biology, or nursing with focus on nurse anesthesia or post-master's certificate from program accredited by Council on Accreditation of Nurse Anesthesia Educational Programs (CANAEP); minimum overall master's degree GPA of 3.0. Additional exam requirements/recommendations for international students: Required—TOEFL (minimum score 560 paper-based; 84 iBT), IELTS (minimum score 6.5). *Application deadline:* For fall admission, 8/1 for domestic students, 5/1 for international students; for winter admission, 11/15 for domestic students, 9/1 for international students; for spring admission, 3/15 for domestic students, 1/1 for international students. Applications are processed on a rolling basis. Application fee: $55. Electronic applications accepted. *Expenses:* Contact institution. *Financial support:* Federal Work-Study, scholarships/grants, and unspecified assistantships available. Support available to part-time students. Financial award application deadline: 3/1; financial award applicants required to submit FAFSA. *Faculty research:* CRNA expected retirement patterns, factors of importance in CENA selection of first job, lidocaine 4% in ETT cuff and reducing in coughing on emergence, orientation of spinal needle benel, length of time to discharge outpatients. *Unit head:* Dr. Shawn Fryzel, Director, 810-257-9264, Fax: 810-760-0839, E-mail: sfryzel@hurleymc.com. *Application contact:* Bradley T. Maki, Director of Graduate Admissions, 810-762-3171, Fax: 810-766-6789, E-mail: bmaki@umflint.edu.
Website: https://www.umflint.edu/pubhealth/graduate-degrees

University of Minnesota, Twin Cities Campus, Graduate School, School of Nursing, Program in Nurse Anesthetist, Minneapolis, MN 55455-0213. Offers MS. *Accreditation:* AANA/CANAEP. *Entrance requirements:* Additional exam requirements/ recommendations for international students: Required—TOEFL (minimum score 586 paper-based).

University of New England, Westbrook College of Health Professions, Program in Nurse Anesthesia, Biddeford, ME 04005-9526. Offers MS. Program affiliated with St. Joseph's Hospital School of Anesthesia for Nurses, RI. *Accreditation:* AANA/CANAEP. *Faculty:* 2 full-time (both women), 2 part-time/adjunct (1 woman). *Students:* 43 full-time (30 women); includes 10 minority (7 Black or African American, non-Hispanic/Latino; 1 Asian, non-Hispanic/Latino; 1 Hispanic/Latino; 1 Two or more races, non-Hispanic/ Latino), 1 international. Average age 34. 77 applicants, 40% accepted, 20 enrolled. In 2015, 30 master's awarded. *Degree requirements:* For master's, thesis, clinical practicum. *Entrance requirements:* For master's, GRE, RN license, 1 year of acute care experience, 3 letters of reference, Advanced Cardiac Life Support Certification, Pediatric Advanced Life Support Certification. *Application deadline:* For fall admission, 11/1 for domestic and international students. Applications are processed on a rolling basis. Electronic applications accepted. Tuition and fees vary according to degree level and program. *Financial support:* Application deadline: 5/1; applicants required to submit FAFSA. *Unit head:* Maribeth Massie, Program Director/Associate Clinical Professor, 207-221-4519, Fax: 207-523-1900, E-mail: mmassie@une.edu. *Application contact:* Scott Steinberg, Dean of University Admission, 207-221-4225, Fax: 207-523-1925, E-mail: ssteinberg@une.edu.
Website: http://www.une.edu/wchp/sna

The University of North Carolina at Charlotte, College of Health and Human Services, School of Nursing, Charlotte, NC 28223-0001. Offers adult-gerontology acute care nurse practitioner (MSN, Post-Master's Certificate); advanced clinical nursing (MSN); community public health nursing (MSN); family nurse practitioner across the lifespan (MSN, Post-Master's Certificate); nurse anesthesia (MSN, Post-Master's Certificate); nurse administrator (MSN, Graduate Certificate); nurse educator (MSN, Graduate Certificate); nursing (DNP); nursing systems/population (MSN). *Accreditation:* AACN. *Program availability:* Part-time, blended/hybrid learning. *Faculty:* 26 full-time (25 women), 4 part-time/adjunct (3 women). *Students:* 109 full-time (89 women), 112 part-time (107 women); includes 46 minority (37 Black or African American, non-Hispanic/ Latino; 3 Asian, non-Hispanic/Latino; 5 Hispanic/Latino; 1 Two or more races, non-Hispanic/Latino). Average age 33. 321 applicants, 34% accepted, 84 enrolled. In 2015, 76 master's, 4 doctorates, 7 other advanced degrees awarded. Terminal master's awarded for partial completion of doctoral program. *Degree requirements:* For master's, practicum, synthesis and integration or thesis, residency, internship (varies by program); for doctorate, thesis/dissertation or alternative, residency; for other advanced degree, practicum. *Entrance requirements:* For master's, GRE General Test, unencumbered license as Registered Nurse in North Carolina; BSN from nationally-accredited program; one year of professional nursing practice in acute/critical care; minimum overall GPA of 3.0 in the last degree and 60 hours of nursing coursework; completion of an undergraduate statistics course with minimum grade of C; statement of purpose; for doctorate, GRE or MAT, master's degree in nursing in an advanced nursing practice specialty from nationally-accredited program; minimum overall GPA of 3.5 in MSN program; current RN licensure in U.S. at time of application with eligibility for NC licensure; for other advanced degree, GRE. Additional exam requirements/ recommendations for international students: Required—TOEFL (minimum score 557 paper-based, 83 iBT) or IELTS (minimum score 6.5). *Application deadline:* For fall admission, 2/1 for domestic and international students; for spring admission, 10/1 priority date for domestic and international students; for summer admission, 4/1 priority date for domestic and international students. Applications are processed on a rolling basis. Application fee: $75. Electronic applications accepted. *Expenses:* Contact institution. *Financial support:* In 2015–16, 9 students received support, including 5 research assistantships (averaging $4,850 per year), 3 teaching assistantships (averaging $2,911 per year); career-related internships or fieldwork, institutionally sponsored loans, scholarships/grants, traineeships, unspecified assistantships, and administrative assistantships also available. Support available to part-time students. Financial award application deadline: 3/1; financial award applicants required to submit FAFSA. *Faculty research:* Improving care outcomes for the elderly; vulnerable populations; symptom management; self management/health promotion strategies of older adults; migration and maternal child health; health disparities, health literacy, and access to healthcare in Latino adults with diabetes; psychiatric nursing. *Total annual research expenditures:* $875,169. *Unit head:* Dr. Dee Baldwin, Associate Dean, 704-687-7952, Fax: 704-687-6017, E-mail: dbaldwi5@uncc.edu. *Application contact:* Kathy B. Giddings, Director of Graduate Admissions, 704-687-5503, Fax: 704-687-1668, E-mail: gradadm@uncc.edu.
Website: http://nursing.uncc.edu/

The University of North Carolina at Greensboro, Graduate School, School of Nursing, Greensboro, NC 27412-5001. Offers adult clinical nurse specialist (MSN, PMC); adult/gerontological nurse practitioner (MSN, PMC); nurse anesthesia (MSN, PMC); nursing (PhD); nursing administration (MSN); nursing education (MSN); MSN/ MBA. *Accreditation:* AACN; AANA/CANAEP; ACEN. *Degree requirements:* For master's, thesis or alternative. *Entrance requirements:* For master's, GRE General Test or MAT, BSN, clinical experience, liability insurance, RN license; for PMC, liability insurance, MSN, RN license. Additional exam requirements/recommendations for international students: Required—TOEFL. Electronic applications accepted.

University of North Dakota, Graduate School, College of Nursing, Department of Nursing, Grand Forks, ND 58202. Offers adult-gerontological nurse practitioner (MSN); advanced public health nurse (MSN); family nurse practitioner (MSN); nurse anesthesia (MSN); nurse educator (MSN); nursing (DNP, PhD); psychiatric and mental health nurse practitioner (MSN).

University of North Florida, Brooks College of Health, School of Nursing, Jacksonville, FL 32224. Offers clinical nurse leader (MSN); clinical nurse specialist (MSN); family nurse practitioner (Certificate); nurse anesthetist (MSN); nursing practice (DNP); primary care nurse practitioner (MSN). *Accreditation:* AACN; AANA/CANAEP. *Program availability:* Part-time. *Faculty:* 23 full-time (17 women), 2 part-time/adjunct (1 woman). *Students:* 108 full-time (90 women), 117 part-time (93 women); includes 54 minority (17 Black or African American, non-Hispanic/Latino; 1 American Indian or Alaska Native, non-Hispanic/Latino; 13 Asian, non-Hispanic/Latino; 17 Hispanic/Latino; 1 Native Hawaiian or other Pacific Islander, non-Hispanic/Latino; 5 Two or more races, non-Hispanic/Latino), 3 international. Average age 36. 136 applicants, 81% accepted, 74 enrolled. In 2015, 46 master's, 6 doctorates awarded. *Degree requirements:* For master's, thesis optional. *Entrance requirements:* For master's, GRE General Test, minimum GPA of 3.0 in last 60 hours of course work, RSN, clinical experience, resume; for doctorate, GRE, master's degree in nursing specialty from nationally-accredited program; national certification in one of the following APRN roles: CNE, CNM, CNS, CRNA, CNP; minimum graduate GPA of 3.3; three letters of reference which address academic ability and clinical skills; active license as registered nurse or advanced practice registered nurse. Additional exam requirements/recommendations for international students: Required—TOEFL (minimum score 500 paper-based; 61 iBT). *Application deadline:* For fall admission, 3/15 for domestic students, 4/1 for international students. Application fee: $30. Electronic applications accepted. *Expenses:* Tuition, state resident: part-time $408.10 per credit hour. Tuition, nonresident: part-time $932.61 per credit hour. *Required fees:* $111.81 per credit hour. Tuition and fees vary according to course load, campus/location and program. *Financial support:* In 2015–16, 35 students received support. Research assistantships available. Financial award application deadline: 4/1; financial award applicants required to submit FAFSA. *Faculty research:* Teen pregnancy, diabetes, ethical decision-making, family caregivers. *Total annual research expenditures:* $39,413. *Unit head:* Dr. Li Loriz, Chair, 904-620-1053, E-mail: lloriz@unf.edu. *Application contact:* Beth Dibble, Assistant Director of Admissions for Nursing and Physical Therapy, 904-620-2684, Fax: 904-620-1832, E-mail: nursingadmissions@unf.edu.
Website: http://www.unf.edu/brooks/nursing

University of Pennsylvania, School of Nursing, Nurse Anesthesia Program, Philadelphia, PA 19104. Offers MSN. *Accreditation:* AANA/CANAEP. *Students:* 50 full-time (34 women), 2 part-time (1 woman); includes 15 minority (4 Black or African American, non-Hispanic/Latino; 4 Asian, non-Hispanic/Latino; 6 Hispanic/Latino; 1 Two or more races, non-Hispanic/Latino). Average age 29. 131 applicants, 18% accepted, 22 enrolled. In 2015, 22 master's awarded. *Expenses:* Tuition, area resident: Full-time $31,068; part-time $5762 per course. *Required fees:* $3200; $336 per course. Full-time tuition and fees vary according to degree level, program and student level. Part-time tuition and fees vary according to course load, degree level and program.

University of Pittsburgh, School of Nursing, Nurse Anesthesia Program, Pittsburgh, PA 15260. Offers MSN, DNP. *Accreditation:* AACN; AANA/CANAEP. *Students:* 109 full-time (80 women), 20 part-time (12 women); includes 13 minority (4 Black or African American, non-Hispanic/Latino; 6 Asian, non-Hispanic/Latino; 3 Hispanic/Latino), 1 international. Average age 28. 181 applicants, 32% accepted, 53 enrolled. In 2015, 45 master's awarded. *Degree requirements:* For master's, comprehensive exam, thesis optional. *Entrance requirements:* For master's, GRE General Test, BSN, RN license, 1-3 years of nursing experience, letters of recommendation, resume, course work in statistics. Additional exam requirements/recommendations for international students: Required—TOEFL (minimum score 600 paper-based; 100 iBT). *Application deadline:* For fall admission, 1/5 for domestic and international students. Application fee: $50. Electronic applications accepted. *Expenses:* $12,464 per term in-state; $14,430 per term out-of-state; $1,016 per credit in-state; $1,179 per credit out-of-state. *Faculty research:* Behavioral management of chronic disorders, patient management in critical care, consumer informatics, genetic applications (molecular genetics and psychosocial implications), technology for nurses and patients to improve care. *Unit head:* John O'Donnell, Director, 412-624-4860, Fax: 412-624-2401, E-mail: jod01@pitt.edu. *Application contact:* Laurie Lapsley, Administrator of Graduate Student Services, 412-624-9670, Fax: 412-624-2409, E-mail: lapsleyl@pitt.edu.
Website: http://www.nursing.pitt.edu/

The University of Scranton, Panuska College of Professional Studies, Department of Nursing, Scranton, PA 18510-4595. Offers family nurse practitioner (MSN, PMC); nurse anesthesia (MSN, PMC); nursing leadership (DNP). Applicants accepted in odd-numbered years only. *Accreditation:* AACN; AANA/CANAEP. *Program availability:* Part-time, evening/weekend. *Students:* 58 full-time (46 women), 22 part-time (all women); includes 16 minority (12 Black or African American, non-Hispanic/Latino; 1 Asian, non-Hispanic/Latino; 2 Hispanic/Latino; 1 Two or more races, non-Hispanic/Latino). Average age 33. 104 applicants, 51% accepted, 45 enrolled. *Degree requirements:* For master's, comprehensive exam (for some programs), thesis (for some programs), capstone experience. *Entrance requirements:* For master's, minimum GPA of 3.0, three letters of reference; for doctorate, RN licensure and evidence of certification in advanced practice nursing specialty. Additional exam requirements/recommendations for international students: Required—TOEFL (minimum score 500 paper-based; 80 iBT), IELTS (minimum score 6.5). *Application deadline:* For fall admission, 9/1 for domestic students, 6/1 for international students; for spring admission, 11/1 for international students; for summer admission, 3/1 for international students. Applications are processed on a rolling basis. Application fee: $0. Electronic applications accepted. *Financial support:* Applicants required to submit FAFSA. *Faculty research:* Home care, doctoral education, health care of women and children, pain, health promotion and adolescence. *Unit head:* Dr. Dona Carpenter, Chair, 570-941-7673, Fax: 570-941-4201, E-mail: dona.carpenter@scranton.edu. *Application contact:* Dr. Mary Jane Hanson, Director, 570-941-4060, Fax: 570-941-4201, E-mail: hansonm2@scranton.edu.
Website: http://www.scranton.edu/academics/pcps/nursing/index.shtml

University of South Carolina, School of Medicine and The Graduate School, Graduate Programs in Medicine, Program in Nurse Anesthesia, Columbia, SC 29208. Offers MNA. *Accreditation:* AACN; AANA/CANAEP. *Degree requirements:* For master's, comprehensive exam, practicum. *Entrance requirements:* For master's, GRE, 1 year of critical care experience, RN license. Electronic applications accepted. *Expenses:*

Contact institution. *Faculty research:* Neuroscience, cardiovascular, hormones, stress, homeostasis.

University of South Florida, College of Nursing, Tampa, FL 33612. Offers advanced pain management (Graduate Certificate); nursing (MS, DNP), including adult gerontology acute care (DNP), adult gerontology acute care nursing (MS), adult gerontology primary care (DNP), adult gerontology primary care nursing (MS), adult gerontology primary care/occupational health nursing (MS), adult gerontology primary care/oncology nursing (MS), clinical nurse leader (MS), family health nursing, nurse anesthesia (MS), nursing education (MS), nursing practice (DNP), occupational health/adult-gerontology (DNP), oncology/adult-gerontology primary care (DNP), pediatric health (DNP), pediatric nurse practitioner (MS); nursing education (Post Master's Certificate); nursing science (PhD). *Accreditation:* AACN; AANA/CANAEP. *Program availability:* Part-time. *Faculty:* 43 full-time (38 women), 7 part-time/adjunct (4 women). *Students:* 159 full-time (135 women), 721 part-time (625 women); includes 292 minority (119 Black or African American, non-Hispanic/Latino; 2 American Indian or Alaska Native, non-Hispanic/Latino; 60 Asian, non-Hispanic/Latino; 90 Hispanic/Latino; 1 Native Hawaiian or other Pacific Islander, non-Hispanic/Latino; 20 Two or more races, non-Hispanic/Latino), 12 international. Average age 35. 636 applicants, 44% accepted, 215 enrolled. In 2015, 333 master's, 18 doctorates awarded. *Degree requirements:* For master's, comprehensive exam, thesis optional; for doctorate, comprehensive exam, thesis/dissertation. *Entrance requirements:* For master's, GRE General Test, bachelor's degree from accredited program with minimum GPA of 3.0 in all upper-division coursework; current license as Registered Nurse; 3 letters of recommendation; personal statement of goals; resume or curriculum vitae; personal interview; for doctorate, GRE General Test (recommended), bachelor's degree in nursing from a CCNA/NLNAC regionally-accredited institution with minimum GPA of 3.0 in all coursework or in all upper-division coursework; current license as Registered Nurse in Florida; undergraduate statistics course with minimum B grade; 3 letters of recommendation; statement of goals; resume; interview. Additional exam requirements/recommendations for international students: Required—TOEFL (minimum score 550 paper-based; 79 iBT). *Application deadline:* For fall admission, 2/15 for domestic students, 1/2 for international students; for spring admission, 10/1 for domestic students, 6/1 for international students. Application fee: $30. Electronic applications accepted. *Financial support:* In 2015–16, 36 students received support, including 7 research assistantships with tuition reimbursements available (averaging $18,935 per year), 29 teaching assistantships with tuition reimbursements available (averaging $30,814 per year); tuition waivers (partial) and unspecified assistantships also available. Financial award application deadline: 2/1; financial award applicants required to submit FAFSA. *Faculty research:* Women's health, palliative and end-of-life care, cardiac rehabilitation, complementary therapies for chronic illness and cancer. *Total annual research expenditures:* $2.6 million. *Unit head:* Dr. Dianne C. Morrison-Beedy, Dean and Professor, College of Nursing, 813-974-9091, Fax: 813-974-5418, E-mail: dmbeedy@health.usf.edu. *Application contact:* Dr. Brian Graves, Assistant Professor/Assistant Dean, 813-974-8054, Fax: 813-974-5418, E-mail: bgraves1@health.usf.edu.
Website: http://health.usf.edu/nursing/index.htm

The University of Tennessee at Chattanooga, School of Nursing, Chattanooga, TN 37403. Offers administration (MSN); certified nurse anesthetist (Post-Master's Certificate); education (MSN); family nurse practitioner (MSN, Post-Master's Certificate); health care informatics (Post-Master's Certificate); nurse anesthesia (MSN); nurse education (Post-Master's Certificate); nursing (DNP). *Accreditation:* AACN; AANA/CANAEP (one or more programs are accredited). *Faculty:* 9 full-time (7 women), 2 part-time/adjunct (1 woman). *Students:* 50 full-time (25 women), 43 part-time (37 women); includes 14 minority (7 Black or African American, non-Hispanic/Latino; 1 American Indian or Alaska Native, non-Hispanic/Latino; 4 Asian, non-Hispanic/Latino; 2 Two or more races, non-Hispanic/Latino). Average age 34. In 2015, 40 master's, 12 doctorates, 1 other advanced degree awarded. *Degree requirements:* For master's, thesis optional, qualifying exams, professional project; for Post-Master's Certificate, thesis or alternative, practicum, seminar. *Entrance requirements:* For master's, GRE General Test, MAT, BSN, minimum GPA of 3.0, eligibility for Tennessee RN license, 1 year of direct patient care experience; for Post-Master's Certificate, GRE General Test, MAT, MSN, minimum GPA of 3.0, eligibility for Tennessee RN license, one year of direct patient care experience. Additional exam requirements/recommendations for international students: Required—TOEFL (minimum score 79 iBT), IELTS (minimum score 6). *Application deadline:* For fall admission, 6/13 priority date for domestic students, 6/1 for international students; for spring admission, 10/15 priority date for domestic students, 10/1 for international students. Applications are processed on a rolling basis. Application fee: $30 ($35 for international students). Electronic applications accepted. *Expenses:* Tuition, state resident: full-time $7938; part-time $441 per credit hour. Tuition, nonresident: full-time $24,056; part-time $1336 per credit hour. *Required fees:* $1732; $253 per credit hour. *Financial support:* Career-related internships or fieldwork and scholarships/grants available. Support available to part-time students. *Faculty research:* Diabetes in women, health care for elderly, alternative medicine, hypertension, nurse anesthesia. *Total annual research expenditures:* $2.6 million. *Unit head:* Dr. Chris Smith, Interim Director, 423-425-1741, Fax: 423-425-4668, E-mail: chris-smith@utc.edu. *Application contact:* Dr. J. Randy Walker, Interim Dean of Graduate Studies, 423-425-4478, Fax: 423-425-5223, E-mail: randy-walker@utc.edu.
Website: http://www.utc.edu/Academic/Nursing

University of Wisconsin–La Crosse, College of Science and Health, Department of Biology, La Crosse, WI 54601-3742. Offers aquatic sciences (MS); biology (MS); cellular and molecular biology (MS); clinical microbiology (MS); microbiology (MS); nurse anesthesia (MS); physiology (MS). *Program availability:* Part-time. *Students:* 19 full-time (12 women), 50 part-time (26 women); includes 4 minority (3 Asian, non-Hispanic/Latino; 1 Hispanic/Latino), 1 international. Average age 29. 44 applicants, 75% accepted, 27 enrolled. In 2015, 27 master's awarded. *Degree requirements:* For master's, comprehensive exam, thesis. *Entrance requirements:* For master's, GRE General Test, minimum GPA of 2.85. Additional exam requirements/recommendations for international students: Required—TOEFL (minimum score 550 paper-based; 79 iBT). *Application deadline:* For fall admission, 2/1 priority date for domestic and international students; for spring admission, 1/4 priority date for domestic and international students. Applications are processed on a rolling basis. Electronic applications accepted. *Financial support:* Research assistantships with partial tuition reimbursements, Federal Work-Study, scholarships/grants, health care benefits, and tuition waivers (partial) available. Support available to part-time students. Financial award application deadline: 3/15; financial award applicants required to submit FAFSA. *Unit head:* Dr. Mark Sandheinrich, Department Chair, 608-785-8261, E-mail: msandheinrich@uwlax.edu. *Application contact:* Brandon Schaller, Senior Graduate Student Status Examiner, 608-785-8941, E-mail: admissions@uwlax.edu.
Website: http://uwlax.edu/biology/

Villanova University, College of Nursing, Villanova, PA 19085-1699. Offers adult nurse practitioner (MSN, Post Master's Certificate); family nurse practitioner (MSN, Post Master's Certificate); nurse anesthetist (MSN, Post Master's Certificate); nursing (PhD); nursing education (MSN, Post Master's Certificate); nursing practice (DNP); pediatric nurse practitioner (MSN, Post Master's Certificate). *Accreditation:* AACN; AANA/CANAEP. *Program availability:* Part-time, online learning. *Faculty:* 16 full-time (15 women), 9 part-time/adjunct (7 women). *Students:* 219 full-time (198 women), 108 part-time (96 women); includes 36 minority (25 Black or African American, non-Hispanic/Latino; 9 Asian, non-Hispanic/Latino; 2 Hispanic/Latino), 16 international. Average age 31. 147 applicants, 78% accepted, 106 enrolled. In 2015, 64 master's, 8 doctorates, 9 other advanced degrees awarded. *Degree requirements:* For master's, comprehensive exam, independent study project; for doctorate, comprehensive exam, thesis/dissertation; for Post Master's Certificate, scholarly project. *Entrance requirements:* For master's, GRE or MAT, BSN, 1 year of recent nursing experience, physical assessment, course work in statistics; for doctorate, GRE, MSN. Additional exam requirements/recommendations for international students: Required—TOEFL (minimum score 540 paper-based; 83 iBT), IELTS (minimum score 6.5). *Application deadline:* For fall admission, 7/1 priority date for domestic students, 7/1 for international students; for spring admission, 11/1 priority date for domestic students, 11/1 for international students; for summer admission, 4/1 priority date for domestic students, 3/1 for international students. Applications are processed on a rolling basis. Application fee: $50. Electronic applications accepted. *Expenses:* $837 per credit (MSN); $1,049 per credit (PhD); $1,375 per credit (DNP). *Financial support:* In 2015–16, 22 students received support, including 5 teaching assistantships with full tuition reimbursements available (averaging $15,475 per year); institutionally sponsored loans, scholarships/grants, traineeships, tuition waivers (full), and unspecified assistantships also available. Financial award application deadline: 7/1; financial award applicants required to submit FAFSA. *Faculty research:* Genetics, ethics, cognitive development of students, women with disabilities, nursing leadership. *Unit head:* Dr. Marguerite K. Schlag, Assistant Dean/Director, Graduate Programs, 610-519-4907, Fax: 610-519-7650, E-mail: marguerite.schlag@villanova.edu. *Application contact:* Rebecca Harold, Administrative Assistant, 610-519-4934, Fax: 610-519-7650, E-mail: rebecca.harold@villanova.edu.
Website: http://www.nursing.villanova.edu/

Virginia Commonwealth University, Graduate School, School of Allied Health Professions, Department of Nurse Anesthesia, Richmond, VA 23284-9005. Offers MSNA, DNAP. *Accreditation:* AANA/CANAEP. *Degree requirements:* For master's, thesis. *Entrance requirements:* For master's, GRE General Test, 1 year experience in acute critical care nursing, current state RN license, minimum GPA of 3.0; for doctorate, GRE General Test, accredited MSNA, CCNA certification, minimum GPA of 3.0. Additional exam requirements/recommendations for international students: Required—TOEFL (minimum score 600 paper-based; 100 iBT); Recommended—IELTS (minimum score 6.5). Electronic applications accepted. *Faculty research:* Obstetrical anesthesia, ambulatory anesthesia, regional anesthesia, practice profiles, clinical practice.

Virginia Commonwealth University, Graduate School, School of Allied Health Professions, Doctoral Program in Health Related Sciences, Richmond, VA 23284-9005. Offers clinical laboratory sciences (PhD); gerontology (PhD); health administration (PhD); nurse anesthesia (PhD); occupational therapy (PhD); physical therapy (PhD); radiation sciences (PhD); rehabilitation leadership (PhD). *Entrance requirements:* For doctorate, GRE General Test or MAT, minimum GPA of 3.3 in master's degree. Additional exam requirements/recommendations for international students: Required—TOEFL (minimum score 600 paper-based; 100 iBT); Recommended—IELTS (minimum score 6.5). Electronic applications accepted.

Wayne State University, Eugene Applebaum College of Pharmacy and Health Sciences, Department of Health Care Sciences, Program in Nurse Anesthesia, Detroit, MI 48202. Offers anesthesia (MS); pediatric anesthesia (Certificate). *Accreditation:* AACN; AANA/CANAEP. *Faculty:* 7. *Students:* 41 full-time (20 women); includes 6 minority (4 Black or African American, non-Hispanic/Latino; 1 Asian, non-Hispanic/Latino; 1 Hispanic/Latino). Average age 30. In 2015, 16 master's awarded. *Entrance requirements:* For master's, GRE General Test, bachelor's degree in nursing or related science with minimum GPA of 3.0 overall and in science, current RN license, CCRN certification, one year of full-time experience in adult ICU, ACLS certification, hospital shadow experience (arranged by department); for Certificate, MS in anesthesia from accredited program, meeting with course coordinators from Children's Hospital of Michigan. Additional exam requirements/recommendations for international students: Required—TOEFL (minimum score 550 paper-based; 79 iBT), Michigan English Language Assessment Battery (minimum score 85); Recommended—IELTS (minimum score 6.5), TWE (minimum score 5.5). *Application deadline:* For fall admission, 7/1 for domestic students, 5/1 priority date for international students. Application fee: $0. Electronic applications accepted. *Expenses:* $16,104 per year resident tuition, $32,401 non-resident tuition; $671 per credit hour resident tuition, $1,350.05 per credit hour non-resident tuition; fees include $47.45 per credit hour student services fee and $274.60 per semester registration fee. *Financial support:* In 2015–16, 20 students received support. Scholarships/grants available. Financial award application deadline: 3/31; financial award applicants required to submit FAFSA. *Faculty research:* Music therapy in pain management, student success/students perspective, pacemaker management-safety, airway devices. *Unit head:* Dr. Prudentia A. Worth, Program Director, 313-993-7168, E-mail: aa1635@wayne.edu.
Website: http://cphs.wayne.edu/nurse-anesthesia/

Webster University, College of Arts and Sciences, Department of Nurse Anesthesia, St. Louis, MO 63119-3194. Offers MS. *Accreditation:* AANA/CANAEP. *Program availability:* Online learning. *Degree requirements:* For master's, thesis. *Entrance requirements:* For master's, 1 year of work-related experience, 75 hours of graduate course work, BSN, interview, minimum GPA of 3.0. Additional exam requirements/recommendations for international students: Required—TOEFL. *Expenses:* Tuition, area resident: Full-time $20,550; part-time $685 per credit hour. Tuition and fees vary according to campus/location and program. *Faculty research:* Clinical anesthesia, substance abuse education in the health professions, technology and education, clinical pharmacology.

Westminster College, School of Nursing and Health Sciences, Salt Lake City, UT 84105-3697. Offers family nurse practitioner (MSN); nurse anesthesia (MSNA); nurse education (MSNED); public health (MPH). *Accreditation:* AACN; AANA/CANAEP. *Faculty:* 15 full-time (9 women), 7 part-time/adjunct (2 women). *Students:* 120 full-time (79 women), 3 part-time (all women); includes 18 minority (1 Black or African American, non-Hispanic/Latino; 3 Asian, non-Hispanic/Latino; 10 Hispanic/Latino; 4 Two or more races, non-Hispanic/Latino), 3 international. Average age 32. 157 applicants, 40% accepted, 45 enrolled. In 2015, 56 master's awarded. *Degree requirements:* For master's, clinical practicum, 504 clinical practice hours. *Entrance requirements:* For master's, GRE, personal statement, resume, 3 professional recommendations, copy of unrestricted Utah license to practice professional nursing, background check, minimum cumulative GPA of 3.0, documentation of current immunizations, physical and mental health certificate signed by primary care provider. Additional exam requirements/recommendations for international students: Required—TOEFL (minimum score 600 paper-based; 100 iBT), IELTS (minimum score 7.5). Application fee: $50. Electronic applications accepted. *Expenses:* Contact institution. *Financial support:* In 2015–16, 8 students received support. Career-related internships or fieldwork, unspecified assistantships, and tuition reimbursements, tuition remission available. Support available to part-time students. Financial award applicants required to submit FAFSA. *Faculty research:* Intellectual empathy, professional boundaries, learned optimism, collaborative testing in nursing: student outcomes and perspectives, implementing new

educational paradigms into pre-licensure nursing curricula. *Unit head:* Dr. Sheryl Steadman, Dean, 801-832-2164, Fax: 801-832-3110, E-mail: ssteadman@westminstercollege.edu. *Application contact:* Dr. John Baworowsky, Vice President of Enrollment Management, 801-832-2200, Fax: 801-832-3101, E-mail: admission@westminstercollege.edu.
Website: http://www.westminstercollege.edu/msn

York College of Pennsylvania, Department of Nursing, York, PA 17405-7199. Offers adult gerontology clinical nurse specialist (MS), including administration, education; adult gerontology nurse practitioner (MS); nurse anesthetist (MS); nurse educator (MS); nursing practice (DNP). *Accreditation:* AACN; AANA/CANAEP. *Program availability:* Part-time, evening/weekend. *Faculty:* 9 full-time (all women), 5 part-time/adjunct (2 women). *Students:* 36 full-time (26 women), 55 part-time (47 women); includes 14 minority (4 Black or African American, non-Hispanic/Latino; 2 American Indian or Alaska Native, non-Hispanic/Latino; 5 Asian, non-Hispanic/Latino; 2 Hispanic/Latino; 1 Two or more races, non-Hispanic/Latino), 1 international. Average age 33. 115 applicants, 28% accepted, 28 enrolled. In 2015, 24 master's, 4 doctorates awarded. *Entrance requirements:* For master's, GRE General Test (for nurse anesthetist program), minimum GPA of 3.0 from CCNE- or NLNAC-accredited institution; for doctorate, master's degree in nursing from a CCNE- or NLNAC-accredited institution; minimum GPA of 3.5. Additional exam requirements/recommendations for international students: Required—TOEFL (minimum score 530 paper-based; 72 iBT). *Application deadline:* Applications are processed on a rolling basis. Application fee: $0. Electronic applications accepted. *Expenses: Tuition, area resident:* Full-time $13,770. *Required fees:* $1750; $380. Tuition and fees vary according to degree level. *Financial support:* Federal Work-Study available. *Faculty research:* Student stress response to simulation versus clinical, evidence-based practice in all clinical settings. *Unit head:* Dr. Kimberly Fenstermacher, Graduate Program Director, 717-815-1383, E-mail: kfenster@ycp.edu. *Application contact:* Allison Malachosky, Administrative Assistant, 717-815-1243, E-mail: amalacho@ycp.edu.
Website: http://www.ycp.edu/academics/academic-departments/nursing/

Nurse Midwifery

Bastyr University, School of Natural Health Arts and Sciences, Kenmore, WA 98028-4966. Offers counseling psychology (MA); holistic landscape design (Certificate); midwifery (MS); nutrition (MS); nutrition and clinical health psychology (MS). *Accreditation:* AND. *Program availability:* Part-time. *Degree requirements:* For master's, thesis optional. *Entrance requirements:* For master's, 1-2 years' basic sciences course work (depending on program). Additional exam requirements/recommendations for international students: Required—TOEFL (minimum score 550 paper-based; 79 iBT). *Faculty research:* Whole-food nutrition for type 2 diabetes; meditation in end-of-life care; stress management; Qi Gong, Tai Chi and yoga for older adults; Echinacea and immunology.

Baylor University, Graduate School, Louise Herrington School of Nursing, Dallas, TX 75246. Offers family nurse practitioner (MSN); neonatal nurse practitioner (MSN); nurse-midwifery (DNP). *Accreditation:* AACN. *Program availability:* Part-time, online learning. *Degree requirements:* For doctorate, comprehensive exam (for some programs), capstone project. *Entrance requirements:* For master's, GRE General Test or MAT; for doctorate, GRE General Test. Additional exam requirements/recommendations for international students: Required—TOEFL. Electronic applications accepted. *Faculty research:* Women and strokes, obesity and pregnancy, educational environmental factors, international undeserved populations, midwifery.

Bethel University, Graduate School, St. Paul, MN 55112-6999. Offers business administration (MBA); child and adolescent mental health (Certificate); classroom management (Certificate); communication (MA); counseling psychology (MA); educational leadership (Ed D); gerontology (MA, Certificate); international baccalaureate teaching and learning (Certificate); K-12 education (MA); leadership foundations (Certificate); literacy education (MA); nurse educator (Certificate); nurse-midwifery (MS); nursing (MS); physician assistant (MS); special education (MA); STEM education (Certificate); strategic leadership (MA); teaching (MA). *Program availability:* Part-time, evening/weekend, 100% online, blended/hybrid learning. *Faculty:* 21 full-time (15 women), 74 part-time/adjunct (38 women). *Students:* 772 full-time (537 women), 372 part-time (232 women); includes 188 minority (94 Black or African American, non-Hispanic/Latino; 3 American Indian or Alaska Native, non-Hispanic/Latino; 43 Asian, non-Hispanic/Latino; 31 Hispanic/Latino; 1 Native Hawaiian or other Pacific Islander, non-Hispanic/Latino; 16 Two or more races, non-Hispanic/Latino), 33 international. Average age 37. 663 applicants, 49% accepted, 232 enrolled. In 2015, 272 master's, 16 doctorates, 65 other advanced degrees awarded. *Degree requirements:* For master's, comprehensive exam (for some programs), thesis (for some programs); for doctorate, comprehensive exam, thesis/dissertation. *Entrance requirements:* Additional exam requirements/recommendations for international students: Required—TOEFL (minimum score 550 paper-based, 80 iBT) or IELTS. *Application deadline:* Applications are processed on a rolling basis. Application fee: $0. Electronic applications accepted. *Expenses:* Contact institution. *Financial support:* In 2015–16, 132 students received support. Teaching assistantships, career-related internships or fieldwork, and scholarships/grants available. Support available to part-time students. Financial award applicants required to submit FAFSA. *Unit head:* Dick Crombie, Vice-President/Dean, 651-635-8000, Fax: 651-635-8004, E-mail: gs@bethel.edu. *Application contact:* Director of Admissions, 651-635-8000, Fax: 651-635-8004, E-mail: gs@bethel.edu.
Website: https://www.bethel.edu/graduate/

Case Western Reserve University, Frances Payne Bolton School of Nursing, Master's Programs in Nursing, Program in Nurse Midwifery, Cleveland, OH 44106. Offers MSN. *Accreditation:* ACNM/ACME. *Students:* 7 full-time (all women), 8 part-time (all women), 1 international. Average age 35. 4 applicants, 50% accepted, 2 enrolled. In 2015, 2 master's awarded. *Degree requirements:* For master's, thesis optional. *Entrance requirements:* For master's, GRE General Test or MAT. Additional exam requirements/recommendations for international students: Required—TOEFL (minimum score 577 paper-based; 90 iBT), IELTS (minimum score 7). *Application deadline:* For fall admission, 6/1 for domestic and international students; for spring admission, 10/1 for domestic and international students. Applications are processed on a rolling basis. Application fee: $75. *Expenses:* $1,891 per credit hour. *Financial support:* Teaching assistantships and scholarships/grants available. Financial award application deadline: 6/30; financial award applicants required to submit FAFSA. *Faculty research:* Clinical nursing, normal childbearing, descriptive studies of care, high risk pregnancy side effects of bed rest, strengthening and expanding nursing services. *Unit head:* Dr. Gretchen Mettler, Head, 216-368-0671, E-mail: ggm@case.edu. *Application contact:* Donna Hassik, Admissions Coordinator, 216-368-5253, Fax: 216-368-0124, E-mail: dmh7@case.edu.
Website: http://fpb.case.edu/MSN/midwifery.shtm

Columbia University, School of Nursing, Program in Nurse Midwifery, New York, NY 10032. Offers MS. *Accreditation:* AACN; ACNM/ACME. *Program availability:* Part-time. *Entrance requirements:* For master's, GRE General Test, NCLEX, BSN, 1 year of clinical experience (preferred). Additional exam requirements/recommendations for international students: Required—TOEFL (minimum score 100 iBT). Electronic applications accepted.

DeSales University, Division of Healthcare, Center Valley, PA 18034-9568. Offers adult-gerontology acute care (Post Master's Certificate); adult-gerontology acute care nurse practitioner (MSN); adult-gerontology acute certified nurse practitioner (Post Master's Certificate); adult-gerontology clinical nurse specialist (MSN, Post Master's Certificate); clinical leadership (DNP); family nurse practitioner (MSN, Post Master's Certificate); general nursing practice (DNP); health care information management (MSIS); network security (MSIS); nurse anesthetists (MSN); nurse educator (Post Master's Certificate, Postbaccalaureate Certificate); nurse midwives (MSN); nurse practitioner (MSN); project management (MSIS); psychiatric-mental health nurse practitioner (MSN, Post Master's Certificate); DNP/MBA. *Accreditation:* ACEN. *Program availability:* Part-time. *Faculty:* 22 full-time (14 women), 37 part-time/adjunct (29 women). *Students:* 244 full-time (178 women), 55 part-time (50 women); includes 24 minority (7 Black or African American, non-Hispanic/Latino; 9 Asian, non-Hispanic/Latino; 6 Hispanic/Latino; 2 Two or more races, non-Hispanic/Latino). Average age 31. 68 applicants, 85% accepted, 52 enrolled. In 2015, 73 master's awarded. *Degree requirements:* For master's, minimum GPA of 3.0, portfolio; for doctorate, minimum GPA of 3.0, scholarly capstone project. *Entrance requirements:* For master's, GRE or MAT (waived if applicant has an undergraduate GPA of 3.0 or higher), BSN from ACEN- or CCNE-accredited program, minimum undergraduate GPA of 3.0, active RN license or eligibility, two letters of recommendation, essay, health care experience, personal interview; for doctorate, BSN or MSN from ACEN- or CCNE-accredited institution, minimum GPA of 3.3 in graduate program, current licensure as an RN. Additional exam requirements/recommendations for international students: Required—TOEFL (minimum score 104 iBT). *Application deadline:* Applications are processed on a rolling basis. Application fee: $50. Electronic applications accepted. *Expenses:* Contact institution. *Financial support:* Applicants required to submit FAFSA. *Unit head:* Fr. Dr. Peter Leonard, OSFS, Dean of Graduate Education, 610-282-1100 Ext. 1289, E-mail: peter.leonard@desales.edu. *Application contact:* Abigail Wernicki, Director of Graduate Admissions, 610-282-1100 Ext. 1768, Fax: 610-282-2869, E-mail: gradadmissions@desales.edu.

Emory University, Nell Hodgson Woodruff School of Nursing, Atlanta, GA 30322-1100. Offers adult nurse practitioner (MSN); emergency nurse practitioner (MSN); family nurse practitioner (MSN); family nurse-midwife (MSN); health systems leadership (MSN); nurse-midwifery (MSN); pediatric nurse practitioner acute and primary care (MSN); women's health care (Title X) (MSN); women's health nurse practitioner (MSN); MSN/MPH. *Accreditation:* AACN; ACNM/ACME (one or more programs are accredited). *Program availability:* Part-time. *Entrance requirements:* For master's, GRE General Test or MAT, minimum GPA of 3.0, BS in nursing from an accredited institution, RN license and additional course work, 3 letters of recommendation. Additional exam requirements/recommendations for international students: Required—TOEFL (minimum score 600 paper-based; 100 iBT). Electronic applications accepted. *Expenses:* Contact institution. *Faculty research:* Older adult falls and injuries, minority health issues, cardiac symptoms and quality of life, bio-ethics and decision-making, menopausal issues.

Frontier Nursing University, Graduate Programs, Hyden, KY 41749. Offers family nurse practitioner (MSN, DNP, Post Master's Certificate); nurse-midwifery (MSN, DNP, Post Master's Certificate); women's health care nurse practitioner (MSN, DNP, Post Master's Certificate). *Accreditation:* ACEN; ACNM. *Degree requirements:* For doctorate, capstone project, practicum.

Georgetown University, Graduate School of Arts and Sciences, School of Nursing and Health Studies, Washington, DC 20057. Offers acute care nurse practitioner (MS); clinical nurse specialist (MS); family nurse practitioner (MS); nurse anesthesia (MS); nurse-midwifery (MS); nursing (DNP); nursing education (MS). *Accreditation:* AACN; AANA/CANAEP (one or more programs are accredited); ACNM/ACME (one or more programs are accredited). *Degree requirements:* For master's, thesis optional. *Entrance requirements:* For master's, GRE General Test or MAT, bachelor's degree in nursing from NLN-accredited school, minimum undergraduate GPA of 3.0. Additional exam requirements/recommendations for international students: Required—TOEFL.

James Madison University, The Graduate School, College of Health and Behavioral Sciences, Program in Nursing, Harrisonburg, VA 22807. Offers adult/gerontology primary care nurse practitioner (MSN); clinical nurse leader (MSN); family nurse practitioner (MSN); nurse administrator (MSN); nurse midwifery (MSN); nursing (MSN, DNP). *Accreditation:* AACN. *Program availability:* Part-time, 100% online, blended/hybrid learning. *Faculty:* 15 full-time (all women), 1 (woman) part-time/adjunct. *Students:* 14 full-time (all women), 54 part-time (43 women); includes 6 minority (2 Black or African American, non-Hispanic/Latino; 1 Asian, non-Hispanic/Latino; 1 Hispanic/Latino; 2 Two or more races, non-Hispanic/Latino), 1 international. Average age 30. 49 applicants, 67% accepted, 31 enrolled. In 2015, 14 master's awarded. Application fee: $55. Electronic applications accepted. *Financial support:* In 2015–16, 2 students received support. Federal Work-Study, unspecified assistantships, and 2 assistantships (averaging $7530) available. Financial award application deadline: 3/1; financial award applicants required to submit FAFSA. *Unit head:* Dr. Julie T. Sanford, Department Head, 540-568-6314, E-mail: sanforjt@jmu.edu. *Application contact:* Lynette D. Michael, Director of Graduate Admissions and Student Records, 540-568-6131 Ext. 6395, Fax: 540-568-7860, E-mail: michaeld@jmu.edu.
Website: http://www.nursing.jmu.edu

Marquette University, Graduate School, College of Nursing, Milwaukee, WI 53201-1881. Offers acute care nurse practitioner (Certificate); adult clinical nurse specialist (Certificate); adult nurse practitioner (Certificate); advanced practice nursing (MSN, DNP), including adult-older adult acute care (DNP), adults (MSN), adults-older adults (DNP), clinical nurse leader (MSN), health care systems leadership (DNP), nurse-midwifery (MSN), older adults (MSN), pediatrics-acute care, pediatrics-primary care, primary care (DNP), systems leadership and healthcare quality (MSN); family nurse practitioner (Certificate); nurse-midwifery (Certificate); nursing (PhD); pediatric acute care (Certificate); pediatric primary care (Certificate); systems leadership and healthcare quality (Certificate). *Accreditation:* AACN. *Faculty:* 35 full-time (all women), 56 part-time/adjunct (55 women). *Students:* 123 full-time (112 women), 242 part-time (220 women); includes 34 minority (9 Black or African American, non-Hispanic/Latino; 12 Asian, non-Hispanic/Latino; 10 Hispanic/Latino; 3 Two or more races, non-Hispanic/Latino), 4 international. Average age 30. 269 applicants, 61% accepted, 98 enrolled. In 2015, 84 master's, 5 doctorates, 22 other advanced degrees awarded. Terminal master's awarded for partial completion of doctoral program. *Degree requirements:* For master's, comprehensive exam, thesis or alternative. *Entrance requirements:* For master's, GRE General Test, BSN, Wisconsin RN license, official transcripts from all current and previous colleges/universities except Marquette, three completed recommendation forms, resume, written statement of professional goals; for doctorate, GRE General Test, official transcripts from all current and previous colleges/universities except Marquette, three letters of recommendation, resume, written statement of professional goals, sample of scholarly writing. Additional exam requirements/recommendations for international students: Required—TOEFL (minimum score 530 paper-based). *Application deadline:* For fall admission, 2/15 for domestic and international students. Electronic applications accepted. *Financial support:* In 2015–16, 41 students received support, including 1 fellowship with partial tuition reimbursement available (averaging $17,500 per year), 2 research assistantships with full tuition reimbursements available (averaging $13,285 per year), 8 teaching assistantships with full tuition reimbursements available (averaging $13,912 per year); career-related internships or fieldwork, Federal Work-Study, scholarships/grants, health care benefits, tuition waivers (partial), and unspecified assistantships also available. Support available to part-time students. Financial award application deadline: 2/15. *Faculty research:* Psychosocial adjustment to chronic illness, gerontology, reminiscence, health policy: uninsured and access, hospital care delivery systems. *Total annual research expenditures:* $480,591. *Unit head:* Dr. Donna McCarthy, Interim Chair, 414-288-3800, Fax: 414-288-1578. *Application contact:* Dr. Maureen O'Brien, Associate Dean/Clinical Associate Professor, 414-288-3823.

Midwives College of Utah, Graduate Program, Salt Lake City, UT 84106. Offers MS. *Accreditation:* MEAC. *Degree requirements:* For master's, comprehensive exam (for some programs), thesis.

National College of Midwifery, Graduate Programs, Taos, NM 87571. Offers MS, PhD. *Accreditation:* MEAC. *Program availability:* Part-time, evening/weekend, online learning. *Degree requirements:* For master's, thesis, publication; for doctorate, thesis/dissertation, presentation, publication. *Entrance requirements:* For master's and doctorate, midwifery license or certification. Electronic applications accepted.

New York University, Rory Meyers College of Nursing, Doctor of Nursing Practice Program, New York, NY 10012-1019. Offers nursing (DNP), including adult acute care, adult primary care, family, mental health nursing, nurse-midwifery, pediatrics. *Program availability:* Part-time, evening/weekend. *Faculty:* 14 full-time (13 women). *Students:* 2 full-time (both women), 32 part-time (27 women); includes 8 minority (3 Black or African American, non-Hispanic/Latino; 4 Asian, non-Hispanic/Latino; 1 Hispanic/Latino), 1 international. Average age 40. 47 applicants, 51% accepted, 16 enrolled. In 2015, 17 doctorates awarded. *Degree requirements:* For doctorate, thesis/dissertation, project. *Entrance requirements:* For doctorate, MAT or GRE (either taken within past 5 years), MS, RN license, interview, Nurse Practitioner Certification, writing sample. Additional exam requirements/recommendations for international students: Required—TOEFL (minimum score 90 iBT), IELTS (minimum score 7). *Application deadline:* For fall admission, 3/1 for domestic and international students. Applications are processed on a rolling basis. Application fee: $80. Electronic applications accepted. *Expenses:* Contact institution. *Financial support:* In 2015–16, 12 students received support. Scholarships/grants available. Support available to part-time students. Financial award application deadline: 2/1; financial award applicants required to submit FAFSA. *Faculty research:* Workforce, LGBT, breast cancer, HIV. *Unit head:* Dr. Rona Levin, Director, 212-998-5319, Fax: 212-995-3143, E-mail: rfl2039@nyu.edu. *Application contact:* Samantha Jaser, Assistant Director, Graduate Student Affairs and Admissions, 212-992-7653, Fax: 212-995-4302, E-mail: saj283@nyu.edu.

New York University, Rory Meyers College of Nursing, Programs in Advanced Practice Nursing, New York, NY 10012-1019. Offers adult-gerontology acute care nurse practitioner (MS, Advanced Certificate); adult-gerontology primary care nurse practitioner (MS, Advanced Certificate); family nurse practitioner (MS, Advanced Certificate); gerontology nurse practitioner (Advanced Certificate); nurse-midwifery (MS, Advanced Certificate); nursing administration (MS, Advanced Certificate); nursing education (MS, Advanced Certificate); nursing informatics (MS, Advanced Certificate); pediatrics nurse practitioner (MS, Advanced Certificate); psychiatric-mental health nurse practitioner (MS, Advanced Certificate); MS/MPH. *Accreditation:* AACN; ACNM/ACME. *Program availability:* Part-time. *Faculty:* 24 full-time (all women), 76 part-time/adjunct (65 women). *Students:* 46 full-time (26 women), 586 part-time (513 women); includes 242 minority (68 Black or African American, non-Hispanic/Latino; 3 American Indian or Alaska Native, non-Hispanic/Latino; 117 Asian, non-Hispanic/Latino; 38 Hispanic/Latino; 3 Native Hawaiian or other Pacific Islander, non-Hispanic/Latino; 13 Two or more races, non-Hispanic/Latino), 23 international. Average age 32. 402 applicants, 69% accepted, 138 enrolled. In 2015, 198 master's, 5 other advanced degrees awarded. *Degree requirements:* For master's, thesis (for some programs). *Entrance requirements:* For master's, BS in nursing, AS in nursing with another BS/BA, interview, RN license, 1 year of clinical experience (3 for the MS in nursing education program); for Advanced Certificate, master's degree. Additional exam requirements/recommendations for international students: Required—TOEFL (minimum score 90 iBT), IELTS (minimum score 7). *Application deadline:* For fall admission, 6/15 for domestic and international students; for spring admission, 12/1 for domestic and international students; for summer admission, 3/1 for domestic and international students. Application fee: $80. Electronic applications accepted. *Expenses:* Contact institution. *Financial support:* In 2015–16, 101 students received support. Career-related internships or fieldwork, Federal Work-Study, and scholarships/grants available. Support available to part-time students. Financial award application deadline: 3/1; financial award applicants required to submit FAFSA. *Faculty research:* Geriatrics, HIV, families and illness, oral systemic connection, symptom management. *Unit head:* Dr. James Pace, Senior Associate Dean for Academic Programs, 212-992-7343, E-mail: james.pace@nyu.edu. *Application contact:* Samantha Jaser, Assistant Director, Graduate Student Affairs and Admissions, 212-992-7653, Fax: 212-995-4302, E-mail: saj283@nyu.edu.

Old Dominion University, College of Health Sciences, School of Nursing, Norfolk, VA 23529. Offers adult gerontology clinical nurse specialist/educator role (MSN); advanced practice nursing (DNP); family nurse practitioner (MSN), including adult-gerontology clinical nurse specialist/educator, neonatal nurse practitioner, pediatric nurse practitioner; nurse anesthesia (MSN); nurse educator (MSN), including neonatal nurse practitioner, pediatric nurse practitioner; nurse executive (MSN), including neonatal nurse practitioner, pediatric nurse practitioner; nurse midwifery (MSN). *Accreditation:* AACN; AANA/CANAEP (one or more programs are accredited). *Program availability:* Part-time, 100% online, blended/hybrid learning. *Faculty:* 6 full-time (5 women), 17 part-time/adjunct (15 women). *Students:* 116 full-time (105 women), 72 part-time (61 women); includes 34 minority (18 Black or African American, non-Hispanic/Latino; 1 American Indian or Alaska Native, non-Hispanic/Latino; 5 Asian, non-Hispanic/Latino; 2

Hispanic/Latino; 8 Two or more races, non-Hispanic/Latino), 7 international. Average age 39. 199 applicants, 42% accepted, 74 enrolled. In 2015, 67 master's, 27 doctorates awarded. *Degree requirements:* For master's, comprehensive exam; for doctorate, capstone project. *Entrance requirements:* For master's, GRE or MAT, BSN, minimum GPA of 3.0 in nursing and overall. Additional exam requirements/recommendations for international students: Required—TOEFL. *Application deadline:* For fall admission, 3/1 for domestic students, 4/15 for international students; for spring admission, 9/15 for domestic students. Application fee: $50. Electronic applications accepted. *Expenses:* Tuition, state resident: full-time $11,136; part-time $464 per credit hour. Tuition, nonresident: full-time $27,840; part-time $1160 per credit hour. *Required fees:* $64 per semester. Tuition and fees vary according to campus/location, program and reciprocity agreements. *Financial support:* In 2015–16, 18 students received support, including 2 research assistantships with partial tuition reimbursements available (averaging $10,000 per year), 1 teaching assistantship (averaging $2,500 per year); career-related internships or fieldwork, scholarships/grants, traineeships, and tuition waivers (partial) also available. Support available to part-time students. Financial award application deadline: 2/15; financial award applicants required to submit FAFSA. *Faculty research:* Health and culture, cardiovascular health, transition of military families, genetics, cultural diversity. *Total annual research expenditures:* $231,117. *Unit head:* Dr. Karen Karlowicz, Chair, 757-683-5262, Fax: 757-683-5253, E-mail: nursgpd@odu.edu. *Application contact:* Sue Parker, Coordinator, Graduate Student Services, 757-683-4298, Fax: 757-683-5253, E-mail: sparker@odu.edu.
Website: http://www.odu.edu/nursing

Oregon Health & Science University, School of Nursing, Program in Nurse Midwifery, Portland, OR 97239-3098. Offers MN, DNP, Post Master's Certificate. *Accreditation:* AACN; ACNM/ACME (one or more programs are accredited). *Degree requirements:* For master's, thesis optional. *Entrance requirements:* For master's, GRE General Test, bachelor's degree in nursing, minimum undergraduate GPA of 3.0, previous course work in statistics; for Post Master's Certificate, master's degree in nursing.

Philadelphia University, College of Science, Health and the Liberal Arts, Program in Midwifery, Philadelphia, PA 19144. Offers midwifery (MS); nurse midwifery (Postbaccalaureate Certificate). *Accreditation:* ACNM/ACME. *Program availability:* Part-time, evening/weekend, online learning. *Entrance requirements:* For master's, GRE or MAT. Additional exam requirements/recommendations for international students: Required—TOEFL (minimum score 550 paper-based; 79 iBT). Electronic applications accepted.

Seattle University, College of Nursing, Program in Advanced Practice Nursing Immersion, Seattle, WA 98122-1090. Offers adult/gerontological nurse practitioner (MSN); advanced community public health nursing (MSN); family nurse practitioner (MSN); family psychiatric mental health nurse practitioner (MSN); nurse midwifery (MSN). *Degree requirements:* For master's, thesis or scholarly project. *Entrance requirements:* For master's, GRE, bachelor's degree, minimum GPA of 3.0, professional resume, two recommendations, letter of intent. Additional exam requirements/recommendations for international students: Required—TOEFL (minimum score 92 iBT), IELTS. Electronic applications accepted.

Shenandoah University, Eleanor Wade Custer School of Nursing, Winchester, VA 22601. Offers family nurse practitioner (MSN, DNP, Post-Graduate Certificate); health informatics (Certificate); health systems leadership (DNP); nurse midwifery (MSN, Post-Graduate Certificate); nursing education (Post-Graduate Certificate); psychiatric mental health nurse practitioner (MSN, DNP, Post-Graduate Certificate). *Accreditation:* AACN; ACNM/ACME. *Faculty:* 10 full-time (all women), 7 part-time/adjunct (4 women). *Students:* 33 full-time (31 women), 62 part-time (57 women); includes 21 minority (17 Black or African American, non-Hispanic/Latino; 3 Asian, non-Hispanic/Latino; 1 Hispanic/Latino). Average age 36. 55 applicants, 87% accepted, 39 enrolled. In 2015, 32 master's, 3 doctorates, 19 other advanced degrees awarded. *Degree requirements:* For master's, research project, clinical hours; for doctorate, scholarly project, clinical hours; for other advanced degree, clinical hours. *Entrance requirements:* For master's, United States RN license; minimum GPA of 3.0; 2080 hours of clinical experience; curriculum vitae; 3 letters of recommendation from a former dean, a faculty member or advisor familiar with the applicant, and a former or current supervisor; two- to three-page essay on a specified topic; for doctorate, MSN, minimum GPA of 3.0, 3 letters of recommendation, 500-word statement, interview, BSN; for other advanced degree, MSN, minimum GPA of 3.0, 2 letters of recommendation, minimum of one year (2080 hours) of clinical nursing experience, interview. Additional exam requirements/recommendations for international students: Required—TOEFL (minimum score 558 paper-based; 83 iBT). *Application deadline:* For fall admission, 1/15 priority date for domestic and international students; for spring admission, 11/1 for domestic and international students; for summer admission, 3/15 for domestic and international students. Application fee: $30. Electronic applications accepted. *Expenses:* Contact institution. *Financial support:* In 2015–16, 13 students received support, including 3 fellowships (averaging $1,000 per year); scholarships/grants and unspecified assistantships also available. Financial award application deadline: 3/15; financial award applicants required to submit FAFSA. *Faculty research:* Primary care providers and their unique position in geriatric, pre-operative education and its effects on post-operative, variables associated with a woman's multidimensional childbirth, interdisciplinary communication, research on health policy. *Unit head:* Kathryn Ganske, PhD, RN, Dean, 540-678-4374, Fax: 540-665-5519, E-mail: kganske@su.edu. *Application contact:* Andrew Woodall, Executive Director of Recruitment and Admissions, 540-665-4581, Fax: 540-665-4627, E-mail: admit@su.edu.
Website: http://www.su.edu/nursing/

State University of New York Downstate Medical Center, College of Nursing, Graduate Program in Nursing, Program in Nurse Midwifery, Brooklyn, NY 11203-2098. Offers MS, Post Master's Certificate. *Accreditation:* ACNM.

Stony Brook University, State University of New York, Stony Brook Medicine, School of Nursing, Program in Nurse Midwifery, Stony Brook, NY 11794. Offers MS, DNP, Certificate. *Accreditation:* AACN; ACNM/ACME. *Program availability:* Part-time, blended/hybrid learning. *Students:* 3 full-time (all women), 21 part-time (all women); includes 6 minority (4 Black or African American, non-Hispanic/Latino; 1 Asian, non-Hispanic/Latino; 1 Hispanic/Latino). 34 applicants, 68% accepted, 12 enrolled. In 2015, 5 master's awarded. *Degree requirements:* For master's, thesis. *Entrance requirements:* For master's, BSN, minimum GPA of 3.0, course work in statistics. Additional exam requirements/recommendations for international students: Required—TOEFL (minimum score 90 iBT). *Application deadline:* For fall admission, 1/15 for domestic students. Application fee: $100. *Expenses:* $24,781 full-time resident tuition and fees, $968 per credit hour; $44,431 full-time nonresident tuition and fees, $1,787 per credit hour. *Financial support:* Fellowships, research assistantships, and teaching assistantships available. Financial award application deadline: 3/15. *Unit head:* Dr. Kelly Caramore Walker, Director, 631-444-3299, Fax: 631-444-3136, E-mail: kelly.walker@stonybrook.edu. *Application contact:* Crystal Garcia, Staff Assistant, 631-632-3392, Fax: 631-444-3136, E-mail: crystal.garcia@stonybrook.edu.
Website: http://www.nursing.stonybrookmedicine.edu/

University of Cincinnati, Graduate School, College of Nursing, Cincinnati, OH 45221-0038. Offers clinical nurse specialist (MSN), including adult health, community health, neonatal, nursing administration, occupational health, pediatric health, psychiatric nursing, women's health; nurse anesthesia (MSN); nurse midwifery (MSN); nurse practitioner (MSN), including acute care, ambulatory care, family, family/psychiatric, women's health; nursing (PhD); MBA/MSN. *Accreditation:* AACN; AANA/CANAEP (one or more programs are accredited); ACNM/ACME. *Program availability:* Part-time, online learning. Terminal master's awarded for partial completion of doctoral program. *Degree requirements:* For master's, thesis or alternative; for doctorate, comprehensive exam, thesis/dissertation. *Entrance requirements:* For master's and doctorate, GRE General Test. Additional exam requirements/recommendations for international students: Required—TOEFL (minimum score 520 paper-based). Electronic applications accepted. *Faculty research:* Substance abuse, injury and violence, symptom management.

University of Colorado Denver, College of Nursing, Aurora, CO 80045. Offers adult clinical nurse specialist (MS); adult nurse practitioner (MS); family nurse practitioner (MS); family psychiatric mental health nurse practitioner (MS); health care informatics (MS); nurse-midwifery (MS); nursing (DNP, PhD); nursing leadership and health care systems (MS); pediatric nurse practitioner (MS); special studies (MS); women's health (MS); MS/PhD. *Accreditation:* ACNM/ACME (one or more programs are accredited). *Program availability:* Part-time, evening/weekend, online learning. *Faculty:* 109 full-time (100 women), 55 part-time/adjunct (50 women). *Students:* 367 full-time (332 women), 141 part-time (118 women); includes 79 minority (16 Black or African American, non-Hispanic/Latino; 2 American Indian or Alaska Native, non-Hispanic/Latino; 8 Asian, non-Hispanic/Latino; 37 Hispanic/Latino; 16 Two or more races, non-Hispanic/Latino), 6 international. Average age 36. 321 applicants, 53% accepted, 145 enrolled. In 2015, 151 master's, 36 doctorates awarded. Terminal master's awarded for partial completion of doctoral program. *Degree requirements:* For master's, thesis optional; for doctorate, comprehensive exam, thesis/dissertation, 42 credits of coursework. *Entrance requirements:* For master's, GRE if cumulative undergraduate GPA is less than 3.0, undergraduate nursing degree from NLNAC- or CCNE-accredited school or university; completion of research and statistics courses with minimum grade of C; copy of current and unencumbered nursing license; for doctorate, GRE, bachelor's and/or master's degrees in nursing from NLN- or CCNE-accredited institution; portfolio; minimum undergraduate GPA of 3.0, graduate 3.5; graduate-level intermediate statistics and master's-level nursing theory courses with minimum B grade; interview. Additional exam requirements/recommendations for international students: Required—TOEFL (minimum score 560 paper-based; 83 iBT). *Application deadline:* For fall admission, 2/15 for domestic students, 1/15 for international students; for spring admission, 7/1 for domestic students, 6/1 for international students. Application fee: $50 ($75 for international students). Electronic applications accepted. *Expenses:* Contact institution. *Financial support:* In 2015–16, 148 students received support. Fellowships, research assistantships, teaching assistantships, Federal Work-Study, institutionally sponsored loans, scholarships/grants, traineeships, and unspecified assistantships available. Support available to part-time students. Financial award application deadline: 4/1; financial award applicants required to submit FAFSA. *Faculty research:* Biological and behavioral phenomena in pregnancy and postpartum; patterns of glycaemia during the insulin resistance of pregnancy; obesity, gestational diabetes, and relationship to neonatal adiposity; men's awareness and knowledge of male breast cancer; cognitive-behavioral therapy for chronic insomnia after breast cancer treatment; massage therapy for the treatment of tension-type headaches. *Total annual research expenditures:* $5.9 million. *Unit head:* Dr. Sarah Thompson, Dean, 303-724-1679, E-mail: sarah.a.thompson@ucdenver.edu. *Application contact:* Judy Campbell, Graduate Programs Coordinator, 303-724-8503, E-mail: judy.campbell@ucdenver.edu. Website: http://www.ucdenver.edu/academics/colleges/nursing/Pages/default.aspx

University of Illinois at Chicago, College of Nursing, Program in Nursing, Chicago, IL 60607-7128. Offers acute care clinical nurse specialist (MS); administrative nursing leadership (Certificate); adult nurse practitioner (MS); adult/geriatric nurse practitioner (MS); advanced community health nurse specialist (MS); family nurse practitioner (MS); geriatric clinical nurse specialist (MS); geriatric nurse practitioner (MS); nurse midwifery (MS); occupational health/advanced community health nurse specialist (MS); occupational health/family nurse practitioner (MS); pediatric nurse practitioner (MS); perinatal clinical nurse specialist (MS); school/advanced community health nurse specialist (MS); school/family nurse practitioner (MS); women's health nurse practitioner (MS). *Accreditation:* AACN. *Program availability:* Part-time. *Faculty:* 100 full-time (93 women), 89 part-time/adjunct (82 women). *Students:* 359 full-time (326 women), 280 part-time (249 women); includes 169 minority (43 Black or African American, non-Hispanic/Latino; 62 Asian, non-Hispanic/Latino; 56 Hispanic/Latino; 1 Native Hawaiian or other Pacific Islander, non-Hispanic/Latino; 7 Two or more races, non-Hispanic/Latino), 12 international. Average age 32. In 2015, 4 other advanced degrees awarded. *Degree requirements:* For master's, thesis or alternative. *Entrance requirements:* For master's, GRE General Test, minimum GPA of 2.75. Additional exam requirements/recommendations for international students: Required—TOEFL. *Application deadline:* For fall admission, 5/15 for domestic students, 2/15 for international students; for spring admission, 11/1 for domestic students, 7/15 for international students. Applications are processed on a rolling basis. Application fee: $60. Electronic applications accepted. *Expenses:* Tuition, state resident: full-time $11,480; part-time $3826 per credit. Tuition, nonresident: full-time $23,720; part-time $7906 per credit. *Required fees:* $1333 per semester. Part-time tuition and fees vary according to course load and program. *Financial support:* Fellowships with full tuition reimbursements, research assistantships with full tuition reimbursements, teaching assistantships with full tuition reimbursements, career-related internships or fieldwork, Federal Work-Study, institutionally sponsored loans, scholarships/grants, traineeships, tuition waivers (full and partial), and unspecified assistantships available. Support available to part-time students. Financial award application deadline: 3/1; financial award applicants required to submit FAFSA. *Unit head:* Dr. Terri E. Weaver, Dean, 312-996-7808, E-mail: teweaver@uic.edu. *Application contact:* Receptionist, 312-413-2550, E-mail: gradcoll@uic.edu. Website: http://www.nursing.uic.edu/academics-admissions/master-science#program-overview

University of Indianapolis, Graduate Programs, School of Nursing, Indianapolis, IN 46227-3697. Offers advanced practice nursing (DNP); family nurse practitioner (MSN); gerontological nurse practitioner (MSN); neonatal nurse practitioner (MSN); nurse-midwifery (MSN); nursing (MSN); nursing and health systems leadership (MSN); nursing education (MSN); women's health nurse practitioner (MSN); MBA/MSN. *Accreditation:* AACN; ACNM. *Entrance requirements:* For master's, minimum GPA of 3.0, interview, letters of recommendation, resume, RN nursing license, 1 year of professional practice; for doctorate, graduate of NLNAC- or CCNE-accredited nursing program; MSN or MA with nursing major and minimum cumulative GPA of 3.25; unencumbered RN license with eligibility for licensure in Indiana; completion of graduate-level statistics course within last 5 years with minimum grade of B; resume; essay; official transcripts from all academic institutions. Additional exam requirements/recommendations for international students: Required—TOEFL (minimum score 550 paper-based). Electronic applications accepted.

The University of Kansas, University of Kansas Medical Center, School of Nursing, Kansas City, KS 66160. Offers adult/gerontological clinical nurse specialist (PMC); adult/gerontological nurse practitioner (PMC); clinical research management (PMC); health care informatics (PMC); health professions educator (PMC); nurse midwife (PMC); nursing (MS, DNP, PhD); organizational leadership (PMC); psychiatric/mental health nurse practitioner (PMC); public health nursing (PMC). *Accreditation:* AACN; ACNM/ACME. *Program availability:* Part-time, 100% online, blended/hybrid learning. *Faculty:* 59. *Students:* 44 full-time (42 women), 261 part-time (238 women); includes 54 minority (22 Black or African American, non-Hispanic/Latino; 1 American Indian or Alaska Native, non-Hispanic/Latino; 12 Asian, non-Hispanic/Latino; 10 Hispanic/Latino; 9 Two or more races, non-Hispanic/Latino), 1 international. Average age 38. 95 applicants, 97% accepted, 74 enrolled. In 2015, 71 master's, 24 doctorates, 6 other advanced degrees awarded. Terminal master's awarded for partial completion of doctoral program. *Degree requirements:* For master's, comprehensive exam, thesis (for some programs), general oral exam; for doctorate, variable foreign language requirement, thesis/dissertation or alternative, comprehensive oral exam (for DNP); comprehensive written and oral exam, or three publications (for PhD). *Entrance requirements:* For master's, bachelor's degree in nursing, minimum GPA of 3.0, 1 year of clinical experience, RN license in KS and MO; for doctorate, GRE General Test (for PhD only), bachelor's degree in nursing, minimum GPA of 3.5, RN license in KS and MO. Additional exam requirements/recommendations for international students: Required—TOEFL. *Application deadline:* For fall admission, 4/1 for domestic and international students; for spring admission, 9/1 for domestic and international students. Application fee: $60. Electronic applications accepted. *Financial support:* Research assistantships with tuition reimbursements, teaching assistantships with tuition reimbursements, scholarships/grants, and traineeships available. Financial award application deadline: 3/1; financial award applicants required to submit FAFSA. *Faculty research:* Breastfeeding practices of teen mothers, national database of nursing quality indicators, caregiving of families of patients using technology in the home, simulation in nursing education, diaphragm fatigue. *Total annual research expenditures:* $4.6 million. *Unit head:* Dr. Sally Maliski, Dean, 913-588-1601, Fax: 913-588-1660, E-mail: smaliski@kumc.edu. *Application contact:* Dr. Pamela K. Barnes, Associate Dean, Student Affairs, 913-588-1619, Fax: 913-588-1615, E-mail: pbarnes2@kumc.edu. Website: http://nursing.kumc.edu

The University of Manchester, School of Nursing, Midwifery and Social Work, Manchester, United Kingdom. Offers nursing (M Phil, PhD); social work (M Phil, PhD).

University of Maryland, Baltimore, Graduate School, School of Nursing, Master's Program in Nursing, Baltimore, MD 21201. Offers community health nursing (MS); gerontological nursing (MS); maternal-child nursing (MS); medical-surgical nursing (MS); nurse-midwifery education (MS); nursing administration (MS); nursing education (MS); nursing health policy (MS); primary care nursing (MS); psychiatric nursing (MS); MS/MBA. MS/MBA offered jointly with University of Baltimore. *Accreditation:* AACN; AANA/CANAEP. *Program availability:* Part-time. *Degree requirements:* For master's, comprehensive exam (for some programs), thesis or alternative. *Entrance requirements:* For master's, minimum GPA of 2.75, course work in statistics, BS in nursing. Additional exam requirements/recommendations for international students: Required—TOEFL (minimum score 550 paper-based; 80 iBT); Recommended—IELTS (minimum score 7). Electronic applications accepted. Tuition and fees vary according to program.

University of Miami, Graduate School, School of Nursing and Health Studies, Coral Gables, FL 33124. Offers acute care (MSN), including acute care nurse practitioner, nurse anesthesia; nursing (PhD); primary care (MSN), including adult nurse practitioner, family nurse practitioner, nurse midwifery, women's health practitioner. *Accreditation:* AACN; AANA/CANAEP; ACNM/ACME (one or more programs are accredited). *Program availability:* Part-time. *Degree requirements:* For master's, thesis optional; for doctorate, thesis/dissertation. *Entrance requirements:* For master's, GRE General Test, BSN, minimum GPA of 3.0, Florida RN license; for doctorate, GRE General Test, BSN or MSN, minimum GPA of 3.0. Additional exam requirements/recommendations for international students: Required—TOEFL (minimum score 550 paper-based). Electronic applications accepted. *Faculty research:* Transcultural nursing, exercise and depression in Alzheimer's disease, infectious diseases/HIV–AIDS, postpartum depression, outcomes assessment.

University of Minnesota, Twin Cities Campus, Graduate School, School of Nursing, Nurse Midwifery Program, Minneapolis, MN 55455-0213. Offers MS. *Accreditation:* ACNM/ACME. *Program availability:* Online learning. *Degree requirements:* For master's, final oral exam, project or thesis. *Entrance requirements:* Additional exam requirements/recommendations for international students: Required—TOEFL (minimum score 586 paper-based).

University of Pennsylvania, School of Nursing, Program in Nurse Midwifery, Philadelphia, PA 19104. Offers MSN. *Accreditation:* AACN; ACNM/ACME. *Program availability:* Part-time. *Students:* 34 full-time (all women), 15 part-time (all women); includes 14 minority (6 Black or African American, non-Hispanic/Latino; 2 Asian, non-Hispanic/Latino; 6 Hispanic/Latino). Average age 30. 38 applicants, 58% accepted, 14 enrolled. In 2015, 17 master's awarded. *Expenses:* Tuition, area resident: Full-time $31,068; part-time $5762 per course. *Required fees:* $3200; $336 per course. Full-time tuition and fees vary according to degree level, program and student level. Part-time tuition and fees vary according to course load, degree level and program.

University of Puerto Rico, Medical Sciences Campus, Graduate School of Public Health, Department of Human Development, Program in Nurse Midwifery, San Juan, PR 00936-5067. Offers MPH, Certificate. *Accreditation:* ACNM/ACME. *Program availability:* Part-time. *Entrance requirements:* For master's, GRE, previous course work in algebra.

University of South Africa, College of Human Sciences, Pretoria, South Africa. Offers adult education (M Ed); African languages (MA, PhD); African politics (MA, PhD); Afrikaans (MA, PhD); ancient history (MA, PhD); ancient Near Eastern studies (MA, PhD); anthropology (MA, PhD); applied linguistics (MA); Arabic (MA, PhD); archaeology (MA); art history (MA); Biblical archaeology (MA); Biblical studies (M Th, D Th, PhD); Christian spirituality (M Th, D Th); church history (M Th, D Th); classical studies (MA, PhD); clinical psychology (MA); communication (MA, PhD); comparative education (M Ed, Ed D); consulting psychology (D Admin, D Com, PhD); curriculum studies (M Ed, Ed D); development studies (M Admin, MA, D Admin, PhD); didactics (M Ed, Ed D); education (M Tech); education management (M Ed, Ed D); educational psychology (M Ed); English (MA); environmental education (M Ed); French (MA, PhD); German (MA, PhD); Greek (MA); guidance and counseling (M Ed); health studies (MA, PhD), including health sciences education (MA), health services management (MA), medical and surgical nursing science (critical care general) (MA), midwifery and neonatal nursing science (MA), trauma and emergency care (MA); history (MA, PhD); history of education (Ed D); inclusive education (M Ed, Ed D); information and communications technology policy and regulation (MA); information science (MA, MIS, PhD); international politics (MA, PhD); Islamic studies (MA, PhD); Italian (MA, PhD); Judaica (MA); linguistics (MA, PhD); mathematical education (M Ed); mathematics education (MA); missiology (M Th, D Th); modern Hebrew (MA, PhD); musicology (MA, MMus, D Mus, PhD); natural science education (M Ed); New Testament (M Th, D Th); Old Testament (D Th); pastoral therapy (M Th, D Th); philosophy (MA); philosophy of education (M Ed, Ed D); politics (MA, PhD); Portuguese (MA, PhD); practical theology (M Th, D Th); psychology (MA, MS, PhD); psychology of education (M Ed, Ed D); public health (MA); religious studies (MA, D Th, PhD); Romance languages (MA); Russian (MA, PhD); Semitic languages (MA, PhD); social behavior studies in HIV/AIDS (MA); social science (mental health) (MA); social science in development studies (MA); social science in psychology

Nurse Midwifery

(MA); social science in social work (MA); social science in sociology (MA); social work (MSW, DSW, PhD); socio-education (M Ed, Ed D); sociolinguistics (MA); sociology (MA, PhD); Spanish (MA, PhD); systematic theology (M Th, D Th); TESOL (teaching English to speakers of other languages) (MA); theological ethics (M Th, D Th); theory of literature (MA, PhD); urban ministries (D Th); urban ministry (M Th).

Vanderbilt University, Vanderbilt University School of Nursing, Nashville, TN 37240. Offers adult-gerontology acute care nurse practitioner (MSN), including hospitalist, intensivist; adult-gerontology primary care nurse practitioner (MSN); emergency nurse practitioner (MSN); family nurse practitioner (MSN); healthcare leadership (MSN); neonatal nurse practitioner (MSN); nurse midwifery (MSN); nurse midwifery/family nurse practitioner (MSN); nursing (Post-Master's Certificate); nursing informatics (MSN); nursing practice (DNP); nursing science (PhD); pediatric acute care nurse practitioner (MSN); pediatric primary care nurse practitioner (MSN); psychiatric-mental health nurse practitioner (MSN); women's health nurse practitioner (MSN); women's health nurse practitioner/adult gerontology primary care nurse practitioner (MSN); MSN/M Div; MSN/MTS. *Accreditation:* ACEN (one or more programs are accredited); ACNM/ACME. *Program availability:* Part-time, 100% online, blended/hybrid learning. *Faculty:* 258 full-time (232 women), 363 part-time/adjunct (271 women). *Students:* 478 full-time (424 women), 342 part-time (317 women); includes 140 minority (36 Black or African American, non-Hispanic/Latino; 3 American Indian or Alaska Native, non-Hispanic/Latino; 24 Asian, non-Hispanic/Latino; 43 Hispanic/Latino; 3 Native Hawaiian or other Pacific Islander, non-Hispanic/Latino; 31 Two or more races, non-Hispanic/Latino), 11 international. Average age 31. 1,268 applicants, 49% accepted, 477 enrolled. In 2015, 343 master's, 55 doctorates awarded. *Degree requirements:* For doctorate, comprehensive exam, thesis/dissertation. *Entrance requirements:* For master's, GRE General Test (taken within the past 5 years), minimum B average in undergraduate course work, 3 letters of recommendation; for doctorate, GRE General Test, interview, 3 letters of recommendation from doctorally-prepared faculty, MSN, essay. Additional exam requirements/recommendations for international students: Required—TOEFL (minimum score 570 paper-based), IELTS (minimum score 6.5). *Application deadline:* For fall admission, 11/1 priority date for domestic and international students. Applications are processed on a rolling basis. Application fee: $50. Electronic applications accepted. *Expenses:* Contact institution. *Financial support:* In 2015–16, 585 students received support. Scholarships/grants available. Financial award application deadline: 3/15; financial award applicants required to submit FAFSA. *Faculty research:* Lymphedema, palliative care and bereavement, health services research including workforce, safety and quality of care, gerontology, better birth outcomes including nutrition. *Total annual research expenditures:* $2 million. *Unit head:* Dr. Linda Norman, Dean, 615-343-8876, Fax: 615-343-7711, E-mail: linda.norman@vanderbilt.edu. *Application contact:* Patricia Peerman, Assistant Dean for Enrollment Management, 615-322-3800, Fax: 615-343-0333, E-mail: vusn-admissions@vanderbilt.edu.
Website: http://www.nursing.vanderbilt.edu

Wayne State University, College of Nursing, Doctor Program of Nursing Practice, Detroit, MI 48202. Offers adult gerontology nurse practitioner - acute care (DNP); adult gerontology nurse practitioner - primary care (DNP); family nurse practitioner (DNP); infant mental health (DNP); neonatal nurse practitioner (DNP); nurse midwifery (DNP); nursing practice (DNP); pediatric nurse practitioner - acute care (DNP); pediatric nurse practitioner - primary care (DNP); psychiatric mental health nurse practitioner (DNP). *Students:* 56 full-time (50 women), 37 part-time (32 women); includes 32 minority (19 Black or African American, non-Hispanic/Latino; 6 Asian, non-Hispanic/Latino; 3 Hispanic/Latino; 4 Two or more races, non-Hispanic/Latino), 6 international. Average age 35. 44 applicants, 66% accepted, 18 enrolled. In 2015, 16 doctorates awarded. *Entrance requirements:* For doctorate, official transcripts, two professional references, curriculum vitae or resume, statement of goals, BSN or MSN, current Michigan RN license, criminal background check, interview, on-site writing example. Additional exam requirements/recommendations for international students: Required—TOEFL (minimum score 600 paper-based; 101 iBT); Recommended—IELTS (minimum score 7). *Application deadline:* For fall admission, 1/31 for domestic and international students. Electronic applications accepted. *Expenses:* $19,325 per year resident tuition, $35,114 non-resident tuition; $805.20 per credit hour resident tuition, $1,463.10 per credit hour non-resident tuition; fees include $47.45 per credit hour student services fee and $274.60 per semester registration fee. *Financial support:* In 2015–16, 22 students received support. Fellowships, research assistantships, teaching assistantships, institutionally sponsored loans, and scholarships/grants available. Financial award applicants required to submit FAFSA. *Unit head:* Dr. Laurie Lauzon Clabo, Dean and

Professor, 313-577-4104, E-mail: laurie.lauzon.clabo@wayne.edu. *Application contact:* Dr. Nancy George, Director of DNP Program, 313-577-8300.
Website: http://nursing.wayne.edu/dnp/index.php

Wayne State University, College of Nursing, Graduate Certificates Program in Clinical Specialties, Detroit, MI 48202. Offers acute care nurse practitioner (Graduate Certificate); nurse midwifery (Graduate Certificate); pediatric nurse practitioner - acute care (Graduate Certificate); pediatric nurse practitioner - primary care (Graduate Certificate); psychiatric mental health nurse practitioner (Graduate Certificate). *Accreditation:* AACN. *Program availability:* Part-time. *Students:* 2 full-time (both women), 7 part-time (all women). Average age 43. 67 applicants, 12% accepted, 5 enrolled. *Entrance requirements:* For degree, master's or doctoral degree in nursing from nationally-accredited institution, current RN license, three letters of reference, personal statement. Additional exam requirements/recommendations for international students: Required—TOEFL (minimum score 600 paper-based; 101 iBT), TWE, Michigan English Language Assessment Battery (minimum score 85); Recommended—IELTS (minimum score 7). *Application deadline:* For fall admission, 6/1 priority date for domestic students, 5/1 priority date for international students; for winter admission, 10/1 priority date for domestic students, 9/1 priority date for international students; for spring admission, 2/1 priority date for domestic students, 1/1 priority date for international students. Application fee: $0. Electronic applications accepted. *Expenses:* $19,325 annual resident tuition, $35,114 non-resident tuition; $805.20 per credit hour resident tuition, $1,463.10 per credit hour non-resident tuition; fees include $47.45 per credit hour student services fee and $274.60 per semester registration fee. *Financial support:* Scholarships/grants available. Financial award application deadline: 3/31; financial award applicants required to submit FAFSA. *Unit head:* Dr. Laurie Lauzon Clabo, Dean and Professor, 313-577-4104, E-mail: laurie.lauzon.clabo@wayne.edu. *Application contact:* Leanne Nantais-Smith, Director, MSN Program and Graduate Certificates, E-mail: ar2446@wayne.edu. Website: http://nursing.wayne.edu/gradcert/specialties.php

Wayne State University, College of Nursing, M.S.N. Program in Clinical Specialties, Detroit, MI 48202. Offers nurse-midwifery (MSN); pediatric nurse practitioner acute care (MSN); psychiatric mental health nurse practitioner (MSN). *Accreditation:* AACN. *Program availability:* Part-time. *Students:* 49 full-time (47 women), 85 part-time (79 women); includes 29 minority (15 Black or African American, non-Hispanic/Latino; 7 Asian, non-Hispanic/Latino; 3 Hispanic/Latino; 4 Two or more races, non-Hispanic/Latino), 5 international. Average age 33. 111 applicants, 20% accepted, 17 enrolled. In 2015, 108 master's awarded. *Degree requirements:* For master's, thesis or alternative. *Entrance requirements:* For master's, BSN from NLN- or CCNE-accredited program with minimum GPA of 3.0; three references; current RN license; personal statement. Additional exam requirements/recommendations for international students: Required—TOEFL (minimum score 600 paper-based; 101 iBT); Recommended—TWE. *Application deadline:* For fall admission, 6/1 for domestic students, 5/1 priority date for international students; for winter admission, 10/1 for domestic students, 9/1 priority date for international students; for spring admission, 2/1 for domestic students, 1/1 priority date for international students. Electronic applications accepted. *Expenses:* $19,325 per resident tuition, $35,114 non-resident tuition; $805.20 per credit hour resident tuition, $1,463.10 per credit hour non-resident tuition; fees include $47.45 per credit hour student services fee and $274.60 per semester registration fee. *Financial support:* In 2015–16, 36 students received support. Fellowships with tuition reimbursements available, research assistantships with tuition reimbursements available, teaching assistantships with tuition reimbursements available, scholarships/grants, traineeships, and unspecified assistantships available. Support available to part-time students. Financial award applicants required to submit FAFSA. *Faculty research:* Smoking risk behaviors in adolescents, sleep disturbances in postmenopausal women, health disparities in urban environments, nurse practitioner interventions, care giving and pain management. *Unit head:* Dr. Laurie Lauzon Clabo, Dean and Professor, 313-577-4104, E-mail: laurie.lauzon.clabo@wayne.edu. *Application contact:* Dr. Leanne Nantais-Smith, Program Director, MSN and Graduate Certificates, 313-577-5934, E-mail: ar2446@wayne.edu.
Website: http://nursing.wayne.edu/msn/specialty.php

West Virginia Wesleyan College, Department of Nursing, Buckhannon, WV 26201. Offers family nurse practitioner (Post Master's Certificate); family nurse practitoner (MS); nurse administrator (MS); nurse educator (MS); nurse-midwifery (MS); nursing administration (Post Master's Certificate); nursing education (Post Master's Certificate); psychiatric mental health nurse practitioner (MS); MSN/MBA. *Accreditation:* ACEN.

Nursing and Healthcare Administration

Adelphi University, College of Nursing and Public Health, Program in Nursing Administration, Garden City, NY 11530-0701. Offers MS, Certificate.

Allen College, Graduate Programs, Waterloo, IA 50703. Offers acute care nurse practitioner (Post-Master's Certificate); adult nurse practitioner (Post-Master's Certificate); adult psychiatric-mental health nurse practitioner (Post-Master's Certificate); adult-gerontology acute care nurse practitioner (MSN); community public health (Post-Master's Certificate); community/public health nursing (MSN); family nurse practitioner (MSN, Post-Master's Certificate); gerontological nurse practitioner (Post-Master's Certificate); health sciences (Ed D); leadership in health care delivery (MSN, Post-Master's Certificate); nursing (DNP); occupational therapy (MS). *Accreditation:* AACN; ACEN. *Program availability:* Part-time, blended/hybrid learning. *Faculty:* 3 full-time (all women), 21 part-time/adjunct (20 women). *Students:* 61 full-time (54 women), 163 part-time (144 women); includes 9 minority (5 Black or African American, non-Hispanic/Latino; 2 Hispanic/Latino; 2 Two or more races, non-Hispanic/Latino), 2 international. Average age 34. 212 applicants, 60% accepted, 94 enrolled. In 2015, 51 master's, 1 doctorate awarded. *Degree requirements:* For master's, thesis optional. *Entrance requirements:* For master's, minimum GPA of 3.0 in the last 60 hours of undergraduate coursework; for doctorate, minimum GPA of 3.25 in graduate coursework. Additional exam requirements/recommendations for international students: Recommended—TOEFL (minimum score 580 paper-based; 92 iBT), IELTS (minimum score 6). *Application deadline:* For fall admission, 2/1 priority date for domestic students; for spring admission, 9/1 priority date for domestic students. Applications are processed on a rolling basis. Application fee: $50. Electronic applications accepted. *Expenses:* $15,940 tuition, $1,240 fees. *Financial support:* Institutionally sponsored loans, scholarships/grants, and traineeships available. Support available to part-time students. Financial award application deadline: 8/15; financial award applicants required to submit FAFSA. *Unit head:* Nancy Kramer, Vice Chancellor for Academic Affairs, 319-226-2040, Fax: 319-226-2070, E-mail: nancy.kramer@allencollege.edu. *Application contact:* Molly Quinn, Administrative Assistant for Student Services, 319-226-2014, Fax: 319-226-

2010, E-mail: admissions@allencollege.edu.
Website: http://www.allencollege.edu/

American International College, School of Health Sciences, Master of Science in Nursing Program, Springfield, MA 01109-3189. Offers family nurse practitioner (MSN); nursing administration (MSN); nursing education (MSN). *Accreditation:* AACN. *Program availability:* Part-time, evening/weekend, online only, blended/hybrid learning. *Faculty:* 1 (woman) full-time, 1 (woman) part-time/adjunct. *Students:* 52 full-time (49 women), 4 part-time (all women); includes 18 minority (12 Black or African American, non-Hispanic/Latino; 1 Asian, non-Hispanic/Latino; 4 Hispanic/Latino; 1 Two or more races, non-Hispanic/Latino). Average age 36. 66 applicants, 53% accepted, 27 enrolled. In 2015, 8 master's awarded. *Entrance requirements:* For master's, BSN, minimum GPA of 3.0. Additional exam requirements/recommendations for international students: Required—TOEFL, IELTS. *Application deadline:* For fall admission, 8/20 for domestic students, 7/1 priority date for international students; for spring admission, 1/4 for domestic students, 12/1 priority date for international students. Applications are processed on a rolling basis. Application fee: $50. Electronic applications accepted. *Expenses:* Contact institution. *Financial support:* Applicants required to submit FAFSA. *Unit head:* Dr. Ellen Furman, Associate Director of Graduate Nursing, 413-205-3918, Fax: 413-654-1430, E-mail: ellen.furman@aic.edu. *Application contact:* Kerry Barnes, Director of Graduate Admissions, 413-205-3703, Fax: 413-205-3051, E-mail: kerry.barnes@aic.edu.
Website: http://www.aic.edu/academics/hs/nursing

Arizona State University at the Tempe campus, College of Nursing and Health Innovation, Phoenix, AZ 85004. Offers advanced nursing practice (DNP); clinical research management (MS); community and public health practice (Graduate Certificate); family mental health nurse practitioner (Graduate Certificate); family nurse practitioner (Graduate Certificate); geriatric nursing (Graduate Certificate); healthcare innovation (MHI); nurse education in academic and practice settings (Graduate Certificate); nurse educator (MS); nursing and healthcare innovation (PhD).

Accreditation: AACN. *Program availability:* Online learning. *Degree requirements:* For master's, comprehensive exam (for some programs), thesis (for some programs), interactive Program of Study (iPOS) submitted before completing 50 percent of required credit hours; for doctorate, comprehensive exam, thesis/dissertation, interactive Program of Study (iPOS) submitted before completing 50 percent of required credit hours. *Entrance requirements:* For master's and doctorate, GRE, minimum GPA of 3.0 or equivalent in last 2 years of work leading to bachelor's degree. Additional exam requirements/recommendations for international students: Required—TOEFL, IELTS, or PTE. Electronic applications accepted. *Expenses:* Contact institution.

Athabasca University, Faculty of Health Disciplines, Athabasca, AB T9S 3A3, Canada. Offers advanced nursing practice (MN, Advanced Diploma); generalist (MN); health studies (MHS). *Program availability:* Part-time, online learning. *Faculty:* 11 full-time (all women), 1 (woman) part-time/adjunct. *Students:* 1,687 part-time. Average age 38. In 2015, 243 master's, 5 other advanced degrees awarded. *Degree requirements:* For master's, comprehensive exam (for some programs). *Entrance requirements:* For master's, bachelor's degree in health-related field and 2 years of professional health service experience (MHS); bachelor's degree in nursing and 2 years' nursing experience (MN); minimum GPA of 3.0 in final 30 credits; for Advanced Diploma, RN license, 2 years of health care experience. *Application deadline:* For fall admission, 3/1 for domestic and international students. Application fee: $80. Electronic applications accepted. *Expenses:* Contact institution. *Unit head:* Dr. Margaret Edwards, Dean, 800-788-9041 Ext. 6381, Fax: 780-675-6468, E-mail: marge@athabascau.ca. *Application contact:* Donna Dunn Hart, Academic Student Advisor, Graduate Programs, 800-788-9041 Ext. 6300, Fax: 780-675-6468, E-mail: donnad@athabascau.ca.
Website: http://fhd.athabascau.ca/

Augusta University, The Graduate School, Clinical Nurse Leader Program, Augusta, GA 30912. Offers MSN. *Entrance requirements:* For master's, GRE General Test or MAT, bachelor's degree or higher in a non-nursing discipline, minimum undergraduate cumulative GPA of 3.0. Additional exam requirements/recommendations for international students: Required—TOEFL (minimum score 550 paper-based; 79 iBT). *Application deadline:* For fall admission, 4/1 for domestic and international students. Application fee: $50. Electronic applications accepted. *Unit head:* Dr. Stephanie Wright, Director, 706-721-9767, Fax: 706-721-8169. *Application contact:* Emily Holsey, Program Manager, 706-721-9767, Fax: 706-721-8169, E-mail: cnl@augusta.edu.
Website: http://www.augusta.edu/nursing/cnl.php

Austin Peay State University, College of Graduate Studies, College of Behavioral and Health Sciences, School of Nursing, Clarksville, TN 37044. Offers family nurse practitioner (MSN); nursing administration (MSN); nursing education (MSN); nursing informatics (MSN). *Program availability:* Part-time, online learning. *Faculty:* 11 full-time (all women), 6 part-time/adjunct (all women). *Students:* 23 full-time (20 women), 142 part-time (125 women); includes 27 minority (19 Black or African American, non-Hispanic/Latino; 4 Hispanic/Latino; 4 Two or more races, non-Hispanic/Latino). Average age 35. 25 applicants, 76% accepted, 14 enrolled. In 2015, 67 master's awarded. *Degree requirements:* For master's, comprehensive exam. *Entrance requirements:* For master's, minimum GPA of 3.0, RN license eligibility, 3 letters of recommendation. Additional exam requirements/recommendations for international students: Required—TOEFL (minimum score 500 paper-based). *Application deadline:* For fall admission, 8/3 priority date for domestic students. Applications are processed on a rolling basis. Application fee: $25. Electronic applications accepted. *Expenses:* Tuition, state resident: full-time $8080; part-time $404 per credit hour. Tuition, nonresident: full-time $21,680; part-time $1084 per credit hour. *Required fees:* $1453; $72.65 per credit hour. *Financial support:* In 2015–16, research assistantships with full tuition reimbursements (averaging $5,184 per year) were awarded; career-related internships or fieldwork, Federal Work-Study, institutionally sponsored loans, scholarships/grants, and unspecified assistantships also available. Support available to part-time students. Financial award application deadline: 3/1; financial award applicants required to submit FAFSA. *Unit head:* Dr. Grace Moodt, Interim Director, 931-221-6290, Fax: 931-221-7595, E-mail: moodtg@apsu.edu. *Application contact:* June D. Lee, Graduate Coordinator, 800-859-4723, Fax: 931-221-7641, E-mail: gradadmissions@apsu.edu.
Website: http://www.apsu.edu/nursing

Barry University, School of Adult and Continuing Education, Division of Nursing, Program in Nursing Administration, Miami Shores, FL 33161-6695. Offers MSN, PhD, Certificate. *Accreditation:* AACN. *Program availability:* Part-time, evening/weekend. *Degree requirements:* For master's, research project or thesis. *Entrance requirements:* For master's, GRE General Test or MAT, BSN, minimum GPA of 3.0, course work in statistics. Electronic applications accepted. *Faculty research:* Power/empowerment, health delivery systems, managed care, employee health and well being.

Barry University, School of Adult and Continuing Education, Division of Nursing and Andreas School of Business, Program in Nursing Administration and Business Administration, Miami Shores, FL 33161-6695. Offers MSN/MBA. *Accreditation:* AACN. *Program availability:* Part-time, evening/weekend. Electronic applications accepted. *Faculty research:* Power/empowerment, health delivery systems, managed care, employee health well-being.

Bellarmine University, Donna and Allan Lansing School of Nursing and Health Sciences, Louisville, KY 40205. Offers family nurse practitioner (MSN); health science (MHS); nursing administration (MSN); nursing education (MSN); nursing practice (DNP); physical therapy (DPT). *Accreditation:* AACN; APTA. *Program availability:* Part-time, evening/weekend. *Faculty:* 27 full-time (24 women), 8 part-time/adjunct (7 women). *Students:* 210 full-time (144 women), 91 part-time (83 women); includes 22 minority (6 Black or African American, non-Hispanic/Latino; 1 American Indian or Alaska Native, non-Hispanic/Latino; 7 Asian, non-Hispanic/Latino; 4 Hispanic/Latino; 4 Two or more races, non-Hispanic/Latino), 2 international. Average age 28. In 2015, 33 master's, 64 doctorates awarded. *Degree requirements:* For doctorate, comprehensive exam, thesis/dissertation. *Entrance requirements:* For master's, GRE General Test, RN license; for doctorate, GRE General Test, Physical Therapist Centralized Application Service (for DPT). Additional exam requirements/recommendations for international students: Required—TOEFL (minimum score 550 paper-based; 80 iBT). Application fee: $40. Electronic applications accepted. *Expenses:* Contact institution. *Financial support:* Career-related internships or fieldwork and scholarships/grants available. *Faculty research:* Nursing: pain, empathy, leadership styles, control; physical therapy: service-learning; exercise in chronic and pre-operative conditions, athletes; women's health; aging. *Unit head:* Dr. Mark Wiegand, Dean, 800-274-4723 Ext. 8368, E-mail: mwiegand@bellarmine.edu. *Application contact:* Julie Armstrong-Binnix, Health Science Recruiter, 800-274-4723 Ext. 8364, E-mail: julieab@bellarmine.edu.
Website: http://www.bellarmine.edu/lansing

Blessing–Rieman College of Nursing and Health Sciences, Master of Science in Nursing Program, Quincy, IL 62305-7005. Offers nursing administration (MSN); nursing education (MSN). *Program availability:* Part-time-only, online only, 100% online. In 2015, 8 master's awarded. *Degree requirements:* For master's, thesis or project. *Entrance requirements:* Additional exam requirements/recommendations for international students: Required—TOEFL (minimum score 500 paper-based; 80 iBT). *Application deadline:* Applications are processed on a rolling basis. Electronic applications accepted. *Expenses:* Contact institution. *Financial support:* In 2015–16,

20,350 students received support. Scholarships/grants available. Financial award application deadline: 4/30; financial award applicants required to submit FAFSA. *Unit head:* Dr. Karen Mayville, Administrative Coordinator, Accreditation, 217-228-5520 Ext. 6968, Fax: 217-223-4661, E-mail: kmayville@brcn.edu. *Application contact:* Heather Mutter, Admissions Counselor, 217-228-5520 Ext. 6964, Fax: 217-223-1781, E-mail: hmutter@brcn.edu.
Website: http://brcn.edu

Bloomsburg University of Pennsylvania, School of Graduate Studies, College of Science and Technology, Department of Nursing, Bloomsburg, PA 17815. Offers adult and family nurse practitioner (MSN); community health (MSN); nurse anesthesia (MSN); nursing (MSN); nursing administration (MSN). *Accreditation:* AACN; AANA/CANAEP. *Degree requirements:* For master's, thesis (for some programs), clinical experience. *Entrance requirements:* For master's, minimum QPA of 3.0, personal statement, 2 letters of recommendation, nursing license. Additional exam requirements/recommendations for international students: Required—TOEFL. Electronic applications accepted.

Bowie State University, Graduate Programs, Department of Nursing, Bowie, MD 20715-9465. Offers administration of nursing services (MS); family nurse practitioner (MS); nursing education (MS). *Accreditation:* ACEN. *Program availability:* Part-time. *Degree requirements:* For master's, comprehensive exam, thesis, research paper. *Entrance requirements:* For master's, minimum GPA of 2.5. Electronic applications accepted. *Expenses:* Tuition, state resident: full-time $9384; part-time $2346 per year. Tuition, nonresident: full-time $16,344; part-time $4086 per year. *Required fees:* $2552; $325 per semester. *Faculty research:* Minority health, women's health, gerontology, leadership management.

Bradley University, Graduate School, College of Education and Health Sciences, Department of Nursing, Peoria, IL 61625-0002. Offers nursing (DNP, Certificate); nursing administration (MSN); nursing education (MSN). *Accreditation:* ACEN. *Program availability:* Part-time, evening/weekend. *Degree requirements:* For master's, comprehensive exam, thesis optional. *Entrance requirements:* For master's, GRE General Test or MAT, interview, Illinois RN license, advanced cardiac life support certification, pediatric advanced life support certification, 3 letters of recommendation. Additional exam requirements/recommendations for international students: Required—TOEFL (minimum score 550 paper-based; 79 iBT), IELTS (minimum score 6.5). Electronic applications accepted.

Brenau University, Sydney O. Smith Graduate School, College of Health and Science, Gainesville, GA 30501. Offers family nurse practitioner (MSN); nurse educator (MSN); nursing management (MSN); occupational therapy (MS); psychology (MS). *Accreditation:* AOTA. *Program availability:* Part-time, evening/weekend. *Degree requirements:* For master's, comprehensive exam (for some programs), thesis (for some programs), clinical practicum hours. *Entrance requirements:* For master's, GRE General Test or MAT (for some programs), interview, writing sample, references (for some programs). Additional exam requirements/recommendations for international students: Required—TOEFL (minimum score 500 paper-based; 61 iBT); Recommended—IELTS (minimum score 5). Electronic applications accepted. *Expenses:* Contact institution.

California State University, Fullerton, Graduate Studies, College of Health and Human Development, Department of Nursing, Fullerton, CA 92834-9480. Offers leadership (MSN); nurse anesthesia (MSN); nurse educator (MSN); nursing (DNP); women's health care (MSN). *Accreditation:* AACN; AANA/CANAEP. *Program availability:* Part-time.

California University of Pennsylvania, School of Graduate Studies and Research, Eberly College of Science and Technology, Program in Business Administration, California, PA 15419-1394. Offers business administration (MBA); business analytics (MBA); entrepreneurship (MBA); nursing administration and leadership (MBA). *Program availability:* Part-time, evening/weekend. *Degree requirements:* For master's, comprehensive exam. *Entrance requirements:* For master's, minimum GPA of 3.0, official transcripts. Additional exam requirements/recommendations for international students: Required—TOEFL (minimum score 550 paper-based). *Application deadline:* For fall admission, 8/1 priority date for domestic and international students; for winter admission, 12/1 priority date for domestic and international students; for spring admission, 5/1 priority date for domestic and international students. Applications are processed on a rolling basis. Application fee: $25. Electronic applications accepted. *Expenses:* Tuition, state resident: full-time $11,280; part-time $5640 per semester. Tuition, nonresident: full-time $16,920; part-time $8460 per semester. *Required fees:* $2876. Tuition and fees vary according to course load, degree level, campus/location and reciprocity agreements. *Financial support:* Career-related internships or fieldwork, scholarships/grants, traineeships, and unspecified assistantships available. Financial award applicants required to submit FAFSA. *Faculty research:* Economics, applied economics, consumer behavior, technology and business, impact of technology. *Unit head:* Dr. Arshad Chawdhry, Graduate Coordinator, 724-938-5990, Fax: 724-938-5908, E-mail: chawdhry@cup.edu. *Application contact:* Suzanne C. Powers, Director of Graduate Admissions and Recruitment, 724-938-4029, Fax: 724-938-5712, E-mail: powers_s@cup.edu.
Website: http://www.calu.edu/academics/graduate-programs/business-administration/

Capella University, School of Public Service Leadership, Master's Programs in Nursing, Minneapolis, MN 55402. Offers diabetes nursing (MSN); general nursing (MSN); gerontology nursing (MSN); health information management (MS); nurse educator (MSN); nursing leadership and administration (MSN).

Capital University, School of Nursing, Columbus, OH 43209-2394. Offers administration (MSN); legal studies (MSN); theological studies (MSN); JD/MSN; MBA/MSN; MSN/MTS. *Accreditation:* AACN. *Program availability:* Part-time, evening/weekend. *Degree requirements:* For master's, thesis or alternative. *Entrance requirements:* For master's, BSN, current RN license, minimum GPA of 3.0, undergraduate courses in statistics and research. Additional exam requirements/recommendations for international students: Required—TOEFL (minimum score 550 paper-based). *Expenses:* Contact institution. *Faculty research:* Bereavement, wellness/health promotion, emergency cardiac care, critical thinking, complementary and alternative healthcare.

Carlow University, College of Health and Wellness, Program in Nursing Leadership and Education, Pittsburgh, PA 15213-3165. Offers MSN. *Program availability:* Part-time, evening/weekend, 100% online, blended/hybrid learning. *Students:* 34 full-time (31 women), 24 part-time (23 women); includes 5 minority (3 Black or African American, non-Hispanic/Latino; 1 Hispanic/Latino; 1 Two or more races, non-Hispanic/Latino). Average age 38. 19 applicants, 100% accepted, 10 enrolled. In 2015, 18 master's awarded. *Degree requirements:* For master's, internship. *Entrance requirements:* For master's, minimum undergraduate GPA of 3.0 from accredited BSN program; current license as RN in Pennsylvania; two professional recommendations; reflective essay of 300 words or less describing career goals and expectations for education. Additional exam requirements/recommendations for international students: Required—TOEFL (minimum score 550 paper-based). *Application deadline:* Applications are processed on a rolling basis. Electronic applications accepted. Application fee is waived when completed online. *Expenses: Tuition, area resident:* Full-time $11,147; part-time $801

Nursing and Healthcare Administration

per credit. Tuition and fees vary according to course load, degree level and program. *Unit head:* Dr. Renee Ingel, PhD, RN, Director, Nursing Leadership and DNP Programs, 412-578-6103, Fax: 412-578-6114, E-mail: rmingel@carlow.edu. *Application contact:* E-mail: gradstudies@carlow.edu.
Website: http://www.carlow.edu/
Master_of_Science_in_Nursing_Concentration_in_Education_and_Leadership.aspx

Cedar Crest College, Program in Nursing, Allentown, PA 18104-6196. Offers nursing administration (MS); nursing education (MS). *Program availability:* Part-time. *Faculty:* 4 full-time (all women), 1 part-time/adjunct (0 women). *Students:* 12 part-time (all women); includes 1 minority (Hispanic/Latino). Average age 35. In 2015, 15 master's awarded. *Application deadline:* Applications are processed on a rolling basis. Electronic applications accepted. *Expenses:* Contact institution. *Unit head:* Dr. Wendy Robb, Director, 610-606-4666, E-mail: wjrobb@cedarcrest.edu. *Application contact:* Mary Ellen Hickes, Director of School of Adult and Graduate Education, 610-606-4666, E-mail: sage@cedarcrest.edu.
Website: http://sage.cedarcrest.edu/degrees/graduate/nursing-science/

Central Methodist University, College of Graduate and Extended Studies, Fayette, MO 65248-1198. Offers clinical counseling (MS); clinical nurse leader (MSN); education (M Ed); music education (MME); nurse educator (MSN). *Program availability:* Part-time, evening/weekend, online learning. *Degree requirements:* For master's, thesis. *Entrance requirements:* For master's, GRE General Test, minimum GPA of 2.75. Electronic applications accepted.

Chatham University, Nursing Programs, Pittsburgh, PA 15232-2826. Offers education/leadership (MSN); nursing (DNP). *Accreditation:* AACN. *Program availability:* Online learning. *Faculty:* 11 full-time (10 women), 23 part-time/adjunct (18 women). *Students:* 64 full-time (58 women), 80 part-time (73 women); includes 50 minority (31 Black or African American, non-Hispanic/Latino; 9 Asian, non-Hispanic/Latino; 5 Hispanic/Latino; 1 Native Hawaiian or other Pacific Islander, non-Hispanic/Latino; 4 Two or more races, non-Hispanic/Latino), 10 international. Average age 44. 181 applicants, 50% accepted, 61 enrolled. In 2015, 9 master's, 76 doctorates awarded. *Entrance requirements:* For master's, RN license, BSN, minimum GPA of 3.0; for doctorate, RN license, MSN. Additional exam requirements/recommendations for international students: Required—TOEFL (minimum score 600 paper-based; 100 iBT), IELTS (minimum score 6.5), TWE. *Application deadline:* For fall admission, 5/1 priority date for domestic and international students. Applications are processed on a rolling basis. Application fee: $0. Electronic applications accepted. *Expenses:* Tuition, area resident: Full-time $15,786; part-time $877 per credit hour. *Required fees:* $468; $26 per credit hour. *Financial support:* Applicants required to submit FAFSA. *Unit head:* Dr. Diane Hunker, Director, 412-365-1738, E-mail: dhunker@chatham.edu. *Application contact:* Patricia Golla, Assistant Director of Graduate Admissions, 412-365-1386, Fax: 412-365-1720, E-mail: pgolla@chatham.edu.
Website: http://www.chatham.edu/nursing

Clarkson College, Master of Science in Nursing Program, Omaha, NE 68131. Offers adult nurse practitioner (MSN, Post-Master's Certificate); family nurse practitioner (MSN, Post-Master's Certificate); nursing education (MSN, Post-Master's Certificate); nursing health care leadership (MSN, Post-Master's Certificate). *Accreditation:* AANA/CANAEP; ACEN. *Program availability:* Part-time, evening/weekend, online learning. *Degree requirements:* For master's, on-campus skills assessment (family nurse practitioner, adult nurse practitioner), comprehensive exam or thesis. *Entrance requirements:* For master's, minimum GPA of 3.0, 2 references, resume. Additional exam requirements/recommendations for international students: Required—TOEFL (minimum score 600 paper-based; 100 iBT). Electronic applications accepted.

Clarkson College, Program in Health Care Administration, Omaha, NE 68131-2739. Offers MHCA. *Program availability:* Part-time, evening/weekend, online learning. *Entrance requirements:* For master's, minimum GPA of 3.0, resume, references. Additional exam requirements/recommendations for international students: Required—TOEFL (minimum score 600 paper-based; 100 iBT). Electronic applications accepted.

College of Mount Saint Vincent, School of Professional and Continuing Studies, Department of Nursing, Riverdale, NY 10471-1093. Offers adult nurse practitioner (MSN, PMC); family nurse practitioner (MSN, PMC); nurse educator (PMC); nursing administration (MSN); nursing for the adult and aged (MSN). *Accreditation:* AACN. *Program availability:* Part-time. *Entrance requirements:* For master's, BSN, interview, RN license, minimum GPA of 3.0, letters of reference. Additional exam requirements/recommendations for international students: Required—TOEFL. *Expenses:* Contact institution.

The College of New Rochelle, Graduate School, Program in Nursing, New Rochelle, NY 10805-2308. Offers acute care nurse practitioner (MS, Certificate); clinical specialist in holistic nursing (MS, Certificate); family nurse practitioner (MS, Certificate); nursing and health care management (MS); nursing education (Certificate). *Accreditation:* AACN. *Program availability:* Part-time. *Faculty:* 3 full-time (2 women), 6 part-time/adjunct (4 women). *Students:* 116 part-time (104 women); includes 79 minority (58 Black or African American, non-Hispanic/Latino; 11 Asian, non-Hispanic/Latino; 10 Hispanic/Latino). Average age 38. In 2015, 25 master's awarded. *Entrance requirements:* For master's, GRE General Test or MAT, BSN, malpractice insurance, minimum GPA of 3.0, RN license. *Application deadline:* For fall admission, 8/15 priority date for domestic students; for spring admission, 12/1 priority date for domestic students. Applications are processed on a rolling basis. Application fee: $35. Electronic applications accepted. *Expenses:* Tuition, area resident: Part-time $894 per credit. *Required fees:* $350 per semester. *Financial support:* Traineeships available. Support available to part-time students. Financial award application deadline: 8/15; financial award applicants required to submit FAFSA. *Unit head:* Dr. H. Michael Dreher, Dean, School of Nursing, 914-654-5441, E-mail: hdreher@cnr.edu. *Application contact:* Michael Petri, Interim Director of Graduate Admissions, 914-654-5256, E-mail: mpetri@cnr.edu.

Columbus State University, Graduate Studies, College of Education and Health Professions, School of Nursing, Columbus, GA 31907-5645. Offers family nurse practitioner (MSN); nursing (MSN), including nurse educator, nurse informatics, nurse leader. Program offered in collaboration with Georgia Southwestern University. *Program availability:* Part-time, online only, 100% online. *Faculty:* 7 full-time (all women), 1 part-time/adjunct (0 women). *Students:* 29 full-time (24 women), 44 part-time (43 women); includes 35 minority (25 Black or African American, non-Hispanic/Latino; 1 Asian, non-Hispanic/Latino; 3 Hispanic/Latino; 6 Two or more races, non-Hispanic/Latino). Average age 36. 66 applicants, 59% accepted, 32 enrolled. In 2015, 6 master's awarded. *Entrance requirements:* For master's, GRE, BSN, minimum undergraduate GPA of 3.0. Additional exam requirements/recommendations for international students: Required—TOEFL (minimum score 550 paper-based; 79 iBT). *Application deadline:* For fall admission, 5/1 for domestic and international students; for spring admission, 11/1 for domestic and international students; for summer admission, 3/1 for domestic and international students. Applications are processed on a rolling basis. Application fee: $50. Electronic applications accepted. *Expenses:* Contact institution. *Financial support:* In 2015–16, 51 students received support. Institutionally sponsored loans available. Financial award application deadline: 5/1; financial award applicants required to submit FAFSA. *Unit head:* Latonya Sanot, Interim Director, 706-507-8576, E-mail:

santo_latonya@columbusstate.edu. *Application contact:* Kristin Williams, Director of International and Graduate Recruitment, 706-507-8848, Fax: 706-568-5091, E-mail: williams_kristin@columbusstate.edu.
Website: http://nursing.columbusstate.edu/

Cox College, Programs in Nursing, Springfield, MO 65802. Offers clinical nurse leader (MSN); family nurse practitioner (MSN); nurse educator (MSN). *Accreditation:* AACN. *Entrance requirements:* For master's, RN license, essay, 2 letters of recommendation, official transcripts. Electronic applications accepted.

Creighton University, College of Nursing, Omaha, NE 68178-0001. Offers adult acute care nurse practitioner (Post-Master's Certificate); adult gerontology acute care nurse practitioner (DNP); adult gerontology nurse practitioner (DNP); clinical nurse leader (MSN, Post-Graduate Certificate); clinical systems administration (MSN, DNP); family nurse practitioner (DNP, Post-Master's Certificate); neonatal nurse practitioner (DNP, Post-Master's Certificate); pediatric acute care nurse practitioner (DNP, Post-Master's Certificate); psychiatric mental health nurse practitioner (DNP). *Accreditation:* AACN. *Program availability:* Part-time, blended/hybrid learning. *Faculty:* 10 full-time (all women), 48 part-time/adjunct (45 women). *Students:* 132 full-time (120 women), 228 part-time (212 women); includes 38 minority (10 Black or African American, non-Hispanic/Latino; 3 American Indian or Alaska Native, non-Hispanic/Latino; 11 Asian, non-Hispanic/Latino; 1 Hispanic/Latino; 2 Native Hawaiian or other Pacific Islander, non-Hispanic/Latino; 11 Two or more races, non-Hispanic/Latino). Average age 31. 66 applicants, 91% accepted, 43 enrolled. In 2015, 54 master's, 17 doctorates, 1 other advanced degree awarded. *Degree requirements:* For master's, capstone project; for doctorate, scholarly project. *Entrance requirements:* For master's and doctorate, BSN from an ACEN- or CCNE-accredited nursing school, minimum cumulative GPA of 3.0, personal statement, current unencumbered RN license with NE eligibility, undergraduate statistics course, physical assessment course or equivalent; for other advanced degree, MSN or MS in nursing, minimum cumulative GPA of 3.0, current unencumbered RN license with NE eligibility. Additional exam requirements/recommendations for international students: Required—TOEFL (minimum score 600 paper-based; 100 iBT). *Application deadline:* For fall admission, 6/15 priority date for domestic and international students; for spring admission, 11/15 priority date for domestic and international students; for summer admission, 4/15 for domestic and international students. Applications are processed on a rolling basis. Application fee: $50. Electronic applications accepted. *Expenses:* $800 per credit hour tuition; $904 per semester full-time fees; $207 per semester part-time fees; $50 one-time drug screen fee. *Financial support:* In 2015–16, 7 students received support. Scholarships/grants available. Financial award applicants required to submit FAFSA. *Faculty research:* Obesity prevention in children, evaluation of simulated clinical experiences, vitamin D3 and calcium for cancer risk education in post menopausal women, online support and education to reduce stress for prenatal patients on bed rest, health literacy, immunization research. *Total annual research expenditures:* $162,085. *Unit head:* Dr. Catherine Todero, Dean, 402-280-2004, Fax: 402-280-2045. *Application contact:* Shannon Cox, Enrollment Specialist, 402-280-2067, Fax: 402-280-2045, E-mail: shannoncox@creighton.edu.
Website: http://nursing.creighton.edu/

Daemen College, Department of Nursing, Amherst, NY 14226-3592. Offers adult nurse practitioner (MS, Post Master's Certificate); nurse executive leadership (Post Master's Certificate); nursing education (MS, Post Master's Certificate); nursing executive leadership (MS); nursing practice (DNP); palliative care nursing (Post Master's Certificate). *Accreditation:* ACEN. *Program availability:* Part-time. *Degree requirements:* For master's, thesis or alternative, degree completed in 4 years; minimum GPA of 3.0; for doctorate, degree completed in 5 years; 500 post-master's clinical hours. *Entrance requirements:* For master's, BN, 1 year medical/surgical experience, RN license and state registration, statistics course with minimum C grade, 3 letters of recommendation, minimum GPA of 3.25, interview; for doctorate, MS in advance nursing practice; New York state RN license; goal statement; resume; interview; statistics course with minimum grade of 'C'; for Post Master's Certificate, master's degree in clinical area; RN license and current registration; one year of clinical experience; statistics course with minimum grade of 'C'; 3 letters of recommendation; interview; letter of intent. Additional exam requirements/recommendations for international students: Required—TOEFL (minimum score 500 paper-based; 63 iBT), IELTS (minimum score 5.5). Electronic applications accepted. *Faculty research:* Professional stress, client behavior, drug therapy, treatment modalities and pulmonary cancers, chemical dependency.

DeSales University, Division of Healthcare, Center Valley, PA 18034-9568. Offers adult-gerontology acute care (Post Master's Certificate); adult-gerontology acute care nurse practitioner (MSN); adult-gerontology acute certified nurse practitioner (Post Master's Certificate); adult-gerontology clinical nurse specialist (MSN, Post Master's Certificate); clinical leadership (DNP); family nurse practitioner (MSN, Post Master's Certificate); general nursing practice (DNP); health care information management (MSIS); network security (MSIS); nurse anesthetists (MSN); nurse educator (Post Master's Certificate, Postbaccalaureate Certificate); nurse midwives (MSN); nurse practitioner (MSN); project management (MSIS); psychiatric-mental health nurse practitioner (MSN, Post Master's Certificate); DNP/MBA. *Accreditation:* ACEN. *Program availability:* Part-time. *Faculty:* 22 full-time (14 women), 37 part-time/adjunct (29 women). *Students:* 244 full-time (178 women), 55 part-time (50 women); includes 24 minority (7 Black or African American, non-Hispanic/Latino; 9 Asian, non-Hispanic/Latino; 6 Hispanic/Latino; 2 Two or more races, non-Hispanic/Latino). Average age 31. 68 applicants, 85% accepted, 52 enrolled. In 2015, 73 master's awarded. *Degree requirements:* For master's, minimum GPA of 3.0, portfolio; for doctorate, minimum GPA of 3.0, scholarly capstone project. *Entrance requirements:* For master's, GRE or MAT (waived if applicant has an undergraduate GPA of 3.0 or higher), BSN from ACEN- or CCNE-accredited program, minimum undergraduate GPA of 3.0, active RN license or eligibility, two letters of recommendation, essay, health care experience, personal interview; for doctorate, BSN or MSN from ACEN- or CCNE-accredited institution, minimum GPA of 3.3 in graduate program, current licensure as an RN. Additional exam requirements/recommendations for international students: Required—TOEFL (minimum score 104 iBT). *Application deadline:* Applications are processed on a rolling basis. Application fee: $50. Electronic applications accepted. *Expenses:* Contact institution. *Financial support:* Applicants required to submit FAFSA. *Unit head:* Fr. Dr. Peter Leonard, OSFS, Dean of Graduate Education, 610-282-1100 Ext. 1289, E-mail: peter.leonard@desales.edu. *Application contact:* Abigail Wernicki, Director of Graduate Admissions, 610-282-1100 Ext 1768, Fax: 610-282-2860, E-mail: gradadmissions@desales.edu.

Drexel University, College of Nursing and Health Professions, Division of Graduate Nursing, Philadelphia, PA 19104-2875. Offers adult acute care (MSN); adult psychiatric/mental health (MSN); advanced practice nursing (MSN); clinical trials research (MSN); family nurse practitioner (MSN); leadership in health systems management (MSN); nursing education (MSN); pediatric primary care (MSN); women's health (MSN). *Accreditation:* AACN. Electronic applications accepted.

Duke University, School of Nursing, Durham, NC 27708-0586. Offers acute care pediatric nurse practitioner (MSN, Post Master's Certificate); adult-gerontology nurse practitioner (MSN, Post Master's Certificate), including acute care, primary care; family

nurse practitioner (MSN, Post Master's Certificate); neonatal nurse practitioner (MSN, Post Master's Certificate); nurse anesthesia (DNP); nurse practitioner (DNP); nursing (PhD); nursing and health care leadership (MSN); nursing education (MSN); nursing informatics (MSN, Post Master's Certificate); pediatric nurse practitioner (MSN, Post Master's Certificate), including primary care; women's health nurse practitioner (MSN, Post Master's Certificate). *Accreditation:* AACN; AANA/CANAEP. *Program availability:* Part-time, evening/weekend, online learning. *Faculty:* 74 full-time (63 women). *Students:* 179 full-time (152 women), 528 part-time (466 women); includes 145 minority (42 Black or African American, non-Hispanic/Latino; 3 American Indian or Alaska Native, non-Hispanic/Latino; 44 Asian, non-Hispanic/Latino; 35 Hispanic/Latino; 1 Native Hawaiian or other Pacific Islander, non-Hispanic/Latino; 20 Two or more races, non-Hispanic/Latino), 7 international. Average age 33. 619 applicants, 46% accepted, 201 enrolled. In 2015, 243 master's, 62 doctorates, 26 other advanced degrees awarded. Terminal master's awarded for partial completion of doctoral program. *Degree requirements:* For master's, thesis optional; for doctorate, capstone project. *Entrance requirements:* For master's, GRE General Test (waived if undergraduate GPA of 3.4 or higher), 1 year of nursing experience (recommended), BSN, minimum GPA of 3.0, previous course work in statistics; for doctorate, GRE General Test (waived if undergraduate GPA of 3.4 or higher), BSN or MSN, minimum GPA of 3.0, portfolio, resume, personal statement, undergraduate statistics course, current licensure as a registered nurse, transcripts from all post-secondary institutions; for Post Master's Certificate, MSN, licensure or eligibility as a professional nurse, transcripts from all post-secondary institutions, previous course work in statistics. Additional exam requirements/recommendations for international students: Required—TOEFL (minimum score 100 iBT), IELTS (minimum score 7). *Application deadline:* For fall admission, 12/1 for domestic and international students; for spring admission, 5/1 for domestic and international students. Application fee: $50. Electronic applications accepted. *Expenses:* Contact institution. *Financial support:* Career-related internships or fieldwork, institutionally sponsored loans, scholarships/grants, traineeships, and tuition waivers (partial) available. Support available to part-time students. Financial award applicants required to submit FAFSA. *Faculty research:* Cardiovascular disease, caregiver skill training, data mining, prostate cancer, neonatal immune system. *Unit head:* Dr. Marion E. Broome, Dean/Vice Chancellor for Nursing Affairs/Associate Vice President for Academic Affairs for Nursing, 919-684-9446, Fax: 919-684-9414, E-mail: marion.broome@duke.edu. *Application contact:* Dr. Ernie Rushing, Director of Admissions and Recruitment, 919-668-6274, Fax: 919-668-4693, E-mail: ernie.rushing@dm.duke.edu.
Website: http://www.nursing.duke.edu/

Eastern Mennonite University, Program in Nursing, Harrisonburg, VA 22802-2462. Offers leadership and management (MSN); leadership and school nursing (MSN). *Accreditation:* AACN. *Program availability:* Part-time, online learning. *Degree requirements:* For master's, leadership project. *Entrance requirements:* For master's, RN license, one year of full-time work experience as RN, minimum GPA of 3.0. Additional exam requirements/recommendations for international students: Required—TOEFL. *Application deadline:* For fall admission, 6/1 for domestic students. Applications are processed on a rolling basis. Application fee: $25. *Expenses: Tuition, area resident:* Part-time $600 per credit hour. *Required fees:* $25 per unit. Part-time tuition and fees vary according to course load and program. *Financial support:* Federal Work-Study and scholarships/grants available. Financial award applicants required to submit FAFSA. *Faculty research:* Community health, international health, effectiveness of the nursing school environment, development of caring ability in nursing students, international nursing students. *Unit head:* Ann Hershberger, Coordinator, 540-432-4192, E-mail: hershbea@emu.edu. *Application contact:* Don A. Yoder, Director of Seminary and Graduate Admissions, 540-432-4257, Fax: 540-432-4598, E-mail: yoderda@emu.edu.

Eastern Michigan University, Graduate School, College of Health and Human Services, School of Health Sciences, Programs in Clinical Research Administration, Ypsilanti, MI 48197. Offers MS, Graduate Certificate. *Program availability:* Part-time, evening/weekend, online learning. *Students:* 7 full-time (6 women), 22 part-time (17 women); includes 3 minority (1 Black or African American, non-Hispanic/Latino; 2 Asian, non-Hispanic/Latino), 16 international. Average age 33. 31 applicants, 77% accepted, 13 enrolled. In 2015, 11 master's awarded. *Entrance requirements:* Additional exam requirements/recommendations for international students: Required—TOEFL. *Application deadline:* Applications are processed on a rolling basis. Application fee: $45. *Financial support:* Fellowships, research assistantships with full tuition reimbursements, teaching assistantships with full tuition reimbursements, career-related internships or fieldwork, Federal Work-Study, institutionally sponsored loans, scholarships/grants, tuition waivers (partial), and unspecified assistantships available. Support available to part-time students. Financial award applicants required to submit FAFSA. *Application contact:* Dr. Stephen Sonstein, Program Director, 734-487-1238, Fax: 734-487-4095, E-mail: stephen.sonstein@emich.edu.

Edgewood College, Henry Predolin School of Nursing, Madison, WI 53711. Offers administration (MSN); education (MSN); nursing (DNP). *Accreditation:* AACN. *Students:* 11 full-time (10 women), 60 part-time (55 women); includes 4 minority (1 Asian, non-Hispanic/Latino; 3 Hispanic/Latino). Average age 39. In 2015, 25 master's, 5 doctorates awarded. *Degree requirements:* For master's, practicum, research project; for doctorate, practicum, capstone project. *Entrance requirements:* For master's, minimum GPA of 3.0, 2 letters of reference, current RN license. Additional exam requirements/recommendations for international students: Required—TOEFL. *Application deadline:* For fall admission, 8/15 priority date for domestic students, 5/1 for international students; for spring admission, 1/8 priority date for domestic students, 11/1 for international students. Applications are processed on a rolling basis. Application fee: $30. Electronic applications accepted. *Unit head:* Dr. Margaret Noreuil, Dean, 608-663-2820, Fax: 608-663-3291, E-mail: mnoreuil@edgewood.edu. *Application contact:* Tracy Kantor, Enrollment and Applications Manager, 608-663-3297, Fax: 608-663-3496, E-mail: gps@edgewood.edu.
Website: http://www.edgewood.edu/Academics/School-of-Nursing

Elms College, School of Nursing, Chicopee, MA 01013-2839. Offers nursing and health services management (MSN); nursing education (MSN). *Accreditation:* AACN. *Program availability:* Part-time, evening/weekend. *Faculty:* 4 full-time (all women), 5 part-time/adjunct (4 women). *Students:* 99 part-time (91 women); includes 6 minority (2 Black or African American, non-Hispanic/Latino; 1 American Indian or Alaska Native, non-Hispanic/Latino; 3 Hispanic/Latino). Average age 40. 43 applicants, 81% accepted, 27 enrolled. In 2015, 16 master's awarded. *Entrance requirements:* Additional exam requirements/recommendations for international students: Required—TOEFL. *Application deadline:* For fall admission, 7/1 priority date for domestic students; for spring admission, 11/1 priority date for domestic students. Applications are processed on a rolling basis. Application fee: $30. *Financial support:* Applicants required to submit FAFSA. *Unit head:* Dr. Kathleen Scoble, Dean, School of Nursing, 413-265-2204, E-mail: scoblek@elms.edu. *Application contact:* Dr. Cynthia L. Dakin, Director of Graduate Nursing Studies, 413-265-2455, Fax: 413-265-2335, E-mail: dakinc@elms.edu.

Emmanuel College, Graduate and Professional Programs, Graduate Program in Nursing, Boston, MA 02115. Offers education (MSN, Graduate Certificate); management (MSN, Graduate Certificate). *Program availability:* Part-time, evening/weekend. *Faculty:* 4 full-time (all women), 7 part-time/adjunct (all women). *Students:* 43 part-time (42 women); includes 3 minority (1 Black or African American, non-Hispanic/Latino; 1 Hispanic/Latino; 1 Two or more races, non-Hispanic/Latino). Average age 44. In 2015, 9 master's awarded. *Degree requirements:* For master's, 36 credits, including 6-credit practicum. *Entrance requirements:* For master's and Graduate Certificate, transcripts from all regionally-accredited institutions attended (showing proof of bachelor's degree completion), proof of RN license, 2 letters of recommendation, essay, resume. *Application deadline:* For fall admission, 7/30 for domestic students. Applications are processed on a rolling basis. Electronic applications accepted. Application fee is waived when completed online. *Expenses:* $2,581 per course. *Financial support:* Applicants required to submit FAFSA. *Unit head:* Diane Shea, Associate Dean for Nursing/Professor of Nursing Practice, 617-732-1604, E-mail: shead@emmanuel.edu. *Application contact:* Helen Muterperl, Assistant Director of Graduate Admissions, 617-735-9700, Fax: 617-507-0434, E-mail: gpp@emmanuel.edu. Website: http://www.emmanuel.edu/graduate-professional-programs/academics/nursing.html

Emory University, Nell Hodgson Woodruff School of Nursing, Atlanta, GA 30322-1100. Offers adult nurse practitioner (MSN); emergency nurse practitioner (MSN); family nurse practitioner (MSN); family nurse-midwife (MSN); health systems leadership (MSN); nurse-midwifery (MSN); pediatric nurse practitioner acute and primary care (MSN); women's health care (Title X) (MSN); women's health nurse practitioner (MSN); MSN/MPH. *Accreditation:* AACN; ACNM/ACME (one or more programs are accredited). *Program availability:* Part-time. *Entrance requirements:* For master's, GRE General Test or MAT, minimum GPA of 3.0, BS in nursing from an accredited institution, RN license and additional course work, 3 letters of recommendation. Additional exam requirements/recommendations for international students: Required—TOEFL (minimum score 600 paper-based; 100 iBT). Electronic applications accepted. *Expenses:* Contact institution. *Faculty research:* Older adult falls and injuries, minority health issues, cardiac symptoms and quality of life, bio-ethics and decision-making, menopausal issues.

Excelsior College, School of Nursing, Albany, NY 12203-5159. Offers nursing (MS); nursing education (MS); nursing informatics (MS); nursing leadership and administration of health care systems (MS). *Accreditation:* ACEN. *Program availability:* Part-time, evening/weekend, online learning. *Faculty:* 18 part-time/adjunct (14 women). *Students:* 938 part-time (770 women); includes 295 minority (166 Black or African American, non-Hispanic/Latino; 8 American Indian or Alaska Native, non-Hispanic/Latino; 36 Asian, non-Hispanic/Latino; 60 Hispanic/Latino; 8 Native Hawaiian or other Pacific Islander, non-Hispanic/Latino; 17 Two or more races, non-Hispanic/Latino), 2 international. Average age 45. In 2015, 200 master's awarded. *Entrance requirements:* For master's, RN license. *Application deadline:* Applications are processed on a rolling basis. Application fee: $110. Electronic applications accepted. *Expenses: Tuition, area resident:* Part-time $645 per credit. *Required fees:* $265 per unit. *Financial support:* Scholarships/grants available. *Unit head:* Dr. Barbara Pieper, Associate Dean, Graduate Program in Nursing, 518-464-8500, Fax: 518-464-8777, E-mail: msn@excelsior.edu. *Application contact:* Admissions Counselor, 518-464-8500, Fax: 518-464-8777, E-mail: admissions@excelsior.edu.

Fairfield University, Marion Peckham Egan School of Nursing and Health Studies, Fairfield, CT 06824. Offers advanced practice (DNP); family nurse practitioner (MSN, DNP); nurse anesthesia (DNP); nursing leadership (MSN); psychiatric nurse practitioner (MSN, DNP). *Accreditation:* AACN; AANA/CANAEP. *Program availability:* Part-time, evening/weekend. *Faculty:* 8 full-time (all women), 9 part-time/adjunct (7 women). *Students:* 43 full-time (35 women), 181 part-time (163 women); includes 52 minority (20 Black or African American, non-Hispanic/Latino; 1 American Indian or Alaska Native, non-Hispanic/Latino; 11 Asian, non-Hispanic/Latino; 16 Hispanic/Latino; 4 Two or more races, non-Hispanic/Latino), 1 international. Average age 36. 103 applicants, 67% accepted, 43 enrolled. In 2015, 12 master's, 21 doctorates awarded. *Degree requirements:* For master's, capstone project. *Entrance requirements:* For master's, minimum QPA of 3.0, RN license, resume, 2 recommendations; for doctorate, MSN (minimum QPA of 3.2) or BSN (minimum QPA of 3.0); critical care nursing experience (for nurse anesthesia DNP candidates). Additional exam requirements/recommendations for international students: Required—TOEFL (minimum score 550 paper-based; 80 iBT) or IELTS (minimum score 6.5). *Application deadline:* For fall admission, 5/15 for international students; for spring admission, 10/15 for international students. Applications are processed on a rolling basis. Application fee: $60. Electronic applications accepted. *Expenses:* $850 per credit hour (for MSN); $900-$1,000 per credit hour (for DNP). *Financial support:* In 2015-16, 51 students received support. Unspecified assistantships available. Financial award applicants required to submit FAFSA. *Faculty research:* Aging, spiritual care, palliative and end of life care, psychiatric mental health, pediatric trauma. *Unit head:* Dr. Meredith Wallace Kazer, Dean, 203-254-4000 Ext. 2701, Fax: 203-254-4126, E-mail: mkazer@fairfield.edu. *Application contact:* Marianne Gumpper, Director of Graduate and Continuing Studies Admission, 203-254-4184, Fax: 203-254-4073, E-mail: gradadmis@fairfield.edu.
Website: http://fairfield.edu/son

Felician University, Doctor of Nursing Practice Program, Lodi, NJ 07644-2117. Offers advanced practice (DNP); executive leadership (DNP). *Program availability:* Evening/weekend, online learning. *Faculty:* 1 (woman) full-time, 1 (woman) part-time/adjunct. *Students:* 16 part-time (14 women); includes 9 minority (5 Black or African American, non-Hispanic/Latino; 2 Asian, non-Hispanic/Latino; 1 Hispanic/Latino; 1 Native Hawaiian or other Pacific Islander, non-Hispanic/Latino). Average age 53. 16 applicants, 75% accepted, 8 enrolled. In 2015, 6 doctorates awarded. *Degree requirements:* For doctorate, scholarly project. *Entrance requirements:* Additional exam requirements/recommendations for international students: Recommended—TOEFL (minimum score 79 iBT). *Application deadline:* Applications are processed on a rolling basis. Application fee: $40. Electronic applications accepted. Application fee is waived when completed online. *Expenses: Tuition, area resident:* Part-time $965 per credit. Tuition and fees vary according to course load and program. *Financial support:* Applicants required to submit FAFSA. *Unit head:* Dr. Ann Tritak, Associate Dean, Department of Graduate Nursing, 201-559-6151, E-mail: tritaka@felician.edu. *Application contact:* Dr. Margaret Smolin, Director, Graduate Admissions, 201-559-1451, E-mail: graduate@felician.edu.

Felician University, Master of Science in Nursing Program, Lodi, NJ 07644-2117. Offers adult-gerontology nurse practitioner (MSN, PMC); executive leadership (MSN, PMC); family nurse practitioner (MSN, PMC); nursing education (MSN, PMC). *Accreditation:* AACN. *Program availability:* Part-time, evening/weekend, online learning. *Faculty:* 11 full-time (9 women), 2 part-time/adjunct (both women). *Students:* 13 full-time, 121 part-time (112 women); includes 60 minority (23 Black or African American, non-Hispanic/Latino; 1 American Indian or Alaska Native, non-Hispanic/Latino; 19 Asian, non-Hispanic/Latino; 17 Hispanic/Latino). Average age 40. 111 applicants, 83% accepted, 52 enrolled. In 2015, 18 master's awarded. *Entrance requirements:* For master's, BS in nursing or equivalent, minimum GPA of 3.0, 2 letters of recommendation, RN license; for PMC, RN license, minimum GPA of 3.0. Additional exam requirements/recommendations for international students: Recommended—TOEFL (minimum score 79 iBT). *Application deadline:* Applications are processed on a rolling basis. Application fee: $40. Electronic applications accepted. Application fee is waived when completed online. *Expenses: Tuition, area resident:* Part-time $965 per

Nursing and Healthcare Administration

credit. Tuition and fees vary according to course load and program. *Financial support:* In 2015–16, 10 students received support. Traineeships available. Financial award applicants required to submit FAFSA. *Faculty research:* Anxiety and fear, curriculum innovation, health promotion. *Unit head:* Dr. Ann Tritak, Associate Dean, Department of Graduate Nursing, 201-201-559-6151, E-mail: tritaka@felician.edu. *Application contact:* Dr. Margaret Smolin, Director, Graduate Admissions, 201-559-1451, E-mail: graduate@felician.edu.

Ferris State University, College of Health Professions, School of Nursing, Big Rapids, MI 49307. Offers nursing (MSN); nursing administration (MSN); nursing education (MSN); nursing informatics (MSN). *Accreditation:* ACEN. *Program availability:* Part-time, evening/weekend, 100% online. *Faculty:* 5 full-time (all women), 2 part-time/adjunct (both women). *Students:* 95 part-time (84 women); includes 11 minority (4 Black or African American, non-Hispanic/Latino; 1 American Indian or Alaska Native, non-Hispanic/Latino; 3 Asian, non-Hispanic/Latino; 1 Hispanic/Latino; 1 Native Hawaiian or other Pacific Islander, non-Hispanic/Latino; 1 Two or more races, non-Hispanic/Latino). Average age 39. 23 applicants, 74% accepted, 13 enrolled. In 2015, 15 master's awarded. *Degree requirements:* For master's, comprehensive exam, practicum, practicum project. *Entrance requirements:* For master's, BS in nursing (for nursing education track); BS in nursing or related field (for nursing administration and nursing informatics tracks); registered nurse license, writing sample, letters of reference, 2 years' clinical experience (recommended). Additional exam requirements/recommendations for international students: Required—TOEFL (minimum score 550 paper-based; 61 iBT). *Application deadline:* For fall admission, 4/15 priority date for domestic students; for spring admission, 10/15 for domestic students. Application fee: $0. Electronic applications accepted. Tuition and fees vary according to degree level and program. *Financial support:* In 2015–16, 3 students received support. Fellowships, research assistantships, teaching assistantships, career-related internships or fieldwork, and scholarships/grants available. Financial award application deadline: 4/15; financial award applicants required to submit FAFSA. *Faculty research:* Nursing education, end of life, leadership/education introverts in nursing. *Unit head:* Dr. Susan Owens, Chair, School of Nursing, 231-591-2267, Fax: 231-591-2325, E-mail: owenss3@ferris.edu. *Application contact:* Debby Buck, Off-Campus Program Secretary, 231-591-2270, Fax: 231-591-3788, E-mail: buckd@ferris.edu.
Website: http://www.ferris.edu/htmls/colleges/alliedhe/Nursing/homepage.htm

Florida Agricultural and Mechanical University, Division of Graduate Studies, Research, and Continuing Education, School of Allied Health Sciences, Tallahassee, FL 32307-3200. Offers health administration (MS); occupational therapy (MOT); physical therapy (DPT). *Degree requirements:* For master's, thesis (for some programs). *Entrance requirements:* For master's, GRE General Test or GMAT, minimum GPA of 3.0. Additional exam requirements/recommendations for international students: Required—TOEFL (minimum score 550 paper-based).

Florida Atlantic University, Christine E. Lynn College of Nursing, Boca Raton, FL 33431. Offers administrative and financial leadership in nursing and health care (Post Master's Certificate); nursing (PhD); nursing practice (DNP). *Accreditation:* AACN. *Program availability:* Part-time. *Degree requirements:* For master's, thesis or alternative; for doctorate, comprehensive exam, thesis/dissertation. *Entrance requirements:* For master's, GRE General Test or MAT, bachelor's degree in nursing, Florida RN license, minimum GPA of 3.0, resume/curriculum vitae, letter of recommendation; for doctorate, GRE General Test or MAT, curriculum vitae, Florida RN license, minimum GPA of 3.5, master's degree in nursing, three letters of recommendation. *Application deadline:* For fall admission, 6/1 for domestic students, 2/15 for international students; for spring admission, 10/1 for domestic students, 7/15 for international students. Applications are processed on a rolling basis. Application fee: $30. *Expenses: Tuition, area resident:* Full-time $7392; part-time $369.82 per credit hour. Tuition, state resident: full-time $7392; part-time $369.82 per credit hour. Tuition, nonresident: full-time $19,432; part-time $1024.81 per credit hour. *Financial support:* Research assistantships with partial tuition reimbursements, teaching assistantships with partial tuition reimbursements, career-related internships or fieldwork, Federal Work-Study, institutionally sponsored loans, scholarships/grants, and traineeships available. Support available to part-time students. *Faculty research:* Econometrics of nurse-patient relationship, Alzheimer's disease, community-based programs, falls, self-healing.
Website: http://nursing.fau.edu/

Florida National University, Program in Nursing, Hialeah, FL 33012. Offers family nurse practitioner (MSN); nurse educator (MSN); nurse leadership and management (MSN). *Degree requirements:* For master's, practicum. *Entrance requirements:* For master's, active registered nurse license, BSN from accredited institution. *Expenses: Tuition, area resident:* Full-time $15,600. *Required fees:* $650.

Florida Southern College, Program in Nursing, Lakeland, FL 33801-5698. Offers adult gerontology clinical nurse specialist (MSN); adult gerontology primary care nurse practitioner (MSN); nurse educator (MSN); nursing administration (MSN). *Accreditation:* AACN. *Program availability:* Part-time, evening/weekend. *Entrance requirements:* For master's, Florida RN license, 3 letters of recommendation, personal statement, minimum GPA of 3.0, resume. Additional exam requirements/recommendations for international students: Required—TOEFL (minimum score 550 paper-based). *Expenses:* Contact institution. *Faculty research:* End of life care, dementia, health promotion.

Florida State University, The Graduate School, College of Nursing, Tallahassee, FL 32306-4310. Offers family nurse practitioner (DNP); nurse educator (MSN, Certificate); nurse leader (MSN); nursing leadership (Certificate). *Accreditation:* AACN. *Program availability:* Part-time, online learning. *Faculty:* 13 full-time (12 women). *Students:* 56 full-time (49 women), 25 part-time (23 women); includes 25 minority (13 Black or African American, non-Hispanic/Latino; 4 Asian, non-Hispanic/Latino; 7 Hispanic/Latino; 1 Two or more races, non-Hispanic/Latino). Average age 38. 90 applicants, 50% accepted, 44 enrolled. In 2015, 2 master's, 20 doctorates awarded. *Degree requirements:* For master's, thesis optional; for doctorate, thesis/dissertation, evidence-based project. *Entrance requirements:* For master's, GRE General Test, MAT, minimum GPA of 3.0, BSN, United States RN license; for doctorate, GRE General Test, MAT, minimum GPA of 3.0, BSN or MSN, Florida RN license. Additional exam requirements/recommendations for international students: Required—TOEFL (minimum score 550 paper-based). *Application deadline:* For fall admission, 4/15 for domestic and international students. Application fee: $30. Electronic applications accepted. *Expenses: Tuition, area resident:* Full-time $7263; part-time $403.50 per credit hour. Tuition, nonresident: full-time $18,087; part-time $1004.85 per credit hour. *Required fees:* $1365; $75.81 per credit hour. $20 per semester. Tuition and fees vary according to campus/location. *Financial support:* In 2015–16, 75 students received support, including fellowships with partial tuition reimbursements available (averaging $6,300 per year), research assistantships with partial tuition reimbursements available (averaging $3,000 per year), 3 teaching assistantships with partial tuition reimbursements available (averaging $3,000 per year); career-related internships or fieldwork, Federal Work-Study, institutionally sponsored loans, scholarships/grants, traineeships, and tuition waivers (partial) also available. Financial award application deadline: 4/15; financial award applicants required to submit FAFSA. *Faculty research:* Cardiac, women's health, health promotion and prevention, educational strategies, infectious diseases. *Unit head:*

Dr. Judith McFetridge-Durdle, Dean, 850-644-6846, Fax: 850-644-7660, E-mail: jdurdle@nursing.fsu.edu. *Application contact:* Carlos Urrutia, Assistant Director for Student Services, 850-644-5638, Fax: 850-645-7249, E-mail: currutia@fsu.edu.
Website: http://nursing.fsu.edu/

Framingham State University, Continuing Education, Program in Nursing, Framingham, MA 01701-9101. Offers nursing education (MSN); nursing leadership (MSN). *Accreditation:* AACN. *Entrance requirements:* For master's, BSN; minimum cumulative undergraduate GPA of 3.0, 3.25 in nursing courses; coursework in statistics; 2 letters of recommendation; interview. Electronic applications accepted.

Franklin Pierce University, Graduate and Professional Studies, Rindge, NH 03461-0060. Offers curriculum and instruction (M Ed); elementary education (MS Ed); emerging network technologies (Graduate Certificate); energy and sustainability studies (MBA, Graduate Certificate); health administration (MBA, Graduate Certificate); human resource management (MBA, Graduate Certificate); information technology (MBA); leadership (MBA); nursing education (MS); nursing leadership (MS); physical therapy (DPT); physician assistant studies (MPAS); special education (M Ed); sports management (MBA). *Accreditation:* APTA. *Program availability:* Part-time, online learning. *Degree requirements:* For master's, concentrated original research projects; student teaching; fieldwork and/or internship; leadership project; PRAXIS I and II (for M Ed); for doctorate, concentrated original research projects, clinical fieldwork and/or internship, leadership project. *Entrance requirements:* For master's, minimum GPA of 2.5, 3 letters of recommendation; competencies in accounting, economics, statistics, and computer skills through life experience or undergraduate coursework (for MBA); certification/e-portfolio, minimum C grade in all education courses (for M Ed); license to practice as RN (for MS in nursing); for doctorate, GRE, BA/BS, 3 letters of recommendation, personal mission statement, interview, writing sample, minimum cumulative GPA of 2.8, master's degree (for DA); 80 hours of observation/work in PT settings, completion of anatomy, chemistry, physics, and statistics, minimum GPA of 3.0 (for DPT). Additional exam requirements/recommendations for international students: Required—TOEFL (minimum score 550 paper-based; 61 iBT). *Application deadline:* Applications are processed on a rolling basis. Application fee: $0. Electronic applications accepted. *Expenses: Tuition, area resident:* Part-time $660 per credit hour. Tuition and fees vary according to program. *Financial support:* Teaching assistantships with tuition reimbursements, career-related internships or fieldwork, and unspecified assistantships available. Support available to part-time students. Financial award applicants required to submit FAFSA. *Faculty research:* Evidence-based practice in sports physical therapy, human resource management in economic crisis, leadership in nursing, innovation in sports facility management, differentiated learning and understanding by design. *Unit head:* Dr. Maria Altobello, Dean, 603-647-3509, Fax: 603-229-4580, E-mail: altobellom@franklinpierce.edu. *Application contact:* Graduate Studies, 800-325-1090, Fax: 603-626-4815, E-mail: cgps@franklinpierce.edu.
Website: http://www.franklinpierce.edu/academics/gradstudies/index.htm

Frostburg State University, Graduate School, College of Liberal Arts and Sciences, Department of Nursing, Frostburg, MD 21532-1099. Offers nursing administration (MSN); nursing education (MSN). *Program availability:* Part-time, online learning.

Gannon University, School of Graduate Studies, Morosky College of Health Professions and Sciences, School of Health Professions, Erie, PA 16541-0001. Offers athletic training (MAT); nursing administration (MSN), including nursing administration; nursing practice (DNP), including nursing; occupational therapy (MS, OTD); physical therapy (DPT); physician assistant science (MPAS); sport and exercise science (MS), including human performance. *Accreditation:* APTA (one or more programs are accredited). *Program availability:* Part-time, evening/weekend, 100% online. *Faculty:* 36 full-time (31 women), 11 part-time/adjunct (8 women). *Students:* 227 full-time (162 women), 4 part-time (all women); includes 8 minority (2 Black or African American, non-Hispanic/Latino; 5 Asian, non-Hispanic/Latino; 1 Hispanic/Latino; 3 international. Average age 24. 239 applicants, 52% accepted, 57 enrolled. In 2015, 83 master's, 42 doctorates awarded. *Degree requirements:* For master's, thesis (for some programs); for doctorate, thesis/dissertation (for some programs), research project. *Entrance requirements:* For master's, GRE, bachelor's degree from accredited institution, letters of recommendation, transcripts, teaching certificate (for some programs); for doctorate, thesis/dissertation. Additional exam requirements/recommendations for international students: Required—TOEFL (minimum score 79 iBT). *Application deadline:* Applications are processed on a rolling basis. Application fee: $25. Electronic applications accepted. *Financial support:* Teaching assistantships, Federal Work-Study, scholarships/grants, and unspecified assistantships available. Financial award application deadline: 7/1; financial award applicants required to submit FAFSA. *Faculty research:* Assistive technology, cervical cancer screening and prevention, ergonomics and cervical dysfunction, thoracic spine mobilization. *Unit head:* Dr. Carolyn Masters, Dean, 814-871-7568, E-mail: masters004@gannon.edu. *Application contact:* Bridget Philip, Director of Graduate Admissions, 814-871-7412, E-mail: graduate@gannon.edu.

Gannon University, School of Graduate Studies, Morosky College of Health Professions and Sciences, Villa Maria School of Nursing, Program in Nursing Administration, Erie, PA 16541-0001. Offers MSN. *Program availability:* Part-time, evening/weekend. *Students:* 1 (woman) full-time, 4 part-time (all women); includes 1 minority (Black or African American, non-Hispanic/Latino), 1 international. Average age 39. *Degree requirements:* For master's, thesis (for some programs), practicum. *Entrance requirements:* For master's, GRE, RN, transcripts, 3 letters of recommendation, evidence of the fulfillment of legal requirements for the practice of nursing in the United States. Additional exam requirements/recommendations for international students: Required—TOEFL (minimum score 79 iBT). *Application deadline:* Applications are processed on a rolling basis. Application fee: $25. Electronic applications accepted. *Financial support:* Federal Work-Study available. *Unit head:* Dr. Kathleen Patterson, Director, 814-871-5547, E-mail: patterso018@gannon.edu. *Application contact:* Bridget Philip, Director of Graduate Admissions, 814-871-7412, E-mail: graduate@gannon.edu.

The George Washington University, School of Nursing, Washington, DC 20052. Offers adult nurse practitioner (MSN, DNP, Post-Master's Certificate); clinical research administration (MSN); family nurse practitioner (MSN, Post-Master's Certificate); health care quality (MSN, Post-Master's Certificate); nursing leadership and management (MSN); nursing practice (DNP), including nursing education; palliative care nurse practitioner (Post-Master's Certificate). *Accreditation:* AACN. *Faculty:* 42 full-time (all women), 71 part-time/adjunct (66 women). *Students:* 52 full-time (48 women), 519 part-time (463 women); includes 162 minority (72 Black or African American, non-Hispanic/Latino; 4 American Indian or Alaska Native, non-Hispanic/Latino; 52 Asian, non-Hispanic/Latino; 31 Hispanic/Latino; 3 Two or more races, non-Hispanic/Latino), 2 international. Average age 37. 465 applicants, 69% accepted, 187 enrolled. In 2015, 121 master's, 35 doctorates, 1 other advanced degree awarded. *Unit head:* Pamela R. Jeffries, Dean, 202-994-3725, E-mail: pjeffries@gwu.edu. *Application contact:* Kristin Williams, Associate Provost for Graduate Enrollment Management, 202-994-0467, Fax: 202-994-0371, E-mail: ksw@gwu.edu.
Website: http://nursing.gwumc.edu/

Georgia State University, Byrdine F. Lewis School of Nursing, Atlanta, GA 30303. Offers adult health clinical nurse specialist/nurse practitioner (MS, Certificate); child

health clinical nurse specialist/pediatric nurse practitioner (MS, Certificate); family nurse practitioner (MS, Certificate); family psychiatric mental health nurse practitioner (MS, Certificate); nursing (PhD); nursing leadership in healthcare innovations (MS), including nursing administration, nursing informatics; nutrition (MS); perinatal clinical nurse specialist/women's health nurse practitioner (MS, Certificate); physical therapy (DPT); respiratory therapy (MS). *Accreditation:* AACN. *Program availability:* Part-time, blended/hybrid learning. *Faculty:* 18 full-time (11 women). *Students:* 275 full-time (195 women), 230 part-time (204 women); includes 192 minority (123 Black or African American, non-Hispanic/Latino; 49 Asian, non-Hispanic/Latino; 12 Hispanic/Latino; 2 Native Hawaiian or other Pacific Islander, non-Hispanic/Latino; 6 Two or more races, non-Hispanic/Latino), 35 international. Average age 33. 240 applicants, 61% accepted, 95 enrolled. In 2015, 115 master's, 40 doctorates, 19 other advanced degrees awarded. *Degree requirements:* For doctorate, comprehensive exam, thesis/dissertation. *Entrance requirements:* For doctorate, GRE. Additional exam requirements/recommendations for international students: Required—TOEFL. *Application deadline:* For fall admission, 2/1 priority date for domestic and international students; for spring admission, 9/15 for domestic and international students. Applications are processed on a rolling basis. Application fee: $50. Electronic applications accepted. *Expenses:* Contact institution. *Financial support:* In 2015–16, research assistantships with tuition reimbursements (averaging $1,666 per year), teaching assistantships with tuition reimbursements (averaging $1,920 per year) were awarded; scholarships/grants, tuition waivers (full and partial), and unspecified assistantships also available. Support available to part-time students. Financial award application deadline: 8/1; financial award applicants required to submit FAFSA. *Faculty research:* Stroke intervention for caregivers, stroke prevention in African-Americans; relationships between psychological distress and health outcomes in parents with a medically ill infant; medically fragile children; nursing expertise and patient outcomes. *Unit head:* Nancy Kropf, Dean of Nursing, 404-413-1101, Fax: 404-413-1090, E-mail: nkropf@gsu.edu.
Website: http://nursing.gsu.edu/

Grand Valley State University, Kirkhof College of Nursing, Allendale, MI 49401-9403. Offers advanced practice (MSN); case management (MSN); nursing administration (MSN); nursing education (MSN); nursing practice (DNP); MSN/MBA. *Accreditation:* AACN. *Program availability:* Part-time. *Faculty:* 17 full-time (16 women), 6 part-time/adjunct (5 women). *Students:* 71 full-time (59 women), 53 part-time (45 women); includes 16 minority (10 Black or African American, non-Hispanic/Latino; 2 Asian, non-Hispanic/Latino; 3 Hispanic/Latino; 1 Two or more races, non-Hispanic/Latino), 3 international. Average age 33. 64 applicants, 94% accepted, 31 enrolled. In 2015, 1 master's, 11 doctorates awarded. *Degree requirements:* For master's, thesis optional. *Entrance requirements:* For master's, GRE, minimum upper-division GPA of 3.0, course work in statistics, Michigan RN license. Additional exam requirements/recommendations for international students: Required—TOEFL. *Application deadline:* For fall admission, 3/15 priority date for domestic students. Applications are processed on a rolling basis. Application fee: $30. Electronic applications accepted. *Financial support:* In 2015–16, 58 students received support, including 39 fellowships (averaging $11,141 per year), 33 research assistantships with tuition reimbursements available (averaging $7,339 per year); career-related internships or fieldwork, Federal Work-Study, institutionally sponsored loans, and traineeships also available. Financial award application deadline: 2/15. *Faculty research:* Multigenerational health promotion, chronic disease prevention, end-of-life issues, nursing workload, family caregiver health. *Total annual research expenditures:* $36,000. *Unit head:* Dr. Cynthia McCurren, Dean, 616-331-7161, Fax: 616-331-7362. *Application contact:* Dr. Cynthia Coviak, Associate Dean of Nursing Research and Faculty Development, 616-331-7170, Fax: 616-331-7362, E-mail: coviakc@gvsu.edu.
Website: http://www.gvsu.edu/kcon/

Grantham University, College of Nursing and Allied Health, Lenexa, KS 66219. Offers case management (MSN); health systems management (MHSM, MSN); healthcare administration (MHA); nursing education (MSN); nursing informatics (MSN); nursing management and organizational leadership (MSN). *Program availability:* Part-time, evening/weekend, online only, 100% online. *Faculty:* 1 (woman) full-time, 15 part-time/adjunct (11 women). *Students:* 59 full-time (42 women), 368 part-time (277 women); includes 181 minority (119 Black or African American, non-Hispanic/Latino; 2 American Indian or Alaska Native, non-Hispanic/Latino; 23 Asian, non-Hispanic/Latino; 21 Hispanic/Latino; 4 Native Hawaiian or other Pacific Islander, non-Hispanic/Latino; 12 Two or more races, non-Hispanic/Latino). Average age 41. 498 applicants, 94% accepted, 427 enrolled. In 2015, 119 master's awarded. *Degree requirements:* For master's, capstone. *Entrance requirements:* For master's, bachelor's degree from accredited degree-granting institution with minimum GPA of 2.5, BSN from accredited nursing program, valid RN license. Additional exam requirements/recommendations for international students: Required—TOEFL (minimum score 71 iBT); Recommended—IELTS (minimum score 6.5), TSE (minimum score 50). *Application deadline:* Applications are processed on a rolling basis. Electronic applications accepted. *Expenses:* Tuition, area resident: Full-time $3900; part-time $325 per credit hour. *Required fees:* $45 per term. One-time fee: $100. *Financial support:* Scholarships/grants available. *Faculty research:* Experimental exploration of the use of human patient simulation in the theory course, simulation education's impact on nursing confidence in the care of patients with Ebola virus, women's health-smoking cessation program for pregnant women, nursing and healthcare administration, business administration in healthcare. *Unit head:* Dana Basara, Dean, College of Nursing and Allied Health, 913-309-4783, Fax: 844-897-6490, E-mail: dbasara@grantham.edu. *Application contact:* Jared Parlette, Vice President of Student Enrollment, 888-947-2684, Fax: 866-908-2360, E-mail: admissions@grantham.edu.
Website: http://www.grantham.edu/colleges-and-schools/college-of-nursing-and-allied-health/

Herzing University Online, Program in Nursing, Menomonee Falls, WI 53051. Offers nursing (MSN); nursing education (MSN); nursing management (MSN). *Accreditation:* AACN. *Program availability:* Online learning.

Holy Family University, Graduate and Professional Programs, School of Nursing and Allied Health Professions, Philadelphia, PA 19114. Offers nursing administration (MSN); nursing education (MSN). *Accreditation:* AACN. *Program availability:* Part-time, evening/weekend. *Faculty:* 7 full-time (all women). *Students:* 42 part-time (39 women); includes 9 minority (4 Black or African American, non-Hispanic/Latino; 4 Asian, non-Hispanic/Latino; 1 Hispanic/Latino). Average age 36. 17 applicants, 82% accepted, 6 enrolled. In 2015, 12 master's awarded. *Degree requirements:* For master's, thesis or alternative, comprehensive portfolio, clinical practicum. *Entrance requirements:* For master's, BSN or RN from appropriately-accredited program, minimum GPA of 3.0, professional references, official transcripts of all college or university work, essay/personal statement, current resume, completion of one undergraduate statistics course with minimum grade of C. Additional exam requirements/recommendations for international students: Required—TOEFL (minimum score 550 paper-based; 79 iBT), IELTS (minimum score 6), or PTE (minimum score 54). *Application deadline:* For fall admission, 7/1 priority date for domestic and international students; for winter admission, 1/1 for domestic students; for spring admission, 11/1 priority date for domestic and international students; for summer admission, 4/1 priority date for domestic and international students. Applications are processed on a rolling basis. Application fee:

$25. Electronic applications accepted. *Financial support:* In 2015–16, 1 student received support. Available to part-time students. Application deadline: 2/15; applicants required to submit FAFSA. *Unit head:* Dr. Ana Maria Catanzaro, Dean, 267-341-3292, Fax: 215-637-6598, E-mail: acatanzaro@holyfamily.edu. *Application contact:* Gidget Matie Montelibano, Associate Director of Graduate Admissions, 267-341-3558, Fax: 215-637-1478, E-mail: gmontelibano@holyfamily.edu.
Website: http://www.holyfamily.edu/choosing-holy-family-u/academics/schools-of-study/school-of-nursing

Holy Names University, Graduate Division, Department of Nursing, Oakland, CA 94619-1699. Offers administration/management (MSN, PMC); clinical faculty (MSN, PMC); community health nursing/case manager (MSN); family nurse practitioner (MSN, PMC); MSN/MA; MSN/MBA. *Accreditation:* AACN. *Program availability:* Part-time, evening/weekend. *Entrance requirements:* For master's, bachelor's degree in nursing or related field; California RN license or eligibility; minimum cumulative GPA of 2.8, 3.0 in nursing courses from baccalaureate program; courses in pathophysiology, statistics, and research at the undergraduate level. Additional exam requirements/recommendations for international students: Required—TOEFL (minimum score 500 paper-based; 79 iBT). Electronic applications accepted. Application fee is waived when completed online. *Expenses:* Tuition, area resident: Full-time $25,272; part-time $936 per credit hour. *Required fees:* $500; $250 per credit hour. *Faculty research:* Women's reproductive health, gerontology, attitudes about aging, schizophrenic families, international health issues.

Immaculata University, College of Graduate Studies, Division of Nursing, Immaculata, PA 19345. Offers nursing administration (MSN); nursing education (MSN). *Accreditation:* AACN. *Program availability:* Part-time, evening/weekend. *Entrance requirements:* For master's, MAT or GRE, BSN, minimum undergraduate GPA of 3.0. Additional exam requirements/recommendations for international students: Required—TOEFL.

Independence University, Program in Nursing, Salt Lake City, UT 84107. Offers community health (MSN); gerontology (MSN); nursing administration (MSN); wellness promotion (MSN).

Indiana State University, College of Graduate and Professional Studies, College of Nursing, Health, and Human Services, Department of Advanced Practice Nursing, Terre Haute, IN 47809. Offers advanced practice nursing (DNP); family nurse practitioner (MS); nursing administration (MS); nursing education (MS). *Accreditation:* ACEN. *Program availability:* Part-time. *Degree requirements:* For master's, thesis or alternative. *Entrance requirements:* For master's, BSN, RN license, minimum undergraduate GPA of 3.0. Electronic applications accepted. *Faculty research:* Nursing faculty-student interactions, clinical evaluation, program evaluation, sexual dysfunction, faculty attitudes.

Indiana University Kokomo, School of Nursing, Kokomo, IN 46904-9003. Offers nurse administrator (MSN); nurse educator (MSN).

Indiana University of Pennsylvania, School of Graduate Studies and Research, College of Health and Human Services, Department of Nursing and Allied Health, Program in Nursing Administration, Indiana, PA 15705-1087. Offers MS. *Accreditation:* AACN. *Program availability:* Part-time. *Faculty:* 12 full-time (11 women). *Students:* 18 full-time (15 women), 9 part-time (8 women), 18 international. Average age 30. 24 applicants, 79% accepted, 10 enrolled. In 2015, 5 master's awarded. *Degree requirements:* For master's, thesis optional, practicum. *Entrance requirements:* Additional exam requirements/recommendations for international students: Required—TOEFL (minimum score 540 paper-based). *Application deadline:* Applications are processed on a rolling basis. Application fee: $50. Electronic applications accepted. *Financial support:* In 2015–16, 2 research assistantships with tuition reimbursements (averaging $4,080 per year) were awarded; career-related internships or fieldwork, Federal Work-Study, scholarships/grants, and unspecified assistantships also available. Financial award application deadline: 4/15; financial award applicants required to submit FAFSA. *Unit head:* Dr. Nashat Zuraikat, Graduate Coordinator, 724-357-3262, E-mail: zuraikat@iup.edu.
Website: http://www.iup.edu/grad/nursing/default.aspx

Indiana University–Purdue University Fort Wayne, College of Health and Human Services, Department of Nursing, Fort Wayne, IN 46805-1499. Offers adult-gerontology primary care nurse practitioner (MS); family nurse practitioner (MS); nurse executive (MS); nursing administration (Certificate); nursing education (MS). *Accreditation:* ACEN. *Program availability:* Part-time. *Faculty:* 8 full-time (all women). *Students:* 6 full-time (all women), 79 part-time (70 women); includes 8 minority (2 Black or African American, non-Hispanic/Latino; 3 Asian, non-Hispanic/Latino; 3 Hispanic/Latino). Average age 36. 14 applicants, 100% accepted, 10 enrolled. In 2015, 17 master's awarded. *Entrance requirements:* For master's, GRE Writing Test (if GPA below 3.0), BS in nursing, eligibility for Indiana RN license, minimum GPA of 3.0, essay, copy of resume, three references, undergraduate course work in research and statistics within last 5 years. Additional exam requirements/recommendations for international students: Required—TOEFL (minimum score 550 paper-based; 79 iBT); Recommended—TWE. *Application deadline:* For fall admission, 5/1 priority date for domestic and international students; for spring admission, 11/15 priority date for domestic students. Applications are processed on a rolling basis. Application fee: $55 ($60 for international students). Electronic applications accepted. *Financial support:* In 2015–16, 12 teaching assistantships with partial tuition reimbursements (averaging $13,522 per year) were awarded; scholarships/grants also available. Support available to part-time students. Financial award application deadline: 3/1; financial award applicants required to submit FAFSA. *Faculty research:* Community engagement, cervical screening, evidence-based practice. *Total annual research expenditures:* $22,966. *Unit head:* Dr. Lee-Ellen Kirkhorn, Chair/Professor, 260-481-6789, Fax: 260-481-5767, E-mail: kirkhorl@ipfw.edu. *Application contact:* Dr. Deb Poling, Director of Graduate Program, 260-481-6276, Fax: 260-481-5767, E-mail: polingd@ipfw.edu.
Website: http://www.ipfw.edu/nursing/

Indiana University–Purdue University Indianapolis, School of Nursing, MSN Program in Nursing, Indianapolis, IN 46202. Offers nursing education (MSN); nursing leadership in health systems (MSN). *Program availability:* Part-time, online learning. *Degree requirements:* For master's, thesis. *Entrance requirements:* For master's, minimum GPA of 3.0, RN license, background check, statistics. Additional exam requirements/recommendations for international students: Required—TOEFL (minimum score 550 paper-based; 79 iBT). *Expenses:* Contact institution. *Faculty research:* Clinical science, health systems.

Indiana Wesleyan University, College of Adult and Professional Studies, Graduate Studies in Business, Marion, IN 46953. Offers accounting (MBA, Graduate Certificate); applied management (MBA); business administration (MBA); health care (MBA, Graduate Certificate); human resources (MBA, Graduate Certificate); management (MS); organizational leadership (MA). *Program availability:* Part-time, evening/weekend, online learning. *Faculty:* 94 full-time (28 women), 6 part-time/adjunct (1 woman). *Students:* 1,564 full-time (980 women), 158 part-time (96 women); includes 715 minority (590 Black or African American, non-Hispanic/Latino; 6 American Indian or Alaska Native, non-Hispanic/Latino; 30 Asian, non-Hispanic/Latino; 57 Hispanic/Latino; 32 Two

Nursing and Healthcare Administration

or more races, non-Hispanic/Latino), 4 international. Average age 36. *Degree requirements:* For master's, applied business or management project. *Entrance requirements:* For master's, minimum GPA of 2.5, 2 years of related work experience. Additional exam requirements/recommendations for international students: Required—TOEFL (minimum score 550 paper-based). *Application deadline:* Applications are processed on a rolling basis. Application fee: $25. Electronic applications accepted. *Financial support:* Available to part-time students. Applicants required to submit FAFSA. *Unit head:* Dr. Paul Richardson, Associate Director, 765-677-2283, Fax: 765-677-1464, E-mail: paul.richardson@indwes.edu. *Application contact:* Graduate School, 866-IWU-4-YOU, Fax: 765-677-2541, E-mail: graduate@indwes.edu. Website: http://caps.indwes.edu/

Indiana Wesleyan University, Graduate School, School of Nursing, Marion, IN 46953-4974. Offers nursing administration (MS); nursing education (MS); primary care nursing (MS); MSN/MBA. *Accreditation:* AACN. *Program availability:* Part-time, online learning. *Students:* 884 full-time (818 women), 27 part-time (all women); includes 148 minority (92 Black or African American, non-Hispanic/Latino; 5 American Indian or Alaska Native, non-Hispanic/Latino; 18 Asian, non-Hispanic/Latino; 16 Hispanic/Latino; 17 Two or more races, non-Hispanic/Latino), 2 international. Average age 38. *Degree requirements:* For master's, capstone project or thesis. *Entrance requirements:* For master's, writing sample, RN license, 1 year of related experience, graduate statistics course. Additional exam requirements/recommendations for international students: Required—TOEFL. *Application deadline:* Applications are processed on a rolling basis. *Expenses:* Contact institution. *Financial support:* Fellowships, career-related internships or fieldwork, scholarships/grants, and traineeships available. Support available to part-time students. Financial award application deadline: 3/15; financial award applicants required to submit FAFSA. *Faculty research:* Primary health care with international emphasis, international nursing. *Unit head:* Dr. Barbara Ihrke, Dean, 765-677-2813, Fax: 765-677-1768, E-mail: barbara.ihrke@indwes.edu. *Application contact:* Graduate School, 866-IWU-4-YOU, Fax: 765-677-2541, E-mail: graduate@indwes.edu. Website: http://graduatenursing.indwes.edu

James Madison University, The Graduate School, College of Health and Behavioral Sciences, Program in Nursing, Harrisonburg, VA 22807. Offers adult/gerontology primary care nurse practitioner (MSN); clinical nurse leader (MSN); family nurse practitioner (MSN); nurse administrator (MSN); nurse midwifery (MSN); nursing (MSN, DNP). *Accreditation:* AACN. *Program availability:* Part-time, 100% online, blended/hybrid learning. *Faculty:* 15 full-time (all women), 1 (woman) part-time/adjunct. *Students:* 14 full-time (all women), 54 part-time (43 women); includes 6 minority (2 Black or African American, non-Hispanic/Latino; 1 Asian, non-Hispanic/Latino; 1 Hispanic/Latino; 2 Two or more races, non-Hispanic/Latino), 1 international. Average age 30. 49 applicants, 67% accepted, 31 enrolled. In 2015, 14 master's awarded. Application fee: $55. Electronic applications accepted. *Financial support:* In 2015–16, 2 students received support. Federal Work-Study, unspecified assistantships, and 2 assistantships (averaging $7530) available. Financial award application deadline: 3/1; financial award applicants required to submit FAFSA. *Unit head:* Dr. Julie T. Sanford, Department Head, 540-568-6314, E-mail: sanforjt@jmu.edu. *Application contact:* Lynette D. Michael, Director of Graduate Admissions and Student Records, 540-568-6131 Ext. 6395, Fax: 540-568-7860, E-mail: michaeld@jmu.edu. Website: http://www.nursing.jmu.edu

Jefferson College of Health Sciences, Program in Nursing, Roanoke, VA 24013. Offers nursing education (MSN); nursing management (MSN). *Accreditation:* AACN. *Program availability:* Part-time. *Degree requirements:* For master's, project. *Entrance requirements:* For master's, MAT. Additional exam requirements/recommendations for international students: Required—TOEFL (minimum score 550 paper-based; 80 iBT). Electronic applications accepted. *Faculty research:* Nursing, teaching and learning techniques, cultural competence, spirituality and nursing.

Kaplan University, Davenport Campus, School of Nursing, Davenport, IA 52807-2095. Offers nurse administrator (MS); nurse educator (MS). *Program availability:* Part-time, evening/weekend, online learning. *Entrance requirements:* For master's, RN. Additional exam requirements/recommendations for international students: Required—TOEFL (minimum score 550 paper-based).

Kean University, College of Natural, Applied and Health Sciences, Program in Nursing, Union, NJ 07083. Offers clinical management (MSN); community health nursing (MSN); school nursing (MSN). *Accreditation:* ACEN. *Program availability:* Part-time. *Faculty:* 9 full-time (all women). *Students:* 10 full-time (all women), 120 part-time (114 women); includes 63 minority (47 Black or African American, non-Hispanic/Latino; 11 Asian, non-Hispanic/Latino; 3 Hispanic/Latino; 2 Two or more races, non-Hispanic/Latino), 1 international. Average age 44. 64 applicants, 63% accepted, 22 enrolled. In 2015, 46 master's awarded. *Degree requirements:* For master's, thesis or alternative, clinical field experience. *Entrance requirements:* For master's, minimum GPA of 3.0; BS in nursing; RN license; 2 letters of recommendation; interview; official transcripts from all institutions attended. Additional exam requirements/recommendations for international students: Required—TOEFL (minimum score 550 paper-based; 79 iBT), IELTS. *Application deadline:* For fall admission, 6/1 for domestic and international students; for spring admission, 12/1 for domestic and international students. Applications are processed on a rolling basis. Application fee: $75 ($150 for international students). Electronic applications accepted. *Expenses:* Tuition, state resident: full-time $12,835; part-time $625 per credit. Tuition, nonresident: full-time $17,396; part-time $766 per credit. *Required fees:* $3235; $147 per credit. Tuition and fees vary according to course level, course load, degree level and program. *Financial support:* In 2015–16, research assistantships with full tuition reimbursements (averaging $3,771 per year) were awarded; scholarships/grants and unspecified assistantships also available. Financial award applicants required to submit FAFSA. *Unit head:* Dr. Portia Johnson, Program Coordinator, 908-737-3386, E-mail: johnsonpo@kean.edu. *Application contact:* Pedro Lopes, Admissions Counselor, 908-737-7100, E-mail: grad-adm@kean.edu. Website: http://grad.kean.edu/masters-programs/nursing-clinical-management

Kean University, College of Natural, Applied and Health Sciences, Program in Nursing Educational Leadership, Union, NJ 07083. Offers PhD. *Accreditation:* ACEN. *Faculty:* 9 full-time (all women). *Students:* 30 part-time (28 women); includes 9 minority (8 Black or African American, non-Hispanic/Latino; 1 Asian, non-Hispanic/Latino). Average age 49. 1 applicant, 100% accepted. *Degree requirements:* For doctorate, comprehensive exam, thesis/dissertation. *Entrance requirements:* For doctorate, GRE, MSN, minimum cumulative GPA of 3.2 in last degree obtained, official transcripts from all institutions attended, valid RN license, three letters of recommendation, professional resume/curriculum vitae, personal statement. *Application deadline:* For fall admission, 5/1 for domestic students; for spring admission, 12/1 for domestic and international students. Application fee: $75 ($150 for international students). Electronic applications accepted. *Expenses:* Contact institution. *Financial support:* Research assistantships with full tuition reimbursements, scholarships/grants, and unspecified assistantships available. *Unit head:* Dr. Virginia Fitzsimons, Coordinator, 609-361-4798, E-mail: vfitzsim@kean.edu. *Application contact:* Pedro Lopes, Admissions Counselor, 908-737-7100, E-mail: grad-adm@kean.edu. Website: http://grad.kean.edu/doctoral-programs/doctor-nursing-educational-leadership

Kent State University, College of Nursing, Kent, OH 44242. Offers advanced nursing practice (DNP), including adult gerontology acute care nurse practitioner (MSN, DNP), adult gerontology clinical nurse specialist (MSN, DNP), family nurse practitioner (MSN, DNP); nursing (MSN, PhD), including adult gerontology acute care nurse practitioner (MSN, DNP), adult gerontology clinical nurse specialist (MSN, DNP), family nurse practitioner (MSN, DNP), nurse educator (MSN), nursing healthcare management (MSN), primary care adult nurse practitioner (MSN), primary care pediatric clinical nurse specialist (MSN), primary care pediatric nurse practitioner (MSN), psychiatric mental health practitioner (MSN), women's health nurse practitioner (MSN); nursing education (Certificate); primary care pediatric nurse practitioner (Certificate); women's health nurse practitioner (Certificate). PhD program offered jointly with The University of Akron. *Accreditation:* AACN. *Program availability:* Part-time, online learning. *Faculty:* 52 full-time (48 women). *Students:* 78 full-time (56 women), 414 part-time (365 women); includes 63 minority (34 Black or African American, non-Hispanic/Latino; 1 American Indian or Alaska Native, non-Hispanic/Latino; 12 Asian, non-Hispanic/Latino; 12 Hispanic/Latino; 4 Two or more races, non-Hispanic/Latino), 16 international. Average age 37. 653 applicants, 54% accepted, 309 enrolled. In 2015, 140 master's, 1 doctorate, 13 other advanced degrees awarded. *Degree requirements:* For master's, thesis optional, practicum; for doctorate, comprehensive exam (for some programs), thesis/dissertation (for some programs), practicum and scholarly project (for DNP programs); for Certificate, practicum. *Entrance requirements:* For master's, minimum GPA of 3.0, transcripts, active unrestricted RN license, essay/goal statement, interview, 3 letters of recommendation; for doctorate, GRE (for PhD), minimum GPA of 3.0, transcripts, 3 letters of recommendation, interview; active unrestricted RN license, clinical experience and hours record (for DNP); goal statement, sample of written work, curriculum vitae, statement of research interests, and eligibility for RN license (for PhD); for Certificate, MSN, minimum GPA of 3.0, transcripts. Additional exam requirements/recommendations for international students: Required—TOEFL (minimum score: paper-based 525, iBT 71), Michigan English Language Assessment Battery (minimum score of 75), IELTS (minimum score of 6.0), PTE Academic (minimum score of 48), or completion of ELS level 112 Intensive Program. *Application deadline:* For fall admission, 2/1 for domestic students; for spring admission, 11/1 for domestic students. Application fee: $45 ($70 for international students). Electronic applications accepted. *Expenses:* Tuition, state resident: full-time $10,864; part-time $495 per credit hour. Tuition, nonresident: full-time $18,380; part-time $837 per credit hour. *Financial support:* Research assistantships with full tuition reimbursements, teaching assistantships with full tuition reimbursements, career-related internships or fieldwork, Federal Work-Study, traineeships, and unspecified assistantships available. Financial award application deadline: 2/1. *Unit head:* Dr. Barbara Broome, Dean, 330-672-3777, E-mail: bbroome1@kent.edu. *Application contact:* Dr. Wendy A. Umberger, Associate Dean for Graduate Programs/Professor, 330-672-8813, E-mail: wlewando@kent.edu. Website: http://www.kent.edu/nursing/

Lamar University, College of Graduate Studies, College of Arts and Sciences, JoAnne Gay Dishman Department of Nursing, Beaumont, TX 77710. Offers nursing administration (MSN); nursing education (MSN); MSN/MBA. *Accreditation:* ACEN. *Program availability:* Part-time, evening/weekend, online learning. *Faculty:* 8 full-time (all women), 2 part-time/adjunct (both women). *Students:* 2 full-time (both women), 73 part-time (64 women); includes 32 minority (17 Black or African American, non-Hispanic/Latino; 7 Asian, non-Hispanic/Latino; 6 Hispanic/Latino; 2 Two or more races, non-Hispanic/Latino). Average age 38. 47 applicants, 77% accepted, 14 enrolled. In 2015, 14 master's awarded. *Degree requirements:* For master's, comprehensive exam, practicum project presentation, evidence-based project. *Entrance requirements:* For master's, GRE General Test, MAT, criminal background check, RN license, NLN-accredited BSN, college course work in statistics in past 5 years, letters of recommendation, minimum undergraduate GPA of 3.0. Additional exam requirements/recommendations for international students: Required—TOEFL (minimum score 550 paper-based; 79 iBT), IELTS (minimum score 6.5). *Application deadline:* For fall admission, 8/10 for domestic students, 7/1 for international students; for spring admission, 1/5 for domestic students, 12/1 for international students. Applications are processed on a rolling basis. Application fee: $25 ($50 for international students). Electronic applications accepted. *Expenses:* Tuition, area resident: Full-time $6720; part-time $4032. Tuition, nonresident: full-time $14,880; part-time $8928. *Required fees:* $1900; $950 $784. *Financial support:* In 2015–16, 3 students received support. Teaching assistantships, scholarships/grants, and traineeships available. Financial award application deadline: 4/1; financial award applicants required to submit FAFSA. *Faculty research:* Student retention, theory, care giving, online course and research. *Unit head:* Cynthia Stinson, Interim Chair, 409-880-8817, Fax: 409-880-8698. *Application contact:* Melissa Gallien, Director, Admissions and Academic Services, 409-880-8888, Fax: 409-880-7419, E-mail: gradmissions@lamar.edu. Website: http://artssciences.lamar.edu/nursing

La Roche College, School of Graduate Studies and Adult Education, Program in Nursing, Pittsburgh, PA 15237-5898. Offers nursing education (MSN); nursing management (MSN). *Accreditation:* AANA/CANAEP; ACEN. *Program availability:* Part-time, evening/weekend, online only, 100% online. *Faculty:* 3 full-time (all women), 1 part-time/adjunct (0 women). *Students:* 14 full-time (all women), 8 part-time (all women), 2 international. Average age 40. 20 applicants, 75% accepted, 11 enrolled. In 2015, 3 master's awarded. *Degree requirements:* For master's, thesis optional, internship, practicum. *Entrance requirements:* For master's, GRE General Test, BSN, nursing license, work experience. Additional exam requirements/recommendations for international students: Recommended—TOEFL (minimum score 550 paper-based). *Application deadline:* For fall admission, 8/15 priority date for domestic students, 8/15 for international students; for spring admission, 12/15 priority date for domestic students, 12/15 for international students. Applications are processed on a rolling basis. Application fee: $50. Electronic applications accepted. *Expenses:* Contact institution. *Financial support:* Application deadline: 3/31; applicants required to submit FAFSA. *Faculty research:* Patient education, perception. *Unit head:* Dr. Terri Liberto, Division Chair, 412-847-1813, Fax: 412-536-1175, E-mail: terri.liberto@laroche.edu. *Application contact:* Hope Schiffgens, Director of Graduate Studies and Adult Education, 412-536-1266, Fax: 412-536-1283, E-mail: schombh1@laroche.edu.

La Salle University, School of Nursing and Health Sciences, Program in Nursing, Philadelphia, PA 19141-1199. Offers adult gerontology primary care nurse practitioner (MSN, Certificate); adult health and illness clinical nurse specialist (MSN); adult-gerontology clinical nurse specialist (MSN, Certificate); clinical nurse leader (MSN); family primary care nurse practitioner (MSN, Certificate); gerontology (Certificate); nurse anesthetist (MSN, Certificate); nursing (MSN, Certificate); nursing administration (MSN, Certificate); nursing education (Certificate); nursing practice (DNP); nursing service administration (MSN); public health nursing (MSN, Certificate); school nursing (Certificate); MSN/MBA; MSN/MPH. *Accreditation:* AANA/CANAEP. *Program availability:* Part-time, evening/weekend, 100% online. *Faculty:* 11 full-time (all women), 9 part-time/adjunct (8 women). *Students:* 368 part-time (56 women); includes 103 minority (62 Black or African American, non-Hispanic/Latino; 1 American Indian or Alaska Native, non-Hispanic/Latino; 26 Asian, non-Hispanic/Latino; 9 Hispanic/Latino; 5 Two or more races, non-Hispanic/Latino), 5 international. Average age 36. 98 applicants, 85% accepted, 53 enrolled. In 2015, 87 master's, 3 doctorates, 10 other

advanced degrees awarded. *Degree requirements:* For doctorate, minimum of 1,000 hours of post baccalaureate clinical practice supervised by preceptors. *Entrance requirements:* For master's, GRE, MAT, or GMAT (for students with BSN GPA of less than 3.2), baccalaureate degree in nursing from an NLNAC- or CCNE-accredited program or an MSN Bridge program; Pennsylvania RN license; 2 letters of reference; resume; statement of philosophy articulating professional values and future educational goal; 1 year of work experience as a registered nurse; for doctorate, GRE (waived for applicants with MSN cumulative GPA of 3.7 or above), MSN from nationally-accredited program or master's degree, MBA or MHA from nationally-accredited program; resume or curriculum vitae; 2 letters of reference; interview; for Certificate, GRE, MAT, or GMAT (for students with BSN GPA of less than 3.2, baccalaureate degree in nursing from an NLNAC- or CCNE-accredited program or an MSN Bridge program; Pennsylvania RN license; 2 letters of reference; resume; statement of philosophy articulating professional values and future educational goal; 1 year of work experience as a registered nurse. Additional exam requirements/recommendations for international students: Required— TOEFL. *Application deadline:* For fall admission, 8/15 priority date for domestic students, 7/15 for international students; for spring admission, 12/15 priority date for domestic students, 11/15 for international students; for summer admission, 4/15 priority date for domestic students, 3/15 for international students. Applications are processed on a rolling basis. Application fee: $35. Electronic applications accepted. Application fee is waived when completed online. *Expenses:* $870 per credit hour (for MSN); $930 per credit hour (for DNP); $150 technology fee full-time, $75 part-time; $135 general university fee. *Financial support:* In 2015–16, 13 students received support. Scholarships/grants and traineeships available. Support available to part-time students. Financial award application deadline: 8/31; financial award applicants required to submit FAFSA. *Unit head:* Dr. Patricia M. Dillon, Director, 215-951-1322, Fax: 215-951-1896, E-mail: manapn@laoallo.odu. *Application contact:* Alison McAnespey Target, Director, Graduate and Adult Enrollment, 215-951-1100, Fax: 215-951-1462, E-mail: reilly@lasalle.edu.
Website: http://www.lasalle.edu/nursing/program-options/

Le Moyne College, Department of Nursing, Syracuse, NY 13214. Offers informatics (MS, CAS); nursing administration (MS, CAS); nursing education (MS, CAS); nursing gerontology (MS, CAS); palliative care (MS, CAS). *Accreditation:* AACN. *Program availability:* Part-time, evening/weekend. *Degree requirements:* For master's, scholarly project. *Entrance requirements:* For master's, bachelor's degree, interview, minimum GPA of 3.0, New York RN license, 2 letters of recommendation, writing sample, transcripts. *Expenses:* Contact institution. *Faculty research:* Inter-profession education, gerontology, utilization of free healthcare services by the insured, health promotion education, innovative undergraduate nursing education models, patient and family education, horizontal violence.

Lenoir-Rhyne University, Graduate Programs, School of Nursing, Program in Nursing, Hickory, NC 28601. Offers nursing administration (MSN); nursing education (MSN). *Program availability:* Online learning. *Faculty:* 7 full-time (all women). *Students:* 4 full-time (all women), 46 part-time (45 women); includes 4 minority (2 Black or African American, non-Hispanic/Latino; 2 Hispanic/Latino). Average age 39. In 2015, 11 master's awarded. *Degree requirements:* For master's, comprehensive exam, thesis optional. *Entrance requirements:* For master's, official transcripts, two recommendations, essay, resume, unrestricted RN license, criminal background check. Additional exam requirements/recommendations for international students: Required— TOEFL (minimum score 600 paper-based). Application fee: $35. Electronic applications accepted. *Expenses:* $550 per credit hour. *Unit head:* Dr. Kerry Thompson, Chair, School of Nursing, 828-328-7282, Fax: 828-328-7368, E-mail: thompsonk@lr.edu. *Application contact:* Mary Ann Gosnell, Director of Graduate Recruiting, 828-328-7300, E-mail: admission@lr.edu.
Website: http://www.lr.edu/academics/programs/nursing-0

Lewis University, College of Nursing and Health Professions, Program in Nursing, Romeoville, IL 60446. Offers adult nurse practitioner (MSN); nursing administration (MSN); nursing education (MSN). *Accreditation:* AACN. *Program availability:* Part-time, evening/weekend, online learning. *Degree requirements:* For master's, clinical practicum. *Entrance requirements:* For master's, minimum undergraduate GPA of 3.0, degree in nursing, RN license, letter of recommendation, interview, resume or curriculum vitae. Additional exam requirements/recommendations for international students: Required—TOEFL (minimum score 550 paper-based; 80 iBT). Electronic applications accepted. *Faculty research:* Cancer prevention, phenomenological methods, public policy analysis.

Liberty University, School of Nursing, Lynchburg, VA 24515. Offers family nurse practitioner (DNP); nurse educator (MSN); nursing administration (MSN). *Program availability:* Part-time, online learning. *Students:* 108 full-time (100 women), 508 part-time (454 women); includes 106 minority (84 Black or African American, non-Hispanic/Latino; 3 American Indian or Alaska Native, non-Hispanic/Latino; 8 Asian, non-Hispanic/Latino; 1 Hispanic/Latino; 10 Two or more races, non-Hispanic/Latino; 7 international. Average age 39. 577 applicants, 30% accepted, 119 enrolled. In 2015, 161 master's awarded. *Entrance requirements:* For master's, minimum cumulative undergraduate GPA of 3.0; for doctorate, minimum GPA of 3.25 in most current nursing program completed. Additional exam requirements/recommendations for international students: Recommended—TOEFL. *Application deadline:* Applications are processed on a rolling basis. Application fee: $50. Electronic applications accepted. *Unit head:* Dr. Deanna Britt, Dean, 434-582-2519, E-mail: dbritt@liberty.edu. *Application contact:* Jay Bridge, Director of Admissions, 800-424-9595, Fax: 800-628-7977, E-mail: gradadmissions@liberty.edu.

Loma Linda University, School of Nursing, Program in Nursing Administration, Loma Linda, CA 92350. Offers MS. *Accreditation:* AACN. *Program availability:* Part-time. *Degree requirements:* For master's, thesis or alternative. *Entrance requirements:* For master's, GRE General Test, BSN, minimum GPA of 3.0, RN license. Additional exam requirements/recommendations for international students: Required—TOEFL. *Application deadline:* For fall admission, 8/1 for domestic and international students; for winter admission, 11/1 for domestic and international students; for spring admission, 2/1 for domestic and international students. Application fee: $60. Electronic applications accepted. *Financial support:* Career-related internships or fieldwork, Federal Work-Study, institutionally sponsored loans, and scholarships/grants available. Financial award application deadline: 6/1. Support available to part-time students. *Faculty research:* Job aspects contributing to satisfaction among leaders in health care institutions, leadership content significant to RN graduates. *Unit head:* Director, 909-824-4360. *Application contact:* Admissions Office, 909-651-5029, Fax: 909-558-4879, E-mail: admissions.app@llu.edu.

Long Island University–LIU Post, College of Liberal Arts and Sciences, Brookville, NY 11548-1300. Offers applied mathematics (MS); behavior analysis (MA); biology (MS); criminal justice (MS); earth science (MS); English (MA); environmental studies (MS); environmental sustainability (MS); genetic counseling (MS); gerontology (Advanced Certificate); health care administration (MPA); history (MA); interdisciplinary studies (MA, MS); mathematics for secondary school teachers (MS); mobile GIS application development (Advanced Certificate); non-profit management (Advanced Certificate); political science (MA); psychology (MA); public administration (MPA). *Program*

availability: Part-time, evening/weekend, online learning. *Faculty:* 77 full-time (35 women), 36 part-time/adjunct (17 women). *Students:* 254 full-time (178 women), 177 part-time (134 women); includes 104 minority (40 Black or African American, non-Hispanic/Latino; 27 Asian, non-Hispanic/Latino; 28 Hispanic/Latino; 1 Native Hawaiian or other Pacific Islander, non-Hispanic/Latino; 8 Two or more races, non-Hispanic/Latino, 44 international. Average age 31. 686 applicants, 47% accepted, 138 enrolled. In 2015, 135 master's awarded. *Degree requirements:* For master's, comprehensive exam (for some programs), thesis (for some programs). *Entrance requirements:* Additional exam requirements/recommendations for international students: Required— TOEFL (minimum score 550 paper-based; 79 iBT), IELTS (minimum score 6.5). *Application deadline:* Applications are processed on a rolling basis. Application fee: $50. Electronic applications accepted. *Expenses:* $1,155 per credit; $934 full-time fees; $442 part-time fees. *Financial support:* In 2015–16, 48 fellowships (averaging $12,637 per year), 5 research assistantships with full tuition reimbursements were awarded; Federal Work-Study and institutionally sponsored loans also available. Support available to part-time students. Financial award application deadline: 2/15; financial award applicants required to submit FAFSA. *Faculty research:* Biology, criminal justice, earth and environmental science, English, health care and public administration, history, mathematics, political science, psychology, Spanish. *Unit head:* Dr. Nicholas J. Ramer, Acting Dean, 516-299-2233, Fax: 516-299-4140, E-mail: nicholas.ramer@liu.edu. *Application contact:* Carol Zerah, Director of Graduate Admissions, 516-299-2900 Ext. 3952, Fax: 516-299-2137, E-mail: enroll@cwpost.liu.edu.
Website: http://liu.edu/CWPost/Academics/Schools/CLAS

Louisiana State University Health Sciences Center, School of Nursing, New Orleans, LA 70112. Offers adult gerontology clinical nurse specialist (Post-Master's Certificate); clinical nurse leader (MSN); executive nurse leader (Post-Master's Certificate); neonatal nurse practitioner (Post-Master's Certificate); nurse anesthesia (Post-Master's Certificate); nurse educator (MSN); nursing (DNS); primary care family nurse practitioner (Post-Master's Certificate); public/community health nursing (Post-Master's Certificate). *Accreditation:* AACN; AANA/CANAEP (one or more programs are accredited). *Program availability:* Part-time. *Faculty:* 22 full-time (19 women), 21 part-time/adjunct (8 women). *Students:* 254 (185 women); includes 68 minority (44 Black or African American, non-Hispanic/Latino; 12 Asian, non-Hispanic/Latino; 12 Hispanic/Latino). Average age 33. 144 applicants, 54% accepted, 73 enrolled. In 2015, 84 master's, 6 doctorates awarded. *Degree requirements:* For master's, thesis optional; for doctorate, thesis/dissertation. *Entrance requirements:* For master's, GRE General Test, MAT, minimum GPA of 3.0; for doctorate, GRE General Test, minimum GPA of 3.5. Additional exam requirements/recommendations for international students: Required— TOEFL (minimum score 550 paper-based; 79 iBT). *Application deadline:* Applications are processed on a rolling basis. Application fee: $250. Electronic applications accepted. *Expenses:* $9,136.50 per year; $19,633.50 per year (for DNP). *Financial support:* Federal Work-Study, institutionally sponsored loans, scholarships/grants, and traineeships available. Financial award applicants required to submit FAFSA. *Faculty research:* Advanced clinical practice, nursing education, health, social support, nursing administration. *Unit head:* Dr. Demetrius James Porche, Dean, 504-568-4106, Fax: 504-599-0573, E-mail: dporch@lsuhsc.edu. *Application contact:* Tracie Gravolet, Director, Office of Student Affairs, 504-568-4114, Fax: 504-568-5711, E-mail: tgravo@lsuhsc.edu.
Website: http://nursing.lsuhsc.edu/

Lourdes University, Graduate School, Sylvania, OH 43560-2898. Offers business (MBA); leadership (M Ed); nurse anesthesia (MSN); nurse educator (MSN); nurse leader (MSN); organizational leadership (MOL); reading (M Ed); teaching and curriculum (M Ed); theology (MA). *Program availability:* Evening/weekend. *Entrance requirements:* Additional exam requirements/recommendations for international students: Required— TOEFL.

Loyola University Chicago, Graduate School, Marcella Niehoff School of Nursing, Maywood, IL 60153. Offers adult gerontology acute care clinical nurse specialist (MSN), including emergency care (MSN, Certificate); adult gerontology acute care nurse practitioner (MSN), including oncology (MSN, Certificate); adult gerontology clinical nurse specialist (MSN), including oncology (MSN, Certificate); adult gerontology nursing (Certificate), including oncology (MSN, Certificate); adult nurse practitioner (Certificate); dietetics (MS); family nurse practitioner (MSN, Certificate), including emergency care; informatics (MSN); leadership (DNP), including healthcare quality using education in safety and technology, infection prevention; nursing science (PhD); women's health nurse practitioner (MSN); women's health nursing (Certificate). *Accreditation:* AACN. *Program availability:* Part-time, blended/hybrid learning. *Faculty:* 27 full-time (25 women), 12 part-time/adjunct (10 women). *Students:* 174 full-time (161 women), 232 part-time (221 women); includes 95 minority (19 Black or African American, non-Hispanic/Latino; 2 American Indian or Alaska Native, non-Hispanic/Latino; 38 Asian, non-Hispanic/Latino; 28 Hispanic/Latino; 2 Native Hawaiian or other Pacific Islander, non-Hispanic/Latino; 6 Two or more races, non-Hispanic/Latino), 3 international. Average age 35. 209 applicants, 52% accepted, 83 enrolled. In 2015, 78 master's, 10 doctorates, 17 other advanced degrees awarded. *Degree requirements:* For master's, comprehensive exam; for doctorate, thesis/dissertation, qualifying examination (for PhD); capstone project (for DNP). *Entrance requirements:* For master's, BSN, minimum nursing GPA of 3.0, Illinois RN license, 3 letters of recommendation, 1000 hours of experience in area of specialty prior to starting clinical rotations, personal statement; for doctorate, GRE General Test (for PhD), BSN or MSN, minimum GPA of 3.0, professional nursing license, 3 letters of recommendation, personal statement. Additional exam requirements/recommendations for international students: Required— TOEFL (minimum score 550 paper-based; 79 iBT), IELTS (minimum score 6.5). *Application deadline:* For fall admission, 6/1 priority date for domestic and international students; for spring admission, 11/15 priority date for domestic and international students; for summer admission, 3/15 priority date for domestic and international students. Applications are processed on a rolling basis. Application fee: $50. Electronic applications accepted. Application fee is waived when completed online. *Expenses:* $1,081 per credit hour. *Financial support:* In 2015–16, 10 students received support, including 3 research assistantships with full tuition reimbursements available (averaging $18,000 per year), 1 teaching assistantship with full tuition reimbursement available (averaging $18,000 per year); scholarships/grants, unspecified assistantships, and nurse faculty loan program also available. Financial award application deadline: 5/1; financial award applicants required to submit FAFSA. *Faculty research:* Epigenetics and social determinants of health, women's health, vitamin D, interprofessional education, prevention and self-management of chronic disease. *Total annual research expenditures:* $649,606. *Unit head:* Dr. Vicky Keough, Dean, 708-216-5448, Fax: 708-216-9555, E-mail: vkeough@luc.edu. *Application contact:* Toni Topalova, Enrollment Advisor, 708-216-3751, Fax: 708-216-9555, E-mail: atopalova@luc.edu.
Website: http://www.luc.edu/nursing/

Lynchburg College, Graduate Studies, MS Program in Nursing, Lynchburg, VA 24501-3199. Offers clinical nurse leader (MS). *Accreditation:* AACN. *Program availability:* Part-time, evening/weekend, online only, 100% online. *Faculty:* 1 (woman) full-time, 2 part-time/adjunct (both women). *Students:* 2 full-time (both women), 32 part-time (30 women); includes 4 minority (3 Black or African American, non-Hispanic/Latino; 1 Hispanic/Latino). Average age 40. In 2015, 6 master's awarded. *Degree requirements:*

Nursing and Healthcare Administration

For master's, practicum. *Entrance requirements:* For master's, GRE or 2 years of professional nursing experience, official transcripts, personal essay, 3 letters of recommendation, current unrestricted registered nurse license in Virginia. Additional exam requirements/recommendations for international students: Required—TOEFL (minimum score 550 paper-based; 79 iBT), IELTS (minimum score 6.5). *Application deadline:* For fall admission, 7/31 for domestic students, 6/1 for international students; for spring admission, 11/30 for domestic students, 10/15 for international students. Applications are processed on a rolling basis. Application fee: $30. Electronic applications accepted. Application fee is waived when completed online. *Expenses:* $8,550. *Financial support:* Federal Work-Study, scholarships/grants, health care benefits, and unspecified assistantships available. Support available to part-time students. Financial award application deadline: 7/31; financial award applicants required to submit FAFSA. *Unit head:* Dr. Jenna Lloyd, Director of MSN Program, 434-544-8461, E-mail: lloyd.j@lynchburg.edu.
Website: http://www.lynchburg.edu/graduate/online-master-of-science-in-nursing/

Madonna University, Program in Nursing, Livonia, MI 48150-1173. Offers adult health: chronic health conditions (MSN); adult nurse practitioner (MSN); nursing administration (MSN); MSN/MSBA. *Accreditation:* AACN. *Program availability:* Part-time. *Degree requirements:* For master's, thesis or alternative. *Entrance requirements:* For master's, GRE General Test, Michigan nursing license. Electronic applications accepted. *Faculty research:* Coping, caring.

Marquette University, Graduate School, College of Nursing, Milwaukee, WI 53201-1881. Offers acute care nurse practitioner (Certificate); adult clinical nurse specialist (Certificate); adult nurse practitioner (Certificate); advanced practice nursing (MSN, DNP), including adult-older adult acute care (DNP), adults (MSN), adults-older adults (DNP), clinical nurse leader (MSN), health care systems leadership (DNP), nurse-midwifery (MSN), older adults (MSN), pediatrics-acute care, pediatrics-primary care, primary care (DNP), systems leadership and healthcare quality (MSN); family nurse practitioner (Certificate); nurse-midwifery (Certificate); nursing (PhD); pediatric acute care (Certificate); pediatric primary care (Certificate); systems leadership and healthcare quality (Certificate). *Accreditation:* AACN. *Faculty:* 35 full-time (all women), 56 part-time/adjunct (55 women). *Students:* 123 full-time (112 women), 242 part-time (220 women); includes 34 minority (9 Black or African American, non-Hispanic/Latino; 12 Asian, non-Hispanic/Latino; 10 Hispanic/Latino; 3 Two or more races, non-Hispanic/Latino), 4 international. Average age 30. 269 applicants, 61% accepted, 98 enrolled. In 2015, 84 master's, 5 doctorates, 22 other advanced degrees awarded. Terminal master's awarded for partial completion of doctoral program. *Degree requirements:* For master's, comprehensive exam, thesis or alternative. *Entrance requirements:* For master's, GRE General Test, BSN, Wisconsin RN license, official transcripts from all current and previous colleges/universities except Marquette, three completed recommendation forms, resume, written statement of professional goals; for doctorate, GRE General Test, official transcripts from all current and previous colleges/universities except Marquette, three letters of recommendation, resume, written statement of professional goals, sample of scholarly writing. Additional exam requirements/recommendations for international students: Required—TOEFL (minimum score 530 paper-based). *Application deadline:* For fall admission, 2/15 for domestic and international students. Electronic applications accepted. *Financial support:* In 2015–16, 41 students received support, including 1 fellowship with partial tuition reimbursement available (averaging $17,500 per year), 2 research assistantships with full tuition reimbursements available (averaging $13,285 per year), 8 teaching assistantships with full tuition reimbursements available (averaging $13,912 per year); career-related internships or fieldwork, Federal Work-Study, scholarships/grants, health care benefits, tuition waivers (partial), and unspecified assistantships also available. Support available to part-time students. Financial award application deadline: 2/15. *Faculty research:* Psychosocial adjustment to chronic illness, gerontology, reminiscence, health policy: uninsured and access, hospital care delivery systems. *Total annual research expenditures:* $480,591. *Unit head:* Dr. Donna McCarthy, Interim Chair, 414-288-3800, Fax: 414-288-1578. *Application contact:* Dr. Maureen O'Brien, Associate Dean/Clinical Associate Professor, 414-288-3823.

McKendree University, Graduate Programs, Master of Science in Nursing Program, Lebanon, IL 62254-1299. Offers nursing education (MSN); nursing management/administration (MSN). *Accreditation:* AACN. *Program availability:* Part-time, evening/weekend, online learning. *Degree requirements:* For master's, research project or thesis. *Entrance requirements:* For master's, resume, references, valid Professional Registered Nurse license. Additional exam requirements/recommendations for international students: Required—TOEFL. Electronic applications accepted.

McNeese State University, Doré School of Graduate Studies, College of Nursing, Department of Graduate Nursing, Nursing Case Management Program, Lake Charles, LA 70609. Offers Postbaccalaureate Certificate. *Degree requirements:* For Postbaccalaureate Certificate, thesis. *Entrance requirements:* For degree, GRE, MSN, eligible for unencumbered licensure as RN in Louisiana.

McNeese State University, Doré School of Graduate Studies, College of Nursing, Department of Graduate Nursing, Nursing Program, Lake Charles, LA 70609. Offers family nurse practitioner (MSN); family psychiatric/mental health nurse practitioner (MSN); nurse educator (MSN); nurse executive (MSN). *Degree requirements:* For master's, comprehensive exam. *Entrance requirements:* For master's, GRE, baccalaureate degree in nursing, minimum overall GPA of 2.7 for all undergraduate coursework, eligibility for unencumbered licensure as Registered Nurse in Louisiana or Texas, course in introductory statistics with minimum C grade, physical assessment skills, two letters of professional reference, 500-word essay, current resume.

Medical University of South Carolina, College of Nursing, Nurse Administrator Program, Charleston, SC 29425. Offers MSN. *Accreditation:* AACN. *Program availability:* Part-time, online learning. *Degree requirements:* For master's, thesis optional. *Entrance requirements:* For master's, BSN, nursing license, minimum GPA of 3.0, current curriculum vitae, essay, three references. Additional exam requirements/recommendations for international students: Required—TOEFL (minimum score 600 paper-based). Electronic applications accepted. *Faculty research:* Hospital billing for nursing intensity.

Mercy College, School of Health and Natural Sciences, Programs in Nursing, Dobbs Ferry, NY 10522-1189. Offers nursing administration (MS); nursing education (MS). *Accreditation:* AACN. *Program availability:* Part-time, evening/weekend, online learning. *Degree requirements:* For master's, comprehensive exam (for some programs), written comprehensive exam or the production of a comprehensive project. *Entrance requirements:* For master's, interview, two letters of reference, bachelor's degree, RN registration in the U.S. Additional exam requirements/recommendations for international students: Required—TOEFL (minimum score 600 paper-based; 100 iBT), IELTS (minimum score 8). Electronic applications accepted. *Expenses: Tuition, area resident:* Full-time $14,904; part-time $828 per credit hour. *Required fees:* $610; $153 per term. $153 per term. Tuition and fees vary according to course load and program.

Metropolitan State University, College of Health, Community and Professional Studies, St. Paul, MN 55106-5000. Offers advanced dental therapy (MS); leadership and management (MSN); nurse educator (MSN); nursing (DNP); psychology (MA).

Accreditation: AACN. *Program availability:* Part-time. *Degree requirements:* For master's, thesis or alternative; for doctorate, thesis/dissertation or alternative. *Entrance requirements:* For master's, GRE General Test, minimum GPA of 3.0, RN license, BS/BA; for doctorate, minimum GPA of 3.0; RN license, MSN. Additional exam requirements/recommendations for international students: Required—TOEFL (minimum score 550 paper-based). *Faculty research:* Women's health, gerontology.

MidAmerica Nazarene University, Post-Licensure and Graduate Nursing Education Program, Olathe, KS 66062-1899. Offers healthcare administration (MSN); healthcare quality management (MSN); nursing education (MSN); public health (MSN); MSN/MBA. *Program availability:* Part-time, 100% online, blended/hybrid learning. *Faculty:* 8 full-time (all women), 6 part-time/adjunct (3 women). *Students:* 9 full-time (8 women), 103 part-time (100 women); includes 23 minority (14 Black or African American, non-Hispanic/Latino; 1 American Indian or Alaska Native, non-Hispanic/Latino; 4 Asian, non-Hispanic/Latino; 4 Hispanic/Latino). 50 applicants, 82% accepted. In 2015, 36 master's awarded. *Degree requirements:* For master's, final project. *Entrance requirements:* For master's, BSN, minimum GPA of 3.0, active unencumbered RN license, undergraduate statistics course. *Application deadline:* Applications are processed on a rolling basis. *Expenses:* $22,065 tuition, $1,186 fee (including technology, carrying and graduation fee). *Financial support:* Unspecified assistantships available. Financial award applicants required to submit FAFSA. *Faculty research:* Technology in education, minority recruitment and retention in nursing programs, faculty views and attitudes on culturally competency, innovative nursing program development, spirituality and holistic health. *Unit head:* Dr. Karen Wiegman, RN, Dean, 913-971-3839, E-mail: kdwiegman@mnu.edu. *Application contact:* E-mail: pgadmissions@mnu.edu.
Website: http://www.mnu.edu/nursing.html

Middle Tennessee State University, College of Graduate Studies, University College, Murfreesboro, TN 37132. Offers advanced studies in teaching and learning (M Ed); human resources leadership (MPS); nursing administration (MSN); nursing education (MSN); strategic leadership (MPS); training and development (MPS). *Program availability:* Part-time, evening/weekend, online learning. *Entrance requirements:* Additional exam requirements/recommendations for international students: Required—TOEFL (minimum score 525 paper-based; 71 iBT) or IELTS (minimum score 6).

Milwaukee School of Engineering, Program in Health Care Systems Management, Milwaukee, WI 53202-3109. Offers MSN. *Faculty:* 1 (woman) full-time, 1 (woman) part-time/adjunct. *Students:* 4 full-time (all women), 6 part-time (all women); includes 2 minority (both Hispanic/Latino). 8 applicants, 75% accepted, 4 enrolled. *Entrance requirements:* For master's, GRE General Test or GMAT if undergraduate GPA less than 3.0, 2 letters of recommendation; BSN. Additional exam requirements/recommendations for international students: Required—TOEFL (minimum score 90 iBT), IELTS (minimum score 6.5). *Application deadline:* Applications are processed on a rolling basis. Electronic applications accepted. Application fee is waived when completed online. *Expenses: Tuition, area resident:* Full-time $34,200; part-time $760 per credit. *Financial support:* In 2015–16, 2 students received support. Scholarships/grants available. Financial award application deadline: 3/15; financial award applicants required to submit FAFSA. *Unit head:* Dr. Debra Jenks, Department Chair, 414-277-4516, E-mail: jenks@msoe.edu. *Application contact:* Ian Dahlinghaus, Graduate Admissions Counselor, 414-277-7208, E-mail: dahlinghaus@msoe.edu.
Website: http://www.msoe.edu/community/academics/nursing/page/2419/ms-in-nursing-healthcare-systems-management

See Display on page 501 and Close-Up on page 533.

Missouri Western State University, Program in Nursing, St. Joseph, MO 64507-2294. Offers health care leadership (MSN); nurse educator (MSN, Graduate Certificate). *Program availability:* Part-time. *Students:* 31 part-time (30 women). Average age 34. 17 applicants, 100% accepted, 14 enrolled. In 2015, 2 master's awarded. *Entrance requirements:* For master's, minimum GPA of 2.75, interview. Additional exam requirements/recommendations for international students: Recommended—TOEFL (minimum score 79 iBT), IELTS (minimum score 6). *Application deadline:* For fall admission, 7/15 for domestic and international students; for spring admission, 11/1 for domestic students, 10/15 for international students; for summer admission, 4/29 for domestic students. Applications are processed on a rolling basis. Application fee: $45 ($50 for international students). Electronic applications accepted. *Expenses:* Tuition, state resident: full-time $6290; part-time $314 per credit hour. Tuition, nonresident: full-time $11,490; part-time $574 per credit hour. *Required fees:* $542; $99 per credit. $176 per semester. One-time fee: $45. Tuition and fees vary according to course load and program. *Financial support:* Scholarships/grants and unspecified assistantships available. Support available to part-time students. *Unit head:* Dr. Carolyn Brose, Associate Professor, 816-271-5912, E-mail: brose@missouriwestern.edu. *Application contact:* Dr. Benjamin D. Caldwell, Dean of the Graduate School, 816-271-4394, Fax: 816-271-4525, E-mail: graduate@missouriwestern.edu.
Website: https://www.missouriwestern.edu/nursing/master-of-science-in-nursing/

Molloy College, Division of Nursing, Rockville Centre, NY 11571-5002. Offers adult-gerontology primary care nurse practitioner (MS); clinical nurse specialist (MS), including adult-gerontology health; clinical nurse specialist: adult-gerontology (Advanced Certificate), including adult-gerontology; family nurse practitioner (MS, Advanced Certificate), including primary care; family psychiatric mental health nurse practitioner (MS); nursing (DNP, PhD); nursing administration (MS), including informatics; nursing education (MS); pediatric nurse practitioner (MS), including primary care (MS, Advanced Certificate). *Accreditation:* AACN. *Program availability:* Part-time, evening/weekend. *Faculty:* 26 full-time (all women), 12 part-time/adjunct (9 women). *Students:* 13 full-time (all women), 550 part-time (515 women); includes 316 minority (169 Black or African American, non-Hispanic/Latino; 1 American Indian or Alaska Native, non-Hispanic/Latino; 88 Asian, non-Hispanic/Latino; 56 Hispanic/Latino; 2 Native Hawaiian or other Pacific Islander, non-Hispanic/Latino). Average age 43. 208 applicants, 69% accepted, 121 enrolled. In 2015, 116 master's, 1 doctorate, 6 other advanced degrees awarded. *Degree requirements:* For master's, thesis optional. *Entrance requirements:* For master's, 3 letters of reference, BS in nursing, minimum undergraduate GPA of 3.0; for Advanced Certificate, 3 letters of reference, master's degree in nursing. Additional exam requirements/recommendations for international students: Required—TOEFL (minimum score 550 paper-based; 79 iBT). *Application deadline:* For fall admission, 9/2 priority date for domestic students; for spring admission, 1/20 priority date for domestic students. Applications are processed on a rolling basis. Application fee: $60. Electronic applications accepted. *Expenses: Tuition, area resident:* Full-time $18,450; part-time $1025 per credit. *Required fees:* $900; $740 per unit. Tuition and fees vary according to course load. *Financial support:* Research assistantships with partial tuition reimbursements, teaching assistantships with partial tuition reimbursements, institutionally sponsored loans, scholarships/grants, and unspecified assistantships available. Support available to part-time students. Financial award application deadline: 4/1; financial award applicants required to submit FAFSA. *Unit head:* Dr. Jeannine Muldoon, Dean of Nursing, 516-323-3651, E-mail: jmuldoon@molloy.edu. *Application contact:* Jaclyn Machowicz, Assistant Director for Admissions, 516-323-4010, E-mail: jmachowicz@molloy.edu.

Monmouth University, Graduate Studies, The Marjorie K. Unterberg School of Nursing and Health Studies, West Long Branch, NJ 07764-1898. Offers adult and gerontological primary care nurse practitioner (MSN); adult-gerontological primary care nurse practitioner (Post-Master's Certificate); family nurse practitioner (MSN, Post-Master's Certificate); family psychiatric and mental health advanced practice nursing (MSN); family psychiatric and mental health nurse practitioner (Post-Master's Certificate); forensic nursing (MSN, Certificate); nursing (MSN); nursing administration (MSN, Post-Master's Certificate); nursing education (MSN, Post-Master's Certificate); nursing practice (DNP); physician assistant (MS); school nursing (MSN, Certificate). *Accreditation:* AACN. *Program availability:* Part-time, evening/weekend, 100% online, blended/hybrid learning. *Faculty:* 14 full-time (13 women), 10 part-time/adjunct (5 women). *Students:* 58 full-time (46 women), 271 part-time (252 women); includes 93 minority (31 Black or African American, non-Hispanic/Latino; 40 Asian, non-Hispanic/Latino; 18 Hispanic/Latino; 1 Native Hawaiian or other Pacific Islander, non-Hispanic/Latino; 3 Two or more races, non-Hispanic/Latino), 1 international. Average age 37. 450 applicants, 32% accepted, 103 enrolled. In 2015, 68 master's, 8 doctorates, 11 other advanced degrees awarded. *Degree requirements:* For master's, practicum (for some tracks); for doctorate, practicum, capstone course. *Entrance requirements:* For master's, GRE General Test (waived for MSN applicants with minimum B grade in each of the first four courses and for MS applicants with master's degree), BSN with minimum GPA of 2.75, current RN license, proof of liability and malpractice policy, personal statement, two letters of recommendation, college course work in health assessment, resume; CASPA application (for MS); for doctorate, accredited master's nursing program degree with minimum GPA of 3.2, graduate research course in statistics, active RN license, national certification as Nurse Practitioner or Nurse Administrator, working knowledge of statistics, statement of goals and vision for change, 2 letters of recommendation (professional or academic), resume, interview. Additional exam requirements/recommendations for international students: Required—TOEFL (minimum score 550 paper-based; 79 iBT), IELTS (minimum score 6) or Michigan English Language Assessment Battery (minimum score 77). *Application deadline:* For fall admission, 7/15 priority date for domestic students, 6/1 for international students; for spring admission, 12/15 priority date for domestic students, 11/1 for international students; for summer admission, 5/1 for domestic students. Applications are processed on a rolling basis. Application fee: $50. Electronic applications accepted. *Expenses:* Contact institution. *Financial support:* In 2015–16, 241 students received support, including 220 fellowships (averaging $3,403 per year), 5 research assistantships (averaging $5,146 per year); career-related internships or fieldwork, scholarships/grants, and unspecified assistantships also available. Support available to part-time students. Financial award applicants required to submit FAFSA. *Faculty research:* School nursing, health policy, and smoking cessation in teens, Multiple Sclerosis; adherence and self-efficacy, aging issues and geriatric care. *Unit head:* Dr. Janet Mahoney, Dean, 732-571-3443, Fax: 732-263-5131, E-mail: jmahoney@monmouth.edu. *Application contact:* Lucia Fedele, Graduate Admission Counselor, 732-571-3452, Fax: 732-263-5123, E-mail: gradadm@monmouth.edu.
Website: http://www.monmouth.edu/school-of-nursing-health/graduate-nursing-programs.aspx

Montana State University, The Graduate School, College of Nursing, Bozeman, MT 59717. Offers clinical nurse leader (MN); family and individual nurse practitioner (DNP); family nurse practitioner (MN, Post-Master's Certificate); nursing education (Certificate, Post-Master's Certificate); psychiatric mental health nurse practitioner (MN); psychiatric/mental health nurse practitioner (DNP). *Accreditation:* AACN. *Program availability:* Part-time, online learning. *Degree requirements:* For master's, comprehensive exam, thesis (for some programs); for doctorate, thesis/dissertation, 1,125 hours in clinical settings. *Entrance requirements:* For master's, GRE General Test, minimum GPA of 3.0 for undergraduate and post-baccalaureate work. Additional exam requirements/recommendations for international students: Required—TOEFL (minimum score 580 paper-based). Electronic applications accepted. *Faculty research:* Rural nursing, health disparities, environmental/public health, oral health, resilience.

Moravian College, Moravian College Comenius Center, St. Luke's School of Nursing, Bethlehem, PA 18018-6650. Offers clinical nurse leader (MS); nurse administrator (MS); nurse educator (MS). *Accreditation:* AACN. *Program availability:* Part-time, evening/weekend. *Degree requirements:* For master's, comprehensive exam (for some programs), evidence-based practice project. *Entrance requirements:* For master's, GRE or MAT. Additional exam requirements/recommendations for international students: Required—TOEFL (minimum score 550 paper-based; 90 iBT).

Mount Carmel College of Nursing, Nursing Program, Columbus, OH 43222. Offers adult gerontology acute care nurse practitioner (MS); adult health clinical nurse specialist (MS); family nurse practitioner (MS); nursing (DNP); nursing administration (MS); nursing education (MS). *Accreditation:* AACN. *Program availability:* Part-time. *Faculty:* 8 full-time (all women), 5 part-time/adjunct (4 women). *Students:* 72 full-time (63 women), 92 part-time (84 women); includes 15 minority (7 Black or African American, non-Hispanic/Latino; 3 Asian, non-Hispanic/Latino; 2 Hispanic/Latino; 3 Two or more races, non-Hispanic/Latino). Average age 37. 140 applicants, 45% accepted, 50 enrolled. In 2015, 50 master's awarded. *Degree requirements:* For master's, professional manuscript; for doctorate, practicum. *Entrance requirements:* For master's, letters of recommendation, statement of purpose, current resume, baccalaureate degree in nursing, current Ohio RN license, minimum cumulative GPA of 3.0; for doctorate, master's degree in nursing from program accredited by either NLNAC/ACEN or CCNE. Additional exam requirements/recommendations for international students: Required—TOEFL (minimum score 550 paper-based; 80 iBT). *Application deadline:* For fall admission, 6/1 priority date for domestic students; for winter admission, 11/1 for domestic students; for spring admission, 10/1 priority date for domestic students; for summer admission, 3/1 for domestic students. Applications are processed on a rolling basis. Application fee: $30. *Expenses: Tuition, area resident:* Full-time $9480; part-time $474 per credit. One-time fee: $120. Tuition and fees vary according to course load, degree level and program. *Financial support:* In 2015–16, 5 students received support. Institutionally sponsored loans and scholarships/grants available. Financial award applicants required to submit FAFSA. *Unit head:* Dr. Jill Kilanowski, 614-234-5237, Fax: 614-234-2875, E-mail: jkilanowski@mccn.edu. *Application contact:* Dr. Kim Campbell, Director of Recruitment and Admissions, 614-234-5144, Fax: 614-234-5427, E-mail: kcampbell@mccn.edu.
Website: http://www.mccn.edu/

Mount Mary University, Graduate Division, Program in Business Administration, Milwaukee, WI 53222-4597. Offers general management (MBA); health systems leadership (MBA). *Program availability:* Part-time, evening/weekend. *Faculty:* 2 full-time (1 woman), 7 part-time/adjunct (1 woman). *Students:* 33 full-time (32 women), 6 part-time (5 women); includes 9 minority (4 Black or African American, non-Hispanic/Latino; 1 Asian, non-Hispanic/Latino; 2 Hispanic/Latino; 2 Two or more races, non-Hispanic/Latino). Average age 32. 19 applicants, 32% accepted, 6 enrolled. In 2015, 22 master's awarded. *Degree requirements:* For master's, terminal project. *Entrance requirements:* For master's, minimum GPA of 2.75. Additional exam requirements/recommendations for international students: Required—TOEFL (minimum score 550 paper-based; 80 iBT); Recommended—IELTS (minimum score 6.5). *Application deadline:* For fall admission, 7/15 for domestic and international students; for winter admission, 9/15 for domestic and

international students; for spring admission, 12/1 for domestic and international students; for summer admission, 5/1 for domestic and international students. Applications are processed on a rolling basis. Application fee: $45. Electronic applications accepted. *Expenses:* $660 per credit. *Financial support:* Career-related internships or fieldwork and Federal Work-Study available. Support available to part-time students. Financial award application deadline: 5/1; financial award applicants required to submit FAFSA. *Unit head:* Dr. Kristen Roche, Director, 414-930-3419, E-mail: rochek@mtmary.edu. *Application contact:* Kirk Heller de Messer, Director, Graduate Admissions, 414-930-3221, E-mail: hellerk@mtmary.edu.
Website: http://www.mtmary.edu/majors-programs/graduate/mba/index.html

Mount Mercy University, Program in Nursing, Cedar Rapids, IA 52402-4797. Offers health advocacy (MSN); nurse administration (MSN); nurse education (MSN). *Program availability:* Evening/weekend. *Degree requirements:* For master's, project/practicum.

Mount St. Joseph University, Master of Science in Nursing Program, Cincinnati, OH 45233-1670. Offers administration (MSN); clinical nurse leader (MSN); education (MSN). *Program availability:* Part-time. *Faculty:* 12 full-time (11 women), 5 part-time/adjunct (all women). *Students:* 53 full-time (all women), 2 part-time (both women); includes 4 minority (all Black or African American, non-Hispanic/Latino). Average age 44. 148 applicants, 68% accepted, 58 enrolled. In 2015, 65 master's awarded. *Entrance requirements:* For master's, essay; BSN from regionally-accredited university; minimum undergraduate GPA of 3.25 or GRE; professional resume; three professional references; interview; 2 years of clinical nursing experience; active RN license; criminal background check. Additional exam requirements/recommendations for international students: Required—TOEFL (minimum score 560 paper-based; 83 iBT). Application fee: $50. Electronic applications accepted. *Expenses: Tuition, area resident:* Full-time $15,255; part-time $565 per credit hour. *Required fees:* $500; $100 per term. $1.00 per semester. Full-time tuition and fees vary according to course load, degree level and program. *Financial support:* In 2015–16, 3 students received support. Application deadline: 3/1; applicants required to submit FAFSA. *Unit head:* Dr. Nancy Hinzman, MSN/DNP Director, 513-244-4325, E-mail: nancy.hinzman@msj.edu. *Application contact:* Mary Brigham, Assistant Director for Graduate Recruitment, 513-244-4233, Fax: 513-244-4629, E-mail: mary.brigham@msj.edu.
Website: http://www.msj.edu/academics/graduate-programs/master-of-science-in-nursing/

Mount Saint Mary College, School of Nursing, Newburgh, NY 12550-3494. Offers adult nurse practitioner (MS, Advanced Certificate), including nursing education (MS); nursing management (MS); clinical nurse specialist-adult health (MS), including nursing education, nursing management; family nurse practitioner (Advanced Certificate). *Accreditation:* AACN. *Program availability:* Part-time, evening/weekend, blended/hybrid learning. *Faculty:* 6 full-time (all women), 1 (woman) part-time/adjunct. *Students:* 5 full-time (4 women), 117 part-time (105 women); includes 42 minority (18 Black or African American, non-Hispanic/Latino; 2 American Indian or Alaska Native, non-Hispanic/Latino; 8 Asian, non-Hispanic/Latino; 12 Hispanic/Latino; 2 Native Hawaiian or other Pacific Islander, non-Hispanic/Latino). Average age 38. 44 applicants, 84% accepted, 25 enrolled. In 2015, 25 master's, 4 other advanced degrees awarded. *Degree requirements:* For master's, research utilization project. *Entrance requirements:* For master's, BSN, minimum GPA of 3.0, RN license. Additional exam requirements/recommendations for international students: Required—TOEFL (minimum score 80 iBT). *Application deadline:* For fall admission, 6/3 priority date for domestic students; for spring admission, 10/31 priority date for domestic students. Applications are processed on a rolling basis. Application fee: $45. Electronic applications accepted. Application fee is waived when completed online. *Expenses: Tuition, area resident:* Part-time $750 per credit. *Required fees:* $40 per semester. *Financial support:* In 2015–16, 14 students received support. Unspecified assistantships available. Financial award application deadline: 4/15; financial award applicants required to submit FAFSA. *Unit head:* Christine Berte, Graduate Coordinator, 845-569-3141, Fax: 845-562-6762, E-mail: christine.berte@msmc.edu. *Application contact:* Lisa Gallina, Director of Admissions for Graduate Programs and Adult Degree Completion, 845-569-3166, Fax: 845-569-3450, E-mail: lisa.gallina@msmc.edu.
Website: http://www.msmc.edu/Academics/Graduate_Programs/Master_of_Science_in_Nursing

National University, Academic Affairs, School of Health and Human Services, La Jolla, CA 92037-1011. Offers clinical affairs (MS); clinical informatics (Certificate); clinical regulatory affairs (MS); health and life science analytics (MS); health coaching (Certificate); health informatics (MS); healthcare administration (MHA); nurse anesthesia (MS); nursing (MS), including forensic nursing, nursing administration, nursing informatics; nursing administration (Certificate); nursing informatics (Certificate); nursing practice (DNP); public health (MPH), including health promotion, healthcare administration, mental health. *Program availability:* Part-time, evening/weekend, 100% online, blended/hybrid learning. *Faculty:* 31 full-time (18 women), 33 part-time/adjunct (20 women). *Students:* 353 full-time (263 women), 136 part-time (87 women); includes 322 minority (111 Black or African American, non-Hispanic/Latino; 1 American Indian or Alaska Native, non-Hispanic/Latino; 105 Asian, non-Hispanic/Latino; 72 Hispanic/Latino; 7 Native Hawaiian or other Pacific Islander, non-Hispanic/Latino; 26 Two or more races, non-Hispanic/Latino), 31 international. Average age 32. In 2015, 103 master's awarded. *Degree requirements:* For master's, thesis (for some programs). *Entrance requirements:* For master's, interview, minimum GPA of 2.5. Additional exam requirements/recommendations for international students: Required—TOEFL (minimum score 550 paper-based; 79 iBT), IELTS (minimum score 6). *Application deadline:* Applications are processed on a rolling basis. Application fee: $60 ($65 for international students). Electronic applications accepted. *Financial support:* Career-related internships or fieldwork, institutionally sponsored loans, scholarships/grants, and tuition waivers (partial) available. Support available to part-time students. Financial award application deadline: 6/30; financial award applicants required to submit FAFSA. *Faculty research:* Nursing education, obesity prevention, workforce diversity. *Unit head:* School of Health and Human Services, 800-628-8648, E-mail: shhs@nu.edu. *Application contact:* Frank Rojas, Vice President for Enrollment Services, 800-628-8648, E-mail: advisor@nu.edu.
Website: http://www.nu.edu/OurPrograms/SchoolOfHealthAndHumanServices.html

Nebraska Methodist College, Program in Nursing, Omaha, NE 68114. Offers nurse educator (MSN); nurse executive (MSN). *Accreditation:* AACN. *Program availability:* Evening/weekend, online learning. *Degree requirements:* For master's, thesis or alternative, Evidence Based Practice (EBP) project. *Entrance requirements:* For master's, interview. Additional exam requirements/recommendations for international students: Required—TOEFL (minimum score 550 paper-based; 80 iBT). *Faculty research:* Spirituality, student outcomes, service-learning, leadership and administration, women's issues.

New Mexico State University, College of Health and Social Services, School of Nursing, Las Cruces, NM 88003. Offers adult/geriatric nursing (DNP); family nurse practitioner (DNP); family/psychiatric mental health nursing (DNP); nursing administration (MSN); nursing science (PhD); public/community health nursing (DNP). *Accreditation:* AACN. *Program availability:* Blended/hybrid learning. *Faculty:* 16 full-time (15 women). *Students:* 24 full-time (18 women), 90 part-time (80 women); includes 49 minority (10 Black or African American, non-Hispanic/Latino; 1 American Indian or

Nursing and Healthcare Administration

Alaska Native, non-Hispanic/Latino; 4 Asian, non-Hispanic/Latino; 32 Hispanic/Latino; 2 Two or more races, non-Hispanic/Latino), 1 international. Average age 43. 40 applicants, 58% accepted, 17 enrolled. In 2015, 6 master's, 11 doctorates awarded. *Degree requirements:* For master's, comprehensive exam, thesis optional, clinical practice; for doctorate, comprehensive exam, thesis/dissertation. *Entrance requirements:* For master's, NCLEX, BSN, minimum GPA of 3.0, course work in statistics, 3 letters of reference, writing sample, RN license, CPR certification, proof of liability, immunizations, criminal background check; for doctorate, NCLEX, MSN, minimum GPA of 3.0, 3 letters of reference, writing sample, RN license, CPR certification, proof of liability, immunizations, criminal background check, statistics course. Additional exam requirements/recommendations for international students: Required—TOEFL (minimum score 550 paper-based; 79 iBT), IELTS (minimum score 6.5). *Application deadline:* For fall admission, 1/15 for domestic students; for spring admission, 1/15 priority date for domestic students; for summer admission, 1/15 for domestic students. Application fee: $40 ($50 for international students). Electronic applications accepted. *Expenses:* $274.50 per credit hour for in-state students, and all students enrolled in six or fewer credits; $839.30 per credit hour for out-of-state and international students enrolled in at least seven hours. *Financial support:* In 2015–16, 23 students received support, including 1 teaching assistantship (averaging $9,473 per year); career-related internships or fieldwork, Federal Work-Study, scholarships/grants, traineeships, health care benefits, and unspecified assistantships also available. Support available to part-time students. Financial award application deadline: 3/1. *Faculty research:* Women's health, community health, health disparities, nursing informatics and health care technologies, health care and nursing administration. *Total annual research expenditures:* $127,778. *Unit head:* Dr. Kathleen Huttlinger, Department Head, 575-646-3812, Fax: 575-646-2167, E-mail: khuttlin@nmsu.edu. *Application contact:* Dr. Teresa Keller, Director of Graduate Studies, 575-646-4370, Fax: 575-646-2167, E-mail: tkeller@nmsu.edu.
Website: http://schoolofnursing.nmsu.edu

Nicholls State University, Graduate Studies, College of Nursing and Allied Health, Thibodaux, LA 70310. Offers family nurse practitioner (MSN); nurse executive (MSN); nursing education (MSN); psychiatric/mental health nurse practitioner (MSN).
Website: http://www.nicholls.edu/cona/

Northeastern University, Bouvé College of Health Sciences, Boston, MA 02115-5096. Offers applied behavior analysis (MS, CAGS); audiology (Au D); biomedical nanotechnology (MS); college student development and counseling (MS, CAGS); counseling psychology (MS, PhD, CAGS); exercise science (MS); health informatics (MS); medicinal chemistry (MS); nurse anesthesia (DNP, CAGS); nursing (MS, PhD, CAGS), including administration (MS), adult-gerontology acute care nurse practitioner (MS, CAGS), adult-gerontology primary care nurse practitioner (MS, CAGS), anesthesia (MS), family nurse practitioner (MS, CAGS), neonatal nurse practitioner (MS, CAGS), pediatric nurse practitioner (MS, CAGS), psychiatric mental health nurse practitioner (MS, CAGS); nursing practice (DNP); personal health informatics (PhD); pharmaceutical sciences (MS, PhD), including interdisciplinary concentration, pharmaceutics and drug delivery systems; pharmacology (MS); pharmacy (Pharm D); physical therapy (Postbaccalaureate Certificate); physician assistant (MS); population health (PhD); school psychology (MS, PhD, CAGS); speech-language pathology (MS); urban health (MPH); MS/MBA. *Accreditation:* ACPE (one or more programs are accredited). *Program availability:* Part-time, evening/weekend, online learning. *Faculty:* 194 full-time (120 women), 169 part-time/adjunct (136 women). *Students:* 1,416 full-time (1,049 women), 310 part-time (248 women). In 2015, 374 master's, 313 doctorates, 37 other advanced degrees awarded. *Degree requirements:* For doctorate, thesis/dissertation (for some programs); for other advanced degree, comprehensive exam. Application fee: $75. Electronic applications accepted. *Expenses:* Contact institution. *Financial support:* Applicants required to submit FAFSA. *Unit head:* John R. Reynolds, Professor and Interim Dean, 617-373-3323, Fax: 617-373-3030. *Application contact:* Molly Schnabel, Senior Director of Graduate Affairs, 617-373-2708, Fax: 617-373-4701, E-mail: bouvegrad@neu.edu.
Website: http://www.northeastern.edu/bouve/

North Park University, School of Nursing, Chicago, IL 60625-4895. Offers advanced practice nursing (MS); leadership and management (MS); MBA/MS; MM/MSN; MS/MHR; MS/MNA. *Accreditation:* AACN. *Program availability:* Part-time, evening/weekend. *Degree requirements:* For master's, thesis. *Entrance requirements:* For master's, GMAT, MAT. *Faculty research:* Aging, consultation roles, critical thinking skills, family breakdown, science of caring.

Northwest Nazarene University, Graduate Studies, Program in Nursing, Nampa, ID 83686-5897. Offers MSN. *Accreditation:* AACN. *Program availability:* Online learning. *Degree requirements:* For master's, internship.

Norwich University, College of Graduate and Continuing Studies, Master of Science in Nursing Program, Northfield, VT 05663. Offers nursing administration (MSN); nursing education (MSN). *Accreditation:* AACN. *Program availability:* Evening/weekend, mostly all online with a week-long residency requirement. *Faculty:* 10 part-time/adjunct (7 women). *Students:* 84 full-time (78 women); includes 11 minority (8 Black or African American, non-Hispanic/Latino; 2 Asian, non-Hispanic/Latino; 1 Hispanic/Latino). Average age 40. 33 applicants, 100% accepted, 29 enrolled. In 2015, 57 master's awarded. *Entrance requirements:* For master's, minimum undergraduate GPA of 3.0. Additional exam requirements/recommendations for international students: Required—TOEFL (minimum score 550 paper-based; 80 iBT), IELTS (minimum score 6.5). *Application deadline:* For fall admission, 8/15 for domestic and international students; for winter admission, 11/14 for domestic and international students; for spring admission, 2/13 for domestic and international students; for summer admission, 5/15 for domestic and international students. Applications are processed on a rolling basis. Electronic applications accepted. *Expenses:* Contact institution. *Financial support:* In 2015–16, 22 students received support. Scholarships/grants available. Financial award application deadline: 8/5; financial award applicants required to submit FAFSA. *Unit head:* Dr. Sharon Richie-Melvan, Director, 802-485-2600, E-mail: srichiem@norwich.edu. *Application contact:* Rija Ramahatra, Associate Program Director, 802-485-2892, Fax: 802-485-2533, E-mail: rramahatr@norwich.edu.
Website: http://online.norwich.edu/degree-programs/masters/master-science-nursing/overview

Ohio University, Graduate College, College of Health Sciences and Professions, School of Nursing, Athens, OH 45701-2979. Offers acute care nurse practitioner (MSN); acute care nurse practitioner and family nurse practitioner (MSN); acute care nurse practitioner and nurse administrator (MSN); acute care nurse practitioner and nurse educator (MSN); family nurse practitioner (MSN); nurse administrator (MSN); nurse administrator and family nurse practitioner (MSN); nurse educator (MSN); nurse educator and family nurse practitioner (MSN); nurse educator and nurse administrator (MSN). *Accreditation:* AACN. *Degree requirements:* For master's, capstone project. *Entrance requirements:* For master's, GRE, bachelor's degree in nursing from an accredited college or university, minimum overall undergraduate GPA of 3.0, official transcripts, statement of goals and objectives, resume, 3 letters of recommendation. Additional exam requirements/recommendations for international students: Required—

TOEFL (minimum score 550 paper-based; 80 iBT) or IELTS (minimum score 6.5). Electronic applications accepted.

Oklahoma Wesleyan University, Professional Studies Division, Bartlesville, OK 74006-6299. Offers nursing administration (MSN); nursing education (MSN); strategic leadership (MS); theology and apologetics (MA).

Old Dominion University, College of Health Sciences, Doctor of Nursing Practice Program, Norfolk, VA 23529. Offers advance practice (DNP); nurse executive (DNP). *Program availability:* Part-time, blended/hybrid learning. *Faculty:* 4 full-time (all women), 3 part-time/adjunct (2 women). *Students:* 19 full-time (18 women), 42 part-time (38 women); includes 9 minority (5 Black or African American, non-Hispanic/Latino; 2 Asian, non-Hispanic/Latino; 2 Two or more races, non-Hispanic/Latino). Average age 46. 55 applicants, 67% accepted, 36 enrolled. In 2015, 27 doctorates awarded. Terminal master's awarded for partial completion of doctoral program. *Degree requirements:* For doctorate, thesis/dissertation, capstone project. *Entrance requirements:* For doctorate, 3 letters of recommendation, essay, resume, transcripts. Additional exam requirements/recommendations for international students: Required—TOEFL. *Application deadline:* For spring admission, 9/15 priority date for domestic students, 4/15 priority date for international students. Applications are processed on a rolling basis. Application fee: $50. Electronic applications accepted. *Expenses:* Tuition, state resident: full-time $11,136; part-time $464 per credit hour. Tuition, nonresident: full-time $27,840; part-time $1160 per credit hour. *Required fees:* $64 per semester. Tuition and fees vary according to campus/location, program and reciprocity agreements. *Financial support:* In 2015–16, 2 fellowships with full tuition reimbursements (averaging $15,000 per year), 1 teaching assistantship with full tuition reimbursement (averaging $15,000 per year) were awarded; scholarships/grants, traineeships, and unspecified assistantships also available. *Faculty research:* Cultural competency, sleep disorders, self-care in HIV positive African-American women, ethical decision-making in pediatric cases. *Unit head:* Dr. Carolyn M. Rutledge, Associate Chair of Graduate Program, 757-683-5009, Fax: 757-683-5253, E-mail: crutledg@odu.edu. *Application contact:* Sue Parker, Graduate Program Coordinator, 757-683-4298, Fax: 757-683-5253, E-mail: sparker@odu.edu.
Website: http://www.odu.edu/academics/programs/doctoral/nursing-practice

Old Dominion University, College of Health Sciences, School of Nursing, Nurse Executive Emphasis, Norfolk, VA 23529. Offers MSN. *Program availability:* Part-time, blended/hybrid learning. *Faculty:* 1 (woman) full-time, 3 part-time/adjunct (2 women). *Students:* 2 full-time (1 woman), 7 part-time (all women); includes 1 minority (Black or African American, non-Hispanic/Latino). Average age 44. 8 applicants, 75% accepted, 5 enrolled. In 2015, 10 degrees awarded. *Degree requirements:* For master's, comprehensive exam. *Entrance requirements:* For master's, GRE or MAT if GPA is below 3.5, 3 letters of recommendation, essay, resume, transcripts. Additional exam requirements/recommendations for international students: Required—TOEFL. *Application deadline:* For fall admission, 4/15 priority date for international students; for spring admission, 9/15 priority date for domestic students. Applications are processed on a rolling basis. Application fee: $50. Electronic applications accepted. *Expenses:* Tuition, state resident: full-time $11,136; part-time $464 per credit hour. Tuition, nonresident: full-time $27,840; part-time $1160 per credit hour. *Required fees:* $64 per semester. Tuition and fees vary according to campus/location, program and reciprocity agreements. *Financial support:* Research assistantships and teaching assistantships available. *Faculty research:* Telehealth, vulnerable populations. *Unit head:* Dr. Carolyn M. Rutledge, Graduate Program Director, 757-683-5009, Fax: 757-683-5253, E-mail: crutledg@odu.edu. *Application contact:* Sue Parker, Graduate Program Coordinator, 757-683-4298, Fax: 757-683-5253, E-mail: sparker@odu.edu.
Website: http://catalog.odu.edu/graduate/collegeofhealthsciences/schoolofnursing/#doctorofnursingpracticednp-advancedpracticepostmasters

Otterbein University, Department of Nursing, Westerville, OH 43081. Offers advanced practice nurse educator (Certificate); clinical nurse leader (MSN); family nurse practitioner (MSN, Certificate); nurse anesthesia (MSN, Certificate); nursing (DNP); nursing service administration (MSN). *Accreditation:* AACN; AANA/CANAEP; ACEN. *Program availability:* Part-time, evening/weekend, online learning. *Degree requirements:* For master's, comprehensive exam (for some programs), thesis (for some programs). *Entrance requirements:* For master's, 2 reference forms, resume; for Certificate, official transcripts, 2 reference forms, essay, resumé. Additional exam requirements/recommendations for international students: Required—TOEFL (minimum score 550 paper-based; 79 iBT). *Faculty research:* Patient education, women's health, trauma curriculum development, administration.

Our Lady of the Lake College, School of Nursing, Program in Nursing, Baton Rouge, LA 70808. Offers administration (MS); education (MS). *Program availability:* Part-time. *Degree requirements:* For master's, capstone project. *Entrance requirements:* For master's, BSN with minimum GPA of 3.0 during the last 60 hours of undergraduate work, 1 year of clinical nursing experience as a registered nurse, current licensure or eligibility to practice as registered nurse in Louisiana, 3 professional references, 3 credit hours of undergraduate statistics with minimum C average.

Pace University, College of Health Professions, Lienhard School of Nursing, New York, NY 10038. Offers family nurse practitioner (MS); nurse education (Advanced Certificate); nursing education (MS); nursing leadership (Advanced Certificate); nursing practice (DNP). *Accreditation:* AACN. *Program availability:* Part-time, evening/weekend, blended/hybrid learning. *Faculty:* 11 full-time (10 women), 31 part-time/adjunct (27 women). *Students:* 3 full-time (all women), 415 part-time (385 women); includes 196 minority (97 Black or African American, non-Hispanic/Latino; 2 American Indian or Alaska Native, non-Hispanic/Latino; 57 Asian, non-Hispanic/Latino; 33 Hispanic/Latino; 7 Two or more races, non-Hispanic/Latino), 2 international. Average age 34. 291 applicants, 69% accepted, 129 enrolled. In 2015, 129 master's, 20 doctorates, 7 other advanced degrees awarded. *Degree requirements:* For doctorate, thesis/dissertation. *Entrance requirements:* For master's, RN license, resume, personal statement, 2 letters of recommendation, official transcripts; for doctorate, RN license, resume, personal statement, 2 letters of recommendation, official transcripts, accredited master's degree in nursing, minimum GPA of 3.3, national certification; for Advanced Certificate, RN license, completion of 2nd degree in nursing. Additional exam requirements/recommendations for international students: Required—TOEFL (minimum score 100 iBT), IELTS or PTE. *Application deadline:* For fall admission, 3/1 for domestic and international students. Applications are processed on a rolling basis. Application fee: $70. Electronic applications accepted. *Financial support:* Research assistantships, teaching assistantships, career-related internships or fieldwork, Federal Work-Study, tuition waivers (partial), and unspecified assistantships available. Support available to part-time students. Financial award application deadline: 2/15; financial award applicants required to submit FAFSA. *Unit head:* Dr. Harriet R. Feldman, Dean, College of Health Professions, 914-773-3341, E-mail: hfeldman@pace.edu. *Application contact:* Susan Ford-Goldschein, Director of Graduate Admissions, 212-346-1531, Fax: 212-346-1585, E-mail: graduateadmission@pace.edu.
Website: http://www.pace.edu/lienhard

Palm Beach Atlantic University, School of Nursing, West Palm Beach, FL 33416-4708. Offers family nurse practitioner (DNP); health systems leadership (MSN). *Program availability:* Part-time. *Faculty:* 5 part-time/adjunct (4 women). *Students:* 43 full-time (37 women), 1 (woman) part-time; includes 22 minority (11 Black or African

American, non-Hispanic/Latino; 2 Asian, non-Hispanic/Latino; 8 Hispanic/Latino; 1 Two or more races, non-Hispanic/Latino). Average age 32. 34 applicants, 100% accepted, 24 enrolled. *Entrance requirements:* For master's, minimum GPA of 3.0; for doctorate, minimum GPA of 3.0; one year of experience as an RN; personal interview. Additional exam requirements/recommendations for international students: Required—TOEFL (minimum score 550 paper-based; 79 iBT). *Application deadline:* Applications are processed on a rolling basis. Application fee: $50. Electronic applications accepted. *Expenses: Tuition, area resident:* Part-time $525 per credit hour. *Financial support:* In 2015–16, 13 students received support. Scholarships/grants and employee education grants available. Financial award application deadline: 5/1; financial award applicants required to submit FAFSA. *Unit head:* Joanne Masella, Dean, 561-803-2827. *Application contact:* Graduate Admissions, 888-468-6722, E-mail: grad@pba.edu.
Website: http://www.pba.edu/school-of-nursing

Pennsylvania College of Health Sciences, Graduate Programs, Lancaster, PA 17602. Offers administration (MSN); education (MSHS, MSN); healthcare administration (MHA). *Degree requirements:* For master's, internship (for MHA, MSN in administration); practicum (for MSHS, MSN in education).

Prairie View A&M University, College of Nursing, Houston, TX 77030. Offers family nurse practitioner (MSN); nursing administration (MSN); nursing education (MSN). *Accreditation:* AACN; ACEN. *Program availability:* Part-time, evening/weekend. *Faculty:* 11 full-time (all women), 7 part-time/adjunct (6 women). *Students:* 65 full-time (58 women), 78 part-time (71 women); includes 128 minority (94 Black or African American, non-Hispanic/Latino; 24 Asian, non-Hispanic/Latino; 9 Hispanic/Latino; 1 Two or more races, non-Hispanic/Latino), 5 international. Average age 35. 84 applicants, 44% accepted, 25 enrolled. In 2015, 63 master's awarded. *Degree requirements:* For master's, comprehensive exam, thesis. *Entrance requirements:* For master's, MAT or GRE, BS in nursing; minimum 1 year of experience as registered nurse, minimum GPA of 2.75, 3 letters of recommendation from professional nurses. Additional exam requirements/recommendations for international students: Required—TOEFL (minimum score 550 paper-based; 79 iBT). *Application deadline:* For fall admission, 7/1 priority date for domestic students, 6/1 priority date for international students; for spring admission, 11/1 priority date for domestic students, 10/1 priority date for international students; for summer admission, 3/1 priority date for domestic students, 2/1 priority date for international students. Applications are processed on a rolling basis. Application fee: $50. Electronic applications accepted. *Expenses: Tuition, state resident:* full-time $4243; part-time $237.29 per credit hour. Tuition, nonresident: full-time $11,798; part-time $657 per credit hour. *Required fees:* $2762; $172.10 per credit hour. *Financial support:* Career-related internships or fieldwork, Federal Work-Study, institutionally sponsored loans, scholarships/grants, and traineeships available. Support available to part-time students. Financial award application deadline: 4/1; financial award applicants required to submit FAFSA. *Faculty research:* Software development and violence prevention, health promotion and disease prevention. *Unit head:* Dr. Betty N. Adams, Dean, 713-797-7009, Fax: 713-797-7013, E-mail: bnadams@pvamu.edu. *Application contact:* Dr. Forest Smith, Director of Student Services and Admissions, 713-797-7031, Fax: 713-797-7012, E-mail: fdsmith@pvamu.edu.
Website: http://www.pvamu.edu/nursing

Purdue University Northwest, Graduate Studies Office, School of Nursing, Hammond, IN 46323-2094. Offers adult health clinical nurse specialist (MS); critical care clinical nurse specialist (MS); family nurse practitioner (MS); nurse executive (MS). *Accreditation:* AACN; ACEN. *Program availability:* Part-time, online learning. *Entrance requirements:* For master's, BSN. Additional exam requirements/recommendations for international students: Required—TOEFL. Electronic applications accepted. *Faculty research:* Adult health, cardiovascular and pulmonary nursing.

Queens University of Charlotte, Presbyterian School of Nursing, Charlotte, NC 28274-0002. Offers clinical nurse leader (MSN); nurse educator (MSN); nursing administrator (MSN). *Accreditation:* AACN. *Degree requirements:* For master's, research project. *Entrance requirements:* For master's, minimum GPA of 3.0. Additional exam requirements/recommendations for international students: Required—TOEFL. Electronic applications accepted. *Expenses:* Contact institution.

Quinnipiac University, School of Nursing, Nursing Leadership Track, Hamden, CT 06518-1940. Offers DNP. *Program availability:* Part-time-only, evening/weekend, online only. *Faculty:* 19 full-time (18 women), 13 part-time/adjunct (9 women). *Students:* 30 part-time (29 women); includes 4 minority (1 Asian, non-Hispanic/Latino; 2 Hispanic/Latino; 1 Two or more races, non-Hispanic/Latino). 22 applicants, 82% accepted, 15 enrolled. *Application deadline:* For fall admission, 7/1 for domestic students. Applications are processed on a rolling basis. Application fee: $45. Electronic applications accepted. *Expenses:* $700 per credit tuition; $40 per credit student fee (not to exceed $360 per semester); $150 per semester (fall/spring) technology and lab fee; $75 per semester summer technology and lab fee. *Financial support:* Federal Work-Study and unspecified assistantships available. Support available to part-time students. Financial award application deadline: 6/1; financial award applicants required to submit FAFSA. *Application contact:* Quinnipiac University Online Admissions, 203-582-3918, E-mail: quonlineadmissions@quinnipiac.edu.
Website: https://quonline.quinnipiac.edu/online-programs/online-doctorate-programs/doctor-of-nursing-practice/nursing-leadership-track.php

Research College of Nursing, Nursing Program, Kansas City, MO 64132. Offers adult-gerontological nurse practitioner (MSN); executive practice and healthcare leadership (MSN); family nurse practitioner (MSN); nursing (MSN). *Accreditation:* AACN. *Program availability:* Part-time, 100% online. *Faculty:* 9 full-time (all women), 5 part-time/adjunct (2 women). *Students:* 4 full-time (2 women), 148 part-time (132 women); includes 15 minority (9 Black or African American, non-Hispanic/Latino; 1 American Indian or Alaska Native, non-Hispanic/Latino; 3 Asian, non-Hispanic/Latino; 1 Native Hawaiian or other Pacific Islander, non-Hispanic/Latino; 1 Two or more races, non-Hispanic/Latino). In 2015, 34 master's awarded. *Degree requirements:* For master's, research project. *Entrance requirements:* For master's, 3 letters of recommendation, official transcripts, resume, personal statement/writing sample. *Application deadline:* Applications are processed on a rolling basis. Application fee: $65. Electronic applications accepted. *Expenses:* $525 per credit hour; $25 per credit hour clinical fee. *Financial support:* Applicants required to submit FAFSA. *Unit head:* Dr. Nancy O. DeBasio, President and Dean, 816-995-2815, Fax: 816-995-2817, E-mail: nancy.debasio@researchcollege.edu. *Application contact:* Leslie Burry, Director of Transfer and Graduate Recruitment, 816-995-2820, Fax: 816-995-2813, E-mail: leslie.burry@researchcollege.edu.

Roberts Wesleyan College, Department of Nursing, Rochester, NY 14624-1997. Offers nursing education (MSN); nursing leadership and administration (MSN). *Accreditation:* AACN. *Program availability:* Evening/weekend, online learning. *Faculty:* 6 full-time (all women), 5 part-time/adjunct (3 women). *Students:* 66 full-time (64 women); includes 9 minority (6 Black or African American, non-Hispanic/Latino; 1 American Indian or Alaska Native, non-Hispanic/Latino; 2 Hispanic/Latino), 9 international. Average age 35. 53 applicants, 83% accepted, 41 enrolled. In 2015, 2 master's awarded. *Degree requirements:* For master's, thesis. *Entrance requirements:* For master's, minimum GPA of 3.0; BS in nursing; interview; RN license; resume; course work in statistics. Additional exam requirements/recommendations for international students: Required—TOEFL (minimum score 90 iBT), IELTS (minimum score 6.5).

Application deadline: Applications are processed on a rolling basis. Application fee: $0. Electronic applications accepted. *Financial support:* In 2015–16, 49 students received support. Scholarships/grants available. Financial award applicants required to submit FAFSA. *Unit head:* Dr. Cheryl B. Crotser, Chairperson/Director of Graduate Program, 585-594-6668, E-mail: crotser_cheryl@roberts.edu. *Application contact:* Brenda Mutton, Admissions Coordinator, 585-594-6686, E-mail: mutton_brenda@roberts.edu.
Website: http://www.roberts.edu/gradnursing

Rush University, College of Nursing, Direct Entry Master's for Non-Nurses: Generalist Entry Master's Clinical Nurse Leader Program, Chicago, IL 60612. Offers MSN. *Faculty:* 52 full-time (49 women), 43 part-time/adjunct (40 women). *Students:* 289 full-time (256 women); includes 86 minority (28 Black or African American, non-Hispanic/Latino; 1 American Indian or Alaska Native, non-Hispanic/Latino; 22 Asian, non-Hispanic/Latino; 35 Hispanic/Latino). Average age 27. 197 applicants, 34% accepted, 49 enrolled. In 2015, 136 master's awarded. *Degree requirements:* For master's, comprehensive exam, capstone project. *Entrance requirements:* For master's, GRE General Test (waived if cumulative GPA is 3.25 or greater), interview, 3 letters of recommendation, personal statement, current resume. Additional exam requirements/recommendations for international students: Required—TOEFL (minimum score 94 iBT). *Application deadline:* For fall admission, 1/5 for domestic students; for spring admission, 8/4 for domestic students; for summer admission, 12/1 for domestic students. Application fee: $100. Electronic applications accepted. *Expenses:* Contact institution. *Financial support:* Research assistantships, Federal Work-Study, scholarships/grants, and health care benefits available. Support available to part-time students. Financial award application deadline: 3/1; financial award applicants required to submit FAFSA. *Faculty research:* Physical activity adherence in African-American women; reduction of health disparities; evidence-based interventions for caregivers; benefit of human milk feedings for low birth weight infants; patient-centered quality assessment of psychiatric inpatient environments. *Unit head:* Dr. Rebecca Hamilton, Director for Generalist Education/Assistant Dean for Academic Affairs, 312-942-7111. *Application contact:* Molly Spurlock, Manager for Admissions and Social Media, 312-942-6222, E-mail: molly_spurlock@rush.edu.
Website: http://www.rushu.rush.edu/servlet/
Satellite?MetaAttrName=meta_university&ParentId=1320160849834&ParentType=RushUnivLevel2Page&c=content_block&cid=1211

Rush University, College of Nursing, MSN for RN's: Clinical Nurse Leader (CNL) Program, Chicago, IL 60612. Offers MSN. *Program availability:* Part-time, online learning. *Faculty:* 43 full-time (40 women), 52 part-time/adjunct (49 women). *Students:* 45 part-time (39 women); includes 13 minority (3 Black or African American, non-Hispanic/Latino; 4 Asian, non-Hispanic/Latino; 6 Hispanic/Latino). Average age 35. 15 applicants, 67% accepted, 9 enrolled. In 2015, 21 master's awarded. *Degree requirements:* For master's, thesis, clinical residency, capstone project. *Entrance requirements:* For master's, GRE (waived if cumulative GPA is 3.25 or greater or if nursing GPA is 3.0 or greater), interview, 3 letters of recommendation, personal statement, current resume. Additional exam requirements/recommendations for international students: Required—TOEFL (minimum score 94 iBT). *Application deadline:* For fall admission, 5/1 for domestic students; for spring admission, 8/4 for domestic students; for summer admission, 12/1 for domestic students. Applications are processed on a rolling basis. Application fee: $100. Electronic applications accepted. *Expenses:* Contact institution. *Financial support:* Research assistantships, Federal Work-Study, scholarships/grants, and health care benefits available. Support available to part-time students. Financial award application deadline: 3/1; financial award applicants required to submit FAFSA. *Faculty research:* Physical activity adherence in African-American women; reduction of health disparities; evidence-based interventions for caregivers; fish oil for HIV-related immunosenescence; BAILA: Being Active, Increasing Latinos Health Aging. *Unit head:* Dr. Rebecca Hamilton, Director of Generalist Education/Assistant Dean for Academic Affairs, 312-942-5587. *Application contact:* Jennifer Thorndyke, Admissions Specialist, 312-563-7526, E-mail: jennifer_thorndyke@rush.edu.
Website: http://www.rushu.rush.edu/servlet/
Satellite?MetaAttrName=meta_university&ParentId=1320160849834&ParentType=RushUnivLevel2Page&c=content_block&cid=1221

Sacred Heart University, Graduate Programs, College of Nursing, Fairfield, CT 06825. Offers clinical nurse leader (MSN); clinical practice (DNP); family nurse practitioner (MSN, Graduate Certificate); leadership (DNP); nurse educator (MSN); nursing management and executive leadership (MSN); patient care services (MSN). *Accreditation:* AACN. *Program availability:* Part-time, evening/weekend, online learning. *Faculty:* 17 full-time (all women), 21 part-time/adjunct (18 women). *Students:* 19 full-time (18 women), 777 part-time (711 women); includes 144 minority (56 Black or African American, non-Hispanic/Latino; 2 American Indian or Alaska Native, non-Hispanic/Latino; 33 Asian, non-Hispanic/Latino; 41 Hispanic/Latino; 2 Native Hawaiian or other Pacific Islander, non-Hispanic/Latino; 10 Two or more races, non-Hispanic/Latino). Average age 38. 116 applicants, 53% accepted, 50 enrolled. In 2015, 192 master's, 13 doctorates awarded. *Degree requirements:* For master's, thesis, 500 clinical hours. *Entrance requirements:* For master's, minimum GPA of 3.0, BSN or RN plus BS (for MSN); for doctorate, minimum GPA of 3.0, MSN or BSN plus MS in related field (for DNP). Additional exam requirements/recommendations for international students: Required—PTE; Recommended—TOEFL (minimum score 570 paper-based; 80 iBT), IELTS (minimum score 6.5). *Application deadline:* For fall admission, 2/15 for domestic and international students. Applications are processed on a rolling basis. Application fee: $75. Electronic applications accepted. *Expenses:* Contact institution. *Financial support:* Unspecified assistantships available. Financial award applicants required to submit FAFSA. *Unit head:* Mary Alice Donius, Dean of Nursing, 203-365-4508, E-mail: donium@sacredheart.edu. *Application contact:* William Sweeney, Director of Graduate Admissions Operations, 203-365-4716, Fax: 203-365-4732, E-mail: gradstudies@sacredheart.edu.
Website: http://www.sacredheart.edu/academics/collegeofhealthprofessions/academicprograms/nursing/nursingprograms/graduateprograms/

Saginaw Valley State University, College of Health and Human Services, Program in Health System Nurse Specialist, University Center, MI 48710. Offers MSN. *Accreditation:* AACN. *Program availability:* Part-time, evening/weekend. In 2015, 2 master's awarded. *Degree requirements:* For master's, thesis optional. *Entrance requirements:* For master's, GRE, minimum GPA of 3.0. Additional exam requirements/recommendations for international students: Required—TOEFL (minimum score 580 paper-based; 92 iBT). *Application deadline:* For fall admission, 7/15 for international students; for winter admission, 11/15 for international students; for spring admission, 4/15 for international students. Applications are processed on a rolling basis. Application fee: $30 ($90 for international students). Electronic applications accepted. *Expenses:* Tuition, state resident: full-time $9515; part-time $514 per credit hour. Tuition, nonresident: full-time $17,899; part-time $980 per credit hour. *Required fees:* $263; $14.60 per credit hour. Tuition and fees vary according to degree level. *Financial support:* Federal Work-Study and scholarships/grants available. Support available to part-time students. Financial award application deadline: 4/1; financial award applicants required to submit FAFSA. *Unit head:* Dr. Sally Decker, Department Chair, 989-964-4098, E-mail: decker@svsu.edu. *Application contact:* Jenna Briggs, Director, Graduate

Nursing and Healthcare Administration

and International Admissions, 989-964-6096, Fax: 989-964-2788, E-mail: gradadm@svsu.edu.

Saint Francis Medical Center College of Nursing, Graduate Programs, Peoria, IL 61603-3783. Offers adult gerontology (MSN); clinical nurse leader (MSN); family nurse practitioner (MSN); family psychiatric mental health nurse practitioner (MSN); neonatal nurse practitioner (MSN); nurse clinician (Post-Graduate Certificate); nurse educator (MSN, Post-Graduate Certificate); nursing (DNP); nursing management leadership (MSN). *Accreditation:* ACEN. *Program availability:* Part-time, 100% online, blended/hybrid learning. *Faculty:* 14 full-time (all women), 5 part-time/adjunct (all women). *Students:* 13 full-time (12 women), 257 part-time (228 women); includes 23 minority (14 Black or African American, non-Hispanic/Latino; 3 Asian, non-Hispanic/Latino; 4 Hispanic/Latino; 2 Two or more races, non-Hispanic/Latino). Average age 37. 86 applicants, 86% accepted, 44 enrolled. In 2015, 61 master's, 6 doctorates awarded. *Degree requirements:* For master's, research experience, portfolio, practicum; for doctorate, practicum hours. *Entrance requirements:* For master's, nursing research, health assessment, graduate course work in statistics, RN license; for doctorate, master's degree in nursing, professional portfolio, graduate statistics, transcripts, RN license. Additional exam requirements/recommendations for international students: Required—TOEFL (minimum score 550 paper-based; 79 iBT). *Application deadline:* For fall admission, 6/1 priority date for domestic and international students; for spring admission, 11/15 priority date for domestic and international students. Applications are processed on a rolling basis. Application fee: $50. *Financial support:* In 2015–16, 18 students received support. Scholarships/grants and tuition waivers (partial) available. Support available to part-time students. Financial award application deadline: 6/15; financial award applicants required to submit FAFSA. *Faculty research:* Outcome and curriculum planning, health promotion, NCLEX-RN results, decision-making program evaluation. *Unit head:* Dr. Patti A. Stockert, President of the College, 309-655-4124, Fax: 309-624-8973, E-mail: patricia.a.stockert@osfhealthcare.org. *Application contact:* Dr. Kim A. Mitchell, Dean, Graduate Program, 309-655-2201, Fax: 309-624-8973, E-mail: kim.a.mitchell@osfhealthcare.org.
Website: http://www.sfmccon.edu/graduate-programs/

Saint Joseph's College of Maine, Master of Science in Nursing Program, Standish, ME 04084. Offers administration (MSN); education (MSN); family nurse practitioner (MSN); nursing administration and leadership (Certificate); nursing and health care education (Certificate). *Accreditation:* AACN. *Program availability:* Part-time, online learning. *Entrance requirements:* For master's, MAT. Electronic applications accepted.

Saint Joseph's University, College of Arts and Sciences, Department of Health Services, Philadelphia, PA 19131-1395. Offers health administration (MS); health education (MS); healthcare ethics (MS); long-term care administration (MS); nurse anesthesia (MS); school nurse certification (MS). *Program availability:* Part-time, evening/weekend. *Entrance requirements:* For master's, GRE (if GPA less than 3.0), 2 letters of recommendation, resume, personal statement, official transcripts. Additional exam requirements/recommendations for international students: Required—TOEFL (minimum score 550 paper-based; 80 iBT), IELTS (minimum score 6.5). Electronic applications accepted.

Saint Joseph's University, College of Arts and Sciences, Program in Gerontological Services, Philadelphia, PA 19131-1395. Offers gerontological services (MS); long-term care administration (MS). *Program availability:* Part-time, evening/weekend. *Entrance requirements:* For master's, 2 letters of recommendation, personal statement, resume. Additional exam requirements/recommendations for international students: Required—TOEFL (minimum score 550 paper-based; 80 iBT). Electronic applications accepted.

Saint Peter's University, School of Nursing, Nursing Program, Jersey City, NJ 07306-5997. Offers adult nurse practitioner (MSN, Certificate); advanced practice (DNP); case management (MSN, DNP). *Accreditation:* AACN. *Program availability:* Part-time, evening/weekend. *Entrance requirements:* Additional exam requirements/recommendations for international students: Required—TOEFL. Electronic applications accepted.

Salem State University, School of Graduate Studies, Program in Nursing, Salem, MA 01970-5353. Offers adult-gerontology primary care nursing (MSN); nursing administration (MSN); nursing education (MSN); MBA/MSN. *Accreditation:* AACN. *Program availability:* Part-time, evening/weekend. *Entrance requirements:* For master's, GRE or MAT. Additional exam requirements/recommendations for international students: Required—TOEFL (minimum score 550 paper-based; 80 iBT) or IELTS (minimum score 5.5).

Salisbury University, DNP in Nursing Program, Salisbury, MD 21801-6837. Offers family nurse practitioner (DNP); nursing (DNP); nursing leadership (DNP). *Accreditation:* AACN. *Program availability:* Part-time. *Faculty:* 7 full-time (5 women). *Students:* 22 full-time (20 women), 1 (woman) part-time; includes 9 minority (7 Black or African American, non-Hispanic/Latino; 1 Hispanic/Latino; 1 Two or more races, non-Hispanic/Latino). Average age 35. 16 applicants, 56% accepted, 6 enrolled. In 2015, 8 doctorates awarded. Terminal master's awarded for partial completion of doctoral program. *Entrance requirements:* For doctorate, undergraduate nursing degree with minimum cumulative GPA of 3.0; current and active United States Registered Nurse license; current resume or curriculum vitae; essay; 3 letters of recommendation. Additional exam requirements/recommendations for international students: Required—TOEFL (minimum score 550 paper-based, 79 iBT) or IELTS (6.5). *Application deadline:* For fall admission, 5/15 priority date for domestic students, 3/15 priority date for international students. Applications are processed on a rolling basis. Application fee: $65. Electronic applications accepted. *Expenses:* $620 per credit hour resident; $787 per credit hour non-resident; $78 per credit hour fees. *Financial support:* In 2015–16, 18 students received support. Career-related internships or fieldwork, institutionally sponsored loans, scholarships/grants, and unspecified assistantships available. Support available to part-time students. Financial award application deadline: 3/1; financial award applicants required to submit FAFSA. *Faculty research:* Intimate partner violence; telehealth; nursing faculty shortage; oral health needs; gerontology. *Unit head:* Dr. Lisa Seldomridge, Graduate Program Director, Nursing (DNP), 410-543-6344, Fax: 410-548-3313, E-mail: laseldomridge@salisbury.edu. *Application contact:* Carmel Boger, Administrative Assistant, 410-543-6420, Fax: 410-548-3313, E-mail: ciboger@salisbury.edu.
Website: http://www.salisbury.edu/gsr/gradstudies/DNPpage.html

Salisbury University, MS in Nursing Program, Salisbury, MD 21801-6837. Offers clinical nurse educator (MS); health care leadership (MS); nursing (MS). *Program availability:* Part-time. *Faculty:* 5 full-time (3 women). *Students:* 6 part-time (5 women); includes 1 minority (Black or African American, non-Hispanic/Latino). Average age 33. 1 applicant. In 2015, 6 master's awarded. *Degree requirements:* For master's, thesis. *Entrance requirements:* For master's, BS in nursing with minimum cumulative GPA of 3.0; current and active United States Registered Nursing license; current resume or curriculum vitae; personal statement; 2 letters of reference; interview. Additional exam requirements/recommendations for international students: Required—TOEFL (minimum score 550 paper-based, 79 iBT) or IELTS (6.5). *Application deadline:* For fall admission, 5/15 priority date for domestic and international students. Applications are processed on a rolling basis. Application fee: $65. Electronic applications accepted. *Expenses:* $620 per credit hour resident; $787 per credit hour non-resident; $78 per credit hour fees. *Financial support:* In 2015–16, 18 students received support, including 1 research

assistantship with full tuition reimbursement available (averaging $8,000 per year); career-related internships or fieldwork, institutionally sponsored loans, scholarships/grants, and unspecified assistantships also available. Support available to part-time students. Financial award application deadline: 3/1; financial award applicants required to submit FAFSA. *Faculty research:* Gerontology; epidemiology; palliative care; global health; depression. *Unit head:* Dr. Lisa Seldomridge, Graduate Program Director, Nursing, 410-543-6344, Fax: 410-548-3313, E-mail: laseldomridge@salisbury.edu. *Application contact:* Carmel Boger, Administrative Assistant, 410-543-6420, Fax: 410-548-3313, E-mail: ciboger@salisbury.edu.
Website: http://www.salisbury.edu/gsr/gradstudies/MSNpage.html

Samford University, Ida V. Moffett School of Nursing, Birmingham, AL 35229. Offers administration (DNP); advanced practice (DNP); family nurse practitioner (MSN); health systems management and leadership (MSN); nurse anesthesia (MSN); nurse educator (MSN). *Accreditation:* AACN; AANA/CANAEP (one or more programs are accredited). *Program availability:* Part-time, blended/hybrid learning. *Faculty:* 19 full-time (all women), 5 part-time/adjunct (1 woman). *Students:* 300 full-time (228 women), 40 part-time (36 women); includes 65 minority (28 Black or African American, non-Hispanic/Latino; 4 American Indian or Alaska Native, non-Hispanic/Latino; 8 Asian, non-Hispanic/Latino; 13 Hispanic/Latino; 12 Two or more races, non-Hispanic/Latino). Average age 35. 69 applicants, 77% accepted, 52 enrolled. In 2015, 98 master's, 16 doctorates awarded. *Degree requirements:* For doctorate, capstone project with oral presentation. *Entrance requirements:* For master's, MAT; GRE (for nurse anesthesia), unencumbered licensure as registered nurse; BSN from CCNE, CNEA, or ACEN (formerly NLNAC) accredited program; minimum cumulative GPA of 3.0 in nursing courses; video submission; one undergraduate course in nursing research with minimum grade of C; for doctorate, unencumbered licensure as registered nurse; master's degree from CCNE, CNEA or ACEN (formerly NLNAC) accredited program in the area of advanced practice or administration; minimum master's degree cumulative GPA of 3.5; video interview submission. Additional exam requirements/recommendations for international students: Required—TOEFL (minimum score 550 paper-based; 80 iBT). *Application deadline:* For fall admission, 6/1 for domestic and international students; for spring admission, 9/1 for domestic and international students. Application fee: $65. Electronic applications accepted. *Expenses:* Tuition, area resident: Full-time $18,673; part-time $766 per credit hour. *Required fees:* $550. Tuition and fees vary according to course load, degree level and student level. *Financial support:* In 2015–16, 56 students received support. Institutionally sponsored loans, scholarships/grants, and traineeships available. Financial award application deadline: 3/1; financial award applicants required to submit FAFSA. *Faculty research:* Issues in rural health care, vulnerable populations, genetics and disabilities in pediatrics, geriatrics, parish nursing research, interprofessional education, global health disparities. *Unit head:* Dr. Nena F. Sanders, Vice Provost, College of Health Sciences/Dean/Professor, 205-726-2612, Fax: 205-726-4179, E-mail: nfsander@samford.edu. *Application contact:* Allyson Maddox, Director of Graduate Student Services, Ida V. Moffett School of Nursing, 205-726-2047, Fax: 205-726-4179, E-mail: amaddox@samford.edu.
Website: http://samford.edu/nursing

Samuel Merritt University, School of Nursing, Oakland, CA 94609. Offers case management (MSN); family nurse practitioner (MSN, Certificate); nurse anesthetist (MSN, Certificate); nursing (DNP). *Accreditation:* AACN; AANA/CANAEP (one or more programs are accredited). *Program availability:* Part-time, evening/weekend, 100% online, blended/hybrid learning. *Faculty:* 47 full-time (40 women), 50 part-time/adjunct (43 women). *Students:* 437 full-time (350 women), 59 part-time (45 women); includes 327 minority (29 Black or African American, non-Hispanic/Latino; 3 American Indian or Alaska Native, non-Hispanic/Latino; 163 Asian, non-Hispanic/Latino; 95 Hispanic/Latino; 9 Native Hawaiian or other Pacific Islander, non-Hispanic/Latino; 28 Two or more races, non-Hispanic/Latino). Average age 33. 392 applicants, 43% accepted, 126 enrolled. In 2015, 31 master's awarded. *Degree requirements:* For master's, thesis or alternative. *Entrance requirements:* For master's, minimum GPA of 2.5 in science, 3.0 overall; previous course work in statistics; current RN license. Additional exam requirements/recommendations for international students: Required—TOEFL (minimum score 100 iBT). *Application deadline:* For fall admission, 1/1 priority date for domestic students; for spring admission, 7/1 for domestic students; for summer admission, 1/1 for domestic students. Applications are processed on a rolling basis. Application fee: $50. Electronic applications accepted. *Expenses:* $61,299 tuition; $240 lab fees; $160 graduation fee. *Financial support:* In 2015–16, 34 students received support. Career-related internships or fieldwork, Federal Work-Study, scholarships/grants, and traineeships available. Support available to part-time students. Financial award application deadline: 3/2; financial award applicants required to submit FAFSA. *Faculty research:* Gerontology, community health, maternal-child health, sexually transmitted diseases, substance abuse, oncology. *Total annual research expenditures:* $35,000. *Unit head:* Dr. Audrey Berman, Graduate Coordinator, 510-869-6733, Fax: 510-869-6525. *Application contact:* Timothy Cranford, Dean of Admission, 510-869-6576, Fax: 510-869-6525, E-mail: admission@samuelmerritt.edu.
Website: http://www.samuelmerritt.edu/nursing

San Francisco State University, Division of Graduate Studies, College of Health and Social Sciences, School of Nursing, San Francisco, CA 94132-1722. Offers adult acute care (MS); clinical nurse specialist (MS); community/public health nursing (MS); family nurse practitioner (MS, Certificate); nursing administration (MS); pediatrics (MS); women's health (MS). *Accreditation:* AACN. *Program availability:* Part-time. *Application deadline:* Applications are processed on a rolling basis. *Expenses:* Tuition, state resident: full-time $6738. Tuition, nonresident: full-time $15,666. *Required fees:* $1004. *Financial support:* Career-related internships or fieldwork available. *Unit head:* Dr. Mary-Ann van Dam, Director, 415-338-1802, Fax: 415-338-0555, E-mail: vandam@sfsu.edu. *Application contact:* Connie Carr, Graduate Coordinator, 415-338-6856, Fax: 415-338-0555, E-mail: ccarr@sfsu.edu.
Website: http://nursing.sfsu.edu

Seattle Pacific University, MS in Nursing Program, Seattle, WA 98119-1997. Offers administration (MSN); adult/gerontology nurse practitioner (MSN); clinical nurse specialist (MSN); family nurse practitioner (MSN, Certificate); informatics (MSN); nurse educator (MSN). *Accreditation:* AACN. *Program availability:* Part-time. *Students:* 39 full-time (36 women), 30 part-time (25 women); includes 14 minority (3 Black or African American, non-Hispanic/Latino; 7 Asian, non-Hispanic/Latino; 3 Hispanic/Latino; 1 Two or more races, non-Hispanic/Latino), 1 international. Average age 38. 60 applicants, 48% accepted, 29 enrolled. In 2015, 23 master's awarded. *Degree requirements:* For master's, thesis. *Entrance requirements:* For master's, personal statement, transcripts, undergraduate nursing degree, proof of undergraduate statistics course with minimum GPA of 2.0, 2 recommendations. *Application deadline:* For fall admission, 1/15 priority date for domestic students; for spring admission, 1/15 for domestic students. Applications are processed on a rolling basis. Application fee: $50. Electronic applications accepted. *Expenses:* Contact institution. *Financial support:* Fellowships and scholarships/grants available. Financial award applicants required to submit FAFSA. *Unit head:* Dr. Christine Hoyle, Associate Dean, 206-281-2469, E-mail: hoylec@spu.edu.
Website: http://spu.edu/depts/health-sciences/grad/index.asp

Seton Hall University, College of Nursing, South Orange, NJ 07079-2697. Offers advanced practice in primary health care (MSN, DNP), including adult/gerontological nurse practitioner, pediatric nurse practitioner; entry into practice (MSN); health systems administration (MSN, DNP); nursing (PhD); nursing case management (MSN); nursing education (MA); school nurse (MSN); MSN/MA. *Accreditation:* AACN. *Program availability:* Part-time, online learning. *Degree requirements:* For master's, research project; for doctorate, dissertation or scholarly project. *Entrance requirements:* For doctorate, GRE (waived for students with GPA of 3.5 or higher). Additional exam requirements/recommendations for international students: Required—TOEFL. Electronic applications accepted. *Faculty research:* Parent/child, adult, and gerontological nursing; breast cancer; families of children with HIV; parish nursing.

Shenandoah University, Eleanor Wade Custer School of Nursing, Winchester, VA 22601. Offers family nurse practitioner (MSN, DNP, Post-Graduate Certificate); health informatics (Certificate); health systems leadership (DNP); nurse midwifery (MSN, Post-Graduate Certificate); nursing education (Post-Graduate Certificate); psychiatric mental health nurse practitioner (MSN, DNP, Post-Graduate Certificate). *Accreditation:* AACN; ACNM/ACME. *Faculty:* 10 full-time (all women), 7 part-time/adjunct (4 women). *Students:* 33 full-time (31 women), 62 part-time (57 women); includes 21 minority (17 Black or African American, non-Hispanic/Latino; 3 Asian, non-Hispanic/Latino; 1 Hispanic/Latino). Average age 36. 55 applicants, 87% accepted, 39 enrolled. In 2015, 32 master's, 3 doctorates, 19 other advanced degrees awarded. *Degree requirements:* For master's, research project, clinical hours; for doctorate, scholarly project, clinical hours; for other advanced degree, clinical hours. *Entrance requirements:* For master's, United States RN license; minimum GPA of 3.0; 2080 hours of clinical experience; curriculum vitae; 3 letters of recommendation from a former dean, a faculty member or advisor familiar with the applicant, and a former or current supervisor; two- to three-page essay on a specified topic; for doctorate, MSN, minimum GPA of 3.0, 3 letters of recommendation, 500-word statement, interview, BSN; for other advanced degree, MSN, minimum GPA of 3.0, 2 letters of recommendation, minimum of one year (2080 hours) of clinical nursing experience, interview. Additional exam requirements/recommendations for international students: Required—TOEFL (minimum score 558 paper-based; 83 iBT). *Application deadline:* For fall admission, 1/15 priority date for domestic and international students; for spring admission, 11/1 for domestic and international students; for summer admission, 3/15 for domestic and international students. Application fee: $30. Electronic applications accepted. *Expenses:* Contact institution. *Financial support:* In 2015–16, 13 students received support, including 3 fellowships (averaging $1,000 per year); scholarships/grants and unspecified assistantships also available. Financial award application deadline: 3/15; financial award applicants required to submit FAFSA. *Faculty research:* Primary care providers and their unique position in geriatric, pre-operative education and its effects on post-operative, variables associated with a woman's multidimensional childbirth, interdisciplinary communication, research on health policy. *Unit head:* Kathryn Ganske, PhD, RN, Dean, 540-678-4374, Fax: 540-665-5519, E-mail: kganske@su.edu. *Application contact:* Andrew Woodall, Executive Director of Recruitment and Admissions, 540-665-4581, Fax: 540-665-4627, E-mail: admit@su.edu.
Website: http://www.su.edu/nursing/

Southern Adventist University, School of Nursing, Collegedale, TN 37315-0370. Offers acute care nurse practitioner (MSN); adult nurse practitioner (MSN); family nurse practitioner (MSN); nurse educator (MSN); MSN/MSBA. *Accreditation:* ACEN. *Program availability:* Part-time. *Degree requirements:* For master's, thesis or project. *Entrance requirements:* For master's, RN license. Additional exam requirements/recommendations for international students: Required—TOEFL (minimum score 600 paper-based). Electronic applications accepted. *Faculty research:* Pain management, ethics, corporate wellness, caring spirituality, stress.

Southern Illinois University Edwardsville, Graduate School, School of Nursing, Program in Health Care and Nursing Administration, Edwardsville, IL 62026. Offers MS, Post-Master's Certificate. *Program availability:* Part-time. *Students:* 31 part-time (27 women); includes 5 minority (3 Black or African American, non-Hispanic/Latino; 2 Two or more races, non-Hispanic/Latino). 10 applicants, 100% accepted. In 2015, 8 master's awarded. *Degree requirements:* For master's, comprehensive exam. *Entrance requirements:* For master's, RN licensure, minimum undergraduate nursing GPA of 3.0, BS from CCNE- or NLNAC-accredited program. Additional exam requirements/recommendations for international students: Required—TOEFL (minimum score 550 paper-based; 79 iBT), IELTS (minimum score 6.5). *Application deadline:* For fall admission, 3/1 for domestic and international students. Application fee: $30. Electronic applications accepted. *Expenses:* Tuition, state resident: full-time $5026; part-time $837 per course. Tuition, nonresident: full-time $12,566; part-time $2094 per course. *Required fees:* $1682; $474 per course. Tuition and fees vary according to course load, campus/location and program. *Financial support:* In 2015–16, 1 teaching assistantship with full tuition reimbursement was awarded; fellowships, research assistantships, institutionally sponsored loans, scholarships/grants, and unspecified assistantships also available. Financial award application deadline: 3/1; financial award applicants required to submit FAFSA. *Unit head:* Dr. Kathy Ketchum, Associate Dean for Graduate Programs, 618-650-3936, E-mail: kketchu@siue.edu. *Application contact:* Bob Skorczewski, Coordinator of International and Graduate Recruitment, 618-650-3705, Fax: 618-650-3618, E-mail: gradadmissions@siue.edu.
Website: http://www.siue.edu/nursing/graduate

Southern Nazarene University, College of Professional and Graduate Studies, School of Nursing, Bethany, OK 73008. Offers nursing education (MS); nursing leadership (MS). *Accreditation:* AACN. *Program availability:* Part-time, evening/weekend. *Degree requirements:* For master's, thesis. *Entrance requirements:* For master's, minimum undergraduate cumulative GPA of 3.0; baccalaureate degree in nursing from nationally-accredited program; current unencumbered registered nurse licensure in Oklahoma or eligibility for same; documentation of basic computer skills; basic statistics course; statement of professional goals; three letters of recommendation. Additional exam requirements/recommendations for international students: Required—TOEFL (minimum score 550 paper-based).

Southern University and Agricultural and Mechanical College, School of Nursing, Baton Rouge, LA 70813. Offers educator/administrator (PhD); family health nursing (MSN); family nurse practitioner (Post Master's Certificate); geriatric nurse practitioner/gerontology (PhD). *Accreditation:* AACN. *Program availability:* Part-time. *Degree requirements:* For master's, comprehensive exam, thesis; for doctorate, comprehensive exam, thesis/dissertation. *Entrance requirements:* For master's, GRE General Test, BSN, minimum GPA of 2.7; for doctorate, GRE General Test; for Post Master's Certificate, MSN. Additional exam requirements/recommendations for international students: Required—TOEFL (minimum score 525 paper-based). *Faculty research:* Health promotions, vulnerable populations, (community-based) cardiovascular participating research, health disparities chronic diseases, care of the elderly.

Spalding University, Graduate Studies, Kosair College of Health and Natural Sciences, School of Nursing, Louisville, KY 40203-2188. Offers adult nurse practitioner (MSN, PMC); family nurse practitioner (MSN, PMC); leadership in nursing and healthcare (MSN); pediatric nurse practitioner (MSN, PMC). *Accreditation:* AACN. *Program availability:* Part-time, evening/weekend. *Faculty:* 10 full-time (9 women), 8 part-time/adjunct (7 women). *Students:* 101 full-time (94 women), 9 part-time (all women); includes 20 minority (14 Black or African American, non-Hispanic/Latino; 3 Asian, non-Hispanic/Latino; 1 Native Hawaiian or other Pacific Islander, non-Hispanic/Latino; 2 Two or more races, non-Hispanic/Latino). Average age 36. 10 applicants, 30% accepted, 2 enrolled. In 2015, 43 master's awarded. *Degree requirements:* For master's, comprehensive exam (for some programs), thesis. *Entrance requirements:* For master's, GRE General Test, BSN or bachelor's degree in related field, RN licensure, autobiographical statement, transcripts, letters of recommendation. Additional exam requirements/recommendations for international students: Required—TOEFL (minimum score 535 paper-based). *Application deadline:* For fall admission, 2/1 priority date for domestic students. Application fee: $30. *Financial support:* Career-related internships or fieldwork, scholarships/grants, and traineeships available. Support available to part-time students. Financial award application deadline: 3/30; financial award applicants required to submit FAFSA. *Faculty research:* Nurse educational administration, gerontology, bioterrorism, healthcare ethics, leadership. *Unit head:* Dr. Patricia Spurr, Chair, 502-873-4304, E-mail: pspurr@spalding.edu. *Application contact:* Dr. Pam King, Program Director, 502-873-4292, E-mail: pking@spalding.edu.
Website: http://www.spalding.edu/nursing/

Spring Hill College, Graduate Programs, Program in Nursing, Mobile, AL 36608-1791. Offers clinical nurse leader (MSN, Post-Master's Certificate). *Accreditation:* AACN. *Program availability:* Part-time, evening/weekend, online learning. *Faculty:* 2 full-time (both women), 1 (woman) part-time/adjunct. *Students:* 13 part-time (12 women); includes 6 minority (5 Black or African American, non-Hispanic/Latino; 1 Hispanic/Latino). Average age 45. In 2015, 8 master's awarded. *Degree requirements:* For master's, comprehensive exam, capstone courses, completion of program within 6 calendar years; for Post-Master's Certificate, 460 clinical integration hours. *Entrance requirements:* For master's, RN license in state where practicing nursing; 1 year of clinical nursing experience; work in clinical setting or access to health care facility for clinical integration/research; 3 written references; employer verification; resume; 500-word essay explaining how becoming a CNL will help applicant achieve personal and professional goals; for Post-Master's Certificate, RN license; master's degree in nursing. Additional exam requirements/recommendations for international students: Required—TOEFL (minimum score 550 paper-based; 80 iBT), IELTS (minimum score 6.5), CPE or CAE (minimum score C), Michigan English Language Assessment Battery (minimum score 90). *Application deadline:* For fall admission, 8/1 priority date for domestic and international students; for spring admission, 12/1 priority date for domestic and international students. Applications are processed on a rolling basis. Application fee: $25 ($35 for international students). Electronic applications accepted. *Expenses:* Contact institution. *Financial support:* Applicants required to submit FAFSA. *Unit head:* Dr. Ola H. Fox, Director, 251-380-4486, Fax: 251-460-4495, E-mail: ofox@shc.edu. *Application contact:* Robert Stewart, Vice President of Enrollment, 251-380-3030, Fax: 251-460-2186, E-mail: rstewart@shc.edu.
Website: http://ug.shc.edu/graduate-degrees/master-science-nursing/

State University of New York Polytechnic Institute, Program in Business Administration in Technology Management, Utica, NY 13504-3050. Offers accounting and finance (MBA); business management (MBA); health services management (MBA); human resource management (MBA); marketing management (MBA). *Program availability:* Part-time, online learning. *Degree requirements:* For master's, capstone course. *Entrance requirements:* For master's, GMAT, resume, one letter of reference. Additional exam requirements/recommendations for international students: Required—TOEFL (minimum score 550 paper-based; 79 iBT), IELTS (minimum score 6.5). Electronic applications accepted. *Faculty research:* Technology management, writing schools, leadership, new products.

Stony Brook University, State University of New York, Stony Brook Medicine, School of Nursing, Program in Nursing Leadership, Stony Brook, NY 11794. Offers MS, Certificate. *Program availability:* Part-time, blended/hybrid learning. *Students:* 73 part-time (61 women); includes 22 minority (9 Black or African American, non-Hispanic/Latino; 5 Asian, non-Hispanic/Latino; 7 Hispanic/Latino; 1 Two or more races, non-Hispanic/Latino). 65 applicants, 95% accepted, 53 enrolled. *Entrance requirements:* Additional exam requirements/recommendations for international students: Required—TOEFL (minimum score 90 iBT). *Application deadline:* For fall admission, 2/25 for domestic students. Application fee: $100. *Expenses:* $24,781 per year full-time resident tuition and fees, $968 per credit hour; $44,431 per year full-time non-resident tuition and fees, $1,787 per credit hour. *Unit head:* Stacey Frawley, Program Director, 631-444-3284, Fax: 631-444-3136, E-mail: stacey.frawley@stonybrook.edu. *Application contact:* Anita Defranco, Staff Assistant, 631-444-3276, Fax: 631-444-3136, E-mail: anita.defranco@stonybrook.edu.

Tarleton State University, College of Graduate Studies, College of Science and Technology, Department of Nursing, Stephenville, TX 76402. Offers nursing administration (MSN); nursing education (MSN). *Program availability:* Part-time, evening/weekend. *Faculty:* 3 full-time (all women). *Students:* 19 part-time (17 women); includes 6 minority (3 Black or African American, non-Hispanic/Latino; 3 Hispanic/Latino). 12 applicants, 83% accepted, 8 enrolled. In 2015, 8 master's awarded. *Degree requirements:* For master's, comprehensive exam. *Entrance requirements:* For master's, GRE General Test, minimum GPA of 3.0. Additional exam requirements/recommendations for international students: Required—TOEFL (minimum score 500 paper-based; 80 iBT). *Application deadline:* For fall admission, 8/15 priority date for domestic students; for spring admission, 1/7 for domestic students. Applications are processed on a rolling basis. Application fee: $45 ($145 for international students). Electronic applications accepted. *Expenses:* Tuition, state resident: part-time $204 per credit hour. Tuition, nonresident: part-time $594 per credit hour. *Required fees:* $1994 per unit. *Financial support:* Career-related internships or fieldwork, Federal Work-Study, and institutionally sponsored loans available. Support available to part-time students. Financial award applicants required to submit FAFSA. *Unit head:* Dr. Susan Rugari, Department Head, 254-968-9139, E-mail: rugari@tarleton.edu. *Application contact:* Information Contact, 254-968-9104, Fax: 254-968-9670, E-mail: gradoffice@tarleton.edu.
Website: http://www.tarleton.edu/nursing/degrees_grad.html

Teachers College, Columbia University, Department of Organization and Leadership, New York, NY 10027-6696. Offers adult education guided intensive study (Ed D); adult learning and leadership (Ed M, MA, ME, Ed D); educational leadership studies (Ed D); higher and post secondary education (MA, ME, Ed D); inquiry educational leadership practice (Ed D); leadership, policy and politics (Ed D); nurse education (MA); nurse executive (MA), including administration studies, professional studies; nurse executive role (MA, Ed D), including nurse executive (Ed D); private school leadership (Ed M, MA, ME); public school building leadership (Ed M, MA, ME); social and organizational psychology (MA); urban education leaders (Ed D); MA/MBA. *Program availability:* Part-time, evening/weekend. *Students:* 285 full-time (173 women), 491 part-time (344 women); includes 333 minority (119 Black or African American, non-Hispanic/Latino; 1 American Indian or Alaska Native, non-Hispanic/Latino; 102 Asian, non-Hispanic/Latino; 97 Hispanic/Latino; 14 Two or more races, non-Hispanic/Latino), 36 international. *Degree requirements:* For doctorate, thesis/dissertation. *Expenses:* Tuition, area resident: Part-time $1454 per credit. *Required fees:* $428 per semester. One-time fee:

Nursing and Healthcare Administration

$475 full-time. Full-time tuition and fees vary according to course load. *Unit head:* Prof. Anna Neumann, Chair, 212-678-3272, Fax: 212-678-3036, E-mail: neumann@tc.columbia.edu. *Application contact:* David Estrella, Director of Admission, E-mail: estrella@tc.columbia.edu.

Tennessee Technological University, Whitson-Hester School of Nursing, Cookeville, TN 38505. Offers family nurse practitioner (MSN); informatics (MSN); nursing administration (MSN); nursing education (MSN). *Program availability:* Part-time, evening/weekend, online learning. *Students:* 21 full-time (20 women), 95 part-time (80 women); includes 5 minority (2 Black or African American, non-Hispanic/Latino; 1 Asian, non-Hispanic/Latino; 1 Hispanic/Latino; 1 Two or more races, non-Hispanic/Latino). 42 applicants, 57% accepted, 15 enrolled. In 2015, 47 master's awarded. *Degree requirements:* For master's, comprehensive exam, thesis or alternative. *Entrance requirements:* Additional exam requirements/recommendations for international students: Required—TOEFL (minimum score 600 paper-based; 100 iBT), IELTS (minimum score 5.5), PTE, or TOEIC (Test of English as an International Communication). *Application deadline:* For fall admission, 8/1 for domestic students, 5/1 for international students; for spring admission, 12/1 for domestic students, 10/1 for international students; for summer admission, 5/1 for domestic students, 2/1 for international students. Applications are processed on a rolling basis. Application fee: $35 ($40 for international students). Electronic applications accepted. *Expenses:* Tuition, state resident: full-time $8961; part-time $6132 per credit hour. Tuition, nonresident: full-time $23,121; part-time $14,608 per credit hour. *Financial support:* Application deadline: 4/1. *Unit head:* Dr. Huey-Ming Tzeng, Dean, 931-372-3547, Fax: 931-372-6244, E-mail: htzeng@tntech.edu. *Application contact:* Shelia K. Kendrick, Coordinator of Graduate Studies, 931-372-3808, Fax: 931-372-3497, E-mail: skendrick@tntech.edu.

Texas A&M University–Corpus Christi, College of Graduate Studies, College of Nursing and Health Sciences, Corpus Christi, TX 78412-5503. Offers family nurse practitioner (MSN); leadership in nursing systems (MSN); nurse educator (MSN). *Accreditation:* AACN. *Program availability:* Part-time, evening/weekend, online only, 100% online. *Students:* 12 full-time (11 women), 375 part-time (322 women); includes 200 minority (20 Black or African American, non-Hispanic/Latino; 1 American Indian or Alaska Native, non-Hispanic/Latino; 27 Asian, non-Hispanic/Latino; 142 Hispanic/Latino; 3 Native Hawaiian or other Pacific Islander, non-Hispanic/Latino; 7 Two or more races, non-Hispanic/Latino), 1 international. Average age 38. 337 applicants, 42% accepted, 128 enrolled. In 2015, 102 master's awarded. *Degree requirements:* For master's, comprehensive exam, thesis (for some programs), capstone - clinical. *Entrance requirements:* For master's, essay, resume, 3 letters of recommendation, minimum GPA of 3.0. Additional exam requirements/recommendations for international students: Required—TOEFL (minimum score 550 paper-based; 79 iBT), IELTS (minimum score 6.5). *Application deadline:* For fall admission, 4/15 priority date for domestic and international students; for spring admission, 1/7 for domestic and international students; for summer admission, 5/27 for domestic and international students. Applications are processed on a rolling basis. Application fee: $50 ($70 for international students). Electronic applications accepted. *Financial support:* Research assistantships, teaching assistantships, career-related internships or fieldwork, Federal Work-Study, institutionally sponsored loans, scholarships/grants, health care benefits, and unspecified assistantships available. Support available to part-time students. Financial award application deadline: 3/15; financial award applicants required to submit FAFSA. *Unit head:* Dr. Mary Jane Hamilton, Dean, 361-825-2469, E-mail: mary.hamilton@tamucc.edu. *Application contact:* Graduate Admissions Coordinator, 361-825-2177, Fax: 361-825-2755, E-mail: gradweb@tamucc.edu.
Website: http://conhs.tamucc.edu/

Texas Christian University, Harris College of Nursing and Health Sciences, Doctor of Nursing Practice Program, Fort Worth, TX 76129. Offers advanced practice registered nurse (DNP); nursing administration (DNP). *Program availability:* Part-time. *Faculty:* 20 full-time (17 women), 2 part-time/adjunct (both women). *Students:* 19 full-time (17 women), 26 part-time (23 women); includes 9 minority (4 Black or African American, non-Hispanic/Latino; 1 American Indian or Alaska Native, non-Hispanic/Latino; 2 Asian, non-Hispanic/Latino; 2 Hispanic/Latino). Average age 46. 24 applicants, 58% accepted, 13 enrolled. In 2015, 24 doctorates awarded. *Degree requirements:* For doctorate, thesis/dissertation or alternative, practicum. *Entrance requirements:* For doctorate, three reference letters, essay, resume, two official transcripts from each institution attended, APRN recognition or MSN with experience in nursing administration. *Application deadline:* For summer admission, 11/15 for domestic and international students. Application fee: $60. Electronic applications accepted. *Expenses:* Tuition, area resident: Full-time $26,640; part-time $1480 per credit hour. *Required fees:* $48; $48 per unit. Tuition and fees vary according to program. *Financial support:* Teaching assistantships and scholarships/grants available. Financial award application deadline: 2/15; financial award applicants required to submit FAFSA. *Faculty research:* Geriatrics, cancer survivorship, health literacy, endothelial cells, clinical simulation outcomes. *Unit head:* Dr. Kenneth Lowrance, Director, Post Master's DNP Program and CNS Program, 817-257-6729, Fax: 817-257-8383, E-mail: k.w.lowrance@tcu.edu. *Application contact:* Mary Jane Allred, Administrative Program Specialist, 817-257-6726, Fax: 817-257-8383, E-mail: m.allred@tcu.edu.
Website: http://dnp.tcu.edu/

Texas Christian University, Harris College of Nursing and Health Sciences, Master's Program in Nursing, Fort Worth, TX 76129. Offers clinical nurse leader (MSN, Certificate); clinical nurse specialist (MSN), including adult/gerontology nursing, pediatrics; nursing education (MSN). *Accreditation:* AACN; AANA/CANAEP (one or more programs are accredited). *Program availability:* Part-time, online only, 100% online. *Faculty:* 20 full-time (17 women), 2 part-time/adjunct (both women). *Students:* 47 full-time (40 women), 24 part-time (all women); includes 19 minority (3 Black or African American, non-Hispanic/Latino; 1 American Indian or Alaska Native, non-Hispanic/Latino; 10 Asian, non-Hispanic/Latino; 2 Hispanic/Latino; 1 Native Hawaiian or other Pacific Islander, non-Hispanic/Latino; 2 Two or more races, non-Hispanic/Latino), 1 international. Average age 39. 34 applicants, 82% accepted, 23 enrolled. In 2015, 14 master's awarded. *Degree requirements:* For master's, thesis or alternative, practicum. *Entrance requirements:* For master's, GRE General Test, 3 letters of reference, essay, resume, two official transcripts from every institution attended. *Application deadline:* For fall admission, 4/1 for domestic and international students; for spring admission, 9/1 for domestic and international students; for summer admission, 2/1 for domestic and international students. Applications are processed on a rolling basis. Application fee: $60. Electronic applications accepted. *Expenses:* $1,415 per semester hour; $112 fee per course. *Financial support:* In 2015–16, 71 students received support. Teaching assistantships and scholarships/grants available. Financial award application deadline: 2/15; financial award applicants required to submit FAFSA. *Faculty research:* Geriatrics, cancer survivorship, health literacy, endothelial cells, clinical simulation outcomes. *Unit head:* Dr. Kathy Baker, Director, Division of Nursing Graduate Studies and Scholarship, 817-257-6726, Fax: 817-257-8383, E-mail: kathy.baker@tcu.edu. *Application contact:* Mary Jane Allred, Administrative Program Specialist, 817-257-6726, Fax: 817-257-8383, E-mail: m.allred@tcu.edu.
Website: http://www.nursing.tcu.edu/graduate.asp

Texas Tech University Health Sciences Center, School of Nursing, Lubbock, TX 79430. Offers acute care nurse practitioner (MSN, Certificate); administration (MSN); advanced practice (DNP); education (MSN); executive leadership (DNP); family nurse practitioner (MSN, Certificate); geriatric nurse practitioner (MSN, Certificate); pediatric nurse practitioner (MSN, Certificate). *Accreditation:* AACN. *Program availability:* Part-time, online learning. *Degree requirements:* For master's, thesis optional. *Entrance requirements:* For master's, minimum GPA of 3.0, 3 letters of reference, BSN, RN license; for Certificate, minimum GPA of 3.0, 3 letters of reference, RN license. Additional exam requirements/recommendations for international students: Required—TOEFL (minimum score 550 paper-based). *Faculty research:* Diabetes/obesity, nurse competency, disease management, intervention and measurements, health disparities.

Texas Woman's University, Graduate School, College of Nursing, Denton, TX 76204-5498. Offers acute care nurse practitioner (MS); adult health clinical nurse specialist (MS); adult health nurse practitioner (MS); child health clinical nurse specialist (MS); clinical nurse leader (MS); family nurse practitioner (MS); health systems management (MS); nursing education (MS); nursing practice (DNP); nursing science (PhD); pediatric nurse practitioner (MS); women's health clinical nurse specialist (MS); women's health nurse practitioner (MS). *Accreditation:* AACN. *Program availability:* Part-time, online learning. *Faculty:* 55 full-time (51 women), 42 part-time/adjunct (35 women). *Students:* 39 full-time (37 women), 958 part-time (888 women); includes 566 minority (226 Black or African American, non-Hispanic/Latino; 8 American Indian or Alaska Native, non-Hispanic/Latino; 221 Asian, non-Hispanic/Latino; 88 Hispanic/Latino; 3 Native Hawaiian or other Pacific Islander, non-Hispanic/Latino; 20 Two or more races, non-Hispanic/Latino), 37 international. Average age 36. 430 applicants, 65% accepted, 193 enrolled. In 2015, 248 master's, 10 doctorates awarded. *Degree requirements:* For master's, comprehensive exam, thesis or alternative; for doctorate, comprehensive exam, thesis/dissertation. *Entrance requirements:* For master's, GRE or MAT, minimum GPA of 3.0 on last 60 hours in undergraduate nursing degree and overall, RN license, BS in nursing, basic statistics course; for doctorate, GRE (preferred minimum score 153 [500 old version] Verbal, 144 [500 old version] Quantitative, 4 Analytical), MS in nursing, minimum preferred GPA of 3.5, RN license, statistics, 2 letters of reference, curriculum vitae, graduate nursing-theory course, graduate research course, statement of professional goals and research interests. Additional exam requirements/recommendations for international students: Required—TOEFL (minimum score 550 paper-based; 79 iBT). *Application deadline:* For fall admission, 5/1 priority date for domestic students, 3/1 for international students; for spring admission, 9/15 priority date for domestic students, 7/1 for international students. Applications are processed on a rolling basis. Application fee: $50 ($75 for international students). Electronic applications accepted. *Expenses:* Tuition, state resident: full-time $4380; part-time $243 per credit hour. Tuition, nonresident: full-time $11,400; part-time $633 per credit hour. *International tuition:* $11,465 full-time. *Required fees:* $1778; $99 per credit hour. $283 per semester. One-time fee: $50. Tuition and fees vary according to course load and program. *Financial support:* In 2015–16, 149 students received support, including 10 research assistantships (averaging $5,600 per year), 1 teaching assistantship (averaging $5,600 per year); career-related internships or fieldwork, Federal Work-Study, institutionally sponsored loans, scholarships/grants, traineeships, health care benefits, and unspecified assistantships also available. Support available to part-time students. Financial award application deadline: 3/1; financial award applicants required to submit FAFSA. *Faculty research:* Screening, prevention, and treatment for intimate partner violence; needs of adolescents during childbirth intervention; a network analysis decision tool for nurse managers (social network analysis); support for adolescents with implantable cardioverter defibrillators; informatics: nurse staffing, safety, quality, and financial data as they relate to patient care outcomes; prevention and treatment of obesity; improving infant outcomes related to premature birth. *Total annual research expenditures:* $1.7 million. *Unit head:* Dr. Anita G. Hufft, Dean, 940-898-2401, Fax: 940-898-2437, E-mail: nursing@twu.edu. *Application contact:* Dr. Samuel Wheeler, Assistant Director of Admissions, 940-898-3188, Fax: 940-898-3081, E-mail: wheelersr@twu.edu.
Website: http://www.twu.edu/nursing/

Union University, School of Nursing, Jackson, TN 38305-3697. Offers executive leadership (DNP); nurse anesthesia (DNP); nurse practitioner (DNP); nursing education (MSN, PMC). *Accreditation:* AACN; AANA/CANAEP. *Degree requirements:* For master's, thesis or alternative. *Entrance requirements:* For master's, GRE, 3 letters of reference, bachelor's degree in nursing, minimum GPA of 3.0. Additional exam requirements/recommendations for international students: Required—TOEFL (minimum score 560 paper-based). Electronic applications accepted. *Faculty research:* Children's health, occupational rehabilitation, informatics, health promotion.

Universidad Metropolitana, School of Health Sciences, Department of Nursing, San Juan, PR 00928-1150. Offers case management (Certificate); nursing (MSN); oncology nursing (Certificate). *Accreditation:* ACEN.

University at Buffalo, the State University of New York, Graduate School, School of Nursing, Buffalo, NY 14214. Offers adult gerontology nurse practitioner (DNP); family nurse practitioner (DNP); health care systems and leadership (MS); nurse anesthetist (DNP); nursing (PhD); nursing education (Certificate); psychiatric/mental health nurse practitioner (DNP). *Accreditation:* AACN; AANA/CANAEP (one or more programs are accredited). *Program availability:* Part-time, 100% online. *Students:* 61 full-time (37 women), 137 part-time (114 women); includes 35 minority (17 Black or African American, non-Hispanic/Latino; 1 American Indian or Alaska Native, non-Hispanic/Latino; 17 Asian, non-Hispanic/Latino), 7 international. Average age 32. 193 applicants, 49% accepted, 75 enrolled. In 2015, 6 master's, 37 doctorates awarded. *Degree requirements:* For master's, thesis optional; for doctorate, comprehensive exam (for some programs), capstone (for DNP), dissertation (for PhD). *Entrance requirements:* For master's, GRE or MAT; for doctorate, GRE or MAT, minimum GPA of 3.0 (for DNP), 3.25 (for PhD); RN license; BS or MS in nursing; 3 references; writing sample; resume; personal statement; for Certificate, interview, minimum GPA of 3.0 or GRE General Test, RN license, MS in nursing, professional certification. Additional exam requirements/recommendations for international students: Required—TOEFL (minimum score 550 paper-based; 79 iBT), IELTS (minimum score 6.5). *Application deadline:* For fall admission, 7/1 for domestic students, 2/1 for international students; for spring admission, 12/1 for domestic students, 10/1 for international students; for summer admission, 2/1 for domestic students. Applications are processed on a rolling basis. Application fee: $75. Electronic applications accepted. *Financial support:* In 2015–16, 80 students received support, including 2 fellowships with tuition reimbursements available (averaging $17,000 per year), 4 research assistantships with tuition reimbursements available (averaging $10,600 per year), 7 teaching assistantships with tuition reimbursements available (averaging $10,600 per year); scholarships/grants, traineeships, health care benefits, and unspecified assistantships also available. Financial award application deadline: 2/1; financial award applicants required to submit FAFSA. *Faculty research:* Oncology, palliative care, gerontology, addictions, mental health, community wellness, sleep, workforce, care of underserved populations, quality and safety, person-centered care, adolescent health. *Total annual research expenditures:* $1.4 million. *Unit head:* Dr. Marsha L. Lewis, Dean and Professor, 716-829-2533, Fax: 716-829-2566, E-mail: ubnursingdean@buffalo.edu. *Application contact:* Jennifer H. VanLaeken, Director of Graduate Student Services, 716-829-3311, Fax: 716-829-2067, E-mail: jhv2@buffalo.edu.
Website: http://nursing.buffalo.edu/

University of Central Arkansas, Graduate School, College of Health and Behavioral Sciences, Department of Nursing, Conway, AR 72035-0001. Offers adult nurse practitioner (PMC); clinical nurse leader (PMC); clinical nurse specialist (MSN); family nurse practitioner (PMC); nurse educator (PMC); nurse practitioner (MSN). *Accreditation:* AACN. *Program availability:* Part-time, evening/weekend, online learning. *Degree requirements:* For master's, comprehensive exam, thesis optional, clinicals. *Entrance requirements:* For master's, GRE General Test, minimum GPA of 2.7. Additional exam requirements/recommendations for international students: Required—TOEFL (minimum score 550 paper-based; 80 iBT). Electronic applications accepted. *Expenses:* Contact institution.

University of Cincinnati, Graduate School, College of Nursing, Cincinnati, OH 45221-0038. Offers clinical nurse specialist (MSN), including adult health, community health, neonatal, nursing administration, occupational health, pediatric health, psychiatric nursing, women's health; nurse anesthesia (MSN); nurse midwifery (MSN); nurse practitioner (MSN), including acute care, ambulatory care, family, family/psychiatric, women's health; nursing (PhD); MBA/MSN. *Accreditation:* AACN; AANA/CANAEP (one or more programs are accredited); ACNM/ACME. *Program availability:* Part-time, online learning. Terminal master's awarded for partial completion of doctoral program. *Degree requirements:* For master's, thesis or alternative; for doctorate, comprehensive exam, thesis/dissertation. *Entrance requirements:* For master's and doctorate, GRE General Test. Additional exam requirements/recommendations for international students: Required—TOEFL (minimum score 520 paper-based). Electronic applications accepted. *Faculty research:* Substance abuse, injury and violence, symptom management.

University of Colorado Denver, College of Nursing, Aurora, CO 80045. Offers adult clinical nurse specialist (MS); adult nurse practitioner (MS); family nurse practitioner (MS); family psychiatric mental health nurse practitioner (MS); health care informatics (MS); nurse-midwifery (MS); nursing (DNP, PhD); nursing leadership and health care systems (MS); pediatric nurse practitioner (MS); special studies (MS); women's health (MS); MS/PhD. *Accreditation:* ACNM/ACME (one or more programs are accredited). *Program availability:* Part-time, evening/weekend, online learning. *Faculty:* 109 full-time (100 women), 55 part-time/adjunct (50 women). *Students:* 367 full-time (332 women), 141 part-time (118 women); includes 79 minority (16 Black or African American, non-Hispanic/Latino; 2 American Indian or Alaska Native, non-Hispanic/Latino; 8 Asian, non-Hispanic/Latino; 37 Hispanic/Latino; 16 Two or more races, non-Hispanic/Latino), 6 international. Average age 36. 321 applicants, 53% accepted, 145 enrolled. In 2015, 151 master's, 36 doctorates awarded. Terminal master's awarded for partial completion of doctoral program. *Degree requirements:* For master's, thesis optional; for doctorate, comprehensive exam, thesis/dissertation, 42 credits of coursework. *Entrance requirements:* For master's, GRE if cumulative undergraduate GPA is less than 3.0, undergraduate nursing degree from NLNAC- or CCNE-accredited school or university; completion of research and statistics courses with minimum grade of C; copy of current and unencumbered nursing license; for doctorate, GRE, bachelor's and/or master's degrees in nursing from NLN- or CCNE-accredited institution; portfolio; minimum undergraduate GPA of 3.0, graduate 3.5; graduate-level intermediate statistics and master's-level nursing theory courses with minimum B grade; interview. Additional exam requirements/recommendations for international students: Required—TOEFL (minimum score 560 paper-based; 83 iBT). *Application deadline:* For fall admission, 2/15 for domestic students, 1/15 for international students; for spring admission, 7/1 for domestic students, 6/1 for international students. Application fee: $50 ($75 for international students). Electronic applications accepted. *Expenses:* Contact institution. *Financial support:* In 2015–16, 148 students received support. Fellowships, research assistantships, teaching assistantships, Federal Work-Study, institutionally sponsored loans, scholarships/grants, traineeships, and unspecified assistantships available. Support available to part-time students. Financial award application deadline: 4/1; financial award applicants required to submit FAFSA. *Faculty research:* Biological and behavioral phenomena in pregnancy and postpartum; patterns of glycaemia during the insulin resistance of pregnancy; obesity, gestational diabetes, and relationship to neonatal adiposity; men's awareness and knowledge of male breast cancer; cognitive-behavioral therapy for chronic insomnia after breast cancer treatment; massage therapy for the treatment of tension-type headaches. *Total annual research expenditures:* $5.9 million. *Unit head:* Dr. Sarah Thompson, Dean, 303-724-1679, E-mail: sarah.a.thompson@ucdenver.edu. *Application contact:* Judy Campbell, Graduate Programs Coordinator, 303-724-8503, E-mail: judy.campbell@ucdenver.edu. Website: http://www.ucdenver.edu/academics/colleges/nursing/Pages/default.aspx

University of Delaware, College of Health Sciences, School of Nursing, Newark, DE 19716. Offers adult nurse practitioner (MSN, PMC); cardiopulmonary clinical nurse specialist (MSN, PMC); cardiopulmonary clinical nurse specialist/adult nurse practitioner (MSN, PMC); family nurse practitioner (MSN, PMC); gerontology clinical nurse specialist (MSN, PMC); gerontology clinical nurse specialist geriatric nurse practitioner (PMC); gerontology clinical nurse specialist/geriatric nurse practitioner (MSN); health services administration (MSN, PMC); nursing of children clinical nurse specialist (MSN, PMC); nursing of children clinical nurse specialist/pediatric nurse practitioner (MSN, PMC); oncology/immune deficiency clinical nurse specialist (MSN, PMC); oncology/immune deficiency clinical nurse specialist/adult nurse practitioner (MSN, PMC); perinatal/women's health clinical nurse specialist (MSN, PMC); perinatal/women's health clinical nurse specialist/women's health nurse practitioner (MSN, PMC); psychiatric nursing clinical nurse specialist (MSN, PMC). *Accreditation:* AACN. *Program availability:* Part-time, evening/weekend, online learning. *Degree requirements:* For master's, thesis optional. *Entrance requirements:* For master's, BSN, interview, RN license. Electronic applications accepted. *Faculty research:* Marriage and chronic illness, health promotion, congestive heart failure patient outcomes, school nursing, diabetes in children, culture, health disparities, cardiovascular, prison nursing, oncology, public policy, child obesity, smoking and teen pregnancy, blood pressure measurements, men's health.

University of Hawaii at Manoa, Graduate Division, School of Nursing and Dental Hygiene, Honolulu, HI 96822. Offers clinical nurse specialist (MS), including adult health, community mental health; nurse practitioner (MS), including adult health, community mental health, family nurse practitioner; nursing (PhD, Graduate Certificate); nursing administration (MS). *Accreditation:* AACN. *Program availability:* Part-time, online learning. *Faculty:* 32 full-time (27 women), 22 part-time/adjunct (11 women). *Students:* 167 full-time (145 women), 118 part-time (104 women); includes 128 minority (3 Black or African American, non-Hispanic/Latino; 1 American Indian or Alaska Native, non-Hispanic/Latino; 57 Asian, non-Hispanic/Latino; 14 Hispanic/Latino; 4 Native Hawaiian or other Pacific Islander, non-Hispanic/Latino; 49 Two or more races, non-Hispanic/Latino), 2 international. Average age 41. 253 applicants, 42% accepted, 88 enrolled. In 2015, 20 master's, 8 doctorates awarded. *Degree requirements:* For master's, thesis optional; for doctorate, comprehensive exam, thesis/dissertation. *Entrance requirements:* For master's, Hawaii RN license. Additional exam requirements/recommendations for international students: Required—TOEFL (minimum score 580 paper-based; 92 iBT), IELTS (minimum score 5). *Application deadline:* For fall admission, 2/1 for domestic and international students. Application fee: $100. *Expenses:* Contact institution. *Financial support:* In 2015–16, 78 fellowships (averaging $1,277 per year), 3 research assistantships (averaging $16,824 per year), 2 teaching assistantships (averaging $14,382 per year) were awarded. *Total annual research expenditures:* $1.8 million. *Unit head:* Mary Boland, Dean, 808-956-8522, Fax: 808-956-3257, E-mail: mgboland@hawaii.edu. *Application contact:* Maureen Shannon, Graduate Chair, 808-956-5201, Fax: 808-956-3257, E-mail: maureens@hawaii.edu. Website: http://www.hawaii.edu/graduatestudies/fields/html/departments/mno/nursing/nursing.htm

University of Houston, School of Nursing, Houston, TX 77204. Offers family nurse practitioner (MSN); nursing administration (MSN); nursing education (MSN). *Accreditation:* AACN. *Entrance requirements:* For master's, GRE or MAT, minimum GPA of 3.0 in last 60 hours of academic course work, valid Texas RN licensure, 2 letters of recommendation. Electronic applications accepted.

University of Illinois at Chicago, College of Nursing, Program in Nursing, Chicago, IL 60607-7128. Offers acute care clinical nurse specialist (MS); administrative nursing leadership (Certificate); adult nurse practitioner (MS); adult/geriatric nurse practitioner (MS); advanced community health nurse specialist (MS); family nurse practitioner (MS); geriatric clinical nurse specialist (MS); geriatric nurse practitioner (MS); nurse midwifery (MS); occupational health/advanced community health nurse specialist (MS); occupational health/family nurse practitioner (MS); pediatric nurse practitioner (MS); perinatal clinical nurse specialist (MS); school/advanced community health nurse specialist (MS); school/family nurse practitioner (MS); women's health nurse practitioner (MS). *Accreditation:* AACN. *Program availability:* Part-time. *Faculty:* 100 full-time (89 women), 89 part-time/adjunct (82 women). *Students:* 359 full-time (326 women), 280 part-time (249 women); includes 169 minority (43 Black or African American, non-Hispanic/Latino; 62 Asian, non-Hispanic/Latino; 56 Hispanic/Latino; 1 Native Hawaiian or other Pacific Islander, non-Hispanic/Latino; 7 Two or more races, non-Hispanic/Latino), 12 international. Average age 32. In 2015, 4 other advanced degrees awarded. *Degree requirements:* For master's, thesis or alternative. *Entrance requirements:* For master's, GRE General Test, minimum GPA of 2.75. Additional exam requirements/recommendations for international students: Required—TOEFL. *Application deadline:* For fall admission, 5/15 for domestic students, 2/15 for international students; for spring admission, 11/1 for domestic students, 7/15 for international students. Applications are processed on a rolling basis. Application fee: $60. Electronic applications accepted. *Expenses:* Tuition, state resident: full-time $11,480; part-time $3826 per credit. Tuition, nonresident: full-time $23,720; part-time $7906 per credit. *Required fees:* $1333 per semester. Part-time tuition and fees vary according to course load and program. *Financial support:* Fellowships with full tuition reimbursements, research assistantships with full tuition reimbursements, teaching assistantships with full tuition reimbursements, career-related internships or fieldwork, Federal Work-Study, institutionally sponsored loans, scholarships/grants, traineeships, tuition waivers (full and partial), and unspecified assistantships available. Support available to part-time students. Financial award application deadline: 3/1; financial award applicants required to submit FAFSA. *Unit head:* Dr. Terri E. Weaver, Dean, 312-996-7808, E-mail: teweaver@uic.edu. *Application contact:* Receptionist, 312-413-2550, E-mail: gradcoll@uic.edu. Website: http://www.nursing.uic.edu/academics-admissions/master-science#program-overview

University of Indianapolis, Graduate Programs, School of Nursing, Indianapolis, IN 46227-3697. Offers advanced practice nursing (DNP); family nurse practitioner (MSN); gerontological nurse practitioner (MSN); neonatal nurse practitioner (MSN); nurse-midwifery (MSN); nursing (MSN); nursing and health systems leadership (MSN); nursing education (MSN); women's health nurse practitioner (MSN); MBA/MSN. *Accreditation:* AACN; ACNM. *Entrance requirements:* For master's, minimum GPA of 3.0, interview, letters of recommendation, resume, IN nursing license, 1 year of professional practice; for doctorate, graduate of NLNAC- or CCNE-accredited nursing program; MSN or MA with nursing major and minimum cumulative GPA of 3.25; unencumbered RN license with eligibility for licensure in Indiana; completion of graduate-level statistics course within last 5 years with minimum grade of B; resume; essay; official transcripts from all academic institutions. Additional exam requirements/recommendations for international students: Required—TOEFL (minimum score 550 paper-based). Electronic applications accepted.

The University of Kansas, University of Kansas Medical Center, School of Nursing, Kansas City, KS 66160. Offers adult/gerontological clinical nurse specialist (PMC); adult/gerontological nurse practitioner (PMC); clinical research management (PMC); health care informatics (PMC); health professions educator (PMC); nurse midwife (PMC); nursing (MS, DNP, PhD); organizational leadership (PMC); psychiatric/mental health nurse practitioner (PMC); public health nursing (PMC). *Accreditation:* AACN; ACNM/ACME. *Program availability:* Part-time, 100% online, blended/hybrid learning. *Faculty:* 59. *Students:* 44 full-time (42 women), 261 part-time (238 women); includes 54 minority (22 Black or African American, non-Hispanic/Latino; 1 American Indian or Alaska Native, non-Hispanic/Latino; 12 Asian, non-Hispanic/Latino; 10 Hispanic/Latino; 9 Two or more races, non-Hispanic/Latino), 1 international. Average age 38. 95 applicants, 97% accepted, 74 enrolled. In 2015, 71 master's, 24 doctorates, 6 other advanced degrees awarded. Terminal master's awarded for partial completion of doctoral program. *Degree requirements:* For master's, comprehensive exam, thesis (for some programs), general oral exam; for doctorate, variable foreign language requirement, thesis/dissertation or alternative, comprehensive oral exam (for DNP); comprehensive written and oral exam, or three publications (for PhD). *Entrance requirements:* For master's, bachelor's degree in nursing, minimum GPA of 3.0, 1 year of clinical experience, RN license in KS and MO; for doctorate, GRE General Test (for PhD only), bachelor's degree in nursing, minimum GPA of 3.5, RN license in KS and MO. Additional exam requirements/recommendations for international students: Required—TOEFL. *Application deadline:* For fall admission, 4/1 for domestic and international students; for spring admission, 9/1 for domestic and international students. Application fee: $60. Electronic applications accepted. *Financial support:* Research assistantships with tuition reimbursements, teaching assistantships with tuition reimbursements, scholarships/grants, and traineeships available. Financial award application deadline: 3/1; financial award applicants required to submit FAFSA. *Faculty research:* Breastfeeding practices of teen mothers, national database of nursing quality indicators, caregiving of families of patients using technology in the home, simulation in nursing education, diaphragm fatigue. *Total annual research expenditures:* $4.6 million. *Unit head:* Dr. Sally Maliski, Dean, 913-588-1601, Fax: 913-588-1660, E-mail: smaliski@kumc.edu. *Application contact:* Dr. Pamela K. Barnes, Associate Dean, Student Affairs, 913-588-1619, Fax: 913-588-1615, E-mail: pbarnes2@kumc.edu. Website: http://nursing.kumc.edu

University of Louisville, Graduate School, School of Nursing, Louisville, KY 40202. Offers adult gerontology nurse practitioner (MSN, DNP); education and administration (MSN); family nurse practitioner (MSN, DNP); neonatal nurse practitioner (MSN, DNP); nursing research (PhD); psychiatric/mental health nurse practitioner (MSN, DNP); women's health nurse practitioner (MSN). *Accreditation:* AACN. *Program availability:* Part-time. *Faculty:* 53 full-time (48 women), 27 part-time/adjunct (23 women). *Students:* 110 full-time (99 women), 33 part-time (29 women); includes 17 minority (11 Black or African American, non-Hispanic/Latino; 1 Asian, non-Hispanic/Latino; 2 Hispanic/Latino; 3 Two or more races, non-Hispanic/Latino), 5 international. Average age 34. 62 applicants, 68% accepted, 40 enrolled. In 2015, 41 master's awarded. *Degree requirements:* For doctorate, comprehensive exam (for some programs), thesis/dissertation (for some programs). *Entrance requirements:* For master's, bachelor's

Nursing and Healthcare Administration

degree in nursing, minimum GPA of 3.0, RN license; for doctorate, GRE General Test (for PhD), 3 letters of professional reference. Additional exam requirements/recommendations for international students: Required—TOEFL (minimum score 560 paper-based; 79 iBT). *Application deadline:* For fall admission, 3/1 priority date for domestic students, 3/1 for international students. Applications are processed on a rolling basis. Application fee: $60. Electronic applications accepted. *Expenses:* Tuition, state resident: full-time $11,664; part-time $649 per credit hour. Tuition, nonresident: full-time $24,274; part-time $1350 per credit hour. *Required fees:* $196. Tuition and fees vary according to program and reciprocity agreements. *Financial support:* In 2015–16, 722,568 students received support, including 10 research assistantships with full tuition reimbursements available (averaging $20,000 per year), 2 teaching assistantships with full tuition reimbursements available (averaging $15,000 per year); fellowships with full tuition reimbursements available, scholarships/grants, and unspecified assistantships also available. Financial award application deadline: 2/15; financial award applicants required to submit FAFSA. *Faculty research:* Children and adolescents with chronic illnesses, women's mental health and parenting, asthma and environmental health, type 2 diabetes self-management in adults, health disparities and community engagement. *Total annual research expenditures:* $722,568. *Unit head:* Dr. Marcia J. Hern, Dean, 502-852-8300, Fax: 502-852-8783, E-mail: m.hern@louisville.edu. *Application contact:* Trish Hart, Assistant Dean for Student Affairs, 502-852-5825, Fax: 502-852-8783, E-mail: trish.hart@louisville.edu.
Website: http://www.louisville.edu/nursing/

University of Mary, School of Health Sciences, Division of Nursing, Bismarck, ND 58504-9652. Offers family nurse practitioner (DNP); nurse administrator (MSN); nursing educator (MSN); MSN/MBA. *Accreditation:* AACN. *Program availability:* Part-time, evening/weekend, online learning. *Degree requirements:* For master's, comprehensive exam (for some programs), thesis (for some programs), internship (family nurse practitioner), teaching practice. *Entrance requirements:* For master's, minimum GPA of 2.75 in nursing, interview, letters of recommendation, criminal background check, immunizations, statement of professional goals. Additional exam requirements/recommendations for international students: Required—TOEFL (minimum score 500 paper-based; 71 iBT). *Application deadline:* Applications are processed on a rolling basis. Application fee: $40. Electronic applications accepted. *Financial support:* Fellowships with partial tuition reimbursements and teaching assistantships with partial tuition reimbursements available. Financial award application deadline: 8/1; financial award applicants required to submit FAFSA. *Faculty research:* Gerontology issues, rural nursing, health policy, primary care, women's health.

University of Mary Hardin-Baylor, Graduate Studies in Nursing, Belton, TX 76513. Offers clinical nurse leader (MSN); family nurse practitioner (MSN, Post-Master's Certificate); nurse educator (Post-Master's Certificate); nursing education (MSN). *Accreditation:* AACN. *Program availability:* Part-time, evening/weekend. *Faculty:* 6 full-time (all women), 3 part-time/adjunct (2 women). *Students:* 54 full-time (47 women), 2 part-time (1 woman); includes 14 minority (10 Black or African American, non-Hispanic/Latino; 3 Hispanic/Latino; 1 Two or more races, non-Hispanic/Latino), 1 international. Average age 32. 46 applicants, 70% accepted, 26 enrolled. In 2015, 47 master's awarded. *Degree requirements:* For master's, practicum. *Entrance requirements:* For master's, full-time RN for 1 year, BSN, minimum GPA of 3.0 in last 60 hours of undergraduate program, two letters of recommendation. Additional exam requirements/recommendations for international students: Required—TOEFL (minimum score 100 iBT), IELTS (minimum score 7). *Application deadline:* For fall admission, 4/15 for domestic students, 4/30 priority date for international students; for spring admission, 11/1 for domestic students, 9/30 priority date for international students. Applications are processed on a rolling basis. Application fee: $35 ($135 for international students). Electronic applications accepted. *Expenses:* Tuition, area resident: Part-time $815 per credit hour. Tuition and fees vary according to course load and degree level. *Financial support:* Applicants required to submit FAFSA. *Unit head:* Dr. Carrie Johnson, Associate Professor/Director, Master of Science in Nursing Programs, 254-295-4178, E-mail: cjohnson@umhb.edu. *Application contact:* Melissa Williams, Director, Graduate Student Services and Engagement, 254-295-4020, Fax: 254-295-5038, E-mail: mwilliams@umhb.edu.
Website: http://graduate.umhb.edu/nursing/

University of Maryland, Baltimore, Graduate School, School of Nursing, Master's Program in Nursing, Baltimore, MD 21201. Offers community health nursing (MS); gerontological nursing (MS); maternal-child nursing (MS); medical-surgical nursing (MS); nurse-midwifery education (MS); nursing administration (MS); nursing education (MS); nursing health policy (MS); primary care nursing (MS); psychiatric nursing (MS); MS/MBA. MS/MBA offered jointly with University of Baltimore. *Accreditation:* AACN; AANA/CANAEP. *Program availability:* Part-time. *Degree requirements:* For master's, comprehensive exam (for some programs), thesis or alternative. *Entrance requirements:* For master's, minimum GPA of 2.75, course work in statistics, BS in nursing. Additional exam requirements/recommendations for international students: Required—TOEFL (minimum score 550 paper-based; 80 iBT); Recommended—IELTS (minimum score 7). Electronic applications accepted. Tuition and fees vary according to program.

University of Massachusetts Amherst, Graduate School, College of Nursing, Amherst, MA 01003. Offers adult gerontology primary care nurse practitioner (DNP); clinical nurse leader (MS); family nurse practitioner (DNP); nursing (PhD); public health nurse leader (DNP). *Accreditation:* AACN. *Program availability:* Part-time, online learning. Terminal master's awarded for partial completion of doctoral program. *Degree requirements:* For master's, thesis optional; for doctorate, comprehensive exam, thesis/dissertation. *Entrance requirements:* Additional exam requirements/recommendations for international students: Required—TOEFL (minimum score 550 paper-based; 80 iBT), IELTS (minimum score 6.5). Electronic applications accepted. *Faculty research:* Health of older adults and their caretakers, mental health of individuals and families, health of children and adolescents, power and decision-making, transcultural health.

University of Massachusetts Medical School, Graduate School of Nursing, Worcester, MA 01655-0115. Offers adult gerontological acute care nurse practitioner (DNP, Post Master's Certificate); adult gerontological primary care nurse practitioner (DNP, Post Master's Certificate); family nursing practitioner (DNP); nurse administrator (DNP); nurse educator (MS, Post Master's Certificate); nursing (PhD); nursing practitioner (DNP); population health (MS). *Accreditation:* AACN. *Faculty:* 18 full-time (15 women), 28 part-time/adjunct (22 women). *Students:* 143 full-time (119 women), 27 part-time (25 women); includes 28 minority (15 Black or African American, non-Hispanic/Latino; 10 Asian, non-Hispanic/Latino; 3 Hispanic/Latino), 1 international. Average age 34. 129 applicants, 68% accepted, 56 enrolled. In 2015, 43 master's, 10 doctorates, 2 other advanced degrees awarded. *Degree requirements:* For doctorate, thesis/dissertation (for some programs), comprehensive exam (for PhD); capstone project and manuscript (for DNP). *Entrance requirements:* For master's, GRE General Test, bachelor's degree in nursing, course work in statistics, unrestricted Massachusetts license as registered nurse; for doctorate, GRE General Test, bachelor's or master's degree; for Post Master's Certificate, GRE General Test, MS in nursing. Additional exam requirements/recommendations for international students: Required—TOEFL. *Application deadline:* For fall admission, 12/1 priority date for domestic students. Applications are processed on a rolling basis. Application fee: $60. Electronic

applications accepted. *Expenses:* $10,994 resident per year; $18,210 non-resident per year. *Financial support:* In 2015–16, 31 students received support. Institutionally sponsored loans, scholarships/grants, traineeships, and tuition waivers (partial) available. Support available to part-time students. Financial award application deadline: 5/16; financial award applicants required to submit FAFSA. *Faculty research:* Health literacy, social justice, HIV prevention, cancer-related decision making, nursing education. *Total annual research expenditures:* $650,993. *Unit head:* Dr. Joan Vitello-Cicciu, Dean, 508-856-5081, Fax: 508-856-6552, E-mail: joan.vitello@umassmed.edu. *Application contact:* Diane Brescia, Admissions Coordinator, 508-856-3488, Fax: 508-856-5851, E-mail: diane.brescia@umassmed.edu.
Website: http://www.umassmed.edu/gsn/

University of Memphis, Loewenberg College of Nursing, Memphis, TN 38152. Offers executive leadership (MSN); family nurse practitioner (MSN); nursing (Graduate Certificate); nursing administration (MSN); nursing education (MSN). *Accreditation:* AACN. *Program availability:* Part-time, evening/weekend, online learning. *Faculty:* 12 full-time (all women), 3 part-time/adjunct (2 women). *Students:* 34 full-time (32 women), 220 part-time (196 women); includes 91 minority (80 Black or African American, non-Hispanic/Latino; 8 Asian, non-Hispanic/Latino; 1 Hispanic/Latino; 2 Two or more races, non-Hispanic/Latino). Average age 36. 165 applicants, 48% accepted, 27 enrolled. In 2015, 73 master's, 3 other advanced degrees awarded. *Degree requirements:* For master's, comprehensive exam, thesis optional, scholarly project; completion of clinical practicum hours. *Entrance requirements:* For master's, NCLEX Exam, interview. Additional exam requirements/recommendations for international students: Required—TOEFL (minimum score 550 paper-based; 79 iBT). *Application deadline:* For fall admission, 2/15 for domestic and international students; for spring admission, 10/1 for domestic and international students. Application fee: $35 ($60 for international students). *Financial support:* In 2015–16, 147 students received support. Federal Work-Study and scholarships/grants available. Financial award application deadline: 2/15; financial award applicants required to submit FAFSA. *Faculty research:* Technology in nursing, nurse retention, cultural competence, health policy, health access. *Total annual research expenditures:* $560,619. *Unit head:* Dr. Robert Koch, Associate Dean, 901-678-3908, Fax: 901-678-4907, E-mail: rakoch@memphis.edu. *Application contact:* Dr. Karen Weddle-West, Information Contact, 901-678-2531, Fax: 901-678-5023, E-mail: gradsch@memphis.edu.
Website: http://www.memphis.edu/nursing

University of Minnesota, Twin Cities Campus, Graduate School, School of Nursing, Program in Nursing and Health Care Systems Administration, Minneapolis, MN 55455-0213. Offers MS. *Accreditation:* AACN. *Program availability:* Part-time. *Degree requirements:* For master's, final oral exam, project or thesis. *Entrance requirements:* Additional exam requirements/recommendations for international students: Required—TOEFL (minimum score 586 paper-based).

University of Missouri, Office of Research and Graduate Studies, Sinclair School of Nursing, Columbia, MO 65211. Offers adult-gerontology clinical nurse specialist (DNP, Certificate); family nurse practitioner (DNP); family psychiatric and mental health nurse practitioner (DNP); nursing (MS, PhD); nursing leadership and innovations in health care (DNP); pediatric clinical nurse specialist (DNP, Certificate); pediatric nurse practitioner (DNP). *Accreditation:* AACN. *Program availability:* Part-time. *Degree requirements:* For master's, thesis optional, oral exam; for doctorate, thesis/dissertation. *Entrance requirements:* For master's, GRE General Test, BSN, minimum GPA of 3.0 during last 60 hours, nursing license. Additional exam requirements/recommendations for international students: Required—TOEFL (minimum score 550 paper-based; 79 iBT). *Application deadline:* For fall admission, 2/1 priority date for domestic and international students. Applications are processed on a rolling basis. Application fee: $55 ($75 for international students). Electronic applications accepted. *Financial support:* Fellowships, research assistantships, teaching assistantships, career-related internships or fieldwork, institutionally sponsored loans, scholarships/grants, traineeships, health care benefits, tuition waivers (full), and unspecified assistantships available. Support available to part-time students.
Website: http://nursing.missouri.edu/

University of Missouri–Kansas City, School of Nursing and Health Studies, Kansas City, MO 64108. Offers adult clinical nurse specialist (MSN), including adult nurse practitioner, women's health nurse practitioner (MSN, DNP); adult clinical nursing practice (DNP), including adult gerontology nurse practitioner, women's health nurse practitioner (MSN, DNP); clinical nursing practice (DNP), including family nurse practitioner; family nurse practitioner (MSN); neonatal nurse practitioner (MSN); nurse educator (MSN); nurse executive (MSN); nursing (PhD); nursing practice (DNP); pediatric clinical nursing practice (DNP), including pediatric nurse practitioner; pediatric nurse practitioner (MSN). *Accreditation:* AACN. *Program availability:* Part-time, online learning. *Faculty:* 44 full-time (40 women), 47 part-time/adjunct (45 women). *Students:* 62 full-time (43 women), 259 part-time (239 women); includes 61 minority (28 Black or African American, non-Hispanic/Latino; 3 American Indian or Alaska Native, non-Hispanic/Latino; 16 Asian, non-Hispanic/Latino; 10 Hispanic/Latino; 4 Two or more races, non-Hispanic/Latino). Average age 35. 102 applicants, 35% accepted, 36 enrolled. In 2015, 116 master's, 23 doctorates awarded. *Degree requirements:* For master's, thesis or alternative. *Entrance requirements:* For master's, minimum undergraduate GPA of 3.2; for doctorate, GRE, 3 letters of reference. Additional exam requirements/recommendations for international students: Required—TOEFL (minimum score 550 paper-based; 80 iBT). *Application deadline:* For fall admission, 2/1 priority date for domestic and international students; for spring admission, 9/1 priority date for domestic and international students. Application fee: $45 ($50 for international students). *Financial support:* In 2015–16, 2 teaching assistantships with partial tuition reimbursements (averaging $6,650 per year) were awarded; fellowships, research assistantships, career-related internships or fieldwork, Federal Work-Study, institutionally sponsored loans, and tuition waivers (full and partial) also available. Support available to part-time students. Financial award application deadline: 3/1; financial award applicants required to submit FAFSA. *Faculty research:* Geriatrics/gerontology, children's pain, neonatology, Alzheimer's care, cancer caregivers. *Unit head:* Dr. Ann Cary, Dean, 816-235-1723, Fax: 816-235-1701, E-mail: caryah@umkc.edu. *Application contact:* Judy Jellison, Coordinator for Admissions and Recruitment, 816-235-1740, Fax: 816-235-1701, E-mail: jellisonj@umkc.edu.
Website: http://nursing.umkc.edu/

The University of North Carolina at Chapel Hill, School of Nursing, Chapel Hill, NC 27599-7460. Offers advanced practice registered nurse (DNP); health care systems (DNP); nursing (MSN, PhD, PMC), including administration (MSN), adult gerontology primary care nurse practitioner (MSN), clinical nurse leader (MSN), education (MSN), informatics (MSN, PMC), nursing leadership (PMC), outcomes management (MSN), primary care family nurse practitioner (MSN), primary care pediatric nurse practitioner (MSN), psychiatric/mental health nurse practitioner (MSN, PMC). *Accreditation:* ACEN (one or more programs are accredited). *Program availability:* Part-time. *Faculty:* 86 full-time (78 women), 44 part-time/adjunct (40 women). *Students:* 208 full-time (186 women), 128 part-time (116 women); includes 109 minority (49 Black or African American, non-Hispanic/Latino; 4 American Indian or Alaska Native, non-Hispanic/Latino; 32 Asian, non-Hispanic/Latino; 7 Hispanic/Latino; 17 Two or more races, non-

Hispanic/Latino), 17 international. Average age 33. 624 applicants, 25% accepted, 150 enrolled. In 2015, 91 master's, 14 doctorates awarded. *Degree requirements:* For master's, comprehensive exam, thesis; for doctorate, thesis/dissertation, 3 exams; for PMC, thesis. *Entrance requirements:* Additional exam requirements/recommendations for international students: Required—TOEFL (minimum score 575 paper-based; 89 iBT), IELTS (minimum score 8). *Application deadline:* For fall admission, 12/15 for domestic and international students. Application fee: $85. Electronic applications accepted. *Financial support:* In 2015–16, 8 fellowships with full tuition reimbursements, 6 research assistantships with partial tuition reimbursements (averaging $8,000 per year), 10 teaching assistantships with partial tuition reimbursements (averaging $8,000 per year) were awarded; scholarships/grants, traineeships, health care benefits, and unspecified assistantships also available. Support available to part-time students. Financial award application deadline: 3/1; financial award applicants required to submit FAFSA. *Faculty research:* Preventing and managing chronic illness, reducing health disparities, Improving healthcare quality and patient outcomes, understanding biobehavioral and genetic bases of health and illness, developing innovative ways to enhance science and its clinical translation. *Unit head:* Donna S. Havens, PhD, RN, Dean/Professor, 919-966-3731, Fax: 919-966-3540, E-mail: dhavens@email.unc.edu. *Application contact:* Emily Sayed, Assistant Director, Graduate Admissions, 919-966-4260, Fax: 919-966-3540, E-mail: sayed@unc.edu.
Website: http://nursing.unc.edu

The University of North Carolina at Charlotte, College of Health and Human Services, School of Nursing, Charlotte, NC 28223-0001. Offers adult-gerontology acute care nurse practitioner (MSN, Post-Master's Certificate); advanced clinical nursing (MSN); community public health nursing (MSN); family nurse practitioner across the lifespan (MSN, Post-Master's Certificate); nurse administrator (MSN, Graduate Certificate); nurse anesthesia (MSN, Post-Master's Certificate); nurse educator (MSN, Graduate Certificate); nursing (DNP); nursing systems/population (MSN). *Accreditation:* AACN. *Program availability:* Part-time, blended/hybrid learning. *Faculty:* 26 full-time (25 women), 4 part-time/adjunct (3 women). *Students:* 109 full-time (89 women), 112 part-time (107 women); includes 46 minority (37 Black or African American, non-Hispanic/Latino; 3 Asian, non-Hispanic/Latino; 5 Hispanic/Latino; 1 Two or more races, non-Hispanic/Latino). Average age 33. 321 applicants, 34% accepted, 84 enrolled. In 2015, 76 master's, 4 doctorates, 7 other advanced degrees awarded. Terminal master's awarded for partial completion of doctoral program. *Degree requirements:* For master's, practicum, synthesis and integration or thesis, residency, internship (varies by program); for doctorate, thesis/dissertation or alternative, residency; for other advanced degree, practicum. *Entrance requirements:* For master's, GRE General Test, unencumbered license as Registered Nurse in North Carolina; BSN from nationally-accredited program; one year of professional nursing practice in acute/critical care; minimum overall GPA of 3.0 in the last degree and 60 hours of nursing coursework; completion of an undergraduate statistics course with minimum grade of C; statement of purpose; for doctorate, GRE or MAT, master's degree in nursing in an advanced nursing practice specialty from nationally-accredited program; minimum overall GPA of 3.5 in MSN program; current RN licensure in U.S. at time of application with eligibility for NC licensure; for other advanced degree, GRE. Additional exam requirements/recommendations for international students: Required—TOEFL (minimum score 557 paper-based, 83 iBT) or IELTS (minimum score 6.5). *Application deadline:* For fall admission, 2/1 for domestic and international students; for spring admission, 10/1 priority date for domestic and international students; for summer admission, 4/1 priority date for domestic and international students. Applications are processed on a rolling basis. Application fee: $75. Electronic applications accepted. *Expenses:* Contact institution. *Financial support:* In 2015–16, 9 students received support, including 5 research assistantships (averaging $4,850 per year), 3 teaching assistantships (averaging $2,911 per year); career-related internships or fieldwork, institutionally sponsored loans, scholarships/grants, traineeships, unspecified assistantships, and administrative assistantships also available. Support available to part-time students. Financial award application deadline: 3/1; financial award applicants required to submit FAFSA. *Faculty research:* Improving care outcomes for the elderly; vulnerable populations; symptom management; self management/health promotion strategies of older adults; migration and maternal child health; health disparities, health literacy, and access to healthcare in Latino adults with diabetes; psychiatric nursing. *Total annual research expenditures:* $875,169. *Unit head:* Dr. Dee Baldwin, Associate Dean, 704-687-7952, Fax: 704-687-6017, E-mail: dbaldwi5@uncc.edu. *Application contact:* Kathy B. Giddings, Director of Graduate Admissions, 704-687-5503, Fax: 704-687-1668, E-mail: gradadm@uncc.edu.
Website: http://nursing.uncc.edu/

The University of North Carolina at Greensboro, Graduate School, School of Nursing, Greensboro, NC 27412-5001. Offers adult clinical nurse specialist (MSN, PMC); adult/gerontological nurse practitioner (MSN, PMC); nurse anesthesia (MSN, PMC); nursing (PhD); nursing administration (MSN); nursing education (MSN); MSN/MBA. *Accreditation:* AACN; AANA/CANAEP; ACEN. *Degree requirements:* For master's, thesis or alternative. *Entrance requirements:* For master's, GRE General Test or MAT, BSN, clinical experience, liability insurance, RN license; for PMC, liability insurance, MSN, RN license. Additional exam requirements/recommendations for international students: Required—TOEFL. Electronic applications accepted.

The University of North Carolina at Pembroke, Graduate School, Department of Nursing, Pembroke, NC 28372-1510. Offers clinical nurse leader (MSN); nurse educator (MSN); rural case manager (MSN). *Program availability:* Part-time. Application fee: $45 ($60 for international students). *Unit head:* Dr. Jennifer W. Twaddell, Interim Chair, 910-775-4142, Fax: 910-521-6751, E-mail: jennifer.twaddell@uncp.edu. *Application contact:* Dr. Jennifer W. Twaddell, Interim Chair, 910-775-4142, Fax: 910-521-6751, E-mail: jennifer.twaddell@uncp.edu.
Website: http://www.uncp.edu/nursing/

University of North Florida, Brooks College of Health, School of Nursing, Jacksonville, FL 32224. Offers clinical nurse leader (MSN); clinical nurse specialist (MSN); family nurse practitioner (Certificate); nurse anesthetist (MSN); nursing practice (DNP); primary care nurse practitioner (MSN). *Accreditation:* AACN; AANA/CANAEP. *Program availability:* Part-time. *Faculty:* 23 full-time (17 women), 2 part-time/adjunct (1 woman). *Students:* 108 full-time (90 women), 117 part-time (93 women); includes 54 minority (17 Black or African American, non-Hispanic/Latino; 1 American Indian or Alaska Native, non-Hispanic/Latino; 13 Asian, non-Hispanic/Latino; 17 Hispanic/Latino; 1 Native Hawaiian or other Pacific Islander, non-Hispanic/Latino; 5 Two or more races, non-Hispanic/Latino), 3 international. Average age 36. 136 applicants, 81% accepted, 74 enrolled. In 2015, 46 master's, 6 doctorates awarded. *Degree requirements:* For master's, thesis optional. *Entrance requirements:* For master's, GRE General Test, minimum GPA of 3.0 in last 60 hours of course work, BSN, clinical experience, resume; for doctorate, GRE, master's degree in nursing specialty from nationally-accredited program; national certification in one of the following APRN roles: CNE, CNM, CNS, CRNA, CNP; minimum graduate GPA of 3.3; three letters of reference which address academic ability and clinical skills; active license as registered nurse or advanced practice registered nurse. Additional exam requirements/recommendations for international students: Required—TOEFL (minimum score 500 paper-based; 61 iBT). *Application deadline:* For fall admission, 3/15 for domestic students, 4/1 for international

students. Application fee: $30. Electronic applications accepted. *Expenses:* Tuition, state resident: part-time $408.10 per credit hour. Tuition, nonresident: part-time $932.61 per credit hour. *Required fees:* $111.81 per credit hour. Tuition and fees vary according to course load, campus/location and program. *Financial support:* In 2015–16, 35 students received support. Research assistantships available. Financial award application deadline: 4/1; financial award applicants required to submit FAFSA. *Faculty research:* Teen pregnancy, diabetes, ethical decision-making, family caregivers. *Total annual research expenditures:* $39,413. *Unit head:* Dr. Li Loriz, Chair, 904-620-1053, E-mail: lloriz@unf.edu. *Application contact:* Beth Dibble, Assistant Director of Admissions for Nursing and Physical Therapy, 904-620-2684, Fax: 904-620-1832, E-mail: nursingadmissions@unf.edu.
Website: http://www.unf.edu/brooks/nursing

University of Pennsylvania, School of Nursing, Health Leadership Program, Philadelphia, PA 19104. Offers MSN. *Accreditation:* AACN. *Program availability:* Part-time. *Students:* 2 full-time (1 woman), 27 part-time (26 women); includes 6 minority (2 Black or African American, non-Hispanic/Latino; 3 Asian, non-Hispanic/Latino; 1 Two or more races, non-Hispanic/Latino). Average age 33. 18 applicants, 78% accepted, 7 enrolled. In 2015, 6 master's awarded. *Expenses: Tuition, area resident:* Full-time $31,068; part-time $5762 per course. *Required fees:* $3200; $336 per course. Full-time tuition and fees vary according to degree level, program and student level. Part-time tuition and fees vary according to course load, degree level and program. *Financial support:* Application deadline: 4/1.

University of Pennsylvania, School of Nursing, Program in Nursing and Health Care Administration, Philadelphia, PA 19104. Offers MSN; MBA/MSN. *Accreditation:* AACN. *Program availability:* Part-time. *Students:* 7 full-time (6 women), 24 part-time (17 women); includes 8 minority (1 Black or African American, non-Hispanic/Latino; 4 Asian, non-Hispanic/Latino; 1 Hispanic/Latino; 2 Two or more races, non-Hispanic/Latino), 1 international. Average age 29. 14 applicants, 86% accepted, 9 enrolled. In 2015, 7 master's awarded. Terminal master's awarded for partial completion of doctoral program. *Expenses: Tuition, area resident:* Full-time $31,068; part-time $5762 per course. *Required fees:* $3200; $336 per course. Full-time tuition and fees vary according to degree level, program and student level. Part-time tuition and fees vary according to course load, degree level and program.

University of Phoenix–Bay Area Campus, College of Nursing, San Jose, CA 95134-1805. Offers education (MHA); gerontology (MHA); health administration (MHA, DHA); informatics (MHA, MSN); nursing (MSN, PhD); nursing/health care education (MSN); MSN/MBA. *Program availability:* Evening/weekend, online learning. *Degree requirements:* For master's, thesis (for some programs). *Entrance requirements:* For master's, minimum undergraduate GPA of 2.5, 3 years of work experience, RN license. Additional exam requirements/recommendations for international students: Required—TOEFL (minimum score 550 paper-based; 79 iBT). Electronic applications accepted.

University of Phoenix–Washington D.C. Campus, College of Nursing, Washington, DC 20001. Offers education (MHA); gerontology (MHA); health administration (MHA, DHA); informatics (MHA, MSN); nursing (MSN, PhD); nursing/health care education (MSN); MSN/MBA; MSN/MHA.

University of Pittsburgh, School of Nursing, Nurse Specialty Role Program, Pittsburgh, PA 15260. Offers clinical nurse leader (MSN); nursing administration (DNP); nursing informatics (MSN). *Accreditation:* AACN. *Program availability:* Part-time. *Students:* 4 full-time (2 women), 67 part-time (54 women); includes 5 minority (3 Black or African American, non-Hispanic/Latino; 2 Asian, non-Hispanic/Latino), 2 international. Average age 36. 24 applicants, 63% accepted, 12 enrolled. In 2015, 14 master's, 11 doctorates awarded. *Degree requirements:* For master's, comprehensive exam, thesis optional. *Entrance requirements:* For master's, GRE or MAT, BSN, RN license, 3 letters of recommendation, personal essay, resume, course work in statistics, 1-3 years of nursing experience; for doctorate, BSN/MSN, RN license, 3 letters of recommendation, personal essay, resume, course work in statistics, 1-3 years of nursing experience. Additional exam requirements/recommendations for international students: Required—TOEFL (minimum score 600 paper-based; 100 iBT). *Application deadline:* For fall admission, 5/1 priority date for domestic students, 2/15 priority date for international students. Application fee: $50. Electronic applications accepted. *Expenses:* Contact institution. *Financial support:* In 2015–16, 1 student received support, including 1 fellowship with tuition reimbursement available (averaging $9,125 per year). Financial award application deadline: 3/15. *Faculty research:* Behavioral management of chronic disorders, patient management in critical care, consumer informatics, genetic applications (molecular genetics and psychosocial implications), technology for nurses and patients to improve care. *Unit head:* Dr. Sandra Engberg, Associate Dean for Clinical Education, 412-624-3835, Fax: 412-624-8521, E-mail: sje1@pitt.edu. *Application contact:* Laurie Lapsley, Administrator of Graduate Student Services, 412-624-9670, Fax: 412-624-2409, E-mail: lapsleyl@pitt.edu.
Website: http://www.nursing.pitt.edu/

University of Rochester, School of Nursing, Rochester, NY 14642. Offers adult gerontological acute care nurse practitioner (MS); clinical nurse leader (MS); family nurse practitioner (MS); family psychiatric mental health nurse practitioner (MS); health care organization management and leadership (MS); health practice research (PhD); nursing (DNP); nursing education (MS); pediatric nurse practitioner (MS); pediatric nurse practitioner/neonatal nurse practitioner (MS). *Accreditation:* AACN. *Program availability:* Part-time, online learning. *Faculty:* 56 full-time (45 women), 63 part-time/adjunct (55 women). *Students:* 21 full-time (20 women), 212 part-time (175 women); includes 35 minority (12 Black or African American, non-Hispanic/Latino; 1 American Indian or Alaska Native, non-Hispanic/Latino; 10 Asian, non-Hispanic/Latino; 7 Hispanic/Latino; 5 Two or more races, non-Hispanic/Latino), 2 international. Average age 35. 111 applicants, 68% accepted, 71 enrolled. In 2015, 52 master's, 9 doctorates awarded. Terminal master's awarded for partial completion of doctoral program. *Degree requirements:* For master's, comprehensive exam (for some programs); for doctorate, thesis/dissertation. *Entrance requirements:* For master's, BS in nursing, minimum GPA of 3.0, course work in statistics; for doctorate, GRE General Test (for PhD), MS in nursing, minimum GPA of 3.5. Additional exam requirements/recommendations for international students: Required—TOEFL (minimum score 560 paper-based; 88 iBT) or IELTS (minimum score 6.5) recommended. *Application deadline:* For fall admission, 4/1 for domestic and international students; for spring admission, 9/1 for domestic and international students; for summer admission, 1/2 for domestic and international students. Application fee: $50. Electronic applications accepted. *Expenses: Tuition, area resident:* Full-time $47,450; part-time $1482 per credit hour. *Required fees:* $528. Tuition and fees vary according to program. *Financial support:* In 2015–16, 52 students received support, including 2 fellowships with tuition reimbursements available (averaging $30,000 per year); scholarships/grants, traineeships, health care benefits, tuition waivers (full and partial), and unspecified assistantships also available. Support available to part-time students. Financial award application deadline: 6/30. *Faculty research:* Symptom assessment and self-management of chronic illness, health promotion and illness prevention, nursing intervention research with vulnerable populations, palliative care, aging. *Total annual research expenditures:* $2.1 million. *Unit head:* Dr. Kathy H. Rideout, Dean, 585-273-8902, Fax: 585-273-1268, E-mail: kathy_rideout@urmc.rochester.edu. *Application contact:* Elaine Andolina, Director of

Nursing and Healthcare Administration

Admissions, 585-275-2375, Fax: 585-756-8299, E-mail: elaine_andolina@urmc.rochester.edu.
Website: http://www.son.rochester.edu

University of St. Francis, Leach College of Nursing, Joliet, IL 60435-6169. Offers family nurse practitioner (MSN, Post-Master's Certificate); family psychology/mental health nurse practitioner (MSN, Post-Master's Certificate); nursing administration (MSN); nursing education (MSN); nursing practice (DNP); teaching in nursing (Certificate). *Accreditation:* AACN. *Program availability:* Part-time, evening/weekend, 100% online. *Faculty:* 7 full-time (all women), 16 part-time/adjunct (13 women). *Students:* 82 full-time (72 women), 356 part-time (325 women); includes 147 minority (62 Black or African American, non-Hispanic/Latino; 1 American Indian or Alaska Native, non-Hispanic/Latino; 27 Asian, non-Hispanic/Latino; 45 Hispanic/Latino; 3 Native Hawaiian or other Pacific Islander, non-Hispanic/Latino; 9 Two or more races, non-Hispanic/Latino). Average age 41. 338 applicants, 42% accepted, 100 enrolled. In 2015, 91 master's, 9 doctorates, 6 other advanced degrees awarded. *Entrance requirements:* Additional exam requirements/recommendations for international students: Required—TOEFL (minimum score 550 paper-based; 79 iBT), IELTS (minimum score 6). *Application deadline:* Applications are processed on a rolling basis. Application fee: $30. Electronic applications accepted. Application fee is waived when completed online. *Expenses:* Contact institution. *Financial support:* In 2015–16, 149 students received support. Career-related internships or fieldwork, scholarships/grants, and tuition waivers (partial) available. Support available to part-time students. Financial award applicants required to submit FAFSA. *Unit head:* Dr. Carol Wilson, Dean, 815-740-3840, Fax: 815-740-4243, E-mail: cwilson@stfrancis.edu. *Application contact:* Sandra Sloka, Director of Admissions for Graduate and Degree Completion Programs, 800-735-7500, Fax: 815-740-3431, E-mail: ssloka@stfrancis.edu.
Website: http://www.stfrancis.edu/academics/college-of-nursing/

University of Saint Mary, Graduate Programs, Program in Nursing, Leavenworth, KS 66048-5082. Offers nurse administrator (MSN); nurse educator (MSN). *Program availability:* Part-time, online only, 100% online. *Students:* 19 full-time (all women), 12 part-time (11 women); includes 5 minority (3 Black or African American, non-Hispanic/Latino; 1 Hispanic/Latino; 1 Two or more races, non-Hispanic/Latino). Average age 41. *Degree requirements:* For master's, practicum. *Entrance requirements:* For master's, BSN from CCNE- or NLNAC-accredited baccalaureate nursing program at regionally-accredited institution. Application fee: $25. *Expenses:* $580 per credit hour. *Unit head:* Karen R. Kidder, Chair, 877-307-4915, Fax: 913-345-2802. *Application contact:* Dr. Linda King, Director, 877-307-4915, Fax: 913-345-2802.
Website: http://online.stmary.edu/msn

University of San Diego, Hahn School of Nursing and Health Science, San Diego, CA 92110-2492. Offers adult-gerontology clinical nurse specialist (MSN); adult-gerontology nurse practitioner/family nurse practitioner (MSN); executive nurse leader (MSN); family nurse practitioner (MSN); family/lifespan psychiatric-mental health nurse practitioner (MSN); healthcare informatics (MS, MSN); nursing (PhD); nursing practice (DNP). *Accreditation:* AACN. *Program availability:* Part-time, evening/weekend. *Faculty:* 27 full-time (23 women), 46 part-time/adjunct (41 women). *Students:* 178 full-time (151 women), 157 part-time (131 women); includes 143 minority (25 Black or African American, non-Hispanic/Latino; 2 American Indian or Alaska Native, non-Hispanic/Latino; 53 Asian, non-Hispanic/Latino; 49 Hispanic/Latino; 4 Native Hawaiian or other Pacific Islander, non-Hispanic/Latino; 10 Two or more races, non-Hispanic/Latino); 5 international. Average age 36. In 2015, 122 master's, 43 doctorates awarded. *Degree requirements:* For doctorate, thesis/dissertation (for some programs), residency (DNP). *Entrance requirements:* For master's, GRE General Test (for entry-level nursing), BSN, current California RN licensure (except for entry-level nursing); minimum GPA of 3.0; for doctorate, minimum GPA of 3.5, MSN, current California RN licensure. Additional exam requirements/recommendations for international students: Required—TOEFL (minimum score 580 paper-based; 83 iBT), TWE. *Application deadline:* Applications are processed on a rolling basis. Application fee: $45. Electronic applications accepted. *Financial support:* In 2015–16, 217 students received support. Scholarships/grants and traineeships available. Support available to part-time students. Financial award application deadline: 4/1; financial award applicants required to submit FAFSA. *Faculty research:* Maternal/neonatal health, palliative and end of life care, adolescent obesity, health disparities, cognitive dysfunction. *Unit head:* Dr. Sally Hardin, Dean, 619-260-4550, Fax: 619-260-6814. *Application contact:* Monica Mahon, Associate Director of Graduate Admissions, 619-260-4524, Fax: 619-260-4158, E-mail: grads@sandiego.edu.
Website: http://www.sandiego.edu/nursing/

University of San Francisco, School of Nursing and Health Professions, Doctoral Programs, San Francisco, CA 94117-1080. Offers executive leadership (DNP); family nurse practitioner (DNP); healthcare systems leadership (DNP); psychiatric mental health nurse practitioner (DNP). *Faculty:* 19 full-time (13 women), 15 part-time/adjunct (11 women). *Students:* 150 full-time (114 women), 54 part-time (46 women); includes 114 minority (25 Black or African American, non-Hispanic/Latino; 1 American Indian or Alaska Native, non-Hispanic/Latino; 56 Asian, non-Hispanic/Latino; 21 Hispanic/Latino; 3 Native Hawaiian or other Pacific Islander, non-Hispanic/Latino; 8 Two or more races, non-Hispanic/Latino), 2 international. Average age 38. 121 applicants, 81% accepted, 70 enrolled. In 2015, 31 doctorates awarded. *Entrance requirements:* For doctorate, nursing bachelor's degree, valid RN license in California. Electronic applications accepted. *Expenses: Tuition, area resident:* Full-time $22,410; part-time $1245 per credit. Tuition and fees vary according to course load, degree level and campus/location. *Financial support:* In 2015–16, 43 students received support. *Unit head:* Dr. Judith Karshmer, Dean, 415-422-6681, Fax: 415-422-6877, E-mail: nursing@usfca.edu. *Application contact:* Ingrid McVanner, Information Contact, 415-422-2746, Fax: 415-422-2217.

University of San Francisco, School of Nursing and Health Professions, Master's Programs, San Francisco, CA 94117-1080. Offers behavioral health (MSBH); clinical nurse leader (MS); public health (MPH). *Faculty:* 33 full-time (27 women), 44 part-time/adjunct (39 women). *Students:* 426 full-time (357 women), 130 part-time (110 women); includes 305 minority (45 Black or African American, non-Hispanic/Latino; 140 Asian, non-Hispanic/Latino; 78 Hispanic/Latino; 14 Native Hawaiian or other Pacific Islander, non-Hispanic/Latino; 28 Two or more races, non-Hispanic/Latino), 23 international. Average age 33. 542 applicants, 59% accepted, 190 enrolled. In 2015, 180 master's awarded. *Application deadline:* For fall admission, 5/15 priority date for domestic students; for spring admission, 11/30 priority date for domestic students. *Expenses: Tuition, area resident:* Full-time $22,410; part-time $1245 per credit. Tuition and fees vary according to course load, degree level and campus/location. *Financial support:* In 2015–16, 99 students received support. *Unit head:* Dr. Michelle Montagno, Director, 415-422-4074, E-mail: mjmontagno@usfca.edu. *Application contact:* Ingrid McVanner, Information Contact, 415-422-2746, Fax: 415-422-2217.

The University of Scranton, Panuska College of Professional Studies, Department of Nursing, Scranton, PA 18510-4595. Offers family nurse practitioner (MSN, PMC); nurse anesthesia (MSN, PMC); nursing leadership (DNP). Applicants accepted in odd-numbered years only. *Accreditation:* AACN; AANA/CANAEP. *Program availability:* Part-time, evening/weekend. *Students:* 58 full-time (46 women), 22 part-time (all women); includes 16 minority (12 Black or African American, non-Hispanic/Latino; 1 Asian, non-Hispanic/Latino; 2 Hispanic/Latino; 1 Two or more races, non-Hispanic/Latino). Average age 33. 104 applicants, 51% accepted, 45 enrolled. *Degree requirements:* For master's, comprehensive exam (for some programs), thesis (for some programs), capstone experience. *Entrance requirements:* For master's, minimum GPA of 3.0, three letters of reference; for doctorate, RN licensure and evidence of certification in advanced practice nursing specialty. Additional exam requirements/recommendations for international students: Required—TOEFL (minimum score 500 paper-based; 80 iBT), IELTS (minimum score 6.5). *Application deadline:* For fall admission, 9/1 for domestic students, 6/1 for international students; for spring admission, 11/1 for international students; for summer admission, 3/1 for international students. Applications are processed on a rolling basis. Application fee: $0. Electronic applications accepted. *Financial support:* Applicants required to submit FAFSA. *Faculty research:* Home care, doctoral education, health care of women and children, pain, health promotion and adolescence. *Unit head:* Dr. Dona Carpenter, Chair, 570-941-7673, Fax: 570-941-4201, E-mail: dona.carpenter@scranton.edu. *Application contact:* Dr. Mary Jane Hanson, Director, 570-941-4060, Fax: 570-941-4201, E-mail: hansonm2@scranton.edu.
Website: http://www.scranton.edu/academics/pcps/nursing/index.shtml

University of South Alabama, College of Nursing, Mobile, AL 36688. Offers nursing (MSN, DNP); nursing administration (Certificate); nursing education (MAIA); nursing practice (Certificate). *Accreditation:* AACN. *Program availability:* Part-time, online learning. *Faculty:* 69 full-time (63 women), 97 part-time/adjunct (89 women). *Students:* 2,489 full-time (2,179 women), 341 part-time (297 women); includes 789 minority (520 Black or African American, non-Hispanic/Latino; 26 American Indian or Alaska Native, non-Hispanic/Latino; 118 Asian, non-Hispanic/Latino; 82 Hispanic/Latino; 9 Native Hawaiian or other Pacific Islander, non-Hispanic/Latino; 34 Two or more races, non-Hispanic/Latino), 7 international. Average age 35. 1,923 applicants, 51% accepted, 722 enrolled. In 2015, 572 master's, 90 doctorates, 79 other advanced degrees awarded. *Degree requirements:* For master's, thesis optional; for doctorate, final project. *Entrance requirements:* For master's, BSN, RN licensure, minimum GPA of 3.0, resume documenting clinical experience, background check, drug screening; for doctorate, MSN, RN licensure, minimum GPA of 3.0; for Certificate, MSN/DN/DNP, RN licensure, minimum GPA of 3.0, resume documenting clinical experience, background check, drug screening. *Application deadline:* For fall admission, 3/15 for domestic students; for spring admission, 7/15 priority date for domestic students; for summer admission, 1/15 priority date for domestic students. Applications are processed on a rolling basis. Application fee: $85. Electronic applications accepted. *Expenses:* Tuition, state resident: full-time $9480; part-time $395 per credit hour. Tuition, nonresident: full-time $18,960; part-time $790 per credit hour. *Financial support:* Fellowships, research assistantships, teaching assistantships, career-related internships or fieldwork, Federal Work-Study, institutionally sponsored loans, scholarships/grants, and unspecified assistantships available. Support available to part-time students. Financial award application deadline: 5/31; financial award applicants required to submit FAFSA. *Unit head:* Dr. Debra Davis, Dean, College of Nursing, 251-445-9400, Fax: 251-445-9416, E-mail: ddavis@southalabama.edu. *Application contact:* Gail Soles, Academic Records Specialist, 251-445-9400, Fax: 251-445-9416, E-mail: gsoles@southalabama.edu.
Website: http://www.southalabama.edu/colleges/con/index.html

University of South Carolina, The Graduate School, College of Nursing, Program in Nursing Administration, Columbia, SC 29208. Offers MSN. *Accreditation:* AACN. *Program availability:* Part-time. *Degree requirements:* For master's, thesis or alternative. *Entrance requirements:* For master's, GRE General Test or MAT, BS in nursing, nursing license. Additional exam requirements/recommendations for international students: Required—TOEFL (minimum score 570 paper-based). Electronic applications accepted. *Faculty research:* System research, evidence based practice, breast cancer, violence.

University of Southern Maine, College of Science, Technology, and Health, School of Nursing, Portland, ME 04103. Offers adult-gerontology primary care nurse practitioner (MS, PMC); education (MS); family nurse practitioner (MS, PMC); family psychiatric/mental health nurse practitioner (MS); management (MS); nursing (CAS, CGS); psychiatric-mental health nurse practitioner (PMC). *Accreditation:* AACN. *Program availability:* Part-time. *Degree requirements:* For master's, thesis optional. *Entrance requirements:* For master's, GRE General Test or MAT, minimum GPA of 3.0; for doctorate, GRE. Additional exam requirements/recommendations for international students: Required—TOEFL (minimum score 550 paper-based). Electronic applications accepted. *Expenses: Tuition, area resident:* Full-time $6840; part-time $380 per credit hour. Tuition, state resident: full-time $10,260; part-time $570 per credit hour. Tuition, nonresident: full-time $18,468; part-time $1026 per credit hour. *Required fees:* $830; $83 per credit hour. Tuition and fees vary according to course load and program. *Faculty research:* Women's health, nursing history, weight control, community services, substance abuse.

University of South Florida, College of Nursing, Tampa, FL 33612. Offers advanced pain management (Graduate Certificate); nursing (MS, DNP), including adult gerontology acute care (DNP), adult gerontology acute care nursing (MS), adult gerontology primary care (DNP), adult gerontology primary care nursing (MS), adult gerontology primary care/occupational health nursing (MS), adult gerontology primary care/oncology nursing (MS), clinical nurse leader (MS), family health nursing, nurse anesthesia (MS), nursing education (MS), nursing practice (DNP), occupational health/adult-gerontology (DNP), oncology/adult-gerontology primary care (DNP), pediatric health (DNP), pediatric nurse practitioner (MS); nursing education (Post Master's Certificate); nursing science (PhD). *Accreditation:* AACN; AANA/CANAEP. *Program availability:* Part-time. *Faculty:* 43 full-time (38 women), 7 part-time/adjunct (4 women). *Students:* 159 full-time (135 women), 721 part-time (625 women); includes 292 minority (119 Black or African American, non-Hispanic/Latino; 2 American Indian or Alaska Native, non-Hispanic/Latino; 60 Asian, non-Hispanic/Latino; 90 Hispanic/Latino; 1 Native Hawaiian or other Pacific Islander, non-Hispanic/Latino; 20 Two or more races, non-Hispanic/Latino), 12 international. Average age 35. 636 applicants, 44% accepted, 215 enrolled. In 2015, 333 master's, 18 doctorates awarded. *Degree requirements:* For master's, comprehensive exam, thesis optional; for doctorate, comprehensive exam, thesis/dissertation. *Entrance requirements:* For master's, GRE General Test, bachelor's degree from accredited program with minimum GPA of 3.0 in all upper-division coursework; current license as Registered Nurse; 3 letters of recommendation; personal statement of goals; resume or curriculum vitae; personal interview; for doctorate, GRE General Test (recommended), bachelor's degree in nursing from a CCNA/NLNAC regionally-accredited institution with minimum GPA of 3.0 in all coursework or in all upper-division coursework; current license as Registered Nurse in Florida; undergraduate statistics course with minimum B grade; 3 letters of recommendation; statement of goals; resume; interview. Additional exam requirements/recommendations for international students: Required—TOEFL (minimum score 550 paper-based; 79 iBT). *Application deadline:* For fall admission, 2/15 for domestic students, 1/2 for international students; for spring admission, 10/1 for domestic students, 6/1 for international students. Application fee: $30. Electronic applications accepted. *Financial support:* In 2015–16, 36 students received support, including 7 research assistantships with tuition reimbursements available (averaging $18,935 per year), 29 teaching assistantships with tuition reimbursements available (averaging $30,814 per year); tuition waivers (partial) and unspecified assistantships also available. Financial award application deadline: 2/1; financial award applicants required to submit FAFSA. *Faculty research:* Women's

health, palliative and end-of-life care, cardiac rehabilitation, complementary therapies for chronic illness and cancer. *Total annual research expenditures:* $2.6 million. *Unit head:* Dr. Dianne C. Morrison-Beedy, Dean and Professor, College of Nursing, 813-974-9091, Fax: 813-974-5418, E-mail: dmbeedy@health.usf.edu. *Application contact:* Dr. Brian Graves, Assistant Professor/Assistant Dean, 813-974-8054, Fax: 813-974-5418, E-mail: bgraves1@health.usf.edu.
Website: http://health.usf.edu/nursing/index.htm

The University of Tennessee at Chattanooga, School of Nursing, Chattanooga, TN 37403. Offers administration (MSN); certified nurse anesthetist (Post-Master's Certificate); education (MSN); family nurse practitioner (MSN, Post-Master's Certificate); health care informatics (Post-Master's Certificate); nurse anesthesia (MSN); nurse education (Post-Master's Certificate); nursing (DNP). *Accreditation:* AACN; AANA/CANAEP (one or more programs are accredited). *Faculty:* 9 full-time (7 women), 2 part-time/adjunct (1 woman). *Students:* 50 full-time (25 women), 43 part-time (37 women); includes 14 minority (7 Black or African American, non-Hispanic/Latino; 1 American Indian or Alaska Native, non-Hispanic/Latino; 4 Asian, non-Hispanic/Latino; 2 Two or more races, non-Hispanic/Latino). Average age 34. In 2015, 40 master's, 12 doctorates, 1 other advanced degree awarded. *Degree requirements:* For master's, thesis optional, qualifying exams, professional project; for Post-Master's Certificate, thesis or alternative, practicum, seminar. *Entrance requirements:* For master's, GRE General Test, MAT, BSN, minimum GPA of 3.0, eligibility for Tennessee RN license, 1 year of direct patient care experience; for Post-Master's Certificate, GRE General Test, MAT, MSN, minimum GPA of 3.0, eligibility for Tennessee RN license, one year of direct patient care experience. Additional exam requirements/recommendations for international students: Required—TOEFL (minimum score 79 iBT), IELTS (minimum score 6). *Application deadline:* For fall admission, 6/13 priority date for domestic students, 6/1 for international students; for spring admission, 10/15 priority date for domestic students, 10/1 for international students. Applications are processed on a rolling basis. Application fee: $30 ($35 for international students). Electronic applications accepted. *Expenses:* Tuition, state resident: full-time $7938; part-time $441 per credit hour. Tuition, nonresident: full-time $24,056; part-time $1336 per credit hour. *Required fees:* $1732; $253 per credit hour. *Financial support:* Career-related internships or fieldwork and scholarships/grants available. Support available to part-time students. *Faculty research:* Diabetes in women, health care for elderly, alternative medicine, hypertension, nurse anesthesia. *Total annual research expenditures:* $2.6 million. *Unit head:* Dr. Chris Smith, Interim Director, 423-425-1741, Fax: 423-425-4668, E-mail: chris-smith@utc.edu. *Application contact:* Dr. J. Randy Walker, Interim Dean of Graduate Studies, 423-425-4478, Fax: 423-425-5223, E-mail: randy-walker@utc.edu.
Website: http://www.utc.edu/Academic/Nursing/

The University of Tennessee Health Science Center, College of Nursing, Memphis, TN 38163. Offers adult-gerontology acute care nurse practitioner (Certificate); advanced practice nursing (DNP); clinical nurse leader (MSN). *Accreditation:* AACN; AANA/CANAEP. *Program availability:* Part-time, online learning. *Degree requirements:* For master's, thesis, portfolio; for doctorate, portfolio. *Entrance requirements:* For master's, minimum GPA of 3.0; for doctorate, RN license, minimum GPA of 3.0; for Certificate, MSN, APN license, minimum GPA of 3.0. Additional exam requirements/recommendations for international students: Required—TOEFL (minimum score 550 paper-based; 80 iBT). Electronic applications accepted. *Expenses:* Contact institution. *Faculty research:* Efficacy of a cognitive behavioral group intervention and its influence on symptoms of depression and anxiety as well as caregiver function; ability of newly-developed assays to aid in the diagnosis of preeclampsia; quality of life and sexual function in women who undergo vulvar surgeries; influence of prenatal and early childhood environments on health and developmental trajectories across childhood; interaction between physical activity, diet, genetics, insulin resistance, and obesity.

The University of Texas at Arlington, Graduate School, College of Nursing, Arlington, TX 76019. Offers nurse practitioner (MSN); nursing administration (MSN); nursing education (MSN); nursing practice (DNP); nursing science (PhD). *Accreditation:* AACN. *Program availability:* Part-time, evening/weekend, online learning. *Degree requirements:* For master's, practicum course; for doctorate, comprehensive exam (for some programs), thesis/dissertation (for some programs), proposal defense dissertation (for PhD); scholarship project (for DNP). *Entrance requirements:* For master's, GRE General Test if GPA less than 3.0, minimum GPA of 3.0, Texas nursing license, minimum C grade in undergraduate statistics course; for doctorate, GRE General Test (waived for MSN-to-PhD applicants), minimum undergraduate, graduate and statistics GPA of 3.0; Texas RN license; interview; written statement of goals. Additional exam requirements/recommendations for international students: Required—TOEFL (minimum score 550 paper-based), IELTS (minimum score 7). *Faculty research:* Simulation in clinical education and practice, cultural diversity, vulnerable populations, substance abuse.

The University of Texas at Austin, Graduate School, School of Nursing, Austin, TX 78712-1111. Offers adult - gerontology clinical nurse specialist (MSN); child health (MSN), including administration, public health nursing, teaching; family nurse practitioner (MSN); family psychiatric/mental health nurse practitioner (MSN); holistic adult health (MSN), including administration, teaching; maternity (MSN), including administration, public health nursing, teaching; nursing (PhD); nursing administration and healthcare systems management (MSN); nursing practice (DNP); pediatric nurse practitioner (MSN); public health nursing (MSN). *Accreditation:* AACN. *Program availability:* Part-time. *Degree requirements:* For master's, thesis optional; for doctorate, thesis/dissertation. *Entrance requirements:* For master's and doctorate, GRE General Test. Additional exam requirements/recommendations for international students: Required—TOEFL (minimum score 550 paper-based). Electronic applications accepted. *Faculty research:* Chronic illness management, memory and aging, health promotion, women's health, adolescent health.

The University of Texas at El Paso, Graduate School, School of Nursing, El Paso, TX 79968-0001. Offers family nurse practitioner (MSN); health care leadership and management (Certificate); interdisciplinary health sciences (PhD); nursing (DNP); nursing education (MSN, Certificate); nursing systems management (MSN). *Accreditation:* AACN. *Program availability:* Online learning. *Degree requirements:* For master's, thesis optional; for doctorate, thesis/dissertation. *Entrance requirements:* For master's, minimum GPA of 3.0, resume; for doctorate, GRE, letters of reference, relevant personal/professional experience; master's degree in nursing (for DNP); for Certificate, bachelor's degree in nursing. Additional exam requirements/recommendations for international students: Required—TOEFL; Recommended—IELTS. Electronic applications accepted.

The University of Texas at Tyler, College of Nursing and Health Sciences, Program in Nursing, Tyler, TX 75799-0001. Offers nurse practitioner (MSN); nursing (PhD); nursing administration (MSN); nursing education (MSN); MSN/MBA. *Accreditation:* AACN. *Program availability:* Part-time, evening/weekend, online learning. *Degree requirements:* For master's, comprehensive exam (for some programs), thesis (for some programs); for doctorate, thesis/dissertation. *Entrance requirements:* For master's, GRE General Test or MAT, GMAT, minimum undergraduate GPA of 3.0, course work in statistics, RN license, BSN. Additional exam requirements/recommendations for international students: Required—TOEFL. Electronic applications accepted. *Faculty research:* Psychosocial adjustment, aging, support/commitment of caregivers, psychological

abuse and violence, hope/hopelessness, professional values, end of life care, suicidology, clinical supervision, workforce retention and issues, global health issues, health promotion.

The University of Texas Health Science Center at San Antonio, School of Nursing, San Antonio, TX 78229-3900. Offers administrative management (MSN); adult-gerontology acute care nurse practitioner (PGC); advanced practice leadership (DNP); clinical nurse leader (MSN); executive administrative management (DNP); family nurse practitioner (MSN, PGC); nursing (MSN, PhD); nursing education (MSN, PGC); pediatric nurse practitioner primary care (PGC); psychiatric mental health nurse practitioner (PGC); public health nurse leader (DNP). *Accreditation:* AACN. *Program availability:* Part-time. Terminal master's awarded for partial completion of doctoral program. *Degree requirements:* For master's, thesis optional; for doctorate, comprehensive exam, thesis/dissertation.

University of the Incarnate Word, School of Graduate Studies and Research, School of Nursing and Health Professions, Program in Nursing, San Antonio, TX 78209-6397. Offers clinical nursing leader (MSN); clinical nursing specialist (MSN); nursing (DNP). *Accreditation:* AACN. *Program availability:* Part-time, evening/weekend. *Faculty:* 7 full-time (all women), 1 (woman) part-time/adjunct. *Students:* 3 full-time (all women), 66 part-time (55 women); includes 42 minority (5 Black or African American, non-Hispanic/Latino; 1 American Indian or Alaska Native, non-Hispanic/Latino; 3 Asian, non-Hispanic/Latino; 31 Hispanic/Latino; 2 Two or more races, non-Hispanic/Latino), 3 international. Average age 39. 7 applicants, 100% accepted, 6 enrolled. In 2015, 10 master's awarded. *Degree requirements:* For master's, capstone, clinical hours. *Entrance requirements:* For master's, baccalaureate degree in nursing from CCNE- or NLN-accredited program including courses in statistics and health assessment; minimum undergraduate cumulative GPA of 2.5, 3.0 in upper-division nursing courses; three professional references; license to practice nursing in Texas or recognized state. Additional exam requirements/recommendations for international students: Required—TOEFL (minimum score 560 paper-based; 83 iBT). *Application deadline:* Applications are processed on a rolling basis. Application fee: $20. Electronic applications accepted. *Expenses: Tuition, area resident:* Part-time $885 per credit hour. *Required fees:* $40 per credit hour. Tuition and fees vary according to course load, degree level, campus/location, program and student level. *Financial support:* Federal Work-Study, scholarships/grants, traineeships, and unspecified assistantships available. Support available to part-time students. Financial award applicants required to submit FAFSA. *Unit head:* Dr. Holly Cassells, Chair, Graduate Programs, 210-829-3977, Fax: 210-829-3174, E-mail: cassells@uiwtx.edu. *Application contact:* Johnny Garcia, Graduate Admissions Counselor, 210-805-3554, Fax: 210-829-3921, E-mail: admis@uiwtx.edu.
Website: http://uiw.edu/nursing/msn-program/

The University of Toledo, College of Graduate Studies, College of Nursing, Department of Population and Community Care, Toledo, OH 43606-3390. Offers clinical nurse leader (MSN); family nurse practitioner (MSN, Certificate); nurse educator (MSN, Certificate); pediatric nurse practitioner (MSN, Certificate). *Program availability:* Part-time. *Degree requirements:* For master's, thesis or alternative. *Entrance requirements:* For master's, GRE, BS in nursing, minimum undergraduate GPA of 3.0, statement of purpose, three letters of recommendation, transcripts from all prior institutions attended, Nursing CAS application, UT supplemental application; for Certificate, BS in nursing, minimum undergraduate GPA of 3.0, statement of purpose, three letters of recommendation, transcripts from all prior institutions attended. Additional exam requirements/recommendations for international students: Required—TOEFL (minimum score 550 paper-based; 80 iBT). Electronic applications accepted.

University of Victoria, Faculty of Graduate Studies, Faculty of Human and Social Development, School of Nursing, Victoria, BC V8W 2Y2, Canada. Offers advanced nursing practice (advanced practice leadership option) (MN); advanced nursing practice (nurse educator option) (MN); advanced nursing practice (nurse practitioner option) (MN); nursing (PhD). *Program availability:* Part-time, online learning. *Entrance requirements:* Additional exam requirements/recommendations for international students: Required—TOEFL (minimum score 575 paper-based), IELTS (minimum score 7). Electronic applications accepted.

University of Virginia, School of Nursing, Charlottesville, VA 22903. Offers acute and specialty care (MSN); acute care nurse practitioner (MSN); clinical nurse leadership (MSN); community-public health leadership (MSN); nursing (DNP, PhD); psychiatric mental health counseling (MSN); MSN/MBA. *Accreditation:* AACN. *Program availability:* Part-time. *Degree requirements:* For doctorate, comprehensive exam (for some programs), capstone project (DNP), dissertation (PhD). *Entrance requirements:* For master's, GRE General Test, MAT; for doctorate, GRE General Test. Additional exam requirements/recommendations for international students: Required—TOEFL, IELTS. Electronic applications accepted. *Expenses:* Contact institution.

University of Washington, Tacoma, Graduate Programs, Program in Nursing, Tacoma, WA 98402-3100. Offers communities, populations and health (MN); leadership in healthcare (MN); nurse educator (MN). *Program availability:* Part-time. *Degree requirements:* For master's, thesis (for some programs), advance fieldwork. *Entrance requirements:* For master's, Washington State NCLEX exam, minimum GPA of 3.0. Additional exam requirements/recommendations for international students: Required—TOEFL (minimum score 580 paper-based; 70 iBT); Recommended—IELTS (minimum score 7). *Faculty research:* Hospice and palliative care; clinical trial decision-making; minority nurse retention; asthma and public health; injustice, suffering, difference; Linking Them to Us; adolescent health.

University of West Florida, College of Education and Professional Studies, Program in Administration, Pensacola, FL 32514-5750. Offers acquisition and contract administration (MSA); database administration (MSA); health care administration (MSA); human performance technology (MSA); leadership (MSA); public administration (MSA); software engineering administration (MSA). *Program availability:* Part-time, evening/weekend, online learning. *Entrance requirements:* For master's, GRE General Test, letter of intent, names of references. Additional exam requirements/recommendations for international students: Required—TOEFL (minimum score 550 paper-based).

University of Wisconsin–Eau Claire, College of Nursing and Health Sciences, Program in Nursing, Eau Claire, WI 54702-4004. Offers adult-gerontological administration (DNP); adult-gerontological clinical nurse specialist (DNP); adult-gerontological education (MSN); adult-gerontological primary care nurse practitioner (DNP); family health administration (DNP); family health in education (MSN); family health nurse practitioner (DNP); nursing (MSN); nursing practice (DNP). *Program availability:* Part-time. Terminal master's awarded for partial completion of doctoral program. *Degree requirements:* For master's, thesis optional, 500-600 hours clinical practicum, oral and written exams. *Entrance requirements:* For master's, Wisconsin RN license, minimum GPA of 3.0, undergraduate statistics, course work in health assessment. Additional exam requirements/recommendations for international students: Required—TOEFL (minimum score 79 iBT). *Expenses:* Contact institution.

University of Wisconsin–Green Bay, Graduate Studies, Program in Nursing Leadership and Management in Health Systems, Green Bay, WI 54311-7001. Offers MSN. *Program availability:* Part-time, evening/weekend, online only, 100% online. *Faculty:* 2 full-time (both women), 1 (woman) part-time/adjunct. *Students:* 23 part-time

Nursing and Healthcare Administration

(19 women); includes 1 minority (Two or more races, non-Hispanic/Latino). Average age 39. 23 applicants, 100% accepted, 18 enrolled. *Degree requirements:* For master's, 9-credit practicum. *Entrance requirements:* For master's, baccalaureate degree in nursing with minimum GPA of 3.0; college-level inferential statistics course with minimum C grade (within past 5 years); statement of interest; official undergraduate and graduate transcripts; three letters of evaluation; curriculum vitae or resume; copy of current, unencumbered RN license; background check. Additional exam requirements/recommendations for international students: Required—TOEFL. *Application deadline:* Applications are processed on a rolling basis. Application fee: $56. Electronic applications accepted. *Expenses:* Tuition, state resident: full-time $7640; part-time $424 per credit hour. Tuition, nonresident: full-time $16,771; part-time $932 per credit hour. *Required fees:* $1526; $85 per credit hour. $85 per semester. Tuition and fees vary according to program and reciprocity agreements. *Financial support:* In 2015–16, 3 students received support. *Unit head:* Dr. Janet Reilly, Director, 920-465-2826, E-mail: reillyj@uwgb.edu. *Application contact:* Mary Valitchka, Graduate Studies Coordinator, 920-465-2123, Fax: 920-465-5043, E-mail: valitchm@uwgb.edu.
Website: http://www.uwgb.edu/nursing/msn/overview.asp

Vanderbilt University, Vanderbilt University School of Nursing, Nashville, TN 37240. Offers adult-gerontology acute care nurse practitioner (MSN), including hospitalist, intensivist; adult-gerontology primary care nurse practitioner (MSN); emergency nurse practitioner (MSN); family nurse practitioner (MSN); healthcare leadership (MSN); neonatal nurse practitioner (MSN); nurse midwifery (MSN); nurse midwifery/family nurse practitioner (MSN); nursing (Post-Master's Certificate); nursing informatics (MSN); nursing practice (DNP); nursing science (PhD); pediatric acute care nurse practitioner (MSN); pediatric primary care nurse practitioner (MSN); psychiatric-mental health nurse practitioner (MSN); women's health nurse practitioner (MSN); women's health nurse practitioner/adult gerontology primary care nurse practitioner (MSN); MSN/M Div; MSN/MTS. *Accreditation:* ACEN (one or more programs are accredited); ACNM/ACME. *Program availability:* Part-time, 100% online, blended/hybrid learning. *Faculty:* 258 full-time (232 women), 363 part-time/adjunct (271 women). *Students:* 478 full-time (424 women), 342 part-time (317 women); includes 140 minority (36 Black or African American, non-Hispanic/Latino; 3 American Indian or Alaska Native, non-Hispanic/Latino; 24 Asian, non-Hispanic/Latino; 43 Hispanic/Latino; 3 Native Hawaiian or other Pacific Islander, non-Hispanic/Latino; 31 Two or more races, non-Hispanic/Latino), 11 international. Average age 31. 1,268 applicants, 49% accepted, 477 enrolled. In 2015, 343 master's, 55 doctorates awarded. *Degree requirements:* For doctorate, comprehensive exam, thesis/dissertation. *Entrance requirements:* For master's, GRE General Test (taken within the past 5 years), minimum B average in undergraduate course work, 3 letters of recommendation; for doctorate, GRE General Test, interview, 3 letters of recommendation from doctorally-prepared faculty, MSN, essay. Additional exam requirements/recommendations for international students: Required—TOEFL (minimum score 570 paper-based), IELTS (minimum score 6.5). *Application deadline:* For fall admission, 11/1 priority date for domestic and international students. Applications are processed on a rolling basis. Application fee: $50. Electronic applications accepted. *Expenses:* Contact institution. *Financial support:* In 2015–16, 585 students received support. Scholarships/grants available. Financial award application deadline: 3/15; financial award applicants required to submit FAFSA. *Faculty research:* Lymphedema, palliative care and bereavement, health services research including workforce, safety and quality of care, gerontology, better birth outcomes including nutrition. *Total annual research expenditures:* $2 million. *Unit head:* Dr. Linda Norman, Dean, 615-343-8876, Fax: 615-343-7711, E-mail: linda.norman@vanderbilt.edu. *Application contact:* Patricia Peerman, Assistant Dean for Enrollment Management, 615-322-3800, Fax: 615-343-0333, E-mail: vusn-admissions@vanderbilt.edu.
Website: http://www.nursing.vanderbilt.edu

Virginia Commonwealth University, Graduate School, School of Nursing, Richmond, VA 23284-9005. Offers adult health acute nursing (MS); adult health primary nursing (MS); biobehavioral clinical research (PhD); child health nursing (MS); clinical nurse leader (MS); family health nursing (MS); nurse educator (MS); nurse practitioner (MS); nursing (Certificate); nursing administration (MS), including clinical nurse manager; psychiatric-mental health nursing (MS); quality and safety in health care (DNP); women's health nursing (MS). *Accreditation:* ACEN (one or more programs are accredited). *Program availability:* Part-time, evening/weekend, online learning. *Degree requirements:* For master's, thesis optional; for doctorate, thesis/dissertation. *Entrance requirements:* For master's, GRE General Test, BSN, minimum GPA of 2.8; for doctorate, GRE General Test. Additional exam requirements/recommendations for international students: Required—TOEFL (minimum score 600 paper-based; 100 iBT). Electronic applications accepted.

Walden University, Graduate Programs, School of Nursing, Minneapolis, MN 55401. Offers adult-gerontology acute care nurse practitioner (MSN); adult-gerontology nurse practitioner (MSN); education (MSN); family nurse practitioner (MSN); informatics (MSN); leadership and management (MSN); nursing (PhD, Post-Master's Certificate), including education (PhD), healthcare administration (PhD), interdisciplinary health (PhD), leadership (PhD), nursing education (Post-Master's Certificate), nursing informatics (Post-Master's Certificate), nursing leadership and management (Post-Master's Certificate), public health policy (PhD); nursing practice (DNP); psychiatric mental health (MSN). *Accreditation:* AACN. *Program availability:* Part-time, evening/weekend, online only, 100% online. *Faculty:* 22 full-time (18 women), 540 part-time/adjunct (487 women). *Students:* 4,320 full-time (3,773 women), 5,250 part-time (4,740 women); includes 3,550 minority (2,360 Black or African American, non-Hispanic/Latino; 29 American Indian or Alaska Native, non-Hispanic/Latino; 523 Asian, non-Hispanic/Latino; 421 Hispanic/Latino; 25 Native Hawaiian or other Pacific Islander, non-Hispanic/Latino; 192 Two or more races, non-Hispanic/Latino), 221 international. Average age 40. 2,057 applicants, 100% accepted, 1507 enrolled. In 2015, 3,022 master's, 86 doctorates, 34 other advanced degrees awarded. *Degree requirements:* For doctorate, thesis/dissertation (for some programs), residency (for some programs), field experience (for some programs). *Entrance requirements:* For master's, bachelor's degree or equivalent in related field or RN; minimum GPA of 2.5; official transcripts; goal statement (for some programs); access to computer and Internet; for doctorate, master's degree or higher; RN; three years of related professional or academic experience; goal statement; access to computer and Internet; for Post-Master's Certificate, relevant work experience; access to computer and Internet. Additional exam requirements/recommendations for international students: Required—TOEFL (minimum score 550 paper-based, 79 iBT), IELTS (minimum score 6.5), Michigan English Language Assessment Battery (minimum score 82), or PTE (minimum score 53). *Application deadline:* Applications are processed on a rolling basis. Application fee: $0. Electronic applications accepted. *Financial support:* Fellowships, Federal Work-Study, scholarships/grants, unspecified assistantships, and family tuition reduction, active duty/veteran tuition reduction, group tuition reduction, interest-free payment plans, employee tuition reduction available. Support available to part-time students. Financial award applicants required to submit FAFSA. *Unit head:* Dr. Andrea Lindell, Dean, 866-492-5336. *Application contact:* Meghan Thomas, Vice President of Enrollment Management, 866-492-5336, E-mail: info@waldenu.edu.
Website: http://www.waldenu.edu/programs/colleges-schools/nursing

Walsh University, Graduate Studies, Gary and Linda Byers School of Nursing, North Canton, OH 44720-3396. Offers academic nurse educator (MSN); clinical nurse leader (MSN); nursing practice (DNP). *Program availability:* Part-time, evening/weekend, online only, 100% online. *Faculty:* 6 full-time (all women), 6 part-time/adjunct (4 women). *Students:* 25 full-time (20 women), 38 part-time (34 women); includes 2 minority (1 Black or African American, non-Hispanic/Latino; 1 Hispanic/Latino). Average age 36. 45 applicants, 71% accepted, 22 enrolled. In 2015, 9 master's, 5 doctorates awarded. *Degree requirements:* For doctorate, scholarly project; residency practicum. *Entrance requirements:* For master's, undergraduate nursing degree, current unencumbered RN license, completion of an undergraduate or graduate statistics course, essay, interview, recommendations; for doctorate, BSN; master's degree; statistics and research courses; essay; interview. Additional exam requirements/recommendations for international students: Required—TOEFL. *Application deadline:* Applications are processed on a rolling basis. Application fee: $25. Electronic applications accepted. *Expenses:* Tuition, area resident: Full-time $11,610; part-time $7740 per credit hour. Full-time tuition and fees vary according to program. *Financial support:* In 2015–16, 1 student received support, including 1 research assistantship (averaging $3,870 per year). Financial award application deadline: 12/31; financial award applicants required to submit FAFSA. *Faculty research:* Faith community nursing, gerontology, women's health, global nursing education, nursing assessment, grief and reconstitution, health needs of psychiatric patients, psychometric testing, nursing education, clinical reasoning. *Unit head:* Dr. Maris Pappas-Rogich, Director of Graduate Nursing Programs, 330-490-7283, Fax: 330-490-7371, E-mail: mpappas@walsh.edu. *Application contact:* Audra Dice, Graduate and Transfer Admissions Counselor, 330-490-7181, Fax: 330-244-4680, E-mail: adice@walsh.edu.
Website: http://www.walsh.edu/master-of-science-in-nursing

Washburn University, School of Nursing, Topeka, KS 66621. Offers clinical nurse leader (MSN); nursing (DNP); psychiatric mental health nurse practitioner (Post-Graduate Certificate). *Accreditation:* AACN. *Program availability:* Part-time. *Students:* 17 full-time (15 women), 110 part-time (96 women). Average age 37. In 2015, 43 master's, 1 doctorate, 11 other advanced degrees awarded. *Entrance requirements:* Additional exam requirements/recommendations for international students: Required—TOEFL (minimum score 550 paper-based). *Application deadline:* For fall admission, 3/15 for domestic and international students. Application fee: $40. *Expenses:* Tuition, state resident: full-time $6426; part-time $357 per credit hour. Tuition, nonresident: full-time $13,086; part-time $727 per credit hour. *Required fees:* $110; $55 per semester. Tuition and fees vary according to degree level and program. *Financial support:* Application deadline: 2/15; applicants required to submit FAFSA. *Unit head:* Dr. Monica S. Scheibmeir, Dean, 785-670-1526, E-mail: monica.scheibmeir@washburn.edu. *Application contact:* Mary V. Allen, Director of Student Services, 785-670-1533, E-mail: mary.allen@washburn.edu.
Website: http://www.washburn.edu/sonu

Washington Adventist University, Program in Nursing - Business Leadership, Takoma Park, MD 20912. Offers MSN. *Program availability:* Part-time. *Entrance requirements:* Additional exam requirements/recommendations for international students: Required—TOEFL (minimum score 550 paper-based), IELTS (minimum score 5).

Waynesburg University, Graduate and Professional Studies, Canonsburg, PA 15370. Offers business (MBA), including energy management, finance, health systems, human resources, leadership, market development; counseling (MA), including addictions counseling, clinical mental health; counselor education and supervision (PhD); criminal investigation (MA); education (M Ed), including autism, curriculum and instruction, educational leadership, online teaching; nursing (MSN), including administration, education, informatics; nursing practice (DNP); special education (M Ed); technology (M Ed); MSN/MBA. *Accreditation:* AACN. *Program availability:* Part-time, evening/weekend. *Degree requirements:* For doctorate, thesis/dissertation. *Entrance requirements:* Additional exam requirements/recommendations for international students: Required—TOEFL. Electronic applications accepted.

Webster University, College of Arts and Sciences, Department of Nursing, St. Louis, MO 63119-3194. Offers nurse educator (MSN); nurse leader (MSN). *Accreditation:* ACEN. *Degree requirements:* For master's, comprehensive exam. *Entrance requirements:* For master's, 1 year of clinical experience, BSN, interview, minimum C+ average in statistics and physical assessment, minimum GPA of 3.0, RN license. Additional exam requirements/recommendations for international students: Required—TOEFL. *Expenses:* Tuition, area resident: Full-time $20,550; part-time $685 per credit hour. Tuition and fees vary according to campus/location and program. *Faculty research:* Health teaching.

Western Governors University, College of Health Professions, Salt Lake City, UT 84107. Offers healthcare management (MBA); leadership and management (MSN); nursing education (MSN). *Program availability:* Evening/weekend. *Degree requirements:* For master's, capstone project. *Entrance requirements:* For master's, Readiness Assessment, transcripts. Additional exam requirements/recommendations for international students: Required—TOEFL (minimum score 450 paper-based; 80 iBT). Electronic applications accepted.

Western University of Health Sciences, College of Graduate Nursing, Master of Science in Nursing Program, Pomona, CA 91766-1854. Offers administrative nurse leader (MSN); ambulatory care (MSN); clinical nurse leader (MSN); family nurse practitioner (MSN); nursing (MSN). *Program availability:* Blended/hybrid learning. *Faculty:* 15 full-time (all women), 13 part-time/adjunct (7 women). *Students:* 243 full-time (206 women), 13 part-time (10 women); includes 155 minority (6 Black or African American, non-Hispanic/Latino; 76 Asian, non-Hispanic/Latino; 54 Hispanic/Latino; 19 Two or more races, non-Hispanic/Latino), 1 international. Average age 30. 467 applicants, 36% accepted, 93 enrolled. In 2015, 97 master's awarded. *Degree requirements:* For master's, comprehensive exam (for some programs), thesis (for some programs), project. *Entrance requirements:* For master's, personal statement, BSN, minimum GPA of 3.0, 3 letters of recommendation, resume/curriculum vitae, official transcripts of all schools attended. Additional exam requirements/recommendations for international students: Required—TOEFL (minimum score 80 iBT). *Application deadline:* For fall admission, 11/1 for domestic and international students. Application fee: $60. Electronic applications accepted. *Expenses:* $1,026 per unit tuition; $1,836 clinical fees; $40 student body fee. *Financial support:* Fellowships, research assistantships, teaching assistantships, and scholarships/grants available. Support available to part-time students. Financial award application deadline: 3/2; financial award applicants required to submit FAFSA. *Unit head:* Dr. Karen J. Hanford, Dean, 909-469-5523, Fax: 909-469-5521, E-mail: khanford@westernu.edu. *Application contact:* Kathryn Ford, Director of Admissions/International Student Advisor, 909-469-5335, Fax: 909-469-5570, E-mail: admissions@westernu.edu.

West Virginia Wesleyan College, Department of Nursing, Buckhannon, WV 26201. Offers family nurse practitioner (Post Master's Certificate); family nurse practitoner (MS); nurse administrator (MS); nurse educator (MS); nurse-midwifery (MS); nursing administration (Post Master's Certificate); nursing education (Post Master's Certificate); psychiatric mental health nurse practitioner (MS); MSN/MBA. *Accreditation:* ACEN.

Wilmington University, College of Health Professions, New Castle, DE 19720-6491. Offers adult nurse practitioner (MSN); family nurse practitioner (MSN); gerontology nurse practitioner (MSN); nursing (MSN); nursing leadership (MSN); nursing practice (DNP). *Accreditation:* AACN. *Program availability:* Part-time. *Degree requirements:* For master's, thesis. *Entrance requirements:* For master's, BSN, RN license, interview, 3 letters of recommendation. Additional exam requirements/recommendations for international students: Required—TOEFL (minimum score 500 paper-based). Electronic applications accepted. *Faculty research:* Outcomes assessment, student writing ability.

Wilson College, Graduate Programs, Chambersburg, PA 17201-1285. Offers accounting (M Acc); choreography and visual art (MFA); education (M Ed); healthcare management for sustainability (MHM); humanities (MA), including art and culture, critical/cultural theory, English language and literature, women's studies; nursing (MSN), including nursing education, nursing leadership and management. *Program availability:* Evening/weekend. *Degree requirements:* For master's, project. *Entrance requirements:* For master's, PRAXIS, minimum undergraduate cumulative GPA of 3.0, 2 letters of recommendation, current certification for eligibility to teach in grades K-12, resume, personal interview. Electronic applications accepted.

Winona State University, College of Nursing and Health Sciences, Winona, MN 55987. Offers adult nurse practitioner (MS, Post Master's Certificate); clinical nurse specialist (MS, Post Master's Certificate); family nurse practitioner (MS, Post Master's Certificate); nurse administrator (MS); nurse educator (MS, Post Master's Certificate); nursing (DNP). *Accreditation:* AACN. *Program availability:* Part-time, online learning. *Degree requirements:* For master's, thesis; for doctorate, capstone. *Entrance requirements:* For master's, GRE (if GPA less than 3.0). Additional exam requirements/recommendations for international students: Required—TOEFL (minimum score 550 paper-based).

Wright State University, School of Graduate Studies, College of Nursing and Health, Program in Nursing, Dayton, OH 45435. Offers acute care nurse practitioner (MS); administration of nursing and health care systems (MS); adult health (MS); child and adolescent health (MS); community health (MS); family nurse practitioner (MS); nurse practitioner (MS); school nurse (MS); MBA/MS. *Accreditation:* AACN. *Program*

availability: Part-time, evening/weekend. *Degree requirements:* For master's, thesis or alternative. *Entrance requirements:* For master's, GRE General Test, BSN from NLN-accredited college, Ohio RN license. Additional exam requirements/recommendations for international students: Required—TOEFL. *Faculty research:* Clinical nursing and health, teaching, caring, pain administration, informatics and technology.

York College of Pennsylvania, Department of Nursing, York, PA 17405-7199. Offers adult gerontology clinical nurse specialist (MS), including administration, education; adult gerontology nurse practitioner (MS); nurse anesthetist (MS); nurse educator (MS); nursing practice (DNP). *Accreditation:* AACN; AANA/CANAEP. *Program availability:* Part-time, evening/weekend. *Faculty:* 9 full-time (all women), 5 part-time/adjunct (2 women). *Students:* 36 full-time (26 women), 55 part-time (47 women); includes 14 minority (4 Black or African American, non-Hispanic/Latino; 2 American Indian or Alaska Native, non-Hispanic/Latino; 5 Asian, non-Hispanic/Latino; 2 Hispanic/Latino; 1 Two or more races, non-Hispanic/Latino), 1 international. Average age 33. 115 applicants, 28% accepted, 28 enrolled. In 2015, 24 master's, 4 doctorates awarded. *Entrance requirements:* For master's, GRE General Test (for nurse anesthetist program), minimum GPA of 3.0 from CCNE- or NLNAC-accredited institution; for doctorate, master's degree in nursing from a CCNE- or NLNAC-accredited institution; minimum GPA of 3.5. Additional exam requirements/recommendations for international students: Required—TOEFL (minimum score 530 paper-based; 72 iBT). *Application deadline:* Applications are processed on a rolling basis. Application fee: $0. Electronic applications accepted. *Expenses: Tuition,* area resident: Full-time $13,770. *Required fees:* $1750; $380. Tuition and fees vary according to degree level. *Financial support:* Federal Work-Study available. *Faculty research:* Student stress response to simulation versus clinical, evidence-based practice in all clinical settings. *Unit head:* Dr. Kimberly Fenstermacher, Graduate Program Director, 717-815-1383, E-mail: kfenster@ycp.edu. *Application contact:* Allison Malachosky, Administrative Assistant, 717-815-1243, E-mail: amalacho@ycp.edu.
Website: http://www.ycp.edu/academics/academic-departments/nursing/

Nursing Education

Albany State University, College of Sciences and Health Professions, Albany, GA 31705-2717. Offers criminal justice (MS), including corrections, forensic science, law enforcement, public administration; mathematics education (M Ed); nursing (MSN), including RN to MSN family nurse practitioner, RN to MSN nurse educator; science education (M Ed). *Accreditation:* ACEN. *Program availability:* Part-time, evening/weekend, online learning. *Degree requirements:* For master's, comprehensive exam, thesis. *Entrance requirements:* For master's, GRE or MAT, official transcript, letters of recommendations, pre-medical/certificate of immunizations. Electronic applications accepted.

American International College, School of Health Sciences, Master of Science in Nursing Program, Springfield, MA 01109-3189. Offers family nurse practitioner (MSN); nursing administration (MSN); nursing education (MSN). *Accreditation:* AACN. *Program availability:* Part-time, evening/weekend, online only, blended/hybrid learning. *Faculty:* 1 (woman) full-time, 1 (woman) part-time/adjunct. *Students:* 52 full-time (49 women), 4 part-time (all women); includes 18 minority (12 Black or African American, non-Hispanic/Latino; 1 Asian, non-Hispanic/Latino; 4 Hispanic/Latino; 1 Two or more races, non-Hispanic/Latino). Average age 36. 66 applicants, 53% accepted, 27 enrolled. In 2015, 8 master's awarded. *Entrance requirements:* For master's, BSN, minimum GPA of 3.0. Additional exam requirements/recommendations for international students: Required—TOEFL, IELTS. *Application deadline:* For fall admission, 8/20 for domestic students, 7/1 priority date for international students; for spring admission, 1/4 for domestic students, 12/1 priority date for international students. Applications are processed on a rolling basis. Application fee: $50. Electronic applications accepted. *Expenses:* Contact institution. *Financial support:* Applicants required to submit FAFSA. *Unit head:* Dr. Ellen Furman, Associate Director of Graduate Nursing, 413-205-3918, Fax: 413-654-1430, E-mail: ellen.furman@aic.edu. *Application contact:* Kerry Barnes, Director of Graduate Admissions, 413-205-3703, Fax: 413-205-3051, E-mail: kerry.barnes@aic.edu.
Website: http://www.aic.edu/academics/hs/nursing

Angelo State University, College of Graduate Studies, Archer College of Health and Human Services, Department of Nursing, San Angelo, TX 76909. Offers family nurse practitioner (MSN); nurse educator (MSN). *Accreditation:* ACEN. *Program availability:* Part-time, evening/weekend, online learning. *Degree requirements:* For master's, comprehensive exam. *Entrance requirements:* For master's, essay, three letters of recommendation. Additional exam requirements/recommendations for international students: Required—TOEFL or IELTS. *Application deadline:* For fall admission, 4/1 priority date for domestic students, 6/10 for international students; for spring admission, 9/1 priority date for domestic students, 11/1 for international students. Applications are processed on a rolling basis. Application fee: $40 ($50 for international students). Electronic applications accepted. *Expenses: Tuition,* area resident: Full-time $3726; part-time $2484 per year. Tuition, state resident: full-time $3726; part-time $2484 per year. Tuition, nonresident: full-time $10,746; part-time $7164 per year. *International tuition:* $10,746 full-time. *Required fees:* $2538; $1702 per unit. *Financial support:* Research assistantships, career-related internships or fieldwork, Federal Work-Study, and scholarships/grants available. Support available to part-time students. Financial award application deadline: 3/1. *Unit head:* Dr. Wrennah L. Gabbert, Chair, 325-942-2224, Fax: 325-942-2236, E-mail: wrennah.gabbert@angelo.edu. *Application contact:* Dr. Molly J. Walker, Graduate Advisor, 325-486-6872, Fax: 325-942-2236, E-mail: molly.walker@angelo.edu.
Website: http://www.angelo.edu/dept/nursing/

Aquinas College, School of Nursing, Nashville, TN 37205-2005. Offers nursing education (MSN).

Arizona State University at the Tempe campus, College of Nursing and Health Innovation, Phoenix, AZ 85004. Offers advanced nursing practice (DNP); clinical research management (MS); community and public health practice (Graduate Certificate); family mental health nurse practitioner (Graduate Certificate); family nurse practitioner (Graduate Certificate); geriatric nursing (Graduate Certificate); healthcare innovation (MHI); nurse education in academic and service settings (Graduate Certificate); nurse educator (MS); nursing and healthcare innovation (PhD). *Accreditation:* AACN. *Program availability:* Online learning. *Degree requirements:* For master's, comprehensive exam (for some programs), thesis (for some programs), interactive Program of Study (iPOS) submitted before completing 50 percent of required credit hours; for doctorate, comprehensive exam, thesis/dissertation, interactive

Program of Study (iPOS) submitted before completing 50 percent of required credit hours. *Entrance requirements:* For master's and doctorate, GRE, minimum GPA of 3.0 or equivalent in last 2 years of work leading to bachelor's degree. Additional exam requirements/recommendations for international students: Required—TOEFL, IELTS, or PTE. Electronic applications accepted. *Expenses:* Contact institution.

Auburn University, Graduate School, School of Nursing, Auburn University, AL 36849. Offers nursing education (MSN); primary care practitioner (MSN). *Accreditation:* AACN. *Faculty:* 21 full-time (18 women). *Students:* 13 full-time (all women), 107 part-time (101 women); includes 21 minority (14 Black or African American, non-Hispanic/Latino; 1 American Indian or Alaska Native, non-Hispanic/Latino; 2 Asian, non-Hispanic/Latino; 1 Hispanic/Latino; 3 Two or more races, non-Hispanic/Latino), 1 international. Average age 34. 78 applicants, 53% accepted, 35 enrolled. In 2015, 32 master's awarded. *Expenses:* Tuition, state resident: full-time $8802; part-time $489 per credit hour. Tuition, nonresident: full-time $26,406; part-time $1467 per credit hour. *Required fees:* $808 per semester. Tuition and fees vary according to degree level and program. *Unit head:* Dr. Gregg Newschwander, Dean, 334-844-3658, E-mail: gen0002@auburn.edu. *Application contact:* Dr. George Flowers, Dean of the Graduate School, 334-844-4700, E-mail: gradadm@auburn.edu.
Website: http://www.auburn.edu/academic/nursing/

Auburn University at Montgomery, College of Nursing and Health Sciences, Montgomery, AL 36124-4023. Offers nurse educator (MSN); nurse practitioner (MSN). *Expenses:* Tuition, state resident: full-time $6462; part-time $359 per credit hour. Tuition, nonresident: full-time $14,526; part-time $807 per credit hour. *Required fees:* $554. *Unit head:* Dr. Jean Leuner, Dean, 334-244-3658, E-mail: jleuner@aum.edu. *Application contact:* Dr. Barbara Wilder, Graduate Program Director, 334-844-6766, E-mail: wildebf@auburn.edu.
Website: http://www.nursing.aum.edu/

Austin Peay State University, College of Graduate Studies, College of Behavioral and Health Sciences, School of Nursing, Clarksville, TN 37044. Offers family nurse practitioner (MSN); nursing administration (MSN); nursing education (MSN); nursing informatics (MSN). *Program availability:* Part-time, online learning. *Faculty:* 11 full-time (all women), 6 part-time/adjunct (all women). *Students:* 23 full-time (20 women), 142 part-time (125 women); includes 27 minority (19 Black or African American, non-Hispanic/Latino; 4 Hispanic/Latino; 4 Two or more races, non-Hispanic/Latino). Average age 35. 25 applicants, 76% accepted, 14 enrolled. In 2015, 67 master's awarded. *Degree requirements:* For master's, comprehensive exam. *Entrance requirements:* For master's, minimum GPA of 3.0, RN license eligibility, 3 letters of recommendation. Additional exam requirements/recommendations for international students: Required—TOEFL (minimum score 500 paper-based). *Application deadline:* For fall admission, 8/3 priority date for domestic students. Applications are processed on a rolling basis. Application fee: $25. Electronic applications accepted. *Expenses:* Tuition, state resident: full-time $8080; part-time $404 per credit hour. Tuition, nonresident: full-time $21,680; part-time $1084 per credit hour. *Required fees:* $1453; $72.65 per credit hour. *Financial support:* In 2015–16, research assistantships with full tuition reimbursements (averaging $5,184 per year) were awarded; career-related internships or fieldwork, Federal Work-Study, institutionally sponsored loans, scholarships/grants, and unspecified assistantships also available. Support available to part-time students. Financial award application deadline: 3/1; financial award applicants required to submit FAFSA. *Unit head:* Dr. Grace Moodt, Interim Director, 931-221-6290, Fax: 931-221-7595, E-mail: moodtg@apsu.edu. *Application contact:* June D. Lee, Graduate Coordinator, 800-859-4723, Fax: 931-221-7641, E-mail: gradadmissions@apsu.edu.
Website: http://www.apsu.edu/nursing

Azusa Pacific University, School of Nursing, Azusa, CA 91702-7000. Offers nursing (MSN); nursing education (PhD). *Accreditation:* AACN. *Program availability:* Part-time, evening/weekend. *Degree requirements:* For master's, thesis optional. *Entrance requirements:* For master's, BSN.

Ball State University, Graduate School, College of Applied Sciences and Technology, School of Nursing, Muncie, IN 47306. Offers adult/gerontology nurse practitioner (Post Master's Certificate); evidence-based clinical practice (Postbaccalaureate Certificate); family nurse practitioner (Post Master's Certificate); family nurse practitioner for the adult nurse practitioner or adult/gerontology nurse practitioner (Post Master's Certificate); nurse educator (Post Master's Certificate); nursing (MS), including family nurse

Nursing Education

practitioner, nurse administrator, nurse educator; nursing education (Postbaccalaureate Certificate); nursing practice (DNP). *Accreditation:* AACN. *Program availability:* Part-time-only, online only, 100% online. *Faculty:* 12 full-time (all women), 7 part-time/adjunct (6 women). *Students:* 9 full-time (8 women), 334 part-time (311 women); includes 23 minority (11 Black or African American, non-Hispanic/Latino; 5 Asian, non-Hispanic/Latino; 6 Hispanic/Latino; 1 Two or more races, non-Hispanic/Latino). Average age 33. 88 applicants, 85% accepted, 63 enrolled. In 2015, 115 master's, 8 doctorates awarded. *Entrance requirements:* For master's, bachelor's degree in nursing, minimum GPA of 3.0, minimum C grade in at least 2 quarter or semester hours in an undergraduate research course, unencumbered license as a registered nurse in state of practice; for doctorate, advanced practice nurse (nurse practitioner, clinical nurse specialist, nurse midwife); master's degree in nursing from accredited program with minimum GPA of 3.2; graduate-level statistics, nursing research, and health assessment courses; unencumbered license as registered nurse in state of practice. Additional exam requirements/recommendations for international students: Required—TOEFL (minimum score 550 paper-based; 79 iBT), IELTS (minimum score 6.5). *Application deadline:* For fall admission, 2/9 for domestic students; for spring admission, 8/9 for domestic students. Applications are processed on a rolling basis. Application fee: $60. Electronic applications accepted. *Expenses:* Contact institution. *Financial support:* Application deadline: 3/1; applicants required to submit FAFSA. *Unit head:* Dr. Linda Siktberg, Director, 765-285-8718, Fax: 765-285-2169, E-mail: lsiktberg@bsu.edu. *Application contact:* Shantelle Estes, Graduate Advisor, 765-285-9130, Fax: 765-285-2169, E-mail: smestes@bsu.edu.
Website: http://www.bsu.edu/nursing/

Barry University, School of Adult and Continuing Education, Division of Nursing, Program in Nursing Education, Miami Shores, FL 33161-6695. Offers MSN, Certificate. *Accreditation:* AACN. *Program availability:* Part-time, evening/weekend. *Degree requirements:* For master's, research project or thesis. *Entrance requirements:* For master's, GRE General Test or MAT, BSN, minimum GPA of 3.0, course work in statistics. Electronic applications accepted. *Faculty research:* HIV/AIDS, gerontology.

Bellarmine University, Donna and Allan Lansing School of Nursing and Health Sciences, Louisville, KY 40205. Offers family nurse practitioner (MSN); health science (MHS); nursing administration (MSN); nursing education (MSN); nursing practice (DNP); physical therapy (DPT). *Accreditation:* AACN; APTA. *Program availability:* Part-time, evening/weekend. *Faculty:* 27 full-time (24 women), 8 part-time/adjunct (7 women). *Students:* 210 full-time (144 women), 91 part-time (83 women); includes 22 minority (6 Black or African American, non-Hispanic/Latino; 1 American Indian or Alaska Native, non-Hispanic/Latino; 7 Asian, non-Hispanic/Latino; 4 Hispanic/Latino; 4 Two or more races, non-Hispanic/Latino), 2 international. Average age 28. In 2015, 33 master's, 64 doctorates awarded. *Degree requirements:* For doctorate, comprehensive exam, thesis/dissertation. *Entrance requirements:* For master's, GRE General Test, RN license; for doctorate, GRE General Test, Physical Therapist Centralized Application Service (for DPT). Additional exam requirements/recommendations for international students: Required—TOEFL (minimum score 550 paper-based; 80 iBT). Application fee: $40. Electronic applications accepted. *Expenses:* Contact institution. *Financial support:* Career-related internships or fieldwork and scholarships/grants available. *Faculty research:* Nursing: pain, empathy, leadership styles, control; physical therapy: service-learning; exercise in chronic and pre-operative conditions, athletes; women's health; aging. *Unit head:* Dr. Mark Wiegand, Dean, 800-274-4723 Ext. 8368, E-mail: mwiegand@bellarmine.edu. *Application contact:* Julie Armstrong-Binnix, Health Science Recruiter, 800-274-4723 Ext. 8364, E-mail: julieab@bellarmine.edu.
Website: http://www.bellarmine.edu/lansing

Bellin College, School of Nursing, Green Bay, WI 54305. Offers family nurse practitioner (MSN); nurse educator (MSN). *Accreditation:* AACN.

Bethel University, Graduate School, St. Paul, MN 55112-6999. Offers business administration (MBA); child and adolescent mental health (Certificate); classroom management (Certificate); communication (MA); counseling psychology (MA); educational leadership (Ed D); gerontology (MA, Certificate); international baccalaureate teaching and learning (Certificate); K-12 education (MA); leadership foundations (Certificate); literacy education (MA); nurse educator (Certificate); nurse-midwifery (MS); nursing (MS); physician assistant (MS); special education (MA); STEM education (Certificate); strategic leadership (MA); teaching (MA). *Program availability:* Part-time, evening/weekend, 100% online, blended/hybrid learning. *Faculty:* 21 full-time (15 women), 74 part-time/adjunct (38 women). *Students:* 772 full-time (537 women), 372 part-time (232 women); includes 188 minority (94 Black or African American, non-Hispanic/Latino; 3 American Indian or Alaska Native, non-Hispanic/Latino; 43 Asian, non-Hispanic/Latino; 31 Hispanic/Latino; 1 Native Hawaiian or other Pacific Islander, non-Hispanic/Latino; 16 Two or more races, non-Hispanic/Latino), 33 international. Average age 37. 663 applicants, 49% accepted, 232 enrolled. In 2015, 272 master's, 16 doctorates, 65 other advanced degrees awarded. *Degree requirements:* For master's, comprehensive exam (for some programs), thesis (for some programs); for doctorate, comprehensive exam, thesis/dissertation. *Entrance requirements:* Additional exam requirements/recommendations for international students: Required—TOEFL (minimum score 550 paper-based, 80 iBT) or IELTS. *Application deadline:* Applications are processed on a rolling basis. Application fee: $0. Electronic applications accepted. *Expenses:* Contact institution. *Financial support:* In 2015–16, 132 students received support. Teaching assistantships, career-related internships or fieldwork, and scholarships/grants available. Support available to part-time students. Financial award applicants required to submit FAFSA. *Unit head:* Dick Crombie, Vice-President/Dean, 651-635-8000, Fax: 651-635-8004, E-mail: gs@bethel.edu. *Application contact:* Director of Admissions, 651-635-8000, Fax: 651-635-8004, E-mail: gs@bethel.edu.
Website: https://www.bethel.edu/graduate/

Blessing–Rieman College of Nursing and Health Sciences, Master of Science in Nursing Program, Quincy, IL 62305-7005. Offers nursing administration (MSN); nursing education (MSN). *Program availability:* Part-time-only, online only, 100% online. In 2015, 8 master's awarded. *Degree requirements:* For master's, thesis or project. *Entrance requirements:* Additional exam requirements/recommendations for international students: Required—TOEFL (minimum score 500 paper-based; 80 iBT). *Application deadline:* Applications are processed on a rolling basis. Electronic applications accepted. *Expenses:* Contact institution. *Financial support:* In 2015–16, 20,350 students received support. Scholarships/grants available. Financial award application deadline: 4/30; financial award applicants required to submit FAFSA. *Unit head:* Dr. Karen Mayville, Administrative Coordinator, Accreditation, 217-228-5520 Ext. 6900, Fax: 217-223-4001, E-mail: kmayville@brcn.edu. *Application contact:* Heather Mutter, Admissions Counselor, 217-228-5520 Ext. 6964, Fax: 217-223-1781, E-mail: hmutter@brcn.edu.
Website: http://brcn.edu

Bowie State University, Graduate Programs, Department of Nursing, Bowie, MD 20715-9465. Offers administration of nursing services (MS); family nurse practitioner (MS); nursing education (MS). *Accreditation:* ACEN. *Program availability:* Part-time. *Degree requirements:* For master's, comprehensive exam, thesis, research paper. *Entrance requirements:* For master's, minimum GPA of 2.5. Electronic applications accepted. *Expenses:* Tuition, state resident: full-time $9384; part-time $2346 per year.

Tuition, nonresident: full-time $16,344; part-time $4086 per year. *Required fees:* $2552; $325 per semester. *Faculty research:* Minority health, women's health, gerontology, leadership management.

Bradley University, Graduate School, College of Education and Health Sciences, Department of Nursing, Peoria, IL 61625-0002. Offers nursing (DNP, Certificate); nursing administration (MSN); nursing education (MSN). *Accreditation:* ACEN. *Program availability:* Part-time, evening/weekend. *Degree requirements:* For master's, comprehensive exam, thesis optional. *Entrance requirements:* For master's, GRE General Test or MAT, interview, Illinois RN license, advanced cardiac life support certification, pediatric advanced life support certification, 3 letters of recommendation. Additional exam requirements/recommendations for international students: Required—TOEFL (minimum score 550 paper-based; 79 iBT), IELTS (minimum score 6.5). Electronic applications accepted.

Brenau University, Sydney O. Smith Graduate School, College of Health and Science, Gainesville, GA 30501. Offers family nurse practitioner (MSN); nurse educator (MSN); nursing management (MSN); occupational therapy (MS); psychology (MS). *Accreditation:* AOTA. *Program availability:* Part-time, evening/weekend. *Degree requirements:* For master's, comprehensive exam (for some programs), thesis (for some programs), clinical practicum hours. *Entrance requirements:* For master's, GRE General Test or MAT (for some programs), interview, writing sample, references (for some programs). Additional exam requirements/recommendations for international students: Required—TOEFL (minimum score 500 paper-based; 61 iBT); Recommended—IELTS (minimum score 5). Electronic applications accepted. *Expenses:* Contact institution.

California Baptist University, Program in Nursing, Riverside, CA 92504-3206. Offers clinical nurse specialist (MSN); family nurse practitioner (MSN); healthcare systems management (MSN); teaching-learning (MSN). *Program availability:* Part-time. *Faculty:* 18 full-time (17 women), 14 part-time/adjunct (11 women). *Students:* 77 full-time (63 women), 143 part-time (117 women); includes 111 minority (26 Black or African American, non-Hispanic/Latino; 3 American Indian or Alaska Native, non-Hispanic/Latino; 38 Asian, non-Hispanic/Latino; 39 Hispanic/Latino; 1 Native Hawaiian or other Pacific Islander, non-Hispanic/Latino; 4 Two or more races, non-Hispanic/Latino), 5 international. Average age 33. 44 applicants, 64% accepted, 23 enrolled. In 2015, 19 master's awarded. *Degree requirements:* For master's, comprehensive exam or directed project thesis; capstone practicum. *Entrance requirements:* For master's, GRE or California Critical Thinking Skills Test; Test of Essential Academic Skills (TEAS), minimum undergraduate GPA of 3.0; completion of prerequisite courses with minimum grade of C; CPR certification; background check clearance; health clearance; drug testing; proof of health insurance; proof of motor vehicle insurance; three letters of recommendation; 1000-word essay; interview. Additional exam requirements/recommendations for international students: Required—TOEFL (minimum score 80 iBT). *Application deadline:* For fall admission, 8/1 priority date for domestic students, 7/1 for international students; for spring admission, 12/1 priority date for domestic students, 11/1 for international students. Applications are processed on a rolling basis. Application fee: $45. Electronic applications accepted. *Expenses:* $742 per unit, $355 per semester fees. *Financial support:* Federal Work-Study and scholarships/grants available. Financial award applicants required to submit CSS PROFILE or FAFSA. *Faculty research:* Qualitative research using Parse methodology, gerontology, disaster preparedness, medical-surgical nursing, maternal-child nursing. *Unit head:* Dr. Geneva Oaks, Dean, School of Nursing, 951-343-4702, E-mail: goaks@calbaptist.edu. *Application contact:* Dr. Rebecca Meyer, Director, Graduate Program in Nursing, 951-343-4952, Fax: 951-343-5095, E-mail: rmeyer@calbaptist.edu.
Website: http://www.calbaptist.edu/explore-cbu/schools-colleges/school-nursing/master-science-nursing/

California State University, Fresno, Division of Graduate Studies, College of Health and Human Services, Department of Nursing, Fresno, CA 93740-8027. Offers nursing (MS), including clinical nurse, primary care nurse practitioner, specialist/nurse educator. *Accreditation:* AACN. *Program availability:* Part-time, evening/weekend. *Degree requirements:* For master's, thesis or alternative. *Entrance requirements:* For master's, GRE General Test, 1 year of clinical practice, previous course work in statistics, BSN, minimum GPA of 3.0 in nursing. Additional exam requirements/recommendations for international students: Required—TOEFL. Electronic applications accepted. *Faculty research:* Training grant, HIV assessment.

California State University, Fullerton, Graduate Studies, College of Health and Human Development, Department of Nursing, Fullerton, CA 92834-9480. Offers leadership (MSN); nurse anesthesia (MSN); nurse educator (MSN); nursing (DNP); women's health care (MSN). *Accreditation:* AACN; AANA/CANAEP. *Program availability:* Part-time.

California State University, Stanislaus, College of Human and Health Sciences, Program in Nursing (MS), Turlock, CA 95382. Offers gerontological nursing (MS); nursing education (MS). *Accreditation:* AACN. *Program availability:* Part-time. *Degree requirements:* For master's, comprehensive exam, thesis or alternative. *Entrance requirements:* For master's, GRE or MAT, minimum GPA of 3.0, 3 letters of reference, RN. Additional exam requirements/recommendations for international students: Required—TOEFL (minimum score 550 paper-based). Electronic applications accepted.

Capella University, School of Public Service Leadership, Doctoral Programs in Nursing, Minneapolis, MN 55402. Offers nursing education (PhD); nursing practice (DNP).

Capella University, School of Public Service Leadership, Master's Programs in Nursing, Minneapolis, MN 55402. Offers diabetes nursing (MSN); general nursing (MSN); gerontology nursing (MSN); health information management (MS); nurse educator (MSN); nursing leadership and administration (MSN).

Carlow University, College of Health and Wellness, Program in Nursing Leadership and Education, Pittsburgh, PA 15213-3165. Offers MSN. *Program availability:* Part-time, evening/weekend, 100% online, blended/hybrid learning. *Students:* 34 full-time (31 women), 24 part-time (23 women); includes 5 minority (3 Black or African American, non-Hispanic/Latino; 1 Hispanic/Latino; 1 Two or more races, non-Hispanic/Latino). Average age 38. 19 applicants, 100% accepted, 10 enrolled. In 2015, 18 master's awarded. *Degree requirements:* For master's, internship. *Entrance requirements:* For master's, minimum undergraduate GPA of 3.0 from accredited BSN program; current license as RN in Pennsylvania; two professional recommendations; reflective essay of 300 words or less describing career goals and expectations for education. Additional exam requirements/recommendations for international students: Required—TOEFL (minimum score 550 paper-based). *Application deadline:* Applications are processed on a rolling basis. Electronic applications accepted. Application fee is waived when completed online. *Expenses: Tuition, area resident:* Full-time $11,147; part-time $801 per credit. Tuition and fees vary according to course load, degree level and program. *Unit head:* Dr. Renee Ingel, PhD, RN, Director, Nursing Leadership and DNP Programs, 412-578-6103, Fax: 412-578-6114, E-mail: rmingel@carlow.edu. *Application contact:* E-mail: gradstudies@carlow.edu.
Website: http://www.carlow.edu/Master_of_Science_in_Nursing_Concentration_in_Education_and_Leadership.aspx

Carson-Newman University, Department of Nursing, Jefferson City, TN 37760. Offers family nurse practitioner (MSN); nurse educator (MSN). *Accreditation:* AACN. *Program availability:* Part-time. *Faculty:* 4 full-time (3 women), 1 (woman) part-time/adjunct. *Students:* 9 full-time (8 women), 34 part-time (31 women); includes 1 minority (Black or African American, non-Hispanic/Latino). Average age 33. 14 applicants, 100% accepted, 9 enrolled. In 2015, 19 master's awarded. *Degree requirements:* For master's, comprehensive exam, thesis optional. *Entrance requirements:* For master's, GRE (minimum score of 290 within ten years of application), minimum GPA of 3.0 for all undergraduate work. Additional exam requirements/recommendations for international students: Recommended—TOEFL (minimum score 79 iBT), IELTS (minimum score 6.5), TSE (minimum score 53). *Application deadline:* For fall admission, 3/15 for domestic students; for spring admission, 10/15 for domestic students. Applications are processed on a rolling basis. Application fee: $50. *Expenses: Tuition, area resident:* Full-time $10,142; part-time $461 per credit hour. *Required fees:* $300; $461 per credit hour. $150 per semester. One-time fee: $150. *Financial support:* Federal Work-Study and tuition waivers (full and partial) available. Financial award applicants required to submit FAFSA. *Unit head:* Dr. Kimberly Bolton, Director, 865-471-4056, E-mail: kbolton@cn.edu. *Application contact:* Nilma Stewart, Graduate Admissions and Services Adviser, 865-471-3230, Fax: 865-471-3875, E-mail: adults@cn.edu.
Website: http://www.cn.edu/adult-graduate-studies/programs/new/nursing

Case Western Reserve University, Frances Payne Bolton School of Nursing, Master's Programs in Nursing, Cleveland, OH 44106. Offers nurse anesthesia (MSN); nurse educator (MSN); nurse midwifery (MSN); nurse practitioner (MSN), including acute care cardiovascular nursing, acute care nurse practitioner, acute care pediatric nurse practitioner, acute care/flight nurse, adult gerontology acute care nurse practitioner, adult gerontology nurse practitioner, adult gerontology oncology and palliative care, family nurse practitioner, family systems psychiatric mental health nursing, neonatal nurse practitioner, pediatric nurse practitioner, women's health nurse practitioner; nursing (MN). *Accreditation:* ACEN. *Program availability:* Part-time, blended/hybrid learning. *Students:* 147 full-time (120 women), 140 part-time (108 women); includes 54 minority (20 Black or African American, non-Hispanic/Latino; 20 Asian, non-Hispanic/Latino; 9 Hispanic/Latino; 5 Two or more races, non-Hispanic/Latino). Average age 35. 174 applicants, 66% accepted, 66 enrolled. In 2015, 125 master's awarded. Terminal master's awarded for partial completion of doctoral program. *Entrance requirements:* For master's, GRE General Test or MAT, CCRN certification (for nurse anesthesia). Additional exam requirements/recommendations for international students: Required—TOEFL (minimum score 577 paper-based; 90 iBT), IELTS (minimum score 7). *Application deadline:* For fall admission, 6/1 for domestic and international students; for spring admission, 10/1 for domestic and international students. Applications are processed on a rolling basis. Application fee: $75. *Expenses:* $1,891 per credit hour. *Financial support:* In 2015–16, 44 students received support, including 17 teaching assistantships with tuition reimbursements available (averaging $17,019 per year); scholarships/grants and traineeships also available. Financial award application deadline: 6/30; financial award applicants required to submit FAFSA. *Faculty research:* Symptom science, family/community care, aging across the lifespan, self-management of health and illness, neuroscience. *Unit head:* Dr. Carol Savrin, Director, 216-368-5304, Fax: 215-368-3542, E-mail: cls18@case.edu. *Application contact:* Donna Hassik, Admissions Coordinator, 216-368-5253, Fax: 216-368-0124, E-mail: dmh7@case.edu.
Website: http://fpb.case.edu/MSN/

Cedar Crest College, Program in Nursing, Allentown, PA 18104-6196. Offers nursing administration (MS); nursing education (MS). *Program availability:* Part-time. *Faculty:* 4 full-time (all women), 1 part-time/adjunct (0 women). *Students:* 12 part-time (all women); includes 1 minority (Hispanic/Latino). Average age 35. In 2015, 15 master's awarded. *Application deadline:* Applications are processed on a rolling basis. Electronic applications accepted. *Expenses:* Contact institution. *Unit head:* Dr. Wendy Robb, Director, 610-606-4666, E-mail: wjrobb@cedarcrest.edu. *Application contact:* Mary Ellen Hickes, Director of School of Adult and Graduate Education, 610-606-4666, E-mail: sage@cedarcrest.edu.
Website: http://sage.cedarcrest.edu/degrees/graduate/nursing-science/

Central Methodist University, College of Graduate and Extended Studies, Fayette, MO 65248-1198. Offers clinical counseling (MS); clinical nurse leader (MSN); education (M Ed); music education (MME); nurse educator (MSN). *Program availability:* Part-time, evening/weekend, online learning. *Degree requirements:* For master's, thesis. *Entrance requirements:* For master's, GRE General Test, minimum GPA of 2.75. Electronic applications accepted.

Chatham University, Nursing Programs, Pittsburgh, PA 15232-2826. Offers education/leadership (MSN); nursing (DNP). *Accreditation:* AACN. *Program availability:* Online learning. *Faculty:* 11 full-time (10 women), 23 part-time/adjunct (18 women). *Students:* 64 full-time (58 women), 80 part-time (73 women); includes 50 minority (31 Black or African American, non-Hispanic/Latino; 9 Asian, non-Hispanic/Latino; 5 Hispanic/Latino; 1 Native Hawaiian or other Pacific Islander, non-Hispanic/Latino; 4 Two or more races, non-Hispanic/Latino), 10 international. Average age 44. 181 applicants, 50% accepted, 61 enrolled. In 2015, 9 master's, 76 doctorates awarded. *Entrance requirements:* For master's, RN license, BSN, minimum GPA of 3.0; for doctorate, RN license, MSN. Additional exam requirements/recommendations for international students: Required—TOEFL (minimum score 600 paper-based; 100 iBT), IELTS (minimum score 6.5), TWE. *Application deadline:* For fall admission, 5/1 priority date for domestic and international students. Applications are processed on a rolling basis. Application fee: $0. Electronic applications accepted. *Expenses: Tuition, area resident:* Full-time $15,786; part-time $877 per credit hour. *Required fees:* $468; $26 per credit hour. *Financial support:* Applicants required to submit FAFSA. *Unit head:* Dr. Diane Hunker, Director, 412-365-1738, E-mail: dhunker@chatham.edu. *Application contact:* Patricia Golla, Assistant Director of Graduate Admissions, 412-365-1386, Fax: 412-365-1720, E-mail: pgolla@chatham.edu.
Website: http://www.chatham.edu/nursing

Clarion University of Pennsylvania, Office of Transfer, Adult and Graduate Admissions, Master of Science in Nursing Program, Clarion, PA 16214. Offers family nurse practitioner (MSN); nurse educator (MSN). Program offered jointly with Slippery Rock University of Pennsylvania. *Accreditation:* ACEN. *Program availability:* Part-time, online learning. *Degree requirements:* For master's, comprehensive exam, thesis. *Entrance requirements:* For master's, minimum QPA of 2.75. Additional exam requirements/recommendations for international students: Required—TOEFL (minimum score 550 paper-based; 80 iBT). Electronic applications accepted.

Clarion University of Pennsylvania, Office of Transfer, Adult and Graduate Admissions, Online Certificate Programs, Clarion, PA 16214. Offers family nurse practitioner (Post-Master's Certificate); library science (CAS); nurse educator (Post-Master's Certificate); public relations (Certificate). *Accreditation:* ALA (one or more programs are accredited at the [master's] level). *Program availability:* Part-time, online learning. *Entrance requirements:* Additional exam requirements/recommendations for international students: Required—TOEFL (minimum score 550 paper-based; 80 iBT), IELTS (minimum score 7). Electronic applications accepted.

Clarkson College, Master of Science in Nursing Program, Omaha, NE 68131. Offers adult nurse practitioner (MSN, Post-Master's Certificate); family nurse practitioner (MSN,

Post-Master's Certificate); nursing education (MSN, Post-Master's Certificate); nursing health care leadership (MSN, Post-Master's Certificate). *Accreditation:* AANA/CANAEP; ACEN. *Program availability:* Part-time, evening/weekend, online learning. *Degree requirements:* For master's, on-campus skills assessment (family nurse practitioner, adult nurse practitioner), comprehensive exam or thesis. *Entrance requirements:* For master's, minimum GPA of 3.0, 2 references, resume. Additional exam requirements/recommendations for international students: Required—TOEFL (minimum score 600 paper-based; 100 iBT). Electronic applications accepted.

Cleveland State University, College of Graduate Studies, College of Education and Human Services, Program in Urban Education, Specialization in Nursing Education, Cleveland, OH 44115. Offers PhD. *Program availability:* Part-time. *Faculty:* 6 full-time (all women). *Students:* 3 part-time (2 women). Average age 55. *Degree requirements:* For doctorate, one foreign language, comprehensive exam, thesis/dissertation. *Entrance requirements:* For doctorate, GRE General Test (minimum score of 297 for combined Verbal and Quantitative exams, 4.0 preferred for Analytical Writing), minimum GPA of 3.25 for MSN, curriculum vitae or resume, personal statement, 2 letters of recommendation. Additional exam requirements/recommendations for international students: Required—TOEFL (minimum score 550 paper-based; 78 iBT), IELTS (minimum score 6). *Application deadline:* For fall admission, 1/15 for domestic and international students. Electronic applications accepted. *Expenses:* Tuition, state resident: full-time $9565. Tuition, nonresident: full-time $17,980. Tuition and fees vary according to program. *Faculty research:* Aspects of educating individuals to function in a complex applied discipline, educating nurses. *Unit head:* Dr. Graham Stead, Program Coordinator, 216-875-9869, E-mail: g.b.stead@csuohio.edu. *Application contact:* Rita M. Grabowski, Administrative Coordinator, 216-687-4697, Fax: 216-875-9697, E-mail: r.grabowski@csuohio.edu.
Website: http://www.csuohio.edu/cehs/doc/specializations-nursing-education

Cleveland State University, College of Graduate Studies, School of Nursing, Cleveland, OH 44115. Offers clinical nurse leader (MSN); forensic nursing (MSN); nursing education (MSN); specialized population (MSN); urban education (PhD), including nursing education; MSN/MBA. *Accreditation:* AACN. *Program availability:* Part-time, 100% online. *Faculty:* 7 full-time (all women). *Students:* 7 full-time (all women), 43 part-time (42 women); includes 14 minority (12 Black or African American, non-Hispanic/Latino; 1 Asian, non-Hispanic/Latino; 1 Hispanic/Latino). Average age 37. 60 applicants, 62% accepted, 26 enrolled. In 2015, 11 master's awarded. *Degree requirements:* For master's, thesis optional, portfolio, capstone practicum project; for doctorate, comprehensive exam, thesis/dissertation. *Entrance requirements:* For master's, RN license in the U.S., BSN with minimum cumulative GPA of 3.0, recent (within last 5 years) course work in statistics; for doctorate, GRE, MSN with minimum cumulative GPA of 3.25. Additional exam requirements/recommendations for international students: Required—TOEFL (minimum score 550 paper-based; 78 iBT), IELTS (minimum score 6). *Application deadline:* For fall admission, 3/1 priority date for domestic and international students. Application fee: $55. Electronic applications accepted. *Expenses:* Tuition, state resident: full-time $9565. Tuition, nonresident: full-time $17,980. Tuition and fees vary according to program. *Financial support:* Tuition waivers (full) and unspecified assistantships available. Financial award application deadline: 5/1; financial award applicants required to submit FAFSA. *Faculty research:* Diabetes management, African-American elders medication compliance, risk in home visiting, suffering, COPD and stress, nursing education, disaster health preparedness. *Total annual research expenditures:* $330,000. *Unit head:* Dr. Vida Lock, Dean, 216-523-7237, Fax: 216-687-3556, E-mail: v.lock@csuohio.edu. *Application contact:* Maureen Mitchell, Assistant Professor and Graduate Program Director, 216-523-7128, Fax: 216-687-3556, E-mail: m.m.mitchell1@csuohio.edu.
Website: http://www.csuohio.edu/nursing/

College of Mount Saint Vincent, School of Professional and Continuing Studies, Department of Nursing, Riverdale, NY 10471-1093. Offers adult nurse practitioner (MSN, PMC); family nurse practitioner (MSN, PMC); nurse educator (PMC); nursing administration (MSN); nursing for the adult and aged (MSN). *Accreditation:* AACN. *Program availability:* Part-time. *Entrance requirements:* For master's, BSN, interview, RN license, minimum GPA of 3.0, letters of reference. Additional exam requirements/recommendations for international students: Required—TOEFL. *Expenses:* Contact institution.

The College of New Rochelle, Graduate School, Program in Nursing, New Rochelle, NY 10805-2308. Offers acute care nurse practitioner (MS, Certificate); clinical specialist in holistic nursing (MS, Certificate); family nurse practitioner (MS, Certificate); nursing and health care management (MS); nursing education (Certificate). *Accreditation:* AACN. *Program availability:* Part-time. *Faculty:* 3 full-time (2 women), 6 part-time/adjunct (4 women). *Students:* 116 part-time (104 women); includes 79 minority (58 Black or African American, non-Hispanic/Latino; 11 Asian, non-Hispanic/Latino; 10 Hispanic/Latino). Average age 38. In 2015, 25 master's awarded. *Entrance requirements:* For master's, GRE General Test or MAT, BSN, malpractice insurance, minimum GPA of 3.0, RN license. *Application deadline:* For fall admission, 8/15 priority date for domestic students; for spring admission, 12/1 priority date for domestic students. Applications are processed on a rolling basis. Application fee: $35. Electronic applications accepted. *Expenses: Tuition, area resident:* Part-time $894 per credit. *Required fees:* $350 per semester. *Financial support:* Traineeships available. Support available to part-time students. Financial award application deadline: 8/15; financial award applicants required to submit FAFSA. *Unit head:* Dr. H. Michael Dreher, Dean, School of Nursing, 914-654-5441, E-mail: hdreher@cnr.edu. *Application contact:* Michael Petri, Interim Director of Graduate Admissions, 914-654-5256, E-mail: mpetri@cnr.edu.

Colorado Mesa University, Department of Health Sciences, Grand Junction, CO 81501-3122. Offers advanced nursing practice (MSN); family nurse practitioner (DNP); health information technology systems (Graduate Certificate); nursing education (MSN). *Program availability:* Part-time, evening/weekend, online learning. *Degree requirements:* For master's and doctorate, Capstone. *Entrance requirements:* For master's and doctorate, Minimum GPA of 3.0 in BSN Program. Additional exam requirements/recommendations for international students: Required—TOEFL (minimum score 550 paper-based). Electronic applications accepted.

Columbus State University, Graduate Studies, College of Education and Health Professions, School of Nursing, Columbus, GA 31907-5645. Offers family nurse practitioner (MSN); nursing (MSN), including nurse educator, nurse informatics, nurse leader. Program offered in collaboration with Georgia Southwestern University. *Program availability:* Part-time, online only, 100% online. *Faculty:* 7 full-time (all women), 1 part-time/adjunct (0 women). *Students:* 29 full-time (24 women), 44 part-time (43 women); includes 35 minority (25 Black or African American, non-Hispanic/Latino; 1 Asian, non-Hispanic/Latino; 3 Hispanic/Latino; 6 Two or more races, non-Hispanic/Latino). Average age 38. 66 applicants, 59% accepted, 32 enrolled. In 2015, 6 master's awarded. *Entrance requirements:* For master's, GRE, BSN, minimum undergraduate GPA of 3.0. Additional exam requirements/recommendations for international students: Required—TOEFL (minimum score 550 paper-based; 79 iBT). *Application deadline:* For fall admission, 5/1 for domestic and international students; for spring admission, 11/1 for domestic and international students; for summer admission, 3/1 for domestic and international students. Applications are processed on a rolling basis. Application fee:

Nursing Education

$50. Electronic applications accepted. *Expenses:* Contact institution. *Financial support:* In 2015–16, 51 students received support. Institutionally sponsored loans available. Financial award application deadline: 5/1; financial award applicants required to submit FAFSA. *Unit head:* Latonya Sanot, Interim Director, 706-507-8576, E-mail: santo_latonya@columbusstate.edu. *Application contact:* Kristin Williams, Director of International and Graduate Recruitment, 706-507-8848, Fax: 706-568-5091, E-mail: williams_kristin@columbusstate.edu.
Website: http://nursing.columbusstate.edu/

Concordia University Wisconsin, Graduate Programs, School of Human Services, Program in Nursing, Mequon, WI 53097-2402. Offers family nurse practitioner (MSN); geriatric nurse practitioner (MSN); nurse educator (MSN). *Accreditation:* AACN. *Program availability:* Online learning. *Degree requirements:* For master's, comprehensive exam, thesis or alternative. *Entrance requirements:* Additional exam requirements/recommendations for international students: Required—TOEFL. *Expenses:* Contact institution.

Cox College, Programs in Nursing, Springfield, MO 65802. Offers clinical nurse leader (MSN); family nurse practitioner (MSN); nurse educator (MSN). *Accreditation:* AACN. *Entrance requirements:* For master's, RN license, essay, 2 letters of recommendation, official transcripts. Electronic applications accepted.

Daemen College, Department of Nursing, Amherst, NY 14226-3592. Offers adult nurse practitioner (MS, Post Master's Certificate); nurse executive leadership (Post Master's Certificate); nursing education (MS, Post Master's Certificate); nursing executive leadership (MS); nursing practice (DNP); palliative care nursing (Post Master's Certificate). *Accreditation:* ACEN. *Program availability:* Part-time. *Degree requirements:* For master's, thesis or alternative, degree completed in 4 years; minimum GPA of 3.0; for doctorate, degree completed in 5 years; 500 post-master's clinical hours. *Entrance requirements:* For master's, BN, 1 year medical/surgical experience, RN license and state registration, statistics course with minimum C grade, 3 letters of recommendation, minimum GPA of 3.25, interview; for doctorate, MS in advance nursing practice; New York state RN license; goal statement; resume; interview; statistics course with minimum grade of 'C'; for Post Master's Certificate, master's degree in clinical area; RN license and current registration; one year of clinical experience; statistics course with minimum grade of 'C'; 3 letters of recommendation; interview; letter of intent. Additional exam requirements/recommendations for international students: Required—TOEFL (minimum score 500 paper-based; 63 iBT), IELTS (minimum score 5.5). Electronic applications accepted. *Faculty research:* Professional stress, client behavior, drug therapy, treatment modalities and pulmonary cancers, chemical dependency.

Delta State University, Graduate Programs, School of Nursing, Cleveland, MS 38733. Offers family nurse practitioner (MSN); nurse administrator (MSN); nurse educator (MSN). *Accreditation:* AACN. *Program availability:* Part-time. *Degree requirements:* For master's, thesis optional. *Entrance requirements:* For master's, GRE General Test. Electronic applications accepted.

DeSales University, Division of Healthcare, Center Valley, PA 18034-9568. Offers adult-gerontology acute care (Post Master's Certificate); adult-gerontology acute care nurse practitioner (MSN); adult-gerontology acute certified nurse practitioner (Post Master's Certificate); adult-gerontology clinical nurse specialist (MSN, Post Master's Certificate); clinical leadership (DNP); family nurse practitioner (MSN, Post Master's Certificate); general nursing practice (DNP); health care information management (MSIS); network security (MSIS); nurse anesthetists (MSN); nurse educator (Post Master's Certificate, Postbaccalaureate Certificate); nurse midwives (MSN); nurse practitioner (MSN); project management (MSIS); psychiatric-mental health nurse practitioner (MSN, Post Master's Certificate); DNP/MBA. *Accreditation:* ACEN. *Program availability:* Part-time. *Faculty:* 22 full-time (14 women), 37 part-time/adjunct (29 women). *Students:* 244 full-time (178 women), 55 part-time (50 women); includes 24 minority (7 Black or African American, non-Hispanic/Latino; 9 Asian, non-Hispanic/Latino; 6 Hispanic/Latino; 2 Two or more races, non-Hispanic/Latino). Average age 31. 68 applicants, 85% accepted, 52 enrolled. In 2015, 73 master's awarded. *Degree requirements:* For master's, minimum GPA of 3.0, portfolio; for doctorate, minimum GPA of 3.0, scholarly capstone project. *Entrance requirements:* For master's, GRE or MAT (waived if applicant has an undergraduate GPA of 3.0 or higher), BSN from ACEN- or CCNE-accredited program, minimum undergraduate GPA of 3.0, active RN license or eligibility, two letters of recommendation, essay, health care experience, personal interview; for doctorate, BSN or MSN from ACEN- or CCNE-accredited institution, minimum GPA of 3.3 in graduate program, current licensure as an RN. Additional exam requirements/recommendations for international students: Required—TOEFL (minimum score 104 iBT). *Application deadline:* Applications are processed on a rolling basis. Application fee: $50. Electronic applications accepted. *Expenses:* Contact institution. *Financial support:* Applicants required to submit FAFSA. *Unit head:* Fr. Dr. Peter Leonard, OSFS, Dean of Graduate Education, 610-282-1100 Ext. 1289, E-mail: peter.leonard@desales.edu. *Application contact:* Abigail Wernicki, Director of Graduate Admissions, 610-282-1100 Ext. 1768, Fax: 610-282-2869, E-mail: gradadmissions@desales.edu.

Drexel University, College of Nursing and Health Professions, Division of Graduate Nursing, Philadelphia, PA 19104-2875. Offers adult acute care (MSN); adult psychiatric/mental health (MSN); advanced practice nursing (MSN); clinical trials research (MSN); family nurse practitioner (MSN); leadership in health systems management (MSN); nursing education (MSN); pediatric primary care (MSN); women's health (MSN). *Accreditation:* AACN. Electronic applications accepted.

Duke University, School of Nursing, Durham, NC 27708-0586. Offers acute care pediatric nurse practitioner (MSN, Post Master's Certificate); adult-gerontology nurse practitioner (MSN, Post Master's Certificate), including acute care, primary care; family nurse practitioner (MSN, Post Master's Certificate); neonatal nurse practitioner (MSN, Post Master's Certificate); nurse anesthesia (DNP); nurse practitioner (DNP); nursing (PhD); nursing and health care leadership (MSN); nursing education (MSN); nursing informatics (MSN, Post Master's Certificate); pediatric nurse practitioner (MSN, Post Master's Certificate), including primary care; women's health nurse practitioner (MSN, Post Master's Certificate). *Accreditation:* AACN; AANA/CANAEP. *Program availability:* Part-time, evening/weekend, online learning. *Faculty:* 74 full-time (63 women). *Students:* 179 full-time (152 women), 528 part-time (466 women); includes 145 minority (42 Black or African American, non-Hispanic/Latino; 3 American Indian or Alaska Native, non-Hispanic/Latino; 44 Asian, non-Hispanic/Latino; 35 Hispanic/Latino; 1 Native Hawaiian or other Pacific Islander, non-Hispanic/Latino; 20 Two or more races, non-Hispanic/Latino), 7 international. Average age 33. 619 applicants, 46% accepted, 201 enrolled. In 2015, 243 master's, 62 doctorates, 26 other advanced degrees awarded. Terminal master's awarded for partial completion of doctoral program. *Degree requirements:* For master's, thesis optional; for doctorate, capstone project. *Entrance requirements:* For master's, GRE General Test (waived if undergraduate GPA of 3.4 or higher), 1 year of nursing experience (recommended), minimum GPA of 3.0, previous course work in statistics; for doctorate, GRE General Test (waived if undergraduate GPA of 3.4 or higher), BSN or MSN, minimum GPA of 3.0, portfolio, resume, personal statement, undergraduate statistics course, current licensure as a registered nurse, transcripts from all post-secondary institutions; for Post Master's Certificate, MSN, licensure or eligibility as a professional nurse, transcripts from all post-secondary institutions, previous course

work in statistics. Additional exam requirements/recommendations for international students: Required—TOEFL (minimum score 100 iBT), IELTS (minimum score 7). *Application deadline:* For fall admission, 12/1 for domestic and international students; for spring admission, 5/1 for domestic and international students. Application fee: $50. Electronic applications accepted. *Expenses:* Contact institution. *Financial support:* Career-related internships or fieldwork, institutionally sponsored loans, scholarships/grants, traineeships, and tuition waivers (partial) available. Support available to part-time students. Financial award applicants required to submit FAFSA. *Faculty research:* Cardiovascular disease, caregiver skill training, data mining, prostate cancer, neonatal immune system. *Unit head:* Dr. Marion E. Broome, Dean/Vice Chancellor for Nursing Affairs/Associate Vice President for Academic Affairs for Nursing, 919-684-9446, Fax: 919-684-9414, E-mail: marion.broome@duke.edu. *Application contact:* Dr. Ernie Rushing, Director of Admissions and Recruitment, 919-668-6274, Fax: 919-668-4693, E-mail: ernie.rushing@dm.duke.edu.
Website: http://www.nursing.duke.edu/

Duquesne University, School of Nursing, Master of Science in Nursing Program, Pittsburgh, PA 15282-0001. Offers family (individual across the life span) nurse practitioner (MSN); forensic nursing (MSN); nursing education (MSN). *Accreditation:* AACN. *Program availability:* Part-time, evening/weekend, minimal on-campus study. *Faculty:* 13 full-time (11 women), 9 part-time/adjunct (all women). *Students:* 91 full-time (84 women), 87 part-time (76 women); includes 31 minority (16 Black or African American, non-Hispanic/Latino; 4 Asian, non-Hispanic/Latino; 7 Hispanic/Latino; 4 Two or more races, non-Hispanic/Latino; 1 international. Average age 34. 280 applicants, 34% accepted, 73 enrolled. In 2015, 39 master's awarded. *Entrance requirements:* For master's, current RN license; BSN with minimum GPA of 3.0; minimum of 1 year of full-time work experience as RN prior to registration in clinical or specialty course. Additional exam requirements/recommendations for international students: Required—TOEFL (minimum score 600 paper-based; 100 iBT). *Application deadline:* For fall admission, 3/1 for domestic and international students. Application fee: $0. Electronic applications accepted. *Expenses:* $1,218 per credit. *Financial support:* In 2015–16, 11 students received support, including 2 research assistantships with partial tuition reimbursements available (averaging $2,200 per year), 7 teaching assistantships with partial tuition reimbursements available (averaging $1,100 per year); scholarships/grants, traineeships, and tuition waivers (partial) also available. Support available to part-time students. Financial award application deadline: 7/1; financial award applicants required to submit FAFSA. *Faculty research:* Vulnerable populations, social justice, cultural competence, health disparities, wellness within chronic illness, forensics. *Total annual research expenditures:* $246,973. *Unit head:* Dr. Alison Colbert, Associate Professor/Associate Dean of Academic Affairs, 412-396-1511, Fax: 412-396-1821, E-mail: colberta@duq.edu. *Application contact:* Susan Hardner, Nurse Recruiter, 412-396-4945, Fax: 412-396-6346, E-mail: nursing@duq.edu.
Website: http://www.duq.edu/academics/schools/nursing/graduate-programs/master-science-nursing

Duquesne University, School of Nursing, Post Master's Certificate Program, Pittsburgh, PA 15282-0001. Offers family (individual across the life span) nurse practitioner (Post-Master's Certificate); forensic nursing (Post-Master's Certificate); nursing education and faculty role (Post-Master's Certificate). *Program availability:* Part-time, evening/weekend, minimal on-campus study. *Faculty:* 3 full-time (all women), 7 part-time/adjunct (all women). *Students:* 2 full-time (both women), 10 part-time (9 women); includes 4 minority (3 Black or African American, non-Hispanic/Latino; 1 Hispanic/Latino). Average age 42. 28 applicants, 36% accepted, 5 enrolled. In 2015, 4 Post-Master's Certificates awarded. *Entrance requirements:* For degree, current RN license, BSN, MSN. Additional exam requirements/recommendations for international students: Required—TOEFL (minimum score 600 paper-based; 100 iBT). *Application deadline:* For fall admission, 3/1 for domestic and international students. Application fee: $0. Electronic applications accepted. *Expenses:* $1,218 per credit. *Financial support:* Teaching assistantships with partial tuition reimbursements, scholarships/grants, traineeships, and tuition waivers (partial) available. Support available to part-time students. Financial award application deadline: 7/1; financial award applicants required to submit FAFSA. *Faculty research:* Vulnerable populations, social justice, cultural competence, health disparities, wellness within chronic illness, forensics. *Total annual research expenditures:* $296,973. *Unit head:* Dr. Alison Colbert, Associate Professor/Associate Dean of Academic Affairs, 412-396-1511, Fax: 412-396-1821, E-mail: colberta@duq.edu. *Application contact:* Susan Hardner, Nurse Recruiter, 412-396-4945, Fax: 412-396-6346, E-mail: nursing@duq.edu.
Website: http://www.duq.edu/academics/schools/nursing/graduate-programs/post-masters-certificates

Eastern Michigan University, Graduate School, College of Health and Human Services, School of Nursing, Ypsilanti, MI 48197. Offers nursing (MSN); teaching in health care systems (MSN, Graduate Certificate). *Accreditation:* AACN. *Program availability:* Part-time, evening/weekend, online learning. *Faculty:* 29 full-time (26 women). *Students:* 6 full-time (5 women), 22 part-time (19 women); includes 8 minority (6 Black or African American, non-Hispanic/Latino; 2 Asian, non-Hispanic/Latino). Average age 41. 24 applicants, 25% accepted, 2 enrolled. In 2015, 12 master's, 9 other advanced degrees awarded. *Degree requirements:* For master's, thesis optional. *Entrance requirements:* For master's, GRE General Test, Michigan RN license. Additional exam requirements/recommendations for international students: Required—TOEFL. *Application deadline:* Applications are processed on a rolling basis. Application fee: $45. *Financial support:* Fellowships, research assistantships with full tuition reimbursements, teaching assistantships with full tuition reimbursements, career-related internships or fieldwork, Federal Work-Study, institutionally sponsored loans, scholarships/grants, tuition waivers (partial), and unspecified assistantships available. Support available to part-time students. Financial award applicants required to submit FAFSA. *Unit head:* Dr. Michael Williams, Director, 734-487-2310, Fax: 734-487-6946, E-mail: mwilliams@emich.edu. *Application contact:* Roberta (Bobbi) Towne, Coordinator, School of Nursing, 734-487-2340, Fax: 734-487-6946, E-mail: rtowne1@emich.edu.
Website: http://www.emich.edu/nursing

Edgewood College, Henry Predolin School of Nursing, Madison, WI 53711. Offers administration (MSN); education (MSN); nursing (DNP). *Accreditation:* AACN. *Students:* 11 full-time (10 women), 60 part-time (55 women); includes 4 minority (1 Asian, non-Hispanic/Latino; 3 Hispanic/Latino). Average age 39. In 2015, 25 master's, 5 doctorates awarded. *Degree requirements:* For master's, practicum, research project; for doctorate, practicum, capstone project. *Entrance requirements:* For master's, minimum GPA of 3.0, 2 letters of reference, current RN license. Additional exam requirements/recommendations for international students: Required—TOEFL. *Application deadline:* For fall admission, 8/15 priority date for domestic students, 5/1 for international students; for spring admission, 1/8 priority date for domestic students, 11/1 for international students. Applications are processed on a rolling basis. Application fee: $30. Electronic applications accepted. *Unit head:* Dr. Margaret Noreuil, Dean, 608-663-2820, Fax: 608-663-3291, E-mail: mnoreuil@edgewood.edu. *Application contact:* Tracy Kantor, Enrollment and Applications Manager, 608-663-3297, Fax: 608-663-3496, E-mail: gps@edgewood.edu.
Website: http://www.edgewood.edu/Academics/School-of-Nursing

Edinboro University of Pennsylvania, Department of Nursing, Edinboro, PA 16444. Offers advanced practice nursing (DNP); family nurse practitioner (MSN); nurse educator (MSN). *Program availability:* Part-time, evening/weekend. *Degree requirements:* For master's, thesis, competency exam. *Entrance requirements:* For master's, GRE or MAT, minimum QPA of 2.5. *Application deadline:* Applications are processed on a rolling basis. Application fee: $30. Electronic applications accepted. *Expenses:* Tuition, state resident: full-time $11,280; part-time $470 per credit hour. Tuition, nonresident: full-time $16,920; part-time $705 per credit hour. *International tuition:* $16,920 full-time. *Required fees:* $3247.20; $135.30 per credit hour. *Financial support:* Research assistantships with tuition reimbursements, career-related internships or fieldwork, Federal Work-Study, scholarships/grants, and unspecified assistantships available. Support available to part-time students. Financial award application deadline: 2/15; financial award applicants required to submit FAFSA. *Unit head:* Dr. Amy McClune, Chair, 814-732-2619, E-mail: amcclune@edinboro.edu. *Application contact:* Dr. Amy McClune, Chair, 814-732-2619, E-mail: amcclune@edinboro.edu.
Website: http://www.edinboro.edu/departments/nursing/nursing.dot

Elms College, School of Nursing, Chicopee, MA 01013-2839. Offers nursing and health services management (MSN); nursing education (MSN). *Accreditation:* AACN. *Program availability:* Part-time, evening/weekend. *Faculty:* 4 full-time (all women), 5 part-time/adjunct (4 women). *Students:* 99 part-time (91 women); includes 6 minority (2 Black or African American, non-Hispanic/Latino; 1 American Indian or Alaska Native, non-Hispanic/Latino; 3 Hispanic/Latino). Average age 40. 43 applicants, 81% accepted, 27 enrolled. In 2015, 16 master's awarded. *Entrance requirements:* Additional exam requirements/recommendations for international students: Required—TOEFL. *Application deadline:* For fall admission, 7/1 priority date for domestic students; for spring admission, 11/1 priority date for domestic students. Applications are processed on a rolling basis. Application fee: $30. *Financial support:* Applicants required to submit FAFSA. *Unit head:* Dr. Kathleen Scoble, Dean, School of Nursing, 413-265-2204, E-mail: scoblek@elms.edu. *Application contact:* Dr. Cynthia L. Dakin, Director of Graduate Nursing Studies, 413-265-2455, Fax: 413-265-2335, E-mail: dakinc@elms.edu.

Emmanuel College, Graduate and Professional Programs, Graduate Program in Nursing, Boston, MA 02115. Offers education (MSN, Graduate Certificate); management (MSN, Graduate Certificate). *Program availability:* Part-time, evening/weekend. *Faculty:* 4 full-time (all women), 7 part-time/adjunct (all women). *Students:* 43 part-time (42 women); includes 3 minority (1 Black or African American, non-Hispanic/Latino; 1 Hispanic/Latino; 1 Two or more races, non-Hispanic/Latino). Average age 44. In 2015, 9 master's awarded. *Degree requirements:* For master's, 36 credits, including 6-credit practicum. *Entrance requirements:* For master's and Graduate Certificate, transcripts from all regionally-accredited institutions attended (showing proof of bachelor's degree completion), proof of RN license, 2 letters of recommendation, essay, resume. *Application deadline:* For fall admission, 7/30 for domestic students. Applications are processed on a rolling basis. Electronic applications accepted. Application fee is waived when completed online. *Expenses:* $2,581 per course. *Financial support:* Applicants required to submit FAFSA. *Unit head:* Diane Shea, Associate Dean for Nursing/Professor of Nursing Practice, 617-732-1604, E-mail: shead@emmanuel.edu. *Application contact:* Helen Muterperl, Assistant Director of Graduate Admissions, 617-735-9700, Fax: 617-507-0434, E-mail: gpp@emmanuel.edu. Website: http://www.emmanuel.edu/graduate-professional-programs/academics/nursing.html

Excelsior College, School of Nursing, Albany, NY 12203-5159. Offers nursing (MS); nursing education (MS); nursing informatics (MS); nursing leadership and administration of health care systems (MS). *Accreditation:* ACEN. *Program availability:* Part-time, evening/weekend, online learning. *Faculty:* 18 part-time/adjunct (14 women). *Students:* 938 part-time (770 women); includes 295 minority (166 Black or African American, non-Hispanic/Latino; 8 American Indian or Alaska Native, non-Hispanic/Latino; 36 Asian, non-Hispanic/Latino; 60 Hispanic/Latino; 8 Native Hawaiian or other Pacific Islander, non-Hispanic/Latino; 17 Two or more races, non-Hispanic/Latino), 2 international. Average age 45. In 2015, 200 master's awarded. *Entrance requirements:* For master's, RN license. *Application deadline:* Applications are processed on a rolling basis. Application fee: $110. Electronic applications accepted. *Expenses:* Tuition, area resident: Part-time $645 per credit. *Required fees:* $265 per unit. *Financial support:* Scholarships/grants available. *Unit head:* Dr. Barbara Pieper, Associate Dean, Graduate Program in Nursing, 518-464-8500, Fax: 518-464-8777, E-mail: msn@excelsior.edu. *Application contact:* Admissions Counselor, 518-464-8500, Fax: 518-464-8777, E-mail: admissions@excelsior.edu.

Felician University, Master of Science in Nursing Program, Lodi, NJ 07644-2117. Offers adult-gerontology nurse practitioner (MSN, PMC); executive leadership (MSN, PMC); family nurse practitioner (MSN, PMC); nursing education (MSN, PMC). *Accreditation:* AACN. *Program availability:* Part-time, evening/weekend, online learning. *Faculty:* 11 full-time (9 women), 2 part-time/adjunct (both women). *Students:* 1 (woman) full-time, 121 part-time (112 women); includes 60 minority (23 Black or African American, non-Hispanic/Latino; 1 American Indian or Alaska Native, non-Hispanic/Latino; 19 Asian, non-Hispanic/Latino; 17 Hispanic/Latino). Average age 40. 111 applicants, 83% accepted, 52 enrolled. In 2015, 18 master's awarded. *Entrance requirements:* For master's, BS in nursing or equivalent, minimum GPA of 3.0, 2 letters of recommendation, RN license; for PMC, RN license, minimum GPA of 3.0. Additional exam requirements/recommendations for international students: Recommended—TOEFL (minimum score 79 iBT). *Application deadline:* Applications are processed on a rolling basis. Application fee: $40. Electronic applications accepted. Application fee is waived when completed online. *Expenses:* Tuition, area resident: Part-time $965 per credit. Tuition and fees vary according to course load and program. *Financial support:* In 2015–16, 10 students received support. Traineeships available. Financial award applicants required to submit FAFSA. *Faculty research:* Anxiety and fear, curriculum innovation, health promotion. *Unit head:* Dr. Ann Tritak, Associate Dean, Department of Graduate Nursing, 201-201-559-6151, E-mail: tritaka@felician.edu. *Application contact:* Dr. Margaret Smolin, Director, Graduate Admissions, 201-559-1451, E-mail: graduate@felician.edu.

Ferris State University, College of Health Professions, School of Nursing, Big Rapids, MI 49307. Offers nursing (MSN); nursing administration (MSN); nursing education (MSN); nursing informatics (MSN). *Accreditation:* ACEN. *Program availability:* Part-time, evening/weekend, 100% online. *Faculty:* 5 full-time (all women), 2 part-time/adjunct (both women). *Students:* 95 part-time (84 women); includes 11 minority (4 Black or African American, non-Hispanic/Latino; 1 American Indian or Alaska Native, non-Hispanic/Latino; 3 Asian, non-Hispanic/Latino; 1 Hispanic/Latino; 1 Native Hawaiian or other Pacific Islander, non-Hispanic/Latino; 1 Two or more races, non-Hispanic/Latino). Average age 39. 23 applicants, 74% accepted, 13 enrolled. In 2015, 15 master's awarded. *Degree requirements:* For master's, comprehensive exam, practicum, practicum project. *Entrance requirements:* For master's, BS in nursing (for nursing education track); BS in nursing or related field (for nursing administration and nursing informatics tracks); registered nurse license, writing sample, letters of reference, 2 years' clinical experience (recommended). Additional exam requirements/

recommendations for international students: Required—TOEFL (minimum score 550 paper-based; 61 iBT). *Application deadline:* For fall admission, 4/15 priority date for domestic students; for spring admission, 10/15 for domestic students. Application fee: $0. Electronic applications accepted. Tuition and fees vary according to degree level and program. *Financial support:* In 2015–16, 3 students received support. Fellowships, research assistantships, teaching assistantships, career-related internships or fieldwork, and scholarships/grants available. Financial award application deadline: 4/15; financial award applicants required to submit FAFSA. *Faculty research:* Nursing education, end of life, leadership/education introverts in nursing. *Unit head:* Dr. Susan Owens, Chair, School of Nursing, 231-591-2267, Fax: 231-591-2325, E-mail: owenss3@ferris.edu. *Application contact:* Debby Buck, Off-Campus Program Secretary, 231-591-2270, Fax: 231-591-3788, E-mail: buckd@ferris.edu.
Website: http://www.ferris.edu/htmls/colleges/alliedhe/Nursing/homepage.htm

Florida National University, Program in Nursing, Hialeah, FL 33012. Offers family nurse practitioner (MSN); nurse educator (MSN); nurse leadership and management (MSN). *Degree requirements:* For master's, practicum. *Entrance requirements:* For master's, active registered nurse license, BSN from accredited institution. *Expenses: Tuition, area resident:* Full-time $15,600. *Required fees:* $650.

Florida Southern College, Program in Nursing, Lakeland, FL 33801-5698. Offers adult gerontology clinical nurse specialist (MSN); adult gerontology primary care nurse practitioner (MSN); nurse educator (MSN); nursing administration (MSN). *Accreditation:* AACN. *Program availability:* Part-time, evening/weekend. *Entrance requirements:* For master's, Florida RN license, 3 letters of recommendation, personal statement, minimum GPA of 3.0, resume. Additional exam requirements/recommendations for international students: Required—TOEFL (minimum score 550 paper-based). *Expenses:* Contact institution. *Faculty research:* End of life care, dementia, health promotion.

Florida State University, The Graduate School, College of Nursing, Tallahassee, FL 32306-4310. Offers family nurse practitioner (DNP); nurse educator (MSN, Certificate); nurse leader (MSN); nursing leadership (Certificate). *Accreditation:* AACN. *Program availability:* Part-time, online learning. *Faculty:* 13 full-time (12 women). *Students:* 56 full-time (49 women), 25 part-time (23 women); includes 25 minority (13 Black or African American, non-Hispanic/Latino; 4 Asian, non-Hispanic/Latino; 7 Hispanic/Latino; 1 Two or more races, non-Hispanic/Latino). Average age 38. 90 applicants, 50% accepted, 44 enrolled. In 2015, 2 master's, 20 doctorates awarded. *Degree requirements:* For master's, thesis optional; for doctorate, thesis/dissertation, evidence-based project. *Entrance requirements:* For master's, GRE General Test, MAT, minimum GPA of 3.0, BSN, United States RN license; for doctorate, GRE General Test, MAT, minimum GPA of 3.0, BSN or MSN, Florida RN license. Additional exam requirements/recommendations for international students: Required—TOEFL (minimum score 550 paper-based). *Application deadline:* For fall admission, 4/15 for domestic and international students. Application fee: $30. Electronic applications accepted. *Expenses: Tuition, area resident:* Full-time $7263; part-time $403.50 per credit hour. Tuition, nonresident: full-time $18,087; part-time $1004.85 per credit hour. *Required fees:* $1365; $75.81 per credit hour. $20 per semester. Tuition and fees vary according to campus/location. *Financial support:* In 2015–16, 75 students received support, including fellowships with partial tuition reimbursements available (averaging $6,300 per year), research assistantships with partial tuition reimbursements available (averaging $3,000 per year), 3 teaching assistantships with partial tuition reimbursements available (averaging $3,000 per year); career-related internships or fieldwork, Federal Work-Study, institutionally sponsored loans, scholarships/grants, traineeships, and tuition waivers (partial) also available. Financial award application deadline: 4/15; financial award applicants required to submit FAFSA. *Faculty research:* Cardiac, women's health, health promotion and prevention, educational strategies, infectious diseases. *Unit head:* Dr. Judith McFetridge-Durdle, Dean, 850-644-6846, Fax: 850-644-7660, E-mail: jdurdle@nursing.fsu.edu. *Application contact:* Carlos Urrutia, Assistant Director for Student Services, 850-644-5638, Fax: 850-645-7249, E-mail: currutia@fsu.edu. Website: http://nursing.fsu.edu/

Framingham State University, Continuing Education, Program in Nursing, Framingham, MA 01701-9101. Offers nursing education (MSN); nursing leadership (MSN). *Accreditation:* AACN. *Entrance requirements:* For master's, BSN; minimum cumulative undergraduate GPA of 3.0, 3.25 in nursing courses; coursework in statistics; 2 letters of recommendation; interview. Electronic applications accepted.

Francis Marion University, Graduate Programs, Department of Nursing, Florence, SC 29502-0547. Offers family nurse practitioner (MSN); family nurse practitioner with nurse educator certificate (MSN); nurse educator (MSN). *Program availability:* Part-time. *Faculty:* 7 full-time (all women). *Students:* 52 full-time (40 women), 28 part-time (23 women); includes 19 minority (16 Black or African American, non-Hispanic/Latino; 1 American Indian or Alaska Native, non-Hispanic/Latino; 1 Asian, non-Hispanic/Latino; 1 Two or more races, non-Hispanic/Latino). Average age 34. 37 applicants, 84% accepted, 27 enrolled. In 2015, 27 master's awarded. *Entrance requirements:* For master's, GRE, official transcripts, two letters of recommendation from professional associates or former professors, written statement of applicant's career goals, current nursing license. Additional exam requirements/recommendations for international students: Required—TOEFL (minimum score 550 paper-based; 79 iBT). *Application deadline:* For fall admission, 3/1 for domestic and international students; for spring admission, 10/1 for domestic and international students. Applications are processed on a rolling basis. Application fee: $37. Electronic applications accepted. *Expenses:* Contact institution. *Financial support:* Available to part-time students. Application deadline: 3/1; applicants required to submit FAFSA. *Unit head:* Dr. Ruth Wittmann-Price, Chair, 843-661-4625, E-mail: rwittmannprice@fmarion.edu. *Application contact:* Jennifer Taylor, Administrative Manager, Provost's Office, 843-661-1286, Fax: 843-661-4688, E-mail: jtaylor@fmarion.edu.

Franklin Pierce University, Graduate and Professional Studies, Rindge, NH 03461-0060. Offers curriculum and instruction (M Ed); elementary education (MS Ed); emerging network technologies (Graduate Certificate); energy and sustainability studies (MBA, Graduate Certificate); health administration (MBA, Graduate Certificate); human resource management (MBA, Graduate Certificate); information technology (MBA); leadership (MBA); nursing education (MS); nursing leadership (MS); physical therapy (DPT); physician assistant studies (MPAS); special education (M Ed); sports management (MBA). *Accreditation:* APTA. *Program availability:* Part-time, online learning. *Degree requirements:* For master's, concentrated original research projects; student teaching; fieldwork and/or internship; leadership project; PRAXIS I and II (for M Ed); for doctorate, concentrated original research projects, clinical fieldwork and/or internship, leadership project. *Entrance requirements:* For master's, minimum GPA of 2.5, 3 letters of recommendation; competencies in accounting, economics, statistics, and computer skills through life experience or undergraduate coursework (for MBA); certification/e-portfolio, minimum C grade in all education courses (for M Ed); license to practice as RN (for MS in nursing); for doctorate, GRE, BA/BS, 3 letters of recommendation, personal mission statement, interview, writing sample, minimum cumulative GPA of 2.8, master's degree (for DA); 80 hours of observation/work in PT settings, completion of anatomy, chemistry, physics, and statistics, minimum GPA of 3.0 (for DPT). Additional exam requirements/recommendations for international students:

Nursing Education

Required—TOEFL (minimum score 550 paper-based; 61 iBT). *Application deadline:* Applications are processed on a rolling basis. Application fee: $0. Electronic applications accepted. *Expenses: Tuition, area resident:* Part-time $660 per credit hour. Tuition and fees vary according to program. *Financial support:* Teaching assistantships with tuition reimbursements, career-related internships or fieldwork, and unspecified assistantships available. Support available to part-time students. Financial award applicants required to submit FAFSA. *Faculty research:* Evidence-based practice in sports physical therapy, human resource management in economic crisis, leadership in nursing, innovation in sports facility management, differentiated learning and understanding by design. *Unit head:* Dr. Maria Altobello, Dean, 603-647-3509, Fax: 603-229-4580, E-mail: altobellom@franklinpierce.edu. *Application contact:* Graduate Studies, 800-325-1090, Fax: 603-626-4815, E-mail: cgps@franklinpierce.edu.
Website: http://www.franklinpierce.edu/academics/gradstudies/index.htm

Frostburg State University, Graduate School, College of Liberal Arts and Sciences, Department of Nursing, Frostburg, MD 21532-1099. Offers nursing administration (MSN); nursing education (MSN). *Program availability:* Part-time, online learning.

Georgetown University, Graduate School of Arts and Sciences, School of Nursing and Health Studies, Washington, DC 20057. Offers acute care nurse practitioner (MS); clinical nurse specialist (MS); family nurse practitioner (MS); nurse anesthesia (MS); nurse-midwifery (MS); nursing (DNP); nursing education (MS). *Accreditation:* AACN; AANA/CANAEP (one or more programs are accredited); ACNM/ACME (one or more programs are accredited). *Degree requirements:* For master's, thesis optional. *Entrance requirements:* For master's, GRE General Test or MAT, bachelor's degree in nursing from NLN-accredited school, minimum undergraduate GPA of 3.0. Additional exam requirements/recommendations for international students: Required—TOEFL.

The George Washington University, School of Nursing, Washington, DC 20052. Offers adult nurse practitioner (MSN, DNP, Post-Master's Certificate); clinical research administration (MSN); family nurse practitioner (MSN, Post-Master's Certificate); health care quality (MSN, Post-Master's Certificate); nursing leadership and management (MSN); nursing practice (DNP), including nursing education; palliative care nurse practitioner (Post-Master's Certificate). *Accreditation:* AACN. *Faculty:* 42 full-time (all women), 71 part-time/adjunct (66 women). *Students:* 52 full-time (48 women), 519 part-time (463 women); includes 162 minority (72 Black or African American, non-Hispanic/Latino; 4 American Indian or Alaska Native, non-Hispanic/Latino; 52 Asian, non-Hispanic/Latino; 31 Hispanic/Latino; 3 Two or more races, non-Hispanic/Latino), 2 international. Average age 37. 465 applicants, 69% accepted, 187 enrolled. In 2015, 121 master's, 35 doctorates, 1 other advanced degree awarded. *Unit head:* Pamela R. Jeffries, Dean, 202-994-3725, E-mail: pjeffries@gwu.edu. *Application contact:* Kristin Williams, Associate Provost for Graduate Enrollment Management, 202-994-0467, Fax: 202-994-0371, E-mail: ksw@gwu.edu.
Website: http://nursing.gwumc.edu/

Georgia Southern University, Jack N. Averitt College of Graduate Studies, College of Health and Human Sciences, School of Nursing, Nurse Educator Certificate Program, Statesboro, GA 30458. Offers Certificate. *Students:* 1 (woman) full-time; minority (Black or African American, non-Hispanic/Latino). Average age 30. 3 applicants, 100% accepted. In 2015, 2 Certificates awarded. *Entrance requirements:* For degree, master's degree in nursing, minimum GPA of 3.0, current RN license. Additional exam requirements/recommendations for international students: Required—TOEFL (minimum score 80 iBT). *Application deadline:* For fall admission, 7/31 for domestic students; for spring admission, 11/30 for domestic students; for summer admission, 3/31 for domestic students. *Expenses:* Tuition, state resident: full-time $7236; part-time $277 per semester hour. Tuition, nonresident: full-time $27,118; part-time $1105 per semester hour. *Required fees:* $2092. *Faculty research:* Promotion of health and quality of life for individuals, families, and communities within a global society. *Unit head:* Dr. Sharon Radzyminski, Department Chair, 912-478-5455, Fax: 912-478-0536, E-mail: sradzyminski@georgiasouthern.edu.

Goldfarb School of Nursing at Barnes-Jewish College, Graduate Programs, St. Louis, MO 63110. Offers adult-gerontology acute care nurse practitioner (MSN); adult-gerontology nurse practitioner (MSN); nurse anesthesia (MSN); nurse educator (MSN); nurse executive (MSN). *Accreditation:* AACN; AANA/CANAEP. *Program availability:* Part-time, online learning. *Faculty:* 51 full-time (47 women), 6 part-time/adjunct (all women). *Students:* 58 full-time (57 women), 29 part-time (24 women); includes 17 minority (11 Black or African American, non-Hispanic/Latino; 2 Asian, non-Hispanic/Latino; 2 Hispanic/Latino; 2 Two or more races, non-Hispanic/Latino). Average age 26. 41 applicants, 22% accepted, 8 enrolled. In 2015, 56 master's awarded. *Degree requirements:* For master's, thesis or alternative. *Entrance requirements:* For master's, 2 references, personal statement, curriculum vitae or resume. Additional exam requirements/recommendations for international students: Required—TOEFL (minimum score 575 paper-based; 85 iBT). *Application deadline:* For fall admission, 2/1 priority date for international students; for spring admission, 10/1 priority date for international students. Applications are processed on a rolling basis. Application fee: $50. *Expenses:* Contact institution. *Financial support:* Fellowships, research assistantships, Federal Work-Study, institutionally sponsored loans, and scholarships/grants available. Support available to part-time students. Financial award applicants required to submit FAFSA. *Faculty research:* HIV stigma, HIV symptom management, palliative care with children and their families, heart disease prevention in Hispanic women, depression in the well elderly, alternative therapies in pre-term infants. *Unit head:* Dr. Gretchen Drinkard, Dean, 314-454-7540, Fax: 314-362-9222, E-mail: gld9643@bjc.org. *Application contact:* Karen Sartorius, Admissions Specialist, 314-454-7057, Fax: 314-362-9250, E-mail: ksartorius@bjc.org.
Website: http://www.barnesjewishcollege.edu/

Graceland University, School of Nursing, Independence, MO 64050-3434. Offers family nurse practitioner (MSN, PMC); nurse educator (MSN, PMC); organizational leadership (DNP). *Program availability:* Part-time, online learning. *Faculty:* 14 full-time (12 women), 21 part-time/adjunct (20 women). *Students:* 489 full-time (441 women); includes 75 minority (41 Black or African American, non-Hispanic/Latino; 5 American Indian or Alaska Native, non-Hispanic/Latino; 15 Asian, non-Hispanic/Latino; 2 Native Hawaiian or other Pacific Islander, non-Hispanic/Latino; 12 Two or more races, non-Hispanic/Latino), 1 international. Average age 39. 140 applicants, 69% accepted, 69 enrolled. In 2015, 137 master's, 11 doctorates awarded. *Degree requirements:* For master's, comprehensive exam (for some programs), thesis optional, scholarly project; for doctorate, capstone project. *Entrance requirements:* For master's, BSN from nationally-accredited program, RN license, minimum GPA of 3.0, satisfactory criminal background check; for doctorate, MSN from nationally-accredited program, RN license, minimum GPA of 3.2, criminal background check. Additional exam requirements/recommendations for international students: Recommended—TOEFL. *Application deadline:* For fall admission, 6/1 priority date for domestic students; for winter admission, 10/1 priority date for domestic students; for spring admission, 10/1 priority date for domestic students; for summer admission, 2/1 priority date for domestic students. Application fee: $50. Electronic applications accepted. *Expenses:* Contact institution. *Financial support:* Institutionally sponsored loans available. Support available to part-time students. Financial award applicants required to submit FAFSA. *Faculty research:* International nursing, family care-giving, health promotion. *Unit head:* Dr. Claudia D. Horton, Dean,

816-423-4670, Fax: 816-423-4753, E-mail: horton@graceland.edu. *Application contact:* Nick Walker, Admissions Representative, 816-423-4717, Fax: 816-833-2990, E-mail: nowalker@graceland.edu.
Website: http://www.graceland.edu/nursing

Grand Canyon University, College of Nursing, Phoenix, AZ 85017-1097. Offers acute care nurse practitioner (MS, PMC); clinical nurse specialist (PMC), including clinical nurse specialist, education; family nurse practitioner (MS); leadership in health care systems (MS); nurse education (MS). *Accreditation:* AACN. *Program availability:* Part-time, evening/weekend, online learning. *Degree requirements:* For master's and PMC, comprehensive exam (for some programs). *Entrance requirements:* For master's, minimum cumulative and science course undergraduate GPA of 3.0. Additional exam requirements/recommendations for international students: Required—TOEFL (minimum score 575 paper-based; 90 iBT), IELTS (minimum score 7).

Grand Valley State University, Kirkhof College of Nursing, Allendale, MI 49401-9403. Offers advanced practice (MSN); case management (MSN); nursing administration (MSN); nursing education (MSN); nursing practice (DNP); MSN/MBA. *Accreditation:* AACN. *Program availability:* Part-time. *Faculty:* 17 full-time (16 women), 6 part-time/adjunct (5 women). *Students:* 71 full-time (59 women), 53 part-time (45 women); includes 16 minority (10 Black or African American, non-Hispanic/Latino; 2 Asian, non-Hispanic/Latino; 3 Hispanic/Latino; 1 Two or more races, non-Hispanic/Latino), 3 international. Average age 33. 64 applicants, 94% accepted, 31 enrolled. In 2015, 1 master's, 11 doctorates awarded. *Degree requirements:* For master's, thesis optional. *Entrance requirements:* For master's, GRE, minimum upper-division GPA of 3.0, course work in statistics, Michigan RN license. Additional exam requirements/recommendations for international students: Required—TOEFL. *Application deadline:* For fall admission, 3/15 priority date for domestic students. Applications are processed on a rolling basis. Application fee: $30. Electronic applications accepted. *Financial support:* In 2015–16, 58 students received support, including 39 fellowships (averaging $11,141 per year), 33 research assistantships with tuition reimbursements available (averaging $7,339 per year); career-related internships or fieldwork, Federal Work-Study, institutionally sponsored loans, and traineeships also available. Financial award application deadline: 2/15. *Faculty research:* Multigenerational health promotion, chronic disease prevention, end-of-life issues, nursing workload, family caregiver health. *Total annual research expenditures:* $36,000. *Unit head:* Dr. Cynthia McCurren, Dean, 616-331-7161, Fax: 616-331-7362. *Application contact:* Dr. Cynthia Coviak, Associate Dean of Nursing Research and Faculty Development, 616-331-7170, Fax: 616-331-7362, E-mail: coviakc@gvsu.edu.
Website: http://www.gvsu.edu/kcon/

Grantham University, College of Nursing and Allied Health, Lenexa, KS 66219. Offers case management (MSN); health systems management (MHSM, MSN); healthcare administration (MHA); nursing education (MSN); nursing informatics (MSN); nursing management and organizational leadership (MSN). *Program availability:* Part-time, evening/weekend, online only, 100% online. *Faculty:* 1 (woman) full-time, 15 part-time/adjunct (11 women). *Students:* 59 full-time (42 women), 368 part-time (277 women); includes 181 minority (119 Black or African American, non-Hispanic/Latino; 2 American Indian or Alaska Native, non-Hispanic/Latino; 23 Asian, non-Hispanic/Latino; 21 Hispanic/Latino; 4 Native Hawaiian or other Pacific Islander, non-Hispanic/Latino; 12 Two or more races, non-Hispanic/Latino). Average age 41. 498 applicants, 94% accepted, 427 enrolled. In 2015, 119 master's awarded. *Degree requirements:* For master's, capstone. *Entrance requirements:* For master's, bachelor's degree from accredited degree-granting institution with minimum GPA of 2.5, BSN from accredited nursing program, valid RN license. Additional exam requirements/recommendations for international students: Required—TOEFL (minimum score 71 iBT); Recommended—IELTS (minimum score 6.5), TSE (minimum score 50). *Application deadline:* Applications are processed on a rolling basis. Electronic applications accepted. *Expenses: Tuition, area resident:* Full-time $3900; part-time $325 per credit hour. *Required fees:* $45 per term. One-time fee: $100. *Financial support:* Scholarships/grants available. *Faculty research:* Experimental exploration of the use of human patient simulation in the theory course, simulation education's impact on nursing confidence in the care of patients with Ebola virus, women's health-smoking cessation program for pregnant women, nursing and healthcare administration, business administration in healthcare. *Unit head:* Dana Basara, Dean, College of Nursing and Allied Health, 913-309-4783, Fax: 844-897-6490, E-mail: dbasara@grantham.edu. *Application contact:* Jared Parlette, Vice President of Student Enrollment, 888-947-2684, Fax: 866-908-2360, E-mail: admissions@grantham.edu.
Website: http://www.grantham.edu/colleges-and-schools/college-of-nursing-and-allied-health/

Gwynedd Mercy University, Frances M. Maguire School of Nursing and Health Professions, Gwynedd Valley, PA 19437-0901. Offers clinical nurse specialist (MSN), including gerontology, oncology, pediatrics; nurse educator (MSN); nurse practitioner (MSN), including adult health, pediatric health; nursing (DNP). *Accreditation:* ACEN. *Program availability:* Part-time, online learning. *Faculty:* 3 full-time (all women), 2 part-time/adjunct (both women). *Students:* 28 full-time (23 women), 68 part-time (62 women); includes 27 minority (18 Black or African American, non-Hispanic/Latino; 7 Asian, non-Hispanic/Latino; 2 Hispanic/Latino). Average age 37. 72 applicants, 25% accepted, 16 enrolled. In 2015, 7 master's awarded. *Degree requirements:* For master's, thesis optional; for doctorate, evidence-based scholarly project. *Entrance requirements:* For master's, GRE General Test or MAT, current nursing experience, physical assessment, course work in statistics, BSN from NLNAC-accredited program, 2 letters of recommendation, personal interview. Additional exam requirements/recommendations for international students: Required—TOEFL (minimum score 575 paper-based). *Application deadline:* For fall admission, 8/1 priority date for domestic students; for winter admission, 12/1 priority date for domestic students. Applications are processed on a rolling basis. Electronic applications accepted. *Expenses:* Contact institution. *Financial support:* In 2015–16, 21 students received support. Scholarships/grants, traineeships, and unspecified assistantships available. Financial award application deadline: 8/30. *Faculty research:* Critical thinking, primary care, domestic violence, multiculturalism, nursing centers. *Unit head:* Dr. Andrea D. Hollingsworth, Dean, 215-646-7300 Ext. 539, Fax: 215-641-5517, E-mail: hollingsworth.a@gmc.edu. *Application contact:* Dr. Barbara A. Jones, Director, 215-646-7300 Ext. 407, Fax: 215-641-5564, E-mail: jones.b@gmc.edu.
Website: http://www.gmercyu.edu/academics/graduate-programs/nursing

Herzing University Online, Program in Nursing, Menomonee Falls, WI 53051. Offers nursing (MSN); nursing education (MSN); nursing management (MSN). *Accreditation:* AACN. *Program availability:* Online learning.

Holy Family University, Graduate and Professional Programs, School of Nursing and Allied Health Professions, Philadelphia, PA 19114. Offers nursing administration (MSN); nursing education (MSN). *Accreditation:* AACN. *Program availability:* Part-time, evening/weekend. *Faculty:* 7 full-time (all women). *Students:* 42 part-time (39 women); includes 9 minority (4 Black or African American, non-Hispanic/Latino; 4 Asian, non-Hispanic/Latino; 1 Hispanic/Latino). Average age 36. 17 applicants, 82% accepted, 6 enrolled. In 2015, 12 master's awarded. *Degree requirements:* For master's, thesis or alternative, comprehensive portfolio, clinical practicum. *Entrance requirements:* For master's, BSN

or RN from appropriately-accredited program, minimum GPA of 3.0, professional references, official transcripts of all college or university work, essay/personal statement, current resume, completion of one undergraduate statistics course with minimum grade of C. Additional exam requirements/recommendations for international students: Required—TOEFL (minimum score 550 paper-based; 79 iBT), IELTS (minimum score 6), or PTE (minimum score 54). *Application deadline:* For fall admission, 7/1 priority date for domestic and international students; for winter admission, 1/1 for domestic students; for spring admission, 11/1 priority date for domestic and international students; for summer admission, 4/1 priority date for domestic and international students. Applications are processed on a rolling basis. Application fee: $25. Electronic applications accepted. *Financial support:* In 2015–16, 1 student received support. Available to part-time students. Application deadline: 2/15; applicants required to submit FAFSA. *Unit head:* Dr. Ana Maria Catanzaro, Dean, 267-341-3292, Fax: 215-637-6598, E-mail: acatanzaro@holyfamily.edu. *Application contact:* Gidget Matie Montelibano, Associate Director of Graduate Admissions, 267-341-3558, Fax: 215-637-1478, E-mail: gmontelibano@holyfamily.edu.
Website: http://www.holyfamily.edu/choosing-holy-family-u/academics/schools-of-study/school-of-nursing

Holy Names University, Graduate Division, Department of Nursing, Oakland, CA 94619-1699. Offers administration/management (MSN, PMC); clinical faculty (MSN, PMC); community health nursing/case manager (MSN); family nurse practitioner (MSN, PMC); MSN/MA; MSN/MBA. *Accreditation:* AACN. *Program availability:* Part-time, evening/weekend. *Entrance requirements:* For master's, bachelor's degree in nursing or related field; California RN license or eligibility; minimum cumulative GPA of 2.8, 3.0 in nursing courses from baccalaureate program; courses in pathophysiology, statistics, and research at the undergraduate level. Additional exam requirements/recommendations for international students: Required—TOEFL (minimum score 500 paper-based; 79 iBT). Electronic applications accepted. Application fee is waived when completed online. *Expenses: Tuition, area resident:* Full-time $25,272; part-time $936 per credit hour. *Required fees:* $500; $250 per credit hour. *Faculty research:* Women's reproductive health, gerontology, attitudes about aging, schizophrenic families, international health issues.

Husson University, Graduate Nursing Program, Bangor, ME 04401-2999. Offers advanced practice psychiatric nursing (MSN, PMC); family and community nurse practitioner (MSN, PMC); nursing education (MSN, PMC). *Accreditation:* AACN. *Program availability:* Part-time. *Faculty:* 6 full-time (all women), 2 part-time/adjunct (1 woman). *Students:* 27 full-time (26 women), 10 part-time (9 women); includes 4 minority (2 Asian, non-Hispanic/Latino; 2 Two or more races, non-Hispanic/Latino). Average age 39. 70 applicants, 27% accepted, 13 enrolled. In 2015, 9 master's awarded. *Degree requirements:* For master's, comprehensive exam (for some programs), research project. *Entrance requirements:* For master's, MAT or GRE, BSN. Additional exam requirements/recommendations for international students: Required—TOEFL (minimum score 550 paper-based; 80 iBT). *Application deadline:* For fall admission, 3/31 for domestic students; for spring admission, 10/30 for domestic students. Application fee: $40. Electronic applications accepted. *Expenses:* Contact institution. *Financial support:* Research assistantships, Federal Work-Study, institutionally sponsored loans, traineeships, and unspecified assistantships available. Financial award application deadline: 3/31; financial award applicants required to submit FAFSA. *Faculty research:* Health disparities and methods to better identify and provide healthcare services to those most in need. *Unit head:* Prof. Mary Jude, Director, Graduate Nursing, 207-941-7769, Fax: 207-941-7198, E-mail: judem@husson.edu. *Application contact:* Kristen Card, Director of Graduate Admissions, 207-404-5660, Fax: 207-941-7935, E-mail: cardk@husson.edu.
Website: http://www.husson.edu/nursing-msn

Immaculata University, College of Graduate Studies, Division of Nursing, Immaculata, PA 19345. Offers nursing administration (MSN); nursing education (MSN). *Accreditation:* AACN. *Program availability:* Part-time, evening/weekend. *Entrance requirements:* For master's, MAT or GRE, BSN, minimum undergraduate GPA of 3.0. Additional exam requirements/recommendations for international students: Required—TOEFL.

Indiana State University, College of Graduate and Professional Studies, College of Nursing, Health, and Human Services, Department of Advanced Practice Nursing, Terre Haute, IN 47809. Offers advanced practice nursing (DNP); family nurse practitioner (MS); nursing administration (MS); nursing education (MS). *Accreditation:* ACEN. *Program availability:* Part-time. *Degree requirements:* For master's, thesis or alternative. *Entrance requirements:* For master's, BSN, RN license, minimum undergraduate GPA of 3.0. Electronic applications accepted. *Faculty research:* Nursing faculty-student interactions, clinical evaluation, program evaluation, sexual dysfunction, faculty attitudes.

Indiana University Kokomo, School of Nursing, Kokomo, IN 46904-9003. Offers nurse administrator (MSN); nurse educator (MSN).

Indiana University of Pennsylvania, School of Graduate Studies and Research, College of Health and Human Services, Department of Nursing and Allied Health, Program in Nursing Education, Indiana, PA 15705-1087. Offers MS. *Program availability:* Part-time. *Faculty:* 12 full-time (11 women). *Students:* 8 full-time (7 women), 23 part-time (21 women), 7 international. Average age 35. 30 applicants, 70% accepted, 11 enrolled. In 2015, 7 master's awarded. *Degree requirements:* For master's, thesis optional, practicum. *Entrance requirements:* Additional exam requirements/recommendations for international students: Required—TOEFL (minimum score 540 paper-based). *Application deadline:* Applications are processed on a rolling basis. Application fee: $50. Electronic applications accepted. *Financial support:* In 2015–16, 2 research assistantships with tuition reimbursements (averaging $2,720 per year) were awarded; career-related internships or fieldwork, Federal Work-Study, scholarships/grants, and unspecified assistantships also available. Financial award application deadline: 4/15; financial award applicants required to submit FAFSA. *Unit head:* Dr. Nashat Zuraikat, Graduate Coordinator, 724-357-3262, E-mail: zuraikat@iup.edu.
Website: http://www.iup.edu/grad/nursing/default.aspx

Indiana University–Purdue University Fort Wayne, College of Health and Human Services, Department of Nursing, Fort Wayne, IN 46805-1499. Offers adult-gerontology primary care nurse practitioner (MS); family nurse practitioner (MS); nurse executive (MS); nursing administration (Certificate); nursing education (MS). *Accreditation:* ACEN. *Program availability:* Part-time. *Faculty:* 8 full-time (all women). *Students:* 6 full-time (all women), 79 part-time (70 women); includes 8 minority (2 Black or African American, non-Hispanic/Latino; 3 Asian, non-Hispanic/Latino; 3 Hispanic/Latino). Average age 36. 14 applicants, 100% accepted, 10 enrolled. In 2015, 17 master's awarded. *Entrance requirements:* For master's, GRE Writing Test (if GPA below 3.0), BS in nursing, eligibility for Indiana RN license, minimum GPA of 3.0, essay, copy of resume, three references, undergraduate course work in research and statistics within last 5 years. Additional exam requirements/recommendations for international students: Required—TOEFL (minimum score 550 paper based; 79 iBT); Recommended—TWE. *Application deadline:* For fall admission, 5/1 priority date for domestic and international students; for spring admission, 11/15 priority date for domestic students. Applications are processed on a rolling basis. Application fee: $55 ($60 for international students). Electronic

applications accepted. *Financial support:* In 2015–16, 12 teaching assistantships with partial tuition reimbursements (averaging $13,522 per year) were awarded; scholarships/grants also available. Support available to part-time students. Financial award application deadline: 3/1; financial award applicants required to submit FAFSA. *Faculty research:* Community engagement, cervical screening, evidence-based practice. *Total annual research expenditures:* $22,966. *Unit head:* Dr. Lee-Ellen Kirkhorn, Chair/Professor, 260-481-6789, Fax: 260-481-5767, E-mail: kirkhorl@ipfw.edu. *Application contact:* Dr. Deb Poling, Director of Graduate Program, 260-481-6276, Fax: 260-481-5767, E-mail: polingd@ipfw.edu.
Website: http://www.ipfw.edu/nursing/

Indiana University–Purdue University Indianapolis, School of Nursing, MSN Program in Nursing, Indianapolis, IN 46202. Offers nursing education (MSN); nursing leadership in health systems (MSN). *Program availability:* Part-time, online learning. *Degree requirements:* For master's, thesis. *Entrance requirements:* For master's, minimum GPA of 3.0, RN license, background check, statistics. Additional exam requirements/recommendations for international students: Required—TOEFL (minimum score 550 paper-based; 79 iBT). *Expenses:* Contact institution. *Faculty research:* Clinical science, health systems.

Indiana Wesleyan University, Graduate School, School of Nursing, Marion, IN 46953-4974. Offers nursing administration (MS); nursing education (MS); primary care nursing (MS); MSN/MBA. *Accreditation:* AACN. *Program availability:* Part-time, online learning. *Students:* 884 full-time (818 women), 27 part-time (all women); includes 148 minority (92 Black or African American, non-Hispanic/Latino; 5 American Indian or Alaska Native, non-Hispanic/Latino; 18 Asian, non-Hispanic/Latino; 16 Hispanic/Latino; 17 Two or more races, non-Hispanic/Latino), 2 international. Average age 38. *Degree requirements:* For master's, capstone project or thesis. *Entrance requirements:* For master's, writing sample, RN license, 1 year of related experience, graduate statistics course. Additional exam requirements/recommendations for international students: Required—TOEFL. *Application deadline:* Applications are processed on a rolling basis. *Expenses:* Contact institution. *Financial support:* Fellowships, career-related internships or fieldwork, scholarships/grants, and traineeships available. Support available to part-time students. Financial award application deadline: 3/15; financial award applicants required to submit FAFSA. *Faculty research:* Primary health care with international emphasis, international nursing. *Unit head:* Dr. Barbara Ihrke, Dean, 765-677-2813, Fax: 765-677-1768, E-mail: barbara.ihrke@indwes.edu. *Application contact:* Graduate School, 866-IWU-4-YOU, Fax: 765-677-2541, E-mail: graduate@indwes.edu.
Website: http://graduatenursing.indwes.edu

Jefferson College of Health Sciences, Program in Nursing, Roanoke, VA 24013. Offers nursing education (MSN); nursing management (MSN). *Accreditation:* AACN. *Program availability:* Part-time. *Degree requirements:* For master's, project. *Entrance requirements:* For master's, MAT. Additional exam requirements/recommendations for international students: Required—TOEFL (minimum score 550 paper-based; 80 iBT). Electronic applications accepted. *Faculty research:* Nursing, teaching and learning techniques, cultural competence, spirituality and nursing.

Kaplan University, Davenport Campus, School of Nursing, Davenport, IA 52807-2095. Offers nurse administrator (MS); nurse educator (MS). *Program availability:* Part-time, evening/weekend, online learning. *Entrance requirements:* For master's, RN. Additional exam requirements/recommendations for international students: Required—TOEFL (minimum score 550 paper-based).

Kent State University, College of Nursing, Kent, OH 44242. Offers advanced nursing practice (DNP), including adult gerontology acute care nurse practitioner (MSN, DNP), adult gerontology clinical nurse specialist (MSN, DNP), family nurse practitioner (MSN, DNP); nursing (MSN, PhD), including adult gerontology acute care nurse practitioner (MSN, DNP), adult gerontology clinical nurse specialist (MSN, DNP), family nurse practitioner (MSN, DNP), nurse educator (MSN), nursing healthcare management (MSN), primary care adult nurse practitioner (MSN), primary care pediatric clinical nurse specialist (MSN), primary care pediatric nurse practitioner (MSN), psychiatric mental health practitioner (MSN), women's health nurse practitioner (MSN); nursing education (Certificate); primary care pediatric nurse practitioner (Certificate); women's health nurse practitioner (Certificate). PhD program offered jointly with The University of Akron. *Accreditation:* AACN. *Program availability:* Part-time, online learning. *Faculty:* 52 full-time (48 women). *Students:* 78 full-time (56 women), 414 part-time (365 women); includes 63 minority (34 Black or African American, non-Hispanic/Latino; 1 American Indian or Alaska Native, non-Hispanic/Latino; 12 Asian, non-Hispanic/Latino; 12 Hispanic/Latino; 4 Two or more races, non-Hispanic/Latino), 16 international. Average age 37. 653 applicants, 54% accepted, 309 enrolled. In 2015, 140 master's, 1 doctorate, 13 other advanced degrees awarded. *Degree requirements:* For master's, thesis optional, practicum; for doctorate, comprehensive exam (for some programs), thesis/dissertation (for some programs), practicum and scholarly project (for DNP programs); for Certificate, practicum. *Entrance requirements:* For master's, minimum GPA of 3.0, transcripts, active unrestricted RN license, essay/goal statement, interview, 3 letters of recommendation; for doctorate, GRE (for PhD), minimum GPA of 3.0, transcripts, 3 letters of recommendation, interview; active unrestricted RN license, clinical experience and hours record (for DNP); goal statement, sample of written work, curriculum vitae, statement of research interests, and eligibility for RN license (for PhD); for Certificate, MSN, minimum GPA of 3.0, transcripts. Additional exam requirements/recommendations for international students: Required—TOEFL (minimum score: paper-based 525, iBT 71), Michigan English Language Assessment Battery (minimum score of 75), IELTS (minimum score 6.0), PTE Academic (minimum score of 48), or completion of ELS level 112 Intensive Program. *Application deadline:* For fall admission, 2/1 for domestic students; for spring admission, 11/1 for domestic students. Application fee: $45 ($70 for international students). Electronic applications accepted. *Expenses:* Tuition, state resident: full-time $10,864; part-time $495 per credit hour. Tuition, nonresident: full-time $18,380; part-time $837 per credit hour. *Financial support:* Research assistantships with full tuition reimbursements, teaching assistantships with full tuition reimbursements, career-related internships or fieldwork, Federal Work-Study, traineeships, and unspecified assistantships available. Financial award application deadline: 2/1. *Unit head:* Dr. Barbara Broome, Dean, 330-672-3777, E-mail: bbroome1@kent.edu. *Application contact:* Dr. Wendy A. Umberger, Associate Dean for Graduate Programs/Professor, 330-672-8813, E-mail: wlewando@kent.edu.
Website: http://www.kent.edu/nursing/

Lamar University, College of Graduate Studies, College of Arts and Sciences, JoAnne Gay Dishman Department of Nursing, Beaumont, TX 77710. Offers nursing administration (MSN); nursing education (MSN); MSN/MBA. *Accreditation:* ACEN. *Program availability:* Part-time, evening/weekend, online learning. *Faculty:* 8 full-time (all women), 2 part-time/adjunct (both women). *Students:* 2 full-time (both women), 73 part-time (64 women); includes 32 minority (17 Black or African American, non-Hispanic/Latino; 7 Asian, non-Hispanic/Latino; 6 Hispanic/Latino; 2 Two or more races, non-Hispanic/Latino). Average age 38. 47 applicants, 77% accepted, 14 enrolled. In 2015, 14 master's awarded. *Degree requirements:* For master's, comprehensive exam, practicum project presentation, evidence-based project. *Entrance requirements:* For master's, GRE General Test, MAT, criminal background check, RN license, NLN-accredited BSN, college course work in statistics in past 5 years, letters of

Nursing Education

recommendation, minimum undergraduate GPA of 3.0. Additional exam requirements/recommendations for international students: Required—TOEFL (minimum score 550 paper-based; 79 iBT), IELTS (minimum score 6.5). *Application deadline:* For fall admission, 8/10 for domestic students, 7/1 for international students; for spring admission, 1/5 for domestic students, 12/1 for international students. Applications are processed on a rolling basis. Application fee: $25 ($50 for international students). Electronic applications accepted. *Expenses: Tuition, area resident:* Full-time $6720; part-time $4032. Tuition, nonresident: full-time $14,880; part-time $8928. *Required fees:* $1900; $950 $784. *Financial support:* In 2015–16, 3 students received support. Teaching assistantships, scholarships/grants, and traineeships available. Financial award application deadline: 4/1; financial award applicants required to submit FAFSA. *Faculty research:* Student retention, theory, care giving, online course and research. *Unit head:* Cynthia Stinson, Interim Chair, 409-880-8817, Fax: 409-880-8698. *Application contact:* Melissa Gallien, Director, Admissions and Academic Services, 409-880-8888, Fax: 409-880-7419, E-mail: gradmissions@lamar.edu.
Website: http://artssciences.lamar.edu/nursing

La Roche College, School of Graduate Studies and Adult Education, Program in Nursing, Pittsburgh, PA 15237-5898. Offers nursing education (MSN); nursing management (MSN). *Accreditation:* AANA/CANAEP; ACEN. *Program availability:* Part-time, evening/weekend, online only, 100% online. *Faculty:* 3 full-time (all women), 1 part-time/adjunct (0 women). *Students:* 14 full-time (all women), 8 part-time (all women), 2 international. Average age 40. 20 applicants, 75% accepted, 11 enrolled. In 2015, 3 master's awarded. *Degree requirements:* For master's, thesis optional, internship, practicum. *Entrance requirements:* For master's, GRE General Test, BSN, nursing license, work experience. Additional exam requirements/recommendations for international students: Recommended—TOEFL (minimum score 550 paper-based). *Application deadline:* For fall admission, 8/15 priority date for domestic students, 8/15 for international students; for spring admission, 12/15 priority date for domestic students, 12/15 for international students. Applications are processed on a rolling basis. Application fee: $50. Electronic applications accepted. *Expenses:* Contact institution. *Financial support:* Application deadline: 3/31; applicants required to submit FAFSA. *Faculty research:* Patient education, perception. *Unit head:* Dr. Terri Liberto, Division Chair, 412-847-1813, Fax: 412-536-1175, E-mail: terri.liberto@laroche.edu. *Application contact:* Hope Schiffgens, Director of Graduate Studies and Adult Education, 412-536-1266, Fax: 412-536-1283, E-mail: schombh1@laroche.edu.

La Salle University, School of Nursing and Health Sciences, Program in Nursing, Philadelphia, PA 19141-1199. Offers adult gerontology primary care nurse practitioner (MSN, Certificate); adult health and illness clinical nurse specialist (MSN); adult-gerontology clinical nurse specialist (MSN, Certificate); clinical nurse leader (MSN); family primary care nurse practitioner (MSN, Certificate); gerontology (Certificate); nurse anesthetist (MSN, Certificate); nursing (MSN, Certificate); nursing administration (MSN, Certificate); nursing education (Certificate); nursing practice (DNP); nursing service administration (MSN); public health nursing (MSN, Certificate); school nursing (Certificate); MSN/MBA; MSN/MPH. *Accreditation:* AANA/CANAEP. *Program availability:* Part-time, evening/weekend, 100% online. *Faculty:* 13 full-time (all women), 9 part-time/adjunct (8 women). *Students:* 368 part-time (56 women); includes 103 minority (62 Black or African American, non-Hispanic/Latino; 1 American Indian or Alaska Native, non-Hispanic/Latino; 26 Asian, non-Hispanic/Latino; 9 Hispanic/Latino; 5 Two or more races, non-Hispanic/Latino), 5 international. Average age 36. 98 applicants, 85% accepted, 53 enrolled. In 2015, 87 master's, 3 doctorates, 10 other advanced degrees awarded. *Degree requirements:* For doctorate, minimum of 1,000 hours of post baccalaureate clinical practice supervised by preceptors. *Entrance requirements:* For master's, GRE, MAT, or GMAT (for students with BSN GPA of less than 3.2), baccalaureate degree in nursing from an NLNAC- or CCNE-accredited program or an MSN Bridge program; Pennsylvania RN license; 2 letters of reference; resume; statement of philosophy articulating professional values and future educational goal; 1 year of work experience as a registered nurse; for doctorate, GRE (waived for applicants with MSN cumulative GPA of 3.7 or above), MSN from nationally-accredited program or master's degree, MBA or MHA from nationally-accredited program; resume or curriculum vitae; 2 letters of reference; interview; for Certificate, GRE, MAT, or GMAT (for students with BSN GPA of less than 3.2, baccalaureate degree in nursing from an NLNAC- or CCNE-accredited program or an MSN Bridge program; Pennsylvania RN license; 2 letters of reference; resume; statement of philosophy articulating professional values and future educational goal; 1 year of work experience as a registered nurse. Additional exam requirements/recommendations for international students: Required—TOEFL. *Application deadline:* For fall admission, 8/15 priority date for domestic students, 7/15 for international students; for spring admission, 12/15 priority date for domestic students, 11/15 for international students; for summer admission, 4/15 priority date for domestic students, 3/15 for international students. Applications are processed on a rolling basis. Application fee: $35. Electronic applications accepted. Application fee is waived when completed online. *Expenses:* $870 per credit hour (for MSN); $930 per credit hour (for DNP); $150 technology fee full-time, $75 part-time; $135 general university fee. *Financial support:* In 2015–16, 13 students received support. Scholarships/grants and traineeships available. Support available to part-time students. Financial award application deadline: 8/31; financial award applicants required to submit FAFSA. *Unit head:* Dr. Patricia M. Dillon, Director, 215-951-1322, Fax: 215-951-1896, E-mail: msnapn@lasalle.edu. *Application contact:* Alison McAnespey Target, Director, Graduate and Adult Enrollment, 215-951-1100, Fax: 215-951-1462, E-mail: reilly@lasalle.edu.
Website: http://www.lasalle.edu/nursing/program-options/

Le Moyne College, Department of Nursing, Syracuse, NY 13214. Offers informatics (MS, CAS); nursing administration (MS, CAS); nursing education (MS, CAS); nursing gerontology (MS, CAS); palliative care (MS, CAS). *Accreditation:* AACN. *Program availability:* Part-time, evening/weekend. *Degree requirements:* For master's, scholarly project. *Entrance requirements:* For master's, bachelor's degree, interview, minimum GPA of 3.0, New York RN license, 2 letters of recommendation, writing sample, transcripts. *Expenses:* Contact institution. *Faculty research:* Inter-profession education, gerontology, utilization of free healthcare services by the insured, health promotion education, innovative undergraduate nursing education models, patient and family education, horizontal violence.

Lenoir-Rhyne University, Graduate Programs, School of Nursing, Program in Nursing, Hickory, NC 28601. Offers nursing administration (MSN); nursing education (MSN). *Program availability:* Online learning. *Faculty:* 7 full-time (all women). *Students:* 4 full-time (all women), 46 part-time (45 women); includes 4 minority (2 Black or African American, non-Hispanic/Latino; 2 Hispanic/Latino). Average age 39. In 2015, 11 master's awarded. *Degree requirements:* For master's, comprehensive exam, thesis optional. *Entrance requirements:* For master's, official transcripts, two recommendations, essay, resume, unrestricted RN license, criminal background check. Additional exam requirements/recommendations for international students: Required—TOEFL (minimum score 600 paper-based). Application fee: $35. Electronic applications accepted. *Expenses:* $550 per credit hour. *Unit head:* Dr. Kerry Thompson, Chair, School of Nursing, 828-328-7282, Fax: 828-328-7368, E-mail: thompsonk@lr.edu. *Application contact:* Mary Ann Gosnell, Director of Graduate Recruiting, 828-328-7300, E-mail: admission@lr.edu.
Website: http://www.lr.edu/academics/programs/nursing-0

Lewis University, College of Nursing and Health Professions, Program in Nursing, Romeoville, IL 60446. Offers adult nurse practitioner (MSN); nursing administration (MSN); nursing education (MSN). *Accreditation:* AACN. *Program availability:* Part-time, evening/weekend, online learning. *Degree requirements:* For master's, clinical practicum. *Entrance requirements:* For master's, minimum undergraduate GPA of 3.0, degree in nursing, RN license, letter of recommendation, interview, resume or curriculum vitae. Additional exam requirements/recommendations for international students: Required—TOEFL (minimum score 550 paper-based; 80 iBT). Electronic applications accepted. *Faculty research:* Cancer prevention, phenomenological methods, public policy analysis.

Liberty University, School of Nursing, Lynchburg, VA 24515. Offers family nurse practitioner (DNP); nurse educator (MSN); nursing administration (MSN). *Program availability:* Part-time, online learning. *Students:* 108 full-time (100 women), 508 part-time (454 women); includes 106 minority (84 Black or African American, non-Hispanic/Latino; 3 American Indian or Alaska Native, non-Hispanic/Latino; 8 Asian, non-Hispanic/Latino; 1 Hispanic/Latino; 10 Two or more races, non-Hispanic/Latino), 7 international. Average age 39. 577 applicants, 30% accepted, 119 enrolled. In 2015, 161 master's awarded. *Entrance requirements:* For master's, minimum cumulative undergraduate GPA of 3.0; for doctorate, minimum GPA of 3.25 in most current nursing program completed. Additional exam requirements/recommendations for international students: Recommended—TOEFL. *Application deadline:* Applications are processed on a rolling basis. Application fee: $50. Electronic applications accepted. *Unit head:* Dr. Deanna Britt, Dean, 434-582-2519, E-mail: dbritt@liberty.edu. *Application contact:* Jay Bridge, Director of Admissions, 800-424-9595, Fax: 800-628-7977, E-mail: gradadmissions@liberty.edu.

Loma Linda University, School of Nursing, Program in Nurse Educator, Loma Linda, CA 92350. Offers adult/gerontology (MS); obstetrics-pediatrics (MS). *Accreditation:* AACN. *Program availability:* Part-time. *Degree requirements:* For master's, thesis or alternative. *Entrance requirements:* For master's, GRE General Test, BSN, minimum GPA of 3.0, RN license. Additional exam requirements/recommendations for international students: Required—TOEFL. *Application deadline:* For fall admission, 8/1 for domestic and international students; for winter admission, 11/1 for domestic and international students; for spring admission, 2/1 for domestic and international students. Application fee: $60. Electronic applications accepted. *Financial support:* Career-related internships or fieldwork, Federal Work-Study, institutionally sponsored loans, and scholarships/grants available. Support available to part-time students. Financial award application deadline: 6/1. *Faculty research:* Coping, integration of research. *Unit head:* Coordinator, 909-824-4360. *Application contact:* Admissions Office, 909-651-5029, Fax: 909-558-4879, E-mail: admissions.app@llu.edu.

Long Island University–LIU Brooklyn, Harriet Rothkopf Heilbrunn School of Nursing, Brooklyn, NY 11201-8423. Offers adult nurse practitioner (MS, Advanced Certificate); family nurse practitioner (MS, Advanced Certificate); nurse educator (MS). *Accreditation:* AACN. *Program availability:* Part-time, evening/weekend, blended/hybrid learning. *Faculty:* 6 full-time (4 women), 5 part-time/adjunct (4 women). *Students:* 1 (woman) full-time, 215 part-time (192 women); includes 136 minority (89 Black or African American, non-Hispanic/Latino; 28 Asian, non-Hispanic/Latino; 13 Hispanic/Latino; 2 Native Hawaiian or other Pacific Islander, non-Hispanic/Latino; 4 Two or more races, non-Hispanic/Latino), 1 international. Average age 43. 167 applicants, 57% accepted, 63 enrolled. In 2015, 23 master's, 5 other advanced degrees awarded. *Entrance requirements:* For master's and Advanced Certificate, New York RN license, two letters of recommendation. Additional exam requirements/recommendations for international students: Required—TOEFL (minimum score 550 paper-based; 79 iBT), IELTS (minimum score 6.5). *Application deadline:* Applications are processed on a rolling basis. Application fee: $50. Electronic applications accepted. *Expenses:* $1,155 per credit tuition; $934 per term full-time fees; $442 per term part-time fees. *Financial support:* In 2015–16, 24 students received support. Scholarships/grants and unspecified assistantships available. Support available to part-time students. Financial award application deadline: 2/15; financial award applicants required to submit FAFSA. *Faculty research:* Cultural competency, high fidelity simulation to improve nursing assessment and increase patient safety, relationship of diabetes to stress, end of life care, geriatric issues, foreign nurse's adaptation to the United States. *Unit head:* Dr. Loretta Knapp, Interim Dean, 718-488-1508, Fax: 718-780-4019, E-mail: lori.knapp@liu.edu. *Application contact:* Richard Sunday, Dean of Admissions, 718-488-1011, Fax: 718-780-6110, E-mail: bkln-admissions@liu.edu.
Website: http://liu.edu/Brooklyn/Academics/Harriet-Rothkopf-Heilbrunn-School-of-Nursing

Long Island University–LIU Post, School of Health Professions and Nursing, Brookville, NY 11548-1300. Offers biomedical sciences (MS), including applied laboratory medicine, cancer biology, medical and molecular immunology, microbiology/infectious diseases; cardiovascular perfusion (MS); dietetic internship (Advanced Certificate); family nurse practitioner (MS); forensic social work (Advanced Certificate); nursing education (MS); social work (MSW). *Program availability:* Part-time, evening/weekend, blended/hybrid learning. *Faculty:* 16 full-time (14 women), 46 part-time/adjunct (33 women). *Students:* 190 full-time (139 women), 181 part-time (157 women); includes 141 minority (51 Black or African American, non-Hispanic/Latino; 46 Asian, non-Hispanic/Latino; 41 Hispanic/Latino; 3 Two or more races, non-Hispanic/Latino), 47 international. Average age 36. 422 applicants, 64% accepted, 141 enrolled. In 2015, 96 master's, 28 other advanced degrees awarded. *Degree requirements:* For master's, comprehensive exam (for some programs), thesis (for some programs). *Entrance requirements:* Additional exam requirements/recommendations for international students: Required—TOEFL, IELTS. *Application deadline:* Applications are processed on a rolling basis. Application fee: $50. Electronic applications accepted. *Expenses:* $1,155 per credit, $934 per term full-time university fee, $442 per term part-time university fee. *Financial support:* In 2015–16, 6 research assistantships with partial tuition reimbursements were awarded; career-related internships or fieldwork, Federal Work-Study, institutionally sponsored loans, tuition waivers (partial), and unspecified assistantships also available. Support available to part-time students. Financial award application deadline: 2/15; financial award applicants required to submit FAFSA. *Faculty research:* Breast cancer, childhood obesity, dietary beverage consumption, emotional distress, histone modification, interprofessional practice, interstitial cystitis, lung cancer, pancreatic cancer, pediatric pain management, post-traumatic growth, poverty, renal nutrition, social ethics, yeast and bacterial drug resistance. *Total annual research expenditures:* $15,000. *Unit head:* Dr. Stacy Gropack, Acting Dean, 516-299-2486, Fax: 516-299-2527, E-mail: post-shpn@liu.edu. *Application contact:* Carol Zerah, Director of Graduate and International Admissions, 516-299-2900 Ext. 3952, Fax: 516-299-2137, E-mail: post-enroll@liu.edu.
Website: http://liu.edu/post/health

Louisiana State University Health Sciences Center, School of Nursing, New Orleans, LA 70112. Offers adult gerontology clinical nurse specialist (Post-Master's Certificate); clinical nurse leader (MSN); executive nurse leader (Post-Master's Certificate); neonatal nurse practitioner (Post-Master's Certificate); nurse anesthesia (Post-Master's Certificate); nurse educator (MSN); nursing (DNS); primary care family nurse practitioner (Post-Master's Certificate); public/community health nursing (Post-Master's

Certificate). *Accreditation:* AACN; AANA/CANAEP (one or more programs are accredited). *Program availability:* Part-time. *Faculty:* 22 full-time (19 women), 21 part-time/adjunct (8 women). *Students:* 254 (185 women); includes 68 minority (44 Black or African American, non-Hispanic/Latino; 12 Asian, non-Hispanic/Latino; 12 Hispanic/Latino). Average age 33. 144 applicants, 54% accepted, 73 enrolled. In 2015, 84 master's, 6 doctorates awarded. *Degree requirements:* For master's, thesis optional; for doctorate, thesis/dissertation. *Entrance requirements:* For master's, GRE General Test, MAT, minimum GPA of 3.0; for doctorate, GRE General Test, minimum GPA of 3.5. Additional exam requirements/recommendations for international students: Required—TOEFL (minimum score 550 paper-based; 79 iBT). *Application deadline:* Applications are processed on a rolling basis. Application fee: $250. Electronic applications accepted. *Expenses:* $9,136.50 per year; $19,633.50 per year (for DNP). *Financial support:* Federal Work-Study, institutionally sponsored loans, scholarships/grants, and traineeships available. Financial award applicants required to submit FAFSA. *Faculty research:* Advanced clinical practice, nursing education, health, social support, nursing administration. *Unit head:* Dr. Demetrius James Porche, Dean, 504-568-4106, Fax: 504-599-0573, E-mail: dporch@lsuhsc.edu. *Application contact:* Tracie Gravolet, Director, Office of Student Affairs, 504-568-4114, Fax: 504-568-5711, E-mail: tgravo@lsuhsc.edu.
Website: http://nursing.lsuhsc.edu/

Lourdes University, Graduate School, Sylvania, OH 43560-2898. Offers business (MBA); leadership (M Ed); nurse anesthesia (MSN); nurse educator (MSN); nurse leader (MSN); organizational leadership (MOL); reading (M Ed); teaching and curriculum (M Ed); theology (MA). *Program availability:* Evening/weekend. *Entrance requirements:* Additional exam requirements/recommendations for international students: Required—TOEFL.

Marian University, School of Nursing and Health Professions, Fond du Lac, WI 54935-4699. Offers adult nurse practitioner (MSN); nurse educator (MSN). *Accreditation:* AACN. *Program availability:* Part-time, evening/weekend. *Faculty:* 6 full-time (all women), 4 part-time/adjunct (2 women). *Students:* 21 full-time (20 women), 95 part-time (85 women); includes 10 minority (6 Black or African American, non-Hispanic/Latino; 2 Asian, non-Hispanic/Latino; 2 Hispanic/Latino). Average age 40. In 2015, 26 master's awarded. *Degree requirements:* For master's, thesis, 675 clinical practicum hours. *Entrance requirements:* For master's, 3 letters of professional recommendation; undergraduate work in nursing research, statistics, health assessment. Additional exam requirements/recommendations for international students: Required—TOEFL (minimum score 525 paper-based; 70 iBT). *Application deadline:* Applications are processed on a rolling basis. Application fee: $50. Electronic applications accepted. *Expenses:* Contact institution. *Financial support:* In 2015–16, 3 students received support. Institutionally sponsored loans and scholarships/grants available. Support available to part-time students. Financial award application deadline: 3/1; financial award applicants required to submit FAFSA. *Unit head:* Dr. Linda Matheson, Dean, 920-923-7668, Fax: 920-923-8770, E-mail: lkmatheson85@marianuniversity.edu. *Application contact:* Selina Scoles, Admissions Counselor, 920-923-8938, Fax: 920-923-8770, E-mail: sascoles30@marianuniversity.edu.
Website: http://www.marianuniversity.edu/nursing/

McKendree University, Graduate Programs, Master of Science in Nursing Program, Lebanon, IL 62254-1299. Offers nursing education (MSN); nursing management/administration (MSN). *Accreditation:* AACN. *Program availability:* Part-time, evening/weekend, online learning. *Degree requirements:* For master's, research project or thesis. *Entrance requirements:* For master's, resume, references, valid Professional Registered Nurse license. Additional exam requirements/recommendations for international students: Required—TOEFL. Electronic applications accepted.

McMurry University, Graduate Studies, Abilene, TX 79697. Offers education (MSN); family nurse practitioner (MSN).

McNeese State University, Doré School of Graduate Studies, College of Nursing, Department of Graduate Nursing, Nursing Program, Lake Charles, LA 70609. Offers family nurse practitioner (MSN); family psychiatric/mental health nurse practitioner (MSN); nurse educator (MSN); nurse executive (MSN). *Degree requirements:* For master's, comprehensive exam. *Entrance requirements:* For master's, GRE, baccalaureate degree in nursing, minimum overall GPA of 2.7 for all undergraduate coursework, eligibility for unencumbered licensure as Registered Nurse in Louisiana or Texas, course in introductory statistics with minimum C grade, physical assessment skills, two letters of professional reference, 500-word essay, current resume.

Medical University of South Carolina, College of Nursing, Nurse Educator Program, Charleston, SC 29425. Offers MSN. *Program availability:* Part-time, evening/weekend, online learning. *Degree requirements:* For master's, thesis optional. *Entrance requirements:* For master's, BSN, course work in statistics, nursing license, minimum GPA of 3.0, current curriculum vitae, essay, three references. Additional exam requirements/recommendations for international students: Required—TOEFL (minimum score 600 paper-based). Electronic applications accepted. *Faculty research:* Prenatal care outcomes, perinatal wellness in Hispanic women, use of personal digital assistants (PDAs) in clinical practice.

Mercy College, School of Health and Natural Sciences, Programs in Nursing, Dobbs Ferry, NY 10522-1189. Offers nursing administration (MS); nursing education (MS). *Accreditation:* AACN. *Program availability:* Part-time, evening/weekend, online learning. *Degree requirements:* For master's, comprehensive exam (for some programs), written comprehensive exam or the production of a comprehensive project. *Entrance requirements:* For master's, interview, two letters of reference, bachelor's degree, RN registration in the U.S. Additional exam requirements/recommendations for international students: Required—TOEFL (minimum score 600 paper-based; 100 iBT), IELTS (minimum score 8). Electronic applications accepted. *Expenses:* Tuition, area resident: Full-time $14,904; part-time $828 per credit hour. *Required fees:* $610; $153 per term. $153 per term. Tuition and fees vary according to course load and program.

Messiah College, Program in Nursing, Mechanicsburg, PA 17055. Offers nurse educator (MSN).

Metropolitan State University, College of Health, Community and Professional Studies, St. Paul, MN 55106-5000. Offers advanced dental therapy (MS); leadership and management (MSN); nurse educator (MSN); nursing (DNP); psychology (MA). *Accreditation:* AACN. *Program availability:* Part-time. *Degree requirements:* For master's, thesis or alternative; for doctorate, thesis/dissertation or alternative. *Entrance requirements:* For master's, GRE General Test, minimum GPA of 3.0, RN license, BS/BA; for doctorate, minimum GPA of 3.0; RN license, MSN. Additional exam requirements/recommendations for international students: Required—TOEFL (minimum score 550 paper-based). *Faculty research:* Women's health, gerontology.

MGH Institute of Health Professions, School of Nursing, Boston, MA 02129. Offers advanced practice nursing (MSN); gerontological nursing (MSN); nursing (DNP); pediatric nursing (MSN); psychiatric nursing (MSN); teaching and learning for health care education (Certificate); women's health nursing (MSN). *Accreditation:* AACN. *Degree requirements:* For master's, thesis or alternative. *Entrance requirements:* For master's, GRE General Test, bachelor's degree from regionally-accredited college or university. Additional exam requirements/recommendations for international students:

Required—TOEFL (minimum score 550 paper-based; 80 iBT). Electronic applications accepted. *Faculty research:* Biobehavioral nursing, HIV/AIDS, gerontological nursing, women's health, vulnerable populations, health systems.

MidAmerica Nazarene University, Post-Licensure and Graduate Nursing Education Program, Olathe, KS 66062-1899. Offers healthcare administration (MSN); healthcare quality management (MSN); nursing education (MSN); public health (MSN); MSN/MBA. *Program availability:* Part-time, 100% online, blended/hybrid learning. *Faculty:* 8 full-time (all women), 6 part-time/adjunct (3 women). *Students:* 9 full-time (8 women), 103 part-time (100 women); includes 23 minority (14 Black or African American, non-Hispanic/Latino; 1 American Indian or Alaska Native, non-Hispanic/Latino; 4 Asian, non-Hispanic/Latino; 4 Hispanic/Latino). 50 applicants, 82% accepted. In 2015, 36 master's awarded. *Degree requirements:* For master's, final project. *Entrance requirements:* For master's, BSN, minimum GPA of 3.0, active unencumbered RN license, undergraduate statistics course. *Application deadline:* Applications are processed on a rolling basis. Electronic applications accepted. *Expenses:* $22,065 tuition, $1,186 fee (including technology, carrying and graduation fee). *Financial support:* Unspecified assistantships available. Financial award applicants required to submit FAFSA. *Faculty research:* Technology in education, minority recruitment and retention in nursing programs, faculty views and attitudes on culturally competency, innovative nursing program development, spirituality and holistic health. *Unit head:* Dr. Karen Wiegman, RN, Dean, 913-971-3839, E-mail: kdwiegman@mnu.edu. *Application contact:* E-mail: pgadmissions@mnu.edu.
Website: http://www.mnu.edu/nursing.html

Middle Tennessee State University, College of Graduate Studies, University College, Murfreesboro, TN 37132. Offers advanced studies in teaching and learning (M Ed); human resources leadership (MPS); nursing administration (MSN); nursing education (MSN); strategic leadership (MPS); training and development (MPS). *Program availability:* Part-time, evening/weekend, online learning. *Entrance requirements:* Additional exam requirements/recommendations for international students: Required—TOEFL (minimum score 525 paper-based; 71 iBT) or IELTS (minimum score 6).

Midwestern State University, Billie Doris McAda Graduate School, Robert D. and Carol Gunn College of Health Sciences and Human Services, Wilson School of Nursing, Wichita Falls, TX 76308. Offers family nurse practitioner (MSN); family psychiatric mental health nurse practitioner (MSN); nurse educator (MSN). *Accreditation:* AACN. *Program availability:* Part-time, evening/weekend. *Degree requirements:* For master's, comprehensive exam, thesis optional. *Entrance requirements:* For master's, GRE General Test or MAT. Additional exam requirements/recommendations for international students: Required—TOEFL (minimum score 550 paper-based). Electronic applications accepted. *Faculty research:* Infant feeding, musculoskeletal disorders, diabetes, community health education, water quality reporting.

Millersville University of Pennsylvania, College of Graduate Studies and Adult Learning, College of Science and Technology, Department of Nursing, Program in Nursing Education, Millersville, PA 17551-0302. Offers MSN. *Program availability:* Part-time, evening/weekend. *Faculty:* 6 full-time (all women), 4 part-time/adjunct (all women). *Students:* 1 (woman) full-time, 8 part-time (all women); includes 1 minority (Black or African American, non-Hispanic/Latino). 2 applicants, 50% accepted, 1 enrolled. In 2015, 4 master's awarded. *Degree requirements:* For master's, internship, scholarly project. *Entrance requirements:* For master's, resume, copy of RN license, minimum GPA of 3.0, all transfer transcripts, interview. Additional exam requirements/recommendations for international students: Required—TOEFL (minimum score 600 paper-based), IELTS (minimum score 6). *Application deadline:* Applications are processed on a rolling basis. Application fee: $40. Electronic applications accepted. *Expenses:* Tuition, state resident: full-time $8460; part-time $470 per credit. Tuition, nonresident: full-time $12,690; part-time $705 per credit. *Required fees:* $2471; $133.75 per credit. Tuition and fees vary according to course load, degree level and program. *Financial support:* Application deadline: 3/15; applicants required to submit FAFSA. *Unit head:* Dr. Kelly A. Kuhns, Chair, 717-871-5276, Fax: 717-871-4877, E-mail: kelly.kuhns@millersville.edu. *Application contact:* Dr. Victor S. DeSantis, Dean of College of Graduate Studies and Adult Learning/Associate Provost for Civic and Community Engagement, 717-871-7619, Fax: 717-871-7954, E-mail: victor.desantis@millersville.edu.
Website: http://www.millersville.edu/nursing/msn/nursing-education.php

Millikin University, School of Nursing, Decatur, IL 62522-2084. Offers entry into nursing practice (MSN); nurse anesthesia (DNP); nurse educator (MSN); nursing practice (DNP). *Accreditation:* AACN; AANA/CANAEP. *Program availability:* Part-time. *Faculty:* 11 full-time (all women), 4 part-time/adjunct (3 women). *Students:* 44 full-time (27 women), 14 part-time (13 women); includes 9 minority (5 Black or African American, non-Hispanic/Latino; 1 American Indian or Alaska Native, non-Hispanic/Latino; 1 Asian, non-Hispanic/Latino; 1 Hispanic/Latino; 1 Two or more races, non-Hispanic/Latino), 1 international. Average age 32. 117 applicants, 29% accepted, 26 enrolled. In 2015, 15 master's awarded. *Degree requirements:* For master's, thesis or alternative, scholarly project; for doctorate, thesis/dissertation or alternative, scholarly project. *Entrance requirements:* For master's, GRE, official academic transcript(s), essay, immunizations, statistics course, 3 letters of recommendation, CPR certification, professional liability/malpractice insurance; for doctorate, GRE (if undergraduate cumulative GPA is below 3.0), official academic transcript(s); undergraduate courses in nursing research, health assessment, inorganic and organic chemistry, intro to statistics; graduate-level statistics; 3 written recommendations; Assessment of Critical Care Skills form; written statement; resume or curriculum vitae. Additional exam requirements/recommendations for international students: Required—TOEFL (minimum score 650 paper-based; 81 iBT). *Application deadline:* For spring admission, 7/1 priority date for domestic and international students; for summer admission, 11/1 priority date for domestic and international students. Applications are processed on a rolling basis. Application fee: $0. Electronic applications accepted. *Expenses:* Contact institution. *Financial support:* Traineeships and unspecified assistantships available. Financial award applicants required to submit FAFSA. *Faculty research:* Quality of life, transcultural nursing issues, teaching/learning strategies, clinical simulation. *Unit head:* Dr. Pamela Lindsey, Director, 217-424-6348, Fax: 217-420-6731, E-mail: plindsey@millikin.edu. *Application contact:* Bonnie Niemeyer, Administrative Assistant, 800-373-7733 Ext. 5034, Fax: 217-420-6677, E-mail: bniemeyer@millikin.edu.
Website: http://www.millikin.edu/grad-nursing

Missouri State University, Graduate College, College of Health and Human Services, Department of Nursing, Springfield, MO 65897. Offers nursing (MSN), including family nurse practitioner, nurse educator, nursing practice (DNP). *Accreditation:* AACN. *Program availability:* 100% online, blended/hybrid learning. *Faculty:* 9 full-time (all women), 16 part-time/adjunct (13 women). *Students:* 27 full-time (23 women), 23 part-time (all women); includes 8 minority (3 Black or African American, non-Hispanic/Latino; 1 American Indian or Alaska Native, non-Hispanic/Latino; 2 Asian, non-Hispanic/Latino; 2 Two or more races, non-Hispanic/Latino). Average age 35. 13 applicants, 46% accepted, 1 enrolled. In 2015, 1 master's, 1 doctorate awarded. *Degree requirements:* For master's, comprehensive exam, thesis or alternative. *Entrance requirements:* For master's, GRE General Test, minimum GPA of 3.0, RN license (for MSN), 1 year of work experience (for MPH). Additional exam requirements/recommendations for international students: Required—TOEFL (minimum score 550 paper-based; 79 iBT), IELTS

Nursing Education

(minimum score 6). *Application deadline:* For fall admission, 12/1 priority date for domestic students, 5/1 for international students. Applications are processed on a rolling basis. Application fee: $35 ($50 for international students). Electronic applications accepted. *Expenses:* Tuition, state resident: full-time $5500. Tuition, nonresident: full-time $10,108. *Required fees:* $1000. *Financial support:* In 2015–16, 2 teaching assistantships with partial tuition reimbursements (averaging $8,600 per year) were awarded; Federal Work-Study, institutionally sponsored loans, scholarships/grants, and unspecified assistantships also available. Financial award application deadline: 3/31; financial award applicants required to submit FAFSA. *Faculty research:* Preconceptual health, women's health, nursing satisfaction, nursing education. *Unit head:* Dr. Kathryn Hope, Head, 417-836-5310, Fax: 417-836-5484, E-mail: nursing@missouristate.edu. *Application contact:* Michael Edwards, Coordinator of Graduate Admissions, 417-836-5330, Fax: 417-836-6200, E-mail: michaeledwards@missouristate.edu.
Website: http://www.missouristate.edu/nursing/

Missouri Western State University, Program in Nursing, St. Joseph, MO 64507-2294. Offers health care leadership (MSN); nurse educator (MSN, Graduate Certificate). *Program availability:* Part-time. *Students:* 31 part-time (30 women). Average age 34. 17 applicants, 100% accepted, 14 enrolled. In 2015, 2 master's awarded. *Entrance requirements:* For master's, minimum GPA of 2.75, interview. Additional exam requirements/recommendations for international students: Recommended—TOEFL (minimum score 79 iBT), IELTS (minimum score 6). *Application deadline:* For fall admission, 7/15 for domestic and international students; for spring admission, 11/1 for domestic students, 10/15 for international students; for summer admission, 4/29 for domestic students. Applications are processed on a rolling basis. Application fee: $45 ($50 for international students). Electronic applications accepted. *Expenses:* Tuition, state resident: full-time $6290; part-time $314 per credit hour. Tuition, nonresident: full-time $11,490; part-time $574 per credit hour. *Required fees:* $542; $99 per credit hour. $176 per semester. One-time fee: $45. Tuition and fees vary according to course load and program. *Financial support:* Scholarships/grants and unspecified assistantships available. Support available to part-time students. *Unit head:* Dr. Carolyn Brose, Associate Professor, 816-271-5912, E-mail: brose@missouriwestern.edu. *Application contact:* Dr. Benjamin D. Caldwell, Dean of the Graduate School, 816-271-4394, Fax: 816-271-4525, E-mail: graduate@missouriwestern.edu.
Website: https://www.missouriwestern.edu/nursing/master-of-science-in-nursing/

Molloy College, Division of Nursing, Rockville Centre, NY 11571-5002. Offers adult-gerontology primary care nurse practitioner (MS); clinical nurse specialist (MS), including adult-gerontology health; clinical nurse specialist: adult-gerontology (Advanced Certificate), including adult-gerontology; family nurse practitioner (MS, Advanced Certificate), including primary care; family psychiatric mental health nurse practitioner (MS); nursing (DNP, PhD); nursing administration (MS), including informatics; nursing education (MS); pediatric nurse practitioner (MS), including primary care (MS, Advanced Certificate). *Accreditation:* AACN. *Program availability:* Part-time, evening/weekend. *Faculty:* 26 full-time (all women), 12 part-time/adjunct (9 women). *Students:* 13 full-time (all women), 550 part-time (515 women); includes 316 minority (169 Black or African American, non-Hispanic/Latino; 1 American Indian or Alaska Native, non-Hispanic/Latino; 88 Asian, non-Hispanic/Latino; 56 Hispanic/Latino; 2 Native Hawaiian or other Pacific Islander, non-Hispanic/Latino). Average age 43. 208 applicants, 69% accepted, 121 enrolled. In 2015, 116 master's, 1 doctorate, 6 other advanced degrees awarded. *Degree requirements:* For master's, thesis optional. *Entrance requirements:* For master's, 3 letters of reference, BS in nursing, minimum undergraduate GPA of 3.0; for Advanced Certificate, 3 letters of reference, master's degree in nursing. Additional exam requirements/recommendations for international students: Required—TOEFL (minimum score 550 paper-based; 79 iBT). *Application deadline:* For fall admission, 9/2 priority date for domestic students; for spring admission, 1/20 priority date for domestic students. Applications are processed on a rolling basis. Application fee: $60. Electronic applications accepted. *Expenses:* Tuition, area resident: Full-time $18,450; part-time $1025 per credit. *Required fees:* $900; $740 per unit. Tuition and fees vary according to course load. *Financial support:* Research assistantships with partial tuition reimbursements, teaching assistantships with partial tuition reimbursements, institutionally sponsored loans, scholarships/grants, and unspecified assistantships available. Support available to part-time students. Financial award application deadline: 4/1; financial award applicants required to submit FAFSA. *Unit head:* Dr. Jeannine Muldoon, Dean of Nursing, 516-323-3651, E-mail: jmuldoon@molloy.edu. *Application contact:* Jaclyn Machowicz, Assistant Director for Admissions, 516-323-4010, E-mail: jmachowicz@molloy.edu.

Monmouth University, Graduate Studies, The Marjorie K. Unterberg School of Nursing and Health Studies, West Long Branch, NJ 07764-1898. Offers adult and gerontological primary care nurse practitioner (MSN); adult-gerontological primary care nurse practitioner (Post-Master's Certificate); family nurse practitioner (MSN, Post-Master's Certificate); family psychiatric and mental health advanced practice nursing (MSN); family psychiatric and mental health nurse practitioner (Post-Master's Certificate); forensic nursing (MSN, Certificate); nursing (MSN); nursing administration (MSN, Post-Master's Certificate); nursing education (MSN, Post-Master's Certificate); nursing practice (DNP); physician assistant (MS); school nursing (MSN, Certificate). *Accreditation:* AACN. *Program availability:* Part-time, evening/weekend, 100% online, blended/hybrid learning. *Faculty:* 14 full-time (13 women), 10 part-time/adjunct (5 women). *Students:* 58 full-time (46 women), 271 part-time (252 women); includes 93 minority (31 Black or African American, non-Hispanic/Latino; 40 Asian, non-Hispanic/Latino; 18 Hispanic/Latino; 1 Native Hawaiian or other Pacific Islander, non-Hispanic/Latino; 3 Two or more races, non-Hispanic/Latino), 1 international. Average age 37. 450 applicants, 32% accepted, 103 enrolled. In 2015, 68 master's, 8 doctorates, 11 other advanced degrees awarded. *Degree requirements:* For master's, practicum (for some tracks); for doctorate, practicum, capstone course. *Entrance requirements:* For master's, GRE General Test (waived for MSN applicants with minimum B grade in each of the first four courses and for MS applicants with master's degree), BSN with minimum GPA of 2.75, current RN license, proof of liability and malpractice policy, personal statement, two letters of recommendation, college course work in health assessment, resume; CASPA application (for MS); for doctorate, accredited master's nursing program degree with minimum GPA of 3.2, graduate research course in statistics, active RN license, national certification as Nurse Practitioner or Nurse Administrator, working knowledge of statistics, statement of goals and vision for change, 2 letters of recommendation (professional or academic), resume, interview. Additional exam requirements/recommendations for international students: Required—TOEFL (minimum score 550 paper-based; 79 iBT), IELTS (minimum score 6) or Michigan English Language Assessment Battery (minimum score 77). *Application deadline:* For fall admission, 7/15 priority date for domestic students, 6/1 for international students; for spring admission, 12/15 priority date for domestic students, 11/1 for international students; for summer admission, 5/1 for domestic students. Applications are processed on a rolling basis. Application fee: $50. Electronic applications accepted. *Expenses:* Contact institution. *Financial support:* In 2015–16, 241 students received support, including 220 fellowships (averaging $3,403 per year), 5 research assistantships (averaging $5,146 per year); career-related internships or fieldwork, scholarships/grants, and unspecified assistantships also available. Support available to part-time students. Financial award applicants required to submit FAFSA. *Faculty research:* School nursing, health policy,

and smoking cessation in teens, Multiple Sclerosis; adherence and self-efficacy, aging issues and geriatric care. *Unit head:* Dr. Janet Mahoney, Dean, 732-571-3443, Fax: 732-263-5131, E-mail: jmahoney@monmouth.edu. *Application contact:* Lucia Fedele, Graduate Admission Counselor, 732-571-3452, Fax: 732-263-5123, E-mail: gradadm@monmouth.edu.
Website: http://www.monmouth.edu/school-of-nursing-health/graduate-nursing-programs.aspx

Montana State University, The Graduate School, College of Nursing, Bozeman, MT 59717. Offers clinical nurse leader (MN); family and individual nurse practitioner (DNP); family nurse practitioner (MN, Post-Master's Certificate); nursing education (Certificate, Post-Master's Certificate); psychiatric mental health nurse practitioner (MN); psychiatric/mental health nurse practitioner (DNP). *Accreditation:* AACN. *Program availability:* Part-time, online learning. *Degree requirements:* For master's, comprehensive exam, thesis (for some programs); for doctorate, thesis/dissertation, 1,125 hours in clinical settings. *Entrance requirements:* For master's, GRE General Test, minimum GPA of 3.0 for undergraduate and post-baccalaureate work. Additional exam requirements/recommendations for international students: Required—TOEFL (minimum score 580 paper-based). Electronic applications accepted. *Faculty research:* Rural nursing, health disparities, environmental/public health, oral health, resilience.

Moravian College, Moravian College Comenius Center, St. Luke's School of Nursing, Bethlehem, PA 18018-6650. Offers clinical nurse leader (MS); nurse administrator (MS); nurse educator (MS). *Accreditation:* AACN. *Program availability:* Part-time, evening/weekend. *Degree requirements:* For master's, comprehensive exam (for some programs), evidence-based practice project. *Entrance requirements:* For master's, GRE or MAT. Additional exam requirements/recommendations for international students: Required—TOEFL (minimum score 550 paper-based; 90 iBT).

Mount Carmel College of Nursing, Nursing Program, Columbus, OH 43222. Offers adult gerontology acute care nurse practitioner (MS); adult health clinical nurse specialist (MS); family nurse practitioner (MS); nursing (DNP); nursing administration (MS); nursing education (MS). *Accreditation:* AACN. *Program availability:* Part-time. *Faculty:* 8 full-time (all women), 5 part-time/adjunct (4 women). *Students:* 72 full-time (63 women), 92 part-time (84 women); includes 15 minority (7 Black or African American, non-Hispanic/Latino; 3 Asian, non-Hispanic/Latino; 2 Hispanic/Latino; 3 Two or more races, non-Hispanic/Latino). Average age 37. 140 applicants, 45% accepted, 50 enrolled. In 2015, 50 master's awarded. *Degree requirements:* For master's, professional manuscript; for doctorate, practicum. *Entrance requirements:* For master's, letters of recommendation, statement of purpose, current resume, baccalaureate degree in nursing, current Ohio RN license, minimum cumulative GPA of 3.0; for doctorate, master's degree in nursing from program accredited by either NLNAC/ACEN or CCNE. Additional exam requirements/recommendations for international students: Required—TOEFL (minimum score 550 paper-based; 80 iBT). *Application deadline:* For fall admission, 6/1 priority date for domestic students; for winter admission, 11/1 for domestic students; for spring admission, 10/1 priority date for domestic students; for summer admission, 3/1 for domestic students. Applications are processed on a rolling basis. Application fee: $30. *Expenses:* Tuition, area resident: Full-time $9480; part-time $474 per credit. One-time fee: $120. Tuition and fees vary according to course load, degree level and program. *Financial support:* In 2015–16, 5 students received support. Institutionally sponsored loans and scholarships/grants available. Financial award applicants required to submit FAFSA. *Unit head:* Dr. Jill Kilanowski, 614-234-5237, Fax: 614-234-2875, E-mail: jkilanowski@mccn.edu. *Application contact:* Dr. Kim Campbell, Director of Recruitment and Admissions, 614-234-5144, Fax: 614-234-5427, E-mail: kcampbell@mccn.edu.
Website: http://www.mccn.edu/

Mount Mercy University, Program in Nursing, Cedar Rapids, IA 52402-4797. Offers health advocacy (MSN); nurse administration (MSN); nurse education (MSN). *Program availability:* Evening/weekend. *Degree requirements:* For master's, project/practicum.

Mount St. Joseph University, Master of Science in Nursing Program, Cincinnati, OH 45233-1670. Offers administration (MSN); clinical nurse leader (MSN); education (MSN). *Program availability:* Part-time. *Faculty:* 12 full-time (11 women), 5 part-time/adjunct (all women). *Students:* 53 full-time (all women), 2 part-time (both women); includes 4 minority (all Black or African American, non-Hispanic/Latino). Average age 44. 148 applicants, 68% accepted, 58 enrolled. In 2015, 65 master's awarded. *Entrance requirements:* For master's, essay, BSN from regionally-accredited university; minimum undergraduate GPA of 3.25 or GRE; professional resume; three professional references; interview; 2 years of clinical nursing experience; active RN license; criminal background check. Additional exam requirements/recommendations for international students: Required—TOEFL (minimum score 560 paper-based; 83 iBT). Application fee: $50. Electronic applications accepted. *Expenses:* Tuition, area resident: Full-time $15,255; part-time $565 per credit hour. *Required fees:* $500; $100 per term. $100 per semester. Full-time tuition and fees vary according to course load, degree level and program. *Financial support:* In 2015–16, 3 students received support. Application deadline: 3/1; applicants required to submit FAFSA. *Unit head:* Dr. Nancy Hinzman, MSN/DNP Director, 513-244-4325, E-mail: nancy.hinzman@msj.edu. *Application contact:* Mary Brigham, Assistant Director for Graduate Recruitment, 513-244-4233, Fax: 513-244-4629, E-mail: mary.brigham@msj.edu.
Website: http://www.msj.edu/academics/graduate-programs/master-of-science-in-nursing/

Mount Saint Mary College, School of Nursing, Newburgh, NY 12550-3494. Offers adult nurse practitioner (MS, Advanced Certificate), including nursing education (MS), nursing management (MS); clinical nurse specialist-adult health (MS), including nursing education, nursing management; family nurse practitioner (Advanced Certificate). *Accreditation:* AACN. *Program availability:* Part-time, evening/weekend, blended/hybrid learning. *Faculty:* 6 full-time (all women), 1 (woman) part-time/adjunct. *Students:* 5 full-time (4 women), 117 part-time (105 women); includes 42 minority (18 Black or African American, non-Hispanic/Latino; 2 American Indian or Alaska Native, non-Hispanic/Latino; 8 Asian, non-Hispanic/Latino; 12 Hispanic/Latino; 2 Native Hawaiian or other Pacific Islander, non-Hispanic/Latino). Average age 38. 44 applicants, 84% accepted, 25 enrolled. In 2015, 25 master's, 4 other advanced degrees awarded. *Degree requirements:* For master's, research utilization project. *Entrance requirements:* For master's, BSN, minimum GPA of 3.0, RN license. Additional exam requirements/recommendations for international students: Required—TOEFL (minimum score 80 iBT). *Application deadline:* For fall admission, 6/3 priority date for domestic students; for spring admission, 10/31 priority date for domestic students. Applications are processed on a rolling basis. Application fee: $45. Electronic applications accepted. Application fee is waived when completed online. *Expenses:* Tuition, area resident: Part-time $750 per credit. *Required fees:* $40 per semester. *Financial support:* In 2015–16, 14 students received support. Unspecified assistantships available. Financial award application deadline: 4/15; financial award applicants required to submit FAFSA. *Unit head:* Christine Berte, Graduate Coordinator, 845-569-3141, Fax: 845-562-6762, E-mail: christine.berte@msmc.edu. *Application contact:* Lisa Gallina, Director of Admissions for Graduate Programs and Adult Degree Completion, 845-569-3166, Fax: 845-569-3450, E-mail: lisa.gallina@msmc.edu.

Website: http://www.msmc.edu/Academics/Graduate_Programs/ Master_of_Science_in_Nursing

Nebraska Methodist College, Program in Nursing, Omaha, NE 68114. Offers nurse educator (MSN); nurse executive (MSN). *Accreditation:* AACN. *Program availability:* Evening/weekend, online learning. *Degree requirements:* For master's, thesis or alternative, Evidence Based Practice (EBP) project. *Entrance requirements:* For master's, interview. Additional exam requirements/recommendations for international students: Required—TOEFL (minimum score 550 paper-based; 80 iBT). *Faculty research:* Spirituality, student outcomes, service-learning, leadership and administration, women's issues.

Neumann University, Program in Nursing, Aston, PA 19014. Offers adult-gerontology nurse practitioner (MS); nurse educator (MS). *Accreditation:* ACEN. *Program availability:* Part-time. *Students:* 18 part-time. *Entrance requirements:* For master's, GRE or MAT. Additional exam requirements/recommendations for international students: Required—TOEFL. *Application deadline:* Applications are processed on a rolling basis. Application fee: $50. *Expenses:* Contact institution. *Financial support:* Available to part-time students. Application deadline: 3/15; applicants required to submit FAFSA. *Unit head:* Dr. Kathleen Hoover, Dean, Division of Nursing and Health Sciences, 610-558-5560, Fax: 610-459-1370, E-mail: hooverk@neumann.edu. *Application contact:* Kittie D. Pain, Associate Director, Graduate and Adult Admissions, 610-558-5613, Fax: 610-558-5652, E-mail: paink@neumann.edu.

New York University, Rory Meyers College of Nursing, Programs in Advanced Practice Nursing, New York, NY 10012-1019. Offers adult-gerontology acute care nurse practitioner (MS, Advanced Certificate); adult-gerontology primary care nurse practitioner (MS, Advanced Certificate); family nurse practitioner (MS, Advanced Certificate); gerontology nurse practitioner (Advanced Certificate); nurse-midwifery (MS, Advanced Certificate); nursing administration (MS, Advanced Certificate); nursing education (MS, Advanced Certificate); nursing informatics (MS, Advanced Certificate); pediatrics nurse practitioner (MS, Advanced Certificate); psychiatric-mental health nurse practitioner (MS, Advanced Certificate); MS/MPH. *Accreditation:* AACN; ACNM/ACME. *Program availability:* Part-time. *Faculty:* 24 full-time (all women), 76 part-time/adjunct (65 women). *Students:* 46 full-time (26 women), 586 part-time (513 women); includes 242 minority (68 Black or African American, non-Hispanic/Latino; 3 American Indian or Alaska Native, non-Hispanic/Latino; 117 Asian, non-Hispanic/Latino; 38 Hispanic/Latino; 3 Native Hawaiian or other Pacific Islander, non-Hispanic/Latino; 13 Two or more races, non-Hispanic/Latino), 23 international. Average age 32. 402 applicants, 69% accepted, 138 enrolled. In 2015, 198 master's, 5 other advanced degrees awarded. *Degree requirements:* For master's, thesis (for some programs). *Entrance requirements:* For master's, BS in nursing, AS in nursing with another BS/BA, interview, RN license, 1 year of clinical experience (3 for the MS in nursing education program); for Advanced Certificate, master's degree. Additional exam requirements/recommendations for international students: Required—TOEFL (minimum score 90 iBT), IELTS (minimum score 7). *Application deadline:* For fall admission, 6/15 for domestic and international students; for spring admission, 12/1 for domestic and international students; for summer admission, 3/1 for domestic and international students. Application fee: $80. Electronic applications accepted. *Expenses:* Contact institution. *Financial support:* In 2015–16, 101 students received support. Career-related internships or fieldwork, Federal Work-Study, and scholarships/grants available. Support available to part-time students. Financial award application deadline: 3/1; financial award applicants required to submit FAFSA. *Faculty research:* Geriatrics, HIV, families and illness, oral systemic connection, symptom management. *Unit head:* Dr. James Pace, Senior Associate Dean for Academic Programs, 212-992-7343, E-mail: james.pace@nyu.edu. *Application contact:* Samantha Jaser, Assistant Director, Graduate Student Affairs and Admissions, 212-992-7653, Fax: 212-995-4302, E-mail: saj283@nyu.edu.

Nicholls State University, Graduate Studies, College of Nursing and Allied Health, Thibodaux, LA 70310. Offers family nurse practitioner (MSN); nurse executive (MSN); nursing education (MSN); psychiatric/mental health nurse practitioner (MSN). Website: http://www.nicholls.edu/cona/

Northeastern State University, College of Science and Health Professions, Department of Health Professions, Program in Nursing Education, Muskogee, OK 74401. Offers MSN. *Faculty:* 3 full-time (all women), 2 part-time/adjunct (both women). *Students:* 1 (woman) full-time, 25 part-time (23 women); includes 12 minority (1 Black or African American, non-Hispanic/Latino; 3 American Indian or Alaska Native, non-Hispanic/Latino; 1 Hispanic/Latino; 7 Two or more races, non-Hispanic/Latino). Average age 41. In 2015, 8 master's awarded. Application fee: $25. *Expenses:* Tuition, state resident: part-time $189.60 per credit hour. Tuition, nonresident: part-time $462.60 per credit hour. *Required fees:* $37.40 per credit hour. *Unit head:* Dr. Heather Fenton, Program Chair, 918-444-5025, E-mail: fentonh@nsuok.edu. *Application contact:* Donna Roberson, Secretary, 918-444-5410, E-mail: robersod@nsuok.edu. Website: http://academics.nsuok.edu/healthprofessions/DegreePrograms/Graduate/ NursingEducationMSN.aspx

Norwich University, College of Graduate and Continuing Studies, Master of Science in Nursing Program, Northfield, VT 05663. Offers nursing administration (MSN); nursing education (MSN). *Accreditation:* AACN. *Program availability:* Evening/weekend, mostly all online with a week-long residency requirement. *Faculty:* 10 part-time/adjunct (7 women). *Students:* 84 full-time (78 women); includes 11 minority (8 Black or African American, non-Hispanic/Latino; 2 Asian, non-Hispanic/Latino; 1 Hispanic/Latino). Average age 40. 33 applicants, 100% accepted, 29 enrolled. In 2015, 57 master's awarded. *Entrance requirements:* For master's, minimum undergraduate GPA of 3.0. Additional exam requirements/recommendations for international students: Required—TOEFL (minimum score 550 paper-based; 80 iBT), IELTS (minimum score 6.5). *Application deadline:* For fall admission, 8/15 for domestic and international students; for winter admission, 11/14 for domestic and international students; for spring admission, 2/13 for domestic and international students; for summer admission, 5/15 for domestic and international students. Applications are processed on a rolling basis. Electronic applications accepted. *Expenses:* Contact institution. *Financial support:* In 2015–16, 22 students received support. Scholarships/grants available. Financial award application deadline: 8/5; financial award applicants required to submit FAFSA. *Unit head:* Dr. Sharon Richie-Melvan, Director, 802-485-2600, E-mail: srichiem@norwich.edu. *Application contact:* Rija Ramahatra, Associate Program Director, 802-485-2892, Fax: 802-485-2533, E-mail: rramahatr@norwich.edu. Website: http://online.norwich.edu/degree-programs/masters/master-science-nursing/ overview

Ohio University, Graduate College, College of Health Sciences and Professions, School of Nursing, Athens, OH 45701-2979. Offers acute care nurse practitioner (MSN); acute care nurse practitioner and family nurse practitioner (MSN); acute care nurse practitioner and nurse administrator (MSN); acute care nurse practitioner and nurse educator (MSN); family nurse practitioner (MSN); nurse administrator (MSN); nurse administrator and family nurse practitioner (MSN); nurse educator (MSN); nurse educator and family nurse practitioner (MSN); nurse educator and nurse administrator (MSN). *Accreditation:* AACN. *Degree requirements:* For master's, capstone project. *Entrance requirements:* For master's, GRE, bachelor's degree in nursing from an accredited college or university, minimum overall undergraduate GPA of 3.0, official

transcripts, statement of goals and objectives, resume, 3 letters of recommendation. Additional exam requirements/recommendations for international students: Required—TOEFL (minimum score 550 paper-based; 80 iBT) or IELTS (minimum score 6.5). Electronic applications accepted.

Oklahoma Baptist University, Program in Nursing, Shawnee, OK 74804. Offers global nursing (MSN); nursing education (MSN). *Accreditation:* AACN.

Oklahoma City University, Kramer School of Nursing, Oklahoma City, OK 73106-1402. Offers clinical nurse leader (MSN); nursing (DNP, PhD); nursing education (MSN). *Accreditation:* ACEN. *Program availability:* Part-time, evening/weekend, online learning. *Faculty:* 11 full-time (all women), 6 part-time/adjunct (5 women). *Students:* 125 full-time (107 women), 30 part-time (29 women); includes 46 minority (13 Black or African American, non-Hispanic/Latino; 11 American Indian or Alaska Native, non-Hispanic/Latino; 10 Asian, non-Hispanic/Latino; 5 Hispanic/Latino; 7 Two or more races, non-Hispanic/Latino), 19 international. Average age 38. 54 applicants, 78% accepted, 31 enrolled. In 2015, 17 master's, 7 doctorates awarded. *Degree requirements:* For master's, thesis, minimum GPA of 3.0; for doctorate, comprehensive exam, thesis/ dissertation, minimum GPA of 3.0. *Entrance requirements:* For master's, registered nurse licensure, minimum undergraduate GPA of 3.0, BSN from nationally-accredited nursing program, completion of courses in health assessment and statistics; for doctorate, GRE, current RN licensure; bachelor's and master's degrees from accredited programs (at least one of which must be in nursing); minimum graduate GPA of 3.5; personal essay; approved scholarly paper or published article/paper in a refereed journal. Additional exam requirements/recommendations for international students: Required—TOEFL (minimum score 550 paper-based; 80 iBT), IELTS (minimum score 6). *Application deadline:* Applications are processed on a rolling basis. Application fee: $50. Electronic applications accepted. *Expenses:* $13,320 tuition and general fee per year for full-time study. *Financial support:* In 2015–16, 89 students received support. Federal Work-Study, institutionally sponsored loans, scholarships/grants, and tuition waivers (full and partial) available. Support available to part-time students. Financial award application deadline: 3/1; financial award applicants required to submit FAFSA. *Unit head:* Dr. Lois Salmeron, Dean, Kramer School of Nursing, 405-208-5900, Fax: 405-208-5914, E-mail: lsalmeron@okcu.edu. *Application contact:* Michael Harrington, Director of Graduate Admissions, 800-633-7242, Fax: 405-208-5916, E-mail: gadmissions@okcu.edu. Website: http://www.okcu.edu/nursing/

Oklahoma Wesleyan University, Professional Studies Division, Bartlesville, OK 74006-6299. Offers nursing administration (MSN); nursing education (MSN); strategic leadership (MS); theology and apologetics (MA).

Old Dominion University, College of Health Sciences, School of Nursing, Nurse Educator Emphasis, Norfolk, VA 23529. Offers neonatal nurse practitioner (MSN); pediatric nurse practitioner (MSN). *Program availability:* Part-time, online learning. *Faculty:* 1 (woman) full-time, 2 part-time/adjunct (both women). *Students:* 9 full-time (7 women), 17 part-time (11 women); includes 5 minority (1 Black or African American, non-Hispanic/Latino; 1 American Indian or Alaska Native, non-Hispanic/Latino; 3 Two or more races, non-Hispanic/Latino), 7 international. Average age 36. In 2015, 7 master's awarded. *Degree requirements:* For master's, comprehensive exam, thesis optional. *Entrance requirements:* For master's, GRE or MAT (waived if GPA is above 3.5), 3 letters of recommendation, essay, resume, transcripts. Additional exam requirements/ recommendations for international students: Required—TOEFL. *Application deadline:* For fall admission, 4/15 priority date for international students. Application fee: $50. *Expenses:* Tuition, state resident: full-time $11,136; part-time $464 per credit hour. Tuition, nonresident: full-time $27,840; part-time $1160 per credit hour. *Required fees:* $64 per semester. Tuition and fees vary according to campus/location, program and reciprocity agreements. *Financial support:* Fellowships, research assistantships, teaching assistantships, and unspecified assistantships available. *Faculty research:* Technology in nursing education, evidence-based instructional strategies, clinical judgment and decision-making. *Total annual research expenditures:* $35,726. *Unit head:* Dr. Kimberly Adams-Tufts, Graduate Program Director, 757-683-5011, E-mail: ktufts@ odu.edu. *Application contact:* Sue Parker, Graduate Program Coordinator, 757-683-4298, Fax: 757-683-5253, E-mail: sparker@odu.edu.

Oregon Health & Science University, School of Nursing, Program in Nursing Education, Portland, OR 97239-3098. Offers MN, MS, Post Master's Certificate.

Otterbein University, Department of Nursing, Westerville, OH 43081. Offers advanced practice nurse educator (Certificate); clinical nurse leader (MSN); family nurse practitioner (MSN, Certificate); nurse anesthesia (MSN, Certificate); nursing (DNP); nursing service administration (MSN). *Accreditation:* AACN; AANA/CANAEP; ACEN. *Program availability:* Part-time, evening/weekend, online learning. *Degree requirements:* For master's, comprehensive exam (for some programs), thesis (for some programs). *Entrance requirements:* For master's, 2 reference forms, resume; for Certificate, official transcripts, 2 reference forms, essay, resumé. Additional exam requirements/ recommendations for international students: Required—TOEFL (minimum score 550 paper-based; 79 iBT). *Faculty research:* Patient education, women's health, trauma curriculum development, administration.

Our Lady of the Lake College, School of Nursing, Program in Nursing, Baton Rouge, LA 70808. Offers administration (MS); education (MS). *Program availability:* Part-time. *Degree requirements:* For master's, capstone project. *Entrance requirements:* For master's, BSN with minimum GPA of 3.0 during the last 60 hours of undergraduate work, 1 year of clinical nursing experience as a registered nurse, current licensure or eligibility to practice as registered nurse in Louisiana, 3 professional references, 3 credit hours of undergraduate statistics with minimum C average.

Pace University, College of Health Professions, Lienhard School of Nursing, New York, NY 10038. Offers family nurse practitioner (MS); nurse education (Advanced Certificate); nursing education (MS); nursing leadership (Advanced Certificate); nursing practice (DNP). *Accreditation:* AACN. *Program availability:* Part-time, evening/weekend, blended/hybrid learning. *Faculty:* 11 full-time (10 women), 31 part-time/adjunct (27 women). *Students:* 3 full-time (all women), 415 part-time (385 women); includes 196 minority (97 Black or African American, non-Hispanic/Latino; 2 American Indian or Alaska Native, non-Hispanic/Latino; 57 Asian, non-Hispanic/Latino; 33 Hispanic/Latino; 7 Two or more races, non-Hispanic/Latino), 2 international. Average age 34. 291 applicants, 69% accepted, 129 enrolled. In 2015, 129 master's, 20 doctorates, 7 other advanced degrees awarded. *Degree requirements:* For doctorate, thesis/dissertation. *Entrance requirements:* For master's, RN license, resume, personal statement, 2 letters of recommendation, official transcripts; for doctorate, RN license, resume, personal statement, 2 letters of recommendation, official transcripts, accredited master's degree in nursing, minimum GPA of 3.3, national certification; for Advanced Certificate, RN license, completion of 2nd degree in nursing. Additional exam requirements/ recommendations for international students: Required—TOEFL (minimum score 100 iBT), IELTS or PTE. *Application deadline:* For fall admission, 3/1 for domestic and international students. Applications are processed on a rolling basis. Application fee: $70. Electronic applications accepted. *Expenses:* Contact institution. *Financial support:* Research assistantships, teaching assistantships, career-related internships or fieldwork, Federal Work-Study, tuition waivers (partial), and unspecified assistantships

Nursing Education

available. Support available to part-time students. Financial award application deadline: 2/15; financial award applicants required to submit FAFSA. *Unit head:* Dr. Harriet R. Feldman, Dean, College of Health Professions, 914-773-3341, E-mail: hfeldman@pace.edu. *Application contact:* Susan Ford-Goldschein, Director of Graduate Admissions, 212-346-1531, Fax: 212-346-1585, E-mail: graduateadmission@pace.edu. Website: http://www.pace.edu/lienhard

Pennsylvania College of Health Sciences, Graduate Programs, Lancaster, PA 17602. Offers administration (MSN); education (MSHS, MSN); healthcare administration (MHA). *Degree requirements:* For master's, internship (for MHA, MSN in administration); practicum (for MSHS, MSN in education).

Prairie View A&M University, College of Nursing, Houston, TX 77030. Offers family nurse practitioner (MSN); nursing administration (MSN); nursing education (MSN). *Accreditation:* AACN; ACEN. *Program availability:* Part-time, evening/weekend. *Faculty:* 11 full-time (all women), 7 part-time/adjunct (6 women). *Students:* 65 full-time (58 women), 78 part-time (71 women); includes 128 minority (94 Black or African American, non-Hispanic/Latino; 24 Asian, non-Hispanic/Latino; 9 Hispanic/Latino; 1 Two or more races, non-Hispanic/Latino), 5 international. Average age 35. 84 applicants, 44% accepted, 25 enrolled. In 2015, 63 master's awarded. *Degree requirements:* For master's, comprehensive exam, thesis. *Entrance requirements:* For master's, MAT or GRE, BS in nursing; minimum 1 year of experience as registered nurse; minimum GPA of 2.75, 3 letters of recommendation from professional nurses. Additional exam requirements/recommendations for international students: Required—TOEFL (minimum score 550 paper-based; 79 iBT). *Application deadline:* For fall admission, 7/1 priority date for domestic students, 6/1 priority date for international students; for spring admission, 11/1 priority date for domestic students, 10/1 priority date for international students; for summer admission, 3/1 priority date for domestic students, 2/1 priority date for international students. Applications are processed on a rolling basis. Application fee: $50. Electronic applications accepted. *Expenses:* Tuition, state resident: full-time $4243; part-time $237.29 per credit hour. Tuition, nonresident: full-time $11,798; part-time $657 per credit hour. *Required fees:* $2762; $172.10 per credit hour. *Financial support:* Career-related internships or fieldwork, Federal Work-Study, institutionally sponsored loans, scholarships/grants, and traineeships available. Support available to part-time students. Financial award application deadline: 4/1; financial award applicants required to submit FAFSA. *Faculty research:* Software development and violence prevention, health promotion and disease prevention. *Unit head:* Dr. Betty N. Adams, Dean, 713-797-7009, Fax: 713-797-7013, E-mail: bnadams@pvamu.edu. *Application contact:* Dr. Forest Smith, Director of Student Services and Admissions, 713-797-7031, Fax: 713-797-7012, E-mail: fdsmith@pvamu.edu. Website: http://www.pvamu.edu/nursing/

Queens University of Charlotte, Presbyterian School of Nursing, Charlotte, NC 28274-0002. Offers clinical nurse leader (MSN); nurse educator (MSN); nursing administrator (MSN). *Accreditation:* AACN. *Degree requirements:* For master's, research project. *Entrance requirements:* For master's, minimum GPA of 3.0. Additional exam requirements/recommendations for international students: Required—TOEFL. Electronic applications accepted. *Expenses:* Contact institution.

Ramapo College of New Jersey, Master of Science in Nursing Program, Mahwah, NJ 07430. Offers nursing education (MSN). *Accreditation:* ACEN. *Program availability:* Part-time. *Faculty:* 3 full-time (all women), 1 part-time/adjunct (0 women). *Students:* 1 full-time (0 women), 49 part-time (43 women); includes 16 minority (4 Black or African American, non-Hispanic/Latino; 8 Asian, non-Hispanic/Latino; 3 Hispanic/Latino; 1 Two or more races, non-Hispanic/Latino). Average age 35. 36 applicants, 81% accepted, 25 enrolled. In 2015, 6 master's awarded. *Entrance requirements:* For master's, official transcript; personal statement; 2 letters of recommendation; resume; current licensure as a Registered Nurse, or eligibility for licensure; evidence of one year of recent experience as RN prior to entry into clinical practicum courses; evidence of undergraduate statistics course; criminal background check. Additional exam requirements/recommendations for international students: Required—TOEFL (minimum score 550 paper-based; 90 iBT); Recommended—IELTS (minimum score 6). *Application deadline:* For fall admission, 5/1 for domestic and international students; for spring admission, 12/1 for domestic and international students. Applications are processed on a rolling basis. Application fee: $60. Electronic applications accepted. *Expenses:* $597.05 per credit tuition, $129.45 per credit fees. *Financial support:* Career-related internships or fieldwork available. Financial award application deadline: 3/1; financial award applicants required to submit FAFSA. *Faculty research:* Learning styles and critical thinking, evidence-based education, outcomes measurement. *Unit head:* Dr. Kathleen M. Burke, Assistant Dean in Charge of Nursing Programs/Professor, 201-684-7737, Fax: 201-684-7954, E-mail: kmburke@ramapo.edu. *Application contact:* Anthony Dovi, Associate Director of Admissions, Adult Learners and Graduate Programs, 201-684-7305, Fax: 201-684-7964, E-mail: adovi@ramapo.edu. Website: http://www.ramapo.edu/msn/

Regis College, School of Nursing and Health Sciences, Weston, MA 02493. Offers applied behavior analysis (MS); biomedical sciences (MS); counseling psychology (MA); health administration (MS); molecular imaging and therapeutics (MS); nurse practitioner (Certificate); nursing (MS, DNP); nursing education (Certificate); occupational therapy (MS). *Accreditation:* ACEN. *Program availability:* Part-time, evening/weekend. *Degree requirements:* For master's, thesis. *Entrance requirements:* For master's, GRE General Test or MAT, minimum GPA of 3.0; for doctorate, MAT or GRE if GPA from master's lower than 3.5. Additional exam requirements/recommendations for international students: Required—TOEFL (minimum score 550 paper-based). *Application deadline:* Applications are processed on a rolling basis. Application fee: $50. Electronic applications accepted. *Financial support:* Research assistantships, Federal Work-Study, scholarships/grants, traineeships, and unspecified assistantships available. Support available to part-time students. Financial award applicants required to submit FAFSA. *Faculty research:* Health policy, education, aging, job satisfaction, psychiatric nursing, critical thinking. *Application contact:* Shelagh Tomaino, Associate Director, Graduate Admission, 781-768-7188, Fax: 781-768-7071, E-mail: shelagh.tomaino@regiscollege.edu.

Regis University, Rueckert-Hartman College for Health Professions, Denver, CO 80221-1099. Offers addictions counseling (Post-Graduate Certificate); advanced practice nurse specialization (DNP); counseling (MA); counseling children and adolescents (Post-Graduate Certificate); counseling military families (Post-Graduate Certificate); depth psychotherapy (Post-Graduate Certificate); family nurse practitioner (MSN); health care business management (Certificate); health care quality and patient safety (Certificate); health industry leadership (MBA); health professions (Postbaccalaureate Certificate); health services administration (MS); marriage and family therapy (MA); neonatal nurse practitioner (MSN); nursing education or leadership (MSN); orthopedic manual physical therapy fellowship (Certificate); pharmacy (Pharm D); physical therapy (DPT). *Program availability:* Part-time, evening/weekend, 100% online, blended/hybrid learning. *Faculty:* 40 full-time (29 women), 116 part-time/adjunct (86 women). *Students:* 1,080 full-time (771 women), 274 part-time (239 women); includes 388 minority (59 Black or African American, non-Hispanic/Latino; 6 American Indian or Alaska Native, non-Hispanic/Latino; 109 Asian, non-Hispanic/Latino; 163 Hispanic/Latino; 1 Native Hawaiian or other Pacific Islander, non-Hispanic/Latino; 50

Two or more races, non-Hispanic/Latino), 7 international. Average age 34. 2,188 applicants, 31% accepted, 303 enrolled. In 2015, 329 master's, 160 doctorates awarded. *Degree requirements:* For master's, thesis (for some programs), internship. *Entrance requirements:* For master's, official transcript reflecting baccalaureate degree awarded from regionally-accredited college or university. Additional exam requirements/recommendations for international students: Required—TOEFL (minimum score 550 paper-based; 82 iBT). *Application deadline:* For fall admission, 8/15 priority date for domestic students; for spring admission, 1/10 priority date for domestic students; for summer admission, 5/1 priority date for domestic students. Applications are processed on a rolling basis. Application fee: $75. Electronic applications accepted. *Expenses:* Contact institution. *Financial support:* In 2015–16, 102 students received support. Federal Work-Study and scholarships/grants available. Financial award application deadline: 4/15; financial award applicants required to submit FAFSA. *Faculty research:* Normal and pathological balance and gait research, normal/pathological upper limb motor control/biomechanics, exercise energy/metabolism research, optical treatment protocols for therapeutic modalities. *Unit head:* Dr. Janet Houser, Academic Dean. *Application contact:* Cate Clark, Director of Admissions, 303-458-4900, Fax: 303-964-5534, E-mail: ruadmissions@regis.edu. Website: http://www.regis.edu/RHCHP.aspx

River University, School of Graduate Studies, Division of Nursing, Nashua, NH 03060. Offers adult psychiatric/mental health practitioner (MS); family nurse practitioner (MS); nursing education (MS). *Accreditation:* ACEN. *Program availability:* Part-time, evening/weekend. *Entrance requirements:* For master's, GRE, MAT. Electronic applications accepted.

Roberts Wesleyan College, Department of Nursing, Rochester, NY 14624-1997. Offers nursing education (MSN); nursing leadership and administration (MSN). *Accreditation:* AACN. *Program availability:* Evening/weekend, online learning. *Faculty:* 6 full-time (all women), 5 part-time/adjunct (3 women). *Students:* 66 full-time (64 women); includes 9 minority (6 Black or African American, non-Hispanic/Latino; 1 American Indian or Alaska Native, non-Hispanic/Latino; 2 Hispanic/Latino), 9 international. Average age 35. 53 applicants, 83% accepted, 41 enrolled. In 2015, 2 master's awarded. *Degree requirements:* For master's, thesis. *Entrance requirements:* For master's, minimum GPA of 3.0; BS in nursing; interview; RN license; resume; course work in statistics. Additional exam requirements/recommendations for international students: Required—TOEFL (minimum score 90 iBT), IELTS (minimum score 6.5). *Application deadline:* Applications are processed on a rolling basis. Application fee: $0. Electronic applications accepted. *Financial support:* In 2015–16, 49 students received support. Scholarships/grants available. Financial award applicants required to submit FAFSA. *Unit head:* Dr. Cheryl B. Crotser, Chairperson/Director of Graduate Program, 585-594-6668, E-mail: crotser_cheryl@roberts.edu. *Application contact:* Brenda Mutton, Admissions Coordinator, 585-594-6686, E-mail: mutton_brenda@roberts.edu. Website: http://www.roberts.edu/gradnursing

Sacred Heart University, Graduate Programs, College of Nursing, Fairfield, CT 06825. Offers clinical nurse leader (MSN); clinical practice (DNP); family nurse practitioner (MSN, Graduate Certificate); leadership (DNP); nurse educator (MSN); nursing management and executive leadership (MSN); patient care services (MSN). *Accreditation:* AACN. *Program availability:* Part-time, evening/weekend, online learning. *Faculty:* 17 full-time (all women), 21 part-time/adjunct (18 women). *Students:* 19 full-time (18 women), 777 part-time (711 women); includes 144 minority (56 Black or African American, non-Hispanic/Latino; 2 American Indian or Alaska Native, non-Hispanic/Latino; 33 Asian, non-Hispanic/Latino; 41 Hispanic/Latino; 2 Native Hawaiian or other Pacific Islander, non-Hispanic/Latino; 10 Two or more races, non-Hispanic/Latino). Average age 38. 116 applicants, 53% accepted, 50 enrolled. In 2015, 192 master's, 13 doctorates awarded. *Degree requirements:* For master's, thesis, 500 clinical hours. *Entrance requirements:* For master's, minimum GPA of 3.0, BSN or RN plus BS (for MSN); for doctorate, minimum GPA of 3.0, MSN or BSN plus MS in related field (for DNP). Additional exam requirements/recommendations for international students: Required—PTE; Recommended—TOEFL (minimum score 570 paper-based; 80 iBT), IELTS (minimum score 6.5). *Application deadline:* For fall admission, 2/15 for domestic and international students. Applications are processed on a rolling basis. Application fee: $75. Electronic applications accepted. *Expenses:* Contact institution. *Financial support:* Unspecified assistantships available. Financial award applicants required to submit FAFSA. *Unit head:* Mary Alice Donius, Dean of Nursing, 203-365-4508, E-mail: doniusm@sacredheart.edu. *Application contact:* William Sweeney, Director of Graduate Admissions Operations, 203-365-4716, Fax: 203-365-4732, E-mail: gradstudies@sacredheart.edu. Website: http://www.sacredheart.edu/academics/collegeofhealthprofessions/academicprograms/nursing/nursingprograms/graduateprograms/

Sage Graduate School, School of Health Sciences, Department of Nursing, Program in Education and Leadership, Troy, NY 12180-4115. Offers DNS. *Program availability:* Part-time-only. *Faculty:* 9 full-time (all women), 27 part-time/adjunct (24 women). *Students:* 41 part-time (39 women); includes 6 minority (1 Black or African American, non-Hispanic/Latino; 2 Asian, non-Hispanic/Latino; 2 Hispanic/Latino; 1 Two or more races, non-Hispanic/Latino), 2 international. Average age 49. 25 applicants, 44% accepted, 8 enrolled. In 2015, 8 doctorates awarded. *Degree requirements:* For doctorate, thesis/dissertation. *Entrance requirements:* For doctorate, master's degree in nursing from accredited institution; minimum GPA of 3.5; official transcripts; academic curriculum vitae; 3 letters of recommendation; 1-2 page personal essay; interview; current registered nurse license. Additional exam requirements/recommendations for international students: Required—TOEFL (minimum score 550 paper-based). Application fee: $40. Electronic applications accepted. *Expenses:* Contact institution. *Financial support:* Fellowships, research assistantships, Federal Work-Study, scholarships/grants, and unspecified assistantships available. Support available to part-time students. *Unit head:* Dr. Theresa Hand, Dean, School of Health Sciences, 518-200-2264, Fax: 518-244-4571, E-mail: handt@sage.edu. *Application contact:* Dr. Kathleen A. Kelly, Associate Professor/Director, Doctor of Nursing Science Program, 518-244-2030, Fax: 518-244-2009, E-mail: kelly5@sage.edu.

St. Catherine University, Graduate Programs, Program in Nursing, St. Paul, MN 55105. Offers adult gerontological nurse practitioner (MS); neonatal nurse practitioner (MS); nurse educator (MS); nursing (DNP); nursing: entry-level (MS); pediatric nurse practitioner (MS). *Accreditation:* ACEN. *Program availability:* Part-time, evening/weekend. *Degree requirements:* For master's, thesis; for doctorate, portfolio, systems change project. *Entrance requirements:* For master's, GRE General Test, bachelor's degree in nursing, current nursing license, 2 years of recent clinical practice; for doctorate, master's degree in nursing, RN license, advanced nursing position. Additional exam requirements/recommendations for international students: Required—TOEFL (minimum score 600 paper-based; 100 iBT). *Expenses:* Contact institution.

Saint Francis Medical Center College of Nursing, Graduate Programs, Peoria, IL 61603-3783. Offers adult gerontology (MSN); clinical nurse leader (MSN); family nurse practitioner (MSN); family psychiatric mental health nurse practitioner (MSN); neonatal nurse practitioner (MSN); nurse clinician (Post-Graduate Certificate); nurse educator (MSN, Post-Graduate Certificate); nursing (DNP); nursing management leadership (MSN). *Accreditation:* ACEN. *Program availability:* Part-time, 100% online, blended/

hybrid learning. *Faculty:* 14 full-time (all women), 5 part-time/adjunct (all women). *Students:* 13 full-time (12 women), 257 part-time (228 women); includes 23 minority (14 Black or African American, non-Hispanic/Latino; 3 Asian, non-Hispanic/Latino; 4 Hispanic/Latino; 2 Two or more races, non-Hispanic/Latino). Average age 37. 86 applicants, 86% accepted, 44 enrolled. In 2015, 61 master's, 6 doctorates awarded. *Degree requirements:* For master's, research experience, portfolio, practicum; for doctorate, practicum hours. *Entrance requirements:* For master's, nursing research, health assessment, graduate course work in statistics, RN license; for doctorate, master's degree in nursing, professional portfolio, graduate statistics, transcripts, RN license. Additional exam requirements/recommendations for international students: Required—TOEFL (minimum score 550 paper-based; 79 iBT). *Application deadline:* For fall admission, 6/1 priority date for domestic and international students; for spring admission, 11/15 priority date for domestic and international students. Applications are processed on a rolling basis. Application fee: $50. *Financial support:* In 2015–16, 18 students received support. Scholarships/grants and tuition waivers (partial) available. Support available to part-time students. Financial award application deadline: 6/15; financial award applicants required to submit FAFSA. *Faculty research:* Outcome and curriculum planning, health promotion, NCLEX-RN results, decision-making program evaluation. *Unit head:* Dr. Patti A. Stockert, President of the College, 309-655-4124, Fax: 309-624-8973, E-mail: patricia.a.stockert@osfhealthcare.org. *Application contact:* Dr. Kim A. Mitchell, Dean, Graduate Program, 309-655-2201, Fax: 309-624-8973, E-mail: kim.a.mitchell@osfhealthcare.org.
Website: http://www.sfmccon.edu/graduate-programs/

Saint Joseph's College of Maine, Master of Science in Nursing Program, Standish, ME 04084. Offers administration (MSN); education (MSN); family nurse practitioner (MSN); nursing administration and leadership (Certificate); nursing and health care education (Certificate). *Accreditation:* AACN. *Program availability:* Part-time, online learning. *Entrance requirements:* For master's, MAT. Electronic applications accepted.

Salem State University, School of Graduate Studies, Program in Nursing, Salem, MA 01970-5353. Offers adult-gerontology primary care nursing (MSN); nursing administration (MSN); nursing education (MSN); MBA/MSN. *Accreditation:* AACN. *Program availability:* Part-time, evening/weekend. *Entrance requirements:* For master's, GRE or MAT. Additional exam requirements/recommendations for international students: Required—TOEFL (minimum score 550 paper-based; 80 iBT) or IELTS (minimum score 5.5).

Salisbury University, MS in Nursing Program, Salisbury, MD 21801-6837. Offers clinical nurse educator (MS); health care leadership (MS); nursing (MS). *Program availability:* Part-time. *Faculty:* 5 full-time (3 women). *Students:* 6 part-time (5 women); includes 1 minority (Black or African American, non-Hispanic/Latino). Average age 33. 1 applicant. In 2015, 6 master's awarded. *Degree requirements:* For master's, thesis. *Entrance requirements:* For master's, BS in nursing with minimum cumulative GPA of 3.0; current and active United States Registered Nursing license; current resume or curriculum vitae; personal statement; 2 letters of reference; interview. Additional exam requirements/recommendations for international students: Required—TOEFL (minimum score 550 paper-based, 79 iBT) or IELTS (6.5). *Application deadline:* For fall admission, 5/15 priority date for domestic and international students. Applications are processed on a rolling basis. Application fee: $65. Electronic applications accepted. *Expenses:* $620 per credit hour resident; $787 per credit hour non-resident; $78 per credit hour fees. *Financial support:* In 2015–16, 18 students received support, including 1 research assistantship with full tuition reimbursement available (averaging $8,000 per year); career-related internships or fieldwork, institutionally sponsored loans, scholarships/grants, and unspecified assistantships also available. Support available to part-time students. Financial award application deadline: 3/1; financial award applicants required to submit FAFSA. *Faculty research:* Gerontology; epidemiology; palliative care; global health; depression. *Unit head:* Dr. Lisa Seldomridge, Graduate Program Director, Nursing, 410-543-6344, Fax: 410-548-3313, E-mail: laseldomridge@salisbury.edu. *Application contact:* Carmel Boger, Administrative Assistant, 410-543-6420, Fax: 410-548-3313, E-mail: ciboger@salisbury.edu.
Website: http://www.salisbury.edu/gsr/gradstudies/MSNpage.html

Samford University, Ida V. Moffett School of Nursing, Birmingham, AL 35229. Offers administration (DNP); advanced practice (DNP); family nurse practitioner (MSN); health systems management and leadership (MSN); nurse anesthesia (MSN); nurse educator (MSN). *Accreditation:* AACN; AANA/CANAEP (one or more programs are accredited). *Program availability:* Part-time, blended/hybrid learning. *Faculty:* 19 full-time (all women), 5 part-time/adjunct (1 woman). *Students:* 300 full-time (228 women), 40 part-time (36 women); includes 65 minority (28 Black or African American, non-Hispanic/Latino; 4 American Indian or Alaska Native, non-Hispanic/Latino; 8 Asian, non-Hispanic/Latino; 13 Hispanic/Latino; 12 Two or more races, non-Hispanic/Latino). Average age 35. 69 applicants, 77% accepted, 52 enrolled. In 2015, 98 master's, 16 doctorates awarded. *Degree requirements:* For doctorate, capstone project with oral presentation. *Entrance requirements:* For master's, MAT; GRE (for nurse anesthesia), unencumbered licensure as registered nurse; BSN from CCNE, CNEA, or ACEN (formerly NLNAC) accredited program; minimum cumulative GPA of 3.0 in nursing courses; video submission; one undergraduate course in nursing research with minimum grade of C; for doctorate, unencumbered licensure as registered nurse; master's degree from CCNE, CNEA or ACEN (formerly NLNAC) accredited program in the area of advanced practice or administration; minimum master's degree cumulative GPA of 3.5; video interview submission. Additional exam requirements/recommendations for international students: Required—TOEFL (minimum score 550 paper-based; 80 iBT). *Application deadline:* For fall admission, 6/1 for domestic and international students; for spring admission, 9/1 for domestic and international students. Application fee: $65. Electronic applications accepted. *Expenses:* Tuition, area resident: Full-time $18,673; part-time $766 per credit hour. *Required fees:* $550. Tuition and fees vary according to course load, degree level and student level. *Financial support:* In 2015–16, 56 students received support. Institutionally sponsored loans, scholarships/grants, and traineeships available. Financial award application deadline: 3/1; financial award applicants required to submit FAFSA. *Faculty research:* Issues in rural health care, vulnerable populations, genetics and disabilities in pediatrics, geriatrics, parish nursing research, interprofessional education, global health disparities. *Unit head:* Dr. Nena F. Sanders, Vice Provost, College of Health Sciences/Dean/Professor, 205-726-2612, Fax: 205-726-4179, E-mail: nfsander@samford.edu. *Application contact:* Allyson Maddox, Director of Graduate Student Services, Ida V. Moffett School of Nursing, 205-726-2047, Fax: 205-726-4179, E-mail: amaddox@samford.edu.
Website: http://samford.edu/nursing

Seattle Pacific University, MS in Nursing Program, Seattle, WA 98119-1997. Offers administration (MSN); adult/gerontology nurse practitioner (MSN); clinical nurse specialist (MSN); family nurse practitioner (MSN, Certificate); informatics (MSN); nurse educator (MSN). *Accreditation:* AACN. *Program availability:* Part-time. *Students:* 39 full-time (36 women), 30 part-time (25 women); includes 14 minority (3 Black or African American, non-Hispanic/Latino; 7 Asian, non-Hispanic/Latino; 3 Hispanic/Latino; 1 Two or more races, non-Hispanic/Latino), 1 international. Average age 38. 60 applicants, 48% accepted, 29 enrolled. In 2015, 23 master's awarded. *Degree requirements:* For master's, thesis. *Entrance requirements:* For master's, personal statement, transcripts,

undergraduate nursing degree, proof of undergraduate statistics course with minimum GPA of 2.0, 2 recommendations. *Application deadline:* For fall admission, 1/15 priority date for domestic students; for spring admission, 1/15 for domestic students. Applications are processed on a rolling basis. Application fee: $50. Electronic applications accepted. *Expenses:* Contact institution. *Financial support:* Fellowships and scholarships/grants available. Financial award applicants required to submit FAFSA. *Unit head:* Dr. Christine Hoyle, Associate Dean, 206-281-2469, E-mail: hoylec@spu.edu.
Website: http://spu.edu/depts/health-sciences/grad/index.asp

Seton Hall University, College of Nursing, South Orange, NJ 07079-2697. Offers advanced practice in primary health care (MSN, DNP), including adult/gerontological nurse practitioner, pediatric nurse practitioner; entry into practice (MSN); health systems administration (MSN, DNP); nursing (PhD); nursing case management (MSN); nursing education (MA); school nurse (MSN); MSN/MA. *Accreditation:* AACN. *Program availability:* Part-time, online learning. *Degree requirements:* For master's, research project; for doctorate, dissertation or scholarly project. *Entrance requirements:* For doctorate, GRE (waived for students with GPA of 3.5 or higher). Additional exam requirements/recommendations for international students: Required—TOEFL. Electronic applications accepted. *Faculty research:* Parent/child, adult, and gerontological nursing; breast cancer; families of children with HIV; parish nursing.

Shenandoah University, Eleanor Wade Custer School of Nursing, Winchester, VA 22601. Offers family nurse practitioner (MSN, DNP, Post-Graduate Certificate); health informatics (Certificate); health systems leadership (DNP); nurse midwifery (MSN, Post-Graduate Certificate); nursing education (Post-Graduate Certificate); psychiatric mental health nurse practitioner (MSN, DNP, Post-Graduate Certificate). *Accreditation:* AACN; ACNM/ACME. *Faculty:* 10 full-time (all women), 7 part-time/adjunct (4 women). *Students:* 33 full-time (31 women), 62 part-time (57 women); includes 21 minority (17 Black or African American, non-Hispanic/Latino; 3 Asian, non-Hispanic/Latino; 1 Hispanic/Latino). Average age 36. 55 applicants, 87% accepted, 39 enrolled. In 2015, 32 master's, 3 doctorates, 19 other advanced degrees awarded. *Degree requirements:* For master's, research project, clinical hours; for doctorate, scholarly project, clinical hours; for other advanced degree, clinical hours. *Entrance requirements:* For master's, United States RN license; minimum GPA of 3.0; 2080 hours of clinical experience; curriculum vitae; 3 letters of recommendation from a former dean, a faculty member or advisor familiar with the applicant, and a former or current supervisor; two- to three-page essay on a specified topic; for doctorate, MSN, minimum GPA of 3.0, 3 letters of recommendation, 500-word statement, interview, BSN; for other advanced degree, MSN, minimum GPA of 3.0, 2 letters of recommendation, minimum of one year (2080 hours) of clinical nursing experience, interview. Additional exam requirements/recommendations for international students: Required—TOEFL (minimum score 558 paper-based; 83 iBT). *Application deadline:* For fall admission, 1/15 priority date for domestic and international students; for spring admission, 11/1 for domestic and international students; for summer admission, 3/15 for domestic and international students. Application fee: $30. Electronic applications accepted. *Expenses:* Contact institution. *Financial support:* In 2015–16, 13 students received support, including 3 fellowships (averaging $1,000 per year); scholarships/grants and unspecified assistantships also available. Financial award application deadline: 3/15; financial award applicants required to submit FAFSA. *Faculty research:* Primary care providers and their unique position in geriatric, pre-operative education and its effects on post-operative, variables associated with a woman's multidimensional childbirth, interdisciplinary communication, research on health policy. *Unit head:* Kathryn Ganske, PhD, RN, Dean, 540-678-4374, Fax: 540-665-5519, E-mail: kganske@su.edu. *Application contact:* Andrew Woodall, Executive Director of Recruitment and Admissions, 540-665-4581, Fax: 540-665-4627, E-mail: admit@su.edu.
Website: http://www.su.edu/nursing/

Southern Connecticut State University, School of Graduate Studies, School of Health and Human Services, Department of Nursing, New Haven, CT 06515-1355. Offers family nurse practitioner (MSN); nursing education (MSN). *Accreditation:* AACN. *Program availability:* Part-time, evening/weekend. *Faculty:* 12 full-time (all women), 2 part-time/adjunct (both women). *Students:* 7 full-time (6 women), 80 part-time (70 women); includes 20 minority (8 Black or African American, non-Hispanic/Latino; 5 Asian, non-Hispanic/Latino; 6 Hispanic/Latino; 1 Two or more races, non-Hispanic/Latino). Average age 36. 112 applicants, 11% accepted, 11 enrolled. In 2015, 15 master's awarded. *Degree requirements:* For master's, thesis. *Entrance requirements:* For master's, GRE, MAT, interview, minimum QPA of 2.8, RN license, minimum 1 year of professional nursing experience. *Application deadline:* For fall admission, 7/15 priority date for domestic students. Applications are processed on a rolling basis. Application fee: $50. Electronic applications accepted. *Expenses:* Tuition, state resident: full-time $4968; part-time $494 per credit hour. Tuition, nonresident: full-time $16,078; part-time $509 per credit hour. *Required fees:* $4632; $55 per semester. Tuition and fees vary according to program. *Financial support:* Career-related internships or fieldwork, scholarships/grants, and unspecified assistantships available. Financial award application deadline: 4/15; financial award applicants required to submit FAFSA. *Unit head:* Dr. Lisa Rebeschi, Chairperson, 203-392-6485, E-mail: rebeschi1@southernct.edu. *Application contact:* Lisa Galvin, Director of Graduate Admissions, 203-392-5240, Fax: 203-392-5235, E-mail: galvinl1@southernct.edu.

Southern Illinois University Edwardsville, Graduate School, School of Nursing, Program in Nurse Educator, Edwardsville, IL 62026. Offers MS, Post-Master's Certificate. *Program availability:* Part-time, evening/weekend. *Students:* 33 part-time (31 women); includes 2 minority (1 Black or African American, non-Hispanic/Latino; 1 Hispanic/Latino). 20 applicants, 100% accepted. In 2015, 9 master's awarded. *Degree requirements:* For master's, comprehensive exam. *Entrance requirements:* For master's, RN licensure, minimum undergraduate nursing GPA of 3.0. Additional exam requirements/recommendations for international students: Required—TOEFL (minimum score 550 paper-based; 79 iBT), IELTS (minimum score 6.5). *Application deadline:* For fall admission, 3/1 for domestic and international students. Application fee: $30. Electronic applications accepted. *Expenses:* Tuition, state resident: full-time $5026; part-time $837 per course. Tuition, nonresident: full-time $12,566; part-time $2094 per course. *Required fees:* $1682; $474 per course. Tuition and fees vary according to course load, campus/location and program. *Financial support:* In 2015–16, 2 teaching assistantships with full tuition reimbursements were awarded; fellowships, research assistantships, institutionally sponsored loans, scholarships/grants, and unspecified assistantships also available. Financial award application deadline: 3/1; financial award applicants required to submit FAFSA. *Unit head:* Dr. Kathy Ketchum, Associate Dean for Graduate Programs, 618-650-3936, E-mail: kketchu@siue.edu. *Application contact:* Bob Skorczewski, Coordinator of International and Graduate Recruitment, 618-650-3705, Fax: 618-650-3618, E-mail: gradadmissions@siue.edu.
Website: http://www.siue.edu/nursing/graduate

Southern Nazarene University, College of Professional and Graduate Studies, School of Nursing, Bethany, OK 73008. Offers nursing education (MS); nursing leadership (MS). *Accreditation:* AACN. *Program availability:* Part-time, evening/weekend. *Degree requirements:* For master's, thesis. *Entrance requirements:* For master's, minimum undergraduate cumulative GPA of 3.0; baccalaureate degree in nursing from nationally-

Nursing Education

accredited program; current unencumbered registered nurse licensure in Oklahoma or eligibility for same; documentation of basic computer skills; basic statistics course; statement of professional goals; three letters of recommendation. Additional exam requirements/recommendations for international students: Required—TOEFL (minimum score 550 paper-based).

Southern University and Agricultural and Mechanical College, School of Nursing, Baton Rouge, LA 70813. Offers educator/administrator (PhD); family health nursing (MSN); family nurse practitioner (Post Master's Certificate); geriatric nurse practitioner/ gerontology (PhD). *Accreditation:* AACN. *Program availability:* Part-time. *Degree requirements:* For master's, comprehensive exam, thesis; for doctorate, comprehensive exam, thesis/dissertation. *Entrance requirements:* For master's, GRE General Test, BSN, minimum GPA of 2.7; for doctorate, GRE General Test; for Post Master's Certificate, MSN. Additional exam requirements/recommendations for international students: Required—TOEFL (minimum score 525 paper-based). *Faculty research:* Health promotions, vulnerable populations, (community-based) cardiovascular participating research, health disparities chronic diseases, care of the elderly.

South University, Graduate Programs, College of Nursing, Savannah, GA 31406. Offers nurse educator (MS).

South University, Program in Nursing, Tampa, FL 33614. Offers adult health nurse practitioner (MS); family nurse practitioner (MS); nurse educator (MS).

State University of New York College of Technology at Delhi, Program in Nursing Education, Delhi, NY 13753. Offers MS.

State University of New York Empire State College, School for Graduate Studies, Program in Nursing Education, Saratoga Springs, NY 12866-4391. Offers MSN. *Program availability:* Online learning. *Degree requirements:* For master's, capstone.

State University of New York Polytechnic Institute, Program in Nursing Education, Utica, NY 13504-3050. Offers MS, CAS. *Program availability:* Part-time, online learning. *Degree requirements:* For master's, culminating internship. *Entrance requirements:* For master's, minimum GPA of 3.0 in last 30 hours of undergraduate work, bachelor's in nursing, 1 year of RN experience, RN license, 2 letters of reference, resume, educational objective; for CAS, master's degree in nursing. Additional exam requirements/recommendations for international students: Required—TOEFL (minimum score 550 paper-based; 79 iBT), IELTS (minimum score 6.5). Electronic applications accepted. *Faculty research:* Nursing faculty shortages, curriculum enhancements, measurement and assessment, evidence-based practice.

Stevenson University, Program in Nursing, Owings Mills, MD 21117. Offers nursing education (MS); nursing leadership/management (MS); population-based care coordination (MS). *Program availability:* Part-time, blended/hybrid learning. *Faculty:* 4 full-time (all women), 7 part-time/adjunct (all women). *Students:* 178 part-time (169 women); includes 67 minority (53 Black or African American, non-Hispanic/Latino; 12 Asian, non-Hispanic/Latino; 2 Hispanic/Latino). Average age 40. 83 applicants, 75% accepted, 44 enrolled. In 2015, 37 master's awarded. *Degree requirements:* For master's, capstone course. *Entrance requirements:* For master's, bachelor's degree from regionally-accredited institution, current registered nurse's license in good standing, official college transcripts from all previous academic work, minimum cumulative GPA of 3.0 in past academic work, personal statement (250-350 words), two professional letters of recommendation, resume. Additional exam requirements/ recommendations for international students: Required—TOEFL (minimum score 550 paper-based), IELTS (minimum score 6.5). *Application deadline:* Applications are processed on a rolling basis. Application fee: $0. Electronic applications accepted. *Expenses:* $625 per credit, $125 per semester. *Financial support:* Applicants required to submit FAFSA. *Unit head:* Judith Feustle, PhD, Associate Dean, 443-352-4292, Fax: 443-394-0538, E-mail: jfeustle@stevenson.edu. *Application contact:* Amanda Courter, Enrollment Counselor, 443-352-4243, Fax: 443-394-0538, E-mail: acourter@ stevenson.edu.
Website: http://www.stevenson.edu

Stony Brook University, State University of New York, Stony Brook Medicine, School of Nursing, Program in Nursing Education, Stony Brook, NY 11794. Offers MS, Certificate. *Program availability:* Part-time, blended/hybrid learning. *Students:* 1 (woman) full-time, 70 part-time (66 women); includes 27 minority (17 Black or African American, non-Hispanic/Latino; 2 Asian, non-Hispanic/Latino; 7 Hispanic/Latino; 1 Two or more races, non-Hispanic/Latino). 33 applicants, 94% accepted, 27 enrolled. *Entrance requirements:* For master's, baccalaureate degree with major in nursing, minimum cumulative GPA of 3.0, current professional RN license, three letters of recommendation. Additional exam requirements/recommendations for international students: Required—TOEFL (minimum score 90 iBT). *Application deadline:* For fall admission, 2/18 for domestic students. Application fee: $100. Electronic applications accepted. *Expenses:* $24,781 per year full-time resident tuition and fees, $968 per credit hour; $44,431 per year full-time out-of-state tuition and fees, $1,787 per credit hour. *Unit head:* Stacey Frawley, Program Director, 631-444-3284, Fax: 631-444-3136, E-mail: stacey.frawley@stonybrook.edu. *Application contact:* Anita Defranco, Staff Assistant, 631-444-3276, Fax: 631-444-3136, E-mail: anita.defranco@stonybrook.edu.
Website: http://www.nursing.stonybrookmedicine.edu/nursingeducationmaster

Tarleton State University, College of Graduate Studies, College of Science and Technology, Department of Nursing, Stephenville, TX 76402. Offers nursing administration (MSN); nursing education (MSN). *Program availability:* Part-time, evening/weekend. *Faculty:* 3 full-time (all women). *Students:* 19 part-time (17 women); includes 6 minority (3 Black or African American, non-Hispanic/Latino; 3 Hispanic/Latino). 12 applicants, 83% accepted, 8 enrolled. In 2015, 8 master's awarded. *Degree requirements:* For master's, comprehensive exam. *Entrance requirements:* For master's, GRE General Test, minimum GPA of 3.0. Additional exam requirements/ recommendations for international students: Required—TOEFL (minimum score 550 paper-based; 80 iBT). *Application deadline:* For fall admission, 8/15 priority date for domestic students; for spring admission, 1/7 for domestic students. Applications are processed on a rolling basis. Application fee: $45 ($145 for international students). Electronic applications accepted. *Expenses:* Tuition, state resident: part-time $204 per credit hour. Tuition, nonresident: part-time $594 per credit hour. *Required fees:* $1994 per unit. *Financial support:* Career-related internships or fieldwork, Federal Work-Study, and institutionally sponsored loans available. Support available to part-time students. Financial award applicants required to submit FAFSA. *Unit head:* Dr. Susan Rugari, Department Head, 254-968-9139, E-mail: rugari@tarleton.edu. *Application contact:* Information Contact, 254-968-9104, Fax: 254-968-9670, E-mail: gradoffice@ tarleton.edu.
Website: http://www.tarleton.edu/nursing/degrees_grad.html

Teachers College, Columbia University, Department of Health and Behavior Studies, New York, NY 10027-6696. Offers applied behavior analysis (MA, PhD); applied educational psychology: school psychology (Ed M, PhD); behavioral nutrition (PhD), including nutrition (Ed D, PhD); community health education (MS); community nutrition education (Ed M), including community nutrition education; education of deaf and hard of hearing (MA, PhD); health education (MA, Ed D); hearing impairment (Ed D); intellectual disability/autism (MA, Ed D, PhD); nursing education (Advanced Certificate); nutrition and education (MS); nutrition and exercise physiology (MS); nutrition and public

health (MS); nutrition education (Ed D), including nutrition (Ed D, PhD); physical disabilities (Ed D); reading specialist (MA); severe or multiple disabilities (MA); special education (Ed M, MA, Ed D); teaching of sign language (MA). *Program availability:* Part-time, evening/weekend. *Students:* 186 full-time (168 women), 362 part-time (319 women); includes 199 minority (50 Black or African American, non-Hispanic/Latino; 1 American Indian or Alaska Native, non-Hispanic/Latino; 73 Asian, non-Hispanic/Latino; 59 Hispanic/Latino; 1 Native Hawaiian or other Pacific Islander, non-Hispanic/Latino; 15 Two or more races, non-Hispanic/Latino), 13 international. Terminal master's awarded for partial completion of doctoral program. *Expenses: Tuition, area resident:* Part-time $1454 per credit. *Required fees:* $428 per semester. One-time fee: $475 full-time. Full-time tuition and fees vary according to course load. *Unit head:* Prof. Stephen T. Peverly, Chair, 212-678-3964, Fax: 212-678-8259, E-mail: stp4@columbia.edu. *Application contact:* David Estrella, Director of Admission, 212-678-3305, E-mail: estrella@ tc.columbia.edu.
Website: http://www.tc.columbia.edu/health-and-behavior-studies/

Teachers College, Columbia University, Department of Organization and Leadership, New York, NY 10027-6696. Offers adult education guided intensive study (Ed D); adult learning and leadership (Ed M, MA, ME, Ed D); educational leadership studies (Ed D); higher and post secondary education (MA, ME, Ed D); inquiry educational leadership practice (Ed D); leadership, policy and politics (Ed D); nurse education (MA); nurse executive (MA), including administration studies, professorial studies; nurse executive role (MA, Ed D), including nurse executive (Ed D); private school leadership (Ed M, MA, ME); public school building leadership (Ed M, MA, ME); social and organizational psychology (MA); urban education leaders (Ed D); MA/MBA. *Program availability:* Part-time, evening/weekend. *Students:* 285 full-time (173 women), 491 part-time (344 women); includes 333 minority (119 Black or African American, non-Hispanic/Latino; 1 American Indian or Alaska Native, non-Hispanic/Latino; 102 Asian, non-Hispanic/Latino; 97 Hispanic/Latino; 14 Two or more races, non-Hispanic/Latino), 36 international. *Degree requirements:* For doctorate, thesis/dissertation. *Expenses: Tuition, area resident:* Part-time $1454 per credit. *Required fees:* $428 per semester. One-time fee: $475 full-time. Full-time tuition and fees vary according to course load. *Unit head:* Prof. Anna Neumann, Chair, 212-678-3272, Fax: 212-678-3036, E-mail: neumann@ tc.columbia.edu. *Application contact:* David Estrella, Director of Admission, E-mail: estrella@tc.columbia.edu.

Tennessee Technological University, Whitson-Hester School of Nursing, Cookeville, TN 38505. Offers family nurse practitioner (MSN); informatics (MSN); nursing administration (MSN); nursing education (MSN). *Program availability:* Part-time, evening/weekend, online learning. *Students:* 21 full-time (20 women), 95 part-time (80 women); includes 5 minority (2 Black or African American, non-Hispanic/Latino; 1 Asian, non-Hispanic/Latino; 1 Hispanic/Latino; 1 Two or more races, non-Hispanic/Latino). 42 applicants, 57% accepted, 15 enrolled. In 2015, 47 master's awarded. *Degree requirements:* For master's, comprehensive exam, thesis or alternative. *Entrance requirements:* Additional exam requirements/recommendations for international students: Required—TOEFL (minimum score 600 paper-based; 100 iBT), IELTS (minimum score 5.5), PTE, or TOEIC (Test of English as an International Communication). *Application deadline:* For fall admission, 8/1 for domestic students, 5/1 for international students; for spring admission, 12/1 for domestic students, 10/1 for international students; for summer admission, 5/1 for domestic students, 2/1 for international students. Applications are processed on a rolling basis. Application fee: $35 ($40 for international students). Electronic applications accepted. *Expenses:* Tuition, state resident: full-time $8961; part-time $6132 per credit hour. Tuition, nonresident: full-time $23,121; part-time $14,608 per credit hour. *Financial support:* Application deadline: 4/1. *Unit head:* Dr. Huey-Ming Tzeng, Dean, 931-372-3547, Fax: 931-372-6244, E-mail: htzeng@tntech.edu. *Application contact:* Shelia K. Kendrick, Coordinator of Graduate Studies, 931-372-3808, Fax: 931-372-3497, E-mail: skendrick@tntech.edu.

Texas A&M University, College of Nursing, Bryan, TX 77807. Offers family nurse practitioner (MSN); nursing education (MSN). *Faculty:* 47. *Students:* 10 full-time (8 women), 27 part-time (23 women); includes 4 minority (2 Black or African American, non-Hispanic/Latino; 1 Asian, non-Hispanic/Latino; 1 Hispanic/Latino). Average age 35. 30 applicants, 100% accepted, 30 enrolled. *Expenses:* Contact institution. *Financial support:* In 2015–16, 4 students received support. Career-related internships or fieldwork, institutionally sponsored loans, scholarships/grants, traineeships, health care benefits, tuition waivers (full and partial), and unspecified assistantships available. Support available to part-time students. Financial award applicants required to submit FAFSA. *Unit head:* Dr. Sharon A. Wilkerson, Founding Dean, 979-436-0111, Fax: 979-436-0098, E-mail: wilkerson@tamhsc.edu. *Application contact:* Jennifer Frank, Program Coordinator for Recruitment and Admission, 979-436-0110, E-mail: conadmissions@ tamhsc.edu.
Website: http://nursing.tamhsc.edu/

Texas A&M University–Corpus Christi, College of Graduate Studies, College of Nursing and Health Sciences, Corpus Christi, TX 78412-5503. Offers family nurse practitioner (MSN); leadership in nursing systems (MSN); nurse educator (MSN). *Accreditation:* AACN. *Program availability:* Part-time, evening/weekend, online only, 100% online. *Students:* 12 full-time (11 women), 375 part-time (322 women); includes 200 minority (20 Black or African American, non-Hispanic/Latino; 1 American Indian or Alaska Native, non-Hispanic/Latino; 27 Asian, non-Hispanic/Latino; 142 Hispanic/Latino; 3 Native Hawaiian or other Pacific Islander, non-Hispanic/Latino; 7 Two or more races, non-Hispanic/Latino), 1 international. Average age 38. 337 applicants, 42% accepted, 128 enrolled. In 2015, 102 master's awarded. *Degree requirements:* For master's, comprehensive exam, thesis (for some programs), capstone - clinical. *Entrance requirements:* For master's, essay, resume, 3 letters of recommendation, minimum GPA of 3.0. Additional exam requirements/recommendations for international students: Required—TOEFL (minimum score 550 paper-based; 79 iBT), IELTS (minimum score 6.5). *Application deadline:* For fall admission, 4/15 priority date for domestic and international students; for spring admission, 1/7 for domestic and international students; for summer admission, 5/27 for domestic and international students. Applications are processed on a rolling basis. Application fee: $50 ($70 for international students). Electronic applications accepted. *Financial support:* Research assistantships, teaching assistantships, career-related internships or fieldwork, Federal Work-Study, institutionally sponsored loans, scholarships/grants, health care benefits, and unspecified assistantships available. Support available to part-time students. Financial award application deadline: 3/15; financial award applicants required to submit FAFSA. *Unit head:* Dr. Mary Jane Hamilton, Dean, 361-825-2469, E-mail: mary.hamilton@ tamucc.edu. *Application contact:* Graduate Admissions Coordinator, 361-825-2177, Fax: 361-825-2755, E-mail: gradweb@tamucc.edu.
Website: http://conhs.tamucc.edu/

Texas Christian University, Harris College of Nursing and Health Sciences, Master's Program in Nursing, Fort Worth, TX 76129. Offers clinical nurse leader (MSN, Certificate); clinical nurse specialist (MSN), including adult/gerontology nursing, pediatrics; nursing education (MSN). *Accreditation:* AACN; AANA/CANAEP (one or more programs are accredited). *Program availability:* Part-time, online only, 100% online. *Faculty:* 20 full-time (17 women), 2 part-time/adjunct (both women). *Students:* 47

full-time (40 women), 24 part-time (all women); includes 19 minority (3 Black or African American, non-Hispanic/Latino; 1 American Indian or Alaska Native, non-Hispanic/Latino; 10 Asian, non-Hispanic/Latino; 2 Hispanic/Latino; 1 Native Hawaiian or other Pacific Islander, non-Hispanic/Latino; 2 Two or more races, non-Hispanic/Latino), 1 international. Average age 39. 34 applicants, 82% accepted, 23 enrolled. In 2015, 14 master's awarded. *Degree requirements:* For master's, thesis or alternative, practicum. *Entrance requirements:* For master's, GRE General Test, 3 letters of reference, essay, resume, two official transcripts from every institution attended. *Application deadline:* For fall admission, 4/1 for domestic and international students; for spring admission, 9/1 for domestic and international students; for summer admission, 2/1 for domestic and international students. Applications are processed on a rolling basis. Application fee: $60. Electronic applications accepted. *Expenses:* $1,415 per semester hour; $112 fee per course. *Financial support:* In 2015–16, 71 students received support. Teaching assistantships and scholarships/grants available. Financial award application deadline: 2/15; financial award applicants required to submit FAFSA. *Faculty research:* Geriatrics, cancer survivorship, health literacy, endothelial cells, clinical simulation outcomes. *Unit head:* Dr. Kathy Baker, Director, Division of Nursing Graduate Studies and Scholarship, 817-257-6726, Fax: 817-257-8383, E-mail: kathy.baker@tcu.edu. *Application contact:* Mary Jane Allred, Administrative Program Specialist, 817-257-6726, Fax: 817-257-8383, E-mail: m.allred@tcu.edu.
Website: http://www.nursing.tcu.edu/graduate.asp

Texas Tech University Health Sciences Center, School of Nursing, Lubbock, TX 79430. Offers acute care nurse practitioner (MSN, Certificate); administration (MSN); advanced practice (DNP); education (MSN); executive leadership (DNP); family nurse practitioner (MSN, Certificate); geriatric nurse practitioner (MSN, Certificate); pediatric nurse practitioner (MSN, Certificate). *Accreditation:* AACN. *Program availability:* Part-time, online learning. *Degree requirements:* For master's, thesis optional. *Entrance requirements:* For master's, minimum GPA of 3.0, 3 letters of reference, BSN, RN license; for Certificate, minimum GPA of 3.0, 3 letters of reference, RN license. Additional exam requirements/recommendations for international students: Required—TOEFL (minimum score 550 paper-based). *Faculty research:* Diabetes/obesity, nurse competency, disease management, intervention and measurements, health disparities.

Texas Woman's University, Graduate School, College of Nursing, Denton, TX 76204-5498. Offers acute care nurse practitioner (MS); adult health clinical nurse specialist (MS); adult health nurse practitioner (MS); child health clinical nurse specialist (MS); clinical nurse leader (MS); family nurse practitioner (MS); health systems management (MS); nursing education (MS); nursing practice (DNP); nursing science (PhD); pediatric nurse practitioner (MS); women's health clinical nurse specialist (MS); women's health nurse practitioner (MS). *Accreditation:* AACN. *Program availability:* Part-time, online learning. *Faculty:* 55 full-time (51 women), 42 part-time/adjunct (35 women). *Students:* 39 full-time (37 women), 958 part-time (888 women); includes 566 minority (226 Black or African American, non-Hispanic/Latino; 8 American Indian or Alaska Native, non-Hispanic/Latino; 221 Asian, non-Hispanic/Latino; 88 Hispanic/Latino; 3 Native Hawaiian or other Pacific Islander, non-Hispanic/Latino; 20 Two or more races, non-Hispanic/Latino), 37 international. Average age 36. 430 applicants, 65% accepted, 193 enrolled. In 2015, 248 master's, 10 doctorates awarded. *Degree requirements:* For master's, comprehensive exam, thesis or alternative; for doctorate, comprehensive exam, thesis/dissertation. *Entrance requirements:* For master's, GRE or MAT, minimum GPA of 3.0 on last 60 hours in undergraduate nursing degree and overall, RN license, BS in nursing, basic statistics course; for doctorate, GRE (preferred minimum score 153 [500 old version] Verbal, 144 [500 old version] Quantitative, 4 Analytical), MS in nursing, minimum preferred GPA of 3.5, RN license, statistics, 2 letters of reference, curriculum vitae, graduate nursing-theory course, graduate research course, statement of professional goals and research interests. Additional exam requirements/recommendations for international students: Required—TOEFL (minimum score 550 paper-based; 79 iBT). *Application deadline:* For fall admission, 5/1 priority date for domestic students, 3/1 for international students; for spring admission, 9/15 priority date for domestic students, 7/1 for international students. Applications are processed on a rolling basis. Application fee: $50 ($75 for international students). Electronic applications accepted. *Expenses:* Tuition, state resident: full-time $4380; part-time $243 per credit hour. Tuition, nonresident: full-time $11,400; part-time $633 per credit hour. *International tuition:* $11,465 full-time. *Required fees:* $1778; $99 per credit hour. $283 per semester. One-time fee: $50. Tuition and fees vary according to course load and program. *Financial support:* In 2015–16, 149 students received support, including 10 research assistantships (averaging $5,600 per year), 1 teaching assistantship (averaging $5,600 per year); career-related internships or fieldwork, Federal Work-Study, institutionally sponsored loans, scholarships/grants, traineeships, health care benefits, and unspecified assistantships also available. Support available to part-time students. Financial award application deadline: 3/1; financial award applicants required to submit FAFSA. *Faculty research:* Screening, prevention, and treatment for intimate partner violence; needs of adolescents during childbirth intervention; a network analysis decision tool for nurse managers (social network analysis); support for adolescents with implantable cardioverter defibrillators; informatics: nurse staffing, safety, quality, and financial data as they relate to patient care outcomes; prevention and treatment of obesity; improving infant outcomes related to premature birth. *Total annual research expenditures:* $1.7 million. *Unit head:* Dr. Anita G. Hufft, Dean, 940-898-2401, Fax: 940-898-2437, E-mail: nursing@twu.edu. *Application contact:* Dr. Samuel Wheeler, Assistant Director of Admissions, 940-898-3188, Fax: 940-898-3081, E-mail: wheelersr@twu.edu.
Website: http://www.twu.edu/nursing/

Thomas Edison State University, W. Cary Edwards School of Nursing, Program in Nurse Educator, Trenton, NJ 08608-1176. Offers Post-Master's Certificate. *Accreditation:* AACN. *Program availability:* Part-time, online learning. *Degree requirements:* For Post-Master's Certificate, nursing education seminar and online practicum. *Entrance requirements:* For degree, master's degree in nursing, RN. Additional exam requirements/recommendations for international students: Required—TOEFL (minimum score 550 paper-based; 79 iBT). Electronic applications accepted.

Towson University, Program in Nursing, Towson, MD 21252-0001. Offers nursing (MS); nursing education (Postbaccalaureate Certificate). *Accreditation:* AACN. *Program availability:* Part-time. *Students:* 12 full-time (10 women), 45 part-time (43 women); includes 19 minority (15 Black or African American, non-Hispanic/Latino; 2 Asian, non-Hispanic/Latino; 1 Hispanic/Latino; 1 Two or more races, non-Hispanic/Latino), 3 international. *Degree requirements:* For master's, thesis optional. *Entrance requirements:* For master's, minimum GPA of 3.0, copy of current nursing license, bachelor's degree in nursing, current resume or curriculum vitae, completion of an elementary statistics and/or nursing research course, completion of an approved physical assessment course; for Postbaccalaureate Certificate, minimum GPA of 3.0, copy of current nursing license, current resume or curriculum vitae, bachelor's degree, completion of an elementary statistics and/or nursing research course, completion of an approved physical assessment course, personal statement. *Application deadline:* Applications are processed on a rolling basis. Application fee: $45. Electronic applications accepted. *Expenses:* Tuition, state resident: full-time $7440; part-time $372 per unit. Tuition, nonresident: full-time $15,400; part-time $770 per unit. *Required fees:* $2360; $118 per year. $354 per term. *Financial support:* Application deadline: 4/1. *Unit*

head: Dr. Nikki Austin, Graduate Program Director, 410-704-4389, E-mail: nursinggradprogram@towson.edu. *Application contact:* Alicia Arkell-Kleis, University Admissions, 410-704-2113, Fax: 410-704-3030, E-mail: grads@towson.edu.
Website: http://grad.towson.edu/program/master/nurs-ms/

Union University, School of Nursing, Jackson, TN 38305-3697. Offers executive leadership (DNP); nurse anesthesia (DNP); nurse practitioner (DNP); nursing education (MSN, PMC). *Accreditation:* AACN; AANA/CANAEP. *Degree requirements:* For master's, thesis or alternative. *Entrance requirements:* For master's, GRE, 3 letters of reference, bachelor's degree in nursing, minimum GPA of 3.0. Additional exam requirements/recommendations for international students: Required—TOEFL (minimum score 560 paper-based). Electronic applications accepted. *Faculty research:* Children's health, occupational rehabilitation, informatics, health promotion.

The University of Alabama in Huntsville, School of Graduate Studies, College of Nursing, Huntsville, AL 35899. Offers family nurse practitioner (Certificate); nursing (MSN, DNP), including adult-gerontology acute care nurse practitioner (MSN), adult-gerontology clinical nurse specialist (MSN), family nurse practitioner (MSN), leadership in health care systems (MSN); nursing education (Certificate). DNP offered jointly with The University of Alabama at Birmingham. *Accreditation:* AACN. *Program availability:* Part-time, evening/weekend, online learning. *Degree requirements:* For master's, comprehensive exam, thesis or alternative, oral and written exams. *Entrance requirements:* For master's, MAT or GRE, Alabama RN license, BSN, minimum GPA of 3.0; for doctorate, master's degree in nursing in an advanced practice area; for Certificate, MAT or GRE, minimum GPA of 3.0. Additional exam requirements/recommendations for international students: Required—TOEFL (minimum score 500 paper-based; 80 iBT), IELTS (minimum score 6.5). *Application deadline:* For fall admission, 7/15 for domestic students, 4/1 for international students; for spring admission, 11/30 for domestic students, 9/1 for international students. Applications are processed on a rolling basis. Application fee: $50. Electronic applications accepted. *Expenses: Tuition, area resident:* Full-time $9548; part-time $547 per credit hour. Tuition, state resident: full-time $9548; part-time $547 per credit hour. Tuition, nonresident: full-time $21,402; part-time $1224 per credit hour. *International tuition:* $21,402 full-time. *Financial support:* Teaching assistantships with full tuition reimbursements, career-related internships or fieldwork, Federal Work-Study, institutionally sponsored loans, scholarships/grants, traineeships, health care benefits, and unspecified assistantships available. Support available to part-time students. Financial award application deadline: 4/1; financial award applicants required to submit FAFSA. *Faculty research:* Health care informatics, chronic illness management, maternal and child health, genetics/genomics, technology and health care. *Unit head:* Dr. Marsha Adams, Dean, 256-824-6345, Fax: 256-824-6026, E-mail: marsha.adams@uah.edu. *Application contact:* Charles Davis, Director of Graduate Admission and Advisement, 256-824-6669, Fax: 256-824-6026, E-mail: charles.davis@uah.edu.
Website: http://www.uah.edu/nursing

University of Central Arkansas, Graduate School, College of Health and Behavioral Sciences, Department of Nursing, Conway, AR 72035-0001. Offers adult nurse practitioner (PMC); clinical nurse leader (PMC); clinical nurse specialist (MSN); family nurse practitioner (PMC); nurse educator (PMC); nurse practitioner (MSN). *Accreditation:* AACN. *Program availability:* Part-time, evening/weekend, online learning. *Degree requirements:* For master's, comprehensive exam, thesis optional, clinicals. *Entrance requirements:* For master's, GRE General Test, minimum GPA of 2.7. Additional exam requirements/recommendations for international students: Required—TOEFL (minimum score 550 paper-based; 80 iBT). Electronic applications accepted. *Expenses:* Contact institution.

University of Detroit Mercy, College of Health Professions, Detroit, MI 48221. Offers clinical nurse leader (MSN); family nurse practitioner (MSN); health services administration (MHSA); health systems management (MSN); nurse anesthesia (MS); nursing (DNP); nursing education (MSN, Certificate); nursing leadership and financial management (Certificate); outcomes performance management (Certificate); physician assistant (MS). *Entrance requirements:* For master's, GRE General Test, minimum GPA of 3.0. Application fee: $30 ($50 for international students). *Expenses: Tuition, area resident:* Full-time $26,802; part-time $1489 per credit. Tuition and fees vary according to course load and program. *Financial support:* Institutionally sponsored loans and tuition waivers (partial) available. Support available to part-time students. Financial award applicants required to submit FAFSA. *Faculty research:* Research design, respiratory physiology, AIDS prevention, adolescent health, community, low income health education. *Unit head:* Dr. Christine M. Pacini, RN, Dean, 313-993-6055, Fax: 313-993-6175.
Website: http://healthprofessions.udmercy.edu/

University of Hartford, College of Education, Nursing, and Health Professions, Program in Nursing, West Hartford, CT 06117-1599. Offers community/public health nursing (MSN); nursing education (MSN); nursing management (MSN). *Accreditation:* AACN. *Program availability:* Part-time, evening/weekend. *Degree requirements:* For master's, research project. *Entrance requirements:* For master's, BSN, Connecticut RN license. Additional exam requirements/recommendations for international students: Required—TOEFL (minimum score 550 paper-based). Electronic applications accepted. *Expenses:* Contact institution. *Faculty research:* Child development, women in doctoral study, applying feminist theory in teaching methods, near death experience, grandmothers as primary care providers.

University of Houston, School of Nursing, Houston, TX 77204. Offers family nurse practitioner (MSN); nursing administration (MSN); nursing education (MSN). *Accreditation:* AACN. *Entrance requirements:* For master's, GRE or MAT, minimum GPA of 3.0 in last 60 hours of academic course work, valid Texas RN licensure, 2 letters of recommendation. Electronic applications accepted.

University of Indianapolis, Graduate Programs, School of Nursing, Indianapolis, IN 46227-3697. Offers advanced practice nursing (DNP); family nurse practitioner (MSN); gerontological nurse practitioner (MSN); neonatal nurse practitioner (MSN); nurse-midwifery (MSN); nursing (MSN); nursing and health systems leadership (MSN); nursing education (MSN); women's health nurse practitioner (MSN); MBA/MSN. *Accreditation:* AACN; ACNM. *Entrance requirements:* For master's, minimum GPA of 3.0, interview, letters of recommendation, resume, IN nursing license, 1 year of professional practice; for doctorate, graduate of NLNAC- or CCNE-accredited nursing program; MSN or MA with nursing major and minimum cumulative GPA of 3.25; unencumbered RN license with eligibility for licensure in Indiana; completion of graduate-level statistics course within last 5 years with minimum grade of B; resume; essay; official transcripts from all academic institutions. Additional exam requirements/recommendations for international students: Required—TOEFL (minimum score 550 paper-based). Electronic applications accepted.

University of Louisville, Graduate School, School of Nursing, Louisville, KY 40202. Offers adult gerontology nurse practitioner (MSN, DNP); education and administration (MSN); family nurse practitioner (MSN, DNP); neonatal nurse practitioner (MSN, DNP); nursing research (PhD); psychiatric/mental health nurse practitioner (MSN, DNP); women's health nurse practitioner (MSN). *Accreditation:* AACN. *Program availability:* Part-time. *Faculty:* 53 full-time (48 women), 27 part-time/adjunct (23 women). *Students:*

Nursing Education

110 full-time (99 women), 33 part-time (29 women); includes 17 minority (11 Black or African American, non-Hispanic/Latino; 1 Asian, non-Hispanic/Latino; 2 Hispanic/Latino; 3 Two or more races, non-Hispanic/Latino), 5 international. Average age 34. 62 applicants, 68% accepted, 40 enrolled. In 2015, 41 master's awarded. *Degree requirements:* For doctorate, comprehensive exam (for some programs), thesis/dissertation (for some programs). *Entrance requirements:* For master's, bachelor's degree in nursing, minimum GPA of 3.0, RN license; for doctorate, GRE General Test (for PhD), 3 letters of professional reference. Additional exam requirements/recommendations for international students: Required—TOEFL (minimum score 560 paper-based; 79 iBT). *Application deadline:* For fall admission, 3/1 priority date for domestic students, 3/1 for international students. Applications are processed on a rolling basis. Application fee: $60. Electronic applications accepted. *Expenses:* Tuition, state resident: full-time $11,664; part-time $649 per credit hour. Tuition, nonresident: full-time $24,274; part-time $1350 per credit hour. *Required fees:* $196. Tuition and fees vary according to program and reciprocity agreements. *Financial support:* In 2015–16, 722,568 students received support, including 10 research assistantships with full tuition reimbursements available (averaging $20,000 per year), 2 teaching assistantships with full tuition reimbursements available (averaging $15,000 per year); fellowships with full tuition reimbursements available, scholarships/grants, and unspecified assistantships also available. Financial award application deadline: 2/15; financial award applicants required to submit FAFSA. *Faculty research:* Children and adolescents with chronic illnesses, women's mental health and parenting, asthma and environmental health, type 2 diabetes self-management in adults, health disparities and community engagement. *Total annual research expenditures:* $722,568. *Unit head:* Dr. Marcia J. Hern, Dean, 502-852-8300, Fax: 502-852-8783, E-mail: m.hern@louisville.edu. *Application contact:* Trish Hart, Assistant Dean for Student Affairs, 502-852-5825, Fax: 502-852-8783, E-mail: trish.hart@louisville.edu.
Website: http://www.louisville.edu/nursing/

University of Maine, Graduate School, College of Natural Sciences, Forestry, and Agriculture, School of Nursing, Orono, ME 04469. Offers individualized (MS); nursing education (CGS); rural health family nurse practitioner (MS, CAS). *Accreditation:* AACN. *Faculty:* 6 full-time (all women), 3 part-time/adjunct (1 woman). *Students:* 12 full-time (10 women), 3 part-time (all women); includes 2 minority (1 American Indian or Alaska Native, non-Hispanic/Latino; 1 Hispanic/Latino). Average age 41. 7 applicants, 43% accepted, 2 enrolled. In 2015, 7 master's, 1 other advanced degree awarded. *Entrance requirements:* For master's, GRE General Test; for other advanced degree, master's degree. Additional exam requirements/recommendations for international students: Required—TOEFL. *Application deadline:* For fall admission, 2/1 for domestic students. Applications are processed on a rolling basis. Application fee: $65. Electronic applications accepted. *Financial support:* In 2015–16, 1 student received support. Career-related internships or fieldwork, Federal Work-Study, institutionally sponsored loans, tuition waivers (full and partial), and unspecified assistantships available. Support available to part-time students. Financial award application deadline: 3/1. *Faculty research:* Work experiences of chief nursing officers, fatigue related to radiation therapy in oncology patients, patients' perceptions of nurses' caring behaviors, health disparities of rural Maine older women. *Unit head:* Dr. Nancy Fishwick, Director, 207-581-2505, Fax: 207-581-2585. *Application contact:* Scott G. Delcourt, Assistant Vice President for Graduate Studies and Senior Associate Dean, 207-581-3291, Fax: 207-581-3232, E-mail: graduate@maine.edu.
Website: http://umaine.edu/nursing/

University of Mary, School of Health Sciences, Division of Nursing, Bismarck, ND 58504-9652. Offers family nurse practitioner (DNP); nurse administrator (MSN); nursing educator (MSN); MSN/MBA. *Accreditation:* AACN. *Program availability:* Part-time, evening/weekend, online learning. *Degree requirements:* For master's, comprehensive exam (for some programs), thesis (for some programs), internship (family nurse practitioner), teaching practice. *Entrance requirements:* For master's, minimum GPA of 2.75 in nursing, interview, letters of recommendation, criminal background check, immunizations, statement of professional goals. Additional exam requirements/recommendations for international students: Required—TOEFL (minimum score 500 paper-based; 71 iBT). *Application deadline:* Applications are processed on a rolling basis. Application fee: $40. Electronic applications accepted. *Financial support:* Fellowships with partial tuition reimbursements and teaching assistantships with partial tuition reimbursements available. Financial award application deadline: 8/1; financial award applicants required to submit FAFSA. *Faculty research:* Gerontology issues, rural nursing, health policy, primary care, women's health.

University of Mary Hardin-Baylor, Graduate Studies in Education, Belton, TX 76513. Offers curriculum and instruction (M Ed); educational administration (M Ed, Ed D), including higher education (Ed D), leadership in nursing education (Ed D), P-12 (Ed D). *Program availability:* Part-time, evening/weekend. *Faculty:* 15 full-time (11 women), 4 part-time/adjunct (2 women). *Students:* 48 full-time (36 women), 69 part-time (52 women); includes 44 minority (19 Black or African American, non-Hispanic/Latino; 1 American Indian or Alaska Native, non-Hispanic/Latino; 1 Asian, non-Hispanic/Latino; 22 Hispanic/Latino; 1 Two or more races, non-Hispanic/Latino), 4 international. Average age 39. 21 applicants, 81% accepted, 13 enrolled. In 2015, 31 master's, 18 doctorates awarded. *Degree requirements:* For master's, comprehensive exam; for doctorate, thesis/dissertation. *Entrance requirements:* For master's, minimum GPA of 3.0, interview; for doctorate, minimum GPA of 3.5, interview, essay, resume, employment verification, employer letter of support, 3 letters of recommendation. Additional exam requirements/recommendations for international students: Required—TOEFL (minimum score 100 iBT), IELTS (minimum score 7). *Application deadline:* For fall admission, 6/1 for domestic students, 3/30 priority date for international students; for spring admission, 11/1 for domestic students, 9/30 priority date for international students. Applications are processed on a rolling basis. Application fee: $35 ($135 for international students). Electronic applications accepted. *Expenses: Tuition, area resident:* Part-time $815 per credit hour. Tuition and fees vary according to course load and degree level. *Financial support:* Federal Work-Study and scholarships for some active duty military personnel available. Support available to part-time students. Financial award application deadline: 6/1; financial award applicants required to submit FAFSA. *Unit head:* Dr. Marlene Zipperlen, Dean, College of Education/Director, Doctor of Education Program, 254-295-4572, Fax: 254-295-4480, E-mail: mzipperlen@umhb.edu. *Application contact:* Melissa Williams, Director, Graduate Student Services and Engagement, 254-295-4020, Fax: 254-295-5038, E-mail: mwilliams@umhb.edu.
Website: http://graduate.umhb.edu/education/

University of Mary Hardin-Baylor, Graduate Studies in Nursing, Belton, TX 76513. Offers clinical nurse leader (MSN); family nurse practitioner (MSN, Post-Master's Certificate); nurse educator (Post-Master's Certificate); nursing education (MSN). *Accreditation:* AACN. *Program availability:* Part-time, evening/weekend. *Faculty:* 6 full-time (all women), 3 part-time/adjunct (2 women). *Students:* 54 full-time (47 women), 2 part-time (1 woman); includes 14 minority (10 Black or African American, non-Hispanic/Latino; 3 Hispanic/Latino; 1 Two or more races, non-Hispanic/Latino), 1 international. Average age 32. 46 applicants, 70% accepted, 26 enrolled. In 2015, 47 master's awarded. *Degree requirements:* For master's, practicum. *Entrance requirements:* For master's, full-time RN for 1 year, BSN, minimum GPA of 3.0 in last 60 hours of undergraduate program, two letters of recommendation. Additional exam requirements/

recommendations for international students: Required—TOEFL (minimum score 100 iBT), IELTS (minimum score 7). *Application deadline:* For fall admission, 4/15 for domestic students, 4/30 priority date for international students; for spring admission, 11/1 for domestic students, 9/30 priority date for international students. Applications are processed on a rolling basis. Application fee: $35 ($135 for international students). Electronic applications accepted. *Expenses: Tuition, area resident:* Part-time $815 per credit hour. Tuition and fees vary according to course load and degree level. *Financial support:* Applicants required to submit FAFSA. *Unit head:* Dr. Carrie Johnson, Associate Professor/Director, Master of Science in Nursing Programs, 254-295-4178, E-mail: cjohnson@umhb.edu. *Application contact:* Melissa Williams, Director, Graduate Student Services and Engagement, 254-295-4020, Fax: 254-295-5038, E-mail: mwilliams@umhb.edu.
Website: http://graduate.umhb.edu/nursing/

University of Maryland, Baltimore, Graduate School, School of Nursing, Master's Program in Nursing, Baltimore, MD 21201. Offers community health nursing (MS); gerontological nursing (MS); maternal-child nursing (MS); medical-surgical nursing (MS); nurse-midwifery education (MS); nursing administration (MS); nursing education (MS); nursing health policy (MS); primary care nursing (MS); psychiatric nursing (MS); MS/MBA. MS/MBA offered jointly with University of Baltimore. *Accreditation:* AACN; AANA/CANAEP. *Program availability:* Part-time. *Degree requirements:* For master's, comprehensive exam (for some programs), thesis or alternative. *Entrance requirements:* For master's, minimum GPA of 2.75, course work in statistics, BS in nursing. Additional exam requirements/recommendations for international students: Required—TOEFL (minimum score 550 paper-based; 80 iBT); Recommended—IELTS (minimum score 7). Electronic applications accepted. Tuition and fees vary according to program.

University of Massachusetts Medical School, Graduate School of Nursing, Worcester, MA 01655-0115. Offers adult gerontological acute care nurse practitioner (DNP, Post Master's Certificate); adult gerontological primary care nurse practitioner (DNP, Post Master's Certificate); family nursing practitioner (DNP); nurse administrator (DNP); nurse educator (MS, Post Master's Certificate); nursing (PhD); nursing practitioner (DNP); population health (MS). *Accreditation:* AACN. *Faculty:* 18 full-time (15 women), 28 part-time/adjunct (22 women). *Students:* 143 full-time (119 women), 27 part-time (25 women); includes 28 minority (15 Black or African American, non-Hispanic/Latino; 10 Asian, non-Hispanic/Latino; 3 Hispanic/Latino), 1 international. Average age 34. 129 applicants, 68% accepted, 56 enrolled. In 2015, 43 master's, 10 doctorates, 2 other advanced degrees awarded. *Degree requirements:* For doctorate, thesis/dissertation (for some programs), comprehensive exam (for PhD); capstone project and manuscript (for DNP). *Entrance requirements:* For master's, GRE General Test, bachelor's degree in nursing, course work in statistics, unrestricted Massachusetts license as registered nurse; for doctorate, GRE General Test, bachelor's or master's degree; for Post Master's Certificate, GRE General Test, MS in nursing. Additional exam requirements/recommendations for international students: Required—TOEFL. *Application deadline:* For fall admission, 12/1 priority date for domestic students. Applications are processed on a rolling basis. Application fee: $60. Electronic applications accepted. *Expenses:* $10,994 resident per year; $18,210 non-resident per year. *Financial support:* In 2015–16, 31 students received support. Institutionally sponsored loans, scholarships/grants, traineeships, and tuition waivers (partial) available. Support available to part-time students. Financial award application deadline: 5/16; financial award applicants required to submit FAFSA. *Faculty research:* Health literacy, social justice, HIV prevention, cancer-related decision making, nursing education. *Total annual research expenditures:* $650,993. *Unit head:* Joan Vitello-Cicciu, Dean, 508-856-5081, Fax: 508-856-6552, E-mail: joan.vitello@umassmed.edu. *Application contact:* Diane Brescia, Admissions Coordinator, 508-856-3488, Fax: 508-856-5851, E-mail: diane.brescia@umassmed.edu.
Website: http://www.umassmed.edu/gsn/

University of Memphis, Loewenberg College of Nursing, Memphis, TN 38152. Offers executive leadership (MSN); family nurse practitioner (MSN); nursing (Graduate Certificate); nursing administration (MSN); nursing education (MSN). *Accreditation:* AACN. *Program availability:* Part-time, evening/weekend, online learning. *Faculty:* 12 full-time (all women), 3 part-time/adjunct (2 women). *Students:* 34 full-time (32 women), 220 part-time (196 women); includes 91 minority (80 Black or African American, non-Hispanic/Latino; 8 Asian, non-Hispanic/Latino; 1 Hispanic/Latino; 2 Two or more races, non-Hispanic/Latino). Average age 36. 165 applicants, 48% accepted, 27 enrolled. In 2015, 73 master's, 3 other advanced degrees awarded. *Degree requirements:* For master's, comprehensive exam, thesis optional, scholarly project; completion of clinical practicum hours. *Entrance requirements:* For master's, NCLEX Exam, interview. Additional exam requirements/recommendations for international students: Required—TOEFL (minimum score 550 paper-based; 79 iBT). *Application deadline:* For fall admission, 2/15 for domestic and international students; for spring admission, 10/1 for domestic and international students. Application fee: $35 ($60 for international students). *Financial support:* In 2015–16, 147 students received support. Federal Work-Study and scholarships/grants available. Financial award application deadline: 2/15; financial award applicants required to submit FAFSA. *Faculty research:* Technology in nursing, nurse retention, cultural competence, health policy, health access. *Total annual research expenditures:* $560,619. *Unit head:* Dr. Robert Koch, Associate Dean, 901-678-3908, Fax: 901-678-4907, E-mail: rakoch@memphis.edu. *Application contact:* Dr. Karen Weddle-West, Information Contact, 901-678-2531, Fax: 901-678-5023, E-mail: gradsch@memphis.edu.
Website: http://www.memphis.edu/nursing

University of Missouri–Kansas City, School of Nursing and Health Studies, Kansas City, MO 64108. Offers adult clinical nurse specialist (MSN), including adult nurse practitioner, women's health nurse practitioner (MSN, DNP); adult clinical nursing practice (DNP), including adult gerontology nurse practitioner, women's health nurse practitioner (MSN, DNP); clinical nursing practice (DNP), including family nurse practitioner; family nurse practitioner (MSN); neonatal nurse practitioner (MSN); nurse educator (MSN); nurse executive (MSN); nursing (PhD); nursing practice (DNP); pediatric clinical nursing practice (DNP), including pediatric nurse practitioner; pediatric nurse practitioner (MSN). *Accreditation:* AACN. *Program availability:* Part-time, online learning. *Faculty:* 44 full-time (40 women), 47 part-time/adjunct (45 women). *Students:* 62 full-time (43 women), 259 part-time (239 women); includes 61 minority (28 Black or African American, non-Hispanic/Latino; 3 American Indian or Alaska Native, non-Hispanic/Latino; 16 Asian, non-Hispanic/Latino; 10 Hispanic/Latino; 4 Two or more races, non-Hispanic/Latino). Average age 35. 102 applicants, 35% accepted, 36 enrolled. In 2015, 118 master's, 23 doctorates awarded. *Degree requirements:* For master's, thesis or alternative. *Entrance requirements:* For master's, minimum undergraduate GPA of 3.2; for doctorate, GRE, 3 letters of reference. Additional exam requirements/recommendations for international students: Required—TOEFL (minimum score 550 paper-based; 80 iBT). *Application deadline:* For fall admission, 2/1 priority date for domestic and international students; for spring admission, 9/1 priority date for domestic and international students. Application fee: $45 ($50 for international students). *Financial support:* In 2015–16, 2 teaching assistantships with partial tuition reimbursements (averaging $6,650 per year) were awarded; fellowships, research assistantships, career-related internships or fieldwork, Federal Work-Study, institutionally sponsored loans, and tuition waivers (full and partial) also available.

Support available to part-time students. Financial award application deadline: 3/1; financial award applicants required to submit FAFSA. *Faculty research:* Geriatrics/ gerontology, children's pain, neonatology, Alzheimer's care, cancer caregivers. *Unit head:* Dr. Ann Cary, Dean, 816-235-1723, Fax: 816-235-1701, E-mail: caryah@ umkc.edu. *Application contact:* Judy Jellison, Coordinator for Admissions and Recruitment, 816-235-1740, Fax: 816-235-1701, E-mail: jellisonj@umkc.edu.
Website: http://nursing.umkc.edu/

University of Missouri–St. Louis, College of Nursing, St. Louis, MO 63121-4400. Offers adult/geriatric nurse practitioner (Post Master's Certificate); family nurse practitioner (Post Master's Certificate); nurse educator (MSN); nurse practitioner (MSN); nursing (DNP, PhD); pediatric nurse practitioner (Post Master's Certificate); psychiatric-mental health nurse practitioner (Post Master's Certificate); women's health nurse practitioner (Post Master's Certificate). *Accreditation:* AACN. *Program availability:* Part-time. *Faculty:* 21 full-time (19 women), 6 part-time/adjunct (5 women). *Students:* 18 full-time (17 women), 227 part-time (215 women); includes 34 minority (22 Black or African American, non-Hispanic/Latino; 8 Asian, non-Hispanic/Latino; 3 Hispanic/Latino; 1 Two or more races, non-Hispanic/Latino), 1 international. Average age 35. 152 applicants, 69% accepted, 83 enrolled. *Degree requirements:* For doctorate, comprehensive exam, thesis/dissertation; for Post Master's Certificate, thesis. *Entrance requirements:* For master's, 2 recommendation letters; minimum GPA of 3.0; BSN; nursing licensure; statement of purpose; course in differential/inferential statistics; for doctorate, GRE, 2 letters of recommendation, MSN, minimum GPA of 3.2, course in differential/inferential statistics; for Post Master's Certificate, 2 recommendation letters; MSN; advanced practice certificate; minimum GPA of 3.0; essay. Additional exam requirements/ recommendations for international students: Recommended—TOEFL (minimum score 550 paper-based; 79 iBT), IELTS (minimum score 6.5). *Application deadline:* For fall admission, 2/15 for domestic and international students. Application fee: $50 ($40 for international students). Electronic applications accepted. *Financial support:* Research assistantships with tuition reimbursements available. Financial award application deadline: 4/1; financial award applicants required to submit FAFSA. *Faculty research:* Health promotion and restoration, family disruption, violence, abuse, battered women, health survey methods. *Unit head:* Dr. Roberta Lavin, Director, 314-516-6066. *Application contact:* 314-516-5458, Fax: 314-516-6996, E-mail: gradadm@umsl.edu.
Website: http://www.umsl.edu/divisions/nursing/

University of New Brunswick Fredericton, School of Graduate Studies, Faculty of Nursing, Fredericton, NB E3B 5A3, Canada. Offers nurse educator (MN); nurse practitioner (MN); nursing (MN). *Program availability:* Part-time, online learning. *Faculty:* 19 full-time (18 women). *Students:* 14 full-time (13 women), 30 part-time (29 women). In 2015, 18 master's awarded. *Degree requirements:* For master's, comprehensive exam (for some programs), thesis (for some programs). *Entrance requirements:* For master's, undergraduate coursework in statistics and nursing research, minimum GPA of 3.3, registration as a nurse (or eligibility) in New Brunswick. Additional exam requirements/ recommendations for international students: Required—TOEFL (minimum score 600 paper-based). *Application deadline:* For winter admission, 1/2 priority date for domestic students. Application fee: $50 Canadian dollars. Electronic applications accepted. *Financial support:* In 2015–16, 7 fellowships, 2 research assistantships were awarded. *Faculty research:* Intimate partner violence; abuse; healthy child development, chronic illness and addiction; rural populations' access to health care and primary healthcare; teaching and learning in the classroom, clinical lab, and by distance; Aboriginal nursing; workplace bullying; eating disorders; women's health; lesbian health; nurse managed primary care clinics; HIV/AIDS; returning to work after depression; adolescent mental health; cancer survivorship. *Unit head:* Kathy Wilson, Assistant Dean of Graduate and Advanced RN Studies, 506-458-7640, Fax: 506-447-3057, E-mail: kewilson@unb.ca. *Application contact:* Francis Perry, Graduate Secretary, 506-451-6844, Fax: 506-447-3057, E-mail: fperry@unb.ca.
Website: http://www.unb.ca/fredericton/nursing/graduate/

The University of North Carolina at Chapel Hill, School of Nursing, Chapel Hill, NC 27599-7460. Offers advanced practice registered nurse (DNP); health care systems (DNP); nursing (MSN, PhD, PMC), including administration (MSN), adult gerontology primary care nurse practitioner (MSN), clinical nurse leader (MSN), education (MSN), informatics (MSN, PMC), nursing leadership (PMC), outcomes management (MSN), primary care family nurse practitioner (MSN), primary care pediatric nurse practitioner (MSN), psychiatric/mental health nurse practitioner (MSN, PMC). *Accreditation:* AACN; ACEN (one or more programs are accredited). *Program availability:* Part-time. *Faculty:* 86 full-time (78 women), 44 part-time/adjunct (40 women). *Students:* 208 full-time (186 women), 128 part-time (116 women); includes 109 minority (49 Black or African American, non-Hispanic/Latino; 4 American Indian or Alaska Native, non-Hispanic/ Latino; 32 Asian, non-Hispanic/Latino; 7 Hispanic/Latino; 17 Two or more races, non-Hispanic/Latino), 17 international. Average age 33. 624 applicants, 25% accepted, 150 enrolled. In 2015, 91 master's, 14 doctorates awarded. *Degree requirements:* For master's, comprehensive exam, thesis; for doctorate, thesis/dissertation, 3 exams; for PMC, thesis. *Entrance requirements:* Additional exam requirements/recommendations for international students: Required—TOEFL (minimum score 575 paper-based; 89 iBT), IELTS (minimum score 8). *Application deadline:* For fall admission, 12/15 for domestic and international students. Application fee: $85. Electronic applications accepted. *Financial support:* In 2015–16, 8 fellowships with full tuition reimbursements, 6 research assistantships with partial tuition reimbursements (averaging $8,000 per year), 10 teaching assistantships with partial tuition reimbursements (averaging $8,000 per year) were awarded; scholarships/grants, traineeships, health care benefits, and unspecified assistantships also available. Support available to part-time students. Financial award application deadline: 3/1; financial award applicants required to submit FAFSA. *Faculty research:* Preventing and managing chronic illness, reducing health disparities, Improving healthcare quality and patient outcomes, understanding biobehavioral and genetic bases of health and illness, developing innovative ways to enhance science and its clinical translation. *Unit head:* Donna S. Havens, PhD, RN, Dean/Professor, 919-966-3731, Fax: 919-966-3540, E-mail: dhavens@email.unc.edu. *Application contact:* Emily Sayed, Assistant Director, Graduate Admissions, 919-966-4260, Fax: 919-966-3540, E-mail: sayed@unc.edu.
Website: http://nursing.unc.edu

The University of North Carolina at Charlotte, College of Health and Human Services, School of Nursing, Charlotte, NC 28223-0001. Offers adult-gerontology acute care nurse practitioner (MSN, Post-Master's Certificate); advanced clinical nursing (MSN); community public health nursing (MSN); family nurse practitioner across the lifespan (MSN, Post-Master's Certificate); nurse administrator (MSN, Graduate Certificate); nurse anesthesia (MSN, Post-Master's Certificate); nurse educator (MSN, Graduate Certificate); nursing (DNP); nursing systems/population (MSN). *Accreditation:* AACN. *Program availability:* Part-time, blended/hybrid learning. *Faculty:* 26 full-time (25 women), 4 part-time/adjunct (3 women). *Students:* 109 full-time (89 women), 112 part-time (107 women); includes 46 minority (37 Black or African American, non-Hispanic/ Latino; 3 Asian, non-Hispanic/Latino; 5 Hispanic/Latino; 1 Two or more races, non-Hispanic/Latino). Average age 33. 321 applicants, 34% accepted, 84 enrolled. In 2015, 76 master's, 4 doctorates, 7 other advanced degrees awarded. Terminal master's awarded for partial completion of doctoral program. *Degree requirements:* For master's, practicum, synthesis and integration or thesis, residency, internship (varies by program);

for doctorate, thesis/dissertation or alternative, residency; for other advanced degree, practicum. *Entrance requirements:* For master's, GRE General Test, unencumbered license as Registered Nurse in North Carolina; BSN from nationally-accredited program; one year of professional nursing practice in acute/critical care; minimum overall GPA of 3.0 in the last degree and 60 hours of nursing coursework; completion of an undergraduate statistics course with minimum grade of C; statement of purpose; for doctorate, GRE or MAT, master's degree in nursing in an advanced nursing practice specialty from nationally-accredited program; minimum overall GPA of 3.5 in MSN program; current RN licensure in U.S. at time of application with eligibility for NC licensure; for other advanced degree, GRE. Additional exam requirements/ recommendations for international students: Required—TOEFL (minimum score 557 paper-based, 83 iBT) or IELTS (minimum score 6.5). *Application deadline:* For fall admission, 2/1 for domestic and international students; for spring admission, 10/1 priority date for domestic and international students; for summer admission, 4/1 priority date for domestic and international students. Applications are processed on a rolling basis. Application fee: $75. Electronic applications accepted. *Expenses:* Contact institution. *Financial support:* In 2015–16, 9 students received support, including 5 research assistantships (averaging $4,850 per year), 3 teaching assistantships (averaging $2,911 per year); career-related internships or fieldwork, institutionally sponsored loans, scholarships/grants, traineeships, unspecified assistantships, and administrative assistantships also available. Support available to part-time students. Financial award application deadline: 3/1; financial award applicants required to submit FAFSA. *Faculty research:* Improving care outcomes for the elderly; vulnerable populations; symptom management; self management/health promotion strategies of older adults; migration and maternal child health; health disparities, health literacy, and access to healthcare in Latino adults with diabetes; psychiatric nursing. *Total annual research expenditures:* $875,169. *Unit head:* Dr. Dee Baldwin, Associate Dean, 704-687-7952, Fax: 704-687-8017, E-mail: dbaldwi5@uncc.edu. *Application contact:* Kathy B. Giddings, Director of Graduate Admissions, 704-687-5503, Fax: 704-687-1668, E-mail: gradadm@uncc.edu.
Website: http://nursing.uncc.edu/

The University of North Carolina at Greensboro, Graduate School, School of Nursing, Greensboro, NC 27412-5001. Offers adult clinical nurse specialist (MSN, PMC); adult/gerontological nurse practitioner (MSN, PMC); nurse anesthesia (MSN, PMC); nursing (PhD); nursing administration (MSN); nursing education (MSN); MSN/ MBA. *Accreditation:* AACN; AANA/CANAEP; ACEN. *Degree requirements:* For master's, thesis or alternative. *Entrance requirements:* For master's, GRE General Test or MAT, BSN, clinical experience, liability insurance, RN license; for PMC, liability insurance, MSN, RN license. Additional exam requirements/recommendations for international students: Required—TOEFL. Electronic applications accepted.

The University of North Carolina at Pembroke, Graduate School, Department of Nursing, Pembroke, NC 28372-1510. Offers clinical nurse leader (MSN); nurse educator (MSN); rural case manager (MSN). *Program availability:* Part-time. Application fee: $45 ($60 for international students). *Unit head:* Dr. Jennifer W. Twaddell, Interim Chair, 910-775-4142, Fax: 910-521-6751, E-mail: jennifer.twaddell@uncp.edu. *Application contact:* Dr. Jennifer W. Twaddell, Interim Chair, 910-775-4142, Fax: 910-521-6751, E-mail: jennifer.twaddell@uncp.edu.
Website: http://www.uncp.edu/nursing/

University of North Dakota, Graduate School, College of Nursing, Department of Nursing, Grand Forks, ND 58202. Offers adult-gerontological nurse practitioner (MSN); advanced public health nurse (MSN); family nurse practitioner (MSN); nurse anesthesia (MSN); nurse educator (MSN); nursing (DNP, PhD); psychiatric and mental health nurse practitioner (MSN).

University of Northern Colorado, Graduate School, College of Natural and Health Sciences, School of Nursing, Greeley, CO 80639. Offers clinical nurse specialist in chronic illness (MS); family nurse practitioner (MS); nursing education (MS, PhD). *Accreditation:* AACN. *Program availability:* Online learning. *Degree requirements:* For master's, comprehensive exam, thesis or alternative; for doctorate, comprehensive exam, thesis/dissertation. *Entrance requirements:* For master's and doctorate, GRE General Test, minimum GPA of 3.0 in last 60 hours, BS in nursing, 2 letters of recommendation. Electronic applications accepted.

University of Phoenix–Atlanta Campus, College of Nursing, Sandy Springs, GA 30350-4147. Offers health administration (MHA); nursing (MSN); nursing/health care education (MSN); MSN/MBA; MSN/MHA. *Program availability:* Evening/weekend, online learning. *Degree requirements:* For master's, thesis (for some programs). *Entrance requirements:* For master's, minimum undergraduate GPA of 2.5, 3 years of work experience. Additional exam requirements/recommendations for international students: Required—TOEFL (minimum score 550 paper-based; 79 iBT). Electronic applications accepted.

University of Phoenix–Augusta Campus, College of Nursing, Augusta, GA 30909-4583. Offers health administration (MHA); nursing (MSN); nursing/health care education (MSN); MSN/MBA; MSN/MHA. *Program availability:* Online learning.

University of Phoenix–Bay Area Campus, College of Nursing, San Jose, CA 95134-1805. Offers education (MHA); gerontology (MHA); health administration (MHA, DHA); informatics (MHA, MSN); nursing (MSN, PhD); nursing/health care education (MSN); MSN/MBA. *Program availability:* Evening/weekend, online learning. *Degree requirements:* For master's, thesis (for some programs). *Entrance requirements:* For master's, minimum undergraduate GPA of 2.5, 3 years of work experience, RN license. Additional exam requirements/recommendations for international students: Required— TOEFL (minimum score 550 paper-based; 79 iBT). Electronic applications accepted.

University of Phoenix–Charlotte Campus, College of Nursing, Charlotte, NC 28273-3409. Offers education (MHA); gerontology (MHA); health administration (MHA); informatics (MHA, MSN); nursing (MSN); nursing/health care education (MSN). *Program availability:* Evening/weekend. *Degree requirements:* For master's, thesis (for some programs). *Entrance requirements:* For master's, minimum undergraduate GPA of 2.5, 3 years work experience. Additional exam requirements/recommendations for international students: Required—TOEFL (minimum score 550 paper-based; 79 iBT). Electronic applications accepted.

University of Phoenix–Hawaii Campus, College of Nursing, Honolulu, HI 96813-3800. Offers education (MHA); family nurse practitioner (MSN); gerontology (MHA); health administration (MHA); nursing (MSN); nursing/health care education (MSN); MSN/MBA. *Program availability:* Evening/weekend. *Degree requirements:* For master's, thesis (for some programs). *Entrance requirements:* For master's, minimum undergraduate GPA of 2.5, 3 years of work experience, RN license. Additional exam requirements/ recommendations for international students: Required—TOEFL (minimum score 550 paper-based; 79 iBT). Electronic applications accepted.

University of Phoenix–New Mexico Campus, College of Nursing, Albuquerque, NM 87113-1570. Offers health administration (MHA); health care education (MSN); nursing (MSN); MSN/MBA. *Program availability:* Evening/weekend. *Degree requirements:* For master's, thesis (for some programs). *Entrance requirements:* For master's, minimum undergraduate GPA of 2.5, 3 years of work experience, RN license. Additional exam

Nursing Education

requirements/recommendations for international students: Required—TOEFL (minimum score 550 paper-based; 79 iBT). Electronic applications accepted.

University of Phoenix–North Florida Campus, College of Nursing, Jacksonville, FL 32216-0959. Offers health administration (MHA); health care education (MSN); nursing (MSN); MSN/MBA; MSN/MHA. *Program availability:* Evening/weekend. *Degree requirements:* For master's, thesis (for some programs). *Entrance requirements:* For master's, minimum undergraduate GPA of 2.5, 3 years work experience, RN license. Additional exam requirements/recommendations for international students: Required—TOEFL (minimum score 550 paper-based; 79 iBT). Electronic applications accepted.

University of Phoenix–Online Campus, College of Health Sciences and Nursing, Phoenix, AZ 85034-7209. Offers family nurse practitioner (Certificate); health care (Certificate); health care education (Certificate); health care informatics (Certificate); informatics (MSN); nursing (MSN); nursing and health care education (MSN); MSN/MBA; MSN/MHA. *Accreditation:* AACN. *Program availability:* Evening/weekend, online learning. *Entrance requirements:* Additional exam requirements/recommendations for international students: Required—TOEFL, TOEIC (Test of English as an International Communication), Berlitz Online English Proficiency Exam, PTE, or IELTS. Electronic applications accepted. *Expenses:* Contact institution.

University of Phoenix–Phoenix Campus, College of Health Sciences and Nursing, Tempe, AZ 85282-2371. Offers family nurse practitioner (MSN, Certificate); gerontology health care (Certificate); health care education (MSN, Certificate); health care informatics (Certificate); informatics (MSN); nursing (MSN); MSN/MHA. *Program availability:* Evening/weekend, online learning. *Entrance requirements:* Additional exam requirements/recommendations for international students: Required—TOEFL, TOEIC (Test of English as an International Communication), Berlitz Online English Proficiency Exam, PTE, or IELTS. Electronic applications accepted. *Expenses:* Contact institution.

University of Phoenix–Sacramento Valley Campus, College of Nursing, Sacramento, CA 95833-4334. Offers family nurse practitioner (MSN); health administration (MHA); health care education (MSN); nursing (MSN); MSN/MBA. *Program availability:* Evening/weekend. *Degree requirements:* For master's, thesis (for some programs). *Entrance requirements:* For master's, RN license, minimum undergraduate GPA of 2.5, 3 years work experience. Additional exam requirements/recommendations for international students: Required—TOEFL (minimum score 550 paper-based; 79 iBT). Electronic applications accepted.

University of Phoenix–San Diego Campus, College of Nursing, San Diego, CA 92123. Offers health care education (MSN); nursing (MSN); MSN/MBA. *Program availability:* Evening/weekend. *Degree requirements:* For master's, thesis (for some programs). *Entrance requirements:* For master's, minimum undergraduate GPA of 2.5, 3 years work experience, RN license. Additional exam requirements/recommendations for international students: Required—TOEFL (minimum score 550 paper-based; 79 iBT). Electronic applications accepted.

University of Phoenix–Southern California Campus, College of Health Sciences and Nursing, Costa Mesa, CA 92626. Offers family nurse practitioner (MSN, Certificate); health care (Certificate); informatics (MSN); nursing (MSN); nursing/health care education (MSN, Certificate); MSN/MBA; MSN/MHA. *Program availability:* Evening/weekend, online learning. *Entrance requirements:* Additional exam requirements/recommendations for international students: Required—TOEFL, TOEIC (Test of English as an International Communication), Berlitz Online English Proficiency Exam, PTE, or IELTS. Electronic applications accepted. *Expenses:* Contact institution.

University of Phoenix–South Florida Campus, College of Nursing, Miramar, FL 33027-4145. Offers health administration (MHA); health care education (MSN); nursing (MSN); MSN/MBA; MSN/MHA. *Program availability:* Evening/weekend. *Degree requirements:* For master's, thesis (for some programs). *Entrance requirements:* For master's, minimum undergraduate GPA of 2.5, 3 years work experience, RN license. Additional exam requirements/recommendations for international students: Required—TOEFL (minimum score 550 paper-based; 79 iBT). Electronic applications accepted.

University of Phoenix–Utah Campus, College of Nursing, Salt Lake City, UT 84123-4642. Offers health care education (MSN); nursing (MSN); MSN/MBA. *Program availability:* Evening/weekend. *Degree requirements:* For master's, thesis (for some programs). *Entrance requirements:* For master's, minimum undergraduate GPA of 2.5, 3 years work experience, RN license. Additional exam requirements/recommendations for international students: Required—TOEFL (minimum score 550 paper-based; 79 iBT). Electronic applications accepted.

University of Phoenix–Washington D.C. Campus, College of Nursing, Washington, DC 20001. Offers education (MHA); gerontology (MHA); health administration (MHA, DHA); informatics (MHA, MSN); nursing (MSN, PhD); nursing/health care education (MSN); MSN/MBA; MSN/MHA.

University of Portland, School of Nursing, Portland, OR 97203. Offers clinical nurse leader (MS); family nurse practitioner (DNP); nurse educator (MS). *Accreditation:* AACN. *Program availability:* Part-time, evening/weekend, online learning. *Entrance requirements:* For master's, GRE General Test or MAT, Oregon RN license, BSN, course work in statistics, resume, letters of recommendation, writing sample; for doctorate, GRE General Test or MAT, Oregon RN license, BSN or MSN, 2 letters of recommendation, resume, writing sample, official transcripts. Additional exam requirements/recommendations for international students: Required—TOEFL (minimum score 550 paper-based; 80 iBT), IELTS (minimum score 7). *Expenses:* Contact institution.

University of Rhode Island, Graduate School, College of Nursing, Kingston, RI 02881. Offers acute care nurse practitioner (MS); adult-gerontological nurse practitioner/clinical nurse specialist (MS); family nurse practitioner (MS); nursing (PhD); nursing education (MS); nursing practice (DNP). *Accreditation:* AACN; ACNM/ACME (one or more programs are accredited). *Program availability:* Part-time. *Faculty:* 11 full-time (all women). *Students:* 51 full-time (41 women), 77 part-time (70 women); includes 18 minority (11 Black or African American, non-Hispanic/Latino; 2 Asian, non-Hispanic/Latino; 4 Hispanic/Latino; 1 Two or more races, non-Hispanic/Latino), 5 international. In 2015, 19 master's, 7 doctorates awarded. *Degree requirements:* For master's, comprehensive exam; for doctorate, comprehensive exam, thesis/dissertation. *Entrance requirements:* For master's, GRE or MAT, 2 letters of recommendation, scholarly papers; for doctorate, GRE, 3 letters of recommendation, scholarly papers. Additional exam requirements/recommendations for international students: Required—TOEFL (minimum score 550 paper-based). *Application deadline:* For fall admission, 2/15 for domestic students, 2/1 for international students; for spring admission, 10/15 for domestic students, 7/15 for international students. Application fee: $65. Electronic applications accepted. *Expenses:* Tuition, state resident: full-time $11,796; part-time $655 per credit. Tuition, nonresident: full-time $24,206; part-time $1345 per credit. *Required fees:* $1546; $44 per credit. One-time fee: $155 full-time; $35 part-time. *Financial support:* In 2015–16, 2 research assistantships (averaging $12,111 per year), 7 teaching assistantships with tuition reimbursements (averaging $13,112 per year) were awarded. Financial award application deadline: 2/15; financial award applicants required to submit FAFSA. *Faculty research:* Group intervention for grieving women in prison, translating best practice in non-drug interventions for postoperative pain management, further development and testing of the pain assessment inventory, preschool motor and functional performance of two cohorts, neuroactivation of brain motor areas in preterm children. *Unit head:* Dr. Mary Sullivan, Interim Dean, 401-874-5339, Fax: 401-874-2061, E-mail: mcsullivan@uri.edu. *Application contact:* Graduate Admission, 401-874-2872, E-mail: gradadm@etal.uri.edu.
Website: http://www.uri.edu/nursing/

University of Rochester, School of Nursing, Rochester, NY 14642. Offers adult gerontological acute care nurse practitioner (MS); clinical nurse leader (MS); family nurse practitioner (MS); family psychiatric mental health nurse practitioner (MS); health care organization management and leadership (MS); health practice research (PhD); nursing (DNP); nursing education (MS); pediatric nurse practitioner (MS); pediatric nurse practitioner/neonatal nurse practitioner (MS). *Accreditation:* AACN. *Program availability:* Part-time, online learning. *Faculty:* 56 full-time (45 women), 63 part-time/adjunct (55 women). *Students:* 21 full-time (20 women), 212 part-time (175 women); includes 35 minority (12 Black or African American, non-Hispanic/Latino; 1 American Indian or Alaska Native, non-Hispanic/Latino; 10 Asian, non-Hispanic/Latino; 7 Hispanic/Latino; 5 Two or more races, non-Hispanic/Latino), 2 international. Average age 35. 111 applicants, 68% accepted, 71 enrolled. In 2015, 52 master's, 9 doctorates awarded. Terminal master's awarded for partial completion of doctoral program. *Degree requirements:* For master's, comprehensive exam (for some programs); for doctorate, thesis/dissertation. *Entrance requirements:* For master's, BS in nursing, minimum GPA of 3.0, course work in statistics; for doctorate, GRE General Test (for PhD), MS in nursing, minimum GPA of 3.5. Additional exam requirements/recommendations for international students: Required—TOEFL (minimum score 560 paper-based; 88 iBT) or IELTS (minimum score 6.5) recommended. *Application deadline:* For fall admission, 4/1 for domestic and international students; for spring admission, 9/1 for domestic and international students; for summer admission, 1/2 for domestic and international students. Application fee: $50. Electronic applications accepted. *Expenses: Tuition, area resident:* Full-time $47,450; part-time $1482 per credit hour. *Required fees:* $528. Tuition and fees vary according to program. *Financial support:* In 2015–16, 52 students received support, including 2 fellowships with tuition reimbursements available (averaging $30,000 per year); scholarships/grants, traineeships, health care benefits, tuition waivers (full and partial), and unspecified assistantships also available. Support available to part-time students. Financial award application deadline: 6/30. *Faculty research:* Symptom assessment and self-management of chronic illness, health promotion and illness prevention, nursing intervention research with vulnerable populations, palliative care, aging. *Total annual research expenditures:* $2.1 million. *Unit head:* Dr. Kathy H. Rideout, Dean, 585-273-8902, Fax: 585-273-1268, E-mail: kathy_rideout@urmc.rochester.edu. *Application contact:* Elaine Andolina, Director of Admissions, 585-275-2375, Fax: 585-756-8299, E-mail: elaine_andolina@urmc.rochester.edu.
Website: http://www.son.rochester.edu

University of St. Francis, Leach College of Nursing, Joliet, IL 60435-6169. Offers family nurse practitioner (MSN, Post-Master's Certificate); family psychology/mental health nurse practitioner (MSN, Post-Master's Certificate); nursing administration (MSN); nursing education (MSN); nursing practice (DNP); teaching in nursing (Certificate). *Accreditation:* AACN. *Program availability:* Part-time, evening/weekend, 100% online. *Faculty:* 7 full-time (all women), 16 part-time/adjunct (13 women). *Students:* 82 full-time (72 women), 356 part-time (325 women); includes 147 minority (62 Black or African American, non-Hispanic/Latino; 1 American Indian or Alaska Native, non-Hispanic/Latino; 27 Asian, non-Hispanic/Latino; 45 Hispanic/Latino; 3 Native Hawaiian or other Pacific Islander, non-Hispanic/Latino; 9 Two or more races, non-Hispanic/Latino). Average age 41. 338 applicants, 42% accepted, 100 enrolled. In 2015, 91 master's, 9 doctorates, 6 other advanced degrees awarded. *Entrance requirements:* Additional exam requirements/recommendations for international students: Required—TOEFL (minimum score 550 paper-based; 79 iBT), IELTS (minimum score 6). *Application deadline:* Applications are processed on a rolling basis. Application fee: $30. Electronic applications accepted. Application fee is waived when completed online. *Expenses:* Contact institution. *Financial support:* In 2015–16, 149 students received support. Career-related internships or fieldwork, scholarships/grants, and tuition waivers (partial) available. Support available to part-time students. Financial award applicants required to submit FAFSA. *Unit head:* Dr. Carol Wilson, Dean, 815-740-3840, Fax: 815-740-4243, E-mail: cwilson@stfrancis.edu. *Application contact:* Sandra Sloka, Director of Admissions for Graduate and Degree Completion Programs, 800-735-7500, Fax: 815-740-3431, E-mail: ssloka@stfrancis.edu.
Website: http://www.stfrancis.edu/academics/college-of-nursing/

University of Saint Joseph, Department of Nursing, West Hartford, CT 06117-2700. Offers family nurse practitioner (MS); family psychiatric/mental health nurse practitioner (MS); nurse educator (MS); nursing practice (DNP). *Accreditation:* AACN. *Program availability:* Part-time, evening/weekend. *Degree requirements:* For master's, thesis. *Entrance requirements:* For master's, 2 letters of recommendation. *Application deadline:* Applications are processed on a rolling basis. Application fee: $50. Electronic applications accepted. Application fee is waived when completed online. *Financial support:* Career-related internships or fieldwork and unspecified assistantships available. Support available to part-time students. Financial award applicants required to submit FAFSA.
Website: http://www.usj.edu/academics/schools/school-of-health-natural-sciences/nursing/

University of Saint Mary, Graduate Programs, Program in Nursing, Leavenworth, KS 66048-5082. Offers nurse administrator (MSN); nurse educator (MSN). *Program availability:* Part-time, online only, 100% online. *Students:* 19 full-time (all women), 12 part-time (11 women); includes 5 minority (3 Black or African American, non-Hispanic/Latino; 1 Hispanic/Latino; 1 Two or more races, non-Hispanic/Latino). Average age 41. *Degree requirements:* For master's, practicum. *Entrance requirements:* For master's, BSN from CCNE- or NLNAC-accredited baccalaureate nursing program at regionally-accredited institution. Application fee: $25. *Expenses:* $580 per credit hour. *Unit head:* Karen R. Kidder, Chair, 877-307-4915, Fax: 913-345-2802. *Application contact:* Dr. Linda King, Director, 877-307-4915, Fax: 913-345-2802.
Website: http://online.stmary.edu/msn

University of South Alabama, College of Nursing, Mobile, AL 36688. Offers nursing (MSN, DNP); nursing administration (Certificate); nursing education (MAIA); nursing practice (Certificate). *Accreditation:* AACN. *Program availability:* Part-time, online learning. *Faculty:* 09 full-time (63 women), 97 part-time/adjunct (89 women). *Students:* 2,489 full-time (2,179 women), 341 part-time (297 women); includes 789 minority (520 Black or African American, non-Hispanic/Latino; 26 American Indian or Alaska Native, non-Hispanic/Latino; 118 Asian, non-Hispanic/Latino; 82 Hispanic/Latino; 9 Native Hawaiian or other Pacific Islander, non-Hispanic/Latino; 34 Two or more races, non-Hispanic/Latino), 7 international. Average age 35. 1,923 applicants, 51% accepted, 722 enrolled. In 2015, 572 master's, 90 doctorates, 79 other advanced degrees awarded. *Degree requirements:* For master's, thesis optional; for doctorate, final project. *Entrance requirements:* For master's, BSN, RN licensure, minimum GPA of 3.0, resume documenting clinical experience, background check, drug screening; for doctorate, MSN, RN licensure, minimum GPA of 3.0; for Certificate, MSN/DN/DNP, RN licensure, minimum GPA of 3.0, resume documenting clinical experience, background check, drug screening. *Application deadline:* For fall admission, 3/15 for domestic students; for spring admission, 7/15 priority date for domestic students; for summer admission, 1/15 priority date for domestic students. Applications are processed on a rolling basis. Application fee: $85. Electronic applications accepted. *Expenses:* Tuition, state resident: full-time $9480; part-time $395 per credit hour. Tuition, nonresident: full-time $18,960; part-time $790 per credit hour. *Financial support:* Fellowships, research assistantships, teaching assistantships, career-related internships or fieldwork, Federal Work-Study, institutionally sponsored loans, scholarships/grants, and unspecified assistantships available. Support available to part-time students. Financial award application deadline: 5/31; financial award applicants required to submit FAFSA. *Unit head:* Dr. Debra Davis, Dean, College of Nursing, 251-445-9400, Fax: 251-445-9416, E-mail: ddavis@southalabama.edu. *Application contact:* Gail Soles, Academic Records Specialist, 251-445-9400, Fax: 251-445-9416, E-mail: gsoles@southalabama.edu. Website: http://www.southalabama.edu/colleges/con/index.html

University of Southern Maine, College of Science, Technology, and Health, School of Nursing, Portland, ME 04103. Offers adult-gerontology primary care nurse practitioner (MS, PMC); education (MS); family nurse practitioner (MS, PMC); family psychiatric/ mental health nurse practitioner (MS); management (MS); nursing (CAS, CGS); psychiatric-mental health nurse practitioner (PMC). *Accreditation:* AACN. *Program availability:* Part-time. *Degree requirements:* For master's, thesis optional. *Entrance requirements:* For master's, GRE General Test or MAT, minimum GPA of 3.0; for doctorate, GRE. Additional exam requirements/recommendations for international students: Required—TOEFL (minimum score 550 paper-based). Electronic applications accepted. *Expenses:* Tuition, area resident: Full-time $6840; part-time $380 per credit hour. Tuition, state resident: full-time $10,260; part-time $570 per credit hour. Tuition, nonresident: full-time $18,468; part-time $1026 per credit hour. *Required fees:* $830; $83 per credit hour. Tuition and fees vary according to course load and program. *Faculty research:* Women's health, nursing history, weight control, community services, substance abuse.

University of South Florida, College of Nursing, Tampa, FL 33612. Offers advanced pain management (Graduate Certificate); nursing (MS, DNP), including adult gerontology acute care (DNP), adult gerontology acute care nursing (MS), adult gerontology primary care (DNP), adult gerontology primary care nursing (MS), adult gerontology primary care/ occupational health nursing (MS), adult gerontology primary care/oncology nursing (MS), clinical nurse leader (MS), family health nursing, nurse anesthesia (MS), nursing education (MS), nursing practice (DNP), occupational health/adult-gerontology (DNP), oncology/adult-gerontology primary care (DNP), pediatric health (DNP), pediatric nurse practitioner (MS); nursing education (Post Master's Certificate); nursing science (PhD). *Accreditation:* AACN; AANA/CANAEP. *Program availability:* Part-time. *Faculty:* 43 full-time (38 women), 7 part-time/adjunct (4 women). *Students:* 159 full-time (135 women), 721 part-time (625 women); includes 292 minority (119 Black or African American, non-Hispanic/Latino; 2 American Indian or Alaska Native, non-Hispanic/Latino; 60 Asian, non-Hispanic/Latino; 90 Hispanic/Latino; 1 Native Hawaiian or other Pacific Islander, non-Hispanic/Latino; 20 Two or more races, non-Hispanic/Latino), 12 international. Average age 35. 636 applicants, 44% accepted, 215 enrolled. In 2015, 333 master's, 18 doctorates awarded. *Degree requirements:* For master's, comprehensive exam, thesis optional; for doctorate, comprehensive exam, thesis/dissertation. *Entrance requirements:* For master's, GRE General Test, bachelor's degree from accredited program with minimum GPA of 3.0 in all upper-division coursework; current license as Registered Nurse; 3 letters of recommendation; personal statement of goals; resume or curriculum vitae; personal interview; for doctorate, GRE General Test (recommended), bachelor's degree in nursing from a CCNA/NLNAC regionally-accredited institution with minimum GPA of 3.0 in all coursework or in all upper-division coursework; current license as Registered Nurse in Florida; undergraduate statistics course with minimum B grade; 3 letters of recommendation; statement of goals; resume; interview. Additional exam requirements/ recommendations for international students: Required—TOEFL (minimum score 550 paper-based; 79 iBT). *Application deadline:* For fall admission, 2/15 for domestic students, 1/2 for international students; for spring admission, 10/1 for domestic students, 6/1 for international students. Application fee: $30. Electronic applications accepted. *Financial support:* In 2015–16, 36 students received support, including 7 research assistantships with tuition reimbursements available (averaging $18,935 per year), 29 teaching assistantships with tuition reimbursements available (averaging $30,814 per year); tuition waivers (partial) and unspecified assistantships also available. Financial award application deadline: 2/1; financial award applicants required to submit FAFSA. *Faculty research:* Women's health, palliative and end-of-life care, cardiac rehabilitation, complementary therapies for chronic illness and cancer. *Total annual research expenditures:* $2.6 million. *Unit head:* Dr. Dianne C. Morrison-Beedy, Dean and Professor, College of Nursing, 813-974-9091, Fax: 813-974-5418, E-mail: dmbeedy@health.usf.edu. *Application contact:* Dr. Brian Graves, Assistant Professor/Assistant Dean, 813-974-8054, Fax: 813-974-5418, E-mail: bgraves1@health.usf.edu. Website: http://health.usf.edu/nursing/index.htm

The University of Tennessee at Chattanooga, School of Nursing, Chattanooga, TN 37403. Offers administration (MSN); certified nurse anesthetist (Post-Master's Certificate); education (MSN); family nurse practitioner (MSN, Post-Master's Certificate); health care informatics (Post-Master's Certificate); nurse anesthesia (MSN); nurse education (Post-Master's Certificate); nursing (DNP). *Accreditation:* AACN; AANA/ CANAEP (one or more programs are accredited). *Faculty:* 9 full-time (7 women), 2 part-time/adjunct (1 woman). *Students:* 50 full-time (25 women), 43 part-time (37 women); includes 14 minority (7 Black or African American, non-Hispanic/Latino; 1 American Indian or Alaska Native, non-Hispanic/Latino; 4 Asian, non-Hispanic/Latino; 2 Two or more races, non-Hispanic/Latino). Average age 34. In 2015, 40 master's, 12 doctorates, 1 other advanced degree awarded. *Degree requirements:* For master's, thesis optional, qualifying exams, professional project; for Post-Master's Certificate, thesis or alternative, practicum, seminar. *Entrance requirements:* For master's, GRE General Test, MAT, BSN, minimum GPA of 3.0, eligibility for Tennessee RN license, 1 year of direct patient care experience; for Post-Master's Certificate, GRE General Test, MAT, MSN, minimum GPA of 3.0, eligibility for Tennessee RN license, one year of direct patient care experience. Additional exam requirements/recommendations for international students: Required—TOEFL (minimum score 79 iBT), IELTS (minimum score 6). *Application deadline:* For fall admission, 6/13 priority date for domestic students, 6/1 for international students; for spring admission, 10/15 priority date for domestic students, 10/1 for international students. Applications are processed on a rolling basis. Application fee: $30 ($35 for international students). Electronic applications accepted. *Expenses:* Tuition, state resident: full-time $7938; part-time $441 per credit hour. Tuition, nonresident: full-time $24,056; part-time $1336 per credit hour. *Required fees:* $1732; $253 per credit hour. *Financial support:* Career-related internships or fieldwork and scholarships/grants available. Support available to part-time students. *Faculty research:* Diabetes in women, health care for elderly, alternative medicine, hypertension, nurse anesthesia. *Total annual research expenditures:* $2.6 million. *Unit head:* Dr. Chris Smith, Interim Director, 423-425-1741, Fax: 423-425-4668, E-mail: chris-smith@utc.edu. *Application contact:* Dr. J. Randy Walker, Interim Dean of Graduate Studies, 423-425-4478, Fax: 423-425-5223, E-mail: randy-walker@utc.edu. Website: http://www.utc.edu/Academic/Nursing/

The University of Texas at Arlington, Graduate School, College of Nursing, Arlington, TX 76019. Offers nurse practitioner (MSN); nursing administration (MSN); nursing education (MSN); nursing practice (DNP); nursing science (PhD). *Accreditation:* AACN. *Program availability:* Part-time, evening/weekend, online learning. *Degree requirements:* For master's, practicum course; for doctorate, comprehensive exam (for some programs), thesis/dissertation (for some programs), proposal defense dissertation (for PhD); scholarship project (for DNP). *Entrance requirements:* For master's, GRE General Test if GPA less than 3.0, minimum GPA of 3.0, Texas nursing license, minimum C grade in undergraduate statistics course; for doctorate, GRE General Test (waived for MSN-to-PhD applicants), minimum undergraduate, graduate and statistics GPA of 3.0; Texas RN license; interview; written statement of goals. Additional exam requirements/ recommendations for international students: Required—TOEFL (minimum score 550 paper-based), IELTS (minimum score 7). *Faculty research:* Simulation in clinical education and practice, cultural diversity, vulnerable populations, substance abuse.

The University of Texas at Austin, Graduate School, School of Nursing, Austin, TX 78712-1111. Offers adult - gerontology clinical nurse specialist (MSN); child health (MSN), including administration, public health nursing, teaching; family nurse practitioner (MSN); family psychiatric/mental health nurse practitioner (MSN); holistic adult health (MSN), including administration, teaching; maternity (MSN), including administration, public health nursing, teaching; nursing (PhD); nursing administration and healthcare systems management (MSN); nursing practice (DNP); pediatric nurse practitioner (MSN); public health nursing (MSN). *Accreditation:* AACN. *Program availability:* Part-time. *Degree requirements:* For master's, thesis optional; for doctorate, thesis/dissertation. *Entrance requirements:* For master's and doctorate, GRE General Test. Additional exam requirements/recommendations for international students: Required—TOEFL (minimum score 550 paper-based). Electronic applications accepted. *Faculty research:* Chronic illness management, memory and aging, health promotion, women's health, adolescent health.

The University of Texas at El Paso, Graduate School, School of Nursing, El Paso, TX 79968-0001. Offers family nurse practitioner (MSN); health care leadership and management (Certificate); interdisciplinary health sciences (PhD); nursing (DNP); nursing education (MSN, Certificate); nursing systems management (MSN). *Accreditation:* AACN. *Program availability:* Online learning. *Degree requirements:* For master's, thesis optional; for doctorate, thesis/dissertation. *Entrance requirements:* For master's, minimum GPA of 3.0, resume; for doctorate, GRE, letters of reference, relevant personal/professional experience; master's degree in nursing (for DNP); for Certificate, bachelor's degree in nursing. Additional exam requirements/ recommendations for international students: Required—TOEFL; Recommended— IELTS. Electronic applications accepted.

The University of Texas at Tyler, College of Nursing and Health Sciences, Program in Nursing, Tyler, TX 75799-0001. Offers nurse practitioner (MSN); nursing (PhD); nursing administration (MSN); nursing education (MSN); MSN/MBA. *Accreditation:* AACN. *Program availability:* Part-time, evening/weekend, online learning. *Degree requirements:* For master's, comprehensive exam (for some programs), thesis (for some programs); for doctorate, thesis/dissertation. *Entrance requirements:* For master's, GRE General Test or MAT, GMAT, minimum undergraduate GPA of 3.0, course work in statistics, RN license, BSN. Additional exam requirements/recommendations for international students: Required—TOEFL. Electronic applications accepted. *Faculty research:* Psychosocial adjustment, aging, support/commitment of caregivers, psychological abuse and violence, hope/hopelessness, professional values, end of life care, suicidology, clinical supervision, workforce retention and issues, global health issues, health promotion.

The University of Texas Health Science Center at San Antonio, School of Nursing, San Antonio, TX 78229-3900. Offers administrative management (MSN); adult-gerontology acute care nurse practitioner (PGC); advanced practice leadership (DNP); clinical nurse leader (MSN); executive administrative management (DNP); family nurse practitioner (MSN, PGC); nursing (MSN, PhD); nursing education (MSN, PGC); pediatric nurse practitioner primary care (PGC); psychiatric mental health nurse practitioner (PGC); public health nurse leader (DNP). *Accreditation:* AACN. *Program availability:* Part-time. Terminal master's awarded for partial completion of doctoral program. *Degree requirements:* For master's, thesis optional; for doctorate, comprehensive exam, thesis/ dissertation.

The University of Toledo, College of Graduate Studies, College of Nursing, Department of Population and Community Care, Toledo, OH 43606-3390. Offers clinical nurse leader (MSN); family nurse practitioner (MSN, Certificate); nurse educator (MSN, Certificate); pediatric nurse practitioner (MSN, Certificate). *Program availability:* Part-time. *Degree requirements:* For master's, thesis or alternative. *Entrance requirements:* For master's, GRE, BS in nursing, minimum undergraduate GPA of 3.0, statement of purpose, three letters of recommendation, transcripts from all prior institutions attended, Nursing CAS application, UT supplemental application; for Certificate, BS in nursing, minimum undergraduate GPA of 3.0, statement of purpose, three letters of recommendation, transcripts from all prior institutions attended. Additional exam requirements/recommendations for international students: Required—TOEFL (minimum score 550 paper-based; 80 iBT). Electronic applications accepted.

University of Victoria, Faculty of Graduate Studies, Faculty of Human and Social Development, School of Nursing, Victoria, BC V8W 2Y2, Canada. Offers advanced nursing practice (advanced practice leadership option) (MN); advanced nursing practice (nurse educator option) (MN); advanced nursing practice (nurse practitioner option) (MN); nursing (PhD). *Program availability:* Part-time, online learning. *Entrance requirements:* Additional exam requirements/recommendations for international students: Required—TOEFL (minimum score 575 paper-based), IELTS (minimum score 7). Electronic applications accepted.

University of Washington, Tacoma, Graduate Programs, Program in Nursing, Tacoma, WA 98402-3100. Offers communities, populations and health (MN); leadership in healthcare (MN); nurse educator (MN). *Program availability:* Part-time. *Degree requirements:* For master's, thesis (for some programs), advance fieldwork. *Entrance requirements:* For master's, Washington State NCLEX exam, minimum GPA of 3.0. Additional exam requirements/recommendations for international students: Required— TOEFL (minimum score 580 paper-based; 70 iBT); Recommended—IELTS (minimum score 7). *Faculty research:* Hospice and palliative care; clinical trial decision-making; minority nurse retention; asthma and public health; injustice, suffering, difference; Linking Them to Us; adolescent health.

University of West Georgia, Tanner Health System School of Nursing, Carrollton, GA 30118. Offers health systems leadership (Post-Master's Certificate); nursing (MSN); nursing education (Ed D, Post-Master's Certificate). *Accreditation:* AACN. *Program availability:* Part-time, evening/weekend, 100% online. *Faculty:* 13 full-time (all women). *Students:* 58 full-time (51 women), 69 part-time (64 women); includes 33 minority (29 Black or African American, non-Hispanic/Latino; 1 Asian, non-Hispanic/Latino; 3 Hispanic/Latino). Average age 42. 78 applicants, 90% accepted, 58 enrolled. In 2015, 32 master's, 1 other advanced degree awarded. *Entrance requirements:* Additional exam requirements/recommendations for international students: Required—TOEFL (minimum score 523 paper-based; 69 iBT); Recommended—IELTS (minimum score

Nursing Education

6.5). *Application deadline:* For fall admission, 2/1 priority date for domestic and international students. Applications are processed on a rolling basis. Application fee: $40. Electronic applications accepted. *Expenses:* Contact institution. *Financial support:* Fellowships, research assistantships, teaching assistantships, career-related internships or fieldwork, Federal Work-Study, institutionally sponsored loans, scholarships/grants, and unspecified assistantships available. Support available to part-time students. Financial award application deadline: 4/1; financial award applicants required to submit FAFSA. *Unit head:* Dr. Jennifer Schuessler, Dean, 678-839-5640, Fax: 678-839-6553, E-mail: jschuess@westga.edu. *Application contact:* Dr. Toby Ziglar, Director of Graduate and International Admissions, 678-839-1390, Fax: 678-839-1395, E-mail: graduate@westga.edu.
Website: http://nursing.westga.edu

University of Wisconsin–Eau Claire, College of Nursing and Health Sciences, Program in Nursing, Eau Claire, WI 54702-4004. Offers adult-gerontological administration (DNP); adult-gerontological clinical nurse specialist (DNP); adult-gerontological education (MSN); adult-gerontological primary care nurse practitioner (DNP); family health administration (DNP); family health in education (MSN); family health nurse practitioner (DNP); nursing (MSN); nursing practice (DNP). *Program availability:* Part-time. Terminal master's awarded for partial completion of doctoral program. *Degree requirements:* For master's, thesis optional, 500-600 hours clinical practicum, oral and written exams. *Entrance requirements:* For master's, Wisconsin RN license, minimum GPA of 3.0, undergraduate statistics, course work in health assessment. Additional exam requirements/recommendations for international students: Required—TOEFL (minimum score 79 iBT). *Expenses:* Contact institution.

Ursuline College, School of Graduate Studies, Programs in Nursing, Pepper Pike, OH 44124-4398. Offers adult nurse practitioner (MSN); adult-gerontology clinical nurse specialist (MSN); family nurse practitioner (MSN); nursing (DNP); nursing education (MSN); palliative care (MSN). *Accreditation:* AACN. *Program availability:* Part-time. *Faculty:* 5 full-time (all women), 26 part-time/adjunct (21 women). *Students:* 150 full-time (141 women), 108 part-time (99 women); includes 66 minority (50 Black or African American, non-Hispanic/Latino; 6 Asian, non-Hispanic/Latino; 6 Hispanic/Latino; 4 Two or more races, non-Hispanic/Latino), 5 international. Average age 37. 115 applicants, 95% accepted, 73 enrolled. In 2015, 69 master's, 2 doctorates awarded. *Degree requirements:* For master's, comprehensive exam. *Entrance requirements:* For master's, minimum undergraduate GPA of 3.0, bachelor's degree in nursing, eligibility for or current Ohio RN license. Additional exam requirements/recommendations for international students: Required—TOEFL (minimum score 500 paper-based). *Application deadline:* For fall admission, 8/1 priority date for domestic students. Applications are processed on a rolling basis. Application fee: $25. Electronic applications accepted. *Expenses:* Tuition, area resident: Full-time $18,036; part-time $6012 per semester. *Required fees:* $290; $210 per credit. $105 per semester. Tuition and fees vary according to program. *Financial support:* In 2015–16, 12 students received support. Scholarships/grants available. Financial award application deadline: 3/1; financial award applicants required to submit FAFSA. *Unit head:* Dr. Janet Baker, Director, 440-864-8172, Fax: 440-684-6053, E-mail: jbaker@ursuline.edu. *Application contact:* Stephanie Pratt McRoberts, Graduate Admission Coordinator, 440-646-8119, Fax: 440-684-6138, E-mail: graduateadmissions@ursuline.edu.

Valparaiso University, Graduate School, College of Nursing and Health Professions, Valparaiso, IN 46383. Offers nursing (DNP); nursing education (MSN, Certificate); public health (MPH); MSN/MHA. *Accreditation:* AACN. *Program availability:* Part-time, evening/weekend, online learning. *Faculty:* 13 part-time/adjunct (all women). *Students:* 52 full-time (43 women), 33 part-time (30 women); includes 9 minority (4 Black or African American, non-Hispanic/Latino; 1 Asian, non-Hispanic/Latino; 4 Hispanic/Latino), 22 international. Average age 33. In 2015, 9 master's, 16 doctorates awarded. *Entrance requirements:* For master's, minimum GPA of 3.0, undergraduate major in nursing, Indiana registered nursing license, undergraduate courses in research and statistics. Additional exam requirements/recommendations for international students: Required—TOEFL (minimum score 550 paper-based; 80 iBT), IELTS (minimum score 6). *Application deadline:* Applications are processed on a rolling basis. Application fee: $30 ($50 for international students). Electronic applications accepted. *Expenses:* Contact institution. *Financial support:* Available to part-time students. Applicants required to submit FAFSA. *Unit head:* Dr. Janet Brown, Dean, 219-464-5289, Fax: 219-464-5425, E-mail: janet.brown@valpo.edu. *Application contact:* Jessica Choquette, Graduate Admissions Specialist, 219-464-6510, Fax: 219-464-5381, E-mail: jessica.choquette@valpo.edu.
Website: http://www.valpo.edu/nursing/

Villanova University, College of Nursing, Villanova, PA 19085-1699. Offers adult nurse practitioner (MSN, Post Master's Certificate); family nurse practitioner (MSN, Post Master's Certificate); nurse anesthetist (MSN, Post Master's Certificate); nursing (PhD); nursing education (MSN, Post Master's Certificate); nursing practice (DNP); pediatric nurse practitioner (MSN, Post Master's Certificate). *Accreditation:* AACN; AANA/CANAEP. *Program availability:* Part-time, online learning. *Faculty:* 16 full-time (15 women), 9 part-time/adjunct (7 women). *Students:* 219 full-time (198 women), 108 part-time (96 women); includes 36 minority (25 Black or African American, non-Hispanic/Latino; 9 Asian, non-Hispanic/Latino; 2 Hispanic/Latino), 16 international. Average age 31. 147 applicants, 78% accepted, 106 enrolled. In 2015, 64 master's, 8 doctorates, 9 other advanced degrees awarded. *Degree requirements:* For master's, independent study project; for doctorate, comprehensive exam, thesis/dissertation; for Post Master's Certificate, scholarly project. *Entrance requirements:* For master's, GRE or MAT, BSN, 1 year of recent nursing experience, physical assessment, course work in statistics; for doctorate, GRE, MSN. Additional exam requirements/recommendations for international students: Required—TOEFL (minimum score 540 paper-based; 83 iBT), IELTS (minimum score 6.5). *Application deadline:* For fall admission, 7/1 priority date for domestic students, 7/1 for international students; for spring admission, 11/1 priority date for domestic students, 11/1 for international students; for summer admission, 4/1 priority date for domestic students, 3/1 for international students. Applications are processed on a rolling basis. Application fee: $50. Electronic applications accepted. *Expenses:* $837 per credit (MSN); $1,049 per credit (PhD); $1,375 per credit (DNP). *Financial support:* In 2015–16, 22 students received support, including 5 teaching assistantships with full tuition reimbursements available (averaging $15,475 per year); institutionally sponsored loans, scholarships/grants, traineeships, tuition waivers (full), and unspecified assistantships also available. Financial award application deadline: 7/1; financial award applicants required to submit FAFSA. *Faculty research:* Genetics, ethics, cognitive development of students, women with disabilities, nursing leadership. *Unit head:* Dr. Marguerite K. Schlag, Assistant Dean/Director, Graduate Programs, 610-519-4907, Fax: 610-519-7650, E-mail: marguerite.schlag@villanova.edu. *Application contact:* Rebecca Harold, Administrative Assistant, 610-519-4934, Fax: 610-519-7650, E-mail: rebecca.harold@villanova.edu.
Website: http://www.nursing.villanova.edu/

Virginia Commonwealth University, Graduate School, School of Nursing, Richmond, VA 23284-9005. Offers adult health acute nursing (MS); adult health primary nursing (MS); biobehavioral clinical research (PhD); child health nursing (MS); clinical nurse leader (MS); family health nursing (MS); nurse educator (MS); nurse practitioner (MS);

nursing (Certificate); nursing administration (MS), including clinical nurse manager; psychiatric-mental health nursing (MS); quality and safety in health care (DNP); women's health nursing (MS). *Accreditation:* ACEN (one or more programs are accredited). *Program availability:* Part-time, evening/weekend, online learning. *Degree requirements:* For master's, thesis optional; for doctorate, thesis/dissertation. *Entrance requirements:* For master's, GRE General Test, BSN, minimum GPA of 2.8; for doctorate, GRE General Test. Additional exam requirements/recommendations for international students: Required—TOEFL (minimum score 600 paper-based; 100 iBT). Electronic applications accepted.

Walden University, Graduate Programs, School of Nursing, Minneapolis, MN 55401. Offers adult-gerontology acute care nurse practitioner (MSN); adult-gerontology nurse practitioner (MSN); education (MSN); family nurse practitioner (MSN); informatics (MSN); leadership and management (MSN); nursing (PhD, Post-Master's Certificate), including education (PhD), healthcare administration (PhD), interdisciplinary health (PhD), leadership (PhD), nursing education (Post-Master's Certificate), nursing informatics (Post-Master's Certificate), nursing leadership and management (Post-Master's Certificate), public health policy (PhD); nursing practice (DNP); psychiatric mental health (MSN). *Accreditation:* AACN. *Program availability:* Part-time, evening/weekend, online only, 100% online. *Faculty:* 22 full-time (18 women), 540 part-time/adjunct (487 women). *Students:* 4,320 full-time (3,773 women), 5,250 part-time (4,740 women); includes 3,550 minority (2,360 Black or African American, non-Hispanic/Latino; 29 American Indian or Alaska Native, non-Hispanic/Latino; 523 Asian, non-Hispanic/Latino; 421 Hispanic/Latino; 25 Native Hawaiian or other Pacific Islander, non-Hispanic/Latino; 192 Two or more races, non-Hispanic/Latino), 221 international. Average age 40. 2,057 applicants, 100% accepted, 1507 enrolled. In 2015, 3,022 master's, 86 doctorates, 34 other advanced degrees awarded. *Degree requirements:* For doctorate, thesis/dissertation (for some programs), residency (for some programs), field experience (for some programs). *Entrance requirements:* For master's, bachelor's degree or equivalent in related field or RN; minimum GPA of 2.5; official transcripts; goal statement (for some programs); access to computer and Internet; for doctorate, master's degree or higher; RN; three years of related professional or academic experience; goal statement; access to computer and Internet; for Post-Master's Certificate, relevant work experience; access to computer and Internet. Additional exam requirements/recommendations for international students: Required—TOEFL (minimum score 550 paper-based, 79 iBT), IELTS (minimum score 6.5), Michigan English Language Assessment Battery (minimum score 82), or PTE (minimum score 53). *Application deadline:* Applications are processed on a rolling basis. Application fee: $0. Electronic applications accepted. *Financial support:* Fellowships, Federal Work-Study, scholarships/grants, unspecified assistantships, and family tuition reduction, active duty/veteran tuition reduction, group tuition reduction, interest-free payment plans, employee tuition reduction available. Support available to part-time students. Financial award applicants required to submit FAFSA. *Unit head:* Dr. Andrea Lindell, Dean, 866-492-5336. *Application contact:* Meghan Thomas, Vice President of Enrollment Management, 866-492-5336, E-mail: info@waldenu.edu.
Website: http://www.waldenu.edu/programs/colleges-schools/nursing

Walsh University, Graduate Studies, Gary and Linda Byers School of Nursing, North Canton, OH 44720-3396. Offers academic nurse educator (MSN); clinical nurse leader (MSN); nursing practice (DNP). *Program availability:* Part-time, evening/weekend, online only, 100% online. *Faculty:* 6 full-time (all women), 6 part-time/adjunct (4 women). *Students:* 25 full-time (20 women), 38 part-time (34 women); includes 2 minority (1 Black or African American, non-Hispanic/Latino; 1 Hispanic/Latino). Average age 36. 45 applicants, 71% accepted, 22 enrolled. In 2015, 9 master's, 5 doctorates awarded. *Degree requirements:* For doctorate, scholarly project; residency practicum. *Entrance requirements:* For master's, undergraduate nursing degree, current unencumbered RN license, completion of an undergraduate or graduate statistics course, essay, interview, recommendations; for doctorate, BSN; master's degree; statistics and research courses; essay; interview. Additional exam requirements/recommendations for international students: Required—TOEFL. *Application deadline:* Applications are processed on a rolling basis. Application fee: $25. Electronic applications accepted. *Expenses:* Tuition, area resident: Full-time $11,610; part-time $7740 per credit hour. Full-time tuition and fees vary according to program. *Financial support:* In 2015–16, 1 student received support, including 1 research assistantship (averaging $3,870 per year). Financial award application deadline: 12/31; financial award applicants required to submit FAFSA. *Faculty research:* Faith community nursing, gerontology, women's health, global nursing education, nursing assessment, grief and reconstitution, health needs of psychiatric patients, psychometric testing, nursing education, clinical reasoning. *Unit head:* Dr. Maris Pappas-Rogich, Director of Graduate Nursing Programs, 330-490-7283, Fax: 330-490-7371, E-mail: mpappas@walsh.edu. *Application contact:* Audra Dice, Graduate and Transfer Admissions Counselor, 330-490-7181, Fax: 330-244-4680, E-mail: adice@walsh.edu.
Website: http://www.walsh.edu/master-of-science-in-nursing

Washington Adventist University, Program in Nursing - Education, Takoma Park, MD 20912. Offers MS. *Program availability:* Part-time. *Entrance requirements:* Additional exam requirements/recommendations for international students: Required—TOEFL (minimum score 550 paper-based), IELTS (minimum score 5).

Waynesburg University, Graduate and Professional Studies, Canonsburg, PA 15370. Offers business (MBA), including energy management, finance, health systems, human resources, leadership, market development; counseling (MA), including addictions counseling, clinical mental health; counselor education and supervision (PhD); criminal investigation (MA); education (M Ed), including autism, curriculum and instruction, educational leadership, online teaching; nursing (MSN), including administration, education, informatics; nursing practice (DNP); special education (M Ed); technology (M Ed); MSN/MBA. *Accreditation:* AACN. *Program availability:* Part-time, evening/weekend. *Degree requirements:* For doctorate, thesis/dissertation. *Entrance requirements:* Additional exam requirements/recommendations for international students: Required—TOEFL. Electronic applications accepted.

Wayne State University, College of Nursing, Program in Nursing Education, Detroit, MI 48202. Offers Graduate Certificate. *Students:* 11 full-time (10 women), 6 part-time (all women); includes 4 minority (2 Black or African American, non-Hispanic/Latino; 2 Asian, non-Hispanic/Latino), 1 international. Average age 35. 4 applicants. In 2015, 8 Graduate Certificates awarded. *Entrance requirements:* For degree, MSN or concurrent enrollment in master's program, current RN license, statement of purpose, three letters of reference. Additional exam requirements/recommendations for international students: Required—TOEFL (minimum score 600 paper-based; 101 iBT); Recommended—TWE (minimum score 7). *Application deadline:* For fall admission, 6/1 priority date for domestic students, 5/1 priority date for international students; for winter admission, 10/1 priority date for domestic students, 9/1 priority date for international students; for spring admission, 2/1 priority date for domestic students, 1/1 priority date for international students. Electronic applications accepted. *Expenses:* $19,325 per year resident tuition, $35,114 non-resident tuition; $805.20 per credit hour resident tuition, $1,463.10 per credit hour non-resident tuition; fees include $47.45 per credit hour student services fee and $274.60 per semester registration fee. *Financial support:* Scholarships/grants available. Financial award application deadline: 7/1; financial award applicants required

to submit FAFSA. *Unit head:* Dr. Barbara Redman, Dean and Professor, 313-577-4104, E-mail: laurie.lauzon.clabo@wayne.edu. *Application contact:* Nancy Artinian, Professor, 313-577-4143, E-mail: n.artinian@wayne.edu.
Website: http://nursing.wayne.edu/gradcert/nursing-education.php

Webster University, College of Arts and Sciences, Department of Nursing, St. Louis, MO 63119-3194. Offers nurse educator (MSN); nurse leader (MSN). *Accreditation:* ACEN. *Degree requirements:* For master's, comprehensive exam. *Entrance requirements:* For master's, 1 year of clinical experience, BSN, interview, minimum C+ average in statistics and physical assessment, minimum GPA of 3.0, RN license. Additional exam requirements/recommendations for international students: Required— TOEFL. *Expenses: Tuition, area resident:* Full-time $20,550; part-time $685 per credit hour. Tuition and fees vary according to campus/location and program. *Faculty research:* Health teaching.

West Chester University of Pennsylvania, College of Health Sciences, Department of Nursing, West Chester, PA 19383. Offers adult-gerontology clinical nurse specialist (MSN); nursing (DNP); nursing education (MSN); school nurse (Certificate). *Accreditation:* AACN. *Program availability:* Part-time, evening/weekend, blended/hybrid learning. *Faculty:* 7 full-time (6 women), 1 (woman) part-time/adjunct. *Students:* 2 full-time (1 woman), 85 part-time (78 women); includes 10 minority (7 Black or African American, non-Hispanic/Latino; 3 Asian, non-Hispanic/Latino). Average age 45. 30 applicants, 90% accepted, 20 enrolled. In 2015, 10 master's, 3 other advanced degrees awarded. *Entrance requirements:* For master's, goals statement; official academic transcript(s) from all colleges and universities attended demonstrating minimum cumulative undergraduate GPA of 2.8 with successful completion of BSN and courses in statistics and physical assessment; documentation of current clinical experience; for doctorate, master's degree in nursing in an advanced nursing specialty from nationally-accredited program; minimum master's GPA of 3.0; licensed Registered Nurse. Additional exam requirements/recommendations for international students: Required— TOEFL or IELTS. *Application deadline:* For fall admission, 5/15 for international students; for spring admission, 10/15 for international students. Applications are processed on a rolling basis. Application fee: $50. Electronic applications accepted. *Expenses:* Tuition, state resident: full-time $8460; part-time $470 per credit. Tuition, nonresident: full-time $12,690; part-time $705 per credit. *Required fees:* $2312; $126.75 per credit. Tuition and fees vary according to campus/location and program. *Financial support:* Scholarships/grants and unspecified assistantships available. Financial award application deadline: 2/15; financial award applicants required to submit FAFSA. *Unit head:* Dr. Charlotte Mackey, Chair, 610-436-3474, Fax: 610-436-3083, E-mail: cmackey@wcupa.edu. *Application contact:* Dr. Cheryl Schlamb, Graduate Coordinator, 610-436-2219, E-mail: cschlamb@wcupa.edu.
Website: http://www.wcupa.edu/_ACADEMICS/HealthSciences/nursing/

Western Connecticut State University, Division of Graduate Studies, School of Professional Studies, Nursing Department, Ed D in Nursing Education Program, Danbury, CT 06810-6885. Offers Ed D. Offered in collaboration with Southern Connecticut State University. *Program availability:* Online learning. *Degree requirements:* For doctorate, thesis/dissertation. *Entrance requirements:* For doctorate, GRE or MAT, official transcripts, current copy of RN license, three letters of reference, curriculum vitae or resume, personal statement. *Expenses:* Tuition, state resident: full-time $6188; part-time $343 per credit hour. Tuition, nonresident: full-time $17,240; part-time $350 per credit hour. *Required fees:* $4399; $173 per credit hour. One-time fee: $60 part-time. Tuition and fees vary according to degree level and program.

Western Governors University, College of Health Professions, Salt Lake City, UT 84107. Offers healthcare management (MBA); leadership and management (MSN); nursing education (MSN). *Program availability:* Evening/weekend. *Degree requirements:* For master's, capstone project. *Entrance requirements:* For master's, Readiness Assessment, transcripts. Additional exam requirements/recommendations for international students: Required—TOEFL (minimum score 450 paper-based; 80 iBT). Electronic applications accepted.

Westminster College, School of Nursing and Health Sciences, Salt Lake City, UT 84105-3697. Offers family nurse practitioner (MSN); nurse anesthesia (MSNA); nurse education (MSNED); public health (MPH). *Accreditation:* AACN; AANA/CANAEP. *Faculty:* 15 full-time (9 women), 7 part-time/adjunct (2 women). *Students:* 120 full-time (79 women), 3 part-time (all women); includes 18 minority (1 Black or African American, non-Hispanic/Latino; 3 Asian, non-Hispanic/Latino; 10 Hispanic/Latino; 4 Two or more races, non-Hispanic/Latino), 3 international. Average age 32. 157 applicants, 40% accepted, 45 enrolled. In 2015, 56 master's awarded. *Degree requirements:* For master's, clinical practicum, 504 clinical practice hours. *Entrance requirements:* For master's, GRE, personal statement, resume, 3 professional recommendations, copy of unrestricted Utah license to practice professional nursing, background check, minimum cumulative GPA of 3.0, documentation of current immunizations, physical and mental health certificate signed by primary care provider. Additional exam requirements/recommendations for international students: Required—TOEFL (minimum score 600 paper-based; 100 iBT), IELTS (minimum score 7.5). Application fee: $50. Electronic applications accepted. *Expenses:* Contact institution. *Financial support:* In 2015–16, 8 students received support. Career-related internships or fieldwork, unspecified assistantships, and tuition reimbursements, tuition remission available. Support available to part-time students. Financial award applicants required to submit FAFSA. *Faculty research:* Intellectual empathy, professional boundaries, learned optimism, collaborative testing in nursing: student outcomes and perspectives, implementing new educational paradigms into pre-licensure nursing curricula. *Unit head:* Dr. Sheryl

Steadman, Dean, 801-832-2164, Fax: 801-832-3110, E-mail: ssteadman@westminstercollege.edu. *Application contact:* Dr. John Baworowsky, Vice President of Enrollment Management, 801-832-2200, Fax: 801-832-3101, E-mail: admission@westminstercollege.edu.
Website: http://www.westminstercollege.edu/msn

West Virginia Wesleyan College, Department of Nursing, Buckhannon, WV 26201. Offers family nurse practitioner (Post Master's Certificate); family nurse practitoner (MS); nurse administrator (MS); nurse educator (MS); nurse-midwifery (MS); nursing administration (Post Master's Certificate); nursing education (Post Master's Certificate); psychiatric mental health nurse practitioner (MS); MSN/MBA. *Accreditation:* ACEN.

Wilson College, Graduate Programs, Chambersburg, PA 17201-1285. Offers accounting (M Acc); choreography and visual art (MFA); education (M Ed); healthcare management for sustainability (MHM); humanities (MA), including art and culture, critical/cultural theory, English language and literature, women's studies; nursing (MSN), including nursing education, nursing leadership and management. *Program availability:* Evening/weekend. *Degree requirements:* For master's, project. *Entrance requirements:* For master's, PRAXIS, minimum undergraduate cumulative GPA of 3.0, 2 letters of recommendation, current certification for eligibility to teach in grades K-12, resume, personal interview. Electronic applications accepted.

Winona State University, College of Nursing and Health Sciences, Winona, MN 55987. Offers adult nurse practitioner (MS, Post Master's Certificate); clinical nurse specialist (MS, Post Master's Certificate); family nurse practitioner (MS, Post Master's Certificate); nurse administrator (MS); nurse educator (MS, Post Master's Certificate); nursing (DNP). *Accreditation:* AACN. *Program availability:* Part-time, online learning. *Degree requirements:* For master's, thesis; for doctorate, capstone. *Entrance requirements:* For master's, GRE (if GPA less than 3.0). Additional exam requirements/recommendations for international students: Required—TOEFL (minimum score 550 paper based).

Winston-Salem State University, Program in Nursing, Winston-Salem, NC 27110-0003. Offers advanced nurse educator (MSN); family nurse practitioner (MSN); nursing (DNP). *Accreditation:* AACN. *Program availability:* Part-time, evening/weekend, online learning. *Entrance requirements:* For master's, GRE, MAT, resume, NC or state compact license, 3 letters of recommendation. Electronic applications accepted. *Faculty research:* Elimination of health care disparities.

Worcester State University, Graduate Studies, Department of Nursing, Program in Nurse Educator, Worcester, MA 01602-2597. Offers MSN. *Accreditation:* AACN. *Program availability:* Part-time. *Faculty:* 4 full-time (all women), 2 part-time/adjunct (1 woman). *Students:* 24 part-time (22 women); includes 2 minority (both Black or African American, non-Hispanic/Latino). Average age 44. 31 applicants, 81% accepted, 11 enrolled. In 2015, 6 master's awarded. *Degree requirements:* For master's, practicum. *Entrance requirements:* For master's, unencumbered license to practice as a Registered Nurse in Massachusetts. Additional exam requirements/recommendations for international students: Required—TOEFL (minimum score 550 paper-based; 79 iBT). *Application deadline:* For fall admission, 6/15 for domestic and international students; for spring admission, 11/1 for domestic and international students; for summer admission, 4/1 for domestic and international students. Applications are processed on a rolling basis. Application fee: $50. Electronic applications accepted. *Expenses:* Tuition, state resident: part-time $150 per credit. Tuition, nonresident: part-time $150 per credit. *Financial support:* Career-related internships or fieldwork, scholarships/grants, and unspecified assistantships available. Financial award application deadline: 3/1; financial award applicants required to submit FAFSA. *Unit head:* Dr. Stephanie Chalupka, Program Coordinator, 508-929-8680, E-mail: schalupka@worcester.edu. *Application contact:* Sara Grady, Associate Dean of Graduate and Continuing Education, 508-929-8787, Fax: 508-929-8100, E-mail: sara.grady@worcester.edu.

York College of Pennsylvania, Department of Nursing, York, PA 17405-7199. Offers adult gerontology clinical nurse specialist (MS), including administration, education; adult gerontology nurse practitioner (MS); nurse anesthetist (MS); nurse educator (MS); nursing practice (DNP). *Accreditation:* AACN; AANA/CANAEP. *Program availability:* Part-time, evening/weekend. *Faculty:* 9 full-time (all women), 5 part-time/adjunct (2 women). *Students:* 36 full-time (26 women), 55 part-time (47 women); includes 14 minority (4 Black or African American, non-Hispanic/Latino; 2 American Indian or Alaska Native, non-Hispanic/Latino; 5 Asian, non-Hispanic/Latino; 2 Hispanic/Latino; 1 Two or more races, non-Hispanic/Latino), 1 international. Average age 33. 115 applicants, 28% accepted, 28 enrolled. In 2015, 24 master's, 4 doctorates awarded. *Entrance requirements:* For master's, GRE General Test (for nurse anesthetist program), minimum GPA of 3.0 from CCNE- or NLNAC-accredited institution; for doctorate, master's degree in nursing from a CCNE- or NLNAC-accredited institution; minimum GPA of 3.5. Additional exam requirements/recommendations for international students: Required—TOEFL (minimum score 530 paper-based; 72 iBT). *Application deadline:* Applications are processed on a rolling basis. Application fee: $0. Electronic applications accepted. *Expenses: Tuition, area resident:* Full-time $13,770. *Required fees:* $1750; $380. Tuition and fees vary according to degree level. *Financial support:* Federal Work-Study available. *Faculty research:* Student stress response to simulation versus clinical, evidence-based practice in all clinical settings. *Unit head:* Dr. Kimberly Fenstermacher, Graduate Program Director, 717-815-1383, E-mail: kfenster@ycp.edu. *Application contact:* Allison Malachosky, Administrative Assistant, 717-815-1243, E-mail: amalacho@ycp.edu.
Website: http://www.ycp.edu/academics/academic-departments/nursing/

Nursing Informatics

Austin Peay State University, College of Graduate Studies, College of Behavioral and Health Sciences, School of Nursing, Clarksville, TN 37044. Offers family nurse practitioner (MSN); nursing administration (MSN); nursing education (MSN); nursing informatics (MSN). *Program availability:* Part-time, online learning. *Faculty:* 11 full-time (all women), 6 part-time/adjunct (all women). *Students:* 23 full-time (20 women), 142 part-time (125 women); includes 27 minority (19 Black or African American, non-Hispanic/Latino; 4 Hispanic/Latino; 4 Two or more races, non-Hispanic/Latino). Average age 35. 25 applicants, 76% accepted, 14 enrolled. In 2015, 67 master's awarded. *Degree requirements:* For master's, comprehensive exam. *Entrance requirements:* For master's, minimum GPA of 3.0, RN license eligibility, 3 letters of recommendation. Additional exam requirements/recommendations for international students: Required— TOEFL (minimum score 500 paper-based). *Application deadline:* For fall admission, 8/3 priority date for domestic students. Applications are processed on a rolling basis. Application fee: $25. Electronic applications accepted. *Expenses:* Tuition, state

resident: full-time $8080; part-time $404 per credit hour. Tuition, nonresident: full-time $21,680; part-time $1084 per credit hour. *Required fees:* $1453; $72.65 per credit hour. *Financial support:* In 2015–16, research assistantships with full tuition reimbursements (averaging $5,184 per year) were awarded; career-related internships or fieldwork, Federal Work-Study, institutionally sponsored loans, scholarships/grants, and unspecified assistantships also available. Support available to part-time students. Financial award application deadline: 3/1; financial award applicants required to submit FAFSA. *Unit head:* Dr. Grace Moodt, Interim Director, 931-221-6290, Fax: 931-221-7595, E-mail: moodtg@apsu.edu. *Application contact:* June D. Lee, Graduate Coordinator, 800-859-4723, Fax: 931-221-7641, E-mail: gradadmissions@apsu.edu.
Website: http://www.apsu.edu/nursing

Columbus State University, Graduate Studies, College of Education and Health Professions, School of Nursing, Columbus, GA 31907-5645. Offers family nurse practitioner (MSN); nursing (MSN), including nurse educator, nurse informatics, nurse

Nursing Informatics

leader. Program offered in collaboration with Georgia Southwestern University. *Program availability:* Part-time, online only, 100% online. *Faculty:* 7 full-time (all women), 1 part-time/adjunct (0 women). *Students:* 29 full-time (24 women), 44 part-time (43 women); includes 35 minority (25 Black or African American, non-Hispanic/Latino; 1 Asian, non-Hispanic/Latino; 3 Hispanic/Latino; 6 Two or more races, non-Hispanic/Latino). Average age 38. 66 applicants, 59% accepted, 32 enrolled. In 2015, 6 master's awarded. *Entrance requirements:* For master's, GRE, BSN, minimum undergraduate GPA of 3.0. Additional exam requirements/recommendations for international students: Required—TOEFL (minimum score 550 paper-based; 79 iBT). *Application deadline:* For fall admission, 5/1 for domestic and international students; for spring admission, 11/1 for domestic and international students; for summer admission, 3/1 for domestic and international students. Applications are processed on a rolling basis. Application fee: $50. Electronic applications accepted. *Expenses:* Contact institution. *Financial support:* In 2015–16, 51 students received support. Institutionally sponsored loans available. Financial award application deadline: 5/1; financial award applicants required to submit FAFSA. *Unit head:* Latonya Sanot, Interim Director, 706-507-8576, E-mail: santo_latonya@columbusstate.edu. *Application contact:* Kristin Williams, Director of International and Graduate Recruitment, 706-507-8848, Fax: 706-568-5091, E-mail: williams_kristin@columbusstate.edu.
Website: http://nursing.columbusstate.edu/

Duke University, School of Nursing, Durham, NC 27708-0586. Offers acute care pediatric nurse practitioner (MSN, Post Master's Certificate); adult-gerontology nurse practitioner (MSN, Post Master's Certificate), including acute care, primary care; family nurse practitioner (MSN, Post Master's Certificate); neonatal nurse practitioner (MSN, Post Master's Certificate); nurse anesthesia (DNP); nurse practitioner (DNP); nursing (PhD); nursing and health care leadership (MSN); nursing education (MSN); nursing informatics (MSN, Post Master's Certificate); pediatric nurse practitioner (MSN, Post Master's Certificate), including primary care; women's health nurse practitioner (MSN, Post Master's Certificate). *Accreditation:* AACN; AANA/CANAEP. *Program availability:* Part-time, evening/weekend, online learning. *Faculty:* 74 full-time (63 women). *Students:* 179 full-time (152 women), 528 part-time (466 women); includes 145 minority (42 Black or African American, non-Hispanic/Latino; 3 American Indian or Alaska Native, non-Hispanic/Latino; 44 Asian, non-Hispanic/Latino; 35 Hispanic/Latino; 1 Native Hawaiian or other Pacific Islander, non-Hispanic/Latino; 20 Two or more races, non-Hispanic/Latino), 7 international. Average age 33. 619 applicants, 46% accepted, 201 enrolled. In 2015, 243 master's, 62 doctorates, 26 other advanced degrees awarded. Terminal master's awarded for partial completion of doctoral program. *Degree requirements:* For master's, thesis optional; for doctorate, capstone project. *Entrance requirements:* For master's, GRE General Test (waived if undergraduate GPA of 3.4 or higher), 1 year of nursing experience (recommended), BSN, minimum GPA of 3.0, previous course work in statistics; for doctorate, GRE General Test (waived if undergraduate GPA of 3.4 or higher), BSN or MSN, minimum GPA of 3.0, portfolio, resume, personal statement, undergraduate statistics course, current licensure as a registered nurse, transcripts from all post-secondary institutions; for Post Master's Certificate, MSN, licensure or eligibility as a professional nurse, transcripts from all post-secondary institutions, previous course work in statistics. Additional exam requirements/recommendations for international students: Required—TOEFL (minimum score 100 iBT), IELTS (minimum score 7). *Application deadline:* For fall admission, 12/1 for domestic and international students; for spring admission, 5/1 for domestic and international students. Application fee: $50. Electronic applications accepted. *Expenses:* Contact institution. *Financial support:* Career-related internships or fieldwork, institutionally sponsored loans, scholarships/grants, traineeships, and tuition waivers (partial) available. Support available to part-time students. Financial award applicants required to submit FAFSA. *Faculty research:* Cardiovascular disease, caregiver skill training, data mining, prostate cancer, neonatal immune system. *Unit head:* Dr. Marion E. Broome, Dean/Vice Chancellor for Nursing Affairs/Associate Vice President for Academic Affairs for Nursing, 919-684-9446, Fax: 919-684-9414, E-mail: marion.broome@duke.edu. *Application contact:* Dr. Ernie Rushing, Director of Admissions and Recruitment, 919-668-6274, Fax: 919-668-4693, E-mail: ernie.rushing@dm.duke.edu.
Website: http://www.nursing.duke.edu/

Emporia State University, Program in Informatics, Emporia, KS 66801-5415. Offers nursing (MS). *Program availability:* Part-time, 100% online. *Faculty:* 9 full-time (5 women). *Students:* 8 part-time (7 women); includes 3 minority (2 Black or African American, non-Hispanic/Latino; 1 Hispanic/Latino). 8 applicants, 100% accepted, 8 enrolled. *Degree requirements:* For master's, practicum. *Entrance requirements:* Additional exam requirements/recommendations for international students: Required—TOEFL. *Application deadline:* Applications are processed on a rolling basis. Application fee: $40. Electronic applications accepted. *Expenses:* Tuition, state resident: full-time $5640; part-time $235 per credit hour. Tuition, nonresident: full-time $17,544; part-time $731 per credit hour. *Required fees:* $1848; $77 per credit hour. *Unit head:* Dr. Mirah Dow, Interim Dean, 620-341-5203, E-mail: mdow@emporia.edu. *Application contact:* April Huddleston, Recruitment and Development Specialist, 800-950-GRAD, Fax: 620-341-5909, E-mail: ahuddles@emporia.edu.

Excelsior College, School of Nursing, Albany, NY 12203-5159. Offers nursing (MS); nursing education (MS); nursing informatics (MS); nursing leadership and administration of health care systems (MS). *Accreditation:* ACEN. *Program availability:* Part-time, evening/weekend, online learning. *Faculty:* 18 part-time/adjunct (14 women). *Students:* 938 part-time (770 women); includes 295 minority (166 Black or African American, non-Hispanic/Latino; 8 American Indian or Alaska Native, non-Hispanic/Latino; 36 Asian, non-Hispanic/Latino; 60 Hispanic/Latino; 8 Native Hawaiian or other Pacific Islander, non-Hispanic/Latino; 17 Two or more races, non-Hispanic/Latino), 2 international. Average age 45. In 2015, 200 master's awarded. *Entrance requirements:* For master's, RN license. *Application deadline:* Applications are processed on a rolling basis. Application fee: $110. Electronic applications accepted. *Expenses: Tuition, area resident:* Part-time $645 per credit. *Required fees:* $265 per unit. *Financial support:* Scholarships/grants available. *Unit head:* Dr. Barbara Pieper, Associate Dean, Graduate Program in Nursing, 518-464-8500, Fax: 518-464-8777, E-mail: msn@excelsior.edu. *Application contact:* Admissions Counselor, 518-464-8500, Fax: 518-464-8777, E-mail: admissions@excelsior.edu.

Ferris State University, College of Health Professions, School of Nursing, Big Rapids, MI 49307. Offers nursing (MSN); nursing administration (MSN); nursing education (MSN); nursing informatics (MSN). *Accreditation:* ACEN. *Program availability:* Part-time, evening/weekend, 100% online. *Faculty:* 5 full-time (all women), 2 part-time/adjunct (both women). *Students:* 95 part-time (84 women); includes 11 minority (4 Black or African American, non-Hispanic/Latino; 1 American Indian or Alaska Native, non-Hispanic/Latino; 3 Asian, non-Hispanic/Latino; 1 Hispanic/Latino; 1 Native Hawaiian or other Pacific Islander, non-Hispanic/Latino; 1 Two or more races, non-Hispanic/Latino). Average age 39. 23 applicants, 74% accepted, 13 enrolled. In 2015, 15 master's awarded. *Degree requirements:* For master's, comprehensive exam, practicum, practicum project. *Entrance requirements:* For master's, BS in nursing (for nursing education track); BS in nursing or related field (for nursing administration and nursing informatics tracks); registered nurse license, writing sample, letters of reference, 2 years' clinical experience (recommended). Additional exam requirements/recommendations for international students: Required—TOEFL (minimum score 550

paper-based; 61 iBT). *Application deadline:* For fall admission, 4/15 priority date for domestic students; for spring admission, 10/15 for domestic students. Application fee: $0. Electronic applications accepted. Tuition and fees vary according to degree level and program. *Financial support:* In 2015–16, 3 students received support. Fellowships, research assistantships, teaching assistantships, career-related internships or fieldwork, and scholarships/grants available. Financial award application deadline: 4/15; financial award applicants required to submit FAFSA. *Faculty research:* Nursing education, end of life, leadership/education introverts in nursing. *Unit head:* Dr. Susan Owens, Chair, School of Nursing, 231-591-2267, Fax: 231-591-2325, E-mail: owenss3@ferris.edu. *Application contact:* Debby Buck, Off-Campus Program Secretary, 231-591-2270, Fax: 231-591-3788, E-mail: buckd@ferris.edu.
Website: http://www.ferris.edu/htmls/colleges/alliedhe/Nursing/homepage.htm

Georgia State University, Byrdine F. Lewis School of Nursing, Atlanta, GA 30303. Offers adult health clinical nurse specialist/nurse practitioner (MS, Certificate); child health clinical nurse specialist/pediatric nurse practitioner (MS, Certificate); family nurse practitioner (MS, Certificate); family psychiatric mental health nurse practitioner (MS, Certificate); nursing (PhD); nursing leadership in healthcare innovations (MS), including nursing administration, nursing informatics; nutrition (MS); perinatal clinical nurse specialist/women's health nurse practitioner (MS, Certificate); physical therapy (DPT); respiratory therapy (MS). *Accreditation:* AACN. *Program availability:* Part-time, blended/hybrid learning. *Faculty:* 18 full-time (11 women). *Students:* 275 full-time (195 women), 230 part-time (204 women); includes 192 minority (123 Black or African American, non-Hispanic/Latino; 49 Asian, non-Hispanic/Latino; 12 Hispanic/Latino; 2 Native Hawaiian or other Pacific Islander, non-Hispanic/Latino; 6 Two or more races, non-Hispanic/Latino), 35 international. Average age 33. 240 applicants, 61% accepted, 95 enrolled. In 2015, 115 master's, 40 doctorates, 19 other advanced degrees awarded. *Degree requirements:* For doctorate, comprehensive exam, thesis/dissertation. *Entrance requirements:* For doctorate, GRE. Additional exam requirements/recommendations for international students: Required—TOEFL. *Application deadline:* For fall admission, 2/1 priority date for domestic and international students; for spring admission, 9/15 for domestic and international students. Applications are processed on a rolling basis. Application fee: $50. Electronic applications accepted. *Expenses:* Contact institution. *Financial support:* In 2015–16, research assistantships with tuition reimbursements (averaging $1,666 per year), teaching assistantships with tuition reimbursements (averaging $1,920 per year) were awarded; scholarships/grants, tuition waivers (full and partial), and unspecified assistantships also available. Support available to part-time students. Financial award application deadline: 8/1; financial award applicants required to submit FAFSA. *Faculty research:* Stroke intervention for caregivers, stroke prevention in African-Americans; relationships between psychological distress and health outcomes in parents with a medically ill infant; medically fragile children; nursing expertise and patient outcomes. *Unit head:* Nancy Kropf, Dean of Nursing, 404-413-1101, Fax: 404-413-1090, E-mail: nkropf@gsu.edu.
Website: http://nursing.gsu.edu/

Grantham University, College of Nursing and Allied Health, Lenexa, KS 66219. Offers case management (MSN); health systems management (MHSM, MSN); healthcare administration (MHA); nursing education (MSN); nursing informatics (MSN); nursing management and organizational leadership (MSN). *Program availability:* Part-time, evening/weekend, online only, 100% online. *Faculty:* 1 (woman) full-time, 15 part-time/adjunct (11 women). *Students:* 59 full-time (42 women), 368 part-time (277 women); includes 181 minority (119 Black or African American, non-Hispanic/Latino; 2 American Indian or Alaska Native, non-Hispanic/Latino; 23 Asian, non-Hispanic/Latino; 21 Hispanic/Latino; 4 Native Hawaiian or other Pacific Islander, non-Hispanic/Latino; 12 Two or more races, non-Hispanic/Latino). Average age 41. 498 applicants, 94% accepted, 427 enrolled. In 2015, 119 master's awarded. *Degree requirements:* For master's, capstone. *Entrance requirements:* For master's, bachelor's degree from accredited degree-granting institution with minimum GPA of 2.5, BSN from accredited nursing program, valid RN license. Additional exam requirements/recommendations for international students: Required—TOEFL (minimum score 71 iBT); Recommended—IELTS (minimum score 6.5), TSE (minimum score 50). *Application deadline:* Applications are processed on a rolling basis. Electronic applications accepted. *Expenses: Tuition, area resident:* Full-time $3900; part-time $325 per credit hour. *Required fees:* $45 per term. One-time fee: $100. *Financial support:* Scholarships/grants available. *Faculty research:* Experimental exploration of the use of human patient simulation in the theory course, simulation education's impact on nursing confidence in the care of patients with Ebola virus, women's health-smoking cessation program for pregnant women, nursing and healthcare administration, business administration in healthcare. *Unit head:* Dana Basara, Dean, College of Nursing and Allied Health, 913-309-4783, Fax: 844-897-6490, E-mail: dbasara@grantham.edu. *Application contact:* Jared Parlette, Vice President of Student Enrollment, 888-947-2684, Fax: 866-908-2360, E-mail: admissions@grantham.edu.
Website: http://www.grantham.edu/colleges-and-schools/college-of-nursing-and-allied-health/

Le Moyne College, Department of Nursing, Syracuse, NY 13214. Offers informatics (MS, CAS); nursing administration (MS, CAS); nursing education (MS, CAS); nursing gerontology (MS, CAS); palliative care (MS, CAS). *Accreditation:* ACEN. *Program availability:* Part-time, evening/weekend. *Degree requirements:* For master's, scholarly project. *Entrance requirements:* For master's, bachelor's degree, interview, minimum GPA of 3.0, New York RN license, 2 letters of recommendation, writing sample, transcripts. *Expenses:* Contact institution. *Faculty research:* Inter-profession education, gerontology, utilization of free healthcare services by the insured, health promotion education, innovative undergraduate nursing education models, patient and family education, horizontal violence.

National University, Academic Affairs, School of Health and Human Services, La Jolla, CA 92037-1011. Offers clinical affairs (MS); clinical informatics (Certificate); clinical regulatory affairs (MS); health and life science analytics (MS); health coaching (Certificate); health informatics (MS); healthcare administration (MHA); nurse anesthesia (MS); nursing (MS), including forensic nursing, nursing administration, nursing informatics; nursing administration (Certificate); nursing informatics (Certificate); nursing practice (DNP); public health (MPH), including health promotion, healthcare administration, mental health. *Program availability:* Part-time, evening/weekend, 100% online, blended/hybrid learning. *Faculty:* 31 full-time (18 women), 33 part-time/adjunct (20 women). *Students:* 353 full-time (263 women), 136 part-time (87 women); includes 322 minority (111 Black or African American, non-Hispanic/Latino; 1 American Indian or Alaska Native, non-Hispanic/Latino; 105 Asian, non-Hispanic/Latino; 72 Hispanic/Latino; 7 Native Hawaiian or other Pacific Islander, non-Hispanic/Latino; 26 Two or more races, non-Hispanic/Latino), 31 international. Average age 32. In 2015, 103 master's awarded. *Degree requirements:* For master's, thesis (for some programs). *Entrance requirements:* For master's, interview, minimum GPA of 2.5. Additional exam requirements/recommendations for international students: Required—TOEFL (minimum score 550 paper-based; 79 iBT), IELTS (minimum score 6). *Application deadline:* Applications are processed on a rolling basis. Application fee: $60 ($65 for international students). Electronic applications accepted. *Financial support:* Career-related internships or fieldwork, institutionally sponsored loans, scholarships/grants, and tuition waivers (partial) available. Support available to part-time students. Financial award application deadline: 6/30; financial award applicants required to submit FAFSA. *Faculty research:* Nursing education, obesity prevention, workforce diversity. *Unit head:* School of Health and Human Services, 800-628-8648, E-mail: shhs@nu.edu. *Application contact:* Frank Rojas, Vice President for Enrollment Services, 800-628-8648, E-mail: advisor@nu.edu. Website: http://www.nu.edu/OurPrograms/SchoolOfHealthAndHumanServices.html

New York University, Rory Meyers College of Nursing, Programs in Advanced Practice Nursing, New York, NY 10012-1019. Offers adult-gerontology acute care nurse practitioner (MS, Advanced Certificate); adult-gerontology primary care nurse practitioner (MS, Advanced Certificate); family nurse practitioner (MS, Advanced Certificate); gerontology nurse practitioner (Advanced Certificate); nurse-midwifery (MS, Advanced Certificate); nursing administration (MS, Advanced Certificate); nursing education (MS, Advanced Certificate); nursing informatics (MS, Advanced Certificate); pediatrics nurse practitioner (MS, Advanced Certificate); psychiatric-mental health nurse practitioner (MS, Advanced Certificate); MS/MPH. *Accreditation:* AACN; ACNM/ACME. *Program availability:* Part-time. *Faculty:* 24 full-time (all women), 76 part-time/adjunct (65 women). *Students:* 46 full-time (26 women), 586 part-time (513 women); includes 242 minority (68 Black or African American, non-Hispanic/Latino; 3 American Indian or Alaska Native, non-Hispanic/Latino; 117 Asian, non-Hispanic/Latino; 38 Hispanic/Latino; 3 Native Hawaiian or other Pacific Islander, non-Hispanic/Latino; 13 Two or more races, non-Hispanic/Latino), 23 international. Average age 32. 402 applicants, 69% accepted, 138 enrolled. In 2015, 198 master's, 5 other advanced degrees awarded. *Degree requirements:* For master's, thesis (for some programs). *Entrance requirements:* For master's, BS in nursing, AS in nursing with another BS/BA, interview, RN license, 1 year of clinical experience (3 for the MS in nursing education program); for Advanced Certificate, master's degree. Additional exam requirements/recommendations for international students: Required—TOEFL (minimum score 90 iBT), IELTS (minimum score 7). *Application deadline:* For fall admission, 6/15 for domestic and international students; for spring admission, 12/1 for domestic and international students; for summer admission, 3/1 for domestic and international students. Application fee: $80. Electronic applications accepted. *Expenses:* Contact institution. *Financial support:* In 2015–16, 101 students received support. Career-related internships or fieldwork, Federal Work-Study, and scholarships/grants available. Support available to part-time students. Financial award application deadline: 3/1; financial award applicants required to submit FAFSA. *Faculty research:* Geriatrics, HIV, families and illness, oral systemic connection, symptom management. *Unit head:* Dr. James Pace, Senior Associate Dean for Academic Programs, 212-992-7343, E-mail: james.pace@nyu.edu. *Application contact:* Samantha Jaser, Assistant Director, Graduate Student Affairs and Admissions, 212-992-7653, Fax: 212-995-4302, E-mail: saj283@nyu.edu.

Rutgers University–Newark, Rutgers School of Nursing, Program in Nursing Informatics - Newark, Newark, NJ 07102. Offers MSN. Program offered jointly with New Jersey Institute of Technology. *Entrance requirements:* Additional exam requirements/recommendations for international students: Required—TOEFL. Electronic applications accepted.

Rutgers University–Newark, Rutgers School of Nursing, Program in Nursing Informatics - Stratford, Newark, NJ 07102. Offers MSN. Program offered jointly with New Jersey Institute of Technology. *Entrance requirements:* Additional exam requirements/recommendations for international students: Required—TOEFL. Electronic applications accepted.

Seattle Pacific University, MS in Nursing Program, Seattle, WA 98119-1997. Offers administration (MSN); adult/gerontology nurse practitioner (MSN); clinical nurse specialist (MSN); family nurse practitioner (MSN, Certificate); informatics (MSN); nurse educator (MSN). *Accreditation:* AACN. *Program availability:* Part-time. *Students:* 39 full-time (36 women), 30 part-time (25 women); includes 14 minority (3 Black or African American, non-Hispanic/Latino; 7 Asian, non-Hispanic/Latino; 3 Hispanic/Latino; 1 Two or more races, non-Hispanic/Latino), 1 international. Average age 38. 60 applicants, 48% accepted, 29 enrolled. In 2015, 23 master's awarded. *Degree requirements:* For master's, thesis. *Entrance requirements:* For master's, personal statement, transcripts, undergraduate nursing degree, proof of undergraduate statistics course with minimum GPA of 2.0, 2 recommendations. *Application deadline:* For fall admission, 1/15 priority date for domestic students; for spring admission, 1/15 for domestic students. Applications are processed on a rolling basis. Application fee: $50. Electronic applications accepted. *Expenses:* Contact institution. *Financial support:* Fellowships and scholarships/grants available. Financial award applicants required to submit FAFSA. *Unit head:* Dr. Christine Hoyle, Associate Dean, 206-281-2469, E-mail: hoylec@spu.edu. Website: http://spu.edu/depts/health-sciences/grad/index.asp

Tennessee Technological University, Whitson-Hester School of Nursing, Cookeville, TN 38505. Offers family nurse practitioner (MSN); informatics (MSN); nursing administration (MSN); nursing education (MSN). *Program availability:* Part-time, evening/weekend, online learning. *Students:* 21 full-time (20 women), 95 part-time (80 women); includes 5 minority (2 Black or African American, non-Hispanic/Latino; 1 Asian, non-Hispanic/Latino; 1 Hispanic/Latino; 1 Two or more races, non-Hispanic/Latino). 42 applicants, 57% accepted, 15 enrolled. In 2015, 47 master's awarded. *Degree requirements:* For master's, comprehensive exam, thesis or alternative. *Entrance requirements:* Additional exam requirements/recommendations for international students: Required—TOEFL (minimum score 600 paper-based; 100 iBT), IELTS (minimum score 5.5), PTE, or TOEIC (Test of English as an International Communication). *Application deadline:* For fall admission, 8/1 for domestic students, 5/1 for international students; for spring admission, 12/1 for domestic students, 10/1 for international students; for summer admission, 5/1 for domestic students, 2/1 for international students. Applications are processed on a rolling basis. Application fee: $35 ($40 for international students). Electronic applications accepted. *Expenses:* Tuition, state resident: full-time $8961; part-time $6132 per credit hour. Tuition, nonresident: full-time $23,121; part-time $14,608 per credit hour. *Financial support:* Application deadline: 4/1. *Unit head:* Dr. Huey-Ming Tzeng, Dean, 931-372-3547, Fax: 931-372-6244, E-mail: htzeng@tntech.edu. *Application contact:* Shelia K. Kendrick, Coordinator of Graduate Studies, 931-372-3808, Fax: 931-372-3497, E-mail: skendrick@tntech.edu.

Troy University, Graduate School, College of Health and Human Services, Program in Nursing, Troy, AL 36082. Offers adult health (MSN); clinical nurse specialist adult health (DNP); clinical nurse specialist maternal infant (DNP); family nurse practitioner (MSN, DNP, PMC); informatics specialist (MSN); maternal infant (MSN). *Accreditation:* ACEN. *Program availability:* Part-time, evening/weekend. *Faculty:* 13 full-time (12 women), 11 part-time/adjunct (all women). *Students:* 75 full-time (62 women), 202 part-time (179 women); includes 91 minority (72 Black or African American, non-Hispanic/Latino; 1 Asian, non-Hispanic/Latino; 8 Hispanic/Latino; 10 Two or more races, non-Hispanic/Latino). Average age 34. 50 applicants, 96% accepted. In 2015, 43 master's, 13 doctorates, 15 other advanced degrees awarded. *Degree requirements:* For master's, comprehensive exam, minimum GPA of 3.0, candidacy; for doctorate, minimum GPA of 3.0, submission of approved comprehensive e-portfolio, completion of residency synthesis project, minimum of 1000 hours of clinical practice, qualifying exam. *Entrance requirements:* For master's, GRE (minimum score of 850 on old exam or 290 on new exam) or MAT (minimum score of 396), minimum GPA of 3.0, BSN, current RN licensure, 2 letters of reference, undergraduate health assessment course; for doctorate, GRE (minimum score of 850 on old exam or 294 on new exam), BSN or MSN, minimum GPA of 3.0, 2 letters of reference, current RN licensure, essay. Additional exam requirements/recommendations for international students: Required—TOEFL (minimum score 523 paper-based; 70 iBT), IELTS (minimum score 6). *Application deadline:* Applications are processed on a rolling basis. Application fee: $50. Electronic applications accepted. *Expenses:* Tuition, state resident: full-time $7146; part-time $397 per credit hour. Tuition, nonresident: full-time $14,292; part-time $794 per credit hour. *Required fees:* $802. Tuition and fees vary according to campus/location and program. *Financial support:* Fellowships, career-related internships or fieldwork, and scholarships/grants available. Support available to part-time students. Financial award applicants required to submit FAFSA. *Unit head:* Dr. Diane Weed, Director, School of Nursing, 334-670-5864, Fax: 334-670-3745, E-mail: lweed@troy.edu. *Application contact:* Crystal G. Bishop, Director of Graduate Admissions, School of Nursing, 334-241-8631, E-mail: cdgodwin@troy.edu.

The University of North Carolina at Chapel Hill, School of Nursing, Chapel Hill, NC 27599-7460. Offers advanced practice registered nurse (DNP); health care systems (DNP); nursing (MSN, PhD, PMC), including administration (MSN), adult gerontology primary care nurse practitioner (MSN), clinical nurse leader (MSN), education (MSN), informatics (MSN, PMC), nursing leadership (PMC), outcomes management (MSN), primary care family nurse practitioner (MSN), primary care pediatric nurse practitioner (MSN), psychiatric/mental health nurse practitioner (MSN, PMC). *Accreditation:* AACN; ACEN (one or more programs are accredited). *Program availability:* Part-time. *Faculty:* 86 full-time (78 women), 44 part-time/adjunct (40 women). *Students:* 208 full-time (186 women), 128 part-time (116 women); includes 109 minority (49 Black or African American, non-Hispanic/Latino; 4 American Indian or Alaska Native, non-Hispanic/Latino; 32 Asian, non-Hispanic/Latino; 7 Hispanic/Latino; 17 Two or more races, non-Hispanic/Latino), 17 international. Average age 33. 624 applicants, 26% accepted, 150 enrolled. In 2015, 91 master's, 14 doctorates awarded. *Degree requirements:* For master's, comprehensive exam, thesis; for doctorate, thesis/dissertation, 3 exams; for PMC, thesis. *Entrance requirements:* Additional exam requirements/recommendations for international students: Required—TOEFL (minimum score 575 paper-based; 89 iBT), IELTS (minimum score 8). *Application deadline:* For fall admission, 12/15 for domestic and international students. Application fee: $85. Electronic applications accepted. *Financial support:* In 2015–16, 8 fellowships with full tuition reimbursements, 6 research assistantships with partial tuition reimbursements (averaging $8,000 per year), 10 teaching assistantships with partial tuition reimbursements (averaging $8,000 per year) were awarded; scholarships/grants, traineeships, health care benefits, and unspecified assistantships also available. Support available to part-time students. Financial award application deadline: 3/1; financial award applicants required to submit FAFSA. *Faculty research:* Preventing and managing chronic illness, reducing health disparities, improving healthcare quality and patient outcomes, understanding biobehavioral and genetic bases of health and illness, developing innovative ways to enhance science and its clinical translation. *Unit head:* Donna S. Havens, PhD, RN, Dean/Professor, 919-966-3731, Fax: 919-966-3540, E-mail: dhavens@email.unc.edu. *Application contact:* Emily Sayed, Assistant Director, Graduate Admissions, 919-966-4260, Fax: 919-966-3540, E-mail: sayed@unc.edu.
Website: http://nursing.unc.edu

University of Phoenix–Bay Area Campus, College of Nursing, San Jose, CA 95134-1805. Offers education (MHA); gerontology (MHA); health administration (MHA, DHA); informatics (MHA, MSN); nursing (MSN, PhD); nursing/health care education (MSN); MSN/MBA. *Program availability:* Evening/weekend, online learning. *Degree requirements:* For master's, thesis (for some programs). *Entrance requirements:* For master's, minimum undergraduate GPA of 2.5, 3 years of work experience, RN license. Additional exam requirements/recommendations for international students: Required—TOEFL (minimum score 550 paper-based; 79 iBT). Electronic applications accepted.

University of Phoenix–Charlotte Campus, College of Nursing, Charlotte, NC 28273-3409. Offers education (MHA); gerontology (MHA); health administration (MHA); informatics (MHA, MSN); nursing (MSN); nursing/health care education (MSN). *Program availability:* Evening/weekend. *Degree requirements:* For master's, thesis (for some programs). *Entrance requirements:* For master's, minimum undergraduate GPA of 2.5, 3 years work experience. Additional exam requirements/recommendations for international students: Required—TOEFL (minimum score 550 paper-based; 79 iBT). Electronic applications accepted.

University of Phoenix–Phoenix Campus, College of Health Sciences and Nursing, Tempe, AZ 85282-2371. Offers family nurse practitioner (MSN, Certificate); gerontology health care (Certificate); health care education (MSN, Certificate); health care informatics (Certificate); informatics (MSN); nursing (MSN); MSN/MHA. *Program availability:* Evening/weekend, online learning. *Entrance requirements:* Additional exam requirements/recommendations for international students: Required—TOEFL, TOEIC (Test of English as an International Communication), Berlitz Online English Proficiency Exam, PTE, or IELTS. Electronic applications accepted. *Expenses:* Contact institution.

University of Phoenix–Southern California Campus, College of Health Sciences and Nursing, Costa Mesa, CA 92626. Offers family nurse practitioner (MSN, Certificate); health care (Certificate); informatics (MSN); nursing (MSN); nursing/health care education (MSN, Certificate); MSN/MBA; MSN/MHA. *Program availability:* Evening/weekend, online learning. *Entrance requirements:* Additional exam requirements/recommendations for international students: Required—TOEFL, TOEIC (Test of English as an International Communication), Berlitz Online English Proficiency Exam, PTE, or IELTS. Electronic applications accepted. *Expenses:* Contact institution.

University of Phoenix–Washington D.C. Campus, College of Nursing, Washington, DC 20001. Offers education (MHA); gerontology (MHA); health administration (MHA, DHA); informatics (MHA, MSN); nursing (MSN, PhD); nursing/health care education (MSN); MSN/MBA; MSN/MHA.

University of Pittsburgh, School of Nursing, Nurse Specialty Role Program, Pittsburgh, PA 15260. Offers clinical nurse leader (MSN); nursing administration (DNP); nursing informatics (MSN). *Accreditation:* AACN. *Program availability:* Part-time. *Students:* 4 full-time (2 women), 67 part-time (54 women); includes 5 minority (3 Black or African American, non-Hispanic/Latino; 2 Asian, non-Hispanic/Latino), 2 international. Average age 36. 24 applicants, 63% accepted, 12 enrolled. In 2015, 14 master's, 11 doctorates awarded. *Degree requirements:* For master's, comprehensive exam, thesis optional. *Entrance requirements:* For master's, GRE or MAT, BSN, RN license, 3 letters of recommendation, personal essay, resume, course work in statistics, 1-3 years of nursing experience; for doctorate, BSN/MSN, RN license, 3 letters of recommendation, personal essay, resume, course work in statistics, 1-3 years of nursing experience. Additional exam requirements/recommendations for international students: Required—TOEFL (minimum score 600 paper-based; 100 iBT). *Application deadline:* For fall admission, 5/1 priority date for domestic students, 2/15 priority date for international students. Application fee: $50. Electronic applications accepted. *Expenses:* Contact institution. *Financial support:* In 2015–16, 1 student received support, including 1 fellowship with tuition reimbursement available (averaging $9,125 per year). Financial award application deadline: 3/15. *Faculty research:* Behavioral management of chronic disorders, patient management in critical care, consumer informatics, genetic

Nursing Informatics

applications (molecular genetics and psychosocial implications), technology for nurses and patients to improve care. *Unit head:* Dr. Sandra Engberg, Associate Dean for Clinical Education, 412-624-3835, Fax: 412-624-8521, E-mail: sje1@pitt.edu. *Application contact:* Laurie Lapsley, Administrator of Graduate Student Services, 412-624-9670, Fax: 412-624-2409, E-mail: lapsleyl@pitt.edu.
Website: http://www.nursing.pitt.edu/

Vanderbilt University, Vanderbilt University School of Nursing, Nashville, TN 37240. Offers adult-gerontology acute care nurse practitioner (MSN), including hospitalist, intensivist; adult-gerontology primary care nurse practitioner (MSN); emergency nurse practitioner (MSN); family nurse practitioner (MSN); healthcare leadership (MSN); neonatal nurse practitioner (MSN); nurse midwifery (MSN); nurse midwifery/family nurse practitioner (MSN); nursing (Post-Master's Certificate); nursing informatics (MSN); nursing practice (DNP); nursing science (PhD); pediatric acute care nurse practitioner (MSN); pediatric primary care nurse practitioner (MSN); psychiatric-mental health nurse practitioner (MSN); women's health nurse practitioner (MSN); women's health nurse practitioner/adult gerontology primary care nurse practitioner (MSN); MSN/M Div; MSN/MTS. *Accreditation:* ACEN (one or more programs are accredited); ACNM/ACME. *Program availability:* Part-time, 100% online, blended/hybrid learning. *Faculty:* 258 full-time (232 women), 363 part-time/adjunct (271 women). *Students:* 478 full-time (424 women), 342 part-time (317 women); includes 140 minority (36 Black or African American, non-Hispanic/Latino; 3 American Indian or Alaska Native, non-Hispanic/Latino; 24 Asian, non-Hispanic/Latino; 43 Hispanic/Latino; 3 Native Hawaiian or other Pacific Islander, non-Hispanic/Latino; 31 Two or more races, non-Hispanic/Latino), 11 international. Average age 31. 1,268 applicants, 49% accepted, 477 enrolled. In 2015, 343 master's, 55 doctorates awarded. *Degree requirements:* For doctorate, comprehensive exam, thesis/dissertation. *Entrance requirements:* For master's, GRE General Test (taken within the past 5 years), minimum B average in undergraduate course work, 3 letters of recommendation; for doctorate, GRE General Test, interview, 3 letters of recommendation from doctorally-prepared faculty, MSN, essay. Additional exam requirements/recommendations for international students: Required—TOEFL (minimum score 570 paper-based), IELTS (minimum score 6.5). *Application deadline:* For fall admission, 11/1 priority date for domestic and international students. Applications are processed on a rolling basis. Application fee: $50. Electronic applications accepted. *Expenses:* Contact institution. *Financial support:* In 2015–16, 585 students received support. Scholarships/grants available. Financial award application deadline: 3/15; financial award applicants required to submit FAFSA. *Faculty research:* Lymphedema, palliative care and bereavement, health services research including workforce, safety and quality of care, gerontology, better birth outcomes including nutrition. *Total annual research expenditures:* $2 million. *Unit head:* Dr. Linda Norman, Dean, 615-343-8876, Fax: 615-343-7711, E-mail: linda.norman@vanderbilt.edu. *Application contact:* Patricia Peerman, Assistant Dean for Enrollment Management, 615-322-3800, Fax: 615-343-0333, E-mail: vusn-admissions@vanderbilt.edu.
Website: http://www.nursing.vanderbilt.edu

Walden University, Graduate Programs, School of Nursing, Minneapolis, MN 55401. Offers adult-gerontology acute care nurse practitioner (MSN); adult-gerontology nurse practitioner (MSN); education (MSN); family nurse practitioner (MSN); informatics (MSN); leadership and management (MSN); nursing (PhD, Post-Master's Certificate), including education (PhD), healthcare administration (PhD), interdisciplinary health (PhD), leadership (PhD), nursing education (Post-Master's Certificate), nursing informatics (Post-Master's Certificate), nursing leadership and management (Post-Master's Certificate), public health policy (PhD); nursing practice (DNP); psychiatric mental health (MSN). *Accreditation:* AACN. *Program availability:* Part-time, evening/weekend, online only, 100% online. *Faculty:* 22 full-time (18 women), 540 part-time/adjunct (487 women). *Students:* 4,320 full-time (3,773 women), 5,250 part-time (4,740 women); includes 3,550 minority (2,360 Black or African American, non-Hispanic/Latino; 29 American Indian or Alaska Native, non-Hispanic/Latino; 523 Asian, non-Hispanic/Latino; 421 Hispanic/Latino; 25 Native Hawaiian or other Pacific Islander, non-Hispanic/Latino; 192 Two or more races, non-Hispanic/Latino), 221 international. Average age 40. 2,057 applicants, 100% accepted, 1507 enrolled. In 2015, 3,022 master's, 86 doctorates, 34 other advanced degrees awarded. *Degree requirements:* For doctorate, thesis/dissertation (for some programs), residency (for some programs), field experience (for some programs). *Entrance requirements:* For master's, bachelor's degree or equivalent in related field or RN; minimum GPA of 2.5; official transcripts; goal statement (for some programs); access to computer and Internet; for doctorate, master's degree or higher; RN; three years of related professional or academic experience; goal statement; access to computer and Internet; for Post-Master's Certificate, relevant work experience; access to computer and Internet. Additional exam requirements/recommendations for international students: Required—TOEFL (minimum score 550 paper-based, 79 iBT), IELTS (minimum score 6.5), Michigan English Language Assessment Battery (minimum score 82), or PTE (minimum score 53). *Application deadline:* Applications are processed on a rolling basis. Application fee: $0. Electronic applications accepted. *Financial support:* Fellowships, Federal Work-Study, scholarships/grants, unspecified assistantships, and family tuition reduction, active duty/veteran tuition reduction, group tuition reduction, interest-free payment plans, employee tuition reduction available. Support available to part-time students. Financial award applicants required to submit FAFSA. *Unit head:* Dr. Andrea Lindell, Dean, 866-492-5336. *Application contact:* Meghan Thomas, Vice President of Enrollment Management, 866-492-5336, E-mail: info@waldenu.edu.
Website: http://www.waldenu.edu/programs/colleges-schools/nursing

Waynesburg University, Graduate and Professional Studies, Canonsburg, PA 15370. Offers business (MBA), including energy management, finance, health systems, human resources, leadership, market development; counseling (MA), including addictions counseling, clinical mental health; counselor education and supervision (PhD); criminal investigation (MA); education (M Ed), including autism, curriculum and instruction, educational leadership, online teaching; nursing (MSN), including administration, education, informatics; nursing practice (DNP); special education (M Ed); technology (M Ed); MSN/MBA. *Accreditation:* AACN. *Program availability:* Part-time, evening/weekend. *Degree requirements:* For doctorate, thesis/dissertation. *Entrance requirements:* Additional exam requirements/recommendations for international students: Required—TOEFL. Electronic applications accepted.

Occupational Health Nursing

Rutgers University–Newark, Rutgers School of Nursing, Newark, NJ 07107-3001. Offers adult health (MSN); adult occupational health (MSN); advanced practice nursing (MSN, Post Master's Certificate); family nurse practitioner (MSN); nurse anesthesia (MSN); nursing (MSN); nursing informatics (MSN); urban health (PhD); women's health practitioner (MSN). *Accreditation:* AANA/CANAEP. *Program availability:* Part-time. *Entrance requirements:* For master's, GRE, RN license; basic life support, statistics, and health assessment experience. Additional exam requirements/recommendations for international students: Required—TOEFL. Electronic applications accepted. *Expenses:* Contact institution. *Faculty research:* HIV/AIDS, diabetes education, learned helplessness, nursing science, psychoeducation.

University of Cincinnati, Graduate School, College of Nursing, Cincinnati, OH 45221-0038. Offers clinical nurse specialist (MSN), including adult health, community health, neonatal, nursing administration, occupational health, pediatric health, psychiatric nursing, women's health; nurse anesthesia (MSN); nurse midwifery (MSN); nurse practitioner (MSN), including acute care, ambulatory care, family, family/psychiatric, women's health; nursing (PhD); MBA/MSN. *Accreditation:* AACN; AANA/CANAEP (one or more programs are accredited); ACNM/ACME. *Program availability:* Part-time, online learning. Terminal master's awarded for partial completion of doctoral program. *Degree requirements:* For master's, thesis or alternative; for doctorate, comprehensive exam, thesis/dissertation. *Entrance requirements:* For master's and doctorate, GRE General Test. Additional exam requirements/recommendations for international students: Required—TOEFL (minimum score 520 paper-based). Electronic applications accepted. *Faculty research:* Substance abuse, injury and violence, symptom management.

University of Illinois at Chicago, College of Nursing, Program in Nursing, Chicago, IL 60607-7128. Offers acute care clinical nurse specialist (MS); administrative nursing leadership (Certificate); adult nurse practitioner (MS); adult/geriatric nurse practitioner (MS); advanced community health nurse specialist (MS); family nurse practitioner (MS); geriatric clinical nurse specialist (MS); geriatric nurse practitioner (MS); nurse midwifery (MS); occupational health/advanced community health nurse specialist (MS); occupational health/family nurse practitioner (MS); pediatric nurse practitioner (MS); perinatal clinical nurse specialist (MS); school/advanced community health nurse specialist (MS); school/family nurse practitioner (MS); women's health nurse practitioner (MS). *Accreditation:* AACN. *Program availability:* Part-time. *Faculty:* 100 full-time (93 women), 89 part-time/adjunct (82 women). *Students:* 359 full-time (326 women), 280 part-time (249 women); includes 169 minority (43 Black or African American, non-Hispanic/Latino; 62 Asian, non-Hispanic/Latino; 56 Hispanic/Latino; 1 Native Hawaiian or other Pacific Islander, non-Hispanic/Latino; 7 Two or more races, non-Hispanic/Latino), 12 international. Average age 32. In 2015, 4 other advanced degrees awarded. *Degree requirements:* For master's, thesis or alternative. *Entrance requirements:* For master's, GRE General Test, minimum GPA of 2.75. Additional exam requirements/recommendations for international students: Required—TOEFL. *Application deadline:* For fall admission, 5/15 for domestic students, 2/15 for international students; for spring admission, 11/1 for domestic students, 7/15 for international students. Applications are processed on a rolling basis. Application fee: $60. Electronic applications accepted. *Expenses:* Tuition, state resident: full-time $11,480; part-time $3826 per credit. Tuition, nonresident: full-time $23,720; part-time $7906 per credit. *Required fees:* $1333 per semester. Part-time tuition and fees vary according to course load and program.

Financial support: Fellowships with full tuition reimbursements, research assistantships with full tuition reimbursements, teaching assistantships with full tuition reimbursements, career-related internships or fieldwork, Federal Work-Study, institutionally sponsored loans, scholarships/grants, traineeships, tuition waivers (full and partial), and unspecified assistantships available. Support available to part-time students. Financial award application deadline: 3/1; financial award applicants required to submit FAFSA. *Unit head:* Dr. Terri E. Weaver, Dean, 312-996-7808, E-mail: teweaver@uic.edu. *Application contact:* Receptionist, 312-413-2550, E-mail: gradcoll@uic.edu.
Website: http://www.nursing.uic.edu/academics-admissions/master-science#program-overview

University of Minnesota, Twin Cities Campus, School of Public Health, Division of Environmental Health Sciences, Area in Occupational Health Nursing, Minneapolis, MN 55455-0213. Offers MPH, MS, PhD, MPH/MS. *Accreditation:* AACN. *Degree requirements:* For doctorate, thesis/dissertation. *Entrance requirements:* For master's and doctorate, GRE General Test. Electronic applications accepted.

The University of North Carolina at Chapel Hill, Graduate School, Gillings School of Global Public Health, Public Health Leadership Program, Chapel Hill, NC 27599. Offers health care and prevention (MPH); leadership (MPH); occupational health nursing (MPH). *Program availability:* Part-time, online learning. *Students:* 157 full-time (105 women); includes 67 minority (27 Black or African American, non-Hispanic/Latino; 16 Asian, non-Hispanic/Latino; 15 Hispanic/Latino; 9 Two or more races, non-Hispanic/Latino), 9 international. Average age 35. 78 applicants, 95% accepted, 54 enrolled. *Degree requirements:* For master's, comprehensive exam, thesis (MS), paper (MPH). *Entrance requirements:* For master's, GRE General Test, minimum GPA of 3.0 (recommended), public health experience. *Financial support:* Career-related internships or fieldwork, institutionally sponsored loans, traineeships, and health care benefits available. Financial award application deadline: 12/10; financial award applicants required to submit FAFSA. *Faculty research:* Occupational health issues, clinical outcomes, prenatal and early childcare, adolescent health, effectiveness of home visiting, issues in occupational health nursing, community-based interventions. *Unit head:* Dr. Anna Schenck, Director, 919-843-8546, E-mail: anna.schenck@unc.edu. *Application contact:* Sue Robeson, Student Services Manager, 919-966-5305, Fax: 919-966-0981, E-mail: robeson@email.unc.edu.
Website: http://www2.sph.unc.edu/phlp/

University of South Florida, College of Nursing, Tampa, FL 33612. Offers advanced pain management (Graduate Certificate); nursing (MS, DNP), including adult gerontology acute care (DNP), adult gerontology acute care nursing (MS), adult gerontology primary care (DNP), adult gerontology primary care nursing (MS), adult gerontology primary care/occupational health nursing (MS), adult gerontology primary care/oncology nursing (MS), clinical nurse leader (MS), family health nursing, nurse anesthesia (MS), nursing education (MS), nursing practice (DNP), occupational health/adult-gerontology (DNP), oncology/adult-gerontology primary care (DNP), pediatric health (DNP), pediatric nurse practitioner (MS); nursing education (Post Master's Certificate); nursing science (PhD). *Accreditation:* AACN; AANA/CANAEP. *Program availability:* Part-time. *Faculty:* 43 full-time (38 women), 7 part-time/adjunct (4 women). *Students:* 159 full-time (135 women), 721 part-time (625 women); includes 292 minority (119 Black or African American, non-Hispanic/Latino; 2 American Indian or Alaska

Native, non-Hispanic/Latino; 60 Asian, non-Hispanic/Latino; 90 Hispanic/Latino; 1 Native Hawaiian or other Pacific Islander, non-Hispanic/Latino; 20 Two or more races, non-Hispanic/Latino; 12 international. Average age 35. 636 applicants, 44% accepted, 215 enrolled. In 2015, 333 master's, 18 doctorates awarded. *Degree requirements:* For master's, comprehensive exam, thesis optional; for doctorate, comprehensive exam, thesis/dissertation. *Entrance requirements:* For master's, GRE General Test, bachelor's degree from accredited program with minimum GPA of 3.0 in all upper-division coursework; current license as Registered Nurse; 3 letters of recommendation; personal statement of goals; resume or curriculum vitae; personal interview; for doctorate, GRE General Test (recommended), bachelor's degree in nursing from a CCNA/NLNAC regionally-accredited institution with minimum GPA of 3.0 in all coursework or in all upper-division coursework; current license as Registered Nurse in Florida; undergraduate statistics course with minimum B grade; 3 letters of recommendation; statement of goals; resume; interview. Additional exam requirements/recommendations for international students: Required—TOEFL (minimum score 550 paper-based; 79 iBT). *Application deadline:* For fall admission, 2/15 for domestic students, 1/2 for international students; for spring admission, 10/1 for domestic students, 6/1 for international students.

Application fee: $30. Electronic applications accepted. *Financial support:* In 2015–16, 36 students received support, including 7 research assistantships with tuition reimbursements available (averaging $18,935 per year), 29 teaching assistantships with tuition reimbursements available (averaging $30,814 per year); tuition waivers (partial) and unspecified assistantships also available. Financial award application deadline: 2/1; financial award applicants required to submit FAFSA. *Faculty research:* Women's health, palliative and end-of-life care, cardiac rehabilitation, complementary therapies for chronic illness and cancer. *Total annual research expenditures:* $2.6 million. *Unit head:* Dr. Dianne C. Morrison-Beedy, Dean and Professor, College of Nursing, 813-974-9091, Fax: 813-974-5418, E-mail: dmbeedy@health.usf.edu. *Application contact:* Dr. Brian Graves, Assistant Professor/Assistant Dean, 813-974-8054, Fax: 813-974-5418, E-mail: bgraves1@health.usf.edu.
Website: http://health.usf.edu/nursing/index.htm

University of the Sacred Heart, Graduate Programs, Department of Natural Sciences, San Juan, PR 00914-0383. Offers occupational health and safety (MS); occupational nursing (MSN). *Program availability:* Part-time, evening/weekend.

Oncology Nursing

Case Western Reserve University, Frances Payne Bolton School of Nursing, Master's Programs in Nursing, Nurse Practitioner Program, Cleveland, OH 44106. Offers acute care cardiovascular nursing (MSN); acute care nurse practitioner (MSN); acute care pediatric nurse practitioner (MSN); acute care/flight nurse (MSN); adult gerontology acute care nurse practitioner (MSN); adult gerontology oncology and palliative care (MSN); adult gerontology primary care nurse practitioner (MSN); family nurse practitioner (MSN); family systems psychiatric mental health nursing (MSN); neonatal nurse practitioner (MSN); pediatric nurse practitioner (MSN); women's health nurse practitioner (MSN). *Accreditation:* ACEN. *Program availability:* Part-time, online learning. *Students:* 52 full-time (45 women), 78 part-time (68 women); includes 31 minority (10 Black or African American, non-Hispanic/Latino; 14 Asian, non-Hispanic/Latino; 7 Hispanic/Latino). Average age 35. 64 applicants, 66% accepted, 29 enrolled. In 2015, 45 master's awarded. *Degree requirements:* For master's, thesis optional. *Entrance requirements:* For master's, GRE General Test or MAT. Additional exam requirements/recommendations for international students: Required—TOEFL (minimum score 577 paper-based; 90 iBT), IELTS (minimum score 7). *Application deadline:* For fall admission, 6/1 for domestic students; for spring admission, 10/1 for domestic students. Applications are processed on a rolling basis. Application fee: $75. *Expenses:* $1,891 per credit hour. *Financial support:* In 2015–16, 54 students received support, including 17 teaching assistantships with partial tuition reimbursements available (averaging $17,019 per year); scholarships/grants and traineeships also available. Financial award application deadline: 6/30; financial award applicants required to submit FAFSA. *Faculty research:* Symptom science, family/community care, aging across the lifespan, self-management of health and illness, neuroscience. *Unit head:* Dr. Carol Savrin, Director, 216-368-5304, Fax: 216-368-3542, E-mail: cls18@case.edu. *Application contact:* Donna Hassik, Admissions Coordinator, 216-368-5253, Fax: 216-368-0124, E-mail: dmh7@case.edu.
Website: http://fpb.cwru.edu/MSN/majors.shtm

Gwynedd Mercy University, Frances M. Maguire School of Nursing and Health Professions, Gwynedd Valley, PA 19437-0901. Offers clinical nurse specialist (MSN), including gerontology, oncology, pediatrics; nurse educator (MSN); nurse practitioner (MSN), including adult health, pediatric health; nursing (DNP). *Accreditation:* ACEN. *Program availability:* Part-time, online learning. *Faculty:* 3 full-time (all women), 2 part-time/adjunct (both women). *Students:* 28 full-time (23 women), 68 part-time (62 women); includes 27 minority (18 Black or African American, non-Hispanic/Latino; 7 Asian, non-Hispanic/Latino; 2 Hispanic/Latino). Average age 37. 72 applicants, 25% accepted, 16 enrolled. In 2015, 7 master's awarded. *Degree requirements:* For master's, thesis optional; for doctorate, evidence-based scholarly project. *Entrance requirements:* For master's, GRE General Test or MAT, current nursing experience, physical assessment, course work in statistics, BSN from NLNAC-accredited program, 2 letters of recommendation, personal interview. Additional exam requirements/recommendations for international students: Required—TOEFL (minimum score 575 paper-based). *Application deadline:* For fall admission, 8/1 priority date for domestic students; for winter admission, 12/1 priority date for domestic students. Applications are processed on a rolling basis. Electronic applications accepted. *Expenses:* Contact institution. *Financial support:* In 2015–16, 21 students received support. Scholarships/grants, traineeships, and unspecified assistantships available. Financial award application deadline: 8/30. *Faculty research:* Critical thinking, primary care, domestic violence, multiculturalism, nursing centers. *Unit head:* Dr. Andrea D. Hollingsworth, Dean, 215-646-7300 Ext. 539, Fax: 215-641-5517, E-mail: hollingsworth.a@gmc.edu. *Application contact:* Dr. Barbara A. Jones, Director, 215-646-7300 Ext. 407, Fax: 215-641-5564, E-mail: jones.b@gmc.edu.
Website: http://www.gmercyu.edu/academics/graduate-programs/nursing

Universidad Metropolitana, School of Health Sciences, Department of Nursing, San Juan, PR 00928-1150. Offers case management (Certificate); nursing (MSN); oncology nursing (Certificate). *Accreditation:* ACEN.

University of Delaware, College of Health Sciences, School of Nursing, Newark, DE 19716. Offers adult nurse practitioner (MSN, PMC); cardiopulmonary clinical nurse specialist (MSN, PMC); cardiopulmonary clinical nurse specialist/adult nurse practitioner (MSN, PMC); family nurse practitioner (MSN, PMC); gerontology clinical nurse specialist (MSN, PMC); gerontology clinical nurse specialist geriatric nurse practitioner (PMC); gerontology clinical nurse specialist/geriatric nurse practitioner (MSN); health services administration (MSN, PMC); nursing of children clinical nurse specialist (MSN, PMC); nursing of children clinical nurse specialist/pediatric nurse practitioner (MSN, PMC); oncology/immune deficiency clinical nurse specialist (MSN, PMC); oncology/immune deficiency clinical nurse specialist/adult nurse practitioner (MSN, PMC); perinatal/women's health clinical nurse specialist (MSN, PMC); perinatal/women's health clinical nurse specialist/women's health nurse practitioner (MSN, PMC); psychiatric nursing clinical nurse specialist (MSN, PMC). *Accreditation:* AACN. *Program availability:* Part-time, evening/weekend, online learning. *Degree requirements:* For master's, thesis optional. *Entrance requirements:* For master's, BSN, interview, RN license. Electronic applications accepted. *Faculty research:* Marriage and chronic illness, health promotion, congestive heart failure patient outcomes, school nursing, diabetes in children, culture, health disparities, cardiovascular, prison nursing, oncology, public policy, child obesity, smoking and teen pregnancy, blood pressure measurements, men's health.

University of South Florida, College of Nursing, Tampa, FL 33612. Offers advanced pain management (Graduate Certificate); nursing (MS, DNP), including adult gerontology acute care (DNP), adult gerontology acute care nursing (MS), adult gerontology primary care (DNP), adult gerontology primary care nursing (MS), adult gerontology primary care/occupational health nursing (MS), adult gerontology primary care/oncology nursing (MS), clinical nurse leader (MS), family health nursing, nurse anesthesia (MS), nursing education (MS), nursing practice (DNP), occupational health/adult-gerontology (DNP), oncology/adult-gerontology primary care (DNP), pediatric health (DNP), pediatric nurse practitioner (MS); nursing education (Post Master's Certificate); nursing science (PhD). *Accreditation:* AACN; AANA/CANAEP. *Program availability:* Part-time. *Faculty:* 43 full-time (38 women), 7 part-time/adjunct (4 women). *Students:* 159 full-time (135 women), 721 part-time (625 women); includes 292 minority (119 Black or African American, non-Hispanic/Latino; 2 American Indian or Alaska Native, non-Hispanic/Latino; 60 Asian, non-Hispanic/Latino; 90 Hispanic/Latino; 1 Native Hawaiian or other Pacific Islander, non-Hispanic/Latino; 20 Two or more races, non-Hispanic/Latino; 12 international. Average age 35. 636 applicants, 44% accepted, 215 enrolled. In 2015, 333 master's, 18 doctorates awarded. *Degree requirements:* For master's, comprehensive exam, thesis optional; for doctorate, comprehensive exam, thesis/dissertation. *Entrance requirements:* For master's, GRE General Test, bachelor's degree from accredited program with minimum GPA of 3.0 in all upper-division coursework; current license as Registered Nurse; 3 letters of recommendation; personal statement of goals; resume or curriculum vitae; personal interview; for doctorate, GRE General Test (recommended), bachelor's degree in nursing from a CCNA/NLNAC regionally-accredited institution with minimum GPA of 3.0 in all coursework or in all upper-division coursework; current license as Registered Nurse in Florida; undergraduate statistics course with minimum B grade; 3 letters of recommendation; statement of goals; resume; interview. Additional exam requirements/recommendations for international students: Required—TOEFL (minimum score 550 paper-based; 79 iBT). *Application deadline:* For fall admission, 2/15 for domestic students, 1/2 for international students; for spring admission, 10/1 for domestic students, 6/1 for international students. Application fee: $30. Electronic applications accepted. *Financial support:* In 2015–16, 36 students received support, including 7 research assistantships with tuition reimbursements available (averaging $18,935 per year), 29 teaching assistantships with tuition reimbursements available (averaging $30,814 per year); tuition waivers (partial) and unspecified assistantships also available. Financial award application deadline: 2/1; financial award applicants required to submit FAFSA. *Faculty research:* Women's health, palliative and end-of-life care, cardiac rehabilitation, complementary therapies for chronic illness and cancer. *Total annual research expenditures:* $2.6 million. *Unit head:* Dr. Dianne C. Morrison-Beedy, Dean and Professor, College of Nursing, 813-974-9091, Fax: 813-974-5418, E-mail: dmbeedy@health.usf.edu. *Application contact:* Dr. Brian Graves, Assistant Professor/Assistant Dean, 813-974-8054, Fax: 813-974-5418, E-mail: bgraves1@health.usf.edu.
Website: http://health.usf.edu/nursing/index.htm

Pediatric Nursing

Augusta University, The Graduate School, Doctor of Nursing Practice Program, Augusta, GA 30912. Offers adult gerontology acute care nurse practitioner (DNP); family nurse practitioner (DNP); nursing (DNP); nursing anesthesia (DNP); pediatric nurse practitioner (DNP); psychiatric mental health nurse practitioner (DNP). *Students:* 40 part-time. *Degree requirements:* For doctorate, thesis/dissertation or alternative. *Entrance requirements:* For doctorate, GRE General Test or MAT, master's degree in nursing or related field, current professional nurse licensure. Additional exam requirements/recommendations for international students: Required—TOEFL (minimum score 600 paper-based; 100 iBT). *Application deadline:* For fall admission, 3/1 for domestic and international students; for spring admission, 7/1 for domestic and international students. Applications are processed on a rolling basis. Application fee: $50. Electronic applications accepted. *Unit head:* Dr. Marguerite Murphy, RN, Director, 706-721-3676, Fax: 706-721-8169. *Application contact:* Karen Sturgill, Program Manager, 706-721-3676, Fax: 706-721-8169, E-mail: dnp@augusta.edu.
Website: http://www.augusta.edu/nursing/dnp_programs.php

Pediatric Nursing

Augusta University, The Graduate School, Pediatric Nurse Practitioner Program, Augusta, GA 30912. Offers MSN, Post-Master's Certificate. *Entrance requirements:* For master's, GRE General Test or MAT, Georgia license as a registered professional nurse. Additional exam requirements/recommendations for international students: Required—TOEFL (minimum score 550 paper-based; 79 iBT). *Application deadline:* For fall admission, 2/1 for domestic and international students; for spring admission, 10/1 for domestic and international students. Application fee: $50. Electronic applications accepted. *Unit head:* Dr. Jean Pawl, Interim Director, 706-721-3676, Fax: 706-721-8169. *Application contact:* Karen Sturgill, Program Manager, 706-721-3676, Fax: 706-721-8169.
Website: http://www.augusta.edu/nursing/

Boston College, William F. Connell School of Nursing, Chestnut Hill, MA 02467. Offers adult-gerontology nursing (MS); family health nursing (MS); forensic nursing (MS); nurse anesthesia (MS); nursing (PhD); pediatric nursing (MS), including pediatric and women's health; psychiatric-mental health nursing (MS); women's health nursing (MS); MBA/MS; MS/MA; MS/PhD. *Accreditation:* AACN; AANA/CANAEP (one or more programs are accredited). *Program availability:* Part-time. *Faculty:* 53 full-time (48 women), 47 part-time/adjunct (44 women). *Students:* 185 full-time (167 women), 66 part-time (56 women); includes 31 minority (10 Black or African American, non-Hispanic/Latino; 12 Asian, non-Hispanic/Latino; 7 Hispanic/Latino; 2 Two or more races, non-Hispanic/Latino), 7 international. Average age 32. 313 applicants, 66% accepted, 91 enrolled. In 2015, 98 master's, 5 doctorates awarded. *Degree requirements:* For master's, comprehensive exam; for doctorate, comprehensive exam, thesis/dissertation, computer literacy exam or foreign language. *Entrance requirements:* For master's, bachelor's degree in nursing; for doctorate, GRE General Test, MS in nursing. Additional exam requirements/recommendations for international students: Required—TOEFL (minimum score 600 paper-based; 100 iBT), IELTS (minimum score 7.5). *Application deadline:* For fall admission, 9/30 for domestic and international students; for winter admission, 1/15 for domestic and international students; for spring admission, 3/15 for domestic and international students. Applications are processed on a rolling basis. Application fee: $40. Electronic applications accepted. *Expenses:* Contact institution. *Financial support:* In 2015–16, 1 fellowship with full tuition reimbursement (averaging $23,700 per year), 25 teaching assistantships (averaging $4,370 per year) were awarded; research assistantships, scholarships/grants, health care benefits, tuition waivers (partial), and unspecified assistantships also available. Support available to part-time students. Financial award application deadline: 3/1; financial award applicants required to submit FAFSA. *Faculty research:* Sexual and reproductive health, health promotion/illness prevention, aging, eating disorders, symptom management. *Total annual research expenditures:* $1 million. *Unit head:* Dr. Susan Gennaro, Dean, 617-552-4251, Fax: 617-552-0931, E-mail: susan.gennaro@bc.edu. *Application contact:* MaryBeth Crowley, Graduate Programs Assistant, 617-552-4928, Fax: 617-552-2121, E-mail: csongrad@bc.edu.
Website: http://www.bc.edu/schools/son/

Caribbean University, Graduate School, Bayamón, PR 00960-0493. Offers administration and supervision (MA Ed); criminal justice (MA); curriculum and instruction (MA Ed, PhD), including elementary education (MA Ed), English education (MA Ed), history education (MA Ed), mathematics education (MA Ed), primary education (MA Ed), science education (MA Ed), Spanish education (MA Ed); educational technology in instructional systems (MA Ed); gerontology (MSN); human resources (MBA); museology, archiving and art history (MA Ed); neonatal pediatrics (MSN); physical education (MA Ed); special education (MA Ed). *Entrance requirements:* For master's, interview, minimum GPA of 2.5.

Case Western Reserve University, Frances Payne Bolton School of Nursing, Master's Programs in Nursing, Nurse Practitioner Program, Cleveland, OH 44106. Offers acute care cardiovascular nursing (MSN); acute care nurse practitioner (MSN); acute care pediatric nurse practitioner (MSN); acute care/flight nurse (MSN); adult gerontology acute care nurse practitioner (MSN); adult gerontology oncology and palliative care (MSN); adult gerontology primary care nurse practitioner (MSN); family nurse practitioner (MSN); family systems psychiatric mental health nursing (MSN); neonatal nurse practitioner (MSN); pediatric nurse practitioner (MSN); women's health nurse practitioner (MSN). *Accreditation:* ACEN. *Program availability:* Part-time, online learning. *Students:* 52 full-time (45 women), 78 part-time (68 women); includes 31 minority (10 Black or African American, non-Hispanic/Latino; 14 Asian, non-Hispanic/Latino; 7 Hispanic/Latino). Average age 35. 64 applicants, 66% accepted, 29 enrolled. In 2015, 45 master's awarded. *Degree requirements:* For master's, thesis optional. *Entrance requirements:* For master's, GRE General Test or MAT. Additional exam requirements/recommendations for international students: Required—TOEFL (minimum score 577 paper-based; 90 iBT), IELTS (minimum score 7). *Application deadline:* For fall admission, 6/1 for domestic students; for spring admission, 10/1 for domestic students. Applications are processed on a rolling basis. Application fee: $75. *Expenses:* $1,891 per credit hour. *Financial support:* In 2015–16, 54 students received support, including 17 teaching assistantships with partial tuition reimbursements available (averaging $17,019 per year); scholarships/grants and traineeships also available. Financial award application deadline: 6/30; financial award applicants required to submit FAFSA. *Faculty research:* Symptom science, family/community care, aging across the lifespan, self-management of health and illness, neuroscience. *Unit head:* Dr. Carol Savrin, Director, 216-368-5304, Fax: 216-368-3542, E-mail: cls18@case.edu. *Application contact:* Donna Hassik, Admissions Coordinator, 216-368-5253, Fax: 216-368-0124, E-mail: dmh7@case.edu.
Website: http://fpb.cwru.edu/MSN/majors.shtm

Columbia University, School of Nursing, Program in Pediatric Nurse Practitioner, New York, NY 10032. Offers MS, Adv C. *Accreditation:* AACN. *Program availability:* Part-time. *Entrance requirements:* For master's, GRE General Test, NCLEX, BSN, 1 year of clinical experience (preferred); for Adv C, MSN. Additional exam requirements/recommendations for international students: Required—TOEFL. Electronic applications accepted.

Creighton University, College of Nursing, Omaha, NE 68178-0001. Offers adult acute care nurse practitioner (Post-Master's Certificate); adult gerontology acute care nurse practitioner (DNP); adult gerontology nurse practitioner (DNP); clinical nurse leader (MSN, Post-Graduate Certificate); clinical systems administration (MSN, DNP); family nurse practitioner (DNP, Post-Master's Certificate); neonatal nurse practitioner (DNP, Post-Master's Certificate); pediatric acute care nurse practitioner (DNP, Post-Master's Certificate); psychiatric mental health nurse practitioner (DNP). *Accreditation:* AACN. *Program availability:* Part-time, blended/hybrid learning. *Faculty:* 10 full-time (all women), 48 part-time/adjunct (45 women). *Students:* 132 full-time (120 women), 228 part-time (212 women); includes 38 minority (10 Black or African American, non-Hispanic/Latino; 3 American Indian or Alaska Native, non-Hispanic/Latino; 11 Asian, non-Hispanic/Latino; 1 Hispanic/Latino; 2 Native Hawaiian or other Pacific Islander, non-Hispanic/Latino; 11 Two or more races, non-Hispanic/Latino). Average age 31. 66 applicants, 91% accepted, 43 enrolled. In 2015, 54 master's, 17 doctorates, 1 other advanced degree awarded. *Degree requirements:* For master's, capstone project; for doctorate, scholarly project. *Entrance requirements:* For master's and doctorate, BSN from an ACEN- or CCNE-accredited nursing school, minimum cumulative GPA of 3.0, personal statement, current unencumbered RN license with NE eligibility, undergraduate statistics course, physical assessment course or equivalent; for other advanced degree, MSN or MS in nursing, minimum cumulative GPA of 3.0, current unencumbered RN license with NE eligibility. Additional exam requirements/recommendations for international students: Required—TOEFL (minimum score 600 paper-based; 100 iBT). *Application deadline:* For fall admission, 6/15 priority date for domestic and international students; for spring admission, 11/15 priority date for domestic and international students; for summer admission, 4/15 for domestic and international students. Applications are processed on a rolling basis. Application fee: $50. Electronic applications accepted. *Expenses:* $800 per credit hour tuition; $904 per semester full-time fees; $207 per semester part-time fees; $50 one-time drug screen fee. *Financial support:* In 2015–16, 7 students received support. Scholarships/grants available. Financial award applicants required to submit FAFSA. *Faculty research:* Obesity prevention in children, evaluation of simulated clinical experiences, vitamin D3 and calcium for cancer risk education in post menopausal women, online support and education to reduce stress for prenatal patients on bed rest, health literacy, immunization research. *Total annual research expenditures:* $162,085. *Unit head:* Dr. Catherine Todero, Dean, 402-280-2004, Fax: 402-280-2045. *Application contact:* Shannon Cox, Enrollment Specialist, 402-280-2067, Fax: 402-280-2045, E-mail: shannoncox@creighton.edu.
Website: http://nursing.creighton.edu/

Drexel University, College of Nursing and Health Professions, Division of Graduate Nursing, Philadelphia, PA 19104-2875. Offers adult acute care (MSN); adult psychiatric/mental health (MSN); advanced practice nursing (MSN); clinical trials research (MSN); family nurse practitioner (MSN); leadership in health systems management (MSN); nursing education (MSN); pediatric primary care (MSN); women's health (MSN). *Accreditation:* AACN. Electronic applications accepted.

Duke University, School of Nursing, Durham, NC 27708-0586. Offers acute care pediatric nurse practitioner (MSN, Post Master's Certificate); adult-gerontology nurse practitioner (MSN, Post Master's Certificate), including acute care, primary care; family nurse practitioner (MSN, Post Master's Certificate); neonatal nurse practitioner (MSN, Post Master's Certificate); nurse anesthesia (DNP); nurse practitioner (DNP); nursing (PhD); nursing and health care leadership (MSN); nursing education (MSN); nursing informatics (MSN, Post Master's Certificate); pediatric nurse practitioner (MSN, Post Master's Certificate), including primary care; women's health nurse practitioner (MSN, Post Master's Certificate). *Accreditation:* AACN; AANA/CANAEP. *Program availability:* Part-time, evening/weekend, online learning. *Faculty:* 74 full-time (63 women). *Students:* 179 full-time (152 women), 528 part-time (466 women); includes 145 minority (42 Black or African American, non-Hispanic/Latino; 3 American Indian or Alaska Native, non-Hispanic/Latino; 44 Asian, non-Hispanic/Latino; 35 Hispanic/Latino; 1 Native Hawaiian or other Pacific Islander, non-Hispanic/Latino; 20 Two or more races, non-Hispanic/Latino), 7 international. Average age 33. 619 applicants, 46% accepted, 201 enrolled. In 2015, 243 master's, 62 doctorates, 26 other advanced degrees awarded. Terminal master's awarded for partial completion of doctoral program. *Degree requirements:* For master's, thesis optional; for doctorate, capstone project. *Entrance requirements:* For master's, GRE General Test (waived if undergraduate GPA of 3.4 or higher), 1 year of nursing experience (recommended), BSN, minimum GPA of 3.0, previous course work in statistics; for doctorate, GRE General Test (waived if undergraduate GPA of 3.4 or higher), BSN or MSN, minimum GPA of 3.0, portfolio, resume, personal statement, undergraduate statistics course, current licensure as a registered nurse, transcripts from all post-secondary institutions; for Post Master's Certificate, MSN, licensure or eligibility as a professional nurse, transcripts from all post-secondary institutions, previous course work in statistics. Additional exam requirements/recommendations for international students: Required—TOEFL (minimum score 100 iBT), IELTS (minimum score 7). *Application deadline:* For fall admission, 12/1 for domestic and international students; for spring admission, 5/1 for domestic and international students. Application fee: $50. Electronic applications accepted. *Expenses:* Contact institution. *Financial support:* Career-related internships or fieldwork, institutionally sponsored loans, scholarships/grants, traineeships, and tuition waivers (partial) available. Support available to part-time students. Financial award applicants required to submit FAFSA. *Faculty research:* Cardiovascular disease, caregiver skill training, data mining, prostate cancer, neonatal immune system. *Unit head:* Dr. Marion E. Broome, Dean/Vice Chancellor for Nursing Affairs/Associate Vice President for Academic Affairs for Nursing, 919-684-9446, Fax: 919-684-9414, E-mail: marion.broome@duke.edu. *Application contact:* Dr. Ernie Rushing, Director of Admissions and Recruitment, 919-668-6274, Fax: 919-668-4693, E-mail: ernie.rushing@dm.duke.edu.
Website: http://www.nursing.duke.edu/

Emory University, Nell Hodgson Woodruff School of Nursing, Atlanta, GA 30322-1100. Offers adult nurse practitioner (MSN); emergency nurse practitioner (MSN); family nurse practitioner (MSN); family nurse-midwife (MSN); health systems leadership (MSN); nurse-midwifery (MSN); pediatric nurse practitioner acute and primary care (MSN); women's health care (Title X) (MSN); women's health nurse practitioner (MSN); MSN/MPH. *Accreditation:* AACN; ACNM/ACME (one or more programs are accredited). *Program availability:* Part-time. *Entrance requirements:* For master's, GRE General Test or MAT, minimum GPA of 3.0, BS in nursing from an accredited institution, RN license and additional course work, 3 letters of recommendation. Additional exam requirements/recommendations for international students: Required—TOEFL (minimum score 600 paper-based; 100 iBT). Electronic applications accepted. *Expenses:* Contact institution. *Faculty research:* Older adult falls and injuries, minority health issues, cardiac symptoms and quality of life, bio-ethics and decision-making, menopausal issues.

Georgia State University, Byrdine F. Lewis School of Nursing, Atlanta, GA 30303. Offers adult health clinical nurse specialist/nurse practitioner (MS, Certificate); child health clinical nurse specialist/pediatric nurse practitioner (MS, Certificate); family nurse practitioner (MS, Certificate); family psychiatric mental health nurse practitioner (MS, Certificate); nursing (PhD); nursing leadership in healthcare innovations (MS), including nursing administration, nursing informatics; nutrition (MS); perinatal clinical nurse specialist/women's health nurse practitioner (MS, Certificate); physical therapy (DPT); respiratory therapy (MS). *Accreditation:* AACN. *Program availability:* Part-time, blended/hybrid learning. *Faculty:* 18 full-time (11 women). *Students:* 275 full-time (195 women), 230 part-time (204 women); includes 192 minority (123 Black or African American, non-Hispanic/Latino; 49 Asian, non-Hispanic/Latino; 12 Hispanic/Latino; 2 Native Hawaiian or other Pacific Islander, non-Hispanic/Latino; 6 Two or more races, non-Hispanic/Latino), 35 international. Average age 33. 240 applicants, 61% accepted, 95 enrolled. In 2015, 115 master's, 40 doctorates, 19 other advanced degrees awarded. *Degree requirements:* For doctorate, comprehensive exam, thesis/dissertation. *Entrance requirements:* For doctorate, GRE. Additional exam requirements/recommendations for international students: Required—TOEFL. *Application deadline:* For fall admission, 2/1 priority date for domestic and international students; for spring admission, 9/15 for domestic and international students. Applications are processed on a rolling basis. Application fee: $50. Electronic applications accepted. *Expenses:* Contact institution. *Financial support:* In 2015–16, research assistantships with tuition reimbursements (averaging $1,666 per year), teaching assistantships with tuition reimbursements (averaging $1,920 per year) were awarded; scholarships/grants, tuition waivers (full and partial), and unspecified assistantships also available. Support available to part-time students. Financial award application deadline: 8/1; financial award applicants required

to submit FAFSA. *Faculty research:* Stroke intervention for caregivers, stroke prevention in African-Americans; relationships between psychological distress and health outcomes in parents with a medically ill infant; medically fragile children; nursing expertise and patient outcomes. *Unit head:* Nancy Kropf, Dean of Nursing, 404-413-1101, Fax: 404-413-1090, E-mail: nkropf@gsu.edu.
Website: http://nursing.gsu.edu/

Gwynedd Mercy University, Frances M. Maguire School of Nursing and Health Professions, Gwynedd Valley, PA 19437-0901. Offers clinical nurse specialist (MSN), including gerontology, oncology, pediatrics; nurse educator (MSN); nurse practitioner (MSN), including adult health, pediatric health; nursing (DNP). *Accreditation:* ACEN. *Program availability:* Part-time, online learning. *Faculty:* 3 full-time (all women), 2 part-time/adjunct (both women). *Students:* 28 full-time (23 women), 68 part-time (62 women); includes 27 minority (18 Black or African American, non-Hispanic/Latino; 7 Asian, non-Hispanic/Latino; 2 Hispanic/Latino). Average age 37. 72 applicants, 25% accepted, 16 enrolled. In 2015, 7 master's awarded. *Degree requirements:* For master's, thesis optional; for doctorate, evidence-based scholarly project. *Entrance requirements:* For master's, GRE General Test or MAT, current nursing experience, physical assessment, course work in statistics, BSN from NLNAC-accredited program, 2 letters of recommendation, personal interview. Additional exam requirements/recommendations for international students: Required—TOEFL (minimum score 575 paper-based). *Application deadline:* For fall admission, 8/1 priority date for domestic students; for winter admission, 12/1 priority date for domestic students. Applications are processed on a rolling basis. Electronic applications accepted. *Expenses:* Contact institution. *Financial support:* In 2015–16, 21 students received support. Scholarships/grants, traineeships, and unspecified assistantships available. Financial award application deadline: 8/30. *Faculty research:* Critical thinking, primary care, domestic violence, multiculturalism, nursing centers. *Unit head:* Dr. Andrea D. Hollingsworth, Dean, 215-646-7300 Ext. 539, Fax: 215-641-5517, E-mail: hollingsworth.a@gmc.edu. *Application contact:* Dr. Barbara A. Jones, Director, 215-646-7300 Ext. 407, Fax: 215-641-5564, E-mail: jones.b@gmc.edu.
Website: http://www.gmercyu.edu/academics/graduate-programs/nursing

Hampton University, School of Nursing, Hampton, VA 23668. Offers advanced adult nursing (MS); community health nursing (MS); community mental health/psychiatric nursing (MS); family nursing (MS); gerontological nursing for the nurse practitioner (MS); nursing (PhD); women's health nursing (MS). *Accreditation:* AACN. *Program availability:* Part-time, online learning. *Degree requirements:* For master's, comprehensive exam, thesis optional; for doctorate, comprehensive exam, thesis/dissertation. *Entrance requirements:* For master's, GRE General Test. Additional exam requirements/recommendations for international students: Required—TOEFL (minimum score 525 paper-based) or IELTS (6.5). Electronic applications accepted. *Expenses: Tuition, area resident:* Full-time $10,263; part-time $522 per credit hour. *Required fees:* $35. Tuition and fees vary according to course load and program. *Faculty research:* African-American stress, HIV education, pediatric obesity, hypertension, breast cancer.

Kent State University, College of Nursing, Kent, OH 44242. Offers advanced nursing practice (DNP), including adult gerontology acute care nurse practitioner (MSN, DNP), adult gerontology clinical nurse specialist (MSN, DNP), family nurse practitioner (MSN, DNP); nursing (MSN, PhD), including adult gerontology acute care nurse practitioner (MSN, DNP), adult gerontology clinical nurse specialist (MSN, DNP), family nurse practitioner (MSN, DNP), nurse educator (MSN), nursing healthcare management (MSN), primary care adult nurse practitioner (MSN), primary care pediatric clinical nurse specialist (MSN), primary care pediatric nurse practitioner (MSN), psychiatric mental health practitioner (MSN), women's health nurse practitioner (MSN); nursing education (Certificate); primary care pediatric nurse practitioner (Certificate); women's health nurse practitioner (Certificate). PhD program offered jointly with The University of Akron. *Accreditation:* AACN. *Program availability:* Part-time, online learning. *Faculty:* 52 full-time (48 women). *Students:* 78 full-time (56 women), 414 part-time (365 women); includes 63 minority (34 Black or African American, non-Hispanic/Latino; 1 American Indian or Alaska Native, non-Hispanic/Latino; 12 Asian, non-Hispanic/Latino; 12 Hispanic/Latino; 4 Two or more races, non-Hispanic/Latino), 16 international. Average age 37. 653 applicants, 54% accepted, 309 enrolled. In 2015, 140 master's, 1 doctorate, 13 other advanced degrees awarded. *Degree requirements:* For master's, thesis optional, practicum; for doctorate, comprehensive exam (for some programs), thesis/dissertation (for some programs), practicum and scholarly project (for DNP programs); for Certificate, practicum. *Entrance requirements:* For master's, minimum GPA of 3.0, transcripts, active unrestricted RN license, essay/goal statement, interview, 3 letters of recommendation; for doctorate, GRE (for PhD), minimum GPA of 3.0, transcripts, 3 letters of recommendation, interview; active unrestricted RN license, clinical experience and hours record (for DNP); goal statement, sample of written work, curriculum vitae, statement of research interests, and eligibility for RN license (for PhD); for Certificate, MSN, minimum GPA of 3.0, transcripts. Additional exam requirements/recommendations for international students: Required—TOEFL (minimum score: paper-based 525, iBT 71), Michigan English Language Assessment Battery (minimum score of 75), IELTS (minimum score of 6.0), PTE Academic (minimum score of 48), or completion of ELS level 112 Intensive Program. *Application deadline:* For fall admission, 2/1 for domestic students; for spring admission, 11/1 for domestic students. Application fee: $45 ($70 for international students). Electronic applications accepted. *Expenses:* Tuition, state resident: full-time $10,864; part-time $495 per credit hour. Tuition, nonresident: full-time $18,380; part-time $837 per credit hour. *Financial support:* Research assistantships with full tuition reimbursements, teaching assistantships with full tuition reimbursements, career-related internships or fieldwork, Federal Work-Study, traineeships, and unspecified assistantships available. Financial award application deadline: 2/1. *Unit head:* Dr. Barbara Broome, Dean, 330-672-3777, E-mail: bbroome1@kent.edu. *Application contact:* Dr. Wendy A. Umberger, Associate Dean for Graduate Programs/Professor, 330-672-8813, E-mail: wlewando@kent.edu.
Website: http://www.kent.edu/nursing/

Lehman College of the City University of New York, School of Natural and Social Sciences, Department of Nursing, Bronx, NY 10468-1589. Offers adult health nursing (MS); nursing of older adults (MS); parent-child nursing (MS); pediatric nurse practitioner (MS). *Accreditation:* AACN. *Program availability:* Part-time, evening/weekend. *Entrance requirements:* For master's, bachelor's degree in nursing, New York RN license.

Loma Linda University, School of Nursing, Program in Nurse Educator, Loma Linda, CA 92350. Offers adult/gerontology (MS); obstetrics-pediatrics (MS). *Accreditation:* AACN. *Program availability:* Part-time. *Degree requirements:* For master's, thesis or alternative. *Entrance requirements:* For master's, GRE General Test, BSN, minimum GPA of 3.0, RN license. Additional exam requirements/recommendations for international students: Required—TOEFL. *Application deadline:* For fall admission, 8/1 for domestic and international students; for winter admission, 11/1 for domestic and international students; for spring admission, 2/1 for domestic and international students. Application fee: $60. Electronic applications accepted. *Financial support:* Career-related internships or fieldwork, Federal Work-Study, institutionally sponsored loans, and scholarships/grants available. Support available to part-time students. Financial award application deadline: 6/1. *Faculty research:* Coping, integration of research. *Unit head:*

Coordinator, 909-824-4360. *Application contact:* Admissions Office, 909-651-5029, Fax: 909-558-4879, E-mail: admissions.app@llu.edu.

Marquette University, Graduate School, College of Nursing, Milwaukee, WI 53201-1881. Offers acute care nurse practitioner (Certificate); adult clinical nurse specialist (Certificate); adult nurse practitioner (Certificate); advanced practice nursing (MSN, DNP), including adult-older adult acute care (DNP), adults (MSN), adults-older adults (DNP), clinical nurse leader (MSN), health care systems leadership (DNP), nurse-midwifery (MSN), older adults (MSN), pediatrics-acute care, pediatrics-primary care, primary care (DNP), systems leadership and healthcare quality (MSN); family nurse practitioner (Certificate); nurse-midwifery (Certificate); nursing (PhD); pediatric acute care (Certificate); pediatric primary care (Certificate); systems leadership and healthcare quality (Certificate). *Accreditation:* AACN. *Faculty:* 35 full-time (all women), 56 part-time/adjunct (55 women). *Students:* 123 full-time (112 women), 242 part-time (220 women); includes 34 minority (9 Black or African American, non-Hispanic/Latino; 12 Asian, non-Hispanic/Latino; 10 Hispanic/Latino; 3 Two or more races, non-Hispanic/Latino), 4 international. Average age 30. 269 applicants, 61% accepted, 98 enrolled. In 2015, 84 master's, 5 doctorates, 22 other advanced degrees awarded. Terminal master's awarded for partial completion of doctoral program. *Degree requirements:* For master's, comprehensive exam, thesis or alternative. *Entrance requirements:* For master's, GRE General Test, BSN, Wisconsin RN license, official transcripts from all current and previous colleges/universities except Marquette, three completed recommendation forms, resume, written statement of professional goals; for doctorate, GRE General Test, official transcripts from all current and previous colleges/ universities except Marquette, three letters of recommendation, resume, written statement of professional goals, sample of scholarly writing. Additional exam requirements/ recommendations for international students: Required—TOEFL (minimum score 530 paper-based). *Application deadline:* For fall admission, 2/15 for domestic and international students. Electronic applications accepted. *Financial support:* In 2015–16, 41 students received support, including 1 fellowship with partial tuition reimbursement available (averaging $17,500 per year), 2 research assistantships with full tuition reimbursements available (averaging $13,285 per year), 8 teaching assistantships with full tuition reimbursements available (averaging $13,912 per year); career-related internships or fieldwork, Federal Work-Study, scholarships/grants, health care benefits, tuition waivers (partial), and unspecified assistantships also available. Support available to part-time students. Financial award application deadline: 2/15. *Faculty research:* Psychosocial adjustment to chronic illness, gerontology, reminiscence, health policy: uninsured and access, hospital care delivery systems. *Total annual research expenditures:* $480,591. *Unit head:* Dr. Donna McCarthy, Interim Chair, 414-288-3800, Fax: 414-288-1578. *Application contact:* Dr. Maureen O'Brien, Associate Dean/Clinical Associate Professor, 414-288-3823.

Maryville University of Saint Louis, Walker College of Health Professions, The Catherine McAuley School of Nursing, St. Louis, MO 63141-7299. Offers acute care nurse practice (MSN); adult gerontology nurse practitioner (MSN); advanced practice nursing (DNP); family nurse practitioner (MSN); pediatric nurse practice (MSN). *Accreditation:* AACN. *Program availability:* 100% online. *Faculty:* 18 full-time (all women), 158 part-time/adjunct (141 women). *Students:* 38 full-time (35 women), 2,802 part-time (2,511 women); includes 681 minority (332 Black or African American, non-Hispanic/Latino; 40 American Indian or Alaska Native, non-Hispanic/Latino; 126 Asian, non-Hispanic/Latino; 126 Hispanic/Latino; 8 Native Hawaiian or other Pacific Islander, non-Hispanic/Latino; 49 Two or more races, non-Hispanic/Latino), 58 international. Average age 37. In 2015, 413 master's, 33 doctorates awarded. *Degree requirements:* For master's, practicum. *Entrance requirements:* For master's, BSN, current licensure, minimum GPA of 3.0, 3 letters of recommendation, curriculum vitae. Additional exam requirements/recommendations for international students: Required—TOEFL (minimum score 550 paper-based). *Application deadline:* Applications are processed on a rolling basis. Electronic applications accepted. Application fee is waived when completed online. *Expenses: Tuition, area resident:* Full-time $25,558; part-time $781 per credit hour. *Required fees:* $2400. Part-time tuition and fees vary according to course load and degree level. *Financial support:* Federal Work-Study and campus employment available. Support available to part-time students. Financial award application deadline: 3/1; financial award applicants required to submit FAFSA. *Unit head:* Dr. Elizabeth Buck, Director, 314-529-9453, Fax: 314-529-9139, E-mail: ebuck@maryville.edu. *Application contact:* Crystal Jacobsmeyer, Assistant Director, Graduate Enrollment Advising, 314-929-9654, Fax: 314-529-9927, E-mail: cjacobsmeyer@maryville.edu.
Website: http://www.maryville.edu/hp/nursing/

MGH Institute of Health Professions, School of Nursing, Boston, MA 02129. Offers advanced practice nursing (MSN); gerontological nursing (MSN); nursing (DNP); pediatric nursing (MSN); psychiatric nursing (MSN); teaching and learning for health care education (Certificate); women's health nursing (MSN). *Accreditation:* AACN. *Degree requirements:* For master's, thesis or alternative. *Entrance requirements:* For master's, GRE General Test, bachelor's degree from regionally-accredited college or university. Additional exam requirements/recommendations for international students: Required—TOEFL (minimum score 550 paper-based; 80 iBT). Electronic applications accepted. *Faculty research:* Biobehavioral nursing, HIV/AIDS, gerontological nursing, women's health, vulnerable populations, health systems.

Molloy College, Division of Nursing, Rockville Centre, NY 11571-5002. Offers adult-gerontology primary care nurse practitioner (MS); clinical nurse specialist (MS), including adult-gerontology health; clinical nurse specialist: adult-gerontology (Advanced Certificate), including adult-gerontology; family nurse practitioner (MS, Advanced Certificate), including primary care; family psychiatric mental health nurse practitioner (MS); nursing (DNP, PhD); nursing administration (MS), including informatics; nursing education (MS); pediatric nurse practitioner (MS), including primary care (MS, Advanced Certificate). *Accreditation:* AACN. *Program availability:* Part-time, evening/weekend. *Faculty:* 26 full-time (all women), 12 part-time/adjunct (9 women). *Students:* 13 full-time (all women), 550 part-time (515 women); includes 316 minority (169 Black or African American, non-Hispanic/Latino; 1 American Indian or Alaska Native, non-Hispanic/Latino; 88 Asian, non-Hispanic/Latino; 56 Hispanic/Latino; 2 Native Hawaiian or other Pacific Islander, non-Hispanic/Latino). Average age 43. 208 applicants, 69% accepted, 121 enrolled. In 2015, 116 master's, 1 doctorate, 6 other advanced degrees awarded. *Degree requirements:* For master's, thesis optional. *Entrance requirements:* For master's, 3 letters of reference, BS in nursing, minimum undergraduate GPA of 3.0; for Advanced Certificate, 3 letters of reference, master's degree in nursing. Additional exam requirements/ recommendations for international students: Required—TOEFL (minimum score 550 paper-based; 79 iBT). *Application deadline:* For fall admission, 9/2 priority date for domestic students; for spring admission, 1/20 priority date for domestic students. Applications are processed on a rolling basis. Application fee: $60. Electronic applications accepted. *Expenses: Tuition, area resident:* Full-time $18,450; part-time $1025 per credit. *Required fees:* $900; $740 per unit. Tuition and fees vary according to course load. *Financial support:* Research assistantships with partial tuition reimbursements, teaching assistantships with partial tuition reimbursements, institutionally sponsored loans, scholarships/grants, and unspecified assistantships available. Support available to part-time students. Financial award application deadline: 4/1; financial award applicants required to submit FAFSA. *Unit head:* Dr. Jeannine Muldoon, Dean of Nursing, 516-323-3651, E-mail: jmuldoon@molloy.edu. *Application contact:* Jaclyn Machowicz, Assistant Director for Admissions, 516-323-4010, E-mail: jmachowicz@molloy.edu.

Pediatric Nursing

New York University, Rory Meyers College of Nursing, Doctor of Nursing Practice Program, New York, NY 10012-1019. Offers nursing (DNP), including adult acute care, adult primary care, family, mental health nursing, nurse-midwifery, pediatrics. *Program availability:* Part-time, evening/weekend. *Faculty:* 14 full-time (13 women). *Students:* 2 full-time (both women), 32 part-time (27 women); includes 8 minority (3 Black or African American, non-Hispanic/Latino; 4 Asian, non-Hispanic/Latino; 1 Hispanic/Latino), 1 international. Average age 40. 47 applicants, 51% accepted, 16 enrolled. In 2015, 17 doctorates awarded. *Degree requirements:* For doctorate, thesis/dissertation, project. *Entrance requirements:* For doctorate, MAT or GRE (either taken within past 5 years), MS, RN license, interview, Nurse Practitioner Certification, writing sample. Additional exam requirements/recommendations for international students: Required—TOEFL (minimum score 90 iBT), IELTS (minimum score 7). *Application deadline:* For fall admission, 3/1 for domestic and international students. Applications are processed on a rolling basis. Application fee: $80. Electronic applications accepted. *Expenses:* Contact institution. *Financial support:* In 2015–16, 12 students received support. Scholarships/grants available. Support available to part-time students. Financial award application deadline: 2/1; financial award applicants required to submit FAFSA. *Faculty research:* Workforce, LGBT, breast cancer, HIV. *Unit head:* Dr. Rona Levin, Director, 212-998-5319, Fax: 212-995-3143, E-mail: rfl2039@nyu.edu. *Application contact:* Samantha Jaser, Assistant Director, Graduate Student Affairs and Admissions, 212-992-7653, Fax: 212-995-4302, E-mail: saj283@nyu.edu.

New York University, Rory Meyers College of Nursing, Programs in Advanced Practice Nursing, New York, NY 10012-1019. Offers adult-gerontology acute care nurse practitioner (MS, Advanced Certificate); adult-gerontology primary care nurse practitioner (MS, Advanced Certificate); family nurse practitioner (MS, Advanced Certificate); gerontology nurse practitioner (Advanced Certificate); nurse-midwifery (MS, Advanced Certificate); nursing administration (MS, Advanced Certificate); nursing education (MS, Advanced Certificate); nursing informatics (MS, Advanced Certificate); pediatrics nurse practitioner (MS, Advanced Certificate); psychiatric-mental health nurse practitioner (MS, Advanced Certificate); MS/MPH. *Accreditation:* AACN; ACNM/ACME. *Program availability:* Part-time. *Faculty:* 24 full-time (all women), 76 part-time/adjunct (65 women). *Students:* 46 full-time (26 women), 586 part-time (513 women); includes 242 minority (68 Black or African American, non-Hispanic/Latino; 3 American Indian or Alaska Native, non-Hispanic/Latino; 117 Asian, non-Hispanic/Latino; 38 Hispanic/Latino; 3 Native Hawaiian or other Pacific Islander, non-Hispanic/Latino; 13 Two or more races, non-Hispanic/Latino), 23 international. Average age 32. 402 applicants, 69% accepted, 138 enrolled. In 2015, 198 master's, 5 other advanced degrees awarded. *Degree requirements:* For master's, thesis (for some programs). *Entrance requirements:* For master's, BS in nursing, AS in nursing with another BS/BA, interview, RN license, 1 year of clinical experience (3 for the MS in nursing education program); for Advanced Certificate, master's degree. Additional exam requirements/recommendations for international students: Required—TOEFL (minimum score 90 iBT), IELTS (minimum score 7). *Application deadline:* For fall admission, 6/15 for domestic and international students; for spring admission, 12/1 for domestic and international students; for summer admission, 3/1 for domestic and international students. Application fee: $80. Electronic applications accepted. *Expenses:* Contact institution. *Financial support:* In 2015–16, 101 students received support. Career-related internships or fieldwork, Federal Work-Study, and scholarships/grants available. Support available to part-time students. Financial award application deadline: 3/1; financial award applicants required to submit FAFSA. *Faculty research:* Geriatrics, HIV, families and illness, oral systemic connection, symptom management. *Unit head:* Dr. James Pace, Senior Associate Dean for Academic Programs, 212-992-7343, E-mail: james.pace@nyu.edu. *Application contact:* Samantha Jaser, Assistant Director, Graduate Student Affairs and Admissions, 212-992-7653, Fax: 212-995-4302, E-mail: saj283@nyu.edu.

Northeastern University, Bouvé College of Health Sciences, Boston, MA 02115-5096. Offers applied behavior analysis (MS, CAGS); audiology (Au D); biomedical nanotechnology (MS); college student development and counseling (MS, CAGS); counseling psychology (MS, PhD, CAGS); exercise science (MS); health informatics (MS); medicinal chemistry (MS); nurse anesthesia (DNP, CAGS); nursing (MS, PhD, CAGS), including administration (MS), adult-gerontology acute care nurse practitioner (MS, CAGS), adult-gerontology primary care nurse practitioner (MS, CAGS), anesthesia (MS), family nurse practitioner (MS, CAGS), neonatal nurse practitioner (MS, CAGS), pediatric nurse practitioner (MS, CAGS), psychiatric mental health nurse practitioner (MS, CAGS); nursing practice (DNP); personal health informatics (MS); pharmaceutical sciences (MS, PhD), including interdisciplinary concentration, pharmaceutics and drug delivery systems; pharmacology (MS); pharmacy (Pharm D); physical therapy (Postbaccalaureate Certificate); physician assistant (MS); population health (PhD); school psychology (MS, PhD, CAGS); speech-language pathology (MS); urban health (MPH); MS/MBA. *Accreditation:* ACPE (one or more programs are accredited). *Program availability:* Part-time, evening/weekend, online learning. *Faculty:* 194 full-time (120 women), 169 part-time/adjunct (136 women). *Students:* 1,416 full-time (1,049 women), 310 part-time (248 women). In 2015, 374 master's, 313 doctorates, 37 other advanced degrees awarded. *Degree requirements:* For doctorate, thesis/dissertation (for some programs); for other advanced degree, comprehensive exam. Application fee: $75. Electronic applications accepted. *Expenses:* Contact institution. *Financial support:* Applicants required to submit FAFSA. *Unit head:* John R. Reynolds, Professor and Interim Dean, 617-373-3323, Fax: 617-373-3030. *Application contact:* Molly Schnabel, Senior Director of Graduate Affairs, 617-373-2708, Fax: 617-373-4701, E-mail: bouvegrad@neu.edu.
Website: http://www.northeastern.edu/bouve/

Old Dominion University, College of Health Sciences, School of Nursing, Family Nurse Practitioner Emphasis, Norfolk, VA 23529. Offers adult-gerontology clinical nurse specialist/educator (MSN); neonatal nurse practitioner (MSN); pediatric nurse practitioner (MSN). *Program availability:* Blended/hybrid learning. *Faculty:* 3 full-time (all women), 9 part-time/adjunct (all women). *Students:* 53 full-time (52 women), 5 part-time (all women); includes 14 minority (9 Black or African American, non-Hispanic/Latino; 2 Asian, non-Hispanic/Latino; 1 Hispanic/Latino; 2 Two or more races, non-Hispanic/Latino). Average age 35. 53 applicants, 66% accepted, 23 enrolled. In 2015, 60 master's awarded. *Degree requirements:* For master's, comprehensive exam. *Entrance requirements:* For master's, GRE or MAT (waived with a GPA above 3.5), 3 letters of recommendation, essay, resume, transcripts. Additional exam requirements/recommendations for international students: Required—TOEFL. *Application deadline:* For fall admission, 3/1 priority date for domestic students, 4/15 priority date for international students. Application fee: $50. Electronic applications accepted. *Expenses:* Tuition, state resident: full-time $11,136; part-time $464 per credit hour. Tuition, nonresident: full-time $27,840; part-time $1160 per credit hour. *Required fees:* $64 per semester. Tuition and fees vary according to campus/location, program and reciprocity agreements. *Financial support:* In 2015–16, research assistantships with partial tuition reimbursements (averaging $10,000 per year) were awarded; career-related internships or fieldwork, scholarships/grants, and traineeships also available. Support available to part-time students. *Faculty research:* Military families, nurse practitioner student reaching modalities, gerontology, pediatrics, ethics. *Unit head:* Dr. Carolyn M. Rutledge, Associate Chair for Graduate Programs, 757-683-5009, Fax: 757-683-5253, E-mail: crutledg@odu.edu. *Application contact:* Sue Parker, Graduate Program Coordinator, 757-683-4298, Fax: 757-683-5253, E-mail: sparker@odu.edu.
Website: http://catalog.odu.edu/graduate/collegeofhealthsciences/schoolofnursing/#masterofscienceinnursing013familynursepractitionerrole

Old Dominion University, College of Health Sciences, School of Nursing, Nurse Educator Emphasis, Norfolk, VA 23529. Offers neonatal nurse practitioner (MSN); pediatric nurse practitioner (MSN). *Program availability:* Part-time, online learning. *Faculty:* 1 (woman) full-time, 2 part-time/adjunct (both women). *Students:* 9 full-time (7 women), 17 part-time (11 women); includes 5 minority (1 Black or African American, non-Hispanic/Latino; 1 American Indian or Alaska Native, non-Hispanic/Latino; 3 Two or more races, non-Hispanic/Latino), 7 international. Average age 36. In 2015, 7 master's awarded. *Degree requirements:* For master's, comprehensive exam, thesis optional. *Entrance requirements:* For master's, GRE or MAT (waived if GPA is above 3.5), 3 letters of recommendation, essay, resume, transcripts. Additional exam requirements/recommendations for international students: Required—TOEFL. *Application deadline:* For fall admission, 4/15 priority date for international students. Application fee: $50. *Expenses:* Tuition, state resident: full-time $11,136; part-time $464 per credit hour. Tuition, nonresident: full-time $27,840; part-time $1160 per credit hour. *Required fees:* $64 per semester. Tuition and fees vary according to campus/location, program and reciprocity agreements. *Financial support:* Fellowships, research assistantships, teaching assistantships, and unspecified assistantships available. *Faculty research:* Technology in nursing education, evidence-based instructional strategies, clinical judgment and decision-making. *Total annual research expenditures:* $35,726. *Unit head:* Dr. Kimberly Adams-Tufts, Graduate Program Director, 757-683-5011, E-mail: ktufts@odu.edu. *Application contact:* Sue Parker, Graduate Program Coordinator, 757-683-4298, Fax: 757-683-5253, E-mail: sparker@odu.edu.

Oregon Health & Science University, School of Nursing, Program in Pediatric Nurse Practitioner, Portland, OR 97239-3098. Offers MN, DNP, PMC.

Queen's University at Kingston, School of Graduate Studies, Faculty of Health Sciences, School of Nursing, Kingston, ON K7L 3N6, Canada. Offers health and chronic illness (M Sc); nurse scientist (PhD); primary health care nurse practitioner (Certificate); women's and children's health (M Sc). *Degree requirements:* For master's, thesis. *Entrance requirements:* For master's, RN license. Additional exam requirements/recommendations for international students: Required—TOEFL. *Faculty research:* Women and children's health, health and chronic illness.

Rush University, College of Nursing, Department of Women, Children, and Family Nursing, Chicago, IL 60612. Offers neonatal clinical nurse specialist (DNP); neonatal nurse practitioner (DNP, Post-Graduate Certificate); nursing science (PhD); pediatric acute care nurse practitioner (DNP, Post-Graduate Certificate); pediatric clinical nurse specialist (DNP); pediatric primary care nurse practitioner (DNP); pediatric primary nurse practitioner (Post-Graduate Certificate); systems leadership (DNP). *Accreditation:* AACN. *Program availability:* Part-time, online learning. *Faculty:* 43 full-time (40 women), 52 part-time/adjunct (49 women). *Students:* 11 full-time (all women), 143 part-time (140 women); includes 20 minority (3 Black or African American, non-Hispanic/Latino; 1 American Indian or Alaska Native, non-Hispanic/Latino; 7 Asian, non-Hispanic/Latino; 9 Hispanic/Latino). Average age 32. 58 applicants, 91% accepted, 40 enrolled. In 2015, 19 doctorates awarded. *Degree requirements:* For doctorate, leadership project (for DNP); dissertation (for PhD). *Entrance requirements:* For doctorate, GRE General Test (waived for DNP if cumulative GPA is 3.25 or greater, nursing GPA is 3.0 or greater, or a completed graduate program GPA is 3.5 or greater), interview, 3 letters of recommendation, personal statement, current resume; for Post-Graduate Certificate, MSN in a clinical discipline, 3 letters of recommendation, personal statement, current resume, interview. Additional exam requirements/recommendations for international students: Required—TOEFL (minimum score 94 iBT). *Application deadline:* For fall admission, 1/2 for domestic students; for winter admission, 10/15 for domestic students; for spring admission, 8/3 for domestic students; for summer admission, 12/1 for domestic students. Applications are processed on a rolling basis. Application fee: $100. Electronic applications accepted. *Expenses:* Contact institution. *Financial support:* Research assistantships, teaching assistantships with tuition reimbursements, Federal Work-Study, scholarships/grants, traineeships, and health care benefits available. Support available to part-time students. Financial award application deadline: 3/1; financial award applicants required to submit FAFSA. *Faculty research:* Reduction of health disparities; benefit of human milk feedings for low birth weight infants; decision-making when living with a BRCA mutation over 5-8 year time period; accelerating adoption of comparative effectiveness research in premature infants. *Unit head:* Dr. Wrenetha Julion, Chairperson, 312-942-7117, E-mail: wrenetha_a_julion@rush.edu. *Application contact:* Jennifer Thorndyke, Admissions Specialist, 312-563-7526, E-mail: jennifer_thorndyke@rush.edu.
Website: http://www.rushu.rush.edu/servlet/Satellite?c=content_block&cid=1320160764996&pagename=CollegeOfNursing%2Fcontent_block%2FContentBlockDetail&rendermod

St. Catherine University, Graduate Programs, Program in Nursing, St. Paul, MN 55105. Offers adult gerontological nurse practitioner (MS); neonatal nurse practitioner (MS); nurse educator (MS); nursing (DNP); nursing: entry-level (MS); pediatric nurse practitioner (MS). *Accreditation:* ACEN. *Program availability:* Part-time, evening/weekend. *Degree requirements:* For master's, thesis; for doctorate, portfolio, systems change project. *Entrance requirements:* For master's, GRE General Test, bachelor's degree in nursing, current nursing license, 2 years of recent clinical practice; for doctorate, master's degree in nursing, RN license, advanced nursing position. Additional exam requirements/recommendations for international students: Required—TOEFL (minimum score 600 paper-based; 100 iBT). *Expenses:* Contact institution.

San Francisco State University, Division of Graduate Studies, College of Health and Social Sciences, School of Nursing, San Francisco, CA 94132-1722. Offers adult acute care (MS); clinical nurse specialist (MS); community/public health nursing (MS); family nurse practitioner (MS, Certificate); nursing administration (MS); pediatrics (MS); women's health (MS). *Accreditation:* AACN. *Program availability:* Part-time. *Application deadline:* Applications are processed on a rolling basis. *Expenses:* Tuition, state resident: full-time $6738. Tuition, nonresident: full-time $15,666. *Required fees:* $1004. *Financial support:* Career-related internships or fieldwork available. *Unit head:* Dr. Mary-Ann van Dam, Director, 415-338-1802, Fax: 415-338-0555, E-mail: vandam@sfsu.edu. *Application contact:* Connie Carr, Graduate Coordinator, 415-338-6856, Fax: 415-338-0555, E-mail: ccarr@sfsu.edu.
Website: http://nursing.sfsu.edu

Seton Hall University, College of Nursing, South Orange, NJ 07079-2697. Offers advanced practice in primary health care (MSN, DNP), including adult/gerontological nurse practitioner, pediatric nurse practitioner; entry into practice (MSN); health systems administration (MSN, DNP); nursing (PhD); nursing case management (MSN); nursing education (MA); school nurse (MSN); MSN/MA. *Accreditation:* AACN. *Program availability:* Part-time, online learning. *Degree requirements:* For master's, research project; for doctorate, dissertation or scholarly project. *Entrance requirements:* For doctorate, GRE (waived for students with GPA of 3.5 or higher). Additional exam requirements/recommendations for international students: Required—TOEFL. Electronic applications accepted. *Faculty research:* Parent/child, adult, and gerontological nursing; breast cancer; families of children with HIV; parish nursing.

Spalding University, Graduate Studies, Kosair College of Health and Natural Sciences, School of Nursing, Louisville, KY 40203-2188. Offers adult nurse practitioner (MSN, PMC); family nurse practitioner (MSN, PMC); leadership in nursing and healthcare (MSN); pediatric nurse practitioner (MSN, PMC). *Accreditation:* AACN. *Program availability:* Part-time, evening/weekend. *Faculty:* 10 full-time (9 women), 8 part-time/adjunct (7 women). *Students:* 101 full-time (94 women), 9 part-time (all women); includes 20 minority (14 Black or African American, non-Hispanic/Latino; 3 Asian, non-Hispanic/Latino; 1 Native Hawaiian or other Pacific Islander, non-Hispanic/Latino; 2 Two or more races, non-Hispanic/Latino). Average age 36. 10 applicants, 30% accepted, 2 enrolled. In 2015, 43 master's awarded. *Degree requirements:* For master's, comprehensive exam (for some programs), thesis. *Entrance requirements:* For master's, GRE General Test, BSN or bachelor's degree in related field, RN licensure, autobiographical statement, transcripts, letters of recommendation. Additional exam requirements/recommendations for international students: Required—TOEFL (minimum score 535 paper-based). *Application deadline:* For fall admission, 2/1 priority date for domestic students. Application fee: $30. *Financial support:* Career-related internships or fieldwork, scholarships/grants, and traineeships available. Support available to part-time students. Financial award application deadline: 3/30; financial award applicants required to submit FAFSA. *Faculty research:* Nurse educational administration, gerontology, bioterrorism, healthcare ethics, leadership. *Unit head:* Dr. Patricia Spurr, Chair, 502-873-4304, E-mail: pspurr@spalding.edu. *Application contact:* Dr. Pam King, Program Director, 502-873-4292, E-mail: pking@spalding.edu.
Website: http://www.spalding.edu/nursing/

Stony Brook University, State University of New York, Stony Brook Medicine, School of Nursing, Program in Child Health Nursing, Stony Brook, NY 11794. Offers child health nurse practitioner (Certificate); child health nursing (MS, DNP). *Accreditation:* AACN. *Program availability:* Part time, blended/hybrid learning. *Students:* 7 full-time (all women), 89 part-time (88 women); includes 24 minority (12 Black or African American, non-Hispanic/Latino; 8 Asian, non-Hispanic/Latino; 4 Hispanic/Latino), 1 international. 46 applicants, 93% accepted, 39 enrolled. In 2015, 24 master's awarded. *Degree requirements:* For master's, thesis. *Entrance requirements:* For master's, BSN, minimum GPA of 3.0, course work in statistics. Additional exam requirements/recommendations for international students: Required—TOEFL (minimum score 90 iBT). *Application deadline:* For fall admission, 12/1 for domestic students. Application fee: $100. *Expenses:* $24,781 full-time resident tuition and fees, $968 per credit hour; $44,431 full-time nonresident tuition and fees, $1,787 per credit hour. *Financial support:* Application deadline: 3/15. *Unit head:* Kammy McLoughlin, Program Director, 631-444-3264, Fax: 631-444-3136, E-mail: kammy.mcloughlin@stonybrook.edu. *Application contact:* Pamela Criscuolo, Staff Assistant, 631-444-3549, Fax: 631-444-3136, E-mail: pamela.criscuolo@stonybrook.edu.
Website: http://www.stonybrook.edu/sb/departments/nursing.shtml

Texas Christian University, Harris College of Nursing and Health Sciences, Master's Program in Nursing, Fort Worth, TX 76129. Offers clinical nurse leader (MSN, Certificate); clinical nurse specialist (MSN), including adult/gerontology nursing, pediatrics; nursing education (MSN). *Accreditation:* AACN; AANA/CANAEP (one or more programs are accredited). *Program availability:* Part-time, online only, 100% online. *Faculty:* 20 full-time (17 women), 2 part-time/adjunct (both women). *Students:* 47 full-time (40 women), 24 part-time (all women); includes 19 minority (3 Black or African American, non-Hispanic/Latino; 1 American Indian or Alaska Native, non-Hispanic/Latino; 10 Asian, non-Hispanic/Latino; 2 Hispanic/Latino; 1 Native Hawaiian or other Pacific Islander, non-Hispanic/Latino; 2 Two or more races, non-Hispanic/Latino), 1 international. Average age 39. 34 applicants, 82% accepted, 23 enrolled. In 2015, 14 master's awarded. *Degree requirements:* For master's, thesis or alternative, practicum. *Entrance requirements:* For master's, GRE General Test, 3 letters of reference, essay, resume, two official transcripts from every institution attended. *Application deadline:* For fall admission, 4/1 for domestic and international students; for spring admission, 9/1 for domestic and international students; for summer admission, 2/1 for domestic and international students. Applications are processed on a rolling basis. Application fee: $60. Electronic applications accepted. *Expenses:* $1,415 per semester hour; $112 fee per course. *Financial support:* In 2015–16, 71 students received support. Teaching assistantships and scholarships/grants available. Financial award application deadline: 2/15; financial award applicants required to submit FAFSA. *Faculty research:* Geriatrics, cancer survivorship, health literacy, endothelial cells, clinical simulation outcomes. *Unit head:* Dr. Kathy Baker, Director, Division of Nursing Graduate Studies and Scholarship, 817-257-6726, Fax: 817-257-8383, E-mail: kathy.baker@tcu.edu. *Application contact:* Mary Jane Allred, Administrative Program Specialist, 817-257-6726, Fax: 817-257-8383, E-mail: m.allred@tcu.edu.
Website: http://www.nursing.tcu.edu/graduate.asp

Texas Tech University Health Sciences Center, School of Nursing, Lubbock, TX 79430. Offers acute care nurse practitioner (MSN, Certificate); administration (MSN); advanced practice (DNP); education (MSN); executive leadership (DNP); family nurse practitioner (MSN, Certificate); geriatric nurse practitioner (MSN, Certificate); pediatric nurse practitioner (MSN, Certificate). *Accreditation:* AACN. *Program availability:* Part-time, online learning. *Degree requirements:* For master's, thesis optional. *Entrance requirements:* For master's, minimum GPA of 3.0, 3 letters of reference, BSN, RN license; for Certificate, minimum GPA of 3.0, 3 letters of reference, RN license. Additional exam requirements/recommendations for international students: Required—TOEFL (minimum score 550 paper-based). *Faculty research:* Diabetes/obesity, nurse competency, disease management, intervention and measurements, health disparities.

Texas Woman's University, Graduate School, College of Nursing, Denton, TX 76204-5498. Offers acute care nurse practitioner (MS); adult health clinical nurse specialist (MS); adult health nurse practitioner (MS); child health clinical nurse specialist (MS); clinical nurse leader (MS); family nurse practitioner (MS); health systems management (MS); nursing education (MS); nursing practice (DNP); nursing science (PhD); pediatric nurse practitioner (MS); women's health clinical nurse specialist (MS); women's health nurse practitioner (MS). *Accreditation:* AACN. *Program availability:* Part-time, online learning. *Faculty:* 55 full-time (51 women), 42 part-time/adjunct (35 women). *Students:* 39 full-time (37 women), 958 part-time (888 women); includes 566 minority (226 Black or African American, non-Hispanic/Latino; 8 American Indian or Alaska Native, non-Hispanic/Latino; 221 Asian, non-Hispanic/Latino; 88 Hispanic/Latino; 3 Native Hawaiian or other Pacific Islander, non-Hispanic/Latino; 20 Two or more races, non-Hispanic/Latino), 37 international. Average age 36. 430 applicants, 65% accepted, 193 enrolled. In 2015, 248 master's, 10 doctorates awarded. *Degree requirements:* For master's, comprehensive exam, thesis or alternative; for doctorate, comprehensive exam, thesis/dissertation. *Entrance requirements:* For master's, GRE or MAT, minimum GPA of 3.0 on last 60 hours in undergraduate nursing degree and overall, RN license, BS in nursing, basic statistics course; for doctorate, GRE (preferred minimum score 153 [500 old version] Verbal, 144 [500 old version] Quantitative, 4 Analytical), MS in nursing, minimum preferred GPA of 3.5, RN license, statistics, 2 letters of reference, curriculum vitae, graduate nursing-theory course, graduate research course, statement of professional goals and research interests. Additional exam requirements/recommendations for international students: Required—TOEFL (minimum score 550 paper-based; 79 iBT). *Application deadline:* For fall admission, 5/1 priority date for domestic students, 3/1 for international students; for spring admission, 9/15 priority date

for domestic students, 7/1 for international students. Applications are processed on a rolling basis. Application fee: $50 ($75 for international students). Electronic applications accepted. *Expenses:* Tuition, state resident: full-time $4380; part-time $243 per credit hour. Tuition, nonresident: full-time $11,400; part-time $633 per credit hour. *International tuition:* $11,465 full-time. *Required fees:* $1778; $99 per credit hour. $283 per semester. One-time fee: $50. Tuition and fees vary according to course load and program. *Financial support:* In 2015–16, 149 students received support, including 10 research assistantships (averaging $5,600 per year), 1 teaching assistantship (averaging $5,600 per year); career-related internships or fieldwork, Federal Work-Study, institutionally sponsored loans, scholarships/grants, traineeships, health care benefits, and unspecified assistantships also available. Support available to part-time students. Financial award application deadline: 3/1; financial award applicants required to submit FAFSA. *Faculty research:* Screening, prevention, and treatment for intimate partner violence; needs of adolescents during childbirth intervention; a network analysis decision tool for nurse managers (social network analysis); support for adolescents with implantable cardioverter defibrillators; informatics: nurse staffing, safety, quality, and financial data as they relate to patient care outcomes; prevention and treatment of obesity; improving infant outcomes related to premature birth. *Total annual research expenditures:* $1.7 million. *Unit head:* Dr. Anita G. Hufft, Dean, 940-898-2401, Fax: 940-898-2437, E-mail: nursing@twu.edu. *Application contact:* Dr. Samuel Wheeler, Assistant Director of Admissions, 940-898-3188, Fax: 940-898-3081, E-mail: wheelersr@twu.edu.
Website: http://www.twu.edu/nursing/

University of Cincinnati, Graduate School, College of Nursing, Cincinnati, OH 45221-0038. Offers clinical nurse specialist (MSN), including adult health, community health, neonatal, nursing administration, occupational health, pediatric health, psychiatric nursing, women's health; nurse anesthesia (MSN); nurse midwifery (MSN); nurse practitioner (MSN), including acute care, ambulatory care, family, family/psychiatric, women's health; nursing (PhD); MBA/MSN. *Accreditation:* AACN; AANA/CANAEP (one or more programs are accredited); ACNM/ACME. *Program availability:* Part-time, online learning. Terminal master's awarded for partial completion of doctoral program. *Degree requirements:* For master's, thesis or alternative; for doctorate, comprehensive exam, thesis/dissertation. *Entrance requirements:* For master's and doctorate, GRE General Test. Additional exam requirements/recommendations for international students: Required—TOEFL (minimum score 520 paper-based). Electronic applications accepted. *Faculty research:* Substance abuse, injury and violence, symptom management.

University of Colorado Denver, College of Nursing, Aurora, CO 80045. Offers adult clinical nurse specialist (MS); adult nurse practitioner (MS); family nurse practitioner (MS); family psychiatric mental health nurse practitioner (MS); health care informatics (MS); nurse-midwifery (MS); nursing (DNP, PhD); nursing leadership and health care systems (MS); pediatric nurse practitioner (MS); special studies (MS); women's health (MS); MS/PhD. *Accreditation:* ACNM/ACME (one or more programs are accredited). *Program availability:* Part-time, evening/weekend, online learning. *Faculty:* 109 full-time (100 women), 55 part-time/adjunct (50 women). *Students:* 367 full-time (332 women), 141 part-time (118 women); includes 79 minority (16 Black or African American, non-Hispanic/Latino; 2 American Indian or Alaska Native, non-Hispanic/Latino; 8 Asian, non-Hispanic/Latino; 37 Hispanic/Latino; 16 Two or more races, non-Hispanic/Latino), 6 international. Average age 36. 321 applicants, 53% accepted, 145 enrolled. In 2015, 151 master's, 36 doctorates awarded. Terminal master's awarded for partial completion of doctoral program. *Degree requirements:* For master's, thesis optional; for doctorate, comprehensive exam, thesis/dissertation, 42 credits of coursework. *Entrance requirements:* For master's, GRE if cumulative undergraduate GPA is less than 3.0, undergraduate nursing degree from NLNAC- or CCNE-accredited school or university; completion of research and statistics courses with minimum grade of C; copy of current and unencumbered nursing license; for doctorate, GRE, bachelor's and/or master's degrees in nursing from NLN- or CCNE-accredited institution; portfolio; minimum undergraduate GPA of 3.0, graduate 3.5; graduate-level intermediate statistics and master's-level nursing theory courses with minimum B grade; interview. Additional exam requirements/recommendations for international students: Required—TOEFL (minimum score 560 paper-based; 83 iBT). *Application deadline:* For fall admission, 2/15 for domestic students, 1/15 for international students; for spring admission, 7/1 for domestic students, 6/1 for international students. Application fee: $50 ($75 for international students). Electronic applications accepted. *Expenses:* Contact institution. *Financial support:* In 2015–16, 148 students received support. Fellowships, research assistantships, teaching assistantships, Federal Work-Study, institutionally sponsored loans, scholarships/grants, traineeships, and unspecified assistantships available. Support available to part-time students. Financial award application deadline: 4/1; financial award applicants required to submit FAFSA. *Faculty research:* Biological and behavioral phenomena in pregnancy and postpartum; patterns of glycaemia during the insulin resistance of pregnancy; obesity, gestational diabetes, and relationship to neonatal adiposity; men's awareness and knowledge of male breast cancer; cognitive-behavioral therapy for chronic insomnia after breast cancer treatment; massage therapy for the treatment of tension-type headaches. *Total annual research expenditures:* $5.9 million. *Unit head:* Dr. Sarah Thompson, Dean, 303-724-1679, E-mail: sarah.a.thompson@ucdenver.edu. *Application contact:* Judy Campbell, Graduate Programs Coordinator, 303-724-8503, E-mail: judy.campbell@ucdenver.edu.
Website: http://www.ucdenver.edu/academics/colleges/nursing/Pages/default.aspx

University of Colorado Denver, School of Medicine, Physician Assistant Program, Aurora, CO 80045. Offers child health associate (MPAS), including global health, leadership, education, advocacy, development, and scholarship, pediatric critical and acute care, rural health, urban/underserved populations. *Accreditation:* ARC-PA. *Students:* 131 full-time (107 women); includes 18 minority (2 Black or African American, non-Hispanic/Latino; 6 Asian, non-Hispanic/Latino; 9 Hispanic/Latino; 1 Two or more races, non-Hispanic/Latino). Average age 28. In 2015, 45 master's awarded. *Degree requirements:* For master's, comprehensive exam. *Entrance requirements:* For master's, GRE General Test, minimum GPA of 2.8; 3 letters of recommendation; prerequisite courses in chemistry, biology, general genetics, psychology and statistics; interview. Additional exam requirements/recommendations for international students: Required—TOEFL (minimum score 550 paper-based; 80 iBT). *Application deadline:* For fall admission, 9/1 for domestic students, 8/15 for international students. Application fee: $170. Electronic applications accepted. *Expenses:* Contact institution. *Financial support:* In 2015–16, 130 students received support. Fellowships, research assistantships, teaching assistantships, career-related internships or fieldwork, Federal Work-Study, institutionally sponsored loans, scholarships/grants, traineeships, and unspecified assistantships available. Financial award application deadline: 3/15; financial award applicants required to submit FAFSA. *Faculty research:* Clinical genetics and genetic counseling, evidence-based medicine, pediatric allergy and asthma, childhood diabetes, standardized patient assessment. *Unit head:* Jonathan Bowser, Program Director, 303-724-1349, E-mail: jonathan.bowser@ucdenver.edu. *Application contact:* Kay Denler, Academic Services Program Manager, 303-724-7963, E-mail: kay.denler@ucdenver.edu.
Website: http://www.ucdenver.edu/academics/colleges/medicalschool/education/degree_programs/PAProgram/Pages/Home.aspx

Pediatric Nursing

University of Delaware, College of Health Sciences, School of Nursing, Newark, DE 19716. Offers adult nurse practitioner (MSN, PMC); cardiopulmonary clinical nurse specialist (MSN, PMC); cardiopulmonary clinical nurse specialist/adult nurse practitioner (MSN, PMC); family nurse practitioner (MSN, PMC); gerontology clinical nurse specialist (MSN, PMC); gerontology clinical nurse specialist geriatric nurse practitioner (PMC); gerontology clinical nurse specialist/geriatric nurse practitioner (MSN); health services administration (MSN, PMC); nursing of children clinical nurse specialist (MSN, PMC); nursing of children clinical nurse specialist/pediatric nurse practitioner (MSN, PMC); oncology/immune deficiency clinical nurse specialist (MSN, PMC); oncology/immune deficiency clinical nurse specialist/adult nurse practitioner (MSN, PMC); perinatal/women's health clinical nurse specialist (MSN, PMC); perinatal/women's health clinical nurse specialist/women's health nurse practitioner (MSN, PMC); psychiatric nursing clinical nurse specialist (MSN, PMC). *Accreditation:* AACN. *Program availability:* Part-time, evening/weekend, online learning. *Degree requirements:* For master's, thesis optional. *Entrance requirements:* For master's, BSN, interview, RN license. Electronic applications accepted. *Faculty research:* Marriage and chronic illness, health promotion, congestive heart failure patient outcomes, school nursing, diabetes in children, culture, health disparities, cardiovascular, prison nursing, oncology, public policy, child obesity, smoking and teen pregnancy, blood pressure measurements, men's health.

University of Illinois at Chicago, College of Nursing, Program in Nursing, Chicago, IL 60607-7128. Offers acute care clinical nurse specialist (MS); administrative nursing leadership (Certificate); adult nurse practitioner (MS); adult/geriatric nurse practitioner (MS); advanced community health nurse specialist (MS); family nurse practitioner (MS); geriatric clinical nurse specialist (MS); geriatric nurse practitioner (MS); nurse midwifery (MS); occupational health/advanced community health nurse specialist (MS); occupational health/family nurse practitioner (MS); pediatric nurse practitioner (MS); perinatal clinical nurse specialist (MS); school/advanced community health nurse specialist (MS); school/family nurse practitioner (MS); women's health nurse practitioner (MS). *Accreditation:* AACN. *Program availability:* Part-time. *Faculty:* 100 full-time (93 women), 89 part-time/adjunct (82 women). *Students:* 359 full-time (326 women), 280 part-time (249 women); includes 169 minority (43 Black or African American, non-Hispanic/Latino; 62 Asian, non-Hispanic/Latino; 56 Hispanic/Latino; 1 Native Hawaiian or other Pacific Islander, non-Hispanic/Latino; 7 Two or more races, non-Hispanic/Latino), 12 international. Average age 32. In 2015, 4 other advanced degrees awarded. *Degree requirements:* For master's, thesis or alternative. *Entrance requirements:* For master's, GRE General Test, minimum GPA of 2.75. Additional exam requirements/recommendations for international students: Required—TOEFL. *Application deadline:* For fall admission, 5/15 for domestic students, 2/15 for international students; for spring admission, 11/1 for domestic students, 7/15 for international students. Applications are processed on a rolling basis. Application fee: $60. Electronic applications accepted. *Expenses:* Tuition, state resident: full-time $11,480; part-time $3826 per credit. Tuition, nonresident: full-time $23,720; part-time $7906 per credit. *Required fees:* $1333 per semester. Part-time tuition and fees vary according to course load and program. *Financial support:* Fellowships with full tuition reimbursements, research assistantships with full tuition reimbursements, teaching assistantships with full tuition reimbursements, career-related internships or fieldwork, Federal Work-Study, institutionally sponsored loans, scholarships/grants, traineeships, tuition waivers (full and partial), and unspecified assistantships available. Support available to part-time students. Financial award application deadline: 3/1; financial award applicants required to submit FAFSA. *Unit head:* Dr. Terri E. Weaver, Dean, 312-996-7808, E-mail: teweaver@uic.edu. *Application contact:* Receptionist, 312-413-2550, E-mail: gradcoll@uic.edu. Website: http://www.nursing.uic.edu/academics-admissions/master-science#program-overview

University of Maryland, Baltimore, Graduate School, School of Nursing, Master's Program in Nursing, Baltimore, MD 21201. Offers community health nursing (MS); gerontological nursing (MS); maternal-child nursing (MS); medical-surgical nursing (MS); nurse-midwifery education (MS); nursing administration (MS); nursing education (MS); nursing health policy (MS); primary care nursing (MS); psychiatric nursing (MS); MS/MBA. MS/MBA offered jointly with University of Baltimore. *Accreditation:* AACN; AANA/CANAEP. *Program availability:* Part-time. *Degree requirements:* For master's, comprehensive exam (for some programs), thesis or alternative. *Entrance requirements:* For master's, minimum GPA of 2.75, course work in statistics, BS in nursing. Additional exam requirements/recommendations for international students: Required—TOEFL (minimum score 550 paper-based; 80 iBT); Recommended—IELTS (minimum score 7). Electronic applications accepted. Tuition and fees vary according to program.

University of Michigan, Rackham Graduate School, School of Nursing, Ann Arbor, MI 48109. Offers acute care pediatric nurse practitioner (MS); nursing (DNP, PhD, Post Master's Certificate). *Accreditation:* AACN; ACNM/ACME (one or more programs are accredited). *Program availability:* Part-time, online learning. Terminal master's awarded for partial completion of doctoral program. *Degree requirements:* For doctorate, thesis/dissertation. *Faculty research:* Preparation of clinical nurse researchers, biobehavior, women's health, health promotion, substance abuse, psychobiology of menopause, fertility, obesity, health care systems. *Unit head:* Dr. Kathleen Potempa, Dean, 734-764-7185, Fax: 734-764-7186. *Application contact:* E-mail: sn-osams@umich.edu. Website: http://www.nursing.umich.edu/

University of Minnesota, Twin Cities Campus, Graduate School, School of Nursing, Children with Special Health Care Needs Program, Minneapolis, MN 55455-0213. Offers MS. *Entrance requirements:* Additional exam requirements/recommendations for international students: Required—TOEFL (minimum score 586 paper-based).

University of Minnesota, Twin Cities Campus, Graduate School, School of Nursing, Pediatric Clinical Nurse Specialist Program, Minneapolis, MN 55455-0213. Offers MS. *Accreditation:* AACN. *Program availability:* Part-time. *Degree requirements:* For master's, final oral exam, project or thesis.

University of Minnesota, Twin Cities Campus, Graduate School, School of Nursing, Pediatric Nurse Practitioner Program, Minneapolis, MN 55455-0213. Offers MS. *Accreditation:* AACN. *Degree requirements:* For master's, final oral exam, project or thesis.

University of Minnesota, Twin Cities Campus, Graduate School, School of Nursing, Program in Adolescent Nursing, Minneapolis, MN 55455-0213. Offers MS. *Accreditation:* AACN. *Program availability:* Part-time. *Degree requirements:* For master's, final oral exam, project or thesis. *Entrance requirements:* Additional exam requirements/recommendations for international students: Required—TOEFL (minimum score 586 paper-based).

University of Missouri, Office of Research and Graduate Studies, Sinclair School of Nursing, Columbia, MO 65211. Offers adult-gerontology clinical nurse specialist (DNP, Certificate); family nurse practitioner (DNP); family psychiatric and mental health nurse practitioner (DNP); nursing (MS, DNP); nursing leadership and innovations in health care (DNP); pediatric clinical nurse specialist (DNP, Certificate); pediatric nurse practitioner (DNP). *Accreditation:* AACN. *Program availability:* Part-time. *Degree requirements:* For master's, thesis optional, oral exam; for doctorate, thesis/dissertation. *Entrance requirements:* For master's, GRE General Test, BSN, minimum GPA of 3.0 during last 60 hours, nursing license. Additional exam requirements/recommendations for

international students: Required—TOEFL (minimum score 550 paper-based; 79 iBT). *Application deadline:* For fall admission, 2/1 priority date for domestic and international students. Applications are processed on a rolling basis. Application fee: $55 ($75 for international students). Electronic applications accepted. *Financial support:* Fellowships, research assistantships, teaching assistantships, career-related internships or fieldwork, institutionally sponsored loans, scholarships/grants, traineeships, health care benefits, tuition waivers (full), and unspecified assistantships available. Support available to part-time students. Website: http://nursing.missouri.edu/

University of Missouri–Kansas City, School of Nursing and Health Studies, Kansas City, MO 64108. Offers adult clinical nurse specialist (MSN), including adult nurse practitioner, women's health nurse practitioner (MSN, DNP); adult clinical nursing practice (DNP), including adult gerontology nurse practitioner, women's health nurse practitioner (MSN, DNP); clinical nursing practice (DNP), including family nurse practitioner; family nurse practitioner (MSN); neonatal nurse practitioner (MSN); nurse educator (MSN); nurse executive (MSN); nursing (PhD); nursing practice (DNP); pediatric clinical nursing practice (DNP), including pediatric nurse practitioner; pediatric nurse practitioner (MSN). *Accreditation:* AACN. *Program availability:* Part-time, online learning. *Faculty:* 44 full-time (40 women), 47 part-time/adjunct (45 women). *Students:* 62 full-time (43 women), 259 part-time (239 women); includes 61 minority (28 Black or African American, non-Hispanic/Latino; 3 American Indian or Alaska Native, non-Hispanic/Latino; 16 Asian, non-Hispanic/Latino; 10 Hispanic/Latino; 4 Two or more races, non-Hispanic/Latino). Average age 35. 102 applicants, 35% accepted, 36 enrolled. In 2015, 116 master's, 23 doctorates awarded. *Degree requirements:* For master's, thesis or alternative. *Entrance requirements:* For master's, minimum undergraduate GPA of 3.2; for doctorate, GRE, 3 letters of reference. Additional exam requirements/recommendations for international students: Required—TOEFL (minimum score 550 paper-based; 80 iBT). *Application deadline:* For fall admission, 2/1 priority date for domestic and international students; for spring admission, 9/1 priority date for domestic and international students. Application fee: $45 ($50 for international students). *Financial support:* In 2015–16, 2 teaching assistantships with partial tuition reimbursements (averaging $6,650 per year) were awarded; fellowships, research assistantships, career-related internships or fieldwork, Federal Work-Study, institutionally sponsored loans, and tuition waivers (full and partial) also available. Support available to part-time students. Financial award application deadline: 3/1; financial award applicants required to submit FAFSA. *Faculty research:* Geriatrics/gerontology, children's pain, neonatology, Alzheimer's care, cancer caregivers. *Unit head:* Dr. Ann Cary, Dean, 816-235-1723, Fax: 816-235-1701, E-mail: caryah@umkc.edu. *Application contact:* Judy Jellison, Coordinator for Admissions and Recruitment, 816-235-1740, Fax: 816-235-1701, E-mail: jellisonj@umkc.edu. Website: http://nursing.umkc.edu/

University of Missouri–St. Louis, College of Nursing, St. Louis, MO 63121-4400. Offers adult/geriatric nurse practitioner (Post Master's Certificate); family nurse practitioner (Post Master's Certificate); nurse educator (MSN); nurse practitioner (MSN); nursing (DNP, PhD); pediatric nurse practitioner (Post Master's Certificate); psychiatric-mental health nurse practitioner (Post Master's Certificate); women's health nurse practitioner (Post Master's Certificate). *Accreditation:* AACN. *Program availability:* Part-time. *Faculty:* 21 full-time (19 women), 6 part-time/adjunct (5 women). *Students:* 18 full-time (17 women), 227 part-time (215 women); includes 34 minority (22 Black or African American, non-Hispanic/Latino; 8 Asian, non-Hispanic/Latino; 3 Hispanic/Latino; 1 Two or more races, non-Hispanic/Latino), 1 international. Average age 35. 152 applicants, 69% accepted, 83 enrolled. *Degree requirements:* For doctorate, comprehensive exam, thesis/dissertation; for Post Master's Certificate, thesis. *Entrance requirements:* For master's, 2 recommendation letters; minimum GPA of 3.0; BSN; nursing licensure; statement of purpose; course in differential/inferential statistics; for doctorate, GRE, 2 letters of recommendation, MSN, minimum GPA of 3.2, course in differential/inferential statistics; for Post Master's Certificate, 2 recommendation letters; MSN; advanced practice certificate; minimum GPA of 3.0; essay. Additional exam requirements/recommendations for international students: Recommended—TOEFL (minimum score 550 paper-based; 79 iBT), IELTS (minimum score 6.5). *Application deadline:* For fall admission, 2/15 for domestic and international students. Application fee: $50 ($40 for international students). Electronic applications accepted. *Financial support:* Research assistantships with tuition reimbursements available. Financial award application deadline: 4/1; financial award applicants required to submit FAFSA. *Faculty research:* Health promotion and restoration, family disruption, violence, abuse, battered women, health survey methods. *Unit head:* Dr. Roberta Lavin, Director, 314-516-6066. *Application contact:* 314-516-5458, Fax: 314-516-6996, E-mail: gradadm@umsl.edu. Website: http://www.umsl.edu/divisions/nursing/

The University of North Carolina at Chapel Hill, School of Nursing, Chapel Hill, NC 27599-7460. Offers advanced practice registered nurse (DNP); health care systems (DNP); nursing (MSN, PhD, PMC), including administration (MSN), adult gerontology primary care nurse practitioner (MSN), clinical nurse leader (MSN), education (MSN), informatics (MSN, PMC), nursing leadership (PMC), outcomes management (MSN), primary care family nurse practitioner (MSN), primary care pediatric nurse practitioner (MSN), psychiatric/mental health nurse practitioner (MSN, PMC). *Accreditation:* AACN; ACEN (one or more programs are accredited). *Program availability:* Part-time. *Faculty:* 86 full-time (78 women), 44 part-time/adjunct (40 women). *Students:* 208 full-time (186 women), 128 part-time (116 women); includes 109 minority (49 Black or African American, non-Hispanic/Latino; 4 American Indian or Alaska Native, non-Hispanic/Latino; 32 Asian, non-Hispanic/Latino; 7 Hispanic/Latino; 17 Two or more races, non-Hispanic/Latino), 17 international. Average age 33. 624 applicants, 25% accepted, 150 enrolled. In 2015, 91 master's, 14 doctorates awarded. *Degree requirements:* For master's, comprehensive exam, thesis; for doctorate, thesis/dissertation, 3 exams; for PMC, thesis. *Entrance requirements:* Additional exam requirements/recommendations for international students: Required—TOEFL (minimum score 575 paper-based; 89 iBT), IELTS (minimum score 8). *Application deadline:* For fall admission, 12/15 for domestic and international students. Application fee: $85. Electronic applications accepted. *Financial support:* In 2015–16, 8 fellowships with full tuition reimbursements, 6 research assistantships with partial tuition reimbursements (averaging $8,000 per year), 10 teaching assistantships with partial tuition reimbursements (averaging $8,000 per year) were awarded; scholarships/grants, traineeships, health care benefits, and unspecified assistantships also available. Support available to part-time students. Financial award application deadline: 3/1; financial award applicants required to submit FAFSA. *Faculty research:* Preventing and managing chronic illness, reducing health disparities, Improving healthcare quality and patient outcomes, understanding biobehavioral and genetic bases of health and illness, developing innovative ways to enhance science and its clinical translation. *Unit head:* Donna S. Havens, PhD, RN, Dean/Professor, 919-966-3731, Fax: 919-966-3540, E-mail: dhavens@email.unc.edu. *Application contact:* Emily Sayed, Assistant Director, Graduate Admissions, 919-966-4260, Fax: 919-966-3540, E-mail: sayed@unc.edu. Website: http://nursing.unc.edu

University of Pennsylvania, School of Nursing, Pediatric Acute Care Nurse Practitioner Program, Philadelphia, PA 19104. Offers MSN. *Accreditation:* AACN. *Program availability:* Part-time, online learning. *Students:* 10 full-time (all women), 37

part-time (all women); includes 11 minority (3 Black or African American, non-Hispanic/Latino; 5 Asian, non-Hispanic/Latino; 1 Hispanic/Latino; 2 Two or more races, non-Hispanic/Latino). Average age 28. 56 applicants, 71% accepted, 24 enrolled. In 2015, 31 master's awarded. *Expenses: Tuition, area resident:* Full-time $31,068; part-time $5762 per course. *Required fees:* $3200; $336 per course. Full-time tuition and fees vary according to degree level, program and student level. Part-time tuition and fees vary according to course load, degree level and program.

University of Pennsylvania, School of Nursing, Pediatric Clinical Nurse Specialist Program, Philadelphia, PA 19104. Offers MSN. *Accreditation:* AACN. *Students:* 3 full-time (all women), 1 (woman) part-time, 1 international. Average age 31. 9 applicants, 89% accepted, 3 enrolled. In 2015, 1 master's awarded. *Expenses: Tuition, area resident:* Full-time $31,068; part-time $5762 per course. *Required fees:* $3200; $336 per course. Full-time tuition and fees vary according to degree level, program and student level. Part-time tuition and fees vary according to course load, degree level and program. *Financial support:* Application deadline: 4/1. *Unit head:* Assistant Dean of Admissions and Financial Aid, 866-867-6877, Fax: 215-573-8439, E-mail: admissions@nursing.upenn.edu. *Application contact:* Judy Verger, Senior Lecturer, 215-898-4271, E-mail: jtv@nursing.upenn.edu.
Website: http://www.nursing.upenn.edu/peds/

University of Pennsylvania, School of Nursing, Pediatric Primary Care Nurse Practitioner Program, Philadelphia, PA 19104. Offers MSN. *Accreditation:* AACN. *Program availability:* Part-time. *Students:* 16 full-time (all women), 14 part-time (13 women); includes 4 minority (3 Asian, non-Hispanic/Latino; 1 Two or more races, non-Hispanic/Latino). Average age 26. 44 applicants, 70% accepted, 24 enrolled. In 2015, 17 master's awarded. *Expenses: Tuition, area resident:* Full-time $31,068; part-time $5762 per course. *Required fees:* $3200; $336 per course. Full-time tuition and fees vary according to degree level, program and student level. Part-time tuition and fees vary according to course load, degree level and program.

University of Pittsburgh, School of Nursing, Nurse Practitioner Program, Pittsburgh, PA 15261. Offers adult-gerontology acute care (DNP); adult-gerontology primary care (DNP); family (individual across the lifespan) (DNP); neonatal (MSN, DNP); pediatric primary care (DNP); psychiatric mental health (DNP). *Accreditation:* AACN. *Program availability:* Part-time. *Students:* 74 full-time (65 women), 59 part-time (51 women); includes 14 minority (5 Black or African American, non-Hispanic/Latino; 2 American Indian or Alaska Native, non-Hispanic/Latino; 6 Asian, non-Hispanic/Latino; 1 Hispanic/Latino). Average age 30. 65 applicants, 55% accepted, 28 enrolled. In 2015, 14 master's, 19 doctorates awarded. *Degree requirements:* For master's, comprehensive exam, thesis optional. *Entrance requirements:* For master's, GRE General Test or MAT, BSN, RN license, letters of recommendation, resume, course work in statistics, 1-3 years of nursing experience; for doctorate, GRE General Test, BSN, RN license, minimum GPA of 3.5, 3 letters of recommendation. Additional exam requirements/recommendations for international students: Required—TOEFL (minimum score 600 paper-based; 100 iBT). *Application deadline:* For fall admission, 5/1 priority date for domestic students, 2/15 priority date for international students. Application fee: $50. Electronic applications accepted. *Expenses:* Contact institution. *Financial support:* In 2015–16, 16 students received support, including 7 fellowships with tuition reimbursements available (averaging $11,278 per year), 9 teaching assistantships with tuition reimbursements available (averaging $10,879 per year); scholarships/grants, traineeships, health care benefits, and unspecified assistantships also available. Support available to part-time students. Financial award application deadline: 3/15. *Faculty research:* Behavioral management of chronic disorders, patient management in critical care, consumer informatics, genetic applications (molecular genetics and psychosocial implications), technology for nurses and patients to improve care. *Unit head:* Dr. Sandra Engberg, Associate Dean for Clinical Education, 412-624-3835, Fax: 412-624-8521, E-mail: sje1@pitt.edu. *Application contact:* Laurie Lapsley, Administrator of Graduate Student Services, 412-624-9670, Fax: 412-624-2409, E-mail: lapsleyl@pitt.edu.
Website: http://www.nursing.pitt.edu

University of Puerto Rico, Medical Sciences Campus, School of Nursing, San Juan, PR 00936-5067. Offers adult and elderly nursing (MSN); child and adolescent nursing (MSN); critical care nursing (MSN); family and community nursing (MSN); family nurse practitioner (MSN); maternity nursing (MSN); mental health and psychiatric nursing (MSN). *Accreditation:* AACN. *Entrance requirements:* For master's, GRE or EXADEP, interview, Puerto Rico RN license or professional license for international students, general and specific point average, article analysis. Electronic applications accepted. *Faculty research:* HIV, health disparities, teen violence, women and violence, neurological disorders.

University of Rochester, School of Nursing, Rochester, NY 14642. Offers adult gerontological acute care nurse practitioner (MS); clinical nurse leader (MS); family nurse practitioner (MS); family psychiatric mental health nurse practitioner (MS); health care organization management and leadership (MS); health practice research (PhD); nursing (DNP); nursing education (MS); pediatric nurse practitioner (MS); pediatric nurse practitioner/neonatal nurse practitioner (MS). *Accreditation:* AACN. *Program availability:* Part-time, online learning. *Faculty:* 56 full-time (45 women), 63 part-time/adjunct (55 women). *Students:* 21 full-time (20 women), 212 part-time (175 women); includes 35 minority (12 Black or African American, non-Hispanic/Latino; 1 American Indian or Alaska Native, non-Hispanic/Latino; 10 Asian, non-Hispanic/Latino; 7 Hispanic/Latino; 5 Two or more races, non-Hispanic/Latino), 2 international. Average age 35. 111 applicants, 68% accepted, 71 enrolled. In 2015, 52 master's, 9 doctorates awarded. Terminal master's awarded for partial completion of doctoral program. *Degree requirements:* For master's, comprehensive exam (for some programs); for doctorate, thesis/dissertation. *Entrance requirements:* For master's, BS in nursing, minimum GPA of 3.0, course work in statistics; for doctorate, GRE General Test (for PhD), MS in nursing, minimum GPA of 3.5. Additional exam requirements/recommendations for international students: Required—TOEFL (minimum score 560 paper-based; 88 iBT) or IELTS (minimum score 6.5) recommended. *Application deadline:* For fall admission, 4/1 for domestic and international students; for spring admission, 9/1 for domestic and international students; for summer admission, 1/2 for domestic and international students. Application fee: $50. Electronic applications accepted. *Expenses: Tuition, area resident:* Full-time $47,450; part-time $1482 per credit hour. *Required fees:* $528. Tuition and fees vary according to program. *Financial support:* In 2015–16, 52 students received support, including 2 fellowships with tuition reimbursements available (averaging $30,000 per year); scholarships/grants, traineeships, health care benefits, tuition waivers (full and partial), and unspecified assistantships also available. Support available to part-time students. Financial award application deadline: 6/30. *Faculty research:* Symptom assessment and self-management of chronic illness, health promotion and illness prevention, nursing intervention research with vulnerable populations, palliative care, aging. *Total annual research expenditures:* $2.1 million. *Unit head:* Dr. Kathy H. Rideout, Dean, 585-273-8902, Fax: 585-273-1268, E-mail: kathy_rideout@urmc.rochester.edu. *Application contact:* Elaine Andolina, Director of Admissions, 585-275-2375, Fax: 585-756-8299, E-mail: elaine_andolina@urmc.rochester.edu.
Website: http://www.son.rochester.edu

University of South Carolina, The Graduate School, College of Nursing, Program in Health Nursing, Columbia, SC 29208. Offers adult nurse practitioner (MSN); community/public health clinical nurse specialist (MSN); family nurse practitioner (MSN); pediatric nurse practitioner (MSN). *Accreditation:* AACN. *Program availability:* Part-time. *Degree requirements:* For master's, thesis or alternative. *Entrance requirements:* For master's, GRE General Test or MAT, BS in nursing, nursing license. Additional exam requirements/recommendations for international students: Required—TOEFL (minimum score 570 paper-based). Electronic applications accepted. *Faculty research:* System research, evidence based practice, breast cancer, violence.

University of South Florida, College of Nursing, Tampa, FL 33612. Offers advanced pain management (Graduate Certificate); nursing (MS, DNP), including adult gerontology acute care (DNP), adult gerontology acute care nursing (MS), adult gerontology primary care (DNP), adult gerontology primary care nursing (MS), adult gerontology primary care/occupational health nursing (MS), adult gerontology primary care/oncology nursing (MS), clinical nurse leader (MS), family health nursing, nurse anesthesia (MS), nursing education (MS), nursing practice (DNP), occupational health/adult-gerontology (DNP), oncology/adult-gerontology primary care (DNP), pediatric health (DNP), pediatric nurse practitioner (MS); nursing education (Post Master's Certificate); nursing science (PhD). *Accreditation:* AACN; AANA/CANAEP. *Program availability:* Part-time. *Faculty:* 43 full-time (38 women), 7 part-time/adjunct (4 women). *Students:* 159 full-time (135 women), 721 part-time (625 women); includes 292 minority (119 Black or African American, non-Hispanic/Latino; 2 American Indian or Alaska Native, non-Hispanic/Latino; 60 Asian, non-Hispanic/Latino; 90 Hispanic/Latino; 1 Native Hawaiian or other Pacific Islander, non-Hispanic/Latino; 20 Two or more races, non-Hispanic/Latino), 12 international. Average age 35. 636 applicants, 44% accepted, 215 enrolled. In 2015, 333 master's, 18 doctorates awarded. *Degree requirements:* For master's, comprehensive exam, thesis optional; for doctorate, comprehensive exam, thesis/dissertation. *Entrance requirements:* For master's, GRE General Test, bachelor's degree from accredited program with minimum GPA of 3.0 in all upper-division coursework; current license as Registered Nurse; 3 letters of recommendation; personal statement of goals; resume or curriculum vitae; personal interview; for doctorate, GRE General Test (recommended), bachelor's degree in nursing from a CCNA/NLNAC regionally-accredited institution with minimum GPA of 3.0 in all coursework or in all upper-division coursework; current license as Registered Nurse in Florida; undergraduate statistics course with minimum B grade; 3 letters of recommendation; statement of goals; resume; interview. Additional exam requirements/recommendations for international students: Required—TOEFL (minimum score 550 paper-based; 79 iBT). *Application deadline:* For fall admission, 2/15 for domestic students, 1/2 for international students; for spring admission, 10/1 for domestic students, 6/1 for international students. Application fee: $30. Electronic applications accepted. *Financial support:* In 2015–16, 36 students received support, including 7 research assistantships with tuition reimbursements available (averaging $18,935 per year), 29 teaching assistantships with tuition reimbursements available (averaging $30,814 per year); tuition waivers (partial) and unspecified assistantships also available. Financial award application deadline: 2/1; financial award applicants required to submit FAFSA. *Faculty research:* Women's health, palliative and end-of-life care, cardiac rehabilitation, complementary therapies for chronic illness and cancer. *Total annual research expenditures:* $2.6 million. *Unit head:* Dr. Dianne C. Morrison-Beedy, Dean and Professor, College of Nursing, 813-974-9091, Fax: 813-974-5418, E-mail: dmbeedy@health.usf.edu. *Application contact:* Dr. Brian Graves, Assistant Professor/Assistant Dean, 813-974-8054, Fax: 813-974-5418, E-mail: bgraves1@health.usf.edu.
Website: http://health.usf.edu/nursing/index.htm

The University of Texas at Austin, Graduate School, School of Nursing, Austin, TX 78712-1111. Offers adult - gerontology clinical nurse specialist (MSN); child health (MSN), including administration, public health nursing, teaching; family nurse practitioner (MSN); family psychiatric/mental health nurse practitioner (MSN); holistic adult health (MSN), including administration, teaching; maternity (MSN), including administration, public health nursing, teaching; nursing (PhD); nursing administration and healthcare systems management (MSN); nursing practice (DNP); pediatric nurse practitioner (MSN); public health nursing (MSN). *Accreditation:* AACN. *Program availability:* Part-time. *Degree requirements:* For master's, thesis optional; for doctorate, thesis/dissertation. *Entrance requirements:* For master's and doctorate, GRE General Test. Additional exam requirements/recommendations for international students: Required—TOEFL (minimum score 550 paper-based). Electronic applications accepted. *Faculty research:* Chronic illness management, memory and aging, health promotion, women's health, adolescent health.

The University of Texas Health Science Center at San Antonio, School of Nursing, San Antonio, TX 78229-3900. Offers administrative management (MSN); adult-gerontology acute care nurse practitioner (PGC); advanced practice leadership (DNP); clinical nurse leader (MSN); executive administrative management (DNP); family nurse practitioner (MSN, PGC); nursing (MSN, PhD); nursing education (MSN, PGC); pediatric nurse practitioner primary care (PGC); psychiatric mental health nurse practitioner (PGC); public health nurse leader (DNP). *Accreditation:* AACN. *Program availability:* Part-time. Terminal master's awarded for partial completion of doctoral program. *Degree requirements:* For master's, thesis optional; for doctorate, comprehensive exam, thesis/dissertation.

The University of Toledo, College of Graduate Studies, College of Nursing, Department of Population and Community Care, Toledo, OH 43606-3390. Offers clinical nurse leader (MSN); family nurse practitioner (MSN, Certificate); nurse educator (MSN, Certificate); pediatric nurse practitioner (MSN, Certificate). *Program availability:* Part-time. *Degree requirements:* For master's, thesis or alternative. *Entrance requirements:* For master's, GRE, BS in nursing, minimum undergraduate GPA of 3.0, statement of purpose, three letters of recommendation, transcripts from all prior institutions attended, Nursing CAS application, UT supplemental application; for Certificate, BS in nursing, minimum undergraduate GPA of 3.0, statement of purpose, three letters of recommendation, transcripts from all prior institutions attended. Additional exam requirements/recommendations for international students: Required—TOEFL (minimum score 550 paper-based; 80 iBT). Electronic applications accepted.

University of Wisconsin–Madison, School of Nursing, Madison, WI 53706-1380. Offers adult/gerontology (DNP); nursing (PhD); pediatrics (DNP); psychiatric mental health (DNP); MS/MPH. *Accreditation:* AACN. *Program availability:* Part-time. *Degree requirements:* For doctorate, comprehensive exam, thesis/dissertation. *Entrance requirements:* For doctorate, GRE General Test, 2 samples of scholarly written work, BS in nursing from an accredited program, minimum undergraduate GPA of 3.0 in last 60 credits (for PhD); licensure as professional nurse (for DNP). Additional exam requirements/recommendations for international students: Required—TOEFL (minimum score 600 paper-based; 100 iBT). Electronic applications accepted. *Expenses:* Tuition, state resident: full-time $5364. Tuition, nonresident: full-time $12,027. *Required fees:* $571. Tuition and fees vary according to campus/location, program and reciprocity agreements. *Faculty research:* Nursing informatics to promote self-care and disease management skills among patients and caregivers; quality of care to frail, vulnerable, and chronically ill populations; study of health-related and health-seeking behaviors; eliminating health disparities; pain and symptom management for patients with cancer.

Pediatric Nursing

Vanderbilt University, Vanderbilt University School of Nursing, Nashville, TN 37240. Offers adult-gerontology acute care nurse practitioner (MSN), including hospitalist, intensivist; adult-gerontology primary care nurse practitioner (MSN); emergency nurse practitioner (MSN); family nurse practitioner (MSN); healthcare leadership (MSN); neonatal nurse practitioner (MSN); nurse midwifery (MSN); nurse midwifery/family nurse practitioner (MSN); nursing (Post-Master's Certificate); nursing informatics (MSN); nursing practice (DNP); nursing science (PhD); pediatric acute care nurse practitioner (MSN); pediatric primary care nurse practitioner (MSN); psychiatric-mental health nurse practitioner (MSN); women's health nurse practitioner (MSN); women's health nurse practitioner/adult gerontology primary care nurse practitioner (MSN); MSN/M Div; MSN/MTS. *Accreditation:* ACEN (one or more programs are accredited); ACNM/ACME. *Program availability:* Part-time, 100% online, blended/hybrid learning. *Faculty:* 258 full-time (232 women), 363 part-time/adjunct (271 women). *Students:* 478 full-time (424 women), 342 part-time (317 women); includes 140 minority (36 Black or African American, non-Hispanic/Latino; 3 American Indian or Alaska Native, non-Hispanic/Latino; 24 Asian, non-Hispanic/Latino; 43 Hispanic/Latino; 3 Native Hawaiian or other Pacific Islander, non-Hispanic/Latino; 31 Two or more races, non-Hispanic/Latino), 11 international. Average age 31. 1,268 applicants, 49% accepted, 477 enrolled. In 2015, 343 master's, 55 doctorates awarded. *Degree requirements:* For doctorate, comprehensive exam, thesis/dissertation. *Entrance requirements:* For master's, GRE General Test (taken within the past 5 years), minimum B average in undergraduate course work, 3 letters of recommendation; for doctorate, GRE General Test, interview, 3 letters of recommendation from doctorally-prepared faculty, MSN, essay. Additional exam requirements/recommendations for international students: Required—TOEFL (minimum score 570 paper-based), IELTS (minimum score 6.5). *Application deadline:* For fall admission, 11/1 priority date for domestic and international students. Applications are processed on a rolling basis. Application fee: $50. Electronic applications accepted. *Expenses:* Contact institution. *Financial support:* In 2015–16, 585 students received support. Scholarships/grants available. Financial award application deadline: 3/15; financial award applicants required to submit FAFSA. *Faculty research:* Lymphedema, palliative care and bereavement, health services research including workforce, safety and quality of care, gerontology, better birth outcomes including nutrition. *Total annual research expenditures:* $2 million. *Unit head:* Dr. Linda Norman, Dean, 615-343-8876, Fax: 615-343-7711, E-mail: linda.norman@vanderbilt.edu. *Application contact:* Patricia Peerman, Assistant Dean for Enrollment Management, 615-322-3800, Fax: 615-343-0333, E-mail: vusn-admissions@vanderbilt.edu.
Website: http://www.nursing.vanderbilt.edu

Villanova University, College of Nursing, Villanova, PA 19085-1699. Offers adult nurse practitioner (MSN, Post Master's Certificate); family nurse practitioner (MSN, Post Master's Certificate); nurse anesthetist (MSN, Post Master's Certificate); nursing (PhD); nursing education (MSN, Post Master's Certificate); nursing practice (DNP); pediatric nurse practitioner (MSN, Post Master's Certificate). *Accreditation:* AACN; AANA/CANAEP. *Program availability:* Part-time, online learning. *Faculty:* 16 full-time (15 women), 9 part-time/adjunct (7 women). *Students:* 219 full-time (198 women), 108 part-time (96 women); includes 36 minority (25 Black or African American, non-Hispanic/Latino; 9 Asian, non-Hispanic/Latino; 2 Hispanic/Latino), 16 international. Average age 31. 147 applicants, 78% accepted, 106 enrolled. In 2015, 64 master's, 8 doctorates, 9 other advanced degrees awarded. *Degree requirements:* For master's, independent study project; for doctorate, comprehensive exam, thesis/dissertation; for Post Master's Certificate, scholarly project. *Entrance requirements:* For master's, GRE or MAT, BSN, 1 year of recent nursing experience, physical assessment, course work in statistics; for doctorate, GRE, MSN. Additional exam requirements/recommendations for international students: Required—TOEFL (minimum score 540 paper-based; 83 iBT), IELTS (minimum score 6.5). *Application deadline:* For fall admission, 7/1 priority date for domestic students, 7/1 for international students; for spring admission, 11/1 priority date for domestic students, 11/1 for international students; for summer admission, 4/1 priority date for domestic students, 3/1 for international students. Applications are processed on a rolling basis. Application fee: $50. Electronic applications accepted. *Expenses:* $837 per credit (MSN); $1,049 per credit (PhD); $1,375 per credit (DNP). *Financial support:* In 2015–16, 22 students received support, including 5 teaching assistantships with full tuition reimbursements available (averaging $15,475 per year); institutionally sponsored loans, scholarships/grants, traineeships, tuition waivers (full), and unspecified assistantships also available. Financial award application deadline: 7/1; financial award applicants required to submit FAFSA. *Faculty research:* Genetics, ethics, cognitive development of students, women with disabilities, nursing leadership. *Unit head:* Dr. Marguerite K. Schlag, Assistant Dean/Director, Graduate Programs, 610-519-4907, Fax: 610-519-7650, E-mail: marguerite.schlag@villanova.edu. *Application contact:* Rebecca Harold, Administrative Assistant, 610-519-4934, Fax: 610-519-7650, E-mail: rebecca.harold@villanova.edu.
Website: http://www.nursing.villanova.edu/

Virginia Commonwealth University, Graduate School, School of Nursing, Richmond, VA 23284-9005. Offers adult health acute nursing (MS); adult health primary nursing (MS); biobehavioral clinical research (PhD); child health nursing (MS); clinical nurse leader (MS); family health nursing (MS); nurse educator (MS); nurse practitioner (MS); nursing (Certificate); nursing administration (MS), including clinical nurse manager; psychiatric-mental health nursing (MS); quality and safety in health care (DNP); women's health nursing (MS). *Accreditation:* ACEN (one or more programs are accredited). *Program availability:* Part-time, evening/weekend, online learning. *Degree requirements:* For master's, thesis optional; for doctorate, thesis/dissertation. *Entrance requirements:* For master's, GRE General Test, BSN, minimum GPA of 2.8; for doctorate, GRE General Test. Additional exam requirements/recommendations for international students: Required—TOEFL (minimum score 600 paper-based; 100 iBT). Electronic applications accepted.

Wayne State University, College of Nursing, Doctor Program of Nursing Practice, Detroit, MI 48202. Offers adult gerontology nurse practitioner - acute care (DNP); adult gerontology nurse practitioner - primary care (DNP); family nurse practitioner (DNP); infant mental health (DNP); neonatal nurse practitioner (DNP); nurse midwifery (DNP); nursing practice (DNP); pediatric nurse practitioner - acute care (DNP); pediatric nurse practitioner - primary care (DNP); psychiatric mental health nurse practitioner (DNP). *Students:* 56 full-time (50 women), 37 part-time (32 women); includes 32 minority (19 Black or African American, non-Hispanic/Latino; 6 Asian, non-Hispanic/Latino; 3 Hispanic/Latino; 4 Two or more races, non-Hispanic/Latino), 6 international. Average age 35. 44 applicants, 66% accepted, 18 enrolled. In 2015, 16 doctorates awarded. *Entrance requirements:* For doctorate, official transcripts, two professional references, curriculum vitae or resume, statement of goals, BSN or MSN, current Michigan RN license, criminal background check, interview, on-site writing example. Additional exam requirements/recommendations for international students: Required—TOEFL (minimum score 600 paper-based; 101 iBT); Recommended—IELTS (minimum score 7). *Application deadline:* For fall admission, 1/31 for domestic and international students. Electronic applications accepted. *Expenses:* $19,325 per year resident tuition, $35,114 non-resident tuition; $805.20 per credit hour resident tuition, $1,463.10 per credit hour non-resident tuition; fees include $47.45 per credit hour student services fee and $274.60 per semester registration fee. *Financial support:* In 2015–16, 22 students

received support. Fellowships, research assistantships, teaching assistantships, institutionally sponsored loans, and scholarships/grants available. Financial award applicants required to submit FAFSA. *Unit head:* Dr. Laurie Lauzon Clabo, Dean and Professor, 313-577-4104, E-mail: laurie.lauzon.clabo@wayne.edu. *Application contact:* Dr. Nancy George, Director of DNP Program, 313-577-8300.
Website: http://nursing.wayne.edu/dnp/index.php

Wayne State University, College of Nursing, Graduate Certificates Program in Clinical Specialties, Detroit, MI 48202. Offers acute care nurse practitioner (Graduate Certificate); nurse midwifery (Graduate Certificate); pediatric nurse practitioner - acute care (Graduate Certificate); pediatric nurse practitioner - primary care (Graduate Certificate); psychiatric mental health nurse practitioner (Graduate Certificate). *Accreditation:* AACN. *Program availability:* Part-time. *Students:* 2 full-time (both women), 7 part-time (all women). Average age 43. 67 applicants, 12% accepted, 5 enrolled. *Entrance requirements:* For degree, master's or doctoral degree in nursing from nationally-accredited institution, current RN license, three letters of reference, personal statement. Additional exam requirements/recommendations for international students: Required—TOEFL (minimum score 600 paper-based; 101 iBT), TWE, Michigan English Language Assessment Battery (minimum score 85); Recommended—IELTS (minimum score 7). *Application deadline:* For fall admission, 6/1 priority date for domestic students, 5/1 priority date for international students; for winter admission, 10/1 priority date for domestic students, 9/1 priority date for international students; for spring admission, 2/1 priority date for domestic students, 1/1 priority date for international students. Application fee: $0. Electronic applications accepted. *Expenses:* $19,325 annual resident tuition, $35,114 non-resident tuition; $805.20 per credit hour resident tuition, $1,463.10 per credit hour non-resident tuition; fees include $47.45 per credit hour student services fee and $274.60 per semester registration fee. *Financial support:* Scholarships/grants available. Financial award application deadline: 3/31; financial award applicants required to submit FAFSA. *Unit head:* Dr. Laurie Lauzon Clabo, Dean and Professor, 313-577-4104, E-mail: laurie.lauzon.clabo@wayne.edu. *Application contact:* Leanne Nantais-Smith, Director, MSN Program and Graduate Certificates, E-mail: ar2446@wayne.edu.
Website: http://nursing.wayne.edu/gradcert/specialties.php

Wayne State University, College of Nursing, M.S.N. Program in Clinical Specialties, Detroit, MI 48202. Offers nurse-midwifery (MSN); pediatric nurse practitioner acute care (MSN); psychiatric mental health nurse practitioner (MSN). *Accreditation:* AACN. *Program availability:* Part-time. *Students:* 49 full-time (47 women), 85 part-time (79 women); includes 29 minority (15 Black or African American, non-Hispanic/Latino; 7 Asian, non-Hispanic/Latino; 3 Hispanic/Latino; 4 Two or more races, non-Hispanic/Latino), 5 international. Average age 33. 111 applicants, 20% accepted, 17 enrolled. In 2015, 108 master's awarded. *Degree requirements:* For master's, thesis or alternative. *Entrance requirements:* For master's, BSN from NLN- or CCNE-accredited program with minimum GPA of 3.0; three references; current RN license; personal statement. Additional exam requirements/recommendations for international students: Required—TOEFL (minimum score 600 paper-based; 101 iBT); Recommended—TWE. *Application deadline:* For fall admission, 6/1 for domestic students, 5/1 priority date for international students; for winter admission, 10/1 for domestic students, 9/1 priority date for international students; for spring admission, 2/1 for domestic students, 1/1 priority date for international students. Electronic applications accepted. *Expenses:* $19,325 per year resident tuition, $35,114 non-resident tuition; $805.20 per credit hour resident tuition, $1,463.10 per credit hour non-resident tuition; fees include $47.45 per credit hour student services fee and $274.60 per semester registration fee. *Financial support:* In 2015–16, 36 students received support. Fellowships with tuition reimbursements available, research assistantships with tuition reimbursements available, teaching assistantships with tuition reimbursements available, scholarships/grants, traineeships, and unspecified assistantships available. Support available to part-time students. Financial award applicants required to submit FAFSA. *Faculty research:* Smoking risk behaviors in adolescents, sleep disturbances in postmenopausal women, health disparities in urban environments, nurse practitioner interventions, care giving and pain management. *Unit head:* Dr. Laurie Lauzon Clabo, Dean and Professor, 313-577-4104, E-mail: laurie.lauzon.clabo@wayne.edu. *Application contact:* Dr. Leanne Nantais-Smith, Program Director, MSN and Graduate Certificates, 313-577-5934, E-mail: ar2446@wayne.edu.
Website: http://nursing.wayne.edu/msn/specialty.php

Wayne State University, College of Nursing, Program in Advanced Practice Nursing with Women, Neonates and Children, Detroit, MI 48202. Offers MSN, DNP. *Accreditation:* AACN. *Program availability:* Part-time. *Degree requirements:* For master's, thesis or alternative. *Entrance requirements:* For master's, BSN from NLN- or CCNE-accredited program with minimum GPA of 3.0; three references; current RN license; personal statement; for doctorate, GRE General Test (for applicants without a master's degree), resume or curriculum vitae; current RN license; goals statement; bachelor's or master's degree in nursing from NLN- or CCNE-accredited program with minimum GPA of 3.0; writing sample and interview (for DNP); reference letters (3 for PhD, 2 for DNP). Additional exam requirements/recommendations for international students: Required—TOEFL (minimum score 101 iBT); Recommended—TWE (minimum score 7). *Application deadline:* For fall admission, 6/1 priority date for domestic students, 5/1 priority date for international students; for winter admission, 10/1 priority date for domestic students, 9/1 priority date for international students; for spring admission, 2/1 priority date for domestic students, 1/1 priority date for international students. Electronic applications accepted. *Expenses:* $19,325 annual resident tuition, $35,114 non-resident tuition; $805.20 per credit hour resident tuition, $1,463.10 per credit hour non-resident tuition; fees include $47.45 per credit hour student services fee and $274.60 per semester registration fee. *Financial support:* Fellowships with tuition reimbursements, research assistantships with tuition reimbursements, teaching assistantships with tuition reimbursements, scholarships/grants, and unspecified assistantships available. Financial award application deadline: 3/31; financial award applicants required to submit FAFSA. *Faculty research:* Acculturation and parenting, domestic violence, evidence-based midwifery practice, pain in children, trauma and community violence. *Unit head:* Dr. Laurie Lauzon Clabo, Dean and Professor, 313-577-4104, E-mail: laurie.lauzon.clabo@wayne.edu. *Application contact:* Dr. Janet Harden, Associate Professor/Interim Dean, Office of Student Affairs, 313-577-4082, E-mail: nursinginfo@wayne.edu.
Website: http://nursing.wayne.edu/programs/index.php

Wayne State University, Eugene Applebaum College of Pharmacy and Health Sciences, Department of Health Care Sciences, Program in Nurse Anesthesia, Detroit, MI 48202. Offers anesthesia (MS); pediatric anesthesia (Certificate). *Accreditation:* AACN; AANA/CANAEP. *Faculty:* 7. *Students:* 41 full-time (20 women); includes 6 minority (4 Black or African American, non-Hispanic/Latino; 1 Asian, non-Hispanic/Latino; 1 Hispanic/Latino). Average age 30. In 2015, 16 master's awarded. *Entrance requirements:* For master's, GRE General Test, bachelor's degree in nursing or related science with minimum GPA of 3.0 overall and in science, current RN license, CCRN certification, one year of full-time experience in adult ICU, ACLS certification, hospital shadow experience (arranged by department); for Certificate, MS in anesthesia from accredited program, meeting with course coordinators from Children's Hospital of Michigan. Additional exam requirements/recommendations for international students: Required—TOEFL (minimum score 550 paper-based; 79 iBT), Michigan English Language Assessment Battery (minimum score 85); Recommended—IELTS (minimum

score 6.5), TWE (minimum score 5.5). *Application deadline:* For fall admission, 7/1 for domestic students, 5/1 priority date for international students. Application fee: $0. Electronic applications accepted. *Expenses:* $16,104 per year resident tuition, $32,401 non-resident tuition; $671 per credit hour resident tuition, $1,350.05 per credit hour non-resident tuition; fees include $47.45 per credit hour student services fee and $274.60 per semester registration fee. *Financial support:* In 2015–16, 20 students received support. Scholarships/grants available. Financial award application deadline: 3/31; financial award applicants required to submit FAFSA. *Faculty research:* Music therapy in pain management, student success/students perspective, pacemaker management-safety, airway devices. *Unit head:* Dr. Prudentia A. Worth, Program Director, 313-993-7168, E-mail: aa1635@wayne.edu.
Website: http://cphs.wayne.edu/nurse-anesthesia/

Wright State University, School of Graduate Studies, College of Nursing and Health, Program in Nursing, Dayton, OH 45435. Offers acute care nurse practitioner (MS); administration of nursing and health care systems (MS); adult health (MS); child and adolescent health (MS); community health (MS); family nurse practitioner (MS); nurse practitioner (MS); school nurse (MS); MBA/MS. *Accreditation:* AACN. *Program availability:* Part-time, evening/weekend. *Degree requirements:* For master's, thesis or alternative. *Entrance requirements:* For master's, GRE General Test, BSN from NLN-accredited college, Ohio RN license. Additional exam requirements/recommendations for international students: Required—TOEFL. *Faculty research:* Clinical nursing and health, teaching, caring, pain administration, informatics and technology.

Psychiatric Nursing

Allen College, Graduate Programs, Waterloo, IA 50703. Offers acute care nurse practitioner (Post-Master's Certificate); adult nurse practitioner (Post-Master's Certificate); adult psychiatric-mental health nurse practitioner (Post-Master's Certificate); adult-gerontology acute care nurse practitioner (MSN); community public health (Post-Master's Certificate); community/public health nursing (MSN); family nurse practitioner (MSN, Post-Master's Certificate); gerontological nurse practitioner (Post-Master's Certificate); health sciences (Ed D); leadership in health care delivery (MSN, Post-Master's Certificate); nursing (DNP); occupational therapy (MS). *Accreditation:* AACN; ACEN. *Program availability:* Part-time, blended/hybrid learning. *Faculty:* 3 full-time (all women), 21 part-time/adjunct (20 women). *Students:* 61 full-time (54 women), 163 part-time (144 women); includes 9 minority (5 Black or African American, non-Hispanic/Latino; 2 Hispanic/Latino; 2 Two or more races, non-Hispanic/Latino), 2 international. Average age 34. 212 applicants, 60% accepted, 94 enrolled. In 2015, 51 master's, 1 doctorate awarded. *Degree requirements:* For master's, thesis optional. *Entrance requirements:* For master's, minimum GPA of 3.0 in the last 60 hours of undergraduate coursework; for doctorate, minimum GPA of 3.25 in graduate coursework. Additional exam requirements/recommendations for international students: Recommended—TOEFL (minimum score 580 paper-based; 92 iBT), IELTS (minimum score 6). *Application deadline:* For fall admission, 2/1 priority date for domestic students; for spring admission, 9/1 priority date for domestic students. Applications are processed on a rolling basis. Application fee: $50. Electronic applications accepted. *Expenses:* $15,940 tuition, $1,240 fees. *Financial support:* Institutionally sponsored loans, scholarships/grants, and traineeships available. Support available to part-time students. Financial award application deadline: 8/15; financial award applicants required to submit FAFSA. *Unit head:* Nancy Kramer, Vice Chancellor for Academic Affairs, 319-226-2040, Fax: 319-226-2070, E-mail: nancy.kramer@allencollege.edu. *Application contact:* Molly Quinn, Administrative Assistant for Student Services, 319-226-2014, Fax: 319-226-2010, E-mail: admissions@allencollege.edu.
Website: http://www.allencollege.edu/

Alverno College, JoAnn McGrath School of Nursing, Milwaukee, WI 53234-3922. Offers clinical nurse specialist (MSN); family nurse practitioner (MSN); mental health nurse practitioner (MSN). *Accreditation:* AACN. *Program availability:* Part-time, evening/weekend. *Faculty:* 8 full-time (all women), 8 part-time/adjunct (4 women). *Students:* 97 full-time (90 women), 87 part-time (82 women); includes 43 minority (18 Black or African American, non-Hispanic/Latino; 11 Asian, non-Hispanic/Latino; 9 Hispanic/Latino; 5 Two or more races, non-Hispanic/Latino), 1 international. Average age 36. 73 applicants, 95% accepted, 45 enrolled. In 2015, 33 master's awarded. *Degree requirements:* For master's, 500 clinical hours, capstone. *Entrance requirements:* For master's, BSN, current license. Additional exam requirements/recommendations for international students: Required—TOEFL. *Application deadline:* For fall admission, 7/15 priority date for domestic and international students; for spring admission, 12/15 priority date for domestic and international students. Applications are processed on a rolling basis. Application fee: $0. Electronic applications accepted. *Expenses:* Contact institution. *Financial support:* In 2015–16, 1 student received support. Federal Work-Study and scholarships/grants available. Support available to part-time students. Financial award applicants required to submit FAFSA. *Faculty research:* Impact of stroke on sexuality, children's asthma management, factors affecting baccalaureate student success. *Unit head:* Margaret Rauschenberger, Interim Dean, 414-382-6276, Fax: 414-382-6354, E-mail: margaret.rauschenberger@alverno.edu. *Application contact:* Dr. Carol Sabel, RN, Graduate Program Director, 414-382-6309, Fax: 414-382-6354, E-mail: carol.sabel@alverno.edu.
Website: http://www.alverno.edu/academics/academicdepartments/joannmcgrathschoolofnursing/

American University of Beirut, Graduate Programs, Rafic Hariri School of Nursing, Beirut, Lebanon. Offers psychiatric mental health nursing (MSN). *Accreditation:* AACN. *Program availability:* Part-time. *Faculty:* 9 full-time (8 women), 13 part-time/adjunct (11 women). *Students:* 2 full-time (both women), 56 part-time (49 women). Average age 29. 22 applicants, 100% accepted, 10 enrolled. In 2015, 11 master's awarded. *Degree requirements:* For master's, one foreign language, comprehensive exam, thesis optional. *Entrance requirements:* For master's, letter of recommendation. Additional exam requirements/recommendations for international students: Required—TOEFL (minimum score 583 paper-based; 97 iBT); Recommended—IELTS. *Application deadline:* For fall admission, 4/1 for domestic and international students; for spring admission, 11/1 for domestic and international students. Applications are processed on a rolling basis. Application fee: $50. Electronic applications accepted. *Expenses:* Contact institution. *Financial support:* In 2015–16, 17 teaching assistantships with partial tuition reimbursements were awarded; unspecified assistantships also available. Financial award application deadline: 12/20. *Faculty research:* Pain management and palliative care, stress and post-traumatic stress disorder, health benefits and chronic illness, health promotion and community interventions. *Unit head:* Dr. Huda Huijer Abu-Saad, Director, 961-1374374 Ext. 5952, Fax: 961-1744476, E-mail: hh35@aub.edu.lb. *Application contact:* Dr. Salim Kanaan, Director, Admissions Office, 961-1350000 Ext. 2594, Fax: 961-1750775, E-mail: sk00@aub.edu.lb.
Website: http://staff.aub.edu.lb/~webson

Arizona State University at the Tempe campus, College of Nursing and Health Innovation, Phoenix, AZ 85004. Offers advanced nursing practice (DNP); clinical research management (MS); community and public health practice (Graduate Certificate); family mental health nurse practitioner (Graduate Certificate); family nurse practitioner (Graduate Certificate); geriatric nursing (Graduate Certificate); healthcare innovation (MHI); nurse education in academic and practice settings (Graduate Certificate); nurse educator (MS); nursing and healthcare innovation (PhD).

Accreditation: AACN. *Program availability:* Online learning. *Degree requirements:* For master's, comprehensive exam (for some programs), thesis (for some programs), interactive Program of Study (iPOS) submitted before completing 50 percent of required credit hours; for doctorate, comprehensive exam, thesis/dissertation, interactive Program of Study (iPOS) submitted before completing 50 percent of required credit hours. *Entrance requirements:* For master's and doctorate, GRE, minimum GPA of 3.0 or equivalent in last 2 years of work leading to bachelor's degree. Additional exam requirements/recommendations for international students: Required—TOEFL, IELTS, or PTE. Electronic applications accepted. *Expenses:* Contact institution.

Augusta University, The Graduate School, Doctor of Nursing Practice Program, Augusta, GA 30912. Offers adult gerontology acute care nurse practitioner (DNP); family nurse practitioner (DNP); nursing (DNP); nursing anesthesia (DNP); pediatric nurse practitioner (DNP); psychiatric mental health nurse practitioner (DNP). *Students:* 40 part-time. *Degree requirements:* For doctorate, thesis/dissertation or alternative. *Entrance requirements:* For doctorate, GRE General Test or MAT, master's degree in nursing or related field, current professional nurse licensure. Additional exam requirements/recommendations for international students: Required—TOEFL (minimum score 600 paper-based; 100 iBT). *Application deadline:* For fall admission, 3/1 for domestic and international students; for spring admission, 7/1 for domestic and international students. Applications are processed on a rolling basis. Application fee: $50. Electronic applications accepted. *Unit head:* Dr. Marguerite Murphy, RN, Director, 706-721-3676, Fax: 706-721-8169. *Application contact:* Karen Sturgill, Program Manager, 706-721-3676, Fax: 706-721-8169, E-mail: dnp@augusta.edu.
Website: http://www.augusta.edu/nursing/dnp_programs.php

Boston College, William F. Connell School of Nursing, Chestnut Hill, MA 02467. Offers adult-gerontology nursing (MS); family health nursing (MS); forensic nursing (MS); nurse anesthesia (MS); nursing (PhD); pediatric nursing (MS), including pediatric and women's health; psychiatric-mental health nursing (MS); women's health nursing (MS); MBA/MS; MS/MA; MS/PhD. *Accreditation:* AACN; AANA/CANAEP (one or more programs are accredited). *Program availability:* Part-time. *Faculty:* 53 full-time (48 women), 47 part-time/adjunct (44 women). *Students:* 185 full-time (167 women), 66 part-time (56 women); includes 31 minority (10 Black or African American, non-Hispanic/Latino; 12 Asian, non-Hispanic/Latino; 7 Hispanic/Latino; 2 Two or more races, non-Hispanic/Latino), 7 international. Average age 32. 313 applicants, 66% accepted, 91 enrolled. In 2015, 98 master's, 5 doctorates awarded. *Degree requirements:* For master's, comprehensive exam; for doctorate, comprehensive exam, thesis/dissertation, computer literacy exam or foreign language. *Entrance requirements:* For master's, bachelor's degree in nursing; for doctorate, GRE General Test, MS in nursing. Additional exam requirements/recommendations for international students: Required—TOEFL (minimum score 600 paper-based; 100 iBT), IELTS (minimum score 7.5). *Application deadline:* For fall admission, 9/30 for domestic and international students; for winter admission, 1/15 for domestic and international students; for spring admission, 3/15 for domestic and international students. Applications are processed on a rolling basis. Application fee: $40. Electronic applications accepted. *Expenses:* Contact institution. *Financial support:* In 2015–16, 1 fellowship with full tuition reimbursement (averaging $23,700 per year), 25 teaching assistantships (averaging $4,370 per year) were awarded; research assistantships, scholarships/grants, health care benefits, tuition waivers (partial), and unspecified assistantships also available. Support available to part-time students. Financial award application deadline: 3/1; financial award applicants required to submit FAFSA. *Faculty research:* Sexual and reproductive health, health promotion/illness prevention, aging, eating disorders, symptom management. *Total annual research expenditures:* $1 million. *Unit head:* Dr. Susan Gennaro, Dean, 617-552-4251, Fax: 617-552-0931, E-mail: susan.gennaro@bc.edu. *Application contact:* MaryBeth Crowley, Graduate Programs Assistant, 617-552-4928, Fax: 617-552-2121, E-mail: csongrad@bc.edu.
Website: http://www.bc.edu/schools/son/

Case Western Reserve University, Frances Payne Bolton School of Nursing, Master's Programs in Nursing, Nurse Practitioner Program, Cleveland, OH 44106. Offers acute care cardiovascular nursing (MSN); acute care nurse practitioner (MSN); acute care pediatric nurse practitioner (MSN); acute care/flight nurse (MSN); adult gerontology acute care nurse practitioner (MSN); adult gerontology oncology and palliative care (MSN); adult gerontology primary care nurse practitioner (MSN); family nurse practitioner (MSN); family systems psychiatric mental health nursing (MSN); neonatal nurse practitioner (MSN); pediatric nurse practitioner (MSN); women's health nurse practitioner (MSN). *Accreditation:* ACEN. *Program availability:* Part-time, online learning. *Students:* 52 full-time (45 women), 78 part-time (68 women); includes 31 minority (10 Black or African American, non-Hispanic/Latino; 14 Asian, non-Hispanic/Latino; 7 Hispanic/Latino). Average age 35. 64 applicants, 66% accepted, 29 enrolled. In 2015, 45 master's awarded. *Degree requirements:* For master's, thesis optional. *Entrance requirements:* For master's, GRE General Test or MAT. Additional exam requirements/recommendations for international students: Required—TOEFL (minimum score 577 paper-based; 90 iBT), IELTS (minimum score 7). *Application deadline:* For fall admission, 6/1 for domestic students; for spring admission, 10/1 for domestic students. Applications are processed on a rolling basis. Application fee: $75. *Expenses:* $1,891 per credit hour. *Financial support:* In 2015–16, 54 students received support, including 17 teaching assistantships with partial tuition reimbursements available (averaging $17,019 per year); scholarships/grants and traineeships also available. Financial award application deadline: 6/30; financial award applicants required to submit FAFSA. *Faculty research:* Symptom science, family/community care, aging across the lifespan, self-management of health and illness, neuroscience. *Unit head:* Dr. Carol Savrin, Director, 216-368-5304, Fax: 216-368-3542, E-mail: cls18@case.edu. *Application contact:* Donna

Psychiatric Nursing

Hassik, Admissions Coordinator, 216-368-5253, Fax: 216-368-0124, E-mail: dmh7@case.edu.
Website: http://fpb.cwru.edu/MSN/majors.shtm

Columbia University, School of Nursing, Program in Psychiatric Mental Health Nursing, New York, NY 10032. Offers MS, Adv C. *Accreditation:* AACN. *Program availability:* Part-time. *Entrance requirements:* For master's, GRE General Test, NCLEX, BSN, 1 year of clinical experience (preferred); for Adv C, MSN. Additional exam requirements/recommendations for international students: Required—TOEFL (minimum score 100 iBT). Electronic applications accepted.

Creighton University, College of Nursing, Omaha, NE 68178-0001. Offers adult acute care nurse practitioner (Post-Master's Certificate); adult gerontology acute care nurse practitioner (DNP); adult gerontology nurse practitioner (DNP); clinical nurse leader (MSN, Post-Graduate Certificate); clinical systems administration (MSN, DNP); family nurse practitioner (DNP, Post-Master's Certificate); neonatal nurse practitioner (DNP, Post-Master's Certificate); pediatric acute care nurse practitioner (DNP, Post-Master's Certificate); psychiatric mental health nurse practitioner (DNP). *Accreditation:* AACN. *Program availability:* Part-time, blended/hybrid learning. *Faculty:* 10 full-time (all women), 48 part-time/adjunct (45 women). *Students:* 132 full-time (120 women), 228 part-time (212 women); includes 38 minority (10 Black or African American, non-Hispanic/Latino; 3 American Indian or Alaska Native, non-Hispanic/Latino; 11 Asian, non-Hispanic/Latino; 1 Hispanic/Latino; 2 Native Hawaiian or other Pacific Islander, non-Hispanic/Latino; 11 Two or more races, non-Hispanic/Latino). Average age 31. 66 applicants, 91% accepted, 43 enrolled. In 2015, 54 master's, 17 doctorates, 1 other advanced degree awarded. *Degree requirements:* For master's, capstone project; for doctorate, scholarly project. *Entrance requirements:* For master's and doctorate, BSN from an ACEN- or CCNE-accredited nursing school, minimum cumulative GPA of 3.0, personal statement, current unencumbered RN license with NE eligibility, undergraduate statistics course, physical assessment course or equivalent; for other advanced degree, MSN or MS in nursing, minimum cumulative GPA of 3.0, current unencumbered RN license with NE eligibility. Additional exam requirements/recommendations for international students: Required—TOEFL (minimum score 600 paper-based; 100 iBT). *Application deadline:* For fall admission, 6/15 priority date for domestic and international students; for spring admission, 11/15 priority date for domestic and international students; for summer admission, 4/15 for domestic and international students. Applications are processed on a rolling basis. Application fee: $50. Electronic applications accepted. *Expenses:* $800 per credit hour tuition; $904 per semester full-time fees; $207 per semester part-time fees; $50 one-time drug screen fee. *Financial support:* In 2015–16, 7 students received support. Scholarships/grants available. Financial award applicants required to submit FAFSA. *Faculty research:* Obesity prevention in children, evaluation of simulated clinical experiences, vitamin D3 and calcium for cancer risk education in post menopausal women, online support and education to reduce stress for prenatal patients on bed rest, health literacy, immunization research. *Total annual research expenditures:* $162,085. *Unit head:* Dr. Catherine Todero, Dean, 402-280-2004, Fax: 402-280-2045. *Application contact:* Shannon Cox, Enrollment Specialist, 402-280-2067, Fax: 402-280-2045, E-mail: shannoncox@creighton.edu.
Website: http://nursing.creighton.edu/

Drexel University, College of Nursing and Health Professions, Division of Graduate Nursing, Philadelphia, PA 19104-2875. Offers adult acute care (MSN); adult psychiatric/mental health (MSN); advanced practice nursing (MSN); clinical trials research (MSN); family nurse practitioner (MSN); leadership in health systems management (MSN); nursing education (MSN); pediatric primary care (MSN); women's health (MSN). *Accreditation:* AACN. Electronic applications accepted.

Fairfield University, Marion Peckham Egan School of Nursing and Health Studies, Fairfield, CT 06824. Offers advanced practice (DNP); family nurse practitioner (MSN, DNP); nurse anesthesia (DNP); nursing leadership (MSN); psychiatric nurse practitioner (MSN, DNP). *Accreditation:* AACN; AANA/CANAEP. *Program availability:* Part-time, evening/weekend. *Faculty:* 8 full-time (all women), 9 part-time/adjunct (7 women). *Students:* 43 full-time (35 women), 181 part-time (163 women); includes 52 minority (20 Black or African American, non-Hispanic/Latino; 1 American Indian or Alaska Native, non-Hispanic/Latino; 11 Asian, non-Hispanic/Latino; 16 Hispanic/Latino; 4 Two or more races, non-Hispanic/Latino), 1 international. Average age 36. 103 applicants, 67% accepted, 43 enrolled. In 2015, 12 master's, 21 doctorates awarded. *Degree requirements:* For master's, capstone project. *Entrance requirements:* For master's, minimum QPA of 3.0, RN license, resume, 2 recommendations; for doctorate, MSN (minimum QPA of 3.2) or BSN (minimum QPA of 3.0); critical care nursing experience (for nurse anesthesia DNP candidates). Additional exam requirements/recommendations for international students: Required—TOEFL (minimum score 550 paper-based; 80 iBT) or IELTS (minimum score 6.5). *Application deadline:* For fall admission, 5/15 for international students; for spring admission, 10/15 for international students. Applications are processed on a rolling basis. Application fee: $60. Electronic applications accepted. *Expenses:* $850 per credit hour (for MSN); $900-$1,000 per credit hour (for DNP). *Financial support:* In 2015–16, 51 students received support. Unspecified assistantships available. Financial award applicants required to submit FAFSA. *Faculty research:* Aging, spiritual care, palliative and end of life care, psychiatric mental health, pediatric trauma. *Unit head:* Dr. Meredith Wallace Kazer, Dean, 203-254-4000 Ext. 2701, Fax: 203-254-4126, E-mail: mkazer@fairfield.edu. *Application contact:* Marianne Gumpper, Director of Graduate and Continuing Studies Admission, 203-254-4184, Fax: 203-254-4073, E-mail: gradadmis@fairfield.edu.
Website: http://fairfield.edu/son

Georgia Southern University, Jack N. Averitt College of Graduate Studies, College of Health and Human Sciences, School of Nursing, Program in Nurse Practitioner, Statesboro, GA 30458. Offers family nurse practitioner (MSN); psychiatric mental health nurse practitioner (MSN). *Program availability:* Part-time, blended/hybrid learning. *Students:* 30 full-time (26 women), 25 part-time (21 women); includes 17 minority (10 Black or African American, non-Hispanic/Latino; 4 Asian, non-Hispanic/Latino; 2 Hispanic/Latino; 1 Two or more races, non-Hispanic/Latino). Average age 38. 58 applicants, 71% accepted, 15 enrolled. In 2015, 19 master's awarded. *Entrance requirements:* For master's, minimum GPA of 3.0, Georgia nursing license, 2 years of clinical experience, CPR certification. Additional exam requirements/recommendations for international students: Required—TOEFL (minimum score 550 paper-based; 80 iBT), IELTS (minimum score 6). *Application deadline:* For fall admission, 7/31 priority date for domestic and international students; for spring admission, 11/30 priority date for domestic students, 11/30 for international students; for summer admission, 3/31 for domestic and international students. Applications are processed on a rolling basis. Application fee: $50. Electronic applications accepted. *Expenses:* Tuition, state resident: full-time $7236; part-time $277 per semester hour. Tuition, nonresident: full-time $27,118; part-time $1105 per semester hour. *Required fees:* $2092. *Financial support:* In 2015–16, 26 students received support, including 5 fellowships with full tuition reimbursements available (averaging $7,750 per year); career-related internships or fieldwork, Federal Work-Study, scholarships/grants, traineeships, tuition waivers (full), and unspecified assistantships also available. Support available to part-time students. Financial award application deadline: 4/15; financial award applicants required

to submit FAFSA. *Faculty research:* Vulnerable populations, breast cancer, diabetes, mellitus, advanced practice nursing issues. *Unit head:* Dr. Deborah Allen, Graduate Program Director, 912-478-5056, Fax: 912-478-5036, E-mail: debbieallen@georgiasouthern.edu.

Georgia State University, Byrdine F. Lewis School of Nursing, Atlanta, GA 30303. Offers adult health clinical nurse specialist/nurse practitioner (MS, Certificate); child health clinical nurse specialist/pediatric nurse practitioner (MS, Certificate); family nurse practitioner (MS, Certificate); family psychiatric mental health nurse practitioner (MS, Certificate); nursing (PhD); nursing leadership in healthcare innovations (MS), including nursing administration, nursing informatics; nutrition (MS); perinatal clinical nurse specialist/women's health nurse practitioner (MS, Certificate); physical therapy (DPT); respiratory therapy (MS). *Accreditation:* AACN. *Program availability:* Part-time, blended/hybrid learning. *Faculty:* 18 full-time (11 women). *Students:* 275 full-time (195 women), 230 part-time (204 women); includes 192 minority (123 Black or African American, non-Hispanic/Latino; 49 Asian, non-Hispanic/Latino; 12 Hispanic/Latino; 2 Native Hawaiian or other Pacific Islander, non-Hispanic/Latino; 6 Two or more races, non-Hispanic/Latino), 35 international. Average age 33. 240 applicants, 61% accepted, 95 enrolled. In 2015, 115 master's, 40 doctorates, 19 other advanced degrees awarded. *Degree requirements:* For doctorate, comprehensive exam, thesis/dissertation. *Entrance requirements:* For doctorate, GRE. Additional exam requirements/recommendations for international students: Required—TOEFL. *Application deadline:* For fall admission, 2/1 priority date for domestic and international students; for spring admission, 9/15 for domestic and international students. Applications are processed on a rolling basis. Application fee: $50. Electronic applications accepted. *Expenses:* Contact institution. *Financial support:* In 2015–16, research assistantships with tuition reimbursements (averaging $1,666 per year), teaching assistantships with tuition reimbursements (averaging $1,920 per year) were awarded; scholarships/grants, tuition waivers (full and partial), and unspecified assistantships also available. Support available to part-time students. Financial award application deadline: 8/1; financial award applicants required to submit FAFSA. *Faculty research:* Stroke intervention for caregivers, stroke prevention in African-Americans; relationships between psychological distress and health outcomes in parents with a medically ill infant; medically fragile children; nursing expertise and patient outcomes. *Unit head:* Nancy Kropf, Dean of Nursing, 404-413-1101, Fax: 404-413-1090, E-mail: nkropf@gsu.edu.
Website: http://nursing.gsu.edu

Hampton University, School of Nursing, Hampton, VA 23668. Offers advanced adult nursing (MS); community health nursing (MS); community mental health/psychiatric nursing (MS); family nursing (MS); gerontological nursing for the nurse practitioner (MS); nursing (PhD); women's health nursing (MS). *Accreditation:* AACN. *Program availability:* Part-time, online learning. *Degree requirements:* For master's, comprehensive exam, thesis optional; for doctorate, comprehensive exam, thesis/dissertation. *Entrance requirements:* For master's, GRE General Test. Additional exam requirements/recommendations for international students: Required—TOEFL (minimum score 525 paper-based) or IELTS (6.5). Electronic applications accepted. *Expenses:* Tuition, area resident: Full-time $10,263; part-time $522 per credit hour. *Required fees:* $35. Tuition and fees vary according to course load and program. *Faculty research:* African-American stress, HIV education, pediatric obesity, hypertension, breast cancer.

Hunter College of the City University of New York, Graduate School, Schools of the Health Professions, Hunter-Bellevue School of Nursing, Program in Psychiatric Nursing, New York, NY 10065-5085. Offers MS, AC. *Accreditation:* AACN. *Program availability:* Part-time. *Students:* 2 full-time (both women), 91 part-time (71 women); includes 42 minority (26 Black or African American, non-Hispanic/Latino; 10 Asian, non-Hispanic/Latino; 6 Hispanic/Latino), 1 international. Average age 43. 34 applicants, 56% accepted, 14 enrolled. In 2015, 23 master's, 11 other advanced degrees awarded. *Degree requirements:* For master's, practicum. *Entrance requirements:* For master's, minimum GPA of 3.0, New York RN license, BSN. Additional exam requirements/recommendations for international students: Required—TOEFL. *Application deadline:* For fall admission, 4/1 for domestic students, 2/1 for international students; for spring admission, 11/1 for domestic students, 9/1 for international students. Applications are processed on a rolling basis. *Financial support:* Federal Work-Study, scholarships/grants, traineeships, and tuition waivers (partial) available. Support available to part-time students. Financial award application deadline: 5/1; financial award applicants required to submit FAFSA. *Faculty research:* Nursing approaches with the homeless, chronic mentally ill, and depressed; power and empathy. *Unit head:* Dr. Kunsook Bernstein, Coordinator, 212-481-4346, Fax: 212-481-5078, E-mail: kbernst@hunter.cuny.edu. *Application contact:* Milena Solo, Director for Graduate Admissions, 212-772-4288, E-mail: admissions@hunter.cuny.edu.
Website: http://www.hunter.cuny.edu/graduateadmissions/program-requirements/nursing/psychiatric-mental-health-nurse-practitioner

Husson University, Graduate Nursing Program, Bangor, ME 04401-2999. Offers advanced practice psychiatric nursing (MSN, PMC); family and community nurse practitioner (MSN, PMC); nursing education (MSN, PMC). *Accreditation:* AACN. *Program availability:* Part-time. *Faculty:* 6 full-time (all women), 2 part-time/adjunct (1 woman). *Students:* 27 full-time (26 women), 10 part-time (9 women); includes 4 minority (2 Asian, non-Hispanic/Latino; 2 Two or more races, non-Hispanic/Latino). Average age 39. 70 applicants, 27% accepted, 13 enrolled. In 2015, 9 master's awarded. *Degree requirements:* For master's, comprehensive exam (for some programs), research project. *Entrance requirements:* For master's, MAT or GRE, BSN. Additional exam requirements/recommendations for international students: Required—TOEFL (minimum score 550 paper-based; 80 iBT). *Application deadline:* For fall admission, 3/31 for domestic students; for spring admission, 10/30 for domestic students. Application fee: $40. Electronic applications accepted. *Expenses:* Contact institution. *Financial support:* Research assistantships, Federal Work-Study, institutionally sponsored loans, traineeships, and unspecified assistantships available. Financial award application deadline: 3/31; financial award applicants required to submit FAFSA. *Faculty research:* Health disparities and methods to better identify and provide healthcare services to those most in need. *Unit head:* Prof. Mary Jude, Director, Graduate Nursing, 207-941-7769, Fax: 207-941-7198, E-mail: judem@husson.edu. *Application contact:* Kristen Card, Director of Graduate Admissions, 207-404-5660, Fax: 207-941-7935, E-mail: cardk@husson.edu.
Website: http://www.husson.edu/nursing-msn

Kent State University, College of Nursing, Kent, OH 44242. Offers advanced nursing practice (DNP), including adult gerontology acute care nurse practitioner (MSN, DNP), adult gerontology clinical nurse specialist (MSN, DNP), family nurse practitioner (MSN, DNP); nursing (MSN, PhD), including adult gerontology acute care nurse practitioner (MSN, DNP), adult gerontology clinical nurse specialist (MSN, DNP), family nurse practitioner (MSN, DNP), nurse educator (MSN), nursing healthcare management (MSN), primary care adult nurse practitioner (MSN), primary care pediatric clinical nurse specialist (MSN), primary care pediatric nurse practitioner (MSN), psychiatric mental health practitioner (MSN), women's health nurse practitioner (MSN); nursing education (Certificate); primary care pediatric nurse practitioner (Certificate); women's health nurse practitioner (Certificate). PhD program offered jointly with The University of Akron. *Accreditation:* AACN. *Program availability:* Part-time, online learning. *Faculty:* 52 full-

time (48 women). *Students:* 78 full-time (56 women), 414 part-time (365 women); includes 63 minority (34 Black or African American, non-Hispanic/Latino; 1 American Indian or Alaska Native, non-Hispanic/Latino; 12 Asian, non-Hispanic/Latino; 12 Hispanic/Latino; 4 Two or more races, non-Hispanic/Latino), 16 international. Average age 37. 653 applicants, 54% accepted, 309 enrolled. In 2015, 140 master's, 1 doctorate, 13 other advanced degrees awarded. *Degree requirements:* For master's, thesis optional, practicum; for doctorate, comprehensive exam (for some programs), thesis/dissertation (for some programs), practicum and scholarly project (for DNP programs); for Certificate, practicum. *Entrance requirements:* For master's, minimum GPA of 3.0, transcripts, active unrestricted RN license, essay/goal statement, interview, 3 letters of recommendation; for doctorate, GRE (for PhD), minimum GPA of 3.0, transcripts, 3 letters of recommendation, interview; active unrestricted RN license, clinical experience and hours record (for DNP); goal statement, sample of written work, curriculum vitae, statement of research interests, and eligibility for RN license (for PhD); for Certificate, MSN, minimum GPA of 3.0, transcripts. Additional exam requirements/recommendations for international students: Required—TOEFL (minimum score: paper-based 525, iBT 71), Michigan English Language Assessment Battery (minimum score of 75), IELTS (minimum score of 6.0), PTE Academic (minimum score of 48), or completion of ELS level 112 Intensive Program. *Application deadline:* For fall admission, 2/1 for domestic students; for spring admission, 11/1 for domestic students. Application fee: $45 ($70 for international students). Electronic applications accepted. *Expenses:* Tuition, state resident: full-time $10,864; part-time $495 per credit hour. Tuition, nonresident: full-time $18,380; part-time $837 per credit hour. *Financial support:* Research assistantships with full tuition reimbursements, teaching assistantships with full tuition reimbursements, career-related internships or fieldwork, Federal Work-Study, traineeships, and unspecified assistantships available. Financial award application deadline: 2/1. *Unit head:* Dr. Barbara Broome, Dean, 330-672-3777, E-mail: bbroome1@kent.edu. *Application contact:* Dr. Wendy A. Umborgor, Associate Dean for Graduate Programs/Professor, 330-672-8813, E-mail: wlewando@kent.edu.
Website: http://www.kent.edu/nursing/

Lincoln Memorial University, Caylor School of Nursing, Harrogate, TN 37752-1901. Offers family nurse practitioner (MSN); nurse anesthesia (MSN); psychiatric mental health nurse practitioner (MSN). *Accreditation:* AANA/CANAEP; ACEN. *Program availability:* Part-time. *Entrance requirements:* For master's, GRE.

McNeese State University, Doré School of Graduate Studies, College of Nursing, Department of Graduate Nursing, Family Psychiatric/Mental Health Nurse Practitioner Program, Lake Charles, LA 70609. Offers PMC. *Degree requirements:* For PMC, thesis. *Entrance requirements:* For degree, GRE, MSN, eligible for unencumbered licensure as RN in Louisiana.

McNeese State University, Doré School of Graduate Studies, College of Nursing, Department of Graduate Nursing, Nursing Program, Lake Charles, LA 70609. Offers family nurse practitioner (MSN); family psychiatric/mental health nurse practitioner (MSN); nurse educator (MSN); nurse executive (MSN). *Degree requirements:* For master's, comprehensive exam. *Entrance requirements:* For master's, GRE, baccalaureate degree in nursing, minimum overall GPA of 2.7 for all undergraduate coursework, eligibility for unencumbered licensure as Registered Nurse in Louisiana or Texas, course in introductory statistics with minimum C grade, physical assessment skills, two letters of professional reference, 500-word essay, current resume.

MGH Institute of Health Professions, School of Nursing, Boston, MA 02129. Offers advanced practice nursing (MSN); gerontological nursing (MSN); nursing (DNP); pediatric nursing (MSN); psychiatric nursing (MSN); teaching and learning for health care education (Certificate); women's health nursing (MSN). *Accreditation:* AACN. *Degree requirements:* For master's, thesis or alternative. *Entrance requirements:* For master's, GRE General Test, bachelor's degree from regionally-accredited college or university. Additional exam requirements/recommendations for international students: Required—TOEFL (minimum score 550 paper-based; 80 iBT). Electronic applications accepted. *Faculty research:* Biobehavioral nursing, HIV/AIDS, gerontological nursing, women's health, vulnerable populations, health systems.

Midwestern State University, Billie Doris McAda Graduate School, Robert D. and Carol Gunn College of Health Sciences and Human Services, Wilson School of Nursing, Wichita Falls, TX 76308. Offers family nurse practitioner (MSN); family psychiatric mental health nurse practitioner (MSN); nurse educator (MSN). *Accreditation:* AACN. *Program availability:* Part-time, evening/weekend. *Degree requirements:* For master's, comprehensive exam, thesis optional. *Entrance requirements:* For master's, GRE General Test or MAT. Additional exam requirements/recommendations for international students: Required—TOEFL (minimum score 550 paper-based). Electronic applications accepted. *Faculty research:* Infant feeding, musculoskeletal disorders, diabetes, community health education, water quality reporting.

Molloy College, Division of Nursing, Rockville Centre, NY 11571-5002. Offers adult-gerontology primary care nurse practitioner (MS); clinical nurse specialist (MS), including adult-gerontology health; clinical nurse specialist: adult-gerontology (Advanced Certificate), including adult-gerontology; family nurse practitioner (MS, Advanced Certificate), including primary care; family psychiatric mental health nurse practitioner (MS); nursing (DNP, PhD); nursing administration (MS), including informatics; nursing education (MS); pediatric nurse practitioner (MS), including primary care (MS, Advanced Certificate). *Accreditation:* AACN. *Program availability:* Part-time, evening/weekend. *Faculty:* 26 full-time (all women), 12 part-time/adjunct (9 women). *Students:* 13 full-time (all women), 550 part-time (515 women); includes 316 minority (169 Black or African American, non-Hispanic/Latino; 1 American Indian or Alaska Native, non-Hispanic/Latino; 88 Asian, non-Hispanic/Latino; 56 Hispanic/Latino; 2 Native Hawaiian or other Pacific Islander, non-Hispanic/Latino). Average age 43. 208 applicants, 69% accepted, 121 enrolled. In 2015, 116 master's, 1 doctorate, 6 other advanced degrees awarded. *Degree requirements:* For master's, 3 letters of reference, BS in nursing, minimum undergraduate GPA of 3.0; for Advanced Certificate, 3 letters of reference, master's degree in nursing. Additional exam requirements/recommendations for international students: Required—TOEFL (minimum score 550 paper-based; 79 iBT). *Application deadline:* For fall admission, 9/2 priority date for domestic students; for spring admission, 1/20 priority date for domestic students. Applications are processed on a rolling basis. Application fee: $60. Electronic applications accepted. *Expenses:* Tuition, area resident: Full-time $18,450; part-time $1025 per credit. *Required fees:* $900; $740 per unit. Tuition and fees vary according to course load. *Financial support:* Research assistantships with partial tuition reimbursements, teaching assistantships with partial tuition reimbursements, institutionally sponsored loans, scholarships/grants, and unspecified assistantships available. Support available to part-time students. Financial award application deadline: 4/1; financial award applicants required to submit FAFSA. *Unit head:* Dr. Jeannine Muldoon, Dean of Nursing, 516-323-3651, E-mail: jmuldoon@molloy.edu. *Application contact:* Jaclyn Machowicz, Assistant Director for Admissions, 516-323-4010, E-mail: jmachowicz@molloy.edu.

Monmouth University, Graduate Studies, The Marjorie K. Unterberg School of Nursing and Health Studies, West Long Branch, NJ 07764-1898. Offers adult and gerontological primary care nurse practitioner (MSN); adult-gerontological primary care nurse practitioner (Post-Master's Certificate); family nurse practitioner (MSN, Post-Master's Certificate); family psychiatric and mental health advanced practice nursing (MSN); family psychiatric and mental health nurse practitioner (Post-Master's Certificate); forensic nursing (MSN, Certificate); nursing (MSN); nursing administration (MSN, Post-Master's Certificate); nursing education (MSN, Post-Master's Certificate); nursing practice (DNP); physician assistant (MS); school nursing (MSN, Certificate). *Accreditation:* AACN. *Program availability:* Part-time, evening/weekend, 100% online, blended/hybrid learning. *Faculty:* 14 full-time (13 women), 10 part-time/adjunct (5 women). *Students:* 58 full-time (46 women), 271 part-time (252 women); includes 93 minority (31 Black or African American, non-Hispanic/Latino; 40 Asian, non-Hispanic/Latino; 18 Hispanic/Latino; 1 Native Hawaiian or other Pacific Islander, non-Hispanic/Latino; 3 Two or more races, non-Hispanic/Latino), 1 international. Average age 37. 450 applicants, 32% accepted, 103 enrolled. In 2015, 68 master's, 8 doctorates, 11 other advanced degrees awarded. *Degree requirements:* For master's, practicum (for some tracks); for doctorate, practicum, capstone course. *Entrance requirements:* For master's, GRE General Test (waived for MSN applicants with minimum B grade in each of the first four courses and for MS applicants with master's degree), BSN with minimum GPA of 2.75, current RN license, proof of liability and malpractice policy, personal statement, two letters of recommendation, college course work in health assessment, resume; CASPA application (for MS); for doctorate, accredited master's nursing program degree with minimum GPA of 3.2, graduate research course in statistics, active RN license, national certification as Nurse Practitioner or Nurse Administrator, working knowledge of statistics, statement of goals and vision for change, 2 letters of recommendation (professional or academic), resume, interview. Additional exam requirements/recommendations for international students: Required—TOEFL (minimum score 550 paper-based; 79 iBT), IELTS (minimum score 6) or Michigan English Language Assessment Battery (minimum score 77). *Application deadline:* For fall admission, 7/15 priority date for domestic students, 6/1 for international students; for spring admission, 12/15 priority date for domestic students, 11/1 for international students; for summer admission, 5/1 for domestic students. Applications are processed on a rolling basis. Application fee: $50. Electronic applications accepted. *Expenses:* Contact institution. *Financial support:* In 2015–16, 241 students received support, including 220 fellowships (averaging $3,403 per year), 5 research assistantships (averaging $5,146 per year); career-related internships or fieldwork, scholarships/grants, and unspecified assistantships also available. Support available to part-time students. Financial award applicants required to submit FAFSA. *Faculty research:* School nursing, health policy, and smoking cessation in teens, Multiple Sclerosis; adherence and self-efficacy, aging issues and geriatric care. *Unit head:* Dr. Janet Mahoney, Dean, 732-571-3443, Fax: 732-263-5131, E-mail: jmahoney@monmouth.edu. *Application contact:* Lucia Fedele, Graduate Admission Counselor, 732-571-3452, Fax: 732-263-5123, E-mail: gradadm@monmouth.edu.
Website: http://www.monmouth.edu/school-of-nursing-health/graduate-nursing-programs.aspx

Montana State University, The Graduate School, College of Nursing, Bozeman, MT 59717. Offers clinical nurse leader (MN); family and individual nurse practitioner (DNP); family nurse practitioner (MN, Post-Master's Certificate); nursing education (Certificate, Post-Master's Certificate); psychiatric mental health nurse practitioner (MN); psychiatric/mental health nurse practitioner (DNP). *Accreditation:* AACN. *Program availability:* Part-time, online learning. *Degree requirements:* For master's, comprehensive exam, thesis (for some programs); for doctorate, thesis/dissertation, 1,125 hours in clinical settings. *Entrance requirements:* For master's, GRE General Test, minimum GPA of 3.0 for undergraduate and post-baccalaureate work. Additional exam requirements/recommendations for international students: Required—TOEFL (minimum score 580 paper-based). Electronic applications accepted. *Faculty research:* Rural nursing, health disparities, environmental/public health, oral health, resilience.

New Mexico State University, College of Health and Social Services, School of Nursing, Las Cruces, NM 88003. Offers adult/geriatric nursing (DNP); family nurse practitioner (DNP); family/psychiatric mental health nursing (DNP); nursing administration (MSN); nursing science (PhD); public/community health nursing (DNP). *Accreditation:* AACN. *Program availability:* Blended/hybrid learning. *Faculty:* 16 full-time (15 women). *Students:* 24 full-time (18 women), 90 part-time (80 women); includes 49 minority (10 Black or African American, non-Hispanic/Latino; 1 American Indian or Alaska Native, non-Hispanic/Latino; 4 Asian, non-Hispanic/Latino; 32 Hispanic/Latino; 2 Two or more races, non-Hispanic/Latino), 1 international. Average age 43. 40 applicants, 58% accepted, 17 enrolled. In 2015, 6 master's, 11 doctorates awarded. *Degree requirements:* For master's, comprehensive exam, thesis optional, clinical practice; for doctorate, comprehensive exam, thesis/dissertation. *Entrance requirements:* For master's, NCLEX, BSN, minimum GPA of 3.0, course work in statistics, 3 letters of reference, writing sample, RN license, CPR certification, proof of liability, immunizations, criminal background check; for doctorate, NCLEX, MSN, minimum GPA of 3.0, 3 letters of reference, writing sample, RN license, CPR certification, proof of liability, immunizations, criminal background check, statistics course. Additional exam requirements/recommendations for international students: Required—TOEFL (minimum score 550 paper-based; 79 iBT), IELTS (minimum score 6.5). *Application deadline:* For fall admission, 1/15 for domestic students; for spring admission, 1/15 priority date for domestic students; for summer admission, 1/15 for domestic students. Application fee: $40 ($50 for international students). Electronic applications accepted. *Expenses:* $274.50 per credit hour for in-state students, and all students enrolled in six or fewer credits; $839.30 per credit hour for out-of-state and international students enrolled in at least seven hours. *Financial support:* In 2015–16, 23 students received support, including 1 teaching assistantship (averaging $9,473 per year); career-related internships or fieldwork, Federal Work-Study, scholarships/grants, traineeships, health care benefits, and unspecified assistantships also available. Support available to part-time students. Financial award application deadline: 3/1. *Faculty research:* Women's health, community health, health disparities, nursing informatics and health care technologies, health care and nursing administration. *Total annual research expenditures:* $127,778. *Unit head:* Dr. Kathleen Huttlinger, Department Head, 575-646-3812, Fax: 575-646-2167, E-mail: khuttlin@nmsu.edu. *Application contact:* Dr. Teresa Keller, Director of Graduate Studies, 575-646-4370, Fax: 575-646-2167, E-mail: tkeller@nmsu.edu.
Website: http://schoolofnursing.nmsu.edu

New York University, Rory Meyers College of Nursing, Doctor of Nursing Practice Program, New York, NY 10012-1019. Offers nursing (DNP), including adult acute care, adult primary care, family, mental health nursing, nurse-midwifery, pediatrics. *Program availability:* Part-time, evening/weekend. *Faculty:* 14 full-time (13 women). *Students:* 2 full-time (both women), 32 part-time (27 women); includes 8 minority (3 Black or African American, non-Hispanic/Latino; 4 Asian, non-Hispanic/Latino; 1 Hispanic/Latino), 1 international. Average age 40. 47 applicants, 51% accepted, 16 enrolled. In 2015, 17 doctorates awarded. *Degree requirements:* For doctorate, thesis/dissertation, project. *Entrance requirements:* For doctorate, MAT or GRE (either taken within past 5 years), MS, RN license, interview, Nurse Practitioner Certification, writing sample. Additional exam requirements/recommendations for international students: Required—TOEFL (minimum score 90 iBT), IELTS (minimum score 7). *Application deadline:* For fall admission, 3/1 for domestic and international students. Applications are processed on a rolling basis. Application fee: $80. Electronic applications accepted. *Expenses:* Contact

Psychiatric Nursing

institution. *Financial support:* In 2015–16, 12 students received support. Scholarships/grants available. Support available to part-time students. Financial award application deadline: 2/1; financial award applicants required to submit FAFSA. *Faculty research:* Workforce, LGBT, breast cancer, HIV. *Unit head:* Dr. Rona Levin, Director, 212-998-5319, Fax: 212-995-3143, E-mail: rfl2039@nyu.edu. *Application contact:* Samantha Jaser, Assistant Director, Graduate Student Affairs and Admissions, 212-992-7653, Fax: 212-995-4302, E-mail: saj283@nyu.edu.

New York University, Rory Meyers College of Nursing, Programs in Advanced Practice Nursing, New York, NY 10012-1019. Offers adult-gerontology acute care nurse practitioner (MS, Advanced Certificate); adult-gerontology primary care nurse practitioner (MS, Advanced Certificate); family nurse practitioner (MS, Advanced Certificate); gerontology nurse practitioner (Advanced Certificate); nurse-midwifery (MS, Advanced Certificate); nursing administration (MS, Advanced Certificate); nursing education (MS, Advanced Certificate); nursing informatics (MS, Advanced Certificate); pediatrics nurse practitioner (MS, Advanced Certificate); psychiatric-mental health nurse practitioner (MS, Advanced Certificate); MS/MPH. *Accreditation:* AACN; ACNM/ACME. *Program availability:* Part-time. *Faculty:* 24 full-time (all women), 76 part-time/adjunct (65 women). *Students:* 46 full-time (26 women), 586 part-time (513 women); includes 242 minority (68 Black or African American, non-Hispanic/Latino; 3 American Indian or Alaska Native, non-Hispanic/Latino; 117 Asian, non-Hispanic/Latino; 38 Hispanic/Latino; 3 Native Hawaiian or other Pacific Islander, non-Hispanic/Latino; 13 Two or more races, non-Hispanic/Latino), 23 international. Average age 32. 402 applicants, 69% accepted, 138 enrolled. In 2015, 198 master's, 5 other advanced degrees awarded. *Degree requirements:* For master's, thesis (for some programs). *Entrance requirements:* For master's, BS in nursing, AS in nursing with another BS/BA, interview, RN license, 1 year of clinical experience (3 for the MS in nursing education program); for Advanced Certificate, master's degree. Additional exam requirements/recommendations for international students: Required—TOEFL (minimum score 90 iBT), IELTS (minimum score 7). *Application deadline:* For fall admission, 6/15 for domestic and international students; for spring admission, 12/1 for domestic and international students; for summer admission, 3/1 for domestic and international students. Application fee: $80. Electronic applications accepted. *Expenses:* Contact institution. *Financial support:* In 2015–16, 101 students received support. Career-related internships or fieldwork, Federal Work-Study, and scholarships/grants available. Support available to part-time students. Financial award application deadline: 3/1; financial award applicants required to submit FAFSA. *Faculty research:* Geriatrics, HIV, families and illness, oral systemic connection, symptom management. *Unit head:* Dr. James Pace, Senior Associate Dean for Academic Programs, 212-992-7343, E-mail: james.pace@nyu.edu. *Application contact:* Samantha Jaser, Assistant Director, Graduate Student Affairs and Admissions, 212-992-7653, Fax: 212-995-4302, E-mail: saj283@nyu.edu.

Nicholls State University, Graduate Studies, College of Nursing and Allied Health, Thibodaux, LA 70310. Offers family nurse practitioner (MSN); nurse executive (MSN); nursing education (MSN); psychiatric/mental health nurse practitioner (MSN). Website: http://www.nicholls.edu/cona/

Northeastern University, Bouvé College of Health Sciences, Boston, MA 02115-5096. Offers applied behavior analysis (MS, CAGS); audiology (Au D); biomedical nanotechnology (MS); college student development and counseling (MS, CAGS); counseling psychology (MS, PhD, CAGS); exercise science (MS); health informatics (MS); medicinal chemistry (MS); nurse anesthesia (DNP, CAGS); nursing (MS, PhD, CAGS), including administration (MS), adult-gerontology acute care nurse practitioner (MS, CAGS), adult-gerontology primary care nurse practitioner (MS, CAGS), anesthesia (MS), family nurse practitioner (MS, CAGS), neonatal nurse practitioner (MS, CAGS), pediatric nurse practitioner (MS, CAGS), psychiatric mental health nurse practitioner (MS, CAGS); nursing practice (DNP); personal health informatics (PhD); pharmaceutical sciences (MS, PhD), including interdisciplinary concentration, pharmaceutics and drug delivery systems; pharmacology (MS); pharmacy (Pharm D); physical therapy (Postbaccalaureate Certificate); physician assistant (MS); population health (PhD); school psychology (MS, PhD, CAGS); speech-language pathology (MS); urban health (MPH); MS/MBA. *Accreditation:* ACPE (one or more programs are accredited). *Program availability:* Part-time, evening/weekend, online learning. *Faculty:* 194 full-time (120 women), 169 part-time/adjunct (136 women). *Students:* 1,416 full-time (1,049 women), 310 part-time (248 women). In 2015, 374 master's, 313 doctorates, 37 other advanced degrees awarded. *Degree requirements:* For doctorate, thesis/dissertation (for some programs); for other advanced degree, comprehensive exam. Application fee: $75. Electronic applications accepted. *Expenses:* Contact institution. *Financial support:* Applicants required to submit FAFSA. *Unit head:* John R. Reynolds, Professor and Interim Dean, 617-373-3323, Fax: 617-373-3030. *Application contact:* Molly Schnabel, Senior Director of Graduate Affairs, 617-373-2708, Fax: 617-373-4701, E-mail: bouvegrad@neu.edu.
Website: http://www.northeastern.edu/bouve/

Oregon Health & Science University, School of Nursing, Program in Mental Health Nursing, Portland, OR 97239-3098. Offers MN, MS, Post Master's Certificate. *Accreditation:* AACN. *Degree requirements:* For master's, thesis optional. *Entrance requirements:* For master's, GRE General Test, bachelor's degree in nursing, minimum undergraduate GPA of 3.0, previous course work in statistics; for Post Master's Certificate, master's degree in nursing.

Point Loma Nazarene University, School of Nursing, San Diego, CA 92106-2899. Offers adult/gerontology nursing (MSN); family/individual health (MSN); general nursing (MSN); nursing (Post-MSN Certificate); pediatric nursing (MSN); psychiatric mental health (MSN). *Accreditation:* AACN. *Program availability:* Part-time. *Faculty:* 6 full-time (5 women), 2 part-time/adjunct (both women). *Students:* 1 (woman) full-time, 74 part-time (61 women); includes 35 minority (4 Black or African American, non-Hispanic/Latino; 15 Asian, non-Hispanic/Latino; 10 Hispanic/Latino; 3 Native Hawaiian or other Pacific Islander, non-Hispanic/Latino; 3 Two or more races, non-Hispanic/Latino), 2 international. Average age 38. 34 applicants, 88% accepted, 18 enrolled. In 2015, 40 master's awarded. *Entrance requirements:* For master's, NCLEX, ADN or BSN in nursing, interview, RN license, essay, letters of recommendation, interview. *Application deadline:* For fall admission, 7/5 priority date for domestic students; for spring admission, 11/1 priority date for domestic students; for summer admission, 3/22 priority date for domestic students. Applications are processed on a rolling basis. Application fee: $50. *Financial support:* Applicants required to submit FAFSA. *Unit head:* Dr. Barb Taylor, Dean of the School of Nursing, 619-849-2766, E-mail: bataylor@pointloma.edu. *Application contact:* Claire Buckley, Director of Graduate Admissions, 619-563 2846, E-mail: clairebuckley@pointloma.edu.
Website: http://www.pointloma.edu/discover/graduate-school/graduate-programs/master-science-nursing-and-post-msn-certification

Pontifical Catholic University of Puerto Rico, College of Sciences, Department of Nursing, Program in Mental Health and Psychiatric Nursing, Ponce, PR 00717-0777. Offers MSN. *Program availability:* Part-time, evening/weekend. *Degree requirements:* For master's, comprehensive exam (for some programs), thesis, clinical research paper. *Entrance requirements:* For master's, GRE General Test, 2 letters of recommendation, interview, minimum GPA of 2.75. Electronic applications accepted.

Rivier University, School of Graduate Studies, Division of Nursing, Nashua, NH 03060. Offers adult psychiatric/mental health practitioner (MS); family nurse practitioner (MS); nursing education (MS). *Accreditation:* ACEN. *Program availability:* Part-time, evening/weekend. *Entrance requirements:* For master's, GRE, MAT. Electronic applications accepted.

Rush University, College of Nursing, Department of Community, Systems, and Mental Health Nursing, Chicago, IL 60612. Offers advanced public health nursing (DNP); family nurse practitioner (DNP); leadership to enhance population health outcomes (DNP); nursing science (PhD); psychiatric mental health nurse practitioner (DNP); systems leadership (DNP). *Accreditation:* AACN. *Program availability:* Part-time, 100% online. *Faculty:* 43 full-time (40 women), 52 part-time/adjunct (49 women). *Students:* 18 full-time (17 women), 341 part-time (314 women); includes 85 minority (38 Black or African American, non-Hispanic/Latino; 2 American Indian or Alaska Native, non-Hispanic/Latino; 21 Asian, non-Hispanic/Latino; 22 Hispanic/Latino; 2 Native Hawaiian or other Pacific Islander, non-Hispanic/Latino). Average age 35. 177 applicants, 62% accepted, 96 enrolled. *Degree requirements:* For doctorate, capstone project (for DNP); dissertation (for PhD). *Entrance requirements:* For doctorate, GRE General Test (waived for DNP if cumulative GPA is 3.25 or greater, nursing GPA is 3.0 or greater, or a completed graduate program GPA is 3.5 or greater), interview, 3 letters of recommendation, personal statement, current resume. Additional exam requirements/recommendations for international students: Required—TOEFL (minimum score 94 iBT). *Application deadline:* For fall admission, 1/2 for domestic students; for winter admission, 10/15 for domestic students; for spring admission, 8/4 for domestic students; for summer admission, 12/1 for domestic students. Applications are processed on a rolling basis. Application fee: $100. Electronic applications accepted. *Expenses:* Contact institution. *Financial support:* Research assistantships, teaching assistantships, Federal Work-Study, scholarships/grants, traineeships, and health care benefits available. Support available to part-time students. Financial award application deadline: 3/1; financial award applicants required to submit FAFSA. *Faculty research:* Reduction of health disparities; evidence-based interventions for caregivers; patient-centered quality assessment of psychiatric inpatient environments; digital delivery of a parent-training program for urban, low-income parents; patient-centered predictors and outcomes of inter-professional care coordination. *Unit head:* Dr. Mona Shattell, Chairperson, 312-942-7117, E-mail: mona_shattell@rush.edu. *Application contact:* Jennifer Thorndyke, Admissions Specialist, 312-563-7526, E-mail: jennifer_thorndyke@rush.edu.
Website: http://www.rushu.rush.edu/servlet/Satellite?c=content_block&cid=1320160764996&pagename=CollegeOfNursing%2Fcontent_block%2FContentBlockDetail&rendermod

Sage Graduate School, School of Health Sciences, Department of Nursing, Program in Family Nurse Practitioner, Troy, NY 12180-4115. Offers adult gerontology acute care (Post Master's Certificate); family nurse practitioner (MS); family psychiatric mental health (Post Master's Certificate). *Accreditation:* AACN. *Program availability:* Part-time, evening/weekend. *Faculty:* 9 full-time (all women), 27 part-time/adjunct (24 women). *Students:* 24 full-time (23 women), 110 part-time (99 women); includes 24 minority (11 Black or African American, non-Hispanic/Latino; 2 American Indian or Alaska Native, non-Hispanic/Latino; 8 Asian, non-Hispanic/Latino; 2 Hispanic/Latino; 1 Two or more races, non-Hispanic/Latino). Average age 34. 114 applicants, 28% accepted, 25 enrolled. In 2015, 4 master's, 6 other advanced degrees awarded. *Degree requirements:* For master's, thesis or alternative. *Entrance requirements:* For master's, currently licensed as registered professional nurse in state of practice; baccalaureate degree in nursing from nationally-accredited program or its international equivalent. Additional exam requirements/recommendations for international students: Required—TOEFL (minimum score 550 paper-based). *Application deadline:* Applications are processed on a rolling basis. Application fee: $40. Electronic applications accepted. *Expenses: Tuition, area resident:* Full-time $12,240; part-time $680 per credit hour. Tuition and fees vary according to degree level and program. *Financial support:* Fellowships, research assistantships, teaching assistantships, Federal Work-Study, scholarships/grants, and unspecified assistantships available. Support available to part-time students. Financial award application deadline: 3/1; financial award applicants required to submit FAFSA. *Unit head:* Dr. Theresa Hand, Dean, School of Health Sciences, 518-244-2264, Fax: 518-244-4571, E-mail: handt@sage.edu. *Application contact:* Dr. Carol Braungart, Co-Director, Graduate Nursing Program, 518-244-2459, Fax: 518-244-2009, E-mail: braunc@sage.edu.

Sage Graduate School, School of Health Sciences, Department of Nursing, Program in Psychiatric Mental Health Nurse Practitioner, Troy, NY 12180-4115. Offers MS, Post Master's Certificate. *Accreditation:* AACN. *Program availability:* Part-time, evening/weekend. *Faculty:* 9 full-time (all women), 27 part-time/adjunct (24 women). *Students:* 11 full-time (10 women), 21 part-time (19 women); includes 1 minority (Black or African American, non-Hispanic/Latino). Average age 40. 23 applicants, 57% accepted, 9 enrolled. In 2015, 3 master's, 1 other advanced degree awarded. *Degree requirements:* For master's, thesis or alternative. *Entrance requirements:* For master's, currently licensed as registered professional nurse in state of practice; baccalaureate degree in nursing from nationally-accredited program or its international equivalent. Additional exam requirements/recommendations for international students: Required—TOEFL (minimum score 550 paper-based). *Application deadline:* Applications are processed on a rolling basis. Application fee: $40. Electronic applications accepted. *Expenses: Tuition, area resident:* Full-time $12,240; part-time $680 per credit hour. Tuition and fees vary according to degree level and program. *Financial support:* Fellowships, research assistantships, teaching assistantships, Federal Work-Study, scholarships/grants, and unspecified assistantships available. Support available to part-time students. Financial award application deadline: 3/1; financial award applicants required to submit FAFSA. *Unit head:* Dr. Theresa Hand, Dean, School of Health Sciences, 518-244-2264, Fax: 518-244-4571, E-mail: handt@sage.edu. *Application contact:* Dr. Carol Braungart, Co-Director, Graduate Nursing Program, 518-244-2459, Fax: 518-244-2009, E-mail: braunc@sage.edu.

Saint Francis Medical Center College of Nursing, Graduate Programs, Peoria, IL 61603-3783. Offers adult gerontology (MSN); clinical nurse leader (MSN); family nurse practitioner (MSN); family psychiatric mental health nurse practitioner (MSN); neonatal nurse practitioner (MSN); nurse clinician (Post-Graduate Certificate); nurse educator (MSN, Post-Graduate Certificate); nursing (DNP); nursing management leadership (MSN). *Accreditation:* ACEN. *Program availability:* Part-time, 100% online, blended/hybrid learning. *Faculty:* 14 full-time (all women), 5 part-time/adjunct (all women). *Students:* 13 full-time (12 women), 257 part-time (228 women); includes 23 minority (14 Black or African American, non-Hispanic/Latino; 3 Asian, non-Hispanic/Latino; 4 Hispanic/Latino; 2 Two or more races, non-Hispanic/Latino). Average age 37. 86 applicants, 86% accepted, 44 enrolled. In 2015, 61 master's, 6 doctorates awarded. *Degree requirements:* For master's, research experience, portfolio, practicum; for doctorate, practicum hours. *Entrance requirements:* For master's, nursing research, health assessment, graduate course work in statistics, RN license; for doctorate, master's degree in nursing, professional portfolio, graduate statistics, transcripts, RN license. Additional exam requirements/recommendations for international students: Required—TOEFL (minimum score 550 paper-based; 79 iBT). *Application deadline:* For fall admission, 6/1 priority date for domestic and international students; for spring admission, 11/15 priority date for domestic and international students. Applications are

processed on a rolling basis. Application fee: $50. *Financial support:* In 2015–16, 18 students received support. Scholarships/grants and tuition waivers (partial) available. Support available to part-time students. Financial award application deadline: 6/15; financial award applicants required to submit FAFSA. *Faculty research:* Outcome and curriculum planning, health promotion, NCLEX-RN results, decision-making program evaluation. *Unit head:* Dr. Patti A. Stockert, President of the College, 309-655-4124, Fax: 309-624-8973, E-mail: patricia.a.stockert@osfhealthcare.org. *Application contact:* Dr. Kim A. Mitchell, Dean, Graduate Program, 309-655-2201, Fax: 309-624-8973, E-mail: kim.a.mitchell@osfhealthcare.org.
Website: http://www.sfmccon.edu/graduate-programs/

Seattle University, College of Nursing, Program in Advanced Practice Nursing Immersion, Seattle, WA 98122-1090. Offers adult/gerontological nurse practitioner (MSN); advanced community public health nursing (MSN); family nurse practitioner (MSN); family psychiatric mental health nurse practitioner (MSN); nurse midwifery (MSN). *Degree requirements:* For master's, thesis or scholarly project. *Entrance requirements:* For master's, GRE, bachelor's degree, minimum GPA of 3.0, professional resume, two recommendations, letter of intent. Additional exam requirements/recommendations for international students: Required—TOEFL (minimum score 92 iBT), IELTS. Electronic applications accepted.

Seattle University, College of Nursing, Program in Nursing, Seattle, WA 98122-1090. Offers adult/gerontological nurse practitioner (MSN); advanced community public health (MSN); psychiatric mental health nurse practitioner (MSN). *Degree requirements:* For master's, thesis or scholarly project. *Entrance requirements:* For master's, GRE, bachelor's degree in nursing or associate degree in nursing with baccalaureate in different major, 5-quarter statistics course, minimum cumulative GPA of 3.0, professional resume, two recommendations, letter of intent, copy of current RN license or ability to obtain RN license in WA state. Additional exam requirements/recommendations for international students: Required—TOEFL (minimum score 92 iBT), IELTS. Electronic applications accepted.

Shenandoah University, Eleanor Wade Custer School of Nursing, Winchester, VA 22601. Offers family nurse practitioner (MSN, DNP, Post-Graduate Certificate); health informatics (Certificate); health systems leadership (DNP); nurse midwifery (MSN, Post-Graduate Certificate); nursing education (Post-Graduate Certificate); psychiatric mental health nurse practitioner (MSN, DNP, Post-Graduate Certificate). *Accreditation:* AACN; ACNM/ACME. *Faculty:* 10 full-time (all women), 7 part-time/adjunct (4 women). *Students:* 33 full-time (31 women), 62 part-time (57 women); includes 21 minority (17 Black or African American, non-Hispanic/Latino; 3 Asian, non-Hispanic/Latino; 1 Hispanic/Latino). Average age 36. 55 applicants, 87% accepted, 39 enrolled. In 2015, 32 master's, 3 doctorates, 19 other advanced degrees awarded. *Degree requirements:* For master's, research project, clinical hours; for doctorate, scholarly project, clinical hours; for other advanced degree, clinical hours. *Entrance requirements:* For master's, United States RN license; minimum GPA of 3.0; 2080 hours of clinical experience; curriculum vitae; 3 letters of recommendation from a former dean, a faculty member or advisor familiar with the applicant, and a former or current supervisor; two- to three-page essay on a specified topic; for doctorate, MSN, minimum GPA of 3.0, 3 letters of recommendation, 500-word statement, interview, BSN; for other advanced degree, MSN, minimum GPA of 3.0, 2 letters of recommendation, minimum of one year (2080 hours) of clinical nursing experience, interview. Additional exam requirements/recommendations for international students: Required—TOEFL (minimum score 558 paper-based; 83 iBT). *Application deadline:* For fall admission, 1/15 priority date for domestic and international students; for spring admission, 11/1 for domestic and international students; for summer admission, 3/15 for domestic and international students. Application fee: $30. Electronic applications accepted. *Expenses:* Contact institution. *Financial support:* In 2015–16, 13 students received support, including 3 fellowships (averaging $1,000 per year); scholarships/grants and unspecified assistantships also available. Financial award application deadline: 3/15; financial award applicants required to submit FAFSA. *Faculty research:* Primary care providers and their unique position in geriatric, pre-operative education and its effects on post-operative, variables associated with a woman's multidimensional childbirth, interdisciplinary communication, research on health policy. *Unit head:* Kathryn Ganske, PhD, RN, Dean, 540-678-4374, Fax: 540-665-5519, E-mail: kganske@su.edu. *Application contact:* Andrew Woodall, Executive Director of Recruitment and Admissions, 540-665-4581, Fax: 540-665-4627, E-mail: admit@su.edu.
Website: http://www.su.edu/nursing/

Southern Arkansas University–Magnolia, School of Graduate Studies, Magnolia, AR 71753. Offers agriculture (MS); business administration (MBA), including agri-business, supply chain management; computer and information sciences (MS); elementary or secondary education (M Ed), including curriculum and instruction, educational administration and supervision, gifted and talented P-8/7-12, instructional specialist 4-12, instructional specialist P-4; higher, adult and lifelong education (M Ed); kinesiology (M Ed), including coaching; library media and information specialist (M Ed); mental health and clinical counseling (MS); public administration (MPA); school counseling K-12 (M Ed); student affairs and college counseling (M Ed); teaching (MAT). *Accreditation:* NCATE. *Program availability:* Part-time, 100% online, blended/hybrid learning. *Faculty:* 33 full-time (17 women), 25 part-time/adjunct (11 women). *Students:* 336 full-time (69 women), 636 part-time (292 women); includes 124 minority (109 Black or African American, non-Hispanic/Latino; 6 American Indian or Alaska Native, non-Hispanic/Latino; 5 Asian, non-Hispanic/Latino; 1 Hispanic/Latino; 3 Two or more races, non-Hispanic/Latino), 554 international. Average age 28. 531 applicants, 88% accepted, 345 enrolled. In 2015, 155 master's awarded. *Degree requirements:* For master's, comprehensive exam (for some programs), thesis optional. *Entrance requirements:* For master's, GRE, MAT or GMAT, minimum GPA of 2.5. Additional exam requirements/recommendations for international students: Required—TOEFL (minimum score 550 paper-based), IELTS (minimum score 6). *Application deadline:* For fall admission, 7/20 for domestic students, 7/5 for international students; for spring admission, 12/1 for domestic students, 11/15 for international students; for summer admission, 6/1 for domestic students, 5/1 for international students. Applications are processed on a rolling basis. Application fee: $25 ($50 for international students). Electronic applications accepted. *Expenses:* Tuition, state resident: part-time $217 per credit hour. Tuition, nonresident: part-time $403 per credit hour. *Required fees:* $769 per semester. Tuition and fees vary according to course load and program. *Financial support:* Career-related internships or fieldwork, Federal Work-Study, scholarships/grants, tuition waivers (full), and unspecified assistantships available. Financial award applicants required to submit FAFSA. *Faculty research:* Alternative certification for teachers, supervision of instruction, instructional leadership, counseling. *Unit head:* Dr. Kim Bloss, Dean, School of Graduate Studies, 870-235-4150, Fax: 870-235-5227, E-mail: kkbloss@saumag.edu. *Application contact:* Shrijana Malakar, Admissions Specialist, 870-235-4150, Fax: 870-235-5227, E-mail: smalakar@saumag.edu.
Website: http://www.saumag.edu/graduate

Stony Brook University, State University of New York, Stony Brook Medicine, School of Nursing, Program in Mental Health/Psychiatric Nursing, Stony Brook, NY 11794. Offers MS, DNP, Certificate. *Accreditation:* AACN. *Program availability:* Part-time, blended/hybrid learning. *Students:* 8 full-time (7 women), 105 part-time (84 women);

includes 43 minority (24 Black or African American, non-Hispanic/Latino; 8 Asian, non-Hispanic/Latino; 8 Hispanic/Latino; 3 Two or more races, non-Hispanic/Latino), 1 international. 109 applicants, 60% accepted, 51 enrolled. In 2015, 29 master's, 11 other advanced degrees awarded. *Degree requirements:* For master's, thesis. *Entrance requirements:* For master's, BSN, minimum GPA of 3.0, course work in statistics. Additional exam requirements/recommendations for international students: Required—TOEFL (minimum score 90 iBT). *Application deadline:* For fall admission, 12/1 for domestic students. Application fee: $100. *Expenses:* $24,781 full-time resident tuition and fees, $968 per credit hour; $44,431 full-time nonresident tuition and fees, $1,787 per credit hour. *Financial support:* Application deadline: 3/15. *Unit head:* Dr. Barbara Sprung, Program Director, 631-444-3292, Fax: 631-444-3136, E-mail: barbara.sprung@stonybrook.edu. *Application contact:* Garcia, Staff Assistant, 631-444-3392, Fax: 631-444-3136, E-mail: crystal.garcia@stonybrook.edu.
Website: http://www.nursing.stonybrookmedicine.edu/

Uniformed Services University of the Health Sciences, Daniel K. Inouye Graduate School of Nursing, Bethesda, MD 20814. Offers adult-gerontology clinical nurse specialist (MSN, DNP); family nurse practitioner (DNP); nurse anesthesia (DNP); nursing science (PhD); psychiatric mental health nurse practitioner (DNP); women's health nurse practitioner (DNP). MSN and DNP programs available to military officers only; PhD to military and DoD students only. *Accreditation:* AACN; AANA/CANAEP. *Faculty:* 38 full-time (22 women), 2 part-time/adjunct (1 woman). *Students:* 51 full-time (29 women); includes 17 minority (8 Black or African American, non-Hispanic/Latino; 4 Asian, non-Hispanic/Latino; 4 Hispanic/Latino; 1 Two or more races, non-Hispanic/Latino). Average age 34. 75 applicants, 68% accepted, 51 enrolled. In 2015, 4 master's, 24 doctorates awarded. *Degree requirements:* For master's, thesis or alternative; for doctorate, thesis/dissertation or alternative. *Entrance requirements:* For master's, GRE, BSN, clinical experience, minimum GPA of 3.0, previous course work in science; for doctorate, GRE, BSN, clinical experience, minimum GPA of 3.0, previous course work in sciences, and writing paper (for DNP); MSN (for PhD). *Application deadline:* For fall admission, 7/1 for domestic students; for winter admission, 2/15 for domestic students. Application fee: $0. Electronic applications accepted. *Faculty research:* Prenatal care, military health care, military readiness, distance learning. *Unit head:* Dr. Diane C. Seibert, Associate Dean for Academic Affairs, 301-295-1080, Fax: 301-295-1707, E-mail: diane.seibert@usuhs.edu. *Application contact:* Terry Lynn Malavakis, Recording Secretary for Admissions Committee/Registrar/Program Analyst, 301-295-1055, Fax: 301-295-1707, E-mail: terry.malavakis@usuhs.edu.
Website: http://www.usuhs.edu/gsn/

University at Buffalo, the State University of New York, Graduate School, School of Nursing, Buffalo, NY 14214. Offers adult gerontology nurse practitioner (DNP); family nurse practitioner (DNP); health care systems and leadership (MS); nurse anesthetist (DNP); nursing (PhD); nursing education (Certificate); psychiatric/mental health nurse practitioner (DNP). *Accreditation:* AACN; AANA/CANAEP (one or more programs are accredited). *Program availability:* Part-time, 100% online. *Students:* 61 full-time (37 women), 137 part-time (114 women); includes 35 minority (17 Black or African American, non-Hispanic/Latino; 1 American Indian or Alaska Native, non-Hispanic/Latino; 17 Asian, non-Hispanic/Latino), 7 international. Average age 32. 193 applicants, 49% accepted, 75 enrolled. In 2015, 6 master's, 37 doctorates awarded. *Degree requirements:* For master's, thesis optional; for doctorate, comprehensive exam (for some programs), capstone (for DNP), dissertation (for PhD). *Entrance requirements:* For master's, GRE or MAT; for doctorate, GRE or MAT, minimum GPA of 3.0 (for DNP), 3.25 (for PhD); RN license; BS or MS in nursing; 3 references; writing sample; resume; personal statement; for Certificate, interview, minimum GPA of 3.0 or GRE General Test, RN license, MS in nursing, professional certification. Additional exam requirements/recommendations for international students: Required—TOEFL (minimum score 550 paper-based; 79 iBT), IELTS (minimum score 6.5). *Application deadline:* For fall admission, 7/1 for domestic students, 2/1 for international students; for spring admission, 12/1 for domestic students, 10/1 for international students; for summer admission, 2/1 for domestic students. Applications are processed on a rolling basis. Application fee: $75. Electronic applications accepted. *Financial support:* In 2015–16, 80 students received support, including 2 fellowships with tuition reimbursements available (averaging $17,000 per year), 4 research assistantships with tuition reimbursements available (averaging $10,600 per year), 7 teaching assistantships with tuition reimbursements available (averaging $10,600 per year); scholarships/grants, traineeships, health care benefits, and unspecified assistantships also available. Financial award application deadline: 2/1; financial award applicants required to submit FAFSA. *Faculty research:* Oncology, palliative care, gerontology, addictions, mental health, community wellness, sleep, workforce, care of underserved populations, quality and safety, person-centered care, adolescent health. *Total annual research expenditures:* $1.4 million. *Unit head:* Dr. Marsha L. Lewis, Dean and Professor, 716-829-2533, Fax: 716-829-2566, E-mail: ubnursingdean@buffalo.edu. *Application contact:* Jennifer H. VanLaeken, Director of Graduate Student Services, 716-829-3311, Fax: 716-829-2067, E-mail: jhv2@buffalo.edu.
Website: http://nursing.buffalo.edu/

University of Cincinnati, Graduate School, College of Nursing, Cincinnati, OH 45221-0038. Offers clinical nurse specialist (MSN), including adult health, community health, neonatal, nursing administration, occupational health, pediatric health, psychiatric nursing, women's health; nurse anesthesia (MSN); nurse midwifery (MSN); nurse practitioner (MSN), including acute care, ambulatory care, family, family/psychiatric, women's health; nursing (PhD); MBA/MSN. *Accreditation:* AACN; AANA/CANAEP (one or more programs are accredited); ACNM/ACME. *Program availability:* Part-time, online learning. Terminal master's awarded for partial completion of doctoral program. *Degree requirements:* For master's, thesis or alternative; for doctorate, comprehensive exam, thesis/dissertation. *Entrance requirements:* For master's and doctorate, GRE General Test. Additional exam requirements/recommendations for international students: Required—TOEFL (minimum score 520 paper-based). Electronic applications accepted. *Faculty research:* Substance abuse, injury and violence, symptom management.

University of Colorado Denver, College of Nursing, Aurora, CO 80045. Offers adult clinical nurse specialist (MS); adult nurse practitioner (MS); family nurse practitioner (MS); family psychiatric mental health nurse practitioner (MS); health care informatics (MS); nurse-midwifery (MS); nursing (DNP, PhD); nursing leadership and health care systems (MS); pediatric nurse practitioner (MS); special studies (MS); women's health (MS); MS/PhD. *Accreditation:* ACNM/ACME (one or more programs are accredited). *Program availability:* Part-time, evening/weekend, online learning. *Faculty:* 109 full-time (100 women), 55 part-time/adjunct (50 women). *Students:* 367 full-time (332 women), 141 part-time (118 women); includes 79 minority (16 Black or African American, non-Hispanic/Latino; 2 American Indian or Alaska Native, non-Hispanic/Latino; 8 Asian, non-Hispanic/Latino; 37 Hispanic/Latino; 16 Two or more races, non-Hispanic/Latino), 6 international. Average age 36. 321 applicants, 53% accepted, 145 enrolled. In 2015, 151 master's, 36 doctorates awarded. Terminal master's awarded for partial completion of doctoral program. *Degree requirements:* For master's, thesis optional; for doctorate, comprehensive exam, thesis/dissertation, 42 credits of coursework. *Entrance requirements:* For master's, GRE if cumulative undergraduate GPA is less than 3.0, undergraduate nursing degree from NLNAC- or CCNE-accredited school or university; completion of research and statistics courses with minimum grade of C; copy of current

Psychiatric Nursing

and unencumbered nursing license; for doctorate, GRE, bachelor's and/or master's degrees in nursing from NLN- or CCNE-accredited institution; portfolio; minimum undergraduate GPA of 3.0, graduate 3.5; graduate-level intermediate statistics and master's-level nursing theory courses with minimum B grade; interview. Additional exam requirements/recommendations for international students: Required—TOEFL (minimum score 560 paper-based; 83 iBT). *Application deadline:* For fall admission, 2/15 for domestic students, 1/15 for international students; for spring admission, 7/1 for domestic students, 6/1 for international students. Application fee: $50 ($75 for international students). Electronic applications accepted. *Expenses:* Contact institution. *Financial support:* In 2015–16, 148 students received support. Fellowships, research assistantships, teaching assistantships, Federal Work-Study, institutionally sponsored loans, scholarships/grants, traineeships, and unspecified assistantships available. Support available to part-time students. Financial award application deadline: 4/1; financial award applicants required to submit FAFSA. *Faculty research:* Biological and behavioral phenomena in pregnancy and postpartum; patterns of glycaemia during the insulin resistance of pregnancy; obesity, gestational diabetes, and relationship to neonatal adiposity; men's awareness and knowledge of male breast cancer; cognitive-behavioral therapy for chronic insomnia after breast cancer treatment; massage therapy for the treatment of tension-type headaches. *Total annual research expenditures:* $5.9 million. *Unit head:* Dr. Sarah Thompson, Dean, 303-724-1679, E-mail: sarah.a.thompson@ucdenver.edu. *Application contact:* Judy Campbell, Graduate Programs Coordinator, 303-724-8503, E-mail: judy.campbell@ucdenver.edu. Website: http://www.ucdenver.edu/academics/colleges/nursing/Pages/default.aspx

University of Delaware, College of Health Sciences, School of Nursing, Newark, DE 19716. Offers adult nurse practitioner (MSN, PMC); cardiopulmonary clinical nurse specialist (MSN, PMC); cardiopulmonary clinical nurse specialist/adult nurse practitioner (MSN, PMC); family nurse practitioner (MSN, PMC); gerontology clinical nurse specialist (MSN, PMC); gerontology clinical nurse specialist geriatric nurse practitioner (PMC); gerontology clinical nurse specialist/geriatric nurse practitioner (MSN); health services administration (MSN, PMC); nursing of children clinical nurse specialist (MSN, PMC); nursing of children clinical nurse specialist/pediatric nurse practitioner (MSN, PMC); oncology/immune deficiency clinical nurse specialist (MSN, PMC); oncology/immune deficiency clinical nurse specialist/adult nurse practitioner (MSN, PMC); perinatal/women's health clinical nurse specialist (MSN, PMC); perinatal/women's health clinical nurse specialist/women's health nurse practitioner (MSN, PMC); psychiatric nursing clinical nurse specialist (MSN, PMC). *Accreditation:* AACN. *Program availability:* Part-time, evening/weekend, online learning. *Degree requirements:* For master's, thesis optional. *Entrance requirements:* For master's, BSN, interview, RN license. Electronic applications accepted. *Faculty research:* Marriage and chronic illness, health promotion, congestive heart failure patient outcomes, school nursing, diabetes in children, culture, health disparities, cardiovascular, prison nursing, oncology, public policy, child obesity, smoking and teen pregnancy, blood pressure measurements, men's health.

The University of Kansas, University of Kansas Medical Center, School of Nursing, Kansas City, KS 66160. Offers adult/gerontological clinical nurse specialist (PMC); adult/gerontological nurse practitioner (PMC); clinical research management (PMC); health care informatics (PMC); health professions educator (PMC); nurse midwife (PMC); nursing (MS, DNP, PhD); organizational leadership (PMC); psychiatric/mental health nurse practitioner (PMC); public health nursing (PMC). *Accreditation:* AACN; ACNM/ACME. *Program availability:* Part-time, 100% online, blended/hybrid learning. *Faculty:* 59. *Students:* 44 full-time (42 women), 261 part-time (238 women); includes 54 minority (22 Black or African American, non-Hispanic/Latino; 1 American Indian or Alaska Native, non-Hispanic/Latino; 12 Asian, non-Hispanic/Latino; 10 Hispanic/Latino; 9 Two or more races, non-Hispanic/Latino), 1 international. Average age 38. 95 applicants, 97% accepted, 74 enrolled. In 2015, 71 master's, 24 doctorates, 6 other advanced degrees awarded. Terminal master's awarded for partial completion of doctoral program. *Degree requirements:* For master's, comprehensive exam, thesis (for some programs), general oral exam; for doctorate, variable foreign language requirement, thesis/dissertation or alternative, comprehensive oral exam (for DNP); comprehensive written and oral exam, or three publications (for PhD). *Entrance requirements:* For master's, bachelor's degree in nursing, minimum GPA of 3.0, 1 year of clinical experience, RN license in KS and MO; for doctorate, GRE General Test (for PhD only), bachelor's degree in nursing, minimum GPA of 3.5, RN license in KS and MO. Additional exam requirements/recommendations for international students: Required—TOEFL. *Application deadline:* For fall admission, 4/1 for domestic and international students; for spring admission, 9/1 for domestic and international students. Application fee: $60. Electronic applications accepted. *Financial support:* Research assistantships with tuition reimbursements, teaching assistantships with tuition reimbursements, scholarships/grants, and traineeships available. Financial award application deadline: 3/1; financial award applicants required to submit FAFSA. *Faculty research:* Breastfeeding practices of teen mothers, national database of nursing quality indicators, caregiving of families of patients using technology in the home, simulation in nursing education, diaphragm fatigue. *Total annual research expenditures:* $4.6 million. *Unit head:* Dr. Sally Maliski, Dean, 913-588-1601, Fax: 913-588-1660, E-mail: smaliski@kumc.edu. *Application contact:* Dr. Pamela K. Barnes, Associate Dean, Student Affairs, 913-588-1619, Fax: 913-588-1615, E-mail: pbarnes2@kumc.edu. Website: http://nursing.kumc.edu

University of Louisville, Graduate School, School of Nursing, Louisville, KY 40202. Offers adult gerontology nurse practitioner (MSN, DNP); education and administration (MSN); family nurse practitioner (MSN, DNP); neonatal nurse practitioner (MSN, DNP); nursing research (PhD); psychiatric/mental health nurse practitioner (MSN, DNP); women's health nurse practitioner (MSN). *Accreditation:* AACN. *Program availability:* Part-time. *Faculty:* 53 full-time (48 women), 27 part-time/adjunct (23 women). *Students:* 110 full-time (99 women), 33 part-time (29 women); includes 17 minority (11 Black or African American, non-Hispanic/Latino; 1 Asian, non-Hispanic/Latino; 2 Hispanic/Latino; 3 Two or more races, non-Hispanic/Latino), 5 international. Average age 34. 62 applicants, 68% accepted, 40 enrolled. In 2015, 41 master's awarded. *Degree requirements:* For doctorate, comprehensive exam (for some programs), thesis/dissertation (for some programs). *Entrance requirements:* For master's, bachelor's degree in nursing, minimum GPA of 3.0, RN license; for doctorate, GRE General Test (for PhD), 3 letters of professional reference. Additional exam requirements/recommendations for international students: Required—TOEFL (minimum score 560 paper-based; 79 iBT). *Application deadline:* For fall admission, 3/1 priority date for domestic students, 3/1 for international students. Applications are processed on a rolling basis. Application fee: $60. Electronic applications accepted. *Expenses:* Tuition, state resident: full-time $11,664; part-time $649 per credit hour. Tuition, nonresident: full-time $24,274; part-time $1350 per credit hour. *Required fees:* $196. Tuition and fees vary according to program and reciprocity agreements. *Financial support:* In 2015–16, 722,568 students received support, including 10 research assistantships with full tuition reimbursements available (averaging $20,000 per year), 2 teaching assistantships with full tuition reimbursements available (averaging $15,000 per year); fellowships with full tuition reimbursements available, scholarships/grants, and unspecified assistantships also available. Financial award application deadline: 2/15; financial award applicants required to submit FAFSA. *Faculty research:* Children and adolescents with chronic illnesses, women's mental health and parenting, asthma and environmental health, type

2 diabetes self-management in adults, health disparities and community engagement. *Total annual research expenditures:* $722,568. *Unit head:* Dr. Marcia J. Hern, Dean, 502-852-8300, Fax: 502-852-8783, E-mail: m.hern@louisville.edu. *Application contact:* Trish Hart, Assistant Dean for Student Affairs, 502-852-5825, Fax: 502-852-8783, E-mail: trish.hart@louisville.edu. Website: http://www.louisville.edu/nursing/

University of Maryland, Baltimore, Graduate School, School of Nursing, Master's Program in Nursing, Baltimore, MD 21201. Offers community health nursing (MS); gerontological nursing (MS); maternal-child nursing (MS); medical-surgical nursing (MS); nurse-midwifery education (MS); nursing administration (MS); nursing education (MS); nursing health policy (MS); primary care nursing (MS); psychiatric nursing (MS); MS/MBA. MS/MBA offered jointly with University of Baltimore. *Accreditation:* AACN; AANA/CANAEP. *Program availability:* Part-time. *Degree requirements:* For master's, comprehensive exam (for some programs), thesis or alternative. *Entrance requirements:* For master's, minimum GPA of 2.75, course work in statistics, BS in nursing. Additional exam requirements/recommendations for international students: Required—TOEFL (minimum score 550 paper-based; 80 iBT); Recommended—IELTS (minimum score 7). Electronic applications accepted. Tuition and fees vary according to program.

University of Michigan–Flint, School of Health Professions and Studies, Program in Nursing, Flint, MI 48502-1950. Offers adult-gerontology acute care (DNP); adult-gerontology primary care (DNP); family nurse practitioner (MSN, DNP); psychiatric mental health (DNP); psychiatric mental health nurse practitioner (Certificate). *Accreditation:* AACN. *Program availability:* Part-time. *Faculty:* 32 full-time (31 women), 77 part-time/adjunct (69 women). *Students:* 131 full-time (114 women), 81 part-time (71 women); includes 59 minority (35 Black or African American, non-Hispanic/Latino; 2 American Indian or Alaska Native, non-Hispanic/Latino; 7 Asian, non-Hispanic/Latino; 7 Hispanic/Latino; 8 Two or more races, non-Hispanic/Latino), 2 international. Average age 38. 108 applicants, 75% accepted, 56 enrolled. In 2015, 16 master's, 29 doctorates awarded. *Degree requirements:* For master's, thesis. *Entrance requirements:* For master's, BSN from accredited college or university with minimum overall undergraduate GPA of 3.2; for doctorate, BSN or MSN (with APRN certification) from accredited college or university; for Certificate, completion of nurse practitioner program with MS from accredited college or university and minimum overall GPA of 3.2; current unencumbered RN license in the United States; current unencumbered license as nurse practitioner. Additional exam requirements/recommendations for international students: Required—TOEFL (minimum score 560 paper-based; 84 iBT), IELTS (minimum score 6.5). *Application deadline:* For fall admission, 8/1 for domestic students, 5/1 for international students; for winter admission, 11/15 for domestic students, 9/1 for international students; for spring admission, 3/15 for domestic students, 1/1 for international students. Applications are processed on a rolling basis. Application fee: $55. Electronic applications accepted. *Financial support:* Federal Work-Study, scholarships/grants, and unspecified assistantships available. Support available to part-time students. Financial award application deadline: 3/1; financial award applicants required to submit FAFSA. *Faculty research:* Family system stress, self breast exam, family roads evaluation, causal model testing for psychosocial development, basic needs. *Unit head:* Dr. Constance J. Creech, Director, 810-762-3420, Fax: 810-766-6851, E-mail: ccreech@umflint.edu. *Application contact:* Bradley T. Maki, Director of Graduate Admissions, 810-762-3171, Fax: 810-766-6789, E-mail: bmaki@umflint.edu. Website: https://www.umflint.edu/nursing

University of Minnesota, Twin Cities Campus, Graduate School, School of Nursing, Program in Psychiatric Mental Health Clinical Nurse Specialist, Minneapolis, MN 55455-0213. Offers MS. *Accreditation:* AACN. *Program availability:* Part-time. *Entrance requirements:* Additional exam requirements/recommendations for international students: Required—TOEFL (minimum score 586 paper-based).

University of Missouri, Office of Research and Graduate Studies, Sinclair School of Nursing, Columbia, MO 65211. Offers adult-gerontology clinical nurse specialist (DNP, Certificate); family nurse practitioner (DNP); family psychiatric and mental health nurse practitioner (DNP); nursing (MS, PhD); nursing leadership and innovations in health care (DNP); pediatric clinical nurse specialist (DNP, Certificate); pediatric nurse practitioner (DNP). *Accreditation:* AACN. *Program availability:* Part-time. *Degree requirements:* For master's, thesis optional, oral exam; for doctorate, thesis/dissertation. *Entrance requirements:* For master's, GRE General Test, BSN, minimum GPA of 3.0 during last 60 hours, nursing license. Additional exam requirements/recommendations for international students: Required—TOEFL (minimum score 550 paper-based; 79 iBT). *Application deadline:* For fall admission, 2/1 priority date for domestic and international students. Applications are processed on a rolling basis. Application fee: $55 ($75 for international students). Electronic applications accepted. *Financial support:* Fellowships, research assistantships, teaching assistantships, career-related internships or fieldwork, institutionally sponsored loans, scholarships/grants, traineeships, health care benefits, tuition waivers (full), and unspecified assistantships available. Support available to part-time students. Website: http://nursing.missouri.edu/

University of Missouri–St. Louis, College of Nursing, St. Louis, MO 63121-4400. Offers adult/geriatric nurse practitioner (Post Master's Certificate); family nurse practitioner (Post Master's Certificate); nurse educator (MSN); nurse practitioner (MSN); nursing (DNP, PhD); pediatric nurse practitioner (Post Master's Certificate); psychiatric-mental health nurse practitioner (Post Master's Certificate); women's health nurse practitioner (Post Master's Certificate). *Accreditation:* AACN. *Program availability:* Part-time. *Faculty:* 21 full-time (19 women), 6 part-time/adjunct (5 women). *Students:* 18 full-time (17 women), 227 part-time (215 women); includes 34 minority (22 Black or African American, non-Hispanic/Latino; 8 Asian, non-Hispanic/Latino; 3 Hispanic/Latino; 1 Two or more races, non-Hispanic/Latino), 1 international. Average age 35. 152 applicants, 69% accepted, 83 enrolled. *Degree requirements:* For doctorate, comprehensive exam, thesis/dissertation; for Post Master's Certificate, thesis. *Entrance requirements:* For master's, 2 recommendation letters; minimum GPA of 3.0; BSN; nursing licensure; statement of purpose; course in differential/inferential statistics; for doctorate, GRE, 2 letters of recommendation, MSN, minimum GPA of 3.2, course in differential/inferential statistics; for Post Master's Certificate, 2 recommendation letters; MSN; advanced practice certificate; minimum GPA of 3.0; essay. Additional exam requirements/recommendations for international students: Recommended—TOEFL (minimum score 550 paper-based; 79 iBT), IELTS (minimum score 6.5). *Application deadline:* For fall admission, 2/15 for domestic and international students. Application fee: $50 ($40 for international students). Electronic applications accepted. *Financial support:* Research assistantships with tuition reimbursements available. Financial award application deadline: 4/1; financial award applicants required to submit FAFSA. *Faculty research:* Health promotion and restoration, family disruption, violence, abuse, battered women, health survey methods. *Unit head:* Dr. Roberta Lavin, Director, 314-516-6066. *Application contact:* 314-516-5458, Fax: 314-516-6996, E-mail: gradadm@umsl.edu. Website: http://www.umsl.edu/divisions/nursing/

The University of North Carolina at Chapel Hill, School of Nursing, Chapel Hill, NC 27599-7460. Offers advanced practice registered nurse (DNP); health care systems (DNP); nursing (MSN, PhD, PMC), including administration (MSN), adult gerontology primary care nurse practitioner (MSN), clinical nurse leader (MSN), education (MSN),

informatics (MSN, PMC), nursing leadership (PMC), outcomes management (MSN), primary care family nurse practitioner (MSN), primary care pediatric nurse practitioner (MSN), psychiatric/mental health nurse practitioner (MSN, PMC). *Accreditation:* AACN; ACEN (one or more programs are accredited). *Program availability:* Part-time. *Faculty:* 86 full-time (78 women), 44 part-time/adjunct (40 women). *Students:* 208 full-time (186 women), 128 part-time (116 women); includes 109 minority (49 Black or African American, non-Hispanic/Latino; 4 American Indian or Alaska Native, non-Hispanic/Latino; 32 Asian, non-Hispanic/Latino; 7 Hispanic/Latino; 17 Two or more races, non-Hispanic/Latino), 17 international. Average age 33. 624 applicants, 25% accepted, 150 enrolled. In 2015, 91 master's, 14 doctorates awarded. *Degree requirements:* For master's, comprehensive exam, thesis; for doctorate, thesis/dissertation, 3 exams; for PMC, thesis. *Entrance requirements:* Additional exam requirements/recommendations for international students: Required—TOEFL (minimum score 575 paper-based; 89 iBT), IELTS (minimum score 8). *Application deadline:* For fall admission, 12/15 for domestic and international students. Application fee: $85. Electronic applications accepted. *Financial support:* In 2015–16, 8 fellowships with full tuition reimbursements, 6 research assistantships with partial tuition reimbursements (averaging $8,000 per year), 10 teaching assistantships with partial tuition reimbursements (averaging $8,000 per year) were awarded; scholarships/grants, traineeships, health care benefits, and unspecified assistantships also available. Support available to part-time students. Financial award application deadline: 3/1; financial award applicants required to submit FAFSA. *Faculty research:* Preventing and managing chronic illness, reducing health disparities, Improving healthcare quality and patient outcomes, understanding biobehavioral and genetic bases of health and illness, developing innovative ways to enhance science and its clinical translation. *Unit head:* Donna S. Havens, PhD, RN, Dean/Professor, 919-966-3731, Fax: 919-966-3540, E-mail: dhavens@email.unc.edu. *Application contact:* Emily Sayed, Assistant Director, Graduate Admissions, 919-966-4260, Fax: 919-966-3540, E mail: oayod@unc.odu.
Website: http://nursing.unc.edu

University of North Dakota, Graduate School, College of Nursing, Department of Nursing, Grand Forks, ND 58202. Offers adult-gerontological nurse practitioner (MSN); advanced public health nurse (MSN); family nurse practitioner (MSN); nurse anesthesia (MSN); nurse educator (MSN); nursing (DNP, PhD); psychiatric and mental health nurse practitioner (MSN).

University of Pennsylvania, School of Nursing, Psychiatric Mental Health Advanced Practice Nurse Program, Philadelphia, PA 19104. Offers adult and special populations (MSN); child and family (MSN); geropsychiatrics (MSN). *Accreditation:* AACN. *Program availability:* Part-time. *Students:* 9 full-time (8 women), 18 part-time (15 women); includes 9 minority (2 Black or African American, non-Hispanic/Latino; 1 Asian, non-Hispanic/Latino; 3 Hispanic/Latino; 3 Two or more races, non-Hispanic/Latino), 1 international. Average age 33. 48 applicants, 38% accepted, 13 enrolled. In 2015, 18 master's awarded. *Expenses: Tuition, area resident:* Full-time $31,068; part-time $5762 per course. *Required fees:* $3200; $336 per course. Full-time tuition and fees vary according to degree level, program and student level. Part-time tuition and fees vary according to course load, degree level and program. *Financial support:* Application deadline: 4/1.

University of Pittsburgh, School of Nursing, Clinical Nurse Specialist Program, Pittsburgh, PA 15260. Offers adult-gerontology (DNP); psychiatric mental health (DNP). *Accreditation:* AACN. *Program availability:* Part-time. *Students:* 1 (woman) full-time, 8 part-time (6 women); includes 2 minority (both Black or African American, non-Hispanic/Latino). Average age 47. 1 applicant, 100% accepted. In 2015, 4 doctorates awarded. *Entrance requirements:* Additional exam requirements/recommendations for international students: Required—TOEFL (minimum score 600 paper-based; 100 iBT). *Application deadline:* For fall admission, 5/1 priority date for domestic students, 2/15 priority date for international students. Application fee: $50. Electronic applications accepted. *Expenses:* Contact institution. *Financial support:* In 2015–16, 2 students received support, including 2 fellowships with tuition reimbursements available (averaging $11,294 per year); research assistantships, teaching assistantships, scholarships/grants, health care benefits, and unspecified assistantships also available. Support available to part-time students. Financial award application deadline: 3/15. *Faculty research:* Behavioral management of chronic disorders, patient management in critical care, consumer informatics, genetic applications (molecular genetics and psychosocial implications), technology for nurses and patients to improve care. *Unit head:* Dr. Sandra Engberg, Associate Dean for Clinical Education, 412-624-3835, Fax: 412-624-8521, E-mail: sje1@pitt.edu. *Application contact:* Laurie Lapsley, Administrator of Graduate Student Services, 412-624-9670, Fax: 412-624-2409, E-mail: lapsleyl@pitt.edu.

University of Pittsburgh, School of Nursing, Nurse Practitioner Program, Pittsburgh, PA 15261. Offers adult-gerontology acute care (DNP); adult-gerontology primary care (DNP); family (individual across the lifespan) (DNP); neonatal (MSN, DNP); pediatric primary care (DNP); psychiatric mental health (DNP). *Accreditation:* AACN. *Program availability:* Part-time. *Students:* 74 full-time (65 women), 59 part-time (51 women); includes 14 minority (5 Black or African American, non-Hispanic/Latino; 2 American Indian or Alaska Native, non-Hispanic/Latino; 6 Asian, non-Hispanic/Latino; 1 Hispanic/Latino). Average age 30. 65 applicants, 55% accepted, 28 enrolled. In 2015, 14 master's, 19 doctorates awarded. *Degree requirements:* For master's, comprehensive exam, thesis optional. *Entrance requirements:* For master's, GRE General Test or MAT, BSN, RN license, letters of recommendation, resume, course work in statistics, 1-3 years of nursing experience; for doctorate, GRE General Test, BSN, RN license, minimum GPA of 3.5, 3 letters of recommendation. Additional exam requirements/recommendations for international students: Required—TOEFL (minimum score 600 paper-based; 100 iBT). *Application deadline:* For fall admission, 5/1 priority date for domestic students, 2/15 priority date for international students. Application fee: $50. Electronic applications accepted. *Expenses:* Contact institution. *Financial support:* In 2015–16, 16 students received support, including 7 fellowships with tuition reimbursements available (averaging $11,278 per year), 9 teaching assistantships with tuition reimbursements available (averaging $10,879 per year); scholarships/grants, traineeships, health care benefits, and unspecified assistantships also available. Support available to part-time students. Financial award application deadline: 3/15. *Faculty research:* Behavioral management of chronic disorders, patient management in critical care, consumer informatics, genetic applications (molecular genetics and psychosocial implications), technology for nurses and patients to improve care. *Unit head:* Dr. Sandra Engberg, Associate Dean for Clinical Education, 412-624-3835, Fax: 412-624-8521, E-mail: sje1@pitt.edu. *Application contact:* Laurie Lapsley, Administrator of Graduate Student Services, 412-624-9670, Fax: 412-624-2409, E-mail: lapsleyl@pitt.edu.
Website: http://www.nursing.pitt.edu

University of Puerto Rico, Medical Sciences Campus, School of Nursing, San Juan, PR 00936-5067. Offers adult and elderly nursing (MSN); child and adolescent nursing (MSN); critical care nursing (MSN); family and community nursing (MSN); family nurse practitioner (MSN); maternity nursing (MSN); mental health and psychiatric nursing (MSN). *Accreditation:* AACN. *Entrance requirements:* For master's, GRE or EXADEP, interview, Puerto Rico RN license or professional license for international students,

general and specific point average, article analysis. Electronic applications accepted. *Faculty research:* HIV, health disparities, teen violence, women and violence, neurological disorders.

University of Rochester, School of Nursing, Rochester, NY 14642. Offers adult gerontological acute care nurse practitioner (MS); clinical nurse leader (MS); family nurse practitioner (MS); family psychiatric mental health nurse practitioner (MS); health care organization management and leadership (MS); health practice research (PhD); nursing (DNP); nursing education (MS); pediatric nurse practitioner (MS); pediatric nurse practitioner/neonatal nurse practitioner (MS). *Accreditation:* AACN. *Program availability:* Part-time, online learning. *Faculty:* 56 full-time (45 women), 63 part-time/adjunct (55 women). *Students:* 81 full-time (20 women), 212 part-time (175 women); includes 35 minority (12 Black or African American, non-Hispanic/Latino; 1 American Indian or Alaska Native, non-Hispanic/Latino; 10 Asian, non-Hispanic/Latino; 7 Hispanic/Latino; 5 Two or more races, non-Hispanic/Latino), 2 international. Average age 35. 111 applicants, 68% accepted, 71 enrolled. In 2015, 52 master's, 9 doctorates awarded. Terminal master's awarded for partial completion of doctoral program. *Degree requirements:* For master's, comprehensive exam (for some programs); for doctorate, thesis/dissertation. *Entrance requirements:* For master's, BS in nursing, minimum GPA of 3.0, course work in statistics; for doctorate, GRE General Test (for PhD), MS in nursing, minimum GPA of 3.5. Additional exam requirements/recommendations for international students: Required—TOEFL (minimum score 560 paper-based; 88 iBT) or IELTS (minimum score 6.5) recommended. *Application deadline:* For fall admission, 4/1 for domestic and international students; for spring admission, 9/1 for domestic and international students; for summer admission, 1/2 for domestic and international students. Application fee: $50. Electronic applications accepted. *Expenses: Tuition, area resident:* Full-time $47,450; part-time $1482 per credit hour. *Required fees:* $528. Tuition and fees vary according to program. *Financial support:* In 2015–16, 52 students received support, including 2 fellowships with tuition reimbursements available (averaging $30,000 per year); scholarships/grants, traineeships, health care benefits, tuition waivers (full and partial), and unspecified assistantships also available. Support available to part-time students. Financial award application deadline: 6/30. *Faculty research:* Symptom assessment and self-management of chronic illness, health promotion and illness prevention, nursing intervention research with vulnerable populations, palliative care, aging. *Total annual research expenditures:* $2.1 million. *Unit head:* Dr. Kathy H. Rideout, Dean, 585-273-8902, Fax: 585-273-1268, E-mail: kathy_rideout@urmc.rochester.edu. *Application contact:* Elaine Andolina, Director of Admissions, 585-275-2375, Fax: 585-756-8299, E-mail: elaine_andolina@urmc.rochester.edu.
Website: http://www.son.rochester.edu

University of St. Francis, Leach College of Nursing, Joliet, IL 60435-6169. Offers family nurse practitioner (MSN, Post-Master's Certificate); family psychology/mental health nurse practitioner (MSN, Post-Master's Certificate); nursing administration (MSN); nursing education (MSN); nursing practice (DNP); teaching in nursing (Certificate). *Accreditation:* AACN. *Program availability:* Part-time, evening/weekend, 100% online. *Faculty:* 7 full-time (all women), 16 part-time/adjunct (13 women). *Students:* 82 full-time (72 women), 356 part-time (325 women); includes 147 minority (62 Black or African American, non-Hispanic/Latino; 1 American Indian or Alaska Native, non-Hispanic/Latino; 27 Asian, non-Hispanic/Latino; 45 Hispanic/Latino; 3 Native Hawaiian or other Pacific Islander, non-Hispanic/Latino; 9 Two or more races, non-Hispanic/Latino). Average age 41. 338 applicants, 42% accepted, 100 enrolled. In 2015, 91 master's, 9 doctorates, 6 other advanced degrees awarded. *Entrance requirements:* Additional exam requirements/recommendations for international students: Required—TOEFL (minimum score 550 paper-based; 79 iBT), IELTS (minimum score 6). *Application deadline:* Applications are processed on a rolling basis. Application fee: $30. Electronic applications accepted. Application fee is waived when completed online. *Expenses:* Contact institution. *Financial support:* In 2015–16, 149 students received support. Career-related internships or fieldwork, scholarships/grants, and tuition waivers (partial) available. Support available to part-time students. Financial award applicants required to submit FAFSA. *Unit head:* Dr. Carol Wilson, Dean, 815-740-3840, Fax: 815-740-4243, E-mail: cwilson@stfrancis.edu. *Application contact:* Sandra Sloka, Director of Admissions for Graduate and Degree Completion Programs, 800-735-7500, Fax: 815-740-3431, E-mail: ssloka@stfrancis.edu.
Website: http://www.stfrancis.edu/academics/college-of-nursing/

University of Saint Joseph, Department of Nursing, West Hartford, CT 06117-2700. Offers family nurse practitioner (MS); family psychiatric/mental health nurse practitioner (MS); nurse educator (MS); nursing practice (DNP). *Accreditation:* AACN. *Program availability:* Part-time, evening/weekend. *Degree requirements:* For master's, thesis. *Entrance requirements:* For master's, 2 letters of recommendation. *Application deadline:* Applications are processed on a rolling basis. Application fee: $50. Electronic applications accepted. Application fee is waived when completed online. *Financial support:* Career-related internships or fieldwork and unspecified assistantships available. Support available to part-time students. Financial award applicants required to submit FAFSA.
Website: http://www.usj.edu/academics/schools/school-of-health-natural-sciences/nursing/

University of San Diego, Hahn School of Nursing and Health Science, San Diego, CA 92110-2492. Offers adult-gerontology clinical nurse specialist (MSN); adult-gerontology nurse practitioner/family nurse practitioner (MSN); executive nurse leader (MSN); family nurse practitioner (MSN); family/lifespan psychiatric-mental health nurse practitioner (MSN); healthcare informatics (MS, MSN); nursing (PhD); nursing practice (DNP). *Accreditation:* AACN. *Program availability:* Part-time, evening/weekend. *Faculty:* 27 full-time (23 women), 46 part-time/adjunct (41 women). *Students:* 178 full-time (151 women), 157 part-time (131 women); includes 143 minority (25 Black or African American, non-Hispanic/Latino; 2 American Indian or Alaska Native, non-Hispanic/Latino; 53 Asian, non-Hispanic/Latino; 49 Hispanic/Latino; 4 Native Hawaiian or other Pacific Islander, non-Hispanic/Latino; 10 Two or more races, non-Hispanic/Latino), 5 international. Average age 36. In 2015, 122 master's, 43 doctorates awarded. *Degree requirements:* For doctorate, thesis/dissertation (for some programs), residency (DNP). *Entrance requirements:* For master's, GRE General Test (for entry-level nursing), BSN, current California RN licensure (except for entry-level nursing); minimum GPA of 3.0; for doctorate, minimum GPA of 3.5, MSN, current California RN licensure. Additional exam requirements/recommendations for international students: Required—TOEFL (minimum score 580 paper-based; 83 iBT), TWE. *Application deadline:* Applications are processed on a rolling basis. Application fee: $45. Electronic applications accepted. *Financial support:* In 2015–16, 217 students received support. Scholarships/grants and traineeships available. Support available to part-time students. Financial award application deadline: 4/1; financial award applicants required to submit FAFSA. *Faculty research:* Maternal/neonatal health, palliative and end of life care, adolescent obesity, health disparities, cognitive dysfunction. *Unit head:* Dr. Sally Hardin, Dean, 619-260-4550, Fax: 619-260-6814. *Application contact:* Monica Mahon, Associate Director of Graduate Admissions, 619-260-4524, Fax: 619-260-4158, E-mail: grads@sandiego.edu.
Website: http://www.sandiego.edu/nursing/

Psychiatric Nursing

University of San Francisco, School of Nursing and Health Professions, Doctoral Programs, San Francisco, CA 94117-1080. Offers executive leadership (DNP); family nurse practitioner (DNP); healthcare systems leadership (DNP); psychiatric mental health nurse practitioner (DNP). *Faculty:* 19 full-time (13 women), 15 part-time/adjunct (11 women). *Students:* 150 full-time (114 women), 54 part-time (46 women); includes 114 minority (25 Black or African American, non-Hispanic/Latino; 1 American Indian or Alaska Native, non-Hispanic/Latino; 56 Asian, non-Hispanic/Latino; 21 Hispanic/Latino; 3 Native Hawaiian or other Pacific Islander, non-Hispanic/Latino; 8 Two or more races, non-Hispanic/Latino), 2 international. Average age 38. 121 applicants, 81% accepted, 70 enrolled. In 2015, 31 doctorates awarded. *Entrance requirements:* For doctorate, nursing bachelor's degree, valid RN license in California. Electronic applications accepted. *Expenses: Tuition,* area resident: Full-time $22,410; part-time $1245 per credit. Tuition and fees vary according to course load, degree level and campus/location. *Financial support:* In 2015–16, 43 students received support. *Unit head:* Dr. Judith Karshmer, Dean, 415-422-6681, Fax: 415-422-6877, E-mail: nursing@usfca.edu. *Application contact:* Ingrid McVanner, Information Contact, 415-422-2746, Fax: 415-422-2217.

University of South Carolina, The Graduate School, College of Nursing, Program in Advanced Practice Nursing in Psychiatric Mental Health, Columbia, SC 29208. Offers MSN, Certificate. *Program availability:* Part-time, online learning. *Entrance requirements:* For master's, master's degree in nursing, RN license; for Certificate, MSN. Additional exam requirements/recommendations for international students: Required—TOEFL (minimum score 570 paper-based). Electronic applications accepted. *Faculty research:* Systems research, evidence based practice, breast cancer, violence.

University of South Carolina, The Graduate School, College of Nursing, Program in Community Mental Health and Psychiatric Health Nursing, Columbia, SC 29208. Offers psychiatric/mental health nurse practitioner (MSN); psychiatric/mental health specialist (MSN). *Accreditation:* AACN. *Program availability:* Part-time. *Degree requirements:* For master's, thesis or alternative. *Entrance requirements:* For master's, GRE General Test, MAT, BS in nursing, nursing license. Additional exam requirements/recommendations for international students: Required—TOEFL (minimum score 570 paper-based). Electronic applications accepted. *Faculty research:* Systems research, evidence based practice, breast cancer, violence.

University of Southern Maine, College of Science, Technology, and Health, School of Nursing, Portland, ME 04103. Offers adult-gerontology primary care nurse practitioner (MS, PMC); education (MS); family nurse practitioner (MS, PMC); family psychiatric/mental health nurse practitioner (MS); management (MS); nursing (CAS, CGS); psychiatric-mental health nurse practitioner (PMC). *Accreditation:* AACN. *Program availability:* Part-time. *Degree requirements:* For master's, thesis optional. *Entrance requirements:* For master's, GRE General Test or MAT, minimum GPA of 3.0; for doctorate, GRE. Additional exam requirements/recommendations for international students: Required—TOEFL (minimum score 550 paper-based). Electronic applications accepted. *Expenses: Tuition,* area resident: Full-time $6840; part-time $380 per credit hour. Tuition, state resident: full-time $10,260; part-time $570 per credit hour. Tuition, nonresident: full-time $18,468; part-time $1026 per credit hour. *Required fees:* $830; $83 per credit hour. Tuition and fees vary according to course load and program. *Faculty research:* Women's health, nursing history, weight control, community services, substance abuse.

University of Southern Mississippi, Graduate School, College of Nursing, Hattiesburg, MS 39406-0001. Offers family nurse practitioner (MSN, Graduate Certificate); family psychiatric-mental health nurse practitioner (Graduate Certificate); nursing (DNP, PhD); psychiatric-mental health nurse practitioner (Graduate Certificate). *Accreditation:* AACN. *Program availability:* Part-time, evening/weekend. *Degree requirements:* For master's, comprehensive exam, thesis optional; for doctorate, comprehensive exam, thesis/dissertation. *Entrance requirements:* For master's, GRE General Test, minimum GPA of 2.75 during last 60 hours, nursing license, BS in nursing; for doctorate, GRE General Test, master's degree in nursing, minimum GPA of 3.5. Additional exam requirements/recommendations for international students: Required—TOEFL, IELTS. Electronic applications accepted. *Faculty research:* Gerontology, caregivers, HIV, bereavement, pain, nursing leadership.

The University of Texas at Austin, Graduate School, School of Nursing, Austin, TX 78712-1111. Offers adult - gerontology clinical nurse specialist (MSN); child health (MSN), including administration, public health nursing, teaching; family nurse practitioner (MSN); family psychiatric/mental health nurse practitioner (MSN); holistic adult health (MSN), including administration, teaching; maternity (MSN), including administration, public health nursing, teaching; nursing (PhD); nursing administration and healthcare systems management (MSN); nursing practice (DNP); pediatric nurse practitioner (MSN); public health nursing (MSN). *Accreditation:* AACN. *Program availability:* Part-time. *Degree requirements:* For master's, thesis optional; for doctorate, thesis/dissertation. *Entrance requirements:* For master's and doctorate, GRE General Test. Additional exam requirements/recommendations for international students: Required—TOEFL (minimum score 550 paper-based). Electronic applications accepted. *Faculty research:* Chronic illness management, memory and aging, health promotion, women's health, adolescent health.

The University of Texas Health Science Center at San Antonio, School of Nursing, San Antonio, TX 78229-3900. Offers administrative management (MSN); adult-gerontology acute care nurse practitioner (PGC); advanced practice leadership (DNP); clinical nurse leader (MSN); executive administrative management (DNP); family nurse practitioner (MSN, PGC); nursing (MSN, PhD); nursing education (MSN, PGC); pediatric nurse practitioner primary care (PGC); psychiatric mental health nurse practitioner (PGC); public health nurse leader (DNP). *Accreditation:* AACN. *Program availability:* Part-time. Terminal master's awarded for partial completion of doctoral program. *Degree requirements:* For master's, thesis optional; for doctorate, comprehensive exam, thesis/dissertation.

University of Virginia, School of Nursing, Charlottesville, VA 22903. Offers acute and specialty care (MSN); acute care nurse practitioner (MSN); clinical nurse leadership (MSN); community-public health leadership (MSN); nursing (DNP, PhD); psychiatric mental health counseling (MSN); MSN/MBA. *Accreditation:* AACN. *Program availability:* Part-time. *Degree requirements:* For doctorate, comprehensive exam (for some programs), capstone project (DNP), dissertation (PhD). *Entrance requirements:* For master's, GRE General Test, MAT; for doctorate, GRE General Test. Additional exam requirements/recommendations for international students: Required—TOEFL, IELTS. Electronic applications accepted. *Expenses:* Contact institution.

University of Wisconsin–Madison, School of Nursing, Madison, WI 53706-1380. Offers adult/gerontology (DNP); nursing (PhD); pediatrics (DNP); psychiatric mental health (DNP); MS/MPH. *Accreditation:* AACN. *Program availability:* Part-time. *Degree requirements:* For doctorate, comprehensive exam, thesis/dissertation. *Entrance requirements:* For doctorate, GRE General Test, 2 samples of scholarly written work, BS in nursing from an accredited program, minimum undergraduate GPA of 3.0 in last 60 credits (for PhD); licensure as professional nurse (for DNP). Additional exam requirements/recommendations for international students: Required—TOEFL (minimum score 600 paper-based; 100 iBT). Electronic applications accepted. *Expenses:* Tuition, state resident: full-time $5364. Tuition, nonresident: full-time $12,027. *Required fees:* $571. Tuition and fees vary according to campus/location, program and reciprocity agreements. *Faculty research:* Nursing informatics to promote self-care and disease management skills among patients and caregivers; quality of care to frail, vulnerable, and chronically ill populations; study of health-related and health-seeking behaviors; eliminating health disparities; pain and symptom management for patients with cancer.

Vanderbilt University, Vanderbilt University School of Nursing, Nashville, TN 37240. Offers adult-gerontology acute care nurse practitioner (MSN), including hospitalist, intensivist; adult-gerontology primary care nurse practitioner (MSN); emergency nurse practitioner (MSN); family nurse practitioner (MSN); healthcare leadership (MSN); neonatal nurse practitioner (MSN); nurse midwifery (MSN); nurse midwifery/family nurse practitioner (MSN); nursing (Post-Master's Certificate); nursing informatics (MSN); nursing practice (DNP); nursing science (PhD); pediatric acute care nurse practitioner (MSN); pediatric primary care nurse practitioner (MSN); psychiatric-mental health nurse practitioner (MSN); women's health nurse practitioner (MSN); women's health nurse practitioner/adult gerontology primary care nurse practitioner (MSN); MSN/M Div; MSN/MTS. *Accreditation:* ACEN (one or more programs are accredited); ACNM/ACME. *Program availability:* Part-time, 100% online, blended/hybrid learning. *Faculty:* 258 full-time (232 women), 363 part-time/adjunct (271 women). *Students:* 478 full-time (424 women), 342 part-time (317 women); includes 140 minority (36 Black or African American, non-Hispanic/Latino; 3 American Indian or Alaska Native, non-Hispanic/Latino; 24 Asian, non-Hispanic/Latino; 43 Hispanic/Latino; 3 Native Hawaiian or other Pacific Islander, non-Hispanic/Latino; 31 Two or more races, non-Hispanic/Latino), 11 international. Average age 31. 1,268 applicants, 49% accepted, 477 enrolled. In 2015, 343 master's, 55 doctorates awarded. *Degree requirements:* For doctorate, comprehensive exam, thesis/dissertation. *Entrance requirements:* For master's, GRE General Test (taken within the past 5 years), minimum B average in undergraduate course work, 3 letters of recommendation; for doctorate, GRE General Test, interview, 3 letters of recommendation from doctorally-prepared faculty, MSN, essay. Additional exam requirements/recommendations for international students: Required—TOEFL (minimum score 570 paper-based), IELTS (minimum score 6.5). *Application deadline:* For fall admission, 11/1 priority date for domestic and international students. Applications are processed on a rolling basis. Application fee: $50. Electronic applications accepted. *Expenses:* Contact institution. *Financial support:* In 2015–16, 585 students received support. Scholarships/grants available. Financial award application deadline: 3/15; financial award applicants required to submit FAFSA. *Faculty research:* Lymphedema, palliative care and bereavement, health services research including workforce, safety and quality of care, gerontology, better birth outcomes including nutrition. *Total annual research expenditures:* $2 million. *Unit head:* Dr. Linda Norman, Dean, 615-343-8876, Fax: 615-343-7711, E-mail: linda.norman@vanderbilt.edu. *Application contact:* Patricia Peerman, Assistant Dean for Enrollment Management, 615-322-3800, Fax: 615-343-0333, E-mail: vusn-admissions@vanderbilt.edu.
Website: http://www.nursing.vanderbilt.edu

Virginia Commonwealth University, Graduate School, School of Nursing, Richmond, VA 23284-9005. Offers adult health acute nursing (MS); adult health primary nursing (MS); biobehavioral clinical research (PhD); child health nursing (MS); clinical nurse leader (MS); family health nursing (MS); nurse educator (MS); nurse practitioner (MS); nursing (Certificate); nursing administration (MS), including clinical nurse manager; psychiatric-mental health nursing (MS); quality and safety in health care (DNP); women's health nursing (MS). *Accreditation:* ACEN (one or more programs are accredited). *Program availability:* Part-time, evening/weekend, online learning. *Degree requirements:* For master's, thesis optional; for doctorate, thesis/dissertation. *Entrance requirements:* For master's, GRE General Test, BSN, minimum GPA of 2.8; for doctorate, GRE General Test. Additional exam requirements/recommendations for international students: Required—TOEFL (minimum score 600 paper-based; 100 iBT). Electronic applications accepted.

Washington State University, College of Nursing, Spokane, WA 99210. Offers advanced population health (MN, DNP); family nurse practitioner (MN, DNP); nursing (PhD); psychiatric/mental health nurse practitioner (DNP); psychiatric/mental health practitioner (MN). Programs offered at the Spokane, Tri-Cities, and Vancouver campuses. *Accreditation:* AACN. *Degree requirements:* For master's, comprehensive exam (for some programs), thesis (for some programs), oral exam, research project. *Entrance requirements:* For master's, minimum GPA of 3.0, Washington state RN license, physical assessment skills, course work in statistics, recommendations, written interview (for nurse practitioner). *Faculty research:* Cardiovascular and Type 2 diabetes in children, evaluation of strategies to increase physical activity in sedentary people.

Wayne State University, College of Nursing, Graduate Certificates Program in Clinical Specialties, Detroit, MI 48202. Offers acute care nurse practitioner (Graduate Certificate); nurse midwifery (Graduate Certificate); pediatric nurse practitioner - acute care (Graduate Certificate); pediatric nurse practitioner - primary care (Graduate Certificate); psychiatric mental health nurse practitioner (Graduate Certificate). *Accreditation:* AACN. *Program availability:* Part-time. *Students:* 2 full-time (both women), 7 part-time (all women). Average age 43. 67 applicants, 12% accepted, 5 enrolled. *Entrance requirements:* For degree, master's or doctoral degree in nursing from nationally-accredited institution, current RN license, three letters of reference, personal statement. Additional exam requirements/recommendations for international students: Required—TOEFL (minimum score 600 paper-based; 101 iBT), TWE, Michigan English Language Assessment Battery (minimum score 85); Recommended—IELTS (minimum score 7). *Application deadline:* For fall admission, 6/1 priority date for domestic students, 5/1 priority date for international students; for winter admission, 10/1 priority date for domestic students, 9/1 priority date for international students; for spring admission, 2/1 priority date for domestic students, 1/1 priority date for international students. Application fee: $0. Electronic applications accepted. *Expenses:* $19,325 annual resident tuition, $35,114 non-resident tuition; $805.20 per credit hour resident tuition, $1,463.10 per credit hour non-resident tuition; fees include $47.45 per credit hour student services fee and $274.60 per semester registration fee. *Financial support:* Scholarships/grants available. Financial award application deadline: 3/31; financial award applicants required to submit FAFSA. *Unit head:* Dr. Laurie Lauzon Clabo, Dean and Professor, 313-577-4104, E-mail: laurie.lauzon.clabo@wayne.edu. *Application contact:* Leanne Nantais-Smith, Director, MSN Program and Graduate Certificates, E-mail: ar2446@wayne.edu. Website: http://nursing.wayne.edu/gradcert/specialties.php

Wayne State University, College of Nursing, M.S.N. Program in Clinical Specialties, Detroit, MI 48202. Offers nurse-midwifery (MSN); pediatric nurse practitioner acute care (MSN); psychiatric mental health nurse practitioner (MSN). *Accreditation:* AACN. *Program availability:* Part-time. *Students:* 49 full-time (47 women), 85 part-time (79 women); includes 29 minority (15 Black or African American, non-Hispanic/Latino; 7 Asian, non-Hispanic/Latino; 3 Hispanic/Latino; 4 Two or more races, non-Hispanic/Latino), 5 international. Average age 33. 111 applicants, 20% accepted, 17 enrolled. In 2015, 108 master's awarded. *Degree requirements:* For master's, thesis or alternative. *Entrance requirements:* For master's, BSN from NLN- or CCNE-accredited program with minimum GPA of 3.0; three references; current RN license; personal statement. Additional exam requirements/recommendations for international students: Required—

TOEFL (minimum score 600 paper-based; 101 iBT); Recommended—TWE. *Application deadline:* For fall admission, 6/1 for domestic students, 5/1 priority date for international students; for winter admission, 10/1 for domestic students, 9/1 priority date for international students; for spring admission, 2/1 for domestic students, 1/1 priority date for international students. Electronic applications accepted. *Expenses:* \$19,325 per year resident tuition, \$35,114 non-resident tuition; \$805.20 per credit hour resident tuition, \$1,463.10 per credit hour non-resident tuition; fees include \$47.45 per credit hour student services fee and \$274.60 per semester registration fee. *Financial support:* In 2015–16, 36 students received support. Fellowships with tuition reimbursements available, research assistantships with tuition reimbursements available, teaching assistantships with tuition reimbursements available, scholarships/grants, traineeships, and unspecified assistantships available. Support available to part-time students. Financial award applicants required to submit FAFSA. *Faculty research:* Smoking risk behaviors in adolescents, sleep disturbances in postmenopausal women, health disparities in urban environments, nurse practitioner interventions, care giving and pain management. *Unit head:* Dr. Laurie Lauzon Clabo, Dean and Professor, 313-577-4104, E-mail: laurie.lauzon.clabo@wayne.edu. *Application contact:* Dr. Leanne Nantais-Smith, Program Director, MSN and Graduate Certificates, 313-577-5934, E-mail: ar2446@wayne.edu. Website: http://nursing.wayne.edu/msn/specialty.php

West Virginia Wesleyan College, Department of Nursing, Buckhannon, WV 26201. Offers family nurse practitioner (Post Master's Certificate); family nurse practitoner (MS); nurse administrator (MS); nurse educator (MS); nurse-midwifery (MS); nursing administration (Post Master's Certificate); nursing education (Post Master's Certificate); psychiatric mental health nurse practitioner (MS); MSN/MBA. *Accreditation:* ACEN.

School Nursing

Cambridge College, School of Education, Cambridge, MA 02138-5304. Offers autism specialist (M Ed); autism/behavior analyst (M Ed); behavior analyst (Post-Master's Certificate); behavioral management (M Ed); early childhood teacher (M Ed); education specialist in curriculum and instruction (CAGS); educational leadership (Ed D); elementary teacher (M Ed); English as a second language (M Ed, Certificate); general science (M Ed); health education (Post-Master's Certificate); health/family and consumer sciences (M Ed); history (M Ed); individualized (M Ed); information technology literacy (M Ed); instructional technology (M Ed); interdisciplinary studies (M Ed); library teacher (M Ed); literacy education (M Ed); mathematics (M Ed); mathematics specialist (Certificate); middle school mathematics and science (M Ed); school administration (M Ed, CAGS); school guidance counselor (M Ed); school nurse education (M Ed); school social worker/school adjustment counselor (M Ed); special education administrator (CAGS); special education/moderate disabilities (M Ed); teaching skills and methodologies (M Ed). *Program availability:* Part-time, evening/ weekend, online learning. *Degree requirements:* For master's, thesis, internship/ practicum (licensure program only); for doctorate, thesis/dissertation; for other advanced degree, thesis. *Entrance requirements:* For master's, interview, resume, documentation of licensure, 2 professional references; for doctorate, official transcripts, interview, resume, documentation of licensure (if any), written personal statement/essay, portfolio of scholarly and professional work, qualifying assessment, 2 professional references, health insurance, immunizations form; for other advanced degree, official transcripts, interview, resume, documentation of licensure (if any), written personal statement/ essay, 2 professional references, health insurance, immunizations form. Additional exam requirements/recommendations for international students: Required—TOEFL (minimum score 550 paper-based; 79 iBT), Michigan English Language Assessment Battery (minimum score 85); Recommended—IELTS (minimum score 6). Electronic applications accepted. *Expenses:* Contact institution. *Faculty research:* Adult education, accelerated learning, mathematics education, brain compatible learning, special education and law.

Eastern Mennonite University, Program in Nursing, Harrisonburg, VA 22802-2462. Offers leadership and management (MSN); leadership and school nursing (MSN). *Accreditation:* AACN. *Program availability:* Part-time, online learning. *Degree requirements:* For master's, leadership project. *Entrance requirements:* For master's, RN license, one year of full-time work experience as RN, minimum GPA of 3.0. Additional exam requirements/recommendations for international students: Required— TOEFL. *Application deadline:* For fall admission, 6/1 for domestic students. Applications are processed on a rolling basis. Application fee: \$25. *Expenses: Tuition, area resident:* Part-time \$600 per credit hour. *Required fees:* \$25 per unit. Part-time tuition and fees vary according to course load and program. *Financial support:* Federal Work-Study and scholarships/grants available. Financial award applicants required to submit FAFSA. *Faculty research:* Community health, international health, effectiveness of the nursing school environment, development of caring ability in nursing students, international nursing students. *Unit head:* Ann Hershberger, Coordinator, 540-432-4192, E-mail: hershbea@emu.edu. *Application contact:* Don A. Yoder, Director of Seminary and Graduate Admissions, 540-432-4257, Fax: 540-432-4598, E-mail: yoderda@emu.edu.

Eastern University, Graduate Education Programs, St. Davids, PA 19087-3696. Offers ESL program specialist (K-12) (Certificate); general supervisor (PreK-12) (Certificate); health and physical education (K-12) (Certificate); middle level (4-8) (Certificate); multicultural education (M Ed); pre K-4 (Certificate); pre K-4 with special education (Certificate); reading (M Ed); reading specialist (K-12) (Certificate); reading supervisor (K-12) (Certificate); school health services (M Ed); school health supervisor (Certificate); school nurse (Certificate); school principalship (K-12) (Certificate); secondary biology education (7-12) (Certificate); secondary chemistry education (7-12) (Certificate); secondary communication education (7-12) (Certificate); secondary education (7-12) (Certificate); secondary English education (7-12) (Certificate); secondary math education (7-12) (Certificate); secondary social studies education (7-12) (Certificate); special education (M Ed); special education (7-12) (Certificate); special education (Pre K-8) (Certificate); special education supervisor (N-12) (Certificate); TESOL (M Ed); world language (Certificate), including French, Spanish. *Program availability:* Part-time, evening/weekend, online learning. *Faculty:* 22 full-time (11 women), 26 part-time/adjunct (18 women). *Students:* 50 full-time (39 women), 96 part-time (75 women); includes 51 minority (32 Black or African American, non-Hispanic/Latino; 2 Asian, non-Hispanic/ Latino; 13 Hispanic/Latino; 4 Two or more races, non-Hispanic/Latino), 2 international. Average age 39. 109 applicants, 95% accepted, 85 enrolled. In 2015, 72 master's awarded. *Entrance requirements:* For master's, minimum GPA of 2.5; for Certificate, minimum GPA of 3.0. Additional exam requirements/recommendations for international students: Required—TOEFL. *Application deadline:* For fall admission, 8/14 for domestic students; for spring admission, 12/20 for domestic students. Applications are processed on a rolling basis. Application fee: \$35. Application fee is waived when completed online. *Financial support:* In 2015–16, 84 students received support, including 6 research assistantships with partial tuition reimbursements available (averaging \$7,710 per year); scholarships/grants and unspecified assistantships also available. Financial award application deadline: 3/15; financial award applicants required to submit FAFSA. *Unit head:* Michael Dziedziak, Executive Director of Enrollment, 800-732-7669, Fax: 610-225-5601, E-mail: gpsadm@eastern.edu. Website: http://www.eastern.edu/academics/programs/loeb-school-education-0

Felician University, Program in Education, Lodi, NJ 07644-2117. Offers education (MA); educational leadership (principal/supervision) (MA); educational supervision (PMC); principal (PMC); school nursing and health education (MA, Certificate). *Accreditation:* Teacher Education Accreditation Council. *Program availability:* Part-time, evening/weekend. *Faculty:* 6 full-time (4 women), 8 part-time/adjunct (4 women). *Students:* 6 full-time (4 women), 72 part-time (66 women); includes 22 minority (5 Black or African American, non-Hispanic/Latino; 6 Asian, non-Hispanic/Latino; 11 Hispanic/ Latino), 3 international. Average age 35. 50 applicants, 72% accepted, 19 enrolled. In 2015, 21 master's awarded. *Degree requirements:* For master's, project. *Entrance requirements:* For master's, MAT, minimum GPA of 3.0, 3 letters of recommendation. Additional exam requirements/recommendations for international students: Recommended—TOEFL (minimum score 79 iBT). *Application deadline:* Applications are processed on a rolling basis. Application fee: \$40. Electronic applications accepted. Application fee is waived when completed online. *Expenses: Tuition,* area resident: Part-time \$965 per credit. Tuition and fees vary according to course load and program. *Financial support:* Federal Work-Study available. Financial award applicants required to submit FAFSA. *Unit head:* Dr. Rose Rudnitski, Dean and Professor, School of Education, 201-559-3551, E-mail: rudnitskir@felician.edu. *Application contact:* Dr. Margaret Smolin, Director, Graduate Admissions, 201-559-1451, E-mail: graduate@ felician.edu.

Kean University, College of Natural, Applied and Health Sciences, Program in Nursing, Union, NJ 07083. Offers clinical management (MSN); community health nursing (MSN); school nursing (MSN). *Accreditation:* ACEN. *Program availability:* Part-time. *Faculty:* 9 full-time (all women). *Students:* 10 full-time (all women), 120 part-time (114 women); includes 63 minority (47 Black or African American, non-Hispanic/Latino; 11 Asian, non-Hispanic/Latino; 3 Hispanic/Latino; 2 Two or more races, non-Hispanic/Latino), 1 international. Average age 44. 64 applicants, 63% accepted, 22 enrolled. In 2015, 46 master's awarded. *Degree requirements:* For master's, thesis or alternative, clinical field experience. *Entrance requirements:* For master's, minimum GPA of 3.0; BS in nursing; RN license; 2 letters of recommendation; interview; official transcripts from all institutions attended. Additional exam requirements/recommendations for international students: Required—TOEFL (minimum score 550 paper-based; 79 iBT), IELTS. *Application deadline:* For fall admission, 6/1 for domestic and international students; for spring admission, 12/1 for domestic and international students. Applications are processed on a rolling basis. Application fee: \$75 (\$150 for international students). Electronic applications accepted. *Expenses:* Tuition, state resident: full-time \$12,835; part-time \$625 per credit. Tuition, nonresident: full-time \$17,396; part-time \$766 per credit. *Required fees:* \$3235; \$147 per credit. Tuition and fees vary according to course level, course load, degree level and program. *Financial support:* In 2015–16, research assistantships with full tuition reimbursements (averaging \$3,771 per year) were awarded; scholarships/grants and unspecified assistantships also available. Financial award applicants required to submit FAFSA. *Unit head:* Dr. Portia Johnson, Program Coordinator, 908-737-3386, E-mail: johnsonpo@kean.edu. *Application contact:* Pedro Lopes, Admissions Counselor, 908-737-7100, E-mail: grad-adm@kean.edu. Website: http://grad.kean.edu/masters-programs/nursing-clinical-management

La Salle University, School of Nursing and Health Sciences, Program in Nursing, Philadelphia, PA 19141-1199. Offers adult gerontology primary care nurse practitioner (MSN, Certificate); adult health and illness clinical nurse specialist (MSN); adult-gerontology clinical nurse specialist (MSN, Certificate); clinical nurse leader (MSN); family primary care nurse practitioner (MSN, Certificate); gerontology (Certificate); nurse anesthetist (MSN, Certificate); nursing (MSN, Certificate); nursing administration (MSN, Certificate); nursing education (Certificate); nursing practice (DNP); nursing service administration (MSN); public health nursing (MSN, Certificate); school nursing (Certificate); MSN/MBA; MSN/MPH. *Accreditation:* AANA/CANAEP. *Program availability:* Part-time, evening/weekend, 100% online. *Faculty:* 13 full-time (all women), 9 part-time/adjunct (8 women). *Students:* 368 part-time (56 women); includes 103 minority (62 Black or African American, non-Hispanic/Latino; 1 American Indian or Alaska Native, non-Hispanic/Latino; 26 Asian, non-Hispanic/Latino; 9 Hispanic/Latino; 5 Two or more races, non-Hispanic/Latino), 5 international. Average age 36. 98 applicants, 85% accepted, 53 enrolled. In 2015, 87 master's, 3 doctorates, 10 other advanced degrees awarded. *Degree requirements:* For doctorate, minimum of 1,000 hours of post baccalaureate clinical practice supervised by preceptors. *Entrance requirements:* For master's, GRE, MAT, or GMAT (for students with BSN GPA of less than 3.2), baccalaureate degree in nursing from an NLNAC- or CCNE-accredited program or an MSN Bridge program; Pennsylvania RN license; 2 letters of reference; resume; statement of philosophy articulating professional values and future educational goal; 1 year of work experience as a registered nurse; for doctorate, GRE (waived for applicants with MSN cumulative GPA of 3.7 or above), MSN from nationally-accredited program or master's degree, MBA or MHA from nationally-accredited program; resume or curriculum vitae; 2 letters of reference; interview; for Certificate, GRE, MAT, or GMAT (for students with BSN GPA of less than 3.2, baccalaureate degree in nursing from an NLNAC- or CCNE-accredited program or an MSN Bridge program; Pennsylvania RN license; 2 letters of reference; resume; statement of philosophy articulating professional values and future educational goal; 1 year of work experience as a registered nurse. Additional exam requirements/recommendations for international students: Required— TOEFL. *Application deadline:* For fall admission, 8/15 priority date for domestic students, 7/15 for international students; for spring admission, 12/15 priority date for domestic students, 11/15 for international students; for summer admission, 4/15 priority date for domestic students, 3/15 for international students. Applications are processed on a rolling basis. Application fee: \$35. Electronic applications accepted. Application fee is waived when completed online. *Expenses:* \$870 per credit hour (for MSN); \$930 per credit hour (for DNP); \$150 technology fee full-time, \$75 part-time; \$135 general university fee. *Financial support:* In 2015–16, 13 students received support. Scholarships/grants and traineeships available. Support available to part-time students. Financial award application deadline: 8/31; financial award applicants required to submit FAFSA. *Unit head:* Dr. Patricia M. Dillon, Director, 215-951-1322, Fax: 215-951-1896,

E-mail: msnapn@lasalle.edu. *Application contact:* Alison McAnespey Target, Director, Graduate and Adult Enrollment, 215-951-1100, Fax: 215-951-1462, E-mail: reilly@lasalle.edu.
Website: http://www.lasalle.edu/nursing/program-options/

Monmouth University, Graduate Studies, The Marjorie K. Unterberg School of Nursing and Health Studies, West Long Branch, NJ 07764-1898. Offers adult and gerontological primary care nurse practitioner (MSN); adult-gerontological primary care nurse practitioner (Post-Master's Certificate); family nurse practitioner (MSN, Post-Master's Certificate); family psychiatric and mental health advanced practice nursing (MSN); family psychiatric and mental health nurse practitioner (Post-Master's Certificate); forensic nursing (MSN, Certificate); nursing (MSN); nursing administration (MSN, Post-Master's Certificate); nursing education (MSN, Post-Master's Certificate); nursing practice (DNP); physician assistant (MS); school nursing (MSN, Certificate). *Accreditation:* AACN. *Program availability:* Part-time, evening/weekend, 100% online, blended/hybrid learning. *Faculty:* 14 full-time (13 women), 10 part-time/adjunct (5 women). *Students:* 58 full-time (46 women), 271 part-time (252 women); includes 93 minority (31 Black or African American, non-Hispanic/Latino; 40 Asian, non-Hispanic/Latino; 18 Hispanic/Latino; 1 Native Hawaiian or other Pacific Islander, non-Hispanic/Latino; 3 Two or more races, non-Hispanic/Latino), 1 international. Average age 37. 450 applicants, 32% accepted, 103 enrolled. In 2015, 68 master's, 8 doctorates, 11 other advanced degrees awarded. *Degree requirements:* For master's, practicum (for some tracks); for doctorate, practicum, capstone course. *Entrance requirements:* For master's, GRE General Test (waived for MSN applicants with minimum B grade in each of the first four courses and for MS applicants with master's degree), BSN with minimum GPA of 2.75, current RN license, proof of liability and malpractice policy, personal statement, two letters of recommendation, college course work in health assessment, resume; CASPA application (for MS); for doctorate, accredited master's nursing program degree with minimum GPA of 3.2, graduate research course in statistics, active RN license, national certification as Nurse Practitioner or Nurse Administrator, working knowledge of statistics, statement of goals and vision for change, 2 letters of recommendation (professional or academic), resume, interview. Additional exam requirements/recommendations for international students: Required—TOEFL (minimum score 550 paper-based; 79 iBT), IELTS (minimum score 6) or Michigan English Language Assessment Battery (minimum score 77). *Application deadline:* For fall admission, 7/15 priority date for domestic students, 6/1 for international students; for spring admission, 12/15 priority date for domestic students, 11/1 for international students; for summer admission, 5/1 for domestic students. Applications are processed on a rolling basis. Application fee: $50. Electronic applications accepted. *Expenses:* Contact institution. *Financial support:* In 2015–16, 241 students received support, including 220 fellowships (averaging $3,403 per year), 5 research assistantships (averaging $5,146 per year); career-related internships or fieldwork, scholarships/grants, and unspecified assistantships also available. Support available to part-time students. Financial award applicants required to submit FAFSA. *Faculty research:* School nursing, health policy, and smoking cessation in teens, Multiple Sclerosis; adherence and self-efficacy, aging issues and geriatric care. *Unit head:* Dr. Janet Mahoney, Dean, 732-571-3443, Fax: 732-263-5131, E-mail: jmahoney@monmouth.edu. *Application contact:* Lucia Fedele, Graduate Admission Counselor, 732-571-3452, Fax: 732-263-5123, E-mail: gradadm@monmouth.edu.
Website: http://www.monmouth.edu/school-of-nursing-health/graduate-nursing-programs.aspx

Rowan University, Graduate School, College of Education, Department of Educational Services and Leadership, Glassboro, NJ 08028-1701. Offers counseling in educational settings (MA); educational leadership (Ed D, CAGS); higher education administration (MA); principal preparation (CAGS); school administration (MA); school and public librarianship (MA); school nursing (Postbaccalaureate Certificate); school psychology (MA, Ed S); supervisor (CAGS). *Accreditation:* NCATE. *Program availability:* Part-time, evening/weekend. *Degree requirements:* For master's, comprehensive exam, thesis; for other advanced degree, thesis or alternative. *Entrance requirements:* For master's and other advanced degree, GRE General Test. Additional exam requirements/recommendations for international students: Required—TOEFL. Electronic applications accepted. *Expenses: Tuition, area resident:* Full-time $8710; part-time $871 per credit. Tuition, state resident: full-time $8710; part-time $871 per credit. Tuition, nonresident: full-time $8710; part-time $871 per credit. *International tuition:* $8710 full-time. *Required fees:* $1510; $151 per credit.

Saint Joseph's University, College of Arts and Sciences, Department of Health Services, Philadelphia, PA 19131-1395. Offers health administration (MS); health education (MS); healthcare ethics (MS); long-term care administration (MS); nurse anesthesia (MS); school nurse certification (MS). *Program availability:* Part-time, evening/weekend. *Entrance requirements:* For master's, GRE (if GPA less than 3.0), 2 letters of recommendation, resume, personal statement, official transcripts. Additional exam requirements/recommendations for international students: Required—TOEFL (minimum score 550 paper-based; 80 iBT), IELTS (minimum score 6.5). Electronic applications accepted.

Seton Hall University, College of Nursing, South Orange, NJ 07079-2697. Offers advanced practice in primary health care (MSN, DNP), including adult/gerontological nurse practitioner, pediatric nurse practitioner; entry into practice (MSN); health systems administration (MSN, DNP); nursing (PhD); nursing case management (MSN); nursing education (MA); school nurse (MSN); MSN/MA. *Accreditation:* AACN. *Program availability:* Part-time, online learning. *Degree requirements:* For master's, research project; for doctorate, dissertation or scholarly project. *Entrance requirements:* For doctorate, GRE (waived for students with GPA of 3.5 or higher). Additional exam requirements/recommendations for international students: Required—TOEFL. Electronic applications accepted. *Faculty research:* Parent/child, adult, and gerontological nursing; breast cancer; families of children with HIV; parish nursing.

University of Illinois at Chicago, College of Nursing, Program in Nursing, Chicago, IL 60607-7128. Offers acute care clinical nurse specialist (MS); administrative nursing leadership (Certificate); adult nurse practitioner (MS); adult/geriatric nurse practitioner (MS); advanced community health nurse specialist (MS); family nurse practitioner (MS); geriatric clinical nurse specialist (MS); geriatric nurse practitioner (MS); nurse midwifery (MS); occupational health/advanced community health nurse specialist (MS); occupational health/family nurse practitioner (MS); pediatric nurse practitioner (MS); perinatal clinical nurse specialist (MS); school/advanced community health nurse specialist (MS); school/family nurse practitioner (MS); women's health nurse practitioner (MS). *Accreditation:* AACN. *Program availability:* Part-time. *Faculty:* 100 full-time (93 women), 89 part-time/adjunct (82 women). *Students:* 359 full-time (326 women), 280 part-time (249 women); includes 169 minority (43 Black or African American, non-Hispanic/Latino; 62 Asian, non-Hispanic/Latino; 56 Hispanic/Latino; 1 Native Hawaiian or other Pacific Islander, non-Hispanic/Latino; 7 Two or more races, non-Hispanic/Latino), 12 international. Average age 32. In 2015, 4 other advanced degrees awarded. *Degree requirements:* For master's, thesis or alternative. *Entrance requirements:* For master's, GRE General Test, minimum GPA of 2.75. Additional exam requirements/recommendations for international students: Required—TOEFL. *Application deadline:* For fall admission, 5/15 for domestic students, 2/15 for international students; for spring admission, 11/1 for domestic students, 7/15 for international students. Applications are processed on a rolling basis. Application fee: $60. Electronic applications accepted. *Expenses:* Tuition, state resident: full-time $11,480; part-time $3826 per credit. Tuition, nonresident: full-time $23,720; part-time $7906 per credit. *Required fees:* $1333 per semester. Part-time tuition and fees vary according to course load and program. *Financial support:* Fellowships with full tuition reimbursements, research assistantships with full tuition reimbursements, teaching assistantships with full tuition reimbursements, career-related internships or fieldwork, Federal Work-Study, institutionally sponsored loans, scholarships/grants, traineeships, tuition waivers (full and partial), and unspecified assistantships available. Support available to part-time students. Financial award application deadline: 3/1; financial award applicants required to submit FAFSA. *Unit head:* Dr. Terri E. Weaver, Dean, 312-996-7808, E-mail: teweaver@uic.edu. *Application contact:* Receptionist, 312-413-2550, E-mail: gradcoll@uic.edu.
Website: http://www.nursing.uic.edu/academics-admissions/master-science#program-overview

West Chester University of Pennsylvania, College of Health Sciences, Department of Nursing, West Chester, PA 19383. Offers adult-gerontology clinical nurse specialist (MSN); nursing (DNP); nursing education (MSN); school nurse (Certificate). *Accreditation:* AACN. *Program availability:* Part-time, evening/weekend, blended/hybrid learning. *Faculty:* 7 full-time (6 women), 1 (woman) part-time/adjunct. *Students:* 2 full-time (1 woman), 85 part-time (78 women); includes 10 minority (7 Black or African American, non-Hispanic/Latino; 3 Asian, non-Hispanic/Latino). Average age 45. 30 applicants, 90% accepted, 20 enrolled. In 2015, 10 master's, 3 other advanced degrees awarded. *Entrance requirements:* For master's, goals statement; official academic transcript(s) from all colleges and universities attended demonstrating minimum cumulative undergraduate GPA of 2.8 with successful completion of BSN and courses in statistics and physical assessment; documentation of current clinical experience; for doctorate, master's degree in nursing in an advanced nursing specialty from nationally-accredited program; minimum master's GPA of 3.0; licensed Registered Nurse. Additional exam requirements/recommendations for international students: Required—TOEFL or IELTS. *Application deadline:* For fall admission, 5/15 for international students; for spring admission, 10/15 for international students. Applications are processed on a rolling basis. Application fee: $50. Electronic applications accepted. *Expenses:* Tuition, state resident: full-time $8460; part-time $470 per credit. Tuition, nonresident: full-time $12,690; part-time $705 per credit. *Required fees:* $2312; $126.75 per credit. Tuition and fees vary according to campus/location and program. *Financial support:* Scholarships/grants and unspecified assistantships available. Financial award application deadline: 2/15; financial award applicants required to submit FAFSA. *Unit head:* Dr. Charlotte Mackey, Chair, 610-436-3474, Fax: 610-436-3083, E-mail: cmackey@wcupa.edu. *Application contact:* Dr. Cheryl Schlamb, Graduate Coordinator, 610-436-2219, E-mail: cschlamb@wcupa.edu.
Website: http://www.wcupa.edu/_ACADEMICS/HealthSciences/nursing/

Wright State University, School of Graduate Studies, College of Nursing and Health, Program in Nursing, Dayton, OH 45435. Offers acute care nurse practitioner (MS); administration of nursing and health care systems (MS); adult health (MS); child and adolescent health (MS); community health (MS); family nurse practitioner (MS); nurse practitioner (MS); school nurse (MS); MBA/MS. *Accreditation:* AACN. *Program availability:* Part-time, evening/weekend. *Degree requirements:* For master's, thesis or alternative. *Entrance requirements:* For master's, GRE General Test, BSN from NLN-accredited college, Ohio RN license. Additional exam requirements/recommendations for international students: Required—TOEFL. *Faculty research:* Clinical nursing and health, teaching, caring, pain administration, informatics and technology.

Transcultural Nursing

Augsburg College, Programs in Nursing, Minneapolis, MN 55454-1351. Offers MA, DNP. *Accreditation:* AACN. *Degree requirements:* For master's, thesis or alternative.

Rutgers University–Newark, Rutgers School of Nursing, Newark, NJ 07107-3001. Offers adult health (MSN); adult occupational health (MSN); advanced practice nursing (MSN, Post Master's Certificate); family nurse practitioner (MSN); nurse anesthesia (MSN); nursing (MSN); nursing informatics (MSN); urban health (PhD); women's health practitioner (MSN). *Accreditation:* AANA/CANAEP. *Program availability:* Part-time. *Entrance requirements:* For master's, GRE, RN license; basic life support, statistics, and health assessment experience. Additional exam requirements/recommendations for international students: Required—TOEFL. Electronic applications accepted. *Expenses:* Contact institution. *Faculty research:* HIV/AIDS, diabetes education, learned helplessness, nursing science, psychoeducation.

Women's Health Nursing

Boston College, William F. Connell School of Nursing, Chestnut Hill, MA 02467. Offers adult-gerontology nursing (MS); family health nursing (MS); forensic nursing (MS); nurse anesthesia (MS); nursing (PhD); pediatric nursing (MS), including pediatric and women's health; psychiatric-mental health nursing (MS); women's health nursing (MS); MBA/MS; MS/MA; MS/PhD. *Accreditation:* AACN; AANA/CANAEP (one or more programs are accredited). *Program availability:* Part-time. *Faculty:* 53 full-time (48 women), 47 part-time/adjunct (44 women). *Students:* 185 full-time (167 women), 66 part-time (56 women); includes 31 minority (10 Black or African American, non-Hispanic/Latino; 12 Asian, non-Hispanic/Latino; 7 Hispanic/Latino; 2 Two or more races, non-Hispanic/Latino), 7 international. Average age 32. 313 applicants, 66% accepted, 91 enrolled. In 2015, 98 master's, 5 doctorates awarded. *Degree requirements:* For master's, comprehensive exam; for doctorate, comprehensive exam, thesis/dissertation, computer literacy exam or foreign language. *Entrance requirements:* For master's, bachelor's degree in nursing; for doctorate, GRE General Test, MS in nursing. Additional exam requirements/recommendations for international students: Required—TOEFL (minimum score 600 paper-based; 100 iBT), IELTS (minimum score 7.5). *Application deadline:* For fall admission, 9/30 for domestic and international students; for winter admission, 1/15 for domestic and international students; for spring admission, 3/15 for domestic and international students. Applications are processed on a rolling basis. Application fee: $40. Electronic applications accepted. *Expenses:* Contact institution. *Financial support:* In 2015–16, 1 fellowship with full tuition reimbursement (averaging $23,700 per year), 25 teaching assistantships (averaging $4,370 per year) were awarded; research assistantships, scholarships/grants, health care benefits, tuition waivers (partial), and unspecified assistantships also available. Support available to part-time students. Financial award application deadline: 3/1; financial award applicants required to submit FAFSA. *Faculty research:* Sexual and reproductive health, health promotion/illness prevention, aging, eating disorders, symptom management. *Total annual research expenditures:* $1 million. *Unit head:* Dr. Susan Gennaro, Dean, 617-552-4251, Fax: 617-552-0931, E-mail: susan.gennaro@bc.edu. *Application contact:* MaryBeth Crowley, Graduate Programs Assistant, 617-552-4928, Fax: 617-552-2121, E-mail: csongrad@bc.edu.
Website: http://www.bc.edu/schools/son/

California State University, Fullerton, Graduate Studies, College of Health and Human Development, Department of Nursing, Fullerton, CA 92834-9480. Offers leadership (MSN); nurse anesthesia (MSN); nurse educator (MSN); nursing (DNP); women's health care (MSN). *Accreditation:* AACN; AANA/CANAEP. *Program availability:* Part-time.

Case Western Reserve University, Frances Payne Bolton School of Nursing, Master's Programs in Nursing, Nurse Practitioner Program, Cleveland, OH 44106. Offers acute care cardiovascular nursing (MSN); acute care nurse practitioner (MSN); acute care pediatric nurse practitioner (MSN); acute care/flight nurse (MSN); adult gerontology acute care nurse practitioner (MSN); adult gerontology oncology and palliative care (MSN); adult gerontology primary care nurse practitioner (MSN); family nurse practitioner (MSN); family systems psychiatric mental health nursing (MSN); neonatal nurse practitioner (MSN); pediatric nurse practitioner (MSN); women's health nurse practitioner (MSN). *Accreditation:* ACEN. *Program availability:* Part-time, online learning. *Students:* 52 full-time (45 women), 78 part-time (68 women); includes 31 minority (10 Black or African American, non-Hispanic/Latino; 14 Asian, non-Hispanic/Latino; 7 Hispanic/Latino). Average age 35. 64 applicants, 66% accepted, 29 enrolled. In 2015, 45 master's awarded. *Degree requirements:* For master's, thesis optional. *Entrance requirements:* For master's, GRE General Test or MAT. Additional exam requirements/recommendations for international students: Required—TOEFL (minimum score 577 paper-based; 90 iBT), IELTS (minimum score 7). *Application deadline:* For fall admission, 6/1 for domestic students; for spring admission, 10/1 for domestic students. Applications are processed on a rolling basis. Application fee: $75. *Expenses:* $1,891 per credit hour. *Financial support:* In 2015–16, 54 students received support, including 17 teaching assistantships with partial tuition reimbursements available (averaging $17,019 per year); scholarships/grants and traineeships also available. Financial award application deadline: 6/30; financial award applicants required to submit FAFSA. *Faculty research:* Symptom science, family/community care, aging across the lifespan, self-management of health and illness, neuroscience. *Unit head:* Dr. Carol Savrin, Director, 216-368-5304, Fax: 216-368-3542, E-mail: cls18@case.edu. *Application contact:* Donna Hassik, Admissions Coordinator, 216-368-5253, Fax: 216-368-0124, E-mail: dmh7@case.edu.
Website: http://fpb.cwru.edu/MSN/majors.shtm

Drexel University, College of Nursing and Health Professions, Division of Graduate Nursing, Philadelphia, PA 19104-2875. Offers adult acute care (MSN); adult psychiatric/mental health (MSN); advanced practice nursing (MSN); clinical trials research (MSN); family nurse practitioner (MSN); leadership in health systems management (MSN); nursing education (MSN); pediatric primary care (MSN); women's health (MSN). *Accreditation:* AACN. Electronic applications accepted.

Duke University, School of Nursing, Durham, NC 27708-0586. Offers acute care pediatric nurse practitioner (MSN, Post Master's Certificate); adult-gerontology nurse practitioner (MSN, Post Master's Certificate), including acute care, primary care; family nurse practitioner (MSN, Post Master's Certificate); neonatal nurse practitioner (MSN, Post Master's Certificate); nurse anesthesia (DNP); nurse practitioner (DNP); nursing (PhD); nursing and health care leadership (MSN); nursing education (MSN); nursing informatics (MSN, Post Master's Certificate); pediatric nurse practitioner (MSN, Post Master's Certificate), including primary care; women's health nurse practitioner (MSN, Post Master's Certificate). *Accreditation:* AACN; AANA/CANAEP. *Program availability:* Part-time, evening/weekend, online learning. *Faculty:* 74 full-time (63 women). *Students:* 179 full-time (152 women), 528 part-time (466 women); includes 145 minority (42 Black or African American, non-Hispanic/Latino; 3 American Indian or Alaska Native, non-Hispanic/Latino; 44 Asian, non-Hispanic/Latino; 35 Hispanic/Latino; 1 Native Hawaiian or other Pacific Islander, non-Hispanic/Latino; 20 Two or more races, non-Hispanic/Latino), 7 international. Average age 33. 619 applicants, 46% accepted, 201 enrolled. In 2015, 243 master's, 62 doctorates, 26 other advanced degrees awarded. Terminal master's awarded for partial completion of doctoral program. *Degree requirements:* For master's, thesis optional; for doctorate, capstone project. *Entrance requirements:* For master's, GRE General Test (waived if undergraduate GPA of 3.4 or higher), 1 year of nursing experience (recommended), BSN, minimum GPA of 3.0, previous course work in statistics; for doctorate, GRE General Test (waived if undergraduate GPA of 3.4 or higher), BSN or MSN, minimum GPA of 3.0, portfolio, resume, personal statement, undergraduate statistics course, current licensure as a registered nurse, transcripts from all post-secondary institutions; for Post Master's Certificate, MSN, licensure or eligibility as a professional nurse, transcripts from all post-secondary institutions, previous course work in statistics. Additional exam requirements/recommendations for international

students: Required—TOEFL (minimum score 100 iBT), IELTS (minimum score 7). *Application deadline:* For fall admission, 12/1 for domestic and international students; for spring admission, 5/1 for domestic and international students. Application fee: $50. Electronic applications accepted. *Expenses:* Contact institution. *Financial support:* Career-related internships or fieldwork, institutionally sponsored loans, scholarships/grants, traineeships, and tuition waivers (partial) available. Support available to part-time students. Financial award applicants required to submit FAFSA. *Faculty research:* Cardiovascular disease, caregiver skill training, data mining, prostate cancer, neonatal immune system. *Unit head:* Dr. Marion E. Broome, Dean/Vice Chancellor for Nursing Affairs/Associate Vice President for Academic Affairs for Nursing, 919-684-9446, Fax: 919-684-9414, E-mail: marion.broome@duke.edu. *Application contact:* Dr. Ernie Rushing, Director of Admissions and Recruitment, 919-668-6274, Fax: 919-668-4693, E-mail: ernie.rushing@dm.duke.edu.
Website: http://www.nursing.duke.edu/

Emory University, Nell Hodgson Woodruff School of Nursing, Atlanta, GA 30322-1100. Offers adult nurse practitioner (MSN); emergency nurse practitioner (MSN); family nurse practitioner (MSN); family nurse-midwife (MSN); health systems leadership (MSN); nurse-midwifery (MSN); pediatric nurse practitioner acute and primary care (MSN); women's health care (Title X) (MSN); women's health nurse practitioner (MSN); MSN/MPH. *Accreditation:* AACN; ACNM/ACME (one or more programs are accredited). *Program availability:* Part-time. *Entrance requirements:* For master's, GRE General Test or MAT, minimum GPA of 3.0, BS in nursing from an accredited institution, RN license and additional course work, 3 letters of recommendation. Additional exam requirements/recommendations for international students: Required—TOEFL (minimum score 600 paper-based; 100 iBT). Electronic applications accepted. *Expenses:* Contact institution. *Faculty research:* Older adult falls and injuries, minority health issues, cardiac symptoms and quality of life, bio-ethics and decision-making, menopausal issues.

Frontier Nursing University, Graduate Programs, Hyden, KY 41749. Offers family nurse practitioner (MSN, DNP, Post Master's Certificate); nurse-midwifery (MSN, DNP, Post Master's Certificate); women's health care nurse practitioner (MSN, DNP, Post Master's Certificate). *Accreditation:* ACEN; ACNM. *Degree requirements:* For doctorate, capstone project, practicum.

Georgia State University, Byrdine F. Lewis School of Nursing, Atlanta, GA 30303. Offers adult health clinical nurse specialist/nurse practitioner (MS, Certificate); child health clinical nurse specialist/pediatric nurse practitioner (MS, Certificate); family nurse practitioner (MS, Certificate); family psychiatric mental health nurse practitioner (MS, Certificate); nursing (PhD); nursing leadership in healthcare innovations (MS), including nursing administration, nursing informatics; nutrition (MS); perinatal clinical nurse specialist/women's health nurse practitioner (MS, Certificate); physical therapy (DPT); respiratory therapy (MS). *Accreditation:* AACN. *Program availability:* Part-time, blended/hybrid learning. *Faculty:* 18 full-time (11 women). *Students:* 275 full-time (195 women), 230 part-time (204 women); includes 192 minority (123 Black or African American, non-Hispanic/Latino; 49 Asian, non-Hispanic/Latino; 12 Hispanic/Latino; 2 Native Hawaiian or other Pacific Islander, non-Hispanic/Latino; 6 Two or more races, non-Hispanic/Latino), 35 international. Average age 33. 240 applicants, 61% accepted, 95 enrolled. In 2015, 115 master's, 40 doctorates, 19 other advanced degrees awarded. *Degree requirements:* For doctorate, comprehensive exam, thesis/dissertation. *Entrance requirements:* For doctorate, GRE. Additional exam requirements/recommendations for international students: Required—TOEFL. *Application deadline:* For fall admission, 2/1 priority date for domestic and international students; for spring admission, 9/15 for domestic and international students. Applications are processed on a rolling basis. Application fee: $50. Electronic applications accepted. *Expenses:* Contact institution. *Financial support:* In 2015–16, research assistantships with tuition reimbursements (averaging $1,666 per year), teaching assistantships with tuition reimbursements (averaging $1,920 per year) were awarded; scholarships/grants, tuition waivers (full and partial), and unspecified assistantships also available. Support available to part-time students. Financial award application deadline: 8/1; financial award applicants required to submit FAFSA. *Faculty research:* Stroke intervention for caregivers, stroke prevention in African-Americans; relationships between psychological distress and health outcomes in parents with a medically ill infant; medically fragile children; nursing expertise and patient outcomes. *Unit head:* Nancy Kropf, Dean of Nursing, 404-413-1101, Fax: 404-413-1090, E-mail: nkropf@gsu.edu.
Website: http://nursing.gsu.edu/

Hampton University, School of Nursing, Hampton, VA 23668. Offers advanced adult nursing (MS); community health nursing (MS); community mental health/psychiatric nursing (MS); family nursing (MS); gerontological nursing for the nurse practitioner (MS); nursing (PhD); women's health nursing (MS). *Accreditation:* AACN. *Program availability:* Part-time, online learning. *Degree requirements:* For master's, comprehensive exam, thesis optional; for doctorate, comprehensive exam, thesis/dissertation. *Entrance requirements:* For master's, GRE General Test. Additional exam requirements/recommendations for international students: Required—TOEFL (minimum score 525 paper-based) or IELTS (6.5). Electronic applications accepted. *Expenses: Tuition, area resident:* Full-time $10,263; part-time $522 per credit hour. *Required fees:* $35. Tuition and fees vary according to course load and program. *Faculty research:* African-American stress, HIV education, pediatric obesity, hypertension, breast cancer.

Kent State University, College of Nursing, Kent, OH 44242. Offers advanced nursing practice (DNP), including adult gerontology acute care nurse practitioner (MSN, DNP), adult gerontology clinical nurse specialist (MSN, DNP), family nurse practitioner (MSN, DNP); nursing (MSN, PhD), including adult gerontology acute care nurse practitioner (MSN, DNP), adult gerontology clinical nurse specialist (MSN, DNP), family nurse practitioner (MSN, DNP), nurse educator (MSN), nursing healthcare management (MSN), primary care adult nurse practitioner (MSN), primary care pediatric clinical nurse specialist (MSN), primary care pediatric nurse practitioner (MSN), psychiatric mental health practitioner (MSN), women's health nurse practitioner (MSN); nursing education (Certificate); primary care pediatric nurse practitioner (Certificate); women's health nurse practitioner (Certificate). PhD program offered jointly with The University of Akron. *Accreditation:* AACN. *Program availability:* Part-time, online learning. *Faculty:* 52 full-time (48 women). *Students:* 78 full-time (56 women), 414 part-time (365 women); includes 63 minority (34 Black or African American, non-Hispanic/Latino; 1 American Indian or Alaska Native, non-Hispanic/Latino; 12 Asian, non-Hispanic/Latino; 12 Hispanic/Latino; 4 Two or more races, non-Hispanic/Latino), 16 international. Average age 37. 653 applicants, 54% accepted, 309 enrolled. In 2015, 140 master's, 1 doctorate, 13 other advanced degrees awarded. *Degree requirements:* For master's, thesis optional, practicum; for doctorate, comprehensive exam (for some programs), thesis/dissertation (for some programs), practicum and scholarly project (for DNP programs); for Certificate, practicum. *Entrance requirements:* For master's, minimum GPA of 3.0, transcripts, active unrestricted RN license, essay/goal statement, interview, 3 letters of

Women's Health Nursing

recommendation; for doctorate, GRE (for PhD), minimum GPA of 3.0, transcripts, 3 letters of recommendation, interview; active unrestricted RN license, clinical experience and hours record (for DNP); goal statement, sample of written work, curriculum vitae, statement of research interests, and eligibility for RN license (for PhD); for Certificate, MSN, minimum GPA of 3.0, transcripts. Additional exam requirements/recommendations for international students: Required—TOEFL (minimum score: paper-based 525, iBT 71), Michigan English Language Assessment Battery (minimum score of 75), IELTS (minimum score of 6.0), PTE Academic (minimum score of 48), or completion of ELS level 112 Intensive Program. Application deadline: For fall admission, 2/1 for domestic students; for spring admission, 11/1 for domestic students. Application fee: $45 ($70 for international students). Electronic applications accepted. Expenses: Tuition, state resident: full-time $10,864; part-time $495 per credit hour. Tuition, nonresident: full-time $18,380; part-time $837 per credit hour. Financial support: Research assistantships with full tuition reimbursements, teaching assistantships with full tuition reimbursements, career-related internships or fieldwork, Federal Work-Study, traineeships, and unspecified assistantships available. Financial award application deadline: 2/1. Unit head: Dr. Barbara Broome, Dean, 330-672-3777, E-mail: bbroome1@kent.edu. Application contact: Dr. Wendy A. Umberger, Associate Dean for Graduate Programs/Professor, 330-672-8813, E-mail: wlewando@kent.edu.
Website: http://www.kent.edu/nursing/

Loyola University Chicago, Graduate School, Marcella Niehoff School of Nursing, Maywood, IL 60153. Offers adult gerontology acute care clinical nurse specialist (MSN), including emergency care (MSN, Certificate); adult gerontology acute care nurse practitioner (MSN), including oncology (MSN, Certificate); adult gerontology clinical nurse specialist (MSN), including oncology (MSN, Certificate); adult gerontology nursing (Certificate), including oncology (MSN, Certificate); adult nurse practitioner (Certificate); dietetics (MS); family nurse practitioner (MSN, Certificate), including emergency care; informatics (MSN); leadership (DNP), including healthcare quality using education in safety and technology, infection prevention; nursing science (PhD); women's health nurse practitioner (MSN); women's health nursing (Certificate). Accreditation: AACN. Program availability: Part-time, blended/hybrid learning. Faculty: 27 full-time (25 women), 12 part-time/adjunct (10 women). Students: 174 full-time (161 women), 232 part-time (221 women); includes 95 minority (19 Black or African American, non-Hispanic/Latino; 2 American Indian or Alaska Native, non-Hispanic/Latino; 38 Asian, non-Hispanic/Latino; 28 Hispanic/Latino; 2 Native Hawaiian or other Pacific Islander, non-Hispanic/Latino; 6 Two or more races, non-Hispanic/Latino), 3 international. Average age 35. 209 applicants, 52% accepted, 83 enrolled. In 2015, 78 master's, 10 doctorates, 17 other advanced degrees awarded. Degree requirements: For master's, comprehensive exam; for doctorate, thesis/dissertation, qualifying examination (for PhD); capstone project (for DNP). Entrance requirements: For master's, BSN, minimum nursing GPA of 3.0, Illinois RN license, 3 letters of recommendation, 1000 hours of experience in area of specialty prior to starting clinical rotations, personal statement; for doctorate, GRE General Test (for PhD), BSN or MSN, minimum GPA of 3.0, professional nursing license, 3 letters of recommendation, personal statement. Additional exam requirements/recommendations for international students: Required—TOEFL (minimum score 550 paper-based; 79 iBT), IELTS (minimum score 6.5). Application deadline: For fall admission, 6/1 priority date for domestic and international students; for spring admission, 11/15 priority date for domestic and international students; for summer admission, 3/15 priority date for domestic and international students. Applications are processed on a rolling basis. Application fee: $50. Electronic applications accepted. Application fee is waived when completed online. Expenses: $1,081 per credit hour. Financial support: In 2015–16, 10 students received support, including 3 research assistantships with full tuition reimbursements available (averaging $18,000 per year), 1 teaching assistantship with full tuition reimbursement available (averaging $18,000 per year); scholarships/grants, unspecified assistantships, and nurse faculty loan program also available. Financial award application deadline: 5/1; financial award applicants required to submit FAFSA. Faculty research: Epigenetics and social determinants of health, women's health, vitamin D, interprofessional education, prevention and self-management of chronic disease. Total annual research expenditures: $649,606. Unit head: Dr. Vicky Keough, Dean, 708-216-5448, Fax: 708-216-9555, E-mail: vkeough@luc.edu. Application contact: Toni Topalova, Enrollment Advisor, 708-216-3751, Fax: 708-216-9555, E-mail: atopalova@luc.edu.
Website: http://www.luc.edu/nursing/

MGH Institute of Health Professions, School of Nursing, Boston, MA 02129. Offers advanced practice nursing (MSN); gerontological nursing (MSN); nursing (DNP); pediatric nursing (MSN); psychiatric nursing (MSN); teaching and learning for health care education (Certificate); women's health nursing (MSN). Accreditation: AACN. Degree requirements: For master's, thesis or alternative. Entrance requirements: For master's, GRE General Test, bachelor's degree from regionally-accredited college or university. Additional exam requirements/recommendations for international students: Required—TOEFL (minimum score 550 paper-based; 80 iBT). Electronic applications accepted. Faculty research: Biobehavioral nursing, HIV/AIDS, gerontological nursing, women's health, vulnerable populations, health systems.

Queen's University at Kingston, School of Graduate Studies, Faculty of Health Sciences, School of Nursing, Kingston, ON K7L 3N6, Canada. Offers health and chronic illness (M Sc); nurse scientist (PhD); primary health care nurse practitioner (Certificate); women's and children's health (M Sc). Degree requirements: For master's, thesis. Entrance requirements: For master's, RN license. Additional exam requirements/recommendations for international students: Required—TOEFL. Faculty research: Women and children's health, health and chronic illness.

Rutgers University–Newark, Rutgers School of Nursing, Newark, NJ 07107-3001. Offers adult health (MSN); adult occupational health (MSN); advanced practice nursing (MSN, Post Master's Certificate); family nurse practitioner (MSN); nurse anesthesia (MSN); nursing (MSN); nursing informatics (MSN); urban health (PhD); women's health practitioner (MSN). Accreditation: AANA/CANAEP. Program availability: Part-time. Entrance requirements: For master's, GRE, RN license; basic life support, statistics, and health assessment experience. Additional exam requirements/recommendations for international students: Required—TOEFL. Electronic applications accepted. Expenses: Contact institution. Faculty research: HIV/AIDS, diabetes education, learned helplessness, nursing science, psychoeducation.

San Francisco State University, Division of Graduate Studies, College of Health and Social Sciences, School of Nursing, San Francisco, CA 94132-1722. Offers adult acute care (MS); clinical nurse specialist (MS); community/public health nursing (MS); family nurse practitioner (MS, Certificate); nursing administration (MS); pediatrics (MS); women's health (MS). Accreditation: AACN. Program availability: Part-time. Application deadline: Applications are processed on a rolling basis. Expenses: Tuition, state resident: full-time $6738. Tuition, nonresident: full-time $15,666. Required fees: $1004. Financial support: Career-related internships or fieldwork available. Unit head: Dr. Mary-Ann van Dam, Director, 415-338-1802, Fax: 415-338-0555, E-mail: vandam@sfsu.edu. Application contact: Connie Carr, Graduate Coordinator, 415-338-6856, Fax: 415-338-0555, E-mail: ccarr@sfsu.edu.
Website: http://nursing.sfsu.edu

Stony Brook University, State University of New York, Stony Brook Medicine, School of Nursing, Program in Perinatal Women's Health Nursing, Stony Brook, NY 11794. Offers MS, DNP, Certificate. Accreditation: AACN. Program availability: Blended/hybrid learning. Students: 1 (woman) full-time, 21 part-time (all women); includes 4 minority (1 Black or African American, non-Hispanic/Latino; 1 American Indian or Alaska Native, non-Hispanic/Latino; 1 Asian, non-Hispanic/Latino; 1 Hispanic/Latino). In 2015, 11 master's awarded. Degree requirements: For master's, thesis. Entrance requirements: For master's, BSN, minimum GPA of 3.0, course work in statistics. Additional exam requirements/recommendations for international students: Required—TOEFL (minimum score 90 iBT). Application deadline: For fall admission, 1/1 for domestic students. Application fee: $100. Expenses: $24,781 full-time resident tuition and fees, $968 per credit hour; $44,431 full-time nonresident tuition and fees, $1,787 per credit hour. Financial support: Application deadline: 3/15. Unit head: Prof. Elizabeth Collins, Director, 631-444-3296, Fax: 631-444-3136, E-mail: elizabeth.collins@stonybrook.edu. Application contact: Crystal Garcia, Staff Assistant, 631-632-3392, Fax: 631-632-3136, E-mail: crystal.garcia@stonybrook.edu.
Website: http://www.nursing.stonybrookmedicine.edu/

Texas Woman's University, Graduate School, College of Nursing, Denton, TX 76204-5498. Offers acute care nurse practitioner (MS); adult health clinical nurse specialist (MS); adult health nurse practitioner (MS); child health clinical nurse specialist (MS); clinical nurse leader (MS); family nurse practitioner (MS); health systems management (MS); nursing education (MS); nursing practice (DNP); nursing science (PhD); pediatric nurse practitioner (MS); women's health clinical nurse specialist (MS); women's health nurse practitioner (MS). Accreditation: AACN. Program availability: Part-time, online learning. Faculty: 55 full-time (51 women), 42 part-time/adjunct (35 women). Students: 39 full-time (37 women), 958 part-time (888 women); includes 566 minority (226 Black or African American, non-Hispanic/Latino; 8 American Indian or Alaska Native, non-Hispanic/Latino; 221 Asian, non-Hispanic/Latino; 88 Hispanic/Latino; 3 Native Hawaiian or other Pacific Islander, non-Hispanic/Latino; 20 Two or more races, non-Hispanic/Latino), 37 international. Average age 36. 430 applicants, 65% accepted, 193 enrolled. In 2015, 248 master's, 10 doctorates awarded. Degree requirements: For master's, comprehensive exam, thesis or alternative; for doctorate, comprehensive exam, thesis/dissertation. Entrance requirements: For master's, GRE or MAT, minimum GPA of 3.0 on last 60 hours in undergraduate nursing degree and overall, RN license, BS in nursing, basic statistics course; for doctorate, GRE (preferred minimum score 153 [500 old version] Verbal, 144 [500 old version] Quantitative, 4 Analytical), MS in nursing, minimum preferred GPA of 3.5, RN license, statistics, 2 letters of reference, curriculum vitae, graduate nursing-theory course, graduate research course, statement of professional goals and research interests. Additional exam requirements/recommendations for international students: Required—TOEFL (minimum score 550 paper-based; 79 iBT). Application deadline: For fall admission, 5/1 priority date for domestic students, 3/1 for international students; for spring admission, 9/15 priority date for domestic students, 7/1 for international students. Applications are processed on a rolling basis. Application fee: $50 ($75 for international students). Electronic applications accepted. Expenses: Tuition, state resident: full-time $4380; part-time $243 per credit hour. Tuition, nonresident: full-time $11,400; part-time $633 per credit hour. International tuition: $11,465 full-time. Required fees: $1778; $99 per credit hour. $283 per semester. One-time fee: $50. Tuition and fees vary according to course load and program. Financial support: In 2015–16, 149 students received support, including 10 research assistantships (averaging $5,600 per year), 1 teaching assistantship (averaging $5,600 per year); career-related internships or fieldwork, Federal Work-Study, institutionally sponsored loans, scholarships/grants, traineeships, health care benefits, and unspecified assistantships also available. Support available to part-time students. Financial award application deadline: 3/1; financial award applicants required to submit FAFSA. Faculty research: Screening, prevention, and treatment for intimate partner violence; needs of adolescents during childbirth intervention; a network analysis decision tool for nurse managers (social network analysis); support for adolescents with implantable cardioverter defibrillators; informatics: nurse staffing, safety, quality, and financial data as they relate to patient care outcomes; prevention and treatment of obesity; improving infant outcomes related to premature birth. Total annual research expenditures: $1.7 million. Unit head: Dr. Anita G. Hufft, Dean, 940-898-2401, Fax: 940-898-2437, E-mail: nursing@twu.edu. Application contact: Dr. Samuel Wheeler, Assistant Director of Admissions, 940-898-3188, Fax: 940-898-3081, E-mail: wheelersr@twu.edu.
Website: http://www.twu.edu/nursing/

Uniformed Services University of the Health Sciences, Daniel K. Inouye Graduate School of Nursing, Bethesda, MD 20814. Offers adult-gerontology clinical nurse specialist (MSN, DNP); family nurse practitioner (DNP); nurse anesthesia (DNP); nursing science (PhD); psychiatric mental health nurse practitioner (DNP); women's health nurse practitioner (DNP). MSN and DNP programs available to military officers only; PhD to military and DoD students only. Accreditation: AACN; AANA/CANAEP. Faculty: 38 full-time (22 women), 2 part-time/adjunct (1 woman). Students: 51 full-time (29 women); includes 17 minority (8 Black or African American, non-Hispanic/Latino; 4 Asian, non-Hispanic/Latino; 4 Hispanic/Latino; 1 Two or more races, non-Hispanic/Latino). Average age 34. 75 applicants, 68% accepted, 51 enrolled. In 2015, 4 master's, 24 doctorates awarded. Degree requirements: For master's, thesis or alternative; for doctorate, thesis/dissertation or alternative. Entrance requirements: For master's, GRE, BSN, clinical experience, minimum GPA of 3.0, previous course work in science; for doctorate, GRE, BSN, clinical experience, minimum GPA of 3.0, previous course work in sciences, and writing paper (for DNP); MSN (for PhD). Application deadline: For fall admission, 7/1 for domestic students; for winter admission, 2/15 for domestic students. Application fee: $0. Electronic applications accepted. Faculty research: Prenatal care, military health care, military readiness, distance learning. Unit head: Dr. Diane C. Seibert, Associate Dean for Academic Affairs, 301-295-1080, Fax: 301-295-1707, E-mail: diane.seibert@usuhs.edu. Application contact: Terry Lynn Malavakis, Recording Secretary for Admissions Committee/Registrar/Program Analyst, 301-295-1055, Fax: 301-295-1707, E-mail: terry.malavakis@usuhs.edu.
Website: http://www.usuhs.edu/gsn/

University of Cincinnati, Graduate School, College of Nursing, Cincinnati, OH 45221-0038. Offers clinical nurse specialist (MSN), including adult health, community health, neonatal, nursing administration, occupational health, pediatric health, psychiatric nursing, women's health; nurse anesthesia (MSN); nurse midwifery (MSN); nurse practitioner (MSN), including acute care, ambulatory care, family, family/psychiatric, women's health; nursing (PhD); MBA/MSN. Accreditation: AACN; AANA/CANAEP (one or more programs are accredited); ACNM/ACME. Program availability: Part-time, online learning. Terminal master's awarded for partial completion of doctoral program. Degree requirements: For master's, thesis or alternative; for doctorate, comprehensive exam, thesis/dissertation. Entrance requirements: For master's and doctorate, GRE General Test. Additional exam requirements/recommendations for international students: Required—TOEFL (minimum score 520 paper-based). Electronic applications accepted. Faculty research: Substance abuse, injury and violence, symptom management.

University of Colorado Denver, College of Nursing, Aurora, CO 80045. Offers adult clinical nurse specialist (MS); adult nurse practitioner (MS); family nurse practitioner (MS); family psychiatric mental health nurse practitioner (MS); health care informatics

(MS); nurse-midwifery (MS); nursing (DNP, PhD); nursing leadership and health care systems (MS); pediatric nurse practitioner (MS); special studies (MS); women's health (MS); MS/PhD. *Accreditation:* ACNM/ACME (one or more programs are accredited). *Program availability:* Part-time, evening/weekend, online learning. *Faculty:* 109 full-time (100 women), 55 part-time/adjunct (50 women). *Students:* 367 full-time (332 women), 141 part-time (118 women); includes 79 minority (16 Black or African American, non-Hispanic/Latino; 2 American Indian or Alaska Native, non-Hispanic/Latino; 8 Asian, non-Hispanic/Latino; 37 Hispanic/Latino; 16 Two or more races, non-Hispanic/Latino), 6 international. Average age 36. 321 applicants, 53% accepted, 145 enrolled. In 2015, 151 master's, 36 doctorates awarded. Terminal master's awarded for partial completion of doctoral program. *Degree requirements:* For master's, thesis optional; for doctorate, comprehensive exam, thesis/dissertation, 42 credits of coursework. *Entrance requirements:* For master's, GRE if cumulative undergraduate GPA is less than 3.0, undergraduate nursing degree from NLNAC- or CCNE-accredited school or university; completion of research and statistics courses with minimum grade of C; copy of current and unencumbered nursing license; for doctorate, GRE, bachelor's and/or master's degrees in nursing from NLN- or CCNE-accredited institution; portfolio; minimum undergraduate GPA of 3.0, graduate 3.5; graduate-level intermediate statistics and master's-level nursing theory courses with minimum B grade; interview. Additional exam requirements/recommendations for international students: Required—TOEFL (minimum score 560 paper-based; 83 iBT). *Application deadline:* For fall admission, 2/15 for domestic students, 1/15 for international students; for spring admission, 7/1 for domestic students, 6/1 for international students. Application fee: $50 ($75 for international students). Electronic applications accepted. *Expenses:* Contact institution. *Financial support:* In 2015–16, 148 students received support. Fellowships, research assistantships, teaching assistantships, Federal Work-Study, institutionally sponsored loans, scholarships/grants, traineeships, and unspecified assistantships available. Support available to part-time students. Financial award application deadline: 4/1; financial award applicants required to submit FAFSA. *Faculty research:* Biological and behavioral phenomena in pregnancy and postpartum; patterns of glycaemia during the insulin resistance of pregnancy; obesity, gestational diabetes, and relationship to neonatal adiposity; men's awareness and knowledge of male breast cancer; cognitive-behavioral therapy for chronic insomnia after breast cancer treatment; massage therapy for the treatment of tension-type headaches. *Total annual research expenditures:* $5.9 million. *Unit head:* Dr. Sarah Thompson, Dean, 303-724-1679, E-mail: sarah.a.thompson@ucdenver.edu. *Application contact:* Judy Campbell, Graduate Programs Coordinator, 303-724-8503, E-mail: judy.campbell@ucdenver.edu.
Website: http://www.ucdenver.edu/academics/colleges/nursing/Pages/default.aspx

University of Delaware, College of Health Sciences, School of Nursing, Newark, DE 19716. Offers adult nurse practitioner (MSN, PMC); cardiopulmonary clinical nurse specialist (MSN, PMC); cardiopulmonary clinical nurse specialist/adult nurse practitioner (MSN, PMC); family nurse practitioner (MSN, PMC); gerontology clinical nurse specialist (MSN, PMC); gerontology clinical nurse specialist geriatric nurse practitioner (PMC); gerontology clinical nurse specialist/geriatric nurse practitioner (MSN); health services administration (MSN, PMC); nursing of children clinical nurse specialist (MSN, PMC); nursing of children clinical nurse specialist/pediatric nurse practitioner (MSN, PMC); oncology/immune deficiency clinical nurse specialist (MSN, PMC); oncology/immune deficiency clinical nurse specialist/adult nurse practitioner (MSN, PMC); perinatal/women's health clinical nurse specialist (MSN, PMC); perinatal/women's health clinical nurse specialist/women's health nurse practitioner (MSN, PMC); psychiatric nursing clinical nurse specialist (MSN, PMC). *Accreditation:* AACN. *Program availability:* Part-time, evening/weekend, online learning. *Degree requirements:* For master's, thesis optional. *Entrance requirements:* For master's, BSN, interview, RN license. Electronic applications accepted. *Faculty research:* Marriage and chronic illness, health promotion, congestive heart failure patient outcomes, school nursing, diabetes in children, culture, health disparities, cardiovascular, prison nursing, oncology, public policy, child obesity, smoking and teen pregnancy, blood pressure measurements, men's health.

University of Illinois at Chicago, College of Nursing, Program in Nursing, Chicago, IL 60607-7128. Offers acute care clinical nurse specialist (MS); administrative nursing leadership (Certificate); adult nurse practitioner (MS); adult/geriatric nurse practitioner (MS); advanced community health nurse specialist (MS); family nurse practitioner (MS); geriatric clinical nurse specialist (MS); geriatric nurse practitioner (MS); nurse midwifery (MS); occupational health/advanced community health nurse specialist (MS); occupational health/family nurse practitioner (MS); pediatric nurse practitioner (MS); perinatal clinical nurse specialist (MS); school/advanced community health nurse specialist (MS); school/family nurse practitioner (MS); women's health nurse practitioner (MS). *Accreditation:* AACN. *Program availability:* Part-time. *Faculty:* 100 full-time (93 women), 89 part-time/adjunct (82 women). *Students:* 359 full-time (326 women), 280 part-time (249 women); includes 169 minority (43 Black or African American, non-Hispanic/Latino; 62 Asian, non-Hispanic/Latino; 56 Hispanic/Latino; 1 Native Hawaiian or other Pacific Islander, non-Hispanic/Latino; 7 Two or more races, non-Hispanic/Latino), 12 international. Average age 32. In 2015, 4 other advanced degrees awarded. *Degree requirements:* For master's, thesis or alternative. *Entrance requirements:* For master's, GRE General Test, minimum GPA of 2.75. Additional exam requirements/recommendations for international students: Required—TOEFL. *Application deadline:* For fall admission, 5/15 for domestic students, 2/15 for international students; for spring admission, 11/1 for domestic students, 7/15 for international students. Applications are processed on a rolling basis. Application fee: $60. Electronic applications accepted. *Expenses:* Tuition, state resident: full-time $11,480; part-time $3826 per credit. Tuition, nonresident: full-time $23,720; part-time $7906 per credit. *Required fees:* $1333 per semester. Part-time tuition and fees vary according to course load and program. *Financial support:* Fellowships with full tuition reimbursements, research assistantships with full tuition reimbursements, teaching assistantships with full tuition reimbursements, career-related internships or fieldwork, Federal Work-Study, institutionally sponsored loans, scholarships/grants, traineeships, tuition waivers (full and partial), and unspecified assistantships available. Support available to part-time students. Financial award application deadline: 3/1; financial award applicants required to submit FAFSA. *Unit head:* Dr. Terri E. Weaver, Dean, 312-996-7808, E-mail: teweaver@uic.edu. *Application contact:* Receptionist, 312-413-2550, E-mail: gradcoll@uic.edu.
Website: http://www.nursing.uic.edu/academics-admissions/master-science#program-overview

University of Indianapolis, Graduate Programs, School of Nursing, Indianapolis, IN 46227-3697. Offers advanced practice nursing (DNP); family nurse practitioner (MSN); gerontological nurse practitioner (MSN); neonatal nurse practitioner (MSN); nurse-midwifery (MSN); nursing (MSN); nursing and health systems leadership (MSN); nursing education (MSN); women's health nurse practitioner (MSN); MBA/MSN. *Accreditation:* AACN; ACNM. *Entrance requirements:* For master's, minimum GPA of 3.0, interview, letters of recommendation, resume, IN nursing license, 1 year of professional practice; for doctorate, graduate of NLNAC- or CCNE-accredited nursing program; MSN or MA with nursing major and minimum cumulative GPA of 3.25; unencumbered RN license with eligibility for licensure in Indiana; completion of graduate-level statistics course within last 5 years with minimum grade of B; resume; essay; official transcripts from all academic institutions. Additional exam requirements/recommendations for international

students: Required—TOEFL (minimum score 550 paper-based). Electronic applications accepted.

University of Louisville, Graduate School, School of Nursing, Louisville, KY 40202. Offers adult gerontology nurse practitioner (MSN, DNP); education and administration (MSN); family nurse practitioner (MSN, DNP); neonatal nurse practitioner (MSN, DNP); nursing research (PhD); psychiatric/mental health nurse practitioner (MSN, DNP); women's health nurse practitioner (MSN). *Accreditation:* AACN. *Program availability:* Part-time. *Faculty:* 53 full-time (48 women), 27 part-time/adjunct (23 women). *Students:* 110 full-time (99 women), 33 part-time (29 women); includes 17 minority (11 Black or African American, non-Hispanic/Latino; 1 Asian, non-Hispanic/Latino; 2 Hispanic/Latino; 3 Two or more races, non-Hispanic/Latino), 5 international. Average age 34. 62 applicants, 68% accepted, 40 enrolled. In 2015, 41 master's awarded. *Degree requirements:* For doctorate, comprehensive exam (for some programs), thesis/dissertation (for some programs). *Entrance requirements:* For master's, bachelor's degree in nursing, minimum GPA of 3.0, RN license; for doctorate, GRE General Test (for PhD), 3 letters of professional reference. Additional exam requirements/recommendations for international students: Required—TOEFL (minimum score 560 paper-based; 79 iBT). *Application deadline:* For fall admission, 3/1 priority date for domestic students, 3/1 for international students. Applications are processed on a rolling basis. Application fee: $60. Electronic applications accepted. *Expenses:* Tuition, state resident: full-time $11,664; part-time $649 per credit hour. Tuition, nonresident: full-time $24,274; part-time $1350 per credit hour. *Required fees:* $196. Tuition and fees vary according to program and reciprocity agreements. *Financial support:* In 2015–16, 722,568 students received support, including 10 research assistantships with full tuition reimbursements available (averaging $20,000 per year), 2 teaching assistantships with full tuition reimbursements available (averaging $15,000 per year); fellowships with full tuition reimbursements available, scholarships/grants, and unspecified assistantships also available. Financial award application deadline: 2/15; financial award applicants required to submit FAFSA. *Faculty research:* Children and adolescents with chronic illnesses, women's mental health and parenting, asthma and environmental health, type 2 diabetes self-management in adults, health disparities and community engagement. *Total annual research expenditures:* $722,568. *Unit head:* Dr. Marcia J. Hern, Dean, 502-852-8300, Fax: 502-852-8783, E-mail: m.hern@louisville.edu. *Application contact:* Trish Hart, Assistant Dean for Student Affairs, 502-852-5825, Fax: 502-852-8783, E-mail: trish.hart@louisville.edu.
Website: http://www.louisville.edu/nursing/

University of Minnesota, Twin Cities Campus, Graduate School, School of Nursing, Program in Women's Health Nurse Practitioner, Minneapolis, MN 55455-0213. Offers MS. *Accreditation:* AACN. *Program availability:* Online learning. *Entrance requirements:* Additional exam requirements/recommendations for international students: Required—TOEFL (minimum score 586 paper-based).

University of Missouri–Kansas City, School of Nursing and Health Studies, Kansas City, MO 64108. Offers adult clinical nurse specialist (MSN), including adult nurse practitioner, women's health nurse practitioner (MSN, DNP); adult clinical nursing practice (DNP), including adult gerontology nurse practitioner, women's health nurse practitioner (MSN, DNP); clinical nursing practice (DNP), including family nurse practitioner; family nurse practitioner (MSN); neonatal nurse practitioner (MSN); nurse educator (MSN); nurse executive (MSN); nursing (PhD); nursing practice (DNP); pediatric clinical nursing practice (DNP), including pediatric nurse practitioner; pediatric nurse practitioner (MSN). *Accreditation:* AACN. *Program availability:* Part-time, online learning. *Faculty:* 44 full-time (40 women), 47 part-time/adjunct (45 women). *Students:* 62 full-time (43 women), 259 part-time (239 women); includes 61 minority (28 Black or African American, non-Hispanic/Latino; 3 American Indian or Alaska Native, non-Hispanic/Latino; 16 Asian, non-Hispanic/Latino; 10 Hispanic/Latino; 4 Two or more races, non-Hispanic/Latino). Average age 35. 102 applicants, 35% accepted, 36 enrolled. In 2015, 116 master's, 23 doctorates awarded. *Degree requirements:* For master's, thesis or alternative. *Entrance requirements:* For master's, minimum undergraduate GPA of 3.2; for doctorate, GRE, 3 letters of reference. Additional exam requirements/recommendations for international students: Required—TOEFL (minimum score 550 paper-based; 80 iBT). *Application deadline:* For fall admission, 2/1 priority date for domestic and international students; for spring admission, 9/1 priority date for domestic and international students. Application fee: $45 ($50 for international students). *Financial support:* In 2015–16, 2 teaching assistantships with partial tuition reimbursements (averaging $6,650 per year) were awarded; fellowships, research assistantships, career-related internships or fieldwork, Federal Work-Study, institutionally sponsored loans, and tuition waivers (full and partial) also available. Support available to part-time students. Financial award application deadline: 3/1; financial award applicants required to submit FAFSA. *Faculty research:* Geriatrics/gerontology, children's pain, neonatology, Alzheimer's care, cancer caregivers. *Unit head:* Dr. Ann Cary, Dean, 816-235-1723, Fax: 816-235-1701, E-mail: caryah@umkc.edu. *Application contact:* Judy Jellison, Coordinator for Admissions and Recruitment, 816-235-1740, Fax: 816-235-1701, E-mail: jellisonj@umkc.edu.
Website: http://nursing.umkc.edu/

University of Missouri–St. Louis, College of Nursing, St. Louis, MO 63121-4400. Offers adult/geriatric nurse practitioner (Post Master's Certificate); family nurse practitioner (Post Master's Certificate); nurse educator (MSN); nurse practitioner (MSN); nursing (DNP, PhD); pediatric nurse practitioner (Post Master's Certificate); psychiatric-mental health nurse practitioner (Post Master's Certificate); women's health nurse practitioner (Post Master's Certificate). *Accreditation:* AACN. *Program availability:* Part-time. *Faculty:* 21 full-time (19 women), 6 part-time/adjunct (5 women). *Students:* 18 full-time (17 women), 227 part-time (215 women); includes 34 minority (22 Black or African American, non-Hispanic/Latino; 8 Asian, non-Hispanic/Latino; 3 Hispanic/Latino; 1 Two or more races, non-Hispanic/Latino), 1 international. Average age 35. 152 applicants, 69% accepted, 83 enrolled. *Degree requirements:* For doctorate, comprehensive exam, thesis/dissertation; for Post Master's Certificate, thesis. *Entrance requirements:* For master's, 2 recommendation letters; minimum GPA of 3.0; BSN; nursing licensure; statement of purpose; course in differential/inferential statistics; for doctorate, GRE, 2 letters of recommendation, MSN, minimum GPA of 3.2, course in differential/inferential statistics; for Post Master's Certificate, 2 recommendation letters; MSN; advanced practice certificate; minimum GPA of 3.0; essay. Additional exam requirements/recommendations for international students: Recommended—TOEFL (minimum score 550 paper-based; 79 iBT), IELTS (minimum score 6.5). *Application deadline:* For fall admission, 2/15 for domestic and international students. Application fee: $50 ($40 for international students). Electronic applications accepted. *Financial support:* Research assistantships with tuition reimbursements available. Financial award application deadline: 4/1; financial award applicants required to submit FAFSA. *Faculty research:* Health promotion and restoration, family disruption, violence, abuse, battered women, health survey methods. *Unit head:* Dr. Roberta Lavin, Director, 314-516-6066. *Application contact:* 314-516-5458, Fax: 314-516-6996, E-mail: gradadm@umsl.edu.
Website: http://www.umsl.edu/divisions/nursing

University of Pennsylvania, School of Nursing, Women's Health/Gender Related Nurse Practitioner Program, Philadelphia, PA 19104. Offers MSN. *Accreditation:* AACN. *Program availability:* Part-time, online learning. *Students:* 8 full-time (all women), 16 part-time (all women); includes 4 minority (2 Asian, non-Hispanic/Latino; 2 Hispanic/Latino). Average age 28. 25 applicants, 72% accepted, 13 enrolled. In 2015, 14 master's awarded. *Expenses: Tuition, area resident:* Full-time $31,068; part-time $5762 per course. *Required fees:* $3200; $336 per course. Full-time tuition and fees vary according to degree level, program and student level. Part-time tuition and fees vary according to course load, degree level and program. *Financial support:* Application deadline: 4/1. Website: http://www.nursing.edu/

University of South Carolina, The Graduate School, College of Nursing, Program in Clinical Nursing, Columbia, SC 29208. Offers acute care clinical specialist (MSN); acute care nurse practitioner (MSN); women's health nurse practitioner (MSN). *Accreditation:* AACN. *Program availability:* Part-time. *Degree requirements:* For master's, thesis or alternative. *Entrance requirements:* For master's, GRE General Test or MAT, BS in nursing, RN licensure. Additional exam requirements/recommendations for international students: Required—TOEFL (minimum score 570 paper-based). Electronic applications accepted. *Faculty research:* Systems research, evidence based practice, breast cancer, violence.

Vanderbilt University, Vanderbilt University School of Nursing, Nashville, TN 37240. Offers adult-gerontology acute care nurse practitioner (MSN), including hospitalist, intensivist; adult-gerontology primary care nurse practitioner (MSN); emergency nurse practitioner (MSN); family nurse practitioner (MSN); healthcare leadership (MSN); neonatal nurse practitioner (MSN); nurse midwifery (MSN); nurse midwifery/family nurse practitioner (MSN); nursing (Post-Master's Certificate); nursing informatics (MSN); nursing practice (DNP); nursing science (PhD); pediatric acute care nurse practitioner (MSN); pediatric primary care nurse practitioner (MSN); psychiatric-mental health nurse practitioner (MSN); women's health nurse practitioner (MSN); women's health nurse practitioner/adult gerontology primary care nurse practitioner (MSN); MSN/M Div; MSN/MTS. *Accreditation:* ACEN (one or more programs are accredited); ACNM/ACME. *Program availability:* Part-time, 100% online, blended/hybrid learning. *Faculty:* 258 full-time (232 women), 363 part-time/adjunct (271 women). *Students:* 478 full-time (424 women), 342 part-time (317 women); includes 140 minority (36 Black or African American, non-Hispanic/Latino; 3 American Indian or Alaska Native, non-Hispanic/Latino; 24 Asian, non-Hispanic/Latino; 43 Hispanic/Latino; 3 Native Hawaiian or other Pacific Islander, non-Hispanic/Latino; 31 Two or more races, non-Hispanic/Latino), 11 international. Average age 31. 1,268 applicants, 49% accepted, 477 enrolled. In 2015, 343 master's, 55 doctorates awarded. *Degree requirements:* For doctorate, comprehensive exam, thesis/dissertation. *Entrance requirements:* For master's, GRE General Test (taken within the past 5 years), minimum B average in undergraduate course work, 3 letters of recommendation; for doctorate, GRE General Test, interview, 3 letters of recommendation from doctorally-prepared faculty, MSN, essay. Additional exam requirements/recommendations for international students: Required—TOEFL (minimum score 570 paper-based), IELTS (minimum score 6.5). *Application deadline:* For fall admission, 11/1 priority date for domestic and international students. Applications are processed on a rolling basis. Application fee: $50. Electronic applications accepted. *Expenses:* Contact institution. *Financial support:* In 2015–16, 585 students received support. Scholarships/grants available. Financial award application deadline: 3/15; financial award applicants required to submit FAFSA. *Faculty research:* Lymphedema, palliative care and bereavement, health services research including workforce, safety and quality of care, gerontology, better birth outcomes including nutrition. *Total annual research expenditures:* $2 million. *Unit head:* Dr. Linda Norman, Dean, 615-343-8876, Fax: 615-343-7711, E-mail: linda.norman@vanderbilt.edu. *Application contact:* Patricia Peerman, Assistant Dean for Enrollment Management, 615-322-3800, Fax: 615-343-0333, E-mail: vusn-admissions@vanderbilt.edu.
Website: http://www.nursing.vanderbilt.edu

Virginia Commonwealth University, Graduate School, School of Nursing, Richmond, VA 23284-9005. Offers adult health acute nursing (MS); adult health primary nursing (MS); biobehavioral clinical research (PhD); child health nursing (MS); clinical nurse leader (MS); family health nursing (MS); nurse educator (MS); nurse practitioner (MS); nursing (Certificate); nursing administration (MS), including clinical nurse manager; psychiatric-mental health nursing (MS); quality and safety in health care (DNP); women's health nursing (MS). *Accreditation:* ACEN (one or more programs are accredited). *Program availability:* Part-time, evening/weekend, online learning. *Degree requirements:* For master's, thesis optional; for doctorate, thesis/dissertation. *Entrance requirements:* For master's, GRE General Test, BSN, minimum GPA of 2.8; for doctorate, GRE General Test. Additional exam requirements/recommendations for international students: Required—TOEFL (minimum score 600 paper-based; 100 iBT). Electronic applications accepted.

Section 24
Public Health

This section contains a directory of institutions offering graduate work in public health, followed by in-depth entries submitted by institutions that chose to prepare detailed program descriptions. Additional information about programs listed in the directory but not augmented by an in-depth entry may be obtained by writing directly to the dean of a graduate school or chair of a department at the address given in the directory.

For programs offering related work, see also in this book *Allied Health; Biological and Biomedical Sciences; Ecology, Environmental Biology, and Evolutionary Biology; Health Services; Microbiological Sciences; Nursing;* and *Nutrition.* In the other guides in this series:

Graduate Programs in the Humanities, Arts & Social Sciences

See *Family and Consumer Sciences (Gerontology)* and *Sociology, Anthropology, and Archaeology (Demography and Population Studies)*

Graduate Programs in the Physical Sciences, Mathematics, Agricultural Sciences, the Environment & Natural Resources

See *Mathematical Sciences* and *Environmental Sciences and Management*

Graduate Programs in Engineering & Applied Sciences

See *Biomedical Engineering and Biotechnology, Civil and Environmental Engineering, Industrial Engineering, Energy and Power Engineering (Nuclear Engineering),* and *Management of Engineering and Technology*

Graduate Programs in Business, Education, Information Studies, Law & Social Work

See *Education.*

CONTENTS

Program Directories

Public Health—General

Adelphi University, College of Nursing and Public Health, Program in Public Health, Garden City, NY 11530-0701. Offers MPH.

Adelphi University, University College, Graduate Certificate in Emergency Management Program, Garden City, NY 11530-0701. Offers Certificate. *Program availability:* Part-time, evening/weekend. Electronic applications accepted. *Faculty research:* Emergency nursing, disaster management, disaster preparedness.

Allen College, Graduate Programs, Waterloo, IA 50703. Offers acute care nurse practitioner (Post-Master's Certificate); adult nurse practitioner (Post-Master's Certificate); adult psychiatric-mental health nurse practitioner (Post-Master's Certificate); adult-gerontology acute care nurse practitioner (MSN); community public health (Post-Master's Certificate); community/public health nursing (MSN); family nurse practitioner (MSN, Post-Master's Certificate); gerontological nurse practitioner (Post-Master's Certificate); health sciences (Ed D); leadership in health care delivery (MSN, Post-Master's Certificate); nursing (DNP); occupational therapy (MS). *Accreditation:* AACN; ACEN. *Program availability:* Part-time, blended/hybrid learning. *Faculty:* 3 full-time (all women), 21 part-time/adjunct (20 women). *Students:* 61 full-time (54 women), 163 part-time (144 women); includes 9 minority (5 Black or African American, non-Hispanic/Latino; 2 Hispanic/Latino; 2 Two or more races, non-Hispanic/Latino), 2 international. Average age 34. 212 applicants, 60% accepted, 94 enrolled. In 2015, 51 master's, 1 doctorate awarded. *Degree requirements:* For master's, thesis optional. *Entrance requirements:* For master's, minimum GPA of 3.0 in the last 60 hours of undergraduate coursework; for doctorate, minimum GPA of 3.25 in graduate coursework. Additional exam requirements/recommendations for international students: Recommended—TOEFL (minimum score 580 paper-based; 92 iBT), IELTS (minimum score 6). *Application deadline:* For fall admission, 2/1 priority date for domestic students; for spring admission, 9/1 priority date for domestic students. Applications are processed on a rolling basis. Application fee: $50. Electronic applications accepted. *Expenses:* $15,940 tuition, $1,240 fees. *Financial support:* Institutionally sponsored loans, scholarships/grants, and traineeships available. Support available to part-time students. Financial award application deadline: 8/15; financial award applicants required to submit FAFSA. *Unit head:* Nancy Kramer, Vice Chancellor for Academic Affairs, 319-226-2040, Fax: 319-226-2070, E-mail: nancy.kramer@allencollege.edu. *Application contact:* Molly Quinn, Administrative Assistant for Student Services, 319-226-2014, Fax: 319-226-2010, E-mail: admissions@allencollege.edu.
Website: http://www.allencollege.edu/

American Public University System, AMU/APU Graduate Programs, Charles Town, WV 25414. Offers accounting (MBA, MS); analytics (MBA); criminal justice (MA), including business administration, emergency and disaster management, general (MA, MS); educational leadership (M Ed); emergency and disaster management (MA); entrepreneurship (MBA); environmental policy and management (MS), including environmental planning, environmental sustainability, fish and wildlife management, general (MA, MS), global environmental management; finance (MBA); general (MBA); global business management (MBA); government contracting and acquisition (MBA); health care administration (MBA); history (MA), including American history, ancient and classical history, European history, global history, public history; homeland security (MA), including business administration, counterterrorism studies, criminal justice, cyber, emergency management and public health, intelligence studies, transportation security; homeland security resource allocation (MBA); humanities (MA); information technology (MS), including digital forensics, enterprise software development, information assurance and security, IT project management; information technology management (MBA); intelligence studies (MA), including criminal intelligence, cyber, general (MA, MS), homeland security, intelligence analysis, intelligence collection, intelligence management, intelligence operations, terrorism studies; international relations and conflict resolution (MA), including comparative and security issues, conflict resolution, international and transnational security issues, peacekeeping; legal studies (MA); management (MA), including strategic consulting; marketing (MBA); military history (MA), including American military history, American Revolution, civil war, war since 1945, World War II; military studies (MA), including joint warfare, strategic leadership; national security studies (MA), including cyber, general (MA, MS), homeland security, regional security studies, security and intelligence analysis, terrorism studies; nonprofit management (MBA); political science (MA), including American politics and government, comparative government and development, general (MA, MS), international relations, public policy; psychology (MA); public administration (MPA), including disaster management, environmental policy, health policy, human resources, national security, organizational management, security management; public health (MPH); reverse logistics management (MA); school counseling (M Ed); security management (MA); space studies (MS), including aerospace science, general (MA, MS), planetary science; sports and health sciences (MS); sports management (MBA); teaching (M Ed), including autism spectrum disorder, curriculum and instruction for elementary teachers, elementary reading, English language learners, instructional leadership, online learning, special education, STEAM (STEM plus the arts); transportation and logistics management (MA). *Program availability:* Part-time, evening/weekend, online only. *Faculty:* 431 full-time (241 women), 1,839 part-time/adjunct (865 women). *Students:* 531 full-time (233 women), 9,094 part-time (3,735 women); includes 3,140 minority (1,679 Black or African American, non-Hispanic/Latino; 55 American Indian or Alaska Native, non-Hispanic/Latino; 252 Asian, non-Hispanic/Latino; 773 Hispanic/Latino; 75 Native Hawaiian or other Pacific Islander, non-Hispanic/Latino; 306 Two or more races, non-Hispanic/Latino), 111 international. Average age 37. In 2015, 3,391 master's awarded. *Degree requirements:* For master's, comprehensive exam or practicum. *Entrance requirements:* For master's, official transcript showing earned bachelor's degree from institution accredited by recognized accrediting body. Additional exam requirements/recommendations for international students: Required—TOEFL (minimum score 550 paper-based), IELTS (minimum score 6.5). *Application deadline:* Applications are processed on a rolling basis. Application fee: $0. Electronic applications accepted. *Expenses: Tuition, area resident:* Part-time $350 per credit hour. *Financial support:* Applicants required to submit FAFSA. *Unit head:* Dr. Karan Powell, Executive Vice President and Provost, 877-468-6268, Fax: 304-724-3780. *Application contact:* Terry Grant, Vice President of Enrollment Management, 877-468-6268, Fax: 304-724-3780, E-mail: info@apus.edu.
Website: http://www.apus.edu

American University of Armenia, Graduate Programs, Yerevan, Armenia. Offers business administration (MBA); computer and information science (MS), including business management, design and manufacturing, energy (ME, MS), industrial engineering and systems management; economics (MS); industrial engineering and systems management (ME), including business, computer aided design/manufacturing, energy (ME, MS), information technology; law (LL M); political science and international affairs (MPSIA); public health (MPH); teaching English as a foreign language (MA).

Program availability: Part-time, evening/weekend. *Degree requirements:* For master's, thesis (for some programs), capstone/project. *Entrance requirements:* For master's, GRE, GMAT, or LSAT. Additional exam requirements/recommendations for international students: Recommended—TOEFL (minimum score 79 iBT), IELTS (minimum score 6.5). *Faculty research:* Microfinance, finance (rural/development, international, corporate), firm life cycle theory, TESOL, language proficiency testing, public policy, administrative law, economic development, cryptography, artificial intelligence, energy efficiency/renewable energy, computer-aided design/manufacturing, health financing, tuberculosis control, mother/child health, preventive ophthalmology, post-earthquake psychopathological investigations, tobacco control, environmental health risk assessments.

Andrews University, School of Health Professions, Department of Nutrition, Berrien Springs, MI 49104. Offers nutrition (MS); nutrition and dietetics (Certificate); public health (MPH). *Program availability:* Part-time. *Faculty:* 1 (woman) full-time/adjunct (2 women). *Students:* 19 full-time (18 women), 22 part-time (19 women); includes 15 minority (5 Black or African American, non-Hispanic/Latino; 2 Asian, non-Hispanic/Latino; 7 Hispanic/Latino; 1 Two or more races, non-Hispanic/Latino), 4 international. Average age 31. 50 applicants, 50% accepted, 25 enrolled. In 2015, 1 master's, 11 other advanced degrees awarded. *Entrance requirements:* For master's, GRE. Additional exam requirements/recommendations for international students: Required—TOEFL (minimum score 550 paper-based). *Application deadline:* Applications are processed on a rolling basis. Application fee: $40. *Faculty research:* Exercise education. *Unit head:* Dr. Sherine Brown-Fraser, Chairperson, 269-471-3370. *Application contact:* Monica Wringer, Supervisor of Graduate Admission, 800-253-2874, Fax: 269-471-6321, E-mail: graduate@andrews.edu.
Website: http://www.andrews.edu/shp/nutrition/

Arcadia University, Graduate Studies, Program in Public Health, Glenside, PA 19038-3295. Offers MPH. *Accreditation:* CEPH. *Students:* 22 full-time (17 women), 27 part-time (23 women); includes 15 minority (7 Black or African American, non-Hispanic/Latino; 6 Asian, non-Hispanic/Latino; 2 Hispanic/Latino). Average age 28. 113 applicants, 90% accepted, 20 enrolled. In 2015, 25 master's awarded. *Expenses: Tuition, area resident:* Full-time $28,364; part-time $720 per credit hour. Tuition and fees vary according to course load and program. *Unit head:* Dr. Andrea Crivelli-Kovach, Coordinator, 215-572-4014. *Application contact:* 215-572-2910, Fax: 215-572-4049, E-mail: admiss@arcadia.edu.
Website: http://www.arcadia.edu/academic/public-health/

Argosy University, Atlanta, College of Health Sciences, Atlanta, GA 30328. Offers public health (MPH).

Argosy University, Chicago, College of Health Sciences, Chicago, IL 60601. Offers public health (MPH).

Argosy University, Dallas, College of Health Sciences, Farmers Branch, TX 75244. Offers public health (MPH).

Argosy University, Denver, College of Health Sciences, Denver, CO 80231. Offers public health (MPH).

Argosy University, Hawai`i, College of Health Sciences, Honolulu, HI 96813. Offers public health (MPH).

Argosy University, Inland Empire, College of Health Sciences, Ontario, CA 91761. Offers public health (MPH).

Argosy University, Los Angeles, College of Health Sciences, Santa Monica, CA 90045. Offers public health (MPH).

Argosy University, Nashville, College of Health Sciences, Nashville, TN 37214. Offers public health (MPH).

Argosy University, Orange County, College of Health Sciences, Orange, CA 92868. Offers public health (MPH).

Argosy University, Phoenix, College of Health Sciences, Phoenix, AZ 85021. Offers public health (MPH).

Argosy University, Salt Lake City, College of Health Sciences, Draper, UT 84020. Offers public health (MPH).

Argosy University, San Diego, College of Health Sciences, San Diego, CA 92108. Offers public health (MPH).

Argosy University, San Francisco Bay Area, College of Health Sciences, Alameda, CA 94501. Offers public health (MPH).

Argosy University, Sarasota, College of Health Sciences, Sarasota, FL 34235. Offers public health (MPH).

Argosy University, Schaumburg, College of Health Sciences, Schaumburg, IL 60173-5403. Offers public health (MPH).

Argosy University, Seattle, College of Health Sciences, Seattle, WA 98121. Offers public health (MPH).

Argosy University, Tampa, College of Health Sciences, Tampa, FL 33607. Offers public health (MPH).

Argosy University, Twin Cities, College of Health Sciences, Eagan, MN 55121. Offers health services management (MS); public health (MPH).

Argosy University, Washington DC, College of Health Sciences, Arlington, VA 22209. Offers public health (MPH).

Arizona State University at the Tempe campus, College of Nursing and Health Innovation, Phoenix, AZ 85004. Offers advanced nursing practice (DNP); clinical research management (MS); community and public health practice (Graduate Certificate); family mental health nurse practitioner (Graduate Certificate); family nurse practitioner (Graduate Certificate); geriatric nursing (Graduate Certificate); healthcare innovation (MHI); nurse education in academic and practice settings (Graduate Certificate); nurse educator (MS); nursing and healthcare innovation (PhD). *Accreditation:* AACN. *Program availability:* Online learning. *Degree requirements:* For master's, comprehensive exam (for some programs), thesis (for some programs), interactive Program of Study (iPOS) submitted before completing 50 percent of required credit hours; for doctorate, comprehensive exam, thesis/dissertation, interactive Program of Study (iPOS) submitted before completing 50 percent of required credit hours. *Entrance requirements:* For master's and doctorate, GRE, minimum GPA of 3.0 or equivalent in last 2 years of work leading to bachelor's degree. Additional exam requirements/recommendations for international students: Required—TOEFL, IELTS, or PTE. Electronic applications accepted. *Expenses:* Contact institution.

Armstrong State University, School of Graduate Studies, Program in Public Health, Savannah, GA 31419-1997. Offers MPH. *Accreditation:* CEPH. *Program availability:* Part-time, evening/weekend, online learning. *Faculty:* 4 full-time (all women), 2 part-time/adjunct (1 woman). *Students:* 46 full-time (37 women), 8 part-time (5 women); includes 29 minority (24 Black or African American, non-Hispanic/Latino; 2 Asian, non-Hispanic/Latino; 2 Hispanic/Latino; 1 Two or more races, non-Hispanic/Latino), 7 international. Average age 28. 25 applicants, 92% accepted, 17 enrolled. In 2015, 34 master's awarded. *Degree requirements:* For master's, comprehensive exam, thesis optional, internship. *Entrance requirements:* For master's, GMAT or GRE General Test, MAT, letters of recommendation, letter of intent, minimum undergraduate GPA of 2.8. Additional exam requirements/recommendations for international students: Required—TOEFL. *Application deadline:* For fall admission, 6/1 priority date for domestic students, 5/1 priority date for international students; for spring admission, 11/15 priority date for domestic students, 9/15 priority date for international students; for summer admission, 4/15 for domestic students, 9/15 priority date for international students. Applications are processed on a rolling basis. Application fee: $30. Electronic applications accepted. *Expenses:* Tuition, state resident: part-time $211 per credit hour. Tuition, nonresident: part-time $782 per credit hour. *Required fees:* $1224 per unit. $612 per semester. Tuition and fees vary according to course load, campus/location and program. *Financial support:* In 2015–16, research assistantships with full tuition reimbursements (averaging $5,000 per year) were awarded; career-related internships or fieldwork, Federal Work-Study, scholarships/grants, tuition waivers (full), and unspecified assistantships also available. Support available to part-time students. Financial award application deadline: 3/15; financial award applicants required to submit FAFSA. *Unit head:* Dr. Robert LeFavi, Interim Department Head, 912-344-3208, Fax: 912-344-3477, E-mail: robert.lefavi@armstrong.edu. *Application contact:* McKenzie Peterman, Assistant Director of Graduate Admissions, 912-344-2503, Fax: 912-344-3417, E-mail: graduate@armstrong.edu.
Website: http://www.armstrong.edu/Health_Professions/Health_Sciences/healthsciences_master_of_public_health

A.T. Still University, College of Graduate Health Studies, Kirksville, MO 63501. Offers dental public health (MPH); health administration (MHA, DHA); health education (DH Ed); health sciences (DH Sc); kinesiology (MS); public health (MPH); school health education (MS). *Program availability:* Part-time, evening/weekend, 100% online, blended/hybrid learning. *Faculty:* 29 full-time (18 women), 89 part-time/adjunct (46 women). *Students:* 456 full-time (271 women), 391 part-time (232 women); includes 291 minority (126 Black or African American, non-Hispanic/Latino; 7 American Indian or Alaska Native, non-Hispanic/Latino; 71 Asian, non-Hispanic/Latino; 80 Hispanic/Latino; 4 Native Hawaiian or other Pacific Islander, non-Hispanic/Latino; 3 Two or more races, non-Hispanic/Latino), 21 international. Average age 37. 286 applicants, 99% accepted, 221 enrolled. In 2015, 130 master's, 74 doctorates awarded. *Degree requirements:* For master's, thesis, integrated terminal project, practicum; for doctorate, thesis/dissertation. *Entrance requirements:* For master's, minimum GPA of 3.0, bachelor's degree or equivalent, background check, essay, three references; for doctorate, minimum GPA of 3.0, master's or terminal degree, background check, essay, three references. Additional exam requirements/recommendations for international students: Required—TOEFL (minimum score 550 paper-based; 80 iBT). *Application deadline:* For fall admission, 5/16 for domestic and international students; for winter admission, 8/1 for domestic and international students; for spring admission, 11/7 for domestic and international students; for summer admission, 1/23 for domestic and international students. Applications are processed on a rolling basis. Application fee: $70. Electronic applications accepted. Application fee is waived when completed online. *Expenses:* Contact institution. *Financial support:* In 2015–16, 30 students received support. Scholarships/grants available. Financial award application deadline: 5/1; financial award applicants required to submit FAFSA. *Faculty research:* Public health: influence of availability of comprehensive wellness resources online, student wellness, oral health care needs assessment of community, oral health knowledge and behaviors of Medicaid-eligible pregnant women and mothers of young children in relations to early childhood caries and tooth decay, alcohol use and alcohol related problems among college students. *Unit head:* Dr. Donald Altman, Interim Dean, Fax: 660-626-2826, E-mail: daltman@atsu.edu. *Application contact:* Amie Waldemer, Associate Director, Online Admissions, 480-219-6146, E-mail: awaldemer@atsu.edu.
Website: http://www.atsu.edu/college-of-graduate-health-studies

Auburn University at Montgomery, College of Public Policy and Justice, Department of Political Science and Public Administration, Montgomery, AL 36124-4023. Offers international relations (MIR); nonprofit management and leadership (Certificate); political science (MPS); public administration (MPA); public administration and public policy (PhD); public health care administration and policy (Certificate). PhD offered jointly with Auburn University. *Accreditation:* NASPAA (one or more programs are accredited). *Program availability:* Part-time, evening/weekend. *Faculty:* 5 full-time (1 woman), 1 part-time/adjunct (0 women). *Students:* 5 full-time (3 women), 44 part-time (30 women); includes 13 minority (10 Black or African American, non-Hispanic/Latino; 2 American Indian or Alaska Native, non-Hispanic/Latino; 1 Hispanic/Latino), 1 international. Average age 29. 32 applicants, 88% accepted, 19 enrolled. In 2015, 15 master's awarded. *Degree requirements:* For master's, comprehensive exam; for doctorate, thesis/dissertation. *Entrance requirements:* For master's, GRE General Test or MAT; for doctorate, GRE General Test. *Application deadline:* Applications are processed on a rolling basis. Electronic applications accepted. *Expenses:* Tuition, state resident: full-time $6462; part-time $359 per credit hour. Tuition, nonresident: full-time $14,526; part-time $807 per credit hour. *Required fees:* $554. *Financial support:* In 2015–16, 1 teaching assistantship was awarded; research assistantships, career-related internships or fieldwork, and scholarships/grants also available. Support available to part-time students. Financial award application deadline: 3/1; financial award applicants required to submit FAFSA. *Unit head:* Dr. Andrew Cortell, Department Head, 334-244-3622, E-mail: acortell@aum.edu.
Website: http://www.cla.auburn.edu/polisci/graduate-programs/phd-in-public-administration-and-public-policy/

Augusta University, College of Allied Health Sciences, Program in Public Health, Augusta, GA 30912. Offers environmental health (MPH); health informatics (MPH); health management (MPH); social and behavioral sciences (MPH). *Program availability:* Part-time. *Degree requirements:* For master's, thesis (for some programs). *Entrance requirements:* For master's, GRE General Test, three letters of recommendation. Additional exam requirements/recommendations for international students: Required—TOEFL. *Application deadline:* For fall admission, 5/1 for domestic and international students. Application fee: $50. Electronic applications accepted. *Financial support:* Federal Work-Study available. Financial award application deadline: 5/31; financial award applicants required to submit FAFSA. *Unit head:* Dr. Andrew Balas, Dean, College of Allied Health Sciences, 706-721-2621, Fax: 706-721-7312. *Application contact:* Dr. Pavani Rangachari, Director, 706-721-4830, E-mail: prangachari@augusta.edu.
Website: http://www.augusta.edu/alliedhealth/cdhs/mph/

Austin Peay State University, College of Graduate Studies, College of Behavioral and Health Sciences, Department of Health and Human Performance, Clarksville, TN 37044. Offers public health education (MS); sports and wellness leadership (MS). *Program*

availability: Part-time, evening/weekend, online learning. *Faculty:* 6 full-time (3 women). *Students:* 15 full-time (5 women), 35 part-time (24 women); includes 17 minority (12 Black or African American, non-Hispanic/Latino; 1 Asian, non-Hispanic/Latino; 2 Hispanic/Latino; 2 Two or more races, non-Hispanic/Latino). Average age 29. 58 applicants, 86% accepted, 34 enrolled. In 2015, 28 master's awarded. *Degree requirements:* For master's, comprehensive exam, thesis optional. *Entrance requirements:* For master's, GRE General Test, 3 letters of recommendation, minimum undergraduate GPA of 2.5. Additional exam requirements/recommendations for international students: Required—TOEFL (minimum score 500 paper-based). *Application deadline:* For fall admission, 8/3 priority date for domestic students. Applications are processed on a rolling basis. Application fee: $25. Electronic applications accepted. *Expenses:* Tuition, state resident: full-time $8080; part-time $404 per credit hour. Tuition, nonresident: full-time $21,680; part-time $1084 per credit hour. *Required fees:* $1453; $72.65 per credit hour. *Financial support:* In 2015–16, research assistantships with full tuition reimbursements (averaging $5,184 per year) were awarded; career-related internships or fieldwork, Federal Work-Study, institutionally sponsored loans, scholarships/grants, and unspecified assistantships also available. Support available to part-time students. Financial award application deadline: 3/1; financial award applicants required to submit FAFSA. *Unit head:* Dr. Marcy Maurer, Chair, 931-221-6105, Fax: 931-221-7040, E-mail: maurerm@apsu.edu. *Application contact:* June D. Lee, Graduate Coordinator, 800-859-4723, Fax: 931-221-7641, E-mail: gradadmissions@apsu.edu.
Website: http://www.apsu.edu/hhp/

Barry University, School of Podiatric Medicine, Podiatric Medicine and Surgery Program, Podiatric Medicine/Public Health Option, Miami Shores, FL 33161-6695. Offers DPM/MPH.

Benedictine University, Graduate Programs, Program in Public Health, Lisle, IL 60532. Offers administration of health care institutions (MPH); dietetics (MPH); disaster management (MPH); health education (MPH); health information systems (MPH); MBA/MPH; MPH/MS. *Accreditation:* CEPH. *Program availability:* Part-time, evening/weekend, online learning. *Entrance requirements:* For master's, MAT, GRE, or GMAT. Additional exam requirements/recommendations for international students: Required—TOEFL (minimum score 550 paper-based).

Boise State University, College of Health Sciences, Boise, ID 83725. Offers MAL, MHS, MK, MSN, MSW, DNP, Graduate Certificate. *Program availability:* Part-time, 100% online. *Faculty:* 72. *Students:* 221 full-time (174 women), 183 part-time (138 women); includes 42 minority (11 Black or African American, non-Hispanic/Latino; 3 Asian, non-Hispanic/Latino; 24 Hispanic/Latino; 1 Native Hawaiian or other Pacific Islander, non-Hispanic/Latino; 3 Two or more races, non-Hispanic/Latino). Average age 35. 246 applicants, 49% accepted, 85 enrolled. In 2015, 151 master's, 13 other advanced degrees awarded. *Degree requirements:* For master's, comprehensive exam (for some programs), thesis (for some programs); for doctorate, thesis/dissertation. *Entrance requirements:* For master's, GRE General Test, GMAT or MAT, minimum GPA of 3.0. Additional exam requirements/recommendations for international students: Required—TOEFL (minimum score 550 paper-based; 80 iBT), IELTS (minimum score 6). *Application deadline:* Applications are processed on a rolling basis. Application fee: $65 ($95 for international students). Electronic applications accepted. *Expenses:* Tuition, state resident: full-time $6058; part-time $358 per credit hour. Tuition, nonresident: full-time $20,108; part-time $608 per credit hour. *Required fees:* $2108. Tuition and fees vary according to program. *Financial support:* In 2015–16, 79 students received support, including 4 research assistantships (averaging $3,510 per year); scholarships/grants and unspecified assistantships also available. Financial award applicants required to submit FAFSA. *Unit head:* Dr. Tim Dunnagan, Dean, 208-426-4150, Fax: 208-426-3469. *Application contact:* Dr. Tedd McDonald, Program Director, 208-426-2425, E-mail: tmcdonal@boisestate.edu.
Website: http://hs.boisestate.edu/

Boston University, Henry M. Goldman School of Dental Medicine, Boston, MA 02118. Offers dental public health (MS, MSD, D Sc D); dentistry (DMD); endodontics (MSD, D Sc D, CAGS); operative dentistry (MSD, D Sc D, CAGS); oral and maxillofacial surgery (MSD, D Sc D, CAGS); oral biology (MSD, D Sc D); orthodontics (MSD, D Sc D); pediatric dentistry (MSD, D Sc D, CAGS); periodontology (MSD, D Sc D, CAGS); prosthodontics (D Sc D). *Accreditation:* ADA (one or more programs are accredited). *Faculty:* 136 full-time (60 women), 90 part-time/adjunct (31 women). *Students:* 812 full-time (428 women), 2 part-time (1 woman); includes 195 minority (12 Black or African American, non-Hispanic/Latino; 127 Asian, non-Hispanic/Latino; 42 Hispanic/Latino; 14 Two or more races, non-Hispanic/Latino), 316 international. Average age 28. 6,681 applicants, 8% accepted, 263 enrolled. In 2015, 23 master's, 204 doctorates, 59 other advanced degrees awarded. *Degree requirements:* For master's and CAGS, thesis; for doctorate, thesis/dissertation (for some programs). *Entrance requirements:* For doctorate, DAT (for DMD), minimum recommended GPA of 3.0 (for DMD); for CAGS, National Board Dental Exam Part 1, dental degree. Additional exam requirements/recommendations for international students: Required—TOEFL. *Application deadline:* For fall admission, 12/1 for domestic and international students. Applications are processed on a rolling basis. Application fee: $75 ($105 for international students). Electronic applications accepted. *Expenses:* Contact institution. *Financial support:* In 2015–16, 125 students received support. Career-related internships or fieldwork, institutionally sponsored loans, scholarships/grants, and stipends available. Financial award application deadline: 4/18; financial award applicants required to submit FAFSA. *Faculty research:* Defense mechanisms, bone-cell regulation, protein biochemistry, molecular biology, biomaterials. *Unit head:* Dr. Jeffrey W. Hutter, Dean, 617-638-4780. *Application contact:* Admissions Representative, 617-638-4787, Fax: 617-638-4798, E-mail: sdmadmis@bu.edu.
Website: http://www.bu.edu/dental

Boston University, School of Public Health, Boston, MA 02118. Offers MA, MPH, MS, Dr PH, PhD, JD/MPH, MBA/MPH, MD/MPH, MPH/MS, MSW/MPH. *Accreditation:* CEPH. *Program availability:* Part-time, evening/weekend. *Faculty:* 153 full-time, 271 part-time/adjunct. *Students:* 607 full-time (488 women), 353 part-time (295 women); includes 263 minority (72 Black or African American, non-Hispanic/Latino; 2 American Indian or Alaska Native, non-Hispanic/Latino; 103 Asian, non-Hispanic/Latino; 57 Hispanic/Latino; 1 Native Hawaiian or other Pacific Islander, non-Hispanic/Latino; 28 Two or more races, non-Hispanic/Latino), 110 international. Average age 27. 2,594 applicants, 43% accepted, 396 enrolled. In 2015, 442 master's, 18 doctorates awarded. *Degree requirements:* For master's, comprehensive exam (for some programs), thesis optional, culminating experience, practicum; for doctorate, thesis/dissertation, comprehensive written and oral exams. *Entrance requirements:* For master's, GRE, GMAT, U.S. bachelor's degree or international equivalent; for doctorate, GRE, GMAT, MPH or equivalent. Additional exam requirements/recommendations for international students: Required—TOEFL (minimum score 600 paper-based; 100 iBT), IELTS (minimum score 7). *Application deadline:* For fall admission, 1/1 priority date for domestic and international students; for spring admission, 10/1 priority date for domestic and international students. Applications are processed on a rolling basis. Application fee: $120. Electronic applications accepted. *Financial support:* In 2015–16, 494 students received support. Fellowships, career-related internships or fieldwork, Federal

Public Health—General

Work-Study, institutionally sponsored loans, scholarships/grants, traineeships, and tuition waivers (partial) available. Support available to part-time students. Financial award application deadline: 5/29; financial award applicants required to submit FAFSA. *Faculty research:* Clinical trials, observational studies, environmental epidemiology, global ecology, environmental sustainability, community health, environmental justice, infectious disease, non-infectious disease, research methods, pharmaceutical assessment, bioethics, health law, human rights, health policy, management, finance and management, family health, disease control in developing countries, child and adolescent health, women's health, health disparities. *Unit head:* Dr. Sandro Galea, Dean, 617-638-4640, Fax: 617-638-5299, E-mail: asksph@bu.edu. *Application contact:* LePhan Quan, Associate Director of Admissions, 617-638-4640, Fax: 617-638-5299, E-mail: asksph@bu.edu.
Website: http://www.bu.edu/sph

Bowling Green State University, Graduate College, College of Health and Human Services, Program in Public Health, Bowling Green, OH 43403. Offers MPH. *Program availability:* Part-time. *Degree requirements:* For master's, thesis or alternative. *Entrance requirements:* For master's, GRE General Test, minimum GPA of 3.0. Additional exam requirements/recommendations for international students: Required—TOEFL. Electronic applications accepted.

Brooklyn College of the City University of New York, School of Natural and Behavioral Sciences, Department of Health and Nutrition Sciences, Program in Public Health, Brooklyn, NY 11210-2889. Offers general public health (MPH); health care policy and administration (MPH). *Accreditation:* CEPH. *Degree requirements:* For master's, thesis or alternative, 46 credits. *Entrance requirements:* For master's, GRE, 2 letters of recommendation, essay, interview. Electronic applications accepted.

Brown University, Graduate School, Division of Biology and Medicine, School of Public Health, Program in Public Health, Providence, RI 02912. Offers MPH. *Accreditation:* CEPH. *Entrance requirements:* For master's, GRE General Test or MCAT. Additional exam requirements/recommendations for international students: Required—TOEFL.

California Baptist University, Program in Public Health, Riverside, CA 92504-3206. Offers health education and promotion (MPH); health policy and administration (MPH). *Program availability:* Part-time, evening/weekend. *Faculty:* 7 full-time (4 women), 3 part-time/adjunct (2 women). *Students:* 41 full-time (36 women), 9 part-time (8 women); includes 33 minority (4 Black or African American, non-Hispanic/Latino; 1 Asian, non-Hispanic/Latino; 26 Hispanic/Latino; 2 Two or more races, non-Hispanic/Latino), 2 international. Average age 25. 41 applicants, 71% accepted, 26 enrolled. *Degree requirements:* For master's, capstone project; practicum. *Entrance requirements:* For master's, minimum undergraduate GPA of 2.75, two recommendations, 500-word essay, resume. Additional exam requirements/recommendations for international students: Required—TOEFL (minimum score 80 iBT). *Application deadline:* For fall admission, 8/1 priority date for domestic students, 7/1 for international students; for spring admission, 12/1 priority date for domestic students, 11/1 for international students. Applications are processed on a rolling basis. Application fee: $45. Electronic applications accepted. *Expenses:* $800 per unit, $355 per semester fees. *Financial support:* Federal Work-Study and scholarships/grants available. Financial award applicants required to submit CSS PROFILE or FAFSA. *Faculty research:* Epidemiology, statistical education, exercise and immunity, obesity and chronic disease. *Unit head:* Dr. David Pearson, Dean, College of Health Science, 951-343-4298, E-mail: dpearson@calbaptist.edu. *Application contact:* Dr. Robert LaChausse, Chair, Department of Public Health Sciences, 951-552-8484, E-mail: rlachausse@calbaptist.edu.
Website: http://www.calbaptist.edu/explore-cbu/schools-colleges/college-allied-health/health-sciences/master-public-health/

California State University, Fresno, Division of Graduate Studies, College of Health and Human Services, Department of Public Health, Fresno, CA 93740-8027. Offers health policy and management (MPH); health promotion (MPH). *Accreditation:* CEPH. *Program availability:* Part-time, evening/weekend. *Degree requirements:* For master's, thesis or alternative. *Entrance requirements:* For master's, GRE General Test, minimum GPA of 2.5. Additional exam requirements/recommendations for international students: Required—TOEFL. Electronic applications accepted. *Faculty research:* Foster parent training, geriatrics, tobacco control.

California State University, Fullerton, Graduate Studies, College of Health and Human Development, Department of Health Science, Fullerton, CA 92834-9480. Offers public health (MPH). *Accreditation:* CEPH. *Program availability:* Part-time. *Entrance requirements:* For master's, minimum GPA of 3.0 in last 60 units attempted.

California State University, Northridge, Graduate Studies, College of Health and Human Development, Department of Health Sciences, Northridge, CA 91330. Offers health administration (MS); public health (MPH). *Accreditation:* CEPH. *Faculty:* 14 full-time (8 women), 47 part-time/adjunct (26 women). *Students:* 107 full-time (83 women), 74 part-time (59 women); includes 63 minority (11 Black or African American, non-Hispanic/Latino; 18 Asian, non-Hispanic/Latino; 30 Hispanic/Latino; 4 Two or more races, non-Hispanic/Latino), 21 international. Average age 30. 258 applicants, 40% accepted, 52 enrolled. *Entrance requirements:* For master's, GRE General Test or minimum GPA of 3.0. Additional exam requirements/recommendations for international students: Required—TOEFL. *Application deadline:* For fall admission, 11/30 for domestic students. Application fee: $55. *Financial support:* Teaching assistantships available. Financial award application deadline: 3/1. *Faculty research:* Labor market needs assessment, health education products, dental hygiene, independent practice prototype. *Unit head:* Anita Slechta, Chair, 818-677-3101.
Website: http://www.csun.edu/hhd/hsci/

California State University, San Bernardino, Graduate Studies, College of Natural Sciences, Program in Public Health, San Bernardino, CA 92407. Offers public health (MPH). *Students:* 2 full-time (both women), 8 part-time (7 women); includes 4 minority (1 Black or African American, non-Hispanic/Latino; 3 Hispanic/Latino), 1 international. 36 applicants, 47% accepted, 6 enrolled. In 2015, 6 master's awarded. *Entrance requirements:* Additional exam requirements/recommendations for international students: Required—TOEFL. *Application deadline:* For fall admission, 5/5 for domestic students. Application fee: $55. *Expenses:* Tuition, state resident: full-time $7843; part-time $5011.20 per year. Tuition and fees vary according to course load, degree level, program and reciprocity agreements. *Unit head:* Dr. Marsha Greer, Chair, 909-537-5341, Fax: 909-537-7037, E-mail: mgreer@csusb.edu. *Application contact:* Dr. Jeffrey Thompson, Dean of Graduate Studies, 909-537-5058, E-mail: jthompso@csusb.edu.

Case Western Reserve University, School of Medicine and School of Graduate Studies, Graduate Programs in Medicine, Department of Epidemiology and Biostatistics, Program in Public Health, Cleveland, OH 44106. Offers MPH. *Accreditation:* CEPH. *Program availability:* Part-time. *Degree requirements:* For master's, essay, field experience, presentation. *Entrance requirements:* For master's, GRE General Test or MCAT, 3 letters of recommendation. Additional exam requirements/recommendations for international students: Required—TOEFL. Electronic applications accepted. *Expenses: Tuition, area resident:* Full-time $41,137; part-time $1714 per credit hour. *Required fees:* $32. Tuition and fees vary according to course load and program. *Faculty*

research: Public policy and aging, statistical modeling, behavioral medicine and evaluation, continuous quality improvement; tobacco cessation and prevention.

Charles R. Drew University of Medicine and Science, College of Science and Health, Los Angeles, CA 90059. Offers urban public health (MPH).

Chicago State University, School of Graduate and Professional Studies, College of Health Sciences, Department of Health Studies, Chicago, IL 60628. Offers public health (MPH).

Claremont Graduate University, Graduate Programs, School of Community and Global Health, Claremont, CA 91773. Offers health promotion science (PhD); public health (MPH). *Accreditation:* CEPH. *Faculty:* 8 full-time (3 women). *Students:* 48 full-time (27 women), 46 part-time (36 women); includes 47 minority (8 Black or African American, non-Hispanic/Latino; 19 Asian, non-Hispanic/Latino; 16 Hispanic/Latino; 4 Two or more races, non-Hispanic/Latino), 14 international. Average age 30. In 2015, 23 master's, 1 doctorate awarded. *Entrance requirements:* For master's and doctorate, GRE. Additional exam requirements/recommendations for international students: Required—TOEFL (minimum score 75 iBT). *Application deadline:* For fall admission, 2/1 priority date for domestic and international students; for spring admission, 11/1 priority date for domestic students. Applications are processed on a rolling basis. Application fee: $80. Electronic applications accepted. *Expenses: Tuition, area resident:* Full-time $43,032; part-time $1793 per unit. *Required fees:* $600; $300 per semester. $300 per semester. Tuition and fees vary according to course load and program. *Financial support:* Fellowships, research assistantships, teaching assistantships, Federal Work-Study, institutionally sponsored loans, and scholarships/grants available. Support available to part-time students. Financial award application deadline: 2/15; financial award applicants required to submit FAFSA. *Unit head:* Stewart Donaldson, Dean, 909-607-8235, E-mail: stewart.donaldson@cgu.edu. *Application contact:* Paige Piontkowsky, Assistant Director of Admissions, 909-607-3240, E-mail: paige.piontkowsky@cgu.edu.
Website: http://www.cgu.edu/pages/5644.asp

Clemson University, Graduate School, College of Behavioral, Social and Health Sciences, Department of Public Health Sciences, Clemson, SC 29634-0745. Offers applied health research and evaluation (MS, PhD); clinical and translational research (Certificate). *Program availability:* Part-time. *Faculty:* 21 full-time (9 women), 7 part-time/adjunct (all women). *Students:* 10 full-time (6 women); includes 2 minority (both Asian, non-Hispanic/Latino). Average age 33. 7 applicants, 29% accepted, 1 enrolled. *Degree requirements:* For doctorate, comprehensive exam, thesis/dissertation. *Entrance requirements:* For master's and Certificate, GRE General Test, curriculum vitae, statement of career goals, letters of recommendation, unofficial transcripts; for doctorate, GRE General Test, MS/MA thesis or publications, curriculum vitae, statement of career goals, letters of recommendation, unofficial transcripts. Additional exam requirements/recommendations for international students: Required—TOEFL (minimum score 80 iBT), IELTS (minimum score 6.5). *Application deadline:* For fall admission, 4/15 for international students; for spring admission, 10/15 for international students. Applications are processed on a rolling basis. Application fee: $80 ($90 for international students). Electronic applications accepted. *Expenses:* $4,060 per semester full-time resident, $8,103 per semester full-time non-resident, $448 per credit hour part-time resident, $898 per credit hour part-time non-resident. *Financial support:* In 2015–16, 3 students received support, including 1 research assistantship with partial tuition reimbursement available (averaging $24,192 per year), 3 teaching assistantships with partial tuition reimbursements available (averaging $12,000 per year). *Faculty research:* Health promotion and behavior, epidemiology and outcomes research, public health informatics, health policy and health services research, global health, evaluation. *Unit head:* Dr. Joel Williams, Director of Graduate Studies/PhD Program Coordinator, 864-656-1017, E-mail: joel2@clemson.edu. *Application contact:* Rebecca Moses, Graduate Student Services Coordinator, 864-656-5502, E-mail: coffey2@clemson.edu.
Website: http://www.clemson.edu/hehd/departments/public-health/academics/graduate-programs/index.html

Cleveland State University, College of Graduate Studies, College of Education and Human Services, Department of Health and Human Performance, Cleveland, OH 44115. Offers community health education (M Ed); exercise science (M Ed); human performance (M Ed); physical education pedagogy (M Ed); public health (MPH); school health education (M Ed); sport and exercise psychology (M Ed); sports management (M Ed). *Program availability:* Part-time. *Faculty:* 7 full-time (4 women), 3 part-time/adjunct (2 women). *Students:* 49 full-time (35 women), 63 part-time (35 women); includes 32 minority (27 Black or African American, non-Hispanic/Latino; 1 Asian, non-Hispanic/Latino; 4 Hispanic/Latino), 15 international. Average age 27. 103 applicants, 72% accepted, 43 enrolled. In 2015, 47 master's awarded. *Degree requirements:* For master's, comprehensive exam, thesis optional. *Entrance requirements:* For master's, GRE General Test or MAT (if undergraduate GPA less than 2.75), minimum undergraduate GPA of 2.75. Additional exam requirements/recommendations for international students: Required—TOEFL (minimum score 550 paper-based; 78 iBT), IELTS (minimum score 6). *Application deadline:* For fall admission, 7/15 priority date for domestic students; for spring admission, 12/15 priority date for domestic students. Applications are processed on a rolling basis. Application fee: $30. Electronic applications accepted. *Expenses:* Tuition, state resident: full-time $9565. Tuition, nonresident: full-time $17,980. Tuition and fees vary according to program. *Financial support:* In 2015–16, 6 research assistantships with tuition reimbursements (averaging $3,480 per year), 1 teaching assistantship with tuition reimbursement (averaging $3,480 per year) were awarded; career-related internships or fieldwork, tuition waivers (full), and unspecified assistantships also available. Financial award application deadline: 3/15; financial award applicants required to submit FAFSA. *Faculty research:* Bone density, marketing fitness centers, motor development of disabled, online learning and survey research. *Unit head:* Dr. Sheila M. Patterson, Chairperson, 216-687-4870, Fax: 216-687-5410, E-mail: s.m.patterson@csuohio.edu. *Application contact:* Deborah L. Brown, Interim Assistant Director, Graduate Admissions, 216-523-7572, Fax: 216-687-5400, E-mail: d.l.brown@csuohio.edu.
Website: http://www.csuohio.edu/cehs/departments/HPERD/hperd_dept.html

Columbia University, Columbia University Mailman School of Public Health, New York, NY 10032. Offers Exec MHA, Exec MPH, MHA, MPH, MS, Dr PH, PhD, DDS/MPH, MBA/MPH, MD/MPH, MPA/MPH, MPH/MIA, MPH/MOT, MPH/MS, MPH/MSN, MPH/MSSW. PhD offered in cooperation with the Graduate School of Arts and Sciences. *Accreditation:* CEPH (one or more programs are accredited). *Program availability:* Part-time, evening/weekend. *Faculty:* 235 full-time (118 women), 233 part-time/adjunct (105 women). *Students:* 521 full-time (359 women), 912 part-time (727 women); includes 505 minority (97 Black or African American, non-Hispanic/Latino; 4 American Indian or Alaska Native, non-Hispanic/Latino; 245 Asian, non-Hispanic/Latino; 123 Hispanic/Latino; 1 Native Hawaiian or other Pacific Islander, non-Hispanic/Latino; 35 Two or more races, non-Hispanic/Latino), 281 international. Average age 28. 2,927 applicants, 58% accepted, 668 enrolled. In 2015, 582 master's, 29 doctorates awarded. *Degree requirements:* For master's, thesis (for some programs); for doctorate, comprehensive exam, thesis/dissertation. *Entrance requirements:* For master's, GRE General Test; for doctorate, GRE General Test, MPH or equivalent (for Dr PH). Additional exam requirements/recommendations for international students: Required—TOEFL (minimum

score 600 paper-based; 100 iBT). *Application deadline:* For fall admission, 12/1 priority date for domestic and international students. Application fee: $120. Electronic applications accepted. *Expenses:* Contact institution. *Financial support:* In 2015–16, 619 students received support. Fellowships, research assistantships, teaching assistantships, career-related internships or fieldwork, Federal Work-Study, and traineeships available. Support available to part-time students. Financial award application deadline: 2/1; financial award applicants required to submit FAFSA. *Unit head:* Dr. Linda P. Fried, Dean/Professor, 212-305-9300, Fax: 212-305-9342, E-mail: lpfried@columbia.edu. *Application contact:* Dr. Joseph Korevec, Senior Director of Admissions and Financial Aid, 212-305-8698, Fax: 212-342-1861, E-mail: ph-admit@columbia.edu.
Website: http://www.mailman.hs.columbia.edu/

Daemen College, Program in Public Health, Amherst, NY 14226-3592. Offers community health education (MPH); epidemiology (MPH); generalist (MPH). *Program availability:* Part-time, online learning. *Degree requirements:* For master's, practicum.

Dartmouth College, The Dartmouth Institute, Program in Public Health, Hanover, NH 03755. Offers MPH. *Accreditation:* CEPH. *Program availability:* Part-time. *Students:* 6 full-time (4 women), 16 part-time (7 women); includes 2 minority (1 Asian, non-Hispanic/Latino; 1 Hispanic/Latino), 2 international. Average age 36. 284 applicants, 54% accepted, 47 enrolled. In 2015, 11 master's awarded. *Degree requirements:* For master's, research project or practicum. *Entrance requirements:* For master's, GRE or MCAT, 3 letters of recommendation. Additional exam requirements/recommendations for international students: Required—TOEFL. *Application deadline:* For fall admission, 1/15 for domestic students. Applications are processed on a rolling basis. Application fee: $50. *Expenses: Tuition, area resident:* Full-time $48,120. *Required fees:* $296. One-time fee: $50 full-time. *Unit head:* Dr. Elliot S. Fisher, Director, 603-653-0802. *Application contact:* Courtney Theroux, Director of Recruitment and Admissions, 603-653-3234, E-mail: courtney.l.theroux@dartmouth.edu.
Website: http://tdi.dartmouth.edu/education/degree-programs/mph-ms

Davenport University, Sneden Graduate School, Grand Rapids, MI 49512. Offers accounting (MBA); business administration (EMBA); finance (MBA); health care management (MBA); human resources (MBA); information assurance (MS); public health (MPH); strategic management (MBA). *Program availability:* Evening/weekend. *Entrance requirements:* For master's, GMAT, minimum undergraduate GPA of 2.75. Additional exam requirements/recommendations for international students: Required—TOEFL. Electronic applications accepted. *Faculty research:* Leadership, management, marketing, organizational culture.

DePaul University, College of Liberal Arts and Social Sciences, Chicago, IL 60614. Offers Arabic (MA); Chinese (MA); English (MA); French (MA); German (MA); history (MA); interdisciplinary studies (MA, MS); international public service (MS); international studies (MA); Italian (MA); Japanese (MA); leadership and policy studies (MS); liberal studies (MA); new media studies (MA); nonprofit management (MNM); public administration (MPA); public health (MPH); public service management (MS); social work (MSW); sociology (MA); Spanish (MA); sustainable urban development (MA); women and gender studies (MA); writing and publishing (MA); writing, rhetoric, and discourse (MA); MA/PhD. *Program availability:* Part-time, evening/weekend, online learning. Terminal master's awarded for partial completion of doctoral program. *Degree requirements:* For master's, variable foreign language requirement, comprehensive exam (for some programs), thesis (for some programs). Electronic applications accepted.

Des Moines University, College of Health Sciences, Program in Public Health, Des Moines, IA 50312-4104. Offers MPH. *Accreditation:* CEPH. *Program availability:* Part-time, evening/weekend. *Entrance requirements:* For master's, minimum GPA of 3.0. Additional exam requirements/recommendations for international students: Required—TOEFL (minimum score 600 paper-based). Electronic applications accepted. *Expenses:* Contact institution. *Faculty research:* Quality improvement, women's health, health promotion, patient education.

Drexel University, School of Public Health, Philadelphia, PA 19104-2875. Offers MPH, MS, PhD, Certificate. *Accreditation:* CEPH. *Entrance requirements:* For master's, GMAT, GRE, LSAT, or MCAT, previous course work in statistics and word processing. Additional exam requirements/recommendations for international students: Required—TOEFL. Electronic applications accepted. *Expenses:* Contact institution. *Faculty research:* Epidemiology, behavioral and social sciences, problem-based learning.

East Carolina University, Brody School of Medicine, Program in Public Health, Greenville, NC 27858-4353. Offers MPH, MD/MPH. *Accreditation:* CEPH. *Program availability:* Part-time. *Students:* 65 full-time (58 women), 17 part-time (15 women); includes 37 minority (21 Black or African American, non-Hispanic/Latino; 1 American Indian or Alaska Native, non-Hispanic/Latino; 8 Asian, non-Hispanic/Latino; 4 Hispanic/Latino; 3 Two or more races, non-Hispanic/Latino), 3 international. Average age 27. 75 applicants, 87% accepted, 38 enrolled. In 2015, 34 master's awarded. *Degree requirements:* For master's, field placement professional paper. *Entrance requirements:* For master's, GRE or MCAT. Additional exam requirements/recommendations for international students: Required—TOEFL (minimum score 550 paper-based). *Application deadline:* For fall admission, 4/15 for domestic and international students; for spring admission, 10/15 for domestic and international students. Application fee: $50. Electronic applications accepted. *Financial support:* Research assistantships with full tuition reimbursements and unspecified assistantships available. Financial award applicants required to submit FAFSA. *Faculty research:* Public health, disparities in public health. *Unit head:* Dr. Maria C. Clay, Chairman, Bioethics, E-mail: clayma@ecu.edu.

East Carolina University, Graduate School, College of Fine Arts and Communication, School of Communication, Greenville, NC 27858-4353. Offers health communication (MA). *Students:* 15 full-time (all women), 22 part-time (17 women); includes 15 minority (10 Black or African American, non-Hispanic/Latino; 1 American Indian or Alaska Native, non-Hispanic/Latino; 3 Hispanic/Latino; 1 Two or more races, non-Hispanic/Latino). Average age 29. 31 applicants, 68% accepted, 17 enrolled. In 2015, 8 master's awarded. *Entrance requirements:* For master's, GRE. *Financial support:* Teaching assistantships available. *Unit head:* Dr. Linda Kean, Director, 252-328-4227, E-mail: keanl@ecu.edu. *Application contact:* Dean of Graduate School, 252-328-6012, Fax: 252-328-6071, E-mail: gradschool@ecu.edu.
Website: http://www.ecu.edu/cs-cfac/comm/graduate/index.cfm

Eastern Virginia Medical School, Master of Public Health Program, Norfolk, VA 23501-1980. Offers MPH. Program offered jointly with Old Dominion University. *Accreditation:* CEPH. *Program availability:* Evening/weekend. *Degree requirements:* For master's, field practicum. *Entrance requirements:* For master's, GRE General Test. Additional exam requirements/recommendations for international students: Required—TOEFL (minimum score 650 paper-based). Electronic applications accepted. *Expenses:* Contact institution.

East Stroudsburg University of Pennsylvania, Graduate College, College of Health Sciences, Department of Health Studies, East Stroudsburg, PA 18301-2999. Offers health education (MS); public health (MPH). *Accreditation:* CEPH (one or more programs are accredited). *Program availability:* Part-time, evening/weekend, online learning. *Degree requirements:* For master's, oral comprehensive exam. *Entrance requirements:* For master's, GRE General Test, minimum GPA of 3.0 in major, 2.8 overall; undergraduate prerequisites in anatomy and physiology; 3 verifiable letters of recommendation; professional resume. Additional exam requirements/recommendations for international students: Required—TOEFL (minimum score 560 paper-based; 83 iBT) or IELTS. *Application deadline:* For fall admission, 7/31 priority date for domestic students, 6/30 priority date for international students; for spring admission, 11/30 for domestic students, 10/31 for international students. Applications are processed on a rolling basis. Application fee: $50. Electronic applications accepted. *Expenses: Tuition, area resident:* Full-time $8460; part-time $5640 per year. Tuition, state resident: full-time $8460; part-time $5640 per year. Tuition, nonresident: full-time $12,690; part-time $8460 per year. *International tuition:* $15,368 full-time. *Required fees:* $2462; $1630 per unit. $815 per semester. Tuition and fees vary according to course load, campus/location and program. *Financial support:* Research assistantships with tuition reimbursements, Federal Work-Study, and institutionally sponsored loans available. Financial award application deadline: 3/1; financial award applicants required to submit FAFSA. *Faculty research:* HIV prevention, wellness, international health issues. *Unit head:* Kim Razzano, Chair, 570-422-3693, Fax: 570-422-3848, E-mail: krazzano@esu.edu. *Application contact:* Dr. Steven Godin, Graduate Coordinator, 570-422-3536, Fax: 570-422-2711, E-mail: sgodin@esu.edu.

East Tennessee State University, School of Graduate Studies, College of Public Health, Department of Public Health, Johnson City, TN 37614. Offers MPH, DPH, Postbaccalaureate Certificate. *Accreditation:* CEPH. *Program availability:* Part-time, online learning. *Faculty:* 37 full-time (13 women), 3 part-time/adjunct (2 women). *Students:* 95 full-time (71 women), 76 part-time (65 women); includes 38 minority (23 Black or African American, non-Hispanic/Latino; 9 Asian, non-Hispanic/Latino; 3 Hispanic/Latino; 3 Two or more races, non-Hispanic/Latino), 21 international. Average age 30. 139 applicants, 73% accepted, 47 enrolled. In 2015, 25 master's, 6 doctorates, 9 other advanced degrees awarded. *Degree requirements:* For master's, comprehensive exam, field experience; for doctorate, thesis/dissertation, practicum. *Entrance requirements:* For master's, GRE General Test, minimum GPA of 2.75, SOPHAS application, three letters of recommendation; for doctorate, GRE General Test, SOPHAS application, three letters of recommendation; for Postbaccalaureate Certificate, minimum GPA of 2.5, three letters of recommendation, resume. Additional exam requirements/recommendations for international students: Required—TOEFL (minimum score 550 paper-based; 79 iBT), IELTS (minimum score 6.5). *Application deadline:* For fall admission, 3/1 for domestic and international students. Application fee: $35 ($45 for international students). Electronic applications accepted. *Financial support:* In 2015–16, 54 students received support, including 51 research assistantships with tuition reimbursements available (averaging $7,175 per year), 3 teaching assistantships with full tuition reimbursements available (averaging $14,000 per year); career-related internships or fieldwork, institutionally sponsored loans, scholarships/grants, and unspecified assistantships also available. Financial award application deadline: 7/1; financial award applicants required to submit FAFSA. *Unit head:* Dr. Randy Wykoff, Dean, 423-439-4243, Fax: 423-439-5238, E-mail: wykoff@etsu.edu. *Application contact:* Mary Duncan, Graduate Specialist, 423-439-4302, Fax: 423-439-5624, E-mail: duncanm@etsu.edu.
Website: http://www.etsu.edu/cph/

Elmhurst College, Graduate Programs, Program in Public Health, Elmhurst, IL 60126-3296. Offers MPH. *Program availability:* Part-time, evening/weekend, online learning. *Faculty:* 1 full-time (0 women), 5 part-time/adjunct (all women). *Students:* 1 (woman) full-time, 35 part-time (31 women); includes 21 minority (13 Black or African American, non-Hispanic/Latino; 5 Asian, non-Hispanic/Latino; 3 Hispanic/Latino), 1 international. Average age 29. 27 applicants, 59% accepted, 14 enrolled. In 2015, 6 master's awarded. *Degree requirements:* For master's, practicum. *Entrance requirements:* For master's, 3 recommendations, resume, statement of purpose. Additional exam requirements/recommendations for international students: Required—TOEFL (minimum score 550 paper-based; 79 iBT). *Application deadline:* Applications are processed on a rolling basis. Application fee: $0. Electronic applications accepted. *Expenses:* $650 per semester hour. *Financial support:* In 2015–16, 19 students received support. Scholarships/grants available. Support available to part-time students. Financial award application deadline: 6/1; financial award applicants required to submit FAFSA. *Application contact:* Timothy J. Panfil, Director of Enrollment Management, School for Professional Studies, 630-617-3300 Ext. 3256, Fax: 630-617-6471, E-mail: panfilt@elmhurst.edu.
Website: http://www.elmhurst.edu/master_public_health

Emory University, Rollins School of Public Health, Atlanta, GA 30322. Offers MPH, MSPH, PhD, JD/MPH, MBA/MPH, MD/MPH, MM Sc/MPH, MSN/MPH. *Accreditation:* CEPH (one or more programs are accredited). *Program availability:* Part-time, evening/weekend, online learning. *Degree requirements:* For master's, variable foreign language requirement, comprehensive exam (for some programs), thesis (for some programs), practicum. *Entrance requirements:* For master's, GRE General Test. Additional exam requirements/recommendations for international students: Required—TOEFL (minimum score 550 paper-based; 80 iBT). Electronic applications accepted. *Expenses:* Contact institution. *Faculty research:* HIV/AIDS prevention, infectious disease, minority health, health disparities, bioterrorism.

Everglades University, Graduate Programs, Program in Public Health Administration, Boca Raton, FL 33431. Offers complementary and alternative medicine (MPH). *Program availability:* Part-time, evening/weekend, 100% online. *Faculty:* 6 full-time (2 women), 10 part-time/adjunct (3 women). *Students:* 72 full-time (59 women), 7 part-time (6 women); includes 27 minority (13 Black or African American, non-Hispanic/Latino; 9 Hispanic/Latino; 5 Two or more races, non-Hispanic/Latino), 1 international. Average age 42. 35 applicants, 32 enrolled. In 2015, 1 master's awarded. *Degree requirements:* For master's, capstone course. *Entrance requirements:* For master's, GMAT (minimum score of 400) or GRE (minimum score of 290), bachelor's or graduate degree from college accredited by an agency recognized by the U.S. Department of Education; minimum cumulative GPA of 2.0 at the baccalaureate level, 3.0 at the master's level. Additional exam requirements/recommendations for international students: Recommended—TOEFL (minimum score 500 paper-based). *Application deadline:* Applications are processed on a rolling basis. Application fee: $50. Electronic applications accepted. *Expenses:* $15,696 tuition; $1,600 fees. *Financial support:* In 2015–16, 4 students received support. Scholarships/grants available. Financial award applicants required to submit FAFSA. *Application contact:* Patricia Ramirez, Director of Admissions, 561-912-1211, Fax: 561-912-1191, E-mail: pramirez@evergladesuniversity.edu.

Excelsior College, School of Health Sciences, Albany, NY 12203-5159. Offers health care informatics (Certificate); health professions education (MSHS); healthcare informatics (MS); public health (MSHS). *Program availability:* Part-time, evening/weekend, online learning. *Faculty:* 9 part-time/adjunct (8 women). *Students:* 256 part-time (183 women); includes 148 minority (83 Black or African American, non-Hispanic/Latino; 2 American Indian or Alaska Native, non-Hispanic/Latino; 18 Asian, non-Hispanic/Latino; 30 Hispanic/Latino; 6 Native Hawaiian or other Pacific Islander, non-Hispanic/Latino; 9 Two or more races, non-Hispanic/Latino), 1 international. Average

Public Health—General

age 39. In 2015, 2 master's awarded. *Entrance requirements:* For degree, bachelor's degree in applicable field. *Application deadline:* Applications are processed on a rolling basis. Application fee: $110. Electronic applications accepted. *Expenses: Tuition, area resident:* Part-time $645 per credit. *Required fees:* $265 per unit. *Financial support:* Scholarships/grants available. *Unit head:* Dr. Deborah Sopczyk, Dean, 518-464-8500, Fax: 518-464-8777. *Application contact:* Admissions Counselor, 518-464-8500, Fax: 518-464-8777, E-mail: admissions@excelsior.edu.

Florida Agricultural and Mechanical University, Division of Graduate Studies, Research, and Continuing Education, College of Pharmacy and Pharmaceutical Sciences, Institute of Public Health, Tallahassee, FL 32307-3200. Offers MPH, DPH. *Accreditation:* CEPH. *Entrance requirements:* Additional exam requirements/recommendations for international students: Required—TOEFL.

Florida International University, Robert Stempel College of Public Health and Social Work, Programs in Public Health, Miami, FL 33199. Offers biostatistics (MPH); environmental and occupational health (MPH, PhD); epidemiology (MPH, PhD); health policy and management (MPH); health promotion and disease prevention (PhD); health promotion and diseases prevention (MPH). Ph D program has fall admissions only; MPH offered jointly with University of Miami. *Accreditation:* CEPH. *Program availability:* Part-time, evening/weekend, online learning. *Faculty:* 27 full-time (12 women), 2 part-time/adjunct (1 woman). *Students:* 126 full-time (80 women), 62 part-time (46 women); includes 129 minority (47 Black or African American, non-Hispanic/Latino; 10 Asian, non-Hispanic/Latino; 69 Hispanic/Latino; 3 Two or more races, non-Hispanic/Latino), 32 international. Average age 30. 298 applicants, 35% accepted, 68 enrolled. In 2015, 67 master's, 10 doctorates awarded. *Degree requirements:* For master's, thesis optional; for doctorate, comprehensive exam, thesis/dissertation. *Entrance requirements:* For master's, minimum GPA of 3.0, letters of recommendation; for doctorate, GRE, resume, minimum GPA of 3.0, letters of recommendation, letter of intent. Additional exam requirements/recommendations for international students: Required—TOEFL (minimum score 550 paper-based; 80 iBT). *Application deadline:* For fall admission, 6/1 for domestic students, 4/1 for international students; for spring admission, 10/1 for domestic students, 9/1 for international students. Applications are processed on a rolling basis. Application fee: $30. Electronic applications accepted. *Expenses:* Contact institution. *Financial support:* Institutionally sponsored loans, scholarships/grants, and tuition waivers (full) available. Financial award application deadline: 3/1; financial award applicants required to submit FAFSA. *Faculty research:* Drugs/AIDS intervention among migrant workers, provision of services for active/recovering drug users with HIV. *Unit head:* Dr. Benjamin C. Amick, III, Chair, 305-348-4903, E-mail: benjamin.amickiii@fiu.edu. *Application contact:* Dr. Vukosava Pekovic, Director, 305-348-1823, Fax: 305-348-4901, E-mail: pekovic@fiu.edu.

Florida State University, The Graduate School, College of Social Sciences and Public Policy, Public Health Program, Tallahassee, FL 32306. Offers MPH. *Accreditation:* CEPH. *Program availability:* Part-time. *Faculty:* 9 full-time (2 women). *Students:* 38 full-time (22 women), 15 part-time (7 women); includes 22 minority (15 Black or African American, non-Hispanic/Latino; 4 Asian, non-Hispanic/Latino; 3 Hispanic/Latino), 6 international. Average age 26. 99 applicants, 71% accepted, 26 enrolled. In 2015, 26 master's awarded. *Degree requirements:* For master's, internship, research paper. *Entrance requirements:* For master's, GRE General Test, minimum GPA of 3.0. Additional exam requirements/recommendations for international students: Required—TOEFL (minimum score 550 paper-based; 80 iBT). *Application deadline:* For fall admission, 7/1 priority date for domestic students, 7/1 for international students; for spring admission, 11/1 for domestic and international students. Applications are processed on a rolling basis. Application fee: $30. Electronic applications accepted. *Expenses: Tuition, area resident:* Full-time $7263; part-time $403.50 per credit hour. Tuition, nonresident: full-time $18,087; part-time $1004.85 per credit hour. *Required fees:* $1365; $75.81 per credit hour. $20 per semester. Tuition and fees vary according to campus/location. *Financial support:* In 2015–16, 3 students received support, including 3 research assistantships with full tuition reimbursements available (averaging $5,000 per year); fellowships with tuition reimbursements available, career-related internships or fieldwork, Federal Work-Study, institutionally sponsored loans, and unspecified assistantships also available. Financial award application deadline: 2/15. *Faculty research:* Health behavior surveillance, long term care policy, long term care evaluation, HMOs, Medicaid. *Total annual research expenditures:* $1 million. *Unit head:* Dr. William G. Weissert, Director, 850-644-4418, Fax: 850-644-1367, E-mail: william.weissert@fsu.edu. *Application contact:* Sam Bandak, Academic Program Specialist, 850-644-4418, E-mail: sbandak@fsu.edu. Website: http://www.coss.fsu.edu/publichealth/

Fort Valley State University, College of Graduate Studies and Extended Education, Program in Public Health, Fort Valley, GA 31030. Offers environmental health (MPH). *Degree requirements:* For master's, thesis. *Entrance requirements:* For master's, GRE General Test. Additional exam requirements/recommendations for international students: Recommended—TOEFL. *Application deadline:* For fall admission, 8/23 for domestic students. Applications are processed on a rolling basis. Application fee: $20. *Financial support:* Federal Work-Study and unspecified assistantships available. Support available to part-time students. *Unit head:* Dr. Oreta Samples, 478-825-6904, E-mail: sampleso@fvsu.edu. *Application contact:* Dr. Oreta Samples, 478-825-6904, E-mail: sampleso@fvsu.edu.

George Mason University, College of Health and Human Services, Department of Global and Community Health, Fairfax, VA 22030. Offers global and community health (Certificate); global health (MS); public health (MPH), including epidemiology. *Accreditation:* CEPH. *Faculty:* 14 full-time (10 women), 18 part-time/adjunct (14 women). *Students:* 62 full-time (56 women), 47 part-time (42 women); includes 50 minority (22 Black or African American, non-Hispanic/Latino; 16 Asian, non-Hispanic/Latino; 9 Hispanic/Latino; 3 Two or more races, non-Hispanic/Latino), 1 international. Average age 27. 121 applicants, 72% accepted, 44 enrolled. In 2015, 56 master's, 6 other advanced degrees awarded. *Degree requirements:* For master's, comprehensive exam (for some programs), thesis or practicum. *Entrance requirements:* For master's, GRE, GMAT (depending on program), 2 official transcripts; expanded goals statement; 3 letters of recommendation; resume; 1 completed course in health science, statistics, natural sciences and social science (for MPH); 6 credits of foreign language if not fluent (for MS); for Certificate, 2 official transcripts; expanded goals statement; 3 letters of recommendation; resume; bachelor's degree from regionally-accredited institution with minimum GPA of 3.0. Additional exam requirements/recommendations for international students: Required—TOEFL (minimum score 570 paper-based; 88 iBT), IELTS (minimum score 6.5), PTE (minimum score 59). *Application deadline:* For fall admission, 2/1 for domestic students. Application fee: $75 ($80 for international students). Electronic applications accepted. *Expenses:* Contact institution. *Financial support:* In 2015–16, 5 students received support, including 9 research assistantships with tuition reimbursements available (averaging $16,472 per year), 1 teaching assistantship with tuition reimbursement available (averaging $9,000 per year); career-related internships or fieldwork, Federal Work-Study, scholarships/grants, unspecified assistantships, and health care benefits (for full-time research or teaching assistantship recipients) also available. Financial award application deadline: 3/1; financial award applicants required to submit FAFSA. *Faculty research:* Health issues and the needs of affected populations

at the regional and global level. *Total annual research expenditures:* $28,950. *Unit head:* Brian Gillette, Director, 703-993-4636, Fax: 703-993-1908, E-mail: bgillett@gmu.edu. *Application contact:* Ali Weinstein, Graduate Program Coordinator, 703-993-9632, Fax: 703-993-1908, E-mail: aweinst2@gmu.edu. Website: http://chhs.gmu.edu/gch/index

Georgetown University, Graduate School of Arts and Sciences, Department of Microbiology and Immunology, Washington, DC 20057. Offers biohazardous threat agents and emerging infectious diseases (MS); biomedical science policy and advocacy (MS); general microbiology and immunology (MS); global infectious diseases (PhD); microbiology and immunology (PhD). *Program availability:* Part-time. *Degree requirements:* For master's, 30 credit hours of coursework; for doctorate, comprehensive exam, thesis/dissertation. *Entrance requirements:* For master's, GRE General Test, 3 letters of reference, bachelor's degree in related field; for doctorate, GRE General Test, 3 letters of reference, MS/BS in related field. Additional exam requirements/recommendations for international students: Required—TOEFL (minimum score 505 paper-based). Electronic applications accepted. *Faculty research:* Pathogenesis and basic biology of the fungus Candida albicans, molecular biology of viral immunopathological mechanisms in Multiple Sclerosis.

The George Washington University, Milken Institute School of Public Health, Department of Global Health, Washington, DC 20052. Offers global health (Dr PH); global health communication (MPH). *Accreditation:* CEPH. *Faculty:* 13 full-time (7 women), 2 part-time/adjunct. *Students:* 3 full-time (1 woman), 23 part-time (19 women); includes 8 minority (5 Black or African American, non-Hispanic/Latino; 2 Asian, non-Hispanic/Latino; 1 Hispanic/Latino), 3 international. Average age 33. In 2015, 29 master's awarded. *Degree requirements:* For master's, case study or special project. *Entrance requirements:* For master's, GMAT, GRE General Test, or MCAT. Additional exam requirements/recommendations for international students: Required—TOEFL. *Application deadline:* For fall admission, 4/15 priority date for domestic students, 4/15 for international students; for spring admission, 11/1 for domestic and international students. Applications are processed on a rolling basis. Application fee: $75. *Financial support:* In 2015–16, 24 students received support. Tuition waivers available. Financial award application deadline: 2/15. *Unit head:* Prof. James Tielsch, Chair, 202-994-4124, Fax: 202-994-1955, E-mail: jtielsch@gwu.edu. *Application contact:* Jane Smith, Director of Admissions, 202-994-0248, Fax: 202-994-1860, E-mail: sphhsinfo@gwumc.edu.

Georgia Southern University, Jack N. Averitt College of Graduate Studies, Jiann-Ping Hsu College of Public Health, Program in Public Health, Statesboro, GA 30460. Offers biostatistics (MPH, Dr PH); community health behavior and education (Dr PH); community health education (MPH); environmental health sciences (MPH); epidemiology (MPH); health policy and management (MPH, Dr PH). *Accreditation:* CEPH. *Program availability:* Part-time. *Students:* 129 full-time (86 women), 41 part-time (32 women); includes 87 minority (67 Black or African American, non-Hispanic/Latino; 6 Asian, non-Hispanic/Latino; 8 Hispanic/Latino; 6 Two or more races, non-Hispanic/Latino), 30 international. Average age 30. 218 applicants, 63% accepted, 41 enrolled. In 2015, 37 master's, 8 doctorates awarded. *Degree requirements:* For master's, thesis optional, practicum; for doctorate, comprehensive exam, thesis/dissertation, practicum. *Entrance requirements:* For master's, GRE General Test, minimum GPA of 2.75, resume, 3 letters of reference; for doctorate, GRE, GMAT, MCAT, LSAT, 3 letters of reference, statement of purpose, resume or curriculum vitae. Additional exam requirements/recommendations for international students: Required—TOEFL (minimum score 550 paper-based; 80 iBT), IELTS (minimum score 6). *Application deadline:* For fall admission, 6/1 priority date for domestic and international students; for spring admission, 10/1 priority date for domestic students, 10/1 for international students. Applications are processed on a rolling basis. Application fee: $50. Electronic applications accepted. *Expenses:* $335 per credit hour. *Financial support:* In 2015–16, 93 students received support, including 23 fellowships with full tuition reimbursements available (averaging $7,750 per year), 1 research assistantship with full tuition reimbursement available (averaging $7,750 per year), 1 teaching assistantship with full tuition reimbursement available (averaging $7,750 per year); career-related internships or fieldwork, Federal Work-Study, scholarships/grants, tuition waivers (full), and unspecified assistantships also available. Support available to part-time students. Financial award application deadline: 4/15; financial award applicants required to submit FAFSA. *Faculty research:* Rural public health best practices, health disparity elimination, community initiatives to enhance public health, cost effectiveness analysis, epidemiology of rural public health, environmental health issues, health care system assessment, rural health care, health policy and healthcare financing, survival analysis, nonparametric statistics and resampling methods, micro-arrays and genomics, data imputation techniques and clinical trial methodology. *Total annual research expenditures:* $281,707. *Unit head:* Dr. Shamia Garrett, Program Coordinator, 912-478-2393, E-mail: sgarrett@georgiasouthern.edu. Website: http://chhs.georgiasouthern.edu/health/

Georgia State University, Andrew Young School of Policy Studies, Department of Public Management and Policy, Atlanta, GA 30303. Offers criminal justice (MPA); disaster management (Certificate); disaster policy (MPA); environmental policy (PhD); health policy (PhD); management and finance (MPA); nonprofit management (MPA, Certificate); nonprofit policy (MPA); planning and economic development (MPP, Certificate); policy analysis and evaluation (MPA), including planning and economic development; public and nonprofit management (PhD); public finance and budgeting (PhD), including science and technology policy, urban and regional economic development; public finance policy (MPA), including social policy; public health (MPA). *Accreditation:* NASPAA (one or more programs are accredited). *Program availability:* Part-time. *Faculty:* 15 full-time (8 women). *Students:* 128 full-time (80 women), 78 part-time (48 women); includes 78 minority (61 Black or African American, non-Hispanic/Latino; 4 Asian, non-Hispanic/Latino; 11 Hispanic/Latino; 2 Two or more races, non-Hispanic/Latino), 31 international. Average age 30. 262 applicants, 63% accepted, 74 enrolled. In 2015, 92 master's, 2 doctorates, 6 other advanced degrees awarded. Terminal master's awarded for partial completion of doctoral program. *Degree requirements:* For master's, thesis optional; for doctorate, comprehensive exam, thesis/dissertation. *Entrance requirements:* For master's and doctorate, GRE. Additional exam requirements/recommendations for international students: Required—TOEFL (minimum score 603 paper-based; 100 iBT) or IELTS (minimum score 7). *Application deadline:* For fall admission, 1/15 for domestic and international students. Application fee: $50. Electronic applications accepted. *Expenses:* Tuition, state resident: full-time $6876; part-time $382 per credit hour. Tuition, nonresident: full-time $22,374; part-time $1243 per credit hour. *Required fees:* $2128; $2128 per term. $1064 per term. Part-time tuition and fees vary according to course load and program. *Financial support:* In 2015–16, fellowships (averaging $8,194 per year), research assistantships (averaging $8,068 per year), teaching assistantships (averaging $3,600 per year) were awarded; institutionally sponsored loans, scholarships/grants, health care benefits, and unspecified assistantships also available. Financial award application deadline: 2/1. *Faculty research:* Public budgeting and finance, public management, nonprofit management, performance measurement and management, urban development. *Unit head:* Dr. Carolyn Bourdeaux, Chair and Professor, 404-413-0013, Fax: 404-413-0104, E-mail: cbourdeaux@gsu.edu. Website: http://aysps.gsu.edu/pmap/

Georgia State University, School of Public Health, Atlanta, GA 30302-3995. Offers MPH, PhD, Certificate. *Accreditation:* CEPH. *Program availability:* Part-time. *Faculty:* 21 full-time (13 women). *Students:* 192 full-time (152 women), 106 part-time (86 women); includes 156 minority (112 Black or African American, non-Hispanic/Latino; 2 American Indian or Alaska Native, non-Hispanic/Latino; 29 Asian, non-Hispanic/Latino; 9 Hispanic/Latino; 4 Two or more races, non-Hispanic/Latino), 38 international. Average age 30. 524 applicants, 41% accepted, 90 enrolled. In 2015, 60 master's, 4 doctorates, 9 other advanced degrees awarded. *Degree requirements:* For master's, thesis, applied practicum; for doctorate, comprehensive exam, thesis/dissertation, applied, research or teaching practicum. *Entrance requirements:* For master's, doctorate, and Certificate, GRE or GMAT. Additional exam requirements/recommendations for international students: Required—TOEFL (minimum score 550 paper-based; 80 iBT). *Application deadline:* For fall admission, 2/1 for domestic and international students; for spring admission, 10/1 for domestic and international students. Application fee: $50. Electronic applications accepted. *Expenses:* Contact institution. *Financial support:* In 2015–16, fellowships (averaging $2,500 per year), research assistantships with full tuition reimbursements (averaging $22,000 per year), teaching assistantships with full tuition reimbursements (averaging $22,000 per year) were awarded; career-related internships or fieldwork, scholarships/grants, health care benefits, unspecified assistantships, and out-of-state tuition waivers also available. *Faculty research:* Infectious and chronic disease epidemiology; environmental health and the built environment; adolescent risk behaviors: tobacco use, alcohol and drug use, and risky sexual behaviors; reduction of health disparities especially among minority populations in urban areas; program evaluation, evidence-based interventions and implementation. *Unit head:* Dr. Michael P. Eriksen, Dean, 404-413-1132, Fax: 404-413-1140, E-mail: meriksen@gsu.edu. *Application contact:* Courtney M. Burton, Graduate Coordinator, 404-413-1143, E-mail: cmburton@gsu.edu.
Website: http://publichealth.gsu.edu/

The Graduate Center, City University of New York, Graduate Studies, Program in Public Health, New York, NY 10016-4039. Offers DPH. *Accreditation:* CEPH. *Program availability:* Part-time. *Degree requirements:* For doctorate, thesis/dissertation, exams, research seminars. *Entrance requirements:* For doctorate, GRE General Test, MPH, 2 letters of recommendation, curriculum vitae or resume.

Grand Canyon University, College of Nursing and Health Sciences, Phoenix, AZ 85017-1097. Offers addiction counseling (MS); health care administration (MS); health care informatics (MS); marriage and family therapy (MS); professional counseling (MS); public health (MS). *Program availability:* Part-time, evening/weekend, online learning. *Entrance requirements:* For master's, undergraduate degree with minimum GPA of 2.8. Additional exam requirements/recommendations for international students: Required—TOEFL (minimum score 575 paper-based; 90 iBT), IELTS (minimum score 7).

Grand Valley State University, College of Health Professions, Public Health Program, Allendale, MI 49401-9403. Offers MPH. *Faculty:* 8 full-time (6 women). *Students:* 103 full-time (75 women), 24 part-time (20 women); includes 26 minority (9 Black or African American, non-Hispanic/Latino; 3 Asian, non-Hispanic/Latino; 6 Hispanic/Latino; 8 Two or more races, non-Hispanic/Latino), 3 international. Average age 26. 73 applicants, 96% accepted, 69 enrolled. In 2015, 24 master's awarded. *Entrance requirements:* For master's, baccalaureate degree, official transcripts, minimum GPA of 3.0, two recommendations. Additional exam requirements/recommendations for international students: Required—TOEFL, IELTS, or Michigan English Language Assessment Battery. *Application deadline:* For fall admission, 2/1 for domestic students. Application fee: $30. *Financial support:* In 2015–16, 13 students received support, including 6 fellowships (averaging $3,508 per year), 7 research assistantships (averaging $8,289 per year). *Unit head:* Ranelle Brew, Director, 616-331-5570, Fax: 616-331-5550,

E-mail: brewr@gvsu.edu. *Application contact:* Darlene Zwart, Student Services Coordinator, 616-331-3958, E-mail: zwartda@gvsu.edu.
Website: http://www.gvsu.edu/grad/mph/

Harvard University, Cyprus International Institute for the Environment and Public Health in Association with Harvard School of Public Health, Cambridge, MA 02138. Offers environmental health (MS); environmental/public health (PhD); epidemiology and biostatistics (MS). *Entrance requirements:* For master's and doctorate, GRE, resume/curriculum vitae, 3 letters of recommendation, BA or BS (including diploma and official transcripts). Additional exam requirements/recommendations for international students: Required—TOEFL, IELTS (minimum score 7). Electronic applications accepted. *Faculty research:* Air pollution, climate change, biostatistics, sustainable development, environmental management.

Harvard University, Harvard T.H. Chan School of Public Health, Master of Public Health Program, Boston, MA 02115-6096. Offers clinical effectiveness (MPH); global health (MPH); health and social behavior (MPH); health management (MPH); health policy (MPH); occupational and environmental health (MPH); quantitative methods (MPH); JD/MPH; MD/MPH. *Program availability:* Part-time. *Students:* 225 full-time (138 women), 230 part-time (110 women); includes 146 minority (22 Black or African American, non-Hispanic/Latino; 85 Asian, non-Hispanic/Latino; 27 Hispanic/Latino; 12 Two or more races, non-Hispanic/Latino), 161 international. Average age 29. 773 applicants, 56% accepted, 346 enrolled. In 2015, 323 master's awarded. *Entrance requirements:* For master's, GRE, MCAT, GMAT, DAT, LSAT. Additional exam requirements/recommendations for international students: Recommended—TOEFL (minimum score 600 paper-based; 100 iBT), IELTS (minimum score 7). *Application deadline:* For fall admission, 12/15 priority date for domestic and international students. Applications are processed on a rolling basis. Application fee: $120. Electronic applications accepted. *Financial support:* Federal Work-Study, scholarships/grants, and unspecified assistantships available. Support available to part-time students. Financial award application deadline: 2/15; financial award applicants required to submit FAFSA. *Faculty research:* Clinical effectiveness, global health, health and social behavior, health care management and policy, law and public health, occupational and environmental health, quantitative methods. *Unit head:* Dr. Murray Mittleman, Chair of the MPH Steering Committee, 617-432-0090, Fax: 617-432-3365, E-mail: mmittlem@hsph.harvard.edu. *Application contact:* Vincent W. James, Director of Admissions, 617-432-1031, Fax: 617-432-7080, E-mail: admissions@hsph.harvard.edu.
Website: http://www.hsph.harvard.edu/master-of-public-health-program/
See Display below and Close-Up on page 849.

Harvard University, Harvard T.H. Chan School of Public Health, PhD Program in Biological Sciences in Public Health, Boston, MA 02115. Offers PhD. *Faculty:* 28 full-time (11 women), 13 part-time/adjunct (2 women). *Students:* 48 full-time (33 women); includes 16 minority (5 Black or African American, non-Hispanic/Latino; 5 Asian, non-Hispanic/Latino; 4 Hispanic/Latino; 2 Two or more races, non-Hispanic/Latino), 9 international. Average age 25. 249 applicants, 14% accepted, 27 enrolled. In 2015, 7 doctorates awarded. *Degree requirements:* For doctorate, qualifying examination, dissertation/defense. *Entrance requirements:* For doctorate, GRE General Test. Additional exam requirements/recommendations for international students: Recommended—TOEFL (minimum score 600 paper-based; 100 iBT), IELTS (minimum score 7). *Application deadline:* For fall admission, 12/8 for domestic students. Electronic applications accepted. *Financial support:* In 2015–16, 48 students received support. Fellowships, research assistantships, teaching assistantships, institutionally sponsored loans, health care benefits, and tuition waivers (full) available. Financial award application deadline: 1/1. *Faculty research:* Nutrition biochemistry, molecular and cellular toxicology, cardiovascular disease, cancer biology, immunology and infectious

Public Health—General

diseases, environmental health physiology. *Unit head:* Carole Knapp, Administrator, 617-432-2932. Website: http://www.hsph.harvard.edu/admissions/degree-programs/doctor-of-philosophy/phd-in-biological-sciences-and-public-health/

See Display on page 789 and Close-Up on page 849.

Hofstra University, School of Health Sciences and Human Services, Programs in Health, Hempstead, NY 11549. Offers community health (MS), including adventure education, strength and conditioning; health administration (MHA); public health (MPH). *Program availability:* Part-time, evening/weekend. *Students:* 145 full-time (98 women), 96 part-time (60 women); includes 104 minority (45 Black or African American, non-Hispanic/Latino; 39 Asian, non-Hispanic/Latino; 16 Hispanic/Latino; 2 Native Hawaiian or other Pacific Islander, non-Hispanic/Latino; 2 Two or more races, non-Hispanic/Latino), 21 international. Average age 28. 174 applicants, 85% accepted, 87 enrolled. In 2015, 59 master's awarded. *Degree requirements:* For master's, internship, minimum GPA of 3.0. *Entrance requirements:* For master's, interview, 2 letters of recommendation, essay, resume. Additional exam requirements/recommendations for international students: Required—TOEFL (minimum score 550 paper-based; 80 iBT). *Application deadline:* Applications are processed on a rolling basis. Application fee: $70 ($75 for international students). Electronic applications accepted. *Financial support:* In 2015–16, 71 students received support, including 40 fellowships with tuition reimbursements available (averaging $4,332 per year), 4 research assistantships with tuition reimbursements available (averaging $8,834 per year); Federal Work-Study, institutionally sponsored loans, scholarships/grants, and tuition waivers (full and partial) also available. Support available to part-time students. Financial award applicants required to submit FAFSA. *Faculty research:* Integrated long term care and policy reform; health care policy; cost benefit analysis; chronic illness management; development and implementation of leadership in sports, physical activity and recreation. *Unit head:* Dr. Jayne Ellinger, Chairperson, 516-463-6952, Fax: 516-463-6275, E-mail: hprjmk@hofstra.edu. *Application contact:* Sunil Samuel, Assistant Vice President of Admissions, 516-463-4723, Fax: 516-463-4664, E-mail: graduateadmission@hofstra.edu.
Website: http://www.hofstra.edu/academics/colleges/healthscienceshumanservices/

Howard University, College of Medicine, Program in Public Health, Washington, DC 20059-0002. Offers MPH.

Hunter College of the City University of New York, Graduate School, Schools of the Health Professions, School of Health Sciences, Programs in Urban Public Health, New York, NY 10065-5085. Offers community health education (MPH); environmental and occupational health sciences (MPH); epidemiology and biostatistics (MPH); health policy management (MPH); nutrition (MPH); MS/MPH. *Accreditation:* CEPH. *Program availability:* Part-time. *Students:* 36 full-time (31 women), 257 part-time (188 women); includes 117 minority (47 Black or African American, non-Hispanic/Latino; 1 American Indian or Alaska Native, non-Hispanic/Latino; 35 Asian, non-Hispanic/Latino; 34 Hispanic/Latino), 10 international. Average age 31. 360 applicants, 55% accepted, 143 enrolled. *Degree requirements:* For master's, comprehensive exam. *Entrance requirements:* For master's, GRE General Test, undergraduate major in natural or social sciences, health studies, or related field; 1 year of work or volunteer experience related to public health, nutrition, environmental health, social services, or community organization. Additional exam requirements/recommendations for international students: Required—TOEFL. *Application deadline:* For fall admission, 4/1 for domestic students, 2/1 for international students; for spring admission, 11/1 for domestic students, 9/1 for international students. *Financial support:* Application deadline: 3/1. *Unit head:* Jack Caravanos, Director, 212-396-7780, Fax: 212-481-5260, E-mail: jcaravan@hunter.cuny.edu. *Application contact:* Milena Solo, Director for Graduate Admissions, 212-772-4288, E-mail: admissions@hunter.cuny.edu.
Website: http://cuny.edu/site/sph/hunter-college/a-programs/graduate.html

Idaho State University, Office of Graduate Studies, College of Education, Department of Educational Foundations, Pocatello, ID 83209-8059. Offers child and family studies (M Ed); curriculum leadership (M Ed); education (M Ed); educational administration (M Ed); educational foundations (5th Year Certificate); elementary education (M Ed), including K-12 education, literacy, secondary education. *Program availability:* Part-time. *Degree requirements:* For master's, comprehensive exam, thesis optional, oral exam, written exam; for 5th Year Certificate, comprehensive exam, thesis (for some programs), oral exam, written exam. *Entrance requirements:* For master's, GRE General Test or MAT, minimum undergraduate GPA of 3.0; for 5th Year Certificate, GRE General Test, minimum undergraduate GPA of 3.0, master's degree. Additional exam requirements/recommendations for international students: Required—TOEFL (minimum score 550 paper-based; 80 iBT). Electronic applications accepted. *Faculty research:* Child and families studies; business education; special education; math, science, and technology education.

Idaho State University, Office of Graduate Studies, Kasiska College of Health Professions, Department of Health and Nutrition Sciences, Program in Public Health, Pocatello, ID 83209-8109. Offers MPH. *Accreditation:* CEPH. *Program availability:* Part-time. *Degree requirements:* For master's, comprehensive exam, thesis. *Entrance requirements:* For master's, GRE General Test, minimum GPA of 3.0 for upper division classes, 2 letters of recommendation. Additional exam requirements/recommendations for international students: Required—TOEFL (minimum score 600 paper-based). Electronic applications accepted.

Independence University, Program in Public Health, Salt Lake City, UT 84107. Offers MPH. *Program availability:* Part-time, evening/weekend, online learning. *Degree requirements:* For master's, final project or thesis.

Indiana University Bloomington, School of Public Health, Department of Applied Health Science, Bloomington, IN 47405. Offers behavioral, social, and community health (MPH); family health (MPH); health behavior (PhD); nutrition science (MS); professional health education (MPH); public health administration (MPH); safety management (MS); school and college health education (MS). *Accreditation:* CEPH (one or more programs are accredited). *Degree requirements:* For master's, thesis optional; for doctorate, comprehensive exam, thesis/dissertation. *Entrance requirements:* For master's, GRE (for MS in nutrition science), 3 recommendations; for doctorate, GRE, 3 recommendations. Additional exam requirements/recommendations for international students: Required—TOEFL (minimum score 550 paper-based; 80 iBT). Electronic applications accepted. *Faculty research:* Cancer education, HIV/AIDS and drug education, public health, parent-child interactions, safety education, obesity, public health policy, public health administration, school health, health education, human development, nutrition, human sexuality, chronic disease, early childhood health.

Indiana University–Purdue University Indianapolis, School of Public Health, Indianapolis, IN 46202. Offers biostatistics (MPH); environmental health science (MPH); epidemiology (MPH, PhD); health administration (MHA); health policy and management (MPH, PhD); social and behavioral sciences (MPH). *Accreditation:* CEPH. *Expenses:* Contact institution.

Johns Hopkins University, Bloomberg School of Public Health, Baltimore, MD 21205. Offers MBE, MHA, MHS, MPH, MPP, MSPH, Sc M, Dr PH, PhD, Sc D, JD/MPH, MBA/MPH, MHS/MA, MSN/MPH, MSW/MPH. *Accreditation:* CEPH (one or more programs

are accredited). *Program availability:* Part-time, online learning. *Degree requirements:* For master's, comprehensive exam (for some programs), thesis (for some programs); for doctorate, comprehensive exam, thesis/dissertation. *Entrance requirements:* Additional exam requirements/recommendations for international students: Required—TOEFL, IELTS. Electronic applications accepted.

Kansas State University, Graduate School, College of Human Ecology, Department of Human Nutrition, Manhattan, KS 66506. Offers human nutrition (MS, PhD); nutritional sciences (PhD); public health nutrition (PhD); public health physical activity (PhD); sensory analysis and consumer behavior (PhD). *Program availability:* Part-time. *Degree requirements:* For master's, thesis or alternative, residency; for doctorate, thesis/dissertation, residency. *Entrance requirements:* For master's, GRE General Test, minimum undergraduate GPA of 3.0; for doctorate, GRE General Test, minimum graduate GPA of 3.0. Additional exam requirements/recommendations for international students: Required—TOEFL (minimum score 550 paper-based; 79 iBT), IELTS (minimum score 6.5). Electronic applications accepted. *Faculty research:* Cancer and immunology, obesity, sensory analysis and consumer behavior, nutrient metabolism, clinical and community interventions.

Kansas State University, Graduate School, College of Veterinary Medicine, Department of Clinical Sciences, Manhattan, KS 66506. Offers MPH, Graduate Certificate. *Degree requirements:* For master's, thesis. *Entrance requirements:* For master's, GRE, DVM. Additional exam requirements/recommendations for international students: Required—TOEFL (minimum score 550 paper-based). Electronic applications accepted. *Faculty research:* Clinical trials, equine gastrointestinal ulceration, leptospirosis, food animal pharmacology, equine immunology, diabetes.

Kent State University, College of Public Health, Kent, OH 44242-0001. Offers MPH, PhD. *Accreditation:* CEPH. *Program availability:* Part-time, evening/weekend, online learning. *Faculty:* 23 full-time (11 women). *Students:* 139 full-time (101 women), 100 part-time (76 women); includes 56 minority (33 Black or African American, non-Hispanic/Latino; 1 American Indian or Alaska Native, non-Hispanic/Latino; 9 Asian, non-Hispanic/Latino; 9 Hispanic/Latino; 1 Native Hawaiian or other Pacific Islander, non-Hispanic/Latino; 3 Two or more races, non-Hispanic/Latino), 22 international. Average age 33. 291 applicants, 65% accepted, 137 enrolled. In 2015, 29 master's, 1 doctorate awarded. *Degree requirements:* For master's, practicum and culminating experience; for doctorate, comprehensive exam, thesis/dissertation. *Entrance requirements:* For master's, minimum GPA of 3.0, transcript, goal statement, resume, 3 letters of recommendation; for doctorate, GRE, minimum GPA of 3.0, transcript, personal statement, resume, interview, 3 letters of recommendation. Additional exam requirements/recommendations for international students: Required—TOEFL (minimum score: paper-based 525, iBT 71), Michigan English Language Assessment Battery (minimum score of 75), IELTS (minimum score of 6.0), PTE Academic (minimum score of 48), or completion of ELS level 112 Intensive Program. *Application deadline:* For fall admission, 7/1 priority date for domestic students; 3/1 for international students; for spring admission, 11/15 priority date for domestic students; for summer admission, 4/15 priority date for domestic students. Applications are processed on a rolling basis. Application fee: $45 ($70 for international students). Electronic applications accepted. *Expenses:* Tuition, state resident: full-time $10,864; part-time $495 per credit hour. Tuition, nonresident: full-time $18,380; part-time $837 per credit hour. *Financial support:* Research assistantships with full tuition reimbursements, teaching assistantships with full tuition reimbursements, career-related internships or fieldwork, Federal Work-Study, and unspecified assistantships available. *Unit head:* Dr. Sonia Alemagno, Dean, 330-672-6500, E-mail: salemagn@kent.edu. *Application contact:* 330-325-6500, E-mail: publichealth@kent.edu.
Website: http://www.kent.edu/publichealth/

Lamar University, College of Graduate Studies, College of Education and Human Development, Department of Health and Kinesiology, Beaumont, TX 77710. Offers public health (MS); science of kinesiology promotion (MS). *Faculty:* 8 full-time (3 women). *Students:* 34 full-time (17 women), 13 part-time (8 women); includes 24 minority (20 Black or African American, non-Hispanic/Latino; 3 Hispanic/Latino; 1 Two or more races, non-Hispanic/Latino), 6 international. Average age 27. 45 applicants, 87% accepted, 22 enrolled. In 2015, 33 master's awarded. *Degree requirements:* For master's, comprehensive exam (for some programs), thesis optional. *Entrance requirements:* For master's, GRE General Test, minimum GPA of 2.5. Additional exam requirements/recommendations for international students: Required—TOEFL (minimum score 550 paper-based; 79 iBT), IELTS (minimum score 6.5). *Application deadline:* For fall admission, 8/10 for domestic students, 7/1 for international students; for spring admission, 1/5 for domestic students, 12/1 for international students. Applications are processed on a rolling basis. Application fee: $25. Electronic applications accepted. *Expenses: Tuition, area resident:* Full-time $6720; part-time $4032. *Tuition, nonresident:* full-time $14,880; part-time $8928. *Required fees:* $1900; $950 $784. *Financial support:* Teaching assistantships available. Financial award application deadline: 4/1; financial award applicants required to submit FAFSA. *Faculty research:* Motor learning, exercise physiology, pedagogy. *Unit head:* Dr. Douglas Boatwright, Chair, 409-880-8711, Fax: 409-880-1761. *Application contact:* Melissa Gallien, Director, Admissions and Academic Services, 409-880-8888, Fax: 409-880-7419, E-mail: gradmissions@lamar.edu.
Website: http://education.lamar.edu/health-and-kinesiology

La Salle University, School of Nursing and Health Sciences, Program in Public Health, Philadelphia, PA 19141-1199. Offers MPH, MPH/MSN. *Program availability:* Part-time, evening/weekend. *Faculty:* 5 full-time (4 women). *Students:* 2 full-time (1 woman), 37 part-time (30 women); includes 23 minority (16 Black or African American, non-Hispanic/Latino; 1 Asian, non-Hispanic/Latino; 3 Hispanic/Latino; 3 Two or more races, non-Hispanic/Latino), 5 international. Average age 33. 37 applicants, 86% accepted, 13 enrolled. In 2015, 10 master's awarded. *Degree requirements:* For master's, capstone project. *Entrance requirements:* For master's, minimum undergraduate GPA of 3.0; curriculum vitae/resume; personal statement; 2 letters of reference; interview; prior academic and professional experience in healthcare (recommended). Additional exam requirements/recommendations for international students: Required—TOEFL. *Application deadline:* For fall admission, 8/15 priority date for domestic students, 8/15 for international students; for spring admission, 12/15 priority date for domestic students, 11/15 for international students; for summer admission, 4/14 priority date for domestic students, 3/15 for international students. Application fee: $35. Electronic applications accepted. Application fee is waived when completed online. *Expenses:* $775 per credit hour; $150 full-time technology fee, $75 part-time; $135 general university fee. *Financial support:* In 2015–16, 3 students received support. Scholarships/grants available. Support available to part-time students. Financial award applicants required to submit FAFSA. *Unit head:* Dr. Jillian Baker, Interim Director, 215-991-2274, Fax: 215-951-1896, E-mail: mph@lasalle.edu. *Application contact:* Alison McAnespey Target, Director, Graduate and Adult Enrollment, 215-951-1100, Fax: 215-951-1462, E-mail: target@lasalle.edu.
Website: http://www.lasalle.edu/master-public-health/

Laurentian University, School of Graduate Studies and Research, Interdisciplinary Program in Rural and Northern Health, Sudbury, ON P3E 2C6, Canada. Offers PhD.

Lenoir-Rhyne University, Graduate Programs, School of Health, Exercise and Sport Science, Program in Public Health, Hickory, NC 28601. Offers MPH. *Faculty:* 3 full-time (2 women). *Students:* 9 full-time (5 women), 30 part-time (25 women); includes 12 minority (7 Black or African American, non-Hispanic/Latino; 2 Asian, non-Hispanic/Latino; 2 Hispanic/Latino; 1 Two or more races, non-Hispanic/Latino), 5 international. Average age 29. In 2015, 1 master's awarded. *Entrance requirements:* For master's, GRE General Test or MAT, essay; resume; minimum GPA of 2.7 undergraduate, 3.0 graduate. Additional exam requirements/recommendations for international students: Required—TOEFL (minimum score 600 paper-based). Application fee: $35. Electronic applications accepted. *Expenses:* $550 per credit hour. *Unit head:* Dr. Amy Wood, Coordinator, 828-328-7728, Fax: 828-328-7368, E-mail: amy.wood@lr.edu. *Application contact:* Mary Ann Gosnell, Director, Graduate Recruiting, 828-328-7111, E-mail: admission@lr.edu.
Website: http://www.lr.edu/academics/programs/master-public-health

Loma Linda University, School of Public Health, Loma Linda, CA 92350. Offers MBA, MPH, MS, Dr PH, PhD. *Accreditation:* CEPH (one or more programs are accredited). *Program availability:* Part-time. *Degree requirements:* For doctorate, thesis/dissertation. *Entrance requirements:* For master's, GRE General Test, baccalaureate degree, minimum 3.0 GPA; for doctorate, GRE General Test, minimum GPA of 3.2. Additional exam requirements/recommendations for international students: Required—TOEFL (minimum score 550 paper-based) or Michigan English Language Assessment Battery. *Application deadline:* Applications are processed on a rolling basis. Application fee: $100. Electronic applications accepted. *Financial support:* Fellowships, research assistantships, teaching assistantships, career-related internships or fieldwork, Federal Work-Study, institutionally sponsored loans, tuition waivers (partial), and unspecified assistantships available. Support available to part-time students. Financial award application deadline: 5/15. *Faculty research:* Lifestyle and health, nutrition and cancer, nutrition and cardiovascular disease, smoking and health, aging and longevity. *Unit head:* Helen Hopp Marshak, Dean, 909-558-4578, Fax: 909-824-4087. *Application contact:* Wendy Genovez, Assistant Dan of Admissions and Records, 909-824-4694, Fax: 909-824-8087, E-mail: wgenovez@llu.edu.
Website: http://publichealth.llu.edu

London Metropolitan University, Graduate Programs, London, United Kingdom. Offers applied psychology (M Sc); architecture (MA); biomedical science (M Sc); blood science (M Sc); cancer pharmacology (M Sc); computer networking and cyber security (M Sc); computing and information systems (M Sc); conference interpreting (MA); counter-terrorism studies (M Sc); creative, digital and professional writing (MA); crime, violence and prevention (M Sc); criminology (M Sc); curating contemporary art (MA); data analytics (M Sc); digital media (MA); early childhood studies (MA); education (MA, Ed D); financial services law, regulation and compliance (LL M); food science (M Sc); forensic psychology (M Sc); health and social care management and policy (M Sc); human nutrition (M Sc); human resource management (MA); human rights and international conflict (MA); information technology (M Sc); intelligence and security studies (M Sc); international oil, gas and energy law (LL M); international relations (MA); interpreting (MA); learning and teaching in higher education (MA); legal practice (LL M); media and entertainment law (LL M); organizational and consumer psychology (M Sc); psychological therapy (M Sc); psychology of mental health (M Sc); public health (M Sc); public policy and management (MPA); security studies (M Sc); social work (M Sc); spatial planning and urban design (MA); sports therapy (M Sc); supporting older children and young people with dyslexia (MA); teaching languages (MA), including Arabic, English; translation (MA); woman and child abuse (MA).

Long Island University–LIU Brooklyn, School of Health Professions, Brooklyn, NY 11201-8423. Offers athletic training and sport sciences (MS); exercise science (MS); occupational therapy (MS); physical therapy (DPT); physician assistant (MS); public health (MPH); social work (MSW). *Faculty:* 36 full-time (26 women), 47 part-time/adjunct (19 women). *Students:* 503 full-time (326 women), 112 part-time (82 women); includes 212 minority (117 Black or African American, non-Hispanic/Latino; 35 Asian, non-Hispanic/Latino; 48 Hispanic/Latino; 12 Two or more races, non-Hispanic/Latino), 59 international. Average age 31. 1,154 applicants, 38% accepted, 227 enrolled. In 2015, 228 master's, 41 doctorates awarded. *Degree requirements:* For master's, comprehensive exam (for some programs), thesis (for some programs), research capstone; for doctorate, comprehensive exam, research capstone. *Entrance requirements:* For master's and doctorate, GRE, two letters of recommendation. Additional exam requirements/recommendations for international students: Required—TOEFL (minimum score 550 paper-based; 79 iBT). *Application deadline:* Applications are processed on a rolling basis. Application fee: $50. Electronic applications accepted. *Expenses:* $1,155 per credit tuition, $934 per term full-time fees, $442 per term part-time fees. *Financial support:* In 2015–16, 10 research assistantships with partial tuition reimbursements (averaging $12,660 per year), 40 teaching assistantships with partial tuition reimbursements (averaging $12,660 per year) were awarded. Financial award application deadline: 2/15; financial award applicants required to submit FAFSA. *Faculty research:* Manual physical therapy, Parkinson's disease response to physical activity, violence in young minority men, LGBT safety. *Unit head:* Dr. Barry S. Eckert, Dean, 718-780-6578, Fax: 718-780-4561, E-mail: barry.eckert@liu.edu. *Application contact:* Richard Sunday, Dean of Admissions, 718-488-1011, Fax: 718-780-6110, E-mail: bkln-admissions@liu.edu.
Website: http://liu.edu/brooklyn/academics/school-of-health-professions

Louisiana State University Health Sciences Center, School of Public Health, New Orleans, LA 70112. Offers behavioral and community health sciences (MPH); biostatistics (MPH, MS, PhD); community health sciences (PhD); environmental and occupational health sciences (MPH); epidemiology (MPH, PhD); health policy and systems management (MPH). *Accreditation:* CEPH. *Program availability:* Part-time. *Entrance requirements:* For master's, GRE General Test.

Louisiana State University in Shreveport, College of Business, Education, and Human Development, Program in Public Health, Shreveport, LA 71115-2399. Offers MPH. Program offered jointly with Louisiana State University Health Sciences Center at Shreveport. *Program availability:* Part-time, evening/weekend. *Students:* 18 full-time (12 women), 11 part-time (9 women); includes 11 minority (10 Black or African American, non-Hispanic/Latino; 1 American Indian or Alaska Native, non-Hispanic/Latino), 1 international. Average age 30. 33 applicants, 100% accepted, 8 enrolled. In 2015, 7 master's awarded. *Degree requirements:* For master's, thesis optional, practicum. *Entrance requirements:* For master's, GRE or MCAT, 3 letters of recommendation, personal interview. Additional exam requirements/recommendations for international students: Required—TOEFL (minimum score 550 paper-based; 61 iBT). *Application deadline:* For fall admission, 6/30 for domestic and international students; for spring admission, 11/30 for domestic and international students; for summer admission, 4/30 for domestic and international students. Applications are processed on a rolling basis. Application fee: $20 ($30 for international students). Electronic applications accepted. *Expenses:* Tuition, state resident: part-time $325 per credit hour. Tuition, nonresident: part-time $1019 per credit hour. *Required fees:* $52 per credit hour. Tuition and fees vary according to program. *Financial support:* Applicants required to submit FAFSA. *Unit head:* Dr. Jill Rush-Kolodzey, MD, Program Director, 318-797-5218, E-mail:

jill.rush-kolodzey@lsus.edu. *Application contact:* David Stanford, Director of Admissions, 318-795-2403, Fax: 318-797-5286, E-mail: david.stanford@lsus.edu.

Loyola University Chicago, Graduate School, Public Health Program, Chicago, IL 60660. Offers MPH. *Program availability:* Part-time, online learning. *Faculty:* 7 full-time (3 women), 1 part-time/adjunct (0 women). *Students:* 39 full-time (30 women), 33 part-time (21 women); includes 29 minority (7 Black or African American, non-Hispanic/Latino; 13 Asian, non-Hispanic/Latino; 6 Hispanic/Latino; 1 Native Hawaiian or other Pacific Islander, non-Hispanic/Latino; 2 Two or more races, non-Hispanic/Latino), 3 international. Average age 30. 73 applicants, 74% accepted, 27 enrolled. In 2015, 20 master's awarded. *Degree requirements:* For master's, comprehensive exam. *Entrance requirements:* For master's, GRE, MCAT. *Application deadline:* For fall admission, 5/15 for domestic and international students; for spring admission, 11/15 for domestic and international students. *Expenses:* Tuition, area resident: Full-time $18,054; part-time $9027 per credit hour. *Required fees:* $832; $284 per credit hour. Part-time tuition and fees vary according to course load, degree level and program. *Financial support:* Career-related internships or fieldwork available. Financial award applicants required to submit FAFSA. *Faculty research:* Genetics of hypertension and obesity, vitamin D metabolism, kidney diseases. *Unit head:* Dr. Samuel Attoh, Dean, 773-508-3459, Fax: 773-508-2460, E-mail: sattoh@luc.edu. *Application contact:* Izlze Berzins, Administrative Coordinator, 708-327-9224, Fax: 708-327-9090, E-mail: iberzin@lumc.edu.

Marshall University, Academic Affairs Division, College of Health Professions, Department of Public Health, Huntington, WV 25755. Offers MPH. *Faculty:* 1 full-time (0 women). *Students:* 18 full-time (12 women), 2 part-time (1 woman); includes 3 minority (1 Black or African American, non-Hispanic/Latino; 2 Asian, non-Hispanic/Latino), 4 international. Average age 26. *Unit head:* William Pewen, Chair, 304-696-3743, E-mail: pewen@marshall.edu. *Application contact:* Information Contact, 304-746-1900, Fax: 304-746-1902, E-mail: services@marshall.edu.
Website: http://www.marshall.edu/cohp/index.php/departments/public-health/

Medical College of Wisconsin, Graduate School of Biomedical Sciences, Department of Population Health, Program in Public Health, Milwaukee, WI 53226-0509. Offers public and community health (PhD); public health (MPH, Graduate Certificate). *Accreditation:* CEPH. *Entrance requirements:* For master's, doctorate, and Graduate Certificate, GRE, official transcripts, three letters of recommendation. Additional exam requirements/recommendations for international students: Required—TOEFL.

Medical College of Wisconsin, Graduate School of Biomedical Sciences, Program in Public and Community Health, Milwaukee, WI 53226-0509. Offers PhD, MD/PhD. *Accreditation:* CEPH. *Degree requirements:* For doctorate, comprehensive exam, thesis/dissertation. *Entrance requirements:* For doctorate, GRE, official transcripts, three letters of recommendation. Additional exam requirements/recommendations for international students: Required—TOEFL (minimum score 580 paper-based; 100 iBT). Electronic applications accepted. *Expenses:* Contact institution. *Faculty research:* Community-academic partnerships, community-based participatory research, injury prevention, health policy, women's health, emergency medical services.

Mercer University, Graduate Studies, Cecil B. Day Campus, College of Health Professions, Atlanta, GA 30341. Offers physical therapy (DPT); physician assistant (MM Sc); public health (MPH). *Faculty:* 27 full-time (19 women), 14 part-time/adjunct (7 women). *Students:* 286 full-time (230 women), 4 part-time (all women); includes 94 minority (69 Black or African American, non-Hispanic/Latino; 14 Asian, non-Hispanic/Latino; 7 Hispanic/Latino; 4 Two or more races, non-Hispanic/Latino), 3 international. Average age 26. In 2015, 80 master's, 32 doctorates awarded. *Expenses:* Contact institution. *Financial support:* Federal Work-Study, traineeships, and unspecified assistantships available. *Faculty research:* Scholarship of teaching and learning, health disparities, clinical outcomes, health promotion. *Unit head:* Dr. Lisa Lundquist, Dean/Clinical Professor, 678-547-6308, E-mail: lundquist_lm@mercer.edu. *Application contact:* Laura Ellison, Director of Admissions and Student Affairs, 678-547-6391, E-mail: ellison_la@mercer.edu.
Website: http://chp.mercer.edu/

Michigan State University, College of Human Medicine and The Graduate School, Graduate Programs in Human Medicine, Program in Public Health, East Lansing, MI 48824. Offers MPH.

MidAmerica Nazarene University, Post-Licensure and Graduate Nursing Education Program, Olathe, KS 66062-1899. Offers healthcare administration (MSN); healthcare quality management (MSN); nursing education (MSN); public health (MSN); MSN/MBA. *Program availability:* Part-time, 100% online, blended/hybrid learning. *Faculty:* 8 full-time (all women), 6 part-time/adjunct (3 women). *Students:* 9 full-time (8 women), 103 part-time (100 women); includes 23 minority (14 Black or African American, non-Hispanic/Latino; 1 American Indian or Alaska Native, non-Hispanic/Latino; 4 Asian, non-Hispanic/Latino; 4 Hispanic/Latino). 50 applicants, 82% accepted. In 2015, 36 master's awarded. *Degree requirements:* For master's, final project. *Entrance requirements:* For master's, BSN, minimum GPA of 3.0, active unencumbered RN license, undergraduate statistics course. *Application deadline:* Applications are processed on a rolling basis. Electronic applications accepted. *Expenses:* $22,065 tuition, $1,186 fee (including technology, carrying and graduation fee). *Financial support:* Unspecified assistantships available. Financial award applicants required to submit FAFSA. *Faculty research:* Technology in education, minority recruitment and retention in nursing programs, faculty views and attitudes on culturally competency, innovative nursing program development, spirituality and holistic health. *Unit head:* Dr. Karen Wiegman, RN, Dean, 913-971-3839, E-mail: kdwiegman@mnu.edu. *Application contact:* E-mail: pgadmissions@mnu.edu.
Website: http://www.mnu.edu/nursing.html

Missouri State University, Graduate College, College of Health and Human Services, Program in Public Health, Springfield, MO 65897. Offers MPH. *Accreditation:* CEPH. *Faculty:* 3 full-time (1 woman). *Students:* 23 full-time (16 women), 16 part-time (14 women); includes 3 minority (1 Asian, non-Hispanic/Latino; 1 Hispanic/Latino; 1 Two or more races, non-Hispanic/Latino), 19 international. Average age 30. 60 applicants, 40% accepted, 12 enrolled. In 2015, 13 master's awarded. *Degree requirements:* For master's, comprehensive exam, thesis or alternative. *Entrance requirements:* For master's, GRE, minimum GPA of 3.0, 1 year of work experience. Additional exam requirements/recommendations for international students: Required—TOEFL (minimum score 550 paper-based; 79 iBT), IELTS (minimum score 6). *Application deadline:* For fall admission, 4/1 priority date for domestic students, 4/1 for international students; for spring admission, 10/1 priority date for domestic students, 10/1 for international students. Applications are processed on a rolling basis. Application fee: $35 ($50 for international students). Electronic applications accepted. *Expenses:* Tuition, state resident: full-time $5500. Tuition, nonresident: full-time $10,108. *Required fees:* $1000. *Financial support:* Federal Work-Study, institutionally sponsored loans, scholarships/grants, and unspecified assistantships available. Financial award application deadline: 3/31; financial award applicants required to submit FAFSA. *Unit head:* Dr. David Claborn, Program Director, 417-836-8945, E-mail: davidclaborn@missouristate.edu. *Application contact:* Michael Edwards, Coordinator of Graduate Admissions, 417-836-5033, Fax: 417-836-6200, E-mail: michaeledwards@missouristate.edu.
Website: http://www.missouristate.edu/mph/

Public Health—General

Monroe College, King Graduate School, Bronx, NY 10468-5407. Offers business management (MBA); criminal justice (MS); executive leadership in hospitality management (MS); public health (MPH). Program also offered in New Rochelle, NY. *Program availability:* Online learning.

Montclair State University, The Graduate School, College of Education and Human Services, Program in Public Health, Montclair, NJ 07043-1624. Offers MPH. *Program availability:* Part-time, evening/weekend. *Students:* 35 full-time (32 women), 12 part-time (10 women); includes 19 minority (7 Black or African American, non-Hispanic/Latino; 4 Asian, non-Hispanic/Latino; 8 Hispanic/Latino), 5 international. Average age 29. 51 applicants, 43% accepted, 22 enrolled. In 2015, 20 master's awarded. *Degree requirements:* For master's, comprehensive exam, thesis or alternative. *Entrance requirements:* For master's, GRE General Test, essay, 2 letters of recommendation. Additional exam requirements/recommendations for international students: Required—TOEFL (minimum score 83 iBT), IELTS (minimum score 6.5). *Application deadline:* Applications are processed on a rolling basis. Application fee: $60. Electronic applications accepted. *Expenses:* Tuition, state resident: part-time $553 per credit. Tuition, nonresident: part-time $854 per credit. *Required fees:* $91 per credit. Tuition and fees vary according to program. *Financial support:* In 2015–16, 4 research assistantships with full tuition reimbursements (averaging $7,000 per year) were awarded; Federal Work-Study, scholarships/grants, and unspecified assistantships also available. Support available to part-time students. Financial award application deadline: 3/1; financial award applicants required to submit FAFSA. *Unit head:* Dr. Eva Goldfarb, Chairperson, 973-655-4154. *Application contact:* Amy Aiello, Executive Director of The Graduate School, 973-655-5147, Fax: 973-655-7869, E-mail: graduate.school@montclair.edu.
Website: http://www.montclair.edu/cehs/academics/departments/hns/academic-programs/ma-public-health/

Morehouse School of Medicine, Master of Public Health Program, Atlanta, GA 30310-1495. Offers MPH. *Accreditation:* CEPH. *Program availability:* Part-time. *Degree requirements:* For master's, thesis, practicum, public health leadership seminar. *Entrance requirements:* For master's, GRE General Test, writing test, public health or human service experience. Additional exam requirements/recommendations for international students: Required—TOEFL (minimum score 550 paper-based). *Application deadline:* For fall admission, 3/1 for domestic and international students. Application fee: $50. Electronic applications accepted. *Expenses:* Contact institution. *Financial support:* Fellowships, research assistantships with partial tuition reimbursements, teaching assistantships, career-related internships or fieldwork, Federal Work-Study, institutionally sponsored loans, scholarships/grants, and unspecified assistantships available. Support available to part-time students. Financial award application deadline: 5/1; financial award applicants required to submit FAFSA. *Faculty research:* Women's and adolescent health, violence prevention, cancer epidemiology/disparities, substance abuse prevention. *Unit head:* Dr. Stephanie Miles-Richardson, Director, 404-752-1944, Fax: 404-752-1051, E-mail: smiles-richardson@msm.edu. *Application contact:* Brandon Hunter, Director of Admissions, 404-752-1650, Fax: 404-752-1512, E-mail: mphadmissions@msm.edu.
Website: http://www.msm.edu/Education/MPH/index.php

Morgan State University, School of Graduate Studies, School of Community Health and Policy, Baltimore, MD 21251. Offers nursing (MS); public health (MPH, Dr PH). *Accreditation:* CEPH. *Degree requirements:* For doctorate, thesis/dissertation. *Entrance requirements:* For doctorate, GRE, minimum GPA of 3.0. Additional exam requirements/recommendations for international students: Required—TOEFL (minimum score 550 paper-based).

National University, Academic Affairs, School of Health and Human Services, La Jolla, CA 92037-1011. Offers clinical affairs (MS); clinical informatics (Certificate); clinical regulatory affairs (MS); health and life science analytics (MS); health coaching (Certificate); health informatics (MS); healthcare administration (MHA); nurse anesthesia (MS); nursing (MS), including forensic nursing, nursing administration, nursing informatics; nursing administration (Certificate); nursing informatics (Certificate); nursing practice (DNP); public health (MPH), including health promotion, healthcare administration, mental health. *Program availability:* Part-time, evening/weekend, 100% online, blended/hybrid learning. *Faculty:* 31 full-time (18 women), 33 part-time/adjunct (20 women). *Students:* 353 full-time (263 women), 136 part-time (87 women); includes 322 minority (111 Black or African American, non-Hispanic/Latino; 1 American Indian or Alaska Native, non-Hispanic/Latino; 105 Asian, non-Hispanic/Latino; 72 Hispanic/Latino; 7 Native Hawaiian or other Pacific Islander, non-Hispanic/Latino; 26 Two or more races, non-Hispanic/Latino), 31 international. Average age 32. In 2015, 103 master's awarded. *Degree requirements:* For master's, thesis (for some programs). *Entrance requirements:* For master's, interview, minimum GPA of 2.5. Additional exam requirements/recommendations for international students: Required—TOEFL (minimum score 550 paper-based; 79 iBT), IELTS (minimum score 6). *Application deadline:* Applications are processed on a rolling basis. Application fee: $60 ($65 for international students). Electronic applications accepted. *Financial support:* Career-related internships or fieldwork, institutionally sponsored loans, scholarships/grants, and tuition waivers (partial) available. Support available to part-time students. Financial award application deadline: 6/30; financial award applicants required to submit FAFSA. *Faculty research:* Nursing education, obesity prevention, workforce diversity. *Unit head:* School of Health and Human Services, 800-628-8648, E-mail: shhs@nu.edu. *Application contact:* Frank Rojas, Vice President for Enrollment Services, 800-628-8648, E-mail: advisor@nu.edu.
Website: http://www.nu.edu/OurPrograms/SchoolOfHealthAndHumanServices.html

New Mexico State University, College of Health and Social Services, Department of Public Health Sciences, Las Cruces, NM 88003-8001. Offers public health (MPH, Graduate Certificate). *Program availability:* Part-time, blended/hybrid learning. *Faculty:* 10 full-time (6 women), 3 part-time/adjunct (1 woman). *Students:* 41 full-time (31 women), 54 part-time (37 women); includes 39 minority (6 Black or African American, non-Hispanic/Latino; 3 American Indian or Alaska Native, non-Hispanic/Latino; 2 Asian, non-Hispanic/Latino; 27 Hispanic/Latino; 1 Two or more races, non-Hispanic/Latino), 11 international. Average age 35. 72 applicants, 72% accepted, 6 enrolled. In 2015, 24 master's, 3 other advanced degrees awarded. *Degree requirements:* For master's, thesis optional. *Entrance requirements:* For master's, GRE. Additional exam requirements/recommendations for international students: Required—TOEFL (minimum score 550 paper-based; 79 iBT), IELTS (minimum score 6.5). *Application deadline:* For fall admission, 2/15 for domestic and international students. Application fee: $40 ($50 for international students). Electronic applications accepted. *Expenses:* $274.50 per credit hour for in-state students, and all students enrolled in six or fewer credits; $839.30 per credit hour for out-of-state and international students enrolled in at least seven hours. *Financial support:* In 2015–16, 16 students received support, including 9 teaching assistantships (averaging $10,367 per year); career-related internships or fieldwork, Federal Work-Study, health care benefits, and unspecified assistantships available. Financial award application deadline: 3/1. *Faculty research:* Community health education, health issues of U.S.-Mexico border, health policy and management, victims of violence, environmental and occupational health issues. *Total annual research expenditures:* $449,037. *Unit head:* Dr. Joe Tomaka, Department Head, 575-646-4300, Fax: 575-646-4343, E-mail: tomaka@nmsu.edu. *Application contact:* Dr. James Robinson, III, Graduate Coordinator, 575-646-7431, Fax: 575-646-4343, E-mail: jrobins3@nmsu.edu.
Website: http://publichealth.nmsu.edu

New York Medical College, School of Health Sciences and Practice, Valhalla, NY 10595-1691. Offers MPH, MS, DPT, Graduate Certificate. *Accreditation:* CEPH. *Expenses: Tuition, area resident:* Full-time $44,355; part-time $1025 per credit. *Required fees:* $500; $95 per year. One-time fee: $140 part-time. Tuition and fees vary according to course load and program.

New York Medical College, School of Health Sciences and Practice, Department of Epidemiology and Community Health, Program in Behavioral Sciences and Health Promotion, Valhalla, NY 10595-1691. Offers behavioral sciences and health promotion (MPH); public health (Graduate Certificate). *Program availability:* Part-time, evening/weekend. *Degree requirements:* For master's, thesis, capstone. *Entrance requirements:* For master's, minimum undergraduate GPA of 3.0. Additional exam requirements/recommendations for international students: Required—TOEFL (minimum score 637 paper-based; 110 iBT), IELTS (minimum score 7). Electronic applications accepted. *Expenses: Tuition, area resident:* Full-time $44,355; part-time $1025 per credit. *Required fees:* $500; $95 per year. One-time fee: $140 part-time. Tuition and fees vary according to course load and program.

New York University, College of Global Public Health, New York, NY 10003. Offers biological basis of public health (PhD); community and international health (MPH); global health leadership (MPH); health systems and health services research (PhD); population and community health (PhD); public health nutrition (MPH); social and behavioral sciences (MPH); socio-behavioral health (PhD). *Program availability:* Part-time, online learning. *Degree requirements:* For master's, thesis (for some programs); for doctorate, thesis/dissertation. *Entrance requirements:* For master's and doctorate, GRE. Additional exam requirements/recommendations for international students: Required—TOEFL. Electronic applications accepted.

North Dakota State University, College of Graduate and Interdisciplinary Studies, College of Health Professions, Fargo, ND 58102. Offers MPH, MS, DNP, PhD, Pharm D, Pharm D/MBA, Pharm D/MPH, Pharm D/PhD. *Program availability:* Part-time. Terminal master's awarded for partial completion of doctoral program. *Degree requirements:* For master's, thesis; for doctorate, thesis/dissertation. *Entrance requirements:* For master's and doctorate, GRE General Test. Additional exam requirements/recommendations for international students: Required—TOEFL. *Application deadline:* Applications are processed on a rolling basis. Application fee: $35. Electronic applications accepted. *Financial support:* Research assistantships with full tuition reimbursements, career-related internships or fieldwork, Federal Work-Study, institutionally sponsored loans, and scholarships/grants available. Financial award application deadline: 4/1. *Unit head:* Dr. Charles D. Peterson, Dean, 701-231-5383, Fax: 701-231-7606. *Application contact:* Dr. Charles D. Peterson, Dean, 701-231-5383, Fax: 701-231-7606.
Website: http://www.ndsu.edu/healthprofessions/

Northeast Ohio Medical University, College of Graduate Studies, Rootstown, OH 44272-0095. Offers bioethics (Certificate); health-system pharmacy administration (MS); integrated pharmaceutical medicine (MS, PhD); public health (MS). *Program availability:* Part-time. *Faculty:* 15 part-time/adjunct (6 women). *Students:* 15 full-time (7 women), 26 part-time (11 women); includes 7 minority (5 Asian, non-Hispanic/Latino; 2 Hispanic/Latino). Average age 27. In 2015, 9 master's, 1 doctorate awarded. *Application deadline:* For fall admission, 9/1 priority date for domestic students; for winter admission, 1/5 priority date for domestic students. Applications are processed on a rolling basis. Electronic applications accepted. *Expenses:* Contact institution. *Financial support:* In 2015–16, 18 students received support. *Unit head:* Dr. Walter E. Horton, Jr., Dean. *Application contact:* Heidi Terry, Executive Director, Enrollment Services, 330-325-6479, E-mail: hterry@neoucom.edu.
Website: http://www.neomed.edu/academics/graduatestudies

Northern Illinois University, Graduate School, College of Health and Human Sciences, School of Nursing and Health Studies, De Kalb, IL 60115-2854. Offers nursing (MS); public health (MPH). *Accreditation:* AACN. *Program availability:* Part-time. *Faculty:* 12 full-time (11 women), 1 (woman) part-time/adjunct. *Students:* 29 full-time (22 women), 200 part-time (179 women); includes 48 minority (12 Black or African American, non-Hispanic/Latino; 21 Asian, non-Hispanic/Latino; 10 Hispanic/Latino; 5 Two or more races, non-Hispanic/Latino), 5 international. Average age 35. 177 applicants, 40% accepted, 36 enrolled. In 2015, 102 master's awarded. *Degree requirements:* For master's, thesis optional, internship. *Entrance requirements:* For master's, minimum GPA of 3.0 in last 60 hours, BA in nursing, nursing license. Additional exam requirements/recommendations for international students: Required—TOEFL (minimum score 550 paper-based). *Application deadline:* For fall admission, 6/1 for domestic students, 5/1 for international students; for spring admission, 11/1 for domestic students, 10/1 for international students. Applications are processed on a rolling basis. Application fee: $40. Electronic applications accepted. *Financial support:* In 2015–16, 1 research assistantship with full tuition reimbursement, 22 teaching assistantships with full tuition reimbursements were awarded; fellowships with full tuition reimbursements, career-related internships or fieldwork, Federal Work-Study, scholarships/grants, tuition waivers (full), and unspecified assistantships also available. Support available to part-time students. Financial award applicants required to submit FAFSA. *Faculty research:* Neonatal intensive care, stress and coping, refugee and immigrant issues, older adults, autoimmune disorders. *Unit head:* Dr. Janice Strom, Chair, 815-753-6550, Fax: 815-753-0814, E-mail: jstrom@niu.edu. *Application contact:* Graduate School Office, 815-753-0395, E-mail: gradsch@niu.edu.
Website: http://www.chhs.niu.edu/nursing/

Northwestern University, Feinberg School of Medicine, Program in Public Health, Evanston, IL 60208. Offers MPH. *Accreditation:* CEPH. *Program availability:* Part-time, evening/weekend. *Entrance requirements:* For master's, GRE General Test. Additional exam requirements/recommendations for international students: Required—TOEFL. *Faculty research:* Cardiovascular epidemiology, cancer epidemiology, nutritional interventions for the prevention of cardiovascular disease and cancer, women's health, outcomes research.

Nova Southeastern University, College of Osteopathic Medicine, Fort Lauderdale, FL 33328. Offers biomedical informatics (MS, Graduate Certificate), including biomedical informatics (MS), clinical informatics (Graduate Certificate), public health informatics (Graduate Certificate); disaster and emergency preparedness (MS); osteopathic medicine (DO); public health (MPH). *Accreditation:* AOsA. *Faculty:* 107 full-time (55 women), 1,235 part-time/adjunct (297 women). *Students:* 1,027 full-time (436 women), 189 part-time (124 women); includes 560 minority (92 Black or African American, non-Hispanic/Latino; 260 Asian, non-Hispanic/Latino; 174 Hispanic/Latino; 1 Native Hawaiian or other Pacific Islander, non-Hispanic/Latino; 33 Two or more races, non-Hispanic/Latino), 45 international. Average age 28. 4,012 applicants, 12% accepted, 246 enrolled. In 2015, 75 master's, 237 doctorates, 4 other advanced degrees awarded. *Entrance requirements:* For master's, GRE; for doctorate, MCAT, biology, chemistry, organic chemistry, physics (all with labs), and English. *Application deadline:* For fall admission, 1/15 for domestic students. Applications are processed on a rolling basis.

Application fee: $50. Electronic applications accepted. *Expenses:* Contact institution. *Financial support:* In 2015–16, 39 students received support, including 24 fellowships (averaging $45,593 per year); research assistantships, teaching assistantships, Federal Work-Study, and scholarships/grants also available. Financial award application deadline: 6/1; financial award applicants required to submit FAFSA. *Faculty research:* Teaching strategies, simulated patient use, HIV/AIDS education, minority health issues, managed care education. *Unit head:* Elaine M. Wallace, DO, Dean, 954-262-1407, E-mail: ewallace@nova.edu. *Application contact:* Monica Sanchez, Admissions Counselor, College of Osteopathic Medicine, 954-262-1110, Fax: 954-262-2282, E-mail: mh1156@nova.edu.
Website: http://www.medicine.nova.edu/

The Ohio State University, College of Public Health, Columbus, OH 43210. Offers MHA, MPH, MS, PhD, DVM/MPH, JD/MHA, MHA/MBA, MHA/MD, MHA/MPA, MHA/MS, MPH/MBA, MPH/MD, MPH/MSW. *Accreditation:* CAHME; CEPH. *Program availability:* Part-time. *Faculty:* 44. *Students:* 268 full-time (189 women), 67 part-time (49 women); includes 73 minority (22 Black or African American, non-Hispanic/Latino; 1 American Indian or Alaska Native, non-Hispanic/Latino; 29 Asian, non-Hispanic/Latino; 12 Hispanic/Latino; 9 Two or more races, non-Hispanic/Latino), 11 international. Average age 28. In 2015, 114 master's, 7 doctorates awarded. Terminal master's awarded for partial completion of doctoral program. *Degree requirements:* For master's, thesis optional, practicum; for doctorate, thesis/dissertation. *Entrance requirements:* For master's and doctorate, GRE. Additional exam requirements/recommendations for international students: Required—TOEFL (minimum score 550 paper-based; 79 iBT); Recommended—IELTS (minimum score 7). *Application deadline:* For fall admission, 12/1 priority date for domestic students, 11/1 priority date for international students. Applications are processed on a rolling basis. Application fee: $60 ($70 for international students). Electronic applications accepted. *Financial support:* Fellowships with tuition reimbursements and research assistantships with tuition reimbursements available. *Unit head:* Dr. William J. Martin, II, Dean and Professor, 614-292-8350, E-mail: martin.3047@osu.edu. *Application contact:* Dr. William J. Martin, II, Dean and Professor, 614-292-8350, E-mail: martin.3047@osu.edu.
Website: http://cph.osu.edu/

Ohio University, Graduate College, College of Health Sciences and Professions, Department of Social and Public Health, Athens, OH 45701-2979. Offers early child development and family life (MS); family studies (MS); health administration (MHA); public health (MPH); social work (MSW). *Accreditation:* CEPH. *Program availability:* Part-time, evening/weekend, online learning. *Degree requirements:* For master's, capstone (MPH). *Entrance requirements:* For master's, GMAT, GRE General Test, previous course work in accounting, management, and statistics, previous public health background (MHA, MPH). Additional exam requirements/recommendations for international students: Required—TOEFL (minimum score 550 paper-based; 80 iBT) or IELTS (minimum score 6.5). Electronic applications accepted. *Expenses:* Contact institution. *Faculty research:* Health care management, health policy, managed care, health behavior, disease prevention.

Oregon State University, College of Public Health and Human Sciences, Program in Public Health, Corvallis, OR 97331. Offers biostatistics (MPH); environmental and occupational health and safety (MPH, PhD); epidemiology (MPH, PhD); health management and policy (MPH); health policy (PhD); health promotion and health behavior (MPH, PhD); international health (MPH). *Accreditation:* CEPH. *Program availability:* Part-time. *Faculty:* 32 full-time (18 women), 3 part-time/adjunct (0 women). *Students:* 123 full-time (91 women), 20 part-time (14 women); includes 43 minority (2 Black or African American, non-Hispanic/Latino; 2 American Indian or Alaska Native, non-Hispanic/Latino; 9 Asian, non-Hispanic/Latino; 18 Hispanic/Latino; 1 Native Hawaiian or other Pacific Islander, non-Hispanic/Latino; 11 Two or more races, non-Hispanic/Latino), 18 international. Average age 31. 276 applicants, 65% accepted, 45 enrolled. In 2015, 59 master's, 6 doctorates awarded. Terminal master's awarded for partial completion of doctoral program. *Degree requirements:* For doctorate, one foreign language, thesis/dissertation. *Entrance requirements:* For master's and doctorate, GRE, minimum GPA of 3.0 in last 90 hours. Additional exam requirements/recommendations for international students: Required—TOEFL (minimum score 80 iBT), IELTS (minimum score 6.5). *Application deadline:* For fall admission, 12/1 priority date for domestic students. Applications are processed on a rolling basis. *Expenses:* $13,851 full-time resident tuition, $23,679 full-time non-resident tuition, $1,572 fees. *Financial support:* Fellowships, research assistantships, teaching assistantships, career-related internships or fieldwork, Federal Work-Study, and institutionally sponsored loans available. Support available to part-time students. Financial award application deadline: 12/1. *Faculty research:* Traffic safety, health safety, injury control, health promotion. *Unit head:* Dr. Sheryl Thorburn, Professor/Co-Director. *Application contact:* Amanda Armington, Public Health Program Manager, 541-737-3825, E-mail: amanda.armington@oregonstate.edu.

Penn State Hershey Medical Center, College of Medicine, Graduate School Programs in the Biomedical Sciences, Graduate Program in Public Health, Hershey, PA 17033. Offers MPH, Dr PH. *Accreditation:* CEPH. *Program availability:* Part-time, evening/weekend. *Students:* 32 full-time (23 women); includes 9 minority (3 Black or African American, non-Hispanic/Latino; 5 Asian, non-Hispanic/Latino; 1 Hispanic/Latino), 3 international. 56 applicants, 73% accepted, 22 enrolled. *Degree requirements:* For master's, thesis or alternative. *Entrance requirements:* For doctorate, master's degree. Additional exam requirements/recommendations for international students: Required—TOEFL (minimum score 550 paper-based; 80 iBT). *Application deadline:* For fall admission, 3/1 for domestic students, 1/15 for international students. Applications are processed on a rolling basis. Application fee: $65. Electronic applications accepted. *Financial support:* Fellowships available. Financial award applicants required to submit FAFSA. *Unit head:* Dr. Wenke Hwang, Director, 717-531-1502, E-mail: whwang@phs.psu.edu. *Application contact:* Farah Kauffman, Deputy Director, 717-531-1502, Fax: 717-531-0608, E-mail: pennstatepublichealth@phs.psu.edu.
Website: http://www2.med.psu.edu/phs/graduate-programs/

Penn State Hershey Medical Center, College of Medicine, Graduate School Programs in the Biomedical Sciences, Graduate Program in Public Health Sciences, Hershey, PA 17033. Offers MS. *Program availability:* Part-time. *Students:* 10 full-time (7 women); includes 1 minority (Asian, non-Hispanic/Latino), 3 international. 26 applicants, 12% accepted, 3 enrolled. In 2015, 9 master's awarded. *Degree requirements:* For master's, thesis or alternative. *Entrance requirements:* Additional exam requirements/recommendations for international students: Required—TOEFL (minimum score 550 paper-based). *Application deadline:* For fall admission, 1/31 priority date for domestic students, 2/1 priority date for international students. Applications are processed on a rolling basis. Application fee: $65. Electronic applications accepted. *Financial support:* Fellowships available. Financial award applicants required to submit FAFSA. *Faculty research:* Clinical trials, statistical methods in genetic epidemiology, genetic factors in nicotine dependence and dementia syndromes, health economics, cancer. *Unit head:* Dr. Douglas Leslie, Director, 717-531-7178, Fax: 717-531-5779, E-mail: hes-grad-hmc@psu.edu. *Application contact:* Mardi Sawyer, Program Administrator, 717-531-7178, Fax: 717-531-5779, E-mail: hes-grad-hmc@psu.edu.

Website: http://www2.med.psu.edu/phs/graduate-programs/master-of-science-in-public-health-sciences-program-ms-phs/

Ponce Health Sciences University, Program in Public Health, Ponce, PR 00732-7004. Offers epidemiology (Dr PH); public health (MPH). *Accreditation:* CEPH. *Degree requirements:* For master's, one foreign language, comprehensive exam, thesis. *Entrance requirements:* For master's, GRE General Test or EXADEP, proficiency in Spanish and English, minimum GPA of 2.7, 3 letters of recommendation; for doctorate, GRE, proficiency in Spanish and English, minimum GPA of 3.0, letter of recommendation.

Portland State University, Graduate Studies, College of Urban and Public Affairs, School of Community Health, Portland, OR 97207-0751. Offers aging (Certificate); community health (PhD); health education (MA, MS); health promotion (MPH); health studies (MPA, MPH), including health administration. MPH offered jointly with Oregon Health & Science University. *Accreditation:* CEPH. *Program availability:* Part-time. *Faculty:* 35 full-time (25 women), 14 part-time/adjunct (6 women). *Students:* 67 full-time (53 women), 61 part-time (54 women); includes 33 minority (2 Black or African American, non-Hispanic/Latino; 6 American Indian or Alaska Native, non-Hispanic/Latino; 5 Asian, non-Hispanic/Latino; 12 Hispanic/Latino; 8 Two or more races, non-Hispanic/Latino), 4 international. Average age 33. 85 applicants, 49% accepted, 33 enrolled. In 2015, 46 master's, 1 doctorate awarded. *Degree requirements:* For master's, comprehensive exam (for some programs), thesis (for some programs), internship/praticum, oral and written exams (depending on program; for doctorate, comprehensive exam, thesis/dissertation. *Entrance requirements:* For master's, GRE (for MPH program), 3 letters of recommendation, minimum GPA of 3.0, resume; for doctorate, GRE, transcripts, personal statement, resume, writing sample, 3 letters of recommendation. Additional exam requirements/recommendations for international students: Required—TOEFL (minimum score 550 paper-based; 80 iBT). *Application deadline:* For fall admission, 2/1 for domestic and international students. Applications are processed on a rolling basis. Application fee: $50. *Expenses:* $11,301 per year. *Financial support:* In 2015–16, 13 research assistantships with tuition reimbursements (averaging $7,336 per year) were awarded; teaching assistantships, career-related internships or fieldwork, Federal Work-Study, scholarships/grants, and unspecified assistantships also available. Support available to part-time students. Financial award application deadline: 3/1; financial award applicants required to submit FAFSA. *Total annual research expenditures:* $1.7 million. *Unit head:* Dr. Carlos J. Crespo, Director, 503-725-5120, Fax: 503-725-5100. *Application contact:* Elizabeth Bull, Assistant to the Director, 503-725-4592, Fax: 503-725-5100, E-mail: bulle@pdx.edu.
Website: http://www.healthed.pdx.edu/

Purdue University, Graduate School, College of Health and Human Sciences, Department of Nutrition Science, West Lafayette, IN 47907. Offers animal health (MS, PhD); biochemical and molecular nutrition (MS, PhD); growth and development (MS, PhD); human and clinical nutrition (MS, PhD); public health and education (MS, PhD). *Degree requirements:* For master's, thesis; for doctorate, thesis/dissertation. *Entrance requirements:* For master's and doctorate, GRE General Test (minimum scores in verbal and quantitative areas of 1000 or 300 on new scoring), minimum undergraduate GPA of 3.0 or equivalent. Additional exam requirements/recommendations for international students: Required—TOEFL (minimum score 600 paper-based; 77 iBT). Electronic applications accepted. *Faculty research:* Nutrient requirements, nutrient metabolism, nutrition and disease prevention.

Purdue University, School of Veterinary Medicine and Graduate School, Graduate Programs in Veterinary Medicine, Department of Comparative Pathobiology, West Lafayette, IN 47907-2027. Offers comparative epidemiology and public health (MS); comparative epidemiology and public heath (PhD); comparative microbiology and immunology (MS, PhD); comparative pathobiology (MS, PhD); interdisciplinary studies (PhD), including microbial pathogenesis, molecular signaling and cancer biology, molecular virology; lab animal medicine (MS); veterinary anatomic pathology (MS); veterinary clinical pathology (MS). Terminal master's awarded for partial completion of doctoral program. *Degree requirements:* For master's, thesis (for some programs); for doctorate, thesis/dissertation. *Entrance requirements:* For master's and doctorate, GRE General Test. Additional exam requirements/recommendations for international students: Required—TOEFL (minimum score 575 paper-based), IELTS (minimum score 6.5), TWE (minimum score 4). Electronic applications accepted.

Queen's University at Kingston, School of Graduate Studies, Faculty of Health Sciences, Department of Community Health and Epidemiology, Kingston, ON K7L 3N6, Canada. Offers epidemiology (PhD); epidemiology and population health (M Sc); health services (M Sc); policy research and clinical epidemiology (M Sc); public health (MPH). *Program availability:* Part-time. *Degree requirements:* For master's, thesis. *Entrance requirements:* For master's, GRE General Test (strongly recommended). Additional exam requirements/recommendations for international students: Required—TOEFL (minimum score 600 paper-based). *Faculty research:* Cancer epidemiology, clinical trials, biostatistics health services research, health policy.

Rutgers University–Camden, School of Public Health, Stratford, NJ 08084. Offers general public health (Certificate); health systems and policy (MPH); DO/MPH. *Accreditation:* CEPH. *Program availability:* Part-time, evening/weekend. *Degree requirements:* For master's, thesis, internship. *Entrance requirements:* For master's, GRE General Test. Additional exam requirements/recommendations for international students: Required—TOEFL. Electronic applications accepted.

Rutgers University–Newark, School of Public Health, Newark, NJ 07107-1709. Offers clinical epidemiology (Certificate); dental public health (MPH); general public health (Certificate); public policy and oral health services administration (Certificate); quantitative methods (MPH); urban health (MPH); DMD/MPH; MD/MPH; MS/MPH. *Accreditation:* CEPH. *Program availability:* Part-time, evening/weekend. *Degree requirements:* For master's, thesis, internship. *Entrance requirements:* For master's, GRE General Test. Additional exam requirements/recommendations for international students: Required—TOEFL. Electronic applications accepted.

Rutgers University–New Brunswick, School of Public Health, Program in Public Health, Piscataway, NJ 08854-8097. Offers MPH, Dr PH, PhD, MBA/MPH, MD/MPH. *Accreditation:* CEPH. *Program availability:* Part-time, evening/weekend. *Degree requirements:* For master's, internship; for doctorate, thesis/dissertation. *Entrance requirements:* For master's, GMAT, GRE General Test; for doctorate, GRE General Test, MPH (for Dr PH). Additional exam requirements/recommendations for international students: Required—TOEFL. *Expenses:* Contact institution. *Faculty research:* Epidemiology, risk perception, statistical research design, health care utilization, health promotion.

St. Catherine University, Graduate Programs, Program in Holistic Health Studies, St. Paul, MN 55105. Offers MA. *Program availability:* Part-time. *Degree requirements:* For master's, thesis optional. *Entrance requirements:* For master's, 1 course in anatomy, physiology and psychology. Additional exam requirements/recommendations for international students: Required—TOEFL (minimum score 600 paper-based; 100 iBT). *Expenses:* Contact institution.

St. John's University, College of Pharmacy and Health Sciences, Graduate Programs in Pharmaceutical Sciences and Division of Library and Information Science, Master of

Public Health—General

Public Health Program, Queens, NY 11439. Offers MPH. *Program availability:* Part-time, evening/weekend. *Degree requirements:* For master's, comprehensive exam, thesis optional, fieldwork. *Entrance requirements:* For master's, GRE, bachelor's degree with pharmacy or related major, minimum GPA of 3.0, 3 letters of recommendation, personal statement. Additional exam requirements/recommendations for international students: Required—TOEFL (minimum score 600 paper-based; 100 iBT), IELTS (minimum score 7). Electronic applications accepted. *Expenses:* Contact institution.

Saint Louis University, Graduate Education, School of Public Health and Graduate Education, Department of Health Management and Policy, St. Louis, MO 63103. Offers health administration (MHA); health policy (MPH); public health studies (PhD). *Accreditation:* CAHME. *Program availability:* Part-time. *Degree requirements:* For master's, comprehensive exam, internship. *Entrance requirements:* For master's, GMAT or GRE General Test, LSAT, MCAT, letters of recommendation, resume. Additional exam requirements/recommendations for international students: Required—TOEFL (minimum score 525 paper-based). *Faculty research:* Management of HIV/AIDS, rural health services, prevention of asthma, genetics and health services use, health insurance and access to care.

Salus University, College of Health Sciences, Elkins Park, PA 19027-1598. Offers physician assistant (MMS); public health (MPH). *Accreditation:* ARC-PA. *Entrance requirements:* For master's, GRE (recommended). Additional exam requirements/recommendations for international students: Required—TOEFL. Electronic applications accepted.

Samford University, School of Public Health, Birmingham, AL 35229. Offers clinical social work (MSW); global community development (MSW); public health (MPH). *Program availability:* Part-time, evening/weekend, 100% online. *Faculty:* 10 full-time (8 women), 1 part-time/adjunct (0 women). *Students:* 36 full-time (35 women), 1 (woman) part-time; includes 9 minority (1 American Indian or Alaska Native, non-Hispanic/Latino; 8 Asian, non-Hispanic/Latino). Average age 27. 19 applicants, 89% accepted, 15 enrolled. *Entrance requirements:* Additional exam requirements/recommendations for international students: Required—TOEFL (minimum score 550 paper-based). *Application deadline:* For fall admission, 6/1 for domestic and international students; for spring admission, 10/1 for domestic and international students. Application fee: $75. Electronic applications accepted. *Expenses: Tuition, area resident:* Full-time $18,673; part-time $766 per credit hour. *Required fees:* $550. Tuition and fees vary according to course load, degree level and student level. *Financial support:* In 2015–16, 15 students received support. Scholarships/grants available. Financial award application deadline: 3/1; financial award applicants required to submit FAFSA. *Unit head:* Dr. Keith Elder, Dean, School of Public Health. *Application contact:* Dr. Marian Carter, Assistant Dean of Enrollment Management and Student Services, 205-726-2611, Fax: 205-726-2666, E-mail: mwcarter@samford.edu.
Website: http://www.samford.edu/publichealth/

San Diego State University, Graduate and Research Affairs, College of Health and Human Services, Graduate School of Public Health, San Diego, CA 92182. Offers environmental health (MPH); epidemiology (MPH, PhD), including biostatistics (MPH); global emergency preparedness and response (MS); global health (PhD); health behavior (PhD); health promotion (MPH); health services administration (MPH); toxicology (MS); MPH/MA; MSW/MPH. *Accreditation:* CAHME (one or more programs are accredited); CEPH (one or more programs are accredited). *Program availability:* Part-time. *Degree requirements:* For master's, comprehensive exam (for some programs), thesis (for some programs); for doctorate, thesis/dissertation. *Entrance requirements:* For master's, GMAT (MPH in health services administration), GRE General Test; for doctorate, GRE General Test. Additional exam requirements/recommendations for international students: Required—TOEFL. *Faculty research:* Evaluation of tobacco, AIDS prevalence and prevention, mammography, infant death project, Alzheimer's in elderly Chinese.

San Francisco State University, Division of Graduate Studies, College of Health and Social Sciences, Department of Health Education, San Francisco, CA 94132-1722. Offers MPH. *Accreditation:* CEPH. *Program availability:* Part-time. *Students:* Average age 36. *Application deadline:* Applications are processed on a rolling basis. *Expenses:* Tuition, state resident: full-time $6738. Tuition, nonresident: full-time $15,666. *Required fees:* $1004. *Unit head:* Dr. Mary Beth Love, Chair, 415-338-1413, Fax: 415-338-0570, E-mail: love@sfsu.edu. *Application contact:* Prof. Sally Geisse, Graduate Coordinator, 415-338-1413, Fax: 415-338-0570, E-mail: sgeisse@sfsu.edu.
Website: http://healthed.sfsu.edu/graduate

San Jose State University, Graduate Studies and Research, College of Applied Sciences and Arts, San Jose, CA 95192-0001. Offers big data (Certificate); California library media teacher services (Certificate); collaborative response to family violence (Certificate); justice studies (MS); kinesiology (MA), including applied sciences and arts (MA, MS), athletic training, exercise physiology, sport management, sport studies; library and information science (MLIS, Certificate); mass communication (MA); master of social work (MSW); nutritional science (MS); occupational therapy (MS); public health (MPH); pupil personnel services (Credential); recreation (MS), including applied sciences and arts (MA, MS), international tourism; Spanish language counseling (Certificate); strategic management of digital assets and services (Certificate). *Program availability:* Part-time, evening/weekend. *Students:* 219 full-time (155 women), 140 part-time (103 women); includes 472 minority (38 Black or African American, non-Hispanic/Latino; 2 American Indian or Alaska Native, non-Hispanic/Latino; 190 Asian, non-Hispanic/Latino; 238 Hispanic/Latino; 4 Native Hawaiian or other Pacific Islander, non-Hispanic/Latino), 28 international. Average age 31. 1,404 applicants, 37% accepted, 360 enrolled. In 2015, 850 master's awarded. *Application deadline:* For fall admission, 6/29 for domestic students; for spring admission, 11/30 for domestic students. Applications are processed on a rolling basis. Application fee: $55. Electronic applications accepted. *Financial support:* Career-related internships or fieldwork, Federal Work-Study, institutionally sponsored loans, and scholarships/grants available. Support available to part-time students. Financial award application deadline: 6/15; financial award applicants required to submit FAFSA. *Unit head:* Dr. Mary Schutten, Dean, 408-924-2900, Fax: 408-924-2901, E-mail: mary.schutten@sjsu.edu. *Application contact:* 408-924-2480, Fax: 408-924-2477.
Website: http://www.sjsu.edu/casa/

Sarah Lawrence College, Graduate Studies, Program in Health Advocacy, Bronxville, NY 10708-5999. Offers MA. *Program availability:* Part-time. *Degree requirements:* For master's, thesis, fieldwork. *Entrance requirements:* For master's, previous course work in biology and microeconomics, minimum B average in undergraduate course work. Additional exam requirements/recommendations for international students: Required—TOEFL (minimum score 600 paper-based). Electronic applications accepted.

Simon Fraser University, Office of Graduate Studies, Faculty of Health Sciences, Burnaby, BC V5A 1S6, Canada. Offers global health (Graduate Diploma); health sciences (M Sc, PhD); public health (MPH). *Degree requirements:* For master's, thesis (for some programs); for doctorate, comprehensive exam, thesis/dissertation. *Entrance requirements:* For master's, minimum GPA of 3.0 (on scale of 4.33), or 3.33 based on last 60 credits of undergraduate courses; for doctorate, minimum GPA of 3.5 (on scale of 4.33); for Graduate Diploma, minimum GPA of 2.5 (on scale of 4.33), or 2.67 based

on the last 60 credits of undergraduate courses. Additional exam requirements/recommendations for international students: Recommended—TOEFL (minimum score 580 paper-based; 93 iBT), IELTS (minimum score 7), TWE (minimum score 5). Electronic applications accepted.

Southern Connecticut State University, School of Graduate Studies, School of Health and Human Services, Department of Public Health, New Haven, CT 06515-1355. Offers MPH. *Accreditation:* CEPH. *Program availability:* Part-time, evening/weekend. *Faculty:* 11 full-time (9 women). *Students:* 43 full-time (33 women), 38 part-time (36 women); includes 26 minority (17 Black or African American, non-Hispanic/Latino; 2 Asian, non-Hispanic/Latino; 5 Hispanic/Latino; 2 Two or more races, non-Hispanic/Latino), 4 international. Average age 32. 141 applicants, 40% accepted, 27 enrolled. In 2015, 22 master's awarded. *Degree requirements:* For master's, thesis or alternative. *Entrance requirements:* For master's, minimum undergraduate QPA of 3.0 in graduate major field or 2.5 overall, interview. *Application deadline:* For fall admission, 3/15 for domestic students. Application fee: $50. Electronic applications accepted. *Expenses:* Tuition, state resident: full-time $4968; part-time $494 per credit hour. Tuition, nonresident: full-time $16,078; part-time $509 per credit hour. *Required fees:* $4632; $55 per semester. Tuition and fees vary according to program. *Financial support:* Career-related internships or fieldwork, scholarships/grants, and unspecified assistantships available. Financial award application deadline: 4/15; financial award applicants required to submit FAFSA. *Unit head:* Dr. Jean Breny, Chairperson, 203-392-5243, Fax: 203-392-6965, E-mail: brenyj1@southernct.edu. *Application contact:* Lisa Galvin, Director of Graduate Admissions, 203-392-5240, Fax: 203-392-5235, E-mail: galvinl1@southernct.edu.

State University of New York Downstate Medical Center, College of Medicine, Program in Public Health, Brooklyn, NY 11203-2098. Offers urban and immigrant health (MPH); MD/MPH. *Accreditation:* CEPH. *Program availability:* Part-time. *Degree requirements:* For master's, practicum. *Entrance requirements:* For master's, GRE, MCAT or OAT, 2 letters of recommendation, minimum undergraduate GPA of 3.0. Additional exam requirements/recommendations for international students: Required—TOEFL (minimum score 550 paper-based).

Stony Brook University, State University of New York, Stony Brook Medicine, School of Medicine, Program in Public Health, Stony Brook, NY 11794. Offers community health (MPH); evaluation sciences (MPH); family violence (MPH); health communication (Certificate); health economics (MPH); population health (MPH); substance abuse (MPH). *Accreditation:* CEPH. *Program availability:* Part-time, evening/weekend. *Students:* 39 full-time (29 women), 18 part-time (16 women); includes 28 minority (5 Black or African American, non-Hispanic/Latino; 12 Asian, non-Hispanic/Latino; 11 Hispanic/Latino), 4 international. Average age 30. 158 applicants, 59% accepted, 34 enrolled. In 2015, 28 master's awarded. *Entrance requirements:* For master's, GRE, 3 references, bachelor's degree from accredited college or university with minimum GPA of 3.0, essays, interview. Additional exam requirements/recommendations for international students: Required—TOEFL (minimum score 85 iBT). *Application deadline:* For fall admission, 6/1 for domestic students, 3/15 for international students. Application fee: $100. Electronic applications accepted. *Expenses:* $12,421 full-time resident tuition and fees, $453 per credit hour; $23,761 full-time nonresident tuition and fees, $952 per credit hour. *Financial support:* Fellowships available. *Faculty research:* Abnormal psychology, academic achievement, broadcast media, communications, communications systems, public health. *Total annual research expenditures:* $102,281. *Unit head:* Dr. Lisa A. Benz Scott, Director, 631-444-9396, Fax: 631-444-3480, E-mail: lisa.benzscott@stonybrook.edu. *Application contact:* Senior Academic Coordinator, 631-444-9396, Fax: 631-444-3480, E-mail: joanmarie.maniaci@stonybrook.edu.
Website: http://publichealth.stonybrookmedicine.edu/

Syracuse University, Maxwell School of Citizenship and Public Affairs, MPH Program in in Public Health, Syracuse, NY 13244. Offers public health (MPH). *Accreditation:* CEPH. *Students:* Average age 32. *Entrance requirements:* For master's, GRE, resume, three letters of recommendation, personal statement, official transcripts. Additional exam requirements/recommendations for international students: Required—TOEFL. *Application deadline:* For fall admission, 4/30 for domestic and international students. Application fee: $75. *Expenses: Tuition, area resident:* Full-time $25,974; part-time $1443 per credit hour. *Required fees:* $802; $50 per course. Tuition and fees vary according to course load and program. *Financial support:* Fellowships, research assistantships, and teaching assistantships available. *Faculty research:* Investigating and managing public health problems, developing innovative methods to improve the health of communities and larger populations. *Unit head:* Dr. David Van Slyke, Associate Dean and Chair, 315-443-8840, E-mail: vanslyke@maxwell.syr.edu. *Application contact:* Christine Omolino, Director, Admission and Financial Aid, 315-443-4000, E-mail: comolino@maxwell.syr.edu.

Tarleton State University, College of Graduate Studies, College of Science and Technology, Department of Medical Laboratory Sciences and Public Health, Fort Worth, TX 76104. Offers medical laboratory sciences (MS). *Program availability:* Part-time, evening/weekend. *Faculty:* 6 full-time (4 women). *Students:* 4 full-time (3 women), 12 part-time (10 women); includes 8 minority (4 Black or African American, non-Hispanic/Latino; 3 Asian, non-Hispanic/Latino; 1 Hispanic/Latino), 3 international. 8 applicants, 50% accepted, 4 enrolled. In 2015, 8 master's awarded. *Degree requirements:* For master's, comprehensive exam, thesis optional. *Entrance requirements:* For master's, GRE, minimum GPA of 3.0. Additional exam requirements/recommendations for international students: Required—TOEFL (minimum score 550 paper-based; 80 iBT). *Application deadline:* For fall admission, 8/15 for domestic students; for spring admission, 1/7 for domestic students. Applications are processed on a rolling basis. Application fee: $45 ($145 for international students). Electronic applications accepted. *Expenses:* Tuition, state resident: part-time $204 per credit hour. Tuition, nonresident: part-time $594 per credit hour. *Required fees:* $1994 per unit. *Financial support:* Career-related internships or fieldwork, Federal Work-Study, and scholarships/grants available. Support available to part-time students. Financial award application deadline: 5/1; financial award applicants required to submit FAFSA. *Unit head:* Sally Lewis, Head, 817-926-1101, E-mail: slewis@tarleton.edu. *Application contact:* Information Contact, 254-968-9104, Fax: 254-968-9670, E-mail: gradoffice@tarleton.edu.
Website: http://www.tarleton.edu/degrees/masters/ms-medical-laboratory-science/

Temple University, College of Public Health, Department of Social and Behavioral Sciences, Philadelphia, PA 19122. Offers social and behavioral science (MPH, PhD). *Accreditation:* CEPH (one or more programs are accredited). *Program availability:* Part-time, evening/weekend. *Faculty:* 18 full-time (9 women), 1 (woman) part-time/adjunct. *Students:* 49 full-time (34 women), 103 part-time (79 women); includes 37 minority (13 Black or African American, non-Hispanic/Latino; 13 Asian, non-Hispanic/Latino; 7 Hispanic/Latino; 4 Two or more races, non-Hispanic/Latino), 9 international. 268 applicants, 49% accepted, 35 enrolled. In 2015, 23 master's, 3 doctorates awarded. Terminal master's awarded for partial completion of doctoral program. *Degree requirements:* For master's, thesis (for some programs), capstone project; for doctorate, comprehensive exam, thesis/dissertation. *Entrance requirements:* For master's, GRE General Test (for MS only); DAT, GMAT, MCAT, OAT, or PCAT (for MPH, Ed M), minimum undergraduate GPA of 3.0, letters of reference, statement of goals, writing sample, resume, interview (only for MS); for doctorate, GRE General Test, minimum undergraduate GPA of 3.0, 3 letters of reference, statement of goals, writing sample,

resume. Additional exam requirements/recommendations for international students: Required—TOEFL (minimum score 550 paper-based; 79 iBT). *Application deadline:* For fall admission, 3/1 for domestic students, 2/1 for international students; for spring admission, 10/15 for domestic students, 8/1 for international students. Applications are processed on a rolling basis. Application fee: $60. Electronic applications accepted. *Expenses:* Contact institution. *Financial support:* Fellowships with tuition reimbursements, research assistantships with tuition reimbursements, teaching assistantships with tuition reimbursements, career-related internships or fieldwork, Federal Work-Study, scholarships/grants, tuition waivers (partial), and unspecified assistantships available. Financial award application deadline: 1/15. *Faculty research:* Smoking cessation, obesity prevention, tobacco policy, community engagement, health communication. *Unit head:* Dr. Stephen Lepore, Department Chair and Professor, 215-204-8726, Fax: 215-204-1854, E-mail: slepore@temple.edu. *Application contact:* Theresa White, Senior Graduate Advisor/Admissions, 215-204-5105, E-mail: theresawhite@temple.edu.
Website: http://cph.temple.edu/publichealth/home

Tennessee State University, The School of Graduate Studies and Research, College of Health Sciences, Department of Public Health, Health Administration and Health Sciences, Nashville, TN 37209-1561. Offers public health (MPH). *Degree requirements:* For master's, capstone project. *Unit head:* Dr. Mohamed Kanu, Chair, 615-963-7326, E-mail: mkanu@tnstate.edu. *Application contact:* Dr. Mohamed Kanu, Chair, 615-963-7326, E-mail: mkanu@tnstate.edu.
Website: http://www.tnstate.edu/phas

Texas A&M University, School of Public Health, College Station, TX 77843. Offers health administration (MHA); health policy and management (MPH); health promotion and community health science (MPH); health services research (PhD) *Accreditation:* CEPH. *Program availability:* Part-time, blended/hybrid learning. *Faculty:* 68. *Students:* 313 full-time (189 women), 71 part-time (41 women); includes 169 minority (40 Black or African American, non-Hispanic/Latino; 38 Asian, non-Hispanic/Latino; 88 Hispanic/Latino; 3 Two or more races, non-Hispanic/Latino), 88 international. Average age 30. 138 applicants, 100% accepted, 126 enrolled. In 2015, 139 master's, 5 doctorates awarded. *Degree requirements:* For master's, thesis optional. *Entrance requirements:* For master's, GRE General Test, 3 letters of recommendation; statement of purpose; current curriculum vitae or resume; official transcripts; for doctorate, GRE General Test, 3 letters of recommendation; statement of purpose; current curriculum vitae or resume; official transcripts; interview (in some cases). Additional exam requirements/recommendations for international students: Required—TOEFL (minimum score 597 paper-based, 95 iBT) or GRE (minimum verbal score 153). *Application deadline:* For fall admission, 8/27 for domestic students; for spring admission, 1/14 for domestic students. Application fee: $120. Electronic applications accepted. *Expenses:* Contact institution. *Financial support:* In 2015–16, 186 students received support, including 2 fellowships with tuition reimbursements available (averaging $17,190 per year), 55 research assistantships with tuition reimbursements available (averaging $5,728 per year), 14 teaching assistantships with tuition reimbursements available (averaging $5,836 per year); career-related internships or fieldwork, institutionally sponsored loans, scholarships/grants, traineeships, health care benefits, tuition waivers (full and partial), and unspecified assistantships also available. Support available to part-time students. Financial award applicants required to submit FAFSA. *Unit head:* Dr. Jay Maddock, Dean, 979-436-9322, Fax: 979-458-1878, E-mail: maddock@tamhsc.edu. *Application contact:* Erin E. Schneider, Associate Director of Admissions and Recruitment, 979-436-9380, E-mail: eschneider@sph.tamhsc.edu.
Website: http://sph.tamhsc.edu/

Thomas Jefferson University, Jefferson School of Population Health, Program in Public Health, Philadelphia, PA 19107. Offers MPH, Certificate. *Accreditation:* CEPH. *Program availability:* Part-time, evening/weekend, online learning. Terminal master's awarded for partial completion of doctoral program. *Degree requirements:* For master's, capstone project or thesis. *Entrance requirements:* For master's, GRE or other graduate examination, 2 letters of recommendation, interview, curriculum vitae. Additional exam requirements/recommendations for international students: Required—TOEFL (minimum score 100 iBT). Electronic applications accepted.

Touro University California, Graduate Programs, Vallejo, CA 94592. Offers education (MA); medical health sciences (MS); osteopathic medicine (DO); pharmacy (Pharm D); public health (MPH). *Accreditation:* AOsA; ARC-PA. *Program availability:* Part-time, evening/weekend. *Degree requirements:* For master's, comprehensive exam, thesis; for doctorate, comprehensive exam. *Entrance requirements:* For doctorate, BS/BA. Electronic applications accepted. *Faculty research:* Cancer, heart disease.

Trident University International, College of Health Sciences, Cypress, CA 90630. Offers MS, PhD, Certificate. *Program availability:* Part-time, evening/weekend, online learning. *Degree requirements:* For doctorate, comprehensive exam, thesis/dissertation. *Entrance requirements:* For master's, minimum GPA of 2.5 (students with GPA 3.0 or greater may transfer up to 30% of graduate level credits); for doctorate, minimum GPA of 3.4. Additional exam requirements/recommendations for international students: Required—TOEFL. Electronic applications accepted.

Trinity Washington University, School of Business and Graduate Studies, Washington, DC 20017-1094. Offers business administration (MBA); communication (MA); international security studies (MA); organizational management (MSA), including federal program management, human resource management, nonprofit management, organizational development, public and community health. *Program availability:* Part-time, evening/weekend. *Degree requirements:* For master's, thesis (for some programs), capstone project (MSA). *Entrance requirements:* For master's, minimum GPA of 2.5. Additional exam requirements/recommendations for international students: Required—TOEFL (minimum score 550 paper-based).

Tufts University, School of Medicine, Public Health and Professional Degree Programs, Boston, MA 02111. Offers biomedical sciences (MS); health communication (MS, Certificate); pain research, education and policy (MS, Certificate); physician assistant (MS); public health (MPH, Dr PH), including behavioral science (MPH), biostatistics (MPH), epidemiology (MPH), health communication (MPH), health services (MPH), management and policy (MPH), nutrition (MPH); DMD/MPH; DVM/MPH; JD/MPH; MD/MPH; MMS/MPH; MS/MBA; MS/MPH. MS programs offered jointly with Emerson College. *Accreditation:* CEPH (one or more programs are accredited). *Program availability:* Part-time, evening/weekend. *Faculty:* 78 full-time (29 women), 42 part-time/adjunct (20 women). *Students:* 457 full-time (266 women), 61 part-time (46 women); includes 187 minority (21 Black or African American, non-Hispanic/Latino; 107 Asian, non-Hispanic/Latino; 37 Hispanic/Latino; 22 Two or more races, non-Hispanic/Latino), 24 international. Average age 27. 1,599 applicants, 48% accepted, 222 enrolled. In 2015, 219 master's awarded. *Degree requirements:* For master's, thesis (for some programs); for doctorate, thesis/dissertation. *Entrance requirements:* For master's, GRE General Test, MCAT, or GMAT; for doctorate, GRE General Test or MCAT. Additional exam requirements/recommendations for international students: Required—TOEFL (minimum score 100 iBT). *Application deadline:* For fall admission, 1/15 priority date for domestic students, 12/15 priority date for international students; for spring admission, 10/25 priority date for domestic and international students. Applications are processed on a rolling basis. Application fee: $70. Electronic applications accepted. *Expenses:*

Contact institution. *Financial support:* In 2015–16, 12 students received support, including 1 fellowship (averaging $3,000 per year), 50 research assistantships (averaging $1,000 per year), 65 teaching assistantships (averaging $2,000 per year); Federal Work-Study and scholarships/grants also available. Support available to part-time students. Financial award application deadline: 2/19; financial award applicants required to submit FAFSA. *Faculty research:* Environmental and occupational health, nutrition, epidemiology, health communication, biostatics, obesity/chronic disease, health policy and health care delivery, global health, health inequality and social determinants of health. *Unit head:* Dr. Aviva Must, Dean, 617-636-0935, Fax: 617-636-0898, E-mail: aviva.must@tufts.edu. *Application contact:* Emily Keily, Director of Admissions, 617-636-0935, Fax: 617-636-0898, E-mail: med-phpd@tufts.edu.
Website: http://publichealth.tufts.edu

Tulane University, School of Public Health and Tropical Medicine, New Orleans, LA 70118-5669. Offers MHA, MPH, MPHTM, MS, MSPH, Dr PH, PhD, Sc D, JD/MHA, JD/MPH, JD/MSPH, MBA/MHA, MD/MPA, MD/MPH, MD/MPHTM, MD/MSPH, MSW/MPH. MS and PhD offered through the Graduate School. *Accreditation:* CAHME (one or more programs are accredited); CEPH (one or more programs are accredited). *Program availability:* Part-time, evening/weekend, online learning. Terminal master's awarded for partial completion of doctoral program. *Degree requirements:* For master's, comprehensive exam (for some programs); for doctorate, comprehensive exam, thesis/dissertation. *Entrance requirements:* For master's and doctorate, GRE General Test. Additional exam requirements/recommendations for international students: Required—TOEFL. *Application deadline:* For fall admission, 4/15 priority date for domestic and international students; for winter admission, 10/15 priority date for domestic and international students. Applications are processed on a rolling basis. Application fee: $40. Electronic applications accepted. *Expenses:* Contact institution. *Financial support:* Fellowships, research assistantships, teaching assistantships, Federal Work-Study, scholarships/grants, and traineeships available. Support available to part-time students. Financial award application deadline: 4/15; financial award applicants required to submit FAFSA.
Website: http://www.sph.tulane.edu/

Uniformed Services University of the Health Sciences, F. Edward Hebert School of Medicine, Graduate Programs in the Biomedical Sciences and Public Health, Bethesda, MD 20814. Offers emerging infectious diseases (PhD); medical and clinical psychology (PhD), including clinical psychology, medical psychology; medicine (MS, PhD), including health professions education; molecular and cell biology (MS, PhD); neuroscience (PhD); preventive medicine and biometrics (MPH, MS, MSPH, MTMH, Dr PH, PhD), including environmental health sciences (PhD), healthcare administration and policy (MS), medical zoology (PhD), public health (MPH, MSPH, Dr PH), tropical medicine and hygiene (MTMH). *Faculty:* 372 full-time (119 women), 4,044 part-time/adjunct (908 women). *Students:* 240 full-time (133 women); includes 40 minority (15 Black or African American, non-Hispanic/Latino; 13 Asian, non-Hispanic/Latino; 12 Hispanic/Latino), 30 international. Average age 25. 598 applicants, 17% accepted, 77 enrolled. In 2015, 19 master's, 50 doctorates awarded. Terminal master's awarded for partial completion of doctoral program. *Degree requirements:* For master's, comprehensive exam, thesis or alternative; for doctorate, comprehensive exam, thesis/dissertation, qualifying exam. *Entrance requirements:* For master's, GRE General Test; for doctorate, GRE General Test, minimum GPA of 3.0. *Application deadline:* For fall admission, 12/15 priority date for domestic students. Applications are processed on a rolling basis. Application fee: $0. Electronic applications accepted. *Financial support:* In 2015–16, 50 fellowships (averaging $43,000 per year) were awarded; research assistantships, career-related internships or fieldwork, scholarships/grants, health care benefits, and tuition waivers (full) also available. *Unit head:* Dr. Gregory Mueller, Associate Dean, 301-295-3507, E-mail: gregory.mueller@usuhs.edu. *Application contact:* Tina Finley, Administrative Officer, 301-295-3642, Fax: 301-295-6772, E-mail: netina.finley@usuhs.edu.
Website: http://www.usuhs.mil/graded

Uniformed Services University of the Health Sciences, F. Edward Hebert School of Medicine, Graduate Programs in the Biomedical Sciences and Public Health, Department of Preventive Medicine and Biometrics, Program in Public Health, Bethesda, MD 20814-4799. Offers MPH, MSPH, Dr PH. *Accreditation:* CEPH (one or more programs are accredited). *Degree requirements:* For master's, comprehensive exam; for doctorate, thesis/dissertation, qualifying exam. *Entrance requirements:* For master's, GRE General Test; for doctorate, GRE General Test, minimum GPA of 3.0. Additional exam requirements/recommendations for international students: Required—TOEFL. *Faculty research:* Epidemiology, biostatistics, health services administration, environmental and occupational health, tropical public health.

Université de Montréal, Faculty of Arts and Sciences, Program in Societies, Public Policies and Health, Montréal, QC H3C 3J7, Canada. Offers DESS.

Université de Montréal, Faculty of Medicine, Program in Communal and Public Health, Montréal, QC H3C 3J7, Canada. Offers community health (M Sc, DESS); public health (PhD). *Accreditation:* CEPH. *Program availability:* Part-time. Terminal master's awarded for partial completion of doctoral program. *Degree requirements:* For master's, thesis; for doctorate, thesis/dissertation, general exam. *Entrance requirements:* For master's and doctorate, proficiency in French, knowledge of English; for DESS, proficiency in French. Electronic applications accepted. *Faculty research:* Epidemiology, health services utilization, health promotion and education, health behaviors, poverty and child health.

University at Albany, State University of New York, School of Public Health, Department of Epidemiology and Biostatistics, Program in Public Health, Rensselaer, NY 12144. Offers MPH, Dr PH. *Degree requirements:* For master's, thesis; for doctorate, thesis/dissertation. *Entrance requirements:* For master's and doctorate, GRE General Test. Additional exam requirements/recommendations for international students: Required—TOEFL (minimum score 550 paper-based). Electronic applications accepted.

University at Buffalo, the State University of New York, Graduate School, School of Public Health and Health Professions, Department of Epidemiology and Environmental Health, Buffalo, NY 14214. Offers epidemiology (MS, PhD); public health (MPH). *Accreditation:* CEPH. *Program availability:* Part-time. *Faculty:* 12 full-time (6 women), 11 part-time/adjunct (5 women). *Students:* 58 full-time (38 women), 20 part-time (15 women); includes 13 minority (3 Black or African American, non-Hispanic/Latino; 10 Asian, non-Hispanic/Latino; 12 international. Average age 29. 201 applicants, 38% accepted, 33 enrolled. In 2015, 29 master's, 4 doctorates awarded. Terminal master's awarded for partial completion of doctoral program. *Degree requirements:* For master's, comprehensive exam, thesis; for doctorate, comprehensive exam, thesis/dissertation. *Entrance requirements:* For master's and doctorate, GRE General Test. Additional exam requirements/recommendations for international students: Required—TOEFL (minimum score 600 paper-based; 100 iBT). *Application deadline:* For fall admission, 1/15 priority date for domestic and international students. Applications are processed on a rolling basis. Application fee: $50. Electronic applications accepted. *Financial support:* In 2015–16, 17 students received support, including 4 fellowships with full tuition reimbursements (averaging $22,000 per year), 5 research assistantships with full tuition reimbursements available (averaging $20,000 per year); teaching assistantships with full tuition reimbursements available, career-related internships or

Public Health—General

fieldwork, Federal Work-Study, institutionally sponsored loans, health care benefits, and unspecified assistantships also available. Financial award application deadline: 2/1; financial award applicants required to submit FAFSA. *Faculty research:* Epidemiology of cancer, nutrition, infectious diseases, epidemiology of environmental, women's health and cardiovascular disease research. *Unit head:* Dr. Jo Freudenheim, Interim Chair, 716-829-5375, Fax: 716-829-2979, E-mail: phhpadv@buffalo.edu. *Application contact:* Dr. Carl Li, Director of Graduate Studies, 716-829-5382, Fax: 716-829-2979, E-mail: carlli@buffalo.edu.
Website: http://sphhp.buffalo.edu/spm/

The University of Akron, Graduate School, College of Health Professions, School of Nursing, Akron, OH 44325-3701. Offers nursing (MSN, PhD); nursing practice (DNP); public health (MPH). PhD offered jointly with Kent State University. *Accreditation:* AACN; AANA/CANAEP (one or more programs are accredited). *Program availability:* Part-time. *Faculty:* 13 full-time (12 women), 37 part-time/adjunct (35 women). *Students:* 40 full-time (27 women), 286 part-time (223 women); includes 45 minority (19 Black or African American, non-Hispanic/Latino; 10 Asian, non-Hispanic/Latino; 10 Hispanic/Latino; 6 Two or more races, non-Hispanic/Latino), 4 international. Average age 37. 140 applicants, 56% accepted, 64 enrolled. In 2015, 101 master's, 2 doctorates awarded. *Degree requirements:* For doctorate, one foreign language, thesis/dissertation, qualifying exam. *Entrance requirements:* For master's, current Ohio state license as registered nurse, three letters of reference, 300-word essay, interview with program coordinator; for doctorate, GRE, minimum GPA of 3.0, MSN, nursing license or eligibility for licensure, writing sample, letters of recommendation, interview, resume, personal statement of research interests and career goals. Additional exam requirements/recommendations for international students: Required—TOEFL (minimum score 550 paper-based; 79 iBT), IELTS (minimum score 6.5). *Application deadline:* For fall admission, 7/15 for domestic and international students. Applications are processed on a rolling basis. Application fee: $45 ($70 for international students). Electronic applications accepted. *Expenses:* Tuition, state resident: full-time $7958; part-time $442 per credit hour. Tuition, nonresident: full-time $13,464; part-time $748 per credit hour. *Required fees:* $1404. *Financial support:* In 2015–16, 11 teaching assistantships with full tuition reimbursements were awarded. *Faculty research:* Health promotion and chronic disease prevention, mental health and psychosocial resilience, gerontological health, trauma and violence, gut oxygenation during shock and trauma, simulation and the pedagogy of teaching and learning. *Total annual research expenditures:* $476,886. *Unit head:* Dr. Marlene Huff, Interim Director, 330-972-5930, E-mail: mhuff@uakron.edu. Website: http://www.uakron.edu/nursing/

The University of Alabama at Birmingham, School of Public Health, Program in Public Health, Birmingham, AL 35294. Offers applied epidemiology and pharmacoepidemiology (MSPH); biostatistics (MPH); clinical and translational science (MSPH); environmental health (MPH); environmental health and toxicology (MSPH); epidemiology (MPH); general theory and practice (MPH); health behavior (MPH); health care organization (MPH); health policy quantitative policy analysis (MPH); industrial hygiene (MPH, MSPH); maternal and child health policy (Dr PH); maternal and child health policy and leadership (MPH); occupational health and safety (MPH); outcomes research (MSPH, Dr PH); public health (PhD); public health management (Dr PH); public health preparedness management (MPH). *Accreditation:* CEPH. *Program availability:* Part-time, online learning. *Degree requirements:* For doctorate, comprehensive exam, thesis/dissertation. *Entrance requirements:* For master's and doctorate, GRE. Additional exam requirements/recommendations for international students: Recommended—TOEFL (minimum score 550 paper-based; 79 iBT), IELTS (minimum score 6.5). Electronic applications accepted. *Expenses:* Tuition, state resident: full-time $7340. Tuition, nonresident: full-time $16,628. Full-time tuition and fees vary according to course load and program.

University of Alaska Anchorage, College of Health, Department of Health Sciences, Anchorage, AK 99508. Offers public health practice (MPH). *Accreditation:* CEPH. *Program availability:* Part-time. *Degree requirements:* For master's, comprehensive exam, thesis. *Entrance requirements:* For master's, writing sample. Additional exam requirements/recommendations for international students: Required—TOEFL (minimum score 550 paper-based).

University of Alberta, School of Public Health, Department of Public Health Sciences, Edmonton, AB T6G 2E1, Canada. Offers clinical epidemiology (M Sc, MPH); environmental and occupational health (MPH); environmental health sciences (M Sc); epidemiology (M Sc); global health (M Sc, MPH); health policy and management (MPH); health policy research (M Sc); health technology assessment (MPH); occupational health (M Sc); population health (M Sc); public health leadership (MPH); public health sciences (PhD); quantitative methods (MPH). *Accreditation:* CEPH (one or more programs are accredited). Terminal master's awarded for partial completion of doctoral program. *Degree requirements:* For master's, thesis (for some programs); for doctorate, thesis/dissertation. *Entrance requirements:* For master's, GMAT or GRE General Test. Additional exam requirements/recommendations for international students: Required—TOEFL (minimum score 550 paper-based) or IELTS (minimum score 6). Electronic applications accepted. *Faculty research:* Biostatistics, health promotion and socio-behavioral health science.

The University of Arizona, Mel and Enid Zuckerman College of Public Health, Program in Public Health, Tucson, AZ 85721. Offers MPH, Dr PH, PhD. *Entrance requirements:* Additional exam requirements/recommendations for international students: Required—TOEFL (minimum score 550 paper-based; 79 iBT). *Application deadline:* For fall admission, 1/1 for domestic and international students. Applications are processed on a rolling basis. Application fee: $75. Electronic applications accepted. *Financial support:* Research assistantships and teaching assistantships available. *Unit head:* Dr. Iman Hakim, Dean, 520-626-7083, E-mail: ihakim@email.arizona.edu. *Application contact:* Amy Clicken, Senior Program Coordinator, 520-626-3201, E-mail: coph-admit@email.arizona.edu.

University of Arkansas for Medical Sciences, College of Public Health, Little Rock, AR 72205-7199. Offers biostatistics (MPH); environmental and occupational health (MPH, Certificate); epidemiology (MPH, PhD); health behavior and health education (MPH); health policy and management (MPH); health promotion and prevention research (PhD); health services administration (MHSA); health systems research (PhD); public health (Certificate); public health leadership (Dr PH). *Program availability:* Part-time. *Degree requirements:* For master's, preceptorship, culminating experience, internship; for doctorate, comprehensive exam, capstone. *Entrance requirements:* For master's, GRE, GMAT, LSAT, PCAT, MCAT, DAT; for doctorate, GRE. Additional exam requirements/recommendations for international students: Required—TOEFL (minimum score 80 iBT), IELTS. Electronic applications accepted. *Expenses:* Contact institution. *Faculty research:* Health systems, tobacco prevention control, obesity prevention, environmental and occupational exposure, cancer prevention.

The University of British Columbia, Faculty of Medicine, School of Population and Public Health, Vancouver, BC V6T 1Z3, Canada. Offers health administration (MHA); health care and epidemiology (MH Sc, PhD); public health (MPH). *Accreditation:* CEPH (one or more programs are accredited). *Program availability:* Online learning. *Degree requirements:* For master's, thesis (for some programs), major paper (MH Sc), research project (MHA); for doctorate, thesis/dissertation. *Entrance requirements:* For master's, GRE General Test or GMAT, PCAT, MCAT (MHA), MD or equivalent (for MH Sc); 4-year undergraduate degree from accredited university with minimum B+ overall academic average and in math or statistics course at undergraduate level (for MPH); 4-year undergraduate degree from accredited university with minimum B+ overall academic average plus work experience (for MHA); for doctorate, master's degree from accredited university with minimum B+ overall academic average and in math or statistics course at undergraduate level. Additional exam requirements/recommendations for international students: Required—TOEFL. Electronic applications accepted. *Faculty research:* Population and public health, clinical epidemiology, epidemiology and biostatistics, global health and vulnerable populations, health care services and systems, occupational and environmental health, public health emerging threats and rapid response, social and life course determinants of health, health administration.

University of California, Berkeley, Graduate Division, Haas School of Business and School of Public Health, Concurrent MBA/MPH Program, Berkeley, CA 94720-1500. Offers MBA/MPH. *Accreditation:* AACSB; CEPH. *Students:* 35 full-time (24 women); includes 10 minority (1 Black or African American, non-Hispanic/Latino; 8 Asian, non-Hispanic/Latino; 1 Hispanic/Latino), 6 international. Average age 28. 87 applicants, 10 enrolled. *Entrance requirements:* Additional exam requirements/recommendations for international students: Required—TOEFL (minimum score 570 paper-based; 90 iBT); Recommended—IELTS (minimum score 7). *Application deadline:* For fall admission, 10/1 for domestic and international students; for winter admission, 1/7 for domestic and international students; for spring admission, 3/31 for domestic students, 3/11 for international students. Application fee: $200. Electronic applications accepted. *Expenses:* Contact institution. *Financial support:* In 2015–16, 11 students received support, including 9 fellowships (averaging $10,556 per year), 2 teaching assistantships with partial tuition reimbursements available (averaging $27,469 per year); research assistantships with partial tuition reimbursements available, career-related internships or fieldwork, institutionally sponsored loans, scholarships/grants, and non-resident tuition waivers for some students, such as veterans also available. Financial award application deadline: 5/18. *Faculty research:* Accounting, business and public policy, economic analysis and public policy, entrepreneurship, finance, management of organizations, marketing, operations and information technology management, real estate. *Unit head:* Prof. Kim MacPherson, Associate Director, Health Services Management Program, 510-642-9175, Fax: 510-643-6659, E-mail: kmacpherson@haas.berkeley.edu. *Application contact:* Morgan Bernstein, Executive Director of Admissions, 510-642-1405, Fax: 510-643-6659, E-mail: mbaadm@haas.berkeley.edu.
Website: http://www.haas.berkeley.edu/

University of California, Berkeley, Graduate Division, School of Public Health, Group in Environmental Health Sciences, Berkeley, CA 94720-1500. Offers MPH, MS, Dr PH, PhD. *Degree requirements:* For master's, comprehensive exam (MPH), project or thesis (MS); for doctorate, thesis/dissertation, departmental and qualifying exams. *Entrance requirements:* For master's, GRE General Test, minimum GPA of 3.0; previous course work in biology, calculus, and chemistry; 3 letters of recommendation; for doctorate, GRE General Test, master's degree in relevant scientific discipline or engineering; minimum GPA of 3.0; previous course work in biology, calculus, and chemistry; 3 letters of recommendation. Additional exam requirements/recommendations for international students: Required—TOEFL. *Faculty research:* Toxicology, industrial hygiene, exposure assessment, risk assessment, ergonomics.

University of California, Berkeley, Graduate Division, School of Public Health, Group in Epidemiology, Berkeley, CA 94720-1500. Offers epidemiology (MS, PhD); infectious diseases (MPH, PhD). *Accreditation:* CEPH (one or more programs are accredited). *Degree requirements:* For master's, comprehensive exam; for doctorate, thesis/dissertation, oral and written exam. *Entrance requirements:* For master's, GRE General Test, minimum GPA of 3.0; MD, DDS, DVM, or PhD in biomedical science (MPH); for doctorate, GRE General Test, minimum GPA of 3.0.

University of California, Berkeley, Graduate Division, School of Public Health, Programs in Public Health, Berkeley, CA 94720-1500. Offers MPH, Dr PH. *Accreditation:* CEPH. *Program availability:* Online learning. *Degree requirements:* For doctorate, thesis/dissertation, exam. *Entrance requirements:* For doctorate, GRE General Test, minimum GPA of 3.0.

University of California, Irvine, Programs in Health Sciences, Program in Public Health, Irvine, CA 92697. Offers MPH, PhD. *Students:* 52 full-time (40 women), 5 part-time (4 women); includes 28 minority (2 Black or African American, non-Hispanic/Latino; 13 Asian, non-Hispanic/Latino; 9 Hispanic/Latino; 4 Two or more races, non-Hispanic/Latino), 10 international. Average age 29. 242 applicants, 48% accepted, 27 enrolled. In 2015, 15 master's awarded. Application fee: $90 ($110 for international students). *Unit head:* Oladele A. Ogunseitan, Chair, 949-824-6350, Fax: 949-824-2056, E-mail: oladele.ogunseitan@uci.edu. *Application contact:* Stephanie Leonard, Director of Student Affairs, 949-824-0546, E-mail: stephapl@uci.edu.
Website: http://publichealth.uci.edu/

University of California, Irvine, School of Social Ecology, Programs in Social Ecology, Irvine, CA 92697. Offers environmental analysis and design (PhD); epidemiology and public health (PhD); social ecology (PhD). *Students:* 11 full-time (9 women), 1 part-time (0 women); includes 1 minority (Hispanic/Latino), 1 international. Average age 32. 14 applicants, 36% accepted, 2 enrolled. In 2015, 1 doctorate awarded. Application fee: $90 ($110 for international students). *Unit head:* Tim-Allen Bruckner, Professor, 949-824-5797, Fax: 949-824-1845, E-mail: tim.bruckner@uci.edu. *Application contact:* Jennnifer Craig, Director of Graduate Student Services, 949-824-5918, Fax: 949-824-1845, E-mail: craigj@uci.edu.
Website: http://socialecology.uci.edu/core/graduate-se-core-programs

University of California, Los Angeles, Graduate Division, School of Public Health, Los Angeles, CA 90095. Offers MPH, MS, D Env, Dr PH, PhD, JD/MPH, MA/MPH, MBA/MPH, MD/MPH, MD/PhD, MSW/MPH. *Accreditation:* CAHME (one or more programs are accredited); CEPH (one or more programs are accredited). *Degree requirements:* For doctorate, thesis/dissertation, oral and written qualifying exams. *Entrance requirements:* For master's, GRE General Test, minimum GPA of 3.0; for doctorate, GRE General Test, minimum undergraduate GPA of 3.0. Electronic applications accepted.

University of California, San Diego, Graduate Division, Program in Public Health, La Jolla, CA 92093. Offers epidemiology (PhD); global health (PhD); health behavior (PhD). Program offered jointly with San Diego State University. *Students:* 16 full-time (13 women), 21 part-time (14 women); includes 11 minority (2 Black or African American, non-Hispanic/Latino; 3 Asian, non-Hispanic/Latino; 6 Hispanic/Latino), 4 international. In 2015, 12 doctorates awarded. *Degree requirements:* For doctorate, thesis/dissertation, 2 semesters/quarters of teaching assistantship. *Entrance requirements:* For doctorate, GRE General Test, minimum GPA of 3.0. Additional exam requirements/recommendations for international students: Required—TOEFL, IELTS. *Application deadline:* For fall admission, 12/15 priority date for domestic students. Electronic applications accepted. *Expenses:* Tuition, state resident: full-time $11,220. Tuition, nonresident: full-time $26,322. *Required fees:* $1800. *Financial support:* Teaching assistantships available. Financial award applicants required to submit FAFSA. *Faculty*

research: Maternal and pediatric HIV/AIDS; healthy aging and gender differences; non-parametric and semi-parametric regression, resampling, and the analysis of high-dimensional data; neighborhood correlates of physical activity in children, teens, adults and older adults; medication safety and medication therapy management through practice-based research networks. *Unit head:* David Strong, Faculty Director, 858-657-5241, E-mail: dstrong@ucsd.edu. *Application contact:* Hollie Ward, Graduate Coordinator, 858-822-2382, E-mail: hcward@ucsd.edu.
Website: http://publichealth.ucsd.edu/jdp/

University of Colorado Denver, Colorado School of Public Health, Program in Public Health, Aurora, CO 80045. Offers community and behavioral health (MPH, Dr PH); environmental and occupational health (MPH); epidemiology (MPH); health systems, management and policy (MPH). *Accreditation:* CEPH. *Program availability:* Part-time, evening/weekend. *Faculty:* 16 full-time (14 women), 1 (woman) part-time/adjunct. *Students:* 379 full-time (293 women), 77 part-time (69 women); includes 111 minority (10 Black or African American, non-Hispanic/Latino; 3 American Indian or Alaska Native, non-Hispanic/Latino; 36 Asian, non-Hispanic/Latino; 47 Hispanic/Latino; 1 Native Hawaiian or other Pacific Islander, non-Hispanic/Latino; 14 Two or more races, non-Hispanic/Latino), 12 international. Average age 31. 785 applicants, 25% accepted, 166 enrolled. In 2015, 144 master's awarded. *Degree requirements:* For master's, thesis or alternative, 42 credit hours; for doctorate, comprehensive exam, thesis/dissertation, 67 credit hours. *Entrance requirements:* For master's, GRE, MCAT, DAT, LSAT, PCAT, GMAT or master's degree from accredited institution, baccalaureate degree or equivalent; minimum GPA of 3.0; transcripts; references; resume; essay; for doctorate, GRE, MCAT, DAT, LSAT, PCAT or GMAT, MPH or master's or higher degree in related field or equivalent; 2 years of previous work experience in public health; essay; resume. Additional exam requirements/recommendations for international students: Required—TOEFL (minimum score 550 paper-based; 80 iBT) *Application deadline:* For fall admission, 12/15 priority date for domestic students, 12/1 priority date for international students. Application fee: $65. Electronic applications accepted. *Expenses:* Contact institution. *Financial support:* In 2015–16, 265 students received support. Fellowships, research assistantships, teaching assistantships, Federal Work-Study, institutionally sponsored loans, scholarships/grants, traineeships, and unspecified assistantships available. Financial award application deadline: 3/15; financial award applicants required to submit FAFSA. *Faculty research:* Cancer prevention by nutrition, cancer survivorship outcomes, social and cultural factors related to health. *Total annual research expenditures:* $302,793. *Unit head:* Dr. Lori Crane, Chair, 303-724-4385, E-mail: lori.crane@ucdenver.edu. *Application contact:* 303-724-4613, E-mail: csph.studentaffairs@ucdenver.edu.
Website: http://www.ucdenver.edu/academics/colleges/PublicHealth/Academics/degreesandprograms/Pages/index.aspx

University of Connecticut Health Center, Graduate School, Program in Public Health, Farmington, CT 06030. Offers MPH, DMD/MPH, MD/MPH. *Accreditation:* CEPH. *Program availability:* Part-time, evening/weekend. *Degree requirements:* For master's, thesis optional. *Entrance requirements:* For master's, GRE. Additional exam requirements/recommendations for international students: Required—TOEFL (minimum score 600 paper-based). Electronic applications accepted. *Faculty research:* Cancer epidemiology, birth defects, gerontology, health manpower, health services.

University of Florida, College of Medicine, Program in Clinical Investigation, Gainesville, FL 32611. Offers clinical investigation (MS); epidemiology (MS); public health (MPH). *Program availability:* Part-time. *Entrance requirements:* For master's, GRE, MD, PhD, DMD/DDS or Pharm D.

University of Florida, Graduate School, College of Public Health and Health Professions, Programs in Public Health, Gainesville, FL 32611. Offers biostatistics (MPH); clinical and translational science (PhD); environmental health (MPH); epidemiology (MPH); health management and policy (MPH); public health (MPH, PhD, Certificate); public health practice (MPH); rehabilitation science (PhD); social and behavioral sciences (MPH); DPT/MPH; DVM/MPH; JD/MPH; MD/MPH; Pharm D/MPH. *Accreditation:* CEPH. *Program availability:* Online learning. *Faculty:* 31. *Students:* 174 full-time (134 women), 59 part-time (42 women); includes 67 minority (27 Black or African American, non-Hispanic/Latino; 1 American Indian or Alaska Native, non-Hispanic/Latino; 25 Asian, non-Hispanic/Latino; 14 Hispanic/Latino), 24 international. Average age 30. 385 applicants, 44% accepted, 75 enrolled. In 2015, 81 master's, 6 doctorates awarded. *Degree requirements:* For master's, internship. *Entrance requirements:* For master's, GRE General Test, minimum GPA of 3.0. Additional exam requirements/recommendations for international students: Required—TOEFL (minimum score 550 paper-based; 80 iBT), IELTS (minimum score 6). *Application deadline:* For fall admission, 7/1 for domestic students, 4/1 for international students. Application fee: $30. *Financial support:* In 2015–16, 5 research assistantships, 10 teaching assistantships were awarded; fellowships also available. Financial award applicants required to submit FAFSA. *Unit head:* Sarah L. McKune, PhD, Program Director, 352-273-0615, Fax: 352-273-6448, E-mail: smckune@ufl.edu. *Application contact:* Telisha Martin, PhD, Associate Director, MPH Program, 352-273-6444, E-mail: martints@ufl.edu.
Website: http://www.mph.ufl.edu/

University of Georgia, College of Public Health, Doctor of Public Health Program, Athens, GA 30602. Offers Dr PH.

University of Hawaii at Manoa, John A. Burns School of Medicine, Department of Public Health Sciences and Epidemiology, Honolulu, HI 96822. Offers epidemiology (PhD); global health and population studies (Graduate Certificate); public health (MPH, MS, Dr PH). *Accreditation:* CEPH. *Program availability:* Part-time. *Faculty:* 57 full-time (23 women). *Students:* 58 full-time, 14 part-time. Average age 36. 95 applicants, 73% accepted, 46 enrolled. In 2015, 18 master's, 1 doctorate, 1 other advanced degree awarded. *Entrance requirements:* Additional exam requirements/recommendations for international students: Required—TOEFL (minimum score 550 paper-based; 79 iBT), IELTS (minimum score 5). *Application deadline:* For fall admission, 3/1 for domestic and international students; for spring admission, 9/1 for domestic and international students. Application fee: $100. *Financial support:* In 2015–16, 28 fellowships, 23 research assistantships, 1 teaching assistantship were awarded. *Unit head:* Dr. Jerris R. Hedges, Dean, 808-692-0881. *Application contact:* Alan Katz, Graduate Chair, 808-956-5741, Fax: 808-956-5818, E-mail: katz@hawaii.edu.

University of Illinois at Chicago, School of Public Health, Chicago, IL 60607-7128. Offers MHA, MPH, MS, Dr PH, PhD, DDS/MPH, MBA/MPH, MD/PhD, MPH/MS. *Accreditation:* CEPH (one or more programs are accredited). *Program availability:* Part-time. *Faculty:* 67 full-time (40 women), 65 part-time/adjunct (33 women). *Students:* 421 full-time (298 women), 384 part-time (284 women); includes 344 minority (115 Black or African American, non-Hispanic/Latino; 1 American Indian or Alaska Native, non-Hispanic/Latino; 118 Asian, non-Hispanic/Latino; 86 Hispanic/Latino; 2 Native Hawaiian or other Pacific Islander, non-Hispanic/Latino; 22 Two or more races, non-Hispanic/Latino), 75 international. Average age 32. 1,134 applicants, 53% accepted, 230 enrolled. In 2015, 206 master's, 24 doctorates awarded. Terminal master's awarded for partial completion of doctoral program. *Degree requirements:* For master's, thesis, field practicum; for doctorate, thesis/dissertation, independent research, internship. *Entrance requirements:* For master's and doctorate, GRE General Test, minimum GPA of 2.75. Additional exam requirements/recommendations for international students: Required—

TOEFL. *Application deadline:* For fall admission, 2/1 for domestic students, 1/1 priority date for international students. Applications are processed on a rolling basis. Application fee: $60. Electronic applications accepted. *Expenses:* Contact institution. *Financial support:* In 2015–16, 4 fellowships with full tuition reimbursements were awarded; research assistantships with full tuition reimbursements, teaching assistantships with full tuition reimbursements, career-related internships or fieldwork, Federal Work-Study, institutionally sponsored loans, scholarships/grants, traineeships, tuition waivers (full), and unspecified assistantships also available. Support available to part-time students. Financial award application deadline: 3/1; financial award applicants required to submit FAFSA. *Faculty research:* Global health, community health, environmental and occupational health, epidemiology and biostatistics, health policy and administration. *Total annual research expenditures:* $30.4 million. *Unit head:* Dr. Paul Brandt-Rauf, Dean, 312-996-6620. *Application contact:* Prof. Babette Neuberger, Associate Dean and Director of Graduate Studies, 312-996-5381, Fax: 312-996-1734, E-mail: bjn@uic.edu.
Website: http://publichealth.uic.edu/

University of Illinois at Springfield, Graduate Programs, College of Public Affairs and Administration, Program in Public Health, Springfield, IL 62703-5407. Offers community health education (Graduate Certificate); emergency preparedness and homeland security (Graduate Certificate); epidemiology (Graduate Certificate); public health (MPH). *Program availability:* Part-time, evening/weekend, 100% online. *Faculty:* 7 full-time (5 women), 1 part-time/adjunct (0 women). *Students:* 41 full-time (23 women), 58 part-time (39 women); includes 25 minority (14 Black or African American, non-Hispanic/Latino; 6 Asian, non-Hispanic/Latino; 3 Hispanic/Latino; 2 Two or more races, non-Hispanic/Latino), 23 international. Average age 32. 87 applicants, 36% accepted, 23 enrolled. In 2015, 30 master's, 19 other advanced degrees awarded. *Degree requirements:* For master's, comprehensive exam, internship. *Entrance requirements:* For master's, GRE, minimum undergraduate GPA of 3.0, 3 letters of recommendation, statement of personal goals. Additional exam requirements/recommendations for international students: Required—TOEFL (minimum score 500 paper-based; 61 iBT). *Application deadline:* Applications are processed on a rolling basis. Application fee: $60 ($75 for international students). Electronic applications accepted. *Expenses:* Tuition, state resident: part-time $329 per credit hour. Tuition, nonresident: part-time $675 per credit hour. *Financial support:* In 2015–16, fellowships with full tuition reimbursements (averaging $9,900 per year), research assistantships with full tuition reimbursements (averaging $9,956 per year), teaching assistantships with full tuition reimbursements (averaging $9,956 per year) were awarded; career-related internships or fieldwork, Federal Work-Study, scholarships/grants, health care benefits, and unspecified assistantships also available. Support available to part-time students. Financial award application deadline: 11/15; financial award applicants required to submit FAFSA. *Unit head:* Dr. Josiah Alamu, Program Administrator, 217-206-7874, Fax: 217-206-7279, E-mail: jalam3@uis.edu. *Application contact:* Dr. Lynn Pardie, Office of Graduate Studies, 800-252-8533, Fax: 217-206-7623, E-mail: lpard1@uis.edu.
Website: http://www.uis.edu/publichealth/

University of Illinois at Urbana–Champaign, Graduate College, College of Applied Health Sciences, Department of Kinesiology and Community Health, Champaign, IL 61820. Offers community health (MS, MSPH, PhD); kinesiology (MS, PhD); public health (MPH); rehabilitation (MS); PhD/MPH.

University of Indianapolis, Graduate Programs, College of Health Sciences, Program in Public Health, Indianapolis, IN 46227-3697. Offers MPH. *Degree requirements:* For master's, capstone.

The University of Iowa, College of Dentistry and Graduate College, Graduate Programs in Dentistry, Department of Preventive and Community Dentistry, Iowa City, IA 52242-1316. Offers dental public health (MS). *Degree requirements:* For master's, thesis. *Entrance requirements:* For master's, GRE, DDS. Additional exam requirements/recommendations for international students: Required—TOEFL.

The University of Iowa, Graduate College, College of Public Health, Iowa City, IA 52242-1316. Offers MHA, MPH, MS, PhD, Certificate, DVM/MPH, JD/MHA, JD/MPH, MBA/MHA, MD/MPH, MHA/MA, MS/MA, MS/MS, Pharm D/MPH. *Accreditation:* CEPH. *Degree requirements:* For master's, exam; for doctorate, comprehensive exam, thesis/dissertation. *Entrance requirements:* For master's and doctorate, GRE General Test, minimum GPA of 3.0. Additional exam requirements/recommendations for international students: Required—TOEFL. Electronic applications accepted. *Expenses:* Contact institution.

The University of Kansas, University of Kansas Medical Center, School of Medicine, Department of Preventive Medicine and Public Health, Kansas City, KS 66160. Offers clinical research (MS); environmental health sciences (MPH); epidemiology (MPH); public health management (MPH); social and behavioral health (MPH); MD/MPH; PhD/MPH. *Program availability:* Part-time. *Faculty:* 70. *Students:* 48 full-time (35 women), 46 part-time (31 women); includes 31 minority (9 Black or African American, non-Hispanic/Latino; 4 American Indian or Alaska Native, non-Hispanic/Latino; 8 Asian, non-Hispanic/Latino; 6 Hispanic/Latino; 4 Two or more races, non-Hispanic/Latino), 8 international. Average age 31. 66 applicants, 68% accepted, 44 enrolled. In 2015, 31 master's awarded. *Degree requirements:* For master's, thesis, capstone practicum defense. *Entrance requirements:* For master's, GRE, MCAT, LSAT, GMAT or other equivalent graduate professional exam. Additional exam requirements/recommendations for international students: Required—TOEFL. *Application deadline:* For fall admission, 3/1 for domestic and international students. Applications are processed on a rolling basis. Application fee: $60. Electronic applications accepted. *Financial support:* In 2015–16, 9 research assistantships (averaging $15,000 per year) were awarded; career-related internships or fieldwork, Federal Work-Study, scholarships/grants, and unspecified assistantships also available. Support available to part-time students. Financial award application deadline: 3/1; financial award applicants required to submit FAFSA. *Faculty research:* Cancer screening and prevention, smoking cessation, obesity and physical activity, health services/outcomes research, health disparities. *Total annual research expenditures:* $6.6 million. *Unit head:* Dr. Edward F. Ellerbeck, Chairman, 913-588-2774, Fax: 913-588-2780, E-mail: eellerbe@kumc.edu. *Application contact:* Tanya Honderick, MPH Director, 913-588-2720, Fax: 913-588-8505, E-mail: thonderick@kumc.edu.
Website: http://www.kumc.edu/school-of-medicine/preventive-medicine-and-public-health.html

University of Kentucky, Graduate School, College of Public Health, Program in Public Health, Lexington, KY 40506-0032. Offers MPH, Dr PH. *Accreditation:* CEPH. *Entrance requirements:* For master's, GRE General Test, minimum undergraduate GPA of 2.75. Additional exam requirements/recommendations for international students: Required—TOEFL (minimum score 550 paper-based). Electronic applications accepted.

University of Louisville, Graduate School, School of Public Health and Information Sciences, Department of Public Health and Information Sciences, Louisville, KY 40202. Offers biostatistics (MS, PhD); clinical investigation (M Sc); epidemiology (MS); health management and systems sciences (MPH); public health sciences (PhD), including environmental health, epidemiology, health management, health promotion; public health sciences - health management (PhD). *Program availability:* Part-time. *Students:* 92 full-time (60 women), 33 part-time (19 women); includes 37 minority (16 Black or

Public Health—General

African American, non-Hispanic/Latino; 12 Asian, non-Hispanic/Latino; 6 Hispanic/Latino; 3 Two or more races, non-Hispanic/Latino), 19 international. Average age 32. 128 applicants, 77% accepted, 56 enrolled. In 2015, 38 master's, 6 doctorates awarded. *Degree requirements:* For master's, thesis optional; for doctorate, comprehensive exam, thesis/dissertation. *Entrance requirements:* For master's and doctorate, GRE General Test. Additional exam requirements/recommendations for international students: Required—TOEFL (minimum score 600 paper-based; 100 iBT). *Application deadline:* For fall admission, 5/1 for domestic and international students. Application fee: $60. Electronic applications accepted. *Expenses:* Tuition, state resident: full-time $11,664; part-time $649 per credit hour. Tuition, nonresident: full-time $24,274; part-time $1350 per credit hour. *Required fees:* $196. Tuition and fees vary according to program and reciprocity agreements. *Financial support:* In 2015–16, 718,988 students received support. Research assistantships with full tuition reimbursements available, scholarships/grants, health care benefits, and unspecified assistantships available. Financial award applicants required to submit FAFSA. *Faculty research:* Department of environmental and occupational health sciences department of health management and systems sciences department of health promotion and behavioral sciences. *Total annual research expenditures:* $2.1 million. *Unit head:* Dr. Craig Blakely, Dean, 502-852-3297, Fax: 502-852-3291, E-mail: chblak01@louisville.edu.
Website: http://louisville.edu/sphis/departments/health-management-systems-science

The University of Manchester, School of Dentistry, Manchester, United Kingdom. Offers basic dental sciences (cancer studies) (M Phil, PhD); basic dental sciences (molecular genetics) (M Phil, PhD); basic dental sciences (stem cell biology) (M Phil, PhD); biomaterials sciences and dental technology (M Phil, PhD); dental public health/community dentistry (M Phil, PhD); dental science (clinical) (PhD); endodontology (M Phil, PhD); fixed and removable prosthodontics (M Phil, PhD); operative dentistry (M Phil, PhD); oral and maxillofacial surgery (M Phil, PhD); oral radiology (M Phil, PhD); orthodontics (M Phil, PhD); restorative dentistry (M Phil, PhD).

University of Maryland, College Park, Academic Affairs, School of Public Health, College Park, MD 20742. Offers MA, MHA, MPH, MS, PhD. *Program availability:* Part-time, evening/weekend. *Degree requirements:* For doctorate, thesis/dissertation. *Entrance requirements:* For master's and doctorate, GRE General Test, minimum GPA of 3.0, 3 letters of recommendation. Additional exam requirements/recommendations for international students: Required—TOEFL. Electronic applications accepted.

University of Massachusetts Amherst, Graduate School, Interdisciplinary Programs, Dual Degree Program in Public Policy and Administration and Public Health, Amherst, MA 01003. Offers MPH/MPPA. *Entrance requirements:* Additional exam requirements/recommendations for international students: Required—TOEFL (minimum score 550 paper-based; 80 iBT), IELTS (minimum score 6.5). Electronic applications accepted.

University of Massachusetts Amherst, Graduate School, School of Public Health and Health Sciences, Department of Public Health, Amherst, MA 01003. Offers biostatistics (MPH, MS, PhD); community health education (MPH, MS, PhD); environmental health sciences (MPH, MS, PhD); epidemiology (MPH, MS, PhD); health policy and management (MPH, MS, PhD); nutrition (MPH, PhD); public health practice (MPH); MPH/MPPA. *Accreditation:* CEPH (one or more programs are accredited). *Program availability:* Part-time, evening/weekend, online learning. Terminal master's awarded for partial completion of doctoral program. *Degree requirements:* For master's, thesis (for some programs); for doctorate, comprehensive exam, thesis/dissertation. *Entrance requirements:* For master's and doctorate, GRE General Test. Additional exam requirements/recommendations for international students: Required—TOEFL (minimum score 550 paper-based; 80 iBT), IELTS (minimum score 6.5). Electronic applications accepted.

University of Memphis, Graduate School, School of Public Health, Memphis, TN 38152. Offers biostatistics (MPH); environmental health (MPH); epidemiology (MPH); health systems management (MPH); public health (MHA); social and behavioral sciences (MPH). *Program availability:* Part-time, evening/weekend, online learning. *Faculty:* 117 full-time (5 women), 5 part-time/adjunct (1 woman). *Students:* 100 full-time (68 women), 48 part-time (35 women); includes 63 minority (33 Black or African American, non-Hispanic/Latino; 20 Asian, non-Hispanic/Latino; 7 Hispanic/Latino; 3 Two or more races, non-Hispanic/Latino), 17 international. Average age 30. 114 applicants, 83% accepted, 37 enrolled. In 2015, 55 master's awarded. *Degree requirements:* For master's, comprehensive exam, thesis. *Entrance requirements:* For master's, GRE, letters of recommendation. Additional exam requirements/recommendations for international students: Required—TOEFL. *Application deadline:* For fall admission, 4/1 for domestic students; for spring admission, 11/1 for domestic students. Application fee: $35 ($60 for international students). Electronic applications accepted. *Financial support:* In 2015–16, 46 students received support. Research assistantships with full tuition reimbursements available, Federal Work-Study, scholarships/grants, and unspecified assistantships available. Financial award application deadline: 2/15; financial award applicants required to submit FAFSA. *Faculty research:* Health and medical savings accounts, adoption rates, health informatics, Telehealth technologies, biostatistics, environmental health, epidemiology, health systems management, social and behavioral sciences. *Unit head:* Dr. Lisa M. Klesges, Director, 901-678-4637, E-mail: lmklsges@memphis.edu. *Application contact:* Dr. Karen Weddle-West, Information Contact, 901-678-2531, Fax: 901-678-5023, E-mail: gradsch@memphis.edu.
Website: http://www.memphis.edu/sph/

University of Miami, Graduate School, Miller School of Medicine, Graduate Programs in Medicine, Department of Epidemiology and Public Health, Coral Gables, FL 33124. Offers epidemiology (PhD); public health (MPH, MSPH); JD/MPH; MD/MPH; MD/PhD; MPA/MPH; MPH/MAIA. *Accreditation:* CEPH (one or more programs are accredited). *Program availability:* Part-time. *Degree requirements:* For master's, thesis (for some programs), project, practicum; for doctorate, comprehensive exam, thesis/dissertation. *Entrance requirements:* For master's, GRE General Test, minimum GPA of 3.0, 3 letters of recommendation; for doctorate, GRE General Test, minimum GPA of 3.0, course work in epidemiology and statistics, 3 letters of recommendation. Additional exam requirements/recommendations for international students: Required—TOEFL (minimum score 550 paper-based; 59 iBT). Electronic applications accepted. *Faculty research:* Behavioral epidemiology, substance abuse, AIDS, cardiovascular diseases, women's health.

University of Michigan, School of Public Health, Ann Arbor, MI 48109. Offers MHSA, MPH, MS, PhD, JD/MHSA, MD/MPH, MHSA/MBA, MHSA/MPP, MHSA/MSIOE, MPH/JD, MPH/MA, MPH/MPP, MPH/MS, MPH/MSW. MS and PhD offered through the Rackham Graduate School. *Accreditation:* CAHME (one or more programs are accredited); CEPH (one or more programs are accredited). *Program availability:* Evening/weekend. *Faculty:* 136 full-time (62 women), 160 part-time/adjunct (70 women). *Students:* 891 full-time (610 women), 28 part-time (18 women); includes 212 minority (44 Black or African American, non-Hispanic/Latino; 116 Asian, non-Hispanic/Latino; 32 Hispanic/Latino; 20 Two or more races, non-Hispanic/Latino), 179 international. Average age 27. 2,956 applicants, 37% accepted, 441 enrolled. In 2015, 402 master's, 51 doctorates awarded. Terminal master's awarded for partial completion of doctoral program. *Degree requirements:* For master's, internship; for doctorate, oral defense of dissertation, preliminary exam. *Entrance requirements:* For master's and doctorate, GRE General Test. Additional exam requirements/recommendations for international

students: Required—TOEFL (minimum score 100 iBT). *Application deadline:* For fall admission, 12/15 priority date for domestic students, 1/15 for international students. Application fee: $75. Electronic applications accepted. *Financial support:* Fellowships, research assistantships with tuition reimbursements, teaching assistantships with tuition reimbursements, career-related internships or fieldwork, Federal Work-Study, institutionally sponsored loans, scholarships/grants, traineeships, health care benefits, and unspecified assistantships available. *Unit head:* Martin Philbert, Dean, 734-763-4523, Fax: 734-763-5455, E-mail: philbert@umich.edu. *Application contact:* Charles Dill, Admissions Coordinator, 734-764-5425, Fax: 734-763-5455, E-mail: sph.inquiries@umich.edu.
Website: http://www.sph.umich.edu/

University of Michigan–Flint, School of Health Professions and Studies, Program in Public Health, Flint, MI 48502-1950. Offers health administration (MPH); health education (MPH). *Program availability:* Part-time. *Faculty:* 6 full-time (2 women), 5 part-time/adjunct (2 women). *Students:* 23 full-time (15 women), 43 part-time (34 women); includes 20 minority (13 Black or African American, non-Hispanic/Latino; 2 American Indian or Alaska Native, non-Hispanic/Latino; 4 Asian, non-Hispanic/Latino; 1 Hispanic/Latino), 11 international. Average age 31. 87 applicants, 64% accepted, 25 enrolled. In 2015, 2 master's awarded. *Entrance requirements:* For master's, bachelor's degree from accredited institution with sufficient preparation in algebra to succeed in epidemiology and biostatistics; minimum overall undergraduate GPA of 3.0. Additional exam requirements/recommendations for international students: Required—TOEFL (minimum score 560 paper-based; 84 iBT), IELTS (minimum score 6.5). *Application deadline:* For fall admission, 8/1 for domestic students, 5/1 for international students; for winter admission, 11/15 for domestic students, 8/15 for international students; for spring admission, 3/15 for domestic students, 1/15 for international students. Applications are processed on a rolling basis. Application fee: $55. Electronic applications accepted. *Financial support:* Federal Work-Study, scholarships/grants, and unspecified assistantships available. Support available to part-time students. Financial award application deadline: 3/1; financial award applicants required to submit FAFSA. *Unit head:* Dr. Suzanne Selig, Director, 810-762-3172, E-mail: sselig@umflint.edu. *Application contact:* Bradley T. Maki, Director of Graduate Admissions, 810-762-3171, Fax: 810-766-6789, E-mail: bmaki@umflint.edu.
Website: http://www.umflint.edu/graduateprograms/public-health-mph

University of Minnesota, Twin Cities Campus, School of Public Health, Minneapolis, MN 55455. Offers MHA, MPH, MS, PhD, Certificate, DVM/MPH, JD/MS, JD/PhD, MD/MPH, MD/PhD, MPH/JD, MPH/MS, MPH/MSN, MPP/MS. *Accreditation:* CEPH (one or more programs are accredited). *Program availability:* Part-time, online learning. Terminal master's awarded for partial completion of doctoral program. *Degree requirements:* For doctorate, thesis/dissertation. *Entrance requirements:* For master's and doctorate, GRE General Test. Additional exam requirements/recommendations for international students: Required—TOEFL. Electronic applications accepted. *Expenses:* Contact institution.

University of Missouri, Office of Research and Graduate Studies, Master of Public Health Program, Columbia, MO 65211. Offers global public health (Graduate Certificate); health promotion and policy (MPH); public health (Graduate Certificate); veterinary public health (MPH); DVM/MPH; MPH/MA; MPH/MPA. *Accreditation:* CEPH. *Entrance requirements:* Additional exam requirements/recommendations for international students: Required—TOEFL (minimum score 550 paper-based; 80 iBT). *Application deadline:* For fall admission, 6/30 priority date for domestic and international students. Applications are processed on a rolling basis. Application fee: $55 ($75 for international students). Electronic applications accepted. *Financial support:* Fellowships with tuition reimbursements, research assistantships with tuition reimbursements, teaching assistantships with tuition reimbursements, scholarships/grants, traineeships, health care benefits, and unspecified assistantships available. Support available to part-time students.
Website: http://publichealth.missouri.edu/

University of Missouri, School of Medicine, Program in Public Health, Columbia, MO 65211. Offers MS, Graduate Certificate. *Accreditation:* CEPH. *Entrance requirements:* For master's, 3 letters of recommendation; personal statement; curriculum vitae or resume; verification from medical school and residency program; official transcripts. Additional exam requirements/recommendations for international students: Required—TOEFL (minimum score 500 paper-based).
Website: http://www.fcm.missouri.edu

University of Montana, Graduate School, College of Health Professions and Biomedical Sciences, School of Public and Community Health Sciences, Missoula, MT 59812-0002. Offers public health (MPH, CPH). *Accreditation:* CEPH. *Program availability:* Part-time, online learning.

University of Nebraska Medical Center, College of Public Health, Omaha, NE 68198-4355. Offers MPH. *Accreditation:* CEPH. *Program availability:* Part-time, online learning. *Degree requirements:* For master's, service-learning capstone course. *Entrance requirements:* Additional exam requirements/recommendations for international students: Required—TOEFL (minimum score 550 paper-based). Electronic applications accepted. *Expenses:* Tuition, state resident: full-time $7830; part-time $3915 per credit hour. Tuition, nonresident: full-time $22,410; part-time $11,205 per credit hour. *Required fees:* $521. *Faculty research:* Ethics, environmental health, cultural influence on health, rural health policy, cancer prevention.

University of Nevada, Las Vegas, Graduate College, School of Community Health Sciences, Department of Environmental and Occupational Health, Las Vegas, NV 89154-3064. Offers public health (MPH, PhD). *Program availability:* Part-time. *Faculty:* 7 full-time (4 women), 1 part-time/adjunct (0 women). *Students:* 46 full-time (32 women), 49 part-time (39 women); includes 36 minority (5 Black or African American, non-Hispanic/Latino; 3 American Indian or Alaska Native, non-Hispanic/Latino; 7 Asian, non-Hispanic/Latino; 11 Hispanic/Latino; 1 Native Hawaiian or other Pacific Islander, non-Hispanic/Latino; 9 Two or more races, non-Hispanic/Latino), 15 international. Average age 33. 51 applicants, 76% accepted, 29 enrolled. In 2015, 19 master's, 6 doctorates awarded. *Degree requirements:* For master's, thesis; for doctorate, comprehensive exam, thesis/dissertation. *Entrance requirements:* For master's, GRE General Test or GMAT (for some programs); for doctorate, GRE General Test. Additional exam requirements/recommendations for international students: Required—TOEFL (minimum score 550 paper-based; 85 iBT), IELTS (minimum score 7). *Application deadline:* For fall admission, 4/1 for domestic students, 5/1 for international students; for spring admission, 11/1 for domestic students, 10/1 for international students. Application fee: $60 ($95 for international students). Electronic applications accepted. *Expenses:* $264 per credit resident full-time and part-time; $6,955 per semester nonresident full-time; $264 per credit; $555 per credit nonresident part-time. *Financial support:* In 2015–16, 13 students received support, including 12 research assistantships with partial tuition reimbursements available (averaging $12,192 per year), 1 teaching assistantship with partial tuition reimbursement available (averaging $13,000 per year); institutionally sponsored loans, scholarships/grants, health care benefits, and unspecified assistantships also available. Financial award application deadline: 3/1. *Faculty research:* Environmental health: micro (mold) to macro (Lake Mead ecosystem). *Total annual research expenditures:* $2.2 million. *Unit head:* Dr. Shawn Gerstenberger, Chair/

Professor, 702-895-1565, E-mail: shawn.gerstenberger@unlv.edu. *Application contact:* Graduate College Admissions Evaluator, 702-895-3367, Fax: 702-895-4180, E-mail: gradadmissions@unlv.edu.
Website: http://publichealth.unlv.edu/EOH_welcome.html

University of Nevada, Reno, Graduate School, Division of Health Sciences, Department of Public Health, Reno, NV 89557. Offers MPH, PhD, MPH/MSN. *Accreditation:* CEPH. Terminal master's awarded for partial completion of doctoral program. *Degree requirements:* For master's, thesis optional, culminating experience; for doctorate, thesis/dissertation. *Entrance requirements:* For master's, GRE General Test, GMAT, LSAT, MCAT or DAT, minimum GPA of 2.75; for doctorate, GRE General Test, GMAT, LSAT, MCAT or DAT, minimum GPA of 3.0. Additional exam requirements/recommendations for international students: Required—TOEFL (minimum score 500 paper-based; 61 iBT), IELTS (minimum score 6). Electronic applications accepted. *Faculty research:* Biomechanics and basic fundamentals of skiing, social psychology in sports and recreation, fitness and aging, elementary physical education, body fat evaluation.

University of New Hampshire, Graduate School, College of Health and Human Services, Department of Health Management and Policy, Durham, NH 03824. Offers public health (MPH, Postbaccalaureate Certificate). *Program availability:* Part-time, evening/weekend. *Entrance requirements:* For master's, GMAT or GRE General Test. Additional exam requirements/recommendations for international students: Required—TOEFL (minimum score 550 paper-based; 80 iBT). *Application deadline:* For fall admission, 6/1 priority date for domestic students, 4/1 for international students; for spring admission, 12/1 for domestic students. Applications are processed on a rolling basis. Application fee: $65. Electronic applications accepted. *Expenses:* Contact institution. *Financial support:* Fellowships, research assistantships, teaching assistantships, and scholarships/grants available. Financial award application deadline: 2/15. *Unit head:* Rosemary M. Caron, Chair, 603-862-5047. *Application contact:* Rosemary M. Caron, Chair, 603-862-5047.
Website: http://chhs.unh.edu/hmp

University of New Hampshire, Graduate School Manchester Campus, Manchester, NH 03101. Offers business administration (MBA); educational administration and supervision (Ed S); educational studies (M Ed); elementary teacher education (M Ed); information technology (MS); public administration (MPA); public health (MPH, Certificate); secondary teacher education (M Ed, MAT); social work (MSW); substance use disorders (Certificate). *Program availability:* Part-time, evening/weekend. *Degree requirements:* For master's, thesis or alternative. *Entrance requirements:* Additional exam requirements/recommendations for international students: Required—TOEFL (minimum score 550 paper-based; 80 iBT). *Application deadline:* For fall admission, 6/1 for domestic students, 4/1 for international students; for spring admission, 12/1 for domestic students. Applications are processed on a rolling basis. Application fee: $65. Electronic applications accepted. *Expenses:* Tuition, state resident: full-time $13,840; part-time $770 per credit hour. Tuition, nonresident: full-time $27,130; part-time $1175 per credit hour. *Required fees:* $2080; $1040. Tuition and fees vary according to degree level and program. *Financial support:* Fellowships, research assistantships, teaching assistantships, Federal Work-Study, scholarships/grants, health care benefits, and unspecified assistantships available. Support available to part-time students. Financial award application deadline: 3/1; financial award applicants required to submit FAFSA. *Unit head:* Candice Morey, Program Coordinator, 603-641-4313, E-mail: unhm.gradcenter@unh.edu. *Application contact:* Candice Morey, Program Coordinator, 603-641-4313, E-mail: unhm.gradcenter@unh.edu.
Website: http://www.gradschool.unh.edu/manchester/

University of New Mexico, Graduate Studies, Health Sciences Center, Program in Public Health, Albuquerque, NM 87131-5196. Offers community health (MPH); epidemiology (MPH); health systems, services and policy (MPH). *Accreditation:* CEPH. *Program availability:* Part-time, online learning. *Faculty:* 9 full-time (7 women), 3 part-time/adjunct (2 women). *Students:* 25 full-time (17 women), 20 part-time (16 women); includes 17 minority (3 Black or African American, non-Hispanic/Latino; 1 American Indian or Alaska Native, non-Hispanic/Latino; 3 Asian, non-Hispanic/Latino; 10 Hispanic/Latino), 1 international. Average age 31. 32 applicants, 63% accepted, 16 enrolled. In 2015, 13 master's awarded. *Degree requirements:* For master's, thesis. *Entrance requirements:* For master's, GRE, MCAT, 2 years of experience in health field. Additional exam requirements/recommendations for international students: Required—TOEFL. *Application deadline:* For fall admission, 2/1 for domestic students. Application fee: $50. *Financial support:* Fellowships, research assistantships with tuition reimbursements, and Federal Work-Study available. Financial award application deadline: 12/15; financial award applicants required to submit FAFSA. *Faculty research:* Epidemiology, rural health, environmental health, Native American health issues. *Unit head:* Dr. Kristine Tollestrup, Director, 505-272-4173, Fax: 505-272-4494, E-mail: ktollestrup@salud.unm.edu. *Application contact:* Gayle Garcia, Education Coordinator, 505-272-3982, Fax: 505-272-4494, E-mail: garciag@salud.unm.edu.
Website: http://fcm.unm.edu/

The University of North Carolina at Chapel Hill, Graduate School, Gillings School of Global Public Health, Chapel Hill, NC 27599. Offers MHA, MPH, MS, MSCR, MSEE, MSPH, Dr PH, PhD, JD/MPH, MBA/MSPH, MD/MPH, MD/MSPH, MHA/MBA, MHA/MCRP, MHA/MSIS, MHA/MSLS, MPH/MCRP, MPH/MSW, MSPH/M Ed, MSPH/MCRP, MSPH/MSIS, MSPH/MSLS, MSPH/MSW, MSPH/PhD, PhD/MD. *Accreditation:* CAHME (one or more programs are accredited); CEPH (one or more programs are accredited). *Program availability:* Part-time, 100% online, blended/hybrid learning. *Faculty:* 252 full-time (141 women). *Students:* 1,382 full-time (985 women); includes 441 minority (126 Black or African American, non-Hispanic/Latino; 2 American Indian or Alaska Native, non-Hispanic/Latino; 138 Asian, non-Hispanic/Latino; 82 Hispanic/Latino; 3 Native Hawaiian or other Pacific Islander, non-Hispanic/Latino; 90 Two or more races, non-Hispanic/Latino), 171 international. Average age 31. 1,893 applicants, 40% accepted, 402 enrolled. In 2015, 395 master's, 114 doctorates awarded. Terminal master's awarded for partial completion of doctoral program. *Degree requirements:* For master's, comprehensive exam, thesis; for doctorate, comprehensive exam, thesis/dissertation. *Entrance requirements:* For master's and doctorate, GRE General Test. Additional exam requirements/recommendations for international students: Required—TOEFL (minimum score 550 paper-based; 79 iBT). *Application deadline:* For fall admission, 12/10 priority date for domestic and international students. Applications are processed on a rolling basis. Application fee: $85. Electronic applications accepted. *Faculty research:* Infectious disease, health promotion and disease prevention, injury prevention, international health, environmental studies, occupational health studies. *Unit head:* Dr. Barbara K. Rimer, Dean, 919-966-3245, Fax: 919-966-7678. *Application contact:* Johnston King, Admissions Coordinator, 919-962-6314, Fax: 919-966-6352, E-mail: sph-osa@unc.edu.
Website: http://www.sph.unc.edu/

The University of North Carolina at Charlotte, College of Health and Human Services, Department of Public Health Sciences, Charlotte, NC 28223-0001. Offers community health (MPH); health administration (MHA); public health (MSPH); public health core concepts (Graduate Certificate); public health sciences (PhD). *Accreditation:* CAHME. *Program availability:* Part-time. *Faculty:* 18 full-time (9 women),

6 part-time/adjunct (4 women). *Students:* 96 full-time (78 women), 22 part-time (18 women); includes 46 minority (26 Black or African American, non-Hispanic/Latino; 1 American Indian or Alaska Native, non-Hispanic/Latino; 11 Asian, non-Hispanic/Latino; 7 Hispanic/Latino; 1 Two or more races, non-Hispanic/Latino), 15 international. Average age 26. 154 applicants, 66% accepted, 55 enrolled. In 2015, 47 master's, 4 other advanced degrees awarded. *Degree requirements:* For master's, thesis (for some programs), thesis or project; internship; for doctorate, thesis/dissertation. *Entrance requirements:* For master's, GRE or MCAT (for MSPH); GRE or GMAT (for MHA); for doctorate, GRE, master's degree in public health or a related field with minimum GPA of 3.5 in all graduate work; statement of purpose detailing why applicant wants to pursue a PhD in public health sciences in the specified concentration at UNC Charlotte; three letters of recommendation (including at least two letters from former professors); for other advanced degree, bachelor's degree from regionally-accredited university; minimum GPA of 2.75 on all post-secondary work attempted; transcripts; personal statement outlining why the applicant seeks admission to the program. Additional exam requirements/recommendations for international students: Required—TOEFL (minimum score 557 paper-based, 83 iBT) or IELTS (minimum score 6.5). *Application deadline:* For fall admission, 1/10 for domestic and international students; for spring admission, 9/15 for domestic and international students; for summer admission, 2/15 for domestic and international students. Applications are processed on a rolling basis. Application fee: $75. Electronic applications accepted. *Expenses:* Contact institution. *Financial support:* In 2015–16, 18 students received support, including 1 fellowship (averaging $42,000 per year), 15 research assistantships (averaging $6,031 per year); career-related internships or fieldwork, Federal Work-Study, institutionally sponsored loans, scholarships/grants, unspecified assistantships, and administrative assistantships also available. Support available to part-time students. Financial award application deadline: 3/1; financial award applicants required to submit FAFSA. *Faculty research:* Pediatric asthma self-management, reproductive epidemiology, social aspects of injury prevention, chronic illness self-care, competency-based professional education, cognitive health, aging and dementia, infant health outcomes, policing and suicide, data mining for health executive decision support, segmentation analyses in identifying patient satisfaction problems in the primary care setting, enhancing community capacity through data sharing. *Total annual research expenditures:* $573,805. *Unit head:* Dr. Susan M. Sell, Interim Chair, 704-687-7191, Fax: 704-687-1644, E-mail: ssell@uncc.edu. *Application contact:* Kathy B. Giddings, Director of Graduate Admissions, 704-687-5503, Fax: 704-687-1668, E-mail: gradadm@uncc.edu.
Website: http://publichealth.uncc.edu/

University of North Dakota, Graduate School, College of Nursing, Department of Nursing, Grand Forks, ND 58202. Offers adult-gerontological nurse practitioner (MSN); advanced public health nurse (MSN); family nurse practitioner (MSN); nurse anesthesia (MSN); nurse educator (MSN); nursing (DNP, PhD); psychiatric and mental health nurse practitioner (MSN).

University of Northern Colorado, Graduate School, College of Natural and Health Sciences, School of Human Sciences, Program in Public Health, Greeley, CO 80639. Offers public health education (MPH). *Accreditation:* CEPH. *Degree requirements:* For master's, comprehensive exam, thesis or alternative. *Entrance requirements:* For master's, GRE General Test, 2 letters of recommendation. Electronic applications accepted.

University of North Florida, Brooks College of Health, Department of Public Health, Jacksonville, FL 32224. Offers aging services (Certificate); community health (MPH); geriatric management (MSH); health administration (MHA); rehabilitation counseling (MS). *Accreditation:* CEPH. *Program availability:* Part-time, evening/weekend. *Faculty:* 19 full-time (14 women), 3 part-time/adjunct (all women). *Students:* 149 full-time (109 women), 59 part-time (40 women); includes 58 minority (28 Black or African American, non-Hispanic/Latino; 10 Asian, non-Hispanic/Latino; 11 Hispanic/Latino; 9 Two or more races, non-Hispanic/Latino), 9 international. Average age 29. 244 applicants, 43% accepted, 75 enrolled. In 2015, 74 master's awarded. *Degree requirements:* For master's, thesis optional. *Entrance requirements:* For master's, GRE General Test (MSH, MS, MPH); GMAT or GRE General Test (MHA), minimum GPA of 3.0 in last 60 hours. Additional exam requirements/recommendations for international students: Required—TOEFL (minimum score 500 paper-based). *Application deadline:* For fall admission, 7/1 for domestic students, 5/1 for international students; for spring admission, 11/1 for domestic students, 10/1 for international students. Application fee: $30. Electronic applications accepted. *Expenses:* Tuition, state resident: part-time $408.10 per credit hour. Tuition, nonresident: part-time $932.61 per credit hour. *Required fees:* $111.81 per credit hour. Tuition and fees vary according to course load, campus/location and program. *Financial support:* In 2015–16, 33 students received support, including 10 teaching assistantships (averaging $1,500 per year); research assistantships, career-related internships or fieldwork, Federal Work-Study, scholarships/grants, and tuition waivers (partial) also available. Support available to part-time students. Financial award application deadline: 4/1; financial award applicants required to submit FAFSA. *Faculty research:* Dietary supplements; alcohol, tobacco, and other drug use prevention; turnover among health professionals; aging; psychosocial aspects of disabilities. *Total annual research expenditures:* $57,986. *Unit head:* Dr. Jeffrey Harrison, Chair, 904-620-1440, Fax: 904-620-2848, E-mail: jeffrey.harrison@unf.edu. *Application contact:* Dr. Heather Kenney, Director of Advising, 904-620-2810, Fax: 904-620-1030, E-mail: heather.kenney@unf.edu.
Website: http://www.unf.edu/brooks/public_health/

University of North Texas Health Science Center at Fort Worth, School of Public Health, Fort Worth, TX 76107-2699. Offers biostatistics (MPH); community health (MPH); disease control and prevention (Dr PH); environmental and occupational health sciences (MPH); epidemiology (MPH); health administration (MHA); health policy and management (MPH, Dr PH); DO/MPH; MS/MPH; MSN/MPH. MPH offered jointly with University of North Texas; DO/MPH with Texas College of Osteopathic Medicine. *Accreditation:* CEPH. *Program availability:* Part-time, evening/weekend. *Degree requirements:* For master's, thesis or alternative, supervised internship; for doctorate, thesis/dissertation, supervised internship. *Entrance requirements:* For master's, GRE General Test. Additional exam requirements/recommendations for international students: Required—TOEFL. Electronic applications accepted.

University of Oklahoma Health Sciences Center, Graduate College, College of Public Health, Program in General Public Health, Oklahoma City, OK 73190. Offers MPH, Dr PH.

University of Oklahoma Health Sciences Center, Graduate College, College of Public Health, Program in Preparedness and Terrorism, Oklahoma City, OK 73190. Offers MPH.

University of Ottawa, Faculty of Graduate and Postdoctoral Studies, Interdisciplinary Programs, Program in Population Health, Ottawa, ON K1N 6N5, Canada. Offers PhD. *Degree requirements:* For doctorate, comprehensive exam, thesis/dissertation. Electronic applications accepted. *Faculty research:* Population health.

University of Pennsylvania, Perelman School of Medicine, Master of Public Health Program, Philadelphia, PA 19104. Offers generalist, global health, environmental health (MPH); DMD/MPH; JD/MPH; MD/MPH; MPH/MBE; MSN/MPH; MSSP/MPH; MSW/

Public Health—General

MPH; PhD/MPH. *Program availability:* Part-time, evening/weekend. *Faculty:* 21 full-time (14 women), 20 part-time/adjunct (15 women). *Students:* 94 full-time (81 women), 68 part-time (54 women); includes 74 minority (30 Black or African American, non-Hispanic/Latino; 31 Asian, non-Hispanic/Latino; 3 Hispanic/Latino; 10 Two or more races, non-Hispanic/Latino), 2 international. Average age 29. 448 applicants, 49% accepted, 79 enrolled. In 2015, 41 master's awarded. *Entrance requirements:* For master's, GRE. Additional exam requirements/recommendations for international students: Required—TOEFL (minimum score 100 iBT). *Application deadline:* For fall admission, 4/15 for domestic and international students. Applications are processed on a rolling basis. Electronic applications accepted. *Expenses: Tuition, area resident:* Full-time $31,068; part-time $5762 per course. *Required fees:* $3200; $336 per course. Full-time tuition and fees vary according to degree level, program and student level. Part-time tuition and fees vary according to course load, degree level and program. *Financial support:* In 2015–16, 31 students received support, including 1 fellowship with partial tuition reimbursement available (averaging $1,000 per year), 7 research assistantships with partial tuition reimbursements available (averaging $18,104 per year), 24 teaching assistantships with partial tuition reimbursements available (averaging $4,526 per year); tuition waivers (partial) also available. Financial award application deadline: 5/15; financial award applicants required to submit FAFSA. *Faculty research:* Health disparities, health behaviors, obesity, global health, epidemiology and prevention research. *Unit head:* Dr. Jennifer Pinto-Martin, Director, 215-898-4726, E-mail: pinto@nursing.upenn.edu. *Application contact:* Moriah Hall, Associate Director, MPH Program, 215-573-8841, E-mail: moriahh@mail.med.upenn.edu.
Website: http://www.publichealth.med.upenn.edu/

University of Pittsburgh, Graduate School of Public Health, Pittsburgh, PA 15260. Offers MHA, MPH, MS, Dr PH, PhD, Certificate, JD/MPH, MD/MPH, MD/PhD, MID/MPH, MPH/MPA, MPH/MSW, MPH/PhD, MS/MPH. *Accreditation:* CEPH (one or more programs are accredited). *Program availability:* Part-time. *Faculty:* 157 full-time (72 women), 131 part-time/adjunct (67 women). *Students:* 387 full-time (261 women), 218 part-time (162 women); includes 119 minority (27 Black or African American, non-Hispanic/Latino; 47 Asian, non-Hispanic/Latino; 27 Hispanic/Latino; 18 Two or more races, non-Hispanic/Latino), 130 international. Average age 28. 1,593 applicants, 49% accepted, 197 enrolled. In 2015, 169 master's, 52 doctorates awarded. Terminal master's awarded for partial completion of doctoral program. *Degree requirements:* For master's, final paper; comprehensive exam (MS); for doctorate, comprehensive exam, thesis/dissertation. *Entrance requirements:* For master's and Certificate, GRE, U.S. bachelor's or equivalent foreign degree; for doctorate, GRE, U.S. graduate, bachelor's, or equivalent foreign degree; MPH (for Dr PH; courses in mathematics and the biological and social sciences (for PhD). Additional exam requirements/recommendations for international students: Required—TOEFL (minimum score 550 paper-based, 80 iBT) or IELTS (minimum score 6.5). *Application deadline:* For fall admission, 1/15 for domestic and international students; for spring admission, 10/15 for domestic students, 8/1 for international students; for summer admission, 3/15 for domestic students, 12/1 for international students. Applications are processed on a rolling basis. Application fee: $120. Electronic applications accepted. *Expenses:* $12,464 per term full-time in-state; $1,016 per credit part-time in-state; $20,502 per term full-time out-of-state; $1,680 per credit part-time out-of-state. *Financial support:* In 2015–16, 152 students received support, including 20 fellowships (averaging $9,838 per year), 124 research assistantships (averaging $20,360 per year), 16 teaching assistantships (averaging $16,339 per year); career-related internships or fieldwork, scholarships/grants, traineeships, health care benefits, and unspecified assistantships also available. Financial award applicants required to submit FAFSA. *Faculty research:* Epidemiology of physical activity and subclinical CVD, biostatistical assessment of occupational health and environmental risk, effects of arsenic levels in water and food, complications of antiretroviral therapy, behavioral interventions improving long-term care. *Total annual research expenditures:* $59.9 million. *Unit head:* Dr. Donald S. Burke, Dean, 412-624-3001, Fax: 412-624-3013, E-mail: bradym1@pitt.edu. *Application contact:* Karrie A. Lukin, Admissions Manager, 412-624-3003, Fax: 412-624-3755, E-mail: presutti@pitt.edu.
Website: http://www.publichealth.pitt.edu/

University of Rochester, School of Medicine and Dentistry, Graduate Programs in Medicine and Dentistry, Department of Community and Preventive Medicine, Programs in Public Health and Clinical Investigation, Rochester, NY 14627. Offers clinical investigation (MS); public health (MPH); MBA/MPH; MD/MPH; MPH/MS; MPH/PhD. *Accreditation:* CEPH. *Entrance requirements:* For master's, GRE General Test. *Expenses: Tuition, area resident:* Full-time $47,450; part-time $1482 per credit hour. *Required fees:* $528. Tuition and fees vary according to program.

University of San Francisco, School of Nursing and Health Professions, Master's Programs, San Francisco, CA 94117-1080. Offers behavioral health (MSBH); clinical nurse leader (MS); public health (MPH). *Faculty:* 33 full-time (27 women), 44 part-time/adjunct (39 women). *Students:* 426 full-time (357 women), 130 part-time (110 women); includes 305 minority (45 Black or African American, non-Hispanic/Latino; 140 Asian, non-Hispanic/Latino; 78 Hispanic/Latino; 14 Native Hawaiian or other Pacific Islander, non-Hispanic/Latino; 28 Two or more races, non-Hispanic/Latino), 23 international. Average age 33. 542 applicants, 59% accepted, 190 enrolled. In 2015, 180 master's awarded. *Application deadline:* For fall admission, 5/15 priority date for domestic students; for spring admission, 11/30 priority date for domestic students. *Expenses: Tuition, area resident:* Full-time $22,410; part-time $1245 per credit. Tuition and fees vary according to course load, degree level and campus/location. *Financial support:* In 2015–16, 99 students received support. *Unit head:* Dr. Michelle Montagno, Director, 415-422-4074, E-mail: mjmontagno@usfca.edu. *Application contact:* Ingrid McVanner, Information Contact, 415-422-2746, Fax: 415-422-2217.

University of South Africa, College of Human Sciences, Pretoria, South Africa. Offers adult education (M Ed); African languages (MA, PhD); African politics (MA, PhD); Afrikaans (MA, PhD); ancient history (MA, PhD); ancient Near Eastern studies (MA, PhD); anthropology (MA, PhD); applied linguistics (MA); Arabic (MA, PhD); archaeology (MA); art history (MA); Biblical archaeology (MA); Biblical studies (M Th, D Th, PhD); Christian spirituality (M Th, D Th); church history (M Th, D Th); classical studies (MA, PhD); clinical psychology (MA); communication (MA, PhD); comparative education (M Ed, Ed D); consulting psychology (D Admin, D Com, PhD); curriculum studies (M Ed, Ed D); development studies (M Admin, MA, D Admin, PhD); didactics (M Ed, Ed D); education (M Tech); education management (M Ed, Ed D); educational psychology (M Ed); English (MA); environmental education (M Ed); French (MA, PhD); German (MA, PhD); Greek (MA); guidance and counseling (M Ed); health studies (MA, PhD), including health sciences education (MA), health services management (MA), medical and surgical nursing science (critical care general) (MA), midwifery and neonatal nursing science (MA), trauma and emergency care (MA); history (MA, PhD); history of education (Ed D); inclusive education (M Ed, Ed D); information and communications technology policy and regulation (MA); information science (MA, MIS, PhD); international politics (MA, PhD); Islamic studies (MA, PhD); Italian (MA, PhD); Judaica (MA, PhD); linguistics (MA, PhD); mathematical education (M Ed); mathematics education (MA); missiology (M Th, D Th); modern Hebrew (MA, PhD); musicology (MA, MMus, D Mus, PhD); natural science education (M Ed); New Testament (M Th, D Th); Old Testament (D Th); pastoral therapy (M Th, D Th); philosophy (MA); philosophy of education (M Ed, Ed D);

politics (MA, PhD); Portuguese (MA, PhD); practical theology (M Th, D Th); psychology (MA, MS, PhD); psychology of education (M Ed, Ed D); public health (MA); religious studies (MA, D Th, PhD); Romance languages (MA); Russian (MA, PhD); Semitic languages (MA, PhD); social behavior studies in HIV/AIDS (MA); social science (mental health) (MA); social science in development studies (MA); social science in psychology (MA); social science in social work (MA); social science in sociology (MA); social work (MSW, DSW, PhD); socio-education (M Ed, Ed D); sociolinguistics (MA); sociology (MA, PhD); Spanish (MA, PhD); systematic theology (M Th, D Th); TESOL (teaching English to speakers of other languages) (MA); theological ethics (M Th, D Th); theory of literature (MA, PhD); urban ministries (D Th); urban ministry (M Th).

University of South Carolina, The Graduate School, Arnold School of Public Health, Program in General Public Health, Columbia, SC 29208. Offers MPH. *Accreditation:* CEPH. *Program availability:* Part-time. *Degree requirements:* For master's, comprehensive exam, practicum. *Entrance requirements:* For master's, DAT or MCAT, GRE General Test, previously earned MD or doctoral degree. Additional exam requirements/recommendations for international students: Required—TOEFL (minimum score 570 paper-based). Electronic applications accepted.

University of South Carolina, The Graduate School, Arnold School of Public Health, Program in Physical Activity and Public Health, Columbia, SC 29208. Offers MPH. *Accreditation:* CEPH. *Program availability:* Part-time. *Degree requirements:* For master's, comprehensive exam, practicum. *Entrance requirements:* For master's, GRE. Additional exam requirements/recommendations for international students: Required—TOEFL (minimum score 570 paper-based). Electronic applications accepted.

University of South Carolina, The Graduate School, College of Nursing, Program in Nursing and Public Health, Columbia, SC 29208. Offers MPH/MSN. *Accreditation:* AACN; CEPH. *Program availability:* Part-time. *Entrance requirements:* Additional exam requirements/recommendations for international students: Required—TOEFL (minimum score 570 paper-based). Electronic applications accepted. *Faculty research:* System research, evidence based practice, breast cancer, violence.

University of Southern California, Keck School of Medicine and Graduate School, Graduate Programs in Medicine, Department of Preventive Medicine, Master of Public Health Program, Los Angeles, CA 91803. Offers biostatistics and epidemiology (MPH); child and family health (MPH); environmental health (MPH); global health leadership (MPH); health communication (MPH); health education and promotion (MPH); public health policy (MPH). *Accreditation:* CEPH. *Program availability:* Part-time, evening/weekend. *Faculty:* 22 full-time (12 women), 3 part-time/adjunct (0 women). *Students:* 182 full-time (142 women), 35 part-time (25 women); includes 120 minority (19 Black or African American, non-Hispanic/Latino; 64 Asian, non-Hispanic/Latino; 37 Hispanic/Latino), 33 international. Average age 24. 236 applicants, 70% accepted, 71 enrolled. In 2015, 99 master's awarded. *Degree requirements:* For master's, practicum, final report, oral presentation. *Entrance requirements:* For master's, GRE General Test, MCAT, GMAT, minimum GPA of 3.0. Additional exam requirements/recommendations for international students: Required—TOEFL (minimum score 600 paper-based; 90 iBT). *Application deadline:* For fall admission, 6/1 priority date for domestic and international students; for spring admission, 10/1 priority date for domestic and international students; for summer admission, 3/1 for domestic and international students. Applications are processed on a rolling basis. Application fee: $85. Electronic applications accepted. *Expenses:* Contact institution. *Financial support:* Career-related internships or fieldwork, Federal Work-Study, institutionally sponsored loans, and scholarships/grants available. Support available to part-time students. Financial award application deadline: 5/4; financial award applicants required to submit CSS PROFILE or FAFSA. *Faculty research:* Substance abuse prevention, cancer and heart disease prevention, mass media and health communication research, health promotion, treatment compliance. *Unit head:* Dr. Louise A. Rohrbach, Director, 323-442-8237, Fax: 323-442-8297, E-mail: rohrbac@usc.edu. *Application contact:* Valerie Burris, Admissions Counselor, 323-442-7257, Fax: 323-442-8297, E-mail: valeriem@usc.edu.
Website: http://mph.usc.edu/

University of Southern California, Keck School of Medicine and Graduate School, Graduate Programs in Medicine, Department of Preventive Medicine, Program in Health Behavior Research, Los Angeles, CA 90032. Offers PhD. *Faculty:* 21 full-time (13 women), 1 (woman) part-time/adjunct. *Students:* 33 full-time (20 women), 1 part-time (0 women); includes 16 minority (2 Black or African American, non-Hispanic/Latino; 9 Asian, non-Hispanic/Latino; 4 Hispanic/Latino; 1 Two or more races, non-Hispanic/Latino), 2 international. Average age 31. 42 applicants, 17% accepted, 4 enrolled. In 2015, 1 doctorate awarded. *Degree requirements:* For doctorate, comprehensive exam, thesis/dissertation. *Entrance requirements:* For doctorate, GRE General Test (minimum preferred score for combined Verbal and Quantitative of 311), minimum GPA of 3.0 (3.5 preferred). Additional exam requirements/recommendations for international students: Required—TOEFL (minimum score 600 paper-based; 100 iBT). *Application deadline:* For fall admission, 12/1 priority date for domestic and international students. Application fee: $85. Electronic applications accepted. *Financial support:* In 2015–16, 30 students received support, including 11 fellowships with full tuition reimbursements available (averaging $32,000 per year), 7 research assistantships with tuition reimbursements available (averaging $32,000 per year), 7 teaching assistantships with tuition reimbursements available (averaging $32,000 per year); institutionally sponsored loans, scholarships/grants, traineeships, health care benefits, and unspecified assistantships also available. Financial award application deadline: 5/12; financial award applicants required to submit CSS PROFILE or FAFSA. *Faculty research:* Obesity prevention; etiology and prevention of substance abuse, other addictive behaviors, and chronic diseases; health disparities; translational research. *Unit head:* Dr. Jennifer Unger, Director, 323-442-8234, E-mail: unger@usc.edu. *Application contact:* Marny Barovich, Program Manager, 323-442-8299, E-mail: barovich@hsc.usc.edu.
Website: http://phdhbr.usc.edu

University of Southern Maine, College of Management and Human Service, Muskie School of Public Service, Program in Health Policy and Management, Portland, ME 04103. Offers MPH, CGS, MBA/MPH. *Accreditation:* CAHME. *Program availability:* Part-time, evening/weekend, online learning. *Degree requirements:* For master's, thesis, capstone project, field experience. *Entrance requirements:* For master's, GRE General Test. Additional exam requirements/recommendations for international students: Required—TOEFL. Electronic applications accepted. *Expenses: Tuition, area resident:* Full-time $6840; part-time $380 per credit hour. Tuition, state resident: full-time $10,260; part-time $570 per credit hour. Tuition, nonresident: full-time $18,468; part-time $1026 per credit hour. *Required fees:* $830; $83 per credit hour. Tuition and fees vary according to course load and program. *Faculty research:* Public health systems, population health and health policy, rural health, patient safety, health services research, aging and disability policy, Medicare and Medicaid policy, mental health policy.

University of Southern Mississippi, Graduate School, College of Health, Department of Public Health, Hattiesburg, MS 39406-0001. Offers epidemiology and biostatistics (MPH); health education (MPH); health policy and administration (MPH). *Accreditation:* CEPH. *Program availability:* Part-time, evening/weekend. *Degree requirements:* For master's, comprehensive exam, thesis (for some programs). *Entrance requirements:* For master's, GRE General Test, minimum GPA of 2.75 in last 60 hours. Additional exam requirements/recommendations for international students: Required—TOEFL, IELTS.

Electronic applications accepted. *Faculty research:* Rural health care delivery, school health, nutrition of pregnant teens, risk factor reduction, sexually transmitted diseases.

⭐ **University of South Florida,** College of Public Health, Tampa, FL 33612. Offers MHA, MPH, MSPH, Dr PH, PhD. *Accreditation:* CEPH (one or more programs are accredited). *Program availability:* Part-time, evening/weekend, online learning. *Degree requirements:* For master's, comprehensive exam, thesis (for some programs); for doctorate, comprehensive exam, thesis/dissertation. *Entrance requirements:* For master's, GRE General Test, minimum GPA of 3.0 in upper-level course work, 3 professional letters of recommendation, resume/curriculum vitae; for doctorate, GRE General Test, minimum GPA of 3.0 in upper-level course work, goal statement letter, three professional letters of recommendation, resume/curriculum vitae, writing sample. Additional exam requirements/recommendations for international students: Required—TOEFL (minimum score 550 paper-based; 79 iBT). Electronic applications accepted.

See Display below and Close-Up on page 853.

University of South Florida, Innovative Education, Tampa, FL 33620-9951. Offers adult, career and higher education (Graduate Certificate), including college teaching, leadership in developing human resources, leadership in higher education; Africana studies (Graduate Certificate), including diasporas and health disparities, genocide and human rights; aging studies (Graduate Certificate), including gerontology; art research (Graduate Certificate), including museum studies; business foundations (Graduate Certificate); chemical and biomedical engineering (Graduate Certificate), including materials science and engineering, water, health and sustainability; child and family studies (Graduate Certificate), including positive behavior support; civil and industrial engineering (Graduate Certificate), including transportation systems analysis; community and family health (Graduate Certificate), including maternal and child health, social marketing and public health, violence and injury: prevention and intervention, women's health; criminology (Graduate Certificate), including criminal justice administration; educational measurement and research (Graduate Certificate), including evaluation; English (Graduate Certificate), including comparative literary studies, creative writing, professional and technical communication; entrepreneurship (Graduate Certificate); environmental health (Graduate Certificate), including safety management; epidemiology and biostatistics (Graduate Certificate), including applied biostatistics, biostatistics, concepts and tools of epidemiology, epidemiology, epidemiology of infectious diseases; geography, environment and planning (Graduate Certificate), including community development, environmental policy and management, geographical information systems; geology (Graduate Certificate), including hydrogeology; global health (Graduate Certificate), including disaster management, global health and Latin American and Caribbean studies, global health practice, humanitarian assistance, infection control; government and international affairs (Graduate Certificate), including Cuban studies, globalization studies; health policy and management (Graduate Certificate), including health management and leadership, public health policy and programs; hearing specialist: early intervention (Graduate Certificate); industrial and management systems engineering (Graduate Certificate), including systems engineering, technology management; information studies (Graduate Certificate), including school library media specialist; information systems/decision sciences (Graduate Certificate), including analytics and business intelligence; instructional technology (Graduate Certificate), including distance education, Florida digital/virtual educator, instructional design, multimedia design, Web design; internal medicine, bioethics and medical humanities (Graduate Certificate), including biomedical ethics; Latin American and Caribbean studies (Graduate Certificate); mass communications (Graduate Certificate), including multimedia journalism; mathematics and statistics (Graduate Certificate), including mathematics; medicine (Graduate

Certificate), including aging and neuroscience, bioinformatics, biotechnology, brain fitness and memory management, clinical investigation, health informatics, health sciences, integrative weight management, intellectual property, medicine and gender, metabolic and nutritional medicine, metabolic cardiology, pharmacy sciences; national and competitive intelligence (Graduate Certificate); psychological and social foundations (Graduate Certificate), including career counseling, college teaching, diversity in education, mental health counseling, school counseling; public affairs (Graduate Certificate), including nonprofit management, public management, research administration; public health (Graduate Certificate), including environmental health, health equity, public health generalist, translational research in adolescent behavioral health; public health practices (Graduate Certificate), including planning for healthy communities; rehabilitation and mental health counseling (Graduate Certificate), including integrative mental health care, marriage and family therapy, rehabilitation technology; secondary education (Graduate Certificate), including ESOL, foreign language education: culture and content, foreign language education: professional; social work (Graduate Certificate), including geriatric social work/clinical gerontology; special education (Graduate Certificate), including autism spectrum disorder, disabilities education: severe/profound; world languages (Graduate Certificate), including teaching English as a second language (TESL) or foreign language. *Unit head:* Kathy Barnes, Interdisciplinary Programs Coordinator, 813-974-8031, Fax: 813-974-7061, E-mail: barnesk@usf.edu. *Application contact:* Karen Tylinski, Metro Initiatives, 813-974-9943, Fax: 813-974-7061, E-mail: ktylinsk@usf.edu.
Website: http://www.usf.edu/innovative-education/

The University of Tennessee, Graduate School, College of Education, Health and Human Sciences, Program in Public Health, Knoxville, TN 37996. Offers community health education (MPH); gerontology (MPH); health planning/administration (MPH); MS/MPH. *Accreditation:* CEPH. *Degree requirements:* For master's, thesis optional. *Entrance requirements:* For master's, minimum GPA of 2.7. Additional exam requirements/recommendations for international students: Required—TOEFL. Electronic applications accepted.

The University of Texas Health Science Center at Houston, The University of Texas School of Public Health, Houston, TX 77030. Offers MPH, MS, Dr PH, PhD, Certificate, JD/MPH, MBA/MPH, MD/MPH, MGPS/MPH, MP Aff/MPH, MS/MPH, MSN/MPH, MSW/MPH, PhD/MPH. Applications to dual degree programs are handled independently between the collaborating institutions. *Accreditation:* CEPH. *Program availability:* Part-time. *Degree requirements:* For master's, thesis (for some programs); for doctorate, comprehensive exam, thesis/dissertation. *Entrance requirements:* For master's and doctorate, GRE General Test. Additional exam requirements/recommendations for international students: Required—TOEFL (minimum score 565 paper-based; 86 iBT). Electronic applications accepted. *Faculty research:* Chronic and infectious disease epidemiology; health promotion and health education; applied and theoretical biostatistics; health management, policy and economics; environmental and occupational health.

The University of Texas Medical Branch, Graduate School of Biomedical Sciences, Department of Preventive Medicine and Community Health, Program in Public Health, Galveston, TX 77555. Offers MPH. *Accreditation:* CEPH. *Degree requirements:* For master's, thesis. *Entrance requirements:* For master's, GRE, United States Medical Licensing Exam (USMLE) or NBE, preventive medicine residency. Additional exam requirements/recommendations for international students: Required—TOEFL (minimum score 550 paper-based). Electronic applications accepted.

University of the Sciences, Program in Public Health, Philadelphia, PA 19104-4495. Offers MPH. *Program availability:* Part-time, evening/weekend, online learning. *Entrance requirements:* Additional exam requirements/recommendations for

Peterson's Graduate Programs in the Biological/Biomedical Sciences & Health-Related Medical Professions 2017

Public Health—General

international students: Required—TOEFL, TWE. *Unit head:* Dr. Amalia M. Issa, Chair/Director, 267-295-7033, E-mail: a.issa@usciences.edu. *Application contact:* Dr. Amalia M. Issa, Chair/Director, 267-295-7033, E-mail: a.issa@usciences.edu.

The University of Toledo, College of Graduate Studies, College of Medicine and Life Sciences, Department of Public Health and Preventative Medicine, Toledo, OH 43606-3390. Offers biostatistics and epidemiology (Certificate); contemporary gerontological practice (Certificate); environmental and occupational health and safety (MPH); epidemiology (Certificate); global public health (Certificate); health promotion and education (MPH); industrial hygiene (MSOH); medical and health science teaching and learning (Certificate); occupational health (Certificate); public health administration (MPH); public health and emergency response (Certificate); public health epidemiology (MPH); public health nutrition (MPH); MD/MPH. *Program availability:* Part-time, evening/weekend. *Degree requirements:* For master's, thesis or alternative. *Entrance requirements:* For master's, GRE, minimum undergraduate GPA of 3.0, three letters of recommendation, statement of purpose, transcripts from all prior institutions attended, resume; for Certificate, minimum undergraduate GPA of 3.0, three letters of recommendation, statement of purpose, transcripts from all prior institutions attended, resume. Additional exam requirements/recommendations for international students: Required—TOEFL (minimum score 550 paper-based; 80 iBT), IELTS (minimum score 6.5). Electronic applications accepted.

University of Toronto, School of Graduate Studies, Department of Public Health Sciences, Toronto, ON M5S 1A1, Canada. Offers biostatistics (M Sc, PhD); community health (M Sc); community nutrition (MPH), including nutrition and dietetics; epidemiology (MPH, PhD); family and community medicine (MPH); occupational and environmental health (MPH); social and behavioral health science (PhD); social and behavioral health sciences (MPH), including health promotion. *Accreditation:* CAHME (one or more programs are accredited); CEPH (one or more programs are accredited). *Program availability:* Part-time. *Degree requirements:* For master's, thesis (for some programs), practicum; for doctorate, comprehensive exam, thesis/dissertation, oral thesis defense. *Entrance requirements:* For master's, 2 letters of reference, relevant professional/research experience, minimum B average in final year; for doctorate, 2 letters of reference, relevant professional/research experience, minimum B+ average. Additional exam requirements/recommendations for international students: Required—TOEFL (minimum score 580 paper-based; 93 iBT), TWE (minimum score 5). Electronic applications accepted. *Expenses:* Contact institution.

University of Utah, School of Medicine and Graduate School, Graduate Programs in Medicine, Programs in Public Health, Salt Lake City, UT 84112-1107. Offers biostatistics (M Stat); public health (MPH, MSPH, PhD). *Accreditation:* CEPH (one or more programs are accredited). *Program availability:* Part-time. *Degree requirements:* For master's, comprehensive exam, thesis or project (MSPH); for doctorate, comprehensive exam, thesis/dissertation. *Entrance requirements:* For master's and doctorate, GRE General Test, 3 letters of reference, in-person interviews, minimum GPA of 3.0. Additional exam requirements/recommendations for international students: Required—TOEFL (minimum score 550 paper-based). Electronic applications accepted. *Faculty research:* Health services, health policy, epidemiology of chronic disease, infectious disease epidemiology, cancer epidemiology.

University of Virginia, School of Medicine, Department of Public Health Sciences, Program in Public Health, Charlottesville, VA 22903. Offers MPH, MPP/MPH. *Accreditation:* CEPH. *Degree requirements:* For master's, written or oral comprehensive exam or thesis. *Entrance requirements:* For master's, GRE, MCAT, LSAT or GMAT, 2 letters of recommendation. Additional exam requirements/recommendations for international students: Required—TOEFL. Electronic applications accepted.

University of Virginia, School of Nursing, Charlottesville, VA 22903. Offers acute and specialty care (MSN); acute care nurse practitioner (MSN); clinical nurse leadership (MSN); community-public health leadership (MSN); nursing (DNP, PhD); psychiatric mental health counseling (MSN); MSN/MBA. *Accreditation:* AACN. *Program availability:* Part-time. *Degree requirements:* For doctorate, comprehensive exam (for some programs), capstone project (DNP), dissertation (PhD). *Entrance requirements:* For master's, GRE General Test, MAT; for doctorate, GRE General Test. Additional exam requirements/recommendations for international students: Required—TOEFL, IELTS. Electronic applications accepted. *Expenses:* Contact institution.

University of Washington, Graduate School, School of Public Health, Executive MPH Program, Seattle, WA 98195. Offers MPH. *Program availability:* Evening/weekend, online learning. *Degree requirements:* For master's, capstone or thesis, practicum. *Entrance requirements:* For master's, GRE General Test or other comparable test scores (unless applicant already has graduate-level degree from accredited U.S. institution). Additional exam requirements/recommendations for international students: Required—TOEFL (minimum score 580 paper-based; 70 iBT). Electronic applications accepted. *Expenses:* Contact institution.

University of Waterloo, Graduate Studies, Faculty of Applied Health Sciences, School of Public Health and Health Systems, Waterloo, ON N2L 3G1, Canada. Offers health evaluation (MHE); health informatics (MHI); health studies and gerontology (M Sc, PhD); public health (MPH). *Program availability:* Part-time. *Degree requirements:* For master's, thesis; for doctorate, comprehensive exam, thesis/dissertation. *Entrance requirements:* For master's, honors degree, minimum B average, resume, writing sample; for doctorate, GRE (recommended), master's degree, minimum B average, resume, writing sample. Additional exam requirements/recommendations for international students: Required—TOEFL, IELTS, PTE. *Application deadline:* For fall admission, 2/1 for domestic and international students. Application fee: $100 Canadian dollars. Electronic applications accepted. *Financial support:* In 2015–16, teaching assistantships (averaging $6,141 per year) were awarded; research assistantships, career-related internships or fieldwork, Federal Work-Study, institutionally sponsored loans, scholarships/grants, and university-sponsored bursaries also available. *Faculty research:* Population health, health promotion and disease prevention, healthy aging, health policy, planning and evaluation, health information management and health informatics, aging, health and well-being, work and health. Website: https://uwaterloo.ca/public-health-and-health-systems/

University of West Florida, College of Science and Engineering, School of Allied Health and Life Sciences, Program in Public Health, Pensacola, FL 32514-5750. Offers MPH. *Accreditation:* CEPH. *Program availability:* Part-time, evening/weekend. *Entrance requirements:* For master's, GRE (minimum score: verbal 450, quantitative 550), GMAT (minimum score 465), or MCAT (minimum score 25), official transcripts; two personal writing samples (e.g., written reports completed by applicant or other representative samples of professional writing skills); basic computer competency; three letters of recommendation. Additional exam requirements/recommendations for international students: Required—TOEFL (minimum score 550 paper-based).

University of Wisconsin–Madison, School of Medicine and Public Health, Master of Public Health Program, Madison, WI 53706-1380. Offers MPH. *Expenses:* Tuition, state resident: full-time $5364. Tuition, nonresident: full-time $12,027. *Required fees:* $571. Tuition and fees vary according to campus/location, program and reciprocity agreements. Website: http://mph.wisc.edu/

University of Wisconsin–Milwaukee, Graduate School, Zilber School of Public Health, Department of Public Health, Milwaukee, WI 53201-0413. Offers community and behavioral health promotion (PhD); public health (MPH, Graduate Certificate). *Students:* 56 full-time (39 women), 17 part-time (13 women); includes 17 minority (6 Black or African American, non-Hispanic/Latino; 6 Asian, non-Hispanic/Latino; 5 Two or more races, non-Hispanic/Latino), 4 international. Average age 31. 113 applicants, 58% accepted, 34 enrolled. In 2015, 10 master's awarded. *Unit head:* Amy Harley, Assistant Professor, 414-229-4342, E-mail: harley@uwm.edu. *Application contact:* Darcie K. G. Warren, Graduate Program Manager, 414-229-5633, E-mail: darcie@uwm.edu.

Valparaiso University, Graduate School, College of Nursing and Health Professions, Valparaiso, IN 46383. Offers nursing (DNP); nursing education (MSN, Certificate); public health (MPH); MSN/MHA. *Accreditation:* AACN. *Program availability:* Part-time, evening/weekend, online learning. *Faculty:* 13 part-time/adjunct (all women). *Students:* 52 full-time (43 women), 33 part-time (30 women); includes 9 minority (4 Black or African American, non-Hispanic/Latino; 1 Asian, non-Hispanic/Latino; 4 Hispanic/Latino), 22 international. Average age 33. In 2015, 9 master's, 16 doctorates awarded. *Entrance requirements:* For master's, minimum GPA 3.0, undergraduate major in nursing, Indiana registered nursing license, undergraduate courses in research and statistics. Additional exam requirements/recommendations for international students: Required—TOEFL (minimum score 550 paper-based; 80 iBT), IELTS (minimum score 6). *Application deadline:* Applications are processed on a rolling basis. Application fee: $30 ($50 for international students). Electronic applications accepted. *Expenses:* Contact institution. *Financial support:* Available to part-time students. Applicants required to submit FAFSA. *Unit head:* Dr. Janet Brown, Dean, 219-464-5289, Fax: 219-464-5425, E-mail: janet.brown@valpo.edu. *Application contact:* Jessica Choquette, Graduate Admissions Specialist, 219-464-6510, Fax: 219-464-5381, E-mail: jessica.choquette@valpo.edu. Website: http://www.valpo.edu/nursing/

Vanderbilt University, Center for Medicine, Health, and Society, Nashville, TN 37240-1001. Offers MA, MD/MA. *Accreditation:* CEPH. *Faculty:* 4 full-time (2 women). *Students:* 6 full-time (3 women); all minorities (4 Black or African American, non-Hispanic/Latino; 1 Asian, non-Hispanic/Latino; 1 Two or more races, non-Hispanic/Latino). Average age 23. 16 applicants, 69% accepted, 10 enrolled. In 2015, 10 master's awarded. *Degree requirements:* For master's, comprehensive exam (for some programs), thesis (for some programs). *Entrance requirements:* Additional exam requirements/recommendations for international students: Required—TOEFL (minimum score 570 paper-based; 88 iBT). *Application deadline:* For fall admission, 1/15 for domestic and international students. Electronic applications accepted. *Financial support:* Federal Work-Study, scholarships/grants, and health care benefits available. Financial award application deadline: 1/15; financial award applicants required to submit CSS PROFILE or FAFSA. *Faculty research:* Cultural history of health and disease, the rise of scientific medicine, scientific and medical constructions of gender and sexuality, integrative medicine, domestic and international public health, healthcare administration. *Unit head:* Dr. Jonathan Metzl, Director, 615-343-0916, Fax: 615-343-8889, E-mail: jonathan.metzl@vanderbilt.edu. *Application contact:* Elisabeth Sandberg, Assistant Director, 615-343-0916, Fax: 615-322-2731, E-mail: elisabeth.sandberg@vanderbilt.edu. Website: http://www.vanderbilt.edu/mhs/

Virginia Commonwealth University, Medical College of Virginia-Professional Programs, School of Medicine, School of Medicine Graduate Programs, Department of Epidemiology and Community Health, Richmond, VA 23284-9005. Offers epidemiology (MPH, PhD); public health practice (MPH); social and behavioral science (MPH); MD/MPH; MSW/MPH. *Accreditation:* CEPH. *Program availability:* Part-time. *Degree requirements:* For doctorate, comprehensive exam, thesis/dissertation. *Entrance requirements:* For master's, GRE; for doctorate, GRE General Test, interview, 3 letters of recommendation, minimum graduate GPA of 3.0, master's degree in public health or related field including epidemiology and biostatistics. Additional exam requirements/recommendations for international students: Required—TOEFL (minimum score 600 paper-based; 100 iBT). Electronic applications accepted. *Faculty research:* Sickle cell anemia, breast cancer, HIV/AIDS, hospital epidemiology, infectious diseases.

Virginia Polytechnic Institute and State University, Virginia-Maryland Regional College of Veterinary Medicine, Blacksburg, VA 24061. Offers biomedical and veterinary sciences (MS, PhD); public health (MPH); research in translational medicine (Certificate); veterinary medicine (DVM). *Accreditation:* AVMA (one or more programs are accredited). *Degree requirements:* For master's, comprehensive exam (for some programs), thesis (for some programs); for doctorate, comprehensive exam (for some programs), thesis/dissertation (for some programs). *Entrance requirements:* For master's and doctorate, GRE/GMAT (may vary by department). Additional exam requirements/recommendations for international students: Required—TOEFL (minimum score 550 paper-based). Electronic applications accepted. *Expenses:* Contact institution.

Walden University, Graduate Programs, School of Counseling, Minneapolis, MN 55401. Offers addiction counseling (MS), including addictions and public health, child and adolescent counseling, family studies and interventions, forensic counseling, general program, military families and culture, trauma and crisis counseling; clinical mental health counseling (MS), including addiction counseling, forensic counseling, military families and culture, trauma and crisis counseling; counselor education and supervision (PhD), including consultation, counseling and social change, forensic mental health counseling, leadership and program evaluation, trauma and crisis; marriage, couple, and family counseling (MS), including addiction counseling, career counseling, forensic counseling, military families and culture, trauma and crisis counseling; school counseling (MS), including addiction counseling, career counseling, crisis and trauma, military families and culture. *Program availability:* Part-time, evening/weekend, online only, 100% online. *Faculty:* 76 full-time (60 women), 155 part-time/adjunct (115 women). *Students:* 1,827 full-time (1,569 women), 1,352 part-time (1,158 women); includes 1,484 minority (1,110 Black or African American, non-Hispanic/Latino; 19 American Indian or Alaska Native, non-Hispanic/Latino; 38 Asian, non-Hispanic/Latino; 189 Hispanic/Latino; 128 Two or more races, non-Hispanic/Latino), 21 international. Average age 38. 711 applicants, 94% accepted, 513 enrolled. In 2015, 531 master's, 14 doctorates awarded. *Degree requirements:* For master's, residency, field experience, professional development plan, licensure plan; for doctorate, thesis/dissertation, residency, practicum, internship. *Entrance requirements:* For master's, bachelor's degree or higher; minimum GPA of 2.5; official transcripts; goal statement (for some programs); access to computer and Internet; for doctorate, master's degree or higher; three years of related professional or academic experience (preferred); minimum GPA of 3.0; goal statement and current resume (for select programs); official transcripts; access to computer and Internet. Additional exam requirements/recommendations for international students: Required—TOEFL (minimum score 550 paper-based, 79 iBT), IELTS (minimum score 6.5), Michigan English Language Assessment Battery (minimum score 82), or PTE (minimum score 53). *Application deadline:* Applications are processed on a rolling basis. Application fee: $0. Electronic applications accepted. *Financial support:* Federal Work-Study, scholarships/grants, unspecified assistantships, and family tuition reduction, active duty/veteran tuition reduction, group tuition reduction, interest-free payment plans, employee tuition reduction available. Support available to part-time students. Financial award applicants required to submit FAFSA. *Unit head:* Dr. Savitri Dixon-Saxon, Dean, 866-492-5336. *Application contact:* Meghan Thomas, Vice President of Enrollment Management, 866-492-5336, E-mail: info@waldenu.edu.

Walden University, Graduate Programs, School of Health Sciences, Minneapolis, MN 55401. Offers clinical research administration (MS, Graduate Certificate); health education and promotion (MS, PhD), including behavioral health (PhD), disease surveillance (PhD), emergency preparedness (MS), general (MHA, MS), global health (PhD), health policy (PhD), health policy and advocacy (MS), population health (PhD); health informatics (MS); health services (PhD), including community health, healthcare administration, leadership, public health policy, self-designed; healthcare administration (MHA), including general (MHA, MS); leadership and organizational development (MHA); public health (MPH, Dr PH, PhD, Graduate Certificate), including community health education (PhD), epidemiology (PhD); systems policy (MHA). *Program availability:* Part-time, evening/weekend, online only, 100% online. *Faculty:* 14 full-time (8 women), 222 part-time/adjunct (121 women). *Students:* 2,487 full-time (1,804 women), 2,282 part-time (1,540 women); includes 2,763 minority (2,129 Black or African American, non-Hispanic/Latino; 30 American Indian or Alaska Native, non-Hispanic/Latino; 237 Asian, non-Hispanic/Latino; 268 Hispanic/Latino; 13 Native Hawaiian or other Pacific Islander, non-Hispanic/Latino; 86 Two or more races, non-Hispanic/Latino), 87 international. Average age 39. 1,205 applicants, 98% accepted, 820 enrolled. In 2015, 641 master's, 147 doctorates, 18 other advanced degrees awarded. *Degree requirements:* For doctorate, thesis/dissertation, residency. *Entrance requirements:* For master's, bachelor's degree or higher; minimum GPA of 2.5; official transcripts; goal statement (for some programs); access to computer and Internet; for doctorate, master's degree or higher; three years of related professional or academic experience (preferred); minimum GPA of 3.0; goal statement and current resume (for select programs); official transcripts; access to computer and Internet; for Graduate Certificate, relevant work experience; access to computer and Internet. Additional exam requirements/recommendations for international students: Required—TOEFL (minimum score 550 paper-based, 79 iBT), IELTS (minimum score 6.5), Michigan English Language Assessment Battery (minimum score 82), or PTE (minimum score 53). *Application deadline:* Applications are processed on a rolling basis. Application fee: $0. Electronic applications accepted. *Financial support:* Fellowships, Federal Work-Study, scholarships/grants, unspecified assistantships, and family tuition reduction, active duty/veteran tuition reduction, group tuition reduction, interest-free payment plans, employee tuition reduction available. Support available to part-time students. Financial award applicants required to submit FAFSA. *Unit head:* Dr. Jorg Westermann, Dean, 866-492-5336. *Application contact:* Meghan Thomas, Vice President of Enrollment Management, 866-492-5336, E-mail: info@waldenu.edu.
Website: http://www.waldenu.edu/colleges-schools/school-of-health-sciences

Walden University, Graduate Programs, School of Nursing, Minneapolis, MN 55401. Offers adult-gerontology acute care nurse practitioner (MSN); adult-gerontology nurse practitioner (MSN); education (MSN); family nurse practitioner (MSN); informatics (MSN); leadership and management (MSN); nursing (PhD, Post-Master's Certificate), including education (PhD), healthcare administration (PhD), interdisciplinary health (PhD), leadership (PhD), nursing education (Post-Master's Certificate), nursing informatics (Post-Master's Certificate), nursing leadership and management (Post-Master's Certificate), public health policy (PhD); nursing practice (DNP); psychiatric mental health (MSN). *Accreditation:* AACN. *Program availability:* Part-time, evening/weekend, online only, 100% online. *Faculty:* 22 full-time (18 women), 540 part-time/adjunct (487 women). *Students:* 4,320 full-time (3,773 women), 5,250 part-time (4,740 women); includes 3,550 minority (2,360 Black or African American, non-Hispanic/Latino; 29 American Indian or Alaska Native, non-Hispanic/Latino; 523 Asian, non-Hispanic/Latino; 421 Hispanic/Latino; 25 Native Hawaiian or other Pacific Islander, non-Hispanic/Latino; 192 Two or more races, non-Hispanic/Latino), 221 international. Average age 40. 2,057 applicants, 100% accepted, 1507 enrolled. In 2015, 3,022 master's, 86 doctorates, 34 other advanced degrees awarded. *Degree requirements:* For doctorate, thesis/dissertation (for some programs), residency (for some programs), field experience (for some programs). *Entrance requirements:* For master's, bachelor's degree or equivalent in related field or RN; minimum GPA of 2.5; official transcripts; goal statement (for some programs); access to computer and Internet; for doctorate, master's degree or higher; RN; three years of related professional or academic experience; goal statement; access to computer and Internet; for Post-Master's Certificate, relevant work experience; access to computer and Internet. Additional exam requirements/recommendations for international students: Required—TOEFL (minimum score 550 paper-based, 79 iBT), IELTS (minimum score 6.5), Michigan English Language Assessment Battery (minimum score 82), or PTE (minimum score 53). *Application deadline:* Applications are processed on a rolling basis. Application fee: $0. Electronic applications accepted. *Financial support:* Fellowships, Federal Work-Study, scholarships/grants, unspecified assistantships, and family tuition reduction, active duty/veteran tuition reduction, group tuition reduction, interest-free payment plans, employee tuition reduction available. Support available to part-time students. Financial award applicants required to submit FAFSA. *Unit head:* Dr. Andrea Lindell, Dean, 866-492-5336. *Application contact:* Meghan Thomas, Vice President of Enrollment Management, 866-492-5336, E-mail: info@waldenu.edu.
Website: http://www.waldenu.edu/programs/colleges-schools/nursing

Washington University in St. Louis, Brown School, St. Louis, MO 63130. Offers affordable housing and mixed-income community management (Certificate); American Indian and Alaska native (MSW); children, youth and families (MSW); health (MSW); individualized (MSW), including health; mental health (MSW); older adults and aging societies (MSW); public health (MPH), including epidemiology/biostatistics, global health, health policy analysis, urban design; public health sciences (PhD); social and economic development (MSW); social work (MSW, PhD), including management (MSW), policy (MSW), research (MSW), sexual health and education (MSW), social entrepreneurship (MSW), system dynamics (MSW); violence and injury prevention (MSW, Certificate); JD/MSW; M Arch/MSW; MPH/MBA; MPH/MS; MSW/M Div; MSW/M Ed; MSW/MAPS; MSW/MBA; MSW/MPH; MUD/MSW. MSW/M Div and MSW/MAPS offered in partnership with Eden Theological Seminary. *Accreditation:* CSWE (one or more programs are accredited). *Faculty:* 54 full-time (31 women), 87 part-time/adjunct (61 women). *Students:* 303 full-time (256 women); includes 125 minority (42 Black or African American, non-Hispanic/Latino; 16 American Indian or Alaska Native, non-Hispanic/Latino; 47 Asian, non-Hispanic/Latino; 9 Hispanic/Latino; 11 Two or more races, non-Hispanic/Latino), 71 international. Average age 26. 923 applicants, 322 enrolled. In 2015, 239 master's, 5 doctorates awarded. *Degree requirements:* For master's, 60 credit hours (for MSW), 52 credit hours (for MPH); practicum; for doctorate, comprehensive exam, thesis/dissertation. *Entrance requirements:* For master's, GRE, GMAT, LSAT, or MCAT (for MPH); for doctorate, GRE, MA or MSW. Additional exam requirements/recommendations for international students: Required—TOEFL (minimum score 100 iBT) or IELTS. *Application deadline:* For fall admission, 12/15 priority date for domestic and international students; for winter admission, 3/1 priority date for domestic and international students. Applications are processed on a rolling basis. Application fee: $50. Electronic applications accepted. *Expenses:* Contact institution. *Financial support:* In 2015–16, 267 students received support. Fellowships, research

assistantships, Federal Work-Study, institutionally sponsored loans, scholarships/grants, health care benefits, tuition waivers (partial), and unspecified assistantships available. Support available to part-time students. Financial award application deadline: 3/1; financial award applicants required to submit FAFSA. *Faculty research:* Mental health services, social development, child welfare, at-risk teens, autism, environmental health, health policy, health communications, obesity, gender and sexuality, violence and injury prevention, chronic disease prevention, poverty, older adults/aging societies, civic engagement, school social work, program evaluation, health disparities. *Unit head:* Jamie L. Adkisson, Director of Admissions and Recruitment, 314-935-3524, Fax: 314-935-4859, E-mail: jadkisson@wustl.edu. *Application contact:* Office of Admissions and Recruitment, 314-935-6676, Fax: 314-935-4859, E-mail: brownadmissions@wustl.ed.
Website: http://brownschool.wustl.edu

Washington University in St. Louis, School of Medicine, Master of Population Health Sciences Program, St. Louis, MO 63110. Offers clinical epidemiology (MPHS); health services (MPHS); psychiatric and behavioral health sciences (MPHS); quantitative methods (MPHS). *Program availability:* Part-time. *Faculty:* 28 part-time/adjunct (18 women). *Students:* 10 full-time (4 women), 9 part-time (6 women); includes 9 minority (5 Asian, non-Hispanic/Latino; 4 Hispanic/Latino). Average age 31. 20 applicants, 100% accepted, 19 enrolled. In 2015, 11 master's awarded. *Entrance requirements:* For master's, possess or currently be in pursuit of a clinical doctorate degree (including but not limited to: MD, PhD, PharmD, DPH, DO, DPT, DNP, OTD, etc.). Additional exam requirements/recommendations for international students: Required—TOEFL. *Application deadline:* For fall admission, 1/15 priority date for domestic and international students. Applications are processed on a rolling basis. *Financial support:* Scholarships/grants, traineeships, and health care benefits available. Support available to part-time students. *Faculty research:* Clinical epidemiology, population health, biostatistics, clinical outcomes research and comparative effectiveness research. *Unit head:* Dr. Graham Colditz, Director, 314-454-7939, E-mail: colditzg@wustl.edu. *Application contact:* Joyce Linn, Program Coordinator, 314-362-5501, E-mail: linnj@wudosis.wustl.edu.
Website: http://www.mphs.wustl.edu/

Wayne State University, School of Medicine, Office of Biomedical Graduate Programs, Department of Family Medicine and Public Health Sciences, Detroit, MI 48202. Offers public health practice (MPH, Graduate Certificate); MD/MPH; MPH/MA. *Faculty:* 17. *Students:* 50 full-time (33 women), 36 part-time (24 women); includes 31 minority (4 Black or African American, non-Hispanic/Latino; 18 Asian, non-Hispanic/Latino; 6 Hispanic/Latino; 3 Two or more races, non-Hispanic/Latino), 18 international. Average age 31. 246 applicants, 27% accepted, 38 enrolled. In 2015, 13 master's awarded. *Degree requirements:* For master's, project. *Entrance requirements:* For master's, GRE, undergraduate work in mathematics, natural sciences, and social sciences; experience in health-related position; minimum undergraduate GPA of 3.0 overall and in mathematics, social sciences, and natural sciences; college-level mathematics; personal statement; three letters of recommendation; for Graduate Certificate, undergraduate work in mathematics, natural sciences, and social sciences; experience in health-related position; minimum undergraduate GPA of 3.0 overall and in mathematics, social sciences, and natural sciences; college-level mathematics; personal statement; three letters of recommendation. Additional exam requirements/recommendations for international students: Required—TOEFL (minimum score 100 iBT), TWE; Recommended—IELTS. *Application deadline:* For fall admission, 3/31 for domestic and international students. Application fee: $0. Electronic applications accepted. *Expenses:* $17,645 annual resident tuition, $33,311 non-resident tuition; $735.20 per credit hour resident tuition, $1,387.95 per credit hour non-resident tuition; fees include $47.45 per credit hour student services fee and $274.60 per semester registration fee. *Financial support:* In 2015–16, 24 students received support. Fellowships with tuition reimbursements available and scholarships/grants available. Financial award application deadline: 3/31; financial award applicants required to submit FAFSA. *Faculty research:* Behavioral science, medical education, occupational/environmental health, practice-based research, community-based research, and epidemiology. *Unit head:* Dr. Kimberly Campbell-Voytal, Program Director, 313-577-9454, E-mail: kvoytal@med.wayne.edu. *Application contact:* 313-577-1051, E-mail: mphprogram@med.wayne.edu.
Website: http://familymedicine.med.wayne.edu/

West Chester University of Pennsylvania, College of Health Sciences, Department of Health, West Chester, PA 19383. Offers community health (MPH); emergency preparedness (Certificate); environmental health (MPH); gerontology (Certificate); health care management (MPH, Certificate); integrative health (Certificate); school health (M Ed). *Accreditation:* CEPH. *Program availability:* Part-time, evening/weekend. *Faculty:* 12 full-time (7 women), 4 part-time/adjunct (3 women). *Students:* 98 full-time (74 women), 85 part-time (59 women); includes 73 minority (60 Black or African American, non-Hispanic/Latino; 8 Asian, non-Hispanic/Latino; 4 Hispanic/Latino; 1 Two or more races, non-Hispanic/Latino), 26 international. Average age 30. 118 applicants, 86% accepted, 60 enrolled. In 2015, 72 master's, 17 other advanced degrees awarded. *Degree requirements:* For master's, thesis or alternative, minimum GPA of 3.0; research report (for M Ed); major project and practicum (for MPH); for Certificate, minimum GPA of 3.0. *Entrance requirements:* For master's, goal statement, two letters of recommendation, undergraduate introduction to statistics course; for Certificate, minimum undergraduate GPA of 2.8 (for gerontology). Additional exam requirements/recommendations for international students: Required—TOEFL or IELTS. *Application deadline:* For fall admission, 5/15 for international students; for spring admission, 10/15 for international students. Applications are processed on a rolling basis. Application fee: $50. Electronic applications accepted. *Expenses:* Tuition, state resident: full-time $8460; part-time $470 per credit. Tuition, nonresident: full-time $12,690; part-time $705 per credit. *Required fees:* $2312; $126.75 per credit. Tuition and fees vary according to campus/location and program. *Financial support:* Scholarships/grants and unspecified assistantships available. Financial award application deadline: 2/15; financial award applicants required to submit FAFSA. *Faculty research:* Healthy school communities, community health issues and evidence-based programs, environment and health, nutrition and health, integrative health. *Unit head:* Dr. Bethann Cinelli, Chair, 610-436-2267, E-mail: bcinelli@wcupa.edu. *Application contact:* Dr. Lynn Carson, Graduate Coordinator, 610-436-2138, E-mail: lcarson@wcupa.edu.
Website: http://www.wcupa.edu/_ACADEMICS/HealthSciences/health/

Western Kentucky University, Graduate Studies, College of Health and Human Services, Department of Public Health, Bowling Green, KY 42101. Offers healthcare administration (MHA); public health (MPH). *Accreditation:* CEPH. *Program availability:* Part-time, evening/weekend. *Degree requirements:* For master's, comprehensive exam, thesis or alternative. *Entrance requirements:* For master's, GRE General Test, minimum GPA of 2.75. Additional exam requirements/recommendations for international students: Required—TOEFL (minimum score 555 paper-based; 79 iBT). *Faculty research:* Health education training, driver traffic safety, community readiness, occupational injuries, local health departments.

Westminster College, School of Nursing and Health Sciences, Salt Lake City, UT 84105-3697. Offers family nurse practitioner (MSN); nurse anesthesia (MSNA); nurse education (MSNED); public health (MPH). *Accreditation:* AACN; AANA/CANAEP.

Faculty: 15 full-time (9 women), 7 part-time/adjunct (2 women). *Students:* 120 full-time (79 women), 3 part-time (all women); includes 18 minority (1 Black or African American, non-Hispanic/Latino; 3 Asian, non-Hispanic/Latino; 10 Hispanic/Latino; 4 Two or more races, non-Hispanic/Latino), 3 international. Average age 32. 157 applicants, 40% accepted, 45 enrolled. In 2015, 56 master's awarded. *Degree requirements:* For master's, clinical practicum, 504 clinical practice hours. *Entrance requirements:* For master's, GRE, personal statement, resume, 3 professional recommendations, copy of unrestricted Utah license to practice professional nursing, background check, minimum cumulative GPA of 3.0, documentation of current immunizations, physical and mental health certificate signed by primary care provider. Additional exam requirements/recommendations for international students: Required—TOEFL (minimum score 600 paper-based; 100 iBT), IELTS (minimum score 7.5). Application fee: $50. Electronic applications accepted. *Expenses:* Contact institution. *Financial support:* In 2015–16, 8 students received support. Career-related internships or fieldwork, unspecified assistantships, and tuition reimbursements, tuition remission available. Support available to part-time students. Financial award applicants required to submit FAFSA. *Faculty research:* Intellectual empathy, professional boundaries, learned optimism, collaborative testing in nursing: student outcomes and perspectives, implementing new educational paradigms into pre-licensure nursing curricula. *Unit head:* Dr. Sheryl Steadman, Dean, 801-832-2164, Fax: 801-832-3110, E-mail: ssteadman@westminstercollege.edu. *Application contact:* Dr. John Baworowsky, Vice President of Enrollment Management, 801-832-2200, Fax: 801-832-3101, E-mail: admission@westminstercollege.edu.
Website: http://www.westminstercollege.edu/msn

West Virginia University, School of Medicine, Department of Community Medicine, Morgantown, WV 26506. Offers public health (MPH), including community health/preventative medicine; public health sciences (PhD). *Accreditation:* CEPH. *Program availability:* Part-time, evening/weekend, online learning. *Degree requirements:* For master's, thesis (for some programs). *Entrance requirements:* For master's, minimum GPA of 3.0. Additional exam requirements/recommendations for international students: Required—TOEFL. *Expenses:* Tuition, state resident: full-time $8568. Tuition, nonresident: full-time $22,140. Tuition and fees vary according to program. *Faculty research:* Adolescent smoking cessation, cardiovascular disease, women's health, worker's health.

West Virginia University, School of Public Health, Morgantown, WV 26506-9190. Offers biostatistics; community health promotion (MS); community health/preventative medicine (MPH); public health sciences (PhD). *Accreditation:* CEPH. *Program availability:* Part-time, online learning. *Faculty:* 37 full-time (17 women), 3 part-time/adjunct (2 women). *Students:* 85 full-time (55 women), 52 part-time (34 women); includes 28 minority (8 Black or African American, non-Hispanic/Latino; 1 American

Indian or Alaska Native, non-Hispanic/Latino; 13 Asian, non-Hispanic/Latino; 3 Hispanic/Latino; 3 Two or more races, non-Hispanic/Latino), 10 international. Average age 31. In 2015, 11 doctorates awarded. *Degree requirements:* For master's, practicum, project. *Entrance requirements:* For master's, GRE General Test, MCAT, medical degree, medical internship. Additional exam requirements/recommendations for international students: Required—TOEFL (minimum score 550 paper-based; 80 iBT). *Application deadline:* For fall admission, 4/15 priority date for domestic students; for spring admission, 12/1 for domestic students. Applications are processed on a rolling basis. Application fee: $60. *Expenses:* Contact institution. *Financial support:* Research assistantships, teaching assistantships, scholarships/grants, and health care benefits available. Financial award application deadline: 2/1; financial award applicants required to submit FAFSA. *Faculty research:* Occupational health, environmental health, clinical epidemiology, health care management, prevention. *Unit head:* Dr. Gregory A. Hand, Dean, School of Public Health, 304-293-2502, Fax: 304-293-6685, E-mail: gahand@hsc.wvu.edu. *Application contact:* Sherry Kuhl, Director, Office of Student Services, 304-293-1795, Fax: 304-293-6685, E-mail: skuhl@hsc.wvu.edu.
Website: http://pubichealth.hsc.wvu.edu

Wright State University, School of Medicine, Program in Public Health, Dayton, OH 45435. Offers health promotion and education (MPH); public health management (MPH); public health nursing (MPH). *Accreditation:* CEPH.

Yale University, School of Medicine, Yale School of Public Health, New Haven, CT 06520. Offers applied biostatistics and epidemiology (APMPH); biostatistics (MPH, MS, PhD), including global health (MPH); chronic disease epidemiology (MPH, PhD), including global health (MPH); environmental health sciences (MPH, PhD), including global health (MPH); epidemiology of microbial diseases (MPH, PhD), including global health (MPH); global health (APMPH); health management (MPH), including global health; health policy (MPH), including global health; health policy and administration (APMPH, PhD); occupational and environmental medicine (APMPH); preventive medicine (APMPH); social and behavioral sciences (APMPH, MPH), including global health (MPH); JD/MPH; M Div/MPH; MBA/MPH; MD/MPH; MEM/MPH; MFS/MPH; MM Sc/MPH; MPH/MA; MSN/MPH. MS and PhD offered through the Graduate School. *Accreditation:* CEPH. *Program availability:* Part-time. Terminal master's awarded for partial completion of doctoral program. *Degree requirements:* For master's, thesis, summer internship; for doctorate, comprehensive exam, thesis/dissertation, residency. *Entrance requirements:* For master's, GMAT, GRE, or MCAT, two years of undergraduate coursework in math and science; for doctorate, GRE General Test. Additional exam requirements/recommendations for international students: Required—TOEFL (minimum score 100 iBT). Electronic applications accepted. *Expenses:* Contact institution. *Faculty research:* Genetic and emerging infections epidemiology, virology, cost/quality, vector biology, quantitative methods, aging, asthma, cancer.

Community Health

Adelphi University, Ruth S. Ammon School of Education, Program in Health Studies, Garden City, NY 11530-0701. Offers community health education (MA, Certificate); school health education (MA). *Program availability:* Part-time, evening/weekend. *Degree requirements:* For master's, internship. *Entrance requirements:* For master's, 3 letters of recommendation, resume, minimum cumulative GPA of 2.75. Additional exam requirements/recommendations for international students: Required—TOEFL (minimum score 550 paper-based; 80 iBT). Electronic applications accepted. *Faculty research:* Alcohol abuse, tobacco cessation, drug abuse, healthy family lives, healthy personal living.

American University of Beirut, Graduate Programs, Faculty of Health Sciences, Beirut, Lebanon. Offers environmental sciences (MS), including environmental health; epidemiology (MS); epidemiology and biostatistics (MPH); health management and policy (MPH); health promotion and community health (MPH). *Program availability:* Part-time. *Faculty:* 30 full-time (21 women), 3 part-time/adjunct (1 woman). *Students:* 49 full-time (38 women), 99 part-time (81 women). Average age 27. 115 applicants, 71% accepted, 40 enrolled. In 2015, 51 master's awarded. *Degree requirements:* For master's, one foreign language, comprehensive exam (for some programs), thesis (for some programs). *Entrance requirements:* For master's, 2 letters of recommendation, personal statement, transcripts. Additional exam requirements/recommendations for international students: Required—TOEFL (minimum score 583 paper-based; 97 iBT), IELTS (minimum score 7). *Application deadline:* For fall admission, 1/4 priority date for domestic and international students; for spring admission, 11/1 for domestic and international students. Application fee: $50. Electronic applications accepted. *Expenses:* Tuition, area resident: Full-time $16,254; part-time $903 per credit. Required fees: $699. Tuition and fees vary according to course load and program. *Financial support:* In 2015–16, 70 students received support. Scholarships/grants, health care benefits, and unspecified assistantships available. Financial award application deadline: 4/1. *Faculty research:* Tobacco control; health of the elderly; youth health; mental health; women's health; reproductive and sexual health, including HIV/AIDS; water quality; health systems; quality in health care delivery; health human resources; health policy; occupational and environmental health; social inequality; social determinants of health; non-communicable diseases; nutrition; refugees health; conflict and health. *Total annual research expenditures:* $2 million. *Unit head:* Iman Adel Nuwayhid, Dean, 961-1759683, Fax: 961-1744470, E-mail: nuwayhid@aub.edu.lb. *Application contact:* Mitra Tauk, Administrative Coordinator, 961-1350000 Ext. 4687, Fax: 961-1744470, E-mail: mt12@aub.edu.lb.

Arcadia University, Graduate Studies, Department of Medical Science and Community Health, Glenside, PA 19038-3295. Offers health education (MA, MSHE); physician assistant (MM Sc); MM Sc/MAHE; MM Sc/MSPH. *Students:* 206 full-time (174 women); includes 36 minority (4 Black or African American, non-Hispanic/Latino; 26 Asian, non-Hispanic/Latino; 4 Hispanic/Latino; 2 Two or more races, non-Hispanic/Latino). Average age 25. 2,449 applicants, 9% accepted, 104 enrolled. In 2015, 93 master's awarded. *Entrance requirements:* For master's, GRE General Test or MCAT. Additional exam requirements/recommendations for international students: Required—TOEFL. *Application deadline:* For fall admission, 1/5 priority date for domestic students. Application fee: $50. *Expenses:* Contact institution. *Financial support:* Tuition waivers (partial) available. *Unit head:* Diana Noller, Chair, 215-517-2376. *Application contact:* 215-572-2910, Fax: 215-572-4041, E-mail: admiss@arcadia.edu.

Arizona State University at the Tempe campus, College of Nursing and Health Innovation, Phoenix, AZ 85004. Offers advanced nursing practice (DNP); clinical research management (MS); community and public health practice (Graduate Certificate); family mental health nurse practitioner (Graduate Certificate); family nurse practitioner (Graduate Certificate); geriatric nursing (Graduate Certificate); healthcare

innovation (MHI); nurse education in academic and practice settings (Graduate Certificate); nurse educator (MS); nursing and healthcare innovation (PhD). *Accreditation:* AACN. *Program availability:* Online learning. *Degree requirements:* For master's, comprehensive exam (for some programs), thesis (for some programs), interactive Program of Study (iPOS) submitted before completing 50 percent of required credit hours; for doctorate, comprehensive exam, thesis/dissertation, interactive Program of Study (iPOS) submitted before completing 50 percent of required credit hours. *Entrance requirements:* For master's and doctorate, GRE, minimum GPA of 3.0 or equivalent in last 2 years of work leading to bachelor's degree. Additional exam requirements/recommendations for international students: Required—TOEFL, IELTS, or PTE. Electronic applications accepted. *Expenses:* Contact institution.

Baylor University, Graduate School, Robbins College of Health and Human Sciences, Department of Health, Human Performance and Recreation, Waco, TX 76798. Offers community health (MPH); exercise physiology (MS); kinesiology, exercise nutrition and health promotion (PhD); sport pedagogy (MS). *Accreditation:* NCATE. *Program availability:* Part-time. *Faculty:* 13 full-time (5 women), 3 part-time/adjunct (1 woman). *Students:* 67 full-time (39 women), 11 part-time (6 women); includes 22 minority (7 Black or African American, non-Hispanic/Latino; 6 Asian, non-Hispanic/Latino; 6 Hispanic/Latino; 3 Two or more races, non-Hispanic/Latino), 6 international. 109 applicants, 59% accepted, 44 enrolled. In 2015, 46 master's, 1 doctorate awarded. *Degree requirements:* For master's, comprehensive exam, thesis optional; for doctorate, comprehensive exam, thesis/dissertation. *Entrance requirements:* For master's and doctorate, GRE General Test. Additional exam requirements/recommendations for international students: Required—TOEFL (minimum score 550 paper-based; 80 iBT). *Application deadline:* For fall admission, 2/1 priority date for domestic students, 2/1 for international students; for spring admission, 10/1 for domestic and international students. Applications are processed on a rolling basis. Application fee: $25. Electronic applications accepted. *Financial support:* In 2015–16, 60 students received support, including 1 research assistantship with full tuition reimbursement available (averaging $12,700 per year), 33 teaching assistantships with full tuition reimbursements available (averaging $7,650 per year); career-related internships or fieldwork, Federal Work-Study, institutionally sponsored loans, scholarships/grants, tuition waivers (full), and unspecified assistantships also available. Financial award application deadline: 2/1. *Faculty research:* Behavior change theory, nutrition and enzyme therapy, exercise testing, health planning. *Unit head:* Dr. Jaeho Shim, Graduate Program Director, 254-710-4009, Fax: 254-710-3527, E-mail: joe_shim@baylor.edu. *Application contact:* Kathy Mirick, Administrative Assistant, 254-710-3526, Fax: 254-710-3527, E-mail: kathy_mirick@baylor.edu.
Website: http://www.baylor.edu/HHPR

Bloomsburg University of Pennsylvania, School of Graduate Studies, College of Science and Technology, Department of Nursing, Bloomsburg, PA 17815. Offers adult and family nurse practitioner (MSN); community health (MSN); nurse anesthesia (MSN); nursing (MSN); nursing administration (MSN). *Accreditation:* AACN; AANA/CANAEP. *Degree requirements:* For master's, thesis (for some programs), clinical experience. *Entrance requirements:* For master's, minimum QPA of 3.0, personal statement, 2 letters of recommendation, nursing license. Additional exam requirements/recommendations for international students: Required—TOEFL. Electronic applications accepted.

Boston University, School of Public Health, Community Health Sciences Department, Boston, MA 02215. Offers MPH, Dr PH. *Program availability:* Part-time, evening/weekend. *Students:* 53 full-time (51 women), 31 part-time (30 women); includes 31 minority (14 Black or African American, non-Hispanic/Latino; 6 Asian, non-Hispanic/Latino; 8 Hispanic/Latino; 3 Two or more races, non-Hispanic/Latino), 3 international.

Average age 27. 576 applicants, 56% accepted, 92 enrolled. In 2015, 58 master's, 3 doctorates awarded. *Degree requirements:* For doctorate, thesis/dissertation. *Entrance requirements:* For master's, GRE, MCAT, GMAT; for doctorate, GRE, GMAT. Additional exam requirements/recommendations for international students: Required—TOEFL (minimum score 600 paper-based; 100 iBT), IELTS (minimum score 7). *Application deadline:* For fall admission, 1/1 priority date for domestic and international students; for spring admission, 10/1 priority date for domestic students. Applications are processed on a rolling basis. Application fee: $115. Electronic applications accepted. *Financial support:* In 2015–16, 10 fellowships were awarded; career-related internships or fieldwork, Federal Work-Study, institutionally sponsored loans, scholarships/grants, traineeships, and tuition waivers (partial) also available. Financial award application deadline: 3/1; financial award applicants required to submit FAFSA. *Faculty research:* Sexual and reproductive health, substance use, mental health, community health, maternal and child health. *Unit head:* Dr. Richard Saitz, Chair, Community Health Sciences, 617-638-5205, E-mail: askmch@bu.edu. *Application contact:* LePhan Quan, Associate Director of Admissions, 617-638-4640, Fax: 617-638-5299, E-mail: asksph@bu.edu.
Website: http://www.bu.edu/sph/chs

Brooklyn College of the City University of New York, School of Natural and Behavioral Sciences, Department of Health and Nutrition Sciences, Program in Community Health, Brooklyn, NY 11210-2889. Offers community health education (MA); thanatology (MA). *Accreditation:* CEPH. *Degree requirements:* For master's, thesis or alternative. *Entrance requirements:* For master's, 2 letters of recommendation, essay. Additional exam requirements/recommendations for international students: Required—TOEFL. Electronic applications accepted. *Faculty research:* Diet restriction, religious practices in bereavement, diabetes, stress management, palliative care.

Brown University, Graduate School, Division of Biology and Medicine, School of Public Health, Providence, RI 02912. Offers behavioral and social sciences intervention (M Sc); biostatistics (AM, Sc M, PhD); epidemiology (Sc M); health services, policy and practice (PhD); public health (MPH); MD/PhD. *Accreditation:* CEPH. *Degree requirements:* For doctorate, thesis/dissertation, preliminary exam. *Entrance requirements:* For master's and doctorate, GRE General Test. Additional exam requirements/recommendations for international students: Required—TOEFL.

Canisius College, Graduate Division, School of Education and Human Services, Office of Professional Studies, Buffalo, NY 14208-1098. Offers applied nutrition (MS, Certificate); community and school health (MS); health and human performance (MS); health information technology (MS); respiratory care (MS). *Program availability:* Part-time, evening/weekend, 100% online, blended/hybrid learning. *Faculty:* 1 full-time (0 women), 11 part-time/adjunct (7 women). *Students:* 23 full-time (14 women), 79 part-time (58 women); includes 13 minority (7 Black or African American, non-Hispanic/Latino; 1 American Indian or Alaska Native, non-Hispanic/Latino; 3 Asian, non-Hispanic/Latino; 2 Hispanic/Latino), 4 international. Average age 35. 62 applicants, 81% accepted, 32 enrolled. In 2015, 37 master's awarded. *Entrance requirements:* For master's, GRE (recommended), bachelor's degree transcript, two letters of recommendation, current licensure (for applied nutrition), minimum GPA of 2.7, current resume. Additional exam requirements/recommendations for international students: Required—TOEFL (minimum score 550 paper-based, 80 iBT), IELTS (minimum score 6.5), or CAEL (minimum score 70). *Application deadline:* Applications are processed on a rolling basis. Application fee: $25. Electronic applications accepted. Application fee is waived when completed online. *Expenses:* $780 per credit hour; $644 per year full-time fees. *Financial support:* Career-related internships or fieldwork, Federal Work-Study, scholarships/grants, tuition waivers (partial), and unspecified assistantships available. Support available to part-time students. Financial award application deadline: 4/30; financial award applicants required to submit FAFSA. *Faculty research:* Nutrition, community and school health; community and health; health and human performance applied; nutrition and respiratory care. *Unit head:* Sandy McKenna, Director, Professional Studies, 716-888-8296, E-mail: mckekkas@canisius.edu. *Application contact:* Kathleen B. Davis, Vice President of Enrollment Management, 716-888-2500, Fax: 716-888-3195, E-mail: daviskb@canisius.edu.
Website: http://www.canisius.edu/graduate/

Columbia University, Columbia University Mailman School of Public Health, Division of Sociomedical Sciences, New York, NY 10032. Offers MPH, MS, Dr PH, PhD. PhD offered in cooperation with the Graduate School of Arts and Sciences. *Accreditation:* CEPH (one or more programs are accredited). *Program availability:* Part-time. *Students:* 58 full-time (45 women), 205 part-time (170 women); includes 107 minority (25 Black or African American, non-Hispanic/Latino; 1 American Indian or Alaska Native, non-Hispanic/Latino; 46 Asian, non-Hispanic/Latino; 27 Hispanic/Latino; 8 Two or more races, non-Hispanic/Latino), 28 international. Average age 26. 517 applicants, 57% accepted, 116 enrolled. In 2015, 104 master's, 10 doctorates awarded. *Degree requirements:* For master's; for doctorate, thesis/dissertation. *Entrance requirements:* For master's, GRE General Test; for doctorate, GRE General Test, MPH or equivalent (for Dr PH). Additional exam requirements/recommendations for international students: Required—TOEFL (minimum score 600 paper-based; 100 iBT). *Application deadline:* For fall admission, 12/1 priority date for domestic and international students. Application fee: $120. Electronic applications accepted. *Financial support:* Research assistantships, teaching assistantships, career-related internships or fieldwork, and Federal Work-Study available. Support available to part-time students. Financial award application deadline: 2/1; financial award applicants required to submit FAFSA. *Faculty research:* Social and cultural factors in health and health care, health services delivery and utilization, health promotion and disease prevention, AIDS. *Unit head:* Dr. Lisa Metsch, Chair, 212-305-5656. *Application contact:* Dr. Joseph Korevec, Senior Director of Admissions and Financial Aid, 212-305-8698, Fax: 212-342-1861, E-mail: ph-admit@columbia.edu.
Website: https://www.mailman.columbia.edu/become-student/departments/sociomedical-sciences

Daemen College, Program in Public Health, Amherst, NY 14226-3592. Offers community health education (MPH); epidemiology (MPH); generalist (MPH). *Program availability:* Part-time, online learning. *Degree requirements:* For master's, practicum.

Dalhousie University, Faculty of Medicine, Department of Community Health and Epidemiology, Halifax, NS B3H 4R2, Canada. Offers M Sc. *Degree requirements:* For master's, thesis. *Entrance requirements:* Additional exam requirements/recommendations for international students: Required—1 of 5 approved tests: TOEFL, IELTS, CANTEST, CAEL, Michigan English Language Assessment Battery. Electronic applications accepted. *Expenses:* Contact institution. *Faculty research:* Population health, health promotion and disease prevention, health services utilization, chronic disease epidemiology.

East Carolina University, Graduate School, Thomas Harriot College of Arts and Sciences, Department of Political Science, Greenville, NC 27858-4353. Offers community health administration (Certificate); public administration (MPA); security studies (Certificate). *Accreditation:* NASPAA. *Program availability:* Part-time, evening/weekend. *Students:* 30 full-time (13 women), 55 part-time (22 women); includes 16 minority (6 Black or African American, non-Hispanic/Latino; 1 American Indian or Alaska Native, non-Hispanic/Latino; 3 Asian, non-Hispanic/Latino; 2 Hispanic/Latino; 4 Two or

more races, non-Hispanic/Latino), 1 international. Average age 31. 43 applicants, 98% accepted, 30 enrolled. In 2015, 20 master's awarded. *Degree requirements:* For master's, one foreign language, comprehensive exam. *Entrance requirements:* For master's, GRE General Test. Additional exam requirements/recommendations for international students: Required—TOEFL. *Application deadline:* For fall admission, 6/1 priority date for domestic students; for spring admission, 10/15 for domestic students. Applications are processed on a rolling basis. Application fee: $50. *Financial support:* Research assistantships with partial tuition reimbursements, teaching assistantships with partial tuition reimbursements, and Federal Work-Study available. Support available to part-time students. Financial award application deadline: 6/1. *Unit head:* Dr. Robert Thompson, Interim Chair, 252-328-5686, E-mail: thompsonro@ecu.edu. *Application contact:* Dean of Graduate School, 252-328-6012, Fax: 252-328-6071, E-mail: gradschool@ecu.edu.
Website: http://www.ecu.edu/polsci/mpa/index.html

Eastern Kentucky University, The Graduate School, College of Health Sciences, Department of Health Promotion and Administration, Richmond, KY 40475-3102. Offers community health (MPH). *Degree requirements:* For master's, comprehensive exam, thesis optional. *Entrance requirements:* For master's, GRE or MAT, letters of recommendation. *Faculty research:* Risk behavior, health systems, injury control, nutrition.

George Mason University, College of Health and Human Services, Department of Global and Community Health, Fairfax, VA 22030. Offers global and community health (Certificate); global health (MS); public health (MPH), including epidemiology. *Accreditation:* CEPH. *Faculty:* 14 full-time (10 women), 18 part-time/adjunct (14 women). *Students:* 62 full-time (56 women), 47 part-time (42 women); includes 50 minority (22 Black or African American, non-Hispanic/Latino; 16 Asian, non-Hispanic/Latino; 9 Hispanic/Latino; 3 Two or more races, non-Hispanic/Latino), 1 international. Average age 27. 121 applicants, 72% accepted, 44 enrolled. In 2015, 56 master's, 6 other advanced degrees awarded. *Degree requirements:* For master's, comprehensive exam (for some programs), thesis or practicum. *Entrance requirements:* For master's, GRE, GMAT (depending on program), 2 official transcripts; expanded goals statement; 3 letters of recommendation; resume; 1 completed course in health science, statistics, natural sciences and social science (for MPH); 6 credits of foreign language if not fluent (for MS); for Certificate, 2 official transcripts; expanded goals statement; 3 letters of recommendation; resume; bachelor's degree from regionally-accredited institution with minimum GPA of 3.0. Additional exam requirements/recommendations for international students: Required—TOEFL (minimum score 570 paper-based; 88 iBT), IELTS (minimum score 6.5), PTE (minimum score 59). *Application deadline:* For fall admission, 2/1 for domestic students. Application fee: $75 ($80 for international students). Electronic applications accepted. *Expenses:* Contact institution. *Financial support:* In 2015–16, 5 students received support, including 9 research assistantships with tuition reimbursements available (averaging $16,472 per year), 1 teaching assistantship with tuition reimbursement available (averaging $9,000 per year); career-related internships or fieldwork, Federal Work-Study, scholarships/grants, unspecified assistantships, and health care benefits (for full-time research or teaching assistantship recipients) also available. Financial award application deadline: 3/1; financial award applicants required to submit FAFSA. *Faculty research:* Health issues and the needs of affected populations at the regional and global level. *Total annual research expenditures:* $28,950. *Unit head:* Brian Gillette, Director, 703-993-4636, Fax: 703-993-1908, E-mail: bgillett@gmu.edu. *Application contact:* Ali Weinstein, Graduate Program Coordinator, 703-993-9632, Fax: 703-993-1908, E-mail: aweinst2@gmu.edu.
Website: http://chhs.gmu.edu/gch/index

The George Washington University, Milken Institute School of Public Health, Department of Prevention and Community Health, Washington, DC 20052. Offers MPH, Dr PH. *Faculty:* 22 full-time (15 women), 22 part-time/adjunct (16 women). *Students:* 41 full-time (31 women), 17 part-time (14 women); includes 15 minority (4 Black or African American, non-Hispanic/Latino; 3 Asian, non-Hispanic/Latino; 5 Hispanic/Latino; 3 Two or more races, non-Hispanic/Latino). Average age 26. 121 applicants, 68% accepted, 28 enrolled. In 2015, 32 master's awarded. *Unit head:* Dr. Lynn Goldman, Dean, 202-994-5179, E-mail: goldmanl@gwu.edu. *Application contact:* Director of Admissions, 202-994-2160, Fax: 202-994-1860, E-mail: sphhsinfo@gwumc.edu.

Georgia Southern University, Jack N. Averitt College of Graduate Studies, Jiann-Ping Hsu College of Public Health, Program in Public Health, Statesboro, GA 30460. Offers biostatistics (MPH, Dr PH); community health behavior and education (Dr PH); community health education (MPH); environmental health sciences (MPH); epidemiology (MPH); health policy and management (MPH, Dr PH). *Accreditation:* CEPH. *Program availability:* Part-time. *Students:* 129 full-time (86 women), 41 part-time (32 women); includes 87 minority (67 Black or African American, non-Hispanic/Latino; 6 Asian, non-Hispanic/Latino; 8 Hispanic/Latino; 6 Two or more races, non-Hispanic/Latino), 30 international. Average age 30. 218 applicants, 63% accepted, 41 enrolled. In 2015, 37 master's, 8 doctorates awarded. *Degree requirements:* For master's, thesis optional, practicum; for doctorate, comprehensive exam, thesis/dissertation, practicum. *Entrance requirements:* For master's, GRE General Test, minimum GPA of 2.75, resume, 3 letters of reference; for doctorate, GRE, GMAT, MCAT, LSAT, 3 letters of reference, statement of purpose, resume or curriculum vitae. Additional exam requirements/recommendations for international students: Required—TOEFL (minimum score 550 paper-based; 80 iBT), IELTS (minimum score 6). *Application deadline:* For fall admission, 6/1 priority date for domestic and international students; for spring admission, 10/1 priority date for domestic students, 10/1 for international students. Applications are processed on a rolling basis. Application fee: $50. Electronic applications accepted. *Expenses:* $335 per credit hour. *Financial support:* In 2015–16, 93 students received support, including 23 fellowships with full tuition reimbursements available (averaging $7,750 per year), 1 research assistantship with full tuition reimbursement available (averaging $7,750 per year), 1 teaching assistantship with full tuition reimbursement available (averaging $7,750 per year); career-related internships or fieldwork, Federal Work-Study, scholarships/grants, tuition waivers (full), and unspecified assistantships also available. Support available to part-time students. Financial award application deadline: 4/15; financial award applicants required to submit FAFSA. *Faculty research:* Rural public health best practices, health disparity elimination, community initiatives to enhance public health, cost effectiveness analysis, epidemiology of rural public health, environmental health issues, health care system assessment, rural health care, health policy and healthcare financing, survival analysis, nonparametric statistics and resampling methods, micro-arrays and genomics, data imputation techniques and clinical trial methodology. *Total annual research expenditures:* $281,707. *Unit head:* Dr. Shamia Garrett, Program Coordinator, 912-478-2393, E-mail: sgarrett@georgiasouthern.edu.
Website: http://chhs.georgiasouthern.edu/health/

Hofstra University, School of Health Sciences and Human Services, Programs in Health, Hempstead, NY 11549. Offers community health (MS), including adventure education, strength and conditioning; health administration (MHA); public health (MPH). *Program availability:* Part-time, evening/weekend. *Students:* 145 full-time (98 women), 96 part-time (60 women); includes 104 minority (45 Black or African American, non-Hispanic/Latino; 39 Asian, non-Hispanic/Latino; 16 Hispanic/Latino; 2 Native Hawaiian

Community Health

or other Pacific Islander, non-Hispanic/Latino; 2 Two or more races, non-Hispanic/Latino), 21 international. Average age 28. 174 applicants, 85% accepted, 87 enrolled. In 2015, 59 master's awarded. *Degree requirements:* For master's, internship, minimum GPA of 3.0. *Entrance requirements:* For master's, interview, 2 letters of recommendation, essay, resume. Additional exam requirements/recommendations for international students: Required—TOEFL (minimum score 550 paper-based; 80 iBT). *Application deadline:* Applications are processed on a rolling basis. Application fee: $70 ($75 for international students). Electronic applications accepted. *Financial support:* In 2015–16, 71 students received support, including 40 fellowships with tuition reimbursements available (averaging $4,332 per year), 4 research assistantships with tuition reimbursements available (averaging $8,834 per year); Federal Work-Study, institutionally sponsored loans, scholarships/grants, and tuition waivers (full and partial) also available. Support available to part-time students. Financial award applicants required to submit FAFSA. *Faculty research:* Integrated long term care and policy reform; health care policy; cost benefit analysis; chronic illness management; development and implementation of leadership in sports, physical activity and recreation. *Unit head:* Dr. Jayne Ellinger, Chairperson, 516-463-6952, Fax: 516-463-6275, E-mail: hprjmk@hofstra.edu. *Application contact:* Sunil Samuel, Assistant Vice President of Admissions, 516-463-4723, Fax: 516-463-4664, E-mail: graduateadmission@hofstra.edu.
Website: http://www.hofstra.edu/academics/colleges/healthscienceshumanservices/

Hunter College of the City University of New York, Graduate School, Schools of the Health Professions, School of Health Sciences, Programs in Urban Public Health, Program in Community Health Education, New York, NY 10065-5085. Offers MPH. *Accreditation:* CEPH. *Program availability:* Part-time, evening/weekend. *Students:* 95 applicants, 63% accepted, 31 enrolled. *Degree requirements:* For master's, comprehensive exam, thesis optional, internship. *Entrance requirements:* For master's, GRE General Test, previous course work in calculus and statistics. Additional exam requirements/recommendations for international students: Required—TOEFL. *Application deadline:* For fall admission, 4/1 for domestic students; for spring admission, 11/1 for domestic students. *Financial support:* In 2015–16, 6 fellowships were awarded; career-related internships or fieldwork, Federal Work-Study, institutionally sponsored loans, and tuition waivers (partial) also available. Support available to part-time students. Financial award application deadline: 3/1. *Unit head:* Nicholas Freudenberg, Director, Center of Community and Urban Health, 212-396-7738, Fax: 212-481-5260, E-mail: nfreuden@hunter.cuny.edu. *Application contact:* Milena Solo, Director of Graduate Admissions, 212-772-4482, Fax: 212-650-3336, E-mail: admissions@hunter.cuny.edu.
Website: http://www.hunter.cuny.edu/uph/grad-test/community-health-education-1

Icahn School of Medicine at Mount Sinai, Graduate School of Biomedical Sciences, New York, NY 10029-6504. Offers biomedical sciences (MS, PhD); clinical research education (MS, PhD); community medicine (MPH); genetic counseling (MS); neurosciences (PhD); MD/PhD. Terminal master's awarded for partial completion of doctoral program. *Degree requirements:* For master's, thesis; for doctorate, comprehensive exam, thesis/dissertation. *Entrance requirements:* For master's, GRE General Test; for doctorate, GRE General Test, GRE Subject Test, 3 years of college pre-med course work. Additional exam requirements/recommendations for international students: Required—TOEFL. Electronic applications accepted. *Faculty research:* Cancer, genetics and genomics, immunology, neuroscience, developmental and stem cell biology, translational research.

Idaho State University, Office of Graduate Studies, Kasiska College of Health Professions, Department of Family Medicine, Pocatello, ID 83209-8357. Offers Post-Master's Certificate. *Degree requirements:* For Post-Master's Certificate, comprehensive exam, thesis optional, 3 year residency program. *Entrance requirements:* For degree, GRE General Test, MD or DO. Additional exam requirements/recommendations for international students: Required—TOEFL (minimum score 600 paper-based). Electronic applications accepted. *Faculty research:* Health disparities in primary care, cardiovascular risk reduction (particularly in dyslipidemia, diabetes, hypertension), health application of geographic information systems, mechanisms for increasing quality in primary care, collaborative care models for improving health.

Independence University, Program in Health Services, Salt Lake City, UT 84107. Offers community health (MSHS); wellness promotion (MSHS). *Program availability:* Part-time, evening/weekend, online learning. *Degree requirements:* For master's, fieldwork, internship, final project (wellness promotion). *Entrance requirements:* For master's, previous course work in psychology.

Indiana University Bloomington, School of Public Health, Department of Applied Health Science, Bloomington, IN 47405. Offers behavioral, social, and community health (MPH); family health (MPH); health behavior (PhD); nutrition science (MS); professional health education (MPH); public health administration (MPH); safety management (MS); school and college health education (MS). *Accreditation:* CEPH (one or more programs are accredited). *Degree requirements:* For master's, thesis optional; for doctorate, comprehensive exam, thesis/dissertation. *Entrance requirements:* For master's, GRE (for MS in nutrition science), 3 recommendations; for doctorate, GRE, 3 recommendations. Additional exam requirements/recommendations for international students: Required—TOEFL (minimum score 550 paper-based; 80 iBT). Electronic applications accepted. *Faculty research:* Cancer education, HIV/AIDS and drug education, public health, parent-child interactions, safety education, obesity, public health policy, public health administration, school health, health education, human development, nutrition, human sexuality, chronic disease, early childhood health.

Indiana University–Purdue University Indianapolis, School of Public Health, Indianapolis, IN 46202. Offers biostatistics (MPH); environmental health science (MPH); epidemiology (MPH, PhD); health administration (MHA); health policy and management (MPH, PhD); social and behavioral sciences (MPH). *Accreditation:* CEPH. *Expenses:* Contact institution.

Johns Hopkins University, Bloomberg School of Public Health, Department of Health, Behavior and Society, Baltimore, MD 21218. Offers genetic counseling (Sc M); health education and health communication (MSPH); social and behavioral sciences (Dr PH, PhD); social factors in health (MHS). *Degree requirements:* For master's, comprehensive exam (for some programs), thesis (for some programs); for doctorate, comprehensive exam, thesis/dissertation. *Entrance requirements:* For master's, GRE, curriculum vitae, 3 letters of recommendation; for doctorate, GRE, transcripts, curriculum vitae, 3 recommendation letters. Additional exam requirements/recommendations for international students: Required—TOEFL (minimum score 600 paper-based; 100 iBT). Electronic applications accepted. *Faculty research:* Social determinants of health and structural and community-level inventions to improve health, communication and health education, behavioral and social aspects of genetic counseling.

Louisiana State University Health Sciences Center, School of Public Health, New Orleans, LA 70112. Offers behavioral and community health sciences (MPH); biostatistics (MPH, MS, PhD); community health sciences (PhD); environmental and occupational health sciences (MPH); epidemiology (MPH, PhD); health policy and

systems management (MPH). *Accreditation:* CEPH. *Program availability:* Part-time. *Entrance requirements:* For master's, GRE General Test.

McGill University, Faculty of Graduate and Postdoctoral Studies, Faculty of Medicine, Department of Epidemiology and Biostatistics, Montréal, QC H3A 2T5, Canada. Offers community health (M Sc); environmental health (M Sc); epidemiology and biostatistics (M Sc, PhD, Diploma); health care evaluation (M Sc); medical statistics (M Sc). *Accreditation:* CEPH (one or more programs are accredited).

Medical College of Wisconsin, Graduate School of Biomedical Sciences, Department of Population Health, Program in Public Health, Milwaukee, WI 53226-0509. Offers public and community health (PhD); public health (MPH, Graduate Certificate). *Accreditation:* CEPH. *Entrance requirements:* For master's, doctorate, and Graduate Certificate, GRE, official transcripts, three letters of recommendation. Additional exam requirements/recommendations for international students: Required—TOEFL.

Medical College of Wisconsin, Graduate School of Biomedical Sciences, Program in Public and Community Health, Milwaukee, WI 53226-0509. Offers PhD, MD/PhD. *Accreditation:* CEPH. *Degree requirements:* For doctorate, comprehensive exam, thesis/dissertation. *Entrance requirements:* For doctorate, GRE, official transcripts, three letters of recommendation. Additional exam requirements/recommendations for international students: Required—TOEFL (minimum score 580 paper-based; 100 iBT). Electronic applications accepted. *Expenses:* Contact institution. *Faculty research:* Community-academic partnerships, community-based participatory research, injury prevention, health policy, women's health, emergency medical services.

Meharry Medical College, School of Graduate Studies, Division of Community Health Sciences, Nashville, TN 37208-9989. Offers occupational medicine (MSPH); public health administration (MSPH). *Accreditation:* CEPH. *Program availability:* Part-time, evening/weekend. *Degree requirements:* For master's, thesis, externship. *Entrance requirements:* For master's, GRE General Test, GMAT. *Application deadline:* For fall admission, 6/1 for domestic students. Applications are processed on a rolling basis. Application fee: $65. *Expenses:* Contact institution. *Financial support:* Career-related internships or fieldwork, Federal Work-Study, institutionally sponsored loans, and scholarships/grants available. Support available to part-time students. Financial award application deadline: 7/15; financial award applicants required to submit FAFSA.

Memorial University of Newfoundland, Faculty of Medicine and School of Graduate Studies, Graduate Programs in Medicine, Division of Community Health and Humanities, St. John's, NL A1C 5S7, Canada. Offers community health (M Sc, PhD, Diploma). *Program availability:* Part-time. *Degree requirements:* For master's, thesis; for doctorate, comprehensive exam, thesis/dissertation, oral defense of thesis. *Entrance requirements:* For master's, MD or B Sc; for doctorate, MD or M Sc; for Diploma, bachelor's degree in health-related field. Additional exam requirements/recommendations for international students: Required—TOEFL. *Expenses: Tuition, area resident:* Full-time $2199 Canadian dollars. *International tuition:* $2859 Canadian dollars full-time. *Faculty research:* Health care delivery and administration, health services, psychosocial, aging.

Merrimack College, School of Science and Engineering, North Andover, MA 01845-5800. Offers civil engineering (MS); community health education (MS); computer science (MS); exercise and sport science (MS); health and wellness management (MS); mechanical engineering (MS), including engineering management. *Program availability:* Part-time. *Faculty:* 18 full-time, 4 part-time/adjunct. *Students:* 62 full-time (25 women), 12 part-time (4 women); includes 5 minority (1 Asian, non-Hispanic/Latino; 4 Hispanic/Latino), 18 international. Average age 24. 141 applicants, 67% accepted, 62 enrolled. In 2015, 12 master's awarded. *Degree requirements:* For master's, comprehensive exam, thesis optional, internship or capstone (for some programs). *Entrance requirements:* For master's, official college transcripts, resume, personal statement, 2 recommendations. Additional exam requirements/recommendations for international students: Required—TOEFL (minimum score 84 iBT), IELTS (minimum score 6.5), PTE (minimum score 56). *Application deadline:* For fall admission, 8/13 for domestic students, 7/13 for international students; for spring admission, 1/10 for domestic and international students; for summer admission, 5/10 for domestic students, 4/10 for international students. Applications are processed on a rolling basis. Application fee: $0. Electronic applications accepted. *Expenses:* Contact institution. *Financial support:* Fellowships with partial tuition reimbursements, career-related internships or fieldwork, scholarships/grants, and health care benefits available. Support available to part-time students. Financial award applicants required to submit FAFSA. *Faculty research:* Geotechnical (civil engineering), smart materials (mechanical engineering), computer graphics and network security (computer science). *Application contact:* Allison Pena, Graduate Admissions Counselor, 978-837-5227, E-mail: penaa@merrimack.edu.
Website: http://www.merrimack.edu/academics/graduate/

Midwestern State University, Billie Doris McAda Graduate School, Robert D. and Carol Gunn College of Health Sciences and Human Services, Department of Criminal Justice and Health Services Administration, Wichita Falls, TX 76308. Offers criminal justice (MA); health information management (MHA); health services administration (Graduate Certificate); medical practice management (MHA); public and community sector health care management (MHA); rural and urban hospital management (MHA). *Program availability:* Part-time, evening/weekend. *Degree requirements:* For master's, comprehensive exam, thesis. *Entrance requirements:* For master's, GRE. Additional exam requirements/recommendations for international students: Required—TOEFL (minimum score 550 paper-based). Electronic applications accepted. *Faculty research:* Universal service policy, telehealth, bullying, healthcare financial management, public health ethics.

Minnesota State University Mankato, College of Graduate Studies and Research, College of Allied Health and Nursing, Department of Health Science, Mankato, MN 56001. Offers community health education (MS); school health education (MS, Postbaccalaureate Certificate). *Program availability:* Part-time. *Degree requirements:* For master's, comprehensive exam, thesis or alternative. *Entrance requirements:* For master's, minimum GPA of 3.0 during previous 2 years; for Postbaccalaureate Certificate, teaching license. Additional exam requirements/recommendations for international students: Required—TOEFL (minimum score 500 paper-based; 61 iBT). Electronic applications accepted. *Faculty research:* Teaching methods, stress prophylaxis and management, effects of alcohol.

New Jersey City University, College of Professional Studies, Department of Health Sciences, Jersey City, NJ 07305-1597. Offers community health education (MS); health administration (MS); school health education (MS). *Program availability:* Part-time, evening/weekend. *Degree requirements:* For master's, thesis or alternative, internship. *Entrance requirements:* Additional exam requirements/recommendations for international students: Required—TOEFL (minimum score 79 iBT). *Application deadline:* For fall admission, 8/1 priority date for domestic students; for spring admission, 12/1 for domestic students. Applications are processed on a rolling basis. Application fee: $0. *Expenses:* Tuition, state resident: part-time $566.55 per credit. Tuition, nonresident: part-time $998.15 per credit. *Required fees:* $108 per credit. Part-time tuition and fees vary according to class time, degree level, campus/location and program. *Financial support:* Career-related internships or fieldwork and unspecified assistantships available.

New York University, College of Global Public Health, New York, NY 10003. Offers biological basis of public health (PhD); community and international health (MPH); global health leadership (MPH); health systems and health services research (PhD); population and community health (PhD); public health nutrition (MPH); social and behavioral sciences (MPH); socio-behavioral health (PhD). *Program availability:* Part-time, online learning. *Degree requirements:* For master's, thesis (for some programs); for doctorate, thesis/dissertation. *Entrance requirements:* For master's and doctorate, GRE. Additional exam requirements/recommendations for international students: Required—TOEFL. Electronic applications accepted.

Northeastern University, Bouvé College of Health Sciences, Boston, MA 02115-5096. Offers applied behavior analysis (MS, CAGS); audiology (Au D); biomedical nanotechnology (MS); college student development and counseling (MS, CAGS); counseling psychology (MS, PhD, CAGS); exercise science (MS); health informatics (MS); medicinal chemistry (MS); nurse anesthesia (DNP, CAGS); nursing (MS, PhD, CAGS), including administration (MS), adult-gerontology acute care nurse practitioner (MS, CAGS), adult-gerontology primary care nurse practitioner (MS, CAGS), anesthesia (MS), family nurse practitioner (MS, CAGS), neonatal nurse practitioner (MS, CAGS), pediatric nurse practitioner (MS, CAGS), psychiatric mental health nurse practitioner (MS, CAGS); nursing practice (DNP); personal health informatics (PhD); pharmaceutical sciences (MS, PhD), including interdisciplinary concentration, pharmaceutics and drug delivery systems; pharmacology (MS); pharmacy (Pharm D); physical therapy (Postbaccalaureate Certificate); physician assistant (MS); population health (PhD); school psychology (MS, PhD, CAGS); speech-language pathology (MS); urban health (MPH); MS/MBA. *Accreditation:* ACPE (one or more programs are accredited). *Program availability:* Part-time, evening/weekend, online learning. *Faculty:* 194 full-time (120 women), 169 part-time/adjunct (136 women). *Students:* 1,416 full-time (1,049 women), 310 part-time (248 women). In 2015, 374 master's, 313 doctorates, 37 other advanced degrees awarded. *Degree requirements:* For doctorate, thesis/dissertation (for some programs); for other advanced degree, comprehensive exam. Application fee: $75. Electronic applications accepted. *Expenses:* Contact institution. *Financial support:* Applicants required to submit FAFSA. *Unit head:* John R. Reynolds, Professor and Interim Dean, 617-373-3323, Fax: 617-373-3030. *Application contact:* Molly Schnabel, Senior Director of Graduate Affairs, 617-373-2708, Fax: 617-373-4701, E-mail: bouvegrad@neu.edu.
Website: http://www.northeastern.edu/bouve/

Old Dominion University, College of Health Sciences, School of Community and Environmental Health, Norfolk, VA 23529. Offers MS. *Program availability:* Part-time, evening/weekend, online learning. *Faculty:* 5 full-time (2 women), 4 part-time/adjunct (2 women). *Students:* 9 full-time (6 women), 15 part-time (8 women); includes 9 minority (7 Black or African American, non-Hispanic/Latino; 1 Hispanic/Latino; 1 Two or more races, non-Hispanic/Latino). Average age 29. 12 applicants, 83% accepted, 8 enrolled. In 2015, 6 master's awarded. *Degree requirements:* For master's, comprehensive exam, oral exam, written exam, practicum or thesis. *Entrance requirements:* For master's, GRE General Test, minimum GPA of 2.75. Additional exam requirements/recommendations for international students: Required—TOEFL (minimum score 650 paper-based). *Application deadline:* For fall admission, 8/1 priority date for domestic students, 7/1 priority date for international students; for winter admission, 11/1 priority date for domestic students, 10/1 priority date for international students; for spring admission, 4/1 priority date for domestic students, 3/1 priority date for international students. Applications are processed on a rolling basis. Application fee: $50. Electronic applications accepted. *Expenses:* Tuition, state resident: full-time $11,136; part-time $464 per credit hour. Tuition, nonresident: full-time $27,840; part-time $1160 per credit hour. *Required fees:* $64 per semester. Tuition and fees vary according to campus/location, program and reciprocity agreements. *Financial support:* In 2015–16, 3 research assistantships with tuition reimbursements (averaging $14,000 per year), 2 teaching assistantships with partial tuition reimbursements (averaging $10,000 per year) were awarded; career-related internships or fieldwork, institutionally sponsored loans, scholarships/grants, and tuition waivers (partial) also available. Financial award applicants required to submit FAFSA. *Faculty research:* Toxicology, occupational health, environmental hazards. *Total annual research expenditures:* $150,133. *Unit head:* Dr. Anna Jeng, Graduate Program Director, 757-683-4594, Fax: 757-683-4410, E-mail: hjeng@odu.edu. *Application contact:* William Heffelfinger, Director of Graduate Admissions, 757-683-5554, Fax: 757-683-3255, E-mail: gradadmit@odu.edu.
Website: http://www.odu.edu/commhealth

Quinnipiac University, School of Nursing, Care of Populations Track, Hamden, CT 06518-1940. Offers DNP. *Program availability:* Part-time-only, evening/weekend, online only. *Faculty:* 19 full-time (18 women), 13 part-time/adjunct (9 women). *Students:* 2 full-time (both women), 28 part-time (26 women); includes 4 minority (3 Black or African American, non-Hispanic/Latino; 1 Hispanic/Latino). 27 applicants, 89% accepted, 19 enrolled. *Entrance requirements:* For doctorate, minimum GPA of 3.0; RN or NCLEX-eligible nurse with bachelor's degree in nursing or another field; master's degree in relevant field; minimum of 1000 hours of field work observation. Additional exam requirements/recommendations for international students: Required—TOEFL (minimum score 575 paper-based; 90 iBT), IELTS (minimum score 6.5). *Application deadline:* Applications are processed on a rolling basis. Application fee: $45. Electronic applications accepted. *Expenses:* $985 per credit tuition; $40 per credit student fees (not to exceed $360 per semester); $150 per semester part-time technology fee, $340 per semester full-time technology fee (fall/spring); $75 technology fee (summer). *Financial support:* Scholarships/grants and unspecified assistantships available. Support available to part-time students. Financial award application deadline: 6/1; financial award applicants required to submit FAFSA. *Application contact:* Quinnipiac University Online Admissions Office, 203-582-3918, E-mail: quonlineadmissions@quinnipiac.edu.
Website: https://quonline.quinnipiac.edu/online-programs/online-doctorate-programs/doctor-of-nursing-practice/care-of-populations-track.php

Saint Louis University, Graduate Education, School of Public Health and Graduate Education, Department of Community Health, St. Louis, MO 63103. Offers MPH, MS, MSPH. *Accreditation:* CEPH. *Program availability:* Part-time, online learning. *Degree requirements:* For master's, comprehensive exam. *Entrance requirements:* For master's, GRE General Test, LSAT, GMAT or MCAT, letters of recommendation, resume. Additional exam requirements/recommendations for international students: Required—TOEFL (minimum score 525 paper-based). Electronic applications accepted. *Faculty research:* Obesity prevention, health disparities, health policy, child health.

Southern Illinois University Carbondale, Graduate School, College of Education and Human Services, Department of Health Education and Recreation, Program in Community Health Education, Carbondale, IL 62901-4701. Offers MPH, MD/MPH, PhD/MPH. *Accreditation:* CEPH. *Faculty:* 7 full-time (4 women). *Students:* 43 full-time (32 women), 5 part-time (4 women); includes 18 minority (16 Black or African American, non-Hispanic/Latino; 1 Asian, non-Hispanic/Latino; 1 Hispanic/Latino), 16 international. 51 applicants, 41% accepted, 24 enrolled. In 2015, 16 master's awarded. *Entrance requirements:* Additional exam requirements/recommendations for international students: Required—TOEFL (minimum score 550 paper-based; 80 iBT). *Application deadline:* For fall admission, 3/7 for domestic and international students; for summer admission, 3/7 for domestic and international students. Application fee: $65. *Financial*

support: In 2015–16, 20 students received support, including 7 research assistantships, 5 teaching assistantships; unspecified assistantships also available. *Unit head:* Dr. Heewon Yang, Chair, 618-453-1841, Fax: 618-453-1829, E-mail: hyang@siu.edu. *Application contact:* Dr. Kathleen Welshimer, Administrative Assistant, 618-453-2777, Fax: 618-453-1829, E-mail: welshime@siu.edu.

Southern New Hampshire University, School of Arts and Sciences, Manchester, NH 03106-1045. Offers community mental health (Graduate Certificate); community mental health and mental health counseling (MS); fiction and nonfiction (MFA); teaching English as a foreign language (MS). *Program availability:* Part-time, evening/weekend. *Degree requirements:* For master's, one foreign language, thesis. *Entrance requirements:* For master's, minimum GPA of 2.75 (for MS in teaching English as a foreign language), 3.0 (for MFA). Additional exam requirements/recommendations for international students: Required—TOEFL (minimum score 550 paper-based; 79 iBT), IELTS (minimum score 6.5), TWE (minimum score 5). Electronic applications accepted. *Expenses:* Contact institution. *Faculty research:* Action research, state of the art practice in behavioral health services, wraparound approaches to working with youth, learning styles.

State University of New York College at Cortland, Graduate Studies, School of Professional Studies, Department of Health, Cortland, NY 13045. Offers community health (MS); health education (MST). *Accreditation:* NCATE. *Program availability:* Part-time, evening/weekend. *Entrance requirements:* Additional exam requirements/recommendations for international students: Required—TOEFL. *Application deadline:* For fall admission, 7/1 for domestic and international students; for spring admission, 12/1 for domestic and international students. Applications are processed on a rolling basis. Application fee: $65. *Financial support:* Career-related internships or fieldwork, Federal Work-Study, tuition waivers (partial), and unspecified assistantships available. Support available to part-time students. Financial award applicants required to submit CSS PROFILE or FAFSA. *Unit head:* Dr. Bonni Hodges, Chair, 607-753-4225, Fax: 607-753-4226, E-mail: bonni.hodges@cortland.edu. *Application contact:* Dr. Bonni Hodges, Chair, 607-753-4225, Fax: 607-753-4226, E-mail: bonni.hodges@cortland.edu.
Website: http://www2.cortland.edu/departments/health/

State University of New York College at Potsdam, School of Education and Professional Studies, Program in Community Health, Potsdam, NY 13676. Offers MS. *Entrance requirements:* For master's, baccalaureate degree from accredited institution, minimum GPA of 3.0 for final 60 credits of baccalaureate work, statement of professional and educational goals, three letters of recommendation, resume or curriculum vitae.

State University of New York Downstate Medical Center, College of Medicine, Program in Public Health, Brooklyn, NY 11203-2098. Offers urban and immigrant health (MPH); MD/MPH. *Accreditation:* CEPH. *Program availability:* Part-time. *Degree requirements:* For master's, practicum. *Entrance requirements:* For master's, GRE, MCAT or OAT, 2 letters of recommendation, minimum undergraduate GPA of 3.0. Additional exam requirements/recommendations for international students: Required—TOEFL (minimum score 550 paper-based).

Stony Brook University, State University of New York, Stony Brook Medicine, School of Medicine, Program in Population Health and Clinical Outcomes Research, Stony Brook, NY 11794. Offers PhD. *Degree requirements:* For doctorate, thesis/dissertation. *Entrance requirements:* For doctorate, GRE, personal or telephone interview, minimum GPA of 3.0 in undergraduate work. Additional exam requirements/recommendations for international students: Required—TOEFL (minimum score 600 paper-based; 90 iBT). *Application deadline:* For fall admission, 1/15 for domestic students. *Expenses:* $12,421 full-time resident tuition and fees, $453 per credit hour; $23,761 full-time nonresident tuition and fees, $925 per credit hour. *Unit head:* Dr. Iris Granek, Chair, 631-444-8811, Fax: 631-444-3480, E-mail: iris.granek@stonybrook.edu. *Application contact:* JoanMarie Maniaci, Graduate Program Coordinator, 631-632-4378, Fax: 631-444-3480, E-mail: joanmarie.maniaci@stonybrook.edu.
Website: https://www.grad.stonybrook.edu/brochure/PHCOR/

Stony Brook University, State University of New York, Stony Brook Medicine, School of Medicine, Program in Public Health, Stony Brook, NY 11794. Offers community health (MPH); evaluation sciences (MPH); family violence (MPH); health communication (Certificate); health economics (MPH); population health (MPH); substance abuse (MPH). *Accreditation:* CEPH. *Program availability:* Part-time, evening/weekend. *Students:* 39 full-time (29 women), 18 part-time (16 women); includes 28 minority (5 Black or African American, non-Hispanic/Latino; 12 Asian, non-Hispanic/Latino; 11 Hispanic/Latino), 4 international. Average age 30. 158 applicants, 59% accepted, 34 enrolled. In 2015, 28 master's awarded. *Entrance requirements:* For master's, GRE, 3 references, bachelor's degree from accredited college or university with minimum GPA of 3.0, essays, interview. Additional exam requirements/recommendations for international students: Required—TOEFL (minimum score 85 iBT). *Application deadline:* For fall admission, 6/1 for domestic students, 3/15 for international students. Application fee: $100. Electronic applications accepted. *Expenses:* $12,421 full-time resident tuition and fees, $453 per credit hour; $23,761 full-time nonresident tuition and fees, $952 per credit hour. *Financial support:* Fellowships available. *Faculty research:* Abnormal psychology, academic achievement, broadcast media, communications, communications systems, public health. *Total annual research expenditures:* $102,281. *Unit head:* Dr. Lisa A. Benz Scott, Director, 631-444-9396, Fax: 631-444-3480, E-mail: lisa.benzscott@stonybrook.edu. *Application contact:* Senior Academic Coordinator, 631-444-9396, Fax: 631-444-3480, E-mail: joanmarie.maniaci@stonybrook.edu.
Website: http://publichealth.stonybrookmedicine.edu/

Teachers College, Columbia University, Department of Health and Behavior Studies, New York, NY 10027-6696. Offers applied behavior analysis (MA, PhD); applied educational psychology: school psychology (Ed M, PhD); behavioral nutrition (PhD), including nutrition (Ed D, PhD); community health education (MS); community nutrition education (Ed M), including community nutrition education; education of deaf and hard of hearing (MA, PhD); health education (MA, Ed D); hearing impairment (Ed D); intellectual disability/autism (MA, Ed D, PhD); nursing education (Advanced Certificate); nutrition and education (MS); nutrition and exercise physiology (MS); nutrition and public health (MS); nutrition education (Ed D), including nutrition (Ed D, PhD); physical disabilities (Ed D); reading specialist (MA); severe or multiple disabilities (MA); special education (Ed M, MA, Ed D); teaching of sign language (MA). *Program availability:* Part-time, evening/weekend. *Students:* 186 full-time (168 women), 362 part-time (319 women); includes 199 minority (50 Black or African American, non-Hispanic/Latino; 1 American Indian or Alaska Native, non-Hispanic/Latino; 73 Asian, non-Hispanic/Latino; 59 Hispanic/Latino; 1 Native Hawaiian or other Pacific Islander, non-Hispanic/Latino; 15 Two or more races, non-Hispanic/Latino), 13 international. Terminal master's awarded for partial completion of doctoral program. *Expenses:* Tuition, area resident: Part-time $1454 per credit. *Required fees:* $428 per semester. One-time fee: $475 full-time. Full-time tuition and fees vary according to course load. *Unit head:* Prof. Stephen T. Peverly, Chair, 212-678-3964, Fax: 212-678-8259, E-mail: stp4@columbia.edu. *Application contact:* David Estrella, Director of Admission, 212-678-3305, E-mail: estrella@tc.columbia.edu.
Website: http://www.tc.columbia.edu/health-and-behavior-studies/

Texas A&M University, School of Public Health, College Station, TX 77843. Offers health administration (MHA); health policy and management (MPH); health promotion

Community Health

and community health sciences (MPH); health services research (PhD). *Accreditation:* CEPH. *Program availability:* Part-time, blended/hybrid learning. *Faculty:* 68. *Students:* 313 full-time (189 women), 71 part-time (41 women); includes 169 minority (40 Black or African American, non-Hispanic/Latino; 38 Asian, non-Hispanic/Latino; 88 Hispanic/Latino; 3 Two or more races, non-Hispanic/Latino), 88 international. Average age 30. 138 applicants, 100% accepted, 126 enrolled. In 2015, 139 master's, 5 doctorates awarded. *Degree requirements:* For master's, thesis optional. *Entrance requirements:* For master's, GRE General Test, 3 letters of recommendation; statement of purpose; current curriculum vitae or resume; official transcripts; for doctorate, GRE General Test, 3 letters of recommendation; statement of purpose; current curriculum vitae or resume; official transcripts; interview (in some cases). Additional exam requirements/recommendations for international students: Required—TOEFL (minimum score 597 paper-based, 95 iBT) or GRE (minimum verbal score 153). *Application deadline:* For fall admission, 8/27 for domestic students; for spring admission, 1/14 for domestic students. Application fee: $120. Electronic applications accepted. *Expenses:* Contact institution. *Financial support:* In 2015–16, 186 students received support, including 2 fellowships with tuition reimbursements available (averaging $17,190 per year), 55 research assistantships with tuition reimbursements available (averaging $5,728 per year), 14 teaching assistantships with tuition reimbursements available (averaging $5,836 per year); career-related internships or fieldwork, institutionally sponsored loans, scholarships/grants, traineeships, health care benefits, tuition waivers (full and partial), and unspecified assistantships also available. Support available to part-time students. Financial award applicants required to submit FAFSA. *Unit head:* Dr. Jay Maddock, Dean, 979-436-9322, Fax: 979-458-1878, E-mail: maddock@tamhsc.edu. *Application contact:* Erin E. Schneider, Associate Director of Admissions and Recruitment, 979-436-9380, E-mail: eschneider@sph.tamhsc.edu.
Website: http://sph.tamhsc.edu/

Tulane University, School of Public Health and Tropical Medicine, Department of Global community Health and Behavioral Sciences, New Orleans, LA 70118-5669. Offers community health sciences (MPH); global community health and behavioral sciences (Dr PH, PhD); JD/MPH; MD/MPH; MSW/MPH. *Program availability:* Part-time. *Degree requirements:* For doctorate, comprehensive exam, thesis/dissertation. *Entrance requirements:* For master's and doctorate, GRE General Test. Additional exam requirements/recommendations for international students: Required—TOEFL. *Application deadline:* For fall admission, 4/15 priority date for domestic and international students; for spring admission, 10/15 for domestic students, 10/15 priority date for international students. Applications are processed on a rolling basis. Electronic applications accepted. *Expenses:* Tuition, area resident: Full-time $47,658; part-time $2648 per credit hour. *Required fees:* $1980; $44.50 per credit hour. $550 per term. Tuition and fees vary according to course load, degree level and program. *Financial support:* Federal Work-Study, scholarships/grants, and traineeships available. Support available to part-time students. Financial award application deadline: 4/15.

Universidad de Ciencias Medicas, Graduate Programs, San Jose, Costa Rica. Offers dermatology (SP); family health (MS); health service center administration (MHA); human anatomy (MS); medical and surgery (MD); occupational medicine (MS); pharmacy (Pharm D). *Program availability:* Part-time. *Degree requirements:* For master's, thesis; for doctorate and SP, comprehensive exam. *Entrance requirements:* For master's, MD or bachelor's degree; for doctorate, admissions test; for SP, admissions test, MD.

Université de Montréal, Faculty of Medicine, Program in Communal and Public Health, Montréal, QC H3C 3J7, Canada. Offers community health (M Sc, DESS); public health (PhD). *Accreditation:* CEPH. *Program availability:* Part-time. Terminal master's awarded for partial completion of doctoral program. *Degree requirements:* For master's, thesis; for doctorate, thesis/dissertation, general exam. *Entrance requirements:* For master's and doctorate, proficiency in French, knowledge of English; for DESS, proficiency in French. Electronic applications accepted. *Faculty research:* Epidemiology, health services utilization, health promotion and education, health behaviors, poverty and child health.

Université Laval, Faculty of Medicine, Graduate Programs in Medicine, Department of Social and Preventive Medicine, Program in Community Health, Québec, QC G1K 7P4, Canada. Offers M Sc, PhD. *Program availability:* Part-time. Terminal master's awarded for partial completion of doctoral program. *Degree requirements:* For master's, thesis (for some programs); for doctorate, comprehensive exam, thesis/dissertation. *Entrance requirements:* For master's, knowledge of French, comprehension of written English; for doctorate, French exam, comprehension of French, written comprehension of English. Electronic applications accepted.

Université Laval, Faculty of Medicine, Post-Professional Programs in Medical Studies, Québec, QC G1K 7P4, Canada. Offers anatomy–pathology (DESS); anesthesiology (DESS); cardiology (DESS); care of older people (Diploma); clinical research (DESS); community health (DESS); dermatology (DESS); diagnostic radiology (DESS); emergency medicine (Diploma); family medicine (DESS); general surgery (DESS); geriatrics (DESS); hematology (DESS); internal medicine (DESS); maternal and fetal medicine (Diploma); medical biochemistry (DESS); medical microbiology and infectious diseases (DESS); medical oncology (DESS); nephrology (DESS); neurology (DESS); neurosurgery (DESS); obstetrics and gynecology (DESS); ophthalmology (DESS); orthopedic surgery (DESS); oto-rhino-laryngology (DESS); palliative medicine (Diploma); pediatrics (DESS); plastic surgery (DESS); psychiatry (DESS); pulmonary medicine (DESS); radiology–oncology (DESS); thoracic surgery (DESS); urology (DESS). *Degree requirements:* For other advanced degree, comprehensive exam. *Entrance requirements:* For degree, knowledge of French. Electronic applications accepted.

University at Buffalo, the State University of New York, Graduate School, School of Public Health and Health Professions, Department of Community Health and Health Behavior, Buffalo, NY 14203. Offers MPH, PhD. *Accreditation:* CEPH. *Program availability:* Part-time. *Faculty:* 9 full-time (5 women), 1 part-time/adjunct (0 women). *Students:* 22 full-time (19 women), 6 part-time (all women); includes 3 minority (2 Black or African American, non-Hispanic/Latino; 1 Asian, non-Hispanic/Latino). Average age 31. 80 applicants, 40% accepted, 17 enrolled. In 2015, 11 master's, 2 doctorates awarded. *Degree requirements:* For master's, thesis; for doctorate, comprehensive exam, thesis/dissertation. *Entrance requirements:* For master's and doctorate, GRE. Additional exam requirements/recommendations for international students: Required—TOEFL (minimum score 79 iBT). *Application deadline:* For fall admission, 1/15 priority date for domestic students, 2/1 priority date for international students. Applications are processed on a rolling basis. Application fee: $50. Electronic applications accepted. *Financial support:* In 2015–16, 6 students received support, including 2 fellowships with full tuition reimbursements available (averaging $4,000 per year), 2 research assistantships with full tuition reimbursements available (averaging $21,000 per year). Financial award application deadline: 3/15; financial award applicants required to submit FAFSA. *Unit head:* Dr. Gary A. Giovino, Chair, 716-829-6952, E-mail: ggiovino@buffalo.edu. *Application contact:* Barbara L. Sen, Graduate Program Coordinator, 716-829-6956, Fax: 716-829-6040, E-mail: bsen@buffalo.edu.
Website: http://sphhp.buffalo.edu/community-health-and-health-behavior.html

The University of Alabama, Graduate School, College of Human Environmental Sciences, Program in Human Environmental Science, Tuscaloosa, AL 35487. Offers interactive technology (MS); quality management (MS); restaurant and meeting management (MS); rural community health (MS); sport management (MS). *Program availability:* Part-time, evening/weekend, online learning. *Students:* 66 full-time (38 women), 99 part-time (52 women); includes 45 minority (34 Black or African American, non-Hispanic/Latino; 2 Asian, non-Hispanic/Latino; 4 Hispanic/Latino; 1 Native Hawaiian or other Pacific Islander, non-Hispanic/Latino; 4 Two or more races, non-Hispanic/Latino), 1 international. Average age 34. 103 applicants, 80% accepted, 83 enrolled. In 2015, 82 master's awarded. *Degree requirements:* For master's, comprehensive exam. *Entrance requirements:* For master's, GRE (for some specializations), minimum GPA of 3.0. Additional exam requirements/recommendations for international students: Required—TOEFL. *Application deadline:* For fall admission, 7/1 for domestic students; for spring admission, 11/1 for domestic students; for summer admission, 4/15 for domestic students. Applications are processed on a rolling basis. Application fee: $50 ($60 for international students). Electronic applications accepted. *Expenses:* Tuition, state resident: full-time $10,170. Tuition, nonresident: full-time $25,950. *Financial support:* In 2015–16, 2 teaching assistantships with full tuition reimbursements were awarded. Financial award application deadline: 7/1. *Faculty research:* Rural health, hospitality management, sport management, interactive technology, consumer quality management, environmental health and safety. *Unit head:* Dr. Milla D. Boschung, Dean, 205-348-6250, Fax: 205-348-1786, E-mail: mboschun@ches.ua.edu. *Application contact:* Dr. Stuart Usdan, Associate Dean, 205-348-6150, Fax: 205-348-3789, E-mail: susdan@ches.ua.edu.
Website: http://www.ches.ua.edu/programs-of-study.html

The University of Alabama at Birmingham, School of Education, Community Health and Human Services Program, Birmingham, AL 35294. Offers MA Ed. *Accreditation:* NCATE. *Faculty:* 4 full-time (2 women). *Students:* 12 full-time (11 women), 12 part-time (9 women); includes 14 minority (13 Black or African American, non-Hispanic/Latino; 1 Hispanic/Latino), 1 international. Average age 33. In 2015, 14 master's awarded. *Degree requirements:* For master's, comprehensive exam (for some programs), thesis optional. *Entrance requirements:* For master's, GRE General Test or MAT, minimum GPA of 3.0, references. *Application deadline:* Applications are processed on a rolling basis. Application fee: $35 ($60 for international students). Electronic applications accepted. *Expenses:* Tuition, state resident: full-time $7340. Tuition, nonresident: full-time $16,628. Full-time tuition and fees vary according to course load and program. *Faculty research:* College student health, minority health disparities/disease, health eating. *Total annual research expenditures:* $10,000. *Unit head:* Dr. Kristi Menear, Chair, 205-975-7409, Fax: 205-975-8040, E-mail: kmenear@uab.edu. *Application contact:* Dr. Retta R. Evans, Program Coordinator, 205-996-2701, Fax: 205-975-8040, E-mail: rrevans@uab.edu.

University of Alberta, School of Public Health, Department of Public Health Sciences, Edmonton, AB T6G 2E1, Canada. Offers clinical epidemiology (M Sc, MPH); environmental and occupational health (MPH); environmental health sciences (M Sc); epidemiology (M Sc); global health (M Sc, MPH); health policy and management (MPH); health policy research (M Sc); health technology assessment (MPH); occupational health (M Sc); population health (M Sc); public health leadership (MPH); public health sciences (PhD); quantitative methods (MPH). *Accreditation:* CEPH (one or more programs are accredited). Terminal master's awarded for partial completion of doctoral program. *Degree requirements:* For master's, thesis (for some programs); for doctorate, thesis/dissertation. *Entrance requirements:* For master's, GMAT or GRE General Test. Additional exam requirements/recommendations for international students: Required—TOEFL (minimum score 550 paper-based) or IELTS (minimum score 6). Electronic applications accepted. *Faculty research:* Biostatistics, health promotion and socio-behavioral health science.

University of Arkansas, Graduate School, College of Education and Health Professions, Department of Health, Human Performance and Recreation, Program in Community Health Promotion, Fayetteville, AR 72701-1201. Offers MS, PhD. *Students:* 8 full-time (7 women), 12 part-time (all women); includes 5 minority (2 Black or African American, non-Hispanic/Latino; 1 American Indian or Alaska Native, non-Hispanic/Latino; 1 Hispanic/Latino; 1 Two or more races, non-Hispanic/Latino). In 2015, 7 master's, 5 doctorates awarded. *Unit head:* Dr. Bart Hammig, Departmental Chairperson, 479-575-2857, Fax: 479-575-5778, E-mail: bhammig@uark.edu. *Application contact:* Dr. Stephen Dittmore, Coordinator of Graduate Studies, 479-575-6625, E-mail: dittmore@uark.edu.
Website: http://chlp.uark.edu

University of Calgary, Cumming School of Medicine and Faculty of Graduate Studies, Department of Community Health Sciences, Calgary, AB T2N 1N4, Canada. Offers M Sc, PhD. *Degree requirements:* For master's, thesis; for doctorate, thesis/dissertation, candidacy exam. *Entrance requirements:* For master's and doctorate, minimum GPA of 3.2. Additional exam requirements/recommendations for international students: Required—TOEFL (minimum score 600 paper-based). Electronic applications accepted. *Faculty research:* Epidemiology, health research, biostatistics, health economics, health policy.

University of California, Los Angeles, Graduate Division, School of Public Health, Department of Community Health Sciences, Los Angeles, CA 90095. Offers public health (MPH, MS, Dr PH, PhD); JD/MPH; MA/MPH; MD/MPH; MSW/MPH. *Degree requirements:* For master's, comprehensive exam or thesis; for doctorate, thesis/dissertation, oral and written qualifying exams. *Entrance requirements:* For master's, GRE General Test, minimum GPA of 3.0; for doctorate, GRE General Test, minimum undergraduate GPA of 3.0. Electronic applications accepted.

University of Colorado Denver, College of Liberal Arts and Sciences, Program in Humanities, Denver, CO 80217. Offers community health science (MSS); humanities (MH); international studies (MSS); philosophy and theory (MH); social justice (MSS); society and the environment (MSS); visual studies (MH); women's and gender studies (MSS). *Program availability:* Part-time, evening/weekend. *Faculty:* 2 full-time (0 women). *Students:* 42 full-time (29 women), 27 part-time (19 women); includes 20 minority (3 Black or African American, non-Hispanic/Latino; 1 American Indian or Alaska Native, non-Hispanic/Latino; 2 Asian, non-Hispanic/Latino; 9 Hispanic/Latino; 5 Two or more races, non-Hispanic/Latino). Average age 35. 19 applicants, 74% accepted, 6 enrolled. In 2015, 13 master's awarded. *Degree requirements:* For master's, 36 credit hours, project or thesis. *Entrance requirements:* For master's, writing sample, statement of purpose/letter of intent, three letters of recommendation. Additional exam requirements/recommendations for international students: Required—TOEFL (minimum score 537 paper-based; 75 iBT); Recommended—IELTS (minimum score 6.5). *Application deadline:* For fall admission, 5/15 for domestic students, 5/15 priority date for international students; for spring admission, 10/15 for domestic students, 10/15 priority date for international students; for summer admission, 3/15 for domestic and international students. Application fee: $50 ($75 for international students). Electronic applications accepted. *Financial support:* In 2015–16, 9 students received support. Fellowships, research assistantships, teaching assistantships, Federal Work-Study, institutionally sponsored loans, scholarships/grants, and traineeships available. Financial award application deadline: 4/1; financial award applicants required to submit

FAFSA. *Faculty research:* Women and gender in the classical Mediterranean, communication theory and democracy, relationship between psychology and philosophy. *Unit head:* Margaret Woodhull, Director of Humanities, 303-315-3568, E-mail: margaret.woodhull@ucdenver.edu. *Application contact:* Angela Beale, Program Assistant, 303-315-3565, E-mail: mastershs@ucdenver.edu.
Website: http://www.ucdenver.edu/academics/colleges/CLAS/Programs/HumanitiesSocialSciences/Programs/Pages/MasterofHumanities.aspx

University of Colorado Denver, Colorado School of Public Health, Program in Public Health, Aurora, CO 80045. Offers community and behavioral health (MPH, Dr PH); environmental and occupational health (MPH); epidemiology (MPH); health systems, management and policy (MPH). *Accreditation:* CEPH. *Program availability:* Part-time, evening/weekend. *Faculty:* 16 full-time (14 women), 1 (woman) part-time/adjunct. *Students:* 379 full-time (293 women), 77 part-time (69 women); includes 111 minority (10 Black or African American, non-Hispanic/Latino; 3 American Indian or Alaska Native, non-Hispanic/Latino; 36 Asian, non-Hispanic/Latino; 47 Hispanic/Latino; 1 Native Hawaiian or other Pacific Islander, non-Hispanic/Latino; 14 Two or more races, non-Hispanic/Latino), 12 international. Average age 31. 785 applicants, 25% accepted, 166 enrolled. In 2015, 144 master's awarded. *Degree requirements:* For master's, thesis or alternative, 42 credit hours; for doctorate, comprehensive exam, thesis/dissertation, 67 credit hours. *Entrance requirements:* For master's, GRE, MCAT, DAT, LSAT, PCAT, GMAT or master's degree from accredited institution, baccalaureate degree or equivalent; minimum GPA of 3.0; transcripts; references; resume; essay; for doctorate, GRE, MCAT, DAT, LSAT, PCAT or GMAT, MPH or master's or higher degree in related field or equivalent; 2 years of previous work experience in public health; essay; resume. Additional exam requirements/recommendations for international students: Required—TOEFL (minimum score 550 paper-based; 80 iBT). *Application deadline:* For fall admission, 12/15 priority date for domestic students, 12/1 priority date for international students. Application fee: $65. Electronic applications accepted. *Expenses:* Contact institution. *Financial support:* In 2015–16, 265 students received support. Fellowships, research assistantships, teaching assistantships, Federal Work-Study, institutionally sponsored loans, scholarships/grants, traineeships, and unspecified assistantships available. Financial award application deadline: 3/15; financial award applicants required to submit FAFSA. *Faculty research:* Cancer prevention by nutrition, cancer survivorship outcomes, social and cultural factors related to health. *Total annual research expenditures:* $302,793. *Unit head:* Dr. Lori Crane, Chair, 303-724-4385, E-mail: lori.crane@ucdenver.edu. *Application contact:* 303-724-4613, E-mail: csph.studentaffairs@ucdenver.edu.
Website: http://www.ucdenver.edu/academics/colleges/PublicHealth/Academics/degreesandprograms/Pages/index.aspx

University of Colorado Denver, School of Medicine, Physician Assistant Program, Aurora, CO 80045. Offers child health associate (MPAS), including global health, leadership, education, advocacy, development, and scholarship, pediatric critical and acute care, rural health, urban/underserved populations. *Accreditation:* ARC-PA. *Students:* 131 full-time (107 women); includes 18 minority (2 Black or African American, non-Hispanic/Latino; 6 Asian, non-Hispanic/Latino; 9 Hispanic/Latino; 1 Two or more races, non-Hispanic/Latino). Average age 28. In 2015, 45 master's awarded. *Degree requirements:* For master's, comprehensive exam. *Entrance requirements:* For master's, GRE General Test, minimum GPA of 2.8; 3 letters of recommendation; prerequisite courses in chemistry, biology, general genetics, psychology and statistics; interview. Additional exam requirements/recommendations for international students: Required—TOEFL (minimum score 550 paper-based; 80 iBT). *Application deadline:* For fall admission, 9/1 for domestic students, 8/15 for international students. Application fee: $170. Electronic applications accepted. *Expenses:* Contact institution. *Financial support:* In 2015–16, 130 students received support. Fellowships, research assistantships, teaching assistantships, career-related internships or fieldwork, Federal Work-Study, institutionally sponsored loans, scholarships/grants, traineeships, and unspecified assistantships available. Financial award application deadline: 3/15; financial award applicants required to submit FAFSA. *Faculty research:* Clinical genetics and genetic counseling, evidence-based medicine, pediatric allergy and asthma, childhood diabetes, standardized patient assessment. *Unit head:* Jonathan Bowser, Program Director, 303-724-1349, E-mail: jonathan.bowser@ucdenver.edu. *Application contact:* Kay Denler, Academic Services Program Manager, 303-724-7963, E-mail: kay.denler@ucdenver.edu.
Website: http://www.ucdenver.edu/academics/colleges/medicalschool/education/degree_programs/PAProgram/Pages/Home.aspx

University of Illinois at Chicago, School of Public Health, Division of Community Health Sciences, Chicago, IL 60607-7128. Offers MPH, MS, Dr PH. *Accreditation:* CEPH (one or more programs are accredited). *Program availability:* Part-time. *Faculty:* 19 full-time (14 women), 7 part-time/adjunct (all women). *Students:* 104 full-time (85 women), 73 part-time (65 women); includes 80 minority (32 Black or African American, non-Hispanic/Latino; 20 Asian, non-Hispanic/Latino; 22 Hispanic/Latino; 1 Native Hawaiian or other Pacific Islander, non-Hispanic/Latino; 5 Two or more races, non-Hispanic/Latino), 6 international. Average age 31. Terminal master's awarded for partial completion of doctoral program. *Degree requirements:* For master's, thesis, field practicum; for doctorate, thesis/dissertation, independent research, internship. *Entrance requirements:* For master's and doctorate, GRE General Test, minimum GPA of 2.75. Additional exam requirements/recommendations for international students: Required—TOEFL. *Application deadline:* For fall admission, 2/1 for domestic students, 1/1 priority date for international students. Applications are processed on a rolling basis. Application fee: $60. Electronic applications accepted. *Expenses:* Contact institution. *Financial support:* Fellowships with full tuition reimbursements, research assistantships with full tuition reimbursements, teaching assistantships with full tuition reimbursements, career-related internships or fieldwork, Federal Work-Study, institutionally sponsored loans, scholarships/grants, traineeships, and unspecified assistantships available. Support available to part-time students. Financial award application deadline: 3/1; financial award applicants required to submit FAFSA. *Faculty research:* Promoting wellness, disease prevention; public health preparedness; public health security capabilities. *Total annual research expenditures:* $629,000. *Unit head:* Prof. Jesus Ramirez-Valles, Director, 312-996-6346, E-mail: valles@uic.edu. *Application contact:* David Brand, Academic Coordinator, 312-996-8940, Fax: 312-996-3551, E-mail: dbrand@uic.edu.
Website: http://publichealth.uic.edu/departments/communityhealthsciences/

University of Illinois at Springfield, Graduate Programs, College of Public Affairs and Administration, Program in Public Health, Springfield, IL 62703-5407. Offers community health education (Graduate Certificate); emergency preparedness and homeland security (Graduate Certificate); epidemiology (Graduate Certificate); public health (MPH). *Program availability:* Part-time, evening/weekend, 100% online. *Faculty:* 7 full-time (5 women), 1 part-time/adjunct (0 women). *Students:* 41 full-time (23 women), 58 part-time (39 women); includes 25 minority (14 Black or African American, non-Hispanic/Latino; 6 Asian, non-Hispanic/Latino; 3 Hispanic/Latino; 2 Two or more races, non-Hispanic/Latino), 23 international. Average age 32. 87 applicants, 36% accepted, 23 enrolled. In 2015, 30 master's, 19 other advanced degrees awarded. *Degree requirements:* For master's, comprehensive exam, internship. *Entrance requirements:* For master's, GRE, minimum undergraduate GPA of 3.0, 3 letters of recommendation, statement of personal goals. Additional exam requirements/recommendations for

international students: Required—TOEFL (minimum score 500 paper-based; 61 iBT). *Application deadline:* Applications are processed on a rolling basis. Application fee: $60 ($75 for international students). Electronic applications accepted. *Expenses:* Tuition, state resident: part-time $329 per credit hour. Tuition, nonresident: part-time $675 per credit hour. *Financial support:* In 2015–16, fellowships with full tuition reimbursements (averaging $9,900 per year), research assistantships with full tuition reimbursements (averaging $9,956 per year), teaching assistantships with full tuition reimbursements (averaging $9,956 per year) were awarded; career-related internships or fieldwork, Federal Work-Study, scholarships/grants, health care benefits, and unspecified assistantships also available. Support available to part-time students. Financial award application deadline: 11/15; financial award applicants required to submit FAFSA. *Unit head:* Dr. Josiah Alamu, Program Administrator, 217-206-7874, Fax: 217-206-7279, E-mail: jalam3@uis.edu. *Application contact:* Dr. Lynn Pardie, Office of Graduate Studies, 800-252-8533, Fax: 217-206-7623, E-mail: lpard1@uis.edu.
Website: http://www.uis.edu/publichealth/

University of Illinois at Urbana–Champaign, Graduate College, College of Applied Health Sciences, Department of Kinesiology and Community Health, Champaign, IL 61820. Offers community health (MS, MSPH, PhD); kinesiology (MS, PhD); public health (MPH); rehabilitation (MS); PhD/MPH.

The University of Iowa, Graduate College, College of Public Health, Department of Community and Behavioral Health, Iowa City, IA 52242-1316. Offers MPH, MS, PhD. *Accreditation:* CEPH. *Degree requirements:* For master's, thesis; for doctorate, comprehensive exam, thesis/dissertation. *Entrance requirements:* For master's and doctorate, GRE General Test, minimum GPA of 3.0. Additional exam requirements/recommendations for international students: Required—TOEFL (minimum score 600 paper-based; 100 iBT). Electronic applications accepted.

University of Louisville, Graduate School, College of Education and Human Development, Department of Health and Sport Sciences, Louisville, KY 40292-0001. Offers community health education (M Ed); exercise physiology (MS), including health and sport sciences, strength and conditioning; health and physical education (MAT); sport administration (MS). *Program availability:* Part-time, evening/weekend. *Students:* 44 full-time (23 women), 12 part-time (11 women); includes 6 minority (3 Black or African American, non-Hispanic/Latino; 1 Hispanic/Latino; 2 Two or more races, non-Hispanic/Latino), 2 international. Average age 27. 80 applicants, 64% accepted, 27 enrolled. In 2015, 30 master's awarded. *Entrance requirements:* For master's, GRE General Test. Additional exam requirements/recommendations for international students: Required—TOEFL (minimum score 560 paper-based; 83 iBT). Application fee: $60. Electronic applications accepted. *Expenses:* Tuition, state resident: full-time $11,664; part-time $649 per credit hour. Tuition, nonresident: full-time $24,274; part-time $1350 per credit hour. *Required fees:* $196. Tuition and fees vary according to program and reciprocity agreements. *Financial support:* In 2015–16, 221,928 students received support. Fellowships, research assistantships, teaching assistantships, career-related internships or fieldwork, Federal Work-Study, scholarships/grants, health care benefits, and unspecified assistantships available. Financial award application deadline: 6/1; financial award applicants required to submit FAFSA. *Faculty research:* Sport administration; exercise physiology; exercise science; physical education; health education. *Total annual research expenditures:* $293,958. *Unit head:* Dr. Margaret Hancock, Interim Co-Chair, 502-852-5040, E-mail: meg.hancock@louisville.edu. *Application contact:* Libby Leggett, Director, Graduate Admissions, 502-852-3101, Fax: 502-852-6536, E-mail: gradadm@louisville.edu.
Website: http://www.louisville.edu/education/departments/hss

University of Manitoba, Faculty of Medicine and Faculty of Graduate Studies, Graduate Programs in Medicine, Department of Community Health Sciences, Winnipeg, MB R3T 2N2, Canada. Offers M Sc, MPH, PhD, G Dip. *Program availability:* Part-time. *Degree requirements:* For master's, thesis; for doctorate, thesis/dissertation. *Entrance requirements:* For master's and doctorate, minimum GPA of 3.0. *Faculty research:* Health services, aboriginal health, health policy, epidemiology, international health.

University of Massachusetts Amherst, Graduate School, School of Public Health and Health Sciences, Department of Public Health, Amherst, MA 01003. Offers biostatistics (MPH, MS, PhD); community health education (MPH, MS, PhD); environmental health sciences (MPH, MS, PhD); epidemiology (MPH, MS, PhD); health policy and management (MPH, MS, PhD); nutrition (MPH, PhD); public health practice (MPH); MPH/MPPA. *Accreditation:* CEPH (one or more programs are accredited). *Program availability:* Part-time, evening/weekend, online learning. Terminal master's awarded for partial completion of doctoral program. *Degree requirements:* For master's, thesis (for some programs); for doctorate, comprehensive exam, thesis/dissertation. *Entrance requirements:* For master's and doctorate, GRE General Test. Additional exam requirements/recommendations for international students: Required—TOEFL (minimum score 550 paper-based; 80 iBT), IELTS (minimum score 6.5). Electronic applications accepted.

University of Massachusetts Medical School, Graduate School of Nursing, Worcester, MA 01655-0115. Offers adult gerontological acute care nurse practitioner (DNP, Post Master's Certificate); adult gerontological primary care nurse practitioner (DNP, Post Master's Certificate); family nursing practitioner (DNP); nurse administrator (DNP); nurse educator (MS, Post Master's Certificate); nursing (PhD); nursing practitioner (DNP); population health (MS). *Accreditation:* AACN. *Faculty:* 18 full-time (15 women), 28 part-time/adjunct (22 women). *Students:* 143 full-time (119 women), 27 part-time (25 women); includes 28 minority (15 Black or African American, non-Hispanic/Latino; 10 Asian, non-Hispanic/Latino; 3 Hispanic/Latino), 1 international. Average age 34. 129 applicants, 68% accepted, 56 enrolled. In 2015, 43 master's, 10 doctorates, 2 other advanced degrees awarded. *Degree requirements:* For doctorate, thesis/dissertation (for some programs), comprehensive exam (for PhD); capstone project and manuscript (for DNP). *Entrance requirements:* For master's, GRE General Test, bachelor's degree in nursing, course work in statistics, unrestricted Massachusetts license as registered nurse; for doctorate, GRE General Test, bachelor's or master's degree; for Post Master's Certificate, GRE General Test, MS in nursing. Additional exam requirements/recommendations for international students: Required—TOEFL. *Application deadline:* For fall admission, 12/1 priority date for domestic students. Applications are processed on a rolling basis. Application fee: $60. Electronic applications accepted. *Expenses:* $10,994 resident per year; $18,210 non-resident per year. *Financial support:* In 2015–16, 31 students received support. Institutionally sponsored loans, scholarships/grants, traineeships, and tuition waivers (partial) available. Support available to part-time students. Financial award application deadline: 5/16; financial award applicants required to submit FAFSA. *Faculty research:* Health literacy, social justice, HIV prevention, cancer-related decision making, nursing education. *Total annual research expenditures:* $650,993. *Unit head:* Dr. Joan Vitello-Cicciu, Dean, 508-856-5081, Fax: 508-856-6552, E-mail: joan.vitello@umassmed.edu. *Application contact:* Diane Brescia, Admissions Coordinator, 508-856-3488, Fax: 508-856-5851, E-mail: diane.brescia@umassmed.edu.
Website: http://www.umassmed.edu/gsn/

University of Miami, Graduate School, School of Education and Human Development, Department of Educational and Psychological Studies, Program in Community Well-Being, Coral Gables, FL 33124. Offers PhD. *Degree requirements:* For doctorate, thesis/

Community Health

dissertation. *Entrance requirements:* For doctorate, GRE General Test. Additional exam requirements/recommendations for international students: Required—TOEFL (minimum score 550 paper-based; 80 iBT); Recommended—IELTS. Electronic applications accepted.

University of Minnesota, Twin Cities Campus, School of Public Health, Major in Community Health Education, Minneapolis, MN 55455-0213. Offers MPH. *Accreditation:* CEPH. *Program availability:* Part-time. *Degree requirements:* For master's, fieldwork, project. *Entrance requirements:* For master's, GRE General Test. Additional exam requirements/recommendations for international students: Required—TOEFL. Electronic applications accepted. *Faculty research:* Assessing population behavior, designing community-wide prevention and treatment, preventing alcohol and drug abuse, influencing health policies.

University of Missouri, School of Medicine and Office of Research and Graduate Studies, Graduate Programs in Medicine, Columbia, MO 65211. Offers family and community medicine (MS); health administration (MS); medical pharmacology and physiology (MS, PhD); molecular microbiology and immunology (MS, PhD); pathology and anatomical sciences (MS). *Program availability:* Part-time. *Degree requirements:* For doctorate, thesis/dissertation. *Entrance requirements:* For master's and doctorate, GRE General Test, minimum GPA of 3.0. Additional exam requirements/recommendations for international students: Required—TOEFL. *Application deadline:* Applications are processed on a rolling basis. Application fee: $55 ($75 for international students). *Expenses:* Contact institution. *Financial support:* Fellowships, research assistantships, teaching assistantships, career-related internships or fieldwork, and institutionally sponsored loans available.
Website: http://som.missouri.edu/departments.shtml

University of Montana, Graduate School, Phyllis J. Washington College of Education and Human Sciences, Department of Health and Human Performance, Missoula, MT 59812-0002. Offers community health (MS); exercise science (MS); health and human performance generalist (MS). *Program availability:* Part-time. *Entrance requirements:* For master's, GRE General Test. Additional exam requirements/recommendations for international students: Required—TOEFL. *Faculty research:* Exercise physiology, performance psychology, nutrition, pre-employment physical screening, program evaluation.

University of Nevada, Las Vegas, Graduate College, School of Community Health Sciences, Las Vegas, NV 89154-3063. Offers MHA, MPH, PhD. *Faculty:* 18 full-time (6 women), 5 part-time/adjunct (4 women). *Students:* 61 full-time (41 women), 69 part-time (51 women); includes 48 minority (7 Black or African American, non-Hispanic/Latino; 3 American Indian or Alaska Native, non-Hispanic/Latino; 11 Asian, non-Hispanic/Latino; 13 Hispanic/Latino; 2 Native Hawaiian or other Pacific Islander, non-Hispanic/Latino; 2 Two or more races, non-Hispanic/Latino), 19 international. Average age 33. 68 applicants, 75% accepted, 35 enrolled. In 2015, 40 master's, 6 doctorates awarded. *Degree requirements:* For master's, thesis (for some programs); for doctorate, comprehensive exam (for some programs), thesis/dissertation. *Entrance requirements:* For master's and doctorate, GRE General Test. Additional exam requirements/recommendations for international students: Required—TOEFL (minimum score 550 paper-based; 85 iBT), IELTS (minimum score 7). *Application deadline:* For fall admission, 4/1 for domestic students, 5/1 for international students; for spring admission, 11/1 for domestic students, 10/1 for international students. Application fee: $60 ($95 for international students). Electronic applications accepted. *Expenses:* $264 per credit resident; $6,955 per semester full-time nonresident; $264 per credit full-time nonresident; $555 per credit part-time nonresident. *Financial support:* In 2015–16, 15 students received support, including 14 research assistantships with partial tuition reimbursements available (averaging $11,879 per year), 1 teaching assistantship (averaging $13,000 per year); institutionally sponsored loans, scholarships/grants, health care benefits, and unspecified assistantships also available. Financial award application deadline: 3/1. *Faculty research:* Environmental health: micro (mold), hospital-acquired infections; health care: health services research, patient-centered outcome research, comparative effectiveness research, health management and policy/health information technology, healthcare disparities; social and behavioral health disease prevention: health equity, asthma, diabetes, cancer, HIV/AIDS, substance abuse, injury; biostatistics and epidemiology: big data, health data analysis and disease patterns among minority populations. *Total annual research expenditures:* $3.7 million. *Unit head:* Dr. Shawn Gerstenberger, Dean, 702-895-1565, Fax: 702-895-5184, E-mail: shawn.gerstenberger@unlv.edu. *Application contact:* Graduate College Admissions Evaluator, 702-895-3367, Fax: 702-895-4180, E-mail: gradadmissions@unlv.edu. Website: http://publichealth.unlv.edu/

University of New Mexico, Graduate Studies, College of Education, Program in Health Education, Albuquerque, NM 87131-2039. Offers community health education (MS). *Accreditation:* NCATE. *Program availability:* Part-time. *Faculty:* 6 full-time (3 women), 1 (woman) part-time/adjunct. *Students:* 19 full-time (17 women), 15 part-time (12 women); includes 18 minority (1 Black or African American, non-Hispanic/Latino; 4 American Indian or Alaska Native, non-Hispanic/Latino; 12 Hispanic/Latino; 1 Native Hawaiian or other Pacific Islander, non-Hispanic/Latino), 1 international. Average age 33. 12 applicants, 75% accepted, 8 enrolled. In 2015, 11 master's awarded. *Degree requirements:* For master's, comprehensive exam, thesis optional. *Entrance requirements:* For master's, 3 letters of reference, resume, minimum cumulative GPA of 3.0 in last 2 years of bachelor's degree, letter of intent. Additional exam requirements/recommendations for international students: Required—TOEFL (minimum score 550 paper-based). *Application deadline:* For fall admission, 6/15 priority date for domestic students; for spring admission, 11/1 priority date for domestic students. Applications are processed on a rolling basis. Application fee: $50. Electronic applications accepted. *Financial support:* Fellowships, teaching assistantships with full tuition reimbursements, career-related internships or fieldwork, institutionally sponsored loans, scholarships/grants, and health care benefits available. Financial award application deadline: 3/1; financial award applicants required to submit FAFSA. *Faculty research:* Alcohol and families, health behaviors and sexuality, multicultural health behavior, health promotion policy, school/community-based prevention, health and aging. *Unit head:* Dr. Elias Duryea, Coordinator, 505-277-5151, Fax: 505-277-6227, E-mail: duryea@unm.edu. *Application contact:* Carol Catania, Graduate Coordinator, 505-277-5151, Fax: 505-277-6227, E-mail: catania@unm.edu.

University of New Mexico, Graduate Studies, Health Sciences Center, Program in Public Health, Albuquerque, NM 87131-5196. Offers community health (MPH); epidemiology (MPH); health systems, services and policy (MPH). *Accreditation:* CEPH. *Program availability:* Part-time, online learning. *Faculty:* 9 full-time (7 women), 3 part-time/adjunct (2 women). *Students:* 25 full-time (17 women), 20 part-time (16 women); includes 17 minority (3 Black or African American, non-Hispanic/Latino; 1 American Indian or Alaska Native, non-Hispanic/Latino; 3 Asian, non-Hispanic/Latino; 10 Hispanic/Latino), 1 international. Average age 31. 32 applicants, 63% accepted, 16 enrolled. In 2015, 13 master's awarded. *Degree requirements:* For master's, thesis. *Entrance requirements:* For master's, GRE, MCAT, 2 years of experience in health field. Additional exam requirements/recommendations for international students: Required—TOEFL. *Application deadline:* For fall admission, 2/1 for domestic students. Application fee: $50. *Financial support:* Fellowships, research assistantships with tuition

reimbursements, and Federal Work-Study available. Financial award application deadline: 12/15; financial award applicants required to submit FAFSA. *Faculty research:* Epidemiology, rural health, environmental health, Native American health issues. *Unit head:* Dr. Kristine Tollestrup, Director, 505-272-4173, Fax: 505-272-4494, E-mail: ktollestrup@salud.unm.edu. *Application contact:* Gayle Garcia, Education Coordinator, 505-272-3982, Fax: 505-272-4494, E-mail: garciag@salud.unm.edu. Website: http://fcm.unm.edu/

The University of North Carolina at Charlotte, College of Health and Human Services, Department of Public Health Sciences, Charlotte, NC 28223-0001. Offers community health (Certificate); health administration (MHA); public health (MSPH); public health core concepts (Graduate Certificate); public health sciences (PhD). *Accreditation:* CAHME. *Program availability:* Part-time. *Faculty:* 18 full-time (9 women), 6 part-time/adjunct (4 women). *Students:* 96 full-time (78 women), 22 part-time (18 women); includes 46 minority (26 Black or African American, non-Hispanic/Latino; 1 American Indian or Alaska Native, non-Hispanic/Latino; 11 Asian, non-Hispanic/Latino; 7 Hispanic/Latino; 1 Two or more races, non-Hispanic/Latino), 15 international. Average age 26. 154 applicants, 66% accepted, 55 enrolled. In 2015, 47 master's, 4 other advanced degrees awarded. *Degree requirements:* For master's, thesis (for some programs), thesis or project; internship; for doctorate, thesis/dissertation. *Entrance requirements:* For master's, GRE or MCAT (for MSPH); GRE or GMAT (for MHA); for doctorate, GRE, master's degree in public health or a related field with minimum GPA of 3.5 in all graduate work; statement of purpose detailing why applicant wants to pursue a PhD in public health sciences in the specified concentration at UNC Charlotte; three letters of recommendation (including at least two letters from former professors); for other advanced degree, bachelor's degree from regionally-accredited university; minimum GPA of 2.75 on all post-secondary work attempted; transcripts; personal statement outlining why the applicant seeks admission to the program. Additional exam requirements/recommendations for international students: Required—TOEFL (minimum score 557 paper-based, 83 iBT) or IELTS (minimum score 6.5). *Application deadline:* For fall admission, 1/10 for domestic and international students; for spring admission, 9/15 for domestic and international students; for summer admission, 2/15 for domestic and international students. Applications are processed on a rolling basis. Application fee: $75. Electronic applications accepted. *Expenses:* Contact institution. *Financial support:* In 2015–16, 18 students received support, including 1 fellowship (averaging $42,000 per year), 15 research assistantships (averaging $6,031 per year); career-related internships or fieldwork, Federal Work-Study, institutionally sponsored loans, scholarships/grants, unspecified assistantships, and administrative assistantships also available. Support available to part-time students. Financial award application deadline: 3/1; financial award applicants required to submit FAFSA. *Faculty research:* Pediatric asthma self-management, reproductive epidemiology, social aspects of injury prevention, chronic illness self-care, competency-based professional education, cognitive health, aging and dementia, infant health outcomes, policing and suicide, data mining for health executive decision support, segmentation analyses in identifying patient satisfaction problems in the primary care setting, enhancing community capacity through data sharing. *Total annual research expenditures:* $573,805. *Unit head:* Dr. Susan M. Sell, Interim Chair, 704-687-7191, Fax: 704-687-1644, E-mail: ssell@uncc.edu. *Application contact:* Kathy B. Giddings, Director of Graduate Admissions, 704-687-5503, Fax: 704-687-1668, E-mail: gradadm@uncc.edu. Website: http://publichealth.uncc.edu/

The University of North Carolina at Greensboro, Graduate School, School of Health and Human Sciences, Department of Public Health Education, Greensboro, NC 27412-5001. Offers community health education (MPH, Dr PH). *Accreditation:* CEPH; NCATE. *Degree requirements:* For master's, comprehensive exam, thesis or alternative. *Entrance requirements:* For master's, GRE General Test or MAT. Additional exam requirements/recommendations for international students: Required—TOEFL. Electronic applications accepted. *Faculty research:* Peer facilitator training, innovative health education approaches.

University of Northern British Columbia, Office of Graduate Studies, Prince George, BC V2N 4Z9, Canada. Offers business administration (Diploma); community health science (M Sc); disability management (MA); education (M Ed); first nations studies (MA); gender studies (MA); history (MA); interdisciplinary studies (MA); international studies (MA); mathematical, computer and physical sciences (M Sc); natural resources and environmental studies (M Sc, MA, MNRES, PhD); political science (MA); psychology (M Sc, PhD); social work (MSW). *Program availability:* Part-time, evening/weekend, online learning. *Degree requirements:* For master's, thesis; for doctorate, thesis/dissertation. *Entrance requirements:* For master's, GRE, minimum B average in undergraduate course work; for doctorate, candidacy exam, minimum A average in graduate course work.

University of Northern Iowa, Graduate College, College of Education, School of Kinesiology, Allied Health and Human Services, MA Program in Health Education, Cedar Falls, IA 50614. Offers community health education (MA); health promotion/fitness management (MA); school health education (MA). *Program availability:* Part-time, evening/weekend. *Students:* 14 full-time (11 women), 12 part-time (8 women); includes 3 minority (2 Black or African American, non-Hispanic/Latino; 1 Hispanic/Latino), 3 international. 20 applicants, 55% accepted, 11 enrolled. In 2015, 6 master's awarded. *Degree requirements:* For master's, comprehensive exam, thesis or alternative. *Entrance requirements:* For master's, minimum GPA of 3.0. Additional exam requirements/recommendations for international students: Required—TOEFL (minimum score 500 paper-based; 61 iBT). *Application deadline:* For fall admission, 8/1 priority date for domestic students. Applications are processed on a rolling basis. Application fee: $50 ($70 for international students). Electronic applications accepted. *Financial support:* Career-related internships or fieldwork, Federal Work-Study, and tuition waivers (full and partial) available. Support available to part-time students. Financial award application deadline: 2/1. *Unit head:* Dr. Susan Roberts-Dobie, Coordinator, 319-273-5930, Fax: 319-273-5958, E-mail: susan.dobie@uni.edu. *Application contact:* Laurie S. Russell, Record Analyst, 319-273-2623, Fax: 319-273-2885, E-mail: laurie.russell@uni.edu.
Website: http://www.uni.edu/coe/departments/school-health-physical-education-leisure-services/health-promotion-and-education

University of North Florida, Brooks College of Health, Department of Public Health, Jacksonville, FL 32224. Offers aging services (Certificate); community health (MPH); geriatric management (MSH); health administration (MHA); rehabilitation counseling (MS). *Accreditation:* CEPH. *Program availability:* Part-time, evening/weekend. *Faculty:* 19 full-time (14 women), 3 part-time/adjunct (all women). *Students:* 149 full-time (109 women), 59 part-time (40 women); includes 58 minority (28 Black or African American, non-Hispanic/Latino; 10 Asian, non-Hispanic/Latino; 11 Hispanic/Latino; 9 Two or more races, non-Hispanic/Latino), 9 international. Average age 29. 244 applicants, 43% accepted, 75 enrolled. In 2015, 74 master's awarded. *Degree requirements:* For master's, thesis optional. *Entrance requirements:* For master's, GRE General Test (MSH, MS, MPH); GMAT or GRE General Test (MHA), minimum GPA of 3.0 in last 60 hours. Additional exam requirements/recommendations for international students: Required—TOEFL (minimum score 500 paper-based). *Application deadline:* For fall admission, 7/1 for domestic students, 5/1 for international students; for spring

admission, 11/1 for domestic students, 10/1 for international students. Application fee: $30. Electronic applications accepted. *Expenses:* Tuition, state resident: part-time $408.10 per credit hour. Tuition, nonresident: part-time $932.61 per credit hour. *Required fees:* $111.81 per credit hour. Tuition and fees vary according to course load, campus/location and program. *Financial support:* In 2015–16, 33 students received support, including 10 teaching assistantships (averaging $1,500 per year); research assistantships, career-related internships or fieldwork, Federal Work-Study, scholarships/grants, and tuition waivers (partial) also available. Support available to part-time students. Financial award application deadline: 4/1; financial award applicants required to submit FAFSA. *Faculty research:* Dietary supplements; alcohol, tobacco, and other drug use prevention; turnover among health professionals; aging; psychosocial aspects of disabilities. *Total annual research expenditures:* $57,986. *Unit head:* Dr. Jeffrey Harrison, Chair, 904-620-1440, Fax: 904-620-2848, E-mail: jeffrey.harrison@unf.edu. *Application contact:* Dr. Heather Kenney, Director of Advising, 904-620-2810, Fax: 904-620-1030, E-mail: heather.kenney@unf.edu.
Website: http://www.unf.edu/brooks/public_health/

University of North Texas Health Science Center at Fort Worth, School of Public Health, Fort Worth, TX 76107-2699. Offers biostatistics (MPH); community health (MPH); disease control and prevention (Dr PH); environmental and occupational health sciences (MPH); epidemiology (MPH); health administration (MHA); health policy and management (MPH, Dr PH); DO/MPH; MS/MPH; MSN/MPH. MPH offered jointly with University of North Texas; DO/MPH with Texas College of Osteopathic Medicine. *Accreditation:* CEPH. *Program availability:* Part-time, evening/weekend. *Degree requirements:* For master's, thesis or alternative, supervised internship; for doctorate, thesis/dissertation, supervised internship. *Entrance requirements:* For master's, GRE General Test. Additional exam requirements/recommendations for international students: Required—TOEFL. Electronic applications accepted.

University of Ottawa, Faculty of Graduate and Postdoctoral Studies, Faculty of Medicine, Department of Epidemiology and Community Medicine, Ottawa, ON K1N 6N5, Canada. Offers epidemiology (M Sc), including health technology assessment. *Degree requirements:* For master's, thesis. *Entrance requirements:* For master's, honors degree or equivalent, minimum B average. Electronic applications accepted. *Faculty research:* Epidemiologic concepts and methods, health technology assessment.

University of Ottawa, Faculty of Graduate and Postdoctoral Studies, Interdisciplinary Programs, Ottawa, ON K1N 6N5, Canada. Offers e-business (Certificate); e-commerce (Certificate); finance (Certificate); health services and policies research (Diploma); population health (PhD); population health risk assessment and management (Certificate); public management and governance (Certificate); systems science (Certificate).

University of Phoenix–Central Valley Campus, College of Nursing, Fresno, CA 93720-1552. Offers education (MHA); gerontology (MHA); health administration (MHA); nursing (MSN); MSN/MBA.

University of Phoenix–Hawaii Campus, College of Nursing, Honolulu, HI 96813-3800. Offers education (MHA); family nurse practitioner (MSN); gerontology (MHA); health administration (MHA); nursing (MSN); nursing/health care education (MSN); MSN/MBA. *Program availability:* Evening/weekend. *Degree requirements:* For master's, thesis (for some programs). *Entrance requirements:* For master's, minimum undergraduate GPA of 2.5, 3 years of work experience, RN license. Additional exam requirements/recommendations for international students: Required—TOEFL (minimum score 550 paper-based; 79 iBT). Electronic applications accepted.

University of Pittsburgh, Graduate School of Public Health, Department of Behavioral and Community Health Sciences, Pittsburgh, PA 15261. Offers applied research and leadership (Dr PH); applied social and behavioral concepts in public health (MPH); community-based participatory research (Certificate); health equity (Certificate); LGBT health and wellness (Certificate); maternal and child health (MPH); program evaluation (Certificate); MID/MPH; MPH/MPA; MPH/MSW; MPH/PhD. *Accreditation:* CAHME (one or more programs are accredited). *Program availability:* Part-time. *Faculty:* 15 full-time (9 women), 15 part-time/adjunct (4 women). *Students:* 48 full-time (38 women), 69 part-time (56 women); includes 29 minority (9 Black or African American, non-Hispanic/Latino; 8 Asian, non-Hispanic/Latino; 7 Hispanic/Latino; 5 Two or more races, non-Hispanic/Latino), 6 international. Average age 28. 311 applicants, 56% accepted, 23 enrolled. In 2015, 26 master's, 4 doctorates awarded. *Degree requirements:* For master's, thesis, 200 contact hour practicum; for doctorate, comprehensive exam, thesis/dissertation, preliminary exam. *Entrance requirements:* For master's, GRE, bachelor's degree; for doctorate, GRE, master's degree in public health or related field; for Certificate, GRE. Additional exam requirements/recommendations for international students: Required—TOEFL (minimum score 550 paper-based; 80 iBT), IELTS (minimum score 6.5). *Application deadline:* For fall admission, 1/15 for domestic and international students; for spring admission, 10/15 for domestic students, 8/1 for international students. Applications are processed on a rolling basis. Application fee: $120. Electronic applications accepted. *Expenses:* $12,834 per term in-state; $20,872 per term out-of-state. *Financial support:* In 2015–16, 14 students received support, including 6 fellowships with partial tuition reimbursements available (averaging $3,775 per year), 8 research assistantships with tuition reimbursements available (averaging $21,922 per year); teaching assistantships with tuition reimbursements available, scholarships/grants, traineeships, and health care benefits also available. Financial award applicants required to submit FAFSA. *Faculty research:* Community-based participatory research, health equity, evaluation science, LGBT health, aging, violence prevention. *Total annual research expenditures:* $3.3 million. *Unit head:* Dr. Steven M. Albert, Chair, 412-624-3102, Fax: 412-648-5975, E-mail: smalbert@pitt.edu. *Application contact:* Miriam P. Fagan, Academic Administrator, 412-624-3107, Fax: 412-624-5510, E-mail: mpfagan@pitt.edu.
Website: http://www.bchs.pitt.edu/

University of Pittsburgh, Graduate School of Public Health, Department of Infectious Diseases and Microbiology, Pittsburgh, PA 15261. Offers infectious disease management, intervention, and community practice (MPH); infectious disease pathogenesis, eradication, and laboratory practice (MPH); infectious diseases and microbiology (MS, PhD). *Program availability:* Part-time. *Faculty:* 19 full-time (5 women), 5 part-time/adjunct (2 women). *Students:* 67 full-time (47 women), 14 part-time (10 women); includes 19 minority (5 Black or African American, non-Hispanic/Latino; 5 Asian, non-Hispanic/Latino; 7 Hispanic/Latino; 2 Two or more races, non-Hispanic/Latino), 11 international. Average age 26. 178 applicants, 65% accepted, 39 enrolled. In 2015, 15 master's, 3 doctorates awarded. *Degree requirements:* For master's, comprehensive exam (for some programs), thesis; for doctorate, comprehensive exam, thesis/dissertation, preliminary exam, dissertation approval. *Entrance requirements:* For master's and doctorate, GRE General Test, MCAT, DAT, or GMAT. Additional exam requirements/recommendations for international students: Required—TOEFL (minimum score 550 paper-based, 80 iBT) or IELTS (minimum score 6.5). *Application deadline:* For fall admission, 1/15 priority date for domestic and international students. Applications are processed on a rolling basis. Application fee: $120. Electronic applications accepted. *Expenses:* $12,464 per semester in-state, $20,502 per semester out-of-state; $450 fees. *Financial support:* In 2015–16, 19 students received support, including 6 fellowships (averaging $19,210 per year), 13 research assistantships

(averaging $16,556 per year); scholarships/grants, traineeships, health care benefits, and unspecified assistantships also available. Financial award applicants required to submit FAFSA. *Faculty research:* HIV, complications of antiretroviral therapy, Hepatitis C, emerging infections, clinical and molecular epidemiology, genetic basis of innate immune response, HIV prevention and care, AIDS education and training. *Total annual research expenditures:* $10.8 million. *Unit head:* Dr. Charles R. Rinaldo, Chair, 412-624-3928, Fax: 412-624-4953, E-mail: rinaldo@pitt.edu. *Application contact:* Meredith Mavero, Student Services Coordinator, 412-624-3331, Fax: 412-383-8926, E-mail: mlm72@pitt.edu.
Website: http://www.idm.pitt.edu/

University of Saskatchewan, College of Medicine, Department of Community Health and Epidemiology, Saskatoon, SK S7N 5A2, Canada. Offers M Sc, PhD. *Degree requirements:* For master's, thesis; for doctorate, thesis/dissertation. *Entrance requirements:* Additional exam requirements/recommendations for international students: Required—TOEFL.

University of South Florida, College of Public Health, Department of Community and Family Health, Tampa, FL 33620-9951. Offers MPH, MSPH, Dr PH, PhD. *Accreditation:* CEPH (one or more programs are accredited). *Program availability:* Part-time, evening/weekend. *Degree requirements:* For master's, comprehensive exam, thesis (for some programs); for doctorate, comprehensive exam, thesis/dissertation. *Entrance requirements:* For master's, GRE General Test, minimum GPA of 3.0 in upper-level course work, goal statement letter, two professional letters of recommendation, resume/curriculum vitae; for doctorate, GRE General Test, minimum GPA of 3.0 in upper-level course work, goal statement letter, three professional letters of recommendation, resume/curriculum vitae, writing sample. Additional exam requirements/recommendations for international students: Required—TOEFL (minimum score 550 paper-based; 79 iBT). Electronic applications accepted. *Faculty research:* Family violence, high-risk infants, medical material and child health, healthy start, social marketing, adolescent health, high-risk behaviors.

University of South Florida, Innovative Education, Tampa, FL 33620-9951. Offers adult, career and higher education (Graduate Certificate), including college teaching, leadership in developing human resources, leadership in higher education; Africana studies (Graduate Certificate), including diasporas and health disparities, genocide and human rights; aging studies (Graduate Certificate), including gerontology; art research (Graduate Certificate), including museum studies; business foundations (Graduate Certificate); chemical and biomedical engineering (Graduate Certificate), including materials science and engineering, water, health and sustainability; child and family studies (Graduate Certificate), including positive behavior support; civil and industrial engineering (Graduate Certificate), including transportation systems analysis; community and family health (Graduate Certificate), including maternal and child health, social marketing and public health, violence and injury: prevention and intervention, women's health; criminology (Graduate Certificate), including criminal justice administration; educational measurement and research (Graduate Certificate), including evaluation; English (Graduate Certificate), including comparative literary studies, creative writing, professional and technical communication; entrepreneurship (Graduate Certificate); environmental health (Graduate Certificate), including safety management; epidemiology and biostatistics (Graduate Certificate), including applied biostatistics, biostatistics, concepts and tools of epidemiology, epidemiology, epidemiology of infectious diseases; geography, environment and planning (Graduate Certificate), including community development, environmental policy and management, geographical information systems; geology (Graduate Certificate), including hydrogeology; global health (Graduate Certificate), including disaster management, global health and Latin American and Caribbean studies, global health practice, humanitarian assistance, infection control; government and international affairs (Graduate Certificate), including Cuban studies, globalization studies; health policy and management (Graduate Certificate), including health management and leadership, public health policy and programs; hearing specialist: early intervention (Graduate Certificate); industrial and management systems engineering (Graduate Certificate), including systems engineering, technology management; information studies (Graduate Certificate), including school library media specialist; information systems/decision sciences (Graduate Certificate), including analytics and business intelligence; instructional technology (Graduate Certificate), including distance education, Florida digital/virtual educator, instructional design, multimedia design, Web design; internal medicine, bioethics and medical humanities (Graduate Certificate), including biomedical ethics; Latin American and Caribbean studies (Graduate Certificate); mass communications (Graduate Certificate), including multimedia journalism; mathematics and statistics (Graduate Certificate), including mathematics; medicine (Graduate Certificate), including aging and neuroscience, bioinformatics, biotechnology, brain fitness and memory management, clinical investigation, health informatics, health sciences, integrative weight management, intellectual property, medicine and gender, metabolic and nutritional medicine, metabolic cardiology, pharmacy sciences; national and competitive intelligence (Graduate Certificate); psychological and social foundations (Graduate Certificate), including career counseling, college teaching, diversity in education, mental health counseling, school counseling; public affairs (Graduate Certificate), including nonprofit management, public management, research administration; public health (Graduate Certificate), including environmental health, health equity, public health generalist, translational research in adolescent behavioral health; public health practices (Graduate Certificate), including planning for healthy communities; rehabilitation and mental health counseling (Graduate Certificate), including integrative mental health care, marriage and family therapy, rehabilitation technology; secondary education (Graduate Certificate), including ESOL, foreign language education: culture and content, foreign language education: professional; social work (Graduate Certificate), including geriatric social work/clinical gerontology; special education (Graduate Certificate), including autism spectrum disorder, disabilities education: severe/profound; world languages (Graduate Certificate), including teaching English as a second language (TESL) or foreign language. *Unit head:* Kathy Barnes, Interdisciplinary Programs Coordinator, 813-974-8031, Fax: 813-974-7061, E-mail: barnesk@usf.edu. *Application contact:* Karen Tylinski, Metro Initiatives, 813-974-9943, Fax: 813-974-7061, E-mail: ktylinsk@usf.edu.
Website: http://www.usf.edu/innovative-education/

The University of Tennessee, Graduate School, College of Education, Health and Human Sciences, Program in Human Ecology, Knoxville, TN 37996. Offers child and family studies (PhD); community health (PhD); nutrition science (PhD); retailing and consumer sciences (PhD); textile science (PhD). *Degree requirements:* For doctorate, thesis/dissertation. *Entrance requirements:* For doctorate, GRE General Test, minimum GPA of 2.7. Additional exam requirements/recommendations for international students: Required—TOEFL. Electronic applications accepted.

The University of Tennessee, Graduate School, College of Education, Health and Human Sciences, Program in Public Health, Knoxville, TN 37996. Offers community health education (MPH); gerontology (MPH); health planning/administration (MPH); MS/MPH. *Accreditation:* CEPH. *Degree requirements:* For master's, thesis optional. *Entrance requirements:* For master's, minimum GPA of 2.7. Additional exam

Community Health

requirements/recommendations for international students: Required—TOEFL. Electronic applications accepted.

The University of Texas Medical Branch, Graduate School of Biomedical Sciences, Department of Preventive Medicine and Community Health, Galveston, TX 77555. Offers population health sciences (MS, PhD); public health (MPH); rehabilitation sciences (PhD). *Accreditation:* CEPH. *Degree requirements:* For master's, thesis; for doctorate, thesis/dissertation. *Entrance requirements:* For master's, GRE General Test or MAT; for doctorate, GRE General Test. Additional exam requirements/recommendations for international students: Required—TOEFL (minimum score 550 paper-based). Electronic applications accepted.

University of Toronto, School of Graduate Studies, Department of Public Health Sciences, Toronto, ON M5S 1A1, Canada. Offers biostatistics (M Sc, PhD); community health (M Sc); community nutrition (MPH), including nutrition and dietetics; epidemiology (MPH, PhD); family and community medicine (MPH); occupational and environmental health (MPH); social and behavioral health science (PhD); social and behavioral health sciences (MPH), including health promotion. *Accreditation:* CAHME (one or more programs are accredited); CEPH (one or more programs are accredited). *Program availability:* Part-time. *Degree requirements:* For master's, thesis (for some programs), practicum; for doctorate, comprehensive exam, thesis/dissertation, oral thesis defense. *Entrance requirements:* For master's, 2 letters of reference, relevant professional/research experience, minimum B average in final year; for doctorate, 2 letters of reference, relevant professional/research experience, minimum B+ average. Additional exam requirements/recommendations for international students: Required—TOEFL (minimum score 580 paper-based; 93 iBT), TWE (minimum score 5). Electronic applications accepted. *Expenses:* Contact institution.

University of Virginia, School of Nursing, Charlottesville, VA 22903. Offers acute and specialty care (MSN); acute care nurse practitioner (MSN); clinical nurse leadership (MSN); community-public health leadership (MSN); nursing (DNP, PhD); psychiatric mental health counseling (MSN); MSN/MBA. *Accreditation:* AACN. *Program availability:* Part-time. *Degree requirements:* For doctorate, comprehensive exam (for some programs), capstone project (DNP), dissertation (PhD). *Entrance requirements:* For master's, GRE General Test, MAT; for doctorate, GRE General Test. Additional exam requirements/recommendations for international students: Required—TOEFL, IELTS. Electronic applications accepted. *Expenses:* Contact institution.

University of Washington, Graduate School, School of Public Health, Department of Health Services, Seattle, WA 98195. Offers clinical research (MS); community-oriented public health practice (MPH); evaluative sciences and statistics (PhD); health behavior and social determinants of health (PhD); health economics (PhD); health informatics and health information management (MHIHIM); health services (MS, PhD); health services administration (EMHA, MHA); health systems and policy (MPH); health systems research (PhD); maternal and child health (MPH); social and behavioral sciences (MPH); JD/MHA; MHA/MBA; MHA/MD; MHA/MPA; MPH/JD; MPH/MD; MPH/MN; MPH/MPA; MPH/MS; MPH/MSD; MPH/MSW; MPH/PhD. *Program availability:* Online learning. Terminal master's awarded for partial completion of doctoral program. *Degree requirements:* For master's, thesis (for some programs), practicum (MPH); for doctorate, comprehensive exam, thesis/dissertation. *Entrance requirements:* For master's and doctorate, GRE General Test, minimum GPA of 3.0. Additional exam requirements/recommendations for international students: Required—TOEFL (minimum score 580 paper-based; 92 iBT), IELTS (minimum score 7). Electronic applications accepted. *Expenses:* Contact institution. *Faculty research:* Public health practice, health promotion and disease prevention, maternal and child health, organizational behavior and culture, health policy.

University of West Florida, College of Education and Professional Studies, Department of Health, Leisure, and Exercise Science, Community Health Education Program, Pensacola, FL 32514-5750. Offers aging studies (MS); health promotion and worksite wellness (MS); psychosocial (MS). *Program availability:* Part-time, evening/weekend. *Degree requirements:* For master's, thesis or alternative. *Entrance requirements:* For master's, GRE or MAT, official transcripts; minimum GPA of 3.0; letter of intent; three personal references. Additional exam requirements/recommendations for international students: Required—TOEFL (minimum score 550 paper-based).

University of Wisconsin–La Crosse, College of Science and Health, Department of Health Education and Health Promotion, Program in Community Health Education, La Crosse, WI 54601-3742. Offers MPH, MS. *Accreditation:* CEPH. *Students:* 21 full-time (18 women), 9 part-time (8 women); includes 4 minority (3 Asian, non-Hispanic/Latino; 1 Hispanic/Latino), 2 international. Average age 29. 18 applicants, 94% accepted, 14 enrolled. In 2015, 11 master's awarded. *Degree requirements:* For master's, thesis. *Entrance requirements:* For master's, GRE General Test, GRE Subject Test (for MPH), 3 letters of recommendation. Additional exam requirements/recommendations for international students: Required—TOEFL (minimum score 550 paper-based; 79 iBT). Electronic applications accepted. *Financial support:* Research assistantships with partial tuition reimbursements, Federal Work-Study, scholarships/grants, health care benefits, and tuition waivers (partial) available. Support available to part-time students. Financial award applicants required to submit FAFSA. *Unit head:* Dr. Gary Gilmore, Director, 608-785-8163, E-mail: gilmore.gary@uwlax.edu. *Application contact:* Brandon Schaller, Senior Graduate Student Status Examiner, 608-785-8941, E-mail: admissions@uwlax.edu.
Website: http://www.uwlax.edu/sah/hehp/

⭐ **University of Wisconsin–Madison,** School of Medicine and Public Health, Population Health and Epidemiology Program, Madison, WI 53726. Offers epidemiology (MS, PhD); population health (MS, PhD). *Accreditation:* CEPH. *Program availability:* Part-time. *Faculty:* 104 full-time (54 women), 2 part-time/adjunct (0 women). *Students:* 52 full-time (43 women), 10 part-time (7 women); includes 15 minority (7 Black or African American, non-Hispanic/Latino; 3 Asian, non-Hispanic/Latino; 4 Hispanic/Latino; 1 Native Hawaiian or other Pacific Islander, non-Hispanic/Latino), 6 international. Average age 31. 84 applicants, 38% accepted, 20 enrolled. In 2015, 11 master's, 8 doctorates awarded. Terminal master's awarded for partial completion of doctoral program. *Degree requirements:* For master's, thesis, thesis defense; for doctorate, comprehensive exam, thesis/dissertation, qualifying exam, preliminary exam, dissertation defense. *Entrance requirements:* For master's and doctorate, GRE taken within the last 5 years (MCAT or LSAT acceptable for those with doctoral degrees), minimum GPA of 3.0, quantitative preparation (calculus, statistics, or other) with minimum B average. Additional exam requirements/recommendations for international students: Required—TOEFL (minimum score 580 paper-based; 92 iBT). *Application deadline:* For fall admission, 1/15 for domestic and international students. Application fee: $56. Electronic applications accepted. *Expenses:* Tuition, state resident: full-time $5364. Tuition, nonresident: full-time $12,027. *Required fees:* $571. Tuition and fees vary according to campus/location, program and reciprocity agreements. *Financial support:* Fellowships with full tuition reimbursements, research assistantships with full tuition reimbursements, teaching assistantships with full tuition reimbursements, scholarships/grants, traineeships, health care benefits, and unspecified assistantships available. Support available to part-time students. *Faculty research:* Epidemiology (cancer, environmental, aging, infectious and genetic disease), determinants of population health, health services research, social and behavioral

health sciences, biostatistics. *Total annual research expenditures:* $11.4 million. *Unit head:* Programs Coordinator, 608-265-8108, Fax: 608-263-2820, E-mail: pophealth@mailplus.wisc.edu. *Application contact:* Assistant Programs Coordinator, 608-263-6583, Fax: 608-263-2820, E-mail: pophealth@mailplus.wisc.edu.
Website: https://pophealth.wisc.edu/grad

See Display on next page and Close-Up on page 855.

University of Wyoming, College of Education, Programs in Counselor Education, Laramie, WY 82071. Offers community mental health (MS); counselor education and supervision (PhD); school counseling (MS); student affairs (MS). *Accreditation:* ACA (one or more programs are accredited). *Degree requirements:* For master's, comprehensive exam (for some programs), thesis optional; for doctorate, thesis/dissertation, video demonstration. *Entrance requirements:* For master's, interview, background check; for doctorate, video tape session, interview, writing sample, master's degree, background check. Additional exam requirements/recommendations for international students: Required—TOEFL. *Faculty research:* Wyoming SAGE photovoice project; accountable school counseling programs; GLBT issues; addictions; play therapy-early childhood mental health.

Virginia Commonwealth University, Medical College of Virginia-Professional Programs, School of Medicine, School of Medicine Graduate Programs, Department of Epidemiology and Community Health, Richmond, VA 23284-9005. Offers epidemiology (MPH, PhD); public health practice (MPH); social and behavioral science (MPH); MD/MPH; MSW/MPH. *Accreditation:* CEPH. *Program availability:* Part-time. *Degree requirements:* For doctorate, comprehensive exam, thesis/dissertation. *Entrance requirements:* For master's, GRE; for doctorate, GRE General Test, interview, 3 letters of recommendation, minimum graduate GPA of 3.0, master's degree in public health or related field including epidemiology and biostatistics. Additional exam requirements/recommendations for international students: Required—TOEFL (minimum score 600 paper-based; 100 iBT). Electronic applications accepted. *Faculty research:* Sickle cell anemia, breast cancer, HIV/AIDS, hospital epidemiology, infectious diseases.

Virginia State University, College of Graduate Studies, College of Natural and Health Sciences, Department of Psychology, Petersburg, VA 23806-0001. Offers behavioral and community health sciences (PhD); clinical health psychology (PhD); clinical psychology (MS); general psychology (MS). *Degree requirements:* For master's, one foreign language, thesis. *Entrance requirements:* For master's, GRE General Test. *Application deadline:* For fall admission, 5/1 priority date for domestic students. Applications are processed on a rolling basis. Application fee: $25. *Financial support:* Fellowships and career-related internships or fieldwork available. Financial award application deadline: 5/1.
Website: http://www.cnhs.vsu.edu/departments/psychology/

Walden University, Graduate Programs, School of Health Sciences, Minneapolis, MN 55401. Offers clinical research administration (MS, Graduate Certificate); health education and promotion (MS, PhD), including behavioral health (PhD), disease surveillance (PhD), emergency preparedness (MS), general (MHA, MS), global health (PhD), health policy (PhD), health policy and advocacy (MS), population health (PhD); health informatics (MS); health services (PhD), including community health, healthcare administration, leadership, public health policy, self-designed; healthcare administration (MHA), including general (MHA, MS); leadership and organizational development (MHA); public health (MPH, Dr PH, PhD, Graduate Certificate), including community health education (PhD), epidemiology (PhD); systems policy (MHA). *Program availability:* Part-time, evening/weekend, online only, 100% online. *Faculty:* 14 full-time (8 women), 222 part-time/adjunct (121 women). *Students:* 2,487 full-time (1,804 women), 2,282 part-time (1,540 women); includes 2,763 minority (2,129 Black or African American, non-Hispanic/Latino; 30 American Indian or Alaska Native, non-Hispanic/Latino; 237 Asian, non-Hispanic/Latino; 268 Hispanic/Latino; 13 Native Hawaiian or other Pacific Islander, non-Hispanic/Latino; 86 Two or more races, non-Hispanic/Latino), 87 international. Average age 39. 1,205 applicants, 98% accepted, 820 enrolled. In 2015, 641 master's, 147 doctorates, 18 other advanced degrees awarded. *Degree requirements:* For doctorate, thesis/dissertation, residency. *Entrance requirements:* For master's, bachelor's degree or higher; minimum GPA of 2.5; official transcripts; goal statement (for some programs); access to computer and Internet; for doctorate, master's degree or higher; three years of related professional or academic experience (preferred); minimum GPA of 3.0; goal statement and current resume (for select programs); official transcripts; access to computer and Internet; for Graduate Certificate, relevant work experience; access to computer and Internet. Additional exam requirements/recommendations for international students: Required—TOEFL (minimum score 550 paper-based, 79 iBT), IELTS (minimum score 6.5), Michigan English Language Assessment Battery (minimum score 82), or PTE (minimum score 53). *Application deadline:* Applications are processed on a rolling basis. Application fee: $0. Electronic applications accepted. *Financial support:* Fellowships, Federal Work-Study, scholarships/grants, unspecified assistantships, and family tuition reduction, active duty/veteran tuition reduction, group tuition reduction, interest-free payment plans, employee tuition reduction available. Support available to part-time students. Financial award applicants required to submit FAFSA. *Unit head:* Dr. Jorg Westermann, Dean, 866-492-5336. *Application contact:* Meghan Thomas, Vice President of Enrollment Management, 866-492-5336, E-mail: info@waldenu.edu.
Website: http://www.waldenu.edu/colleges-schools/school-of-health-sciences

Washington State University, College of Nursing, Spokane, WA 99210. Offers advanced population health (MN, DNP); family nurse practitioner (MN, DNP); nursing (PhD); psychiatric/mental health nurse practitioner (DNP); psychiatric/mental health practitioner (MN). Programs offered at the Spokane, Tri-Cities, and Vancouver campuses. *Accreditation:* AACN. *Degree requirements:* For master's, comprehensive exam (for some programs), thesis (for some programs), oral exam, research project. *Entrance requirements:* For master's, minimum GPA of 3.0, Washington state RN license, physical assessment skills, course work in statistics, recommendations, written interview (for nurse practitioner). *Faculty research:* Cardiovascular and Type 2 diabetes in children, evaluation of strategies to increase physical activity in sedentary people.

West Chester University of Pennsylvania, College of Health Sciences, Department of Health, West Chester, PA 19383. Offers community health (MPH); emergency preparedness (Certificate); environmental health (MPH); gerontology (Certificate); health care management (MPH, Certificate); integrative health (Certificate); school health (M Ed). *Accreditation:* CEPH. *Program availability:* Part-time, evening/weekend. *Faculty:* 12 full-time (7 women), 4 part-time/adjunct (3 women). *Students:* 98 full-time (74 women), 85 part-time (59 women); includes 73 minority (60 Black or African American, non-Hispanic/Latino; 8 Asian, non-Hispanic/Latino; 4 Hispanic/Latino; 1 Two or more races, non-Hispanic/Latino), 26 international. Average age 30. 118 applicants, 86% accepted, 60 enrolled. In 2015, 72 master's, 17 other advanced degrees awarded. *Degree requirements:* For master's, thesis or alternative, minimum GPA of 3.0; research report (for M Ed); major project and practicum (for MPH); for Certificate, minimum GPA of 3.0. *Entrance requirements:* For master's, goal statement, two letters of recommendation, undergraduate introduction to statistics course; for Certificate, minimum undergraduate GPA of 2.8 (for gerontology). Additional exam requirements/recommendations for international students: Required—TOEFL or IELTS. *Application*

deadline: For fall admission, 5/15 for international students; for spring admission, 10/15 for international students. Applications are processed on a rolling basis. Application fee: $50. Electronic applications accepted. *Expenses:* Tuition, state resident: full-time $8460; part-time $470 per credit. Tuition, nonresident: full-time $12,690; part-time $705 per credit. *Required fees:* $2312; $126.75 per credit. Tuition and fees vary according to campus/location and program. *Financial support:* Scholarships/grants and unspecified assistantships available. Financial award application deadline: 2/15; financial award applicants required to submit FAFSA. *Faculty research:* Healthy school communities, community health issues and evidence-based programs, environment and health, nutrition and health, integrative health. *Unit head:* Dr. Bethann Cinelli, Chair, 610-436-2267, E-mail: bcinelli@wcupa.edu. *Application contact:* Dr. Lynn Carson, Graduate Coordinator, 610-436-2138, E-mail: lcarson@wcupa.edu.
Website: http://www.wcupa.edu/_ACADEMICS/HealthSciences/health/

West Virginia University, School of Medicine, Department of Community Medicine, Morgantown, WV 26506. Offers public health (MPH), including community health/preventative medicine; public health sciences (PhD). *Accreditation:* CEPH. *Program availability:* Part-time, evening/weekend, online learning. *Degree requirements:* For master's, thesis (for some programs). *Entrance requirements:* For master's, minimum GPA of 3.0. Additional exam requirements/recommendations for international students: Required—TOEFL. *Expenses:* Tuition, state resident: full-time $8568. Tuition, nonresident: full-time $22,140. Tuition and fees vary according to program. *Faculty research:* Adolescent smoking cessation, cardiovascular disease, women's health, worker's health.

West Virginia University, School of Public Health, Morgantown, WV 26506-9190. Offers biostatistics; community health promotion (MS); community health/preventative medicine (MPH); public health sciences (PhD). *Accreditation:* CEPH. *Program availability:* Part-time, online learning. *Faculty:* 37 full-time (17 women), 3 part-time/adjunct (2 women). *Students:* 85 full-time (55 women), 52 part-time (34 women);

includes 28 minority (8 Black or African American, non-Hispanic/Latino; 1 American Indian or Alaska Native, non-Hispanic/Latino; 13 Asian, non-Hispanic/Latino; 3 Hispanic/Latino; 3 Two or more races, non-Hispanic/Latino), 10 international. Average age 31. In 2015, 11 doctorates awarded. *Degree requirements:* For master's, practicum, project. *Entrance requirements:* For master's, GRE General Test, MCAT, medical degree, medical internship. Additional exam requirements/recommendations for international students: Required—TOEFL (minimum score 550 paper-based; 80 iBT). *Application deadline:* For fall admission, 4/15 priority date for domestic students; for spring admission, 12/1 for domestic students. Applications are processed on a rolling basis. Application fee: $60. *Expenses:* Contact institution. *Financial support:* Research assistantships, teaching assistantships, scholarships/grants, and health care benefits available. Financial award application deadline: 2/1; financial award applicants required to submit FAFSA. *Faculty research:* Occupational health, environmental health, clinical epidemiology, health care management, prevention. *Unit head:* Dr. Gregory A. Hand, Dean, School of Public Health, 304-293-2502, Fax: 304-293-6685, E-mail: gahand@hsc.wvu.edu. *Application contact:* Sherry Kuhl, Director, Office of Student Services, 304-293-1795, Fax: 304-293-6685, E-mail: skuhl@hsc.wvu.edu.
Website: http://publichealth.hsc.wvu.edu

William James College, Graduate Programs, Newton, MA 02459. Offers applied psychology in higher education student personnel administration (MA); clinical psychology (Psy D); counseling psychology (MA); counseling psychology and community mental health (MA); counseling psychology and global mental health (MA); executive coaching (Graduate Certificate); forensic and counseling psychology (MA); leadership psychology (Psy D); organizational psychology (MA); primary care psychology (MA); respecialization in clinical psychology (Certificate); school psychology (Psy D); MA/CAGS. *Accreditation:* APA. *Degree requirements:* For master's, comprehensive exam (for some programs); for doctorate, thesis/dissertation (for some programs). Electronic applications accepted.

Environmental and Occupational Health

American University of Beirut, Graduate Programs, Faculty of Health Sciences, Beirut, Lebanon. Offers environmental sciences (MS), including environmental health; epidemiology (MS); epidemiology and biostatistics (MPH); health management and policy (MPH); health promotion and community health (MPH). *Program availability:* Part-time. *Faculty:* 30 full-time (21 women), 3 part-time/adjunct (1 woman). *Students:* 49 full-time (38 women), 99 part-time (81 women). Average age 27. 115 applicants, 71% accepted, 40 enrolled. In 2015, 51 master's awarded. *Degree requirements:* For master's, one foreign language, comprehensive exam (for some programs), thesis (for some programs). *Entrance requirements:* For master's, 2 letters of recommendation, personal statement, transcripts. Additional exam requirements/recommendations for international students: Required—TOEFL (minimum score 583 paper-based; 97 iBT), IELTS (minimum score 7). *Application deadline:* For fall admission, 1/4 priority date for domestic and international students; for spring admission, 11/1 for domestic and international students. Application fee: $50. Electronic applications accepted. *Expenses:* Tuition, area resident: Full-time $16,254; part-time $903 per credit. *Required fees:* $699. Tuition and fees vary according to course load and program. *Financial support:* In

2015–16, 70 students received support. Scholarships/grants, health care benefits, and unspecified assistantships available. Financial award application deadline: 4/1. *Faculty research:* Tobacco control; health of the elderly; youth health; mental health; women's health; reproductive and sexual health, including HIV/AIDS; water quality; health systems; quality in health care delivery; health human resources; health policy; occupational and environmental health; social inequality; social determinants of health; non-communicable diseases; nutrition; refugees health; conflict and health. *Total annual research expenditures:* $2 million. *Unit head:* Iman Adel Nuwayhid, Dean, 961-1759683, Fax: 961-1744470, E-mail: nuwayhid@aub.edu.lb. *Application contact:* Mitra Tauk, Administrative Coordinator, 961-1350000 Ext. 4687, Fax: 961-1744470, E-mail: mt12@aub.edu.lb.

Anna Maria College, Graduate Division, Program in Occupational and Environmental Health and Safety, Paxton, MA 01612. Offers MS. *Program availability:* Part-time, evening/weekend. *Degree requirements:* For master's, thesis. *Entrance requirements:* For master's, minimum GPA of 2.7. Additional exam requirements/recommendations for

Environmental and Occupational Health

international students: Required—TOEFL (minimum score 500 paper-based). Electronic applications accepted.

Augusta University, College of Allied Health Sciences, Program in Public Health, Augusta, GA 30912. Offers environmental health (MPH); health informatics (MPH); health management (MPH); social and behavioral sciences (MPH). *Program availability:* Part-time. *Degree requirements:* For master's, thesis (for some programs). *Entrance requirements:* For master's, GRE General Test, three letters of recommendation. Additional exam requirements/recommendations for international students: Required—TOEFL. *Application deadline:* For fall admission, 5/1 for domestic and international students. Application fee: $50. Electronic applications accepted. *Financial support:* Federal Work-Study available. Financial award application deadline: 5/31; financial award applicants required to submit FAFSA. *Unit head:* Dr. Andrew Balas, Dean, College of Allied Health Sciences, 706-721-2621, Fax: 706-721-7312. *Application contact:* Dr. Pavani Rangachari, Director, 706-721-4830, E-mail: prangachari@augusta.edu.
Website: http://www.augusta.edu/alliedhealth/cdhs/mph/

Boise State University, College of Health Sciences, Department of Community and Environmental Health, Boise, ID 83712-1835. Offers community and environmental health (MHS); health science (MHS), including health policy, health promotion, health services leadership; health services leadership (Graduate Certificate). *Faculty:* 11. *Students:* 20 full-time (18 women), 38 part-time (33 women); includes 7 minority (1 Asian, non-Hispanic/Latino; 5 Hispanic/Latino; 1 Two or more races, non-Hispanic/Latino). Average age 36. 38 applicants, 50% accepted, 11 enrolled. In 2015, 21 master's, 13 Graduate Certificates awarded. *Entrance requirements:* For master's, writing assessment, minimum GPA of 3.0. Additional exam requirements/recommendations for international students: Required—TOEFL (minimum score 550 paper-based; 80 iBT), IELTS (minimum score 6). *Application deadline:* For fall admission, 3/15 for domestic and international students; for spring admission, 10/15 for domestic and international students. Application fee: $65 ($95 for international students). Electronic applications accepted. *Expenses:* Tuition, state resident: full-time $6058; part-time $358 per credit hour. Tuition, nonresident: full-time $20,108; part-time $608 per credit hour. *Required fees:* $2108. Tuition and fees vary according to program. *Financial support:* In 2015–16, 10 students received support, including 2 research assistantships (averaging $2,937 per year); scholarships/grants and unspecified assistantships also available. Financial award application deadline: 3/15; financial award applicants required to submit FAFSA. *Unit head:* Dr. Dale Stephenson, Department Chair, 208-426-3795, E-mail: dalestephenson@boisestate.edu. *Application contact:* Dr. Sarah Toevs, Director, Master of Health Science Program, 208-426-2452, E-mail: stoevs@boisestate.edu.
Website: http://hs.boisestate.edu/ceh/

Boston University, School of Public Health, Environmental Health Department, Boston, MA 02215. Offers MPH, MS, PhD. *Accreditation:* CEPH (one or more programs are accredited). *Program availability:* Part-time, evening/weekend. *Faculty:* 14 full-time, 20 part-time/adjunct. *Students:* 23 full-time (20 women), 21 part-time (17 women); includes 10 minority (2 Black or African American, non-Hispanic/Latino; 4 Asian, non-Hispanic/Latino; 4 Hispanic/Latino), 1 international. Average age 27. 138 applicants, 45% accepted, 18 enrolled. In 2015, 12 master's, 3 doctorates awarded. *Degree requirements:* For master's, comprehensive exam (for some programs), thesis (for some programs); for doctorate, one foreign language, thesis/dissertation, comprehensive written and oral exams. *Entrance requirements:* For master's, GRE, GMAT, or MCAT, U.S. bachelor's degree or foreign equivalent; for doctorate, GRE, MPH or equivalent. Additional exam requirements/recommendations for international students: Required—TOEFL (minimum score 600 paper-based; 100 iBT) or IELTS (minimum score 6). *Application deadline:* For fall admission, 12/1 priority date for domestic and international students; for spring admission, 10/1 priority date for domestic students. Applications are processed on a rolling basis. Application fee: $115. Electronic applications accepted. *Financial support:* Career-related internships or fieldwork, Federal Work-Study, institutionally sponsored loans, and scholarships/grants available. Support available to part-time students. Financial award application deadline: 3/1; financial award applicants required to submit FAFSA. *Faculty research:* Exposure assessment, GIS, toxicology. *Unit head:* Dr. Roberta White, Chair, 617-638-4620, E-mail: envhlth@bu.edu. *Application contact:* LePhan Quan, Associate Director of Admissions, 617-638-4640, Fax: 617-638-5299, E-mail: asksph@bu.edu.
Website: http://www.bu.edu/sph/eh

California State University, Northridge, Graduate Studies, College of Health and Human Development, Department of Environmental and Occupational Health, Northridge, CA 91330. Offers environmental and occupational health (MS); industrial hygiene (MS). *Faculty:* 7 full-time (5 women), 9 part-time/adjunct (all women). *Students:* 26 full-time (19 women), 35 part-time (19 women); includes 37 minority (6 Black or African American, non-Hispanic/Latino; 19 Asian, non-Hispanic/Latino; 10 Hispanic/Latino; 2 Two or more races, non-Hispanic/Latino), 4 international. Average age 31. 52 applicants, 52% accepted, 19 enrolled. *Degree requirements:* For master's, seminar, field experience, comprehensive exam or thesis. *Entrance requirements:* For master's, GRE General Test or minimum GPA of 3.0. Additional exam requirements/recommendations for international students: Required—TOEFL. *Application deadline:* For fall admission, 11/30 for domestic students. Application fee: $55. *Financial support:* Application deadline: 3/1. *Unit head:* Peter Bellin, Chair, 818-677-7476.
Website: http://www.csun.edu/hhd/eoh/

Capella University, School of Public Service Leadership, Doctoral Programs in Healthcare, Minneapolis, MN 55402. Offers criminal justice (PhD); emergency management (PhD); epidemiology (Dr PH); general health administration (DHA); general public administration (DPA); health advocacy and leadership (Dr PH); health care administration (PhD); health care leadership (DHA); health policy advocacy (DHA); multidisciplinary human services (PhD); nonprofit management and leadership (PhD); public safety leadership (PhD); social and community services (PhD).

Capella University, School of Public Service Leadership, Master's Programs in Healthcare, Minneapolis, MN 55402. Offers criminal justice (MS); emergency management (MS); general public health (MPH); gerontology (MS); health administration (MHA); health care operations (MHA); health management policy (MPH); health policy (MHA); homeland security (MS); multidisciplinary human services (MS); public administration (MPA); public safety leadership (MS); social and community services (MS); social behavioral sciences (MPH); MS/MPA.

Clemson University, Graduate School, College of Engineering, Computing and Applied Sciences, Department of Environmental Engineering and Earth Sciences, Program in Environmental Health Physics, Anderson, SC 29625. Offers MS. Terminal master's awarded for partial completion of doctoral program. *Degree requirements:* For master's, thesis optional. *Entrance requirements:* For master's, GRE General Test, unofficial transcripts, letters of recommendation, statement of purpose. Additional exam requirements/recommendations for international students: Required—TOEFL (minimum score 80 iBT), IELTS (minimum score 6.5). *Application deadline:* For fall admission, 2/15 for domestic and international students. Applications are processed on a rolling basis. Application fee: $85 ($90 for international students). Electronic applications accepted. *Expenses:* $4,610 per semester full-time resident, $9,203 per semester full-time non-

resident, $582 per credit hour part-time resident, $1,166 per credit hour part-time non-resident. *Financial support:* Application deadline: 2/15. *Faculty research:* Nuclear forensics, environmental radiochemistry, actinide biogeochemistry, environmental mineralogy, computational materials science. *Unit head:* Dr. Tanju Karanfil, Department Chair, 864-656-1005, Fax: 864-656-0672, E-mail: tkaranf@clemson.edu. *Application contact:* Dr. Timothy Devol, Graduate Student Services Coordinator, 864-656-3278, Fax: 864-656-0672, E-mail: ehp-l@clemson.edu.
Website: http://www.clemson.edu/ces/eees/gradprog/ehp/

Colorado State University, College of Veterinary Medicine and Biomedical Sciences, Department of Environmental and Radiological Health Sciences, Fort Collins, CO 80523-1681. Offers environmental health (MS, PhD); radiological health sciences (MS, PhD); toxicology (MS, PhD). *Program availability:* Part-time. *Faculty:* 31 full-time (13 women), 6 part-time/adjunct (3 women). *Students:* 100 full-time (48 women), 40 part-time (21 women); includes 20 minority (2 Black or African American, non-Hispanic/Latino; 1 American Indian or Alaska Native, non-Hispanic/Latino; 4 Asian, non-Hispanic/Latino; 12 Hispanic/Latino; 1 Two or more races, non-Hispanic/Latino), 9 international. Average age 29. 117 applicants, 83% accepted, 69 enrolled. In 2015, 35 master's, 5 doctorates awarded. Terminal master's awarded for partial completion of doctoral program. *Degree requirements:* For master's, comprehensive exam (for some programs), thesis (for some programs); for doctorate, comprehensive exam, thesis/dissertation. *Entrance requirements:* For master's, GRE, minimum GPA of 3.0; for doctorate, GRE, minimum GPA of 3.0, MS or proof of research. Additional exam requirements/recommendations for international students: Recommended—TOEFL (minimum score 550 paper-based; 80 iBT), IELTS (minimum score 6.5). *Application deadline:* For fall admission, 7/1 for domestic students, 5/1 for international students; for spring admission, 7/1 for domestic students, 5/1 for international students. Applications are processed on a rolling basis. Application fee: $60 ($70 for international students). Electronic applications accepted. *Expenses:* Contact institution. *Financial support:* In 2015–16, 4 students received support, including 16 fellowships with full tuition reimbursements available (averaging $48,116 per year), 21 research assistantships with full tuition reimbursements available (averaging $21,807 per year), 3 teaching assistantships with full tuition reimbursements available (averaging $13,680 per year); scholarships/grants, traineeships, unspecified assistantships, and hourly employment positions also available. Financial award application deadline: 2/1. *Faculty research:* Chromosomes and telomeres in cancer and other human disease states, ambient environmental exposures, radiation physics and dosimetry, cellular toxicity, noise exposure assessment. *Total annual research expenditures:* $8.4 million. *Unit head:* Dr. Jac A. Nickoloff, Professor/Department Head, 970-491-6674, Fax: 970-491-0623, E-mail: j.nickoloff@colostate.edu. *Application contact:* Jeanne A. Brockway, Graduate Program Coordinator, 970-491-5003, Fax: 970-491-2940, E-mail: jeanne.brockway@colostate.edu.
Website: http://csu-cvmbs.colostate.edu/academics/erhs/Pages/graduate-studies.aspx

Columbia Southern University, College of Safety and Emergency Services, Orange Beach, AL 36561. Offers criminal justice administration (MS); emergency services management (MS); occupational safety and health (MS), including environmental management. *Program availability:* Part-time, evening/weekend, online learning. *Entrance requirements:* For master's, bachelor's degree from accredited/approved institution. Additional exam requirements/recommendations for international students: Required—TOEFL. Electronic applications accepted.

Columbia University, Columbia University Mailman School of Public Health, Department of Environmental Health Sciences, New York, NY 10032. Offers MPH, Dr PH, PhD. PhD offered in cooperation with the Graduate School of Arts and Sciences. *Accreditation:* CEPH (one or more programs are accredited). *Program availability:* Part-time. *Students:* 46 full-time (40 women), 20 part-time (16 women); includes 25 minority (4 Black or African American, non-Hispanic/Latino; 12 Asian, non-Hispanic/Latino; 7 Hispanic/Latino; 2 Two or more races, non-Hispanic/Latino), 13 international. Average age 27. 157 applicants, 47% accepted, 27 enrolled. In 2015, 29 master's, 3 doctorates awarded. *Degree requirements:* For master's, thesis optional; for doctorate, thesis/dissertation. *Entrance requirements:* For master's, GRE General Test, 1 year of course work in biology, general chemistry, organic chemistry, and mathematics; for doctorate, GRE General Test, MPH or equivalent (for Dr PH). Additional exam requirements/recommendations for international students: Required—TOEFL (minimum score 600 paper-based; 100 iBT). *Application deadline:* For fall admission, 12/1 priority date for domestic and international students. Applications are processed on a rolling basis. Application fee: $120. Electronic applications accepted. *Financial support:* Research assistantships, teaching assistantships, career-related internships or fieldwork, and Federal Work-Study available. Support available to part-time students. Financial award application deadline: 2/1; financial award applicants required to submit FAFSA. *Faculty research:* Health effects of environmental and occupational exposure to chemicals and radiation, molecular epidemiology, risk assessment, molecular toxicology, environmental policy. *Unit head:* Dr. Andrea Baccarelli, Chair, 212-305-3466, Fax: 212-305-4012. *Application contact:* Dr. Joseph Korevec, Senior Director of Admissions and Financial Aid, 212-305-8698, Fax: 212-342-1861, E-mail: ph-admit@columbia.edu.
Website: https://www.mailman.columbia.edu/become-student/departments/environmental-health-sciences

Duke University, Graduate School, Integrated Toxicology and Environmental Health Program, Durham, NC 27708. Offers Certificate. *Entrance requirements:* Additional exam requirements/recommendations for international students: Required—TOEFL (minimum score 577 paper-based; 90 iBT) or IELTS (minimum score 7). Electronic applications accepted.

East Carolina University, Graduate School, College of Health and Human Performance, Department of Health Education and Promotion, Greenville, NC 27858-4353. Offers environmental health (MS); health education (MA Ed); health education and promotion (MA). *Accreditation:* NCATE. *Students:* 29 full-time (21 women), 60 part-time (43 women); includes 22 minority (18 Black or African American, non-Hispanic/Latino; 1 Asian, non-Hispanic/Latino; 2 Hispanic/Latino; 1 Two or more races, non-Hispanic/Latino). Average age 30. 54 applicants, 81% accepted, 41 enrolled. In 2015, 24 master's awarded. *Degree requirements:* For master's, comprehensive exam, thesis optional. *Entrance requirements:* For master's, GRE General Test or MAT. Additional exam requirements/recommendations for international students: Required—TOEFL. *Application deadline:* For fall admission, 6/1 priority date for domestic students. Applications are processed on a rolling basis. Application fee: $50. *Financial support:* Fellowships, research assistantships, teaching assistantships, and career-related internships or fieldwork available. Support available to part-time students. Financial award application deadline: 6/1. *Faculty research:* Community health education, worksite health promotion, school health education, environmental health. *Unit head:* Dr. J. Don Chaney, Chair, 252-737-4942, E-mail: chaneyj@ecu.edu.
Website: http://www.ecu.edu/hlth/

East Carolina University, Graduate School, Thomas Harriot College of Arts and Sciences, Department of Psychology, Greenville, NC 27858-4353. Offers health psychology (PhD), including clinical health psychology, occupational health psychology, pediatric school psychology; industrial and organizational psychology (MA); MA/CAS. *Program availability:* Part-time, evening/weekend. *Students:* 89 full-time (68 women), 19

part-time (11 women); includes 14 minority (6 Black or African American, non-Hispanic/Latino; 1 Asian, non-Hispanic/Latino; 5 Hispanic/Latino; 2 Two or more races, non-Hispanic/Latino), 1 international. Average age 25. 316 applicants, 21% accepted, 33 enrolled. In 2015, 9 master's, 3 doctorates awarded. *Degree requirements:* For master's, one foreign language, comprehensive exam, thesis. *Entrance requirements:* For master's, GRE General Test, GRE Subject Test. Additional exam requirements/recommendations for international students: Required—TOEFL. *Application deadline:* Applications are processed on a rolling basis. Application fee: $50. *Financial support:* Research assistantships with partial tuition reimbursements, teaching assistantships with partial tuition reimbursements, Federal Work-Study, and traineeships available. Support available to part-time students. Financial award application deadline: 6/1. *Unit head:* Dr. Susan L. McCammon, Chair, 252-328-6357, E-mail: mccammons@ecu.edu. *Application contact:* Dean of Graduate School, 252-328-6012, Fax: 252-328-6071, E-mail: gradschool@ecu.edu.
Website: http://www.ecu.edu/psyc/

Eastern Kentucky University, The Graduate School, College of Health Sciences, Department of Clinical Laboratory Science/Environmental Health Science, Richmond, KY 40475-3102. Offers environmental health science (MPH). *Accreditation:* CEPH. *Degree requirements:* For master's, comprehensive exam, thesis optional, practicum, capstone course. *Entrance requirements:* For master's, GRE. *Faculty research:* Water quality, food safety, occupational health, air quality.

East Tennessee State University, School of Graduate Studies, College of Public Health, Department of Environmental Health, Johnson City, TN 37614. Offers MSEH, PhD. *Program availability:* Part-time. *Faculty:* 6 full-time (1 woman), 1 (woman) part-time/adjunct. *Students:* 5 full-time (2 women), 1 part-time (0 women), 3 international. Average age 31. 8 applicants, 38% accepted, 3 enrolled. In 2015, 1 master's awarded. *Degree requirements:* For master's, comprehensive exam, research project or thesis; environmental health practice; seminar; for doctorate, comprehensive exam, thesis/dissertation, environmental health practice, seminar. *Entrance requirements:* For master's, GRE General Test, 30 hours of course work in natural and physical sciences, minimum GPA of 3.0, SOPHAS application, three letters of recommendation; for doctorate, GRE General Test, MPH or MS in related field of study with research-based thesis, SOPHAS application, three letters of recommendation, curriculum vitae or resume. Additional exam requirements/recommendations for international students: Required—TOEFL (minimum score 550 paper-based; 79 iBT). *Application deadline:* For fall admission, 6/1 for domestic students, 4/30 for international students; for spring admission, 11/1 for domestic students, 9/30 for international students. Application fee: $35 ($45 for international students). Electronic applications accepted. *Financial support:* In 2015–16, 3 students received support, including 3 research assistantships with full tuition reimbursements available (averaging $14,000 per year); career-related internships or fieldwork, institutionally sponsored loans, scholarships/grants, and unspecified assistantships also available. Financial award application deadline: 7/1; financial award applicants required to submit FAFSA. *Faculty research:* Water quality, ecotoxicology, occupational health, indoor air quality, community-focused environmental health. *Unit head:* Dr. Kurt Maier, Chair, 423-439-5251, Fax: 423-439-5230, E-mail: maier@etsu.edu. *Application contact:* Mary Duncan, Graduate Specialist, 423-439-4302, Fax: 423-439-5624, E-mail: duncanm@etsu.edu.
Website: http://www.etsu.edu/cph/eh/

Embry-Riddle Aeronautical University–Prescott, Department of Behavioral and Safety Sciences, Prescott, AZ 86301-3720. Offers aviation safety (MSSS); occupational health and safety (MSSS). *Program availability:* Part-time. *Faculty:* 5 full-time (0 women). *Students:* 28 full-time (5 women), 7 part-time (0 women); includes 6 minority (1 Black or African American, non-Hispanic/Latino; 2 Hispanic/Latino; 3 Two or more races, non-Hispanic/Latino), 10 international. Average age 31. 32 applicants, 59% accepted, 8 enrolled. In 2015, 10 master's awarded. *Degree requirements:* For master's, research project or thesis. *Entrance requirements:* Additional exam requirements/recommendations for international students: Required—TOEFL (minimum score 550 paper-based, 79 iBT) or IELTS (6). *Application deadline:* Applications are processed on a rolling basis. Application fee: $50. Electronic applications accepted. *Expenses: Tuition, area resident:* Full-time $15,972; part-time $7986 per credit hour. *Required fees:* $1200; $600 per semester. *Financial support:* In 2015–16, 12 students received support, including 6 research assistantships (averaging $5,666 per year); career-related internships or fieldwork and unspecified assistantships also available. Financial award application deadline: 3/15; financial award applicants required to submit FAFSA. *Faculty research:* Service quality in aviation, engineering psychology, accident investigation and analysis, occupational safety/biomechanics, crash management/response/survivability. *Unit head:* Erin E. Bowen, PhD, Department Chair/Associate Professor, Safety Science, 928-777-6960, E-mail: erin.bowen@erau.edu. *Application contact:* Graduate Admissions, 928-777-6600, E-mail: prescottgradinfo@erau.edu.
Website: http://prescott.erau.edu/degrees/master/safety-science/index.html

Embry-Riddle Aeronautical University–Worldwide, Department of Aeronautics, Graduate Studies, Daytona Beach, FL 32114-3900. Offers aeronautical science (MAS); aviation maintenance (MS); human factors (MS); occupational safety management (MS); unmanned systems (MS). *Program availability:* Part-time, evening/weekend, 100% online, blended/hybrid learning, EagleVision Classroom (between classrooms), EagleVision Home (faculty and students at home), and a blend of Classroom or Home. *Students:* 882 full-time (145 women), 1,072 part-time (163 women); includes 435 minority (163 Black or African American, non-Hispanic/Latino; 9 American Indian or Alaska Native, non-Hispanic/Latino; 58 Asian, non-Hispanic/Latino; 68 Hispanic/Latino; 6 Native Hawaiian or other Pacific Islander, non-Hispanic/Latino; 131 Two or more races, non-Hispanic/Latino), 114 international. Average age 37. In 2015, 691 master's awarded. *Degree requirements:* For master's, comprehensive exam (for some programs), thesis optional, thesis or capstone project. *Entrance requirements:* Additional exam requirements/recommendations for international students: Required—TOEFL (minimum score 550 paper-based, 79 iBT) or IELTS (6). *Application deadline:* Applications are processed on a rolling basis. Application fee: $50. Electronic applications accepted. *Expenses: Tuition, area resident:* Full-time $6960; part-time $580 per credit hour. Tuition and fees vary according to degree level and program. *Financial support:* Career-related internships or fieldwork available. Financial award applicants required to submit FAFSA. *Faculty research:* Aerodynamics statistical design and educational development. *Unit head:* Dr. Ian McAndrew, Professor and Chair, Aeronautics, 011-441638542916, E-mail: ian.mcandrew@erau.edu. *Application contact:* Admissions Department, 800-522-6787, Fax: 386-226-6894, E-mail: worldwide@erau.edu.
Website: http://worldwide.erau.edu/degrees-programs/colleges/aeronautics/department-of-graduate-studies/index.html

Emory University, Rollins School of Public Health, Department of Environmental Health, Atlanta, GA 30322-1100. Offers environmental health (MPH); environmental health and epidemiology (MSPH); environmental health sciences (PhD); global environmental health (MPH). *Accreditation:* CEPH. *Program availability:* Part-time. *Degree requirements:* For master's, thesis, practicum. *Entrance requirements:* For master's, GRE General Test. Additional exam requirements/recommendations for international students: Required—TOEFL. Electronic applications accepted.

Florida International University, Robert Stempel College of Public Health and Social Work, Programs in Public Health, Miami, FL 33199. Offers biostatistics (MPH); environmental and occupational health (MPH, PhD); epidemiology (MPH, PhD); health policy and management (MPH); health promotion and disease prevention (PhD); health promotion and diseases prevention (MPH). Ph D program has fall admissions only; MPH offered jointly with University of Miami. *Accreditation:* CEPH. *Program availability:* Part-time, evening/weekend, online learning. *Faculty:* 27 full-time (12 women), 2 part-time/adjunct (1 woman). *Students:* 126 full-time (80 women), 62 part-time (46 women); includes 129 minority (47 Black or African American, non-Hispanic/Latino; 10 Asian, non-Hispanic/Latino; 69 Hispanic/Latino; 3 Two or more races, non-Hispanic/Latino), 32 international. Average age 30. 298 applicants, 35% accepted, 68 enrolled. In 2015, 67 master's, 10 doctorates awarded. *Degree requirements:* For master's, thesis optional; for doctorate, comprehensive exam, thesis/dissertation. *Entrance requirements:* For master's, minimum GPA of 3.0, letters of recommendation; for doctorate, GRE, resume, minimum GPA of 3.0, letters of recommendation, letter of intent. Additional exam requirements/recommendations for international students: Required—TOEFL (minimum score 550 paper-based; 80 iBT). *Application deadline:* For fall admission, 6/1 for domestic students, 4/1 for international students; for spring admission, 10/1 for domestic students, 9/1 for international students. Applications are processed on a rolling basis. Application fee: $30. Electronic applications accepted. *Expenses:* Contact institution. *Financial support:* Institutionally sponsored loans, scholarships/grants, and tuition waivers (full) available. Financial award application deadline: 3/1; financial award applicants required to submit FAFSA. *Faculty research:* Drugs/AIDS intervention among migrant workers, provision of services for active/recovering drug users with HIV. *Unit head:* Dr. Benjamin C. Amick, III, Chair, 305-348-4903, E-mail: benjamin.amickiii@fiu.edu. *Application contact:* Dr. Vukosava Pekovic, Director, 305-348-1823, Fax: 305-348-4901, E-mail: pekovic@fiu.edu.

Fort Valley State University, College of Graduate Studies and Extended Education, Program in Public Health, Fort Valley, GA 31030. Offers environmental health (MPH). *Degree requirements:* For master's, thesis. *Entrance requirements:* For master's, GRE General Test. Additional exam requirements/recommendations for international students: Recommended—TOEFL. *Application deadline:* For fall admission, 8/23 for domestic students. Applications are processed on a rolling basis. Application fee: $20. *Financial support:* Federal Work-Study and unspecified assistantships available. Support available to part-time students. *Unit head:* Dr. Oreta Samples, 478-825-6904, E-mail: sampleso@fvsu.edu. *Application contact:* Dr. Oreta Samples, 478-825-6904, E-mail: sampleso@fvsu.edu.

Gannon University, School of Graduate Studies, College of Engineering and Business, School of Engineering and Computer Science, Program in Environmental Science and Engineering, Erie, PA 16541-0001. Offers environmental health and engineering (MS). *Program availability:* Part-time, evening/weekend. *Students:* 6 full-time (3 women), 3 international. Average age 26. 80 applicants, 26% accepted, 4 enrolled. In 2015, 5 master's awarded. *Degree requirements:* For master's, thesis (for some programs), research paper or project (for some programs). *Entrance requirements:* For master's, GRE, bachelor's degree in science or engineering from an accredited college or university. Additional exam requirements/recommendations for international students: Required—TOEFL (minimum score 79 iBT). *Application deadline:* Applications are processed on a rolling basis. Application fee: $25. Electronic applications accepted. Application fee is waived when completed online. *Financial support:* Federal Work-Study and unspecified assistantships available. Financial award application deadline: 7/1; financial award applicants required to submit FAFSA. *Unit head:* Dr. Harry Diz, Chair, 814-871-7633, E-mail: diz001@gannon.edu. *Application contact:* Bridget Philip, Director of Graduate Admissions, 814-871-7412, E-mail: graduate@gannon.edu.

The George Washington University, Milken Institute School of Public Health, Department of Environmental and Occupational Health, Washington, DC 20052. Offers Dr PH. *Accreditation:* CEPH. *Faculty:* 12 full-time (6 women), 9 part-time/adjunct (7 women). *Students:* 4 full-time (3 women), 7 part-time (5 women); includes 4 minority (1 Black or African American, non-Hispanic/Latino; 2 Asian, non-Hispanic/Latino; 1 Hispanic/Latino), 2 international. Average age 34. 20 applicants, 40% accepted, 5 enrolled. In 2015, 1 doctorate awarded. *Entrance requirements:* Additional exam requirements/recommendations for international students: Required—TOEFL. *Application deadline:* For fall admission, 4/15 priority date for domestic students, 4/15 for international students; for spring admission, 11/1 for domestic and international students. Applications are processed on a rolling basis. Application fee: $75. *Financial support:* In 2015–16, 7 students received support. Tuition waivers available. Financial award application deadline: 2/15. *Unit head:* Dr. Melissa Perry, Director, 202-994-1734, E-mail: mperry@gwu.edu. *Application contact:* Jane Smith, Director of Admissions, 202-994-0248, Fax: 202-994-1860, E-mail: sphhsinfo@gwumc.edu.

Georgia Southern University, Jack N. Averitt College of Graduate Studies, Allen E. Paulson College of Engineering and Information Technology, Department of Mechanical Engineering, Program in Occupational Safety and Environmental Compliance, Statesboro, GA 30458. Offers Graduate Certificate. *Students:* 2 applicants, 100% accepted. In 2015, 4 Graduate Certificates awarded. *Entrance requirements:* Additional exam requirements/recommendations for international students: Required—TOEFL (minimum score 550 paper-based; 80 iBT), IELTS (minimum score 6). *Application deadline:* For fall admission, 3/1 priority date for domestic students; for spring admission, 11/1 priority date for domestic students. Applications are processed on a rolling basis. Application fee: $50. Electronic applications accepted. *Expenses:* Tuition, state resident: full-time $7236; part-time $277 per semester hour. Tuition, nonresident: full-time $27,118; part-time $1105 per semester hour. *Required fees:* $2092. *Financial support:* Applicants required to submit FAFSA. *Faculty research:* Mechatronics, mechanical engineering, electronic systems, electrical systems, energy science. *Unit head:* Dr. Frank Goforth, Chair, 912-478-7583, Fax: 912-478-1455, E-mail: fgoforth@georgiasouthern.edu.

Georgia Southern University, Jack N. Averitt College of Graduate Studies, Jiann-Ping Hsu College of Public Health, Program in Public Health, Statesboro, GA 30460. Offers biostatistics (MPH, Dr PH); community health behavior and education (Dr PH); community health education (MPH); environmental health sciences (MPH); epidemiology (MPH); health policy and management (MPH, Dr PH). *Accreditation:* CEPH. *Program availability:* Part-time. *Students:* 129 full-time (86 women), 41 part-time (32 women); includes 87 minority (67 Black or African American, non-Hispanic/Latino; 6 Asian, non-Hispanic/Latino; 8 Hispanic/Latino; 6 Two or more races, non-Hispanic/Latino), 30 international. Average age 30. 218 applicants, 63% accepted, 41 enrolled. In 2015, 37 master's, 8 doctorates awarded. *Degree requirements:* For master's, thesis optional, practicum; for doctorate, comprehensive exam, thesis/dissertation, practicum. *Entrance requirements:* For master's, GRE General Test, minimum GPA of 2.75, resume, 3 letters of reference; for doctorate, GRE, GMAT, MCAT, LSAT, 3 letters of reference, statement of purpose, resume or curriculum vitae. Additional exam requirements/recommendations for international students: Required—TOEFL (minimum score 550 paper-based; 80 iBT), IELTS (minimum score 6). *Application deadline:* For fall admission, 6/1 priority date for domestic and international students; for spring admission, 10/1 priority date for domestic students, 10/1 for international students. Applications are processed on a rolling basis. Application fee: $50. Electronic

Environmental and Occupational Health

applications accepted. *Expenses:* $335 per credit hour. *Financial support:* In 2015–16, 93 students received support, including 23 fellowships with full tuition reimbursements available (averaging $7,750 per year), 1 research assistantship with full tuition reimbursement available (averaging $7,750 per year), 1 teaching assistantship with full tuition reimbursement available (averaging $7,750 per year); career-related internships or fieldwork, Federal Work-Study, scholarships/grants, tuition waivers (full), and unspecified assistantships also available. Support available to part-time students. Financial award application deadline: 4/15; financial award applicants required to submit FAFSA. *Faculty research:* Rural public health best practices, health disparity elimination, community initiatives to enhance public health, cost effectiveness analysis, epidemiology of rural public health, environmental health issues, health care system assessment, rural health care, health policy and healthcare financing, survival analysis, nonparametric statistics and resampling methods, micro-arrays and genomics, data imputation techniques and clinical trial methodology. *Total annual research expenditures:* $281,707. *Unit head:* Dr. Shamia Garrett, Program Coordinator, 912-478-2393, E-mail: sgarrett@georgiasouthern.edu.
Website: http://chhs.georgiasouthern.edu/health/

Harvard University, Cyprus International Institute for the Environment and Public Health in Association with Harvard School of Public Health, Cambridge, MA 02138. Offers environmental health (MS); environmental/public health (PhD); epidemiology and biostatistics (MS). *Entrance requirements:* For master's and doctorate, GRE, resume/curriculum vitae, 3 letters of recommendation, BA or BS (including diploma and official transcripts). Additional exam requirements/recommendations for international students: Required—TOEFL, IELTS (minimum score 7). Electronic applications accepted. *Faculty research:* Air pollution, climate change, biostatistics, sustainable development, environmental management.

Harvard University, Harvard T.H. Chan School of Public Health, Department of Environmental Health, Boston, MA 02115-6096. Offers environmental health (SM, PhD, SD); exposure, epidemiology, and risk (SM, SD); occupational health (SM, SD); physiology (PhD, SD). *Program availability:* Part-time. *Faculty:* 44 full-time (10 women), 20 part-time/adjunct (5 women). *Students:* 79 full-time (49 women); includes 11 minority (1 Black or African American, non-Hispanic/Latino; 6 Asian, non-Hispanic/Latino; 3 Hispanic/Latino; 1 Two or more races, non-Hispanic/Latino), 45 international. Average age 28. 126 applicants, 35% accepted, 34 enrolled. In 2015, 20 master's, 12 doctorates awarded. *Degree requirements:* For doctorate, thesis/dissertation, qualifying exam. *Entrance requirements:* For master's, GRE, MCAT; for doctorate, GRE. Additional exam requirements/recommendations for international students: Recommended—TOEFL (minimum score 600 paper-based; 100 iBT), IELTS (minimum score 7). *Application deadline:* For fall admission, 12/15 for domestic and international students. Application fee: $120. Electronic applications accepted. *Financial support:* Fellowships, research assistantships, teaching assistantships, career-related internships or fieldwork, Federal Work-Study, scholarships/grants, traineeships, and unspecified assistantships available. Support available to part-time students. Financial award application deadline: 2/15; financial award applicants required to submit FAFSA. *Faculty research:* Exposure assessment, epidemiology, risk assessment, environmental epidemiology, ergonomics and safety, environmental exposure assessment, occupational hygiene, industrial hygiene and occupational safety, population genetics, indoor and outdoor air pollution, cell and molecular biology of the lungs, infectious diseases. *Unit head:* Dr. Douglas Dockery, Chairman, 617-432-1270, Fax: 617-432-6913. *Application contact:* Vincent W. James, Director of Admissions, 617-432-1031, Fax: 617-432-7080, E-mail: admissions@hsph.harvard.edu.
Website: http://www.hsph.harvard.edu/environmental-health/

Hunter College of the City University of New York, Graduate School, Schools of the Health Professions, School of Health Sciences, Programs in Urban Public Health, Program in Environmental and Occupational Health Sciences, New York, NY 10065-5085. Offers MPH, MS. *Accreditation:* ABET (one or more programs are accredited); CEPH. *Program availability:* Part-time, evening/weekend. *Students:* 2 full-time (1 woman), 20 part-time (7 women); includes 12 minority (6 Black or African American, non-Hispanic/Latino; 5 Asian, non-Hispanic/Latino; 1 Hispanic/Latino). Average age 30. 27 applicants, 63% accepted, 12 enrolled. *Degree requirements:* For master's, comprehensive exam, thesis optional, internship. *Entrance requirements:* For master's, GRE General Test, previous course work in calculus and statistics. Additional exam requirements/recommendations for international students: Required—TOEFL. *Application deadline:* For fall admission, 4/1 for domestic students, 2/1 for international students; for spring admission, 11/1 for domestic students, 9/1 for international students. *Financial support:* In 2015–16, 6 fellowships were awarded; career-related internships or fieldwork, Federal Work-Study, institutionally sponsored loans, and tuition waivers (partial) also available. Support available to part-time students. Financial award application deadline: 3/1. *Faculty research:* Hazardous waste, asbestos, lead exposures, worker training, public employees. *Unit head:* Jack Caravanos, Director, 212-396-7780. *Application contact:* Milena Solo, Director for Graduate Admissions, 212-772-4280, E-mail: admissions@hunter.cuny.edu.
Website: http://cuny.edu/site/sph/hunter-college/a-programs/graduate/eohs/eohs-mph.html

Indiana State University, College of Graduate and Professional Studies, College of Technology, Department of Built Environment, Terre Haute, IN 47809. Offers occupational safety management (MS).

Indiana University Bloomington, School of Public Health, Department of Environmental Health, Bloomington, IN 47405. Offers MPH, PhD. *Degree requirements:* For doctorate, comprehensive exam, thesis/dissertation. *Entrance requirements:* For master's, GRE if cumulative GPA less than 2.8; for doctorate, GRE. Additional exam requirements/recommendations for international students: Required—TOEFL (minimum score 550 paper-based; 80 iBT). Electronic applications accepted. *Faculty research:* Toxicology, environmental health, oxidative stress, cancer biology.

Indiana University of Pennsylvania, School of Graduate Studies and Research, College of Health and Human Services, Department of Safety Sciences, MS Program in Safety Sciences, Indiana, PA 15705-1087. Offers MS. *Program availability:* Part-time, online learning. *Faculty:* 8 full-time (2 women). *Students:* 15 full-time (1 woman), 44 part-time (11 women); includes 7 minority (2 Black or African American, non-Hispanic/Latino; 1 Asian, non-Hispanic/Latino; 4 Hispanic/Latino), 3 international. Average age 30. 70 applicants, 54% accepted, 21 enrolled. In 2015, 33 master's awarded. *Degree requirements:* For master's, thesis optional. *Entrance requirements:* For master's, 2 letters of recommendation. Additional exam requirements/recommendations for international students: Required—TOEFL (minimum score 540 paper-based). *Application deadline:* For fall admission, 4/1 priority date for domestic students. Applications are processed on a rolling basis. Application fee: $50. Electronic applications accepted. *Financial support:* In 2015–16, 5 fellowships with full tuition reimbursements (averaging $781 per year), 6 research assistantships with tuition reimbursements (averaging $5,830 per year) were awarded; teaching assistantships, career-related internships or fieldwork, Federal Work-Study, scholarships/grants, and unspecified assistantships also available. Financial award application deadline: 4/15; financial award applicants required to submit FAFSA. *Unit head:* Dr. Chris Janicak,

Graduate Coordinator, 724-357-3274, E-mail: cjanicak@iup.edu.
Website: http://www.iup.edu/grad/safety/default.aspx

Indiana University of Pennsylvania, School of Graduate Studies and Research, College of Health and Human Services, Department of Safety Sciences, PhD Program in Safety Sciences, Indiana, PA 15705-1087. Offers PhD. *Program availability:* Online learning. *Faculty:* 8 full-time (0 women), 34 part-time (9 women); includes 8 minority (5 Black or African American, non-Hispanic/Latino; 3 Hispanic/Latino), 1 international. Average age 46. 58 applicants, 43% accepted, 17 enrolled. *Degree requirements:* For doctorate, thesis/dissertation. *Entrance requirements:* For doctorate, GRE, master's degree in safety sciences or closely-related field such as industrial hygiene, environmental health, or ergonomics; minimum graduate GPA of 3.0; official transcripts; three letters of recommendation; statement of goals; resume; sample of written work. Additional exam requirements/recommendations for international students: Required—TOEFL (minimum score 540 paper-based). Application fee: $50. *Financial support:* In 2015–16, 2 fellowships with full tuition reimbursements (averaging $1,138 per year), 1 research assistantship with tuition reimbursement (averaging $3,515 per year), 2 teaching assistantships with partial tuition reimbursements (averaging $17,479 per year) were awarded; unspecified assistantships also available. *Unit head:* Dr. Chris Janicak, Coordinator, 724-357-3274, E-mail: cjanicak@iup.edu.
Website: http://www.iup.edu/safetysciences/grad/safety-sciences-phd/

Indiana University–Purdue University Indianapolis, School of Public and Environmental Affairs, Indianapolis, IN 46202. Offers criminal justice and public safety (MS); homeland security and emergency management (Graduate Certificate); library management (Graduate Certificate); nonprofit management (Graduate Certificate); public affairs (MPA); public management (Graduate Certificate); social entrepreneurship: nonprofit and public benefit organizations (Graduate Certificate); JD/MPA; MLS/NMC; MLS/PMC; MPA/MA. *Accreditation:* CAHME (one or more programs are accredited); NASPAA. *Program availability:* Part-time, evening/weekend, online learning. *Entrance requirements:* For master's, GRE General Test, GMAT or LSAT, minimum GPA of 3.0 (preferred). Additional exam requirements/recommendations for international students: Required—TOEFL (minimum score 93 iBT), IELTS (minimum score 6.5). Electronic applications accepted. *Faculty research:* Nonprofit and public management, public policy, urban policy, sustainability policy, disaster preparedness and recovery, vehicular safety, homicide, offender rehabilitation and re-entry.

Indiana University–Purdue University Indianapolis, School of Public Health, Indianapolis, IN 46202. Offers biostatistics (MPH); environmental health science (MPH); epidemiology (MPH, PhD); health administration (MHA); health policy and management (MPH, PhD); social and behavioral sciences (MPH). *Accreditation:* CEPH. *Expenses:* Contact institution.

Johns Hopkins University, Bloomberg School of Public Health, Department of Environmental Health Sciences, Baltimore, MD 21218. Offers environmental health engineering (PhD); environmental health sciences (MHS, Dr PH); occupational and environmental health (PhD); physiology (PhD); toxicology (PhD). *Program availability:* Online learning. *Degree requirements:* For master's, essay, presentation; for doctorate, comprehensive exam, thesis/dissertation, 1-year full-time residency, oral and written exams. *Entrance requirements:* For master's, GRE General Test or MCAT, 3 letters of recommendation, transcripts; for doctorate, GRE General Test or MCAT, 3 letters of recommendation. Additional exam requirements/recommendations for international students: Required—TOEFL (minimum score 600 paper-based). Electronic applications accepted. *Faculty research:* Chemical carcinogenesis/toxicology, lung disease, occupational and environmental health, nuclear imaging, molecular epidemiology.

Keene State College, School of Professional and Graduate Studies, Keene, NH 03435. Offers curriculum and instruction (M Ed); education leadership (PMC); educational leadership (M Ed); safety and occupational health applied science (MS); school counselor (M Ed, PMC); special education (M Ed). *Accreditation:* NCATE. *Program availability:* Part-time, evening/weekend. *Faculty:* 11 full-time (6 women), 9 part-time/adjunct (5 women). *Students:* 28 full-time (22 women), 67 part-time (47 women); includes 5 minority (3 Hispanic/Latino; 2 Two or more races, non-Hispanic/Latino). Average age 32. 40 applicants, 75% accepted, 24 enrolled. In 2015, 38 master's awarded. *Degree requirements:* For master's, thesis (for some programs). *Entrance requirements:* For master's, PRAXIS I, 3 references; official transcripts; minimum GPA of 2.5; interview; essay; teacher/educator certificate; work/internship experience. Additional exam requirements/recommendations for international students: Required—TOEFL (minimum score 550 paper-based; 61 iBT). *Application deadline:* For fall admission, 4/1 for domestic and international students; for spring admission, 11/1 for domestic and international students; for summer admission, 3/1 for domestic and international students. Applications are processed on a rolling basis. Application fee: $50. Electronic applications accepted. *Expenses:* Tuition, state resident: full-time $4500; part-time $500 per credit. Tuition, nonresident: full-time $4905; part-time $545 per credit. *Required fees:* $909; $101 per credit. Tuition and fees vary according to course load. *Financial support:* In 2015–16, 27 students received support. Career-related internships or fieldwork, Federal Work-Study, institutionally sponsored loans, scholarships/grants, and unspecified assistantships available. Support available to part-time students. Financial award application deadline: 3/1; financial award applicants required to submit FAFSA. *Unit head:* Dr. Rebecca Lytle, Dean of Professional and Graduate Studies, 603-358-2220, E-mail: rebecca.lytle@keene.edu. *Application contact:* Graduate Studies Office, 603-358-2497, E-mail: kscgraduatestudies@keene.edu.
Website: http://www.keene.edu/academics/graduate/

Lewis University, College of Arts and Sciences, Program in Public Safety Administration, Romeoville, IL 60446. Offers MS. *Program availability:* Part-time, evening/weekend, online learning. *Entrance requirements:* For master's, bachelor's degree, 2 letters of recommendation. Additional exam requirements/recommendations for international students: Required—TOEFL (minimum score 500 paper-based; 80 iBT). Electronic applications accepted.

Loma Linda University, School of Public Health, Program in Environmental and Occupational Health, Loma Linda, CA 92350. Offers MPH. *Accreditation:* CEPH. *Entrance requirements:* Additional exam requirements/recommendations for international students: Required—Michigan English Language Assessment Battery or TOEFL. *Application deadline:* Applications are processed on a rolling basis. Application fee: $100. *Financial support:* Application deadline: 5/15. *Faculty research:* Human exposure to toxins, smog. *Unit head:* Robin Smith, Director, 909-824-4918, Fax: 909-824-4087, E-mail: rdsmith@llu.edu. *Application contact:* Wendy Genovez, Assistant Dean of Admissions and Records, 909-824-4694, Fax: 909-824-8087, E-mail: wgenovez@llu.edu.

Louisiana State University Health Sciences Center, School of Public Health, New Orleans, LA 70112. Offers behavioral and community health sciences (MPH); biostatistics (MPH, MS, PhD); community health sciences (PhD); environmental and occupational health sciences (MPH); epidemiology (MPH, PhD); health policy and systems management (MPH). *Accreditation:* CEPH. *Program availability:* Part-time. *Entrance requirements:* For master's, GRE General Test.

McGill University, Faculty of Graduate and Postdoctoral Studies, Faculty of Medicine, Department of Epidemiology and Biostatistics, Montréal, QC H3A 2T5, Canada. Offers community health (M Sc); environmental health (M Sc); epidemiology and biostatistics (M Sc, PhD, Diploma); health care evaluation (M Sc); medical statistics (M Sc). *Accreditation:* CEPH (one or more programs are accredited).

McGill University, Faculty of Graduate and Postdoctoral Studies, Faculty of Medicine and Department of Epidemiology and Biostatistics, Department of Occupational Health, Montréal, QC H3A 2T5, Canada. Offers M Sc, PhD.

Meharry Medical College, School of Graduate Studies, Division of Community Health Sciences, Nashville, TN 37208-9989. Offers occupational medicine (MSPH); public health administration (MSPH). *Accreditation:* CEPH. *Program availability:* Part-time, evening/weekend. *Degree requirements:* For master's, thesis, externship. *Entrance requirements:* For master's, GRE General Test, GMAT. *Application deadline:* For fall admission, 6/1 for domestic students. Applications are processed on a rolling basis. Application fee: $65. *Expenses:* Contact institution. *Financial support:* Career-related internships or fieldwork, Federal Work-Study, institutionally sponsored loans, and scholarships/grants available. Support available to part-time students. Financial award application deadline: 7/15; financial award applicants required to submit FAFSA.

Mercer University, Graduate Studies, Cecil B. Day Campus, Penfield College, Atlanta, GA 30341. Offers certified rehabilitation counseling (MS); clinical mental health (MS); counselor education and supervision (PhD); human services (MS), including child and adolescent services, gerontology services; organizational leadership (MS); public safety leadership (MS); school counseling (MS). *Program availability:* Part-time, evening/weekend, 100% online, blended/hybrid learning. *Faculty:* 17 full-time (9 women), 22 part-time/adjunct (18 women). *Students:* 132 full-time (109 women), 249 part-time (211 women); includes 212 minority (173 Black or African American, non-Hispanic/Latino; 3 American Indian or Alaska Native, non-Hispanic/Latino; 14 Asian, non-Hispanic/Latino; 17 Hispanic/Latino; 2 Native Hawaiian or other Pacific Islander, non-Hispanic/Latino; 3 Two or more races, non-Hispanic/Latino), 4 international. Average age 32. 300 applicants, 45% accepted, 114 enrolled. In 2015, 115 master's, 3 doctorates awarded. *Degree requirements:* For master's, comprehensive exam (for some programs), thesis (for some programs); for doctorate, thesis/dissertation. *Entrance requirements:* For master's, GRE or MAT, Georgia Professional Standards Commission (GPSC) Certification at the SC-5 level; for doctorate, GRE or MAT. Additional exam requirements/recommendations for international students: Recommended—TOEFL (minimum score 550 paper-based; 80 iBT), IELTS (minimum score 6.5). *Application deadline:* For fall admission, 7/1 priority date for domestic and international students; for spring admission, 11/1 priority date for domestic and international students; for summer admission, 4/1 priority date for domestic and international students. Application fee: $35. Electronic applications accepted. Application fee is waived when completed online. *Expenses:* $560 per credit hour (for master's-level courses); $689 per credit hour (for doctorate-level courses). *Financial support:* In 2015–16, 32 students received support. Federal Work-Study, scholarships/grants, and unspecified assistantships available. Financial award applicants required to submit FAFSA. *Faculty research:* Marriage and families issues, leadership and ethics, cyber-bullying, trauma, narrative counseling and theory. *Total annual research expenditures:* $85,000. *Unit head:* Dr. Priscilla R. Danheiser, Dean, 678-547-6028, Fax: 678-547-6008, E-mail: danheiser_p@mercer.edu. *Application contact:* Carmen C. Jones, Director of Graduate Admissions, 678-547-6346, E-mail: jones_c@mercer.edu.
Website: http://penfield.mercer.edu/programs/graduate-professional/

Murray State University, College of Health Sciences and Human Services, Program in Occupational Safety and Health, Murray, KY 42071. Offers environmental science (MS); industrial hygiene (MS); safety management (MS). *Accreditation:* ABET. *Program availability:* Part-time. *Degree requirements:* For master's, comprehensive exam, thesis optional, professional internship. Electronic applications accepted. *Faculty research:* Light effects on plant growth, ergonomics, toxic effects of pets' pesticides, traffic safety.

New York Medical College, School of Health Sciences and Practice, Department of Environmental Health Science, Program in Environmental Health Science, Valhalla, NY 10595-1691. Offers MPH, Graduate Certificate. *Expenses: Tuition, area resident:* Full-time $44,355; part-time $1025 per year. *Required fees:* $500; $95 per year. One-time fee: $140 part-time. Tuition and fees vary according to course load and program.

★ **New York University,** Graduate School of Arts and Science, Department of Environmental Medicine, New York, NY 10012-1019. Offers environmental health sciences (MS, PhD), including biostatistics (PhD), environmental hygiene (MS), epidemiology (PhD), ergonomics and biomechanics (PhD), exposure assessment and health effects (PhD), molecular toxicology/carcinogenesis (PhD), toxicology. *Program availability:* Part-time. Terminal master's awarded for partial completion of doctoral program. *Degree requirements:* For master's, thesis or alternative; for doctorate, one foreign language, thesis/dissertation, oral and written exams. *Entrance requirements:* For master's and doctorate, GRE General Test, minimum GPA of 3.0; bachelor's degree in biological, physical, or engineering science. Additional exam requirements/recommendations for international students: Required—TOEFL.

See Close-Up on page 851.

North Carolina Agricultural and Technical State University, School of Graduate Studies, School of Technology, Department of Construction Management and Occupational Safety and Health, Greensboro, NC 27411. Offers construction management (MSTM); environmental and occupational safety (MSTM); occupational safety and health (MSTM).

Northeastern State University, College of Business and Technology, Program in Environmental, Health, and Safety Management, Tahlequah, OK 74464. Offers MEHS. *Program availability:* Part-time, evening/weekend. *Faculty:* 6 full-time (2 women). *Students:* 5 full-time (3 women), 18 part-time (4 women); includes 14 minority (3 Black or African American, non-Hispanic/Latino; 7 American Indian or Alaska Native, non-Hispanic/Latino; 1 Asian, non-Hispanic/Latino; 1 Hispanic/Latino; 2 Two or more races, non-Hispanic/Latino), 2 international. Average age 35. In 2015, 5 master's awarded. *Degree requirements:* For master's, synergistic experience. *Entrance requirements:* For master's, GRE, MAT, minimum GPA of 2.5. Additional exam requirements/recommendations for international students: Required—TOEFL. *Application deadline:* For fall admission, 6/1 priority date for domestic students. Applications are processed on a rolling basis. Application fee: $25. Electronic applications accepted. *Expenses:* Tuition, state resident: part-time $189.60 per credit hour. Tuition, nonresident: part-time $462.60 per credit hour. *Required fees:* $37.40 per credit hour. *Financial support:* Teaching assistantships and Federal Work-Study available. Financial award application deadline: 3/1. *Unit head:* Dr. Benjamin Ofili, Department Chair, 918-444-2940, E-mail: ofili@nsuok.edu. *Application contact:* Robin Hunter, Department Secretary, 918-444-3086, E-mail: hixrr@nsouk.edu.
Website: http://academics.nsuok.edu/businesstechnology/Graduate/MEHS.aspx

Oakland University, Graduate Study and Lifelong Learning, School of Health Sciences, Environmental Health and Safety Program, Rochester, MI 48309-4401. Offers safety management (MS). *Faculty:* 1 full-time (0 women), 1 part-time/adjunct (0 women).

Students: 1 full-time (0 women), 14 part-time (4 women); includes 3 minority (2 Black or African American, non-Hispanic/Latino; 1 American Indian or Alaska Native, non-Hispanic/Latino). Average age 36. 11 applicants, 36% accepted, 3 enrolled. In 2015, 8 master's awarded. *Application deadline:* For fall admission, 8/1 for domestic students; for winter admission, 12/1 for domestic students; for spring admission, 4/1 for domestic students. Application fee: $0. *Expenses: Tuition, area resident:* Part-time $655 per credit. Tuition and fees vary according to program. *Unit head:* Dr. Charles McGlothlin, Special Instructor/Program Director, 248-364-8651, E-mail: mcglothl@oakland.edu.

Oregon State University, College of Public Health and Human Sciences, Program in Public Health, Corvallis, OR 97331. Offers biostatistics (MPH); environmental and occupational health and safety (MPH, PhD); epidemiology (MPH, PhD); health management and policy (MPH); health policy (PhD); health promotion and health behavior (MPH, PhD); international health (MPH). *Accreditation:* CEPH. *Program availability:* Part-time. *Faculty:* 32 full-time (18 women), 3 part-time/adjunct (0 women). *Students:* 123 full-time (91 women), 20 part-time (14 women); includes 43 minority (2 Black or African American, non-Hispanic/Latino; 2 American Indian or Alaska Native, non-Hispanic/Latino; 9 Asian, non-Hispanic/Latino; 18 Hispanic/Latino; 1 Native Hawaiian or other Pacific Islander, non-Hispanic/Latino; 11 Two or more races, non-Hispanic/Latino), 18 international. Average age 31. 276 applicants, 65% accepted, 45 enrolled. In 2015, 59 master's, 6 doctorates awarded. Terminal master's awarded for partial completion of doctoral program. *Degree requirements:* For doctorate, one foreign language, thesis/dissertation. *Entrance requirements:* For master's and doctorate, GRE, minimum GPA of 3.0 in last 90 hours. Additional exam requirements/recommendations for international students: Required—TOEFL (minimum score 80 iBT), IELTS (minimum score 6.5). *Application deadline:* For fall admission, 12/1 priority date for domestic students. Applications are processed on a rolling basis. *Expenses:* $13,851 full-time resident tuition, $23,679 full-time non-resident tuition, $1,572 fees. *Financial support:* Fellowships, research assistantships, teaching assistantships, career-related internships or fieldwork, Federal Work-Study, and institutionally sponsored loans available. Support available to part-time students. Financial award application deadline: 12/1. *Faculty research:* Traffic safety, health safety, injury control, health promotion. *Unit head:* Dr. Sheryl Thorburn, Professor/Co-Director. *Application contact:* Amanda Armington, Public Health Program Manager, 541-737-3825, E-mail: amanda.armington@oregonstate.edu.

Purdue University, Graduate School, College of Health and Human Sciences, School of Health Sciences, West Lafayette, IN 47907. Offers health physics (MS, PhD); medical physics (MS, PhD); occupational and environmental health science (MS, PhD), including aerosol deposition and lung disease, ergonomics, exposure and risk assessment, indoor air quality and bioaerosols (PhD), liver/lung toxicology; radiation biology (PhD); toxicology (PhD); MS/PhD. *Program availability:* Part-time. *Degree requirements:* For master's, thesis optional; for doctorate, one foreign language, thesis/dissertation. *Entrance requirements:* For master's and doctorate, GRE General Test, minimum undergraduate GPA of 3.0 or equivalent. Additional exam requirements/recommendations for international students: Required—TOEFL (minimum score 550 paper-based; 77 iBT); Recommended—TWE. Electronic applications accepted. *Faculty research:* Environmental toxicology, industrial hygiene, radiation dosimetry.

Rochester Institute of Technology, Graduate Enrollment Services, College of Applied Science and Technology, School of Engineering Technology, MS Program in Environmental, Health and Safety Management, Rochester, NY 14623. Offers MS. *Program availability:* Part-time, evening/weekend, 100% online, blended/hybrid learning. *Students:* 16 full-time (8 women), 12 part-time (3 women); includes 5 minority (1 Black or African American, non-Hispanic/Latino; 2 Asian, non-Hispanic/Latino; 1 Hispanic/Latino; 1 Two or more races, non-Hispanic/Latino), 10 international. Average age 29. 48 applicants, 48% accepted, 16 enrolled. In 2015, 19 master's awarded. *Degree requirements:* For master's, thesis or alternative. *Entrance requirements:* For master's, minimum GPA of 3.0 (recommended). Additional exam requirements/recommendations for international students: Required—PTE (minimum score 58), TOEFL (minimum score 550 paper-based, 79 iBT) or IELTS (minimum score 6.5). *Application deadline:* Applications are processed on a rolling basis. Application fee: $60. Electronic applications accepted. *Expenses: Tuition, area resident:* Full-time $41,084; part-time $1742 per credit hour. *Required fees:* $274. Tuition and fees vary according to course load and program. *Financial support:* In 2015–16, 19 students received support. Research assistantships with partial tuition reimbursements available, teaching assistantships with partial tuition reimbursements available, career-related internships or fieldwork, scholarships/grants, and unspecified assistantships available. Support available to part-time students. Financial award applicants required to submit FAFSA. *Faculty research:* Air emissions, wastewater, solid and hazardous waste, occupational safety and occupational health (industrial hygiene), integrated environmental, health and safety management systems in industry. *Unit head:* Joseph Rosenbeck, Graduate Program Director, 585-475-6469, E-mail: jmrcem@rit.edu. *Application contact:* Diane Ellison, Associate Vice President, Graduate Enrollment Services, 585-475-2229, Fax: 585-475-7164, E-mail: gradinfo@rit.edu.
Website: http://www.rit.edu/cast/cetems/ms-environmental-health-safety-management

Rutgers University–New Brunswick, School of Public Health, Piscataway, NJ 08854. Offers biostatistics (MPH, MS, Dr PH, PhD); clinical epidemiology (Certificate); environmental and occupational health (MPH, Dr PH, PhD, Certificate); epidemiology (MPH, Dr PH, PhD); general public health (Certificate); health education and behavioral science (MPH, Dr PH, PhD); health systems and policy (MPH, PhD); public health (MPH, Dr PH, PhD); public health preparedness (Certificate); DO/MPH; JD/MPH; MBA/MPH; MD/MPH; MPH/MBA; MPH/MSPA; MS/MPH; Psy D/MPH. *Accreditation:* CEPH. *Program availability:* Part-time, evening/weekend. *Degree requirements:* For master's, thesis, internship; for doctorate, comprehensive exam, thesis/dissertation. *Entrance requirements:* For master's, GRE General Test; for doctorate, GRE General Test, MPH (Dr PH), MA, MPH, or MS (PhD). Additional exam requirements/recommendations for international students: Required—TOEFL. Electronic applications accepted.

Saint Joseph's University, College of Arts and Sciences, Programs in Environmental Protection and Safety Management, Philadelphia, PA 19131-1395. Offers MS. *Program availability:* Part-time, evening/weekend. *Entrance requirements:* For master's, GRE (if GPA less than 2.75), minimum GPA of 2.75, 2 letters of recommendation, resume. Additional exam requirements/recommendations for international students: Required—TOEFL (minimum score 550 paper-based; 80 iBT). Electronic applications accepted.

Saint Joseph's University, College of Arts and Sciences, Programs in Public Safety and Management, Philadelphia, PA 19131-1395. Offers homeland security (MS); public safety management (MS). *Program availability:* Part-time, evening/weekend, online learning. *Entrance requirements:* For master's, GRE (if GPA less than 3.0), 2 letters of recommendation, resume, personal statement, official transcripts. Additional exam requirements/recommendations for international students: Required—TOEFL (minimum score 550 paper-based; 80 iBT). Electronic applications accepted.

Saint Mary's University of Minnesota, Schools of Graduate and Professional Programs, Graduate School of Business and Technology, Public Safety Administration Program, Winona, MN 55987-1399. Offers MA. Tuition and fees vary according to degree level and program. *Unit head:* Lora Setter, Program Director, E-mail: lsetter@smumn.edu. *Application contact:* James Callinan, Director of Admissions for Graduate

Environmental and Occupational Health

and Professional Programs, 612-728-5185, Fax: 612-728-5121, E-mail: jcallina@smumn.edu.
Website: http://www.smumn.edu/graduate-home/areas-of-study/graduate-school-of-business-technology/ma-in-public-safety-administration

San Diego State University, Graduate and Research Affairs, College of Health and Human Services, Graduate School of Public Health, San Diego, CA 92182. Offers environmental health (MPH); epidemiology (MPH, PhD), including biostatistics (MPH); global emergency preparedness and response (MS); global health (PhD); health behavior (PhD); health promotion (MPH); health services administration (MPH); toxicology (MS); MPH/MA; MSW/MPH. *Accreditation:* CAHME (one or more programs are accredited); CEPH (one or more programs are accredited). *Program availability:* Part-time. *Degree requirements:* For master's, comprehensive exam (for some programs), thesis (for some programs); for doctorate, thesis/dissertation. *Entrance requirements:* For master's, GMAT (MPH in health services administration), GRE General Test; for doctorate, GRE General Test. Additional exam requirements/recommendations for international students: Required—TOEFL. *Faculty research:* Evaluation of tobacco, AIDS prevalence and prevention, mammography, infant death project, Alzheimer's in elderly Chinese.

Southeastern Oklahoma State University, School of Arts and Sciences, Durant, OK 74701-0609. Offers biology (MT); computer information systems (MT); occupational safety and health (MT). *Program availability:* Part-time, evening/weekend. *Degree requirements:* For master's, thesis optional. *Entrance requirements:* For master's, minimum GPA of 3.0 in last 60 hours or 2.75 overall. Additional exam requirements/recommendations for international students: Required—TOEFL (minimum score 550 paper-based; 79 iBT). Electronic applications accepted.

Syracuse University, College of Engineering and Computer Science, CAS in Environmental Health Program, Syracuse, NY 13244. Offers environmental health (CAS). *Program availability:* Part-time. *Entrance requirements:* For degree, three letters of recommendation, resume, personal statement, official transcripts. *Application deadline:* For fall admission, 7/1 for domestic students, 6/1 for international students; for spring admission, 11/15 for domestic students, 10/15 for international students. Applications are processed on a rolling basis. Application fee: $75. Electronic applications accepted. *Expenses: Tuition, area resident:* Full-time $25,974; part-time $1443 per credit hour. *Required fees:* $802; $50 per course. Tuition and fees vary according to course load and program. *Financial support:* Fellowships, research assistantships, teaching assistantships, and tuition waivers available. Financial award application deadline: 1/1. *Faculty research:* Environmental health engineering, hazardous waste management, industrial hygiene, risk assessment, toxicology. *Unit head:* Dr. Sam Salem, Department Chair, 315-443-2311, E-mail: omsalem@syr.edu. *Application contact:* Kathleen Joyce, Assistant Dean, 315-443-2219, E-mail: topgrads@syr.edu.

Towson University, Program in Occupational Science, Towson, MD 21252-0001. Offers Sc D. *Program availability:* Part-time, evening/weekend. *Students:* 4 full-time (3 women), 8 part-time (6 women); includes 4 minority (2 Black or African American, non-Hispanic/Latino; 1 Asian, non-Hispanic/Latino; 1 Two or more races, non-Hispanic/Latino), 1 international. *Degree requirements:* For doctorate, thesis/dissertation. *Entrance requirements:* For doctorate, master's degree with minimum GPA of 3.25, interview, 3 letters of recommendation, letter of intent. Additional exam requirements/recommendations for international students: Required—TOEFL (minimum score 600 paper-based). *Application deadline:* For fall admission, 8/15 for domestic and international students; for winter admission, 11/15 for domestic and international students; for spring admission, 1/15 for domestic and international students. Applications are processed on a rolling basis. Application fee: $45. Electronic applications accepted. *Expenses: Tuition,* state resident: full-time $7440; part-time $372 per unit. Tuition, nonresident: full-time $15,400; part-time $770 per unit. *Required fees:* $2360; $118 per year. $354 per term. *Financial support:* Application deadline: 4/1. *Unit head:* Dr. Beth Merryman, Graduate Program Director, 410-704-3499, E-mail: bmerryman@towson.edu. *Application contact:* Alicia Arkell-Kleis, University Admissions, 410-704-2113, Fax: 410-704-3030, E-mail: grads@towson.edu.
Website: http://grad.towson.edu/program/doctoral/osc-scd

Trident University International, College of Health Sciences, Program in Health Sciences, Cypress, CA 90630. Offers clinical research administration (MS, Certificate); emergency and disaster management (MS, Certificate); environmental health science (Certificate); health care administration (PhD); health care management (MS), including health informatics; health education (MS, Certificate); health informatics (Certificate); health sciences (PhD); international health (MS); international health: educator or researcher option (PhD); international health: practitioner option (PhD); law and expert witness studies (MS, Certificate); public health (MS); quality assurance (Certificate). *Program availability:* Part-time, evening/weekend, online learning. *Degree requirements:* For doctorate, comprehensive exam, thesis/dissertation, defense of dissertation. *Entrance requirements:* For master's, minimum GPA of 2.5 (students with GPA 3.0 or greater may transfer up to 30% of graduate level credits); for doctorate, minimum GPA of 3.4, curriculum vitae, course work in research methods or statistics. Additional exam requirements/recommendations for international students: Required—TOEFL. Electronic applications accepted.

Tufts University, Cummings School of Veterinary Medicine, Program in Conservation Medicine, Medford, MA 02155. Offers MS. *Degree requirements:* For master's, case study, preceptorship. *Entrance requirements:* For master's, GRE, official transcripts, curriculum vitae. Additional exam requirements/recommendations for international students: Required—TOEFL or IELTS. Electronic applications accepted. *Expenses: Tuition, area resident:* Full-time $48,412; part-time $1210 per credit hour. *Required fees:* $806. Full-time tuition and fees vary according to degree level, program and student level. Part-time tuition and fees vary according to course load. *Faculty research:* Non-invasive saliva collection techniques for free-ranging mountain gorillas and captive eastern gorillas, animal sentinels for infectious diseases.

Tufts University, School of Engineering, Department of Civil and Environmental Engineering, Medford, MA 02155. Offers bioengineering (ME, MS), including environmental technology; civil engineering (ME, MS, PhD), including geotechnical engineering, structural engineering, water diplomacy (PhD); environmental engineering (ME, MS, PhD), including environmental engineering and environmental sciences, environmental geotechnology, environmental health, environmental science and management, hazardous materials management, water diplomacy (PhD), water resources engineering. *Program availability:* Part-time. Terminal master's awarded for partial completion of doctoral program. *Degree requirements:* For master's, thesis or alternative; for doctorate, thesis/dissertation. *Entrance requirements:* For master's and doctorate, GRE General Test. Additional exam requirements/recommendations for international students: Required—TOEFL (minimum score 550 paper-based; 80 iBT), IELTS (minimum score 6.5). Electronic applications accepted. *Expenses: Tuition, area resident:* Full-time $48,412; part-time $1210 per credit hour. *Required fees:* $806. Full-time tuition and fees vary according to degree level, program and student level. Part-time tuition and fees vary according to course load. *Faculty research:* Environmental and water resources engineering, environmental health, geotechnical and geoenvironmental engineering, structural engineering and mechanics, water diplomacy.

Tulane University, School of Public Health and Tropical Medicine, Department of Global Environmental Health Sciences, New Orleans, LA 70118-5669. Offers MPH, MSPH, PhD, JD/MPH, MD/MPH, MSW/MPH. *Accreditation:* ABET (one or more programs are accredited); CEPH (one or more programs are accredited). *Degree requirements:* For doctorate, comprehensive exam, thesis/dissertation. *Entrance requirements:* For master's and doctorate, GRE General Test. Additional exam requirements/recommendations for international students: Required—TOEFL. *Application deadline:* For fall admission, 4/15 priority date for domestic and international students; for spring admission, 10/15 priority date for domestic and international students. Applications are processed on a rolling basis. Application fee: $40. Electronic applications accepted. *Expenses: Tuition,* area resident: Full-time $47,658; part-time $2648 per credit hour. *Required fees:* $1980; $44.50 per credit hour. $550 per term. Tuition and fees vary according to course load, degree level and program. *Financial support:* Federal Work-Study, scholarships/grants, and traineeships available. Support available to part-time students. Financial award application deadline: 4/15.

Uniformed Services University of the Health Sciences, F. Edward Hebert School of Medicine, Graduate Programs in the Biomedical Sciences and Public Health, Bethesda, MD 20814. Offers emerging infectious diseases (PhD); medical and clinical psychology (PhD), including clinical psychology, medical psychology; medicine (MS, PhD), including health professions education; molecular and cell biology (MS, PhD); neuroscience (PhD); preventive medicine and biometrics (MPH, MS, MSPH, MTMH, Dr PH, PhD), including environmental health sciences (PhD), healthcare administration and policy (MS), medical zoology (PhD); public health (MPH, MSPH, Dr PH); tropical medicine and hygiene (MTMH). *Faculty:* 372 full-time (119 women), 4,044 part-time/adjunct (908 women). *Students:* 240 full-time (133 women); includes 40 minority (15 Black or African American, non-Hispanic/Latino; 13 Asian, non-Hispanic/Latino; 12 Hispanic/Latino), 30 international. Average age 25. 598 applicants, 17% accepted, 77 enrolled. In 2015, 19 master's, 50 doctorates awarded. Terminal master's awarded for partial completion of doctoral program. *Degree requirements:* For master's, comprehensive exam, thesis or alternative; for doctorate, comprehensive exam, thesis/dissertation, qualifying exam. *Entrance requirements:* For master's, GRE General Test; for doctorate, GRE General Test, minimum GPA of 3.0. *Application deadline:* For fall admission, 12/15 priority date for domestic students. Applications are processed on a rolling basis. Application fee: $0. Electronic applications accepted. *Financial support:* In 2015–16, 50 fellowships (averaging $43,000 per year) were awarded; research assistantships, career-related internships or fieldwork, scholarships/grants, health care benefits, and tuition waivers (full) also available. *Unit head:* Dr. Gregory Mueller, Associate Dean, 301-295-3507, E-mail: gregory.mueller@usuhs.edu. *Application contact:* Tina Finley, Administrative Officer, 301-295-3642, Fax: 301-295-6772, E-mail: netina.finley@usuhs.edu.
Website: http://www.usuhs.mil/graded

Uniformed Services University of the Health Sciences, F. Edward Hebert School of Medicine, Graduate Programs in the Biomedical Sciences and Public Health, Department of Preventive Medicine and Biometrics, Program in Environmental Health Sciences, Bethesda, MD 20814-4799. Offers PhD. *Accreditation:* CEPH. *Degree requirements:* For doctorate, comprehensive exam, thesis/dissertation, qualifying exam. *Entrance requirements:* For doctorate, GRE, minimum GPA of 3.0. Additional exam requirements/recommendations for international students: Required—TOEFL.

Universidad Autonoma de Guadalajara, Graduate Programs, Guadalajara, Mexico. Offers administrative law and justice (LL M); advertising and corporate communications (MA); architecture (M Arch); business (MBA); computational science (MCC); education (Ed M, Ed D); English-Spanish translation (MA); entrepreneurship and management (MBA); integrated management of digital animation (MA); international business (MIB); international corporate law (LL M); internet technologies (MS); manufacturing systems (MMS); occupational health (MS); philosophy (MA, PhD); power electronics (MS); quality systems (MQS); renewable energy (MS); social evaluation of projects (MBA); strategic market research (MBA); tax law (MA); teaching mathematics (MA).

Universidad de Ciencias Medicas, Graduate Programs, San Jose, Costa Rica. Offers dermatology (SP); family health (MS); health service center administration (MHA); human anatomy (MS); medical and surgery (MD); occupational medicine (MS); pharmacy (Pharm D). *Program availability:* Part-time. *Degree requirements:* For master's, thesis; for doctorate and SP, comprehensive exam. *Entrance requirements:* For master's, MD or bachelor's degree; for doctorate, admissions test; for SP, admissions test, MD.

Université de Montréal, Faculty of Medicine, Department of Environmental and Occupational Health, Montréal, QC H3C 3J7, Canada. Offers M Sc. *Accreditation:* CEPH. *Degree requirements:* For master's, thesis. *Entrance requirements:* For master's, proficiency in French, knowledge of English. Electronic applications accepted. *Faculty research:* Metabolism of chemical substances, toxicity, biological surveillance, risk analysis.

Université du Québec à Montréal, Graduate Programs, Program in Ergonomics in Occupational Health and Safety, Montréal, QC H3C 3P8, Canada. Offers Diploma. *Program availability:* Part-time. *Entrance requirements:* For degree, appropriate bachelor's degree or equivalent, proficiency in French.

Université Laval, Faculty of Medicine, Graduate Programs in Medicine, Department of Social and Preventive Medicine, Program in Accident Prevention and Occupational Health and Safety Management, Québec, QC G1K 7P4, Canada. Offers Diploma. *Program availability:* Part-time. *Entrance requirements:* For degree, knowledge of French. Electronic applications accepted.

University at Albany, State University of New York, School of Public Health, Department of Environmental Health Sciences, Albany, NY 12222-0001. Offers environmental and occupational health (MS, PhD); environmental chemistry (MS, PhD); toxicology (MS, PhD). *Degree requirements:* For master's, thesis; for doctorate, comprehensive exam, thesis/dissertation. *Entrance requirements:* For master's and doctorate, GRE General Test, GRE Subject Test, 3 letters of reference. Additional exam requirements/recommendations for international students: Required—TOEFL (minimum score 600 paper-based). Electronic applications accepted. *Faculty research:* Xenobiotic metabolism, neurotoxicity of halogenated hydrocarbons, pharmac/toxicogenomics, environmental analytical chemistry.

The University of Alabama at Birmingham, School of Public Health, Program in Environmental Health Sciences, Birmingham, AL 35294. Offers environmental health sciences research (PhD); industrial hygiene (MS). *Degree requirements:* For doctorate, comprehensive exam, thesis/dissertation. *Entrance requirements:* For doctorate, GRE General Test. Additional exam requirements/recommendations for international students: Recommended—TOEFL, IELTS. Electronic applications accepted. *Expenses:* Tuition, state resident: full-time $7340. Tuition, nonresident: full-time $16,628. Full-time tuition and fees vary according to course load and program. *Faculty research:* Aquatic toxicology, virology.

The University of Alabama at Birmingham, School of Public Health, Program in Public Health, Birmingham, AL 35294. Offers applied epidemiology and pharmacoepidemiology (MSPH); biostatistics (MPH); clinical and translational science (MSPH); environmental health (MPH); environmental health and toxicology (MSPH); epidemiology (MPH); general theory and practice (MPH); health behavior (MPH); health care organization (MPH); health policy quantitative policy analysis (MPH); industrial hygiene (MPH, MSPH); maternal and child health policy (Dr PH); maternal and child health policy and leadership (MPH); occupational health and safety (MPH); outcomes research (MSPH, Dr PH); public health (PhD); public health management (Dr PH); public health preparedness management (MPH). *Accreditation:* CEPH. *Program availability:* Part-time, online learning. *Degree requirements:* For doctorate, comprehensive exam, thesis/dissertation. *Entrance requirements:* For master's and doctorate, GRE. Additional exam requirements/recommendations for international students: Recommended—TOEFL (minimum score 550 paper-based; 79 iBT), IELTS (minimum score 6.5). Electronic applications accepted. *Expenses:* Tuition, state resident: full-time $7340. Tuition, nonresident: full-time $16,628. Full-time tuition and fees vary according to course load and program.

University of Alberta, School of Public Health, Department of Public Health Sciences, Edmonton, AB T6G 2E1, Canada. Offers clinical epidemiology (M Sc, MPH); environmental and occupational health (MPH); environmental health sciences (M Sc); epidemiology (M Sc); global health (M Sc, MPH); health policy and management (MPH); health policy research (M Sc); health technology assessment (MPH); occupational health (M Sc); population health (M Sc); public health leadership (MPH); public health sciences (PhD); quantitative methods (MPH). *Accreditation:* CEPH (one or more programs are accredited). Terminal master's awarded for partial completion of doctoral program. *Degree requirements:* For master's (for some programs); for doctorate, thesis/dissertation. *Entrance requirements:* For master's, GMAT or GRE General Test. Additional exam requirements/recommendations for international students: Required—TOEFL (minimum score 550 paper-based) or IELTS (minimum score 6). Electronic applications accepted. *Faculty research:* Biostatistics, health promotion and socio-behavioral health science.

University of Arkansas for Medical Sciences, College of Public Health, Little Rock, AR 72205-7199. Offers biostatistics (MPH); environmental and occupational health (MPH, Certificate); epidemiology (MPH, PhD); health behavior and health education (MPH); health policy and management (MPH); health promotion and prevention research (PhD); health services administration (MHSA); health systems research (PhD); public health (Certificate); public health leadership (Dr PH). *Program availability:* Part-time. *Degree requirements:* For master's, preceptorship, culminating experience, internship; for doctorate, comprehensive exam, capstone. *Entrance requirements:* For master's, GRE, GMAT, LSAT, PCAT, MCAT, DAT; for doctorate, GRE. Additional exam requirements/recommendations for international students: Required—TOEFL (minimum score 80 iBT), IELTS. Electronic applications accepted. *Expenses:* Contact institution. *Faculty research:* Health systems, tobacco prevention control, obesity prevention, environmental and occupational exposure, cancer prevention.

The University of British Columbia, School of Environmental Health, Vancouver, BC V6T 1Z1, Canada. Offers M Sc, PhD. *Program availability:* Part-time. *Degree requirements:* For master's, comprehensive exam (for some programs), thesis optional; for doctorate, comprehensive exam, thesis/dissertation. *Entrance requirements:* For master's and doctorate, GRE. Additional exam requirements/recommendations for international students: Required—TOEFL (minimum score 600 paper-based; 100 iBT); Recommended—TWE. Electronic applications accepted. *Faculty research:* Acoustics, exposure assessment and epidemiology, occupational and environmental respiratory disease, occupational and environmental policy.

University of California, Berkeley, Graduate Division, School of Public Health, Group in Environmental Health Sciences, Berkeley, CA 94720-1500. Offers MPH, MS, Dr PH, PhD. *Degree requirements:* For master's, comprehensive exam (MPH), project or thesis (MS); for doctorate, thesis/dissertation, departmental and qualifying exams. *Entrance requirements:* For master's, GRE General Test, minimum GPA of 3.0; previous course work in biology, calculus, and chemistry; 3 letters of recommendation; for doctorate, GRE General Test, master's degree in relevant scientific discipline or engineering; minimum GPA of 3.0; previous course work in biology, calculus, and chemistry; 3 letters of recommendation. Additional exam requirements/recommendations for international students: Required—TOEFL. *Faculty research:* Toxicology, industrial hygiene, exposure assessment, risk assessment, ergonomics.

University of California, Irvine, School of Medicine, Program in Environmental Health Sciences, Irvine, CA 92697. Offers environmental health sciences (MS); environmental toxicology (PhD); exposure sciences and risk assessment (PhD). *Students:* 11 full-time (6 women); includes 2 minority (1 Asian, non-Hispanic/Latino; 1 Two or more races, non-Hispanic/Latino), 1 international. Average age 32. 15 applicants, 40% accepted, 5 enrolled. In 2015, 1 master's awarded. Terminal master's awarded for partial completion of doctoral program. *Degree requirements:* For master's, comprehensive exam; for doctorate, comprehensive exam, thesis/dissertation. *Entrance requirements:* For master's and doctorate, GRE General Test, GRE Subject Test, minimum GPA of 3.0. Additional exam requirements/recommendations for international students: Required—TOEFL (minimum score 550 paper-based). *Application deadline:* For fall admission, 1/15 for domestic students. Applications are processed on a rolling basis. Application fee: $90 ($110 for international students). Electronic applications accepted. *Financial support:* Fellowships, research assistantships with full tuition reimbursements, teaching assistantships, institutionally sponsored loans, traineeships, health care benefits, and unspecified assistantships available. Financial award application deadline: 12/15; financial award applicants required to submit FAFSA. *Faculty research:* Inhalation/pulmonary toxicology, environmental carcinogenesis, biochemical neurotoxicology, toxicokinetics, chemical pathology. *Unit head:* Dr. Ulrike Luderer, Director, 949-824-8848, E-mail: uluderer@uci.edu. *Application contact:* Armando Villalpando, Student Affairs Officer, 949-824-8848, E-mail: afvillal@uci.edu.
Website: http://www.medicine.uci.edu/occupational/graduate.asp

University of California, Los Angeles, Graduate Division, School of Public Health, Department of Environmental Health Sciences, Los Angeles, CA 90095. Offers environmental health sciences (MS, PhD); environmental science and engineering (D Env); molecular toxicology (PhD); JD/MPH. *Accreditation:* ABET (one or more programs are accredited). *Degree requirements:* For master's, comprehensive exam or thesis; for doctorate, thesis/dissertation, oral and written qualifying exams. *Entrance requirements:* For master's, GRE General Test, minimum GPA of 3.0; for doctorate, GRE General Test, minimum undergraduate GPA of 3.0. Electronic applications accepted.

University of Central Missouri, The Graduate School, Warrensburg, MO 64093. Offers accountancy (MA); accounting (MBA); applied mathematics (MS); aviation safety (MA); biology (MS); business administration (MBA); career and technical education leadership (MS); college student personnel administration (MS); communication (MA); computer science (MS); counseling (MS); criminal justice (MS); educational leadership (Ed D); educational technology (MS); elementary and early childhood education (MSE); English (MA); environmental studies (MA); finance (MBA); history (MA); human services/educational technology (Ed S); human services/learning resources (Ed S); human services/professional counseling (Ed S); industrial hygiene (MS); industrial management (MS); information systems (MBA); information technology (MS); kinesiology (MS); library science and information services (MS); literacy education (MSE); marketing (MBA); mathematics (MS); music (MA); occupational safety management (MS); psychology (MS); rural family nursing (MS); school administration (MSE); social gerontology (MS);

sociology (MA); special education (MSE); speech language pathology (MS); superintendency (Ed S); teaching (MAT); teaching English as a second language (MA); technology (MS); technology management (PhD); theatre (MA). *Program availability:* Part-time, 100% online, blended/hybrid learning. *Faculty:* 336 full-time (145 women), 39 part-time/adjunct (25 women). *Students:* 2,161 full-time (723 women), 2,077 part-time (1,061 women); includes 188 minority (93 Black or African American, non-Hispanic/Latino; 4 American Indian or Alaska Native, non-Hispanic/Latino; 15 Asian, non-Hispanic/Latino; 32 Hispanic/Latino; 1 Native Hawaiian or other Pacific Islander, non-Hispanic/Latino; 43 Two or more races, non-Hispanic/Latino), 2,514 international. Average age 28. 3,454 applicants, 68% accepted, 1632 enrolled. In 2015, 1,530 master's, 53 other advanced degrees awarded. *Degree requirements:* For master's and Ed S, comprehensive exam (for some programs), thesis (for some programs). *Entrance requirements:* Additional exam requirements/recommendations for international students: Required—TOEFL (minimum score 550 paper-based; 79 iBT). *Application deadline:* For fall admission, 6/1 priority date for domestic and international students; for spring admission, 10/1 priority date for domestic and international students; for summer admission, 4/1 priority date for domestic and international students. Applications are processed on a rolling basis. Application fee: $30 ($75 for international students). Electronic applications accepted. *Expenses:* Tuition, state resident: full-time $6683; part-time $278.45 per credit hour. Tuition, nonresident: full-time $13,366; part-time $556.90 per credit hour. *Required fees:* $701; $29.20 per credit hour. Tuition and fees vary according to degree level and campus/location. *Financial support:* In 2015–16, 97 students received support, including 146 research assistantships with partial tuition reimbursements available (averaging $7,500 per year), 73 teaching assistantships with partial tuition reimbursements available (averaging $7,500 per year); career-related internships or fieldwork, Federal Work-Study, scholarships/grants, and administrative and laboratory assistantships also available. Support available to part-time students. Financial award application deadline: 3/1; financial award applicants required to submit FAFSA. *Unit head:* Tina Church-Hockett, Director of Graduate School and International Admissions, 660-543-4621, Fax: 660-543-4778, E-mail: church@ucmo.edu. *Application contact:* Brittany Lawrence, Graduate Student Services Coordinator, 660-543-4621, Fax: 660-543-4778, E-mail: gradinfo@ucmo.edu.
Website: http://www.ucmo.edu/graduate/

University of Cincinnati, Graduate School, College of Medicine, Graduate Programs in Biomedical Sciences, Department of Environmental Health, Cincinnati, OH 45221. Offers environmental and industrial hygiene (MS, PhD); environmental and occupational medicine (MS); environmental genetics and molecular toxicology (MS, PhD); epidemiology and biostatistics (MS, PhD); occupational safety and ergonomics (MS, PhD). *Accreditation:* ABET (one or more programs are accredited). Terminal master's awarded for partial completion of doctoral program. *Degree requirements:* For master's, thesis; for doctorate, thesis/dissertation, qualifying exam. *Entrance requirements:* For master's, GRE General Test, bachelor's degree in science; for doctorate, GRE General Test. Additional exam requirements/recommendations for international students: Required—TOEFL (minimum score 600 paper-based; 100 iBT). Electronic applications accepted. *Faculty research:* Carcinogens and mutagenesis, pulmonary studies, reproduction and development.

University of Colorado Denver, College of Liberal Arts and Sciences, Department of Geography and Environmental Sciences, Denver, CO 80217. Offers environmental sciences (MS), including air quality, ecosystems, environmental health, environmental science education, geospatial analysis, urban agriculture, water quality. *Program availability:* Part-time, evening/weekend. *Faculty:* 12 full-time (4 women), 2 part-time/adjunct (1 woman). *Students:* 46 full-time (26 women), 12 part-time (5 women); includes 11 minority (1 Black or African American, non-Hispanic/Latino; 1 Asian, non-Hispanic/Latino; 6 Hispanic/Latino; 3 Two or more races, non-Hispanic/Latino), 3 international. Average age 30. 75 applicants, 61% accepted, 24 enrolled. In 2015, 11 master's awarded. *Degree requirements:* For master's, thesis or alternative, 30 credits including 21 of core requirements and 9 of environmental science electives. *Entrance requirements:* For master's, GRE General Test, BA in one of the natural/physical sciences or engineering (or equivalent background); prerequisite coursework in calculus and physics (one semester each), general chemistry with lab and general biology with lab (two semesters each); three letters of recommendation. Additional exam requirements/recommendations for international students: Required—TOEFL (minimum score 537 paper-based; 75 iBT); Recommended—IELTS (minimum score 6.5). *Application deadline:* For fall admission, 1/20 for domestic and international students; for spring admission, 10/1 for domestic and international students. Application fee: $50 ($75 for international students). Electronic applications accepted. *Financial support:* In 2015–16, 8 students received support. Fellowships, research assistantships, teaching assistantships, Federal Work-Study, institutionally sponsored loans, scholarships/grants, and traineeships available. Financial award application deadline: 4/1; financial award applicants required to submit FAFSA. *Faculty research:* Air quality, environmental health, ecosystems, hazardous waste, water quality, geo-spatial analysis and environmental science education. *Unit head:* Anne Chinn, Director of MS in Environmental Sciences Program, 303-556-3958, E-mail: ges@ucdenver.edu. *Application contact:* Sue Eddleman, Program Assistant, 303-352-3698, E-mail: sue.eddleman@ucdenver.edu.
Website: http://www.ucdenver.edu/academics/colleges/CLAS/Departments/ges/Programs/MasterofScience/Pages/MasterofScience.aspx

University of Colorado Denver, Colorado School of Public Health, Program in Public Health, Aurora, CO 80045. Offers community and behavioral health (MPH, Dr PH); environmental and occupational health (MPH); epidemiology (MPH); health systems, management and policy (MPH). *Accreditation:* CEPH. *Program availability:* Part-time, evening/weekend. *Faculty:* 16 full-time (14 women), 1 (woman) part-time/adjunct. *Students:* 379 full-time (293 women), 77 part-time (69 women); includes 111 minority (10 Black or African American, non-Hispanic/Latino; 3 American Indian or Alaska Native, non-Hispanic/Latino; 36 Asian, non-Hispanic/Latino; 47 Hispanic/Latino; 1 Native Hawaiian or other Pacific Islander, non-Hispanic/Latino; 14 Two or more races, non-Hispanic/Latino), 12 international. Average age 31. 785 applicants, 25% accepted, 166 enrolled. In 2015, 144 master's awarded. *Degree requirements:* For master's, thesis or alternative, 42 credit hours; for doctorate, comprehensive exam, thesis/dissertation, 67 credit hours. *Entrance requirements:* For master's, GRE, MCAT, DAT, LSAT, PCAT, GMAT or master's degree from accredited institution, baccalaureate degree or equivalent; minimum GPA of 3.0; transcripts; references; resume; essay; for doctorate, GRE, MCAT, DAT, LSAT, PCAT or GMAT, MPH or master's or higher degree in related field or equivalent; 2 years of previous work experience in public health; essay; resume. Additional exam requirements/recommendations for international students: Required—TOEFL (minimum score 550 paper-based; 80 iBT). *Application deadline:* For fall admission, 12/15 priority date for domestic students, 12/1 priority date for international students. Application fee: $65. Electronic applications accepted. *Expenses:* Contact institution. *Financial support:* In 2015–16, 265 students received support. Fellowships, research assistantships, teaching assistantships, Federal Work-Study, institutionally sponsored loans, scholarships/grants, traineeships, and unspecified assistantships available. Financial award application deadline: 3/15; financial award applicants required to submit FAFSA. *Faculty research:* Cancer prevention by nutrition, cancer survivorship outcomes, social and cultural factors related to health. *Total annual research*

Environmental and Occupational Health

expenditures: $302,793. Unit head: Dr. Lori Crane, Chair, 303-724-4385, E-mail: lori.crane@ucdenver.edu. Application contact: 303-724-4613, E-mail: csph.studentaffairs@ucdenver.edu. Website: http://www.ucdenver.edu/academics/colleges/PublicHealth/Academics/degreesandprograms/Pages/index.aspx

University of Connecticut, Graduate School, eCampus, Program in Occupational Safety and Health Management, Storrs, CT 06269. Offers Certificate.

University of Florida, Graduate School, College of Public Health and Health Professions, Department of Environmental and Global Health, Gainesville, FL 32611. Offers environmental health (PhD); one health (MHS, PhD). Faculty: 5 full-time, 1 part-time/adjunct. Students: 10 full-time (8 women), 2 part-time (both women); includes 1 minority (Black or African American, non-Hispanic/Latino), 1 international. Average age 28. 7 applicants, 57% accepted, 4 enrolled. In 2015, 2 master's awarded. Entrance requirements: For master's and doctorate, GRE, minimum GPA of 3.0. Additional exam requirements/recommendations for international students: Required—TOEFL (minimum score 550 paper-based; 80 iBT), IELTS (minimum score 6). Application deadline: For fall admission, 1/1 for domestic students. Application fee: $30. Financial support: In 2015–16, 2 fellowships, 12 research assistantships, 7 teaching assistantships were awarded. Financial award applicants required to submit FAFSA. Total annual research expenditures: $2.1 million. Unit head: Dr. Gregory C. Gray, MD, Chair, 352-273-9449, E-mail: gcgray@phhp.ufl.edu. Application contact: Office of Admissions, 352-392-1365, E-mail: webrequests@admissions.ufl.edu. Website: http://egh.phhp.ufl.edu/

University of Florida, Graduate School, College of Public Health and Health Professions, Programs in Public Health, Gainesville, FL 32611. Offers biostatistics (MPH); clinical and translational science (PhD); environmental health (MPH); epidemiology (MPH); health management and policy (MPH); public health (MPH, PhD, Certificate); public health practice (MPH); rehabilitation science (PhD); social and behavioral sciences (MPH); DPT/MPH; DVM/MPH; JD/MPH; MD/MPH; Pharm D/MPH. Accreditation: CEPH. Program availability: Online learning. Faculty: 51. Students: 174 full-time (134 women), 59 part-time (42 women); includes 67 minority (27 Black or African American, non-Hispanic/Latino; 1 American Indian or Alaska Native, non-Hispanic/Latino; 25 Asian, non-Hispanic/Latino; 14 Hispanic/Latino), 24 international. Average age 30. 385 applicants, 44% accepted, 75 enrolled. In 2015, 81 master's, 6 doctorates awarded. Degree requirements: For master's, internship. Entrance requirements: For master's, GRE General Test, minimum GPA of 3.0. Additional exam requirements/recommendations for international students: Required—TOEFL (minimum score 550 paper-based; 80 iBT), IELTS (minimum score 6). Application deadline: For fall admission, 7/1 for domestic students, 4/1 for international students. Application fee: $30. Financial support: In 2015–16, 5 research assistantships, 10 teaching assistantships were awarded; fellowships also available. Financial award applicants required to submit FAFSA. Unit head: Sarah L. McKune, PhD, Program Director, 352-328-0615, Fax: 352-273-6448, E-mail: smckune@ufl.edu. Application contact: Telisha Martin, PhD, Associate Director, MPH Program, 352-273-6444, E-mail: martints@ufl.edu. Website: http://www.mph.ufl.edu/

University of Georgia, College of Public Health, Department of Environmental Health Science, Athens, GA 30602. Offers MPH, MSEH. Accreditation: CEPH. Terminal master's awarded for partial completion of doctoral program. Degree requirements: For master's, thesis. Entrance requirements: For master's, GRE General Test. Additional exam requirements/recommendations for international students: Required—TOEFL. Electronic applications accepted. Faculty research: Risk assessment, environmental toxicology, water quality, air quality.

University of Illinois at Chicago, School of Public Health, Division of Environmental and Occupational Health Sciences, Chicago, IL 60607-7128. Offers MPH, MS, Dr PH, PhD. Accreditation: ABET (one or more programs are accredited); CEPH (one or more programs are accredited). Program availability: Part-time. Faculty: 11 full-time (7 women), 16 part-time/adjunct (6 women). Students: 52 full-time (28 women), 10 part-time (8 women); includes 27 minority (12 Black or African American, non-Hispanic/Latino; 4 Asian, non-Hispanic/Latino; 9 Hispanic/Latino; 2 Two or more races, non-Hispanic/Latino), 15 international. Average age 31. Terminal master's awarded for partial completion of doctoral program. Degree requirements: For master's, thesis, field practicum; for doctorate, thesis/dissertation, independent research, internship. Entrance requirements: For master's and doctorate, GRE General Test, minimum GPA of 2.75. Additional exam requirements/recommendations for international students: Required—TOEFL. Application deadline: For fall admission, 2/1 for domestic students, 1/1 priority date for international students. Application fee: $60. Electronic applications accepted. Expenses: Contact institution. Financial support: Fellowships with full tuition reimbursements, research assistantships with full tuition reimbursements, teaching assistantships with full tuition reimbursements, career-related internships or fieldwork, Federal Work-Study, institutionally sponsored loans, scholarships/grants, traineeships, and unspecified assistantships available. Support available to part-time students. Financial award application deadline: 3/1; financial award applicants required to submit FAFSA. Faculty research: Workers compensation, injury and illness surveillance, and disparities in occupational health; emergency/disaster management and continuity planning; water quality; air pollution; environmental chemistry; industrial hygiene; occupational medicine; hazardous substances management; toxicology; occupational safety, environmental epidemiology, and policy. Unit head: Prof. Linda Forst, Director, 312-355-3826, E-mail: forst-l@uic.edu. Website: http://publichealth.uic.edu/departments/environmentalandoccupationalhealthsciences/

The University of Iowa, Graduate College, Department of Occupational and Environmental Health, Iowa City, IA 52242-1316. Offers agricultural safety and health (MS, PhD); ergonomics (MPH); industrial hygiene (MS, PhD); occupational and environmental health (MPH, MS, PhD, Certificate); MS/MA; MS/MS. Accreditation: ABET (one or more programs are accredited); CEPH. Degree requirements: For master's, thesis optional, exam; for doctorate, comprehensive exam, thesis/dissertation. Entrance requirements: For master's and doctorate, GRE General Test, minimum GPA of 3.0. Additional exam requirements/recommendations for international students: Required—TOEFL (minimum score 600 paper-based; 100 iBT). Electronic applications accepted.

The University of Kansas, University of Kansas Medical Center, School of Medicine, Department of Preventive Medicine and Public Health, Kansas City, KS 66160. Offers clinical research (MS); environmental health sciences (MPH); epidemiology (MPH); public health management (MPH); social and behavioral health (MPH); MD/MPH; PhD/MPH. Program availability: Part-time. Faculty: 70. Students: 48 full-time (35 women), 46 part-time (31 women); includes 31 minority (9 Black or African American, non-Hispanic/Latino; 4 American Indian or Alaska Native, non-Hispanic/Latino; 8 Asian, non-Hispanic/Latino; 6 Hispanic/Latino; 4 Two or more races, non-Hispanic/Latino), 8 international. Average age 31. 66 applicants, 68% accepted, 44 enrolled. In 2015, 31 master's awarded. Degree requirements: For master's, thesis, capstone practicum defense. Entrance requirements: For master's, GRE, MCAT, LSAT, GMAT or other equivalent graduate professional exam. Additional exam requirements/recommendations for international students: Required—TOEFL. Application deadline: For fall admission, 3/1

for domestic and international students. Applications are processed on a rolling basis. Application fee: $60. Electronic applications accepted. Financial support: In 2015–16, 9 research assistantships (averaging $15,000 per year) were awarded; career-related internships or fieldwork, Federal Work-Study, scholarships/grants, and unspecified assistantships also available. Support available to part-time students. Financial award application deadline: 3/1; financial award applicants required to submit FAFSA. Faculty research: Cancer screening and prevention, smoking cessation, obesity and physical activity, health services/outcomes research, health disparities. Total annual research expenditures: $6.6 million. Unit head: Dr. Edward F. Ellerbeck, Chairman, 913-588-2774, Fax: 913-588-2780, E-mail: eellerbe@kumc.edu. Application contact: Tanya Honderick, MPH Director, 913-588-2720, Fax: 913-588-8505, E-mail: thonderick@kumc.edu. Website: http://www.kumc.edu/school-of-medicine/preventive-medicine-and-public-health.html

University of Louisville, Graduate School, School of Public Health and Information Sciences, Department of Public Health and Information Sciences, Louisville, KY 40202. Offers biostatistics (MS, PhD); clinical investigation (M Sc); epidemiology (MS); health management and systems sciences (MPH); public health sciences (PhD), including environmental health, epidemiology, health management, health promotion; public health sciences - health management (PhD). Program availability: Part-time. Students: 92 full-time (60 women), 33 part-time (19 women); includes 37 minority (16 Black or African American, non-Hispanic/Latino; 12 Asian, non-Hispanic/Latino; 6 Hispanic/Latino; 3 Two or more races, non-Hispanic/Latino), 19 international. Average age 32. 128 applicants, 77% accepted, 56 enrolled. In 2015, 38 master's, 6 doctorates awarded. Degree requirements: For master's, thesis optional; for doctorate, comprehensive exam, thesis/dissertation. Entrance requirements: For master's and doctorate, GRE General Test. Additional exam requirements/recommendations for international students: Required—TOEFL (minimum score 600 paper-based; 100 iBT). Application deadline: For fall admission, 5/1 for domestic and international students. Application fee: $60. Electronic applications accepted. Expenses: Tuition, state resident: full-time $11,664; part-time $649 per credit hour. Tuition, nonresident: full-time $24,274; part-time $1350 per credit hour. Required fees: $196. Tuition and fees vary according to program and reciprocity agreements. Financial support: In 2015–16, 718,988 students received support. Research assistantships with full tuition reimbursements available, scholarships/grants, health care benefits, and unspecified assistantships available. Financial award applicants required to submit FAFSA. Faculty research: Department of environmental and occupational health sciences department of health management and systems sciences department of health promotion and behavioral sciences. Total annual research expenditures: $2.1 million. Unit head: Dr. Craig Blakely, Dean, 502-852-3297, Fax: 502-852-3291, E-mail: chblak01@louisville.edu. Website: http://louisville.edu/sphis/departments/health-management-systems-science

University of Maryland, College Park, Academic Affairs, School of Public Health, Maryland Institute for Applied Environmental Health, College Park, MD 20742. Offers environmental health sciences (MPH). Entrance requirements: For master's, GRE General Test, 3 letters of recommendation, minimum undergraduate GPA of 3.0, undergraduate transcripts, statement of goals and interests. Electronic applications accepted.

University of Massachusetts Amherst, Graduate School, School of Public Health and Health Sciences, Department of Public Health, Amherst, MA 01003. Offers biostatistics (MPH, MS, PhD); community health education (MPH, MS, PhD); environmental health sciences (MPH, MS, PhD); epidemiology (MPH, MS, PhD); health policy and management (MPH, MS, PhD); nutrition (MPH, MS, PhD); public health practice (MPH); MPH/MPPA. Accreditation: CEPH (one or more programs are accredited). Program availability: Part-time, evening/weekend, online learning. Terminal master's awarded for partial completion of doctoral program. Degree requirements: For master's, thesis (for some programs); for doctorate, comprehensive exam, thesis/dissertation. Entrance requirements: For master's and doctorate, GRE General Test. Additional exam requirements/recommendations for international students: Required—TOEFL (minimum score 550 paper-based; 80 iBT), IELTS (minimum score 6.5). Electronic applications accepted.

University of Memphis, Graduate School, School of Public Health, Memphis, TN 38152. Offers biostatistics (MPH); environmental health (MPH); epidemiology (MPH); health systems management (MPH); public health (MHA); social and behavioral sciences (MPH). Program availability: Part-time, evening/weekend, online learning. Faculty: 117 full-time (5 women), 5 part-time/adjunct (1 woman). Students: 100 full-time (68 women), 48 part-time (35 women); includes 63 minority (33 Black or African American, non-Hispanic/Latino; 20 Asian, non-Hispanic/Latino; 7 Hispanic/Latino; 3 Two or more races, non-Hispanic/Latino), 17 international. Average age 30. 114 applicants, 83% accepted, 37 enrolled. In 2015, 55 master's awarded. Degree requirements: For master's, comprehensive exam, thesis. Entrance requirements: For master's, GRE, letters of recommendation. Additional exam requirements/recommendations for international students: Required—TOEFL. Application deadline: For fall admission, 4/1 for domestic students; for spring admission, 11/1 for domestic students. Application fee: $35 ($60 for international students). Electronic applications accepted. Financial support: In 2015–16, 46 students received support. Research assistantships with full tuition reimbursements available, Federal Work-Study, scholarships/grants, and unspecified assistantships available. Financial award application deadline: 2/15; financial award applicants required to submit FAFSA. Faculty research: Health and medical savings accounts, adoption rates, health informatics, Telehealth technologies, biostatistics, environmental health, epidemiology, health systems management, social and behavioral sciences. Unit head: Dr. Lisa M. Klesges, Director, 901-678-4637, E-mail: lmklsges@memphis.edu. Application contact: Dr. Karen Weddle-West, Information Contact, 901-678-2531, Fax: 901-678-5023, E-mail: gradsch@memphis.edu. Website: http://www.memphis.edu/sph/

University of Miami, Graduate School, College of Engineering, Department of Industrial Engineering, Program in Occupational Ergonomics and Safety, Coral Gables, FL 33124. Offers environmental health and safety (MS); occupational ergonomics and safety (MSOES). Program availability: Part-time. Degree requirements: For master's, thesis optional. Entrance requirements: For master's, GRE General Test, minimum GPA of 3.0. Additional exam requirements/recommendations for international students: Required—TOEFL (minimum score 550 paper-based). Electronic applications accepted. Faculty research: Noise, heat stress, water pollution.

University of Michigan, School of Public Health, Department of Environmental Health Sciences, Ann Arbor, MI 48109. Offers environmental health sciences (MS, PhD); environmental quality and health (MPH); industrial hygiene (MPH, MS); occupational and environmental epidemiology (MPH); toxicology (MPH, MS, PhD). Accreditation: CEPH (one or more programs are accredited). Program availability: Part-time. Faculty: 22 full-time (7 women), 28 part-time/adjunct (9 women). Students: 76 full-time (53 women), 3 part-time (all women); includes 13 minority (4 Black or African American, non-Hispanic/Latino; 5 Asian, non-Hispanic/Latino; 2 Hispanic/Latino; 2 Two or more races, non-Hispanic/Latino), 12 international. Average age 27. 263 applicants, 39% accepted, 39 enrolled. In 2015, 50 master's, 8 doctorates awarded. Terminal master's awarded for partial completion of doctoral program. Degree requirements: For master's, thesis (for some programs); for doctorate, thesis/dissertation, preliminary exam, oral defense of dissertation. *Entrance requirements:* For master's and doctorate, GRE General Test and/or MCAT. Additional exam requirements/recommendations for international students: Required—TOEFL (minimum score 100 iBT). *Application deadline:* For fall admission, 12/15 priority date for domestic students, 1/15 for international students. Applications are processed on a rolling basis. Application fee: $75. Electronic applications accepted. *Financial support:* Fellowships, research assistantships, teaching assistantships, career-related internships or fieldwork, Federal Work-Study, institutionally sponsored loans, scholarships/grants, traineeships, health care benefits, and unspecified assistantships available. Financial award application deadline: 12/15. *Faculty research:* Toxicology, occupational hygiene, environmental exposure sciences, environmental epidemiology. *Unit head:* Dr. Craig Harris, Chair, 734-939-3397, E-mail: charris@umich.edu. *Application contact:* Susan Crawford, Student Administrative Coordinator, 734-764-3018, E-mail: sph.inquiries@umich.edu. Website: http://www.sph.umich.edu/ehs/

University of Minnesota, Twin Cities Campus, School of Public Health, Division of Environmental Health Sciences, Area in Environmental Health Policy, Minneapolis, MN 55455-0213. Offers MPH, MS, PhD. *Accreditation:* CEPH (one or more programs are accredited). *Degree requirements:* For doctorate, thesis/dissertation. *Entrance requirements:* For master's and doctorate, GRE General Test. Electronic applications accepted.

University of Minnesota, Twin Cities Campus, School of Public Health, Division of Environmental Health Sciences, Area in Occupational Medicine, Minneapolis, MN 55455-0213. Offers MPH. *Accreditation:* CEPH. *Entrance requirements:* For master's, GRE General Test. Electronic applications accepted.

University of Minnesota, Twin Cities Campus, School of Public Health, Major in Public Health Practice, Minneapolis, MN 55455-0213. Offers core concepts (Certificate); food safety and biosecurity (Certificate); occupational health and safety (Certificate); preparedness, response and recovery (Certificate); public health practice (MPH); DVM/MPH; MD/MPH. *Program availability:* Part-time, online learning. *Degree requirements:* For master's, thesis. *Entrance requirements:* For master's, GRE, MCAT, United States Medical Licensing Exam. Additional exam requirements/recommendations for international students: Required—TOEFL (minimum score 600 paper-based). Electronic applications accepted.

University of Nebraska Medical Center, Program in Environmental Health, Occupational Health and Toxicology, Omaha, NE 68198. Offers PhD. *Faculty:* 9 full-time (1 woman). *Students:* 4 full-time (1 woman), 2 part-time (1 woman); includes 1 minority (Asian, non-Hispanic/Latino), 2 international. Average age 40. 7 applicants, 57% accepted, 4 enrolled. In 2015, 3 doctorates awarded. *Degree requirements:* For doctorate, comprehensive exam (for some programs), thesis/dissertation. *Entrance requirements:* For doctorate, GRE General Test, BS in chemistry, biology, biochemistry or related area. Additional exam requirements/recommendations for international students: Required—TOEFL (minimum score 550 paper-based; 80 iBT). *Application deadline:* For fall admission, 4/1 for domestic and international students; for spring admission, 8/1 for domestic and international students; for summer admission, 1/1 for domestic and international students. Applications are processed on a rolling basis. Application fee: $45. Electronic applications accepted. *Expenses:* Tuition, state resident: full-time $7830; part-time $3915 per credit hour. Tuition, nonresident: full-time $22,410; part-time $11,205 per credit hour. *Required fees:* $521. *Financial support:* In 2015–16, fellowships with full tuition reimbursements (averaging $23,100 per year), 1 research assistantship with full tuition reimbursement (averaging $23,100 per year) was awarded; teaching assistantships and scholarships/grants also available. Support available to part-time students. Financial award application deadline: 2/15; financial award applicants required to submit FAFSA. *Faculty research:* Mechanisms of carcinogenesis, alcohol and metal toxicity, DNA damage, human molecular genetics, agrochemicals in soil and water. *Unit head:* Dr. Chandran Achutan, Associate Professor, 402-559-8599, E-mail: cachutan@unmc.edu. *Application contact:* Sherry Cherek, Coordinator, 402-559-8924, Fax: 402-559-8068, E-mail: scherek@unmc.edu. Website: http://www.unmc.edu/publichealth/programs/phdprograms/phdenviromental.html

University of Nevada, Reno, Graduate School, Interdisciplinary Program in Environmental Sciences and Health, Reno, NV 89557. Offers MS, PhD. Terminal master's awarded for partial completion of doctoral program. *Degree requirements:* For master's, thesis; for doctorate, thesis/dissertation. *Entrance requirements:* For master's, GRE General Test, minimum GPA of 2.75; for doctorate, GRE General Test, minimum GPA of 3.0. Additional exam requirements/recommendations for international students: Required—TOEFL (minimum score 500 paper-based; 61 iBT), IELTS (minimum score 6). Electronic applications accepted. *Faculty research:* Environmental chemistry, environmental toxicology, ecological toxicology.

University of New Haven, Graduate School, College of Arts and Sciences, Program in Environmental Science, West Haven, CT 06516-1916. Offers environmental ecology (MS); environmental education (MS); environmental geoscience (MS); environmental health and management (MS); environmental science (MS); geographical information systems (MS, Graduate Certificate). *Program availability:* Part-time, evening/weekend. *Students:* 20 full-time (10 women), 6 part-time (5 women); includes 2 minority (1 Black or African American, non-Hispanic/Latino; 1 Hispanic/Latino), 5 international. Average age 26. 25 applicants, 88% accepted, 13 enrolled. In 2015, 19 master's awarded. *Degree requirements:* For master's, thesis optional, research project. *Entrance requirements:* Additional exam requirements/recommendations for international students: Required—TOEFL (minimum score 80 iBT), IELTS, PTE. *Application deadline:* For fall admission, 5/31 for international students; for winter admission, 10/15 for international students; for spring admission, 1/15 for international students. Applications are processed on a rolling basis. Application fee: $75. Electronic applications accepted. Application fee is waived when completed online. *Expenses:* Tuition, area resident: Full-time $15,282; part-time $849 per credit hour. *Required fees:* $150; $60 per term. Tuition and fees vary according to program. *Financial support:* Research assistantships with partial tuition reimbursements, teaching assistantships with partial tuition reimbursements, career-related internships or fieldwork, Federal Work-Study, scholarships/grants, and unspecified assistantships available. Support available to part-time students. Financial award applicants required to submit FAFSA. *Unit head:* Dr. Roman Zajac, Coordinator, 203-932-7114, E-mail: rzajac@newhaven.edu. *Application contact:* Michelle Mason, Director of Graduate Enrollment, 203-932-7067, E-mail: mmason@newhaven.edu. Website: http://www.newhaven.edu/4728/

University of North Alabama, College of Arts and Sciences, Department of Interdisciplinary and Professional Studies, Florence, AL 35632. Offers community development (MPS); information technology (MPS); security and safety leadership (MPS). *Program availability:* Part-time. *Students:* 17 full-time (9 women), 42 part-time (28 women); includes 10 minority (all Black or African American, non-Hispanic/Latino), 10 international. Average age 36. 25 applicants, 84% accepted, 15 enrolled. In 2015, 9 master's awarded. *Degree requirements:* For master's, thesis optional. *Entrance requirements:* For master's, ETS PPI, baccalaureate degree from accredited institution; minimum cumulative GPA of 2.75 or 3.0 in last 60 hours of undergraduate study; personal statement. Additional exam requirements/recommendations for international

students: Required—TOEFL (minimum score 79 iBT), IELTS (minimum score 6), PTE (minimum score 54). *Application deadline:* Applications are processed on a rolling basis. Application fee: $50 ($100 for international students). Electronic applications accepted. *Expenses:* Tuition, state resident: full-time $2286; part-time $1524 per semester. Tuition, nonresident: full-time $4572; part-time $3048 per semester. *Required fees:* $801; $579 per semester. Tuition and fees vary according to course load. *Financial support:* Application deadline: 12/1; applicants required to submit FAFSA. *Unit head:* Dr. Craig T. Robertson, Director, 256-765-5003, E-mail: ctrobertson@una.edu. *Application contact:* Hillary N. Coats, Graduate Admissions Coordinator, 256-765-4447, E-mail: graduate@una.edu. Website: https://www.una.edu/interdisciplinary-studies/

The University of North Carolina at Chapel Hill, Graduate School, Gillings School of Global Public Health, Department of Environmental Sciences and Engineering, Chapel Hill, NC 27599. Offers air, radiation and industrial hygiene (MPH, MS, MSEE, MSPH, PhD); aquatic and atmospheric sciences (MPH, MS, MSPH, PhD); environmental engineering (MPH, MS, MSEE, MSPH, PhD); environmental health sciences (MPH, MS, MSPH, PhD); environmental management and policy (MPH, MS, MSPH, PhD). *Students:* 112 full-time (68 women); includes 20 minority (11 Asian, non-Hispanic/Latino; 4 Hispanic/Latino; 5 Two or more races, non-Hispanic/Latino), 31 international. Average age 28. 178 applicants, 37% accepted, 39 enrolled. Terminal master's awarded for partial completion of doctoral program. *Degree requirements:* For master's, comprehensive exam, thesis (for some programs), research paper; for doctorate, comprehensive exam, thesis/dissertation. *Entrance requirements:* For master's and doctorate, GRE General Test, minimum GPA of 3.0 (recommended). Additional exam requirements/recommendations for international students: Required—TOEFL. *Application deadline:* For fall admission, 12/10 priority date for domestic and international students; for spring admission, 9/10 for domestic students. Applications are processed on a rolling basis. Application fee: $85. Electronic applications accepted. *Financial support:* Fellowships with tuition reimbursements, research assistantships with tuition reimbursements, teaching assistantships with tuition reimbursements, career-related internships or fieldwork, Federal Work-Study, traineeships, health care benefits, and unspecified assistantships available. Support available to part-time students. Financial award application deadline: 12/10; financial award applicants required to submit FAFSA. *Faculty research:* Air, radiation and industrial hygiene, aquatic and atmospheric sciences, environmental health sciences, environmental management and policy, water resources engineering. *Unit head:* Dr. Michael Aitken, Chair, 919-966-1024, Fax: 919-966-7911, E-mail: mike_aitken@unc.edu. *Application contact:* Jack Whaley, Registrar, 919-966-3844, Fax: 919-966-7911, E-mail: jack_whaley@unc.edu. Website: http://www2.sph.unc.edu/envr/

University of North Texas Health Science Center at Fort Worth, School of Public Health, Fort Worth, TX 76107-2699. Offers biostatistics (MPH); community health (MPH); disease control and prevention (Dr PH); environmental and occupational health sciences (MPH); epidemiology (MPH); health administration (MHA); health policy and management (MPH, Dr PH); DO/MPH; MS/MPH; MSN/MPH. MPH offered jointly with University of North Texas; DO/MPH with Texas College of Osteopathic Medicine. *Accreditation:* CEPH. *Program availability:* Part-time, evening/weekend. *Degree requirements:* For master's, thesis or alternative, supervised internship; for doctorate, thesis/dissertation, supervised internship. *Entrance requirements:* For master's, GRE General Test. Additional exam requirements/recommendations for international students: Required—TOEFL. Electronic applications accepted.

University of Oklahoma Health Sciences Center, Graduate College, College of Public Health, Department of Occupational and Environmental Health, Oklahoma City, OK 73190. Offers MPH, MS, Dr PH, PhD, JD/MPH, JD/MS. JD/MPH, JD/MS offered jointly with University of Oklahoma. *Accreditation:* ABET (one or more programs are accredited); CEPH (one or more programs are accredited). *Program availability:* Part-time. *Degree requirements:* For master's, comprehensive exam, thesis (for some programs); for doctorate, comprehensive exam, thesis/dissertation. *Entrance requirements:* For master's, GRE General Test (for all except occupational medicine), 3 letters of recommendation, resume; for doctorate, GRE (for all except occupational medicine), 3 letters of recommendation, resume. Additional exam requirements/recommendations for international students: Required—TOEFL (minimum score 570 paper-based). *Faculty research:* Environmental safety, accident prevention and injury control.

University of Pennsylvania, Perelman School of Medicine, Master of Public Health Program, Philadelphia, PA 19104. Offers generalist, global health, environmental health (MPH); DMD/MPH; JD/MPH; MD/MPH; MPH/MBE; MSN/MPH; MSSP/MPH; MSW/MPH; PhD/MPH. *Program availability:* Part-time, evening/weekend. *Faculty:* 21 full-time (14 women), 20 part-time/adjunct (15 women). *Students:* 94 full-time (81 women), 68 part-time (54 women); includes 74 minority (30 Black or African American, non-Hispanic/Latino; 31 Asian, non-Hispanic/Latino; 3 Hispanic/Latino; 10 Two or more races, non-Hispanic/Latino), 2 international. Average age 29. 448 applicants, 49% accepted, 79 enrolled. In 2015, 41 master's awarded. *Entrance requirements:* For master's, GRE. Additional exam requirements/recommendations for international students: Required—TOEFL (minimum score 100 iBT). *Application deadline:* For fall admission, 4/15 for domestic and international students. Applications are processed on a rolling basis. Electronic applications accepted. *Expenses: Tuition, area resident:* Full-time $31,068; part-time $5762 per course. *Required fees:* $3200; $336 per course. Full-time tuition and fees vary according to degree level, program and student level. Part-time tuition and fees vary according to course load, degree level and program. *Financial support:* In 2015–16, 31 students received support, including 1 fellowship with partial tuition reimbursement available (averaging $1,000 per year), 7 research assistantships with partial tuition reimbursements available (averaging $18,104 per year), 24 teaching assistantships with partial tuition reimbursements available (averaging $4,526 per year); tuition waivers (partial) also available. Financial award application deadline: 5/15; financial award applicants required to submit FAFSA. *Faculty research:* Health disparities, health behaviors, obesity, global health, epidemiology and prevention research. *Unit head:* Dr. Jennifer Pinto-Martin, Director, 215-898-4726, E-mail: pinto@nursing.upenn.edu. *Application contact:* Moriah Hall, Associate Director, MPH Program, 215-573-8841, E-mail: moriahh@mail.med.upenn.edu. Website: http://www.publichealth.med.upenn.edu/

University of Pittsburgh, Graduate School of Public Health, Department of Environmental and Occupational Health, Pittsburgh, PA 15219. Offers environmental and occupational health (MPH, Dr PH). *Accreditation:* CEPH (one or more programs are accredited). *Program availability:* Part-time. *Faculty:* 23 full-time (6 women), 14 part-time/adjunct (4 women). *Students:* 28 full-time (19 women), 13 part-time (10 women); includes 8 minority (3 Black or African American, non-Hispanic/Latino; 2 Asian, non-Hispanic/Latino; 2 Hispanic/Latino; 1 Two or more races, non-Hispanic/Latino), 13 international. Average age 27. 64 applicants, 58% accepted, 16 enrolled. In 2015, 10 master's, 6 doctorates awarded. Terminal master's awarded for partial completion of doctoral program. *Degree requirements:* For master's, comprehensive exam, thesis, practica; for doctorate, comprehensive exam, thesis/dissertation, preliminary exams, journal club. *Entrance requirements:* For master's, GRE General Test, transcripts,

Environmental and Occupational Health

recommendation letters, personal statement; for doctorate, GRE General Test, minimum GPA of 3.4; background in biology, physics, chemistry and calculus. Additional exam requirements/recommendations for international students: Required—TOEFL (minimum score 550 paper-based, 80 iBT) or IELTS (minimum score 6.5). *Application deadline:* For fall admission, 1/15 for domestic and international students; for spring admission, 10/15 for domestic students, 8/1 for international students. Applications are processed on a rolling basis. Application fee: $120. *Expenses:* $12,464 per term in-state; $20,502 per term out-of-state; $1,016 per credit in-state; $1,680 per credit out-of-state. *Financial support:* In 2015–16, 13 students received support, including 13 research assistantships (averaging $14,270 per year); fellowships, teaching assistantships, Federal Work-Study, institutionally sponsored loans, scholarships/grants, and health care benefits also available. Financial award application deadline: 4/15; financial award applicants required to submit FAFSA. *Faculty research:* Interactions of reactive oxygen, nitrogen, and radiation with mitochondria; understandings of combined health effects of social stressors and air pollution exposures; cellular mechanisms by which various environmental agents contribute to organ dysfunction during toxicity; impact of metals on cardiovascular health and reproductive status of women; mutational pathways that link environmental chemicals to cancer. *Total annual research expenditures:* $8.4 million. *Unit head:* Dr. Bruce R. Pitt, Chair, 412-624-8300, Fax: 412-383-7658, E-mail: brucep@pitt.edu. *Application contact:* Eileen Penny Weiss, Associate Administrator, Payroll and Student Affairs, 412-383-7297, Fax: 412-383-7658, E-mail: pweiss@pitt.edu. Website: http://www.eoh.pitt.edu/

University of Puerto Rico, Medical Sciences Campus, Graduate School of Public Health, Department of Environmental Health, Doctoral Program in Environmental Health, San Juan, PR 00936-5067. Offers MS, Dr PH. *Program availability:* Part-time. *Expenses:* Contact institution.

University of Saint Francis, Graduate School, Keith Busse School of Business and Entrepreneurial Leadership, Fort Wayne, IN 46808-3994. Offers business administration (MBA); environmental health (MEH); healthcare administration (MHA); sustainability (MBA). *Accreditation:* ACBSP. *Program availability:* Part-time, evening/weekend, online learning. *Entrance requirements:* For master's, minimum cumulative GPA of 2.75. Additional exam requirements/recommendations for international students: Required—TOEFL or IELTS. Electronic applications accepted. *Expenses:* Contact institution.

University of Saint Francis, Graduate School, Program in Environmental Health, Fort Wayne, IN 46808-3994. Offers MEH. *Program availability:* Part-time, online learning. *Degree requirements:* For master's, professional e-portfolio. *Entrance requirements:* For master's, bachelor's degree or higher from regionally-accredited institution, minimum cumulative GPA of 2.75, letter of recommendation.

University of South Alabama, Graduate School, Program in Environmental Toxicology, Mobile, AL 36688. Offers MS. *Faculty:* 1 full-time (0 women). *Students:* 5 full-time (4 women), 4 part-time (3 women); includes 1 minority (both Black or African American, non-Hispanic/Latino). Average age 26. 12 applicants, 25% accepted, 2 enrolled. In 2015, 5 master's awarded. *Degree requirements:* For master's, comprehensive exam, research project or thesis. *Entrance requirements:* For master's, GRE, BA/BS in related discipline, minimum undergraduate GPA of 3.0. Additional exam requirements/recommendations for international students: Required—TOEFL (minimum score 525 paper-based; 71 iBT). *Application deadline:* For fall admission, 7/15 for domestic students, 6/15 for international students; for spring admission, 12/1 for domestic students, 11/1 for international students. Application fee: $35. Electronic applications accepted. *Expenses:* Tuition, state resident: full-time $9480; part-time $395 per credit hour. Tuition, nonresident: full-time $18,960; part-time $790 per credit hour. *Financial support:* Fellowships, research assistantships, teaching assistantships, career-related internships or fieldwork, Federal Work-Study, institutionally sponsored loans, scholarships/grants, and unspecified assistantships available. Support available to part-time students. Financial award application deadline: 5/31; financial award applicants required to submit FAFSA. *Unit head:* Dr. B. Keith Harrison, Dean and Senior Vice President for Academic Affairs, 251-460-6310, E-mail: gradschool@southalabama.edu. *Application contact:* Dr. David Forbes, Chair, Chemistry, 251-460-6181, E-mail: dforbes@southalabama.edu. Website: http://www.southalabama.edu/graduatemajors/etox/index.html

University of South Carolina, The Graduate School, Arnold School of Public Health, Department of Environmental Health Sciences, Program in Environmental Quality, Columbia, SC 29208. Offers MPH, MS, MSPH, PhD. *Accreditation:* CEPH (one or more programs are accredited). *Program availability:* Part-time. *Degree requirements:* For master's, comprehensive exam, thesis (for some programs), practicum (MPH); for doctorate, one foreign language, comprehensive exam, thesis/dissertation. *Entrance requirements:* For master's and doctorate, GRE General Test. Additional exam requirements/recommendations for international students: Required—TOEFL (minimum score 570 paper-based). Electronic applications accepted. *Faculty research:* Environmental assessment and planning; environmental toxicology; ecosystems analysis; air quality monitoring and modeling.

University of Southern California, Keck School of Medicine and Graduate School, Graduate Programs in Medicine, Department of Preventive Medicine, Master of Public Health Program, Los Angeles, CA 91803. Offers biostatistics and epidemiology (MPH); child and family health (MPH); environmental health (MPH); global health leadership (MPH); health communication (MPH); health education and promotion (MPH); public health policy (MPH). *Accreditation:* CEPH. *Program availability:* Part-time, evening/weekend. *Faculty:* 22 full-time (12 women), 3 part-time/adjunct (0 women). *Students:* 182 full-time (142 women), 35 part-time (25 women); includes 120 minority (19 Black or African American, non-Hispanic/Latino; 64 Asian, non-Hispanic/Latino; 37 Hispanic/Latino), 33 international. Average age 24. 236 applicants, 70% accepted, 71 enrolled. In 2015, 99 master's awarded. *Degree requirements:* For master's, practicum, final report, oral presentation. *Entrance requirements:* For master's, GRE General Test, MCAT, GMAT, minimum GPA of 3.0. Additional exam requirements/recommendations for international students: Required—TOEFL (minimum score 600 paper-based; 90 iBT). *Application deadline:* For fall admission, 6/1 priority date for domestic and international students; for spring admission, 10/1 priority date for domestic and international students; for summer admission, 3/1 for domestic and international students. Applications are processed on a rolling basis. Application fee: $85. Electronic applications accepted. *Expenses:* Contact institution. *Financial support:* Career-related internships or fieldwork, Federal Work-Study, institutionally sponsored loans, and scholarships/grants available. Support available to part-time students. Financial award application deadline: 5/4; financial award applicants required to submit CSS PROFILE or FAFSA. *Faculty research:* Substance abuse prevention, cancer and heart disease prevention, mass media and health communication research, health promotion, treatment compliance. *Unit head:* Dr. Louise A. Rohrbach, Director, 323-442-8237, Fax: 323-442-8297, E-mail: rohrbac@usc.edu. *Application contact:* Valerie Burris, Admissions Counselor, 323-442-7257, Fax: 323-442-8297, E-mail: valeriem@usc.edu. Website: http://mph.usc.edu/

University of South Florida, College of Public Health, Department of Environmental and Occupational Health, Tampa, FL 33620-9951. Offers MPH, MSPH, PhD. *Accreditation:* ABET (one or more programs are accredited); CEPH (one or more programs are accredited). *Program availability:* Part-time, evening/weekend. *Degree requirements:* For master's, comprehensive exam, thesis (for some programs); for doctorate, comprehensive exam, thesis/dissertation. *Entrance requirements:* For master's, GRE General Test, minimum GPA of 3.0 in upper-level course work, goal statement letter, two professional letters of recommendation, resume/curriculum vitae; for doctorate, GRE General Test, minimum GPA of 3.0 in upper-level course work, goal statement letter, three professional letters of recommendation, resume/curriculum vitae, writing sample. Additional exam requirements/recommendations for international students: Required—TOEFL (minimum score 550 paper-based; 79 iBT). Electronic applications accepted. *Faculty research:* Biomedical assessment/stress test, risk impact, nitrobenzes on mammalism glutathion transferases, lysimeter research management, independent hygiene development.

University of South Florida, Innovative Education, Tampa, FL 33620-9951. Offers adult, career and higher education (Graduate Certificate), including college teaching, leadership in developing human resources, leadership in higher education; Africana studies (Graduate Certificate), including diasporas and health disparities, genocide and human rights; aging studies (Graduate Certificate), including gerontology; art research (Graduate Certificate), including museum studies; business foundations (Graduate Certificate); chemical and biomedical engineering (Graduate Certificate), including materials science and engineering, water, health and sustainability; child and family studies (Graduate Certificate), including positive behavior support; civil and industrial engineering (Graduate Certificate), including transportation systems analysis; community and family health (Graduate Certificate), including maternal and child health, social marketing and public health, violence and injury: prevention and intervention, women's health; criminology (Graduate Certificate), including criminal justice administration; educational measurement and research (Graduate Certificate), including evaluation; English (Graduate Certificate), including comparative literary studies, creative writing, professional and technical communication; entrepreneurship (Graduate Certificate); environmental health (Graduate Certificate), including safety management; epidemiology and biostatistics (Graduate Certificate), including applied biostatistics, biostatistics, concepts and tools of epidemiology, epidemiology, epidemiology of infectious diseases; geography, environment and planning (Graduate Certificate), including community development, environmental policy and management, geographical information systems; geology (Graduate Certificate), including hydrogeology; global health (Graduate Certificate), including disaster management, global health and Latin American and Caribbean studies, global health practice, humanitarian assistance, infection control; government and international affairs (Graduate Certificate), including Cuban studies, globalization studies; health policy and management (Graduate Certificate), including health management and leadership, public health policy and programs; hearing specialist: early intervention (Graduate Certificate); industrial and management systems engineering (Graduate Certificate), including systems engineering, technology management; information studies (Graduate Certificate), including school library media specialist; information systems/decision sciences (Graduate Certificate), including analytics and business intelligence; instructional technology (Graduate Certificate), including distance education, Florida digital/virtual educator, instructional design, multimedia design, Web design; internal medicine, bioethics and medical humanities (Graduate Certificate), including biomedical ethics; Latin American and Caribbean studies (Graduate Certificate); mass communications (Graduate Certificate), including multimedia journalism; mathematics and statistics (Graduate Certificate), including mathematics; medicine (Graduate Certificate), including aging and neuroscience, bioinformatics, biotechnology, brain fitness and memory management, clinical investigation, health informatics, health sciences, integrative weight management, intellectual property, medicine and gender, metabolic and nutritional medicine, metabolic cardiology, pharmacy sciences; national and competitive intelligence (Graduate Certificate); psychological and social foundations (Graduate Certificate), including career counseling, college teaching, diversity in education, mental health counseling, school counseling; public affairs (Graduate Certificate), including nonprofit management, public management, research administration; public health (Graduate Certificate), including environmental health, health equity, public health generalist, translational research in adolescent behavioral health; public health practices (Graduate Certificate), including planning for healthy communities; rehabilitation and mental health counseling (Graduate Certificate), including integrative mental health care, marriage and family therapy, rehabilitation technology; secondary education (Graduate Certificate), including ESOL, foreign language education: culture and content, foreign language education: professional; social work (Graduate Certificate), including geriatric social work/clinical gerontology; special education (Graduate Certificate), including autism spectrum disorder, disabilities education: severe/profound; world languages (Graduate Certificate), including teaching English as a second language (TESL) or foreign language. *Unit head:* Kathy Barnes, Interdisciplinary Programs Coordinator, 813-974-8031, Fax: 813-974-7061, E-mail: barnesk@usf.edu. *Application contact:* Karen Tylinski, Metro Initiatives, 813-974-9943, Fax: 813-974-7061, E-mail: ktylinsk@usf.edu. Website: http://www.usf.edu/innovative-education/

The University of Texas at Tyler, College of Engineering and Computer Science, Department of Civil Engineering, Tyler, TX 75799-0001. Offers environmental engineering (MS); industrial safety (MS); structural engineering (MS); transportation engineering (MS); water resources engineering (MS). *Program availability:* Part-time, evening/weekend. *Degree requirements:* For master's, thesis optional. *Entrance requirements:* For master's, GRE General Test, bachelor's degree in engineering, associated science degree. Additional exam requirements/recommendations for international students: Required—TOEFL. *Faculty research:* Non-destructive strength testing, indoor air quality, transportation routing and signaling, pavement replacement criteria, flood water routing, construction and long-term behavior of innovative geotechnical foundation and embankment construction used in highway construction, engineering education.

University of the Sacred Heart, Graduate Programs, Department of Natural Sciences, Program in Occupational Health and Safety, San Juan, PR 00914-0383. Offers MS.

The University of Toledo, College of Graduate Studies, College of Medicine and Life Sciences, Department of Public Health and Preventative Medicine, Toledo, OH 43606-3390. Offers biostatistics and epidemiology (Certificate); contemporary gerontological practice (Certificate); environmental and occupational health and safety (MPH); epidemiology (Certificate); global public health (Certificate); health promotion and education (MPH); industrial hygiene (MSOH); medical and health science teaching and learning (Certificate); occupational health (Certificate); public health administration (MPH); public health and emergency response (Certificate); public health epidemiology (MPH); public health nutrition (MPH); MD/MPH. *Program availability:* Part-time, evening/weekend. *Degree requirements:* For master's, thesis or alternative. *Entrance requirements:* For master's, GRE, minimum undergraduate GPA of 3.0, three letters of recommendation, statement of purpose, transcripts from all prior institutions attended, resume; for Certificate, minimum undergraduate GPA of 3.0, three letters of recommendation, statement of purpose, transcripts from all prior institutions attended, resume. Additional exam requirements/recommendations for international students: Required—TOEFL (minimum score 550 paper-based; 80 iBT), IELTS (minimum score 6.5). Electronic applications accepted.

University of Toronto, School of Graduate Studies, Department of Public Health Sciences, Toronto, ON M5S 1A1, Canada. Offers biostatistics (M Sc, PhD); community health (M Sc); community nutrition (MPH), including nutrition and dietetics; epidemiology (MPH, PhD); family and community medicine (MPH); occupational and environmental health (MPH); social and behavioral health science (PhD); social and behavioral health sciences (MPH), including health promotion. *Accreditation:* CAHME (one or more programs are accredited); CEPH (one or more programs are accredited). *Program availability:* Part-time. *Degree requirements:* For master's, thesis (for some programs), practicum; for doctorate, comprehensive exam, thesis/dissertation, oral thesis defense. *Entrance requirements:* For master's, 2 letters of reference, relevant professional/research experience, minimum B average in final year; for doctorate, 2 letters of reference, relevant professional/research experience, minimum B+ average. Additional exam requirements/recommendations for international students: Required—TOEFL (minimum score 580 paper-based; 93 iBT), TWE (minimum score 5). Electronic applications accepted. *Expenses:* Contact institution.

University of Washington, Graduate School, School of Public Health, Department of Environmental and Occupational Health Sciences, Seattle, WA 98195. Offers environmental and occupational health (MPH); environmental and occupational hygiene (PhD); environmental health (MS); occupational and environmental exposure sciences (MS); occupational and environmental medicine (MPH); toxicology (MS, PhD); MPH/MPA; MS/MPA. *Program availability:* Part-time. Terminal master's awarded for partial completion of doctoral program. *Degree requirements:* For master's, comprehensive exam, thesis (for some programs), project or thesis; for doctorate, comprehensive exam, thesis/dissertation. *Entrance requirements:* For master's, GRE General Test, one year each of physics, general chemistry, and biology; two quarters of organic chemistry; one quarter of calculus; for doctorate, GRE General Test, minimum GPA of 3.0, prerequisite course work in biology, chemistry, physics, calculus. Additional exam requirements/recommendations for international students: Required—TOEFL (minimum score 580 paper-based; 92 iBT). Electronic applications accepted. *Expenses:* Contact institution. *Faculty research:* Developmental and behavioral toxicology, biochemical toxicology, exposure assessment, hazardous waste, industrial chemistry.

University of West Florida, College of Education and Professional Studies, Department of Health, Leisure, and Exercise Science, Community Health Education Program, Pensacola, FL 32514-5750. Offers aging studies (MS); health promotion and worksite wellness (MS); psychosocial (MS). *Program availability:* Part-time, evening/weekend. *Degree requirements:* For master's, thesis or alternative. *Entrance requirements:* For master's, GRE or MAT, official transcripts; minimum GPA of 3.0; letter of intent; three personal references. Additional exam requirements/recommendations for international students: Required—TOEFL (minimum score 550 paper-based).

University of Wisconsin–Milwaukee, Graduate School, Zilber School of Public Health, Department of Environmental and Occupational Health, Milwaukee, WI 53201-0413. Offers PhD. *Students:* 3 full-time (2 women), 1 (woman) part-time. Average age 38. 7 applicants, 29% accepted, 1 enrolled. In 2015, 3 doctorates awarded. *Unit head:* Darcie Galowitch, Representative, 414-229-3264, E-mail: darcie@uwm.edu. *Application contact:* Darcie K. G. Warren, Graduate Program Manager, 414-229-5633, E-mail: darcie@uwm.edu.

University of Wisconsin–Whitewater, School of Graduate Studies, College of Education and Professional Studies, Department of Occupational and Environmental Safety, Whitewater, WI 53190-1790. Offers safety (MS). *Program availability:* Part-time, evening/weekend, online learning. *Degree requirements:* For master's, thesis or alternative. *Entrance requirements:* For master's, 2 letters of recommendation. Additional exam requirements/recommendations for international students: Required—TOEFL (minimum score 550 paper-based; 80 iBT), IELTS (minimum score 6). *Application deadline:* For fall admission, 7/15 priority date for domestic and international students; for spring admission, 12/1 priority date for domestic and international students. Applications are processed on a rolling basis. Application fee: $56. Electronic applications accepted. *Expenses:* Tuition, state resident: full-time $9008. Tuition, nonresident: full-time $18,600. *Financial support:* Research assistantships, Federal Work-Study, unspecified assistantships, and out-of-state fee waivers available. Support

available to part-time students. Financial award application deadline: 3/15; financial award applicants required to submit FAFSA.

West Chester University of Pennsylvania, College of Health Sciences, Department of Health, West Chester, PA 19383. Offers community health (MPH); emergency preparedness (Certificate); environmental health (MPH); gerontology (Certificate); health care management (MPH, Certificate); integrative health (Certificate); school health (M Ed). *Accreditation:* CEPH. *Program availability:* Part-time, evening/weekend. *Faculty:* 12 full-time (7 women), 4 part-time/adjunct (3 women). *Students:* 98 full-time (74 women), 85 part-time (59 women); includes 73 minority (60 Black or African American, non-Hispanic/Latino; 8 Asian, non-Hispanic/Latino; 4 Hispanic/Latino; 1 Two or more races, non-Hispanic/Latino), 26 international. Average age 30. 118 applicants, 86% accepted, 60 enrolled. In 2015, 72 master's, 17 other advanced degrees awarded. *Degree requirements:* For master's, thesis or alternative, minimum GPA of 3.0; research report (for M Ed); major project and practicum (for MPH); for Certificate, minimum GPA of 3.0. *Entrance requirements:* For master's, goal statement, two letters of recommendation, undergraduate introduction to statistics course; for Certificate, minimum undergraduate GPA of 2.8 (for gerontology). Additional exam requirements/recommendations for international students: Required—TOEFL or IELTS. *Application deadline:* For fall admission, 5/15 for international students; for spring admission, 10/15 for international students. Applications are processed on a rolling basis. Application fee: $50. Electronic applications accepted. *Expenses:* Tuition, state resident: full-time $8460; part-time $470 per credit. Tuition, nonresident: full-time $12,690; part-time $705 per credit. *Required fees:* $2312; $126.75 per credit. Tuition and fees vary according to campus/location and program. *Financial support:* Scholarships/grants and unspecified assistantships available. Financial award application deadline: 2/15; financial award applicants required to submit FAFSA. *Faculty research:* Healthy school communities, community health issues and evidence-based programs, environment and health, nutrition and health, integrative health. *Unit head:* Dr. Bethann Cinelli, Chair, 610-436-2267, E-mail: bcinelli@wcupa.edu. *Application contact:* Dr. Lynn Carson, Graduate Coordinator, 610-436-2138, E-mail: lcarson@wcupa.edu.
Website: http://www.wcupa.edu/_ACADEMICS/HealthSciences/health/

West Virginia University, Statler College of Engineering and Mineral Resources, Department of Industrial and Management Systems Engineering, Program in Occupational Safety and Health, Morgantown, WV 26506. Offers PhD. *Program availability:* Part-time, online learning. *Degree requirements:* For doctorate, comprehensive exam, thesis/dissertation. *Entrance requirements:* For doctorate, GRE General Test, Minimum GPA of 3.5. Additional exam requirements/recommendations for international students: Required—TOEFL. *Expenses:* Tuition, state resident: full-time $8568. Tuition, nonresident: full-time $22,140. Tuition and fees vary according to program. *Faculty research:* Safety management, ergonomics and workplace design, safety and health training, construction safety.

Yale University, School of Medicine, Yale School of Public Health, New Haven, CT 06520. Offers applied biostatistics and epidemiology (APMPH); biostatistics (MPH, MS, PhD), including global health (MPH); chronic disease epidemiology (MPH, PhD), including global health (MPH); environmental health sciences (MPH, PhD), including global health (MPH); epidemiology of microbial diseases (MPH, PhD), including global health (MPH); global health (APMPH); health management (MPH), including global health; health policy (MPH), including global health; health policy and administration (APMPH, PhD); occupational and environmental medicine (APMPH); preventive medicine (APMPH); social and behavioral sciences (APMPH, MPH), including global health (MPH); JD/MPH; M Div/MPH; MBA/MPH; MD/MPH; MEM/MPH; MFS/MPH; MM Sc/MPH; MPH/MA; MSN/MPH. MS and PhD offered through the Graduate School. *Accreditation:* CEPH. *Program availability:* Part-time. Terminal master's awarded for partial completion of doctoral program. *Degree requirements:* For master's, thesis, summer internship; for doctorate, comprehensive exam, thesis/dissertation, residency. *Entrance requirements:* For master's, GMAT, GRE, or MCAT, two years of undergraduate coursework in math and science; for doctorate, GRE General Test. Additional exam requirements/recommendations for international students: Required—TOEFL (minimum score 100 iBT). Electronic applications accepted. *Expenses:* Contact institution. *Faculty research:* Genetic and emerging infections epidemiology, virology, cost/quality, vector biology, quantitative methods, aging, asthma, cancer.

Epidemiology

American University of Beirut, Graduate Programs, Faculty of Health Sciences, Beirut, Lebanon. Offers environmental sciences (MS), including environmental health; epidemiology (MS); epidemiology and biostatistics (MPH); health management and policy (MPH); health promotion and community health (MPH). *Program availability:* Part-time. *Faculty:* 30 full-time (21 women), 3 part-time/adjunct (1 woman). *Students:* 49 full-time (38 women), 99 part-time (81 women). Average age 27. 115 applicants, 71% accepted, 40 enrolled. In 2015, 51 master's awarded. *Degree requirements:* For master's, one foreign language, comprehensive exam (for some programs), thesis (for some programs). *Entrance requirements:* For master's, 2 letters of recommendation, personal statement, transcripts. Additional exam requirements/recommendations for international students: Required—TOEFL (minimum score 583 paper-based; 97 iBT), IELTS (minimum score 7). *Application deadline:* For fall admission, 1/4 priority date for domestic and international students; for spring admission, 11/1 for domestic and international students. Application fee: $50. Electronic applications accepted. *Expenses: Tuition, area resident:* Full-time $16,254; part-time $903 per credit. *Required fees:* $699. Tuition and fees vary according to course load and program. *Financial support:* In 2015–16, 70 students received support. Scholarships/grants, health care benefits, and unspecified assistantships available. Financial award application deadline: 4/1. *Faculty research:* Tobacco control; health of the elderly; youth health; mental health; women's health; reproductive and sexual health, including HIV/AIDS; water quality; health systems; quality in health care delivery; health human resources; health policy; occupational and environmental health; social inequality; social determinants of health; non-communicable diseases; nutrition; refugees health; conflict and health. *Total annual research expenditures:* $2 million. *Unit head:* Iman Adel Nuwayhid, Dean, 961-1759683, Fax: 961-1744470, E-mail: nuwayhid@aub.edu.lb. *Application contact:* Mitra Tauk, Administrative Coordinator, 961-1350000 Ext. 4687, Fax: 961-1744470, E-mail: mt12@aub.edu.lb.

Boston University, School of Public Health, Epidemiology Department, Boston, MA 02215. Offers MPH, MS, PhD. *Accreditation:* CEPH (one or more programs are accredited). *Program availability:* Part-time, evening/weekend. *Faculty:* 25 full-time, 60 part-time/adjunct. *Students:* 146 full-time (108 women), 79 part-time (64 women); includes 57 minority (13 Black or African American, non-Hispanic/Latino; 26 Asian, non-

Hispanic/Latino; 13 Hispanic/Latino; 5 Two or more races, non-Hispanic/Latino), 28 international. Average age 27. 565 applicants, 36% accepted, 65 enrolled. In 2015, 114 master's, 9 doctorates awarded. *Degree requirements:* For master's, comprehensive exam (for some programs), thesis (for some programs); for doctorate, comprehensive exam, thesis/dissertation. *Entrance requirements:* For master's, GRE, GMAT, or MCAT, U.S. bachelor's degree or foreign equivalent; for doctorate, GRE, MPH or equivalent. Additional exam requirements/recommendations for international students: Required—TOEFL (minimum score 600 paper-based; 100 iBT), IELTS (minimum score 7). *Application deadline:* For fall admission, 12/1 priority date for domestic students, 1/1 priority date for international students; for spring admission, 10/1 priority date for domestic students. Applications are processed on a rolling basis. Application fee: $115. Electronic applications accepted. *Financial support:* Career-related internships or fieldwork, Federal Work-Study, institutionally sponsored loans, and scholarships/grants available. Support available to part-time students. Financial award application deadline: 3/1; financial award applicants required to submit FAFSA. *Faculty research:* Infectious disease, chronic disease, reproductive epidemiology, social epidemiology, research methods. *Unit head:* Dr. Martha M. Werler, Chair, 617- 638-7775, E-mail: epi@bu.edu. *Application contact:* LePhan Quan, Associate Director of Admissions, 617-638-4640, Fax: 617-638-5299, E-mail: asksph@bu.edu.
Website: http://www.bu.edu/sph/epi

Brown University, Graduate School, Division of Biology and Medicine, School of Public Health, Department of Epidemiology, Providence, RI 02912. Offers Sc M, PhD. *Degree requirements:* For doctorate, thesis/dissertation, preliminary exam. *Entrance requirements:* For master's and doctorate, GRE General Test.

Capella University, School of Public Service Leadership, Doctoral Programs in Healthcare, Minneapolis, MN 55402. Offers criminal justice (PhD); emergency management (PhD); epidemiology (Dr PH); general health administration (DHA); general public administration (DPA); health advocacy and leadership (Dr PH); health care administration (PhD); health care leadership (DHA); health policy advocacy (DHA); multidisciplinary human services (PhD); nonprofit management and leadership (PhD); public safety leadership (PhD); social and community services (PhD).

Epidemiology

Case Western Reserve University, School of Medicine and School of Graduate Studies, Graduate Programs in Medicine, Department of Epidemiology and Biostatistics, Program in Epidemiology, Cleveland, OH 44106. Offers MS, PhD. *Accreditation:* CEPH. *Program availability:* Part-time. Terminal master's awarded for partial completion of doctoral program. *Degree requirements:* For master's, comprehensive exam, thesis; for doctorate, comprehensive exam, thesis/dissertation. *Entrance requirements:* For master's, GRE General Test or MCAT, 3 recommendations; for doctorate, GRE General Test, 3 recommendations. Additional exam requirements/recommendations for international students: Required—TOEFL (minimum score 550 paper-based). Electronic applications accepted. *Expenses: Tuition,* area resident: Full-time $41,137; part-time $1714 per credit hour. *Required fees:* $32. Tuition and fees vary according to course load and program. *Faculty research:* Cardiovascular epidemiology, cancer risk factors, HIV in underserved populations, effectiveness studies in Medicare patients.

Case Western Reserve University, School of Medicine and School of Graduate Studies, Graduate Programs in Medicine, Department of Epidemiology and Biostatistics, Program in Genetic and Molecular Epidemiology, Cleveland, OH 44106. Offers MS, PhD. *Degree requirements:* For master's, comprehensive exam, thesis; for doctorate, comprehensive exam, thesis/dissertation. *Entrance requirements:* For master's and doctorate, GRE. Additional exam requirements/recommendations for international students: Required—TOEFL (minimum score 550 paper-based). *Expenses: Tuition,* area resident: Full-time $41,137; part-time $1714 per credit hour. *Required fees:* $32. Tuition and fees vary according to course load and program.

Columbia University, Columbia University Mailman School of Public Health, Department of Epidemiology, New York, NY 10032. Offers MPH, MS, Dr PH. PhD offered in cooperation with the Graduate School of Arts and Sciences. *Accreditation:* CEPH (one or more programs are accredited). *Program availability:* Part-time, evening/weekend. *Students:* 242 full-time (191 women), 156 part-time (109 women); includes 151 minority (34 Black or African American, non-Hispanic/Latino; 2 American Indian or Alaska Native, non-Hispanic/Latino; 69 Asian, non-Hispanic/Latino; 32 Hispanic/Latino; 14 Two or more races, non-Hispanic/Latino), 80 international. Average age 28. 729 applicants, 62% accepted, 164 enrolled. In 2015, 144 master's, 10 doctorates awarded. *Degree requirements:* For master's, thesis; for doctorate, thesis/dissertation. *Entrance requirements:* For master's, GRE General Test; for doctorate, GRE General Test, MPH or equivalent (for Dr PH). Additional exam requirements/recommendations for international students: Required—TOEFL (minimum score 600 paper-based; 100 iBT). *Application deadline:* For fall admission, 12/1 priority date for domestic and international students. Application fee: $120. Electronic applications accepted. *Financial support:* Research assistantships, teaching assistantships, career-related internships or fieldwork, and Federal Work-Study available. Support available to part-time students. Financial award application deadline: 2/1; financial award applicants required to submit FAFSA. *Faculty research:* Infectious disease epidemiology, chronic disease epidemiology, social epidemiology, psychiatric epidemiology, neurological epidemiology. *Unit head:* Dr. Guohua Li, Interim Chairperson, 212-305-8486. *Application contact:* Dr. Joseph Korevec, Senior Director of Admissions and Financial Aid, 212-305-8698, Fax: 212-342-1861, E-mail: ph-admit@columbia.edu. Website: https://www.mailman.columbia.edu/become-student/departments/epidemiology

Cornell University, Graduate School, Graduate Fields of Comparative Biomedical Sciences, Field of Comparative Biomedical Sciences, Ithaca, NY 14853-0001. Offers cellular and molecular medicine (MS, PhD); developmental and reproductive biology (MS, PhD); infectious diseases (MS, PhD); population medicine and epidemiology (MS, PhD); structural and functional biology (MS, PhD). *Degree requirements:* For master's, thesis; for doctorate, comprehensive exam, thesis/dissertation. *Entrance requirements:* For master's and doctorate, GRE General Test, 2 letters of recommendation. Additional exam requirements/recommendations for international students: Required—TOEFL (minimum score 550 paper-based; 77 iBT). Electronic applications accepted. *Faculty research:* Receptors and signal transduction, viral and bacterial infectious diseases, tumor metastasis, clinical sciences/nutritional disease, developmental/neurological disorders.

Daemen College, Program in Public Health, Amherst, NY 14226-3592. Offers community health education (MPH); epidemiology (MPH); generalist (MPH). *Program availability:* Part-time, online learning. *Degree requirements:* For master's, practicum.

Dalhousie University, Faculty of Medicine, Department of Community Health and Epidemiology, Halifax, NS B3H 4R2, Canada. Offers M Sc. *Degree requirements:* For master's, thesis. *Entrance requirements:* Additional exam requirements/recommendations for international students: Required—1 of 5 approved tests: TOEFL, IELTS, CANTEST, CAEL, Michigan English Language Assessment Battery. Electronic applications accepted. *Expenses:* Contact institution. *Faculty research:* Population health, health promotion and disease prevention, health services utilization, chronic disease epidemiology.

Drexel University, School of Public Health, Department of Epidemiology and Biostatistics, Philadelphia, PA 19104-2875. Offers biostatistics (MS); epidemiology (PhD); epidemiology and biostatistics (Certificate).

Emory University, Rollins School of Public Health, Department of Environmental Health, Atlanta, GA 30322-1100. Offers environmental health (MPH); environmental health and epidemiology (MSPH); environmental health sciences (PhD); global environmental health (MPH). *Accreditation:* CEPH. *Program availability:* Part-time. *Degree requirements:* For master's, thesis, practicum. *Entrance requirements:* For master's, GRE General Test. Additional exam requirements/recommendations for international students: Required—TOEFL. Electronic applications accepted.

Emory University, Rollins School of Public Health, Department of Epidemiology, Atlanta, GA 30322-1100. Offers MPH, MSPH, PhD. *Accreditation:* CEPH. *Program availability:* Part-time. *Degree requirements:* For master's, thesis, practicum. *Entrance requirements:* For master's, GRE General Test. Additional exam requirements/recommendations for international students: Required—TOEFL (minimum score 550 paper-based; 80 iBT). Electronic applications accepted. *Expenses:* Contact institution. *Faculty research:* Cancer, infectious diseases, epidemiological methods, environmental/occupational health, women's and children's health.

Emory University, Rollins School of Public Health, Online Program in Public Health, Atlanta, GA 30322-1100. Offers applied epidemiology (MPH); applied public health informatics (MPH); prevention science (MPH). *Program availability:* Part-time, evening/weekend, online learning. *Degree requirements:* For master's, thesis, practicum. *Entrance requirements:* For master's, GRE. Additional exam requirements/recommendations for international students: Required—TOEFL (minimum score 550 paper-based; 80 iBT). Electronic applications accepted.

Florida International University, Robert Stempel College of Public Health and Social Work, Programs in Public Health, Miami, FL 33199. Offers biostatistics (MPH); environmental and occupational health (MPH, PhD); epidemiology (MPH, PhD); health policy and management (MPH); health promotion and disease prevention (PhD); health promotion and diseases prevention (MPH). Ph D program has fall admissions only; MPH offered jointly with University of Miami. *Accreditation:* CEPH. *Program availability:* Part-time, evening/weekend, online learning. *Faculty:* 27 full-time (12 women), 2 part-time/

adjunct (1 woman). *Students:* 126 full-time (80 women), 62 part-time (46 women); includes 129 minority (47 Black or African American, non-Hispanic/Latino; 10 Asian, non-Hispanic/Latino; 69 Hispanic/Latino; 3 Two or more races, non-Hispanic/Latino), 32 international. Average age 30. 298 applicants, 35% accepted, 68 enrolled. In 2015, 67 master's, 10 doctorates awarded. *Degree requirements:* For master's, thesis optional; for doctorate, comprehensive exam, thesis/dissertation. *Entrance requirements:* For master's, minimum GPA of 3.0, letters of recommendation; for doctorate, GRE, resume, minimum GPA of 3.0, letters of recommendation, letter of intent. Additional exam requirements/recommendations for international students: Required—TOEFL (minimum score 550 paper-based; 80 iBT). *Application deadline:* For fall admission, 6/1 for domestic students, 4/1 for international students; for spring admission, 10/1 for domestic students, 9/1 for international students. Applications are processed on a rolling basis. Application fee: $30. Electronic applications accepted. *Expenses:* Contact institution. *Financial support:* Institutionally sponsored loans, scholarships/grants, and tuition waivers (full) available. Financial award application deadline: 3/1; financial award applicants required to submit FAFSA. *Faculty research:* Drugs/AIDS intervention among migrant workers, provision of services for active/recovering drug users with HIV. *Unit head:* Dr. Benjamin C. Amick, III, Chair, 305-348-4903, E-mail: benjamin.amickiii@fiu.edu. *Application contact:* Dr. Vukosava Pekovic, Director, 305-348-1823, Fax: 305-348-4901, E-mail: pekovic@fiu.edu.

George Mason University, College of Health and Human Services, Department of Global and Community Health, Fairfax, VA 22030. Offers global and community health (Certificate); global health (MS); public health (MPH), including epidemiology. *Accreditation:* CEPH. *Faculty:* 14 full-time (10 women), 18 part-time/adjunct (14 women). *Students:* 62 full-time (56 women), 47 part-time (42 women); includes 50 minority (22 Black or African American, non-Hispanic/Latino; 16 Asian, non-Hispanic/Latino; 9 Hispanic/Latino; 3 Two or more races, non-Hispanic/Latino), 1 international. Average age 27. 121 applicants, 72% accepted, 44 enrolled. In 2015, 56 master's, 6 other advanced degrees awarded. *Degree requirements:* For master's, comprehensive exam (for some programs), thesis or practicum. *Entrance requirements:* For master's, GRE, GMAT (depending on program), 2 official transcripts; expanded goals statement; 3 letters of recommendation; resume; 1 completed course in health science, statistics, natural sciences and social science (for MPH); 6 credits of foreign language if not fluent (for MS); for Certificate, 2 official transcripts; expanded goals statement; 3 letters of recommendation; resume; bachelor's degree from regionally-accredited institution with minimum GPA of 3.0. Additional exam requirements/recommendations for international students: Required—TOEFL (minimum score 570 paper-based; 88 iBT), IELTS (minimum score 6.5), PTE (minimum score 59). *Application deadline:* For fall admission, 2/1 for domestic students. Application fee: $75 ($80 for international students). Electronic applications accepted. *Expenses:* Contact institution. *Financial support:* In 2015–16, 5 students received support, including 9 research assistantships with tuition reimbursements available (averaging $16,472 per year), 1 teaching assistantship with tuition reimbursement available (averaging $9,000 per year); career-related internships or fieldwork, Federal Work-Study, scholarships/grants, unspecified assistantships, and health care benefits (for full-time research or teaching assistantship recipients) also available. Financial award application deadline: 3/1; financial award applicants required to submit FAFSA. *Faculty research:* Health issues and the needs of affected populations at the regional and global level. *Total annual research expenditures:* $28,950. *Unit head:* Brian Gillette, Director, 703-993-4636, Fax: 703-993-1908, E-mail: bgillett@gmu.edu. *Application contact:* Ali Weinstein, Graduate Program Coordinator, 703-993-9632, Fax: 703-993-1908, E-mail: aweinst2@gmu.edu. Website: http://chhs.gmu.edu/gch/index

Georgetown University, Graduate School of Arts and Sciences, Department of Biostatistics, Bioinformatics and Biomathematics, Washington, DC 20057-1484. Offers biostatistics (MS, Certificate), including bioinformatics (MS); epidemiology (MS); epidemiology (Certificate). *Entrance requirements:* For master's, GRE General Test. Additional exam requirements/recommendations for international students: Required—TOEFL. *Faculty research:* Occupation epidemiology, cancer.

The George Washington University, Milken Institute School of Public Health, Department of Epidemiology and Biostatistics, Washington, DC 20052. Offers biostatistics (MPH); epidemiology (MPH); microbiology and emerging infectious diseases (MSPH). *Faculty:* 30 full-time (20 women), 9 part-time/adjunct (7 women). *Students:* 65 full-time (49 women), 70 part-time (54 women); includes 40 minority (12 Black or African American, non-Hispanic/Latino; 15 Asian, non-Hispanic/Latino; 8 Hispanic/Latino; 5 Two or more races, non-Hispanic/Latino), 12 international. Average age 29. 493 applicants, 55% accepted, 47 enrolled. In 2015, 56 master's awarded. *Degree requirements:* For master's, case study or special project. *Entrance requirements:* For master's, GMAT, GRE General Test, or MCAT. Additional exam requirements/recommendations for international students: Required—TOEFL. *Application deadline:* For fall admission, 4/15 priority date for domestic students, 4/15 for international students; for spring admission, 11/1 for domestic and international students. Applications are processed on a rolling basis. Application fee: $75. *Financial support:* In 2015–16, 6 students received support. Tuition waivers available. Financial award application deadline: 2/15. *Unit head:* Dr. Alan E. Greenberg, Chair, 202-994-0612, E-mail: aeg1@gwu.edu. *Application contact:* Jane Smith, Director of Admissions, 202-994-0248, Fax: 202-994-1860, E-mail: sphhsinfo@gwumc.edu.

Georgia Southern University, Jack N. Averitt College of Graduate Studies, Jiann-Ping Hsu College of Public Health, Program in Public Health, Statesboro, GA 30460. Offers biostatistics (MPH, Dr PH); community health behavior and education (Dr PH); community health education (MPH); environmental health sciences (MPH); epidemiology (MPH); health policy and management (MPH, Dr PH). *Accreditation:* CEPH. *Program availability:* Part-time. *Students:* 129 full-time (86 women), 41 part-time (32 women); includes 87 minority (67 Black or African American, non-Hispanic/Latino; 6 Asian, non-Hispanic/Latino; 8 Hispanic/Latino; 6 Two or more races, non-Hispanic/Latino), 30 international. Average age 30. 218 applicants, 63% accepted, 41 enrolled. In 2015, 37 master's, 8 doctorates awarded. *Degree requirements:* For master's, thesis optional, practicum; for doctorate, comprehensive exam, thesis/dissertation, practicum. *Entrance requirements:* For master's, GRE General Test, minimum GPA of 2.75, resume, 3 letters of reference; for doctorate, GRE, GMAT, MCAT, LSAT, 3 letters of reference, statement of purpose, resume or curriculum vitae. Additional exam requirements/recommendations for international students: Required—TOEFL (minimum score 550 paper-based; 80 iBT), IELTS (minimum score 6). *Application deadline:* For fall admission, 6/1 priority date for domestic and international students; for spring admission, 10/1 priority date for domestic students, 10/1 for international students. Applications are processed on a rolling basis. Application fee: $50. Electronic applications accepted. *Expenses:* $335 per credit hour. *Financial support:* In 2015–16, 93 students received support, including 23 fellowships with full tuition reimbursements available (averaging $7,750 per year), 1 research assistantship with full tuition reimbursement available (averaging $7,750 per year), 1 teaching assistantship with full tuition reimbursement available (averaging $7,750 per year); career-related internships or fieldwork, Federal Work-Study, scholarships/grants, tuition waivers (full), and unspecified assistantships also available. Support available to part-time students. Financial award application deadline: 4/15; financial award applicants required to submit FAFSA. *Faculty research:* Rural public health best practices, health disparity elimination, community initiatives to enhance public health, cost effectiveness analysis, epidemiology of rural public health, environmental health issues, health care system assessment, rural health care, health policy and healthcare financing, survival analysis, nonparametric statistics and resampling methods, micro-arrays and genomics, data imputation techniques and clinical trial methodology. *Total annual research expenditures:* $281,707. *Unit head:* Dr. Shamia Garrett, Program Coordinator, 912-478-2393, E-mail: sgarrett@georgiasouthern.edu. Website: http://chhs.georgiasouthern.edu/health/

Harvard University, Cyprus International Institute for the Environment and Public Health in Association with Harvard School of Public Health, Cambridge, MA 02138. Offers environmental health (MS); environmental/public health (PhD); epidemiology and biostatistics (MS). *Entrance requirements:* For master's and doctorate, GRE, resume/curriculum vitae, 3 letters of recommendation, BA or BS (including diploma and official transcripts). Additional exam requirements/recommendations for international students: Required—TOEFL, IELTS (minimum score 7). Electronic applications accepted. *Faculty research:* Air pollution, climate change, biostatistics, sustainable development, environmental management.

Harvard University, Harvard T.H. Chan School of Public Health, Department of Epidemiology, Boston, MA 02115-6096. Offers cancer epidemiology (SM); cardiovascular epidemiology (SM, SD); clinical epidemiology (SM, SD); environmental and occupational epidemiology (SM, SD); epidemiologic methods (SD); epidemiology of aging (SM, SD); genetic epidemiology and statistical genetics (SD); infectious disease epidemiology (SM, SD); neuroepidemiology (SD); pharmacoepidemiology (SM, SD); psychiatric epidemiology (SM); reproductive epidemiology (SM, SD). *Program availability:* Part-time. *Faculty:* 97 full-time (47 women), 39 part-time/adjunct (11 women). *Students:* 152 full-time (101 women), 230 part-time (110 women); includes 98 minority (7 Black or African American, non-Hispanic/Latino; 62 Asian, non-Hispanic/Latino; 21 Hispanic/Latino; 8 Two or more races, non-Hispanic/Latino), 145 international. Average age 28. 494 applicants, 20% accepted, 57 enrolled. In 2015, 138 master's, 19 doctorates awarded. *Degree requirements:* For doctorate, thesis/dissertation, qualifying exam. *Entrance requirements:* For master's, GRE, MCAT; for doctorate, GRE. Additional exam requirements/recommendations for international students: Recommended—TOEFL (minimum score 600 paper-based; 100 iBT), IELTS (minimum score 7). *Application deadline:* For fall admission, 12/15 for domestic and international students. Application fee: $120. Electronic applications accepted. *Financial support:* Fellowships, research assistantships, teaching assistantships, Federal Work-Study, scholarships/grants, traineeships, and unspecified assistantships available. Support available to part-time students. Financial award application deadline: 2/15; financial award applicants required to submit FAFSA. *Faculty research:* Cancer prevention and epidemiology; epidemiologic methods; epidemiology of aging; infectious diseases; pharmacoepidemiology; cardiovascular, clinical, environmental and occupational, molecular/genetic, neuropsychiatric, nutritional, psychiatric, reproductive, perinatal, and pediatric epidemiology. *Unit head:* Dr. Michelle A. Williams, Chair, 617-432-6477, Fax: 617-432-7805, E-mail: mawilliams@hsph.harvard.edu. *Application contact:* Vincent W. James, Director of Admissions, 617-432-1031, Fax: 617-432-7080, E-mail: admissions@hsph.harvard.edu. Website: http://www.hsph.harvard.edu/epidemiology/

Harvard University, Harvard T.H. Chan School of Public Health, Department of Nutrition, Boston, MA 02115-6096. Offers nutrition (SD); nutritional epidemiology (SD); public health nutrition (SD). *Faculty:* 28 full-time (10 women), 16 part-time/adjunct (6 women). *Students:* 22 full-time (13 women), 3 part-time (2 women); includes 6 minority (1 Black or African American, non-Hispanic/Latino; 1 Asian, non-Hispanic/Latino; 1 Hispanic/Latino; 3 Two or more races, non-Hispanic/Latino), 11 international. Average age 30. 46 applicants, 11% accepted, 5 enrolled. In 2015, 8 doctorates awarded. *Degree requirements:* For doctorate, thesis/dissertation, qualifying exam. *Entrance requirements:* For doctorate, GRE. Additional exam requirements/recommendations for international students: Recommended—TOEFL (minimum score 600 paper-based; 100 iBT), IELTS (minimum score 7). *Application deadline:* For fall admission, 12/15 for domestic and international students. Application fee: $120. Electronic applications accepted. *Financial support:* Fellowships, research assistantships, teaching assistantships, Federal Work-Study, scholarships/grants, traineeships, and unspecified assistantships available. Support available to part-time students. Financial award application deadline: 2/15; financial award applicants required to submit FAFSA. *Faculty research:* Dietary and genetic factors affecting heart diseases in humans; interactions among nutrition, immunity, and infection; role of diet and lifestyle in preventing macrovascular complications in diabetics. *Unit head:* Dr. Walter Willett, Chair, 617-432-1333, Fax: 617-432-2435, E-mail: walter.willett@channing.harvard.edu. *Application contact:* Vincent W. James, Director of Admissions, 617-432-1031, Fax: 617-432-7080, E-mail: admissions@hsph.harvard.edu. Website: http://www.hsph.harvard.edu/nutrition/

Hunter College of the City University of New York, Graduate School, Schools of the Health Professions, School of Health Sciences, Programs in Urban Public Health, Program in Epidemiology and Biostatistics, New York, NY 10065-5085. Offers MPH. *Accreditation:* CEPH. *Program availability:* Part-time, evening/weekend. *Students:* 75 applicants, 55% accepted, 21 enrolled. *Degree requirements:* For master's, comprehensive exam, thesis optional, internship. *Entrance requirements:* For master's, GRE General Test, previous course work in calculus and statistics. Additional exam requirements/recommendations for international students: Required—TOEFL. *Application deadline:* For fall admission, 4/1 for domestic students; for spring admission, 11/1 for domestic students. *Financial support:* In 2015–16, 6 fellowships were awarded; career-related internships or fieldwork, Federal Work-Study, institutionally sponsored loans, and tuition waivers (partial) also available. Support available to part-time students. Financial award application deadline: 3/1. *Unit head:* Prof. Lorna Thorpe, Program Director, 212-396-7746, Fax: 212-481-5260, E-mail: lthor@hunter.cuny.edu. *Application contact:* Milena Solo, Director for Graduate Admissions, 212-772-4288, Fax: 212-650-3336, E-mail: milena.solo@hunter.cuny.edu. Website: http://cuny.edu/site/sph/hunter-college/a-programs/graduate/eb-mph.html

Indiana University Bloomington, School of Public Health, Department of Epidemiology and Biostatistics, Bloomington, IN 47405. Offers biostatistics (MPH); epidemiology (MPH, PhD). *Degree requirements:* For master's, thesis or alternative; for doctorate, comprehensive exam, thesis/dissertation. *Entrance requirements:* For master's, GRE (for applicants with cumulative undergraduate GPA less than 2.8); for doctorate, GRE. Additional exam requirements/recommendations for international students: Required—TOEFL (minimum score 550 paper-based; 80 iBT). Electronic applications accepted. *Faculty research:* Nutritional epidemiology, cancer epidemiology, global health, biostatistics.

Indiana University–Purdue University Indianapolis, School of Public Health, Indianapolis, IN 46202. Offers biostatistics (MPH); environmental health science (MPH); epidemiology (MPH, PhD); health administration (MHA); health policy and management (MPH, PhD); social and behavioral sciences (MPH). *Accreditation:* CEPH. *Expenses:* Contact institution.

Johns Hopkins University, Bloomberg School of Public Health, Department of Epidemiology, Baltimore, MD 21205. Offers cancer etiology and prevention (MHS, Sc M,

PhD, Sc D); cardiovascular diseases (MHS, Sc M, PhD, Sc D); clinical epidemiology (MHS, Sc M, PhD, Sc D); clinical trials (PhD, Sc D); epidemiology (MHS, Sc M, Dr PH, PhD, Sc D); epidemiology of aging (MHS, Sc M, PhD, Sc D); genetic epidemiology (MHS, Sc M, PhD, Sc D); infectious disease epidemiology (MHS, Sc M, PhD, Sc D); occupational and environmental epidemiology (MHS, Sc M, PhD, Sc D). *Program availability:* Part-time. *Degree requirements:* For master's, comprehensive exam, thesis, 1-year full-time residency; for doctorate, comprehensive exam, thesis/dissertation, 2 years' full-time residency, oral and written exams, student teaching. *Entrance requirements:* For master's, GRE General Test or MCAT, 3 letters of recommendation, curriculum vitae; for doctorate, GRE General Test, minimum 1 year of work experience, 3 letters of recommendation, curriculum vitae, academic records from all schools. Additional exam requirements/recommendations for international students: Required—TOEFL (minimum score 600 paper-based; 100 iBT); Recommended—IELTS (minimum score 7.5), TWE. Electronic applications accepted. *Faculty research:* Cancer and congenital malformations, nutritional epidemiology, AIDS, tuberculosis, cardiovascular disease, risk assessment.

Johns Hopkins University, Bloomberg School of Public Health, Department of International Health, Baltimore, MD 21205. Offers global disease epidemiology and control (MHS, PhD); health systems (MHS, PhD); human nutrition (MHS, PhD); international health (MSPH, Dr PH); registered dietician (MSPH); social and behavioral interventions (MHS, PhD). *Degree requirements:* For master's, comprehensive exam, thesis (for some programs), 1-year full-time residency, 4-9 month internship; for doctorate, comprehensive exam, thesis/dissertation or alternative, 1.5 years' full-time residency, oral and written exams. *Entrance requirements:* For master's, GRE General Test or MCAT, 3 letters of recommendation, resume; for doctorate, GRE General Test or MCAT, 3 letters of recommendation, resume, transcripts. Additional exam requirements/recommendations for international students: Required—TOEFL (minimum score 600 paper-based; 100 iBT); Recommended—IELTS (minimum score 7), Electronic applications accepted. *Faculty research:* Nutrition, infectious diseases, health systems, health economics, humanitarian emergencies.

Loma Linda University, School of Public Health, Programs in Epidemiology and Biostatistics, Loma Linda, CA 92350. Offers biostatistics (MPH); epidemiology (MPH, Dr PH, PhD). *Entrance requirements:* Additional exam requirements/recommendations for international students: Required—Michigan English Language Assessment Battery or TOEFL. *Application deadline:* Applications are processed on a rolling basis. Application fee: $100. *Financial support:* Application deadline: 5/15. *Unit head:* Khaled Bahjri, Director, 909-824-4590, Fax: 909-824-4087, E-mail: kbahjri@llu.edu. *Application contact:* Wendy Genovez, Assistant Dean of Admissions and Records, 909-824-4694, Fax: 909-824-8087, E-mail: wgenovez@llu.edu.

Louisiana State University Health Sciences Center, School of Public Health, New Orleans, LA 70112. Offers behavioral and community health sciences (MPH); biostatistics (MPH, MS, PhD); community health sciences (PhD); environmental and occupational health sciences (MPH); epidemiology (MPH, PhD); health policy and systems management (MPH). *Accreditation:* CEPH. *Program availability:* Part-time. *Entrance requirements:* For master's, GRE General Test.

McGill University, Faculty of Graduate and Postdoctoral Studies, Faculty of Medicine, Department of Epidemiology and Biostatistics, Montréal, QC H3A 2T5, Canada. Offers community health (M Sc); environmental health (M Sc); epidemiology and biostatistics (M Sc, PhD, Diploma); health care evaluation (M Sc); medical statistics (M Sc). *Accreditation:* CEPH (one or more programs are accredited).

Medical College of Wisconsin, Graduate School of Biomedical Sciences, Department of Population Health, Milwaukee, WI 53226-0509. Offers biostatistics (PhD); epidemiology (MS); public health (MPH, PhD, Graduate Certificate), including public and community health (PhD), public health (MPH, Graduate Certificate). *Entrance requirements:* For master's, doctorate, and Graduate Certificate, GRE, official transcripts, three letters of recommendation. Additional exam requirements/recommendations for international students: Required—TOEFL.

Medical University of South Carolina, College of Graduate Studies, Division of Biostatistics and Epidemiology, Charleston, SC 29425. Offers biostatistics (MS, PhD); epidemiology (MS, PhD); DMD/PhD; MD/PhD. Terminal master's awarded for partial completion of doctoral program. *Degree requirements:* For master's, comprehensive exam, thesis (for some programs); for doctorate, comprehensive exam, oral and written exams. *Entrance requirements:* For master's, GRE General Test, two semesters of college-level calculus; for doctorate, GRE General Test, interview, minimum GPA of 3.0, two semesters of college-level calculus. Additional exam requirements/recommendations for international students: Required—TOEFL (minimum score 600 paper-based; 100 iBT). Electronic applications accepted. *Faculty research:* Health disparities, central nervous system injuries, radiation exposure, analysis of clinical trial data, biomedical information.

Memorial University of Newfoundland, Faculty of Medicine and School of Graduate Studies, Graduate Programs in Medicine, Division of Clinical Epidemiology, St. John's, NL A1C 5S7, Canada. Offers M Sc, PhD, Diploma. *Expenses:* Tuition, area resident: Full-time $2199 Canadian dollars. *International tuition:* $2859 Canadian dollars full-time.

Michigan State University, College of Human Medicine and The Graduate School, Graduate Programs in Human Medicine, Department of Epidemiology, East Lansing, MI 48824. Offers MS, PhD. *Degree requirements:* For master's, oral thesis defense. *Entrance requirements:* Additional exam requirements/recommendations for international students: Required—TOEFL. Electronic applications accepted.

New York Medical College, School of Health Sciences and Practice, Department of Epidemiology and Community Health, Program in Epidemiology, Valhalla, NY 10595-1691. Offers MPH. *Accreditation:* CEPH. *Program availability:* Part-time, evening/weekend. *Degree requirements:* For master's, thesis, capstone. *Entrance requirements:* For master's, minimum undergraduate GPA of 3.0. Additional exam requirements/recommendations for international students: Required—TOEFL (minimum score 600 paper-based; 96 iBT), IELTS (minimum score 7). Electronic applications accepted. *Expenses:* Tuition, area resident: Full-time $44,355; part-time $1025 per credit. *Required fees:* $500; $95 per year. One-time fee: $140 part-time. Tuition and fees vary according to course load and program.

★ **New York University,** Graduate School of Arts and Science, Department of Environmental Medicine, New York, NY 10012-1019. Offers environmental health sciences (MS, PhD), including biostatistics (PhD), environmental hygiene (MS), epidemiology (PhD), ergonomics and biomechanics (PhD), exposure assessment and health effects (PhD), molecular toxicology/carcinogenesis (PhD), toxicology (PhD). *Program availability:* Part-time. Terminal master's awarded for partial completion of doctoral program. *Degree requirements:* For master's, thesis or alternative; for doctorate, one foreign language, thesis/dissertation, oral and written exams. *Entrance requirements:* For master's and doctorate, GRE General Test, minimum GPA of 3.0; bachelor's degree in biological, physical, or engineering science. Additional exam requirements/recommendations for international students: Required—TOEFL.

See Close-Up on page 851.

Epidemiology

North Carolina State University, College of Veterinary Medicine, Program in Comparative Biomedical Sciences, Raleigh, NC 27695. Offers cell biology (MS, PhD); infectious disease (MS, PhD); pathology (MS, PhD); pharmacology (MS, PhD); population medicine (MS, PhD). *Program availability:* Part-time. *Degree requirements:* For master's, thesis; for doctorate, thesis/dissertation. *Entrance requirements:* For master's and doctorate, GRE General Test. Additional exam requirements/recommendations for international students: Required—TOEFL (minimum score 550 paper-based). Electronic applications accepted. *Expenses:* Contact institution. *Faculty research:* Infectious diseases, cell biology, pharmacology and toxicology, genomics, pathology and population medicine.

Northwestern University, Feinberg School of Medicine and Interdepartmental Programs, Integrated Graduate Programs in the Life Sciences, Chicago, IL 60611. Offers biostatistics (PhD); epidemiology (PhD); health and biomedical informatics (PhD); health services and outcomes research (PhD); healthcare quality and patient safety (PhD); translational outcomes in science (PhD). *Degree requirements:* For doctorate, comprehensive exam, thesis/dissertation, written and oral qualifying exams. *Entrance requirements:* For doctorate, GRE General Test. Additional exam requirements/recommendations for international students: Required—TOEFL (minimum score 600 paper-based). Electronic applications accepted.

Oregon State University, College of Public Health and Human Sciences, Program in Public Health, Corvallis, OR 97331. Offers biostatistics (MPH); environmental and occupational health and safety (MPH, PhD); epidemiology (MPH, PhD); health management and policy (MPH); health policy (PhD); health promotion and health behavior (MPH, PhD); international health (MPH). *Accreditation:* CEPH. *Program availability:* Part-time. *Faculty:* 32 full-time (18 women), 3 part-time/adjunct (0 women). *Students:* 123 full-time (91 women), 20 part-time (14 women); includes 43 minority (2 Black or African American, non-Hispanic/Latino; 2 American Indian or Alaska Native, non-Hispanic/Latino; 9 Asian, non-Hispanic/Latino; 18 Hispanic/Latino; 1 Native Hawaiian or other Pacific Islander, non-Hispanic/Latino; 11 Two or more races, non-Hispanic/Latino), 18 international. Average age 31. 276 applicants, 65% accepted, 45 enrolled. In 2015, 59 master's, 6 doctorates awarded. Terminal master's awarded for partial completion of doctoral program. *Degree requirements:* For doctorate, one foreign language, thesis/dissertation. *Entrance requirements:* For master's and doctorate, GRE, minimum GPA of 3.0 in last 90 hours. Additional exam requirements/recommendations for international students: Required—TOEFL (minimum score 80 iBT), IELTS (minimum score 6.5). *Application deadline:* For fall admission, 12/1 priority date for domestic students. Applications are processed on a rolling basis. *Expenses:* $13,851 full-time resident tuition, $23,679 full-time non-resident tuition, $1,572 fees. *Financial support:* Fellowships, research assistantships, teaching assistantships, career-related internships or fieldwork, Federal Work-Study, and institutionally sponsored loans available. Support available to part-time students. Financial award application deadline: 12/1. *Faculty research:* Traffic safety, health safety, injury control, health promotion. *Unit head:* Dr. Sheryl Thorburn, Professor/Co-Director. *Application contact:* Amanda Armington, Public Health Program Manager, 541-737-3825, E-mail: amanda.armington@oregonstate.edu.

Ponce Health Sciences University, Program in Public Health, Ponce, PR 00732-7004. Offers epidemiology (Dr PH); public health (MPH). *Accreditation:* CEPH. *Degree requirements:* For master's, one foreign language, comprehensive exam, thesis. *Entrance requirements:* For master's, GRE General Test or EXADEP, proficiency in Spanish and English, minimum GPA of 2.7, 3 letters of recommendation; for doctorate, GRE, proficiency in Spanish and English, minimum GPA of 3.0, letter of recommendation.

Purdue University, School of Veterinary Medicine and Graduate School, Graduate Programs in Veterinary Medicine, Department of Comparative Pathobiology, West Lafayette, IN 47907-2027. Offers comparative epidemiology and public health (MS); comparative epidemiology and public heath (PhD); comparative microbiology and immunology (MS, PhD); comparative pathobiology (MS, PhD); interdisciplinary studies (PhD), including microbial pathogenesis, molecular signaling and cancer biology, molecular virology; lab animal medicine (MS); veterinary anatomic pathology (MS); veterinary clinical pathology (MS). Terminal master's awarded for partial completion of doctoral program. *Degree requirements:* For master's, thesis (for some programs); for doctorate, thesis/dissertation. *Entrance requirements:* For master's and doctorate, GRE General Test. Additional exam requirements/recommendations for international students: Required—TOEFL (minimum score 575 paper-based), IELTS (minimum score 6.5), TWE (minimum score 4). Electronic applications accepted.

Queen's University at Kingston, School of Graduate Studies, Faculty of Health Sciences, Department of Community Health and Epidemiology, Kingston, ON K7L 3N6, Canada. Offers epidemiology (PhD); epidemiology and population health (M Sc); health services (M Sc); policy research and clinical epidemiology (M Sc); public health (MPH). *Program availability:* Part-time. *Degree requirements:* For master's, thesis. *Entrance requirements:* For master's, GRE General Test (strongly recommended). Additional exam requirements/recommendations for international students: Required—TOEFL (minimum score 600 paper-based). *Faculty research:* Cancer epidemiology, clinical trials, biostatistics health services research, health policy.

Rutgers University–Newark, School of Public Health, Newark, NJ 07107-1709. Offers clinical epidemiology (Certificate); dental public health (MPH); general public health (Certificate); public policy and oral health services administration (Certificate); quantitative methods (MPH); urban health (MPH); DMD/MPH; MD/MPH; MS/MPH. *Accreditation:* CEPH. *Program availability:* Part-time, evening/weekend. *Degree requirements:* For master's, thesis, internship. *Entrance requirements:* For master's, GRE General Test. Additional exam requirements/recommendations for international students: Required—TOEFL. Electronic applications accepted.

Rutgers University–New Brunswick, School of Public Health, Piscataway, NJ 08854. Offers biostatistics (MPH, MS, Dr PH, PhD); clinical epidemiology (Certificate); environmental and occupational health (MPH, Dr PH, PhD, Certificate); epidemiology (MPH, Dr PH, PhD); general public health (Certificate); health education and behavioral science (MPH, Dr PH, PhD); health systems and policy (MPH, PhD); public health (MPH, Dr PH, PhD); public health preparedness (Certificate); DO/MPH; JD/MPH; MBA/MPH; MD/MPH; MPH/MBA; MPH/MSPA; MS/MPH; Psy D/MPH. *Accreditation:* CEPH. *Program availability:* Part-time, evening/weekend. *Degree requirements:* For master's, thesis, internship; for doctorate, comprehensive exam, thesis/dissertation. *Entrance requirements:* For master's, GRE General Test; for doctorate, GRE General Test, MPH (Dr PH); MA, MPH, or MS (PhD). Additional exam requirements/recommendations for international students: Required—TOEFL. Electronic applications accepted.

San Diego State University, Graduate and Research Affairs, College of Health and Human Services, Graduate School of Public Health, San Diego, CA 92182. Offers environmental health (MPH); epidemiology (MPH, PhD), including biostatistics (MPH); global emergency preparedness and response (MS); global health (PhD); health behavior (PhD); health promotion (MPH); health services administration (MPH); toxicology (MS); MPH/MA; MSW/MPH. *Accreditation:* CAHME (one or more programs are accredited); CEPH (one or more programs are accredited). *Program availability:* Part-time. *Degree requirements:* For master's, comprehensive exam (for some programs), thesis (for some programs); for doctorate, thesis/dissertation. *Entrance requirements:* For master's, GMAT (MPH in health services administration), GRE General Test; for doctorate, GRE General Test. Additional exam requirements/recommendations for international students: Required—TOEFL. *Faculty research:* Evaluation of tobacco, AIDS prevalence and prevention, mammography, infant death project, Alzheimer's in elderly Chinese.

Stanford University, School of Medicine, Graduate Programs in Medicine, Department of Health Research and Policy, Program in Epidemiology and Clinical Research, Stanford, CA 94305-9991. Offers MS, PhD. *Degree requirements:* For master's, thesis; for doctorate, thesis/dissertation, qualifying examinations. *Entrance requirements:* For doctorate, GRE General Test or MCAT. Additional exam requirements/recommendations for international students: Required—TOEFL. Electronic applications accepted. *Expenses: Tuition, area resident:* Full-time $45,729. *Required fees:* $591.

Thomas Edison State University, School of Applied Science and Technology, Program in Clinical Trials Management, Trenton, NJ 08608-1176. Offers Graduate Certificate. *Program availability:* Part-time, online learning. *Entrance requirements:* Additional exam requirements/recommendations for international students: Required—TOEFL (minimum score 550 paper-based; 79 iBT). Electronic applications accepted.

Tufts University, Graduate School of Arts and Sciences, Graduate Certificate Programs, Program in Epidemiology, Medford, MA 02155. Offers Certificate. *Program availability:* Part-time. *Expenses: Tuition, area resident:* Full-time $48,412; part-time $1210 per credit hour. *Required fees:* $806. Full-time tuition and fees vary according to degree level, program and student level. Part-time tuition and fees vary according to course load.

Tufts University, Sackler School of Graduate Biomedical Sciences, Clinical and Translational Science Program, Medford, MA 02155. Offers MS, PhD, Certificate. *Faculty:* 34 full-time (10 women). *Students:* 20 full-time (13 women), 1 part-time; includes 4 minority (1 Black or African American, non-Hispanic/Latino; 3 Asian, non-Hispanic/Latino), 4 international. Average age 37. 34 applicants, 47% accepted, 11 enrolled. In 2015, 3 master's, 3 doctorates, 4 other advanced degrees awarded. *Degree requirements:* For master's, thesis; for doctorate, comprehensive exam, thesis/dissertation. *Entrance requirements:* For master's, MD or PhD, strong clinical research background. Additional exam requirements/recommendations for international students: Required—TOEFL (minimum score 600 paper-based; 100 iBT). *Application deadline:* For fall admission, 4/15 for domestic and international students. Applications are processed on a rolling basis. Application fee: $90. Electronic applications accepted. *Expenses:* $26,964 per year tuition and fees. *Faculty research:* Clinical study design, mathematical modeling, meta analysis, epidemiologic research, coronary heart disease. *Unit head:* Dr. David Kent, Program Director, 617-636-3234, Fax: 617-636-8023, E-mail: dkent@tuftsmedicalcenter.edu. *Application contact:* Kellie Melchin, Associate Director of Admissions, 617-636-6767, Fax: 617-636-0375, E-mail: sackler-school@tufts.edu. Website: http://sackler.tufts.edu/Academics/Degree-Programs/Clinical-and-Translational-Science

Tufts University, School of Medicine, Public Health and Professional Degree Programs, Boston, MA 02111. Offers biomedical sciences (MS); health communication (MS, Certificate); pain research, education and policy (MS, Certificate); physician assistant (MS); public health (MPH, Dr PH), including behavioral science (MPH), biostatistics (MPH), epidemiology (MPH), health communication (MPH), health services (MPH), management and policy (MPH), nutrition (MPH); DMD/MPH; DVM/MPH; JD/MPH; MD/MPH; MMS/MPH; MS/MBA; MS/MPH. MS programs offered jointly with Emerson College. *Accreditation:* CEPH (one or more programs are accredited). *Program availability:* Part-time, evening/weekend. *Faculty:* 78 full-time (29 women), 42 part-time/adjunct (20 women). *Students:* 457 full-time (266 women), 61 part-time (46 women); includes 187 minority (21 Black or African American, non-Hispanic/Latino; 107 Asian, non-Hispanic/Latino; 37 Hispanic/Latino; 22 Two or more races, non-Hispanic/Latino), 24 international. Average age 27. 1,599 applicants, 48% accepted, 222 enrolled. In 2015, 219 master's awarded. *Degree requirements:* For master's, thesis (for some programs); for doctorate, thesis/dissertation. *Entrance requirements:* For master's, GRE General Test, MCAT, or GMAT; for doctorate, GRE General Test or MCAT. Additional exam requirements/recommendations for international students: Required—TOEFL (minimum score 100 iBT). *Application deadline:* For fall admission, 1/15 priority date for domestic students, 12/15 priority date for international students; for spring admission, 10/25 priority date for domestic and international students. Applications are processed on a rolling basis. Application fee: $70. Electronic applications accepted. *Expenses:* Contact institution. *Financial support:* In 2015–16, 12 students received support, including 1 fellowship (averaging $3,000 per year), 50 research assistantships (averaging $1,000 per year), 65 teaching assistantships (averaging $2,000 per year); Federal Work-Study and scholarships/grants also available. Support available to part-time students. Financial award application deadline: 2/19; financial award applicants required to submit FAFSA. *Faculty research:* Environmental and occupational health, nutrition, epidemiology, health communication, biostatics, obesity/chronic disease, health policy and health care delivery, global health, health inequality and social determinants of health. *Unit head:* Dr. Aviva Must, Dean, 617-636-0935, Fax: 617-636-0898, E-mail: aviva.must@tufts.edu. *Application contact:* Emily Keily, Director of Admissions, 617-636-0935, Fax: 617-636-0898, E-mail: med-phpd@tufts.edu. Website: http://publichealth.tufts.edu

Tulane University, School of Public Health and Tropical Medicine, Department of Epidemiology, New Orleans, LA 70118-5669. Offers MPH, MS, Dr PH, PhD, MD/MPH. MS and PhD offered through the Graduate School. *Accreditation:* CEPH (one or more programs are accredited). *Program availability:* Part-time. *Degree requirements:* For doctorate, comprehensive exam, thesis/dissertation. *Entrance requirements:* For master's and doctorate, GRE General Test. Additional exam requirements/recommendations for international students: Required—TOEFL. *Application deadline:* For fall admission, 4/15 priority date for domestic and international students; for spring admission, 10/15 priority date for domestic and international students. Applications are processed on a rolling basis. Application fee: $40. Electronic applications accepted. *Expenses: Tuition, area resident:* Full-time $47,658; part-time $2648 per credit hour. *Required fees:* $1980; $44.50 per credit hour. $550 per term. Tuition and fees vary according to course load, degree level and program. *Financial support:* Research assistantships, teaching assistantships, Federal Work-Study, scholarships/grants, and traineeships available. Support available to part-time students. Financial award application deadline: 4/15. *Faculty research:* Environment, cancer, cardiovascular epidemiology, women's health.

Université Laval, Faculty of Medicine, Graduate Programs in Medicine, Department of Medicine, Programs in Epidemiology, Québec, QC G1K 7P4, Canada. Offers M Sc, PhD. Terminal master's awarded for partial completion of doctoral program. *Degree requirements:* For master's, thesis; for doctorate, comprehensive exam, thesis/dissertation. *Entrance requirements:* For master's and doctorate, knowledge of French, comprehension of written English. Electronic applications accepted.

University at Albany, State University of New York, School of Public Health, Department of Epidemiology and Biostatistics, Albany, NY 12222-0001. Offers epidemiology and biostatistics (MS, PhD); public health (MPH, Dr PH). *Degree*

requirements: For master's, thesis; for doctorate, thesis/dissertation. *Entrance requirements:* For master's and doctorate, GRE General Test. Additional exam requirements/recommendations for international students: Required—TOEFL (minimum score 550 paper-based). Electronic applications accepted.

University at Buffalo, the State University of New York, Graduate School, School of Public Health and Health Professions, Department of Epidemiology and Environmental Health, Buffalo, NY 14214. Offers epidemiology (MS, PhD); public health (MPH). *Accreditation:* CEPH. *Program availability:* Part-time. *Faculty:* 12 full-time (6 women), 11 part-time/adjunct (5 women). *Students:* 58 full-time (38 women), 20 part-time (15 women); includes 13 minority (3 Black or African American, non-Hispanic/Latino; 10 Asian, non-Hispanic/Latino), 12 international. Average age 29. 201 applicants, 38% accepted, 33 enrolled. In 2015, 29 master's, 4 doctorates awarded. Terminal master's awarded for partial completion of doctoral program. *Degree requirements:* For master's, comprehensive exam, thesis; for doctorate, comprehensive exam, thesis/dissertation. *Entrance requirements:* For master's and doctorate, GRE General Test. Additional exam requirements/recommendations for international students: Required—TOEFL (minimum score 600 paper-based; 100 iBT). *Application deadline:* For fall admission, 1/15 priority date for domestic and international students. Applications are processed on a rolling basis. Application fee: $50. Electronic applications accepted. *Financial support:* In 2015–16, 17 students received support, including 4 fellowships with full tuition reimbursements available (averaging $22,000 per year), 5 research assistantships with full tuition reimbursements available (averaging $20,000 per year); teaching assistantships with full tuition reimbursements available, career-related internships or fieldwork, Federal Work-Study, institutionally sponsored loans, health care benefits, and unspecified assistantships also available. Financial award application deadline: 2/1; financial award applicants required to submit FAFSA. *Faculty research:* Epidemiology of cancer, nutrition, infectious diseases, epidemiology of environmental, women's health and cardiovascular disease research. *Unit head:* Dr. Jo Freudenheim, Interim Chair, 716-829-5375, Fax: 716-829-2979, E-mail: phhpadv@buffalo.edu. *Application contact:* Dr. Carl Li, Director of Graduate Studies, 716-829-5382, Fax: 716-829-2979, E-mail: carlli@buffalo.edu.
Website: http://sphhp.buffalo.edu/spm/

The University of Alabama at Birmingham, School of Public Health, Program in Epidemiology, Birmingham, AL 35294. Offers PhD. *Degree requirements:* For doctorate, comprehensive exam, thesis/dissertation, teaching practicum. *Entrance requirements:* For doctorate, GRE General Test, MPH or MSPH. Additional exam requirements/recommendations for international students: Recommended—TOEFL, IELTS. *Expenses:* Tuition, state resident: full-time $7340. Tuition, nonresident: full-time $16,628. Full-time tuition and fees vary according to course load and program. *Faculty research:* Biometry.

The University of Alabama at Birmingham, School of Public Health, Program in Public Health, Birmingham, AL 35294. Offers applied epidemiology and pharmacoepidemiology (MSPH); biostatistics (MPH); clinical and translational science (MSPH); environmental health (MPH); environmental health and toxicology (MSPH); epidemiology (MPH); general theory and practice (MPH); health behavior (MPH); health care organization (MPH); health policy quantitative policy analysis (MPH); industrial hygiene (MPH, MSPH); maternal and child health policy (Dr PH); maternal and child health policy and leadership (MPH); occupational health and safety (MPH); outcomes research (MSPH, Dr PH); public health (PhD); public health management (Dr PH); public health preparedness management (MPH). *Accreditation:* CEPH. *Program availability:* Part-time, online learning. *Degree requirements:* For doctorate, comprehensive exam, thesis/dissertation. *Entrance requirements:* For master's and doctorate, GRE. Additional exam requirements/recommendations for international students: Recommended—TOEFL (minimum score 550 paper-based; 79 iBT), IELTS (minimum score 6.5). Electronic applications accepted. *Expenses:* Tuition, state resident: full-time $7340. Tuition, nonresident: full-time $16,628. Full-time tuition and fees vary according to course load and program.

University of Alberta, School of Public Health, Department of Public Health Sciences, Edmonton, AB T6G 2E1, Canada. Offers clinical epidemiology (M Sc, MPH); environmental and occupational health (MPH); environmental health sciences (M Sc); epidemiology (M Sc); global health (M Sc, MPH); health policy and management (MPH); health policy research (M Sc); health technology assessment (MPH); occupational health (M Sc); population health (M Sc); public health leadership (MPH); public health sciences (PhD); quantitative methods (MPH). *Accreditation:* CEPH (one or more programs are accredited). Terminal master's awarded for partial completion of doctoral program. *Degree requirements:* For master's, thesis (for some programs); for doctorate, thesis/dissertation. *Entrance requirements:* For master's, GMAT or GRE General Test. Additional exam requirements/recommendations for international students: Required—TOEFL (minimum score 550 paper-based) or IELTS (minimum score 6). Electronic applications accepted. *Faculty research:* Biostatistics, health promotion and socio-behavioral health science.

The University of Arizona, Mel and Enid Zuckerman College of Public Health, Program in Epidemiology, Tucson, AZ 85721. Offers MS, PhD. In 2015, 4 doctorates awarded. *Entrance requirements:* Additional exam requirements/recommendations for international students: Required—TOEFL (minimum score 550 paper-based; 79 iBT). *Application deadline:* For fall admission, 1/1 for domestic and international students. Applications are processed on a rolling basis. Application fee: $75. Electronic applications accepted. *Financial support:* Research assistantships and teaching assistantships available. *Unit head:* Dr. Elizabeth Jacobs, Director, 520-626-0641. *Application contact:* Amy Glicken, Special Assistant to the Dean, 520-626-3201, E-mail: pbaldewi@ag.arizona.edu.

University of Arkansas for Medical Sciences, College of Public Health, Little Rock, AR 72205-7199. Offers biostatistics (MPH); environmental and occupational health (MPH, Certificate); epidemiology (MPH, PhD); health behavior and health education (MPH); health policy and management (MPH); health promotion and prevention research (PhD); health services administration (MHSA); health systems research (PhD); public health (Certificate); public health leadership (Dr PH). *Program availability:* Part-time. *Degree requirements:* For master's, preceptorship, culminating experience, internship; for doctorate, comprehensive exam, capstone. *Entrance requirements:* For master's, GRE, GMAT, LSAT, PCAT, MCAT, DAT; for doctorate, GRE. Additional exam requirements/recommendations for international students: Required—TOEFL (minimum score 80 iBT), IELTS. Electronic applications accepted. *Expenses:* Contact institution. *Faculty research:* Health systems, tobacco prevention control, obesity prevention, environmental and occupational exposure, cancer prevention.

The University of British Columbia, Faculty of Medicine, School of Population and Public Health, Vancouver, BC V6T 1Z3, Canada. Offers health administration (MHA); health care and epidemiology (MH Sc, PhD); public health (MPH). *Accreditation:* CEPH (one or more programs are accredited). *Program availability:* Online learning. *Degree requirements:* For master's, thesis (for some programs), major paper (MH Sc), research project (MHA); for doctorate, thesis/dissertation. *Entrance requirements:* For master's, GRE General Test or GMAT, PCAT, MCAT (MHA), MD or equivalent (for MH Sc); 4-year undergraduate degree from accredited university with minimum B+ overall academic average and in math or statistics course at undergraduate level (for MPH); 4-year undergraduate degree from accredited university with minimum B+ overall academic average plus work experience (for MHA); for doctorate, master's degree from accredited university with minimum B+ overall academic average and in math or statistics course at undergraduate level. Additional exam requirements/recommendations for international students: Required—TOEFL. Electronic applications accepted. *Faculty research:* Population and public health, clinical epidemiology, epidemiology and biostatistics, global health and vulnerable populations, health care services and systems, occupational and environmental health, public health emerging threats and rapid response, social and life course determinants of health, health administration.

University of California, Berkeley, Graduate Division, School of Public Health, Group in Epidemiology, Berkeley, CA 94720-1500. Offers epidemiology (MS, PhD); infectious diseases (MPH, PhD). *Accreditation:* CEPH (one or more programs are accredited). *Degree requirements:* For master's, comprehensive exam; for doctorate, thesis/dissertation, oral and written exam. *Entrance requirements:* For master's, GRE General Test, minimum GPA of 3.0; MD, DDS, DVM, or PhD in biomedical science (MPH); for doctorate, GRE General Test, minimum GPA of 3.0.

University of California, Davis, Graduate Studies, Graduate Group in Epidemiology, Davis, CA 95616. Offers MS, PhD. Terminal master's awarded for partial completion of doctoral program. *Degree requirements:* For master's, comprehensive exam (for some programs), thesis (for some programs); for doctorate, thesis/dissertation. *Entrance requirements:* For master's and doctorate, GRE General Test, GRE Subject Test (biology), minimum GPA of 3.25. Additional exam requirements/recommendations for international students: Required—TOEFL (minimum score 550 paper-based). Electronic applications accepted. *Faculty research:* Environmental/occupational wildlife, reproductive and veterinary epidemiology, infectious/chronic disease epidemiology, public health

University of California, Irvine, School of Medicine, Department of Epidemiology, Irvine, CA 92697. Offers MS, PhD. *Students:* 10 full-time (7 women), 1 (woman) part-time; includes 6 minority (1 Black or African American, non-Hispanic/Latino; 3 Asian, non-Hispanic/Latino; 2 Hispanic/Latino). Average age 31. 19 applicants, 11% accepted, 1 enrolled. In 2015, 2 master's awarded. Terminal master's awarded for partial completion of doctoral program. *Degree requirements:* For master's, comprehensive exam, thesis; for doctorate, comprehensive exam, thesis/dissertation, 72 quarter units. *Entrance requirements:* For master's, GRE, minimum GPA of 3.0, letters of recommendation; for doctorate, GRE, minimum GPA of 3.0, personal statement, letters of recommendation. Additional exam requirements/recommendations for international students: Required—TOEFL (minimum score 550 paper-based; 80 iBT), IELTS (minimum score 7). *Application deadline:* For fall admission, 1/15 priority date for domestic and international students. Application fee: $90 ($110 for international students). Electronic applications accepted. *Financial support:* In 2015–16, fellowships with full tuition reimbursements (averaging $25,000 per year), research assistantships with full tuition reimbursements (averaging $46,000 per year), teaching assistantships with full tuition reimbursements (averaging $33,000 per year) were awarded; Federal Work-Study, institutionally sponsored loans, scholarships/grants, traineeships, health care benefits, and unspecified assistantships also available. Financial award application deadline: 1/15; financial award applicants required to submit FAFSA. *Faculty research:* Genetic/molecular epidemiology, cancer epidemiology, biostatistics, environmental health, occupational health. *Total annual research expenditures:* $15 million. *Unit head:* Dr. Hoda Anton-Culver, Chair, 949-824-7401, Fax: 949-824-4773, E-mail: hantoncu@uci.edu. *Application contact:* Julie Strope, Departmental Administrator, 949-824-0306, Fax: 949-824-4773, E-mail: jstrope@uci.edu.
Website: http://www.epi.uci.edu/

University of California, Irvine, School of Social Ecology, Programs in Social Ecology, Irvine, CA 92697. Offers environmental analysis and design (PhD); epidemiology and public health (PhD); social ecology (PhD). *Students:* 11 full-time (9 women), 1 part-time (0 women); includes 1 minority (Hispanic/Latino), 1 international. Average age 32. 14 applicants, 36% accepted, 2 enrolled. In 2015, 1 doctorate awarded. Application fee: $90 ($110 for international students). *Unit head:* Tim-Allen Bruckner, Professor, 949-824-5797, Fax: 949-824-1845, E-mail: tim.bruckner@uci.edu. *Application contact:* Jennnifer Craig, Director of Graduate Student Services, 949-824-5918, Fax: 949-824-1845, E-mail: craigj@uci.edu.
Website: http://socialecology.uci.edu/core/graduate-se-core-programs

University of California, Los Angeles, Graduate Division, School of Public Health, Department of Epidemiology, Los Angeles, CA 90095. Offers MPH, MS, Dr PH, PhD, MD/MPH. *Degree requirements:* For master's, comprehensive exam or thesis; for doctorate, thesis/dissertation, oral and written qualifying exams. *Entrance requirements:* For master's, GRE General Test, minimum GPA of 3.0; for doctorate, GRE General Test, minimum undergraduate GPA of 3.0. Electronic applications accepted.

University of California, San Diego, Graduate Division, Program in Public Health, La Jolla, CA 92093. Offers epidemiology (PhD); health behavior (PhD). Program offered jointly with San Diego State University. *Students:* 16 full-time (13 women), 21 part-time (14 women); includes 11 minority (2 Black or African American, non-Hispanic/Latino; 3 Asian, non-Hispanic/Latino; 6 Hispanic/Latino), 4 international. In 2015, 12 doctorates awarded. *Degree requirements:* For doctorate, thesis/dissertation, 2 semesters/quarters of teaching assistantship. *Entrance requirements:* For doctorate, GRE General Test, minimum GPA of 3.0. Additional exam requirements/recommendations for international students: Required—TOEFL, IELTS. *Application deadline:* For fall admission, 12/15 priority date for domestic students. Electronic applications accepted. *Expenses:* Tuition, state resident: full-time $11,220. Tuition, nonresident: full-time $26,322. *Required fees:* $1800. *Financial support:* Teaching assistantships available. Financial award applicants required to submit FAFSA. *Faculty research:* Maternal and pediatric HIV/AIDS; healthy aging and gender differences; non-parametric and semi-parametric regression, resampling, and the analysis of high-dimensional data; neighborhood correlates of physical activity in children, teens, adults and older adults; medication safety and medication therapy management through practice-based research networks. *Unit head:* David Strong, Faculty Director, 858-657-5241, E-mail: dstrong@ucsd.edu. *Application contact:* Hollie Ward, Graduate Coordinator, 858-822-2382, E-mail: hcward@ucsd.edu.
Website: http://publichealth.ucsd.edu/jdp/

University of Cincinnati, Graduate School, College of Medicine, Graduate Programs in Biomedical Sciences, Department of Environmental Health, Cincinnati, OH 45221. Offers environmental and industrial hygiene (MS, PhD); environmental and occupational medicine (MS); environmental genetics and molecular toxicology (MS, PhD); epidemiology and biostatistics (MS, PhD); occupational safety and ergonomics (MS, PhD). *Accreditation:* ABET (one or more programs are accredited). Terminal master's awarded for partial completion of doctoral program. *Degree requirements:* For master's, thesis; for doctorate, thesis/dissertation, qualifying exam. *Entrance requirements:* For master's, GRE General Test, bachelor's degree in science; for doctorate, GRE General Test. Additional exam requirements/recommendations for international students: Required—TOEFL (minimum score 600 paper-based; 100 iBT). Electronic applications accepted. *Faculty research:* Carcinogens and mutagenesis, pulmonary studies, reproduction and development.

Epidemiology

University of Colorado Denver, Colorado School of Public Health, Department of Epidemiology, Aurora, CO 80045. Offers MS, PhD. *Program availability:* Part-time. *Faculty:* 14 full-time (12 women), 2 part-time/adjunct (1 woman). *Students:* 19 full-time (15 women), 6 part-time (4 women); includes 6 minority (1 Black or African American, non-Hispanic/Latino; 1 American Indian or Alaska Native, non-Hispanic/Latino; 1 Asian, non-Hispanic/Latino; 1 Hispanic/Latino; 2 Two or more races, non-Hispanic/Latino). Average age 28. 51 applicants, 12% accepted, 6 enrolled. In 2015, 4 master's, 2 doctorates awarded. *Degree requirements:* For master's, thesis, 38 credit hours; for doctorate, comprehensive exam, thesis/dissertation, 67 credit hours. *Entrance requirements:* For master's, GRE General Test, baccalaureate degree in scientific field, minimum GPA of 3.0, math course work through integral calculus, two official copies of all academic transcripts, four letters of recommendation/reference, essays describing the applicant's career goals and reasons for applying to the program, resume; for doctorate, GRE or MCAT, bachelor's, master's, or higher degree; minimum undergraduate and graduate GPA of 3.0; coursework in calculus, organic chemistry, epidemiology, biological sciences, and public health; 2 official copies of all academic transcripts; 4 letters of reference; essays. Additional exam requirements/recommendations for international students: Required—TOEFL (minimum score 550 paper-based; 80 iBT). *Application deadline:* For fall admission, 2/1 priority date for domestic students, 1/15 priority date for international students. Application fee: $65. Electronic applications accepted. *Expenses:* Contact institution. *Financial support:* In 2015–16, 25 students received support. Fellowships, research assistantships, teaching assistantships, Federal Work-Study, institutionally sponsored loans, scholarships/grants, traineeships, and unspecified assistantships available. Financial award application deadline: 3/1; financial award applicants required to submit FAFSA. *Faculty research:* Public health practice and practice-based research, reproductive and perinatal epidemiology, obesity, infectious disease epidemiology, diabetes. *Unit head:* Dr. Jill Norris, Chair, 303-724-4428, E-mail: jill.norris@ucdenver.edu. *Application contact:* Melodie Proffitt, Department Assistant, 303-724-4488, E-mail: melodie.proffitt@ucdenver.edu.
Website: http://www.ucdenver.edu/academics/colleges/PublicHealth/departments/Epidemiology/Pages/welcome.aspx

University of Colorado Denver, Colorado School of Public Health, Program in Public Health, Aurora, CO 80045. Offers community and behavioral health (MPH, Dr PH); environmental and occupational health (MPH); epidemiology (MPH); health systems, management and policy (MPH). *Accreditation:* CEPH. *Program availability:* Part-time, evening/weekend. *Faculty:* 16 full-time (14 women), 1 (woman) part-time/adjunct. *Students:* 379 full-time (293 women), 77 part-time (69 women); includes 111 minority (10 Black or African American, non-Hispanic/Latino; 3 American Indian or Alaska Native, non-Hispanic/Latino; 36 Asian, non-Hispanic/Latino; 47 Hispanic/Latino; 1 Native Hawaiian or other Pacific Islander, non-Hispanic/Latino; 14 Two or more races, non-Hispanic/Latino), 12 international. Average age 31. 785 applicants, 25% accepted, 166 enrolled. In 2015, 144 master's awarded. *Degree requirements:* For master's, thesis or alternative, 42 credit hours; for doctorate, comprehensive exam, thesis/dissertation, 67 credit hours. *Entrance requirements:* For master's, GRE, MCAT, DAT, LSAT, PCAT, GMAT or master's degree from accredited institution, baccalaureate degree or equivalent; minimum GPA of 3.0; transcripts; references; resume; essay; for doctorate, GRE, MCAT, DAT, LSAT, PCAT or GMAT, MPH or master's or higher degree in related field or equivalent; 2 years of previous work experience in public health; essay; resume. Additional exam requirements/recommendations for international students: Required—TOEFL (minimum score 550 paper-based; 80 iBT). *Application deadline:* For fall admission, 12/15 priority date for domestic students, 12/1 priority date for international students. Electronic applications accepted. *Expenses:* Contact institution. *Financial support:* In 2015–16, 265 students received support. Fellowships, research assistantships, teaching assistantships, Federal Work-Study, institutionally sponsored loans, scholarships/grants, traineeships, and unspecified assistantships available. Financial award application deadline: 3/15; financial award applicants required to submit FAFSA. *Faculty research:* Cancer prevention by nutrition, cancer survivorship outcomes, social and cultural factors related to health. *Total annual research expenditures:* $302,793. *Unit head:* Dr. Lori Crane, Chair, 303-724-4385, E-mail: lori.crane@ucdenver.edu. *Application contact:* 303-724-4613, E-mail: csph.studentaffairs@ucdenver.edu.
Website: http://www.ucdenver.edu/academics/colleges/PublicHealth/Academics/degreesandprograms/Pages/index.aspx

University of Florida, College of Medicine, Program in Clinical Investigation, Gainesville, FL 32611. Offers clinical investigation (MS); epidemiology (MS); public health (MPH). *Program availability:* Part-time. *Entrance requirements:* For master's, GRE, MD, PhD, DMD/DDS or Pharm D.

University of Florida, Graduate School, College of Public Health and Health Professions, Department of Epidemiology, Gainesville, FL 32611. Offers clinical and translational science (PhD); epidemiology (MS, PhD). *Faculty:* 5 full-time. *Students:* 28 full-time (17 women), 4 part-time (2 women); includes 8 minority (4 Black or African American, non-Hispanic/Latino; 3 Asian, non-Hispanic/Latino; 1 Hispanic/Latino), 13 international. Average age 29. 53 applicants, 32% accepted, 9 enrolled. In 2015, 1 master's, 5 doctorates awarded. *Degree requirements:* For master's, thesis; for doctorate, thesis/dissertation. *Entrance requirements:* For master's and doctorate, GRE (minimum score verbal/quantitative combined 300), minimum GPA of 3.0. Additional exam requirements/recommendations for international students: Required—TOEFL (minimum score 550 paper-based; 80 iBT), IELTS (minimum score 6). *Application deadline:* For fall admission, 2/1 for domestic and international students. Application fee: $30. *Financial support:* In 2015–16, 6 fellowships, 9 research assistantships, 11 teaching assistantships were awarded. Financial award applicants required to submit FAFSA. *Faculty research:* Substance abuse, psychiatric epidemiology, cancer epidemiology, infectious disease epidemiology, bioinformatics. *Total annual research expenditures:* $3.5 million. *Unit head:* Linda Cottler, PhD, Chair, 352-273-5468, E-mail: lbcottler@ufl.edu. *Application contact:* Betsy Jones, Program Assistant, 352-273-5961, E-mail: bjcop@ufl.edu.
Website: http://epidemiology.phhp.ufl.edu/

University of Florida, Graduate School, College of Public Health and Health Professions, Programs in Public Health, Gainesville, FL 32611. Offers biostatistics (MPH); clinical and translational science (PhD); environmental health (MPH); epidemiology (MPH); health management and policy (MPH); public health (MPH, PhD, Certificate); public health practice (MPH); rehabilitation science (PhD); social and behavioral sciences (MPH); DPT/MPH; DVM/MPH; JD/MPH; MD/MPH; Pharm D/MPH. *Accreditation:* CEPH. *Program availability:* Online learning. *Faculty:* 31. *Students:* 174 full-time (134 women), 59 part-time (42 women); includes 67 minority (27 Black or African American, non-Hispanic/Latino; 1 American Indian or Alaska Native, non-Hispanic/Latino; 25 Asian, non-Hispanic/Latino; 14 Hispanic/Latino), 24 international. Average age 30. 385 applicants, 44% accepted, 75 enrolled. In 2015, 81 master's, 6 doctorates awarded. *Degree requirements:* For master's, internship. *Entrance requirements:* For master's, GRE General Test, minimum GPA of 3.0. Additional exam requirements/recommendations for international students: Required—TOEFL (minimum score 550 paper-based; 80 iBT), IELTS (minimum score 6). *Application deadline:* For fall admission, 7/1 for domestic students, 4/1 for international students. Application fee: $30.

Financial support: In 2015–16, 5 research assistantships, 10 teaching assistantships were awarded; fellowships also available. Financial award applicants required to submit FAFSA. *Unit head:* Sarah L. McKune, PhD, Program Director, 352-328-0615, Fax: 352-273-6448, E-mail: smckune@ufl.edu. *Application contact:* Telisha Martin, PhD, Associate Director, MPH Program, 352-273-6444, E-mail: martints@ufl.edu.
Website: http://www.mph.ufl.edu/

University of Guelph, Ontario Veterinary College and Graduate Studies, Graduate Programs in Veterinary Sciences, Department of Population Medicine, Guelph, ON N1G 2W1, Canada. Offers epidemiology (M Sc, DV Sc, PhD); health management (DV Sc); population medicine and health management (M Sc); swine health management (M Sc); theriogenology (M Sc, DV Sc). *Degree requirements:* For master's, thesis; for doctorate, comprehensive exam, thesis/dissertation. *Entrance requirements:* Additional exam requirements/recommendations for international students: Required—TOEFL.

University of Hawaii at Manoa, John A. Burns School of Medicine, Department of Public Health Sciences and Epidemiology, Program in Epidemiology, Honolulu, HI 96822. Offers PhD. *Program availability:* Part-time. *Faculty:* 21 full-time (7 women). *Students:* 8 full-time (4 women), 6 part-time (all women); includes 7 minority (5 Asian, non-Hispanic/Latino; 1 Hispanic/Latino; 1 Two or more races, non-Hispanic/Latino), 1 international. Average age 38. 4 applicants, 75% accepted, 2 enrolled. In 2015, 1 doctorate awarded. *Degree requirements:* For doctorate, comprehensive exam, thesis/dissertation. *Entrance requirements:* For doctorate, GRE General Test. Additional exam requirements/recommendations for international students: Required—TOEFL (minimum score 600 paper-based; 100 iBT), IELTS (minimum score 7). *Application deadline:* For fall admission, 3/1 for domestic and international students; for spring admission, 9/1 for domestic and international students. Application fee: $100. *Financial support:* In 2015–16, 2 fellowships (averaging $4,250 per year), 2 research assistantships (averaging $22,050 per year) were awarded. *Unit head:* Dr. Jerris R. Hedges, Dean, 808-692-0881. *Application contact:* Eric Hurwitz, Graduate Chair, 808-956-6867, Fax: 808-956-1979, E-mail: ehurwitz@hawaii.edu.

University of Illinois at Chicago, School of Public Health, Epidemiology and Biostatistics Division, Chicago, IL 60607-7128. Offers biostatistics (MPH, MS, PhD); epidemiology (MPH, MS, PhD). *Program availability:* Part-time. *Faculty:* 17 full-time (7 women), 12 part-time/adjunct (5 women). *Students:* 132 full-time (93 women), 58 part-time (43 women); includes 50 minority (12 Black or African American, non-Hispanic/Latino; 26 Asian, non-Hispanic/Latino; 10 Hispanic/Latino; 2 Two or more races, non-Hispanic/Latino), 32 international. Average age 30. Terminal master's awarded for partial completion of doctoral program. *Degree requirements:* For master's, thesis, field practicum; for doctorate, thesis/dissertation, independent research, internship. *Entrance requirements:* For master's and doctorate, GRE General Test, minimum GPA of 2.75. Additional exam requirements/recommendations for international students: Required—TOEFL. *Application deadline:* For fall admission, 2/1 for domestic students, 1/1 priority date for international students. Application fee: $60. Electronic applications accepted. *Expenses:* Contact institution. *Financial support:* In 2015–16, 17 students received support. Fellowships with full tuition reimbursements available, research assistantships with full tuition reimbursements available, teaching assistantships with full tuition reimbursements available, career-related internships or fieldwork, Federal Work-Study, institutionally sponsored loans, scholarships/grants, traineeships, tuition waivers (full), and unspecified assistantships available. Support available to part-time students. Financial award application deadline: 3/1; financial award applicants required to submit FAFSA. *Faculty research:* Quantitative methods. *Unit head:* Dr. Ronald Hershow, Division Director, 312-996-4759, E-mail: rchersho@uic.edu.
Website: http://publichealth.uic.edu/departments/epidemiologyandbiostatistics/

University of Illinois at Springfield, Graduate Programs, College of Public Affairs and Administration, Program in Public Health, Springfield, IL 62703-5407. Offers community health education (Graduate Certificate); emergency preparedness and homeland security (Graduate Certificate); epidemiology (Graduate Certificate); public health (MPH). *Program availability:* Part-time, evening/weekend, 100% online. *Faculty:* 7 full-time (5 women), 1 part-time/adjunct (0 women). *Students:* 41 full-time (23 women), 58 part-time (39 women); includes 25 minority (14 Black or African American, non-Hispanic/Latino; 6 Asian, non-Hispanic/Latino; 3 Hispanic/Latino; 2 Two or more races, non-Hispanic/Latino), 23 international. Average age 32. 87 applicants, 36% accepted, 23 enrolled. In 2015, 30 master's, 19 other advanced degrees awarded. *Degree requirements:* For master's, comprehensive exam, internship. *Entrance requirements:* For master's, GRE, minimum undergraduate GPA of 3.0, 3 letters of recommendation, statement of personal goals. Additional exam requirements/recommendations for international students: Required—TOEFL (minimum score 500 paper-based; 61 iBT). *Application deadline:* Applications are processed on a rolling basis. Application fee: $60 ($75 for international students). Electronic applications accepted. *Expenses:* Tuition, state resident: part-time $329 per credit hour. Tuition, nonresident: part-time $675 per credit hour. *Financial support:* In 2015–16, fellowships with full tuition reimbursements (averaging $9,900 per year), research assistantships with full tuition reimbursements (averaging $9,956 per year), teaching assistantships with full tuition reimbursements (averaging $9,956 per year) were awarded; career-related internships or fieldwork, Federal Work-Study, scholarships/grants, health care benefits, and unspecified assistantships also available. Support available to part-time students. Financial award application deadline: 11/15; financial award applicants required to submit FAFSA. *Unit head:* Dr. Josiah Alamu, Program Administrator, 217-206-7874, Fax: 217-206-7279, E-mail: jalam3@uis.edu. *Application contact:* Dr. Lynn Pardie, Office of Graduate Studies, 800-252-8533, Fax: 217-206-7623, E-mail: lpard1@uis.edu.
Website: http://www.uis.edu/publichealth/

The University of Iowa, Graduate College, College of Public Health, Department of Epidemiology, Iowa City, IA 52242-1316. Offers clinical investigation (MS); epidemiology (MPH, MS, PhD). *Accreditation:* CEPH. *Degree requirements:* For master's, thesis optional, exam; for doctorate, comprehensive exam, thesis/dissertation. *Entrance requirements:* For master's and doctorate, GRE General Test, minimum GPA of 3.0. Additional exam requirements/recommendations for international students: Required—TOEFL (minimum score 600 paper-based; 100 iBT). Electronic applications accepted.

The University of Kansas, University of Kansas Medical Center, School of Medicine, Department of Preventive Medicine and Public Health, Kansas City, KS 66160. Offers clinical research (MS); environmental health sciences (MPH); epidemiology (MPH); public health management (MPH); social and behavioral health (MPH); MD/MPH; PhD/MPH. *Program availability:* Part-time. *Faculty:* 70. *Students:* 48 full-time (35 women), 46 part-time (31 women); includes 31 minority (9 Black or African American, non-Hispanic/Latino; 4 American Indian or Alaska Native, non-Hispanic/Latino; 8 Asian, non-Hispanic/Latino; 6 Hispanic/Latino; 4 Two or more races, non-Hispanic/Latino), 8 international. Average age 31. 66 applicants, 68% accepted, 44 enrolled. In 2015, 31 master's awarded. *Degree requirements:* For master's, thesis, capstone practicum defense. *Entrance requirements:* For master's, GRE, MCAT, LSAT, GMAT or other equivalent graduate professional exam. Additional exam requirements/recommendations for international students: Required—TOEFL. *Application deadline:* For fall admission, 3/1 for domestic and international students. Applications are processed on a rolling basis. Application fee: $60. Electronic applications accepted. *Financial support:* In 2015–16, 9 research assistantships (averaging $15,000 per year) were awarded; career-related

internships or fieldwork, Federal Work-Study, scholarships/grants, and unspecified assistantships also available. Support available to part-time students. Financial award application deadline: 3/1; financial award applicants required to submit FAFSA. *Faculty research:* Cancer screening and prevention, smoking cessation, obesity and physical activity, health services/outcomes research, health disparities. *Total annual research expenditures:* $6.6 million. *Unit head:* Dr. Edward F. Ellerbeck, Chairman, 913-588-2774, Fax: 913-588-2780, E-mail: eellerbe@kumc.edu. *Application contact:* Tanya Honderick, MPH Director, 913-588-2720, Fax: 913-588-8505, E-mail: thonderick@kumc.edu.
Website: http://www.kumc.edu/school-of-medicine/preventive-medicine-and-public-health.html

University of Kentucky, Graduate School, College of Public Health, Program in Epidemiology and Biostatistics, Lexington, KY 40506-0032. Offers PhD.

University of Louisville, Graduate School, School of Public Health and Information Sciences, Department of Epidemiology and Population Health, Louisville, KY 40292-0001. Offers epidemiology (MPH, MS, PhD). *Program availability:* Part-time. *Students:* 5 full-time (4 women), 16 part-time (13 women); includes 4 minority (2 Black or African American, non-Hispanic/Latino; 2 Asian, non-Hispanic/Latino), 1 international. Average age 33. 13 applicants, 85% accepted, 7 enrolled. In 2015, 8 master's awarded. Terminal master's awarded for partial completion of doctoral program. *Degree requirements:* For master's, thesis; for doctorate, comprehensive exam, thesis/dissertation. *Entrance requirements:* For master's, GRE General Test; for doctorate, GRE General Test, master's degree in related field. Additional exam requirements/recommendations for international students: Required—TOEFL. *Application deadline:* For fall admission, 2/1 for domestic students, 1/2 priority date for international students. Applications are processed on a rolling basis. Application fee: $60. Electronic applications accepted. *Expenses:* Tuition, state resident: full-time $11,664; part-time $649 per credit hour. Tuition, nonresident: full-time $24,274; part-time $1350 per credit hour. *Required fees:* $196. Tuition and fees vary according to program and reciprocity agreements. *Financial support:* In 2015–16, 99,941 students received support, including fellowships with full tuition reimbursements available (averaging $20,000 per year), research assistantships with full tuition reimbursements available (averaging $20,000 per year), teaching assistantships, scholarships/grants, traineeships, health care benefits, and unspecified assistantships also available. Financial award applicants required to submit FAFSA. *Faculty research:* Breast cancer in minority populations, health policy, clinical trials, chronic disease, genetic epidemiology, Cystic Fibrosis, breast cancer and longevity, Alzheimer's, Parkinson's and microbiomes, lead exposure and Army work, autism and the environment. *Total annual research expenditures:* $1.5 million. *Unit head:* Dr. Richard Baumgartner, Professor and Chair, 502-852-2038, E-mail: rnbaum01@gwise.louisville.edu. *Application contact:* Vicki Lewis, Administrative Assistant, 502-852-1798, Fax: 502-852-3294, E-mail: vicki.lewis@louisville.edu.
Website: http://louisville.edu/sphis/departments/epidemiology-population-health

University of Louisville, Graduate School, School of Public Health and Information Sciences, Department of Public Health and Information Sciences, Louisville, KY 40202. Offers biostatistics (MS, PhD); clinical investigation (M Sc); epidemiology (MS); health management and systems sciences (MPH); public health sciences (PhD), including environmental health, epidemiology, health management, health promotion; public health sciences - health management (PhD). *Program availability:* Part-time. *Students:* 92 full-time (60 women), 33 part-time (19 women); includes 37 minority (16 Black or African American, non-Hispanic/Latino; 12 Asian, non-Hispanic/Latino; 6 Hispanic/Latino; 3 Two or more races, non-Hispanic/Latino), 19 international. Average age 32. 128 applicants, 77% accepted, 56 enrolled. In 2015, 38 master's, 6 doctorates awarded. *Degree requirements:* For master's, thesis optional; for doctorate, comprehensive exam, thesis/dissertation. *Entrance requirements:* For master's and doctorate, GRE General Test. Additional exam requirements/recommendations for international students: Required—TOEFL (minimum score 600 paper-based; 100 iBT). *Application deadline:* For fall admission, 5/1 for domestic and international students. Application fee: $60. Electronic applications accepted. *Expenses:* Tuition, state resident: full-time $11,664; part-time $649 per credit hour. Tuition, nonresident: full-time $24,274; part-time $1350 per credit hour. *Required fees:* $196. Tuition and fees vary according to program and reciprocity agreements. *Financial support:* In 2015–16, 718,988 students received support. Research assistantships with full tuition reimbursements available, scholarships/grants, health care benefits, and unspecified assistantships available. Financial award applicants required to submit FAFSA. *Faculty research:* Department of environmental and occupational health sciences department of health management and systems sciences department of health promotion and behavioral sciences. *Total annual research expenditures:* $2.1 million. *Unit head:* Dr. Craig Blakely, Dean, 502-852-3297, Fax: 502-852-3291, E-mail: chblak01@louisville.edu.
Website: http://louisville.edu/sphis/departments/health-management-systems-science

University of Maryland, Baltimore, Graduate School, Graduate Program in Life Sciences, Baltimore, MD 21201. Offers biochemistry and molecular biology (MS, PhD), including biochemistry; epidemiology (PhD); gerontology (PhD); molecular medicine (MS, PhD), including cancer biology (PhD), cell and molecular physiology (PhD), human genetics and genomic medicine (PhD), molecular medicine (MS), molecular toxicology and pharmacology (PhD); molecular microbiology and immunology (PhD); neuroscience (PhD); physical rehabilitation science (PhD); toxicology (MS, PhD); MD/MS; MD/PhD. *Degree requirements:* For master's, comprehensive exam (for some programs), thesis (for some programs); for doctorate, comprehensive exam, thesis/dissertation. *Entrance requirements:* For master's and doctorate, GRE. Additional exam requirements/recommendations for international students: Required—TOEFL (minimum score 550 paper-based; 80 iBT); Recommended—IELTS (minimum score 7). Electronic applications accepted. Tuition and fees vary according to program. *Faculty research:* Cancer, reproduction, cardiovascular, immunology.

University of Maryland, Baltimore, Graduate School, Graduate Programs in Pharmacy, Department of Pharmaceutical Health Service Research, Baltimore, MD 21201. Offers epidemiology (MS); pharmacy administration (PhD); Pharm D/PhD. *Degree requirements:* For doctorate, comprehensive exam, thesis/dissertation. *Entrance requirements:* For doctorate, GRE General Test. Additional exam requirements/recommendations for international students: Required—TOEFL, IELTS. Electronic applications accepted. Tuition and fees vary according to program. *Faculty research:* Pharmacoeconomics, outcomes research, public health policy, drug therapy and aging.

University of Maryland, Baltimore, School of Medicine, Department of Epidemiology and Public Health, Baltimore, MD 21201. Offers biostatistics (MS); clinical research (MS); epidemiology and preventive medicine (MPH, MS, PhD); gerontology (PhD); human genetics and genomic medicine (MS, PhD); molecular epidemiology (MS, PhD); toxicology (MS, PhD); JD/MS; MD/PhD; MS/PhD. *Accreditation:* CEPH. *Program availability:* Part-time. *Students:* 73 full-time (58 women), 56 part-time (44 women); includes 45 minority (23 Black or African American, non-Hispanic/Latino; 12 Asian, non-Hispanic/Latino; 5 Hispanic/Latino; 5 Two or more races, non-Hispanic/Latino), 17 international. Average age 31. In 2015, 34 master's, 17 doctorates awarded. *Degree requirements:* For doctorate, comprehensive exam, thesis/dissertation. *Entrance requirements:* For master's and doctorate, GRE General Test. Additional exam

requirements/recommendations for international students: Required—TOEFL (minimum score 550 paper-based; 80 iBT); Recommended—IELTS (minimum score 7). *Application deadline:* For fall admission, 1/15 for domestic and international students. Application fee: $75. Electronic applications accepted. *Expenses:* Contact institution. *Financial support:* In 2015–16, research assistantships with partial tuition reimbursements (averaging $26,000 per year) were awarded; fellowships, Federal Work-Study, scholarships/grants, and unspecified assistantships also available. Financial award application deadline: 3/1; financial award applicants required to submit FAFSA. *Unit head:* Dr. Laura Hungerford, Program Director, 410-706-8492, Fax: 410-706-4225. *Application contact:* Jessica Kelley, Program Coordinator, 410-706-8492, Fax: 410-706-4225, E-mail: jkelley@som.umaryland.edu.
Website: http://lifesciences.umaryland.edu/epidemiology/

University of Maryland, Baltimore County, The Graduate School, College of Arts, Humanities and Social Sciences, Department of Emergency Health Services, Baltimore, MD 21250. Offers administration, planning, and policy (MS); education (MS); emergency health services (MS); emergency management (Postbaccalaureate Certificate); preventive medicine and epidemiology (MS). *Program availability:* Part-time, evening/weekend, 100% online, blended/hybrid learning. *Faculty:* 3 full-time (1 woman), 8 part-time/adjunct (2 women). *Students:* 24 full-time (14 women), 11 part-time (9 women); includes 8 minority (2 Black or African American, non-Hispanic/Latino; 3 Asian, non-Hispanic/Latino; 3 Hispanic/Latino), 14 international. Average age 26. 18 applicants, 56% accepted, 7 enrolled. In 2015, 13 master's awarded. *Degree requirements:* For master's, comprehensive exam, thesis (for some programs), capstone project. *Entrance requirements:* For master's, GRE General Test, minimum GPA of 3.2. Additional exam requirements/recommendations for international students: Required—TOEFL (minimum score 85 iBT) or IELTS. *Application deadline:* For fall admission, 6/15 for domestic students, 3/1 for international students; for spring admission, 11/1 for domestic students, 10/1 for international students. Applications are processed on a rolling basis. Application fee: $50. Electronic applications accepted. *Expenses:* Tuition, state resident: full-time $12,816. Tuition, nonresident: full-time $19,710. *Financial support:* In 2015–16, 2 students received support, including 1 fellowship with tuition reimbursement available (averaging $70,000 per year), 1 research assistantship with tuition reimbursement available (averaging $26,800 per year); career-related internships or fieldwork, Federal Work-Study, scholarships/grants, health care benefits, and unspecified assistantships also available. Financial award application deadline: 5/30; financial award applicants required to submit FAFSA. *Faculty research:* EMS management, disaster health services, emergency management, risk profiles. *Total annual research expenditures:* $50,000. *Unit head:* Dr. Bruce J. Walz, Chairman, 410-455-3216, Fax: 410-455-3045, E-mail: walz@umbc.edu. *Application contact:* Dr. Rick Bissell, Program Director, 410-455-3776, Fax: 410-455-3045, E-mail: bissell@umbc.edu.
Website: http://ehs.umbc.edu/

University of Maryland, College Park, Academic Affairs, School of Public Health, Department of Epidemiology and Biostatistics, College Park, MD 20742. Offers biostatistics (MPH); epidemiology (MPH, PhD).

University of Massachusetts Amherst, Graduate School, School of Public Health and Health Sciences, Department of Public Health, Amherst, MA 01003. Offers biostatistics (MPH, MS, PhD); community health education (MPH, MS, PhD); environmental health sciences (MPH, MS, PhD); epidemiology (MPH, MS, PhD); health policy and management (MPH, MS, PhD); nutrition (MPH, PhD); public health practice (MPH); MPH/MPPA. *Accreditation:* CEPH (one or more programs are accredited). *Program availability:* Part-time, evening/weekend, online learning. Terminal master's awarded for partial completion of doctoral program. *Degree requirements:* For master's, thesis (for some programs); for doctorate, comprehensive exam, thesis/dissertation. *Entrance requirements:* For master's and doctorate, GRE General Test. Additional exam requirements/recommendations for international students: Required—TOEFL (minimum score 550 paper-based; 80 iBT), IELTS (minimum score 6.5). Electronic applications accepted.

University of Memphis, Graduate School, School of Public Health, Memphis, TN 38152. Offers biostatistics (MPH); environmental health (MPH); epidemiology (MPH); health systems management (MPH); public health (MHA); social and behavioral sciences (MPH). *Program availability:* Part-time, evening/weekend, online learning. *Faculty:* 117 full-time (5 women), 5 part-time/adjunct (1 woman). *Students:* 100 full-time (68 women), 48 part-time (35 women); includes 63 minority (33 Black or African American, non-Hispanic/Latino; 20 Asian, non-Hispanic/Latino; 7 Hispanic/Latino; 3 Two or more races, non-Hispanic/Latino), 17 international. Average age 30. 114 applicants, 83% accepted, 37 enrolled. In 2015, 55 master's awarded. *Degree requirements:* For master's, comprehensive exam, thesis. *Entrance requirements:* For master's, GRE, letters of recommendation. Additional exam requirements/recommendations for international students: Required—TOEFL. *Application deadline:* For fall admission, 4/1 for domestic students; for spring admission, 11/1 for domestic students. Application fee: $35 ($60 for international students). Electronic applications accepted. *Financial support:* In 2015–16, 46 students received support. Research assistantships with full tuition reimbursements available, Federal Work-Study, scholarships/grants, and unspecified assistantships available. Financial award application deadline: 2/15; financial award applicants required to submit FAFSA. *Faculty research:* Health and medical savings accounts, adoption rates, health informatics, Telehealth technologies, biostatistics, environmental health, epidemiology, health systems management, social and behavioral sciences. *Unit head:* Dr. Lisa M. Klesges, Director, 901-678-4637, E-mail: lmklsges@memphis.edu. *Application contact:* Dr. Karen Weddle-West, Information Contact, 901-678-2531, Fax: 901-678-5023, E-mail: gradsch@memphis.edu.
Website: http://www.memphis.edu/sph/

University of Miami, Graduate School, Miller School of Medicine, Graduate Programs in Medicine, Department of Epidemiology and Public Health, Coral Gables, FL 33124. Offers epidemiology (PhD); public health (MPH, MSPH); JD/MPH; MD/MPH; MD/PhD; MPA/MPH; MPH/MAIA. *Accreditation:* CEPH (one or more programs are accredited). *Program availability:* Part-time. *Degree requirements:* For master's, thesis (for some programs), project, practicum; for doctorate, comprehensive exam, thesis/dissertation. *Entrance requirements:* For master's, GRE General Test, minimum GPA of 3.0, 3 letters of recommendation; for doctorate, GRE General Test, minimum GPA of 3.0, course work in epidemiology and statistics, 3 letters of recommendation. Additional exam requirements/recommendations for international students: Required—TOEFL (minimum score 550 paper-based; 59 iBT). Electronic applications accepted. *Faculty research:* Behavioral epidemiology, substance abuse, AIDS, cardiovascular diseases, women's health.

University of Michigan, School of Public Health, Department of Epidemiology, Ann Arbor, MI 48109-2029. Offers epidemiological science (PhD); general epidemiology (MPH); global health epidemiology (MPH); hospital and molecular epidemiology (MPH); occupational and environmental epidemiology (MPH). PhD and MS offered through the Rackham Graduate School. *Accreditation:* CEPH (one or more programs are accredited). *Faculty:* 31 full-time (17 women), 41 part-time/adjunct (22 women). *Students:* 220 full-time (161 women), 2 part-time (1 woman); includes 30 minority (8 Black or African American, non-Hispanic/Latino; 9 Asian, non-Hispanic/Latino; 8 Hispanic/Latino; 5 Two or more races, non-Hispanic/Latino), 41 international. Average

Epidemiology

age 27. 821 applicants, 38% accepted, 128 enrolled. In 2015, 85 master's, 12 doctorates awarded. Terminal master's awarded for partial completion of doctoral program. *Degree requirements:* For master's, thesis (for some programs); for doctorate, comprehensive exam, thesis/dissertation, oral defense of dissertation, preliminary exam. *Entrance requirements:* For master's and doctorate, GRE General Test, MCAT. Additional exam requirements/recommendations for international students: Required— TOEFL (minimum score 100 iBT). *Application deadline:* For fall admission, 12/15 priority date for domestic students, 1/15 for international students. Applications are processed on a rolling basis. Application fee: $75. Electronic applications accepted. *Financial support:* Fellowships, research assistantships, teaching assistantships, career-related internships or fieldwork, Federal Work-Study, institutionally sponsored loans, scholarships/grants, traineeships, health care benefits, and unspecified assistantships available. Financial award application deadline: 12/15. *Faculty research:* Molecular virology, infectious diseases, women's health, genetics, social epidemiology. *Unit head:* Dr. Joseph Eisenberg, Chair, 734-764-5435, Fax: 734-764-3192. *Application contact:* Nancy Francis, Student Services Coordinator, 734-763-0274, Fax: 734-763-3192, E-mail: nhellner@umich.edu.
Website: http://www.sph.umich.edu/epid/

University of Minnesota, Twin Cities Campus, School of Public Health, Division of Environmental Health Sciences, Area in Environmental and Occupational Epidemiology, Minneapolis, MN 55455-0213. Offers MPH, MS, PhD. *Accreditation:* CEPH (one or more programs are accredited). *Degree requirements:* For doctorate, thesis/dissertation. *Entrance requirements:* For master's and doctorate, GRE General Test. Electronic applications accepted.

University of Minnesota, Twin Cities Campus, School of Public Health, Major in Epidemiology, Minneapolis, MN 55455-0213. Offers MPH, PhD. *Accreditation:* CEPH (one or more programs are accredited). *Program availability:* Part-time. Terminal master's awarded for partial completion of doctoral program. *Degree requirements:* For master's, fieldwork, project; for doctorate, comprehensive exam, thesis/dissertation. *Entrance requirements:* For master's, GRE General Test; for doctorate, GRE General Test, master's degree in related field. Additional exam requirements/recommendations for international students: Required—TOEFL. Electronic applications accepted. *Expenses:* Contact institution. *Faculty research:* Prevention of cardiovascular disease, nutrition, genetic epidemiology, behavioral interventions, research methods.

University of Nebraska Medical Center, Department of Epidemiology, Omaha, NE 68198. Offers PhD. *Program availability:* Part-time. *Faculty:* 11 full-time (6 women), 5 part-time/adjunct (2 women). *Students:* 17 full-time (14 women), 3 part-time (0 women); includes 4 minority (all Asian, non-Hispanic/Latino), 10 international. Average age 31. 21 applicants, 24% accepted, 5 enrolled. *Degree requirements:* For doctorate, comprehensive exam, thesis/dissertation. *Entrance requirements:* For doctorate, GRE, master's degree in epidemiology or related field. Additional exam requirements/ recommendations for international students: Required—TOEFL (minimum score 550 paper-based; 80 iBT). *Application deadline:* For fall admission, 6/1 for domestic students, 3/1 for international students. Application fee: $45. Electronic applications accepted. *Expenses:* Tuition, state resident: full-time $7830; part-time $3915 per credit hour. Tuition, nonresident: full-time $22,410; part-time $11,205 per credit hour. *Required fees:* $521. *Financial support:* In 2015–16, 1 teaching assistantship with full tuition reimbursement (averaging $23,100 per year) was awarded; research assistantships with full tuition reimbursements, scholarships/grants, and unspecified assistantships also available. Financial award applicants required to submit FAFSA. *Faculty research:* Arsenic in drinking water and diabetes, environmental tobacco smoke exposure, injuries in pork processing, cancer-related disparities in Northern Plains American Indian communities, pandemic flu preparedness in Nebraska nursing homes. *Unit head:* Dr. Shinobu Watanabe-Galloway, Associate Professor, 402-559-5387, E-mail: swatanabe@unmc.edu. *Application contact:* Parwin Ibrahim, Coordinator, 402-559-4248, E-mail: parwin.ibrahim@unmc.edu.
Website: http://www.unmc.edu/publichealth/departments/epidemiology/

University of New Mexico, Graduate Studies, Health Sciences Center, Program in Public Health, Albuquerque, NM 87131-5196. Offers community health (MPH); epidemiology (MPH); health systems, services and policy (MPH). *Accreditation:* CEPH. *Program availability:* Part-time, online learning. *Faculty:* 9 full-time (7 women), 3 part-time/adjunct (2 women). *Students:* 25 full-time (17 women), 20 part-time (16 women); includes 17 minority (3 Black or African American, non-Hispanic/Latino; 1 American Indian or Alaska Native, non-Hispanic/Latino; 3 Asian, non-Hispanic/Latino; 10 Hispanic/ Latino), 1 international. Average age 31. 32 applicants, 63% accepted, 16 enrolled. In 2015, 13 master's awarded. *Degree requirements:* For master's, thesis. *Entrance requirements:* For master's, GRE, MCAT, 2 years of experience in health field. Additional exam requirements/recommendations for international students: Required— TOEFL. *Application deadline:* For fall admission, 2/1 for domestic students. Application fee: $50. *Financial support:* Fellowships, research assistantships with tuition reimbursements, and Federal Work-Study available. Financial award application deadline: 12/15; financial award applicants required to submit FAFSA. *Faculty research:* Epidemiology, rural health, environmental health, Native American health issues. *Unit head:* Dr. Kristine Tollestrup, Director, 505-272-4173, Fax: 505-272-4494, E-mail: ktollestrup@salud.unm.edu. *Application contact:* Gayle Garcia, Education Coordinator, 505-272-3982, Fax: 505-272-4494, E-mail: garciag@salud.unm.edu.
Website: http://fcm.unm.edu/

The University of North Carolina at Chapel Hill, Graduate School, Gillings School of Global Public Health, Department of Epidemiology, Chapel Hill, NC 27599. Offers MPH, MSCR, PhD. *Accreditation:* CEPH (one or more programs are accredited). *Students:* 212 full-time (164 women); includes 81 minority (21 Black or African American, non-Hispanic/ Latino; 1 American Indian or Alaska Native, non-Hispanic/Latino; 26 Asian, non-Hispanic/ Latino; 15 Hispanic/Latino; 1 Native Hawaiian or other Pacific Islander, non-Hispanic/ Latino; 17 Two or more races, non-Hispanic/Latino), 20 international. Average age 31. 278 applicants, 26% accepted, 35 enrolled. Terminal master's awarded for partial completion of doctoral program. *Degree requirements:* For master's, comprehensive exam, major paper; for doctorate, comprehensive exam, thesis/dissertation. *Entrance requirements:* For master's and doctorate, GRE General Test, minimum GPA of 3.0 (recommended). Additional exam requirements/recommendations for international students: Required— TOEFL. *Application deadline:* For fall admission, 12/10 priority date for domestic and international students. Applications are processed on a rolling basis. Application fee: $85. Electronic applications accepted. *Financial support:* Fellowships with tuition reimbursements, research assistantships with tuition reimbursements, teaching assistantships with tuition reimbursements, career-related internships or fieldwork, Federal Work-Study, institutionally sponsored loans, scholarships/grants, traineeships, and health care benefits available. Support available to part-time students. Financial award application deadline: 12/10; financial award applicants required to submit FAFSA. *Faculty research:* Chronic disease: cancer, cardiovascular, nutritional; environmental/occupational injury; infectious diseases; reproductive diseases; healthcare. *Unit head:* Dr. Andrew Olshan, Interim Chair, 919-966-7458, Fax: 919-966-2089, E-mail: andy_olshan@unc.edu. *Application contact:* Carmen Woody, Student Services Manager, 919-966-7458, Fax: 919-966-2089, E-mail: carmen_woody@unc.edu.
Website: http://www2.sph.unc.edu/epid/

The University of North Carolina at Chapel Hill, School of Dentistry and Graduate School, Graduate Programs in Dentistry, Chapel Hill, NC 27599. Offers dental hygiene (MS); endodontics (MS); epidemiology (PhD); operative dentistry (MS); oral and maxillofacial pathology (MS); oral and maxillofacial radiology (MS); oral biology (PhD); orthodontics (MS); pediatric dentistry (MS); periodontology (MS); prosthodontics (MS). *Degree requirements:* For master's, thesis; for doctorate, thesis/dissertation. *Entrance requirements:* For master's, GRE General Test (for orthodontics and oral biology only); National Dental Board Part I (Part II if available), dental degree (for all except dental hygiene); for doctorate, GRE General Test. Additional exam requirements/ recommendations for international students: Required—TOEFL (minimum score 550 paper-based; 79 iBT). Electronic applications accepted. *Expenses:* Contact institution. *Faculty research:* Clinical research, inflammation, immunology, neuroscience, molecular biology.

University of North Texas Health Science Center at Fort Worth, School of Public Health, Fort Worth, TX 76107-2699. Offers biostatistics (MPH); community health (MPH); disease control and prevention (Dr PH); environmental and occupational health sciences (MPH); epidemiology (MPH); health administration (MHA); health policy and management (MPH, Dr PH); DO/MPH; MS/MPH; MSN/MPH. MPH offered jointly with University of North Texas; DO/MPH with Texas College of Osteopathic Medicine. *Accreditation:* CEPH. *Program availability:* Part-time, evening/weekend. *Degree requirements:* For master's, thesis or alternative, supervised internship; for doctorate, thesis/dissertation, supervised internship. *Entrance requirements:* For master's, GRE General Test. Additional exam requirements/recommendations for international students: Required—TOEFL. Electronic applications accepted.

University of Oklahoma Health Sciences Center, Graduate College, College of Public Health, Program in Biostatistics and Epidemiology, Oklahoma City, OK 73190. Offers biostatistics (MPH, MS, Dr PH, PhD); epidemiology (MPH, MS, Dr PH, PhD). *Accreditation:* CEPH (one or more programs are accredited). *Program availability:* Part-time. *Degree requirements:* For master's, comprehensive exam, thesis (for some programs); for doctorate, comprehensive exam, thesis/dissertation. *Entrance requirements:* For master's, 3 letters of recommendation, resume; for doctorate, GRE General Test, letters of recommendation. Additional exam requirements/ recommendations for international students: Required—TOEFL (minimum score 570 paper-based), TWE. *Faculty research:* Statistical methodology, applied statistics, acute and chronic disease epidemiology.

University of Ottawa, Faculty of Graduate and Postdoctoral Studies, Faculty of Medicine, Department of Epidemiology and Community Medicine, Ottawa, ON K1N 6N5, Canada. Offers epidemiology (M Sc), including health technology assessment. *Degree requirements:* For master's, thesis. *Entrance requirements:* For master's, honors degree or equivalent, minimum B average. Electronic applications accepted. *Faculty research:* Epidemiologic concepts and methods, health technology assessment.

University of Pennsylvania, Perelman School of Medicine, Center for Clinical Epidemiology and Biostatistics, Philadelphia, PA 19104. Offers clinical epidemiology (MSCE), including bioethics, clinical trials, human genetics, patient centered outcome research, pharmacoepidemiology. *Accreditation:* CEPH. *Program availability:* Part-time. *Faculty:* 97 full-time (47 women), 90 part-time/adjunct (27 women). *Students:* 94 full-time (63 women), 2 part-time (1 woman); includes 34 minority (6 Black or African American, non-Hispanic/Latino; 17 Asian, non-Hispanic/Latino; 11 Hispanic/Latino). Average age 35. 40 applicants, 95% accepted, 33 enrolled. In 2015, 36 master's awarded. *Degree requirements:* For master's, comprehensive exam, thesis. *Entrance requirements:* For master's, GRE General Test or MCAT, advanced degree, clinical experience. Additional exam requirements/recommendations for international students: Required—TOEFL. *Application deadline:* For fall admission, 12/1 priority date for domestic students, 12/1 for international students. Application fee: $0. *Expenses:* Contact institution. *Financial support:* In 2015–16, 60 students received support, including 65 fellowships with tuition reimbursements available (averaging $45,500 per year); career-related internships or fieldwork, scholarships/grants, health care benefits, and unspecified assistantships also available. Financial award application deadline: 12/1. *Faculty research:* Health services research, pharmacoepidemiology, women's health, cancer epidemiology, genetic epidemiology. Total annual research expenditures: $38.7 million. *Unit head:* Dr. Harold I. Feldman, Director, 215-573-0901, E-mail: hfeldman@mail.med.upenn.edu. *Application contact:* Jennifer Kuklinski, Program Coordinator, 215-573-2382, E-mail: jkuklins@ mail.med.upenn.edu.
Website: http://www.cceb.upenn.edu/

University of Pittsburgh, Graduate School of Public Health, Department of Epidemiology, Pittsburgh, PA 15261. Offers theory and research methods (Dr PH); MD/ PhD. *Accreditation:* CEPH (one or more programs are accredited). *Program availability:* Part-time. *Faculty:* 43 full-time (28 women), 21 part-time/adjunct (10 women). *Students:* 91 full-time (67 women), 27 part-time (19 women); includes 16 minority (4 Black or African American, non-Hispanic/Latino; 6 Asian, non-Hispanic/Latino; 3 Hispanic/Latino; 3 Two or more races, non-Hispanic/Latino), 42 international. Average age 29. 449 applicants, 37% accepted, 21 enrolled. In 2015, 28 master's, 18 doctorates awarded. Terminal master's awarded for partial completion of doctoral program. *Degree requirements:* For master's, internship experience (for MPH); comprehensive exam and thesis (for MS); for doctorate, comprehensive exam, thesis/dissertation, teaching practicum. *Entrance requirements:* For master's, GRE General Test, DAT, or MCAT, 3 credits each of course work in human biology and algebra or higher mathematics, 6 in behavioral science (MPH); for doctorate, GRE General Test, DAT, or MCAT, 3 credits of course work in biology and math. Additional exam requirements/recommendations for international students: Required—TOEFL (minimum score 550 paper-based, 80 iBT) or IELTS (minimum score 6.5). *Application deadline:* For fall admission, 1/15 for domestic and international students. Applications are processed on a rolling basis. Application fee: $120. Electronic applications accepted. *Expenses:* $12,464 full-time per term in-state; $20,502 full-time per term out-of-state; $400 full-time fees per term. *Financial support:* In 2015–16, 28 students received support, including 3 fellowships (averaging $3,700 per year), 25 research assistantships (averaging $24,998 per year), 1 teaching assistantship (averaging $21,742 per year). Financial award applicants required to submit FAFSA. *Faculty research:* Cardiovascular and diabetes epidemiology; clinical trials and methods; molecular and genetic epidemiology; environmental epidemiology; global health epidemiology. Total annual research expenditures: $25 million. *Unit head:* Dr. Anne B. Newman, Chair, 412-624-3056, Fax: 412-624-7397, E-mail: newmana@ edc.pitt.edu. *Application contact:* Lori Sarracino Smith, Student Services Manager/ Program Administrator, 412-383-5269, Fax: 412-383-5325, E-mail: smithl@edc.pitt.edu.
Website: http://www.epidemiology.pitt.edu/

University of Prince Edward Island, Atlantic Veterinary College, Graduate Program in Veterinary Medicine, Charlottetown, PE C1A 4P3, Canada. Offers anatomy (M Sc, PhD); bacteriology (M Sc, PhD); clinical pharmacology (M Sc, PhD); clinical sciences (M Sc, PhD); epidemiology (M Sc, PhD), including reproduction; fish health (M Sc, PhD); food animal nutrition (M Sc, PhD); immunology (M Sc, PhD); microanatomy (M Sc, PhD); parasitology (M Sc, PhD); pathology (M Sc, PhD); pharmacology (M Sc, PhD); physiology (M Sc, PhD); toxicology (M Sc, PhD); veterinary science (M Vet Sc); virology (M Sc, PhD). *Program availability:* Part-time. *Degree requirements:* For master's, thesis; for doctorate, thesis/dissertation. *Entrance requirements:* For master's, DVM, B Sc honors degree, or equivalent; for doctorate, M Sc. Additional exam requirements/recommendations for international students: Required—TOEFL (minimum score 550 paper-based; 80 iBT). *Expenses:* Contact institution. *Faculty research:* Animal health management, infectious diseases, fin fish and shellfish health, basic biomedical sciences, ecosystem health.

University of Puerto Rico, Medical Sciences Campus, Graduate School of Public Health, Department of Social Sciences, Program in Epidemiology, San Juan, PR 00936-5067. Offers MPH, MS. *Accreditation:* CEPH (one or more programs are accredited). *Program availability:* Part-time. *Entrance requirements:* For master's, GRE, previous course work in biology, chemistry, physics, mathematics, and social sciences. *Expenses:* Contact institution.

University of Rochester, School of Medicine and Dentistry, Graduate Programs in Medicine and Dentistry, Department of Community and Preventive Medicine, Program in Epidemiology, Rochester, NY 14627. Offers PhD. *Degree requirements:* For doctorate, thesis/dissertation, qualifying exam. *Entrance requirements:* For doctorate, GRE General Test. *Expenses:* Tuition, area resident: Full-time $47,450; part-time $1482 per credit hour. *Required fees:* $528. Tuition and fees vary according to program.

University of Saskatchewan, College of Medicine, Department of Community Health and Epidemiology, Saskatoon, SK S7N 5A2, Canada. Offers M Sc, PhD. *Degree requirements:* For master's, thesis; for doctorate, thesis/dissertation. *Entrance requirements:* Additional exam requirements/recommendations for international students: Required—TOEFL.

University of South Carolina, The Graduate School, Arnold School of Public Health, Department of Epidemiology and Biostatistics, Program in Epidemiology, Columbia, SC 29208. Offers MPH, MSPH, Dr PH, PhD. *Accreditation:* CEPH (one or more programs are accredited). *Program availability:* Part-time. *Degree requirements:* For master's, comprehensive exam, thesis (for some programs), practicum (MPH); for doctorate, comprehensive exam, thesis/dissertation (for some programs), practicum. *Entrance requirements:* For master's, GRE General Test; for doctorate, GRE General Test, master's degree. Additional exam requirements/recommendations for international students: Required—TOEFL (minimum score 570 paper-based; 88 iBT). Electronic applications accepted. *Faculty research:* Cancer epidemiology, mental health epidemiology, health effects of physical activity, environmental epidemiology, genetic epidemiology, asthma epidemiology.

University of Southern California, Keck School of Medicine and Graduate School, Graduate Programs in Medicine, Department of Preventive Medicine, Division of Biostatistics, Los Angeles, CA 90089. Offers applied biostatistics and epidemiology (MS); biostatistics (MS, PhD); epidemiology (PhD); molecular epidemiology (MS). *Faculty:* 47 full-time (8 women), 7 part-time/adjunct (3 women). *Students:* 122 full-time (69 women); includes 22 minority (2 Black or African American, non-Hispanic/Latino; 1 American Indian or Alaska Native, non-Hispanic/Latino; 13 Asian, non-Hispanic/Latino; 4 Hispanic/Latino; 2 Native Hawaiian or other Pacific Islander, non-Hispanic/Latino), 76 international. Average age 29. 116 applicants, 51% accepted, 36 enrolled. In 2015, 21 master's, 13 doctorates awarded. Terminal master's awarded for partial completion of doctoral program. *Degree requirements:* For master's, thesis; for doctorate, thesis/dissertation. *Entrance requirements:* For master's, GRE General Test (minimum scores of 150 each on Verbal and Quantitative sections), minimum GPA of 3.0; for doctorate, GRE General Test (minimum scores of 160 each on Verbal and Quantitative sections), minimum GPA of 3.5. Additional exam requirements/recommendations for international students: Required—TOEFL (minimum score 600 paper-based; 100 iBT), IELTS (minimum score 7). *Application deadline:* For fall admission, 12/1 priority date for domestic and international students; for winter admission, 5/15 priority date for domestic and international students; for spring admission, 11/1 priority date for domestic and international students; for summer admission, 3/1 priority date for domestic and international students. Applications are processed on a rolling basis. Application fee: $85. Electronic applications accepted. *Expenses:* Contact institution. *Financial support:* In 2015–16, 38 students received support, including 10 fellowships with full tuition reimbursements available (averaging $32,000 per year), 36 research assistantships with tuition reimbursements available (averaging $32,000 per year), 15 teaching assistantships with tuition reimbursements available (averaging $32,000 per year); career-related internships or fieldwork, Federal Work-Study, institutionally sponsored loans, scholarships/grants, traineeships, health care benefits, and unspecified assistantships also available. Financial award application deadline: 12/1; financial award applicants required to submit CSS PROFILE or FAFSA. *Faculty research:* Clinical trials in ophthalmology and cancer research, methods of analysis for epidemiological studies, genetic epidemiology. *Total annual research expenditures:* $1.3 million. *Unit head:* Dr. Kiros Berhane, Director, Graduate Programs in Biostatistics and Epidemiology, 323-442-1994, Fax: 323-442-2993, E-mail: kiros@usc.edu. *Application contact:* Mary L. Trujillo, Student Advisor/Program Manager, 323-442-2633, Fax: 323-442-2993, E-mail: mtrujill@usc.edu.
Website: https://biostatepi.usc.edu/

University of Southern California, Keck School of Medicine and Graduate School, Graduate Programs in Medicine, Department of Preventive Medicine, Master of Public Health Program, Los Angeles, CA 91803. Offers biostatistics and epidemiology (MPH); child and family health (MPH); environmental health (MPH); global health leadership (MPH); health communication (MPH); health education and promotion (MPH); public health policy (MPH). *Accreditation:* CEPH. *Program availability:* Part-time, evening/weekend. *Faculty:* 22 full-time (12 women), 3 part-time/adjunct (0 women). *Students:* 182 full-time (142 women), 35 part-time (25 women); includes 120 minority (19 Black or African American, non-Hispanic/Latino; 64 Asian, non-Hispanic/Latino; 37 Hispanic/Latino), 33 international. Average age 24. 236 applicants, 70% accepted, 71 enrolled. In 2015, 99 master's awarded. *Degree requirements:* For master's, practicum, final report, oral presentation. *Entrance requirements:* For master's, GRE General Test, MCAT, GMAT, minimum GPA of 3.0. Additional exam requirements/recommendations for international students: Required—TOEFL (minimum score 600 paper-based; 90 iBT). *Application deadline:* For fall admission, 6/1 priority date for domestic and international students; for spring admission, 10/1 priority date for domestic and international students; for summer admission, 3/1 for domestic and international students. Applications are processed on a rolling basis. Application fee: $85. Electronic applications accepted. *Expenses:* Contact institution. *Financial support:* Career-related internships or fieldwork, Federal Work-Study, institutionally sponsored loans, and scholarships/grants available. Support available to part-time students. Financial award application deadline: 5/4; financial award applicants required to submit CSS PROFILE or FAFSA. *Faculty research:* Substance abuse prevention, cancer and heart disease prevention, mass media and health communication research, health promotion, treatment compliance. *Unit head:* Dr. Louise A. Rohrbach, Director, 323-442-8237, Fax: 323-442-8297, E-mail: rohrbac@usc.edu. *Application contact:* Valerie Burris, Admissions Counselor, 323-442-7257, Fax: 323-442-8297, E-mail: valeriem@usc.edu.
Website: http://mph.usc.edu/

University of Southern Mississippi, Graduate School, College of Health, Department of Public Health, Hattiesburg, MS 39406-0001. Offers epidemiology and biostatistics (MPH); health education (MPH); health policy and administration (MPH). *Accreditation:* CEPH. *Program availability:* Part-time, evening/weekend. *Degree requirements:* For

master's, comprehensive exam, thesis (for some programs). *Entrance requirements:* For master's, GRE General Test, minimum GPA of 2.75 in last 60 hours. Additional exam requirements/recommendations for international students: Required—TOEFL, IELTS. Electronic applications accepted. *Faculty research:* Rural health care delivery, school health, nutrition of pregnant teens, risk factor reduction, sexually transmitted diseases.

University of South Florida, College of Public Health, Department of Epidemiology and Biostatistics, Tampa, FL 33620-9951. Offers MPH, MSPH, PhD. *Accreditation:* CEPH (one or more programs are accredited). *Program availability:* Part-time, evening/weekend. *Degree requirements:* For master's, comprehensive exam, thesis (for some programs); for doctorate, comprehensive exam, thesis/dissertation. *Entrance requirements:* For master's, GRE General Test, minimum GPA of 3.0 in upper-level course work, goal statement letter, two professional letters of recommendation, resume/curriculum vitae; for doctorate, GRE General Test, minimum GPA of 3.0 in upper-level course work, 3 professional letters of recommendation, resume/curriculum vitae, writing sample. Additional exam requirements/recommendations for international students: Required—TOEFL (minimum score 550 paper-based; 79 iBT). Electronic applications accepted. *Faculty research:* Dementia, mental illness, mental health preventative trails, rural health outreach, clinical and administrative studies.

University of South Florida, Innovative Education, Tampa, FL 33620-9951. Offers adult, career and higher education (Graduate Certificate), including college teaching, leadership in developing human resources, leadership in higher education; Africana studies (Graduate Certificate), including diasporas and health disparities, genocide and human rights; aging studies (Graduate Certificate), including gerontology; art research (Graduate Certificate), including museum studies; business foundations (Graduate Certificate); chemical and biomedical engineering (Graduate Certificate), including materials science and engineering, water, health and sustainability; child and family studies (Graduate Certificate), including positive behavior support; civil and industrial engineering (Graduate Certificate), including transportation systems analysis; community and family health (Graduate Certificate), including maternal and child health, social marketing and public health, violence and injury: prevention and intervention, women's health; criminology (Graduate Certificate), including criminal justice administration; educational measurement and research (Graduate Certificate), including evaluation; English (Graduate Certificate), including comparative literary studies, creative writing, professional and technical communication; entrepreneurship (Graduate Certificate); environmental health (Graduate Certificate), including safety management; epidemiology and biostatistics (Graduate Certificate), including applied biostatistics, biostatistics, concepts and tools of epidemiology, epidemiology, epidemiology of infectious diseases; geography, environment and planning (Graduate Certificate), including community development, environmental policy and management, geographical information systems; geology (Graduate Certificate), including hydrogeology; global health (Graduate Certificate), including disaster management, global health and Latin American and Caribbean studies, global health practice, humanitarian assistance, infection control; government and international affairs (Graduate Certificate), including Cuban studies, globalization studies; health policy and management (Graduate Certificate), including health management and leadership, public health policy and programs; hearing specialist: early intervention (Graduate Certificate); industrial and management systems engineering (Graduate Certificate), including systems engineering, technology management; information studies (Graduate Certificate), including school library media specialist; information systems/decision sciences (Graduate Certificate), including analytics and business intelligence; instructional technology (Graduate Certificate), including distance education, Florida digital/virtual educator, instructional design, multimedia design, Web design; internal medicine, bioethics and medical humanities (Graduate Certificate), including biomedical ethics; Latin American and Caribbean studies (Graduate Certificate); mass communications (Graduate Certificate), including multimedia journalism; mathematics and statistics (Graduate Certificate), including mathematics; medicine (Graduate Certificate), including aging and neuroscience, bioinformatics, biotechnology, brain fitness and memory management, clinical investigation, health informatics, health sciences, integrative weight management, intellectual property, medicine and gender, metabolic and nutritional medicine, metabolic cardiology, pharmacy sciences; national and competitive intelligence (Graduate Certificate); psychological and social foundations (Graduate Certificate), including career counseling, college teaching, diversity in education, mental health counseling, school counseling; public affairs (Graduate Certificate), including nonprofit management, public management, research administration; public health (Graduate Certificate), including environmental health, health equity, public health generalist, translational research in adolescent behavioral health; public health practices (Graduate Certificate), including planning for healthy communities; rehabilitation and mental health counseling (Graduate Certificate), including integrative mental health care, marriage and family therapy, rehabilitation technology; secondary education (Graduate Certificate), including ESOL, foreign language education: culture and content, foreign language education: professional; social work (Graduate Certificate), including geriatric social work/clinical gerontology; special education (Graduate Certificate), including autism spectrum disorder, disabilities education: severe/profound; world languages (Graduate Certificate), including teaching English as a second language (TESL) or foreign language. *Unit head:* Kathy Barnes, Interdisciplinary Programs Coordinator, 813-974-8031, Fax: 813-974-7061, E-mail: barnesk@usf.edu. *Application contact:* Karen Tylinski, Metro Initiatives, 813-974-9943, Fax: 813-974-7061, E-mail: ktylinsk@usf.edu.
Website: http://www.usf.edu/innovative-education/

University of South Florida, Morsani College of Medicine and College of Graduate Studies, Graduate Programs in Medical Sciences, Tampa, FL 33620-9951. Offers advanced athletic training (MS); athletic training (MS); bioinformatics and computational biology (MSBCB); biotechnology (MSB); health informatics (MSHI); medical sciences (MSMS, PhD), including aging and neuroscience (MSMS), allergy, immunology and infectious disease (PhD), anatomy, athletic training (MSMS), clinical and translational research, health informatics (MSMS), health science (MSMS), interdisciplinary medical sciences (MSMS), medical microbiology and immunology (MSMS), metabolic and nutritional medicine (MSMS), molecular medicine, molecular pharmacology and physiology (PhD), neurology (PhD), pathology and laboratory medicine (PhD), pharmacology and therapeutics (PhD), physiology and biophysics (PhD), women's health (MSMS). *Students:* 510 full-time (261 women), 318 part-time (208 women); includes 360 minority (108 Black or African American, non-Hispanic/Latino; 3 American Indian or Alaska Native, non-Hispanic/Latino; 101 Asian, non-Hispanic/Latino; 124 Hispanic/Latino; 1 Native Hawaiian or other Pacific Islander, non-Hispanic/Latino; 23 Two or more races, non-Hispanic/Latino), 52 international. Average age 26. 6,567 applicants, 13% accepted, 469 enrolled. In 2015, 216 master's awarded. Terminal master's awarded for partial completion of doctoral program. *Degree requirements:* For master's, comprehensive exam, thesis; for doctorate, comprehensive exam, thesis/dissertation. *Entrance requirements:* For master's, GRE General Test or GMAT, bachelor's degree or equivalent from regionally-accredited university with minimum GPA of 3.0 in upper-division sciences coursework; prerequisites in general biology, general chemistry, general physics, organic chemistry, quantitative analysis, and integral and differential calculus; for doctorate, GRE General Test, bachelor's degree from regionally-accredited university with minimum GPA of 3.0 in upper-division sciences

Epidemiology

coursework; 3 letters of recommendation; personal interview; 1-2 page personal statement; prerequisites in biology, chemistry, physics, organic chemistry, quantitative analysis, and integral/differential calculus. Additional exam requirements/recommendations for international students: Required—TOEFL (minimum score 550 paper-based; 79 iBT) or IELTS (minimum score 6.5). *Application deadline:* For fall admission, 2/15 for domestic students, 1/2 for international students. Application fee: $30. *Expenses:* Contact institution. *Faculty research:* Anatomy, biochemistry, cancer biology, cardiovascular disease, cell biology, immunology, microbiology, molecular biology, neuroscience, pharmacology, physiology. *Unit head:* Dr. Michael Barber, Professor/Associate Dean for Graduate and Postdoctoral Affairs, 813-974-9908, Fax: 813-974-4317, E-mail: mbarber@health.usf.edu. *Application contact:* Dr. Eric Bennett, Graduate Director, PhD Program in Medical Sciences, 813-974-1545, Fax: 813-974-4317, E-mail: esbennet@health.usf.edu.
Website: http://health.usf.edu/nocms/medicine/graduatestudies/

The University of Tennessee Health Science Center, College of Graduate Health Sciences, Memphis, TN 38163-0002. Offers biomedical engineering (MS, PhD); biomedical sciences (PhD); dental sciences (MDS); epidemiology (MS); health outcomes and policy research (PhD); laboratory research and management (MS); nursing science (PhD); pharmaceutical sciences (PhD); pharmacology (MS); speech and hearing science (PhD); DDS/PhD; DNP/PhD; MD/PhD; Pharm D/PhD. Terminal master's awarded for partial completion of doctoral program. *Degree requirements:* For master's, comprehensive exam, thesis; for doctorate, comprehensive exam, thesis/dissertation, oral and written preliminary and comprehensive exams. *Entrance requirements:* For master's and doctorate, GRE General Test, minimum GPA of 3.0. Additional exam requirements/recommendations for international students: Required—TOEFL (minimum score 79 iBT); Recommended—IELTS (minimum score 6.5). Electronic applications accepted.

The University of Toledo, College of Graduate Studies, College of Medicine and Life Sciences, Department of Public Health and Preventative Medicine, Toledo, OH 43606-3390. Offers biostatistics and epidemiology (Certificate); contemporary gerontological practice (Certificate); environmental and occupational health and safety (MPH); epidemiology (Certificate); global public health (Certificate); health promotion and education (MPH); industrial hygiene (MSOH); medical and health science teaching and learning (Certificate); occupational health (Certificate); public health administration (MPH); public health and emergency response (Certificate); public health epidemiology (MPH); public health nutrition (MPH); MD/MPH. *Program availability:* Part-time, evening/weekend. *Degree requirements:* For master's, thesis or alternative. *Entrance requirements:* For master's, GRE, minimum undergraduate GPA of 3.0, three letters of recommendation, statement of purpose, transcripts from all prior institutions attended, resume; for Certificate, minimum undergraduate GPA of 3.0, three letters of recommendation, statement of purpose, transcripts from all prior institutions attended, resume. Additional exam requirements/recommendations for international students: Required—TOEFL (minimum score 550 paper-based; 80 iBT), IELTS (minimum score 6.5). Electronic applications accepted.

University of Toronto, School of Graduate Studies, Department of Public Health Sciences, Toronto, ON M5S 1A1, Canada. Offers biostatistics (M Sc, PhD); community health (M Sc); community nutrition (MPH), including nutrition and dietetics; epidemiology (MPH, PhD); family and community medicine (MPH); occupational and environmental health (MPH); social and behavioral health science (PhD); social and behavioral health sciences (MPH), including health promotion. *Accreditation:* CAHME (one or more programs are accredited); CEPH (one or more programs are accredited). *Program availability:* Part-time. *Degree requirements:* For master's, thesis (for some programs), practicum; for doctorate, comprehensive exam, thesis/dissertation, oral thesis defense. *Entrance requirements:* For master's, 2 letters of reference, relevant professional/research experience, minimum B average in final year; for doctorate, 2 letters of reference, relevant professional/research experience, minimum B+ average. Additional exam requirements/recommendations for international students: Required—TOEFL (minimum score 580 paper-based; 93 iBT), TWE (minimum score 5). Electronic applications accepted. *Expenses:* Contact institution.

University of Washington, Graduate School, School of Public Health, Department of Epidemiology, Seattle, WA 98195. Offers clinical research (MS); epidemiology (MPH, MS, PhD); global health (MPH); maternal/child health (MPH); MPH/MPA. *Accreditation:* CEPH (one or more programs are accredited). *Degree requirements:* For master's, comprehensive exam (for some programs), thesis, formal thesis proposal; for doctorate, comprehensive exam, thesis/dissertation, general exam, dissertation proposals, final exam (dissertation defense). *Entrance requirements:* For master's, GRE (except for those holding PhD, MD, DDS, DVM, DO or equivalent from U.S. institutions); for doctorate, GRE. Additional exam requirements/recommendations for international students: Required—TOEFL (minimum score 580 paper-based; 92 iBT), IELTS (minimum score 7), or PTE (minimum score of 65). Electronic applications accepted. *Expenses:* Contact institution. *Faculty research:* Chronic disease, health disparities and social determinants of health, aging and neuroepidemiology, maternal and child health, molecular and genetic epidemiology.

The University of Western Ontario, Faculty of Graduate Studies, Biosciences Division, Department of Epidemiology and Biostatistics, London, ON N6A 5B8, Canada. Offers M Sc, PhD. *Accreditation:* CEPH (one or more programs are accredited). *Program availability:* Part-time. *Degree requirements:* For master's, thesis; for doctorate, comprehensive exam, thesis proposal defense. *Entrance requirements:* For master's, BA or B Sc honors degree, minimum B+ average in last 10 courses; for doctorate, M Sc or equivalent, minimum B+ average in last 10 courses. *Faculty research:* Chronic disease epidemiology, clinical epidemiology.

★ **University of Wisconsin–Madison,** School of Medicine and Public Health, Population Health and Epidemiology Program, Madison, WI 53726. Offers epidemiology (MS, PhD); population health (MS, PhD). *Accreditation:* CEPH. *Program availability:* Part-time. *Faculty:* 104 full-time (54 women), 2 part-time/adjunct (0 women). *Students:* 52 full-time (43 women), 10 part-time (7 women); includes 15 minority (7 Black or African American, non-Hispanic/Latino; 3 Asian, non-Hispanic/Latino; 4 Hispanic/Latino; 1 Native Hawaiian or other Pacific Islander, non-Hispanic/Latino), 6 international. Average age 31. 84 applicants, 38% accepted, 20 enrolled. In 2015, 11 master's, 8 doctorates awarded. Terminal master's awarded for partial completion of doctoral program. *Degree requirements:* For master's, thesis, thesis defense; for doctorate, comprehensive exam, thesis/dissertation, qualifying exam, preliminary exam, dissertation defense. *Entrance requirements:* For master's and doctorate, GRE taken within the last 5 years (MCAT or LSAT acceptable for those with doctoral degrees), minimum GPA of 3.0, quantitative preparation (calculus, statistics, or other) with minimum B average. Additional exam requirements/recommendations for international students: Required—TOEFL (minimum score 580 paper-based; 92 iBT). *Application deadline:* For fall admission, 1/15 for domestic and international students. Application fee: $56. Electronic applications accepted. *Expenses:* Tuition, state resident: full-time $5364. Tuition, nonresident: full-time $12,027. *Required fees:* $571. Tuition and fees vary according to campus/location, program and reciprocity agreements. *Financial support:* Fellowships with full tuition reimbursements, research assistantships with full tuition reimbursements, teaching assistantships with full tuition reimbursements, scholarships/grants, traineeships, health care benefits, and unspecified assistantships available. Support available to part-time students. *Faculty research:* Epidemiology (cancer, environmental, aging, infectious and genetic disease), determinants of population health, health services research, social and behavioral health sciences, biostatistics. *Total annual research expenditures:* $11.4 million. *Unit head:* Programs Coordinator, 608-265-8108, Fax: 608-263-2820, E-mail: pophealth@mailplus.wisc.edu. *Application contact:* Assistant Programs Coordinator, 608-263-6583, Fax: 608-263-2820, E-mail: pophealth@mailplus.wisc.edu.
Website: https://pophealth.wisc.edu/grad

See Display on page 813 and Close-Up on page 855.

Virginia Commonwealth University, Medical College of Virginia-Professional Programs, School of Medicine, School of Medicine Graduate Programs, Department of Epidemiology and Community Health, Richmond, VA 23284-9005. Offers epidemiology (MPH, PhD); public health practice (MPH); social and behavioral science (MPH); MD/MPH; MSW/MPH. *Accreditation:* CEPH. *Program availability:* Part-time. *Degree requirements:* For doctorate, comprehensive exam, thesis/dissertation. *Entrance requirements:* For master's, GRE; for doctorate, GRE General Test, interview, 3 letters of recommendation, minimum graduate GPA of 3.0, master's degree in public health or related field including epidemiology and biostatistics. Additional exam requirements/recommendations for international students: Required—TOEFL (minimum score 600 paper-based; 100 iBT). Electronic applications accepted. *Faculty research:* Sickle cell anemia, breast cancer, HIV/AIDS, hospital epidemiology, infectious diseases.

Walden University, Graduate Programs, School of Health Sciences, Minneapolis, MN 55401. Offers clinical research administration (MS, Graduate Certificate); health education and promotion (MS, PhD), including behavioral health (PhD), disease surveillance (PhD), emergency preparedness (MS), general (MHA, MS), global health (PhD), health policy (PhD), health policy and advocacy (MS), population health (PhD); health informatics (MS); health services (PhD), including community health, healthcare administration, leadership, public health policy, self-designed; healthcare administration (MHA), including general (MHA, MS), leadership and organizational development (MHA); public health (MPH, Dr PH, PhD, Graduate Certificate), including community health education (PhD), epidemiology (PhD); systems policy (MHA). *Program availability:* Part-time, evening/weekend, online only, 100% online. *Faculty:* 14 full-time (8 women), 222 part-time/adjunct (121 women). *Students:* 2,487 full-time (1,804 women), 2,282 part-time (1,540 women); includes 2,763 minority (2,129 Black or African American, non-Hispanic/Latino; 30 American Indian or Alaska Native, non-Hispanic/Latino; 237 Asian, non-Hispanic/Latino; 268 Hispanic/Latino; 13 Native Hawaiian or other Pacific Islander, non-Hispanic/Latino; 86 Two or more races, non-Hispanic/Latino), 87 international. Average age 39. 1,205 applicants, 98% accepted, 820 enrolled. In 2015, 641 master's, 147 doctorates, 18 other advanced degrees awarded. *Degree requirements:* For doctorate, thesis/dissertation, residency. *Entrance requirements:* For master's, bachelor's degree or higher; minimum GPA of 2.5; official transcripts; goal statement (for some programs); access to computer and Internet; for doctorate, master's degree or higher; three years of related professional or academic experience (preferred); minimum GPA of 3.0; goal statement and current resume (for select programs); official transcripts; access to computer and Internet; for Graduate Certificate, relevant work experience; access to computer and Internet. Additional exam requirements/recommendations for international students: Required—TOEFL (minimum score 550 paper-based, 79 iBT), IELTS (minimum score 6.5), Michigan English Language Assessment Battery (minimum score 82), or PTE (minimum score 53). *Application deadline:* Applications are processed on a rolling basis. Application fee: $0. Electronic applications accepted. *Financial support:* Fellowships, Federal Work-Study, scholarships/grants, unspecified assistantships, and family tuition reduction, active duty/veteran tuition reduction, group tuition reduction, interest-free payment plans, employee tuition reduction available. Support available to part-time students. Financial award applicants required to submit FAFSA. *Unit head:* Dr. Jorg Westermann, Dean, 866-492-5336. *Application contact:* Meghan Thomas, Vice President of Enrollment Management, 866-492-5336, E-mail: info@waldenu.edu.
Website: http://www.waldenu.edu/colleges-schools/school-of-health-sciences

Washington State University, College of Veterinary Medicine, Program in Immunology and Infectious Diseases, Pullman, WA 99164. Offers veterinary science (MS, PhD). *Faculty:* 22 full-time (7 women), 43 part-time/adjunct (19 women). *Students:* 39 full-time (26 women); includes 5 minority (2 Black or African American, non-Hispanic/Latino; 1 Asian, non-Hispanic/Latino; 2 Hispanic/Latino), 14 international. Average age 31. 47 applicants, 11% accepted, 5 enrolled. In 2015, 1 master's, 8 doctorates awarded. Terminal master's awarded for partial completion of doctoral program. *Degree requirements:* For master's, thesis, oral exam; for doctorate, thesis/dissertation, oral exam. *Entrance requirements:* For master's and doctorate, minimum GPA of 3.0. Additional exam requirements/recommendations for international students: Required—TOEFL (minimum score 550 paper-based; 80 iBT). *Application deadline:* Applications are processed on a rolling basis. Application fee: $75. Electronic applications accepted. *Financial support:* In 2015–16, 17 fellowships, 20 research assistantships, 2 teaching assistantships were awarded; institutionally sponsored loans, scholarships/grants, traineeships, health care benefits, and unspecified assistantships also available. Financial award application deadline: 3/1. *Faculty research:* Microbial pathogenesis, veterinary and wildlife parasitology, laboratory animal pathology, immune responses to infectious diseases. *Unit head:* Dr. Michele E. Hardy, Chair, 509-335-6030, Fax: 509-335-8529, E-mail: mhardy@vetmed.wsu.edu. *Application contact:* Sue Zumwalt, Graduate Coordinator, 509-335-6027, Fax: 509-335-8529, E-mail: szumwalt@vetmed.wsu.edu.
Website: http://vmp.vetmed.wsu.edu/graduate-programs/master-phd

Washington University in St. Louis, Brown School, St. Louis, MO 63130. Offers affordable housing and mixed-income community management (Certificate); American Indian and Alaska native (MSW); children, youth and families (MSW); health (MSW); individualized (MSW), including health; mental health (MSW); older adults and aging societies (MSW); public health (MPH), including epidemiology/biostatistics, global health, health policy analysis, urban design; public health sciences (PhD); social and economic development (MSW); social work (MSW, PhD), including management (MSW), policy (MSW), research (MSW), sexual health and education (MSW), social entrepreneurship (MSW), system dynamics (MSW); violence and injury prevention (MSW, Certificate); JD/MSW; M Arch/MSW; MPH/MBA; MPH/MS; MSW/M Div; MSW/M Ed; MSW/MAPS; MSW/MBA; MSW/MPH; MUD/MSW. MSW/M Div and MSW/MAPS offered in partnership with Eden Theological Seminary. *Accreditation:* CSWE (one or more programs are accredited). *Faculty:* 54 full-time (31 women), 87 part-time/adjunct (61 women). *Students:* 303 full-time (256 women); includes 125 minority (42 Black or African American, non-Hispanic/Latino; 16 American Indian or Alaska Native, non-Hispanic/Latino; 47 Asian, non-Hispanic/Latino; 9 Hispanic/Latino; 11 Two or more races, non-Hispanic/Latino), 71 international. Average age 26. 923 applicants, 322 enrolled. In 2015, 239 master's, 5 doctorates awarded. *Degree requirements:* For master's, 60 credit hours (for MSW), 52 credit hours (for MPH); practicum; for doctorate, comprehensive exam, thesis/dissertation. *Entrance requirements:* For master's, GRE, GMAT, LSAT, or MCAT (for MPH); for doctorate, GRE, MA or MSW. Additional exam requirements/recommendations for international students: Required—TOEFL (minimum score 100 iBT) or IELTS. *Application deadline:* For fall admission, 12/15 priority date for domestic and international students; for winter admission, 3/1 priority date for domestic and international students. Applications are processed on a rolling basis. Application fee: $50. Electronic applications accepted. *Expenses:* Contact institution. *Financial support:* In 2015–16, 267 students received support. Fellowships, research assistantships, Federal Work-Study, institutionally sponsored loans, scholarships/grants, health care benefits, tuition waivers (partial), and unspecified assistantships available. Support available to part-time students. Financial award application deadline: 3/1; financial award applicants required to submit FAFSA. *Faculty research:* Mental health services, social development, child welfare, at-risk teens, autism, environmental health, health policy, health communications, obesity, gender and sexuality, violence and injury prevention, chronic disease prevention, poverty, older adults/aging societies, civic engagement, school social work, program evaluation, health disparities. *Unit head:* Jamie L. Adkisson, Director of Admissions and Recruitment, 314-935-3524, Fax: 314-935-4859, E-mail: jadkisson@wustl.edu. *Application contact:* Office of Admissions and Recruitment, 314-935-6676, Fax: 314-935-4859, E-mail: brownadmissions@wustl.ed. Website: http://brownschool.wustl.edu

Weill Cornell Medicine, Weill Cornell Graduate School of Medical Sciences, Program in Clinical Epidemiology and Health Services Research, New York, NY 10021. Offers MS. *Degree requirements:* For master's, thesis. *Entrance requirements:* For master's, 3 years of work experience, MD or RN certificate. *Faculty research:* Research

methodology, biostatistical techniques, data management, decision analysis, health economics.

Yale University, School of Medicine, Yale School of Public Health, New Haven, CT 06520. Offers applied biostatistics and epidemiology (APMPH); biostatistics (MPH, MS, PhD), including global health (MPH); chronic disease epidemiology (MPH, PhD), including global health (MPH); environmental health sciences (MPH, PhD), including global health (MPH); epidemiology of microbial diseases (MPH, PhD), including global health (MPH); global health (APMPH); health management (MPH), including global health; health policy (MPH), including global health; health policy and administration (APMPH, PhD); occupational and environmental medicine (APMPH); preventive medicine (APMPH); social and behavioral sciences (APMPH, MPH), including global health (MPH); JD/MPH; M Div/MPH; MBA/MPH; MD/MPH; MEM/MPH; MFS/MPH; MM Sc/MPH; MPH/MA; MSN/MPH. MS and PhD offered through the Graduate School. *Accreditation:* CEPH. *Program availability:* Part-time. Terminal master's awarded for partial completion of doctoral program. *Degree requirements:* For master's, thesis, summer internship; for doctorate, comprehensive exam, thesis/dissertation, residency. *Entrance requirements:* For master's, GMAT, GRE, or MCAT, two years of undergraduate coursework in math and science; for doctorate, GRE General Test. Additional exam requirements/recommendations for international students: Required—TOEFL (minimum score 100 iBT). Electronic applications accepted. *Expenses:* Contact institution. *Faculty research:* Genetic and emerging infections epidemiology, virology, cost/quality, vector biology, quantitative methods, aging, asthma, cancer.

Health Promotion

American University, College of Arts and Sciences, Department of Health Studies, Program in Health Promotion Management, Washington, DC 22016-8030. Offers health promotion management (MS). *Students:* 22 full-time (15 women), 18 part-time (15 women); includes 11 minority (8 Black or African American, non-Hispanic/Latino; 1 Asian, non-Hispanic/Latino; 2 Hispanic/Latino), 4 international. Average age 27. 30 applicants, 97% accepted, 16 enrolled. In 2015, 12 master's awarded. *Degree requirements:* For master's, comprehensive exam, thesis or alternative. *Entrance requirements:* For master's, GRE, interview (recommended), statement of purpose, transcripts, 2 letters of recommendation, resume. Additional exam requirements/recommendations for international students: Required—TOEFL (minimum score 100 iBT), IELTS (minimum score 7), PTE (minimum score 68). *Application deadline:* For fall admission, 2/1 priority date for domestic students; for spring admission, 11/1 for domestic students. Application fee: $55. *Expenses:* Tuition, area resident: Full-time $27,468; part-time $1526 per credit hour. *Required fees:* $430. Tuition and fees vary according to course level and program. *Unit head:* Sarah Irvine-Belson, Department Chair, Health Studies, 202-885-6278, Fax: 202-885-1187, E-mail: stacey@american.edu. *Application contact:* Kathleen Clowery, Associate Director, Graduate Enrollment Management, 202-885-3620, Fax: 202-885-1344, E-mail: clowery@american.edu. Website: http://www.american.edu/cas/seth/health/index.cfm

American University of Beirut, Graduate Programs, Faculty of Health Sciences, Beirut, Lebanon. Offers environmental sciences (MS), including environmental health; epidemiology (MS); epidemiology and biostatistics (MPH); health management and policy (MPH); health promotion and community health (MPH). *Program availability:* Part-time. *Faculty:* 30 full-time (21 women), 3 part-time/adjunct (1 woman). *Students:* 49 full-time (38 women), 99 part-time (81 women). Average age 27. 115 applicants, 71% accepted, 40 enrolled. In 2015, 51 master's awarded. *Degree requirements:* For master's, one foreign language, comprehensive exam (for some programs), thesis (for some programs). *Entrance requirements:* For master's, 2 letters of recommendation, personal statement, transcripts. Additional exam requirements/recommendations for international students: Required—TOEFL (minimum score 583 paper-based; 97 iBT), IELTS (minimum score 7). *Application deadline:* For fall admission, 1/4 priority date for domestic and international students; for spring admission, 11/1 for domestic and international students. Application fee: $50. Electronic applications accepted. *Expenses:* Tuition, area resident: Full-time $16,254; part-time $903 per credit. *Required fees:* $699. Tuition and fees vary according to course load and program. *Financial support:* In 2015–16, 70 students received support. Scholarships/grants, health care benefits, and unspecified assistantships available. Financial award application deadline: 4/1. *Faculty research:* Tobacco control; health of the elderly; youth health; mental health; women's health; reproductive and sexual health, including HIV/AIDS; water quality; health systems; quality in health care delivery; health human resources; health policy; occupational and environmental health; social inequality; social determinants of health; non-communicable diseases; nutrition; refugees health; conflict and health. *Total annual research expenditures:* $2 million. *Unit head:* Iman Adel Nuwayhid, Dean, 961-1759683, Fax: 961-1744470, E-mail: nuwayhid@aub.edu.lb. *Application contact:* Mitra Tauk, Administrative Coordinator, 961-1350000 Ext. 4687, Fax: 961-1744470, E-mail: mt12@aub.edu.lb.

Arizona State University at the Tempe campus, College of Health Solutions, School of Nutrition and Health Promotion, Tempe, AZ 85287. Offers clinical exercise physiology (MS); exercise and wellness (MS); nutrition (MS), including dietetics, human nutrition; obesity prevention and management (MS); physical activity, nutrition and wellness (PhD).

Auburn University, Graduate School, College of Education, Department of Kinesiology, Auburn University, AL 36849. Offers exercise science (M Ed, MS, PhD); health promotion (M Ed, MS); kinesiology (PhD); physical education/teacher education (M Ed, MS, Ed D, Ed S). *Accreditation:* NCATE. *Program availability:* Part-time. *Faculty:* 19 full-time (9 women), 1 part-time/adjunct (0 women). *Students:* 107 full-time (63 women), 31 part-time (18 women); includes 27 minority (17 Black or African American, non-Hispanic/Latino; 6 Hispanic/Latino; 4 Two or more races, non-Hispanic/Latino), 9 international. Average age 26. 157 applicants, 73% accepted, 68 enrolled. In 2015, 52 master's, 9 doctorates awarded. *Degree requirements:* For master's, thesis (for some programs); for doctorate, thesis/dissertation; for Ed S, exam, field project. *Entrance requirements:* For master's, GRE General Test; for doctorate and Ed S, GRE General Test, interview, master's degree. *Application deadline:* Applications are processed on a rolling basis. Application fee: $50 ($60 for international students). Electronic applications accepted. *Expenses:* Tuition, state resident: full-time $8802; part-time $489 per credit hour. Tuition, nonresident: full-time $26,406; part-time $1467 per credit hour. *Required fees:* $808 per semester. Tuition and fees vary according to degree level and program. *Financial support:* Research assistantships, teaching assistantships, and Federal Work-Study available. Support available to part-time students. Financial award application deadline: 3/15; financial award applicants required to submit FAFSA. *Faculty research:*

Biomechanics, exercise physiology, motor skill learning, school health, curriculum development. *Unit head:* Dr. Mary E. Rudisill, Head, 334-844-1458. *Application contact:* Dr. George Flowers, Dean of the Graduate School, 334-844-2125.

Ball State University, Graduate School, College of Applied Sciences and Technology, School of Kinesiology, Interdepartmental Program in Wellness Management, Muncie, IN 47306. Offers MA, MS. *Students:* 13 full-time (10 women), 3 part-time (all women), 2 international. Average age 26. 10 applicants, 80% accepted, 8 enrolled. In 2015, 3 master's awarded. *Entrance requirements:* For master's, GRE General Test, interview. Application fee: $25 ($35 for international students). *Expenses:* Tuition, area resident: Full-time $6948; part-time $2316 per semester. Tuition, state resident: full-time $10,422; part-time $3474 per semester. Tuition, nonresident: full-time $19,062; part-time $6354 per semester. *Required fees:* $651 per semester. Tuition and fees vary according to campus/location, program and reciprocity agreements. *Financial support:* In 2015–16, 11 students received support, including 9 research assistantships with partial tuition reimbursements available (averaging $9,800 per year), 2 teaching assistantships with partial tuition reimbursements available (averaging $11,187 per year); unspecified assistantships also available. Financial award application deadline: 3/1. *Unit head:* Dr. Jane Ellery, Head, 765-285-8119, E-mail: jellery@bsu.edu. *Application contact:* Dr. Robert Morris, Associate Provost for Research and Dean of the Graduate School, 765-285-5723, Fax: 765-285-1328, E-mail: rmorris@bsu.edu. Website: http://www.bsu.edu/wellness

Baylor University, Graduate School, Robbins College of Health and Human Sciences, Department of Health, Human Performance and Recreation, Waco, TX 76798. Offers community health (MPH); exercise physiology (MS); kinesiology, exercise nutrition and health promotion (PhD); sport pedagogy (MS). *Accreditation:* NCATE. *Program availability:* Part-time. *Faculty:* 13 full-time (5 women), 3 part-time/adjunct (1 woman). *Students:* 67 full-time (39 women), 11 part-time (6 women); includes 22 minority (7 Black or African American, non-Hispanic/Latino; 6 Asian, non-Hispanic/Latino; 6 Hispanic/Latino; 3 Two or more races, non-Hispanic/Latino), 6 international. 109 applicants, 59% accepted, 44 enrolled. In 2015, 46 master's, 1 doctorate awarded. *Degree requirements:* For master's, comprehensive exam, thesis optional; for doctorate, comprehensive exam, thesis/dissertation. *Entrance requirements:* For master's and doctorate, GRE General Test. Additional exam requirements/recommendations for international students: Required—TOEFL (minimum score 550 paper-based; 80 iBT). *Application deadline:* For fall admission, 2/1 priority date for domestic students, 2/1 for international students; for spring admission, 10/1 for domestic and international students. Applications are processed on a rolling basis. Application fee: $25. Electronic applications accepted. *Financial support:* In 2015–16, 60 students received support, including 1 research assistantship with full tuition reimbursement available (averaging $12,700 per year), 33 teaching assistantships with full tuition reimbursements available (averaging $7,650 per year); career-related internships or fieldwork, Federal Work-Study, institutionally sponsored loans, scholarships/grants, tuition waivers (full), and unspecified assistantships also available. Financial award application deadline: 2/1. *Faculty research:* Behavior change theory, nutrition and enzyme therapy, exercise testing, health planning. *Unit head:* Dr. Jaeho Shim, Graduate Program Director, 254-710-4009, Fax: 254-710-3527, E-mail: joe_shim@baylor.edu. *Application contact:* Kathy Mirick, Administrative Assistant, 254-710-3526, Fax: 254-710-3527, E-mail: kathy_mirick@baylor.edu. Website: http://www.baylor.edu/HHPR/

Benedictine University, Graduate Programs, Program in Nutrition and Wellness, Lisle, IL 60532. Offers MS. *Entrance requirements:* Additional exam requirements/recommendations for international students: Required—TOEFL (minimum score 550 paper-based). Electronic applications accepted. *Faculty research:* Community and corporate wellness risk assessment, health behavior change, self-efficacy, evaluation of health program impact and effectiveness.

Boise State University, College of Health Sciences, Department of Community and Environmental Health, Boise, ID 83712-1835. Offers community and environmental health (MHS); health science (MHS), including health policy, health promotion, health services leadership; health services leadership (Graduate Certificate). *Faculty:* 11. *Students:* 20 full-time (18 women), 38 part-time (33 women); includes 7 minority (1 Asian, non-Hispanic/Latino; 5 Hispanic/Latino; 1 Two or more races, non-Hispanic/Latino). Average age 36. 38 applicants, 50% accepted, 11 enrolled. In 2015, 21 master's, 13 Graduate Certificates awarded. *Entrance requirements:* For master's, writing assessment, minimum GPA of 3.0. Additional exam requirements/recommendations for international students: Required—TOEFL (minimum score 550 paper-based; 80 iBT), IELTS (minimum score 6). *Application deadline:* For fall admission, 3/15 for domestic and international students; for spring admission, 10/15 for domestic and international students. Application fee: $65 ($95 for international students). Electronic applications accepted. *Expenses:* Tuition, state resident: full-time $6058; part-time $358 per credit hour. Tuition, nonresident: full-time $20,108; part-time $608 per credit hour. *Required fees:* $2108. Tuition and fees vary according to program.

Health Promotion

Financial support: In 2015–16, 10 students received support, including 2 research assistantships (averaging $2,937 per year); scholarships/grants and unspecified assistantships also available. Financial award application deadline: 3/15; financial award applicants required to submit FAFSA. *Unit head:* Dr. Dale Stephenson, Department Chair, 208-426-3795, E-mail: dalestephenson@boisestate.edu. *Application contact:* Dr. Sarah Toevs, Director, Master of Health Science Program, 208-426-2452, E-mail: stoevs@boisestate.edu.
Website: http://hs.boisestate.edu/ceh/

Bridgewater State University, College of Graduate Studies, School of Education and Allied Studies, Department of Movement Arts, Health Promotion, and Leisure Studies, Program in Health Promotion, Bridgewater, MA 02325-0001. Offers M Ed. *Program availability:* Part-time, evening/weekend. *Entrance requirements:* For master's, GRE General Test.

Brigham Young University, Graduate Studies, College of Life Sciences, Department of Exercise Sciences, Provo, UT 84602. Offers athletic training (MS); exercise physiology (MS, PhD); exercise sciences (MS); health promotion (MS, PhD); physical medicine and rehabilitation (PhD). *Faculty:* 21 full-time (3 women). *Students:* 18 full-time (9 women), 26 part-time (13 women); includes 6 minority (3 Asian, non-Hispanic/Latino; 1 Hispanic/Latino; 2 Two or more races, non-Hispanic/Latino). Average age 29. 18 applicants, 56% accepted, 9 enrolled. In 2015, 8 master's, 2 doctorates awarded. *Degree requirements:* For master's, thesis, oral defense; for doctorate, comprehensive exam, thesis/dissertation, oral defense, oral and written exams. *Entrance requirements:* For master's, GRE General Test, minimum GPA of 3.2 in last 60 hours of course work; for doctorate, GRE General Test, minimum GPA of 3.5 in last 60 hours of course work. Additional exam requirements/recommendations for international students: Required—TOEFL (minimum score 580 paper-based; 85 iBT), IELTS (minimum score 7). *Application deadline:* For fall admission, 2/1 for domestic and international students. Application fee: $50. Electronic applications accepted. *Financial support:* In 2015–16, 36 students received support, including 25 research assistantships (averaging $4,570 per year), 28 teaching assistantships (averaging $6,413 per year); fellowships, career-related internships or fieldwork, institutionally sponsored loans, scholarships/grants, unspecified assistantships, and 9 PhD full-tuition scholarships also available. Financial award application deadline: 3/1. *Faculty research:* Injury prevention and rehabilitation, human skeletal muscle adaptation, cardiovascular health and fitness, lifestyle modification and health promotion. *Total annual research expenditures:* $54,646. *Unit head:* Dr. Gary Mack, Chair, 801-422-2466, Fax: 801-422-0555, E-mail: gary_mack@byu.edu. *Application contact:* Dr. J. William Myrer, Graduate Coordinator, 801-422-2690, Fax: 801-422-0555, E-mail: bill_myrer@byu.edu.
Website: http://exsc.byu.edu/

California Baptist University, Program in Public Health, Riverside, CA 92504-3206. Offers health education and promotion (MPH); health policy and administration (MPH). *Program availability:* Part-time, evening/weekend. *Faculty:* 7 full-time (4 women), 3 part-time/adjunct (2 women). *Students:* 41 full-time (36 women), 9 part-time (8 women); includes 33 minority (4 Black or African American, non-Hispanic/Latino; 1 Asian, non-Hispanic/Latino; 26 Hispanic/Latino; 2 Two or more races, non-Hispanic/Latino), 2 international. Average age 25. 41 applicants, 71% accepted, 26 enrolled. *Degree requirements:* For master's, capstone project; practicum. *Entrance requirements:* For master's, minimum undergraduate GPA of 2.75, two recommendations, 500-word essay, resume. Additional exam requirements/recommendations for international students: Required—TOEFL (minimum score 80 iBT). *Application deadline:* For fall admission, 8/1 priority date for domestic students, 7/1 for international students; for spring admission, 12/1 priority date for domestic students, 11/1 for international students. Applications are processed on a rolling basis. *Expenses:* $800 per unit, $355 per semester fees. *Financial support:* Federal Work-Study and scholarships/grants available. Financial award applicants required to submit CSS PROFILE or FAFSA. *Faculty research:* Epidemiology, statistical education, exercise and immunity, obesity and chronic disease. *Unit head:* Dr. David Pearson, Dean, College of Health Science, 951-343-4298, E-mail: dpearson@calbaptist.edu. *Application contact:* Dr. Robert LaChausse, Chair, Department of Public Health Sciences, 951-552-8484, E-mail: rlachausse@calbaptist.edu.
Website: http://www.calbaptist.edu/explore-cbu/schools-colleges/college-allied-health/health-sciences/master-public-health/

California State University, Fresno, Division of Graduate Studies, College of Health and Human Services, Department of Public Health, Fresno, CA 93740-8027. Offers health policy and management (MPH); health promotion (MPH). *Accreditation:* CEPH. *Program availability:* Part-time, evening/weekend. *Degree requirements:* For master's, thesis or alternative. *Entrance requirements:* For master's, GRE General Test, minimum GPA of 2.5. Additional exam requirements/recommendations for international students: Required—TOEFL. Electronic applications accepted. *Faculty research:* Foster parent training, geriatrics, tobacco control.

Claremont Graduate University, Graduate Programs, School of Community and Global Health, Claremont, CA 91773. Offers health promotion science (PhD); public health (MPH). *Accreditation:* CEPH. *Faculty:* 8 full-time (3 women). *Students:* 48 full-time (27 women), 46 part-time (36 women); includes 47 minority (8 Black or African American, non-Hispanic/Latino; 19 Asian, non-Hispanic/Latino; 16 Hispanic/Latino; 4 Two or more races, non-Hispanic/Latino), 14 international. Average age 30. In 2015, 23 master's, 1 doctorate awarded. *Entrance requirements:* For master's and doctorate, GRE. Additional exam requirements/recommendations for international students: Required—TOEFL (minimum score 75 iBT). *Application deadline:* For fall admission, 2/1 priority date for domestic and international students; for spring admission, 11/1 priority date for domestic students. Applications are processed on a rolling basis. Application fee: $80. Electronic applications accepted. *Expenses: Tuition, area resident:* Full-time $43,032; part-time $1793 per unit. *Required fees:* $600; $300 per semester. $300 per semester. Tuition and fees vary according to course load and program. *Financial support:* Fellowships, research assistantships, teaching assistantships, Federal Work-Study, institutionally sponsored loans, and scholarships/grants available. Support available to part-time students. Financial award application deadline: 2/15; financial award applicants required to submit FAFSA. *Unit head:* Stewart Donaldson, Dean, 909-607-8235, E-mail: stewart.donaldson@cgu.edu. *Application contact:* Paige Piontkowsky, Assistant Director of Admissions, 909-607-3240, E-mail: paige.piontkowsky@cgu.edu.
Website: http://www.cgu.edu/pages/5644.asp

Cleveland University–Kansas City, Program in Health Promotion, Overland Park, KS 66210. Offers MSHP. *Program availability:* Part-time. *Entrance requirements:* Additional exam requirements/recommendations for international students: Required—TOEFL (minimum score 550 paper-based; 79 iBT). Electronic applications accepted. *Expenses:* Contact institution.

Concord University, Graduate Studies, Athens, WV 24712-1000. Offers educational leadership and supervision (M Ed); geography (M Ed); health promotion (MA); reading specialist (M Ed); social work (MSW); special education (M Ed); teaching (MAT). *Program availability:* Part-time, evening/weekend, online learning. *Faculty:* 20 full-time (13 women), 5 part-time/adjunct (3 women). *Students:* 109 full-time (91 women), 256 part-time (195 women); includes 28 minority (26 Black or African American, non-Hispanic/Latino; 1 American Indian or Alaska Native, non-Hispanic/Latino; 1 Hispanic/Latino), 2 international. Average age 34. *Degree requirements:* For master's, thesis (for some programs). *Entrance requirements:* For master's, GRE or MAT, baccalaureate degree with minimum GPA of 2.5 from regionally-accredited institution; teaching license; 2 letters of recommendation; completed disposition assessment form. *Application deadline:* Applications are processed on a rolling basis. Application fee: $25. Electronic applications accepted. *Expenses:* Tuition, state resident: full-time $3619; part-time $2418 per semester. Tuition, nonresident: full-time $6311; part-time $4206 per semester. Tuition and fees vary according to course load. *Financial support:* Tuition waivers and unspecified assistantships available. Financial award applicants required to submit FAFSA. *Unit head:* Dr. Cheryl Barnes, Director, 304-384-6306, E-mail: cbarnes@concord.edu. *Application contact:* Debra Moore, Special Events Assistant, 304-384-5113, E-mail: dlm@concord.edu.
Website: http://www.concord.edu/graduate

East Carolina University, Graduate School, College of Health and Human Performance, Department of Health Education and Promotion, Greenville, NC 27858-4353. Offers environmental health (MS); health education (MA Ed); health education and promotion (MA). *Accreditation:* NCATE. *Students:* 29 full-time (21 women), 60 part-time (43 women); includes 22 minority (18 Black or African American, non-Hispanic/Latino; 1 Asian, non-Hispanic/Latino; 2 Hispanic/Latino; 1 Two or more races, non-Hispanic/Latino). Average age 30. 54 applicants, 81% accepted, 41 enrolled. In 2015, 24 master's awarded. *Degree requirements:* For master's, comprehensive exam, thesis optional. *Entrance requirements:* For master's, GRE General Test or MAT. Additional exam requirements/recommendations for international students: Required—TOEFL. *Application deadline:* For fall admission, 6/1 priority date for domestic students. Applications are processed on a rolling basis. Application fee: $50. *Financial support:* Fellowships, research assistantships, teaching assistantships, and career-related internships or fieldwork available. Support available to part-time students. Financial award application deadline: 6/1. *Faculty research:* Community health education, worksite health promotion, school health education, environmental health. *Unit head:* Dr. J. Don Chaney, Chair, 252-737-4942, E-mail: chaneyj@ecu.edu.
Website: http://www.ecu.edu/hlth/

Eastern Kentucky University, The Graduate School, College of Health Sciences, Department of Exercise and Sport Science, Richmond, KY 40475-3102. Offers exercise and sport science (MS); exercise and wellness (MS); sports administration (MS). *Program availability:* Part-time. *Entrance requirements:* For master's, GRE General Test (minimum score 700 verbal and quantitative), minimum GPA of 2.5 (for most), minimum GPA of 3.0 (analytical writing). *Faculty research:* Nutrition and exercise.

Eastern Michigan University, Graduate School, College of Health and Human Services, School of Health Promotion and Human Performance, Ypsilanti, MI 48197. Offers MS, Graduate Certificate. *Program availability:* Part-time, evening/weekend, online learning. *Faculty:* 35 full-time (19 women). *Students:* 115 full-time (72 women), 90 part-time (49 women); includes 30 minority (18 Black or African American, non-Hispanic/Latino; 3 Asian, non-Hispanic/Latino; 4 Hispanic/Latino; 5 Two or more races, non-Hispanic/Latino), 8 international. Average age 29. 210 applicants, 52% accepted, 68 enrolled. In 2015, 66 master's, 1 other advanced degree awarded. *Entrance requirements:* For master's, MAT (for orthotics and prosthetics). Additional exam requirements/recommendations for international students: Required—TOEFL. *Application deadline:* For fall admission, 8/1 for domestic students, 5/1 for international students; for winter admission, 12/1 for domestic students, 10/1 for international students; for spring admission, 4/15 for domestic students, 3/1 for international students. Applications are processed on a rolling basis. Application fee: $45. *Financial support:* Fellowships, research assistantships with full tuition reimbursements, teaching assistantships with full tuition reimbursements, career-related internships or fieldwork, Federal Work-Study, institutionally sponsored loans, scholarships/grants, tuition waivers (partial), and unspecified assistantships available. Support available to part-time students. Financial award applicants required to submit FAFSA. *Unit head:* Dr. Christopher Herman, Director, 734-487-2185, Fax: 734-487-2024, E-mail: cherman2@emich.edu. *Application contact:* Dr. Linda Jermone, HPHP Academic Advisor, 734-487-0092, Fax: 734-487-2024, E-mail: ljerme@emich.edu.

Emory University, Rollins School of Public Health, Online Program in Public Health, Atlanta, GA 30322-1100. Offers applied epidemiology (MPH); applied public health informatics (MPH); prevention science (MPH). *Program availability:* Part-time, evening/weekend, online learning. *Degree requirements:* For master's, thesis, practicum. *Entrance requirements:* For master's, GRE. Additional exam requirements/recommendations for international students: Required—TOEFL (minimum score 550 paper-based; 80 iBT). Electronic applications accepted.

Fairmont State University, Programs in Education, Fairmont, WV 26554. Offers digital media, new literacies and learning (M Ed); education (MAT); exercise science, fitness and wellness (M Ed); online learning (M Ed); professional studies (M Ed); reading (M Ed); special education (M Ed). *Accreditation:* NCATE. *Program availability:* Part-time, evening/weekend, online learning. *Faculty:* 22 part-time/adjunct (14 women). *Students:* 59 full-time (37 women), 103 part-time (80 women); includes 8 minority (4 Black or African American, non-Hispanic/Latino; 2 Hispanic/Latino; 2 Two or more races, non-Hispanic/Latino). Average age 32. 85 applicants, 79% accepted, 50 enrolled. In 2015, 58 master's awarded. *Entrance requirements:* For master's, GRE. Additional exam requirements/recommendations for international students: Required—TOEFL. *Application deadline:* For fall admission, 5/1 for domestic and international students. Applications are processed on a rolling basis. Application fee: $40. Electronic applications accepted. *Expenses:* Tuition, state resident: full-time $7148; part-time $385 per credit hour. Tuition, nonresident: full-time $15,296; part-time $837 per credit hour. Part-time tuition and fees vary according to course load. *Financial support:* In 2015–16, 25 students received support. Applicants required to submit FAFSA. *Unit head:* Dr. Carolyn Crislip-Tacy, Interim Dean, School of Education, 304-367-4143, Fax: 304-367-4599, E-mail: carolyn.crislip-tacy@fairmontstate.edu. *Application contact:* Jack Kirby, Director of Graduate Studies, 304-367-4101, E-mail: jack.kirby@fairmontstate.edu.
Website: http://www.fairmontstate.edu/graduatestudies/

Florida Atlantic University, College of Education, Department of Exercise Science and Health Promotion, Boca Raton, FL 33431-0991. Offers MS. *Program availability:* Part-time, evening/weekend. *Degree requirements:* For master's, comprehensive exam, thesis optional. *Entrance requirements:* For master's, GRE General Test, minimum GPA of 3.0 during last 60 hours of course work. Additional exam requirements/recommendations for international students: Required—TOEFL (minimum score 500 paper-based; 61 iBT), IELTS (minimum score 6). *Application deadline:* For fall admission, 7/1 priority date for domestic students, 2/15 for international students; for spring admission, 11/1 priority date for domestic students, 7/15 for international students. Applications are processed on a rolling basis. Application fee: $30. *Expenses:* Tuition, area resident: Full-time $7392; part-time $369.82 per credit hour. Tuition, state resident: full-time $7392; part-time $369.82 per credit hour. Tuition, nonresident: full-time $19,432; part-time $1024.81 per credit hour. *Financial support:* Research assistantships with partial tuition reimbursements, teaching assistantships with partial tuition reimbursements, and career-related internships or fieldwork available. *Faculty*

research: Pulmonary limitations during exercise, metabolism regulation, determinants of performance, age-related change in functional mobility and geriatric exercise, behavioral change aimed at promoting active lifestyles. *Unit head:* Dr. Robert Zoeller, 561-297-2549, E-mail: rzoeller@fau.edu. *Application contact:* Dr. Robert Zoeller, 561-297-2549, E-mail: rzoeller@fau.edu.
Website: http://www.coe.fau.edu/academicdepartments/eshp/

Florida International University, Robert Stempel College of Public Health and Social Work, Programs in Public Health, Miami, FL 33199. Offers biostatistics (MPH); environmental and occupational health (MPH, PhD); epidemiology (MPH, PhD); health policy and management (MPH); health promotion and disease prevention (PhD); health promotion and diseases prevention (MPH). Ph D program has fall admissions only; MPH offered jointly with University of Miami. *Accreditation:* CEPH. *Program availability:* Part-time, evening/weekend, online learning. *Faculty:* 27 full-time (12 women), 2 part-time/adjunct (1 woman). *Students:* 126 full-time (80 women), 62 part-time (46 women); includes 129 minority (47 Black or African American, non-Hispanic/Latino; 10 Asian, non-Hispanic/Latino; 69 Hispanic/Latino; 3 Two or more races, non-Hispanic/Latino), 32 international. Average age 30. 298 applicants, 35% accepted, 68 enrolled. In 2015, 67 master's, 10 doctorates awarded. *Degree requirements:* For master's, thesis optional; for doctorate, comprehensive exam, thesis/dissertation. *Entrance requirements:* For master's, minimum GPA of 3.0, letters of recommendation; for doctorate, GRE, resume, minimum GPA of 3.0, letters of recommendation, letter of intent. Additional exam requirements/recommendations for international students: Required—TOEFL (minimum score 550 paper-based; 80 iBT). *Application deadline:* For fall admission, 6/1 for domestic students, 4/1 for international students; for spring admission, 10/1 for domestic students, 9/1 for international students. Applications are processed on a rolling basis. Application fee: $30. Electronic applications accepted. *Expenses:* Contact institution. *Financial support:* Institutionally sponsored loans, scholarships/grants, and tuition waivers (full) available. Financial award application deadline: 3/1; financial award applicants required to submit FAFSA. *Faculty research:* Drugs/AIDS intervention among migrant workers, provision of services for active/recovering drug users with HIV. *Unit head:* Dr. Benjamin C. Amick, III, Chair, 305-348-4903, E-mail: benjamin.amickiii@fiu.edu. *Application contact:* Dr. Vukosava Pekovic, Director, 305-348-1823, Fax: 305-348-4901, E-mail: pekovic@fiu.edu.

George Mason University, College of Education and Human Development, School of Recreation, Health and Tourism, Manassas, VA 20110. Offers exercise, fitness, and health promotion (MS), including advanced practitioner. *Faculty:* 15 full-time (6 women), 36 part-time/adjunct (15 women). *Students:* 32 full-time (19 women), 22 part-time (11 women); includes 8 minority (4 Black or African American, non-Hispanic/Latino; 2 Asian, non-Hispanic/Latino; 1 Hispanic/Latino; 1 Two or more races, non-Hispanic/Latino), 3 international. Average age 27. 64 applicants, 63% accepted, 22 enrolled. In 2015, 11 master's awarded. *Degree requirements:* For master's, thesis (for some programs). *Entrance requirements:* For master's, GRE General Test or MAT, 3 letters of recommendation; official transcripts; expanded goals statement; undergraduate course in statistics and minimum GPA of 3.0 in last 60 credit hours and overall (for MS in sport and recreation studies); baccalaureate degree related to kinesiology, exercise science or athletic training (for MS in exercise, fitness and health promotion). Additional exam requirements/recommendations for international students: Required—TOEFL (minimum score 575 paper-based; 88 iBT), IELTS (minimum score 6.5), PTE (minimum score 59). *Application deadline:* For spring admission, 11/1 priority date for domestic and international students. Application fee: $75 ($80 for international students). Electronic applications accepted. *Financial support:* In 2015–16, 7 students received support, including 3 fellowships (averaging $13,763 per year), 3 research assistantships with tuition reimbursements available (averaging $8,650 per year), 1 teaching assistantship (averaging $2,562 per year); career-related internships or fieldwork, Federal Work-Study, scholarships/grants, unspecified assistantships, and health care benefits (for full-time research or teaching assistantship recipients) also available. Support available to part-time students. Financial award application deadline: 3/1; financial award applicants required to submit FAFSA. *Faculty research:* Informing policy; promoting economic development; advocating stewardship of natural resources; improving the quality of life of individuals, families, and communities at the local, national and international levels. *Total annual research expenditures:* $1.1 million. *Unit head:* David Wiggins, Director, 703-993-2057, Fax: 703-993-2025, E-mail: dwiggin1@gmu.edu. *Application contact:* Lindsey Olson, Office Assistant, 703-993-2098, Fax: 703-993-2025, E-mail: lolson7@gmu.edu.
Website: http://rht.gmu.edu/

Georgetown University, Graduate School of Arts and Sciences, Department of Microbiology and Immunology, Washington, DC 20057. Offers biohazardous threat agents and emerging infectious diseases (MS); biomedical science policy and advocacy (MS); general microbiology and immunology (MS); global infectious diseases (PhD); microbiology and immunology (PhD). *Program availability:* Part-time. *Degree requirements:* For master's, 30 credit hours of coursework; for doctorate, comprehensive exam, thesis/dissertation. *Entrance requirements:* For master's, GRE General Test, 3 letters of reference, bachelor's degree in related field; for doctorate, GRE General Test, 3 letters of reference, MS/BS in related field. Additional exam requirements/recommendations for international students: Required—TOEFL (minimum score 505 paper-based). Electronic applications accepted. *Faculty research:* Pathogenesis and basic biology of the fungus Candida albicans, molecular biology of viral immunopathological mechanisms in Multiple Sclerosis.

Georgia College & State University, Graduate School, College of Health Sciences, School of Health and Human Performance, Milledgeville, GA 31061. Offers health and human performance (MS), including health performance, health promotion; kinesiology/health education (MAT). *Accreditation:* NCATE (one or more programs are accredited). *Program availability:* Part-time, evening/weekend, 100% online. *Students:* 27 full-time (11 women), 14 part-time (12 women); includes 7 minority (4 Black or African American, non-Hispanic/Latino; 1 Asian, non-Hispanic/Latino; 2 Two or more races, non-Hispanic/Latino). Average age 29. 20 applicants, 100% accepted, 13 enrolled. In 2015, 22 master's awarded. *Degree requirements:* For master's, thesis or alternative, completed in 6 years with minimum GPA of 3.0, thesis or project (for MS); minimum GPA of 3.0, GACE Exam and Assessment, and electronic teaching portfolio (for MAT). *Entrance requirements:* For master's, GRE General Test or MAT (for MAT), resume, 2 professional references; minimum GPA of 2.75 in upper-level undergraduate courses and undergraduate statistics course (for MS); minimum GPA of 2.75 on upper-division major courses (for MAT). Additional exam requirements/recommendations for international students: Recommended—TOEFL (minimum score 550 paper-based; 79 iBT). *Application deadline:* For fall admission, 7/1 priority date for domestic students, 4/1 priority date for international students; for spring admission, 11/1 priority date for domestic students, 9/1 priority date for international students; for summer admission, 4/1 priority date for domestic students. Applications are processed on a rolling basis. Application fee: $40. Electronic applications accepted. *Expenses:* $7,174 per year full-time in-state tuition, $20,476 out-of-state (for MAT and MS program in human performance); $7,670 (for online MS). *Financial support:* Unspecified assistantships available. Support available to part-time students. Financial award application deadline: 3/1; financial award applicants required to submit FAFSA. *Unit head:* Dr. Lisa Griffin,

Director, School of Health and Human Performance, 478-445-4072, Fax: 478-445-4074, E-mail: lisa.griffin@gcsu.edu.
Website: http://www.gcsu.edu/health/shhp

Goddard College, Graduate Division, Master of Arts in Health Arts and Sciences Program, Plainfield, VT 05667-9432. Offers MA. *Degree requirements:* For master's, thesis. *Entrance requirements:* For master's, 3 letters of recommendation, interview. *Application deadline:* Applications are processed on a rolling basis. Application fee: $65. Electronic applications accepted. *Financial support:* Scholarships/grants available. Financial award applicants required to submit FAFSA. *Unit head:* Ruth Farmer, Program Director, 802-454-8311, Fax: 802-454-1029, E-mail: ruth.farmer@goddard.edu. *Application contact:* Chip Cummings, 800-906-8312 Ext. 221, Fax: 802-454-1029, E-mail: chip.cummings@goddard.edu.
Website: http://www.goddard.edu/academics/ma/master-arts-health-arts-sciences/

Harvard University, Harvard T.H. Chan School of Public Health, Department of Social and Behavioral Sciences, Boston, MA 02115-6096. Offers SM, SD. *Program availability:* Part-time. *Faculty:* 31 full-time (15 women), 16 part-time/adjunct (8 women). *Students:* 77 full-time (62 women), 13 part-time (all women); includes 33 minority (8 Black or African American, non-Hispanic/Latino; 11 Asian, non-Hispanic/Latino; 4 Hispanic/Latino; 1 Native Hawaiian or other Pacific Islander, non-Hispanic/Latino; 9 Two or more races, non-Hispanic/Latino), 4 international. Average age 26. 157 applicants, 27% accepted, 32 enrolled. In 2015, 31 master's, 4 doctorates awarded. *Degree requirements:* For doctorate, thesis/dissertation, qualifying exam. *Entrance requirements:* For master's, GRE, MCAT; for doctorate, GRE. Additional exam requirements/recommendations for international students: Recommended—TOEFL (minimum score 600 paper-based; 100 iBT), IELTS (minimum score 7). *Application deadline:* For fall admission, 12/15 for domestic and international students. Application fee: $120. Electronic applications accepted. *Financial support:* Fellowships, research assistantships, teaching assistantships, Federal Work-Study, scholarships/grants, traineeships, and unspecified assistantships available. Support available to part-time students. Financial award application deadline: 2/15; financial award applicants required to submit FAFSA. *Faculty research:* Social determinants of health, program design and planned social change, health and social policy, heath care and community-based interventions, health effects and prevention of gender-based violence. *Unit head:* Dr. Ichiro Kawachi, Chair, 617-432-1135, Fax: 617-432-3123, E-mail: ikawachi@hsph.harvard.edu. *Application contact:* Vincent W. James, Director of Admissions, 617-432-1031, Fax: 617-432-7080, E-mail: admissions@hsph.harvard.edu.
Website: http://www.hsph.harvard.edu/social-and-behavioral-sciences/

Immaculata University, College of Graduate Studies, Program in Nutrition Education, Immaculata, PA 19345. Offers nutrition education for the registered dietitian (MA); nutrition education with dietetic internship (MA); nutrition education with wellness promotion (MA). *Program availability:* Part-time, evening/weekend. *Degree requirements:* For master's, comprehensive exam, thesis optional. *Entrance requirements:* For master's, GRE or MAT, minimum GPA of 3.0. Additional exam requirements/recommendations for international students: Required—TOEFL. Electronic applications accepted. *Faculty research:* Sports nutrition, pediatric nutrition, changes in food consumption patterns in weight loss, nutritional counseling.

Independence University, Program in Health Services, Salt Lake City, UT 84107. Offers community health (MSHS); wellness promotion (MSHS). *Program availability:* Part-time, evening/weekend, online learning. *Degree requirements:* For master's, fieldwork, internship, final project (wellness promotion). *Entrance requirements:* For master's, previous course work in psychology.

Independence University, Program in Nursing, Salt Lake City, UT 84107. Offers community health (MSN); gerontology (MSN); nursing administration (MSN); wellness promotion (MSN).

Indiana University Bloomington, School of Public Health, Department of Kinesiology, Bloomington, IN 47405. Offers applied sport science (MS); athletic administration/sport management (MS); athletic training (MS); biomechanics (MS); ergonomics (MS); exercise physiology (MS); human performance (PhD), including biomechanics, exercise physiology, motor learning/control, sport management; motor learning/control (MS); physical activity (MPH); physical activity, fitness and wellness (MS). *Program availability:* Part-time. Terminal master's awarded for partial completion of doctoral program. *Degree requirements:* For master's, thesis optional; for doctorate, variable foreign language requirement, comprehensive exam, thesis/dissertation. *Entrance requirements:* For master's, GRE General Test, minimum GPA of 2.8; for doctorate, GRE General Test, minimum graduate GPA of 3.5, undergraduate 3.0. Additional exam requirements/recommendations for international students: Required—TOEFL (minimum score 80 iBT). *Faculty research:* Exercise physiology and biochemistry, sports biomechanics, human motor control, adaptation of fitness and exercise to special populations.

Instituto Tecnologico de Santo Domingo, Graduate School, Area of Health Sciences, Santo Domingo, Dominican Republic. Offers bioethics (M Bioethics); clinical bioethics (Certificate); clinical nutrition (Certificate); comprehensive health and the adolescent (Certificate); comrehensive adoescent health (MS); health and social security (M Mgmt).

Kent State University, College of Education, Health and Human Services, School of Health Sciences, Program in Health Education and Promotion, Kent, OH 44242-0001. Offers M Ed, PhD. *Accreditation:* NCATE. *Degree requirements:* For doctorate, comprehensive exam, thesis/dissertation. *Entrance requirements:* For master's, 2 letters of reference, goals statement; for doctorate, GRE General Test, goals statement, resume, interview. Additional exam requirements/recommendations for international students: Required—TOEFL (minimum score 550 paper-based; 80 iBT). Electronic applications accepted. *Expenses:* Tuition, state resident: full-time $10,864; part-time $495 per credit hour. Tuition, nonresident: full-time $18,380; part-time $837 per credit hour. *Faculty research:* Substance use/abuse, sexuality, community health assessment, epidemiology, HIV/AIDS.

Lehman College of the City University of New York, School of Natural and Social Sciences, Department of Health Sciences, Program in Health Education and Promotion, Bronx, NY 10468-1589. Offers MA. *Accreditation:* CEPH; NCATE. *Program availability:* Part-time, evening/weekend. *Degree requirements:* For master's, thesis or alternative. *Entrance requirements:* For master's, minimum GPA of 2.7.

Liberty University, School of Behavioral Sciences, Lynchburg, VA 24515. Offers advanced clinical skills (MA); clinical mental health counseling (MA); counselor education and supervision (PhD); human services counseling (MA), including addictions and recovery, business, child and family law, Christian ministries, criminal justice, crisis response and trauma, executive leadership, health and wellness, life coaching, marriage and family, military resilience; marriage and family therapy (MA); military resilience (Certificate); professional counseling (MA). *Program availability:* Part-time, online learning. *Students:* 2,717 full-time (2,135 women), 5,745 part-time (4,465 women); includes 2,407 minority (2,049 Black or African American, non-Hispanic/Latino; 33 American Indian or Alaska Native, non-Hispanic/Latino; 77 Hispanic/Latino; 8 Native Hawaiian or other Pacific Islander, non-Hispanic/Latino; 187 Two or more races, non-Hispanic/Latino), 170 international. Average age 39. 6,318

Health Promotion

applicants, 47% accepted, 1620 enrolled. In 2015, 2,601 master's, 11 doctorates, 2 other advanced degrees awarded. *Application deadline:* Applications are processed on a rolling basis. Application fee: $50. Electronic applications accepted. *Financial support:* Applicants required to submit FAFSA. *Unit head:* Dr. Ronald Hawkins, Founding Dean, School of Behavioral Sciences. *Application contact:* Jay Bridge, Director of Admissions, 800-424-9595, Fax: 800-628-7977, E-mail: gradadmissions@liberty.edu.

Liberty University, School of Health Sciences, Lynchburg, VA 24515. Offers biomedical sciences (MS); global health (MPH); health promotion (MPH); healthcare management (Certificate); nutrition (MPH). *Program availability:* Part-time, online learning. *Students:* 435 full-time (342 women); 609 part-time (489 women); includes 301 minority (238 Black or African American, non-Hispanic/Latino; 6 American Indian or Alaska Native, non-Hispanic/Latino; 25 Asian, non-Hispanic/Latino; 12 Hispanic/Latino; 1 Native Hawaiian or other Pacific Islander, non-Hispanic/Latino; 19 Two or more races, non-Hispanic/Latino), 71 international. Average age 33. 1,433 applicants, 43% accepted, 295 enrolled. In 2015, 50 master's, 8 other advanced degrees awarded. *Degree requirements:* For master's, thesis (for some programs). *Entrance requirements:* Additional exam requirements/recommendations for international students: Required—TOEFL (minimum score 600 paper-based; 100 iBT). Application fee: $50. *Unit head:* Dr. Ralph Linstra, Dean. *Application contact:* Jay Bridge, Director of Admissions, 800-424-9595, Fax: 800-628-7977, E-mail: gradadmissions@liberty.edu.

Lindenwood University, Graduate Programs, School of Sport, Recreation, and Exercise Sciences, St. Charles, MO 63301-1695. Offers human performance (MS). *Program availability:* Part-time, evening/weekend. *Faculty:* 8 full-time (4 women), 1 (woman) part-time/adjunct. *Students:* 42 full-time (15 women), 5 part-time (3 women); includes 4 minority (2 Asian, non-Hispanic/Latino; 1 Hispanic/Latino; 1 Two or more races, non-Hispanic/Latino), 6 international. Average age 25. 46 applicants, 48% accepted, 22 enrolled. In 2015, 20 master's awarded. *Degree requirements:* For master's, comprehensive exam (for some programs), thesis (for some programs), minimum cumulative GPA of 3.0. *Entrance requirements:* For master's, current CPR certification, interview, anatomy and physiology, exercise physiology with lab in past 5 years, minimum undergraduate cumulative GPA of 3.0. Additional exam requirements/recommendations for international students: Required—TOEFL (minimum score 550 paper-based; 80 iBT); Recommended—IELTS (minimum score 6.5). *Application deadline:* For fall admission, 8/22 priority date for domestic and international students; for spring admission, 1/9 priority date for domestic and international students; for summer admission, 5/16 priority date for domestic and international students. Applications are processed on a rolling basis. Application fee: $30 ($100 for international students). Electronic applications accepted. *Expenses: Tuition, area resident:* Full-time $15,672; part-time $453 per credit hour. *Required fees:* $205 per semester. Tuition and fees vary according to course level, course load and degree level. *Financial support:* In 2015–16, 40 students received support. Career-related internships or fieldwork, institutionally sponsored loans, scholarships/grants, tuition waivers (partial), and unspecified assistantships available. Financial award application deadline: 6/30; financial award applicants required to submit FAFSA. *Unit head:* Dr. Cynthia Schroeder, Dean, School of Sport, Recreation, and Exercise Sciences, 636-949-4318, E-mail: cschroeder@lindenwood.edu. *Application contact:* Tyler Kostich, Director, Evening and Graduate Admissions, 636-949-4138, Fax: 636-949-4109, E-mail: adultadmissions@lindenwood.edu.
Website: http://www.lindenwood.edu/sres/

Lock Haven University of Pennsylvania, College of Natural, Behavioral and Health Sciences, Lock Haven, PA 17745-2390. Offers actuarial science (PSM); athletic training (MS); health promotion/education (MHS); healthcare management (MHS); physician assistant (MHS). Program also offered at the Clearfield, Coudersport, and Harrisburg campuses. *Accreditation:* ARC-PA. *Entrance requirements:* For master's, minimum undergraduate GPA of 3.0. Additional exam requirements/recommendations for international students: Required—TOEFL. *Application deadline:* Applications are processed on a rolling basis. Application fee: $25. Electronic applications accepted. *Expenses: Tuition, state resident:* part-time $470 per credit hour. Tuition, nonresident: part-time $705 per credit hour. *Required fees:* $203 per credit hour. $40 per semester. Tuition and fees vary according to program. *Financial support:* Research assistantships available. Financial award application deadline: 8/1. *Unit head:* Dr. Scott Carnicom, Dean, 570-484-2204, E-mail: carnicom@lhup.edu. *Application contact:* Cherie Dolan, Secretary to the Dean, 570-484-2204, Fax: 570-484-2734, E-mail: cdolan1@lhup.edu.
Website: http://www.lhup.edu/colleges/natural_behavioral_health/

Manhattanville College, School of Education, Program in Physical Education and Sport Pedagogy, Purchase, NY 10577-2132. Offers health and wellness specialist (Advanced Certificate); physical education and sport pedagogy (MAT). *Program availability:* Part-time, evening/weekend. *Students:* 30 applicants, 90% accepted, 22 enrolled. In 2015, 29 master's, 1 other advanced degree awarded. *Degree requirements:* For master's, comprehensive exam (for some programs), thesis (for some programs), student teaching, research seminars, portfolios, internships, writing assessment; for Advanced Certificate, comprehensive exam (for some programs). *Entrance requirements:* For master's, GRE or MAT, minimum undergraduate GPA of 3.0, 2 letters of recommendation. Additional exam requirements/recommendations for international students: Required—TOEFL (minimum score 300 paper-based; 85 iBT); Recommended—IELTS. *Application deadline:* For fall admission, 7/1 priority date for domestic and international students; for spring admission, 11/1 priority date for domestic and international students; for summer admission, 4/1 priority date for domestic and international students. Applications are processed on a rolling basis. Application fee: $75. Electronic applications accepted. *Expenses:* $895 per credit. *Financial support:* Teaching assistantships, career-related internships or fieldwork, Federal Work-Study, institutionally sponsored loans, scholarships/grants, and unspecified assistantships available. Financial award applicants required to submit FAFSA. *Faculty research:* Early teaching practices (late 1700s through 1800s), sociocultural examination of games and children's play. *Unit head:* Rhonda Clements, Director of Physical Education, 914-323-5327, Fax: 914-694-2386, E-mail: rhonda.clements@mville.edu. *Application contact:* Jeanine Pardey-Levine, Director of Graduate Enrollment Management, 914-373-3208, Fax: 914-694-1732, E-mail: edschool@mville.edu.
Website: http://www.mville.edu/programs/physical-education-and-sports-pedagogy

Marymount University, School of Health Professions, Program in Health Education and Promotion, Arlington, VA 22207-4299. Offers MS. *Program availability:* Part-time, evening/weekend. *Faculty:* 2 full-time (1 woman), 1 (woman) part-time/adjunct. *Students:* 5 full-time (all women), 10 part-time (9 women); includes 4 minority (all Black or African American, non-Hispanic/Latino). Average age 29. 11 applicants, 100% accepted, 7 enrolled. In 2015, 6 master's awarded. *Entrance requirements:* For master's, GRE or MAT, 2 letters of recommendation, interview, resume. Additional exam requirements/recommendations for international students: Required—TOEFL (minimum score 600 paper-based; 96 iBT), IELTS (minimum score 6.5). *Application deadline:* For fall admission, 7/1 for international students. Applications are processed on a rolling basis. Application fee: $40. Electronic applications accepted. *Expenses: Tuition, area resident:* Part-time $910 per credit hour. *Required fees:* $10 per credit hour. One-time fee: $230 part-time. Tuition and fees vary according to program. *Financial support:* In

2015–16, 4 students received support, including 3 research assistantships with tuition reimbursements available; career-related internships or fieldwork, Federal Work-Study, scholarships/grants, and unspecified assistantships also available. Support available to part-time students. Financial award applicants required to submit FAFSA. *Unit head:* Dr. Michelle Walters-Edwards, Chair, 703-526-1597, Fax: 703-284-3819, E-mail: michelle.walters-edwards@marymount.edu. *Application contact:* Francesca Reed, Director, Graduate Admissions, 703-284-5901, Fax: 703-527-3815, E-mail: grad.admissions@marymount.edu.
Website: http://www.marymount.edu/Academics/Malek-School-of-Health-Professions/Graduate-Programs/Health-Education-Promotion-(M-S-)

McNeese State University, Doré School of Graduate Studies, Burton College of Education, Department of Health and Human Performance, Lake Charles, LA 70609. Offers exercise physiology (MS); health promotion (MS); nutrition and wellness (MS). *Accreditation:* NCATE. *Program availability:* Evening/weekend. *Entrance requirements:* For master's, GRE, undergraduate major or minor in health and human performance or related field of study.

Merrimack College, School of Science and Engineering, North Andover, MA 01845-5800. Offers civil engineering (MS); community health education (MS); computer science (MS); exercise and sport science (MS); health and wellness management (MS); mechanical engineering (MS), including engineering management. *Program availability:* Part-time. *Faculty:* 18 full-time, 4 part-time/adjunct. *Students:* 62 full-time (25 women), 12 part-time (4 women); includes 5 minority (1 Asian, non-Hispanic/Latino; 4 Hispanic/Latino), 18 international. Average age 24. 141 applicants, 67% accepted, 62 enrolled. In 2015, 12 master's awarded. *Degree requirements:* For master's, comprehensive exam, thesis optional, internship or capstone (for some programs). *Entrance requirements:* For master's, official college transcripts, resume, personal statement, 2 recommendations. Additional exam requirements/recommendations for international students: Required—TOEFL (minimum score 84 iBT), IELTS (minimum score 6.5), PTE (minimum score 56). *Application deadline:* For fall admission, 8/13 for domestic students, 7/13 for international students; for spring admission, 1/10 for domestic and international students; for summer admission, 5/10 for domestic students, 4/10 for international students. Applications are processed on a rolling basis. Application fee: $0. Electronic applications accepted. *Expenses:* Contact institution. *Financial support:* Fellowships with partial tuition reimbursements, career-related internships or fieldwork, scholarships/grants, and health care benefits available. Support available to part-time students. Financial award applicants required to submit FAFSA. *Faculty research:* Geotechnical (civil engineering), smart materials (mechanical engineering), computer graphics and network security (computer science). *Application contact:* Allison Pena, Graduate Admissions Counselor, 978-837-5227, E-mail: penaa@merrimack.edu.
Website: http://www.merrimack.edu/academics/graduate/

Mississippi State University, College of Agriculture and Life Sciences, Department of Food Science, Nutrition and Health Promotion, Mississippi State, MS 39762. Offers food science and technology (MS); food science and technology (PhD); health promotion (MS); nutrition (MS, PhD). *Program availability:* Online learning. *Faculty:* 18 full-time (6 women), 2 part-time/adjunct (both women). *Students:* 55 full-time (40 women), 40 part-time (33 women); includes 25 minority (16 Black or African American, non-Hispanic/Latino; 2 Asian, non-Hispanic/Latino; 6 Hispanic/Latino; 1 Two or more races, non-Hispanic/Latino), 25 international. Average age 28. 105 applicants, 47% accepted, 29 enrolled. In 2015, 27 master's, 6 doctorates awarded. *Degree requirements:* For master's, comprehensive exam, thesis; for doctorate, comprehensive exam, thesis/dissertation. *Entrance requirements:* For master's, GRE General Test, minimum GPA of 2.75; for doctorate, GRE General Test, minimum GPA of 2.75 undergraduate, 3.0 graduate. Additional exam requirements/recommendations for international students: Required—TOEFL (minimum score 550 paper-based; 79 iBT); Recommended—IELTS (minimum score 6.5). *Application deadline:* For fall admission, 7/1 for domestic students, 5/1 for international students; for spring admission, 11/1 for domestic students, 9/1 for international students. Applications are processed on a rolling basis. Application fee: $60. Electronic applications accepted. *Expenses: Tuition, area resident:* Full-time $7502; part-time $833.74 per credit hour. Tuition, nonresident: full-time $20,142; part-time $2238.24 per credit hour. *Financial support:* In 2015–16, 17 research assistantships with full tuition reimbursements (averaging $15,465 per year), 4 teaching assistantships with full tuition reimbursements (averaging $11,861 per year) were awarded; Federal Work-Study, institutionally sponsored loans, scholarships/grants, and unspecified assistantships also available. Financial award application deadline: 4/1; financial award applicants required to submit FAFSA. *Faculty research:* Food preservation, food chemistry, food safety, food processing, product development. *Unit head:* Dr. Will Evans, Professor and Head, 662-325-5055, Fax: 662-325-8728, E-mail: mwe59@msstate.edu. *Application contact:* Marina Hunt, Admissions Assistant, 662-325-5188, E-mail: mhunt@grad.msstate.edu.
Website: http://www.fsnhp.msstate.edu

Mount St. Joseph University, Graduate Program in Religious Studies, Cincinnati, OH 45233-1670. Offers pastoral administration (Certificate); religious studies (MA); spirituality and wellness (Certificate). *Program availability:* Part-time, evening/weekend. *Faculty:* 2 full-time (1 woman), 2 part-time/adjunct (1 woman). *Students:* 1 (woman) full-time, 10 part-time (all women); includes 1 minority (Black or African American, non-Hispanic/Latino). Average age 42. 3 applicants, 67% accepted, 3 enrolled. In 2015, 4 master's awarded. *Degree requirements:* For master's, integrating project, field experience. *Entrance requirements:* For master's, 3 letters of recommendation, interview, minimum GPA of 3.0, academic transcripts, essay. Additional exam requirements/recommendations for international students: Required—TOEFL (minimum score 560 paper-based; 83 iBT). *Application deadline:* Applications are processed on a rolling basis. Application fee: $50. Electronic applications accepted. *Expenses: Tuition, area resident:* Full-time $15,255; part-time $565 per credit hour. *Required fees:* $500; $100 per term. $100 per semester. Full-time tuition and fees vary according to course load, degree level and program. *Financial support:* In 2015–16, 6 students received support. Scholarships/grants available. Financial award application deadline: 3/1; financial award applicants required to submit FAFSA. *Faculty research:* Contextual/cultural/systematic theology, historical/spiritual theology, business/economics ethics, social justice, Biblical/cultural/pastoral theology. *Unit head:* Dr. John Trokan, Chair of Religious/Pastoral Studies, 513-244-4272, Fax: 513-244-4222, E-mail: john.trokan@msj.edu. *Application contact:* Mary Brigham, Assistant Director of Graduate Recruitment, 513-244-4233, Fax: 513-244-4629, E-mail: mary.brigham@msj.edu.
Website: http://www.msj.edu/academics/graduate-programs/religious-studies-programs/

National University, Academic Affairs, School of Health and Human Services, La Jolla, CA 92037-1011. Offers clinical affairs (MS); clinical informatics (Certificate); clinical regulatory affairs (MS); health and life science analytics (MS); health coaching (Certificate); health informatics (MS); healthcare administration (MHA); nurse anesthesia (MS); nursing (MS), including forensic nursing, nursing administration, nursing informatics; nursing administration (Certificate); nursing informatics (Certificate); nursing practice (DNP); public health (MPH), including health promotion, healthcare administration, mental health. *Program availability:* Part-time, evening/weekend, 100% online, blended/hybrid learning. *Faculty:* 31 full-time (18 women), 33 part-time/adjunct (20 women). *Students:* 353 full-time (263 women), 136 part-time (87 women); includes

322 minority (111 Black or African American, non-Hispanic/Latino; 1 American Indian or Alaska Native, non-Hispanic/Latino; 105 Asian, non-Hispanic/Latino; 72 Hispanic/Latino; 7 Native Hawaiian or other Pacific Islander, non-Hispanic/Latino; 26 Two or more races, non-Hispanic/Latino), 31 international. Average age 32. In 2015, 103 master's awarded. *Degree requirements:* For master's, thesis (for some programs). *Entrance requirements:* For master's, interview, minimum GPA of 2.5. Additional exam requirements/recommendations for international students: Required—TOEFL (minimum score 550 paper-based; 79 iBT), IELTS (minimum score 6). *Application deadline:* Applications are processed on a rolling basis. Application fee: $60 ($65 for international students). Electronic applications accepted. *Financial support:* Career-related internships or fieldwork, institutionally sponsored loans, scholarships/grants, and tuition waivers (partial) available. Support available to part-time students. Financial award application deadline: 6/30; financial award applicants required to submit FAFSA. *Faculty research:* Nursing education, obesity prevention, workforce diversity. *Unit head:* School of Health and Human Services, 800-628-8648, E-mail: shhs@nu.edu. *Application contact:* Frank Rojas, Vice President for Enrollment Services, 800-628-8648, E-mail: advisor@nu.edu. Website: http://www.nu.edu/OurPrograms/SchoolOfHealthAndHumanServices.html

Nebraska Methodist College, Program in Health Promotion Management, Omaha, NE 68114. Offers MS. *Program availability:* Part-time, evening/weekend, online learning. *Degree requirements:* For master's, thesis or alternative, capstone project. *Entrance requirements:* For master's, interview. Additional exam requirements/recommendations for international students: Required—TOEFL (minimum score 550 paper-based; 80 iBT). *Faculty research:* Congregational health promotion, fitness testing with elderly, educational assessment, statistics instruction, resilience.

New York Medical College, School of Health Sciences and Practice, Department of Epidemiology and Community Health, Program in Behavioral Sciences and Health Promotion, Valhalla, NY 10595-1691. Offers behavioral sciences and health promotion (MPH); public health (Graduate Certificate). *Program availability:* Part-time, evening/weekend. *Degree requirements:* For master's, thesis, capstone. *Entrance requirements:* For master's, minimum undergraduate GPA of 3.0. Additional exam requirements/recommendations for international students: Required—TOEFL (minimum score 637 paper-based; 110 iBT), IELTS (minimum score 7). Electronic applications accepted. *Expenses:* Tuition, area resident: Full-time $44,355; part-time $1025 per credit. *Required fees:* $500; $95 per year. One-time fee: $140 part-time. Tuition and fees vary according to course load and program.

New York University, Steinhardt School of Culture, Education, and Human Development, Department of Applied Psychology, Programs in Counseling, New York, NY 10003. Offers counseling and guidance (MA, Advanced Certificate), including bilingual school counseling K-12 (MA), school counseling K-12 (MA); counseling for mental health and wellness (MA); counseling psychology (PhD); LGBT health, education, and social services (Advanced Certificate); Advanced Certificate/MPH; MA/ Advanced Certificate. *Accreditation:* APA (one or more programs are accredited). *Program availability:* Part-time. *Degree requirements:* For master's, thesis (for some programs); for doctorate, thesis/dissertation. *Entrance requirements:* For doctorate, GRE General Test, interview. Additional exam requirements/recommendations for international students: Required—TOEFL (minimum score 100 iBT). Electronic applications accepted. *Faculty research:* Sexual and gender identities, group dynamics, psychopathy and personality, multicultural assessment, working people's lives.

North Dakota State University, College of Graduate and Interdisciplinary Studies, College of Human Development and Education, Department of Health, Nutrition, and Exercise Sciences, Fargo, ND 58102. Offers athletic training (MAT, MS); dietetics (MS); exercise science and nutrition (PhD); exercise/nutrition science (MS); health promotion (MPH); leadership in physical education and sport (MS). *Program availability:* Part-time, evening/weekend, online learning. *Degree requirements:* For master's, thesis (for some programs). *Entrance requirements:* For master's, minimum GPA of 3.0. Additional exam requirements/recommendations for international students: Required—TOEFL (minimum score 525 paper-based; 71 iBT). *Application deadline:* For fall admission, 3/1 priority date for domestic and international students. Applications are processed on a rolling basis. Application fee: $35. Electronic applications accepted. *Financial support:* Teaching assistantships with full tuition reimbursements available. Financial award application deadline: 3/31. *Faculty research:* Biomechanics, sport specialization, recreation, nutrition, athletic training. *Unit head:* Dr. Yeong Rhee, Head, 701-231-7476, Fax: 701-231-8872, E-mail: yeong.rhee@ndsu.edu. *Application contact:* Nancy Moberg, Academic Assistant, 701-231-7474, Fax: 701-231-6524. Website: http://www.ndsu.edu/hnes/

Old Dominion University, Darden College of Education, Program in Physical Education, Exercise and Wellness Emphasis, Norfolk, VA 23529. Offers MS Ed. *Program availability:* Part-time, evening/weekend. *Faculty:* 8 full-time (3 women). *Students:* 16 full-time (12 women), 5 part-time (2 women); includes 8 minority (2 Black or African American, non-Hispanic/Latino; 5 Hispanic/Latino; 1 Two or more races, non-Hispanic/Latino), 1 international. Average age 25. 32 applicants, 69% accepted, 15 enrolled. In 2015, 11 master's awarded. *Degree requirements:* For master's, comprehensive exam, thesis or alternative, internship, research project. *Entrance requirements:* For master's, GRE, minimum GPA 2.8 overall, 3.0 in major. Additional exam requirements/recommendations for international students: Required—TOEFL (minimum score 550 paper-based; 79 iBT). *Application deadline:* For fall admission, 3/1 for domestic students. Application fee: $50. Electronic applications accepted. *Expenses:* $478 per credit hour in-state, $1,195 per credit hour out-of-state; $300 per year fees. *Financial support:* In 2015–16, 1 research assistantship (averaging $9,000 per year), 2 teaching assistantships (averaging $9,000 per year) were awarded; unspecified assistantships also available. Financial award application deadline: 4/15. *Faculty research:* Diabetes, exercise prescription, nutrition, lower extremity biomechanics, vascular function. *Total annual research expenditures:* $613,790. *Unit head:* Dr. Lynn Ridinger, Chair, 757-683-4353, E-mail: lridinge@odu.edu. *Application contact:* William Heffelfinger, Director of Graduate Admissions, 757-683-5554, Fax: 757-683-3255, E-mail: gradadmit@odu.edu. Website: https://www.odu.edu/academics/programs/masters/exercise-science-wellness

Oregon State University, College of Public Health and Human Sciences, Program in Public Health, Corvallis, OR 97331. Offers biostatistics (MPH); environmental and occupational health and safety (MPH, PhD); epidemiology (MPH, PhD); health management and policy (MPH); health policy (PhD); health promotion and health behavior (MPH, PhD); international health (MPH). *Accreditation:* CEPH. *Program availability:* Part-time. *Faculty:* 32 full-time (18 women), 3 part-time/adjunct (0 women). *Students:* 123 full-time (91 women), 20 part-time (14 women); includes 43 minority (2 Black or African American, non-Hispanic/Latino; 2 American Indian or Alaska Native, non-Hispanic/Latino; 9 Asian, non-Hispanic/Latino; 18 Hispanic/Latino; 1 Native Hawaiian or other Pacific Islander, non-Hispanic/Latino; 11 Two or more races, non-Hispanic/Latino), 18 international. Average age 31. 276 applicants, 65% accepted, 45 enrolled. In 2015, 59 master's, 6 doctorates awarded. Terminal master's awarded for partial completion of doctoral program. *Degree requirements:* For doctorate, one foreign language, thesis/dissertation. *Entrance requirements:* For master's and doctorate, GRE, minimum GPA of 3.0 in last 90 hours. Additional exam requirements/recommendations for international students: Required—TOEFL (minimum score 80 iBT), IELTS (minimum

score 6.5). *Application deadline:* For fall admission, 12/1 priority date for domestic students. Applications are processed on a rolling basis. *Expenses:* $13,851 full-time resident tuition, $23,679 full-time non-resident tuition, $1,572 fees. *Financial support:* Fellowships, research assistantships, teaching assistantships, career-related internships or fieldwork, Federal Work-Study, and institutionally sponsored loans available. Support available to part-time students. Financial award application deadline: 12/1. *Faculty research:* Traffic safety, health safety, injury control, health promotion. *Unit head:* Dr. Sheryl Thorburn, Professor/Co-Director. *Application contact:* Amanda Armington, Public Health Program Manager, 541-737-3825, E-mail: amanda.armington@oregonstate.edu.

Plymouth State University, Program in Personal and Organizational Wellness, Plymouth, NH 03264-1595. Offers MA.

Portland State University, Graduate Studies, College of Urban and Public Affairs, School of Community Health, Portland, OR 97207-0751. Offers aging (Certificate); community health (PhD); health education (MA, MS); health promotion (MPH); health studies (MPA, MPH), including health administration. MPH offered jointly with Oregon Health & Science University. *Accreditation:* CEPH. *Program availability:* Part-time. *Faculty:* 35 full-time (25 women), 14 part-time/adjunct (6 women). *Students:* 67 full-time (53 women), 61 part-time (54 women); includes 33 minority (2 Black or African American, non-Hispanic/Latino; 6 American Indian or Alaska Native, non-Hispanic/Latino; 5 Asian, non-Hispanic/Latino; 12 Hispanic/Latino; 8 Two or more races, non-Hispanic/Latino), 4 international. Average age 33. 85 applicants, 49% accepted, 33 enrolled. In 2015, 46 master's, 1 doctorate awarded. *Degree requirements:* For master's, comprehensive exam (for some programs), thesis (for some programs), internship/praticum, oral and written exams (depending on program; for doctorate, comprehensive exam, thesis/dissertation. *Entrance requirements:* For master's, GRE (for MPH program), 3 letters of recommendation, minimum GPA of 3.0, resume; for doctorate, GRE, transcripts, personal statement, resume, writing sample, 3 letters of recommendation. Additional exam requirements/recommendations for international students: Required—TOEFL (minimum score 550 paper-based; 80 iBT). *Application deadline:* For fall admission, 2/1 for domestic and international students. Applications are processed on a rolling basis. Application fee: $50. *Expenses:* $11,301 per year. *Financial support:* In 2015–16, 13 research assistantships with tuition reimbursements (averaging $7,336 per year) were awarded; teaching assistantships, career-related internships or fieldwork, Federal Work-Study, scholarships/grants, and unspecified assistantships also available. Support available to part-time students. Financial award application deadline: 3/1; financial award applicants required to submit FAFSA. *Total annual research expenditures:* $1.7 million. *Unit head:* Dr. Carlos J. Crespo, Director, 503-725-5120, Fax: 503-725-5100. *Application contact:* Elizabeth Bull, Assistant to the Director, 503-725-4592, Fax: 503-725-5100, E-mail: bulle@pdx.edu. Website: http://www.healthed.pdx.edu/

Rosalind Franklin University of Medicine and Science, College of Health Professions, Department of Nutrition, North Chicago, IL 60064-3095. Offers clinical nutrition (MS); health promotion and wellness (MS); nutrition education (MS). *Program availability:* Part-time, evening/weekend, online learning. *Degree requirements:* For master's, thesis optional, portfolio. *Entrance requirements:* For master's, minimum GPA of 2.75, registered dietitian (RD), professional certificate or license. Additional exam requirements/recommendations for international students: Required—TOEFL. *Expenses:* Contact institution. *Faculty research:* Nutrition education, distance learning, computer-based graduate education, childhood obesity, nutrition medical education.

Rowan University, Graduate School, School of Biomedical Science and Health Professions, Department of Health and Exercise Science, Glassboro, NJ 08028-1701. Offers wellness and lifestyle management (MA). *Degree requirements:* For master's, comprehensive exam, thesis. *Entrance requirements:* For master's, GRE General Test, GRE Subject Test, interview, minimum GPA of 2.8. Additional exam requirements/recommendations for international students: Required—TOEFL. Electronic applications accepted. *Expenses:* Tuition, area resident: Full-time $8710; part-time $871 per credit. Tuition, state resident: full-time $8710; part-time $871 per credit. Tuition, nonresident: full-time $8710; part-time $871 per credit. *International tuition:* $8710 full-time. *Required fees:* $1510; $151 per credit.

San Diego State University, Graduate and Research Affairs, College of Health and Human Services, Graduate School of Public Health, San Diego, CA 92182. Offers environmental health (MPH); epidemiology (MPH, PhD), including biostatistics (MPH); global emergency preparedness and response (MS); global health (PhD); health behavior (PhD); health promotion (MPH); health services administration (MPH); toxicology (MS); MPH/MA; MSW/MPH. *Accreditation:* CAHME (one or more programs are accredited); CEPH (one or more programs are accredited). *Program availability:* Part-time. *Degree requirements:* For master's, comprehensive exam (for some programs), thesis (for some programs); for doctorate, thesis/dissertation. *Entrance requirements:* For master's, GMAT (MPH in health services administration), GRE General Test; for doctorate, GRE General Test. Additional exam requirements/recommendations for international students: Required—TOEFL. *Faculty research:* Evaluation of tobacco, AIDS prevalence and prevention, mammography, infant death project, Alzheimer's in elderly Chinese.

Simmons College, School of Nursing and Health Sciences, Boston, MA 02115. Offers didactic dietetics (Certificate); dietetic internship (Certificate); health education profession (PhD); health professions education (CAGS); nursing (MS), including family nurse practitioner; nursing practice (DNP); nutrition and health promotion (MS); physical therapy (DPT); sports nutrition (Certificate). *Program availability:* Part-time, blended/ hybrid learning. *Faculty:* 21 full-time (17 women), 171 part-time/adjunct (157 women). *Students:* 333 full-time (305 women), 889 part-time (813 women); includes 250 minority (88 Black or African American, non-Hispanic/Latino; 3 American Indian or Alaska Native, non-Hispanic/Latino; 65 Asian, non-Hispanic/Latino; 67 Hispanic/Latino; 2 Native Hawaiian or other Pacific Islander, non-Hispanic/Latino; 25 Two or more races, non-Hispanic/Latino), 9 international. Average age 33. 846 applicants, 66% accepted, 441 enrolled. In 2015, 70 master's, 45 doctorates awarded. *Entrance requirements:* For doctorate, GRE. Additional exam requirements/recommendations for international students: Required—TOEFL (minimum score 570 paper-based; 88 iBT). *Application deadline:* For fall admission, 6/1 for international students. Application fee: $50. Electronic applications accepted. *Expenses:* Contact institution. *Financial support:* In 2015–16, 12 research assistantships (averaging $6,000 per year) were awarded; scholarships/grants and unspecified assistantships also available. *Unit head:* Dr. Judy Beal, Dean, 617-521-2139. *Application contact:* Brett DiMarzo, Director of Graduate Admission, 617-521-2651, Fax: 617-521-3137, E-mail: brett.dimarzo@simmons.edu. Website: http://www.simmons.edu/snhs/

Sonoma State University, School of Science and Technology, Department of Kinesiology, Rohnert Park, CA 94928. Offers adapted physical education (MA); interdisciplinary (MA); interdisciplinary pre-occupational therapy (MA); lifetime physical activity (MA), including coach education, fitness and wellness; physical education (MA); pre-physical therapy (MA). *Program availability:* Part-time. *Degree requirements:* For master's, thesis, oral exam. *Entrance requirements:* For master's, minimum GPA of 2.8. Additional exam requirements/recommendations for international students: Required—TOEFL (minimum score 500 paper-based).

Springfield College, Graduate Programs, Programs in Exercise Science and Sport Studies, Springfield, MA 01109-3797. Offers athletic training (MS); exercise physiology (MS); health promotion and disease prevention (MS); sport and exercise psychology (MS). *Program availability:* Part-time. Terminal master's awarded for partial completion of doctoral program. *Degree requirements:* For master's, comprehensive exam, research project or thesis; for doctorate, comprehensive exam, thesis/dissertation. *Entrance requirements:* For master's and doctorate, GRE General Test. Additional exam requirements/recommendations for international students: Required—TOEFL (minimum score 550 paper-based); Recommended—IELTS (minimum score 6). Electronic applications accepted.

Tennessee Technological University, College of Graduate Studies, College of Education, Department of Exercise Science, Physical Education and Wellness, Cookeville, TN 38505. Offers adapted physical education (MA); elementary/middle school physical education (MA); lifetime wellness (MA); sport management (MA). *Accreditation:* NCATE. *Program availability:* Part-time, online learning. *Faculty:* 7 full-time (0 women). *Students:* 26 full-time (10 women), 35 part-time (14 women); includes 8 minority (6 Black or African American, non-Hispanic/Latino; 2 Hispanic/Latino), 1 international. Average age 27. 31 applicants, 74% accepted, 20 enrolled. In 2015, 13 master's awarded. *Degree requirements:* For master's, comprehensive exam, thesis or alternative. *Entrance requirements:* For master's, MAT or GRE. Additional exam requirements/recommendations for international students: Required—TOEFL (minimum score 520 paper-based; 71 iBT), IELTS (minimum 5.5), PTE (minimum score 48), or TOEIC (Test of English as an International Communication). *Application deadline:* For fall admission, 8/1 for domestic students, 5/1 for international students; for spring admission, 12/1 for domestic students, 10/1 for international students; for summer admission, 5/1 for domestic students, 2/1 for international students. Applications are processed on a rolling basis. Application fee: $35 ($40 for international students). Electronic applications accepted. *Expenses:* Tuition, state resident: full-time $8961; part-time $6132 per credit hour. Tuition, nonresident: full-time $23,121; part-time $14,608 per credit hour. *Financial support:* In 2015–16, fellowships (averaging $8,000 per year), 3 research assistantships (averaging $4,000 per year), 4 teaching assistantships (averaging $4,000 per year) were awarded; career-related internships or fieldwork also available. Financial award application deadline: 4/1. *Unit head:* Dr. Christy Killman, Chairperson, 931-372-3467, Fax: 931-372-6319, E-mail: ckillman@tntech.edu. *Application contact:* Shelia K. Kendrick, Coordinator of Graduate Studies, 931-372-3808, Fax: 931-372-3497, E-mail: skendrick@tntech.edu.

Texas A&M University, School of Public Health, College Station, TX 77843. Offers health administration (MHA); health policy and management (MPH); health promotion and community health sciences (MPH); health services research (PhD). *Accreditation:* CEPH. *Program availability:* Part-time, blended/hybrid learning. *Faculty:* 68. *Students:* 313 full-time (189 women), 71 part-time (41 women); includes 169 minority (40 Black or African American, non-Hispanic/Latino; 38 Asian, non-Hispanic/Latino; 88 Hispanic/Latino; 3 Two or more races, non-Hispanic/Latino), 88 international. Average age 30. 138 applicants, 100% accepted, 126 enrolled. In 2015, 139 master's, 5 doctorates awarded. *Degree requirements:* For master's, thesis optional. *Entrance requirements:* For master's, GRE General Test, 3 letters of recommendation; statement of purpose; current curriculum vitae or resume; official transcripts; for doctorate, GRE General Test, 3 letters of recommendation; statement of purpose; current curriculum vitae or resume; official transcripts; interview (in some cases). Additional exam requirements/recommendations for international students: Required—TOEFL (minimum score 597 paper-based, 95 iBT) or GRE (minimum verbal score 153). *Application deadline:* For fall admission, 8/27 for domestic students; for spring admission, 1/14 for domestic students. Application fee: $120. Electronic applications accepted. *Expenses:* Contact institution. *Financial support:* In 2015–16, 186 students received support, including 2 fellowships with tuition reimbursements available (averaging $17,190 per year), 55 research assistantships with tuition reimbursements available (averaging $5,728 per year), 14 teaching assistantships with tuition reimbursements available (averaging $5,836 per year); career-related internships or fieldwork, institutionally sponsored loans, scholarships/grants, traineeships, health care benefits, tuition waivers (full and partial), and unspecified assistantships also available. Support available to part-time students. Financial award applicants required to submit FAFSA. *Unit head:* Dr. Jay Maddock, Dean, 979-436-9322, Fax: 979-458-1878, E-mail: maddock@tamhsc.edu. *Application contact:* Erin E. Schneider, Associate Director of Admissions and Recruitment, 979-436-9380, E-mail: eschneider@sph.tamhsc.edu.
Website: http://sph.tamhsc.edu/

Union Institute & University, Individualized Master of Arts Program, Cincinnati, OH 45206. Offers creativity studies (MA); health and wellness (MA); history and culture (MA); leadership, public policy, and social issues (MA); literature and writing (MA). *Program availability:* Part-time, online only, 100% online. *Faculty:* 2 full-time (both women), 9 part-time/adjunct (7 women). *Students:* 9 full-time (7 women), 70 part-time (56 women); includes 33 minority (22 Black or African American, non-Hispanic/Latino; 1 American Indian or Alaska Native, non-Hispanic/Latino; 6 Hispanic/Latino; 4 Two or more races, non-Hispanic/Latino). Average age 40. In 2015, 45 master's awarded. *Degree requirements:* For master's, thesis. *Entrance requirements:* For master's, transcript, essay, 3 letters of recommendation, resume. Additional exam requirements/recommendations for international students: Required—TOEFL. *Application deadline:* For spring admission, 3/13 for domestic students. Applications are processed on a rolling basis. Application fee: $50. Electronic applications accepted. *Expenses:* Contact institution. *Financial support:* Career-related internships or fieldwork and tuition waivers available. Financial award applicants required to submit FAFSA. *Application contact:* Director of Admissions, 800-861-6400.
Website: https://www.myunion.edu/academics/masters-programs/master-of-arts/

Universidad del Turabo, Graduate Programs, Programs in Education, Program in Wellness, Gurabo, PR 00778-3030. Offers MPHE.

The University of Alabama, Graduate School, College of Human Environmental Sciences, Department of Health Science, Tuscaloosa, AL 35487-0311. Offers health education and promotion (PhD); health studies (MA). *Program availability:* Part-time, online learning. *Faculty:* 12 full-time (7 women). *Students:* 72 full-time (58 women), 111 part-time (90 women); includes 69 minority (46 Black or African American, non-Hispanic/Latino; 2 American Indian or Alaska Native, non-Hispanic/Latino; 3 Asian, non-Hispanic/Latino; 13 Hispanic/Latino; 1 Native Hawaiian or other Pacific Islander, non-Hispanic/Latino; 4 Two or more races, non-Hispanic/Latino), 2 international. Average age 33. 110 applicants, 75% accepted, 65 enrolled. In 2015, 81 master's, 4 doctorates awarded. *Degree requirements:* For master's, comprehensive exam, thesis optional; for doctorate, one foreign language, comprehensive exam, thesis/dissertation. *Entrance requirements:* For master's, minimum GPA of 3.0; for doctorate, GRE General Test, minimum GPA of 3.0, prerequisites in health education. Additional exam requirements/recommendations for international students: Required—TOEFL. *Application deadline:* For fall admission, 3/15 priority date for domestic students, 3/15 for international students. Applications are processed on a rolling basis. Application fee: $50 ($60 for international students). Electronic applications accepted. *Expenses:* Tuition, state resident: full-time $10,170. Tuition, nonresident: full-time $25,950. *Financial support:* In 2015–16, 2 research assistantships with full tuition reimbursements (averaging $10,500 per year), 6 teaching assistantships with full tuition reimbursements (averaging $10,500 per year) were awarded; career-related internships or fieldwork, Federal Work-Study, institutionally sponsored loans, health care benefits, and unspecified assistantships also available. Financial award application deadline: 4/14. *Faculty research:* Program planning, substance abuse prevention, obesity prevention, nutrition, physical activity, athletic training, osteoporosis, health behavior. *Total annual research expenditures:* $500. *Unit head:* Dr. Lori W. Turner, Department Head and Professor, 205-348-2956, Fax: 205-348-7568, E-mail: lwturner@ches.ua.edu. *Application contact:* Dr. Stuart Usdan, Associate Professor and Doctoral Program Coordinator, 205-348-8373, Fax: 205-348-7568, E-mail: susdan@ches.ua.edu.
Website: http://ches.ua.edu/

The University of Alabama at Birmingham, School of Education, Program in Health Education and Promotion, Birmingham, AL 35294. Offers PhD. Program offered jointly with School of Public Health, School of Health Professions, and The University of Alabama (Tuscaloosa). *Accreditation:* NCATE. *Degree requirements:* For doctorate, thesis/dissertation. *Entrance requirements:* For doctorate, GRE General Test (preferred minimum scores of 156 for each section), minimum GPA of 3.0, letters of recommendation. Electronic applications accepted. *Expenses:* Tuition, state resident: full-time $7340. Tuition, nonresident: full-time $16,628. Full-time tuition and fees vary according to course load and program.

The University of Alabama at Birmingham, School of Public Health, Program in Health Education and Promotion, Birmingham, AL 35294. Offers PhD. Program offered jointly with the School of Education and The University of Alabama (Tuscaloosa). *Degree requirements:* For doctorate, comprehensive exam, thesis/dissertation, research internship. *Entrance requirements:* For doctorate, GRE, letters of recommendation. Additional exam requirements/recommendations for international students: Recommended—TOEFL, IELTS. *Expenses:* Tuition, state resident: full-time $7340. Tuition, nonresident: full-time $16,628. Full-time tuition and fees vary according to course load and program.

University of Alberta, School of Public Health, Centre for Health Promotion Studies, Edmonton, AB T6G 2E1, Canada. Offers health promotion (M Sc, Postgraduate Diploma). *Program availability:* Part-time, online learning.

University of Arkansas, Graduate School, College of Education and Health Professions, Department of Health, Human Performance and Recreation, Program in Community Health Promotion, Fayetteville, AR 72701-1201. Offers MS, PhD. *Students:* 8 full-time (7 women), 12 part-time (all women); includes 5 minority (2 Black or African American, non-Hispanic/Latino; 1 American Indian or Alaska Native, non-Hispanic/Latino; 1 Hispanic/Latino; 1 Two or more races, non-Hispanic/Latino). In 2015, 7 master's, 5 doctorates awarded. *Unit head:* Dr. Bart Hammig, Departmental Chairperson, 479-575-2857, Fax: 479-575-5778, E-mail: bhammig@uark.edu. *Application contact:* Dr. Stephen Dittmore, Coordinator of Graduate Studies, 479-575-6625, E-mail: dittmore@uark.edu.
Website: http://chlp.uark.edu

University of Arkansas for Medical Sciences, College of Public Health, Little Rock, AR 72205-7199. Offers biostatistics (MPH); environmental and occupational health (MPH, Certificate); epidemiology (MPH, PhD); health behavior and health education (MPH); health policy and management (MPH); health promotion and prevention research (PhD); health services administration (MHSA); health systems research (PhD); public health (Certificate); public health leadership (Dr PH). *Program availability:* Part-time. *Degree requirements:* For master's, preceptorship, culminating experience, internship; for doctorate, comprehensive exam, capstone. *Entrance requirements:* For master's, GRE, GMAT, LSAT, PCAT, MCAT, DAT; for doctorate, GRE. Additional exam requirements/recommendations for international students: Required—TOEFL (minimum score 80 iBT), IELTS. Electronic applications accepted. *Expenses:* Contact institution. *Faculty research:* Health systems, tobacco prevention control, obesity prevention, environmental and occupational exposure, cancer prevention.

University of Central Oklahoma, The Jackson College of Graduate Studies, College of Education and Professional Studies, Department of Kinesiology and Health Studies, Edmond, OK 73034-5209. Offers athletic training (MS); wellness management (MS), including exercise science, health studies. *Degree requirements:* For master's, comprehensive exam (for some programs), thesis (for some programs). *Entrance requirements:* For master's, GRE. Additional exam requirements/recommendations for international students: Required—TOEFL (minimum score 550 paper-based; 79 iBT), IELTS (minimum score 6.5). Electronic applications accepted.

University of Chicago, Division of the Biological Sciences, Program in Public Health Sciences, Chicago, IL 60637. Offers MS, PhD. *Program availability:* Part-time. *Students:* 15 full-time (7 women), 24 part-time (13 women); includes 13 minority (3 Black or African American, non-Hispanic/Latino; 8 Asian, non-Hispanic/Latino; 2 Hispanic/Latino), 6 international. Average age 35. 75 applicants, 33% accepted, 22 enrolled. In 2015, 6 master's, 1 doctorate awarded. Terminal master's awarded for partial completion of doctoral program. *Degree requirements:* For master's, thesis; for doctorate, comprehensive exam, thesis/dissertation, ethics class, 2 teaching assistantships. *Entrance requirements:* For master's, MCAT or GRE, doctoral-level clinical degree or completed pre-clinical training at accredited medical school; for doctorate, GRE General Test. Additional exam requirements/recommendations for international students: Required—TOEFL (minimum score 600 paper-based; 104 iBT), IELTS (minimum score 7). *Application deadline:* For fall admission, 12/1 for domestic and international students. Application fee: $90. Electronic applications accepted. *Financial support:* In 2015–16, 13 students received support. Fellowships with tuition reimbursements available, research assistantships with tuition reimbursements available, institutionally sponsored loans, scholarships/grants, traineeships, and health care benefits available. Financial award applicants required to submit FAFSA. *Unit head:* Diane Sperling Lauderdale, PhD, Chair, 773-834-1242, Fax: 773-702-1979, E-mail: thisted@health.bsd.uchicago.edu. *Application contact:* Michele Thompson, Education Program Manager, 773-834-1836, E-mail: mthompso@health.bsd.uchicago.edu.
Website: http://health.bsd.uchicago.edu/

University of Delaware, College of Health Sciences, Department of Behavioral Health and Nutrition, Newark, DE 19716. Offers health promotion (MS); human nutrition (MS). *Program availability:* Part-time. *Degree requirements:* For master's, thesis. *Entrance requirements:* For master's, GRE General Test, interview, minimum GPA of 3.0. Additional exam requirements/recommendations for international students: Required—TOEFL (minimum score 550 paper-based). Electronic applications accepted. *Faculty research:* Sport biomechanics, rehabilitation biomechanics, vascular dynamics.

University of Georgia, College of Public Health, Department of Health Promotion and Behavior, Athens, GA 30602. Offers MPH, PhD. *Accreditation:* CEPH; NCATE (one or more programs are accredited). *Degree requirements:* For master's, thesis (MA); for doctorate, thesis/dissertation. *Entrance requirements:* For master's, GRE General Test or MAT; for doctorate, GRE General Test. Electronic applications accepted.

University of Kentucky, Graduate School, College of Education, Program in Kinesiology and Health Promotion, Lexington, KY 40506-0032. Offers biomechanics (MS); exercise physiology (MS, PhD); exercise science (PhD); health promotion (MS, Ed D); physical education training (Ed D); sport leadership (MS); teaching and coaching

(MS). Terminal master's awarded for partial completion of doctoral program. *Degree requirements:* For master's, comprehensive exam, thesis optional; for doctorate, comprehensive exam, thesis/dissertation. *Entrance requirements:* For master's, GRE General Test, minimum undergraduate GPA of 2.75; for doctorate, GRE General Test, minimum graduate GPA of 3.0. Additional exam requirements/recommendations for international students: Required—TOEFL (minimum score 550 paper-based). Electronic applications accepted.

University of Louisville, Graduate School, School of Public Health and Information Sciences, Department of Public Health and Information Sciences, Louisville, KY 40202. Offers biostatistics (MS, PhD); clinical investigation (M Sc); epidemiology (MS); health management and systems sciences (MPH); public health sciences (PhD), including environmental health, epidemiology, health management, health promotion; public health sciences - health management (PhD). *Program availability:* Part-time. *Students:* 92 full-time (60 women), 33 part-time (19 women); includes 37 minority (16 Black or African American, non-Hispanic/Latino; 12 Asian, non-Hispanic/Latino; 6 Hispanic/Latino; 3 Two or more races, non-Hispanic/Latino), 19 international. Average age 32. 128 applicants, 77% accepted, 56 enrolled. In 2015, 38 master's, 6 doctorates awarded. *Degree requirements:* For master's, thesis optional; for doctorate, comprehensive exam, thesis/dissertation. *Entrance requirements:* For master's and doctorate, GRE General Test. Additional exam requirements/recommendations for international students: Required—TOEFL (minimum score 600 paper-based; 100 iBT). *Application deadline:* For fall admission, 5/1 for domestic and international students. Application fee: $60. Electronic applications accepted. *Expenses:* Tuition, state resident: full-time $11,664; part-time $649 per credit hour. Tuition, nonresident: full-time $24,274; part-time $1350 per credit hour. *Required fees:* $196. Tuition and fees vary according to program and reciprocity agreements. *Financial support:* In 2015–16, 718,988 students received support. Research assistantships with full tuition reimbursements available, scholarships/grants, health care benefits, and unspecified assistantships available. Financial award applicants required to submit FAFSA. *Faculty research:* Department of environmental and occupational health sciences department of health management and systems sciences department of health promotion and behavioral sciences. *Total annual research expenditures:* $2.1 million. *Unit head:* Dr. Craig Blakely, Dean, 502-852-3297, Fax: 502-852-3291, E-mail: chblak01@louisville.edu.
Website: http://louisville.edu/sphis/departments/health-management-systems-science

University of Massachusetts Lowell, College of Health Sciences, School of Nursing, PhD Program in Nursing, Lowell, MA 01854. Offers PhD. *Accreditation:* AACN. *Degree requirements:* For doctorate, thesis/dissertation, qualifying examination. *Entrance requirements:* For doctorate, GRE General Test, master's degree in nursing with minimum GPA of 3.3, current MA RN license, 2 years of professional nursing experience, 3 letters of recommendation. *Application deadline:* For fall admission, 4/1 priority date for domestic students; for spring admission, 10/1 for domestic students. Applications are processed on a rolling basis. Application fee: $20 ($35 for international students). *Expenses:* Tuition, state resident: full-time $14,304. Tuition, nonresident: full-time $25,853. *Required fees:* $375. Full-time tuition and fees vary according to campus/location and reciprocity agreements. *Financial support:* Fellowships with full tuition reimbursements, research assistantships with full tuition reimbursements, teaching assistantships with full tuition reimbursements, career-related internships or fieldwork, Federal Work-Study, institutionally sponsored loans, scholarships/grants, and traineeships available. Support available to part-time students. Financial award application deadline: 4/1.
Website: http://www.uml.edu/Health-Sciences/Nursing/Programs/phd-nursing.aspx

University of Michigan, School of Public Health, Department of Health Behavior and Health Education, Ann Arbor, MI 48109. Offers MPH, PhD, MPH/MSW. PhD offered through the Rackham Graduate School. *Accreditation:* CEPH (one or more programs are accredited). *Faculty:* 23 full-time (11 women), 29 part-time/adjunct (18 women). *Students:* 159 full-time (139 women), 3 part-time (all women); includes 58 minority (21 Black or African American, non-Hispanic/Latino; 16 Asian, non-Hispanic/Latino; 14 Hispanic/Latino; 7 Two or more races, non-Hispanic/Latino), 5 international. Average age 26. 592 applicants, 42% accepted, 84 enrolled. In 2015, 77 master's, 9 doctorates awarded. Terminal master's awarded for partial completion of doctoral program. *Degree requirements:* For doctorate, oral defense of dissertation, preliminary exam. *Entrance requirements:* For master's, GRE General Test (preferred); MCAT; for doctorate, GRE General Test. Additional exam requirements/recommendations for international students: Required—TOEFL (minimum score 100 iBT). *Application deadline:* For fall admission, 12/15 priority date for domestic students, 1/15 for international students. Applications are processed on a rolling basis. Application fee: $75. Electronic applications accepted. *Financial support:* Fellowships, research assistantships, teaching assistantships, career-related internships or fieldwork, Federal Work-Study, institutionally sponsored loans, scholarships/grants, traineeships, health care benefits, and unspecified assistantships available. Financial award application deadline: 12/1; financial award applicants required to submit FAFSA. *Faculty research:* Empowerment theory; structure, culture, and health; health disparities; community-based participatory research; health and medical decision-making. *Unit head:* Dr. Cathleen Connell, Chair, 734-764-9494. *Application contact:* Jackie Cormany, Student Services Coordinator, 734-763-9938, Fax: 734-763-7379, E-mail: sph.hbhe.inquiries@umich.edu.
Website: http://www.sph.umich.edu/hbhe/

University of Mississippi, Graduate School, School of Applied Sciences, University, MS 38677. Offers communicative disorders (MS); criminal justice (MCJ); exercise science (MS); food and nutrition services (MS); health and kinesiology (PhD); health promotion (MS); park and recreation management (MA); social work (MSW). *Faculty:* 65 full-time (36 women), 32 part-time/adjunct (23 women). *Students:* 192 full-time (148 women), 43 part-time (23 women); includes 47 minority (37 Black or African American, non-Hispanic/Latino; 2 Asian, non-Hispanic/Latino; 7 Hispanic/Latino; 1 Two or more races, non-Hispanic/Latino), 12 international. In 2015, 99 master's, 3 doctorates awarded. *Entrance requirements:* For master's, GRE General Test, minimum GPA of 3.0. Additional exam requirements/recommendations for international students: Required—TOEFL. *Application deadline:* For fall admission, 4/1 for domestic students; for spring admission, 10/1 for domestic students. Applications are processed on a rolling basis. Application fee: $40. Electronic applications accepted. *Financial support:* Scholarships/grants available. Financial award application deadline: 3/1; financial award applicants required to submit FAFSA. *Unit head:* Dr. Velmer Stanley Burton, Dean, 662-915-1081, Fax: 662-915-5717, E-mail: applsci@olemiss.edu. *Application contact:* Dr. Christy M. Wyandt, Associate Dean of Graduate School, 662-915-7474, Fax: 662-915-7577, E-mail: cwyandt@olemiss.edu.

University of Missouri, Office of Research and Graduate Studies, Master of Public Health Program, Columbia, MO 65211. Offers global public health (Graduate Certificate); health promotion and policy (MPH); public health (Graduate Certificate); veterinary public health (MPH); DVM/MPH; MPH/MA; MPH/MPA. *Accreditation:* CEPH. *Entrance requirements:* Additional exam requirements/recommendations for international students: Required—TOEFL (minimum score 550 paper-based; 80 iBT). *Application deadline:* For fall admission, 6/30 priority date for domestic and international students. Applications are processed on a rolling basis. Application fee: $55 ($75 for international students). Electronic applications accepted. *Financial support:* Fellowships

with tuition reimbursements, research assistantships with tuition reimbursements, teaching assistantships with tuition reimbursements, scholarships/grants, traineeships, health care benefits, and unspecified assistantships available. Support available to part-time students.
Website: http://publichealth.missouri.edu/

University of Nebraska–Lincoln, Graduate College, College of Education and Human Sciences, Department of Nutrition and Health Sciences, Lincoln, NE 68588. Offers community nutrition and health promotion (MS); nutrition (MS, PhD); nutrition and exercise (MS); nutrition and health sciences (MS, PhD). *Degree requirements:* For master's, thesis optional. *Entrance requirements:* For master's, GRE General Test. Additional exam requirements/recommendations for international students: Required—TOEFL (minimum score 550 paper-based). Electronic applications accepted. *Faculty research:* Foods/food service administration, community nutrition science, diet-health relationships.

University of Nebraska Medical Center, Department of Health Promotion, Social and Behavioral Health, Omaha, NE 68198. Offers health promotion and disease prevention research (PhD). *Program availability:* Part-time. *Faculty:* 13 full-time (9 women), 1 (woman) part-time/adjunct. *Students:* 11 full-time (6 women), 2 part-time (both women); includes 2 minority (1 Black or African American, non-Hispanic/Latino; 1 Asian, non-Hispanic/Latino), 2 international. Average age 35. 12 applicants, 33% accepted, 4 enrolled. In 2015, 2 doctorates awarded. *Degree requirements:* For doctorate, comprehensive exam, thesis/dissertation, teaching experience. *Entrance requirements:* For doctorate, GRE, official transcripts, master's or other advanced degree, written statement of career goals, three letters of recommendation. Additional exam requirements/recommendations for international students: Required—TOEFL (minimum score 550 paper-based; 80 iBT). *Application deadline:* For fall admission, 4/1 for domestic and international students. Application fee: $45. Electronic applications accepted. *Expenses:* Tuition, state resident: full-time $7830; part-time $3915 per credit hour. Tuition, nonresident: full-time $22,410; part-time $11,205 per credit hour. *Required fees:* $521. *Financial support:* In 2015–16, research assistantships with full tuition reimbursements (averaging $23,100 per year) were awarded; scholarships/grants also available. Support available to part-time students. Financial award application deadline: 2/15; financial award applicants required to submit FAFSA. *Unit head:* Dr. Ghada Soliman, Graduate Program Director, 402-559-5157, E-mail: ghada.soliman@unmc.edu. *Application contact:* Kate Kusnerik, Coordinator, 402-559-4325, E-mail: kate.kusnerik@unmc.edu.
Website: http://www.unmc.edu/publichealth/departments/healthpromotion/

University of North Alabama, College of Education, Department of Health, Physical Education, and Recreation, Florence, AL 35632. Offers health and human performance (MS), including exercise science, kinesiology, wellness and health promotion. *Program availability:* Part-time. *Faculty:* 4 full-time (1 woman), 1 part-time/adjunct (0 women). *Students:* 5 full-time (0 women), 9 part-time (5 women). Average age 24. 13 applicants, 77% accepted, 6 enrolled. In 2015, 15 master's awarded. *Degree requirements:* For master's, comprehensive exam (for some programs), thesis optional. *Entrance requirements:* For master's, MAT or GRE, 3 letters of recommendation, essay. Additional exam requirements/recommendations for international students: Required—TOEFL (minimum score 79 iBT), IELTS (minimum score 6), PTE (minimum score 54). *Application deadline:* Applications are processed on a rolling basis. Application fee: $50 ($100 for international students). Electronic applications accepted. *Expenses:* Tuition, state resident: full-time $2286; part-time $1524 per semester. Tuition, nonresident: full-time $4572; part-time $3048 per semester. *Required fees:* $801; $579 per semester. Tuition and fees vary according to course load. *Financial support:* In 2015–16, 3 students received support. Scholarships/grants and unspecified assistantships available. Financial award application deadline: 2/1; financial award applicants required to submit FAFSA. *Unit head:* Dr. Thomas E. Coates, Chair, 256-765-4377. *Application contact:* Hillary N. Coats, Graduate Admissions Coordinator, 256-765-4447, E-mail: graduate@una.edu.
Website: https://www.una.edu/hper/index.html

The University of North Carolina at Chapel Hill, Graduate School, Gillings School of Global Public Health, Public Health Leadership Program, Chapel Hill, NC 27599. Offers health care and prevention (MPH); leadership (MPH); occupational health nursing (MPH). *Program availability:* Part-time, online learning. *Students:* 157 full-time (105 women); includes 67 minority (27 Black or African American, non-Hispanic/Latino; 16 Asian, non-Hispanic/Latino; 15 Hispanic/Latino; 9 Two or more races, non-Hispanic/Latino), 9 international. Average age 35. 78 applicants, 95% accepted, 54 enrolled. *Degree requirements:* For master's, comprehensive exam, thesis (MS), paper (MPH). *Entrance requirements:* For master's, GRE General Test, minimum GPA of 3.0 (recommended), public health experience. *Financial support:* Career-related internships or fieldwork, institutionally sponsored loans, traineeships, and health care benefits available. Financial award application deadline: 12/10; financial award applicants required to submit FAFSA. *Faculty research:* Occupational health issues, clinical outcomes, prenatal and early childcare, adolescent health, effectiveness of home visiting, issues in occupational health nursing, community-based interventions. *Unit head:* Dr. Anna Schenck, Director, 919-843-8580, E-mail: anna.schenck@unc.edu. *Application contact:* Sue Robeson, Student Services Manager, 919-966-5305, Fax: 919-966-0981, E-mail: robeson@email.unc.edu.
Website: http://www2.sph.unc.edu/phlp/

University of Northern Iowa, Graduate College, College of Education, School of Kinesiology, Allied Health and Human Services, MA Program in Health Education, Cedar Falls, IA 50614. Offers community health education (MA); health promotion/fitness management (MA); school health education (MA). *Program availability:* Part-time, evening/weekend. *Students:* 14 full-time (11 women), 12 part-time (8 women); includes 3 minority (2 Black or African American, non-Hispanic/Latino; 1 Hispanic/Latino), 3 international. 20 applicants, 55% accepted, 11 enrolled. In 2015, 6 master's awarded. *Degree requirements:* For master's, comprehensive exam, thesis or alternative. *Entrance requirements:* For master's, minimum GPA of 3.0. Additional exam requirements/recommendations for international students: Required—TOEFL (minimum score 500 paper-based; 61 iBT). *Application deadline:* For fall admission, 8/1 priority date for domestic students. Applications are processed on a rolling basis. Application fee: $50 ($70 for international students). Electronic applications accepted. *Financial support:* Career-related internships or fieldwork, Federal Work-Study, and tuition waivers (full and partial) available. Support available to part-time students. Financial award application deadline: 2/1. *Unit head:* Dr. Susan Roberts-Dobie, Coordinator, 319-273-5930, Fax: 319-273-5958, E-mail: susan.dobie@uni.edu. *Application contact:* Laurie S. Russell, Record Analyst, 319-273-2623, Fax: 319-273-2885, E-mail: laurie.russell@uni.edu.
Website: http://www.uni.edu/coe/departments/school-health-physical-education-leisure-services/health-promotion-and-education

University of Oklahoma, College of Arts and Sciences, Department of Health and Exercise Science, Norman, OK 73019. Offers exercise physiology (PhD); health and exercise science (MS); health promotion (MS, PhD). *Faculty:* 13 full-time (6 women). *Students:* 38 full-time (19 women), 12 part-time (8 women); includes 9 minority (2 Black or African American, non-Hispanic/Latino; 1 American Indian or Alaska Native, non-

Health Promotion

Hispanic/Latino; 3 Hispanic/Latino; 3 Two or more races, non-Hispanic/Latino), 7 international. Average age 27. 31 applicants, 65% accepted, 19 enrolled. In 2015, 18 master's, 1 doctorate awarded. Terminal master's awarded for partial completion of doctoral program. *Degree requirements:* For master's, comprehensive exam (for some programs), thesis; for doctorate, comprehensive exam, thesis/dissertation. *Entrance requirements:* For master's and doctorate, GRE. Additional exam requirements/recommendations for international students: Required—TOEFL (minimum score 80 iBT). *Application deadline:* For fall and spring admission, 2/1 for domestic and international students. Applications are processed on a rolling basis. Application fee: $50 ($100 for international students). Electronic applications accepted. *Expenses:* Tuition, state resident: full-time $4577; part-time $190.70 per credit hour. Tuition, nonresident: full-time $17,758; part-time $739.90 per credit hour. *Required fees:* $3060; $115.70 per credit hour. $141.50 per semester. *Financial support:* In 2015–16, 48 students received support, including 45 teaching assistantships with full tuition reimbursements available (averaging $12,716 per year); health care benefits, tuition waivers (full), and unspecified assistantships also available. Financial award application deadline: 6/1; financial award applicants required to submit FAFSA. *Faculty research:* Health promotion, neuromuscular exercise physiology, aging, endocrine and bone metabolism, behavioral science. *Total annual research expenditures:* $38,778. *Unit head:* Dr. Michael G. Bemben, Professor/Chair, 405-325-2717, Fax: 405-325-0594, E-mail: mgbemben@ou.edu. *Application contact:* Dr. Paul Branscum, Assistant Professor/Graduate Liaison, 405-325-9028, Fax: 405-325-0594, E-mail: pbranscum@ou.edu.
Website: http://cas.ou.edu/hes

University of Oklahoma Health Sciences Center, Graduate College, College of Public Health, Department of Health Promotion Sciences, Oklahoma City, OK 73190. Offers MPH, MS, Dr PH, PhD. *Accreditation:* CEPH (one or more programs are accredited). *Program availability:* Part-time. *Degree requirements:* For master's, comprehensive exam, thesis (for some programs); for doctorate, 2 foreign languages, comprehensive exam, thesis/dissertation. *Entrance requirements:* For master's, letters of recommendation, resume; for doctorate, GRE, letters of recommendation. Additional exam requirements/recommendations for international students: Required—TOEFL (minimum score 570 paper-based). *Faculty research:* Health education, school health, health behavior, American Indian health.

University of Puerto Rico, Medical Sciences Campus, Graduate School of Public Health, Department of Human Development, Program in School Health Promotion, San Juan, PR 00936-5067. Offers Certificate.

University of South Carolina, The Graduate School, Arnold School of Public Health, Department of Health Promotion, Education, and Behavior, Columbia, SC 29208. Offers health education (MAT); health promotion, education, and behavior (MPH, MS, MSPH, Dr PH, PhD); school health education (Certificate); MSW/MPH. MAT offered in cooperation with the College of Education. *Accreditation:* CEPH (one or more programs are accredited); NCATE (one or more programs are accredited). *Program availability:* Part-time. *Degree requirements:* For master's, comprehensive exam, thesis or alternative, practicum (MPH), project (MS); for doctorate, comprehensive exam, thesis/dissertation. *Entrance requirements:* For master's and doctorate, GRE General Test. Additional exam requirements/recommendations for international students: Required—TOEFL (minimum score 570 paper-based; 75 iBT). Electronic applications accepted. *Faculty research:* Health disparities and inequalities in communities, global health and nutrition, cancer and HIV/AIDS prevention, health communication, policy and program design.

University of South Carolina, The Graduate School, Arnold School of Public Health, Program in Physical Activity and Public Health, Columbia, SC 29208. Offers MPH. *Accreditation:* CEPH. *Program availability:* Part-time. *Degree requirements:* For master's, comprehensive exam, practicum. *Entrance requirements:* For master's, GRE. Additional exam requirements/recommendations for international students: Required—TOEFL (minimum score 570 paper-based). Electronic applications accepted.

University of Southern California, Keck School of Medicine and Graduate School, Graduate Programs in Medicine, Department of Preventive Medicine, Master of Public Health Program, Los Angeles, CA 91803. Offers biostatistics and epidemiology (MPH); child and family health (MPH); environmental health (MPH); global health leadership (MPH); health communication (MPH); health education and promotion (MPH); public health policy (MPH). *Accreditation:* CEPH. *Program availability:* Part-time, evening/weekend. *Faculty:* 22 full-time (12 women), 3 part-time/adjunct (0 women). *Students:* 182 full-time (142 women), 35 part-time (25 women); includes 120 minority (19 Black or African American, non-Hispanic/Latino; 64 Asian, non-Hispanic/Latino; 37 Hispanic/Latino), 33 international. Average age 24. 236 applicants, 70% accepted, 71 enrolled. In 2015, 99 master's awarded. *Degree requirements:* For master's, practicum, final report, oral presentation. *Entrance requirements:* For master's, GRE General Test, MCAT, GMAT, minimum GPA of 3.0. Additional exam requirements/recommendations for international students: Required—TOEFL (minimum score 600 paper-based; 90 iBT). *Application deadline:* For fall admission, 6/1 priority date for domestic and international students; for spring admission, 10/1 priority date for domestic and international students; for summer admission, 3/1 for domestic and international students. Applications are processed on a rolling basis. Application fee: $85. Electronic applications accepted. *Expenses:* Contact institution. *Financial support:* Career-related internships or fieldwork, Federal Work-Study, institutionally sponsored loans, and scholarships/grants available. Support available to part-time students. Financial award application deadline: 5/4; financial award applicants required to submit CSS PROFILE or FAFSA. *Faculty research:* Substance abuse prevention, cancer and heart disease prevention, mass media and health communication research, health promotion, treatment compliance. *Unit head:* Dr. Louise A. Rohrbach, Director, 323-442-8237, Fax: 323-442-8297, E-mail: rohrbac@usc.edu. *Application contact:* Valerie Burris, Admissions Counselor, 323-442-7257, Fax: 323-442-8297, E-mail: valeriem@usc.edu.
Website: http://mph.usc.edu/

The University of Tennessee, Graduate School, College of Education, Health and Human Sciences, Program in Health Promotion and Health Education, Knoxville, TN 37996. Offers MS. *Accreditation:* CEPH. *Program availability:* Part-time. *Degree requirements:* For master's, thesis optional. *Entrance requirements:* For master's, minimum GPA of 2.7. Additional exam requirements/recommendations for international students: Required—TOEFL. Electronic applications accepted.

University of the Incarnate Word, School of Graduate Studies and Research, School of Mathematics, Science, and Engineering, Program in Nutrition, San Antonio, TX 78209-6397. Offers administration (MS); nutrition education and health promotion (MS). *Program availability:* Part-time, evening/weekend. *Faculty:* 8 full-time (4 women), 1 (woman) part-time/adjunct. *Students:* 8 full-time (all women), 22 part-time (19 women); includes 18 minority (1 Asian, non-Hispanic/Latino; 17 Hispanic/Latino), 1 international. Average age 26. 46 applicants, 89% accepted, 14 enrolled. In 2015, 5 master's awarded. *Degree requirements:* For master's, comprehensive exam, thesis or alternative. *Entrance requirements:* For master's, two letters of recommendation. Additional exam requirements/recommendations for international students: Required—TOEFL (minimum score 560 paper-based; 83 iBT). *Application deadline:* Applications are processed on a rolling basis. Application fee: $20. Electronic applications accepted.

Expenses: Tuition, area resident: Part-time $885 per credit hour. *Required fees:* $40 per credit hour. Tuition and fees vary according to course load, degree level, campus/location, program and student level. *Financial support:* In 2015–16, research assistantships (averaging $5,000 per year) were awarded; Federal Work-Study and scholarships/grants also available. Financial award applicants required to submit FAFSA. *Faculty research:* Nutrition. *Unit head:* Dr. Beth Senne-Duff, Associate Professor, 210-829-3165, Fax: 210-829-3153, E-mail: beths@uiwtx.edu. *Application contact:* Johnny Garcia, Assistant Director of Graduate Admissions, 210-805-3554, Fax: 210-829-3921, E-mail: admis@uiwtx.edu.
Website: http://www.uiw.edu/nutrition/nutrition3.htm

The University of Toledo, College of Graduate Studies, College of Medicine and Life Sciences, Department of Public Health and Preventative Medicine, Toledo, OH 43606-3390. Offers biostatistics and epidemiology (Certificate); contemporary gerontological practice (Certificate); environmental and occupational health and safety (MPH); epidemiology (Certificate); global public health (Certificate); health promotion and education (MPH); industrial hygiene (MSOH); medical and health science teaching and learning (Certificate); occupational health (Certificate); public health administration (MPH); public health and emergency response (Certificate); public health epidemiology (MPH); public health nutrition (MPH); MD/MPH. *Program availability:* Part-time, evening/weekend. *Degree requirements:* For master's, thesis or alternative. *Entrance requirements:* For master's, GRE, minimum undergraduate GPA of 3.0, three letters of recommendation, statement of purpose, transcripts from all prior institutions attended, resume; for Certificate, minimum undergraduate GPA of 3.0, three letters of recommendation, statement of purpose, transcripts from all prior institutions attended, resume. Additional exam requirements/recommendations for international students: Required—TOEFL (minimum score 550 paper-based; 80 iBT), IELTS (minimum score 6.5). Electronic applications accepted.

The University of Toledo, College of Graduate Studies, College of Nursing, Department of Health Promotions, Outcomes, Systems, and Policy, Toledo, OH 43606-3390. Offers MSN, DNP. *Accreditation:* CEPH. *Program availability:* Online learning. *Degree requirements:* For doctorate, thesis/dissertation or alternative, evidence-based project. *Entrance requirements:* For doctorate, GRE (taken within the past 5 years), personal statement, resume/curriculum vitae, letters of recommendation, documented supervised clinical hours in master's program, Nursing CAS application, UT supplemental application. Additional exam requirements/recommendations for international students: Required—TOEFL (minimum score 550 paper-based; 80 iBT). Electronic applications accepted.

University of Toronto, School of Graduate Studies, Department of Public Health Sciences, Toronto, ON M5S 1A1, Canada. Offers biostatistics (M Sc, PhD); community health (M Sc); community nutrition (MPH), including nutrition and dietetics; epidemiology (MPH, PhD); family and community medicine (MPH); occupational and environmental health (MPH); social and behavioral health science (PhD); social and behavioral health sciences (MPH), including health promotion. *Accreditation:* CAHME (one or more programs are accredited); CEPH (one or more programs are accredited). *Program availability:* Part-time. *Degree requirements:* For master's, thesis (for some programs), practicum; for doctorate, comprehensive exam, thesis/dissertation, oral thesis defense. *Entrance requirements:* For master's, 2 letters of reference, relevant professional/research experience, minimum B average in final year; for doctorate, 2 letters of reference, relevant professional/research experience, minimum B+ average. Additional exam requirements/recommendations for international students: Required—TOEFL (minimum score 580 paper-based; 93 iBT), TWE (minimum score 5). Electronic applications accepted. *Expenses:* Contact institution.

University of Utah, Graduate School, College of Health, Department of Health Promotion and Education, Salt Lake City, UT 84112. Offers M Phil, MS, Ed D, PhD. *Program availability:* Part-time. *Faculty:* 2 full-time (1 woman), 9 part-time/adjunct (5 women). *Students:* 36 full-time (29 women), 17 part-time (11 women); includes 8 minority (1 American Indian or Alaska Native, non-Hispanic/Latino; 3 Asian, non-Hispanic/Latino; 2 Hispanic/Latino; 2 Two or more races, non-Hispanic/Latino), 5 international. Average age 30. 37 applicants, 76% accepted, 23 enrolled. In 2015, 13 master's, 3 doctorates awarded. Terminal master's awarded for partial completion of doctoral program. *Degree requirements:* For master's, comprehensive exam, thesis or alternative, field experience; for doctorate, comprehensive exam, thesis/dissertation, field experience. *Entrance requirements:* For master's, GRE (for thesis option), minimum GPA of 3.0; for doctorate, GRE, minimum GPA of 3.2. Additional exam requirements/recommendations for international students: Required—TOEFL (minimum score 550 paper-based; 80 iBT). *Application deadline:* For fall admission, 2/1 for domestic and international students; for spring admission, 2/15 for domestic and international students; for summer admission, 2/1 for domestic and international students. Application fee: $55 ($65 for international students). Electronic applications accepted. *Expenses:* $1,930 per year in-state. *Financial support:* In 2015–16, 9 students received support, including 2 research assistantships with full tuition reimbursements available (averaging $14,000 per year), 4 teaching assistantships with full tuition reimbursements available (averaging $14,000 per year); health care benefits and unspecified assistantships also available. Financial award application deadline: 3/1; financial award applicants required to submit FAFSA. *Faculty research:* Health behavior and counseling, health service administration, evaluation of health programs. *Unit head:* Leslie K. Chatelain, Interim Department Chair, 801-581-4512, Fax: 801-585-3646, E-mail: les.chatelain@utah.edu. *Application contact:* Dr. Glenn E. Richardson, Director of Graduate Studies, 801-581-8039, Fax: 801-585-3646, E-mail: glenn.richardson@health.utah.edu.
Website: http://www.health.utah.edu/healthed/index.htm

University of Wisconsin–Milwaukee, Graduate School, Zilber School of Public Health, Department of Public Health, Milwaukee, WI 53201-0413. Offers community and behavioral health promotion (PhD); public health (MPH, Graduate Certificate). *Students:* 56 full-time (39 women), 17 part-time (13 women); includes 17 minority (6 Black or African American, non-Hispanic/Latino; 6 Asian, non-Hispanic/Latino; 5 Two or more races, non-Hispanic/Latino), 4 international. Average age 31. 113 applicants, 58% accepted, 34 enrolled. In 2015, 10 master's awarded. *Unit head:* Amy Harley, Assistant Professor, 414-229-4342, E-mail: harley@uwm.edu. *Application contact:* Darcie K. G. Warren, Graduate Program Manager, 414-229-5633, E-mail: darcie@uwm.edu.

University of Wisconsin–Stevens Point, College of Professional Studies, School of Health Promotion and Human Development, Stevens Point, WI 54481-3897. Offers human and community resources (MS); nutritional sciences (MS). *Program availability:* Part-time. *Degree requirements:* For master's, thesis or alternative. *Entrance requirements:* For master's, minimum GPA of 2.75.

University of Wyoming, College of Health Sciences, Division of Kinesiology and Health, Laramie, WY 82071. Offers MS. *Accreditation:* NCATE. *Program availability:* Part-time, online learning. *Degree requirements:* For master's, comprehensive exam (for some programs), thesis (for some programs). *Entrance requirements:* For master's, GRE General Test, minimum GPA of 3.0. Additional exam requirements/recommendations for international students: Required—TOEFL. Electronic applications accepted. *Faculty research:* Teacher effectiveness, effects of exercising on heart function, physiological responses of overtraining, psychological benefits of physical activity, health behavior.

Walden University, Graduate Programs, School of Health Sciences, Minneapolis, MN 55401. Offers clinical research administration (MS, Graduate Certificate); health education and promotion (MS, PhD), including behavioral health (PhD); disease surveillance (PhD), emergency preparedness (MS), general (MHA, MS), global health (PhD), health policy (PhD), health policy and advocacy (MS), population health (PhD); health informatics (MS); health services (PhD), including community health, healthcare administration, leadership, public health policy, self-designed; healthcare administration (MHA), including general (MHA, MS); leadership and organizational development (MHA); public health (MPH, Dr PH, PhD, Graduate Certificate), including community health education (PhD), epidemiology (PhD); systems policy (MHA). *Program availability:* Part-time, evening/weekend, online only, 100% online. *Faculty:* 14 full-time (8 women), 222 part-time/adjunct (121 women). *Students:* 2,487 full-time (1,804 women), 2,282 part-time (1,540 women); includes 2,763 minority (2,129 Black or African American, non-Hispanic/Latino; 30 American Indian or Alaska Native, non-Hispanic/Latino; 237 Asian, non-Hispanic/Latino; 268 Hispanic/Latino; 13 Native Hawaiian or other Pacific Islander, non-Hispanic/Latino; 86 Two or more races, non-Hispanic/Latino), 87 international. Average age 39. 1,205 applicants, 98% accepted, 820 enrolled. In 2015, 641 master's, 147 doctorates, 18 other advanced degrees awarded. *Degree requirements:* For doctorate, thesis/dissertation, residency. *Entrance requirements:* For master's, bachelor's degree or higher; minimum GPA of 2.5; official transcripts; goal statement (for some programs); access to computer and Internet; for doctorate, master's degree or higher; three years of related professional or academic experience (preferred); minimum GPA of 3.0; goal statement and current resume (for select programs); official transcripts; access to computer and Internet; for Graduate Certificate, relevant work experience; access to computer and Internet. Additional exam requirements/recommendations for international students: Required—TOEFL (minimum score 550 paper-based, 79 iBT), IELTS (minimum score 6.5), Michigan English Language Assessment Battery (minimum score 82), or PTE (minimum score 53). *Application deadline:* Applications are processed on a rolling basis. Application fee: $0. Electronic applications accepted. *Financial support:* Fellowships, Federal Work-Study, scholarships/grants, unspecified assistantships, and family tuition reduction, active duty/veteran tuition reduction, group tuition reduction, interest-free payment plans, employee tuition reduction available. Support available to part-time students. Financial award applicants required to submit FAFSA. *Unit head:* Dr. Jorg Westermann, Dean, 866-492-5336. *Application contact:* Meghan Thomas, Vice President of Enrollment Management, 866-492-5336, E-mail: info@waldenu.edu.
Website: http://www.waldenu.edu/colleges-schools/school-of-health-sciences

West Virginia University, School of Medicine, Department of Community Medicine, Morgantown, WV 26506. Offers public health (MPH), including community health/preventative medicine; public health sciences (PhD). *Accreditation:* CEPH. *Program availability:* Part-time, evening/weekend, online learning. *Degree requirements:* For master's, thesis (for some programs). *Entrance requirements:* For master's, minimum GPA of 3.0. Additional exam requirements/recommendations for international students: Required—TOEFL. *Expenses:* Tuition, state resident: full-time $8568. Tuition, nonresident: full-time $22,140. Tuition and fees vary according to program. *Faculty research:* Adolescent smoking cessation, cardiovascular disease, women's health, worker's health.

Wilfrid Laurier University, Faculty of Graduate and Postdoctoral Studies, Faculty of Science, Department of Kinesiology and Physical Education, Waterloo, ON N2L 3C5, Canada. Offers physical activity and health (M Sc). *Degree requirements:* For master's, thesis. *Entrance requirements:* For master's, honours degree in kinesiology, health, physical education with a minimum B+ in kinesiology and health-related courses. Additional exam requirements/recommendations for international students: Required—TOEFL (minimum score 89 iBT). Electronic applications accepted. *Faculty research:* Biomechanics, health, exercise physiology, motor control, sport psychology.

Wright State University, School of Medicine, Program in Public Health, Dayton, OH 45435. Offers health promotion and education (MPH); public health management (MPH); public health nursing (MPH). *Accreditation:* CEPH.

Industrial Hygiene

California State University, Northridge, Graduate Studies, College of Health and Human Development, Department of Environmental and Occupational Health, Northridge, CA 91330. Offers environmental and occupational health (MS); industrial hygiene (MS). *Faculty:* 7 full-time (5 women), 9 part-time/adjunct (all women). *Students:* 26 full-time (19 women), 35 part-time (19 women); includes 37 minority (6 Black or African American, non-Hispanic/Latino; 19 Asian, non-Hispanic/Latino; 10 Hispanic/Latino; 2 Two or more races, non-Hispanic/Latino), 4 international. Average age 31. 52 applicants, 52% accepted, 19 enrolled. *Degree requirements:* For master's, seminar, field experience, comprehensive exam or thesis. *Entrance requirements:* For master's, GRE General Test or minimum GPA of 3.0. Additional exam requirements/recommendations for international students: Required—TOEFL. *Application deadline:* For fall admission, 11/30 for domestic students. Application fee: $55. *Financial support:* Application deadline: 3/1. *Unit head:* Peter Bellin, Chair, 818-677-7476.
Website: http://www.csun.edu/hhd/eoh/

Montana Tech of The University of Montana, Graduate School, Department of Industrial Hygiene, Butte, MT 59701-8997. Offers MS. *Accreditation:* ABET. *Program availability:* Part-time, online learning. *Faculty:* 7 full-time (2 women). *Students:* 2 full-time (both women), 79 part-time (29 women); includes 10 minority (2 Black or African American, non-Hispanic/Latino; 1 Asian, non-Hispanic/Latino; 6 Hispanic/Latino; 1 Native Hawaiian or other Pacific Islander, non-Hispanic/Latino). 31 applicants, 32% accepted, 10 enrolled. In 2015, 23 master's awarded. *Degree requirements:* For master's, comprehensive exam (for some programs), thesis. *Entrance requirements:* For master's, GRE or 5 years' work experience (for online program), minimum GPA of 3.0. Additional exam requirements/recommendations for international students: Required—TOEFL (minimum score 545 paper-based; 78 iBT), IELTS (minimum score 6.5). *Application deadline:* For fall admission, 4/1 priority date for domestic students; for spring admission, 10/1 priority date for domestic students. Applications are processed on a rolling basis. Application fee: $50. Electronic applications accepted. *Expenses:* Tuition, state resident: full-time $2901; part-time $1450.68 per degree program. Tuition, nonresident: full-time $8432; part-time $4215.84 per degree program. *Required fees:* $668; $354 per degree program. Tuition and fees vary according to course load and program. *Financial support:* In 2015–16, 15 students received support, including 9 teaching assistantships with partial tuition reimbursements available (averaging $2,400 per year); research assistantships with partial tuition reimbursements available, career-related internships or fieldwork, institutionally sponsored loans, and tuition waivers (full and partial) also available. Financial award application deadline: 4/1; financial award applicants required to submit FAFSA. *Faculty research:* Ergonomics, metal bioavailability, aerosols, particulate sizing, respiration protection. *Unit head:* Dr. Terry Spear, Head, 406-496-4445, Fax: 406-496-4650, E-mail: tspear@mtech.edu. *Application contact:* Daniel Stirling, Administrator, Graduate School, 406-496-4304, Fax: 406-496-4710, E-mail: gradschool@mtech.edu.
Website: http://www.mtech.edu/academics/gradschool/degreeprograms/degrees-industrial-hygiene.htm

Murray State University, College of Health Sciences and Human Services, Program in Occupational Safety and Health, Murray, KY 42071. Offers environmental science (MS); industrial hygiene (MS); safety management (MS). *Accreditation:* ABET. *Program availability:* Part-time. *Degree requirements:* For master's, comprehensive exam, thesis optional, professional internship. Electronic applications accepted. *Faculty research:* Light effects on plant growth, ergonomics, toxic effects of pets' pesticides, traffic safety.

New York Medical College, School of Health Sciences and Practice, Department of Environmental Health Science, Graduate Certificate Program in Industrial Hygiene, Valhalla, NY 10595-1691. Offers Graduate Certificate. *Expenses: Tuition, area resident:* Full-time $44,355; part-time $1025 per credit. *Required fees:* $500; $95 per year. One-time fee: $140 part-time. Tuition and fees vary according to course load and program.

The University of Alabama at Birmingham, School of Public Health, Program in Environmental Health Sciences, Birmingham, AL 35294. Offers environmental health sciences research (PhD); industrial hygiene (PhD). *Degree requirements:* For doctorate, comprehensive exam, thesis/dissertation. *Entrance requirements:* For doctorate, GRE General Test. Additional exam requirements/recommendations for international students: Recommended—TOEFL, IELTS. Electronic applications accepted. *Expenses:* Tuition, state resident: full-time $7340. Tuition, nonresident: full-time $16,628. Full-time tuition and fees vary according to course load and program. *Faculty research:* Aquatic toxicology, virology.

The University of Alabama at Birmingham, School of Public Health, Program in Public Health, Birmingham, AL 35294. Offers applied epidemiology and pharmacoepidemiology (MSPH); biostatistics (MPH); clinical and translational science (MSPH); environmental health (MPH); environmental health and toxicology (MSPH); epidemiology (MPH); general theory and practice (MPH); health behavior (MPH); health care organization (MPH); health policy quantitative policy analysis (MPH); industrial hygiene (MPH, MSPH); maternal and child health policy (Dr PH); maternal and child health policy and leadership (MPH); occupational health and safety (MPH); outcomes research (MSPH, Dr PH); public health (PhD); public health management (Dr PH); public health preparedness management (MPH). *Accreditation:* CEPH. *Program availability:* Part-time, online learning. *Degree requirements:* For doctorate, comprehensive exam, thesis/dissertation. *Entrance requirements:* For master's and doctorate, GRE. Additional exam requirements/recommendations for international students: Recommended—TOEFL (minimum score 550 paper-based; 79 iBT), IELTS (minimum score 6.5). Electronic applications accepted. *Expenses:* Tuition, state resident: full-time $7340. Tuition, nonresident: full-time $16,628. Full-time tuition and fees vary according to course load and program.

University of Central Missouri, The Graduate School, Warrensburg, MO 64093. Offers accountancy (MA); accounting (MBA); applied mathematics (MS); aviation safety (MA); biology (MS); business administration (MBA); career and technical education leadership (MS); college student personnel administration (MS); communication (MA); computer science (MS); counseling (MS); criminal justice (MS); educational leadership (Ed D); educational technology (MS); elementary and early childhood education (MSE); English (MA); environmental studies (MA); finance (MBA); history (MA); human services/educational technology (Ed S); human services/learning resources (Ed S); human services/professional counseling (Ed S); industrial hygiene (MS); industrial management (MS); information systems (MBA); information technology (MS); kinesiology (MS); library science and information services (MS); literacy education (MSE); marketing (MBA); mathematics (MS); music (MA); occupational safety management (MS); psychology (MS); rural family nursing (MS); school administration (MSE); social gerontology (MS); sociology (MA); special education (MSE); speech language pathology (MS); superintendency (Ed S); teaching (MAT); teaching English as a second language (MS); technology (MS); technology management (PhD); theatre (MA). *Program availability:* Part-time, 100% online, blended/hybrid learning. *Faculty:* 336 full-time (145 women), 39 part-time/adjunct (25 women). *Students:* 2,161 full-time (723 women), 2,077 part-time (1,061 women); includes 188 minority (93 Black or African American, non-Hispanic/Latino; 4 American Indian or Alaska Native, non-Hispanic/Latino; 15 Asian, non-Hispanic/Latino; 32 Hispanic/Latino; 1 Native Hawaiian or other Pacific Islander, non-Hispanic/Latino; 43 Two or more races, non-Hispanic/Latino), 2,514 international. Average age 28. 3,454 applicants, 68% accepted, 1632 enrolled. In 2015, 1,530 master's, 53 other advanced degrees awarded. *Degree requirements:* For master's and Ed S, comprehensive exam (for some programs), thesis (for some programs). *Entrance requirements:* Additional exam requirements/recommendations for international students: Required—TOEFL (minimum score 550 paper-based; 79 iBT). *Application deadline:* For fall admission, 6/1 priority date for domestic and international students; for spring admission, 10/1 priority date for domestic and international students; for summer admission, 4/1 priority date for domestic and international students. Applications are processed on a rolling basis. Application fee: $30 ($75 for international students). Electronic applications accepted. *Expenses:* Tuition, state resident: full-time $6683; part-time $278.45 per credit hour. Tuition, nonresident: full-time $13,366; part-time $556.90 per credit hour. *Required fees:* $701; $29.20 per credit hour. Tuition and fees vary according to degree level and campus/location. *Financial support:* In 2015–16, 97 students received support, including 146 research assistantships with partial tuition reimbursements available (averaging $7,500 per year), 73 teaching assistantships with partial tuition reimbursements available (averaging $7,500 per year); career-related internships or fieldwork, Federal Work-Study, scholarships/grants, and administrative and laboratory assistantships also available. Support available to part-time students. Financial award application deadline: 3/1; financial award applicants required to submit FAFSA. *Unit head:* Tina Church-Hockett, Director of Graduate School and International Admissions, 660-543-4621, Fax: 660-543-4778, E-mail: church@ucmo.edu. *Application contact:* Brittany Lawrence, Graduate Student Services Coordinator, 660-543-4621, Fax: 660-543-4778, E-mail: gradinfo@ucmo.edu.
Website: http://www.ucmo.edu/graduate/

Industrial Hygiene

University of Cincinnati, Graduate School, College of Medicine, Graduate Programs in Biomedical Sciences, Department of Environmental Health, Cincinnati, OH 45221. Offers environmental and industrial hygiene (MS, PhD); environmental and occupational medicine (MS); environmental genetics and molecular toxicology (MS, PhD); epidemiology and biostatistics (MS, PhD); occupational safety and ergonomics (MS, PhD). *Accreditation:* ABET (one or more programs are accredited). Terminal master's awarded for partial completion of doctoral program. *Degree requirements:* For master's, thesis; for doctorate, thesis/dissertation, qualifying exam. *Entrance requirements:* For master's, GRE General Test, bachelor's degree in science; for doctorate, GRE General Test. Additional exam requirements/recommendations for international students: Required—TOEFL (minimum score 600 paper-based; 100 iBT). Electronic applications accepted. *Faculty research:* Carcinogens and mutagenesis, pulmonary studies, reproduction and development.

The University of Iowa, Graduate College, College of Public Health, Department of Occupational and Environmental Health, Iowa City, IA 52242-1316. Offers agricultural safety and health (MS, PhD); ergonomics (MPH); industrial hygiene (MS, PhD); occupational and environmental health (MPH, MS, PhD, Certificate); MS/MA; MS/MS. *Accreditation:* ABET (one or more programs are accredited); CEPH. *Degree requirements:* For master's, thesis optional, exam; for doctorate, comprehensive exam, thesis/dissertation. *Entrance requirements:* For master's and doctorate, GRE General Test, minimum GPA of 3.0. Additional exam requirements/recommendations for international students: Required—TOEFL (minimum score 600 paper-based; 100 iBT). Electronic applications accepted.

University of Michigan, School of Public Health, Department of Environmental Health Sciences, Ann Arbor, MI 48109. Offers environmental health sciences (MS, PhD); environmental quality and health (MPH); industrial hygiene (MPH, MS); occupational and environmental epidemiology (MPH); toxicology (MPH, MS, PhD). *Accreditation:* CEPH (one or more programs are accredited). *Program availability:* Part-time. *Faculty:* 22 full-time (7 women), 28 part-time/adjunct (9 women). *Students:* 76 full-time (53 women), 3 part-time (all women); includes 13 minority (4 Black or African American, non-Hispanic/Latino; 5 Asian, non-Hispanic/Latino; 2 Hispanic/Latino; 2 Two or more races, non-Hispanic/Latino), 12 international. Average age 27. 263 applicants, 39% accepted, 39 enrolled. In 2015, 50 master's, 8 doctorates awarded. Terminal master's awarded for partial completion of doctoral program. *Degree requirements:* For master's, thesis (for some programs); for doctorate, thesis/dissertation, preliminary exam, oral defense of dissertation. *Entrance requirements:* For master's and doctorate, GRE General Test and/or MCAT. Additional exam requirements/recommendations for international students: Required—TOEFL (minimum score 100 iBT). *Application deadline:* For fall admission, 12/15 priority date for domestic students, 1/15 for international students. Applications are processed on a rolling basis. Application fee: $75. Electronic applications accepted. *Financial support:* Fellowships, research assistantships, teaching assistantships, career-related internships or fieldwork, Federal Work-Study, institutionally sponsored loans, scholarships/grants, traineeships, health care benefits, and unspecified assistantships available. Financial award application deadline: 12/15. *Faculty research:* Toxicology, occupational hygiene, environmental exposure sciences, environmental epidemiology. *Unit head:* Dr. Craig Harris, Chair, 734-939-3397, E-mail: charris@umich.edu. *Application contact:* Susan Crawford, Student Administrative Coordinator, 734-764-3018, E-mail: sph.inquiries@umich.edu. Website: http://www.sph.umich.edu/ehs/

University of Minnesota, Twin Cities Campus, School of Public Health, Division of Environmental Health Sciences, Area in Industrial Hygiene, Minneapolis, MN 55455-0213. Offers MPH, MS, PhD. *Accreditation:* ABET (one or more programs are accredited); CEPH (one or more programs are accredited). *Degree requirements:* For doctorate, thesis/dissertation. *Entrance requirements:* For master's and doctorate, GRE General Test. Electronic applications accepted.

The University of North Carolina at Chapel Hill, Graduate School, Gillings School of Global Public Health, Department of Environmental Sciences and Engineering, Chapel Hill, NC 27599. Offers air, radiation and industrial hygiene (MPH, MS, MSEE, MSPH, PhD); aquatic and atmospheric sciences (MPH, MS, MSPH, PhD); environmental engineering (MPH, MS, MSEE, MSPH, PhD); environmental health sciences (MPH, MS, MSPH, PhD); environmental management and policy (MPH, MS, MSPH, PhD). *Students:* 112 full-time (68 women); includes 20 minority (11 Asian, non-Hispanic/Latino; 4 Hispanic/Latino; 5 Two or more races, non-Hispanic/Latino), 31 international. Average age 28. 178 applicants, 37% accepted, 39 enrolled. Terminal master's awarded for partial completion of doctoral program. *Degree requirements:* For master's, comprehensive exam, thesis (for some programs), research paper; for doctorate, comprehensive exam, thesis/dissertation. *Entrance requirements:* For master's and

doctorate, GRE General Test, minimum GPA of 3.0 (recommended). Additional exam requirements/recommendations for international students: Required—TOEFL. *Application deadline:* For fall admission, 12/10 priority date for domestic and international students; for spring admission, 9/10 for domestic students. Applications are processed on a rolling basis. Application fee: $85. Electronic applications accepted. *Financial support:* Fellowships with tuition reimbursements, research assistantships with tuition reimbursements, teaching assistantships with tuition reimbursements, career-related internships or fieldwork, Federal Work-Study, traineeships, health care benefits, and unspecified assistantships available. Support available to part-time students. Financial award application deadline: 12/10; financial award applicants required to submit FAFSA. *Faculty research:* Air, radiation and industrial hygiene, aquatic and atmospheric sciences, environmental health sciences, environmental management and policy, water resources engineering. *Unit head:* Dr. Michael Aitken, Chair, 919-966-1024, Fax: 919-966-7911, E-mail: mike_aitken@unc.edu. *Application contact:* Jack Whaley, Registrar, 919-966-3844, Fax: 919-966-7911, E-mail: jack_whaley@unc.edu.
Website: http://www2.sph.unc.edu/envr/

University of Puerto Rico, Medical Sciences Campus, Graduate School of Public Health, Department of Environmental Health, Program in Industrial Hygiene, San Juan, PR 00936-5067. Offers MS. *Program availability:* Part-time. *Degree requirements:* For master's, thesis. *Entrance requirements:* For master's, GRE, previous course work in biology, chemistry, mathematics, and physics. *Expenses:* Contact institution.

University of South Carolina, The Graduate School, Arnold School of Public Health, Department of Environmental Health Sciences, Program in Industrial Hygiene, Columbia, SC 29208. Offers MPH, MSPH, PhD. *Accreditation:* CEPH (one or more programs are accredited). *Degree requirements:* For master's, comprehensive exam, thesis (for some programs), practicum (MPH); for doctorate, one foreign language, comprehensive exam, thesis/dissertation. *Entrance requirements:* Additional exam requirements/recommendations for international students: Required—TOEFL (minimum score 570 paper-based). Electronic applications accepted. *Faculty research:* Sampling and calibration method development, exposure and risk assessment, respirator and dermal protective equipment, ergonomics, air cleaning methods and devices.

The University of Toledo, College of Graduate Studies, College of Medicine and Life Sciences, Department of Public Health and Preventative Medicine, Toledo, OH 43606-3390. Offers biostatistics and epidemiology (Certificate); contemporary gerontological practice (Certificate); environmental and occupational health and safety (MPH); epidemiology (Certificate); global public health (Certificate); health promotion and education (MPH); industrial hygiene (MSOH); medical and health science teaching and learning (Certificate); occupational health (Certificate); public health administration (MPH); public health and emergency response (Certificate); public health epidemiology (MPH); public health nutrition (MPH); MD/MPH. *Program availability:* Part-time, evening/weekend. *Degree requirements:* For master's, thesis or alternative. *Entrance requirements:* For master's, GRE, minimum undergraduate GPA of 3.0, three letters of recommendation, statement of purpose, transcripts from all prior institutions attended, resume; for Certificate, minimum undergraduate GPA of 3.0, three letters of recommendation, statement of purpose, transcripts from all prior institutions attended, resume. Additional exam requirements/recommendations for international students: Required—TOEFL (minimum score 550 paper-based; 80 iBT), IELTS (minimum score 6.5). Electronic applications accepted.

University of Wisconsin–Stout, Graduate School, College of Management, Program in Risk Control, Menomonie, WI 54751. Offers MS. *Program availability:* Part-time. *Degree requirements:* For master's, thesis. *Entrance requirements:* For master's, minimum GPA of 3.0. Additional exam requirements/recommendations for international students: Required—TOEFL (minimum score 500 paper-based; 61 iBT). Electronic applications accepted. *Faculty research:* Environmental microbiology, water supply safety, facilities planning, industrial ventilation, bioterrorist.

West Virginia University, Statler College of Engineering and Mineral Resources, Department of Industrial and Management Systems Engineering, Program in Industrial Hygiene, Morgantown, WV 26506. Offers MS. *Accreditation:* ABET. *Program availability:* Part-time. *Degree requirements:* For master's, thesis or alternative. *Entrance requirements:* For master's, GRE General Test, minimum GPA of 3.0. Additional exam requirements/recommendations for international students: Required—TOEFL. *Expenses:* Tuition, state resident: full-time $8568. Tuition, nonresident: full-time $22,140. Tuition and fees vary according to program. *Faculty research:* Safety management, ergonomics and workplace design, safety and health training, construction safety.

International Health

Arizona State University at the Tempe campus, College of Liberal Arts and Sciences, School of Human Evolution and Social Change, Tempe, AZ 85287-2402. Offers anthropology (MA, PhD), including anthropology (PhD), archaeology (PhD), bioarchaeology (PhD), evolutionary (PhD), museum studies (MA), sociocultural (PhD); applied mathematics for the life and social sciences (PhD); environmental social science (PhD), including environmental social science, urbanism; global health (MA, PhD), including complex adaptive systems science (PhD), evolutionary global health sciences (PhD), health and culture (PhD), urbanism (PhD); immigration studies (Graduate Certificate). Terminal master's awarded for partial completion of doctoral program. *Degree requirements:* For master's, thesis or alternative, interactive Program of Study (iPOS) submitted before completing 50 percent of required credit hours; for doctorate, comprehensive exam, thesis/dissertation, interactive Program of Study (iPOS) submitted before completing 50 percent of required credit hours. *Entrance requirements:* For master's and doctorate, GRE, minimum GPA of 3.0 or equivalent in last 2 years of work leading to bachelor's degree. Additional exam requirements/recommendations for international students: Required—TOEFL, IELTS, or PTE. Electronic applications accepted.

Boston University, School of Public Health, Global Health Department, Boston, MA 02215. Offers MPH, Dr PH. *Accreditation:* CEPH (one or more programs are accredited). *Program availability:* Part-time, evening/weekend. *Faculty:* 29 full-time, 37 part-time/adjunct. *Students:* 142 full-time (119 women), 57 part-time (50 women); includes 56 minority (15 Black or African American, non-Hispanic/Latino; 24 Asian, non-Hispanic/Latino; 10 Hispanic/Latino; 1 Native Hawaiian or other Pacific Islander, non-Hispanic/Latino; 6 Two or more races, non-Hispanic/Latino), 27 international. Average age 26. 656 applicants, 54% accepted, 108 enrolled. *Degree requirements:* For doctorate, thesis/dissertation. *Entrance requirements:* For master's, GRE, MCAT,

GMAT; for doctorate, GRE, GMAT. Additional exam requirements/recommendations for international students: Required—TOEFL (minimum score 600 paper-based; 100 iBT), IELTS (minimum score 7). *Application deadline:* For fall admission, 1/1 priority date for domestic and international students; for spring admission, 10/1 priority date for domestic students. Applications are processed on a rolling basis. Application fee: $115. Electronic applications accepted. *Financial support:* Career-related internships or fieldwork, Federal Work-Study, institutionally sponsored loans, and scholarships/grants available. Financial award application deadline: 3/1; financial award applicants required to submit FAFSA. *Faculty research:* Pharmaceutical assessment, monitoring and evaluation, program management, capacity building, program assessment. *Unit head:* Dr. Frank Richard Feeley, Interim Chair, 617-638-5234, E-mail: gh@bu.edu. *Application contact:* LePhan Quan, Associate Director of Admissions, 617-638-4640, Fax: 617-638-5299, E-mail: asksph@bu.edu.
Website: http://www.bu.edu/sph/academics/departments/global-health

Brandeis University, The Heller School for Social Policy and Management, Program in International Health Policy and Management, Waltham, MA 02454-9110. Offers MS. *Entrance requirements:* For master's, 3 letters of recommendation, curriculum vitae or resume, 5 years of international health experience. Additional exam requirements/recommendations for international students: Required—TOEFL (minimum score 600 paper-based; 100 iBT). Electronic applications accepted. *Faculty research:* International development, health financing, and health systems.

Brandeis University, The Heller School for Social Policy and Management, Program in Social Policy, Waltham, MA 02454-9110. Offers assets and inequalities (PhD); children, youth and families (PhD); global health and development (PhD); health and behavioral health (PhD). *Degree requirements:* For doctorate, comprehensive exam, thesis/dissertation, qualifying paper, 2-year residency. *Entrance requirements:* For doctorate,

GRE General Test, 3 letters of recommendation, statement of purpose, writing sample, at least 3-5 years of professional experience. Additional exam requirements/recommendations for international students: Required—TOEFL (minimum score 600 paper-based; 100 iBT). Electronic applications accepted. *Faculty research:* Health; mental health; substance abuse; children, youth, and families; aging; international and community development; disabilities; work and inequality; hunger and poverty.

Cedarville University, Graduate Programs, Cedarville, OH 45314-0601. Offers business administration (MBA); curriculum (M Ed); educational administration (M Ed); family nurse practitioner (MSN); global health ministries (MSN); instruction (M Ed); ministry (M Min); pharmacy (Pharm D). *Program availability:* Part-time, evening/weekend, online learning. *Faculty:* 61 full-time (26 women), 7 part-time/adjunct (2 women). *Students:* 201 full-time (116 women), 100 part-time (71 women); includes 53 minority (32 Black or African American, non-Hispanic/Latino; 3 American Indian or Alaska Native, non-Hispanic/Latino; 15 Asian, non-Hispanic/Latino; 2 Hispanic/Latino; 1 Native Hawaiian or other Pacific Islander, non-Hispanic/Latino), 5 international. Average age 30. 142 applicants, 58% accepted, 57 enrolled. In 2015, 41 degrees awarded. *Degree requirements:* For master's, thesis. *Entrance requirements:* For master's, GRE, 2 professional recommendations; for doctorate, PCAT, professional recommendation from a practicing pharmacist or current employer/supervisor, resume, essay, interview. Additional exam requirements/recommendations for international students: Required—TOEFL (minimum score 550 paper-based; 80 iBT). *Application deadline:* For fall admission, 5/1 priority date for domestic and international students; for spring admission, 11/1 priority date for domestic and international students. Applications are processed on a rolling basis. Application fee: $0. Electronic applications accepted. *Expenses:* Contact institution. *Financial support:* In 2015–16, 129 students received support. Scholarships/grants and unspecified assistantships available. Support available to part-time students. Financial award applicants required to submit FAFSA. *Unit head:* Dr. Mark McClain, Dean of Graduate Studies, 937-766-7700, E-mail: mcclain@cedarville.edu. *Application contact:* Roscoe Smith, Associate Vice President for University Admissions, 937-766-7700, Fax: 937-766-7575, E-mail: smithr@cedarville.edu.
Website: http://www.cedarville.edu/academics/graduate/

Central Michigan University, Central Michigan University Global Campus, Program in Health Administration, Mount Pleasant, MI 48859. Offers health administration (DHA); international health (Certificate); nutrition and dietetics (MS). *Program availability:* Part-time, evening/weekend, online learning. Electronic applications accepted.

Duke University, Graduate School, Duke Global Health Institute, Durham, NC 27708. Offers MS. *Degree requirements:* For master's, thesis. *Entrance requirements:* For master's, GRE General Test or MCAT. Additional exam requirements/recommendations for international students: Required—TOEFL (minimum score 577 paper-based; 90 iBT) or IELTS (minimum score 7).

Emory University, Rollins School of Public Health, Hubert Department of Global Health, Atlanta, GA 30322-1100. Offers global health (MPH); public nutrition (MSPH). *Accreditation:* CEPH. *Degree requirements:* For master's, thesis, practicum. *Entrance requirements:* For master's, GRE General Test. Additional exam requirements/recommendations for international students: Required—TOEFL (minimum score 550 paper-based; 80 iBT). Electronic applications accepted.

George Mason University, College of Health and Human Services, Department of Global and Community Health, Fairfax, VA 22030. Offers global and community health (Certificate); global health (MS); public health (MPH), including epidemiology. *Accreditation:* CEPH. *Faculty:* 14 full-time (10 women), 18 part-time/adjunct (14 women). *Students:* 62 full-time (56 women), 47 part-time (42 women); includes 50 minority (22 Black or African American, non-Hispanic/Latino; 16 Asian, non-Hispanic/Latino; 9 Hispanic/Latino; 3 Two or more races, non-Hispanic/Latino), 1 international. Average age 27. 121 applicants, 72% accepted, 44 enrolled. In 2015, 56 master's, 6 other advanced degrees awarded. *Degree requirements:* For master's, comprehensive exam (for some programs), thesis or practicum. *Entrance requirements:* For master's, GRE, GMAT (depending on program), 2 official transcripts; expanded goals statement; 3 letters of recommendation; resume; 1 completed course in health science, statistics, natural sciences and social science (for MPH); 6 credits of foreign language if not fluent (for MS); for Certificate, 2 official transcripts; expanded goals statement; 3 letters of recommendation; resume; bachelor's degree from regionally-accredited institution with minimum GPA of 3.0. Additional exam requirements/recommendations for international students: Required—TOEFL (minimum score 570 paper-based; 88 iBT), IELTS (minimum score 6.5), PTE (minimum score 59). *Application deadline:* For fall admission, 2/1 for domestic students. Application fee: $75 ($80 for international students). Electronic applications accepted. *Expenses:* Contact institution. *Financial support:* In 2015–16, 5 students received support, including 9 research assistantships with tuition reimbursements available (averaging $16,472 per year), 1 teaching assistantship with tuition reimbursement available (averaging $9,000 per year); career-related internships or fieldwork, Federal Work-Study, scholarships/grants, unspecified assistantships, and health care benefits (for full-time research or teaching assistantship recipients) also available. Financial award application deadline: 3/1; financial award applicants required to submit FAFSA. *Faculty research:* Health issues and the needs of affected populations at the regional and global level. *Total annual research expenditures:* $28,950. *Unit head:* Brian Gillette, Director, 703-993-4636, Fax: 703-993-1908, E-mail: bgillett@gmu.edu. *Application contact:* Ali Weinstein, Graduate Program Coordinator, 703-993-1908, E-mail: aweinst2@gmu.edu.
Website: http://chhs.gmu.edu/gch/index

George Mason University, College of Humanities and Social Sciences, Program in Global Affairs, Fairfax, VA 22030. Offers MA. *Faculty:* 18 full-time (7 women), 4 part-time/adjunct (2 women). *Students:* 28 full-time (16 women), 23 part-time (15 women); includes 19 minority (6 Black or African American, non-Hispanic/Latino; 3 Asian, non-Hispanic/Latino; 10 Hispanic/Latino), 5 international. Average age 28. 62 applicants, 68% accepted, 20 enrolled. In 2015, 30 master's awarded. *Degree requirements:* For master's, capstone seminar. *Entrance requirements:* For master's, GRE, expanded goals statement, 2 letters of recommendation, evidence of professional competency in a second language tested through Language Testing International or other means approved by the department. Additional exam requirements/recommendations for international students: Required—TOEFL (minimum score 575 paper-based; 88 iBT), IELTS (minimum score 6.5), PTE (minimum score 59). *Application deadline:* For fall admission, 3/15 for domestic students. Application fee: $75 ($80 for international students). Electronic applications accepted. *Financial support:* Career-related internships or fieldwork, Federal Work-Study, and scholarships/grants available. Financial award application deadline: 3/1; financial award applicants required to submit FAFSA. *Faculty research:* Social movements, globalization, law and economics, comparative politics, global environmentalism and governance, international business and economic development. *Unit head:* Lisa Breglia, Director, 703-993-9184, Fax: 703-993-1244, E-mail: lbreglia@gmu.edu. *Application contact:* Erin McSherry, Academic Advisor, 703-993-5639, Fax: 703-993-1244, E-mail: emcsherr@gmu.edu.
Website: http://globalaffairs.gmu.edu

Georgetown University, Law Center, Washington, DC 20001. Offers environmental law (LL M); global health law (LL M); global health law and international institutions (LL M); individualized study (LL M); international business and economic law (LL M); law (JD, SJD); national security law (LL M); securities and financial regulation (LL M); taxation (LL M); JD/LL M; JD/MA; JD/MBA; JD/MPH; JD/PhD. *Accreditation:* ABA. *Program availability:* Part-time, evening/weekend. *Degree requirements:* For master's, thesis; for doctorate, thesis/dissertation (for some programs). *Entrance requirements:* For master's, JD, LL B, or first law degree earned in country of origin; for doctorate, LSAT (for JD). Additional exam requirements/recommendations for international students: Required—TOEFL. *Expenses:* Contact institution. *Faculty research:* Constitutional law, legal history, jurisprudence.

The George Washington University, Milken Institute School of Public Health, Department of Global Health, Washington, DC 20052. Offers global health (Dr PH); global health communication (MPH). *Accreditation:* CEPH. *Faculty:* 13 full-time (7 women), 2 part-time/adjunct. *Students:* 3 full-time (1 woman), 23 part-time (19 women); includes 8 minority (5 Black or African American, non-Hispanic/Latino; 2 Asian, non-Hispanic/Latino; 1 Hispanic/Latino), 3 international. Average age 33. In 2015, 29 master's awarded. *Degree requirements:* For master's, case study or special project. *Entrance requirements:* For master's, GMAT, GRE General Test, or MCAT. Additional exam requirements/recommendations for international students: Required—TOEFL. *Application deadline:* For fall admission, 4/15 priority date for domestic students, 4/15 for international students; for spring admission, 11/1 for domestic and international students. Applications are processed on a rolling basis. Application fee: $75. *Financial support:* In 2015–16, 24 students received support. Tuition waivers available. Financial award application deadline: 2/15. *Unit head:* Prof. James Tielsch, Chair, 202-994-4124, Fax: 202-994-1955, E-mail: jtielsch@gwu.edu. *Application contact:* Jane Smith, Director of Admissions, 202-994-0248, Fax: 202-994-1860, E-mail: sphhsinfo@gwumc.edu.

Harvard University, Harvard T.H. Chan School of Public Health, Department of Global Health and Population, Boston, MA 02115. Offers SM, SD. *Program availability:* Part-time. *Faculty:* 61 full-time (20 women), 19 part-time/adjunct (5 women). *Students:* 114 full-time (80 women), 12 part-time (8 women); includes 31 minority (3 Black or African American, non-Hispanic/Latino; 19 Asian, non-Hispanic/Latino; 6 Hispanic/Latino; 3 Two or more races, non-Hispanic/Latino), 51 international. Average age 27. 428 applicants, 26% accepted, 78 enrolled. In 2015, 43 master's, 8 doctorates awarded. *Degree requirements:* For master's, thesis; for doctorate, thesis/dissertation, qualifying exam. *Entrance requirements:* For master's, GRE, MCAT; for doctorate, GRE. Additional exam requirements/recommendations for international students: Recommended—TOEFL (minimum score 600 paper-based; 100 iBT), IELTS (minimum score 7). *Application deadline:* For fall admission, 12/15 for domestic and international students. Application fee: $120. Electronic applications accepted. *Financial support:* Fellowships, research assistantships, teaching assistantships, Federal Work-Study, scholarships/grants, traineeships, and unspecified assistantships available. Support available to part-time students. Financial award application deadline: 2/15; financial award applicants required to submit FAFSA. *Faculty research:* Health systems, international health policy, economics, population and reproductive health, ecology. *Unit head:* Dr. Wafaie W. Fawzi, Chair, 617-432-1232, Fax: 617-432-2435, E-mail: mina@hsph.harvard.edu. *Application contact:* Vincent W. James, Director of Admissions, 617-432-1031, Fax: 617-432-7080, E-mail: admissions@hsph.harvard.edu.
Website: http://www.hsph.harvard.edu/global-health-and-population/

Johns Hopkins University, Bloomberg School of Public Health, Department of International Health, Baltimore, MD 21205. Offers global disease epidemiology and control (MHS, PhD); health systems (MHS, PhD); human nutrition (MHS, PhD); international health (MSPH, Dr PH); registered dietician (MSPH); social and behavioral interventions (MHS, PhD). *Degree requirements:* For master's, comprehensive exam, thesis (for some programs), 1-year full-time residency, 4-9 month internship; for doctorate, comprehensive exam, thesis/dissertation or alternative, 1.5 years' full-time residency, oral and written exams. *Entrance requirements:* For master's, GRE General Test or MCAT, 3 letters of recommendation, resume; for doctorate, GRE General Test or MCAT, 3 letters of recommendation, resume, transcripts. Additional exam requirements/recommendations for international students: Required—TOEFL (minimum score 600 paper-based; 100 iBT); Recommended—IELTS (minimum score 7). Electronic applications accepted. *Faculty research:* Nutrition, infectious diseases, health systems, health economics, humanitarian emergencies.

Liberty University, School of Health Sciences, Lynchburg, VA 24515. Offers biomedical sciences (MS); global health (MPH); health promotion (MPH); healthcare management (Certificate); nutrition (MPH). *Program availability:* Part-time, online learning. *Students:* 435 full-time (342 women), 609 part-time (489 women); includes 301 minority (238 Black or African American, non-Hispanic/Latino; 6 American Indian or Alaska Native, non-Hispanic/Latino; 25 Asian, non-Hispanic/Latino; 12 Hispanic/Latino; 1 Native Hawaiian or other Pacific Islander, non-Hispanic/Latino; 19 Two or more races, non-Hispanic/Latino), 71 international. Average age 33. 1,433 applicants, 43% accepted, 295 enrolled. In 2015, 50 master's, 8 other advanced degrees awarded. *Degree requirements:* For master's, thesis (for some programs). *Entrance requirements:* Additional exam requirements/recommendations for international students: Required—TOEFL (minimum score 600 paper-based; 100 iBT). Application fee: $50. *Unit head:* Dr. Ralph Linstra, Dean. *Application contact:* Jay Bridge, Director of Admissions, 800-424-9595, Fax: 800-628-7977, E-mail: gradadmissions@liberty.edu.

Loma Linda University, School of Public Health, Program in Global Health, Loma Linda, CA 92350. Offers MPH. *Accreditation:* CEPH. *Entrance requirements:* Additional exam requirements/recommendations for international students: Required—Michigan English Language Assessment Battery or TOEFL. *Application deadline:* Applications are processed on a rolling basis. Application fee: $100. *Expenses:* $880 per unit. *Financial support:* Application deadline: 5/15. *Unit head:* Donn Gaede, Director, 909-824-4902, E-mail: dgaede@llu.edu. *Application contact:* Wendy Genovez, Assistant Dean of Admissions and Records, 909-824-4694, Fax: 909-824-8087, E-mail: wgenovez@llu.edu.

Medical University of South Carolina, College of Health Professions, Program in Health Administration-Global, Charleston, SC 29425. Offers MHA. *Entrance requirements:* Additional exam requirements/recommendations for international students: Required—TOEFL.

New York Medical College, School of Health Sciences and Practice, Department of Health Policy and Management, Graduate Certificate Program in Global Health, Valhalla, NY 10595-1691. Offers Graduate Certificate. *Accreditation:* CEPH. *Program availability:* Part-time, evening/weekend. *Entrance requirements:* Additional exam requirements/recommendations for international students: Required—TOEFL (minimum score 637 paper-based; 96 iBT), IELTS (minimum score 7). Electronic applications accepted. *Expenses:* Tuition, area resident: Full-time $44,355; part-time $1025 per credit. *Required fees:* $500; $95 per year. One-time fee: $140 part-time. Tuition and fees vary according to course load and program.

New York University, College of Global Public Health, New York, NY 10003. Offers biological basis of public health (PhD); community and international health (MPH); global health leadership (MPH); health systems and health services research (PhD); population and community health (PhD); public health nutrition (MPH); social and behavioral sciences (MPH); socio-behavioral health (PhD). *Program availability:* Part-

International Health

time, online learning. *Degree requirements:* For master's, thesis (for some programs); for doctorate, thesis/dissertation. *Entrance requirements:* For master's and doctorate, GRE. Additional exam requirements/recommendations for international students: Required—TOEFL. Electronic applications accepted.

Northwestern University, School of Professional Studies, Program in Global Health, Evanston, IL 60208. Offers MS. Program offered in partnership with Northwestern University Feinberg School of Medicine?s Center for Global Health. *Program availability:* Online learning. *Degree requirements:* For master's, practicum.

Oregon State University, College of Public Health and Human Sciences, Program in Public Health, Corvallis, OR 97331. Offers biostatistics (MPH); environmental and occupational health and safety (MPH, PhD); epidemiology (MPH, PhD); health management and policy (MPH); health policy (PhD); health promotion and health behavior (MPH, PhD); international health (MPH). *Accreditation:* CEPH. *Program availability:* Part-time. *Faculty:* 32 full-time (18 women), 3 part-time/adjunct (0 women). *Students:* 123 full-time (91 women), 20 part-time (14 women); includes 43 minority (2 Black or African American, non-Hispanic/Latino; 2 American Indian or Alaska Native, non-Hispanic/Latino; 9 Asian, non-Hispanic/Latino; 18 Hispanic/Latino; 1 Native Hawaiian or other Pacific Islander, non-Hispanic/Latino; 11 Two or more races, non-Hispanic/Latino), 18 international. Average age 31. 276 applicants, 65% accepted, 45 enrolled. In 2015, 59 master's, 6 doctorates awarded. Terminal master's awarded for partial completion of doctoral program. *Degree requirements:* For doctorate, one foreign language, thesis/dissertation. *Entrance requirements:* For master's and doctorate, GRE, minimum GPA of 3.0 in last 90 hours. Additional exam requirements/recommendations for international students: Required—TOEFL (minimum score 80 iBT), IELTS (minimum score 6.5). *Application deadline:* For fall admission, 12/1 priority date for domestic students. Applications are processed on a rolling basis. *Expenses:* $13,851 full-time resident tuition, $23,679 full-time non-resident tuition, $1,572 fees. *Financial support:* Fellowships, research assistantships, teaching assistantships, career-related internships or fieldwork, Federal Work-Study, and institutionally sponsored loans available. Support available to part-time students. Financial award application deadline: 12/1. *Faculty research:* Traffic safety, health safety, injury control, health promotion. *Unit head:* Dr. Sheryl Thorburn, Professor/Co-Director. *Application contact:* Amanda Armington, Public Health Program Manager, 541-737-3825, E-mail: amanda.armington@oregonstate.edu.

Park University, School of Graduate and Professional Studies, Kansas City, MO 54105. Offers adult education (M Ed); business and government leadership (Graduate Certificate); business, government, and global society (MPA); communication and leadership (MA); creative and life writing (Graduate Certificate); disaster and emergency management (MPA, Graduate Certificate); educational leadership (M Ed); finance (MBA, Graduate Certificate); general business (MBA); global business (Graduate Certificate); healthcare administration (MHA); healthcare services management and leadership (Graduate Certificate); international business (MBA); language and literacy (M Ed), including English for speakers of other languages, special reading teacher/literacy coach; leadership of international healthcare organizations (Graduate Certificate); management information systems (MBA, Graduate Certificate); music performance (ADP, Graduate Certificate), including cello (MM, ADP), piano (MM, ADP), viola (MM, ADP), violin (MM, ADP); nonprofit and community services management (MPA); nonprofit leadership (Graduate Certificate); performance (MM), including cello (MM, ADP), piano (MM, ADP), viola (MM, ADP), violin (MM, ADP); public management (MPA); social work (MSW); teacher leadership (M Ed), including curriculum and assessment, instructional leader. *Program availability:* Part-time, evening/weekend, online learning. *Degree requirements:* For master's, comprehensive exam (for some programs), thesis (for some programs), internship (for some programs); exam (for some programs). *Entrance requirements:* For master's, GRE or GMAT (for some programs), teacher certification (for some M Ed programs), letters of recommendation, essay, resume (for some programs). Additional exam requirements/recommendations for international students: Required—TOEFL (minimum score 550 paper-based; 79 iBT), IELTS (minimum score 6). Electronic applications accepted.

San Diego State University, Graduate and Research Affairs, College of Health and Human Services, Graduate School of Public Health, San Diego, CA 92182. Offers environmental health (MPH); epidemiology (MPH, PhD), including biostatistics (MPH); global emergency preparedness and response (MS); global health (PhD); health behavior (PhD); health promotion (MPH); health services administration (MPH); toxicology (MS); MPH/MA; MSW/MPH. *Accreditation:* CAHME (one or more programs are accredited); CEPH (one or more programs are accredited). *Program availability:* Part-time. *Degree requirements:* For master's, comprehensive exam (for some programs), thesis (for some programs); for doctorate, thesis/dissertation. *Entrance requirements:* For master's, GMAT (MPH in health services administration), GRE General Test; for doctorate, GRE General Test. Additional exam requirements/recommendations for international students: Required—TOEFL. *Faculty research:* Evaluation of tobacco, AIDS prevalence and prevention, mammography, infant death project, Alzheimer's in elderly Chinese.

Seton Hall University, School of Diplomacy and International Relations, South Orange, NJ 07079-2697. Offers diplomacy and international relations (MA); global health management (Graduate Certificate); post-conflict state reconstruction and sustainability (Graduate Certificate); United Nations studies (Graduate Certificate); JD/MA; MA/MA; MBA/MA; MPA/MA. *Program availability:* Part-time, evening/weekend, 100% online, blended/hybrid learning. *Faculty:* 17 full-time, 10 part-time/adjunct. *Students:* 110. Average age 26. *Degree requirements:* For master's, thesis (for some programs), 45 credits; for Graduate Certificate, 15 credits. *Entrance requirements:* For master's, GRE, GMAT, or LSAT. Additional exam requirements/recommendations for international students: Required—TOEFL. *Application deadline:* For fall admission, 3/31 priority date for domestic students; for spring admission, 10/30 priority date for domestic students. Applications are processed on a rolling basis. Application fee: $75. Electronic applications accepted. *Expenses:* Contact institution. *Financial support:* In 2015–16, fellowships with partial tuition reimbursements (averaging $6,810 per year), research assistantships with partial tuition reimbursements (averaging $13,620 per year) were awarded; career-related internships or fieldwork, scholarships/grants, and unspecified assistantships also available. *Faculty research:* International economics and development, global health, United Nations, conflict negotiation, foreign policy analysis, international security, energy politics, Eastern and Central Europe, Latin America, Africa, peacemaking, genocide prevention, international organizations, international political economy, U.S.-China relations, democratization, international law, research methods. *Application contact:* Daniel Kristo, Director of Graduate Admissions, 973-275-2142, Fax: 973-275-2519, E-mail: daniel.kristo@shu.edu.
Website: http://diplomacy.shu.edu/

Simon Fraser University, Office of Graduate Studies, Faculty of Health Sciences, Burnaby, BC V5A 1S6, Canada. Offers global health (Graduate Diploma); health sciences (M Sc, PhD); public health (MPH). *Degree requirements:* For master's, thesis (for some programs); for doctorate, comprehensive exam, thesis/dissertation. *Entrance requirements:* For master's, minimum GPA of 3.0 (on scale of 4.33), or 3.33 based on last 60 credits of undergraduate courses; for doctorate, minimum GPA of 3.5 (on scale of 4.33); for Graduate Diploma, minimum GPA of 2.5 (on scale of 4.33), or 2.67 based

on the last 60 credits of undergraduate courses. Additional exam requirements/recommendations for international students: Recommended—TOEFL (minimum score 580 paper-based; 93 iBT), IELTS (minimum score 7), TWE (minimum score 5). Electronic applications accepted.

Syracuse University, David B. Falk College of Sport and Human Dynamics, MS Program in Global Health, Syracuse, NY 13244. Offers global health (MS). *Program availability:* Part-time. *Entrance requirements:* For master's, GRE, personal statement, official transcripts, letters of recommendation, resume. Additional exam requirements/recommendations for international students: Required—TOEFL (minimum score 100 iBT). *Application deadline:* For fall admission, 2/15 priority date for domestic and international students; for spring admission, 11/15 priority date for domestic and international students. Electronic applications accepted. *Expenses: Tuition, area resident:* Full-time $25,974; part-time $1443 per credit hour. *Required fees:* $802; $50 per course. Tuition and fees vary according to course load and program. *Financial support:* Fellowships, research assistantships, teaching assistantships, and career-related internships or fieldwork available. Financial award application deadline: 1/1. *Faculty research:* Cardiovascular disease risk in children, environmental toxicants, health disparities and socioeconomic status, stress and health. *Unit head:* Dr. Brooks Gump, Graduate Program Director, 315-443-2208, E-mail: bbgump@syr.edu. *Application contact:* Felicia Otero, Director of College Admissions, 315-443-5555, Fax: 315-443-2562, E-mail: falk@syr.edu.
Website: http://falk.syr.edu/HealthWellness/GlobalHealth_CAS.aspx

Trident University International, College of Health Sciences, Program in Health Sciences, Cypress, CA 90630. Offers clinical research administration (MS, Certificate); emergency and disaster management (MS, Certificate); environmental health science (Certificate); health care administration (PhD); health care management (MS), including health informatics; health education (MS, Certificate); health informatics (Certificate); health sciences (PhD); international health (MS); international health: educator or researcher option (PhD); international health: practitioner option (PhD); law and expert witness studies (MS, Certificate); public health (MS); quality assurance (Certificate). *Program availability:* Part-time, evening/weekend, online learning. *Degree requirements:* For doctorate, comprehensive exam, thesis/dissertation, defense of dissertation. *Entrance requirements:* For master's, minimum GPA of 2.5 (students with GPA 3.0 or greater may transfer up to 30% of graduate level credits); for doctorate, minimum GPA of 3.4, curriculum vitae, course work in research methods or statistics. Additional exam requirements/recommendations for international students: Required—TOEFL. Electronic applications accepted.

Tufts University, The Fletcher School of Law and Diplomacy, Medford, MA 02155. Offers LL M, MA, MALD, MIB, PhD, DVM/MA, JD/MALD, MALD/MA, MALD/MBA, MALD/MS, MD/MA. *Program availability:* Online learning. *Degree requirements:* For master's, one foreign language, thesis; for doctorate, one foreign language, comprehensive exam, thesis/dissertation, dissertation defense. *Entrance requirements:* For master's and doctorate, GMAT or GRE General Test. Additional exam requirements/recommendations for international students: Required—TOEFL (minimum score 600 paper-based; 100 iBT), IELTS (minimum score 7). Electronic applications accepted. *Expenses:* Contact institution. *Faculty research:* Negotiation and conflict resolution, international organizations, international business and economic law, security studies, development economics.

Tulane University, School of Public Health and Tropical Medicine, Department of Global community Health and Behavioral Sciences, New Orleans, LA 70118-5669. Offers community health sciences (MPH); global community health and behavioral sciences (Dr PH, PhD); JD/MPH; MD/MPH; MSW/MPH. *Program availability:* Part-time. *Degree requirements:* For doctorate, comprehensive exam, thesis/dissertation. *Entrance requirements:* For master's and doctorate, GRE General Test. Additional exam requirements/recommendations for international students: Required—TOEFL. *Application deadline:* For fall admission, 4/15 priority date for domestic and international students; for spring admission, 10/15 for domestic students, 10/15 priority date for international students. Applications are processed on a rolling basis. Electronic applications accepted. *Expenses: Tuition, area resident:* Full-time $47,658; part-time $2648 per credit hour. *Required fees:* $1980; $44.50 per credit hour. $550 per term. Tuition and fees vary according to course load, degree level and program. *Financial support:* Federal Work-Study, scholarships/grants, and traineeships available. Support available to part-time students. Financial award application deadline: 4/15.

Tulane University, School of Public Health and Tropical Medicine, Department of Global Environmental Health Sciences, New Orleans, LA 70118-5669. Offers MPH, MSPH, PhD, JD/MPH, MD/MPH, MSW/MPH. *Accreditation:* ABET (one or more programs are accredited); CEPH (one or more programs are accredited). *Degree requirements:* For doctorate, comprehensive exam, thesis/dissertation. *Entrance requirements:* For master's and doctorate, GRE General Test. Additional exam requirements/recommendations for international students: Required—TOEFL. *Application deadline:* For fall admission, 4/15 priority date for domestic and international students; for spring admission, 10/15 priority date for domestic and international students. Applications are processed on a rolling basis. Application fee: $40. Electronic applications accepted. *Expenses: Tuition, area resident:* Full-time $47,658; part-time $2648 per credit hour. *Required fees:* $1980; $44.50 per credit hour. $550 per term. Tuition and fees vary according to course load, degree level and program. *Financial support:* Federal Work-Study, scholarships/grants, and traineeships available. Support available to part-time students. Financial award application deadline: 4/15.

Tulane University, School of Public Health and Tropical Medicine, Department of Global Health Management and Policy, New Orleans, LA 70118-5669. Offers MHA, MPH, PhD, Sc D, JD/MHA, MBA/MHA, MD/MPH, MSW/MPH. *Accreditation:* CAHME (one or more programs are accredited). *Degree requirements:* For doctorate, comprehensive exam, thesis/dissertation. *Entrance requirements:* For master's, GMAT, GRE General Test; for doctorate, GRE General Test. Additional exam requirements/recommendations for international students: Required—TOEFL. *Application deadline:* For fall admission, 4/15 priority date for domestic and international students; for spring admission, 10/15 priority date for domestic and international students. Applications are processed on a rolling basis. Application fee: $40. Electronic applications accepted. *Expenses: Tuition, area resident:* Full-time $47,658; part-time $2648 per credit hour. *Required fees:* $1980; $44.50 per credit hour. $550 per term. Tuition and fees vary according to course load, degree level and program. *Financial support:* Fellowships with tuition reimbursements, Federal Work-Study, scholarships/grants, traineeships, and tuition waivers (partial) available. Support available to part-time students. Financial award application deadline: 4/15. *Faculty research:* Health policy, organizational governance, international health administration.

Uniformed Services University of the Health Sciences, F. Edward Hebert School of Medicine, Graduate Programs in the Biomedical Sciences and Public Health, Bethesda, MD 20814. Offers emerging infectious diseases (PhD); medical and clinical psychology (PhD), including clinical psychology, medical psychology; medicine (MS, PhD), including health professions education; molecular and cell biology (MS, PhD); neuroscience (PhD); preventive medicine and biometrics (MPH, MS, MSPH, MTMH, Dr PH, PhD), including environmental health sciences (PhD), healthcare administration and policy (MS), medical zoology (PhD), public health (MPH, MSPH, Dr PH), tropical medicine and hygiene (MTMH). *Faculty:* 372 full-time (119 women), 4,044 part-time/adjunct (908 women). *Students:* 240 full-time (133 women); includes 40 minority (15 Black or African American, non-Hispanic/Latino; 13 Asian, non-Hispanic/Latino; 12 Hispanic/Latino), 30 international. Average age 25. 598 applicants, 17% accepted, 77 enrolled. In 2015, 19 master's, 50 doctorates awarded. Terminal master's awarded for partial completion of doctoral program. *Degree requirements:* For master's, comprehensive exam, thesis or alternative; for doctorate, comprehensive exam, thesis/dissertation, qualifying exam. *Entrance requirements:* For master's, GRE General Test; for doctorate, GRE General Test, minimum GPA of 3.0. *Application deadline:* For fall admission, 12/15 priority date for domestic students. Applications are processed on a rolling basis. Application fee: $0. Electronic applications accepted. *Financial support:* In 2015–16, 50 fellowships (averaging $43,000 per year) were awarded; research assistantships, career-related internships or fieldwork, scholarships/grants, health care benefits, and tuition waivers (full) also available. *Unit head:* Dr. Gregory Mueller, Associate Dean, 301-295-3507, E-mail: gregory.mueller@usuhs.edu. *Application contact:* Tina Finley, Administrative Officer, 301-295-3642, Fax: 301-295-6772, E-mail: netina.finley@usuhs.edu. Website: http://www.usuhs.mil/graded

Uniformed Services University of the Health Sciences, F. Edward Hebert School of Medicine, Graduate Programs in the Biomedical Sciences and Public Health, Department of Preventive Medicine and Biometrics, Program in Tropical Medicine and Hygiene, Bethesda, MD 20814-4799. Offers MTMH. *Accreditation:* CEPH. *Degree requirements:* For master's, comprehensive exam. *Entrance requirements:* For master's, GRE General Test, MD, U.S. citizenship. *Faculty research:* Epidemiology, biostatistics, tropical public health.

University of Alberta, School of Public Health, Department of Public Health Sciences, Edmonton, AB T6G 2E1, Canada. Offers clinical epidemiology (M Sc, MPH); environmental and occupational health (MPH); environmental health sciences (M Sc); epidemiology (M Sc); global health (M Sc, MPH); health policy and management (MPH); health policy research (M Sc); health technology assessment (MPH); occupational health (M Sc); population health (M Sc); public health leadership (MPH); public health sciences (PhD); quantitative methods (MPH). *Accreditation:* CEPH (one or more programs are accredited). Terminal master's awarded for partial completion of doctoral program. *Degree requirements:* For master's, thesis (for some programs); for doctorate, thesis/dissertation. *Entrance requirements:* For master's, GMAT or GRE General Test. Additional exam requirements/recommendations for international students: Required—TOEFL (minimum score 550 paper-based) or IELTS (minimum score 6). Electronic applications accepted. *Faculty research:* Biostatistics, health promotion and socio-behavioral health science.

University of California, San Diego, Graduate Division, Program in Public Health, La Jolla, CA 92093. Offers epidemiology (PhD); global health (PhD); health behavior (PhD). Program offered jointly with San Diego State University. *Students:* 16 full-time (13 women), 21 part-time (14 women); includes 11 minority (2 Black or African American, non-Hispanic/Latino; 3 Asian, non-Hispanic/Latino; 6 Hispanic/Latino), 4 international. In 2015, 12 doctorates awarded. *Degree requirements:* For doctorate, thesis/dissertation, 2 semesters/quarters of teaching assistantship. *Entrance requirements:* For doctorate, GRE General Test, minimum GPA of 3.0. Additional exam requirements/recommendations for international students: Required—TOEFL, IELTS. *Application deadline:* For fall admission, 12/15 priority date for domestic students. Electronic applications accepted. *Expenses:* Tuition, state resident: full-time $11,220. Tuition, nonresident: full-time $26,322. *Required fees:* $1800. *Financial support:* Teaching assistantships available. Financial award applicants required to submit FAFSA. *Faculty research:* Maternal and pediatric HIV/AIDS; healthy aging and gender differences; non-parametric and semi-parametric regression, resampling, and the analysis of high-dimensional data; neighborhood correlates of physical activity in children, teens, adults and older adults; medication safety and medication therapy management through practice-based research networks. *Unit head:* David Strong, Faculty Director, 858-657-5241, E-mail: dstrong@ucsd.edu. *Application contact:* Hollie Ward, Graduate Coordinator, 858-822-2382, E-mail: hcward@ucsd.edu. Website: http://publichealth.ucsd.edu/jdp/

University of Colorado Denver, Business School, Master of Business Administration Program, Denver, CO 80217. Offers bioinnovation and entrepreneurship (MBA); business intelligence (MBA); business strategy (MBA); business to business marketing (MBA); business to consumer marketing (MBA); change management (MBA); corporate financial management (MBA); enterprise technology management (MBA); entrepreneurship (MBA); health administration (MBA), including financial management, health administration, health information technologies, international health management and policy; human resources management (MBA); international business (MBA); investment management (MBA); managing for sustainability (MBA); sports and entertainment management (MBA). *Accreditation:* AACSB. *Program availability:* Part-time, evening/weekend, 100% online, blended/hybrid learning. *Students:* 541 full-time (211 women), 135 part-time (41 women); includes 82 minority (16 Black or African American, non-Hispanic/Latino; 2 American Indian or Alaska Native, non-Hispanic/Latino; 29 Asian, non-Hispanic/Latino; 30 Hispanic/Latino; 5 Two or more races, non-Hispanic/Latino), 24 international. Average age 33. 330 applicants, 75% accepted, 175 enrolled. In 2015, 290 master's awarded. *Degree requirements:* For master's, 48 semester hours, including 30 of core courses, 3 in international business, and 15 in electives from over 50 other graduate business courses. *Entrance requirements:* For master's, GMAT, resume, official transcripts, essay, two letters of recommendation, financial statements (for international applicants). Additional exam requirements/recommendations for international students: Required—TOEFL (minimum score 560 paper-based; 83 iBT); Recommended—IELTS (minimum score 6.5). *Application deadline:* For fall admission, 4/15 priority date for domestic students, 3/15 priority date for international students; for spring admission, 10/15 priority date for domestic students, 9/15 priority date for international students; for summer admission, 2/15 priority date for domestic students, 1/15 priority date for international students. Applications are processed on a rolling basis. Application fee: $50 ($75 for international students). Electronic applications accepted. *Expenses:* Contact institution. *Financial support:* In 2015–16, 202 students received support. Fellowships, research assistantships, teaching assistantships, Federal Work-Study, institutionally sponsored loans, scholarships/grants, traineeships, and unspecified assistantships available. Financial award application deadline: 4/1; financial award applicants required to submit FAFSA. *Faculty research:* Marketing, management, entrepreneurship, finance, health administration. *Unit head:* Woodrow Eckard, MBA Director, 303-315-8470, E-mail: woody.eckard@ucdenver.edu. *Application contact:* Shelly Townley, Admissions Director, Graduate Programs, 303-315-8202, E-mail: shelly.townley@ucdenver.edu. Website: http://www.ucdenver.edu/academics/colleges/business/degrees/mba/Pages/MBA.aspx

University of Colorado Denver, School of Medicine, Physician Assistant Program, Aurora, CO 80045. Offers child health associate (MPAS), including global health, leadership, education, advocacy, development, and scholarship, pediatric critical and acute care, rural health, urban/underserved populations. *Accreditation:* ARC-PA. *Students:* 131 full-time (107 women); includes 18 minority (2 Black or African American, non-Hispanic/Latino; 6 Asian, non-Hispanic/Latino; 9 Hispanic/Latino; 1 Two or more

races, non-Hispanic/Latino). Average age 28. In 2015, 45 master's awarded. *Degree requirements:* For master's, comprehensive exam. *Entrance requirements:* For master's, GRE General Test, minimum GPA of 2.8; 3 letters of recommendation; prerequisite courses in chemistry, biology, and general genetics, psychology and statistics; interview. Additional exam requirements/recommendations for international students: Required—TOEFL (minimum score 550 paper-based; 80 iBT). *Application deadline:* For fall admission, 9/1 for domestic students, 8/15 for international students. Application fee: $170. Electronic applications accepted. *Expenses:* Contact institution. *Financial support:* In 2015–16, 130 students received support. Fellowships, research assistantships, teaching assistantships, career-related internships or fieldwork, Federal Work-Study, institutionally sponsored loans, scholarships/grants, traineeships, and unspecified assistantships available. Financial award application deadline: 3/15; financial award applicants required to submit FAFSA. *Faculty research:* Clinical genetics and genetic counseling, evidence-based medicine, pediatric allergy and asthma, childhood diabetes, standardized patient assessment. *Unit head:* Jonathan Bowser, Program Director, 303-724-1349, E-mail: jonathan.bowser@ucdenver.edu. *Application contact:* Kay Denler, Academic Services Program Manager, 303-724-7963, E-mail: kay.denler@ucdenver.edu. Website: http://www.ucdenver.edu/academics/colleges/medicalschool/education/degree_programs/PAProgram/Pages/Home.aspx

University of Denver, Josef Korbel School of International Studies, Denver, CO 80208. Offers conflict resolution (MA); global business and corporate social responsibility (Certificate); global finance, trade and economic integration (MA); global health affairs (Certificate); homeland security (Certificate); humanitarian assistance (Certificate); international administration (MA); international development (MA); international human rights (MA); international security (MA); international studies (MA, PhD); religion and international affairs (Certificate). *Program availability:* Part-time. *Faculty:* 42 full-time (15 women), 20 part-time/adjunct (7 women). *Students:* 406 full-time (238 women), 26 part-time (13 women); includes 82 minority (11 Black or African American, non-Hispanic/Latino; 14 Asian, non-Hispanic/Latino; 46 Hispanic/Latino; 11 Two or more races, non-Hispanic/Latino), 42 international. Average age 27. 724 applicants, 89% accepted, 185 enrolled. In 2015, 203 master's, 2 doctorates, 38 other advanced degrees awarded. *Degree requirements:* For master's, one foreign language, thesis (for some programs); for doctorate, one foreign language, comprehensive exam, thesis/dissertation, two extended research papers. *Entrance requirements:* For master's, GRE General Test, bachelor's degree, transcripts, two letters of recommendation, statement of purpose, resume or curriculum vitae; for doctorate, GRE General Test, master's degree, transcripts, three letters of recommendation, statement of purpose, resume or curriculum vitae, writing sample; for Certificate, bachelor's degree, transcripts, two letters of recommendation, statement of purpose, resume or curriculum vitae. Additional exam requirements/recommendations for international students: Required—TOEFL (minimum score 587 paper-based; 95 iBT). *Application deadline:* For fall admission, 1/15 priority date for domestic and international students; for winter admission, 11/1 for domestic and international students. Applications are processed on a rolling basis. Application fee: $65. Electronic applications accepted. *Expenses:* $45,621. *Financial support:* In 2015–16, 275 students received support, including 2 research assistantships with tuition reimbursements available (averaging $7,250 per year), 4 teaching assistantships with tuition reimbursements available (averaging $1,488 per year); career-related internships or fieldwork, Federal Work-Study, institutionally sponsored loans, scholarships/grants, and unspecified assistantships also available. Support available to part-time students. Financial award application deadline: 2/15; financial award applicants required to submit FAFSA. *Faculty research:* Human rights and international security, international politics and economics, economic-social and political development, international technology analysis and management. *Unit head:* Christopher R. Hill, Dean, 303-871-2359, Fax: 303-871-2456, E-mail: christopher.r.hill@du.edu. *Application contact:* Brad Miller, Director of Graduate Admissions, 303-871-2989, Fax: 303-871-2124, E-mail: brad.miller@du.edu. Website: http://www.du.edu/korbel

University of Florida, Graduate School, College of Public Health and Health Professions, Department of Environmental and Global Health, Gainesville, FL 32611. Offers environmental health (PhD); one health (MHS, PhD). *Faculty:* 5 full-time, 1 part-time/adjunct. *Students:* 10 full-time (8 women), 2 part-time (both women); includes 1 minority (Black or African American, non-Hispanic/Latino), 1 international. Average age 28. 7 applicants, 57% accepted, 4 enrolled. In 2015, 2 master's awarded. *Entrance requirements:* For master's and doctorate, GRE, minimum GPA of 3.0. Additional exam requirements/recommendations for international students: Required—TOEFL (minimum score 550 paper-based; 80 iBT), IELTS (minimum score 6). *Application deadline:* For fall admission, 1/1 for domestic students. Application fee: $30. *Financial support:* In 2015–16, 2 fellowships, 12 research assistantships, 7 teaching assistantships were awarded. Financial award applicants required to submit FAFSA. *Total annual research expenditures:* $2.1 million. *Unit head:* Dr. Gregory C. Gray, MD, Chair, 352-273-9449, E-mail: gcgray@phhp.ufl.edu. *Application contact:* Office of Admissions, 352-392-1365, E-mail: webrequests@admissions.ufl.edu. Website: http://egh.phhp.ufl.edu/

University of Michigan, School of Public Health, Department of Epidemiology, Ann Arbor, MI 48109-2029. Offers epidemiological science (PhD); general epidemiology (MPH); global health epidemiology (MPH); hospital and molecular epidemiology (MPH); occupational and environmental epidemiology (MPH). PhD and MS offered through the Rackham Graduate School. *Accreditation:* CEPH (one or more programs are accredited). *Faculty:* 31 full-time (17 women), 41 part-time/adjunct (22 women). *Students:* 220 full-time (161 women), 2 part-time (1 woman); includes 30 minority (8 Black or African American, non-Hispanic/Latino; 9 Asian, non-Hispanic/Latino; 8 Hispanic/Latino; 5 Two or more races, non-Hispanic/Latino), 41 international. Average age 27. 821 applicants, 38% accepted, 128 enrolled. In 2015, 85 master's, 12 doctorates awarded. Terminal master's awarded for partial completion of doctoral program. *Degree requirements:* For master's, thesis (for some programs); for doctorate, comprehensive exam, thesis/dissertation, oral defense of dissertation, preliminary exam. *Entrance requirements:* For master's and doctorate, GRE General Test, MCAT. Additional exam requirements/recommendations for international students: Required—TOEFL (minimum score 100 iBT). *Application deadline:* For fall admission, 12/15 priority date for domestic students, 1/15 for international students. Applications are processed on a rolling basis. Application fee: $75. Electronic applications accepted. *Financial support:* Fellowships, research assistantships, teaching assistantships, career-related internships or fieldwork, Federal Work-Study, institutionally sponsored loans, scholarships/grants, traineeships, health care benefits, and unspecified assistantships available. Financial award application deadline: 12/15. *Faculty research:* Molecular virology, infectious diseases, women's health, genetics, social epidemiology. *Unit head:* Dr. Joseph Eisenberg, Chair, 734-764-5435, Fax: 734-764-3192. *Application contact:* Nancy Francis, Student Services Coordinator, 734-763-0274, Fax: 734-763-3192, E-mail: nhellner@umich.edu. Website: http://www.sph.umich.edu/epid

University of Minnesota, Twin Cities Campus, School of Public Health, Division of Environmental Health Sciences, Minneapolis, MN 55455-0213. Offers environmental and occupational epidemiology (MPH, MS, PhD); environmental chemistry (MS, PhD);

International Health

environmental health policy (MPH, MS, PhD); environmental infectious diseases (MPH, MS, PhD); environmental toxicology (MPH, MS, PhD); exposure sciences (MS); general environmental health (MPH, MS); global environmental health (MPH, MS, PhD); industrial hygiene (MPH, MS, PhD); occupational health nursing (MPH, MS, PhD); occupational medicine (MPH); MPH/MS. *Accreditation:* CEPH (one or more programs are accredited). *Program availability:* Part-time. *Degree requirements:* For master's, thesis optional; for doctorate, thesis/dissertation. *Entrance requirements:* For master's and doctorate, GRE General Test. Additional exam requirements/recommendations for international students: Required—TOEFL (minimum score 600 paper-based; 100 iBT). Electronic applications accepted. *Faculty research:* Behavior/measurement of airborne particles, toxicity mechanisms of environmental contaminants, health and safety interventions, foodborne disease surveillance, measuring pesticide exposures in children.

University of Missouri, Office of Research and Graduate Studies, Master of Public Health Program, Columbia, MO 65211. Offers global public health (Graduate Certificate); health promotion and policy (MPH); public health (Graduate Certificate); veterinary public health (MPH); DVM/MPH; MPH/MA; MPH/MPA. *Accreditation:* CEPH. *Entrance requirements:* Additional exam requirements/recommendations for international students: Required—TOEFL (minimum score 550 paper-based; 80 iBT). *Application deadline:* For fall admission, 6/30 priority date for domestic and international students. Applications are processed on a rolling basis. Application fee: $55 ($75 for international students). Electronic applications accepted. *Financial support:* Fellowships with tuition reimbursements, research assistantships with tuition reimbursements, teaching assistantships with tuition reimbursements, scholarships/grants, traineeships, health care benefits, and unspecified assistantships available. Support available to part-time students.
Website: http://publichealth.missouri.edu/

University of Pennsylvania, Perelman School of Medicine, Master of Public Health Program, Philadelphia, PA 19104. Offers generalist, global health, environmental health (MPH); DMD/MPH; JD/MPH; MD/MPH; MPH/MBE; MSN/MPH; MSSP/MPH; MSW/MPH; PhD/MPH. *Program availability:* Part-time, evening/weekend. *Faculty:* 21 full-time (14 women), 20 part-time/adjunct (15 women). *Students:* 94 full-time (81 women), 68 part-time (54 women); includes 74 minority (30 Black or African American, non-Hispanic/Latino; 31 Asian, non-Hispanic/Latino; 3 Hispanic/Latino; 10 Two or more races, non-Hispanic/Latino), 2 international. Average age 29. 448 applicants, 49% accepted, 79 enrolled. In 2015, 41 master's awarded. *Entrance requirements:* For master's, GRE. Additional exam requirements/recommendations for international students: Required—TOEFL (minimum score 100 iBT). *Application deadline:* For fall admission, 4/15 for domestic and international students. Applications are processed on a rolling basis. Electronic applications accepted. *Expenses: Tuition, area resident:* Full-time $31,068; part-time $5762 per course. *Required fees:* $3200; $336 per course. Full-time tuition and fees vary according to degree level, program and student level. Part-time tuition and fees vary according to course load, degree level and program. *Financial support:* In 2015–16, 31 students received support, including 1 fellowship with partial tuition reimbursement available (averaging $1,000 per year), 7 research assistantships with partial tuition reimbursements available (averaging $18,104 per year), 24 teaching assistantships with partial tuition reimbursements available (averaging $4,526 per year); tuition waivers (partial) also available. Financial award application deadline: 5/15; financial award applicants required to submit FAFSA. *Faculty research:* Health disparities, health behaviors, obesity, global health, epidemiology and prevention research. *Unit head:* Dr. Jennifer Pinto-Martin, Director, 215-898-4726, E-mail: pinto@nursing.upenn.edu. *Application contact:* Moriah Hall, Associate Director, MPH Program, 215-573-8841, E-mail: moriahh@mail.med.upenn.edu.
Website: http://www.publichealth.med.upenn.edu/

University of Southern California, Keck School of Medicine and Graduate School, Graduate Programs in Medicine, Department of Preventive Medicine, Master of Public Health Program, Los Angeles, CA 91803. Offers biostatistics and epidemiology (MPH); child and family health (MPH); environmental health (MPH); global health leadership (MPH); health communication (MPH); health education and promotion (MPH); public health policy (MPH). *Accreditation:* CEPH. *Program availability:* Part-time, evening/weekend. *Faculty:* 22 full-time (12 women), 3 part-time/adjunct (0 women). *Students:* 182 full-time (142 women), 35 part-time (25 women); includes 120 minority (19 Black or African American, non-Hispanic/Latino; 64 Asian, non-Hispanic/Latino; 37 Hispanic/Latino), 33 international. Average age 24. 236 applicants, 70% accepted, 71 enrolled. In 2015, 99 master's awarded. *Degree requirements:* For master's, practicum, final report, oral presentation. *Entrance requirements:* For master's, GRE General Test, MCAT, GMAT, minimum GPA of 3.0. Additional exam requirements/recommendations for international students: Required—TOEFL (minimum score 600 paper-based; 90 iBT). *Application deadline:* For fall admission, 6/1 priority date for domestic and international students; for spring admission, 10/1 priority date for domestic and international students; for summer admission, 3/1 for domestic and international students. Applications are processed on a rolling basis. Application fee: $85. Electronic applications accepted. *Expenses:* Contact institution. *Financial support:* Career-related internships or fieldwork, Federal Work-Study, institutionally sponsored loans, and scholarships/grants available. Support available to part-time students. Financial award application deadline: 5/4; financial award applicants required to submit CSS PROFILE or FAFSA. *Faculty research:* Substance abuse prevention, cancer and heart disease prevention, mass media and health communication research, health promotion, treatment compliance. *Unit head:* Dr. Louise A. Rohrbach, Director, 323-442-8237, Fax: 323-442-8297, E-mail: rohrbac@usc.edu. *Application contact:* Valerie Burris, Admissions Counselor, 323-442-7257, Fax: 323-442-8297, E-mail: valeriem@usc.edu.
Website: http://mph.usc.edu/

University of Southern California, Keck School of Medicine and Graduate School, Graduate Programs in Medicine, Program in Global Medicine, Los Angeles, CA 90089. Offers MS, Certificate. *Program availability:* Part-time. *Students:* 129 full-time (79 women), 3 part-time (2 women); includes 81 minority (12 Black or African American, non-Hispanic/Latino; 1 American Indian or Alaska Native, non-Hispanic/Latino; 52 Asian, non-Hispanic/Latino; 12 Hispanic/Latino; 2 Native Hawaiian or other Pacific Islander, non-Hispanic/Latino; 2 Two or more races, non-Hispanic/Latino), 9 international. Average age 24. In 2015, 97 master's awarded. *Entrance requirements:* For master's and Certificate, GRE, MCAT, or DAT. Additional exam requirements/recommendations for international students: Required—TOEFL (minimum score 100 iBT), TOEFL (minimum score 100 iBT), IELTS, or PTE. *Application deadline:* For fall admission, 6/1 for domestic and international students; for spring admission, 10/31 for domestic and international students. Applications are processed on a rolling basis. Application fee: $85. Electronic applications accepted. *Expenses:* Contact institution. *Unit head:* Dr. Elahe Nezami, Program Director, 323-442-3141, E-mail: nezami@usc.edu. *Application contact:* Farah Zerehi, Student Services Advisor, 323-442-3141, E-mail: fzerehi@usc.edu.
Website: http://msgm.usc.edu

University of South Florida, College of Public Health, Department of Global Health, Tampa, FL 33620-9951. Offers MPH, MSPH, Dr PH, PhD. *Program availability:* Part-time, evening/weekend. *Degree requirements:* For master's, comprehensive exam,

thesis (for some programs), minimum GPA of 3.0; for doctorate, comprehensive exam, thesis/dissertation. *Entrance requirements:* For master's, GRE General Test, minimum GPA of 3.0 in upper-level course work, goal statement letter, two professional letters of recommendation, resume/curriculum vitae; for doctorate, GRE General Test, minimum GPA of 3.0 in upper-level course work, goal statement letter, three professional letters of recommendation, resume/curriculum vitae, writing sample. Additional exam requirements/recommendations for international students: Required—TOEFL (minimum score 550 paper-based; 79 iBT). Electronic applications accepted.

University of South Florida, Innovative Education, Tampa, FL 33620-9951. Offers adult, career and higher education (Graduate Certificate), including college teaching, leadership in developing human resources, leadership in higher education; Africana studies (Graduate Certificate), including diasporas and health disparities, genocide and human rights; aging studies (Graduate Certificate), including gerontology; art research (Graduate Certificate), including museum studies; business foundations (Graduate Certificate); chemical and biomedical engineering (Graduate Certificate), including materials science and engineering, water, health and sustainability; child and family studies (Graduate Certificate), including positive behavior support; civil and industrial engineering (Graduate Certificate), including transportation systems analysis; community and family health (Graduate Certificate), including maternal and child health, social marketing and public health, violence and injury: prevention and intervention, women's health; criminology (Graduate Certificate), including criminal justice administration; educational measurement and research (Graduate Certificate), including evaluation; English (Graduate Certificate), including comparative literary studies, creative writing, professional and technical communication; entrepreneurship (Graduate Certificate); environmental health (Graduate Certificate), including safety management; epidemiology and biostatistics (Graduate Certificate), including applied biostatistics, biostatistics, concepts and tools of epidemiology, epidemiology, epidemiology of infectious diseases; geography, environment and planning (Graduate Certificate), including community development, environmental policy and management, geographical information systems; geology (Graduate Certificate), including hydrogeology; global health (Graduate Certificate), including disaster management, global health and Latin American and Caribbean studies, global health practice, humanitarian assistance, infection control; government and international affairs (Graduate Certificate), including Cuban studies, globalization studies; health policy and management (Graduate Certificate), including health management and leadership, public health policy and programs; hearing specialist: early intervention (Graduate Certificate); industrial and management systems engineering (Graduate Certificate), including systems engineering, technology management; information studies (Graduate Certificate), including school library media specialist; information systems/decision sciences (Graduate Certificate), including analytics and business intelligence; instructional technology (Graduate Certificate), including distance education, Florida digital/virtual educator, instructional design, multimedia design, Web design; internal medicine, bioethics and medical humanities (Graduate Certificate), including biomedical ethics; Latin American and Caribbean studies (Graduate Certificate); mass communications (Graduate Certificate), including multimedia journalism; mathematics and statistics (Graduate Certificate), including mathematics; medicine (Graduate Certificate), including aging and neuroscience, bioinformatics, biotechnology, brain fitness and memory management, clinical investigation, health informatics, health sciences, integrative weight management, intellectual property, medicine and gender, metabolic and nutritional medicine, metabolic cardiology, pharmacy sciences; national and competitive intelligence (Graduate Certificate); psychological and social foundations (Graduate Certificate), including career counseling, college teaching, diversity in education, mental health counseling, school counseling; public affairs (Graduate Certificate), including nonprofit management, public management, research administration; public health (Graduate Certificate), including environmental health, health equity, public health generalist, translational research in adolescent behavioral health; public health practices (Graduate Certificate), including planning for healthy communities; rehabilitation and mental health counseling (Graduate Certificate), including integrative mental health care, marriage and family therapy, rehabilitation technology; secondary education (Graduate Certificate), including ESOL, foreign language education: culture and content, foreign language education: professional; social work (Graduate Certificate), including geriatric social work/clinical gerontology; special education (Graduate Certificate), including autism spectrum disorder, disabilities education: severe/profound; world languages (Graduate Certificate), including teaching English as a second language (TESL) or foreign language. *Unit head:* Kathy Barnes, Interdisciplinary Programs Coordinator, 813-974-8031, Fax: 813-974-7061, E-mail: barnesk@usf.edu. *Application contact:* Karen Tylinski, Metro Initiatives, 813-974-9943, Fax: 813-974-7061, E-mail: ktylinsk@usf.edu.
Website: http://www.usf.edu/innovative-education/

The University of Toledo, College of Graduate Studies, College of Medicine and Life Sciences, Department of Public Health and Preventative Medicine, Toledo, OH 43606-3390. Offers biostatistics and epidemiology (Certificate); contemporary gerontological practice (Certificate); environmental and occupational health and safety (MPH); epidemiology (Certificate); global public health (Certificate); health promotion and education (MPH); industrial hygiene (MSOH); medical and health science teaching and learning (Certificate); occupational health (Certificate); public health administration (MPH); public health and emergency response (Certificate); public health epidemiology (MPH); public health nutrition (MPH); MD/MPH. *Program availability:* Part-time, evening/weekend. *Degree requirements:* For master's, thesis or alternative. *Entrance requirements:* For master's, GRE, minimum undergraduate GPA of 3.0, three letters of recommendation, statement of purpose, transcripts from all prior institutions attended, resume; for Certificate, minimum undergraduate GPA of 3.0, three letters of recommendation, statement of purpose, transcripts from all prior institutions attended, resume. Additional exam requirements/recommendations for international students: Required—TOEFL (minimum score 550 paper-based; 80 iBT), IELTS (minimum score 6.5). Electronic applications accepted.

University of Washington, Graduate School, School of Public Health, Department of Epidemiology, Seattle, WA 98195. Offers clinical research (MS); epidemiology (MPH, MS, PhD); global health (MPH); maternal/child health (MPH); MPH/MPA. *Accreditation:* CEPH (one or more programs are accredited). *Degree requirements:* For master's, comprehensive exam (for some programs), thesis, formal thesis proposal; for doctorate, comprehensive exam, thesis/dissertation, general exam, dissertation proposals, final exam (dissertation defense). *Entrance requirements:* For master's, GRE (except for those holding PhD, MD, DDS, DVM, DO or equivalent from U.S. institutions); for doctorate, GRE. Additional exam requirements/recommendations for international students: Required—TOEFL (minimum score 580 paper-based, 92 iBT), IELTS (minimum score 7), or PTE (minimum score of 65). Electronic applications accepted. *Expenses:* Contact institution. *Faculty research:* Chronic disease, health disparities and social determinants of health, aging and neuroepidemiology, maternal and child health, molecular and genetic epidemiology.

University of Washington, Graduate School, School of Public Health, Department of Global Health, Seattle, WA 98195. Offers global health (MPH); global health metrics and implementation science (PhD); health metrics and evaluation (MPH); leadership, policy and management (MPH); pathobiology (PhD); MPH/MAIS; MPH/MD; MPH/MN; MPH/

MPA; MPH/MSW; MPH/PhD. Terminal master's awarded for partial completion of doctoral program. *Degree requirements:* For master's, thesis, practicum; for doctorate, comprehensive exam, thesis/dissertation. *Entrance requirements:* For master's, GRE. Additional exam requirements/recommendations for international students: Required—TOEFL (minimum score 500 paper-based; 61 iBT), IELTS (minimum score 6). Electronic applications accepted. *Expenses:* Contact institution. *Faculty research:* AIDS and sexually-transmitted diseases, international health, reproductive health, tuberculosis, infectious disease.

Walden University, Graduate Programs, School of Health Sciences, Minneapolis, MN 55401. Offers clinical research administration (MS, Graduate Certificate); health education and promotion (MS, PhD), including behavioral health (PhD), disease surveillance (PhD), emergency preparedness (MS), general (MHA, MS), global health (PhD), health policy (PhD), health policy and advocacy (MS), population health (PhD); health informatics (MS); health services (PhD), including community health, healthcare administration, leadership, public health policy, self-designed; healthcare administration (MHA), including general (MHA, MS); leadership and organizational development (MHA); public health (MPH, Dr PH, PhD, Graduate Certificate), including community health education (PhD), epidemiology (PhD); systems policy (MHA). *Program availability:* Part-time, evening/weekend, online only, 100% online. *Faculty:* 14 full-time (8 women), 222 part-time/adjunct (121 women). *Students:* 2,487 full-time (1,804 women), 2,282 part-time (1,540 women); includes 2,763 minority (2,129 Black or African American, non-Hispanic/Latino; 30 American Indian or Alaska Native, non-Hispanic/Latino; 237 Asian, non-Hispanic/Latino; 268 Hispanic/Latino; 13 Native Hawaiian or other Pacific Islander, non-Hispanic/Latino; 86 Two or more races, non-Hispanic/Latino), 87 international. Average age 39. 1,205 applicants, 98% accepted, 820 enrolled. In 2015, 641 master's, 147 doctorates, 18 other advanced degrees awarded. *Degree requirements:* For doctorate, thesis/dissertation, residency. *Entrance requirements:* For master's, bachelor's degree or higher; minimum GPA of 2.5; official transcripts; goal statement (for some programs); access to computer and Internet; for doctorate, master's degree or higher; three years of related professional or academic experience (preferred); minimum GPA of 3.0; goal statement and current resume (for select programs); official transcripts; access to computer and Internet; for Graduate Certificate, relevant work experience; access to computer and Internet. Additional exam requirements/recommendations for international students: Required—TOEFL (minimum score 550 paper-based, 79 iBT), IELTS (minimum score 6.5), Michigan English Language Assessment Battery (minimum score 82), or PTE (minimum score 53). *Application deadline:* Applications are processed on a rolling basis. Application fee: $0. Electronic applications accepted. *Financial support:* Fellowships, Federal Work-Study, scholarships/grants, unspecified assistantships, and family tuition reduction, active duty/veteran tuition reduction, group tuition reduction, interest-free payment plans, employee tuition reduction available. Support available to part-time students. Financial award applicants required to submit FAFSA. *Unit head:* Dr. Jorg Westermann, Dean, 866-492-5336. *Application contact:* Meghan Thomas, Vice President of Enrollment Management, 866-492-5336, E-mail: info@waldenu.edu.
Website: http://www.waldenu.edu/colleges-schools/school-of-health-sciences

Washington University in St. Louis, Brown School, St. Louis, MO 63130. Offers affordable housing and mixed-income community management (Certificate); American Indian and Alaska native (MSW); children, youth and families (MSW); health (MSW); individualized (MSW), including health; mental health (MSW); older adults and aging societies (MSW); public health (MPH), including epidemiology/biostatistics, global health, health policy analysis, urban design; public health sciences (PhD); social and economic development (MSW); social work (MSW, PhD), including management (MSW), policy (MSW), research (MSW), sexual health and education (MSW), social entrepreneurship (MSW), system dynamics (MSW); violence and injury prevention (MSW, Certificate); JD/MSW; M Arch/MSW; MPH/MBA; MPH/MS; MSW/M Div; MSW/M Ed; MSW/MAPS; MSW/MBA; MSW/MPH; MUD/MSW. MSW/M Div and MSW/MAPS offered in partnership with Eden Theological Seminary. *Accreditation:* CSWE (one or more programs are accredited). *Faculty:* 54 full-time (31 women), 87 part-time/adjunct (61 women). *Students:* 303 full-time (256 women); includes 125 minority (42 Black or African American, non-Hispanic/Latino; 16 American Indian or Alaska Native, non-Hispanic/Latino; 47 Asian, non-Hispanic/Latino; 9 Hispanic/Latino; 11 Two or more races, non-Hispanic/Latino), 71 international. Average age 26. 923 applicants, 322 enrolled. In 2015, 239 master's, 5 doctorates awarded. *Degree requirements:* For master's, 60 credit hours (for MSW), 52 credit hours (for MPH); practicum; for doctorate, comprehensive exam, thesis/dissertation. *Entrance requirements:* For master's, GRE, GMAT, LSAT, or MCAT (for MPH); for doctorate, GRE, MA or MSW. Additional exam requirements/recommendations for international students: Required—TOEFL (minimum score 100 iBT) or IELTS. *Application deadline:* For fall admission, 12/15 priority date for domestic and international students; for winter admission, 3/1 priority date for domestic and international students. Applications are processed on a rolling basis. Application fee: $50. Electronic applications accepted. *Expenses:* Contact institution. *Financial support:* In 2015–16, 267 students received support. Fellowships, research assistantships, Federal Work-Study, institutionally sponsored loans, scholarships/grants, health care benefits, tuition waivers (partial), and unspecified assistantships available. Support available to part-time students. Financial award application deadline: 3/1; financial award applicants required to submit FAFSA. *Faculty research:* Mental health services, social development, child welfare, at-risk teens, autism, environmental health, health policy, health communications, obesity, gender and sexuality, violence and injury prevention, chronic disease prevention, poverty, older adults/aging societies, civic engagement, school social work, program evaluation, health disparities. *Unit head:* Jamie L. Adkisson, Director of Admissions and Recruitment, 314-935-3524, Fax: 314-935-4859, E-mail: jadkisson@wustl.edu. *Application contact:* Office of Admissions and Recruitment, 314-935-6676, Fax: 314-935-4859, E-mail: brownadmissions@wustl.ed.
Website: http://brownschool.wustl.edu

William James College, Graduate Programs, Newton, MA 02459. Offers applied psychology in higher education student personnel administration (MA); clinical psychology (Psy D); counseling psychology (MA); counseling psychology and community mental health (MA); counseling psychology and global mental health (MA); executive coaching (Graduate Certificate); forensic and counseling psychology (MA); leadership psychology (Psy D); organizational psychology (MA); primary care psychology (MA); respecialization in clinical psychology (Certificate); school psychology (Psy D); MA/CAGS. *Accreditation:* APA. *Degree requirements:* For master's, comprehensive exam (for some programs); for doctorate, thesis/dissertation (for some programs). Electronic applications accepted.

Yale University, School of Medicine, Yale School of Public Health, New Haven, CT 06520. Offers applied biostatistics and epidemiology (APMPH); biostatistics (MPH, MS, PhD), including global health (MPH); chronic disease epidemiology (MPH, PhD), including global health (MPH); environmental health sciences (MPH, PhD), including global health (MPH); epidemiology of microbial diseases (MPH, PhD), including global health (MPH); global health (APMPH); health management (MPH), including global health; health policy (MPH), including global health; health policy and administration (APMPH, PhD); occupational and environmental medicine (APMPH); preventive medicine (APMPH); social and behavioral sciences (APMPH, MPH), including global health (MPH); JD/MPH; M Div/MPH; MBA/MPH; MD/MPH; MEM/MPH; MFS/MPH; MM Sc/MPH; MPH/MA; MSN/MPH. MS and PhD offered through the Graduate School. *Accreditation:* CEPH. *Program availability:* Part-time. Terminal master's awarded for partial completion of doctoral program. *Degree requirements:* For master's, thesis, summer internship; for doctorate, comprehensive exam, thesis/dissertation, residency. *Entrance requirements:* For master's, GMAT, GRE, or MCAT, two years of undergraduate coursework in math and science; for doctorate, GRE General Test. Additional exam requirements/recommendations for international students: Required—TOEFL (minimum score 100 iBT). Electronic applications accepted. *Expenses:* Contact institution. *Faculty research:* Genetic and emerging infections epidemiology, virology, cost/quality, vector biology, quantitative methods, aging, asthma, cancer.

Maternal and Child Health

Bank Street College of Education, Graduate School, Program in Child Life, New York, NY 10025. Offers MS. *Degree requirements:* For master's, thesis. *Entrance requirements:* For master's, interview, essays, 100 hours of volunteer experience in a child life setting. Additional exam requirements/recommendations for international students: Required—TOEFL (minimum score 600 paper-based; 100 iBT), IELTS (minimum score 7). *Faculty research:* Therapeutic play in child life setting, child advocacy, psychosocial and educational intervention with care of sick children.

Bank Street College of Education, Graduate School, Program in Infant and Family Development and Early Intervention, New York, NY 10025. Offers infant and family development (MS Ed); infant and family early childhood special and general education (MS Ed); infant and family/early childhood special education (Ed M). *Degree requirements:* For master's, thesis. *Entrance requirements:* For master's, interview, essays. Additional exam requirements/recommendations for international students: Required—TOEFL (minimum score 600 paper-based; 100 iBT), IELTS (minimum score 7). Electronic applications accepted. *Faculty research:* Early intervention, early attachment practice in infant and toddler childcare, parenting skills in adolescents.

Columbia University, Columbia University Mailman School of Public Health, Department of Population and Family Health, New York, NY 10032. Offers MPH, Dr PH. *Accreditation:* CEPH (one or more programs are accredited). *Program availability:* Part-time. *Students:* 27 full-time (25 women), 118 part-time (107 women); includes 50 minority (9 Black or African American, non-Hispanic/Latino; 17 Asian, non-Hispanic/Latino; 20 Hispanic/Latino; 4 Two or more races, non-Hispanic/Latino), 13 international. Average age 28. 332 applicants, 58% accepted, 75 enrolled. In 2015, 68 master's awarded. *Entrance requirements:* For master's, GRE General Test; for doctorate, GRE General Test, MPH or equivalent (for Dr PH). Additional exam requirements/recommendations for international students: Required—TOEFL (minimum score 600 paper-based; 100 iBT). *Application deadline:* For fall admission, 12/1 priority date for domestic and international students. Application fee: $120. *Financial support:* Research assistantships, career-related internships or fieldwork, and Federal Work-Study available. Financial award application deadline: 2/1; financial award applicants required to submit FAFSA. *Faculty research:* Child and adolescent health, global health systems, health and human rights, humanitarian disasters, sexual and reproductive health. *Unit head:* Dr. John Santelli, Chairperson, 212-304-5200. *Application contact:* Dr. Joseph Korevec, Senior Director of Admissions and Financial Aid, 212-305-8698, Fax: 212-342-1861, E-mail: ph-admit@columbia.edu.

Website: https://www.mailman.columbia.edu/become-student/departments/population-and-family-health

East Carolina University, Graduate School, Thomas Harriot College of Arts and Sciences, Department of Psychology, Greenville, NC 27858-4353. Offers health psychology (PhD), including clinical health psychology, occupational health psychology, pediatric school psychology; industrial and organizational psychology (MA); MA/CAS. *Program availability:* Part-time, evening/weekend. *Students:* 89 full-time (68 women), 19 part-time (11 women); includes 14 minority (6 Black or African American, non-Hispanic/Latino; 1 Asian, non-Hispanic/Latino; 5 Hispanic/Latino; 2 Two or more races, non-Hispanic/Latino), 1 international. Average age 25. 316 applicants, 21% accepted, 33 enrolled. In 2015, 9 master's, 3 doctorates awarded. *Degree requirements:* For master's, one foreign language, comprehensive exam, thesis. *Entrance requirements:* For master's, GRE General Test, GRE Subject Test. Additional exam requirements/recommendations for international students: Required—TOEFL. *Application deadline:* Applications are processed on a rolling basis. Application fee: $50. *Financial support:* Research assistantships with partial tuition reimbursements, teaching assistantships with partial tuition reimbursements, Federal Work-Study, and traineeships available. Support available to part-time students. Financial award application deadline: 6/1. *Unit head:* Dr. Susan L. McCammon, Chair, 252-328-6357, E-mail: mccammons@ecu.edu. *Application contact:* Dean of Graduate School, 252-328-6012, Fax: 252-328-6071, E-mail: gradschool@ecu.edu.
Website: http://www.ecu.edu/psyc/

Instituto Tecnologico de Santo Domingo, Graduate School, Area of Health Sciences, Santo Domingo, Dominican Republic. Offers bioethics (M Bioethics); clinical bioethics (Certificate); clinical nutrition (Certificate); comprehensive health and the adolescent (Certificate); comprehensive adolescent health (MS); health and social security (M Mgmt).

Oakland University, Graduate Study and Lifelong Learning, School of Health Sciences, Program in Physical Therapy, Rochester, MI 48309-4401. Offers clinical exercise science (Dr Sc PT); complementary medicine and wellness (Dr Sc PT); corporate worksite wellness (Dr Sc PT); exercise science (Dr Sc PT); neurological rehabilitation (Dr Sc PT, TDPT); orthopedic manual physical therapy (Dr Sc PT, TDPT, Graduate Certificate); orthopedic physical therapy (Graduate Certificate); orthopedics (Dr Sc PT, TDPT); pediatric rehabilitation (Dr Sc PT, TDPT); physical therapy (DPT); teaching and learning for rehabilitation professionals (Dr Sc PT, TDPT). *Accreditation:* APTA. *Faculty:* 12 full-time (9 women), 1 part-time/adjunct (0 women). *Students:* 138 full-time (100

Maternal and Child Health

women), 19 part-time (13 women); includes 8 minority (4 Asian, non-Hispanic/Latino; 4 Two or more races, non-Hispanic/Latino), 3 international. Average age 25. 604 applicants, 7% accepted, 42 enrolled. In 2015, 41 doctorates, 15 other advanced degrees awarded. *Entrance requirements:* For doctorate, GRE General Test. Additional exam requirements/recommendations for international students: Required—TOEFL (minimum score 550 paper-based). *Application deadline:* For fall admission, 10/15 for domestic and international students. Application fee: $0. *Expenses:* Contact institution. *Financial support:* Federal Work-Study, institutionally sponsored loans, and tuition waivers (full) available. Financial award application deadline: 3/1; financial award applicants required to submit FAFSA. *Unit head:* Dr. Kristine A. Thompson, Physical Therapy Program Director/Special Instructor, 248-364-8662, E-mail: kathomps@oakland.edu.
Website: http://www.oakland.edu/shs/pt/

Troy University, Graduate School, College of Health and Human Services, Program in Nursing, Troy, AL 36082. Offers adult health (MSN); clinical nurse specialist adult health (DNP); clinical nurse specialist maternal infant (DNP); family nurse practitioner (MSN, DNP, PMC); informatics specialist (MSN); maternal infant (MSN). *Accreditation:* ACEN. *Program availability:* Part-time, evening/weekend. *Faculty:* 13 full-time (12 women), 11 part-time/adjunct (all women). *Students:* 75 full-time (62 women), 202 part-time (179 women); includes 91 minority (72 Black or African American, non-Hispanic/Latino; 1 Asian, non-Hispanic/Latino; 8 Hispanic/Latino; 10 Two or more races, non-Hispanic/Latino). Average age 34. 50 applicants, 96% accepted. In 2015, 43 master's, 13 doctorates, 15 other advanced degrees awarded. *Degree requirements:* For master's, comprehensive exam, minimum GPA of 3.0, candidacy; for doctorate, minimum GPA of 3.0, submission of approved comprehensive e-portfolio, completion of residency synthesis project, minimum of 1000 hours of clinical practice, qualifying exam. *Entrance requirements:* For master's, GRE (minimum score of 850 on old exam or 290 on new exam) or MAT (minimum score of 396), minimum GPA of 3.0, BSN, current RN licensure, 2 letters of reference, undergraduate health assessment course; for doctorate, GRE (minimum score of 850 on old exam or 294 on new exam), BSN or MSN, minimum GPA of 3.0, 2 letters of reference, current RN licensure, essay. Additional exam requirements/recommendations for international students: Required—TOEFL (minimum score 523 paper-based; 70 iBT), IELTS (minimum score 6). *Application deadline:* Applications are processed on a rolling basis. Application fee: $50. Electronic applications accepted. *Expenses:* Tuition, state resident: full-time $7146; part-time $397 per credit hour. Tuition, nonresident: full-time $14,292; part-time $794 per credit hour. *Required fees:* $802. Tuition and fees vary according to campus/location and program. *Financial support:* Fellowships, career-related internships or fieldwork, and scholarships/grants available. Support available to part-time students. Financial award applicants required to submit FAFSA. *Unit head:* Dr. Diane Weed, Director, School of Nursing, 334-670-5864, Fax: 334-670-3745, E-mail: lweed@troy.edu. *Application contact:* Crystal G. Bishop, Director of Graduate Admissions, School of Nursing, 334-241-8631, E-mail: cdgodwin@troy.edu.

The University of Alabama at Birmingham, School of Public Health, Program in Public Health, Birmingham, AL 35294. Offers applied epidemiology and pharmacoepidemiology (MSPH); biostatistics (MPH); clinical and translational science (MSPH); environmental health (MPH); environmental health and toxicology (MSPH); epidemiology (MPH); general theory and practice (MPH); health behavior (MPH); health care organization (MPH); health policy quantitative policy analysis (MPH); industrial hygiene (MPH, MSPH); maternal and child health policy (Dr PH); maternal and child health policy and leadership (MPH); occupational health and safety (MPH); outcomes research (MSPH, Dr PH); public health (PhD); public health management (Dr PH); public health preparedness management (MPH). *Accreditation:* CEPH. *Program availability:* Part-time, online learning. *Degree requirements:* For doctorate, comprehensive exam, thesis/dissertation. *Entrance requirements:* For master's and doctorate, GRE. Additional exam requirements/recommendations for international students: Recommended—TOEFL (minimum score 550 paper-based; 79 iBT), IELTS (minimum score 6.5). Electronic applications accepted. *Expenses:* Tuition, state resident: full-time $7340. Tuition, nonresident: full-time $16,628. Full-time tuition and fees vary according to course load and program.

University of California, Davis, Graduate Studies, Program in Maternal and Child Nutrition, Davis, CA 95616. Offers MAS. *Degree requirements:* For master's, comprehensive exam. *Entrance requirements:* Additional exam requirements/recommendations for international students: Required—TOEFL (minimum score 550 paper-based).

University of Maryland, College Park, Academic Affairs, School of Public Health, Department of Family Science, College Park, MD 20742. Offers family studies (PhD); marriage and family therapy (MS); maternal and child health (PhD). *Accreditation:* AAMFT/COAMFTE. *Program availability:* Part-time, evening/weekend. *Degree requirements:* For master's, thesis or alternative; for doctorate, comprehensive exam, thesis/dissertation, oral defense. *Entrance requirements:* For master's, GRE General Test, minimum GPA of 3.0, 3 letters of recommendation; for doctorate, GRE General Test, minimum GPA of 3.0, 3 letters of recommendation, research sample. Electronic applications accepted. *Faculty research:* Family life quality, interracial couples, child support, homeless families, family and child well-being.

University of Minnesota, Twin Cities Campus, School of Public Health, Major in Maternal and Child Health, Minneapolis, MN 55455-0213. Offers MPH. *Accreditation:* CEPH. *Program availability:* Part-time. *Degree requirements:* For master's, fieldwork, project. *Entrance requirements:* For master's, GRE General Test, 1 year of relevant experience. Additional exam requirements/recommendations for international students: Required—TOEFL. Electronic applications accepted. *Expenses:* Contact institution. *Faculty research:* Reproductive and perinatal health, family planning, child adolescent and family health, risk reduction and resiliency, child and family adaptation to chronic health conditions.

The University of North Carolina at Chapel Hill, Graduate School, Gillings School of Global Public Health, Department of Maternal and Child Health, Chapel Hill, NC 27599. Offers MPH, MSPH, Dr PH, PhD, MD/MSPH, MPH/MSW, MSPH/M Ed, MSPH/MSW. *Accreditation:* CEPH (one or more programs are accredited). *Students:* 89 full-time (83 women), 8 part-time (all women); includes 30 minority (9 Black or African American, non-Hispanic/Latino; 9 Asian, non-Hispanic/Latino; 7 Hispanic/Latino; 5 Two or more races, non-Hispanic/Latino), 9 international. Average age 29. 117 applicants, 62% accepted, 40 enrolled. *Degree requirements:* For master's, comprehensive exam, major paper; for doctorate, comprehensive exam, thesis/dissertation. *Entrance requirements:* For master's, GRE General Test or MCAT, minimum GPA of 3.0 (recommended), at least one year of post-BA maternal health/child health-related work experience; for doctorate, GRE General Test, minimum GPA of 3.0, at least one year of post-BA maternal health/child health-related work experience. Additional exam requirements/recommendations for international students: Required—TOEFL. *Application deadline:* For fall admission, 12/10 priority date for domestic and international students. Applications are processed on a rolling basis. Application fee: $85. Electronic applications accepted. *Financial support:* Fellowships with tuition reimbursements, research assistantships with tuition reimbursements, teaching assistantships with tuition reimbursements, career-related internships or fieldwork, Federal Work-Study,

institutionally sponsored loans, scholarships/grants, traineeships, health care benefits, and unspecified assistantships available. Financial award application deadline: 12/10; financial award applicants required to submit FAFSA. *Faculty research:* Women's health, prenatal health, family planning, program evaluation, child health policy and priorities. *Unit head:* Dr. Carolyn Halpern, Chair, 919-966-5981, E-mail: carolyn_halpern@unc.edu. *Application contact:* Carrie Aldrich, Student Services Manager, 919-966-2018, Fax: 919-966-0458, E-mail: carrie_aldrich@unc.edu.

University of Puerto Rico, Medical Sciences Campus, Graduate School of Public Health, Department of Human Development, Program in Maternal and Child Health, San Juan, PR 00936-5067. Offers MPH. *Program availability:* Part-time, evening/weekend. *Entrance requirements:* For master's, GRE, previous course work in algebra.

University of South Florida, Innovative Education, Tampa, FL 33620-9951. Offers adult, career and higher education (Graduate Certificate), including college teaching, leadership in developing human resources, leadership in higher education; Africana studies (Graduate Certificate), including diasporas and health disparities, genocide and human rights; aging studies (Graduate Certificate), including gerontology; art research (Graduate Certificate), including museum studies; business foundations (Graduate Certificate); chemical and biomedical engineering (Graduate Certificate), including materials science and engineering, water, health and sustainability; child and family studies (Graduate Certificate), including positive behavior support; civil and industrial engineering (Graduate Certificate), including transportation systems analysis; community and family health (Graduate Certificate), including maternal and child health, social marketing and public health, violence and injury: prevention and intervention, women's health; criminology (Graduate Certificate), including criminal justice administration; educational measurement and research (Graduate Certificate), including evaluation; English (Graduate Certificate), including comparative literary studies, creative writing, professional and technical communication; entrepreneurship (Graduate Certificate); environmental health (Graduate Certificate), including safety management; epidemiology and biostatistics (Graduate Certificate), including applied biostatistics, biostatistics, concepts and tools of epidemiology, epidemiology, epidemiology of infectious diseases; geography, environment and planning (Graduate Certificate), including community development, environmental policy and management, geographical information systems; geology (Graduate Certificate), including hydrogeology; global health (Graduate Certificate), including disaster management, global health and Latin American and Caribbean studies, global health practice, humanitarian assistance, infection control; government and international affairs (Graduate Certificate), including Cuban studies, globalization studies; health policy and management (Graduate Certificate), including health management and leadership, public health policy and programs; hearing specialist: early intervention (Graduate Certificate); industrial and management systems engineering (Graduate Certificate), including systems engineering, technology management; information studies (Graduate Certificate), including school library media specialist; information systems/decision sciences (Graduate Certificate), including analytics and business intelligence; instructional technology (Graduate Certificate), including distance education, Florida digital/virtual educator, instructional design, multimedia design, Web design; internal medicine, bioethics and medical humanities (Graduate Certificate), including biomedical ethics; Latin American and Caribbean studies (Graduate Certificate); mass communications (Graduate Certificate), including multimedia journalism; mathematics and statistics (Graduate Certificate), including mathematics; medicine (Graduate Certificate), including aging and neuroscience, bioinformatics, biotechnology, brain fitness and memory management, clinical investigation, health informatics, health sciences, integrative weight management, intellectual property, medicine and gender, metabolic and nutritional medicine, metabolic cardiology, pharmacy sciences; national and competitive intelligence (Graduate Certificate); psychological and social foundations (Graduate Certificate), including career counseling, college teaching, diversity in education, mental health counseling, school counseling; public affairs (Graduate Certificate), including nonprofit management, public management, research administration; public health (Graduate Certificate), including environmental health, health equity, public health generalist, translational research in adolescent behavioral health; public health practices (Graduate Certificate), including planning for healthy communities; rehabilitation and mental health counseling (Graduate Certificate), including integrative mental health care, marriage and family therapy, rehabilitation technology; secondary education (Graduate Certificate), including ESOL, foreign language education: culture and content, foreign language education: professional; social work (Graduate Certificate), including geriatric social work/clinical gerontology; special education (Graduate Certificate), including autism spectrum disorder, disabilities education: severe/profound; world languages (Graduate Certificate), including teaching English as a second language (TESL) or foreign language. *Unit head:* Kathy Barnes, Interdisciplinary Programs Coordinator, 813-974-8031, Fax: 813-974-7061, E-mail: barnesk@usf.edu. *Application contact:* Karen Tylinski, Metro Initiatives, 813-974-9943, Fax: 813-974-7061, E-mail: ktylinsk@usf.edu.
Website: http://www.usf.edu/innovative-education/

University of Washington, Graduate School, School of Public Health, Department of Epidemiology, Seattle, WA 98195. Offers clinical research (MS); epidemiology (MPH, MS, PhD); global health (MPH); maternal/child health (MPH); MPH/MPA. *Accreditation:* CEPH (one or more programs are accredited). *Degree requirements:* For master's, comprehensive exam (for some programs), thesis, formal thesis proposal; for doctorate, comprehensive exam, thesis/dissertation, general exam, dissertation proposals, final exam (dissertation defense). *Entrance requirements:* For master's, GRE (except for those holding PhD, MD, DDS, DVM, DO or equivalent from U.S. institutions); for doctorate, GRE. Additional exam requirements/recommendations for international students: Required—TOEFL (minimum score 580 paper-based, 92 iBT), IELTS (minimum score 7), or PTE (minimum score of 65). Electronic applications accepted. *Expenses:* Contact institution. *Faculty research:* Chronic disease, health disparities and social determinants of health, aging and neuroepidemiology, maternal and child health, molecular and genetic epidemiology.

University of Washington, Graduate School, School of Public Health, Department of Health Services, Seattle, WA 98195. Offers clinical research (MS); community-oriented public health practice (MPH); evaluative sciences and statistics (PhD); health behavior and social determinants of health (PhD); health economics (PhD); health informatics and health information management (MHIHIM); health services (MS, PhD); health services administration (EMHA, MHA); health systems and policy (MPH); health systems research (PhD); maternal and child health (MPH); social and behavioral sciences (MPH); JD/MHA; MHA/MBA; MHA/MPA; MHA/MPA; MPH/JD; MPH/MD; MPH/MN; MPH/MPA; MPH/MS; MPH/MSD; MPH/MSW; MPH/PhD. *Program availability:* Online learning. Terminal master's awarded for partial completion of doctoral program. *Degree requirements:* For master's, thesis (for some programs), practicum (MPH); for doctorate, comprehensive exam, thesis/dissertation. *Entrance requirements:* For master's and doctorate, GRE General Test, minimum GPA of 3.0. Additional exam requirements/recommendations for international students: Required—TOEFL (minimum score 580 paper-based; 92 iBT), IELTS (minimum score 7). Electronic applications accepted. *Expenses:* Contact institution. *Faculty research:* Public health practice, health promotion and disease prevention, maternal and child health, organizational behavior and culture, health policy.

HARVARD UNIVERSITY
T. H. Chan School of Public Health

Programs of Study

The Harvard T. H. Chan School of Public Health offers programs leading to the graduate degrees of Master of Public Health (M.P.H.), Master in Health Care Management (M.H.C.M.), Doctor of Public Health (Dr.P.H.), and Master of Science in a specified field (S.M. in that field). Doctor of Philosophy (Ph.D.) degrees are offered in specific fields of study through the Graduate School of Arts and Sciences. Programs are offered in biostatistics; computational biology and quantitative genetics; environmental health; epidemiology; genetics and complex diseases; global health and population; health decision science; health policy and management; immunology and infectious diseases; nutrition; population health sciences, and social and behavioral sciences. Some programs are designed for physicians, lawyers, managers, and other health-care professionals; some for college graduates who wish to train for health careers; and others for individuals who hold graduate degrees in medicine, law, business, government, education, and other fields who wish to apply their special skills to public health problems. Special programs include the M.P.H./M.S.N. in maternal and child health nursing, administered jointly by Harvard Chan and Simmons College; the combined M.D./M.P.H. program, offered in conjunction with accredited U.S. medical schools; the M.P.H./M.U.P. in environmental health and urban planning offered in conjunction with Harvard Graduate School of Design; and the J.D./M.P.H. joint-degree program offered by Harvard Chan and Harvard Law Schools. The School offers residency training leading to certification by the American Board of Preventive Medicine in occupational medicine.

Research Facilities

The main buildings of the School are the Sebastian S. Kresge Educational Facilities Building at 677 Huntington Avenue, the François-Xavier Bagnoud Building at 651 Huntington Avenue, and the Health Sciences Laboratories at 665 Huntington Avenue. The School maintains well-equipped research laboratories containing sophisticated instrumentation and supporting animal facilities. Computing and data processing resources are also available to students through the Instructional Computing Facility. The Francis A. Countway Library serves the library needs of the School. It holds more than 630,000 volumes, subscribes to 3,500 current journal titles, and houses over 10,000 noncurrent biomedical journal titles in addition to its extensive collection of historical materials, making it the largest library in the country serving a medical and health-related school.

Financial Aid

Financial aid at the Harvard Chan School can come from a variety of sources. Some departments have training grants that offer students full tuition plus a stipend. Through need-based and merit-based programs at the School and University levels, other students are offered grants that range from half to full tuition. To supplement other aid, many students borrow through one or more of the federal educational loan programs and work at part-time jobs at Harvard and in the community.

Cost of Study

Master's program students are assessed tuition at $1,072–$1,264 per credit. Students in a one-year master's program are required to take a minimum of 45 credits at $56,880, while students in multiple-year master's programs typically take 40 credits their first year at $42,880. Doctoral students are assessed a flat tuition rate. The full-time rate for 2016–17 for students in their first or second year is $42,880. Health insurance and health services fee are required, which total $3,718. Books and supplies cost approximately $2,079 in 2016–17.

Living and Housing Costs

For the academic year 2016–17, it is estimated that a single student needs a minimum of $24,640 for housing and living costs: $15,070 for rent and utilities and $9,570 for other expenses. Limited housing is available in the Shattuck International House, with preference given to international students. Most students arrange for housing in the adjacent communities.

Student Group

There were 1,224 graduate students (729 women and 495 men) enrolled in 2015–16. Seventy nations are represented.

Student Outcomes

Graduates of the Harvard T. H. Chan School of Public Health find employment in a variety of settings. It depends in part upon their previous experience and in part upon department and degree programs from which they graduate. Recent graduates have found positions in research institutes, with pharmaceutical companies and governmental and nongovernmental agencies, within the health-care industry, and as faculty members of universities.

Location

Boston is a heterogeneous metropolis rich in history and charm. Athletic, cultural, and recreational activities are abundant. The School is within walking distance of museums, colleges and universities, waterways, and parks.

The University and The School

Harvard College was founded in 1636; until the establishment of professorships in medicine in 1782, it composed the whole of the institution now called Harvard University. In addition to the college, eleven graduate schools are now part of the University.

Harvard Chan School recently celebrated its centennial. In September 1913, the new Harvard-MIT School for Health Officers welcomed its class of 8 students. From those modest beginnings emerged Harvard Chan School and its long record of accomplishments. More information can be found at http://www.hsph.harvard.edu/centennial. The primary mission of the School is to carry out teaching and research aimed at improving the health of population groups throughout the world. The School emphasizes not only the development and implementation of disease prevention and treatment programs but also the planning and management of systems involved in the delivery of health services in this country and abroad. The School cooperates with the Medical School in teaching and research and has close ties with other Harvard faculties. The School has more than 480 full-time and part-time faculty members and nine academic departments representing major biomedical and social disciplines.

Applying

Harvard Chan School participates in the SOPHAS, which is the centralized application service for schools and programs of public health. Students should visit the SOPHAS website at http://www.sophas.org for more specific information and for access to the application for admission. All applicants to the School are required to submit scores from the GRE (ETS school code: 3456); applicants are urged to take the test no later than November, since applications are not considered without the scores. Applicants may submit the DAT, GMAT, LSAT, or MCAT, as appropriate to the applicant's background, in lieu of the GRE. In addition, applicants must persuade the Committee on Admissions and Degrees of their ability to meet academic standards and of their overall qualifications to undertake advanced study at a graduate level. Students should visit the School's website (http://www.hsph.harvard.edu/admissions) for information concerning the deadline to apply for admission and to apply online.

As a matter of policy, law, and commitment, the Harvard Chan School does not discriminate against any person on the basis of race, color, sexual orientation, gender identity, religion, age, national or ethnic origin, political beliefs, veteran status, or disability in admission to, access to, treatment in, or employment in its programs and activities. Members of minority groups are strongly encouraged to apply.

Correspondence and Information

Harvard T. H. Chan School of Public Health Admissions Office
158 Longwood Avenue
Boston, Massachusetts 02115-5810
United States
Phone: 617-432-1031
Fax: 617-432-7080
E-mail: admissions@hsph.harvard.edu
Website: http://www.hsph.harvard.edu/admissions

Counseling and program information:
Vincent W. James, Director
Kerri Noonan, Associate Director
Kelly Latendresse, Assistant Director
Ania Grandbois
Megan O'Neil
Priti Thareja
Ruth Thompson

Harvard University

FACULTY CHAIRS AND DEPARTMENTAL ACTIVITIES

Biostatistics (617-432-1056, biostat_admissions@hsph.harvard.edu)
Chair: Xihong Lin, Ph.D. The program combines both theory and application of statistical science to analyze public health problems and further biomedical research. Students are prepared for academic and private-sector research careers. Current departmental research on statistical and computing methods for observational studies and clinical trials includes survival analysis, missing-data problems, and causal inference. Other areas of investigation include environmental research; statistical aspects of the study of AIDS and cancer; quantitative problems in health-risk analysis, technology assessment, and clinical decision making; statistical methodology in psychiatric research and in genetic studies; and statistical genetics and computational biology.

Environmental Health (617-432-1270, envhlth@hsph.harvard.edu)
Chair: Russ Hauser, M.D., Sc.D., M.P.H. The mission of the Department of Environmental Health is to advance the health of all people around the world through research and training in environmental health. The department emphasizes the role of air, water, the built environment, and the workplace as critical determinants of health. Teaching and research activities of the department are carried out through three concentrations: exposure, epidemiology, and risk; occupational health; and molecular and integrative physiological sciences.

Epidemiology (617-432-1050, elfurxhi@hsph.harvard.edu)
Chair: Albert Hofman, M.D., Ph.D. Epidemiology, the study of the frequency, distribution, and determinants of disease in humans, is a fundamental science of public health. Epidemiologists use many approaches, but the ultimate aim of epidemiologic research is the prevention or effective control of human disease. Current research involves the role of viruses in the etiology of cancer; the connection between diet and risk of cancer, cardiovascular disease, and other major chronic diseases; the relationship between exposure to chemicals in the workplace and the development of cancer; the epidemiology of infectious disease; factors in early life predisposing individuals to chronic diseases; and the health effects of drugs and medical devices.

Genetics and Complex Diseases
(617-432-0054, aepshtei@hsph.harvard.edu)
Chair: Gökhan Hotamisligil, M.D., Ph.D. The complex interplay of biological processes with environmental factors as they apply to chronic, multigenic, and multifactorial diseases is the emphasis of the Department of Genetics and Complex Diseases. Research programs in the department focus on molecular mechanisms of adaptive responses to environmental signals to elucidate the mechanisms underlying the intricate interaction between genetic determinants and their divergent responses to stress signals.

Global Health and Population
(617-432-2253, bheil@hsph.harvard.edu)
Chair: Wafaie Fawzi, M.B.B.S., Dr.P.H. The department seeks to improve global health through education, research, and service from a population-based perspective. Research interests span a wide spectrum of topics, including social and economic development, health policy, and demography; design and financing of health-care systems; women's health and children's health; and prevention and control of infectious and chronic diseases. The department has a special concern with questions of health equity and human rights, particularly in relation to health and population issues in developing countries.

Health Policy and Management
(617-432-4324, jmoltoni@hsph.harvard.edu)
Chair: Arnold Epstein, M.D. The department is mission oriented in its concern with improving the health-care delivery system and mitigating public health risks in the United States and abroad. It is dedicated to resolving major management and health policy problems through original research, advanced training, and dispute resolution. Research priorities are organized into seven broad areas: decision science, health care management, health economics, law and public health, quality and access, political policy, and public health policy.

Immunology and Infectious Diseases
(617-432-1023, asabarof@hsph.harvard.edu)
Chair: Dyann Wirth, Ph.D. The department focuses on the biological, immunological, epidemiological, and ecological aspects of viral, bacterial, protozoan, and helminthic diseases of animals and humans and the vectors that transmit some of these infectious agents. Emphasis is on research identifying basic pathogenic mechanisms that may lead to better diagnostic tools and the development of vaccines as well as the identification of new targets for antiviral and antiparasitic drugs.

Nutrition (617-432-1528, sdean@hsph.harvard.edu)
Chair: Walter C. Willett, M.D., M.P.H., D.P.H. The department's mission is to improve human health through research aimed at understanding how diet influences health, the dissemination of new knowledge about nutrition to health professionals and the public, the development of nutritional strategies, and the education of researchers and practitioners. Department research ranges from molecular biology to human studies of cancer and heart disease, including the conduct of population-based intervention trials.

Social and Behavioral Sciences
(617-432-3761, esolomon@hsph.harvard.edu)
Chair: Ichiro Kawachi, M.D., Ph.D. The mission of the Department of Social and Behavioral Sciences is to improve health throughout the lifespan, including a special emphasis on children and adolescents. This mission is achieved through research to identify the social and behavioral determinants of health, development and evaluation of interventions and policies leading to the improvement of population health, and the preparation of professionals and researchers who fill leadership positions in advocacy and public service.

Master of Public Health Program
(617-432-0090, mph@hsph.harvard.edu)
Director: Murray Mittleman, M.D.C.M., M.P.H., D.P.H. The program is designed to provide both a general background and flexibility of specialization in public health. The seven areas of concentration are clinical effectiveness, global health, health and social behavior, health management, health policy, occupational and environmental health, and quantitative methods. There is also an online and on-campus M.P.H. E.P.I. program.

Doctor of Public Health Program (617-432-5008, drph@hsph.harvard.edu)
Director: Peter Berman, M.Sc., Ph.D. The Doctor of Public Health degree is for exceptional individuals with proven potential who want to accelerate their careers, lead organizations, and have an important impact on people's health and lives. Students will enjoy unique opportunities to engage with Harvard's world-renowned faculty through rigorous teaching, interactive learning, case discussions, simulations, and field experiences in a variety of major public health organizations. This innovative, transformative educational experience has been designed so that no prior public health degree is required.

Division of Biological Sciences
(617-432-4470, bph@hsph.harvard.edu)
Director: Brendan Manning, Ph.D. The Division of Biological Sciences is an umbrella organization encompassing the Harvard Chan School Departments of Environmental Health, Genetics and Complex Diseases, Immunology and Infectious Diseases, and Nutrition. The Ph.D. program in Biological Sciences in Public Health trains students in individual fields of biological research with a focus on understanding, preventing, and treating diseases affecting large populations. The Ph.D. programs are offered under the aegis of the Harvard Graduate School of Arts and Sciences and administered by the Harvard Chan School Division of Biological Sciences.

Population Health Sciences (phdphs@hsph.harvard.edu)
Director: S. (Subu) V. Subramanian, Ph.D. The program offers advanced doctoral-level research training that builds on multiple disciplinary perspectives to understand origins and determinants of health and disease across populations. Population Health Sciences is an umbrella organization encompassing the HSPH Departments of Environmental Health, Epidemiology, Global Health and Population, Nutrition, and Social and Behavioral Sciences. In these departments, the doctoral degree offered is the Doctor of Philosophy (Ph.D.). The Ph.D. programs are offered under the aegis of the Harvard Graduate School of Arts and Sciences and administered by the Harvard Chan School Program in Population Health Sciences.

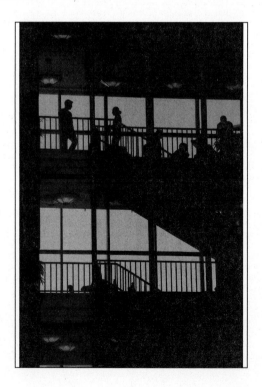

NEW YORK UNIVERSITY
Department of Environmental Medicine

 For more information, visit http://petersons.to/nyu_environmentalsciences

Programs of Study

The Department of Environmental Medicine at New York University (NYU) offers both Master of Science (M.S.) and Doctor of Philosophy (Ph.D.) degrees in environmental health sciences. These programs provide students with advanced training in scientific disciplines related to environmental health, focusing on major health problems such as cancer, respiratory illness, cardiovascular diseases, and musculoskeletal ailments.

Students also acquire specialized knowledge in several environmental health areas including biostatistics, epidemiology, ergonomics and biomechanics, exposure assessment and health effects, molecular toxicology/carcinogenesis, and toxicology.

The **Master of Science (M.S.) in Environmental Health Sciences program** is ideal for individuals who are seeking career opportunities in occupational health and safety, health hazard communication, health risk assessment, and environmental analysis of toxicants. It has two main areas of study: environmental toxicology and occupational and environmental hygiene.

The program, which can be pursued on a full- or part-time basis, focuses on teaching students how to use scientific methodology to find solutions to real-world environmental problems. Students acquire fundamental knowledge about environmental pollution, toxicology, and biostatistics and gain the ability to present scientific data and interpret scientific reports.

Because the program gives students the opportunity to develop individualized courses of study, they may take relevant courses in other schools within New York University such as environment management and planning, environmental law, and risk assessment.

Graduates of the program complete 36 points of course work, at least 24 of which are to be accumulated while in residence at the Graduate School of Arts and Sciences. They must also complete a special project that is either a library thesis or a thesis that is based on a faculty-supervised laboratory project.

Students also attend departmental seminars and participate in journal clubs. In addition, they can complete laboratory rotations in consultation with their academic advisers.

Additional information about the M.S. degree program can be found online at http://www.med.nyu.edu/environmentalmedicine/graduate-program/ms-program.

The **Ph.D. in Environmental Health Sciences program** prepares students for active and productive careers in research and professional service. The instructive component of the program focuses on providing students with a solid foundation in basic sciences. In addition, a research component gives students hands-on experience designing, conducting, and interpreting studies that address scientific issues in environmental health. Areas of study include Molecular Toxicology/Carcinogenesis, Toxicology (Inhalation or Aquatic), and Exposure Assessment and Health Effects.

Doctoral students earn 72 credits that include at least 48 credits of didactic courses. They also attend department seminars and journal clubs as well as write and defend a doctoral dissertation.

First-year students also participate in laboratory rotations that are based on their interests. Students can choose specific courses of study that reflect their educational and career backgrounds, interests, and career goals.

More information about the Ph.D. program is available at http://www.med.nyu.edu/environmentalmedicine/graduate-program/phd-program.

Training Program in Environmental Toxicology: Predoctoral students and post-doctoral fellows in the environmental toxicology program at New York University may be eligible to receive training grant support from the National Institute of Environmental Health Sciences. Grant recipients receive research training in pulmonary or molecular toxicology.

Research

The major mission of the Department of Environmental Medicine is to conduct cutting edge research in Environmental Health Sciences. This is accomplished by obtaining funded grants from The National Institute of Health, The United States' EPA, and other government and non-government funding agencies. Some major areas of research include chemical carcinogenesis, epigenetics, health effects of particulate air pollution, epidemiology of cancer susceptibility and causation, and environmental etiology of cardiovascular disease and diabetes. Students have access to more than 14 labs associated with NYU.

The NYU Department of Environmental Medicine is designated as a center of excellence by the National Institutes of Health, National Institute of Environmental Health Sciences. This designation is through a funded Center Grant from NIH that supports facility cores and is the engine that drives Environmental Health Sciences research at NYU.

Many members of the department are also members of the NCI-funded NYU cancer center. Research programs include exposure assessment and health effects, molecular toxicology/carcinogenesis, and pulmonary toxicology.

The department's Community Outreach and Education Core (COEC) is designed to help the public understand more about environmental health issues and to reduce misconceptions about toxic chemicals in the air, water, and homes. Once accurately informed, individuals can make better decisions regarding prevention and unintentional exposures. Students who are interested in getting more involved in environmental health science can also participate in NYU's "Science in Action" student programs and laboratory mentoring initiatives.

Financial Aid

Successful full-time M.S. applicants are automatically considered for graduate assistantships that cover living costs while at New York University as well as tuition and fees.

Predoctoral trainees receive tuition waivers and a generous annual stipend for the first two years. All full-time doctoral students in the Environmental Health Sciences program at New York University are eligible for assistantships that cover the cost of tuition and fees and also include a generous stipend.

All full-time Ph.D. students, and M.S. students in laboratory research programs, receive graduate assistant stipends plus full tuition and fees. In the 2016–17 academic year, stipends were $31,500 for Ph.D. students and $15,000 for M.S. students.

New York University

The Faculty

Faculty members are dedicated to providing comprehensive education in environmental health sciences and conducting cutting-edge research in the field. They conduct research in a wide variety of areas including chemical carcinogenesis, epigenetics, health effects of particulate air pollution, and epidemiology of cancer susceptibility.

The chair of the Department of Environmental Medicine, Dr. Max Costa's current research interests include molecular and epigenetic mechanisms of metal carcinogenesis. He holds a Ph.D. in pharmacology and began his extensive research and publishing career in 1976.

More information on the department's faculty members and their areas of research can be found online at http://www.med.nyu.edu/environmentalmedicine/graduate-program/faculty-research.

Student Outcomes

Graduates of the Environmental Health Sciences program are well-regarded in the government, business, and education sectors. They have acquired top-tier positions in numerous businesses, private and non-profit organizations, and governmental agencies including Abbott Laboratories, Brown University, Dow Corning Corporation, the New York City Department of Health, the U.S. EPA, U.S. FDA, and U.S. Army Corps of Engineers.

Location

Located in New York City in the northeastern region of the United States, NYU is one of the largest private universities in the country. Diverse in nature, it educates more than 40,000 students per year and consists of 18 schools and colleges located at five major centers in Manhattan (a borough of New York City) as well as sites in Africa, Asia, Europe, and South America.

The university's location in vibrant and culturally-diverse New York City offers students a wealth of work, entertainment, and cultural options such as the American Museum of Natural History, Broadway, Central Park, and Times Square.

The University

Founded in 1831, the prestigious New York University is ranked 36th on *U.S. News & World Report's* "Best Colleges 2017" list. It is also one of only 60 colleges and universities in the United States to become a member of the distinguished Association of American Universities.

Admissions Requirements and Applying

The admissions process for the Environmental Health Sciences program at New York University involves submitting GRE and TOEFL scores, an online or hard copy application that includes academic transcripts from undergraduate and graduate schools attended, and three letters of recommendations.

The following documents are required: NYU Graduate School of Arts and Science (GSAS) application form; official academic transcripts from all undergraduate and graduate institutions attended; three letters of recommendation; and scores on the GRE General Examination.

International students must submit scores on the TOEFL.

Applicants to the M.S. and Ph.D. Graduate Programs in Environmental Health Sciences must use the online admissions application that is available at gsas.nyu.edu/page/grad.admissionsapplication, except for Ph.D. applicants in the Biostatistics and Epidemiology areas of study who should apply at http://www.med.nyu.edu/sackler/phd-program/admissions.

Applications and supporting documents must be received by December 12 of each year. Decisions on GSAS admissions are made by April 15.

Correspondence and Information

Dr. Max Costa, Chair
Dr. Jerome Solomon, Director of Graduate Studies
Dr. Catherine B. Klein, Director of Masters Program
Department of Environmental Medicine
Graduate School of Arts and Science
New York University
70 Washington Square South
New York, New York 10012-1019
United States
Phone: 845-731-3661
Fax: 845-351-4510
E-mail: ehs@env.med.nyu.edu
Website: http://www.med.nyu.edu/environmentalmedicine/graduate-program

UNIVERSITY OF SOUTH FLORIDA
College of Public Health

 For more information, visit http://petersons.to/usf-public-health

our
practice
is
our **passion.**

University of South Florida
College of Public Health

Programs of Study

A founding member of the Association of Schools and Programs of Public Health, the University of South Florida (USF) College of Public Health (COPH) is ranked by *U.S. News & World Report* at #1 in the state of Florida, #2 in the southeast, and #16 nationally among Council on Education for Public Health accredited public health schools and colleges.

The College offers Master of Public Health (M.P.H.), Master of Science in Public Health (M.S.P.H.), Master of Health Administration (M.H.A.), Doctor of Philosophy (Ph.D.), and Doctor of Public Health (Dr.P.H.) degrees. Via five academic departments, graduate students may choose from more than 20 concentrations including:

- Behavioral health
- Biostatistics
- Community and family health
- Environmental and occupational health
- Environmental health
- Epidemiology
- Epidemiology (online)
- Epidemiology and biostatistics
- Epidemiology and global communicable diseases
- Epidemiology and global health practice
- Epidemiology and maternal and child health
- Food safety
- Genetic counseling
- Global communicable diseases
- Global disaster management, humanitarian relief, and homeland security (online)
- Global health practice
- Health care organizations and management
- Health policies and programs
- Health services research
- Health, safety and environment (online)
- Industrial hygiene
- Infection control (online)
- Maternal and child health
- Nutrition and dietetics
- Occupational health
- Occupational health for health professionals
- Occupational health for nurses
- Occupational medicine residency
- Occupational safety
- Public health administration (online)
- Public health education
- Public health practice (online)
- Social marketing (online)
- Toxicology and risk assessment

Dual degrees include the M.P.H. or Ph.D. and anthropology (M.A. or Ph.D.), M.P.H. and health administration (M.H.A.), M.P.H. and law (J.D.), M.P.H. and medicine (M.D.), M.P.H. and nursing (M.S.), M.P.H. and physical therapy (D.P.T.), and the M.P.H. and social work (M.S.W.).

In addition, COPH offers more than 20 certificate options, including some offered fully online.

The average duration to complete the master's degree is two years and three to five years for the doctoral degree.

The COPH curriculum prepares students to improve the health of communities locally and globally. Service-learning opportunities are woven throughout the curriculum at the undergraduate and graduate level. This, paired with opportunities to practice what they've learned in the field, provides the foundation for students to improve the public's health as practitioners, researchers, analysts and policymakers with hospitals and health care providers; NGOs and other nonprofits; academia; military; consulting firms; health insurance companies; and, of course, local, state, and federal government.

Research is encouraged, if not expected, of all students. Under the mentorship of faculty, students conduct research on the major public health challenges and engage in active community-based research and service learning—recognizing that it is not only through discovery and learning, but through the direct translation and application of that knowledge to policies and programs that one succeeds in improving the public's health.

Students continually present their award-winning research and practice at local, state, national, and international professional meetings, and are published in numerous peer-reviewed journals.

Research Facilities

The COPH is home to more than ten internationally recognized centers and institutes addressing areas of public health importance. Within the primary COPH building there are labs that support research and training in environmental health, industrial hygiene, physiology, water and air quality, immunology, toxicology, parasitology, risk management, ergonomics, heat stress, occupational safety, infectious diseases, and microbiology.

USF's Interdisciplinary Research Building is home to the Center for Global Health Infectious Disease with approximately 26,000 square feet of BSL-2 and BSL-3 laboratories. Neglected diseases are researched using drug and vaccine discovery methods with functional genomics and computational biology analysis.

The USF Library provides access to more than 1.3 million books and print and electronic resources including 52,000 e-journal subscriptions, 443,000 e-books, and over 800 databases. Additional facilities include the Shimberg Health Sciences Library, Louis de la Parte Florida Mental Health Institute Research Library, and libraries on the USF St. Petersburg and Sarasota-Manatee campuses.

Financial Aid

Students are the COPH's greatest asset and inspiration. As such, the College makes a variety of funding vehicles available to degree-seeking students. In 2014–15, COPH provided more than $2.7 million in student financial aid support via scholarships, graduate assistantships, and tuition waivers. For this same time period, 80 percent of COPH undergraduates and graduate students reported receiving some sort of financial aid. In addition, the College participates in the federal work-study program. Additional information is available at http://health.usf.edu/publichealth/FinAid.html.

Cost of Study

For the 2015–16 academic year, Florida resident graduate students paid $11,628 for tuition and fees, while nonresidents paid $22,326 for the same. The most up-to-date information regarding costs is available at http://www.usf.edu/financial-aid/cost-of-attendance/.

Other considerations include a reduced-rate program for out-of-state online students and the Academic Common Market tuition-savings program. More details on these programs can be found at http://health.usf.edu/publichealth/financial.html.

Living and Housing Costs

USF offers three building styles: traditional college halls, suite-style halls, and full-kitchen apartments. Graduate students may live in any hall open to upperclassmen. The local area offers a variety of communal living arrangements.

Living expenses for graduate students were estimated $14,650 for the 2015–16 academic year. This estimate includes housing, meals, entertainment, health care, clothing, etc. Additional information on housing costs is available online at http://www.usf.edu/student-affairs/housing.

Student Group

Prospective students should view themselves as a catalyst for health and plan to be fully engaged in research, volunteer in the community, and hone skills via service-learning. Applicants with insufficient training in health/science may need prerequisites. Basic computer competency is expected.

In the fall 2015 semester, the 1,704 students in the COPH broke down as follows: 839 bachelor's degree students, 743 master's degree students, 122 doctoral students; 706 part-time and 998 full-time students; 1,261 women and 443 men; 47 percent underrepresented minorities; 78 percent Florida residents; and 16 percent international students.

Student Outcomes

COPH alumni are improving the public's health as practitioners, researchers, analysts, and policymakers with hospitals and health care providers, NGOs and other nonprofits, academia, military, consulting firms, health insurance companies, and, of course, local, state and federal government.

Alumni practice public health throughout the U.S. and in remote areas around the world. Outside of Florida, the largest concentrations of alumni work in metro Atlanta with CDC-related organizations and in metro Washington, D.C.

University of South Florida

Location

Students can enjoy the outdoors year-round in this major metropolis on Florida's west coast. The region offers plenty of sunshine, arts and entertainment, shopping and dining, professional sports, and an annual average temperature of 72 degrees. Tampa International Airport is only 17 miles from campus and provides service from more than 15 major airlines. Students ride free on the campus and regional buses.

The University and The College

"Our practice is our passion" is more than a tagline for the COPH. Every day students, faculty, alumni, and staff work tirelessly to improve the health of the population in Tampa and around the world. By experiencing public health firsthand, students help find solutions to pressing health issues and understand the human, financial, and other resources needed to make it happen.

The COPH joins the Colleges of Medicine, Nursing, and Pharmacy; School of Physical Therapy and Rehabilitation Sciences; and the USF Physicians Group to form USF Health, whose mission is to envision and implement the future of health.

The COPH was founded in statute by the Florida Legislature in 1984 as the first school of public health in the state. A nationally recognized leader in community health, online education, maternal and child health, social marketing, and global infectious disease research, the COPH is leading a national movement that transforms the M.P.H. curriculum to meet today's public health needs.

As the largest metropolitan research university and the third-largest in total enrollment in the State University System of Florida, USF serves more than 48,000 students. A high-impact, global research university dedicated to student success, USF is a top 25 research university among public institutions nationwide in total research expenditures.

The University and College are accredited by the Commission on Colleges of the Southern Association of Colleges and Schools (USF), the Council on Education for Public Health (COPH), the Applied Science Accreditation Commission of ABET (M.P.S.H. in industrial hygiene), and the Commission on Accreditation Healthcare Management Education (M.H.A.).

The Faculty and Their Research

Committed to the college's mission to improve the public's health through advancing discovery, learning, and service, COPH faculty as a whole are:

- Dedicated to excellence in teaching, scholarship, and mentoring of students
- Developing leaders in health sciences who meet the needs of diverse populations
- Involved in active funded research and are engaged in nationally recognized research programs
- United around improving the health and lives of the poorest people on the planet
- Preparing managers and researchers for leadership positions in health-related organizations

The COPH has 170 faculty members with regular, adjunct, and affiliate appointments, including six who earned the designation of Distinguished University Professor or Distinguished University Health Professor. In 2015, the College's faculty generated more than $25 million in external grants and contracts.

The faculty serve across five academic departments:

Community and Family Health

William M. Sappenfield, M.D., M.P.H., C.P.H.; Professor and Chair. The department focuses on the improved health of women, children, and families; prevention of injuries and family violence; and prevention of sexually transmitted infections and unintended pregnancies. Research and advocacy approaches include behavioral health, social marketing, health literacy, and health education and promotion.

Environmental and Occupational Health

Thomas E. Bernard, Ph.D.; Professor and Chair. The department focuses on measurement and risk assessment of environmental and occupational exposures to chemical, physical, and biological agents.

Epidemiology and Biostatistics

Kathleen O'Rourke, Ph.D.; Professor and Chair. The department employs the use of epidemiological and biostatistical techniques to address maternal child health, diabetes, and cardiovascular disease; PTSD among veteran populations; environmental and global health; the effect of sleep; plus, pharmacoepidemiology, cancer epidemiology, clinical trials, and biostatistics and data analytic methods.

Global Health

Thomas Unnasch, Ph.D., Distinguished University Health Professor and Chair. The department utilizes the application of genomics to address infectious and chronic human disease; ecology and development of drugs, vaccines, and other interventions to prevent, cure, and eliminate vector-borne pathogens; and infection control.

Health Policy and Management

John P. Petrila, J.D., L.L.M.; Professor and Chair. The department engages in health outcomes services research; health economics; public health law and policies; trauma and emergency medicine systems; Medicaid and managed care; healthcare disparities by race/ethnicity, gender, and age; and genomics and law.

Applying

Graduate applicants are required to submit the SOPHAS application and fee. Once verified by SOPHAS, COPH emails applicant with USF application link and the applicant then submits the completed USF application and fee and COPH reviews the applications for the desired term. More details are available at http://health.usf.edu/publichealth/apply/graduate-admissions.

Correspondence and Information

To learn more about programs of study and the 1,700 students who commit to passionately solve problems and create conditions that allow every person the universal right to health and well-being, interested applicants are encouraged to contact a COPH admissions representative.

College of Public Health
University of South Florida
13201 Bruce B. Downs Blvd, MDC 56 (mailing address)
3010 USF Banyan Circle (physical address)
Tampa, Florida 33612
Phone: 813-974-6505 or 888-USF-COPH (toll-free)
Website: www.publichealth.usf.edu

Kamala Dontamsetti, MBA, M.A., Assistant Director of Graduate Admissions
Phone: 813-974-8874
Fax: 813-974-8121
E-mail: cophinfo@health.usf.edu
Website: http://health.usf.edu/publichealth/apply/graduate-admissions

COPH students strike a bullish pose with Dean Donna Petersen.

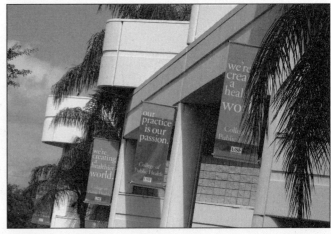

Students with a passion for public health find the USF College of Public Health a great place to build their future.

UNIVERSITY OF WISCONSIN–MADISON

Department of Population Health Sciences

 For more information, visit http://petersons.to/uw-madison_populationhealth

Programs of Study

The Population Health Sciences graduate and professional degree programs at the University of Wisconsin–Madison offer the unusual combination of an integrated school model and an interdisciplinary approach, with degree flexibility and personal attention for students in addition to world-class university resources, learning beyond the classroom, and the pleasure of life in vibrant and beautiful Madison, Wisconsin.

In 2005, the University of Wisconsin Medical School became the University of Wisconsin School of Medicine and Public Health, signaling the development a revolutionary new model of education, research, and service that unites public health and medicine. The vision with this model has been to create a superior education, research, and community engagement enterprise that integrates biomedical sciences, care of individual patients, and the health of diverse populations. This new integrated approach addresses the evolving health and health care needs of Wisconsin and beyond, and in so doing, serves as a national model to solve America's most pressing health issues.

The graduate degree programs at the Department of Population Health Sciences for the University of Wisconsin–Madison are well-suited for those wanting to become excellent, well-rounded health practitioners and/or researchers. Students studying in these programs explore the fields of epidemiology, public health, health policy, social and behavioral health, health services research, biostatistics, environmental health, and others. The school takes pride in preparing its students in a very holistic way for the various aspects of public and population health work. In this way, students come to have a more complete understanding of various public health issues and how to initiate prevention efforts effectively or conduct quality research.

The programs in the Department of Population Health Sciences—which include a Master of Science (M.S.) or Doctor of Philosophy (Ph.D.) degree program in Population Health, an M.S. or Ph.D. degree program in Epidemiology, and a Master of Public Health (M.P.H.) degree program—can be tailored to a student's specific health interests due to the flexibility of the curriculum. All students complete a set of core courses, but beyond these required courses students are afforded great latitude in course selection towards electives related to their own specific interests. Depending on the particular degree program, the University also offers areas of concentration, dual degrees, and certificate options to further enhance students' educational goals and provide degree specialization.

Degree programs offered by the Department include:

Master of Public Health (M.P.H.): This degree program provides a practice-oriented, interdisciplinary focused education for students seeking to gain competence in public health practice and for health professional students who wish to strengthen their knowledge and skills in public health. This 42-credit program includes course work in the five core public health areas, opportunities to choose elective courses from across the campus, and a required 400-hour field experience. The M.P.H. program collaborates with several other health professions programs across campus through its dual degree programs. Additional information about the program is available at http://pophealth.wisc.edu/mph/about.

Population Health Sciences Graduate Programs: The Population Health Sciences programs focus on training tomorrow's leaders in interdisciplinary research. The University offers an M.S. and Ph.D. in Population Health and an M.S. and Ph.D. in Epidemiology. The programs prepare students to conduct, communicate, and share research aimed at the protection, promotion, and restoration of health in human populations. More details can be found online at http://pophealth.wisc.edu/grad/futureStudents/about.

Research

The work of students is valued, as evidenced by their entries in the annual department poster session, participation in public health symposia, authorship of publications, and involvement in community/research projects. The Population Health Sciences Department conducts research in the following fields: biostatistics; clinical research; environmental health; epidemiology; global health; health policy; health services research; public health systems; and social and behavioral health sciences.

Financial Aid

Students admitted to UW–Madison degree programs are automatically considered for any available scholarships, traineeships, or graduate assistant positions in the department. However, students are also encouraged to explore their own funding opportunities. Unlike many departments, the Department of Population Health Sciences does not have a policy of admitting only students for whom initial funding is available. The Department makes every effort to help students finance their education and are most successful with providing funding to Ph.D. admits. Potential funding opportunities are considered during the admissions review process but funding decisions continue to be made throughout the spring and summer. Further information is available at http://pophealth.wisc.edu/grad/finance.

Cost of Study

The most current tuition and fee information is available at https://registrar.wisc.edu/tuition_&_fees.htm.

The Faculty

Students have the advantage of learning from people who practice public health. A number of faculty members in the department have been identified in state and community public health agencies, and these individuals actively contribute their knowledge and skills to the degree programs and students. These faculty members often serve as guest lecturers, discussion group leaders, and preceptors. The field experience requirement of the M.P.H. professional degree program helps students gain additional hands-on experience and provides them the opportunity to serve and benefit the community by applying their classroom knowledge to real world public health issues. Research scientists in the department lead efforts on campus in the creation, consolidation, and translation of new and existing knowledge into community-based practice to improve healthcare delivery and outcomes.

The faculty members, staff members, and community colleagues in the Department are committed to serving students, and are friendly and accessible. Students have the benefit of daily dialogues and personalized training from renowned faculty. In addition, seminars and integrated discussion groups allow for increased interaction with core faculty members and community lecturers. After entering one of the graduate or professional degree programs in the Department of Population Health Science, students are each matched with a faculty adviser. The adviser will help students hone their interests, assist with identifying field experience and research projects, provide support for career development, and link students to the greater campus community. A complete listing of faculty members in the Department and their areas of research can be found at http://pophealth.wisc.edu/grad/faculty.

Location

Built on an Isthmus between Lake Monona and Lake Mendota, Madison offers incredible natural beauty, stimulating cultural opportunities, and a plethora of restaurants, shops, and attractions. The campus rolls along Lake Mendota, with wooded hills and the busy city streets of downtown Madison. Madison is small enough to navigate easily, but it offers cultural resources and amenities that rival those of cities many times its size. As the state capital of Wisconsin, Madison provides a vibrant downtown area and also a wealth of recreational resources, such as the five area lakes, over 200 parks, and numerous biking trails. Healthcare is another of Madison's strengths with five general hospitals, more than 20 major medical clinics, and UW–Madison's medical, nursing, and pharmacy schools. The city's location in south central Wisconsin also makes for convenient access to Milwaukee, Chicago, and Minneapolis. Madison continues to rank high on numerous lists as one of the top communities in which to live, work, play, and raise a family.

Admission and Applying

Applications are welcome from students with diverse academic backgrounds. Students who have strong academic preparation in the biological/medical sciences, quantitative analysis, or population health–related social sciences are strongly encouraged to apply. Historically, many applicants who have succeeded in the programs have come with backgrounds in fields as diverse as microbiology, genetics, nutritional sciences, medicine, nursing, pharmacy, veterinary medicine, environmental sciences, political sciences, business, sociology, education, engineering, psychology, economics, and actuarial science, among others.

Applicants to the **M.P.H. program** must hold a baccalaureate degree (B.A. or B.S.) from a regionally accredited U.S. institution. Official transcripts from all college and graduate work must be submitted. An undergraduate GPA of 3.0 or higher is expected. At minimum, candidates must have successfully completed at least one semester of college level mathematics that includes algebra and/or calculus or a college-level statistics class. In addition, candidates must have taken at minimum, one semester of a college-level science course such as biology, chemistry, or physics. Applicants must submit official test scores from the Graduate Record Exam (GRE) taken within the last five years.

Public health–related experience is highly recommended. This includes, but is not limited to, working in public health departments, volunteer organizations, and health care organizations that do not focus solely on patient care. Clinical care alone does not constitute as public health experience.

In addition to the required M.P.H. application materials, international applicants are required to submit official scores from the Test of English as a Foreign Language (TOEFL) taken within the last five years. Applicants who attended a post-secondary institution outside of the U.S. must have their academic records evaluated by a NACES member credential evaluation service. An official evaluation report from a NACES member organization must also be received for the application to be considered complete.

A non-refundable fee of $56 paid electronically via debit or credit card is required before your application will be reviewed.

For 2017–18 admission consideration, all materials must be received by February 1, 2017. Late applications are not accepted and will not be reviewed. Additional details regarding the application process and requirements can be found at http://mph.wisc.edu/mph/apply.

Applicants to the **Population Health and Epidemiology M.S. and Ph.D. programs** must meet both the departmental admission requirements and the Graduate School admission requirements. The Admissions Committee considers many aspects of the application including grades, GRE scores, quantitative preparation, letters of recommendation, statement of purpose, and prior research and/or professional experience.

Applicants should have a minimum undergraduate G.P.A. of 3.0 (on a 4.0 scale), although successful applicants generally have G.P.A.s above 3.0. GRE scores are required for admission. The scores must be no more than 5 years old at the time of application. Applicants whose native language or language of study was not English must submit official scores from an English proficiency test (TOEFL or the IELTS). Scores must be no more than 5 years old at the start of semester for which the student is applying.

Applicants for the M.S./Ph.D. in Population Health programs should have at least one semester of advanced quantitative preparation (e.g., calculus, statistics, or other) with a grade of B or better.

Applicants for the M.S./Ph.D. in Epidemiology programs must have at least one semester of calculus with a grade of B or better. College-level biology is also required.

For 2017–18 admission consideration, all materials must be received by January 15, 2017. Late applications are not accepted and will not be reviewed. Additional details regarding the application process and requirements can be found at http://pophealth.wisc.edu/grad/apply.

Correspondence and Information

Department of Population Health Sciences
707 WARF Building
University of Wisconsin–Madison
610 N. Walnut Street
Madison, Wisconsin 53726
United States
Phone: 608-263-2880
Fax: 608-263-2820
E-mail: pophealth@mailplus.wisc.edu
Website: https://pophealth.wisc.edu/Home

ACADEMIC AND PROFESSIONAL PROGRAMS IN THE MEDICAL PROFESSIONS AND SCIENCES

Section 25
Acupuncture and Oriental Medicine

This section contains a directory of institutions offering graduate work in acupuncture and oriental medicine. Additional information about programs listed in the directory but not augmented by an in-depth entry may be obtained by writing directly to the dean of a graduate school or chair of a department at the address given in the directory.

CONTENTS

Program Directory

Acupuncture and Oriental Medicine

Academy for Five Element Acupuncture, Graduate Program, Gainesville, FL 32601. Offers M Ac. *Accreditation:* ACAOM.

Academy of Chinese Culture and Health Sciences, Program in Traditional Chinese Medicine, Oakland, CA 94612. Offers MS. *Accreditation:* ACAOM. *Program availability:* Part-time, evening/weekend. *Degree requirements:* For master's, comprehensive exam, thesis. *Entrance requirements:* Additional exam requirements/recommendations for international students: Required—TOEFL (minimum score 500 paper-based). *Faculty research:* Herbs, acupuncture.

Acupuncture & Integrative Medicine College, Berkeley, Program in Oriental Medicine, Berkeley, CA 94704. Offers MS. *Accreditation:* ACAOM. *Program availability:* Part-time. *Faculty:* 29 part-time/adjunct (17 women). *Students:* 61 full-time (48 women), 43 part-time (36 women); includes 30 minority (4 Black or African American, non-Hispanic/Latino; 9 Asian, non-Hispanic/Latino; 8 Hispanic/Latino; 1 Native Hawaiian or other Pacific Islander, non-Hispanic/Latino; 8 Two or more races, non-Hispanic/Latino), 5 international. Average age 37. 40 applicants, 85% accepted, 29 enrolled. In 2015, 33 master's awarded. *Degree requirements:* For master's, comprehensive exam, 350 clinic treatments. *Entrance requirements:* For master's, interview, minimum GPA of 3.0, 60 semester units of course work at the baccalaureate level. Additional exam requirements/recommendations for international students: Required—TOEFL (minimum score 61 iBT). *Application deadline:* For fall admission, 3/15 priority date for domestic and international students; for winter admission, 7/15 priority date for domestic and international students; for spring admission, 11/15 priority date for domestic and international students. Application fee: $100 ($200 for international students). Electronic applications accepted. *Expenses:* $263 per didactic unit; $525 per clinic unit. *Financial support:* Federal Work-Study available. Support available to part-time students. Financial award application deadline: 7/31; financial award applicants required to submit FAFSA. *Faculty research:* Stimulus therapy, oxygen hemoglobin, acupuncture needling, classical Chinese medicine. *Unit head:* Yasou Tanaka, President, 510-666-8248, Fax: 510-666-0111, E-mail: ytanaka@aimc.edu. *Application contact:* Julie Scheff.

Acupuncture and Massage College, Program in Oriental Medicine, Miami, FL 33176. Offers MOM. *Accreditation:* ACAOM.

American College of Acupuncture and Oriental Medicine, Graduate Studies, Houston, TX 77063. Offers MAOM. *Accreditation:* ACAOM. *Program availability:* Part-time. *Entrance requirements:* For master's, 60 undergraduate credit hours. Additional exam requirements/recommendations for international students: Required—TOEFL.

AOMA Graduate School of Integrative Medicine, Doctor of Acupuncture and Oriental Medicine Program, Austin, TX 78757. Offers DAOM. *Degree requirements:* For doctorate, comprehensive exam, clinical internship, clinical externship, capstone research project, portfolio. *Entrance requirements:* For doctorate, master's degree from ACAOM-accredited program in acupuncture and Oriental medicine; minimum GPA of 3.0 in master's studies; current license or eligibility to obtain a license to practice acupuncture in the state of Texas. Additional exam requirements/recommendations for international students: Required—TOEFL (minimum score 508 paper-based; 87 iBT), IELTS (minimum score 6.5). Electronic applications accepted. *Faculty research:* Allergy, cancer, women's health.

AOMA Graduate School of Integrative Medicine, Master of Acupuncture and Oriental Medicine Program, Austin, TX 78757. Offers MAcOM. *Accreditation:* ACAOM. *Degree requirements:* For master's, comprehensive exam, clinical rotations (40.5 credits), portfolio. *Entrance requirements:* For master's, BA or higher or minimum of 90 credits at baccalaureate level from regionally-accredited institution with 30 credits of general education coursework; minimum GPA of 2.5. Additional exam requirements/recommendations for international students: Required—TOEFL (minimum score 508 paper-based; 87 iBT), IELTS. Electronic applications accepted. *Faculty research:* Acupuncture, Chinese herbal medicine, integrative medicine, pulse diagnosis.

Arizona School of Acupuncture and Oriental Medicine, Graduate Programs, Tucson, AZ 85716. Offers M Ac, M Ac OM. *Accreditation:* ACAOM. *Unit head:* Tim Dunn, Admissions Director, 520-795-0787 Ext. 104, Fax: 877-222-4606, E-mail: admissions@asaom.edu.

Atlantic Institute of Oriental Medicine, Graduate Program, Fort Lauderdale, FL 33301. Offers MS, DAOM. *Accreditation:* ACAOM. *Program availability:* Evening/weekend. *Faculty:* 7 full-time (1 woman), 15 part-time/adjunct (6 women). *Students:* 142 full-time (109 women); includes 23 minority (3 Black or African American, non-Hispanic/Latino; 7 Asian, non-Hispanic/Latino; 13 Hispanic/Latino), 7 international. *Entrance requirements:* For master's, official transcripts, professional resume, essay, two letters of reference. Additional exam requirements/recommendations for international students: Required—TOEFL (minimum score 500 paper-based). *Application deadline:* For fall admission, 7/1 for domestic students, 5/1 for international students; for spring admission, 11/30 for domestic students, 2/28 for international students. Applications are processed on a rolling basis. Application fee: $20 ($30 for international students). *Expenses:* Tuition, area resident: Full-time $17,000. *Required fees:* $250. One-time fee: $450 full-time. *Unit head:* Dr. Johanna C. Yen, President, 954-763-9840 Ext. 202, Fax: 954-763-9844, E-mail: president@atom.edu. *Application contact:* Milagros Ferreira, Registrar, 954-763-9840 Ext. 207, Fax: 954-763-9844, E-mail: registrar@atom.edu.

Bastyr University, School of Acupuncture and Oriental Medicine, Kenmore, WA 98028-4966. Offers MS, DAOM, Certificate. *Accreditation:* ACAOM. *Program availability:* Evening/weekend. *Entrance requirements:* For master's, course work in biology, chemistry, intermediate algebra and psychology; for doctorate, MS in acupuncture or certificate and 10 years of clinical experience. Additional exam requirements/recommendations for international students: Required—TOEFL (minimum score 550 paper-based; 79 iBT). Electronic applications accepted. *Faculty research:* Integrative oncology, acupuncture and chemotherapy-induced peripheral neuropathy (CIPN), traditional Chinese medicine and stroke rehabilitation, acupuncture and prevention and wellness, electroacupuncture.

California Institute of Integral Studies, American College of Traditional Chinese Medicine, San Francisco, CA 94107. Offers acupuncture and Chinese medicine (DACM, tDACM); acupuncture and Oriental medicine (DAOM); traditional Chinese medicine (MSTCM). *Students:* 170 full-time (127 women), 64 part-time (44 women); includes 91 minority (5 Black or African American, non-Hispanic/Latino; 2 American Indian or Alaska Native, non-Hispanic/Latino; 66 Asian, non-Hispanic/Latino; 12 Hispanic/Latino; 6 Native Hawaiian or other Pacific Islander, non-Hispanic/Latino), 8 international. Average age 37. 55 applicants, 91% accepted, 34 enrolled. *Entrance requirements:* Additional exam requirements/recommendations for international students: Required—TOEFL (minimum score 550 paper-based; 213 iBT). *Application deadline:* For fall admission, 8/1 priority date for domestic students. Application fee: $65. Electronic applications accepted. *Unit head:* Dr. Bingzen Zou, Academic Dean, 415-8287600, E-mail: bingzou@actcm.edu. *Application contact:* Yuwen Chiu, Associate Director of Admissions, 415-828-7600, E-mail: yuwenchiu@actcm.edu. Website: https://www.actcm.edu

Canadian Memorial Chiropractic College, Certificate Programs, Toronto, ON M2H 3J1, Canada. Offers chiropractic clinical sciences (Certificate); chiropractic radiology (Certificate); chiropractic sports sciences (Certificate); clinical acupuncture (Certificate). *Degree requirements:* For Certificate, thesis. *Entrance requirements:* For degree, DC, board certification. *Faculty research:* Theories and concepts of chiropractic, sciences related to chiropractic, assessments of the efficacy and efficiency of chiropractic.

Colorado School of Traditional Chinese Medicine, Graduate Programs, Denver, CO 80206-2127. Offers acupuncture (MS); traditional Chinese medicine (MS). *Accreditation:* ACAOM. *Program availability:* Part-time. *Faculty:* 52 part-time/adjunct (20 women). *Students:* 92 full-time (67 women). Average age 33. 72 applicants, 88% accepted, 60 enrolled. In 2015, 1 master's awarded. *Entrance requirements:* For master's, 60 semester credits or 90 quarter credits from an accredited college, essay, current curriculum vitae/resume. Additional exam requirements/recommendations for international students: Required—TOEFL (minimum score 61 iBT) or IELTS (minimum score 6). *Application deadline:* For fall admission, 8/19 for domestic and international students; for winter admission, 12/23 for domestic and international students; for summer admission, 4/22 for domestic and international students. Applications are processed on a rolling basis. Application fee: $50. *Expenses:* Tuition, area resident: Full-time $17,000; part-time $9000 per year. *Required fees:* $450; $1020 per unit. $340 per trimester. Part-time tuition and fees vary according to course load and program. *Financial support:* Scholarships/grants available. Financial award applicants required to submit FAFSA. *Unit head:* Vladimir Dibrigida, Administrative Director, 303-329-6355 Ext. 11, Fax: 303-388-8165, E-mail: director@cstcm.edu. *Application contact:* Chris Duxbury-Edwards, Recruiting Director, 303-329-6355 Ext. 21, Fax: 303-388-8165, E-mail: recruiting@cstcm.edu. Website: http://www.cstcm.edu

Dongguk University Los Angeles, Program in Oriental Medicine, Los Angeles, CA 90020. Offers MS. *Accreditation:* ACAOM. *Program availability:* Part-time, evening/weekend.

East West College of Natural Medicine, Graduate Programs, Sarasota, FL 34234. Offers MSOM. *Accreditation:* ACAOM.

Emperor's College of Traditional Oriental Medicine, Graduate Programs, Santa Monica, CA 90403. Offers MTOM, DAOM. *Accreditation:* ACAOM. *Program availability:* Part-time, evening/weekend. *Entrance requirements:* For master's, minimum 2 years of undergraduate course work, interview; for doctorate, CA acupuncture licensure. *Faculty research:* Menopause, dysmenorrhea.

Five Branches University, Graduate School of Traditional Chinese Medicine, Santa Cruz, CA 95062. Offers acupuncture (M Ac); acupuncture and Oriental medicine (DAOM); traditional Chinese medicine (MTCM, PhD). *Accreditation:* ACAOM. *Faculty:* 10 full-time (5 women), 90 part-time/adjunct (45 women). *Students:* 400 full-time (320 women). Average age 35. *Degree requirements:* For master's, comprehensive exam. *Entrance requirements:* For master's, 6 units in anatomy and physiology, 9 units in basic sciences, minimum GPA of 2.5. Additional exam requirements/recommendations for international students: Required—TOEFL, IELTS. *Application deadline:* For fall admission, 6/1 priority date for domestic students; for spring admission, 11/1 priority date for domestic students. Applications are processed on a rolling basis. Application fee: $30. Electronic applications accepted. *Expenses:* Tuition, area resident: Full-time $16,000; part-time $9600 per credit. *Required fees:* $200; $200 per credit. $50 per trimester. Tuition and fees vary according to degree level. *Financial support:* In 2015–16, 80 students received support. Career-related internships or fieldwork and scholarships/grants available. Financial award application deadline: 4/15; financial award applicants required to submit FAFSA. *Unit head:* Joanna Zhao, Vice President, Academic Affairs, 831-476-9424 Ext. 42, Fax: 831-476-8928, E-mail: dean@fivebranches.edu. *Application contact:* Eleonor Mendelson, Admissions Director, 831-476-9424, Fax: 831-476-8928, E-mail: tcm@fivebranches.com. Website: http://www.fivebranches.edu/

Florida College of Integrative Medicine, Graduate Program, Orlando, FL 32809. Offers MSOM. *Accreditation:* ACAOM. *Program availability:* Evening/weekend. *Entrance requirements:* For master's, minimum 60 semester hours of undergraduate coursework. Electronic applications accepted.

Institute of Clinical Acupuncture and Oriental Medicine, Program in Oriental Medicine, Honolulu, HI 96817. Offers MSOM. *Accreditation:* ACAOM.

Maryland University of Integrative Health, Chinese Herb Certificate Program, Laurel, MD 20723. Offers Certificate. *Program availability:* Part-time, evening/weekend. *Entrance requirements:* Additional exam requirements/recommendations for international students: Required—TOEFL.

Maryland University of Integrative Health, Program in Acupuncture, Laurel, MD 20723. Offers M Ac. *Accreditation:* ACAOM. *Degree requirements:* For master's, comprehensive exam, 500 clinical hours, oral exams. *Entrance requirements:* Additional exam requirements/recommendations for international students: Required—TOEFL. *Faculty research:* Philosophical roots of oriental medicine, meridian pathways, points, pulses.

Maryland University of Integrative Health, Program in Applied Healing Arts, Laurel, MD 20723. Offers MA. *Entrance requirements:* Additional exam requirements/recommendations for international students: Required—TOEFL. *Faculty research:* Healing habits of mind and heart, an expanded vision, bringing of one's vision and practices to a special arena.

Maryland University of Integrative Health, Program in Herbal Medicine, Laurel, MD 20723. Offers MS. *Entrance requirements:* Additional exam requirements/recommendations for international students: Required—TOEFL. *Faculty research:* Philosophical roots of holistic healing, botany, herbal pharmacology, materia medica, holistic healing.

MCPHS University, New England School of Acupuncture, Boston, MA 02115-5896. Offers acupuncture (M Ac); acupuncture and Oriental medicine (MAOM). *Accreditation:* ACAOM (one or more programs are accredited). *Program availability:* Part-time. *Degree requirements:* For master's, comprehensive exam. *Entrance requirements:* For master's, previous course work in anatomy, biology, physiology, and psychology. Additional exam requirements/recommendations for international students: Required—TOEFL (minimum score 550 paper-based). *Faculty research:* Acupuncture and women's health, acupuncture and stroke rehabilitation, tai chi and cardiovascular health, tai chi and balance, cancer.

Midwest College of Oriental Medicine, Graduate Programs, Racine, WI 53403-9747. Offers acupuncture (Certificate); oriental medicine (MSOM). *Accreditation:* ACAOM. *Program availability:* Part-time, evening/weekend. *Degree requirements:* For master's and Certificate, comprehensive exam, thesis. *Entrance requirements:* For master's and Certificate, 60 semester credit hours from accredited school, 2 letters of recommendation, interview. Additional exam requirements/recommendations for international students: Required—TOEFL. *Faculty research:* Pharmacology.

Midwest College of Oriental Medicine, Graduate Programs-Chicago, Chicago, IL 60613. Offers acupuncture (Certificate); oriental medicine (MSOM). *Accreditation:* ACAOM. *Program availability:* Part-time, evening/weekend. *Degree requirements:* For master's and Certificate, comprehensive exam, thesis. *Entrance requirements:* For master's and Certificate, 60 semester credit hours from accredited school, 2 letters of recommendation, interview. Additional exam requirements/recommendations for international students: Required—TOEFL.

National College of Natural Medicine, School of Classical Chinese Medicine, Portland, OR 97201. Offers M Ac, MSOM. *Accreditation:* ACAOM. *Program availability:* Evening/weekend. *Degree requirements:* For master's, thesis. *Entrance requirements:* Additional exam requirements/recommendations for international students: Recommended—TOEFL. *Expenses:* Contact institution. *Faculty research:* Cases on herbs and acupuncture for asthma, diabetes, depression associated with menopause; Qi Gong to maintain weight loss.

New York Chiropractic College, Finger Lakes School of Acupuncture and Oriental Medicine, Seneca Falls, NY 13148-0800. Offers acupuncture (MS); acupuncture and Oriental medicine (MS). *Accreditation:* ACAOM. *Degree requirements:* For master's, clinical internship. *Entrance requirements:* For master's, interview, three written references. Additional exam requirements/recommendations for international students: Recommended—TOEFL (minimum score 550 paper-based). Electronic applications accepted. *Faculty research:* Chinese herbal medicine, traditional Chinese medicine, cancer, gait and posture, obesity.

New York College of Health Professions, Graduate School of Oriental Medicine, Syosset, NY 11791-4413. Offers acupuncture (MS); Oriental medicine (MS). *Accreditation:* ACAOM. *Program availability:* Part-time. *Degree requirements:* For master's, thesis. *Entrance requirements:* For master's, minimum GPA of 2.5, 60 semester credits in undergraduate course work. Additional exam requirements/recommendations for international students: Required—TOEFL. *Faculty research:* Breast cancer, diabetic neuropathy hemolysis.

New York College of Traditional Chinese Medicine, Graduate Programs, Mineola, NY 11501. Offers oriental medicine (MAOM). *Accreditation:* ACAOM.

Northwestern Health Sciences University, College of Acupuncture and Oriental Medicine, Bloomington, MN 55431-1599. Offers acupuncture (M Ac); Oriental medicine (MOM). *Accreditation:* ACAOM. *Entrance requirements:* For master's, 60 semester credits of course work with minimum GPA of 2.5. Additional exam requirements/recommendations for international students: Required—TOEFL (minimum score 540 paper-based; 76 iBT). Electronic applications accepted.

Oregon College of Oriental Medicine, Graduate Program in Acupuncture and Oriental Medicine, Portland, OR 97216. Offers M Ac OM, MAcOM, DAOM. *Accreditation:* ACAOM. *Program availability:* Part-time. *Entrance requirements:* For master's, minimum 3 years of college; course work in chemistry, biology, and psychology; for doctorate, documentation of clinical practice, 3 years of clinical experience. Additional exam requirements/recommendations for international students: Required—TOEFL (minimum score 550 paper-based).

Pacific College of Oriental Medicine, Graduate Program, San Diego, CA 92108. Offers MSTOM, DAOM. *Accreditation:* ACAOM. *Program availability:* Part-time, evening/weekend. *Entrance requirements:* For master's, 2 letters of reference, interviews, minimum GPA of 3.0. *Faculty research:* PMS, acupuncture, herbs, Tai Ji Quan, sports medicine.

Pacific College of Oriental Medicine–Chicago, Graduate Program, Chicago, IL 60601. Offers MTOM. *Accreditation:* ACAOM. *Program availability:* Part-time, evening/weekend. *Entrance requirements:* For master's, 2 letters of reference, interview, minimum GPA of 3.0. *Faculty research:* AIDS, cancer, mental health, clinical counseling.

Pacific College of Oriental Medicine-New York, Graduate Program, New York, NY 10010. Offers MSTOM. *Accreditation:* ACAOM. *Program availability:* Part-time, evening/weekend. *Entrance requirements:* For master's, 2 letters of reference, interview, minimum GPA of 3.0. *Faculty research:* Energy medicine, acupuncture in the treatment of neurological disorders.

Seattle Institute of Oriental Medicine, Graduate Program, Seattle, WA 98115. Offers M Ac OM. *Accreditation:* ACAOM. *Degree requirements:* For master's, one foreign language, comprehensive exam. *Entrance requirements:* For master's, course work in biology, psychology, chemistry, anatomy, physiology; CPR/first aid certification; 3 years (90 semester credits) post secondary coursework. Additional exam requirements/

recommendations for international students: Recommended—TOEFL (minimum score 500 paper-based).

South Baylo University, Program in Oriental Medicine and Acupuncture, Anaheim, CA 92801-1701. Offers MS. *Accreditation:* ACAOM. *Program availability:* Evening/weekend. *Degree requirements:* For master's, 3 foreign languages, comprehensive exam. *Entrance requirements:* Additional exam requirements/recommendations for international students: Required—TOEFL (minimum score 500 paper-based). Electronic applications accepted. *Faculty research:* Effectiveness of acupuncture therapy.

Southern California University of Health Sciences, College of Eastern Medicine, Whittier, CA 90609-1166. Offers MAOM, DAOM. *Accreditation:* ACAOM. *Program availability:* Part-time, evening/weekend. *Degree requirements:* For master's and doctorate, comprehensive exam. *Entrance requirements:* For master's, 60 semester hours or 90 quarter credits of undergraduate course work, interview. Additional exam requirements/recommendations for international students: Required—TOEFL (minimum score 500 paper-based). Electronic applications accepted. *Faculty research:* Stress study.

Southwest Acupuncture College, Program in Oriental Medicine, Boulder Campus, Boulder, CO 80301. Offers MS. *Accreditation:* ACAOM. *Program availability:* Part-time. *Entrance requirements:* For master's, minimum 2 years of college general education.

Southwest Acupuncture College, Program in Oriental Medicine, Santa Fe Campus, Santa Fe, NM 87505. Offers MS. *Accreditation:* ACAOM. *Program availability:* Part-time. *Entrance requirements:* For master's, minimum 2 years of college general education. Additional exam requirements/recommendations for international students: Required—TOEFL (minimum score 500 paper-based). Electronic applications accepted.

Swedish Institute, College of Health Sciences, Graduate Program, New York, NY 10001-6700. Offers acupuncture (MS). *Accreditation:* ACAOM. *Program availability:* Part-time, evening/weekend. *Entrance requirements:* Additional exam requirements/recommendations for international students: Required—TOEFL (minimum score 72 iBT).

Tri-State College of Acupuncture, Graduate Programs, New York, NY 10011. Offers acupuncture (MS); Chinese herbology (Certificate); Oriental medicine (MS). *Accreditation:* ACAOM. *Program availability:* Evening/weekend. *Faculty:* 5 full-time (2 women), 32 part-time/adjunct (24 women). *Students:* 95 full-time (65 women), 17 part-time (11 women); includes 16 minority (1 Black or African American, non-Hispanic/Latino; 13 Asian, non-Hispanic/Latino; 2 Hispanic/Latino). *Entrance requirements:* Additional exam requirements/recommendations for international students: Recommended—TOEFL. *Application deadline:* For fall admission, 6/15 priority date for domestic students. Applications are processed on a rolling basis. Application fee: $50. *Expenses: Tuition, area resident:* Full-time $23,600; part-time $11,800 per semester. *Required fees:* $395; $395 per year. *Financial support:* Application deadline: 7/15; applicants required to submit FAFSA. *Application contact:* Sandra Turner, Admissions Office, 212-242-2255, Fax: 212-242-2920, E-mail: sandra.turner@tsca.edu. Website: http://www.tsca.edu

University of Bridgeport, Acupuncture Institute, Bridgeport, CT 06604. Offers MS. *Accreditation:* ACAOM. *Program availability:* Part-time. *Entrance requirements:* Additional exam requirements/recommendations for international students: Recommended—TOEFL (minimum score 550 paper-based; 80 iBT), IELTS (minimum score 6.5). *Application deadline:* For fall admission, 8/1 priority date for domestic students, 8/1 for international students; for spring admission, 12/1 priority date for domestic students, 12/1 for international students. Applications are processed on a rolling basis. Application fee: $50. Electronic applications accepted. *Expenses:* Contact institution.

WON Institute of Graduate Studies, Acupuncture Studies Program, Glenside, PA 19038. Offers M Ac. *Accreditation:* ACAOM. *Entrance requirements:* For master's, 6 prerequisite credits in anatomy and physiology, 2 letters of recommendation, essay, bachelor's degree, 3 credits of basic science (chemistry, biology, physics or botany). Additional exam requirements/recommendations for international students: Required—TOEFL (minimum score 550 paper-based; 79 iBT). Electronic applications accepted. *Faculty research:* Meditation and pulse taking, acupuncture and apprehension.

WON Institute of Graduate Studies, Program in Chinese Herbal Medicine, Glenside, PA 19038. Offers Certificate. *Entrance requirements:* Additional exam requirements/recommendations for international students: Required—TOEFL (minimum score 550 paper-based; 79 iBT). Electronic applications accepted.

World Medicine Institute, Program in Acupuncture and Oriental Medicine, Honolulu, HI 96821. Offers M Ac OM. *Accreditation:* ACAOM. *Program availability:* Part-time, evening/weekend. *Entrance requirements:* For master's, minimum 60 college credits.

Yo San University of Traditional Chinese Medicine, Program in Acupuncture and Traditional Chinese Medicine, Los Angeles, CA 90066. Offers MATCM. *Accreditation:* ACAOM. *Program availability:* Part-time, online learning. *Degree requirements:* For master's, observation and practice internships, exam. *Entrance requirements:* For master's, minimum 2 years of college, interview, minimum GPA of 2.5.

Section 26
Chiropractic

This section contains a directory of institutions offering graduate work in chiropractic. Additional information about programs listed in the directory but not augmented by an in-depth entry may be obtained by writing directly to the dean of a graduate school or chair of a department at the address given in the directory.

CONTENTS

Chiropractic

Canadian Memorial Chiropractic College, Certificate Programs, Toronto, ON M2H 3J1, Canada. Offers chiropractic clinical sciences (Certificate); chiropractic radiology (Certificate); chiropractic sports sciences (Certificate); clinical acupuncture (Certificate). *Degree requirements:* For Certificate, thesis. *Entrance requirements:* For degree, DC, board certification. *Faculty research:* Theories and concepts of chiropractic, sciences related to chiropractic, assessments of the efficacy and efficiency of chiropractic.

Canadian Memorial Chiropractic College, Professional Program, Toronto, ON M2H 3J1, Canada. Offers DC. *Entrance requirements:* For doctorate, 3 full years of university (15 full courses or 90 hours). *Faculty research:* Theories and concepts of chiropractic, sciences related to chiropractic, assessment of the efficacy and efficiency of chiropractic.

Cleveland University–Kansas City, Professional Program, Overland Park, KS 66210. Offers DC. *Accreditation:* CCE. *Program availability:* Part-time. *Degree requirements:* For doctorate, comprehensive exam. *Entrance requirements:* For doctorate, 90 semester hours of pre-professional study. Additional exam requirements/recommendations for international students: Required—TOEFL (minimum score 550 paper-based; 79 iBT). Electronic applications accepted. *Faculty research:* Effectiveness and efficacy of chiropractic care.

D'Youville College, Department of Chiropractic, Buffalo, NY 14201-1084. Offers DC. *Accreditation:* CCE. *Students:* 80 full-time (32 women), 3 part-time (1 woman); includes 5 minority (1 Black or African American, non-Hispanic/Latino; 1 Asian, non-Hispanic/Latino; 3 Hispanic/Latino), 22 international. Average age 26. 74 applicants, 77% accepted, 28 enrolled. In 2015, 27 doctorates awarded. *Entrance requirements:* For doctorate, minimum GPA of 2.5, 90 undergraduate credits. *Application deadline:* Applications are processed on a rolling basis. Electronic applications accepted. *Expenses:* Contact institution. *Faculty research:* Radiology diagnosis, chiropractic treatment and diagnosis. *Unit head:* Dr. Jeffrey Ware, Acting Executive Director, Chiropractic Department, 716-829-8448, Fax: 716-829-7893. *Application contact:* Mark Pavone, Graduate Admissions Director, 716-829-8400, Fax: 716-829-7900, E-mail: graduateadmissions@dyc.edu.

Institut Franco-Europen de Chiropraxie, Professional Program, 94200 Ivry-sur-Seine, France. Offers DC.

Life Chiropractic College West, Professional Program, Hayward, CA 94545. Offers DC. *Accreditation:* CCE. *Entrance requirements:* For doctorate, minimum GPA of 3.0. Additional exam requirements/recommendations for international students: Required—TOEFL (minimum score 550 paper-based). Electronic applications accepted. *Faculty research:* Imaging, ergonomics, upper cervical adjusting, academics.

Life University, College of Chiropractic, Marietta, GA 30060-2903. Offers DC. *Accreditation:* CCE. *Program availability:* Part-time. *Faculty:* 103 full-time (47 women), 33 part-time/adjunct (13 women). *Students:* 1,686 full-time (788 women), 97 part-time (49 women); includes 494 minority (196 Black or African American, non-Hispanic/Latino; 10 American Indian or Alaska Native, non-Hispanic/Latino; 45 Asian, non-Hispanic/Latino; 243 Hispanic/Latino), 64 international. Average age 28. In 2015, 346 doctorates awarded. *Degree requirements:* For doctorate, comprehensive exam, thesis/dissertation or alternative. *Entrance requirements:* For doctorate, minimum of 3 years of college; course work in biology, chemistry, physics, humanities, psychology, and English; minimum GPA of 2.75. Additional exam requirements/recommendations for international students: Required—TOEFL (minimum score 500 paper-based). *Application deadline:* Applications are processed on a rolling basis. Application fee: $50. Electronic applications accepted. *Expenses:* Contact institution. *Financial support:* Research assistantships, Federal Work-Study, institutionally sponsored loans, scholarships/grants, and tuition waivers (partial) available. Support available to part-time students. Financial award application deadline: 9/1; financial award applicants required to submit FAFSA. *Faculty research:* Chiropractic clinical trial, spinal modeling, biomechanics, clinical evaluation studies, chiropractic technique development, sports performance. *Unit head:* Dr. Leslie King, Dean, 770-426-2713, E-mail: lesliek@life.edu. *Application contact:* Jana Holwick, Director of Enrollment, 770-426-2889, Fax: 770-426-2895, E-mail: jana.holwick@life.edu.
Website: http://www.life.edu/academics/chiropractic/

Logan University, College of Chiropractic, Chesterfield, MO 63017. Offers DC. *Accreditation:* CCE. *Faculty:* 50 full-time (21 women), 38 part-time/adjunct (16 women). *Students:* 743 full-time (289 women), 1 (woman) part-time; includes 71 minority (25 Black or African American, non-Hispanic/Latino; 4 American Indian or Alaska Native, non-Hispanic/Latino; 21 Asian, non-Hispanic/Latino; 13 Hispanic/Latino; 8 Two or more races, non-Hispanic/Latino), 11 international. Average age 26. 169 applicants, 73% accepted, 124 enrolled. In 2015, 221 doctorates awarded. *Degree requirements:* For doctorate, comprehensive exam. *Entrance requirements:* For doctorate, 90 hours of pre-chiropractic including biology, chemistry, physics, and social sciences; minimum GPA of 3.0. Additional exam requirements/recommendations for international students: Required—TOEFL (minimum score 500 paper-based; 79 iBT); Recommended—IELTS (minimum score 6.5). *Application deadline:* Applications are processed on a rolling basis. Application fee: $50. Electronic applications accepted. *Financial support:* In 2015–16, 129 students received support. Federal Work-Study and scholarships/grants available. Financial award applicants required to submit FAFSA. *Faculty research:* Effects of injury on proprioception as measured by joint position sense, interventions for older adults with low back pain, interventions affecting heart rate variability, finite element computer modeling of spinal biomechanics, electrophysiological diagnosis of common neuromusculoskeletal conditions, the effects of spinal manipulation on posture and postural control. *Unit head:* Dr. Vincent DeBono, Dean of the College of Chiropractic, 636-227-2100 Ext. 2701, Fax: 636-207-2431, E-mail: vincent.debono@logan.edu. *Application contact:* Caitlin Mueller, Assistant Director of Admissions, 636-227-2100 Ext. 1709, Fax: 636-207-2425, E-mail: admissions@logan.edu.
Website: http://www.logan.edu/academics/doctor-of-chiropractic

Logan University, College of Health Sciences, Chesterfield, MO 63017. Offers health informatics (MS); health professionals education (DHPE); nutrition and human performance (MS); sports science and rehabilitation (MS). *Program availability:* Part-time, 100% online, blended/hybrid learning. *Faculty:* 3 full-time (2 women), 14 part-time/adjunct (5 women). *Students:* 19 full-time (15 women), 96 part-time (60 women); includes 12 minority (6 Black or African American, non-Hispanic/Latino; 1 Asian, non-Hispanic/Latino; 4 Hispanic/Latino; 1 Two or more races, non-Hispanic/Latino). Average age 31. 74 applicants, 85% accepted, 63 enrolled. In 2015, 95 master's awarded.

Entrance requirements: For master's, minimum GPA of 2.5. Additional exam requirements/recommendations for international students: Required—TOEFL (minimum score 500 paper-based; 79 iBT); Recommended—IELTS (minimum score 6.5). *Application deadline:* Applications are processed on a rolling basis. Application fee: $50. Electronic applications accepted. *Expenses:* Contact institution. *Financial support:* In 2015–16, 4 students received support. Federal Work-Study and scholarships/grants available. Support available to part-time students. Financial award applicants required to submit FAFSA. *Faculty research:* Ankle injury prevention in high school athletes, low back pain in college football players, short arc banding and low back pain, the effects of enzymes on inflammatory blood markers, gait analysis in high school and college athletes. *Unit head:* Dr. Sherri Cole, Dean, College of Health Sciences, 636-227-2100 Ext. 2702, Fax: 636-207-2418, E-mail: sherri.cole@logan.edu. *Application contact:* Jordan LaMarca, Assistant Director of Admissions, 636-227-2100 Ext. 1973, Fax: 636-207-2425, E-mail: admissions@logan.edu.
Website: http://www.logan.edu

National University of Health Sciences, Graduate Programs, Lombard, IL 60148-4583. Offers MS, MSAC, MSOM, DC, ND.

New York Chiropractic College, Doctor of Chiropractic Program, Seneca Falls, NY 13148-0800. Offers DC. *Accreditation:* CCE. *Degree requirements:* For doctorate, internship in health center. *Entrance requirements:* For doctorate, 24 credit hours of course work in science; 90 credit hours with minimum GPA of 2.5; references; interview. Additional exam requirements/recommendations for international students: Recommended—TOEFL (minimum score 550 paper-based). Electronic applications accepted. *Faculty research:* Anatomy, pathophysiology, neurophysiology biomechanics, musculoskeletal pain syndrome, nutrition.

See Display on next page and Close-Up on page 867.

Northwestern Health Sciences University, College of Chiropractic, Bloomington, MN 55431-1599. Offers DC. *Accreditation:* CCE. *Entrance requirements:* For doctorate, 90 semester hours of course work in health or science, minimum GPA of 2.75. Additional exam requirements/recommendations for international students: Required—TOEFL (minimum score 540 paper-based; 76 iBT). Electronic applications accepted. *Faculty research:* Headache, low back pain, neck pain, sciatica, rehabilitative exercise.

Palmer College of Chiropractic, Professional Program, Davenport, IA 52803-5287. Offers DC. *Accreditation:* CCE. *Program availability:* Part-time. *Entrance requirements:* For doctorate, minimum GPA of 2.5, 90 hours of prerequisite coursework. Additional exam requirements/recommendations for international students: Required—TOEFL (minimum score 500 paper-based; 61 iBT). *Application deadline:* Applications are processed on a rolling basis. Application fee: $50. Electronic applications accepted. *Financial support:* Career-related internships or fieldwork, Federal Work-Study, and scholarships/grants available. Support available to part-time students. Financial award application deadline: 4/1; financial award applicants required to submit FAFSA. *Faculty research:* Studies to advance the understanding of chiropractic. *Unit head:* Dr. Dennis Marchiori, Chancellor, 563-884-5466, Fax: 563-884-5624, E-mail: marchiori_d@palmer.edu. *Application contact:* Karen Eden, Senior Director of Admissions, 563-884-5656, Fax: 563-884-5414, E-mail: pcadmit@palmer.edu.

Palmer College of Chiropractic, Professional Program–Florida Campus, Port Orange, FL 32129. Offers DC. *Accreditation:* CCE. *Program availability:* Part-time. *Degree requirements:* For doctorate, clinical internship. *Entrance requirements:* For doctorate, minimum GPA of 2.5, 90 hours of prerequisite coursework. Additional exam requirements/recommendations for international students: Recommended—TOEFL (minimum score 500 paper-based; 61 iBT). Application fee: $50. *Financial support:* Career-related internships or fieldwork, Federal Work-Study, and scholarships/grants available. Support available to part-time students. Financial award application deadline: 4/1; financial award applicants required to submit FAFSA. *Unit head:* Dr. Dennis Marchiori, Chancellor, 563-884-5511, Fax: 563-884-5409, E-mail: marchiori_d@palmer.edu. *Application contact:* Admissions Representative, 866-585-9677, Fax: 386-763-2620, E-mail: pcaf_admiss@palmer.edu.

Palmer College of Chiropractic, Professional Program–West Campus, San Jose, CA 95134-1617. Offers DC. *Accreditation:* CCE. *Program availability:* Part-time. *Degree requirements:* For doctorate, clinical internship. *Entrance requirements:* For doctorate, minimum GPA of 2.5. Additional exam requirements/recommendations for international students: Required—TOEFL. *Application deadline:* Applications are processed on a rolling basis. Application fee: $50. Electronic applications accepted. *Financial support:* Career-related internships or fieldwork, Federal Work-Study, and scholarships/grants available. Support available to part-time students. Financial award application deadline: 4/1; financial award applicants required to submit FAFSA. *Faculty research:* Low back pain complaints, spinal manipulation therapy, cervical biomechanics, clinical trials, practice guidelines. *Application contact:* Julie Behn, Campus Enrollment Director, 408-944-6121, Fax: 408-944-6032, E-mail: julie.behn@palmer.edu.

Parker University, Doctor of Chiropractic Program, Dallas, TX 75229-5668. Offers DC. *Accreditation:* CCE. *Program availability:* Part-time. *Entrance requirements:* For doctorate, minimum GPA of 2.65. Additional exam requirements/recommendations for international students: Required—TOEFL (minimum score 550 paper-based). Electronic applications accepted. *Faculty research:* Arterial tonometry, bioenergetics, outcome assessment for clinical care.

★ **Sherman College of Chiropractic,** Professional Program, Spartanburg, SC 29304-1452. Offers DC. *Accreditation:* CCE. *Entrance requirements:* For doctorate, two letters of recommendation, official transcripts. *Application deadline:* For fall admission, 8/22 for domestic students, 4/3 for international students; for spring admission, 2/15 for domestic students; for summer admission, 5/30 for domestic students, 1/25 for international students. Applications are processed on a rolling basis. Application fee: $50. Electronic applications accepted. *Expenses:* Tuition, area resident: Full-time $31,064; part-time $7766 per quarter. *Financial support:* Career-related internships or fieldwork, Federal Work-Study, institutionally sponsored loans, and scholarships/grants available. Support available to part-time students. Financial award applicants required to submit FAFSA. *Faculty research:* Chiropractic effect of immune response, biomechanics, video fluoroscopy, dynamic motion. *Application contact:* Dr. Robert Irwin, Provost, 864-578-8770 Ext. 223, Fax: 864-599-4860, E-mail: admissions@sherman.edu.
Website: http://www.sherman.edu

See Display below and Close-Up on page 869.

Southern California University of Health Sciences, Los Angeles College of Chiropractic, Whittier, CA 90609-1166. Offers DC. *Accreditation:* CCE. *Degree requirements:* For doctorate, comprehensive exam, clinical internship. *Entrance requirements:* For doctorate, minimum GPA of 2.5, 90 incoming units in prerequisite coursework. Additional exam requirements/recommendations for international students: Required—TOEFL (minimum score 500 paper-based). Electronic applications accepted. *Faculty research:* Sports medicine.

Texas Chiropractic College, Professional Program, Pasadena, TX 77505-1699. Offers DC. *Accreditation:* CCE. *Entrance requirements:* For doctorate, 90 semester hours at regionally-accredited college or university, minimum GPA of 3.0 (24 hours of life and physical sciences, half of which have a lab component). Additional exam requirements/recommendations for international students: Required—TOEFL. *Faculty research:* Range of motion comparison male vs. female student stress levels.

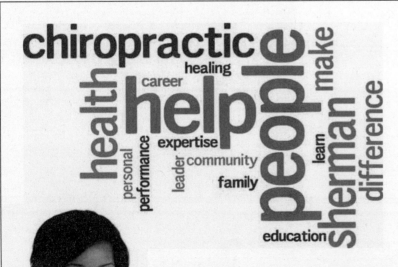

Chiropractic

Université du Québec à Trois-Rivières, Graduate Programs, Program in Chiropractic, Trois-Rivières, QC G9A 5H7, Canada. Offers DC.

University of Bridgeport, College of Chiropractic, Bridgeport, CT 06604. Offers DC. *Accreditation:* CCE. *Degree requirements:* For doctorate, thesis/dissertation, National Board of Chiropractic Exam Parts I and II. *Entrance requirements:* Additional exam requirements/recommendations for international students: Recommended—TOEFL (minimum score 550 paper-based; 80 iBT), IELTS (minimum score 6.5). *Application deadline:* For fall admission, 4/1 priority date for domestic and international students; for spring admission, 11/1 priority date for domestic and international students. Applications are processed on a rolling basis. Application fee: $75. Electronic applications accepted. *Expenses:* Contact institution. *Financial support:* Federal Work-Study and institutionally sponsored loans available. Support available to part-time students. Financial award application deadline: 6/1; financial award applicants required to submit FAFSA.

 University of Western States, Professional Program, Portland, OR 97230-3099. Offers DC. *Accreditation:* CCE. *Degree requirements:* For doctorate, comprehensive exam, internship. *Entrance requirements:* For doctorate, 3 years of pre-chiropractic study in biological sciences, minimum GPA of 2.5. *Faculty research:* Low back pain.

See Display on this page and Close-Up on page 871.

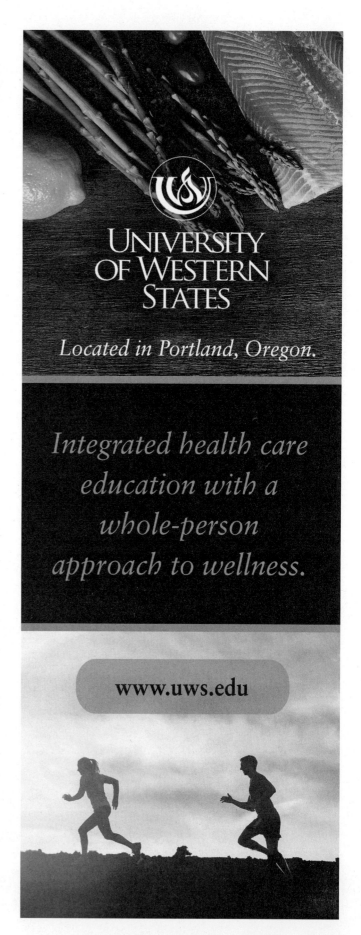

NEW YORK CHIROPRACTIC COLLEGE
Doctor of Chiropractic Program

Programs of Study

New York Chiropractic College (NYCC) offers a rigorous but highly rewarding program leading to the degree of Doctor of Chiropractic (D.C.) and prepares students for a professional career in chiropractic health care as well as in related research and teaching. The program is ten trimesters in length and takes five academic years to complete. New York Chiropractic College offers classes year-round, and students generally complete the program in forty months of continuous study. The program is open only to full-time students. It includes three trimesters of internship at one of the College's three health centers.

Several 3+1 joint-degree B.S./D.C. programs, which enable the student to save a year in the completion of the two degrees, are offered. NYCC's Postgraduate Division offers continuing education for chiropractors to further their professional development and to satisfy the license renewal requirements of various states.

Research Facilities

NYCC research department activity encompasses a wide variety of research interests. The research programs incorporate sports medicine and chiropractic geriatric studies, biomechanics, nutrition, and pathophysiology. The College supports three primary research laboratories: a biochemistry laboratory; a biodynamics laboratory, where sports chiropractic and related ergonomic and neurophysiology research is conducted; and a biomechanical/gait research laboratory. All laboratories are equipped with state-of-the-art technology capable of supporting extensive research activity in those respective areas. The laboratories are housed in an 8,000-square-foot research facility that contains administrative offices as well as a bone histology and microscopy laboratory and several computer graphics and data analysis workstations.

Financial Aid

Financial aid is generally available on the basis of need, as evidenced by information supplied on the FAFSA as well as an institutional application. Federal sources of aid include Federal Perkins Loans, Federal Work-Study, and veterans' benefits to eligible students. Limited grants are available under New York State's Tuition Assistance Program (TAP). Students may obtain Federal Stafford Student Loans and may compete for scholarships offered by chiropractic associations, private foundations, and NYCC.

Cost of Study

Only full-time students are admitted into the doctoral program. For 2015–16, tuition was $11,275 per trimester; tuition and fees for the calendar year (three trimesters) from September 2015 through summer 2016 were estimated at $33,825. The estimated cost of textbooks, equipment, and supplies is an additional $1,400 per trimester.

Living and Housing Costs

NYCC offers excellent on-campus housing in eight residence halls. The cost of a suite for married students is $3,234 (these are trimester rates). Meal plans are additional and range from $450 to $950 per trimester. Off-campus housing is available and comparatively priced. The cost of living in the area is substantially lower than that of urban areas.

Student Group

New York Chiropractic College's 700 students (including senior interns) come from more than twenty states and several other countries. The majority are residents of the Northeast. Students range in age from 21 to over 55, with the largest age group consisting of those in their mid-20s. Thirty percent of the students are women, and 80 percent of all students hold a baccalaureate or higher degree. Many students participate in intramural sports and student government as well as in the more than thirty student organizations that include special interests such as nutrition, sports injuries, publications, and research. Numerous technique clubs (e.g., Applied Kinesiology, Gonstead) are active on campus.

Location

New York Chiropractic College is located in Seneca Falls, New York, in the scenic wine-growing region of the Finger Lakes, a popular vacation spot less than a 45-minute drive from Syracuse, Rochester, and Ithaca. Outpatient clinics are located in Buffalo, Seneca Falls, and Levittown (Long Island). The 286-acre campus has 250 feet of frontage property on Cayuga Lake, the largest of the Finger Lakes. The College borders a state park and has a nine-hole, par 3 golf course on the campus.

The College

Established in 1919 in New York City as Columbia Institute of Chiropractic, the College is the oldest chiropractic institution in the Northeast. In 1976, it moved to Nassau County on suburban Long Island and moved again to a larger campus in upstate New York in 1991. The College is accredited by the Middle States Association of Colleges and Schools and by the Council on Chiropractic Education. It holds an Absolute Charter from the Board of Regents of the University of the State of New York.

Applying

Applications for admission should be submitted via the online application Information and application forms may be obtained by visiting NYCC's website or by calling 800-234-6922 (toll-free). Admission is a continuous process; there are entering classes in September, January, and May of each year. Approximately 300 students are admitted for each year, and applicants are encouraged to apply ten to twelve months in advance of their desired entrance date. Reference forms are supplied upon receipt of an application.

Correspondence and Information

Admissions Office
New York Chiropractic College
2360 Route 89
Seneca Falls, New York 13148-0800
United States
Phone: 315-568-3040
         800-234-6922 (toll-free)
E-mail: Enrollnow@nycc.edu
Website: http://www.nycc.edu

THE FACULTY

Anatomy
M. Elizabeth Bedford, Ph.D., Kent State, 1994.
Andrew S. Choi, D.C., New York Chiropractic, 2000.
Michael L. Lentini, D.C., National Chiropractic, 1991.
Raj J. Philomin, Ph.D., Madras Medical College (India), 1986.

New York Chiropractic College

Maria Thomadaki, D.C., New York Chiropractic, 1994.
Robert A. Walker, Ph.D., Kent State, 1989.
Michael P. Zumpano, Ph.D., SUNY at Buffalo, 1997.

Physiopathology
David S. Aberant, M.S., LIU, C.W. Post, 1970.
Mary E. Balliett, D.C., New York Chiropractic, 1988.
Deborah A. Barr, Sc.D., Boston University, 1988.
Scott Coon, D.C., New York Chiropractic, 1994.
Chithambaram S. Philomin, M.B.B.S., Stanley Medical College, 1989.
Carolyn M. Pover, Ph.D., Bristol, 1986.
Veronica M. Sciotti, Ph.D., SUNY at Buffalo, 1988.
Lee C. VanDusen, D.C., National Chiropractic, 1985.

Diagnosis and Clinical Practice
Lisa K. Bloom, D.C., New York Chiropractic, 1990.
Susan E. Conley, D.C., New York Chiropractic, 1995.
Christine M. Cunningham, M.S., SUNY at Stony Brook, 1988.
Paul E. Dougherty, D.C., Logan Chiropractic, 1990.
Margaret M. Finn, D.C., New York Chiropractic, 1992.
Fiona Jarrett-Thelwell, D.C., New York Chiropractic, 1994.
Stephen J. Mesiti, D.C., New York Chiropractic, 1997.
Joseph A. Miller, D.C., National Chiropractic, 1991.
Michael J. O'Connor, D.C., New York Chiropractic, 1982.
Julie A. Plezbert, D.C., National Chiropractic, 1986.
Robert Ruddy, D.C., New York Chiropractic, 1996.
Fred L. SanFilipo, D.C., New York Chiropractic, 1982.
Judy M. Silvestrone, D.C., Palmer Chiropractic, 1984.
John A. M. Taylor, D.C., Canadian Memorial Chiropractic, 1979.
Meghan B. VanLoon, D.C., Northwestern Chiropractic, 1991.
Jeneen L. Wallace, D.C., New York Chiropractic, 1997.

Technique and Principles
Karen A. Bobak, D.C., National Chiropractic, 1986.
Brian M. Cunningham, D.C., New York Chiropractic, 1986.
John L. DeCicco, D.C., New York Chiropractic, 1982.
James R. Ebbets, D.C., New York Chiropractic, 1992.
Lillian M. Ford, D.C., New York Chiropractic, 1985.
Christopher J. Good, D.C., Palmer Chiropractic, 1982.
Sandra Hartwell-Ford, D.C., New York Chiropractic, 1996.
Lloyd E. Henby, D.C., National Chiropractic, 1952.
Michael E. Howard, D.C., Life Chiropractic, 1981.
Thomas McCloughan, D.C., New York Chiropractic, 1993.
Hunter A. Mollin, D.C., New York Chiropractic, 1980.
David F. Petters, D.C., New York Chiropractic, 1986.
Christopher P. Ryan, D.C., New York Chiropractic, 1987.
Paul W. Ryan, D.C., New York Chiropractic, 1989.
Eileen C. Santipadri, D.C., Palmer Chiropractic, 1981.
David A. Shinherr, D.C., New York Chiropractic, 1995.
Edward J. Sullivan, D.C., Northwestern Chiropractic, 1991.
Michael S. Young, D.C., New York Chiropractic, 1996.

Research
JeanMarie Burke, Ph.D., Indiana, 1991.

Depew Health Center
Margaret M. Anticola, D.C., Life Chiropractic, 1986.
Charles D. Coyle, D.C., National Chiropractic, 1988.
Mark A. Dux, D.C., Western States Chiropractic, 1980.
Daniel R. Johnson, D.C., Logan Chiropractic, 1981.
Sherri L. LaShomb, D.C., Palmer Chiropractic, 1988.
David L. Ribakove, D.C., New York Chiropractic, 1992.

Mark D. Sokolowski, D.C., Palmer Chiropractic, 1985.
Mercedes M. Trzcinski, D.C., Palmer Chiropractic, 1981.

Levittown Health Center
Patricia M. Flynn, D.C., National Chiropractic, 1996.
Charles A. Hemsey, D.C., Life Chiropractic, 1981.
Lloyd H. Kupferman, D.C., New York Chiropractic, 1981.
Frank S. Lizzio, D.C., New York Chiropractic, 1980.
Mariangela Penna, D.C., New York Chiropractic, 1986.
Michael G. Perillo, D.C., National Chiropractic, 1978.
Joseph E. Pfeifer, D.C., New York Chiropractic, 1984.
Lana K. Slinkard, D.C., National Chiropractic, 1985.
Veronica A. Wicks, D.C., New York Chiropractic, 1988.

Seneca Falls Health Center
Steven Feldman, D.C., New York Chiropractic, 1981.
Dennis M. Homack, D.C., New York Chiropractic, 1997.
Wendy L. Maneri, D.C., New York Chiropractic, 1999.
William H. Sherwood, D.C., National Chiropractic, 1990.

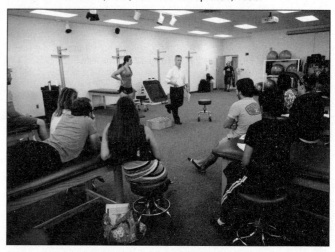

Dr. Chris Marchese instructing students in an active care class.

An NYCC student working on adjusting skills in an open lab class.

SHERMAN COLLEGE OF CHIROPRACTIC
Doctor of Chiropractic Program

 For more information, visit http://petersons.to/shermancollege_chiropractic

Program of Study

Sherman College of Chiropractic provides students with a comprehensive chiropractic education, preparing them to enter the field as doctors of chiropractic who are highly skilled, compassionate, ethical, and successful. On its 80-acre campus in South Carolina, Sherman offers a first professional degree program unique in its approach to health care and known globally for the skill and art of chiropractic delivered by graduates.

Sherman's balanced curriculum offers the knowledge students need in areas like basic science, chiropractic technique and philosophy, and practice management. Courses are hands-on from the first quarter, and students are well-prepared for a smooth transition to chiropractic practice throughout the 1.5-year clinical internship experience.

The program is demanding, including a minimum of 4,956 clock hours in a set course sequence over 14 quarters or 3½ calendar years—comparable to that of the other Doctor of Chiropractic programs in North America, which range from 4,220 to 5,265 contact hours.

Students spend as many as 35 hours per week in class and will need to allow for additional study time, especially in quarters where they prepare to take National Board Exams.

During the first six quarters of the program, students study basic sciences and chiropractic philosophy. They start with gross anatomy, studying each body system, as well as technique, X-ray, and diagnostic courses. In their eighth quarter, students enroll in Pre-Clinic concurrently with supporting technique and analysis courses to put the knowledge into practice.

In the clinical program, students practice every aspect of patient care including case histories, physical and spinal examinations, X-ray, diagnosis, report of findings, chiropractic adjustments, and case management. Students are encouraged to work with the research department to advance the profession with evidence-based study.

Interns practice chiropractic skills on student patients both in the classroom and in the student clinic under the supervision of licensed doctors of chiropractic. After completing student clinic, they advance and see patients as interns in the college's on-campus Chiropractic Health Center, which serves the public by providing excellent, affordable chiropractic care for local residents. While completing their internship and during the remainder of the clinical program, students also finish any remaining clinical science and business practices courses.

Sherman College remains a leader in the profession because of its commitment to education, chiropractic research, and service to the community. Its progressive approach to education is evidenced by such investments as implementing Apple technology for teaching and learning throughout the campus and its use of digital X-rays in both the curriculum and the services in its health center.

Chiropractic student interns serve the local community through health talks, spinal screenings, pro bono care for local student athletes, and free/discounted care for community members in financial need—all this in addition to serving more than 30,000 patient visits each year at the College's on-campus Chiropractic Health Center.

Financial Aid

Sherman College offers Federal Perkins Loans, unsubsidized Stafford Student Loans, and Graduate Plus Loans through federal financial aid services. The College participates in the Federal Work-Study program as well as the Post-9/11 Veterans Educational Assistance Act of the Yellow Ribbon Program. The College also offers numerous scholarships and institutional discounts. A complete listing is available on the College's website at www.sherman.edu/scholarships.

Tuition

Tuition from April 2016–March 2017 is $7,766 per quarter. Total annual tuition is $31,064. Books are estimated at an additional $300 per quarter.

Living and Housing Costs

Sherman College does not provide housing; however, there are numerous housing options available in the nearby area. The cost of living in Spartanburg, South Carolina is approximately 9.6 percent below the national average. An estimated cost of attendance can be found on the College's website at www.sherman.edu/tuition.

Student Group

As of January 2016, the College has just fewer than 400 students, with 54 percent being male and 46 percent female. Students range in age from 19 to 60 years old, with the largest number of students in the 21 to 29 age bracket. Approximately 27 percent of the student body is married. Forty-six states/territories are represented in the student body, and 6 percent of Sherman College students are international.

Sherman College of Chiropractic

Location

Spartanburg is a suburban college town with great weather, plenty of outdoor activities, and a low cost of living. Located in the Upstate of South Carolina, Spartanburg is the sixth largest city in the state with the highest per capita college student population of any major city in South Carolina, making it South Carolina's "College Town." More than 14,000 college students live in Spartanburg, as seven colleges are located in town. The College's location in the foothills of the Blue Ridge Mountains makes for a mild climate, with four distinct seasons, perfect for outdoor activities year-round.

The College

Established January 11, 1973, Sherman College was founded by Thom Gelardi, D.C. He embraced the philosophy of chiropractic and wanted to ensure that its principles prospered and were preserved for future generations. Sherman College is known for its family atmosphere—everyone knows students' names, even the president. Classes are small, with individual attention and mentoring from instructors. Faculty members are experts in their fields of study, and they treat students like colleagues. Hands-on instruction begins in the first quarter of study at Sherman.

The Faculty

A complete listing of Sherman College of Chiropractic faculty can be found at www.sherman.edu/directory.

Applying

Applicants must have at least 90 semester hours of undergraduate study with a minimum grade point average of 3.0 or higher. Of the 90 hours required for traditional admission, 24 must be life and/or physical sciences with corresponding labs for half, and 15 hours must be in the humanities. The deadline to apply is six weeks prior to the start of the quarter. The College enrolls new students in January, April, July, and October.

Correspondence and Information

Tarsha Hamilton, Admission Counselor
Sherman College of Chiropractic
2020 Springfield Road
Spartanburg, South Carolina 29316
United States
Phone: 800-849-8771, Ext. 294
Fax: 864-599-4859
E-mail: thamilton@sherman.edu
Website: www.sherman.edu

Chiropractors take a natural, preventative approach to health care, without the invasive use of drugs or surgery, helping patients enjoy a greater potential for health and optimal human performance.

Sherman College of Chiropractic offers a first professional degree program that is unique in its approach to health care and known globally for the skill and art of chiropractic delivered by its graduates.

UNIVERSITY OF WESTERN STATES
Graduate Programs

UNIVERSITY of WESTERN STATES
Integrating Health and Science

 For more information, visit http://petersons.to/uws-chiropractic

Programs of Study

University of Western States (UWS) is the nation's second oldest Doctor of Chiropractic program, with deep roots in integrating health sciences. With a focus on patient-centered, preventative health care, the University honors the profession's historical foundation and traditions to inspire an enduring spirit of curiosity, imagination, and discovery.

Founded in 1904, in Portland, Oregon, UWS is an integrated health sciences university that emphasizes hands-on learning and focuses education on the body as a whole, versus simply learning to treat symptoms.

Renowned for a high-quality, science-based education in a variety of health and wellness disciplines, UWS offers degrees in the areas of integrative medicine, lifestyle counseling, chiropractic care, exercise and sport science, nutrition and functional medicine, sport and performance psychology, dietary guidance and health promotion.

UWS has an enduring commitment to educating health care professionals with a passion for patient care. This pursuit guides every aspect of the institution and positions UWS to fulfill the mission of improving the health of society through conservative, patient-centered care.

UWS believes the future of health care will focus on integrating disciplines, preparing competent professionals, providing effective care, and promoting health and wellness. UWS graduates exemplify the skills and attributes necessary to meet the individual and collective responsibilities to society.

Doctor of Chiropractic (DC)—On-campus in Portland, Oregon: The Doctor of Chiropractic program is a rigorous 12 academic-quarter, first-professional doctorate program that focuses on evidence-informed, science-based education. The program offers a strong clinical component, allowing students to receive hands-on experience in the evaluation and care of patients.

Human Nutrition and Functional Medicine (HNFM)—Programs available are a fully online Master of Science degree and graduate certificate options. Functional medicine is a science-based, patient-centered and systems-oriented approach to helping people achieve and maintain excellent health. This is accomplished primarily through natural methods, with diet and nutrition as a central focus. Students learn how to treat the root cause, instead of just symptoms with this clinically-oriented HNFM program.

Exercise and Sport Science (ESS): This 100 percent online Master of Science degree program is regionally accredited and prepares graduates to provide expert education, guidance, and services as leaders in sport, exercise, and wellness disciplines. Taught by world-class faculty with extensive athletic industry experience, the evidence-informed curriculum is comprehensive and prepares students with first-hand knowledge needed to succeed in this diverse field. Concentrations in nutrition and health and wellness promotion are available.

Sport and Performance Psychology (SPP): Fully online Master of Science, doctoral degree, and graduate certificate options are available. The SPP program is designed to help students develop the mental essentials to enhance performance and increase human potential. The curriculum is designed specifically to help students become certified sport psychology consultants.

Massage Therapy Certificate Program (MT): The accredited massage therapy program at UWS is a one-year, science-based program that blends a strong foundation of human anatomy and physiology with massage techniques focused on helping patients achieve optimal wellness and function, as well as specialized training for work with injuries, illness, and chronic conditions. Students gain the technical skills, business savvy, and ethical knowledge necessary for a successful career in integrated health care, and cultivate a compassionate approach to massage therapy as a healing art.

Research Facilities

Every chiropractic medicine student participates in a full human cadaver dissection in our world-class anatomy lab during the first three terms of the program.

The W. A. Budden Library provides access to one of the largest health sciences collections in the Pacific Northwest and includes a vast assortment of resources, including anatomical models, DVDs, and textbooks. Online databases, electronic journals, eBooks and research guides are available 24/7 through the library website.

UWS's research department, The Center for Outcomes Studies (COS), has placed the University at the forefront of chiropractic research for more than two decades. In 1994, UWS (then Western States Chiropractic College) became the first chiropractic college ever awarded a federal grant for research. The nearly million dollar grant from the Department of Health and Human Services (HRSA) funded a collaborative study with Oregon Health Science University's Department of Family Medicine. Since then, the Center for Outcome Studies has received additional grants from HRSA and four grants from the National Center for Complementary and Alternative Medicine at the National Institutes of Health.

Under the direction of Mitchell Haas, DC, associate vice president of research, COS activities are currently focused on the efficacy of chiropractic care. Work is proceeding on identifying the dose-response relationship between the number of chiropractic treatments and clinical outcomes for chronic low back pain and headaches. In addition to conducting its own research agenda, the COS continues to participate in projects with local and national collaborators.

Financial Aid

University of Western States students typically use a combination of federal student aid programs to meet their financial needs for their chosen program of study. Some scholarships are also available. The office of financial aid works with students to bring the cost of a UWS education within reach.

Cost of Study

Tuition costs vary by program. The most current information is available online at www.uws.edu/admissionstuition-and-financial-aid/.

Living and Housing Costs

University of Western States is located in a quiet and affordable residential neighborhood just 20 minutes from downtown Portland. UWS does not offer on-campus housing; however, the Office of Student Services helps provide students with housing resources for Portland and surrounding areas near the university.

Student Group

Because of the small, close-knit student body at UWS, students don't just learn with their classmates, they also share experiences and activities that will shape their futures. The paths to these adventures can be found in a myriad of ways: serving as a student body officer, volunteering on a committee, joining an intramural sport team, or participating in one of the many clubs available to students.

University of Western States

The Faculty

A complete listing of faculty members and their areas of expertise can be found on the University's website at www.uws.edu/about/directory.

The directors or deans of the various graduate programs are as follows:

Doctor of Chiropractic Program: Dean, William Borman, Ph.D.
Human Nutrition and Functional Medicine: Director, Daniel Redwood, D.C.
Sport and Performance Psychology: Director, Conrad Woolsey, Ph.D.
Exercise and Sport Science: Director, Tiffany Reiss, Ph.D.
Massage Therapy Certificate Program: Director, Eric Polgar, MBA.

Location

UWS is located in Portland, Oregon, a city that is home to 10,000 acres of public parks, food carts, local coffee, craft breweries and donuts at every corner, and a vibrant bike scene. The people, culture, and atmosphere make it a truly one-of-a kind city and a place that enthusiastically welcomes health and wellness professionals.

The University

The mission of University of Western States is to advance the science and art of integrated health care through excellence in education and patient care. Founded in 1904, UWS is the second oldest chiropractic physician program in the world. It has since evolved into a leading institution for an evidence-informed, science-based education, with a focus on health and wellness. UWS is institutionally accredited by the Northwest Commission on Colleges and Universities (NWCCU).

UWS has cultivated several key community partnerships and is a founding member of the Oregon Collaborative for Integrative Medicine (OCIM). This collaborative provides students, faculty, and staff the opportunity be a part of interdisciplinary education, research, and advocacy for patients in support of integrated care.

Applying

The goal of the admissions process is to recruit and admit candidates who are most likely to succeed in the UWS educational programs, will go on to pass licensing exams, and will succeed as health care professionals. The application process is designed to afford maximum opportunity for prospective students to present the fullest picture of themselves.

UWS encourages practitioners to be aware of their licensure requirements and scopes of practice within each state.

UWS admission requirements reflect institutional expectations of candidates. Requirements vary by program and specific details can be found on the University's website at **www.uws.edu/apply/**.

Correspondence and Information

Admissions Office
University of Western States
2900 NE 132nd Avenue
Portland, Oregon 97230
United States
Phone: 800-641-5641 (toll-free)
E-mail: admissions@uws.edu
Website: www.uws.edu
Facebook: www.facebook.com/UniversityofWesternStates
Twitter: www.twitter.com/UWS_news
YouTube: www.youtube.com/user/UnivWesternStates

Anatomical Sciences Building

Chiropractic student working on an athlete.

Section 27
Dentistry and Dental Sciences

This section contains a directory of institutions offering graduate work in dentistry and dental sciences, followed by an in-depth entry submitted by an institution that chose to prepare a detailed program description. Additional information about programs listed in the directory but not augmented by an in-depth entry may be obtained by writing directly to the dean of a graduate school or chair of a department at the address given in the directory.

For programs offering related work, see also in this book *Allied Health*.

CONTENTS

Dentistry

A.T. Still University, Missouri School of Dentistry and Oral Health, Kirksville, MO 63501. Offers dental medicine (DMD). *Accreditation:* ADA. *Faculty:* 11 full-time (4 women), 34 part-time/adjunct (8 women). *Students:* 126 full-time (75 women); includes 32 minority (1 Black or African American, non-Hispanic/Latino; 1 American Indian or Alaska Native, non-Hispanic/Latino; 21 Asian, non-Hispanic/Latino; 7 Hispanic/Latino; 2 Two or more races, non-Hispanic/Latino). Average age 26. 1,269 applicants, 8% accepted, 42 enrolled. *Degree requirements:* For doctorate, National Board exams 1 and 2. *Entrance requirements:* For doctorate, DAT, minimum GPA of 2.5 overall and science. *Application deadline:* For fall admission, 12/1 for domestic students; for summer admission, 12/1 for domestic students. Applications are processed on a rolling basis. Application fee: $70. Electronic applications accepted. Application fee is waived when completed online. *Financial support:* In 2015–16, 19 students received support. Federal Work-Study and scholarships/grants available. Financial award application deadline: 5/1; financial award applicants required to submit FAFSA. *Faculty research:* Oral perception, dental education assessments, dental ethics, practice-based research, adverse events of dentistry, maxillary arterial variation in the dental anesthesia. *Unit head:* Dr. Christopher G. Halliday, Dean, 660-626-2800. *Application contact:* Donna Sparks, Associate Director for Admissions, 660-626-2237, Fax: 660-626-2969, E-mail: admissions@atsu.edu.
Website: http://www.atsu.edu/mosdoh/

Augusta University, The Dental College of Georgia, Augusta, GA 30912. Offers DMD, DMD/MS, DMD/PhD. *Faculty:* 53 full-time (10 women), 14 part-time/adjunct (4 women). *Students:* 320 full-time (140 women), 2 part-time (1 woman); includes 103 minority (39 Black or African American, non-Hispanic/Latino; 1 American Indian or Alaska Native, non-Hispanic/Latino; 35 Asian, non-Hispanic/Latino; 17 Hispanic/Latino; 11 Two or more races, non-Hispanic/Latino). Average age 26. 309 applicants, 26% accepted, 70 enrolled. *Degree requirements:* For doctorate, comprehensive exam. *Entrance requirements:* For doctorate, DAT, previous course work in biology, English, organic chemistry, and general chemistry; 1 semester of course work in physics. Additional exam requirements/recommendations for international students: Required—TOEFL (minimum score 100 iBT). *Application deadline:* For fall admission, 10/15 for domestic students. Application fee: $30. Electronic applications accepted. *Expenses:* Contact institution. *Financial support:* Federal Work-Study and scholarships/grants available. Financial award application deadline: 5/1; financial award applicants required to submit FAFSA. *Faculty research:* Biocompatibility, dentin bonding, oral cancer, ceramic strengthening, resin polymerization. *Total annual research expenditures:* $1.2 million. *Unit head:* Dr. Carol Lefebvre, Dean, 706-721-2117, Fax: 706-723-0237, E-mail: clefebvr@augusta.edu. *Application contact:* Dr. Carole M. Hanes, Associate Dean for Students, Admissions, and Alumni, 706-721-2813, Fax: 706-723-0237, E-mail: chanes@augusta.edu.
Website: http://www.augusta.edu/dentalmedicine/

Case Western Reserve University, School of Dental Medicine, Professional Program in Dentistry, Cleveland, OH 44106. Offers DMD. *Accreditation:* ADA. *Degree requirements:* For doctorate, thesis/dissertation. *Entrance requirements:* For doctorate, DAT. Additional exam requirements/recommendations for international students: Required—TOEFL (minimum score 550 paper-based). *Expenses:* Contact institution. *Faculty research:* Periodontal disease; overall health; natural antibodies; obesity and periodontal disease; 3D cone beam computerized tomography.

Columbia University, College of Dental Medicine, Professional Program in Dental and Oral Surgery, New York, NY 10032. Offers DDS, DDS/MBA, DDS/MPH. *Accreditation:* ADA. *Entrance requirements:* For doctorate, DAT, previous course work in biology, organic chemistry, inorganic chemistry, physics, and English.

Creighton University, School of Dentistry, Omaha, NE 68178-0001. Offers DDS. *Accreditation:* ADA. *Entrance requirements:* For doctorate, DAT. *Expenses:* Contact institution. *Faculty research:* Dental implants, bone calcification, dental materials, laser usage in dentistry.

East Carolina University, School of Dental Medicine, Greenville, NC 27858-4353. Offers DMD. *Accreditation:* ADA. *Unit head:* Dr. Greg Chadwick, Dean, 252-737-7030. *Application contact:* Student Admissions, E-mail: sodmadmissions@ecu.edu.
Website: http://www.ecu.edu/dental/

Harvard University, School of Dental Medicine, Advanced Graduate Programs in Dentistry, Cambridge, MA 02138. Offers advanced general dentistry (Certificate); dental public health (Certificate); endodontics (Certificate); general practice residency (Certificate); oral biology (M Med Sc, D Med Sc); oral implantology (Certificate); oral medicine (Certificate); oral pathology (Certificate); oral surgery (Certificate); orthodontics (Certificate); pediatric dentistry (Certificate); periodontics (Certificate); prosthodontics (Certificate).

Harvard University, School of Dental Medicine, Professional Program in Dental Medicine, Cambridge, MA 02138. Offers DMD. *Accreditation:* ADA. *Entrance requirements:* For doctorate, DAT, 1 year each: biology, general chemistry, organic chemistry, physics, calculus, English.

Howard University, College of Dentistry, Washington, DC 20059-0002. Offers advanced education program general dentistry (Certificate); dentistry (DDS); general dentistry (Certificate); oral and maxillofacial surgery (Certificate); orthodontics (Certificate); pediatric dentistry (Certificate). *Accreditation:* ADA (one or more programs are accredited). *Degree requirements:* For doctorate, comprehensive exam, didactic and clinical exams. *Entrance requirements:* For doctorate, DAT, 8 semester hours of course work in each biology, inorganic chemistry, organic chemistry. *Expenses:* Contact institution. *Faculty research:* Epidemiological, biomaterial, molecular genetic, behavioral modification, and clinical trial studies.

Idaho State University, Office of Graduate Studies, Kasiska College of Health Professions, Department of Dental Sciences, Pocatello, ID 83209-8088. Offers advanced general dentistry (Post-Doctoral Certificate). First year of Idaho Dental Education Program available in conjunction with Creighton University's School of Dentistry. *Degree requirements:* For Post-Doctoral Certificate, comprehensive exam, thesis optional, 1-year residency. *Entrance requirements:* For degree, DAT, 3 dental application forms. Additional exam requirements/recommendations for international students: Required—TOEFL (minimum score 600 paper-based). Electronic applications accepted. *Expenses:* Contact institution.

Indiana University–Purdue University Indianapolis, School of Dentistry, Indianapolis, IN 46202. Offers MS, MSD, DDS, PhD, Certificate. *Accreditation:* ADA (one or more programs are accredited). *Degree requirements:* For master's, thesis or manuscript, qualifying exam; for doctorate, thesis/dissertation, minimum GPA of 3.0 and qualifying examination (for PhD); minimum GPA of 2.0 and Part I and II of National Board of Dental Examinations (for DDS); for Certificate, thesis, minimum GPA of 3.0. *Entrance*

requirements: For master's, GRE (orthodontics); National Board Dental Exam Part I (periodontics), Parts I and II (endodontics); for doctorate, GRE (for PhD); DAT (for DDS). Additional exam requirements/recommendations for international students: Required—TOEFL (minimum score 550 paper-based; 79 iBT). Electronic applications accepted. *Expenses:* Contact institution. *Faculty research:* Caries research: early caries detection and management, secondary caries, remineralization, oral biofilms, fluoride, dental erosion; oral biology: molecular biology and immunobiology of streptococcus mutans, oral biofilms, infection control, actinobaccillus actinomycetemcomitans; orthodontics and oral facial genetics: orthodontics biomechanics; oral pathology and immunology: chronic inflammation and autoimmunity, innate immunity in oral pathology; periodontal disease and implants.

Loma Linda University, School of Dentistry, Loma Linda, CA 92350. Offers MS, DDS, Certificate, DDS/MS, DDS/PhD, MS/Certificate. *Accreditation:* ADA. *Entrance requirements:* For master's, GRE, minimum GPA of 3.0; for doctorate, DAT. Additional exam requirements/recommendations for international students: Required—TOEFL (minimum score 550 paper-based). *Application deadline:* Applications are processed on a rolling basis. Application fee: $75. *Expenses:* Contact institution. *Financial support:* Fellowships, career-related internships or fieldwork, Federal Work-Study, and institutionally sponsored loans available. *Unit head:* Dr. Ronald J. Dailey, Dean, 909-558-4683, Fax: 909-824-4211. *Application contact:* Admissions Office, 909-651-5029, Fax: 909-558-4879, E-mail: admissions.app@llu.edu.
Website: http://dentistry.llu.edu

Louisiana State University Health Sciences Center, School of Dentistry, New Orleans, LA 70112-2223. Offers DDS. *Accreditation:* ADA. *Entrance requirements:* For doctorate, DAT, interview. *Expenses:* Contact institution. *Faculty research:* HIV/AIDS, implants, metallurgy, lipids, DNA.

Marquette University, School of Dentistry, Professional Program in Dentistry, Milwaukee, WI 53201-1881. Offers DDS. *Accreditation:* ADA. *Faculty:* 44 full-time (11 women), 141 part-time/adjunct (40 women). *Students:* 385 full-time (191 women); includes 100 minority (11 Black or African American, non-Hispanic/Latino; 3 American Indian or Alaska Native, non-Hispanic/Latino; 43 Asian, non-Hispanic/Latino; 32 Hispanic/Latino; 11 Two or more races, non-Hispanic/Latino), 3 international. Average age 24. 2,266 applicants, 5% accepted, 100 enrolled. *Degree requirements:* For doctorate, National Board Dental Exam Part 1 and 2, regional licensure exam. *Entrance requirements:* For doctorate, DAT, 1 year of course work each in biology, inorganic chemistry, organic chemistry, physics, and English. Additional exam requirements/recommendations for international students: Required—TOEFL. *Application deadline:* For fall admission, 1/1 for domestic and international students. Applications are processed on a rolling basis. Application fee: $50. *Expenses:* Contact institution. *Financial support:* In 2015–16, 292 students received support. Institutionally sponsored loans and scholarships/grants available. Financial award applicants required to submit FAFSA. *Faculty research:* Biomaterials, wound healing, diabetes, biocompatibility, cancer, aging, lasers. *Unit head:* Dr. William K. Lobb, Dean and Professor, 414-288-7485. *Application contact:* Dr. T. Gerry Bradley.
Website: http://www.marquette.edu/dentistry

McGill University, Faculty of Graduate and Postdoctoral Studies, Faculty of Dentistry, Montréal, QC H3A 2T5, Canada. Offers forensic dentistry (Certificate); oral and maxillofacial surgery (M Sc, PhD).

McGill University, Professional Program in Dentistry, Montréal, QC H3A 2T5, Canada. Offers DMD. *Accreditation:* ADA. Electronic applications accepted.

Medical University of South Carolina, College of Dental Medicine, Charleston, SC 29425. Offers DMD, DMD/PhD. *Accreditation:* ADA. *Degree requirements:* For doctorate, National Board of Dental Examinations Part I and II. *Entrance requirements:* For doctorate, DAT, interview, 52 hours of specific pre-dental course work. Additional exam requirements/recommendations for international students: Required—TOEFL (minimum score 600 paper-based). Electronic applications accepted. *Expenses:* Contact institution. *Faculty research:* South Carolina oral health, genetics, health disparities, chlamydia, oral cancer.

Meharry Medical College, School of Dentistry, Nashville, TN 37208-9989. Offers DDS, PhD. *Accreditation:* ADA. *Entrance requirements:* For doctorate, DAT. *Application deadline:* For winter admission, 1/15 for domestic and international students. Applications are processed on a rolling basis. Application fee: $65. *Financial support:* Career-related internships or fieldwork, Federal Work-Study, and institutionally sponsored loans available. Financial award application deadline: 4/15; financial award applicants required to submit FAFSA.

Midwestern University, Downers Grove Campus, College of Dental Medicine-Illinois, Downers Grove, IL 60515-1235. Offers DMD. *Accreditation:* ADA. *Entrance requirements:* For doctorate, DAT, bachelor's degree, minimum overall GPA of 2.75, three letters of recommendation.

Midwestern University, Glendale Campus, College of Dental Medicine, Glendale, AZ 85308. Offers DMD. *Accreditation:* ADA.

New York University, College of Dentistry, Advanced Placement DDS Program, New York, NY 10010. Offers DDS. *Accreditation:* ADA. *Entrance requirements:* For doctorate, National Dental Board Exam. Additional exam requirements/recommendations for international students: Required—TOEFL (minimum score 90 iBT). Electronic applications accepted.

New York University, College of Dentistry, Professional Program in Dentistry, New York, NY 10010. Offers DDS. *Accreditation:* ADA. *Entrance requirements:* For doctorate, DAT, BA or 90-credit equivalent. Additional exam requirements/recommendations for international students: Required—TOEFL (minimum score 100 iBT). Electronic applications accepted.

Nova Southeastern University, College of Dental Medicine, Fort Lauderdale, FL 33328. Offers dental medicine (DMD); dentistry (MS). *Accreditation:* ADA. *Faculty:* 106 full-time (38 women), 163 part-time/adjunct (31 women). *Students:* 597 full-time (308 women), 5 part-time (0 women); includes 275 minority (9 Black or African American, non-Hispanic/Latino; 120 Asian, non-Hispanic/Latino; 130 Hispanic/Latino; 16 Two or more races, non-Hispanic/Latino), 86 international. Average age 28. 2,274 applicants, 11% accepted, 124 enrolled. In 2015, 15 master's, 129 doctorates awarded. *Median time to degree:* Of those who began their doctoral program in fall 2007, 99% received their degree in 8 years or less. *Degree requirements:* For master's, thesis. *Entrance requirements:* For doctorate, DAT, minimum GPA of 3.25. Additional exam requirements/recommendations for international students: Required—TOEFL (minimum score 550 paper-based), IELTS (minimum score 6), PTE (minimum score 54). *Application deadline:* For fall admission, 12/31 for domestic students, 1/1 for international students. Applications are processed on a rolling basis. Application fee: $50. Electronic applications accepted. *Expenses:* Contact institution. *Financial support:* In 2015–16, 54 students received support. Application deadline: 4/15; applicants required to submit FAFSA. *Faculty research:* Tissue engineering, dental materials, clinical trials for oral health care products, school based preventive dental programs. *Unit head:* Dr. Linda C. Niessen, Dean, 954-262-7334, Fax: 954-262-3293, E-mail: lniessen@nova.edu. *Application contact:* Su-Ann Zarrett, Associate Director of HPD Admissions, 954-262-1108, Fax: 954-262-2282, E-mail: zarrett@nsu.nova.edu.

The Ohio State University, College of Dentistry, Columbus, OH 43210. Offers dental anesthesiology (MS); dental hygiene (MDH); dentistry (DDS); endodontics (MS); oral and maxillofacial pathology (MS); oral and maxillofacial surgery (MS); oral biology (PhD); orthodontics (MS); pediatric dentistry (MS); periodontology (MS); prosthodontics (MS); DDS/PhD. *Accreditation:* ADA (one or more programs are accredited). *Faculty:* 77. *Students:* 520 full-time (219 women), 5 part-time (4 women); includes 95 minority (12 Black or African American, non-Hispanic/Latino; 2 American Indian or Alaska Native, non-Hispanic/Latino; 49 Asian, non-Hispanic/Latino; 18 Hispanic/Latino; 14 Two or more races, non-Hispanic/Latino), 28 international. Average age 26. In 2015, 31 master's, 112 doctorates awarded. Terminal master's awarded for partial completion of doctoral program. *Degree requirements:* For master's, thesis; for doctorate, thesis/dissertation (for some programs). *Entrance requirements:* For master's, GRE General Test (for all applicants with cumulative GPA below 3.0); for doctorate, DAT (for DDS); GRE General Test, GRE Subject Test in biology recommended (for PhD). Additional exam requirements/recommendations for international students: Required—TOEFL (minimum score 550 paper-based; 79 iBT), IELTS (minimum score 7), Michigan English Language Assessment Battery (minimum score 82). *Application deadline:* For fall admission, 10/1 for domestic and international students; for summer admission, 4/11 for domestic students, 3/10 for international students. Applications are processed on a rolling basis. Electronic applications accepted. *Expenses:* Contact institution. *Financial support:* Fellowships with tuition reimbursements, research assistantships with tuition reimbursements, teaching assistantships with tuition reimbursements, Federal Work-Study, institutionally sponsored loans, and health care benefits available. Financial award application deadline: 2/15. *Faculty research:* Neurobiology, inflammation and immunity, materials science, bone biology. *Unit head:* Dr. Patrick M. Lloyd, Dean, 614-292-9755, E-mail: lloyd.256@osu.edu.
Website: http://www.dentistry.osu.edu/

Oregon Health & Science University, School of Dentistry, Professional Program in Dentistry, Portland, OR 97239-3098. Offers dentistry (DMD); oral and maxillofacial surgery (Certificate); MD/DMD. *Accreditation:* ADA. *Entrance requirements:* For doctorate, DAT. Electronic applications accepted. *Faculty research:* Dentin permeability, tooth sensations, fluoride metabolism, immunology of periodontal disease, craniofacial growth.

Roseman University of Health Sciences, College of Dental Medicine - Henderson Campus, Henderson, NV 89014. Offers business administration (MBA); dental medicine (Post-Doctoral Certificate). *Faculty:* 5 full-time (2 women), 9 part-time/adjunct (1 woman). *Students:* 30 full-time (11 women); includes 14 minority (13 Asian, non-Hispanic/Latino; 1 Two or more races, non-Hispanic/Latino). Average age 30. 125 applicants, 13% accepted, 10 enrolled. In 2015, 11 other advanced degrees awarded. *Degree requirements:* For master's, comprehensive exam, thesis or alternative. *Entrance requirements:* For master's, National Board Dental Examination 1 and 2, graduation from U.S. or Canadian dental school, Nevada dental license. *Application deadline:* For fall admission, 9/15 for domestic students. Applications are processed on a rolling basis. Application fee: $50. *Expenses:* Contact institution. *Financial support:* In 2015–16, 1 student received support. Scholarships/grants, health care benefits, and stipends available. Financial award application deadline: 5/1; financial award applicants required to submit FAFSA. *Unit head:* Dr. Jaleh Pourhamidi, Dean, 702-968-1652, Fax: 702-968-5277, E-mail: jpourhamidi@roseman.edu. *Application contact:* Rochelle Sharp, Administrative Assistant to the Dean, 702-968-1682, E-mail: rsharp@roseman.edu.
Website: http://www.roseman.edu

Roseman University of Health Sciences, College of Dental Medicine - South Jordan, Utah Campus, South Jordan, UT 84095. Offers DMD. *Accreditation:* ADA. *Faculty:* 38 full-time (5 women), 37 part-time/adjunct (2 women). *Students:* 320 full-time (114 women); includes 103 minority (1 American Indian or Alaska Native, non-Hispanic/Latino; 87 Asian, non-Hispanic/Latino; 10 Hispanic/Latino; 5 Two or more races, non-Hispanic/Latino), 7 international. Average age 28. 1,785 applicants, 10% accepted, 82 enrolled. In 2015, 64 doctorates awarded. *Degree requirements:* For doctorate, comprehensive exam, thesis/dissertation or alternative, National Board Dental Examinations (NBDE). *Entrance requirements:* For doctorate, DAT. *Application deadline:* For fall admission, 12/1 for domestic and international students. Applications are processed on a rolling basis. Application fee: $75. Electronic applications accepted. *Expenses:* Contact institution. *Financial support:* In 2015–16, 13 students received support. Federal Work-Study and scholarships/grants available. Financial award application deadline: 5/1; financial award applicants required to submit FAFSA. *Unit head:* Dr. Frank W. Licari, Dean, College of Dental Medicine, 801-878-1400, E-mail: flicari@roseman.edu. *Application contact:* Alicia Spittle, Admissions Coordinator, 801-878-1405, E-mail: aspittle@roseman.edu.
Website: http://www.roseman.edu/dental

Rutgers University–Newark, Rutgers School of Dental Medicine, Newark, NJ 07101-1709. Offers dental science (MS); dentistry (DMD); endodontics (Certificate); oral medicine (Certificate); orthodontics (Certificate); pediatric dentistry (Certificate); periodontics (Certificate); prosthodontics (Certificate); DMD/MPH; DMD/PhD; MD/Certificate; MS/Certificate. DMD/MPH offered jointly with New Jersey Institute of Technology, Rutgers, The State University of New Jersey, Camden. *Accreditation:* ADA (one or more programs are accredited). *Entrance requirements:* For doctorate, DAT. Electronic applications accepted. *Expenses:* Contact institution.

Saint Louis University, Graduate Education, Center for Advanced Dental Education, St. Louis, MO 63103. Offers endodontics (MSD); orthodontics (MSD); periodontics (MSD). *Degree requirements:* For master's, comprehensive exam, thesis, teaching practicum. *Entrance requirements:* For master's, GRE General Test, NBDE (National Board Dental Exam), DDS or DMD, interview, letters of recommendation. Additional exam requirements/recommendations for international students: Required—TOEFL (minimum score 525 paper-based). Electronic applications accepted. *Faculty research:* Craniofacial growth.

Southern Illinois University Edwardsville, School of Dental Medicine, Alton, IL 62002. Offers DMD. *Accreditation:* ADA. *Faculty:* 15 full-time (5 women). *Students:* 547 applicants, 15% accepted. In 2015, 45 doctorates awarded. *Entrance requirements:* For doctorate, DAT. *Application deadline:* For fall admission, 6/1 priority date for domestic and international students. Electronic applications accepted. *Expenses:* Contact institution. *Financial support:* Application deadline: 3/1; applicants required to submit FAFSA. *Unit head:* Dr. Bruce Rotter, Dean, 618-474-7000, Fax: 618-474-7249, E-mail: sdmapps@siue.edu.
Website: http://www.siue.edu/dentalmedicine

Stony Brook University, State University of New York, Stony Brook Medicine, School of Dental Medicine, Professional Program in Dental Medicine, Stony Brook, NY 11794. Offers dental medicine (DDS); endodontics (Certificate); orthodontics (Certificate); periodontics (Certificate). *Accreditation:* ADA (one or more programs are accredited). *Faculty:* 33 full-time (17 women), 70 part-time/adjunct (20 women). *Students:* 190 full-time (99 women); includes 48 minority (3 Black or African American, non-Hispanic/Latino; 34 Asian, non-Hispanic/Latino; 10 Hispanic/Latino; 1 Two or more races, non-Hispanic/Latino), 2 international. 1,422 applicants, 8% accepted, 52 enrolled. In 2015, 39 doctorates, 15 Certificates awarded. *Entrance requirements:* For doctorate, DAT. *Application deadline:* For fall admission, 1/15 for domestic students. Application fee: $100. *Expenses:* $32,960 per year full-time resident tuition and fees, $62,950 per year full-time non-resident tuition and fees. *Financial support:* Research assistantships, teaching assistantships, and Federal Work-Study available. Support available to part-time students. *Unit head:* Dr. Mary R. Truhlar, Dean, 631-632-8950, Fax: 631-632-9105. *Application contact:* Patricia Berry, Acting Director of Admissions, 631-632-8871, Fax: 631-632-7130, E-mail: patricia.berry@stonybrook.edu.
Website: http://dentistry.stonybrookmedicine.edu/

Temple University, Kornberg School of Dentistry, Professional Program in Dentistry, Philadelphia, PA 19122-6096. Offers DMD, DMD/MBA. *Accreditation:* ADA. *Entrance requirements:* For doctorate, DAT, 6 credits of course work in each biology, chemistry, organic chemistry, physics, and English. *Expenses:* Contact institution.

Texas A&M University, Baylor College of Dentistry, Dallas, TX 75246. Offers MS, DDS, PhD, Certificate. *Accreditation:* ADA; SACS/CC. *Faculty:* 286. *Enrollment:* 495 full-time matriculated graduate/professional students (245 women), 36 part-time matriculated graduate/professional students (11 women). *Students:* 495 full-time (245 women), 36 part-time (11 women); includes 267 minority (61 Black or African American, non-Hispanic/Latino; 2 American Indian or Alaska Native, non-Hispanic/Latino; 111 Asian, non-Hispanic/Latino; 89 Hispanic/Latino; 1 Native Hawaiian or other Pacific Islander, non-Hispanic/Latino; 3 Two or more races, non-Hispanic/Latino), 20 international. Average age 31. 109 applicants, 100% accepted, 140 enrolled. In 2015, 22 master's, 3 doctorates, 106 other advanced degrees awarded. *Entrance requirements:* Additional exam requirements/recommendations for international students: Required—TOEFL (minimum score 550 paper-based; 79 iBT). Application fee: $35. Electronic applications accepted. *Expenses:* Contact institution. *Financial support:* In 2015–16, 268 students received support, including 31 research assistantships with tuition reimbursements available (averaging $4,414 per year), 35 teaching assistantships with tuition reimbursements available (averaging $28,751 per year); career-related internships or fieldwork, institutionally sponsored loans, scholarships/grants, traineeships, health care benefits, tuition waivers (full and partial), and unspecified assistantships also available. Support available to part-time students. Financial award applicants required to submit FAFSA. *Unit head:* Dr. Lawrence E. Wolinsky, Dean, 214-828-8300, E-mail: wolinsky@bcd.tamhsc.edu. *Application contact:* Dr. Jack L. Long, Associate Dean for Student Affairs, 214-828-8232, Fax: 214-874-4572, E-mail: jlong@bcd.tamhsc.edu.
Website: http://www.bcd.tamhsc.edu

Tufts University, School of Dental Medicine, International Student Program in Dental Medicine, Medford, MA 02155. Offers DMD. *Accreditation:* ADA. *Entrance requirements:* For doctorate, National Dental Hygiene Board Exam Part I, BDS, DDS, or equivalent. Additional exam requirements/recommendations for international students: Required—TOEFL. *Expenses: Tuition, area resident:* Full-time $48,412; part-time $1210 per credit hour. *Required fees:* $806. Full-time tuition and fees vary according to degree level, program and student level. Part-time tuition and fees vary according to course load.

Tufts University, School of Dental Medicine, Professional Program in Dental Medicine, Medford, MA 02155. Offers DMD, DMD/PhD. *Accreditation:* ADA. *Entrance requirements:* For doctorate, DAT. *Expenses: Tuition, area resident:* Full-time $48,412; part-time $1210 per credit hour. *Required fees:* $806. Full-time tuition and fees vary according to degree level, program and student level. Part-time tuition and fees vary according to course load.

Universidad Central del Este, School of Dentistry, San Pedro de Macoris, Dominican Republic. Offers DMD.

Universidad Iberoamericana, Graduate School, Santo Domingo D.N., Dominican Republic. Offers business administration (MBA, PMBA); constitutional law (LL M); dentistry (DMD); educational management (MA); integrated marketing communication (MA); psychopedagogical intervention (M Ed); real estate law (LL M); strategic management of human talent (MM).

Universidad Nacional Pedro Henriquez Urena, School of Dentistry, Santo Domingo, Dominican Republic. Offers DDS.

Université Laval, Faculty of Dentistry, Professional Programs in Dentistry, Québec, QC G1K 7P4, Canada. Offers DMD. *Accreditation:* ADA. *Entrance requirements:* For doctorate, visual perception exam, manual dexterity exam, interview, knowledge of French. Electronic applications accepted.

University at Buffalo, the State University of New York, Graduate School, School of Dental Medicine, Professional Program in Dental Medicine, Buffalo, NY 14260. Offers DDS. *Accreditation:* ADA. *Degree requirements:* For doctorate, National Dental Board Exams. *Entrance requirements:* For doctorate, DAT, GRE. Additional exam requirements/recommendations for international students: Required—TOEFL (minimum score 500 paper-based; 79 iBT).

The University of Alabama at Birmingham, School of Dentistry, Professional Program in Dentistry, Birmingham, AL 35294. Offers DMD. *Accreditation:* ADA. *Faculty:* 34 full-time (10 women), 29 part-time/adjunct (8 women). *Students:* 241 full-time (117 women); includes 58 minority (20 Black or African American, non-Hispanic/Latino; 2 American Indian or Alaska Native, non-Hispanic/Latino; 21 Asian, non-Hispanic/Latino; 3 Hispanic/Latino; 4 Native Hawaiian or other Pacific Islander, non-Hispanic/Latino; 8 Two or more races, non-Hispanic/Latino), 1 international. Average age 25. 825 applicants, 11% accepted, 60 enrolled. In 2015, 53 doctorates awarded. *Degree requirements:* For doctorate, comprehensive exam. *Entrance requirements:* For doctorate, DAT, letters of recommendation, interview. Additional exam requirements/recommendations for international students: Required—TOEFL (minimum score 94 iBT), National Boards Part I. *Application deadline:* For fall admission, 11/1 for domestic students; for spring admission, 5/31 for international students. Application fee: $75 ($175 for international students). Electronic applications accepted. *Expenses:* Contact institution. *Financial support:* In 2015–16, 13 students received support. Scholarships/grants available. Financial award application deadline: 6/30; financial award applicants required to submit FAFSA. *Faculty research:* Etiology and pathogenesis of dental diseases, dental biomaterials, therapy of dental diseases, practice-based dental, dental implantology. *Total annual research expenditures:* $14 million. *Unit head:* Dr. Michael S. Reddy, Dean, 205-934-4720, Fax: 205-934-9283. *Application contact:* Dr. Steven J. Filler, Director of Dentistry Admissions, 205-934-3387, Fax: 205-934-0209, E-mail: sfiller@uab.edu.
Website: https://www.dental.uab.edu

University of Alberta, Faculty of Medicine and Dentistry, Department of Dentistry, Professional Program in Dentistry, Edmonton, AB T6G 2E1, Canada. Offers DDS. *Accreditation:* ADA. *Entrance requirements:* For doctorate, DAT (Canadian version),

Dentistry

interview. Additional exam requirements/recommendations for international students: Required—TOEFL. Electronic applications accepted. *Faculty research:* Oral biology, biochemistry of connective tissues, preventive dentistry, applied clinical orthodontics, biomaterials.

The University of British Columbia, Faculty of Dentistry, Professional Program in Dentistry, Vancouver, BC V6T 1Z1, Canada. Offers DMD. *Accreditation:* ADA. *Entrance requirements:* For doctorate, DAT, ACFD Eligibility Exam, interview, psychomotor assessment. Additional exam requirements/recommendations for international students: Required—IELTS. Electronic applications accepted. *Expenses:* Contact institution.

University of California, Los Angeles, School of Dentistry, Professional Program in Dentistry, Los Angeles, CA 90095. Offers DDS, Certificate, DDS/MS, DDS/PhD, MS/Certificate, PhD/Certificate. *Accreditation:* ADA (one or more programs are accredited). *Entrance requirements:* For doctorate, DAT, interview. Additional exam requirements/recommendations for international students: Required—TOEFL. Electronic applications accepted. *Expenses:* Contact institution.

University of California, San Francisco, School of Dentistry, San Francisco, CA 94143-0150. Offers DDS. *Accreditation:* ADA. *Entrance requirements:* For doctorate, DAT. *Expenses:* Contact institution.

University of Colorado Denver, School of Dental Medicine, Aurora, CO 80045. Offers dental surgery (DDS); orthodontics (MS); periodontics (MS). *Accreditation:* ADA. *Faculty:* 89 full-time (34 women), 48 part-time/adjunct (14 women). *Students:* 449 full-time (212 women); includes 123 minority (7 Black or African American, non-Hispanic/Latino; 2 American Indian or Alaska Native, non-Hispanic/Latino; 61 Asian, non-Hispanic/Latino; 42 Hispanic/Latino; 11 Two or more races, non-Hispanic/Latino), 15 international. Average age 27. In 2015, 25 master's, 116 doctorates awarded. *Entrance requirements:* For master's, GRE, National Board Dental Exam Part I and II, three letters of recommendation, personal essay; for doctorate, DAT, prerequisite courses in microbiology, general biochemistry and English composition (1 semester each); general chemistry/lab, organic chemistry/lab, general biology/lab and general physics/lab (2 semesters each); interview; letters of recommendation; essay. Additional exam requirements/recommendations for international students: Required—TOEFL (minimum score 580 paper-based; 80 iBT); Recommended—IELTS (minimum score 6.8). *Application deadline:* For fall admission, 12/31 for domestic students, 12/15 for international students. Application fee: $50 ($75 for international students). Electronic applications accepted. *Expenses:* Contact institution. *Financial support:* In 2015–16, 159 students received support. Fellowships, research assistantships, teaching assistantships, Federal Work-Study, institutionally sponsored loans, scholarships/grants, and traineeships available. Financial award application deadline: 4/1; financial award applicants required to submit FAFSA. *Faculty research:* Pain control, materials research, geriatric dentistry, restorative dentistry, periodontics. *Total annual research expenditures:* $4.2 million. *Unit head:* Dr. Denise K. Kassebaum, Dean, 303-724-7100, Fax: 303-724-7109, E-mail: denise.kassebaum@ucdenver.edu. *Application contact:* Graduate Student Admissions, 303-724-7122, Fax: 303-724-7109, E-mail: ddsadmissioninquiries@ucdenver.edu.
Website: http://www.ucdenver.edu/academics/colleges/dentalmedicine/Pages/DentalMedicine.aspx

University of Connecticut Health Center, School of Dental Medicine, Professional Program in Dental Medicine, Farmington, CT 06030. Offers DMD, Certificate. *Accreditation:* ADA. *Entrance requirements:* For doctorate, National Board Dental Examination. Additional exam requirements/recommendations for international students: Required—TOEFL (minimum score 550 paper-based).

University of Detroit Mercy, School of Dentistry, Detroit, MI 48208. Offers MS, DDS, Certificate. *Accreditation:* ADA (one or more programs are accredited). *Degree requirements:* For master's, thesis. *Entrance requirements:* For master's, DDS or DMD; for doctorate, DAT; for Certificate, DAT, DDS or DMD. Application fee: $50. *Expenses:* Contact institution. *Financial support:* Career-related internships or fieldwork, Federal Work-Study, and stipends available. Financial award application deadline: 4/15. *Faculty research:* HIV and periodontal disease, chemotherapeutic management of periodontal disease, oral analgesics, sterilization/disinfection, prosthodontic materials. *Unit head:* Dr. Mert N. Aksu, Dean, 313-494-6621.
Website: http://dental.udmercy.edu

University of Florida, College of Dentistry, Professional Programs in Dentistry, Gainesville, FL 32611. Offers dentistry (DMD); foreign trained dentistry (Certificate). *Degree requirements:* For Certificate, National Dental Boards Parts I and II. *Entrance requirements:* For doctorate, DAT, interview; for Certificate, interview. Additional exam requirements/recommendations for international students: Required—TOEFL (minimum score 550 paper-based). *Faculty research:* Actinobacillus, critical thinking, DNA adenine, methylase, LJP.

University of Illinois at Chicago, College of Dentistry, Professional Program in Dentistry, Chicago, IL 60607-7128. Offers DDS, DDS/MPH, DDS/PhD. *Accreditation:* ADA. *Faculty:* 96 full-time (35 women), 109 part-time/adjunct (47 women). *Students:* 387 full-time (198 women), 2 part-time (1 woman); includes 184 minority (21 Black or African American, non-Hispanic/Latino; 116 Asian, non-Hispanic/Latino; 42 Hispanic/Latino; 1 Native Hawaiian or other Pacific Islander, non-Hispanic/Latino; 4 Two or more races, non-Hispanic/Latino), 10 international. Average age 28. *Entrance requirements:* For doctorate, DAT. Additional exam requirements/recommendations for international students: Required—TOEFL. *Application deadline:* For fall admission, 12/1 for domestic and international students. Applications are processed on a rolling basis. Application fee: $85 ($50 for international students). Electronic applications accepted. *Expenses:* Contact institution. *Financial support:* Fellowships, research assistantships, and teaching assistantships available. *Faculty research:* Oral cancer, wound healing, public health, craniofacial and oral heath, cariology. *Unit head:* Dr. Clark Stanford, Dean, 312-996-1040, Fax: 312-996-1022, E-mail: cmstan60@uic.edu. *Application contact:* Jackie Perry, Graduate College Receptionist, 312-413-2550, Fax: 312-413-0185, E-mail: gradcoll@uic.edu.
Website: http://dentistry.uic.edu

The University of Iowa, College of Dentistry and Graduate College, Graduate Programs in Dentistry, Iowa City, IA 52242-1316. Offers endodontics (MS, Certificate); operative dentistry (MS, Certificate); oral and maxillofacial surgery (MS, PhD, Certificate); oral pathology, radiology and medicine (MS, PhD, Certificate); oral science (MS, PhD); orthodontics (MS, Certificate); pediatric dentistry (Certificate); periodontics (MS, Certificate); preventive and community dontiatry (MS), including dental public health; prosthodontics (MS, Certificate). *Accreditation:* ADA. *Degree requirements:* For master's, thesis; for doctorate, thesis/dissertation. *Entrance requirements:* For master's, GRE, DDS; for Certificate, DDS. Additional exam requirements/recommendations for international students: Required—TOEFL. *Expenses:* Contact institution.

The University of Iowa, College of Dentistry, Professional Program in Dentistry, Iowa City, IA 52242-1316. Offers DDS. *Accreditation:* ADA. *Entrance requirements:* For doctorate, DAT, minimum 90 semester hours with minimum GPA of 2.5.

University of Kentucky, College of Dentistry, Lexington, KY 40536-0297. Offers DMD. *Accreditation:* ADA. *Faculty:* 63 full-time (22 women), 53 part-time/adjunct (20 women).

Students: 252 full-time (128 women); includes 64 minority (9 Black or African American, non-Hispanic/Latino; 1 American Indian or Alaska Native, non-Hispanic/Latino; 25 Asian, non-Hispanic/Latino; 13 Hispanic/Latino; 16 Two or more races, non-Hispanic/Latino), 3 international. Average age 26. 1,839 applicants, 7% accepted, 65 enrolled. In 2015, 53 doctorates awarded. *Entrance requirements:* For doctorate, DAT. *Application deadline:* For fall admission, 12/1 priority date for domestic students. Applications are processed on a rolling basis. Application fee: $75. Electronic applications accepted. *Expenses:* $31,088 per year in-state, $63,472 out-of-state. *Financial support:* In 2015–16, 207 students received support. Fellowships, research assistantships, teaching assistantships, career-related internships or fieldwork, Federal Work-Study, institutionally sponsored loans, and scholarships/grants available. Support available to part-time students. Financial award application deadline: 4/15; financial award applicants required to submit FAFSA. *Faculty research:* Herpes virus biology, chronic oral infection and inflammation of periodontal disease, oral disease prevention and control programs, orofacial pain, craniofacial bone biology. *Total annual research expenditures:* $2.4 million. *Unit head:* Dr. Stephanos Kyrkanides, Dean, 859-323-1884, Fax: 859-323-1042, E-mail: stephanos@uky.edu. *Application contact:* Melissa D. Shelton, Admissions Coordinator, 859-323-6071, Fax: 859-257-5550, E-mail: missy.shelton@uky.edu.
Website: https://dentistry.uky.edu/

University of Louisville, School of Dentistry, Louisville, KY 40202. Offers dentistry (DMD); oral biology (MS). *Accreditation:* ADA (one or more programs are accredited). *Program availability:* Part-time. *Faculty:* 71 full-time (23 women), 81 part-time/adjunct (20 women). *Students:* 518 full-time (220 women), 19 part-time (10 women); includes 118 minority (22 Black or African American, non-Hispanic/Latino; 2 American Indian or Alaska Native, non-Hispanic/Latino; 55 Asian, non-Hispanic/Latino; 24 Hispanic/Latino; 15 Two or more races, non-Hispanic/Latino), 26 international. Average age 26. 176 applicants, 93% accepted, 146 enrolled. In 2015, 2 master's, 115 doctorates awarded. *Degree requirements:* For master's, thesis; for doctorate, National Board exams. *Entrance requirements:* For master's, DAT, GRE General Test, or National Board Dental Exam, minimum GPA of 2.75; for doctorate, DAT, 32 hours of course work in science. Additional exam requirements/recommendations for international students: Required—TOEFL (minimum score 100 iBT). *Application deadline:* For fall admission, 1/1 for domestic and international students. Applications are processed on a rolling basis. Application fee: $60. Electronic applications accepted. *Expenses:* Contact institution. *Financial support:* In 2015–16, 646,062 students received support, including 1 research assistantship with full tuition reimbursement available (averaging $20,000 per year). Financial award application deadline: 3/15; financial award applicants required to submit FAFSA. *Faculty research:* Inflammation and periodontitis, birth defects and developmental biology, biomaterials, oral infections, digital imaging. *Total annual research expenditures:* $5.1 million. *Unit head:* Dr. John J. Sauk, Dean, 502-852-1304, Fax: 502-852-3364, E-mail: jjsauk01@louisville.edu. *Application contact:* Robin Benningfield, Admissions Counselor, 502-852-5081, Fax: 502-852-1210, E-mail: dmdadms@louisville.edu.
Website: http://louisville.edu/dental/

The University of Manchester, School of Dentistry, Manchester, United Kingdom. Offers basic dental sciences (cancer studies) (M Phil, PhD); basic dental sciences (molecular genetics) (M Phil, PhD); basic dental sciences (stem cell biology) (M Phil, PhD); biomaterials sciences and dental technology (M Phil, PhD); dental public health/community dentistry (M Phil, PhD); dental science (clinical) (PhD); endodontology (M Phil, PhD); fixed and removable prosthodontics (M Phil, PhD); operative dentistry (M Phil, PhD); oral and maxillofacial surgery (M Phil, PhD); oral radiology (M Phil, PhD); orthodontics (M Phil, PhD); restorative dentistry (M Phil, PhD).

University of Manitoba, Faculty of Dentistry, Professional Program in Dentistry, Winnipeg, MB R3T 2N2, Canada. Offers DMD. *Accreditation:* ADA. *Entrance requirements:* For doctorate, DAT, interview. *Faculty research:* Oral physiology, microbiology, and biochemistry of the oral cavity in health and disease; application of clinical research.

University of Maryland, Baltimore, Professional and Advanced Education Programs in Dentistry, Baltimore, MD 21201-1627. Offers advanced general dentistry (Certificate); dentistry (DDS); endodontics (Certificate); oral-maxillofacial surgery (Certificate); orthodontics (Certificate); pediatric dentistry (Certificate); periodontics (Certificate); prosthodontics (Certificate); DDS/MBA; DDS/PhD. *Accreditation:* ADA. *Students:* 581 full-time (301 women), 4 part-time (2 women); includes 236 minority (55 Black or African American, non-Hispanic/Latino; 115 Asian, non-Hispanic/Latino; 41 Hispanic/Latino; 1 Native Hawaiian or other Pacific Islander, non-Hispanic/Latino; 24 Two or more races, non-Hispanic/Latino), 32 international. Average age 26. 506 applicants, 89% accepted, 135 enrolled. In 2015, 127 doctorates, 27 Certificates awarded. *Entrance requirements:* For doctorate, DAT, coursework in science; for Certificate, National Dental Board Exams, DDS. Additional exam requirements/recommendations for international students: Required—TOEFL (minimum score 550 paper-based; 80 iBT). *Application deadline:* Applications are processed on a rolling basis. Application fee: $85. Electronic applications accepted. *Expenses:* $31,566 in-state tuition and fees, $61,331 out-of-state. *Financial support:* Career-related internships or fieldwork, Federal Work-Study, scholarships/grants, and traineeships available. Financial award application deadline: 3/1; financial award applicants required to submit FAFSA. *Faculty research:* Pain/neuroscience, oncology/molecular and cell biology, infectious disease/microbiology, biomaterial studies, health promotion and disparities. *Unit head:* Dr. Mark A. Reynolds, Dean, 410-706-7461. *Application contact:* Dr. Judith A. Porter, Assistant Dean for Admissions and Recruitment, 410-706-7472, Fax: 410-706-0945, E-mail: ddsadmissions@umaryland.edu.
Website: http://www.dental.umaryland.edu/

University of Michigan, School of Dentistry, Professional Program in Dentistry, Ann Arbor, MI 48109. Offers DDS. *Accreditation:* ADA. *Students:* 505 full-time (228 women); includes 132 minority (8 Black or African American, non-Hispanic/Latino; 100 Asian, non-Hispanic/Latino; 13 Hispanic/Latino; 11 Two or more races, non-Hispanic/Latino), 33 international. Average age 24. 1,874 applicants, 10% accepted, 104 enrolled. In 2015, 111 doctorates awarded. *Entrance requirements:* For doctorate, DAT, 6 credits of course work in English; 8 credits of course work each in chemistry, organic chemistry, biology, and physics; 3 credits each of biochemistry, microbiology, psychology, and sociology. *Application deadline:* For fall admission, 10/15 for domestic students. Applications are processed on a rolling basis. Application fee: $75. Electronic applications accepted. *Expenses:* $152,748 resident tuition, $221,272 nonresident tuition. *Unit head:* Dr. Renee Duff, Assistant Dean for Student Services, 734-763-3313, Fax: 734-764-1922, E-mail: ddsadmissions@umich.edu. *Application contact:* Patricia Katcher, Associate Director of Admissions, 734-763-3316, Fax: 734-764-1922, E-mail: ddsadmissions@umich.edu.
Website: http://www.dent.umich.edu

University of Minnesota, Twin Cities Campus, School of Dentistry, Professional Program in Dentistry, Minneapolis, MN 55455-0213. Offers DDS. *Accreditation:* ADA. *Entrance requirements:* For doctorate, DAT. Additional exam requirements/recommendations for international students: Required—TOEFL.

University of Mississippi Medical Center, School of Dentistry, Jackson, MS 39216-4505. Offers MS, DMD, PhD. *Accreditation:* ADA. *Entrance requirements:* For doctorate, DAT (for DMD). *Expenses:* Contact institution. *Faculty research:* Bone growth factors, salivary markers of disease, biomaterial synthesis and evaluation, metabolic bone disease, periodontal disease.

University of Missouri–Kansas City, School of Dentistry, Kansas City, MO 64110-2499. Offers advanced education in dentistry (Graduate Dental Certificate); dental hygiene education (MS); dentistry (DDS); endodontics (Graduate Dental Certificate); oral and maxillofacial surgery (Graduate Dental Certificate); oral biology (MS, PhD); orthodontics and dentofacial orthopedics (Graduate Dental Certificate); periodontics (Graduate Dental Certificate). PhD (interdisciplinary) offered through the School of Graduate Studies. *Accreditation:* ADA (one or more programs are accredited). *Faculty:* 84 full-time (38 women), 56 part-time/adjunct (16 women). *Students:* 432 full-time (184 women), 54 part-time (26 women); includes 99 minority (12 Black or African American, non-Hispanic/Latino; 3 American Indian or Alaska Native, non-Hispanic/Latino; 46 Asian, non-Hispanic/Latino; 28 Hispanic/Latino; 10 Two or more races, non-Hispanic/Latino), 3 international. Average age 27. 793 applicants, 17% accepted, 129 enrolled. In 2015, 7 master's, 107 doctorates, 17 other advanced degrees awarded. *Degree requirements:* For master's, thesis; for doctorate, thesis/dissertation (for some programs). *Entrance requirements:* For master's, DAT, letters of evaluation, personal interview; for doctorate, DAT (for DDS); for Graduate Dental Certificate, DDS. Additional exam requirements/recommendations for international students: Required—TOEFL (minimum score 550 paper-based; 80 iBT). *Application deadline:* For fall admission, 2/1 for domestic and international students. Application fee: $45 ($50 for international students). *Expenses:* Contact institution. *Financial support:* In 2015–16, 1 research assistantship (averaging $22,000 per year) was awarded; career-related internships or fieldwork, Federal Work-Study, institutionally sponsored loans, and tuition waivers (full and partial) also available. Support available to part-time students. Financial award application deadline: 3/1; financial award applicants required to submit FAFSA. *Faculty research:* Biomaterials, dental use of lasers, effectiveness of periodontal treatments, temporomandibular joint dysfunction. *Unit head:* Dr. Marsha Pyle, Dean, 816-235-2010, E-mail: pylem@umkc.edu. *Application contact:* Richard Bigham, Assistant Dean for Student Programs, 816-235-2082, E-mail: bighamr@umkc.edu.
Website: http://dentistry.umkc.edu/

University of Nevada, Las Vegas, School of Dental Medicine, Las Vegas, NV 89154. Offers dental medicine (DMD); oral biology (MS). *Accreditation:* ADA. *Faculty:* 63 full-time (23 women), 28 part-time/adjunct (6 women). *Students:* 97 full-time (43 women); includes 50 minority (1 Black or African American, non-Hispanic/Latino; 1 American Indian or Alaska Native, non-Hispanic/Latino; 39 Asian, non-Hispanic/Latino; 9 Hispanic/Latino), 3 international. Average age 28. 1,930 applicants, 10% accepted, 82 enrolled. In 2015, 4 master's, 1 doctorate awarded. *Degree requirements:* For doctorate, comprehensive exam. *Entrance requirements:* For master's, National Dental Boards Examination (Parts 1 & 2), DMD/DDS; for doctorate, DAT, National Board of Dental Examination Part 1 and 2 (for international dentists). Additional exam requirements/recommendations for international students: Required—TOEFL (minimum score 550 paper-based; 80 iBT), IELTS (minimum score 7). *Application deadline:* For fall admission, 1/1 for domestic and international students. Applications are processed on a rolling basis. Application fee: $50. *Expenses:* Contact institution. *Financial support:* In 2015–16, 13 students received support. Application deadline: 2/1; applicants required to submit FAFSA. *Faculty research:* Oral cancer, public health, orthodontic biomechanics, forensic dentistry, nutrition, geriatric dentistry, dental pulp-stem cells, behavioral dentistry, literacyoral cancer. *Total annual research expenditures:* $581,932. *Unit head:* Karen West, Dean, 702-774-2500, E-mail: karen.west@unlv.edu. *Application contact:* Dr. Christine Ancajas, Assistant Dean for Admissions and Student Affairs, 702-774-2520, E-mail: christine.ancajas@unlv.edu.
Website: http://www.unlv.edu/dental

University of New England, College of Dental Medicine, Biddeford, ME 04005-9526. Offers DMD. *Accreditation:* ADA. *Entrance requirements:* For doctorate, DAT, minimum 30 hours of clinical experience in dental setting. Electronic applications accepted. Tuition and fees vary according to degree level and program.

The University of North Carolina at Chapel Hill, School of Dentistry, Professional Program in Dentistry, Chapel Hill, NC 27599-7450. Offers DDS, DDS/PhD. *Accreditation:* ADA. *Entrance requirements:* For doctorate, DAT, interview. Additional exam requirements/recommendations for international students: Required—TOEFL (minimum score 550 paper-based). Electronic applications accepted. *Expenses:* Contact institution.

University of Oklahoma Health Sciences Center, College of Dentistry, Advanced Education in General Dentistry Program, Oklahoma City, OK 73190. Offers Certificate. *Accreditation:* ADA. Electronic applications accepted.

University of Oklahoma Health Sciences Center, College of Dentistry, Professional Program in Dentistry, Oklahoma City, OK 73190. Offers DDS. *Accreditation:* ADA. *Degree requirements:* For doctorate, National Board Dental Exam Part I and Part II. *Entrance requirements:* For doctorate, DAT, minimum GPA of 2.5; course work in English, general psychology, biology, general chemistry, organic chemistry, physics, and biochemistry. Additional exam requirements/recommendations for international students: Required—TOEFL (minimum score 570 paper-based). Electronic applications accepted. *Faculty research:* Dental caries, microwave sterilization, dental care delivery systems, dental materials, oral health of Native Americans.

University of Pennsylvania, School of Dental Medicine, Philadelphia, PA 19104. Offers DMD, DMD/MS Ed. *Accreditation:* ADA. *Entrance requirements:* For doctorate, DAT. *Expenses:* Contact institution. *Faculty research:* Bone, teeth and extracellular matrix; craniofacial genetic anomalies; infection and host response; periodontal diseases; stem cells; improvement of temporomandibular function.

University of Pittsburgh, School of Dental Medicine, Predoctoral Program in Dental Medicine, Pittsburgh, PA 15260. Offers DMD. *Accreditation:* ADA. *Entrance requirements:* For doctorate, DAT (Academic Average of 19), minimum GPA of 3.2 (science and non-science). Additional exam requirements/recommendations for international students: Recommended—TOEFL (minimum score 100 iBT). Electronic applications accepted. *Expenses:* Contact institution. *Faculty research:* Human genetics, tissue engineering, public health, periodontal disease, cariology.

University of Pittsburgh, School of Dental Medicine, Residency Programs in Dental Medicine, Advanced Education Program in General Practice Residency, Pittsburgh, PA 15260. Offers Certificate. *Accreditation:* ADA. Electronic applications accepted. Tuition and fees vary according to program.

University of Pittsburgh, School of Dental Medicine, Residency Programs in Dental Medicine, Department of Pediatric Dentistry, Pittsburgh, PA 15260. Offers MDS, Certificate. *Accreditation:* ADA. *Degree requirements:* For Certificate, clinical research project. *Entrance requirements:* For degree, National Dental Board Exam Parts I and II, U.S. or Canadian dental degree. Electronic applications accepted. Tuition and fees vary according to program. *Faculty research:* Sports dentistry, behavior management, special needs populations, adolescent oral health, infant oral health, genetics, and cariology.

University of Pittsburgh, School of Dental Medicine, Residency Programs in Dental Medicine, Program in Advanced Education in General Dentistry, Pittsburgh, PA 15260. Offers Certificate. *Accreditation:* ADA. *Entrance requirements:* For degree, National Dental Board Parts I and II, American or Canadian DDS or DMD. Electronic applications accepted. Tuition and fees vary according to program.

University of Puerto Rico, Medical Sciences Campus, School of Dental Medicine, Professional Program in Dentistry, San Juan, PR 00936-5067. Offers DMD. *Accreditation:* ADA. *Entrance requirements:* For doctorate, DAT, interview. *Expenses:* Contact institution. *Faculty research:* Analgesic drugs, anti-inflammatory drugs, saliva cytoanalysis, dental material and cariology, oral health condition of school-age population.

University of Saskatchewan, College of Dentistry, Saskatoon, SK S7N 5A2, Canada. Offers DMD. *Accreditation:* ADA. *Entrance requirements:* For doctorate, DAT. Additional exam requirements/recommendations for international students: Required—TOEFL (minimum score 550 paper-based; 80 iBT), IELTS (minimum score 6.5), Michigan English Language Assessment Battery (85); CanTEST (4.0); CAEL (60); CPE (C). Electronic applications accepted. *Expenses:* Contact institution. *Faculty research:* Protein structure, oral cavity, immunology, bone densitometry, biological sciences.

University of Southern California, Graduate School, Herman Ostrow School of Dentistry, Professional Program in Dentistry, Los Angeles, CA 90089. Offers DDS, DDS/MBA, DDS/MS. *Accreditation:* ADA (one or more programs are accredited).

The University of Tennessee Health Science Center, College of Dentistry, Memphis, TN 38163-0002. Offers DDS. *Accreditation:* ADA. *Entrance requirements:* For doctorate, DAT, interview, pre-professional evaluation. Additional exam requirements/recommendations for international students: Required—TOEFL. Electronic applications accepted. *Expenses:* Contact institution. *Faculty research:* Oral cancer, proteomics, inflammation mechanisms, defensins, periopathogens, dental material.

The University of Texas Health Science Center at Houston, The University of Texas School of Dentistry at Houston, Houston, TX 77225-0036. Offers MS, DDS. *Accreditation:* ADA. *Faculty:* 118 full-time (48 women), 105 part-time/adjunct (47 women). *Students:* 399 full-time (214 women); includes 191 minority (18 Black or African American, non-Hispanic/Latino; 2 American Indian or Alaska Native, non-Hispanic/Latino; 80 Asian, non-Hispanic/Latino; 86 Hispanic/Latino; 5 Two or more races, non-Hispanic/Latino). Average age 25. 1,379 applicants, 10% accepted, 101 enrolled. In 2015, 86 doctorates awarded. *Entrance requirements:* For doctorate, DAT, 90 semester hours of prerequisite courses. *Application deadline:* For fall admission, 9/30 for domestic students. Applications are processed on a rolling basis. Application fee: $150. Electronic applications accepted. *Financial support:* In 2015–16, 318 students received support. Institutionally sponsored loans and scholarships/grants available. Financial award application deadline: 3/1; financial award applicants required to submit FAFSA. *Faculty research:* Salivary diagnostics, autoimmune disease, mucosal immunity, craniofacial anomalies, molecular imaging, bioengineering. *Unit head:* Dr. John A. Valenza, Dean, 713-486-4021, Fax: 713-486-4089. *Application contact:* Dr. H. Philip Pierpont, Associate Dean for Student and Alumni Affairs, 713-486-4151, Fax: 713-486-4425.
Website: http://dentistry.uth.edu

The University of Texas Health Science Center at San Antonio, Graduate School of Biomedical Sciences, Program in Dental Science, San Antonio, TX 78229-3900. Offers MS. *Degree requirements:* For master's, thesis.

The University of Texas Health Science Center at San Antonio, School of Dentistry, San Antonio, TX 78229-3900. Offers MS, DDS, Certificate, DDS/PhD. *Accreditation:* ADA (one or more programs are accredited). *Faculty:* 100 full-time (37 women), 97 part-time/adjunct (22 women). *Students:* 497 full-time (244 women), 41 part-time (20 women); includes 228 minority (16 Black or African American, non-Hispanic/Latino; 100 Asian, non-Hispanic/Latino; 99 Hispanic/Latino; 1 Native Hawaiian or other Pacific Islander, non-Hispanic/Latino; 12 Two or more races, non-Hispanic/Latino), 35 international. Average age 26. 1,462 applicants, 21% accepted, 190 enrolled. In 2015, 25 master's, 104 doctorates, 46 other advanced degrees awarded. *Degree requirements:* For master's, thesis; for doctorate, comprehensive exam. *Entrance requirements:* For master's, GRE General Test, DDS; for doctorate, DAT; for Certificate, National Board Part 1 and Part 2, DDS. Additional exam requirements/recommendations for international students: Required—TOEFL (minimum score 92 iBT). *Application deadline:* For fall admission, 10/1 for domestic students, 10/31 for international students. Applications are processed on a rolling basis. Application fee: $150. Electronic applications accepted. *Expenses:* Contact institution. *Financial support:* In 2015–16, 121 students received support, including 7 research assistantships (averaging $3,080 per year) 83 teaching assistantships (averaging $14,550 per year); Federal Work-Study and institutionally sponsored loans also available. Financial award application deadline: 3/1; financial award applicants required to submit FAFSA. *Faculty research:* Neuropharmacology, periodontal disease, biomaterials, bone mineralization. *Total annual research expenditures:* $5.9 million. *Unit head:* Dr. Adriana Segura, Associate Dean for Student Affairs, 210-567-3180, Fax: 210-567-4776, E-mail: seguraa@uthscsa.edu. *Application contact:* E-mail: dsadmissions@uthscsa.edu.
Website: http://dental.uthscsa.edu/

University of the Pacific, Arthur A. Dugoni School of Dentistry, Stockton, CA 95211-0197. Offers MSD, DDS, Certificate. *Accreditation:* ADA (one or more programs are accredited). *Degree requirements:* For master's, comprehensive exam, thesis. *Entrance requirements:* For master's, GRE General Test; for doctorate, National Board Dental Exam Part I, DAT, foreign dental degree (for international students); for Certificate, DDS/DMD. Additional exam requirements/recommendations for international students: Required—TOEFL. Electronic applications accepted. *Expenses:* Contact institution. *Faculty research:* Cell kinetics, cell membrane transport, orthodontics, virus cell membrane fusion, bioenergy transduction.

University of Toronto, School of Graduate Studies, Faculty of Dentistry, Professional Program in Dentistry, Toronto, ON M5S 1A1, Canada. Offers DDS. *Accreditation:* ADA. *Entrance requirements:* For doctorate, Canadian DAT or equivalent, minimum GPA of 3.0; completion of at least 2 courses in life sciences and 1 course in humanities or social sciences. Additional exam requirements/recommendations for international students: Required—TOEFL (minimum score 600 paper-based; 100 iBT), TWE (minimum score 5). Electronic applications accepted. *Expenses:* Contact institution.

University of Utah, School of Dentistry, Salt Lake City, UT 84112. Offers DDS. *Accreditation:* ADA. *Faculty:* 3 full-time (2 women), 30 part-time/adjunct (4 women). *Students:* 71 full-time (22 women); includes 13 minority (1 Asian, non-Hispanic/Latino; 10 Hispanic/Latino; 2 Two or more races, non-Hispanic/Latino). Average age 26. 775 applicants, 3% accepted, 20 enrolled. *Entrance requirements:* For doctorate, DAT, minimum overall and science GPA of 3.3. *Application deadline:* For fall admission, 12/31 priority date for domestic students, 12/31 for international students. Application fee: $75. Electronic applications accepted. *Expenses:* Contact institution. *Financial support:* Application deadline: 4/1; applicants required to submit FAFSA. *Unit head:* Glen R. Hanson, PhD, Interim Dean, 801-581-3174, Fax: 801-585-6485, E-mail: glen.hanson@hsc.utah.edu. *Application contact:* Gary W. Lowder, DDS, Office of Admissions, 801-581-8951, Fax: 801-585-6485, E-mail: dental.admissions@hsc.utah.edu.
Website: http://dentistry.utah.edu/

Dentistry

University of Washington, Graduate School, School of Dentistry, Program in Dental Surgery, Seattle, WA 98195. Offers DDS. *Accreditation:* ADA. *Entrance requirements:* For doctorate, DAT.

The University of Western Ontario, Schulich School of Medicine and Dentistry, Graduate and Professional Programs in Dentistry, Professional Program in Dentistry, London, ON N6A 5B8, Canada. Offers DDS. *Accreditation:* ADA. *Entrance requirements:* For doctorate, DAT (Canadian version), minimum B average.

Virginia Commonwealth University, Medical College of Virginia-Professional Programs, School of Dentistry, Richmond, VA 23284-9005. Offers MS, DDS, DDS/MS, DDS/PhD. *Accreditation:* ADA. *Entrance requirements:* For master's, National Board Dental Exam; for doctorate, DAT. Electronic applications accepted. *Expenses:* Contact institution.

Western University of Health Sciences, College of Dental Medicine, Pomona, CA 91766-1854. Offers DMD. *Accreditation:* ADA. *Faculty:* 35 full-time (15 women), 21 part-time/adjunct (8 women). *Students:* 273 full-time (133 women); includes 166 minority (2 Black or African American, non-Hispanic/Latino; 3 American Indian or Alaska Native, non-Hispanic/Latino; 104 Asian, non-Hispanic/Latino; 33 Hispanic/Latino; 1 Native Hawaiian or other Pacific Islander, non-Hispanic/Latino; 23 Two or more races, non-Hispanic/Latino), 7 international. Average age 28. 2,576 applicants, 7% accepted, 68 enrolled. In 2015, 74 doctorates awarded. *Degree requirements:* For doctorate, comprehensive exam. *Entrance requirements:* For doctorate, DAT, minimum of 90

semester or 135 quarter units of undergraduate/graduate course work; minimum 30 hours of dental-related work experience; complete all prerequisite coursework with minimum grade of C; letters of recommendation. Additional exam requirements/recommendations for international students: Required—TOEFL (minimum score 79 iBT). *Application deadline:* For fall admission, 12/1 for domestic and international students. Application fee: $60. Electronic applications accepted. *Expenses:* $66,878 tuition; $40 student body fees; $5,742 dental instrument and supply fee; $463 digital media fee. *Financial support:* Scholarships/grants available. Financial award application deadline: 3/2; financial award applicants required to submit FAFSA. *Total annual research expenditures:* $2.3 million. *Unit head:* Dr. Steven Friedrichsen, 909-706-3911, E-mail: sfriedrichsen@westernu.edu. *Application contact:* Marie Anderson, Director of Admissions, 909-469-5335, Fax: 909-469-5570, E-mail: admissions@westernu.edu.
Website: http://www.westernu.edu/dentistry/

West Virginia University, School of Dentistry, Professional Program in Dentistry, Morgantown, WV 26506. Offers DDS. *Accreditation:* ADA. *Degree requirements:* For doctorate, comprehensive exam. *Entrance requirements:* For doctorate, DAT, letters of recommendation, interview. Additional exam requirements/recommendations for international students: Required—TOEFL (minimum score 500 paper-based). *Expenses:* Tuition, state resident: full-time $8568. Tuition, nonresident: full-time $22,140. Tuition and fees vary according to program.

Oral and Dental Sciences

A.T. Still University, Arizona School of Dentistry and Oral Health, Mesa, AZ 85206. Offers dental medicine (DMD); orthodontics (Certificate). *Faculty:* 58 full-time (29 women), 132 part-time/adjunct (88 women). *Students:* 316 full-time (152 women), 2 part-time (both women); includes 117 minority (8 Black or African American, non-Hispanic/Latino; 3 American Indian or Alaska Native, non-Hispanic/Latino; 73 Asian, non-Hispanic/Latino; 23 Hispanic/Latino; 2 Native Hawaiian or other Pacific Islander, non-Hispanic/Latino; 8 Two or more races, non-Hispanic/Latino), 3 international. Average age 28. 2,696 applicants, 5% accepted, 76 enrolled. In 2015, 69 doctorates, 5 Certificates awarded. *Degree requirements:* For doctorate, National Board Exams I and II. *Entrance requirements:* For doctorate, DAT, minimum GPA of 2.5 overall and in science. Additional exam requirements/recommendations for international students: Recommended—TOEFL. *Application deadline:* For fall admission, 11/15 for domestic and international students; for summer admission, 11/15 for domestic and international students. Applications are processed on a rolling basis. Application fee: $70. Electronic applications accepted. Application fee is waived when completed online. *Expenses:* Contact institution. *Financial support:* In 2015–16, 30 students received support. Federal Work-Study and scholarships/grants available. Financial award application deadline: 5/1; financial award applicants required to submit FAFSA. *Faculty research:* Evidence-based dentistry in clinical practice; xerostomia and malnutrition in assisted living settings; medical screenings in the dental office: patient attitudes; rapid oral HIV screening in the dental setting; dental public health: early childhood caries, self-efficacy and oral health. *Total annual research expenditures:* $1,427. *Unit head:* Dr. Jack Dillenberg, Dean, 480-219-6000, Fax: 480-219-6110, E-mail: jdillenberg@atsu.edu. *Application contact:* Donna Sparks, Associate Director, Admissions Processing, 660-626-2117, Fax: 660-626-2969, E-mail: admissions@atsu.edu.
Website: http://www.atsu.edu/asdoh

A.T. Still University, College of Graduate Health Studies, Kirksville, MO 63501. Offers dental public health (MPH); health administration (MHA, DHA); health education (DH Ed); health sciences (DH Sc); kinesiology (MS); public health (MPH); school health education (MS). *Program availability:* Part-time, evening/weekend, 100% online, blended/hybrid learning. *Faculty:* 29 full-time (18 women), 89 part-time/adjunct (46 women). *Students:* 456 full-time (271 women), 391 part-time (232 women); includes 291 minority (126 Black or African American, non-Hispanic/Latino; 7 American Indian or Alaska Native, non-Hispanic/Latino; 71 Asian, non-Hispanic/Latino; 80 Hispanic/Latino; 4 Native Hawaiian or other Pacific Islander, non-Hispanic/Latino; 3 Two or more races, non-Hispanic/Latino), 21 international. Average age 37. 286 applicants, 99% accepted, 221 enrolled. In 2015, 130 master's, 74 doctorates awarded. *Degree requirements:* For master's, thesis, integrated terminal project, practicum; for doctorate, thesis/dissertation. *Entrance requirements:* For master's, minimum GPA of 3.0, bachelor's degree or equivalent, background check, essay, three references; for doctorate, minimum GPA of 3.0, master's or terminal degree, background check, essay, three references. Additional exam requirements/recommendations for international students: Required—TOEFL (minimum score 550 paper-based; 80 iBT). *Application deadline:* For fall admission, 5/16 for domestic and international students; for winter admission, 8/1 for domestic and international students; for spring admission, 11/7 for domestic and international students; for summer admission, 1/23 for domestic and international students. Applications are processed on a rolling basis. Application fee: $70. Electronic applications accepted. Application fee is waived when completed online. *Expenses:* Contact institution. *Financial support:* In 2015–16, 30 students received support. Scholarships/grants available. Financial award application deadline: 5/1; financial award applicants required to submit FAFSA. *Faculty research:* Public health: influence of availability of comprehensive wellness resources online, student wellness, oral health care needs assessment of community, oral health knowledge and behaviors of Medicaid-eligible pregnant women and mothers of young children in relations to early childhood caries and tooth decay, alcohol use and alcohol related problems among college students. *Unit head:* Dr. Donald Altman, Interim Dean, 660-626-2820, Fax: 660-626-2826, E-mail: daltman@atsu.edu. *Application contact:* Amie Waldemer, Associate Director, Online Admissions, 480-219-6146, E-mail: awaldemer@atsu.edu.
Website: http://www.atsu.edu/college-of-graduate-health-studies

Augusta University, The Graduate School, Program in Oral Biology and Maxillofacial Pathology, Augusta, GA 30912. Offers MS, PhD. *Program availability:* Part-time. *Degree requirements:* For master's, thesis; for doctorate, thesis/dissertation. *Entrance requirements:* For master's and doctorate, GRE General Test or DAT, DDS, DMD, or equivalent degree. Additional exam requirements/recommendations for international students: Required—TOEFL (minimum score 550 paper-based; 79 iBT). *Application deadline:* For fall admission, 5/1 for domestic students, 3/1 for international students. Application fee: $50. Electronic applications accepted. *Financial support:* Federal Work-Study, institutionally sponsored loans, scholarships/grants, and tuition waivers available. Support available to part-time students. Financial award application deadline: 5/31; financial award applicants required to submit FAFSA. *Faculty research:* Oral cancer and chemoprevention, properties of biomaterials including oxidative stress, mechanical stress and shear stress responses, taurine and blood pressure in diabetes, bone and

dentin biology, induction of periodontal regeneration. *Unit head:* Dr. Regina Messer, Director, 706-721-2991, Fax: 706-721-3392.
Website: http://www.augusta.edu/dentalmedicine/oralbio/

Boston University, Henry M. Goldman School of Dental Medicine, Boston, MA 02118. Offers dental public health (MS, MSD, D Sc D); dentistry (DMD); endodontics (MSD, D Sc D, CAGS); operative dentistry (MSD, D Sc D, CAGS); oral and maxillofacial surgery (MSD, D Sc D, CAGS); oral biology (MSD, D Sc D); orthodontics (MSD, D Sc D); pediatric dentistry (MSD, D Sc D, CAGS); periodontology (MSD, D Sc D, CAGS); prosthodontics (D Sc D). *Accreditation:* ADA (one or more programs are accredited). *Faculty:* 136 full-time (60 women), 90 part-time/adjunct (31 women). *Students:* 812 full-time (428 women), 2 part-time (1 woman); includes 195 minority (12 Black or African American, non-Hispanic/Latino; 127 Asian, non-Hispanic/Latino; 42 Hispanic/Latino; 14 Two or more races, non-Hispanic/Latino), 316 international. Average age 28. 6,681 applicants, 8% accepted, 263 enrolled. In 2015, 23 master's, 204 doctorates, 59 other advanced degrees awarded. *Degree requirements:* For master's and CAGS, thesis; for doctorate, thesis/dissertation (for some programs). *Entrance requirements:* For doctorate, DAT (for DMD), minimum recommended GPA of 3.0 (for DMD); for CAGS, National Board Dental Exam Part 1, dental degree. Additional exam requirements/recommendations for international students: Required—TOEFL. *Application deadline:* For fall admission, 12/1 for domestic and international students. Applications are processed on a rolling basis. Application fee: $75 ($105 for international students). Electronic applications accepted. *Expenses:* Contact institution. *Financial support:* In 2015–16, 125 students received support. Career-related internships or fieldwork, institutionally sponsored loans, scholarships/grants, and stipends available. Financial award application deadline: 4/18; financial award applicants required to submit FAFSA. *Faculty research:* Defense mechanisms, bone-cell regulation, protein biochemistry, molecular biology, biomaterials. *Unit head:* Dr. Jeffrey W. Hutter, Dean, 617-638-4780. *Application contact:* Admissions Representative, 617-638-4787, Fax: 617-638-4798, E-mail: sdmadmis@bu.edu.
Website: http://www.bu.edu/dental

Boston University, School of Medicine, Division of Graduate Medical Sciences, Program in Oral Biology, Boston, MA 02215. Offers PhD. *Degree requirements:* For doctorate, thesis/dissertation. *Application deadline:* For fall admission, 1/15 priority date for domestic students; for spring admission, 10/15 for domestic students. *Unit head:* Dr. Phillip Trackman, Director, 617-638-4942, E-mail: trackman@bu.edu. *Application contact:* GMS Admissions Office, 617-638-5255, Fax: 617-638-5740, E-mail: natashah@bu.edu.
Website: http://www.bu.edu/dental-research/student-research/phd-in-oral-biology/

Boston University, School of Medicine, Division of Graduate Medical Sciences, Program in Oral Health Sciences, Boston, MA 02118. Offers MS. *Degree requirements:* For master's, capstone project or thesis. *Entrance requirements:* For master's, DAT. Electronic applications accepted. *Unit head:* Dr. Theresa A. Davies, Director, 618-638-5242, E-mail: tdavies@bu.edu. *Application contact:* GMS Office of Admissions, 617-638-5255, E-mail: askgms@bu.edu.
Website: http://www.bumc.bu.edu/gms/oral-health-masters/

Case Western Reserve University, School of Dental Medicine and School of Graduate Studies, Advanced Specialty Education Programs in Dentistry, Cleveland, OH 44106. Offers advanced general dentistry (Certificate); endodontics (MSD, Certificate); oral surgery (Certificate); orthodontics (MSD, Certificate); pedodontics (MSD, Certificate); periodontics (MSD, Certificate). *Degree requirements:* For master's, thesis. *Entrance requirements:* For master's, National Dental Board Exam, DDS, minimum GPA of 3.0; for Certificate, DDS. Additional exam requirements/recommendations for international students: Required—TOEFL (minimum score 550 paper-based; 79 iBT). *Expenses:* Contact institution. *Faculty research:* Natural antibiotics, obesity and periodontal disease, perioninfection and CV disease, periodontal disease and overall health, 3D cone beam computerized tomography.

Columbia University, College of Dental Medicine and Graduate School of Arts and Sciences, Programs in Dental Specialties, New York, NY 10027. Offers advanced education in general dentistry (Certificate); biomedical informatics (MA, PhD); endodontics (Certificate); orthodontics (MS, Certificate); periodontics (MS, Certificate); prosthodontics (MS, Certificate); science education (MA). *Degree requirements:* For master's, thesis, presentation of seminar. *Entrance requirements:* For master's, GRE General Test, DDS or equivalent. *Expenses:* Contact institution. *Faculty research:* Analysis of growth/form, pulpal microcirculation, implants, microbiology of oral environment, calcified tissues.

Dalhousie University, Faculty of Dentistry, Department of Oral and Maxillofacial Surgery, Halifax, NS B3H 3J5, Canada. Offers MD/M Sc. Electronic applications accepted. *Expenses:* Contact institution. *Faculty research:* Cleft lip/palate, jaw biomechanics.

Harvard University, Graduate School of Arts and Sciences, Program in Biological Sciences in Dental Medicine, Cambridge, MA 02138. Offers PhD.

Harvard University, School of Dental Medicine, Advanced Graduate Programs in Dentistry, Cambridge, MA 02138. Offers advanced general dentistry (Certificate); dental public health (Certificate); endodontics (Certificate); general practice residency (Certificate); oral biology (M Med Sc, D Med Sc); oral implantology (Certificate); oral medicine (Certificate); oral pathology (Certificate); oral surgery (Certificate); orthodontics (Certificate); pediatric dentistry (Certificate); periodontics (Certificate); prosthodontics (Certificate).

Howard University, College of Dentistry, Washington, DC 20059-0002. Offers advanced education program general dentistry (Certificate); dentistry (DDS); general dentistry (Certificate); oral and maxillofacial surgery (Certificate); orthodontics (Certificate); pediatric dentistry (Certificate). *Accreditation:* ADA (one or more programs are accredited). *Degree requirements:* For doctorate, comprehensive exam, didactic and clinical exams. *Entrance requirements:* For doctorate, DAT, 8 semester hours of course work in each biology, inorganic chemistry, organic chemistry. *Expenses:* Contact institution. *Faculty research:* Epidemiological, biomaterial, molecular genetic, behavioral modification, and clinical trial studies.

Idaho State University, Office of Graduate Studies, Kasiska College of Health Professions, Department of Dental Sciences, Pocatello, ID 83209-8088. Offers advanced general dentistry (Post-Doctoral Certificate). First year of Idaho Dental Education Program available in conjunction with Creighton University's School of Dentistry. *Degree requirements:* For Post-Doctoral Certificate, comprehensive exam, thesis optional, 1-year residency. *Entrance requirements:* For degree, DAT, 3 dental application forms. Additional exam requirements/recommendations for international students: Required—TOEFL (minimum score 600 paper-based). Electronic applications accepted. *Expenses:* Contact institution.

Jacksonville University, School of Orthodontics, Jacksonville, FL 32211. Offers Certificate. *Entrance requirements:* For degree, curriculum vitae, official transcripts. Additional exam requirements/recommendations for international students: Required—TOEFL. *Application deadline:* For fall admission, 9/30 for domestic students. Applications are processed on a rolling basis. Application fee: $175. *Expenses:* Contact institution. *Unit head:* Dr. Laurance Jerrold, Dean, 904-256-7847, E-mail: ljerrol@ju.edu. *Application contact:* Marisol Preston, Chief Admissions Officer, 904-256-7000, E-mail: admissions@ju.edu.
Website: http://www.ju.edu/orthodontics/Pages/default.aspx

Loma Linda University, School of Dentistry, Program in Endodontics, Loma Linda, CA 92350. Offers MS, Certificate, MS/Certificate. *Faculty:* 4 part-time/adjunct. *Degree requirements:* For master's, thesis. *Entrance requirements:* For master's, GRE General Test, DDS or DMD, minimum GPA of 3.0, National Boards. Additional exam requirements/recommendations for international students: Required—TOEFL (minimum score 550 paper-based). *Application deadline:* For fall admission, 10/15 for domestic students. Application fee: $75. *Unit head:* Dr. Leif K. Bakland, Chair, 909-824-4681. *Application contact:* Admissions Office, 909-651-5029, Fax: 909-558-4879, E-mail: admissions.app@llu.edu.

Loma Linda University, School of Dentistry, Program in Implant Dentistry, Loma Linda, CA 92350. Offers MS, Certificate, MS/Certificate. *Degree requirements:* For master's, thesis. *Entrance requirements:* For master's, GRE General Test, DDS or DMD, minimum GPA of 3.0. *Application deadline:* For spring admission, 9/15 for domestic students. Application fee: $40. *Unit head:* Dr. Jaime Lozada, Coordinator, 909-558-1000. *Application contact:* Admissions Office, 909-651-5029, Fax: 909-558-4879, E-mail: admissions.app@llu.edu.

Loma Linda University, School of Dentistry, Program in Oral and Maxillofacial Surgery, Loma Linda, CA 92350. Offers MS, Certificate, MS/Certificate. *Faculty:* 1 part-time/adjunct. *Degree requirements:* For master's, thesis. *Entrance requirements:* For master's, GRE General Test, DDS or DMD, minimum GPA of 3.0. *Application deadline:* For fall admission, 10/15 for domestic students. Application fee: $40. *Unit head:* Dr. Alan S. Herford, Chair, 909-824-4671. *Application contact:* Admissions Office, 909-651-5029, Fax: 909-558-4879, E-mail: admissions.app@llu.edu.

Loma Linda University, School of Dentistry, Program in Orthodontics and Dentofacial Orthopedics, Loma Linda, CA 92350. Offers MS, Certificate, MS/Certificate. *Faculty:* 1 part-time/adjunct. *Degree requirements:* For master's, thesis. *Entrance requirements:* For master's, GRE General Test, DDS or DMD, minimum GPA of 3.0. Additional exam requirements/recommendations for international students: Required—TOEFL (minimum score 550 paper-based). *Application deadline:* For fall admission, 8/1 for domestic students. Application fee: $40. *Unit head:* Dr. Joseph Caruso, Head, 909-558-4604. *Application contact:* Admissions Office, 909-651-5029, Fax: 909-558-4879, E-mail: admissions.app@llu.edu.

Loma Linda University, School of Dentistry, Program in Periodontics, Loma Linda, CA 92350. Offers MS. *Degree requirements:* For master's, thesis. *Entrance requirements:* For master's, GRE General Test, DDS or DMD, minimum GPA of 3.0. Additional exam requirements/recommendations for international students: Required—TOEFL (minimum score 550 paper-based). *Application deadline:* For fall admission, 9/15 for domestic students. Application fee: $40. *Unit head:* Dr. Robert D. Kiger, Head, 909-824-4643. *Application contact:* Admissions Office, 909-651-5029, Fax: 909-558-4879, E-mail: admissions.app@llu.edu.

Marquette University, School of Dentistry and Graduate School, Graduate Programs in Dentistry, Program in Advanced Training in General Dentistry, Milwaukee, WI 53201-1881. Offers MS, Certificate. *Faculty:* 2 full-time (1 woman), 2 part-time/adjunct (0 women). *Students:* 4 full-time (3 women). Average age 31. 57 applicants, 7% accepted, 4 enrolled. *Entrance requirements:* For master's, National Board Dental Exams I and II, DDS or equivalent. Additional exam requirements/recommendations for international students: Required—TOEFL. *Application deadline:* For fall admission, 10/1 for domestic students, 9/1 for international students. Application fee: $50. *Financial support:* In 2015–16, fellowships with partial tuition reimbursements (averaging $35,000 per year) were awarded; institutionally sponsored loans also available. Financial award application deadline: 9/1; financial award applicants required to submit FAFSA. *Unit head:* Dr. T. Gerry Bradley, Professor and Chair, 414-288-5480. *Application contact:* Dr. Joseph Vitolo, Clinical Associate Professor/Director, 414-288-3640.
Website: http://www.marquette.edu/dentistry/admissions/AEGD.shtml

Marquette University, School of Dentistry and Graduate School, Graduate Programs in Dentistry, Program in Dental Biomaterials, Milwaukee, WI 53201-1881. Offers MS. *Program availability:* Part-time. *Faculty:* 1 full-time (0 women). *Students:* 1 (woman) full-time, 3 part-time (2 women); includes 1 minority (Hispanic/Latino), 2 international. Average age 31. 8 applicants, 50% accepted. In 2015, 2 master's awarded. *Degree requirements:* For master's, thesis. *Entrance requirements:* For master's, GRE General Test. Additional exam requirements/recommendations for international students: Required—TOEFL. *Application deadline:* For spring admission, 3/1 priority date for domestic and international students. Applications are processed on a rolling basis. Application fee: $50. *Financial support:* Fellowships, career-related internships or fieldwork, institutionally sponsored loans, and tuition waivers (partial) available.

Financial award application deadline: 9/1. *Faculty research:* Metallurgy, ceramics, polymers, mechanical behavior, cements. Total annual research expenditures: $3,442. *Unit head:* Dr. T. Gerry Bradley, Professor and Chair, 414-288-5480. *Application contact:* Dr. David Berzins, Associate Professor and Director, 414-288-5690.
Website: http://www.marquette.edu/dentistry/admissions/DentalBiomaterials.shtml

Marquette University, School of Dentistry and Graduate School, Graduate Programs in Dentistry, Program in Endodontics, Milwaukee, WI 53201-1881. Offers MS, Certificate. *Faculty:* 1 full-time (0 women), 4 part-time/adjunct (0 women). *Students:* 6 full-time (1 woman); includes 1 minority (Asian, non-Hispanic/Latino), 1 international. Average age 30. 36 applicants, 8% accepted. In 2015, 3 master's awarded. *Degree requirements:* For master's, research thesis or acceptance of a paper in a peer-reviewed journal. *Entrance requirements:* For master's, National Board Dental Exams I and II, DDS or equivalent. Additional exam requirements/recommendations for international students: Required—TOEFL. *Application deadline:* For fall admission, 9/1 priority date for domestic and international students. Application fee: $50. *Expenses:* Contact institution. *Financial support:* Fellowships, institutionally sponsored loans, and tuition waivers (partial) available. Financial award application deadline: 9/1; financial award applicants required to submit FAFSA. *Faculty research:* Properties of NiTi files, prevention of post-endodontic pain. *Unit head:* Dr. T. Gerry Bradley, Professor and Chair, 414-288-5480. *Application contact:* Dr. Sheila Stover, Clinical Associate Professor, 414-288-8393.
Website: http://www.marquette.edu/dentistry/admissions/Endodontics.shtml

Marquette University, School of Dentistry and Graduate School, Graduate Programs in Dentistry, Program in Orthodontics, Milwaukee, WI 53201-1881. Offers MS, Certificate. *Faculty:* 1 full-time (0 women), 10 part-time/adjunct (0 women). *Students:* 9 full-time (2 women), 1 (woman) part-time. Average age 27. 94 applicants, 5% accepted. In 2015, 3 master's awarded. *Degree requirements:* For master's, thesis. *Entrance requirements:* For master's, National Board Dental Exams I and II, DDS or equivalent. Additional exam requirements/recommendations for international students. Required—TOEFL. *Application deadline:* For fall admission, 9/1 priority date for domestic and international students. Application fee: $50. *Expenses:* Contact institution. *Financial support:* Fellowships, institutionally sponsored loans, and tuition waivers (partial) available. Financial award application deadline: 9/1; financial award applicants required to submit FAFSA. *Faculty research:* In vitro and in vivo behavior of orthodontic wires, effect of orthodontic treatment on facial esthetics. Total annual research expenditures: $63,875. *Unit head:* Dr. T. Gerry Bradley, Professor and Chair, 414-288-5480, Fax: 414-288-3586, E-mail: thomas.bradley@marquette.edu. *Application contact:* Dr. David (Dawei) Liu.
Website: http://www.marquette.edu/dentistry/admissions/Mission_000.shtml

Marquette University, School of Dentistry and Graduate School, Graduate Programs in Dentistry, Program in Prosthodontics, Milwaukee, WI 53201-1881. Offers MS, Certificate. *Faculty:* 1 (woman) full-time, 2 part-time/adjunct (0 women). *Students:* 5 full-time (1 woman), 1 part-time (0 women); includes 2 minority (1 Asian, non-Hispanic/Latino; 1 Hispanic/Latino), 3 international. Average age 28. 4 applicants, 75% accepted. In 2015, 2 master's awarded. *Degree requirements:* For master's, thesis or alternative. *Entrance requirements:* For master's, National Board Dental Exams I and II, DDS or equivalent. Additional exam requirements/recommendations for international students: Required—TOEFL. *Application deadline:* For fall admission, 9/1 priority date for domestic and international students. Application fee: $50. *Financial support:* Fellowships, institutionally sponsored loans, and tuition waivers (partial) available. Financial award application deadline: 9/1; financial award applicants required to submit FAFSA. *Faculty research:* Properties of ceramic materials. *Unit head:* Dr. T. Gerry Bradley, Professor and Chair, 414-288-5480. *Application contact:* Dr. Geoffrey Thompson, Assistant Professor and Director, 414-288-8415, E-mail: arthur.hefti@marquette.edu.
Website: http://www.marquette.edu/dentistry/admissions/Prosthodontics.shtml

McGill University, Faculty of Graduate and Postdoctoral Studies, Faculty of Dentistry, Montréal, QC H3A 2T5, Canada. Offers forensic dentistry (Certificate); oral and maxillofacial surgery (M Sc, PhD).

Metropolitan State University, College of Health, Community and Professional Studies, St. Paul, MN 55106-5000. Offers advanced dental therapy (MS); leadership and management (MSN); nurse educator (MSN); nursing (DNP); psychology (MA). *Accreditation:* AACN. *Program availability:* Part-time. *Degree requirements:* For master's, thesis or alternative; for doctorate, thesis/dissertation or alternative. *Entrance requirements:* For master's, GRE General Test, minimum GPA of 3.0, RN license, BS/BA; for doctorate, minimum GPA of 3.0; RN license, MSN. Additional exam requirements/recommendations for international students: Required—TOEFL (minimum score 550 paper-based). *Faculty research:* Women's health, gerontology.

New York University, College of Dentistry and College of Dentistry, Department of Biomaterials and Biomimetics, New York, NY 10012-1019. Offers biomaterials science (MS). *Degree requirements:* For master's, thesis. *Entrance requirements:* For master's, GRE. Additional exam requirements/recommendations for international students: Required—TOEFL. *Faculty research:* Calcium phosphate, composite restoratives, surfactants, dental metallurgy, impression materials.

New York University, College of Dentistry, Postgraduate Programs in Dentistry, New York, NY 10010. Offers endodontics (Advanced Certificate); oral and maxillofacial surgery (Advanced Certificate); orthodontics (Advanced Certificate); pediatric dentistry (Advanced Certificate); periodontics (Advanced Certificate); prosthodontics (Advanced Certificate). *Entrance requirements:* For degree, National Dental Boards Exam Part I, DDS. Additional exam requirements/recommendations for international students: Required—TOEFL (minimum score 587 paper-based; 95 iBT). Electronic applications accepted.

New York University, Graduate School of Arts and Science, Department of Biology, New York, NY 10012-1019. Offers biology (PhD); biomedical journalism (MS); cancer and molecular biology (PhD); computational biology (PhD); computers in biological research (MS); developmental genetics (PhD); general biology (MS); immunology and microbiology (PhD); molecular genetics (PhD); neurobiology (MS); oral biology (MS); plant biology (PhD); recombinant DNA technology (MS); MS/MBA. *Program availability:* Part-time. Terminal master's awarded for partial completion of doctoral program. *Degree requirements:* For master's, thesis or alternative, qualifying paper; for doctorate, comprehensive exam, thesis/dissertation. *Entrance requirements:* For master's and doctorate, GRE General Test. Additional exam requirements/recommendations for international students: Required—TOEFL. *Faculty research:* Genomics, molecular and cell biology, development and molecular genetics, molecular evolution of plants and animals.

The Ohio State University, College of Dentistry, Columbus, OH 43210. Offers dental anesthesiology (MS); dental hygiene (MDH); dentistry (DDS); endodontics (MS); oral and maxillofacial pathology (MS); oral and maxillofacial surgery (MS); oral biology (PhD); orthodontics (MS); pediatric dentistry (MS); periodontology (MS); prosthodontics (MS); DDS/PhD. *Accreditation:* ADA (one or more programs are accredited). *Faculty:* 77. *Students:* 520 full-time (219 women), 5 part-time (4 women); includes 95 minority (12 Black or African American, non-Hispanic/Latino; 2 American Indian or Alaska Native, non-Hispanic/Latino; 49 Asian, non-Hispanic/Latino; 18 Hispanic/Latino; 14 Two or more

Oral and Dental Sciences

races, non-Hispanic/Latino), 28 international. Average age 26. In 2015, 31 master's, 112 doctorates awarded. Terminal master's awarded for partial completion of doctoral program. *Degree requirements:* For master's, thesis; for doctorate, thesis/dissertation (for some programs). *Entrance requirements:* For master's, GRE General Test (for all applicants with cumulative GPA below 3.0); for doctorate, DAT (for DDS); GRE General Test, GRE Subject Test in biology recommended (for PhD). Additional exam requirements/recommendations for international students: Required—TOEFL (minimum score 550 paper-based; 79 iBT), IELTS (minimum score 7), Michigan English Language Assessment Battery (minimum score 82). *Application deadline:* For fall admission, 10/1 for domestic and international students; for summer admission, 4/11 for domestic students, 3/10 for international students. Applications are processed on a rolling basis. Electronic applications accepted. *Expenses:* Contact institution. *Financial support:* Fellowships with tuition reimbursements, research assistantships with tuition reimbursements, teaching assistantships with tuition reimbursements, Federal Work-Study, institutionally sponsored loans, and health care benefits available. Financial award application deadline: 2/15. *Faculty research:* Neurobiology, inflammation and immunity, materials science, bone biology. *Unit head:* Dr. Patrick M. Lloyd, Dean, 614-292-9755, E-mail: lloyd.256@osu.edu. Website: http://www.dentistry.osu.edu/

Oregon Health & Science University, School of Dentistry, Graduate Programs in Dentistry, Department of Endodontics, Portland, OR 97239-3098. Offers Certificate. *Entrance requirements:* For degree, GRE General Test. Additional exam requirements/recommendations for international students: Required—TOEFL.

Oregon Health & Science University, School of Dentistry, Graduate Programs in Dentistry, Department of Orthodontics, Portland, OR 97239-3098. Offers MS, Certificate. *Degree requirements:* For master's, thesis. *Entrance requirements:* For master's and Certificate, GRE General Test, DMD/DDS. Additional exam requirements/recommendations for international students: Required—TOEFL.

Oregon Health & Science University, School of Dentistry, Graduate Programs in Dentistry, Department of Pediatric Dentistry, Portland, OR 97239-3098. Offers Certificate.

Oregon Health & Science University, School of Dentistry, Graduate Programs in Dentistry, Department of Periodontology, Portland, OR 97239-3098. Offers MS, Certificate. *Degree requirements:* For master's, thesis. *Entrance requirements:* For master's and Certificate, GRE General Test, DMD/DDS. Additional exam requirements/recommendations for international students: Required—TOEFL.

Oregon Health & Science University, School of Dentistry, Graduate Programs in Dentistry, Department of Restorative Dentistry, Division of Biomaterials and Biomechanics, Portland, OR 97239-3098. Offers MS.

Oregon Health & Science University, School of Dentistry, Graduate Programs in Dentistry, Program in Oral Molecular Biology, Portland, OR 97239-3098. Offers MS.

Oregon Health & Science University, School of Dentistry, Professional Program in Dentistry, Portland, OR 97239-3098. Offers dentistry (DMD); oral and maxillofacial surgery (Certificate); MD/DMD. *Accreditation:* ADA. *Entrance requirements:* For doctorate, DAT. Electronic applications accepted. *Faculty research:* Dentin permeability, tooth sensations, fluoride metabolism, immunology of periodontal disease, craniofacial growth.

Rutgers University–Newark, Rutgers School of Dental Medicine, Newark, NJ 07101-1709. Offers dental science (MS); dentistry (DMD); endodontics (Certificate); oral medicine (Certificate); orthodontics (Certificate); pediatric dentistry (Certificate); periodontics (Certificate); prosthodontics (Certificate); DMD/MPH; DMD/PhD; MD/Certificate; MS/Certificate. DMD/MPH offered jointly with New Jersey Institute of Technology, Rutgers, The State University of New Jersey, Camden. *Accreditation:* ADA (one or more programs are accredited). *Entrance requirements:* For doctorate, DAT. Electronic applications accepted. *Expenses:* Contact institution.

Saint Louis University, Graduate Education, Center for Advanced Dental Education, St. Louis, MO 63103. Offers endodontics (MSD); orthodontics (MSD); periodontics (MSD). *Degree requirements:* For master's, comprehensive exam, thesis, teaching practicum. *Entrance requirements:* For master's, GRE General Test, NBDE (National Board Dental Exam), DDS or DMD, interview, letters of recommendation. Additional exam requirements/recommendations for international students: Required—TOEFL (minimum score 525 paper-based). Electronic applications accepted. *Faculty research:* Craniofacial growth.

Seton Hill University, Program in Orthodontics, Greensburg, PA 15601. Offers MS, Certificate. *Entrance requirements:* For degree, U.S. National Dental Board Exams (Part 1 & 2), eligibility for PA licensure, DDS/DMD, minimum GPA of 3.0, transcripts, personal statement. Additional exam requirements/recommendations for international students: Required—TOEFL (minimum score 650 paper-based; 114 iBT), IELTS (minimum score 7). *Application deadline:* For fall admission, 9/15 priority date for domestic students, 9/15 for international students. *Expenses: Tuition,* area resident: Part-time $704 per credit. *Financial support:* Application deadline: 5/15; applicants required to submit FAFSA. Website: http://www.setonhill.edu/academics/graduate_programs/orthodontics

Stony Brook University, State University of New York, Stony Brook Medicine, School of Dental Medicine and Graduate School, Department of Oral Biology and Pathology, Stony Brook, NY 11794. Offers MS, PhD. *Faculty:* 10 full-time (5 women), 1 (woman) part-time/adjunct. *Students:* 4 full-time (all women); includes 1 minority (Asian, non-Hispanic/Latino), 1 international. Average age 34. 6 applicants, 67% accepted, 1 enrolled. *Degree requirements:* For doctorate, thesis/dissertation. *Entrance requirements:* For doctorate, GRE General Test. Additional exam requirements/recommendations for international students: Required—TOEFL. *Application deadline:* For fall admission, 1/15 for domestic students; for spring admission, 10/1 for domestic students. Application fee: $100. *Expenses:* $12,421 per year full-time resident tuition and fees, $453 per credit hour; $23,761 per year full-time non-resident tuition and fees, $925 per credit hour. *Financial support:* Fellowships, research assistantships, teaching assistantships, and Federal Work-Study available. Financial award application deadline: 3/15. *Faculty research:* Oral biology, oral diseases, dentistry, pathology, dental health and hygiene. Total annual research expenditures: $1 million. *Unit head:* Dr. Maria E. Ryan, Chair, 631-632-9529, E-mail: maria.ryan@stonybrook.edu. *Application contact:* Marguerite Baldwin, Coordinator, 631-632-9189, Fax: 631-632-9707, E-mail: marguerite.baldwin@stonybrook.edu. Website: http://www.stonybrookmedicalcenter.org/dental/oralbiology

Stony Brook University, State University of New York, Stony Brook Medicine, School of Dental Medicine, Professional Program in Dental Medicine, Stony Brook, NY 11794. Offers dental medicine (DDS); endodontics (Certificate); orthodontics (Certificate); periodontics (Certificate). *Accreditation:* ADA (one or more programs are accredited). *Faculty:* 33 full-time (17 women), 70 part-time/adjunct (20 women). *Students:* 190 full-time (99 women); includes 48 minority (3 Black or African American, non-Hispanic/Latino; 34 Asian, non-Hispanic/Latino; 10 Hispanic/Latino; 1 Two or more races, non-Hispanic/Latino), 2 international. 1,422 applicants, 8% accepted, 52 enrolled. In 2015, 39 doctorates, 15 Certificates awarded. *Entrance requirements:* For doctorate, DAT.

Application deadline: For fall admission, 1/15 for domestic students. Application fee: $100. *Expenses:* $32,960 per year full-time resident tuition and fees, $62,950 per year full-time non-resident tuition and fees. *Financial support:* Research assistantships, teaching assistantships, and Federal Work-Study available. Support available to part-time students. *Unit head:* Dr. Mary R. Truhlar, Dean, 631-632-8950, Fax: 631-632-9105. *Application contact:* Patricia Berry, Acting Director of Admissions, 631-632-8871, Fax: 631-632-7130, E-mail: patricia.berry@stonybrook.edu. Website: http://dentistry.stonybrookmedicine.edu/

Temple University, Kornberg School of Dentistry and Graduate School, Graduate Programs in Dentistry, Philadelphia, PA 19122-6096. Offers advanced education in general dentistry (Certificate); endodontology (Certificate); oral biology (MS); orthodontics (Certificate); periodontology (Certificate). *Degree requirements:* For master's, thesis; for Certificate, comprehensive exam. *Entrance requirements:* For master's, GRE; for Certificate, National Boards Parts I and II, DMD or DDS, 3 letters of recommendation. Additional exam requirements/recommendations for international students: Required—TOEFL (minimum score 650 paper-based). *Expenses:* Contact institution. *Faculty research:* Saliva and salivary glands, implantology, material science, periodontal disease, geriatric dentistry.

Tufts University, School of Dental Medicine, Advanced Education Programs in Dental Medicine, Medford, MA 02155. Offers dentistry (Certificate), including endodontics, oral and maxillofacial surgery, orthodontics, pediatric dentistry, periodontology, prosthodontics. *Entrance requirements:* Additional exam requirements/recommendations for international students: Required—TOEFL. *Expenses:* Contact institution.

Tufts University, School of Dental Medicine, Graduate Programs in Dental Medicine, Medford, MA 02155. Offers MS. *Degree requirements:* For master's, thesis. *Entrance requirements:* For master's, DDS, DMD, or equivalent; minimum B average. Additional exam requirements/recommendations for international students: Required—TOEFL. *Expenses:* Contact institution. *Faculty research:* Periodontal research, dental materials, salivary research, epidemiology, bone biology.

Université de Montréal, Faculty of Dental Medicine, Program in Multidisciplinary Residency, Montréal, QC H3C 3J7, Canada. Offers Certificate. Electronic applications accepted.

Université de Montréal, Faculty of Dental Medicine, Program in Oral and Dental Sciences, Montréal, QC H3C 3J7, Canada. Offers M Sc. Electronic applications accepted.

Université de Montréal, Faculty of Dental Medicine, Program in Orthodontics, Montréal, QC H3C 3J7, Canada. Offers M Sc. Electronic applications accepted.

Université de Montréal, Faculty of Dental Medicine, Program in Pediatric Dentistry, Montréal, QC H3C 3J7, Canada. Offers M Sc. Electronic applications accepted.

Université de Montréal, Faculty of Dental Medicine, Program in Prosthodontics Rehabilitation, Montréal, QC H3C 3J7, Canada. Offers M Sc. Electronic applications accepted.

Université Laval, Faculty of Dentistry, Diploma Program in Buccal and Maxillofacial Surgery, Québec, QC G1K 7P4, Canada. Offers DESS. *Degree requirements:* For DESS, comprehensive exam. *Entrance requirements:* For degree, interview, knowledge of French. Electronic applications accepted.

Université Laval, Faculty of Dentistry, Diploma Program in Gerodontology, Québec, QC G1K 7P4, Canada. Offers DESS. *Program availability:* Part-time. *Entrance requirements:* For degree, interview, good knowledge of French. Electronic applications accepted.

Université Laval, Faculty of Dentistry, Diploma Program in Multidisciplinary Dentistry, Québec, QC G1K 7P4, Canada. Offers DESS. *Entrance requirements:* For degree, interview, knowledge of French. Electronic applications accepted.

Université Laval, Faculty of Dentistry, Diploma Program in Periodontics, Québec, QC G1K 7P4, Canada. Offers DESS. *Entrance requirements:* For degree, interview, knowledge of French. Electronic applications accepted.

Université Laval, Faculty of Dentistry, Graduate Program in Dentistry, Québec, QC G1K 7P4, Canada. Offers M Sc. *Degree requirements:* For master's, thesis (for some programs). Electronic applications accepted.

University at Buffalo, the State University of New York, Graduate School, School of Dental Medicine, Graduate Programs in Dental Medicine, Department of Oral Biology, Buffalo, NY 14260. Offers PhD. *Degree requirements:* For doctorate, thesis/dissertation. *Entrance requirements:* For doctorate, GRE General Test. Additional exam requirements/recommendations for international students: Required—TOEFL (minimum score 550 paper-based; 79 iBT). Electronic applications accepted. *Faculty research:* Oral immunology and microbiology, bone physiology, biochemistry, molecular genetics, neutrophil biology.

University at Buffalo, the State University of New York, Graduate School, School of Dental Medicine, Graduate Programs in Dental Medicine, Department of Orthodontics, Buffalo, NY 14260. Offers MS, Certificate. *Degree requirements:* For master's, thesis. *Entrance requirements:* For master's, GRE General Test, National Board Dental Exam, DDS or equivalent. Additional exam requirements/recommendations for international students: Required—TOEFL (minimum score 550 paper-based; 79 iBT). Electronic applications accepted. *Faculty research:* Stem cell, clinical respiration, growth and development.

University at Buffalo, the State University of New York, Graduate School, School of Dental Medicine, Graduate Programs in Dental Medicine, Program in Biomaterials, Buffalo, NY 14260. Offers MS. *Program availability:* Part-time. *Degree requirements:* For master's, thesis. *Entrance requirements:* For master's, GRE General Test. Additional exam requirements/recommendations for international students: Required—TOEFL (minimum score 550 paper-based; 79 iBT). Electronic applications accepted. *Faculty research:* Orofacial pain, surface science, bioadhesion, ontology, oral medicine.

University at Buffalo, the State University of New York, Graduate School, School of Dental Medicine, Graduate Programs in Dental Medicine, Program in Oral Sciences, Buffalo, NY 14260. Offers MS. *Degree requirements:* For master's, thesis. *Entrance requirements:* For master's, DDS, DMD or equivalent foreign degree. Additional exam requirements/recommendations for international students: Required—TOEFL (minimum score 550 paper-based; 79 iBT). Electronic applications accepted. *Faculty research:* Oral biology and pathology, behavioral sciences, neuromuscular physiology, facial pain, oral microbiology.

The University of Alabama at Birmingham, School of Dentistry, Graduate Programs in Dentistry, Birmingham, AL 35294. Offers MS. *Degree requirements:* For master's, thesis. *Expenses:* Tuition, state resident: full-time $7340. Tuition, nonresident: full-time $16,628. Full-time tuition and fees vary according to course load and program.

University of Alberta, Faculty of Medicine and Dentistry, Department of Dentistry, Program in Orthodontics, Edmonton, AB T6G 2E1, Canada. Offers M Sc, PhD. *Degree requirements:* For master's, thesis; for doctorate, thesis/dissertation. *Entrance requirements:* Additional exam requirements/recommendations for international students: Required—TOEFL (minimum score 580 paper-based). Electronic applications accepted.

The University of British Columbia, Faculty of Dentistry and Faculty of Graduate Studies, Graduate/Postgraduate and Professional Specialty Programs in Dentistry, Vancouver, BC V6T 1Z1, Canada. Offers dental science (M Sc, PhD); periodontics (Diploma). *Degree requirements:* For master's, thesis; for doctorate, comprehensive exam, thesis/dissertation. *Entrance requirements:* For degree, dental license, interview. Additional exam requirements/recommendations for international students: Required—TOEFL (minimum score 580 paper-based). Electronic applications accepted. *Expenses:* Contact institution. *Faculty research:* Cell biology, oral physiology, microbiology, immunology, biomaterials.

University of California, Los Angeles, Graduate Division, College of Letters and Science and David Geffen School of Medicine, UCLA ACCESS to Programs in the Molecular, Cellular and Integrative Life Sciences, Los Angeles, CA 90095. Offers biochemistry and molecular biology (PhD); biological chemistry (PhD); cellular and molecular pathology (PhD); human genetics (PhD); microbiology, immunology, and molecular genetics (PhD); molecular biology (PhD); molecular toxicology (PhD); molecular, cellular and integrative physiology (PhD); neurobiology (PhD); oral biology (PhD); physiology (PhD). *Degree requirements:* For doctorate, thesis/dissertation, oral and written qualifying exams. *Entrance requirements:* For doctorate, GRE General Test, bachelor's degree; minimum undergraduate GPA of 3.0 (or its equivalent if letter grade system not used). Additional exam requirements/recommendations for international students: Required—TOEFL. Electronic applications accepted.

University of California, Los Angeles, School of Dentistry and Graduate Division, Graduate Programs in Dentistry, Program in Oral Biology, Los Angeles, CA 90095. Offers MS, PhD, DDS/MS, DDS/PhD, MD/PhD, MS/Certificate, PhD/Certificate. *Degree requirements:* For master's, thesis; for doctorate, thesis/dissertation, oral and written qualifying exams; 1 quarter of teaching experience. *Entrance requirements:* For master's and doctorate, GRE General Test, bachelor's degree; minimum undergraduate GPA of 3.0 (or its equivalent if letter grade system not used). Additional exam requirements/recommendations for international students: Required—TOEFL. Electronic applications accepted.

University of California, San Francisco, Graduate Division, Program in Oral and Craniofacial Sciences, San Francisco, CA 94143. Offers MS, PhD. Terminal master's awarded for partial completion of doctoral program. *Degree requirements:* For master's, thesis; for doctorate, thesis/dissertation. *Entrance requirements:* For master's and doctorate, GRE General Test.

University of Colorado Denver, School of Dental Medicine, Aurora, CO 80045. Offers dental surgery (DDS); orthodontics (MS); periodontics (MS). *Accreditation:* ADA. *Faculty:* 89 full-time (34 women), 48 part-time/adjunct (14 women). *Students:* 449 full-time (212 women); includes 123 minority (7 Black or African American, non-Hispanic/Latino; 2 American Indian or Alaska Native, non-Hispanic/Latino; 61 Asian, non-Hispanic/Latino; 42 Hispanic/Latino; 11 Two or more races, non-Hispanic/Latino), 15 international. Average age 27. In 2015, 25 master's, 116 doctorates awarded. *Entrance requirements:* For master's, GRE, National Board Dental Exam Part I and II, three letters of recommendation, personal essay; for doctorate, DAT, prerequisite courses in microbiology, general biochemistry and English composition (1 semester each); general chemistry/lab, organic chemistry/lab, general biology/lab and general physics/lab (2 semesters each); interview; letters of recommendation; essay. Additional exam requirements/recommendations for international students: Required—TOEFL (minimum score 580 paper-based; 80 iBT); Recommended—IELTS (minimum score 6.8). *Application deadline:* For fall admission, 12/31 for domestic students, 12/15 for international students. Application fee: $50 ($75 for international students). Electronic

applications accepted. *Expenses:* Contact institution. *Financial support:* In 2015–16, 159 students received support. Fellowships, research assistantships, teaching assistantships, Federal Work-Study, institutionally sponsored loans, scholarships/grants, and traineeships available. Financial award application deadline: 4/1; financial award applicants required to submit FAFSA. *Faculty research:* Pain control, materials research, geriatric dentistry, restorative dentistry, periodontics. *Total annual research expenditures:* $4.2 million. *Unit head:* Dr. Denise K. Kassebaum, Dean, 303-724-7100, Fax: 303-724-7109, E-mail: denise.kassebaum@ucdenver.edu. *Application contact:* Graduate Student Admissions, 303-724-7122, Fax: 303-724-7109, E-mail: ddsadmissioninquiries@ucdenver.edu.
Website: http://www.ucdenver.edu/academics/colleges/dentalmedicine/Pages/DentalMedicine.aspx

University of Connecticut Health Center, Graduate School, Programs in Biomedical Sciences, Combined Degree Programs in Oral Biology, Farmington, CT 06030. Offers DMD/PhD. *Entrance requirements:* Additional exam requirements/recommendations for international students: Required—TOEFL (minimum score 600 paper-based).

★ **University of Connecticut Health Center,** Graduate School, Programs in Biomedical Sciences, Program in Skeletal, Craniofacial and Oral Biology, Farmington, CT 06030. Offers PhD, DMD/PhD, MD/PhD. *Degree requirements:* For doctorate, comprehensive exam, thesis/dissertation. *Entrance requirements:* For doctorate, GRE General Test. Additional exam requirements/recommendations for international students: Required—TOEFL (minimum score 600 paper-based). Electronic applications accepted. *Faculty research:* Skeletal development and patterning, bone biology, connective tissue biology, neurophysiology of taste and smell, microbiological aspects of caries.
See Display below and Close-Up on page 887.

University of Connecticut Health Center, School of Dental Medicine, Program in Dental Science, Farmington, CT 06030. Offers MDS. *Program availability:* Part-time. *Degree requirements:* For master's, comprehensive exam, thesis. *Entrance requirements:* For master's, National Board Dental Examination Parts I and II. *Expenses:* Contact institution.

University of Detroit Mercy, School of Dentistry, Detroit, MI 48208. Offers MS, DDS, Certificate. *Accreditation:* ADA (one or more programs are accredited). *Degree requirements:* For master's, thesis. *Entrance requirements:* For master's, DDS or DMD; for doctorate, DAT; for Certificate, DAT, DDS or DMD. Application fee: $50. *Expenses:* Contact institution. *Financial support:* Career-related internships or fieldwork, Federal Work-Study, and stipends available. Financial award application deadline: 4/15. *Faculty research:* HIV and periodontal disease, chemotherapeutic management of periodontal disease, oral analgesics, sterilization/disinfection, prosthodontic materials. *Unit head:* Dr. Mert N. Aksu, Dean, 313-494-6621.
Website: http://dental.udmercy.edu

University of Florida, College of Dentistry and Graduate School, Graduate Programs in Dentistry, Department of Endodontics, Gainesville, FL 32611. Offers MS, Certificate. *Entrance requirements:* For master's, DAT, GRE General Test, National Board Dental Examination Parts I and II, minimum GPA of 3.0, interview; for Certificate, DAT. Additional exam requirements/recommendations for international students: Required—TOEFL (minimum score 550 paper-based). *Faculty research:* Canal cleanliness, antibiotics, resilon, lasers, microbes.

University of Florida, College of Dentistry and Graduate School, Graduate Programs in Dentistry, Department of Oral Biology, Gainesville, FL 32611. Offers PhD. *Degree requirements:* For doctorate, thesis/dissertation. *Entrance requirements:* For doctorate, GRE General Test, minimum GPA of 3.0. Additional exam requirements/

Oral and Dental Sciences

recommendations for international students: Required—TOEFL. Electronic applications accepted. *Faculty research:* Bacterial genetics, cell adhesion, salivary glands, cell proliferation.

University of Florida, College of Dentistry and Graduate School, Graduate Programs in Dentistry, Department of Orthodontics, Gainesville, FL 32611. Offers MS, Certificate. *Degree requirements:* For master's, thesis. *Entrance requirements:* For master's, DAT, GRE General Test, National Board Dental Examination Parts I and II, minimum GPA of 3.0, interview. Additional exam requirements/recommendations for international students: Required—TOEFL (minimum score 550 paper-based). *Faculty research:* Bone biology, osteoclasts, clinical research, root resorption, pain control.

University of Florida, College of Dentistry and Graduate School, Graduate Programs in Dentistry, Department of Periodontology, Gainesville, FL 32611. Offers MS, Certificate. *Degree requirements:* For master's, thesis. *Entrance requirements:* For master's, DAT, GRE General Test, National Board Dental Examination Parts I and II, minimum GPA of 3.0, interview. Additional exam requirements/recommendations for international students: Required—TOEFL (minimum score 550 paper-based). *Faculty research:* Gingival grafting, periodontal plastic surgery, regenerative periodontal surgery, dental implant complications, osteogenic fibroma.

University of Florida, College of Dentistry and Graduate School, Graduate Programs in Dentistry, Department of Prosthodontics, Gainesville, FL 32611. Offers MS, Certificate. *Degree requirements:* For master's, thesis. *Entrance requirements:* For master's, DAT, GRE General Test, National Board Dental Examination Parts I and II, minimum GPA of 3.0, interview. Additional exam requirements/recommendations for international students: Required—TOEFL (minimum score 550 paper-based). *Faculty research:* Computer panograph, dental implants, resin provisional materials wear rate, implant surface variation, Sjorgen's Syndrome.

University of Illinois at Chicago, College of Dentistry and Graduate College, Graduate Programs in Oral Sciences, Chicago, IL 60607-7128. Offers MS, PhD. *Faculty:* 25 full-time (6 women), 41 part-time/adjunct (15 women). *Students:* 4 full-time (3 women), 11 part-time (9 women); includes 7 minority (4 Black or African American, non-Hispanic/Latino; 1 Asian, non-Hispanic/Latino; 2 Hispanic/Latino), 3 international. Average age 28. *Degree requirements:* For master's, thesis. *Entrance requirements:* For master's, GRE General Test, DDS, DVM, or MD. Additional exam requirements/recommendations for international students: Required—TOEFL. *Application deadline:* For fall admission, 5/15 for domestic students, 2/15 for international students; for spring admission, 11/15 for domestic students, 7/15 for international students. Application fee: $85. Electronic applications accepted. *Expenses:* Contact institution. *Financial support:* Fellowships, research assistantships with full tuition reimbursements, teaching assistantships with full tuition reimbursements, Federal Work-Study, scholarships/grants, traineeships, health care benefits, tuition waivers (full), and unspecified assistantships available. Financial award application deadline: 3/1. *Faculty research:* Medical anthropology and ethnopharmacology research associated with plants and other natural products used for oral medicine conditions, pains and pathologies, craniofacial genetics, genomics, mechanisms of biomineralization, oral microbiology. *Unit head:* Dr. Katherine Bedran-Russo, Director, 312-996-2465, E-mail: bedran@uic.edu. *Application contact:* Jackie Perry, Graduate College Receptionist, 312-413-2550, Fax: 312-413-0185, E-mail: gradcoll@uic.edu.

The University of Iowa, College of Dentistry and Graduate College, Graduate Programs in Dentistry, Department of Endodontics, Iowa City, IA 52242-1316. Offers MS, Certificate. *Degree requirements:* For master's, thesis. *Entrance requirements:* For master's, GRE, DDS; for Certificate, DDS. Additional exam requirements/recommendations for international students: Required—TOEFL.

The University of Iowa, College of Dentistry and Graduate College, Graduate Programs in Dentistry, Department of Operative Dentistry, Iowa City, IA 52242-1316. Offers MS, Certificate. *Degree requirements:* For master's, thesis. *Entrance requirements:* For master's, GRE, DDS; for Certificate, DDS. Additional exam requirements/recommendations for international students: Required—TOEFL.

The University of Iowa, College of Dentistry and Graduate College, Graduate Programs in Dentistry, Department of Oral and Maxillofacial Surgery, Iowa City, IA 52242-1316. Offers MS, PhD, Certificate. *Degree requirements:* For master's, thesis. *Entrance requirements:* For master's, GRE, DDS; for Certificate, DDS.

The University of Iowa, College of Dentistry and Graduate College, Graduate Programs in Dentistry, Department of Oral Pathology, Radiology and Medicine, Iowa City, IA 52242-1316. Offers MS, PhD, Certificate. *Degree requirements:* For master's, thesis. *Entrance requirements:* For master's, GRE, DDS, minimum GPA of 2.7. Additional exam requirements/recommendations for international students: Required—TOEFL.

The University of Iowa, College of Dentistry and Graduate College, Graduate Programs in Dentistry, Department of Orthodontics, Iowa City, IA 52242-1316. Offers MS, Certificate. *Degree requirements:* For master's, thesis. *Entrance requirements:* For master's, GRE, DDS; for Certificate, DDS. Additional exam requirements/recommendations for international students: Required—TOEFL.

The University of Iowa, College of Dentistry and Graduate College, Graduate Programs in Dentistry, Department of Pediatric Dentistry, Iowa City, IA 52242-1316. Offers Certificate. *Entrance requirements:* For degree, DDS. Additional exam requirements/recommendations for international students: Required—TOEFL.

The University of Iowa, College of Dentistry and Graduate College, Graduate Programs in Dentistry, Department of Periodontics, Iowa City, IA 52242-1316. Offers MS, Certificate. *Degree requirements:* For master's, thesis. *Entrance requirements:* For master's, GRE, DDS; for Certificate, DDS. Additional exam requirements/recommendations for international students: Required—TOEFL.

The University of Iowa, College of Dentistry and Graduate College, Graduate Programs in Dentistry, Department of Preventive and Community Dentistry, Iowa City, IA 52242-1316. Offers dental public health (MS). *Degree requirements:* For master's, thesis. *Entrance requirements:* For master's, GRE, DDS. Additional exam requirements/recommendations for international students: Required—TOEFL.

The University of Iowa, College of Dentistry and Graduate College, Graduate Programs in Dentistry, Department of Prosthodontics, Iowa City, IA 52242-1316. Offers MS, Certificate. *Degree requirements:* For master's, thesis. *Entrance requirements:* For master's, GRE, DDS; for Certificate, DDS. Additional exam requirements/recommendations for international students: Required—TOEFL.

The University of Iowa, College of Dentistry and Graduate College, Graduate Programs in Dentistry, Oral Science Graduate Program, Iowa City, IA 52242-1316. Offers MS, PhD. *Degree requirements:* For master's, thesis; for doctorate, thesis/dissertation. *Entrance requirements:* For master's, GRE, DDS. Additional exam requirements/recommendations for international students: Required—TOEFL.

University of Kentucky, Graduate School, Graduate Program in Dentistry, Lexington, KY 40506-0032. Offers MS. *Degree requirements:* For master's, comprehensive exam, thesis. *Entrance requirements:* For master's, GRE General Test, minimum undergraduate GPA of 2.5. Additional exam requirements/recommendations for

international students: Required—TOEFL (minimum score 550 paper-based). Electronic applications accepted.

University of Louisville, School of Dentistry, Louisville, KY 40202. Offers dentistry (DMD); oral biology (MS). *Accreditation:* ADA (one or more programs are accredited). *Program availability:* Part-time. *Faculty:* 71 full-time (23 women), 81 part-time/adjunct (20 women). *Students:* 518 full-time (220 women), 19 part-time (10 women); includes 118 minority (22 Black or African American, non-Hispanic/Latino; 2 American Indian or Alaska Native, non-Hispanic/Latino; 55 Asian, non-Hispanic/Latino; 24 Hispanic/Latino; 15 Two or more races, non-Hispanic/Latino), 26 international. Average age 26. 176 applicants, 93% accepted, 146 enrolled. In 2015, 2 master's, 115 doctorates awarded. *Degree requirements:* For master's, thesis; for doctorate, National Board exams. *Entrance requirements:* For master's, DAT, GRE General Test, or National Board Dental Exam, minimum GPA of 2.75; for doctorate, DAT, 32 hours of course work in science. Additional exam requirements/recommendations for international students: Required—TOEFL (minimum score 100 iBT). *Application deadline:* For fall admission, 1/1 for domestic and international students. Applications are processed on a rolling basis. Application fee: $60. Electronic applications accepted. *Expenses:* Contact institution. *Financial support:* In 2015–16, 646,062 students received support, including 1 research assistantship with full tuition reimbursement available (averaging $20,000 per year). Financial award application deadline: 3/15; financial award applicants required to submit FAFSA. *Faculty research:* Inflammation and periodontitis, birth defects and developmental biology, biomaterials, oral infections, digital imaging. *Total annual research expenditures:* $5.1 million. *Unit head:* Dr. John J. Sauk, Dean, 502-852-1304, Fax: 502-852-3364, E-mail: jjsauk01@louisville.edu. *Application contact:* Robin Benningfield, Admissions Counselor, 502-852-5081, Fax: 502-852-1210, E-mail: dmdadms@louisville.edu.
Website: http://louisville.edu/dental/

The University of Manchester, School of Dentistry, Manchester, United Kingdom. Offers basic dental sciences (cancer studies) (M Phil, PhD); basic dental sciences (molecular genetics) (M Phil, PhD); basic dental sciences (stem cell biology) (M Phil, PhD); biomaterials sciences and dental technology (M Phil, PhD); dental public health/community dentistry (M Phil, PhD); dental science (clinical) (PhD); endodontology (M Phil, PhD); fixed and removable prosthodontics (M Phil, PhD); operative dentistry (M Phil, PhD); oral and maxillofacial surgery (M Phil, PhD); oral radiology (M Phil, PhD); orthodontics (M Phil, PhD); restorative dentistry (M Phil, PhD).

University of Manitoba, Faculty of Dentistry and Faculty of Graduate Studies, Graduate Programs in Dentistry, Department of Dental Diagnostic and Surgical Sciences, Winnipeg, MB R3T 2N2, Canada. Offers oral and maxillofacial surgery (M Dent); periodontology (M Dent). *Entrance requirements:* For master's, dental degree. *Faculty research:* Implantology, clinical trials, tobacco use, periodontal disease.

University of Manitoba, Faculty of Dentistry and Faculty of Graduate Studies, Graduate Programs in Dentistry, Department of Oral Biology, Winnipeg, MB R3T 2N2, Canada. Offers M Sc, PhD. *Degree requirements:* For master's, thesis; for doctorate, comprehensive exam, thesis/dissertation. *Entrance requirements:* For master's, B Sc or pre-M Sc. Additional exam requirements/recommendations for international students: Required—TOEFL. *Faculty research:* Oral bacterial ecology and metabolism, biofilms, saliva and oral health, secretory mechanisms.

University of Manitoba, Faculty of Dentistry and Faculty of Graduate Studies, Graduate Programs in Dentistry, Department of Preventive Dental Science, Winnipeg, MB R3T 2N2, Canada. Offers orthodontics (M Sc). *Degree requirements:* For master's, thesis. *Entrance requirements:* For master's, dental degree. Electronic applications accepted.

University of Maryland, Baltimore, Graduate School, Graduate Programs in Dentistry, Department of Oral Pathology, Baltimore, MD 21201. Offers PhD. *Degree requirements:* For doctorate, comprehensive exam, thesis/dissertation. *Entrance requirements:* For doctorate, GRE General Test, DDS, DMD. Additional exam requirements/recommendations for international students: Required—TOEFL (minimum score 550 paper-based; 80 iBT); Recommended—IELTS (minimum score 7). Electronic applications accepted. Tuition and fees vary according to program. *Faculty research:* Histopathology, epidemiology of oral lesions, embryology.

University of Maryland, Baltimore, Graduate School, Graduate Programs in Dentistry, Graduate Program in Biomedical Sciences, Baltimore, MD 21201. Offers MS, PhD, DDS/PhD. *Degree requirements:* For master's, thesis optional; for doctorate, comprehensive exam, thesis/dissertation. *Entrance requirements:* For master's and doctorate, GRE General Test. Additional exam requirements/recommendations for international students: Required—TOEFL (minimum score 550 paper-based; 80 iBT); Recommended—IELTS (minimum score 7). Electronic applications accepted. Tuition and fees vary according to program. *Faculty research:* Neuroscience, molecular and cell biology, infectious diseases.

University of Maryland, Baltimore, Professional and Advanced Education Programs in Dentistry, Baltimore, MD 21201-1627. Offers advanced general dentistry (Certificate); dentistry (DDS); endodontics (Certificate); oral-maxillofacial surgery (Certificate); orthodontics (Certificate); pediatric dentistry (Certificate); periodontics (Certificate); prosthodontics (Certificate); DDS/MBA; DDS/PhD. *Accreditation:* ADA. *Students:* 581 full-time (301 women), 4 part-time (2 women); includes 236 minority (55 Black or African American, non-Hispanic/Latino; 115 Asian, non-Hispanic/Latino; 41 Hispanic/Latino; 1 Native Hawaiian or other Pacific Islander, non-Hispanic/Latino; 24 Two or more races, non-Hispanic/Latino), 32 international. Average age 26. 506 applicants, 89% accepted, 135 enrolled. In 2015, 127 doctorates, 27 Certificates awarded. *Entrance requirements:* For doctorate, DAT, coursework in science; for Certificate, National Dental Board Exams, DDS. Additional exam requirements/recommendations for international students: Required—TOEFL (minimum score 550 paper-based; 80 iBT). *Application deadline:* Applications are processed on a rolling basis. Application fee: $85. Electronic applications accepted. *Expenses:* $31,566 in-state tuition and fees, $61,331 out-of-state. *Financial support:* Career-related internships or fieldwork, Federal Work-Study, scholarships/grants, and traineeships available. Financial award application deadline: 3/1; financial award applicants required to submit FAFSA. *Faculty research:* Pain/neuroscience, oncology/molecular and cell biology, infectious disease/microbiology, biomaterial studies, health promotion and disparities. *Unit head:* Dr. Mark A. Reynolds, Dean, 410-706-7461. *Application contact:* Dr. Judith A. Porter, Assistant Dean for Admissions and Recruitment, 410-706-7472, Fax: 410-706-0945, E-mail: ddsadmissions@umaryland.edu.
Website: http://www.dental.umaryland.edu/

University of Michigan, School of Dentistry and Rackham Graduate School, Graduate Programs in Dentistry, Endodontics Program, Ann Arbor, MI 48109-1078. Offers MS. *Students:* 11 full-time (5 women); includes 1 minority (Hispanic/Latino), 3 international. 32 applicants, 13% accepted, 4 enrolled. In 2015, 3 master's awarded. *Degree requirements:* For master's, thesis. *Entrance requirements:* For master's, DDS. Additional exam requirements/recommendations for international students: Required—TOEFL (minimum score 84 iBT). *Application deadline:* For fall admission, 7/15 for domestic and international students. Applications are processed on a rolling basis. Application fee: $75 ($90 for international students). Electronic applications accepted.

Expenses: $70,026 resident full-time, $121,146 nonresident full-time. *Unit head:* Dr. Neville McDonald, Program Director, E-mail: somerled@umich.edu. *Application contact:* Patricia Katcher, Associate Admissions Director, 734-763-3316, Fax: 734-764-1922, E-mail: graddentinquiry@umich.edu.
Website: http://www.dent.umich.edu/crse/graduateprogram/endodontics

University of Michigan, School of Dentistry and Rackham Graduate School, Graduate Programs in Dentistry, Orthodontics Program, Ann Arbor, MI 48109-1078. Offers MS. *Students:* 21 full-time (12 women); includes 3 minority (1 Black or African American, non-Hispanic/Latino; 1 Asian, non-Hispanic/Latino; 1 Hispanic/Latino), 3 international. 227 applicants, 3% accepted, 7 enrolled. In 2015, 7 master's awarded. *Degree requirements:* For master's, thesis. *Entrance requirements:* For master's, GRE, National Dental Board Exam, DDS. Additional exam requirements/recommendations for international students: Required—TOEFL (minimum score 84 iBT). *Application deadline:* For fall admission, 8/17 for domestic and international students. Application fee: $75 ($90 for international students). Electronic applications accepted. *Expenses:* $70,026 resident full-time, $121,146 non-resident full time. *Unit head:* Dr. Hera Kim-Berman, Program Director, 734-764-1080, E-mail: bermanh@umich.edu. *Application contact:* Patricia Katcher, Associate Admissions Director, 734-763-3316, Fax: 734-764-1922, E-mail: graddentinquiry@umich.edu.
Website: http://www.dent.umich.edu/opd/graduateprograms/ortho/about

University of Michigan, School of Dentistry and Rackham Graduate School, Graduate Programs in Dentistry, Pediatric Dentistry Program, Ann Arbor, MI 48109-1078. Offers MS. *Students:* 19 full-time (18 women); includes 8 minority (1 Black or African American, non-Hispanic/Latino; 4 Asian, non-Hispanic/Latino; 2 Hispanic/Latino; 1 Two or more races, non-Hispanic/Latino), 2 international. 125 applicants, 5% accepted, 6 enrolled. In 2015, 6 master's awarded. *Degree requirements:* For master's, thesis. *Entrance requirements:* For master's, National Dental Board Exam, DDS. Additional exam requirements/recommendations for international students: Required—TOEFL (minimum score 84 iBT). *Application deadline:* For fall admission, 9/15 for domestic students, 10/1 for international students. Application fee: $75 ($90 for international students). Electronic applications accepted. *Expenses:* $35,926 resident full-time, $61,296 nonresident full-time. *Unit head:* Dr. James Boynton, Program Director, 734-764-1522, E-mail: jboynton@umich.edu. *Application contact:* Patricia Katcher, Associate Admissions Director, 734-763-3316, Fax: 734-764-1922, E-mail: graddentinquiry@umich.edu.
Website: http://www.dent.umich.edu/opd/graduateprograms/ped/aboutus

University of Michigan, School of Dentistry and Rackham Graduate School, Graduate Programs in Dentistry, Periodontics Program, Ann Arbor, MI 48109-1078. Offers MS. *Students:* 13 full-time (5 women); includes 1 minority (Asian, non-Hispanic/Latino), 8 international. 50 applicants, 8% accepted, 4 enrolled. In 2015, 1 master's awarded. *Degree requirements:* For master's, thesis. *Entrance requirements:* For master's, DDS. Additional exam requirements/recommendations for international students: Required—TOEFL (minimum score 84 iBT). *Application deadline:* For fall admission, 7/15 for domestic and international students. Applications are processed on a rolling basis. Application fee: $75 ($90 for international students). Electronic applications accepted. *Expenses:* $70,026 resident full-time, $121,146 nonresident full-time. *Unit head:* Dr. Hom-Lay Wang, Program Director, 734-764-1948, E-mail: homlay@umich.edu. *Application contact:* Patricia Katcher, Associate Admissions Director, 734-763-3316, Fax: 734-764-1922, E-mail: graddentinquiry@umich.edu.
Website: http://www.dent.umich.edu/pom/academics/gradprograms#perio

University of Michigan, School of Dentistry and Rackham Graduate School, Graduate Programs in Dentistry, Prosthodontics Program, Ann Arbor, MI 48109-1078. Offers MS. *Students:* 12 full-time (5 women); includes 2 minority (1 Asian, non-Hispanic/Latino; 1 Hispanic/Latino), 5 international. 71 applicants, 14% accepted, 4 enrolled. In 2015, 6 master's awarded. *Degree requirements:* For master's, thesis. *Entrance requirements:* For master's, DDS. Additional exam requirements/recommendations for international students: Required—TOEFL (minimum score 84 iBT). *Application deadline:* For fall admission, 9/1 for domestic and international students. Applications are processed on a rolling basis. Application fee: $75 ($90 for international students). Electronic applications accepted. *Expenses:* $70,026 resident full-time, $121,146 nonresident full-time. *Unit head:* Dr. Michael Razzoog, Program Director, 734-647-1369, E-mail: merim@umich.edu. *Application contact:* Patricia Katcher, Associate Admissions Director, 734-763-3316, Fax: 734-764-1922, E-mail: graddentinquiry@umich.edu.
Website: http://www.dent.umich.edu/bms/gradstudentsprosgradprog

University of Michigan, School of Dentistry and Rackham Graduate School, Graduate Programs in Dentistry, Restorative Dentistry Program, Ann Arbor, MI 48109-1078. Offers MS. *Students:* 13 full-time (8 women); includes 2 minority (1 Black or African American, non-Hispanic/Latino; 1 Hispanic/Latino), 10 international. 31 applicants, 16% accepted, 4 enrolled. In 2015, 3 master's awarded. *Degree requirements:* For master's, thesis. *Entrance requirements:* For master's, DDS. Additional exam requirements/recommendations for international students: Required—TOEFL (minimum score 84 iBT). *Application deadline:* For fall admission, 9/1 for domestic and international students. Applications are processed on a rolling basis. Application fee: $75 ($90 for international students). Electronic applications accepted. *Expenses:* $70,026 resident full-time, $121,146 nonresident full-time. *Unit head:* Dr. Peter Yaman, Program Director, 734-647-3722, E-mail: pyam@umich.edu. *Application contact:* Patricia Katcher, Associate Admissions Director, 734-763-3316, Fax: 734-764-1922, E-mail: graddentinquiry@umich.edu.
Website: http://www.dent.umich.edu/crse/graduateprograms/restorativedentistry

University of Michigan, School of Dentistry, Oral Health Sciences PhD Program, Ann Arbor, MI 48109-1078. Offers PhD. *Faculty:* 35 full-time (11 women). *Students:* 11 full-time (6 women); includes 3 minority (all Asian, non-Hispanic/Latino), 4 international. Average age 27. 37 applicants, 19% accepted. In 2015, 2 doctorates awarded. *Degree requirements:* For doctorate, thesis/dissertation, preliminary exam, oral defense of dissertation. *Entrance requirements:* For doctorate, GRE. Additional exam requirements/recommendations for international students: Required—TOEFL (minimum score 560 paper-based, 84 iBT) or IELTS (6.5). *Application deadline:* For fall admission, 12/5 for domestic and international students. Applications are processed on a rolling basis. Application fee: $75 ($90 for international students). Electronic applications accepted. *Expenses:* Contact institution. *Financial support:* In 2015–16, 4 students received support, including fellowships with full tuition reimbursements available (averaging $26,000 per year), research assistantships with full tuition reimbursements available (averaging $28,000 per year); scholarships/grants and health care benefits also available. Financial award application deadline: 12/5. *Faculty research:* Craniofacial development, oral and pharyngeal cancer, mineralized tissue biology and musculoskeletal disorders, tissue engineering and regeneration, oral infectious and immunologic diseases, oral sensory systems and central circuits. *Total annual research expenditures:* $17.7 million. *Unit head:* Dr. Jan Hu, Director, 734-615-1970, E-mail: dent-ohsphd@umich.edu. *Application contact:* Kimberly G. Smith, Senior Administrative Assistant, 734-615-1970, E-mail: dent-ohsphd@umich.edu.
Website: http://dent.umich.edu/phd

University of Minnesota, Twin Cities Campus, School of Dentistry and Graduate School, Graduate Programs in Dentistry, Advanced Education Program in Periodontology, Minneapolis, MN 55455-0213. Offers MS. *Degree requirements:* For master's, comprehensive exam, thesis. *Entrance requirements:* For master's, DDS/DMD, letter from Dental Dean, specific GGP/class rank, two letters of recommendation. Additional exam requirements/recommendations for international students: Required—TOEFL (minimum score 590 paper-based). *Faculty research:* Periodontitis, risk factors, regenerating, diabetes immunology.

University of Minnesota, Twin Cities Campus, School of Dentistry and Graduate School, Graduate Programs in Dentistry, Division of Endodontics, Minneapolis, MN 55455-0213. Offers MS, Certificate. *Degree requirements:* For master's, thesis. *Entrance requirements:* Additional exam requirements/recommendations for international students: Required—TOEFL. *Faculty research:* Pain, inflammation, neuropharmacology, neuropeptides, cytokines.

University of Minnesota, Twin Cities Campus, School of Dentistry and Graduate School, Graduate Programs in Dentistry, Division of Orthodontics, Minneapolis, MN 55455-0213. Offers MS. *Degree requirements:* For master's, thesis. *Entrance requirements:* Additional exam requirements/recommendations for international students: Required—TOEFL (minimum score 587 paper-based). *Faculty research:* Bone biology, 3-D imaging.

University of Minnesota, Twin Cities Campus, School of Dentistry and Graduate School, Graduate Programs in Dentistry, Division of Pediatric Dentistry, Minneapolis, MN 55455-0213. Offers MS. *Degree requirements:* For master's, thesis. *Entrance requirements:* Additional exam requirements/recommendations for international students: Required—TOEFL. *Faculty research:* Molecular genetics of facial growth, dental material/adhesion, expanded functions dental auxiliary utilization.

University of Minnesota, Twin Cities Campus, School of Dentistry and Graduate School, Graduate Programs in Dentistry, Division of Prosthodontics, Minneapolis, MN 55455-0213. Offers MS. *Degree requirements:* For master's, thesis, clinical. *Entrance requirements:* Additional exam requirements/recommendations for international students: Required—TOEFL.

University of Minnesota, Twin Cities Campus, School of Dentistry and Graduate School, Graduate Programs in Dentistry, Program in Oral Biology, Minneapolis, MN 55455-0213. Offers MS, PhD. *Degree requirements:* For master's, thesis. *Faculty research:* Microbiology, neuroscience, biomaterials, biochemistry, cancer biology.

University of Minnesota, Twin Cities Campus, School of Dentistry and Graduate School, Graduate Programs in Dentistry, Program in Oral Health Services for Older Adults (Geriatrics), Minneapolis, MN 55455-0213. Offers MS, Certificate. *Degree requirements:* For master's, thesis (for some programs). *Entrance requirements:* For master's, DDS degree or equivalent. Additional exam requirements/recommendations for international students: Required—TOEFL (minimum score 560 paper-based). Electronic applications accepted. *Faculty research:* Geriatrics dental care, long-term care dental services, oral-systemic health relationships, utilization of care by older adults.

University of Minnesota, Twin Cities Campus, School of Dentistry and Graduate School, Graduate Programs in Dentistry, Program in Temporomandibular Joint Disorders, Minneapolis, MN 55455-0213. Offers MS. *Degree requirements:* For master's, comprehensive exam, thesis. *Entrance requirements:* Additional exam requirements/recommendations for international students: Required—TOEFL. Electronic applications accepted. *Faculty research:* Clinical trials, TMJ mechanicals, diagnostic criteria, biomarkers, genetics.

University of Mississippi Medical Center, School of Dentistry, Department of Craniofacial and Dental Research, Jackson, MS 39216-4505. Offers MS, PhD.

University of Missouri–Kansas City, School of Dentistry, Kansas City, MO 64110-2499. Offers advanced education in dentistry (Graduate Dental Certificate); dental hygiene education (MS); dentistry (DDS); endodontics (Graduate Dental Certificate); oral and maxillofacial surgery (Graduate Dental Certificate); oral biology (MS, PhD); orthodontics and dentofacial orthopedics (Graduate Dental Certificate); periodontics (Graduate Dental Certificate). PhD (interdisciplinary) offered through the School of Graduate Studies. *Accreditation:* ADA (one or more programs are accredited). *Faculty:* 84 full-time (38 women), 56 part-time/adjunct (16 women). *Students:* 432 full-time (184 women), 54 part-time (26 women); includes 99 minority (12 Black or African American, non-Hispanic/Latino; 3 American Indian or Alaska Native, non-Hispanic/Latino; 46 Asian, non-Hispanic/Latino; 28 Hispanic/Latino; 10 Two or more races, non-Hispanic/Latino), 3 international. Average age 27. 793 applicants, 17% accepted, 129 enrolled. In 2015, 7 master's, 107 doctorates, 17 other advanced degrees awarded. *Degree requirements:* For master's, thesis; for doctorate, thesis/dissertation (for some programs). *Entrance requirements:* For master's, DAT, letters of evaluation, personal interview; for doctorate, DAT (for DDS); for Graduate Dental Certificate, DDS. Additional exam requirements/recommendations for international students: Required—TOEFL (minimum score 550 paper-based; 80 iBT). *Application deadline:* For fall admission, 2/1 for domestic and international students. Application fee: $45 ($50 for international students). *Expenses:* Contact institution. *Financial support:* In 2015–16, 1 research assistantship (averaging $22,000 per year) was awarded; career-related internships or fieldwork, Federal Work-Study, institutionally sponsored loans, and tuition waivers (full and partial) also available. Support available to part-time students. Financial award application deadline: 3/1; financial award applicants required to submit FAFSA. *Faculty research:* Biomaterials, dental use of lasers, effectiveness of periodontal treatments, temporomandibular joint dysfunction. *Unit head:* Dr. Marsha Pyle, Dean, 816-235-2010, E-mail: pylem@umkc.edu. *Application contact:* Richard Bigham, Assistant Dean for Student Programs, 816-235-2082, E-mail: bighamr@umkc.edu.
Website: http://dentistry.umkc.edu/

University of Missouri–Kansas City, School of Graduate Studies, Kansas City, MO 64110-2499. Offers interdisciplinary studies (PhD), including art history, cell biology and biophysics, chemistry, computer and electrical engineering, computer science and informatics, economics, education, engineering, English, entrepreneurship and innovation, geosciences, history, mathematics and statistics, molecular biology and biochemistry, music education, oral and craniofacial sciences, pharmaceutical sciences, pharmacology, physics, political science, public affairs and administration, religious studies, social science, telecommunications and computer networking; PMBA/MHA. *Students:* 73 full-time (22 women), 287 part-time (110 women); includes 41 minority (17 Black or African American, non-Hispanic/Latino; 8 Asian, non-Hispanic/Latino; 13 Hispanic/Latino; 3 Two or more races, non-Hispanic/Latino), 151 international. Average age 35. 238 applicants, 33% accepted, 66 enrolled. In 2015, 47 doctorates awarded. *Degree requirements:* For doctorate, comprehensive exam, thesis/dissertation, residency. *Entrance requirements:* For doctorate, GRE General Test, minimum GPA of 2.75 (undergraduate), 3.0 (graduate). Additional exam requirements/recommendations for international students: Required—TOEFL (minimum score 550 paper-based; 80 iBT), TWE (minimum score 4). *Application deadline:* For fall admission, 1/15 priority date for domestic and international students. Applications are processed on a rolling basis. Application fee: $45 ($50 for international students). Electronic applications accepted. *Financial support:* Career-related internships or fieldwork, Federal Work-Study, tuition waivers (partial), and unspecified assistantships available. Support available to part-time students. Financial award application deadline: 3/1; financial award applicants required to submit FAFSA. *Unit head:* Dr. Denis M. Medeiros, Dean, 816-235-1301, Fax: 816-

Oral and Dental Sciences

235-1310, E-mail: medeirosd@umkc.edu. *Application contact:* Quincy Bennett Johnson, Coordinator of Admissions and Recruitment, Interdisciplinary PhD Program, 816-235-1559, Fax: 816-235-1310, E-mail: bennettq@umkc.edu.
Website: http://sgs.umkc.edu/

University of Nevada, Las Vegas, School of Dental Medicine, Las Vegas, NV 89154. Offers dental medicine (DMD); oral biology (MS). *Accreditation:* ADA. *Faculty:* 63 full-time (23 women), 28 part-time/adjunct (6 women). *Students:* 97 full-time (43 women); includes 50 minority (1 Black or African American, non-Hispanic/Latino; 1 American Indian or Alaska Native, non-Hispanic/Latino; 39 Asian, non-Hispanic/Latino; 9 Hispanic/Latino), 3 international. Average age 28. 1,930 applicants, 10% accepted, 82 enrolled. In 2015, 4 master's, 1 doctorate awarded. *Degree requirements:* For doctorate, comprehensive exam. *Entrance requirements:* For master's, National Dental Boards Examination (Parts 1 & 2), DMD/DDS; for doctorate, DAT, National Board of Dental Examination Part 1 and 2 (for international dentists). Additional exam requirements/recommendations for international students: Required—TOEFL (minimum score 550 paper-based; 80 iBT), IELTS (minimum score 7). *Application deadline:* For fall admission, 1/1 for domestic and international students. Applications are processed on a rolling basis. Application fee: $50. *Expenses:* Contact institution. *Financial support:* In 2015–16, 13 students received support. Application deadline: 2/1; applicants required to submit FAFSA. *Faculty research:* Oral cancer, public health, orthodontic biomechanics, forensic dentistry, nutrition, geriatric dentistry, dental pulp-stem cells, behavioral dentistry, literacyoral cancer. *Total annual research expenditures:* $581,932. *Unit head:* Karen West, Dean, 702-774-2500, E-mail: karen.west@unlv.edu. *Application contact:* Dr. Christine Ancajas, Assistant Dean for Admissions and Student Affairs, 702-774-2520, E-mail: christine.ancajas@unlv.edu.
Website: http://www.unlv.edu/dental

The University of North Carolina at Chapel Hill, School of Dentistry and Graduate School, Graduate Programs in Dentistry, Chapel Hill, NC 27599. Offers dental hygiene (MS); endodontics (MS); epidemiology (PhD); operative dentistry (MS); oral and maxillofacial pathology (MS); oral and maxillofacial radiology (MS); oral biology (PhD); orthodontics (MS); pediatric dentistry (MS); periodontics (MS); prosthodontics (MS). *Degree requirements:* For master's, thesis; for doctorate, thesis/dissertation. *Entrance requirements:* For master's, GRE General Test (for orthodontics and oral biology only); National Dental Board Part I (Part II if available), dental degree (for all except dental hygiene); for doctorate, GRE General Test. Additional exam requirements/recommendations for international students: Required—TOEFL (minimum score 550 paper-based; 79 iBT). Electronic applications accepted. *Expenses:* Contact institution. *Faculty research:* Clinical research, inflammation, immunology, neuroscience, molecular biology.

University of Oklahoma Health Sciences Center, College of Dentistry and Graduate College, Graduate Programs in Dentistry, Department of Orthodontics, Oklahoma City, OK 73190. Offers MS. *Degree requirements:* For master's, thesis. *Entrance requirements:* For master's, minimum GPA of 3.0, DDS/DMD. Additional exam requirements/recommendations for international students: Required—TOEFL. Electronic applications accepted. *Faculty research:* Craniofacial growth and development, biomechanical principles in orthodontics.

University of Oklahoma Health Sciences Center, College of Dentistry and Graduate College, Graduate Programs in Dentistry, Department of Periodontics, Oklahoma City, OK 73190. Offers MS. *Degree requirements:* For master's, thesis. *Entrance requirements:* For master's, DDS/DMD, minimum GPA of 3.0. Additional exam requirements/recommendations for international students: Required—TOEFL (minimum score 550 paper-based). Electronic applications accepted.

University of Pittsburgh, School of Dental Medicine, Residency Programs in Dental Medicine, Advanced Education Program in Oral and Maxillofacial Pathology, Pittsburgh, PA 15260. Offers Advanced Certificate. *Entrance requirements:* For degree, National Board Dental Exam Parts 1 and 2 (recommended), GRE, three letters of recommendation, official transcripts, current curriculum vitae, one-page personal statement. Additional exam requirements/recommendations for international students: Recommended—TOEFL. *Expenses:* Contact institution. *Faculty research:* Salivary gland neoplasms, dental school patient demographics, data mining of the electronic dental record, clinical oral pathology treatment.

University of Pittsburgh, School of Dental Medicine, Residency Programs in Dental Medicine, Advanced Education Program in Prosthodontics, Pittsburgh, PA 15261. Offers MDS, Certificate. *Degree requirements:* For master's, comprehensive exam, thesis. *Entrance requirements:* Additional exam requirements/recommendations for international students: Required—TOEFL. Electronic applications accepted. Tuition and fees vary according to program. *Faculty research:* Implant dentistry, occlusion, biomechanics, genetics, biomaterials.

University of Pittsburgh, School of Dental Medicine, Residency Programs in Dental Medicine, Department of Dental Anesthesia, Pittsburgh, PA 15260. Offers Certificate. *Entrance requirements:* For degree, National Board Dental Exam Parts I and II, DMD or DDS. Electronic applications accepted. Tuition and fees vary according to program. *Faculty research:* Clinical pharmacology and random controlled trials.

University of Pittsburgh, School of Dental Medicine, Residency Programs in Dental Medicine, Department of Endodontics, Pittsburgh, PA 15260. Offers MDS, Certificate. *Degree requirements:* For master's, comprehensive exam, thesis. *Entrance requirements:* For master's and Certificate, National Dental Board Exams Part 1 and 2. Tuition and fees vary according to program. *Faculty research:* Pulpal neurobiology, root canal therapy, root fracture/resorption repair, osseous grafts related to endodontics, endodontic surge.

University of Pittsburgh, School of Dental Medicine, Residency Programs in Dental Medicine, Department of Oral and Maxillofacial Surgery, Pittsburgh, PA 15260. Offers Certificate. *Degree requirements:* For Certificate, comprehensive exam. *Entrance requirements:* For degree, National Boards Part I, U.S. or Canadian dental degree (DDS or DMD). Electronic applications accepted. *Expenses:* Contact institution. *Faculty research:* Clefts, craniofacial anomalies, facial trauma, head and neck cancer, pain management.

University of Pittsburgh, School of Dental Medicine, Residency Programs in Dental Medicine, Department of Oral Biology, Pittsburgh, PA 15260. Offers MS, PhD. *Program availability:* Part-time. Terminal master's awarded for partial completion of doctoral program. *Degree requirements:* For master's, comprehensive exam, thesis, 36 credits of core classes and electives; for doctorate, comprehensive exam, thesis/dissertation, 76 credits of core classes and electives, teaching practicum. *Entrance requirements:* For master's and doctorate, GRE, science BS or equivalent (DDS, DMD, BS/MS in hygiene); minimum QPA of 3.0, sponsorship from a research faculty in the department (recommended). Additional exam requirements/recommendations for international students: Required—TOEFL, IELTS. Electronic applications accepted. *Expenses:* Contact institution. *Faculty research:* Bone tissue engineering, craniofacial genetics, craniofacial anomalies, growth and development, craniofacial development.

University of Pittsburgh, School of Dental Medicine, Residency Programs in Dental Medicine, Department of Orthodontics and Dentofacial Orthopedics, Pittsburgh, PA

15261. Offers orthodontics (MDS, Certificate). *Degree requirements:* For master's, comprehensive exam, thesis; for Certificate, comprehensive exam. *Entrance requirements:* For master's and Certificate, National Boards Parts I and II. Tuition and fees vary according to program. *Faculty research:* Facial form, orthodontic outcomes.

University of Pittsburgh, School of Dental Medicine, Residency Programs in Dental Medicine, Department of Periodontics, Pittsburgh, PA 15261. Offers MDS, Certificate. *Degree requirements:* For master's, comprehensive exam, thesis. *Entrance requirements:* For degree, DMD, DDS. Electronic applications accepted. *Expenses:* Contact institution. *Faculty research:* Implantology, osteoporosis, perio systemic disease, regeneration.

University of Puerto Rico, Medical Sciences Campus, School of Dental Medicine, Graduate Programs in Dentistry, San Juan, PR 00936-5067. Offers general dentistry (Certificate); oral and maxillofacial surgery (Certificate); orthodontics (Certificate); pediatric dentistry (Certificate); prosthodontics (Certificate). *Degree requirements:* For Certificate, comprehensive exam (for some programs). *Entrance requirements:* For degree, National Board Dental Exam I, National Board Dental Exam II, DDS or DMD, interview. Electronic applications accepted. *Expenses:* Contact institution. *Faculty research:* Analgesic drugs, anti-inflammatory drugs, saliva cytoanalysis, dental materials, oral epidemiology and dental caries.

University of Rochester, School of Medicine and Dentistry, Graduate Programs in Medicine and Dentistry, Center for Oral Biology, Rochester, NY 14627. Offers dental science (MS). *Degree requirements:* For master's, thesis. *Entrance requirements:* For master's, GRE General Test, DDS or equivalent. *Expenses:* Tuition, area resident: Full-time $47,450; part-time $1482 per credit hour. *Required fees:* $528. Tuition and fees vary according to program.

University of Southern California, Graduate School, Herman Ostrow School of Dentistry and Graduate School, Department of Craniofacial Biology, Los Angeles, CA 90089. Offers MS, PhD, Graduate Certificate. Terminal master's awarded for partial completion of doctoral program. *Degree requirements:* For master's, comprehensive exam, thesis; for doctorate, comprehensive exam, thesis/dissertation. *Entrance requirements:* For master's and doctorate, GRE, undergraduate degree. Additional exam requirements/recommendations for international students: Required—TOEFL. Electronic applications accepted. *Faculty research:* Orthodontics, periodontics, tooth development, oral biology, stem cell biology.

The University of Tennessee Health Science Center, College of Graduate Health Sciences, Memphis, TN 38163-0002. Offers biomedical engineering (MS, PhD); biomedical sciences (PhD); dental sciences (MDS); epidemiology (MS); health outcomes and policy research (PhD); laboratory research and management (MS); nursing science (PhD); pharmaceutical sciences (PhD); pharmacology (MS); speech and hearing science (PhD); DDS/PhD; DNP/PhD; MD/PhD; Pharm D/PhD. Terminal master's awarded for partial completion of doctoral program. *Degree requirements:* For master's, comprehensive exam, thesis; for doctorate, comprehensive exam, thesis/dissertation, oral and written preliminary and comprehensive exams. *Entrance requirements:* For master's and doctorate, GRE General Test, minimum GPA of 3.0. Additional exam requirements/recommendations for international students: Required—TOEFL (minimum score 79 iBT); Recommended—IELTS (minimum score 6.5). Electronic applications accepted.

The University of Toledo, College of Graduate Studies, College of Medicine and Life Sciences, Department of Surgery, Toledo, OH 43606-3390. Offers oral biology (MSBS). *Degree requirements:* For master's, thesis or alternative. *Entrance requirements:* For master's, DAT, minimum undergraduate GPA of 3.0, three letters of recommendation, statement of purpose, transcripts from all prior institutions attended, acceptance into Pediatric Dental Residency Program at UT. Additional exam requirements/recommendations for international students: Required—TOEFL (minimum score 550 paper-based; 80 iBT). Electronic applications accepted. *Faculty research:* Oral biology-tissue cultures.

University of Toronto, School of Graduate Studies, Faculty of Dentistry, Graduate Programs in Dentistry, Toronto, ON M5S 1A1, Canada. Offers M Sc, PhD. *Program availability:* Part-time. Terminal master's awarded for partial completion of doctoral program. *Degree requirements:* For master's, thesis; for doctorate, thesis/dissertation. *Entrance requirements:* For master's, honors B Sc, minimum B average, 2 letters of reference; for doctorate, M Sc, minimum B+ average. Additional exam requirements/recommendations for international students: Required—Michigan English Language Assessment Battery, IELTS, TOEFL, or COPE. Electronic applications accepted. *Expenses:* Contact institution. *Faculty research:* Plaque, periodontal biology, biomaterials/dental implants, community dentistry, growth and development.

University of Toronto, School of Graduate Studies, Faculty of Dentistry, Specialty Master's Programs, Toronto, ON M5S 1A1, Canada. Offers dental public health (M Sc); endodontics (M Sc); oral and maxillofacial radiology (M Sc); oral and maxillofacial surgery (M Sc); oral medicine (M Sc); orthodontics and dentofacial orthopedics (M Sc); pediatric dentistry (M Sc); periodontics (M Sc). *Degree requirements:* For master's, thesis. *Entrance requirements:* For master's, completion of professional degree of DDS/BDS, DMD, minimum B average, 2 letters of reference. Additional exam requirements/recommendations for international students: Required—TOEFL (minimum score 600 paper-based; 100 iBT), TWE (minimum score 5). *Expenses:* Contact institution. *Faculty research:* Plaque and periodontal biology, biomaterials/dental implants, community dentistry, growth development, neurophysiology.

University of Washington, Graduate School, School of Dentistry and Graduate School, Graduate Programs in Dentistry, Department of Endodontics, Seattle, WA 98195. Offers MSD, Certificate.

University of Washington, Graduate School, School of Dentistry and Graduate School, Graduate Programs in Dentistry, Department of Orthodontics, Seattle, WA 98195. Offers MSD, Certificate.

University of Washington, Graduate School, School of Dentistry, Program in Dental Surgery, Seattle, WA 98195. Offers DDS. *Accreditation:* ADA. *Entrance requirements:* For doctorate, DAT.

The University of Western Ontario, Schulich School of Medicine and Dentistry, Graduate and Professional Programs in Dentistry, Program in Graduate Orthodontics, London, ON N6A 5B8, Canada. Offers M Cl D. *Degree requirements:* For master's, thesis. *Entrance requirements:* For master's, GRE General Test, minimum B average, 1 year of general practice preferred. Additional exam requirements/recommendations for international students: Required—TOEFL (minimum score 600 paper-based).

West Virginia University, School of Dentistry, Division of Dental Hygiene, Morgantown, WV 26506. Offers MS. *Program availability:* Part-time. *Degree requirements:* For master's, thesis. *Entrance requirements:* For master's, GRE, MAT, BS in dental hygiene or equivalent, minimum GPA of 2.75. Additional exam requirements/recommendations for international students: Required—TOEFL. *Expenses:* Tuition, state resident: full-time $8568. Tuition, nonresident: full-time $22,140. Tuition and fees vary according to program. *Faculty research:* Curriculum and instruction, infection control, special patient care, diversity and cultural sensitivity, oral health disparities.

West Virginia University, School of Dentistry, Graduate Programs in Dentistry, Morgantown, WV 26506. Offers endodontics (MS); orthodontics (MS); prosthodontics (MS). *Degree requirements:* For master's, thesis. *Entrance requirements:* For master's, National Dental Board Exam Parts I and II, DDS/DMD from accredited U.S. or Canadian Dental School, minimum GPA of 3.0. Additional exam requirements/recommendations for international students: Required—TOEFL. *Expenses:* Contact institution. *Faculty research:* Growth and development, cephalographics, endodontic interpretation and therapy.

UCONN HEALTH
Skeletal Biology and Regeneration Program

 For more information, visit http://petersons.to/uconnhealth_skeletalbiology

Programs of Study

The Skeletal Biology and Regeneration program is focused on the study of the basic biological properties of skeletal, craniofacial, and oral tissues and regeneration of connective tissues. Research in this area is problem-oriented and multidisciplinary, incorporating contemporary research techniques of cellular and molecular biology and biochemistry. There are approximately 35 faculty members in the Skeletal Biology and Regeneration program, representing a number of schools, departments, institutes, and centers. This interdisciplinary group of scientists is engaged in advancing understanding of the biology of bone, cartilage, teeth, oral tissues, and skin and exploring development, maintenance, disease, and the potential for regeneration of these tissues. A Ph.D. in the Skeletal Biology and Regeneration program can be combined with D.M.D. or M.D. training leading to D.M.D./Ph.D. and M.D./Ph.D. degrees. It may also be combined with dental clinical specialty training.

Particular areas of research strength include oral and craniofacial biology (immunology, infection and disease, cancer, development, and stem cells); skeletal biology (development, homeostasis, aging, cancer, disease, and stem cells); and regenerative engineering of skeletal tissues (biomaterials, stem cells, and tissue engineering).

Research Facilities

The University complex provides excellent physical facilities for research in both basic and clinical sciences. The Lyman Maynard Stowe Library is well equipped with extensive journal and book holdings and rapid electronic access to database searching, Internet, and library holdings. The library also contains the Computer Education Center and the End User Support Center. The Center for Laboratory Animal Care contains a transgenic mouse production facility fully equipped for gene targeting studies and with special facilities for housing immunodeficient animals. Facilities include the Center for Biomaterials, the General Clinical Research Center, the Center for Cell Analysis and Modeling (confocal microscopy, low light level microscopy, two photon microscopy), the Center for Bone Histology and Histomorphometry; the Molecular Imaging Laboratory, the Fluorescence Flow Cytometry Facility, the Electron Microscopy Facility, Gene Targeting and Transgenic Facility, the Microarray Core Facility, the Molecular Core Facility, NMR Structural Biology Facility, National Resource for Cell Analysis and Modeling, and the Center for Molecular Medicine (laser capture microdissection).

Financial Aid

Support for doctoral students engaged in full-time degree programs at UConn Health is provided on a competitive basis. Graduate research assistantships for 2016–17 provide a stipend of $29,000 per year, which includes a waiver of tuition/most University fees for the fall and spring semesters and the option of participating in a student health-insurance plan. While financial aid is offered competitively, the UConn Health makes every possible effort to address the financial needs of all students during their period of training.

Cost of Study

For 2016–17, tuition is $14,310 per year for full-time students who are Connecticut residents and $35,346 per year for full-time students who are out-of-state residents. General University fees are added to the cost of tuition for students who do not receive a tuition waiver. These costs are usually met by traineeships or research assistantships for doctoral students.

Living and Housing Costs

There is a wide range of affordable housing options in the Greater Hartford area within easy commuting distance of the campus, including an extensive complex that is adjacent to UConn Health. Costs range from $700 to $1,000 per month for a one-bedroom unit; two or more students sharing an apartment usually pay less. University housing is not available on the campus.

Student Group

The Program in Skeletal Biology and Regeneration has approximately 20 trainees. At UConn Health there are about 500 students in the Schools of Medicine and Dental Medicine, 150 Ph.D. students, and about 50 postdoctoral fellows. Graduate students are represented on various administrative committees concerned with curricular affairs. A graduate student organization fosters social contact among graduate students at UConn Health and represents graduate students' needs and concerns to the faculty and administration.

Location

UConn Health is located in the historic town of Farmington, Connecticut. Set in the beautiful New England countryside, on a hill overlooking the Farmington Valley, it is close to ski areas, hiking trails, and facilities for boating, fishing, and swimming. Connecticut's capital city of Hartford, 7 miles east of Farmington, is the center of an urban region of approximately 800,000 people. The beaches of the Long Island Sound are about 50 minutes away to the south, and the beautiful Berkshires are a short drive to the northwest. New York City and Boston can be reached within 2½ hours by car.

Hartford is the home of the acclaimed Hartford Stage Company, TheatreWorks, the Hartford Symphony and Chamber orchestras, two ballet companies, an opera company, the Wadsworth Atheneum (the oldest public art museum in the nation), the Mark Twain House, the Hartford Civic Center, and many other interesting cultural and recreational facilities. The area is also home to several branches of the University of Connecticut, Trinity College, and the University of Hartford, which includes the Hartt School of Music. Bradley International Airport (about 30 minutes from campus) serves the Hartford/Springfield area with frequent airline connections to major cities in this country and abroad. Frequent bus and rail service is also available from Hartford.

The UConn Health Campus

The 200-acre UConn Health campus at Farmington houses a division of the University of Connecticut Graduate School, as well as the Schools of Medicine and Dental Medicine. The campus also includes the John Dempsey Hospital, associated clinics, and extensive medical research facilities, all in a centralized facility with more than 1 million square feet of floor space. The Academic Research Building, built in 1999, is an impressive eleven-story structure providing 170,000 square feet of laboratory space and renovations are underway in the main Laboratory building, converting existing lab space to state-of-the-art open lab areas. In addition, The Jackson Laboratory for Genomic Medicine opened its 189,000-square-foot facility on the UConn Health Campus in fall 2014. The faculty includes more than 260 full-time members. The institution has a strong commitment to graduate study within an environment that promotes social and intellectual interaction among the various educational programs. Graduate students are represented on various administrative committees concerned with curricular affairs, and the Graduate Student Organization (GSO) represents graduate students' needs and concerns to the faculty and administration, in addition to fostering social contact among graduate students at UConn Health.

Applying

Applications for admission should be submitted via the online application system and should be filed together with transcripts, three letters of recommendation, a personal statement, and recent results from the General Test of the Graduate Record Examinations. International students must take the Test of English as a Foreign Language (TOEFL) to satisfy Graduate School requirements.

The deadline for completed applications and receipt of all supplemental materials is **December 1**. Please note that GRE and TOEFL exams taken after the due date will not be accepted for consideration for admission.

Deadlines and application procedures for combined programs vary depending on the program. For further information on combined programs, prospective students should contact Dr. Mina Mina in the Department of Reconstructive Sciences.

In accordance with the laws of the state of Connecticut and of the United States, UConn Health does not discriminate against any person in its educational and employment activities on the grounds of race, color, creed, national origin, sex, age, or physical disability.

Correspondence and Information

Graduate Admissions Office
Skeletal Biology and Regeneration Program
UConn Health
263 Farmington Ave., MC 3906
Farmington, Connecticut 06030-3906
United States
Phone: 860-679-4509
E-mail: BiomedSciAdmissions@uchc.edu
Website: http://health.uconn.edu/graduate-school/academics/programs/
   ph-d-biomedical-science

UConn Health

THE FACULTY AND THEIR RESEARCH

Andrew Arnold, Professor of Medicine and Murray-Heilig Chair in Molecular Medicine; M.D., Harvard. The molecular genetic underpinnings of tumors of the endocrine glands, role of the cyclin D1 oncogene, animal modeling of hyperparathyroidism.

Dashzeveg Bayarsaihan, Associate Professor; Ph.D. TFII-I family proteins.

Ernesto Canalis, Professor of Orthopaedic Surgery and Medicine; M.D., Universidad Peruana Cayetano Heredia. Skeletal growth factors; insulin-like growth factors; hormonal action in bone; mechanisms of glucocorticoid action in bone; anabolic agents and osteoporosis.

I-Ping Chen, Assistant Professor, Oral Health and Diagnostic Sciences, D.D.S., Ph.D. Connecticut Health Center. Generation of induced pluripotent stem (iPS) cells from craniometaphyseal dysplasia (CMD) patients; investigation of osteoclast biology in the human stem cell system as well as in CMD mouse models.

Justin Cotney, Assistant Professor; Ph.D., Emory. Determining how gene regulatory elements, namely enhancers, control gene expression during mammalian development.

Caroline N. Dealy, Associate Professor of Reconstructive Sciences, Center for Regenerative Medicine and Skeletal Development; Ph.D., Connecticut. Roles of various growth factors and signaling molecules, particularly IGF-I and insulin, in the regulation of chick limb development.

Anne Delany, Associate Professor of Medicine; Ph.D., Dartmouth. Study of noncollagenous matrix proteins and metalloproteinases important in bone remodeling, including investigation of function and posttranscriptional regulation of osteonectin or SPARC in bone and function and regulation of the metastasis-associated metalloproteinase, stromelysyin-3, in bone.

Patricia I. Diaz, Assistant Professor; Ph.D., Adelaide (Australia); D.D.S., Universidad CES (Colombia). Interspecies interactions in oral microbial communities that determine oral biofilm formation; shifts in the oral microbiome composition associated with oral diseases such as mucositis during cancer chemotherapy and periodontal diseases; interaction of oral microbial communities with the host.

Anna Dongari-Bagtzoglou, Professor, Department of Oral Health and Diagnostic Sciences, Division of Periodontology; D.D.S., Ph.D., Texas Health Science Center at San Antonio. Host-pathogen interactions, with emphasis on the pathogenesis of inflammation and the innate immune functions of oral mucosal cells.

Hicham Drissi, Associate Professor of Orthopaedic Surgery; Ph.D., University of Paris V. Molecular pathways of bone and cartilage repair.

Paul M. Epstein, Associate Professor of Cell Biology; Ph.D., Yeshiva (Einstein). Second messengers and signal transduction, with particular focus on cyclic nucleotide metabolism and protein phosphorylation, with emphasis on analysis of cyclic nucleotide phosphodiesterase (PDE).

Marion Frank, Professor of Oral Health and Diagnostic Sciences and Director, Center for Neurosciences; Ph.D., Brown. Study of the sense of taste, using basic and clinical research; development of a fundamental understanding of gustatory systems in mammals at all levels from receptors to cerebral cortex; application of basic knowledge of gustatory systems to the diagnosis and treatment of taste disorders in humans.

A. Jon Goldberg, Professor of Reconstructive Sciences, Center for Regenerative Medicine and Skeletal Development; Ph.D., Michigan. Biomaterials, with studies involving structure-property relationships, development of novel systems, clinical evaluations, and surface analysis.

Rosaria Guzzo, Assistant Professor; Ph.D., Ottowa. Identification of key epigenetic mechanisms that modulate the cartilage-forming potential of human iPS cells.

Marc Hansen, Professor of Medicine, Center for Molecular Medicine; Ph.D., Cincinnati. Molecular genetics of osteosarcoma and related bone diseases.

Marja M. Hurley, Professor of Medicine; M.D., Connecticut. Molecular mechanisms regulating the expression of fibroblast growth factors in bone, mechanisms of signal transduction by growth factors in bone cells, and role of fibroblast growth factors in bone remodeling.

Ivo Kalajzic, Assistant Professor, Department of Reconstructive Sciences and Department of Genetics and Developmental Biology; M.D., Zagreb (Croatia); Ph.D., Split (Croatia). Bone biology, differentiation of the osteoblast lineage cells.

Yusuf Khan, Assistant Professor of Orthopaedic Surgery and Chemical, Materials, and Biomolecular Engineering; Ph.D. Drexel. Strategies to synthesize scaffolds that are also capable of delivering proteins and growth factors essential for complete and adequate healing of bone defects through the use of biodegradable polymers alone and in combination with ceramic materials.

Barbara E. Kream, Professor of Medicine; Ph.D., Yale. Hormonal regulation of bone remodeling.

Liisa T. Kuhn, Associate Professor of Reconstructive Sciences, Center for Regenerative Medicine and Skeletal Development; Ph.D., California, Santa Barbara. Biomaterials for drug delivery and bone regeneration and repair.

Sangamesh Kumbar, Assistant Professor of Orthopedic Surgery; Ph.D., Karnatak (India). Synthesis and characterization of novel biomaterials/polymers for tissue engineering and drug delivery applications.

Marc Lalande, Professor and Head, Department of Genetics and Developmental Biology; Ph.D., Toronto. Genomic imprinting of human chromosome 15q.

Cato Laurencin, Professor Orthopaedic Surgery, School of Medicine, M.D., Ph.D. Regenerative engineering using scaffolds of appropriate physical and chemical cues to differentiate stem cells to complex tissue type.

Sun-Kyeong Lee, Assistant Professor of Medicine; Ph.D., Connecticut. Osteoclast biology and molecular and cellular regulation by cytokines in osteoclastogenesis.

Alexander Lichtler, Associate Professor of Reconstructive Sciences, Center for Regenerative Medicine and Skeletal Development; Ph.D., Florida. Hormone regulation of bone collagen synthesis.

Alan G. Lurie, Professor of Oral Health and Diagnostic Sciences and Chairperson, Division of Oral and Maxillofacial Radiology; D.D.S., UCLA; Ph.D., Rochester. Actions and interactions of radiation and chemical carcinogens during epithelial carcinogenesis, DNA mutagenesis and repair by gamma radiation in lymphoblasts from both normal and ataxia telangiectatic humans, clinical research digital imaging.

Peter Maye, Assistant Professor of Reconstructive Sciences, Ph.D., Wesleyan. Isolation, characterization, and differentiation of embryonic and adult skeletal stem cells down the osteogenic lineage.

Mina Mina, Professor of Craniofacial Sciences; Chairperson, Division of Pediatric Dentistry; and Director, Skeletal, Craniofacial, and Oral Biology Graduate Program; D.M.D., National University of Iran; Ph.D., Connecticut Health Center. Development of the mandibular arch, including the elongation and polarized outgrowth of the mandibular primordia and subsequent differentiation of the skeletal tissues in spatially defined patterns; characterization of genetic and epigenetic influences involved in the pattern formation and skeletogenesis of the chick mandible and mouse tooth germ; regulation of patterning in the developing mandible and developing teeth by mandibular epithelium, extracellular matrix molecules, growth factors, and transcription factors.

Lakshmi Nair, Assistant Professor of Orthopedic Surgery and Chemical, Materials, and Biomolecular Engineering; Ph.D., SCTIMST (India). Design and development of regenerative biomaterials to favorably modulate the responses of a variety of cell types involved in tissue regeneration and repair.

Syam P. Nukavarapu, Assistant Professor of Orthopaedic Surgery and Chemical, Materials, and Biomolecular Engineering. Ph.D, Indian Institute of Science. Scaffold-based bone-tissue engineering.

Carol C. Pilbeam, Professor of Medicine; Ph.D., Yale. Mechanisms of regulation of bone formation and resorption.

Ernst Reichenberger, Associate Professor of Reconstructive Sciences, Center for Regenerative Medicine and Skeletal Development; Ph.D., Erlangen (Germany). Study of complex processes required for generating and maintaining the skin and bones through characterization of human genetic disorders in which they are disrupted, including aplasia cutis congenita (ACC), cherubism, and craniometaphyseal dysplasia (CMD).

Blanka Rogina, Associate Professor of Genetics and Developmental Biology; Ph.D., Zagreb (Croatia). Molecular and genetic mechanisms underlying aging and cost of reproduction.

David W. Rowe, Professor of Reconstructive Sciences and Director, Center for Regenerative Medicine and Skeletal Development; M.D., Vermont. Genetic and hormonal control of type I collagen production, development of strategies for somatic gene therapy for heritable diseases of bone built upon the structural and regulatory principles of collagen production.

Archana Sanjay, Assistant Professor of Orthopaedic Surgery, School of Medicine; Ph.D. Regulation of bone remodeling; examining signaling pathways that regulate osteoblast and osteoclast differentiation and function.

Section 28
Medicine

This section contains a directory of institutions offering graduate work in medicine. Additional information about programs listed in the directory may be obtained by writing directly to the dean of a graduate school or chair of a department at the address given in the directory.

CONTENTS

Program Directories

Allopathic Medicine

Albany Medical College, Professional Program, Albany, NY 12208-3479. Offers MD. *Accreditation:* LCME/AMA. *Degree requirements:* For doctorate, United States Medical Licensing Exam Steps 1 and 2, clinical skills. *Entrance requirements:* For doctorate, MCAT, letters of recommendation, interview. Electronic applications accepted. *Expenses:* Contact institution.

Albert Einstein College of Medicine, Professional Program in Medicine, Bronx, NY 10461. Offers MD, MD/PhD. *Accreditation:* LCME/AMA. *Degree requirements:* For doctorate, independent scholars project. *Entrance requirements:* For doctorate, MCAT, interview. *Faculty research:* Cancer, diabetes mellitus, liver disease, infectious disease, neuroscience.

American University of Beirut, Graduate Programs, Faculty of Medicine, Beirut, Lebanon. Offers anatomy, cell biology and human morphology (MS); biochemistry and medical genetics (MS); biomedical sciences (PhD); experimental pathology, immunology and microbiology (MS); medicine (MD); neuroscience (MS); pharmacology and toxicology (MS). *Program availability:* Part-time. *Faculty:* 302 full-time (95 women), 64 part-time/adjunct (11 women). *Students:* 381 full-time (173 women), 61 part-time (51 women). Average age 23. In 2015, 14 master's awarded. *Degree requirements:* For master's, one foreign language, comprehensive exam, thesis (for some programs); for doctorate, one foreign language, comprehensive exam, thesis/dissertation. *Entrance requirements:* For master's, letter of recommendation; for doctorate, MCAT, bachelor's degree. Additional exam requirements/recommendations for international students: Required—TOEFL (minimum score 600 paper-based; 100 iBT), IELTS (minimum score 7.5). *Application deadline:* For fall admission, 4/30 for domestic and international students; for spring admission, 11/1 for domestic and international students. Application fee: $50. Electronic applications accepted. *Expenses: Tuition, area resident:* Full-time $16,254; part-time $903 per credit. *Required fees:* $699. Tuition and fees vary according to course load and program. *Financial support:* In 2015–16, 273 students received support, including 45 teaching assistantships (averaging $9,000 per year); career-related internships or fieldwork, institutionally sponsored loans, scholarships/grants, health care benefits, and unspecified assistantships also available. Financial award application deadline: 2/2. *Faculty research:* Cancer research (targeted therapy, mechanisms of leukemogenesis, tumor cell extravasation and metastasis, cancer stem cells), stem cell research (regenerative medicine, drug discovery), genetic research (neurogenetics, hereditary cardiomyopathy, hemoglobinopathies, pharmacogenomics, proteomics), neuroscience research (pain, neurodegenerative disorder), metabolism (inflammation and metabolism, metabolic disorder, diabetes mellitus), vascular and renal biology, signal transduction. *Total annual research expenditures:* $2.6 million. *Unit head:* Dr. Mohamed Sayegh, Dean, 961-1350000 Ext. 4700, Fax: 961-1744464, E-mail: msayegh@aub.edu.lb. *Application contact:* Dr. Salim Kanaan, Director, Admissions Office, 961-1350000 Ext. 2594, Fax: 961-1750775, E-mail: sk00@aub.edu.lb. Website: http://www.aub.edu.lb/fm/fm_home/Pages/index.aspx

Augusta University, Medical College of Georgia, Augusta, GA 30912. Offers MD, MD/PhD. *Accreditation:* LCME/AMA. *Degree requirements:* For doctorate, comprehensive exam. *Entrance requirements:* For doctorate, MCAT, minimum GPA of 3.6 in sciences, 3.64 overall. *Application deadline:* For fall admission, 8/14 for domestic students. Applications are processed on a rolling basis. Application fee: $0. *Expenses:* Contact institution. *Financial support:* Fellowships with tuition reimbursements, career-related internships or fieldwork, Federal Work-Study, institutionally sponsored loans, and scholarships/grants available. Support available to part-time students. Financial award application deadline: 5/1; financial award applicants required to submit FAFSA. *Faculty research:* Cancer, cardiovascular diseases, diabetes, neurological diseases, infection and inflammation. *Unit head:* Dr. Peter Buckley, Dean, 706-721-2231, Fax: 706-721-7035, E-mail: pbuckley@gru.edu. *Application contact:* Esther Holland, Director of Admissions, 706-721-3186, Fax: 706-721-0959, E-mail: eholland@augusta.edu. Website: http://www.augusta.edu/mcg/

Baylor College of Medicine, Medical School, Professional Program in Medicine, Houston, TX 77030-3498. Offers MD. *Accreditation:* LCME/AMA. *Entrance requirements:* For doctorate, MCAT, 90 hours of pre-med course work. Electronic applications accepted. *Expenses:* Contact institution.

Boston University, School of Medicine, Professional Program in Medicine, Boston, MA 02215. Offers MD, MD/Certificate, MD/JD, MD/MA, MD/MACI, MD/MBA, MD/MPH, MD/PhD. *Accreditation:* LCME/AMA. *Students:* 683 full-time (329 women), 19 part-time (11 women); includes 362 minority (23 Black or African American, non-Hispanic/Latino; 198 Asian, non-Hispanic/Latino; 90 Hispanic/Latino; 4 Native Hawaiian or other Pacific Islander, non-Hispanic/Latino; 47 Two or more races, non-Hispanic/Latino; 47 international. Average age 26. In 2015, 166 doctorates awarded. *Application deadline:* For fall admission, 11/1 for domestic students. Application fee: $95. *Expenses:* Contact institution. *Financial support:* Federal Work-Study available. Support available to part-time students. *Unit head:* Dr. Karen H. Antman, Dean/Provost, 617-638-5300. *Application contact:* Dr. Robert Witzburg, Associate Dean for Admissions, 617-638-4630.

Brown University, Graduate School, Division of Biology and Medicine, Program in Medicine, Providence, RI 02912. Offers MD, MD/PhD. *Accreditation:* LCME/AMA. *Expenses:* Contact institution.

Case Western Reserve University, School of Medicine, Professional Program in Medicine, Cleveland, OH 44106. Offers MD, MD/JD, MD/MA, MD/MBA, MD/MPH, MD/MS, MD/PhD. *Accreditation:* LCME/AMA. *Entrance requirements:* For doctorate, MCAT, interview. Electronic applications accepted. *Expenses: Tuition, area resident:* Full-time $41,137; part-time $1714 per credit hour. *Required fees:* $32. Tuition and fees vary according to course load and program.

Charles R. Drew University of Medicine and Science, Professional Program in Medicine, Los Angeles, CA 90059. Offers MD. *Entrance requirements:* For doctorate, MCAT.

Columbia University, College of Physicians and Surgeons, Professional Program in Medicine, New York, NY 10032. Offers MD, MD/DDS, MD/MPH, MD/MS, MD/PhD. *Accreditation:* LCME/AMA. *Program availability:* Part-time. *Entrance requirements:* For doctorate, MCAT.

Columbia University, School of Continuing Education, Program in Narrative Medicine, New York, NY 10027. Offers MS. Electronic applications accepted.

Creighton University, School of Medicine, Professional Program in Medicine, Omaha, NE 68178-0001. Offers MD, MD/PhD. *Accreditation:* LCME/AMA. *Entrance requirements:* For doctorate, MCAT. Electronic applications accepted. *Expenses: Tuition, area resident:* Full-time $14,400; part-time $800 per credit hour. *Required fees:* $158 per semester. Tuition and fees vary according to course load, campus/location,

program, reciprocity agreements and student's religious affiliation. *Faculty research:* Hereditary cancer, osteoporosis, diabetes, immunology, microbiology.

Dalhousie University, Faculty of Medicine, Halifax, NS B3H 4H7, Canada. Offers M Sc, MD, PhD, M Sc/PhD, MD/M Sc, MD/PhD. *Accreditation:* LCME/AMA. *Entrance requirements:* For master's, MCAT; for doctorate, MCAT (for MD). Electronic applications accepted.

Dartmouth College, Geisel School of Medicine, Hanover, NH 03755. Offers MD, MD/MBA, MD/MPH, MD/MS, MD/PhD. *Accreditation:* LCME/AMA. *Faculty:* 251 full-time (106 women), 88 part-time/adjunct (42 women). *Students:* 363 full-time (212 women), 6 part-time (2 women); includes 166 minority (29 Black or African American, non-Hispanic/Latino; 6 American Indian or Alaska Native, non-Hispanic/Latino; 73 Asian, non-Hispanic/Latino; 1 Native Hawaiian or other Pacific Islander, non-Hispanic/Latino; 4 Two or more races, non-Hispanic/Latino), 42 international. Average age 26. 6,112 applicants, 5% accepted, 92 enrolled. In 2015, 88 doctorates awarded. *Entrance requirements:* For doctorate, one year (8 semester hours or equivalent) of general biology and general physics; two years (16 semester hours or equivalent) of chemistry, which must include one semester each or equivalent of organic chemistry and biochemistry; one half-year (3 semester hours or equivalent) of college-level mathematics. *Application deadline:* For fall admission, 11/1 for domestic students. Application fee: $130. Electronic applications accepted. *Expenses: Tuition, area resident:* Full-time $48,120. *Required fees:* $296. One-time fee: $50 full-time. *Financial support:* Institutionally sponsored loans and scholarships/grants available. *Unit head:* Dr. Leslie Henderson, Senior Associate Dean for Faculty Affairs, 603-650-1312, E-mail: leslie.p.henderson@dartmouth.edu. *Application contact:* Andrew Welch, Director, DMS Admissions, 603-650-1505, Fax: 603-650-1560, E-mail: geisel.admissions@dartmouth.edu. Website: http://dms.dartmouth.edu/

Drexel University, College of Medicine, Professional Program in Medicine, Philadelphia, PA 19104-2875. Offers MD, MD/PhD. *Accreditation:* LCME/AMA. *Degree requirements:* For doctorate, National Board Exam Parts I and II. *Entrance requirements:* For doctorate, MCAT. Electronic applications accepted.

Duke University, School of Medicine, Professional Program in Medicine, Durham, NC 27708-0586. Offers MD, MD/JD, MD/MALS, MD/MBA, MD/MHS, MD/MLS, MD/MMCi, MD/MPH, MD/MPP, MD/MS, MD/MSIS, MD/PhD. *Accreditation:* LCME/AMA. *Faculty:* 1,420 full-time (468 women). *Students:* 452 full-time (211 women); includes 222 minority (47 Black or African American, non-Hispanic/Latino; 13 American Indian or Alaska Native, non-Hispanic/Latino; 148 Asian, non-Hispanic/Latino; 14 Hispanic/Latino), 13 international. Average age 26. 7,015 applicants, 4% accepted, 115 enrolled. In 2015, 89 doctorates awarded. *Entrance requirements:* For doctorate, MCAT. *Application deadline:* For fall admission, 10/15 for domestic students. Application fee: $85. Electronic applications accepted. *Financial support:* In 2015–16, 287 students received support. Scholarships/grants available. Financial award application deadline: 5/1; financial award applicants required to submit FAFSA. *Unit head:* Dr. Edward G. Buckley, Vice Dean of Medical Education, 919-668-3381, Fax: 919-660-7040, E-mail: buckl002@mc.duke.edu. *Application contact:* Andrea Lanahan, Director of Admissions, 919-684-2985, Fax: 919-684-8893, E-mail: medadm@mc.duke.edu. Website: http://www.dukemed.duke.edu/

East Carolina University, Brody School of Medicine, Professional Program in Medicine, Greenville, NC 27858-4353. Offers MD. *Accreditation:* LCME/AMA. *Entrance requirements:* For doctorate, MCAT, pre-med courses, interviews, faculty evaluations. *Application deadline:* For fall admission, 11/1 for domestic students. Applications are processed on a rolling basis. Application fee: $70. Electronic applications accepted. *Financial support:* Institutionally sponsored loans and scholarships/grants available. *Faculty research:* Diabetes, cardiovascular disease, cancer, neurological disorders. *Unit head:* Dr. Paul Cunningham, Dean, 252-744-2201, E-mail: cunninghamp@ecu.edu. *Application contact:* Contact Center, 252-744-1020, E-mail: somadmissions@ecu.edu. Website: http://www.ecu.edu/cs-dhs/med/md.cfm

Eastern Virginia Medical School, Professional Program in Medicine, Norfolk, VA 23501-1980. Offers MD, MD/MPH. *Accreditation:* LCME/AMA. *Entrance requirements:* For doctorate, MCAT, bachelor's degree or equivalent, course work in sciences. Electronic applications accepted.

East Tennessee State University, James H. Quillen College of Medicine, Professional Programs in Medicine, Johnson City, TN 37614. Offers MD. *Accreditation:* LCME/AMA. *Faculty:* 115 full-time (36 women), 35 part-time/adjunct (8 women). *Students:* 284 full-time (119 women); includes 44 minority (8 Black or African American, non-Hispanic/Latino; 3 American Indian or Alaska Native, non-Hispanic/Latino; 23 Asian, non-Hispanic/Latino; 8 Hispanic/Latino; 2 Two or more races, non-Hispanic/Latino). Average age 26. 1,144 applicants, 9% accepted, 60 enrolled. In 2015, 68 doctorates awarded. *Entrance requirements:* For doctorate, MCAT. Additional exam requirements/recommendations for international students: Required—TOEFL (minimum score 550 paper-based). *Application deadline:* For fall admission, 12/1 for domestic students. Applications are processed on a rolling basis. Application fee: $25. *Financial support:* Career-related internships or fieldwork, Federal Work-Study, institutionally sponsored loans, and scholarships/grants available. Financial award application deadline: 5/10; financial award applicants required to submit FAFSA. *Total annual research expenditures:* $2 million. *Unit head:* Dr. Robert T. Means, Jr., Dean, 423-439-6316, Fax: 423-439-8090, E-mail: deanofmedicine@etsu.edu. *Application contact:* E. Doug Taylor, Assistant Dean for Admissions and Records, 423-439-2033, Fax: 423-439-2110, E-mail: dougt@etsu.edu.

Emory University, School of Medicine, Professional Program in Medicine, Atlanta, GA 30322-4510. Offers MD, MD/MA, MD/MPH, MD/MSCR, MD/PhD. *Accreditation:* LCME/AMA. *Degree requirements:* For doctorate, United States Medical Licensing Exam Step 1 and 2. *Entrance requirements:* For doctorate, MCAT, AMCAS application, supplemental application, interview (by invitation only). Electronic applications accepted. *Expenses:* Contact institution. *Faculty research:* Immunology and pathogenesis of chronic viral infections, immunological memory and vaccine development, development of antiviral agents to treat infections caused by human immunodeficiency and hepatitis viruses, development of therapeutic and diagnostic approaches to improve outcomes after transplantation genetic mechanisms of neuropsychiatric disease, Fragile X Syndrome, immune system ontogeny and phylogeny.

Florida International University, Herbert Wertheim College of Medicine, Miami, FL 33199. Offers MPA, MD, PhD. *Accreditation:* LCME/AMA. *Faculty:* 66 full-time (29 women), 69 part-time/adjunct (23 women). *Students:* 532 full-time (273 women); includes 316 minority (35 Black or African American, non-Hispanic/Latino; 95 Asian, non-Hispanic/Latino; 172 Hispanic/Latino; 14 Two or more races, non-Hispanic/Latino),

10 international. Average age 25. 4,966 applicants, 7% accepted, 170 enrolled. In 2015, 80 doctorates awarded. *Entrance requirements:* For doctorate, MCAT (minimum score of 25), minimum overall GPA of 3.0; 3 letters of recommendation, 2 from basic science faculty (biology, chemistry, physics, math) and 1 from any other faculty member. *Application deadline:* For fall admission, 12/15 for domestic students. Application fee: $160. Electronic applications accepted. *Expenses:* Contact institution. *Financial support:* Institutionally sponsored loans and scholarships/grants available. Financial award application deadline: 3/1; financial award applicants required to submit FAFSA. *Unit head:* Dr. John Rock, Dean, 305-348-0570, E-mail: med.admissions@fiu.edu. *Application contact:* Nanett Rojas, Manager, Admissions Operations, 305-348-7464, Fax: 305-348-7441, E-mail: gradadm@fiu.edu.
Website: http://medicine.fiu.edu/

Georgetown University, School of Medicine, Washington, DC 20057. Offers MD, MD/MBA, MD/PhD. *Accreditation:* LCME/AMA. *Entrance requirements:* For doctorate, MCAT, minimum 90 credit hours with 1 year of course work in biology, organic chemistry, inorganic chemistry, physics, mathematics, and English. *Expenses:* Contact institution.

The George Washington University, School of Medicine and Health Sciences, Professional Program in Medicine, Washington, DC 20052. Offers MD. *Accreditation:* LCME/AMA. *Faculty:* 17 full-time (4 women), 16 part-time/adjunct (10 women). *Students:* 727 full-time (411 women), 1 part-time (0 women); includes 314 minority (58 Black or African American, non-Hispanic/Latino; 2 American Indian or Alaska Native, non-Hispanic/Latino; 195 Asian, non-Hispanic/Latino; 50 Hispanic/Latino; 3 Native Hawaiian or other Pacific Islander, non-Hispanic/Latino; 6 Two or more races, non-Hispanic/Latino), 28 international. Average age 26. *Entrance requirements:* For doctorate, MCAT, minimum of 90 undergraduate semester hours, specific pre-med courses equal to 38 semester hours. *Application deadline:* For fall admission, 12/1 for domestic students. Applications are processed on a rolling basis. Application fee: $80. *Financial support:* Career-related internships or fieldwork, Federal Work-Study, and institutionally sponsored loans available. *Unit head:* Dr. Alan Wasserman, Chair, 202-741-2302. *Application contact:* Diane P. McQuail, Director of Admissions, 202-994-3507, E-mail: maeve@gwu.edu.

Harvard University, Harvard Medical School, Professional Program in Medicine, Cambridge, MA 02138. Offers MD, PhD, MD/MBA, MD/MM Sc, MD/MPH, MD/MPP, MD/PhD. *Accreditation:* LCME/AMA. Electronic applications accepted.

Hofstra University, School of Medicine, Hempstead, NY 11549. Offers medicine (MD); molecular basis of medicine (PhD); MD/PhD. *Accreditation:* LCME/AMA. *Faculty:* 12 full-time (6 women), 9 part-time/adjunct (5 women). *Students:* 277 full-time (130 women); includes 104 minority (14 Black or African American, non-Hispanic/Latino; 50 Asian, non-Hispanic/Latino; 30 Hispanic/Latino; 2 Native Hawaiian or other Pacific Islander, non-Hispanic/Latino; 8 Two or more races, non-Hispanic/Latino), 1 international. Average age 25. 6,199 applicants, 4% accepted, 99 enrolled. *Entrance requirements:* For doctorate, MCAT. Additional exam requirements/recommendations for international students: Required—TOEFL (minimum score 600 paper-based; 100 iBT). *Application deadline:* For fall admission, 12/1 priority date for domestic students. Application fee: $100. Electronic applications accepted. *Expenses:* Contact institution. *Financial support:* In 2015–16, 239 students received support, including 222 fellowships with tuition reimbursements available (averaging $23,020 per year); research assistantships with tuition reimbursements available, Federal Work-Study, institutionally sponsored loans, scholarships/grants, and tuition waivers (full and partial) also available. Support available to part-time students. Financial award applicants required to submit FAFSA. *Faculty research:* Pathogenesis of sepsis, pathogenesis of autoimmune disease, pathogenesis of schizophrenia and movement disorders, population health, healthcare quality and effectiveness. *Unit head:* Dr. Veronica Catanese, Vice Dean, 516-463-7517, Fax: 516-463-7543, E-mail: medvmc@hofstra.edu. *Application contact:* Sunil Samuel, Assistant Vice President of Admissions, 516-463-4723, Fax: 516-463-4664.
Website: http://medicine.hofstra.edu/index.html

Howard University, College of Medicine, Professional Program in Medicine, Washington, DC 20059-0002. Offers MD, PhD, MD/PhD. *Accreditation:* LCME/AMA. *Faculty research:* Infectious diseases, protein modeling, neuropsychopharmacology.

Icahn School of Medicine at Mount Sinai, Department of Medical Education, New York, NY 10029-6504. Offers MD, MD/PhD. *Accreditation:* LCME/AMA. *Degree requirements:* For doctorate, comprehensive exam, United States Medical Licensing Examination Steps 1 and 2. *Entrance requirements:* For doctorate, MCAT. Additional exam requirements/recommendations for international students: Required—TOEFL. Electronic applications accepted. *Expenses:* Contact institution. *Faculty research:* Academic medicine, translational research.

Indiana University–Purdue University Indianapolis, Indiana University School of Medicine, Indianapolis, IN 46202-5114. Offers MS, MD, PhD, MD/MA, MD/MBA, MD/MS, MD/PhD. *Accreditation:* LCME/AMA. *Degree requirements:* For doctorate, thesis/dissertation (for some programs). *Entrance requirements:* For master's, GRE General Test; for doctorate, GRE General Test (for PhD); MCAT (for MD). Additional exam requirements/recommendations for international students: Required—TOEFL. *Expenses:* Contact institution.

Instituto Tecnologico de Santo Domingo, School of Medicine, Santo Domingo, Dominican Republic. Offers M Bioethics, MD.

Johns Hopkins University, School of Medicine, Professional Program in Medicine, Baltimore, MD 21218. Offers MD, MD/PhD. *Accreditation:* LCME/AMA. *Entrance requirements:* For doctorate, MCAT. Electronic applications accepted.

Loma Linda University, School of Medicine, Loma Linda, CA 92350. Offers MS, MD, PhD. *Accreditation:* LCME/AMA. *Degree requirements:* For master's, thesis optional; for doctorate, thesis/dissertation (for some programs). *Entrance requirements:* For doctorate, MCAT (for MD). Additional exam requirements/recommendations for international students: Required—TOEFL (minimum score 550 paper-based). *Application deadline:* For fall admission, 11/15 for domestic students. Application fee: $100. *Expenses:* Contact institution. *Financial support:* Fellowships, research assistantships, teaching assistantships, career-related internships or fieldwork, Federal Work-Study, institutionally sponsored loans, and tuition waivers (full and partial) available. Support available to part-time students. *Unit head:* Dr. Roger Hadley, Dean, 909-558-4481, Fax: 909-824-4146. *Application contact:* Admissions Office, 909-651-5029, Fax: 909-558-4879, E-mail: admissions.app@llu.edu.
Website: http://medicine.llu.edu

Louisiana State University Health Sciences Center, School of Medicine in New Orleans, New Orleans, LA 70112-2223. Offers MPH, MD, MD/PhD. Open only to Louisiana residents. *Accreditation:* LCME/AMA. *Entrance requirements:* For doctorate, MCAT. Electronic applications accepted. *Expenses:* Contact institution. *Faculty research:* Medical and basic sciences.

Louisiana State University Health Sciences Center at Shreveport, School of Medicine, Shreveport, LA 71130-3932. Offers MD, MD/PhD. *Accreditation:* LCME/AMA. *Entrance requirements:* For doctorate, MCAT. *Expenses:* Contact institution. *Faculty research:* Biomedical science, molecular biology, cardiovascular science.

Marshall University, Joan C. Edwards School of Medicine, Professional Program in Medicine, Huntington, WV 25755. Offers MD. *Accreditation:* LCME/AMA. *Degree requirements:* For doctorate, U.S. Medical Licensing Exam, Steps 1 and 2. *Entrance requirements:* For doctorate, MCAT, 1 year of course work in biology, physics, chemistry, organic chemistry, English, and social or behavioral sciences. *Expenses:* Contact institution.

Mayo Medical School, Professional Program, Rochester, MN 55905. Offers MD, MD/Certificate, MD offered through the Mayo Foundation's Division of Education; MD/PhD, MD/Certificate with Mayo Graduate School. *Accreditation:* LCME/AMA. *Entrance requirements:* For doctorate, MCAT, previous undergraduate course work in biology, chemistry, physics, and biochemistry. Electronic applications accepted.

McGill University, Faculty of Graduate and Postdoctoral Studies, Faculty of Medicine, Department of Surgery, Montréal, QC H3A 2T5, Canada. Offers M Sc, PhD.

McGill University, Professional Program in Medicine, Montréal, QC H3A 2T5, Canada. Offers MD/CM, MD/MBA, MD/PhD. *Accreditation:* LCME/AMA.

Medical College of Wisconsin, Medical School, Professional Program in Medicine, Milwaukee, WI 53226-0509. Offers MD, MD/MA, MD/MS, MD/PhD. *Accreditation:* LCME/AMA. *Entrance requirements:* For doctorate, GRE, official transcripts, three letters of recommendation. Additional exam requirements/recommendations for international students: Required—TOEFL.

Medical University of South Carolina, College of Medicine, Charleston, SC 29425. Offers MD, MD/MBA, MD/MHA, MD/MPH, MD/MSCR, MD/PhD. *Accreditation:* LCME/AMA. *Degree requirements:* For doctorate, Steps 1 and 2 of Clinical Performance Exam and U.S. Medical Licensing Examination. *Entrance requirements:* For doctorate, MCAT, interview. Electronic applications accepted. *Expenses:* Contact institution. *Faculty research:* Cardiovascular proteomics, translational cancer research, diabetes mellitus, neurodegenerative diseases, addiction.

Meharry Medical College, School of Medicine, Nashville, TN 37208-9989. Offers MD. *Accreditation:* LCME/AMA. *Entrance requirements:* For doctorate, MCAT. *Application deadline:* For fall admission, 12/15 for domestic students. Applications are processed on a rolling basis. Application fee: $65. Electronic applications accepted. *Financial support:* Federal Work-Study, institutionally sponsored loans, and tuition waivers (partial) available. Financial award applicants required to submit FAFSA.

Mercer University, School of Medicine, Macon, GA 31207. Offers MFT, MPH, MSA, MD. *Accreditation:* AAMFT/COAMFTE; LCME/AMA (one or more programs are accredited). *Entrance requirements:* Additional exam requirements/recommendations for international students: Required—TOEFL. Tuition and fees vary according to campus/location and program. *Faculty research:* Anatomy, biochemistry/nutrition, genetics, microbiology/immunology, neuroscience.

Michigan State University, College of Human Medicine, Professional Program in Human Medicine, East Lansing, MI 48824. Offers human medicine (MD); human medicine/medical scientist training program (MD). *Accreditation:* LCME/AMA. *Entrance requirements:* Additional exam requirements/recommendations for international students: Required—TOEFL, Michigan State University ELT (minimum score 85), Michigan Michigan English Language Assessment Battery (minimum score 83). Electronic applications accepted.

Morehouse School of Medicine, Professional Program, Atlanta, GA 30310-1495. Offers MD, MD/MPH. *Accreditation:* LCME/AMA. *Degree requirements:* For doctorate, U.S. Medical Licensing Exam Steps 1 and 2. *Entrance requirements:* For doctorate, MCAT. *Application deadline:* For fall admission, 12/1 for domestic students. Applications are processed on a rolling basis. Application fee: $50. Electronic applications accepted. *Expenses:* Contact institution. *Financial support:* Career-related internships or fieldwork, Federal Work-Study, institutionally sponsored loans, and scholarships/grants available. Financial award application deadline: 5/1; financial award applicants required to submit FAFSA. *Faculty research:* Cardiovascular disease and related sequela, infectious diseases/HIV-AIDS, neurological diseases, cancer. *Unit head:* Dr. Ngozi Anachebe, Associate Dean for Admissions and Student Affairs, 404-752-1650, Fax: 404-752-1594. *Application contact:* Brandon Hunter, Director of Admissions, 404-752-1650, Fax: 404-752-1512, E-mail: mdadmission@msm.edu.
Website: http://www.msm.edu/Education/mdProgram/index.php

New York Medical College, School of Medicine, Valhalla, NY 10595-1691. Offers MD, MD/MPH, MD/PhD. *Accreditation:* LCME/AMA. *Faculty:* 982 full-time (375 women), 1,269 part-time/adjunct (416 women). *Students:* 823 full-time (392 women); includes 349 minority (67 Black or African American, non-Hispanic/Latino; 173 Asian, non-Hispanic/Latino; 92 Hispanic/Latino; 17 Two or more races, non-Hispanic/Latino), 11 international. Average age 25. 13,235 applicants, 4% accepted, 202 enrolled. In 2015, 204 doctorates awarded. *Entrance requirements:* For doctorate, MCAT, 2 semesters of course work in general biology, general chemistry, organic chemistry, physics, and English. *Application deadline:* For fall admission, 1/31 for domestic and international students. Applications are processed on a rolling basis. Application fee: $120. Electronic applications accepted. *Expenses:* $52,200 per year tuition, $2,546 per year fees. *Financial support:* In 2015–16, 417 students received support. Research assistantships, Federal Work-Study, institutionally sponsored loans, and scholarships/grants available. Financial award application deadline: 4/30; financial award applicants required to submit FAFSA. *Faculty research:* Cardiovascular diseases, cancer, infectious diseases, neurosciences, renal diseases, pulmonary diseases. *Total annual research expenditures:* $17.7 million. *Unit head:* Jennifer Koestler, MD, Senior Associate Dean for Medical Education, 914-594-4500, E-mail: jennifer_koestler@nymc.edu. *Application contact:* Fern Juster, MD, Associate Dean of Admissions, 914-594-4507, Fax: 914-594-4613, E-mail: mdadmit@nymc.edu.
Website: http://www.nymc.edu/

New York University, School of Medicine, New York, NY 10016. Offers MS, MD, PhD, MD/MA, MD/MBA, MD/MPA, MD/MPH, MD/MS, MD/PhD. *Accreditation:* LCME/AMA (one or more programs are accredited). *Degree requirements:* For master's, comprehensive exam, thesis; for doctorate, comprehensive exam (for some programs), thesis/dissertation (for some programs). *Entrance requirements:* For doctorate, MCAT (for MD). *Expenses:* Contact institution. *Faculty research:* AIDS, cancer, neuroscience, molecular biology, neuroscience, cell biology and molecular genetics, structural biology, microbial pathogenesis and host defense, pharmacology, molecular oncology and immunology.

Northeast Ohio Medical University, College of Medicine, Rootstown, OH 44272-0095. Offers MD. *Accreditation:* LCME/AMA. *Faculty:* 462 full-time (172 women), 1,724 part-time/adjunct (484 women). *Students:* 596 full-time (280 women); includes 238 minority (13 Black or African American, non-Hispanic/Latino; 1 American Indian or Alaska Native, non-Hispanic/Latino; 196 Asian, non-Hispanic/Latino; 12 Hispanic/Latino; 1 Native Hawaiian or other Pacific Islander, non-Hispanic/Latino; 15 Two or more races, non-Hispanic/Latino). Average age 24. 3,105 applicants, 8% accepted, 160 enrolled. In 2015, 128 doctorates awarded. *Degree requirements:* For doctorate, U. S. Medical Licensing Exam Step 1. *Entrance requirements:* For doctorate, MCAT, 2 semesters of course work in organic chemistry and physics. *Application deadline:* For fall admission, 8/1 priority date for domestic students; for winter admission, 10/1 for domestic students.

Allopathic Medicine

Applications are processed on a rolling basis. Application fee: $40. Electronic applications accepted. *Expenses:* Contact institution. *Financial support:* In 2015–16, 599 students received support. Institutionally sponsored loans and scholarships/grants available. Financial award application deadline: 4/15; financial award applicants required to submit FAFSA. *Faculty research:* Auditory neuroscience, musculoskeletal biology, antiviral and immunomodulatory vaccine development, cellular and molecular mechanisms of thermogenesis associated with diabetes and obesity, cellular and molecular regulation of cardiac remodeling. *Unit head:* Dr. Jeffrey L. Susman, Dean, 330-325-6254. *Application contact:* Heidi Terry, Executive Director, Enrollment Services, 330-325-6479, E-mail: hterry@neoucom.edu.
Website: http://www.neomed.edu/academics/medicine

Northwestern University, Feinberg School of Medicine, Combined MD/PhD Medical Scientist Training Program, Evanston, IL 60208. Offers MD/PhD. Application must be made to both The Graduate School and the Medical School. *Accreditation:* LCME/AMA. Electronic applications accepted. *Faculty research:* Cardiovascular epidemiology, cancer epidemiology, nutritional interventions for the prevention of cardiovascular disease and cancer, women's health, outcomes research.

The Ohio State University, College of Medicine, Professional Program in Medicine, Columbus, OH 43210. Offers MD, MD/PhD. *Accreditation:* LCME/AMA. *Entrance requirements:* For doctorate, MCAT. Electronic applications accepted. *Faculty research:* Molecular genetics, stress and the immune system, molecular cardiology, transplantation biology.

Oregon Health & Science University, School of Medicine, Professional Program in Medicine, Portland, OR 97239-3098. Offers MD, MD/MPH, MD/PhD. *Accreditation:* LCME/AMA. *Faculty:* 1,737. *Students:* 556 full-time (282 women), 9 part-time; includes 126 minority (8 Black or African American, non-Hispanic/Latino; 3 American Indian or Alaska Native, non-Hispanic/Latino; 68 Asian, non-Hispanic/Latino; 25 Hispanic/Latino; 22 Two or more races, non-Hispanic/Latino). Average age 28. 6,049 applicants, 4% accepted, 146 enrolled. *Degree requirements:* For doctorate, National Board Exam Parts I and II. *Entrance requirements:* For doctorate, MCAT, 1 year of course work in biology, English, social science and physics; 2 years of course work in chemistry and genetics. *Application deadline:* For fall admission, 10/15 for domestic students. Applications are processed on a rolling basis. Application fee: $100. Electronic applications accepted. *Financial support:* Fellowships, research assistantships, Federal Work-Study, institutionally sponsored loans, scholarships/grants, and health care benefits available. Financial award application deadline: 3/1; financial award applicants required to submit FAFSA. *Unit head:* Dr. Tracy Bumsted, Associate Dean for Medical Education, 503-494-5646, Fax: 503-494-3400. *Application contact:* Debbie Melton, Director of Admissions, 503-494-8220, Fax: 503-494-3400.
Website: http://www.ohsu.edu/som/

Penn State Hershey Medical Center, College of Medicine, Hershey, PA 17033. Offers MPAS, MPH, MS, Dr PH, MD, PhD, MD/PhD, PhD/MBA. *Accreditation:* LCME/AMA. Terminal master's awarded for partial completion of doctoral program. *Degree requirements:* For master's, thesis optional; for doctorate, comprehensive exam (for some programs), thesis/dissertation (for some programs), minimum GPA of 3.0 (for PhD). *Entrance requirements:* For master's, GRE; for doctorate, GRE (for PhD); MCAT (for MD). Additional exam requirements/recommendations for international students: Required—TOEFL (minimum score 560 paper-based). *Application deadline:* Applications are processed on a rolling basis. Application fee: $65. Electronic applications accepted. *Expenses:* Contact institution. *Financial support:* In 2015–16, 99 students received support, including research assistantships with full tuition reimbursements available (averaging $22,260 per year); fellowships with full tuition reimbursements available, career-related internships or fieldwork, scholarships/grants, health care benefits, and unspecified assistantships also available. *Unit head:* Dr. A. Craig Hillemeier, Dean, 717-531-8323, Fax: 717-531-0786, E-mail: grad-hmc@psu.edu. *Application contact:* Dr. Sheila L. Vrana, Interim Vice Dean for Research and Graduate Studies, 717-531-7199, Fax: 717-531-0786, E-mail: grad-hmc@psu.edu.
Website: http://www.pennstatehershey.org/web/gsa/home

Ponce Health Sciences University, Professional Program, Ponce, PR 00732-7004. Offers MD. *Accreditation:* LCME/AMA. *Degree requirements:* For doctorate, one foreign language, comprehensive exam, United States Medical Licensing Exam. *Entrance requirements:* For doctorate, MCAT, coursework in Spanish language, proficiency in Spanish/English (highly recommended).

Pontificia Universidad Catolica Madre y Maestra, Department of Medicine, Santiago, Dominican Republic. Offers MD.

Queen's University at Kingston, School of Medicine, Professional Program in Medicine, Kingston, ON K7L 3N6, Canada. Offers MD. *Accreditation:* LCME/AMA. *Entrance requirements:* For doctorate, MCAT.

Quinnipiac University, Frank H. Netter MD School of Medicine, MD Program, Hamden, CT 06518-1940. Offers MD. *Accreditation:* LCME/AMA. *Faculty:* 27 full-time (9 women), 4 part-time/adjunct (3 women). *Students:* 240 full-time (100 women); includes 88 minority (8 Black or African American, non-Hispanic/Latino; 67 Asian, non-Hispanic/Latino; 13 Hispanic/Latino). Average age 25. 7,462 applicants, 5% accepted, 91 enrolled. *Degree requirements:* For doctorate, capstone project. *Entrance requirements:* For doctorate, MCAT. *Application deadline:* For fall admission, 12/31 for domestic students. Applications are processed on a rolling basis. Application fee: $100. Electronic applications accepted. *Expenses:* $54,360. *Financial support:* In 2015–16, 208 students received support. Institutionally sponsored loans and scholarships/grants available. Financial award application deadline: 3/1; financial award applicants required to submit FAFSA. *Unit head:* Dr. Bruce Koeppen, Dean, 203-582-5301, E-mail: brucedean.koeppen@quinnipiac.edu. *Application contact:* Michael Cole, Director of Admissions Operations, 203-582-6562, E-mail: michael.cole@quinnipiac.edu.
Website: http://www.quinnipiac.edu/academics/colleges-schools-and-departments/school-of-medicine/academics/md-program/

Rosalind Franklin University of Medicine and Science, Chicago Medical School, North Chicago, IL 60064-3095. Offers MD, MD/MS, MD/PhD. *Accreditation:* LCME/AMA. *Degree requirements:* For doctorate, clerkship, step 1 and step 2 exams. *Entrance requirements:* For doctorate, MCAT, 3 years of course work with lab in biology, physics, inorganic chemistry, and organic chemistry. *Expenses:* Contact institution. *Faculty research:* Neurosciences, structural biology, cancer biology, cell biology, developmental biology.

Rush University, Rush Medical College, Chicago, IL 60612. Offers MD. *Accreditation:* LCME/AMA. *Faculty:* 659 full-time (307 women), 173 part-time/adjunct (74 women). *Students:* 509 full-time (261 women); includes 198 minority (29 Black or African American, non-Hispanic/Latino; 4 American Indian or Alaska Native, non-Hispanic/Latino; 118 Asian, non-Hispanic/Latino; 44 Hispanic/Latino; 3 Native Hawaiian or other Pacific Islander, non-Hispanic/Latino). Average age 26. 6,982 applicants, 4% accepted, 128 enrolled. In 2015, 132 doctorates awarded. *Entrance requirements:* For doctorate, MCAT, in-person interview. *Application deadline:* For fall admission, 11/1 for domestic students. Applications are processed on a rolling basis. Application fee: $100. Electronic applications accepted. *Expenses:* Contact institution. *Financial support:* In 2015–16, 314 students received support. Federal Work-Study, institutionally sponsored loans, and

scholarships/grants available. Financial award application deadline: 3/1; financial award applicants required to submit FAFSA. *Unit head:* Dr. Cynthia E. Boyd, Assistant Dean, Admissions and Recruitment, 312-942-6915, Fax: 312-942-6840, E-mail: rmc_admissions@rush.edu. *Application contact:* Jill M. Volk, Director of Admissions and Recruitment, 312-942-6915, Fax: 312-942-6840, E-mail: rmc_admissions@rush.edu.
Website: http://www.rushu.rush.edu/medcol

Rutgers University–Newark, New Jersey Medical School, Newark, NJ 07101-1709. Offers MD, MD/Certificate, MD/JD, MD/MBA, MD/MPH, MD/PhD. *Accreditation:* LCME/AMA. *Entrance requirements:* For doctorate, MCAT. Additional exam requirements/recommendations for international students: Required—TOEFL. Electronic applications accepted. *Expenses:* Contact institution.

Rutgers University–New Brunswick, Robert Wood Johnson Medical School, Piscataway, NJ 08822. Offers MD, MD/JD, MD/MBA, MD/MPH, MD/MS, MD/MSJ, MD/PhD. *Accreditation:* LCME/AMA (one or more programs are accredited). *Entrance requirements:* For doctorate, MCAT. Additional exam requirements/recommendations for international students: Required—TOEFL. Electronic applications accepted. *Expenses:* Contact institution.

Saint Louis University, Graduate Education, School of Medicine, Program in Medicine, St. Louis, MO 63103. Offers MD. *Accreditation:* LCME/AMA. *Degree requirements:* For doctorate, U.S. Medical Licensing Exam Steps 1 and 2. *Entrance requirements:* For doctorate, MCAT, photograph, letters of recommendation, interview. Additional exam requirements/recommendations for international students: Required—TOEFL (minimum score 525 paper-based). Electronic applications accepted. *Expenses:* Contact institution. *Faculty research:* Geriatric medicine, organ transplantation, chronic disease prevention, vaccine research.

Stanford University, School of Medicine, Professional Program in Medicine, Stanford, CA 94305-9991. Offers MD, MD/PhD. *Accreditation:* LCME/AMA. *Entrance requirements:* For doctorate, MCAT. Electronic applications accepted. *Expenses:* Contact institution.

State University of New York Downstate Medical Center, College of Medicine, Brooklyn, NY 11203-2098. Offers MPH, MD, MD/MPH, MD/PhD. *Accreditation:* LCME/AMA. *Entrance requirements:* For doctorate, MCAT. *Expenses:* Contact institution. *Faculty research:* AIDS epidemiology, virus/host interaction, molecular genetics, developmental neurobiology, prostate cancer.

State University of New York Downstate Medical Center, School of Graduate Studies, MD/PhD Program, Brooklyn, NY 11203-2098. Offers MD/PhD. *Accreditation:* LCME/AMA. *Entrance requirements:* Additional exam requirements/recommendations for international students: Recommended—TOEFL.

State University of New York Upstate Medical University, College of Medicine, Syracuse, NY 13210-2334. Offers MD, MD/PhD. *Accreditation:* LCME/AMA. *Degree requirements:* For doctorate, comprehensive exam. *Entrance requirements:* For doctorate, MCAT. Additional exam requirements/recommendations for international students: Required—TOEFL. Electronic applications accepted. *Expenses:* Contact institution.

Stony Brook University, State University of New York, Stony Brook Medicine, School of Medicine, Medical Scientist Training Program, Stony Brook, NY 11794. Offers MD/PhD. *Entrance requirements:* Additional exam requirements/recommendations for international students: Required—TOEFL. *Application deadline:* For fall admission, 1/15 for domestic students. *Expenses:* Tuition, state resident: full-time $10,870; part-time $453 per credit hour. Tuition, nonresident: full-time $22,210; part-time $925 per credit hour. *Financial support:* Tuition waivers (full) available. *Unit head:* Dr. Michael A. Frohman, Director, Medical Scientist Training Program, 631-444-3219, Fax: 631-444-6229, E-mail: michael.frohman@stonybrook.edu. *Application contact:* Carron Allen, Program Administrator, 631-444-3219, Fax: 631-444-3492, E-mail: carron.kaufman@stonybrook.edu.
Website: http://www.pharm.stonybrook.edu/mstp/

Stony Brook University, State University of New York, Stony Brook Medicine, School of Medicine, Professional Program in Medicine, Stony Brook, NY 11794. Offers MD, MD/PhD. *Accreditation:* LCME/AMA. *Faculty:* 580 full-time (222 women), 72 part-time/adjunct (42 women). *Students:* 516 full-time (235 women); includes 228 minority (29 Black or African American, non-Hispanic/Latino; 161 Asian, non-Hispanic/Latino; 30 Hispanic/Latino; 8 Two or more races, non-Hispanic/Latino), 12 international. Average age 26. 5,255 applicants, 7% accepted, 132 enrolled. In 2015, 123 doctorates awarded. *Entrance requirements:* For doctorate, MCAT, interview. Application fee: $100. *Expenses:* $38,250 full-time in-state tuition, $63,260 full-time out-of-state tuition. *Financial support:* Fellowships and teaching assistantships available. *Total annual research expenditures:* $39.9 million. *Unit head:* Dr. Kenneth Kaushansky, Dean and Senior Vice President of Health Sciences, 631-444-2113, Fax: 631-444-6032, E-mail: somadmissions@stonybrook.edu. *Application contact:* Committee on Admissions, 631-444-2113, Fax: 631-444-6032, E-mail: somadmissions@stonybrookmedicine.edu.
Website: http://www.stonybrookmedicalcenter.org/som/

Temple University, School of Medicine, Doctor of Medicine Program, Philadelphia, PA 19140. Offers MD, MD/MA, MD/MBA, MD/MPH, MD/PhD. *Accreditation:* LCME/AMA. *Degree requirements:* For doctorate, United States Medical Licensing Exam Step 1, Step 2CK, Step 2CS. *Entrance requirements:* For doctorate, MCAT. Electronic applications accepted. *Expenses:* Contact institution. *Faculty research:* Translational medicine, molecular biology and immunology of autoimmune diseases and cancer, cardiovascular and pulmonary disease pathophysiology, biology of substance abuse, causes and consequences of obesity, molecular mechanisms of neurological dysfunction.

Texas Tech University Health Sciences Center, School of Medicine, Lubbock, TX 79430-0002. Offers MD, JD/MD, MD/MBA, MD/PhD. Open only to residents of Texas, eastern New Mexico, and southwestern Oklahoma; MD/PhD offered jointly with Texas Tech University; JD/MD with School of Law. *Accreditation:* LCME/AMA. *Entrance requirements:* For doctorate, MCAT. Additional exam requirements/recommendations for international students: Required—TOEFL. Electronic applications accepted. *Expenses:* Contact institution.

Thomas Jefferson University, Jefferson College of Biomedical Sciences, MD/PhD Program, Philadelphia, PA 19107. Offers MD/PhD. *Students:* 17 full-time (9 women); includes 3 minority (1 Asian, non-Hispanic/Latino; 2 Native Hawaiian or other Pacific Islander, non-Hispanic/Latino), 2 international. 170 applicants, 5% accepted, 5 enrolled. *Entrance requirements:* Additional exam requirements/recommendations for international students: Required—TOEFL (minimum score 100 iBT) or IELTS (7.0). *Application deadline:* For fall admission, 11/1 for domestic and international students. Applications are processed on a rolling basis. Electronic applications accepted. *Financial support:* In 2015–16, 16 fellowships with full tuition reimbursements were awarded; Federal Work-Study and institutionally sponsored loans also available. Financial award application deadline: 5/1; financial award applicants required to submit FAFSA. *Faculty research:* Signal transduction, tumorigenesis, apoptosis, molecular immunology, structural biology. *Unit head:* Dr. Scott A. Waldman, Academic Director, 215-955-6086, Fax: 215-955-5681, E-mail: scott.waldman@jefferson.edu. *Application

contact: Marc E. Stearns, Director of Admissions, 215-503-0155, Fax: 215-503-3433, E-mail: jgsbs-info@jefferson.edu.
Website: http://www.jefferson.edu/university/skmc/programs/md-phd.html

Thomas Jefferson University, Sidney Kimmel Medical College, Philadelphia, PA 19107-5083. Offers MD, MD/PhD. *Accreditation:* LCME/AMA. *Faculty:* 1,165 full-time (417 women), 75 part-time/adjunct (39 women). *Students:* 1,056 full-time (526 women); includes 323 minority (20 Black or African American, non-Hispanic/Latino; 4 American Indian or Alaska Native, non-Hispanic/Latino; 218 Asian, non-Hispanic/Latino; 81 Hispanic/Latino), 40 international. Average age 23. 10,504 applicants, 4% accepted, 267 enrolled. In 2015, 281 doctorates awarded. *Entrance requirements:* For doctorate, MCAT. *Application deadline:* For fall admission, 11/15 for domestic and international students. Applications are processed on a rolling basis. Application fee: $80. Electronic applications accepted. *Expenses:* $52,266 tuition, $416 IT fee, $312 library fee. *Financial support:* In 2015–16, 445 students received support. Federal Work-Study, institutionally sponsored loans, and scholarships/grants available. Financial award application deadline: 3/1; financial award applicants required to submit FAFSA. *Faculty research:* Neuroscience, Alzheimer's research, pancreatic cancer, oncology and endocrinology. *Total annual research expenditures:* $54.1 million. *Unit head:* Dr. Mark Tykowcinski, Dean, 215-955-6980, Fax: 215-923-6939, E-mail: mark.tykowcinski@jefferson.edu. *Application contact:* Dr. Clara Callahan, Dean for Students and Admissions, 215-955-4077, Fax: 215-955-5151, E-mail: clara.callahan@jefferson.edu.
Website: http://www.jefferson.edu/university/skmc.html

Tufts University, School of Medicine, Professional Program in Medicine, Medford, MA 02155. Offers MD, MD/MA, MD/MBA, MD/MPH, MD/PhD. MD/PhD offered jointly with Sackler School of Graduate Biomedical Sciences; MD/MBA with Brandeis University. *Accreditation:* LCME/AMA. *Students:* 816 full-time (431 women), 3 part-time (1 woman); includes 267 minority (28 Black or African American, non-Hispanic/Latino; 2 American Indian or Alaska Native, non-Hispanic/Latino; 155 Asian, non-Hispanic/Latino; 43 Hispanic/Latino; 1 Native Hawaiian or other Pacific Islander, non-Hispanic/Latino; 38 Two or more races, non-Hispanic/Latino), 1 international. Average age 26. 9,333 applicants, 6% accepted, 201 enrolled. In 2015, 186 doctorates awarded. *Entrance requirements:* For doctorate, MCAT. *Application deadline:* For fall admission, 1/15 for domestic students. Applications are processed on a rolling basis. Application fee: $105. Electronic applications accepted. *Expenses:* Contact institution. *Financial support:* Federal Work-Study, institutionally sponsored loans, and scholarships/grants available. Financial award application deadline: 3/26; financial award applicants required to submit FAFSA. *Unit head:* Dr. Harris Berman, Dean, 617-636-6565. *Application contact:* John Matias, Associate Dean of Admissions, 617-636-6571, E-mail: med-admissions@tufts.edu.
Website: http://medicine.tufts.edu/

Tulane University, School of Medicine, Professional Programs in Medicine, New Orleans, LA 70118-5669. Offers MD, MD/MBA, MD/MPH, MD/MPHTM, MD/MSPH, MD/PhD. *Accreditation:* LCME/AMA. *Entrance requirements:* For doctorate, MCAT. *Expenses:* Tuition, area resident: Full-time $47,658; part-time $2648 per credit hour. *Required fees:* $1980; $44.50 per credit hour. $550 per term. Tuition and fees vary according to course load, degree level and program.

Universidad Autonoma de Guadalajara, School of Medicine, Guadalajara, Mexico. Offers MD.

Universidad Central del Caribe, School of Medicine, Bayamón, PR 00960-6032. Offers MA, MS, MD, PhD. *Accreditation:* LCME/AMA. *Degree requirements:* For doctorate, variable foreign language requirement. *Entrance requirements:* For doctorate, MCAT (for MD). *Faculty research:* Membrane neurotransmitter receptors, brain neurotransmission, cocaine toxicology, membrane transport, antimetabolite pharmacology.

Universidad Central del Este, Medical School, San Pedro de Macoris, Dominican Republic. Offers MD.

Universidad de Ciencias Medicas, Graduate Programs, San Jose, Costa Rica. Offers dermatology (SP); family health (MS); health service center administration (MHA); human anatomy (MS); medical and surgery (MD); occupational medicine (MS); pharmacy (Pharm D). *Program availability:* Part-time. *Degree requirements:* For master's, thesis; for doctorate and SP, comprehensive exam. *Entrance requirements:* For master's, MD or bachelor's degree; for doctorate, admissions test; for SP, admissions test, MD.

Universidad de Iberoamerica, Graduate School, San Jose, Costa Rica. Offers clinical neuropsychology (PhD); clinical psychology (M Psych); educational psychology (M Psych); forensic psychology (M Psych); hospital management (MHA); intensive care nursing (MN); medicine (MD).

Universidad Iberoamericana, School of Medicine, Santo Domingo D.N., Dominican Republic. Offers MD.

Universidad Nacional Pedro Henriquez Urena, School of Medicine, Santo Domingo, Dominican Republic. Offers MD.

Université de Montréal, Faculty of Medicine, Professional Program in Medicine, Montréal, QC H3C 3J7, Canada. Offers MD. Open only to Canadian residents. *Accreditation:* LCME/AMA. *Entrance requirements:* For doctorate, proficiency in French. Electronic applications accepted.

Université de Sherbrooke, Faculty of Medicine and Health Sciences, Professional Program in Medicine, Sherbrooke, QC J1K 2R1, Canada. Offers MD. *Accreditation:* LCME/AMA. Electronic applications accepted.

Université Laval, Faculty of Medicine, Post-Professional Programs in Medical Studies, Québec, QC G1K 7P4, Canada. Offers anatomy–pathology (DESS); anesthesiology (DESS); cardiology (DESS); care of older people (Diploma); clinical research (DESS); community health (DESS); dermatology (DESS); diagnostic radiology (DESS); emergency medicine (Diploma); family medicine (DESS); general surgery (DESS); geriatrics (DESS); hematology (DESS); internal medicine (DESS); maternal and fetal medicine (Diploma); medical biochemistry (DESS); medical microbiology and infectious diseases (DESS); medical oncology (DESS); nephrology (DESS); neurology (DESS); neurosurgery (DESS); obstetrics and gynecology (DESS); ophthalmology (DESS); orthopedic surgery (DESS); oto-rhino-laryngology (DESS); palliative medicine (Diploma); pediatrics (DESS); plastic surgery (DESS); psychiatry (DESS); pulmonary medicine (DESS); radiology–oncology (DESS); thoracic surgery (DESS); urology (DESS). *Degree requirements:* For other advanced degree, comprehensive exam. *Entrance requirements:* For degree, knowledge of French. Electronic applications accepted.

Université Laval, Faculty of Medicine, Professional Program in Medicine, Québec, QC G1K 7P4, Canada. Offers MD. *Accreditation:* LCME/AMA. *Entrance requirements:* For doctorate, interview, proficiency in French. Electronic applications accepted.

University at Buffalo, the State University of New York, Graduate School, School of Medicine and Biomedical Sciences, Professional Program in Medicine, Buffalo, NY 14260. Offers MD, MD/MBA, MD/MPH, MD/PhD. *Accreditation:* LCME/AMA. *Students:* 573 full-time (253 women); includes 189 minority (15 Black or African American, non-Hispanic/Latino; 1 American Indian or Alaska Native, non-Hispanic/Latino; 89 Asian, non-Hispanic/Latino; 56 Hispanic/Latino; 28 Two or more races, non-Hispanic/Latino). Average age 25. 4,362 applicants, 7% accepted, 144 enrolled. In 2015, 138 doctorates awarded. *Entrance requirements:* For doctorate, MCAT, interview. *Application deadline:* For fall admission, 11/15 for domestic students. Applications are processed on a rolling basis. Application fee: $65. Electronic applications accepted. *Expenses:* $40,417 resident full-time, $65,427 nonresident full-time. *Financial support:* In 2015–16, 101 students received support. Career-related internships or fieldwork, Federal Work-Study, institutionally sponsored loans, and scholarships/grants available. Financial award application deadline: 3/1; financial award applicants required to submit FAFSA. *Faculty research:* Microbial pathogenesis, neuronal plasticity, structural biology of ion channels, structural development, cell biology of development. *Unit head:* Dr. Charles Severin, Dean for Admissions, 716-829-2803, Fax: 716-829-2798, E-mail: severin@buffalo.edu. *Application contact:* James J. Rosso, Admissions Advisor, 716-829-3466, Fax: 716-829-3849, E-mail: jjrosso@buffalo.edu.
Website: http://medicine.buffalo.edu/education/md.html

The University of Alabama at Birmingham, School of Medicine, Birmingham, AL 35294. Offers MD, MD/PhD. *Accreditation:* LCME/AMA (one or more programs are accredited). *Students:* 780 full-time (346 women); includes 177 minority (33 Black or African American, non-Hispanic/Latino; 6 American Indian or Alaska Native, non-Hispanic/Latino; 71 Asian, non-Hispanic/Latino; 3 Hispanic/Latino; 64 Two or more races, non-Hispanic/Latino). Average age 25. 3,768 applicants, 7% accepted, 186 enrolled. In 2015, 181 doctorates awarded. *Entrance requirements:* For doctorate, MCAT (minimum score of 24), AMCAS application, letters of recommendation, interview, U.S. citizenship or permanent residency. *Application deadline:* For fall admission, 11/1 for domestic students. Application fee: $80. Electronic applications accepted. *Expenses:* Contact institution. *Financial support:* In 2015–16, 233 students received support. Career-related internships or fieldwork and scholarships/grants available. Financial award application deadline: 5/1; financial award applicants required to submit FAFSA. *Unit head:* Dr. Selwyn M. Vickers, Senior Vice President/Dean, School of Medicine, 205-934-1111, Fax: 205-934-0333. *Application contact:* 205-934-2433, Fax: 205-934-8740, E-mail: medschool@uab.edu.
Website: http://www.uab.edu/medicine/home/

The University of Arizona, College of Medicine, Professional Programs in Medicine, Tucson, AZ 85721. Offers MD, PhD. MD program open only to state residents. *Accreditation:* LCME/AMA. *Entrance requirements:* For doctorate, MCAT, previous course work in general chemistry, organic chemistry, biology/zoology, physics, and English. Application fee: $0. *Financial support:* Fellowships, research assistantships, teaching assistantships, career-related internships or fieldwork, Federal Work-Study, institutionally sponsored loans, and tuition waivers (full and partial) available. *Faculty research:* Developmental biology, cellular structure and function, immunology, clinical cancer research, heart and respiratory disease.
Website: http://medicine.arizona.edu/

The University of Arizona, College of Medicine, Program in Medical Sciences, Tucson, AZ 85721. Offers MS, PhD. *Accreditation:* LCME/AMA. *Degree requirements:* For doctorate, comprehensive exam, thesis/dissertation. *Application deadline:* For fall admission, 5/5 for domestic students. Application fee: $75. *Financial support:* Traineeships, health care benefits, and unspecified assistantships available. *Unit head:* Dr. Charles B. Cairns, Interim Dean, 520-626-3972, E-mail: dposkus@surgery.arizona.edu. *Application contact:* Kathy Detloff, Associate Dean for Admissions, 520-626-4555, E-mail: lupeo@email.arizona.edu.
Website: http://surgery.arizona.edu/education/medical-sciences-graduate-program

University of Arkansas for Medical Sciences, College of Medicine, Little Rock, AR 72205-7199. Offers MD, MD/PhD. *Accreditation:* LCME/AMA. *Entrance requirements:* For doctorate, MCAT. Electronic applications accepted. *Expenses:* Contact institution.

The University of British Columbia, Faculty of Medicine, Department of Surgery, Vancouver, BC V6T 1Z1, Canada. Offers M Sc. *Program availability:* Part-time. *Degree requirements:* For master's, thesis. *Entrance requirements:* Additional exam requirements/recommendations for international students: Required—TOEFL. Electronic applications accepted. *Faculty research:* Photodynamic therapy, transplantation immunobiology, isolated cell culture, neurophysiology.

The University of British Columbia, Faculty of Medicine, Professional Program in Medicine, Vancouver, BC V6T 1Z1, Canada. Offers MD, MD/PhD. *Accreditation:* LCME/AMA. *Entrance requirements:* For doctorate, MCAT.

University of Calgary, Cumming School of Medicine, MD Program, Calgary, AB T2N 4N1, Canada. Offers MD. *Accreditation:* LCME/AMA. *Entrance requirements:* For doctorate, MCAT. Electronic applications accepted.

University of California, Berkeley, Graduate Division, School of Public Health, Group in Health and Medical Sciences, Berkeley, CA 94720-1500. Offers MD/MS. Program offered jointly with University of California, San Francisco.

University of California, Davis, School of Medicine, Sacramento, CA 95817. Offers MD, MD/MBA, MD/MPH, MD/MS, MD/PhD. *Accreditation:* LCME/AMA. *Degree requirements:* For doctorate, comprehensive exam. *Entrance requirements:* For doctorate, MCAT, 1 year each of English, biological science (lower-division with lab), general chemistry (with lab), organic chemistry (with lab), physics, and college-level math, plus 1/2 year upper-division biology. Electronic applications accepted. *Expenses:* Contact institution. *Faculty research:* Cancer biology, cardiovascular disease, clinical and translational research, neuroscience, regenerative medicine.

University of California, Irvine, School of Medicine, Professional Program in Medicine, Irvine, CA 92697. Offers MD, MD/MBA, MD/MPH, MD/PhD. *Accreditation:* LCME/AMA. *Students:* 425 full-time (215 women), 38 part-time (19 women); includes 42 minority (1 Black or African American, non-Hispanic/Latino; 2 American Indian or Alaska Native, non-Hispanic/Latino; 23 Asian, non-Hispanic/Latino; 16 Hispanic/Latino), 1 international. Average age 26. In 2015, 93 doctorates awarded. *Entrance requirements:* For doctorate, MCAT. Additional exam requirements/recommendations for international students: Required—TOEFL (minimum score 550 paper-based). *Application deadline:* For fall admission, 11/1 for domestic students. Application fee: $90 ($110 for international students). Electronic applications accepted. *Financial support:* Fellowships, institutionally sponsored loans, traineeships, health care benefits, and unspecified assistantships available. Financial award application deadline: 3/1; financial award applicants required to submit FAFSA. *Unit head:* Ellena Peterson, Associate Dean, 949-824-4169, Fax: 949-824-2160, E-mail: ellena.peterson@uci.edu. *Application contact:* Frances Stephens, Admissions Counselor, 949-824-4614, E-mail: fran.stephens@uci.edu.
Website: http://www.som.uci.edu/graduate-studies/education/md-degree.asp

University of California, Los Angeles, David Geffen School of Medicine, Professional Program in Medicine, Los Angeles, CA 90095. Offers MD, MD/MBA, MD/PhD. *Accreditation:* LCME/AMA. *Entrance requirements:* For doctorate, MCAT, interview. *Expenses:* Contact institution.

University of California, San Diego, School of Medicine, Professional Program in Medicine, La Jolla, CA 92093. Offers MD, MD/PhD. *Accreditation:* LCME/AMA.

Allopathic Medicine

Students: 505 full-time (247 women). *Entrance requirements:* For doctorate, MCAT. *Application deadline:* For fall admission, 11/1 for domestic students. Application fee: $90. *Expenses:* Contact institution. *Unit head:* Dr. Carolyn J. Kelly, MD, Associate Dean, Admissions and Student Affairs. *Application contact:* 858-534-3880, E-mail: somadmissions@ucsd.edu.

University of California, San Francisco, School of Medicine, San Francisco, CA 94143-0410. Offers MD, PhD, MD/MPH, MD/MS, MD/PhD. *Accreditation:* LCME/AMA (one or more programs are accredited). *Faculty:* 2,035 full-time (871 women), 368 part-time/adjunct (195 women). *Students:* 647 full-time (330 women); includes 354 minority (47 Black or African American, non-Hispanic/Latino; 2 American Indian or Alaska Native, non-Hispanic/Latino; 156 Asian, non-Hispanic/Latino; 94 Hispanic/Latino; 9 Native Hawaiian or other Pacific Islander, non-Hispanic/Latino; 46 Two or more races, non-Hispanic/Latino). Average age 24. 7,453 applicants, 4% accepted, 149 enrolled. In 2015, 163 doctorates awarded. *Entrance requirements:* For doctorate, MCAT (for MD), interview (for MD). *Application deadline:* For fall admission, 10/15 for domestic students. Applications are processed on a rolling basis. Application fee: $80 ($100 for international students). Electronic applications accepted. *Expenses:* $32,751 in-state tuition, $44,996 out-of-state tuition, $4,593 student fees. *Financial support:* In 2015–16, 517 students received support. Federal Work-Study, institutionally sponsored loans, scholarships/grants, and tuition waivers (partial) available. Financial award application deadline: 2/1; financial award applicants required to submit FAFSA. *Faculty research:* Neurosciences, human genetics, developmental biology, social/behavioral/policy sciences, immunology. *Total annual research expenditures:* $495.6 million. *Unit head:* Dr. Talmadge E. King, Jr., Dean, 415-476-2342, Fax: 415-476-0689. *Application contact:* Hallen Chung, Director of Admissions, 415-476-8090, Fax: 415-476-5490, E-mail: hallen.chung@ucsf.edu.
Website: http://medschool.ucsf.edu/

University of Central Florida, College of Medicine, Orlando, FL 32816. Offers MS, MD, PhD. *Accreditation:* LCME/AMA. *Expenses:* Tuition, state resident: part-time $288.16 per credit hour. Tuition, nonresident: part-time $1071.31 per credit hour. *Financial support:* Fellowships, research assistantships and teaching assistantships available. *Unit head:* Dr. Deborah C. German, Vice President for Medical Affairs/Dean, 407-266-1000, E-mail: deborah.german@ucf.edu. *Application contact:* Director, Admissions and Registration, 407-823-2766, Fax: 407-823-6442, E-mail: gradadmissions@ucf.edu.
Website: http://www.med.ucf.edu

University of Chicago, Pritzker School of Medicine, Chicago, IL 60637-1513. Offers MD, MD/PhD. *Accreditation:* LCME/AMA. *Entrance requirements:* For doctorate, MCAT, one year of each with lab: chemistry, physics, biology and organic chemistry. Electronic applications accepted. *Faculty research:* Human genetics, diabetes, developmental biology, structural biology, neurobiology.

University of Cincinnati, Graduate School, College of Medicine, Physician Scientist Training Program, Cincinnati, OH 45221. Offers MD/PhD. *Entrance requirements:* Additional exam requirements/recommendations for international students: Required—TOEFL. Electronic applications accepted.

University of Cincinnati, Graduate School, College of Medicine, Professional Program in Medicine, Cincinnati, OH 45221. Offers MD. *Accreditation:* LCME/AMA. *Entrance requirements:* For doctorate, MCAT. Electronic applications accepted. *Faculty research:* Molecular genetics, environmental health, neuroscience and cell biology, cardiovascular science, developmental biology.

University of Colorado Denver, School of Medicine, Professional Program in Medicine, Aurora, CO 80045. Offers MD, MD/MBA, MD/PhD. *Students:* 664 full-time (312 women); includes 127 minority (12 Black or African American, non-Hispanic/Latino; 1 American Indian or Alaska Native, non-Hispanic/Latino; 65 Asian, non-Hispanic/Latino; 39 Hispanic/Latino; 10 Two or more races, non-Hispanic/Latino). Average age 27. In 2015, 159 doctorates awarded. *Entrance requirements:* For doctorate, MCAT, AMCAS application, essay, interviews, prerequisite coursework in biology (with lab), general chemistry (with lab), organic chemistry (with lab), general physics (with lab), English literature/composition, college-level mathematics (algebra and above). Additional exam requirements/recommendations for international students: Required—TOEFL (minimum score 550 paper-based; 80 iBT). *Application deadline:* For fall admission, 11/1 for domestic students, 10/1 for international students. Application fee: $100 ($125 for international students). Electronic applications accepted. *Expenses:* Contact institution. *Financial support:* In 2015–16, 563 students received support. Fellowships, research assistantships, teaching assistantships, Federal Work-Study, institutionally sponsored loans, scholarships/grants, traineeships, health care benefits, and unspecified assistantships available. Financial award application deadline: 4/1; financial award applicants required to submit FAFSA. *Unit head:* Dr. John Reilly, Jr., Dean of the School of Medicine, 303-724-5375, E-mail: john.reillyjr@ucdenver.edu. *Application contact:* Ashley Ehlers, Office of Admissions Medical Program Assistant, 303-724-8025, E-mail: somadmin@ucdenver.edu.
Website: http://www.ucdenver.edu/academics/colleges/medicalschool/Pages/somWelcome.aspx

University of Connecticut Health Center, School of Medicine, Farmington, CT 06030. Offers MD, MD/MBA, MD/MPH, MD/PhD. *Accreditation:* LCME/AMA. *Entrance requirements:* For doctorate, MCAT. Electronic applications accepted. *Expenses:* Contact institution.

University of Florida, College of Medicine, Professional Program in Medicine, Gainesville, FL 32611. Offers MD, MD/PhD. *Accreditation:* LCME/AMA. *Entrance requirements:* For doctorate, MCAT, 8 semester hours of course work in biology, general chemistry, and general physics; 4 semester hours of course work in geochemistry and organic chemistry. Electronic applications accepted. *Faculty research:* Neurobiology, gene therapy and genetic imaging technologies, diabetes and autoimmune diseases, transplantation.

University of Hawaii at Manoa, John A. Burns School of Medicine, Professional Program in Medicine, Honolulu, HI 96822. Offers MD. *Accreditation:* LCME/AMA. *Entrance requirements:* For doctorate, MCAT. Electronic applications accepted. *Expenses:* Contact institution.

University of Illinois at Chicago, College of Medicine, Professional Program in Medicine, Chicago, IL 60607-7128. Offers MD, MD/MS, MD/PhD. *Program availability:* Part-time. *Faculty:* 357 full-time (148 women), 145 part-time/adjunct (43 women). *Students:* 1,252 full-time (570 women), 96 part-time (48 women); includes 723 minority (123 Black or African American, non-Hispanic/Latino; 3 American Indian or Alaska Native, non-Hispanic/Latino; 315 Asian, non-Hispanic/Latino; 235 Hispanic/Latino; 2 Native Hawaiian or other Pacific Islander, non-Hispanic/Latino; 45 Two or more races, non-Hispanic/Latino), 1 international. Average age 26. *Entrance requirements:* For doctorate, MCAT. *Application deadline:* For fall admission, 12/15 for domestic students. Applications are processed on a rolling basis. Application fee: $160. Electronic applications accepted. *Expenses:* Tuition, state resident: full-time $11,480; part-time $3826 per credit. Tuition, nonresident: full-time $23,720; part-time $7906 per credit. *Required fees:* $1333 per semester. Part-time tuition and fees vary according to course load and program. *Financial support:* Fellowships, research assistantships, and teaching assistantships available. *Faculty research:* Biomedical and clinical sciences.

Total annual research expenditures: $72 million. *Unit head:* Dr. Dimitri T. Azar, Dean, 312-996-3500, Fax: 312-996-9006, E-mail: dazar@uic.edu. *Application contact:* Jackie Perry, Graduate College Receptionist, 312-413-2550, Fax: 312-413-0185, E-mail: gradcoll@uic.edu.

University of Illinois at Urbana–Champaign, Graduate College, Medical Scholars Program, Urbana, IL 61801. Offers MD/MBA, MD/PhD. Electronic applications accepted. *Expenses:* Contact institution.

The University of Iowa, Roy J. and Lucille A. Carver College of Medicine and Graduate College, Medical Scientist Training Program, Iowa City, IA 52242-1316. Offers MD/PhD. Electronic applications accepted. Application fee is waived when completed online. *Faculty research:* Structure and function of ion channels, molecular genetics of human disease, neurobiology of pain, viral immunology and immunopathology, epidemiology of aging and cancer, human learning and memory, structural enzymology.

The University of Iowa, Roy J. and Lucille A. Carver College of Medicine, Professional Program in Medicine, Iowa City, IA 52242-1316. Offers MD, MD/JD, MD/MBA, MD/MPH, MD/PhD. *Accreditation:* LCME/AMA. *Degree requirements:* For doctorate, U.S. Medical Licensing Examination Steps 1 and 2. *Entrance requirements:* For doctorate, MCAT, course work in biology, chemistry, organic chemistry, biochemistry, physics, mathematics, English, and social sciences; bachelor's degree. Electronic applications accepted. Application fee is waived when completed online. *Expenses:* Contact institution.

The University of Kansas, University of Kansas Medical Center, School of Medicine, MD/PhD Program, Kansas City, KS 66160. Offers MD/PhD. *Students:* 27 full-time (11 women); includes 7 minority (2 Black or African American, non-Hispanic/Latino; 3 Asian, non-Hispanic/Latino; 1 Hispanic/Latino; 1 Two or more races, non-Hispanic/Latino). Average age 28. 80 applicants, 8% accepted, 2 enrolled. *Application deadline:* For fall admission, 10/15 priority date for domestic students. Applications are processed on a rolling basis. Application fee: $50. Electronic applications accepted. *Financial support:* Fellowships with full tuition reimbursements, research assistantships with full tuition reimbursements, and teaching assistantships with full tuition reimbursements available. Financial award application deadline: 3/1; financial award applicants required to submit FAFSA. *Unit head:* Dr. Timothy A. Fields, Director, 913-588-7169, E-mail: tfields@kumc.edu. *Application contact:* Janice Fletcher, Administrative Manager, 913-588-5241, Fax: 913-945-6848, E-mail: jfletcher@kumc.edu.
Website: http://www.kumc.edu/md-phd-program.html

The University of Kansas, University of Kansas Medical Center, School of Medicine, MD Program, Kansas City, KS 66160. Offers MD. *Students:* 827 full-time (372 women); includes 198 minority (14 Black or African American, non-Hispanic/Latino; 3 American Indian or Alaska Native, non-Hispanic/Latino; 73 Asian, non-Hispanic/Latino; 52 Hispanic/Latino; 56 Two or more races, non-Hispanic/Latino). Average age 26. 3,557 applicants, 7% accepted, 211 enrolled. In 2015, 189 doctorates awarded. *Degree requirements:* For doctorate, comprehensive exam. *Entrance requirements:* For doctorate, MCAT, bachelor's degree. *Application deadline:* For fall admission, 10/15 for domestic students. Applications are processed on a rolling basis. Application fee: $50. Electronic applications accepted. *Expenses:* Contact institution. *Financial support:* Scholarships/grants available. Financial award application deadline: 3/1; financial award applicants required to submit FAFSA. *Faculty research:* Reproductive biology (fertility, ovulation, embryo implantation, pregnancy maintenance), multidisciplinary research on the basic mechanisms of cancer, renal research, neurological research, liver research. *Unit head:* Dr. Robert Simari, Executive Dean. *Application contact:* Jason Edwards, Director of Admissions and Premedical Programs, 913-588-5280, Fax: 913-588-5259, E-mail: premedinfo@kumc.edu.
Website: http://www.kumc.edu/school-of-medicine.html

University of Kentucky, College of Medicine, Lexington, KY 40536-0298. Offers MD, MD/MBA, MD/MPH, MD/PhD. *Accreditation:* LCME/AMA. *Students:* 521 full-time (217 women); includes 105 minority (30 Black or African American, non-Hispanic/Latino; 1 American Indian or Alaska Native, non-Hispanic/Latino; 67 Asian, non-Hispanic/Latino; 7 Hispanic/Latino), 29 international. Average age 24. *Degree requirements:* For doctorate, comprehensive exam (for some programs), thesis/dissertation (for some programs). *Entrance requirements:* For doctorate, MCAT (for MD). *Application deadline:* For fall admission, 11/1 for domestic students. Applications are processed on a rolling basis. Application fee: $50. Electronic applications accepted. *Expenses:* Contact institution. *Financial support:* Institutionally sponsored loans available. Financial award applicants required to submit FAFSA. *Faculty research:* Aging, cancer, cardiovascular disease, infectious disease, women's maternal and child health. *Unit head:* Dr. Carol L. Elam, Associate Dean for Admissions, 859-323-6161. *Application contact:* Kimberly Scott, Assistant Director of Admissions, 859-323-6161, E-mail: kymedap@uky.edu.
Website: http://http://med.uky.edu/

University of Louisville, School of Medicine, Professional Programs in Medicine, Louisville, KY 40292-0001. Offers MD, MD/MBA, MD/MS, MD/PhD. *Accreditation:* LCME/AMA. *Students:* 631 full-time (259 women), 4 part-time (1 woman); includes 136 minority (38 Black or African American, non-Hispanic/Latino; 70 Asian, non-Hispanic/Latino; 13 Hispanic/Latino; 15 Two or more races, non-Hispanic/Latino). Average age 26. 3,643 applicants, 7% accepted, 158 enrolled. In 2015, 151 doctorates awarded. *Entrance requirements:* For doctorate, MCAT. Additional exam requirements/recommendations for international students: Required—TOEFL (minimum score 550 paper-based; 79 iBT). *Application deadline:* For fall admission, 1/28 for domestic students. Applications are processed on a rolling basis. Application fee: $60. Electronic applications accepted. *Expenses:* Tuition, state resident: full-time $11,664; part-time $649 per credit hour. Tuition, nonresident: full-time $24,274; part-time $1350 per credit hour. *Required fees:* $196. Tuition and fees vary according to program and reciprocity agreements. *Faculty research:* Environmental effects on the cardiovascular system, diabetes, obesity and metabolics, molecular targets for cancer chemotherapy, plasticity of neural tissue, stem cells in repair of damaged cardiovascular tissue. *Total annual research expenditures:* $32.4 million. *Unit head:* Dr. Toni M. Ganzel, Dean, 502-852-1499, Fax: 502-852-1484, E-mail: meddean@louisville.edu. *Application contact:* Director of Admissions, 502-852-5793, Fax: 502-852-6849.
Website: http://louisville.edu/medicine/departments

University of Maryland, Baltimore, School of Medicine, Professional Program in Medicine, Baltimore, MD 21201. Offers MD, MD/PhD. *Accreditation:* LCME/AMA. *Students:* 641 full-time (370 women), 10 part-time (7 women); includes 246 minority (34 Black or African American, non-Hispanic/Latino; 1 American Indian or Alaska Native, non-Hispanic/Latino; 174 Asian, non-Hispanic/Latino; 25 Hispanic/Latino; 12 Two or more races, non-Hispanic/Latino), 5 international. Average age 25. 5,263 applicants, 7% accepted, 174 enrolled. In 2015, 157 doctorates awarded. *Entrance requirements:* For doctorate, MCAT, AMCAS application, science coursework. *Application deadline:* For fall admission, 11/1 for domestic students. Applications are processed on a rolling basis. Application fee: $70. Electronic applications accepted. *Expenses:* Contact institution. *Financial support:* Federal Work-Study and scholarships/grants available. Financial award application deadline: 3/15; financial award applicants required to submit FAFSA. *Unit head:* Dr. E. Albert Reece, Dean and Vice President for Medical Affairs, 410-706-7410, Fax: 410-706-0235, E-mail: deanmed@som.umaryland.edu. *Application contact:*

Dr. Milford M. Foxwell, Jr., Associate Dean for Admissions, 410-706-7478, Fax: 410-706-0467, E-mail: admissions@som.umaryland.edu.

University of Massachusetts Medical School, School of Medicine, Worcester, MA 01655-0115. Offers MD. *Accreditation:* LCME/AMA. *Faculty:* 1,339 full-time (521 women), 301 part-time/adjunct (189 women). *Students:* 515 full-time (274 women); includes 149 minority (24 Black or African American, non-Hispanic/Latino; 1 American Indian or Alaska Native, non-Hispanic/Latino; 105 Asian, non-Hispanic/Latino; 19 Hispanic/Latino). Average age 27. 1,266 applicants, 17% accepted, 125 enrolled. In 2015, 123 doctorates awarded. *Degree requirements:* For doctorate, U.S. Medical Licensing Examination Step 1 and Step 2 (CS and CK). *Entrance requirements:* For doctorate, MCAT, state residency; bachelor's degree. *Application deadline:* For fall admission, 12/15 for domestic students. Applications are processed on a rolling basis. Application fee: $100. Electronic applications accepted. *Expenses:* $25,510 per year. *Financial support:* In 2015–16, 444 students received support. Institutionally sponsored loans, scholarships/grants, health care benefits, tuition waivers (partial), and unspecified assistantships available. Financial award application deadline: 4/1; financial award applicants required to submit FAFSA. *Faculty research:* RNA interference, cell dynamics, immunology and virology, chemical biology, stem cell research. *Total annual research expenditures:* $250.3 million. *Unit head:* Dr. Terence R. Flotte, Dean/Provost/Executive Deputy Chancellor, 508-856-8000, E-mail: terry.flotte@umassmed.edu. *Application contact:* Dr. Mariann M. Manno, Associate Dean for Admissions, 508-856-2323, Fax: 508-856-3629, E-mail: mariann.manno@umassmed.edu.
Website: http://www.umassmed.edu/som

University of Miami, Graduate School, Miller School of Medicine, Professional Program in Medicine, Coral Gables, FL 33124. Offers MD. *Accreditation:* LCME/AMA. *Entrance requirements:* For doctorate, MCAT, 90 pre-med semester hours. Electronic applications accepted. *Faculty research:* AIDS, cancer, diabetes, neuroscience, wound healing.

University of Michigan, Medical School and Rackham Graduate School, Medical Scientist Training Program, Ann Arbor, MI 48109. Offers MD/PhD. *Accreditation:* LCME/AMA. *Students:* 92 full-time (39 women); includes 44 minority (2 Black or African American, non-Hispanic/Latino; 1 American Indian or Alaska Native, non-Hispanic/Latino; 38 Asian, non-Hispanic/Latino; 3 Hispanic/Latino). 337 applicants, 11% accepted, 10 enrolled. *Application deadline:* For fall admission, 10/15 for domestic students. Applications are processed on a rolling basis. Application fee: $160. Electronic applications accepted. *Financial support:* In 2015–16, 92 students received support, including 81 fellowships with full tuition reimbursements available (averaging $29,025 per year), 7 research assistantships with full tuition reimbursements available (averaging $29,025 per year), 4 teaching assistantships with full tuition reimbursements available (averaging $29,025 per year); scholarships/grants, traineeships, and health care benefits also available. *Unit head:* Dr. Ronald J. Koenig, Director, 734-764-6176, Fax: 734-764-8180, E-mail: rkoenig@umich.edu. *Application contact:* Laurie Koivupalo, Administrative Associate, 734-764-6176, Fax: 734-764-8180, E-mail: lkoivupl@umich.edu.
Website: http://www.med.umich.edu/medschool/mstp/

University of Michigan, Medical School, Professional Program in Medicine, Ann Arbor, MI 48109. Offers MD, MD/MA Edu, MD/MBA, MD/MPH, MD/MPP, MD/MS, MD/MSI, MD/PhD. *Accreditation:* LCME/AMA. *Faculty:* 2,235 full-time (1,434 women), 1,290 part-time/adjunct (663 women). *Students:* 732 full-time (372 women); includes 261 minority (44 Black or African American, non-Hispanic/Latino; 3 American Indian or Alaska Native, non-Hispanic/Latino; 90 Asian, non-Hispanic/Latino; 51 Hispanic/Latino; 73 Native Hawaiian or other Pacific Islander, non-Hispanic/Latino). Average age 26. 5,726 applicants, 7% accepted, 170 enrolled. In 2015, 169 doctorates awarded. *Entrance requirements:* For doctorate, MCAT. *Application deadline:* For fall admission, 9/30 for domestic students. Applications are processed on a rolling basis. Application fee: $85. Electronic applications accepted. *Expenses:* Contact institution. *Financial support:* In 2015–16, 458 students received support. Institutionally sponsored loans and scholarships/grants available. Financial award application deadline: 3/31; financial award applicants required to submit FAFSA. *Unit head:* Dr. James O. Woolliscroft, Dean, 734-764-8175, Fax: 734-763-4936, E-mail: woolli@umich.edu. *Application contact:* Carol Teener, Director of Admissions, 734-764-6317, Fax: 734-936-3510, E-mail: cteener@umich.edu.
Website: http://medicine.umich.edu/medschool/

University of Minnesota, Duluth, Medical School, Professional Program in Medicine, Duluth, MN 55812-2496. Offers MD. Program offered jointly with University of Minnesota, Twin Cities Campus. *Entrance requirements:* For doctorate, MCAT. Electronic applications accepted.

University of Minnesota, Twin Cities Campus, Medical School, Minneapolis, MN 55455-0213. Offers MA, MS, DPT, MD, PhD, JD/MD, MD/MBA, MD/MHI, MD/MPH, MD/MS, MD/PhD. *Accreditation:* LCME/AMA. *Program availability:* Part-time, evening/weekend. *Expenses:* Contact institution.

University of Mississippi Medical Center, School of Medicine, Jackson, MS 39216-4505. Offers MD, MD/PhD. *Accreditation:* LCME/AMA. *Program availability:* Part-time. *Entrance requirements:* For doctorate, MCAT. Electronic applications accepted.

University of Missouri, School of Medicine, Professional Program in Medicine, Columbia, MO 65211. Offers MD, MD/PhD. *Accreditation:* LCME/AMA. *Entrance requirements:* For doctorate, MCAT, minimum GPA of 3.49. *Faculty research:* Basic and clinical biomedical sciences.

University of Missouri–Kansas City, School of Medicine, Kansas City, MO 64110-2499. Offers anesthesia (MS); bioinformatics (MS); health professions education (MS); medicine (MD); physician assistant (MMS); MD/PhD. *Accreditation:* LCME/AMA. *Faculty:* 41 full-time (15 women), 15 part-time/adjunct (7 women). *Students:* 483 full-time (255 women), 39 part-time (25 women); includes 254 minority (34 Black or African American, non-Hispanic/Latino; 3 American Indian or Alaska Native, non-Hispanic/Latino; 172 Asian, non-Hispanic/Latino; 16 Hispanic/Latino; 1 Native Hawaiian or other Pacific Islander, non-Hispanic/Latino; 28 Two or more races, non-Hispanic/Latino), 10 international. Average age 24. 1,004 applicants, 13% accepted, 104 enrolled. In 2015, 22 master's, 119 doctorates awarded. *Degree requirements:* For doctorate, one foreign language, United States Medical Licensing Exam Step 1 and 2. *Entrance requirements:* For doctorate, interview. *Application deadline:* For fall admission, 11/15 for domestic and international students. Application fee: $50. *Expenses:* Contact institution. *Financial support:* In 2015–16, 3 fellowships (averaging $38,566 per year), 4 research assistantships (averaging $13,200 per year) were awarded; career-related internships or fieldwork, Federal Work-Study, institutionally sponsored loans, scholarships/grants, and tuition waivers (partial) also available. Financial award application deadline: 3/1; financial award applicants required to submit FAFSA. *Faculty research:* Cardiovascular disease, women's and children's health, trauma and infectious diseases, neurological, metabolic disease. *Unit head:* Dr. Steven L. Kanter, MD, Dean, 816-235-1803, E-mail: kantersl@umkc.edu. *Application contact:* Janine Kluckhohn, Admissions Coordinator, 816-235-1870, Fax: 816-235-6579, E-mail: kluckhohnj@umkc.edu.
Website: http://www.med.umkc.edu/

University of Nebraska Medical Center, College of Medicine, Omaha, NE 68198-5527. Offers MD, Certificate, MD/MPH, MD/PhD. *Accreditation:* LCME/AMA. *Faculty:* 725 full-time, 146 part-time/adjunct. *Students:* 503 full-time (199 women); includes 72 minority (17 Black or African American, non-Hispanic/Latino; 1 American Indian or Alaska Native, non-Hispanic/Latino; 43 Asian, non-Hispanic/Latino; 11 Hispanic/Latino). Average age 24. 1,838 applicants, 9% accepted, 127 enrolled. In 2015, 121 doctorates awarded. *Entrance requirements:* For doctorate, MCAT. *Application deadline:* For fall admission, 11/1 for domestic students. Applications are processed on a rolling basis. Application fee: $70. Electronic applications accepted. *Expenses:* Contact institution. *Financial support:* Career-related internships or fieldwork, Federal Work-Study, institutionally sponsored loans, and tuition waivers (full and partial) available. Financial award application deadline: 4/1; financial award applicants required to submit FAFSA. *Unit head:* Dr. Bradley E. Britigan, Dean, 402-559-4283, Fax: 402-559-4148, E-mail: bradley.britigan@unmc.edu. *Application contact:* Gigi R. Rogers, Program Coordinator, 402-559-2259, Fax: 402-559-6840, E-mail: comadmissions@unmc.edu.
Website: https://www.unmc.edu/com/prospective/admissions/index.html

University of New Mexico, School of Medicine, Professional Program in Medicine, Albuquerque, NM 87131-2039. Offers MD. *Degree requirements:* For doctorate, comprehensive exam, research. *Entrance requirements:* For doctorate, MCAT, general biology, general chemistry, organic chemistry, biochemistry and physics; minimum GPA of 3.0. Electronic applications accepted. *Expenses:* Contact institution. *Faculty research:* Cancer, infectious disease, brain and behavioral illness, children's health, cardiovascular and metabolic disease.

The University of North Carolina at Chapel Hill, School of Medicine, Professional Program in Medicine, Chapel Hill, NC 27599. Offers MD, MD/MPH, MD/PhD. *Accreditation:* LCME/AMA. *Entrance requirements:* For doctorate, MCAT.

University of North Dakota, School of Medicine and Health Sciences, Professional Program in Medicine, Grand Forks, ND 58202. Offers MD, MD/PhD. *Accreditation:* LCME/AMA. *Entrance requirements:* For doctorate, MCAT, minimum GPA of 3.0. Additional exam requirements/recommendations for international students: Required—TOEFL (minimum score 550 paper-based; 79 iBT), IELTS (minimum score 6.5). Electronic applications accepted.

University of Oklahoma Health Sciences Center, College of Medicine, Professional Program in Medicine, Oklahoma City, OK 73190. Offers MD, MD/PhD. *Accreditation:* LCME/AMA. *Entrance requirements:* For doctorate, MCAT. *Faculty research:* Behavior and drugs, structure and function of endothelium, genetics and behavior, gene structure and function, action of antibiotics.

University of Ottawa, Faculty of Graduate and Postdoctoral Studies, Faculty of Medicine, Ottawa, ON K1N 6N5, Canada. Offers M Sc, M, PhD. *Accreditation:* LCME/AMA. *Degree requirements:* For master's, thesis; for doctorate, thesis/dissertation (for some programs). *Entrance requirements:* For master's, honors degree or equivalent, minimum B average. Electronic applications accepted.

University of Pennsylvania, Perelman School of Medicine, Professional Program in Medicine, Philadelphia, PA 19104. Offers MD, MD/JD, MD/MBA, MD/MBE, MD/MS, MD/MSCE, MD/PhD. *Accreditation:* LCME/AMA. *Faculty:* 2,924 full-time (1,173 women), 1,197 part-time/adjunct (538 women). *Students:* 772 full-time (337 women); includes 337 minority (35 Black or African American, non-Hispanic/Latino; 166 Asian, non-Hispanic/Latino; 97 Hispanic/Latino; 39 Two or more races, non-Hispanic/Latino), 38 international. Average age 27. 5,436 applicants, 4% accepted, 156 enrolled. *Entrance requirements:* For doctorate, MCAT. Additional exam requirements/recommendations for international students: Required—TOEFL. *Application deadline:* For fall admission, 10/15 for domestic and international students. Application fee: $80. Electronic applications accepted. *Expenses: Tuition, area resident:* Full-time $31,068; part-time $5762 per course. *Required fees:* $3200; $336 per course. Full-time tuition and fees vary according to degree level, program and student level. Part-time tuition and fees vary according to course load, degree level and program. *Financial support:* In 2015–16, 360 students received support. Fellowships, research assistantships, teaching assistantships, career-related internships or fieldwork, Federal Work-Study, institutionally sponsored loans, and scholarships/grants available. Financial award application deadline: 5/1; financial award applicants required to submit FAFSA. *Unit head:* Dr. Gail Morrison, MD, Senior Vice Dean for Education, 215-898-8034, E-mail: morrisog@mail.med.upenn.edu. *Application contact:* Gaye Sheffler, Director, Admissions, 215-898-8000, E-mail: sheffler@mail.med.upenn.edu.

University of Pittsburgh, School of Medicine, Professional Program in Medicine, Pittsburgh, PA 15261. Offers MD. *Accreditation:* LCME/AMA. *Faculty:* 2,227 full-time (828 women), 94 part-time/adjunct (54 women). *Students:* 583 full-time (273 women); includes 270 minority (46 Black or African American, non-Hispanic/Latino; 3 American Indian or Alaska Native, non-Hispanic/Latino; 168 Asian, non-Hispanic/Latino; 32 Hispanic/Latino; 21 Two or more races, non-Hispanic/Latino), 8 international. Average age 26. 5,371 applicants, 7% accepted, 148 enrolled. In 2015, 150 doctorates awarded. *Degree requirements:* For doctorate, comprehensive exam, U.S. Medical Licensing Examination Steps 1 and 2, scholarly project. *Entrance requirements:* For doctorate, MCAT, undergraduate degree including at least one year of post secondary education in the United States or Canada; one year of course work each in biology (with lab), general or inorganic chemistry (with lab), organic chemistry (with lab), physics (with lab), and English. Additional exam requirements/recommendations for international students: Required—TOEFL (minimum score 600 paper-based; 100 iBT), IELTS (minimum score 7). *Application deadline:* For fall admission, 10/15 for domestic and international students. Applications are processed on a rolling basis. Application fee: $85. Electronic applications accepted. *Expenses:* Contact institution. *Financial support:* In 2015–16, 331 students received support. Institutionally sponsored loans and scholarships/grants available. Financial award application deadline: 4/15; financial award applicants required to submit FAFSA. *Faculty research:* Organ transplantation/immunology; cancer research and therapy; bioinformatics and computational biology; psychiatry, neurobiology, and systems neuroscience. *Total annual research expenditures:* $470.5 million. *Unit head:* Dr. Beth Piraino, Associate Dean of Admissions and Financial Aid, 412-648-9891, Fax: 412-648-8768, E-mail: piraino@pitt.edu. *Application contact:* Cynthia May Bonetti, Executive Director for Admissions and Financial Aid, 412-648-9891, Fax: 412-648-8768, E-mail: cmb103@pitt.edu.
Website: http://www.medschool.pitt.edu/

University of Puerto Rico, Medical Sciences Campus, School of Medicine, Professional Program in Medicine, San Juan, PR 00936-5067. Offers MD. *Accreditation:* LCME/AMA. *Degree requirements:* For doctorate, one foreign language. *Entrance requirements:* For doctorate, MCAT, minimum GPA of 2.5, computer literacy.

University of Rochester, School of Medicine and Dentistry, Professional Program in Medicine, Rochester, NY 14627. Offers MD, MD/MPH, MD/MS, MD/PhD. *Accreditation:* LCME/AMA. *Entrance requirements:* For doctorate, MCAT. *Expenses: Tuition, area resident:* Full-time $47,450; part-time $1482 per credit hour. *Required fees:* $528. Tuition and fees vary according to program.

University of Saskatchewan, College of Medicine, Professional Program in Medicine, Saskatoon, SK S7N 5A2, Canada. Offers MD. *Accreditation:* LCME/AMA.

University of South Alabama, College of Medicine, Professional Program in Medicine, Mobile, AL 36688. Offers MD. *Accreditation:* LCME/AMA. *Faculty:* 167 full-time (52

Allopathic Medicine

women), 17 part-time/adjunct (6 women). *Students:* 298 full-time (119 women); includes 71 minority (27 Black or African American, non-Hispanic/Latino; 1 American Indian or Alaska Native, non-Hispanic/Latino; 36 Asian, non-Hispanic/Latino; 2 Hispanic/Latino; 1 Native Hawaiian or other Pacific Islander, non-Hispanic/Latino; 4 Two or more races, non-Hispanic/Latino). Average age 25. In 2015, 74 doctorates awarded. *Degree requirements:* For doctorate, residency. *Entrance requirements:* For doctorate, MCAT. *Application deadline:* For fall admission, 11/15 for domestic and international students. *Application fee:* $75. Electronic applications accepted. *Expenses:* Tuition, state resident: full-time $9480; part-time $395 per credit hour. Tuition, nonresident: full-time $18,960; part-time $790 per credit hour. *Financial support:* Fellowships, research assistantships, teaching assistantships, career-related internships or fieldwork, Federal Work-Study, institutionally sponsored loans, scholarships/grants, and unspecified assistantships available. Support available to part-time students. Financial award application deadline: 5/31; financial award applicants required to submit FAFSA. *Unit head:* Mark Scott, Director, USA College of Medicine Admissions, 251-460-7176, Fax: 251-460-6278, E-mail: mscott@southalabama.edu. *Application contact:* Jonathan Scammell, Assistant Dean for Admissions, 251-460-7176, Fax: 251-460-6278, E-mail: jscammell@southalabama.edu.
Website: http://www.usahealthsystem.com/doctor-of-medicine

University of South Carolina, School of Medicine, Professional Program in Medicine, Columbia, SC 29208. Offers MD, MD/MPH, MD/PhD. *Accreditation:* LCME/AMA. *Entrance requirements:* For doctorate, MCAT. Electronic applications accepted. *Faculty research:* Cardiovascular diseases, oncology, reproductive biology, vision, neuroscience.

The University of South Dakota, Graduate School, Sanford School of Medicine, Professional Program in Medicine, Vermillion, SD 57069-2390. Offers MD. *Accreditation:* LCME/AMA. In 2015, 52 doctorates awarded. *Degree requirements:* For doctorate, U. S. Medical Licensing Exam-Step 1 and 2. *Entrance requirements:* For doctorate, MCAT, previous course work in biology, chemistry, organic chemistry, mathematics and physics. *Application deadline:* For fall admission, 11/15 for domestic and international students. Applications are processed on a rolling basis. Application fee: $35. Electronic applications accepted. *Financial support:* In 2015–16, 199 students received support. Institutionally sponsored loans and scholarships/grants available. *Unit head:* 605-357-1300, Fax: 605-375-1311, E-mail: med@usd.edu.
Website: http://www.usd.edu/med/

University of Southern California, Keck School of Medicine, Professional Program in Medicine, Los Angeles, CA 90089. Offers MD, MD/MBA, MD/MPH, MD/PhD. *Accreditation:* LCME/AMA. *Students:* 736 full-time (353 women); includes 394 minority (43 Black or African American, non-Hispanic/Latino; 2 American Indian or Alaska Native, non-Hispanic/Latino; 285 Asian, non-Hispanic/Latino; 63 Hispanic/Latino; 1 Native Hawaiian or other Pacific Islander, non-Hispanic/Latino), 1 international. Average age 24. 8,189 applicants, 5% accepted, 186 enrolled. In 2015, 168 doctorates awarded. *Entrance requirements:* For doctorate, MCAT, baccalaureate degree, or its equivalent, from accredited college or university. *Application deadline:* For fall admission, 11/1 for domestic and international students. Applications are processed on a rolling basis. Application fee: $100. Electronic applications accepted. *Expenses:* Contact institution. *Financial support:* In 2015–16, 127 students received support, including 16 research assistantships (averaging $27,500 per year); institutionally sponsored loans and scholarships/grants also available. Financial award application deadline: 4/15; financial award applicants required to submit FAFSA. *Unit head:* Dr. Raquel Arias, Associate Dean for Admissions, 323-442-2552, Fax: 323-442-2433, E-mail: medadmit@usc.edu. *Application contact:* Susan Wong, Admissions Coordinator, 323-442-2552, Fax: 323-442-2433, E-mail: medadmit@usc.edu.
Website: http://keck.usc.edu/

University of South Florida, Morsani College of Medicine, Tampa, FL 33620-9951. Offers MS, MSB, MSBCB, MSHI, MSMS, DPT, MD, PhD, DPT/MPH, PhD/MD. *Accreditation:* LCME/AMA. *Program availability:* Part-time. *Faculty:* 94 full-time (31 women), 15 part-time/adjunct (5 women). *Students:* 652 full-time (357 women), 1,011 part-time (508 women); includes 672 minority (144 Black or African American, non-Hispanic/Latino; 10 American Indian or Alaska Native, non-Hispanic/Latino; 287 Asian, non-Hispanic/Latino; 200 Hispanic/Latino; 1 Native Hawaiian or other Pacific Islander, non-Hispanic/Latino; 30 Two or more races, non-Hispanic/Latino), 52 international. Average age 28. 8,060 applicants, 14% accepted, 703 enrolled. In 2015, 330 master's, 241 doctorates awarded. Terminal master's awarded for partial completion of doctoral program. *Degree requirements:* For master's, comprehensive exam, thesis; for doctorate, comprehensive exam (for some programs), thesis/dissertation (for some programs). *Entrance requirements:* For master's, GRE General Test or GMAT, BA or equivalent degree from regionally-accredited university with minimum GPA of 3.0 in upper-division coursework; for doctorate, GRE General Test, BA or equivalent degree from regionally-accredited university with minimum GPA of 3.0 in upper-division sciences coursework; three letters of recommendation; personal interview; one- to two-page personal statement. Additional exam requirements/recommendations for international students: Required—TOEFL (minimum score 550 paper-based; 79 iBT). *Application deadline:* For fall admission, 2/15 for domestic students, 1/2 for international students. Application fee: $30. Electronic applications accepted. *Faculty research:* Allergy, immunology, and infectious diseases; cancer biology; cardiovascular research; neuroscience research; biomedical engineering; nanomedicine; neuromusculoskeletal disorders; pharmacogenomics; regenerative medicine; sport's medicine; women's health. *Total annual research expenditures:* $4.1 million. *Unit head:* Dr. Charles J. Lockwood, Dean, 813-974-0533, Fax: 813-974-4990, E-mail: cjlockwood@health.usf.edu. *Application contact:* Dr. Michael Barber, Associate Dean/Professor, 813-974-9702, Fax: 813-974-4990, E-mail: mbarber@health.usf.edu.
Website: http://health.usf.edu/medicine/index.htm

The University of Tennessee Health Science Center, College of Medicine, Memphis, TN 38163-0002. Offers MD, MD/PhD. *Accreditation:* LCME/AMA. *Entrance requirements:* For doctorate, MCAT. *Expenses:* Contact institution.

The University of Texas Health Science Center at Houston, University of Texas Medical School at Houston, Houston, TX 77225-0036. Offers MD, MD/MPH, MD/PhD. *Accreditation:* LCME/AMA. *Entrance requirements:* For doctorate, MCAT. Electronic applications accepted. *Expenses:* Contact institution. *Faculty research:* Stroke, infectious diseases, cardiovascular disease, neoplastic disease (cancer), molecular medicine for the prevention of diseases.

The University of Texas Health Science Center at San Antonio, School of Medicine, San Antonio, TX 78229-3900. Offers deaf education and hearing (MS); medicine (MD); MPH/MD. *Accreditation:* LCME/AMA. *Degree requirements:* For master's, comprehensive exam, practicum assignments. *Entrance requirements:* For master's, minimum GPA of 3.0, interview, 3 professional letters of recommendation; for doctorate, MCAT. Electronic applications accepted. *Expenses:* Contact institution. *Faculty research:* Geriatrics, diabetes, cancer, AIDS, obesity.

The University of Texas Medical Branch, School of Medicine, Galveston, TX 77555. Offers MD. *Accreditation:* LCME/AMA. *Entrance requirements:* For doctorate, MCAT. *Expenses:* Contact institution.

The University of Texas Rio Grande Valley, School of Medicine, Edinburg, TX 78539. Offers MD. *Program availability:* Part-time, evening/weekend, online learning. Tuition and fees vary according to course load and program.

The University of Texas Southwestern Medical Center, Southwestern Medical School, Dallas, TX 75390. Offers MD, MD/PhD. *Accreditation:* LCME/AMA. *Entrance requirements:* For doctorate, MCAT. Electronic applications accepted. *Expenses:* Contact institution. *Faculty research:* Endocrinology, molecular biology, immunology, cancer biology, neuroscience.

University of Toronto, Faculty of Medicine, Toronto, ON M5S 1A1, Canada. Offers M Sc, M Sc BMC, M Sc OT, M Sc PT, MH Sc, MD, PhD, MD/PhD. *Accreditation:* LCME/AMA. *Entrance requirements:* For doctorate, MCAT (for MD). Electronic applications accepted. *Expenses:* Contact institution.

University of Utah, School of Medicine, MD/PhD Program in Medicine, Salt Lake City, UT 84112-1107. Offers MD/PhD. *Program availability:* Part-time. Electronic applications accepted. *Faculty research:* Molecular biology, biochemistry, cell biology, immunology, bioengineering.

University of Utah, School of Medicine, Professional Program in Medicine, Salt Lake City, UT 84112-1107. Offers MD. *Accreditation:* LCME/AMA. *Entrance requirements:* For doctorate, MCAT, 2 years chemistry with lab, 1 year physics with lab, writing/speech, 2 courses biology, 1 course cell biology or biochemistry, 1 course humanities, 1 course diversity, 1 course social science. Electronic applications accepted. *Expenses:* Contact institution. *Faculty research:* Molecular biology, genetics, immunology, cardiology, endocrinology.

University of Virginia, School of Medicine, Charlottesville, VA 22903. Offers MPH, MS, MD, PhD, JD/MD, JD/MPH, MD/JD, MD/MBA, MD/PhD, MPP/MPH. *Accreditation:* LCME/AMA. *Entrance requirements:* For doctorate, MCAT (for MD). Additional exam requirements/recommendations for international students: Required—TOEFL. Electronic applications accepted.

University of Washington, Graduate School, School of Medicine, Professional Program in Medicine, Seattle, WA 98195. Offers MD, MD/MPH, MD/PhD. *Accreditation:* LCME/AMA. *Entrance requirements:* For doctorate, MCAT or GRE, minimum 3 years of college. Electronic applications accepted.

The University of Western Ontario, Faculty of Graduate Studies, Biosciences Division, Department of Family Medicine, London, ON N6A 5B8, Canada. Offers M Cl Sc. *Accreditation:* LCME/AMA. *Program availability:* Part-time, online learning. *Degree requirements:* For master's, thesis. *Entrance requirements:* For master's, medical degree, minimum B average. Additional exam requirements/recommendations for international students: Required—TOEFL. *Faculty research:* Family medicine education, dietary counseling, alcohol problems, palliative care support, multicultural health care.

The University of Western Ontario, Schulich School of Medicine and Dentistry, Professional Program in Medicine, London, ON N6A 5B8, Canada. Offers MD. *Accreditation:* LCME/AMA.

University of Wisconsin–Madison, School of Medicine and Public Health, Doctor of Medicine Program, Madison, WI 53705. Offers MD. *Accreditation:* LCME/AMA. *Faculty:* 1,310 full-time (496 women), 223 part-time/adjunct (120 women). *Students:* 727 full-time (358 women); includes 186 minority (27 Black or African American, non-Hispanic/Latino; 4 American Indian or Alaska Native, non-Hispanic/Latino; 108 Asian, non-Hispanic/Latino; 27 Hispanic/Latino; 20 Two or more races, non-Hispanic/Latino). Average age 25. 5,034 applicants, 5% accepted, 176 enrolled. *Entrance requirements:* For doctorate, MCAT. *Application deadline:* For fall admission, 11/1 for domestic students. Application fee: $56. *Expenses:* $13,369.60 resident tuition, $18,577.65 non-resident tuition, $571.20 campus fees. *Financial support:* In 2015–16, 250 students received support, including 5 fellowships with full tuition reimbursements available (averaging $18,378 per year), 13 research assistantships with full tuition reimbursements available (averaging $20,565 per year); institutionally sponsored loans, scholarships/grants, and tuition waivers (full and partial) also available. Support available to part-time students. Financial award applicants required to submit FAFSA. *Faculty research:* Biomedical research: population health, medical ethics, cancer research, neurosciences. *Total annual research expenditures:* $559 million. *Unit head:* Dr. Robert N. Golden, Dean, 608-263-4910, Fax: 608-265-3286, E-mail: rngolden@wisc.edu. *Application contact:* Becky Duffy, MD Admissions Advisor, 608-263-8228, Fax: 608-262-4226, E-mail: rlduffy@wisc.edu.
Website: http://www.med.wisc.edu/education/main/100

Vanderbilt University, School of Medicine, Nashville, TN 37240-1001. Offers MDE, MMP, MS, MSCI, Au D, DMP, MD, PhD, MD/PhD. *Accreditation:* LCME/AMA (one or more programs are accredited). *Students:* Average age 20. *Entrance requirements:* For doctorate, MCAT (for MD). *Application deadline:* For fall admission, 11/15 for domestic and international students. Application fee: $50. *Expenses:* Contact institution. *Financial support:* Institutionally sponsored loans and scholarships/grants available. Financial award application deadline: 3/1; financial award applicants required to submit FAFSA. *Unit head:* Dr. Jeffrey R. Balser, Dean, School of Medicine, 615-936-3030, E-mail: jeffrey.balser@vanderbilt.edu.
Website: http://www.mc.vanderbilt.edu/medschool/

Virginia Commonwealth University, Medical College of Virginia-Professional Programs, School of Medicine, Professional Program in Medicine, Richmond, VA 23284-9005. Offers MD, MD/MHA, MD/MPH, MD/PhD. *Accreditation:* LCME/AMA. *Entrance requirements:* For doctorate, MCAT. Electronic applications accepted. *Expenses:* Contact institution.

Wake Forest University, School of Medicine, Professional Program in Medicine, Winston-Salem, NC 27109. Offers MD, MD/MA, MD/MBA, MD/MS, MD/PhD. *Accreditation:* LCME/AMA. *Entrance requirements:* For doctorate, MCAT, 32 hours of course work in science. Electronic applications accepted. *Faculty research:* Cancer, stroke, infectious diseases, membrane biology, nutrition.

Washington University in St. Louis, School of Medicine, Professional Program in Medicine, St. Louis, MO 63130-4899. Offers MD, MD/MA, MD/MS, MD/PhD. *Accreditation:* LCME/AMA. *Degree requirements:* For doctorate, thesis/dissertation (for some programs). *Entrance requirements:* For doctorate, MCAT (for MD). Electronic applications accepted. *Expenses:* Contact institution.

Wayne State University, School of Medicine, Professional Program in Medicine, Detroit, MI 48202. Offers MD, MD/PhD. *Accreditation:* LCME/AMA. *Students:* 1,195 full-time (513 women), 63 part-time (34 women); includes 327 minority (45 Black or African American, non-Hispanic/Latino; 2 American Indian or Alaska Native, non-Hispanic/Latino; 251 Asian, non-Hispanic/Latino; 17 Hispanic/Latino; 12 Two or more races, non-Hispanic/Latino), 94 international. Average age 25. 4,701 applicants, 11% accepted, 290 enrolled. In 2015, 283 doctorates awarded. *Degree requirements:* For doctorate, National Board examinations Step 1 and 2. *Entrance requirements:* For doctorate, MCAT, bachelor's degree or equivalent, strong background in basic sciences, 2 semesters each of inorganic chemistry with labs, biology/zoology with labs, college English, organic chemistry with labs, physics with labs. Additional exam requirements/recommendations for international students: Required—TOEFL, TWE. *Application deadline:* For fall admission, 12/15 for domestic and international students. Application fee: $100. Electronic applications accepted. *Expenses:* $31,603 per year resident tuition, $64,640 non-residents tuition; fees include $22.50 per credit hour student services fee and $823 annual student support fee. *Financial support:* In 2015–16, 872 students received support. Scholarships/grants available. Financial award application deadline: 3/1; financial award applicants required to submit FAFSA. *Unit head:* Dr. Jack Sobel, Dean, 313-577-1335, Fax: 313-577-8777, E-mail: officeofthedean@med.wayne.edu. *Application contact:* Dr. Kevin Sprague, Interim Associate Dean for Admissions, 313-577-1466, Fax: 313-577-9420, E-mail: mdadmissions@wayne.edu. Website: http://home.med.wayne.edu/

West Virginia University, School of Medicine, Professional Program in Medicine, Morgantown, WV 26506. Offers MD, MD/PhD. *Accreditation:* LCME/AMA. *Entrance requirements:* For doctorate, MCAT. *Expenses:* Tuition, state resident: full-time $8568. Tuition, nonresident: full-time $22,140. Tuition and fees vary according to program.

Wright State University, School of Medicine, Professional Program in Medicine, Dayton, OH 45435. Offers MD. *Accreditation:* LCME/AMA. *Entrance requirements:* For doctorate, MCAT.

Yale University, School of Medicine, Professional Program in Medicine, New Haven, CT 06510. Offers MD. *Accreditation:* LCME/AMA. *Degree requirements:* For doctorate, thesis/dissertation. *Entrance requirements:* For doctorate, MCAT. Electronic applications accepted.

Bioethics

Albany Medical College, Alden March Bioethics Institute, Albany, NY 12208. Offers bioethics (MS, DPS); clinical ethics (Certificate); clinical ethics consultation (Certificate). *Program availability:* Part-time, evening/weekend, online learning. *Degree requirements:* For master's, thesis. *Entrance requirements:* For master's and Certificate, GRE, GMAT, LSAT, or MCAT (if no graduate degree), essay, official transcripts, 2 letters of reference. Additional exam requirements/recommendations for international students: Recommended—TOEFL. Electronic applications accepted. *Expenses:* Contact institution. *Faculty research:* Ethics in nanotechnology, ethics in genetics, ethics in transplants, philosophy and bioethics, the states and bioethics.

Case Western Reserve University, School of Medicine and School of Graduate Studies, Graduate Programs in Medicine, Department of Bioethics, Cleveland, OH 44106. Offers MA, JD/MA, MA/MD, MA/MPH, MA/PhD, MSN/MA, MSSA/MA. *Entrance requirements:* For master's, GRE General Test or MCAT or MAT or LSAT or GMAT. Additional exam requirements/recommendations for international students: Required—TOEFL (minimum score 550 paper-based). Electronic applications accepted. *Expenses: Tuition, area resident:* Full-time $41,137; part-time $1714 per credit hour. *Required fees:* $32. Tuition and fees vary according to course load and program. *Faculty research:* Ethical issues in genetics, conflicts of interest, organ donation, end-of-life decision making, clinical ethics consultation.

Clarkson University, Graduate School, Program in Bioethics, Potsdam, NY 13699. Offers bioethics (MS, AC), including bioethics policy (MS), clinical ethics, health policy and law (AC), research ethics. *Program availability:* Part-time, evening/weekend, 100% online, blended/hybrid learning. *Faculty:* 1 full-time (0 women), 8 part-time/adjunct (6 women). *Students:* 32 part-time (30 women); includes 5 minority (2 Black or African American, non-Hispanic/Latino; 1 Asian, non-Hispanic/Latino; 2 Two or more races, non-Hispanic/Latino), 3 international. Average age 43. In 2015, 14 master's, 7 other advanced degrees awarded. *Entrance requirements:* For master's, letters of recommendation. Additional exam requirements/recommendations for international students: Required—TOEFL (minimum score 550 paper-based). *Application deadline:* Applications are processed on a rolling basis. Application fee: $60. Electronic applications accepted. *Expenses:* Contact institution. *Financial support:* Federal Work-Study, scholarships/grants, health care benefits, and tuition waivers (partial) available. Support available to part-time students. Financial award applicants required to submit FAFSA. *Faculty research:* Bioethics education, clinical ethics consultation, research ethics, history of biomedical ethics, international bioethics/research ethics. *Unit head:* Dr. Sean Philpott, Director, 518-631-9860, Fax: 518-631-9903, E-mail: sphilpott@clarkson.edu. *Application contact:* Ann Nolte, Assistant Director, 518-631-9860, Fax: 518-631-9903, E-mail: anolte@clarkson.edu.
Website: http://bioethics.clarkson.edu/

Cleveland State University, College of Graduate Studies, College of Liberal Arts and Social Sciences, Department of Philosophy and Comparative Religion, Cleveland, OH 44115. Offers bioethics (MA, Certificate), including bioethics (MA); philosophy (MA), including philosophy. *Program availability:* Part-time, evening/weekend. *Faculty:* 4 full-time (all women), 2 part-time/adjunct (1 woman). *Students:* 6 full-time (1 woman), 3 part-time (2 women); includes 1 minority (Hispanic/Latino). Average age 38. 5 applicants, 100% accepted, 5 enrolled. In 2015, 6 master's, 1 other advanced degree awarded. *Degree requirements:* For master's, comprehensive exam, thesis optional, 32 credit hours of coursework; for Certificate, 12 credit hours of coursework. *Entrance requirements:* For master's and Certificate, BA, BS, or equivalent degree with minimum GPA of 2.75. Additional exam requirements/recommendations for international students: Required—TOEFL (minimum score 550 paper-based; 78 iBT). *Application deadline:* For fall admission, 7/1 priority date for domestic students, 5/15 priority date for international students; for spring admission, 11/15 for domestic students, 11/1 for international students; for summer admission, 4/1 for domestic students, 3/15 for international students. Applications are processed on a rolling basis. Application fee: $30. Electronic applications accepted. *Expenses:* Tuition, state resident: full-time $9565. Tuition, nonresident: full-time $17,980. Tuition and fees vary according to program. *Financial support:* In 2015–16, 5 students received support, including 5 teaching assistantships with full tuition reimbursements available (averaging $4,000 per year); health care benefits, tuition waivers (full), and unspecified assistantships also available. Support available to part-time students. *Faculty research:* Ethics, early modern philosophy, bioethics, social and political philosophy, history of women philosophers. *Unit head:* Dr. Mary Ellen Waithe, Chairperson, 216-687-3900, Fax: 216-523-7482, E-mail: m.waithe@csuohio.edu. *Application contact:* Deborah L. Brown, Interim Assistant Director, Graduate Admissions, 216-523-7572, Fax: 216-687-5400, E-mail: d.l.brown@csuohio.edu.
Website: http://www.csuohio.edu/class/philosophy-religion/philosophy-religion

Columbia University, School of Continuing Education, Program in Bioethics, New York, NY 10027. Offers MS. *Program availability:* Part-time. *Degree requirements:* For master's, thesis. Electronic applications accepted.

Duke University, Graduate School, Program in Bioethics and Science Policy, Durham, NC 27708-0141. Offers MA. *Entrance requirements:* For master's, GRE General Test. Additional exam requirements/recommendations for international students: Required—TOEFL (minimum score 577 paper-based; 90 iBT) or IELTS (minimum score 7).

Duquesne University, Graduate School of Liberal Arts, Center for Healthcare Ethics, Pittsburgh, PA 15282-0001. Offers MA, DHCE, PhD, Certificate. *Program availability:* Part-time, 100% online. *Faculty:* 3 full-time (0 women). *Students:* 47 full-time (24 women), 4 part-time (all women); includes 9 minority (6 Black or African American, non-Hispanic/Latino; 3 Asian, non-Hispanic/Latino), 16 international. Average age 38. 21 applicants, 67% accepted, 10 enrolled. In 2015, 8 doctorates awarded. Terminal

master's awarded for partial completion of doctoral program. *Degree requirements:* For doctorate, 2 foreign languages, comprehensive exam, thesis/dissertation. *Entrance requirements:* For master's, GRE General Test; for doctorate, GRE General Test, master's degree in health care ethics. Additional exam requirements/recommendations for international students: Required—TOEFL. *Application deadline:* For fall admission, 8/1 for domestic students, 5/1 for international students. Application fee: $0. Electronic applications accepted. *Expenses:* $1,189 per credit. *Financial support:* In 2015–16, 6 teaching assistantships (averaging $18,000 per year) were awarded; Federal Work-Study and tuition waivers (full and partial) also available. Support available to part-time students. Financial award application deadline: 5/1. *Unit head:* Dr. Henk Ten Have, Director, 412-396-1585, E-mail: tenhaveh@duq.edu. *Application contact:* Linda Rendulic, Assistant to the Dean, 412-396-6400, Fax: 412-396-5197, E-mail: rendulic@duq.edu.
Website: http://www.duq.edu/academics/schools/liberal-arts/graduate-school/programs/healthcare-ethics

Emory University, Laney Graduate School, Emory Center for Ethics, Atlanta, GA 30322-1100. Offers bioethics (MA). Terminal master's awarded for partial completion of doctoral program. *Degree requirements:* For master's, practicum experience, capstone project. *Entrance requirements:* Additional exam requirements/recommendations for international students: Recommended—TOEFL. Electronic applications accepted.

Icahn School of Medicine at Mount Sinai, The Bioethics Program, New York, NY 10029-6504. Offers MS. Program offered jointly with Union Graduate College.

Indiana University–Purdue University Indianapolis, School of Liberal Arts, Department of Philosophy, Indianapolis, IN 46202. Offers American philosophy (Certificate); bioethics (Certificate); philosophy (MA); JD/MA; MD/MA. *Program availability:* Part-time. *Degree requirements:* For master's, thesis optional. *Entrance requirements:* For master's, GRE. Additional exam requirements/recommendations for international students: Required—TOEFL. Electronic applications accepted. *Faculty research:* American philosophy, Peirce bioethics, metaphysics, ethical theory.

Instituto Tecnologico de Santo Domingo, Graduate School, Area of Health Sciences, Santo Domingo, Dominican Republic. Offers bioethics (M Bioethics); clinical bioethics (Certificate); clinical nutrition (Certificate); comprehensive health and the adolescent (Certificate); comrehensive adloescent health (MS); health and social security (M Mgmt).

Johns Hopkins University, Bloomberg School of Public Health, Berman Institute of Bioethics, Baltimore, MD 21218. Offers MBE. *Degree requirements:* For master's, thesis, practicum.

Johns Hopkins University, Bloomberg School of Public Health, Department of Health Policy and Management, Baltimore, MD 21205-1996. Offers bioethics and policy (PhD); health and public policy (PhD); health care management and leadership (Dr PH); health economics (MHS); health economics and policy (PhD); health finance and management (MHA); health policy (MSPH); health services research and policy (PhD); public policy (MPP). *Accreditation:* CAHME (one or more programs are accredited). *Program availability:* Part-time. *Degree requirements:* For master's, thesis (for some programs), internship (for some programs); for doctorate, comprehensive exam, thesis/dissertation, 1-year full-time residency (for some programs), oral and written exams. *Entrance requirements:* For master's, GRE General Test or GMAT, 3 letters of recommendation, curriculum vitae/resume; for doctorate, GRE General Test or GMAT, 3 letters of recommendation, curriculum vitae, transcripts. Additional exam requirements/recommendations for international students: Recommended—TOEFL (minimum score 600 paper-based; 100 iBT), IELTS. Electronic applications accepted. *Faculty research:* Quality of care and health outcomes, health care finance and technology, health disparities and vulnerable populations, injury prevention, health policy and health care policy.

Kansas City University of Medicine and Biosciences, College of Biosciences, Kansas City, MO 64106-1453. Offers bioethics (MA); biomedical sciences (MS). *Program availability:* Part-time. *Degree requirements:* For master's, comprehensive exam, thesis (for some programs). *Entrance requirements:* For master's, MCAT, GRE.

Loma Linda University, School of Religion, Program in Bioethics, Loma Linda, CA 92350. Offers MA, Certificate. *Degree requirements:* For master's, comprehensive exam, thesis optional. *Entrance requirements:* For master's, GRE General Test, baccalaureate degree. Additional exam requirements/recommendations for international students: Required—TOEFL. *Application deadline:* For fall admission, 8/1 for domestic and international students; for winter admission, 11/1 for domestic and international students; for spring admission, 2/1 for domestic and international students. Application fee: $60. Electronic applications accepted. *Unit head:* Dr. Jon Paulien, Dean, 909-824-4536. *Application contact:* Admissions Officer, 909-651-5029, Fax: 909-558-4879, E-mail: admissions.app@llu.edu.

Loyola Marymount University, College of Liberal Arts, The Bioethics Institute, Program in Bioethics, Los Angeles, CA 90045. Offers MA. *Program availability:* Part-time. *Faculty:* 1 full-time (0 women). *Students:* 11 full-time (7 women), 2 part-time (1 woman); includes 3 minority (2 Hispanic/Latino; 1 Two or more races, non-Hispanic/Latino), 3 international. Average age 36. 8 applicants, 100% accepted, 7 enrolled. In 2015, 2 master's awarded. *Entrance requirements:* For master's, GRE or MAT, personal statement, interview, letters of recommendation. Additional exam requirements/recommendations for international students: Required—TOEFL (minimum score 600 paper-based; 100 iBT). *Application deadline:* For fall admission, 3/1 for domestic students; for spring admission, 10/1 for domestic students. Applications are processed on a rolling basis. Application fee: $50. Electronic applications accepted. *Financial*

Bioethics

support: In 2015–16, 11 students received support. Scholarships/grants and unspecified assistantships available. Support available to part-time students. Financial award application deadline: 6/1; financial award applicants required to submit FAFSA. *Unit head:* Dr. Roberto Dell'Oro, Director, Bioethics Institute, 310-338-2752, E-mail: rdelloro@lmu.edu. *Application contact:* Chake H. Kouyoumjian, Associate Dean of Graduate Studies, 310-338-2721, E-mail: ckouyoum@lmu.edu.
Website: http://bellarmine.lmu.edu/bioethics

Loyola University Chicago, Graduate School, Neiswanger Institute for Bioethics, Chicago, IL 60660. Offers D Be, Certificate, MD/MA. *Program availability:* Online learning. *Students:* 25 full-time (13 women), 91 part-time (53 women); includes 24 minority (12 Black or African American, non-Hispanic/Latino; 4 Asian, non-Hispanic/Latino; 6 Hispanic/Latino; 1 Native Hawaiian or other Pacific Islander, non-Hispanic/Latino; 1 Two or more races, non-Hispanic/Latino). Average age 48. 21 applicants, 86% accepted, 17 enrolled. In 2015, 10 doctorates, 13 Certificates awarded. *Expenses: Tuition, area resident:* Full-time $18,054; part-time $9027 per credit hour. *Required fees:* $832; $284 per credit hour. Part-time tuition and fees vary according to course load, degree level and program. *Financial support:* Scholarships/grants available. *Unit head:* Dr. Samuel Attoh, Dean, 773-508-8948, Fax: 773-508-2460, E-mail: sattoh@luc.edu. *Application contact:* Ron Martin, Assistant Director of Enrollment Management, 312-915-8950, Fax: 312-915-8905, E-mail: gradapp@luc.edu.

Loyola University Chicago, Graduate School, Program in Bioethics, Chicago, IL 60660. Offers D Be. *Program availability:* Online learning. *Entrance requirements:* For doctorate, master's degree in bioethics or health care ethics. *Expenses: Tuition, area resident:* Full-time $18,054; part-time $9027 per credit hour. *Required fees:* $832; $284 per credit hour. Part-time tuition and fees vary according to course load, degree level and program. *Unit head:* Dr. Samuel Attoh, Dean, 773-508-8948, Fax: 773-508-2460, E-mail: sattoh@luc.edu. *Application contact:* Ron Martin, Assistant Director of Enrollment Management, 312-915-8950, Fax: 312-915-8905, E-mail: gradapp@luc.edu.

McGill University, Faculty of Graduate and Postdoctoral Studies, Faculty of Arts, Department of Philosophy, Montréal, QC H3A 2T5, Canada. Offers bioethics (MA); philosophy (PhD).

McGill University, Faculty of Graduate and Postdoctoral Studies, Faculty of Law, Montréal, QC H3A 2T5, Canada. Offers air and space law (LL M, DCL, Graduate Certificate); bioethics (LL M); comparative law (LL M, DCL, Graduate Certificate); law (LL M, DCL). Applications for LL M with specialization in bioethics are made initially through the Biomedical Ethics Unit in the Faculty of Medicine.

McGill University, Faculty of Graduate and Postdoctoral Studies, Faculty of Medicine, Department of Medicine, Montréal, QC H3A 2T5, Canada. Offers experimental medicine (M Sc, PhD), including bioethics (M Sc), experimental medicine.

Medical College of Wisconsin, Graduate School of Biomedical Sciences, Center for Bioethics and Medical Humanities, Milwaukee, WI 53226-0509. Offers bioethics (MA); clinical bioethics (Graduate Certificate); research ethics (Graduate Certificate). *Program availability:* Part-time. *Degree requirements:* For master's, thesis. *Entrance requirements:* For master's and Graduate Certificate, GRE, official transcripts, three letters of recommendation. Additional exam requirements/recommendations for international students: Required—TOEFL. *Faculty research:* Ethics committees and consultation, ethics of managed care, discussion of code status by physicians.

New York University, Graduate School of Arts and Science, Program in Bioethics, New York, NY 10012-1019. Offers MA. *Program availability:* Part-time. *Entrance requirements:* For master's, one foreign language. *Entrance requirements:* For master's, GRE General Test. Additional exam requirements/recommendations for international students: Required—TOEFL.

Northeast Ohio Medical University, College of Graduate Studies, Rootstown, OH 44272-0095. Offers bioethics (Certificate); health-system pharmacy administration (MS); integrated pharmaceutical medicine (MS, PhD); public health (MS). *Program availability:* Part-time. *Faculty:* 15 part-time/adjunct (6 women). *Students:* 15 full-time (7 women), 26 part-time (11 women); includes 7 minority (5 Asian, non-Hispanic/Latino; 2 Hispanic/Latino). Average age 27. In 2015, 9 master's, 1 doctorate awarded. *Application deadline:* For fall admission, 9/1 priority date for domestic students; for winter admission, 1/5 priority date for domestic students. Applications are processed on a rolling basis. Electronic applications accepted. *Expenses:* Contact institution. *Financial support:* In 2015–16, 18 students received support. *Unit head:* Dr. Walter E. Horton, Jr., Dean. *Application contact:* Heidi Terry, Executive Director, Enrollment Services, 330-325-6479, E-mail: hterry@neoucom.edu.
Website: http://www.neomed.edu/academics/graduatestudies

Oregon State University, College of Liberal Arts, Program in Applied Ethics, Corvallis, OR 97331. Offers art and morality (MA); bioethics (MA); environmental ethics (MA). *Program availability:* Part-time. *Faculty:* 10 full-time (4 women), 1 (woman) part-time/adjunct. *Students:* 8 full-time (6 women), 3 part-time (0 women); includes 3 minority (all Hispanic/Latino). Average age 29. 14 applicants, 57% accepted, 6 enrolled. In 2015, 1 master's awarded. *Entrance requirements:* For master's, writing sample of 5-7 pages. Additional exam requirements/recommendations for international students: Required—TOEFL (minimum score 80 iBT), IELTS (minimum score 6.5). *Application deadline:* For fall admission, 1/15 priority date for domestic and international students. Application fee: $75 ($85 for international students). *Expenses: Tuition, state resident:* full-time $12,150; part-time $450 per credit. *Tuition, nonresident:* full-time $20,952; part-time $776 per credit. *Required fees:* $1572; $1443 per unit. *One-time fee:* $350. Tuition and fees vary according to course load, campus/location and program. *Unit head:* Dr. Ben Mutschler, Director. *Application contact:* Dr. Allen Thompson, Director of Graduate Studies, 541-737-5654, E-mail: allen.thompson@oregonstate.edu.
Website: http://liberalarts.oregonstate.edu/shpr/philosophy

Saint Louis University, Graduate Education, Center for Health Care Ethics, St. Louis, MO 63103. Offers clinical health care ethics (Certificate); health care ethics (PhD). *Degree requirements:* For doctorate, comprehensive exam, thesis/dissertation. *Entrance requirements:* For doctorate, GRE General Test, master's degree in ethics or a field related to health care, basic competencies in philosophical and applied ethics, transcripts. Additional exam requirements/recommendations for international students: Required—TOEFL (minimum score 525 paper-based). Electronic applications accepted. *Faculty research:* Health policy, clinical ethics, research ethics, empirical bioethics, ethics education and assessment.

Stony Brook University, State University of New York, Stony Brook Medicine, School of Medicine, Center for Medical Humanities, Compassionate Care, and Bioethics, Stony Brook, NY 11794. Offers MD/MA. *Students:* 11 full-time (6 women), 5 part-time (3 women); includes 1 minority (Asian, non-Hispanic/Latino). Average age 28. 18 applicants, 83% accepted, 12 enrolled. *Entrance requirements:* Additional exam requirements/recommendations for international students: Required—TOEFL. *Application deadline:* For fall admission, 7/1 for domestic students, 5/15 for international students; for spring admission, 11/1 for domestic students, 10/1 for international students. Application fee: $100. *Expenses:* $12,421 per year full-time resident tuition and fees, $453 per credit hour; $23,761 per year full-time out-of-state tuition and fees, $925 per credit hour. *Financial support:* Fellowships available. *Unit head:* Dr. Stephen

G. Post, Director, 631-444-9797, E-mail: stephen.post@stonybrookmedicine.edu. *Application contact:* Michael Ortega, Program Coordinator, 631-444-8029, E-mail: michael.ortega@stonybrookmedicine.edu.
Website: http://www.stonybrook.edu/bioethics/index.shtml

Trinity International University, Trinity Graduate School, Deerfield, IL 60015-1284. Offers bioethics (MA); communication and culture (MA); counseling psychology (MA); instructional leadership (M Ed); teaching (MA). *Program availability:* Part-time, evening/weekend, online learning. *Degree requirements:* For master's, comprehensive exam. *Entrance requirements:* For master's, GRE General Test or MAT, minimum undergraduate GPA of 3.0. Additional exam requirements/recommendations for international students: Required—TOEFL (minimum score 580 paper-based), TWE (minimum score 4). Electronic applications accepted.

Université de Montréal, Faculty of Medicine, Programs in Bioethics, Montréal, QC H3C 3J7, Canada. Offers MA, DESS. Electronic applications accepted.

Université de Montréal, Faculty of Theology and Sciences of Religions, Montréal, QC H3C 3J7, Canada. Offers health, spirituality and bioethics (DESS); practical theology (MA, PhD); religious sciences (MA, PhD); theology (MA, D Th, PhD, L Th); theology-Biblical studies (PhD). *Degree requirements:* For master's, one foreign language; for doctorate, 2 foreign languages, thesis/dissertation, general exam. Electronic applications accepted.

University of Mary, School of Health Sciences, Program in Bioethics, Bismarck, ND 58504-9652. Offers MS. *Degree requirements:* For master's, practicum, capstone project. *Application deadline:* For fall admission, 6/15 priority date for domestic students. Website: http://www.umary.edu/academics/programs/ms-bioethics.php

University of Pennsylvania, Perelman School of Medicine, Department of Medical Ethics and Health Policy, Philadelphia, PA 19104. Offers MBE, MSME, DMD/MBE, JD/MBE, LL M/MBE, MD/MBE, MPA/MBE, MS Ed/MBE, MSN/MBE, MSW/MBE, PhD/MBE. *Program availability:* Part-time, evening/weekend. *Faculty:* 12 full-time (4 women), 10 part-time/adjunct (4 women). *Students:* 22 full-time (5 women), 100 part-time (64 women); includes 37 minority (6 Black or African American, non-Hispanic/Latino; 15 Asian, non-Hispanic/Latino; 3 Hispanic/Latino; 13 Two or more races, non-Hispanic/Latino). Average age 31. 80 applicants, 86% accepted, 60 enrolled. In 2015, 37 master's awarded. *Degree requirements:* For master's, thesis. *Entrance requirements:* For master's, transcript, essay. *Application deadline:* Applications are processed on a rolling basis. Application fee: $70. *Expenses: Tuition, area resident:* Full-time $31,068; part-time $5762 per course. *Required fees:* $3200; $336 per course. Full-time tuition and fees vary according to degree level, program and student level. Part-time tuition and fees vary according to course load, degree level and program. *Financial support:* Teaching assistantships, career-related internships or fieldwork, Federal Work-Study, institutionally sponsored loans, scholarships/grants, health care benefits, and unspecified assistantships available. *Unit head:* Dr. Autumn Fiester, Director of Education, 215-573-2602, Fax: 215-573-3036, E-mail: fiester@mail.med.upenn.edu. *Application contact:* Tiffany Albright, Program Coordinator, 215-573-4042.
Website: http://medicalethics.med.upenn.edu/

University of Pittsburgh, Dietrich School of Arts and Sciences, Center for Bioethics and Health Law, Pittsburgh, PA 15260. Offers bioethics (MA). *Program availability:* Part-time. *Faculty:* 11 full-time (3 women), 1 (woman) part-time/adjunct. *Students:* 3 full-time (all women), 3 part-time (2 women). Average age 29. 5 applicants, 60% accepted, 2 enrolled. In 2015, 3 master's awarded. *Degree requirements:* For master's, thesis. *Entrance requirements:* For master's, GRE General Test, MCAT, LSAT, letters of recommendation, writing sample, personal statement. Additional exam requirements/recommendations for international students: Required—TOEFL (minimum score 550 paper-based), IELTS (minimum score 7). *Application deadline:* For fall admission, 3/1 priority date for domestic and international students. Applications are processed on a rolling basis. Application fee: $50. Electronic applications accepted. Tuition and fees vary according to program. *Financial support:* Scholarships/grants and tuition waivers (partial) available. Financial award application deadline: 3/1. *Faculty research:* Ethics and genetics, research ethics, palliative care, mental health and ethics. *Unit head:* Lisa S. Parker, Director of Graduate Studies, 412-648-7007, Fax: 412-648-2649, E-mail: lisap@pitt.edu. *Application contact:* Beth Ann Pischke, Administrator, 412-648-7007, Fax: 412-648-2649, E-mail: pischke@pitt.edu.
Website: http://www.bioethics.pitt.edu

University of South Florida, Innovative Education, Tampa, FL 33620-9951. Offers adult, career and higher education (Graduate Certificate), including college teaching, leadership in developing human resources, leadership in higher education; Africana studies (Graduate Certificate), including diasporas and health disparities, genocide and human rights; aging studies (Graduate Certificate), including gerontology; art research (Graduate Certificate), including museum studies; business foundations (Graduate Certificate); chemical and biomedical engineering (Graduate Certificate), including materials science and engineering, water, health and sustainability; child and family studies (Graduate Certificate), including positive behavior support; civil and industrial engineering (Graduate Certificate), including transportation systems analysis; community and family health (Graduate Certificate), including maternal and child health, social marketing and public health, violence and injury: prevention and intervention, women's health; criminology (Graduate Certificate), including criminal justice administration; educational measurement and research (Graduate Certificate), including evaluation; English (Graduate Certificate), including comparative literary studies, creative writing, professional and technical communication; entrepreneurship (Graduate Certificate); environmental health (Graduate Certificate), including safety management; epidemiology and biostatistics (Graduate Certificate), including applied biostatistics, biostatistics, concepts and tools of epidemiology, epidemiology, epidemiology of infectious diseases; geography, environment and planning (Graduate Certificate), including community development, environmental policy and management, geographical information systems; geology (Graduate Certificate), including hydrogeology; global health (Graduate Certificate), including disaster management, global health and Latin American and Caribbean studies, global health practice, humanitarian assistance, infection control; government and international affairs (Graduate Certificate), including Cuban studies, globalization studies; health policy and management (Graduate Certificate), including health management and leadership, public health policy and programs; hearing specialist: early intervention (Graduate Certificate); industrial and management systems engineering (Graduate Certificate), including systems engineering, technology management; information studies (Graduate Certificate), including school library media specialist; information systems/decision sciences (Graduate Certificate), including analytics and business intelligence; instructional technology (Graduate Certificate), including distance education, Florida digital/virtual educator, instructional design, multimedia design, Web design; internal medicine, bioethics and medical humanities (Graduate Certificate), including biomedical ethics; Latin American and Caribbean studies (Graduate Certificate); mass communications (Graduate Certificate), including multimedia journalism; mathematics and statistics (Graduate Certificate), including mathematics; medicine (Graduate Certificate), including aging and neuroscience, bioinformatics, biotechnology, brain fitness and memory management, clinical investigation, health informatics, health sciences, integrative weight management, intellectual property, medicine and gender,

metabolic and nutritional medicine, metabolic cardiology, pharmacy sciences; national and competitive intelligence (Graduate Certificate); psychological and social foundations (Graduate Certificate), including career counseling, college teaching, diversity in education, mental health counseling, school counseling; public affairs (Graduate Certificate), including nonprofit management, public management, research administration; public health (Graduate Certificate), including environmental health, health equity, public health generalist, translational research in adolescent behavioral health; public health practices (Graduate Certificate), including planning for healthy communities; rehabilitation and mental health counseling (Graduate Certificate), including integrative mental health care, marriage and family therapy, rehabilitation technology; secondary education (Graduate Certificate), including ESOL, foreign language education: culture and content, foreign language education: professional; social work (Graduate Certificate), including geriatric social work/clinical gerontology; special education (Graduate Certificate), including autism spectrum disorder, disabilities education: severe/profound; world languages (Graduate Certificate), including teaching English as a second language (TESL) or foreign language. *Unit head:* Kathy Barnes, Interdisciplinary Programs Coordinator, 813-974-8031, Fax: 813-974-7061, E-mail: barnesk@usf.edu. *Application contact:* Karen Tylinski, Metro Initiatives, 813-974-9943, Fax: 813-974-7061, E-mail: ktylinsk@usf.edu.
Website: http://www.usf.edu/innovative-education/

The University of Tennessee, Graduate School, College of Arts and Sciences, Department of Philosophy, Knoxville, TN 37996. Offers medical ethics (MA, PhD); philosophy (MA, PhD); religious studies (MA). *Program availability:* Part-time. *Degree requirements:* For master's, thesis or alternative; for doctorate, one foreign language, thesis/dissertation. *Entrance requirements:* For master's and doctorate, GRE General Test, minimum GPA of 2.7. Additional exam requirements/recommendations for international students: Required—TOEFL. Electronic applications accepted.

University of Toronto, Faculty of Medicine, Institute of Medical Science, Toronto, ON M5S 1A1, Canada. Offers bioethics (MH Sc); biomedical communications (M Sc BMC); medical radiation science (MH Sc); medical science (PhD). *Degree requirements:* For master's, thesis; for doctorate, thesis/dissertation, thesis defense. *Entrance requirements:* For master's, minimum GPA of 3.7 in 3 of 4 years (M Sc), interview; for doctorate, M Sc or equivalent, defended thesis, minimum A- average, interview. Additional exam requirements/recommendations for international students: Required—TOEFL (minimum score 600 paper-based; 93 iBT), TWE (minimum score 5). Electronic applications accepted.

University of Washington, Graduate School, School of Medicine, Graduate Programs in Medicine, Department of Medical History and Ethics, Seattle, WA 98195. Offers bioethics (MA).

Washington State University, College of Arts and Sciences, School of Politics, Philosophy and Public Affairs, Pullman, WA 99164-4880. Offers bioethics (Graduate Certificate); political science (MA, PhD); public affairs (MPA). MPA, MA, and PhD programs also offered at the Vancouver campus; Graduate Certificate offered through Global (online) campus. *Program availability:* Online learning. Terminal master's awarded for partial completion of doctoral program. *Degree requirements:* For master's, comprehensive exam (for some programs), thesis, oral exam; for doctorate, comprehensive exam, thesis/dissertation, oral exam, written exam. *Entrance requirements:* For master's, GRE General Test, minimum GPA of 3.0; for doctorate, GRE General Test, minimum GPA of 3.5. Additional exam requirements/recommendations for international students: Required—TOEFL. Electronic applications accepted. *Faculty research:* Political psychology and image theory, grass roots environmental policy, federal juvenile policy.

Washington University in St. Louis, School of Medicine, Program in Clinical Investigation, St. Louis, MO 63130-4899. Offers clinical investigation (MS), including bioethics, entrepreneurship, genetics/genomics, translational medicine. *Program availability:* Part-time, evening/weekend. *Faculty:* 61 full-time (14 women), 2 part-time/ adjunct (both women). *Students:* 15 full-time (5 women), 39 part-time (19 women); includes 15 minority (3 Black or African American, non-Hispanic/Latino; 8 Asian, non-Hispanic/Latino; 2 Hispanic/Latino; 2 Two or more races, non-Hispanic/Latino), 3 international. Average age 32. 34 applicants, 65% accepted, 22 enrolled. In 2015, 35 master's awarded. *Degree requirements:* For master's, thesis. *Entrance requirements:* For master's, doctoral-level degree or in process of obtaining doctoral-level degree. *Application deadline:* For fall admission, 5/15 for domestic students; for spring admission, 10/15 for domestic students. Application fee: $0. Electronic applications accepted. *Financial support:* In 2015–16, 4 students received support. Tuition waivers (partial) available. Financial award application deadline: 12/12. *Faculty research:* Anesthesiology, infectious diseases, neurology, obstetrics and gynecology, orthopedic surgery. *Unit head:* Dr. David Warren, Associate Professor of Medicine, 314-454-8225, Fax: 314-454-8279, E-mail: dwarren@wustl.edu. *Application contact:* Suzie Fragale, Curriculum and Evaluation Coordinator, 314-454-8936, Fax: 314-454-8279, E-mail: fragale@wustl.edu.
Website: http://crtc.wustl.edu/

Naturopathic Medicine

Bastyr University, School of Naturopathic Medicine, Kenmore, WA 98028-4966. Offers ND. *Accreditation:* CNME; MEAC. *Program availability:* Part-time. *Degree requirements:* For doctorate, comprehensive exam. *Entrance requirements:* For doctorate, 1 year of course work each in biology, chemistry, organic chemistry and physics. Additional exam requirements/recommendations for international students: Required—TOEFL (minimum score 550 paper-based; 79 iBT). Electronic applications accepted. *Faculty research:* Integrative oncology, integrative care for neurodegenerative diseases, vitamin D supplementation, sauna (hyperthermia-based) detoxification, intranasal glutathione (nasal spray) for Parkinson's disease.

Canadian College of Naturopathic Medicine, Bachelor of Naturopathy Program, Toronto, ON M2K 1E2, Canada. Offers BN. *Accreditation:* CNME. *Degree requirements:* For BN, 12-month internship. *Entrance requirements:* For degree, 1 year of course work in general biology, humanities and physiology; 1 semester of course work in organic chemistry and psychology. Additional exam requirements/recommendations for international students: Recommended—TOEFL (minimum score 580 paper-based; 86 iBT), IELTS (minimum score 6.5). Electronic applications accepted. *Faculty research:* Natural health products for lung cancer; the use of habanero chili pepper for cancer; melatonin as an anticancer agent with and without chemotherapy; interactions between natural health products and pharmaceuticals; the use of selenium for patients with HIV/AIDS.

National College of Natural Medicine, School of Naturopathic Medicine, Portland, OR 97201. Offers integrative medicine research (MS); naturopathic medicine (ND). *Accreditation:* CNME. *Entrance requirements:* For master's, GRE. Additional exam requirements/recommendations for international students: Recommended—TOEFL. *Faculty research:* Diet and diabetes, whole practice research, cruciferous vegetables and cancer, natural medicine and immune function, taraxacum and diuretics.

Southwest College of Naturopathic Medicine and Health Sciences, Program in Naturopathic Medicine, Tempe, AZ 85282. Offers ND. *Accreditation:* CNME. *Faculty:* 21 full-time (10 women), 59 part-time/adjunct (41 women). *Students:* 367 full-time (271 women), 18 part-time (16 women); includes 136 minority (37 Black or African American, non-Hispanic/Latino; 3 American Indian or Alaska Native, non-Hispanic/Latino; 32 Asian, non-Hispanic/Latino; 45 Hispanic/Latino; 2 Native Hawaiian or other Pacific Islander, non-Hispanic/Latino; 17 Two or more races, non-Hispanic/Latino), 29 international. Average age 30. 179 applicants, 72% accepted, 83 enrolled. In 2015, 96 doctorates awarded. *Entrance requirements:* For doctorate, minimum GPA of 3.0, letters of recommendation, in-person interview. Additional exam requirements/recommendations for international students: Required—TOEFL (minimum score 637 paper-based; 110 iBT). *Application deadline:* For fall admission, 3/1 priority date for domestic and international students; for spring admission, 12/1 priority date for domestic and international students. Applications are processed on a rolling basis. Application fee: $115. Electronic applications accepted. *Expenses: Tuition, area resident:* Full-time $32,651; part-time $317 per credit. *Required fees:* $1740. One-time fee: $935 full-time. Tuition and fees vary according to course load, program and student level. *Financial support:* In 2015–16, 169 students received support. Federal Work-Study and scholarships/grants available. Financial award application deadline: 5/1; financial award applicants required to submit FAFSA. *Faculty research:* Antimicrobials, anticancer, immune modulation, botanicals. *Unit head:* Dr. Margot Gregory, Chief Academic Officer, 480-858-9100 Ext. 207, E-mail: m.gregory@scnm.edu. *Application contact:* Eve Adams, Director of Admissions, 480-858-9100 Ext. 213, Fax: 480-222-9413, E-mail: e.adams@scnm.edu.
Website: http://www.scnm.edu

Universidad del Turabo, Graduate Programs, School of Health Sciences, Program in Naturopathy, Gurabo, PR 00778-3030. Offers ND.

University of Bridgeport, College of Naturopathic Medicine, Bridgeport, CT 06604. Offers ND. *Accreditation:* CNME. *Degree requirements:* For doctorate, NPLEX Part I. *Entrance requirements:* For doctorate, minimum GPA of 2.5. Additional exam requirements/recommendations for international students: Recommended—TOEFL (minimum score 550 paper-based; 80 iBT), IELTS. *Application deadline:* For fall admission, 8/1 priority date for domestic and international students; for spring admission, 12/1 for domestic students, 2/1 priority date for international students. Applications are processed on a rolling basis. Application fee: $75. Electronic applications accepted. *Financial support:* Federal Work-Study, institutionally sponsored loans, and scholarships/grants available. Financial award application deadline: 4/1; financial award applicants required to submit FAFSA.

Osteopathic Medicine

A.T. Still University, Kirksville College of Osteopathic Medicine, Kirksville, MO 63501. Offers biomedical sciences (MS); osteopathic medicine (DO). *Accreditation:* AOsA. *Faculty:* 40 full-time (7 women), 32 part-time/adjunct (4 women). *Students:* 724 full-time (302 women), 7 part-time (1 woman); includes 129 minority (18 Black or African American, non-Hispanic/Latino; 2 American Indian or Alaska Native, non-Hispanic/Latino; 49 Asian, non-Hispanic/Latino; 31 Hispanic/Latino; 29 Two or more races, non-Hispanic/Latino), 3 international. Average age 26. 5,061 applicants, 8% accepted, 188 enrolled. In 2015, 12 master's, 156 doctorates awarded. *Degree requirements:* For master's, thesis; for doctorate, Level 1 and 2 COMLEX-PE and CE exams. *Entrance requirements:* For master's, GRE, MCAT, or DAT, minimum undergraduate GPA of 2.65 (cumulative and science); for doctorate, MCAT, bachelor's degree with minimum GPA of 2.8 (cumulative and science) or 90 semester hours with minimum GPA of 3.5 (cumulative and science). Additional exam requirements/recommendations for international students: Recommended—TOEFL. *Application deadline:* For fall admission, 2/1 for domestic students; for summer admission, 2/1 for domestic students. Applications are processed on a rolling basis. Application fee: $70. Electronic applications accepted. Application fee is waived when completed online. *Expenses:* Contact institution. *Financial support:* In 2015–16, 243 students received support, including 25 fellowships with full tuition reimbursements available (averaging $52,320 per year); Federal Work-Study and scholarships/grants also available. Financial award application deadline: 5/1; financial award applicants required to submit FAFSA. *Faculty research:* Practice-based research network, antibiotic resistance, staphylococcus aureus, bacterial virulence and environmental survival, excitability of the exercise pressor reflex, clinical trials. *Total annual research expenditures:* $164,130. *Unit head:* Dr. Margaret Wilson, Dean, 660-626-2354, Fax: 660-626-2080, E-mail: mwilson@atsu.edu. *Application contact:* Donna Sparks, Associate Director, Admissions Processing, 660-626-2117, Fax: 660-626-2969, E-mail: admissions@atsu.edu.
Website: http://www.atsu.edu/kcom/

Osteopathic Medicine

A.T. Still University, School of Osteopathic Medicine in Arizona, Mesa, AZ 85206. Offers DO. *Accreditation:* AOsA. *Faculty:* 39 full-time (18 women), 34 part-time/adjunct (10 women). *Students:* 428 full-time (211 women), 1 (woman) part-time; includes 204 minority (6 Black or African American, non-Hispanic/Latino; 1 American Indian or Alaska Native, non-Hispanic/Latino; 138 Asian, non-Hispanic/Latino; 34 Hispanic/Latino; 25 Two or more races, non-Hispanic/Latino). Average age 27. 5,978 applicants, 4% accepted, 108 enrolled. In 2015, 104 doctorates awarded. *Degree requirements:* For doctorate, Level 1 and 2 COMPLEX-PE and CE exams. *Entrance requirements:* For doctorate, MCAT, minimum undergraduate GPA of 2.8 (cumulative and science) with bachelor's degree. *Application deadline:* For fall admission, 3/1 for domestic students; for summer admission, 3/1 for domestic students. Applications are processed on a rolling basis. Application fee: $70. Electronic applications accepted. Application fee is waived when completed online. *Financial support:* In 2015–16, 30 students received support, including 2 fellowships (averaging $48,600 per year); Federal Work-Study and scholarships/grants also available. Financial award application deadline: 5/1; financial award applicants required to submit FAFSA. *Faculty research:* Medical education research, osteopathic medicine research, practice-based research network, QI within community health centers. *Total annual research expenditures:* $4,935. *Unit head:* Dr. Kay Kalousek, Dean, 480-219-6000, Fax: 480-219-6110, E-mail: kkalousek@atsu.edu. *Application contact:* Donna Sparks, Associate Director for Admissions, 660-626-2117, Fax: 660-626-2969, E-mail: admissions@atsu.edu.
Website: http://www.atsu.edu/soma

Des Moines University, College of Osteopathic Medicine, Des Moines, IA 50312-4104. Offers DO. *Accreditation:* AOsA. *Degree requirements:* For doctorate, National Board of Osteopathic Medical Examiners Exam Level 1 and 2. *Entrance requirements:* For doctorate, MCAT, minimum GPA of 3.0; 8 hours of course work in biology, chemistry, organic chemistry, and physics; 3 hours of biochemistry; 6 hours of course work in English; interview. Electronic applications accepted. *Expenses:* Contact institution. *Faculty research:* Cardiovascular, infectious disease, cancer immunology, cell signaling nociception.

Edward Via College of Osteopahtic Medicine–Virginia Campus, Graduate Program, Blacksburg, VA 24060. Offers DO. *Accreditation:* AOsA. *Degree requirements:* For doctorate, thesis/dissertation. *Entrance requirements:* For doctorate, MCAT, 8 hours of biology, general chemistry, and organic chemistry; 6 hours each of additional science and English; minimum overall science GPA of 2.75. *Faculty research:* Nanobiology of aging, calcium transport regulation, prescription drug abuse, oxidative stress and inflammation, immune protection.

Edward Via College of Osteopathic Medicine–Carolinas Campus, Graduate Program, Spartanburg, SC 29303. Offers DO. *Accreditation:* AOsA.

Georgia Campus–Philadelphia College of Osteopathic Medicine, Doctor of Osteopathic Medicine Program, Suwanee, GA 30024. Offers DO. *Accreditation:* AOsA. *Students:* 526 full-time (261 women); includes 280 minority (65 Black or African American, non-Hispanic/Latino; 62 Asian, non-Hispanic/Latino; 16 Hispanic/Latino; 137 Two or more races, non-Hispanic/Latino), 6 international. 4,919 applicants, 5% accepted, 135 enrolled. In 2015, 77 doctorates awarded. *Degree requirements:* For doctorate, comprehensive exam. *Entrance requirements:* For doctorate, MCAT. Additional exam requirements/recommendations for international students: Required—TOEFL (minimum score 79 iBT). *Application deadline:* For fall admission, 3/1 for domestic and international students. Applications are processed on a rolling basis. Application fee: $75. Electronic applications accepted. *Expenses:* Contact institution. *Financial support:* Application deadline: 3/15; applicants required to submit FAFSA. *Application contact:* Deborah Benvenger, Chief Admissions Officer, 678-225-7500.
Website: http://www.pcom.edu/academics/programs-and-degrees/doctor-of-osteopathic-medicine-georgia-campus/

Kansas City University of Medicine and Biosciences, College of Osteopathic Medicine, Kansas City, MO 64106-1453. Offers DO, DO/MA, DO/MBA. *Accreditation:* AOsA. *Degree requirements:* For doctorate, comprehensive exam, National Board Exam - COMPLEX. *Entrance requirements:* For doctorate, MCAT, on-campus interview. *Faculty research:* 2-Chloroadenine in DNA use in controlling leukemia, dietary isoprenoids role in tumor cell control, preventive medicine and public health research of maternal and child health, nonenzymatic glycosylation in cardiac tissue.

Lake Erie College of Osteopathic Medicine, Professional Programs, Erie, PA 16509-1025. Offers biomedical sciences (Postbaccalaureate Certificate); medical education (MS); osteopathic medicine (DO); pharmacy (Pharm D). *Accreditation:* ACPE; AOsA. *Degree requirements:* For doctorate, comprehensive exam, National Osteopathic Medical Licensing Exam, Levels 1 and 2; for Postbaccalaureate Certificate, comprehensive exam, North American Pharmacist Licensure Examination (NAPLEX). *Entrance requirements:* For doctorate, MCAT, minimum GPA of 3.2, letters of recommendation; for Postbaccalaureate Certificate, PCAT, letters of recommendation, minimum GPA of 3.5. Electronic applications accepted. *Faculty research:* Cardiac smooth and skeletal muscle mechanics, chemotherapeutics and vitamins, osteopathic manipulation.

Liberty University, College of Osteopathic Medicine, Lynchburg, VA 24515. Offers DO. *Accreditation:* AOsA. *Students:* 317 full-time (153 women); includes 19 minority (3 Black or African American, non-Hispanic/Latino; 9 Asian, non-Hispanic/Latino; 2 Hispanic/Latino; 5 Two or more races, non-Hispanic/Latino), 16 international. Average age 26. 3,959 applicants, 4% accepted, 161 enrolled. *Entrance requirements:* For doctorate, MCAT (minimum cumulative score of 22). *Application deadline:* Applications are processed on a rolling basis. Electronic applications accepted. *Expenses:* Contact institution. *Unit head:* Dr. Ronnie B. Martin, Dean, 434-592-6400. *Application contact:* Jay Bridge, Director of Admissions, 800-424-9595, Fax: 800-628-7977, E-mail: gradadmissions@liberty.edu.
Website: http://www.liberty.edu/lucom/

Lincoln Memorial University, DeBusk College of Osteopathic Medicine, Harrogate, TN 37752-1901. Offers DO. *Accreditation:* AOsA. *Entrance requirements:* For doctorate, MCAT. Additional exam requirements/recommendations for international students: Required—TOEFL (minimum score 600 paper-based; 100 iBT).

Marian University, College of Osteopathic Medicine, Indianapolis, IN 46222-1997. Offers DO. *Accreditation:* AOsA. *Faculty:* 29 full-time (8 women), 1 part-time/adjunct (0 women). *Students:* 472 full-time (225 women); includes 93 minority (9 Black or African American, non-Hispanic/Latino; 58 Asian, non-Hispanic/Latino; 18 Hispanic/Latino; 8 Two or more races, non-Hispanic/Latino), 12 international. Average age 25. 4,339 applicants, 8% accepted, 162 enrolled. *Degree requirements:* For doctorate, comprehensive exam, cognitive and performance evaluations. *Entrance requirements:* For doctorate, MCAT. Additional exam requirements/recommendations for international students: Required—TOEFL. *Application deadline:* For fall admission, 3/1 for domestic and international students. Applications are processed on a rolling basis. Application fee: $100. Electronic applications accepted. *Expenses:* $46,300 full-time tuition; $1,500 fees. *Financial support:* Applicants required to submit FAFSA. *Faculty research:* Immunologic impact, anatomy and physiology, genetic and molecular analysis, neurosensory functions, pharmacology, pathogenesis. *Unit head:* Dr. Donald Sefcik, Vice President of Health Professions/Dean of the College of Osteopathic Medicine, 317-

955-6289, E-mail: dsefcik@marian.edu. *Application contact:* Bryan Moody, Director of Enrollment Management, 317-955-6284, E-mail: bmoody@marian.edu.
Website: http://www.marian.edu/osteopathic-medical-school

Michigan State University, College of Osteopathic Medicine, Professional Program in Osteopathic Medicine, East Lansing, MI 48824. Offers DO. *Accreditation:* AOsA. Electronic applications accepted.

Midwestern University, Downers Grove Campus, Chicago College of Osteopathic Medicine, Downers Grove, IL 60515-1235. Offers DO. *Accreditation:* AOsA. *Entrance requirements:* For doctorate, MCAT, 1 year course work each in organic chemistry, general chemistry, biology, physics, and English. *Expenses:* Contact institution. *Faculty research:* Cadmium toxicity, amino acid transport, metabolic actions of vanadium, diabetes and obesity.

Midwestern University, Glendale Campus, Arizona College of Osteopathic Medicine, Glendale, AZ 85308. Offers DO. *Accreditation:* AOsA. *Entrance requirements:* For doctorate, MCAT. Electronic applications accepted. *Expenses:* Contact institution.

New York Institute of Technology, College of Osteopathic Medicine, Old Westbury, NY 11568-8000. Offers medical/healthcare simulation (MS); osteopathic medicine (DO); DO/MS. *Accreditation:* AOsA. *Faculty:* 69 full-time (25 women), 24 part-time/adjunct (10 women). *Students:* 1,227 full-time (598 women), 3 part-time (1 woman); includes 538 minority (39 Black or African American, non-Hispanic/Latino; 1 American Indian or Alaska Native, non-Hispanic/Latino; 466 Asian, non-Hispanic/Latino; 27 Hispanic/Latino; 1 Native Hawaiian or other Pacific Islander, non-Hispanic/Latino; 4 Two or more races, non-Hispanic/Latino). Average age 27. 6,515 applicants, 7% accepted, 272 enrolled. In 2015, 15 master's, 269 doctorates awarded. *Degree requirements:* For doctorate, comprehensive exam. *Entrance requirements:* For doctorate, MCAT (within past 3 years), minimum grade of C in following prerequisite courses: 6 semester hours of English; 8 semester hours each of biology, general chemistry, organic chemistry, and physics. *Application deadline:* For fall admission, 2/1 for domestic students. Applications are processed on a rolling basis. Application fee: $80. Electronic applications accepted. *Expenses:* Contact institution. *Financial support:* Fellowships with partial tuition reimbursements and tuition waivers (full and partial) available. Financial award application deadline: 4/1; financial award applicants required to submit FAFSA. *Faculty research:* Cardiovascular physiology and pathophysiology, renal physiology and pathophysiology, paleontology and comparative anatomy, Parkinson's disease: basic mechanisms to therapies, osteopathic manipulative medicine. *Unit head:* Dr. Wolfgang Gilliar, Dean, 516-686-3722, Fax: 516-686-3830, E-mail: wgilliar@nyit.edu. *Application contact:* Edward Dettling, Acting Director of Admissions, 516-686-3747, Fax: 516-686-3831, E-mail: comadm@nyit.edu.
Website: http://www.nyit.edu/medicine

Nova Southeastern University, College of Osteopathic Medicine, Fort Lauderdale, FL 33328. Offers biomedical informatics (MS, Graduate Certificate), including biomedical informatics (MS), clinical informatics (Graduate Certificate), public health informatics (Graduate Certificate); disaster and emergency preparedness (MS); osteopathic medicine (DO); public health (MPH). *Accreditation:* AOsA. *Faculty:* 107 full-time (55 women), 1,235 part-time/adjunct (297 women). *Students:* 1,027 full-time (436 women), 189 part-time (124 women); includes 560 minority (92 Black or African American, non-Hispanic/Latino; 260 Asian, non-Hispanic/Latino; 174 Hispanic/Latino; 1 Native Hawaiian or other Pacific Islander, non-Hispanic/Latino; 33 Two or more races, non-Hispanic/Latino), 45 international. Average age 28. 4,012 applicants, 12% accepted, 246 enrolled. In 2015, 75 master's, 237 doctorates, 4 other advanced degrees awarded. *Entrance requirements:* For master's, GRE; for doctorate, MCAT, biology, chemistry, organic chemistry, physics (all with labs), and English. *Application deadline:* For fall admission, 1/15 for domestic students. Applications are processed on a rolling basis. Application fee: $50. Electronic applications accepted. *Expenses:* Contact institution. *Financial support:* In 2015–16, 39 students received support, including 24 fellowships (averaging $45,593 per year); research assistantships, teaching assistantships, Federal Work-Study, and scholarships/grants also available. Financial award application deadline: 6/1; financial award applicants required to submit FAFSA. *Faculty research:* Teaching strategies, simulated patient use, HIV/AIDS education, minority health issues, managed care education. *Unit head:* Elaine M. Wallace, DO, Dean, 954-262-1407, E-mail: ewallace@nova.edu. *Application contact:* Monica Sanchez, Admissions Counselor, College of Osteopathic Medicine, 954-262-1110, Fax: 954-262-2282, E-mail: mh1156@nova.edu.
Website: http://www.medicine.nova.edu/

Ohio University, Heritage College of Osteopathic Medicine, Athens, OH 45701-2979. Offers DO, DO/MBA, DO/MPH, DO/MS, DO/PhD. Applicants must be U.S. residents to apply. *Accreditation:* AOsA. *Faculty:* 98 full-time (45 women), 35 part-time/adjunct (15 women). *Students:* 716 full-time (333 women); includes 166 minority (62 Black or African American, non-Hispanic/Latino; 3 American Indian or Alaska Native, non-Hispanic/Latino; 61 Asian, non-Hispanic/Latino; 30 Hispanic/Latino; 10 Two or more races, non-Hispanic/Latino). Average age 26. 5,088 applicants, 7% accepted, 240 enrolled. In 2015, 125 doctorates awarded. *Degree requirements:* For doctorate, comprehensive exam, National Board Exam Parts I and II, COMPLEX-PE. *Entrance requirements:* For doctorate, MCAT, interview; course work in English, physics, biology, general chemistry, organic chemistry, and behavioral sciences with minimum grade of C. *Application deadline:* For fall admission, 2/1 for domestic students. Applications are processed on a rolling basis. Application fee: $60. Electronic applications accepted. *Expenses:* Contact institution. *Financial support:* In 2015–16, 187 students received support, including 17 fellowships with full tuition reimbursements available (averaging $13,236 per year); Federal Work-Study, institutionally sponsored loans, scholarships/grants, and tuition waivers (partial) also available. Financial award applicants required to submit FAFSA. *Faculty research:* Primary care, diabetes, healthy aging, pain management, neuroscience. *Total annual research expenditures:* $3.4 million. *Unit head:* Dr. Kenneth Johnson, Executive Dean, 740-593-9350, Fax: 740-593-0761, E-mail: wilcox@ohio.edu. *Application contact:* Jill Harman, Director of Admissions, 740-593-2147, Fax: 740-593-2256, E-mail: harmanj@ohio.edu.
Website: https://www.ohio.edu/medicine/index.cfm

Oklahoma State University Center for Health Sciences, College of Osteopathic Medicine, Tulsa, OK 74114. Offers DO, DO/MBA, DO/MPH, DO/MS, DO/PhD. *Accreditation:* AOsA. *Faculty:* 102 full-time (23 women), 813 part-time/adjunct (196 women). *Students:* 441 full-time (194 women); includes 135 minority (20 Black or African American, non-Hispanic/Latino; 20 American Indian or Alaska Native, non-Hispanic/Latino; 43 Asian, non-Hispanic/Latino; 23 Hispanic/Latino; 32 Two or more races, non-Hispanic/Latino). Average age 27. 2,278 applicants, 5% accepted, 97 enrolled. In 2015, 87 doctorates awarded. *Degree requirements:* For doctorate, COMLEX Board exams. *Entrance requirements:* For doctorate, MCAT (minimum score 492), interview; minimum 90 hours of college course work; minimum cumulative GPA of 3.0, science 2.75. *Application deadline:* For fall admission, 2/1 for domestic students. Applications are processed on a rolling basis. Application fee: $65. Electronic applications accepted. *Financial support:* In 2015–16, 189 students received support. Federal Work-Study, institutionally sponsored loans, scholarships/grants, and tuition waivers available. Financial award application deadline: 4/1; financial award applicants required to submit FAFSA. *Faculty research:* Neuroscience, artificial vision, mechanisms of hormone action, vaccines and immunotherapy, pathogenic free-living amoebae. *Total annual research expenditures:* $1.7 million. *Unit head:* Dr. Kayse M. Shrum, Provost and Dean, Center for Health Sciences, 918-561-8201, Fax: 918-561-8413, E-mail: amy.green@okstate.edu. *Application contact:* Maghin Abernathy, Director of Admissions, 800-677-1972, Fax: 918-561-8243, E-mail: maghin.abernathy@okstate.edu. Website: http://www.healthsciences.okstate.edu/index.php

Philadelphia College of Osteopathic Medicine, Graduate and Professional Programs, Doctor of Osteopathic Medicine Program (Philadelphia Campus), Philadelphia, PA 19131-1694. Offers DO, DO/MA, DO/MBA, DO/MPH, DO/MS, DO/PhD. *Accreditation:* AOsA. *Entrance requirements:* For doctorate, MCAT, minimum GPA of 3.2; premedical prerequisite coursework; biochemistry (recommended). Additional exam requirements/recommendations for international students: Required—TOEFL (minimum score 79 iBT). Electronic applications accepted. *Faculty research:* Neuroscience and neurodegenerative disorders, inflammation and allergic response to food allergens, cardiovascular function and disease, bone and joint disorders, cancer biology.

Rocky Vista University, College of Osteopathic Medicine, Parker, CO 80134. Offers DO.

Rowan University, School of Osteopathic Medicine, Stratford, NJ 08084-1501. Offers DO, DO/MA, DO/MBA, DO/MPH, DO/MS, DO/PhD, JD/DO. *Accreditation:* AOsA. *Degree requirements:* For doctorate, comprehensive exam. *Entrance requirements:* For doctorate, MCAT. Electronic applications accepted. *Expenses:* Contact institution.

Touro University California, Graduate Programs, Vallejo, CA 94592. Offers education (MA); medical health sciences (MS); osteopathic medicine (DO); pharmacy (Pharm D); public health (MPH). *Accreditation:* AOsA; ARC-PA. *Program availability:* Part-time, evening/weekend. *Degree requirements:* For master's, comprehensive exam, thesis; for doctorate, comprehensive exam. *Entrance requirements:* For doctorate, BS/BA. Electronic applications accepted. *Faculty research:* Cancer, heart disease.

University of North Texas Health Science Center at Fort Worth, Texas College of Osteopathic Medicine, Fort Worth, TX 76107-2699. Offers osteopathic medicine (DO); physician assistant studies (MPAS); DO/MPH; DO/MS; DO/PhD; MPAS/MPH. DO/MPH offered jointly with University of North Texas. *Accreditation:* AOsA. *Entrance requirements:* For doctorate, MCAT, 1 year course work in each biology, physics and English; 2 years course work in chemistry. Electronic applications accepted. *Faculty research:* Tuberculosis, aging, cardiovascular disease, cancer.

University of Pikeville, Kentucky College of Osteopathic Medicine, Pikeville, KY 41501. Offers DO. *Accreditation:* AOsA. *Faculty:* 25 full-time (9 women), 37 part-time/adjunct (14 women). *Students:* 532 full-time (229 women); includes 59 minority (8 Black or African American, non-Hispanic/Latino; 10 American Indian or Alaska Native, non-Hispanic/Latino; 21 Asian, non-Hispanic/Latino; 19 Hispanic/Latino; 1 Native Hawaiian or other Pacific Islander, non-Hispanic/Latino), 2 international. Average age 25. 3,982 applicants, 5% accepted, 135 enrolled. In 2015, 67 doctorates awarded. *Degree requirements:* For doctorate, COMLEX Level 1 and COMLEX Level 2CE and 2PE. *Entrance requirements:* For doctorate, MCAT. *Application deadline:* For fall admission, 5/1 for domestic students. Applications are processed on a rolling basis. Application fee: $75. *Expenses:* $41,320 per year. *Financial support:* In 2015–16, 7 students received support, including 7 fellowships with full tuition reimbursements available (averaging $41,320 per year); scholarships/grants also available. Financial award application deadline: 8/1; financial award applicants required to submit FAFSA. *Faculty research:* Primary care in rural and medically underserved areas. *Unit head:* Dr. Boyd Buser, Dean, 606-218-5410, Fax: 606-218-8442, E-mail: boydbuser@upike.edu. *Application contact:* Dr. Linda Dunatov, Associate Dean for Student Affairs, 606-218-5408, Fax: 606-218-5442, E-mail: lindadunatov@upike.edu. Website: http://www.upike.edu/College-of-Osteopathic-Medicine

Western University of Health Sciences, College of Osteopathic Medicine of the Pacific, Pomona, CA 91766-1854. Offers DO. *Accreditation:* AOsA. *Faculty:* 64 full-time (29 women), 26 part-time/adjunct (7 women). *Students:* 1,333 full-time (614 women); includes 574 minority (18 Black or African American, non-Hispanic/Latino; 1 American Indian or Alaska Native, non-Hispanic/Latino; 391 Asian, non-Hispanic/Latino; 73 Hispanic/Latino; 3 Native Hawaiian or other Pacific Islander, non-Hispanic/Latino; 88 Two or more races, non-Hispanic/Latino), 18 international. Average age 27. 10,315 applicants, 7% accepted, 325 enrolled. In 2015, 322 doctorates awarded. *Degree requirements:* For doctorate, comprehensive exam (for some programs). *Entrance requirements:* For doctorate, MCAT, minimum GPA of 3.3, interview, two letters of recommendation. *Application deadline:* For fall admission, 2/1 for domestic and international students. Applications are processed on a rolling basis. Application fee: $65. Electronic applications accepted. *Expenses:* $53,570 tuition; $40 fees. *Financial support:* Scholarships/grants and unspecified assistantships available. Financial award application deadline: 3/2; financial award applicants required to submit FAFSA. *Total annual research expenditures:* $422,264. *Unit head:* Dr. Paula Crone, Dean, 541-259-0206, Fax: 541-259-0201, E-mail: pcrone@westernu.edu. *Application contact:* Susan Hanson, Director of Admissions, 909-469-5335, Fax: 909-469-5570, E-mail: admissions@westernu.edu. Website: http://www.westernu.edu/osteopathy/

West Virginia School of Osteopathic Medicine, Professional Program, Lewisburg, WV 24901-1196. Offers DO. *Accreditation:* AOsA. *Degree requirements:* For doctorate, comprehensive exam, Comlex Level 1 and 2 (PE and CE). *Entrance requirements:* For doctorate, MCAT, 3 hours of English; 8 hours each of biology, physics, inorganic chemistry, and organic chemistry. Electronic applications accepted. *Faculty research:* OMT response bio-markers, linking muscle energy use to power production in primates.

Podiatric Medicine

Barry University, School of Podiatric Medicine, Podiatric Medicine and Surgery Program, Miami Shores, FL 33161-6695. Offers DPM, DPM/MBA, DPM/MPH. *Accreditation:* APMA. *Entrance requirements:* For doctorate, MCAT, GRE General Test, previous course work in science and English. Additional exam requirements/recommendations for international students: Required—TOEFL. Electronic applications accepted. *Expenses:* Contact institution.

California School of Podiatric Medicine at Samuel Merritt University, Professional Program, Oakland, CA 94609. Offers DPM. *Accreditation:* APMA. *Entrance requirements:* For doctorate, MCAT (less than 3 years old), at least 90 semester hours of undergraduate course work; 1 year of course work in organic chemistry or biochemistry, inorganic chemistry, physics, biological sciences (all courses must come with a lab), and English/communications. *Expenses:* Contact institution. *Faculty research:* Glycation in diabetes and protein dysfunction, lower extremity biomechanics, diabetic wound care, plantar warts among HIV-infected patients, interdisciplinary equity and inclusion issues.

Des Moines University, College of Podiatric Medicine and Surgery, Des Moines, IA 50312-4104. Offers DPM. *Accreditation:* APMA. *Entrance requirements:* For doctorate, MCAT, interview; minimum GPA of 2.5; 1 year of organic chemistry, inorganic chemistry, physics, biology, and English. Electronic applications accepted. *Expenses:* Contact institution. *Faculty research:* Physics of equines, gait analysis.

Kent State University, College of Podiatric Medicine, Kent, OH 44242-0001. Offers DPM. *Accreditation:* APMA. *Degree requirements:* For doctorate, comprehensive exam, clinical competencies; NBPME Boards 1 & 2. *Entrance requirements:* For doctorate, MCAT, satisfactory course work in biology, chemistry, English and physics; background check, drug test. Additional exam requirements/recommendations for international students: Recommended—TOEFL (minimum score 81 iBT). Electronic applications accepted. *Expenses:* Tuition, state resident: full-time $10,864; part-time $495 per credit hour. Tuition, nonresident: full-time $18,380; part-time $837 per credit hour. *Faculty research:* Diabetic foot ulcers, plantar shear stresses, nonvisual foot examinations, treatment modalities for onychomycosis.

Midwestern University, Glendale Campus, College of Health Sciences, Arizona Campus, Program in Podiatric Medicine, Glendale, AZ 85308. Offers DPM. *Accreditation:* APMA. *Entrance requirements:* For doctorate, MCAT or PCAT, 90 semester hours at an accredited college or university, minimum GPA of 2.75. *Expenses:* Contact institution.

New York College of Podiatric Medicine, Professional Program, New York, NY 10035. Offers DPM, DPM/MPH. *Accreditation:* APMA. *Degree requirements:* For doctorate, comprehensive exam. *Entrance requirements:* For doctorate, MCAT or DAT, 1 year course work in biology, physics, English, and general and organic chemistry. Additional exam requirements/recommendations for international students: Required—TOEFL.

Rosalind Franklin University of Medicine and Science, Dr. William M. Scholl College of Podiatric Medicine, North Chicago, IL 60064-3095. Offers DPM. *Accreditation:* APMA. *Entrance requirements:* For doctorate, MCAT (or GRE on approval), 12 semester hours of biology; 8 semester hours of inorganic chemistry, organic chemistry and physics; 6 semester hours of English. Additional exam requirements/recommendations for international students: Required—TOEFL.

Temple University, School of Podiatric Medicine, Philadelphia, PA 19107-2496. Offers DPM, DPM/MBA, DPM/PhD. DPM/PhD offered jointly with Drexel University, University of Pennsylvania. *Accreditation:* APMA. *Degree requirements:* For doctorate, National Board Exam. *Entrance requirements:* For doctorate, MCAT, GRE, or DAT, interview, 8 hours of organic chemistry, inorganic chemistry, physics, biology. *Faculty research:* Gait analysis, infectious diseases, diabetic neuropathy, peripheral vascular disease.

Section 29
Optometry and Vision Sciences

This section contains a directory of institutions offering graduate work in optometry and vision sciences. Additional information about programs listed in the directory may be obtained by writing directly to the dean of a graduate school or chair of a department at the address given in the directory.

In the other guides in this series:

Graduate Programs in the Humanities, Arts & Social Sciences
See *Psychology and Counseling*

Graduate Programs in the Physical Sciences, Mathematics, Agricultural Sciences, the Environment & Natural Resources
See *Physics*

Graduate Programs in Engineering & Applied Sciences
See *Biomedical Engineering* and *Biotechnology*

CONTENTS

Program Directories

Optometry

Ferris State University, Michigan College of Optometry, Big Rapids, MI 49307. Offers OD. *Accreditation:* AOA. *Faculty:* 19 full-time (7 women), 143 part-time/adjunct (51 women). *Students:* 146 full-time (79 women); includes 14 minority (1 Black or African American, non-Hispanic/Latino; 3 Asian, non-Hispanic/Latino; 8 Hispanic/Latino; 2 Two or more races, non-Hispanic/Latino), 2 international. Average age 24. 264 applicants, 23% accepted, 38 enrolled. In 2015, 37 doctorates awarded. *Degree requirements:* For doctorate, comprehensive exam, research project. *Entrance requirements:* For doctorate, OAT, Optomcas application. Additional exam requirements/recommendations for international students: Recommended—TOEFL (minimum score 500 paper-based; 61 iBT). *Application deadline:* For fall admission, 2/15 for domestic and international students. Applications are processed on a rolling basis. Application fee: $155. Electronic applications accepted. *Expenses:* Contact institution. *Financial support:* In 2015–16, 68 students received support. Career-related internships or fieldwork, Federal Work-Study, and scholarships/grants available. Financial award application deadline: 3/15; financial award applicants required to submit FAFSA. *Faculty research:* Corneal reshaping, spatial vision and vision science, reading disabilities, vision development, vision care access, contact lens studies. *Unit head:* Dr. David Damari, Dean, 231-591-3706, Fax: 231-591-2394, E-mail: damarid@ferris.edu. *Application contact:* Amy Parks, Health College Administrative Specialist, 231-591-3703, Fax: 231-591-2394, E-mail: amyparks@ferris.edu.
Website: http://www.ferris.edu/mco/

Illinois College of Optometry, Professional Program, Chicago, IL 60616-3878. Offers OD. *Accreditation:* AOA. *Entrance requirements:* For doctorate, OAT. Electronic applications accepted. *Faculty research:* Eye disease treatment, binocular vision, cataract development, pediatric vision, genetic eye disease.

Indiana University Bloomington, School of Optometry, Bloomington, IN 47405-3680. Offers MS, OD, PhD. *Accreditation:* AOA (one or more programs are accredited). Terminal master's awarded for partial completion of doctoral program. *Degree requirements:* For master's, thesis; for doctorate, comprehensive exam, thesis/dissertation. *Entrance requirements:* For master's, GRE, BA in science; for doctorate, GRE; OAT (for OD), BA in science (master's degree preferred). Additional exam requirements/recommendations for international students: Required—TOEFL (minimum score 550 paper-based; 80 iBT). Electronic applications accepted. *Expenses:* Contact institution. *Faculty research:* Corneal physiology, contact lenses, adaptive optics, dry eye, low vision, refractive anomalies, ophthalmic imaging, glaucoma, ocular physiology, infant vision, retinal disease.

Inter American University of Puerto Rico School of Optometry, Professional Program, Bayamn, PR 00957. Offers OD. *Accreditation:* AOA. *Degree requirements:* For doctorate, thesis/dissertation, research project. *Entrance requirements:* For doctorate, OAT, interview, minimum GPA of 2.5, 2 letters of recommendation. Electronic applications accepted. *Expenses:* Contact institution. *Faculty research:* Visual characteristics of special populations, contact lenses, refraction and diabetes.

Marshall B. Ketchum University, Graduate and Professional Programs, Fullerton, CA 92831-1615. Offers optometry (OD); vision science (MS). *Accreditation:* AOA. *Degree requirements:* For doctorate, thesis/dissertation. *Entrance requirements:* For doctorate, OAT. Electronic applications accepted. *Faculty research:* Structure and function of the human visual system.

Midwestern University, Glendale Campus, Arizona College of Optometry, Glendale, AZ 85308. Offers OD. *Accreditation:* AOA. *Entrance requirements:* For doctorate, OAT, bachelor's degree, minimum overall cumulative and science GPA of 2.75, 2 letters of recommendation.

New England College of Optometry, Graduate and Professional Programs, Boston, MA 02115-1100. Offers optometry (OD); vision science (MS). *Accreditation:* AOA. *Entrance requirements:* For doctorate, OAT. Electronic applications accepted.

Northeastern State University, College of Optometry, Tahlequah, OK 74464. Offers OD. Applicants must be a resident of Oklahoma, Arkansas, Kansas, Colorado, New Mexico, Missouri, Texas, or Nebraska. *Accreditation:* AOA. *Faculty:* 32 full-time (13 women), 17 part-time/adjunct (7 women). *Students:* 113 full-time (64 women); includes 33 minority (2 Black or African American, non-Hispanic/Latino; 16 American Indian or Alaska Native, non-Hispanic/Latino; 5 Asian, non-Hispanic/Latino; 6 Hispanic/Latino; 4 Two or more races, non-Hispanic/Latino). Average age 25. In 2015, 28 doctorates awarded. *Degree requirements:* For doctorate, research project. *Entrance requirements:* For doctorate, OAT. *Application deadline:* For fall admission, 2/1 for domestic students. Applications are processed on a rolling basis. Application fee: $45. Electronic applications accepted. *Expenses:* Contact institution. *Financial support:* Federal Work-Study, institutionally sponsored loans, scholarships/grants, tuition waivers (partial), and residencies available. Financial award application deadline: 5/1; financial award applicants required to submit FAFSA. *Unit head:* Dr. Douglas Penisten, Dean of Oklahoma College of Optometry, 918-444-4025, E-mail: penisten@nsuok.edu. *Application contact:* Sandy Medearis, Director of Optometry Student Affairs, 918-444-4006, Fax: 918-458-2104, E-mail: medearis@nsuok.edu.
Website: http://optometry.nsuok.edu

Nova Southeastern University, College of Optometry, Fort Lauderdale, FL 33328. Offers MS, OD. *Accreditation:* AOA. *Program availability:* Online learning. *Students:* 446 full-time (304 women), 2 part-time (both women); includes 186 minority (31 Black or African American, non-Hispanic/Latino; 76 Asian, non-Hispanic/Latino; 67 Hispanic/Latino; 12 Two or more races, non-Hispanic/Latino), 52 international. Average age 26. In 2015, 2 master's, 95 doctorates awarded. *Degree requirements:* For master's, comprehensive exam (for some programs), thesis; for doctorate, comprehensive exam. *Entrance requirements:* For master's, OAT or GRE, BA; for doctorate, OAT, minimum GPA of 3.0. Additional exam requirements/recommendations for international students: Required—TOEFL (minimum score 79 iBT). *Application deadline:* For fall admission, 4/1 for domestic and international students. Applications are processed on a rolling basis. Application fee: $50. Electronic applications accepted. *Expenses:* Contact institution. *Financial support:* In 2015–16, 52 students received support. Federal Work-Study, institutionally sponsored loans, and scholarships/grants available. Support available to part-time students. Financial award application deadline: 4/15; financial award applicants required to submit FAFSA. *Faculty research:* Retinal disease, low vision, binocular vision, contact lenses, accommodation. *Unit head:* Dr. David Loshin, Dean, 954-262-1404, Fax: 954-262-1818. *Application contact:* Juan Saavedra, Admissions Counselor, 954-262-1132, Fax: 954-262-2282, E-mail: jsaavedra@nova.edu.
Website: http://optometry.nova.edu/

The Ohio State University, College of Optometry, Columbus, OH 43210. Offers optometry (OD); vision science (MS, PhD); OD/MS. *Accreditation:* AOA (one or more programs are accredited). *Faculty:* 34. *Students:* 263 full-time (181 women); includes 33

minority (4 Black or African American, non-Hispanic/Latino; 19 Asian, non-Hispanic/Latino; 5 Hispanic/Latino; 5 Two or more races, non-Hispanic/Latino), 2 international. Average age 25. In 2015, 9 master's, 66 doctorates awarded. *Degree requirements:* For master's, thesis; for doctorate, thesis/dissertation. *Entrance requirements:* For master's, GRE; for doctorate, GRE (for PhD); OAT (for OD). Additional exam requirements/recommendations for international students: Required—TOEFL (minimum score 550 paper-based, 79 iBT), Michigan English Language Assessment Battery (minimum score 82), IELTS (minimum score 7) for MS and PhD; TOEFL (minimum score 577 paper-based; 90 iBT), Michigan English Language Assessment Battery (minimum score 84), IELTS (minimum score 7.5) for OD. *Application deadline:* For fall admission, 3/31 for domestic and international students; for spring admission, 12/1 for domestic students, 11/1 for international students. Applications are processed on a rolling basis. Application fee: $60 ($70 for international students). Electronic applications accepted. *Expenses:* Contact institution. *Financial support:* Research assistantships with full tuition reimbursements, teaching assistantships with full tuition reimbursements, institutionally sponsored loans, and scholarships/grants available. Financial award application deadline: 2/15; financial award applicants required to submit FAFSA. *Unit head:* Dr. Karla Zadnik, Dean, 614-292-6603, E-mail: zadnik.4@osu.edu. *Application contact:* Office of Student Affairs, College of Optometry, 614-292-2647, Fax: 614-292-7493, E-mail: admissions@optometry.osu.edu.
Website: http://www.optometry.osu.edu/

Pacific University, College of Optometry, Forest Grove, OR 97116-1797. Offers optometry (OD); vision science (MS, PhD). *Accreditation:* AOA (one or more programs are accredited). *Degree requirements:* For doctorate, thesis/dissertation optional. *Entrance requirements:* For master's, GRE General Test, course work in natural sciences; for doctorate, OAT, 30 hours OD observation; course work in natural sciences, math, psychology, English, letters of recommendation. Additional exam requirements/recommendations for international students: Required—TOEFL (minimum score 600 paper-based). Electronic applications accepted. *Expenses:* Contact institution. *Faculty research:* Sports vision, infant vision care, visual training, contact lenses, ocular pathology.

Salus University, College of Optometry, Elkins Park, PA 19027-1598. Offers OD, OD/MS. *Accreditation:* AOA. *Degree requirements:* For doctorate, comprehensive exam (for some programs). *Entrance requirements:* For doctorate, OAT, interview. Additional exam requirements/recommendations for international students: Required—TOEFL. Electronic applications accepted. *Faculty research:* Vision research, visual perception, ocular motility, electrodiagnosis, photobiology glaucoma, myopia, keratoconus.

Southern College of Optometry, Professional Program, Memphis, TN 38104-2222. Offers OD. *Accreditation:* AOA. *Degree requirements:* For doctorate, clinical experience. *Entrance requirements:* For doctorate, OAT, 3 years of undergraduate pre-optometry course work.

State University of New York College of Optometry, Professional Program, New York, NY 10036. Offers OD, OD/MS, OD/PhD. *Accreditation:* AOA. *Entrance requirements:* For doctorate, OAT. Additional exam requirements/recommendations for international students: Required—TOEFL (minimum score 550 paper-based; 80 iBT). Electronic applications accepted. *Faculty research:* Optometry, vision research.

Université de Montréal, School of Optometry, Professional Program in Optometry, Montréal, QC H3C 3J7, Canada. Offers OD. Open only to Canadian residents. *Accreditation:* AOA. *Degree requirements:* For doctorate, thesis/dissertation. Electronic applications accepted.

The University of Alabama at Birmingham, School of Optometry, Professional Program in Optometry, Birmingham, AL 35294. Offers OD. *Students:* 179 full-time (123 women); includes 43 minority (15 Black or African American, non-Hispanic/Latino; 2 American Indian or Alaska Native, non-Hispanic/Latino; 25 Asian, non-Hispanic/Latino; 1 Two or more races, non-Hispanic/Latino), 2 international. Average age 25. 291 applicants, 35% accepted, 44 enrolled. In 2015, 44 doctorates awarded. *Entrance requirements:* For doctorate, OAT, composite evaluation or letters of recommendation, interview. Additional exam requirements/recommendations for international students: Required—TOEFL. Electronic applications accepted. *Expenses:* Tuition, state resident: full-time $7340. Tuition, nonresident: full-time $16,628. Full-time tuition and fees vary according to course load and program. *Financial support:* In 2015–16, 23 students received support. Scholarships/grants and out-of-state tuition offsets available. Financial award application deadline: 5/1. *Unit head:* Dr. Robert Kleinstein, Interim Chair/Director of Professional Program, 205-934-6757, E-mail: vista@uab.edu. *Application contact:* Dr. Gerald Simon, Director, Optometry Student Affairs, 205-975-0739, Fax: 205-934-6758, E-mail: admissions@icare.opt.uab.edu.

University of California, Berkeley, School of Optometry, Berkeley, CA 94720-1500. Offers OD, Certificate. *Accreditation:* AOA. *Entrance requirements:* For doctorate, OAT. Additional exam requirements/recommendations for international students: Required—TOEFL (minimum score 570 paper-based). Electronic applications accepted. *Faculty research:* Low vision, spatial vision, psychophysics of vision, clinical optics, patient care.

University of Houston, College of Optometry, Professional Program in Optometry, Houston, TX 77204. Offers OD. *Accreditation:* AOA. *Faculty research:* Refractive error development, corneal physiology, low vision, binocular vision.

The University of Manchester, Faculty of Life Sciences, Manchester, United Kingdom. Offers adaptive organismal biology (M Phil, PhD); animal biology (M Phil, PhD); biochemistry (M Phil, PhD); bioinformatics (M Phil, PhD); biomolecular sciences (M Phil, PhD); biotechnology (M Phil, PhD); cell biology (M Phil, PhD); cell matrix research (M Phil, PhD); channels and transporters (M Phil, PhD); developmental biology (M Phil, PhD); Egyptology (M Phil, PhD); environmental biology (M Phil, PhD); evolutionary biology (M Phil, PhD); gene expression (M Phil, PhD); genetics (M Phil, PhD); history of science, technology and medicine (M Phil, PhD); immunology (M Phil, PhD); integrative neurobiology and behavior (M Phil, PhD); membrane trafficking (M Phil, PhD); microbiology (M Phil, PhD); molecular and cellular neuroscience (M Phil, PhD); molecular biology (M Phil, PhD); molecular cancer studies (M Phil, PhD); neuroscience (M Phil, PhD); ophthalmology (M Phil, PhD); optometry (M Phil, PhD); organelle function (M Phil, PhD); pharmacology (M Phil, PhD); physiology (M Phil, PhD); plant sciences (M Phil, PhD); stem cell research (M Phil, PhD); structural biology (M Phil, PhD); systems neuroscience (M Phil, PhD); toxicology (M Phil, PhD).

University of Missouri–St. Louis, College of Optometry, Professional Program in Optometry, St. Louis, MO 63121. Offers OD. *Accreditation:* AOA. *Faculty:* 3 full-time (0 women), 2 part-time/adjunct (0 women). *Students:* 175 full-time (107 women); includes 19 minority (6 Black or African American, non-Hispanic/Latino; 1 American Indian or Alaska Native, non-Hispanic/Latino; 12 Asian, non-Hispanic/Latino), 3 international. Average age 23. 403 applicants, 26% accepted, 45 enrolled. *Entrance requirements:*

For doctorate, OAT, 90 hours of undergraduate course work. *Application deadline:* For fall admission, 2/15 for domestic and international students. Applications are processed on a rolling basis. Application fee: $50. Electronic applications accepted. *Financial support:* Research assistantships, teaching assistantships, Federal Work-Study, institutionally sponsored loans, and scholarships/grants available. Financial award application deadline: 2/15; financial award applicants required to submit FAFSA. *Faculty research:* Visual psychophysics and perception, noninvasive assessment of visual processing, aging and Alzheimer's disease, orthokeratology. *Unit head:* Nick Palisch, Director, Student Services, 314-516-6263, Fax: 314-516-6708, E-mail: optstuaff@umsl.edu. *Application contact:* Linda Stein, Student Support Specialist I, 314-516-5905, Fax: 314-516-6708, E-mail: linda_stein@umsl.edu.
Website: http://www.umsl.edu/divisions/optometry/Academic%20Programs/opt_curric.html

University of the Incarnate Word, Rosenberg School of Optometry, San Antonio, TX 78209-6397. Offers OD. *Accreditation:* AOA. *Faculty:* 15 full-time (5 women), 2 part-time/adjunct (both women). *Students:* 261 full-time (157 women); includes 136 minority (8 Black or African American, non-Hispanic/Latino; 1 American Indian or Alaska Native, non-Hispanic/Latino; 82 Asian, non-Hispanic/Latino; 42 Hispanic/Latino; 1 Native Hawaiian or other Pacific Islander, non-Hispanic/Latino; 2 Two or more races, non-Hispanic/Latino), 8 international. Average age 25. In 2015, 58 doctorates awarded. *Degree requirements:* For doctorate, clinical contact hours. *Entrance requirements:* For doctorate, OAT, 90 credit hours of prerequisite course work; letters of recommendation; interview. Additional exam requirements/recommendations for international students: Required—TOEFL (minimum score 560 paper-based; 83 iBT). *Application deadline:* For fall admission, 5/1 for domestic students. Application fee: $50. Electronic applications accepted. *Expenses:* Contact institution. *Financial support:* In 2015–16, 5 fellowships (averaging $4,000 per year) were awarded; Federal Work-Study and scholarships/grants also available. Financial award applicants required to submit FAFSA. *Faculty research:* Computer-based color vision, contrast sensitivity, and Amsler grid testing; response time in color deficiency; binocular enhancement of color vision; interactive instructional tools for teaching gross anatomy. *Unit head:* Dr. Timothy Wingert, Dean, 210-883-1195, Fax: 210-283-6890, E-mail: twingert@uiwtx.edu. *Application contact:* Kristine Benne, Assistant Dean of Student Affairs, 210-883-1190, Fax: 210-883-1191, E-mail: benne@uiwtx.edu.
Website: http://optometry.uiw.edu/

University of Waterloo, Graduate Studies, Faculty of Science, School of Optometry and Vision Science, Waterloo, ON N2L 3G1, Canada. Offers optometry (OD); vision science (M Sc, PhD). *Accreditation:* AOA. *Program availability:* Part-time. *Degree requirements:* For master's, thesis; for doctorate, thesis/dissertation. *Entrance requirements:* For master's: honors degree, minimum B average; for doctorate, master's degree, minimum B average. Additional exam requirements/recommendations for international students: Required—TOEFL, IELTS, PTE. *Application deadline:* Applications are processed on a rolling basis. Application fee: $100 Canadian dollars. Electronic applications accepted. *Financial support:* In 2015–16, 1 fellowship was awarded; research assistantships, teaching assistantships, career-related internships or fieldwork, institutionally sponsored loans, scholarships/grants, and health care benefits also available. *Faculty research:* Vision science, fundamental and clinical vision, physiological optics, psycho-physics, perception.
Website: https://uwaterloo.ca/optometry-vision-science/

Western University of Health Sciences, College of Optometry, Pomona, CA 91766-1854. Offers OD. *Accreditation:* AOA. *Faculty:* 31 full-time (14 women), 4 part-time/adjunct (3 women). *Students:* 337 full-time (240 women); includes 218 minority (13 Black or African American, non-Hispanic/Latino; 1 American Indian or Alaska Native, non-Hispanic/Latino; 129 Asian, non-Hispanic/Latino; 40 Hispanic/Latino; 35 Two or more races, non-Hispanic/Latino), 21 international. Average age 27. 855 applicants, 25% accepted, 85 enrolled. In 2015, 80 doctorates awarded. *Degree requirements:* For doctorate, comprehensive exam (for some programs), thesis/dissertation (for some programs). *Entrance requirements:* For doctorate, OAT, letters of recommendation; BS or BA (recommended). Additional exam requirements/recommendations for international students: Required—TOEFL (minimum score 550 paper-based; 79 iBT). *Application deadline:* For fall admission, 5/1 for domestic and international students. Application fee: $65. Electronic applications accepted. *Expenses:* $36,140 tuition; $40 student body fees. *Financial support:* Career-related internships or fieldwork, scholarships/grants, and traineeships available. Financial award application deadline: 3/2; financial award applicants required to submit FAFSA. *Total annual research expenditures:* $95,982. *Unit head:* Dr. Elizabeth Hoppe, Dean, 909-706-3497, E-mail: ehoppe@westernu.edu. *Application contact:* Marie Anderson, Director of Admissions, 909-469-5335, Fax: 909-469-5570, E-mail: admissions@westernu.edu.
Website: http://www.westernu.edu/optometry/

Vision Sciences

Eastern Virginia Medical School, Ophthalmic Technology Program, Norfolk, VA 23501-1980. Offers Certificate. Electronic applications accepted. *Expenses:* Contact institution.

Marshall B. Ketchum University, Graduate and Professional Programs, Fullerton, CA 92831-1615. Offers optometry (OD); vision science (MS). *Accreditation:* AOA. *Degree requirements:* For doctorate, thesis/dissertation. *Entrance requirements:* For doctorate, OAT. Electronic applications accepted. *Faculty research:* Structure and function of the human visual system.

New England College of Optometry, Graduate and Professional Programs, Boston, MA 02115-1100. Offers optometry (OD); vision science (MS). *Accreditation:* AOA. *Entrance requirements:* For doctorate, OAT. Electronic applications accepted.

Pacific University, College of Optometry, Forest Grove, OR 97116-1797. Offers optometry (OD); vision science (MS, PhD). *Accreditation:* AOA (one or more programs are accredited). *Degree requirements:* For doctorate, thesis/dissertation optional. *Entrance requirements:* For master's, GRE General Test, course work in natural sciences; for doctorate, OAT, 30 hours OD observation; course work in natural sciences, math, psychology, English, letters of recommendation. Additional exam requirements/recommendations for international students: Required—TOEFL (minimum score 600 paper-based). Electronic applications accepted. *Expenses:* Contact institution. *Faculty research:* Sports vision, infant vision care, visual training, contact lenses, ocular pathology.

Salus University, College of Education and Rehabilitation, Elkins Park, PA 19027-1598. Offers education of children and youth with visual and multiple impairments (M Ed, Certificate); low vision rehabilitation (MS, Certificate); orientation and mobility therapy (MS, Certificate); vision rehabilitation therapy (MS, Certificate); OD/MS. *Program availability:* Part-time, online learning. *Entrance requirements:* For master's, GRE or MAT, letters of reference (3), interviews (2). Additional exam requirements/recommendations for international students: Required—TOEFL, TWE. *Expenses:* Contact institution. *Faculty research:* Knowledge utilization, technology transfer.

State University of New York College of Optometry, Graduate Programs, New York, NY 10036. Offers PhD, OD/MS, OD/PhD. *Program availability:* Part-time. Terminal master's awarded for partial completion of doctoral program. *Degree requirements:* For doctorate, comprehensive exam, thesis/dissertation, specialty exam. *Entrance requirements:* For doctorate, GRE General Test. Additional exam requirements/recommendations for international students: Required—TOEFL (minimum score 550 paper-based; 80 iBT). *Expenses:* Contact institution. *Faculty research:* Oculomotor systems, perception, physiological optics, ocular biochemistry, accommodation, color and motion.

Université de Montréal, School of Optometry, Graduate Programs in Optometry, Montréal, QC H3C 3J7, Canada. Offers vision sciences (M Sc); visual impairment intervention-orientation and mobility (DESS); visual impairment intervention-readaptation (DESS). *Program availability:* Part-time. *Degree requirements:* For master's, thesis. *Entrance requirements:* For master's, OD or appropriate bachelor's degree, minimum GPA of 2.7. Electronic applications accepted. *Faculty research:* Binocular vision, visual electrophysiology, eye movements, corneal metabolism, glare sensitivity.

The University of Alabama at Birmingham, School of Optometry, Graduate Program in Vision Science, Birmingham, AL 35294. Offers sensory impairment (PhD); vision science (MS, PhD). Terminal master's awarded for partial completion of doctoral program. *Degree requirements:* For master's, thesis; for doctorate, thesis/dissertation. *Entrance requirements:* For master's, GRE General Test (minimum combined verbal and quantitative score of 270), minimum GPA of 3.0, letters of recommendation, interview; for doctorate, GRE General Test (minimum combined verbal and quantitative score of 300), interview. Additional exam requirements/recommendations for international students: Required—TOEFL (minimum score 570 paper-based). Electronic applications accepted. *Expenses:* Tuition, state resident: full-time $7340. Tuition,

nonresident: full-time $16,628. Full-time tuition and fees vary according to course load and program.

University of Alberta, Faculty of Medicine and Dentistry and Faculty of Graduate Studies and Research, Graduate Programs in Medicine, Department of Ophthalmology, Edmonton, AB T6G 2E1, Canada. Offers M Sc, PhD. *Program availability:* Part-time. Terminal master's awarded for partial completion of doctoral program. *Degree requirements:* For master's, thesis; for doctorate, comprehensive exam, thesis/dissertation. *Faculty research:* Ocular genetics.

University of California, Berkeley, Graduate Division, Group in Vision Science, Berkeley, CA 94720-1500. Offers MS, PhD. *Degree requirements:* For master's, thesis; for doctorate, thesis/dissertation. *Entrance requirements:* For master's and doctorate, GRE General Test, GRE Subject Test, minimum GPA of 3.0, 3 letters of recommendation. *Faculty research:* Visual neuroscience, bioengineering, computational vision, molecular cell biology, basic and clinical psychophysics.

University of Guelph, Ontario Veterinary College and Graduate Studies, Graduate Programs in Veterinary Sciences, Department of Clinical Studies, Guelph, ON N1G 2W1, Canada. Offers anesthesiology (M Sc, DV Sc); cardiology (DV Sc, Diploma); clinical studies (Diploma); dermatology (M Sc); diagnostic imaging (M Sc, DV Sc); emergency/critical care (M Sc, DV Sc, Diploma); medicine (M Sc, DV Sc); neurology (M Sc, DV Sc); ophthalmology (M Sc, DV Sc); surgery (M Sc, DV Sc). *Degree requirements:* For master's, thesis; for doctorate, comprehensive exam, thesis/dissertation. *Entrance requirements:* Additional exam requirements/recommendations for international students: Required—TOEFL (minimum score 550 paper-based), IELTS (minimum score 6.5). Electronic applications accepted. *Faculty research:* Orthopedics, respirology, oncology, exercise physiology, cardiology.

University of Houston, College of Optometry, Program in Physiological Optics/Vision Science, Houston, TX 77204. Offers physiological optics (MS, PhD). *Faculty research:* Space perception, amblyopia, binocular vision, development of visual skills, strabismus, visual cell biology, refractive error.

The University of Manchester, Faculty of Life Sciences, Manchester, United Kingdom. Offers adaptive organismal biology (M Phil, PhD); animal biology (M Phil, PhD); biochemistry (M Phil, PhD); bioinformatics (M Phil, PhD); biomolecular sciences (M Phil, PhD); biotechnology (M Phil, PhD); cell biology (M Phil, PhD); cell matrix research (M Phil, PhD); channels and transporters (M Phil, PhD); developmental biology (M Phil, PhD); Egyptology (M Phil, PhD); environmental biology (M Phil, PhD); evolutionary biology (M Phil, PhD); gene expression (M Phil, PhD); genetics (M Phil, PhD); history of science, technology and medicine (M Phil, PhD); immunology (M Phil, PhD); integrative neurobiology and behavior (M Phil, PhD); membrane trafficking (M Phil, PhD); microbiology (M Phil, PhD); molecular and cellular neuroscience (M Phil, PhD); molecular biology (M Phil, PhD); molecular cancer studies (M Phil, PhD); neuroscience (M Phil, PhD); ophthalmology (M Phil, PhD); optometry (M Phil, PhD); organelle function (M Phil, PhD); pharmacology (M Phil, PhD); physiology (M Phil, PhD); plant sciences (M Phil, PhD); stem cell research (M Phil, PhD); structural biology (M Phil, PhD); systems neuroscience (M Phil, PhD); toxicology (M Phil, PhD).

University of Massachusetts Boston, Graduate School of Global Inclusion and Social Development, Program in Vision Studies, Boston, MA 02125-3393. Offers M Ed. *Students:* 1 (woman) full-time, 105 part-time (92 women). 57 applicants, 98% accepted, 50 enrolled. In 2015, 31 master's awarded. *Expenses:* Tuition, state resident: full-time $2590. Tuition, nonresident: full-time $9758. *Required fees:* $13,525. *Unit head:* Dr. Kristy Alster, Associate Provost, 617-287-5700, Fax: 617-287-5699, E-mail: kristine.alster@umb.edu. *Application contact:* Peggy Roldan Patel, Graduate Admissions Coordinator, 617-287-6400, Fax: 617-287-6236, E-mail: bos.gadm@dpc.umassp.edu.

University of Pittsburgh, School of Education, Department of Instruction and Learning, Program in Special Education, Pittsburgh, PA 15260. Offers applied behavior analysis (M Ed); early intervention (M Ed, PhD); general special education (M Ed, Ed D); special education teacher preparation (M Ed); vision studies (M Ed, PhD). *Program availability:*

Vision Sciences

Part-time, evening/weekend. *Degree requirements:* For master's, thesis; for doctorate, thesis/dissertation. *Entrance requirements:* For master's, PRAXIS I; for doctorate, GRE General Test. Additional exam requirements/recommendations for international students: Required—TOEFL. Tuition and fees vary according to program.

University of Waterloo, Graduate Studies, Faculty of Science, School of Optometry and Vision Science, Waterloo, ON N2L 3G1, Canada. Offers optometry (OD); vision science (M Sc, PhD). *Accreditation:* AOA. *Program availability:* Part-time. *Degree requirements:* For master's, thesis; for doctorate, thesis/dissertation. *Entrance requirements:* For master's, honors degree, minimum B average; for doctorate, master's degree, minimum B average. Additional exam requirements/recommendations for international students: Required—TOEFL, IELTS, PTE. *Application deadline:* Applications are processed on a rolling basis. Application fee: $100 Canadian dollars. Electronic applications accepted. *Financial support:* In 2015–16, 1 fellowship was awarded; research assistantships, teaching assistantships, career-related internships or fieldwork, institutionally sponsored loans, scholarships/grants, and health care benefits also available. *Faculty research:* Vision science, fundamental and clinical vision, physiological optics, psycho-physics, perception.
Website: https://uwaterloo.ca/optometry-vision-science/

Section 30
Pharmacy and Pharmaceutical Sciences

This section contains a directory of institutions offering graduate work in pharmacy and pharmaceutical sciences, followed by in-depth entries submitted by institutions that chose to prepare detailed program descriptions. Additional information about programs listed in the directory but not augmented by an in-depth entry may be obtained by writing directly to the dean of a graduate school or chair of a department at the address given in the directory.

For programs offering related work, see also in this book *Allied Health, Biochemistry, Biological and Biomedical Sciences, Nutrition, Pharmacology and Toxicology,* and *Physiology.* In the other guides in this series:

Graduate Programs in the Physical Sciences, Mathematics, Agricultural Sciences, the Environment & Natural Resources

See *Chemistry*

Graduate Programs in Engineering & Applied Sciences

See *Biomedical Engineering and Biotechnology,* and *Chemical Engineering*

CONTENTS

Program Directories

Displays and Close-Up1

See also:

Medicinal and Pharmaceutical Chemistry

Duquesne University, Mylan School of Pharmacy, Graduate School of Pharmaceutical Sciences, Program in Medicinal Chemistry, Pittsburgh, PA 15282-0001. Offers MS, PhD. *Faculty:* 5 full-time (0 women). *Students:* 20 full-time (8 women), 18 international. Average age 27. 28 applicants, 11% accepted. In 2015, 1 master's, 4 doctorates awarded. *Degree requirements:* For master's, thesis; for doctorate, comprehensive exam, thesis/dissertation. *Entrance requirements:* For master's and doctorate, GRE General Test. Additional exam requirements/recommendations for international students: Required—TOEFL (minimum score 100 iBT). *Application deadline:* For fall admission, 2/1 priority date for domestic and international students; for spring admission, 10/1 priority date for domestic and international students. Applications are processed on a rolling basis. Application fee: $50. Electronic applications accepted. Application fee is waived when completed online. *Expenses:* $1,432 per credit. *Financial support:* In 2015–16, 19 students received support, including 8 research assistantships with full tuition reimbursements available, 11 teaching assistantships with full tuition reimbursements available. *Unit head:* Dr. Aleem Gangjee, Head, 412-396-6070. *Application contact:* Information Contact, 412-396-1172, E-mail: gsps-adm@duq.edu. Website: http://www.duq.edu/academics/schools/pharmacy/graduate-school-of-pharmaceutical-sciences

Florida Agricultural and Mechanical University, Division of Graduate Studies, Research, and Continuing Education, College of Pharmacy and Pharmaceutical Sciences, Graduate Programs in Pharmaceutical Sciences, Tallahassee, FL 32307-3200. Offers environmental toxicology (PhD); health outcomes research and pharmacoeconomics (PhD); medicinal chemistry (MS, PhD); pharmaceutics (MS, PhD); pharmacology/toxicology (MS, PhD); pharmacy administration (MS). *Accreditation:* CEPH. *Degree requirements:* For master's, comprehensive exam, thesis, publishable paper; for doctorate, comprehensive exam, thesis/dissertation, publishable paper. *Entrance requirements:* For master's and doctorate, GRE General Test, minimum GPA of 3.0 in last 60 hours. Additional exam requirements/recommendations for international students: Required—TOEFL. *Faculty research:* Anticancer agents, anti-inflammatory drugs, chronopharmacology, neuroendocrinology, microbiology.

Idaho State University, Office of Graduate Studies, College of Pharmacy, Department of Biomedical and Pharmaceutical Sciences, Pocatello, ID 83209-8334. Offers biopharmaceutical analysis (PhD); drug delivery (PhD); medicinal chemistry (PhD); pharmaceutical sciences (MS); pharmacology (PhD). *Program availability:* Part-time. *Degree requirements:* For master's, one foreign language, comprehensive exam, thesis, thesis research, classes in speech and technical writing; for doctorate, comprehensive exam, thesis/dissertation, written and oral exams, classes in speech and technical writing. *Entrance requirements:* For master's, GRE General Test, minimum GPA of 3.0, 3 letters of recommendation; for doctorate, GRE General Test, BS in pharmacy or related field, minimum GPA of 3.0, 3 letters of recommendation. Additional exam requirements/recommendations for international students: Required—TOEFL (minimum score 550 paper-based; 80 iBT). Electronic applications accepted. *Expenses:* Contact institution. *Faculty research:* Metabolic toxicity of heavy metals, neuroendocrine pharmacology, cardiovascular pharmacology, cancer biology, immunopharmacology.

Medical University of South Carolina, College of Graduate Studies, Department of Pharmaceutical and Biomedical Sciences, Charleston, SC 29425. Offers cell injury and repair (PhD); drug discovery (PhD); medicinal chemistry (PhD); toxicology (PhD); DMD/PhD; MD/PhD; Pharm D/PhD. *Degree requirements:* For doctorate, thesis/dissertation, oral and written exams, teaching and research seminar. *Entrance requirements:* For doctorate, GRE General Test, interview, minimum GPA of 3.0. Additional exam requirements/recommendations for international students: Required—TOEFL (minimum score 600 paper-based; 100 iBT). Electronic applications accepted. *Faculty research:* Drug discovery, toxicology, metabolomics, cell stress and injury.

New Jersey Institute of Technology, College of Science and Liberal Arts, Newark, NJ 07102. Offers applied mathematics (MS); applied physics (M Sc, PhD); applied statistics (MS, Certificate); biology (MS, PhD); biostatistics (MS); chemistry (MS, PhD); computational biology (MS); environmental science (MS, PhD); history (MA, MAT); materials science and engineering (MS, PhD); mathematical and computational finance (MS); mathematics science (PhD); pharmaceutical chemistry (MS); practice of technical communications (Certificate); professional and technical communications (MS). *Program availability:* Part-time, evening/weekend. *Faculty:* 153 full-time (35 women), 100 part-time/adjunct (40 women). *Students:* 212 full-time (82 women), 94 part-time (37 women); includes 72 minority (22 Black or African American, non-Hispanic/Latino; 25 Asian, non-Hispanic/Latino; 19 Hispanic/Latino; 6 Two or more races, non-Hispanic/Latino), 164 international. Average age 29. 519 applicants, 62% accepted, 104 enrolled. In 2015, 98 master's, 21 doctorates, 3 other advanced degrees awarded. Terminal master's awarded for partial completion of doctoral program. *Degree requirements:* For master's, thesis optional; for doctorate, thesis/dissertation. *Entrance requirements:* For master's, GRE General Test; for doctorate, GRE General Test, minimum graduate GPA of 3.5. Additional exam requirements/recommendations for international students: Required—TOEFL (minimum score 550 paper-based; 79 iBT). *Application deadline:* For fall admission, 6/1 priority date for domestic students, 5/1 priority date for international students; for spring admission, 11/15 priority date for domestic and international students. Applications are processed on a rolling basis. Application fee: $75. Electronic applications accepted. *Expenses:* $28,800 per year non-resident full-time. *Financial support:* In 2015–16, 56 research assistantships with full tuition reimbursements (averaging $17,711 per year), 52 teaching assistantships with full tuition reimbursements (averaging $17,914 per year) were awarded; fellowships with full tuition reimbursements also available. Financial award application deadline: 1/15. *Total annual research expenditures:* $23.1 million. *Unit head:* Dr. Kevin Belfield, Dean, 973-596-3676, Fax: 973-565-0586, E-mail: kevin.d.belfield@njit.edu. *Application contact:* Stephen Eck, Director of Admissions, 973-596-3300, Fax: 973-596-3461, E-mail: admissions@njit.edu. Website: http://csla.njit.edu/

Northeastern University, Bouvé College of Health Sciences, Boston, MA 02115-5096. Offers applied behavior analysis (MS, CAGS); audiology (Au D); biomedical nanotechnology (MS); college student development and counseling (MS, CAGS); counseling psychology (MS, PhD, CAGS); exercise science (MS); health informatics (MS); medicinal chemistry (MS); nurse anesthesia (DNP, CAGS); nursing (MS, PhD, CAGS), including administration (MS), adult-gerontology acute care nurse practitioner (MS, CAGS), adult-gerontology primary care nurse practitioner (MS, CAGS), anesthesia (MS), family nurse practitioner (MS, CAGS), neonatal nurse practitioner (MS, CAGS), pediatric nurse practitioner (MS, CAGS), psychiatric mental health nurse practitioner (MS, CAGS); nursing practice (DNP); personal health informatics (PhD); pharmaceutical sciences (MS, PhD), including interdisciplinary concentration, pharmaceutics and drug delivery systems; pharmacology (MS); pharmacy (Pharm D); physical therapy (Postbaccalaureate Certificate); physician assistant (MS); population health (PhD);

school psychology (MS, PhD, CAGS); speech-language pathology (MS); urban health (MPH); MS/MBA. *Accreditation:* ACPE (one or more programs are accredited). *Program availability:* Part-time, evening/weekend, online learning. *Faculty:* 194 full-time (120 women), 169 part-time/adjunct (136 women). *Students:* 1,416 full-time (1,049 women), 310 part-time (248 women). In 2015, 374 master's, 313 doctorates, 37 other advanced degrees awarded. *Degree requirements:* For doctorate, thesis/dissertation (for some programs); for other advanced degree, comprehensive exam. Application fee: $75. Electronic applications accepted. *Expenses:* Contact institution. *Financial support:* Applicants required to submit FAFSA. *Unit head:* John R. Reynolds, Professor and Interim Dean, 617-373-3323, Fax: 617-373-3030. *Application contact:* Molly Schnabel, Senior Director of Graduate Affairs, 617-373-2708, Fax: 617-373-4701, E-mail: bouvegrad@neu.edu. Website: http://www.northeastern.edu/bouve/

Oregon State University, College of Pharmacy, Program in Pharmaceutical Sciences, Corvallis, OR 97331. Offers medicinal chemistry (MS, PhD); natural products chemistry (MS, PhD); pharmaceutics (MS, PhD); pharmacoeconomics (MS, PhD); pharmacokinetics (MS, PhD); pharmacology (MS, PhD); toxicology (MS, PhD). *Program availability:* Part-time. *Faculty:* 30 full-time (15 women). *Students:* 29 full-time (10 women); includes 2 minority (1 Asian, non-Hispanic/Latino; 1 Hispanic/Latino), 16 international. Average age 29. 79 applicants, 10% accepted, 5 enrolled. In 2015, 4 doctorates awarded. *Entrance requirements:* For master's and doctorate, GRE. Additional exam requirements/recommendations for international students: Required—TOEFL (minimum score 80 iBT), IELTS (minimum score 6.5). *Application deadline:* For fall admission, 1/1 for domestic students. Application fee: $75 ($85 for international students). *Expenses:* Tuition, state resident: full-time $12,150; part-time $450 per credit. Tuition, nonresident: full-time $20,952; part-time $776 per credit. *Required fees:* $1572; $1443 per unit. One-time fee: $350. Tuition and fees vary according to course load, campus/location and program. *Unit head:* Dr. Mark Zabriskie, Dean and Professor, 541-737-5781, E-mail: mark.zabriskie@oregonstate.edu. *Application contact:* Debra Peters, Pharmacy Advisor, 541-737-8743, E-mail: debra.peters@oregonstate.edu. Website: http://pharmacy.oregonstate.edu/

Purdue University, College of Pharmacy and Pharmacal Sciences and Graduate School, Graduate Programs in Pharmacy and Pharmacal Sciences, Department of Medicinal Chemistry and Molecular Pharmacology, West Lafayette, IN 47907. Offers biophysical and computational chemistry (PhD); cancer research (PhD); immunology and infectious disease (PhD); medicinal biochemistry and molecular biology (PhD); medicinal chemistry and chemical biology (PhD); molecular pharmacology (PhD); neuropharmacology, neurodegeneration, and neurotoxicity (PhD); systems biology and functional genomics (PhD). *Degree requirements:* For doctorate, thesis/dissertation. *Entrance requirements:* For doctorate, GRE General Test; GRE Subject Test in biology, biochemistry, and chemistry (recommended), minimum undergraduate GPA of 3.0. Additional exam requirements/recommendations for international students: Required—TOEFL (minimum score 550 paper-based; 77 iBT); Recommended—TWE. Electronic applications accepted. *Faculty research:* Drug design and development, cancer research, drug synthesis and analysis, chemical pharmacology, environmental toxicology.

Rutgers University–New Brunswick, Ernest Mario School of Pharmacy, Program in Medicinal Chemistry, Piscataway, NJ 08854-8097. Offers MS, PhD. *Program availability:* Part-time. *Degree requirements:* For master's, comprehensive exam, thesis; for doctorate, comprehensive exam, thesis/dissertation. *Entrance requirements:* For master's and doctorate, GRE General Test. Additional exam requirements/recommendations for international students: Required—TOEFL (minimum score 600 paper-based; 90 iBT). Electronic applications accepted. *Faculty research:* Synthesis and design of anticancer drugs, synthesis of pro-drugs for prostate cancer, natural product synthesis, natural product isolation and structure elucidation, computational chemistry.

Temple University, School of Pharmacy, Department of Pharmaceutical Sciences, Philadelphia, PA 19122. Offers medicinal chemistry (MS, PhD); pharmaceutics (MS, PhD); pharmacodynamics (MS, PhD); quality assurance/regulatory affairs (MS). *Program availability:* Part-time, online learning. *Faculty:* 12 full-time (2 women), 1 part-time/adjunct (0 women). *Students:* 48 full-time (28 women), 11 part-time (7 women); includes 1 minority (Asian, non-Hispanic/Latino), 42 international. 75 applicants, 32% accepted, 21 enrolled. In 2015, 4 master's, 1 doctorate awarded. *Degree requirements:* For master's, comprehensive exam (for some programs), thesis (for some programs); for doctorate, 2 foreign languages, comprehensive exam, thesis/dissertation. *Entrance requirements:* For master's, GRE General Test, minimum undergraduate GPA of 3.0; for doctorate, GRE General Test, minimum GPA of 3.0. Additional exam requirements/recommendations for international students: Required—TOEFL (minimum score 550 paper-based; 82 iBT). *Application deadline:* For fall admission, 1/15 for domestic students, 12/15 for international students. Application fee: $60. Electronic applications accepted. *Expenses:* Contact institution. *Financial support:* In 2015–16, 2 fellowships with full tuition reimbursements (averaging $23,000 per year), 6 research assistantships with full tuition reimbursements (averaging $22,000 per year), 11 teaching assistantships with full tuition reimbursements (averaging $22,000 per year) were awarded. Financial award application deadline: 1/15; financial award applicants required to submit FAFSA. *Faculty research:* Pharmacokinetics, synthesis of medicinals, protein research, biopharma-formulation. *Unit head:* Dr. Daniel Canney, Director of Graduate Studies, 215-707-4948, E-mail: phscgrad@temple.edu. *Application contact:* Sophon Din, Administrative Assistant, 215-204-4948, E-mail: tuspgrad@temple.edu.

University at Buffalo, the State University of New York, Graduate School, College of Arts and Sciences, Department of Chemistry, Buffalo, NY 14260. Offers chemistry (MA, PhD); medicinal chemistry (MS, PhD). *Program availability:* Part-time. *Faculty:* 30 full-time (5 women), 2 part-time/adjunct (both women). *Students:* 149 full-time (60 women); includes 21 minority (8 Black or African American, non-Hispanic/Latino; 2 American Indian or Alaska Native, non-Hispanic/Latino; 3 Asian, non-Hispanic/Latino; 8 Hispanic/Latino), 38 international. Average age 26. 268 applicants, 28% accepted, 28 enrolled. In 2015, 12 master's, 20 doctorates awarded. Terminal master's awarded for partial completion of doctoral program. *Degree requirements:* For master's, thesis or alternative, project; for doctorate, thesis/dissertation, synopsis proposal. *Entrance requirements:* For master's and doctorate, GRE General Test. Additional exam requirements/recommendations for international students: Required—TOEFL (minimum score 550 paper-based; 79 iBT). *Application deadline:* For fall admission, 3/1 priority date for domestic students, 3/1 for international students; for spring admission, 11/1 priority date for domestic students. Applications are processed on a rolling basis. Application fee: $75. Electronic applications accepted. *Expenses:* $22,210; $925 per credit hour. *Financial support:* In 2015–16, 7 students received support, including 8 fellowships with full tuition reimbursements available (averaging $22,080 per year), 24 research assistantships with full tuition reimbursements available (averaging $22,080 per year), 98 teaching assistantships with full tuition reimbursements available (averaging $23,000 per year); Federal Work-Study, institutionally sponsored loans, and unspecified assistantships also available. Financial award application deadline: 6/15; financial award applicants required to submit FAFSA. *Faculty research:* Synthesis, measurements, structure theory, translation. *Total annual research expenditures:* $8 million. *Unit head:* Dr. Michael R. Detty, Chairman, 716-645-6824, Fax: 716-645-6963, E-mail: chechair@buffalo.edu. *Application contact:* Dr. Diana S. Aga, Director of Graduate Studies, 716-645-4220, Fax: 716-645-6963, E-mail: dianaaga@buffalo.edu. Website: http://www.chemistry.buffalo.edu/

University of California, Irvine, Programs in Health Sciences, Program in Medicinal Chemistry and Pharmacology, Irvine, CA 92697. Offers PhD. *Students:* 6 full-time (4 women); includes 3 minority (1 Black or African American, non-Hispanic/Latino; 1 Asian, non-Hispanic/Latino; 1 Hispanic/Latino), 1 international. Average age 26. 66 applicants, 26% accepted, 8 enrolled. Application fee: $90 ($110 for international students). *Unit head:* Stephen Hanessian, Director, 949-824-5449, Fax: 949-824-9920, E-mail: shanessi@uci.edu. *Application contact:* Geneva Lopez-Sandoval, Student Affairs Office, 949-824-0878, E-mail: lopezg@uci.edu. Website: http://www.pharmsci.uci.edu/graduate/index.php

University of California, San Francisco, School of Pharmacy and Graduate Division, Chemistry and Chemical Biology Graduate Program, San Francisco, CA 94143. Offers PhD. *Degree requirements:* For doctorate, thesis/dissertation. *Entrance requirements:* For doctorate, GRE General Test, minimum GPA of 3.0, bachelor's degree. Additional exam requirements/recommendations for international students: Required—TOEFL (minimum score 550 paper-based; 80 iBT). Electronic applications accepted. *Faculty research:* Macromolecular structure function and dynamics, computational chemistry and biology, biological chemistry and synthetic biology, chemical biology and molecular design, nanomolecular design.

University of Connecticut, Graduate School, School of Pharmacy, Department of Pharmaceutical Sciences, Program in Medicinal Chemistry, Storrs, CT 06269. Offers MS, PhD. Terminal master's awarded for partial completion of doctoral program. *Degree requirements:* For master's, comprehensive exam, thesis; for doctorate, thesis/dissertation. *Entrance requirements:* Additional exam requirements/recommendations for international students: Required—TOEFL (minimum score 550 paper-based). *Application deadline:* For fall admission, 2/1 priority date for domestic and international students; for spring admission, 11/1 for domestic students, 10/1 for international students. Applications are processed on a rolling basis. Application fee: $55. Electronic applications accepted. *Financial support:* Fellowships, research assistantships with full tuition reimbursements, teaching assistantships with full tuition reimbursements, Federal Work-Study, scholarships/grants, traineeships, health care benefits, and unspecified assistantships available. Financial award application deadline: 2/1; financial award applicants required to submit FAFSA. Website: http://www.pharmacy.uconn.edu/

University of Florida, Graduate School, College of Pharmacy and Graduate School, Graduate Programs in Pharmacy, Department of Medicinal Chemistry, Gainesville, FL 32611. Offers clinical toxicology (MSP); forensic DNA and serology (MSP); forensic drug chemistry (MSP); forensic science (MSP); medicinal chemistry (MSP, PhD); pharmaceutical chemistry (MSP). *Program availability:* Part-time, evening/weekend, online learning. *Faculty:* 3 full-time. *Students:* 77 full-time (54 women), 335 part-time (232 women); includes 83 minority (31 Black or African American, non-Hispanic/Latino; 4 American Indian or Alaska Native, non-Hispanic/Latino; 18 Asian, non-Hispanic/Latino; 30 Hispanic/Latino), 31 international. Average age 33. 64 applicants, 16% accepted, 8 enrolled. In 2015, 132 master's awarded. Terminal master's awarded for partial completion of doctoral program. *Degree requirements:* For master's, thesis optional; for doctorate, comprehensive exam, thesis/dissertation. *Entrance requirements:* For master's and doctorate, GRE General Test, minimum GPA of 3.0. Additional exam requirements/recommendations for international students: Required—TOEFL (minimum score 550 paper-based; 80 iBT), IELTS (minimum score 6). *Application deadline:* For fall admission, 1/31 priority date for domestic students, 1/31 for international students; for winter admission, 10/1 for domestic and international students; for spring admission, 11/16 for domestic and international students. Applications are processed on a rolling basis. Application fee: $30. Electronic applications accepted. *Financial support:* In 2015–16, 9 research assistantships, 13 teaching assistantships were awarded; fellowships also available. Financial award application deadline: 4/15; financial award applicants required to submit CSS PROFILE or FAFSA. *Faculty research:* Drug metabolism and toxicology, discovery of biologically active natural products, chelator chemistry and biochemistry, anti-cancer drug and pro-drug discovery, discovery of anti-infective drugs and biosynthetic engineering. *Total annual research expenditures:* $1.9 million. *Unit head:* Dr. Margaret O. James, Professor and Chair, 352-273-7707, Fax: 352-392-9455, E-mail: mojames@ufl.edu. *Application contact:* Hendrik Luesch, PhD, Graduate Coordinator, 352-273-7738, Fax: 352-392-9455, E-mail: luesch@cop.ufl.edu. Website: http://pharmacy.ufl.edu/mc/

The University of Iowa, College of Pharmacy, Iowa City, IA 52242-1316. Offers clinical pharmaceutical sciences (PhD); medicinal and natural products chemistry (PhD); pharamaceutics (PhD); pharmaceutical socioeconomics (PhD); pharmaceutics (MS); pharmacy (Pharm D); Pharm D/MPH. *Accreditation:* ACPE (one or more programs are accredited). *Degree requirements:* For master's, thesis optional, exam; for doctorate, comprehensive exam, thesis/dissertation. *Entrance requirements:* For master's and doctorate, GRE General Test, minimum GPA of 3.0. Additional exam requirements/recommendations for international students: Required—TOEFL (minimum score 550 paper-based; 81 iBT). Electronic applications accepted.

The University of Kansas, Graduate Studies, School of Pharmacy, Department of Medicinal Chemistry, Lawrence, KS 66045. Offers MS, PhD. *Students:* 28 full-time (12 women); includes 1 minority (Two or more races, non-Hispanic/Latino), 12 international. Average age 27. 74 applicants, 11% accepted, 4 enrolled. In 2015, 7 master's, 4 doctorates awarded. Terminal master's awarded for partial completion of doctoral program. *Entrance requirements:* For master's and doctorate, GRE General Test. Additional exam requirements/recommendations for international students: Required—TOEFL. *Application deadline:* For fall admission, 2/1 for domestic and international students. Application fee: $65 ($85 for international students). Electronic applications accepted. *Financial support:* Fellowships, research assistantships, teaching assistantships, health care benefits, and unspecified assistantships available. Financial award application deadline: 3/1. *Faculty research:* Cancer, neuroscience, synthetic methods, natural products, biochemistry. *Unit head:* Dr. Thomas Prisinzano, Chair, 785-864-3267, E-mail: prisinza@ku.edu. *Application contact:* Norma Henley, Administrative Associate, 785-864-4495, E-mail: medchem@ku.edu. Website: http://www.medchem.ku.edu/

The University of Kansas, Graduate Studies, School of Pharmacy, Department of Pharmaceutical Chemistry, Lawrence, KS 66047. Offers MS, PhD. *Program availability:* Part-time, evening/weekend, online learning. *Students:* 36 full-time (14 women), 17 part-time (9 women); includes 11 minority (1 Black or African American, non-Hispanic/Latino; 7 Asian, non-Hispanic/Latino; 2 Hispanic/Latino; 1 Two or more races, non-Hispanic/Latino), 21 international. Average age 29. 71 applicants, 20% accepted, 11 enrolled. In

2015, 9 master's, 8 doctorates awarded. Terminal master's awarded for partial completion of doctoral program. *Entrance requirements:* For master's, GRE General Test, bachelor's degree in biological sciences, chemical engineering, chemistry, or pharmacy; official transcripts from all universities/institutions in which the applicant has studied; personal statement; resume; for doctorate, GRE General Test, official transcripts from all universities/institutions in which the applicant has studied, personal statement, resume. Additional exam requirements/recommendations for international students: Required—TOEFL. *Application deadline:* For fall admission, 1/15 for domestic and international students. Application fee: $65 ($85 for international students). Electronic applications accepted. *Financial support:* Fellowships, research assistantships, career-related internships or fieldwork, scholarships/grants, traineeships, and unspecified assistantships available. Financial award application deadline: 1/15. *Faculty research:* Physical pharmacy, biotechnology, bioanalytical chemistry, biopharmaceutics and pharmacokinetics, nanotechnology. *Unit head:* Dr. Christian Schoneich, Chair, 785-864-4880, E-mail: schoneic@ku.edu. *Application contact:* Nancy Helm, Administrative Associate, 785-864-4822, E-mail: nhelm@ku.edu. Website: http://www.pharmchem.ku.edu/

University of Michigan, College of Pharmacy and University of Michigan, Department of Medicinal Chemistry, Ann Arbor, MI 48109. Offers PhD. *Faculty:* 11 full-time (2 women), 3 part-time/adjunct (0 women). *Students:* 45 full-time (19 women); includes 5 minority (1 Black or African American, non-Hispanic/Latino; 2 Asian, non-Hispanic/Latino; 1 Hispanic/Latino; 1 Two or more races, non-Hispanic/Latino), 5 international. Average age 27. 71 applicants, 14% accepted, 4 enrolled. In 2015, 8 doctorates awarded. *Degree requirements:* For doctorate, thesis/dissertation, oral defense of dissertation, preliminary exam. *Entrance requirements:* For doctorate, GRE. Additional exam requirements/recommendations for international students: Required—TOEFL (minimum score 560 paper-based; 84 iBT) or IELTS (minimum score 6.5). *Application deadline:* For fall admission, 12/31 for domestic and international students. Application fee: $75 ($90 for international students). Electronic applications accepted. *Expenses:* Contact institution. *Financial support:* In 2015–16, 39 students received support, including 9 fellowships (averaging $48,037 per year), 5 research assistantships (averaging $48,037 per year), 17 teaching assistantships (averaging $48,037 per year); career-related internships or fieldwork, institutionally sponsored loans, scholarships/grants, traineeships, health care benefits, and unspecified assistantships also available. *Unit head:* Dr. George A. Garcia, Chair, 734-764-2202, Fax: 734-647-8430, E-mail: gagarcia@med.umich.edu. *Application contact:* Sarah Lloyd, Executive Secretary, 734-647-8429, Fax: 734-647-8430, E-mail: sarlloyd@med.umich.edu. Website: https://pharmacy.umich.edu/medchem

University of Minnesota, Twin Cities Campus, College of Pharmacy and Graduate School, Graduate Programs in Pharmacy, Graduate Program in Medicinal Chemistry, Minneapolis, MN 55455. Offers MS, PhD. *Faculty:* 27 full-time (4 women), 6 part-time/adjunct (2 women). *Students:* 53 full-time (14 women); includes 4 minority (1 Black or African American, non-Hispanic/Latino; 2 Asian, non-Hispanic/Latino; 1 Two or more races, non-Hispanic/Latino), 11 international. Average age 26. 70 applicants, 27% accepted, 10 enrolled. In 2015, 3 master's, 6 doctorates awarded. Terminal master's awarded for partial completion of doctoral program. *Degree requirements:* For master's, comprehensive exam, thesis; for doctorate, comprehensive exam, thesis/dissertation. *Entrance requirements:* For doctorate, GRE General Test, BS in biology, chemistry, or pharmacy. Additional exam requirements/recommendations for international students: Required—TOEFL (minimum score 550 paper-based). *Application deadline:* For fall admission, 1/5 priority date for domestic and international students. Application fee: $75 ($95 for international students). Electronic applications accepted. *Financial support:* In 2015–16, 30 students received support, including 36 fellowships with full tuition reimbursements available (averaging $9,500 per year), 26 research assistantships with full tuition reimbursements available (averaging $26,234 per year), 7 teaching assistantships with full tuition reimbursements available (averaging $16,669 per year); health care benefits and unspecified assistantships also available. Financial award application deadline: 1/5. *Faculty research:* Drug design and synthesis, molecular modeling, chemical aspects of drug metabolism and toxicity. *Total annual research expenditures:* $5.1 million. *Unit head:* Dr. Gunda I. Georg, Department Head of Medicinal Chemistry, 612-626-6320, Fax: 612-626-3114, E-mail: georg@umn.edu. *Application contact:* Information Contact, 612-625-3014, Fax: 612-625-6002, E-mail: gsquest@umn.edu. Website: http://www.pharmacy.umn.edu/medchem/graduate/

University of Montana, Graduate School, College of Health Professions and Biomedical Sciences, Skaggs School of Pharmacy, Department of Biomedical and Pharmaceutical Sciences, Missoula, MT 59812-0002. Offers biomedical sciences (PhD); medicinal chemistry (MS, PhD); molecular and cellular toxicology (MS, PhD); neuroscience (PhD); pharmaceutical sciences (MS). *Accreditation:* ACPE. *Degree requirements:* For master's, oral defense of thesis; for doctorate, research dissertation defense. *Entrance requirements:* For master's and doctorate, GRE General Test. Additional exam requirements/recommendations for international students: Required—TOEFL (minimum score 540 paper-based). Electronic applications accepted. *Faculty research:* Cardiovascular pharmacology, medicinal chemistry, neurosciences, environmental toxicology, pharmacogenetics, cancer.

University of Rhode Island, Graduate School, College of Pharmacy, Department of Biomedical and Pharmaceutical Sciences, Kingston, RI 02881. Offers medicinal chemistry and pharmacognosy (MS, PhD); pharmaceutics and pharmacokinetics (MS, PhD); pharmacology and toxicology (MS, PhD). *Program availability:* Part-time. *Faculty:* 15 full-time (4 women), 4 part-time/adjunct (2 women). *Students:* 39 full-time (14 women), 10 part-time (3 women); includes 3 minority (1 Black or African American, non-Hispanic/Latino; 2 Asian, non-Hispanic/Latino), 24 international. In 2015, 4 master's, 10 doctorates awarded. *Entrance requirements:* For master's and doctorate, GRE (minimum old/new format scores: Verbal 350/143; Quantitative 550/146; Analytical 3.0), 2 letters of recommendation. Additional exam requirements/recommendations for international students: Required—TOEFL (minimum score 550 paper-based). *Application deadline:* For fall admission, 7/15 for domestic students, 2/1 for international students. Application fee: $65. Electronic applications accepted. *Expenses:* Tuition, state resident: full-time $11,796; part-time $655 per credit. Tuition, nonresident: full-time $24,206; part-time $1345 per credit. *Required fees:* $1546; $44 per credit. One-time fee: $155 full-time; $35 part-time. *Financial support:* In 2015–16, 6 research assistantships with tuition reimbursements (averaging $14,828 per year), 18 teaching assistantships with tuition reimbursements (averaging $14,851 per year) were awarded. Financial award application deadline: 2/1; financial award applicants required to submit FAFSA. *Faculty research:* Chemical carcinogenesis with a major emphasis on the structural and synthetic aspects of DNA-adduct formation, drug-drug/herb interaction, drug-genetic interaction, signaling of nuclear receptors, transcriptional regulation, oncogenesis. *Total annual research expenditures:* $5.8 million. *Unit head:* Dr. Bingfang Yan, Chair, 401-874-5032, Fax: 401-874-2181, E-mail: byan@uri.edu. *Application contact:* Graduate Admissions, 401-874-2872, E-mail: gradadm@etal.uri.edu. Website: http://www.uri.edu/pharmacy/departments/bps/index.shtml

The University of Texas at Austin, Graduate School, College of Pharmacy, Graduate Programs in Pharmacy, Austin, TX 78712-1111. Offers health outcomes and pharmacy practice (PhD); health outcomes and pharmacy practice (MS); medicinal chemistry (PhD); pharmaceutics (PhD); pharmacology and toxicology (PhD); pharmacotherapy (MS, PhD); translational science (PhD). PhD in translational science offered jointly with The University of Texas Health Science Center at San Antonio and The University of Texas at San Antonio. *Degree requirements:* For master's, thesis; for doctorate, thesis/dissertation. *Entrance requirements:* For master's and doctorate, GRE General Test. Electronic applications accepted. *Faculty research:* Synthetic medical chemistry, synthetic molecular biology, bio-organic chemistry, pharmacoeconomics, pharmacy practice.

University of the Sciences, Program in Chemistry, Biochemistry and Pharmacognosy, Philadelphia, PA 19104-4495. Offers biochemistry (MS, PhD); chemistry (MS, PhD); pharmacognosy (MS, PhD). *Program availability:* Part-time. *Degree requirements:* For master's, thesis, qualifying exams; for doctorate, comprehensive exam, thesis/dissertation, qualifying exams. *Entrance requirements:* For master's and doctorate, GRE General Test, GRE Subject Test. Additional exam requirements/recommendations for international students: Required—TOEFL, TWE. *Application deadline:* For fall admission, 5/1 for international students; for winter admission, 10/1 for international students; for spring admission, 3/1 for international students. Applications are processed on a rolling basis. Application fee: $50. *Expenses:* Contact institution. *Financial support:* Fellowships with full tuition reimbursements, research assistantships with full tuition reimbursements, teaching assistantships with full tuition reimbursements, institutionally sponsored loans, scholarships/grants, and tuition waivers (full) available. Financial award application deadline: 5/1. *Unit head:* Dr. James R. McKee, Director, 215-596-8847, E-mail: j.mckee@usciences.edu. *Application contact:* Dr. James R. McKee, Director, 215-596-8847, E-mail: j.mckee@usciences.edu.

The University of Toledo, College of Graduate Studies, College of Pharmacy and Pharmaceutical Sciences, Program in Medicinal and Biological Chemistry, Toledo, OH 43606-3390. Offers MS, PhD. Terminal master's awarded for partial completion of doctoral program. *Degree requirements:* For master's, thesis; for doctorate, thesis/dissertation. *Entrance requirements:* For master's and doctorate, GRE General Test. Additional exam requirements/recommendations for international students: Required—TOEFL (minimum score 550 paper-based; 80 iBT). Electronic applications accepted. *Faculty research:* Neuroscience, molecular modeling, immunotoxicology, organic synthesis, peptide biochemistry.

University of Utah, Graduate School, College of Pharmacy, Department of Medicinal Chemistry, Salt Lake City, UT 84112-5820. Offers MS, PhD. *Faculty:* 10 full-time (3 women), 4 part-time/adjunct (2 women). *Students:* 11 full-time (5 women), 7 international. Average age 29. 12 applicants, 33% accepted, 4 enrolled. In 2015, 1 master's, 6 doctorates awarded. *Degree requirements:* For doctorate, thesis/dissertation. *Entrance requirements:* For doctorate, GRE, minimum GPA of 3.0. Additional exam requirements/recommendations for international students: Required—TOEFL (minimum score 550 paper-based; 80 iBT), IELTS (minimum score 6.5). *Application deadline:* For fall admission, 12/15 for domestic and international students. Application fee: $55 ($65 for international students). Electronic applications accepted. *Expenses:* $3,861.48 per semester; $12,334.93 per semester (international); $2,000 per year health insurance. *Financial support:* In 2015–16, 11 students received support, including fellowships with full tuition reimbursements available (averaging $27,000 per year), research assistantships with full tuition reimbursements available (averaging $27,500 per year), 1 teaching assistantship with full tuition reimbursement available (averaging $27,000 per year); health care benefits, tuition waivers (full), and unspecified assistantships also available. Financial award application deadline: 12/15. *Faculty research:* Anticancer and anti-infective drug discovery, assays for high-throughput screening, neuroactive peptides, bioinorganic chemistry, structure-based drug design and modeling. *Total annual research expenditures:* $3.5 million. *Unit head:* Dr. Darrell R. Davis, Chair, 801-581-7063, Fax: 801-585-6208, E-mail: darrell.davis@utah.edu. *Application contact:* Dr. Thomas E. Cheatham, Director of Graduate Studies, 801-587-9652, Fax: 801-585-6208, E-mail: tom.cheatham@pharm.utah.edu. Website: http://www.pharmacy.utah.edu/medchem/

University of Utah, Graduate School, College of Pharmacy, Department of Pharmaceutics and Pharmaceutical Chemistry, Salt Lake City, UT 84112. Offers PhD. *Faculty:* 10 full-time (1 woman), 4 part-time/adjunct (1 woman). *Students:* 16 full-time (6 women), 5 part-time (4 women); includes 3 minority (1 Black or African American, non-Hispanic/Latino; 2 Asian, non-Hispanic/Latino), 13 international. Average age 28. 41 applicants, 7% accepted, 3 enrolled. In 2015, 6 doctorates awarded. Terminal master's awarded for partial completion of doctoral program. *Degree requirements:* For doctorate, comprehensive exam, thesis/dissertation, peer-reviewed scientific publications and oral presentations. *Entrance requirements:* For doctorate, GRE. Additional exam requirements/recommendations for international students: Required—TOEFL (minimum score 550 paper-based). *Application deadline:* For fall admission, 12/1 priority date for domestic and international students. Applications are processed on a rolling basis. Application fee: $55 ($65 for international students). Electronic applications accepted. *Expenses:* $3,861.48 per semester; $12,334.93 per semester (international); $2,000 per year health insurance. *Financial support:* In 2015–16, 20 students received support, including 21 research assistantships (averaging $25,000 per year); scholarships/grants, health care benefits, tuition waivers (full), and unspecified assistantships also available.

Faculty research: Delivery of therapeutic genes, trafficking mechanisms for drugs within cells, combination devices and local drug release from implants, anti-cancer polymer-based therapeutics and vaccines, nanotechnology for drug carriers. *Total annual research expenditures:* $924,131. *Unit head:* Dr. David W. Grainger, Chairperson, 801-581-7831, Fax: 801-581-3674, E-mail: david.grainger@utah.edu. *Application contact:* Dion Duffin, Academic Program Manager, 801-585-0070, E-mail: dion.duffin@pharm.utah.edu.
Website: http://www.pharmacy.utah.edu/pharmaceutics/

University of Washington, School of Pharmacy, Department of Medicinal Chemistry, Seattle, WA 98195. Offers PhD. *Degree requirements:* For doctorate, thesis/dissertation. *Entrance requirements:* For doctorate, GRE General Test, minimum GPA of 3.0, 3 letters of recommendation, statement of purpose, transcripts, resume. Additional exam requirements/recommendations for international students: Required—TOEFL. Electronic applications accepted. *Faculty research:* Chemical and molecular aspects of drug action, metabolism and drug toxicity, theoretical studies on protein folding, nuclear magnetic resonance (NMR) of macromolecules and biomedical mass spectrometry.

Virginia Commonwealth University, Medical College of Virginia-Professional Programs, School of Pharmacy, Department of Pharmaceutics, Richmond, VA 23284-9005. Offers medicinal chemistry (MS); pharmaceutical sciences (PhD); pharmaceutics (MS); pharmacotherapy and pharmacy administration (MS). Terminal master's awarded for partial completion of doctoral program. *Degree requirements:* For master's, thesis; for doctorate, thesis/dissertation. *Entrance requirements:* For master's and doctorate, GRE General Test. Additional exam requirements/recommendations for international students: Required—TOEFL. Electronic applications accepted. *Faculty research:* Drug delivery systems, drug development.

Wayne State University, Eugene Applebaum College of Pharmacy and Health Sciences, Department of Pharmaceutical Sciences, Detroit, MI 48202. Offers medicinal chemistry (MS, PhD); pharmaceutics (MS, PhD), including medicinal chemistry (PhD); pharmacology/toxicology (MS, PhD). *Accreditation:* ACPE (one or more programs are accredited). *Faculty:* 17 full-time (3 women). *Students:* 26 full-time (14 women), 3 part-time (1 woman); includes 3 minority (1 Black or African American, non-Hispanic/Latino; 1 American Indian or Alaska Native, non-Hispanic/Latino; 1 Asian, non-Hispanic/Latino), 23 international. Average age 26. 184 applicants, 15% accepted, 10 enrolled. In 2015, 9 master's, 102 doctorates awarded. *Degree requirements:* For master's, thesis; for doctorate, thesis/dissertation. *Entrance requirements:* For master's, GRE General Test, bachelor's degree; adequate background in biology, physics, calculus, and chemistry; three letters of recommendation; personal statement; for doctorate, GRE General Test, bachelor's or master's degree in one of the behavioral, biological, pharmaceutical or physical sciences; three letters of recommendation. Additional exam requirements/recommendations for international students: Required—TOEFL (minimum score 550 paper-based; 79 iBT), Michigan English Language Assessment Battery (minimum score 85; Recommended—IELTS (minimum score 6.5), TWE (minimum score 5.5). *Application deadline:* For fall admission, 12/1 priority date for domestic and international students. Applications are processed on a rolling basis. Application fee: $0. Electronic applications accepted. *Expenses:* $16,104 per year resident tuition, $32,401 non-resident tuition; $671 per credit hour resident tuition, $1,350.05 per credit hour non-resident tuition; fees include $47.45 per credit hour student services fee and $274.60 per semester registration fee. *Financial support:* In 2015–16, 15 students received support, including 2 fellowships with tuition reimbursements available (averaging $24,179 per year), 10 research assistantships with full tuition reimbursements available (averaging $24,595 per year); teaching assistantships, scholarships/grants, health care benefits, and unspecified assistantships also available. Financial award application deadline: 3/31; financial award applicants required to submit FAFSA. *Faculty research:* Design of new anthracyclines, genetic and epigenetic effects of extracellular inducers, cellular injury and cell death, drug metabolism and nutrition, anti-infective agents, carcinogenesis, diabetes research, theragnostic nanomedicines, neurotoxicity, drug discovery, insulin resistance. *Unit head:* Dr. George Corcoran, Chair and Professor, 313-577-1737, E-mail: corcoran@wayne.edu. *Application contact:* 313-577-5415, Fax: 313-577-2033, E-mail: pscgrad@wayne.edu.
Website: http://cphs.wayne.edu/sciences/index.php

West Virginia University, School of Pharmacy, Program in Pharmaceutical and Pharmacological Sciences, Morgantown, WV 26506. Offers administrative pharmacy (PhD); behavioral pharmacy (MS, PhD); biopharmaceutics/pharmacokinetics (MS, PhD); industrial pharmacy (MS); medicinal chemistry (MS, PhD); pharmaceutical chemistry (MS, PhD); pharmaceutics (MS, PhD); pharmacology and toxicology (MS); pharmacy (MS); pharmacy administration (MS). *Program availability:* Part-time. Terminal master's awarded for partial completion of doctoral program. *Degree requirements:* For master's, thesis; for doctorate, one foreign language, comprehensive exam, thesis/dissertation. *Entrance requirements:* For master's and doctorate, GRE General Test, minimum GPA of 2.75. Additional exam requirements/recommendations for international students: Required—TOEFL; Recommended—TWE. Electronic applications accepted. *Expenses:* Contact institution. *Faculty research:* Pharmaceutics, medicinal chemistry, biopharmaceutics/pharmacokinetics, health outcomes research.

Pharmaceutical Administration

Columbia University, Graduate School of Business, MBA Program, New York, NY 10027. Offers accounting (MBA); decision, risk, and operations (MBA); entrepreneurship (MBA); finance and economics (MBA); healthcare and pharmaceutical management (MBA); human resource management (MBA); international business (MBA); leadership and ethics (MBA); management (MBA); marketing (MBA); media (MBA); private equity (MBA); real estate (MBA); social enterprise (MBA); value investing (MBA); DDS/MBA; JD/MBA; MBA/MIA; MBA/MPH; MBA/MS; MD/MBA. *Entrance requirements:* For master's, GMAT, 2 letters of recommendation. Additional exam requirements/recommendations for international students: Required—TOEFL. Electronic applications accepted. *Expenses:* Contact institution. *Faculty research:* Human decision making and behavioral research; real estate market and mortgage defaults; financial crisis and corporate governance; international business; security analysis and accounting.

Duquesne University, Mylan School of Pharmacy, Graduate School of Pharmaceutical Sciences, Program in Pharmacy Administration, Pittsburgh, PA 15282-0001. Offers MS. *Faculty:* 5 full-time (2 women). *Students:* 8 full-time (4 women), 5 international. Average age 28. 17 applicants, 12% accepted, 2 enrolled. *Degree requirements:* For master's, thesis. *Entrance requirements:* For master's, GRE General Test. Additional exam requirements/recommendations for international students: Required—TOEFL (minimum

score 100 iBT). *Application deadline:* For fall admission, 2/1 priority date for domestic and international students. Applications are processed on a rolling basis. Application fee: $50. Electronic applications accepted. Application fee is waived when completed online. *Expenses:* $1,432 per credit. *Financial support:* In 2015–16, 5 students received support, including 5 teaching assistantships with full tuition reimbursements available. *Unit head:* Dr. Khalid Kamal, Head, 412-396-1926. *Application contact:* Information Contact, 412-396-1172, E-mail: gsps-adm@duq.edu.
Website: http://www.duq.edu/academics/schools/pharmacy/graduate-school-of-pharmaceutical-sciences

Fairleigh Dickinson University, Metropolitan Campus, Silberman College of Business, Program in Pharmaceutical Studies, Teaneck, NJ 07666-1914. Offers chemical studies (Certificate); pharmaceutical studies (MBA, Certificate).

Florida Agricultural and Mechanical University, Division of Graduate Studies, Research, and Continuing Education, College of Pharmacy and Pharmaceutical Sciences, Graduate Programs in Pharmaceutical Sciences, Tallahassee, FL 32307-3200. Offers environmental toxicology (PhD); health outcomes research and pharmacoeconomics (PhD); medicinal chemistry (MS, PhD); pharmaceutics (MS, PhD); pharmacology/toxicology (MS, PhD); pharmacy administration (MS). *Accreditation:*

CEPH. *Degree requirements:* For master's, comprehensive exam, thesis, publishable paper; for doctorate, comprehensive exam, thesis/dissertation, publishable paper. *Entrance requirements:* For master's and doctorate, GRE General Test, minimum GPA of 3.0 in last 60 hours. Additional exam requirements/recommendations for international students: Required—TOEFL. *Faculty research:* Anticancer agents, anti-inflammatory drugs, chronopharmacology, neuroendocrinology, microbiology.

Idaho State University, Office of Graduate Studies, College of Pharmacy, Department of Pharmacy Practice and Administrative Sciences, Pocatello, ID 83209-8333. Offers pharmacy (Pharm D); pharmacy administration (MS, PhD). *Accreditation:* ACPE (one or more programs are accredited). *Program availability:* Part-time. *Degree requirements:* For master's, one foreign language, comprehensive exam, thesis, thesis research, speech and technical writing classes; for doctorate, comprehensive exam, thesis/ dissertation, oral and written exams, speech and technical writing classes. *Entrance requirements:* For master's, GRE General Test, minimum GPA of 3.0, 3 letters of recommendation; for doctorate, GRE General Test, BS in pharmacy or related field, minimum GPA of 3.0, 3 letters of recommendation. Additional exam requirements/ recommendations for international students: Required—TOEFL (minimum score 550 paper-based; 80 iBT). Electronic applications accepted. *Expenses:* Contact institution. *Faculty research:* Pharmaceutical care outcomes, drug use review, pharmacoeconomics.

New Jersey Institute of Technology, Newark College of Engineering, Newark, NJ 07102. Offers biomedical engineering (MS, PhD); chemical engineering (MS, PhD); computer engineering (MS, PhD); electrical engineering (MS, PhD); engineering management (MS); environmental engineering (PhD); healthcare systems management (MS); industrial engineering (MS, PhD); Internet engineering (MS); manufacturing engineering (MS); mechanical engineering (MS, PhD); occupational safety and health engineering (MS); pharmaceutical bioprocessing (MS); pharmaceutical engineering (MS); pharmaceutical systems management (MS); power and energy systems (MS); telecommunications (MS); transportation (MS, PhD). *Program availability:* Part-time, evening/weekend. *Faculty:* 139 full-time (22 women), 152 part-time/adjunct (18 women). *Students:* 946 full-time (226 women), 580 part-time (122 women); includes 397 minority (93 Black or African American, non-Hispanic/Latino; 136 Asian, non-Hispanic/Latino; 145 Hispanic/Latino; 23 Two or more races, non-Hispanic/Latino; 808 international. Average age 28. 3,111 applicants, 62% accepted, 591 enrolled. In 2015, 570 master's, 31 doctorates awarded. Terminal master's awarded for partial completion of doctoral program. *Degree requirements:* For master's, thesis optional; for doctorate, thesis/ dissertation. *Entrance requirements:* For master's, GRE General Test; for doctorate, GRE General Test, minimum graduate GPA of 3.5. Additional exam requirements/ recommendations for international students: Required—TOEFL (minimum score 550 paper-based; 79 iBT). *Application deadline:* For fall admission, 6/1 priority date for domestic students, 5/1 priority date for international students; for spring admission, 11/ 15 priority date for domestic and international students. Applications are processed on a rolling basis. Application fee: $75. Electronic applications accepted. *Expenses:* $28,800 per year non-resident full-time. *Financial support:* In 2015–16, fellowships with partial tuition reimbursements (averaging $3,900 per year), 68 research assistantships with partial tuition reimbursements (averaging $18,120 per year), 68 teaching assistantships with partial tuition reimbursements (averaging $13,325 per year) were awarded. Financial award application deadline: 1/15. *Total annual research expenditures:* $41.3 million. *Unit head:* Dr. Moshe Kam, Dean, 973-596-5534, E-mail: moshe.kam@njit.edu. *Application contact:* Stephen Eck, Director of Admissions, 973-596-3300, Fax: 973-596-3461, E-mail: admissions@njit.edu.
Website: http://engineering.njit.edu/

Northeast Ohio Medical University, College of Graduate Studies, Rootstown, OH 44272-0095. Offers bioethics (Certificate); health-system pharmacy administration (MS); integrated pharmaceutical medicine (MS, PhD); public health (MS). *Program availability:* Part-time. *Faculty:* 15 part-time/adjunct (6 women). *Students:* 15 full-time (7 women), 26 part-time (11 women); includes 7 minority (5 Asian, non-Hispanic/Latino; 2 Hispanic/ Latino). Average age 27. In 2015, 9 master's, 1 doctorate awarded. *Application deadline:* For fall admission, 9/1 priority date for domestic students; for winter admission, 1/5 priority date for domestic students. Applications are processed on a rolling basis. Electronic applications accepted. *Expenses:* Contact institution. *Financial support:* In 2015–16, 18 students received support. *Unit head:* Dr. Walter E. Horton, Jr., Dean. *Application contact:* Heidi Terry, Executive Director, Enrollment Services, 330-325-6479, E-mail: hterry@neoucom.edu.
Website: http://www.neomed.edu/academics/graduatestudies

Nova Southeastern University, College of Pharmacy, Fort Lauderdale, FL 33328. Offers drug development (pharmaceutics) (PhD); molecular medicine and pharmacogenomics (PhD); pharmacy (Pharm D); social and administrative pharmacy (PhD); Pharm D/MBA; Pharm D/MPH. *Accreditation:* ACPE. *Faculty:* 67 full-time (31 women), 3 part-time/adjunct (1 woman). *Students:* 971 full-time (655 women), 25 part-time (12 women); includes 705 minority (57 Black or African American, non-Hispanic/ Latino; 177 Asian, non-Hispanic/Latino; 451 Hispanic/Latino; 1 Native Hawaiian or other Pacific Islander, non-Hispanic/Latino; 19 Two or more races, non-Hispanic/Latino), 96 international. Average age 27. 1,024 applicants, 41% accepted, 255 enrolled. In 2015, 226 doctorates awarded. *Degree requirements:* For doctorate, comprehensive exam (for some programs), thesis/dissertation (for some programs). *Entrance requirements:* For doctorate, PCAT (for Pharm D); GRE (for PhD). Additional exam requirements/ recommendations for international students: Required—TOEFL (minimum score 550 paper-based, 80 iBT) or IELTS (minimum score 6.0). *Application deadline:* For fall admission, 3/15 for domestic students, 2/1 for international students. Applications are processed on a rolling basis. Application fee: $50. Electronic applications accepted. *Expenses:* Contact institution. *Financial support:* In 2015–16, 131 students received support, including 11 teaching assistantships with full tuition reimbursements available (averaging $18,000 per year); career-related internships or fieldwork, Federal Work-Study, institutionally sponsored loans, and scholarships/grants also available. Financial award application deadline: 4/15; financial award applicants required to submit FAFSA. *Faculty research:* Cancer, health care delivery, pharmacoeconomics, cardiovascular/ metabolic diseases, autism. *Total annual research expenditures:* $446,267. *Unit head:* Dr. Lisa Deziel, Dean, 954-262-1304, Fax: 954-262-2278, E-mail: copdean@nova.edu. *Application contact:* Jeffrey Jurkas, Coordinator of Admissions and Recruitment, 954-262-1240, Fax: 954-262-2282, E-mail: nsupharmacyinfo@nova.edu.
Website: http://pharmacy.nova.edu/

See Display on page 923 and Close-Up on page 933.

The Ohio State University, College of Pharmacy, Columbus, OH 43210. Offers MS, PhD, Pharm D, Pharm D/MBA, Pharm D/MPH, Pharm D/PhD. *Accreditation:* ACPE (one or more programs are accredited). *Faculty:* 50. *Students:* 574 full-time (315 women); includes 142 minority (26 Black or African American, non-Hispanic/Latino; 1 American Indian or Alaska Native, non-Hispanic/Latino; 93 Asian, non-Hispanic/Latino; 17 Hispanic/Latino; 1 Native Hawaiian or other Pacific Islander, non-Hispanic/Latino; 4 Two or more races, non-Hispanic/Latino), 53 international. Average age 25. In 2015, 17 master's, 132 doctorates awarded. Terminal master's awarded for partial completion of doctoral program. *Degree requirements:* For doctorate, comprehensive exam (for some programs), thesis/dissertation (for some programs). *Entrance requirements:* For

master's, GRE General Test, minimum GPA of 3.0; for doctorate, GRE General Test; PCAT (for PharmD), minimum GPA of 3.0. Additional exam requirements/ recommendations for international students: Required—TOEFL (minimum score 600 paper-based, 100 iBT) for MS and PhD; TOEFL (minimum score 577 paper-based; 90 iBT), Michigan English Language Assessment Battery (minimum score 84), IELTS (minimum score 7.5) for PharmD. *Application deadline:* For fall admission, 12/15 for domestic and international students. Application fee: $60 ($70 for international students). Electronic applications accepted. *Expenses:* Contact institution. *Financial support:* Fellowships with full tuition reimbursements, research assistantships with full tuition reimbursements, teaching assistantships with full tuition reimbursements, career-related internships or fieldwork, Federal Work-Study, institutionally sponsored loans, scholarships/grants, and traineeships available. *Unit head:* Dr. Henry J. Mann, Dean and Professor, 614-292-5711, Fax: 614-292-2588, E-mail: mann.414@osu.edu. *Application contact:* Dr. Henry J. Mann, Dean and Professor, 614-292-5711, Fax: 614-292-2588, E-mail: mann.414@osu.edu.
Website: http://www.pharmacy.osu.edu

Purdue University, College of Pharmacy and Pharmacal Sciences and Graduate School, Graduate Programs in Pharmacy and Pharmacal Sciences, Department of Industrial and Physical Pharmacy, West Lafayette, IN 47907. Offers pharmaceutics (PhD); regulatory quality compliance (MS, Certificate). *Degree requirements:* For doctorate, thesis/dissertation. *Entrance requirements:* For master's, minimum GPA of 3.0; for doctorate, GRE General Test, minimum GPA of 3.0. Additional exam requirements/recommendations for international students: Required—TOEFL (minimum score 580 paper-based; 77 iBT). Electronic applications accepted. *Faculty research:* Controlled drug delivery systems, liposomes, antacids, coating technology.

Rutgers University–Newark, Rutgers Business School–Newark and New Brunswick, Program in Pharmaceutical Management, Newark, NJ 07102. Offers MBA.

St. John's University, College of Pharmacy and Health Sciences, Graduate Programs in Pharmaceutical Sciences, Program in Pharmacy Administration, Queens, NY 11439. Offers MS. *Program availability:* Part-time, evening/weekend, online learning. *Degree requirements:* For master's, comprehensive exam, thesis optional, one-year residency. *Entrance requirements:* For master's, GRE General Test, bachelor's degree in pharmacy, minimum GPA of 3.0, 2 letters of recommendation. Additional exam requirements/recommendations for international students: Required—TOEFL (minimum score 600 paper-based; 100 iBT), IELTS (minimum score 7). Electronic applications accepted. *Expenses:* Contact institution.

San Diego State University, Graduate and Research Affairs, College of Sciences, Program in Regulatory Affairs, San Diego, CA 92182. Offers MS. *Degree requirements:* For master's, thesis. *Entrance requirements:* For master's, GRE General Test, 3 letters of recommendation, employment/volunteer experience list. Additional exam requirements/recommendations for international students: Required—TOEFL. Electronic applications accepted.

Temple University, Fox School of Business, MBA Programs, Philadelphia, PA 19122-6096. Offers accounting (MBA); business management (MBA); financial management (MBA); healthcare and life sciences innovation (MBA); human resource management (MBA); international business (IMBA); IT management (MBA); marketing management (MBA); pharmaceutical management (MBA); strategic management (EMBA, MBA). EMBA offered in Philadelphia, PA and Tokyo, Japan. *Accreditation:* AACSB. *Program availability:* Part-time, evening/weekend, online learning. *Entrance requirements:* For master's, GMAT, minimum undergraduate GPA of 3.0. Additional exam requirements/ recommendations for international students: Required—TOEFL (minimum score 600 paper-based; 100 iBT), IELTS (minimum score 7.5).

University of Florida, Graduate School, College of Pharmacy and Graduate School, Graduate Programs in Pharmacy, Department of Pharmaceutical Outcomes and Policy, Gainesville, FL 32611. Offers MSP, PhD. *Program availability:* Part-time, online learning. *Faculty:* 4 full-time, 3 part-time/adjunct. *Students:* 30 full-time (19 women), 135 part-time (85 women); includes 64 minority (37 Black or African American, non-Hispanic/ Latino; 2 American Indian or Alaska Native, non-Hispanic/Latino; 15 Asian, non-Hispanic/Latino; 10 Hispanic/Latino), 25 international. Average age 38. 95 applicants, 41% accepted, 34 enrolled. In 2015, 71 master's, 4 doctorates awarded. *Degree requirements:* For doctorate, thesis/dissertation. *Entrance requirements:* For master's and doctorate, GRE General Test, minimum GPA of 3.0. Additional exam requirements/ recommendations for international students: Required—TOEFL (minimum score 550 paper-based; 80 iBT), IELTS (minimum score 6). *Application deadline:* For fall admission, 1/1 priority date for domestic students, 1/1 for international students; for spring admission, 11/15 for domestic and international students. Applications are processed on a rolling basis. Application fee: $30. Electronic applications accepted. *Financial support:* In 2015–16, 2 fellowships, 2 research assistantships, 14 teaching assistantships were awarded; tuition waivers (full) also available. Financial award applicants required to submit FAFSA. *Faculty research:* Phamacoepidemiology, patient safety and program evaluation, sociology-behavioral issues in medication use, medication safety, pharmacoeconomics, medication therapy management. *Total annual research expenditures:* $1.2 million. *Unit head:* Richard Segal, PhD, Chair, 352-273-6265, Fax: 352-273-6270, E-mail: segal@cop.health.ufl.edu. *Application contact:* Almut Winterstein, PhD, Professor and Graduate Program Director, 352-273-6258, Fax: 352-273-6270, E-mail: almut@cop.ufl.edu.
Website: http://pop.pharmacy.ufl.edu/

University of Georgia, College of Pharmacy, Department of Clinical and Administrative Pharmacy, Athens, GA 30602. Offers clinical and experimental therapeutics (PhD); pharmacy care administration (PhD).

University of Houston, College of Pharmacy, Houston, TX 77204. Offers pharmaceutics (MSPHR, PhD); pharmacology (MSPHR, PhD); pharmacy (Pharm D); pharmacy administration (MSPHR, PhD). *Accreditation:* ACPE. *Program availability:* Part-time. Terminal master's awarded for partial completion of doctoral program. *Entrance requirements:* For doctorate, PCAT (for Pharm D). Additional exam requirements/recommendations for international students: Required—TOEFL. Electronic applications accepted. *Faculty research:* Drug screening and design, cardiovascular pharmacology, infectious disease, asthma research, herbal medicine.

University of Illinois at Chicago, College of Pharmacy and Graduate College, Graduate Programs in Pharmacy, Chicago, IL 60607-7128. Offers forensic science (MS), including forensic toxicology; medicinal chemistry (MS); pharmacognosy (MS, PhD); pharmacy administration (MS, PhD). *Faculty:* 237 full-time (137 women), 60 part-time/adjunct (32 women). *Students:* 110 full-time (62 women), 17 part-time (8 women); includes 26 minority (7 Black or African American, non-Hispanic/Latino; 15 Asian, non-Hispanic/Latino; 4 Hispanic/Latino), 54 international. Average age 28. Terminal master's awarded for partial completion of doctoral program. *Degree requirements:* For master's, variable foreign language requirement, thesis; for doctorate, variable foreign language requirement, thesis/dissertation. *Entrance requirements:* For master's and doctorate, GRE General Test. Additional exam requirements/recommendations for international students: Required—TOEFL. *Application deadline:* For fall admission, 2/1 for domestic students. Applications are processed on a rolling basis. Application fee: $60. Electronic applications accepted. *Expenses:* Tuition, state resident: full-time $11,480; part-time

Pharmaceutical Administration

$3826 per credit. Tuition, nonresident: full-time $23,720; part-time $7906 per credit. *Required fees:* $1333 per semester. Part-time tuition and fees vary according to course load and program. *Financial support:* In 2015–16, 2 fellowships with full tuition reimbursements were awarded; research assistantships with full tuition reimbursements, teaching assistantships with full tuition reimbursements, career-related internships or fieldwork, Federal Work-Study, institutionally sponsored loans, traineeships, tuition waivers (full), and unspecified assistantships also available. Financial award application deadline: 3/1; financial award applicants required to submit FAFSA. *Faculty research:* Biopharmaceutical science, forensic science, forensic toxicology, medicinal chemistry, pharmacognosy. *Unit head:* Prof. Joanna Burdette, Associate Dean for Research and Graduate Education, 312-996-6153, E-mail: joannab@uic.edu. *Application contact:* Jackie Perry, Graduate College Receptionist, 312-413-2550, Fax: 312-413-0185, E-mail: gradcoll@uic.edu.
Website: http://www.uic.edu/pharmacy/education/graduatePrograms.php

University of Maryland, Baltimore, Graduate School, Graduate Programs in Pharmacy, Department of Pharmaceutical Health Service Research, Baltimore, MD 21201. Offers epidemiology (MS); pharmacy administration (PhD); Pharm D/PhD. *Degree requirements:* For doctorate, comprehensive exam, thesis/dissertation. *Entrance requirements:* For doctorate, GRE General Test. Additional exam requirements/recommendations for international students: Required—TOEFL, IELTS. Electronic applications accepted. Tuition and fees vary according to program. *Faculty research:* Pharmacoeconomics, outcomes research, public health policy, drug therapy and aging.

University of Maryland, Baltimore, Graduate School, Graduate Programs in Pharmacy, Program in Regulatory Science, Baltimore, MD 21201. Offers MS. Tuition and fees vary according to program.

University of Michigan, College of Pharmacy and Rackham Graduate School, Department of Clinical Pharmacy, Ann Arbor, MI 48109. Offers PhD. *Faculty:* 2 full-time (1 woman), 1 part-time/adjunct (0 women). *Students:* 5 full-time (3 women), 4 international. Average age 28. In 2015, 1 doctorate awarded. Terminal master's awarded for partial completion of doctoral program. *Degree requirements:* For doctorate, thesis/dissertation, oral defense of dissertation, preliminary exam. *Entrance requirements:* For doctorate, GRE. Additional exam requirements/recommendations for international students: Required—TOEFL (minimum score 560 paper-based; 84 iBT) or IELTS (minimum score 6.5). Application fee: $75 ($90 for international students). *Expenses:* Contact institution. *Financial support:* In 2015–16, 4 students received support, including 2 fellowships (averaging $48,037 per year), 1 research assistantship (averaging $48,037 per year), 1 teaching assistantship (averaging $48,037 per year); career-related internships or fieldwork, institutionally sponsored loans, scholarships/grants, traineeships, health care benefits, tuition waivers, and unspecified assistantships also available. *Unit head:* Dr. Karen Farris, Chair, 734-763-6629, Fax: 734-763-4480, E-mail: kfarris@med.umich.edu. *Application contact:* Antoinette Hopper, Student Affairs Program Manager, 734-615-6326, Fax: 734-763-4480, E-mail: acast@med.umich.edu. Website: https://pharmacy.umich.edu/cp

University of Minnesota, Twin Cities Campus, College of Pharmacy and Graduate School, Graduate Programs in Pharmacy, Graduate Program in Social and Administrative Pharmacy, Minneapolis, MN 55455-0213. Offers MS, PhD. *Program availability:* Part-time. Terminal master's awarded for partial completion of doctoral program. *Degree requirements:* For master's, thesis (for some programs); for doctorate, thesis/dissertation. *Entrance requirements:* For master's, GRE General Test, BS in science; for doctorate, GRE General Test or Pharm D. Additional exam requirements/recommendations for international students: Required—TOEFL (minimum score 100 iBT). Electronic applications accepted. *Faculty research:* Pharmaceutical economics, pharmaceutical policy, pharmaceutical social/behavioral sciences.

The University of North Carolina at Chapel Hill, Eshelman School of Pharmacy, Chapel Hill, NC 27599. Offers health system pharmacy administration (MS); pharmacy (PhD). *Accreditation:* ACPE (one or more programs are accredited). *Faculty:* 112 full-time (45 women), 362 part-time/adjunct (188 women). *Students:* 104 full-time (50 women); includes 30 minority (4 Black or African American, non-Hispanic/Latino; 1 American Indian or Alaska Native, non-Hispanic/Latino; 10 Asian, non-Hispanic/Latino; 4 Hispanic/Latino; 2 Native Hawaiian or other Pacific Islander, non-Hispanic/Latino; 9 Two or more races, non-Hispanic/Latino), 16 international. Average age 26. 268 applicants, 9% accepted, 25 enrolled. In 2015, 8 master's, 13 doctorates awarded. Terminal master's awarded for partial completion of doctoral program. *Degree requirements:* For master's, comprehensive exam, thesis or alternative; for doctorate, comprehensive exam, thesis/dissertation. *Entrance requirements:* For master's and doctorate, GRE General Test, minimum GPA of 3.0. Additional exam requirements/recommendations for international students: Required—TOEFL (minimum score 550 paper-based). *Application deadline:* For fall admission, 12/7 priority date for domestic students, 12/15 priority date for international students. Applications are processed on a rolling basis. Application fee: $85. Electronic applications accepted. *Expenses:* Contact institution. *Financial support:* In 2015–16, 11 students received support, including 18 fellowships with full tuition reimbursements available (averaging $27,500 per year), 56 research assistantships with full tuition reimbursements available (averaging $27,500 per year), teaching assistantships with full tuition reimbursements available (averaging $27,500 per year); career-related internships or fieldwork, Federal Work-Study, institutionally sponsored loans, scholarships/grants, traineeships, health care benefits, tuition waivers (full), and unspecified assistantships also available. Financial award application deadline: 12/15. *Faculty research:* Health services research, pharmacokinetics, molecular modeling, infectious disease, genomics and proteomics, translational research. *Total annual research expenditures:* $15.5 million. *Unit head:* Dr. Robert A. Blouin, Dean, 919-966-1122, Fax: 919-966-6919, E-mail: bob_blouin@unc.edu. *Application contact:* Mimi Lewis, Coordinator of Admissions, 919-962-0097, Fax: 919-966-9428, E-mail: mimi_lewis@unc.edu.
Website: http://pharmacy.unc.edu/

University of Southern California, Graduate School, School of Pharmacy, Program in Healthcare Decision Analysis, Los Angeles, CA 90089. Offers MS. *Program availability:* Part-time, online learning.

University of the Sciences, Program in Pharmaceutical and Healthcare Business, Philadelphia, PA 19104-4495. Offers MBA. *Program availability:* Part-time, evening/weekend, online learning. *Entrance requirements:* Additional exam requirements/recommendations for international students: Required—TOEFL, TWE. *Application deadline:* For fall admission, 5/1 for international students; for winter admission, 10/1 for international students; for spring admission, 3/1 for international students. Applications are processed on a rolling basis. Application fee: $50. *Expenses:* Contact institution. *Financial support:* Tuition waivers (partial) available. *Unit head:* Robert Mueller, Director, 215-596-8879, E-mail: r.mueller@usciences.edu. *Application contact:* Robert Mueller, Director, 215-596-8879, E-mail: r.mueller@usciences.edu.

University of the Sciences, Program in Pharmacy Administration, Philadelphia, PA 19104-4495. Offers MS. *Program availability:* Part-time. *Entrance requirements:* Additional exam requirements/recommendations for international students: Required—TOEFL, TWE. *Application deadline:* For fall admission, 5/1 for international students; for winter admission, 10/1 for international students; for spring admission, 3/1 for international students. Applications are processed on a rolling basis. Application fee: $50. *Expenses:* Contact institution. *Financial support:* Research assistantships with full tuition reimbursements, teaching assistantships, institutionally sponsored loans, traineeships, tuition waivers (partial), and unspecified assistantships available. Financial award application deadline: 5/1. *Unit head:* Dr. William F. McGhan, Director, 215-596-8852, E-mail: w.mcghan@usciences.edu. *Application contact:* Dr. William F. McGhan, Director, 215-596-8852, E-mail: w.mcghan@usciences.edu.

The University of Toledo, College of Graduate Studies, College of Pharmacy and Pharmaceutical Sciences, Program in Pharmaceutical Sciences, Toledo, OH 43606-3390. Offers administrative pharmacy (MSPS); industrial pharmacy (MSPS); pharmacology toxicology (MSPS). *Degree requirements:* For master's, thesis. *Entrance requirements:* For master's, GRE General Test. Additional exam requirements/recommendations for international students: Required—TOEFL (minimum score 550 paper-based; 80 iBT). Electronic applications accepted.

University of Utah, Graduate School, College of Pharmacy, Department of Pharmacotherapy, Salt Lake City, UT 84112. Offers health system pharmacy administration (MS); outcomes research and health policy (PhD). *Faculty:* 6 full-time (4 women), 26 part-time/adjunct (18 women). *Students:* 8 full-time (5 women), 5 part-time (3 women), 5 international. Average age 28. 26 applicants, 19% accepted, 4 enrolled. In 2015, 3 master's awarded. Terminal master's awarded for partial completion of doctoral program. *Degree requirements:* For master's, comprehensive exam, thesis or alternative, project; for doctorate, comprehensive exam, thesis/dissertation. *Entrance requirements:* For doctorate, GRE. Additional exam requirements/recommendations for international students: Required—TOEFL (minimum score 550 paper-based; 80 iBT). *Application deadline:* For fall admission, 1/10 for domestic students, 12/15 for international students. Application fee: $55 ($65 for international students). *Financial support:* In 2015–16, 7 students received support, including 9 research assistantships with full tuition reimbursements available (averaging $21,400 per year); health care benefits also available. Financial award application deadline: 12/15. *Faculty research:* Outcomes in pharmacy, pharmacotherapy. *Total annual research expenditures:* $131,217. *Unit head:* Dr. Diana I. Brixner, Department Chair and Professor, 801-581-6731. *Application contact:* Sara Ray, Academic Program Manager, 801-581-5984, Fax: 801-585-6160, E-mail: sara.ray@pharm.utah.edu.
Website: http://www.pharmacy.utah.edu/pharmacotherapy/

University of Wisconsin–Madison, School of Pharmacy and Graduate School, Graduate Programs in Pharmacy, Madison, WI 53706-1380. Offers pharmaceutical sciences (PhD); social and administrative sciences in pharmacy (MS, PhD). Terminal master's awarded for partial completion of doctoral program. *Degree requirements:* For master's, thesis (for some programs); for doctorate, comprehensive exam (for some programs), thesis/dissertation. *Entrance requirements:* For master's and doctorate, GRE. Additional exam requirements/recommendations for international students: Required—TOEFL. Electronic applications accepted. *Expenses:* Contact institution.

Virginia Commonwealth University, Medical College of Virginia-Professional Programs, School of Pharmacy, Department of Pharmaceutics, Richmond, VA 23284-9005. Offers medicinal chemistry (MS); pharmaceutical sciences (PhD); pharmaceutics (MS); pharmacotherapy and pharmacy administration (MS). Terminal master's awarded for partial completion of doctoral program. *Degree requirements:* For master's, thesis; for doctorate, thesis/dissertation. *Entrance requirements:* For master's and doctorate, GRE General Test. Additional exam requirements/recommendations for international students: Required—TOEFL. Electronic applications accepted. *Faculty research:* Drug delivery systems, drug development.

West Virginia University, School of Pharmacy, Program in Pharmaceutical and Pharmacological Sciences, Morgantown, WV 26506. Offers administrative pharmacy (PhD); behavioral pharmacy (MS, PhD); biopharmaceutics/pharmacokinetics (MS, PhD); industrial pharmacy (MS); medicinal chemistry (MS, PhD); pharmaceutical chemistry (MS, PhD); pharmaceutics (MS, PhD); pharmacology and toxicology (MS); pharmacy (MS); pharmacy administration (MS). *Program availability:* Part-time. Terminal master's awarded for partial completion of doctoral program. *Degree requirements:* For master's, thesis; for doctorate, one foreign language, comprehensive exam, thesis/dissertation. *Entrance requirements:* For master's and doctorate, GRE General Test, minimum GPA of 2.75. Additional exam requirements/recommendations for international students: Required—TOEFL; Recommended—TWE. Electronic applications accepted. *Expenses:* Contact institution. *Faculty research:* Pharmaceutics, medicinal chemistry, biopharmaceutics/pharmacokinetics, health outcomes research.

Pharmaceutical Sciences

Albany College of Pharmacy and Health Sciences, School of Pharmacy and Pharmaceutical Sciences, Albany, NY 12208. Offers health outcomes research (MS); pharmaceutical sciences (MS), including pharmaceutics, pharmacology; pharmacy (Pharm D). *Accreditation:* ACPE. *Degree requirements:* For master's, thesis; for doctorate, practice experience. *Entrance requirements:* For master's, GRE, minimum GPA of 3.0; for doctorate, PCAT, minimum GPA of 2.5. Additional exam requirements/recommendations for international students: Required—TOEFL (minimum score 84

iBT). Electronic applications accepted. *Faculty research:* Therapeutic use of drugs, pharmacokinetics, drug delivery and design.

Auburn University, Harrison School of Pharmacy and Graduate School, Graduate Program in Pharmacy, Auburn University, AL 36849. Offers pharmacal sciences (MS, PhD); pharmaceutical sciences (PhD); pharmacy care systems (MS, PhD). *Program availability:* Part-time. *Faculty:* 54 full-time (32 women), 1 (woman) part-time/adjunct. *Students:* 40 full-time (15 women), 6 part-time (3 women); includes 5 minority (3 Black or African American, non-Hispanic/Latino; 1 Hispanic/Latino; 1 Two or more races, non-

Hispanic/Latino), 29 international. Average age 28. 117 applicants, 21% accepted, 12 enrolled. In 2015, 1 master's, 2 doctorates awarded. *Degree requirements:* For master's, thesis; for doctorate, thesis/dissertation. *Entrance requirements:* For master's and doctorate, GRE General Test. *Application deadline:* Applications are processed on a rolling basis. Application fee: $50 ($60 for international students). Electronic applications accepted. *Expenses:* Tuition, state resident: full-time $8802; part-time $489 per credit hour. Tuition, nonresident: full-time $26,406; part-time $1467 per credit hour. *Required fees:* $808 per semester. Tuition and fees vary according to degree level and program. *Financial support:* Fellowships, research assistantships, and teaching assistantships available. *Faculty research:* Communications, facilities design, substance abuse. *Unit head:* Dr. R. Lee Evans, Dean/Professor, Harrison School of Pharmacy, 334-844-8348, Fax: 334-844-8353. *Application contact:* Dr. George Flowers, Dean of the Graduate School, 334-844-2125.

Boston University, School of Medicine, Division of Graduate Medical Sciences, Department of Pharmacology and Experimental Therapeutics, Boston, MA 02118. Offers MA, PhD, MD/PhD. Terminal master's awarded for partial completion of doctoral program. *Degree requirements:* For master's, thesis; for doctorate, thesis/dissertation. *Application deadline:* For fall admission, 1/15 for domestic students; for spring admission, 10/15 for domestic students. *Unit head:* Dr. David H. Farb, Chairman, 617-638-4300, Fax: 617-638-4329, E-mail: dfarb@bu.edu. *Application contact:* GMS Admissions Office, 617-638-5255, E-mail: askgms@bu.edu.
Website: http://www.bumc.bu.edu/busm-pm/

Butler University, College of Pharmacy and Health Sciences, Indianapolis, IN 46208-3485. Offers pharmaceutical science (MS); pharmacy (Pharm D); physician assistant studies (MS). *Accreditation:* ACPE (one or more programs are accredited). *Faculty:* 63 full-time (44 women). *Students:* 310 full-time (219 women), 5 part-time (3 women); includes 25 minority (1 Black or African American, non-Hispanic/Latino; 1 American Indian or Alaska Native, non-Hispanic/Latino; 14 Asian, non-Hispanic/Latino; 6 Hispanic/Latino; 3 Two or more races, non-Hispanic/Latino), 8 international. Average age 24. 42 applicants, 2% accepted. In 2015, 59 master's, 132 doctorates awarded. *Degree requirements:* For master's, thesis (for some programs), research paper or thesis; for doctorate, research paper or thesis. *Entrance requirements:* For master's, GRE General Test, CASPA application, official transcripts, baccalaureate degree from accredited institution (for physician assistant studies). Additional exam requirements/recommendations for international students: Required—TOEFL (minimum score 550 paper-based; 79 iBT). *Application deadline:* For fall admission, 5/1 for domestic and international students. Electronic applications accepted. Application fee is waived when completed online. *Expenses:* Contact institution. *Financial support:* Applicants required to submit FAFSA. *Faculty research:* Cancer research; molecular pharmacology; pharmaceutics; drug delivery and targeting; neuropharmacology. *Total annual research expenditures:* $50,000. *Unit head:* Dr. Mary Graham, Dean, 317-940-8056, E-mail: mandritz@butler.edu. *Application contact:* Diane Dubord, Graduate Student Services Specialist, 317-940-8107, E-mail: ddubord@butler.edu.
Website: http://www.butler.edu/academics/graduate-cophs/

Campbell University, Graduate and Professional Programs, College of Pharmacy and Health Sciences, Buies Creek, NC 27506. Offers clinical research (MS); pharmaceutical sciences (MS); pharmacy (Pharm D); physician assistant (MPAP); public health (MS). *Accreditation:* ACPE. *Program availability:* Part-time, evening/weekend. *Entrance requirements:* For master's, MCAT, PCAT, GRE, bachelor's degree in health sciences or related field; for doctorate, PCAT. Additional exam requirements/recommendations for international students: Required—TOEFL (minimum score 550 paper-based; 79 iBT). Electronic applications accepted. *Expenses:* Contact institution. *Faculty research:* Immunology, medicinal chemistry, pharmaceutics, applied pharmacology.

Chapman University, School of Pharmacy, Orange, CA 92866. Offers pharmaceutical sciences (MS); pharmacy (Pharm D). *Faculty:* 20 full-time (8 women), 1 part-time/adjunct (0 women). *Students:* 94 full-time (57 women), 1 (woman) part-time; includes 53 minority (5 Black or African American, non-Hispanic/Latino; 39 Asian, non-Hispanic/Latino; 7 Hispanic/Latino; 2 Two or more races, non-Hispanic/Latino), 8 international. Average age 28. *Degree requirements:* For master's, thesis; for doctorate, capstone project. *Entrance requirements:* For doctorate, PCAT. Additional exam requirements/recommendations for international students: Required—TOEFL (minimum score 550 paper-based; 80 iBT), IELTS (minimum score 6.5), PTE (minimum score 53). *Application deadline:* For fall admission, 3/1 for domestic students. Applications are processed on a rolling basis. Electronic applications accepted. *Expenses:* Contact institution. *Financial support:* Fellowships, research assistantships, Federal Work-Study, and scholarships/grants available. *Unit head:* Ronald P. Jordan, Dean, 714-516-5486, E-mail: rpjordan@chapman.edu. *Application contact:* Dr. Lawrence Brown, Associate Dean of Student and Academic Affairs, 714-516-5600, E-mail: pharmacyadmissions@chapman.edu.
Website: http://www.chapman.edu/pharmacy/

Creighton University, School of Medicine and Graduate School, Graduate Programs in Medicine, Department of Pharmacology, Omaha, NE 68178-0001. Offers pharmaceutical sciences (MS); pharmacology (MS, PhD); Pharm D/MS. Terminal master's awarded for partial completion of doctoral program. *Degree requirements:* For master's, comprehensive exam, thesis; for doctorate, comprehensive exam, thesis/dissertation, oral and written preliminary exams. *Entrance requirements:* For master's and doctorate, GRE General Test, minimum GPA of 3.0, undergraduate degree in sciences. Additional exam requirements/recommendations for international students: Required—TOEFL. Electronic applications accepted. *Expenses:* Tuition, area resident: Full-time $14,400; part-time $800 per credit hour. *Required fees:* $158 per semester. Tuition and fees vary according to course load, campus/location, program, reciprocity agreements and student's religious affiliation. *Faculty research:* Pharmacology secretion, cardiovascular-renal pharmacology, adrenergic receptors, signal transduction, genetic regulation of receptors.

Creighton University, School of Pharmacy and Health Professions and Department of Pharmacology, Program in Pharmaceutical Sciences, Omaha, NE 68178-0001. Offers MS, Pharm D/MS. *Degree requirements:* For master's, thesis. *Entrance requirements:* For master's, GRE, three recommendations. Additional exam requirements/recommendations for international students: Required—TOEFL (minimum score 550 paper-based; 80 iBT). Electronic applications accepted. *Expenses: Tuition, area resident:* Full-time $14,400; part-time $800 per credit hour. *Required fees:* $158 per semester. Tuition and fees vary according to course load, campus/location, program, reciprocity agreements and student's religious affiliation.

Drexel University, College of Medicine, Biomedical Graduate Programs, Program in Drug Discovery and Development, Philadelphia, PA 19104-2875. Offers MS. *Degree requirements:* For master's, thesis.

Duquesne University, Mylan School of Pharmacy, Graduate School of Pharmaceutical Sciences, Program in Pharmaceutics, Pittsburgh, PA 15282-0001. Offers MS, PhD, MBA/MS. *Faculty:* 6 full-time (1 woman). *Students:* 20 full-time (8 women), 1 part-time (0 women); includes 2 minority (1 Asian, non-Hispanic/Latino; 1 Hispanic/Latino), 14 international. Average age 27. 42 applicants, 19% accepted, 4 enrolled. In 2015, 4 doctorates awarded. *Degree requirements:* For master's, thesis; for doctorate,

comprehensive exam, thesis/dissertation. *Entrance requirements:* For master's and doctorate, GRE General Test. Additional exam requirements/recommendations for international students: Required—TOEFL (minimum score 100 iBT). *Application deadline:* For fall admission, 2/1 priority date for domestic and international students; for spring admission, 10/1 priority date for domestic and international students. Applications are processed on a rolling basis. Application fee: $50. Electronic applications accepted. Application fee is waived when completed online. *Expenses:* $1,432 per credit. *Financial support:* In 2015–16, 19 students received support, including 5 research assistantships with full tuition reimbursements available, 14 teaching assistantships with full tuition reimbursements available; unspecified assistantships also available. *Unit head:* Dr. Wilson S. Meng, Head, 412-396-6366. *Application contact:* Information Contact, 412-396-1172, E-mail: gsps-adm@duq.edu.
Website: http://www.duq.edu/academics/schools/pharmacy/graduate-school-of-pharmaceutical-sciences

East Tennessee State University, James H. Quillen College of Medicine, Department of Biomedical Sciences, Johnson City, TN 37614. Offers anatomy (PhD); biochemistry (PhD); microbiology (PhD); pharmaceutical sciences (PhD); pharmacology (PhD); physiology (PhD); quantitative biosciences (PhD). *Faculty:* 30 full-time (6 women). *Students:* 35 full-time (17 women), 2 part-time (1 woman); includes 13 minority (9 Black or African American, non-Hispanic/Latino; 4 Asian, non-Hispanic/Latino), 13 international. Average age 29. 53 applicants, 17% accepted, 8 enrolled. In 2015, 8 doctorates awarded. *Degree requirements:* For doctorate, thesis/dissertation, comprehensive qualifying exam. *Entrance requirements:* For doctorate, GRE General Test, GRE Subject Test, 3 letters of recommendation. Additional exam requirements/recommendations for international students: Required—TOEFL (minimum score 550 paper-based; 79 iBT). *Application deadline:* For fall admission, 3/15 priority date for domestic students, 3/1 priority date for international students). Application fee: $35 ($45 for international students). Electronic applications accepted. *Expenses:* Contact institution. *Financial support:* In 2015–16, 30 students received support, including 27 research assistantships with full tuition reimbursements available (averaging $20,000 per year); career-related internships or fieldwork, institutionally sponsored loans, scholarships/grants, and unspecified assistantships also available. Financial award application deadline: 7/1; financial award applicants required to submit FAFSA. *Faculty research:* Cardiovascular, infectious disease, neurosciences, cancer, immunology. *Unit head:* Dr. Mitchell E. Robinson, Associate Dean/Program Director, 423-439-2031, Fax: 423-439-2140, E-mail: robinson@etsu.edu. *Application contact:* Shella Bennett, Graduate Specialist, 423-439-4708, Fax: 423-439-5624, E-mail: bennetsg@etsu.edu.
Website: http://www.etsu.edu/com/dbms/

Florida Agricultural and Mechanical University, Division of Graduate Studies, Research, and Continuing Education, College of Pharmacy and Pharmaceutical Sciences, Graduate Programs in Pharmaceutical Sciences, Tallahassee, FL 32307-3200. Offers environmental toxicology (PhD); health outcomes research and pharmacoeconomics (PhD); medicinal chemistry (MS, PhD); pharmaceutics (MS, PhD); pharmacology/toxicology (MS, PhD); pharmacy administration (MS). *Accreditation:* CEPH. *Degree requirements:* For master's, comprehensive exam, thesis, publishable paper; for doctorate, comprehensive exam, thesis/dissertation, publishable paper. *Entrance requirements:* For master's and doctorate, GRE General Test, minimum GPA of 3.0 in last 60 hours. Additional exam requirements/recommendations for international students: Required—TOEFL. *Faculty research:* Anticancer agents, anti-inflammatory drugs, chronopharmacology, neuroendocrinology, microbiology.

Idaho State University, Office of Graduate Studies, College of Pharmacy, Department of Biomedical and Pharmaceutical Sciences, Pocatello, ID 83209-8334. Offers biopharmaceutical analysis (PhD); drug delivery (PhD); medicinal chemistry (PhD); pharmaceutical sciences (MS); pharmacology (PhD). *Program availability:* Part-time. *Degree requirements:* For master's, one foreign language, comprehensive exam, thesis, thesis research, classes in speech and technical writing; for doctorate, comprehensive exam, thesis/dissertation, written and oral exams, classes in speech and technical writing. *Entrance requirements:* For master's, GRE General Test, minimum GPA of 3.0, 3 letters of recommendation; for doctorate, GRE General Test, BS in pharmacy or related field, minimum GPA of 3.0, 3 letters of recommendation. Additional exam requirements/recommendations for international students: Required—TOEFL (minimum score 550 paper-based; 80 iBT). Electronic applications accepted. *Expenses:* Contact institution. *Faculty research:* Metabolic toxicity of heavy metals, neuroendocrine pharmacology, cardiovascular pharmacology, cancer biology, immunopharmacology.

Irell & Manella Graduate School of Biological Sciences, Graduate Program, Duarte, CA 91010. Offers brain metastatic cancer (PhD); cancer and stem cell metabolism (PhD); cancer biology (PhD); cancer biology and developmental therapeutics (PhD); cell biology (PhD); chemical biology (PhD); chromosomal break repair (PhD); diabetes and pancreatic progenitor cell biology (PhD); DNA repair and cancer biology (PhD); germline epigenetic remodeling and endocrine disruptors (PhD); hematology and hematopoietic cell transplantation (PhD); hematology and immunology (PhD); inflammation and cancer (PhD); micrornas and gene regulation in cardiovascular disease (PhD); mixed chimrism for reversal of autoimmunity (PhD); molecular and cellular biology (PhD); molecular biology and genetics (PhD); nanoparticle mediated twist1 silencing in metastatic cancer (PhD); neuro-oncology and stem cell biology (PhD); neuroscience (PhD); rna directed therapies for hiv-1 (PhD); small rna-induced transcriptional gene activation (PhD); stem cell regulation by the microenvironment (PhD); translational oncology and pharmaceutical sciences (PhD); tumor biology (PhD). *Faculty:* 70 full-time (18 women). *Students:* 75 full-time (40 women); includes 28 minority (2 Black or African American, non-Hispanic/Latino; 10 Asian, non-Hispanic/Latino; 10 Hispanic/Latino; 2 Native Hawaiian or other Pacific Islander, non-Hispanic/Latino; 4 Two or more races, non-Hispanic/Latino), 15 international. Average age 26. 197 applicants, 12% accepted, 19 enrolled. In 2015, 12 doctorates awarded. *Degree requirements:* For doctorate, comprehensive exam, thesis/dissertation, qualifying exams, two advanced courses. *Entrance requirements:* For doctorate, GRE General Test; GRE Subject Test (recommended), 2 years of course work in chemistry (general and organic); 1 year of course work each in biochemistry, general biology, and general physics; 2 semesters of course work in mathematics; significant research laboratory experience. Additional exam requirements/recommendations for international students: Required—TOEFL. *Application deadline:* For fall admission, 1/1 priority date for domestic and international students. Application fee: $0. Electronic applications accepted. Full-time tuition and fees vary according to class time, course level, course load, degree level, campus/location, program and student level. *Financial support:* In 2015–16, 12 students received support, including 35 fellowships with full tuition reimbursements available (averaging $32,000 per year); teaching assistantships, health care benefits, and tuition waivers (full) also available. Financial award applicants required to submit FAFSA. *Faculty research:* Cancer biology, diabetes, stem cell biology, neuroscience, immunology. *Unit head:* Dr. John J. Rossi, Dean, 877-715-GRAD, Fax: 626-471-3901, E-mail: gradschool@coh.org. *Application contact:* Dr. Kate Sleeth, Interim Associate Dean of Administration and Student Development, 626-218-1742, Fax: 626-471-3901, E-mail: gradschool@coh.org.
Website: http://cityofhope.org/gradschool

See Display on page 66 and Close-Up on page 111.

Pharmaceutical Sciences

Johns Hopkins University, Zanvyl Krieger School of Arts and Sciences, Advanced Academic Programs, Program in Regulatory Science, Washington, DC 20036. Offers MS. *Program availability:* Part-time, evening/weekend, online learning. *Degree requirements:* For master's, practicum. *Entrance requirements:* For master's, undergraduate degree in the life sciences or engineering with minimum GPA of 3.0 from a four-year college. Additional exam requirements/recommendations for international students: Required—TOEFL (minimum score 100 iBT).

Long Island University–Hudson at Rockland, Graduate School, Orangeburg, NY 10962. Offers adolescence education (MS Ed); business (MBA); early childhood education (Advanced Certificate); early childhood/childhood education (MS Ed); early childhood/literacy b-6 (MS); early childhood/special education (MS Ed, Advanced Certificate); educational leadership (MS Ed); long term care (Advanced Certificate); mental health counseling (MS); pharmaceutics (MS); public administration (MPA); school counseling (Advanced Certificate). *Program availability:* Part-time, evening/weekend, online learning. *Faculty:* 3 full-time (2 women). *Students:* 90 full-time (71 women), 176 part-time (134 women); includes 63 minority (26 Black or African American, non-Hispanic/Latino; 10 Asian, non-Hispanic/Latino; 24 Hispanic/Latino; 3 Two or more races, non-Hispanic/Latino). Average age 34. 140 applicants, 96% accepted, 103 enrolled. In 2015, 89 master's, 17 other advanced degrees awarded. *Entrance requirements:* Additional exam requirements/recommendations for international students: Required—TOEFL (minimum score 550 paper-based; 79 iBT). *Application deadline:* Applications are processed on a rolling basis. Application fee: $50. Electronic applications accepted. *Expenses:* $1,155 per credit; $884 per term full-time fees, $442 per term part-time fees. *Financial support:* Scholarships/grants available. *Unit head:* Dr. Sylvia Blake, Dean and Chief Operating Officer, 845-450-5437, Fax: 845-359-7248, E-mail: sylvia.blake@liu.edu. *Application contact:* Jeffrey McDowell, Recruitment Manager, 845-450-5414, Fax: 845-359-7248, E-mail: jeffrey.mcdowell@liu.edu.

Long Island University–LIU Brooklyn, Arnold and Marie Schwartz College of Pharmacy and Health Sciences, Brooklyn, NY 11201-8423. Offers drug regulatory affairs (MS); pharmaceutics (MS, PhD), including cosmetic science (MS), industrial pharmacy (MS); pharmacology and toxicology (MS); pharmacy (Pharm D). *Accreditation:* ACPE. *Program availability:* Part-time. *Faculty:* 49 full-time (25 women), 20 part-time/adjunct (9 women). *Students:* 579 full-time (346 women), 29 part-time (14 women); includes 191 minority (24 Black or African American, non-Hispanic/Latino; 1 American Indian or Alaska Native, non-Hispanic/Latino; 144 Asian, non-Hispanic/Latino; 19 Hispanic/Latino; 3 Two or more races, non-Hispanic/Latino; 193 international. Average age 27. 350 applicants, 63% accepted, 65 enrolled. In 2015, 114 master's, 206 doctorates awarded. *Degree requirements:* For master's, comprehensive exam (for some programs), thesis optional; for doctorate, comprehensive exam, thesis/dissertation. *Entrance requirements:* For master's and doctorate, GRE, minimum GPA of 3.0. Additional exam requirements/recommendations for international students: Required—TOEFL (minimum score 550 paper-based; 79 iBT), IELTS (minimum score 6.5). *Application deadline:* Applications are processed on a rolling basis. Application fee: $50. Electronic applications accepted. *Expenses:* Contact institution. *Financial support:* In 2015–16, 185 students received support, including 6 fellowships with full tuition reimbursements available (averaging $12,800 per year), 28 teaching assistantships with full tuition reimbursements available (averaging $6,000 per year); Federal Work-Study, institutionally sponsored loans, and scholarships/grants also available. Support available to part-time students. Financial award application deadline: 2/15; financial award applicants required to submit FAFSA. *Faculty research:* Pharmaceutics, pharmacodynamics, pharmacology, pharmacometrics, pharmacotherapeutics. *Unit head:* Dr. John M. Pezzuto, Dean, 718-488-1004, Fax: 718-488-0628, E-mail: john.pezzuto@liu.edu. *Application contact:* Dr. Anait Levinson, Associate Dean of Research and Graduate Studies, 718-246-6323, E-mail: anait.levenson@liu.edu. Website: http://liu.edu/Pharmacy

MCPHS University, Graduate Studies, Program in Pharmaceutics/Industrial Pharmacy, Boston, MA 02115-5896. Offers MS, PhD. Terminal master's awarded for partial completion of doctoral program. *Degree requirements:* For master's, thesis, oral defense of thesis; for doctorate, one foreign language, comprehensive exam, thesis/dissertation, oral defense of dissertation, qualifying exam. *Entrance requirements:* For master's and doctorate, GRE General Test, minimum QPA of 3.0. Additional exam requirements/recommendations for international students: Required—TOEFL (minimum score 550 paper-based; 79 iBT). *Faculty research:* Pharmacokinetics and drug metabolism, pharmaceutics and physical pharmacy, dosage forms.

Memorial University of Newfoundland, School of Graduate Studies, School of Pharmacy, St. John's, NL A1C 5S7, Canada. Offers MSCPharm, PhD. *Program availability:* Part-time. *Degree requirements:* For master's, thesis, seminar; for doctorate, comprehensive exam, thesis/dissertation, oral defense of thesis. *Entrance requirements:* For master's, B Sc in pharmacy or related area; for doctorate, master's degree in pharmacy or closely-related field. *Application deadline:* For fall admission, 2/28 priority date for domestic and international students; for winter admission, 7/31 priority date for domestic and international students. Applications are processed on a rolling basis. Application fee: $50 Canadian dollars ($100 Canadian dollars for international students). Electronic applications accepted. *Expenses: Tuition, area resident:* Full-time $2199 Canadian dollars. *International tuition:* $2859 Canadian dollars full-time. *Financial support:* Fellowships and research assistantships available. *Faculty research:* Pharmaceutics, medicinal chemistry, physical pharmacy, pharmacology, toxicology. *Unit head:* Dr. Carlo Marra, Dean, 709-777-6571, Fax: 709-777-7044. *Application contact:* Dr. John Weber, Graduate Officer, 709-777-7022, Fax: 709-777-7044, E-mail: jweber@mun.ca.

Mercer University, Graduate Studies, Cecil B. Day Campus, College of Pharmacy, Atlanta, GA 30341. Offers pharmaceutical sciences (PhD); pharmacology (PhD); pharmacy (Pharm D); Pharm D/MBA; Pharm D/PhD. *Accreditation:* ACPE (one or more programs are accredited). *Faculty:* 24 full-time (14 women). *Students:* 667 full-time (418 women), 3 part-time (1 woman); includes 355 minority (133 Black or African American, non-Hispanic/Latino; 2 American Indian or Alaska Native, non-Hispanic/Latino; 170 Asian, non-Hispanic/Latino; 22 Hispanic/Latino; 28 Two or more races, non-Hispanic/Latino), 42 international. Average age 26. 1,895 applicants, 18% accepted, 176 enrolled. In 2015, 151 doctorates awarded. *Degree requirements:* For doctorate, comprehensive exam (for some programs), thesis/dissertation (for some programs). *Entrance requirements:* For doctorate, GRE; PCAT (for Pharm D), Pharm D or BS in pharmacy or science, minimum GPA of 3.0. Additional exam requirements/recommendations for international students: Required—TOEFL. *Application deadline:* Applications are processed on a rolling basis. Electronic applications accepted. *Expenses:* Contact institution. *Financial support:* In 2015–16, 350 students received support. Teaching assistantships with tuition reimbursements available, career-related internships or fieldwork, Federal Work-Study, institutionally sponsored loans, scholarships/grants, tuition waivers, and unspecified assistantships available. Support available to part-time students. Financial award application deadline: 5/1; financial award applicants required to submit FAFSA. *Faculty research:* Stability and compatibility of steroids, synthesis of antihypertensive, disposition of cyclosporine, synthesis of enzyme inhibitors. *Unit head:* Dr. Hewitt W. Matthews, Dean, 678-547-6306, Fax: 678-547-6315, E-mail:

matthews_h@mercer.edu. *Application contact:* Dr. James W. Bartling, Associate Dean for Student Affairs and Admissions, 678-547-6181, Fax: 678-547-6518, E-mail: bartling_jw@mercer.edu. Website: http://pharmacy.mercer.edu/

Northeastern University, Bouvé College of Health Sciences, Boston, MA 02115-5096. Offers applied behavior analysis (MS, CAGS); audiology (Au D); biomedical nanotechnology (MS); college student development and counseling (MS, CAGS); counseling psychology (MS, PhD, CAGS); exercise science (MS); health informatics (MS); medicinal chemistry (MS); nurse anesthesia (DNP, CAGS); nursing (MS, PhD, CAGS), including administration (MS), adult-gerontology acute care nurse practitioner (MS, CAGS), adult-gerontology primary care nurse practitioner (MS, CAGS), anesthesia (MS), family nurse practitioner (MS, CAGS), neonatal nurse practitioner (MS, CAGS), pediatric nurse practitioner (MS, CAGS), psychiatric mental health nurse practitioner (MS, CAGS); nursing practice (DNP); personal health informatics (MS); pharmaceutical sciences (MS, PhD), including interdisciplinary concentration, pharmaceutics and drug delivery systems; pharmacology (MS); pharmacy (Pharm D); physical therapy (Postbaccalaureate Certificate); physician assistant (MS); population health (PhD); school psychology (MS, PhD, CAGS); speech-language pathology (MS); urban health (MPH); MS/MBA. *Accreditation:* ACPE (one or more programs are accredited). *Program availability:* Part-time, evening/weekend, online learning. *Faculty:* 194 full-time (120 women), 169 part-time/adjunct (136 women). *Students:* 1,416 full-time (1,049 women), 310 part-time (248 women). In 2015, 374 master's, 313 doctorates, 37 other advanced degrees awarded. *Degree requirements:* For doctorate, thesis/dissertation (for some programs); for other advanced degree, comprehensive exam. Application fee: $75. Electronic applications accepted. *Expenses:* Contact institution. *Financial support:* Applicants required to submit FAFSA. *Unit head:* John R. Reynolds, Professor and Interim Dean, 617-373-3323, Fax: 617-373-3030. *Application contact:* Molly Schnabel, Senior Director of Graduate Affairs, 617-373-2708, Fax: 617-373-4701, E-mail: bouvegrad@neu.edu. Website: http://www.northeastern.edu/bouve/

Northeast Ohio Medical University, College of Graduate Studies, Rootstown, OH 44272-0095. Offers bioethics (Certificate); health-system pharmacy administration (MS); integrated pharmaceutical medicine (MS, PhD); public health (MS). *Program availability:* Part-time. *Faculty:* 15 part-time/adjunct (6 women). *Students:* 15 full-time (7 women), 26 part-time (11 women); includes 7 minority (5 Asian, non-Hispanic/Latino; 2 Hispanic/Latino). Average age 27. In 2015, 9 master's, 1 doctorate awarded. *Application deadline:* For fall admission, 9/1 priority date for domestic students; for winter admission, 1/5 priority date for domestic students. Applications are processed on a rolling basis. Electronic applications accepted. *Expenses:* Contact institution. *Financial support:* In 2015–16, 18 students received support. *Unit head:* Dr. Walter E. Horton, Jr., Dean. *Application contact:* Heidi Terry, Executive Director, Enrollment Services, 330-325-6479, E-mail: hterry@neoucom.edu. Website: http://www.neomed.edu/academics/graduatestudies

Oregon State University, College of Pharmacy, Program in Pharmaceutical Sciences, Corvallis, OR 97331. Offers medicinal chemistry (MS, PhD); natural products chemistry (MS, PhD); pharmaceutics (MS, PhD); pharmacoeconomics (MS, PhD); pharmacokinetics (MS, PhD); pharmacology (MS, PhD); toxicology (MS, PhD). *Program availability:* Part-time. *Faculty:* 30 full-time (15 women). *Students:* 29 full-time (10 women); includes 2 minority (1 Asian, non-Hispanic/Latino; 1 Hispanic/Latino), 16 international. Average age 29. 79 applicants, 10% accepted, 5 enrolled. In 2015, 4 doctorates awarded. *Entrance requirements:* For master's and doctorate, GRE. Additional exam requirements/recommendations for international students: Required—TOEFL (minimum score 80 iBT), IELTS (minimum score 6.5). *Application deadline:* For fall admission, 1/1 for domestic students. Application fee: $75 ($85 for international students). *Expenses:* Tuition, state resident: full-time $12,150; part-time $450 per credit. Tuition, nonresident: full-time $20,952; part-time $776 per credit. *Required fees:* $1572; $1443 per unit. One-time fee: $350. Tuition and fees vary according to course load, campus/location and program. *Unit head:* Dr. Mark Zabriskie, Dean and Professor, 541-737-5781, E-mail: mark.zabriskie@oregonstate.edu. *Application contact:* Debra Peters, Pharmacy Advisor, 541-737-8743, E-mail: debra.peters@oregonstate.edu. Website: http://pharmacy.oregonstate.edu/

Purdue University, College of Pharmacy and Pharmacal Sciences and Graduate School, Graduate Programs in Pharmacy and Pharmacal Sciences, Department of Pharmacy Practice, West Lafayette, IN 47907. Offers clinical pharmacy (MS, PhD); pharmacy administration (MS, PhD). Terminal master's awarded for partial completion of doctoral program. *Degree requirements:* For master's, thesis optional; for doctorate, thesis/dissertation. *Entrance requirements:* For master's, GRE General Test, minimum undergraduate GPA of 3.0 or equivalent; for doctorate, GRE General Test, minimum undergraduate GPA of 3.0 or equivalent; master's degree with minimum GPA of 3.0 or equivalent. Additional exam requirements/recommendations for international students: Required—TOEFL (minimum score 550 paper-based; 77 iBT), TWE (recommended for MS, required for PhD). Electronic applications accepted. *Faculty research:* Clinical drug studies, pharmacy education advancement, administrative studies.

Queen's University at Kingston, School of Graduate Studies, Faculty of Health Sciences, Department of Anatomy and Cell Biology, Kingston, ON K7L 3N6, Canada. Offers biology of reproduction (M Sc, PhD); cancer (M Sc, PhD); cardiovascular pathophysiology (M Sc, PhD); cell and molecular biology (M Sc, PhD); drug metabolism (M Sc, PhD); endocrinology (M Sc, PhD); motor control (M Sc, PhD); neural regeneration (M Sc, PhD); neurophysiology (M Sc, PhD). *Program availability:* Part-time. *Degree requirements:* For master's, thesis; for doctorate, one foreign language, comprehensive exam, thesis/dissertation. *Entrance requirements:* Additional exam requirements/recommendations for international students: Required—TOEFL. Electronic applications accepted. *Faculty research:* Human kinetics, neuroscience, reproductive biology, cardiovascular.

Rowan University, Graduate School, College of Science and Mathematics, Program in Pharmaceutical Sciences, Glassboro, NJ 08028-1701. Offers MS. Electronic applications accepted. *Expenses: Tuition, area resident:* Full-time $8710; part-time $871 per credit. Tuition, state resident: full-time $8710; part-time $871 per credit. Tuition, nonresident: full-time $8710; part-time $871 per credit. *International tuition:* $8710 full-time. *Required fees:* $1510; $151 per credit.

Rush University, Graduate College, Division of Pharmacology, Chicago, IL 60612-3832. Offers clinical research (MS); pharmacology (MS, PhD); MD/PhD. Terminal master's awarded for partial completion of doctoral program. *Degree requirements:* For master's, thesis; for doctorate, thesis/dissertation. *Entrance requirements:* For master's and doctorate, GRE General Test, interview. Additional exam requirements/recommendations for international students: Required—TOEFL (minimum score 550 paper-based). *Faculty research:* Dopamine neurobiology and Parkinson's disease; cardiac electrophysiology and clinical pharmacology; neutrophil motility, apoptosis, and adhesion; angiogenesis; pulmonary vascular physiology.

Rutgers University–New Brunswick, Ernest Mario School of Pharmacy, Program in Pharmaceutical Science, Piscataway, NJ 08854-8097. Offers MS, PhD. *Program availability:* Part-time. Terminal master's awarded for partial completion of doctoral program. *Degree requirements:* For master's, thesis; for doctorate, thesis/dissertation. *Entrance requirements:* For master's and doctorate, GRE General Test, 3 letters of recommendation. Additional exam requirements/recommendations for international students: Required—TOEFL (minimum score 550 paper-based; 83 iBT). Electronic applications accepted. *Faculty research:* Drug delivery, drug transport and drug metabolism; pharmacokinetics and pharmacodynamics; cancer chemoprevention and dietary phytochemicals; pharmacogenomics and personalized medicine; bioinformatics and computational pharmaceutical sciences.

St. John's University, College of Pharmacy and Health Sciences, Graduate Programs in Pharmaceutical Sciences, Program in Pharmaceutical Sciences, Queens, NY 11439. Offers MS, PhD. *Program availability:* Part-time, evening/weekend. Terminal master's awarded for partial completion of doctoral program. *Degree requirements:* For master's, comprehensive exam, thesis optional, one-year residency; for doctorate, comprehensive exam, thesis/dissertation, qualifying exams, residency. *Entrance requirements:* For master's, GRE General Test, minimum GPA of 3.0, 2 letters of recommendation, statement of goals; for doctorate, GRE General Test, minimum GPA of 3.5 (undergraduate), 3.0 (graduate); 2 letters of recommendation. Additional exam requirements/recommendations for international students: Required—TOEFL (minimum score 600 paper-based; 100 iBT), IELTS (minimum score 7). Electronic applications accepted. *Expenses:* Contact institution. *Faculty research:* Neurotoxicology, biochemical toxicology, molecular pharmacology, neuropharmacology, intermediary metabolism.

South Dakota State University, Graduate School, College of Pharmacy, Department of Pharmaceutical Sciences, Brookings, SD 57007. Offers biological science (MS); pharmaceutical sciences (PhD). *Degree requirements:* For master's, thesis, oral exam; for doctorate, comprehensive exam, thesis/dissertation, oral exam. *Entrance requirements:* For master's and doctorate, GRE General Test. Additional exam requirements/recommendations for international students: Required—TOEFL (minimum score 550 paper-based). *Faculty research:* Drugs of abuse, anti-cancer drugs, sustained drug delivery, drug metabolism.

Stevens Institute of Technology, Graduate School, Charles V. Schaefer Jr. School of Engineering, Department of Mechanical Engineering, Program in Pharmaceutical Manufacturing, Hoboken, NJ 07030. Offers M Eng, MS, Certificate. *Program availability:* Part-time, evening/weekend. *Students:* 46 full-time (21 women), 29 part-time (9 women); includes 12 minority (11 Asian, non-Hispanic/Latino; 1 Two or more races, non-Hispanic/Latino), 34 international. Average age 29. 74 applicants, 55% accepted, 24 enrolled. In 2015, 62 master's, 40 other advanced degrees awarded. *Entrance requirements:* Additional exam requirements/recommendations for international students: Required—TOEFL (minimum score 74 iBT). *Application deadline:* For fall admission, 6/1 for domestic students, 4/15 for international students; for spring admission, 11/30 for domestic students, 11/1 for international students. Applications are processed on a rolling basis. Application fee: $60. Electronic applications accepted. *Expenses:* Tuition, area resident: Full-time $32,200; part-time $1450 per credit. *Required fees:* $1150; $550 per unit. $275 per semester. *Financial support:* Fellowships, research assistantships, teaching assistantships, career-related internships or fieldwork, Federal Work-Study, scholarships/grants, and unspecified assistantships available. Financial award application deadline: 2/15; financial award applicants required to submit FAFSA. *Unit head:* Dr. Frank Fisher, Interim Department Director, 201-216-8913, Fax: 201-216-8315, E-mail: ffisher@stevens.edu. *Application contact:* Graduate Admissions, 888-783-8367, Fax: 888-511-1306, E-mail: graduate@stevens.edu.

Stevens Institute of Technology, Graduate School, School of Business, Program in Business Administration, Hoboken, NJ 07030. Offers business intelligence and analytics (MBA); engineering management (MBA); finance (MBA); information systems (MBA); innovation and entrepreneurship (MBA); marketing (MBA); pharmaceutical management (MBA); project management (MBA, Certificate); technology management (MBA); telecommunications management (MBA). *Program availability:* Part-time, evening/weekend. *Students:* 23 full-time (12 women), 90 part-time (27 women); includes 35 minority (3 Black or African American, non-Hispanic/Latino; 1 American Indian or Alaska Native, non-Hispanic/Latino; 24 Asian, non-Hispanic/Latino; 6 Hispanic/Latino; 1 Two or more races, non-Hispanic/Latino), 22 international. Average age 35. 62 applicants, 73% accepted, 29 enrolled. In 2015, 42 master's awarded. *Entrance requirements:* Additional exam requirements/recommendations for international students: Required—TOEFL (minimum score 74 iBT). *Application deadline:* For fall admission, 6/1 for domestic students, 4/15 for international students; for spring admission, 11/30 for domestic students, 11/1 for international students. Applications are processed on a rolling basis. Application fee: $60. Electronic applications accepted. *Expenses:* Tuition, area resident: Full-time $32,200; part-time $1450 per credit. *Required fees:* $1150; $550 per unit. $275 per semester. *Financial support:* Fellowships, research assistantships, teaching assistantships, career-related internships or fieldwork, Federal Work-Study, scholarships/grants, and unspecified assistantships available. Financial award application deadline: 2/15; financial award applicants required to submit FAFSA. *Unit head:* Dr. Gregory Prastacos, Dean, 201-216-8366, E-mail: gprastac@stevens.edu. *Application contact:* Graduate Admissions, 888-783-8367, Fax: 888-511-1306, E-mail: graduate@stevens.edu. Website: https://www.stevens.edu/school-business/masters-programs/mbaemba

Temple University, School of Pharmacy, Department of Pharmaceutical Sciences, Philadelphia, PA 19122. Offers medicinal chemistry (MS, PhD); pharmaceutics (MS, PhD); pharmacodynamics (MS, PhD); quality assurance/regulatory affairs (MS). *Program availability:* Part-time, online learning. *Faculty:* 12 full-time (2 women), 1 part-time/adjunct (0 women). *Students:* 48 full-time (28 women), 11 part-time (7 women); includes 1 minority (Asian, non-Hispanic/Latino), 42 international. 75 applicants, 32% accepted, 21 enrolled. In 2015, 4 master's, 1 doctorate awarded. *Degree requirements:* For master's, comprehensive exam (for some programs); thesis (for some programs); for doctorate, 2 foreign languages, comprehensive exam, thesis/dissertation. *Entrance requirements:* For master's, GRE General Test, minimum undergraduate GPA of 3.0; for doctorate, GRE General Test, minimum GPA of 3.0. Additional exam requirements/recommendations for international students: Required—TOEFL (minimum score 550 paper-based; 82 iBT). *Application deadline:* For fall admission, 1/15 for domestic students, 12/15 for international students. Application fee: $60. Electronic applications accepted. *Expenses:* Contact institution. *Financial support:* In 2015–16, 2 fellowships with full tuition reimbursements (averaging $23,000 per year), 6 research assistantships with full tuition reimbursements (averaging $22,000 per year), 11 teaching assistantships with full tuition reimbursements (averaging $22,000 per year) were awarded. Financial award application deadline: 1/15; financial award applicants required to submit FAFSA. *Faculty research:* Pharmacokinetics, synthesis of medicinals, protein research, biopharma-formulation. *Unit head:* Dr. Daniel Canney, Director of Graduate Studies, 215-707-4948, E-mail: phscgrad@temple.edu. *Application contact:* Sophon Din, Administrative Assistant, 215-204-4948, E-mail: tusprgad@temple.edu.

Texas Southern University, College of Pharmacy and Health Sciences, Department of Pharmaceutical Sciences, Houston, TX 77004-4584. Offers MS, PhD. *Program availability:* Online learning. *Entrance requirements:* For master's, PCAT; for doctorate, GRE General Test. Electronic applications accepted.

Texas Tech University Health Sciences Center, Graduate School of Biomedical Sciences, Program in Pharmaceutical Sciences, Lubbock, TX 79430. Offers MS, PhD.

Accreditation: ACPE. Terminal master's awarded for partial completion of doctoral program. *Degree requirements:* For master's, thesis; for doctorate, thesis/dissertation. *Entrance requirements:* For master's and doctorate, GRE General Test, minimum GPA of 3.0. Additional exam requirements/recommendations for international students: Required—TOEFL (minimum score 550 paper-based; 79 iBT). Electronic applications accepted. *Faculty research:* Drug design and delivery, pharmacology, pharmacokinetics, drug receptor modeling, molecular and reproductive biology.

Université de Montréal, Faculty of Pharmacy, Montréal, QC H3C 3J7, Canada. Offers drugs development (DESS); pharmaceutical care (DESS); pharmaceutical practice (M Sc); pharmaceutical sciences (M Sc, PhD); pharmacist-supervisor teacher (DESS). *Program availability:* Part-time. Terminal master's awarded for partial completion of doctoral program. *Degree requirements:* For master's, thesis; for doctorate, thesis/dissertation. *Entrance requirements:* For master's and doctorate, proficiency in French. Electronic applications accepted. *Faculty research:* Novel drug delivery systems, immunoassay development, medicinal chemistry of CNS compounds, pharmacokinetics and biopharmaceutical compounds.

Université Laval, Faculty of Pharmacy, Program in Hospital Pharmacy, Québec, QC G1K 7P4, Canada. Offers M Sc. *Entrance requirements:* For master's, knowledge of French, interview. Electronic applications accepted.

Université Laval, Faculty of Pharmacy, Programs in Community Pharmacy, Québec, QC G1K 7P4, Canada. Offers DESS. *Program availability:* Part-time. *Entrance requirements:* For degree, knowledge of French. Electronic applications accepted.

Université Laval, Faculty of Pharmacy, Programs in Pharmacy, Québec, QC G1K 7P4, Canada. Offers M Sc, PhD. *Program availability:* Part-time. Terminal master's awarded for partial completion of doctoral program. *Degree requirements:* For master's, thesis; for doctorate, comprehensive exam, thesis/dissertation. *Entrance requirements:* For master's and doctorate, knowledge of French. Electronic applications accepted.

University at Buffalo, the State University of New York, Graduate School, School of Pharmacy and Pharmaceutical Sciences, Department of Pharmaceutical Sciences, Buffalo, NY 14260. Offers MS, PhD, Pharm D/MS, Pharm D/PhD. *Faculty:* 17 full-time (6 women), 2 part-time/adjunct (0 women). *Students:* 77 full-time (37 women), 6 part-time (3 women); includes 14 minority (1 Black or African American, non-Hispanic/Latino; 13 Asian, non-Hispanic/Latino), 33 international. Average age 27. 272 applicants, 11% accepted, 20 enrolled. In 2015, 9 master's, 7 doctorates awarded. Terminal master's awarded for partial completion of doctoral program. *Degree requirements:* For master's, comprehensive exam (for some programs), thesis optional, project; for doctorate, comprehensive exam, thesis/dissertation. *Entrance requirements:* For master's, GRE, BS, B Eng, or Pharm D; for doctorate, GRE, BS, MS, B Eng, M Eng, or Pharm D. Additional exam requirements/recommendations for international students: Required—TOEFL (minimum score 550 paper-based; 79 iBT); Recommended—IELTS, TSE. *Application deadline:* For fall admission, 2/15 for domestic and international students. Applications are processed on a rolling basis. Application fee: $50. Electronic applications accepted. *Expenses:* Contact institution. *Financial support:* In 2015–16, 45 students received support, including 45 research assistantships with full tuition reimbursements available (averaging $33,994 per year); fellowships also available. Financial award application deadline: 3/1; financial award applicants required to submit FAFSA. *Faculty research:* Pharmacokinetics/pharmacodynamics, bioanalysis, pharmacogenomics, drug delivery, pharmacodynamics, drug metabolism and transport, cancer therapeutics, and protein therapeutics. *Total annual research expenditures:* $4 million. *Unit head:* Dr. William J. Jusko, Chair, 716-645-2855 Ext. 225, Fax: 716-645-3693, E-mail: wjjusko@acsu.buffalo.edu. *Application contact:* Dr. Murali Ramanathan, Director of Graduate Studies, 716-645-4846, Fax: 716-645-3690, E-mail: murali@buffalo.edu. Website: http://pharmacy.buffalo.edu/departments-offices/pharmaceutical-sciences.html

University of Alberta, Faculty of Graduate Studies and Research, Department of Pharmacy and Pharmaceutical Sciences, Edmonton, AB T6G 2E1, Canada. Offers M Sc, PhD. Terminal master's awarded for partial completion of doctoral program. *Degree requirements:* For master's, thesis; for doctorate, thesis/dissertation. *Entrance requirements:* Additional exam requirements/recommendations for international students: Required—Michigan English Language Assessment Battery or IELTS. Electronic applications accepted. *Faculty research:* Radiopharmacy, pharmacokinetics, bionucleonics, medicinal chemistry, microbiology.

The University of Arizona, College of Pharmacy, Program in Pharmaceutical Sciences, Tucson, AZ 85721. Offers medicinal and natural products chemistry (MS, PhD); pharmaceutical economics (MS, PhD); pharmaceutics and pharmacokinetics (MS, PhD). *Degree requirements:* For master's, thesis; for doctorate, one foreign language, thesis/dissertation. *Entrance requirements:* For master's, GRE General Test, 3 letters of recommendation, bachelor's degree in related field; for doctorate, GRE General Test, 3 letters of recommendation, statement of purpose, bachelor's degree in related field. Additional exam requirements/recommendations for international students: Required—TOEFL (minimum score 550 paper-based; 79 iBT). *Application deadline:* For fall admission, 1/1 for domestic students, 12/1 for international students. Applications are processed on a rolling basis. Application fee: $75. Electronic applications accepted. *Financial support:* Research assistantships, scholarships/grants, health care benefits, tuition waivers (full), and unspecified assistantships available. Financial award application deadline: 3/1. *Faculty research:* Drug design, natural products isolation, biological applications of NMR and mass spectrometry, drug formulation and delivery, pharmacokinetics. *Unit head:* Nathan J. Cherrington, Director, 520-626-0219, Fax: 520-626-4063. *Application contact:* Sonya M. Flores-Basurto, Information Contact, 520-626-7265, Fax: 520-626-2466, E-mail: basurto@pharmacy.arizona.edu. Website: http://grad.arizona.edu/live/programs/description/129

The University of British Columbia, Faculty of Pharmaceutical Sciences, Vancouver, BC V6T 1Z3, Canada. Offers M Sc, PhD, Pharm D. *Degree requirements:* For master's, thesis, seminar; for doctorate, comprehensive exam, thesis/dissertation, seminar. *Entrance requirements:* Additional exam requirements/recommendations for international students: Required—TOEFL (minimum score 600 paper-based; 100 iBT), IELTS (minimum score 6.5). Electronic applications accepted. *Faculty research:* Pharmacology and cellular pharmacology, neuropharmacology, toxicology, nanomedicines and drug delivery, pharmacogenomics and personalized medicine, health outcomes research and evaluation, pharmacoepidemiology, and medicinal chemistry.

University of California, Irvine, School of Medicine, Program in Pharmacological Sciences, Irvine, CA 92697. Offers PhD, MD/PhD. *Students:* 9 full-time (2 women), 1 part-time (0 women); includes 8 minority (5 Asian, non-Hispanic/Latino; 1 Hispanic/Latino; 2 Two or more races, non-Hispanic/Latino), 2 international. Average age 29. In 2015, 3 degrees awarded. *Degree requirements:* For doctorate, thesis/dissertation. *Entrance requirements:* For doctorate, GRE General Test, GRE Subject Test, minimum GPA of 3.0. Additional exam requirements/recommendations for international students: Required—TOEFL (minimum score 550 paper-based). *Application deadline:* For fall admission, 1/15 priority date for domestic students, 1/15 for international students. Applications are processed on a rolling basis. Application fee: $80 ($100 for international students). Electronic applications accepted. *Financial support:* Fellowships, research assistantships, teaching assistantships, institutionally sponsored loans, traineeships,

Pharmaceutical Sciences

and unspecified assistantships available. Financial award application deadline: 3/1; financial award applicants required to submit FAFSA. *Unit head:* Dr. Olivier Civelli, Chair, 949-924-2522, Fax: 949-824-4855, E-mail: ocivelli@uci.edu. Website: http://www.pharmacology.uci.edu/graduate-program/

★ **University of California, San Francisco,** School of Pharmacy and Graduate Division, Pharmaceutical Sciences and Pharmacogenomics Program, San Francisco, CA 94158-0775. Offers PhD. *Degree requirements:* For doctorate, comprehensive exam, thesis/dissertation. *Entrance requirements:* For doctorate, GRE General Test, bachelor's degree, 3 letters of recommendation, personal statement. Additional exam requirements/recommendations for international students: Required—TOEFL. Electronic applications accepted. *Faculty research:* Drug development sciences, molecular pharmacology, therapeutic bioengineering, pharmacogenomics and functional genomics, quantitative and systems pharmacology, computational genomics.

See Display on page 926 and Close-Up on page 937.

University of Cincinnati, James L. Winkle College of Pharmacy, Division of Pharmaceutical Sciences, Cincinnati, OH 45221. Offers MS, PhD. *Degree requirements:* For master's, thesis; for doctorate, thesis/dissertation. *Entrance requirements:* For master's and doctorate, GRE General Test, minimum GPA of 3.0. Additional exam requirements/recommendations for international students: Required—TOEFL.

University of Colorado Denver, School of Pharmacy, Doctor of Pharmacy Program, Aurora, CO 80045. Offers Pharm D. *Program availability:* Online learning. *Students:* 627 full-time (384 women), 145 part-time (99 women); includes 300 minority (48 Black or African American, non-Hispanic/Latino; 5 American Indian or Alaska Native, non-Hispanic/Latino; 182 Asian, non-Hispanic/Latino; 58 Hispanic/Latino; 1 Native Hawaiian or other Pacific Islander, non-Hispanic/Latino; 6 Two or more races, non-Hispanic/Latino), 25 international. Average age 30. 201 applicants, 86% accepted, 153 enrolled. In 2015, 190 doctorates awarded. *Degree requirements:* For doctorate, final-year experience in pharmacy setting. *Entrance requirements:* For doctorate, PCAT, minimum GPA of 2.5, 2.75 in the sciences; prerequisite coursework in general chemistry with lab, organic chemistry with lab, general biology with lab, microbiology with lab, biochemistry, human anatomy and physiology with lab, general physics, calculus, English composition, public speaking, and microeconomics. Additional exam requirements/recommendations for international students: Required—TOEFL (minimum score 550 paper-based; 80 iBT). *Application deadline:* For fall admission, 12/1 for domestic students, 11/1 for international students. Application fee: $150. Electronic applications accepted. *Expenses:* Contact institution. *Financial support:* In 2015–16, 451 students received support. Fellowships, research assistantships, teaching assistantships, career-related internships or fieldwork, Federal Work-Study, institutionally sponsored loans, scholarships/grants, traineeships, and unspecified assistantships available. Financial award application deadline: 3/15; financial award applicants required to submit FAFSA. *Faculty research:* Mechanistic studies of viral assembly, synthetic gene delivery systems for use in gene therapy, mechanisms of toxicity, pulmonary drug delivery. *Unit head:* Douglas Fish, Chair of Pharm D Program, 303-724-2615, E-mail: doug.fish@ucdenver.edu. *Application contact:* Admissions, 303-724-2882, E-mail: pharmd.info@ucdenver.edu.
Website: http://www.ucdenver.edu/academics/colleges/pharmacy/AcademicPrograms/PharmDProgram/Pages/PharmDProgram.aspx

University of Colorado Denver, School of Pharmacy, Program in Pharmaceutical Sciences, Aurora, CO 80045. Offers clinical pharmaceutical sciences (PhD); pharmaceutical biotechnology (PhD); pharmaceutical outcomes research (PhD). *Students:* 21 full-time (8 women), 1 part-time (0 women); includes 6 minority (1 Black or African American, non-Hispanic/Latino; 5 Asian, non-Hispanic/Latino), 9 international. Average age 30. 44 applicants, 16% accepted, 6 enrolled. In 2015, 3 doctorates awarded. *Degree requirements:* For doctorate, comprehensive exam, thesis/dissertation, minimum 60 credit hours of upper-level courses, 30 of which are thesis research, research rotations and thesis defense. *Entrance requirements:* For doctorate, GRE, minimum undergraduate GPA of 3.0; prior coursework in general chemistry, organic chemistry, calculus, biology, and physics. Additional exam requirements/recommendations for international students: Required—TOEFL (minimum score 550 paper-based; 80 iBT). *Application deadline:* For fall admission, 1/15 for domestic students, 12/15 for international students. Application fee: $50 ($75 for international students). Electronic applications accepted. *Expenses:* Contact institution. *Financial support:* In 2015–16, 20 students received support. Fellowships, research assistantships, teaching assistantships, Federal Work-Study, institutionally sponsored loans, scholarships/grants, traineeships, health care benefits, tuition waivers (full), and unspecified assistantships available. Financial award application deadline: 3/15; financial award applicants required to submit FAFSA. *Faculty research:* Pharmaceutical biotechnology, molecular toxicology, cancer pharmacology, drug discovery, clinical and translational sciences. *Unit head:* Dr. David Ross, Chair/Professor of Toxicology, 303-724-7265, E-mail: david.ross@ucdenver.edu. *Application contact:* Jackie Milowski, Graduate Admissions, 303-724-7263, E-mail: jackie.milowski@ucdenver.edu.
Website: http://www.ucdenver.edu/academics/colleges/pharmacy/AcademicPrograms/PhDPrograms/PhDPharmaceuticalSciences/Pages/PhDPharmaceuticalSciences.aspx

University of Connecticut, Graduate School, School of Pharmacy, Department of Pharmaceutical Sciences, Program in Pharmaceutics, Storrs, CT 06269. Offers MS, PhD. Terminal master's awarded for partial completion of doctoral program. *Degree requirements:* For master's, comprehensive exam, thesis; for doctorate, thesis/dissertation. *Entrance requirements:* For master's and doctorate, GRE General Test. Additional exam requirements/recommendations for international students: Required—TOEFL (minimum score 550 paper-based). *Application deadline:* For fall admission, 2/1 priority date for domestic and international students; for spring admission, 11/1 for domestic students, 10/1 for international students. Applications are processed on a rolling basis. Application fee: $55. Electronic applications accepted. *Financial support:* Fellowships, research assistantships with full tuition reimbursements, teaching assistantships with full tuition reimbursements, Federal Work-Study, scholarships/grants, health care benefits, and unspecified assistantships available. Financial award application deadline: 2/1; financial award applicants required to submit FAFSA. Website: http://www.pharmacy.uconn.edu/

University of Florida, Graduate School, College of Pharmacy and Graduate School, Graduate Programs in Pharmacy, Department of Pharmaceutics, Gainesville, FL 32611. Offers clinical and translational sciences (PhD); pharmaceutical sciences (MSP, PhD); pharmacy (MSP, PhD). *Faculty:* 2 full-time, 1 part-time/adjunct. *Students:* 30 full-time (14 women), 1 (woman) part-time; includes 1 minority (Asian, non-Hispanic/Latino), 24 international. Average age 29. 182 applicants, 57% accepted, 92 enrolled. In 2015, 4 doctorates awarded. *Degree requirements:* For doctorate, comprehensive exam, thesis/dissertation. *Entrance requirements:* For master's and doctorate, GRE General Test, minimum GPA of 3.0. Additional exam requirements/recommendations for international students: Required—TOEFL (minimum score 550 paper-based; 80 iBT), IELTS (minimum score 6). *Application deadline:* For fall admission, 2/1 priority date for domestic students, 2/1 for international students; for spring admission, 10/5 for domestic and international students. Applications are processed on a rolling basis. Application

fee: $30. Electronic applications accepted. *Financial support:* In 2015–16, 3 research assistantships, 19 teaching assistantships were awarded; tuition waivers (full) and unspecified assistantships also available. Financial award applicants required to submit FAFSA. *Faculty research:* Basic, applied, and clinical investigations in pharmacokinetics/biopharmaceutics; pharmaceutical analysis, pharmaceutical biotechnology and drug delivery; herbal medicine. *Total annual research expenditures:* $2.2 million. *Unit head:* Hartmut Derendorf, PhD, Professor and Chair, 352-273-7856, Fax: 352-392-4447, E-mail: hartmut@ufl.edu. *Application contact:* Dr. Anthony Palmieri, III, Graduate Coordinator, 352-273-7868, E-mail: palmieri@cop.ufl.edu.
Website: http://www.cop.ufl.edu/pc/

University of Florida, Graduate School, College of Pharmacy and Graduate School, Graduate Programs in Pharmacy, Department of Pharmacotherapy and Translational Research, Gainesville, FL 32611. Offers clinical pharmaceutical sciences (PhD); clinical pharmacy (MSP). *Faculty:* 3 full-time, 2 part-time/adjunct. *Students:* 4 full-time (2 women), 5 international. Average age 33. *Entrance requirements:* For master's and doctorate, GRE General Test, minimum GPA of 3.0. Additional exam requirements/recommendations for international students: Required—TOEFL (minimum score 550 paper-based; 80 iBT), IELTS (minimum score 6). *Application deadline:* For fall admission, 1/15 for domestic and international students. Application fee: $30. Electronic applications accepted. *Financial support:* In 2015–16, 1 fellowship, 3 teaching assistantships were awarded. Financial award application deadline: 1/15; financial award applicants required to submit FAFSA. *Faculty research:* Understanding genetic and non-genetic factors that contribute to variability in drug response in various therapeutic areas as cardiology, transplant/immunology, asthma/pulmonary, psychiatry, oncology, clinical pharmacology/drug metabolism. *Total annual research expenditures:* $4.3 million. *Unit head:* Dr. Reginald F. Frye, Professor and Chair, 352-273-5453, Fax: 352-273-6242, E-mail: frye@cop.ufl.edu. *Application contact:* Dr. Taimour Langaee, Associate Research Professor/Graduate Coordinator, 352-273-6357, Fax: 352-273-6242, E-mail: langaee@cop.ufl.edu.
Website: http://ptr.pharmacy.ufl.edu/

University of Georgia, College of Pharmacy, Department of Pharmaceutical and Biomedical Sciences, Athens, GA 30602. Offers PhD. *Degree requirements:* For doctorate, one foreign language, thesis/dissertation. *Entrance requirements:* For doctorate, GRE General Test, minimum GPA of 3.0. Additional exam requirements/recommendations for international students: Required—TOEFL. Electronic applications accepted. *Faculty research:* Cancer and infectious diseases, drug delivery, neuropharmacology, cardiovascular pharmacology, bioanalytical chemistry, structural biology.

★ **University of Hawaii at Hilo,** Program in Pharmaceutical Sciences, Hilo, HI 96720-4091. Offers PhD. *Entrance requirements:* Additional exam requirements/recommendations for international students: Required—TOEFL. Electronic applications accepted.

See Display on next page and Close-Up on page 939.

University of Houston, College of Pharmacy, Houston, TX 77204. Offers pharmaceutics (MSPHR, PhD); pharmacology (MSPHR, PhD); pharmacy (Pharm D); pharmacy administration (MSPHR, PhD). *Accreditation:* ACPE. *Program availability:* Part-time. Terminal master's awarded for partial completion of doctoral program. *Entrance requirements:* For doctorate, PCAT (for Pharm D). Additional exam requirements/recommendations for international students: Required—TOEFL. Electronic applications accepted. *Faculty research:* Drug screening and design, cardiovascular pharmacology, infectious disease, asthma research, herbal medicine.

University of Illinois at Chicago, College of Pharmacy and Graduate College, Graduate Programs in Pharmacy, Chicago, IL 60607-7128. Offers forensic science (MS), including forensic toxicology; medicinal chemistry (MS); pharmacognosy (MS, PhD); pharmacy administration (MS, PhD). *Faculty:* 237 full-time (137 women), 60 part-time/adjunct (32 women). *Students:* 110 full-time (62 women), 17 part-time (8 women); includes 26 minority (7 Black or African American, non-Hispanic/Latino; 15 Asian, non-Hispanic/Latino; 4 Hispanic/Latino), 54 international. Average age 28. Terminal master's awarded for partial completion of doctoral program. *Degree requirements:* For master's, variable foreign language requirement, thesis; for doctorate, variable foreign language requirement, thesis/dissertation. *Entrance requirements:* For master's and doctorate, GRE General Test. Additional exam requirements/recommendations for international students: Required—TOEFL. *Application deadline:* For fall admission, 2/1 for domestic students. Applications are processed on a rolling basis. Application fee: $60. Electronic applications accepted. *Expenses:* Tuition, state resident: full-time $11,480; part-time $3826 per credit. Tuition, nonresident: full-time $23,720; part-time $7906 per credit. *Required fees:* $1333 per semester. Part-time tuition and fees vary according to course load and program. *Financial support:* In 2015–16, 2 fellowships with full tuition reimbursements were awarded; research assistantships with full tuition reimbursements, teaching assistantships with full tuition reimbursements, career-related internships or fieldwork, Federal Work-Study, institutionally sponsored loans, traineeships, tuition waivers (full), and unspecified assistantships also available. Financial award application deadline: 3/1; financial award applicants required to submit FAFSA. *Faculty research:* Biopharmaceutical science, forensic science, forensic toxicology, medicinal chemistry, pharmacognosy. *Unit head:* Prof. Joanna Burdette, Associate Dean for Research and Graduate Education, 312-996-6153, E-mail: joannab@uic.edu. *Application contact:* Jackie Perry, Graduate College Receptionist, 312-413-2550, Fax: 312-413-0185, E-mail: gradcoll@uic.edu.
Website: http://www.uic.edu/pharmacy/education/graduatePrograms.php

The University of Iowa, College of Pharmacy, Iowa City, IA 52242-1316. Offers clinical pharmaceutical sciences (PhD); medicinal and natural products chemistry (PhD); pharamaceutics (PhD); pharmaceutical socioeconomics (PhD); pharmaceutics (MS); pharmacy (Pharm D); Pharm D/MPH. *Accreditation:* ACPE (one or more programs are accredited). *Degree requirements:* For master's, thesis optional, exam; for doctorate, comprehensive exam, thesis/dissertation. *Entrance requirements:* For master's and doctorate, GRE General Test, minimum GPA of 3.0. Additional exam requirements/recommendations for international students: Required—TOEFL (minimum score 550 paper-based; 81 iBT). Electronic applications accepted.

The University of Kansas, Graduate Studies, School of Pharmacy, Department of Pharmacy Practice, Lawrence, KS 66047. Offers MS. *Students:* 3 full-time (0 women), 5 part-time (4 women); includes 1 minority (Asian, non-Hispanic/Latino). Average age 26. 4 applicants, 100% accepted, 3 enrolled. In 2015, 3 master's awarded. *Entrance requirements:* For master's, GRE General Test, Pharm D, Kansas pharmacy license. Additional exam requirements/recommendations for international students: Recommended—TOEFL. *Application deadline:* For fall admission, 2/1 priority date for domestic students. Application fee: $65 ($85 for international students). Electronic applications accepted. *Financial support:* Fellowships, health care benefits, and residencies available. Financial award application deadline: 2/15. *Faculty research:* Drug trials, drug stability, pharmacoeconomics, education, outcomes. *Unit head:* David Henry, Chair, 785-864-6066, E-mail: dhenry@ku.edu. *Application contact:* Sandy Urish, Graduate Admissions Contact, 785-864-4882, E-mail: surish@ku.edu.
Website: http://pharmpractice.ku.edu/

University of Kentucky, Graduate School, Graduate Programs in Pharmaceutical Sciences, Lexington, KY 40506-0032. Offers MS, PhD. Terminal master's awarded for partial completion of doctoral program. *Degree requirements:* For master's, thesis optional; for doctorate, comprehensive exam, thesis/dissertation. *Entrance requirements:* For master's, GRE General Test, minimum undergraduate GPA of 3.2; for doctorate, GRE General Test, minimum graduate GPA of 3.2. Additional exam requirements/recommendations for international students: Required—TOEFL (minimum score 550 paper-based; 79 iBT). Electronic applications accepted. *Faculty research:* Drug development, biotechnology, medicinal chemistry, cardiology, pharmacokinetics, CNS pharmacology, clinical pharmacology, pharmacotherapy and health outcomes, pharmaceutical policy.

The University of Manchester, School of Pharmacy and Pharmaceutical Sciences, Manchester, United Kingdom. Offers M Phil, PhD.

University of Manitoba, Faculty of Graduate Studies, Faculty of Pharmacy, Winnipeg, MB R3T 2N2, Canada. Offers M Sc, PhD. *Degree requirements:* For master's, one foreign language, thesis.

University of Maryland, Baltimore, Graduate School, Graduate Programs in Pharmacy, Department of Pharmaceutical Sciences, Baltimore, MD 21201. Offers PhD. *Degree requirements:* For doctorate, comprehensive exam, thesis/dissertation. *Entrance requirements:* For doctorate, GRE General Test. Additional exam requirements/recommendations for international students: Required—TOEFL (minimum score 600 paper-based), IELTS. Electronic applications accepted. Tuition and fees vary according to program. *Faculty research:* Drug delivery, cellular and biological chemistry, clinical pharmaceutical sciences, biopharmaceutics, neuroscience.

University of Michigan, College of Pharmacy and Rackham Graduate School, Department of Pharmaceutical Sciences, Ann Arbor, MI 48109. Offers PhD. *Faculty:* 11 full-time (3 women), 2 part-time/adjunct (0 women). *Students:* 47 full-time (24 women); includes 7 minority (1 Black or African American, non-Hispanic/Latino; 6 Asian, non-Hispanic/Latino), 13 international. Average age 25. 99 applicants, 11% accepted, 7 enrolled. In 2015, 10 doctorates awarded. Terminal master's awarded for partial completion of doctoral program. *Degree requirements:* For doctorate, thesis/dissertation, oral defense of dissertation, preliminary exam. *Entrance requirements:* For doctorate, GRE. Additional exam requirements/recommendations for international students: Required—TOEFL (minimum score 560 paper-based; 84 iBT) or IELTS (minimum score 6.5). *Application deadline:* For fall admission, 1/6 for domestic and international students. Applications are processed on a rolling basis. Application fee: $75 ($90 for international students). Electronic applications accepted. *Expenses:* Contact institution. *Financial support:* In 2015–16, 43 students received support, including 21 fellowships (averaging $48,037 per year), 11 research assistantships (averaging $48,037 per year), 9 teaching assistantships (averaging $48,037 per year); career-related internships or fieldwork, institutionally sponsored loans, scholarships/grants, traineeships, health care benefits, and unspecified assistantships also available. *Faculty research:* New drug design, new drug delivery systems, new biotechnology, pharmacy and the public sector. *Unit head:* Dr. Steven P. Schwedeman, Chair, 734-647-8339, Fax: 734-615-6162, E-mail: schwende@med.umich.edu. *Application contact:* Patrina Hardy, Executive Secretary, 734-615-3749, Fax: 734-615-6162, E-mail: thardy@med.umich.edu.
Website: https://pharmacy.umich.edu/pharmsci

University of Minnesota, Twin Cities Campus, College of Pharmacy and Graduate School, Graduate Programs in Pharmacy, Graduate Program in Experimental and Clinical Pharmacology, Minneapolis, MN 55455-0213. Offers MS, PhD. *Degree requirements:* For doctorate, thesis/dissertation.

University of Minnesota, Twin Cities Campus, College of Pharmacy and Graduate School, Graduate Programs in Pharmacy, Graduate Program in Pharmaceutics, Minneapolis, MN 55455. Offers MS, PhD. *Faculty:* 9 full-time (2 women), 11 part-time/adjunct (2 women). *Students:* 23 full-time (12 women); includes 4 minority (all Asian, non-Hispanic/Latino), 17 international. Average age 26. 85 applicants, 8% accepted, 6 enrolled. In 2015, 1 master's, 4 doctorates awarded. Terminal master's awarded for partial completion of doctoral program. *Degree requirements:* For master's, comprehensive exam, thesis; for doctorate, comprehensive exam, thesis/dissertation. *Entrance requirements:* For master's and doctorate, GRE General Test (preferred minimum score: Analytical Writing 3.5), bachelor's degree. Additional exam requirements/recommendations for international students: Required—TOEFL (minimum score 600 paper-based; 100 iBT), IELTS (minimum score 6.5). *Application deadline:* For fall admission, 12/31 for domestic and international students. Application fee: $75 ($95 for international students). Electronic applications accepted. *Expenses:* Contact institution. *Financial support:* In 2015–16, 19 students received support, including 5 fellowships with full tuition reimbursements available (averaging $22,500 per year), 10 research assistantships with full tuition reimbursements available (averaging $22,500 per year), 4 teaching assistantships with full tuition reimbursements available (averaging $22,500 per year); career-related internships or fieldwork, health care benefits, unspecified assistantships, and summer internships with pharmaceutical companies also available. Financial award application deadline: 12/31. *Faculty research:* Drug delivery, drug metabolism, molecular biopharmaceutics, pharmacokinetics and pharmacodynamics, crystal engineering, biophysical chemistry. *Unit head:* Prof. Jayanth Panyam, PhD, Professor/Head of the Department, 612-624-0951, Fax: 612-626-2125, E-mail: jpanyam@umn.edu. *Application contact:* Katie James, Assistant to the Director of Graduate Studies, 612-624-5153, Fax: 612-626-2125.
Website: http://www.pharmacy.umn.edu/pharmaceutics/

University of Missouri–Kansas City, School of Pharmacy, Kansas City, MO 64110-2499. Offers pharmaceutical sciences (PhD); pharmacology and toxicology (PhD); pharmacy (Pharm D). PhD offered through School of Graduate Studies. *Accreditation:* ACPE (one or more programs are accredited). *Program availability:* Online learning. *Faculty:* 49 full-time (26 women), 6 part-time/adjunct (2 women). *Students:* 447 full-time (276 women); includes 103 minority (24 Black or African American, non-Hispanic/Latino; 1 American Indian or Alaska Native, non-Hispanic/Latino; 53 Asian, non-Hispanic/Latino; 12 Hispanic/Latino; 13 Two or more races, non-Hispanic/Latino), 2 international. Average age 25. 414 applicants, 33% accepted, 133 enrolled. In 2015, 125 doctorates awarded. *Degree requirements:* For doctorate, comprehensive exam (for some programs), thesis/dissertation (for some programs). *Entrance requirements:* For doctorate, PCAT (for Pharm D). Additional exam requirements/recommendations for international students: Required—TOEFL (minimum score 550 paper-based; 80 iBT). *Application deadline:* For fall admission, 3/1 for domestic and international students. Applications are processed on a rolling basis. Application fee: $45 ($50 for international students). Electronic applications accepted. *Expenses:* Contact institution. *Financial support:* In 2015–16, 4 fellowships (averaging $40,082 per year), 14 research assistantships with tuition reimbursements (averaging $13,117 per year), 26 teaching assistantships with full tuition reimbursements (averaging $14,724 per year) were awarded; career-related internships or fieldwork, Federal Work-Study, institutionally sponsored loans, tuition waivers (full and partial), and unspecified assistantships also available. Financial award application deadline: 3/1; financial award applicants required to submit FAFSA. *Faculty research:* Bio-organic and medicinal chemistry, drug delivery, pharmaceutics, molecular neurobiology, neurology. *Unit head:* Dr. Russell B. Melchert, Dean, 816-235-1609, Fax: 816-235-5190, E-mail: melchertr@umkc.edu.

University of Hawai`i at Hilo

Daniel K. Inouye College of Pharmacy (DKICP)

Ph.D. PROGRAM IN PHARMACEUTICAL SCIENCES

Utilizing the extraordinary intellectual, biological, physical and cultural diversity of its geographic region as a focus of investigation and study, the Daniel K. Inouye College of Pharmacy (DKICP) at the University of Hawaii at Hilo is proud to offer a Ph.D. program in the Pharmaceutical Sciences.

This program, which is the only program of its type in the Pacific region, is aimed at students with B.S., M.S., or Pharm.D. degrees and those currently working in the field. It provides graduate training in the Pharmaceutical Sciences including:

- Cancer Research
- Drug Discovery
- Medicinal Chemistry
- Pharmacology
- Pharmaceutics
- Pharmacognosy

For more information, contact:
pharmacy@hawaii.edu

http://pharmacy.uhh.hawaii.edu/academics/graduate/

Pharmaceutical Sciences

Application contact: Shelly M. Janasz, Director, Student Services, 816-235-2400, Fax: 816-235-5190, E-mail: janaszs@umkc.edu.
Website: http://pharmacy.umkc.edu/

University of Montana, Graduate School, College of Health Professions and Biomedical Sciences, Skaggs School of Pharmacy, Department of Biomedical and Pharmaceutical Sciences, Missoula, MT 59812-0002. Offers biomedical sciences (PhD); medicinal chemistry (MS, PhD); molecular and cellular toxicology (MS, PhD); neuroscience (PhD); pharmaceutical sciences (MS). *Accreditation:* ACPE. *Degree requirements:* For master's, oral defense of thesis; for doctorate, research dissertation defense. *Entrance requirements:* For master's and doctorate, GRE General Test. Additional exam requirements/recommendations for international students: Required—TOEFL (minimum score 540 paper-based). Electronic applications accepted. *Faculty research:* Cardiovascular pharmacology, medicinal chemistry, neurosciences, environmental toxicology, pharmacogenetics, cancer.

University of Nebraska Medical Center, Department of Pharmaceutical Sciences, Omaha, NE 68198. Offers MS, PhD. *Faculty:* 20 full-time (3 women), 1 part-time/adjunct (0 women). *Students:* 55 full-time (25 women), 1 part-time (0 women), 48 international. Average age 27. 57 applicants, 26% accepted, 15 enrolled. In 2015, 4 doctorates awarded. Terminal master's awarded for partial completion of doctoral program. *Degree requirements:* For master's, thesis; for doctorate, comprehensive exam, thesis/dissertation. *Entrance requirements:* For master's, GRE General Test; for doctorate, GRE. Additional exam requirements/recommendations for international students: Required—TOEFL (minimum score 550 paper-based; 80 iBT). *Application deadline:* For fall admission, 4/1 priority date for domestic and international students; for spring admission, 10/1 for domestic students, 8/1 for international students. Applications are processed on a rolling basis. Application fee: $45. Electronic applications accepted. *Expenses:* Tuition, state resident: full-time $7830; part-time $3915 per credit hour. Tuition, nonresident: full-time $22,410; part-time $11,205 per credit hour. *Required fees:* $521. *Financial support:* In 2015–16, 2 fellowships with full tuition reimbursements (averaging $23,100 per year), 10 research assistantships with full tuition reimbursements (averaging $23,000 per year), teaching assistantships with full tuition reimbursements (averaging $23,000 per year) were awarded; scholarships/grants also available. Support available to part-time students. Financial award application deadline: 3/1; financial award applicants required to submit FAFSA. *Faculty research:* Pharmaceutics, medicinal chemistry, toxicology, chemical carcinogenesis, pharmacokinetics. *Unit head:* Dr. David Oupicky, Chair, Pharmaceutical Sciences Graduate Program Committee, 402-559-9363, E-mail: david.oupicky@unmc.edu. *Application contact:* Katina Winters, Office Associate, 402-559-5320, E-mail: kwinters@unmc.edu.
Website: http://www.unmc.edu/pharmacy/faculty/pharmaceutical-sciences/

University of New Mexico, Graduate Studies, College of Pharmacy, Graduate Programs in Pharmaceutical Sciences, Albuquerque, NM 87131-2039. Offers MS, PhD. *Program availability:* Part-time. *Degree requirements:* For master's, comprehensive exam, thesis; for doctorate, comprehensive exam, thesis/dissertation. *Entrance requirements:* For master's and doctorate, GRE General Test (for some concentrations), 3 letters of recommendation, letter of intent, resume. Additional exam requirements/recommendations for international students: Required—TOEFL (minimum score 580 paper-based; 93 iBT). Electronic applications accepted. *Faculty research:* Pharmaceutical research, cancer research, pharmacy administration, radiopharmacy, toxicology.

The University of North Carolina at Chapel Hill, Eshelman School of Pharmacy, Chapel Hill, NC 27599. Offers health system pharmacy administration (MS); pharmacy (PhD). *Accreditation:* ACPE (one or more programs are accredited). *Faculty:* 112 full-time (45 women), 362 part-time/adjunct (188 women). *Students:* 104 full-time (50 women); includes 30 minority (4 Black or African American, non-Hispanic/Latino; 1 American Indian or Alaska Native, non-Hispanic/Latino; 10 Asian, non-Hispanic/Latino; 4 Hispanic/Latino; 2 Native Hawaiian or other Pacific Islander, non-Hispanic/Latino; 9 Two or more races, non-Hispanic/Latino), 16 international. Average age 26. 268 applicants, 9% accepted, 25 enrolled. In 2015, 8 master's, 13 doctorates awarded. Terminal master's awarded for partial completion of doctoral program. *Degree requirements:* For master's, comprehensive exam, thesis or alternative; for doctorate, comprehensive exam, thesis/dissertation. *Entrance requirements:* For master's and doctorate, GRE General Test, minimum GPA of 3.0. Additional exam requirements/recommendations for international students: Required—TOEFL (minimum score 550 paper-based). *Application deadline:* For fall admission, 12/7 priority date for domestic students, 12/15 priority date for international students. Applications are processed on a rolling basis. Application fee: $85. Electronic applications accepted. *Expenses:* Contact institution. *Financial support:* In 2015–16, 11 students received support, including 18 fellowships with full tuition reimbursements available (averaging $27,500 per year), 56 research assistantships with full tuition reimbursements available (averaging $27,500 per year), teaching assistantships with full tuition reimbursements available (averaging $27,500 per year); career-related internships or fieldwork, Federal Work-Study, institutionally sponsored loans, scholarships/grants, traineeships, health care benefits, tuition waivers (full), and unspecified assistantships also available. Financial award application deadline: 12/15. *Faculty research:* Health services research, pharmacokinetics, molecular modeling, infectious disease, genomics and proteomics, translational research. *Total annual research expenditures:* $15.5 million. *Unit head:* Dr. Robert A. Blouin, Dean, 919-966-1122, Fax: 919-966-6919, E-mail: bob_blouin@unc.edu. *Application contact:* Mimi Lewis, Coordinator of Admissions, 919-962-0097, Fax: 919-966-9428, E-mail: mimi_lewis@unc.edu.
Website: http://pharmacy.unc.edu/

University of Oklahoma Health Sciences Center, College of Pharmacy and Graduate College, Graduate Programs in Pharmacy, Oklahoma City, OK 73190. Offers MS, PhD, MS/MBA. MS/MBA offered jointly with Oklahoma State University and University of Oklahoma. Terminal master's awarded for partial completion of doctoral program. *Degree requirements:* For master's, comprehensive exam, thesis; for doctorate, comprehensive exam, thesis/dissertation. *Entrance requirements:* For master's and doctorate, GRE General Test. Additional exam requirements/recommendations for international students: Required—TOEFL. *Faculty research:* Medicinal chemistry, pharmacokinetics/biopharmaceutics, nuclear pharmacy, pharmacy administration, pharmacodynamics and toxicology.

University of Pittsburgh, School of Pharmacy, Graduate Program in Pharmaceutical Sciences, Pittsburgh, PA 15261. Offers pharmaceutical sciences (MS, PhD), including biochemical pharmacology, clinical pharmaceutical scientist, medicinal chemistry, pharmaceutical outcomes and research policy, pharmaceutics. *Program availability:* Part-time. *Faculty:* 33 full-time (9 women), 2 part-time/adjunct (1 woman). *Students:* 67 full-time (36 women), 1 part-time (0 women); includes 5 minority (1 Black or African American, non-Hispanic/Latino; 4 Asian, non-Hispanic/Latino), 50 international. Average age 28. 103 applicants, 36% accepted, 20 enrolled. In 2015, 29 master's, 8 doctorates awarded. Terminal master's awarded for partial completion of doctoral program. *Degree requirements:* For master's, comprehensive exam (for some programs), thesis (for some programs), 34 credits (for non-thesis), 30 credits (for thesis); for doctorate, comprehensive exam, thesis/dissertation, 72 credits. *Entrance requirements:* For

master's and doctorate, GRE General Test. Additional exam requirements/recommendations for international students: Required—TOEFL (minimum score 100 iBT), IELTS (minimum score 7). *Application deadline:* For fall admission, 1/5 priority date for domestic and international students. Application fee: $150. Electronic applications accepted. *Expenses:* $24,928 per year; mandatory fees $800 per year. *Financial support:* In 2015–16, 51 students received support, including 1 fellowship with full tuition reimbursement available (averaging $16,885 per year), 15 research assistantships with full tuition reimbursements available (averaging $27,540 per year), 38 teaching assistantships with full tuition reimbursements available (averaging $26,856 per year); scholarships/grants, health care benefits, tuition waivers (full), and unspecified assistantships also available. Financial award application deadline: 1/5. *Faculty research:* Vaginal, cervical and rectal drug delivery in infectious disease; computational and molecular biology; transcriptional regulation of enzymes and transporters; pharmaceutical outcomes and pharmacoepidemiology. *Total annual research expenditures:* $13.3 million. *Unit head:* Dr. Samuel M. Poloyac, Associate Dean for Graduate and Postdoctoral Programs, 412-624-4595, E-mail: poloyac@pitt.edu. *Application contact:* Lori M. Altenbaugh, Graduate Program Coordinator, 412-648-1014, Fax: 412-383-9996, E-mail: schmotze@pitt.edu.
Website: http://www.pharmacy.pitt.edu/Programs/GradProgram

University of Puerto Rico, Medical Sciences Campus, School of Pharmacy, San Juan, PR 00936-5067. Offers industrial pharmacy (MS); pharmaceutical sciences (MS); pharmacy (Pharm D). *Accreditation:* ACPE. *Program availability:* Part-time, evening/weekend. *Degree requirements:* For master's, thesis; for doctorate, portfolio, research project. *Entrance requirements:* For master's, GRE, interview; for doctorate, PCAT, interview. Electronic applications accepted. *Expenses:* Contact institution. *Faculty research:* Controlled release, solid dosage form, screening of anti-HIV drugs, pharmacokinetic/pharmacodynamic of drugs.

University of Rhode Island, Graduate School, College of Pharmacy, Department of Biomedical and Pharmaceutical Sciences, Kingston, RI 02881. Offers medicinal chemistry and pharmacognosy (MS, PhD); pharmaceutics and pharmacokinetics (MS, PhD); pharmacology and toxicology (MS, PhD). *Program availability:* Part-time. *Faculty:* 15 full-time (4 women), 4 part-time/adjunct (2 women). *Students:* 39 full-time (14 women), 10 part-time (3 women); includes 3 minority (1 Black or African American, non-Hispanic/Latino; 2 Asian, non-Hispanic/Latino), 24 international. In 2015, 4 master's, 10 doctorates awarded. *Entrance requirements:* For master's and doctorate, GRE (minimum old/new format scores: Verbal 350/143; Quantitative 550/146; Analytical 3.0), 2 letters of recommendation. Additional exam requirements/recommendations for international students: Required—TOEFL (minimum score 550 paper-based). *Application deadline:* For fall admission, 7/15 for domestic students, 2/1 for international students. Application fee: $65. Electronic applications accepted. *Expenses:* Tuition, state resident: full-time $11,796; part-time $655 per credit. Tuition, nonresident: full-time $24,206; part-time $1345 per credit. *Required fees:* $1546; $44 per credit. One-time fee: $155 full-time; $35 part-time. *Financial support:* In 2015–16, 6 research assistantships with tuition reimbursements (averaging $14,828 per year), 18 teaching assistantships with tuition reimbursements (averaging $14,851 per year) were awarded. Financial award application deadline: 2/1; financial award applicants required to submit FAFSA. *Faculty research:* Chemical carcinogenesis with a major emphasis on the structural and synthetic aspects of DNA-adduct formation, drug-drug/herb interaction, drug-genetic interaction, signaling of nuclear receptors, transcriptional regulation, oncogenesis. *Total annual research expenditures:* $5.8 million. *Unit head:* Dr. Bingfang Yan, Chair, 401-874-5032, Fax: 401-874-2181, E-mail: byan@uri.edu. *Application contact:* Graduate Admissions, 401-874-2872, E-mail: gradadm@etal.uri.edu.
Website: http://www.uri.edu/pharmacy/departments/bps/index.shtml

University of Saskatchewan, College of Graduate Studies and Research, College of Pharmacy and Nutrition, Saskatoon, SK S7N 5A2, Canada. Offers M Sc, PhD. *Degree requirements:* For master's, thesis; for doctorate, thesis/dissertation. *Entrance requirements:* Additional exam requirements/recommendations for international students: Required—TOEFL.

University of South Carolina, South Carolina College of Pharmacy and The Graduate School, Department of Basic Pharmaceutical Sciences, Columbia, SC 29208. Offers MS, PhD. PhD offered jointly with Medical University of South Carolina. *Program availability:* Part-time. Terminal master's awarded for partial completion of doctoral program. *Degree requirements:* For master's, one foreign language, comprehensive exam, thesis; for doctorate, one foreign language, comprehensive exam, thesis/dissertation. *Entrance requirements:* For master's, GRE General Test, BS in biology, chemistry, pharmacy, or related field; for doctorate, GRE General Test, BS in biology, chemistry, or related field. Additional exam requirements/recommendations for international students: Required—TOEFL. Electronic applications accepted. *Faculty research:* Cancer treatment and prevention, Ion channels, DNA damage repair, inflammation.

University of Southern California, Graduate School, School of Pharmacy, Department of Pharmacology and Pharmaceutical Sciences, Los Angeles, CA 90089. Offers MS, PhD. Terminal master's awarded for partial completion of doctoral program. *Degree requirements:* For master's, comprehensive exam, thesis, 24 units of formal course work, excluding research and seminar courses; for doctorate, comprehensive exam, thesis/dissertation, 24 units of formal course work, excluding research and seminar courses. *Entrance requirements:* For master's and doctorate, GRE. Additional exam requirements/recommendations for international students: Required—TOEFL (minimum score 603 paper-based; 100 iBT). Electronic applications accepted. *Faculty research:* Drug design, drug delivery, pharmaceutical sciences.

University of Southern California, Graduate School, School of Pharmacy, Graduate Programs in Pharmaceutical Economics and Policy, Los Angeles, CA 90033. Offers MS, PhD. Terminal master's awarded for partial completion of doctoral program. *Degree requirements:* For master's, comprehensive exam, thesis, 24 units of formal course work, excluding research and seminar courses; for doctorate, comprehensive exam, thesis/dissertation, 24 units of formal course work, excluding research and seminar courses. *Entrance requirements:* For master's and doctorate, GRE. Additional exam requirements/recommendations for international students: Required—TOEFL (minimum score 603 paper-based; 100 iBT). Electronic applications accepted. *Faculty research:* Cost-effective analyses/modeling, retrospective data analysis of comparative effectiveness, quality of life measurement, competitive pricing systems in health care.

University of Southern California, Graduate School, School of Pharmacy, Program in Clinical and Experimental Therapeutics, Los Angeles, CA 90089. Offers PhD. Terminal master's awarded for partial completion of doctoral program. *Degree requirements:* For doctorate, comprehensive exam, thesis/dissertation, 24 units of course work, excluding research and dissertation courses. *Entrance requirements:* For doctorate, GRE, minimum overall GPA of 3.0, three letters of recommendation. Additional exam requirements/recommendations for international students: Required—TOEFL (minimum score 625 paper-based; 100 iBT). Electronic applications accepted. *Faculty research:* Pharmacology and therapeutics: inflammation, tissue regeneration, myelosuppression, bacterial resistance and virulence, alcoholism, CNS disorders, metabolomics and lipidomics.

University of Southern California, Graduate School, School of Pharmacy, Regulatory Science Programs, Los Angeles, CA 90089. Offers clinical research design and management (Graduate Certificate); food safety (Graduate Certificate); patient and product safety (Graduate Certificate); preclinical drug development (Graduate Certificate); regulatory and clinical affairs (Graduate Certificate); regulatory science (MS, DRSc). *Program availability:* Part-time, evening/weekend, online learning. Terminal master's awarded for partial completion of doctoral program. *Degree requirements:* For master's, thesis optional; for doctorate, comprehensive exam, thesis/dissertation. *Entrance requirements:* For master's, GRE. Additional exam requirements/recommendations for international students: Required—TOEFL (minimum score 603 paper-based; 100 iBT). Electronic applications accepted.

University of South Florida, College of Pharmacy, Tampa, FL 33620-9951. Offers pharmaceutical nanotechnology (MS); pharmacy (Pharm D). *Accreditation:* ACPE. *Faculty:* 4 full-time (0 women). *Students:* 344 full-time (191 women); includes 146 minority (30 Black or African American, non-Hispanic/Latino; 53 Asian, non-Hispanic/Latino; 54 Hispanic/Latino; 3 Native Hawaiian or other Pacific Islander, non-Hispanic/Latino; 6 Two or more races, non-Hispanic/Latino). Average age 26. 678 applicants, 25% accepted, 92 enrolled. In 2015, 49 doctorates awarded. *Degree requirements:* For master's, comprehensive exam, thesis optional. *Entrance requirements:* For master's, GRE, MCAT or DAT, minimum GPA of 3.0, letters of reference, resume; for doctorate, PCAT, minimum GPA of 2.75 overall (preferred); completion of 72 prerequisite credit hours; U.S. citizenship or permanent resident. Additional exam requirements/recommendations for international students: Required—TOEFL (minimum score 550 paper-based; 79 iBT), IELTS (minimum score 6.5). *Total annual research expenditures:* $140,853. *Unit head:* Dr. Kevin Sneed, Dean, 813-974-5699, E-mail: ksneed@health.usf.edu. *Application contact:* Dr. Amy Schwartz, Associate Dean, 813-974-2251, E-mail: aschwar1@health.usf.edu.

The University of Tennessee Health Science Center, College of Graduate Health Sciences, Memphis, TN 38163-0002. Offers biomedical engineering (MS, PhD); biomedical sciences (PhD); dental sciences (MDS); epidemiology (MS); health outcomes and policy research (PhD); laboratory research and management (MS); nursing science (PhD); pharmaceutical sciences (PhD); pharmacology (MS); speech and hearing science (PhD); DDS/PhD; DNP/PhD; MD/PhD; Pharm D/PhD. Terminal master's awarded for partial completion of doctoral program. *Degree requirements:* For master's, comprehensive exam, thesis; for doctorate, comprehensive exam, thesis/dissertation, oral and written preliminary and comprehensive exams. *Entrance requirements:* For master's and doctorate, GRE General Test, minimum GPA of 3.0. Additional exam requirements/recommendations for international students: Required—TOEFL (minimum score 79 iBT); Recommended—IELTS (minimum score 6.5). Electronic applications accepted.

The University of Texas at Austin, Graduate School, College of Pharmacy, Graduate Programs in Pharmacy, Austin, TX 78712-1111. Offers health outcomes and pharmacy practice (PhD); health outcomes and pharmacy practice (MS); medicinal chemistry (PhD); pharmaceutics (PhD); pharmacology and toxicology (PhD); pharmacotherapy (MS, PhD); translational science (PhD). PhD in translational science offered jointly with The University of Texas Health Science Center at San Antonio and The University of Texas at San Antonio. *Degree requirements:* For master's, thesis; for doctorate, thesis/dissertation. *Entrance requirements:* For master's and doctorate, GRE General Test. Electronic applications accepted. *Faculty research:* Synthetic medical chemistry, synthetic molecular biology, bio-organic chemistry, pharmacoeconomics, pharmacy practice.

University of the Pacific, Thomas J. Long School of Pharmacy and Health Sciences, Pharmaceutical and Chemical Sciences Graduate Program, Stockton, CA 95211-0197. Offers MS, PhD. *Entrance requirements:* Additional exam requirements/recommendations for international students: Required—TOEFL (minimum score 475 paper-based).

University of the Sciences, Program in Pharmaceutics, Philadelphia, PA 19104-4495. Offers MS, PhD. *Program availability:* Part-time. Terminal master's awarded for partial completion of doctoral program. *Degree requirements:* For master's, thesis (for some programs); for doctorate, comprehensive exam, thesis/dissertation, oral defense. *Entrance requirements:* For master's and doctorate, GRE General Test. Additional exam requirements/recommendations for international students: Required—TOEFL, TWE. *Application deadline:* For fall admission, 5/1 for international students; for winter admission, 10/1 for international students; for spring admission, 3/1 for international students. Applications are processed on a rolling basis. Application fee: $50. *Financial support:* Fellowships with full tuition reimbursements, research assistantships with full tuition reimbursements, teaching assistantships with full tuition reimbursements, institutionally sponsored loans, and tuition waivers (full and partial) available. Financial award application deadline: 3/1. *Unit head:* Dr. Steven Neau, Director, 215-596-8825, E-mail: s.neau@usciences.edu. *Application contact:* Dr. Steven Neau, Director, 215-596-8825, E-mail: s.neau@usciences.edu.

The University of Toledo, College of Graduate Studies, College of Pharmacy and Pharmaceutical Sciences, Program in Pharmaceutical Sciences, Toledo, OH 43606-3390. Offers administrative pharmacy (MSPS); industrial pharmacy (MSPS); pharmacology toxicology (MSPS). *Degree requirements:* For master's, thesis. *Entrance requirements:* For master's, GRE General Test. Additional exam requirements/recommendations for international students: Required—TOEFL (minimum score 550 paper-based; 80 iBT). Electronic applications accepted.

University of Toronto, School of Graduate Studies, Leslie Dan Faculty of Pharmacy, Toronto, ON M5S 1A1, Canada. Offers M Sc, PhD, Pharm D. *Program availability:* Part-time. *Degree requirements:* For master's, thesis, poster presentation, oral thesis defense; for doctorate, thesis/dissertation (for some programs). *Entrance requirements:* For master's, minimum B average in last 2 years of full-time study, 3 letters of reference, resume. Additional exam requirements/recommendations for international students: Required—TOEFL (minimum score 600 paper-based), Michigan English Language Assessment Battery (minum score 88) or IELTS (minimum score 7). Electronic applications accepted.

University of Utah, Graduate School, College of Pharmacy, Department of Pharmacotherapy, Salt Lake City, UT 84112. Offers health system pharmacy administration (MS); outcomes research and health policy (PhD). *Faculty:* 6 full-time (4 women), 26 part-time/adjunct (18 women). *Students:* 8 full-time (5 women), 5 part-time (3 women), 5 international. Average age 28. 26 applicants, 19% accepted, 4 enrolled. In 2015, 3 master's awarded. Terminal master's awarded for partial completion of doctoral program. *Degree requirements:* For master's, comprehensive exam, thesis or alternative, project; for doctorate, comprehensive exam, thesis/dissertation. *Entrance requirements:* For doctorate, GRE. Additional exam requirements/recommendations for international students: Required—TOEFL (minimum score 550 paper-based; 80 iBT). *Application deadline:* For fall admission, 1/10 for domestic students, 12/15 for international students. Application fee: $55 ($65 for international students). *Financial support:* In 2015–16, 7 students received support, including 9 research assistantships with full tuition reimbursements available (averaging $21,400 per year); health care benefits also available. Financial award application deadline: 12/15. *Faculty research:*

Outcomes in pharmacy, pharmacotherapy. *Total annual research expenditures:* $131,217. *Unit head:* Dr. Diana I. Brixner, Department Chair and Professor, 801-581-6731. *Application contact:* Sara Ray, Academic Program Manager, 801-581-5984, Fax: 801-585-6160, E-mail: sara.ray@pharm.utah.edu.
Website: http://www.pharmacy.utah.edu/pharmacotherapy/

University of Washington, School of Pharmacy, Department of Pharmaceutics, Seattle, WA 98195. Offers MS, PhD, Pharm D/PhD. Terminal master's awarded for partial completion of doctoral program. *Degree requirements:* For master's, thesis; for doctorate, thesis/dissertation. *Entrance requirements:* For master's and doctorate, GRE General Test. Additional exam requirements/recommendations for international students: Required—TOEFL. Electronic applications accepted. *Faculty research:* Pharmacokinetics, drug delivery, drug metabolism, pharmacogenetics, transporters.

University of Wisconsin–Madison, School of Pharmacy and Graduate School, Graduate Programs in Pharmacy, Pharmaceutical Sciences Division, Madison, WI 53705. Offers PhD. *Faculty:* 23 full-time (4 women), 4 part-time/adjunct (2 women). *Students:* 41 full-time (19 women); includes 32 minority (2 Black or African American, non-Hispanic/Latino; 27 Asian, non-Hispanic/Latino; 3 Hispanic/Latino), 31 international. Average age 27. 219 applicants, 11% accepted, 7 enrolled. In 2015, 6 doctorates awarded. Terminal master's awarded for partial completion of doctoral program. *Degree requirements:* For doctorate, comprehensive exam, thesis/dissertation. *Entrance requirements:* For doctorate, GRE. Additional exam requirements/recommendations for international students: Required—TOEFL. *Application deadline:* 12/30 for domestic and international students. Application fee: $56. Electronic applications accepted. *Expenses:* Tuition, state resident: full-time $5364. Tuition, nonresident: full-time $12,027. *Required fees:* $571. Tuition and fees vary according to campus/location, program and reciprocity agreements. *Financial support:* In 2015–16, 38 students received support, including 15 fellowships with full tuition reimbursements available (averaging $24,000 per year), 14 research assistantships with full tuition reimbursements available (averaging $24,000 per year), 21 teaching assistantships with full tuition reimbursements available (averaging $24,000 per year); traineeships and unspecified assistantships also available. Financial award application deadline: 12/30. *Faculty research:* Drug action, drug delivery, drug discovery. *Unit head:* Dr. Ron Burnette, Chair, 608-262-3814, E-mail: ronald.burnette@wisc.edu. *Application contact:* Ken Niemeyer, Graduate Program Coordinator, 608-262-4257, E-mail: kenneth.niemeyer@wisc.edu.
Website: http://www.pharmacy.wisc.edu/pharmsci/

University of Wisconsin–Madison, School of Pharmacy and Graduate School, Graduate Programs in Pharmacy, Social and Administrative Sciences in Pharmacy Division, Madison, WI 53706-1380. Offers MS, PhD. Terminal master's awarded for partial completion of doctoral program. *Degree requirements:* For master's, comprehensive exam (for some programs), thesis optional; for doctorate, comprehensive exam, thesis/dissertation. *Entrance requirements:* For master's and doctorate, GRE. Additional exam requirements/recommendations for international students: Required—TOEFL. Electronic applications accepted. *Expenses:* Tuition, state resident: full-time $5364. Tuition, nonresident: full-time $12,027. *Required fees:* $571. Tuition and fees vary according to campus/location, program and reciprocity agreements. *Faculty research:* Patient-provider communication, economics, patient care systems.

Virginia Commonwealth University, Medical College of Virginia-Professional Programs, School of Pharmacy, Department of Pharmaceutics, Richmond, VA 23284-9005. Offers medicinal chemistry (MS); pharmaceutical sciences (PhD); pharmaceutics (MS); pharmacotherapy and pharmacy administration (MS). Terminal master's awarded for partial completion of doctoral program. *Degree requirements:* For master's, thesis; for doctorate, thesis/dissertation. *Entrance requirements:* For master's and doctorate, GRE General Test. Additional exam requirements/recommendations for international students: Required—TOEFL. Electronic applications accepted. *Faculty research:* Drug delivery systems, drug development.

Wayne State University, Eugene Applebaum College of Pharmacy and Health Sciences, Department of Pharmaceutical Sciences, Detroit, MI 48202. Offers medicinal chemistry (MS, PhD); pharmaceutics (MS, PhD), including medicinal chemistry (PhD); pharmacology/toxicology (MS, PhD). *Accreditation:* ACPE (one or more programs are accredited). *Faculty:* 17 full-time (3 women). *Students:* 26 full-time (14 women), 3 part-time (1 woman); includes 3 minority (1 Black or African American, non-Hispanic/Latino; 1 American Indian or Alaska Native, non-Hispanic/Latino; 1 Asian, non-Hispanic/Latino), 23 international. Average age 26. 184 applicants, 15% accepted, 10 enrolled. In 2015, 9 master's, 102 doctorates awarded. *Degree requirements:* For master's, thesis; for doctorate, thesis/dissertation. *Entrance requirements:* For master's, GRE General Test, bachelor's degree; adequate background in biology, physics, calculus, and chemistry; three letters of recommendation; personal statement; for doctorate, GRE General Test, bachelor's or master's degree in one of the behavioral, biological, pharmaceutical or physical sciences; three letters of recommendation. Additional exam requirements/recommendations for international students: Required—TOEFL (minimum score 550 paper-based; 79 iBT), Michigan English Language Assessment Battery (minimum score 85); Recommended—IELTS (minimum score 6.5), TWE (minimum score 5.5). *Application deadline:* For fall admission, 12/1 priority date for domestic and international students. Applications are processed on a rolling basis. Application fee: $0. Electronic applications accepted. *Expenses:* $16,104 per year resident tuition, $32,401 non-resident tuition; $671 per credit hour resident tuition, $1,350.05 per credit hour non-resident tuition; fees include $47.45 per credit hour student services fee and $274.60 per semester registration fee. *Financial support:* In 2015–16, 15 students received support, including 2 fellowships with tuition reimbursements available (averaging $24,179 per year), 10 research assistantships with full tuition reimbursements available (averaging $24,595 per year); teaching assistantships, scholarships/grants, health care benefits, and unspecified assistantships also available. Financial award application deadline: 3/31; financial award applicants required to submit FAFSA. *Faculty research:* Design of new anthracyclines, genetic and epigenetic effects of extracellular inducers, cellular injury and cell death, drug metabolism and nutrition, anti-infective agents, carcinogenesis, diabetes research, theragnostic nanomedicines, neurotoxicity, drug discovery, insulin resistance. *Unit head:* Dr. George Corcoran, Chair and Professor, 313-577-1737, E-mail: corcoran@wayne.edu. *Application contact:* 313-577-5415, Fax: 313-577-2033, E-mail: pscgrad@wayne.edu.
Website: http://cphs.wayne.edu/sciences/index.php

Western University of Health Sciences, College of Pharmacy, Program in Pharmaceutical Sciences, Pomona, CA 91766-1854. Offers MS. *Faculty:* 12 full-time (4 women). *Students:* 10 full-time (5 women), 6 part-time (2 women); includes 7 minority (1 American Indian or Alaska Native, non-Hispanic/Latino; 3 Asian, non-Hispanic/Latino; 3 Hispanic/Latino), 5 international. Average age 26. 38 applicants, 13% accepted, 5 enrolled. In 2015, 6 master's awarded. *Entrance requirements:* For master's, GRE, minimum overall GPA of 2.5; BS in pharmacy, chemistry, biology or related scientific area; letters of recommendation; curriculum vitae. Additional exam requirements/recommendations for international students: Required—TOEFL (minimum score 89 iBT), IELTS (minimum score 6.5). *Application deadline:* For fall admission, 4/1 for domestic and international students; for spring admission, 9/1 for domestic and international students. Application fee: $40. Electronic applications accepted. *Expenses:*

Pharmaceutical Sciences

$14,500, $725 per unit. *Financial support:* In 2015–16, 24 students received support. Teaching assistantships available. Financial award application deadline: 3/2; financial award applicants required to submit FAFSA. *Faculty research:* Thrombosis and platelet biology; immune regulation of heart failure; defining the role of endogenous opiod peptides in actions of drug abuse; novel strategies for cancer prevention and therapy; novel dosage forms. *Unit head:* Jeffrey Wang, Chair, 909-469-5413, Fax: 909-469-5539, E-mail: jwang@westernu.edu. *Application contact:* Kathryn Ford, Director of Admissions, 909-469-5335, Fax: 909-469-5570, E-mail: admissions@westernu.edu. Website: http://www.westernu.edu/pharmacy-dpp_message

West Virginia University, School of Medicine, Graduate Programs at the Health Sciences Center, Interdisciplinary Graduate Programs in Biomedical Sciences, Program in Pharmaceutical and Pharmacological Sciences, Morgantown, WV 26506. Offers MS, PhD, MD/PhD. *Degree requirements:* For doctorate, comprehensive exam, thesis/dissertation. *Entrance requirements:* For doctorate, GRE General Test, minimum GPA of 3.0. Additional exam requirements/recommendations for international students: Required—TOEFL. Electronic applications accepted. *Expenses:* Tuition, state resident:

full-time $8568. Tuition, nonresident: full-time $22,140. Tuition and fees vary according to program. *Faculty research:* Medicinal chemistry, pharmacokinetics, nano-pharmaceutics, polymer-based drug delivery, molecular therapeutics.

West Virginia University, School of Pharmacy, Program in Pharmaceutical and Pharmacological Sciences, Morgantown, WV 26506. Offers administrative pharmacy (PhD); behavioral pharmacy (MS, PhD); biopharmaceutics/pharmacokinetics (MS, PhD); industrial pharmacy (MS); medicinal chemistry (MS, PhD); pharmaceutical chemistry (MS, PhD); pharmaceutics (MS, PhD); pharmacology and toxicology (MS); pharmacy (MS); pharmacy administration (MS). *Program availability:* Part-time. Terminal master's awarded for partial completion of doctoral program. *Degree requirements:* For master's, thesis; for doctorate, one foreign language, comprehensive exam, thesis/dissertation. *Entrance requirements:* For master's and doctorate, GRE General Test, minimum GPA of 2.75. Additional exam requirements/recommendations for international students: Required—TOEFL; Recommended—TWE. Electronic applications accepted. *Expenses:* Contact institution. *Faculty research:* Pharmaceutics, medicinal chemistry, biopharmaceutics/pharmacokinetics, health outcomes research.

Pharmacy

Albany College of Pharmacy and Health Sciences, School of Pharmacy and Pharmaceutical Sciences, Albany, NY 12208. Offers health outcomes research (MS); pharmaceutical sciences (MS), including pharmaceutics, pharmacology; pharmacy (Pharm D). *Accreditation:* ACPE. *Degree requirements:* For master's, thesis; for doctorate, practice experience. *Entrance requirements:* For master's, GRE, minimum GPA of 3.0; for doctorate, PCAT, minimum GPA of 2.5. Additional exam requirements/recommendations for international students: Required—TOEFL (minimum score 84 iBT). Electronic applications accepted. *Faculty research:* Therapeutic use of drugs, pharmacokinetics, drug delivery and design.

Appalachian College of Pharmacy, Doctor of Pharmacy Program, Oakwood, VA 24631. Offers Pharm D. *Accreditation:* ACPE.

Auburn University, Harrison School of Pharmacy, Professional Program in Pharmacy, Auburn University, AL 36849. Offers Pharm D. *Accreditation:* ACPE. *Program availability:* Part-time. *Faculty:* 54 full-time (32 women), 1 (woman) part-time/adjunct. *Students:* 583 full-time (397 women), 5 part-time (4 women); includes 117 minority (49 Black or African American, non-Hispanic/Latino; 7 American Indian or Alaska Native, non-Hispanic/Latino; 41 Asian, non-Hispanic/Latino; 8 Hispanic/Latino; 2 Native Hawaiian or other Pacific Islander, non-Hispanic/Latino; 10 Two or more races, non-Hispanic/Latino), 2 international. Average age 25. 460 applicants, 60% accepted, 148 enrolled. In 2015, 142 doctorates awarded. Application fee: $0. *Expenses:* Contact institution. *Financial support:* Federal Work-Study available. Support available to part-time students. Financial award applicants required to submit FAFSA. *Unit head:* Dr. R. Lee Evans, Dean/Professor, Harrison School of Pharmacy, 334-844-8348, Fax: 334-844-8353. *Application contact:* Dr. George Flowers, Dean of the Graduate School, 334-844-2125.

Belmont University, College of Pharmacy, Nashville, TN 37212-3757. Offers Pharm D. *Accreditation:* ACPE. *Faculty:* 25 full-time (16 women), 4 part-time/adjunct (3 women). *Students:* 290 full-time (165 women); includes 56 minority (18 Black or African American, non-Hispanic/Latino; 31 Asian, non-Hispanic/Latino; 4 Hispanic/Latino; 3 Two or more races, non-Hispanic/Latino), 2 international. Average age 25. *Degree requirements:* For doctorate, comprehensive exam. *Entrance requirements:* For doctorate, PCAT. Additional exam requirements/recommendations for international students: Required—TOEFL. *Application deadline:* For fall admission, 8/31 priority date for domestic students; for spring admission, 3/1 for domestic students. Applications are processed on a rolling basis. Application fee: $50. Electronic applications accepted. *Financial support:* Applicants required to submit FAFSA. *Faculty research:* Academic innovation, cultural competency, medication errors, patient safety. *Unit head:* Dr. Phil Johnston, Dean, 615-460-6746, Fax: 615-460-6741, E-mail: phil.johnston@belmont.edu. *Application contact:* Dr. Elinor Gray, Dean of Enrollment Services, 615-460-6747, Fax: 615-460-6741, E-mail: elinor.gray@belmont.edu. Website: http://www.belmont.edu/pharmacy

Butler University, College of Pharmacy and Health Sciences, Indianapolis, IN 46208-3485. Offers pharmaceutical science (MS); pharmacy (Pharm D); physician assistant studies (MS). *Accreditation:* ACPE (one or more programs are accredited). *Faculty:* 63 full-time (44 women). *Students:* 310 full-time (219 women), 5 part-time (3 women); includes 25 minority (1 Black or African American, non-Hispanic/Latino; 1 American Indian or Alaska Native, non-Hispanic/Latino; 14 Asian, non-Hispanic/Latino; 6 Hispanic/Latino; 3 Two or more races, non-Hispanic/Latino), 8 international. Average age 24. 42 applicants, 2% accepted. In 2015, 59 master's, 132 doctorates awarded. *Degree requirements:* For master's, thesis (for some programs), research paper or thesis; for doctorate, research paper or thesis. *Entrance requirements:* For master's, GRE General Test, CASPA application, official transcripts, baccalaureate degree from accredited institution (for physician assistant studies). Additional exam requirements/recommendations for international students: Required—TOEFL (minimum score 550 paper-based; 79 iBT). *Application deadline:* For fall admission, 5/1 for domestic and international students. Electronic applications accepted. Application fee is waived when completed online. *Expenses:* Contact institution. *Financial support:* Applicants required to submit FAFSA. *Faculty research:* Cancer research; molecular pharmacology; pharmaceutics; drug delivery and targeting; neuropharmacology. *Total annual research expenditures:* $50,000. *Unit head:* Dr. Mary Graham, Dean, 317-940-8056, E-mail: mandritz@butler.edu. *Application contact:* Diane Dubord, Graduate Student Services Specialist, 317-940-8107, E-mail: ddubord@butler.edu. Website: http://www.butler.edu/academics/graduate-cophs/

Campbell University, Graduate and Professional Programs, College of Pharmacy and Health Sciences, Buies Creek, NC 27506. Offers clinical research (MS); pharmaceutical sciences (MS); pharmacy (Pharm D); physician assistant (MPAP); public health (MS). *Accreditation:* ACPE. *Program availability:* Part-time, evening/weekend. *Entrance requirements:* For master's, MCAT, PCAT, GRE, bachelor's degree in health sciences or related field; for doctorate, PCAT. Additional exam requirements/recommendations for international students: Required—TOEFL (minimum score 550 paper-based; 79 iBT). Electronic applications accepted. *Expenses:* Contact institution. *Faculty research:* Immunology, medicinal chemistry, pharmaceutics, applied pharmacology.

Cedarville University, Graduate Programs, Cedarville, OH 45314-0601. Offers business administration (MBA); curriculum (M Ed); educational administration (M Ed); family nurse practitioner (MSN); global health ministries (MSN); instruction (M Ed); ministry (M Min); pharmacy (Pharm D). *Program availability:* Part-time, evening/

weekend, online learning. *Faculty:* 61 full-time (26 women), 7 part-time/adjunct (2 women). *Students:* 201 full-time (116 women), 100 part-time (71 women); includes 53 minority (32 Black or African American, non-Hispanic/Latino; 3 American Indian or Alaska Native, non-Hispanic/Latino; 15 Asian, non-Hispanic/Latino; 2 Hispanic/Latino; 1 Native Hawaiian or other Pacific Islander, non-Hispanic/Latino), 5 international. Average age 30. 142 applicants, 58% accepted, 57 enrolled. In 2015, 41 degrees awarded. *Degree requirements:* For master's, thesis. *Entrance requirements:* For master's, GRE, 2 professional recommendations; for doctorate, PCAT, professional recommendation from a practicing pharmacist or current employer/supervisor, resume, essay, interview. Additional exam requirements/recommendations for international students: Required—TOEFL (minimum score 550 paper-based; 80 iBT). *Application deadline:* For fall admission, 5/1 priority date for domestic and international students; for spring admission, 11/1 priority date for domestic and international students. Applications are processed on a rolling basis. Application fee: $0. Electronic applications accepted. *Expenses:* Contact institution. *Financial support:* In 2015–16, 129 students received support. Scholarships/grants and unspecified assistantships available. Support available to part-time students. Financial award applicants required to submit FAFSA. *Unit head:* Dr. Mark McClain, Dean of Graduate Studies, 937-766-7700, E-mail: mcclain@cedarville.edu. *Application contact:* Roscoe Smith, Associate Vice President for University Admissions, 937-766-7700, Fax: 937-766-7575, E-mail: smithr@cedarville.edu. Website: http://www.cedarville.edu/academics/graduate/

Chapman University, School of Pharmacy, Orange, CA 92866. Offers pharmaceutical sciences (MS); pharmacy (Pharm D). *Faculty:* 20 full-time (8 women), 1 part-time/adjunct (0 women). *Students:* 94 full-time (57 women), 1 (woman) part-time; includes 53 minority (5 Black or African American, non-Hispanic/Latino; 39 Asian, non-Hispanic/Latino; 7 Hispanic/Latino; 2 Two or more races, non-Hispanic/Latino), 8 international. Average age 28. *Degree requirements:* For master's, thesis; for doctorate, capstone project. *Entrance requirements:* For doctorate, PCAT. Additional exam requirements/recommendations for international students: Required—TOEFL (minimum score 550 paper-based; 80 iBT), IELTS (minimum score 6.5), PTE (minimum score 53). *Application deadline:* For fall admission, 3/1 for domestic students. Applications are processed on a rolling basis. Electronic applications accepted. *Expenses:* Contact institution. *Financial support:* Fellowships, research assistantships, Federal Work-Study, and scholarships/grants available. *Unit head:* Ronald P. Jordan, Dean, 714-516-5486, E-mail: rpjordan@chapman.edu. *Application contact:* Dr. Lawrence Brown, Associate Dean of Student and Academic Affairs, 714-516-5600, E-mail: pharmacyadmissions@chapman.edu. Website: http://www.chapman.edu/pharmacy/

Chicago State University, College of Pharmacy, Chicago, IL 60628. Offers Pharm D. *Accreditation:* ACPE. *Entrance requirements:* For doctorate, PCAT, minimum cumulative GPA of 2.5.

Creighton University, School of Pharmacy and Health Professions, Professional Program in Pharmacy, Omaha, NE 68178-0001. Offers Pharm D. *Accreditation:* ACPE. *Program availability:* Online learning. *Entrance requirements:* For doctorate, PCAT. Additional exam requirements/recommendations for international students: Required—TOEFL. Electronic applications accepted. *Expenses: Tuition, area resident:* Full-time $14,400; part-time $800 per credit hour. *Required fees:* $158 per semester. Tuition and fees vary according to course load, campus/location, program, reciprocity agreements and student's religious affiliation. *Faculty research:* Patient safety in health services research, health information technology and health services research, nanotechnology and drug development, pharmacy practice outcomes research, cross-cultural care of patients in pharmacy practice.

Drake University, College of Pharmacy and Health Sciences, Des Moines, IA 50311-4516. Offers pharmacy (Pharm D); Pharm D/JD; Pharm D/MBA; Pharm D/MPA. *Accreditation:* ACPE. *Faculty:* 36 full-time (18 women). *Students:* 432 full-time (285 women), 4 part-time (1 woman); includes 62 minority (4 Black or African American, non-Hispanic/Latino; 1 American Indian or Alaska Native, non-Hispanic/Latino; 46 Asian, non-Hispanic/Latino; 5 Hispanic/Latino; 6 Two or more races, non-Hispanic/Latino), 1 international. Average age 22. 54 applicants, 31% accepted, 17 enrolled. In 2015, 122 doctorates awarded. *Degree requirements:* For doctorate, rotations. *Entrance requirements:* For doctorate, PCAT, interview. Additional exam requirements/recommendations for international students: Required—TOEFL. *Application deadline:* For fall admission, 2/1 priority date for domestic students. Application fee: $135. Electronic applications accepted. *Expenses:* Contact institution. *Financial support:* In 2015–16, 10 teaching assistantships (averaging $3,200 per year) were awarded; career-related internships or fieldwork, Federal Work-Study, institutionally sponsored loans, and scholarships/grants also available. Support available to part-time students. Financial award application deadline: 3/1; financial award applicants required to submit FAFSA. *Faculty research:* Cost-benefit and cost-analysis of pharmaceutical products and services, patient satisfaction, community health planning and development, nutrition, ambulatory care. *Total annual research expenditures:* $163,164. *Unit head:* Dr. Renae Chesnut, Dean, 515-271-3018, Fax: 515-271-4171, E-mail: renae.chesnut@drake.edu. Website: http://pharmacy.drake.edu/

Duquesne University, Mylan School of Pharmacy, Professional Program in Pharmacy, Pittsburgh, PA 15282. Offers Pharm D. Students enter program as first-year

undergraduates. *Accreditation:* ACPE. *Program availability:* Evening/weekend. *Faculty:* 48 full-time (22 women), 4 part-time/adjunct (0 women). *Students:* 707 full-time (440 women), 40 part-time (22 women); includes 64 minority (17 Black or African American, non-Hispanic/Latino; 30 Asian, non-Hispanic/Latino; 9 Hispanic/Latino; 8 Two or more races, non-Hispanic/Latino), 9 international. Average age 23. 308 applicants, 60% accepted, 171 enrolled. In 2015, 169 doctorates awarded. *Entrance requirements:* For doctorate, PCAT (for professional phase). Additional exam requirements/recommendations for international students: Required—TOEFL. *Application deadline:* For fall admission, 12/1 priority date for domestic and international students. Applications are processed on a rolling basis. Application fee: $100. Electronic applications accepted. *Expenses:* $1,336 per credit tuition, $1,402 (for Weekend Path). *Financial support:* In 2015–16, 870 students received support. Federal Work-Study and scholarships/grants available. Financial award application deadline: 5/1; financial award applicants required to submit FAFSA. *Unit head:* Dr. Janet K. Astle, Assistant Dean for Professional Programs, 412-396-6393, E-mail: astle@duq.edu.
Website: http://www.duq.edu/academics/schools/pharmacy/become-a-student/doctor-of-pharmacy

D'Youville College, School of Pharmacy, Buffalo, NY 14201-1084. Offers Pharm D. *Accreditation:* ACPE. *Faculty:* 29 full-time (13 women), 2 part-time/adjunct (1 woman). *Students:* 281 full-time (143 women), 4 part-time (3 women); includes 45 minority (6 Black or African American, non-Hispanic/Latino; 1 American Indian or Alaska Native, non-Hispanic/Latino; 26 Asian, non-Hispanic/Latino; 4 Hispanic/Latino; 8 Two or more races, non-Hispanic/Latino), 29 international. Average age 23. 523 applicants, 23% accepted, 76 enrolled. In 2015, 60 doctorates awarded. *Entrance requirements:* For doctorate, PCAT, PharmCAS application, official transcripts from all colleges previously attended, three letters of recommendation. *Application deadline:* For fall admission, 3/1 for domestic and international students. Applications are processed on a rolling basis. Electronic applications accepted. *Expenses:* Contact institution. *Financial support:* In 2015–16, 62 students received support. Application deadline: 4/15; applicants required to submit FAFSA. *Faculty research:* Investigating anticancer properties of aspirin and other compounds; design, development, implementation and analysis of inter-professional educational programs, medication adherence and polypharmacy; geriatrics, medication reconciliation; buccal/transmucosal drug delivery, application of herbal medicine in cancer; acute care of internal medicine. *Unit head:* Dr. Canio Marasco, Assistant Dean of Faculty and Student Affairs, 716-829-7846, Fax: 716-829-7760, E-mail: pharmacyadmissions@dyc.edu. *Application contact:* Kathryn Stricker, School of Pharmacy Admission Counselor, 716-829-8324, Fax: 716-829-7904, E-mail: pharmacyadmissions@dyc.edu.
Website: http://www.dyc.edu/academics/pharmacy/

East Tennessee State University, Bill Gatton College of Pharmacy, Johnson City, TN 37614. Offers Pharm D. *Accreditation:* ACPE. *Program availability:* Part-time. *Students:* 323 full-time (164 women); includes 26 minority (9 Black or African American, non-Hispanic/Latino; 10 Asian, non-Hispanic/Latino; 4 Hispanic/Latino; 3 Two or more races, non-Hispanic/Latino). Average age 25. 630 applicants, 27% accepted, 78 enrolled. In 2015, 76 doctorates awarded. *Unit head:* Dr. Larry D. Calhoun, Dean, 423-439-2068, Fax: 423-439-6310, E-mail: calhoun@etsu.edu. *Application contact:* Admissions and Records Office, 423-439-6300, Fax: 423-439-6320, E-mail: pharmacy@etsu.edu.
Website: http://www.etsu.edu/pharmacy/

Ferris State University, College of Pharmacy, Big Rapids, MI 49307. Offers Pharm D. *Accreditation:* ACPE. *Faculty:* 35 full-time (24 women), 4 part-time/adjunct (2 women). *Students:* 580 full-time (321 women), 18 part-time (9 women); includes 40 minority (6 Black or African American, non-Hispanic/Latino; 2 American Indian or Alaska Native, non-Hispanic/Latino; 9 Asian, non-Hispanic/Latino; 17 Hispanic/Latino; 6 Two or more races, non-Hispanic/Latino), 20 international. Average age 24. 468 applicants, 39% accepted, 152 enrolled. In 2015, 126 doctorates awarded. *Degree requirements:* For doctorate, 6 clerkships during 4th professional year which equals 1,740 hours of clerkship. *Entrance requirements:* For doctorate, PCAT, 3 years or more of pre-pharmacy course work. *Application deadline:* For fall admission, 2/2 for domestic and international students. Application fee: $150. *Expenses:* Contact institution. *Financial support:* Career-related internships or fieldwork, Federal Work-Study, institutionally sponsored loans, and scholarships/grants available. Financial award applicants required to submit FAFSA. *Faculty research:* Diabetes, rural health education, managed care practice, antimicrobial pharmacotherapy, medicinal flora. *Unit head:* Dr. Stephen Durst, Dean, 231-591-2254, Fax: 231-591-3829, E-mail: dursts@ferris.edu. *Application contact:* Tara M. Lee, Administrative Specialist, Admissions, 231-591-3780, Fax: 231-591-3829, E-mail: leet@ferris.edu.
Website: http://www.ferris.edu/colleges/pharmacy/

Florida Agricultural and Mechanical University, Division of Graduate Studies, Research, and Continuing Education, College of Pharmacy and Pharmaceutical Sciences, Professional Program in Pharmacy and Pharmaceutical Sciences, Tallahassee, FL 32307-3200. Offers Pharm D. *Accreditation:* ACPE. *Entrance requirements:* Additional exam requirements/recommendations for international students: Required—TOEFL.

Georgia Campus–Philadelphia College of Osteopathic Medicine, School of Pharmacy, Suwanee, GA 30024. Offers Pharm D. *Faculty:* 29 full-time (12 women), 174 part-time/adjunct (99 women). *Students:* 405 full-time (216 women); includes 270 minority (85 Black or African American, non-Hispanic/Latino; 17 Asian, non-Hispanic/Latino; 1 Hispanic/Latino; 167 Two or more races, non-Hispanic/Latino), 17 international. Average age 27. 931 applicants, 23% accepted, 103 enrolled. In 2015, 78 doctorates awarded. *Degree requirements:* For doctorate, capstone. *Entrance requirements:* For doctorate, PCAT. Additional exam requirements/recommendations for international students: Required—TOEFL (minimum score 79 iBT). *Application deadline:* For fall admission, 3/1 for domestic students. Applications are processed on a rolling basis. Electronic applications accepted. *Expenses:* Contact institution. *Financial support:* Federal Work-Study, institutionally sponsored loans, and scholarships/grants available. Financial award application deadline: 3/15; financial award applicants required to submit FAFSA. *Total annual research expenditures:* $533,489. *Unit head:* Dr. Mark Okamoto, Dean, 678-407-7330, Fax: 678-407-7339. *Application contact:* Marsha Williams, Associate Director of Admissions, 215-871-6700, E-mail: marshawi@pcom.edu.
Website: http://www.pcom.edu/academics/programs-and-degrees//doctor-of-pharmacy/pharmd_curriculum.html

See Display on this page and Close-Up on page 931.

Hampton University, School of Pharmacy, Hampton, VA 23668. Offers Pharm D. *Accreditation:* ACPE. *Entrance requirements:* For doctorate, PCAT. *Expenses:* Tuition, area resident: Full-time $10,263; part-time $522 per credit hour. *Required fees:* $35. Tuition and fees vary according to course load and program. *Faculty research:* Signal transduction pathways in pulmonary fibrosis, molecular mechanisms in cancer cell biology, design and synthesis of new receptor ligands, design and synthesis of novel biomaterials for drug delivery, cytotoxic effects of organophosphates, drugs of abuse-behavioral and molecular pharmacology.

Pharmacy

Harding University, College of Pharmacy, Searcy, AR 72147-2230. Offers Pharm D. *Accreditation:* ACPE. *Faculty:* 34 full-time (18 women), 1 part-time/adjunct (0 women). *Students:* 221 full-time (134 women), 3 part-time (2 women); includes 65 minority (22 Black or African American, non-Hispanic/Latino; 4 American Indian or Alaska Native, non-Hispanic/Latino; 35 Asian, non-Hispanic/Latino; 4 Hispanic/Latino), 8 international. Average age 27. 208 applicants, 37% accepted, 48 enrolled. In 2015, 43 doctorates awarded. *Degree requirements:* For doctorate, licensure as a pharmacy intern in AR, completion of 300 hours of introductory pharmacy practice experience and 1,440 hours of advanced pharmacy practice experience. *Entrance requirements:* For doctorate, PCAT, 90 semester hours of undergraduate work. Additional exam requirements/ recommendations for international students: Required—TOEFL (minimum score 550 paper-based). *Application deadline:* For fall admission, 3/1 priority date for domestic and international students. Applications are processed on a rolling basis. Application fee: $50. Electronic applications accepted. *Expenses:* Contact institution. *Financial support:* In 2015–16, 35 students received support. Scholarships/grants available. Financial award applicants required to submit FAFSA. *Faculty research:* Field stable molecular diagnostics reagent development; the impact of UGT2B17 genetic polymorphisms on the disposition and action exemestane in healthy volunteers; optimization of 5-FU cancer chemotherapy, evaluation of issues associated with pediatric dosing; exploration of the physiologic impact of salmonella toxins; clinical study evaluating a novel point of care device as compared to the current industry standard for measurement of prothrombin time. *Total annual research expenditures:* $53,000. *Unit head:* Dr. Julie Ann Hixson-Wallace, Vice Provost, 501-279-5205, Fax: 501-279-5525, E-mail: jahixson@ harding.edu. *Application contact:* Carol Jones, Director of Admissions, 501-279-5523, Fax: 501-279-5525, E-mail: ccjones@harding.edu.
Website: http://www.harding.edu/pharmacy/

Howard University, College of Pharmacy, Washington, DC 20059-0002. Offers Pharm D, Pharm D/MBA. *Accreditation:* ACPE. *Program availability:* Online learning. *Degree requirements:* For doctorate, comprehensive exam. *Entrance requirements:* For doctorate, PCAT, minimum GPA of 2.5. Electronic applications accepted. *Expenses:* Contact institution. *Faculty research:* Kinetics of drug absorption, stealth liposomes, synthesis, opiate analgesics.

Husson University, School of Pharmacy, Bangor, ME 04401-2999. Offers Pharm D. *Accreditation:* ACPE. *Faculty:* 30 full-time (10 women), 1 part-time/adjunct (0 women). *Students:* 213 full-time (117 women); includes 83 minority (36 Black or African American, non-Hispanic/Latino; 2 American Indian or Alaska Native, non-Hispanic/ Latino; 37 Asian, non-Hispanic/Latino; 5 Hispanic/Latino; 1 Native Hawaiian or other Pacific Islander, non-Hispanic/Latino; 2 Two or more races, non-Hispanic/Latino), 8 international. Average age 27. 268 applicants, 31% accepted, 44 enrolled. In 2015, 65 doctorates awarded. *Entrance requirements:* For doctorate, PCAT, PharmCAS application. Additional exam requirements/recommendations for international students: Required—TOEFL (minimum score 550 paper-based; 80 iBT). *Application deadline:* For fall admission, 3/1 for domestic students. Application fee: $50 ($0 for international students). *Expenses:* $34,758 per year. *Financial support:* Federal Work-Study, scholarships/grants, and unspecified assistantships available. Financial award application deadline: 3/1; financial award applicants required to submit FAFSA. *Faculty research:* Development of nanoparticles for noninvasive delivery of therapeutic agents; clinical implications in anti-infective resistance; using stochastic modeling to determine appropriate antibiotic selection, infectious diseases surveillance and epidemiology; impaired healing in individuals with diabetes; assessment of pharmaceutical needs in rural settings in the midst of the changing health care environment. *Total annual research expenditures:* $45,000. *Unit head:* Dr. Rodney A. Larson, Dean, 207-941-7122, E-mail: larsonr@husson.edu. *Application contact:* Kristen Card, Director of Graduate Admissions, 207-404-5660, E-mail: cardk@husson.edu.
Website: http://www.husson.edu/pharmacy

Idaho State University, Office of Graduate Studies, College of Pharmacy, Department of Pharmacy Practice and Administrative Sciences, Pocatello, ID 83209-8333. Offers pharmacy (Pharm D); pharmacy administration (MS, PhD). *Accreditation:* ACPE (one or more programs are accredited). *Program availability:* Part-time. *Degree requirements:* For master's, one foreign language, comprehensive exam, thesis, thesis research, speech and technical writing classes; for doctorate, comprehensive exam, thesis/ dissertation, oral and written exams, speech and technical writing classes. *Entrance requirements:* For master's, GRE General Test, minimum GPA of 3.0, 3 letters of recommendation; for doctorate, GRE General Test, BS in pharmacy or related field, minimum GPA of 3.0, 3 letters of recommendation. Additional exam requirements/ recommendations for international students: Required—TOEFL (minimum score 550 paper-based; 80 iBT). Electronic applications accepted. *Expenses:* Contact institution. *Faculty research:* Pharmaceutical care outcomes, drug use review, pharmacoeconomics.

Keck Graduate Institute, KGI School of Pharmacy, Claremont, CA 91711. Offers Pharm D.

Lake Erie College of Osteopathic Medicine, Professional Programs, Erie, PA 16509-1025. Offers biomedical sciences (Postbaccalaureate Certificate); medical education (MS); osteopathic medicine (DO); pharmacy (Pharm D). *Accreditation:* ACPE; AOsA. *Degree requirements:* For doctorate, comprehensive exam, National Osteopathic Medical Licensing Exam, Levels 1 and 2; for Postbaccalaureate Certificate, comprehensive exam, North American Pharmacist Licensure Examination (NAPLEX). *Entrance requirements:* For doctorate, MCAT, minimum GPA of 3.2, letters of recommendation; for Postbaccalaureate Certificate, PCAT, letters of recommendation, minimum GPA of 3.5. Electronic applications accepted. *Faculty research:* Cardiac smooth and skeletal muscle mechanics, chemotherapeutics and vitamins, osteopathic manipulation.

Lebanese American University, School of Pharmacy, Beirut, Lebanon. Offers Pharm D. *Accreditation:* ACPE.

Lipscomb University, College of Pharmacy, Nashville, TN 37204-3951. Offers healthcare informatics (MS); Pharm D/MS. *Accreditation:* ACPE. *Faculty:* 32 full-time (16 women), 5 part-time/adjunct (1 woman). *Students:* 292 full-time (167 women), 5 part-time (3 women); includes 70 minority (22 Black or African American, non-Hispanic/ Latino; 4 American Indian or Alaska Native, non-Hispanic/Latino; 31 Asian, non-Hispanic/Latino; 7 Hispanic/Latino; 2 Native Hawaiian or other Pacific Islander, non-Hispanic/Latino; 4 Two or more races, non-Hispanic/Latino). Average age 27. In 2015, 3 master's, 78 doctorates awarded. *Degree requirements:* For master's, capstone project; for doctorate, comprehensive exam. *Entrance requirements:* For master's, GRE, 2 references, transcripts, resume, personal statement, eligibility documentation (degree and/or experience in related area); for doctorate, PCAT (minimum 45th percentile), 66 pre-professional semester hours, minimum GPA of 2.5, interview, PharmCAS application (for international students). Additional exam requirements/recommendations for international students: Required—TOEFL (minimum score 550 paper-based; 80 iBT). *Application deadline:* For fall admission, 2/7 for domestic students. Applications are processed on a rolling basis. Application fee: $50 ($75 for international students). Electronic applications accepted. *Expenses:* $37,938 per year (for Pharm D); $1,000 per credit hour (for MS in health care informatics). *Financial support:* Application deadline: 2/15; applicants required to submit FAFSA. *Unit head:* Dr. Roger Davis, Dean/Professor

of Pharmacy Practice, 615-966-7161. *Application contact:* Laura Ward, Director of Admissions and Student Affairs, 615-966-7173, E-mail: laura.ward@lipscomb.edu.
Website: http://lipscomb.edu/pharmacy

Loma Linda University, School of Pharmacy, Loma Linda, CA 92350. Offers Pharm D. *Accreditation:* ACPE. *Degree requirements:* For doctorate, intern pharmacist license. Application fee: $75. *Unit head:* Dr. Marilyn M. Herrmann, Interim Dean, 909-558-4745, Fax: 909-558-7973. *Application contact:* Admissions Office, 909-651-5029, Fax: 909-558-4879, E-mail: admissions.app@llu.edu.
Website: http://pharmacy.llu.edu

Long Island University–LIU Brooklyn, Arnold and Marie Schwartz College of Pharmacy and Health Sciences, Brooklyn, NY 11201-8423. Offers drug regulatory affairs (MS); pharmaceutics (MS, PhD), including cosmetic science (MS), industrial pharmacy (MS); pharmacology and toxicology (MS); pharmacy (Pharm D). *Accreditation:* ACPE. *Program availability:* Part-time. *Faculty:* 49 full-time (25 women), 20 part-time/adjunct (9 women). *Students:* 579 full-time (346 women), 29 part-time (14 women); includes 191 minority (24 Black or African American, non-Hispanic/Latino; 1 American Indian or Alaska Native, non-Hispanic/Latino; 144 Asian, non-Hispanic/Latino; 19 Hispanic/Latino; 3 Two or more races, non-Hispanic/Latino), 193 international. Average age 27. 350 applicants, 63% accepted, 65 enrolled. In 2015, 114 master's, 206 doctorates awarded. *Degree requirements:* For master's, comprehensive exam (for some programs), thesis optional; for doctorate, comprehensive exam, thesis/ dissertation. *Entrance requirements:* For master's and doctorate, GRE, minimum GPA of 3.0. Additional exam requirements/recommendations for international students: Required—TOEFL (minimum score 550 paper-based; 79 iBT), IELTS (minimum score 6.5). *Application deadline:* Applications are processed on a rolling basis. Application fee: $50. Electronic applications accepted. *Expenses:* Contact institution. *Financial support:* In 2015–16, 185 students received support, including 6 fellowships with full tuition reimbursements available (averaging $12,800 per year), 28 teaching assistantships with full tuition reimbursements available (averaging $6,000 per year); Federal Work-Study, institutionally sponsored loans, and scholarships/grants also available. Support available to part-time students. Financial award application deadline: 2/15; financial award applicants required to submit FAFSA. *Faculty research:* Pharmaceutics, pharmacodynamics, pharmacology, pharmacometrics, pharmacotherapeutics. *Unit head:* Dr. John M. Pezzuto, Dean, 718-488-1004, Fax: 718-488-0628, E-mail: john.pezzuto@liu.edu. *Application contact:* Dr. Anait Levinson, Associate Dean of Research and Graduate Studies, 718-246-6323, E-mail: anait.levenson@liu.edu.
Website: http://liu.edu/Pharmacy

Manchester University, Doctor of Pharmacy Program, Fort Wayne, IN 46845. Offers Pharm D. *Faculty:* 34 full-time (19 women). *Students:* 271 full-time (166 women), 6 part-time (4 women); includes 120 minority (41 Black or African American, non-Hispanic/ Latino; 2 American Indian or Alaska Native, non-Hispanic/Latino; 71 Asian, non-Hispanic/Latino; 6 Hispanic/Latino). Average age 25. 667 applicants, 21% accepted, 72 enrolled. *Degree requirements:* For doctorate, service learning, portfolio, competency assessments. *Entrance requirements:* For doctorate, minimum GPA of 2.5 (cumulative and prerequisites), minimum C grade on all prerequisite courses, U.S. citizenship or permanent residency, PharmCAS and supplemental application, 3 letters of recommendation. *Application deadline:* For fall admission, 3/1 for domestic students. Application fee: $180. *Expenses:* $38,800. *Unit head:* Dr. Joseph K. Bonnarens, Associate Dean for Student Affairs, 260-470-2655, E-mail: jkbonnarens@ manchester.edu.
Website: http://pharmacy.manchester.edu/

Marshall University, Academic Affairs Division, School of Pharmacy, Huntington, WV 25755. Offers Pharm D. *Faculty:* 10 full-time (5 women). *Students:* 303 part-time (159 women); includes 60 minority (19 Black or African American, non-Hispanic/Latino; 1 American Indian or Alaska Native, non-Hispanic/Latino; 28 Asian, non-Hispanic/Latino; 5 Hispanic/Latino; 7 Two or more races, non-Hispanic/Latino), 3 international. Average age 26. *Unit head:* Dr. Kevin W. Yingling, Founding Dean, 304-696-7302, E-mail: pharmacy@marshall.edu. *Application contact:* Dr. Tammy Johnson, Graduate Admissions, 304-746-1900, Fax: 304-746-1902, E-mail: services@marshall.edu.
Website: http://www.marshall.edu/wpmu/pharmacy/

MCPHS University, Graduate Studies, Doctoral Programs in Pharmacy–Boston, Doctor of Pharmacy Program - Boston, Boston, MA 02115-5896. Offers Pharm D. Students enter program as undergraduates. *Program availability:* Online learning. *Entrance requirements:* For doctorate, SAT (if fewer than 30 semester hours completed), minimum GPA of 2.5, interview. Additional exam requirements/recommendations for international students: Required—TOEFL (minimum score 550 paper-based; 79 iBT). Electronic applications accepted.

MCPHS University, Graduate Studies, Doctoral Programs in Pharmacy–Boston, Postbaccalaureate Doctor of Pharmacy Pathway Program, Boston, MA 02115-5896. Offers Pharm D. *Program availability:* Part-time, online learning. *Entrance requirements:* For doctorate, registered pharmacist status in the U.S.; working at or have access to a site that provides opportunities to practice pharmaceutical care; curriculum vitae; letter of recommendation. Additional exam requirements/recommendations for international students: Required—TOEFL (minimum score 550 paper-based; 79 iBT). Electronic applications accepted.

MCPHS University, School of Pharmacy–Worcester/Manchester, Boston, MA 02115-5896. Offers Pharm D. *Entrance requirements:* Additional exam requirements/ recommendations for international students: Required—TOEFL (minimum score 550 paper-based; 79 iBT).

Medical University of South Carolina, South Carolina College of Pharmacy, Charleston, SC 29425. Offers Pharm D. *Accreditation:* ACPE. *Entrance requirements:* For doctorate, PCAT, 2 years of pre-professional course work, interview, minimum GPA of 2.5. Additional exam requirements/recommendations for international students: Required—TOEFL (minimum score 550 paper-based). Electronic applications accepted. *Expenses:* Contact institution. *Faculty research:* Rational and computer aided drug design; drug metabolism and transport; molecular immunology and cellular toxicology; cell injury, death and regeneration; outcome sciences.

Mercer University, Graduate Studies, Cecil B. Day Campus, College of Pharmacy, Atlanta, GA 30341. Offers pharmaceutical sciences (PhD); pharmacology (PhD); pharmacy (Pharm D); Pharm D/MBA; Pharm D/PhD. *Accreditation:* ACPE (one or more programs are accredited). *Faculty:* 24 full-time (14 women). *Students:* 667 full-time (418 women), 3 part-time (1 woman); includes 355 minority (133 Black or African American, non-Hispanic/Latino; 2 American Indian or Alaska Native, non-Hispanic/Latino; 170 Asian, non-Hispanic/Latino; 22 Hispanic/Latino; 28 Two or more races, non-Hispanic/ Latino), 42 international. Average age 26. 1,895 applicants, 18% accepted, 176 enrolled. In 2015, 151 doctorates awarded. *Degree requirements:* For doctorate, comprehensive exam (for some programs), thesis/dissertation (for some programs). *Entrance requirements:* For doctorate, GRE; PCAT (for Pharm D), Pharm D or BS in pharmacy or science, minimum GPA of 3.0. Additional exam requirements/recommendations for international students: Required—TOEFL. *Application deadline:* Applications are processed on a rolling basis. Electronic applications accepted. *Expenses:* Contact institution. *Financial support:* In 2015–16, 350 students received support. Teaching

assistantships with tuition reimbursements available, career-related internships or fieldwork, Federal Work-Study, institutionally sponsored loans, scholarships/grants, tuition waivers, and unspecified assistantships available. Support available to part-time students. Financial award application deadline: 5/1; financial award applicants required to submit FAFSA. *Faculty research:* Stability and compatibility of steroids, synthesis of antihypertensive, disposition of cyclosporine, synthesis of enzyme inhibitors. *Unit head:* Dr. Hewitt W. Matthews, Dean, 678-547-6306, Fax: 678-547-6315, E-mail: matthews_h@mercer.edu. *Application contact:* Dr. James W. Bartling, Associate Dean for Student Affairs and Admissions, 678-547-6181, Fax: 678-547-6518, E-mail: bartling_jw@mercer.edu.
Website: http://pharmacy.mercer.edu/

Midwestern University, Downers Grove Campus, Chicago College of Pharmacy, Downers Grove, IL 60515-1235. Offers Pharm D. *Accreditation:* ACPE. *Program availability:* Part-time, online learning. *Entrance requirements:* For doctorate, PCAT. *Expenses:* Contact institution.

Midwestern University, Glendale Campus, College of Pharmacy-Glendale, Glendale, AZ 85308. Offers Pharm D. *Accreditation:* ACPE. *Entrance requirements:* For doctorate, PCAT. *Expenses:* Contact institution.

North Dakota State University, College of Graduate and Interdisciplinary Studies, College of Health Professions, School of Pharmacy, Fargo, ND 58102. Offers MS, PhD, Pharm D, Pharm D/MBA, Pharm D/MPH, Pharm D/PhD. *Accreditation:* ACPE. *Program availability:* Part-time. Terminal master's awarded for partial completion of doctoral program. *Degree requirements:* For master's, thesis; for doctorate, thesis/dissertation. *Entrance requirements:* For master's and doctorate, GRE General Test. Additional exam requirements/recommendations for international students: Required—TOEFL. *Application deadline:* For fall admission, 3/15 priority date for domestic students; for spring admission, 11/15 priority date for domestic students. Applications are processed on a rolling basis. Application fee: $35. Electronic applications accepted. *Financial support:* Research assistantships with full tuition reimbursements and institutionally sponsored loans available. Financial award application deadline: 4/15. *Faculty research:* Subcellular pharmacokinetics, cancer, cardiovascular drug design, iontophonesis, neuropharmacology. *Unit head:* Dr. Jagdish Singh, Chair, Department of Pharmaceutical Sciences, 701-231-7943, E-mail: jagdish.singh@ndsu.edu. *Application contact:* Dr. Jagdish Singh, Chair, Department of Pharmaceutical Sciences, 701-231-7943, E-mail: jagdish.singh@ndsu.edu.
Website: http://www.ndsu.edu/pharmacy/

Northeastern University, Bouvé College of Health Sciences, Boston, MA 02115-5096. Offers applied behavior analysis (MS, CAGS); audiology (Au D); biomedical nanotechnology (MS); college student development and counseling (MS, CAGS); counseling psychology (MS, PhD, CAGS); exercise science (MS); health informatics (MS); medicinal chemistry (MS); nurse anesthesia (DNP, CAGS); nursing (MS, PhD, CAGS), including administration (MS); adult-gerontology acute care nurse practitioner (MS, CAGS), adult-gerontology primary care nurse practitioner (MS, CAGS), anesthesia (MS), family nurse practitioner (MS, CAGS), neonatal nurse practitioner (MS, CAGS), pediatric nurse practitioner (MS, CAGS), psychiatric mental health nurse practitioner (MS, CAGS); nursing practice (DNP); personal health informatics (PhD); pharmaceutical sciences (MS, PhD), including interdisciplinary concentration, pharmaceutics and drug delivery systems; pharmacology (MS); pharmacy (Pharm D); physical therapy (Postbaccalaureate Certificate); physician assistant (MS); population health (PhD); school psychology (MS, PhD, CAGS); speech-language pathology (MS); urban health (MPH); MS/MBA. *Accreditation:* ACPE (one or more programs are accredited). *Program availability:* Part-time, evening/weekend, online learning. *Faculty:* 194 full-time (120 women), 169 part-time/adjunct (136 women). *Students:* 1,416 full-time (1,049 women),

310 part-time (248 women). In 2015, 374 master's, 313 doctorates, 37 other advanced degrees awarded. *Degree requirements:* For doctorate, thesis/dissertation (for some programs); for other advanced degree, comprehensive exam. Application fee: $75. Electronic applications accepted. *Expenses:* Contact institution. *Financial support:* Applicants required to submit FAFSA. *Unit head:* John R. Reynolds, Professor and Interim Dean, 617-373-3323, Fax: 617-373-3030. *Application contact:* Molly Schnabel, Senior Director of Graduate Affairs, 617-373-2708, Fax: 617-373-4701, E-mail: bouvegrad@neu.edu.
Website: http://www.northeastern.edu/bouve/

Northeast Ohio Medical University, College of Pharmacy, Rootstown, OH 44272-0095. Offers Pharm D. *Accreditation:* ACPE. *Faculty:* 51 full-time (20 women), 463 part-time/adjunct (258 women). *Students:* 299 full-time (173 women); includes 51 minority (14 Black or African American, non-Hispanic/Latino; 28 Asian, non-Hispanic/Latino; 5 Hispanic/Latino; 4 Two or more races, non-Hispanic/Latino). Average age 26. 315 applicants, 46% accepted, 75 enrolled. In 2015, 61 doctorates awarded. *Entrance requirements:* For doctorate, PCAT. *Application deadline:* For fall admission, 9/1 priority date for domestic students; for winter admission, 1/5 for domestic students. Applications are processed on a rolling basis. Application fee: $50. Electronic applications accepted. *Expenses:* Contact institution. *Financial support:* In 2015–16, 300 students received support. Scholarships/grants available. Financial award application deadline: 4/15; financial award applicants required to submit FAFSA. *Total annual research expenditures:* $869,327. *Unit head:* Dr. Charles Taylor, Dean, 330-325-6461, Fax: 330-325-5930. *Application contact:* Heidi Terry, Executive Director, Enrollment Services, 330-325-6479, E-mail: hterry@neoucom.edu.
Website: http://www.neomed.edu/academics/pharmacy

Nova Southeastern University, College of Pharmacy, Fort Lauderdale, FL 33328. Offers drug development (pharmaceutics) (PhD); molecular medicine and pharmacogenomics (PhD); pharmacy (Pharm D); social and administrative pharmacy (PhD); Pharm D/MBA; Pharm D/MPH. *Accreditation:* ACPE. *Faculty:* 67 full-time (31 women), 3 part-time/adjunct (1 woman). *Students:* 971 full-time (655 women), 25 part-time (12 women); includes 705 minority (57 Black or African American, non-Hispanic/Latino; 177 Asian, non-Hispanic/Latino; 451 Hispanic/Latino; 1 Native Hawaiian or other Pacific Islander, non-Hispanic/Latino; 19 Two or more races, non-Hispanic/Latino), 96 international. Average age 27. 1,024 applicants, 41% accepted, 255 enrolled. In 2015, 226 doctorates awarded. *Degree requirements:* For doctorate, comprehensive exam (for some programs), thesis/dissertation (for some programs). *Entrance requirements:* For doctorate, PCAT (for Pharm D); GRE (for PhD). Additional exam requirements/recommendations for international students: Required—TOEFL (minimum score 550 paper-based, 80 iBT) or IELTS (minimum score 6.0). *Application deadline:* For fall admission, 3/15 for domestic students, 2/1 for international students. Applications are processed on a rolling basis. Application fee: $50. Electronic applications accepted. *Expenses:* Contact institution. *Financial support:* In 2015–16, 131 students received support, including 11 teaching assistantships with full tuition reimbursements available (averaging $18,000 per year); career-related internships or fieldwork, Federal Work-Study, institutionally sponsored loans, and scholarships/grants also available. Financial award application deadline: 4/15; financial award applicants required to submit FAFSA. *Faculty research:* Cancer, health care delivery, pharmacoeconomics, cardiovascular/metabolic diseases, autism. *Total annual research expenditures:* $446,267. *Unit head:* Dr. Lisa Deziel, Dean, 954-262-1304, Fax: 954-262-2278, E-mail: copdean@nova.edu. *Application contact:* Jeffrey Jurkas, Coordinator of Admissions and Recruitment, 954-262-1240, Fax: 954-262-2282, E-mail: nsupharmacyinfo@nova.edu.
Website: http://pharmacy.nova.edu/

See Display below and Close-Up on page 933.

Pharmacy

Ohio Northern University, Raabe College of Pharmacy, Ada, OH 45810-1599. Offers Pharm D. Students enter the program as undergraduates. *Accreditation:* ACPE. *Faculty:* 26 full-time (12 women), 3 part-time/adjunct (2 women). *Students:* 750 full-time (500 women), 1 (woman) part-time; includes 69 minority (14 Black or African American, non-Hispanic/Latino; 26 Asian, non-Hispanic/Latino; 8 Hispanic/Latino; 21 Two or more races, non-Hispanic/Latino), 26 international. Average age 22. 656 applicants, 45% accepted, 176 enrolled. In 2015, 164 doctorates awarded. *Degree requirements:* For doctorate, 9 clinical rotations, capstone course. *Entrance requirements:* For doctorate, ACT or SAT. Additional exam requirements/recommendations for international students: Required—TOEFL (minimum score 550 paper-based; 80 iBT). *Expenses:* Contact institution. *Financial support:* Federal Work-Study, institutionally sponsored loans, and scholarships/grants available. Financial award applicants required to submit FAFSA. *Faculty research:* Alcohol and substance abuse, women in pharmacy, non-traditional educations, continuing pharmaceutical education, medicinal chemistry. *Unit head:* Dr. Tom Kier, Interim Dean, 419-772-2282, Fax: 419-772-2282, E-mail: t-kier@onu.edu. *Application contact:* Dr. Kelly Shields, Assistant Dean of Student Services, 419-772-2752, Fax: 419-772-2752, E-mail: k-shields@onu.edu.
Website: http://www.onu.edu/pharmacy/

The Ohio State University, College of Pharmacy, Columbus, OH 43210. Offers MS, PhD, Pharm D, Pharm D/MBA, Pharm D/MPH, Pharm D/PhD. *Accreditation:* ACPE (one or more programs are accredited). *Faculty:* 50. *Students:* 574 full-time (315 women); includes 142 minority (26 Black or African American, non-Hispanic/Latino; 1 American Indian or Alaska Native, non-Hispanic/Latino; 93 Asian, non-Hispanic/Latino; 17 Hispanic/Latino; 1 Native Hawaiian or other Pacific Islander, non-Hispanic/Latino; 4 Two or more races, non-Hispanic/Latino), 53 international. Average age 25. In 2015, 17 master's, 132 doctorates awarded. Terminal master's awarded for partial completion of doctoral program. *Degree requirements:* For doctorate, comprehensive exam (for some programs), thesis/dissertation (for some programs). *Entrance requirements:* For master's, GRE General Test, minimum GPA of 3.0; for doctorate, GRE General Test, PCAT (for PharmD), minimum GPA of 3.0. Additional exam requirements/recommendations for international students: Required—TOEFL (minimum score 600 paper-based, 100 iBT) for MS and PhD; TOEFL (minimum score 577 paper-based; 90 iBT), Michigan English Language Assessment Battery (minimum score 84), IELTS (minimum score 7.5) for PharmD. *Application deadline:* For fall admission, 12/15 for domestic and international students. Application fee: $60 ($70 for international students). Electronic applications accepted. *Expenses:* Contact institution. *Financial support:* Fellowships with full tuition reimbursements, research assistantships with full tuition reimbursements, teaching assistantships with full tuition reimbursements, career-related internships or fieldwork, Federal Work-Study, institutionally sponsored loans, scholarships/grants, and traineeships available. *Unit head:* Dr. Henry J. Mann, Dean and Professor, 614-292-5711, Fax: 614-292-2588, E-mail: mann.414@osu.edu. *Application contact:* Dr. Henry J. Mann, Dean and Professor, 614-292-5711, Fax: 614-292-2588, E-mail: mann.414@osu.edu.
Website: http://www.pharmacy.osu.edu

Oregon State University, College of Pharmacy, Pharmacy Doctoral Program, Corvallis, OR 97331. Offers Pharm D. *Faculty:* 30 full-time (15 women). *Students:* 342 full-time (189 women), 14 part-time (11 women); includes 173 minority (6 Black or African American, non-Hispanic/Latino; 1 American Indian or Alaska Native, non-Hispanic/Latino; 130 Asian, non-Hispanic/Latino; 15 Hispanic/Latino; 1 Native Hawaiian or other Pacific Islander, non-Hispanic/Latino; 20 Two or more races, non-Hispanic/Latino), 8 international. Average age 27. In 2015, 83 doctorates awarded. *Application deadline:* For fall admission, 11/1 priority date for domestic students. Applications are processed on a rolling basis. *Expenses:* $21,384 full-time resident tuition; $36,828 full-time non-resident tuition; $1,572 fees. *Unit head:* Dr. Mark Zabriskie, Dean and Professor. *Application contact:* Angela Austin Haney, Director of Student Services/Head Advisor, 541-737-5784, E-mail: angela.austinhaney@oregonstate.edu.
Website: http://pharmacy.oregonstate.edu/

Pacific University, School of Pharmacy, Forest Grove, OR 97116-1797. Offers Pharm D. *Accreditation:* ACPE. *Entrance requirements:* Additional exam requirements/recommendations for international students: Required—TOEFL (minimum score 600 paper-based). Electronic applications accepted. *Expenses:* Contact institution. *Faculty research:* Informatics, enzyme metabolism, apostosis/cell cycle, neurophysiology of chronic pain, neurophysiology of Alzheimer's.

Palm Beach Atlantic University, Gregory School of Pharmacy, West Palm Beach, FL 33416-4708. Offers Pharm D. *Accreditation:* ACPE. *Faculty:* 25 full-time (17 women), 6 part-time/adjunct (3 women). *Students:* 293 full-time (168 women), 21 part-time (13 women); includes 178 minority (45 Black or African American, non-Hispanic/Latino; 2 American Indian or Alaska Native, non-Hispanic/Latino; 47 Asian, non-Hispanic/Latino; 69 Hispanic/Latino; 2 Native Hawaiian or other Pacific Islander, non-Hispanic/Latino; 13 Two or more races, non-Hispanic/Latino), 8 international. Average age 26. 552 applicants, 30% accepted, 76 enrolled. In 2015, 67 doctorates awarded. *Entrance requirements:* For doctorate, PCAT, minimum GPA of 2.75. Additional exam requirements/recommendations for international students: Required—TOEFL (minimum score 550 paper-based; 79 iBT). *Application deadline:* For fall admission, 3/1 priority date for domestic and international students. Applications are processed on a rolling basis. Application fee: $150. Electronic applications accepted. *Expenses:* Contact institution. *Financial support:* In 2015–16, 49 students received support. Scholarships/grants and employee education grants available. Financial award application deadline: 5/1; financial award applicants required to submit FAFSA. *Unit head:* Dr. Scott Mohrland, Interim Dean, 561-803-2701, E-mail: scott_mohrland@pba.edu. *Application contact:* Lucas Whittaker, Director of Pharmacy Admissions, 561-803-2751, E-mail: lucas_whittaker@pba.edu.
Website: http://www.pba.edu/school-of-pharmacy

Purdue University, College of Pharmacy and Pharmacal Sciences, Professional Program in Pharmacy and Pharmacal Sciences, West Lafayette, IN 47907. Offers Pharm D. *Accreditation:* ACPE. *Entrance requirements:* For doctorate, minimum 2 years of pre-pharmacy course work, interview. *Expenses:* Contact institution. *Faculty research:* Medicinal chemistry, pharmacology, pharmaceutics, clinical pharmacy, pharmacy administration.

Regis University, Rueckert-Hartman College for Health Professions, Denver, CO 80221-1099. Offers addictions counseling (Post-Graduate Certificate); advanced practice nurse specialization (DNP); counseling (MA); counseling children and adolescents (Post-Graduate Certificate); counseling military families (Post-Graduate Certificate); depth psychotherapy (Post-Graduate Certificate); family nurse practitioner (MSN); health care business management (Certificate); health care quality and patient safety (Certificate); health industry leadership (MBA); health professions (Postbaccalaureate Certificate); health services administration (MS); marriage and family therapy (MA); neonatal nurse practitioner (MSN); nursing education or leadership (MSN); orthopedic manual physical therapy fellowship (Certificate); pharmacy (Pharm D); physical therapy (DPT). *Program availability:* Part-time, evening/weekend, 100% online, blended/hybrid learning. *Faculty:* 40 full-time (29 women), 116 part-time/adjunct (86 women). *Students:* 1,080 full-time (771 women), 274 part-time (239 women); includes 388 minority (59 Black or African American, non-Hispanic/Latino; 6 American

Indian or Alaska Native, non-Hispanic/Latino; 109 Asian, non-Hispanic/Latino; 163 Hispanic/Latino; 1 Native Hawaiian or other Pacific Islander, non-Hispanic/Latino; 50 Two or more races, non-Hispanic/Latino), 7 international. Average age 34. 2,188 applicants, 31% accepted, 303 enrolled. In 2015, 329 master's, 160 doctorates awarded. *Degree requirements:* For master's, thesis (for some programs), internship. *Entrance requirements:* For master's, official transcript reflecting baccalaureate degree awarded from regionally-accredited college or university. Additional exam requirements/recommendations for international students: Required—TOEFL (minimum score 550 paper-based; 82 iBT). *Application deadline:* For fall admission, 8/15 priority date for domestic students; for spring admission, 1/10 priority date for domestic students; for summer admission, 5/1 priority date for domestic students. Applications are processed on a rolling basis. Application fee: $75. Electronic applications accepted. *Expenses:* Contact institution. *Financial support:* In 2015–16, 102 students received support. Federal Work-Study and scholarships/grants available. Financial award application deadline: 4/15; financial award applicants required to submit FAFSA. *Faculty research:* Normal and pathological balance and gait research, normal/pathological upper limb motor control/biomechanics, exercise energy/metabolism research, optical treatment protocols for therapeutic modalities. *Unit head:* Dr. Janet Houser, Academic Dean. *Application contact:* Cate Clark, Director of Admissions, 303-458-4900, Fax: 303-964-5534, E-mail: ruadmissions@regis.edu.
Website: http://www.regis.edu/RHCHP.aspx

Roosevelt University, Graduate Division, College of Pharmacy, Chicago, IL 60605. Offers Pharm D. *Accreditation:* ACPE.

Rosalind Franklin University of Medicine and Science, College of Pharmacy, North Chicago, IL 60064-3095. Offers Pharm D. *Accreditation:* ACPE.

Roseman University of Health Sciences, College of Pharmacy, Henderson, NV 89014. Offers Pharm D. *Accreditation:* ACPE. *Faculty:* 49 full-time (23 women), 12 part-time/adjunct (5 women). *Students:* 741 full-time (404 women); includes 407 minority (38 Black or African American, non-Hispanic/Latino; 2 American Indian or Alaska Native, non-Hispanic/Latino; 284 Asian, non-Hispanic/Latino; 37 Hispanic/Latino; 10 Native Hawaiian or other Pacific Islander, non-Hispanic/Latino; 36 Two or more races, non-Hispanic/Latino), 8 international. Average age 28. 658 applicants, 60% accepted, 252 enrolled. In 2015, 260 doctorates awarded. *Degree requirements:* For doctorate, comprehensive exam. *Entrance requirements:* For doctorate, PCAT. *Application deadline:* For fall admission, 2/1 for domestic and international students. Applications are processed on a rolling basis. Application fee: $60. *Expenses:* Contact institution. *Financial support:* In 2015–16, 34 students received support. Federal Work-Study and scholarships/grants available. Financial award application deadline: 5/1; financial award applicants required to submit FAFSA. *Unit head:* Dr. Scott Stolte, Dean, 702-968-5944, Fax: 702-990-4435, E-mail: sstolte@roseman.edu. *Application contact:* Dr. Helen Park, Director of Admissions and Student Affairs, 702-968-5248, Fax: 702-968-1644, E-mail: hpark@roseman.edu.
Website: http://www.roseman.edu

Rutgers University–New Brunswick, Ernest Mario School of Pharmacy, Piscataway, NJ 08854-8097. Offers medicinal chemistry (MS, PhD); pharmaceutical science (MS, PhD); pharmacy (Pharm D). *Accreditation:* ACPE. *Degree requirements:* For doctorate, variable foreign language requirement. *Entrance requirements:* For doctorate, SAT or PCAT (for Pharm D), interview, criminal background check (for Pharm D). Additional exam requirements/recommendations for international students: Recommended—TOEFL (minimum score 550 paper-based). Electronic applications accepted. *Expenses:* Contact institution. *Faculty research:* Pharmacokinetics, cancer prevention, cardiology, neurology, pharmacodynamics.

St. John Fisher College, Wegmans School of Pharmacy, Doctor of Pharmacy Program, Rochester, NY 14618-3597. Offers Pharm D. *Accreditation:* ACPE. *Faculty:* 32 full-time (20 women), 1 part-time/adjunct (0 women). *Students:* 331 full-time (197 women), 2 part-time (0 women); includes 64 minority (14 Black or African American, non-Hispanic/Latino; 2 American Indian or Alaska Native, non-Hispanic/Latino; 34 Asian, non-Hispanic/Latino; 9 Hispanic/Latino; 5 Two or more races, non-Hispanic/Latino), 7 international. Average age 25. 571 applicants, 25% accepted, 87 enrolled. In 2015, 69 doctorates awarded. *Degree requirements:* For doctorate, advanced pharmacy practice experience. *Entrance requirements:* For doctorate, PCAT, 2 letters of recommendation, interview, minimum of 62 credit hours of specific undergraduate courses. Additional exam requirements/recommendations for international students: Required—TOEFL (minimum score 575 paper-based; 80 iBT). *Application deadline:* For fall admission, 3/1 for domestic students. Applications are processed on a rolling basis. Electronic applications accepted. *Expenses:* $18,582.50 per semester. *Financial support:* Scholarships/grants available. Financial award applicants required to submit FAFSA. *Faculty research:* Opioid pharmacology, heavy metal toxicology. *Unit head:* Dr. Christine Birnie, Interim Dean of the School of Pharmacy, 585-385-7202, E-mail: cbirnie@sjfc.edu. *Application contact:* Rebecca Norman, Associate Director of Transfer and Graduate Admissions, 585-385-8064, E-mail: rnorman@sjfc.edu.
Website: http://www.sjfc.edu/pharmacy

★ **St. Louis College of Pharmacy,** Professional Program, St. Louis, MO 63110-1088. Offers Pharm D. *Accreditation:* ACPE. *Faculty:* 78 full-time (46 women), 25 part-time/adjunct (18 women). *Students:* 937 full-time (558 women), 16 part-time (7 women); includes 277 minority (46 Black or African American, non-Hispanic/Latino; 5 American Indian or Alaska Native, non-Hispanic/Latino; 202 Asian, non-Hispanic/Latino; 8 Hispanic/Latino; 2 Native Hawaiian or other Pacific Islander, non-Hispanic/Latino; 14 Two or more races, non-Hispanic/Latino), 24 international. Average age 22. 204 applicants, 12% accepted, 10 enrolled. In 2015, 204 doctorates awarded. *Entrance requirements:* For doctorate, PCAT. Additional exam requirements/recommendations for international students: Required—TOEFL (minimum score 550 paper-based). Application fee: $55. Electronic applications accepted. *Expenses:* Tuition, area resident: Full-time $30,976; part-time $1033 per credit hour. *Required fees:* $498; $498 per unit. *Financial support:* In 2015–16, 547 students received support. Federal Work-Study and scholarships/grants available. Financial award application deadline: 12/1; financial award applicants required to submit FAFSA. *Unit head:* Dr. Bruce Canaday, Dean of Pharmacy. *Application contact:* Chase Davis, Director of Admissions, 314-446-8140, Fax: 314-446-8309, E-mail: chase.davis@stlcop.edu.

See Display on next page and Close-Up on page 935.

Samford University, McWhorter School of Pharmacy, Birmingham, AL 35229. Offers Pharm D. *Accreditation:* ACPE. *Faculty:* 40 full-time (23 women), 2 part-time/adjunct (1 woman). *Students:* 495 full-time (308 women), 7 part-time (2 women); includes 95 minority (47 Black or African American, non-Hispanic/Latino; 1 American Indian or Alaska Native, non-Hispanic/Latino; 36 Asian, non-Hispanic/Latino; 5 Hispanic/Latino; 6 Two or more races, non-Hispanic/Latino), 9 international. Average age 25. 451 applicants, 42% accepted, 146 enrolled. In 2015, 119 doctorates awarded. *Entrance requirements:* For doctorate, PCAT, minimum GPA of 2.75. Additional exam requirements/recommendations for international students: Required—TOEFL (minimum score 550 paper-based; 80 iBT). *Application deadline:* For spring admission, 3/1 for domestic and international students. Applications are processed on a rolling basis.

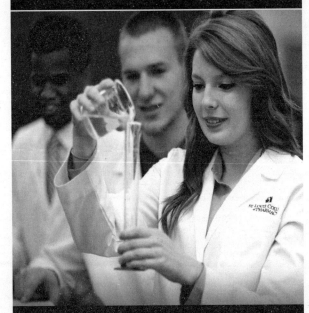
Application fee: $25. Electronic applications accepted. *Expenses: Tuition, area resident:* Full-time $18,673; part-time $766 per credit hour. *Required fees:* $550. Tuition and fees vary according to course load, degree level and student level. *Financial support:* In 2015–16, 187 students received support. Research assistantships, teaching assistantships, Federal Work-Study, institutionally sponsored loans, and scholarships/grants available. Financial award application deadline: 3/1; financial award applicants required to submit FAFSA. *Faculty research:* Biotechnology, transdermal drug delivery, vaccines, human skin models, genetic mapping of disease, determination of pharmacokinetics of new drug candidates, impact of herbal supplements on administered chemotherapeutic drugs, stability of compounded drug formulations, novel ophthalmic drug delivery systems, ion channel, cystic fibrosis novel drug discovery (protein misfolding). *Total annual research expenditures:* $45,000. *Unit head:* Dr. Michael A. Crouch, Dean/Professor, 205-726-2820, Fax: 205-726-2759, E-mail: macrouch@samford.edu. *Application contact:* Jon M. Parker, Assistant Director of Pharmacy Admissions, 205-726-4242, Fax: 205-726-4141, E-mail: jmparker@samford.edu.
Website: http://pharmacy.samford.edu

Shenandoah University, Bernard J. Dunn School of Pharmacy, Winchester, VA 22602. Offers Pharm D. *Accreditation:* ACPE. *Program availability:* Part-time, evening/weekend, online learning. *Faculty:* 39 full-time (26 women), 11 part-time/adjunct (6 women). *Students:* 403 full-time (266 women), 162 part-time (107 women); includes 264 minority (88 Black or African American, non-Hispanic/Latino; 2 American Indian or Alaska Native, non-Hispanic/Latino; 147 Asian, non-Hispanic/Latino; 21 Hispanic/Latino; 6 Two or more races, non-Hispanic/Latino), 25 international. Average age 31. 481 applicants, 51% accepted, 136 enrolled. In 2015, 122 doctorates awarded. *Degree requirements:* For doctorate, 142 credit hours in the didactic and experiential curriculum (not including prerequisite courses) with minimum cumulative GPA of 2.0. *Entrance requirements:* For doctorate, PCAT, BS in pharmacy (or foreign equivalent), essay, interview, minimum GPA of 2.5, 3 letters of recommendation. Additional exam requirements/recommendations for international students: Required—TOEFL (minimum score 550 paper-based; 79 iBT). *Application deadline:* For fall admission, 3/1 for domestic and international students. Application fee: $30. Electronic applications accepted. *Expenses:* $130,080 tuition, $5,960 fees (inclduing technology fee, NT Pharmacy fee, pharmacy clinical fee, and student services fee). *Financial support:* In 2015–16, 11 students received support. Career-related internships or fieldwork, scholarships/grants, and unspecified assistantships available. Support available to part-time students. Financial award application deadline: 3/15; financial award applicants required to submit FAFSA. *Faculty research:* Pharmacogenomics, pharmaceutics, clinical pharmacy. *Unit head:* Alan McKay, PhD, Dean, 540-665-1282, Fax: 540-665-1283, E-mail: amckay@su.edu. *Application contact:* Andrew Woodall, Executive Director of Recruitment and Admissions, 540-665-4581, Fax: 540-665-4627, E-mail: admit@su.edu.
Website: http://www.pharmacy.su.edu

South Dakota State University, Graduate School, College of Pharmacy, Professional Program in Pharmacy, Brookings, SD 57007. Offers Pharm D. *Accreditation:* ACPE. *Entrance requirements:* For doctorate, ACT or PCAT, bachelor's degree in pharmacy. Additional exam requirements/recommendations for international students: Required—TOEFL (minimum score 550 paper-based). *Faculty research:* Geriatric medicine, drugs of abuse, anti-cancer drugs, drug metabolism, sustained drug delivery.

Southern Illinois University Edwardsville, School of Pharmacy, Edwardsville, IL 62026. Offers pharmacy education (Pharm D); pharmacy pediatrics (Pharm D). *Accreditation:* ACPE. *Faculty:* 40 full-time (23 women). *Students:* 220 applicants, 46% accepted. In 2015, 76 doctorates awarded. *Entrance requirements:* For doctorate, PCAT. *Application deadline:* For fall admission, 2/1 for domestic and international students. Application fee: $40. Electronic applications accepted. *Expenses:* Tuition, state resident: full-time $5026; part-time $837 per course. Tuition, nonresident: full-time $12,566; part-time $2094 per course. *Required fees:* $1682; $474 per course. Tuition and fees vary according to course load, campus/location and program. *Financial support:* Career-related internships or fieldwork, Federal Work-Study, institutionally sponsored loans, scholarships/grants, and traineeships available. Support available to part-time students. Financial award application deadline: 3/1; financial award applicants required to submit FAFSA. *Unit head:* Dr. Gireesh V. Gupchup, Dean, 618-650-5150, Fax: 618-650-5152, E-mail: pharmacy@siue.edu. *Application contact:* Connie Stamper-Carr, Director of Student Affairs, 618-650-5150, Fax: 618-650-5152, E-mail: pharmacy@siue.edu.
Website: http://www.siue.edu/pharmacy

South University, Graduate Programs, School of Pharmacy, Savannah, GA 31406. Offers Pharm D/MBA. *Accreditation:* ACPE.

South University, Program in Pharmacy, Columbia, SC 29203. Offers Pharm D.

Southwestern Oklahoma State University, College of Pharmacy, Weatherford, OK 73096-3098. Offers Pharm D. *Accreditation:* ACPE. *Entrance requirements:* For doctorate, PCAT.

Texas A&M University, Irma Lerma Rangel College of Pharmacy, Kingsville, TX 78363. Offers pharmacy (Pharm D). *Accreditation:* ACPE. *Faculty:* 46. *Students:* 406 full-time (215 women), 1 (woman) part-time; includes 312 minority (24 Black or African American, non-Hispanic/Latino; 1 American Indian or Alaska Native, non-Hispanic/Latino; 141 Asian, non-Hispanic/Latino; 136 Hispanic/Latino; 1 Native Hawaiian or other Pacific Islander, non-Hispanic/Latino; 9 Two or more races, non-Hispanic/Latino), 1 international. Average age 26. 126 applicants, 100% accepted, 118 enrolled. *Entrance requirements:* For doctorate, PCAT, transcripts from each college/university attended; 3 PharmCAS recommendations. Additional exam requirements/recommendations for international students: Required—TOEFL (minimum score 550 paper-based; 80 iBT). *Application deadline:* For fall admission, 11/3 for domestic students. Application fee: $100. Electronic applications accepted. *Expenses:* Contact institution. *Financial support:* In 2015–16, 189 students received support. Career-related internships or fieldwork, institutionally sponsored loans, scholarships/grants, traineeships, health care benefits, tuition waivers (full and partial), and unspecified assistantships available. Support available to part-time students. Financial award applicants required to submit FAFSA. *Unit head:* Dr. Indra K. Reddy, Dean, 361-593-4273, Fax: 361-593-4929, E-mail: ireddy@pharmacy.tamhsc.edu. *Application contact:* Maria de Leon, Director of Admission, 361-221-0642, E-mail: mdeleon@tamhsc.edu.
Website: http://pharmacy.tamhsc.edu/

Texas Southern University, College of Pharmacy and Health Sciences, Department of Pharmacy Practice, Houston, TX 77004-4584. Offers Pharm D. *Program availability:* Online learning. *Entrance requirements:* For doctorate, GRE General Test, PCAT. Electronic applications accepted.

Thomas Jefferson University, Jefferson School of Pharmacy, Philadelphia, PA 19107. Offers Pharm D. *Accreditation:* ACPE. *Students:* 267 full-time (162 women), 10 part-time (4 women); includes 27 minority (13 Black or African American, non-Hispanic/Latino; 1 American Indian or Alaska Native, non-Hispanic/Latino; 8 Asian, non-Hispanic/Latino; 5 Hispanic/Latino). Average age 26. 617 applicants, 29% accepted, 85 enrolled. In 2015, 89 doctorates awarded. *Entrance requirements:* For doctorate, PCAT. Additional exam

requirements/recommendations for international students: Required—TOEFL. *Application deadline:* For fall admission, 3/1 for domestic and international students. Applications are processed on a rolling basis. Application fee: $25. Electronic applications accepted. *Expenses:* Contact institution. *Financial support:* In 2015–16, 161 students received support. Federal Work-Study, institutionally sponsored loans, and scholarships/grants available. Financial award application deadline: 4/1; financial award applicants required to submit FAFSA. *Unit head:* Dr. Rebecca S. Finley, Dean, 215-955-6300. *Application contact:* Niki M. Kelley, Associate Director of Admissions, 215-503-1041, E-mail: niki.kelley@jefferson.edu.
Website: http://www.jefferson.edu/pharmacy.

Touro University California, Graduate Programs, Vallejo, CA 94592. Offers education (MA); medical health sciences (MS); osteopathic medicine (DO); pharmacy (Pharm D); public health (MPH). *Accreditation:* AOsA; ARC-PA. *Program availability:* Part-time, evening/weekend. *Degree requirements:* For master's, comprehensive exam, thesis; for doctorate, comprehensive exam. *Entrance requirements:* For doctorate, BS/BA. Electronic applications accepted. *Faculty research:* Cancer, heart disease.

Universidad de Ciencias Medicas, Graduate Programs, San Jose, Costa Rica. Offers dermatology (SP); family health (MS); health service center administration (MHA); human anatomy (MS); medical and surgery (MD); occupational medicine (MS); pharmacy (Pharm D). *Program availability:* Part-time. *Degree requirements:* For master's, thesis; for doctorate and SP, comprehensive exam. *Entrance requirements:* For master's, MD or bachelor's degree; for doctorate, admissions test; for SP, admissions test, MD.

University at Buffalo, the State University of New York, Graduate School, School of Pharmacy and Pharmaceutical Sciences, Professional Program in Pharmacy, Buffalo, NY 14214. Offers Pharm D, Pharm D/JD, Pharm D/MBA, Pharm D/MPH, Pharm D/MS, Pharm D/PhD. *Accreditation:* ACPE. *Faculty:* 25 full-time (10 women), 7 part-time/adjunct (3 women). *Students:* 499 full-time (293 women), 3 part-time (1 woman); includes 202 minority (21 Black or African American, non-Hispanic/Latino; 1 American Indian or Alaska Native, non-Hispanic/Latino; 172 Asian, non-Hispanic/Latino; 8 Hispanic/Latino), 19 international. Average age 24. 600 applicants, 36% accepted, 137 enrolled. In 2015, 131 doctorates awarded. *Degree requirements:* For doctorate, project. *Entrance requirements:* For doctorate, PCAT. Additional exam requirements/recommendations for international students: Required—TOEFL (minimum score 550 paper-based; 79 iBT); Recommended—IELTS, TSE. *Application deadline:* For fall admission, 2/1 priority date for domestic and international students. Applications are processed on a rolling basis. Application fee: $50. Electronic applications accepted. *Expenses:* Contact institution. *Financial support:* In 2015–16, 313 students received support, including 4 fellowships (averaging $43,000 per year); scholarships/grants and health care benefits also available. Financial award application deadline: 3/1; financial award applicants required to submit FAFSA. *Faculty research:* Pharmacokinetics/pharmacodynamics, HIV/AIDS, oncology, health outcomes research, translational research. *Total annual research expenditures:* $4.8 million. *Unit head:* Dr. Edward M. Bednarczyk, Chairman, 716-645-2828 Ext. 357, Fax: 716-829-6568, E-mail: eb@buffalo.edu. *Application contact:* Dr. Jennifer M. Hess, Associate Dean, 716-645-2825 Ext. 1, Fax: 716-829-6568, E-mail: prepharm@buffalo.edu.
Website: http://pharmacy.buffalo.edu/academic-programs/pharmd.html

University of Alberta, Faculty of Graduate Studies and Research, Department of Pharmacy and Pharmaceutical Sciences, Edmonton, AB T6G 2E1, Canada. Offers M Sc, PhD. Terminal master's awarded for partial completion of doctoral program. *Degree requirements:* For master's, thesis; for doctorate, thesis/dissertation. *Entrance requirements:* Additional exam requirements/recommendations for international students: Required—Michigan English Language Assessment Battery or IELTS.

Electronic applications accepted. *Faculty research:* Radiopharmacy, pharmacokinetics, bionucleonics, medicinal chemistry, microbiology.

The University of Arizona, College of Pharmacy, Pharmacy Professional Program, Tucson, AZ 85721. Offers Pharm D. *Accreditation:* ACPE. *Program availability:* Part-time. *Entrance requirements:* For doctorate, PCAT, 4-6 months of pharmacy experience. Additional exam requirements/recommendations for international students: Required—TOEFL (minimum score 550 paper-based; 79 iBT). Electronic applications accepted. *Faculty research:* Health/service administrative pharmacy education, geriatric pharmacy, social and behavioral pharmacy management and economics.

University of Arkansas for Medical Sciences, College of Pharmacy, Little Rock, AR 72205-7199. Offers MS, Pharm D. *Accreditation:* ACPE (one or more programs are accredited). *Degree requirements:* For master's, thesis. *Entrance requirements:* For master's, GRE; for doctorate, PCAT. Additional exam requirements/recommendations for international students: Recommended—TOEFL. Electronic applications accepted. *Expenses:* Contact institution.

The University of British Columbia, Faculty of Pharmaceutical Sciences, Vancouver, BC V6T 1Z3, Canada. Offers M Sc, PhD. *Degree requirements:* For master's, thesis, seminar; for doctorate, comprehensive exam, thesis/dissertation, seminar. *Entrance requirements:* Additional exam requirements/recommendations for international students: Required—TOEFL (minimum score 600 paper-based; 100 iBT), IELTS (minimum score 6.5). Electronic applications accepted. *Faculty research:* Pharmacology and cellular pharmacology, neuropharmacology, toxicology, nanomedicines and drug delivery, pharmacogenomics and personalized medicine, health outcomes research and evaluation, pharmacoepidemiology, and medicinal chemistry.

University of California, San Diego, School of Pharmacy and Pharmaceutical Sciences, La Jolla, CA 92093. Offers Pharm D. *Accreditation:* ACPE. *Faculty:* 33. *Students:* 249 full-time (171 women). *Application deadline:* For fall admission, 11/2 for domestic students. Application fee: $90. *Expenses:* Tuition, state resident: full-time $11,220. Tuition, nonresident: full-time $26,322. *Required fees:* $1800. *Unit head:* Dr. James McKerrow, Dean. *Application contact:* 858-822-4900, Fax: 858-822-5591, E-mail: sppsadmissions@ucsd.edu.
Website: http://www.pharmacy.ucsd.edu/

 University of California, San Francisco, School of Pharmacy, Program in Pharmacy, San Francisco, CA 94143. Offers Pharm D. *Accreditation:* ACPE. *Degree requirements:* For doctorate, comprehensive exam, supervised practice experience. *Entrance requirements:* For doctorate, 2 years of preparatory course work in basic sciences. Electronic applications accepted. *Faculty research:* Drug delivery, drug metabolism and chemical toxicology, macromolecular structure, molecular parasitology, pharmacokinetics.

See Display below and Close-Up on page 937.

University of Charleston, School of Pharmacy, Charleston, WV 25304-1099. Offers Pharm D. *Accreditation:* ACPE. *Students:* 291 full-time (152 women), 5 part-time (2 women); includes 96 minority (41 Black or African American, non-Hispanic/Latino; 2 American Indian or Alaska Native, non-Hispanic/Latino; 39 Asian, non-Hispanic/Latino; 9 Hispanic/Latino; 1 Native Hawaiian or other Pacific Islander, non-Hispanic/Latino; 4 Two or more races, non-Hispanic/Latino), 9 international. Average age 26. *Degree requirements:* For doctorate, minimum cumulative GPA of 2.3 for all courses. *Entrance requirements:* For doctorate, PCAT (taken within 3 years of the date of application), criminal background check, proof of health insurance, immunizations and health clearance, minimum undergraduate GPA of 2.75, two letters of recommendation, interview. Additional exam requirements/recommendations for international students:

Required—TOEFL. *Application deadline:* For fall admission, 2/1 for domestic and international students. Applications are processed on a rolling basis. Electronic applications accepted. *Expenses: Tuition, area resident:* Full-time $20,602; part-time $425 per credit. *Required fees:* $200. *Financial support:* Career-related internships or fieldwork and scholarships/grants available. Financial award application deadline: 3/1; financial award applicants required to submit FAFSA. *Unit head:* Dr. Michelle Easton, Dean, 304-357-4889, Fax: 304-357-4868, E-mail: michelleeaston@ucwv.edu. *Application contact:* Jamie Bero, Director of Recruitment and Admissions, 304-357-4889, E-mail: staciegeise@ucwv.edu.
Website: http://www.ucwv.edu/Pharmacy/

University of Cincinnati, James L. Winkle College of Pharmacy, Division of Pharmacy Practice, Cincinnati, OH 45221. Offers Pharm D. *Accreditation:* ACPE. *Entrance requirements:* For doctorate, GRE General Test, BS in pharmacy or equivalent, minimum GPA of 3.0. Additional exam requirements/recommendations for international students: Required—TOEFL.

University of Connecticut, Graduate School, School of Pharmacy, Professional Program in Pharmacy, Storrs, CT 06269. Offers Pharm D.
Website: http://www.pharmacy.uconn.edu/

The University of Findlay, Office of Graduate Admissions, Findlay, OH 45840-3653. Offers athletic training (MAT); business (MBA), including health care management, hospitality management, organizational leadership, public management; education (MA Ed), including administration, children's literature, early childhood, human resource development, reading, science, special education, technology; environmental, safety and health management (MSEM); health informatics (MS); occupational therapy (MOT); pharmacy (Pharm D); physical therapy (DPT); physician assistant (MPA); rhetoric and writing (MA); teaching English to speakers of other languages (TESOL) and bilingual education (MA). *Program availability:* Part-time, evening/weekend, online learning. *Degree requirements:* For master's, thesis, cumulative project, capstone project. *Entrance requirements:* For master's, GRE/GMAT, bachelor's degree from accredited institution, minimum undergraduate GPA of 2.5 in last 64 hours of course work; for doctorate, GRE, minimum cumulative GPA of 3.0. Additional exam requirements/recommendations for international students: Required—TOEFL (minimum score 80 iBT). Electronic applications accepted.

University of Florida, Graduate School, College of Pharmacy and Graduate School, Graduate Programs in Pharmacy, Department of Pharmaceutics, Gainesville, FL 32611. Offers clinical and translational sciences (PhD); pharmaceutical sciences (MSP, PhD); pharmacy (MSP, PhD). *Faculty:* 2 full-time, 1 part-time/adjunct. *Students:* 30 full-time (14 women), 1 (woman) part-time; includes 1 minority (Asian, non-Hispanic/Latino), 24 international. Average age 29. 182 applicants, 57% accepted, 92 enrolled. In 2015, 4 doctorates awarded. *Degree requirements:* For doctorate, comprehensive exam, thesis/dissertation. *Entrance requirements:* For master's and doctorate, GRE General Test, minimum GPA of 3.0. Additional exam requirements/recommendations for international students: Required—TOEFL (minimum score 550 paper-based; 80 iBT), IELTS (minimum score 6). *Application deadline:* For fall admission, 2/1 priority date for domestic students, 2/1 for international students; for spring admission, 10/5 for domestic and international students. Applications are processed on a rolling basis. Application fee: $30. Electronic applications accepted. *Financial support:* In 2015–16, 3 research assistantships, 19 teaching assistantships were awarded; tuition waivers (full) and unspecified assistantships also available. Financial award applicants required to submit FAFSA. *Faculty research:* Basic, applied, and clinical investigations in pharmacokinetics/biopharmaceutics; pharmaceutical analysis, pharmaceutical biotechnology and drug delivery; herbal medicine. *Total annual research expenditures:* $2.2 million. *Unit head:* Hartmut Derendorf, PhD, Professor and Chair, 352-273-7856, Fax: 352-392-4447, E-mail: hartmut@ufl.edu. *Application contact:* Dr. Anthony Palmieri, III, Graduate Coordinator, 352-273-7868, E-mail: palmieri@cop.ufl.edu.
Website: http://www.cop.ufl.edu/pc/

University of Florida, Graduate School, College of Pharmacy, Professional Program in Pharmacy, Gainesville, FL 32611. Offers Pharm D, MBA/Pharm D, Pharm D/MPH, Pharm D/PhD. *Accreditation:* ACPE. *Program availability:* Part-time, online learning. *Faculty:* 12. *Entrance requirements:* For doctorate, PCAT, minimum GPA of 2.5. Additional exam requirements/recommendations for international students: Required—TOEFL. *Application deadline:* For fall admission, 3/1 for domestic and international students. Applications are processed on a rolling basis. Application fee: $30. Electronic applications accepted. *Financial support:* Federal Work-Study and institutionally sponsored loans available. Support available to part-time students. Financial award applicants required to submit FAFSA. *Faculty research:* Drug discovery, drug delivery, pharmacodynamics, socioeconomics of pharmacy, neurobiology of aging. *Unit head:* Michael W. McKenzie, PhD, Associate Dean for Professional Affairs, 352-273-6217, Fax: 352-273-6219, E-mail: mckenzie@cop.ufl.edu. *Application contact:* Mary Beth Yokomi, Admissions Coordinator, 352-273-6216, E-mail: yokomi@cop.ufl.edu.
Website: http://pharmacy.ufl.edu/education/doctor-of-pharmacy-degree-pharmd/

University of Georgia, College of Pharmacy, Athens, GA 30602. Offers MS, PhD, Pharm D, Certificate. *Accreditation:* ACPE (one or more programs are accredited). *Degree requirements:* For doctorate, variable foreign language requirement, thesis/dissertation (for some programs). *Entrance requirements:* For master's, GRE General Test, minimum GPA of 3.0; for doctorate, GRE General Test (for PhD), minimum GPA of 3.0 (for PhD). Additional exam requirements/recommendations for international students: Required—TOEFL (minimum score 80 iBT). Electronic applications accepted. *Expenses:* Contact institution.

University of Hawaii at Hilo, Program in Pharmacy, Hilo, HI 96720-4091. Offers Pharm D. *Accreditation:* ACPE. Electronic applications accepted.

University of Houston, College of Pharmacy, Houston, TX 77204. Offers pharmaceutics (MSPHR, PhD); pharmacology (MSPHR, PhD); pharmacy (Pharm D); pharmacy administration (MSPHR, PhD). *Accreditation:* ACPE. *Program availability:* Part-time. Terminal master's awarded for partial completion of doctoral program. *Entrance requirements:* For doctorate, PCAT (for Pharm D). Additional exam requirements/recommendations for international students: Required—TOEFL. Electronic applications accepted. *Faculty research:* Drug screening and design, cardiovascular pharmacology, infectious disease, asthma research, herbal medicine.

University of Illinois at Chicago, College of Pharmacy, Department of Biopharmaceutical Sciences, Chicago, IL 60607-7173. Offers MS, PhD. *Faculty:* 13 full-time (4 women), 12 part-time/adjunct (2 women). *Students:* 31 full-time (19 women), 1 (woman) part-time; includes 4 minority (3 Asian, non-Hispanic/Latino; 1 Hispanic/Latino), 18 international. Average age 26. *Expenses: Tuition, state resident:* full-time $11,480; part-time $3826 per credit. *Tuition, nonresident:* full-time $23,720; part-time $7906 per credit. *Required fees:* $1333 per semester. Part-time tuition and fees vary according to course level and program. *Faculty research:* Lipid and polymer-based drug delivery systems, targeted drug delivery, pharmacokinetic membrane transport and absorption, behavioral and cardiovascular pharmacology; neuropharmacology, environmental toxicology, cancer chemotherapy. *Unit head:* Prof. William T. Beck, Head, 312-996-0888, Fax: 312-996-0098, E-mail: wtbeck@uic.edu.
Website: http://www.uic.edu/pharmacy/depts/Biopharmaceutical_Sciences/index.php

University of Illinois at Chicago, College of Pharmacy, Professional Program in Pharmacy, Chicago, IL 60607-7128. Offers Pharm D. *Accreditation:* ACPE. *Faculty:* 237 full-time (137 women), 60 part-time/adjunct (32 women). *Students:* 784 full-time (470 women), 5 part-time (3 women); includes 408 minority (44 Black or African American, non-Hispanic/Latino; 1 American Indian or Alaska Native, non-Hispanic/Latino; 292 Asian, non-Hispanic/Latino; 45 Hispanic/Latino; 3 Native Hawaiian or other Pacific Islander, non-Hispanic/Latino; 23 Two or more races, non-Hispanic/Latino), 26 international. Average age 26. *Entrance requirements:* For doctorate, PCAT. Application fee: $60 ($50 for international students). *Expenses:* Contact institution. *Financial support:* Fellowships available. *Unit head:* Dr. Jerry Bauman, Dean, 312-996-7240, E-mail: jbauman@uic.edu. *Application contact:* Jackie Perry, Graduate College Receptionist, 312-413-2550, Fax: 312-413-0185, E-mail: gradcoll@uic.edu.
Website: http://www.uic.edu/pharmacy/education/professional_degree_prog.php

The University of Iowa, College of Pharmacy, Iowa City, IA 52242-1316. Offers clinical pharmaceutical sciences (PhD); medicinal and natural products chemistry (PhD); pharmaceutics (PhD); pharmaceutical socioeconomics (PhD); pharmaceutics (MS); pharmacy (Pharm D); Pharm D/MPH. *Accreditation:* ACPE (one or more programs are accredited). *Degree requirements:* For master's, thesis optional, exam; for doctorate, comprehensive exam, thesis/dissertation. *Entrance requirements:* For master's and doctorate, GRE General Test, minimum GPA of 3.0. Additional exam requirements/recommendations for international students: Required—TOEFL (minimum score 550 paper-based; 81 iBT). Electronic applications accepted.

University of Kentucky, Graduate School, Professional Program in Pharmacy, Lexington, KY 40506-0032. Offers Pharm D. *Accreditation:* ACPE. *Entrance requirements:* For doctorate, PCAT, interview, minimum GPA of 2.5. Additional exam requirements/recommendations for international students: Required—TOEFL (minimum score 527 paper-based). Electronic applications accepted. *Expenses:* Contact institution. *Faculty research:* Innovations in pharmacy practice and education, policy and outcomes research; drug discovery and development; drug delivery and nanotechnology; natural products and computational chemistry.

University of Louisiana at Monroe, Graduate School, College of Health and Pharmaceutical Sciences, School of Pharmacy, Monroe, LA 71209-0001. Offers pharmacy (PhD, Pharm D); toxicology (PhD). *Accreditation:* ACPE. *Degree requirements:* For doctorate, comprehensive exam, thesis/dissertation. *Entrance requirements:* For doctorate, GRE General Test, minimum undergraduate GPA of 2.5. Additional exam requirements/recommendations for international students: Required—TOEFL (minimum score 500 paper-based; 61 iBT). Electronic applications accepted.

The University of Manchester, School of Pharmacy and Pharmaceutical Sciences, Manchester, United Kingdom. Offers M Phil, PhD.

University of Maryland, Baltimore, Graduate School, Graduate Programs in Pharmacy, Baltimore, MD 21201. Offers pharmaceutical health service research (MS, PhD), including epidemiology (MS), pharmacy administration (PhD); pharmaceutical sciences (PhD); Pharm D/PhD. *Accreditation:* ACPE (one or more programs are accredited). *Degree requirements:* For doctorate, comprehensive exam, thesis/dissertation. *Entrance requirements:* For doctorate, GRE General Test. Additional exam requirements/recommendations for international students: Required—TOEFL (minimum score 550 paper-based), IELTS. Electronic applications accepted. Tuition and fees vary according to program. *Faculty research:* Drug discovery, pharmacokinetics, drug delivery, pharmaceutical outcomes and policy, pharmaceutical sciences.

University of Maryland, Baltimore, Professional Program in Pharmacy, Baltimore, MD 21201. Offers Pharm D, JD/Pharm D, Pharm D/MBA, Pharm D/MPH, Pharm D/PhD. *Accreditation:* ACPE. *Entrance requirements:* For doctorate, PCAT, 65 hours in pre-pharmacy course work, on-site interview. Additional exam requirements/recommendations for international students: Required—TOEFL (minimum score 550 paper-based; 80 iBT). Electronic applications accepted. Tuition and fees vary according to program. *Faculty research:* Pharmaceutics, molecular biology, pharmacology, pharmacoepidemiology, pharmacoeconomics.

University of Michigan, College of Pharmacy, Professional Program in Pharmacy, Ann Arbor, MI 48109. Offers Pharm D, Pharm D/PhD. *Accreditation:* ACPE. *Entrance requirements:* For doctorate, PCAT. *Application deadline:* For fall admission, 2/1 for domestic students. *Financial support:* Applicants required to submit FAFSA. *Unit head:* James T. Dalton, Dean, 734-764-7144, Fax: 734-763-2022, E-mail: cop.deansoffice@med.umich.edu. *Application contact:* Mark S. Nelson, Director, Admissions and Student Counseling Services, 734-764-7312, E-mail: mnelson@med.umich.edu.
Website: https://pharmacy.umich.edu/pharmd

University of Minnesota, Duluth, Medical School, Department of Biochemistry, Molecular Biology and Biophysics, Duluth, MN 55812-2496. Offers biochemistry, molecular biology and biophysics (MS); biology and biophysics (PhD); social, administrative, and clinical pharmacy (MS, PhD); toxicology (MS, PhD). Terminal master's awarded for partial completion of doctoral program. *Degree requirements:* For master's, comprehensive exam, thesis; for doctorate, comprehensive exam, thesis/dissertation. *Entrance requirements:* For master's and doctorate, GRE General Test. Additional exam requirements/recommendations for international students: Required—TOEFL. Electronic applications accepted. *Faculty research:* Intestinal cancer biology; hepatotoxins and mitochondriopathies; toxicology; cell cycle regulation in stem cells; neurobiology of brain development, trace metal function and blood-brain barrier; hibernation biology.

University of Minnesota, Twin Cities Campus, College of Pharmacy, Professional Program in Pharmacy, Minneapolis, MN 55455-0213. Offers Pharm D. *Accreditation:* ACPE. *Degree requirements:* For doctorate, paper and seminar presentation. *Entrance requirements:* For doctorate, 2 years of pharmacy-related course work.

University of Mississippi, Graduate School, School of Pharmacy, University, MS 39677. Offers MS, PhD, Pharm D. *Accreditation:* ACPE (one or more programs are accredited). *Program availability:* Part-time. *Faculty:* 57 full-time (26 women), 15 part-time/adjunct (6 women). *Students:* 410 full-time (250 women), 12 part-time (4 women); includes 77 minority (26 Black or African American, non-Hispanic/Latino; 3 American Indian or Alaska Native, non-Hispanic/Latino; 37 Asian, non-Hispanic/Latino; 5 Hispanic/Latino; 1 Native Hawaiian or other Pacific Islander, non-Hispanic/Latino; 5 Two or more races, non-Hispanic/Latino), 70 international. In 2015, 22 master's, 49 doctorates awarded. Terminal master's awarded for partial completion of doctoral program. *Degree requirements:* For master's, thesis; for doctorate, thesis/dissertation (for some programs). *Entrance requirements:* For master's, GRE General Test, minimum GPA of 3.0; for doctorate, GRE General Test (for PhD). Additional exam requirements/recommendations for international students: Required—TOEFL. *Application deadline:* For fall admission, 4/1 for domestic students; for spring admission, 10/1 for domestic students. Applications are processed on a rolling basis. Application fee: $40. Electronic applications accepted. *Financial support:* Fellowships, research assistantships, teaching assistantships, career-related internships or fieldwork, Federal Work-Study, institutionally sponsored loans, scholarships/grants, tuition waivers (full), and unspecified assistantships available. Financial award application deadline: 3/1; financial award applicants required to submit FAFSA. *Unit head:* Dr. David D. Allen, II, Dean,

Pharmacy

662-915-7265, Fax: 662-915-5118, E-mail: sopdean@olemiss.edu. Website: http://www.pharmacy.olemiss.edu/

University of Missouri–Kansas City, School of Pharmacy, Kansas City, MO 64110-2499. Offers pharmaceutical sciences (PhD); pharmacology and toxicology (PhD); pharmacy (Pharm D). PhD offered through School of Graduate Studies. *Accreditation:* ACPE (one or more programs are accredited). *Program availability:* Online learning. *Faculty:* 49 full-time (26 women), 6 part-time/adjunct (2 women). *Students:* 447 full-time (276 women); includes 103 minority (24 Black or African American, non-Hispanic/Latino; 1 American Indian or Alaska Native, non-Hispanic/Latino; 53 Asian, non-Hispanic/Latino; 12 Hispanic/Latino; 13 Two or more races, non-Hispanic/Latino), 2 international. Average age 25. 414 applicants, 33% accepted, 133 enrolled. In 2015, 125 doctorates awarded. *Degree requirements:* For doctorate, comprehensive exam (for some programs), thesis/dissertation (for some programs). *Entrance requirements:* For doctorate, PCAT (for Pharm D). Additional exam requirements/recommendations for international students: Required—TOEFL (minimum score 550 paper-based; 80 iBT). *Application deadline:* For fall admission, 3/1 for domestic and international students. Applications are processed on a rolling basis. Application fee: $45 ($50 for international students). Electronic applications accepted. *Expenses:* Contact institution. *Financial support:* In 2015–16, 4 fellowships (averaging $40,082 per year), 14 research assistantships with tuition reimbursements (averaging $13,117 per year), 26 teaching assistantships with full tuition reimbursements (averaging $14,724 per year) were awarded; career-related internships or fieldwork, Federal Work-Study, institutionally sponsored loans, tuition waivers (full and partial), and unspecified assistantships also available. Financial award application deadline: 3/1; financial award applicants required to submit FAFSA. *Faculty research:* Bio-organic and medicinal chemistry, drug delivery, pharmaceutics, molecular neurobiology, neurology. *Unit head:* Dr. Russell B. Melchert, Dean, 816-235-1609, Fax: 816-235-5190, E-mail: melchertr@umkc.edu. *Application contact:* Shelly M. Janasz, Director, Student Services, 816-235-2400, Fax: 816-235-5190, E-mail: janaszs@umkc.edu. Website: http://pharmacy.umkc.edu/

University of Montana, Graduate School, College of Health Professions and Biomedical Sciences, Skaggs School of Pharmacy, Missoula, MT 59812-0002. Offers biomedical and pharmaceutical sciences (MS, PhD), including biomedical sciences (PhD), medicinal chemistry, molecular and cellular toxicology, neuroscience (PhD), pharmaceutical sciences (MS); pharmacy (Pharm D). Electronic applications accepted. *Faculty research:* Neuroendocrinology, neuropharmacology, molecular biochemistry, cardiovascular pharmacology, pharmacognosy.

University of Nebraska Medical Center, College of Pharmacy, Omaha, NE 68198-6000. Offers Pharm D. *Accreditation:* ACPE. *Entrance requirements:* For doctorate, PCAT, 90 semester hours of pre-pharmacy work. Electronic applications accepted. *Expenses:* Contact institution. *Faculty research:* Biopharmaceutics, nanomedicine, drug design, pharmaceutics, pharmacokinetics.

University of New England, College of Pharmacy, Portland, ME 04103. Offers Pharm D. *Accreditation:* ACPE. *Faculty:* 28 full-time (9 women), 4 part-time/adjunct (0 women). *Students:* 393 full-time (238 women); includes 137 minority (34 Black or African American, non-Hispanic/Latino; 3 American Indian or Alaska Native, non-Hispanic/Latino; 80 Asian, non-Hispanic/Latino; 11 Hispanic/Latino; 2 Native Hawaiian or other Pacific Islander, non-Hispanic/Latino; 7 Two or more races, non-Hispanic/Latino), 4 international. Average age 26. 570 applicants, 34% accepted, 99 enrolled. In 2015, 90 doctorates awarded. *Entrance requirements:* For doctorate, PCAT. *Application deadline:* For fall admission, 3/1 for domestic students. Applications are processed on a rolling basis. Electronic applications accepted. Tuition and fees vary according to degree level and program. *Financial support:* Application deadline: 5/1; applicants required to submit FAFSA. *Unit head:* Dr. Gayle A. Brazeau, Dean, College of Pharmacy, 207-221-4500, Fax: 207-523-1927, E-mail: gbrazeau@une.edu. *Application contact:* Scott Steinberg, Dean of University Admission, 207-221-4225, Fax: 207-523-1925, E-mail: ssteinberg@une.edu. Website: http://www.une.edu/pharmacy/

University of New Mexico, Graduate Studies, College of Pharmacy, Professional Program in Pharmacy, Albuquerque, NM 87131-2039. Offers Pharm D. *Accreditation:* ACPE. *Entrance requirements:* For doctorate, PCAT, 3 letters of recommendation, interview, 91 credit hours of prerequisites, letter of intent, Pharmcas application. Electronic applications accepted. *Expenses:* Contact institution.

University of Oklahoma Health Sciences Center, College of Pharmacy, Professional Program in Pharmacy, Oklahoma City, OK 73190. Offers Pharm D. *Accreditation:* ACPE.

University of Pittsburgh, School of Pharmacy, Professional Program in Pharmacy, Pittsburgh, PA 15261. Offers Pharm D. *Accreditation:* ACPE. *Faculty:* 72 full-time (37 women), 8 part-time/adjunct (3 women). *Students:* 447 full-time (286 women); includes 95 minority (12 Black or African American, non-Hispanic/Latino; 1 American Indian or Alaska Native, non-Hispanic/Latino; 71 Asian, non-Hispanic/Latino; 5 Hispanic/Latino; 6 Two or more races, non-Hispanic/Latino), 6 international. Average age 22. 537 applicants, 27% accepted, 114 enrolled. In 2015, 108 doctorates awarded. *Entrance requirements:* For doctorate, PCAT. Additional exam requirements/recommendations for international students: Required—TOEFL (minimum score 100 iBT), IELTS (minimum score 7), PCAT. *Application deadline:* For fall admission, 12/1 for domestic and international students. Applications are processed on a rolling basis. Application fee: $205. Electronic applications accepted. *Expenses:* $29,604 per year, $1,144 per credit in-state; $33,002 per year, $1,274 per credit out-of-state. *Financial support:* In 2015–16, 180 students received support. Federal Work-Study, institutionally sponsored loans, and scholarships/grants available. Financial award application deadline: 10/1. *Faculty research:* Drug delivery and targeting; neuroendocrine pharmacology; genomics, proteomics, and drug discovery; clinical pharmaceutical sciences. *Unit head:* Dr. Sharon Corey, Dean, 412-648-9157, Fax: 412-383-9996, E-mail: coreys@pitt.edu. *Application contact:* Marcia L. Borrelli, Director of Student Services, 412-383-9000, Fax: 412-383-9996, E-mail: rxschool@pitt.edu. Website: http://www.pharmacy.pitt.edu

University of Puerto Rico, Medical Sciences Campus, School of Pharmacy, San Juan, PR 00936-5067. Offers industrial pharmacy (MS); pharmaceutical sciences (MS); pharmacy (Pharm D). *Accreditation:* ACPE. *Program availability:* Part-time, evening/weekend. *Degree requirements:* For master's, thesis; for doctorate, portfolio, research project. *Entrance requirements:* For master's, GRE, interview; for doctorate, PCAT, interview. Electronic applications accepted. *Expenses:* Contact institution. *Faculty research:* Controlled release, solid dosage form, screening of anti-HIV drugs, pharmacokinetic/pharmacodynamic of drugs.

University of Rhode Island, Graduate School, College of Pharmacy, Department of Pharmacy Practice, Kingston, RI 02881. Offers pharmacoepidemiology and pharmacoeconomics (MS, PhD); pharmacy practice (Pharm D); Pharm D/MBA; Pharm D/MS. *Accreditation:* ACPE. *Faculty:* 11 full-time (8 women), 1 (woman) part-time/adjunct. *Students:* 753 full-time (501 women), 2 part-time (1 woman); includes 131 minority (11 Black or African American, non-Hispanic/Latino; 66 Asian, non-Hispanic/Latino; 37 Hispanic/Latino; 17 Two or more races, non-Hispanic/Latino), 39

international. In 2015, 114 doctorates awarded. *Entrance requirements:* For master's and doctorate, 2 letters of recommendation. Additional exam requirements/recommendations for international students: Required—TOEFL (minimum score 550 paper-based). *Application deadline:* For fall admission, 2/1 for domestic and international students. Application fee: $65. Electronic applications accepted. *Expenses:* Tuition, state resident: full-time $11,796; part-time $655 per credit. Tuition, nonresident: full-time $24,206; part-time $1345 per credit. *Required fees:* $1546; $44 per credit. One-time fee: $155 full-time; $35 part-time. *Financial support:* Application deadline: 2/1; applicants required to submit FAFSA. *Faculty research:* Treatment, virulence inhibition (toxin and biofilm), colonization and control of methicillin-resistant staphylococcus aureus (MRSA), investigating activity of catheter lock solutions against biofilm producing bacteria. *Unit head:* Dr. Marilyn Barbour, Chair, 401-874-5842, Fax: 401-874-2181, E-mail: mbarbourri@aol.com. Website: http://www.uri.edu/pharmacy/departments/php/index.shtml

University of Saint Joseph, School of Pharmacy, West Hartford, CT 06117-2700. Offers Pharm D. *Application deadline:* Applications are processed on a rolling basis. Electronic applications accepted. *Financial support:* Career-related internships or fieldwork available. Website: http://www.usj.edu/academics/schools/school-of-pharmacy/

University of South Carolina, South Carolina College of Pharmacy, Professional Program in Pharmacy, Columbia, SC 29208. Offers Pharm D. *Degree requirements:* For doctorate, one foreign language. *Entrance requirements:* For doctorate, PCAT, 2 years of preprofessional study, interview. Electronic applications accepted. *Faculty research:* Cancer treatment and prevention, Ion channels, DNA damage repair, inflammation.

University of Southern California, Graduate School, School of Pharmacy, Professional Program in Pharmacy, Los Angeles, CA 90089. Offers Pharm D, Pharm D/MBA, Pharm D/MS, Pharm D/PhD. *Accreditation:* ACPE. Electronic applications accepted. *Faculty research:* Infectious diseases, health services research, geriatric pharmacology, clinical psychopharmacology.

University of South Florida, College of Engineering, Department of Chemical and Biomedical Engineering, Tampa, FL 33620. Offers biomedical engineering (MSBE, PhD), including biomedical engineering (MSBE); pharmacy (MSBE); chemical engineering (M Ch E, PhD), including biomedical and biotechnology, manufacturing (PhD); MSBE/MS; PhD/MD. *Program availability:* Part-time. *Faculty:* 15 full-time (2 women). *Students:* 84 full-time (34 women), 22 part-time (9 women); includes 21 minority (4 Black or African American, non-Hispanic/Latino; 1 American Indian or Alaska Native, non-Hispanic/Latino; 3 Asian, non-Hispanic/Latino; 10 Hispanic/Latino; 3 Two or more races, non-Hispanic/Latino), 49 international. Average age 28. 135 applicants, 39% accepted, 28 enrolled. In 2015, 30 master's, 9 doctorates awarded. Terminal master's awarded for partial completion of doctoral program. *Degree requirements:* For master's, comprehensive exam, thesis (for some programs); for doctorate, comprehensive exam, thesis/dissertation. *Entrance requirements:* For master's, GRE General Test, undergraduate degree in engineering, science, or chemical engineering with minimum GPA of 3.0; at least two letters of recommendation; current resume; statement of research interests (for students who wish to pursue thesis option); for doctorate, GRE General Test, undergraduate degree in engineering, science, or chemical engineering with minimum GPA of 3.0; three letters of recommendation; current resume; statement of research interests. Additional exam requirements/recommendations for international students: Required—TOEFL (minimum score 550 paper-based; 79 iBT) or IELTS (minimum score 6.5). *Application deadline:* For fall admission, 2/15 for domestic students, 1/2 priority date for international students; for spring admission, 10/15 for domestic students, 6/1 priority date for international students. Application fee: $30. Electronic applications accepted. *Financial support:* In 2015–16, 41 students received support, including 29 research assistantships with tuition reimbursements available (averaging $13,171 per year), 12 teaching assistantships with tuition reimbursements available (averaging $14,017 per year); unspecified assistantships also available. Financial award applicants required to submit FAFSA. *Faculty research:* Neuroengineering, tissue engineering, biomedicine and biotechnology, engineering education, functional materials and nanotechnology, energy, environment/sustainability. *Total annual research expenditures:* $950,677. *Unit head:* Dr. Venkat R. Bhethanabotla, Professor and Department Chair, 813-974-3997, E-mail: bhethana@usf.edu. *Application contact:* Dr. Robert Frisina, Jr., Professor and Graduate Program Director, 813-974-4013, Fax: 813-974-3651, E-mail: rfrisina@usf.edu. Website: http://che.eng.usf.edu/

University of South Florida, College of Pharmacy, Tampa, FL 33620-9951. Offers pharmaceutical nanotechnology (MS); pharmacy (Pharm D). *Accreditation:* ACPE. *Faculty:* 4 full-time (0 women). *Students:* 344 full-time (191 women); includes 146 minority (30 Black or African American, non-Hispanic/Latino; 53 Asian, non-Hispanic/Latino; 54 Hispanic/Latino; 3 Native Hawaiian or other Pacific Islander, non-Hispanic/Latino; 6 Two or more races, non-Hispanic/Latino). Average age 26. 678 applicants, 25% accepted, 92 enrolled. In 2015, 49 doctorates awarded. *Degree requirements:* For master's, comprehensive exam, thesis optional. *Entrance requirements:* For master's, GRE, MCAT or DAT, minimum GPA of 3.0, letters of reference, resume; for doctorate, PCAT, minimum GPA of 2.75 overall (preferred); completion of 72 prerequisite credit hours; U.S. citizenship or permanent resident. Additional exam requirements/recommendations for international students: Required—TOEFL (minimum score 550 paper-based; 79 iBT), IELTS (minimum score 6.5). *Total annual research expenditures:* $140,853. *Unit head:* Dr. Kevin Sneed, Dean, 813-974-5699, E-mail: ksneed@health.usf.edu. *Application contact:* Dr. Amy Schwartz, Associate Dean, 813-974-2251, E-mail: aschwar1@health.usf.edu.

University of South Florida, Innovative Education, Tampa, FL 33620-9951. Offers adult, career and higher education (Graduate Certificate), including college teaching, leadership in developing human resources, leadership in higher education; Africana studies (Graduate Certificate), including diasporas and health disparities, genocide and human rights; aging studies (Graduate Certificate), including gerontology; art research (Graduate Certificate), including museum studies; business foundations (Graduate Certificate); chemical and biomedical engineering (Graduate Certificate), including materials science and engineering, water, health and sustainability; child and family studies (Graduate Certificate), including positive behavior support; civil and industrial engineering (Graduate Certificate), including transportation systems analysis; community and family health (Graduate Certificate), including maternal and child health, social marketing and public health, violence and injury: prevention and intervention, women's health; criminology (Graduate Certificate), including criminal justice administration; educational measurement and research (Graduate Certificate), including evaluation; English (Graduate Certificate), including comparative literary studies, creative writing, professional and technical communication; entrepreneurship (Graduate Certificate); environmental health (Graduate Certificate), including safety management; epidemiology and biostatistics (Graduate Certificate), including applied biostatistics, biostatistics, concepts and tools of epidemiology, epidemiology, epidemiology of infectious diseases; geography, environment and planning (Graduate Certificate), including community development, environmental policy and management, geographical information systems; geology (Graduate Certificate), including hydrogeology; global health (Graduate Certificate), including disaster management,

global health and Latin American and Caribbean studies, global health practice, humanitarian assistance, infection control; government and international affairs (Graduate Certificate), including Cuban studies, globalization studies; health policy and management (Graduate Certificate), including health management and leadership, public health policy and programs; hearing specialist: early intervention (Graduate Certificate); industrial and management systems engineering (Graduate Certificate), including systems engineering, technology management; information studies (Graduate Certificate), including school library media specialist; information systems/decision sciences (Graduate Certificate), including analytics and business intelligence; instructional technology (Graduate Certificate), including distance education, Florida digital/virtual educator, instructional design, multimedia design, Web design; internal medicine, bioethics and medical humanities (Graduate Certificate), including biomedical ethics; Latin American and Caribbean studies (Graduate Certificate); mass communications (Graduate Certificate), including multimedia journalism; mathematics and statistics (Graduate Certificate), including mathematics; medicine (Graduate Certificate), including aging and neuroscience, bioinformatics, biotechnology, brain fitness and memory management, clinical investigation, health informatics, health sciences, integrative weight management, intellectual property, medicine and gender, metabolic and nutritional medicine, metabolic cardiology, pharmacy sciences; national and competitive intelligence (Graduate Certificate); psychological and social foundations (Graduate Certificate), including career counseling, college teaching, diversity in education, mental health counseling, school counseling; public affairs (Graduate Certificate), including nonprofit management, public management, research administration; public health (Graduate Certificate), including environmental health, health equity, public health generalist, translational research in adolescent behavioral health; public health practices (Graduate Certificate), including planning for healthy communities; rehabilitation and mental health counseling (Graduate Certificate), including integrative mental health care, marriage and family therapy, rehabilitation technology; secondary education (Graduate Certificate), including ESOL, foreign language education: culture and content, foreign language education: professional; social work (Graduate Certificate), including geriatric social work/clinical gerontology; special education (Graduate Certificate), including autism spectrum disorder, disabilities education: severe/profound; world languages (Graduate Certificate), including teaching English as a second language (TESL) or foreign language. *Unit head:* Kathy Barnes, Interdisciplinary Programs Coordinator, 813-974-8031, Fax: 813-974-7061, E-mail: barnesk@usf.edu. *Application contact:* Karen Tylinski, Metro Initiatives, 813-974-9943, Fax: 813-974-7061, E-mail: ktylinsk@usf.edu.
Website: http://www.usf.edu/innovative-education/

The University of Tennessee Health Science Center, College of Pharmacy, Memphis, TN 38163. Offers MS, PhD, Pharm D, Pharm D/PhD. *Accreditation:* ACPE (one or more programs are accredited). Terminal master's awarded for partial completion of doctoral program. *Degree requirements:* For master's, thesis; for doctorate, thesis/dissertation (for some programs). *Entrance requirements:* For master's, GRE; for doctorate, PCAT (for Pharm D); GRE (for PhD). Additional exam requirements/recommendations for international students: Required—TOEFL. Electronic applications accepted. *Expenses:* Contact institution. *Faculty research:* Detection and quantification of molecular entities of biological and pharmaceutical interest; design, synthesis, and biologic evaluation of new medications; quantitative assessment of drug disposition and effects using mathematical models; design, development, and evaluation of drug delivery systems.

The University of Texas at Austin, Graduate School, College of Pharmacy, Professional Program in Pharmacy, Austin, TX 78712-1111. Offers Pharm D, Pharm D/PhD. Program offered jointly with The University of Texas Health Science Center at San Antonio. *Accreditation:* ACPE. *Entrance requirements:* For doctorate, GRE General Test.

University of the Incarnate Word, Feik School of Pharmacy, San Antonio, TX 78209-6397. Offers Pharm D. *Accreditation:* ACPE. *Faculty:* 27 full-time (17 women), 1 (woman) part-time/adjunct. *Students:* 370 full-time (244 women), 14 part-time (11 women); includes 248 minority (23 Black or African American, non-Hispanic/Latino; 77 Asian, non-Hispanic/Latino; 137 Hispanic/Latino; 1 Native Hawaiian or other Pacific Islander, non-Hispanic/Latino; 10 Two or more races, non-Hispanic/Latino), 6 international. Average age 26. In 2015, 95 doctorates awarded. *Entrance requirements:* For doctorate, PCAT, 80 hours of documented pharmacy observational experience; minimum GPA of 2.5; 64 hours (71 hours for financial aid) in accredited pre-pharmacy course. Additional exam requirements/recommendations for international students: Required—TOEFL (minimum score 560 paper-based; 83 iBT). *Application deadline:* For fall admission, 12/1 for domestic and international students. Application fee: $50. Electronic applications accepted. *Expenses:* $35,500 per year; $995 per credit hour; $5,420 per clinical rotation. *Financial support:* Research assistantships, Federal Work-Study, scholarships/grants, and unspecified assistantships available. Financial award applicants required to submit FAFSA. *Unit head:* Dr. Arcelia Johnson-Fannin, Founding Dean, 210-883-1015, Fax: 210-822-1516, E-mail: johnsonf@uiwtx.edu. *Application contact:* Dr. Amy Diepenbrock, Assistant Dean, Student Affairs, 210-883-1060, Fax: 210-822-1521, E-mail: diepenbr@uiwtx.edu.
Website: http://www.uiw.edu/pharmacy

University of the Pacific, Thomas J. Long School of Pharmacy and Health Sciences, Professional Program in Pharmacy, Stockton, CA 95211-0197. Offers Pharm D. *Accreditation:* ACPE. *Entrance requirements:* Additional exam requirements/recommendations for international students: Required—TOEFL.

University of the Sciences, Philadelphia College of Pharmacy, Philadelphia, PA 19104-4495. Offers Pharm D. *Accreditation:* ACPE. *Entrance requirements:* Additional exam requirements/recommendations for international students: Required—TOEFL, TWE. *Application deadline:* For fall admission, 4/15 for domestic students; for spring admission, 10/24 for domestic students. Application fee: $50. *Financial support:* Fellowships, research assistantships, teaching assistantships, and career-related internships or fieldwork available. Support available to part-time students. Financial award application deadline: 4/15; financial award applicants required to submit FAFSA. Website: http://www.usciences.edu/academics/collegesDepts/pcp

University of Utah, Graduate School, College of Pharmacy, Professional Program in Pharmacy, Salt Lake City, UT 84112-5820. Offers Pharm D. *Accreditation:* ACPE. *Faculty:* 37 full-time (11 women), 46 part-time/adjunct (21 women). *Students:* 234 full-time (110 women), 1 part-time (0 women); includes 64 minority (2 Black or African American, non-Hispanic/Latino; 44 Asian, non-Hispanic/Latino; 11 Hispanic/Latino; 7 Two or more races, non-Hispanic/Latino), 3 international. Average age 28. 198 applicants, 39% accepted, 59 enrolled. In 2015, 58 doctorates awarded. *Entrance requirements:* For doctorate, PCAT. Additional exam requirements/recommendations for international students: Required—TOEFL (minimum score 80 iBT), IELTS (minimum score 6.5). *Application deadline:* For fall admission, 12/1 for domestic and international students. Application fee: $55 ($65 for international students). Electronic applications accepted. *Expenses:* Contact institution. *Financial support:* In 2015–16, 96 students received support, including 31 teaching assistantships (averaging $1,500 per year); Federal Work-Study, institutionally sponsored loans, and scholarships/grants also available. Financial award application deadline: 2/4; financial award applicants required

to submit FAFSA. *Faculty research:* Drug discovery, development, metabolism and toxicology; molecular and cellular neuroscience; nanomedicine; precision medicine; and outcomes research. *Total annual research expenditures:* $15.9 million. *Unit head:* Dr. James N. Herron, Executive Associate Dean for Professional Education, 801-581-6731, E-mail: james.herron@utah.edu.
Website: http://www.pharmacy.utah.edu/

University of Washington, School of Pharmacy and Graduate School, Department of Pharmacy, Seattle, WA 98195-7630. Offers biomedical regulatory affairs (MS); pharmacy (MS, PhD). *Degree requirements:* For master's, thesis; for doctorate, thesis/dissertation. *Entrance requirements:* For master's and doctorate, GRE General Test. Additional exam requirements/recommendations for international students: Required—TOEFL. Electronic applications accepted. *Faculty research:* Pharmacoeconomics, pharmacoepidemiology, drug policy, outcomes research.

University of Washington, School of Pharmacy, Professional Program in Pharmacy, Seattle, WA 98195-7631. Offers Pharm D, Pharm D/Certificate, Pharm D/MS. *Accreditation:* ACPE. *Entrance requirements:* For doctorate, PCAT. Additional exam requirements/recommendations for international students: Required—TOEFL (minimum score 100 iBT). Electronic applications accepted.

University of Wisconsin–Madison, School of Pharmacy, Professional Program in Pharmacy, Madison, WI 53706-1380. Offers Pharm D. *Accreditation:* ACPE. *Expenses:* Tuition, state resident: full-time $5364. Tuition, nonresident: full-time $12,027. *Required fees:* $571. Tuition and fees vary according to campus/location, program and reciprocity agreements.

University of Wyoming, College of Health Sciences, School of Pharmacy, Laramie, WY 82071. Offers health services administration (MS); pharmacy (Pharm D). *Accreditation:* ACPE (one or more programs are accredited). *Program availability:* Online learning. *Entrance requirements:* For doctorate, PCAT. Additional exam requirements/recommendations for international students: Required—TOEFL.

Virginia Commonwealth University, Medical College of Virginia-Professional Programs, School of Pharmacy, Professional Program in Pharmacy, Richmond, VA 23284-9005. Offers Pharm D, Pharm D/MBA, Pharm D/MPH, Pharm D/PhD. *Accreditation:* ACPE. *Program availability:* Part-time. *Degree requirements:* For doctorate, research project. *Entrance requirements:* For doctorate, PCAT. Electronic applications accepted. *Faculty research:* Oncology, cardiology, infectious diseases, epilepsy, connective tissue.

Washington State University, College of Pharmacy, Spokane, WA 99210-1495. Offers health policy and administration (MHPA); nutrition and exercise physiology (MS); pharmacy (Pharm D). Programs offered at the Spokane campus. *Accreditation:* ACPE (one or more programs are accredited). *Degree requirements:* For master's, comprehensive exam, thesis, oral exam; for doctorate, comprehensive exam, thesis/dissertation, oral exam (for PhD). *Entrance requirements:* For master's, GRE General Test, minimum GPA of 3.0, interview; for doctorate, GRE General Test, minimum GPA of 3.0, interview, minimum 60 hours of documented pharmacy experience. *Faculty research:* Hormonal carcinogenesis, drug metabolism/transport, toxicology of chlorinated compounds, alcohol effects on immune system, effects of cocaine on neuronal function.

Wayne State University, Eugene Applebaum College of Pharmacy and Health Sciences, Department of Pharmaceutical Sciences, Detroit, MI 48202. Offers medicinal chemistry (MS, PhD); pharmaceutics (MS, PhD), including medicinal chemistry (PhD); pharmacology/toxicology (MS, PhD). *Accreditation:* ACPE (one or more programs are accredited). *Faculty:* 17 full-time (3 women). *Students:* 26 full-time (14 women), 3 part-time (1 woman); includes 3 minority (1 Black or African American, non-Hispanic/Latino; 1 American Indian or Alaska Native, non-Hispanic/Latino; 1 Asian, non-Hispanic/Latino), 23 international. Average age 26. 184 applicants, 15% accepted, 10 enrolled. In 2015, 9 master's, 102 doctorates awarded. *Degree requirements:* For master's, thesis; for doctorate, thesis/dissertation. *Entrance requirements:* For master's, GRE General Test, bachelor's degree; adequate background in biology, physics, calculus, and chemistry; three letters of recommendation; personal statement; for doctorate, GRE General Test, bachelor's or master's degree in one of the behavioral, biological, pharmaceutical or physical sciences; three letters of recommendation. Additional exam requirements/recommendations for international students: Required—TOEFL (minimum score 550 paper-based; 79 iBT), Michigan English Language Assessment Battery (minimum score 85); Recommended—IELTS (minimum score 6.5), TWE (minimum score 5.5). *Application deadline:* For fall admission, 12/1 priority date for domestic and international students. Applications are processed on a rolling basis. Application fee: $0. Electronic applications accepted. *Expenses:* $16,104 per year resident tuition; $32,401 non-resident tuition; $671 per credit hour resident tuition, $1,350.05 per credit hour non-resident tuition; fees include $47.45 per credit hour student services fee and $274.60 per semester registration fee. *Financial support:* In 2015–16, 15 students received support, including 2 fellowships with tuition reimbursements available (averaging $24,179 per year), 10 research assistantships with full tuition reimbursements available (averaging $24,595 per year); teaching assistantships, scholarships/grants, health care benefits, and unspecified assistantships also available. Financial award application deadline: 3/31; financial award applicants required to submit FAFSA. *Faculty research:* Design of new anthracyclines, genetic and epigenetic effects of extracellular inducers, cellular injury and cell death, drug metabolism and nutrition, anti-infective agents, carcinogenesis, diabetes research, theragnostic nanomedicines, neurotoxicity, drug discovery, insulin resistance. *Unit head:* Dr. George Corcoran, Chair and Professor, 313-577-1737, E-mail: corcoran@wayne.edu. *Application contact:* 313-577-5415, Fax: 313-577-2033, E-mail: pscgrad@wayne.edu.
Website: http://cphs.wayne.edu/sciences/index.php

Wayne State University, Eugene Applebaum College of Pharmacy and Health Sciences, Doctor of Pharmacy Program, Detroit, MI 48202. Offers Pharm D, Pharm D/PhD. *Faculty:* 26 full-time (16 women), 1 part-time/adjunct (0 women). *Students:* 360 full-time (214 women), 25 part-time (17 women); includes 58 minority (4 Black or African American, non-Hispanic/Latino; 1 American Indian or Alaska Native, non-Hispanic/Latino; 47 Asian, non-Hispanic/Latino; 3 Hispanic/Latino; 3 Two or more races, non-Hispanic/Latino), 26 international. Average age 24. 335 applicants, 41% accepted, 99 enrolled. In 2015, 102 doctorates awarded. *Entrance requirements:* For doctorate, PCAT, PharmCAS application, interview, criminal background check, minimum GPA of 3.0 in required preprofessional courses and overall, work experience, community service, leadership abilities. Additional exam requirements/recommendations for international students: Required—TOEFL (minimum score 550 paper-based; 79 iBT), Michigan English Language Assessment Battery (minimum score 85); Recommended—IELTS (minimum score 6.5), TWE (minimum score 5.5). *Application deadline:* For fall admission, 11/1 for domestic and international students. Electronic applications accepted. *Expenses:* $20,801 per year resident tuition; $41,852 non-resident tuition; $671 per credit hour resident tuition, $1,350.05 per credit hour non-resident tuition; fees include $47.45 per credit hour student services fee and $274.60 per semester registration fee. *Financial support:* In 2015–16, 103 students received support. Scholarships/grants available. Financial award application deadline: 3/31; financial award applicants required to submit FAFSA. *Unit head:* Dr. Brian L. Crabtree, Chair and

Pharmacy

Professor, 313-577-0824, E-mail: brian.crabtree@wayne.edu. *Application contact:* 313-577-6823, E-mail: cphsinfo@wayne.edu.
Website: http://cphs.wayne.edu/practice/pharmd.php

West Coast University, Graduate Programs, North Hollywood, CA 91606. Offers advanced generalist (MSN); family nurse practitioner (MSN); health administration (MHA); occupational therapy (MS); pharmacy (Pharm D); physical therapy (DPT).

Western New England University, College of Pharmacy, Springfield, MA 01119. Offers Pharm D, Pharm D/MBA. *Accreditation:* ACPE. *Faculty:* 29 full-time (13 women), 2 part-time/adjunct (both women). *Students:* 297 full-time (178 women); includes 41 minority (8 Black or African American, non-Hispanic/Latino; 26 Asian, non-Hispanic/Latino; 7 Hispanic/Latino), 3 international. Average age 24. 397 applicants, 34% accepted, 75 enrolled. In 2015, 68 doctorates awarded. *Entrance requirements:* For doctorate, PCAT, PharmCAS application, college transcripts, two letters of recommendation. Additional exam requirements/recommendations for international students: Required—TOEFL (minimum score 80 iBT). *Application deadline:* For fall admission, 3/1 for domestic students. Applications are processed on a rolling basis. Application fee: $150. Electronic applications accepted. *Expenses:* $39,060 tuition per year; $2,246 fees per year. *Financial support:* Scholarships/grants available. Financial award application deadline: 4/15; financial award applicants required to submit FAFSA. *Unit head:* Dr. Evan T. Robinson, Dean, 413-796-2323, E-mail: erobinson@wne.edu. *Application contact:* Bonnie Mannix, Director of Pharmacy Admissions and Recruitment, 413-796-2300, Fax: 413-796-2266, E-mail: rxadmissions@wne.edu.
Website: http://www1.wne.edu/pharmacy/index.cfm?selection-doc.8399

Western University of Health Sciences, College of Pharmacy, Program in Pharmacy, Pomona, CA 91766-1854. Offers Pharm D. *Accreditation:* ACPE. *Faculty:* 26 full-time (12 women). *Students:* 514 full-time (350 women); includes 353 minority (16 Black or African American, non-Hispanic/Latino; 1 American Indian or Alaska Native, non-Hispanic/Latino; 282 Asian, non-Hispanic/Latino; 30 Hispanic/Latino; 24 Two or more races, non-Hispanic/Latino), 13 international. Average age 28. 1,205 applicants, 28% accepted, 128 enrolled. In 2015, 137 doctorates awarded. *Degree requirements:* For doctorate, comprehensive exam (for some programs). *Entrance requirements:* For doctorate, minimum GPA of 2.75, interview, letters of recommendation; BS in pharmacy or equivalent (recommended). Additional exam requirements/recommendations for international students: Required—TOEFL (minimum score 79 iBT). *Application deadline:* For fall admission, 9/8 priority date for domestic and international students. Application fee: $65. Electronic applications accepted. *Expenses:* $47,405 tuition; $40 fees. *Financial support:* Scholarships/grants available. Financial award application deadline: 3/2; financial award applicants required to submit FAFSA. *Unit head:* Dr. Daniel Robinson, Dean, 909-469-5533, Fax: 909-469-5539, E-mail: drobinson@westernu.edu. *Application contact:* Kathryn Ford, Admission Director, 909-469-5335, Fax: 909-469-5570, E-mail: admissions@westernu.edu.
Website: http://www.westernu.edu/pharmacy-dpp_message

West Virginia University, School of Pharmacy, Professional Program in Pharmacy, Morgantown, WV 26506. Offers clinical pharmacy (Pharm D). Students enter program as undergraduates. *Accreditation:* ACPE. *Degree requirements:* For doctorate, 100 hours of community service. *Entrance requirements:* For doctorate, PCAT, minimum GPA of 3.1. Electronic applications accepted. *Expenses:* Tuition, state resident: full-time $8568. Tuition, nonresident: full-time $22,140. Tuition and fees vary according to program.

West Virginia University, School of Pharmacy, Program in Pharmaceutical and Pharmacological Sciences, Morgantown, WV 26506. Offers administrative pharmacy (PhD); behavioral pharmacy (MS, PhD); biopharmaceutics/pharmacokinetics (MS, PhD); industrial pharmacy (MS); medicinal chemistry (MS, PhD); pharmaceutical chemistry (MS, PhD); pharmaceutics (MS, PhD); pharmacology and toxicology (MS); pharmacy (MS); pharmacy administration (MS). *Program availability:* Part-time. Terminal master's awarded for partial completion of doctoral program. *Degree requirements:* For master's, thesis; for doctorate, one foreign language, comprehensive exam, thesis/dissertation. *Entrance requirements:* For master's and doctorate, GRE General Test, minimum GPA of 2.75. Additional exam requirements/recommendations for international students: Required—TOEFL; Recommended—TWE. Electronic applications accepted. *Application contact:* Contact institution. *Faculty research:* Pharmaceutics, medicinal chemistry, biopharmaceutics/pharmacokinetics, health outcomes research.

Wilkes University, College of Graduate and Professional Studies, Nesbitt School of Pharmacy, Wilkes-Barre, PA 18766-0002. Offers Pharm D. *Accreditation:* ACPE. *Program availability:* Part-time, evening/weekend. *Students:* 284 full-time (179 women), 1 part-time (0 women); includes 25 minority (4 Black or African American, non-Hispanic/Latino; 7 Asian, non-Hispanic/Latino; 6 Hispanic/Latino; 8 Two or more races, non-Hispanic/Latino), 1 international. Average age 23. In 2015, 71 doctorates awarded. *Entrance requirements:* Additional exam requirements/recommendations for international students: Required—TOEFL (minimum score 79 iBT). *Application deadline:* Applications are processed on a rolling basis. *Expenses:* Contact institution. *Financial support:* Federal Work-Study and unspecified assistantships available. Financial award application deadline: 3/1; financial award applicants required to submit FAFSA. *Unit head:* Dr. Bernard Graham, Dean, 570-408-4280, Fax: 570-408-7828, E-mail: bernard.graham@wilkes.edu. *Application contact:* Joanne Thomas, Director of Graduate Enrollment, 570-408-4234, Fax: 570-408-7846, E-mail: joanne.thomas1@wilkes.edu.
Website: http://www.wilkes.edu/academics/colleges/nesbitt-college-of-pharmacy/index.aspx

Wingate University, School of Pharmacy, Wingate, NC 28174. Offers Pharm D. *Accreditation:* ACPE. *Degree requirements:* For doctorate, comprehensive exam. *Entrance requirements:* For doctorate, PCAT. Electronic applications accepted. *Expenses:* Contact institution. *Faculty research:* Stress response in aging, arthritis therapy educational processes, professional development, sarcopenia in aging, geriatric-psych drug therapy.

Xavier University of Louisiana, College of Pharmacy, New Orleans, LA 70125-1098. Offers Pharm D. *Accreditation:* ACPE. *Entrance requirements:* Additional exam requirements/recommendations for international students: Required—TOEFL. Electronic applications accepted. *Expenses:* Contact institution.

NOVA SOUTHEASTERN UNIVERSITY
College of Pharmacy

Programs of Study

Nova Southeastern University (NSU) offers an innovative program of graduate study and research leading to the Doctor of Philosophy degree (Ph.D.). Students can choose to pursue the Ph.D. degree in one of three distinct sequences: Molecular Medicine and Pharmacogenomics (Drug Discovery), Drug Development (Pharmaceutics), or Social and Administrative Pharmacy (Determinants of Drug Use). Typically, the first year of study involves course work and rotations through several research laboratories. Upon completion of the first year, students will select their major adviser. During the second years, area-specific course work will be taken and the student will begin their research. The third and subsequent years are largely devoted to research. A variety of research areas are available including cancer research, neuroscience, cardiovascular research, and novel drug delivery systems.

At the completion of the Ph.D. sequences, students are able to demonstrate the knowledge base expected at the Ph.D. level in a pharmacy specialty; design and conduct independent research that adds to the understanding of their pharmacy specialty; prepare and defend rational and structured proposals seeking support for research efforts; and prepare and present lucid reports on their own research.

Programs in the College of Pharmacy (COP) are taught primarily by multilingual, multicultural, full-time faculty members. Clinical and applied research is delivered at sites in Fort Lauderdale and Palm Beach, Florida, and San Juan, Puerto Rico. Both live and online lectures are used.

Research Facilities

The research laboratories in the COP occupy approximately 3,000 square feet of the Library/Research Building in the Health Professions Division (HPD). Each individual laboratory space ranges from 300 to 750 square feet and is equipped with general biochemistry and/or tissue culture equipment. Some laboratories include specialized equipment for pharmaceutical preparations, radioligand binding assays, molecular biological applications, and proteomics applications. There are also common laboratory facilities for shared equipment. Two FluorChem E digital darkroom systems are available for use, along with a fully equipped darkroom and a fully equipped laboratory designed for studies using radioactive materials. All common use laboratories are located in close proximity to the College of Pharmacy laboratories and are fully accessible to all HPD researchers. Additional research lab space will become available in 2016 with the planned opening of the Center for Collaborative Research (CCR).

The animal facility is located within the research facilities of the Library/Laboratory Building and it complies with the minimum standards for use of rats and mice. The College of Pharmacy also has access to an OLAW approved animal facility at the Rumbaugh-Goodwin Institute for Cancer Research (RGICR), located near the main campus. This facility has two holding rooms to house rodents and separate cage wash and storage areas. The RGICR animal facility is maintained by a full-time caretaker who also oversees the animal rooms in the HPD Library and Research Building. Both facilities are governed by an Institutional Animal Care and Use Committee (IACUC). The RGICR facility is fully compliant with OLAW standards and is available for use by all NSU researchers. A consulting veterinarian is responsible for oversight of the health of animals in both facilities.

NSU maintains an extensive information technology network for teaching, learning, research, and administrative computing. Comprehensive fiber-optic and wireless networks provide connectivity for user access. A dedicated wide area network (WAN) supports high-speed connections from all campuses. The research facility has computers for data collection, processing, and analysis. COP researchers all have access to modern computers in their offices as well as in their laboratories, equipped with the necessary software for word processing, routine data analysis, and photo processing. Researchers also have easy access to NSU's four computer labs that house more than 200 Pentium 200 MHz PCs with ready access to the Internet and Ovid online database. When the CCR opens in 2016, researchers will have access to a supercomputer (IBM Power 8 Supercomputer).

Financial Aid

Top candidates are eligible for scholarships, which consist of a tuition waiver and teaching assistantships. Non-scholarship students can apply for a variety of loans.

Cost of Study

Tuition for 2016–17 is $26,265 (subject to change by the board of trustees without notice). An HPD general access fee of $145 is required each year. An NSU student services fee of $1,050 is also required annually.

Living and Housing Costs

The Rolling Hills Graduate Apartments, are about 1 mile west of the NSU main campus and offer housing for approximately 373 students. Rooms are fully furnished and include a kitchen, bathroom, and living room. Married housing is also available. Costs range from $3,390 to $6,513 per semester or from $8,165 to $15,691 for a twelve-month contract. Unlimited laundry, NSU-secured wi-fi, furnishings, utilities, air conditioning, cable TV, and local telephone service are included. More information about student housing is available at http://www.nova.edu/housing/.

Student Group

The current enrollment in all three sequences is approximately 50 students and roughly 96 percent of these students have scholarships or fellowships. The student population is comprised of about 20 percent women and about 80 percent are international students. The desired background of students is a degree in pharmacy or areas related to one of the three sequences.

Student Outcomes

Graduates of the program are prepared for employment by the pharmaceutical industry, governmental regulatory agencies, biomedical sciences profession, and academic positions. Most of the graduates from the Ph.D. program have or expect to obtain academic positions.

Location

Davie, a city of more than 95,000, maintains a sense of small-town intimacy while located near both an international airport and a seaport. The area is famous for its wide expanses of sandy beaches and its tropical climate. Nearby Fort Lauderdale is home to numerous museums, art galleries, and a performing arts center.

The College of Pharmacy also has branch campuses in Palm Beach, Florida and San Juan, Puerto Rico.

The University

Founded in 1964 as Nova University, the institution merged with Southeastern University of the Health Sciences in 1994, creating Nova Southeastern University. NSU offers a wide range of undergraduate, graduate, and professional degree programs to more than 29,000 students every year. It is the seventh-largest independent institution in the nation and the largest independent not-for-profit university in the Southeast. NSU is experiencing a sustained period of academic and fiscal growth and is committed to preparing students to meet the challenges of the twenty-first century.

Applying

Application materials that must be submitted include GRE results (NSU code 5522), proof of proficiency in English, transcripts received directly from the degree-granting institution (international applicants must have course work evaluated by World Education Services, Josef Silney & Associates, or Educational Credential Evaluators, Inc.), a formal application form, three letters of reference, and a brief written essay on the goals of the applicant.

Applications and a $50 nonrefundable fee must be submitted to Enrollment Processing Services (EPS), College of Pharmacy, Office of Admissions, 3301 College Ave, P.O. Box 299000, Ft. Lauderdale, Florida 33329-9905 prior to March 1. Applicants may also have an application mailed to them upon request.

Correspondence and Information

Dr. Peter M. Gannett
Associate Dean, Research and Graduate Education
Health Professions Division
College of Pharmacy
Nova Southeastern University
3200 South University Drive
Fort Lauderdale, Florida 33328
United States
E-mail: copphd@nova.edu

Health Professions Admissions Office
Attention: Thomas Bouchard, Jr.
Nova Southeastern University
Phone: 954-262-1112
        877-640-0218 (toll-free)
Website: http://www.nova.edu

Nova Southeastern University

THE FACULTY AND THEIR RESEARCH

Drug Development and Molecular Medicine and Pharmacogenomics (Drug Discovery) Sequences

Michelle A. Clark, Interim Associate Dean, Research and Graduate Education; Associate Professor and Chairperson, Department of Pharmaceutical Sciences; Ph.D., South Florida, 1996. Central signaling pathways for blood pressure regulation and control, role of the central renin angiotensin system in the regulation of cardiovascular and other diseases.

Rais A. Ansari, Assistant Professor, Pharmaceutical Sciences; Ph.D., Kanpur (India), 1985. Mechanism of alcohol-mediated hypertension, transcriptional regulation of human angiotensinogen gene after ethanol and environmental toxicants exposure.

Ana Maria Castejon, Associate Professor, Pharmaceutical Sciences; Ph.D., Central University (Venezuela), 1997. Oxidative stress and autism, diabetes mellitus, effects of statins in vascular smooth muscle cells, genetics of salt sensitivity in human subjects.

Luigi Cubeddu, Professor, Pharmaceutical Sciences; M.D., Central University (Venezuela); Ph.D., Colorado. Mechanisms and treatment of hypertension associated with obesity, salt-sensitive hypertension, early detection of insulin resistance and abnormalities in glucose metabolism, statin withdrawal syndrome.

Richard C. Deth, Professor, Pharmaceutical Sciences, Ph.D., Miami (Florida), 1975. Role of redox and methylation status in neurodevelopmental disorders.

Young M. Kwon, Assistant Professor, Pharmaceutical Sciences, Ph.D., Utah, 2003. Targeted delivery and triggered release system for therapeutic macromolecules; bioconjugate chemistry and PEGylation; nonviral gene carriers and intracellular drug delivery; protein stability and release from biodegradable polymer.

Jean J. Latimer, Associate Professor, Pharmaceutical Sciences; Ph.D., Buffalo, SUNY, 1989. Loss of DNA repair as causative factor in cancer formation; breast tissue engineering; ancestral disparity in breast cancer development and pharmacogenomics; drug resistance (via cancer stem cells) in childhood leukemia.

Anastasios Lymperopoulos, Assistant Professor, Pharmaceutical Sciences; Ph.D., Patras (Greece), 2004. Cardiovascular biology/pharmacology and gene therapy, with a focus on adrenergic system regulation in heart failure; novel roles of G-protein coupled receptor kinases and their cofactors, beta-arrestins, in regulation of various important cardiovascular G-protein coupled receptors; roles of G-protein coupled receptor kinases and their cofactors, beta-arrestins, in adrenal gland physiology and biology.

David J. Mastropietro, Assistant Professor, Pharmaceutical Sciences; Ph.D., Nova Southeastern, 2014. Formulation and laboratory assessment of abuse deterrent pharmaceutical dosage forms, personalized medicine through the art and science of pharmacy compounding.

Enrique A. Nieves, Assistant Professor, Pharmaceutical Sciences; Ph.D., Florida, 1982. Applications of nanotechnology in drug product development and pharmaceutical process designs, development of co-excipients for improved drug formulations, nanotechnology applications in the extraction and isolation of new drugs from natural sources.

Hamid Omidian, Associate Professor, Pharmaceutical Sciences; Ph.D., Brunel (London), 1997. Hydrogels for pharmaceutical and biomedical applications, hydrogel-based controlled delivery systems and technologies, hydrogel-based gastroretentive drug delivery platforms, hydrogel-based platforms for cell culture and proliferation.

Mutasem Rawas-Qalaji, Associate Professor, Pharmaceutical Sciences; Ph.D., Manitoba (Canada), 2006. Enhancing the permeability and the relative bioavailability of poorly absorbed drugs by nanotechnology, formulation and delivery of drug-loaded nanoparticles through noninvasive and user-friendly routes of administration, formulation and evaluation of sublingual ODT tablets as an alternative noninvasive dosage form.

Syed A. A. Rizvi, Assistant Professor, Pharmaceutical Sciences; Ph.D., Mercer, 2010. Cocrystallization and formulation strategies for low bioavailability drugs; micellar electrokinetic chromatography.

Robert C. Speth, Professor, Pharmaceutical Sciences; Ph.D., Vanderbilt, 1976. Brain renin-angiotensin system pharmacology and functionality.

Malav S. Trivedi, Assistant Professor, Pharmaceutical Sciences, Ph.D., Northeastern, 2013. Investigating the effect of environmental insults and dietary interventions on nuclear and mitochondrial epigenetic changes, and characterizing its contribution in neurodevelopmental and neurodegenerative diseases as well as tumor biology and drug targeting.

Social and Administrative Pharmacy (Determinants of Drug Use) Sequence

Barry A. Bleidt, Professor, Sociobehavioral and Administrative Pharmacy; Pharm.D., Xavier of Louisiana, 1994; Ph.D., Florida, 1982. Cultural competency/diversity/health disparities; assessment of student achievement; faculty workload and performance measures; peer teaching evaluation strategies; Internet, technology and medical information; and pharmacoeconomics.

Manuel J. Carvajal, Professor and Chairperson, Department of Sociobehavioral and Administrative Pharmacy; Ph.D., Florida, 1974. Applied econometrics geared to problem solving; various areas of human capital including fertility, migration, poverty, and discrimination; gender and ethnic differences in labor market outcomes and job satisfaction.

Catherine A. Harrington, Associate Professor, Sociobehavioral and Administrative Pharmacy; Ph.D., Michigan, 1993; Pharm.D., Michigan, 1987. Developing databases and information systems that assist in evaluation of drug therapy, use of meta-analysis techniques to obtain evidence from literature.

Nile M. Khanfar, Assistant Professor, Sociobehavioral and Administrative Pharmacy; Ph.D., Louisiana at Monroe, 2005; M.B.A., Louisiana at Monroe, 2001. Management leadership, strategic management/ marketing business cases, direct-to-consumer advertising of prescription medication and its influence on consumer behavior.

L. Leanne Lai, Professor, Sociobehavioral and Administrative Pharmacy; Ph.D., Maryland, Baltimore, 1996. Pharmacoeconomics and outcomes research, pharmacoepidemiology and secondary data analysis, international education.

Ioana Popovici, Assistant Professor, Sociobehavioral and Administrative Pharmacy; Ph.D., Florida International, 2007. Economic evaluation of substance abuse treatment interventions, relationship between addictive substance use or abuse and its economic consequences.

Sylvia E. Rabionet, Associate Professor, Sociobehavioral and Administrative Pharmacy; Ed.D., Harvard, 2002. Health disparities, public health issues.

Jesus Sanchez, Assistant Professor, Sociobehavioral and Administrative Pharmacy; Ph.D., Miami (Florida), 2001. HIV reduction among high-risk migrant workers; building capacity and infrastructure in the migrant farm worker communities in South Florida; prevalence of HIV, hepatitis B and C, and associated risk factors among Hispanic injection drug users.

Georgina Silva-Suárez, Assistant Professor, Sociobehavioral and Administrative Pharmacy; Ph.D., Florida International, 2014. Adherence to ART, HIV prevention, adolescent health, human sexuality and sex education.

PHILADELPHIA COLLEGE OF OSTEOPATHIC MEDICINE

School of Pharmacy–Georgia Campus

 For more information, visit http://petersons.to/pcompharmacygeorgia

Program of Study

The Philadelphia College of Osteopathic Medicine (PCOM) School of Pharmacy–Georgia Campus offers a four-year Doctor of Pharmacy (Pharm.D.) degree program. The program prepares generalist, entry-level pharmacists capable of delivering high-quality pharmaceutical care. The PCOM School of Pharmacy–Georgia Campus's mission is to educate caring, proactive pharmacists according to a model of patient-centered care, a practice of pharmacy in which the practitioner assumes responsibility for a patient's medication-related needs and is held accountable for this commitment.

While preparing pharmacy practitioners is the primary mission of the Pharm.D. program, it also provides an avenue by which students may explore a broad range of career opportunities. The program is designed to prepare a well-rounded student who is able to practice in many areas of pharmacy. The program also aspires to develop analytical and life-long learning skills to help students excel after graduation in the rapidly changing and evolving field of health care. Each student in the program is assigned to a group of peers for team- and case-based learning to foster team-building skills in clinical case discussions. Each student is also assigned a faculty adviser to assist with their academic needs and guide them as they progress through the curriculum and prepare for a career in pharmacy.

Research Facilities and Library Resources

Georgia Campus–Philadelphia College of Osteopathic Medicine (GA–PCOM) features teaching and research laboratories, and an Information Commons which integrates library and student computer lab functions.

Faculty members conduct research in basic, clinical, and administrative sciences, sharing their experience and scholarly expertise with students. GA–PCOM has more than 6,500 square feet of research space in addition to an animal-care facility research laboratory that houses shared common equipment such as -80° C freezers and centrifuges. There are multiple storage spaces outside of the labs for supplies and areas that store cell culture equipment and laboratory gases.

The PCOM Digital Library provides access to a wealth of licensed Internet resources, including over 10,000 full-text e-journals, electronic textbooks, bibliographic databases, streaming videos, clinical simulations, diagnostic decision support programs, and evidence-based clinical information systems, as well as subject access to selected Internet resources. Print subscriptions to a number of core journals are also available in the Information Commons. The PCOM library electronically provides articles from any print-only titles in its collection to GA–PCOM users. GA–PCOM and the School of Pharmacy are committed to the advancement of knowledge and intellectual growth through teaching and research, and to the well-being of the community through leadership and service.

Financial Aid

GA–PCOM's Office of Financial Aid provides comprehensive assistance to all admitted students. Financial assistance can be provided through the Federal Direct Loan program, institutional grants, and various alternative private loan programs.

Cost of Study

Tuition and fees for the Pharm.D. program for the 2016–17 academic year are $37,278.

Living and Housing Costs

Suwanee and the neighboring communities of Lawrenceville and Duluth offer a less hurried lifestyle with an abundance of amenities and easy access to all Atlanta has to offer: shopping, professional sports, the arts, and more. There is no on-campus housing so students live off-campus. Room and board costs vary based on each student's arrangements.

Student Group

PCOM School of Pharmacy–Georgia Campus enrolled 79 students in its inaugural class in August, 2010. For the 2015–16 academic year, the School of Pharmacy enrolled 103 new students with a diverse cultural makeup. Current enrollment projections call for approximately 100 new students to be admitted to the Pharm.D. program each year.

Location

The GA–PCOM campus is located in Gwinnett County, approximately 30 minutes north of Atlanta. A welcoming community with a nationally recognized public school system, an award-winning parks and recreation department, and ample entertainment options, Gwinnett is home to a minor league sports team, and numerous shopping and dining opportunities. The campus is close to a myriad of outdoor recreational opportunities, including Stone Mountain Park, the North Georgia mountains, and scenic Lake Lanier which offers boating, fishing, water parks, canoeing, and horseback riding.

The College

PCOM is one of the largest of 30 osteopathic colleges in the United States, with campuses in Philadelphia and suburban Atlanta. GA–PCOM was chartered in 2005, and is committed to educating responsive medical professionals prepared to practice in the 21st century. Supported by advanced medical and educational technology, Georgia Campus shares the PCOM mission and also seeks to improve the quality of life for residents of Georgia and the Southeast by preparing healthcare practitioners and professionals to address the social, economic, and healthcare needs of the region. Since joining the established community of students, faculty, and staff in Georgia in 2010, the School of Pharmacy's focus has been to train students for entry-level careers with the right combination of skills, knowledge, and attitudes to develop and grow in the ever-changing field.

Applying

Admission to the Pharm.D. program is competitive and selective. Students are evaluated on a variety of criteria. Academic performance in science courses, as well as overall academic performance as determined by grade point average (GPA), are the major criteria used by the Admissions Committee. Competitive scores on the Pharmacy College Admissions Test (PCAT) are also considered. Professional preparedness, motivation, decision-making skills, and written and verbal communication skills are also evaluated. Prior degrees earned and previous pharmacy-related

Philadelphia College of Osteopathic Medicine

work experiences are additional considerations. Qualified applicants who have satisfactorily completed all prerequisite coursework, but have not earned a bachelor's degree can apply and enroll at PCOM School of Pharmacy–Georgia Campus. Qualified applicants may also apply and be offered admission without having completed all prerequisite course work. However, all applicants must successfully complete prerequisite coursework before matriculating to the School of Pharmacy. Note also, that while a bachelor's degree is not required, the Admissions Committee gives preference to those students who have earned a bachelor's degree.

PCOM School of Pharmacy–Georgia Campus participates in the PharmCAS application service (http://www.pharmcas.org). The School participates in the Early Decision program, with a primary application deadline in early September. The application deadline for regular decision candidates is early March. Supplemental applications are due in early April.

Prospective students can find additional information about the application process, including prerequisite coursework requirements, at http://admissions.pcom.edu/app-process/pharmacy-pharmd/.

Correspondence and Information

Office of Admissions
Georgia Campus–Philadelphia College of Osteopathic Medicine
625 Old Peachtree Road NW
Suwanee, Georgia 30024
Phone: 678-225-7500
          866-282-4544 (toll-free)
Fax: 678-225-7509
E-mail: pharmdadmissions@pcom.edu
Website: http://www.pcom.edu
Twitter: @PCOMAdmissions

THE FACULTY

Shari Allen, Pharm.D., Assistant Professor of Pharmacy Practice.
Yun Bai, Ph.D., Assistant Professor of Pharmaceutical Sciences.
Vishakha Bhave, Ph.D., Assistant Professor of Pharmaceutical Sciences.
Drew Cates, Pharm.D., Assistant Professor of Pharmacy Practice.
Caroline Champion, Pharm.D., Assistant Professor of Pharmacy Practice.
Jennifer Elliot, Pharm.D., Assistant Professor of Pharmacy Practice.
Naushad Khan Ghilzai, Ph.D., Associate Dean for Academics and Assessment, Professor of Pharmaceutical Sciences.
Adina Hirsch, Pharm.D., Assistant Professor of Pharmacy Practice.
Christopher (Shawn) Holaway, Pharm.D., Assistant Professor of Pharmacy Practice.
Yue-Qiao (George) Huang, Ph.D., Assistant Professor of Pharmaceutical Sciences.
Samuel M. John, Pharm.D., Assistant Professor of Pharmacy Practice.
Michael Lee, Ph.D., Assistant Dean of Professional and Student Affairs, Associate Professor of Pharmaceutical Sciences.
Dusty Lisi, Pharm.D., Assistant Professor of Pharmacy Practice.
Edo-abasi McGee, Pharm.D., Assistant Professor of Pharmacy Practice.
Candis McGraw, Pharm.D., Assistant Professor of Pharmacy Practice.
Vicky Mody, Ph.D., Associate Professor of Pharmaceutical Sciences.
Amanda Naujelis, Pharm.D., Assistant Professor of Pharmacy Practice.
Mark Okamoto, Pharm.D., Dean & Chief Academic Officer, Professor of Pharmacy.

Harish S. Parihar, R.Ph., Ph.D., Associate Professor of Pharmacy Practice.
Sonia Patel, Pharm.D., Assistant Professor of Pharmacy Practice.
Srujana Rayalam, Ph.D., Assistant Professor of Pharmaceutical Sciences.
Mandy Reece, Pharm.D., BC-ADM, CDE, Associate Professor of Pharmacy Practice.
Brent Rollins, R.Ph., Ph.D., Assistant Professor of Pharmacy Administration.
Rangaiah Shashidharamurthy, Ph.D., Assistant Professor of Pharmaceutical Sciences.
Avadhesh C. Sharma, Pharm.D., Ph.D., Chair and Professor, Department of Pharmaceutical Science.
Gregory Smallwood, Pharm.D., Chair and Associate Professor, Department of Pharmacy Practice.
LeAnne Honeycutt Varner, Pharm.D., Clinical Coordinator of Experiential Education, Assistant Professor of Pharmacy Practice.
Desuo Wang, Ph.D., Associate Professor of Pharmaceutical Sciences.
Xinyu (Eric) Wang, Ph.D., Assistant Professor of Pharmaceutical Sciences.
Julie Wickman, Pharm.D., Assistant Dean for Experiential Education, Associate Professor of Pharmacy Practice.
Zhiqian (James) Wu, Ph.D., Associate Professor of Pharmaceutical Sciences.

The PCOM School of Pharmacy–Georgia Campus provides students with a collaborative learning environment.

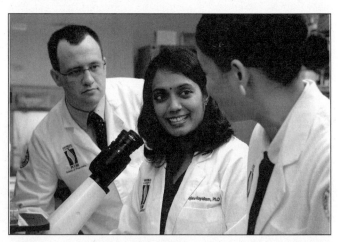

Pharmacy students learn pharmaceutical and clinical skills in modern lab facilities.

ST. LOUIS COLLEGE OF PHARMACY
Doctor of Pharmacy (Pharm.D.) Program

 For more information, visit http://petersons.to/slcp-grad

Program of Study

The St. Louis College of Pharmacy's (STLCOP) academic program includes three years of undergraduate work followed by a four-year professional program leading to a Doctor of Pharmacy (Pharm.D.) degree with an integrated Bachelor of Science degree. The curriculum prepares students to take on the expanding role of pharmacists on patient-centered, health care teams and includes significant preparation in the sciences. The program provides an innovative teaching model, which integrates course work across foundational subject areas to improve learning and advance patient care. Students can also incorporate specialty areas into their studies to help prepare them for a wide range of career options available to pharmacists.

Students are primarily admitted directly from high school, and, after three years of undergraduate coursework, advance into the professional program without additional testing (provided all progression requirements are met). Transfer opportunities are also available during the undergraduate and first professional years.

The College's Doctor of Pharmacy (Pharm.D.) program prepares students for the expanding role of pharmacists in patient-centered, interprofessional health care teams. STLCOP is one of only a few colleges of pharmacy to use an innovative organ-based model in the curriculum, where students learn about each organ system in the body. Students apply their interprofessional skills and knowledge in state-of-the-art labs and during patient-care experiences in a variety of real-world practice settings. At the College, students are enabled to take on a vital role in today's health care industry.

After graduation, many pursue a career in a variety of health care professions or a pharmacy residency program. Residents at the College receive additional experience and specialization while opening doors to new career paths and opportunities.

During the final year of the curriculum, students complete eight, five-week rotations and have the opportunity to gain first-hand experience in hospitals, outpatient HIV/AIDS clinics, develop pharmacy assistant programs, or choose from more than 600 other settings. Settings have included the U.S. Food and Drug Administration, Pfizer, Walgreens, Bristol-Myers Squibb, Alaska Native Medical Center, North Texas Medical Center and Tampa General Hospital. In each of these settings and in many of their electives/specialty rotations, student pharmacists work closely with others to provide health care services as part of an interprofessional team.

St. Louis College of Pharmacy students have the opportunity to participate in Advanced Pharmacy Practice Experiences (APPE) and international programs in 15 different countries.

Through the international service learning courses students have given many hours of service in countries such as Costa Rica, Guatemala, Poland, Romania and Macedonia. Students also volunteer in the local community each year for events such as the College's Asthma-Friendly Pharmacies program, the St. Louis Medication Disposal Initiative, and Boo Fest, a sugar-free Halloween event for children with Type 1 diabetes and their families.

Research Opportunities

St. Louis College of Pharmacy's location in one of the world's preeminent medical centers offers unparalleled opportunities for research and collaboration. Its location among Washington University School of Medicine, Barnes-Jewish Hospital, St. Louis Children's Hospital, and Siteman Cancer Center is a setting that few colleges of pharmacy can rival. The College is involved in education, research, and practice programs with all of its neighboring institutions, and collaborates with them to advance health care in St. Louis and around the world. Faculty and students are involved in several College research centers and initiatives.

Among STLCOP's newest research centers, The Center for Clinical Pharmacology is housed on the sixth floor of the new Academic and Research Building. It was established in collaboration with Washington University School of Medicine in St. Louis' Department of Anesthesiology and is Washington University's first shared research center with another higher education institution. The center will bring together resources and researchers to deepen the understanding of the mechanisms of action of drugs and identify strategies for the development and application of new treatments.

The Center for Interprofessional Education (CIPE) creates opportunities for St. Louis College of Pharmacy students to serve on interprofessional, patient-centered health care teams from Washington University School of Medicine and Goldfarb School of Nursing. The center also provides professional development opportunities for practicing pharmacists to develop skills as an active member on collaborative health care teams.

The Center for Patient Education and Health Literacy targets the gap between health information and patient practices and collaborates with other researchers through the Institute of Clinical and Translational Sciences.

The Office for Research on Aging examines the physiological aspects of aging as well as the psychological, social, and cultural aspects of growing older through basic scientific and clinical research.

STLCOP is also involved with basic science research, examining drugs and their effects in a laboratory setting. Rapid changes in technology and health care call for constant evolution in drug therapies, and the College is responding by bringing to bear faculty and educational resources to strengthen this type of research.

Financial Aid

Earning a pharmacy degree is an investment in the future. Students may apply for merit and need-based institutional, state, and federal financial aid. Almost all STLCOP students receive financial aid. Most students who attend St. Louis College of Pharmacy receive more than one type of financial aid, creating a financial aid package designed to cover tuition, fees, and housing costs. The College participates in all applicable federal and state financial aid programs. Scholarships, grants, loans, and student employment are offered to help qualified students pay for college expenses.

St. Louis College of Pharmacy's Financial Aid Office assists students by performing a holistic evaluation of students' academic achievement, financial need, community service, and leadership experience. All students are encouraged to follow the steps for

St. Louis College of Pharmacy

applying for financial aid to ensure that they maximize their financial aid eligibility. Admissions applications serve as students' scholarship applications. Completing admissions applications early maximizes scholarship opportunities.

Costs

For the 2016–17 academic year, professional program tuition and fees were $16,247 per semester. The individual rate of $1,084 per credit hour applies to courses in excess of 18 credit hours, less than 12 credit hours and summer session courses. Additional costs, including books, student activity fees, student health fees, professional program fees, and new student program fees vary each year but average $1,360 per semester.

Faculty

STLCOP faculty research programs contribute significantly to health care and the practice of pharmacy. With a wide variety of research interests, STLCOP's faculty members are experts in areas ranging from drug discovery and health literacy to public health and infectious disease. A complete listing of faculty members and their areas of expertise is available online at https://www.stlcop.edu/about/directory/index.html.

Campus Facilities

St. Louis College of Pharmacy is undergoing a physical transformation to better meet the needs of students, faculty, and staff. Construction is underway on a new, seven-story Recreation and Student Center scheduled for completion in early 2017. As it is currently planned, the new 193,000-square-foot building will house a second residence hall, dining hall, competition and intramural gymnasiums, indoor track, and spaces for residential life offices. In 2015, the state-of-the-art Academic and Research Building (ARB) opened. The ARB features a welcome center, classrooms, teaching and research labs, auditorium, library, and study spaces accessible to students 24/7.

Jones Hall has been a part of the College's campus since it was constructed in 1927 and is home to several large classrooms, all of the basic science laboratories, as well as offices for faculty and staff. The current Residence Hall is at the center of campus and houses 265 students and 10 resident assistants. Living on campus provides students with a supportive environment that emphasizes community and personal development. Residence Life staff organizes social and educational activities designed to help students be successful at St. Louis College of Pharmacy and in life outside of the College. Support is offered in many ways, including individual counseling, tutoring, individual coaching, student-to-student mentoring, and disability accommodations.

Location

St. Louis College of Pharmacy is located on nine acres in the heart of one of the world's finest biomedical and patient-care centers. The campus is located in St. Louis' Central West End, one of the city's oldest and most historic neighborhoods. It showcases many grand private residences built at the turn of the 20th century. Dining, nightlife, shopping and entertainment venues are plentiful in this pedestrian-friendly area, particularly along Euclid Avenue, which boasts more than 125 shops, boutiques, galleries, cafes, bistros, pubs, bars, salons, and other businesses. Students are often seen studying at one of the neighborhood's many sidewalk cafes and coffeehouses. Local businesses frequently host special events, art openings, musical performances, and other activities. The College is located adjacent to Forest Park, one of the nation's largest and most visited urban parks.

Applying

All prospective students may apply for admission to any of the undergraduate years and the first year of the professional program. Admission to the College is selective, and applicants are encouraged to apply early. Questions may be directed to the Office of Admissions at 314-446-8328 or admissions@stlcop.edu.

The College's direct-entry program means that students are admitted for the program's duration, assuming all academic requirements are met. There is no need to apply for a pre-pharmacy curriculum and then apply again for entrance into the professional portion of the program. More information is available at stlcop.edu/apply.

Correspondence and Information

Director of Admissions
St. Louis College of Pharmacy
4588 Parkview Place
St. Louis, Missouri 63110-1088
United States
Phone: 314-446-8328
       800-278-5267 Ext. 8328 (toll-free)
E-mail: admissions@stlcop.edu
Website: stlcop.edu/apply
Facebook: facebook.com/stlcop
Twitter: twitter.com/stlcopedu

UNIVERSITY OF CALIFORNIA, SAN FRANCISCO
Doctor of Pharmacy Program

 For more information, visit http://petersons.to/ucsf-pharmacy

Programs of Study

The Doctor of Pharmacy (Pharm.D.) curriculum at University of California, San Francisco (UCSF) is a 12-quarter, full-time course of study designed to graduate pharmacists who think critically; advocate for patient-centered care; work collaboratively alongside physicians, nurses, and other health care colleagues; and lead the profession in assuming new responsibilities related to the management of medicines.

The UCSF Pharm.D. curriculum offers a science-focused curriculum to prepare graduates to be medication experts. The curriculum provides extensive direct patient care experiences that allow students to apply their clinical knowledge and skills to deliver pharmacy services that improve medication safety and patient health outcomes. At UCSF, students learn from renowned scientists and clinicians who are leaders and innovators in science and health care.

The Doctor of Pharmacy curriculum consists of four years of full-time study to prepare students to be leaders and innovators in pharmacy practice. All students complete a required core curriculum and select an emphasis in one of three pathways: Pharmaceutical Care, Health Services and Policy Research, or Pharmaceutical Sciences. The UCSF Doctor of Pharmacy curriculum prepares graduates to demonstrate competence in patient and population-based care, scientific and clinical foundations, practice-based learning and improvement, interpersonal and communication skills, professionalism, and systems-based practice. However, a new curriculum is being developed for the program and will be introduced for entering students in 2018. Information regarding the changes is available on the UCSF website at http://pharmd.ucsf.edu/curriculum.

Opportunities abound at UCSF for students to focus their Pharm.D. education on their specific professional interests. Whether it is a focus on patient populations and policy development, global health, or expanded scientific and clinical research, UCSF offers students the chance to engage with faculty and students who are committed to advancing scientific discovery, solving complex health problems, and exploring new frontiers in patient care.

The UCSF Interprofessional Health Post-Baccalaureate Certificate Program is a comprehensive educational opportunity designed for individuals seeking to improve their academic foundation for pharmacy school. Through a combination of advanced science coursework, collaborative study, and personalized support in preparing for the professional school application process, participants are able to distinguish themselves as competitive candidates for pharmacy school. More details are available at http://pharmd.ucsf.edu/admissions/postbacc.

University of California San Francisco School of Pharmacy's Doctor of Pharmacy program is accredited by the Accreditation Council for Pharmacy Education, 135 South LaSalle Street, Suite 4100, Chicago, Illinois 60603; 312-664-3575; www.acpe-accredit.org.

Interprofessional Education

Pharm.D. students learn alongside students from UCSF programs in dentistry, medicine, nursing and physical therapy. Through the Center for Innovation in Interprofessional Education, faculty leaders across the UCSF campus create opportunities for students from different fields to interact and learn in a way that prepares them for the seamless teamwork of interprofessional, collaborative practice that successful modern patient care delivery requires. Interprofessional education represents an exciting and important dimension of pharmacy education at UCSF. Additional information regarding this aspect of the program can be found at https://www.ucsf.edu/about/education-overview.

Research

UCSF School of Pharmacy faculty discoveries significantly impact the lives of the world's patients, with research that encompasses the full spectrum, from understanding molecules to ensuring the right patient receives the right medication. The University's scientists reveal the basic biochemical mechanisms of health and disease and explore molecular targets for new drugs. They both develop and share the leading technologies that enable their science. They drive the development of new medicines, medical devices, and diagnostic tests. And they investigate methodologies toward the safest, individualized, and most effective use of affordable, accessible medications for all patients. The School of Pharmacy has been the recipient of more National Institutes of Health research funding than any other pharmacy school in the United States, every year since 1979.

Areas of Research

Department of Bioengineering and Therapeutic Sciences
- Therapeutic Bioengineering
- Pharmacogenomics and Genomics
- Computational Biology and Systems Pharmacology
- Drug Development and Regulatory Sciences

Department of Clinical Pharmacy
- Clinical Research
- Education Research
- Health Services and Policy Research

Department of Pharmaceutical Chemistry
- Chemical Biology and Medicinal Chemistry
- Computational Chemistry and Biology
- Physical Biology
- Protein and Cellular Engineering

Research Services and Facilities

Department of Bioengineering and Therapeutic Sciences
- Biomedical Micro and Nanotechnology Core (BMNC)
- Drug Studies Unit (DSU)

Department of Clinical Pharmacy
- Drug Research Unit (DRU)

Department of Pharmaceutical Chemistry
- Antibiome Center
- National Bio-organic Biomedical Mass Spectrometry Resource Center
- Nuclear Magnetic Resonance Facility (NMR)
- Resource for Biocomputing, Visualization, and Informatics (RBVI)
- Sequence Analysis and Consulting Service (SACS)
- Small Molecule Discovery Center (SMDC)

Further information about the School of Pharmacy's research programs is available online at https://pharmacy.ucsf.edu/research.

Cost of Study

For the 2016–17 academic year, tuition and fees total $38,154 for years 1–3 of the Pharm.D. program. Year 4 is estimated at $38,083. There is also a nonresident supplemental tuition of $12,245 per year. There are additional charges for books and supplies. Actual tuition, fees, and charges are subject to change by the Regents of the University of California and could be affected by increases or reductions in State funding, or other developments. The most current information regarding tuition and fees is available on the University's website at https://finaid.ucsf.edu/newly-admitted-students/cost-attendance.

Student Group

Though the nearly 500 student pharmacists in the Pharm.D. program represent diverse backgrounds and experiences, they share a common commitment to patient care and to gaining as much as they can from their pharmacy education. Students' active involvement in student organizations and in the community creates a rich and vibrant environment for learning and professional development. Students contribute to a culture of collaboration both inside and outside the classroom and a thriving student life.

All students are eligible for pharmacist licensure upon graduation, and more than 99 percent pass the licensure examinations. About 60 to 70 percent of the graduates pursue, and are highly competitive for, postgraduate training or education in the form of residencies, fellowships, or advanced degrees. Additional details can be found at https://pharmd.ucsf.edu/about/student-life.

Faculty

The Pharm.D. program is delivered by faculty members from across UCSF and primarily by those in the School of Pharmacy. A complete list of faculty members affiliated with the School can be found at http://pharmacy.ucsf.edu/faculty.

Location

Located in the heart of San Francisco, the vibrant city allows our students to learn to embrace diversity and inclusion as a source of innovation, lifelong learning and personal fulfillment. More information is available at https://pharmacy.ucsf.edu/about/locations.

The University

UCSF's four professional schools—Dentistry, Medicine, Nursing, and Pharmacy—and the Graduate Division consistently rank as top programs nationwide in their fields and attract the world's most talented students.

University of California, San Francisco

Training takes place in some of the finest "classrooms" in the nation, including UCSF Medical Center, Zuckerberg San Francisco General Hospital and Trauma Center, the San Francisco VA Medical Center and numerous clinics throughout Northern California. In each of the four schools, students become part of a highly collaborative, solutions-driven culture; each graduating class is expected to set a higher standard for the next when it comes to health leadership.

UCSF is leading revolutions in health—and those revolutions often start in the lab. From basic science to clinical research, the University's researchers are constantly pushing scientific boundaries and earning worldwide recognition for their discoveries. A key element of UCSF's research success is its deeply ingrained culture of collaboration. Scientists regularly reach across disciplines and beyond the borders of UCSF to advance knowledge in basic science and formulate new strategies for treating disease—insights that would be elusive in laboratories focused only on a single research approach. The caliber of UCSF's research is world renowned. Faculty members have won nearly every leading prize in the health sciences, from Nobel Prizes to National Medals of Science. For nearly a decade, UCSF has earned its place as the top-funded public academic institution by the National Institutes of Health. Further information about UCSF can be found at https://www.ucsf.edu/.

Applying

Each year, the School accepts about 122 students from a pool that has ranged as high as 1,200 applicants. The School seeks to admit students who have diverse cultural, educational, economic, and social backgrounds. Although grade point average is an important factor, it is not the sole reason for acceptance. In addition to intellectual and academic competence, the School's admissions committee considers communication skills, leadership ability, community service, and health care related experience. More information about the School's admitted students is available at http://pharmd.ucsf.edu/about/students.

In order to have application materials accepted for review, applicants must be able to verify that they meet certain minimum eligibility requirements. Applicants who do not meet these requirements, or who are unable to provide the verification necessary, will not be considered for admission and their applications will be administratively canceled.

Applicants must have a minimum, cumulative undergraduate GPA of 2.80. The Pharmacy College Admissions Test (PCAT) is required for applicants applying for entry in 2017 and beyond. The PCAT exam must be taken in time for scores to be delivered by the November 1 application deadline.

All prerequisites must be satisfied with course work approved by the Office of Student and Curricular Affairs and must be completed prior to September 1 of the year of entry into the program. It is the applicant's responsibility to verify if their course work is approved to meet UCSF's prerequisites. The process varies according to the type of institution where the course work was completed.

Applicants must have basic skills using a computer. If offered admission, students must be able to secure and maintain a valid intern pharmacist license with the California Board of Pharmacy.

The application consists of 2 parts, the Pharmacy College Application Service (PharmCAS) application and a supplemental application. Both parts are required. Applicants must submit official copies of transcripts.

An interview is also part of the application process. The primary purpose of the interview is to assess the applicant's communication skills, but also to assess problem-solving and critical-thinking skills. Interviews are by invitation only. They are scheduled from late January through mid-February and are held at UCSF. Invitations are mailed beginning in mid-December. The invitations will include instructions for accepting or declining the offer. All applicants are notified of their application status by the end of January.

Correspondence and Information

Office of Student and Curricular Affairs
Medical Sciences Box 0150
513 Parnassus Avenue, Room S960
San Francisco, California 94143
United States
Phone: 415-476-2732
Fax: 415-476-6805
E-mail: osaca@pharmacy.ucsf.edu
Website: http://pharmd.ucsf.edu/

UNIVERSITY OF HAWAI'I AT HILO
Daniel K. Inouye College of Pharmacy (DKICP)
Ph.D. in Pharmaceutical Sciences

 For more information, visit http://petersons.to/uhawaii-hilo_pharm-phd

Programs of Study

The Daniel K. Inouye College of Pharmacy (DKICP) at the University of Hawai'i at Hilo (UH Hilo) is the only institution in the central Pacific to offer the Ph.D. in Pharmaceutical Sciences degree program.

Using the extraordinary intellectual, biological, physical, and cultural diversity of its geographic region as a focus of investigation and study, the Ph.D. in Pharmaceutical Sciences program provides graduate training in the pharmaceutical sciences, including medicinal chemistry, pharmacology, pharmaceutics, and pharmacognosy, with an emphasis on natural products discovery and development and their importance in pharmacy and healthcare in general.

The Ph.D. degree program is aimed at students with B.S., M.S., or Pharm.D. degrees, and those currently working in the field. The program is designed to foster student development as critical thinkers, team players, self-directed interdisciplinary scholars, and communicators.

Students are prepared for senior leadership positions in the pharmaceutical sciences in academia, research, education, government, industry, and related fields, and become leaders who can identify, research, and solve problems related to the pharmaceutical sciences.

The program utilizes the extraordinary intellectual, biological, physical, and cultural diversity on the Island of Hawaii, and within both the State and Asia-Pacific Region, as a focus of investigation and study.

The University of Hawai'i at Hilo's Doctor of Pharmacy (Pharm.D.) program is accredited by the Accreditation Council for Pharmacy Education (ACPE).

DKICP also offers the Doctor of Pharmacy (Pharm.D.) degree program and the Master of Science (M.S.) degree program in Clinical Psychopharmacology.

Research Facilities

The research facilities are located on the main UH Hilo campus and at the Waiakea research facility a few miles away. These facilities house all the scientific equipment and instruments needed for molecular isolation and structural analyses, including 400 MHz multinuclear NMR spectrometers, LC-MC systems with ESI and APCI interfaces, LC-qTOF high mass accuracy mass spectrometer, GC-triple quadrupole mass spectrometer, X-ray diffractometer, polarimeter, FT-IR, several UV-VIS spectrophotometers, and HPLC systems (analytical and preparative). Pharmaceutics equipment includes a NiComp 380 particle analyzer and a Nano DeBEE

homogenizer while a microwave reactor is available for chemical synthesis. Equipment for cellular analysis and molecular biology includes a Perkin Elmer Operetta high content imaging system, Leica confocal microscopes, flow cytometers, multiple research grade upright, inverted and stereo microscopes, centrifuges (high speed, ultra- and microcentrifuges), a GenePix microarray scanner, real-time qPCR cyclers, and a variety of microplate readers with state-of-the-art detection technologies based on photometry, fluorometry, luminometry, time-resolved fluorescence and fluorescence polarization. All of the University's BSL-2 labs are equipped for the growth of microbes and mammalian cells in culture.

The Daniel K. Inouye College of Pharmacy also has strong research programs in cancer biology and natural product drug discovery.

UH Hilo—DKICP students also have access to a specialized pharmacy library. Students utilize information systems that serve as a foundation for their ability to use concepts and evidence-based medicine to answer drug information questions and compare therapeutic alternatives.

Financial Aid

Qualified applicants are eligible to apply for a Graduate Assistantship. Students may also submit the free application for Federal Student Aid (FAFSA) in January and indicate the University of Hawai'i at Hilo (UH Hilo); code number 001611, however, applicants must be accepted for admission before a financial aid award can be issued.

More information can be found on the UH Hilo Financial Aid Office's website at http://hilo.hawaii.edu/financialaid/.

Cost of Study

For the 2016–17 academic year, resident tuition for the Ph.D. in Pharmaceutical Sciences program is $479 per credit hour or $5,748 per semester for full-time students. Tuition for nonresidents is $1,097 per credit hour or $13,164 for full-time students.

The most recent information on tuition, fees, and living and housing costs can be found at http://hilo.hawaii.edu/uhh/bo/cashier/tuition_schedule.php.

The Faculty

The faculty includes cancer researchers, Dr. Linda Connelly (role of inflammation in tumor progression and metastasis), Dr. Aaron Jacobs (cell signaling and characterization of novel heat shock-induced gene products), Dr. Dana-Lynn Koomoa-Lange (calcium signaling changes in disease states), and Dr. Ingo Koomoa-Lange (cancer cell biology).

University of Hawai'i at Hilo

Faculty members who are medicinal chemists include Dr. Dianqing Sun (organic synthesis of anticancer and antimicrobial drugs) and Dr. Daniela Gündisch (organic synthesis of central nervous system drugs and development of in vivo tracers for imaging).

Dr. Leng Chee Chang's work on phytochemistry centers on the isolation of novel molecules from plants with anticancer and other biological activities. Dr. Ghee Tan's multidisciplinary drug discovery work focuses on the identification and mechanistic evaluation of anticancer and antimalarial natural products from terrestrial and marine sources. Dr. Susan Jarvi studies host genetics in resistance to avian malaria and is actively involved in rat lung worm disease. Dr. Mahavir Chougule focuses on targeted therapies for lung cancer and asthma utilizing nanoparticles as a drug delivery system. Dr. Supakit Wongwiwatthananukit is involved in mathematical analysis of health care outcomes.

A complete listing of DKICP faculty and staff is available online at http://pharmacy.uhh.hawaii.edu/cop/.

Location

UH Hilo is located on the windward side of the Big Island of Hawai'i in the bayside town of Hilo. With a population of approximately 40,000, Hilo has small-town charm, but is large enough to support 3 shopping centers and to provide needed services. The island of Hawai`i offers many natural attractions, including Hawai`i Volcanoes National Park, white sand beaches, plunging waterfalls, and scenic Waipio valley.

The University

The University of Hawai`i, with a student population of about 4,000, is a multicultural comprehensive university, offering a wide range of baccalaureate degrees and graduate degrees in a few selected disciplines. While UH Hilo is a state university, the atmosphere is that of a private college, with small class sizes, a low faculty-to-student ratio, and opportunities for research, and hands-on learning.

As a public university, the University of Hawai`i at Hilo has a unique position in the State—and country—by offering a rigorous and engaging curriculum at an affordable tuition rate. The admission requirements are moderately selective, allowing above-average students the opportunity to enjoy the benefits of a small school experience.

UH Hilo is accredited by the Accrediting Commission for Senior Colleges and Universities of the Western Association of Schools and Colleges.

Applying

Acceptance is granted at the discretion of the Pharmaceutical Science Ph.D. Admissions Committee. Applicants must: complete the application process; hold a baccalaureate degree or graduate degree from a regionally accredited U.S. college or university, or its equivalent from a recognized non–U.S. institution of learning; have a minimum GPA of 3.0 out of 4.0 or the equivalent in the last 60 semester credits of undergraduate and in all post-baccalaureate work; submit a personal statement of objectives which includes applicant's background, professional goals, and academic and research interests; submit a resume; provide official GRE scores; submit three letters of recommendation using the "Ph.D. Letter of Recommendation Form" from people who can speak to the applicant's educational ability, motivation, and character, and/or leadership experiences, including a professor of one of the natural or physical sciences; complete a SKYPE or equivalent electronic interview; and submit a $50 application fee.

Applicants are also recommended to have successfully completed the following courses with a grade of C or higher: General Biology I and II for science majors with labs, General Chemistry I and II for science majors with labs, Organic Chemistry I and II for science majors with labs, and Calculus 1 or Advanced Calculus. Students may have to take additional courses if proficiency cannot be demonstrated.

Foreign applicants must also submit official TOEFL score report unless the degree was conferred by an institution whose language of instruction is English, and the International Graduate Student Supplemental Information form. .

Further information on the details of fulfilling admissions requirements are available from the Ph.D. Program Admissions Office pharmacy@hawaii.edu, and on the DKICP Graduate Admissions website. All documents can be found online at http://pharmacy.uhh.hawaii.edu/academics/graduate/admissions.php.

Applications are accepted and reviewed on a rolling basis until all spots are filled for the following fall semester. The final application deadline is May 15.

Correspondence and Information
Ph.D. Program Admissions
Office of Student Services
The Daniel K. Inouye College of Pharmacy (DKICP)
University of Hawaii at Hilo
200 W. Kawili Street
Hilo, Hawaii 96720
United States
Fax: 808-933-3889
E-mail: pharmacy@hawaii.edu
Website: http://pharmacy.uhh.hawaii.edu/academics/graduate/

Section 31
Veterinary Medicine and Sciences

This section contains a directory of institutions offering graduate work in veterinary medicine and sciences. Additional information about programs listed in the directory may be obtained by writing directly to the dean of a graduate school or chair of a department at the address given in the directory.

For programs offering related work, see also in this book *Biological and Biomedical Sciences* and *Zoology*. In the other guides in this series:

Graduate Programs in the Humanities, Arts & Social Sciences
See *Economics (Agricultural Economics and Agribusiness)*
Graduate Programs in the Physical Sciences, Mathematics, Agricultural Sciences, the Environment & Natural Resources
See *Agricultural and Food Sciences, Marine Sciences and Oceanography,* and *Natural Resources*
Graduate Programs in Engineering & Applied Sciences
See *Agricultural Engineering and Bioengineering* and *Biomedical Engineering and Biotechnology*

CONTENTS

Program Directories

Veterinary Medicine

Auburn University, College of Veterinary Medicine, Professional Program in Veterinary Medicine, Auburn University, AL 36849. Offers DVM, DVM/MS. *Accreditation:* AVMA. *Faculty:* 97 full-time (40 women), 4 part-time/adjunct (2 women). *Students:* 482 full-time (379 women), 33 part-time (26 women); includes 39 minority (7 Black or African American, non-Hispanic/Latino; 1 American Indian or Alaska Native, non-Hispanic/Latino; 7 Asian, non-Hispanic/Latino; 15 Hispanic/Latino; 9 Two or more races, non-Hispanic/Latino). Average age 25. 1,158 applicants, 17% accepted, 120 enrolled. In 2015, 113 doctorates awarded. *Degree requirements:* For doctorate, preceptorship. *Application deadline:* Applications are processed on a rolling basis. Application fee: $50 ($60 for international students). *Expenses:* Contact institution. *Financial support:* Fellowships available. Financial award application deadline: 3/15; financial award applicants required to submit FAFSA. *Unit head:* Dr. Calvin Johnson, Dean, 334-844-4546. *Application contact:* Dr. George Flowers, Interim Dean of the Graduate School, 334-844-2125.

Colorado State University, College of Veterinary Medicine and Biomedical Sciences, Professional Program in Veterinary Medicine, Fort Collins, CO 80523-1601. Offers DVM, DVM/MPH, DVM/MS, DVM/MST, DVM/PhD, MBA/DVM. *Accreditation:* AVMA. *Students:* 551 full-time (453 women); includes 106 minority (1 Black or African American, non-Hispanic/Latino; 2 American Indian or Alaska Native, non-Hispanic/Latino; 37 Asian, non-Hispanic/Latino; 44 Hispanic/Latino; 22 Two or more races, non-Hispanic/Latino), 3 international. Average age 27. 1,452 applicants, 11% accepted, 149 enrolled. In 2015, 126 doctorates awarded. *Degree requirements:* For doctorate, comprehensive exam, thesis/dissertation. *Entrance requirements:* For doctorate, GRE General Test, transcripts, VMCAS (Veterinary Medical College Application Service), three letters of recommendation, interview. Additional exam requirements/recommendations for international students: Required—TOEFL (minimum score 550 paper-based; 80 iBT), IELTS (minimum score 6.5). *Application deadline:* For fall admission, 9/15 priority date for domestic and international students. Application fee: $60 ($70 for international students). Electronic applications accepted. *Expenses:* Contact institution. *Financial support:* In 2015–16, 3 fellowships (averaging $48,667 per year) were awarded; research assistantships, teaching assistantships, and scholarships/grants also available. Financial award application deadline: 9/15; financial award applicants required to submit FAFSA. *Faculty research:* Animal reproduction, infectious diseases, cancer biology, musculoskeletal research, neurobiology. *Total annual research expenditures:* $119,399. *Unit head:* Dr. Melinda Frye, Associate Dean, 970-491-2009, Fax: 970-491-2250, E-mail: melinda.frye@colostate.edu. *Application contact:* Janet Janke, Director, Admissions Operations, 970-491-7052, Fax: 970-491-2250, E-mail: janet.janke@colostate.edu.
Website: http://csu-cvmbs.colostate.edu/dvm-program/Pages/default.aspx

Cornell University, College of Veterinary Medicine, Ithaca, NY 14853-0001. Offers DVM. *Accreditation:* AVMA. *Faculty:* 185 full-time (84 women). *Students:* 398 full-time (320 women); includes 79 minority (12 Black or African American, non-Hispanic/Latino; 3 American Indian or Alaska Native, non-Hispanic/Latino; 26 Asian, non-Hispanic/Latino; 31 Hispanic/Latino; 7 Two or more races, non-Hispanic/Latino), 7 international. Average age 26. 948 applicants, 16% accepted, 102 enrolled. In 2015, 95 doctorates awarded. *Entrance requirements:* For doctorate, GRE General Test or MCAT, animal or veterinary experience, letters of recommendation. Additional exam requirements/recommendations for international students: Required—TOEFL (minimum score 600 paper-based; 100 iBT). *Application deadline:* For fall admission, 9/15 for domestic and international students. Electronic applications accepted. *Expenses:* Contact institution. *Financial support:* In 2015–16, 326 students received support. Federal Work-Study, institutionally sponsored loans, and scholarships/grants available. Financial award application deadline: 2/1; financial award applicants required to submit CSS PROFILE or FAFSA. *Faculty research:* Biomedical research, comparative cancer, infectious diseases/host response, reproductive biology, genetics/epigenetics. *Total annual research expenditures:* $45.2 million. *Unit head:* Dr. Lorin Warnick, Interim Dean, 607-253-3771, Fax: 607-253-3701. *Application contact:* Jennifer A. Mailey, Director of Admissions, 607-253-3700, Fax: 607-253-3709, E-mail: jam333@cornell.edu.
Website: http://www.vet.cornell.edu/

Iowa State University of Science and Technology, Department of Veterinary Diagnostic and Production Animal Medicine, Ames, IA 50011. Offers veterinary preventative medicine (MS). *Accreditation:* AVMA. *Degree requirements:* For master's, thesis or alternative. *Entrance requirements:* For master's, GRE General Test. Additional exam requirements/recommendations for international students: Required—TOEFL (minimum score 550 paper-based; 79 iBT), IELTS (minimum score 6.5). Electronic applications accepted.

Kansas State University, Graduate School, College of Veterinary Medicine, Professional Program in Veterinary Medicine, Manhattan, KS 66506. Offers DVM. *Accreditation:* AVMA. *Entrance requirements:* Additional exam requirements/recommendations for international students: Required—TOEFL. *Expenses:* Contact institution. *Faculty research:* Surgery and medicine, epithelial function, infectious disease of animals, neuroscience, analytical pharmacology.

Louisiana State University and Agricultural & Mechanical College, School of Veterinary Medicine, Professional Program in Veterinary Medicine, Baton Rouge, LA 70803. Offers DVM.

Michigan State University, College of Veterinary Medicine, Professional Program in Veterinary Medicine, East Lansing, MI 48824. Offers veterinary medicine (DVM); veterinary medicine/medical scientist training program (DVM). *Accreditation:* AVMA. *Entrance requirements:* Additional exam requirements/recommendations for international students: Required—TOEFL. Electronic applications accepted. *Expenses:* Contact institution.

Mississippi State University, College of Veterinary Medicine, Professional Program in Veterinary Medicine, Mississippi State, MS 39762. Offers DVM. *Accreditation:* AVMA. *Faculty:* 48 full-time (18 women), 3 part-time/adjunct (0 women). *Students:* 332 full-time (251 women); includes 26 minority (8 Black or African American, non-Hispanic/Latino; 3 American Indian or Alaska Native, non-Hispanic/Latino; 3 Asian, non-Hispanic/Latino; 10 Hispanic/Latino; 2 Two or more races, non-Hispanic/Latino). Average age 25. 92 applicants, 100% accepted, 88 enrolled. *Entrance requirements:* For doctorate, GRE, minimum overall GPA of 2.8. Additional exam requirements/recommendations for international students: Required—TOEFL. *Application deadline:* For fall admission, 10/1 for domestic students. Application fee: $60. Electronic applications accepted. *Expenses:* Contact institution. *Faculty research:* Veterinary education, advancing research in veterinary medicine and biomedical fields. *Unit head:* Dr. Margaret Kern, Associate Dean for Academic Affairs, 662-325-1326, Fax: 662-325-8714, E-mail: kern@cvm.msstate.edu. *Application contact:* Missy Hadaway, Admissions Coordinator, 662-

325-9065, Fax: 662-325-8714, E-mail: hadaway@cvm.msstate.edu.
Website: http://www.cvm.msstate.edu/

North Carolina State University, College of Veterinary Medicine, Professional Program, Raleigh, NC 27695. Offers DVM. *Entrance requirements:* For doctorate, GRE. Additional exam requirements/recommendations for international students: Required—TOEFL.

North Carolina State University, College of Veterinary Medicine, Program in Specialized Veterinary Medicine, Raleigh, NC 27695. Offers MSpVM. *Accreditation:* AVMA. *Degree requirements:* For master's, thesis optional. *Entrance requirements:* For master's, GRE General Test. Additional exam requirements/recommendations for international students: Required—TOEFL (minimum score 550 paper-based). Electronic applications accepted. *Faculty research:* Cell biology, infectious diseases, pharmacology and toxicology, genomics, pathology and population medicine.

North Carolina State University, College of Veterinary Medicine, Program in Veterinary Public Health, Raleigh, NC 27695. Offers MVPH. *Degree requirements:* For master's, thesis optional. Electronic applications accepted.

Oklahoma State University, Center for Veterinary Health Sciences, Professional Program in Veterinary Medicine, Stillwater, OK 74078. Offers DVM. *Accreditation:* AVMA. *Entrance requirements:* For doctorate, GRE General Test, GRE Subject Test (biology). Electronic applications accepted. *Expenses:* Tuition, state resident: full-time $3528; part-time $196 per credit hour. Tuition, nonresident: full-time $14,144; part-time $785.75 per credit hour. *Required fees:* $1895; $105.25 per credit hour. Tuition and fees vary according to campus/location. *Faculty research:* Infectious diseases, physiology, toxicology, biomedical lasers, clinical studies.

Oregon State University, College of Veterinary Medicine, Veterinary Medicine Professional Program, Corvallis, OR 97331. Offers DVM. Program admissions open only to residents of Oregon and other states participating in the Western Interstate Commission for Higher Education. *Accreditation:* AVMA. *Faculty:* 41 full-time (18 women), 3 part-time/adjunct (2 women). *Students:* 221 full-time (186 women), 2 part-time (both women); includes 26 minority (1 American Indian or Alaska Native, non-Hispanic/Latino; 8 Asian, non-Hispanic/Latino; 11 Hispanic/Latino; 6 Two or more races, non-Hispanic/Latino), 1 international. Average age 27. In 2015, 57 doctorates awarded. *Entrance requirements:* For doctorate, GRE. *Application deadline:* For fall admission, 9/15 for domestic students. *Expenses:* $21,084 full-time resident tuition; $42,174 full-time non-resident tuition; $1,572 fees. *Unit head:* Dr. Susan J. Tornquist, Dean. *Application contact:* Admissions, 541-737-2098, E-mail: cvmproginfo@oregonstate.edu.
Website: http://vetmed.oregonstate.edu/

Purdue University, School of Veterinary Medicine, Professional Program in Veterinary Medicine, West Lafayette, IN 47907. Offers DVM, DVM/MS, DVM/PhD. *Accreditation:* AVMA. *Entrance requirements:* For doctorate, GRE General Test. Additional exam requirements/recommendations for international students: Required—TOEFL. Electronic applications accepted.

Texas A&M University, College of Veterinary Medicine and Biomedical Sciences, College Station, TX 77843. Offers MS, DVM, PhD. *Accreditation:* AVMA. *Program availability:* Part-time. *Faculty:* 134. *Students:* 791 full-time (584 women), 50 part-time (34 women); includes 170 minority (21 Black or African American, non-Hispanic/Latino; 1 American Indian or Alaska Native, non-Hispanic/Latino; 43 Asian, non-Hispanic/Latino; 89 Hispanic/Latino; 1 Native Hawaiian or other Pacific Islander, non-Hispanic/Latino; 15 Two or more races, non-Hispanic/Latino), 60 international. Average age 29. 241 applicants, 89% accepted, 206 enrolled. In 2015, 63 master's, 13 doctorates awarded. Terminal master's awarded for partial completion of doctoral program. *Entrance requirements:* For master's and doctorate, GRE General Test. Additional exam requirements/recommendations for international students: Required—TOEFL (minimum score 550 paper-based; 80 iBT), IELTS (minimum score 6), PTE (minimum score 53). *Application deadline:* For fall admission, 10/1 for domestic and international students. Application fee: $50 ($90 for international students). *Expenses:* Contact institution. *Financial support:* In 2015–16, 763 students received support, including 24 fellowships with tuition reimbursements available (averaging $11,758 per year), 106 research assistantships with tuition reimbursements available (averaging $7,379 per year), 25 teaching assistantships with tuition reimbursements available (averaging $6,754 per year); career-related internships or fieldwork, institutionally sponsored loans, scholarships/grants, traineeships, health care benefits, tuition waivers (full and partial), unspecified assistantships, and clinical associateships also available. Support available to part-time students. Financial award application deadline: 3/15; financial award applicants required to submit FAFSA. *Faculty research:* Physiology, pharmacology, anatomy, microbiology, parasitology. *Unit head:* Dr. Eleanor M. Green, Dean, 979-845-5053, Fax: 979-845-5088, E-mail: emgreen@tamu.edu. *Application contact:* Graduate Admissions, 979-845-1044, E-mail: admissions@tamu.edu.
Website: http://vetmed.tamu.edu/

Tufts University, Cummings School of Veterinary Medicine, North Grafton, MA 01536. Offers animals and public policy (MS); biomedical sciences (PhD), including digestive diseases, infectious diseases, neuroscience and reproductive biology, pathology; conservation medicine (MS); veterinary medicine (DVM); DVM/MPH; DVM/MS. *Accreditation:* AVMA (one or more programs are accredited). *Degree requirements:* For master's, thesis (for some programs); for doctorate, comprehensive exam, thesis/dissertation (for some programs). *Entrance requirements:* For master's and doctorate, GRE General Test. Additional exam requirements/recommendations for international students: Required—TOEFL or IELTS. Electronic applications accepted. *Expenses:* Contact institution. *Faculty research:* Oncology, veterinary ethics, international veterinary medicine, veterinary genomics, pathogenesis of Clostridium difficile, wildlife fertility control.

Tuskegee University, Graduate Programs, College of Veterinary Medicine, Nursing and Allied Health, School of Veterinary Medicine, Tuskegee, AL 36088. Offers MS, DVM. *Degree requirements:* For master's, thesis. *Entrance requirements:* For master's, GRE General Test; for doctorate, VCAT. Additional exam requirements/recommendations for international students: Required—TOEFL (minimum score 500 paper-based).

Université de Montréal, Faculty of Veterinary Medicine, Professional Program in Veterinary Medicine, Montréal, QC H3C 3J7, Canada. Offers DES. Open only to Canadian residents. *Accreditation:* AVMA. *Program availability:* Part-time. Electronic applications accepted. *Faculty research:* Animal reproduction, infectious diseases of swine, physiology of exercise in horses, viral diseases of cattle, health management and epidemiology.

University of California, Davis, School of Veterinary Medicine, Program in Veterinary Medicine, Davis, CA 95616. Offers DVM, DVM/MPVM. *Accreditation:* AVMA. *Entrance* *requirements:* For doctorate, GRE General Test. Additional exam requirements/recommendations for international students: Required—TOEFL. Electronic applications accepted.

University of Florida, College of Veterinary Medicine, Professional Program in Veterinary Medicine, Gainesville, FL 32611. Offers DVM. *Accreditation:* AVMA. *Entrance requirements:* For doctorate, GRE General Test.

University of Georgia, College of Veterinary Medicine, Athens, GA 30602. Offers MAM, MFAM, MS, DVM, PhD. *Accreditation:* AVMA (one or more programs are accredited). *Degree requirements:* For doctorate, variable foreign language requirement, thesis/dissertation (for some programs). *Entrance requirements:* For master's, GRE General Test; for doctorate, GRE General Test; GRE Subject Test in biology (for DVM). Electronic applications accepted. *Expenses:* Contact institution.

University of Guelph, Ontario Veterinary College and Graduate Studies, Graduate Programs in Veterinary Sciences, Department of Clinical Studies, Guelph, ON N1G 2W1, Canada. Offers anesthesiology (M Sc, DV Sc); cardiology (DV Sc, Diploma); clinical studies (Diploma); dermatology (M Sc); diagnostic imaging (M Sc, DV Sc); emergency/critical care (M Sc, DV Sc, Diploma); medicine (M Sc, DV Sc); neurology (M Sc, DV Sc); ophthalmology (M Sc, DV Sc); surgery (M Sc, DV Sc). *Degree requirements:* For master's, thesis; for doctorate, comprehensive exam, thesis/dissertation. *Entrance requirements:* Additional exam requirements/recommendations for international students: Required—TOEFL (minimum score 550 paper-based), IELTS (minimum score 6.5). Electronic applications accepted. *Faculty research:* Orthopedics, respirology, oncology, exercise physiology, cardiology.

University of Illinois at Urbana–Champaign, College of Veterinary Medicine, Professional Program in Veterinary Medicine, Champaign, IL 61820. Offers veterinary medical science (DVM). *Accreditation:* AVMA. *Expenses:* Contact institution.

University of Maryland, College Park, Academic Affairs, College of Agriculture and Natural Resources, Maryland Campus of VA/MD Regional College of Veterinary Medicine, Professional Program in Veterinary Medicine, College Park, MD 20742. Offers DVM. *Degree requirements:* For doctorate, thesis/dissertation, oral exam, public seminar.

University of Minnesota, Twin Cities Campus, College of Veterinary Medicine, Professional Program in Veterinary Medicine, Minneapolis, MN 55455-0213. Offers DVM, DVM/PhD. *Accreditation:* AVMA. *Entrance requirements:* For doctorate, GRE General Test. Electronic applications accepted. *Expenses:* Contact institution. *Faculty research:* Infectious toxic diseases of animals, zoonotic animal models of human disease, epidemiologic and preventive medicine.

University of Missouri, College of Veterinary Medicine and Office of Research and Graduate Studies, Graduate Programs in Veterinary Medicine, Department of Biomedical Sciences, Columbia, MO 65211. Offers biomedical sciences (MS, PhD); comparative medicine (MS); veterinary medicine and surgery (MS); DVM/PhD. *Degree requirements:* For master's, thesis; for doctorate, comprehensive exam, thesis/dissertation. *Entrance requirements:* For master's, GRE General Test, minimum GPA of 3.0; 10 hrs biology, 3 hrs physics, 3 hrs biochemistry, 10 hrs chemistry, 3 hrs calculus; for doctorate, GRE General Test (V+B = 300 if taken after 8/1/11); 3.5 analytical, minimum GPA of 3.0; 10 hrs biology, 3 hrs physics, 3 hrs biochemistry, 10 hrs chemistry, 3 hrs calculus. Additional exam requirements/recommendations for international students: Required—TOEFL (minimum score 600 paper-based; 100 iBT). *Application deadline:* For fall admission, 2/1 for domestic and international students; for winter admission, 9/1 for domestic and international students. Application fee: $65 ($90 for international students). Electronic applications accepted. *Financial support:* Fellowships with full tuition reimbursements, research assistantships with full tuition reimbursements, teaching assistantships with full tuition reimbursements, institutionally sponsored loans, scholarships/grants, traineeships, health care benefits, and unspecified assistantships available. Support available to part-time students. Financial award applicants required to submit FAFSA. *Faculty research:* Anatomy (gross or microscopic); physiology/pharmacology (molecular, cellular and integrative); biochemistry/molecular biology; endocrinology; toxicology; exercise biology including cardiac, vascular and muscle biology; cardiovascular biology including neuroendocrine regulation; membrane transport biology including cystic fibrosis and cardiac disease; reproductive biology. Website: http://biomed.missouri.edu/

University of Missouri, College of Veterinary Medicine, Professional Program in Veterinary Medicine, Columbia, MO 65211. Offers DVM. *Accreditation:* AVMA. *Entrance requirements:* For doctorate, VCAT, minimum GPA of 2.5 (for state residents), 3.0 (for nonresidents). *Application deadline:* For fall admission, 11/1 for domestic students. Electronic applications accepted. *Financial support:* Fellowships, research assistantships, career-related internships or fieldwork, institutionally sponsored loans, tuition waivers (full), and research associateships available. *Faculty research:* Cardiovascular physiology, food safety, infectious diseases, laboratory animal medicine, ophthalmology. Website: http://vetmed.missouri.edu/

University of Pennsylvania, School of Veterinary Medicine, Philadelphia, PA 19104. Offers VMD, VMD/MBA, VMD/PhD. *Accreditation:* AVMA. *Faculty:* 107 full-time (57 women), 32 part-time/adjunct (13 women). *Students:* 481 full-time (395 women), 9 part-time (6 women); includes 58 minority (7 Black or African American, non-Hispanic/Latino; 29 Asian, non-Hispanic/Latino; 17 Hispanic/Latino; 5 Two or more races, non-Hispanic/Latino), 2 international. Average age 26. 1,190 applicants, 14% accepted, 120 enrolled. In 2015, 119 doctorates awarded. *Expenses: Tuition, area resident:* Full-time $31,068; part-time $5762 per course. *Required fees:* $3200; $336 per course. Full-time tuition and fees vary according to degree level, program and student level. Part-time tuition and fees vary according to course load, degree level and program.

University of Prince Edward Island, Atlantic Veterinary College, Professional Program in Veterinary Medicine, Charlottetown, PE C1A 4P3, Canada. Offers DVM. *Accreditation:* AVMA. *Entrance requirements:* For doctorate, GRE. Additional exam requirements/recommendations for international students: Required—TOEFL (minimum score 550 paper-based; 80 iBT), Canadian Academic English Language Assessment, Michigan English Language Assessment Battery, Canadian Test of English for Scholars and Trainees). *Faculty research:* Shellfish toxicology, animal nutrition, fish health, toxicology, animal health management.

University of Saskatchewan, Western College of Veterinary Medicine and College of Graduate Studies and Research, Graduate Programs in Veterinary Medicine, Department of Large Animal Clinical Sciences, Saskatoon, SK S7N 5A2, Canada. Offers

M Sc, M Vet Sc, PhD. *Degree requirements:* For master's, thesis (for some programs); for doctorate, comprehensive exam (for some programs), thesis/dissertation. *Entrance requirements:* Additional exam requirements/recommendations for international students: Required—TOEFL (minimum score 80 iBT); Recommended—IELTS (minimum score 6.5). Electronic applications accepted. *Faculty research:* Reproduction, infectious diseases, epidemiology, food safety.

University of Saskatchewan, Western College of Veterinary Medicine and College of Graduate Studies and Research, Graduate Programs in Veterinary Medicine, Department of Small Animal Clinical Sciences, Saskatoon, SK S7N 5A2, Canada. Offers small animal clinical sciences (M Sc, PhD); veterinary anesthesiology, radiology and surgery (M Vet Sc); veterinary internal medicine (M Vet Sc). *Degree requirements:* For master's, thesis (for some programs); for doctorate, comprehensive exam (for some programs), thesis/dissertation. *Entrance requirements:* Additional exam requirements/recommendations for international students: Required—TOEFL (minimum score 80 iBT); Recommended—IELTS (minimum score 6.5). Electronic applications accepted. *Faculty research:* Orthopedics, wildlife, cardiovascular exercise/myelopathy, ophthalmology.

University of Saskatchewan, Western College of Veterinary Medicine, Professional Program in Veterinary Medicine, Saskatoon, SK S7N 5A2, Canada. Offers DVM. *Accreditation:* AVMA. *Degree requirements:* For doctorate, thesis/dissertation.

The University of Tennessee, Graduate School, College of Veterinary Medicine, Knoxville, TN 37996. Offers DVM. *Accreditation:* AVMA. *Entrance requirements:* For doctorate, VCAT, interview, minimum GPA of 2.7. Additional exam requirements/recommendations for international students: Required—TOEFL. *Expenses:* Contact institution.

University of Wisconsin–Madison, School of Veterinary Medicine, Madison, WI 53706-1380. Offers MS, DVM, PhD. *Accreditation:* AVMA (one or more programs are accredited). Terminal master's awarded for partial completion of doctoral program. *Degree requirements:* For master's, thesis; for doctorate, thesis/dissertation (for some programs). *Entrance requirements:* For doctorate, GRE General Test (for DVM). *Expenses:* Contact institution. *Faculty research:* Infectious disease, ophthalmology, orthopedics, food animal production, oncology, cardio-respiratory.

Virginia Polytechnic Institute and State University, Virginia-Maryland Regional College of Veterinary Medicine, Blacksburg, VA 24061. Offers biomedical and veterinary sciences (MS, PhD); public health (MPH); research in translational medicine (Certificate); veterinary medicine (DVM). *Accreditation:* AVMA (one or more programs are accredited). *Degree requirements:* For master's, comprehensive exam (for some programs), thesis (for some programs); for doctorate, comprehensive exam (for some programs), thesis/dissertation (for some programs). *Entrance requirements:* For master's and doctorate, GRE/GMAT (may vary by department). Additional exam requirements/recommendations for international students: Required—TOEFL (minimum score 550 paper-based). Electronic applications accepted. *Expenses:* Contact institution.

Washington State University, College of Veterinary Medicine, Professional Program in Veterinary Medicine, Pullman, WA 99164. Offers DVM, DVM/MS, DVM/PhD. *Accreditation:* AVMA. *Faculty:* 37 full-time (8 women), 43 part-time/adjunct (10 women). *Students:* 516 full-time (386 women); includes 53 minority (1 Black or African American, non-Hispanic/Latino; 4 American Indian or Alaska Native, non-Hispanic/Latino; 7 Asian, non-Hispanic/Latino; 10 Hispanic/Latino; 1 Native Hawaiian or other Pacific Islander, non-Hispanic/Latino; 30 Two or more races, non-Hispanic/Latino), 1 international. Average age 24. 1,236 applicants, 19% accepted, 137 enrolled. In 2015, 99 doctorates awarded. Terminal master's awarded for partial completion of doctoral program. *Entrance requirements:* For doctorate, GRE General Test. Additional exam requirements/recommendations for international students: Required—TOEFL (minimum score 550 paper-based; 80 iBT). *Application deadline:* For fall admission, 9/15 for domestic and international students. Application fee: $60. Electronic applications accepted. *Financial support:* In 2015–16, 446 students received support, including 28 fellowships with full tuition reimbursements available, 87 research assistantships with full tuition reimbursements available (averaging $23,000 per year), 34 teaching assistantships with full tuition reimbursements available (averaging $22,000 per year); career-related internships or fieldwork, Federal Work-Study, institutionally sponsored loans, scholarships/grants, traineeships, health care benefits, and unspecified assistantships also available. Support available to part-time students. Financial award application deadline: 2/15; financial award applicants required to submit FAFSA. *Faculty research:* Biotechnology, immunology, pathology, neurosciences, clinical sciences. *Unit head:* Dr. Patricia Talcott, Director of Admissions, 509-355-1532. *Application contact:* Barbara Hodson, Program Coordinator, 509-335-1532, Fax: 509-335-6133, E-mail: bhodson@vetmed.wsu.edu. Website: http://www.vetmed.wsu.edu/

Western University of Health Sciences, College of Veterinary Medicine, Pomona, CA 91766-1854. Offers DVM. *Accreditation:* AVMA. *Faculty:* 53 full-time (25 women), 7 part-time/adjunct (2 women). *Students:* 423 full-time (334 women); includes 165 minority (13 Black or African American, non-Hispanic/Latino; 1 American Indian or Alaska Native, non-Hispanic/Latino; 60 Asian, non-Hispanic/Latino; 70 Hispanic/Latino; 1 Native Hawaiian or other Pacific Islander, non-Hispanic/Latino; 20 Two or more races, non-Hispanic/Latino), 6 international. Average age 27. 800 applicants, 30% accepted, 102 enrolled. In 2015, 109 doctorates awarded. *Degree requirements:* For doctorate, comprehensive exam (for some programs), thesis/dissertation (for some programs). *Entrance requirements:* For doctorate, MCAT or GRE General Test, minimum GPA of 2.75, three letters of recommendation, BA or BS (recommended), 500 hours of hands-on animal-related experience. Additional exam requirements/recommendations for international students: Required—TOEFL (minimum score 550 paper-based; 79 iBT). *Application deadline:* For fall admission, 11/1 for domestic and international students. Application fee: $50. Electronic applications accepted. *Expenses:* $50,735 tuition; $40 fees. *Financial support:* Institutionally sponsored loans, scholarships/grants, and veterans' educational benefits available. Financial award application deadline: 3/2; financial award applicants required to submit FAFSA. *Total annual research expenditures:* $184,505. *Unit head:* Dr. Phil Nelson, Dean, 909-469-5661, Fax: 909-469-5635, E-mail: pnelson@westernu.edu. *Application contact:* Karen Hutton-Lopez, Director of Admissions, 909-469-5335, Fax: 909-469-5570, E-mail: admissions@westernu.edu. Website: http://www.westernu.edu/veterinary

Veterinary Sciences

Auburn University, College of Veterinary Medicine and Graduate School, Graduate Programs in Veterinary Medicine, Auburn University, AL 36849. Offers biomedical sciences (MS, PhD), including anatomy, physiology and pharmacology (MS), biomedical sciences (PhD), clinical sciences (MS), large animal surgery and medicine (MS), pathobiology (MS), radiology (MS), small animal surgery and medicine (MS); DVM/MS. *Program availability:* Part-time. *Faculty:* 97 full-time (40 women), 4 part-time/adjunct (2 women). *Students:* 19 full-time (11 women), 54 part-time (34 women); includes 10 minority (2 Black or African American, non-Hispanic/Latino; 2 American Indian or Alaska Native, non-Hispanic/Latino; 2 Asian, non-Hispanic/Latino; 4 Hispanic/Latino), 23 international. Average age 31. 39 applicants, 59% accepted, 14 enrolled. In 2015, 12 master's, 6 doctorates awarded. *Degree requirements:* For doctorate, thesis/dissertation. *Entrance requirements:* For master's, GRE General Test; for doctorate, GRE General Test, GRE Subject Test. *Application deadline:* Applications are processed on a rolling basis. Application fee: $50 ($60 for international students). Electronic applications accepted. *Expenses:* Tuition, state resident: full-time $8802; part-time $489 per credit hour. Tuition, nonresident: full-time $26,406; part-time $1467 per credit hour. *Required fees:* $808 per semester. Tuition and fees vary according to degree level and program. *Financial support:* Research assistantships, teaching assistantships, and Federal Work-Study available. Support available to part-time students. Financial award application deadline: 3/15; financial award applicants required to submit FAFSA. *Unit head:* Dr. Calvin Johnson, Acting Dean, 334-844-2650. *Application contact:* Dr. George Flowers, Dean of the Graduate School, 334-844-2125.

Clemson University, Graduate School, College of Agriculture, Forestry and Life Sciences, Department of Animal and Veterinary Sciences, Clemson, SC 29634-0311. Offers animal and veterinary sciences (MS, PhD). *Program availability:* Part-time. *Faculty:* 16 full-time (9 women), 1 part-time/adjunct (0 women). *Students:* 17 full-time (10 women), 7 part-time (4 women); includes 2 minority (1 Hispanic/Latino; 1 Two or more races, non-Hispanic/Latino), 4 international. Average age 29. 9 applicants, 78% accepted, 7 enrolled. In 2015, 5 master's, 1 doctorate awarded. *Degree requirements:* For master's, thesis (for some programs); for doctorate, comprehensive exam, thesis/dissertation. *Entrance requirements:* For master's and doctorate, GRE General Test, unofficial transcripts, letters of recommendation. Additional exam requirements/recommendations for international students: Required—TOEFL, IELTS (minimum score 7). *Application deadline:* For fall admission, 4/15 for domestic and international students; for spring admission, 10/15 for domestic students, 9/15 for international students. Applications are processed on a rolling basis. Application fee: $80 ($90 for international students). Electronic applications accepted. *Expenses:* $4,060 per semester full-time resident, $8,103 per semester full-time non-resident, $448 per credit hour part-time resident, $898 per credit hour part-time non-resident. *Financial support:* In 2015–16, 25 students received support, including 1 fellowship with partial tuition reimbursement available (averaging $5,000 per year), 12 research assistantships with partial tuition reimbursements available (averaging $13,792 per year), 12 teaching assistantships with partial tuition reimbursements available (averaging $10,714 per year); career-related internships or fieldwork and health care benefits also available. Financial award application deadline: 4/15. *Total annual research expenditures:* $265,131. *Unit head:* Dr. James Strickland, Department Chair, 864-656-3138, E-mail: jrstric@clemson.edu. *Application contact:* Dr. Peter Skewes, Graduate Program Coordinator, 864-656-4026, E-mail: pskewes@clemson.edu.

Colorado State University, College of Veterinary Medicine and Biomedical Sciences, Department of Clinical Sciences, Fort Collins, CO 80523-1678. Offers MS, PhD. *Program availability:* Part-time, evening/weekend. *Faculty:* 91 full-time (47 women), 12 part-time/adjunct (6 women). *Students:* 22 full-time (14 women), 50 part-time (36 women); includes 6 minority (2 Asian, non-Hispanic/Latino; 3 Hispanic/Latino; 1 Two or more races, non-Hispanic/Latino), 23 international. Average age 32. 23 applicants, 96% accepted, 22 enrolled. In 2015, 13 master's, 5 doctorates awarded. Terminal master's awarded for partial completion of doctoral program. *Degree requirements:* For master's, comprehensive exam (for some programs), thesis (for some programs); for doctorate, comprehensive exam, thesis/dissertation, preliminary examination, publication. *Entrance requirements:* For master's and doctorate, minimum overall GPA of 3.0. Additional exam requirements/recommendations for international students: Required—TOEFL (minimum score 550 paper-based; 80 iBT). *Application deadline:* For fall admission, 4/1 priority date for domestic and international students; for spring admission, 9/1 priority date for domestic and international students. Application fee: $60 ($70 for international students). Electronic applications accepted. *Expenses:* Tuition, state resident: full-time $9348. Tuition, nonresident: full-time $22,916. *Required fees:* $2174; $473.72 per credit hour. $236.86 per semester. Tuition and fees vary according to course load and program. *Financial support:* In 2015–16, 50 students received support, including 56 fellowships with full tuition reimbursements available (averaging $35,576 per year), 12 research assistantships with partial tuition reimbursements available (averaging $20,940 per year); teaching assistantships with partial tuition reimbursements available, career-related internships or fieldwork, and scholarships/grants also available. Financial award application deadline: 4/1. *Faculty research:* Epidemiology, musculoskeletal biology, pharmacology, cardiology, microbiology and immunology. *Total annual research expenditures:* $4.7 million. *Unit head:* Dr. Wayne Jensen, Professor and Interim Department Head, 970-297-4284, Fax: 970-297-1275, E-mail: wayne.jensen@colostate.edu. *Application contact:* Morna J. Mynard, Graduate Coordinator, 970-297-4030, Fax: 970-297-1275, E-mail: morna.mynard@colostate.edu. Website: http://csu-cvmbs.colostate.edu/academics/clinsci/graduate-programs/Pages/default.aspx

Drexel University, College of Medicine, Biomedical Graduate Programs, Program in Laboratory Animal Science, Philadelphia, PA 19104-2875. Offers MLAS. *Program availability:* Part-time. *Degree requirements:* For master's, comprehensive exam. *Entrance requirements:* For master's, GRE General Test, minimum GPA of 3.0. Additional exam requirements/recommendations for international students: Required—TOEFL. Electronic applications accepted. *Faculty research:* Laboratory animal medicine, experimental surgery, development of animal models for human diseases.

Iowa State University of Science and Technology, Department of Veterinary Clinical Sciences, Ames, IA 50011. Offers MS. *Degree requirements:* For master's, thesis or alternative. *Entrance requirements:* For master's, GRE. Additional exam requirements/recommendations for international students: Required—TOEFL (minimum score 550 paper-based; 79 iBT), IELTS (minimum score 6.5). Electronic applications accepted. *Faculty research:* Theriogenology, veterinary medicine, veterinary surgery, extracorporeal shock waves, therapy, orthopedic research in animals.

Iowa State University of Science and Technology, Department of Veterinary Microbiology and Preventive Medicine, Ames, IA 50011. Offers veterinary microbiology (MS, PhD). *Entrance requirements:* For master's and doctorate, GRE General Test. Additional exam requirements/recommendations for international students: Required—

TOEFL (minimum score 550 paper-based; 79 iBT), IELTS (minimum score 6.5). Electronic applications accepted. *Faculty research:* Bacteriology, immunology, virology, public health and food safety.

Kansas State University, Graduate School, College of Veterinary Medicine, Department of Clinical Sciences, Manhattan, KS 66506. Offers MPH, Graduate Certificate. *Degree requirements:* For master's, thesis. *Entrance requirements:* For master's, GRE, DVM. Additional exam requirements/recommendations for international students: Required—TOEFL (minimum score 550 paper-based). Electronic applications accepted. *Faculty research:* Clinical trials, equine gastrointestinal ulceration, leptospirosis, food animal pharmacology, equine immunology, diabetes.

Louisiana State University and Agricultural & Mechanical College, School of Veterinary Medicine and Graduate School, Department of Comparative Biomedical Sciences, Baton Rouge, LA 70803. Offers MS, PhD.

Louisiana State University and Agricultural & Mechanical College, School of Veterinary Medicine and Graduate School, Department of Pathobiological Sciences, Baton Rouge, LA 70803. Offers MS, PhD.

Louisiana State University and Agricultural & Mechanical College, School of Veterinary Medicine and Graduate School, Department of Veterinary Clinical Sciences, Baton Rouge, LA 70803. Offers MS, PhD.

Michigan State University, College of Veterinary Medicine and The Graduate School, Graduate Programs in Veterinary Medicine, East Lansing, MI 48824. Offers comparative medicine and integrative biology (MS, PhD), including comparative medicine and integrative biology, comparative medicine and integrative biology–environmental toxicology (PhD); food safety and toxicology (MS), including food safety; integrative toxicology (PhD), including animal science–environmental toxicology, biochemistry and molecular biology–environmental toxicology, chemistry–environmental toxicology, crop and soil sciences–environmental toxicology, environmental engineering–environmental toxicology, environmental geosciences–environmental toxicology, fisheries and wildlife–environmental toxicology, food science–environmental toxicology, forestry–environmental toxicology, genetics–environmental toxicology, human nutrition–environmental toxicology, microbiology–environmental toxicology, pharmacology and toxicology–environmental toxicology, zoology–environmental toxicology; large animal clinical sciences (MS, PhD); microbiology and molecular genetics (MS, PhD), including industrial microbiology, microbiology, microbiology and molecular genetics, microbiology–environmental toxicology (PhD); pathobiology and diagnostic investigation (MS, PhD), including pathology, pathology–environmental toxicology (PhD); pharmacology and toxicology (MS, PhD); pharmacology and toxicology–environmental toxicology (PhD); physiology (MS, PhD); small animal clinical sciences (MS). Electronic applications accepted. *Faculty research:* Molecular genetics, food safety/toxicology, comparative orthopedics, airway disease, population medicine.

Mississippi State University, College of Veterinary Medicine, Office of Research and Graduate Studies, Mississippi State, MS 39762. Offers environmental toxicology (PhD); veterinary medical sciences (MS, PhD). *Program availability:* Part-time. *Faculty:* 85 full-time (30 women), 46 part-time/adjunct (16 women). *Students:* 39 full-time (19 women), 27 part-time (16 women); includes 5 minority (2 Black or African American, non-Hispanic/Latino; 1 Asian, non-Hispanic/Latino; 1 Native Hawaiian or other Pacific Islander, non-Hispanic/Latino; 1 Two or more races, non-Hispanic/Latino), 24 international. Average age 31. 15 applicants, 67% accepted, 9 enrolled. In 2015, 6 master's, 6 doctorates awarded. Terminal master's awarded for partial completion of doctoral program. *Degree requirements:* For master's, thesis (for some programs); for doctorate, thesis/dissertation. *Entrance requirements:* For master's, minimum undergraduate GPA of 3.0, bachelor's degree; for doctorate, minimum undergraduate GPA of 3.0. Additional exam requirements/recommendations for international students: Required—TOEFL (minimum score 550 paper-based; 79 iBT); Recommended—IELTS (minimum score 6.5). *Application deadline:* For fall admission, 7/1 priority date for domestic students, 5/1 priority date for international students; for spring admission, 11/1 priority date for domestic students, 9/1 priority date for international students; for summer admission, 4/1 priority date for domestic students, 3/1 priority date for international students. Applications are processed on a rolling basis. Application fee: $60. Electronic applications accepted. *Expenses: Tuition, area resident:* Full-time $7502; part-time $833.74 per credit hour. Tuition, nonresident: full-time $20,142; part-time $2238.24 per credit hour. *Financial support:* In 2015–16, 35 students received support, including 35 research assistantships with full tuition reimbursements available (averaging $20,107 per year); career-related internships or fieldwork, institutionally sponsored loans, scholarships/grants, and unspecified assistantships also available. Financial award application deadline: 4/1; financial award applicants required to submit FAFSA. *Faculty research:* Food animal health (poultry and warm-water aquaculture) using immunology, microbiology, molecular biology, parasitology, pathology, pharmacology, and environmental toxicology. *Total annual research expenditures:* $5.7 million. *Unit head:* Dr. Mark L. Lawrence, Associate Dean of Research and Graduate Studies, 662-325-1205, Fax: 662-325-1193, E-mail: lawrence@cvm.msstate.edu. *Application contact:* Tia H. Perkins, Coordinator, Graduate Studies, 662-325-1417, Fax: 662-325-1193, E-mail: tia.perkins@msstate.edu. Website: http://www.cvm.msstate.edu/index.php/academics/degree-programs-research/office-of-research-graduate-studies-orgs

North Carolina State University, College of Veterinary Medicine, Program in Comparative Biomedical Sciences, Raleigh, NC 27695. Offers cell biology (MS, PhD); infectious disease (MS, PhD); pathology (MS, PhD); pharmacology (MS, PhD); population medicine (MS, PhD). *Program availability:* Part-time. *Degree requirements:* For master's, thesis; for doctorate, thesis/dissertation. *Entrance requirements:* For master's and doctorate, GRE General Test. Additional exam requirements/recommendations for international students: Required—TOEFL (minimum score 550 paper-based). Electronic applications accepted. *Expenses:* Contact institution. *Faculty research:* Infectious diseases, cell biology, pharmacology and toxicology, genomics, pathology and population medicine.

The Ohio State University, College of Veterinary Medicine, Program in Comparative and Veterinary Medicine, Columbus, OH 43210. Offers MS, PhD. *Faculty:* 105. *Students:* 78 full-time (50 women), 13 part-time (9 women); includes 6 minority (1 Black or African American, non-Hispanic/Latino; 2 Asian, non-Hispanic/Latino; 3 Hispanic/Latino), 30 international. Average age 31. In 2015, 26 master's, 13 doctorates awarded. *Entrance requirements:* For master's and doctorate, GRE. Additional exam requirements/recommendations for international students: Required—TOEFL (minimum score 550 paper-based; 79 iBT), Michigan English Language Assessment Battery (minimum score 82); Recommended—IELTS (minimum score 7). *Application deadline:* For fall admission, 12/15 priority date for domestic students, 11/30 priority date for international students; for spring admission, 10/15 for domestic students, 9/15 for

international students; for summer admission, 3/15 for domestic students, 2/15 for international students. Applications are processed on a rolling basis. Application fee: $60 ($70 for international students). Electronic applications accepted. *Unit head:* Dr. Rustin M. Moore, Dean/Chair/Professor, 614-688-8749, Fax: 614-292-3544, E-mail: moore.66@osu.edu. *Application contact:* Graduate and Professional Admissions, 614-292-6031, Fax: 614-292-3656, E-mail: gpadmissions@osu.edu.
Website: http://vet.osu.edu/education/graduate-programs

Oklahoma State University, Center for Veterinary Health Sciences and Graduate College, Graduate Program in Veterinary Biomedical Sciences, Stillwater, OK 74078. Offers MS, PhD. *Program availability:* Online learning. Terminal master's awarded for partial completion of doctoral program. *Degree requirements:* For master's, thesis; for doctorate, comprehensive exam, thesis/dissertation. *Entrance requirements:* For master's and doctorate, GRE General Test. Additional exam requirements/recommendations for international students: Required—TOEFL (minimum score 80 iBT). Electronic applications accepted. *Expenses:* Contact institution. *Faculty research:* Infectious and parasitic diseases, physiology, toxicology, biomedical lasers, clinical studies.

Penn State Hershey Medical Center, College of Medicine, Graduate School Programs in the Biomedical Sciences, Graduate Program in Laboratory Animal Medicine, Hershey, PA 17033. Offers MS. *Students:* 4 full-time (3 women); includes 1 minority (Black or African American, non-Hispanic/Latino). 2 applicants, 100% accepted, 2 enrolled. In 2015, 1 master's awarded. *Degree requirements:* For master's, thesis or alternative. *Entrance requirements:* For master's, GRE, DVM. Additional exam requirements/recommendations for international students: Required—TOEFL (minimum score 550 paper-based). *Application deadline:* For fall admission, 1/31 priority date for domestic students, 2/1 priority date for international students. Applications are processed on a rolling basis. Application fee: $65. Electronic applications accepted. *Financial support:* In 2015–16, 2 students received support. Fellowships with full tuition reimbursements available, research assistantships with full tuition reimbursements available, scholarships/grants, traineeships, health care benefits, and unspecified assistantships available. Financial award applicants required to submit FAFSA. *Faculty research:* Veterinary pathology; pain, analgesia and anesthesia of lab animals; genetically modified animal models of cancer; transgenic animals. *Unit head:* Dr. Ronald P. Wilson, Chair, 717-531-8460, Fax: 717-531-5001, E-mail: grad-hmc@psu.edu. *Application contact:* Nannette Kirst, Program Aide, 717-531-8460, Fax: 717-531-5001, E-mail: nkirst@psu.edu.
Website: http://www.pennstatehershey.org/web/comparativemedicine/programs

Purdue University, School of Veterinary Medicine and Graduate School, Graduate Programs in Veterinary Medicine, Department of Basic Medical Sciences, West Lafayette, IN 47907. Offers anatomy (MS, PhD); pharmacology (MS, PhD); physiology (MS, PhD). *Program availability:* Part-time. Terminal master's awarded for partial completion of doctoral program. *Degree requirements:* For master's, thesis; for doctorate, thesis/dissertation. *Entrance requirements:* For master's and doctorate, GRE General Test. Additional exam requirements/recommendations for international students: Required—TOEFL. Electronic applications accepted. *Faculty research:* Development and regeneration, tissue injury and shock, biomedical engineering, ovarian function, bone and cartilage biology, cell and molecular biology.

Purdue University, School of Veterinary Medicine and Graduate School, Graduate Programs in Veterinary Medicine, Department of Comparative Pathobiology, West Lafayette, IN 47907-2027. Offers comparative epidemiology and public health (MS); comparative epidemiology and public heath (PhD); comparative microbiology and immunology (MS, PhD); comparative pathobiology (MS, PhD); interdisciplinary studies (PhD), including microbial pathogenesis, molecular signaling and cancer biology, molecular virology; lab animal medicine (MS); veterinary anatomic pathology (MS); veterinary clinical pathology (MS). Terminal master's awarded for partial completion of doctoral program. *Degree requirements:* For master's, thesis (for some programs); for doctorate, thesis/dissertation. *Entrance requirements:* For master's and doctorate, GRE General Test. Additional exam requirements/recommendations for international students: Required—TOEFL (minimum score 575 paper-based), IELTS (minimum score 6.5), TWE (minimum score 4). Electronic applications accepted.

Purdue University, School of Veterinary Medicine and Graduate School, Graduate Programs in Veterinary Medicine, Department of Veterinary Clinical Sciences, West Lafayette, IN 47907. Offers MS, PhD. Degrees offered are post-DVM. Terminal master's awarded for partial completion of doctoral program. *Degree requirements:* For master's, thesis (for some programs); for doctorate, thesis/dissertation. *Entrance requirements:* For master's and doctorate, DVM. *Faculty research:* Flow cytometry, chemotherapy, biologic response modifiers, broncho-alveolar lavage, lithotripsy.

South Dakota State University, Graduate School, College of Agriculture and Biological Sciences, Department of Veterinary and Biomedical Sciences, Brookings, SD 57007. Offers biological sciences (MS, PhD). *Program availability:* Part-time, evening/weekend. *Degree requirements:* For master's, thesis (for some programs), oral exam; for doctorate, comprehensive exam, thesis/dissertation, preliminary oral and written exams. *Entrance requirements:* Additional exam requirements/recommendations for international students: Required—TOEFL (minimum score 525 paper-based; 71 iBT). *Faculty research:* Infectious disease, food animal, virology, immunology.

Texas A&M University, College of Veterinary Medicine and Biomedical Sciences, College Station, TX 77843. Offers MS, DVM, PhD. *Accreditation:* AVMA. *Program availability:* Part-time. *Faculty:* 134. *Students:* 791 full-time (584 women), 50 part-time (34 women); includes 170 minority (21 Black or African American, non-Hispanic/Latino; 1 American Indian or Alaska Native, non-Hispanic/Latino; 43 Asian, non-Hispanic/Latino; 89 Hispanic/Latino; 1 Native Hawaiian or other Pacific Islander, non-Hispanic/Latino; 15 Two or more races, non-Hispanic/Latino), 60 international. Average age 29. 241 applicants, 89% accepted, 206 enrolled. In 2015, 63 master's, 13 doctorates awarded. Terminal master's awarded for partial completion of doctoral program. *Entrance requirements:* For master's and doctorate, GRE General Test. Additional exam requirements/recommendations for international students: Required—TOEFL (minimum score 550 paper-based; 80 iBT), IELTS (minimum score 6), PTE (minimum score 53). *Application deadline:* For fall admission, 10/1 for domestic and international students. Application fee: $50 ($90 for international students). *Expenses:* Contact institution. *Financial support:* In 2015–16, 763 students received support, including 24 fellowships with tuition reimbursements available (averaging $11,758 per year), 106 research assistantships with tuition reimbursements available (averaging $7,379 per year), 25 teaching assistantships with tuition reimbursements available (averaging $6,754 per year); career-related internships or fieldwork, institutionally sponsored loans, scholarships/grants, traineeships, health care benefits, tuition waivers (full and partial), unspecified assistantships, and clinical associateships also available. Support available to part-time students. Financial award application deadline: 3/15; financial award applicants required to submit FAFSA. *Faculty research:* Physiology, pharmacology, anatomy, microbiology, parasitology. *Unit head:* Dr. Eleanor M. Green, Dean, 979-845-5053, Fax: 979-845-5088, E-mail: emgreen@tamu.edu. *Application contact:* Graduate Admissions, 979-845-1044, E-mail: admissions@tamu.edu.
Website: http://vetmed.tamu.edu/

Tuskegee University, Graduate Programs, College of Veterinary Medicine, Nursing and Allied Health, School of Veterinary Medicine, Tuskegee, AL 36088. Offers MS, DVM. *Degree requirements:* For master's, thesis. *Entrance requirements:* For master's, GRE General Test; for doctorate, VCAT. Additional exam requirements/recommendations for international students: Required—TOEFL (minimum score 500 paper-based).

Université de Montréal, Faculty of Veterinary Medicine and Faculty of Graduate Studies, Graduate Programs in Veterinary Sciences, Montréal, QC H3C 3J7, Canada. Offers M Sc, PhD. *Degree requirements:* For master's, one foreign language, thesis optional. Electronic applications accepted. *Faculty research:* Animal reproduction, infectious diseases of swine, physiology of exercise in horses, viral diseases of cattle, health management and epidemiology.

University of California, Davis, School of Veterinary Medicine and Graduate Studies, Program in Preventive Veterinary Medicine, Davis, CA 95616. Offers MPVM, DVM/MPVM. *Program availability:* Part-time. *Degree requirements:* For master's, thesis. *Entrance requirements:* For master's, DVM or equivalent. Additional exam requirements/recommendations for international students: Required—TOEFL (minimum score 550 paper-based). *Faculty research:* Epidemiology, zoonoses, veterinary public health, wildlife and ecosystem health.

University of California, Davis, School of Veterinary Medicine, Residency Training Program, Davis, CA 95616. Offers Certificate. *Entrance requirements:* For degree, DVM or equivalent, 1 year of related experience. *Faculty research:* Small animal and large animal medicine, surgery, infectious diseases, pathology.

University of Florida, College of Veterinary Medicine, Graduate Program in Veterinary Medical Sciences, Gainesville, FL 32611. Offers forensic toxicology (Certificate); veterinary medical sciences (MS, PhD), including forensic toxicology (MS). *Program availability:* Online learning. Terminal master's awarded for partial completion of doctoral program. *Degree requirements:* For master's, thesis; for doctorate, thesis/dissertation. *Entrance requirements:* For master's and doctorate, GRE General Test, minimum GPA of 3.0. Additional exam requirements/recommendations for international students: Required—TOEFL (minimum score 550 paper-based). Electronic applications accepted. *Expenses:* Contact institution.

University of Georgia, College of Veterinary Medicine, Department of Large Animal Medicine, Athens, GA 30602. Offers MS. Application fee is waived when completed online.

University of Georgia, College of Veterinary Medicine, Department of Population Health, Athens, GA 30602. Offers food animal medicine (MFAM); population health (MAM). *Entrance requirements:* For master's, GRE General Test. Electronic applications accepted.

University of Georgia, College of Veterinary Medicine, Department of Small Animal Medicine and Surgery, Athens, GA 30602. Offers MS.

University of Guelph, Ontario Veterinary College and Graduate Studies, Graduate Programs in Veterinary Sciences, Guelph, ON N1G 2W1, Canada. Offers M Sc, DV Sc, PhD, Diploma. *Accreditation:* AVMA (one or more programs are accredited). *Degree requirements:* For master's, thesis; for doctorate, comprehensive exam, thesis/dissertation. *Entrance requirements:* Additional exam requirements/recommendations for international students: Required—TOEFL. *Faculty research:* Veterinary and comparative medicine, biomedical sciences, population medicine, pathology, microbiology.

University of Idaho, College of Graduate Studies, College of Agricultural and Life Sciences, Department of Animal and Veterinary Science, Moscow, ID 83844-2330. Offers animal physiology (PhD); animal science (MS), including production. *Faculty:* 3 full-time. *Students:* 8 full-time, 8 part-time. Average age 30. In 2015, 6 master's, 1 doctorate awarded. *Degree requirements:* For doctorate, thesis/dissertation. *Entrance requirements:* For master's, GRE General Test, minimum GPA of 2.8; for doctorate, minimum undergraduate GPA of 2.8, graduate 3.0. *Application deadline:* For fall admission, 8/1 for domestic students; for spring admission, 12/15 for domestic students. Applications are processed on a rolling basis. Application fee: $60. Electronic applications accepted. *Expenses:* Tuition, state resident: full-time $6205; part-time $399 per credit hour. Tuition, nonresident: full-time $20,209; part-time $1177 per credit hour. *Required fees:* $2017; $58 per credit hour. Full-time tuition and fees vary according to course load and reciprocity agreements. *Financial support:* Research assistantships and teaching assistantships available. Financial award applicants required to submit FAFSA. *Faculty research:* Reproductive biology, muscle and growth physiology, meat science, aquaculture, ruminant nutrition. *Unit head:* Dr. Amin Ahmadzadeh, Interim Department Co-Chair, 208-885-6345, E-mail: avs-students@uidaho.edu. *Application contact:* Sean Scoggin, Graduate Recruitment Coordinator, 208-885-4001, Fax: 208-885-4406, E-mail: graduateadmissions@uidaho.edu.
Website: http://www.uidaho.edu/cals/avs

University of Illinois at Urbana–Champaign, College of Veterinary Medicine, Department of Comparative Biosciences, Urbana, IL 61802. Offers MS, PhD, DVM/PhD. *Degree requirements:* For doctorate, thesis/dissertation.

University of Illinois at Urbana–Champaign, College of Veterinary Medicine, Department of Pathobiology, Urbana, IL 61802. Offers MS, PhD, DVM/PhD. Terminal master's awarded for partial completion of doctoral program. *Degree requirements:* For doctorate, thesis/dissertation.

University of Illinois at Urbana–Champaign, College of Veterinary Medicine, Department of Veterinary Clinical Medicine, Urbana, IL 61801. Offers MS, PhD, DVM/PhD. *Degree requirements:* For doctorate, thesis/dissertation.

University of Kentucky, Graduate School, College of Agriculture, Food and Environment, Program in Veterinary Science, Lexington, KY 40506-0032. Offers MS, PhD. *Degree requirements:* For master's, comprehensive exam, thesis; for doctorate, comprehensive exam, thesis/dissertation. *Entrance requirements:* For master's, GRE General Test, minimum undergraduate GPA of 2.75; for doctorate, GRE General Test, minimum graduate GPA of 3.0. Additional exam requirements/recommendations for international students: Required—TOEFL (minimum score 550 paper-based). Electronic applications accepted. *Faculty research:* Microbiology, reproductive physiology, genetics, pharmacology/toxicology, parasitology.

University of Maryland, College Park, Academic Affairs, College of Agriculture and Natural Resources, Maryland Campus of VA/MD Regional College of Veterinary Medicine, Veterinary Medical Sciences Program, College Park, MD 20742. Offers MS, PhD. *Degree requirements:* For master's, thesis, oral exam; for doctorate, thesis/dissertation, oral exam, public seminar. *Entrance requirements:* For doctorate, GRE General Test. Electronic applications accepted.

University of Minnesota, Twin Cities Campus, College of Veterinary Medicine and Graduate School, Graduate Programs in Veterinary Medicine, Program in Comparative and Molecular Bioscience, Minneapolis, MN 55455-0213. Offers MS, PhD, DVM/PhD. Terminal master's awarded for partial completion of doctoral program. *Degree requirements:* For master's, comprehensive exam, thesis; for doctorate, comprehensive exam, thesis/dissertation. *Entrance requirements:* For master's and doctorate, GRE.

SECTION 31: VETERINARY MEDICINE AND SCIENCES

Veterinary Sciences

Additional exam requirements/recommendations for international students: Required—TOEFL (minimum score 550 paper-based; 79 iBT). Electronic applications accepted. *Faculty research:* Molecular regulation of immunity; mechanisms of bacterial, viral, and parasite pathogenesis; structural and functional comparative physiology and pathology.

University of Minnesota, Twin Cities Campus, College of Veterinary Medicine and Graduate School, Graduate Programs in Veterinary Medicine, Program in Veterinary Medicine, Minneapolis, MN 55455-0213. Offers MS, PhD, DVM/PhD. Terminal master's awarded for partial completion of doctoral program. *Degree requirements:* For master's, comprehensive exam, thesis; for doctorate, comprehensive exam, thesis/dissertation. *Entrance requirements:* Additional exam requirements/recommendations for international students: Required—TOEFL (minimum score 550 paper-based; 79 iBT). Electronic applications accepted. *Faculty research:* Infectious diseases, internal medicine, population medicine, surgery/radiology/anesthesiology, theriogenology.

University of Missouri, College of Veterinary Medicine and Office of Research and Graduate Studies, Graduate Programs in Veterinary Medicine, Department of Veterinary Medicine and Surgery, Columbia, MO 65211. Offers MS. *Degree requirements:* For master's, thesis. *Entrance requirements:* For master's, GRE General Test, minimum GPA of 3.0; 2 letters of recommendation; departmental application. Additional exam requirements/recommendations for international students: Required—TOEFL (minimum score 550 paper-based; 80 iBT). *Application deadline:* Applications are processed on a rolling basis. Application fee: $65 ($90 for international students). Electronic applications accepted. *Financial support:* Fellowships, research assistantships with full tuition reimbursements, teaching assistantships with full tuition reimbursements, institutionally sponsored loans, scholarships/grants, traineeships, health care benefits, and unspecified assistantships available. Support available to part-time students. Financial award applicants required to submit FAFSA. *Faculty research:* Anesthesiology, comparative cardiology, equine, food animal and companion animal medicine and surgery, neurology, oncology, comparative ophthalmology, radiation oncology, radiology, nutrition, theriogenology.
Website: http://www.vms.missouri.edu/vmsgraduateprogram.html

University of Nebraska–Lincoln, Graduate College, College of Agricultural Sciences and Natural Resources, School of Veterinary Medicine and Biomedical Sciences, Lincoln, NE 68588. Offers veterinary science (MS). MS, PhD offered jointly with University of Nebraska Medical Center. *Program availability:* Online learning. *Degree requirements:* For master's, thesis optional; for doctorate, comprehensive exam, thesis/dissertation. *Entrance requirements:* For master's, GRE General Test; for doctorate, GRE General Test, MCAT, or VCAT. Additional exam requirements/recommendations for international students: Required—TOEFL (minimum score 550 paper-based). Electronic applications accepted. *Faculty research:* Virology, immunobiology, molecular biology, mycotoxins, ocular degeneration.

University of Prince Edward Island, Atlantic Veterinary College, Graduate Program in Veterinary Medicine, Charlottetown, PE C1A 4P3, Canada. Offers anatomy (M Sc, PhD); bacteriology (M Sc, PhD); clinical pharmacology (M Sc, PhD); clinical sciences (M Sc, PhD); epidemiology (M Sc, PhD), including reproduction; fish health (M Sc, PhD); food animal nutrition (M Sc, PhD); immunology (M Sc, PhD); microanatomy (M Sc, PhD); parasitology (M Sc, PhD); pathology (M Sc, PhD); pharmacology (M Sc, PhD); physiology (M Sc, PhD); toxicology (M Sc, PhD); veterinary science (M Vet Sc); virology (M Sc, PhD). *Program availability:* Part-time. *Degree requirements:* For master's, thesis; for doctorate, thesis/dissertation. *Entrance requirements:* For master's, DVM, B Sc honors degree, or equivalent; for doctorate, M Sc. Additional exam requirements/recommendations for international students: Required—TOEFL (minimum score 550 paper-based; 80 iBT). *Expenses:* Contact institution. *Faculty research:* Animal health management, infectious diseases, fin fish and shellfish health, basic biomedical sciences, ecosystem health.

University of Saskatchewan, Western College of Veterinary Medicine and College of Graduate Studies and Research, Graduate Programs in Veterinary Medicine, Saskatoon, SK S7N 5A2, Canada. Offers large animal clinical sciences (M Sc, M Vet Sc, PhD); small animal clinical sciences (M Sc, M Vet Sc, PhD), including small animal clinical sciences (M Sc, PhD), veterinary anesthesiology, radiology and surgery (M Vet Sc), veterinary internal medicine (M Vet Sc); veterinary biomedical sciences (M Sc, M Vet Sc, PhD), including veterinary anatomy (M Sc), veterinary biomedical sciences (M Vet Sc), veterinary physiological sciences (M Sc, PhD); veterinary medicine (M Sc, PhD); veterinary microbiology (M Sc, M Vet Sc, PhD); veterinary pathology (M Sc, M Vet Sc, PhD). *Degree requirements:* For master's, comprehensive exam, thesis (for some programs); for doctorate, comprehensive exam, thesis/dissertation. *Entrance requirements:* Additional exam requirements/recommendations for international students: Required—TOEFL (minimum score 80 iBT) or IELTS (minimum score 6.5). Electronic applications accepted. *Expenses:* Contact institution. *Faculty research:* Reproduction, toxicology, wildlife diseases, food animal medicine, equine health.

University of Washington, Graduate School, School of Medicine, Graduate Programs in Medicine, Department of Comparative Medicine, Seattle, WA 98195. Offers MS.

University of Wisconsin–Madison, School of Veterinary Medicine, Madison, WI 53706-1380. Offers MS, DVM, PhD. *Accreditation:* AVMA (one or more programs are accredited). Terminal master's awarded for partial completion of doctoral program. *Degree requirements:* For master's, thesis; for doctorate, thesis/dissertation (for some programs). *Entrance requirements:* For doctorate, GRE General Test (for DVM). *Expenses:* Contact institution. *Faculty research:* Infectious disease, ophthalmology, orthopedics, food animal production, oncology, cardio-respiratory.

Utah State University, School of Graduate Studies, College of Agriculture, Department of Animal, Dairy and Veterinary Sciences, Logan, UT 84322. Offers animal science (MS, PhD); bioveterinary science (MS, PhD); dairy science (MS). *Program availability:* Part-time. *Degree requirements:* For master's, thesis (for some programs); for doctorate, comprehensive exam, thesis/dissertation. *Entrance requirements:* For master's and doctorate, GRE General Test, minimum GPA of 3.0. Additional exam requirements/recommendations for international students: Required—TOEFL. Electronic applications accepted. *Faculty research:* Monoclonal antibodies, antiviral chemotherapy, management systems, biotechnology, rumen fermentation manipulation.

Virginia Polytechnic Institute and State University, Virginia-Maryland Regional College of Veterinary Medicine, Blacksburg, VA 24061. Offers biomedical and veterinary sciences (MS, PhD); public health (MPH); research in translational medicine (Certificate); veterinary medicine (DVM). *Accreditation:* AVMA (one or more programs are accredited). *Degree requirements:* For master's, comprehensive exam (for some programs), thesis (for some programs); for doctorate, comprehensive exam (for some programs), thesis/dissertation (for some programs). *Entrance requirements:* For master's and doctorate, GRE/GMAT (may vary by department). Additional exam requirements/recommendations for international students: Required—TOEFL (minimum score 550 paper-based). Electronic applications accepted. *Expenses:* Contact institution.

Washington State University, College of Veterinary Medicine, Program in Veterinary Clinical Sciences, Pullman, WA 99164. Offers MS, PhD. *Program availability:* Part-time. *Faculty:* 36 full-time (18 women). *Students:* 10 full-time (8 women), 18 part-time (11 women), 13 international. Average age 30. 10 applicants, 100% accepted, 10 enrolled. In 2015, 6 master's awarded. *Degree requirements:* For master's, thesis, oral exam; for doctorate, thesis/dissertation, oral exam. *Entrance requirements:* For master's and doctorate, minimum GPA of 3.0, DVM or equivalent. Additional exam requirements/recommendations for international students: Required—TOEFL. *Application deadline:* For fall admission, 3/31 priority date for domestic and international students. Application fee: $75. Electronic applications accepted. *Financial support:* In 2015–16, 23 research assistantships with full tuition reimbursements (averaging $30,084 per year) were awarded. Financial award application deadline: 3/1. *Faculty research:* Oncology, mastitis, nuclear medicine, neuroanesthesia, exercise physiology. *Total annual research expenditures:* $500,000. *Unit head:* Dr. William Dernell, Chair, 509-335-0738, Fax: 509-335-0880. *Application contact:* Kathy L. Dahmen, Administrative Manager, 509-335-4156, Fax: 509-335-0880, E-mail: dahmen@vetmed.wsu.edu.
Website: http://graduate.vetmed.wsu.edu/

APPENDIXES

Institutional Changes
Since the 2016 Edition

Following is an alphabetical listing of institutions that have recently closed, merged with other institutions, or changed their names or status. In the case of a name change, the former name appears first, followed by the new name.

American Baptist College of American Baptist Theological Seminary (Nashville, TN): *no longer offers graduate degrees*

American College of Traditional Chinese Medicine (San Francisco, CA): *merged with California Institute of Integral Studies (San Francisco, CA)*

Augustana College (Sioux Falls, SD): *name changed to Augustana University*

Bainbridge Graduate Institute (Bainbridge Island, WA): *name changed to Pinchot University*

Benedictine University at Springfield (Springfield, IL): *degree programs now offered through Benedictine University's National Moser Center for Adult Learning*

The Boston Conservatory (Boston, MA): *merged with Berklee College of Music (Boston, MA)*

Burlington College (Burlington, VT): *closed*

Cabrini College (Radnor, PA): *name changed to Cabrini University*

Carolina Evangelical Divinity School (High Point, NC): *name changed to Carolina Graduate School of Divinity*

Castleton State College (Castleton, VT): *name changed to Castleton University*

Charles Drew University of Medicine and Science (Los Angeles, CA): *name changed to Charles R. Drew University of Medicine and Science*

The Chicago School of Professional Psychology at Westwood (Los Angeles, CA): *closed*

Concordia University (Irvine, CA): *name changed to Concordia University Irvine*

Concordia University College of Alberta (Edmonton, AB, Canada): *name changed to Concordia University of Edmonton*

The Criswell College (Dallas, TX): *name changed to Criswell College*

DeVry University (Louisville, KY): *closed*

DeVry University (Bethesda, MD): *closed*

DeVry University (Sandy, UT): *closed*

Doane College (Crete, NE): *name changed to Doane University*

Dowling College (Oakdale, NY): *closed*

Emmanuel Christian Seminary (Johnson City, TN): *merged with Milligan College (Milligan College, TN)*

Everest University (Jacksonville, FL): *closed*

Everest University (Melbourne, FL): *closed*

Everest University (Orlando, FL): *closed*

Everest University (Pompano Beach, FL): *closed*

Felician College (Lodi, NJ): *name changed to Felician University*

Five Branches University: Graduate School of Traditional Chinese Medicine (Santa Cruz, CA): *name changed to Five Branches University*

Georgia Regents University (Augusta, GA): *name changed to Augusta University*

Golden Gate Baptist Theological Seminary (Mill Valley, CA): *name changed to Gateway Seminary*

Gooding Institute of Nurse Anesthesia (Panama City, FL): *closed*

Hawaii College of Oriental Medicine (Kamuela, HI): *closed*

Institut Franco-Européen de Chiropratique (94200 Ivry-sur-Seine, France): *name changed to Institut Franco-Européen de Chiropraxie*

King's University (Southlake, TX): *name changed to The King's University*

Lakeland College (Plymouth, WI): *name changed to Lakeland University*

Laurel University (High Point, NC): *name changed to John Wesley University*

Lutheran Theological Southern Seminary (Columbia, SC): *merged with Lenoir-Rhyne University (Hickory, NC)*

Massachusetts School of Professional Psychology (Boston, MA): *name changed to William James College*

Middlebury Institute of International Studies (Monterey, CA): *name changed to Middlebury Institute of International Studies at Monterey*

Midway College (Midway, KY): *name changed to Midway University*

Nashotah House (Nashotah, WI): *name changed to Nashotah House Theological Seminary*

The New England College of Optometry (Boston, MA): *name changed to New England College of Optometry*

New England School of Acupuncture (Newton, MA): *merged with MCPHS University (Boston, MA)*

Northern Baptist Theological Seminary (Lombard, IL): *name changed to Northern Seminary*

Northwest Institute of Literary Arts (Freeland, WA): *closed*

Our Lady of Holy Cross College (New Orleans, LA): *name changed to University of Holy Cross*

Penn State Dickinson School of Law (University Park, PA): *name changed to Penn State University–Dickinson Law*

Purdue University Calumet (Hammond, IN): *name changed to Purdue University Northwest*

Purdue University North Central (Westville, IN): *name changed to Purdue University Northwest*

Rutgers, The State University of New Jersey, Camden (Camden, NJ): *name changed to Rutgers University–Camden*

Rutgers, The State University of New Jersey, Newark (Newark, NJ): *name changed to Rutgers University–Newark*

Rutgers, The State University of New Jersey, New Brunswick (Piscataway, NJ): *name changed to Rutgers University–New Brunswick*

St. Catharine College (St. Catharine, KY): *closed*

Samra University of Oriental Medicine (Los Angeles, CA): *closed*

The School of Professional Psychology at Forest Institute (Springfield, MO): *closed*

Skidmore College (Saratoga Springs, NY): *no longer offers graduate degrees*

Southern Baptist Theological Seminary (Louisville, KY): *name changed to The Southern Baptist Theological Seminary*

Southern Polytechnic State University (Marietta, GA): *merged with Kennesaw State University (Kennesaw, GA)*

South Texas College of Law (Houston, TX): *name changed to Houston College of Law*

Stevens-Henager College–Salt Lake City/Murray (Salt Lake City, UT): *name changed to Stevens-Henager College*

Taft Law School (Santa Ana, CA): *merged into a single entry for Taft University System (Denver, CO)*

Temple Baptist Seminary (Chattanooga, TN): *merged with Piedmont International University (Winston-Salem, NC)*

Texas A&M Health Science Center (College Station, TX): *merged into a single entry for Texas A&M University (College Station, TX)*

Thomas Edison State College (Trenton, NJ): *name changed to Thomas Edison State University*

Thunderbird School of Global Management (Glendale, AZ): *merged with Arizona State University at the Tempe campus (Tempe, AZ)*

Touro University (Vallejo, CA): *name changed to Touro University California*

Toyota Technological Institute of Chicago (Chicago, IL): *name changed to Toyota Technological Institute at Chicago*

Trinity International University, South Florida Campus (Davie, FL): *name changed to Trinity International University Florida*

Union Graduate College (Schenectady, NY): *merged with Clarkson University (Potsdam, NY)*

United States International University (Nairobi, Kenya): *name changed to United States International University–Africa*

United States University (Cypress, CA): *closed*

University of Massachusetts Worcester (Worcester, MA): *name changed to University of Massachusetts Medical School*

The University of Montana (Missoula, MT): *name changed to University of Montana*

University of Phoenix–Austin Campus (Austin, TX): *closed*

University of Phoenix–Birmingham Campus (Birmingham, AL): *closed*

University of Phoenix–Boston Campus (Braintree, MA): *closed*

University of Phoenix–Chicago Campus (Schaumburg, IL): *closed*

University of Phoenix–Cleveland Campus (Beachwood, OH): *closed*

University of Phoenix–Columbia Campus (Columbia, SC): *closed*

University of Phoenix–Des Moines Campus (Des Moines, IA): *closed*

University of Phoenix–Idaho Campus (Meridian, ID): *closed*

University of Phoenix–Indianapolis Campus (Indianapolis, IN): *closed*

University of Phoenix–Kansas City Campus (Kansas City, MO): *closed*

University of Phoenix–Little Rock Campus (Little Rock, AR): *closed*

University of Phoenix–Louisville Campus (Louisville, KY): *closed*

University of Phoenix–Maryland Campus (Columbia, MD): *closed*

University of Phoenix–Memphis Campus (Cordova, TN): *closed*

University of Phoenix–Milwaukee Campus (Milwaukee, WI): *closed*

University of Phoenix–Minneapolis/St. Paul Campus (St. Louis Park, MN): *closed*

University of Phoenix–Nashville Campus (Nashville, TN): *closed*

University of Phoenix–Oklahoma City Campus (Oklahoma City, OK): *closed*

University of Phoenix–Oregon Campus (Tigard, OR): *closed*

University of Phoenix–Philadelphia Campus (Wayne, PA): *closed*

University of Phoenix–Puerto Rico Campus (Guaynabo, PR): *closed*

University of Phoenix–Richmond-Virginia Beach Campus (Glen Allen, VA): *closed*

University of Phoenix–St. Louis Campus (St. Louis, MO): *closed*

University of Phoenix–Savannah Campus (Savannah, GA): *closed*

University of Southernmost Florida (Jacksonville, FL): *closed*

The University of Texas at Brownsville (Brownsville, TX): *merged with The University of Texas–Pan American to become The University of Texas Rio Grande Valley (Edinburg, TX)*

The University of Texas–Pan American (Edinburg, TX): *merged with The University of Texas at Brownsville to become The University of Texas Rio Grande Valley (Edinburg, TX)*

Washington College (Chestertown, MD): *no longer offers graduate degrees*

Weill Cornell Medical College (New York, NY): *name changed to Weill Cornell Medicine*

Western Michigan University Cooley Law School (Lansing, MI): *name changed to Western Michigan University Thomas M. Cooley Law School*

William Howard Taft University (Santa Ana, CA): *merged into a single entry for Taft University System (Denver, CO)*

William Mitchell College of Law (St. Paul, MN): *merged with Hamline University School of Law, a unit of Hamline University (St. Paul, MN)*

Abbreviations Used in the Guides

The following list includes abbreviations of degree names used in the profiles in the 2016 edition of the guides. Because some degrees (e.g., Doctor of Education) can be abbreviated in more than one way (e.g., D.Ed. or Ed.D.), and because the abbreviations used in the guides reflect the preferences of the individual colleges and universities, the list may include two or more abbreviations for a single degree.

DEGREES

A Mus D	Doctor of Musical Arts
AC	Advanced Certificate
AD	Artist's Diploma
	Doctor of Arts
ADP	Artist's Diploma
Adv C	Advanced Certificate
AGC	Advanced Graduate Certificate
AGSC	Advanced Graduate Specialist Certificate
ALM	Master of Liberal Arts
AM	Master of Arts
AMBA	Accelerated Master of Business Administration
AMRS	Master of Arts in Religious Studies
APC	Advanced Professional Certificate
APMPH	Advanced Professional Master of Public Health
App Sc	Applied Scientist
App Sc D	Doctor of Applied Science
AstE	Astronautical Engineer
ATC	Advanced Training Certificate
Au D	Doctor of Audiology
B Th	Bachelor of Theology
BN	Bachelor of Naturopathy
CAES	Certificate of Advanced Educational Specialization
CAGS	Certificate of Advanced Graduate Studies
CAL	Certificate in Applied Linguistics
CAPS	Certificate of Advanced Professional Studies
CAS	Certificate of Advanced Studies
CASPA	Certificate of Advanced Study in Public Administration
CASR	Certificate in Advanced Social Research
CATS	Certificate of Achievement in Theological Studies
CBHS	Certificate in Basic Health Sciences
CCJA	Certificate in Criminal Justice Administration
CCTS	Certificate in Clinical and Translational Science
CE	Civil Engineer
CEM	Certificate of Environmental Management
CET	Certificate in Educational Technologies
CGS	Certificate of Graduate Studies
Ch E	Chemical Engineer
Clin Sc D	Doctor of Clinical Science
CM	Certificate in Management
CMH	Certificate in Medical Humanities
CMM	Master of Church Ministries
CMS	Certificate in Ministerial Studies
CNM	Certificate in Nonprofit Management
CPASF	Certificate Program for Advanced Study in Finance
CPC	Certificate in Professional Counseling
	Certificate in Publication and Communication
CPH	Certificate in Public Health
CPM	Certificate in Public Management
CPS	Certificate of Professional Studies
CScD	Doctor of Clinical Science
CSD	Certificate in Spiritual Direction
CSS	Certificate of Special Studies
CTS	Certificate of Theological Studies
CURP	Certificate in Urban and Regional Planning
D Admin	Doctor of Administration
D Arch	Doctor of Architecture
D Be	Doctor in Bioethics
D Com	Doctor of Commerce
D Couns	Doctor of Counseling
D Des	Doctorate of Design
D Div	Doctor of Divinity
D Ed	Doctor of Education
D Ed Min	Doctor of Educational Ministry
D Eng	Doctor of Engineering
D Engr	Doctor of Engineering
D Ent	Doctor of Enterprise
D Env	Doctor of Environment
D Law	Doctor of Law
D Litt	Doctor of Letters
D Med Sc	Doctor of Medical Science
D Min	Doctor of Ministry
D Miss	Doctor of Missiology
D Mus	Doctor of Music
D Mus A	Doctor of Musical Arts
D Phil	Doctor of Philosophy
D Prof	Doctor of Professional Studies
D Ps	Doctor of Psychology
D Sc	Doctor of Science
D Sc D	Doctor of Science in Dentistry
D Sc IS	Doctor of Science in Information Systems
D Sc PA	Doctor of Science in Physician Assistant Studies
D Th	Doctor of Theology
D Th P	Doctor of Practical Theology
DA	Doctor of Accounting
	Doctor of Arts
DAH	Doctor of Arts in Humanities
DAOM	Doctorate in Acupuncture and Oriental Medicine
DAT	Doctorate of Athletic Training
	Professional Doctor of Art Therapy
DBA	Doctor of Business Administration
DBH	Doctor of Behavioral Health
DBL	Doctor of Business Leadership
DC	Doctor of Chiropractic
DCC	Doctor of Computer Science
DCD	Doctor of Communications Design
DCL	Doctor of Civil Law
	Doctor of Comparative Law
DCM	Doctor of Church Music
DCN	Doctor of Clinical Nutrition
DCS	Doctor of Computer Science
DDN	Diplôme du Droit Notarial
DDS	Doctor of Dental Surgery
DE	Doctor of Education
	Doctor of Engineering
DED	Doctor of Economic Development
DEIT	Doctor of Educational Innovation and Technology
DEL	Doctor of Executive Leadership
DEM	Doctor of Educational Ministry
DEPD	Diplôme Études Spécialisées
DES	Doctor of Engineering Science
DESS	Diplôme Études Supérieures Spécialisées
DET	Doctor of Educational Technology
DFA	Doctor of Fine Arts
DGP	Diploma in Graduate and Professional Studies
DH Ed	Doctor of Health Education

DH Sc	Doctor of Health Sciences
DHA	Doctor of Health Administration
DHCE	Doctor of Health Care Ethics
DHL	Doctor of Hebrew Letters
DHPE	Doctorate of Health Professionals Education
DHS	Doctor of Health Science
DHSc	Doctor of Health Science
Dip CS	Diploma in Christian Studies
DIT	Doctor of Industrial Technology
	Doctor of Information Technology
DJS	Doctor of Jewish Studies
DLS	Doctor of Liberal Studies
DM	Doctor of Management
	Doctor of Music
DMA	Doctor of Musical Arts
DMD	Doctor of Dental Medicine
DME	Doctor of Manufacturing Management
	Doctor of Music Education
DMEd	Doctor of Music Education
DMFT	Doctor of Marital and Family Therapy
DMH	Doctor of Medical Humanities
DML	Doctor of Modern Languages
DMP	Doctorate in Medical Physics
DMPNA	Doctor of Management Practice in Nurse Anesthesia
DN Sc	Doctor of Nursing Science
DNAP	Doctor of Nurse Anesthesia Practice
DNP	Doctor of Nursing Practice
DNP-A	Doctor of Nursing Practice - Anesthesia
DNS	Doctor of Nursing Science
DO	Doctor of Osteopathy
DOT	Doctor of Occupational Therapy
DPA	Doctor of Public Administration
DPDS	Doctor of Planning and Development Studies
DPH	Doctor of Public Health
DPM	Doctor of Plant Medicine
	Doctor of Podiatric Medicine
DPPD	Doctor of Policy, Planning, and Development
DPS	Doctor of Professional Studies
DPT	Doctor of Physical Therapy
DPTSc	Doctor of Physical Therapy Science
Dr DES	Doctor of Design
Dr NP	Doctor of Nursing Practice
Dr OT	Doctor of Occupational Therapy
Dr PH	Doctor of Public Health
Dr Sc PT	Doctor of Science in Physical Therapy
DrAP	Doctor of Anesthesia Practice
DRSc	Doctor of Regulatory Science
DS	Doctor of Science
DS Sc	Doctor of Social Science
DSJS	Doctor of Science in Jewish Studies
DSL	Doctor of Strategic Leadership
DSS	Doctor of Strategic Security
DSW	Doctor of Social Work
DTL	Doctor of Talmudic Law
	Doctor of Transformational Leadership
DV Sc	Doctor of Veterinary Science
DVM	Doctor of Veterinary Medicine
DWS	Doctor of Worship Studies
EAA	Engineer in Aeronautics and Astronautics
EASPh D	Engineering and Applied Science Doctor of Philosophy
ECS	Engineer in Computer Science
Ed D	Doctor of Education
Ed DCT	Doctor of Education in College Teaching
Ed L D	Doctor of Education Leadership
Ed M	Master of Education
Ed S	Specialist in Education
Ed Sp	Specialist in Education

EDB	Executive Doctorate in Business
EDBA	Executive Doctor of Business Administration
EDM	Executive Doctorate in Management
EE	Electrical Engineer
EJD	Executive Juris Doctor
EMBA	Executive Master of Business Administration
EMFA	Executive Master of Forensic Accounting
EMHA	Executive Master of Health Administration
EMIB	Executive Master of International Business
EML	Executive Master of Leadership
EMPA	Executive Master of Public Administration
EMPL	Executive Master in Public Leadership
EMS	Executive Master of Science
EMTM	Executive Master of Technology Management
Eng	Engineer
Eng Sc D	Doctor of Engineering Science
Engr	Engineer
Exec M Tax	Executive Master of Taxation
Exec MAC	Executive Master of Accounting
Exec Ed D	Executive Doctor of Education
Exec MBA	Executive Master of Business Administration
Exec MPA	Executive Master of Public Administration
Exec MPH	Executive Master of Public Health
Exec MS	Executive Master of Science
Executive Fellows MBA	Executive Fellows Master of Business Administration
G Dip	Graduate Diploma
GBC	Graduate Business Certificate
GDM	Graduate Diploma in Management
GDPA	Graduate Diploma in Public Administration
GDRE	Graduate Diploma in Religious Education
GEMBA	Global Executive Master of Business Administration
GMBA	Global Master of Business Administration
GP LL M	Global Professional Master of Laws
GPD	Graduate Performance Diploma
GSS	Graduate Special Certificate for Students in Special Situations
IEMBA	International Executive Master of Business Administration
IMA	Interdisciplinary Master of Arts
IMBA	International Master of Business Administration
IMES	International Master's in Environmental Studies
Ingeniero	Engineer
JCD	Doctor of Canon Law
JCL	Licentiate in Canon Law
JD	Juris Doctor
JM	Juris Master
JSD	Doctor of Juridical Science
	Doctor of Jurisprudence
	Doctor of the Science of Law
JSM	Master of the Science of Law
L Th	Licenciate in Theology
LL B	Bachelor of Laws
LL CM	Master of Comparative Law
LL D	Doctor of Laws
LL M	Master of Laws
LL M in Tax	Master of Laws in Taxation
LL M CL	Master of Laws in Common Law
M Ac	Master of Accountancy
	Master of Accounting
	Master of Acupuncture
M Ac OM	Master of Acupuncture and Oriental Medicine
M Acc	Master of Accountancy
	Master of Accounting
M Acct	Master of Accountancy
	Master of Accounting

M Accy	Master of Accountancy
M Actg	Master of Accounting
M Acy	Master of Accountancy
M Ad	Master of Administration
M Ad Ed	Master of Adult Education
M Adm	Master of Administration
M Adm Mgt	Master of Administrative Management
M Admin	Master of Administration
M ADU	Master of Architectural Design and Urbanism
M Adv	Master of Advertising
M AEST	Master of Applied Environmental Science and Technology
M Ag	Master of Agriculture
M Ag Ed	Master of Agricultural Education
M Agr	Master of Agriculture
M Anesth Ed	Master of Anesthesiology Education
M App Comp Sc	Master of Applied Computer Science
M App St	Master of Applied Statistics
M Appl Stat	Master of Applied Statistics
M Aq	Master of Aquaculture
M Arc	Master of Architecture
M Arch	Master of Architecture
M Arch I	Master of Architecture I
M Arch II	Master of Architecture II
M Arch E	Master of Architectural Engineering
M Arch H	Master of Architectural History
M Bioethics	Master in Bioethics
M Biomath	Master of Biomathematics
M Ch E	Master of Chemical Engineering
M Chem	Master of Chemistry
M Cl D	Master of Clinical Dentistry
M Cl Sc	Master of Clinical Science
M Comp	Master of Computing
M Comp Sc	Master of Computer Science
M Coun	Master of Counseling
M Dent	Master of Dentistry
M Dent Sc	Master of Dental Sciences
M Des	Master of Design
M Des S	Master of Design Studies
M Div	Master of Divinity
M E Sci	Master of Earth Science
M Ec	Master of Economics
M Econ	Master of Economics
M Ed	Master of Education
M Ed T	Master of Education in Teaching
M En	Master of Engineering
M En S	Master of Environmental Sciences
M Eng	Master of Engineering
M Eng Mgt	Master of Engineering Management
M Engr	Master of Engineering
M Ent	Master of Enterprise
M Env	Master of Environment
M Env Des	Master of Environmental Design
M Env E	Master of Environmental Engineering
M Env Sc	Master of Environmental Science
M Fin	Master of Finance
M FSc	Master of Fisheries Science
M Geo E	Master of Geological Engineering
M Geoenv E	Master of Geoenvironmental Engineering
M Geog	Master of Geography
M Hum	Master of Humanities
M IDST	Master's in Interdisciplinary Studies
M Kin	Master of Kinesiology
M Land Arch	Master of Landscape Architecture
M Litt	Master of Letters
M Mat SE	Master of Material Science and Engineering
M Math	Master of Mathematics
M Mech E	Master of Mechanical Engineering
M Med Sc	Master of Medical Science
M Mgmt	Master of Management
M Mgt	Master of Management
M Min	Master of Ministries
M Mtl E	Master of Materials Engineering
M Mu	Master of Music
M Mus	Master of Music
M Mus Ed	Master of Music Education
M Music	Master of Music
M Nat Sci	Master of Natural Science
M Pet E	Master of Petroleum Engineering
M Pharm	Master of Pharmacy
M Phil	Master of Philosophy
M Phil F	Master of Philosophical Foundations
M Pl	Master of Planning
M Plan	Master of Planning
M Pol	Master of Political Science
M Pr Met	Master of Professional Meteorology
M Prob S	Master of Probability and Statistics
M Psych	Master of Psychology
M Pub	Master of Publishing
M Rel	Master of Religion
M Sc	Master of Science
M Sc A	Master of Science (Applied)
M Sc AC	Master of Science in Applied Computing
M Sc AHN	Master of Science in Applied Human Nutrition
M Sc BMC	Master of Science in Biomedical Communications
M Sc CS	Master of Science in Computer Science
M Sc E	Master of Science in Engineering
M Sc Eng	Master of Science in Engineering
M Sc Engr	Master of Science in Engineering
M Sc F	Master of Science in Forestry
M Sc FE	Master of Science in Forest Engineering
M Sc Geogr	Master of Science in Geography
M Sc N	Master of Science in Nursing
M Sc OT	Master of Science in Occupational Therapy
M Sc P	Master of Science in Planning
M Sc Pl	Master of Science in Planning
M Sc PT	Master of Science in Physical Therapy
M Sc T	Master of Science in Teaching
M SEM	Master of Sustainable Environmental Management
M Serv Soc	Master of Social Service
M Soc	Master of Sociology
M Sp Ed	Master of Special Education
M St	Master of Studies
M Stat	Master of Statistics
M Sys E	Master of Systems Engineering
M Sys Sc	Master of Systems Science
M Tax	Master of Taxation
M Tech	Master of Technology
M Th	Master of Theology
M Tox	Master of Toxicology
M Trans E	Master of Transportation Engineering
M U Ed	Master of Urban Education
M Urb	Master of Urban Planning
M Vet Sc	Master of Veterinary Science
MA	Master of Accounting
	Master of Administration
	Master of Arts
MA Comm	Master of Arts in Communication
MA Ed	Master of Arts in Education
MA Ed/HD	Master of Arts in Education and Human Development
MA Ext	Master of Agricultural Extension
MA Min	Master of Arts in Ministry
MA Past St	Master of Arts in Pastoral Studies
MA Ph	Master of Arts in Philosophy

MA Psych	Master of Arts in Psychology		Master of Arts in Education
MA Sc	Master of Applied Science		Master of Arts in English
MA Sp	Master of Arts (Spirituality)	MAEd	Master of Arts Education
MA Th	Master of Arts in Theology	MAEL	Master of Arts in Educational Leadership
MA-R	Master of Arts (Research)	MAEM	Master of Arts in Educational Ministries
MAA	Master of Administrative Arts	MAEP	Master of Arts in Economic Policy
	Master of Applied Anthropology		Master of Arts in Educational Psychology
	Master of Applied Arts	MAES	Master of Arts in Environmental Sciences
	Master of Arts in Administration	MAET	Master of Arts in English Teaching
MAAA	Master of Arts in Arts Administration	MAF	Master of Arts in Finance
MAAAP	Master of Arts Administration and Policy	MAFE	Master of Arts in Financial Economics
MAAD	Master of Advanced Architectural Design	MAFLL	Master of Arts in Foreign Language and Literature
MAAE	Master of Arts in Art Education	MAFM	Master of Accounting and Financial Management
MAAPPS	Master of Arts in Asia Pacific Policy Studies		
MAAS	Master of Arts in Aging and Spirituality	MAFS	Master of Arts in Family Studies
MAASJ	Master of Arts in Applied Social Justice	MAG	Master of Applied Geography
MAAT	Master of Arts in Applied Theology	MAGS	Master of Arts in Global Service
	Master of Arts in Art Therapy	MAGU	Master of Urban Analysis and Management
MAB	Master of Agribusiness	MAH	Master of Arts in Humanities
MABC	Master of Arts in Biblical Counseling	MAHA	Master of Arts in Humanitarian Assistance
MABE	Master of Arts in Bible Exposition	MAHCM	Master of Arts in Health Care Mission
MABL	Master of Arts in Biblical Languages	MAHG	Master of American History and Government
MABM	Master of Agribusiness Management	MAHL	Master of Arts in Hebrew Letters
MABS	Master of Arts in Biblical Studies	MAHN	Master of Applied Human Nutrition
MABT	Master of Arts in Bible Teaching	MAHR	Master of Applied Historical Research
MAC	Master of Accountancy	MAHS	Master of Arts in Human Services
	Master of Accounting	MAHSR	Master in Applied Health Services Research
	Master of Arts in Communication	MAIA	Master of Arts in International Administration
	Master of Arts in Counseling		Master of Arts in International Affairs
MACC	Master of Arts in Christian Counseling	MAIDM	Master of Arts in Interior Design and Merchandising
	Master of Arts in Clinical Counseling		
MACCT	Master of Accounting	MAIH	Master of Arts in Interdisciplinary Humanities
MACD	Master of Arts in Christian Doctrine	MAIOP	Master of Applied Industrial/Organizational Psychology
MACE	Master of Arts in Christian Education		
MACH	Master of Arts in Church History	MAIPCR	Master of Arts in International Peace and Conflict Management
MACI	Master of Arts in Curriculum and Instruction		
MACIS	Master of Accounting and Information Systems	MAIS	Master of Arts in Intercultural Studies
MACJ	Master of Arts in Criminal Justice		Master of Arts in Interdisciplinary Studies
MACL	Master of Arts in Christian Leadership		Master of Arts in International Studies
	Master of Arts in Community Leadership	MAIT	Master of Administration in Information Technology
MACM	Master of Arts in Christian Ministries		
	Master of Arts in Christian Ministry	MAJ	Master of Arts in Journalism
	Master of Arts in Church Music	MAJ Ed	Master of Arts in Jewish Education
	Master of Arts in Counseling Ministries	MAJCS	Master of Arts in Jewish Communal Service
MACN	Master of Arts in Counseling	MAJE	Master of Arts in Jewish Education
MACO	Master of Arts in Counseling	MAJPS	Master of Arts in Jewish Professional Studies
MAcOM	Master of Acupuncture and Oriental Medicine	MAJS	Master of Arts in Jewish Studies
MACP	Master of Arts in Christian Practice	MAL	Master in Agricultural Leadership
	Master of Arts in Church Planting	MALA	Master of Arts in Liberal Arts
	Master of Arts in Counseling Psychology	MALD	Master of Arts in Law and Diplomacy
MACS	Master of Applied Computer Science	MALER	Master of Arts in Labor and Employment Relations
	Master of Arts in Catholic Studies		
	Master of Arts in Christian Studies	MALL	Master of Arts in Language Learning
MACSE	Master of Arts in Christian School Education	MALP	Master of Arts in Language Pedagogy
MACT	Master of Arts in Communications and Technology	MALS	Master of Arts in Liberal Studies
		MAM	Master of Acquisition Management
MAD	Master in Educational Institution Administration		Master of Agriculture and Management
			Master of Applied Mathematics
	Master of Art and Design		Master of Arts in Management
MADR	Master of Arts in Dispute Resolution		Master of Arts in Ministry
MADS	Master of Animal and Dairy Science		Master of Arts Management
	Master of Applied Disability Studies		Master of Avian Medicine
MAE	Master of Aerospace Engineering	MAMB	Master of Applied Molecular Biology
	Master of Agricultural Economics	MAMC	Master of Arts in Mass Communication
	Master of Agricultural Education		Master of Arts in Ministry and Culture
	Master of Applied Economics		Master of Arts in Ministry for a Multicultural Church
	Master of Architectural Engineering		
	Master of Art Education		Master of Arts in Missional Christianity
		MAME	Master of Arts in Missions/Evangelism

MAMFC	Master of Arts in Marriage and Family Counseling		Master's in Administration of Telecommunications
MAMFT	Master of Arts in Marriage and Family Therapy	Mat E	Materials Engineer
MAMHC	Master of Arts in Mental Health Counseling	MATCM	Master of Acupuncture and Traditional Chinese Medicine
MAMS	Master of Applied Mathematical Sciences	MATDE	Master of Arts in Theology, Development, and Evangelism
	Master of Applied Meditation Studies		
	Master of Arts in Ministerial Studies	MATDR	Master of Territorial Management and Regional Development
	Master of Arts in Ministry and Spirituality		
MAMT	Master of Arts in Mathematics Teaching	MATE	Master of Arts for the Teaching of English
MAN	Master of Applied Nutrition	MATESL	Master of Arts in Teaching English as a Second Language
MANT	Master of Arts in New Testament		
MAOL	Master of Arts in Organizational Leadership	MATESOL	Master of Arts in Teaching English to Speakers of Other Languages
MAOM	Master of Acupuncture and Oriental Medicine		
MAOT	Master of Arts in Old Testament	MATF	Master of Arts in Teaching English as a Foreign Language/Intercultural Studies
MAP	Master of Applied Politics		
	Master of Applied Psychology	MATFL	Master of Arts in Teaching Foreign Language
	Master of Arts in Planning	MATH	Master of Arts in Therapy
	Master of Psychology	MATI	Master of Administration of Information Technology
	Master of Public Administration		
MAP Min	Master of Arts in Pastoral Ministry	MATL	Master of Arts in Teacher Leadership
MAPA	Master of Arts in Public Administration		Master of Arts in Teaching of Languages
MAPC	Master of Arts in Pastoral Counseling		Master of Arts in Transformational Leadership
MAPE	Master of Arts in Physics Education	MATM	Master of Arts in Teaching of Mathematics
	Master of Arts in Political Economy	MATS	Master of Arts in Theological Studies
MAPM	Master of Arts in Pastoral Ministry		Master of Arts in Transforming Spirituality
	Master of Arts in Pastoral Music	MATSL	Master of Arts in Teaching a Second Language
	Master of Arts in Practical Ministry	MAUA	Master of Arts in Urban Affairs
MAPP	Master of Arts in Public Policy	MAUD	Master of Arts in Urban Design
MAPS	Master of Arts in Pastoral Studies	MAURP	Master of Arts in Urban and Regional Planning
	Master of Arts in Public Service	MAW	Master of Arts in Worship
MAPT	Master of Practical Theology	MAWSHP	Master of Arts in Worship
MAPW	Master of Arts in Professional Writing	MAYM	Master of Arts in Youth Ministry
MAR	Master of Arts in Reading	MB	Master of Bioinformatics
	Master of Arts in Religion	MBA	Master of Business Administration
Mar Eng	Marine Engineer	MBA-AM	Master of Business Administration in Aviation Management
MARC	Master of Arts in Rehabilitation Counseling		
MARE	Master of Arts in Religious Education	MBA-EP	Master of Business Administration–Experienced Professionals
MARL	Master of Arts in Religious Leadership		
MARS	Master of Arts in Religious Studies	MBAA	Master of Business Administration in Aviation
MAS	Master of Accounting Science	MBAE	Master of Biological and Agricultural Engineering
	Master of Actuarial Science		
	Master of Administrative Science		Master of Biosystems and Agricultural Engineering
	Master of Advanced Study		
	Master of Aeronautical Science	MBAH	Master of Business Administration in Health
	Master of American Studies	MBAi	Master of Business Administration–International
	Master of Animal Science		
	Master of Applied Science	MBAICT	Master of Business Administration in Information and Communication Technology
	Master of Applied Statistics		
	Master of Archival Studies	MBATM	Master of Business Administration in Technology Management
MASA	Master of Advanced Studies in Architecture		
MASD	Master of Arts in Spiritual Direction	MBC	Master of Building Construction
MASE	Master of Arts in Special Education	MBE	Master of Bilingual Education
MASF	Master of Arts in Spiritual Formation		Master of Bioengineering
MASJ	Master of Arts in Systems of Justice		Master of Bioethics
MASLA	Master of Advanced Studies in Landscape Architecture		Master of Biomedical Engineering
			Master of Business Economics
MASM	Master of Aging Services Management		Master of Business Education
	Master of Arts in Specialized Ministries	MBEE	Master in Biotechnology Enterprise and Entrepreneurship
MASP	Master of Applied Social Psychology		
	Master of Arts in School Psychology	MBET	Master of Business, Entrepreneurship and Technology
MASPAA	Master of Arts in Sports and Athletic Administration		
		MBID	Master of Biomedical Innovation and Development
MASS	Master of Applied Social Science		
	Master of Arts in Social Science	MBIOT	Master of Biotechnology
MAST	Master of Arts in Science Teaching	MBiotech	Master of Biotechnology
MAT	Master of Arts in Teaching	MBL	Master of Business Law
	Master of Arts in Theology		Master of Business Leadership
	Master of Athletic Training	MBLE	Master in Business Logistics Engineering
		MBME	Master's in Biomedical Engineering
		MBMSE	Master of Business Management and Software Engineering

MBOE	Master of Business Operational Excellence	
MBS	Master of Biblical Studies	
	Master of Biological Science	
	Master of Biomedical Sciences	
	Master of Bioscience	
	Master of Building Science	
	Master of Business and Science	
MBST	Master of Biostatistics	
MBT	Master of Biomedical Technology	
	Master of Biotechnology	
	Master of Business Taxation	
MBV	Master of Business for Veterans	
MC	Master of Communication	
	Master of Counseling	
	Master of Cybersecurity	
MC Ed	Master of Continuing Education	
MC Sc	Master of Computer Science	
MCA	Master in Collegiate Athletics	
	Master of Commercial Aviation	
	Master of Criminology (Applied)	
MCAM	Master of Computational and Applied Mathematics	
MCC	Master of Computer Science	
MCD	Master of Communications Disorders	
	Master of Community Development	
MCE	Master in Electronic Commerce	
	Master of Christian Education	
	Master of Civil Engineering	
	Master of Control Engineering	
MCEM	Master of Construction Engineering Management	
MCHE	Master of Chemical Engineering	
MCIS	Master of Communication and Information Studies	
	Master of Computer and Information Science	
	Master of Computer Information Systems	
MCIT	Master of Computer and Information Technology	
MCJ	Master of Criminal Justice	
MCL	Master in Communication Leadership	
	Master of Canon Law	
	Master of Comparative Law	
MCM	Master of Christian Ministry	
	Master of Church Music	
	Master of City Management	
	Master of Communication Management	
	Master of Community Medicine	
	Master of Construction Management	
	Master of Contract Management	
MCMin	Master of Christian Ministry	
MCMP	Master of City and Metropolitan Planning	
MCMS	Master of Clinical Medical Science	
MCN	Master of Clinical Nutrition	
MCOL	Master of Arts in Community and Organizational Leadership	
MCP	Master of City Planning	
	Master of Community Planning	
	Master of Counseling Psychology	
	Master of Cytopathology Practice	
	Master of Science in Quality Systems and Productivity	
MCPC	Master of Arts in Chaplaincy and Pastoral Care	
MCPD	Master of Community Planning and Development	
MCR	Master in Clinical Research	
MCRP	Master of City and Regional Planning	
	Master of Community and Regional Planning	
MCRS	Master of City and Regional Studies	
MCS	Master of Chemical Sciences	
	Master of Christian Studies	

	Master of Clinical Science	
	Master of Combined Sciences	
	Master of Communication Studies	
	Master of Computer Science	
	Master of Consumer Science	
MCSE	Master of Computer Science and Engineering	
MCSL	Master of Catholic School Leadership	
MCSM	Master of Construction Science and Management	
MCTM	Master of Clinical Translation Management	
MCTP	Master of Communication Technology and Policy	
MCTS	Master of Clinical and Translational Science	
MCVS	Master of Cardiovascular Science	
MD	Doctor of Medicine	
MDA	Master of Dietetic Administration	
MDB	Master of Design-Build	
MDE	Master of Developmental Economics	
	Master of Distance Education	
	Master of the Education of the Deaf	
MDH	Master of Dental Hygiene	
MDM	Master of Design Methods	
	Master of Digital Media	
MDP	Master in Sustainable Development Practice	
	Master of Development Practice	
MDR	Master of Dispute Resolution	
MDS	Master of Dental Surgery	
	Master of Design Studies	
	Master of Digital Sciences	
ME	Master of Education	
	Master of Engineering	
	Master of Entrepreneurship	
ME Sc	Master of Engineering Science	
ME-PD	Master of Education–Professional Development	
MEA	Master of Educational Administration	
	Master of Engineering Administration	
MEAE	Master of Entertainment Arts and Engineering	
MEAP	Master of Environmental Administration and Planning	
MEB	Master of Energy Business	
MEBD	Master in Environmental Building Design	
MEBT	Master in Electronic Business Technologies	
MEC	Master of Electronic Commerce	
Mech E	Mechanical Engineer	
MED	Master of Education of the Deaf	
MEDS	Master of Environmental Design Studies	
MEE	Master in Education	
	Master of Electrical Engineering	
	Master of Energy Engineering	
	Master of Environmental Engineering	
MEEM	Master of Environmental Engineering and Management	
MEENE	Master of Engineering in Environmental Engineering	
MEEP	Master of Environmental and Energy Policy	
MEERM	Master of Earth and Environmental Resource Management	
MEH	Master in Humanistic Studies	
	Master of Environmental Health	
	Master of Environmental Horticulture	
MEHS	Master of Environmental Health and Safety	
MEIM	Master of Entertainment Industry Management	
	Master of Equine Industry Management	
MEL	Master of Educational Leadership	
	Master of English Literature	
MELP	Master of Environmental Law and Policy	
MEM	Master of Engineering Management	
	Master of Environmental Management	
	Master of Marketing	

MEME	Master of Engineering in Manufacturing Engineering
	Master of Engineering in Mechanical Engineering
MENR	Master of Environment and Natural Resources
MENVEGR	Master of Environmental Engineering
MEP	Master of Engineering Physics
MEPC	Master of Environmental Pollution Control
MEPD	Master of Environmental Planning and Design
MER	Master of Employment Relations
MERE	Master of Entrepreneurial Real Estate
MERL	Master of Energy Regulation and Law
MES	Master of Education and Science
	Master of Engineering Science
	Master of Environment and Sustainability
	Master of Environmental Science
	Master of Environmental Studies
	Master of Environmental Systems
	Master of Special Education
MESM	Master of Environmental Science and Management
MET	Master of Educational Technology
	Master of Engineering Technology
	Master of Entertainment Technology
	Master of Environmental Toxicology
METM	Master of Engineering and Technology Management
MEVE	Master of Environmental Engineering
MF	Master of Finance
	Master of Forestry
MFA	Master of Fine Arts
MFALP	Master of Food and Agriculture Law and Policy
MFAM	Master's of Food Animal Medicine
MFAS	Master of Fisheries and Aquatic Science
MFAW	Master of Fine Arts in Writing
MFC	Master of Forest Conservation
MFCS	Master of Family and Consumer Sciences
MFE	Master of Financial Economics
	Master of Financial Engineering
	Master of Forest Engineering
MFES	Master of Fire and Emergency Services
MFG	Master of Functional Genomics
MFHD	Master of Family and Human Development
MFM	Master of Financial Management
	Master of Financial Mathematics
MFPE	Master of Food Process Engineering
MFR	Master of Forest Resources
MFRC	Master of Forest Resources and Conservation
MFRE	Master of Food and Resource Economics
MFS	Master of Food Science
	Master of Forensic Sciences
	Master of Forest Science
	Master of Forest Studies
	Master of French Studies
MFST	Master of Food Safety and Technology
MFT	Master of Family Therapy
	Master of Food Technology
MFWB	Master of Fishery and Wildlife Biology
MFWCB	Master of Fish, Wildlife and Conservation Biology
MFWS	Master of Fisheries and Wildlife Sciences
MFYCS	Master of Family, Youth and Community Sciences
MG	Master of Genetics
MGA	Master of Global Affairs
	Master of Government Administration
	Master of Governmental Administration
MGC	Master of Genetic Counseling
MGD	Master of Graphic Design

MGE	Master of Geotechnical Engineering
MGEM	Master of Global Entrepreneurship and Management
MGIS	Master of Geographic Information Science
	Master of Geographic Information Systems
MGM	Master of Global Management
MGP	Master of Gestion de Projet
MGPS	Master of Global Policy Studies
MGREM	Master of Global Real Estate Management
MGS	Master of Gerontological Studies
	Master of Global Studies
MGsc	Master of Geoscience
MH	Master of Humanities
MH Sc	Master of Health Sciences
MHA	Master of Health Administration
	Master of Healthcare Administration
	Master of Hospital Administration
	Master of Hospitality Administration
MHB	Master of Human Behavior
MHC	Master of Mental Health Counseling
MHCA	Master of Health Care Administration
MHCD	Master of Health Care Design
MHCI	Master of Human-Computer Interaction
MHCL	Master of Health Care Leadership
MHE	Master of Health Education
	Master of Human Ecology
MHE Ed	Master of Home Economics Education
MHEA	Master of Higher Education Administration
MHHS	Master of Health and Human Services
MHI	Master of Health Informatics
	Master of Healthcare Innovation
MHIHIM	Master of Health Informatics and Health Information Management
MHIIM	Master of Health Informatics and Information Management
MHIS	Master of Health Information Systems
MHK	Master of Human Kinetics
MHM	Master of Healthcare Management
MHMS	Master of Health Management Systems
MHP	Master of Health Physics
	Master of Heritage Preservation
	Master of Historic Preservation
MHPA	Master of Heath Policy and Administration
MHPE	Master of Health Professions Education
MHR	Master of Human Resources
MHRD	Master in Human Resource Development
MHRIR	Master of Human Resources and Industrial Relations
MHRLR	Master of Human Resources and Labor Relations
MHRM	Master of Human Resources Management
MHS	Master of Health Science
	Master of Health Sciences
	Master of Health Studies
	Master of Hispanic Studies
	Master of Human Services
	Master of Humanistic Studies
MHSA	Master of Health Services Administration
MHSE	Master of Health Science Education
MHSM	Master of Health Systems Management
MI	Master of Information
	Master of Instruction
MI Arch	Master of Interior Architecture
MIA	Master of Interior Architecture
	Master of International Affairs
MIAA	Master of International Affairs and Administration
MIAM	Master of International Agribusiness Management

MIAPD	Master of Interior Architecture and Product Design
MIB	Master of International Business
MIBA	Master of International Business Administration
MICM	Master of International Construction Management
MID	Master of Industrial Design
	Master of Industrial Distribution
	Master of Interior Design
	Master of International Development
MIDA	Master of International Development Administration
MIDC	Master of Integrated Design and Construction
MIDP	Master of International Development Policy
MIE	Master of Industrial Engineering
MIHTM	Master of International Hospitality and Tourism Management
MIJ	Master of International Journalism
MILR	Master of Industrial and Labor Relations
MIM	Master in Ministry
	Master of Information Management
	Master of International Management
MIMLAE	Master of International Management for Latin American Executives
MIMS	Master of Information Management and Systems
	Master of Integrated Manufacturing Systems
MIP	Master of Infrastructure Planning
	Master of Intellectual Property
	Master of International Policy
MIPA	Master of International Public Affairs
MIPD	Master of Integrated Product Design
MIPM	Master of International Policy Management
MIPP	Master of International Policy and Practice
	Master of International Public Policy
MIPS	Master of International Planning Studies
MIR	Master of Industrial Relations
	Master of International Relations
MIRHR	Master of Industrial Relations and Human Resources
MIS	Master of Imaging Science
	Master of Industrial Statistics
	Master of Information Science
	Master of Information Systems
	Master of Integrated Science
	Master of Interdisciplinary Studies
	Master of International Service
	Master of International Studies
MISE	Master of Industrial and Systems Engineering
MISKM	Master of Information Sciences and Knowledge Management
MISM	Master of Information Systems Management
MISW	Master of Indigenous Social Work
MIT	Master in Teaching
	Master of Industrial Technology
	Master of Information Technology
	Master of Initial Teaching
	Master of International Trade
	Master of Internet Technology
MITA	Master of Information Technology Administration
MITM	Master of Information Technology and Management
MJ	Master of Journalism
	Master of Jurisprudence
MJ Ed	Master of Jewish Education
MJA	Master of Justice Administration
MJM	Master of Justice Management
MJS	Master of Judicial Studies

	Master of Juridical Studies
MK	Master of Kinesiology
MKM	Master of Knowledge Management
ML	Master of Latin
ML Arch	Master of Landscape Architecture
MLA	Master of Landscape Architecture
	Master of Liberal Arts
MLAS	Master of Laboratory Animal Science
	Master of Liberal Arts and Sciences
MLAUD	Master of Landscape Architecture in Urban Development
MLD	Master of Leadership Development
	Master of Leadership Studies
MLE	Master of Applied Linguistics and Exegesis
MLER	Master of Labor and Employment Relations
MLI Sc	Master of Library and Information Science
MLIS	Master of Library and Information Science
	Master of Library and Information Studies
MLM	Master of Leadership in Ministry
MLPD	Master of Land and Property Development
MLRHR	Master of Labor Relations and Human Resources
MLS	Master of Leadership Studies
	Master of Legal Studies
	Master of Liberal Studies
	Master of Library Science
	Master of Life Sciences
MLSCM	Master of Logistics and Supply Chain Management
MLSP	Master of Law and Social Policy
MLT	Master of Language Technologies
MLTCA	Master of Long Term Care Administration
MLW	Master of Studies in Law
MLWS	Master of Land and Water Systems
MM	Master of Management
	Master of Ministry
	Master of Missiology
	Master of Music
MM Ed	Master of Music Education
MM Sc	Master of Medical Science
MM St	Master of Museum Studies
MMA	Master of Marine Affairs
	Master of Media Arts
	Master of Ministry Administration
	Master of Musical Arts
MMAL	Master of Maritime Administration and Logistics
MMAS	Master of Military Art and Science
MMB	Master of Microbial Biotechnology
MMC	Master of Manufacturing Competitiveness
	Master of Mass Communications
	Master of Music Conducting
MMCM	Master of Music in Church Music
MMCSS	Master of Mathematical Computational and Statistical Sciences
MME	Master of Manufacturing Engineering
	Master of Mathematics Education
	Master of Mathematics for Educators
	Master of Mechanical Engineering
	Master of Mining Engineering
	Master of Music Education
MMF	Master of Mathematical Finance
MMFT	Master of Marriage and Family Therapy
MMH	Master of Management in Hospitality
	Master of Medical Humanities
MMI	Master of Management of Innovation
MMIS	Master of Management Information Systems
MML	Master of Managerial Logistics
MMM	Master of Manufacturing Management

	Master of Marine Management		Master of Physician Assistant
	Master of Medical Management		Master of Professional Accountancy
MMP	Master of Management Practice		Master of Professional Accounting
	Master of Marine Policy		Master of Public Administration
	Master of Medical Physics		Master of Public Affairs
	Master of Music Performance	MPAC	Master of Professional Accounting
MMPA	Master of Management and Professional Accounting	MPAID	Master of Public Administration and International Development
MMQM	Master of Manufacturing Quality Management	MPAP	Master of Physician Assistant Practice
MMR	Master of Marketing Research		Master of Public Administration and Policy
MMRM	Master of Marine Resources Management		Master of Public Affairs and Politics
MMS	Master of Management Science	MPAS	Master of Physician Assistant Science
	Master of Management Studies		Master of Physician Assistant Studies
	Master of Manufacturing Systems	MPC	Master of Professional Communication
	Master of Marine Studies		Master of Professional Counseling
	Master of Materials Science	MPD	Master of Product Development
	Master of Mathematical Sciences		Master of Public Diplomacy
	Master of Medical Science	MPDS	Master of Planning and Development Studies
	Master of Medieval Studies	MPE	Master of Physical Education
MMSE	Master of Manufacturing Systems Engineering	MPEM	Master of Project Engineering and Management
MMSM	Master of Music in Sacred Music		
MMT	Master in Marketing	MPH	Master of Public Health
	Master of Music Teaching	MPHE	Master of Public Health Education
	Master of Music Therapy	MPHM	Master in Plant Health Management
	Master's in Marketing Technology	MPHS	Master of Population Health Sciences
MMus	Master of Music	MPHTM	Master of Public Health and Tropical Medicine
MN	Master of Nursing	MPI	Master of Product Innovation
	Master of Nutrition	MPIA	Master of Public and International Affairs
MN NP	Master of Nursing in Nurse Practitioner	MPM	Master of Pastoral Ministry
MNA	Master of Nonprofit Administration		Master of Pest Management
	Master of Nurse Anesthesia		Master of Policy Management
MNAL	Master of Nonprofit Administration and Leadership		Master of Practical Ministries
			Master of Project Management
MNAS	Master of Natural and Applied Science		Master of Public Management
MNCM	Master of Network and Communications Management	MPNA	Master of Public and Nonprofit Administration
		MPNL	Master of Philanthropy and Nonprofit Leadership
MNE	Master of Nuclear Engineering		
MNL	Master in International Business for Latin America	MPO	Master of Prosthetics and Orthotics
		MPOD	Master of Positive Organizational Development
MNM	Master of Nonprofit Management	MPP	Master of Public Policy
MNO	Master of Nonprofit Organization	MPPA	Master of Public Policy Administration
MNPL	Master of Not-for-Profit Leadership		Master of Public Policy and Administration
MNpS	Master of Nonprofit Studies	MPPAL	Master of Public Policy, Administration and Law
MNR	Master of Natural Resources	MPPM	Master of Public and Private Management
MNRD	Master of Natural Resources Development		Master of Public Policy and Management
MNRES	Master of Natural Resources and Environmental Studies	MPPPM	Master of Plant Protection and Pest Management
MNRM	Master of Natural Resource Management	MPRTM	Master of Parks, Recreation, and Tourism Management
MNRMG	Master of Natural Resource Management and Geography		
		MPS	Master of Pastoral Studies
MNRS	Master of Natural Resource Stewardship		Master of Perfusion Science
MNS	Master of Natural Science		Master of Planning Studies
MO	Master of Oceanography		Master of Political Science
MOD	Master of Organizational Development		Master of Preservation Studies
MOGS	Master of Oil and Gas Studies		Master of Prevention Science
MOL	Master of Organizational Leadership		Master of Professional Studies
MOM	Master of Organizational Management		Master of Public Service
	Master of Oriental Medicine	MPSA	Master of Public Service Administration
MOR	Master of Operations Research	MPSG	Master of Population and Social Gerontology
MOT	Master of Occupational Therapy	MPSIA	Master of Political Science and International Affairs
MP	Master of Physiology		
	Master of Planning	MPSL	Master of Public Safety Leadership
MP Ac	Master of Professional Accountancy	MPSRE	Master of Professional Studies in Real Estate
MP Acc	Master of Professional Accountancy	MPT	Master of Pastoral Theology
	Master of Professional Accounting		Master of Physical Therapy
	Master of Public Accounting		Master of Practical Theology
MP Aff	Master of Public Affairs	MPVM	Master of Preventive Veterinary Medicine
MP Th	Master of Pastoral Theology	MPW	Master of Professional Writing
MPA	Master of Performing Arts		Master of Public Works

MQM	Master of Quality Management		Master of Science in Agriculture
MQS	Master of Quality Systems		Master of Science in Analytics
MR	Master of Recreation		Master of Science in Anesthesia
	Master of Retailing		Master of Science in Architecture
MRA	Master in Research Administration		Master of Science in Aviation
MRC	Master of Rehabilitation Counseling		Master of Sports Administration
MRCP	Master of Regional and City Planning		Master of Surgical Assisting
	Master of Regional and Community Planning	MSAA	Master of Science in Astronautics and Aeronautics
MRD	Master of Rural Development	MSAAE	Master of Science in Aeronautical and Astronautical Engineering
MRE	Master of Real Estate		
	Master of Religious Education	MSABE	Master of Science in Agricultural and Biological Engineering
MRED	Master of Real Estate Development		
MREM	Master of Resource and Environmental Management	MSAC	Master of Science in Acupuncture
		MSACC	Master of Science in Accounting
MRLS	Master of Resources Law Studies	MSACS	Master of Science in Applied Computer Science
MRM	Master of Resources Management	MSAE	Master of Science in Aeronautical Engineering
MRP	Master of Regional Planning		Master of Science in Aerospace Engineering
MRRD	Master in Recreation Resource Development		Master of Science in Applied Economics
MRS	Master of Religious Studies		Master of Science in Applied Engineering
MRSc	Master of Rehabilitation Science		Master of Science in Architectural Engineering
MRTP	Master of Rural and Town Planning	MSAEM	Master of Science in Aerospace Engineering and Mechanics
MS	Master of Science		
MS Cmp E	Master of Science in Computer Engineering	MSAF	Master of Science in Aviation Finance
MS Kin	Master of Science in Kinesiology	MSAG	Master of Science in Applied Geosciences
MS Acct	Master of Science in Accounting	MSAH	Master of Science in Allied Health
MS Accy	Master of Science in Accountancy	MSAL	Master of Sport Administration and Leadership
MS Aero E	Master of Science in Aerospace Engineering	MSAM	Master of Science in Applied Mathematics
MS Ag	Master of Science in Agriculture	MSANR	Master of Science in Agriculture and Natural Resources
MS Arch	Master of Science in Architecture		
MS Arch St	Master of Science in Architectural Studies	MSAPM	Master of Security Analysis and Portfolio Management
MS Bio E	Master of Science in Bioengineering		
MS Bm E	Master of Science in Biomedical Engineering	MSAS	Master of Science in Applied Statistics
MS Ch E	Master of Science in Chemical Engineering		Master of Science in Architectural Studies
MS Cp E	Master of Science in Computer Engineering	MSAT	Master of Science in Accounting and Taxation
MS Eco	Master of Science in Economics		Master of Science in Advanced Technology
MS Econ	Master of Science in Economics		Master of Science in Athletic Training
MS Ed	Master of Science in Education	MSB	Master of Science in Biotechnology
MS El	Master of Science in Educational Leadership and Administration		Master of Sustainable Business
		MSBA	Master of Science in Business Administration
MS En E	Master of Science in Environmental Engineering		Master of Science in Business Analysis
		MSBAE	Master of Science in Biological and Agricultural Engineering
MS Eng	Master of Science in Engineering		
MS Engr	Master of Science in Engineering		Master of Science in Biosystems and Agricultural Engineering
MS Env E	Master of Science in Environmental Engineering		
		MSBC	Master of Science in Building Construction
MS Exp Surg	Master of Science in Experimental Surgery		Master of Science in Business Communication
MS Mat E	Master of Science in Materials Engineering	MSBCB	Master's in Bioinformatics and Computational Biology
MS Mat SE	Master of Science in Material Science and Engineering		
		MSBE	Master of Science in Biological Engineering
MS Met E	Master of Science in Metallurgical Engineering		Master of Science in Biomedical Engineering
MS Mgt	Master of Science in Management	MSBENG	Master of Science in Bioengineering
MS Min	Master of Science in Mining	MSBH	Master of Science in Behavioral Health
MS Min E	Master of Science in Mining Engineering	MSBIT	Master of Science in Business Information Technology
MS Mt E	Master of Science in Materials Engineering		
MS Otol	Master of Science in Otolaryngology	MSBM	Master of Sport Business Management
MS Pet E	Master of Science in Petroleum Engineering	MSBME	Master of Science in Biomedical Engineering
MS Sc	Master of Social Science	MSBMS	Master of Science in Basic Medical Science
MS Sp Ed	Master of Science in Special Education	MSBS	Master of Science in Biomedical Sciences
MS Stat	Master of Science in Statistics	MSBTM	Master of Science in Biotechnology and Management
MS Surg	Master of Science in Surgery		
MS Tax	Master of Science in Taxation	MSC	Master of Science in Commerce
MS Tc E	Master of Science in Telecommunications Engineering		Master of Science in Communication
			Master of Science in Computers
MS-R	Master of Science (Research)		Master of Science in Counseling
MSA	Master of School Administration		Master of Science in Criminology
	Master of Science in Accountancy		Master of Strategic Communication
	Master of Science in Accounting	MSCC	Master of Science in Community Counseling
	Master of Science in Administration	MSCD	Master of Science in Communication Disorders
	Master of Science in Aeronautics		Master of Science in Community Development

MSCE	Master of Science in Civil Engineering		Master of Science in Environmental Management
	Master of Science in Clinical Epidemiology	MSENE	Master of Science in Environmental Engineering
	Master of Science in Computer Engineering		
	Master of Science in Continuing Education	MSEO	Master of Science in Electro-Optics
MSCEE	Master of Science in Civil and Environmental Engineering	MSEP	Master of Science in Economic Policy
		MSES	Master of Science in Embedded Software Engineering
MSCF	Master of Science in Computational Finance		
MSCH	Master of Science in Chemical Engineering		Master of Science in Engineering Science
MSChE	Master of Science in Chemical Engineering		Master of Science in Environmental Science
MSCI	Master of Science in Clinical Investigation		Master of Science in Environmental Studies
MSCIS	Master of Science in Computer and Information Science		Master of Science in Exercise Science
		MSET	Master of Science in Educational Technology
	Master of Science in Computer and Information Systems		Master of Science in Engineering Technology
	Master of Science in Computer Information Science	MSEV	Master of Science in Environmental Engineering
	Master of Science in Computer Information Systems	MSF	Master of Science in Finance
			Master of Science in Forestry
MSCIT	Master of Science in Computer Information Technology		Master of Spiritual Formation
MSCJ	Master of Science in Criminal Justice	MSFA	Master of Science in Financial Analysis
MSCJA	Master of Science in Criminal Justice Administration	MSFCS	Master of Science in Family and Consumer Science
MSCJS	Master of Science in Crime and Justice Studies	MSFE	Master of Science in Financial Engineering
MSCLS	Master of Science in Clinical Laboratory Studies	MSFM	Master of Sustainable Forest Management
MSCM	Master of Science in Church Management	MSFOR	Master of Science in Forestry
	Master of Science in Conflict Management	MSFP	Master of Science in Financial Planning
	Master of Science in Construction Management	MSFS	Master of Science in Financial Sciences
	Master of Supply Chain Management		Master of Science in Forensic Science
MSCNU	Master of Science in Clinical Nutrition	MSFSB	Master of Science in Financial Services and Banking
MSCP	Master of Science in Clinical Psychology		
	Master of Science in Community Psychology	MSFT	Master of Science in Family Therapy
	Master of Science in Computer Engineering	MSGC	Master of Science in Genetic Counseling
	Master of Science in Counseling Psychology	MSH	Master of Science in Health
MSCPE	Master of Science in Computer Engineering		Master of Science in Hospice
MSCPharm	Master of Science in Pharmacy	MSHA	Master of Science in Health Administration
MSCR	Master of Science in Clinical Research	MSHCA	Master of Science in Health Care Administration
MSCRP	Master of Science in City and Regional Planning		
		MSHCI	Master of Science in Human Computer Interaction
	Master of Science in Community and Regional Planning	MSHCPM	Master of Science in Health Care Policy and Management
MSCS	Master of Science in Clinical Science		
	Master of Science in Computer Science	MSHE	Master of Science in Health Education
	Master of Science in Cyber Security	MSHES	Master of Science in Human Environmental Sciences
MSCSD	Master of Science in Communication Sciences and Disorders		
		MSHFID	Master of Science in Human Factors in Information Design
MSCSE	Master of Science in Computer Science and Engineering	MSHFS	Master of Science in Human Factors and Systems
MSCTE	Master of Science in Career and Technical Education	MSHI	Master of Science in Health Informatics
		MSHP	Master of Science in Health Professions
MSD	Master of Science in Dentistry		Master of Science in Health Promotion
	Master of Science in Design	MSHR	Master of Science in Human Resources
	Master of Science in Dietetics	MSHRL	Master of Science in Human Resource Leadership
MSE	Master of Science Education		
	Master of Science in Economics	MSHRM	Master of Science in Human Resource Management
	Master of Science in Education		
	Master of Science in Engineering	MSHROD	Master of Science in Human Resources and Organizational Development
	Master of Science in Engineering Management		
	Master of Software Engineering	MSHS	Master of Science in Health Science
	Master of Special Education		Master of Science in Health Services
	Master of Structural Engineering		Master of Science in Homeland Security
MSECE	Master of Science in Electrical and Computer Engineering	MSI	Master of Science in Information
			Master of Science in Instruction
MSED	Master of Sustainable Economic Development		Master of System Integration
MSEE	Master of Science in Electrical Engineering	MSIA	Master of Science in Industrial Administration
	Master of Science in Environmental Engineering		Master of Science in Information Assurance
		MSIB	Master of Science in International Business
MSEH	Master of Science in Environmental Health	MSIDM	Master of Science in Interior Design and Merchandising
MSEL	Master of Science in Educational Leadership		
MSEM	Master of Science in Engineering Management	MSIE	Master of Science in Industrial Engineering
	Master of Science in Engineering Mechanics		Master of Science in International Economics

MSIEM	Master of Science in Information Engineering and Management	MSMS	Master of Science in Management Science
			Master of Science in Marine Science
MSIID	Master of Science in Information and Instructional Design		Master of Science in Medical Sciences
		MSMSE	Master of Science in Manufacturing Systems Engineering
MSIM	Master of Science in Information Management		
	Master of Science in International Management		Master of Science in Material Science and Engineering
MSIMC	Master of Science in Integrated Marketing Communications		Master of Science in Mathematics and Science Education
MSIR	Master of Science in Industrial Relations	MSMT	Master of Science in Management and Technology
MSIS	Master of Science in Information Science		
	Master of Science in Information Studies	MSMus	Master of Sacred Music
	Master of Science in Information Systems	MSN	Master of Science in Nursing
	Master of Science in Interdisciplinary Studies	MSNA	Master of Science in Nurse Anesthesia
MSISE	Master of Science in Infrastructure Systems Engineering	MSNE	Master of Science in Nuclear Engineering
		MSNED	Master of Science in Nurse Education
MSISM	Master of Science in Information Systems Management	MSNM	Master of Science in Nonprofit Management
		MSNS	Master of Science in Natural Science
MSISPM	Master of Science in Information Security Policy and Management		Master of Science in Nutritional Science
		MSOD	Master of Science in Organization Development
MSIST	Master of Science in Information Systems Technology		Master of Science in Organizational Development
MSIT	Master of Science in Industrial Technology	MSOEE	Master of Science in Outdoor and Environmental Education
	Master of Science in Information Technology		
	Master of Science in Instructional Technology	MSOES	Master of Science in Occupational Ergonomics and Safety
MSITM	Master of Science in Information Technology Management	MSOH	Master of Science in Occupational Health
		MSOL	Master of Science in Organizational Leadership
MSJ	Master of Science in Journalism	MSOM	Master of Science in Operations Management
	Master of Science in Jurisprudence		Master of Science in Oriental Medicine
MSJC	Master of Social Justice and Criminology	MSOR	Master of Science in Operations Research
MSJE	Master of Science in Jewish Education	MSOT	Master of Science in Occupational Technology
MSJFP	Master of Science in Juvenile Forensic Psychology		Master of Science in Occupational Therapy
		MSP	Master of Science in Pharmacy
MSJJ	Master of Science in Juvenile Justice		Master of Science in Planning
MSJPS	Master of Science in Justice and Public Safety		Master of Speech Pathology
MSJS	Master of Science in Jewish Studies	MSPA	Master of Science in Physician Assistant
MSL	Master of School Leadership		Master of Science in Professional Accountancy
	Master of Science in Leadership	MSPAS	Master of Science in Physician Assistant Studies
	Master of Science in Limnology	MSPC	Master of Science in Professional Communications
	Master of Strategic Leadership		
	Master of Studies in Law	MSPE	Master of Science in Petroleum Engineering
MSLA	Master of Science in Legal Administration	MSPH	Master of Science in Public Health
MSLFS	Master of Science in Life Sciences	MSPHR	Master of Science in Pharmacy
MSLP	Master of Speech-Language Pathology	MSPM	Master of Science in Professional Management
MSLS	Master of Science in Library Science		Master of Science in Project Management
MSLSCM	Master of Science in Logistics and Supply Chain Management	MSPNGE	Master of Science in Petroleum and Natural Gas Engineering
MSLT	Master of Second Language Teaching	MSPO	Master of Science in Prosthetics and Orthotics
MSM	Master of Sacred Ministry	MSPPM	Master of Science in Public Policy and Management
	Master of Sacred Music		
	Master of School Mathematics	MSPS	Master of Science in Pharmaceutical Science
	Master of Science in Management		Master of Science in Political Science
	Master of Science in Medicine		Master of Science in Psychological Services
	Master of Science in Organization Management	MSPT	Master of Science in Physical Therapy
	Master of Security Management	MSpVM	Master of Specialized Veterinary Medicine
MSMA	Master of Science in Marketing Analysis	MSR	Master of Science in Radiology
MSMAE	Master of Science in Materials Engineering		Master of Science in Reading
MSMC	Master of Science in Mass Communications	MSRA	Master of Science in Recreation Administration
MSME	Master of Science in Mathematics Education	MSRE	Master of Science in Real Estate
	Master of Science in Mechanical Engineering		Master of Science in Religious Education
MSMFT	Master of Science in Marriage and Family Therapy	MSRED	Master of Science in Real Estate Development
			Master of Sustainable Real Estate Development
MSMHC	Master of Science in Mental Health Counseling	MSRLS	Master of Science in Recreation and Leisure Studies
MSMIS	Master of Science in Management Information Systems		
		MSRM	Master of Science in Risk Management
MSMIT	Master of Science in Management and Information Technology	MSRMP	Master of Science in Radiological Medical Physics
MSMLS	Master of Science in Medical Laboratory Science	MSRS	Master of Science in Radiological Sciences
MSMOT	Master of Science in Management of Technology		Master of Science in Rehabilitation Science
MSMP	Master of Science in Medical Physics		

MSS	Master of Security Studies	MTHM	Master of Tourism and Hospitality Management
	Master of Social Science	MTI	Master of Information Technology
	Master of Social Services	MTID	Master of Tangible Interaction Design
	Master of Software Systems	MTL	Master of Talmudic Law
	Master of Sports Science	MTM	Master of Technology Management
	Master of Strategic Studies		Master of Telecommunications Management
	Master's in Statistical Science		Master of the Teaching of Mathematics
MSSA	Master of Science in Social Administration	MTMH	Master of Tropical Medicine and Hygiene
MSSCM	Master of Science in Supply Chain Management	MTMS	Master in Teaching Mathematics and Science
MSSD	Master of Arts in Software Driven Systems Design	MTOM	Master of Traditional Oriental Medicine
	Master of Science in Sustainable Design	MTPC	Master of Technical and Professional Communication
MSSE	Master of Science in Software Engineering	MTR	Master of Translational Research
	Master of Science in Special Education	MTS	Master of Theatre Studies
MSSEM	Master of Science in Systems and Engineering Management		Master of Theological Studies
		MTWM	Master of Trust and Wealth Management
MSSI	Master of Science in Security Informatics	MTX	Master of Taxation
	Master of Science in Strategic Intelligence	MUA	Master of Urban Affairs
MSSL	Master of Science in School Leadership	MUCD	Master of Urban and Community Design
	Master of Science in Strategic Leadership	MUD	Master of Urban Design
MSSLP	Master of Science in Speech-Language Pathology	MUDS	Master of Urban Design Studies
		MUEP	Master of Urban and Environmental Planning
MSSM	Master of Science in Sports Medicine	MUP	Master of Urban Planning
MSSP	Master of Science in Social Policy	MUPDD	Master of Urban Planning, Design, and Development
MSSPA	Master of Science in Student Personnel Administration		
		MUPP	Master of Urban Planning and Policy
MSSS	Master of Science in Safety Science	MUPRED	Master of Urban Planning and Real Estate Development
	Master of Science in Systems Science		
MSST	Master of Science in Security Technologies	MURP	Master of Urban and Regional Planning
MSSW	Master of Science in Social Work		Master of Urban and Rural Planning
MSSWE	Master of Science in Software Engineering	MUS	Master of Urban Studies
MST	Master of Science and Technology	MUSA	Master of Urban Spatial Analytics
	Master of Science in Taxation	MVP	Master of Voice Pedagogy
	Master of Science in Teaching	MVPH	Master of Veterinary Public Health
	Master of Science in Technology	MVS	Master of Visual Studies
	Master of Science in Telecommunications	MWC	Master of Wildlife Conservation
	Master of Science Teaching	MWM	Master of Water Management
MSTC	Master of Science in Technical Communication	MWPS	Master of Wood and Paper Science
	Master of Science in Telecommunications	MWR	Master of Water Resources
MSTCM	Master of Science in Traditional Chinese Medicine	MWS	Master of Women's Studies
			Master of Worship Studies
MSTE	Master of Science in Telecommunications Engineering	MWSc	Master of Wildlife Science
		MZS	Master of Zoological Science
	Master of Science in Transportation Engineering	Nav Arch	Naval Architecture
		Naval E	Naval Engineer
MSTL	Master of Science in Teacher Leadership	ND	Doctor of Naturopathic Medicine
MSTM	Master of Science in Technology Management	NE	Nuclear Engineer
	Master of Science in Transfusion Medicine	Nuc E	Nuclear Engineer
MSTOM	Master of Science in Traditional Oriental Medicine	OD	Doctor of Optometry
		OTD	Doctor of Occupational Therapy
MSUASE	Master of Science in Unmanned and Autonomous Systems Engineering	PBME	Professional Master of Biomedical Engineering
		PC	Performer's Certificate
MSUD	Master of Science in Urban Design	PD	Professional Diploma
MSUS	Master of Science in Urban Studies	PGC	Post-Graduate Certificate
MSW	Master of Social Work	PGD	Postgraduate Diploma
MSWE	Master of Software Engineering	Ph L	Licentiate of Philosophy
MSWREE	Master of Science in Water Resources and Environmental Engineering	Pharm D	Doctor of Pharmacy
		PhD	Doctor of Philosophy
MT	Master of Taxation	PhD Otol	Doctor of Philosophy in Otolaryngology
	Master of Teaching	PhD Surg	Doctor of Philosophy in Surgery
	Master of Technology	PhDEE	Doctor of Philosophy in Electrical Engineering
	Master of Textiles	PMBA	Professional Master of Business Administration
MTA	Master of Tax Accounting	PMC	Post Master Certificate
	Master of Teaching Arts	PMD	Post-Master's Diploma
	Master of Tourism Administration	PMS	Professional Master of Science
MTCM	Master of Traditional Chinese Medicine		Professional Master's
MTD	Master of Training and Development	Post-Doctoral MS	Post-Doctoral Master of Science
MTE	Master in Educational Technology	Post-MSN Certificate	Post-Master of Science in Nursing Certificate
MTESOL	Master in Teaching English to Speakers of Other Languages	PPDPT	Postprofessional Doctor of Physical Therapy

Pro-MS	Professional Science Master's
Professional MA	Professional Master of Arts
Professional MBA	Professional Master of Business Administration
Professional MS	Professional Master of Science
PSM	Professional Master of Science
	Professional Science Master's
Psy D	Doctor of Psychology
Psy M	Master of Psychology
Psy S	Specialist in Psychology
Psya D	Doctor of Psychoanalysis
S Psy S	Specialist in Psychological Services
Sc D	Doctor of Science
Sc M	Master of Science
SCCT	Specialist in Community College Teaching
ScDPT	Doctor of Physical Therapy Science
SD	Doctor of Science
	Specialist Degree
SJD	Doctor of Juridical Sciences
SLPD	Doctor of Speech-Language Pathology
SM	Master of Science
SM Arch S	Master of Science in Architectural Studies

SMACT	Master of Science in Art, Culture and Technology
SMBT	Master of Science in Building Technology
SP	Specialist Degree
Sp Ed	Specialist in Education
Sp LIS	Specialist in Library and Information Science
SPA	Specialist in Arts
Spec	Specialist's Certificate
Spec M	Specialist in Music
Spt	Specialist Degree
SSP	Specialist in School Psychology
STB	Bachelor of Sacred Theology
STD	Doctor of Sacred Theology
STL	Licentiate of Sacred Theology
STM	Master of Sacred Theology
TDPT	Transitional Doctor of Physical Therapy
Th D	Doctor of Theology
Th M	Master of Theology
TOTD	Transitional Doctor of Occupational Therapy
VMD	Doctor of Veterinary Medicine
WEMBA	Weekend Executive Master of Business Administration
XMA	Executive Master of Arts

INDEXES

Displays and Close-Ups

Directories and Subject Areas

Following is an alphabetical listing of directories and subject areas. Also listed are cross-references for subject area names not used in the directory structure of the guides, for example, "City and Regional Planning (*see* Urban and Regional Planning)."

Graduate Programs in the Humanities, Arts & Social Sciences

Addictions/Substance Abuse Counseling
Administration (*see* Arts Administration; Public Administration)
African-American Studies
African Languages and Literatures (*see* African Studies)
African Studies
Agribusiness (*see* Agricultural Economics and Agribusiness)
Agricultural Economics and Agribusiness
Alcohol Abuse Counseling (*see* Addictions/Substance Abuse Counseling)
American Indian/Native American Studies
American Studies
Anthropology
Applied Arts and Design—General
Applied Behavior Analysis
Applied Economics
Applied History (*see* Public History)
Applied Psychology
Applied Social Research
Arabic (*see* Near and Middle Eastern Languages)
Arab Studies (*see* Near and Middle Eastern Studies)
Archaeology
Architectural History
Architecture
Archives Administration (*see* Public History)
Area and Cultural Studies (*see* African-American Studies; African Studies; American Indian/Native American Studies; American Studies; Asian-American Studies; Asian Studies; Canadian Studies; Cultural Studies; East European and Russian Studies; Ethnic Studies; Folklore; Gender Studies; Hispanic Studies; Holocaust Studies; Jewish Studies; Latin American Studies; Near and Middle Eastern Studies; Northern Studies; Pacific Area/Pacific Rim Studies; Western European Studies; Women's Studies)
Art/Fine Arts
Art History
Arts Administration
Arts Journalism
Art Therapy
Asian-American Studies
Asian Languages
Asian Studies
Behavioral Sciences (*see* Psychology)
Bible Studies (*see* Religion; Theology)
Biological Anthropology
Black Studies (*see* African-American Studies)
Broadcasting (*see* Communication; Film, Television, and Video Production)
Broadcast Journalism
Building Science
Canadian Studies
Celtic Languages
Ceramics (*see* Art/Fine Arts)
Child and Family Studies
Child Development
Chinese
Chinese Studies (*see* Asian Languages; Asian Studies)
Christian Studies (*see* Missions and Missiology; Religion; Theology)
Cinema (*see* Film, Television, and Video Production)
City and Regional Planning (*see* Urban and Regional Planning)
Classical Languages and Literatures (*see* Classics)
Classics

Clinical Psychology
Clothing and Textiles
Cognitive Psychology (*see* Psychology—General; Cognitive Sciences)
Cognitive Sciences
Communication—General
Community Affairs (*see* Urban and Regional Planning; Urban Studies)
Community Planning (*see* Architecture; Environmental Design; Urban and Regional Planning; Urban Design; Urban Studies)
Community Psychology (*see* Social Psychology)
Comparative and Interdisciplinary Arts
Comparative Literature
Composition (*see* Music)
Computer Art and Design
Conflict Resolution and Mediation/Peace Studies
Consumer Economics
Corporate and Organizational Communication
Corrections (*see* Criminal Justice and Criminology)
Counseling (*see* Counseling Psychology; Pastoral Ministry and Counseling)
Counseling Psychology
Crafts (*see* Art/Fine Arts)
Creative Arts Therapies (*see* Art Therapy; Therapies—Dance, Drama, and Music)
Criminal Justice and Criminology
Cultural Anthropology
Cultural Studies
Dance
Decorative Arts
Demography and Population Studies
Design (*see* Applied Arts and Design; Architecture; Art/Fine Arts; Environmental Design; Graphic Design; Industrial Design; Interior Design; Textile Design; Urban Design)
Developmental Psychology
Diplomacy (*see* International Affairs)
Disability Studies
Drama Therapy (*see* Therapies—Dance, Drama, and Music)
Dramatic Arts (*see* Theater)
Drawing (*see* Art/Fine Arts)
Drug Abuse Counseling (*see* Addictions/Substance Abuse Counseling)
Drug and Alcohol Abuse Counseling (*see* Addictions/Substance Abuse Counseling)
East Asian Studies (*see* Asian Studies)
East European and Russian Studies
Economic Development
Economics
Educational Theater (*see* Theater; Therapies—Dance, Drama, and Music)
Emergency Management
English
Environmental Design
Ethics
Ethnic Studies
Ethnomusicology (*see* Music)
Experimental Psychology
Family and Consumer Sciences—General
Family Studies (*see* Child and Family Studies)
Family Therapy (*see* Child and Family Studies; Clinical Psychology; Counseling Psychology; Marriage and Family Therapy)
Filmmaking (*see* Film, Television, and Video Production)
Film Studies (*see* Film, Television, and Video Production)
Film, Television, and Video Production
Film, Television, and Video Theory and Criticism
Fine Arts (*see* Art/Fine Arts)
Folklore
Foreign Languages (*see* specific language)
Foreign Service (*see* International Affairs; International Development)
Forensic Psychology
Forensic Sciences
Forensics (*see* Speech and Interpersonal Communication)
French
Gender Studies
General Studies (*see* Liberal Studies)

Genetic Counseling
Geographic Information Systems
Geography
German
Gerontology
Graphic Design
Greek (*see* Classics)
Health Communication
Health Psychology
Hebrew (*see* Near and Middle Eastern Languages)
Hebrew Studies (*see* Jewish Studies)
Hispanic and Latin American Languages
Hispanic Studies
Historic Preservation
History
History of Art (*see* Art History)
History of Medicine
History of Science and Technology
Holocaust and Genocide Studies
Home Economics (*see* Family and Consumer Sciences—General)
Homeland Security
Household Economics, Sciences, and Management (*see* Family and Consumer Sciences—General)
Human Development
Humanities
Illustration
Industrial and Labor Relations
Industrial and Organizational Psychology
Industrial Design
Interdisciplinary Studies
Interior Design
International Affairs
International Development
International Economics
International Service (*see* International Affairs; International Development)
International Trade Policy
Internet and Interactive Multimedia
Interpersonal Communication (*see* Speech and Interpersonal Communication)
Interpretation (*see* Translation and Interpretation)
Islamic Studies (*see* Near and Middle Eastern Studies; Religion)
Italian
Japanese
Japanese Studies (*see* Asian Languages; Asian Studies; Japanese)
Jewelry (*see* Art/Fine Arts)
Jewish Studies
Journalism
Judaic Studies (*see* Jewish Studies; Religion)
Labor Relations (*see* Industrial and Labor Relations)
Landscape Architecture
Latin American Studies
Latin (*see* Classics)
Law Enforcement (*see* Criminal Justice and Criminology)
Liberal Studies
Lighting Design
Linguistics
Literature (*see* Classics; Comparative Literature; specific language)
Marriage and Family Therapy
Mass Communication
Media Studies
Medical Illustration
Medieval and Renaissance Studies
Metalsmithing (*see* Art/Fine Arts)
Middle Eastern Studies (*see* Near and Middle Eastern Studies)
Military and Defense Studies
Mineral Economics
Ministry (*see* Pastoral Ministry and Counseling; Theology)
Missions and Missiology
Motion Pictures (*see* Film, Television, and Video Production)
Museum Studies
Music
Musicology (*see* Music)
Music Therapy (*see* Therapies—Dance, Drama, and Music)
National Security

Native American Studies (*see* American Indian/Native American Studies)
Near and Middle Eastern Languages
Near and Middle Eastern Studies
Near Environment (*see* Family and Consumer Sciences)
Northern Studies
Organizational Psychology (*see* Industrial and Organizational Psychology)
Oriental Languages (*see* Asian Languages)
Oriental Studies (*see* Asian Studies)
Pacific Area/Pacific Rim Studies
Painting (*see* Art/Fine Arts)
Pastoral Ministry and Counseling
Philanthropic Studies
Philosophy
Photography
Playwriting (*see* Theater; Writing)
Policy Studies (*see* Public Policy)
Political Science
Population Studies (*see* Demography and Population Studies)
Portuguese
Printmaking (*see* Art/Fine Arts)
Product Design (*see* Industrial Design)
Psychoanalysis and Psychotherapy
Psychology—General
Public Administration
Public Affairs
Public History
Public Policy
Public Speaking (*see* Mass Communication; Rhetoric; Speech and Interpersonal Communication)
Publishing
Regional Planning (*see* Architecture; Urban and Regional Planning; Urban Design; Urban Studies)
Rehabilitation Counseling
Religion
Renaissance Studies (*see* Medieval and Renaissance Studies)
Rhetoric
Romance Languages
Romance Literatures (*see* Romance Languages)
Rural Planning and Studies
Rural Sociology
Russian
Scandinavian Languages
School Psychology
Sculpture (*see* Art/Fine Arts)
Security Administration (*see* Criminal Justice and Criminology)
Slavic Languages
Slavic Studies (*see* East European and Russian Studies; Slavic Languages)
Social Psychology
Social Sciences
Sociology
Southeast Asian Studies (*see* Asian Studies)
Soviet Studies (*see* East European and Russian Studies; Russian)
Spanish
Speech and Interpersonal Communication
Sport Psychology
Studio Art (*see* Art/Fine Arts)
Substance Abuse Counseling (*see* Addictions/Substance Abuse Counseling)
Survey Methodology
Sustainable Development
Technical Communication
Technical Writing
Telecommunications (*see* Film, Television, and Video Production)
Television (*see* Film, Television, and Video Production)
Textile Design
Textiles (*see* Clothing and Textiles; Textile Design)
Thanatology
Theater
Theater Arts (*see* Theater)
Theology
Therapies—Dance, Drama, and Music
Translation and Interpretation
Transpersonal and Humanistic Psychology

Urban and Regional Planning
Urban Design
Urban Planning (*see* Architecture; Urban and Regional Planning; Urban Design; Urban Studies)
Urban Studies
Video (*see* Film, Television, and Video Production)
Visual Arts (*see* Applied Arts and Design; Art/Fine Arts; Film, Television, and Video Production; Graphic Design; Illustration; Photography)
Western European Studies
Women's Studies
World Wide Web (*see* Internet and Interactive Multimedia)
Writing

Graduate Programs in the Biological/ Biomedical Sciences & Health-Related Medical Professions

Acupuncture and Oriental Medicine
Acute Care/Critical Care Nursing Administration (*see* Health Services Management and Hospital Administration; Nursing and Healthcare Administration; Pharmaceutical Administration)
Adult Nursing
Advanced Practice Nursing (*see* Family Nurse Practitioner Studies)
Allied Health—General
Allied Health Professions (*see* Clinical Laboratory Sciences/Medical Technology; Clinical Research; Communication Disorders; Dental Hygiene; Emergency Medical Services; Occupational Therapy; Physical Therapy; Physician Assistant Studies; Rehabilitation Sciences)
Allopathic Medicine
Anatomy
Anesthesiologist Assistant Studies
Animal Behavior
Bacteriology
Behavioral Sciences (*see* Biopsychology; Neuroscience; Zoology)
Biochemistry
Bioethics
Biological and Biomedical Sciences—General Biological Chemistry (*see* Biochemistry)
Biological Oceanography (*see* Marine Biology)
Biophysics
Biopsychology
Botany
Breeding (*see* Botany; Plant Biology; Genetics)
Cancer Biology/Oncology
Cardiovascular Sciences
Cell Biology
Cellular Physiology (*see* Cell Biology; Physiology)
Child-Care Nursing (*see* Maternal and Child/Neonatal Nursing)
Chiropractic
Clinical Laboratory Sciences/Medical Technology
Clinical Research
Community Health
Community Health Nursing
Computational Biology
Conservation (*see* Conservation Biology; Environmental Biology)
Conservation Biology
Crop Sciences (*see* Botany; Plant Biology)
Cytology (*see* Cell Biology)
Dental and Oral Surgery (*see* Oral and Dental Sciences)
Dental Assistant Studies (*see* Dental Hygiene)
Dental Hygiene
Dental Services (*see* Dental Hygiene)
Dentistry
Developmental Biology Dietetics (*see* Nutrition)
Ecology
Embryology (*see* Developmental Biology)
Emergency Medical Services
Endocrinology (*see* Physiology)
Entomology
Environmental Biology

Environmental and Occupational Health
Epidemiology
Evolutionary Biology
Family Nurse Practitioner Studies
Foods (*see* Nutrition)
Forensic Nursing
Genetics
Genomic Sciences
Gerontological Nursing
Health Physics/Radiological Health
Health Promotion
Health-Related Professions (*see* individual allied health professions)
Health Services Management and Hospital Administration
Health Services Research
Histology (*see* Anatomy; Cell Biology)
HIV/AIDS Nursing
Hospice Nursing
Hospital Administration (*see* Health Services Management and Hospital Administration)
Human Genetics
Immunology
Industrial Hygiene
Infectious Diseases
International Health
Laboratory Medicine (*see* Clinical Laboratory Sciences/Medical Technology; Immunology; Microbiology; Pathology)
Life Sciences (*see* Biological and Biomedical Sciences)
Marine Biology
Maternal and Child Health
Maternal and Child/Neonatal Nursing
Medical Imaging
Medical Microbiology
Medical Nursing (*see* Medical/Surgical Nursing)
Medical Physics
Medical/Surgical Nursing
Medical Technology (*see* Clinical Laboratory Sciences/Medical Technology)
Medical Sciences (*see* Biological and Biomedical Sciences)
Medical Science Training Programs (*see* Biological and Biomedical Sciences)
Medicinal and Pharmaceutical Chemistry
Medicinal Chemistry (*see* Medicinal and Pharmaceutical Chemistry)
Medicine (*see* Allopathic Medicine; Naturopathic Medicine; Osteopathic Medicine; Podiatric Medicine)
Microbiology
Midwifery (*see* Nurse Midwifery)
Molecular Biology
Molecular Biophysics
Molecular Genetics
Molecular Medicine
Molecular Pathogenesis
Molecular Pathology
Molecular Pharmacology
Molecular Physiology
Molecular Toxicology
Naturopathic Medicine
Neural Sciences (*see* Biopsychology; Neurobiology; Neuroscience)
Neurobiology
Neuroendocrinology (*see* Biopsychology; Neurobiology; Neuroscience; Physiology)
Neuropharmacology (*see* Biopsychology; Neurobiology; Neuroscience; Pharmacology)
Neurophysiology (*see* Biopsychology; Neurobiology; Neuroscience; Physiology)
Neuroscience
Nuclear Medical Technology (*see* Clinical Laboratory Sciences/ Medical Technology)
Nurse Anesthesia
Nurse Midwifery
Nurse Practitioner Studies (*see* Family Nurse Practitioner Studies)
Nursing Administration (*see* Nursing and Healthcare Administration)
Nursing and Healthcare Administration
Nursing Education
Nursing—General
Nursing Informatics
Nutrition

Occupational Health (*see* Environmental and Occupational Health; Occupational Health Nursing)
Occupational Health Nursing
Occupational Therapy
Oncology (*see* Cancer Biology/Oncology)
Oncology Nursing
Optometry
Oral and Dental Sciences
Oral Biology (*see* Oral and Dental Sciences)
Oral Pathology (*see* Oral and Dental Sciences)
Organismal Biology (*see* Biological and Biomedical Sciences; Zoology)
Oriental Medicine and Acupuncture (*see* Acupuncture and Oriental Medicine)
Orthodontics (*see* Oral and Dental Sciences)
Osteopathic Medicine
Parasitology
Pathobiology
Pathology
Pediatric Nursing
Pedontics (*see* Oral and Dental Sciences)
Perfusion
Pharmaceutical Administration
Pharmaceutical Chemistry (*see* Medicinal and Pharmaceutical Chemistry)
Pharmaceutical Sciences
Pharmacology
Pharmacy
Photobiology of Cells and Organelles (*see* Botany; Cell Biology; Plant Biology)
Physical Therapy
Physician Assistant Studies
Physiological Optics (*see* Vision Sciences)
Podiatric Medicine
Preventive Medicine (*see* Community Health and Public Health)
Physiological Optics (*see* Physiology)
Physiology
Plant Biology
Plant Molecular Biology
Plant Pathology
Plant Physiology
Pomology (*see* Botany; Plant Biology)
Psychiatric Nursing
Public Health—General
Public Health Nursing (*see* Community Health Nursing)
Psychiatric Nursing
Psychobiology (*see* Biopsychology)
Psychopharmacology (*see* Biopsychology; Neuroscience; Pharmacology)
Radiation Biology
Radiological Health (*see* Health Physics/Radiological Health)
Rehabilitation Nursing
Rehabilitation Sciences
Rehabilitation Therapy (*see* Physical Therapy)
Reproductive Biology
School Nursing
Sociobiology (*see* Evolutionary Biology)
Structural Biology
Surgical Nursing (*see* Medical/Surgical Nursing)
Systems Biology
Teratology
Therapeutics
Theoretical Biology (*see* Biological and Biomedical Sciences)
Therapeutics (*see* Pharmaceutical Sciences; Pharmacology; Pharmacy)
Toxicology
Transcultural Nursing
Translational Biology
Tropical Medicine (*see* Parasitology)
Veterinary Medicine
Veterinary Sciences
Virology
Vision Sciences
Wildlife Biology (*see* Zoology)
Women's Health Nursing
Zoology

Graduate Programs in the Physical Sciences, Mathematics, Agricultural Sciences, the Environment & Natural Resources

Acoustics
Agricultural Sciences
Agronomy and Soil Sciences
Analytical Chemistry
Animal Sciences
Applied Mathematics
Applied Physics
Applied Statistics
Aquaculture
Astronomy
Astrophysical Sciences (*see* Astrophysics; Atmospheric Sciences; Meteorology; Planetary and Space Sciences)
Astrophysics
Atmospheric Sciences
Biological Oceanography (*see* Marine Affairs; Marine Sciences; Oceanography)
Biomathematics
Biometry
Biostatistics
Chemical Physics
Chemistry
Computational Sciences
Condensed Matter Physics
Dairy Science (*see* Animal Sciences)
Earth Sciences (*see* Geosciences)
Environmental Management and Policy
Environmental Sciences
Environmental Studies (*see* Environmental Management and Policy)
Experimental Statistics (*see* Statistics)
Fish, Game, and Wildlife Management
Food Science and Technology
Forestry
General Science (*see* specific topics)
Geochemistry
Geodetic Sciences
Geological Engineering (*see* Geology)
Geological Sciences (*see* Geology)
Geology
Geophysical Fluid Dynamics (*see* Geophysics)
Geophysics
Geosciences
Horticulture
Hydrogeology
Hydrology
Inorganic Chemistry
Limnology
Marine Affairs
Marine Geology
Marine Sciences
Marine Studies (*see* Marine Affairs; Marine Geology; Marine Sciences; Oceanography)
Mathematical and Computational Finance
Mathematical Physics
Mathematical Statistics (*see* Applied Statistics; Statistics)
Mathematics
Meteorology
Mineralogy
Natural Resource Management (*see* Environmental Management and Policy; Natural Resources)
Natural Resources
Nuclear Physics (*see* Physics)
Ocean Engineering (*see* Marine Affairs; Marine Geology; Marine Sciences; Oceanography)
Oceanography
Optical Sciences
Optical Technologies (*see* Optical Sciences)
Optics (*see* Applied Physics; Optical Sciences; Physics)
Organic Chemistry

Paleontology
Paper Chemistry (*see* Chemistry)
Photonics
Physical Chemistry
Physics
Planetary and Space Sciences
Plant Sciences
Plasma Physics
Poultry Science (*see* Animal Sciences)
Radiological Physics (*see* Physics)
Range Management (*see* Range Science)
Range Science
Resource Management (*see* Environmental Management and Policy; Natural Resources)
Solid-Earth Sciences (*see* Geosciences)
Space Sciences (*see* Planetary and Space Sciences)
Statistics
Theoretical Chemistry
Theoretical Physics
Viticulture and Enology
Water Resources

Graduate Programs in Engineering & Applied Sciences

Aeronautical Engineering (*see* Aerospace/Aeronautical Engineering)
Aerospace/Aeronautical Engineering
Aerospace Studies (*see* Aerospace/Aeronautical Engineering)
Agricultural Engineering
Applied Mechanics (*see* Mechanics)
Applied Science and Technology
Architectural Engineering
Artificial Intelligence/Robotics
Astronautical Engineering (*see* Aerospace/Aeronautical Engineering)
Automotive Engineering
Aviation
Biochemical Engineering
Bioengineering
Bioinformatics
Biological Engineering (*see* Bioengineering)
Biomedical Engineering
Biosystems Engineering
Biotechnology
Ceramic Engineering (*see* Ceramic Sciences and Engineering)
Ceramic Sciences and Engineering
Ceramics (*see* Ceramic Sciences and Engineering)
Chemical Engineering
Civil Engineering
Computer and Information Systems Security
Computer Engineering
Computer Science
Computing Technology (*see* Computer Science)
Construction Engineering
Construction Management
Database Systems
Electrical Engineering
Electronic Materials
Electronics Engineering (*see* Electrical Engineering)
Energy and Power Engineering
Energy Management and Policy
Engineering and Applied Sciences
Engineering and Public Affairs (*see* Technology and Public Policy)
Engineering and Public Policy (*see* Energy Management and Policy; Technology and Public Policy)
Engineering Design
Engineering Management
Engineering Mechanics (*see* Mechanics)
Engineering Metallurgy (*see* Metallurgical Engineering and Metallurgy)
Engineering Physics
Environmental Design (*see* Environmental Engineering)
Environmental Engineering
Ergonomics and Human Factors
Financial Engineering

Fire Protection Engineering
Food Engineering (*see* Agricultural Engineering)
Game Design and Development
Gas Engineering (*see* Petroleum Engineering)
Geological Engineering
Geophysics Engineering (*see* Geological Engineering)
Geotechnical Engineering
Hazardous Materials Management
Health Informatics
Health Systems (*see* Safety Engineering; Systems Engineering)
Highway Engineering (*see* Transportation and Highway Engineering)
Human-Computer Interaction
Human Factors (*see* Ergonomics and Human Factors)
Hydraulics
Hydrology (*see* Water Resources Engineering)
Industrial Engineering (*see* Industrial/Management Engineering)
Industrial/Management Engineering
Information Science
Internet Engineering
Macromolecular Science (*see* Polymer Science and Engineering)
Management Engineering (*see* Engineering Management; Industrial/Management Engineering)
Management of Technology
Manufacturing Engineering
Marine Engineering (*see* Civil Engineering)
Materials Engineering
Materials Sciences
Mechanical Engineering
Mechanics
Medical Informatics
Metallurgical Engineering and Metallurgy
Metallurgy (*see* Metallurgical Engineering and Metallurgy)
Mineral/Mining Engineering
Modeling and Simulation
Nanotechnology
Nuclear Engineering
Ocean Engineering
Operations Research
Paper and Pulp Engineering
Petroleum Engineering
Pharmaceutical Engineering
Plastics Engineering (*see* Polymer Science and Engineering)
Polymer Science and Engineering
Public Policy (*see* Energy Management and Policy; Technology and Public Policy)
Reliability Engineering
Robotics (*see* Artificial Intelligence/Robotics)
Safety Engineering
Software Engineering
Solid-State Sciences (*see* Materials Sciences)
Structural Engineering
Surveying Science and Engineering
Systems Analysis (*see* Systems Engineering)
Systems Engineering
Systems Science
Technology and Public Policy
Telecommunications
Telecommunications Management
Textile Sciences and Engineering
Textiles (*see* Textile Sciences and Engineering)
Transportation and Highway Engineering
Urban Systems Engineering (*see* Systems Engineering)
Waste Management (*see* Hazardous Materials Management)
Water Resources Engineering

Graduate Programs in Business, Education, Information Studies, Law & Social Work

Accounting
Actuarial Science
Adult Education

Advertising and Public Relations
Agricultural Education
Alcohol Abuse Counseling (*see* Counselor Education)
Archival Management and Studies
Art Education
Athletics Administration (*see* Kinesiology and Movement Studies)
Athletic Training and Sports Medicine
Audiology (*see* Communication Disorders)
Aviation Management
Banking (*see* Finance and Banking)
Business Administration and Management—General
Business Education
Communication Disorders
Community College Education
Computer Education
Continuing Education (*see* Adult Education)
Counseling (*see* Counselor Education)
Counselor Education
Curriculum and Instruction
Developmental Education
Distance Education Development
Drug Abuse Counseling (*see* Counselor Education)
Early Childhood Education
Educational Leadership and Administration
Educational Measurement and Evaluation
Educational Media/Instructional Technology
Educational Policy
Educational Psychology
Education—General
Education of the Blind (*see* Special Education)
Education of the Deaf (*see* Special Education)
Education of the Gifted
Education of the Hearing Impaired (*see* Special Education)
Education of the Learning Disabled (*see* Special Education)
Education of the Mentally Retarded (*see* Special Education)
Education of the Physically Handicapped (*see* Special Education)
Education of Students with Severe/Multiple Disabilities
Education of the Visually Handicapped (*see* Special Education)
Electronic Commerce
Elementary Education
English as a Second Language
English Education
Entertainment Management
Entrepreneurship
Environmental Education
Environmental Law
Exercise and Sports Science
Exercise Physiology (*see* Kinesiology and Movement Studies)
Facilities and Entertainment Management
Finance and Banking
Food Services Management (*see* Hospitality Management)
Foreign Languages Education
Foundations and Philosophy of Education
Guidance and Counseling (*see* Counselor Education)
Health Education
Health Law
Hearing Sciences (*see* Communication Disorders)
Higher Education
Home Economics Education
Hospitality Management
Hotel Management (*see* Travel and Tourism)
Human Resources Development
Human Resources Management
Human Services
Industrial Administration (*see* Industrial and Manufacturing Management)
Industrial and Manufacturing Management
Industrial Education (*see* Vocational and Technical Education)
Information Studies
Instructional Technology (*see* Educational Media/Instructional Technology)
Insurance
Intellectual Property Law
International and Comparative Education
International Business
International Commerce (*see* International Business)

International Economics (*see* International Business)
International Trade (*see* International Business)
Investment and Securities (*see* Business Administration and Management; Finance and Banking; Investment Management)
Investment Management
Junior College Education (*see* Community College Education)
Kinesiology and Movement Studies
Law
Legal and Justice Studies
Leisure Services (*see* Recreation and Park Management)
Leisure Studies
Library Science
Logistics
Management (*see* Business Administration and Management)
Management Information Systems
Management Strategy and Policy
Marketing
Marketing Research
Mathematics Education
Middle School Education
Movement Studies (*see* Kinesiology and Movement Studies)
Multilingual and Multicultural Education
Museum Education
Music Education
Nonprofit Management
Nursery School Education (*see* Early Childhood Education)
Occupational Education (*see* Vocational and Technical Education)
Organizational Behavior
Organizational Management
Parks Administration (*see* Recreation and Park Management)
Personnel (*see* Human Resources Development; Human Resources Management; Organizational Behavior; Organizational Management; Student Affairs)
Philosophy of Education (*see* Foundations and Philosophy of Education)
Physical Education
Project Management
Public Relations (*see* Advertising and Public Relations)
Quality Management
Quantitative Analysis
Reading Education
Real Estate
Recreation and Park Management
Recreation Therapy (*see* Recreation and Park Management)
Religious Education
Remedial Education (*see* Special Education)
Restaurant Administration (*see* Hospitality Management)
Science Education
Secondary Education
Social Sciences Education
Social Studies Education (*see* Social Sciences Education)
Social Work
Special Education
Speech-Language Pathology and Audiology (*see* Communication Disorders)
Sports Management
Sports Medicine (*see* Athletic Training and Sports Medicine)
Sports Psychology and Sociology (*see* Kinesiology and Movement Studies)
Student Affairs
Substance Abuse Counseling (*see* Counselor Education)
Supply Chain Management
Sustainability Management
Systems Management (*see* Management Information Systems)
Taxation
Teacher Education (*see* specific subject areas)
Teaching English as a Second Language (*see* English as a Second Language)
Technical Education (*see* Vocational and Technical Education)
Transportation Management
Travel and Tourism
Urban Education
Vocational and Technical Education
Vocational Counseling (*see* Counselor Education)

Directories and Subject Areas in This Book